PDR for all of your drug i s.

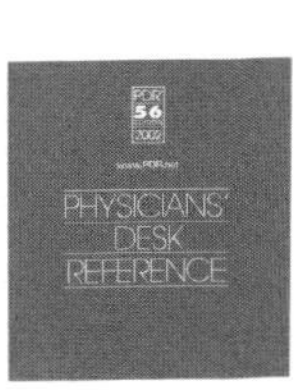

Physicians' Desk Reference®

Physicians have turned to the PDR for the latest word on prescription drugs for more than 55 years. Today, PDR is still considered the standard prescription drug reference and can be found in virtually every physician's office, hospital and pharmacy in the United States. You can search the more than 4,000 drugs by using one of many indices and look at more than 2,100 full-color photos of drugs cross-referenced to the label information. More than 3,000 pages—our largest ever!

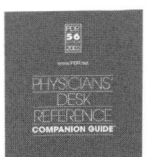

PDR® Companion Guide

This unique 1,900-page all-in-one clinical companion to the PDR assures safe, appropriate drug selection with ten critical checkpoint indices including *Indications, Side Effects, Interactions, Off-Label Treatment* and much more.

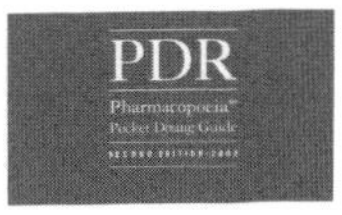

PDR® Pharmacopoeia Pocket Dosing Guide - Second Edition 2002

This pocket dosing guide brings important dispensing information to the practitioner's fingertips. Organized in tabular format, this small, 280-page quick reference is easy to navigate and gives important FDA approved dosing information, black box warning summaries and much more, whenever it is needed. Based on the PDR information, this guide proves that other Dosing Guides just don't measure up!

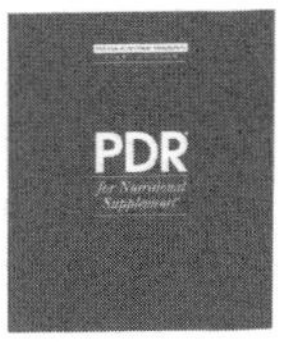

PDR® for Nutritional Supplements™- 1st Edition

The definitive information source for more than 300 nutritional supplements. This first, comprehensive, unbiased source of solid, evidence based information about nutritional and dietary supplements provides practitioners with more than 700 pages of the most current and reliable information available.

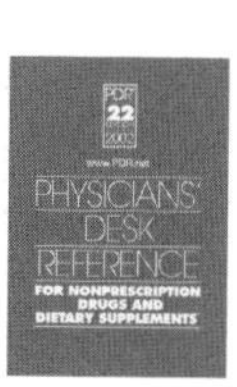

PDR for Nonprescription Drugs and Dietary Supplements™

This acknowledged authority offers full FDA-approved descriptions of the most commonly used OTC medicines in four separate indices within more than 400 pages. Plus, it includes a section on supplements, vitamins and Herbal remedies.

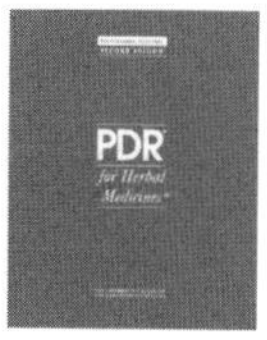

PDR® for Herbal Medicines™ - 2nd Edition

This guide, the most comprehensive reference on Herbal remedies, is based upon the work by Germany's Commission E and Jöerg Grüenwald, Ph. D. a botanist and renowned expert on herbal medicines. This detailed guide provides more than 1,100 pages of thorough descriptions on over 600 botanical remedies; the plant and the derived compounds.

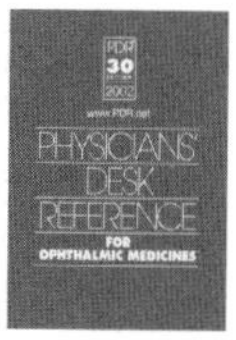

PDR for Ophthalmic Medicines™

The definitive reference for the eye-care professional offers 230 pages of detailed information on drugs and equipment used in the fields of ophthalmology and optometry. With five full indices and information on specialized instruments, lenses and much more, this guide is the most comprehensive of its kind.

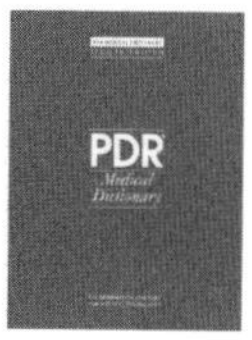

PDR® Medical Dictionary™ - 2nd Edition

This fully updated second edition with more than 2,100 pages, includes a complete medical etymology section on medical/scientific word formation as well as a complete cross-reference table of generic and brand name pharmaceuticals and manufacturers and much more!

Complete Your 2002 PDR® Library NOW! Enclose payment and save shipping costs.

101501	______ copies **2002 Physicians' Desk Reference®**	$89.95 ea.	$ ______
101519	______ copies **2002 PDR® Companion Guide**	$64.95 ea.	$ ______
101584	______ copies **PDR Pharmacopoeia Pocket Dosing Guide***	$9.95 ea.	$ ______
101568	______ copies **PDR® for Nutritional Supplements™, 1st EDITION!**	$59.95 ea.	$ ______
101527	______ copies **2002 PDR for Nonprescription Drugs and Dietary Supplements™**	$55.95 ea.	$ ______
101550	______ copies **PDR® for Herbal Medicines™, 2nd EDITION!**	$59.95 ea.	$ ______
101535	______ copies **2002 PDR for Ophthalmic Medicines™**	$61.95 ea.	$ ______
101543	______ copies **PDR® Medical Dictionary™, 2nd EDITION!**	$49.95 ea.	$ ______

Shipping & Handling (Add $9.95 S&H per book if paying later*) $ ______

Sales Tax (FL, GA, IA, & NJ) $ ______

Total Amount of Order $ ______

(*Shipping and handling is $1.95 for PDR Pharmacopoeia)

Mail this order form to: **PDR**, P.O. Box 10689, Des Moines, IA 50336-0689
e-mail: customer.service@medec.com

For Faster Service—FAX YOUR ORDER (515) 284-6714
or CALL TOLL-FREE (888) 859-8053
Do not mail a confirmation order in addition to this fax.

Valid for 2002 editions only, prices and shipping & handling higher outside U.S.

SAVE TIME AND MONEY EVERY YEAR AS A STANDING ORDER SUBSCRIBER

☐ Check here to enter your standing order for future editions of publications ordered. They will be shipped to you automatically, after advance notice. As a standing order subscriber, you are **guaranteed** our lowest price offer, earliest delivery and FREE shipping and handling. 756395

PLEASE INDICATE METHOD OF PAYMENT:

Payment Enclosed (shipping & handling FREE)

☐ Check payable to PDR

☐ VISA ☐ MasterCard

☐ Discover ☐ American Express

Account No. ______

Exp. Date ______

Telephone No. ______

Signature ______

Name ______

Address ______

City ______

State/Zip ______

☐ **Bill me later**

(Add $9.95 per book for shipping and handling*)

PDR® for Herbal Medicines™

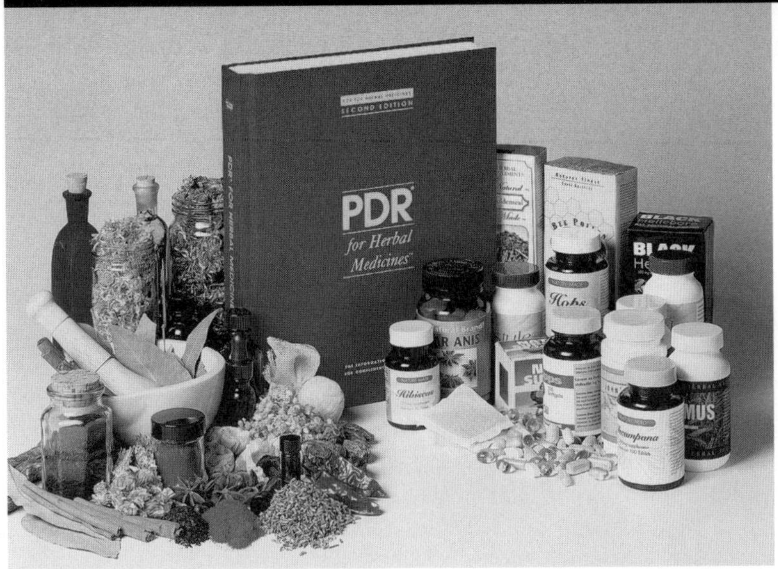

The most scientific assessment of herbal remedies ever published.

The PDR® for Herbal Medicines,™ First Edition was our first comprehensive resource in the field—and an instant best-seller. But we've worked to make the Second Edition even more useful and valuable to our readers. Just look at all the new information and important improvements you get!

- ◆ **NEW!** Monographs on over 100 additional plants — for coverage of nearly 700 herbs.
- ◆ **NEW!** Organized by common name — enabling you to more easily find the herb you're interested in.
- ◆ **NEW!** Extensive new research data on safety and efficacy.
- ◆ **NEW!** Expanded side effects and indications indices.
- ◆ **NEW!** Asian and homeopathic herbs indices — rapid reference for practitioners in these specialty areas.
- ◆ **NEW!** Safety Guide — covering 139 different herbs to be avoided during pregnancy and breastfeeding, or used only under professional supervision.
- ◆ **NEW!** Expanded Drug/Herb Interaction Guide — example: St. Johns Wort can significantly decrease digoxin levels resulting in reduced efficacy of digoxin.
- ◆ **NEW!** Daily dosage information — for unprocessed herbs and commercially available products.
- ◆ **NEW!** Manufacturers' Index — including name, address, contact information, and products sold.
- ◆ **NEW!** Trade names — added to the monographs for available products.
- ◆ **NEW!** Expanded Therapeutic Category Index — example: look up "sexual dysfunction." Find l-arginine, avena sativa, muira puama, niacin, nettles, cayenne pepper, and more.

The newest PDR® to meet a growing need!

PDR® for Nutritional Supplements™

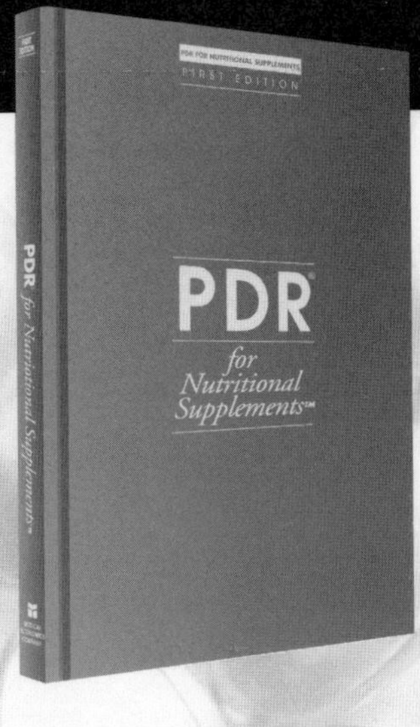

The latest figures show that 75% of Americans are currently using nutritional supplements on a regular basis. These supplements include:

- ■ Vitamins
- ■ Minerals
- ■ Sports nutritional products
- ■ Amino acids
- ■ Probiotics
- ■ Metabolites
- ■ Hormones
- ■ Enzymes
- ■ Cartilage products

That makes it more important than ever for you to know the facts about these supplements: How real are their benefits? What are their side effects? What are the potential interactions with prescription and OTC drugs, food, alcohol and tobacco? What dosages are appropriate?

Now healthcare professionals can have the facts at their fingertips with the *PDR for Nutritional Supplements,* the first comprehensive, unbiased source of solid, evidence-based information covering a full range of nutritional supplements. A detailed analysis of each supplement, including a clinical research summary, is presented in a clear, easy-to-read format.

The *PDR for Nutritional Supplements* provides practitioners with the most current and reliable information to help them assist their patients in making more educated choices.

The science behind the supplements

"In a part of the health field not known for its devotion to rigorous science, Dr. Hendler brings to the practitioner and the curious patient a wealth of hard facts. Easy reading, well referenced. A welcome addition to the classic PDR."

Roger Guillemin, M.D., Ph.D.
Nobel Laureate in Physiology and Medicine

"Assaulted from every angle by strident nutritional claims, today's wary consumer is in greater need of reliable information than ever before. This important new volume supplies the unbiased facts quickly, concisely, with authority…A beacon in the shadowy world of nutritional quackery and hype and an invaluable guide to the supplements that really work."

Susan Calvert Finn, Ph.D., R.D., F.A.D.A.
Past President, American Dietetic Association
Clinical Professor, Ohio State University

"This book is a timely and superbly written exploration of the dynamic field of supplements…A brilliant presentation of complex information in a logical and appropriately critical manner."

Walter H. Glinsmann, M.D.
Past Associate Director for Clinical Nutrition, FDA Center for Food Safety and Applied Nutrition
Fellow & Adjunct Professor, Center for Food and Nutrition Policy, Georgetown University

FOREWORD

Welcome to the 2002 edition of the *PDR Companion Guide*™, the unique handbook that, in conjunction with *Physicians' Desk Reference*®, provides you with a complete drug selection system. From its Indications Index, which permits you to instantly identify the full range of alternatives, to its Contraindications Index, which just as swiftly singles out alternatives to avoid, the Guide is designed to make safe, effective prescribing as fast, easy, and accurate as possible. Whether the challenge is identification of an unknown tablet or capsule, detecting the source of an adverse reaction, or avoiding a negative interaction, the *PDR Companion Guide* provides the tools you need to quickly find the answer. Here's a brief overview of the many facilities the Guide offers:

Interactions Index. In this section you'll find an entry for each product described in *PDR* and its companion volumes. Listed are generic compounds and dietary items that may interact with the product, as well as the specific brands containing each generic ingredient. A brief description of the interaction also appears. (Because product labeling varies in the scope of its interaction reporting, be sure to check the listing for each product in the patient's regimen.)

Food Interactions Cross-Reference. If you suspect an interaction with a specific dietary item, turn to this section. There you will find potential drug/food and drug/alcohol interactions cross-referenced alphabetically by the name or type of food. Each entry includes a list of implicated drugs and a brief description of each interaction.

Side Effects Index. When a multi-drug regimen masks the source of a side effect, this section provides the solution. It contains an alphabetical list of the more than 3,600 distinct reactions cited throughout *PDR* and its companion volumes. Each entry includes an alphabetical list of the brands that have been associated with the problem. To help target the most likely offenders, incidence data are included whenever found in the official labeling.

Indications Index. If you need to locate an alternative to a problem medication—or simply want to review the full range of options for a particular diagnosis—turn to this part of the book. Here each indication found in *PDR* and its companions is listed alphabetically, with a cross-reference to all brands approved for that purpose. For easy comparison, the listings include the generic name and manufacturer of each product. (Only FDA-approved indications are referenced.)

Off-Label Treatment Guide. This section picks up where *PDR's* comprehensive index of approved indications leaves off. It identifies medications routinely used—but never formally approved—for treatment of nearly 1,000 specific medical problems. If, for any reason, none of the products approved for a particular indication meet your needs, this guide will quickly inform you of the most common off-label alternatives. The entries have been restricted to legitimate uses well-documented in the peer-reviewed literature, so you can be confident you're considering only the most commonly accepted alternatives.

Contraindications Index. When therapy is complicated by other medical conditions, this convenient index will enable you to quickly eliminate contraindicated drugs from consideration. Here each contraindication cited in *PDR* is listed alphabetically, together with the drugs to avoid in its presence.

International Drug Name Index. This section enables you to quickly determine a U.S. equivalent when you're confronted with a foreign medication. The index gives you the product's country of origin, the closest domestic generic equivalent, all associated *PDR* brand-name entries, and the *PDR* page number of each. Included are over 33,000 entries covering products from 20 nations, including five countries new to the index this year. Prescribing a U.S. substitute has never been easier!

Generic Availability Guide. If you've ever had trouble remembering whether there's a generic alternative for a particular brand, you're sure to appreciate this handy guide. It alerts you to the existence of alternatives, *form by form, and strength by strength.* Included are all prescription drugs described in *PDR* and *PDR For Ophthalmic Medicines*™.

Imprint Identification Guide. This comprehensive table permits you to quickly establish the identity of virtually any unknown tablet or capsule. Organized alphabetically by imprint, it supplies the brand or generic name of the drug, its strength and manufacturer, and, to confirm its identity, its color, form, and shape.

Based on the FDA-approved labeling in the 2002 editions of *Physicians' Desk Reference*® and *PDR for Ophthalmic Medicines*™ and the 2001 edition of *PDR for Nonprescription Drugs and Dietary Supplements*™—and augmented with a wealth of authoritative data from such *PDR* affiliates as *Red Book*® and Micromedex, Inc.—the entries in the *PDR Companion Guide* cover some 2,900 domestic drug products. Please note, however, that because the entries in the Indications, Contraindications, Interactions, and Side Effects indices are derived directly from the FDA-sanctioned prescribing information published by *PDR*, only products described in *Physicians' Desk Reference* and its main companion volumes are cited in these sections.

Please note, too, that the publisher cannot guarantee that all entries are totally accurate or complete, nor is the publisher responsible for misuse of a product due to typographical error. Remember that important qualifications of the information listed in these indices may reside in the underlying text. Use this guide as a convenient cross-reference; but consult the *PDR* text, as well as the medical literature, when more detailed information is needed.

Other Prescribing Aids from PDR

For those times when all you need is quick confirmation of a particular dosage, you'll appreciate the convenience of the *PDR Pharmacopoeia™ Pocket Dosing Guide*. This handy little book can accompany you wherever you need to go, around the office or on rounds. Only slightly larger than an index card and a half-inch thick, it fits easily into any pocket, while providing you with FDA-approved dosing recommendations for over 1,500 drugs. Unlike other condensed drug references, it's drawn almost exclusively from the FDA-approved drug labeling published in *Physicians' Desk Reference*. And its tabular presentation makes lookups a breeze. At $9.95 a copy, it's a tool you really can't afford to be without.

Recently, the use of over-the-counter nutritional supplements has sky-rocketed, and *PDR* has responded with a brand new medical reference covering this unfamiliar—even exotic—set of agents. Entitled *PDR® for Nutritional Supplements™*, it offers the latest scientific consensus on hundreds of popular supplement products, including an array of amino acids, co-factors, fatty acids, probiotics, phytoestrogens, phytosterols, over-the-counter hormones, hormonal precursors, and much more. Focused on the scientific evidence for each supplement's claims, this unique reference offers you today's most detailed, informed, and objective overview of a burgeoning new area in the field of self-treatment. To protect your patients from bogus remedies and steer them towards truly beneficial products, this book is a must.

For counseling patients who favor herbal remedies, another *PDR* reference may prove equally valuable. Now in its second edition, *PDR® for Herbal Medicines™* provides you with the latest science-based assessment of some 700 botanicals. Indexed by scientific, common, and brand names (as well as Western, Asian, and homeopathic indications) this volume also includes a Side Effects Index, a Drug/Herb Interactions Guide, an Herb Identification Guide with nearly 400 color photos, and a Safety Guide that lists herbs to be avoided during pregnancy and nursing and herbs to be used only under professional supervision. Although botanical products are not officially regulated or monitored in the United States, *PDR for Herbal Medicines* provides you the closest analog to FDA-approved labeling—the findings of the German Regulatory Authority's herbal watchdog agency, Commission E.

PDR and its major companion volumes are also found in the *PDR® Electronic Library™* on CD-ROM, now used in over 100,000 practices. This Windows-compatible disc provides users with a complete database of *PDR* prescribing information, electronically searchable for instant retrieval. A standard subscription includes *PDR's* sophisticated search software and an extensive file of chemical structures, illustrations, and full-color product photographs. Optional enhancements include the complete contents of *The Merck Manual Seventeenth Edition, Stedman's Medical Dictionary*, and *Stedman's Spellchecker*. For anyone who wants to run a fast double check on a proposed prescription, there's also the *PDR® Drug Interactions and Side Effects System™*—software capable of automatically screening a 20-drug regimen for conflicts, then proposing alternatives for any problematic medication. This unique decision-making tool comes free with the *PDR Electronic Library*.

Remember, too, that the contents of *PDR* and its main companion volumes can always be found on the Internet at **www.pdr.net**. For more information on these or any other members of the growing family of *PDR* products, please call, toll-free, 1-800-232-7379 or fax 201-573-4956.

SECTION 1

INTERACTIONS INDEX

Cataloged in this section are all interactions found during a review of the labeling published in *PDR®*, *PDR For Nonprescription Drugs and Dietary Supplements™*, and *PDR For Ophthalmic Medicines™*. The list is arranged alphabetically by brand or, when applicable, generic name.

Whenever appropriate, each brand-name heading is followed by a summary of the major pharmaceutical categories with which the product is said to interact. Beneath this summary is an alphabetical list of the compounds in these categories, each followed by a brief notation regarding the results of concurrent administration with the brand in question. After each notation is an alphabetical list of the brands of the compound found in *PDR®* and its companion volumes. Page numbers refer to the 2002 editions of *PDR®* and *PDR for Ophthalmic Medicines™* and the 2001 edition of *PDR for Nonprescription Drugs and Dietary Supplements™*, which is published later each year. A key to the symbols denoting the companion volumes appears in the bottom margin of every other page.

Following the list of interactive drugs is a similar list of foods. Note that interactions with alcohol are listed here as well.

This index lists only interactions cited in official prescribing information as published by *PDR®*. Because product labeling varies in the scope of its interaction reporting, the most prudent course is to check each product in the patient's regimen. Note also that cross-sensitivity reactions and effects on laboratory results are not included in the listings.

8-MOP CAPSULES
(Methoxsalen) 1727
May interact with phenothiazines, sulfonamides, tetracyclines, thiazides, and certain other agents. Compounds in these categories include:

Anthralin (Concomitant therapy, either topically or systemically, with photosensitizing agents requires special care). Products include:
- Psoriatec Cream 3247

Bendroflumethiazide (Concomitant therapy, either topically or systemically, with photosensitizing agents requires special care). Products include:
- Corzide 40/5 Tablets 2247
- Corzide 80/5 Tablets 2247

Chlorothiazide (Concomitant therapy, either topically or systemically, with photosensitizing agents requires special care). Products include:
- Aldoclor Tablets 2035
- Diuril Oral 2087

Chlorothiazide Sodium (Concomitant therapy, either topically or systemically, with photosensitizing agents requires special care). Products include:
- Diuril Sodium Intravenous 2086

Chlorpromazine (Concomitant therapy, either topically or systemically, with photosensitizing agents requires special care). Products include:
- Thorazine Suppositories 1656

Chlorpromazine Hydrochloride (Concomitant therapy, either topically or systemically, with photosensitizing agents requires special care). Products include:
- Thorazine 1656

Chlorpropamide (Concomitant therapy, either topically or systemically, with photosensitizing agents requires special care). Products include:
- Diabinese Tablets 2680

Coal Tar (Concomitant therapy, either topically or systemically, with photosensitizing agents requires special care). Products include:
- Tegrin Dandruff Shampoo - Extra Conditioning .... ▣623
- Tegrin Dandruff Shampoo - Fresh Herbal .... ▣624
- Tegrin Skin Cream .... ▣624

Demeclocycline Hydrochloride (Concomitant therapy, either topically or systemically, with photosensitizing agents requires special care). Products include:
- Declomycin Tablets 1855

Doxycycline Calcium (Concomitant therapy, either topically or systemically, with photosensitizing agents requires special care). Products include:
- Vibramycin Calcium Oral Suspension Syrup 2735

Doxycycline Hyclate (Concomitant therapy, either topically or systemically, with photosensitizing agents requires special care). Products include:
- Doryx Coated Pellet Filled Capsules 3357
- Periostat Tablets 1208
- Vibramycin Hyclate Capsules 2735
- Vibramycin Hyclate Intravenous 2737
- Vibra-Tabs Film Coated Tablets 2735

Doxycycline Monohydrate (Concomitant therapy, either topically or systemically, with photosensitizing agents requires special care). Products include:
- Monodox Capsules 2442
- Vibramycin Monohydrate for Oral Suspension 2735

Fluphenazine Decanoate (Concomitant therapy, either topically or systemically, with photosensitizing agents requires special care).
No products indexed under this heading.

Fluphenazine Enanthate (Concomitant therapy, either topically or systemically, with photosensitizing agents requires special care).
No products indexed under this heading.

Fluphenazine Hydrochloride (Concomitant therapy, either topically or systemically, with photosensitizing agents requires special care).
No products indexed under this heading.

Glipizide (Concomitant therapy, either topically or systemically, with photosensitizing agents requires special care). Products include:
- Glucotrol Tablets 2692
- Glucotrol XL Extended Release Tablets 2693

Glyburide (Concomitant therapy, either topically or systemically, with photosensitizing agents requires special care). Products include:
- DiaBeta Tablets 741
- Glucovance Tablets 1086

Griseofulvin (Concomitant therapy, either topically or systemically, with photosensitizing agents requires special care). Products include:
- Grifulvin V Tablets Microsize and Oral Suspension Microsize 2518
- Gris-PEG Tablets 2661

Hydrochlorothiazide (Concomitant therapy, either topically or systemically, with photosensitizing agents requires special care). Products include:
- Accuretic Tablets 2614
- Aldoril Tablets 2039
- Atacand HCT Tablets 597
- Avalide Tablets 1070
- Diovan HCT Tablets 2338
- Dyazide Capsules 1515
- HydroDIURIL Tablets 2108
- Hyzaar 2109
- Inderide Tablets 3517
- Inderide LA Long-Acting Capsules 3519
- Lotensin HCT Tablets 2367
- Maxzide 1008
- Micardis HCT Tablets 1051
- Microzide Capsules 3414
- Moduretic Tablets 2138
- Monopril HCT 1094
- Prinzide Tablets 2168
- Timolide Tablets 2187
- Uniretic Tablets 3178
- Vaseretic Tablets 2204
- Zestoretic Tablets 695
- Ziac Tablets 1887

Hydroflumethiazide (Concomitant therapy, either topically or systemically, with photosensitizing agents requires special care). Products include:
- Diucardin Tablets 3494

Mesoridazine Besylate (Concomitant therapy, either topically or systemically, with photosensitizing agents requires special care). Products include:
- Serentil 1057

Methacycline Hydrochloride (Concomitant therapy, either topically or systemically, with photosensitizing agents requires special care).
No products indexed under this heading.

Methotrimeprazine (Concomitant therapy, either topically or systemically, with photosensitizing agents

requires special care).
No products indexed under this heading.

Methyclothiazide (Concomitant therapy, either topically or systemically, with photosensitizing agents requires special care).
No products indexed under this heading.

Methylene Blue (Concomitant therapy, either topically or systemically, with photosensitizing agents requires special care). Products include:
Prosed/DS Tablets 3268
Urimax Tablets 1769
Urised Tablets 2876

Minocycline Hydrochloride (Concomitant therapy, either topically or systemically, with photosensitizing agents requires special care). Products include:
Dynacin Capsules 2019
Minocin Intravenous 1862
Minocin Oral Suspension 1865
Minocin Pellet-Filled Capsules 1863

Nalidixic Acid (Concomitant therapy, either topically or systemically, with photosensitizing agents requires special care).
No products indexed under this heading.

Oxytetracycline Hydrochloride (Concomitant therapy, either topically or systemically, with photosensitizing agents requires special care). Products include:
Terra-Cortril Ophthalmic Suspension 2716
Urobiotic-250 Capsules 2731

Perphenazine (Concomitant therapy, either topically or systemically, with photosensitizing agents requires special care). Products include:
Etrafon 3115
Trilafon 3160

Polythiazide (Concomitant therapy, either topically or systemically, with photosensitizing agents requires special care). Products include:
Minizide Capsules 2700
Renese Tablets 2712

Prochlorperazine (Concomitant therapy, either topically or systemically, with photosensitizing agents requires special care). Products include:
Compazine 1505

Promethazine Hydrochloride (Concomitant therapy, either topically or systemically, with photosensitizing agents requires special care). Products include:
Mepergan Injection 3539
Phenergan Injection 3553
Phenergan 3556
Phenergan Syrup 3554
Phenergan with Codeine Syrup 3557
Phenergan with Dextromethorphan Syrup 3559
Phenergan VC Syrup 3560
Phenergan VC with Codeine Syrup .. 3561

Rose Bengal (Concomitant therapy, either topically or systemically, with photosensitizing agents requires special care).
No products indexed under this heading.

Sulfacytine (Concomitant therapy, either topically or systemically, with photosensitizing agents requires special care).
No products indexed under this heading.

Sulfamethizole (Concomitant therapy, either topically or systemically, with photosensitizing agents requires special care). Products include:
Urobiotic-250 Capsules 2731

Sulfamethoxazole (Concomitant therapy, either topically or systemically, with photosensitizing agents requires special care). Products include:
Bactrim 2949
Septra Suspension 2265
Septra Tablets 2265
Septra DS Tablets 2265

Sulfasalazine (Concomitant therapy, either topically or systemically, with photosensitizing agents requires special care). Products include:
Azulfidine EN-tabs Tablets 2775

Sulfinpyrazone (Concomitant therapy, either topically or systemically, with photosensitizing agents requires special care).
No products indexed under this heading.

Sulfisoxazole (Concomitant therapy, either topically or systemically, with photosensitizing agents requires special care).
No products indexed under this heading.

Sulfisoxazole Acetyl (Concomitant therapy, either topically or systemically, with photosensitizing agents requires special care). Products include:
Pediazole Suspension 3050

Sulfisoxazole Diolamine (Concomitant therapy, either topically or systemically, with photosensitizing agents requires special care).
No products indexed under this heading.

Tetracycline Hydrochloride (Concomitant therapy, either topically or systemically, with photosensitizing agents requires special care).
No products indexed under this heading.

Thioridazine Hydrochloride (Concomitant therapy, either topically or systemically, with photosensitizing agents requires special care). Products include:
Thioridazine Hydrochloride Tablets 2289

Tolazamide (Concomitant therapy, either topically or systemically, with photosensitizing agents requires special care).
No products indexed under this heading.

Tolbutamide (Concomitant therapy, either topically or systemically, with photosensitizing agents requires special care).
No products indexed under this heading.

Trifluoperazine Hydrochloride (Concomitant therapy, either topically or systemically, with photosensitizing agents requires special care). Products include:
Stelazine 1640

A + D ORIGINAL OINTMENT

(Lanolin, Petrolatum) .... ▣733
None cited in PDR database.

A + D OINTMENT WITH ZINC OXIDE

(Dimethicone, Zinc Oxide) .... ▣733
None cited in PDR database.

ABELCET INJECTION

(Amphotericin B) 1273
May interact with aminoglycosides, antineoplastics, corticosteroids, curariform skeletal muscle relaxants, cardiac glycosides, imidazoles, and certain other agents. Compounds in these categories include:

ACTH (Concurrent use may potentiate hypokalemia which could predispose the patient to cardiac dysfunction).
No products indexed under this heading.

Altretamine (Concurrent use may enhance the potential for renal toxicity, bronchospasm, and hypotension). Products include:
Hexalen Capsules 2226

Amikacin Sulfate (Concurrent use may enhance the potential for drug-induced renal toxicity).
No products indexed under this heading.

Anastrozole (Concurrent use may enhance the potential for renal toxicity, bronchospasm, and hypotension). Products include:
Arimidex Tablets 659

Asparaginase (Concurrent use may enhance the potential for renal toxicity, bronchospasm, and hypotension). Products include:
Elspar for Injection 2092

Atracurium Besylate (Amphotericin B-induced hypokalemia may enhance the curariform effect of skeletal relaxants).
No products indexed under this heading.

Betamethasone Acetate (Concurrent use may potentiate hypokalemia which could predispose the patient to cardiac dysfunction). Products include:
Celestone Soluspan Injectable Suspension 3097

Betamethasone Sodium Phosphate (Concurrent use may potentiate hypokalemia which could predispose the patient to cardiac dysfunction). Products include:
Celestone Soluspan Injectable Suspension 3097

Bicalutamide (Concurrent use may enhance the potential for renal toxicity, bronchospasm, and hypotension). Products include:
Casodex Tablets 662

Bleomycin Sulfate (Concurrent use may enhance the potential for renal toxicity, bronchospasm, and hypotension).
No products indexed under this heading.

Busulfan (Concurrent use may enhance the potential for renal toxicity, bronchospasm, and hypotension). Products include:
Myleran Tablets 1603

Carboplatin (Concurrent use may enhance the potential for renal toxicity, bronchospasm, and hypotension). Products include:
Paraplatin for Injection 1126

Carmustine (BCNU) (Concurrent use may enhance the potential for renal toxicity, bronchospasm, and hypotension). Products include:
Gliadel Wafer 1723

Chlorambucil (Concurrent use may enhance the potential for renal toxicity, bronchospasm, and hypotension). Products include:
Leukeran Tablets 1591

Cisplatin (Concurrent use may enhance the potential for renal toxicity, bronchospasm, and hypotension).
No products indexed under this heading.

Clotrimazole (Antagonism between amphotericin B and imidazole derivatives, which inhibit ergosterol synthesis, has been reported; clinical significance of this finding has not been determined). Products include:
Gyne-Lotrimin 3, 3-Day Cream .... ▣741
Lotrimin AF Cream, Lotion, Solution, and Jock Itch Cream .... ▣742
Lotrimin 3128
Lotrisone 3129
Mycelex Troche 573
Mycelex-7 Combination-Pack Vaginal Inserts & External Vulvar Cream .... ▣614
Mycelex-7 Vaginal Cream .... ▣614
Mycelex-7 Vaginal Cream with 7 Disposable Applicators .... ▣614

Cortisone Acetate (Concurrent use may potentiate hypokalemia which could predispose the patient to cardiac dysfunction). Products include:
Cortone Acetate Injectable Suspension 2059
Cortone Acetate Tablets 2061

Cyclophosphamide (Concurrent use may enhance the potential for renal toxicity, bronchospasm, and hypotension).
No products indexed under this heading.

Cyclosporine (Concurrent initiation of cyclosporine and Abelcet within several days of bone marrow ablation may be associated with increased nephrotoxicity). Products include:
Gengraf Capsules 457
Neoral Soft Gelatin Capsules 2380
Neoral Oral Solution 2380
Sandimmune 2388

Dacarbazine (Concurrent use may enhance the potential for renal toxicity, bronchospasm, and hypotension). Products include:
DTIC-Dome 902

Daunorubicin Citrate (Concurrent use may enhance the potential for renal toxicity, bronchospasm, and hypotension). Products include:
DaunoXome Injection 1442

Daunorubicin Hydrochloride (Concurrent use may enhance the potential for renal toxicity, bronchospasm, and hypotension). Products include:
Cerubidine for Injection 947

Denileukin Diftitox (Concurrent use may enhance the potential for renal toxicity, bronchospasm, and hypotension).
No products indexed under this heading.

Deslanoside (Concurrent use may induce hypokalemia and may potentiate digitalis toxicity).
No products indexed under this heading.

Dexamethasone (Concurrent use may potentiate hypokalemia which could predispose the patient to cardiac dysfunction). Products include:
Decadron Elixir 2078
Decadron Tablets 2079
TobraDex Ophthalmic Ointment 542
TobraDex Ophthalmic Suspension .. 541

Dexamethasone Acetate (Concurrent use may potentiate hypokalemia which could predispose the patient to cardiac dysfunction).
No products indexed under this heading.

Dexamethasone Sodium Phosphate (Concurrent use may potentiate hypokalemia which could predispose the patient to cardiac dysfunction). Products include:
Decadron Phosphate Injection 2081
Decadron Phosphate Sterile Ophthalmic Ointment 2083
Decadron Phosphate Sterile Ophthalmic Solution 2084
NeoDecadron Sterile Ophthalmic Solution 2144

Digitoxin (Concurrent use may induce hypokalemia and may potentiate digitalis toxicity).
No products indexed under this heading.

Digoxin (Concurrent use may induce hypokalemia and may potentiate digitalis toxicity). Products include:
Digitek Tablets 1003
Lanoxicaps Capsules 1574
Lanoxin Injection 1581
Lanoxin Tablets 1587
Lanoxin Elixir Pediatric 1578
Lanoxin Injection Pediatric 1584

Docetaxel (Concurrent use may enhance the potential for renal toxicity, bronchospasm, and hypotension). Products include:
Taxotere for Injection Concentrate 778

Doxorubicin Hydrochloride (Concurrent use may enhance the potential for renal toxicity, bronchospasm, and hypotension). Products include:
Adriamycin PFS/RDF Injection 2767
Doxil Injection 566

Epirubicin Hydrochloride (Concurrent use may enhance the potential for renal toxicity, bronchospasm, and hypotension). Products include:
Ellence Injection 2806

Estramustine Phosphate Sodium (Concurrent use may enhance the potential for renal toxicity, bronchospasm, and hypotension). Products include:
Emcyt Capsules 2810

Etoposide (Concurrent use may enhance the potential for renal toxicity, bronchospasm, and hypotension).
No products indexed under this heading.

Exemestane (Concurrent use may enhance the potential for renal toxicity, bronchospasm, and hypotension). Products include:
Aromasin Tablets 2769

Floxuridine (Concurrent use may enhance the potential for renal toxicity, bronchospasm, and hypotension). Products include:
Sterile FUDR 2974

Fluconazole (Antagonism between amphotericin B and imidazole derivatives, which inhibit ergosterol synthesis, has been reported; clinical significance of this finding has not been determined). Products include:
Diflucan Tablets, Injection, and Oral Suspension 2681

Flucytosine (Concurrent use may increase the toxicity of flucytosine by possibly increasing its cellular uptake and/or impairing its renal excretion). Products include:
Ancobon Capsules 1730

Fludrocortisone Acetate (Concurrent use may potentiate hypokalemia which could predispose the patient to cardiac dysfunction). Products include:
Florinef Acetate Tablets 2250

Fluorouracil (Concurrent use may enhance the potential for renal toxicity, bronchospasm, and hypotension). Products include:
Carac Cream 1222
Efudex 1733
Fluoroplex 552

Flutamide (Concurrent use may enhance the potential for renal toxicity, bronchospasm, and hypotension). Products include:
Eulexin Capsules 3118

Gemcitabine Hydrochloride (Concurrent use may enhance the potential for renal toxicity, bronchospasm, and hypotension). Products include:
Gemzar for Injection 1919

Gentamicin Sulfate (Concurrent use may enhance the potential for drug-induced renal toxicity). Products include:
Genoptic Ophthalmic Ointment .... ⊙239
Genoptic Sterile Ophthalmic Solution .... ⊙239
Pred-G Ophthalmic Suspension .... ⊙247
Pred-G Sterile Ophthalmic Ointment .... ⊙248

Hydrocortisone (Concurrent use may potentiate hypokalemia which could predispose the patient to cardiac dysfunction). Products include:
Anusol-HC Cream 2.5% 2237
Cipro HC Otic Suspension 540
Cortaid Intensive Therapy Cream .... ▣717
Cortaid Maximum Strength Cream .... ▣717
Cortisporin Ophthalmic Suspension Sterile .... ⊙297
Cortizone•5 .... ▣699
Cortizone•10 .... ▣699
Cortizone•10 Plus Creme .... ▣700
Cortizone for Kids Creme .... ▣699
Hydrocortone Tablets 2106
Massengill Medicated Soft Cloth Towelette .... ▣753
VōSoL HC Otic Solution 3356

Hydrocortisone Acetate (Concurrent use may potentiate hypokalemia which could predispose the patient to cardiac dysfunction). Products include:
Analpram-HC 1338
Anusol HC-1 Hydrocortisone Anti-Itch Cream .... ▣689
Anusol-HC Suppositories 2238
Cortaid .... ▣717
Cortifoam Rectal Foam 3170
Cortisporin-TC Otic Suspension 2246
Hydrocortone Acetate Injectable Suspension 2103
Pramosone 1343
Proctocort Suppositories 2264
ProctoFoam-HC 3177
Terra-Cortril Ophthalmic Suspension 2716

Hydrocortisone Sodium Phosphate (Concurrent use may potentiate hypokalemia which could predispose the patient to cardiac dysfunction). Products include:
Hydrocortone Phosphate Injection, Sterile 2105

Hydrocortisone Sodium Succinate (Concurrent use may potentiate hypokalemia which could predispose the patient to cardiac dysfunction).
No products indexed under this heading.

Hydroxyurea (Concurrent use may enhance the potential for renal toxicity, bronchospasm, and hypotension). Products include:
Mylocel Tablets 2227

Idarubicin Hydrochloride (Concurrent use may enhance the potential for renal toxicity, bronchospasm, and hypotension). Products include:
Idamycin PFS Injection 2825

Ifosfamide (Concurrent use may enhance the potential for renal toxicity, bronchospasm, and hypotension). Products include:
Ifex for Injection 1123

Interferon alfa-2A, Recombinant (Concurrent use may enhance the potential for renal toxicity, bronchospasm, and hypotension). Products include:
Roferon-A Injection 2996

Interferon alfa-2B, Recombinant (Concurrent use may enhance the potential for renal toxicity, bronchospasm, and hypotension). Products include:
Intron A for Injection 3120
Rebetron Combination Therapy 3153

Irinotecan Hydrochloride (Concurrent use may enhance the potential for renal toxicity, bronchospasm, and hypotension).
No products indexed under this heading.

Kanamycin Sulfate (Concurrent use may enhance the potential for drug-induced renal toxicity).
No products indexed under this heading.

Ketoconazole (Antagonism between amphotericin B and imidazole derivatives, which inhibit ergosterol synthesis, has been reported; clinical significance of this finding has not been determined). Products include:
Nizoral 2% Cream 3620
Nizoral A-D Shampoo 2008
Nizoral 2% Shampoo 2007
Nizoral Tablets 1791

Leukocyte Transfusions (Concurrent use has resulted in acute pulmonary toxicity; concurrent use should be avoided).

Levamisole Hydrochloride (Concurrent use may enhance the potential for renal toxicity, bronchospasm, and hypotension). Products include:
Ergamisol Tablets 1789

Lomustine (CCNU) (Concurrent use may enhance the potential for renal toxicity, bronchospasm, and hypotension).
No products indexed under this heading.

Mechlorethamine Hydrochloride (Concurrent use may enhance the potential for renal toxicity, bronchospasm, and hypotension). Products include:
Mustargen for Injection 2142

Megestrol Acetate (Concurrent use may enhance the potential for renal toxicity, bronchospasm, and hypotension). Products include:
Megace Oral Suspension 1124

Melphalan (Concurrent use may enhance the potential for renal toxicity, bronchospasm, and hypotension). Products include:
Alkeran Tablets 1466

Mercaptopurine (Concurrent use may enhance the potential for renal toxicity, bronchospasm, and hypotension). Products include:
Purinethol Tablets 1615

Methotrexate Sodium (Concurrent use may enhance the potential for renal toxicity, bronchospasm, and hypotension).
No products indexed under this heading.

Methylprednisolone Acetate (Concurrent use may potentiate hypokalemia which could predispose the patient to cardiac dysfunction). Products include:
Depo-Medrol Injectable Suspension 2795

Methylprednisolone Sodium Succinate (Concurrent use may potentiate hypokalemia which could predispose the patient to cardiac dysfunction). Products include:
Solu-Medrol Sterile Powder 2855

Miconazole (Antagonism between amphotericin B and imidazole derivatives, which inhibit ergosterol synthesis, has been reported; clinical significance of this finding has not been determined).
No products indexed under this heading.

Miconazole Nitrate (Antagonism between amphotericin B and imidazole derivatives, which inhibit ergosterol synthesis, has been reported; clinical significance of this finding has not been determined). Products include:
Desenex .... ▣668
Desenex Jock Itch Spray Powder .... ▣668
Lotrimin AF Spray Powder, Spray Liquid, Spray Deodorant Powder, Shaker Powder and Jock Itch Spray Powder .... ▣742

Mitomycin (Mitomycin-C) (Concurrent use may enhance the potential for renal toxicity, bronchospasm, and hypotension).
No products indexed under this heading.

Mitotane (Concurrent use may enhance the potential for renal toxicity, bronchospasm, and hypotension).
No products indexed under this heading.

Mitoxantrone Hydrochloride (Concurrent use may enhance the potential for renal toxicity, bronchospasm, and hypotension). Products include:
Novantrone for Injection 1760

Mivacurium Chloride (Amphotericin B-induced hypokalemia may enhance the curariform effect of skeletal relaxants).
No products indexed under this heading.

Paclitaxel (Concurrent use may enhance the potential for renal toxicity, bronchospasm, and hypotension). Products include:
Taxol Injection 1129

Pancuronium Bromide (Amphotericin B-induced hypokalemia may enhance the curariform effect of skeletal relaxants).
No products indexed under this heading.

Pentamidine Isethionate (Concurrent use may enhance the potential for drug-induced renal toxicity).
No products indexed under this heading.

Prednisolone Acetate (Concurrent use may potentiate hypokalemia which could predispose the patient to cardiac dysfunction). Products include:
Blephamide Ophthalmic Ointment 547
Blephamide Ophthalmic Suspension 548
Poly-Pred Liquifilm Ophthalmic Suspension .... ⊙245
Pred Forte Ophthalmic Suspension .... ⊙246
Pred Mild Sterile Ophthalmic Suspension .... ⊙249
Pred-G Ophthalmic Suspension .... ⊙247
Pred-G Sterile Ophthalmic Ointment .... ⊙248

Prednisolone Sodium Phosphate (Concurrent use may potentiate hypokalemia which could predispose the patient to cardiac dysfunction). Products include:
Pediapred Oral Solution 1170

Prednisolone Tebutate (Concurrent use may potentiate hypokalemia which could predispose the patient to cardiac dysfunction).
No products indexed under this heading.

Prednisone (Concurrent use may potentiate hypokalemia which could predispose the patient to cardiac dysfunction). Products include:
Prednisone 3064

Procarbazine Hydrochloride (Concurrent use may enhance the potential for renal toxicity, bronchospasm, and hypotension). Products include:
Matulane Capsules 3246

Rapacuronium Bromide (Amphotericin B-induced hypokalemia may enhance the curariform effect of skeletal relaxants).
No products indexed under this heading.

Rocuronium Bromide (Amphotericin B-induced hypokalemia may enhance the curariform effect of skeletal relaxants). Products include:
Zemuron Injection 2491

Streptomycin Sulfate (Concurrent use may enhance the potential for drug-induced renal toxicity). Products include:
Streptomycin Sulfate Injection 2714

Streptozocin (Concurrent use may enhance the potential for renal toxicity, bronchospasm, and hypotension).
No products indexed under this heading.

Tamoxifen Citrate (Concurrent use may enhance the potential for renal toxicity, bronchospasm, and hypotension). Products include:
Nolvadex Tablets 678

Teniposide (Concurrent use may enhance the potential for renal toxicity, bronchospasm, and hypotension).
No products indexed under this heading.

Thioguanine (Concurrent use may enhance the potential for renal toxicity, bronchospasm, and hypotension). Products include:
Tabloid Tablets 1642

Thiotepa (Concurrent use may enhance the potential for renal toxicity, bronchospasm, and hypotension). Products include:
Thioplex for Injection 1765

Tobramycin (Concurrent use may enhance the potential for drug-induced renal toxicity). Products include:
TOBI Solution for Inhalation 1206
TobraDex Ophthalmic Ointment 542
TobraDex Ophthalmic Suspension 541
Tobrex Ophthalmic Ointment .... ⊙220
Tobrex Ophthalmic Solution .... ⊙221

Tobramycin Sulfate (Concurrent use may enhance the potential for drug-induced renal toxicity). Products include:
- Nebcin Vials, Hyporets & ADD-Vantage 1955

Topotecan Hydrochloride (Concurrent use may enhance the potential for renal toxicity, bronchospasm, and hypotension). Products include:
- Hycamtin for Injection 1546

Toremifene Citrate (Concurrent use may enhance the potential for renal toxicity, bronchospasm, and hypotension). Products include:
- Fareston Tablets 3237

Triamcinolone (Concurrent use may potentiate hypokalemia which could predispose the patient to cardiac dysfunction).
No products indexed under this heading.

Triamcinolone Acetonide (Concurrent use may potentiate hypokalemia which could predispose the patient to cardiac dysfunction). Products include:
- Azmacort Inhalation Aerosol 728
- Nasacort Nasal Inhaler 750
- Nasacort AQ Nasal Spray 752
- Tri-Nasal Spray 2274

Triamcinolone Diacetate (Concurrent use may potentiate hypokalemia which could predispose the patient to cardiac dysfunction).
No products indexed under this heading.

Triamcinolone Hexacetonide (Concurrent use may potentiate hypokalemia which could predispose the patient to cardiac dysfunction).
No products indexed under this heading.

Tubocurarine Chloride (Amphotericin B-induced hypokalemia may enhance the curariform effect of skeletal muscle relaxants).
No products indexed under this heading.

Valrubicin (Concurrent use may enhance the potential for renal toxicity, bronchospasm, and hypotension). Products include:
- Valstar Sterile Solution for Intravesical Instillation 1175

Vecuronium Bromide (Amphotericin B-induced hypokalemia may enhance the curariform effect of skeletal muscle relaxants). Products include:
- Norcuron for Injection 2478

Vincristine Sulfate (Concurrent use may enhance the potential for renal toxicity, bronchospasm, and hypotension).
No products indexed under this heading.

Vinorelbine Tartrate (Concurrent use may enhance the potential for renal toxicity, bronchospasm, and hypotension). Products include:
- Navelbine Injection 1604

Zidovudine (Potential for increased myelotoxicity and nephrotoxicity). Products include:
- Combivir Tablets 1502
- Retrovir 1625
- Retrovir IV Infusion 1629
- Trizivir Tablets 1669

ABREVA CREAM

(Docosanol) .... ▣744
None cited in PDR database.

ACCOLATE TABLETS

(Zafirlukast) 657
May interact with dihydropyridine calcium channel blockers, erythromycin, phenytoin, theophylline, and certain other agents. Compounds in these categories include:

Aminophylline (Rare cases of patients experiencing increased theophylline levels with or without clinical signs or symptoms of theophylline toxicity after addition of zafirlukast to an existing theophylline regimen have been reported; co-administration with liquid theophylline products has resulted in a decrease in the mean plasma levels of zafirlukast by approximately 30%).
No products indexed under this heading.

Amlodipine Besylate (Zafirlukast is known inhibitor of CYP3A4 in vitro; co-administration with other drugs known to be metabolized by this isoenzyme, such as dihydropyridine calcium channel blockers, should be undertaken with reasonable clinical monitoring; no formal interaction studies have been conducted). Products include:
- Lotrel Capsules 2370
- Norvasc Tablets 2704

Aspirin (Co-administration has resulted in mean increased plasma levels of zafirlukast by approximately 45%). Products include:
- Aggrenox Capsules 1026
- Alka-Seltzer .... ▣603
- Alka-Seltzer Lemon Lime Antacid and Pain Reliever Effervescent Tablets .... ▣603
- Alka-Seltzer Extra Strength Antacid and Pain Reliever Effervescent Tablets .... ▣603
- Alka-Seltzer PM Effervescent Tablets .... ▣605
- Genuine Bayer Tablets, Caplets and Gelcaps .... ▣606
- Extra Strength Bayer Caplets and Gelcaps .... ▣610
- Aspirin Regimen Bayer Children's Chewable Tablets (Orange or Cherry Flavored) .... ▣607
- Bayer, Aspirin Regimen .... ▣606
- Aspirin Regimen Bayer 81 mg Caplets with Calcium .... ▣607
- Genuine Bayer Professional Labeling (Aspirin Regimen Bayer) .... ▣608
- Extra Strength Bayer Arthritis Caplets .... ▣610
- Extra Strength Bayer Plus Caplets .... ▣610
- Extra Strength Bayer PM Caplets .... ▣611
- BC Powder .... ▣619
- BC Allergy Sinus Cold Powder .... ▣619
- Arthritis Strength BC Powder .... ▣619
- BC Sinus Cold Powder .... ▣619
- Darvon Compound-65 Pulvules 1910
- Ecotrin Enteric Coated Aspirin Low, Regular and Maximum Strength Tablets 1715
- Excedrin Extra-Strength Tablets, Caplets, and Geltabs .... ▣629
- Excedrin Migraine 1070
- Goody's Body Pain Formula Powder .... ▣620
- Goody's Extra Strength Headache Powder .... ▣620
- Goody's Extra Strength Pain Relief Tablets .... ▣620
- Percodan Tablets 1327
- Robaxisal Tablets 2939
- Soma Compound Tablets 3354
- Soma Compound w/Codeine Tablets 3355
- Vanquish Caplets .... ▣617

Astemizole (Zafirlukast is known inhibitor of CYP3A4 in vitro; co-administration with other drugs known to be metabolized by this isoenzyme, such as astemizole, should be undertaken with reasonable clinical monitoring; no formal interaction studies have been conducted).
No products indexed under this heading.

Carbamazepine (Zafirlukast is inhibitor of the cytochrome P4502C9 isoenzyme; co-administration with other drugs known to be metabolized by this isoenzyme, such as carbamazepine, should be undertaken with caution; no formal interaction studies have been conducted). Products include:
- Carbatrol Capsules 3234
- Tegretol/Tegretol-XR 2404

Cisapride (Zafirlukast is known inhibitor of CYP3A4 in vitro; co-administration with other drugs known to be metabolized by this isoenzyme, such as cisapride, should be undertaken with reasonable clinical monitoring; no formal interaction studies have been conducted).
No products indexed under this heading.

Cyclosporine (Zafirlukast is known inhibitor of CYP3A4 in vitro; co-administration with other drugs known to be metabolized by this isoenzyme, such as cyclosporine, should be undertaken with reasonable clinical monitoring; no formal interaction studies have been conducted). Products include:
- Gengraf Capsules 457
- Neoral Soft Gelatin Capsules 2380
- Neoral Oral Solution 2380
- Sandimmune 2388

Dyphylline (Rare cases of patients experiencing increased theophylline levels with or without clinical signs or symptoms of theophylline toxicity after addition of zafirlukast to an existing theophylline regimen have been reported; co-administration with liquid theophylline products has resulted in a decrease in the mean plasma levels of zafirlukast by approximately 30%). Products include:
- Lufyllin Tablets 3347
- Lufyllin-400 Tablets 3347
- Lufyllin-GG Elixir 3348
- Lufyllin-GG Tablets 3348

Erythromycin (Co-administration results in a decrease in the mean plasma levels of zafirlukast by approximately 40% due to decrease in zafirlukast bioavailability). Products include:
- Emgel 2% Topical Gel 1285
- Ery-Tab Tablets 448
- Erythromycin Base Filmtab Tablets . 454
- Erythromycin Delayed-Release Capsules, USP 455
- PCE Dispertab Tablets 498

Erythromycin Estolate (Co-administration results in a decrease in the mean plasma levels of zafirlukast by approximately 40% due to decrease in zafirlukast bioavailability).
No products indexed under this heading.

Erythromycin Ethylsuccinate (Co-administration results in a decrease in the mean plasma levels of zafirlukast by approximately 40% due to decrease in zafirlukast bioavailability). Products include:
- E.E.S. 450
- EryPed 446
- Pediazole Suspension 3050

Erythromycin Gluceptate (Co-administration results in a decrease in the mean plasma levels of zafirlukast by approximately 40% due to decrease in zafirlukast bioavailability).
No products indexed under this heading.

Erythromycin Stearate (Co-administration results in a decrease in the mean plasma levels of zafirlukast by approximately 40% due to decrease in zafirlukast bioavailability). Products include:
- Erythrocin Stearate Filmtab Tablets 452

Felodipine (Zafirlukast is known inhibitor of CYP3A4 in vitro; co-administration with other drugs known to be metabolized by this isoenzyme, such as dihydropyridine calcium channel blockers, should be undertaken with reasonable clinical monitoring; no formal interaction studies have been conducted). Products include:
- Lexxel Tablets 608
- Plendil Extended-Release Tablets ... 623

Fosphenytoin Sodium (Zafirlukast is known inhibitor of the cytochrome P4502C9 isoenzyme; co-administration with other drugs known to be metabolized by this isoenzyme, such as phenytoin, should be undertaken with caution; no formal interaction studies have been conducted). Products include:
- Cerebyx Injection 2619

Isradipine (Zafirlukast is known inhibitor of CYP3A4 in vitro; co-administration with other drugs known to be metabolized by this isoenzyme, such as dihydropyridine calcium channel blockers, should be undertaken with reasonable clinical monitoring; no formal interaction studies have been conducted). Products include:
- DynaCirc Capsules 2921
- DynaCirc CR Tablets 2923

Nicardipine Hydrochloride (Zafirlukast is known inhibitor of CYP3A4 in vitro; co-administration with other drugs known to be metabolized by this isoenzyme, such as dihydropyridine calcium channel blockers, should be undertaken with reasonable clinical monitoring; no formal interaction studies have been conducted). Products include:
- Cardene I.V. 3485

Nifedipine (Zafirlukast is known inhibitor of CYP3A4 in vitro; co-administration with other drugs known to be metabolized by this isoenzyme, such as dihydropyridine calcium channel blockers, should be undertaken with reasonable clinical monitoring; no formal interaction studies have been conducted). Products include:
- Adalat CC Tablets 877
- Procardia Capsules 2708
- Procardia XL Extended Release Tablets 2710

Nimodipine (Zafirlukast is known inhibitor of CYP3A4 in vitro; co-administration with other drugs known to be metabolized by this isoenzyme, such as dihydropyridine calcium channel blockers, should be undertaken with reasonable clinical monitoring; no formal interaction studies have been conducted). Products include:
- Nimotop Capsules 904

Phenytoin (Zafirlukast is known inhibitor of the cytochrome P4502C9 isoenzyme; co-administration with other drugs known to be metabolized by this isoenzyme, such as phenytoin, should be undertaken with caution; no formal interaction studies have been conducted). Products include:
- Dilantin Infatabs 2624
- Dilantin-125 Oral Suspension 2625

Phenytoin Sodium (Zafirlukast is known inhibitor of the cytochrome P4502C9 isoenzyme; co-administration with other drugs known to be metabolized by this isoenzyme, such as phenytoin, should be undertaken with caution; no formal interaction studies have been conducted). Products include:
- Dilantin Kapseals 2622

Terfenadine (Co-administration results in a decrease in the mean Cmax (-66%) and AUC (-54%) of zafirlukast; no effect of zafirlukast on terfenadine plasma concentrations or ECG parameters).
No products indexed under this heading.

Theophylline (Rare cases of patients experiencing increased theophylline levels with or without clinical signs or symptoms of theophylline toxicity after addition of zafirlukast to an existing theophylline regimen have been reported; co-administration with liquid theophylline products has resulted in a decrease in the mean plasma levels of zafirlukast by approximately 30%). Products include:

Aerolate 1361
Theo-Dur Extended-Release Tablets 1835
Uni-Dur Extended-Release Tablets .. 1841
Uniphyl 400 mg and 600 mg Tablets 2903

Theophylline Calcium Salicylate (Rare cases of patients experiencing increased theophylline levels with or without clinical signs or symptoms of theophylline toxicity after addition of zafirlukast to an existing theophylline regimen have been reported; co-administration with liquid theophylline products has resulted in a decrease in the mean plasma levels of zafirlukast by approximately 30%).
No products indexed under this heading.

Theophylline Sodium Glycinate (Rare cases of patients experiencing increased theophylline levels with or without clinical signs or symptoms of theophylline toxicity after addition of zafirlukast to an existing theophylline regimen have been reported; co-administration with liquid theophylline products has resulted in a decrease in the mean plasma levels of zafirlukast by approximately 30%).
No products indexed under this heading.

Tolbutamide (Zafirlukast is inhibitor of the cytochrome P4502C9 isoenzyme; co-administration with other drugs known to be metabolized by this isoenzyme, such as tolbutamide, should be undertaken with caution; no formal interaction studies have been conducted).
No products indexed under this heading.

Warfarin Sodium (Co-administration results in a significant increase in the mean AUC and half-life of S-warfarin producing a clinically significant increase in prothrombin time). Products include:
Coumadin for Injection 1243
Coumadin Tablets 1243
Warfarin Sodium Tablets, USP 3302

Food Interactions

Food, unspecified (Co-administration with food reduces mean bioavailability by approximately 40%; patients should be instructed to take Accolate at least 1 hour before or 2 hours after meals).

ACCUNEB INHALATION SOLUTION

(Albuterol Sulfate) 1230
May interact with beta blockers, monoamine oxidase inhibitors, potassium-depleting diuretics, sympathomimetics, tricyclic antidepressants, and certain other agents. Compounds in these categories include:

Acebutolol Hydrochloride (Co-administration with beta blockers inhibits the effects of each other). Products include:
Sectral Capsules 3589

Albuterol (Co-administration with other sympathomimetic agents increases the risk of adverse cardiovascular effects). Products include:
Proventil Inhalation Aerosol 3142
Ventolin Inhalation Aerosol and Refill 1679

Amitriptyline Hydrochloride (Co-administration with tricyclic antidepressants can potentiate the action of albuterol on the cardiovascular system). Products include:
Etrafon 3115
Limbitrol 1738

Amoxapine (Co-administration with tricyclic antidepressants can potentiate the action of albuterol on the cardiovascular system).
No products indexed under this heading.

Atenolol (Co-administration with beta blockers inhibits the effects of each other). Products include:
Tenoretic Tablets 690
Tenormin I.V. Injection 692

Bendroflumethiazide (Co-administration with non-potassium sparing diuretics can result in acute worsening of ECG changes and/or hypokalemia, especially when recommended dose of the beta agonist is exceeded; clinical significance of this interaction is unknown). Products include:
Corzide 40/5 Tablets 2247
Corzide 80/5 Tablets 2247

Betaxolol Hydrochloride (Co-administration with beta blockers inhibits the effects of each other). Products include:
Betoptic S Ophthalmic Suspension 537

Bisoprolol Fumarate (Co-administration with beta blockers inhibits the effects of each other). Products include:
Zebeta Tablets 1885
Ziac Tablets 1887

Bumetanide (Co-administration with non-potassium sparing diuretics can result in acute worsening of ECG changes and/or hypokalemia, especially when recommended dose of the beta agonist is exceeded; clinical significance of this interaction is unknown).
No products indexed under this heading.

Carteolol Hydrochloride (Co-administration with beta blockers inhibits the effects of each other). Products include:
Carteolol Hydrochloride Ophthalmic Solution USP, 1% ..... ⊙ 258
Ocupress Ophthalmic Solution, 1% Sterile .... ⊙ 303

Chlorothiazide (Co-administration with non-potassium sparing diuretics can result in acute worsening of ECG changes and/or hypokalemia, especially when recommended dose of the beta agonist is exceeded; clinical significance of this interaction is unknown). Products include:
Aldoclor Tablets 2035
Diuril Oral 2087

Chlorothiazide Sodium (Co-administration with non-potassium sparing diuretics can result in acute worsening of ECG changes and/or hypokalemia, especially when recommended dose of the beta agonist is exceeded; clinical significance of this interaction is unknown). Products include:
Diuril Sodium Intravenous 2086

Clomipramine Hydrochloride (Co-administration with tricyclic antidepressants can potentiate the action of albuterol on the cardiovascular system).
No products indexed under this heading.

Desipramine Hydrochloride (Co-administration with tricyclic antidepressants can potentiate the action of albuterol on the cardiovascular system). Products include:
Norpramin Tablets 755

Digoxin (Mean decreases of 16% to 22% in serum digoxin levels were demonstrated after single dose IV and oral albuterol, respectively; the clinical significance of this interaction is unknown). Products include:
Digitek Tablets 1003
Lanoxicaps Capsules 1574
Lanoxin Injection 1581
Lanoxin Tablets 1587
Lanoxin Elixir Pediatric 1578
Lanoxin Injection Pediatric 1584

Dobutamine Hydrochloride (Co-administration with other sympathomimetic agents increases the risk of adverse cardiovascular effects). Products include:
Dobutrex Solution Vials 1914

Dopamine Hydrochloride (Co-administration with other sympathomimetic agents increases the risk of adverse cardiovascular effects).
No products indexed under this heading.

Doxepin Hydrochloride (Co-administration with tricyclic antidepressants can potentiate the action of albuterol on the cardiovascular system). Products include:
Sinequan 2713

Ephedrine Hydrochloride (Co-administration with other sympathomimetic agents increases the risk of adverse cardiovascular effects). Products include:
Primatene Tablets .... ▣ 780

Ephedrine Sulfate (Co-administration with other sympathomimetic agents increases the risk of adverse cardiovascular effects).
No products indexed under this heading.

Ephedrine Tannate (Co-administration with other sympathomimetic agents increases the risk of adverse cardiovascular effects). Products include:
Rynatuss Pediatric Suspension 3353
Rynatuss Tablets 3353

Epinephrine (Co-administration with other sympathomimetic agents increases the risk of adverse cardiovascular effects). Products include:
Epifrin Sterile Ophthalmic Solution .... ⊙ 235
EpiPen 1236
Primatene Mist .... ▣ 779
Xylocaine with Epinephrine Injection 653

Epinephrine Bitartrate (Co-administration with other sympathomimetic agents increases the risk of adverse cardiovascular effects). Products include:
Sensorcaine 643

Epinephrine Hydrochloride (Co-administration with other sympathomimetic agents increases the risk of adverse cardiovascular effects).
No products indexed under this heading.

Esmolol Hydrochloride (Co-administration with beta blockers inhibits the effects of each other). Products include:
Brevibloc Injection 858

Ethacrynic Acid (Co-administration with non-potassium sparing diuretics can result in acute worsening of ECG changes and/or hypokalemia, especially when recommended dose of the beta agonist is exceeded; clinical significance of this interaction is unknown). Products include:
Edecrin Tablets 2091

Furosemide (Co-administration with non-potassium sparing diuretics can result in acute worsening of ECG changes and/or hypokalemia, especially when recommended dose of the beta agonist is exceeded; clinical significance of this interaction is unknown). Products include:
Furosemide Tablets 2284

Hydrochlorothiazide (Co-administration with non-potassium sparing diuretics can result in acute worsening of ECG changes and/or hypokalemia, especially when recommended dose of the beta agonist is exceeded; clinical significance of this interaction is unknown). Products include:
Accuretic Tablets 2614
Aldoril Tablets 2039
Atacand HCT Tablets 597
Avalide Tablets 1070
Diovan HCT Tablets 2338
Dyazide Capsules 1515
HydroDIURIL Tablets 2108
Hyzaar 2109
Inderide Tablets 3517
Inderide LA Long-Acting Capsules .. 3519
Lotensin HCT Tablets 2367
Maxzide 1008
Micardis HCT Tablets 1051
Microzide Capsules 3414
Moduretic Tablets 2138
Monopril HCT 1094
Prinzide Tablets 2168
Timolide Tablets 2187
Uniretic Tablets 3178
Vaseretic Tablets 2204
Zestoretic Tablets 695
Ziac Tablets 1887

Hydroflumethiazide (Co-administration with non-potassium sparing diuretics can result in acute worsening of ECG changes and/or hypokalemia, especially when recommended dose of the beta agonist is exceeded; clinical significance of this interaction is unknown). Products include:
Diucardin Tablets 3494

Imipramine Hydrochloride (Co-administration with tricyclic antidepressants can potentiate the action of albuterol on the cardiovascular system).
No products indexed under this heading.

Imipramine Pamoate (Co-administration with tricyclic antidepressants can potentiate the action of albuterol on the cardiovascular system).
No products indexed under this heading.

Isocarboxazid (Co-administration with MAO inhibitors can potentiate the action of albuterol on the cardiovascular system).
No products indexed under this heading.

Isoproterenol Hydrochloride (Co-administration with other sympathomimetic agents increases the risk of adverse cardiovascular effects).
No products indexed under this heading.

Isoproterenol Sulfate (Co-administration with other sympathomimetic agents increases the risk of adverse cardiovascular effects).
No products indexed under this heading.

Labetalol Hydrochloride (Co-administration with beta blockers inhibits the effects of each other). Products include:
Normodyne Injection 3135
Normodyne Tablets 3137

Levalbuterol Hydrochloride (Co-administration with other sympathomimetic agents increases the risk of adverse cardiovascular effects). Products include:
Xopenex Inhalation Solution 3207

Levobunolol Hydrochloride (Co-administration with beta blockers inhibits the effects of each other). Products include:
Betagan .... ⊙ 228

Maprotiline Hydrochloride (Co-administration with tricyclic antidepressants can potentiate the action of albuterol on the cardiovascular system).
No products indexed under this heading.

Metaproterenol Sulfate (Co-administration with other sympathomimetic agents increases the risk of adverse cardiovascular effects). Products include:
Alupent 1029

Metaraminol Bitartrate (Co-administration with other sympathomimetic agents increases the risk of adverse cardiovascular effects). Products include:
Aramine Injection 2043

Methoxamine Hydrochloride (Co-administration with other sympathomimetic agents increases the risk of adverse cardiovascular effects).
No products indexed under this heading.

Methyclothiazide (Co-administration with non-potassium

sparing diuretics can result in acute worsening of ECG changes and/or hypokalemia, especially when recommended dose of the beta agonist is exceeded; clinical significance of this interaction is unknown).
No products indexed under this heading.

Metipranolol Hydrochloride (Co-administration with beta blockers inhibits the effects of each other).
No products indexed under this heading.

Metoprolol Succinate (Co-administration with beta blockers inhibits the effects of each other). Products include:
Toprol-XL Tablets 651

Metoprolol Tartrate (Co-administration with beta blockers inhibits the effects of each other).
No products indexed under this heading.

Moclobemide (Co-administration with MAO inhibitors can potentiate the action of albuterol on the cardiovascular system).
No products indexed under this heading.

Nadolol (Co-administration with beta blockers inhibits the effects of each other). Products include:
Corgard Tablets 2245
Corzide 40/5 Tablets 2247
Corzide 80/5 Tablets 2247
Nadolol Tablets 2288

Norepinephrine Bitartrate (Co-administration with other sympathomimetic agents increases the risk of adverse cardiovascular effects).
No products indexed under this heading.

Nortriptyline Hydrochloride (Co-administration with tricyclic antidepressants can potentiate the action of albuterol on the cardiovascular system).
No products indexed under this heading.

Pargyline Hydrochloride (Co-administration with MAO inhibitors can potentiate the action of albuterol on the cardiovascular system).
No products indexed under this heading.

Penbutolol Sulfate (Co-administration with beta blockers inhibits the effects of each other).
No products indexed under this heading.

Phenelzine Sulfate (Co-administration with MAO inhibitors can potentiate the action of albuterol on the cardiovascular system). Products include:
Nardil Tablets 2653

Phenylephrine Bitartrate (Co-administration with other sympathomimetic agents increases the risk of adverse cardiovascular effects).
No products indexed under this heading.

Phenylephrine Hydrochloride (Co-administration with other sympathomimetic agents increases the risk of adverse cardiovascular effects). Products include:
Afrin Nasal Decongestant Children's Pump Mist .... ■ 734
Extendryl 1361
Hycomine Compound Tablets 1317
Neo-Synephrine .... ■ 614
Phenergan VC Syrup 3560
Phenergan VC with Codeine Syrup . 3561
Preparation H Cream .... ■ 778
Preparation H Cooling Gel .... ■ 778
Preparation H .... ■ 778
Vicks Sinex Nasal Spray and Ultra Fine Mist .... ■ 729

Phenylephrine Tannate (Co-administration with other sympathomimetic agents increases the risk of adverse cardiovascular effects). Products include:
Ryna-12 S Suspension 3351
Reformulated Rynatan Pediatric Suspension 3352
Rynatuss Pediatric Suspension 3353
Rynatuss Tablets 3353

Phenylpropanolamine Hydrochloride (Co-administration with other sympathomimetic agents increases the risk of adverse cardiovascular effects).
No products indexed under this heading.

Pindolol (Co-administration with beta blockers inhibits the effects of each other).
No products indexed under this heading.

Pirbuterol Acetate (Co-administration with other sympathomimetic agents increases the risk of adverse cardiovascular effects). Products include:
Maxair Autohaler 1981
Maxair Inhaler 1984

Polythiazide (Co-administration with non-potassium sparing diuretics can result in acute worsening of ECG changes and/or hypokalemia, especially when recommended dose of the beta agonist is exceeded; clinical significance of this interaction is unknown). Products include:
Minizide Capsules 2700
Renese Tablets 2712

Procarbazine Hydrochloride (Co-administration with MAO inhibitors can potentiate the action of albuterol on the cardiovascular system). Products include:
Matulane Capsules 3246

Propranolol Hydrochloride (Co-administration with beta blockers inhibits the effects of each other). Products include:
Inderal 3513
Inderal LA Long-Acting Capsules 3516
Inderide Tablets 3517
Inderide LA Long-Acting Capsules .. 3519

Protriptyline Hydrochloride (Co-administration with tricyclic antidepressants can potentiate the action of albuterol on the cardiovascular system). Products include:
Vivactil Tablets 2446
Vivactil Tablets 2217

Pseudoephedrine Hydrochloride (Co-administration with other sympathomimetic agents increases the risk of adverse cardiovascular effects). Products include:
Actifed Cold & Allergy Tablets .... ■ 688
Actifed Cold & Sinus Caplets and Tablets .... ■ 688
Advil Cold and Sinus Caplets .... ■ 771
Advil Cold and Sinus Tablets .... ■ 771
Advil Flu & Body Ache Caplets .... ■ 772
Aleve Cold & Sinus Caplets .... ■ 603
Alka-Seltzer Plus Liqui-Gels .... ■ 604
Alka-Seltzer Plus Cold & Flu Medicine Liqui-Gels .... ■ 604
Alka-Seltzer Plus Cold & Sinus Medicine Liqui-Gels .... ■ 604
Allegra-D Extended-Release Tablets 714
BC Cold Powder .... ■ 619
Benadryl Allergy/Cold Tablets .... ■ 691
Benadryl Allergy/Congestion Tablets .... ■ 692
Benadryl Allergy & Sinus Liquid .... ■ 693
Benadryl Allergy & Sinus Fastmelt Tablets .... ■ 693
Benadryl Allergy Sinus Headache Caplets & Gelcaps .... ■ 693
Benadryl Severe Allergy & Sinus Headache Caplets .... ■ 694
Benadryl Children's Allergy/Cold Fastmelt Tablets .... ■ 692
Benylin Multi-Symptom Liquid .... ■ 697
Bromfed Capsules (Extended-Release) 2269
Bromfed-PD Capsules (Extended-Release) 2269
Children's Cēpacol Sore Throat .... ■ 788
Comtrex Acute Head Cold & Sinus Pressure Relief Tablets .... ■ 627
Comtrex Deep Chest Cold & Congestion Relief Softgels .... ■ 627
Comtrex Flu Therapy & Fever Relief Daytime Caplets .... ■ 628
Comtrex Flu Therapy & Fever Relief Nighttime Tablets .... ■ 628
Comtrex Maximum Strength Multi-Symptom Cold & Cough Relief Tablets and Caplets .... ■ 626
Contac Non-Drowsy 12 Hour Cold Caplets .... ■ 745
Contac Non-Drowsy Timed Release 12 Hour Cold Caplets ... ■ 746
Contac Severe Cold and Flu Caplets Maximum Strength .... ■ 746
Contac Severe Cold and Flu Caplets Non-Drowsy .... ■ 746
Dimetapp Elixir .... ■ 777
Dimetapp Cold and Fever Suspension .... ■ 775
Dimetapp DM Cold & Cough Elixir . ■ 775
Dimetapp Nighttime Flu Liquid .... ■ 776
Dimetapp Non-Drowsy Flu Syrup ... ■ 777
Dimetapp Infant Drops Decongestant .... ■ 775
Dimetapp Infant Drops Decongestant Plus Cough .... ■ 776
Guaifed 2272
Kronofed-A 1341
Children's Motrin Cold Oral Suspension 2007
Motrin Sinus Headache Caplets 2005
PediaCare Cough-Cold Liquid .... ■ 719
PediaCare Infants' Drops Decongestant .... ■ 719
PediaCare Infants' Drops Decongestant Plus Cough .... ■ 719
PediaCare NightRest Cough-Cold Liquid .... ■ 719
Robitussin Cold Caplets Cold & Congestion .... ■ 780
Robitussin Cold Softgels Cold & Congestion .... ■ 780
Robitussin Cold Caplets Multi-Symptom Cold & Flu .... ■ 781
Robitussin Cold Softgels Multi-Symptom Cold & Flu .... ■ 781
Robitussin Cold Softgels Severe Congestion .... ■ 782
Robitussin Cough & Cold Infant Drops .... ■ 782
Robitussin Maximum Strength Cough & Cold Liquid .... ■ 785
Robitussin Pediatric Cough & Cold Formula Liquid .... ■ 785
Robitussin Multi Symptom Honey Flu Liquid .... ■ 785
Robitussin Nighttime Honey Flu Liquid .... ■ 786
Robitussin-CF Liquid .... ■ 783
Robitussin-DAC Syrup 2942
Robitussin-PE Liquid .... ■ 782
Ryna .... ■ 768
Semprex-D Capsules 1172
Singlet Caplets .... ■ 761
Sinutab Non-Drying Liquid Caps .... ■ 706
Sinutab Sinus Allergy Medication, Maximum Strength Formula, Tablets & Caplets .... ■ 707
Sinutab Sinus Medication, Maximum Strength Without Drowsiness Formula, Tablets & Caplets .... ■ 707
Sudafed 12 Hour Tablets .... ■ 708
Sudafed 24 Hour Tablets .... ■ 708
Children's Sudafed Cold & Cough Liquid .... ■ 709
Children's Sudafed Nasal Decongestant Chewables .... ■ 711
Children's Sudafed Nasal Decongestant Liquid Medication .... ■ 711
Sudafed Cold & Allergy Tablets .... ■ 708
Sudafed Cold & Cough Liquid Caps .... ■ 709
Sudafed Cold & Sinus Liquid Caps .... ■ 710
Sudafed Nasal Decongestant Tablets .... ■ 710
Sudafed Non-Drying Sinus Liquid Caps .... ■ 712
Sudafed Severe Cold .... ■ 711
Sudafed Sinus Headache Caplets .... ■ 712
Sudafed Sinus Headache Tablets .... ■ 712
Tavist Sinus Non-Drowsy Coated Caplets .... ■ 676
TheraFlu Regular Strength Cold & Cough Night Time Hot Liquid .... ■ 676
TheraFlu Regular Strength Cold & Sore Throat Night Time Hot Liquid .... ■ 676
TheraFlu Maximum Strength Flu & Congestion Non-Drowsy Hot Liquid .... ■ 677
TheraFlu Maximum Strength Flu & Cough Night Time Hot Liquid .... ■ 678
TheraFlu Maximum Strength Flu & Sore Throat Night Time Hot Liquid .... ■ 677
TheraFlu Maximum Strength Severe Cold & Congestion Night Time Caplets .... ■ 678
TheraFlu Maximum Strength Severe Cold & Congestion Night Time Hot Liquid .... ■ 678
TheraFlu Maximum Strength Severe Cold & Congestion Non-Drowsy .... ■ 679
Triaminic Allergy Congestion Liquid .... ■ 680
Triaminic Chest Congestion Liquid .... ■ 680
Triaminic Cold & Allergy Liquid .... ■ 681
Triaminic Cold & Allergy Softchews .... ■ 683
Triaminic Cold & Cough Liquid .... ■ 681
Triaminic Cold & Cough Softchews .... ■ 683
Triaminic Cold & Night Time Cough Liquid .... ■ 681
Triaminic Cold, Cough & Fever Liquid .... ■ 681
Triaminic Cough Liquid .... ■ 682
Triaminic Cough & Congestion Liquid .... ■ 682
Triaminic Cough & Sore Throat Liquid .... ■ 682
Triaminic Cough & Sore Throat Softchews .... ■ 684
Children's Tylenol Allergy-D Liquid ... 2014
Children's Tylenol Cold Suspension Liquid and Chewable Tablets 2015
Children's Tylenol Cold Plus Cough Suspension Liquid and Chewable Tablets 2015
Children's Tylenol Flu Suspension Liquid 2015
Children's Tylenol Sinus Suspension Liquid 2017
Infants' Tylenol Cold Decongestant and Fever Reducer Concentrated Drops 2015
Infants' Tylenol Cold Decongestant and Fever Reducer Concentrated Drops Plus Cough .. 2015
Tylenol Allergy Sinus 2010
Multi-Symptom Tylenol Cold Complete Formula Caplets 2010
Multi-Symptom Tylenol Cold Non-Drowsy Caplets and Gelcaps 2010
Multi-Symptom Tylenol Cold Severe Congestion Non-Drowsy Caplets 2011
Maximum Strength Tylenol Flu NightTime Gelcaps 2011
Maximum Strength Tylenol Flu NightTime Liquid 2011
Maximum Strength Tylenol Flu Non-Drowsy Gelcaps 2011
Maximum Strength Tylenol Sinus NightTime Caplets 2012
Maximum Strength Tylenol Sinus Non-Drowsy Geltabs, Gelcaps, Caplets, and Tablets 2012
Vicks 44D Cough & Head Congestion Relief Liquid .... ■ 724
Vicks 44M Cough, Cold & Flu Relief Liquid .... ■ 725
Pediatric Vicks 44m Cough & Cold Relief .... ■ 728
Vicks DayQuil LiquiCaps/Liquid Multi-Symptom Cold/Flu Relief ... ■ 727
Children's Vicks NyQuil Cold/Cough Relief .... ■ 726
Vicks NyQuil LiquiCaps/Liquid Multi-Symptom Cold/Flu Relief, Original and Cherry Flavors .... ■ 727
Zephrex Tablets 3091
Zephrex LA Tablets 3092
Zyrtec-D 12 Hour Extended Relief Tablets 2758

Pseudoephedrine Sulfate (Co-administration with other sympathomimetic agents increases the risk of adverse cardiovascular effects). Products include:
Chlor-Trimeton Allergy/Decongestant Tablets .... ■ 736
Claritin-D 12 Hour Extended Release Tablets 3102
Claritin-D 24 Hour Extended Release Tablets 3104
Coricidin 'D' Cold, Flu & Sinus Tablets .... ■ 737
Drixoral Allergy/Sinus Extended-Release Tablets .... ■ 741
Drixoral Cold & Allergy Sustained-Action Tablets .... ■ 740
Drixoral Cold & Flu Extended-Release Tablets .... ■ 740
Drixoral Nasal Decongestant Long-Acting Non-Drowsy Tablets .... ■ 740
Rynatan Tablets 3351

Salmeterol Xinafoate (Co-administration with other sympatho-

mimetic agents increases the risk of adverse cardiovascular effects). Products include:

- Advair Diskus 100/50 1448
- Advair Diskus 250/50 1448
- Advair Diskus 500/50 1448
- Serevent Diskus 1637
- Serevent Inhalation Aerosol 1633

Selegiline Hydrochloride (Co-administration with MAO inhibitors can potentiate the action of albuterol on the cardiovascular system). Products include:

- Eldepryl Capsules 3266

Sotalol Hydrochloride (Co-administration with beta blockers inhibits the effects of each other). Products include:

- Betapace Tablets 950
- Betapace AF Tablets 954

Terbutaline Sulfate (Co-administration with other sympathomimetic agents increases the risk of adverse cardiovascular effects). Products include:

- Brethine Ampuls 2314
- Brethine Tablets 2313

Timolol Hemihydrate (Co-administration with beta blockers inhibits the effects of each other). Products include:

- Betimol Ophthalmic Solution .... ⊙ 324

Timolol Maleate (Co-administration with beta blockers inhibits the effects of each other). Products include:

- Blocadren Tablets 2046
- Cosopt Sterile Ophthalmic Solution 2065
- Timolide Tablets 2187
- Timolol GFS .... ⊙ 266
- Timoptic in Ocudose 2192
- Timoptic Sterile Ophthalmic Solution 2190
- Timoptic-XE Sterile Ophthalmic Gel Forming Solution 2194

Torsemide (Co-administration with non-potassium sparing diuretics can result in acute worsening of ECG changes and/or hypokalemia, especially when recommended dose of the beta agonist is exceeded; clinical significance of this interaction is unknown). Products include:

- Demadex Tablets and Injection 2965

Tranylcypromine Sulfate (Co-administration with MAO inhibitors can potentiate the action of albuterol on the cardiovascular system). Products include:

- Parnate Tablets 1607

Trimipramine Maleate (Co-administration with tricyclic antidepressants can potentiate the action of albuterol on the cardiovascular system). Products include:

- Surmontil Capsules 3595

ACCUPRIL TABLETS

(Quinapril Hydrochloride) 2611

May interact with diuretics, lithium preparations, potassium preparations, potassium sparing diuretics, tetracyclines, and certain other agents. Compounds in these categories include:

Amiloride Hydrochloride (Occasional excessive reduction of blood pressure; potential for hyperkalemia). Products include:

- Midamor Tablets 2136
- Moduretic Tablets 2138

Bendroflumethiazide (Occasional excessive reduction of blood pressure). Products include:

- Corzide 40/5 Tablets 2247
- Corzide 80/5 Tablets 2247

Bumetanide (Occasional excessive reduction of blood pressure).

No products indexed under this heading.

Chlorothiazide (Occasional excessive reduction of blood pressure). Products include:

- Aldoclor Tablets 2035
- Diuril Oral 2087

Chlorothiazide Sodium (Occasional excessive reduction of blood pressure). Products include:

- Diuril Sodium Intravenous 2086

Chlorthalidone (Occasional excessive reduction of blood pressure). Products include:

- Clorpres Tablets 1002
- Combipres Tablets 1040
- Tenoretic Tablets 690

Demeclocycline Hydrochloride (Simultaneous administration of tetracyclines and Accupril reduces the oral absorption of tetracycline by approximately 28% to 37%, possibly due to high magnesium content in Accupril tablets). Products include:

- Declomycin Tablets 1855

Doxycycline Calcium (Simultaneous administration of tetracyclines and Accupril reduces the oral absorption of tetracycline by approximately 28% to 37%, possibly due to high magnesium content in Accupril tablets). Products include:

- Vibramycin Calcium Oral Suspension Syrup 2735

Doxycycline Hyclate (Simultaneous administration of tetracyclines and Accupril reduces the oral absorption of tetracycline by approximately 28% to 37%, possibly due to high magnesium content in Accupril tablets). Products include:

- Doryx Coated Pellet Filled Capsules 3357
- Periostat Tablets 1208
- Vibramycin Hyclate Capsules 2735
- Vibramycin Hyclate Intravenous 2737
- Vibra-Tabs Film Coated Tablets 2735

Doxycycline Monohydrate (Simultaneous administration of tetracyclines and Accupril reduces the oral absorption of tetracycline by approximately 28% to 37%, possibly due to high magnesium content in Accupril tablets). Products include:

- Monodox Capsules 2442
- Vibramycin Monohydrate for Oral Suspension 2735

Ethacrynic Acid (Occasional excessive reduction of blood pressure). Products include:

- Edecrin Tablets 2091

Furosemide (Occasional excessive reduction of blood pressure). Products include:

- Furosemide Tablets 2284

Hydrochlorothiazide (Occasional excessive reduction of blood pressure). Products include:

- Accuretic Tablets 2614
- Aldoril Tablets 2039
- Atacand HCT Tablets 597
- Avalide Tablets 1070
- Diovan HCT Tablets 2338
- Dyazide Capsules 1515
- HydroDIURIL Tablets 2108
- Hyzaar 2109
- Inderide Tablets 3517
- Inderide LA Long-Acting Capsules 3519
- Lotensin HCT Tablets 2367
- Maxzide 1008
- Micardis HCT Tablets 1051
- Microzide Capsules 3414
- Moduretic Tablets 2138
- Monopril HCT 1094
- Prinzide Tablets 2168
- Timolide Tablets 2187
- Uniretic Tablets 3178
- Vaseretic Tablets 2204
- Zestoretic Tablets 695
- Ziac Tablets 1887

Hydroflumethiazide (Occasional excessive reduction of blood pressure). Products include:

- Diucardin Tablets 3494

Indapamide (Occasional excessive reduction of blood pressure). Products include:

- Indapamide Tablets 2286

Lithium Carbonate (Increased serum lithium levels and symptoms of lithium toxicity). Products include:

- Eskalith 1527
- Lithium Carbonate 3061
- Lithobid Slow-Release Tablets 3255

Lithium Citrate (Increased serum lithium levels and symptoms of lithium toxicity). Products include:

- Lithium Citrate Syrup 3061

Methacycline Hydrochloride (Simultaneous administration of tetracyclines and Accupril reduces the oral absorption of tetracycline by approximately 28% to 37%, possibly due to high magnesium content in Accupril tablets).

No products indexed under this heading.

Methyclothiazide (Occasional excessive reduction of blood pressure).

No products indexed under this heading.

Metolazone (Occasional excessive reduction of blood pressure). Products include:

- Mykrox Tablets 1168
- Zaroxolyn Tablets 1177

Minocycline Hydrochloride (Simultaneous administration of tetracyclines and Accupril reduces the oral absorption of tetracycline by approximately 28% to 37%, possibly due to high magnesium content in Accupril tablets). Products include:

- Dynacin Capsules 2019
- Minocin Intravenous 1862
- Minocin Oral Suspension 1865
- Minocin Pellet-Filled Capsules 1863

Oxytetracycline Hydrochloride (Simultaneous administration of tetracyclines and Accupril reduces the oral absorption of tetracycline by approximately 28% to 37%, possibly due to high magnesium content in Accupril tablets). Products include:

- Terra-Cortril Ophthalmic Suspension 2716
- Urobiotic-250 Capsules 2731

Polythiazide (Occasional excessive reduction of blood pressure). Products include:

- Minizide Capsules 2700
- Renese Tablets 2712

Potassium Acid Phosphate (Potential for hyperkalemia). Products include:

- K-Phos Original (Sodium Free) Tablets 947

Potassium Bicarbonate (Potential for hyperkalemia).

No products indexed under this heading.

Potassium Chloride (Potential for hyperkalemia). Products include:

- Chlor-3 1361
- Colyte with Flavor Packs for Oral Solution 3170
- GoLYTELY and Pineapple Flavor GoLYTELY for Oral Solution 1068
- K-Dur Microburst Release System ER Tablets 1832
- Klor-Con M20/Klor-Con M10 Tablets 3329
- K-Lor Powder Packets 469
- K-Tab Filmtab Tablets 470
- Micro-K 3311
- NuLYTELY, Cherry Flavor, Lemon-Lime Flavor, and Orange Flavor NuLYTELY for Oral Solution 1068
- Rum-K 1363

Potassium Citrate (Potential for hyperkalemia). Products include:

- Urocit-K Tablets 2232

Potassium Gluconate (Potential for hyperkalemia).

No products indexed under this heading.

Potassium Phosphate (Potential for hyperkalemia). Products include:

- K-Phos Neutral Tablets 946

Spironolactone (Occasional excessive reduction of blood pressure; potential for hyperkalemia).

No products indexed under this heading.

Tetracycline Hydrochloride (Simultaneous administration of tetracyclines and Accupril reduces the oral absorption of tetracycline by approximately 28% to 37%, possibly due to high magnesium content in Accupril tablets).

No products indexed under this heading.

Torsemide (Occasional excessive reduction of blood pressure). Products include:

- Demadex Tablets and Injection 2965

Triamterene (Occasional excessive reduction of blood pressure; potential for hyperkalemia). Products include:

- Dyazide Capsules 1515
- Dyrenium Capsules 3458
- Maxzide 1008

Food Interactions

Diet, high-lipid (Rate and extent of quinapril absorption are diminished moderately).

ACCURETIC TABLETS

(Hydrochlorothiazide, Quinapril Hydrochloride) 2614

May interact with barbiturates, corticosteroids, oral hypoglycemic agents, insulin, lithium preparations, narcotic analgesics, nondepolarizing neuromuscular blocking agents, nonsteroidal anti-inflammatory agents, potassium preparations, potassium sparing diuretics, tetracyclines, and certain other agents. Compounds in these categories include:

Acarbose (Thiazides can cause hyperglycemia; dosage adjustments of the antidiabetic drug may be required). Products include:

- Precose Tablets 906

ACTH (Co-administration of thiazide diuretics with ACTH can lead to intensified electrolyte depletion, particularly hypokalemia).

No products indexed under this heading.

Alfentanil Hydrochloride (May potentiate orthostatic hypotension).

No products indexed under this heading.

Amiloride Hydrochloride (Co-administration can increase the risk of hyperkalemia). Products include:

- Midamor Tablets 2136
- Moduretic Tablets 2138

Aprobarbital (May potentiate orthostatic hypotension).

No products indexed under this heading.

Atracurium Besylate (Possible increased responsiveness to the muscle relaxant).

No products indexed under this heading.

Betamethasone Acetate (Co-administration of thiazide diuretics with corticosteroids can lead to intensified electrolyte depletion, particularly hypokalemia). Products include:

- Celestone Soluspan Injectable Suspension 3097

Betamethasone Sodium Phosphate (Co-administration of thiazide diuretics with corticosteroids can lead to intensified electrolyte depletion, particularly hypokalemia). Products include:

- Celestone Soluspan Injectable Suspension 3097

Buprenorphine Hydrochloride (May potentiate orthostatic hypotension). Products include:

- Buprenex Injectable 2918

Butabarbital (May potentiate orthostatic hypotension).

No products indexed under this heading.

Butalbital (May potentiate orthostatic hypotension). Products include:

- Phrenilin 578
- Sedapap Tablets 50 mg/650 mg 2225

Celecoxib (Co-administration of thiazide diuretics with non-steroidal

anti-inflammatory agents can lead to reduced diuretic, natriuretic, antihypertensive effects of thiazides). Products include:
- Celebrex Capsules 2676
- Celebrex Capsules 2780

Chlorpropamide (Thiazides can cause hyperglycemia; dosage adjustments of the antidiabetic drug may be required). Products include:
- Diabinese Tablets 2680

Cholestyramine (Co-administration of hydrochlorothiazide with cholestyramine can impair absorption of hydrochlorothiazide and reduces the absorption from gastrointestinal tract by up to 85%).
No products indexed under this heading.

Cisatracurium Besylate (Possible increased responsiveness to the muscle relaxant).
No products indexed under this heading.

Codeine Phosphate (May potentiate orthostatic hypotension). Products include:
- Phenergan with Codeine Syrup 3557
- Phenergan VC with Codeine Syrup . 3561
- Robitussin A-C Syrup 2942
- Robitussin-DAC Syrup 2942
- Ryna-C Liquid .... ▣768
- Soma Compound w/Codeine Tablets 3355
- Tussi-Organidin NR Liquid 3350
- Tussi-Organidin-S NR Liquid 3350
- Tylenol with Codeine 2595

Colestipol Hydrochloride (Co-administration of hydrochlorothiazide with colestipol can impair absorption of hydrochlorothiazide and reduces the absorption from gastrointestinal tract by up to 43%). Products include:
- Colestid Tablets 2791

Cortisone Acetate (Co-administration of thiazide diuretics with corticosteroids can lead to intensified electrolyte depletion, particularly hypokalemia). Products include:
- Cortone Acetate Injectable Suspension 2059
- Cortone Acetate Tablets 2061

Demeclocycline Hydrochloride (Simultaneous administration of oral tetracycline and quinapril reduced the absorption of tetracycline by approximately 28% to 37%, possibly due to the high magnesium content of quinapril tablets). Products include:
- Declomycin Tablets 1855

Dexamethasone (Co-administration of thiazide diuretics with corticosteroids can lead to intensified electrolyte depletion, particularly hypokalemia). Products include:
- Decadron Elixir 2078
- Decadron Tablets 2079
- TobraDex Ophthalmic Ointment 542
- TobraDex Ophthalmic Suspension .. 541

Dexamethasone Acetate (Co-administration of thiazide diuretics with corticosteroids can lead to intensified electrolyte depletion, particularly hypokalemia).
No products indexed under this heading.

Dexamethasone Sodium Phosphate (Co-administration of thiazide diuretics with corticosteroids can lead to intensified electrolyte depletion, particularly hypokalemia). Products include:
- Decadron Phosphate Injection 2081
- Decadron Phosphate Sterile Ophthalmic Ointment 2083
- Decadron Phosphate Sterile Ophthalmic Solution 2084
- NeoDecadron Sterile Ophthalmic Solution 2144

Dezocine (May potentiate orthostatic hypotension).
No products indexed under this heading.

Diclofenac Potassium (Co-administration of thiazide diuretics with non-steroidal anti-inflammatory agents can lead to reduced diuretic, natriuretic, antihypertensive effects of thiazides). Products include:
- Cataflam Tablets 2315

Diclofenac Sodium (Co-administration of thiazide diuretics with non-steroidal anti-inflammatory agents can lead to reduced diuretic, natriuretic, antihypertensive effects of thiazides). Products include:
- Arthrotec Tablets 3195
- Voltaren Ophthalmic Sterile Ophthalmic Solution .... ⊙312
- Voltaren Tablets 2315
- Voltaren-XR Tablets 2315

Doxycycline Calcium (Simultaneous administration of oral tetracycline and quinapril reduced the absorption of tetracycline by approximately 28% to 37%, possibly due to the high magnesium content of quinapril tablets). Products include:
- Vibramycin Calcium Oral Suspension Syrup 2735

Doxycycline Hyclate (Simultaneous administration of oral tetracycline and quinapril reduced the absorption of tetracycline by approximately 28% to 37%, possibly due to the high magnesium content of quinapril tablets). Products include:
- Doryx Coated Pellet Filled Capsules 3357
- Periostat Tablets 1208
- Vibramycin Hyclate Capsules 2735
- Vibramycin Hyclate Intravenous 2737
- Vibra-Tabs Film Coated Tablets 2735

Doxycycline Monohydrate (Simultaneous administration of oral tetracycline and quinapril reduced the absorption of tetracycline by approximately 28% to 37%, possibly due to the high magnesium content of quinapril tablets). Products include:
- Monodox Capsules 2442
- Vibramycin Monohydrate for Oral Suspension 2735

Etodolac (Co-administration of thiazide diuretics with non-steroidal anti-inflammatory agents can lead to reduced diuretic, natriuretic, antihypertensive effects of thiazides). Products include:
- Lodine 3528
- Lodine XL Extended-Release Tablets 3530

Fenoprofen Calcium (Co-administration of thiazide diuretics with non-steroidal anti-inflammatory agents can lead to reduced diuretic, natriuretic, antihypertensive effects of thiazides).
No products indexed under this heading.

Fentanyl (May potentiate orthostatic hypotension). Products include:
- Duragesic Transdermal System 1786

Fentanyl Citrate (May potentiate orthostatic hypotension). Products include:
- Actiq 1184

Fludrocortisone Acetate (Co-administration of thiazide diuretics with corticosteroids can lead to intensified electrolyte depletion, particularly hypokalemia). Products include:
- Florinef Acetate Tablets 2250

Flurbiprofen (Co-administration of thiazide diuretics with non-steroidal anti-inflammatory agents can lead to reduced diuretic, natriuretic, antihypertensive effects of thiazides).
No products indexed under this heading.

Glimepiride (Thiazides can cause hyperglycemia; dosage adjustments of the antidiabetic drug may be required). Products include:
- Amaryl Tablets 717

Glipizide (Thiazides can cause hyperglycemia; dosage adjustments of the antidiabetic drug may be required). Products include:
- Glucotrol Tablets 2692
- Glucotrol XL Extended Release Tablets 2693

Glyburide (Thiazides can cause hyperglycemia; dosage adjustments of the antidiabetic drug may be required). Products include:
- DiaBeta Tablets 741
- Glucovance Tablets 1086

Hydrocodone Bitartrate (May potentiate orthostatic hypotension). Products include:
- Hycodan 1316
- Hycomine Compound Tablets 1317
- Hycotuss Expectorant Syrup 1318
- Lortab 3319
- Lortab Elixir 3317
- Maxidone Tablets CIII 3399
- Norco 5/325 Tablets CIII 3424
- Norco 7.5/325 Tablets CIII 3425
- Norco 10/325 Tablets CIII 3427
- Norco 10/325 Tablets CIII 3425
- Vicodin Tablets 516
- Vicodin ES Tablets 517
- Vicodin HP Tablets 518
- Vicodin Tuss Expectorant 519
- Vicoprofen Tablets 520
- Zydone Tablets 1330

Hydrocodone Polistirex (May potentiate orthostatic hypotension). Products include:
- Tussionex Pennkinetic Extended-Release Suspension 1174

Hydrocortisone (Co-administration of thiazide diuretics with corticosteroids can lead to intensified electrolyte depletion, particularly hypokalemia). Products include:
- Anusol-HC Cream 2.5% 2237
- Cipro HC Otic Suspension 540
- Cortaid Intensive Therapy Cream . ▣717
- Cortaid Maximum Strength Cream .... ▣717
- Cortisporin Ophthalmic Suspension Sterile .... ⊙297
- Cortizone•5 .... ▣699
- Cortizone•10 .... ▣699
- Cortizone•10 Plus Creme .... ▣700
- Cortizone for Kids Creme .... ▣699
- Hydrocortone Tablets 2106
- Massengill Medicated Soft Cloth Towelette .... ▣753
- VōSoL HC Otic Solution 3356

Hydrocortisone Acetate (Co-administration of thiazide diuretics with corticosteroids can lead to intensified electrolyte depletion, particularly hypokalemia). Products include:
- Analpram-HC 1338
- Anusol HC-1 Hydrocortisone Anti-Itch Cream .... ▣689
- Anusol-HC Suppositories 2238
- Cortaid .... ▣717
- Cortifoam Rectal Foam 3170
- Cortisporin-TC Otic Suspension 2246
- Hydrocortone Acetate Injectable Suspension 2103
- Pramosone 1343
- Proctocort Suppositories 2264
- ProctoFoam-HC 3177
- Terra-Cortril Ophthalmic Suspension 2716

Hydrocortisone Sodium Phosphate (Co-administration of thiazide diuretics with corticosteroids can lead to intensified electrolyte depletion, particularly hypokalemia). Products include:
- Hydrocortone Phosphate Injection, Sterile 2105

Hydrocortisone Sodium Succinate (Co-administration of thiazide diuretics with corticosteroids can lead to intensified electrolyte depletion, particularly hypokalemia).
No products indexed under this heading.

Hydromorphone Hydrochloride (May potentiate orthostatic hypotension). Products include:
- Dilaudid 441
- Dilaudid Oral Liquid 445
- Dilaudid Powder 441
- Dilaudid Rectal Suppositories 441
- Dilaudid Tablets 441
- Dilaudid Tablets - 8 mg 445
- Dilaudid-HP 443

Ibuprofen (Co-administration of thiazide diuretics with non-steroidal anti-inflammatory agents can lead to reduced diuretic, natriuretic, antihypertensive effects of thiazides). Products include:
- Advil .... ▣771
- Children's Advil Oral Suspension ... ▣773
- Children's Advil Chewable Tablets . ▣773
- Advil Cold and Sinus Caplets .... ▣771
- Advil Cold and Sinus Tablets .... ▣771
- Advil Flu & Body Ache Caplets .... ▣772
- Infants' Advil Drops .... ▣773
- Junior Strength Advil Tablets .... ▣773
- Junior Strength Advil Chewable Tablets .... ▣773
- Advil Migraine Liquigels .... ▣772
- Children's Motrin Oral Suspension and Chewable Tablets 2006
- Children's Motrin Cold Oral Suspension 2007
- Children's Motrin Oral Suspension .... ▣643
- Motrin Suspension, Oral Drops, Chewable Tablets, and Caplets 2002
- Infants' Motrin Concentrated Drops 2006
- Junior Strength Motrin Caplets and Chewable Tablets 2006
- Motrin IB Tablets, Caplets, and Gelcaps 2002
- Motrin Migraine Pain Caplets 2005
- Motrin Sinus Headache Caplets 2005
- Vicoprofen Tablets 520

Indomethacin (Co-administration of thiazide diuretics with non-steroidal anti-inflammatory agents can lead to reduced diuretic, natriuretic, antihypertensive effects of thiazides). Products include:
- Indocin 2112

Indomethacin Sodium Trihydrate (Co-administration of thiazide diuretics with non-steroidal anti-inflammatory agents can lead to reduced diuretic, natriuretic, antihypertensive effects of thiazides). Products include:
- Indocin I.V. 2115

Insulin, Human, Zinc Suspension (Thiazides can cause hyperglycemia; dosage adjustments of the antidiabetic drug may be required). Products include:
- Humulin L, 100 Units 1937
- Humulin U, 100 Units 1943
- Novolin L Human Insulin 10 ml Vials 2422

Insulin, Human NPH (Thiazides can cause hyperglycemia; dosage adjustments of the antidiabetic drug may be required). Products include:
- Humulin N, 100 Units 1939
- Humulin N NPH Pen 1940
- Novolin N Human Insulin 10 ml Vials 2422
- Novolin N PenFill 2423
- Novolin N Prefilled Syringe Disposable Insulin Delivery System 2425

Insulin, Human Regular (Thiazides can cause hyperglycemia; dosage adjustments of the antidiabetic drug may be required). Products include:
- Humulin R Regular (U-500) 1943
- Humulin R, 100 Units 1941
- Novolin R Human Insulin 10 ml Vials 2423
- Novolin R PenFill 2423
- Novolin R Prefilled Syringe Disposable Insulin Delivery System 2425
- Velosulin BR Human Insulin 10 ml Vials 2435

Insulin, Human Regular and Human NPH Mixture (Thiazides can cause hyperglycemia; dosage adjustments of the antidiabetic drug may be required). Products include:
- Humulin 50/50, 100 Units 1934
- Humulin 70/30, 100 Units 1935
- Humulin 70/30 Pen 1936
- Novolin 70/30 Human Insulin 10 ml Vials 2421
- Novolin 70/30 PenFill 2423

Novolin 70/30 Prefilled Disposable Insulin Delivery System 2425

Insulin, NPH (Thiazides can cause hyperglycemia; dosage adjustments of the antidiabetic drug may be required). Products include:
Iletin II, NPH (Pork), 100 Units 1946

Insulin, Regular (Thiazides can cause hyperglycemia; dosage adjustments of the antidiabetic drug may be required). Products include:
Iletin II, Regular (Pork), 100 Units ... 1947

Insulin, Zinc Crystals (Thiazides can cause hyperglycemia; dosage adjustments of the antidiabetic drug may be required).
No products indexed under this heading.

Insulin, Zinc Suspension (Thiazides can cause hyperglycemia; dosage adjustments of the antidiabetic drug may be required). Products include:
Iletin II, Lente (Pork), 100 Units 1945

Insulin Aspart, Human Regular (Thiazides can cause hyperglycemia; dosage adjustments of the antidiabetic drug may be required).
No products indexed under this heading.

Insulin glargine (Thiazides can cause hyperglycemia; dosage adjustments of the antidiabetic drug may be required). Products include:
Lantus Injection 742

Insulin Lispro, Human (Thiazides can cause hyperglycemia; dosage adjustments of the antidiabetic drug may be required). Products include:
Humalog 1926
Humalog Mix 75/25 Pen 1928

Insulin Lispro Protamine, Human (Thiazides can cause hyperglycemia; dosage adjustments of the antidiabetic drug may be required). Products include:
Humalog Mix 75/25 Pen 1928

Ketoprofen (Co-administration of thiazide diuretics with non-steroidal anti-inflammatory agents can lead to reduced diuretic, natriuretic, antihypertensive effects of thiazides). Products include:
Orudis Capsules 3548
Orudis KT Tablets .... ■□778
Oruvail Capsules 3548

Ketorolac Tromethamine (Co-administration of thiazide diuretics with non-steroidal anti-inflammatory agents can lead to reduced diuretic, natriuretic, antihypertensive effects of thiazides). Products include:
Acular Ophthalmic Solution 544
Acular PF Ophthalmic Solution 544
Toradol 3018

Levorphanol Tartrate (May potentiate orthostatic hypotension). Products include:
Levo-Dromoran 1734
Levorphanol Tartrate Tablets 3059

Lithium Carbonate (Co-administration of ACE inhibitors and lithium increases serum lithium levels and symptoms of lithium toxicity; renal clearance of lithium is reduced by thiazides raising the risk of lithium toxicity). Products include:
Eskalith 1527
Lithium Carbonate 3061
Lithobid Slow-Release Tablets 3255

Lithium Citrate (Co-administration of ACE inhibitors and lithium increases serum lithium levels and symptoms of lithium toxicity; renal clearance of lithium is reduced by thiazides raising the risk of lithium toxicity). Products include:
Lithium Citrate Syrup 3061

Meclofenamate Sodium (Co-administration of thiazide diuretics with non-steroidal anti-inflammatory agents can lead to reduced diuretic, natriuretic, antihypertensive effects of thiazides).
No products indexed under this heading.

Mefenamic Acid (Co-administration of thiazide diuretics with non-steroidal anti-inflammatory agents can lead to reduced diuretic, natriuretic, antihypertensive effects of thiazides). Products include:
Ponstel Capsules 1356

Meloxicam (Co-administration of thiazide diuretics with non-steroidal anti-inflammatory agents can lead to reduced diuretic, natriuretic, antihypertensive effects of thiazides). Products include:
Mobic Tablets 1054

Meperidine Hydrochloride (May potentiate orthostatic hypotension). Products include:
Demerol 3079
Mepergan Injection 3539

Mephobarbital (May potentiate orthostatic hypotension).
No products indexed under this heading.

Metformin Hydrochloride (Thiazides can cause hyperglycemia; dosage adjustments of the antidiabetic drug may be required). Products include:
Glucophage Tablets 1080
Glucophage XR Tablets 1080
Glucovance Tablets 1086

Methacycline Hydrochloride (Simultaneous administration of oral tetracycline and quinapril reduced the absorption of tetracycline by approximately 28% to 37%, possibly due to the high magnesium content of quinapril tablets).
No products indexed under this heading.

Methadone Hydrochloride (May potentiate orthostatic hypotension). Products include:
Dolophine Hydrochloride Tablets 3056

Methylprednisolone Acetate (Co-administration of thiazide diuretics with corticosteroids can lead to intensified electrolyte depletion, particularly hypokalemia). Products include:
Depo-Medrol Injectable Suspension 2795

Methylprednisolone Sodium Succinate (Co-administration of thiazide diuretics with corticosteroids can lead to intensified electrolyte depletion, particularly hypokalemia). Products include:
Solu-Medrol Sterile Powder 2855

Metocurine Iodide (Possible increased responsiveness to the muscle relaxant).
No products indexed under this heading.

Miglitol (Thiazides can cause hyperglycemia; dosage adjustments of the antidiabetic drug may be required). Products include:
Glyset Tablets 2821

Minocycline Hydrochloride (Simultaneous administration of oral tetracycline and quinapril reduced the absorption of tetracycline by approximately 28% to 37%, possibly due to the high magnesium content of quinapril tablets). Products include:
Dynacin Capsules 2019
Minocin Intravenous 1862
Minocin Oral Suspension 1865
Minocin Pellet-Filled Capsules 1863

Mivacurium Chloride (Possible increased responsiveness to the muscle relaxant).
No products indexed under this heading.

Morphine Sulfate (May potentiate orthostatic hypotension). Products include:
Astramorph/PF Injection, USP (Preservative-Free) 594
Duramorph Injection 1312
Infumorph 200 and Infumorph 500 Sterile Solutions 1314
Kadian Capsules 1335
MS Contin Tablets 2896
MSIR 2898
Oramorph SR Tablets 3062
Roxanol 3066

Nabumetone (Co-administration of thiazide diuretics with non-steroidal anti-inflammatory agents can lead to reduced diuretic, natriuretic, antihypertensive effects of thiazides). Products include:
Relafen Tablets 1617

Naproxen (Co-administration of thiazide diuretics with non-steroidal anti-inflammatory agents can lead to reduced diuretic, natriuretic, antihypertensive effects of thiazides). Products include:
EC-Naprosyn Delayed-Release Tablets 2967
Naprosyn Suspension 2967
Naprosyn Tablets 2967

Naproxen Sodium (Co-administration of thiazide diuretics with non-steroidal anti-inflammatory agents can lead to reduced diuretic, natriuretic, antihypertensive effects of thiazides). Products include:
Aleve Tablets, Caplets and Gelcaps .... ■□602
Aleve Cold & Sinus Caplets .... ■□603
Anaprox Tablets 2967
Anaprox DS Tablets 2967
Naprelan Tablets 1293

Norepinephrine Bitartrate (Possible decreased response to pressor amine).
No products indexed under this heading.

Oxaprozin (Co-administration of thiazide diuretics with non-steroidal anti-inflammatory agents can lead to reduced diuretic, natriuretic, antihypertensive effects of thiazides).
No products indexed under this heading.

Oxycodone Hydrochloride (May potentiate orthostatic hypotension). Products include:
OxyContin Tablets 2912
OxyFast Oral Concentrate Solution 2916
OxyIR Capsules 2916
Percocet Tablets 1326
Percodan Tablets 1327
Percolone Tablets 1327
Roxicodone 3067
Tylox Capsules 2597

Oxytetracycline Hydrochloride (Simultaneous administration of oral tetracycline and quinapril reduced the absorption of tetracycline by approximately 28% to 37%, possibly due to the high magnesium content of quinapril tablets). Products include:
Terra-Cortril Ophthalmic Suspension 2716
Urobiotic-250 Capsules 2731

Pancuronium Bromide (Possible increased responsiveness to the muscle relaxant).
No products indexed under this heading.

Pentobarbital Sodium (May potentiate orthostatic hypotension). Products include:
Nembutal Sodium Solution 485

Phenobarbital (May potentiate orthostatic hypotension). Products include:
Arco-Lase Plus Tablets 592
Donnatal 2929
Donnatal Extentabs 2930

Phenylbutazone (Co-administration of thiazide diuretics with non-steroidal anti-inflammatory agents can lead to reduced diuretic, natriuretic, antihypertensive effects of thiazides).
No products indexed under this heading.

Pioglitazone Hydrochloride (Thiazides can cause hyperglycemia; dosage adjustments of the antidiabetic drug may be required). Products include:
Actos Tablets 3275

Piroxicam (Co-administration of thiazide diuretics with non-steroidal anti-inflammatory agents can lead to reduced diuretic, natriuretic, antihypertensive effects of thiazides). Products include:
Feldene Capsules 2685

Potassium Acid Phosphate (Co-administration can increase the risk of hyperkalemia). Products include:
K-Phos Original (Sodium Free) Tablets 947

Potassium Bicarbonate (Co-administration can increase the risk of hyperkalemia).
No products indexed under this heading.

Potassium Chloride (Co-administration can increase the risk of hyperkalemia). Products include:
Chlor-3 1361
Colyte with Flavor Packs for Oral Solution 3170
GoLYTELY and Pineapple Flavor GoLYTELY for Oral Solution 1068
K-Dur Microburst Release System ER Tablets 1832
Klor-Con M20/Klor-Con M10 Tablets 3329
K-Lor Powder Packets 469
K-Tab Filmtab Tablets 470
Micro-K 3311
NuLYTELY, Cherry Flavor, Lemon-Lime Flavor, and Orange Flavor NuLYTELY for Oral Solution 1068
Rum-K 1363

Potassium Citrate (Co-administration can increase the risk of hyperkalemia). Products include:
Urocit-K Tablets 2232

Potassium Gluconate (Co-administration can increase the risk of hyperkalemia).
No products indexed under this heading.

Potassium Phosphate (Co-administration can increase the risk of hyperkalemia). Products include:
K-Phos Neutral Tablets 946

Prednisolone Acetate (Co-administration of thiazide diuretics with corticosteroids can lead to intensified electrolyte depletion, particularly hypokalemia). Products include:
Blephamide Ophthalmic Ointment 547
Blephamide Ophthalmic Suspension 548
Poly-Pred Liquifilm Ophthalmic Suspension .... ⊙245
Pred Forte Ophthalmic Suspension .... ⊙246
Pred Mild Sterile Ophthalmic Suspension .... ⊙249
Pred-G Ophthalmic Suspension .... ⊙247
Pred-G Sterile Ophthalmic Ointment .... ⊙248

Prednisolone Sodium Phosphate (Co-administration of thiazide diuretics with corticosteroids can lead to intensified electrolyte depletion, particularly hypokalemia). Products include:
Pediapred Oral Solution 1170

Prednisolone Tebutate (Co-administration of thiazide diuretics with corticosteroids can lead to intensified electrolyte depletion, particularly hypokalemia).
No products indexed under this heading.

Prednisone (Co-administration of thiazide diuretics with corticosteroids can lead to intensified electrolyte depletion, particularly hypokalemia). Products include:
Prednisone 3064

Propoxyphene Hydrochloride (May potentiate orthostatic hypotension). Products include:
Darvon Pulvules 1909
Darvon Compound-65 Pulvules 1910

Propoxyphene Napsylate (May potentiate orthostatic hypotension). Products include:
Darvon-N/Darvocet-N 1907
Darvon-N Tablets 1912

Rapacuronium Bromide (Possible increased responsiveness to the muscle relaxant).
No products indexed under this heading.

Remifentanil Hydrochloride (May potentiate orthostatic hypotension).
No products indexed under this heading.

Repaglinide (Thiazides can cause hyperglycemia; dosage adjustments of the antidiabetic drug may be required). Products include:
Prandin Tablets (0.5, 1, and 2 mg) 2432

Rocuronium Bromide (Possible increased responsiveness to the muscle relaxant). Products include:
Zemuron Injection 2491

Rofecoxib (Co-administration of thiazide diuretics with non-steroidal anti-inflammatory agents can lead to reduced diuretic, natriuretic, antihypertensive effects of thiazides). Products include:
Vioxx 2213

Rosiglitazone Maleate (Thiazides can cause hyperglycemia; dosage adjustments of the antidiabetic drug may be required). Products include:
Avandia Tablets 1490

Secobarbital Sodium (May potentiate orthostatic hypotension).
No products indexed under this heading.

Spironolactone (Co-administration can increase the risk of hyperkalemia).
No products indexed under this heading.

Sufentanil Citrate (May potentiate orthostatic hypotension).
No products indexed under this heading.

Sulindac (Co-administration of thiazide diuretics with non-steroidal anti-inflammatory agents can lead to reduced diuretic, natriuretic, antihypertensive effects of thiazides). Products include:
Clinoril Tablets 2053

Tetracycline Hydrochloride (Simultaneous administration of oral tetracycline and quinapril reduced the absorption of tetracycline by approximately 28% to 37%, possibly due to the high magnesium content of quinapril tablets).
No products indexed under this heading.

Thiamylal Sodium (May potentiate orthostatic hypotension).
No products indexed under this heading.

Tolazamide (Thiazides can cause hyperglycemia; dosage adjustments of the antidiabetic drug may be required).
No products indexed under this heading.

Tolbutamide (Thiazides can cause hyperglycemia; dosage adjustments of the antidiabetic drug may be required).
No products indexed under this heading.

Tolmetin Sodium (Co-administration of thiazide diuretics with non-steroidal anti-inflammatory agents can lead to reduced diuretic, natriuretic, antihypertensive effects of thiazides). Products include:
Tolectin 2589

Triamcinolone (Co-administration of thiazide diuretics with corticosteroids can lead to intensified electrolyte depletion, particularly hypokalemia).
No products indexed under this heading.

Triamcinolone Acetonide (Co-administration of thiazide diuretics with corticosteroids can lead to intensified electrolyte depletion, particularly hypokalemia). Products include:
Azmacort Inhalation Aerosol 728
Nasacort Nasal Inhaler 750
Nasacort AQ Nasal Spray 752
Tri-Nasal Spray 2274

Triamcinolone Diacetate (Co-administration of thiazide diuretics with corticosteroids can lead to intensified electrolyte depletion, particularly hypokalemia).
No products indexed under this heading.

Triamcinolone Hexacetonide (Co-administration of thiazide diuretics with corticosteroids can lead to intensified electrolyte depletion, particularly hypokalemia).
No products indexed under this heading.

Triamterene (Co-administration can increase the risk of hyperkalemia). Products include:
Dyazide Capsules 1515
Dyrenium Capsules 3458
Maxzide 1008

Troglitazone (Thiazides can cause hyperglycemia; dosage adjustments of the antidiabetic drug may be required).
No products indexed under this heading.

Tubocurarine Chloride (Possible increased responsiveness to the muscle relaxant).
No products indexed under this heading.

Vecuronium Bromide (Possible increased responsiveness to the muscle relaxant). Products include:
Norcuron for Injection 2478

Food Interactions

Alcohol (May potentiate orthostatic hypotension).

Food, unspecified (The rate of quinapril absorption was reduced by 14% and hydrochlorothiazide absorption by 12%, when Accuretic was administered with a high-fat meal compared to fasting, while extent of absorption was not affected; Accuretic can be given without regard to food).

ACCUTANE CAPSULES

(Isotretinoin) 2944
May interact with tetracyclines and certain other agents. Compounds in these categories include:

Demeclocycline Hydrochloride (Concomitant treatment with Accutane and tetracyclines should be avoided because Accutane is associated with a number of cases of pseudotumor cerebri, some of which involved concomitant use of tetracyclines). Products include:
Declomycin Tablets 1855

Doxycycline Calcium (Concomitant treatment with Accutane and tetracyclines should be avoided because Accutane is associated with a number of cases of pseudotumor cerebri, some of which involved concomitant use of tetracyclines). Products include:
Vibramycin Calcium Oral Suspension Syrup 2735

Doxycycline Hyclate (Concomitant treatment with Accutane and tetracyclines should be avoided because Accutane is associated with a number of cases of pseudotumor cerebri, some of which involved concomitant use of tetracyclines). Products include:
Doryx Coated Pellet Filled Capsules 3357
Periostat Tablets 1208
Vibramycin Hyclate Capsules 2735
Vibramycin Hyclate Intravenous 2737
Vibra-Tabs Film Coated Tablets 2735

Doxycycline Monohydrate (Concomitant treatment with Accutane and tetracyclines should be avoided because Accutane is associated with a number of cases of pseudotumor cerebri, some of which involved concomitant use of tetracyclines). Products include:
Monodox Capsules 2442
Vibramycin Monohydrate for Oral Suspension 2735

Methacycline Hydrochloride (Concomitant treatment with Accutane and tetracyclines should be avoided because Accutane is associated with a number of cases of pseudotumor cerebri, some of which involved concomitant use of tetracyclines).
No products indexed under this heading.

Minocycline Hydrochloride (Concomitant treatment with Accutane and tetracyclines should be avoided because Accutane is associated with a number of cases of pseudotumor cerebri, some of which involved concomitant use of tetracyclines). Products include:
Dynacin Capsules 2019
Minocin Intravenous 1862
Minocin Oral Suspension 1865
Minocin Pellet-Filled Capsules 1863

Norethindrone (Microdosed progesterone preparations (minipills) may be an inadequate method of contraception during Accutane therapy). Products include:
Brevicon 28-Day Tablets 3380
Micronor Tablets 2543
Modicon 2563
Necon 3415
Norinyl 1 +35 28-Day Tablets 3380
Norinyl 1 + 50 28-Day Tablets 3380
Nor-QD Tablets 3423
Ortho-Novum 2563
Ortho-Novum 1/50□28 Tablets 2556
Ovcon 3364
Tri-Norinyl-28 Tablets 3433

Oxytetracycline Hydrochloride (Concomitant treatment with Accutane and tetracyclines should be avoided because Accutane is associated with a number of cases of pseudotumor cerebri, some of which involved concomitant use of tetracyclines). Products include:
Terra-Cortril Ophthalmic Suspension 2716
Urobiotic-250 Capsules 2731

Tetracycline Hydrochloride (Concomitant treatment with Accutane and tetracyclines should be avoided because Accutane is associated with a number of cases of pseudotumor cerebri, some of which involved concomitant use of tetracyclines).
No products indexed under this heading.

Vitamin A (Additive Vitamin A toxicity). Products include:
Aquasol A Parenteral 593
Beta-C Tablets .... ▣811
Centrum Focused Formulas Prostate Softgels .... ▣816

ACCUZYME DEBRIDING OINTMENT

(Papain, Urea) 1725
None cited in PDR database.

ACEL-IMUNE

(Diphtheria & Tetanus Toxoids and Acellular Pertussis Vaccine Adsorbed) 1851
May interact with alkylating agents, anticoagulants, corticosteroids, cytotoxic drugs, immunosuppressive agents, and certain other agents. Compounds in these categories include:

Ardeparin Sodium (Caution should be exercised).
No products indexed under this heading.

Azathioprine (Reduces response to active immunization procedures).
No products indexed under this heading.

Basiliximab (Reduces response to active immunization procedures). Products include:
Simulect for Injection 2399

Betamethasone Acetate (Reduces response to active immunization procedures). Products include:
Celestone Soluspan Injectable Suspension 3097

Betamethasone Sodium Phosphate (Reduces response to active immunization procedures). Products include:
Celestone Soluspan Injectable Suspension 3097

Bleomycin Sulfate (Reduces response to active immunization procedures).
No products indexed under this heading.

Busulfan (Reduces response to active immunization procedures). Products include:
Myleran Tablets 1603

Carmustine (BCNU) (Reduces response to active immunization procedures). Products include:
Gliadel Wafer 1723

Chlorambucil (Reduces response to active immunization procedures). Products include:
Leukeran Tablets 1591

Cortisone Acetate (Reduces response to active immunization procedures). Products include:
Cortone Acetate Injectable Suspension 2059
Cortone Acetate Tablets 2061

Cyclophosphamide (Reduces response to active immunization procedures).
No products indexed under this heading.

Cyclosporine (Reduces response to active immunization procedures). Products include:
Gengraf Capsules 457
Neoral Soft Gelatin Capsules 2380
Neoral Oral Solution 2380
Sandimmune 2388

Dacarbazine (Reduces response to active immunization procedures). Products include:
DTIC-Dome 902

Dalteparin Sodium (Caution should be exercised). Products include:
Fragmin Injection 2814

Danaparoid Sodium (Caution should be exercised). Products include:
Orgaran Injection 2480

Daunorubicin Hydrochloride (Reduces response to active immunization procedures). Products include:
Cerubidine for Injection 947

Dexamethasone (Reduces response to active immunization procedures). Products include:
Decadron Elixir 2078
Decadron Tablets 2079
TobraDex Ophthalmic Ointment 542
TobraDex Ophthalmic Suspension 541

Dexamethasone Acetate (Reduces response to active immunization procedures).
No products indexed under this heading.

Dexamethasone Sodium Phosphate (Reduces response to active immunization procedures). Products include:
Decadron Phosphate Injection 2081
Decadron Phosphate Sterile Ophthalmic Ointment 2083
Decadron Phosphate Sterile Ophthalmic Solution 2084
NeoDecadron Sterile Ophthalmic Solution 2144

Dicumarol (Caution should be exercised).
- No products indexed under this heading.

Doxorubicin Hydrochloride (Reduces response to active immunization procedures). Products include:
- Adriamycin PFS/RDF Injection 2767
- Doxil Injection 566

Enoxaparin (Caution should be exercised). Products include:
- Lovenox Injection 746

Epirubicin Hydrochloride (Reduces response to active immunization procedures). Products include:
- Ellence Injection 2806

Fludrocortisone Acetate (Reduces response to active immunization procedures). Products include:
- Florinef Acetate Tablets 2250

Fluorouracil (Reduces response to active immunization procedures). Products include:
- Carac Cream 1222
- Efudex 1733
- Fluoroplex 552

Heparin Sodium (Caution should be exercised). Products include:
- Heparin Lock Flush Solution 3509
- Heparin Sodium Injection 3511

Hydrocortisone (Reduces response to active immunization procedures). Products include:
- Anusol-HC Cream 2.5% 2237
- Cipro HC Otic Suspension 540
- Cortaid Intensive Therapy Cream .... ▣717
- Cortaid Maximum Strength Cream .... ▣717
- Cortisporin Ophthalmic Suspension Sterile .... ⊙297
- Cortizone•5 .... ▣699
- Cortizone•10 .... ▣699
- Cortizone•10 Plus Creme .... ▣700
- Cortizone for Kids Creme .... ▣699
- Hydrocortone Tablets 2106
- Massengill Medicated Soft Cloth Towelette .... ▣753
- VōSoL HC Otic Solution 3356

Hydrocortisone Acetate (Reduces response to active immunization procedures). Products include:
- Analpram-HC 1338
- Anusol HC-1 Hydrocortisone Anti-Itch Cream .... ▣689
- Anusol-HC Suppositories 2238
- Cortaid .... ▣717
- Cortifoam Rectal Foam 3170
- Cortisporin-TC Otic Suspension 2246
- Hydrocortone Acetate Injectable Suspension 2103
- Pramosone 1343
- Proctocort Suppositories 2264
- ProctoFoam-HC 3177
- Terra-Cortril Ophthalmic Suspension 2716

Hydrocortisone Sodium Phosphate (Reduces response to active immunization procedures). Products include:
- Hydrocortone Phosphate Injection, Sterile 2105

Hydrocortisone Sodium Succinate (Reduces response to active immunization procedures).
- No products indexed under this heading.

Hydroxyurea (Reduces response to active immunization procedures). Products include:
- Mylocel Tablets 2227

Immune Globulin Intravenous (Human) (Reduces response to active immunization procedures).
- No products indexed under this heading.

Lomustine (CCNU) (Reduces response to active immunization procedures).
- No products indexed under this heading.

Mechlorethamine Hydrochloride (Reduces response to active immunization procedures). Products include:
- Mustargen for Injection 2142

Melphalan (Reduces response to active immunization procedures). Products include:
- Alkeran Tablets 1466

Methotrexate Sodium (Reduces response to active immunization procedures).
- No products indexed under this heading.

Methylprednisolone Acetate (Reduces response to active immunization procedures). Products include:
- Depo-Medrol Injectable Suspension 2795

Methylprednisolone Sodium Succinate (Reduces response to active immunization procedures). Products include:
- Solu-Medrol Sterile Powder 2855

Mitotane (Reduces response to active immunization procedures).
- No products indexed under this heading.

Mitoxantrone Hydrochloride (Reduces response to active immunization procedures). Products include:
- Novantrone for Injection 1760

Muromonab-CD3 (Reduces response to active immunization procedures). Products include:
- Orthoclone OKT3 Sterile Solution 2498

Mycophenolate Mofetil (Reduces response to active immunization procedures). Products include:
- CellCept Capsules 2951
- CellCept Oral Suspension 2951
- CellCept Tablets 2951

Prednisolone Acetate (Reduces response to active immunization procedures). Products include:
- Blephamide Ophthalmic Ointment 547
- Blephamide Ophthalmic Suspension 548
- Poly-Pred Liquifilm Ophthalmic Suspension .... ⊙245
- Pred Forte Ophthalmic Suspension .... ⊙246
- Pred Mild Sterile Ophthalmic Suspension .... ⊙249
- Pred-G Ophthalmic Suspension .... ⊙247
- Pred-G Sterile Ophthalmic Ointment .... ⊙248

Prednisolone Sodium Phosphate (Reduces response to active immunization procedures). Products include:
- Pediapred Oral Solution 1170

Prednisolone Tebutate (Reduces response to active immunization procedures).
- No products indexed under this heading.

Prednisone (Reduces response to active immunization procedures). Products include:
- Prednisone 3064

Procarbazine Hydrochloride (Reduces response to active immunization procedures). Products include:
- Matulane Capsules 3246

Sirolimus (Reduces response to active immunization procedures). Products include:
- Rapamune Oral Solution and Tablets 3584

Tacrolimus (Reduces response to active immunization procedures). Products include:
- Prograf 1393
- Protopic Ointment 1397

Tamoxifen Citrate (Reduces response to active immunization procedures). Products include:
- Nolvadex Tablets 678

Thiotepa (Reduces response to active immunization procedures). Products include:
- Thioplex for Injection 1765

Tinzaparin sodium (Caution should be exercised). Products include:
- Innohep Injection 1248

Triamcinolone (Reduces response to active immunization procedures).
- No products indexed under this heading.

Triamcinolone Acetonide (Reduces response to active immunization procedures). Products include:
- Azmacort Inhalation Aerosol 728
- Nasacort Nasal Inhaler 750
- Nasacort AQ Nasal Spray 752
- Tri-Nasal Spray 2274

Triamcinolone Diacetate (Reduces response to active immunization procedures).
- No products indexed under this heading.

Triamcinolone Hexacetonide (Reduces response to active immunization procedures).
- No products indexed under this heading.

Vincristine Sulfate (Reduces response to active immunization procedures).
- No products indexed under this heading.

Warfarin Sodium (Caution should be exercised). Products include:
- Coumadin for Injection 1243
- Coumadin Tablets 1243
- Warfarin Sodium Tablets, USP 3302

ACEON TABLETS (2 MG, 4 MG, 8 MG)

(Perindopril Erbumine) 3249

May interact with diuretics, lithium preparations, potassium preparations, potassium sparing diuretics, and certain other agents. Compounds in these categories include:

Amiloride Hydrochloride (Co-administration of perindopril with potassium-sparing diuretics may increase the risk of hyperkalemia). Products include:
- Midamor Tablets 2136
- Moduretic Tablets 2138

Bendroflumethiazide (Patients on diuretics, and especially those started recently, may occasionally experience an excessive reduction in blood pressure after initiation of perindopril therapy; co-administration has resulted in reduced bioavailability of perindopril). Products include:
- Corzide 40/5 Tablets 2247
- Corzide 80/5 Tablets 2247

Bumetanide (Patients on diuretics, and especially those started recently, may occasionally experience an excessive reduction in blood pressure after initiation of perindopril therapy; co-administration has resulted in reduced bioavailability of perindopril).
- No products indexed under this heading.

Chlorothiazide (Patients on diuretics, and especially those started recently, may occasionally experience an excessive reduction in blood pressure after initiation of perindopril therapy; co-administration has resulted in reduced bioavailability of perindopril). Products include:
- Aldoclor Tablets 2035
- Diuril Oral 2087

Chlorothiazide Sodium (Patients on diuretics, and especially those started recently, may occasionally experience an excessive reduction in blood pressure after initiation of perindopril therapy; co-administration has resulted in reduced bioavailability of perindopril). Products include:
- Diuril Sodium Intravenous 2086

Chlorthalidone (Patients on diuretics, and especially those started recently, may occasionally experience an excessive reduction in blood pressure after initiation of perindopril therapy; co-administration has resulted in reduced bioavailability of perindopril). Products include:
- Clorpres Tablets 1002
- Combipres Tablets 1040
- Tenoretic Tablets 690

Cyclosporine (Co-administration of perindopril with other drugs capable of increasing serum potassium, such as cyclosporine, may increase the risk of hyperkalemia). Products include:
- Gengraf Capsules 457
- Neoral Soft Gelatin Capsules 2380
- Neoral Oral Solution 2380
- Sandimmune 2388

Ethacrynic Acid (Patients on diuretics, and especially those started recently, may occasionally experience an excessive reduction in blood pressure after initiation of perindopril therapy; co-administration has resulted in reduced bioavailability of perindopril). Products include:
- Edecrin Tablets 2091

Furosemide (Patients on diuretics, and especially those started recently, may occasionally experience an excessive reduction in blood pressure after initiation of perindopril therapy; co-administration has resulted in reduced bioavailability of perindopril). Products include:
- Furosemide Tablets 2284

Gentamicin Sulfate (Animal data have suggested the possibility of interaction between gentamicin and perindopril; co-administration should proceed with caution.). Products include:
- Genoptic Ophthalmic Ointment .... ⊙239
- Genoptic Sterile Ophthalmic Solution .... ⊙239
- Pred-G Ophthalmic Suspension .... ⊙247
- Pred-G Sterile Ophthalmic Ointment .... ⊙248

Heparin Sodium (Co-administration of perindopril with other drugs capable of increasing serum potassium, such as heparin, may increase the risk of hyperkalemia). Products include:
- Heparin Lock Flush Solution 3509
- Heparin Sodium Injection 3511

Hydrochlorothiazide (Patients on diuretics, and especially those started recently, may occasionally experience an excessive reduction in blood pressure after initiation of perindopril therapy; co-administration has resulted in reduced bioavailability of perindopril). Products include:
- Accuretic Tablets 2614
- Aldoril Tablets 2039
- Atacand HCT Tablets 597
- Avalide Tablets 1070
- Diovan HCT Tablets 2338
- Dyazide Capsules 1515
- HydroDIURIL Tablets 2108
- Hyzaar 2109
- Inderide Tablets 3517
- Inderide LA Long-Acting Capsules 3519
- Lotensin HCT Tablets 2367
- Maxzide 1008
- Micardis HCT Tablets 1051
- Microzide Capsules 3414
- Moduretic Tablets 2138
- Monopril HCT 1094
- Prinzide Tablets 2168
- Timolide Tablets 2187
- Uniretic Tablets 3178
- Vaseretic Tablets 2204
- Zestoretic Tablets 695
- Ziac Tablets 1887

Hydroflumethiazide (Patients on diuretics, and especially those started recently, may occasionally experience an excessive reduction in blood pressure after initiation of perindopril therapy; co-administration has resulted in reduced bioavailability of perindopril). Products include:
- Diucardin Tablets 3494

Indapamide (Patients on diuretics, and especially those started recently, may occasionally experience an excessive reduction in blood pressure after initiation of perindopril therapy; co-administration has resulted in reduced bioavailability of perindopril). Products include:

Indapamide Tablets 2286

Indomethacin (Co-administration of perindopril with other drugs capable of increasing serum potassium, such as indomethacin, may increase the risk of hyperkalemia). Products include:

Indocin 2112

Lithium Carbonate (Co-administration of ACE inhibitors and lithium has resulted in increased serum lithium levels and symptoms of lithium toxicity). Products include:

Eskalith 1527
Lithium Carbonate 3061
Lithobid Slow-Release Tablets 3255

Lithium Citrate (Co-administration of ACE inhibitors and lithium has resulted in increased serum lithium levels and symptoms of lithium toxicity). Products include:

Lithium Citrate Syrup 3061

Methyclothiazide (Patients on diuretics, and especially those started recently, may occasionally experience an excessive reduction in blood pressure after initiation of perindopril therapy; co-administration has resulted in reduced bioavailability of perindopril).

No products indexed under this heading.

Metolazone (Patients on diuretics, and especially those started recently, may occasionally experience an excessive reduction in blood pressure after initiation of perindopril therapy; co-administration has resulted in reduced bioavailability of perindopril). Products include:

Mykrox Tablets 1168
Zaroxolyn Tablets 1177

Polythiazide (Patients on diuretics, and especially those started recently, may occasionally experience an excessive reduction in blood pressure after initiation of perindopril therapy; co-administration has resulted in reduced bioavailability of perindopril). Products include:

Minizide Capsules 2700
Renese Tablets 2712

Potassium Acid Phosphate (Co-administration of perindopril with potassium supplements may increase the risk of hyperkalemia). Products include:

K-Phos Original (Sodium Free) Tablets 947

Potassium Bicarbonate (Co-administration of perindopril with potassium supplements may increase the risk of hyperkalemia).

No products indexed under this heading.

Potassium Chloride (Co-administration of perindopril with potassium supplements may increase the risk of hyperkalemia). Products include:

Chlor-3 1361
Colyte with Flavor Packs for Oral Solution 3170
GoLYTELY and Pineapple Flavor GoLYTELY for Oral Solution 1068
K-Dur Microburst Release System ER Tablets 1832
Klor-Con M20/Klor-Con M10 Tablets 3329
K-Lor Powder Packets 469
K-Tab Filmtab Tablets 470
Micro-K 3311
NuLYTELY, Cherry Flavor, Lemon-Lime Flavor, and Orange Flavor NuLYTELY for Oral Solution 1068
Rum-K 1363

Potassium Citrate (Co-administration of perindopril with potassium supplements may increase the risk of hyperkalemia). Products include:

Urocit-K Tablets 2232

Potassium Gluconate (Co-administration of perindopril with potassium supplements may increase the risk of hyperkalemia).

No products indexed under this heading.

Potassium Phosphate (Co-administration of perindopril with potassium supplements may increase the risk of hyperkalemia). Products include:

K-Phos Neutral Tablets 946

Spironolactone (Co-administration of perindopril with potassium-sparing diuretics may increase the risk of hyperkalemia).

No products indexed under this heading.

Torsemide (Patients on diuretics, and especially those started recently, may occasionally experience an excessive reduction in blood pressure after initiation of perindopril therapy; co-administration has resulted in reduced bioavailability of perindopril). Products include:

Demadex Tablets and Injection 2965

Triamterene (Co-administration of perindopril with potassium-sparing diuretics may increase the risk of hyperkalemia). Products include:

Dyazide Capsules 1515
Dyrenium Capsules 3458
Maxzide 1008

Food Interactions

Food, unspecified (The presence of food in the GI tract does not affect the rate or extent of absorption of perindopril but reduces bioavailability of perindoprilat by about 35%; in clinical trials, perindopril was generally administered in a non-fasting state).

ACI-JEL THERAPEUTIC VAGINAL JELLY

(Acetic Acid, Oxyquinoline Sulfate) ... 2525
None cited in PDR database.

ACIPHEX TABLETS

(Rabeprazole Sodium) 1783
May interact with iron containing oral preparations and certain other agents. Compounds in these categories include:

Bacampicillin Hydrochloride (Rabeprazole produces sustained inhibition of gastric acid secretion; rabeprazole may interfere with the absorption of certain drugs, such as bacampicillin, where gastric pH is an important determinant of the bioavailability).

No products indexed under this heading.

Digoxin (Co-administration has resulted in an increase in the AUC and Cmax for digoxin of 19% and 29% respectively). Products include:

Digitek Tablets 1003
Lanoxicaps Capsules 1574
Lanoxin Injection 1581
Lanoxin Tablets 1587
Lanoxin Elixir Pediatric 1578
Lanoxin Injection Pediatric 1584

Ferrous Fumarate (Rabeprazole produces sustained inhibition of gastric acid secretion; rabeprazole may interfere with the absorption of certain drugs, such as iron salts, where gastric pH is an important determinant of the bioavailability). Products include:

New Formulation Chromagen OB Capsules 3094
Loestrin Fe Tablets 2642
NataChew Tablets 3364

Ferrous Gluconate (Rabeprazole produces sustained inhibition of gastric acid secretion; rabeprazole may interfere with the absorption of certain drugs, such as iron salts, where gastric pH is an important determinant of the bioavailability). Products include:

Fergon Iron Tablets .... ■802

Ferrous Sulfate (Rabeprazole produces sustained inhibition of gastric acid secretion; rabeprazole may interfere with the absorption of certain drugs, such as iron salts, where gastric pH is an important determinant of the bioavailability). Products include:

Feosol Tablets 1717
Slow Fe Tablets .... ■827
Slow Fe with Folic Acid Tablets ..... ■828

Iron (Rabeprazole produces sustained inhibition of gastric acid secretion; rabeprazole may interfere with the absorption of certain drugs, such as iron salts, where gastric pH is an important determinant of the bioavailability).

No products indexed under this heading.

Ketoconazole (Co-administration has resulted in an approximately 30% decrease in the bioavailability of ketoconazole and increase in the AUC). Products include:

Nizoral 2% Cream 3620
Nizoral A-D Shampoo 2008
Nizoral 2% Shampoo 2007
Nizoral Tablets 1791

Polysaccharide-Iron Complex (Rabeprazole produces sustained inhibition of gastric acid secretion; rabeprazole may interfere with the absorption of certain drugs, such as iron salts, where gastric pH is an important determinant of the bioavailability). Products include:

Niferex 3176
Niferex-150 Capsules 3176
Nu-Iron 150 Capsules 2224

ACIPHEX TABLETS

(Rabeprazole Sodium) 1267
May interact with iron containing oral preparations and certain other agents. Compounds in these categories include:

Bacampicillin Hydrochloride (Rabeprazole produces sustained inhibition of gastric acid secretion; rabeprazole may interfere with the absorption of certain drugs, such as bacampicillin, where gastric pH is an important determinant of the bioavailability).

No products indexed under this heading.

Digoxin (Co-administration has resulted in an increase in the AUC and Cmax for digoxin of 19% and 29% respectively). Products include:

Digitek Tablets 1003
Lanoxicaps Capsules 1574
Lanoxin Injection 1581
Lanoxin Tablets 1587
Lanoxin Elixir Pediatric 1578
Lanoxin Injection Pediatric 1584

Ferrous Fumarate (Rabeprazole produces sustained inhibition of gastric acid secretion; rabeprazole may interfere with the absorption of certain drugs, such as iron salts, where gastric pH is an important determinant of the bioavailability). Products include:

New Formulation Chromagen OB Capsules 3094
Loestrin Fe Tablets 2642
NataChew Tablets 3364

Ferrous Gluconate (Rabeprazole produces sustained inhibition of gastric acid secretion; rabeprazole may interfere with the absorption of certain drugs, such as iron salts, where gastric pH is an important determinant of the bioavailability). Products include:

Fergon Iron Tablets .... ■802

Ferrous Sulfate (Rabeprazole produces sustained inhibition of gastric acid secretion; rabeprazole may interfere with the absorption of certain drugs, such as iron salts, where gastric pH is an important determinant of the bioavailability). Products include:

Feosol Tablets 1717
Slow Fe Tablets .... ■827
Slow Fe with Folic Acid Tablets ..... ■828

Iron (Rabeprazole produces sustained inhibition of gastric acid secretion; rabeprazole may interfere with the absorption of certain drugs, such as iron salts, where gastric pH is an important determinant of the bioavailability).

No products indexed under this heading.

Ketoconazole (Co-administration has resulted in an approximately 30% decrease in the bioavailability of ketoconazole and increase in the AUC). Products include:

Nizoral 2% Cream 3620
Nizoral A-D Shampoo 2008
Nizoral 2% Shampoo 2007
Nizoral Tablets 1791

Polysaccharide-Iron Complex (Rabeprazole produces sustained inhibition of gastric acid secretion; rabeprazole may interfere with the absorption of certain drugs, such as iron salts, where gastric pH is an important determinant of the bioavailability). Products include:

Niferex 3176
Niferex-150 Capsules 3176
Nu-Iron 150 Capsules 2224

ACLOVATE CREAM

(Alclometasone Dipropionate) 1275
None cited in PDR database.

ACLOVATE OINTMENT

(Alclometasone Dipropionate) 1275
None cited in PDR database.

ACTHIB VACCINE

(Haemophilus B Conjugate Vaccine) 798
May interact with alkylating agents, anticoagulants, corticosteroids, cytotoxic drugs, and immunosuppressive agents. Compounds in these categories include:

Ardeparin Sodium (Use with caution).

No products indexed under this heading.

Azathioprine (May reduce the immune response to vaccine).

No products indexed under this heading.

Basiliximab (May reduce the immune response to vaccine). Products include:

Simulect for Injection 2399

Betamethasone Acetate (Corticosteroids, when used in greater than physiologic doses, may reduce the immune response to vaccine). Products include:

Celestone Soluspan Injectable Suspension 3097

Betamethasone Sodium Phosphate (Corticosteroids, when used in greater than physiologic doses, may reduce the immune response to vaccine). Products include:

Celestone Soluspan Injectable Suspension 3097

Bleomycin Sulfate (May reduce the immune response to vaccine).

No products indexed under this heading.

Busulfan (May reduce the immune response to vaccine). Products include:

Myleran Tablets 1603

Carmustine (BCNU) (May reduce the immune response to vaccine). Products include:

Gliadel Wafer 1723

Chlorambucil (May reduce the immune response to vaccine). Products include:

Leukeran Tablets 1591

Cortisone Acetate (Corticosteroids, when used in greater than physiologic doses, may reduce the immune response to vaccine). Products include:

Cortone Acetate Injectable Suspension 2059
Cortone Acetate Tablets 2061

Cyclophosphamide (May reduce the immune response to vaccine).
No products indexed under this heading.

Cyclosporine (May reduce the immune response to vaccine). Products include:
Gengraf Capsules 457
Neoral Soft Gelatin Capsules 2380
Neoral Oral Solution 2380
Sandimmune 2388

Dacarbazine (May reduce the immune response to vaccine). Products include:
DTIC-Dome 902

Dalteparin Sodium (Use with caution). Products include:
Fragmin Injection 2814

Danaparoid Sodium (Use with caution). Products include:
Orgaran Injection 2480

Daunorubicin Hydrochloride (May reduce the immune response to vaccine). Products include:
Cerubidine for Injection 947

Dexamethasone (Corticosteroids, when used in greater than physiologic doses, may reduce the immune response to vaccine). Products include:
Decadron Elixir 2078
Decadron Tablets 2079
TobraDex Ophthalmic Ointment 542
TobraDex Ophthalmic Suspension 541

Dexamethasone Acetate (Corticosteroids, when used in greater than physiologic doses, may reduce the immune response to vaccine).
No products indexed under this heading.

Dexamethasone Sodium Phosphate (Corticosteroids, when used in greater than physiologic doses, may reduce the immune response to vaccine). Products include:
Decadron Phosphate Injection 2081
Decadron Phosphate Sterile Ophthalmic Ointment 2083
Decadron Phosphate Sterile Ophthalmic Solution 2084
NeoDecadron Sterile Ophthalmic Solution 2144

Dicumarol (Use with caution).
No products indexed under this heading.

Doxorubicin Hydrochloride (May reduce the immune response to vaccine). Products include:
Adriamycin PFS/RDF Injection 2767
Doxil Injection 566

Enoxaparin (Use with caution). Products include:
Lovenox Injection 746

Epirubicin Hydrochloride (May reduce the immune response to vaccine). Products include:
Ellence Injection 2806

Fludrocortisone Acetate (Corticosteroids, when used in greater than physiologic doses, may reduce the immune response to vaccine). Products include:
Florinef Acetate Tablets 2250

Fluorouracil (May reduce the immune response to vaccine). Products include:
Carac Cream 1222
Efudex 1733
Fluoroplex 552

Heparin Sodium (Use with caution). Products include:
Heparin Lock Flush Solution 3509
Heparin Sodium Injection 3511

Hydrocortisone (Corticosteroids, when used in greater than physiologic doses, may reduce the immune response to vaccine). Products include:
Anusol-HC Cream 2.5% 2237
Cipro HC Otic Suspension 540
Cortaid Intensive Therapy Cream .... ▣717
Cortaid Maximum Strength Cream .... ▣717
Cortisporin Ophthalmic Suspension Sterile .... ⊙297
Cortizone•5 .... ▣699
Cortizone•10 .... ▣699
Cortizone•10 Plus Creme .... ▣700
Cortizone for Kids Creme .... ▣699
Hydrocortone Tablets 2106
Massengill Medicated Soft Cloth Towelette .... ▣753
VōSoL HC Otic Solution 3356

Hydrocortisone Acetate (Corticosteroids, when used in greater than physiologic doses, may reduce the immune response to vaccine). Products include:
Analpram-HC 1338
Anusol HC-1 Hydrocortisone Anti-Itch Cream .... ▣689
Anusol-HC Suppositories 2238
Cortaid .... ▣717
Cortifoam Rectal Foam 3170
Cortisporin-TC Otic Suspension 2246
Hydrocortone Acetate Injectable Suspension 2103
Pramosone 1343
Proctocort Suppositories 2264
ProctoFoam-HC 3177
Terra-Cortril Ophthalmic Suspension 2716

Hydrocortisone Sodium Phosphate (Corticosteroids, when used in greater than physiologic doses, may reduce the immune response to vaccine). Products include:
Hydrocortone Phosphate Injection, Sterile 2105

Hydrocortisone Sodium Succinate (Corticosteroids, when used in greater than physiologic doses, may reduce the immune response to vaccine).
No products indexed under this heading.

Hydroxyurea (May reduce the immune response to vaccine). Products include:
Mylocel Tablets 2227

Lomustine (CCNU) (May reduce the immune response to vaccine).
No products indexed under this heading.

Mechlorethamine Hydrochloride (May reduce the immune response to vaccine). Products include:
Mustargen for Injection 2142

Melphalan (May reduce the immune response to vaccine). Products include:
Alkeran Tablets 1466

Methotrexate Sodium (May reduce the immune response to vaccine).
No products indexed under this heading.

Methylprednisolone Acetate (Corticosteroids, when used in greater than physiologic doses, may reduce the immune response to vaccine). Products include:
Depo-Medrol Injectable Suspension 2795

Methylprednisolone Sodium Succinate (Corticosteroids, when used in greater than physiologic doses, may reduce the immune response to vaccine). Products include:
Solu-Medrol Sterile Powder 2855

Mitotane (May reduce the immune response to vaccine).
No products indexed under this heading.

Mitoxantrone Hydrochloride (May reduce the immune response to vaccine). Products include:
Novantrone for Injection 1760

Muromonab-CD3 (May reduce the immune response to vaccine). Products include:
Orthoclone OKT3 Sterile Solution 2498

Mycophenolate Mofetil (May reduce the immune response to vaccine). Products include:
CellCept Capsules 2951
CellCept Oral Suspension 2951
CellCept Tablets 2951

Prednisolone Acetate (Corticosteroids, when used in greater than physiologic doses, may reduce the immune response to vaccine). Products include:
Blephamide Ophthalmic Ointment 547
Blephamide Ophthalmic Suspension 548
Poly-Pred Liquifilm Ophthalmic Suspension .... ⊙245
Pred Forte Ophthalmic Suspension .... ⊙246
Pred Mild Sterile Ophthalmic Suspension .... ⊙249
Pred-G Ophthalmic Suspension .... ⊙247
Pred-G Sterile Ophthalmic Ointment .... ⊙248

Prednisolone Sodium Phosphate (Corticosteroids, when used in greater than physiologic doses, may reduce the immune response to vaccine). Products include:
Pediapred Oral Solution 1170

Prednisolone Tebutate (Corticosteroids, when used in greater than physiologic doses, may reduce the immune response to vaccine).
No products indexed under this heading.

Prednisone (Corticosteroids, when used in greater than physiologic doses, may reduce the immune response to vaccine). Products include:
Prednisone 3064

Procarbazine Hydrochloride (May reduce the immune response to vaccine). Products include:
Matulane Capsules 3246

Sirolimus (May reduce the immune response to vaccine). Products include:
Rapamune Oral Solution and Tablets 3584

Tacrolimus (May reduce the immune response to vaccine). Products include:
Prograf 1393
Protopic Ointment 1397

Tamoxifen Citrate (May reduce the immune response to vaccine). Products include:
Nolvadex Tablets 678

Thiotepa (May reduce the immune response to vaccine). Products include:
Thioplex for Injection 1765

Tinzaparin sodium (Use with caution). Products include:
Innohep Injection 1248

Triamcinolone (Corticosteroids, when used in greater than physiologic doses, may reduce the immune response to vaccine).
No products indexed under this heading.

Triamcinolone Acetonide (Corticosteroids, when used in greater than physiologic doses, may reduce the immune response to vaccine). Products include:
Azmacort Inhalation Aerosol 728
Nasacort Nasal Inhaler 750
Nasacort AQ Nasal Spray 752
Tri-Nasal Spray 2274

Triamcinolone Diacetate (Corticosteroids, when used in greater than physiologic doses, may reduce the immune response to vaccine).
No products indexed under this heading.

Triamcinolone Hexacetonide (Corticosteroids, when used in greater than physiologic doses, may reduce the immune response to vaccine).
No products indexed under this heading.

Vincristine Sulfate (May reduce the immune response to vaccine).
No products indexed under this heading.

Warfarin Sodium (Use with caution). Products include:
Coumadin for Injection 1243
Coumadin Tablets 1243
Warfarin Sodium Tablets, USP 3302

ACTHREL FOR INJECTION

(Corticorelin Ovine Triflutate) 3629
May interact with dexamethasone and certain other agents. Compounds in these categories include:

Dexamethasone (The plasma ACTH response to corticorelin injection is inhibited or blunted in normal subjects pretreated with dexamethasone). Products include:
Decadron Elixir 2078
Decadron Tablets 2079
TobraDex Ophthalmic Ointment 542
TobraDex Ophthalmic Suspension 541

Dexamethasone Acetate (The plasma ACTH response to corticorelin injection is inhibited or blunted in normal subjects pretreated with dexamethasone).
No products indexed under this heading.

Dexamethasone Sodium Phosphate (The plasma ACTH response to corticorelin injection is inhibited or blunted in normal subjects pretreated with dexamethasone). Products include:
Decadron Phosphate Injection 2081
Decadron Phosphate Sterile Ophthalmic Ointment 2083
Decadron Phosphate Sterile Ophthalmic Solution 2084
NeoDecadron Sterile Ophthalmic Solution 2144

Heparin Sodium (A possible interaction between corticorelin and heparin may be associated with a major hypotensive reaction; use of heparin to maintain i.v. canula patency during corticorelin test is not recommended). Products include:
Heparin Lock Flush Solution 3509
Heparin Sodium Injection 3511

ACTICIN CREAM

(Permethrin) 998
None cited in PDR database.

ACTIFED COLD & ALLERGY TABLETS

(Pseudoephedrine Hydrochloride, Triprolidine Hydrochloride) .... ▣688
May interact with hypnotics and sedatives, monoamine oxidase inhibitors, tranquilizers, and certain other agents. Compounds in these categories include:

Alprazolam (May increase drowsiness effect). Products include:
Xanax Tablets 2865

Buspirone Hydrochloride (May increase drowsiness effect).
No products indexed under this heading.

Chlordiazepoxide (May increase drowsiness effect). Products include:
Limbitrol 1738

Chlordiazepoxide Hydrochloride (May increase drowsiness effect). Products include:
Librium Capsules 1736
Librium for Injection 1737

Chlorpromazine (May increase drowsiness effect). Products include:
Thorazine Suppositories 1656

Chlorpromazine Hydrochloride (May increase drowsiness effect). Products include:
Thorazine 1656

Chlorprothixene (May increase drowsiness effect).
No products indexed under this heading.

Chlorprothixene Hydrochloride (May increase drowsiness effect).
No products indexed under this heading.

Clorazepate Dipotassium (May increase drowsiness effect). Products include:
Tranxene ... 511
Diazepam (May increase drowsiness effect). Products include:
Valium Injectable ... 3026
Valium Tablets ... 3047
Droperidol (May increase drowsiness effect).
No products indexed under this heading.
Estazolam (May increase drowsiness effect). Products include:
ProSom Tablets ... 500
Ethchlorvynol (May increase drowsiness effect).
No products indexed under this heading.
Ethinamate (May increase drowsiness effect).
No products indexed under this heading.
Fluphenazine Decanoate (May increase drowsiness effect).
No products indexed under this heading.
Fluphenazine Enanthate (May increase drowsiness effect).
No products indexed under this heading.
Fluphenazine Hydrochloride (May increase drowsiness effect).
No products indexed under this heading.
Flurazepam Hydrochloride (May increase drowsiness effect).
No products indexed under this heading.
Glutethimide (May increase drowsiness effect).
No products indexed under this heading.
Haloperidol (May increase drowsiness effect). Products include:
Haldol Injection, Tablets and Concentrate ... 2533
Haloperidol Decanoate (May increase drowsiness effect). Products include:
Haldol Decanoate ... 2535
Hydroxyzine Hydrochloride (May increase drowsiness effect). Products include:
Atarax Tablets & Syrup ... 2667
Vistaril Intramuscular Solution ... 2738
Isocarboxazid (Concurrent and/or sequential use is not recommended).
No products indexed under this heading.
Lorazepam (May increase drowsiness effect). Products include:
Ativan Injection ... 3478
Ativan Tablets ... 3482
Loxapine Hydrochloride (May increase drowsiness effect).
No products indexed under this heading.
Loxapine Succinate (May increase drowsiness effect). Products include:
Loxitane Capsules ... 3398
Meprobamate (May increase drowsiness effect). Products include:
Miltown Tablets ... 3349
Mesoridazine Besylate (May increase drowsiness effect). Products include:
Serentil ... 1057
Midazolam Hydrochloride (May increase drowsiness effect). Products include:
Versed Injection ... 3027
Versed Syrup ... 3033
Moclobemide (Concurrent and/or sequential use is not recommended).
No products indexed under this heading.
Molindone Hydrochloride (May increase drowsiness effect). Products include:
Moban ... 1320
Oxazepam (May increase drowsiness effect).
No products indexed under this heading.
Pargyline Hydrochloride (Concurrent and/or sequential use is not recommended).
No products indexed under this heading.
Perphenazine (May increase drowsiness effect). Products include:
Etrafon ... 3115
Trilafon ... 3160
Phenelzine Sulfate (Concurrent and/or sequential use is not recommended). Products include:
Nardil Tablets ... 2653
Prazepam (May increase drowsiness effect).
No products indexed under this heading.
Procarbazine Hydrochloride (Concurrent and/or sequential use is not recommended). Products include:
Matulane Capsules ... 3246
Prochlorperazine (May increase drowsiness effect). Products include:
Compazine ... 1505
Promethazine Hydrochloride (May increase drowsiness effect). Products include:
Mepergan Injection ... 3539
Phenergan Injection ... 3553
Phenergan ... 3556
Phenergan Syrup ... 3554
Phenergan with Codeine Syrup ... 3557
Phenergan with Dextromethorphan Syrup ... 3559
Phenergan VC Syrup ... 3560
Phenergan VC with Codeine Syrup . 3561
Propofol (May increase drowsiness effect). Products include:
Diprivan Injectable Emulsion ... 667
Quazepam (May increase drowsiness effect).
No products indexed under this heading.
Secobarbital Sodium (May increase drowsiness effect).
No products indexed under this heading.
Selegiline Hydrochloride (Concurrent and/or sequential use is not recommended). Products include:
Eldepryl Capsules ... 3266
Temazepam (May increase drowsiness effect).
No products indexed under this heading.
Thioridazine Hydrochloride (May increase drowsiness effect). Products include:
Thioridazine Hydrochloride Tablets ... 2289
Thiothixene (May increase drowsiness effect). Products include:
Navane Capsules ... 2701
Thiothixene Capsules ... 2290
Tranylcypromine Sulfate (Concurrent and/or sequential use is not recommended). Products include:
Parnate Tablets ... 1607
Triazolam (May increase drowsiness effect). Products include:
Halcion Tablets ... 2823
Trifluoperazine Hydrochloride (May increase drowsiness effect). Products include:
Stelazine ... 1640
Zaleplon (May increase drowsiness effect). Products include:
Sonata Capsules ... 3591
Zolpidem Tartrate (May increase drowsiness effect). Products include:
Ambien Tablets ... 3191

Food Interactions

Alcohol (May increase drowsiness effect).

ACTIFED COLD & SINUS CAPLETS AND TABLETS
(Acetaminophen, Chlorpheniramine Maleate, Pseudoephedrine Hydrochloride) ... ■688
May interact with hypnotics and sedatives, monoamine oxidase inhibitors, tranquilizers, and certain other agents. Compounds in these categories include:
Alprazolam (May increase drowsiness effect). Products include:
Xanax Tablets ... 2865
Buspirone Hydrochloride (May increase drowsiness effect).
No products indexed under this heading.
Chlordiazepoxide (May increase drowsiness effect). Products include:
Limbitrol ... 1738
Chlordiazepoxide Hydrochloride (May increase drowsiness effect). Products include:
Librium Capsules ... 1736
Librium for Injection ... 1737
Chlorpromazine (May increase drowsiness effect). Products include:
Thorazine Suppositories ... 1656
Chlorpromazine Hydrochloride (May increase drowsiness effect). Products include:
Thorazine ... 1656
Chlorprothixene (May increase drowsiness effect).
No products indexed under this heading.
Chlorprothixene Hydrochloride (May increase drowsiness effect).
No products indexed under this heading.
Clorazepate Dipotassium (May increase drowsiness effect). Products include:
Tranxene ... 511
Diazepam (May increase drowsiness effect). Products include:
Valium Injectable ... 3026
Valium Tablets ... 3047
Droperidol (May increase drowsiness effect).
No products indexed under this heading.
Estazolam (May increase drowsiness effect). Products include:
ProSom Tablets ... 500
Ethchlorvynol (May increase drowsiness effect).
No products indexed under this heading.
Ethinamate (May increase drowsiness effect).
No products indexed under this heading.
Fluphenazine Decanoate (May increase drowsiness effect).
No products indexed under this heading.
Fluphenazine Enanthate (May increase drowsiness effect).
No products indexed under this heading.
Fluphenazine Hydrochloride (May increase drowsiness effect).
No products indexed under this heading.
Flurazepam Hydrochloride (May increase drowsiness effect).
No products indexed under this heading.
Glutethimide (May increase drowsiness effect).
No products indexed under this heading.
Haloperidol (May increase drowsiness effect). Products include:
Haldol Injection, Tablets and Concentrate ... 2533
Haloperidol Decanoate (May increase drowsiness effect). Products include:
Haldol Decanoate ... 2535
Hydroxyzine Hydrochloride (May increase drowsiness effect). Products include:
Atarax Tablets & Syrup ... 2667
Vistaril Intramuscular Solution ... 2738
Isocarboxazid (Concurrent and/or sequential use with MAO inhibitors is not recommended).
No products indexed under this heading.
Lorazepam (May increase drowsiness effect). Products include:
Ativan Injection ... 3478
Ativan Tablets ... 3482
Loxapine Hydrochloride (May increase drowsiness effect).
No products indexed under this heading.
Loxapine Succinate (May increase drowsiness effect). Products include:
Loxitane Capsules ... 3398
Meprobamate (May increase drowsiness effect). Products include:
Miltown Tablets ... 3349
Mesoridazine Besylate (May increase drowsiness effect). Products include:
Serentil ... 1057
Midazolam Hydrochloride (May increase drowsiness effect). Products include:
Versed Injection ... 3027
Versed Syrup ... 3033
Moclobemide (Concurrent and/or sequential use with MAO inhibitors is not recommended).
No products indexed under this heading.
Molindone Hydrochloride (May increase drowsiness effect). Products include:
Moban ... 1320
Oxazepam (May increase drowsiness effect).
No products indexed under this heading.
Pargyline Hydrochloride (Concurrent and/or sequential use with MAO inhibitors is not recommended).
No products indexed under this heading.
Perphenazine (May increase drowsiness effect). Products include:
Etrafon ... 3115
Trilafon ... 3160
Phenelzine Sulfate (Concurrent and/or sequential use with MAO inhibitors is not recommended). Products include:
Nardil Tablets ... 2653
Prazepam (May increase drowsiness effect).
No products indexed under this heading.
Procarbazine Hydrochloride (Concurrent and/or sequential use with MAO inhibitors is not recommended). Products include:
Matulane Capsules ... 3246
Prochlorperazine (May increase drowsiness effect). Products include:
Compazine ... 1505
Promethazine Hydrochloride (May increase drowsiness effect). Products include:
Mepergan Injection ... 3539
Phenergan Injection ... 3553
Phenergan ... 3556
Phenergan Syrup ... 3554
Phenergan with Codeine Syrup ... 3557
Phenergan with Dextromethorphan Syrup ... 3559
Phenergan VC Syrup ... 3560
Phenergan VC with Codeine Syrup . 3561
Propofol (May increase drowsiness effect). Products include:
Diprivan Injectable Emulsion ... 667
Quazepam (May increase drowsiness effect).
No products indexed under this heading.

Secobarbital Sodium (May increase drowsiness effect).
No products indexed under this heading.

Selegiline Hydrochloride (Concurrent and/or sequential use with MAO inhibitors is not recommended). Products include:
Eldepryl Capsules 3266

Temazepam (May increase drowsiness effect).
No products indexed under this heading.

Thioridazine Hydrochloride (May increase drowsiness effect). Products include:
Thioridazine Hydrochloride Tablets 2289

Thiothixene (May increase drowsiness effect). Products include:
Navane Capsules 2701
Thiothixene Capsules 2290

Tranylcypromine Sulfate (Concurrent and/or sequential use with MAO inhibitors is not recommended). Products include:
Parnate Tablets 1607

Triazolam (May increase drowsiness effect). Products include:
Halcion Tablets 2823

Trifluoperazine Hydrochloride (May increase drowsiness effect). Products include:
Stelazine 1640

Zaleplon (May increase drowsiness effect). Products include:
Sonata Capsules 3591

Zolpidem Tartrate (May increase drowsiness effect). Products include:
Ambien Tablets 3191

Food Interactions

Alcohol (May increase drowsiness effect; patients consuming 3 or more alcoholic beverages a day should consult a physician for advice on when and how they should take this medication).

ACTIMMUNE

(Interferon Gamma-1B) 1772
May interact with:

Bone Marrow Depressants, unspecified (Caution should be exercised when administering with other potentially myelosuppressive agents).

ACTIQ

(Fentanyl Citrate) 1184
May interact with antihistamines, central nervous system depressants, erythromycin, general anesthetics, hypnotics and sedatives, monoamine oxidase inhibitors, narcotic analgesics, phenothiazines, tranquilizers, and certain other agents. Compounds in these categories include:

Acrivastine (Co-administration may result in increased depressant effects). Products include:
Semprex-D Capsules 1172

Alfentanil Hydrochloride (Co-administration may result in increased depressant effects; hypoventilation, hypotension, and profound sedation may occur).
No products indexed under this heading.

Alprazolam (Co-administration may result in increased depressant effects; hypoventilation, hypotension, and profound sedation may occur). Products include:
Xanax Tablets 2865

Aprobarbital (Co-administration may result in increased depressant effects; hypoventilation, hypotension, and profound sedation may occur).
No products indexed under this heading.

Astemizole (Co-administration may result in increased depressant effects).
No products indexed under this heading.

Azatadine Maleate (Co-administration may result in increased depressant effects). Products include:
Rynatan Tablets 3351

Bromodiphenhydramine Hydrochloride (Co-administration may result in increased depressant effects).
No products indexed under this heading.

Brompheniramine Maleate (Co-administration may result in increased depressant effects). Products include:
Bromfed Capsules (Extended-Release) 2269
Bromfed-PD Capsules (Extended-Release) 2269
Comtrex Acute Head Cold & Sinus Pressure Relief Tablets 627
Dimetapp Elixir 777
Dimetapp Cold and Fever Suspension 775
Dimetapp DM Cold & Cough Elixir 775
Dimetapp Nighttime Flu Liquid 776

Buprenorphine Hydrochloride (Co-administration may result in increased depressant effects; hypoventilation, hypotension, and profound sedation may occur). Products include:
Buprenex Injectable 2918

Buspirone Hydrochloride (Co-administration may result in increased depressant effects; hypoventilation, hypotension, and profound sedation may occur).
No products indexed under this heading.

Butabarbital (Co-administration may result in increased depressant effects; hypoventilation, hypotension, and profound sedation may occur).
No products indexed under this heading.

Butalbital (Co-administration may result in increased depressant effects; hypoventilation, hypotension, and profound sedation may occur). Products include:
Phrenilin 578
Sedapap Tablets 50 mg/650 mg 2225

Cetirizine Hydrochloride (Co-administration may result in increased depressant effects). Products include:
Zyrtec 2756
Zyrtec-D 12 Hour Extended Relief Tablets 2758

Chlordiazepoxide (Co-administration may result in increased depressant effects; hypoventilation, hypotension, and profound sedation may occur). Products include:
Limbitrol 1738

Chlordiazepoxide Hydrochloride (Co-administration may result in increased depressant effects; hypoventilation, hypotension, and profound sedation may occur). Products include:
Librium Capsules 1736
Librium for Injection 1737

Chlorpheniramine Maleate (Co-administration may result in increased depressant effects). Products include:
Actifed Cold & Sinus Caplets and Tablets 688
Alka-Seltzer Plus Liqui-Gels 604
BC Allergy Sinus Cold Powder 619
Chlor-Trimeton Allergy Tablets 735
Chlor-Trimeton Allergy/Decongestant Tablets 736
Comtrex Flu Therapy & Fever Relief Nighttime Tablets 628
Comtrex Maximum Strength Multi-Symptom Cold & Cough Relief Tablets and Caplets 626
Contac Severe Cold and Flu Caplets Maximum Strength 746
Coricidin 'D' Cold, Flu & Sinus Tablets 737
Coricidin/Coricidin D 738
Coricidin HBP Maximum Strength Flu Tablets 738
Extendryl 1361
Hycomine Compound Tablets 1317
Kronofed-A 1341
PediaCare Cough-Cold Liquid 719
PediaCare NightRest Cough-Cold Liquid 719
Robitussin Nighttime Honey Flu Liquid 786
Ryna 768
Singlet Caplets 761
Sinutab Sinus Allergy Medication, Maximum Strength Formula, Tablets & Caplets 707
Sudafed Cold & Allergy Tablets 708
TheraFlu Regular Strength Cold & Cough Night Time Hot Liquid 676
TheraFlu Regular Strength Cold & Sore Throat Night Time Hot Liquid 676
TheraFlu Maximum Strength Flu & Cough Night Time Hot Liquid 678
TheraFlu Maximum Strength Flu & Sore Throat Night Time Hot Liquid 677
TheraFlu Maximum Strength Severe Cold & Congestion Night Time Caplets 678
TheraFlu Maximum Strength Severe Cold & Congestion Night Time Hot Liquid 678
Triaminic Cold & Allergy Liquid 681
Triaminic Cold & Allergy Softchews 683
Triaminic Cold & Cough Liquid 681
Triaminic Cold & Cough Softchews 683
Triaminic Cold & Night Time Cough Liquid 681
Triaminic Cold, Cough & Fever Liquid 681
Children's Tylenol Cold Suspension Liquid and Chewable Tablets 2015
Children's Tylenol Cold Plus Cough Suspension Liquid and Chewable Tablets 2015
Children's Tylenol Flu Suspension Liquid 2015
Maximum Strength Tylenol Allergy Sinus Caplets, Gelcaps, and Geltabs 2010
Multi-Symptom Tylenol Cold Complete Formula Caplets 2010
Vicks 44M Cough, Cold & Flu Relief Liquid 725
Pediatric Vicks 44m Cough & Cold Relief 728
Children's Vicks NyQuil Cold/Cough Relief 726

Chlorpheniramine Polistirex (Co-administration may result in increased depressant effects). Products include:
Tussionex Pennkinetic Extended-Release Suspension 1174

Chlorpheniramine Tannate (Co-administration may result in increased depressant effects). Products include:
Reformulated Rynatan Pediatric Suspension 3352
Rynatuss Pediatric Suspension 3353
Rynatuss Tablets 3353
Tussi-12 S Suspension 3356
Tussi-12 Tablets 3356

Chlorpromazine (Co-administration may result in increased depressant effects; hypoventilation, hypotension, and profound sedation may occur). Products include:
Thorazine Suppositories 1656

Chlorpromazine Hydrochloride (Co-administration may result in increased depressant effects; hypoventilation, hypotension, and profound sedation may occur). Products include:
Thorazine 1656

Chlorprothixene (Co-administration may result in increased depressant effects; hypoventilation, hypotension, and profound sedation may occur).
No products indexed under this heading.

Chlorprothixene Hydrochloride (Co-administration may result in increased depressant effects; hypoventilation, hypotension, and profound sedation may occur).
No products indexed under this heading.

Chlorprothixene Lactate (Co-administration may result in increased depressant effects; hypoventilation, hypotension, and profound sedation may occur).
No products indexed under this heading.

Clemastine Fumarate (Co-administration may result in increased depressant effects). Products include:
Tavist 12 Hour Allergy Tablets 676

Clorazepate Dipotassium (Co-administration may result in increased depressant effects; hypoventilation, hypotension, and profound sedation may occur). Products include:
Tranxene 511

Clozapine (Co-administration may result in increased depressant effects; hypoventilation, hypotension, and profound sedation may occur). Products include:
Clozaril Tablets 2319

Codeine Phosphate (Co-administration may result in increased depressant effects; hypoventilation, hypotension, and profound sedation may occur). Products include:
Phenergan with Codeine Syrup 3557
Phenergan VC with Codeine Syrup 3561
Robitussin A-C Syrup 2942
Robitussin-DAC Syrup 2942
Ryna-C Liquid 768
Soma Compound w/Codeine Tablets 3355
Tussi-Organidin NR Liquid 3350
Tussi-Organidin-S NR Liquid 3350
Tylenol with Codeine 2595

Cyproheptadine Hydrochloride (Co-administration may result in increased depressant effects). Products include:
Periactin Tablets 2155

Desflurane (Co-administration may result in increased depressant effects; hypoventilation, hypotension, and profound sedation may occur). Products include:
Suprane Liquid for Inhalation 874

Dexchlorpheniramine Maleate (Co-administration may result in increased depressant effects).
No products indexed under this heading.

Dezocine (Co-administration may result in increased depressant effects; hypoventilation, hypotension, and profound sedation may occur).
No products indexed under this heading.

Diazepam (Co-administration may result in increased depressant effects; hypoventilation, hypotension, and profound sedation may occur). Products include:
Valium Injectable 3026
Valium Tablets 3047

Diphenhydramine Citrate (Co-administration may result in increased depressant effects). Products include:
Alka-Seltzer PM Effervescent Tablets 605
Benadryl Allergy & Sinus Fastmelt Tablets 693
Benadryl Children's Allergy/Cold Fastmelt Tablets 692
Excedrin PM Tablets, Caplets, and Geltabs 631
Goody's PM Powder 621

Diphenhydramine Hydrochloride (Co-administration may result in increased depressant effects). Products include:

Extra Strength Bayer PM Caplets ■611
Benadryl Allergy Chewables ■689
Benadryl Allergy ■691
Benadryl Allergy Liquid ■690
Benadryl Allergy/Cold Tablets ■691
Benadryl Allergy/Congestion Tablets ■692
Benadryl Allergy & Sinus Liquid ■693
Benadryl Allergy Sinus Headache Caplets & Gelcaps ■693
Benadryl Severe Allergy & Sinus Headache Caplets ■694
Benadryl Dye-Free Allergy Liquid ■690
Benadryl Dye-Free Allergy Liqui-Gels Softgels ■690
Benadryl Itch Relief Stick Extra Strength ■695
Benadryl Cream ■695
Benadryl Gel ■695
Benadryl Spray ■696
Benadryl Parenteral 2617
Coricidin HBP Night-Time Cold & Flu Tablets ■738
Nytol QuickCaps Caplets ■622
Maximum Strength Nytol QuickGels Softgels ■621
Extra Strength Percogesic Aspirin-Free Coated Caplets ■665
Simply Sleep Caplets 2008
Sominex Original Formula Tablets ■761
Children's Tylenol Allergy-D Liquid 2014
Maximum Strength Tylenol Allergy Sinus NightTime Caplets 2010
Tylenol Severe Allergy Caplets 2010
Maximum Strength Tylenol Flu NightTime Gelcaps 2011
Extra Strength Tylenol PM Caplets, Geltabs, and Gelcaps 2012
Unisom Maximum Strength SleepGels ■713

Diphenylpyraline Hydrochloride (Co-administration may result in increased depressant effects).
No products indexed under this heading.

Droperidol (Co-administration may result in increased depressant effects; hypoventilation, hypotension, and profound sedation may occur).
No products indexed under this heading.

Enflurane (Co-administration may result in increased depressant effects; hypoventilation, hypotension, and profound sedation may occur).
No products indexed under this heading.

Erythromycin (Co-administration with potent inhibitors of CYP4503A4 isoform, such as erythromycin, may increase the bioavailability of swallowed fentanyl by decreasing intestinal and hepatic first pass metabolism and may decrease the systemic clearance resulting in increased or prolonged opioid effects). Products include:
Emgel 2% Topical Gel 1285
Ery-Tab Tablets 448
Erythromycin Base Filmtab Tablets 454
Erythromycin Delayed-Release Capsules, USP 455
PCE Dispertab Tablets 498

Erythromycin Estolate (Co-administration with potent inhibitors of CYP4503A4 isoform, such as erythromycin, may increase the bioavailability of swallowed fentanyl by decreasing intestinal and hepatic first pass metabolism and may decrease the systemic clearance resulting in increased or prolonged opioid effects).
No products indexed under this heading.

Erythromycin Ethylsuccinate (Co-administration with potent inhibitors of CYP4503A4 isoform, such as erythromycin, may increase the bioavailability of swallowed fentanyl by decreasing intestinal and hepatic first pass metabolism and may decrease the systemic clearance resulting in increased or prolonged opioid effects). Products include:
E.E.S. 450
EryPed 446
Pediazole Suspension 3050

Erythromycin Gluceptate (Co-administration with potent inhibitors of CYP4503A4 isoform, such as erythromycin, may increase the bioavailability of swallowed fentanyl by decreasing intestinal and hepatic first pass metabolism and may decrease the systemic clearance resulting in increased or prolonged opioid effects).
No products indexed under this heading.

Erythromycin Stearate (Co-administration with potent inhibitors of CYP4503A4 isoform, such as erythromycin, may increase the bioavailability of swallowed fentanyl by decreasing intestinal and hepatic first pass metabolism and may decrease the systemic clearance resulting in increased or prolonged opioid effects). Products include:
Erythrocin Stearate Filmtab Tablets 452

Estazolam (Co-administration may result in increased depressant effects; hypoventilation, hypotension, and profound sedation may occur). Products include:
ProSom Tablets 500

Ethchlorvynol (Co-administration may result in increased depressant effects; hypoventilation, hypotension, and profound sedation may occur).
No products indexed under this heading.

Ethinamate (Co-administration may result in increased depressant effects; hypoventilation, hypotension, and profound sedation may occur).
No products indexed under this heading.

Fentanyl (Co-administration may result in increased depressant effects; hypoventilation, hypotension, and profound sedation may occur). Products include:
Duragesic Transdermal System 1786

Fexofenadine Hydrochloride (Co-administration may result in increased depressant effects). Products include:
Allegra 712
Allegra-D Extended-Release Tablets 714

Fluphenazine Decanoate (Co-administration may result in increased depressant effects; hypoventilation, hypotension, and profound sedation may occur).
No products indexed under this heading.

Fluphenazine Enanthate (Co-administration may result in increased depressant effects; hypoventilation, hypotension, and profound sedation may occur).
No products indexed under this heading.

Fluphenazine Hydrochloride (Co-administration may result in increased depressant effects; hypoventilation, hypotension, and profound sedation may occur).
No products indexed under this heading.

Flurazepam Hydrochloride (Co-administration may result in increased depressant effects; hypoventilation, hypotension, and profound sedation may occur).
No products indexed under this heading.

Glutethimide (Co-administration may result in increased depressant effects; hypoventilation, hypotension, and profound sedation may occur).
No products indexed under this heading.

Haloperidol (Co-administration may result in increased depressant effects; hypoventilation, hypotension, and profound sedation may occur). Products include:
Haldol Injection, Tablets and Concentrate 2533

Haloperidol Decanoate (Co-administration may result in increased depressant effects; hypoventilation, hypotension, and profound sedation may occur). Products include:
Haldol Decanoate 2535

Hydrocodone Bitartrate (Co-administration may result in increased depressant effects; hypoventilation, hypotension, and profound sedation may occur). Products include:
Hycodan 1316
Hycomine Compound Tablets 1317
Hycotuss Expectorant Syrup 1318
Lortab 3319
Lortab Elixir 3317
Maxidone Tablets CIII 3399
Norco 5/325 Tablets CIII 3424
Norco 7.5/325 Tablets CIII 3425
Norco 10/325 Tablets CIII 3427
Norco 10/325 Tablets CIII 3425
Vicodin Tablets 516
Vicodin ES Tablets 517
Vicodin HP Tablets 518
Vicodin Tuss Expectorant 519
Vicoprofen Tablets 520
Zydone Tablets 1330

Hydrocodone Polistirex (Co-administration may result in increased depressant effects; hypoventilation, hypotension, and profound sedation may occur). Products include:
Tussionex Pennkinetic Extended-Release Suspension 1174

Hydromorphone Hydrochloride (Co-administration may result in increased depressant effects; hypoventilation, hypotension, and profound sedation may occur). Products include:
Dilaudid 441
Dilaudid Oral Liquid 445
Dilaudid Powder 441
Dilaudid Rectal Suppositories 441
Dilaudid Tablets 441
Dilaudid Tablets - 8 mg 445
Dilaudid-HP 443

Hydroxyzine Hydrochloride (Co-administration may result in increased depressant effects; hypoventilation, hypotension, and profound sedation may occur). Products include:
Atarax Tablets & Syrup 2667
Vistaril Intramuscular Solution 2738

Isocarboxazid (Concurrent and/or sequential use with MAO inhibitors is not recommended; potential for severe and unpredictable potentiation of MAO inhibitors has been reported with opioid analgesics).
No products indexed under this heading.

Isoflurane (Co-administration may result in increased depressant effects; hypoventilation, hypotension, and profound sedation may occur).
No products indexed under this heading.

Itraconazole (Co-administration with potent inhibitors of CYP4503A4 isoform, such as azole antifungal itraconazole, may increase the bioavailability of swallowed fentanyl by decreasing intestinal and hepatic first pass metabolism and may decrease the systemic clearance resulting in increased or prolonged opioid effects). Products include:
Sporanox Capsules 1800
Sporanox Injection 1804
Sporanox Injection 2509
Sporanox Oral Solution 1808
Sporanox Oral Solution 2512

Ketamine Hydrochloride (Co-administration may result in increased depressant effects; hypoventilation, hypotension, and profound sedation may occur).
No products indexed under this heading.

Ketoconazole (Co-administration with potent inhibitors of CYP4503A4 isoform, such as azole antifungal ketoconazole, may increase the bioavailability of swallowed fentanyl by decreasing intestinal and hepatic first pass metabolism and may decrease the systemic clearance resulting in increased or prolonged opioid effects). Products include:
Nizoral 2% Cream 3620
Nizoral A-D Shampoo 2008
Nizoral 2% Shampoo 2007
Nizoral Tablets 1791

Levomethadyl Acetate Hydrochloride (Co-administration may result in increased depressant effects; hypoventilation, hypotension, and profound sedation may occur).
No products indexed under this heading.

Levorphanol Tartrate (Co-administration may result in increased depressant effects; hypoventilation, hypotension, and profound sedation may occur). Products include:
Levo-Dromoran 1734
Levorphanol Tartrate Tablets 3059

Loratadine (Co-administration may result in increased depressant effects). Products include:
Claritin 3100
Claritin-D 12 Hour Extended Release Tablets 3102
Claritin-D 24 Hour Extended Release Tablets 3104

Lorazepam (Co-administration may result in increased depressant effects; hypoventilation, hypotension, and profound sedation may occur). Products include:
Ativan Injection 3478
Ativan Tablets 3482

Loxapine Hydrochloride (Co-administration may result in increased depressant effects; hypoventilation, hypotension, and profound sedation may occur).
No products indexed under this heading.

Loxapine Succinate (Co-administration may result in increased depressant effects; hypoventilation, hypotension, and profound sedation may occur). Products include:
Loxitane Capsules 3398

Meperidine Hydrochloride (Co-administration may result in increased depressant effects; hypoventilation, hypotension, and profound sedation may occur). Products include:
Demerol 3079
Mepergan Injection 3539

Mephobarbital (Co-administration may result in increased depressant effects; hypoventilation, hypotension, and profound sedation may occur).
No products indexed under this heading.

Meprobamate (Co-administration may result in increased depressant effects; hypoventilation, hypotension, and profound sedation may occur). Products include:
Miltown Tablets 3349

Mesoridazine Besylate (Co-administration may result in increased depressant effects; hypoventilation, hypotension, and profound sedation may occur). Products include:
Serentil 1057

Methadone Hydrochloride (Co-administration may result in increased depressant effects; hypo-

ventilation, hypotension, and profound sedation may occur). Products include:

Dolophine Hydrochloride Tablets 3056

Methdilazine Hydrochloride (Co-administration may result in increased depressant effects).

No products indexed under this heading.

Methohexital Sodium (Co-administration may result in increased depressant effects; hypoventilation, hypotension, and profound sedation may occur). Products include:

Brevital Sodium for Injection, USP .. 1815

Methotrimeprazine (Co-administration may result in increased depressant effects; hypoventilation, hypotension, and profound sedation may occur).

No products indexed under this heading.

Methoxyflurane (Co-administration may result in increased depressant effects; hypoventilation, hypotension, and profound sedation may occur).

No products indexed under this heading.

Midazolam Hydrochloride (Co-administration may result in increased depressant effects; hypoventilation, hypotension, and profound sedation may occur). Products include:

Versed Injection 3027
Versed Syrup 3033

Moclobemide (Concurrent and/or sequential use with MAO inhibitors is not recommended; potential for severe and unpredictable potentiation of MAO inhibitors has been reported with opioid analgesics).

No products indexed under this heading.

Molindone Hydrochloride (Co-administration may result in increased depressant effects; hypoventilation, hypotension, and profound sedation may occur). Products include:

Moban 1320

Morphine Sulfate (Co-administration may result in increased depressant effects; hypoventilation, hypotension, and profound sedation may occur). Products include:

Astramorph/PF Injection, USP (Preservative-Free)........................ 594
Duramorph Injection 1312
Infumorph 200 and Infumorph 500 Sterile Solutions........................ 1314
Kadian Capsules 1335
MS Contin Tablets 2896
MSIR 2898
Oramorph SR Tablets 3062
Roxanol 3066

Olanzapine (Co-administration may result in increased depressant effects; hypoventilation, hypotension, and profound sedation may occur). Products include:

Zyprexa Tablets 1973
Zyprexa ZYDIS Orally Disintegrating Tablets.................. 1973

Oxazepam (Co-administration may result in increased depressant effects; hypoventilation, hypotension, and profound sedation may occur).

No products indexed under this heading.

Oxycodone Hydrochloride (Co-administration may result in increased depressant effects; hypoventilation, hypotension, and profound sedation may occur). Products include:

OxyContin Tablets 2912
OxyFast Oral Concentrate Solution . 2916
OxyIR Capsules 2916
Percocet Tablets 1326
Percodan Tablets 1327
Percolone Tablets 1327
Roxicodone 3067
Tylox Capsules 2597

Pargyline Hydrochloride (Concurrent and/or sequential use with MAO inhibitors is not recommended; potential for severe and unpredictable potentiation of MAO inhibitors has been reported with opioid analgesics).

No products indexed under this heading.

Pentobarbital Sodium (Co-administration may result in increased depressant effects; hypoventilation, hypotension, and profound sedation may occur). Products include:

Nembutal Sodium Solution 485

Perphenazine (Co-administration may result in increased depressant effects; hypoventilation, hypotension, and profound sedation may occur). Products include:

Etrafon 3115
Trilafon 3160

Phenelzine Sulfate (Concurrent and/or sequential use with MAO inhibitors is not recommended; potential for severe and unpredictable potentiation of MAO inhibitors has been reported with opioid analgesics). Products include:

Nardil Tablets 2653

Phenobarbital (Co-administration may result in increased depressant effects; hypoventilation, hypotension, and profound sedation may occur). Products include:

Arco-Lase Plus Tablets 592
Donnatal 2929
Donnatal Extentabs 2930

Prazepam (Co-administration may result in increased depressant effects; hypoventilation, hypotension, and profound sedation may occur).

No products indexed under this heading.

Procarbazine Hydrochloride (Concurrent and/or sequential use with MAO inhibitors is not recommended; potential for severe and unpredictable potentiation of MAO inhibitors has been reported with opioid analgesics). Products include:

Matulane Capsules 3246

Prochlorperazine (Co-administration may result in increased depressant effects; hypoventilation, hypotension, and profound sedation may occur). Products include:

Compazine 1505

Promethazine Hydrochloride (Co-administration may result in increased depressant effects). Products include:

Mepergan Injection 3539
Phenergan Injection 3553
Phenergan 3556
Phenergan Syrup 3554
Phenergan with Codeine Syrup 3557
Phenergan with Dextromethorphan Syrup... 3559
Phenergan VC Syrup 3560
Phenergan VC with Codeine Syrup .. 3561

Propofol (Co-administration may result in increased depressant effects; hypoventilation, hypotension, and profound sedation may occur). Products include:

Diprivan Injectable Emulsion 667

Propoxyphene Hydrochloride (Co-administration may result in increased depressant effects; hypoventilation, hypotension, and profound sedation may occur). Products include:

Darvon Pulvules 1909
Darvon Compound-65 Pulvules 1910

Propoxyphene Napsylate (Co-administration may result in increased depressant effects; hypoventilation, hypotension, and profound sedation may occur). Products include:

Darvon-N/Darvocet-N 1907
Darvon-N Tablets 1912

Pyrilamine Maleate (Co-administration may result in increased depressant effects). Products include:

Maximum Strength Midol Menstrual Caplets and Gelcaps.............................. 612
Maximum Strength Midol PMS Caplets and Gelcaps.................. 613

Pyrilamine Tannate (Co-administration may result in increased depressant effects). Products include:

Ryna-12 S Suspension 3351

Quazepam (Co-administration may result in increased depressant effects; hypoventilation, hypotension, and profound sedation may occur).

No products indexed under this heading.

Quetiapine Fumarate (Co-administration may result in increased depressant effects; hypoventilation, hypotension, and profound sedation may occur). Products include:

Seroquel Tablets 684

Remifentanil Hydrochloride (Co-administration may result in increased depressant effects; hypoventilation, hypotension, and profound sedation may occur).

No products indexed under this heading.

Risperidone (Co-administration may result in increased depressant effects; hypoventilation, hypotension, and profound sedation may occur). Products include:

Risperdal 1796

Ritonavir (Co-administration with potent inhibitors of CYP4503A4 isoform, such as protease inhibitor ritonavir, may increase the bioavailability of swallowed fentanyl by decreasing intestinal and hepatic first pass metabolism and may decrease the systemic clearance resulting in increased or prolonged opioid effects). Products include:

Kaletra Capsules 471
Kaletra Oral Solution 471
Norvir Capsules 487
Norvir Oral Solution 487

Secobarbital Sodium (Co-administration may result in increased depressant effects; hypoventilation, hypotension, and profound sedation may occur).

No products indexed under this heading.

Selegiline Hydrochloride (Concurrent and/or sequential use with MAO inhibitors is not recommended; potential for severe and unpredictable potentiation of MAO inhibitors has been reported with opioid analgesics). Products include:

Eldepryl Capsules 3266

Sevoflurane (Co-administration may result in increased depressant effects; hypoventilation, hypotension, and profound sedation may occur).

No products indexed under this heading.

Sufentanil Citrate (Co-administration may result in increased depressant effects; hypoventilation, hypotension, and profound sedation may occur).

No products indexed under this heading.

Temazepam (Co-administration may result in increased depressant effects; hypoventilation, hypotension, and profound sedation may occur).

No products indexed under this heading.

Terfenadine (Co-administration may result in increased depressant effects).

No products indexed under this heading.

Thiamylal Sodium (Co-administration may result in increased depressant effects; hypoventilation, hypotension, and profound sedation may occur).

No products indexed under this heading.

Thioridazine Hydrochloride (Co-administration may result in increased depressant effects; hypoventilation, hypotension, and profound sedation may occur). Products include:

Thioridazine Hydrochloride Tablets... 2289

Thiothixene (Co-administration may result in increased depressant effects; hypoventilation, hypotension, and profound sedation may occur). Products include:

Navane Capsules 2701
Thiothixene Capsules 2290

Tranylcypromine Sulfate (Concurrent and/or sequential use with MAO inhibitors is not recommended; potential for severe and unpredictable potentiation of MAO inhibitors has been reported with opioid analgesics). Products include:

Parnate Tablets 1607

Triazolam (Co-administration may result in increased depressant effects; hypoventilation, hypotension, and profound sedation may occur). Products include:

Halcion Tablets 2823

Trifluoperazine Hydrochloride (Co-administration may result in increased depressant effects; hypoventilation, hypotension, and profound sedation may occur). Products include:

Stelazine 1640

Trimeprazine Tartrate (Co-administration may result in increased depressant effects).

No products indexed under this heading.

Tripelennamine Hydrochloride (Co-administration may result in increased depressant effects).

No products indexed under this heading.

Triprolidine Hydrochloride (Co-administration may result in increased depressant effects). Products include:

Actifed Cold & Allergy Tablets 688

Zaleplon (Co-administration may result in increased depressant effects; hypoventilation, hypotension, and profound sedation may occur). Products include:

Sonata Capsules 3591

Ziprasidone Hydrochloride (Co-administration may result in increased depressant effects; hypoventilation, hypotension, and profound sedation may occur). Products include:

Geodon Capsules 2688

Zolpidem Tartrate (Co-administration may result in increased depressant effects; hypoventilation, hypotension, and profound sedation may occur). Products include:

Ambien Tablets 3191

Food Interactions

Alcohol (Concurrent use with alcoholic beverages may result in increased depressant effects; hypoventilation, hypotension, and profound sedation may occur).

ACTIVASE I.V.

(Alteplase, Recombinant) 1410

May interact with vitamin K antagonists and certain other agents. Compounds in these categories include:

Abciximab (Drugs that alter platelet function, such as abciximab, may

increase the risk of bleeding if administered prior to or after alteplase therapy). Products include:

ReoPro Vials 1958

Aspirin (Drugs that alter platelet function, such as aspirin, may increase the risk of bleeding if administered prior to or after alteplase therapy). Products include:

Aggrenox Capsules 1026
Alka-Seltzer ◘603
Alka-Seltzer Lemon Lime Antacid and Pain Reliever Effervescent Tablets ◘603
Alka-Seltzer Extra Strength Antacid and Pain Reliever Effervescent Tablets ◘603
Alka-Seltzer PM Effervescent Tablets ◘605
Genuine Bayer Tablets, Caplets and Gelcaps ◘606
Extra Strength Bayer Caplets and Gelcaps ◘610
Aspirin Regimen Bayer Children's Chewable Tablets (Orange or Cherry Flavored) ◘607
Bayer, Aspirin Regimen ◘606
Aspirin Regimen Bayer 81 mg Caplets with Calcium ◘607
Genuine Bayer Professional Labeling (Aspirin Regimen Bayer) ◘608
Extra Strength Bayer Arthritis Caplets ◘610
Extra Strength Bayer Plus Caplets ◘610
Extra Strength Bayer PM Caplets ◘611
BC Powder ◘619
BC Allergy Sinus Cold Powder ◘619
Arthritis Strength BC Powder ◘619
BC Sinus Cold Powder ◘619
Darvon Compound-65 Pulvules 1910
Ecotrin Enteric Coated Aspirin Low, Regular and Maximum Strength Tablets 1715
Excedrin Extra-Strength Tablets, Caplets, and Geltabs ◘629
Excedrin Migraine 1070
Goody's Body Pain Formula Powder ◘620
Goody's Extra Strength Headache Powder ◘620
Goody's Extra Strength Pain Relief Tablets ◘620
Percodan Tablets 1327
Robaxisal Tablets 2939
Soma Compound Tablets 3354
Soma Compound w/Codeine Tablets 3355
Vanquish Caplets ◘617

Clopidogrel Bisulfate (Drugs that alter platelet function, such as clopidogrel, may increase the risk of bleeding if administered prior to or after alteplase therapy). Products include:

Plavix Tablets 1097
Plavix Tablets 3084

Dicumarol (Co-administration increases the risk of bleeding).

No products indexed under this heading.

Dipyridamole (Drugs that alter platelet function, such as dipyridamole, may increase the risk of bleeding if administered prior to or after alteplase therapy). Products include:

Aggrenox Capsules 1026
Persantine Tablets 1057

Eptifibatide (Drugs that alter platelet function, such as eptifibatide, may increase the risk of bleeding if administered prior to or after alteplase therapy). Products include:

Integrilin Injection 1213
Integrilin Injection 1828

Heparin Sodium (Co-administration increases the risk of bleeding). Products include:

Heparin Lock Flush Solution 3509
Heparin Sodium Injection 3511

Ticlopidine Hydrochloride (Drugs that alter platelet function, such as ticlopidine, may increase the risk of bleeding if administered prior to or after alteplase therapy). Products include:

Ticlid Tablets 3015

Tirofiban Hydrochloride (Drugs that alter platelet function, such as tirofiban, may increase the risk of bleeding if administered prior to or after alteplase therapy). Products include:

Aggrastat 2031

Warfarin Sodium (Co-administration increases the risk of bleeding). Products include:

Coumadin for Injection 1243
Coumadin Tablets 1243
Warfarin Sodium Tablets, USP 3302

ACTIVE CALCIUM TABLETS

(Calcium Citrate, Vitamin D) 3335
None cited in PDR database.

ACTIVELLA TABLETS

(Estradiol, Norethindrone Acetate) 2764
None cited in PDR database.

ACTONEL TABLETS

(Risedronate Sodium) 2879
May interact with antacids containing aluminum, calcium and magnesium, calcium preparations, and certain other agents. Compounds in these categories include:

Aluminum Carbonate (Antacids may interfere with the absorption of Actonel; antacids should be taken at a different time of the day).

No products indexed under this heading.

Aluminum Hydroxide (Antacids may interfere with the absorption of Actonel; antacids should be taken at a different time of the day). Products include:

Amphojel Suspension (Mint Flavor) ◘789
Gaviscon Extra Strength Liquid ◘751
Gaviscon Extra Strength Tablets ◘751
Gaviscon Regular Strength Liquid ◘751
Gaviscon Regular Strength Tablets ◘750
Maalox Antacid/Anti-Gas Oral Suspension ◘673
Maalox Max Maximum Strength Antacid/Anti-Gas Liquid 2300
Maalox Regular Strength Antacid/Antigas Liquid 2300
Mylanta 1813
Vanquish Caplets ◘617

Aspirin (The incidence of gastrointestinal adverse events is, in general, higher with co-administration; caution should be used). Products include:

Aggrenox Capsules 1026
Alka-Seltzer ◘603
Alka-Seltzer Lemon Lime Antacid and Pain Reliever Effervescent Tablets ◘603
Alka-Seltzer Extra Strength Antacid and Pain Reliever Effervescent Tablets ◘603
Alka-Seltzer PM Effervescent Tablets ◘605
Genuine Bayer Tablets, Caplets and Gelcaps ◘606
Extra Strength Bayer Caplets and Gelcaps ◘610
Aspirin Regimen Bayer Children's Chewable Tablets (Orange or Cherry Flavored) ◘607
Bayer, Aspirin Regimen ◘606
Aspirin Regimen Bayer 81 mg Caplets with Calcium ◘607
Genuine Bayer Professional Labeling (Aspirin Regimen Bayer) ◘608
Extra Strength Bayer Arthritis Caplets ◘610
Extra Strength Bayer Plus Caplets ◘610
Extra Strength Bayer PM Caplets ◘611
BC Powder ◘619
BC Allergy Sinus Cold Powder ◘619
Arthritis Strength BC Powder ◘619
BC Sinus Cold Powder ◘619
Darvon Compound-65 Pulvules 1910
Ecotrin Enteric Coated Aspirin Low, Regular and Maximum Strength Tablets 1715
Excedrin Extra-Strength Tablets, Caplets, and Geltabs ◘629
Excedrin Migraine 1070
Goody's Body Pain Formula Powder ◘620
Goody's Extra Strength Headache Powder ◘620
Goody's Extra Strength Pain Relief Tablets ◘620
Percodan Tablets 1327
Robaxisal Tablets 2939
Soma Compound Tablets 3354
Soma Compound w/Codeine Tablets 3355
Vanquish Caplets ◘617

Calcium Carbonate (Calcium-containing preparations may interfere with the absorption of Actonel; calcium preparations should be taken at a different time of the day). Products include:

Aspirin Regimen Bayer 81 mg Caplets with Calcium ◘607
Extra Strength Bayer Plus Caplets ◘610
Caltrate 600 Tablets ◘814
Caltrate 600 PLUS ◘815
Caltrate 600 + D Tablets ◘814
Caltrate 600 + Soy Tablets ◘814
D-Cal Chewable Caplets ◘794
Florical Capsules and Tablets 2223
Quick Dissolve Maalox Max Maximum Strength Antacid/Antigas Tablets 2301
Quick Dissolve Maalox Regular Strength Antacid Tablets 2301
Marblen Suspension ◘633
Monocal Tablets 2223
Mylanta Fast-Acting 1813
Mylanta Calci Tabs ◘636
One-A-Day Bedtime & Rest Tablets ◘805
One-A-Day Calcium Plus Chewable Tablets ◘805
Os-Cal Chewable Tablets ◘838
Pepcid Complete Chewable Tablets 1815
ReSource Wellness CalciWise Soft Chews ◘824
Rolaids Tablets ◘706
Extra Strength Rolaids Tablets ◘706
Slow-Mag Tablets ◘835
Titralac ◘640
3M Titralac Plus Antacid Tablets ◘640
Tums ◘763

Calcium Chloride (Calcium-containing preparations may interfere with the absorption of Actonel; calcium preparations should be taken at a different time of the day).

No products indexed under this heading.

Calcium Citrate (Calcium-containing preparations may interfere with the absorption of Actonel; calcium preparations should be taken at a different time of the day). Products include:

Active Calcium Tablets 3335
Citracal Liquitab Tablets ◘823
Citracal Tablets 2231
Citracal Caplets + D ◘823

Calcium Glubionate (Calcium-containing preparations may interfere with the absorption of Actonel; calcium preparations should be taken at a different time of the day).

No products indexed under this heading.

Magaldrate (Antacids may interfere with the absorption of Actonel; antacids should be taken at a different time of the day).

No products indexed under this heading.

Magnesium Hydroxide (Antacids may interfere with the absorption of Actonel; antacids should be taken at a different time of the day). Products include:

Ex•Lax Milk of Magnesia Liquid ◘670
Maalox Antacid/Anti-Gas Oral Suspension ◘673
Maalox Max Maximum Strength Antacid/Anti-Gas Liquid 2300
Maalox Regular Strength Antacid/Antigas Liquid 2300
Mylanta Fast-Acting 1813
Mylanta 1813
Pepcid Complete Chewable Tablets 1815
Phillips' Chewable Tablets ◘615
Phillips' Milk of Magnesia Liquid (Original, Cherry, & Mint) ◘616
Rolaids Tablets ◘706
Extra Strength Rolaids Tablets ◘706
Vanquish Caplets ◘617

Magnesium Oxide (Antacids may interfere with the absorption of Actonel; antacids should be taken at a different time of the day). Products include:

Beelith Tablets 946
Mag-Ox 400 Tablets 1024
Uro-Mag Capsules 1024

Food Interactions

Food, unspecified (Mean oral bioavailability is decreased when risedronate is administered with food; Actonel is effective when administered at least 30 minutes before breakfast).

ACTOS TABLETS

(Pioglitazone Hydrochloride) 3275
May interact with:

Ethinyl Estradiol (Co-administration of another thiazolidinedione with an oral contraceptive containing ethinyl estradiol and norethindrone has reduced the plasma concentrations of both hormones; the pharmacokinetics between an oral contraceptive and pioglitazone has not been evaluated, therefore, additional caution regarding contraception is advised). Products include:

Alesse-21 Tablets 3468
Alesse-28 Tablets 3473
Brevicon 28-Day Tablets 3380
Cyclessa Tablets 2450
Desogen Tablets 2458
Estinyl Tablets 3112
Estrostep 2627
femhrt Tablets 2635
Levlen 962
Levlite 21 Tablets 962
Levlite 28 Tablets 962
Levora Tablets 3389
Loestrin 21 Tablets 2642
Loestrin Fe Tablets 2642
Lo/Ovral Tablets 3532
Lo/Ovral-28 Tablets 3538
Low-Ogestrel-28 Tablets 3392
Microgestin Fe 1.5/30 Tablets 3407
Microgestin Fe 1/20 Tablets 3400
Mircette Tablets 2470
Modicon 2563
Necon 3415
Nordette-28 Tablets 2257
Norinyl 1 +35 28-Day Tablets 3380
Ogestrel 0.5/50-28 Tablets 3428
Ortho-Cept 21 Tablets 2546
Ortho-Cept 28 Tablets 2546
Ortho-Cyclen/Ortho Tri-Cyclen 2573
Ortho-Novum 2563
Ovcon 3364
Ovral Tablets 3551
Ovral-28 Tablets 3552
Tri-Levlen 962
Tri-Norinyl-28 Tablets 3433
Triphasil-21 Tablets 3600
Triphasil-28 Tablets 3605
Trivora Tablets 3439
Yasmin 28 Tablets 980
Zovia 3449

Ketoconazole (In vitro, ketoconazole appears to significantly inhibit metabolism of pioglitazone). Products include:

Nizoral 2% Cream 3620
Nizoral A-D Shampoo 2008
Nizoral 2% Shampoo 2007
Nizoral Tablets 1791

ACTOTHERM CAPLETS

(Herbals with Vitamins & Minerals) ◘794
None cited in PDR database.

ACULAR OPHTHALMIC SOLUTION

(Ketorolac Tromethamine) 544
None cited in PDR database.

ACULAR PF OPHTHALMIC SOLUTION

(Ketorolac Tromethamine) 544
May interact with:

Warfarin Sodium (Potential for increased bleeding time; concurrent

use with other agents which prolong bleeding time requires caution). Products include:

Coumadin for Injection 1243
Coumadin Tablets 1243
Warfarin Sodium Tablets, USP 3302

ADAGEN INJECTION

(Pegademase Bovine) 1331
May interact with:

Vidarabine Monohydrate (Concomitant use can substantially alter activities of Adagen).
No products indexed under this heading.

ADALAT CC TABLETS

(Nifedipine) 877
May interact with beta blockers, oral anticoagulants, cardiac glycosides, narcotic analgesics, and certain other agents. Compounds in these categories include:

Acebutolol Hydrochloride (Combination of nifedipine and beta blocker may increase the likelihood of congestive heart failure, severe hypotension, or exacerbation of angina). Products include:
Sectral Capsules 3589

Alfentanil Hydrochloride (Potential for severe hypotension and/or increased fluid volume requirements cannot be ruled out when nifedipine is co-administered with beta blocker and narcotic analgesic).
No products indexed under this heading.

Atenolol (Combination of nifedipine and beta blocker may increase the likelihood of congestive heart failure, severe hypotension, or exacerbation of angina). Products include:
Tenoretic Tablets 690
Tenormin I.V. Injection 692

Betaxolol Hydrochloride (Combination of nifedipine and beta blocker may increase the likelihood of congestive heart failure, severe hypotension, or exacerbation of angina). Products include:
Betoptic S Ophthalmic Suspension 537

Bisoprolol Fumarate (Combination of nifedipine and beta blocker may increase the likelihood of congestive heart failure, severe hypotension, or exacerbation of angina). Products include:
Zebeta Tablets 1885
Ziac Tablets 1887

Buprenorphine Hydrochloride (Potential for severe hypotension and/or increased fluid volume requirements cannot be ruled out when nifedipine is co-administered with beta blocker and narcotic analgesic). Products include:
Buprenex Injectable 2918

Carteolol Hydrochloride (Combination of nifedipine and beta blocker may increase the likelihood of congestive heart failure, severe hypotension, or exacerbation of angina). Products include:
Carteolol Hydrochloride Ophthalmic Solution USP, 1% ..... ⊙258
Ocupress Ophthalmic Solution, 1% Sterile .... ⊙303

Cimetidine (Both the peak plasma level of nifedipine and AUC may increase in the presence of cimetidine). Products include:
Tagamet HB 200 Suspension .... ■762
Tagamet HB 200 Tablets .... ■761
Tagamet Tablets 1644

Cimetidine Hydrochloride (Both the peak plasma level of nifedipine and AUC may increase in the presence of cimetidine). Products include:
Tagamet 1644

Codeine Phosphate (Potential for severe hypotension and/or increased fluid volume requirements cannot be ruled out when nifedipine is co-administered with beta blocker and narcotic analgesic). Products include:
Phenergan with Codeine Syrup 3557
Phenergan VC with Codeine Syrup .. 3561
Robitussin A-C Syrup 2942
Robitussin-DAC Syrup 2942
Ryna-C Liquid .... ■768
Soma Compound w/Codeine Tablets 3355
Tussi-Organidin NR Liquid 3350
Tussi-Organidin-S NR Liquid 3350
Tylenol with Codeine 2595

Deslanoside (Potential of elevated digoxin levels).
No products indexed under this heading.

Dezocine (Potential for severe hypotension and/or increased fluid volume requirements cannot be ruled out when nifedipine is co-administered with beta blocker and narcotic analgesic).
No products indexed under this heading.

Dicumarol (Rare reports of increased prothrombin time).
No products indexed under this heading.

Digitoxin (Potential of elevated digoxin levels).
No products indexed under this heading.

Digoxin (Potential of elevated digoxin levels). Products include:
Digitek Tablets 1003
Lanoxicaps Capsules 1574
Lanoxin Injection 1581
Lanoxin Tablets 1587
Lanoxin Elixir Pediatric 1578
Lanoxin Injection Pediatric 1584

Esmolol Hydrochloride (Combination of nifedipine and beta blocker may increase the likelihood of congestive heart failure, severe hypotension, or exacerbation of angina). Products include:
Brevibloc Injection 858

Fentanyl (Potential for severe hypotension and/or increased fluid volume requirements cannot be ruled out when nifedipine is co-administered with beta blocker, narcotic analgesic and high dose fentanyl anesthesia). Products include:
Duragesic Transdermal System 1786

Fentanyl Citrate (Potential for severe hypotension and/or increased fluid volume requirements cannot be ruled out when nifedipine is co-administered with beta blocker, narcotic analgesic and high-dose fentanyl anesthesia). Products include:
Actiq 1184

Hydrocodone Bitartrate (Potential for severe hypotension and/or increased fluid volume requirements cannot be ruled out when nifedipine is co-administered with beta blocker and narcotic analgesic). Products include:
Hycodan 1316
Hycomine Compound Tablets 1317
Hycotuss Expectorant Syrup 1318
Lortab 3319
Lortab Elixir 3317
Maxidone Tablets CIII 3399
Norco 5/325 Tablets CIII 3424
Norco 7.5/325 Tablets CIII 3425
Norco 10/325 Tablets CIII 3427
Norco 10/325 Tablets CIII 3425
Vicodin Tablets 516
Vicodin ES Tablets 517
Vicodin HP Tablets 518
Vicodin Tuss Expectorant 519
Vicoprofen Tablets 520
Zydone Tablets 1330

Hydrocodone Polistirex (Potential for severe hypotension and/or increased fluid volume requirements cannot be ruled out when nifedipine is co-administered with beta blocker and narcotic analgesic). Products include:
Tussionex Pennkinetic Extended-Release Suspension 1174

Hydromorphone Hydrochloride (Potential for severe hypotension and/or increased fluid volume requirements cannot be ruled out when nifedipine is co-administered with beta blocker and narcotic analgesic). Products include:
Dilaudid 441
Dilaudid Oral Liquid 445
Dilaudid Powder 441
Dilaudid Rectal Suppositories 441
Dilaudid Tablets 441
Dilaudid Tablets - 8 mg 445
Dilaudid-HP 443

Labetalol Hydrochloride (Combination of nifedipine and beta blocker may increase the likelihood of congestive heart failure, severe hypotension, or exacerbation of angina). Products include:
Normodyne Injection 3135
Normodyne Tablets 3137

Levobunolol Hydrochloride (Combination of nifedipine and beta blocker may increase the likelihood of congestive heart failure, severe hypotension, or exacerbation of angina). Products include:
Betagan .... ⊙228

Levorphanol Tartrate (Potential for severe hypotension and/or increased fluid volume requirements cannot be ruled out when nifedipine is co-administered with beta blocker and narcotic analgesic). Products include:
Levo-Dromoran 1734
Levorphanol Tartrate Tablets 3059

Meperidine Hydrochloride (Potential for severe hypotension and/or increased fluid volume requirements cannot be ruled out when nifedipine is co-administered with beta blocker and narcotic analgesic). Products include:
Demerol 3079
Mepergan Injection 3539

Methadone Hydrochloride (Potential for severe hypotension and/or increased fluid volume requirements cannot be ruled out when nifedipine is co-administered with beta blocker and narcotic analgesic). Products include:
Dolophine Hydrochloride Tablets 3056

Metipranolol Hydrochloride (Combination of nifedipine and beta blocker may increase the likelihood of congestive heart failure, severe hypotension, or exacerbation of angina).
No products indexed under this heading.

Metoprolol Succinate (Combination of nifedipine and beta blocker may increase the likelihood of congestive heart failure, severe hypotension, or exacerbation of angina). Products include:
Toprol-XL Tablets 651

Metoprolol Tartrate (Combination of nifedipine and beta blocker may increase the likelihood of congestive heart failure, severe hypotension, or exacerbation of angina).
No products indexed under this heading.

Morphine Sulfate (Potential for severe hypotension and/or increased fluid volume requirements cannot be ruled out when nifedipine is co-administered with beta blocker and narcotic analgesic). Products include:
Astramorph/PF Injection, USP (Preservative-Free) 594
Duramorph Injection 1312
Infumorph 200 and Infumorph 500 Sterile Solutions 1314
Kadian Capsules 1335
MS Contin Tablets 2896
MSIR 2898
Oramorph SR Tablets 3062
Roxanol 3066

Nadolol (Combination of nifedipine and beta blocker may increase the likelihood of congestive heart failure, severe hypotension, or exacerbation of angina). Products include:
Corgard Tablets 2245
Corzide 40/5 Tablets 2247
Corzide 80/5 Tablets 2247
Nadolol Tablets 2288

Oxycodone Hydrochloride (Potential for severe hypotension and/or increased fluid volume requirements cannot be ruled out when nifedipine is co-administered with beta blocker and narcotic analgesic). Products include:
OxyContin Tablets 2912
OxyFast Oral Concentrate Solution . 2916
OxyIR Capsules 2916
Percocet Tablets 1326
Percodan Tablets 1327
Percolone Tablets 1327
Roxicodone 3067
Tylox Capsules 2597

Penbutolol Sulfate (Combination of nifedipine and beta blocker may increase the likelihood of congestive heart failure, severe hypotension, or exacerbation of angina).
No products indexed under this heading.

Pindolol (Combination of nifedipine and beta blocker may increase the likelihood of congestive heart failure, severe hypotension, or exacerbation of angina).
No products indexed under this heading.

Propoxyphene Hydrochloride (Potential for severe hypotension and/or increased fluid volume requirements cannot be ruled out when nifedipine is co-administered with beta blocker and narcotic analgesic). Products include:
Darvon Pulvules 1909
Darvon Compound-65 Pulvules 1910

Propoxyphene Napsylate (Potential for severe hypotension and/or increased fluid volume requirements cannot be ruled out when nifedipine is co-administered with beta blocker and narcotic analgesic). Products include:
Darvon-N/Darvocet-N 1907
Darvon-N Tablets 1912

Propranolol Hydrochloride (Combination of nifedipine and beta blocker may increase the likelihood of congestive heart failure, severe hypotension, or exacerbation of angina). Products include:
Inderal 3513
Inderal LA Long-Acting Capsules 3516
Inderide Tablets 3517
Inderide LA Long-Acting Capsules .. 3519

Quinidine Gluconate (Rare reports of decreased plasma level of quinidine). Products include:
Quinaglute Dura-Tabs Tablets 978

Quinidine Polygalacturonate (Rare reports of decreased plasma level of quinidine).
No products indexed under this heading.

Quinidine Sulfate (Rare reports of decreased plasma level of quinidine). Products include:
Quinidex Extentabs 2933

Ranitidine Hydrochloride (Produces smaller, non-significant increases in peak nifedipine plasma levels and AUC). Products include:
Zantac 1690
Zantac Injection 1688
Zantac 75 Tablets .... ■717

Remifentanil Hydrochloride (Potential for severe hypotension and/or increased fluid volume requirements cannot be ruled out when nifedipine is co-administered with beta blocker and narcotic analgesic).
No products indexed under this heading.

Sotalol Hydrochloride (Combination of nifedipine and beta blocker may increase the likelihood of congestive heart failure, severe hypotension, or exacerbation of angina). Products include:
- Betapace Tablets 950
- Betapace AF Tablets 954

Sufentanil Citrate (Potential for severe hypotension and/or increased fluid volume requirements cannot be ruled out when nifedipine is co-administered with beta blocker and narcotic analgesic).
No products indexed under this heading.

Timolol Hemihydrate (Combination of nifedipine and beta blocker may increase the likelihood of congestive heart failure, severe hypotension, or exacerbation of angina). Products include:
- Betimol Ophthalmic Solution .... ⊙324

Timolol Maleate (Combination of nifedipine and beta blocker may increase the likelihood of congestive heart failure, severe hypotension, or exacerbation of angina). Products include:
- Blocadren Tablets 2046
- Cosopt Sterile Ophthalmic Solution 2065
- Timolide Tablets 2187
- Timolol GFS .... ⊙266
- Timoptic in Ocudose 2192
- Timoptic Sterile Ophthalmic Solution 2190
- Timoptic-XE Sterile Ophthalmic Gel Forming Solution 2194

Warfarin Sodium (Rare reports of increased prothrombin time). Products include:
- Coumadin for Injection 1243
- Coumadin Tablets 1243
- Warfarin Sodium Tablets, USP 3302

Food Interactions

Diet, high-lipid (High fat meal increases peak plasma nifedipine concentrations by 60%, a prolongation in the time to peak concentration, but no significant change in the AUC; administer on an empty stomach).

Grapefruit Juice (Co-administration of nifedipine with grapefruit juice results in up to a 2-fold increase in AUC and Cmax, due to inhibition of CYP3A4 related first pass metabolism; co-administration should be avoided).

ADDERALL TABLETS

(Amphetamine Aspartate, Amphetamine Sulfate, Dextroamphetamine Saccharate, Dextroamphetamine Sulfate) 3231

See Adderall XR Capsules

ADDERALL XR CAPSULES

(Amphetamine Aspartate, Amphetamine Sulfate, Dextroamphetamine Saccharate, Dextroamphetamine Sulfate)
May interact with:

Acebutolol Hydrochloride (Adrenergic blockers are inhibited by amphetamines; amphetamines may antagonize the hypotensive effects of antihypertensives). Products include:
- Sectral Capsules 3589

Acetazolamide (Co-administration with urinary alkalinizing agents, such as acetazolamide, increase the concentration of the non-ionized species of the amphetamine molecule, thereby decreasing urinary excretion resulting in increased blood levels and potentiate the actions of amphetamines). Products include:
- Diamox Sequels Sustained Release Capsules .... ⊙270
- Diamox Tablets .... ⊙269

Acetazolamide Sodium (Co-administration with urinary alkalinizing agents, such as acetazolamide, increase the concentration of the non-ionized species of the amphetamine molecule, thereby decreasing urinary excretion resulting in increased blood levels and potentiate the actions of amphetamines). Products include:
- Diamox Intravenous .... ⊙269

Acrivastine (Amphetamines may counteract the sedative effect of antihistamines). Products include:
- Semprex-D Capsules 1172

Aluminum Carbonate (Co-administration with gastrointestinal alkalinizing agents, such as antacids, may increase the absorption of amphetamines; concurrent use should be avoided).
No products indexed under this heading.

Aluminum Hydroxide (Co-administration with gastrointestinal alkalinizing agents, such as antacids, may increase the absorption of amphetamines; concurrent use should be avoided). Products include:
- Amphojel Suspension (Mint Flavor) .... ■789
- Gaviscon Extra Strength Liquid .... ■751
- Gaviscon Extra Strength Tablets .... ■751
- Gaviscon Regular Strength Liquid .... ■751
- Gaviscon Regular Strength Tablets .... ■750
- Maalox Antacid/Anti-Gas Oral Suspension .... ■673
- Maalox Max Maximum Strength Antacid/Anti-Gas Liquid 2300
- Maalox Regular Strength Antacid/Antigas Liquid 2300
- Mylanta 1813
- Vanquish Caplets .... ■617

Amitriptyline Hydrochloride (Enhanced activity of tricyclic antidepressants or sympathomimetics; possible increases in d-amphetamine resulting in potentiation of cardiovascular effects). Products include:
- Etrafon 3115
- Limbitrol 1738

Amlodipine Besylate (Amphetamines may antagonize the hypotensive effects of antihypertensives). Products include:
- Lotrel Capsules 2370
- Norvasc Tablets 2704

Ammonium Chloride (Co-administration with urinary acidifying agents increases the concentration of the ionized species of the amphetamine molecule, thereby increasing urinary excretion resulting in reduced blood levels and efficacy of amphetamines).
No products indexed under this heading.

Amoxapine (Enhanced activity of tricyclic antidepressants or sympathomimetics; possible increases in d-amphetamine resulting in potentiation of cardiovascular effects).
No products indexed under this heading.

Astemizole (Amphetamines may counteract the sedative effect of antihistamines).
No products indexed under this heading.

Atenolol (Adrenergic blockers are inhibited by amphetamines; amphetamines may antagonize the hypotensive effects of antihypertensives). Products include:
- Tenoretic Tablets 690
- Tenormin I.V. Injection 692

Azatadine Maleate (Amphetamines may counteract the sedative effect of antihistamines). Products include:
- Rynatan Tablets 3351

Benazepril Hydrochloride (Amphetamines may antagonize the hypotensive effects of antihypertensives). Products include:
- Lotensin Tablets 2365
- Lotensin HCT Tablets 2367
- Lotrel Capsules 2370

Bendroflumethiazide (Co-administration with urinary alkalinizing agents, such as certain thiazides, increase the concentration of the non-ionized species of the amphetamine molecule, thereby decreasing urinary excretion resulting in increased blood levels and potentiation ofactions of amphetamines; amphetamines may antagonize the hypotensive effects of antihypertensives). Products include:
- Corzide 40/5 Tablets 2247
- Corzide 80/5 Tablets 2247

Betaxolol Hydrochloride (Adrenergic blockers are inhibited by amphetamines; amphetamines may antagonize the hypotensive effects of antihypertensives). Products include:
- Betoptic S Ophthalmic Suspension 537

Bisoprolol Fumarate (Adrenergic blockers are inhibited by amphetamines; amphetamines may antagonize the hypotensive effects of antihypertensives). Products include:
- Zebeta Tablets 1885
- Ziac Tablets 1887

Bromodiphenhydramine Hydrochloride (Amphetamines may counteract the sedative effect of antihistamines).
No products indexed under this heading.

Brompheniramine Maleate (Amphetamines may counteract the sedative effect of antihistamines). Products include:
- Bromfed Capsules (Extended-Release) 2269
- Bromfed-PD Capsules (Extended-Release) 2269
- Comtrex Acute Head Cold & Sinus Pressure Relief Tablets .... ■627
- Dimetapp Elixir .... ■777
- Dimetapp Cold and Fever Suspension .... ■775
- Dimetapp DM Cold & Cough Elixir .... ■775
- Dimetapp Nighttime Flu Liquid .... ■776

Candesartan Cilexetil (Amphetamines may antagonize the hypotensive effects of antihypertensives). Products include:
- Atacand Tablets 595
- Atacand HCT Tablets 597

Captopril (Amphetamines may antagonize the hypotensive effects of antihypertensives). Products include:
- Captopril Tablets 2281

Carteolol Hydrochloride (Adrenergic blockers are inhibited by amphetamines; amphetamines may antagonize the hypotensive effects of antihypertensives). Products include:
- Carteolol Hydrochloride Ophthalmic Solution USP, 1% .... ⊙258
- Ocupress Ophthalmic Solution, 1% Sterile .... ⊙303

Cetirizine Hydrochloride (Amphetamines may counteract the sedative effect of antihistamines). Products include:
- Zyrtec 2756
- Zyrtec-D 12 Hour Extended Relief Tablets 2758

Chlorothiazide (Co-administration with urinary alkalinizing agents, such as certain thiazides, increase the concentration of the non-ionized species of the amphetamine molecule, thereby decreasing urinary excretion resulting in increased blood levels and potentiation ofactions of amphetamines; amphetamines may antagonize the hypotensive effects of antihypertensives). Products include:
- Aldoclor Tablets 2035
- Diuril Oral 2087

Chlorothiazide Sodium (Co-administration with urinary alkalinizing agents, such as certain thiazides, increase the concentration of the non-ionized species of the amphetamine molecule, thereby decreasing urinary excretion resulting in increased blood levels and potentiation ofactions of amphetamines; amphetamines may antagonize the hypotensive effects of antihypertensives). Products include:
- Diuril Sodium Intravenous 2086

Chlorpheniramine Maleate (Amphetamines may counteract the sedative effect of antihistamines). Products include:
- Actifed Cold & Sinus Caplets and Tablets .... ■688
- Alka-Seltzer Plus Liqui-Gels .... ■604
- BC Allergy Sinus Cold Powder .... ■619
- Chlor-Trimeton Allergy Tablets .... ■735
- Chlor-Trimeton Allergy/Decongestant Tablets .... ■736
- Comtrex Flu Therapy & Fever Relief Nighttime Tablets .... ■628
- Comtrex Maximum Strength Multi-Symptom Cold & Cough Relief Tablets and Caplets .... ■626
- Contac Severe Cold and Flu Caplets Maximum Strength .... ■746
- Coricidin 'D' Cold, Flu & Sinus Tablets .... ■737
- Coricidin/Coricidin D .... ■738
- Coricidin HBP Maximum Strength Flu Tablets .... ■738
- Extendryl 1361
- Hycomine Compound Tablets 1317
- Kronofed-A 1341
- PediaCare Cough-Cold Liquid .... ■719
- PediaCare NightRest Cough-Cold Liquid .... ■719
- Robitussin Nighttime Honey Flu Liquid .... ■786
- Ryna .... ■768
- Singlet Caplets .... ■761
- Sinutab Sinus Allergy Medication, Maximum Strength Formula, Tablets & Caplets .... ■707
- Sudafed Cold & Allergy Tablets .... ■708
- TheraFlu Regular Strength Cold & Cough Night Time Hot Liquid .... ■676
- TheraFlu Regular Strength Cold & Sore Throat Night Time Hot Liquid .... ■676
- TheraFlu Maximum Strength Flu & Cough Night Time Hot Liquid .... ■678
- TheraFlu Maximum Strength Flu & Sore Throat Night Time Hot Liquid .... ■677
- TheraFlu Maximum Strength Severe Cold & Congestion Night Time Caplets .... ■678
- TheraFlu Maximum Strength Severe Cold & Congestion Night Time Hot Liquid .... ■678
- Triaminic Cold & Allergy Liquid .... ■681
- Triaminic Cold & Allergy Softchews .... ■683
- Triaminic Cold & Cough Liquid .... ■681
- Triaminic Cold & Cough Softchews .... ■683
- Triaminic Cold & Night Time Cough Liquid .... ■681
- Triaminic Cold, Cough & Fever Liquid .... ■681
- Children's Tylenol Cold Suspension Liquid and Chewable Tablets 2015
- Children's Tylenol Cold Plus Cough Suspension Liquid and Chewable Tablets 2015
- Children's Tylenol Flu Suspension Liquid 2015
- Maximum Strength Tylenol Allergy Sinus Caplets, Gelcaps, and Geltabs 2010
- Multi-Symptom Tylenol Cold Complete Formula Caplets 2010
- Vicks 44M Cough, Cold & Flu Relief Liquid .... ■725
- Pediatric Vicks 44m Cough & Cold Relief .... ■728
- Children's Vicks NyQuil Cold/Cough Relief .... ■726

Chlorpheniramine Polistirex (Amphetamines may counteract the sedative effect of antihistamines). Products include:
- Tussionex Pennkinetic Extended-Release Suspension 1174

Chlorpheniramine Tannate (Amphetamines may counteract the sedative effect of antihistamines). Products include:
- Reformulated Rynatan Pediatric Suspension 3352
- Rynatuss Pediatric Suspension 3353
- Rynatuss Tablets 3353

Tussi-12 S Suspension 3356
Tussi-12 Tablets 3356

Chlorpromazine (Blocks the dopamine and norepinephrine receptors, thus inhibiting the central stimulant effects of amphetamines). Products include:
Thorazine Suppositories 1656

Chlorpromazine Hydrochloride (Blocks the dopamine and norepinephrine receptors, thus inhibiting the central stimulant effects of amphetamines). Products include:
Thorazine 1656

Chlorthalidone (Amphetamines may antagonize the hypotensive effects of antihypertensives). Products include:
Clorpres Tablets 1002
Combipres Tablets 1040
Tenoretic Tablets 690

Clemastine Fumarate (Amphetamines may counteract the sedative effect of antihistamines). Products include:
Tavist 12 Hour Allergy Tablets 676

Clomipramine Hydrochloride (Enhanced activity of tricyclic antidepressants or sympathomimetics; possible increases in d-amphetamine resulting in potentiation of cardiovascular effects).
No products indexed under this heading.

Clonidine (Amphetamines may antagonize the hypotensive effects of antihypertensives). Products include:
Catapres-TTS 1038

Clonidine Hydrochloride (Amphetamines may antagonize the hypotensive effects of antihypertensives). Products include:
Catapres Tablets 1037
Clorpres Tablets 1002
Combipres Tablets 1040
Duraclon Injection 3057

Cryptenamine Preparations (Amphetamines inhibit the hypotensive effect of veratrum alkaloids).
No products indexed under this heading.

Cyproheptadine Hydrochloride (Amphetamines may counteract the sedative effect of antihistamines). Products include:
Periactin Tablets 2155

Deserpidine (Amphetamines may antagonize the hypotensive effects of antihypertensives).
No products indexed under this heading.

Desipramine Hydrochloride (Enhanced activity of tricyclic antidepressants or sympathomimetics; possible increases in d-amphetamine resulting in potentiation of cardiovascular effects). Products include:
Norpramin Tablets 755

Dexchlorpheniramine Maleate (Amphetamines may counteract the sedative effect of antihistamines).
No products indexed under this heading.

Diazoxide (Amphetamines may antagonize the hypotensive effects of antihypertensives).
No products indexed under this heading.

Diltiazem Hydrochloride (Amphetamines may antagonize the hypotensive effects of antihypertensives). Products include:
Cardizem Injectable 1018
Cardizem Lyo-Ject Syringe 1018
Cardizem Monovial 1018
Cardizem CD Capsules 1016
Tiazac Capsules 1378

Diphenhydramine Citrate (Amphetamines may counteract the sedative effect of antihistamines). Products include:
Alka-Seltzer PM Effervescent Tablets 605
Benadryl Allergy & Sinus Fastmelt Tablets 693
Benadryl Children's Allergy/Cold Fastmelt Tablets 692
Excedrin PM Tablets, Caplets, and Geltabs 631
Goody's PM Powder 621

Diphenhydramine Hydrochloride (Amphetamines may counteract the sedative effect of antihistamines). Products include:
Extra Strength Bayer PM Caplets 611
Benadryl Allergy Chewables 689
Benadryl Allergy 691
Benadryl Allergy Liquid 690
Benadryl Allergy/Cold Tablets 691
Benadryl Allergy/Congestion Tablets 692
Benadryl Allergy & Sinus Liquid 693
Benadryl Allergy Sinus Headache Caplets & Gelcaps 693
Benadryl Severe Allergy & Sinus Headache Caplets 694
Benadryl Dye-Free Allergy Liquid 690
Benadryl Dye-Free Allergy Liqui-Gels Softgels 690
Benadryl Itch Relief Stick Extra Strength 695
Benadryl Cream 695
Benadryl Gel 695
Benadryl Spray 696
Benadryl Parenteral 2617
Coricidin HBP Night-Time Cold & Flu Tablets 738
Nytol QuickCaps Caplets 622
Maximum Strength Nytol QuickGels Softgels 621
Extra Strength Percogesic Aspirin-Free Coated Caplets 665
Simply Sleep Caplets 2008
Sominex Original Formula Tablets 761
Children's Tylenol Allergy-D Liquid 2014
Maximum Strength Tylenol Allergy Sinus NightTime Caplets 2010
Tylenol Severe Allergy Caplets 2010
Maximum Strength Tylenol Flu NightTime Gelcaps 2011
Extra Strength Tylenol PM Caplets, Geltabs, and Gelcaps 2012
Unisom Maximum Strength SleepGels 713

Diphenylpyraline Hydrochloride (Amphetamines may counteract the sedative effect of antihistamines).
No products indexed under this heading.

Doxazosin Mesylate (Amphetamines may antagonize the hypotensive effects of antihypertensives). Products include:
Cardura Tablets 2668

Doxepin Hydrochloride (Enhanced activity of tricyclic antidepressants or sympathomimetics; possible increases in d-amphetamine resulting in potentiation of cardiovascular effects). Products include:
Sinequan 2713

Enalapril Maleate (Amphetamines may antagonize the hypotensive effects of antihypertensives). Products include:
Lexxel Tablets 608
Vaseretic Tablets 2204
Vasotec Tablets 2210

Enalaprilat (Amphetamines may antagonize the hypotensive effects of antihypertensives). Products include:
Enalaprilat Injection 863
Vasotec I.V. Injection 2207

Eprosartan Mesylate (Amphetamines may antagonize the hypotensive effects of antihypertensives). Products include:
Teveten Tablets 3327

Esmolol Hydrochloride (Adrenergic blockers are inhibited by amphetamines; amphetamines may antagonize the hypotensive effects of antihypertensives). Products include:
Brevibloc Injection 858

Ethosuximide (Amphetamines may delay intestinal absorption of ethosuximide). Products include:
Zarontin Capsules 2659
Zarontin Syrup 2660

Felodipine (Amphetamines may antagonize the hypotensive effects of antihypertensives). Products include:
Lexxel Tablets 608
Plendil Extended-Release Tablets 623

Fexofenadine Hydrochloride (Amphetamines may counteract the sedative effect of antihistamines). Products include:
Allegra 712
Allegra-D Extended-Release Tablets 714

Fosinopril Sodium (Amphetamines may antagonize the hypotensive effects of antihypertensives). Products include:
Monopril Tablets 1091
Monopril HCT 1094

Fosphenytoin Sodium (Amphetamines may delay intestinal absorption of phenytoin; co-administration may produce a synergistic anticonvulsant action). Products include:
Cerebyx Injection 2619

Furazolidone (Concurrent use with metabolite of furazolidone may result in hypertensive crises; may slow the metabolism of amphetamines with resultant increase in their effect on release of norepinephrine and other monoamines from adrenergic nerve ending; this can cause headaches and other signs of hypertensice crises).
No products indexed under this heading.

Furosemide (Amphetamines may antagonize the hypotensive effects of antihypertensives). Products include:
Furosemide Tablets 2284

Glutamic Acid Hydrochloride (Co-administration with gastrointestinal acidifying agents, such as glutamic acid, lowers absorption of amphetamines resulting in reduced blood levels and efficacy of amphetamines).
No products indexed under this heading.

Guanabenz Acetate (Amphetamines may antagonize the hypotensive effects of antihypertensives).
No products indexed under this heading.

Guanethidine Monosulfate (Co-administration with gastrointestinal acidifying agents, such as guanethidine, lowers absorption of amphetamines resulting in reduced blood levels and efficacy of amphetamines; amphetamines may antagonize the hypotensive effects of antihypertensives).
No products indexed under this heading.

Haloperidol (Blocks the dopamine receptors, thus inhibiting the central stimulant effects of amphetamines). Products include:
Haldol Injection, Tablets and Concentrate 2533

Haloperidol Decanoate (Blocks the dopamine receptors, thus inhibiting the central stimulant effects of amphetamines). Products include:
Haldol Decanoate 2535

Hydralazine Hydrochloride (Amphetamines may antagonize the hypotensive effects of antihypertensives).
No products indexed under this heading.

Hydrochlorothiazide (Co-administration with urinary alkalinizing agents, such as certain thiazides, increase the concentration of the non-ionized species of the amphetamine molecule, thereby decreasing urinary excretion resulting in increased blood levels and potentiation ofactions of amphetamines; amphetamines may antagonize the hypotensive effects of antihypertensives). Products include:
Accuretic Tablets 2614
Aldoril Tablets 2039
Atacand HCT Tablets 597
Avalide Tablets 1070
Diovan HCT Tablets 2338
Dyazide Capsules 1515
HydroDIURIL Tablets 2108
Hyzaar 2109
Inderide Tablets 3517
Inderide LA Long-Acting Capsules 3519
Lotensin HCT Tablets 2367
Maxzide 1008
Micardis HCT Tablets 1051
Microzide Capsules 3414
Moduretic Tablets 2138
Monopril HCT 1094
Prinzide Tablets 2168
Timolide Tablets 2187
Uniretic Tablets 3178
Vaseretic Tablets 2204
Zestoretic Tablets 695
Ziac Tablets 1887

Hydroflumethiazide (Co-administration with urinary alkalinizing agents, such as certain thiazides, increase the concentration of the non-ionized species of the amphetamine molecule, thereby decreasing urinary excretion resulting in increased blood levels and potentiation ofactions of amphetamines; amphetamines may antagonize the hypotensive effects of antihypertensives). Products include:
Diucardin Tablets 3494

Imipramine Hydrochloride (Enhanced activity of tricyclic antidepressants or sympathomimetics; possible increases in d-amphetamine resulting in potentiation of cardiovascular effects).
No products indexed under this heading.

Imipramine Pamoate (Enhanced activity of tricyclic antidepressants or sympathomimetics; possible increases in d-amphetamine resulting in potentiation of cardiovascular effects).
No products indexed under this heading.

Indapamide (Amphetamines may antagonize the hypotensive effects of antihypertensives). Products include:
Indapamide Tablets 2286

Irbesartan (Amphetamines may antagonize the hypotensive effects of antihypertensives). Products include:
Avalide Tablets 1070
Avapro Tablets 1074
Avapro Tablets 3076

Isocarboxazid (Concurrent and/or sequential use may result in hypertensive crises; MAOI may slow the metabolism of amphetamines with resultant increase in their effect on release of norepinephrine and other monoamines from adrenergic nerve ending; this can cause headaches and other signs of hypertensive crises; concurrent and/or sequential use is contraindicated).
No products indexed under this heading.

Isradipine (Amphetamines may antagonize the hypotensive effects of antihypertensives). Products include:
DynaCirc Capsules 2921
DynaCirc CR Tablets 2923

Labetalol Hydrochloride (Adrenergic blockers are inhibited by amphetamines; amphetamines may antagonize the hypotensive effects of antihypertensives). Products include:
Normodyne Injection 3135
Normodyne Tablets 3137

Levobunolol Hydrochloride (Adrenergic blockers are inhibited by amphetamines; amphetamines may

antagonize the hypotensive effects of antihypertensives). Products include:

Betagan .... ⊙ 228

Lisinopril (Amphetamines may antagonize the hypotensive effects of antihypertensives). Products include:

Prinivil Tablets 2164
Prinzide Tablets 2168
Zestoretic Tablets 695
Zestril Tablets 698

Lithium Carbonate (Anorectic and stimulatory effects of amphetamines may be inhibited by lithium carbonate). Products include:

Eskalith 1527
Lithium Carbonate 3061
Lithobid Slow-Release Tablets 3255

Loratadine (Amphetamines may counteract the sedative effect of antihistamines). Products include:

Claritin 3100
Claritin-D 12 Hour Extended Release Tablets 3102
Claritin-D 24 Hour Extended Release Tablets 3104

Losartan Potassium (Amphetamines may antagonize the hypotensive effects of antihypertensives). Products include:

Cozaar Tablets 2067
Hyzaar 2109

Magaldrate (Co-administration with gastrointestinal alkalinizing agents, such as antacids, may increase the absorption of amphetamines; concurrent use should be avoided).

No products indexed under this heading.

Magnesium Hydroxide (Co-administration with gastrointestinal alkalinizing agents, such as antacids, may increase the absorption of amphetamines; concurrent use should be avoided). Products include:

Ex•Lax Milk of Magnesia Liquid .... ▣ 670
Maalox Antacid/Anti-Gas Oral Suspension .... ▣ 673
Maalox Max Maximum Strength Antacid/Anti-Gas Liquid 2300
Maalox Regular Strength Antacid/Antigas Liquid 2300
Mylanta Fast-Acting 1813
Mylanta 1813
Pepcid Complete Chewable Tablets 1815
Phillips' Chewable Tablets .... ▣ 615
Phillips' Milk of Magnesia Liquid (Original, Cherry, & Mint) .... ▣ 616
Rolaids Tablets .... ▣ 706
Extra Strength Rolaids Tablets .... ▣ 706
Vanquish Caplets .... ▣ 617

Magnesium Oxide (Co-administration with gastrointestinal alkalinizing agents, such as antacids, may increase the absorption of amphetamines; concurrent use should be avoided). Products include:

Beelith Tablets 946
Mag-Ox 400 Tablets 1024
Uro-Mag Capsules 1024

Maprotiline Hydrochloride (Enhanced activity of tricyclic antidepressants or sympathomimetics; possible increases in d-amphetamine resulting in potentiation of cardiovascular effects).

No products indexed under this heading.

Mecamylamine Hydrochloride (Amphetamines may antagonize the hypotensive effects of antihypertensives). Products include:

Inversine Tablets 1850

Meperidine Hydrochloride (Amphetamines potentiate the analgesic effect of meperidine). Products include:

Demerol 3079
Mepergan Injection 3539

Methdilazine Hydrochloride (Amphetamines may counteract the sedative effect of antihistamines).

No products indexed under this heading.

Methenamine (Urinary excretion of amphetamines is increased, and efficacy is reduced by acidifying agents used in methenamine therapy). Products include:

Prosed/DS Tablets 3268
Urimax Tablets 1769
Urised Tablets 2876

Methenamine Hippurate (Urinary excretion of amphetamines is increased, and efficacy is reduced by acidifying agents used in methenamine therapy).

No products indexed under this heading.

Methenamine Mandelate (Urinary excretion of amphetamines is increased, and efficacy is reduced by acidifying agents used in methenamine therapy). Products include:

Uroqid-Acid No. 2 Tablets 947

Methyclothiazide (Co-administration with urinary alkalinizing agents, such as certain thiazides, increase the concentration of the non-ionized species of the amphetamine molecule, thereby decreasing urinary excretion resulting in increased blood levels and potentiation ofactions of amphetamines; amphetamines may antagonize the hypotensive effects of antihypertensives).

No products indexed under this heading.

Methyldopa (Amphetamines may antagonize the hypotensive effects of antihypertensives). Products include:

Aldoclor Tablets 2035
Aldomet Tablets 2037
Aldoril Tablets 2039

Methyldopate Hydrochloride (Amphetamines may antagonize the hypotensive effects of antihypertensives).

No products indexed under this heading.

Metipranolol Hydrochloride (Adrenergic blockers are inhibited by amphetamines; amphetamines may antagonize the hypotensive effects of antihypertensives).

No products indexed under this heading.

Metolazone (Amphetamines may antagonize the hypotensive effects of antihypertensives). Products include:

Mykrox Tablets 1168
Zaroxolyn Tablets 1177

Metoprolol Succinate (Adrenergic blockers are inhibited by amphetamines; amphetamines may antagonize the hypotensive effects of antihypertensives). Products include:

Toprol-XL Tablets 651

Metoprolol Tartrate (Adrenergic blockers are inhibited by amphetamines; amphetamines may antagonize the hypotensive effects of antihypertensives).

No products indexed under this heading.

Metyrosine (Amphetamines may antagonize the hypotensive effects of antihypertensives). Products include:

Demser Capsules 2085

Mibefradil Dihydrochloride (Amphetamines may antagonize the hypotensive effects of antihypertensives).

No products indexed under this heading.

Minoxidil (Amphetamines may antagonize the hypotensive effects of antihypertensives). Products include:

Rogaine Extra Strength for Men Topical Solution .... ▣ 721
Rogaine for Women Topical Solution .... ▣ 721

Moclobemide (Concurrent and/or sequential use may result in hypertensive crises; MAOI may slow the metabolism of amphetamines with resultant increase in their effect on release of norepinephrine and other monoamines from adrenergic nerve ending; this can cause headaches and other signs of hypertensive crises; concurrent and/or sequential use is contraindicated).

No products indexed under this heading.

Moexipril Hydrochloride (Amphetamines may antagonize the hypotensive effects of antihypertensives). Products include:

Uniretic Tablets 3178
Univasc Tablets 3181

Nadolol (Adrenergic blockers are inhibited by amphetamines; amphetamines may antagonize the hypotensive effects of antihypertensives). Products include:

Corgard Tablets 2245
Corzide 40/5 Tablets 2247
Corzide 80/5 Tablets 2247
Nadolol Tablets 2288

Nicardipine Hydrochloride (Amphetamines may antagonize the hypotensive effects of antihypertensives). Products include:

Cardene I.V. 3485

Nifedipine (Amphetamines may antagonize the hypotensive effects of antihypertensives). Products include:

Adalat CC Tablets 877
Procardia Capsules 2708
Procardia XL Extended Release Tablets 2710

Nisoldipine (Amphetamines may antagonize the hypotensive effects of antihypertensives). Products include:

Sular Tablets 688

Nitroglycerin (Amphetamines may antagonize the hypotensive effects of antihypertensives). Products include:

Nitro-Dur Transdermal Infusion System 3134
Nitro-Dur Transdermal Infusion System 1834
Nitrolingual Pumpspray 1355
Nitrostat Tablets 2658

Norepinephrine Bitartrate (Amphetamines enhance the adrenergic effect of norepinephrine).

No products indexed under this heading.

Nortriptyline Hydrochloride (Enhanced activity of tricyclic antidepressants or sympathomimetics; possible increases in d-amphetamine resulting in potentiation of cardiovascular effects).

No products indexed under this heading.

Pargyline Hydrochloride (Concurrent and/or sequential use may result in hypertensive crises; MAOI may slow the metabolism of amphetamines with resultant increase in their effect on release of norepinephrine and other monoamines from adrenergic nerve ending; this can cause headaches and other signs of hypertensive crises; concurrent and/or sequential use is contraindicated).

No products indexed under this heading.

Penbutolol Sulfate (Adrenergic blockers are inhibited by amphetamines; amphetamines may antagonize the hypotensive effects of antihypertensives).

No products indexed under this heading.

Perindopril Erbumine (Amphetamines may antagonize the hypotensive effects of antihypertensives). Products include:

Aceon Tablets (2 mg, 4 mg, 8 mg) 3249

Phenelzine Sulfate (Concurrent and/or sequential use may result in hypertensive crises; MAOI may slow the metabolism of amphetamines with resultant increase in their effect on release of norepinephrine and other monoamines from adrenergic nerve ending; this can cause headaches and other signs of hypertensive crises; concurrent and/or sequential use is contraindicated). Products include:

Nardil Tablets 2653

Phenobarbital (Amphetamines may delay intestinal absorption of phenobarbital; co-administration may produce a synergistic anticonvulsant action). Products include:

Arco-Lase Plus Tablets 592
Donnatal 2929
Donnatal Extentabs 2930

Phenoxybenzamine Hydrochloride (Amphetamines may antagonize the hypotensive effects of antihypertensives). Products include:

Dibenzyline Capsules 3457

Phentolamine Mesylate (Amphetamines may antagonize the hypotensive effects of antihypertensives).

No products indexed under this heading.

Phenytoin (Amphetamines may delay intestinal absorption of phenytoin; co-administration may produce a synergistic anticonvulsant action). Products include:

Dilantin Infatabs 2624
Dilantin-125 Oral Suspension 2625

Phenytoin Sodium (Amphetamines may delay intestinal absorption of phenytoin; co-administration may produce a synergistic anticonvulsant action). Products include:

Dilantin Kapseals 2622

Pindolol (Adrenergic blockers are inhibited by amphetamines; amphetamines may antagonize the hypotensive effects of antihypertensives).

No products indexed under this heading.

Polythiazide (Co-administration with urinary alkalinizing agents, such as certain thiazides, increase the concentration of the non-ionized species of the amphetamine molecule, thereby decreasing urinary excretion resulting in increased blood levels and potentiation ofactions of amphetamines; amphetamines may antagonize the hypotensive effects of antihypertensives). Products include:

Minizide Capsules 2700
Renese Tablets 2712

Potassium Citrate (Co-administration with urinary acidifying agents increases the concentration of the ionized species of the amphetamine molecule, thereby increasing urinary excretion resulting in reduced blood levels and efficacy of amphetamines). Products include:

Urocit-K Tablets 2232

Prazosin Hydrochloride (Amphetamines may antagonize the hypotensive effects of antihypertensives). Products include:

Minipress Capsules 2699
Minizide Capsules 2700

Procarbazine Hydrochloride (Concurrent and/or sequential use may result in hypertensive crises; MAOI may slow the metabolism of amphetamines with resultant increase in their effect on release of norepinephrine and other monoamines from adrenergic nerve ending; this can cause headaches and other signs of hypertensive crises; concurrent and/or sequential use is contraindicated). Products include:

Matulane Capsules 3246

Promethazine Hydrochloride (Amphetamines may counteract the sedative effect of antihistamines). Products include:
- Mepergan Injection 3539
- Phenergan Injection 3553
- Phenergan 3556
- Phenergan Syrup 3554
- Phenergan with Codeine Syrup 3557
- Phenergan with Dextromethorphan Syrup 3559
- Phenergan VC Syrup 3560
- Phenergan VC with Codeine Syrup .. 3561

Propoxyphene Hydrochloride (In cases of propoxyphene overdosage, amphetamine CNS stimulation is potentiated and fatal convulsions can occur). Products include:
- Darvon Pulvules 1909
- Darvon Compound-65 Pulvules 1910

Propoxyphene Napsylate (In cases of propoxyphene overdosage, amphetamine CNS stimulation is potentiated and fatal convulsions can occur). Products include:
- Darvon-N/Darvocet-N 1907
- Darvon-N Tablets 1912

Propranolol Hydrochloride (Adrenergic blockers are inhibited by amphetamines; amphetamines may antagonize the hypotensive effects of antihypertensives). Products include:
- Inderal 3513
- Inderal LA Long-Acting Capsules 3516
- Inderide Tablets 3517
- Inderide LA Long-Acting Capsules .. 3519

Protriptyline Hydrochloride (Enhanced activity of tricyclic antidepressants or sympathomimetics; possible increases in d-amphetamine resulting in potentiation of cardiovascular effects). Products include:
- Vivactil Tablets 2446
- Vivactil Tablets 2217

Pyrilamine Maleate (Amphetamines may counteract the sedative effect of antihistamines). Products include:
- Maximum Strength Midol Menstrual Caplets and Gelcaps .... ▣612
- Maximum Strength Midol PMS Caplets and Gelcaps .... ▣613

Pyrilamine Tannate (Amphetamines may counteract the sedative effect of antihistamines). Products include:
- Ryna-12 S Suspension 3351

Quinapril Hydrochloride (Amphetamines may antagonize the hypotensive effects of antihypertensives). Products include:
- Accupril Tablets 2611
- Accuretic Tablets 2614

Ramipril (Amphetamines may antagonize the hypotensive effects of antihypertensives). Products include:
- Altace Capsules 2233

Rauwolfia serpentina (Amphetamines may antagonize the hypotensive effects of antihypertensives).
No products indexed under this heading.

Rescinnamine (Amphetamines may antagonize the hypotensive effects of antihypertensives).
No products indexed under this heading.

Reserpine (Co-administration with gastrointestinal acidifying agents, such as reserpine, lowers absorption of amphetamines resulting in reduced blood levels and efficacy of amphetamines; amphetamines may antagonize the hypotensive effects of antihypertensives).
No products indexed under this heading.

Selegiline Hydrochloride (Concurrent and/or sequential use may result in hypertensive crises; MAOI may slow the metabolism of amphetamines with resultant increase in their effect on release of norepinephrine and other monoamines from adrenergic nerve ending; this can cause headaches and other signs of hypertensive crises; concurrent and/or sequential use is contraindicated). Products include:
- Eldepryl Capsules 3266

Sodium Bicarbonate (Co-administration with gastrointestinal alkalinizing agents, such as systemic disodium bicarbonate, increases the absorption of amphetamines). Products include:
- Alka-Seltzer .... ▣603
- Alka-Seltzer Lemon Lime Antacid and Pain Reliever Effervescent Tablets .... ▣603
- Alka-Seltzer Extra Strength Antacid and Pain Reliever Effervescent Tablets .... ▣603
- Alka-Seltzer Heartburn Relief Tablets .... ▣604
- Ceo-Two Evacuant Suppository .... ▣618
- Colyte with Flavor Packs for Oral Solution 3170
- GoLYTELY and Pineapple Flavor GoLYTELY for Oral Solution 1068
- NuLYTELY, Cherry Flavor, Lemon-Lime Flavor, and Orange Flavor NuLYTELY for Oral Solution 1068

Sodium Citrate (Co-administration with urinary acidifying agents increases the concentration of the ionized species of the amphetamine molecule, thereby increasing urinary excretion resulting in reduced blood levels and efficacy of amphetamines).
No products indexed under this heading.

Sodium Nitroprusside (Amphetamines may antagonize the hypotensive effects of antihypertensives).
No products indexed under this heading.

Sotalol Hydrochloride (Adrenergic blockers are inhibited by amphetamines; amphetamines may antagonize the hypotensive effects of antihypertensives). Products include:
- Betapace Tablets 950
- Betapace AF Tablets 954

Spirapril Hydrochloride (Amphetamines may antagonize the hypotensive effects of antihypertensives).
No products indexed under this heading.

Telmisartan (Amphetamines may antagonize the hypotensive effects of antihypertensives). Products include:
- Micardis Tablets 1049
- Micardis HCT Tablets 1051

Terazosin Hydrochloride (Amphetamines may antagonize the hypotensive effects of antihypertensives). Products include:
- Hytrin Capsules 464

Terfenadine (Amphetamines may counteract the sedative effect of antihistamines).
No products indexed under this heading.

Timolol Hemihydrate (Adrenergic blockers are inhibited by amphetamines; amphetamines may antagonize the hypotensive effects of antihypertensives). Products include:
- Betimol Ophthalmic Solution .... ⊙324

Timolol Maleate (Adrenergic blockers are inhibited by amphetamines; amphetamines may antagonize the hypotensive effects of antihypertensives). Products include:
- Blocadren Tablets 2046
- Cosopt Sterile Ophthalmic Solution 2065
- Timolide Tablets 2187
- Timolol GFS .... ⊙266
- Timoptic in Ocudose 2192
- Timoptic Sterile Ophthalmic Solution 2190
- Timoptic-XE Sterile Ophthalmic Gel Forming Solution 2194

Torsemide (Amphetamines may antagonize the hypotensive effects of antihypertensives). Products include:
- Demadex Tablets and Injection 2965

Trandolapril (Amphetamines may antagonize the hypotensive effects of antihypertensives). Products include:
- Mavik Tablets 478
- Tarka Tablets 508

Tranylcypromine Sulfate (Concurrent and/or sequential use may result in hypertensive crises; MAOI may slow the metabolism of amphetamines with resultant increase in their effect on release of norepinephrine and other monoamines from adrenergic nerve ending; this can cause headaches and other signs of hypertensive crises; concurrent and/or sequential use is contraindicated). Products include:
- Parnate Tablets 1607

Trimeprazine Tartrate (Amphetamines may counteract the sedative effect of antihistamines).
No products indexed under this heading.

Trimethaphan Camsylate (Amphetamines may antagonize the hypotensive effects of antihypertensives).
No products indexed under this heading.

Trimipramine Maleate (Enhanced activity of tricyclic antidepressants or sympathomimetics; possible increases in d-amphetamine resulting in potentiation of cardiovascular effects). Products include:
- Surmontil Capsules 3595

Tripelennamine Hydrochloride (Amphetamines may counteract the sedative effect of antihistamines).
No products indexed under this heading.

Triprolidine Hydrochloride (Amphetamines may counteract the sedative effect of antihistamines). Products include:
- Actifed Cold & Allergy Tablets .... ▣688

Valsartan (Amphetamines may antagonize the hypotensive effects of antihypertensives). Products include:
- Diovan Capsules 2337
- Diovan HCT Tablets 2338

Verapamil Hydrochloride (Amphetamines may antagonize the hypotensive effects of antihypertensives). Products include:
- Covera-HS Tablets 3199
- Isoptin SR Tablets 467
- Tarka Tablets 508
- Verelan Capsules 3184
- Verelan PM Capsules 3186

Vitamin C (Co-administration with gastrointestinal acidifying agents, such as vitamin C, lowers absorption of amphetamines resulting in reduced blood levels and efficacy of amphetamines). Products include:
- Beta-C Tablets .... ▣811
- C-Grams Caplets .... ▣795
- Halls Defense Drops .... ▣687
- Peridin-C Tablets .... ▣618

Food Interactions

Food, unspecified (Concurrent use with food prolongs T_{max} by 2.5 hours, however, food does not affect the extent of absorption).

ADENOCARD INJECTION

(Adenosine) 1380

May interact with cardiac glycosides, theophylline, and certain other agents. Compounds in these categories include:

Aminophylline (The effects of adenosine are antagonized by co-administration with methylxanthines, such as theophylline; larger doses of adenosine may be required or adenosine may not be effective).
No products indexed under this heading.

Caffeine (The effects of adenosine are antagonized by co-administration with methylxanthines, such as caffeine; larger doses of adenosine may be required or adenosine may not be effective). Products include:
- BC Powder .... ▣619
- Arthritis Strength BC Powder .... ▣619
- Darvon Compound-65 Pulvules 1910
- Aspirin Free Excedrin Caplets and Geltabs .... ▣628
- Excedrin Extra-Strength Tablets, Caplets, and Geltabs .... ▣629
- Excedrin Migraine 1070
- Goody's Extra Strength Headache Powder .... ▣620
- Goody's Extra Strength Pain Relief Tablets .... ▣620
- Hycomine Compound Tablets 1317
- Maximum Strength Midol Menstrual Caplets and Gelcaps .... ▣612
- Vanquish Caplets .... ▣617
- Vivarin .... ▣763

Carbamazepine (Adenosine decreases the conduction through AV node, higher degrees of heart block may be produced in the presence of carbamazepine). Products include:
- Carbatrol Capsules 3234
- Tegretol/Tegretol-XR 2404

Deslanoside (The use of adenosine in patients receiving digitalis may be rarely associated with ventricular fibrillation).
No products indexed under this heading.

Digitoxin (The use of adenosine in patients receiving digitalis may be rarely associated with ventricular fibrillation).
No products indexed under this heading.

Digoxin (The use of adenosine in patients receiving digitalis may be rarely associated with ventricular fibrillation). Products include:
- Digitek Tablets 1003
- Lanoxicaps Capsules 1574
- Lanoxin Injection 1581
- Lanoxin Tablets 1587
- Lanoxin Elixir Pediatric 1578
- Lanoxin Injection Pediatric 1584

Dipyridamole (Adenosine effects are potentiated by dipyridamole; smaller doses of adenosine may be effective with concurrent use). Products include:
- Aggrenox Capsules 1026
- Persantine Tablets 1057

Dyphylline (The effects of adenosine are antagonized by co-administration with methylxanthines, such as theophylline; larger doses of adenosine may be required or adenosine may not be effective). Products include:
- Lufyllin Tablets 3347
- Lufyllin-400 Tablets 3347
- Lufyllin-GG Elixir 3348
- Lufyllin-GG Tablets 3348

Theophylline (The effects of adenosine are antagonized by co-administration with methylxanthines, such as theophylline; larger doses of adenosine may be required or adenosine may not be effective). Products include:
- Aerolate 1361
- Theo-Dur Extended-Release Tablets 1835
- Uni-Dur Extended-Release Tablets .. 1841
- Uniphyl 400 mg and 600 mg Tablets 2903

Theophylline Calcium Salicylate (The effects of adenosine are antagonized by co-administration with methylxanthines, such as theophylline; larger doses of adenosine may be required or adenosine may not be effective).
No products indexed under this heading.

Theophylline Sodium Glycinate (The effects of adenosine are antag-

onized by co-administration with methylxanthines, such as theophylline; larger doses of adenosine may be required or adenosine may not be effective).
No products indexed under this heading.

Verapamil Hydrochloride (Digoxin and verapamil use may be rarely associated with ventricular fibrillation when combined with adenosine; potential for additive or synergistic depressant effects on the SA and AV nodes). Products include:
Covera-HS Tablets 3199
Isoptin SR Tablets 467
Tarka Tablets 508
Verelan Capsules 3184
Verelan PM Capsules 3186

ADENOSCAN
(Adenosine) 1381
May interact with adenosine receptor antagonists, beta blockers, calcium channel blockers, cardiac glycosides, and nucleoside transport inhibitors. Compounds in these categories include:

Acebutolol Hydrochloride (Potential for additive or synergistic depressant effects on the SA or AV nodes; adenosine should be used with caution in the presence of these agents; no adverse interactions have been reported when co-administered). Products include:
Sectral Capsules 3589

Aminophylline (The vasoactive effects of adenosine are inhibited by adenosine receptor antagonists such as alkylxanthines).
No products indexed under this heading.

Amlodipine Besylate (Potential for additive or synergistic depressant effects on the SA or AV nodes; adenosine should be used with caution in the presence of these agents; no adverse interactions have been reported when co-administered). Products include:
Lotrel Capsules 2370
Norvasc Tablets 2704

Atenolol (Potential for additive or synergistic depressant effects on the SA or AV nodes; adenosine should be used with caution in the presence of these agents; no adverse interactions have been reported when co-administered). Products include:
Tenoretic Tablets 690
Tenormin I.V. Injection 692

Bepridil Hydrochloride (Potential for additive or synergistic depressant effects on the SA or AV nodes; adenosine should be used with caution in the presence of these agents; no adverse interactions have been reported when co-administered). Products include:
Vascor Tablets 2602

Betaxolol Hydrochloride (Potential for additive or synergistic depressant effects on the SA or AV nodes; adenosine should be used with caution in the presence of these agents; no adverse interactions have been reported when co-administered). Products include:
Betoptic S Ophthalmic Suspension 537

Bisoprolol Fumarate (Potential for additive or synergistic depressant effects on the SA or AV nodes; adenosine should be used with caution in the presence of these agents; no adverse interactions have been reported when co-administered). Products include:
Zebeta Tablets 1885
Ziac Tablets 1887

Caffeine (The vasoactive effects of adenosine are inhibited by adenosine receptor antagonists such as alkylxanthines). Products include:
BC Powder .... ▣619
Arthritis Strength BC Powder .... ▣619
Darvon Compound-65 Pulvules 1910
Aspirin Free Excedrin Caplets and Geltabs .... ▣628
Excedrin Extra-Strength Tablets, Caplets, and Geltabs .... ▣629
Excedrin Migraine 1070
Goody's Extra Strength Headache Powder .... ▣620
Goody's Extra Strength Pain Relief Tablets .... ▣620
Hycomine Compound Tablets 1317
Maximum Strength Midol Menstrual Caplets and Gelcaps .... ▣612
Vanquish Caplets .... ▣617
Vivarin .... ▣763

Carteolol Hydrochloride (Potential for additive or synergistic depressant effects on the SA or AV nodes; adenosine should be used with caution in the presence of these agents; no adverse interactions have been reported when co-administered). Products include:
Carteolol Hydrochloride Ophthalmic Solution USP, 1% .... ⊙258
Ocupress Ophthalmic Solution, 1% Sterile .... ⊙303

Deslanoside (Potential for additive or synergistic depressant effects on the SA or AV nodes; adenosine should be used with caution in the presence of these agents; no adverse interactions have been reported when co-administered).
No products indexed under this heading.

Digitoxin (Potential for additive or synergistic depressant effects on the SA or AV nodes; adenosine should be used with caution in the presence of these agents; no adverse interactions have been reported when co-administered).
No products indexed under this heading.

Digoxin (Potential for additive or synergistic depressant effects on the SA or AV nodes; adenosine should be used with caution in the presence of these agents; no adverse interactions have been reported when co-administered). Products include:
Digitek Tablets 1003
Lanoxicaps Capsules 1574
Lanoxin Injection 1581
Lanoxin Tablets 1587
Lanoxin Elixir Pediatric 1578
Lanoxin Injection Pediatric 1584

Diltiazem Hydrochloride (Potential for additive or synergistic depressant effects on the SA or AV nodes; adenosine should be used with caution in the presence of these agents; no adverse interactions have been reported when co-administered). Products include:
Cardizem Injectable 1018
Cardizem Lyo-Ject Syringe 1018
Cardizem Monovial 1018
Cardizem CD Capsules 1016
Tiazac Capsules 1378

Dipyridamole (Vasoactive effects of adenosine are potentiated by nucleoside transport inhibitors). Products include:
Aggrenox Capsules 1026
Persantine Tablets 1057

Dyphylline (The vasoactive effects of adenosine are inhibited by adenosine receptor antagonists such as alkylxanthines). Products include:
Lufyllin Tablets 3347
Lufyllin-400 Tablets 3347
Lufyllin-GG Elixir 3348
Lufyllin-GG Tablets 3348

Esmolol Hydrochloride (Potential for additive or synergistic depressant effects on the SA or AV nodes; adenosine should be used with caution in the presence of these agents; no adverse interactions have been reported when co-administered). Products include:
Brevibloc Injection 858

Felodipine (Potential for additive or synergistic depressant effects on the SA or AV nodes; adenosine should be used with caution in the presence of these agents; no adverse interactions have been reported when co-administered). Products include:
Lexxel Tablets 608
Plendil Extended-Release Tablets 623

Isradipine (Potential for additive or synergistic depressant effects on the SA or AV nodes; adenosine should be used with caution in the presence of these agents; no adverse interactions have been reported when co-administered). Products include:
DynaCirc Capsules 2921
DynaCirc CR Tablets 2923

Labetalol Hydrochloride (Potential for additive or synergistic depressant effects on the SA or AV nodes; adenosine should be used with caution in the presence of these agents; no adverse interactions have been reported when co-administered). Products include:
Normodyne Injection 3135
Normodyne Tablets 3137

Levobunolol Hydrochloride (Potential for additive or synergistic depressant effects on the SA or AV nodes; adenosine should be used with caution in the presence of these agents; no adverse interactions have been reported when co-administered). Products include:
Betagan .... ⊙228

Metipranolol Hydrochloride (Potential for additive or synergistic depressant effects on the SA or AV nodes; adenosine should be used with caution in the presence of these agents; no adverse interactions have been reported when co-administered).
No products indexed under this heading.

Metoprolol Succinate (Potential for additive or synergistic depressant effects on the SA or AV nodes; adenosine should be used with caution in the presence of these agents; no adverse interactions have been reported when co-administered). Products include:
Toprol-XL Tablets 651

Metoprolol Tartrate (Potential for additive or synergistic depressant effects on the SA or AV nodes; adenosine should be used with caution in the presence of these agents; no adverse interactions have been reported when co-administered).
No products indexed under this heading.

Mibefradil Dihydrochloride (Potential for additive or synergistic depressant effects on the SA or AV nodes; adenosine should be used with caution in the presence of these agents; no adverse interactions have been reported when co-administered).
No products indexed under this heading.

Nadolol (Potential for additive or synergistic depressant effects on the SA or AV nodes; adenosine should be used with caution in the presence of these agents; no adverse interactions have been reported when co-administered). Products include:
Corgard Tablets 2245
Corzide 40/5 Tablets 2247
Corzide 80/5 Tablets 2247
Nadolol Tablets 2288

Nicardipine Hydrochloride (Potential for additive or synergistic depressant effects on the SA or AV nodes; adenosine should be used with caution in the presence of these agents; no adverse interactions have been reported when co-administered). Products include:
Cardene I.V. 3485

Nifedipine (Potential for additive or synergistic depressant effects on the SA or AV nodes; adenosine should be used with caution in the presence of these agents; no adverse interactions have been reported when co-administered). Products include:
Adalat CC Tablets 877
Procardia Capsules 2708
Procardia XL Extended Release Tablets 2710

Nimodipine (Potential for additive or synergistic depressant effects on the SA or AV nodes; adenosine should be used with caution in the presence of these agents; no adverse interactions have been reported when co-administered). Products include:
Nimotop Capsules 904

Nisoldipine (Potential for additive or synergistic depressant effects on the SA or AV nodes; adenosine should be used with caution in the presence of these agents; no adverse interactions have been reported when co-administered). Products include:
Sular Tablets 688

Penbutolol Sulfate (Potential for additive or synergistic depressant effects on the SA or AV nodes; adenosine should be used with caution in the presence of these agents; no adverse interactions have been reported when co-administered).
No products indexed under this heading.

Pindolol (Potential for additive or synergistic depressant effects on the SA or AV nodes; adenosine should be used with caution in the presence of these agents; no adverse interactions have been reported when co-administered).
No products indexed under this heading.

Propranolol Hydrochloride (Potential for additive or synergistic depressant effects on the SA or AV nodes; adenosine should be used with caution in the presence of these agents; no adverse interactions have been reported when co-administered). Products include:
Inderal 3513
Inderal LA Long-Acting Capsules 3516
Inderide Tablets 3517
Inderide LA Long-Acting Capsules 3519

Sotalol Hydrochloride (Potential for additive or synergistic depressant effects on the SA or AV nodes; adenosine should be used with caution in the presence of these agents; no adverse interactions have been reported when co-administered). Products include:
Betapace Tablets 950
Betapace AF Tablets 954

Theophylline (The vasoactive effects of adenosine are inhibited by adenosine receptor antagonists such as alkylxanthines). Products include:
Aerolate 1361
Theo-Dur Extended-Release Tablets 1835
Uni-Dur Extended-Release Tablets 1841
Uniphyl 400 mg and 600 mg Tablets 2903

Theophylline Calcium Salicylate (The vasoactive effects of adenosine are inhibited by adenosine receptor antagonists such as alkylxanthines).
No products indexed under this heading.

Theophylline Sodium Glycinate (The vasoactive effects of adenosine are inhibited by adenosine receptor

antagonists such as alkylxanthines).
No products indexed under this heading.

Timolol Hemihydrate (Potential for additive or synergistic depressant effects on the SA or AV nodes; adenosine should be used with caution in the presence of these agents; no adverse interactions have been reported when co-administered). Products include:
Betimol Ophthalmic Solution .... ⊙ 324

Timolol Maleate (Potential for additive or synergistic depressant effects on the SA or AV nodes; adenosine should be used with caution in the presence of these agents; no adverse interactions have been reported when co-administered). Products include:
Blocadren Tablets 2046
Cosopt Sterile Ophthalmic Solution.. 2065
Timolide Tablets 2187
Timolol GFS .... ⊙ 266
Timoptic in Ocudose 2192
Timoptic Sterile Ophthalmic Solution 2190
Timoptic-XE Sterile Ophthalmic Gel Forming Solution 2194

Verapamil Hydrochloride (Potential for additive or synergistic depressant effects on the SA or AV nodes; adenosine should be used with caution in the presence of these agents; no adverse interactions have been reported when co-administered). Products include:
Covera-HS Tablets 3199
Isoptin SR Tablets 467
Tarka Tablets 508
Verelan Capsules 3184
Verelan PM Capsules 3186

ADIPEX-P CAPSULES

(Phentermine Hydrochloride) 1406
See Adipex-P Tablets

ADIPEX-P TABLETS

(Phentermine Hydrochloride) 1406
May interact with insulin, monoamine oxidase inhibitors, selective serotonin reuptake inhibitors, and certain other agents. Compounds in these categories include:

Citalopram Hydrobromide (The safety and efficacy of combination therapy with phentermine and any other drug products for weight loss, including selective serotonin reuptake inhibitors, have not been established; co-administration of these products for weight loss is not recommended). Products include:
Celexa 1365

Dexfenfluramine Hydrochloride (Co-administration has resulted in primary pulmonary hypertension, a rare, frequently fatal disease of the lungs and serious regurgitant cardiac valvular disease).
No products indexed under this heading.

Fenfluramine Hydrochloride (Co-administration has resulted in primary pulmonary hypertension, a rare, frequently fatal disease of the lungs and serious regurgitant cardiac valvular disease).
No products indexed under this heading.

Fluoxetine Hydrochloride (The safety and efficacy of combination therapy with phentermine and any other drug products for weight loss, including selective serotonin reuptake inhibitors, have not been established; co-administration of these products for weight loss is not recommended). Products include:
Prozac Pulvules, Liquid, and Weekly Capsules 1238
Sarafem Pulvules 1962

Fluvoxamine Maleate (The safety and efficacy of combination therapy with phentermine and any other drug products for weight loss, including selective serotonin reuptake inhibitors, have not been established; co-administration of these products for weight loss is not recommended). Products include:
Luvox Tablets (25, 50, 100 mg) 3256

Guanethidine Monosulfate (Decreased hypotensive effect of guanethidine).
No products indexed under this heading.

Insulin, Human, Zinc Suspension (Insulin requirement may be altered). Products include:
Humulin L, 100 Units 1937
Humulin U, 100 Units 1943
Novolin L Human Insulin 10 ml Vials.. 2422

Insulin, Human NPH (Insulin requirement may be altered). Products include:
Humulin N, 100 Units 1939
Humulin N NPH Pen 1940
Novolin N Human Insulin 10 ml Vials 2422
Novolin N PenFill 2423
Novolin N Prefilled Syringe Disposable Insulin Delivery System 2425

Insulin, Human Regular (Insulin requirement may be altered). Products include:
Humulin R Regular (U-500) 1943
Humulin R, 100 Units 1941
Novolin R Human Insulin 10 ml Vials 2423
Novolin R PenFill 2423
Novolin R Prefilled Syringe Disposable Insulin Delivery System 2425
Velosulin BR Human Insulin 10 ml Vials 2435

Insulin, Human Regular and Human NPH Mixture (Insulin requirement may be altered). Products include:
Humulin 50/50, 100 Units 1934
Humulin 70/30, 100 Units 1935
Humulin 70/30 Pen 1936
Novolin 70/30 Human Insulin 10 ml Vials 2421
Novolin 70/30 PenFill 2423
Novolin 70/30 Prefilled Disposable Insulin Delivery System 2425

Insulin, NPH (Insulin requirement may be altered). Products include:
Iletin II, NPH (Pork), 100 Units 1946

Insulin, Regular (Insulin requirement may be altered). Products include:
Iletin II, Regular (Pork), 100 Units ... 1947

Insulin, Zinc Crystals (Insulin requirement may be altered).
No products indexed under this heading.

Insulin, Zinc Suspension (Insulin requirement may be altered). Products include:
Iletin II, Lente (Pork), 100 Units 1945

Insulin Aspart, Human Regular (Insulin requirement may be altered).
No products indexed under this heading.

Insulin glargine (Insulin requirement may be altered). Products include:
Lantus Injection 742

Insulin Lispro, Human (Insulin requirement may be altered). Products include:
Humalog 1926
Humalog Mix 75/25 Pen 1928

Insulin Lispro Protamine, Human (Insulin requirement may be altered). Products include:
Humalog Mix 75/25 Pen 1928

Isocarboxazid (Concurrent and/or sequential administration with MAO inhibitors may result in hypertensive crises; co-administration is contraindicated).
No products indexed under this heading.

Moclobemide (Concurrent and/or sequential administration with MAO inhibitors may result in hypertensive crises; co-administration is contraindicated).
No products indexed under this heading.

Pargyline Hydrochloride (Concurrent and/or sequential administration with MAO inhibitors may result in hypertensive crises; co-administration is contraindicated).
No products indexed under this heading.

Paroxetine Hydrochloride (The safety and efficacy of combination therapy with phentermine and any other drug products for weight loss, including selective serotonin reuptake inhibitors, have not been established; co-administration of these products for weight loss is not recommended). Products include:
Paxil 1609

Phenelzine Sulfate (Concurrent and/or sequential administration with MAO inhibitors may result in hypertensive crises; co-administration is contraindicated). Products include:
Nardil Tablets 2653

Procarbazine Hydrochloride (Concurrent and/or sequential administration with MAO inhibitors may result in hypertensive crises; co-administration is contraindicated). Products include:
Matulane Capsules 3246

Selegiline Hydrochloride (Concurrent and/or sequential administration with MAO inhibitors may result in hypertensive crises; co-administration is contraindicated). Products include:
Eldepryl Capsules 3266

Sertraline Hydrochloride (The safety and efficacy of combination therapy with phentermine and any other drug products for weight loss, including selective serotonin reuptake inhibitors, have not been established; co-administration of these products for weight loss is not recommended). Products include:
Zoloft 2751

Tranylcypromine Sulfate (Concurrent and/or sequential administration with MAO inhibitors may result in hypertensive crises; co-administration is contraindicated). Products include:
Parnate Tablets 1607

Food Interactions

Alcohol (May result in adverse drug interaction).

ADRIAMYCIN PFS/RDF INJECTION

(Doxorubicin Hydrochloride) 2767
May interact with calcium channel blockers, antineoplastics, phenytoin, and certain other agents. Compounds in these categories include:

Altretamine (Doxorubicin may potentiate the toxicity of other anticancer therapies). Products include:
Hexalen Capsules 2226

Amlodipine Besylate (Co-administration of doxorubicin and calcium channel entry blockers may increase the risk of doxorubicin cardiotoxicity). Products include:
Lotrel Capsules 2370
Norvasc Tablets 2704

Anastrozole (Doxorubicin may potentiate the toxicity of other anticancer therapies). Products include:
Arimidex Tablets 659

Asparaginase (Doxorubicin may potentiate the toxicity of other anticancer therapies). Products include:
Elspar for Injection 2092

Bepridil Hydrochloride (Co-administration of doxorubicin and calcium channel entry blockers may increase the risk of doxorubicin cardiotoxicity). Products include:
Vascor Tablets 2602

Bicalutamide (Doxorubicin may potentiate the toxicity of other anticancer therapies). Products include:
Casodex Tablets 662

Bleomycin Sulfate (Doxorubicin may potentiate the toxicity of other anticancer therapies).
No products indexed under this heading.

Busulfan (Doxorubicin may potentiate the toxicity of other anticancer therapies). Products include:
Myleran Tablets 1603

Carboplatin (Doxorubicin may potentiate the toxicity of other anticancer therapies). Products include:
Paraplatin for Injection 1126

Carmustine (BCNU) (Doxorubicin may potentiate the toxicity of other anticancer therapies). Products include:
Gliadel Wafer 1723

Chlorambucil (Doxorubicin may potentiate the toxicity of other anticancer therapies). Products include:
Leukeran Tablets 1591

Cisplatin (Doxorubicin may potentiate the toxicity of other anticancer therapies).
No products indexed under this heading.

Cyclophosphamide (Co-administration of doxorubicin with cyclophosphamide has resulted in exacerbation of cyclophosphamide-induced hemorrhagic cystitis; cardiac toxicity may occur at lower cumulative doses in patients who are receiving cyclophosphamide).
No products indexed under this heading.

Cyclosporine (Co-administration of doxorubicin may result in increases in AUC for both doxorubicin and doxorubicinol possibly due to a decrease in clearance of parent drug and a decrease in metabolism of doxorubicin; potential for more profound and prolonged hematologic toxicity is associated with combined use; coma and seizures have also been reported). Products include:
Gengraf Capsules 457
Neoral Soft Gelatin Capsules 2380
Neoral Oral Solution 2380
Sandimmune 2388

Cytarabine (Combination therapy results in necrotizing colitis, typhilitis, bloody stools and severe infections).
No products indexed under this heading.

Dacarbazine (Doxorubicin may potentiate the toxicity of other anticancer therapies). Products include:
DTIC-Dome 902

Daunorubicin Citrate (Doxorubicin may potentiate the toxicity of other anticancer therapies). Products include:
DaunoXome Injection 1442

Daunorubicin Hydrochloride (Doxorubicin may potentiate the toxicity of other anticancer therapies). Products include:
Cerubidine for Injection 947

Denileukin Diftitox (Doxorubicin may potentiate the toxicity of other anticancer therapies).
No products indexed under this heading.

Diltiazem Hydrochloride (Co-administration of doxorubicin and calcium channel entry blockers may increase the risk of doxorubicin cardiotoxicity). Products include:
Cardizem Injectable 1018
Cardizem Lyo-Ject Syringe 1018
Cardizem Monovial 1018
Cardizem CD Capsules 1016

Tiazac Capsules 1378

Docetaxel (Doxorubicin may potentiate the toxicity of other anticancer therapies). Products include:
Taxotere for Injection Concentrate 778

Epirubicin Hydrochloride (Doxorubicin may potentiate the toxicity of other anticancer therapies). Products include:
Ellence Injection 2806

Estramustine Phosphate Sodium (Doxorubicin may potentiate the toxicity of other anticancer therapies). Products include:
Emcyt Capsules 2810

Etoposide (Doxorubicin may potentiate the toxicity of other anticancer therapies).
No products indexed under this heading.

Exemestane (Doxorubicin may potentiate the toxicity of other anticancer therapies). Products include:
Aromasin Tablets 2769

Felodipine (Co-administration of doxorubicin and calcium channel entry blockers may increase the risk of doxorubicin cardiotoxicity). Products include:
Lexxel Tablets 608
Plendil Extended-Release Tablets 623

Floxuridine (Doxorubicin may potentiate the toxicity of other anticancer therapies). Products include:
Sterile FUDR 2974

Fluorouracil (Doxorubicin may potentiate the toxicity of other anticancer therapies). Products include:
Carac Cream 1222
Efudex 1733
Fluoroplex 552

Flutamide (Doxorubicin may potentiate the toxicity of other anticancer therapies). Products include:
Eulexin Capsules 3118

Fosphenytoin Sodium (Co-administration may result in decreased phenytoin levels). Products include:
Cerebyx Injection 2619

Gemcitabine Hydrochloride (Doxorubicin may potentiate the toxicity of other anticancer therapies). Products include:
Gemzar for Injection 1919

Hydroxyurea (Doxorubicin may potentiate the toxicity of other anticancer therapies). Products include:
Mylocel Tablets 2227

Idarubicin Hydrochloride (Doxorubicin may potentiate the toxicity of other anticancer therapies; concurrent use is contraindicated in patients who have received previous treatment with complete cumulative doses of idarubicin). Products include:
Idamycin PFS Injection 2825

Ifosfamide (Doxorubicin may potentiate the toxicity of other anticancer therapies). Products include:
Ifex for Injection 1123

Interferon alfa-2A, Recombinant (Doxorubicin may potentiate the toxicity of other anticancer therapies). Products include:
Roferon-A Injection 2996

Interferon alfa-2B, Recombinant (Doxorubicin may potentiate the toxicity of other anticancer therapies). Products include:
Intron A for Injection 3120
Rebetron Combination Therapy 3153

Irinotecan Hydrochloride (Doxorubicin may potentiate the toxicity of other anticancer therapies).
No products indexed under this heading.

Isradipine (Co-administration of doxorubicin and calcium channel entry blockers may increase the risk of doxorubicin cardiotoxicity). Products include:
DynaCirc Capsules 2921
DynaCirc CR Tablets 2923

Levamisole Hydrochloride (Doxorubicin may potentiate the toxicity of other anticancer therapies). Products include:
Ergamisol Tablets 1789

Live Virus Vaccines (Administration of live vaccine to immunocompromised patients, including those undergoing cytotoxic chemotherapy, may be hazardous).

Lomustine (CCNU) (Doxorubicin may potentiate the toxicity of other anticancer therapies).
No products indexed under this heading.

Mechlorethamine Hydrochloride (Doxorubicin may potentiate the toxicity of other anticancer therapies). Products include:
Mustargen for Injection 2142

Medroxyprogesterone Acetate (Co-administration of intravenous progesterone to patients with advanced malignancies at high doses with conventional formulation of fixed doxorubicin dose via bolus enhances doxorubicin-induced neutropenia and thrombocytopenia). Products include:
Depo-Provera Contraceptive Injection 2798
Lunelle Monthly Injection 2827
Premphase Tablets 3572
Prempro Tablets 3572
Provera Tablets 2853

Megestrol Acetate (Doxorubicin may potentiate the toxicity of other anticancer therapies). Products include:
Megace Oral Suspension 1124

Melphalan (Doxorubicin may potentiate the toxicity of other anticancer therapies). Products include:
Alkeran Tablets 1466

Mercaptopurine (Co-administration of doxorubicin with 6-mercaptopurine has resulted in enhancement of hepatotoxicity of 6-mercaptopurine). Products include:
Purinethol Tablets 1615

Methotrexate Sodium (Doxorubicin may potentiate the toxicity of other anticancer therapies).
No products indexed under this heading.

Mibefradil Dihydrochloride (Co-administration of doxorubicin and calcium channel entry blockers may increase the risk of doxorubicin cardiotoxicity).
No products indexed under this heading.

Mitomycin (Mitomycin-C) (Doxorubicin may potentiate the toxicity of other anticancer therapies).
No products indexed under this heading.

Mitotane (Doxorubicin may potentiate the toxicity of other anticancer therapies).
No products indexed under this heading.

Mitoxantrone Hydrochloride (Doxorubicin may potentiate the toxicity of other anticancer therapies). Products include:
Novantrone for Injection 1760

Nicardipine Hydrochloride (Co-administration of doxorubicin and calcium channel entry blockers may increase the risk of doxorubicin cardiotoxicity). Products include:
Cardene I.V. 3485

Nifedipine (Co-administration of doxorubicin and calcium channel entry blockers may increase the risk of doxorubicin cardiotoxicity). Products include:
Adalat CC Tablets 877
Procardia Capsules 2708
Procardia XL Extended Release Tablets 2710

Nimodipine (Co-administration of doxorubicin and calcium channel entry blockers may increase the risk of doxorubicin cardiotoxicity). Products include:
Nimotop Capsules 904

Nisoldipine (Co-administration of doxorubicin and calcium channel entry blockers may increase the risk of doxorubicin cardiotoxicity). Products include:
Sular Tablets 688

Paclitaxel (Administration of paclitaxel infused over 24 hours followed by conventional formulation of doxorubicin administered over 48 hours resulted in a significant decrease in doxorubicin clearance with more profound neutropenic and stomatitis episodes than the reverse sequence of administration). Products include:
Taxol Injection 1129

Phenobarbital (Increases the elimination of doxorubicin). Products include:
Arco-Lase Plus Tablets 592
Donnatal 2929
Donnatal Extentabs 2930

Phenytoin (Co-administration may result in decreased phenytoin levels). Products include:
Dilantin Infatabs 2624
Dilantin-125 Oral Suspension 2625

Phenytoin Sodium (Co-administration may result in decreased phenytoin levels). Products include:
Dilantin Kapseals 2622

Procarbazine Hydrochloride (Doxorubicin may potentiate the toxicity of other anticancer therapies). Products include:
Matulane Capsules 3246

Progesterone (Co-administration of intravenous progesterone to patients with advanced malignancies at high doses with conventional formulation of fixed doxorubicin dose via bolus enhances doxorubicin-induced neutropenia and thrombocytopenia). Products include:
Crinone 3213
Prometrium Capsules (100 mg, 200 mg) 3261

Streptozocin (May inhibit the hepatic metabolism; doxorubicin may potentiate the toxicity of other anticancer therapies).
No products indexed under this heading.

Tamoxifen Citrate (Doxorubicin may potentiate the toxicity of other anticancer therapies). Products include:
Nolvadex Tablets 678

Teniposide (Doxorubicin may potentiate the toxicity of other anticancer therapies).
No products indexed under this heading.

Thioguanine (Doxorubicin may potentiate the toxicity of other anticancer therapies). Products include:
Tabloid Tablets 1642

Thiotepa (Doxorubicin may potentiate the toxicity of other anticancer therapies). Products include:
Thioplex for Injection 1765

Topotecan Hydrochloride (Doxorubicin may potentiate the toxicity of other anticancer therapies). Products include:
Hycamtin for Injection 1546

Toremifene Citrate (Doxorubicin may potentiate the toxicity of other anticancer therapies). Products include:
Fareston Tablets 3237

Valrubicin (Doxorubicin may potentiate the toxicity of other anticancer therapies). Products include:
Valstar Sterile Solution for Intravesical Instillation 1175

Verapamil Hydrochloride (Co-administration of doxorubicin in animal study has resulted in higher initial peak concentrations of doxorubicin in the heart with a higher incidence and severity of degenerative changes in cardiac tissue resulting in a shorter survival). Products include:
Covera-HS Tablets 3199
Isoptin SR Tablets 467
Tarka Tablets 508
Verelan Capsules 3184
Verelan PM Capsules 3186

Vincristine Sulfate (Doxorubicin may potentiate the toxicity of other anticancer therapies).
No products indexed under this heading.

Vinorelbine Tartrate (Doxorubicin may potentiate the toxicity of other anticancer therapies). Products include:
Navelbine Injection 1604

ADVAIR DISKUS 100/50

(Fluticasone Propionate, Salmeterol Xinafoate) 1448
May interact with tricyclic antidepressants and certain other agents. Compounds in these categories include:

Acebutolol Hydrochloride (Co-administration with beta blockers not only blocks the pulmonary effect of beta-agonists, such as salmeterol, but may produce severe bronchospasm in patients with asthma). Products include:
Sectral Capsules 3589

Amitriptyline Hydrochloride (Concurrent and/or sequential administration with tricyclic antidepressants may potentiate the action of salmeterol on the vascular system). Products include:
Etrafon 3115
Limbitrol 1738

Amoxapine (Concurrent and/or sequential administration with tricyclic antidepressants may potentiate the action of salmeterol on the vascular system).
No products indexed under this heading.

Atenolol (Co-administration with beta blockers not only blocks the pulmonary effect of beta-agonists, such as salmeterol, but may produce severe bronchospasm in patients with asthma). Products include:
Tenoretic Tablets 690
Tenormin I.V. Injection 692

Bendroflumethiazide (The ECG changes and/or hypokalemia that may result from the administration of non-potassium sparing diuretics can be acutely worsened by beta-agonists, especially when the recommended dose of beta-agonist is exceeded). Products include:
Corzide 40/5 Tablets 2247
Corzide 80/5 Tablets 2247

Betaxolol Hydrochloride (Co-administration with beta blockers not only blocks the pulmonary effect of beta-agonists, such as salmeterol, but may produce severe bronchospasm in patients with asthma). Products include:
Betoptic S Ophthalmic Suspension 537

Bisoprolol Fumarate (Co-administration with beta blockers not only blocks the pulmonary effect of beta-agonists, such as salmeterol, but may produce severe bronchospasm in patients with asthma). Products include:
Zebeta Tablets 1885
Ziac Tablets 1887

Bumetanide (The ECG changes and/or hypokalemia that may result from the administration of non-potassium sparing diuretics can be acutely worsened by beta-agonists,

especially when the recommended dose of beta-agonist is exceeded).
No products indexed under this heading.

Carteolol Hydrochloride (Co-administration with beta blockers not only blocks the pulmonary effect of beta-agonists, such as salmeterol, but may produce severe bronchospasm in patients with asthma). Products include:
Carteolol Hydrochloride Ophthalmic Solution USP, 1% ..... ⊙258
Ocupress Ophthalmic Solution, 1% Sterile ..... ⊙303

Chlorothiazide (The ECG changes and/or hypokalemia that may result from the administration of non-potassium sparing diuretics can be acutely worsened by beta-agonists, especially when the recommended dose of beta-agonist is exceeded). Products include:
Aldoclor Tablets 2035
Diuril Oral 2087

Chlorothiazide Sodium (The ECG changes and/or hypokalemia that may result from the administration of non-potassium sparing diuretics can be acutely worsened by beta-agonists, especially when the recommended dose of beta-agonist is exceeded). Products include:
Diuril Sodium Intravenous 2086

Clomipramine Hydrochloride (Concurrent and/or sequential administration with tricyclic antidepressants may potentiate the action of salmeterol on the vascular system).
No products indexed under this heading.

Desipramine Hydrochloride (Concurrent and/or sequential administration with tricyclic antidepressants may potentiate the action of salmeterol on the vascular system). Products include:
Norpramin Tablets 755

Doxepin Hydrochloride (Concurrent and/or sequential administration with tricyclic antidepressants may potentiate the action of salmeterol on the vascular system). Products include:
Sinequan 2713

Esmolol Hydrochloride (Co-administration with beta blockers not only blocks the pulmonary effect of beta-agonists, such as salmeterol, but may produce severe bronchospasm in patients with asthma). Products include:
Brevibloc Injection 858

Ethacrynic Acid (The ECG changes and/or hypokalemia that may result from the administration of non-potassium sparing diuretics can be acutely worsened by beta-agonists, especially when the recommended dose of beta-agonist is exceeded). Products include:
Edecrin Tablets 2091

Furosemide (The ECG changes and/or hypokalemia that may result from the administration of non-potassium sparing diuretics can be acutely worsened by beta-agonists, especially when the recommended dose of beta-agonist is exceeded). Products include:
Furosemide Tablets 2284

Hydrochlorothiazide (The ECG changes and/or hypokalemia that may result from the administration of non-potassium sparing diuretics can be acutely worsened by beta-agonists, especially when the recommended dose of beta-agonist is exceeded). Products include:
Accuretic Tablets 2614
Aldoril Tablets 2039
Atacand HCT Tablets 597
Avalide Tablets 1070
Diovan HCT Tablets 2338
Dyazide Capsules 1515
HydroDIURIL Tablets 2108
Hyzaar 2109
Inderide Tablets 3517
Inderide LA Long-Acting Capsules .. 3519
Lotensin HCT Tablets 2367
Maxzide 1008
Micardis HCT Tablets 1051
Microzide Capsules 3414
Moduretic Tablets 2138
Monopril HCT 1094
Prinzide Tablets 2168
Timolide Tablets 2187
Uniretic Tablets 3178
Vaseretic Tablets 2204
Zestoretic Tablets 695
Ziac Tablets 1887

Hydroflumethiazide (The ECG changes and/or hypokalemia that may result from the administration of non-potassium sparing diuretics can be acutely worsened by beta-agonists, especially when the recommended dose of beta-agonist is exceeded). Products include:
Diucardin Tablets 3494

Imipramine Hydrochloride (Concurrent and/or sequential administration with tricyclic antidepressants may potentiate the action of salmeterol on the vascular system).
No products indexed under this heading.

Imipramine Pamoate (Concurrent and/or sequential administration with tricyclic antidepressants may potentiate the action of salmeterol on the vascular system).
No products indexed under this heading.

Isocarboxazid (Concurrent and/or sequential administration with MAO inhibitors may potentiate the action of salmeterol on the vascular system).
No products indexed under this heading.

Ketoconazole (Co-administration of a single dose of fluticasone with multiple doses of ketoconazole to steady state has resulted in increased mean fluticasone concentrations, a reduction in plasma cortisol AUC and no effect on urinary excretion of cortisol). Products include:
Nizoral 2% Cream 3620
Nizoral A-D Shampoo 2008
Nizoral 2% Shampoo 2007
Nizoral Tablets 1791

Labetalol Hydrochloride (Co-administration with beta blockers not only blocks the pulmonary effect of beta-agonists, such as salmeterol, but may produce severe bronchospasm in patients with asthma). Products include:
Normodyne Injection 3135
Normodyne Tablets 3137

Levobunolol Hydrochloride (Co-administration with beta blockers not only blocks the pulmonary effect of beta-agonists, such as salmeterol, but may produce severe bronchospasm in patients with asthma). Products include:
Betagan ..... ⊙228

Maprotiline Hydrochloride (Concurrent and/or sequential administration with tricyclic antidepressants may potentiate the action of salmeterol on the vascular system).
No products indexed under this heading.

Methyclothiazide (The ECG changes and/or hypokalemia that may result from the administration of non-potassium sparing diuretics can be acutely worsened by beta-agonists, especially when the recommended dose of beta-agonist is exceeded).
No products indexed under this heading.

Metipranolol Hydrochloride (Co-administration with beta blockers not only blocks the pulmonary effect of beta-agonists, such as salmeterol, but may produce severe bronchospasm in patients with asthma).
No products indexed under this heading.

Metoprolol Succinate (Co-administration with beta blockers not only blocks the pulmonary effect of beta-agonists, such as salmeterol, but may produce severe bronchospasm in patients with asthma). Products include:
Toprol-XL Tablets 651

Metoprolol Tartrate (Co-administration with beta blockers not only blocks the pulmonary effect of beta-agonists, such as salmeterol, but may produce severe bronchospasm in patients with asthma).
No products indexed under this heading.

Moclobemide (Concurrent and/or sequential administration with MAO inhibitors may potentiate the action of salmeterol on the vascular system).
No products indexed under this heading.

Nadolol (Co-administration with beta blockers not only blocks the pulmonary effect of beta-agonists, such as salmeterol, but may produce severe bronchospasm in patients with asthma). Products include:
Corgard Tablets 2245
Corzide 40/5 Tablets 2247
Corzide 80/5 Tablets 2247
Nadolol Tablets 2288

Nortriptyline Hydrochloride (Concurrent and/or sequential administration with tricyclic antidepressants may potentiate the action of salmeterol on the vascular system).
No products indexed under this heading.

Pargyline Hydrochloride (Concurrent and/or sequential administration with MAO inhibitors may potentiate the action of salmeterol on the vascular system).
No products indexed under this heading.

Penbutolol Sulfate (Co-administration with beta blockers not only blocks the pulmonary effect of beta-agonists, such as salmeterol, but may produce severe bronchospasm in patients with asthma).
No products indexed under this heading.

Phenelzine Sulfate (Concurrent and/or sequential administration with MAO inhibitors may potentiate the action of salmeterol on the vascular system). Products include:
Nardil Tablets 2653

Pindolol (Co-administration with beta blockers not only blocks the pulmonary effect of beta-agonists, such as salmeterol, but may produce severe bronchospasm in patients with asthma).
No products indexed under this heading.

Polythiazide (The ECG changes and/or hypokalemia that may result from the administration of non-potassium sparing diuretics can be acutely worsened by beta-agonists, especially when the recommended dose of beta-agonist is exceeded). Products include:
Minizide Capsules 2700
Renese Tablets 2712

Procarbazine Hydrochloride (Concurrent and/or sequential administration with MAO inhibitors may potentiate the action of salmeterol on the vascular system). Products include:
Matulane Capsules 3246

Propranolol Hydrochloride (Co-administration with beta blockers not only blocks the pulmonary effect of beta-agonists, such as salmeterol, but may produce severe bronchospasm in patients with asthma). Products include:
Inderal 3513
Inderal LA Long-Acting Capsules 3516
Inderide Tablets 3517
Inderide LA Long-Acting Capsules .. 3519

Protriptyline Hydrochloride (Concurrent and/or sequential administration with tricyclic antidepressants may potentiate the action of salmeterol on the vascular system). Products include:
Vivactil Tablets 2446
Vivactil Tablets 2217

Selegiline Hydrochloride (Concurrent and/or sequential administration with MAO inhibitors may potentiate the action of salmeterol on the vascular system). Products include:
Eldepryl Capsules 3266

Sotalol Hydrochloride (Co-administration with beta blockers not only blocks the pulmonary effect of beta-agonists, such as salmeterol, but may produce severe bronchospasm in patients with asthma). Products include:
Betapace Tablets 950
Betapace AF Tablets 954

Timolol Hemihydrate (Co-administration with beta blockers not only blocks the pulmonary effect of beta-agonists, such as salmeterol, but may produce severe bronchospasm in patients with asthma). Products include:
Betimol Ophthalmic Solution ..... ⊙324

Timolol Maleate (Co-administration with beta blockers not only blocks the pulmonary effect of beta-agonists, such as salmeterol, but may produce severe bronchospasm in patients with asthma). Products include:
Blocadren Tablets 2046
Cosopt Sterile Ophthalmic Solution 2065
Timolide Tablets 2187
Timolol GFS ..... ⊙266
Timoptic in Ocudose 2192
Timoptic Sterile Ophthalmic Solution 2190
Timoptic-XE Sterile Ophthalmic Gel Forming Solution 2194

Torsemide (The ECG changes and/or hypokalemia that may result from the administration of non-potassium sparing diuretics can be acutely worsened by beta-agonists, especially when the recommended dose of beta-agonist is exceeded). Products include:
Demadex Tablets and Injection 2965

Tranylcypromine Sulfate (Concurrent and/or sequential administration with MAO inhibitors may potentiate the action of salmeterol on the vascular system). Products include:
Parnate Tablets 1607

Trimipramine Maleate (Concurrent and/or sequential administration with tricyclic antidepressants may potentiate the action of salmeterol on the vascular system). Products include:
Surmontil Capsules 3595

ADVAIR DISKUS 250/50

(Fluticasone Propionate, Salmeterol Xinafoate) 1448
See Advair Diskus 100/50

ADVAIR DISKUS 500/50

(Fluticasone Propionate, Salmeterol Xinafoate) 1448
See Advair Diskus 100/50

ADVANTIN CAPSULES

(Herbals, Multiple) ..... ▣794
None cited in PDR database.

ADVIL CAPLETS

(Ibuprofen) ..... ▣771
See Advil Tablets

IMPORTANT NOTE: Always consult each drug listing in the patient's regimen for possible interactions.

ADVIL GEL CAPLETS
(Ibuprofen) ▣ 771
See Advil Tablets

ADVIL LIQUI-GELS
(Ibuprofen) ▣ 771
See Advil Tablets

ADVIL TABLETS
(Ibuprofen) ▣ 771
May interact with:

Acetaminophen (Concurrent administration should not be undertaken without physician's direction). Products include:
Actifed Cold & Sinus Caplets and Tablets ▣ 688
Alka-Seltzer Plus Liqui-Gels ▣ 604
Alka-Seltzer Plus Cold & Flu Medicine Liqui-Gels ▣ 604
Alka-Seltzer Plus Cold & Sinus Medicine Liqui-Gels ▣ 604
Benadryl Allergy/Cold Tablets ▣ 691
Benadryl Allergy Sinus Headache Caplets & Gelcaps ▣ 693
Benadryl Severe Allergy & Sinus Headache Caplets ▣ 694
Children's Cēpacol Sore Throat ▣ 788
Comtrex Acute Head Cold & Sinus Pressure Relief Tablets ▣ 627
Comtrex Deep Chest Cold & Congestion Relief Softgels ▣ 627
Comtrex Flu Therapy & Fever Relief Daytime Caplets ▣ 628
Comtrex Flu Therapy & Fever Relief Nighttime Tablets ▣ 628
Comtrex Maximum Strength Multi-Symptom Cold & Cough Relief Tablets and Caplets ▣ 626
Contac Severe Cold and Flu Caplets Maximum Strength ▣ 746
Contac Severe Cold and Flu Caplets Non-Drowsy ▣ 746
Coricidin 'D' Cold, Flu & Sinus Tablets ▣ 737
Coricidin HBP Cold & Flu Tablets ▣ 738
Coricidin HBP Maximum Strength Flu Tablets ▣ 738
Coricidin HBP Night-Time Cold & Flu Tablets ▣ 738
Darvon-N/Darvocet-N 1907
Dimetapp Cold and Fever Suspension ▣ 775
Dimetapp Nighttime Flu Liquid ▣ 776
Dimetapp Non-Drowsy Flu Syrup ▣ 777
Drixoral Allergy/Sinus Extended-Release Tablets ▣ 741
Drixoral Cold & Flu Extended-Release Tablets ▣ 740
Aspirin Free Excedrin Caplets and Geltabs ▣ 628
Excedrin Extra-Strength Tablets, Caplets, and Geltabs ▣ 629
Excedrin Migraine 1070
Excedrin PM Tablets, Caplets, and Geltabs ▣ 631
Goody's Body Pain Formula Powder ▣ 620
Goody's Extra Strength Headache Powder ▣ 620
Goody's Extra Strength Pain Relief Tablets ▣ 620
Goody's PM Powder ▣ 621
Hycomine Compound Tablets 1317
Lortab 3319
Lortab Elixir 3317
Maxidone Tablets CIII 3399
Maximum Strength Midol Menstrual Caplets and Gelcaps ▣ 612
Maximum Strength Midol PMS Caplets and Gelcaps ▣ 613
Maximum Strength Midol Teen Caplets ▣ 612
Midrin Capsules 3464
Norco 5/325 Tablets CIII 3424
Norco 7.5/325 Tablets CIII 3425
Norco 10/325 Tablets CIII 3427
Norco 10/325 Tablets CIII 3425
Percocet Tablets 1326
Percogesic Aspirin-Free Coated Tablets ▣ 667
Extra Strength Percogesic Aspirin-Free Coated Caplets ▣ 665
Phrenilin 578
Robitussin Cold Caplets Multi-Symptom Cold & Flu ▣ 781
Robitussin Cold Softgels Multi-Symptom Cold & Flu ▣ 781
Robitussin Multi Symptom Honey Flu Liquid ▣ 785
Robitussin Nighttime Honey Flu Liquid ▣ 786
Sedapap Tablets 50 mg/650 mg 2225
Singlet Caplets ▣ 761
Sinutab Sinus Allergy Medication, Maximum Strength Formula, Tablets & Caplets ▣ 707
Sinutab Sinus Medication, Maximum Strength Without Drowsiness Formula, Tablets & Caplets ▣ 707
Sudafed Cold & Cough Liquid Caps ▣ 709
Sudafed Cold & Sinus Liquid Caps ▣ 710
Sudafed Severe Cold ▣ 711
Sudafed Sinus Headache Caplets ▣ 712
Sudafed Sinus Headache Tablets ▣ 712
Tavist Sinus Non-Drowsy Coated Caplets ▣ 676
TheraFlu Regular Strength Cold & Cough Night Time Hot Liquid ▣ 676
TheraFlu Regular Strength Cold & Sore Throat Night Time Hot Liquid ▣ 676
TheraFlu Maximum Strength Flu & Congestion Non-Drowsy Hot Liquid ▣ 677
TheraFlu Maximum Strength Flu & Cough Night Time Hot Liquid ▣ 678
TheraFlu Maximum Strength Flu & Sore Throat Night Time Hot Liquid ▣ 677
TheraFlu Maximum Strength Severe Cold & Congestion Night Time Caplets ▣ 678
TheraFlu Maximum Strength Severe Cold & Congestion Night Time Hot Liquid ▣ 678
TheraFlu Maximum Strength Severe Cold & Congestion Non-Drowsy ▣ 679
Triaminic Cold, Cough & Fever Liquid ▣ 681
Triaminic Cough & Sore Throat Liquid ▣ 682
Triaminic Cough & Sore Throat Softchews ▣ 684
Tylenol, Children's 2014
Children's Tylenol Allergy-D Liquid 2014
Children's Tylenol Cold Suspension Liquid and Chewable Tablets 2015
Children's Tylenol Cold Plus Cough Suspension Liquid and Chewable Tablets 2015
Children's Tylenol Flu Suspension Liquid 2015
Children's Tylenol Sinus Suspension Liquid 2017
Infants' Tylenol Cold Decongestant and Fever Reducer Concentrated Drops 2015
Infants' Tylenol Cold Decongestant and Fever Reducer Concentrated Drops Plus Cough 2015
Junior Strength Tylenol Soft Chews Chewable Tablets 2014
Tylenol 2009
Tylenol Allergy Sinus 2010
Tylenol Severe Allergy Caplets 2010
Multi-Symptom Tylenol Cold Complete Formula Caplets 2010
Multi-Symptom Tylenol Cold Non-Drowsy Caplets and Gelcaps 2010
Multi-Symptom Tylenol Cold Severe Congestion Non-Drowsy Caplets 2011
Maximum Strength Tylenol Flu NightTime Gelcaps 2011
Maximum Strength Tylenol Flu NightTime Liquid 2011
Maximum Strength Tylenol Flu Non-Drowsy Gelcaps 2011
Extra Strength Tylenol PM Caplets, Geltabs, and Gelcaps 2012
Maximum Strength Tylenol Sinus NightTime Caplets 2012
Maximum Strength Tylenol Sinus Non-Drowsy Geltabs, Gelcaps, Caplets, and Tablets 2012
Maximum Strength Tylenol Sore Throat Adult Liquid 2013
Tylenol with Codeine 2595
Women's Tylenol Menstrual Relief Caplets 2013
Tylox Capsules 2597
Ultracet Tablets 2597
Vanquish Caplets ▣ 617
Vicks 44M Cough, Cold & Flu Relief Liquid ▣ 725
Vicks DayQuil LiquiCaps/Liquid Multi-Symptom Cold/Flu Relief ▣ 727
Vicks NyQuil LiquiCaps/Liquid Multi-Symptom Cold/Flu Relief, Original and Cherry Flavors ▣ 727
Vicodin Tablets 516
Vicodin ES Tablets 517
Vicodin HP Tablets 518
Zydone Tablets 1330

Aspirin (Concurrent administration should not be undertaken without physician's direction). Products include:
Aggrenox Capsules 1026
Alka-Seltzer ▣ 603
Alka-Seltzer Lemon Lime Antacid and Pain Reliever Effervescent Tablets ▣ 603
Alka-Seltzer Extra Strength Antacid and Pain Reliever Effervescent Tablets ▣ 603
Alka-Seltzer PM Effervescent Tablets ▣ 605
Genuine Bayer Tablets, Caplets and Gelcaps ▣ 606
Extra Strength Bayer Caplets and Gelcaps ▣ 610
Aspirin Regimen Bayer Children's Chewable Tablets (Orange or Cherry Flavored) ▣ 607
Bayer, Aspirin Regimen ▣ 606
Aspirin Regimen Bayer 81 mg Caplets with Calcium ▣ 607
Genuine Bayer Professional Labeling (Aspirin Regimen Bayer) ▣ 608
Extra Strength Bayer Arthritis Caplets ▣ 610
Extra Strength Bayer Plus Caplets ▣ 610
Extra Strength Bayer PM Caplets ▣ 611
BC Powder ▣ 619
BC Allergy Sinus Cold Powder ▣ 619
Arthritis Strength BC Powder ▣ 619
BC Sinus Cold Powder ▣ 619
Darvon Compound-65 Pulvules 1910
Ecotrin Enteric Coated Aspirin Low, Regular and Maximum Strength Tablets 1715
Excedrin Extra-Strength Tablets, Caplets, and Geltabs ▣ 629
Excedrin Migraine 1070
Goody's Body Pain Formula Powder ▣ 620
Goody's Extra Strength Headache Powder ▣ 620
Goody's Extra Strength Pain Relief Tablets ▣ 620
Percodan Tablets 1327
Robaxisal Tablets 2939
Soma Compound Tablets 3354
Soma Compound w/Codeine Tablets 3355
Vanquish Caplets ▣ 617

Food Interactions

Alcohol (Chronic heavy alcohol users, 3 or more drinks per day, should consult their physicians for advice on when and how they should take pain relievers/fever reducers including ibuprofen).

CHILDREN'S ADVIL ORAL SUSPENSION
(Ibuprofen) ▣ 773
None cited in PDR database.

CHILDREN'S ADVIL CHEWABLE TABLETS
(Ibuprofen) ▣ 773
None cited in PDR database.

ADVIL COLD AND SINUS CAPLETS
(Ibuprofen, Pseudoephedrine Hydrochloride) ▣ 771
See Advil Cold and Sinus Tablets

ADVIL COLD AND SINUS TABLETS
(Ibuprofen, Pseudoephedrine Hydrochloride) ▣ 771
May interact with monoamine oxidase inhibitors and certain other agents. Compounds in these categories include:

Isocarboxazid (Concurrent and/or sequential use with MAO inhibitors is not recommended).
No products indexed under this heading.

Moclobemide (Concurrent and/or sequential use with MAO inhibitors is not recommended).
No products indexed under this heading.

Pargyline Hydrochloride (Concurrent and/or sequential use with MAO inhibitors is not recommended).
No products indexed under this heading.

Phenelzine Sulfate (Concurrent and/or sequential use with MAO inhibitors is not recommended). Products include:
Nardil Tablets 2653

Procarbazine Hydrochloride (Concurrent and/or sequential use with MAO inhibitors is not recommended). Products include:
Matulane Capsules 3246

Selegiline Hydrochloride (Concurrent and/or sequential use with MAO inhibitors is not recommended). Products include:
Eldepryl Capsules 3266

Tranylcypromine Sulfate (Concurrent and/or sequential use with MAO inhibitors is not recommended). Products include:
Parnate Tablets 1607

Food Interactions

Alcohol (Chronic heavy alcohol users, 3 or more drinks per day, should consult their physician for advice on when and how they should take pain relievers/fever reducers including ibuprofen).

ADVIL FLU & BODY ACHE CAPLETS
(Ibuprofen, Pseudoephedrine Hydrochloride) ▣ 772
May interact with monoamine oxidase inhibitors and certain other agents. Compounds in these categories include:

Isocarboxazid (Concurrent and/or sequential use with MAO inhibitors is not recommended).
No products indexed under this heading.

Moclobemide (Concurrent and/or sequential use with MAO inhibitors is not recommended).
No products indexed under this heading.

Pargyline Hydrochloride (Concurrent and/or sequential use with MAO inhibitors is not recommended).
No products indexed under this heading.

Phenelzine Sulfate (Concurrent and/or sequential use with MAO inhibitors is not recommended). Products include:
Nardil Tablets 2653

Procarbazine Hydrochloride (Concurrent and/or sequential use with MAO inhibitors is not recommended). Products include:
Matulane Capsules 3246

Selegiline Hydrochloride (Concurrent and/or sequential use with MAO inhibitors is not recommended). Products include:
Eldepryl Capsules 3266

Tranylcypromine Sulfate (Concurrent and/or sequential use with MAO inhibitors is not recommended). Products include:
Parnate Tablets 1607

Food Interactions

Alcohol (Chronic heavy alcohol users, 3 or more drinks per day, should consult their physican for advice on when and how they should take pain relievers/fever reducers including ibuprofen).

INFANTS' ADVIL DROPS
(Ibuprofen) ▣ 773
None cited in PDR database.

JUNIOR STRENGTH ADVIL TABLETS
(Ibuprofen) ▣ 773
None cited in PDR database.

JUNIOR STRENGTH ADVIL CHEWABLE TABLETS
(Ibuprofen) .... ▣773
None cited in PDR database.

ADVIL MIGRAINE LIQUIGELS
(Ibuprofen) .... ▣772

Food Interactions

Alcohol (Chronic heavy alcohol users, 3 or more drinks per day, should consult their physician for advice on when and how they should take pain relievers/fever reducers including ibuprofen).

AEROBID INHALER SYSTEM
(Flunisolide) 1363
None cited in PDR database.

AEROBID-M INHALER SYSTEM
(Flunisolide) 1363
None cited in PDR database.

AEROLATE LIQUID
(Theophylline) 1361
None cited in PDR database.

AEROLATE JR. T.D. CAPSULES
(Theophylline) 1361
None cited in PDR database.

AEROLATE SR. T.D. CAPSULES
(Theophylline) 1361
None cited in PDR database.

AFLEXA TABLETS
(Glucosamine) 1997
None cited in PDR database.

AFRIN NASAL DECONGESTANT CHILDREN'S PUMP MIST
(Phenylephrine Hydrochloride) .... ▣734
None cited in PDR database.

AFRIN ORIGINAL NASAL SPRAY
(Oxymetazoline Hydrochloride) .... ▣733
None cited in PDR database.

AFRIN EXTRA MOISTURIZING NASAL SPRAY
(Oxymetazoline Hydrochloride) .... ▣733
None cited in PDR database.

AFRIN SEVERE CONGESTION NASAL SPRAY
(Oxymetazoline Hydrochloride) .... ▣733
None cited in PDR database.

AFRIN SINUS NASAL SPRAY
(Oxymetazoline Hydrochloride) .... ▣733
None cited in PDR database.

AFRIN NO DRIP ORIGINAL NASAL SPRAY
(Oxymetazoline Hydrochloride) .... ▣735
None cited in PDR database.

AFRIN NO DRIP EXTRA MOISTURIZING NASAL SPRAY
(Oxymetazoline Hydrochloride) .... ▣735
None cited in PDR database.

AFRIN NO DRIP SEVERE CONGESTION NASAL SPRAY
(Oxymetazoline Hydrochloride) .... ▣735
None cited in PDR database.

AFRIN NO DRIP SINUS NASAL SPRAY
(Oxymetazoline Hydrochloride) .... ▣735
None cited in PDR database.

AFRIN ORIGINAL PUMP MIST
(Oxymetazoline Hydrochloride) .... ▣733
None cited in PDR database.

AFRIN SALINE AROMATIC MIST
(Menthol, Sodium Chloride) .... ▣734
None cited in PDR database.

AFRIN EXTRA MOISTURIZING SALINE MIST
(Sodium Chloride) .... ▣734
None cited in PDR database.

AGENERASE CAPSULES
(Amprenavir) 1454
See Agenerase Oral Solution

AGENERASE ORAL SOLUTION
(Amprenavir) 1459
May interact with antacids containing aluminum, calcium and magnesium, calcium channel blockers, dexamethasone, ergot-containing drugs, oral hypoglycemic agents, insulin, phenytoin, protease inhibitors, quinidine, and certain other agents. Compounds in these categories include:

Acarbose (New onset diabetes mellitus, exacerbation of pre-existing diabetes mellitus, and hyperglycemia have been reported in HIV-infected patients receiving protease inhibitors; some patients may require dose adjustments). Products include:
- Precose Tablets 906

Alprazolam (Increased benzodiazepine plasma concentrations; clinical significance is unknown; however, a decrease in benzodiazepine dose may be needed). Products include:
- Xanax Tablets 2865

Aluminum Carbonate (Antacids decrease amprenavir plasma concentrations; Agenerase should be taken at least one hour before or after antacids).
No products indexed under this heading.

Aluminum Hydroxide (Antacids decrease amprenavir plasma concentrations; Agenerase should be taken at least one hour before or after antacids). Products include:
- Amphojel Suspension (Mint Flavor) .... ▣789
- Gaviscon Extra Strength Liquid .... ▣751
- Gaviscon Extra Strength Tablets .... ▣751
- Gaviscon Regular Strength Liquid .... ▣751
- Gaviscon Regular Strength Tablets .... ▣750
- Maalox Antacid/Anti-Gas Oral Suspension .... ▣673
- Maalox Max Maximum Strength Antacid/Anti-Gas Liquid 2300
- Maalox Regular Strength Antacid/Antigas Liquid 2300
- Mylanta 1813
- Vanquish Caplets .... ▣617

Amiodarone Hydrochloride (Increases antiarrhythmics plasma concentrations). Products include:
- Cordarone Intravenous 3491
- Cordarone Tablets 3487
- Pacerone Tablets 3331

Amitriptyline Hydrochloride (Increase in tricyclic antidepressant plasma concentrations). Products include:
- Etrafon 3115
- Limbitrol 1738

Amlodipine Besylate (Increased calcium channel blockers plasma concentrations). Products include:
- Lotrel Capsules 2370
- Norvasc Tablets 2704

Amoxapine (Co-administration could result in serious and/or life threatening drug interactions).
No products indexed under this heading.

Astemizole (Co-administration of amprenavir is contraindicated with drugs that are highly dependant of CYP3A4 for clearance and for which elevated plasma concentrations are associated with serious and/or life-threatening events such as cardiac arrhythmias).
No products indexed under this heading.

Atorvastatin Calcium (Increased atorvastatin plasma concentrations). Products include:
- Lipitor Tablets 2639
- Lipitor Tablets 2696

Bepridil Hydrochloride (Increases bepridil plasma concentrations; increased bepridil exposure may be associated with life-threatening reactions such as cardiac arrhythmias). Products include:
- Vascor Tablets 2602

Carbamazepine (Decreases amprenavir plasma concentrations potentially reducing effectiveness of amprenavir). Products include:
- Carbatrol Capsules 3234
- Tegretol/Tegretol-XR 2404

Cerivastatin Sodium (Increased cerivastatin plasma concentrations). Products include:
- Baycol Tablets 883

Chlorpropamide (New onset diabetes mellitus, exacerbation of pre-existing diabetes mellitus, and hyperglycemia have been reported in HIV-infected patients receiving protease inhibitors; some patients may require dose adjustments). Products include:
- Diabinese Tablets 2680

Cisapride (Co-administration of amprenavir is contraindicated with drugs that are highly dependant of CYP3A4 for clearance and for which elevated plasma concentrations are associated with serious and/or life-threatening events).
No products indexed under this heading.

Clarithromycin (Co-administration has resulted in 15% increase in Cmax, 18% increase in AUC, and 39% increase in Cmin of amprenavir; 10% decrease in clarithromycin Cmax was reported). Products include:
- Biaxin/Biaxin XL 403
- PREVPAC 3298

Clomipramine Hydrochloride (Co-administration could result in serious and/or life-threatening drug interactions).
No products indexed under this heading.

Clorazepate Dipotassium (Increased benzodiazepine plasma concentrations; clinical significance is unknown; however, a decrease in benzodiazepine dose may be needed). Products include:
- Tranxene 511

Clozapine (May result in increased plasma concentrations of clozapine). Products include:
- Clozaril Tablets 2319

Cyclosporine (Increased immunosuppressant plasma concentrations). Products include:
- Gengraf Capsules 457
- Neoral Soft Gelatin Capsules 2380
- Neoral Oral Solution 2380
- Sandimmune 2388

Dapsone (Co-administration with dapsone may result in increased plasma concentrations of dapsone). Products include:
- Dapsone Tablets USP 1780

Delavirdine Mesylate (Co-administration with NNRTIs, such as delavirdine, may have potential to increase serum concentrations of amprenavir). Products include:
- Rescriptor Tablets 526

Dexamethasone (Decreases amprenavir plasma concentrations potentially reducing effectiveness of amprenavir). Products include:
- Decadron Elixir 2078
- Decadron Tablets 2079
- TobraDex Ophthalmic Ointment 542
- TobraDex Ophthalmic Suspension 541

Dexamethasone Acetate (Decreases amprenavir plasma concentrations potentially reducing effectiveness of amprenavir).
No products indexed under this heading.

Dexamethasone Sodium Phosphate (Decreases amprenavir plasma concentrations potentially reducing effectiveness of amprenavir). Products include:
- Decadron Phosphate Injection 2081
- Decadron Phosphate Sterile Ophthalmic Ointment 2083
- Decadron Phosphate Sterile Ophthalmic Solution 2084
- NeoDecadron Sterile Ophthalmic Solution 2144

Diazepam (Increased benzodiazepine plasma concentrations; clinical significance is unknown; however, a decrease in benzodiazepine dose may be needed). Products include:
- Valium Injectable 3026
- Valium Tablets 3047

Didanosine (Didanosine secondary to the antacid content has not been specifically studied, however, based upon data with other protease inhibitors, it is advisable that antacids not be taken at the same time as amprenavir because of potential interference with absorption; it is recommended that their administration be separated by at least an hour). Products include:
- Videx 1138
- Videx EC Capsules 1143

Dihydroergotamine Mesylate (Co-administration of amprenavir is contraindicated with drugs that are highly dependant of CYP3A4, such as ergot derivatives, for clearance and for which elevated plasma concentrations are associated with serious and/or life-threatening events such as acute ergot toxicity characterized by peripheral vasospasm, and ischemia of the extremities and other tissues). Products include:
- D.H.E. 45 Injection 2334
- Migranal Nasal Spray 2376

Diltiazem Hydrochloride (Increased calcium channel blockers plasma concentrations). Products include:
- Cardizem Injectable 1018
- Cardizem Lyo-Ject Syringe 1018
- Cardizem Monovial 1018
- Cardizem CD Capsules 1016
- Tiazac Capsules 1378

Disulfiram (Agenerase Oral Solution contains a large amount of propylene glycol and because of the potential risk of toxicity from the large amount of this excipient, co-administration with disulfiram is contraindicated). Products include:
- Antabuse Tablets 2444
- Antabuse Tablets 3474

Efavirenz (Co-administration with NNRTIs, such as efavirenz, may have the potential to decrease serum concentrations of amprenavir). Products include:
- Sustiva Capsules 1258

Ergonovine Maleate (Co-administration of amprenavir is contraindicated with drugs that are highly dependant of CYP3A4, such as ergot derivatives, for clearance and for which elevated plasma concentrations are associated with serious and/or life-threatening events such as acute ergot toxicity characterized by peripheral vasospasm, and ischemia of the extremities and other tissues).

No products indexed under this heading.

Ergotamine Tartrate (Co-administration of amprenavir is contraindicated with drugs that are highly dependant of CYP3A4, such as ergot derivatives, for clearance and for which elevated plasma concentrations are associated with serious and/or life-threatening events such as acute ergot toxicity characterized by peripheral vasospasm, and ischemia of the extremities and other tissues).
No products indexed under this heading.

Ethinyl Estradiol (Alternative or additional contraceptive measures should be used when estrogen-based oral contraceptives are used concurrently). Products include:
Alesse-21 Tablets ... 3468
Alesse-28 Tablets ... 3473
Brevicon 28-Day Tablets ... 3380
Cyclessa Tablets ... 2450
Desogen Tablets ... 2458
Estinyl Tablets ... 3112
Estrostep ... 2627
femhrt Tablets ... 2635
Levlen ... 962
Levlite 21 Tablets ... 962
Levlite 28 Tablets ... 962
Levora Tablets ... 3389
Loestrin 21 Tablets ... 2642
Loestrin Fe Tablets ... 2642
Lo/Ovral Tablets ... 3532
Lo/Ovral-28 Tablets ... 3538
Low-Ogestrel-28 Tablets ... 3392
Microgestin Fe 1.5/30 Tablets ... 3407
Microgestin Fe 1/20 Tablets ... 3400
Mircette Tablets ... 2470
Modicon ... 2563
Necon ... 3415
Nordette-28 Tablets ... 2257
Norinyl 1 +35 28-Day Tablets ... 3380
Ogestrel 0.5/50-28 Tablets ... 3428
Ortho-Cept 21 Tablets ... 2546
Ortho-Cept 28 Tablets ... 2546
Ortho-Cyclen/Ortho Tri-Cyclen ... 2573
Ortho-Novum ... 2563
Ovcon ... 3364
Ovral Tablets ... 3551
Ovral-28 Tablets ... 3552
Tri-Levlen ... 962
Tri-Norinyl-28 Tablets ... 3433
Triphasil-21 Tablets ... 3600
Triphasil-28 Tablets ... 3605
Trivora Tablets ... 3439
Yasmin 28 Tablets ... 980
Zovia ... 3449

Felodipine (Increased calcium channel blockers plasma concentrations). Products include:
Lexxel Tablets ... 608
Plendil Extended-Release Tablets ... 623

Flurazepam Hydrochloride (Increased benzodiazepine plasma concentrations; clinical significance is unknown; however, a decrease in benzodiazepine dose may be needed).
No products indexed under this heading.

Fosphenytoin Sodium (Decreases amprenavir plasma concentrations potentially reducing effectiveness of amprenavir). Products include:
Cerebyx Injection ... 2619

Glimepiride (New onset diabetes mellitus, exacerbation of pre-existing diabetes mellitus, and hyperglycemia have been reported in HIV-infected patients receiving protease inhibitors; some patients may require dose adjustments). Products include:
Amaryl Tablets ... 717

Glipizide (New onset diabetes mellitus, exacerbation of pre-existing diabetes mellitus, and hyperglycemia have been reported in HIV-infected patients receiving protease inhibitors; some patients may require dose adjustments). Products include:
Glucotrol Tablets ... 2692
Glucotrol XL Extended Release Tablets ... 2693

Glyburide (New onset diabetes mellitus, exacerbation of pre-existing diabetes mellitus, and hyperglycemia have been reported in HIV-infected patients receiving protease inhibitors; some patients may require dose adjustments). Products include:
DiaBeta Tablets ... 741
Glucovance Tablets ... 1086

Hypericum (Co-administration of amprenavir and St. John's Wort or products containing St. John's Wort is expected to substantially decrease protease inhibitor concentrations and may result in suboptimal levels of amprenavir and lead to loss of virologic response and possible resistance to amprenavir; concurrent use is not recommended). Products include:
Brite-Life Caplets ... ▣795
Centrum St. John's Wort Softgels ... ▣853
Metabolic Nutrition System ... ▣798
Movana Tablets ... ▣832
One-A-Day Tension & Mood Softgels ... ▣808
ReSource Wellness StayCalm Caplets ... ▣826
Satiete Tablets ... ▣846

Imipramine Hydrochloride (Increase in tricyclic antidepressant plasma concentrations).
No products indexed under this heading.

Imipramine Pamoate (Increase in tricyclic antidepressant plasma concentrations).
No products indexed under this heading.

Indinavir Sulfate (Increases amprenavir plasma concentrations). Products include:
Crixivan Capsules ... 2070

Insulin, Human, Zinc Suspension (New onset diabetes mellitus, exacerbation of pre-existing diabetes mellitus, and hyperglycemia have been reported in HIV-infected patients receiving protease inhibitors; some patients may require dose adjustments). Products include:
Humulin L, 100 Units ... 1937
Humulin U, 100 Units ... 1943
Novolin L Human Insulin 10 ml Vials ... 2422

Insulin, Human NPH (New onset diabetes mellitus, exacerbation of pre-existing diabetes mellitus, and hyperglycemia have been reported in HIV-infected patients receiving protease inhibitors; some patients may require dose adjustments). Products include:
Humulin N, 100 Units ... 1939
Humulin N NPH Pen ... 1940
Novolin N Human Insulin 10 ml Vials ... 2422
Novolin N PenFill ... 2423
Novolin N Prefilled Syringe Disposable Insulin Delivery System ... 2425

Insulin, Human Regular (New onset diabetes mellitus, exacerbation of pre-existing diabetes mellitus, and hyperglycemia have been reported in HIV-infected patients receiving protease inhibitors; some patients may require dose adjustments). Products include:
Humulin R Regular (U-500) ... 1943
Humulin R, 100 Units ... 1941
Novolin R Human Insulin 10 ml Vials ... 2423
Novolin R PenFill ... 2423
Novolin R Prefilled Syringe Disposable Insulin Delivery System ... 2425
Velosulin BR Human Insulin 10 ml Vials ... 2435

Insulin, Human Regular and Human NPH Mixture (New onset diabetes mellitus, exacerbation of pre-existing diabetes mellitus, and hyperglycemia have been reported in HIV-infected patients receiving protease inhibitors; some patients may require dose adjustments). Products include:
Humulin 50/50, 100 Units ... 1934
Humulin 70/30, 100 Units ... 1935
Humulin 70/30 Pen ... 1936
Novolin 70/30 Human Insulin 10 ml Vials ... 2421
Novolin 70/30 PenFill ... 2423
Novolin 70/30 Prefilled Disposable Insulin Delivery System ... 2425

Insulin, NPH (New onset diabetes mellitus, exacerbation of pre-existing diabetes mellitus, and hyperglycemia have been reported in HIV-infected patients receiving protease inhibitors; some patients may require dose adjustments). Products include:
Iletin II, NPH (Pork), 100 Units ... 1946

Insulin, Regular (New onset diabetes mellitus, exacerbation of pre-existing diabetes mellitus, and hyperglycemia have been reported in HIV-infected patients receiving protease inhibitors; some patients may require dose adjustments). Products include:
Iletin II, Regular (Pork), 100 Units ... 1947

Insulin, Zinc Crystals (New onset diabetes mellitus, exacerbation of pre-existing diabetes mellitus, and hyperglycemia have been reported in HIV-infected patients receiving protease inhibitors; some patients may require dose adjustments).
No products indexed under this heading.

Insulin, Zinc Suspension (New onset diabetes mellitus, exacerbation of pre-existing diabetes mellitus, and hyperglycemia have been reported in HIV-infected patients receiving protease inhibitors; some patients may require dose adjustments). Products include:
Iletin II, Lente (Pork), 100 Units ... 1945

Insulin Aspart, Human Regular (New onset diabetes mellitus, exacerbation of pre-existing diabetes mellitus, and hyperglycemia have been reported in HIV-infected patients receiving protease inhibitors; some patients may require dose adjustments).
No products indexed under this heading.

Insulin glargine (New onset diabetes mellitus, exacerbation of pre-existing diabetes mellitus, and hyperglycemia have been reported in HIV-infected patients receiving protease inhibitors; some patients may require dose adjustments). Products include:
Lantus Injection ... 742

Insulin Lispro, Human (New onset diabetes mellitus, exacerbation of pre-existing diabetes mellitus, and hyperglycemia have been reported in HIV-infected patients receiving protease inhibitors; some patients may require dose adjustments). Products include:
Humalog ... 1926
Humalog Mix 75/25 Pen ... 1928

Insulin Lispro Protamine, Human (New onset diabetes mellitus, exacerbation of pre-existing diabetes mellitus, and hyperglycemia have been reported in HIV-infected patients receiving protease inhibitors; some patients may require dose adjustments). Products include:
Humalog Mix 75/25 Pen ... 1928

Isradipine (Increased calcium channel blockers plasma concentrations). Products include:
DynaCirc Capsules ... 2921
DynaCirc CR Tablets ... 2923

Itraconazole (Increased itraconazole plasma concentrations; dose reduction of itraconazole may be needed for patients receiving more than 400 mg itraconazole per day). Products include:
Sporanox Capsules ... 1800
Sporanox Injection ... 1804
Sporanox Injection ... 2509
Sporanox Oral Solution ... 1808
Sporanox Oral Solution ... 2512

Ketoconazole (Increased ketoconazole plasma concentrations; dose reduction of ketoconazole may be needed for patients receiving more than 400 mg ketoconazole per day). Products include:
Nizoral 2% Cream ... 3620
Nizoral A-D Shampoo ... 2008
Nizoral 2% Shampoo ... 2007
Nizoral Tablets ... 1791

Lidocaine Hydrochloride (Increases antiarrhythmics plasma concentrations). Products include:
Bactine First Aid Liquid ... ▣611
Xylocaine Injections ... 653

Lopinavir (Increases amprenavir plasma concentrations). Products include:
Kaletra Capsules ... 471
Kaletra Oral Solution ... 471

Loratadine (May result in increased plasma concentrations of loratadine). Products include:
Claritin ... 3100
Claritin-D 12 Hour Extended Release Tablets ... 3102
Claritin-D 24 Hour Extended Release Tablets ... 3104

Lovastatin (Co-administration increases the serum concentrations of lovastatin resulting in increased activity as well as toxicity such as myopathy and rhabdomyolysis; concurrent use is not recommended). Products include:
Mevacor Tablets ... 2132

Magaldrate (Antacids decrease amprenavir plasma concentrations; Agenerase should be taken at least one hour before or after antacids).
No products indexed under this heading.

Magnesium Hydroxide (Antacids decrease amprenavir plasma concentrations; Agenerase should be taken at least one hour before or after antacids). Products include:
Ex•Lax Milk of Magnesia Liquid ... ▣670
Maalox Antacid/Anti-Gas Oral Suspension ... ▣673
Maalox Max Maximum Strength Antacid/Anti-Gas Liquid ... 2300
Maalox Regular Strength Antacid/Antigas Liquid ... 2300
Mylanta Fast-Acting ... 1813
Mylanta ... 1813
Pepcid Complete Chewable Tablets ... 1815
Phillips' Chewable Tablets ... ▣615
Phillips' Milk of Magnesia Liquid (Original, Cherry, & Mint) ... ▣616
Rolaids Tablets ... ▣706
Extra Strength Rolaids Tablets ... ▣706
Vanquish Caplets ... ▣617

Magnesium Oxide (Antacids decrease amprenavir plasma concentrations; Agenerase should be taken at least one hour before or after antacids). Products include:
Beelith Tablets ... 946
Mag-Ox 400 Tablets ... 1024
Uro-Mag Capsules ... 1024

Metformin Hydrochloride (New onset diabetes mellitus, exacerbation of pre-existing diabetes mellitus, and hyperglycemia have been reported in HIV-infected patients receiving protease inhibitors; some patients may require dose adjustments). Products include:
Glucophage Tablets ... 1080
Glucophage XR Tablets ... 1080
Glucovance Tablets ... 1086

Methylergonovine Maleate (Co-administration of amprenavir is contraindicated with drugs that are highly dependant of CYP3A4, such as ergot derivatives, for clearance and for which elevated plasma concentrations are associated with serious

and/or life-threatening events such as acute ergot toxicity characterized by peripheral vasospasm, and ischemia of the extremities and other tissues).
No products indexed under this heading.

Methysergide Maleate (Co-administration of amprenavir is contraindicated with drugs that are highly dependant of CYP3A4, such as ergot derivatives, for clearance and for which elevated plasma concentrations are associated with serious and/or life-threatening events such as acute ergot toxicity characterized by peripheral vasospasm, and ischemia of the extremities and other tissues).
No products indexed under this heading.

Metronidazole (Agenerase Oral Solution contains a large amount of propylene glycol and because of the potential risk of toxicity from the large amount of this excipient, co-administration with metronidazole is contraindicated). Products include:
MetroCream 1404
MetroGel 1405
MetroGel-Vaginal Gel 1986
MetroLotion 1405
Noritate Cream 1224

Metronidazole Hydrochloride (Agenerase Oral Solution contains a large amount of propylene glycol and because of the potential risk of toxicity from the large amount of this excipient, co-administration with metronidazole is contraindicated).
No products indexed under this heading.

Mibefradil Dihydrochloride (Increased calcium channel blockers plasma concentrations).
No products indexed under this heading.

Midazolam Hydrochloride (Co-administration of amprenavir is contraindicated with drugs that are highly dependant of CYP3A4 for clearance and for which elevated plasma concentrations are associated with serious and/or life-threatening events such as prolonged or increased sedation or respiratory depression). Products include:
Versed Injection 3027
Versed Syrup 3033

Miglitol (New onset diabetes mellitus, exacerbation of pre-existing diabetes mellitus, and hyperglycemia have been reported in HIV-infected patients receiving protease inhibitors; some patients may require dose adjustments). Products include:
Glyset Tablets 2821

Nelfinavir Mesylate (Increases amprenavir plasma concentrations). Products include:
Viracept 532

Nevirapine (Co-administration with NNRTIs, such as nevirapine, may have the potential to decrease serum concentrations of amprenavir). Products include:
Viramune Oral Suspension 1060
Viramune Tablets 1060

Nicardipine Hydrochloride (Increased calcium channel blockers plasma concentrations). Products include:
Cardene I.V. 3485

Nifedipine (Increased calcium channel blockers plasma concentrations). Products include:
Adalat CC Tablets 877
Procardia Capsules 2708
Procardia XL Extended Release Tablets 2710

Nimodipine (Increased calcium channel blockers plasma concentrations). Products include:
Nimotop Capsules 904

Nisoldipine (Increased calcium channel blockers plasma concentrations). Products include:
Sular Tablets 688

Phenobarbital (Decreases amprenavir plasma concentrations potentially reducing effectiveness of amprenavir). Products include:
Arco-Lase Plus Tablets 592
Donnatal 2929
Donnatal Extentabs 2930

Phenytoin (Decreases amprenavir plasma concentrations potentially reducing effectiveness of amprenavir). Products include:
Dilantin Infatabs 2624
Dilantin-125 Oral Suspension 2625

Phenytoin Sodium (Decreases amprenavir plasma concentrations potentially reducing effectiveness of amprenavir). Products include:
Dilantin Kapseals 2622

Pimozide (Co-administration of amprenavir is contraindicated with drugs that are highly dependant of CYP3A4 for clearance and for which elevated plasma concentrations are associated with serious and/or life-threatening events such as cardiac arrhythmias). Products include:
Orap Tablets 1407

Pioglitazone Hydrochloride (New onset diabetes mellitus, exacerbation of pre-existing diabetes mellitus, and hyperglycemia have been reported in HIV-infected patients receiving protease inhibitors; some patients may require dose adjustments). Products include:
Actos Tablets 3275

Pravastatin Sodium (Co-administration increases the serum concentrations of pravastatin resulting in increased activity as well as toxicity such as myopathy and rhabdomyolysis; caution should be exercised if used concurrently). Products include:
Pravachol Tablets 1099

Protriptyline Hydrochloride (Co-administration could result in serious and/or life threatening drug interactions). Products include:
Vivactil Tablets 2446
Vivactil Tablets 2217

Quinidine Gluconate (Increases quinidine plasma concentrations; caution is warranted and therapeutic monitoring is recommended). Products include:
Quinaglute Dura-Tabs Tablets 978

Quinidine Polygalacturonate (Increases quinidine plasma concentrations; caution is warranted and therapeutic monitoring is recommended).
No products indexed under this heading.

Quinidine Sulfate (Increases quinidine plasma concentrations; caution is warranted and therapeutic monitoring is recommended). Products include:
Quinidex Extentabs 2933

Rapamycin (Increased immunosuppressant plasma concentrations).
No products indexed under this heading.

Repaglinide (New onset diabetes mellitus, exacerbation of pre-existing diabetes mellitus, and hyperglycemia have been reported in HIV-infected patients receiving protease inhibitors; some patients may require dose adjustments). Products include:
Prandin Tablets (0.5, 1, and 2 mg) 2432

Rifabutin (Increased rifabutin and rifabutin metabolite plasma concentrations; dosage reduction of rifabutin to at least half the recommended dose is required when used concurrently). Products include:
Mycobutin Capsules 2838

Rifampin (Co-administration may lead to loss of virologic response and possible resistance to amprenavir or the class of protease inhibitors). Products include:
Rifadin 765
Rifamate Capsules 767
Rifater Tablets 769

Ritonavir (Increases amprenavir plasma concentrations). Products include:
Kaletra Capsules 471
Kaletra Oral Solution 471
Norvir Capsules 487
Norvir Oral Solution 487

Rosiglitazone Maleate (New onset diabetes mellitus, exacerbation of pre-existing diabetes mellitus, and hyperglycemia have been reported in HIV-infected patients receiving protease inhibitors; some patients may require dose adjustments). Products include:
Avandia Tablets 1490

Saquinavir (Decreases amprenavir plasma concentrations). Products include:
Fortovase Capsules 2970

Saquinavir Mesylate (Decreases amprenavir plasma concentrations). Products include:
Invirase Capsules 2979

Sildenafil Citrate (Increase in sildenafil plasma concentrations; use with caution at reduced doses of 25 mg every 48 hours with increased monitoring for adverse events). Products include:
Viagra Tablets 2732

Simvastatin (Co-administration increases the serum concentrations of simvastatin resulting in increased activity as well as toxicity such as myopathy and rhabdomyolysis; concurrent use is not recommended). Products include:
Zocor Tablets 2219

Tacrolimus (Increased immunosuppressant plasma concentrations). Products include:
Prograf 1393
Protopic Ointment 1397

Terfenadine (Co-administration of amprenavir is contraindicated with drugs that are highly dependant of CYP3A4 for clearance and for which elevated plasma concentrations are associated with serious and/or life-threatening events such as cardiac arrhythmias).
No products indexed under this heading.

Tolazamide (New onset diabetes mellitus, exacerbation of pre-existing diabetes mellitus, and hyperglycemia have been reported in HIV-infected patients receiving protease inhibitors; some patients may require dose adjustments).
No products indexed under this heading.

Tolbutamide (New onset diabetes mellitus, exacerbation of pre-existing diabetes mellitus, and hyperglycemia have been reported in HIV-infected patients receiving protease inhibitors; some patients may require dose adjustments).
No products indexed under this heading.

Triazolam (Co-administration of amprenavir is contraindicated with drugs that are highly dependant of CYP3A4 for clearance and for which elevated plasma concentrations are associated with serious and/or life-threatening events such as prolonged or increased sedation or respiratory depression). Products include:
Halcion Tablets 2823

Trimipramine Maleate (Co-administration could result in serious and/or life-threatening drug interactions). Products include:
Surmontil Capsules 3595

Troglitazone (New onset diabetes mellitus, exacerbation of pre-existing diabetes mellitus, and hyperglycemia have been reported in HIV-infected patients receiving protease inhibitors; some patients may require dose adjustments).
No products indexed under this heading.

Verapamil Hydrochloride (Increased calcium channel blockers plasma concentrations). Products include:
Covera-HS Tablets 3199
Isoptin SR Tablets 467
Tarka Tablets 508
Verelan Capsules 3184
Verelan PM Capsules 3186

Vitamin E (Amprenavir formulations contain large amounts of vitamin E; high vitamin E doses may exacerbate the blood coagulation defect of vitamin K deficiency caused by anticoagulant therapy; concurrent use with additional vitamin E should be avoided). Products include:
Nutr-E-Sol Liquid 526
One-A-Day Cholesterol Health Tablets 805
One-A-Day Menopause Health Tablets 808
StePHan Bio-Nutritional Daytime Hydrating Creme 770
StePHan Feminine Capsules 848
Unique E Vitamin E Capsules 1723

Warfarin Sodium (Concentrations of warfarin may be affected with concurrent use; monitor INR). Products include:
Coumadin for Injection 1243
Coumadin Tablets 1243
Warfarin Sodium Tablets, USP 3302

Zidovudine (Co-administration has resulted in 13% increase in AUC of amprenavir; 40% increase in Cmax and 31% increase in AUC for zidovudine has been reported). Products include:
Combivir Tablets 1502
Retrovir 1625
Retrovir IV Infusion 1629
Trizivir Tablets 1669

Food Interactions

Alcohol (Concurrent use of Agenerase Oral Solution with alcoholic beverages is not recommended).

Food, unspecified (High fat meals may decrease the absorption of Agenerase and should be avoided; Agenerase may be taken with meals of normal fat content).

AGGRASTAT INJECTION

(Tirofiban Hydrochloride) 2031
May interact with glycoprotein (GP) IIb/IIIa inhibitors and certain other agents. Compounds in these categories include:

Abciximab (Concomitant use with another parenteral GP IIb/IIIa inhibitor is contraindicated). Products include:
ReoPro Vials 1958

Aspirin (The use of tirofiban in combination with aspirin has been associated with an increase in bleeding compared to aspirin alone). Products include:
Aggrenox Capsules 1026
Alka-Seltzer 603
Alka-Seltzer Lemon Lime Antacid and Pain Reliever Effervescent Tablets 603
Alka-Seltzer Extra Strength Antacid and Pain Reliever Effervescent Tablets 603
Alka-Seltzer PM Effervescent Tablets 605
Genuine Bayer Tablets, Caplets and Gelcaps 606
Extra Strength Bayer Caplets and Gelcaps 610

Aspirin Regimen Bayer Children's Chewable Tablets (Orange or Cherry Flavored) ▣607
Bayer, Aspirin Regimen ▣606
Aspirin Regimen Bayer 81 mg Caplets with Calcium ▣607
Genuine Bayer Professional Labeling (Aspirin Regimen Bayer) ▣608
Extra Strength Bayer Arthritis Caplets ▣610
Extra Strength Bayer Plus Caplets ▣610
Extra Strength Bayer PM Caplets ▣611
BC Powder ▣619
BC Allergy Sinus Cold Powder ▣619
Arthritis Strength BC Powder ▣619
BC Sinus Cold Powder ▣619
Darvon Compound-65 Pulvules 1910
Ecotrin Enteric Coated Aspirin Low, Regular and Maximum Strength Tablets 1715
Excedrin Extra-Strength Tablets, Caplets, and Geltabs ▣629
Excedrin Migraine 1070
Goody's Body Pain Formula Powder ▣620
Goody's Extra Strength Headache Powder ▣620
Goody's Extra Strength Pain Relief Tablets ▣620
Percodan Tablets 1327
Robaxisal Tablets 2939
Soma Compound Tablets 3354
Soma Compound w/Codeine Tablets 3355
Vanquish Caplets ▣617

Eptifibatide (Concomitant use with another parenteral GP IIb/IIIa inhibitor is contraindicated). Products include:
Integrilin Injection 1213
Integrilin Injection 1828

Heparin Sodium (The use of tirofiban in combination with heparin has been associated with an increase in bleeding compared to heparin alone). Products include:
Heparin Lock Flush Solution 3509
Heparin Sodium Injection 3511

Levothyroxine Sodium (Co-administration has resulted in a higher rate of clearance of tirofiban; the clinical significance of this is unknown). Products include:
Levothroid Tablets 1373
Levoxyl Tablets 1819
Synthroid 505
Unithroid Tablets 3445

Omeprazole (Co-administration has resulted in a higher rate of clearance of tirofiban; the clinical significance of this is unknown). Products include:
Prilosec Delayed-Release Capsules 628

AGGRASTAT INJECTION PREMIXED

(Tirofiban Hydrochloride) 2031
See Aggrastat Injection

AGGRENOX CAPSULES

(Aspirin, Dipyridamole) 1026
May interact with ACE inhibitors, anticholinesterase drugs, beta blockers, anticoagulants, diuretics, oral hypoglycemic agents, non-steroidal anti-inflammatory agents, phenytoin, valproate, and certain other agents. Compounds in these categories include:

Acarbose (Moderate doses of aspirin may increase the effectiveness of renal hypoglycemic drugs, leading to hypoglycemia). Products include:
Precose Tablets 906

Acebutolol Hydrochloride (The hypertensive effects of beta blockers may be diminished by the concomitant administration of aspirin due to inhibition of renal prostaglandins, leading to decreased renal blood flow and salt and fluid retention). Products include:
Sectral Capsules 3589

Acetazolamide (Co-administration can lead to high serum concentrations of acetazolamide (and toxicity) due to competition at the renal tube for secretion). Products include:
Diamox Sequels Sustained Release Capsules ⊙270
Diamox Tablets ⊙269

Acetazolamide Sodium (Co-administration can lead to high serum concentrations of acetazolamide (and toxicity) due to competition at the renal tube for secretion). Products include:
Diamox Intravenous ⊙269

Adenosine (Dipyridamole has been reported to increase the plasma levels and cardiovascular effects of adenosine). Products include:
Adenocard Injection 1380
Adenoscan 1381

Amiloride Hydrochloride (The effectiveness of diuretics in patients with underlying renal or cardiovascular disease may be diminished by co-administration of aspirin due to inhibition of renal prostaglandins, leading to decreased renal blood flow and salt and fluid retention). Products include:
Midamor Tablets 2136
Moduretic Tablets 2138

Ardeparin Sodium (Patients on anticoagulation therapy are at risk for bleeding).
No products indexed under this heading.

Atenolol (The hypertensive effects of beta blockers may be diminished by the concomitant administration of aspirin due to inhibition of renal prostaglandins, leading to decreased renal blood flow and salt and fluid retention). Products include:
Tenoretic Tablets 690
Tenormin I.V. Injection 692

Benazepril Hydrochloride (Co-administration can result in diminished hypotensive and hyponatremic effects of ACE inhibitors due to the effect of aspirin on the renin-angiotensin conversion pathway). Products include:
Lotensin Tablets 2365
Lotensin HCT Tablets 2367
Lotrel Capsules 2370

Bendroflumethiazide (The effectiveness of diuretics in patients with underlying renal or cardiovascular disease may be diminished by co-administration of aspirin due to inhibition of renal prostaglandins, leading to decreased renal blood flow and salt and fluid retention). Products include:
Corzide 40/5 Tablets 2247
Corzide 80/5 Tablets 2247

Betaxolol Hydrochloride (The hypertensive effects of beta blockers may be diminished by the concomitant administration of aspirin due to inhibition of renal prostaglandins, leading to decreased renal blood flow and salt and fluid retention). Products include:
Betoptic S Ophthalmic Suspension 537

Bisoprolol Fumarate (The hypertensive effects of beta blockers may be diminished by the concomitant administration of aspirin due to inhibition of renal prostaglandins, leading to decreased renal blood flow and salt and fluid retention). Products include:
Zebeta Tablets 1885
Ziac Tablets 1887

Bumetanide (The effectiveness of diuretics in patients with underlying renal or cardiovascular disease may be diminished by co-administration of aspirin due to inhibition of renal prostaglandins, leading to decreased renal blood flow and salt and fluid retention).
No products indexed under this heading.

Captopril (Co-administration can result in diminished hypotensive and hyponatremic effects of ACE inhibitors due to the effect of aspirin on the renin-angiotensin conversion pathway). Products include:
Captopril Tablets 2281

Carteolol Hydrochloride (The hypertensive effects of beta blockers may be diminished by the concomitant administration of aspirin due to inhibition of renal prostaglandins, leading to decreased renal blood flow and salt and fluid retention). Products include:
Carteolol Hydrochloride Ophthalmic Solution USP, 1% ⊙258
Ocupress Ophthalmic Solution, 1% Sterile ⊙303

Celecoxib (Co-administration of non-steroidal anti-inflammatory with aspirin may increase bleeding or lead to decreased renal function). Products include:
Celebrex Capsules 2676
Celebrex Capsules 2780

Chlorothiazide (The effectiveness of diuretics in patients with underlying renal or cardiovascular disease may be diminished by co-administration of aspirin due to inhibition of renal prostaglandins, leading to decreased renal blood flow and salt and fluid retention). Products include:
Aldoclor Tablets 2035
Diuril Oral 2087

Chlorothiazide Sodium (The effectiveness of diuretics in patients with underlying renal or cardiovascular disease may be diminished by co-administration of aspirin due to inhibition of renal prostaglandins, leading to decreased renal blood flow and salt and fluid retention). Products include:
Diuril Sodium Intravenous 2086

Chlorpropamide (Moderate doses of aspirin may increase the effectiveness of renal hypoglycemic drugs, leading to hypoglycemia). Products include:
Diabinese Tablets 2680

Chlorthalidone (The effectiveness of diuretics in patients with underlying renal or cardiovascular disease may be diminished by co-administration of aspirin due to inhibition of renal prostaglandins, leading to decreased renal blood flow and salt and fluid retention). Products include:
Clorpres Tablets 1002
Combipres Tablets 1040
Tenoretic Tablets 690

Dalteparin Sodium (Patients on anticoagulation therapy are at risk for bleeding). Products include:
Fragmin Injection 2814

Danaparoid Sodium (Patients on anticoagulation therapy are at risk for bleeding). Products include:
Orgaran Injection 2480

Diclofenac Potassium (Co-administration of non-steroidal anti-inflammatory with aspirin may increase bleeding or lead to decreased renal function). Products include:
Cataflam Tablets 2315

Diclofenac Sodium (Co-administration of non-steroidal anti-inflammatory with aspirin may increase bleeding or lead to decreased renal function). Products include:
Arthrotec Tablets 3195
Voltaren Ophthalmic Sterile Ophthalmic Solution ⊙312
Voltaren Tablets 2315
Voltaren-XR Tablets 2315

Dicumarol (Patients on anticoagulation therapy are at risk for bleeding).
No products indexed under this heading.

Divalproex Sodium (Salicylic acid can displace protein-bound valproic acid leading to an increase in serum valproic acid levels). Products include:
Depakote Sprinkle Capsules 426
Depakote Tablets 430
Depakote ER Tablets 436

Donepezil Hydrochloride (Dipyridamole may counteract the anticholinesterase effect of cholinesterase inhibitors, thereby potentially aggravating myasthenia gravis). Products include:
Aricept Tablets 1270
Aricept Tablets 2665

Enalapril Maleate (Co-administration can result in diminished hypotensive and hyponatremic effects of ACE inhibitors due to the effect of aspirin on the renin-angiotensin conversion pathway). Products include:
Lexxel Tablets 608
Vaseretic Tablets 2204
Vasotec Tablets 2210

Enalaprilat (Co-administration can result in diminished hypotensive and hyponatremic effects of ACE inhibitors due to the effect of aspirin on the renin-angiotensin conversion pathway). Products include:
Enalaprilat Injection 863
Vasotec I.V. Injection 2207

Enoxaparin (Patients on anticoagulation therapy are at risk for bleeding). Products include:
Lovenox Injection 746

Esmolol Hydrochloride (The hypertensive effects of beta blockers may be diminished by the concomitant administration of aspirin due to inhibition of renal prostaglandins, leading to decreased renal blood flow and salt and fluid retention). Products include:
Brevibloc Injection 858

Ethacrynic Acid (The effectiveness of diuretics in patients with underlying renal or cardiovascular disease may be diminished by co-administration of aspirin due to inhibition of renal prostaglandins, leading to decreased renal blood flow and salt and fluid retention). Products include:
Edecrin Tablets 2091

Etodolac (Co-administration of non-steroidal anti-inflammatory with aspirin may increase bleeding or lead to decreased renal function). Products include:
Lodine 3528
Lodine XL Extended-Release Tablets 3530

Fenoprofen Calcium (Co-administration of non-steroidal anti-inflammatory with aspirin may increase bleeding or lead to decreased renal function).
No products indexed under this heading.

Flurbiprofen (Co-administration of non-steroidal anti-inflammatory with aspirin may increase bleeding or lead to decreased renal function).
No products indexed under this heading.

Fosinopril Sodium (Co-administration can result in diminished hypotensive and hyponatremic effects of ACE inhibitors due to the effect of aspirin on the renin-angiotensin conversion pathway). Products include:
Monopril Tablets 1091
Monopril HCT 1094

Fosphenytoin Sodium (Salicylic acid can displace protein-bound phenytoin leading to a decrease in the total concentration of phenytoin). Products include:
Cerebyx Injection 2619

Furosemide (The effectiveness of diuretics in patients with underlying

renal or cardiovascular disease may be diminished by co-administration of aspirin due to inhibition of renal prostaglandins, leading to decreased renal blood flow and salt and fluid retention). Products include:

Furosemide Tablets 2284

Galantamine Hydrobromide (Dipyridamole may counteract the anticholinesterase effect of cholinesterase inhibitors, thereby potentially aggravating myasthenia gravis). Products include:

Reminyl Oral Solution 1792
Reminyl Tablets 1792

Glimepiride (Moderate doses of aspirin may increase the effectiveness of renal hypoglycemic drugs, leading to hypoglycemia). Products include:

Amaryl Tablets 717

Glipizide (Moderate doses of aspirin may increase the effectiveness of renal hypoglycemic drugs, leading to hypoglycemia). Products include:

Glucotrol Tablets 2692
Glucotrol XL Extended Release Tablets 2693

Glyburide (Moderate doses of aspirin may increase the effectiveness of renal hypoglycemic drugs, leading to hypoglycemia). Products include:

DiaBeta Tablets 741
Glucovance Tablets 1086

Heparin Sodium (Aspirin can increase the anticoagulant activity of heparin, icreasing bleeding risk). Products include:

Heparin Lock Flush Solution 3509
Heparin Sodium Injection 3511

Hydrochlorothiazide (The effectiveness of diuretics in patients with underlying renal or cardiovascular disease may be diminished by co-administration of aspirin due to inhibition of renal prostaglandins, leading to decreased renal blood flow and salt and fluid retention). Products include:

Accuretic Tablets 2614
Aldoril Tablets 2039
Atacand HCT Tablets 597
Avalide Tablets 1070
Diovan HCT Tablets 2338
Dyazide Capsules 1515
HydroDIURIL Tablets 2108
Hyzaar 2109
Inderide Tablets 3517
Inderide LA Long-Acting Capsules .. 3519
Lotensin HCT Tablets 2367
Maxzide 1008
Micardis HCT Tablets 1051
Microzide Capsules 3414
Moduretic Tablets 2138
Monopril HCT 1094
Prinzide Tablets 2168
Timolide Tablets 2187
Uniretic Tablets 3178
Vaseretic Tablets 2204
Zestoretic Tablets 695
Ziac Tablets 1887

Hydroflumethiazide (The effectiveness of diuretics in patients with underlying renal or cardiovascular disease may be diminished by co-administration of aspirin due to inhibition of renal prostaglandins, leading to decreased renal blood flow and salt and fluid retention). Products include:

Diucardin Tablets 3494

Ibuprofen (Co-administration of non-steroidal anti-inflammatory with aspirin may increase bleeding or lead to decreased renal function). Products include:

Advil .... ■771
Children's Advil Oral Suspension ... ■773
Children's Advil Chewable Tablets . ■773
Advil Cold and Sinus Caplets .... ■771
Advil Cold and Sinus Tablets .... ■771
Advil Flu & Body Ache Caplets ...... ■772
Infants' Advil Drops .... ■773
Junior Strength Advil Tablets .... ■773
Junior Strength Advil Chewable Tablets .... ■773
Advil Migraine Liquigels .... ■772
Children's Motrin Oral Suspension and Chewable Tablets 2006
Children's Motrin Cold Oral Suspension 2007
Children's Motrin Oral Suspension .... ■643
Motrin Suspension, Oral Drops, Chewable Tablets, and Caplets 2002
Infants' Motrin Concentrated Drops 2006
Junior Strength Motrin Caplets and Chewable Tablets 2006
Motrin IB Tablets, Caplets, and Gelcaps 2002
Motrin Migraine Pain Caplets 2005
Motrin Sinus Headache Caplets 2005
Vicoprofen Tablets 520

Indapamide (The effectiveness of diuretics in patients with underlying renal or cardiovascular disease may be diminished by co-administration of aspirin due to inhibition of renal prostaglandins, leading to decreased renal blood flow and salt and fluid retention). Products include:

Indapamide Tablets 2286

Indomethacin (Co-administration of non-steroidal anti-inflammatory with aspirin may increase bleeding or lead to decreased renal function). Products include:

Indocin 2112

Indomethacin Sodium Trihydrate (Co-administration of non-steroidal anti-inflammatory with aspirin may increase bleeding or lead to decreased renal function). Products include:

Indocin I.V. 2115

Ketoprofen (Co-administration of non-steroidal anti-inflammatory with aspirin may increase bleeding or lead to decreased renal function). Products include:

Orudis Capsules 3548
Orudis KT Tablets .... ■778
Oruvail Capsules 3548

Ketorolac Tromethamine (Co-administration of non-steroidal anti-inflammatory with aspirin may increase bleeding or lead to decreased renal function). Products include:

Acular Ophthalmic Solution 544
Acular PF Ophthalmic Solution 544
Toradol 3018

Labetalol Hydrochloride (The hypertensive effects of beta blockers may be diminished by the concomitant administration of aspirin due to inhibition of renal prostaglandins, leading to decreased renal blood flow and salt and fluid retention). Products include:

Normodyne Injection 3135
Normodyne Tablets 3137

Levobunolol Hydrochloride (The hypertensive effects of beta blockers may be diminished by the concomitant administration of aspirin due to inhibition of renal prostaglandins, leading to decreased renal blood flow and salt and fluid retention). Products include:

Betagan .... ⊙228

Lisinopril (Co-administration can result in diminished hypotensive and hyponatremic effects of ACE inhibitors due to the effect of aspirin on the renin-angiotensin conversion pathway). Products include:

Prinivil Tablets 2164
Prinzide Tablets 2168
Zestoretic Tablets 695
Zestril Tablets 698

Meclofenamate Sodium (Co-administration of non-steroidal anti-inflammatory with aspirin may increase bleeding or lead to decreased renal function).

No products indexed under this heading.

Mefenamic Acid (Co-administration of non-steroidal anti-inflammatory with aspirin may increase bleeding or lead to decreased renal function). Products include:

Ponstel Capsules 1356

Meloxicam (Co-administration of non-steroidal anti-inflammatory with aspirin may increase bleeding or lead to decreased renal function). Products include:

Mobic Tablets 1054

Metformin Hydrochloride (Moderate doses of aspirin may increase the effectiveness of renal hypoglycemic drugs, leading to hypoglycemia). Products include:

Glucophage Tablets 1080
Glucophage XR Tablets 1080
Glucovance Tablets 1086

Methotrexate Sodium (Salicylic acid can inhibit renal clearance of methotrexate, leading to bone marrow toxicity, especially in the elderly or renal impaired).

No products indexed under this heading.

Methyclothiazide (The effectiveness of diuretics in patients with underlying renal or cardiovascular disease may be diminished by co-administration of aspirin due to inhibition of renal prostaglandins, leading to decreased renal blood flow and salt and fluid retention).

No products indexed under this heading.

Metipranolol Hydrochloride (The hypertensive effects of beta blockers may be diminished by the concomitant administration of aspirin due to inhibition of renal prostaglandins, leading to decreased renal blood flow and salt and fluid retention).

No products indexed under this heading.

Metolazone (The effectiveness of diuretics in patients with underlying renal or cardiovascular disease may be diminished by co-administration of aspirin due to inhibition of renal prostaglandins, leading to decreased renal blood flow and salt and fluid retention). Products include:

Mykrox Tablets 1168
Zaroxolyn Tablets 1177

Metoprolol Succinate (The hypertensive effects of beta blockers may be diminished by the concomitant administration of aspirin due to inhibition of renal prostaglandins, leading to decreased renal blood flow and salt and fluid retention). Products include:

Toprol-XL Tablets 651

Metoprolol Tartrate (The hypertensive effects of beta blockers may be diminished by the concomitant administration of aspirin due to inhibition of renal prostaglandins, leading to decreased renal blood flow and salt and fluid retention).

No products indexed under this heading.

Miglitol (Moderate doses of aspirin may increase the effectiveness of renal hypoglycemic drugs, leading to hypoglycemia). Products include:

Glyset Tablets 2821

Moexipril Hydrochloride (Co-administration can result in diminished hypotensive and hyponatremic effects of ACE inhibitors due to the effect of aspirin on the renin-angiotensin conversion pathway). Products include:

Uniretic Tablets 3178
Univasc Tablets 3181

Nabumetone (Co-administration of non-steroidal anti-inflammatory with aspirin may increase bleeding or lead to decreased renal function). Products include:

Relafen Tablets 1617

Nadolol (The hypertensive effects of beta blockers may be diminished by the concomitant administration of aspirin due to inhibition of renal prostaglandins, leading to decreased renal blood flow and salt and fluid retention). Products include:

Corgard Tablets 2245
Corzide 40/5 Tablets 2247
Corzide 80/5 Tablets 2247
Nadolol Tablets 2288

Naproxen (Co-administration of non-steroidal anti-inflammatory with aspirin may increase bleeding or lead to decreased renal function). Products include:

EC-Naprosyn Delayed-Release Tablets 2967
Naprosyn Suspension 2967
Naprosyn Tablets 2967

Naproxen Sodium (Co-administration of non-steroidal anti-inflammatory with aspirin may increase bleeding or lead to decreased renal function). Products include:

Aleve Tablets, Caplets and Gelcaps .... ■602
Aleve Cold & Sinus Caplets .... ■603
Anaprox Tablets 2967
Anaprox DS Tablets 2967
Naprelan Tablets 1293

Neostigmine Bromide (Dipyridamole may counteract the anticholinesterase effect of cholinesterase inhibitors, thereby potentially aggravating myasthenia gravis). Products include:

Prostigmin Tablets 1744

Neostigmine Methylsulfate (Dipyridamole may counteract the anticholinesterase effect of cholinesterase inhibitors, thereby potentially aggravating myasthenia gravis). Products include:

Prostigmin Injectable 1744

Oxaprozin (Co-administration of non-steroidal anti-inflammatory with aspirin may increase bleeding or lead to decreased renal function).

No products indexed under this heading.

Penbutolol Sulfate (The hypertensive effects of beta blockers may be diminished by the concomitant administration of aspirin due to inhibition of renal prostaglandins, leading to decreased renal blood flow and salt and fluid retention).

No products indexed under this heading.

Perindopril Erbumine (Co-administration can result in diminished hypotensive and hyponatremic effects of ACE inhibitors due to the effect of aspirin on the renin-angiotensin conversion pathway). Products include:

Aceon Tablets (2 mg, 4 mg, 8 mg) 3249

Phenylbutazone (Co-administration of non-steroidal anti-inflammatory with aspirin may increase bleeding or lead to decreased renal function).

No products indexed under this heading.

Phenytoin (Salicylic acid can displace protein-bound phenytoin leading to a decrease in the total concentration of phenytoin). Products include:

Dilantin Infatabs 2624
Dilantin-125 Oral Suspension 2625

Phenytoin Sodium (Salicylic acid can displace protein-bound phenytoin leading to a decrease in the total concentration of phenytoin). Products include:

Dilantin Kapseals 2622

Pindolol (The hypertensive effects of beta blockers may be diminished by the concomitant administration of aspirin due to inhibition of renal prostaglandins, leading to decreased renal blood flow and salt and fluid

retention).
No products indexed under this heading.

Pioglitazone Hydrochloride (Moderate doses of aspirin may increase the effectiveness of renal hypoglycemic drugs, leading to hypoglycemia). Products include:
Actos Tablets ... 3275

Piroxicam (Co-administration of non-steroidal anti-inflammatory with aspirin may increase bleeding or lead to decreased renal function). Products include:
Feldene Capsules ... 2685

Polythiazide (The effectiveness of diuretics in patients with underlying renal or cardiovascular disease may be diminished by co-administration of aspirin due to inhibition of renal prostaglandins, leading to decreased renal blood flow and salt and fluid retention). Products include:
Minizide Capsules ... 2700
Renese Tablets ... 2712

Probenecid (Salicylates antagonize the uricosuric action of uricosuric agents, such as probenecid).
No products indexed under this heading.

Propranolol Hydrochloride (The hypertensive effects of beta blockers may be diminished by the concomitant administration of aspirin due to inhibition of renal prostaglandins, leading to decreased renal blood flow and salt and fluid retention). Products include:
Inderal ... 3513
Inderal LA Long-Acting Capsules ... 3516
Inderide Tablets ... 3517
Inderide LA Long-Acting Capsules ... 3519

Pyridostigmine Bromide (Dipyridamole may counteract the anticholinesterase effect of cholinesterase inhibitors, thereby potentially aggravating myasthenia gravis). Products include:
Mestinon ... 1740

Quinapril Hydrochloride (Co-administration can result in diminished hypotensive and hyponatremic effects of ACE inhibitors due to the effect of aspirin on the renin-angiotensin conversion pathway). Products include:
Accupril Tablets ... 2611
Accuretic Tablets ... 2614

Ramipril (Co-administration can result in diminished hypotensive and hyponatremic effects of ACE inhibitors due to the effect of aspirin on the renin-angiotensin conversion pathway). Products include:
Altace Capsules ... 2233

Repaglinide (Moderate doses of aspirin may increase the effectiveness of renal hypoglycemic drugs, leading to hypoglycemia). Products include:
Prandin Tablets (0.5, 1, and 2 mg) ... 2432

Rivastigmine Tartrate (Dipyridamole may counteract the anticholinesterase effect of cholinesterase inhibitors, thereby potentially aggravating myasthenia gravis). Products include:
Exelon Capsules ... 2342
Exelon Oral Solution ... 2345

Rofecoxib (Co-administration of non-steroidal anti-inflammatory with aspirin may increase bleeding or lead to decreased renal function). Products include:
Vioxx ... 2213

Rosiglitazone Maleate (Moderate doses of aspirin may increase the effectiveness of renal hypoglycemic drugs, leading to hypoglycemia). Products include:
Avandia Tablets ... 1490

Sotalol Hydrochloride (The hypertensive effects of beta blockers may be diminished by the concomitant administration of aspirin due to inhibition of renal prostaglandins, leading to decreased renal blood flow and salt and fluid retention). Products include:
Betapace Tablets ... 950
Betapace AF Tablets ... 954

Spirapril Hydrochloride (Co-administration can result in diminished hypotensive and hyponatremic effects of ACE inhibitors due to the effect of aspirin on the renin-angiotensin conversion pathway).
No products indexed under this heading.

Spironolactone (The effectiveness of diuretics in patients with underlying renal or cardiovascular disease may be diminished by co-administration of aspirin due to inhibition of renal prostaglandins, leading to decreased renal blood flow and salt and fluid retention).
No products indexed under this heading.

Sulfinpyrazone (Salicylates antagonize the uricosuric action of uricosuric agents, such as sulfinpyrazone).
No products indexed under this heading.

Sulindac (Co-administration of non-steroidal anti-inflammatory with aspirin may increase bleeding or lead to decreased renal function). Products include:
Clinoril Tablets ... 2053

Tacrine Hydrochloride (Dipyridamole may counteract the anticholinesterase effect of cholinesterase inhibitors, thereby potentially aggravating myasthenia gravis). Products include:
Cognex Capsules ... 1351

Timolol Hemihydrate (The hypertensive effects of beta blockers may be diminished by the concomitant administration of aspirin due to inhibition of renal prostaglandins, leading to decreased renal blood flow and salt and fluid retention). Products include:
Betimol Ophthalmic Solution ... ⊙324

Timolol Maleate (The hypertensive effects of beta blockers may be diminished by the concomitant administration of aspirin due to inhibition of renal prostaglandins, leading to decreased renal blood flow and salt and fluid retention). Products include:
Blocadren Tablets ... 2046
Cosopt Sterile Ophthalmic Solution ... 2065
Timolide Tablets ... 2187
Timolol GFS ... ⊙266
Timoptic in Ocudose ... 2192
Timoptic Sterile Ophthalmic Solution ... 2190
Timoptic-XE Sterile Ophthalmic Gel Forming Solution ... 2194

Tinzaparin sodium (Patients on anticoagulation therapy are at risk for bleeding). Products include:
Innohep Injection ... 1248

Tolazamide (Moderate doses of aspirin may increase the effectiveness of renal hypoglycemic drugs, leading to hypoglycemia).
No products indexed under this heading.

Tolbutamide (Moderate doses of aspirin may increase the effectiveness of renal hypoglycemic drugs, leading to hypoglycemia).
No products indexed under this heading.

Tolmetin Sodium (Co-administration of non-steroidal anti-inflammatory with aspirin may increase bleeding or lead to decreased renal function). Products include:
Tolectin ... 2589

Torsemide (The effectiveness of diuretics in patients with underlying renal or cardiovascular disease may be diminished by co-administration of aspirin due to inhibition of renal prostaglandins, leading to decreased renal blood flow and salt and fluid retention). Products include:
Demadex Tablets and Injection ... 2965

Trandolapril (Co-administration can result in diminished hypotensive and hyponatremic effects of ACE inhibitors due to the effect of aspirin on the renin-angiotensin conversion pathway). Products include:
Mavik Tablets ... 478
Tarka Tablets ... 508

Triamterene (The effectiveness of diuretics in patients with underlying renal or cardiovascular disease may be diminished by co-administration of aspirin due to inhibition of renal prostaglandins, leading to decreased renal blood flow and salt and fluid retention). Products include:
Dyazide Capsules ... 1515
Dyrenium Capsules ... 3458
Maxzide ... 1008

Troglitazone (Moderate doses of aspirin may increase the effectiveness of renal hypoglycemic drugs, leading to hypoglycemia).
No products indexed under this heading.

Valproate Sodium (Salicylic acid can displace protein-bound valproic acid leading to an increase in serum valproic acid levels). Products include:
Depacon Injection ... 416

Valproic Acid (Salicylic acid can displace protein-bound valproic acid leading to an increase in serum valproic acid levels). Products include:
Depakene ... 421

Warfarin Sodium (Aspirin can displace warfarin from protein binding sites, leading to a prolongation of both the prothrombin time and the bleeding time). Products include:
Coumadin for Injection ... 1243
Coumadin Tablets ... 1243
Warfarin Sodium Tablets, USP ... 3302

Food Interactions

Alcohol (Patients who consume three or more alcoholic drinks every day should be counseled about the bleeding risks involved with chronic, heavy alcohol use while taking aspirin).

AGRYLIN CAPSULES
(Anagrelide Hydrochloride) ... 3232
None cited in PDR database.

AK-FLUOR INJECTION 10% AND 25%
(Fluorescein Sodium) ... ⊙202
None cited in PDR database.

AKINETON INJECTION
(Biperiden Hydrochloride) ... 402
May interact with antihistamines, antipsychotic agents, phenothiazines, tricyclic antidepressants, and certain other agents. Compounds in these categories include:

Acrivastine (Central anticholinergic syndrome). Products include:
Semprex-D Capsules ... 1172

Amitriptyline Hydrochloride (Central anticholinergic syndrome). Products include:
Etrafon ... 3115
Limbitrol ... 1738

Amoxapine (Central anticholinergic syndrome).
No products indexed under this heading.

Astemizole (Central anticholinergic syndrome).
No products indexed under this heading.

Azatadine Maleate (Central anticholinergic syndrome). Products include:
Rynatan Tablets ... 3351

Bromodiphenhydramine Hydrochloride (Central anticholinergic syndrome).
No products indexed under this heading.

Brompheniramine Maleate (Central anticholinergic syndrome). Products include:
Bromfed Capsules (Extended-Release) ... 2269
Bromfed-PD Capsules (Extended-Release) ... 2269
Comtrex Acute Head Cold & Sinus Pressure Relief Tablets ... ▣627
Dimetapp Elixir ... ▣777
Dimetapp Cold and Fever Suspension ... ▣775
Dimetapp DM Cold & Cough Elixir ... ▣775
Dimetapp Nighttime Flu Liquid ... ▣776

Cetirizine Hydrochloride (Central anticholinergic syndrome). Products include:
Zyrtec ... 2756
Zyrtec-D 12 Hour Extended Relief Tablets ... 2758

Chlorpheniramine Maleate (Central anticholinergic syndrome). Products include:
Actifed Cold & Sinus Caplets and Tablets ... ▣688
Alka-Seltzer Plus Liqui-Gels ... ▣604
BC Allergy Sinus Cold Powder ... ▣619
Chlor-Trimeton Allergy Tablets ... ▣735
Chlor-Trimeton Allergy/Decongestant Tablets ... ▣736
Comtrex Flu Therapy & Fever Relief Nighttime Tablets ... ▣628
Comtrex Maximum Strength Multi-Symptom Cold & Cough Relief Tablets and Caplets ... ▣626
Contac Severe Cold and Flu Caplets Maximum Strength ... ▣746
Coricidin 'D' Cold, Flu & Sinus Tablets ... ▣737
Coricidin/Coricidin D ... ▣738
Coricidin HBP Maximum Strength Flu Tablets ... ▣738
Extendryl ... 1361
Hycomine Compound Tablets ... 1317
Kronofed-A ... 1341
PediaCare Cough-Cold Liquid ... ▣719
PediaCare NightRest Cough-Cold Liquid ... ▣719
Robitussin Nighttime Honey Flu Liquid ... ▣786
Ryna ... ▣768
Singlet Caplets ... ▣761
Sinutab Sinus Allergy Medication, Maximum Strength Formula, Tablets & Caplets ... ▣707
Sudafed Cold & Allergy Tablets ... ▣708
TheraFlu Regular Strength Cold & Cough Night Time Hot Liquid ... ▣676
TheraFlu Regular Strength Cold & Sore Throat Night Time Hot Liquid ... ▣676
TheraFlu Maximum Strength Flu & Cough Night Time Hot Liquid ... ▣678
TheraFlu Maximum Strength Flu & Sore Throat Night Time Hot Liquid ... ▣677
TheraFlu Maximum Strength Severe Cold & Congestion Night Time Caplets ... ▣678
TheraFlu Maximum Strength Severe Cold & Congestion Night Time Hot Liquid ... ▣678
Triaminic Cold & Allergy Liquid ... ▣681
Triaminic Cold & Allergy Softchews ... ▣683
Triaminic Cold & Cough Liquid ... ▣681
Triaminic Cold & Cough Softchews ... ▣683
Triaminic Cold & Night Time Cough Liquid ... ▣681
Triaminic Cold, Cough & Fever Liquid ... ▣681
Children's Tylenol Cold Suspension Liquid and Chewable Tablets ... 2015
Children's Tylenol Cold Plus Cough Suspension Liquid and Chewable Tablets ... 2015
Children's Tylenol Flu Suspension Liquid ... 2015
Maximum Strength Tylenol Allergy Sinus Caplets, Gelcaps, and Geltabs ... 2010
Multi-Symptom Tylenol Cold Complete Formula Caplets ... 2010

Vicks 44M Cough, Cold & Flu Relief Liquid .... ▣725
Pediatric Vicks 44m Cough & Cold Relief .... ▣728
Children's Vicks NyQuil Cold/Cough Relief .... ▣726

Chlorpheniramine Polistirex (Central anticholinergic syndrome). Products include:
Tussionex Pennkinetic Extended-Release Suspension 1174

Chlorpheniramine Tannate (Central anticholinergic syndrome). Products include:
Reformulated Rynatan Pediatric Suspension 3352
Rynatuss Pediatric Suspension 3353
Rynatuss Tablets 3353
Tussi-12 S Suspension 3356
Tussi-12 Tablets 3356

Chlorpromazine (Central anticholinergic syndrome). Products include:
Thorazine Suppositories 1656

Chlorpromazine Hydrochloride (Central anticholinergic syndrome). Products include:
Thorazine 1656

Chlorprothixene (Central anticholinergic syndrome).
No products indexed under this heading.

Chlorprothixene Hydrochloride (Central anticholinergic syndrome).
No products indexed under this heading.

Clemastine Fumarate (Central anticholinergic syndrome). Products include:
Tavist 12 Hour Allergy Tablets .... ▣676

Clomipramine Hydrochloride (Central anticholinergic syndrome).
No products indexed under this heading.

Clorazepate Dipotassium (Central anticholinergic syndrome). Products include:
Tranxene 511

Clozapine (Central anticholinergic syndrome). Products include:
Clozaril Tablets 2319

Cyproheptadine Hydrochloride (Central anticholinergic syndrome). Products include:
Periactin Tablets 2155

Desipramine Hydrochloride (Central anticholinergic syndrome). Products include:
Norpramin Tablets 755

Dexchlorpheniramine Maleate (Central anticholinergic syndrome).
No products indexed under this heading.

Diphenhydramine Citrate (Central anticholinergic syndrome). Products include:
Alka-Seltzer PM Effervescent Tablets .... ▣605
Benadryl Allergy & Sinus Fastmelt Tablets .... ▣693
Benadryl Children's Allergy/Cold Fastmelt Tablets .... ▣692
Excedrin PM Tablets, Caplets, and Geltabs .... ▣631
Goody's PM Powder .... ▣621

Diphenhydramine Hydrochloride (Central anticholinergic syndrome). Products include:
Extra Strength Bayer PM Caplets .... ▣611
Benadryl Allergy Chewables .... ▣689
Benadryl Allergy .... ▣691
Benadryl Allergy Liquid .... ▣690
Benadryl Allergy/Cold Tablets .... ▣691
Benadryl Allergy/Congestion Tablets .... ▣692
Benadryl Allergy & Sinus Liquid ..... ▣693
Benadryl Allergy Sinus Headache Caplets & Gelcaps .... ▣693
Benadryl Severe Allergy & Sinus Headache Caplets .... ▣694
Benadryl Dye-Free Allergy Liquid ... ▣690
Benadryl Dye-Free Allergy Liqui-Gels Softgels .... ▣690
Benadryl Itch Relief Stick Extra Strength .... ▣695
Benadryl Cream .... ▣695
Benadryl Gel .... ▣695
Benadryl Spray .... ▣696
Benadryl Parenteral 2617
Coricidin HBP Night-Time Cold & Flu Tablets .... ▣738
Nytol QuickCaps Caplets .... ▣622
Maximum Strength Nytol QuickGels Softgels .... ▣621
Extra Strength Percogesic Aspirin-Free Coated Caplets .... ▣665
Simply Sleep Caplets 2008
Sominex Original Formula Tablets . ▣761
Children's Tylenol Allergy-D Liquid ... 2014
Maximum Strength Tylenol Allergy Sinus NightTime Caplets 2010
Tylenol Severe Allergy Caplets 2010
Maximum Strength Tylenol Flu NightTime Gelcaps 2011
Extra Strength Tylenol PM Caplets, Geltabs, and Gelcaps 2012
Unisom Maximum Strength SleepGels .... ▣713

Diphenylpyraline Hydrochloride (Central anticholinergic syndrome).
No products indexed under this heading.

Doxepin Hydrochloride (Central anticholinergic syndrome). Products include:
Sinequan 2713

Fexofenadine Hydrochloride (Central anticholinergic syndrome). Products include:
Allegra 712
Allegra-D Extended-Release Tablets 714

Fluphenazine Decanoate (Central anticholinergic syndrome).
No products indexed under this heading.

Fluphenazine Enanthate (Central anticholinergic syndrome).
No products indexed under this heading.

Fluphenazine Hydrochloride (Central anticholinergic syndrome).
No products indexed under this heading.

Haloperidol (Central anticholinergic syndrome). Products include:
Haldol Injection, Tablets and Concentrate 2533

Haloperidol Decanoate (Central anticholinergic syndrome). Products include:
Haldol Decanoate 2535

Imipramine Hydrochloride (Central anticholinergic syndrome).
No products indexed under this heading.

Imipramine Pamoate (Central anticholinergic syndrome).
No products indexed under this heading.

Lithium Carbonate (Central anticholinergic syndrome). Products include:
Eskalith 1527
Lithium Carbonate 3061
Lithobid Slow-Release Tablets 3255

Lithium Citrate (Central anticholinergic syndrome). Products include:
Lithium Citrate Syrup 3061

Loratadine (Central anticholinergic syndrome). Products include:
Claritin 3100
Claritin-D 12 Hour Extended Release Tablets 3102
Claritin-D 24 Hour Extended Release Tablets 3104

Loxapine Hydrochloride (Central anticholinergic syndrome).
No products indexed under this heading.

Loxapine Succinate (Central anticholinergic syndrome). Products include:
Loxitane Capsules 3398

Maprotiline Hydrochloride (Central anticholinergic syndrome).
No products indexed under this heading.

Meperidine Hydrochloride (Central anticholinergic syndrome). Products include:
Demerol 3079
Mepergan Injection 3539

Mesoridazine Besylate (Central anticholinergic syndrome). Products include:
Serentil 1057

Methdilazine Hydrochloride (Central anticholinergic syndrome).
No products indexed under this heading.

Methotrimeprazine (Central anticholinergic syndrome).
No products indexed under this heading.

Molindone Hydrochloride (Central anticholinergic syndrome). Products include:
Moban 1320

Nortriptyline Hydrochloride (Central anticholinergic syndrome).
No products indexed under this heading.

Olanzapine (Central anticholinergic syndrome). Products include:
Zyprexa Tablets 1973
Zyprexa ZYDIS Orally Disintegrating Tablets 1973

Perphenazine (Central anticholinergic syndrome). Products include:
Etrafon 3115
Trilafon 3160

Pimozide (Central anticholinergic syndrome). Products include:
Orap Tablets 1407

Prochlorperazine (Central anticholinergic syndrome). Products include:
Compazine 1505

Promethazine Hydrochloride (Central anticholinergic syndrome). Products include:
Mepergan Injection 3539
Phenergan Injection 3553
Phenergan 3556
Phenergan Syrup 3554
Phenergan with Codeine Syrup 3557
Phenergan with Dextromethorphan Syrup 3559
Phenergan VC Syrup 3560
Phenergan VC with Codeine Syrup .. 3561

Protriptyline Hydrochloride (Central anticholinergic syndrome). Products include:
Vivactil Tablets 2446
Vivactil Tablets 2217

Pyrilamine Maleate (Central anticholinergic syndrome). Products include:
Maximum Strength Midol Menstrual Caplets and Gelcaps .... ▣612
Maximum Strength Midol PMS Caplets and Gelcaps .... ▣613

Pyrilamine Tannate (Central anticholinergic syndrome). Products include:
Ryna-12 S Suspension 3351

Quetiapine Fumarate (Central anticholinergic syndrome). Products include:
Seroquel Tablets 684

Quinidine Gluconate (Central anticholinergic syndrome). Products include:
Quinaglute Dura-Tabs Tablets 978

Quinidine Polygalacturonate (Central anticholinergic syndrome).
No products indexed under this heading.

Quinidine Sulfate (Central anticholinergic syndrome). Products include:
Quinidex Extentabs 2933

Risperidone (Central anticholinergic syndrome). Products include:
Risperdal 1796

Terfenadine (Central anticholinergic syndrome).
No products indexed under this heading.

Thioridazine Hydrochloride (Central anticholinergic syndrome). Products include:
Thioridazine Hydrochloride Tablets 2289

Thiothixene (Central anticholinergic syndrome). Products include:
Navane Capsules 2701
Thiothixene Capsules 2290

Trifluoperazine Hydrochloride (Central anticholinergic syndrome). Products include:
Stelazine 1640

Trimeprazine Tartrate (Central anticholinergic syndrome).
No products indexed under this heading.

Trimipramine Maleate (Central anticholinergic syndrome). Products include:
Surmontil Capsules 3595

Tripelennamine Hydrochloride (Central anticholinergic syndrome).
No products indexed under this heading.

Triprolidine Hydrochloride (Central anticholinergic syndrome). Products include:
Actifed Cold & Allergy Tablets .... ▣688

Ziprasidone Hydrochloride (Central anticholinergic syndrome). Products include:
Geodon Capsules 2688

AKINETON TABLETS

(Biperiden Hydrochloride) 402
See Akineton Injection

ALAMAST OPHTHALMIC SOLUTION

(Pemirolast Potassium) 3092
None cited in PDR database.

ALBALON OPHTHALMIC SOLUTION

(Naphazoline Hydrochloride) .... ⊙225
May interact with monoamine oxidase inhibitors, tricyclic antidepressants, and certain other agents. Compounds in these categories include:

Amitriptyline Hydrochloride (May potentiate the pressor effect of naphazoline). Products include:
Etrafon 3115
Limbitrol 1738

Amoxapine (May potentiate the pressor effect of naphazoline).
No products indexed under this heading.

Clomipramine Hydrochloride (May potentiate the pressor effect of naphazoline).
No products indexed under this heading.

Desipramine Hydrochloride (May potentiate the pressor effect of naphazoline). Products include:
Norpramin Tablets 755

Doxepin Hydrochloride (May potentiate the pressor effect of naphazoline). Products include:
Sinequan 2713

Imipramine Hydrochloride (May potentiate the pressor effect of naphazoline).
No products indexed under this heading.

Imipramine Pamoate (May potentiate the pressor effect of naphazoline).
No products indexed under this heading.

Isocarboxazid (Severe hypertensive crisis).
No products indexed under this heading.

Maprotiline Hydrochloride (May potentiate the pressor effect of naphazoline).
No products indexed under this heading.

Moclobemide (Severe hypertensive crisis).
No products indexed under this heading.

Nortriptyline Hydrochloride (May potentiate the pressor effect of

naphazoline).
No products indexed under this heading.

Pargyline Hydrochloride (Severe hypertensive crisis).
No products indexed under this heading.

Phenelzine Sulfate (Severe hypertensive crisis). Products include:
Nardil Tablets 2653

Procarbazine Hydrochloride (Severe hypertensive crisis). Products include:
Matulane Capsules 3246

Protriptyline Hydrochloride (May potentiate the pressor effect of naphazoline). Products include:
Vivactil Tablets 2446
Vivactil Tablets 2217

Selegiline Hydrochloride (Severe hypertensive crisis). Products include:
Eldepryl Capsules 3266

Tranylcypromine Sulfate (Severe hypertensive crisis). Products include:
Parnate Tablets 1607

Trimipramine Maleate (May potentiate the pressor effect of naphazoline). Products include:
Surmontil Capsules 3595

ALBENZA TABLETS

(Albendazole) 1463
May interact with:

Cimetidine (Co-administration has resulted in increased albendazole sulfoxide concentrations in bile and cystic fluid in hydatid cyst). Products include:
Tagamet HB 200 Suspension .... ▣ 762
Tagamet HB 200 Tablets .... ▣ 761
Tagamet Tablets 1644

Cimetidine Hydrochloride (Co-administration has resulted in increased albendazole sulfoxide concentrations in bile and cystic fluid in hydatid cyst). Products include:
Tagamet 1644

Dexamethasone (Co-administration has resulted in higher steady-state trough concentrations of albendazole sulfoxide). Products include:
Decadron Elixir 2078
Decadron Tablets 2079
TobraDex Ophthalmic Ointment 542
TobraDex Ophthalmic Suspension .. 541

Dexamethasone Acetate (Co-administration has resulted in higher steady-state trough concentrations of albendazole sulfoxide).
No products indexed under this heading.

Dexamethasone Sodium Phosphate (Co-administration has resulted in higher steady-state trough concentrations of albendazole sulfoxide). Products include:
Decadron Phosphate Injection 2081
Decadron Phosphate Sterile Ophthalmic Ointment 2083
Decadron Phosphate Sterile Ophthalmic Solution 2084
NeoDecadron Sterile Ophthalmic Solution 2144

Praziquantel (Co-administration has resulted in increased mean maximum plasma concentration and area under the curve of albendazole sulfoxide). Products include:
Biltricide Tablets 887

Food Interactions

Diet, high-lipid (Oral bioavailability appears to be enhanced when albendazole is co-administered with a fatty meal).

ALBUMIN (HUMAN) 5%

(Albumin (human)) 838
None cited in PDR database.

ALBUMIN (HUMAN) 25%

(Albumin (human)) 839
None cited in PDR database.

ALBUMINAR-5, U.S.P.

(Albumin (human)) 785
None cited in PDR database.

ALBUMINAR-25, U.S.P.

(Albumin (human)) 786
None cited in PDR database.

ALDARA CREAM, 5%

(Imiquimod) 1978
None cited in PDR database.

ALDOCLOR TABLETS

(Chlorothiazide, Methyldopa) 2035
May interact with antihypertensives and barbiturates. Compounds in these categories include:

Acarbose (Dosage adjustment of the antidiabetic drug may be required). Products include:
Precose Tablets 906

Acebutolol Hydrochloride (Potentiation of antihypertensive effect). Products include:
Sectral Capsules 3589

ACTH (Hypokalemia may result).
No products indexed under this heading.

Alfentanil Hydrochloride (Aggravates orthostatic hypotension).
No products indexed under this heading.

Amlodipine Besylate (Potentiation of antihypertensive effect). Products include:
Lotrel Capsules 2370
Norvasc Tablets 2704

Aprobarbital (Aggravates orthostatic hypotension).
No products indexed under this heading.

Atenolol (Potentiation of antihypertensive effect). Products include:
Tenoretic Tablets 690
Tenormin I.V. Injection 692

Benazepril Hydrochloride (Potentiation of antihypertensive effect). Products include:
Lotensin Tablets 2365
Lotensin HCT Tablets 2367
Lotrel Capsules 2370

Bendroflumethiazide (Potentiation of antihypertensive effect). Products include:
Corzide 40/5 Tablets 2247
Corzide 80/5 Tablets 2247

Betamethasone Acetate (Hypokalemia may result). Products include:
Celestone Soluspan Injectable Suspension 3097

Betamethasone Sodium Phosphate (Hypokalemia may result). Products include:
Celestone Soluspan Injectable Suspension 3097

Betaxolol Hydrochloride (Potentiation of antihypertensive effect). Products include:
Betoptic S Ophthalmic Suspension 537

Bisoprolol Fumarate (Potentiation of antihypertensive effect). Products include:
Zebeta Tablets 1885
Ziac Tablets 1887

Buprenorphine Hydrochloride (Aggravates orthostatic hypotension). Products include:
Buprenex Injectable 2918

Butabarbital (Aggravates orthostatic hypotension).
No products indexed under this heading.

Butalbital (Aggravates orthostatic hypotension). Products include:
Phrenilin 578
Sedapap Tablets 50 mg/650 mg ... 2225

Candesartan Cilexetil (Potentiation of antihypertensive effect). Products include:
Atacand Tablets 595
Atacand HCT Tablets 597

Captopril (Potentiation of antihypertensive effect). Products include:
Captopril Tablets 2281

Carteolol Hydrochloride (Potentiation of antihypertensive effect). Products include:
Carteolol Hydrochloride Ophthalmic Solution USP, 1% ..... ⊙ 258
Ocupress Ophthalmic Solution, 1% Sterile .... ⊙ 303

Celecoxib (May result in reduced diuretic effect). Products include:
Celebrex Capsules 2676
Celebrex Capsules 2780

Chlorothiazide Sodium (Potentiation of antihypertensive effect). Products include:
Diuril Sodium Intravenous 2086

Chlorpropamide (Dosage adjustment of the antidiabetic drug may be required). Products include:
Diabinese Tablets 2680

Chlorthalidone (Potentiation of antihypertensive effect). Products include:
Clorpres Tablets 1002
Combipres Tablets 1040
Tenoretic Tablets 690

Cholestyramine (Cholestyramine resin has the potential of binding thiazide diuretics and reducing absorption from the gastrointestinal tract).
No products indexed under this heading.

Clonidine (Potentiation of antihypertensive effect). Products include:
Catapres-TTS 1038

Clonidine Hydrochloride (Potentiation of antihypertensive effect). Products include:
Catapres Tablets 1037
Clorpres Tablets 1002
Combipres Tablets 1040
Duraclon Injection 3057

Codeine Phosphate (Aggravates orthostatic hypotension). Products include:
Phenergan with Codeine Syrup 3557
Phenergan VC with Codeine Syrup . 3561
Robitussin A-C Syrup 2942
Robitussin-DAC Syrup 2942
Ryna-C Liquid .... ▣ 768
Soma Compound w/Codeine Tablets 3355
Tussi-Organidin NR Liquid 3350
Tussi-Organidin-S NR Liquid 3350
Tylenol with Codeine 2595

Colestipol Hydrochloride (Colestipole resin has the potential of binding thiazide diuretics and reducing absorption from the gastrointestinal tract). Products include:
Colestid Tablets 2791

Cortisone Acetate (Hypokalemia may result). Products include:
Cortone Acetate Injectable Suspension 2059
Cortone Acetate Tablets 2061

Deserpidine (Potentiation of antihypertensive effect).
No products indexed under this heading.

Deslanoside (Thiazide-induced hypokalemia may cause cardiac arrhythmia and may also sensitize or exaggerate the response of the heart to the toxic effects of digitalis).
No products indexed under this heading.

Dexamethasone (Hypokalemia may result). Products include:
Decadron Elixir 2078
Decadron Tablets 2079
TobraDex Ophthalmic Ointment 542
TobraDex Ophthalmic Suspension .. 541

Dexamethasone Acetate (Hypokalemia may result).
No products indexed under this heading.

Dexamethasone Sodium Phosphate (Hypokalemia may result). Products include:
Decadron Phosphate Injection 2081
Decadron Phosphate Sterile Ophthalmic Ointment 2083
Decadron Phosphate Sterile Ophthalmic Solution 2084
NeoDecadron Sterile Ophthalmic Solution 2144

Dezocine (Aggravates orthostatic hypotension).
No products indexed under this heading.

Diazoxide (Potentiation of antihypertensive effect).
No products indexed under this heading.

Diclofenac Potassium (May result in reduced diuretic effect). Products include:
Cataflam Tablets 2315

Diclofenac Sodium (May result in reduced diuretic effect). Products include:
Arthrotec Tablets 3195
Voltaren Ophthalmic Sterile Ophthalmic Solution .... ⊙ 312
Voltaren Tablets 2315
Voltaren-XR Tablets 2315

Digitoxin (Thiazide-induced hypokalemia may cause cardiac arrhythmia and may also sensitize or exaggerate the response of the heart to the toxic effects of digitalis).
No products indexed under this heading.

Digoxin (Thiazide-induced hypokalemia may cause cardiac arrhythmia and may also sensitize or exaggerate the response of the heart to the toxic effects of digitalis). Products include:
Digitek Tablets 1003
Lanoxicaps Capsules 1574
Lanoxin Injection 1581
Lanoxin Tablets 1587
Lanoxin Elixir Pediatric 1578
Lanoxin Injection Pediatric 1584

Diltiazem Hydrochloride (Potentiation of antihypertensive effect). Products include:
Cardizem Injectable 1018
Cardizem Lyo-Ject Syringe 1018
Cardizem Monovial 1018
Cardizem CD Capsules 1016
Tiazac Capsules 1378

Doxazosin Mesylate (Potentiation of antihypertensive effect). Products include:
Cardura Tablets 2668

Enalapril Maleate (Potentiation of antihypertensive effect). Products include:
Lexxel Tablets 608
Vaseretic Tablets 2204
Vasotec Tablets 2210

Enalaprilat (Potentiation of antihypertensive effect). Products include:
Enalaprilat Injection 863
Vasotec I.V. Injection 2207

Enflurane (May require reduced dose of anesthetics).
No products indexed under this heading.

Eprosartan Mesylate (Potentiation of antihypertensive effect). Products include:
Teveten Tablets 3327

Esmolol Hydrochloride (Potentiation of antihypertensive effect). Products include:
Brevibloc Injection 858

Etodolac (May result in reduced diuretic effect). Products include:
Lodine 3528
Lodine XL Extended-Release Tablets 3530

Felodipine (Potentiation of antihypertensive effect). Products include:
Lexxel Tablets 608
Plendil Extended-Release Tablets ... 623

Fenoprofen Calcium (May result in reduced diuretic effect).
No products indexed under this heading.

Fentanyl (Aggravates orthostatic hypotension). Products include:
Duragesic Transdermal System 1786

Fentanyl Citrate (Aggravates orthostatic hypotension). Products include:
- Actiq 1184

Ferrous Gluconate (Co-administration results in a decrease in the bioavailability of methyldopa; this may adversely affect blood pressure control in patients treated with methyldopa; concurrent use is not recommended). Products include:
- Fergon Iron Tablets .... ▣802

Ferrous Sulfate (Co-administration results in a decrease in the bioavailability of methyldopa; this may adversely affect blood pressure control in patients treated with methyldopa; concurrent use is not recommended). Products include:
- Feosol Tablets 1717
- Slow Fe Tablets .... ▣827
- Slow Fe with Folic Acid Tablets .... ▣828

Fludrocortisone Acetate (Hypokalemia may result). Products include:
- Florinef Acetate Tablets 2250

Flurbiprofen (May result in reduced diuretic effect).
- No products indexed under this heading.

Fosinopril Sodium (Potentiation of antihypertensive effect). Products include:
- Monopril Tablets 1091
- Monopril HCT 1094

Furosemide (Potentiation of antihypertensive effect). Products include:
- Furosemide Tablets 2284

Glimepiride (Dosage adjustment of the antidiabetic drug may be required). Products include:
- Amaryl Tablets 717

Glipizide (Dosage adjustment of the antidiabetic drug may be required). Products include:
- Glucotrol Tablets 2692
- Glucotrol XL Extended Release Tablets 2693

Glyburide (Dosage adjustment of the antidiabetic drug may be required). Products include:
- DiaBeta Tablets 741
- Glucovance Tablets 1086

Guanabenz Acetate (Potentiation of antihypertensive effect).
- No products indexed under this heading.

Guanethidine Monosulfate (Potentiation of antihypertensive effect).
- No products indexed under this heading.

Hydralazine Hydrochloride (Potentiation of antihypertensive effect).
- No products indexed under this heading.

Hydrochlorothiazide (Potentiation of antihypertensive effect). Products include:
- Accuretic Tablets 2614
- Aldoril Tablets 2039
- Atacand HCT Tablets 597
- Avalide Tablets 1070
- Diovan HCT Tablets 2338
- Dyazide Capsules 1515
- HydroDIURIL Tablets 2108
- Hyzaar 2109
- Inderide Tablets 3517
- Inderide LA Long-Acting Capsules 3519
- Lotensin HCT Tablets 2367
- Maxzide 1008
- Micardis HCT Tablets 1051
- Microzide Capsules 3414
- Moduretic Tablets 2138
- Monopril HCT 1094
- Prinzide Tablets 2168
- Timolide Tablets 2187
- Uniretic Tablets 3178
- Vaseretic Tablets 2204
- Zestoretic Tablets 695
- Ziac Tablets 1887

Hydrocodone Bitartrate (Aggravates orthostatic hypotension). Products include:
- Hycodan 1316
- Hycomine Compound Tablets 1317
- Hycotuss Expectorant Syrup 1318
- Lortab 3319
- Lortab Elixir 3317
- Maxidone Tablets CIII 3399
- Norco 5/325 Tablets CIII 3424
- Norco 7.5/325 Tablets CIII 3425
- Norco 10/325 Tablets CIII 3427
- Norco 10/325 Tablets CIII 3425
- Vicodin Tablets 516
- Vicodin ES Tablets 517
- Vicodin HP Tablets 518
- Vicodin Tuss Expectorant 519
- Vicoprofen Tablets 520
- Zydone Tablets 1330

Hydrocodone Polistirex (Aggravates orthostatic hypotension). Products include:
- Tussionex Pennkinetic Extended-Release Suspension 1174

Hydrocortisone (Hypokalemia may result). Products include:
- Anusol-HC Cream 2.5% 2237
- Cipro HC Otic Suspension 540
- Cortaid Intensive Therapy Cream .... ▣717
- Cortaid Maximum Strength Cream .... ▣717
- Cortisporin Ophthalmic Suspension Sterile .... ⊙297
- Cortizone•5 .... ▣699
- Cortizone•10 .... ▣699
- Cortizone•10 Plus Creme .... ▣700
- Cortizone for Kids Creme .... ▣699
- Hydrocortone Tablets 2106
- Massengill Medicated Soft Cloth Towelette .... ▣753
- VōSoL HC Otic Solution 3356

Hydrocortisone Acetate (Hypokalemia may result). Products include:
- Analpram-HC 1338
- Anusol HC-1 Hydrocortisone Anti-Itch Cream .... ▣689
- Anusol-HC Suppositories 2238
- Cortaid .... ▣717
- Cortifoam Rectal Foam 3170
- Cortisporin-TC Otic Suspension 2246
- Hydrocortone Acetate Injectable Suspension 2103
- Pramosone 1343
- Proctocort Suppositories 2264
- ProctoFoam-HC 3177
- Terra-Cortril Ophthalmic Suspension 2716

Hydrocortisone Sodium Phosphate (Hypokalemia may result). Products include:
- Hydrocortone Phosphate Injection, Sterile 2105

Hydrocortisone Sodium Succinate (Hypokalemia may result).
- No products indexed under this heading.

Hydroflumethiazide (Potentiation of antihypertensive effect). Products include:
- Diucardin Tablets 3494

Hydromorphone Hydrochloride (Aggravates orthostatic hypotension). Products include:
- Dilaudid 441
- Dilaudid Oral Liquid 445
- Dilaudid Powder 441
- Dilaudid Rectal Suppositories 441
- Dilaudid Tablets 441
- Dilaudid Tablets - 8 mg 445
- Dilaudid-HP 443

Ibuprofen (May result in reduced diuretic effect). Products include:
- Advil .... ▣771
- Children's Advil Oral Suspension .... ▣773
- Children's Advil Chewable Tablets .... ▣773
- Advil Cold and Sinus Caplets .... ▣771
- Advil Cold and Sinus Tablets .... ▣771
- Advil Flu & Body Ache Caplets .... ▣772
- Infants' Advil Drops .... ▣773
- Junior Strength Advil Tablets .... ▣773
- Junior Strength Advil Chewable Tablets .... ▣773
- Advil Migraine Liquigels .... ▣772
- Children's Motrin Oral Suspension and Chewable Tablets 2006
- Children's Motrin Cold Oral Suspension 2007
- Children's Motrin Oral Suspension .... ▣643
- Motrin Suspension, Oral Drops, Chewable Tablets, and Caplets 2002
- Infants' Motrin Concentrated Drops 2006
- Junior Strength Motrin Caplets and Chewable Tablets 2006
- Motrin IB Tablets, Caplets, and Gelcaps 2002
- Motrin Migraine Pain Caplets 2005
- Motrin Sinus Headache Caplets 2005
- Vicoprofen Tablets 520

Indapamide (Potentiation of antihypertensive effect). Products include:
- Indapamide Tablets 2286

Indomethacin (May result in reduced diuretic effect). Products include:
- Indocin 2112

Indomethacin Sodium Trihydrate (May result in reduced diuretic effect). Products include:
- Indocin I.V. 2115

Insulin, Human, Zinc Suspension (May alter insulin requirements). Products include:
- Humulin L, 100 Units 1937
- Humulin U, 100 Units 1943
- Novolin L Human Insulin 10 ml Vials 2422

Insulin, Human NPH (May alter insulin requirements). Products include:
- Humulin N, 100 Units 1939
- Humulin N NPH Pen 1940
- Novolin N Human Insulin 10 ml Vials 2422
- Novolin N PenFill 2423
- Novolin N Prefilled Syringe Disposable Insulin Delivery System 2425

Insulin, Human Regular (May alter insulin requirements). Products include:
- Humulin R Regular (U-500) 1943
- Humulin R, 100 Units 1941
- Novolin R Human Insulin 10 ml Vials 2423
- Novolin R PenFill 2423
- Novolin R Prefilled Syringe Disposable Insulin Delivery System 2425
- Velosulin BR Human Insulin 10 ml Vials 2435

Insulin, Human Regular and Human NPH Mixture (May alter insulin requirements). Products include:
- Humulin 50/50, 100 Units 1934
- Humulin 70/30, 100 Units 1935
- Humulin 70/30 Pen 1936
- Novolin 70/30 Human Insulin 10 ml Vials 2421
- Novolin 70/30 PenFill 2423
- Novolin 70/30 Prefilled Disposable Insulin Delivery System 2425

Insulin, NPH (May alter insulin requirements). Products include:
- Iletin II, NPH (Pork), 100 Units 1946

Insulin, Regular (May alter insulin requirements). Products include:
- Iletin II, Regular (Pork), 100 Units 1947

Insulin, Zinc Crystals (May alter insulin requirements).
- No products indexed under this heading.

Insulin, Zinc Suspension (May alter insulin requirements). Products include:
- Iletin II, Lente (Pork), 100 Units 1945

Insulin Aspart, Human Regular (May alter insulin requirements).
- No products indexed under this heading.

Insulin glargine (May alter insulin requirements). Products include:
- Lantus Injection 742

Insulin Lispro, Human (May alter insulin requirements). Products include:
- Humalog 1926
- Humalog Mix 75/25 Pen 1928

Insulin Lispro Protamine, Human (May alter insulin requirements). Products include:
- Humalog Mix 75/25 Pen 1928

Irbesartan (Potentiation of antihypertensive effect). Products include:
- Avalide Tablets 1070
- Avapro Tablets 1074
- Avapro Tablets 3076

Isocarboxazid (Concurrent use is contraindicated).
- No products indexed under this heading.

Isoflurane (May require reduced dose of anesthetics).
- No products indexed under this heading.

Isradipine (Potentiation of antihypertensive effect). Products include:
- DynaCirc Capsules 2921
- DynaCirc CR Tablets 2923

Ketamine Hydrochloride (May require reduced dose of anesthetics).
- No products indexed under this heading.

Ketoprofen (May result in reduced diuretic effect). Products include:
- Orudis Capsules 3548
- Orudis KT Tablets .... ▣778
- Oruvail Capsules 3548

Ketorolac Tromethamine (May result in reduced diuretic effect). Products include:
- Acular Ophthalmic Solution 544
- Acular PF Ophthalmic Solution 544
- Toradol 3018

Labetalol Hydrochloride (Potentiation of antihypertensive effect). Products include:
- Normodyne Injection 3135
- Normodyne Tablets 3137

Levorphanol Tartrate (Aggravates orthostatic hypotension). Products include:
- Levo-Dromoran 1734
- Levorphanol Tartrate Tablets 3059

Lisinopril (Potentiation of antihypertensive effect). Products include:
- Prinivil Tablets 2164
- Prinzide Tablets 2168
- Zestoretic Tablets 695
- Zestril Tablets 698

Lithium Carbonate (High risk of lithium toxicity). Products include:
- Eskalith 1527
- Lithium Carbonate 3061
- Lithobid Slow-Release Tablets 3255

Lithium Citrate (High risk of lithium toxicity). Products include:
- Lithium Citrate Syrup 3061

Losartan Potassium (Potentiation of antihypertensive effect). Products include:
- Cozaar Tablets 2067
- Hyzaar 2109

Mecamylamine Hydrochloride (Potentiation of antihypertensive effect). Products include:
- Inversine Tablets 1850

Meclofenamate Sodium (May result in reduced diuretic effect).
- No products indexed under this heading.

Mefenamic Acid (May result in reduced diuretic effect). Products include:
- Ponstel Capsules 1356

Meloxicam (May result in reduced diuretic effect). Products include:
- Mobic Tablets 1054

Meperidine Hydrochloride (Aggravates orthostatic hypotension). Products include:
- Demerol 3079
- Mepergan Injection 3539

Mephobarbital (Aggravates orthostatic hypotension).
- No products indexed under this heading.

Metformin Hydrochloride (Dosage adjustment of the antidiabetic drug may be required). Products include:
- Glucophage Tablets 1080
- Glucophage XR Tablets 1080
- Glucovance Tablets 1086

Methadone Hydrochloride (Aggravates orthostatic hypotension). Products include:
- Dolophine Hydrochloride Tablets 3056

IMPORTANT NOTE: Always consult each drug listing in the patient's regimen for possible interactions.

Methohexital Sodium (May require reduced dose of anesthetics). Products include:
Brevital Sodium for Injection, USP .. 1815

Methoxyflurane (May require reduced dose of anesthetics).
No products indexed under this heading.

Methyclothiazide (Potentiation of antihypertensive effect).
No products indexed under this heading.

Methyldopate Hydrochloride (Potentiation of antihypertensive effect).
No products indexed under this heading.

Methylprednisolone Acetate (Hypokalemia may result). Products include:
Depo-Medrol Injectable Suspension 2795

Methylprednisolone Sodium Succinate (Hypokalemia may result). Products include:
Solu-Medrol Sterile Powder 2855

Metolazone (Potentiation of antihypertensive effect). Products include:
Mykrox Tablets 1168
Zaroxolyn Tablets 1177

Metoprolol Succinate (Potentiation of antihypertensive effect). Products include:
Toprol-XL Tablets 651

Metoprolol Tartrate (Potentiation of antihypertensive effect).
No products indexed under this heading.

Metyrosine (Potentiation of antihypertensive effect). Products include:
Demser Capsules 2085

Mibefradil Dihydrochloride (Potentiation of antihypertensive effect).
No products indexed under this heading.

Miglitol (Dosage adjustment of the antidiabetic drug may be required). Products include:
Glyset Tablets 2821

Minoxidil (Potentiation of antihypertensive effect). Products include:
Rogaine Extra Strength for Men Topical Solution .... ▣721
Rogaine for Women Topical Solution .... ▣721

Moclobemide (Concurrent use is contraindicated).
No products indexed under this heading.

Moexipril Hydrochloride (Potentiation of antihypertensive effect). Products include:
Uniretic Tablets 3178
Univasc Tablets 3181

Morphine Sulfate (Aggravates orthostatic hypotension). Products include:
Astramorph/PF Injection, USP (Preservative-Free) 594
Duramorph Injection 1312
Infumorph 200 and Infumorph 500 Sterile Solutions 1314
Kadian Capsules 1335
MS Contin Tablets 2896
MSIR 2898
Oramorph SR Tablets 3062
Roxanol 3066

Nabumetone (May result in reduced diuretic effect). Products include:
Relafen Tablets 1617

Nadolol (Potentiation of antihypertensive effect). Products include:
Corgard Tablets 2245
Corzide 40/5 Tablets 2247
Corzide 80/5 Tablets 2247
Nadolol Tablets 2288

Naproxen (May result in reduced diuretic effect). Products include:
EC-Naprosyn Delayed-Release Tablets 2967
Naprosyn Suspension 2967
Naprosyn Tablets 2967

Naproxen Sodium (May result in reduced diuretic effect). Products include:
Aleve Tablets, Caplets and Gelcaps .... ▣602
Aleve Cold & Sinus Caplets .... ▣603
Anaprox Tablets 2967
Anaprox DS Tablets 2967
Naprelan Tablets 1293

Nicardipine Hydrochloride (Potentiation of antihypertensive effect). Products include:
Cardene I.V. 3485

Nifedipine (Potentiation of antihypertensive effect). Products include:
Adalat CC Tablets 877
Procardia Capsules 2708
Procardia XL Extended Release Tablets 2710

Nisoldipine (Potentiation of antihypertensive effect). Products include:
Sular Tablets 688

Nitroglycerin (Potentiation of antihypertensive effect). Products include:
Nitro-Dur Transdermal Infusion System 3134
Nitro-Dur Transdermal Infusion System 1834
Nitrolingual Pumpspray 1355
Nitrostat Tablets 2658

Norepinephrine Bitartrate (May decrease arterial responsiveness to norepinephrine).
No products indexed under this heading.

Oxaprozin (May result in reduced diuretic effect).
No products indexed under this heading.

Oxycodone Hydrochloride (Aggravates orthostatic hypotension). Products include:
OxyContin Tablets 2912
OxyFast Oral Concentrate Solution .. 2916
OxyIR Capsules 2916
Percocet Tablets 1326
Percodan Tablets 1327
Percolone Tablets 1327
Roxicodone 3067
Tylox Capsules 2597

Pargyline Hydrochloride (Concurrent use is contraindicated).
No products indexed under this heading.

Penbutolol Sulfate (Potentiation of antihypertensive effect).
No products indexed under this heading.

Pentobarbital Sodium (Aggravates orthostatic hypotension). Products include:
Nembutal Sodium Solution 485

Perindopril Erbumine (Potentiation of antihypertensive effect). Products include:
Aceon Tablets (2 mg, 4 mg, 8 mg) 3249

Phenelzine Sulfate (Concurrent use is contraindicated). Products include:
Nardil Tablets 2653

Phenobarbital (Aggravates orthostatic hypotension). Products include:
Arco-Lase Plus Tablets 592
Donnatal 2929
Donnatal Extentabs 2930

Phenoxybenzamine Hydrochloride (Potentiation of antihypertensive effect). Products include:
Dibenzyline Capsules 3457

Phentolamine Mesylate (Potentiation of antihypertensive effect).
No products indexed under this heading.

Phenylbutazone (May result in reduced diuretic effect).
No products indexed under this heading.

Pindolol (Potentiation of antihypertensive effect).
No products indexed under this heading.

Pioglitazone Hydrochloride (Dosage adjustment of the antidiabetic drug may be required). Products include:
Actos Tablets 3275

Piroxicam (May result in reduced diuretic effect). Products include:
Feldene Capsules 2685

Polythiazide (Potentiation of antihypertensive effect). Products include:
Minizide Capsules 2700
Renese Tablets 2712

Prazosin Hydrochloride (Potentiation of antihypertensive effect). Products include:
Minipress Capsules 2699
Minizide Capsules 2700

Prednisolone Acetate (Hypokalemia may result). Products include:
Blephamide Ophthalmic Ointment 547
Blephamide Ophthalmic Suspension 548
Poly-Pred Liquifilm Ophthalmic Suspension .... ⊙245
Pred Forte Ophthalmic Suspension .... ⊙246
Pred Mild Sterile Ophthalmic Suspension .... ⊙249
Pred-G Ophthalmic Suspension .... ⊙247
Pred-G Sterile Ophthalmic Ointment .... ⊙248

Prednisolone Sodium Phosphate (Hypokalemia may result). Products include:
Pediapred Oral Solution 1170

Prednisolone Tebutate (Hypokalemia may result).
No products indexed under this heading.

Prednisone (Hypokalemia may result). Products include:
Prednisone 3064

Procarbazine Hydrochloride (Concurrent use is contraindicated). Products include:
Matulane Capsules 3246

Propofol (May require reduced dose of anesthetics). Products include:
Diprivan Injectable Emulsion 667

Propoxyphene Hydrochloride (Aggravates orthostatic hypotension). Products include:
Darvon Pulvules 1909
Darvon Compound-65 Pulvules 1910

Propoxyphene Napsylate (Aggravates orthostatic hypotension). Products include:
Darvon-N/Darvocet-N 1907
Darvon-N Tablets 1912

Propranolol Hydrochloride (Potentiation of antihypertensive effect). Products include:
Inderal 3513
Inderal LA Long-Acting Capsules 3516
Inderide Tablets 3517
Inderide LA Long-Acting Capsules .. 3519

Quinapril Hydrochloride (Potentiation of antihypertensive effect). Products include:
Accupril Tablets 2611
Accuretic Tablets 2614

Ramipril (Potentiation of antihypertensive effect). Products include:
Altace Capsules 2233

Rauwolfia serpentina (Potentiation of antihypertensive effect).
No products indexed under this heading.

Remifentanil Hydrochloride (Aggravates orthostatic hypotension).
No products indexed under this heading.

Repaglinide (Dosage adjustment of the antidiabetic drug may be required). Products include:
Prandin Tablets (0.5, 1, and 2 mg) 2432

Rescinnamine (Potentiation of antihypertensive effect).
No products indexed under this heading.

Reserpine (Potentiation of antihypertensive effect).
No products indexed under this heading.

Rofecoxib (May result in reduced diuretic effect). Products include:
Vioxx 2213

Rosiglitazone Maleate (Dosage adjustment of the antidiabetic drug may be required). Products include:
Avandia Tablets 1490

Secobarbital Sodium (Aggravates orthostatic hypotension).
No products indexed under this heading.

Selegiline Hydrochloride (Concurrent use is contraindicated). Products include:
Eldepryl Capsules 3266

Sevoflurane (May require reduced dose of anesthetics).
No products indexed under this heading.

Sodium Nitroprusside (Potentiation of antihypertensive effect).
No products indexed under this heading.

Sotalol Hydrochloride (Potentiation of antihypertensive effect). Products include:
Betapace Tablets 950
Betapace AF Tablets 954

Spirapril Hydrochloride (Potentiation of antihypertensive effect).
No products indexed under this heading.

Sufentanil Citrate (Aggravates orthostatic hypotension).
No products indexed under this heading.

Sulindac (May result in reduced diuretic effect). Products include:
Clinoril Tablets 2053

Telmisartan (Potentiation of antihypertensive effect). Products include:
Micardis Tablets 1049
Micardis HCT Tablets 1051

Terazosin Hydrochloride (Potentiation of antihypertensive effect). Products include:
Hytrin Capsules 464

Thiamylal Sodium (Aggravates orthostatic hypotension).
No products indexed under this heading.

Timolol Maleate (Potentiation of antihypertensive effect). Products include:
Blocadren Tablets 2046
Cosopt Sterile Ophthalmic Solution 2065
Timolide Tablets 2187
Timolol GFS .... ⊙266
Timoptic in Ocudose 2192
Timoptic Sterile Ophthalmic Solution 2190
Timoptic-XE Sterile Ophthalmic Gel Forming Solution 2194

Tolazamide (Dosage adjustment of the antidiabetic drug may be required).
No products indexed under this heading.

Tolbutamide (Dosage adjustment of the antidiabetic drug may be required).
No products indexed under this heading.

Tolmetin Sodium (May result in reduced diuretic effect). Products include:
Tolectin 2589

Torsemide (Potentiation of antihypertensive effect). Products include:
Demadex Tablets and Injection 2965

Trandolapril (Potentiation of antihypertensive effect). Products include:
Mavik Tablets 478
Tarka Tablets 508

Tranylcypromine Sulfate (Concurrent use is contraindicated). Products include:
Parnate Tablets 1607

Triamcinolone (Hypokalemia may result).
No products indexed under this heading.

Triamcinolone Acetonide (Hypokalemia may result). Products include:
Azmacort Inhalation Aerosol 728
Nasacort Nasal Inhaler 750
Nasacort AQ Nasal Spray 752
Tri-Nasal Spray 2274

Triamcinolone Diacetate (Hypokalemia may result).
No products indexed under this heading.

Triamcinolone Hexacetonide (Hypokalemia may result).
No products indexed under this heading.

Trimethaphan Camsylate (Potentiation of antihypertensive effect).
No products indexed under this heading.

Troglitazone (Dosage adjustment of the antidiabetic drug may be required).
No products indexed under this heading.

Tubocurarine Chloride (Increased responsiveness to tubocurarine).
No products indexed under this heading.

Valsartan (Potentiation of antihypertensive effect). Products include:
Diovan Capsules 2337
Diovan HCT Tablets 2338

Verapamil Hydrochloride (Potentiation of antihypertensive effect). Products include:
Covera-HS Tablets 3199
Isoptin SR Tablets 467
Tarka Tablets 508
Verelan Capsules 3184
Verelan PM Capsules 3186

Food Interactions

Alcohol (Aggravates orthostatic hypotension).

ALDOMET TABLETS

(Methyldopa) 2037
May interact with antihypertensives, general anesthetics, lithium preparations, monoamine oxidase inhibitors, and certain other agents. Compounds in these categories include:

Acebutolol Hydrochloride (Potentiation of antihypertensive effect). Products include:
Sectral Capsules 3589

Amlodipine Besylate (Potentiation of antihypertensive effect). Products include:
Lotrel Capsules 2370
Norvasc Tablets 2704

Atenolol (Potentiation of antihypertensive effect). Products include:
Tenoretic Tablets 690
Tenormin I.V. Injection 692

Benazepril Hydrochloride (Potentiation of antihypertensive effect). Products include:
Lotensin Tablets 2365
Lotensin HCT Tablets 2367
Lotrel Capsules 2370

Bendroflumethiazide (Potentiation of antihypertensive effect). Products include:
Corzide 40/5 Tablets 2247
Corzide 80/5 Tablets 2247

Betaxolol Hydrochloride (Potentiation of antihypertensive effect). Products include:
Betoptic S Ophthalmic Suspension 537

Bisoprolol Fumarate (Potentiation of antihypertensive effect). Products include:
Zebeta Tablets 1885
Ziac Tablets 1887

Candesartan Cilexetil (Potentiation of antihypertensive effect). Products include:
Atacand Tablets 595
Atacand HCT Tablets 597

Captopril (Potentiation of antihypertensive effect). Products include:
Captopril Tablets 2281

Carteolol Hydrochloride (Potentiation of antihypertensive effect). Products include:
Carteolol Hydrochloride Ophthalmic Solution USP, 1% ..... ⊙258
Ocupress Ophthalmic Solution, 1% Sterile .... ⊙303

Chlorothiazide (Potentiation of antihypertensive effect). Products include:
Aldoclor Tablets 2035
Diuril Oral 2087

Chlorothiazide Sodium (Potentiation of antihypertensive effect). Products include:
Diuril Sodium Intravenous 2086

Chlorthalidone (Potentiation of antihypertensive effect). Products include:
Clorpres Tablets 1002
Combipres Tablets 1040
Tenoretic Tablets 690

Clonidine (Potentiation of antihypertensive effect). Products include:
Catapres-TTS 1038

Clonidine Hydrochloride (Potentiation of antihypertensive effect). Products include:
Catapres Tablets 1037
Clorpres Tablets 1002
Combipres Tablets 1040
Duraclon Injection 3057

Deserpidine (Potentiation of antihypertensive effect).
No products indexed under this heading.

Diazoxide (Potentiation of antihypertensive effect).
No products indexed under this heading.

Diltiazem Hydrochloride (Potentiation of antihypertensive effect). Products include:
Cardizem Injectable 1018
Cardizem Lyo-Ject Syringe 1018
Cardizem Monovial 1018
Cardizem CD Capsules 1016
Tiazac Capsules 1378

Doxazosin Mesylate (Potentiation of antihypertensive effect). Products include:
Cardura Tablets 2668

Enalapril Maleate (Potentiation of antihypertensive effect). Products include:
Lexxel Tablets 608
Vaseretic Tablets 2204
Vasotec Tablets 2210

Enalaprilat (Potentiation of antihypertensive effect). Products include:
Enalaprilat Injection 863
Vasotec I.V. Injection 2207

Enflurane (May require reduced dose of anesthetics).
No products indexed under this heading.

Eprosartan Mesylate (Potentiation of antihypertensive effect). Products include:
Teveten Tablets 3327

Esmolol Hydrochloride (Potentiation of antihypertensive effect). Products include:
Brevibloc Injection 858

Felodipine (Potentiation of antihypertensive effect). Products include:
Lexxel Tablets 608
Plendil Extended-Release Tablets 623

Ferrous Gluconate (Co-administration decreases the bioavailability of methyldopa; this may adversely affect blood pressure control in patients treated with methyldopa; concurrent use is not recommended). Products include:
Fergon Iron Tablets .... ▣802

Ferrous Sulfate (Co-administration decreases the bioavailability of methyldopa; this may adversely affect blood pressure control in patients treated with methyldopa; concurrent use is not recommended). Products include:
Feosol Tablets 1717
Slow Fe Tablets .... ▣827
Slow Fe with Folic Acid Tablets ...... ▣828

Fosinopril Sodium (Potentiation of antihypertensive effect). Products include:
Monopril Tablets 1091
Monopril HCT 1094

Furosemide (Potentiation of antihypertensive effect). Products include:
Furosemide Tablets 2284

Guanabenz Acetate (Potentiation of antihypertensive effect).
No products indexed under this heading.

Guanethidine Monosulfate (Potentiation of antihypertensive effect).
No products indexed under this heading.

Hydralazine Hydrochloride (Potentiation of antihypertensive effect).
No products indexed under this heading.

Hydrochlorothiazide (Potentiation of antihypertensive effect). Products include:
Accuretic Tablets 2614
Aldoril Tablets 2039
Atacand HCT Tablets 597
Avalide Tablets 1070
Diovan HCT Tablets 2338
Dyazide Capsules 1515
HydroDIURIL Tablets 2108
Hyzaar 2109
Inderide Tablets 3517
Inderide LA Long-Acting Capsules .. 3519
Lotensin HCT Tablets 2367
Maxzide 1008
Micardis HCT Tablets 1051
Microzide Capsules 3414
Moduretic Tablets 2138
Monopril HCT 1094
Prinzide Tablets 2168
Timolide Tablets 2187
Uniretic Tablets 3178
Vaseretic Tablets 2204
Zestoretic Tablets 695
Ziac Tablets 1887

Hydroflumethiazide (Potentiation of antihypertensive effect). Products include:
Diucardin Tablets 3494

Indapamide (Potentiation of antihypertensive effect). Products include:
Indapamide Tablets 2286

Irbesartan (Potentiation of antihypertensive effect). Products include:
Avalide Tablets 1070
Avapro Tablets 1074
Avapro Tablets 3076

Isocarboxazid (Concurrent use is contraindicated).
No products indexed under this heading.

Isoflurane (May require reduced dose of anesthetics).
No products indexed under this heading.

Isradipine (Potentiation of antihypertensive effect). Products include:
DynaCirc Capsules 2921
DynaCirc CR Tablets 2923

Ketamine Hydrochloride (May require reduced dose of anesthetics).
No products indexed under this heading.

Labetalol Hydrochloride (Potentiation of antihypertensive effect). Products include:
Normodyne Injection 3135
Normodyne Tablets 3137

Lisinopril (Potentiation of antihypertensive effect). Products include:
Prinivil Tablets 2164
Prinzide Tablets 2168
Zestoretic Tablets 695
Zestril Tablets 698

Lithium Carbonate (Potential for lithium toxicity). Products include:
Eskalith 1527
Lithium Carbonate 3061
Lithobid Slow-Release Tablets 3255

Lithium Citrate (Potential for lithium toxicity). Products include:
Lithium Citrate Syrup 3061

Losartan Potassium (Potentiation of antihypertensive effect). Products include:
Cozaar Tablets 2067
Hyzaar 2109

Mecamylamine Hydrochloride (Potentiation of antihypertensive effect). Products include:
Inversine Tablets 1850

Methohexital Sodium (May require reduced dose of anesthetics). Products include:
Brevital Sodium for Injection, USP .. 1815

Methoxyflurane (May require reduced dose of anesthetics).
No products indexed under this heading.

Methyclothiazide (Potentiation of antihypertensive effect).
No products indexed under this heading.

Methyldopate Hydrochloride (Potentiation of antihypertensive effect).
No products indexed under this heading.

Metolazone (Potentiation of antihypertensive effect). Products include:
Mykrox Tablets 1168
Zaroxolyn Tablets 1177

Metoprolol Succinate (Potentiation of antihypertensive effect). Products include:
Toprol-XL Tablets 651

Metoprolol Tartrate (Potentiation of antihypertensive effect).
No products indexed under this heading.

Metyrosine (Potentiation of antihypertensive effect). Products include:
Demser Capsules 2085

Mibefradil Dihydrochloride (Potentiation of antihypertensive effect).
No products indexed under this heading.

Minoxidil (Potentiation of antihypertensive effect). Products include:
Rogaine Extra Strength for Men Topical Solution .... ▣721
Rogaine for Women Topical Solution .... ▣721

Moclobemide (Concurrent use is contraindicated).
No products indexed under this heading.

Moexipril Hydrochloride (Potentiation of antihypertensive effect). Products include:
Uniretic Tablets 3178
Univasc Tablets 3181

Nadolol (Potentiation of antihypertensive effect). Products include:
Corgard Tablets 2245
Corzide 40/5 Tablets 2247
Corzide 80/5 Tablets 2247
Nadolol Tablets 2288

Nicardipine Hydrochloride (Potentiation of antihypertensive effect). Products include:
Cardene I.V. 3485

Nifedipine (Potentiation of antihypertensive effect). Products include:
Adalat CC Tablets 877
Procardia Capsules 2708
Procardia XL Extended Release Tablets 2710

Nisoldipine (Potentiation of antihypertensive effect). Products include:
Sular Tablets 688

Nitroglycerin (Potentiation of antihypertensive effect). Products include:
Nitro-Dur Transdermal Infusion System 3134
Nitro-Dur Transdermal Infusion System 1834
Nitrolingual Pumpspray 1355
Nitrostat Tablets 2658

IMPORTANT NOTE: Always consult each drug listing in the patient's regimen for possible interactions.

Pargyline Hydrochloride (Concurrent use is contraindicated).
No products indexed under this heading.

Penbutolol Sulfate (Potentiation of antihypertensive effect).
No products indexed under this heading.

Perindopril Erbumine (Potentiation of antihypertensive effect). Products include:
Aceon Tablets (2 mg, 4 mg, 8 mg) ... 3249

Phenelzine Sulfate (Concurrent use is contraindicated). Products include:
Nardil Tablets ... 2653

Phenoxybenzamine Hydrochloride (Potentiation of antihypertensive effect). Products include:
Dibenzyline Capsules ... 3457

Phentolamine Mesylate (Potentiation of antihypertensive effect).
No products indexed under this heading.

Pindolol (Potentiation of antihypertensive effect).
No products indexed under this heading.

Polythiazide (Potentiation of antihypertensive effect). Products include:
Minizide Capsules ... 2700
Renese Tablets ... 2712

Prazosin Hydrochloride (Potentiation of antihypertensive effect). Products include:
Minipress Capsules ... 2699
Minizide Capsules ... 2700

Procarbazine Hydrochloride (Concurrent use is contraindicated). Products include:
Matulane Capsules ... 3246

Propofol (May require reduced dose of anesthetics). Products include:
Diprivan Injectable Emulsion ... 667

Propranolol Hydrochloride (Potentiation of antihypertensive effect). Products include:
Inderal ... 3513
Inderal LA Long-Acting Capsules ... 3516
Inderide Tablets ... 3517
Inderide LA Long-Acting Capsules ... 3519

Quinapril Hydrochloride (Potentiation of antihypertensive effect). Products include:
Accupril Tablets ... 2611
Accuretic Tablets ... 2614

Ramipril (Potentiation of antihypertensive effect). Products include:
Altace Capsules ... 2233

Rauwolfia serpentina (Potentiation of antihypertensive effect).
No products indexed under this heading.

Rescinnamine (Potentiation of antihypertensive effect).
No products indexed under this heading.

Reserpine (Potentiation of antihypertensive effect).
No products indexed under this heading.

Selegiline Hydrochloride (Concurrent use is contraindicated). Products include:
Eldepryl Capsules ... 3266

Sevoflurane (May require reduced dose of anesthetics).
No products indexed under this heading.

Sodium Nitroprusside (Potentiation of antihypertensive effect).
No products indexed under this heading.

Sotalol Hydrochloride (Potentiation of antihypertensive effect). Products include:
Betapace Tablets ... 950
Betapace AF Tablets ... 954

Spirapril Hydrochloride (Potentiation of antihypertensive effect).
No products indexed under this heading.

Telmisartan (Potentiation of antihypertensive effect). Products include:
Micardis Tablets ... 1049
Micardis HCT Tablets ... 1051

Terazosin Hydrochloride (Potentiation of antihypertensive effect). Products include:
Hytrin Capsules ... 464

Timolol Maleate (Potentiation of antihypertensive effect). Products include:
Blocadren Tablets ... 2046
Cosopt Sterile Ophthalmic Solution ... 2065
Timolide Tablets ... 2187
Timolol GFS ... ⊙266
Timoptic in Ocudose ... 2192
Timoptic Sterile Ophthalmic Solution ... 2190
Timoptic-XE Sterile Ophthalmic Gel Forming Solution ... 2194

Torsemide (Potentiation of antihypertensive effect). Products include:
Demadex Tablets and Injection ... 2965

Trandolapril (Potentiation of antihypertensive effect). Products include:
Mavik Tablets ... 478
Tarka Tablets ... 508

Tranylcypromine Sulfate (Concurrent use is contraindicated). Products include:
Parnate Tablets ... 1607

Trimethaphan Camsylate (Potentiation of antihypertensive effect).
No products indexed under this heading.

Valsartan (Potentiation of antihypertensive effect). Products include:
Diovan Capsules ... 2337
Diovan HCT Tablets ... 2338

Verapamil Hydrochloride (Potentiation of antihypertensive effect). Products include:
Covera-HS Tablets ... 3199
Isoptin SR Tablets ... 467
Tarka Tablets ... 508
Verelan Capsules ... 3184
Verelan PM Capsules ... 3186

ALDORIL TABLETS

(Hydrochlorothiazide, Methyldopa) ... 2039

May interact with antihypertensives, barbiturates, corticosteroids, general anesthetics, cardiac glycosides, oral hypoglycemic agents, insulin, lithium preparations, monoamine oxidase inhibitors, narcotic analgesics, non-steroidal anti-inflammatory agents, and certain other agents. Compounds in these categories include:

Acarbose (Dosage adjustment of the antidiabetic drug may be required). Products include:
Precose Tablets ... 906

Acebutolol Hydrochloride (Potentiation of antihypertensive effect). Products include:
Sectral Capsules ... 3589

ACTH (Hypokalemia may result).
No products indexed under this heading.

Alfentanil Hydrochloride (Aggravates orthostatic hypotension).
No products indexed under this heading.

Amlodipine Besylate (Potentiation of antihypertensive effect). Products include:
Lotrel Capsules ... 2370
Norvasc Tablets ... 2704

Aprobarbital (Aggravates orthostatic hypotension).
No products indexed under this heading.

Atenolol (Potentiation of antihypertensive effect). Products include:
Tenoretic Tablets ... 690
Tenormin I.V. Injection ... 692

Benazepril Hydrochloride (Potentiation of antihypertensive effect). Products include:
Lotensin Tablets ... 2365
Lotensin HCT Tablets ... 2367
Lotrel Capsules ... 2370

Bendroflumethiazide (Potentiation of antihypertensive effect). Products include:
Corzide 40/5 Tablets ... 2247
Corzide 80/5 Tablets ... 2247

Betamethasone Acetate (Hypokalemia may result). Products include:
Celestone Soluspan Injectable Suspension ... 3097

Betamethasone Sodium Phosphate (Hypokalemia may result). Products include:
Celestone Soluspan Injectable Suspension ... 3097

Betaxolol Hydrochloride (Potentiation of antihypertensive effect). Products include:
Betoptic S Ophthalmic Suspension ... 537

Bisoprolol Fumarate (Potentiation of antihypertensive effect). Products include:
Zebeta Tablets ... 1885
Ziac Tablets ... 1887

Buprenorphine Hydrochloride (Aggravates orthostatic hypotension). Products include:
Buprenex Injectable ... 2918

Butabarbital (Aggravates orthostatic hypotension).
No products indexed under this heading.

Butalbital (Aggravates orthostatic hypotension). Products include:
Phrenilin ... 578
Sedapap Tablets 50 mg/650 mg ... 2225

Candesartan Cilexetil (Potentiation of antihypertensive effect). Products include:
Atacand Tablets ... 595
Atacand HCT Tablets ... 597

Captopril (Potentiation of antihypertensive effect). Products include:
Captopril Tablets ... 2281

Carteolol Hydrochloride (Potentiation of antihypertensive effect). Products include:
Carteolol Hydrochloride Ophthalmic Solution USP, 1% ... ⊙258
Ocupress Ophthalmic Solution, 1% Sterile ... ⊙303

Celecoxib (May result in reduced diuretic effect). Products include:
Celebrex Capsules ... 2676
Celebrex Capsules ... 2780

Chlorothiazide (Potentiation of antihypertensive effect). Products include:
Aldoclor Tablets ... 2035
Diuril Oral ... 2087

Chlorothiazide Sodium (Potentiation of antihypertensive effect). Products include:
Diuril Sodium Intravenous ... 2086

Chlorpropamide (Dosage adjustment of the antidiabetic drug may be required). Products include:
Diabinese Tablets ... 2680

Chlorthalidone (Potentiation of antihypertensive effect). Products include:
Clorpres Tablets ... 1002
Combipres Tablets ... 1040
Tenoretic Tablets ... 690

Cholestyramine (Binds the hydrochlorothiazide and reduces its absorption from gastrointestinal tract by up to 85%).
No products indexed under this heading.

Clonidine (Potentiation of antihypertensive effect). Products include:
Catapres-TTS ... 1038

Clonidine Hydrochloride (Potentiation of antihypertensive effect). Products include:
Catapres Tablets ... 1037
Clorpres Tablets ... 1002
Combipres Tablets ... 1040
Duraclon Injection ... 3057

Codeine Phosphate (Aggravates orthostatic hypotension). Products include:
Phenergan with Codeine Syrup ... 3557
Phenergan VC with Codeine Syrup ... 3561
Robitussin A-C Syrup ... 2942
Robitussin-DAC Syrup ... 2942
Ryna-C Liquid ... [nonprescription symbol]768
Soma Compound w/Codeine Tablets ... 3355
Tussi-Organidin NR Liquid ... 3350
Tussi-Organidin-S NR Liquid ... 3350
Tylenol with Codeine ... 2595

Colestipol Hydrochloride (Binds the hydrochlorothiazide and reduces its absorption from gastrointestinal tract by up to 43%). Products include:
Colestid Tablets ... 2791

Cortisone Acetate (Hypokalemia may result). Products include:
Cortone Acetate Injectable Suspension ... 2059
Cortone Acetate Tablets ... 2061

Deserpidine (Potentiation of antihypertensive effect).
No products indexed under this heading.

Deslanoside (Hypokalemia may exaggerate cardiac toxicity of digitalis).
No products indexed under this heading.

Dexamethasone (Hypokalemia may result). Products include:
Decadron Elixir ... 2078
Decadron Tablets ... 2079
TobraDex Ophthalmic Ointment ... 542
TobraDex Ophthalmic Suspension ... 541

Dexamethasone Acetate (Hypokalemia may result).
No products indexed under this heading.

Dexamethasone Sodium Phosphate (Hypokalemia may result). Products include:
Decadron Phosphate Injection ... 2081
Decadron Phosphate Sterile Ophthalmic Ointment ... 2083
Decadron Phosphate Sterile Ophthalmic Solution ... 2084
NeoDecadron Sterile Ophthalmic Solution ... 2144

Dezocine (Aggravates orthostatic hypotension).
No products indexed under this heading.

Diazoxide (Potentiation of antihypertensive effect).
No products indexed under this heading.

Diclofenac Potassium (May result in reduced diuretic effect). Products include:
Cataflam Tablets ... 2315

Diclofenac Sodium (May result in reduced diuretic effect). Products include:
Arthrotec Tablets ... 3195
Voltaren Ophthalmic Sterile Ophthalmic Solution ... ⊙312
Voltaren Tablets ... 2315
Voltaren-XR Tablets ... 2315

Digitoxin (Hypokalemia may exaggerate cardiac toxicity of digitalis).
No products indexed under this heading.

Digoxin (Hypokalemia may exaggerate cardiac toxicity of digitalis). Products include:
Digitek Tablets ... 1003
Lanoxicaps Capsules ... 1574
Lanoxin Injection ... 1581
Lanoxin Tablets ... 1587
Lanoxin Elixir Pediatric ... 1578
Lanoxin Injection Pediatric ... 1584

Diltiazem Hydrochloride (Potentiation of antihypertensive effect). Products include:
Cardizem Injectable ... 1018
Cardizem Lyo-Ject Syringe ... 1018
Cardizem Monovial ... 1018
Cardizem CD Capsules ... 1016
Tiazac Capsules ... 1378

Doxazosin Mesylate (Potentiation of antihypertensive effect). Products include:
Cardura Tablets ... 2668

Enalapril Maleate (Potentiation of antihypertensive effect). Products include:
- Lexxel Tablets ... 608
- Vaseretic Tablets ... 2204
- Vasotec Tablets ... 2210

Enalaprilat (Potentiation of antihypertensive effect). Products include:
- Enalaprilat Injection ... 863
- Vasotec I.V. Injection ... 2207

Enflurane (May require reduced dose of anesthetics).
- No products indexed under this heading.

Eprosartan Mesylate (Potentiation of antihypertensive effect). Products include:
- Teveten Tablets ... 3327

Esmolol Hydrochloride (Potentiation of antihypertensive effect). Products include:
- Brevibloc Injection ... 858

Etodolac (May result in reduced diuretic effect). Products include:
- Lodine ... 3528
- Lodine XL Extended-Release Tablets ... 3530

Felodipine (Potentiation of antihypertensive effect). Products include:
- Lexxel Tablets ... 608
- Plendil Extended-Release Tablets ... 623

Fenoprofen Calcium (May result in reduced diuretic effect).
- No products indexed under this heading.

Fentanyl (Aggravates orthostatic hypotension). Products include:
- Duragesic Transdermal System ... 1786

Fentanyl Citrate (Aggravates orthostatic hypotension). Products include:
- Actiq ... 1184

Ferrous Gluconate (Co-administration results in a decrease in the bioavailability of methyldopa; this may adversely affect blood pressure control in patients treated with methlydopa; concurrent use is not recommended). Products include:
- Fergon Iron Tablets ... ▣802

Ferrous Sulfate (Co-administration results in a decrease in the bioavailability of methyldopa; this may adversely affect blood pressure control in patients treated with methlydopa; concurrent use is not recommended). Products include:
- Feosol Tablets ... 1717
- Slow Fe Tablets ... ▣827
- Slow Fe with Folic Acid Tablets ... ▣828

Fludrocortisone Acetate (Hypokalemia may result). Products include:
- Florinef Acetate Tablets ... 2250

Flurbiprofen (May result in reduced diuretic effect).
- No products indexed under this heading.

Fosinopril Sodium (Potentiation of antihypertensive effect). Products include:
- Monopril Tablets ... 1091
- Monopril HCT ... 1094

Furosemide (Potentiation of antihypertensive effect). Products include:
- Furosemide Tablets ... 2284

Glimepiride (Dosage adjustment of the antidiabetic drug may be required). Products include:
- Amaryl Tablets ... 717

Glipizide (Dosage adjustment of the antidiabetic drug may be required). Products include:
- Glucotrol Tablets ... 2692
- Glucotrol XL Extended Release Tablets ... 2693

Glyburide (Dosage adjustment of the antidiabetic drug may be required). Products include:
- DiaBeta Tablets ... 741
- Glucovance Tablets ... 1086

Guanabenz Acetate (Potentiation of antihypertensive effect).
- No products indexed under this heading.

Guanethidine Monosulfate (Potentiation of antihypertensive effect).
- No products indexed under this heading.

Hydralazine Hydrochloride (Potentiation of antihypertensive effect).
- No products indexed under this heading.

Hydrocodone Bitartrate (Aggravates orthostatic hypotension). Products include:
- Hycodan ... 1316
- Hycomine Compound Tablets ... 1317
- Hycotuss Expectorant Syrup ... 1318
- Lortab ... 3319
- Lortab Elixir ... 3317
- Maxidone Tablets CIII ... 3399
- Norco 5/325 Tablets CIII ... 3424
- Norco 7.5/325 Tablets CIII ... 3425
- Norco 10/325 Tablets CIII ... 3427
- Norco 10/325 Tablets CIII ... 3425
- Vicodin Tablets ... 516
- Vicodin ES Tablets ... 517
- Vicodin HP Tablets ... 518
- Vicodin Tuss Expectorant ... 519
- Vicoprofen Tablets ... 520
- Zydone Tablets ... 1330

Hydrocodone Polistirex (Aggravates orthostatic hypotension). Products include:
- Tussionex Pennkinetic Extended-Release Suspension ... 1174

Hydrocortisone (Hypokalemia may result). Products include:
- Anusol-HC Cream 2.5% ... 2237
- Cipro HC Otic Suspension ... 540
- Cortaid Intensive Therapy Cream ... ▣717
- Cortaid Maximum Strength Cream ... ▣717
- Cortisporin Ophthalmic Suspension Sterile ... ⊙297
- Cortizone•5 ... ▣699
- Cortizone•10 ... ▣699
- Cortizone•10 Plus Creme ... ▣700
- Cortizone for Kids Creme ... ▣699
- Hydrocortone Tablets ... 2106
- Massengill Medicated Soft Cloth Towelette ... ▣753
- VōSoL HC Otic Solution ... 3356

Hydrocortisone Acetate (Hypokalemia may result). Products include:
- Analpram-HC ... 1338
- Anusol HC-1 Hydrocortisone Anti-Itch Cream ... ▣689
- Anusol-HC Suppositories ... 2238
- Cortaid ... ▣717
- Cortifoam Rectal Foam ... 3170
- Cortisporin-TC Otic Suspension ... 2246
- Hydrocortone Acetate Injectable Suspension ... 2103
- Pramosone ... 1343
- Proctocort Suppositories ... 2264
- ProctoFoam-HC ... 3177
- Terra-Cortril Ophthalmic Suspension ... 2716

Hydrocortisone Sodium Phosphate (Hypokalemia may result). Products include:
- Hydrocortone Phosphate Injection, Sterile ... 2105

Hydrocortisone Sodium Succinate (Hypokalemia may result).
- No products indexed under this heading.

Hydroflumethiazide (Potentiation of antihypertensive effect). Products include:
- Diucardin Tablets ... 3494

Hydromorphone Hydrochloride (Aggravates orthostatic hypotension). Products include:
- Dilaudid ... 441
- Dilaudid Oral Liquid ... 445
- Dilaudid Powder ... 441
- Dilaudid Rectal Suppositories ... 441
- Dilaudid Tablets ... 441
- Dilaudid Tablets - 8 mg ... 445
- Dilaudid-HP ... 443

Ibuprofen (May result in reduced diuretic effect). Products include:
- Advil ... ▣771
- Children's Advil Oral Suspension ... ▣773
- Children's Advil Chewable Tablets ... ▣773
- Advil Cold and Sinus Caplets ... ▣771
- Advil Cold and Sinus Tablets ... ▣771
- Advil Flu & Body Ache Caplets ... ▣772
- Infants' Advil Drops ... ▣773
- Junior Strength Advil Tablets ... ▣773
- Junior Strength Advil Chewable Tablets ... ▣773
- Advil Migraine Liquigels ... ▣772
- Children's Motrin Oral Suspension and Chewable Tablets ... 2006
- Children's Motrin Cold Oral Suspension ... 2007
- Children's Motrin Oral Suspension ... ▣643
- Motrin Suspension, Oral Drops, Chewable Tablets, and Caplets ... 2002
- Infants' Motrin Concentrated Drops ... 2006
- Junior Strength Motrin Caplets and Chewable Tablets ... 2006
- Motrin IB Tablets, Caplets, and Gelcaps ... 2002
- Motrin Migraine Pain Caplets ... 2005
- Motrin Sinus Headache Caplets ... 2005
- Vicoprofen Tablets ... 520

Indapamide (Potentiation of antihypertensive effect). Products include:
- Indapamide Tablets ... 2286

Indomethacin (May result in reduced diuretic effect). Products include:
- Indocin ... 2112

Indomethacin Sodium Trihydrate (May result in reduced diuretic effect). Products include:
- Indocin I.V. ... 2115

Insulin, Human, Zinc Suspension (Insulin requirement may be altered). Products include:
- Humulin L, 100 Units ... 1937
- Humulin U, 100 Units ... 1943
- Novolin L Human Insulin 10 ml Vials ... 2422

Insulin, Human NPH (Insulin requirement may be altered). Products include:
- Humulin N, 100 Units ... 1939
- Humulin N NPH Pen ... 1940
- Novolin N Human Insulin 10 ml Vials ... 2422
- Novolin N PenFill ... 2423
- Novolin N Prefilled Syringe Disposable Insulin Delivery System ... 2425

Insulin, Human Regular (Insulin requirement may be altered). Products include:
- Humulin R Regular (U-500) ... 1943
- Humulin R, 100 Units ... 1941
- Novolin R Human Insulin 10 ml Vials ... 2423
- Novolin R PenFill ... 2423
- Novolin R Prefilled Syringe Disposable Insulin Delivery System ... 2425
- Velosulin BR Human Insulin 10 ml Vials ... 2435

Insulin, Human Regular and Human NPH Mixture (Insulin requirement may be altered). Products include:
- Humulin 50/50, 100 Units ... 1934
- Humulin 70/30, 100 Units ... 1935
- Humulin 70/30 Pen ... 1936
- Novolin 70/30 Human Insulin 10 ml Vials ... 2421
- Novolin 70/30 PenFill ... 2423
- Novolin 70/30 Prefilled Disposable Insulin Delivery System ... 2425

Insulin, NPH (Insulin requirement may be altered). Products include:
- Iletin II, NPH (Pork), 100 Units ... 1946

Insulin, Regular (Insulin requirement may be altered). Products include:
- Iletin II, Regular (Pork), 100 Units ... 1947

Insulin, Zinc Crystals (Insulin requirement may be altered).
- No products indexed under this heading.

Insulin, Zinc Suspension (Insulin requirement may be altered). Products include:
- Iletin II, Lente (Pork), 100 Units ... 1945

Insulin Aspart, Human Regular (Insulin requirement may be altered).
- No products indexed under this heading.

Insulin glargine (Insulin requirement may be altered). Products include:
- Lantus Injection ... 742

Insulin Lispro, Human (Insulin requirement may be altered). Products include:
- Humalog ... 1926
- Humalog Mix 75/25 Pen ... 1928

Insulin Lispro Protamine, Human (Insulin requirement may be altered). Products include:
- Humalog Mix 75/25 Pen ... 1928

Irbesartan (Potentiation of antihypertensive effect). Products include:
- Avalide Tablets ... 1070
- Avapro Tablets ... 1074
- Avapro Tablets ... 3076

Isocarboxazid (Concurrent use is contraindicated).
- No products indexed under this heading.

Isoflurane (May require reduced dose of anesthetics).
- No products indexed under this heading.

Isradipine (Potentiation of antihypertensive effect). Products include:
- DynaCirc Capsules ... 2921
- DynaCirc CR Tablets ... 2923

Ketamine Hydrochloride (May require reduced dose of anesthetics).
- No products indexed under this heading.

Ketoprofen (May result in reduced diuretic effect). Products include:
- Orudis Capsules ... 3548
- Orudis KT Tablets ... ▣778
- Oruvail Capsules ... 3548

Ketorolac Tromethamine (May result in reduced diuretic effect). Products include:
- Acular Ophthalmic Solution ... 544
- Acular PF Ophthalmic Solution ... 544
- Toradol ... 3018

Labetalol Hydrochloride (Potentiation of antihypertensive effect). Products include:
- Normodyne Injection ... 3135
- Normodyne Tablets ... 3137

Levorphanol Tartrate (Aggravates orthostatic hypotension). Products include:
- Levo-Dromoran ... 1734
- Levorphanol Tartrate Tablets ... 3059

Lisinopril (Potentiation of antihypertensive effect). Products include:
- Prinivil Tablets ... 2164
- Prinzide Tablets ... 2168
- Zestoretic Tablets ... 695
- Zestril Tablets ... 698

Lithium Carbonate (High risk of lithium toxicity). Products include:
- Eskalith ... 1527
- Lithium Carbonate ... 3061
- Lithobid Slow-Release Tablets ... 3255

Lithium Citrate (High risk of lithium toxicity). Products include:
- Lithium Citrate Syrup ... 3061

Losartan Potassium (Potentiation of antihypertensive effect). Products include:
- Cozaar Tablets ... 2067
- Hyzaar ... 2109

Mecamylamine Hydrochloride (Potentiation of antihypertensive effect). Products include:
- Inversine Tablets ... 1850

Meclofenamate Sodium (May result in reduced diuretic effect).
- No products indexed under this heading.

Mefenamic Acid (May result in reduced diuretic effect). Products include:
- Ponstel Capsules ... 1356

Meloxicam (May result in reduced diuretic effect). Products include:
- Mobic Tablets ... 1054

Meperidine Hydrochloride (Aggravates orthostatic hypotension). Products include:
- Demerol ... 3079
- Mepergan Injection ... 3539

IMPORTANT NOTE: Always consult each drug listing in the patient's regimen for possible interactions.

Mephobarbital (Aggravates orthostatic hypotension).
No products indexed under this heading.

Metformin Hydrochloride (Dosage adjustment of the antidiabetic drug may be required). Products include:
Glucophage Tablets 1080
Glucophage XR Tablets 1080
Glucovance Tablets 1086

Methadone Hydrochloride (Aggravates orthostatic hypotension). Products include:
Dolophine Hydrochloride Tablets 3056

Methohexital Sodium (May require reduced dose of anesthetics). Products include:
Brevital Sodium for Injection, USP .. 1815

Methoxyflurane (May require reduced dose of anesthetics).
No products indexed under this heading.

Methyclothiazide (Potentiation of antihypertensive effect).
No products indexed under this heading.

Methyldopate Hydrochloride (Potentiation of antihypertensive effect).
No products indexed under this heading.

Methylprednisolone Acetate (Hypokalemia may result). Products include:
Depo-Medrol Injectable Suspension 2795

Methylprednisolone Sodium Succinate (Hypokalemia may result). Products include:
Solu-Medrol Sterile Powder 2855

Metolazone (Potentiation of antihypertensive effect). Products include:
Mykrox Tablets 1168
Zaroxolyn Tablets 1177

Metoprolol Succinate (Potentiation of antihypertensive effect). Products include:
Toprol-XL Tablets 651

Metoprolol Tartrate (Potentiation of antihypertensive effect).
No products indexed under this heading.

Metyrosine (Potentiation of antihypertensive effect). Products include:
Demser Capsules 2085

Mibefradil Dihydrochloride (Potentiation of antihypertensive effect).
No products indexed under this heading.

Miglitol (Dosage adjustment of the antidiabetic drug may be required). Products include:
Glyset Tablets 2821

Minoxidil (Potentiation of antihypertensive effect). Products include:
Rogaine Extra Strength for Men Topical Solution .... ■721
Rogaine for Women Topical Solution .... ■721

Moclobemide (Concurrent use is contraindicated).
No products indexed under this heading.

Moexipril Hydrochloride (Potentiation of antihypertensive effect). Products include:
Uniretic Tablets 3178
Univasc Tablets 3181

Morphine Sulfate (Aggravates orthostatic hypotension). Products include:
Astramorph/PF Injection, USP (Preservative-Free) 594
Duramorph Injection 1312
Infumorph 200 and Infumorph 500 Sterile Solutions 1314
Kadian Capsules 1335
MS Contin Tablets 2896
MSIR 2898
Oramorph SR Tablets 3062
Roxanol 3066

Nabumetone (May result in reduced diuretic effect). Products include:
Relafen Tablets 1617

Nadolol (Potentiation of antihypertensive effect). Products include:
Corgard Tablets 2245
Corzide 40/5 Tablets 2247
Corzide 80/5 Tablets 2247
Nadolol Tablets 2288

Naproxen (May result in reduced diuretic effect). Products include:
EC-Naprosyn Delayed-Release Tablets 2967
Naprosyn Suspension 2967
Naprosyn Tablets 2967

Naproxen Sodium (May result in reduced diuretic effect). Products include:
Aleve Tablets, Caplets and Gelcaps .... ■602
Aleve Cold & Sinus Caplets .... ■603
Anaprox Tablets 2967
Anaprox DS Tablets 2967
Naprelan Tablets 1293

Nicardipine Hydrochloride (Potentiation of antihypertensive effect). Products include:
Cardene I.V. 3485

Nifedipine (Potentiation of antihypertensive effect). Products include:
Adalat CC Tablets 877
Procardia Capsules 2708
Procardia XL Extended Release Tablets 2710

Nisoldipine (Potentiation of antihypertensive effect). Products include:
Sular Tablets 688

Nitroglycerin (Potentiation of antihypertensive effect). Products include:
Nitro-Dur Transdermal Infusion System 3134
Nitro-Dur Transdermal Infusion System 1834
Nitrolingual Pumpspray 1355
Nitrostat Tablets 2658

Norepinephrine Bitartrate (Decreased arterial responsiveness to norepinephrine).
No products indexed under this heading.

Oxaprozin (May result in reduced diuretic effect).
No products indexed under this heading.

Oxycodone Hydrochloride (Aggravates orthostatic hypotension). Products include:
OxyContin Tablets 2912
OxyFast Oral Concentrate Solution . 2916
OxyIR Capsules 2916
Percocet Tablets 1326
Percodan Tablets 1327
Percolone Tablets 1327
Roxicodone 3067
Tylox Capsules 2597

Pargyline Hydrochloride (Concurrent use is contraindicated).
No products indexed under this heading.

Penbutolol Sulfate (Potentiation of antihypertensive effect).
No products indexed under this heading.

Pentobarbital Sodium (Aggravates orthostatic hypotension). Products include:
Nembutal Sodium Solution 485

Perindopril Erbumine (Potentiation of antihypertensive effect). Products include:
Aceon Tablets (2 mg, 4 mg, 8 mg) 3249

Phenelzine Sulfate (Concurrent use is contraindicated). Products include:
Nardil Tablets 2653

Phenobarbital (Aggravates orthostatic hypotension). Products include:
Arco-Lase Plus Tablets 592
Donnatal 2929
Donnatal Extentabs 2930

Phenoxybenzamine Hydrochloride (Potentiation of antihypertensive effect). Products include:
Dibenzyline Capsules 3457

Phentolamine Mesylate (Potentiation of antihypertensive effect).
No products indexed under this heading.

Phenylbutazone (May result in reduced diuretic effect).
No products indexed under this heading.

Pindolol (Potentiation of antihypertensive effect).
No products indexed under this heading.

Pioglitazone Hydrochloride (Dosage adjustment of the antidiabetic drug may be required). Products include:
Actos Tablets 3275

Piroxicam (May result in reduced diuretic effect). Products include:
Feldene Capsules 2685

Polythiazide (Potentiation of antihypertensive effect). Products include:
Minizide Capsules 2700
Renese Tablets 2712

Prazosin Hydrochloride (Potentiation of antihypertensive effect). Products include:
Minipress Capsules 2699
Minizide Capsules 2700

Prednisolone Acetate (Hypokalemia may result). Products include:
Blephamide Ophthalmic Ointment .. 547
Blephamide Ophthalmic Suspension 548
Poly-Pred Liquifilm Ophthalmic Suspension .... ⊙245
Pred Forte Ophthalmic Suspension .... ⊙246
Pred Mild Sterile Ophthalmic Suspension .... ⊙249
Pred-G Ophthalmic Suspension ..... ⊙247
Pred-G Sterile Ophthalmic Ointment .... ⊙248

Prednisolone Sodium Phosphate (Hypokalemia may result). Products include:
Pediapred Oral Solution 1170

Prednisolone Tebutate (Hypokalemia may result).
No products indexed under this heading.

Prednisone (Hypokalemia may result). Products include:
Prednisone 3064

Procarbazine Hydrochloride (Concurrent use is contraindicated). Products include:
Matulane Capsules 3246

Propofol (May require reduced dose of anesthetics). Products include:
Diprivan Injectable Emulsion 667

Propoxyphene Hydrochloride (Aggravates orthostatic hypotension). Products include:
Darvon Pulvules 1909
Darvon Compound-65 Pulvules 1910

Propoxyphene Napsylate (Aggravates orthostatic hypotension). Products include:
Darvon-N/Darvocet-N 1907
Darvon-N Tablets 1912

Propranolol Hydrochloride (Potentiation of antihypertensive effect). Products include:
Inderal 3513
Inderal LA Long-Acting Capsules 3516
Inderide Tablets 3517
Inderide LA Long-Acting Capsules .. 3519

Quinapril Hydrochloride (Potentiation of antihypertensive effect). Products include:
Accupril Tablets 2611
Accuretic Tablets 2614

Ramipril (Potentiation of antihypertensive effect). Products include:
Altace Capsules 2233

Rauwolfia serpentina (Potentiation of antihypertensive effect).
No products indexed under this heading.

Remifentanil Hydrochloride (Aggravates orthostatic hypotension).
No products indexed under this heading.

Repaglinide (Dosage adjustment of the antidiabetic drug may be required). Products include:
Prandin Tablets (0.5, 1, and 2 mg) 2432

Rescinnamine (Potentiation of antihypertensive effect).
No products indexed under this heading.

Reserpine (Potentiation of antihypertensive effect).
No products indexed under this heading.

Rofecoxib (May result in reduced diuretic effect). Products include:
Vioxx 2213

Rosiglitazone Maleate (Dosage adjustment of the antidiabetic drug may be required). Products include:
Avandia Tablets 1490

Secobarbital Sodium (Aggravates orthostatic hypotension).
No products indexed under this heading.

Selegiline Hydrochloride (Concurrent use is contraindicated). Products include:
Eldepryl Capsules 3266

Sevoflurane (May require reduced dose of anesthetics).
No products indexed under this heading.

Sodium Nitroprusside (Potentiation of antihypertensive effect).
No products indexed under this heading.

Sotalol Hydrochloride (Potentiation of antihypertensive effect). Products include:
Betapace Tablets 950
Betapace AF Tablets 954

Spirapril Hydrochloride (Potentiation of antihypertensive effect).
No products indexed under this heading.

Sufentanil Citrate (Aggravates orthostatic hypotension).
No products indexed under this heading.

Sulindac (May result in reduced diuretic effect). Products include:
Clinoril Tablets 2053

Telmisartan (Potentiation of antihypertensive effect). Products include:
Micardis Tablets 1049
Micardis HCT Tablets 1051

Terazosin Hydrochloride (Potentiation of antihypertensive effect). Products include:
Hytrin Capsules 464

Thiamylal Sodium (Aggravates orthostatic hypotension).
No products indexed under this heading.

Timolol Maleate (Potentiation of antihypertensive effect). Products include:
Blocadren Tablets 2046
Cosopt Sterile Ophthalmic Solution 2065
Timolide Tablets 2187
Timolol GFS .... ⊙266
Timoptic in Ocudose 2192
Timoptic Sterile Ophthalmic Solution 2190
Timoptic-XE Sterile Ophthalmic Gel Forming Solution 2194

Tolazamide (Dosage adjustment of the antidiabetic drug may be required).
No products indexed under this heading.

Tolbutamide (Dosage adjustment of the antidiabetic drug may be required).
No products indexed under this heading.

Tolmetin Sodium (May result in reduced diuretic effect). Products include:
Tolectin 2589

Torsemide (Potentiation of antihypertensive effect). Products include:
Demadex Tablets and Injection 2965

Trandolapril (Potentiation of antihypertensive effect). Products include:
Mavik Tablets 478
Tarka Tablets 508

Tranylcypromine Sulfate (Concurrent use is contraindicated). Products include:
Parnate Tablets 1607

Triamcinolone (Hypokalemia may result).
No products indexed under this heading.

Triamcinolone Acetonide (Hypokalemia may result). Products include:
Azmacort Inhalation Aerosol 728
Nasacort Nasal Inhaler 750
Nasacort AQ Nasal Spray 752
Tri-Nasal Spray 2274

Triamcinolone Diacetate (Hypokalemia may result).
No products indexed under this heading.

Triamcinolone Hexacetonide (Hypokalemia may result).
No products indexed under this heading.

Trimethaphan Camsylate (Potentiation of antihypertensive effect).
No products indexed under this heading.

Troglitazone (Dosage adjustment of the antidiabetic drug may be required).
No products indexed under this heading.

Tubocurarine Chloride (Increased responsiveness to tubocurarine).
No products indexed under this heading.

Valsartan (Potentiation of antihypertensive effect). Products include:
Diovan Capsules 2337
Diovan HCT Tablets 2338

Verapamil Hydrochloride (Potentiation of antihypertensive effect). Products include:
Covera-HS Tablets 3199
Isoptin SR Tablets 467
Tarka Tablets 508
Verelan Capsules 3184
Verelan PM Capsules 3186

Food Interactions

Alcohol (Aggravates orthostatic hypotension).

ALESSE-21 TABLETS

(Ethinyl Estradiol, Levonorgestrel) 3468
May interact with barbiturates, phenytoin, tetracyclines, and certain other agents. Compounds in these categories include:

Ampicillin (Potential for reduced efficacy and increased incidence of breakthrough bleeding and menstrual irregularities with concomitant use).
No products indexed under this heading.

Ampicillin Sodium (Potential for reduced efficacy and increased incidence of breakthrough bleeding and menstrual irregularities with concomitant use). Products include:
Unasyn for Injection 2728

Aprobarbital (Potential for reduced efficacy and increased incidence of breakthrough bleeding and menstrual irregularities with concomitant use).
No products indexed under this heading.

Butabarbital (Potential for reduced efficacy and increased incidence of breakthrough bleeding and menstrual irregularities with concomitant use).
No products indexed under this heading.

Butalbital (Potential for reduced efficacy and increased incidence of breakthrough bleeding and menstrual irregularities with concomitant use). Products include:
Phrenilin 578
Sedapap Tablets 50 mg/650 mg ... 2225

Demeclocycline Hydrochloride (Potential for reduced efficacy and increased incidence of breakthrough bleeding and menstrual irregularities with concomitant use). Products include:
Declomycin Tablets 1855

Doxycycline Calcium (Potential for reduced efficacy and increased incidence of breakthrough bleeding and menstrual irregularities with concomitant use). Products include:
Vibramycin Calcium Oral Suspension Syrup 2735

Doxycycline Hyclate (Potential for reduced efficacy and increased incidence of breakthrough bleeding and menstrual irregularities with concomitant use). Products include:
Doryx Coated Pellet Filled Capsules 3357
Periostat Tablets 1208
Vibramycin Hyclate Capsules 2735
Vibramycin Hyclate Intravenous 2737
Vibra-Tabs Film Coated Tablets 2735

Doxycycline Monohydrate (Potential for reduced efficacy and increased incidence of breakthrough bleeding and menstrual irregularities with concomitant use). Products include:
Monodox Capsules 2442
Vibramycin Monohydrate for Oral Suspension 2735

Fosphenytoin Sodium (Potential for reduced efficacy and increased incidence of breakthrough bleeding and menstrual irregularities with concomitant use). Products include:
Cerebyx Injection 2619

Griseofulvin (Potential for reduced efficacy and increased incidence of breakthrough bleeding and menstrual irregularities with concomitant use). Products include:
Grifulvin V Tablets Microsize and Oral Suspension Microsize 2518
Gris-PEG Tablets 2661

Mephobarbital (Potential for reduced efficacy and increased incidence of breakthrough bleeding and menstrual irregularities with concomitant use).
No products indexed under this heading.

Methacycline Hydrochloride (Potential for reduced efficacy and increased incidence of breakthrough bleeding and menstrual irregularities with concomitant use).
No products indexed under this heading.

Minocycline Hydrochloride (Potential for reduced efficacy and increased incidence of breakthrough bleeding and menstrual irregularities with concomitant use). Products include:
Dynacin Capsules 2019
Minocin Intravenous 1862
Minocin Oral Suspension 1865
Minocin Pellet-Filled Capsules 1863

Oxytetracycline Hydrochloride (Potential for reduced efficacy and increased incidence of breakthrough bleeding and menstrual irregularities with concomitant use). Products include:
Terra-Cortril Ophthalmic Suspension 2716
Urobiotic-250 Capsules 2731

Pentobarbital Sodium (Potential for reduced efficacy and increased incidence of breakthrough bleeding and menstrual irregularities with concomitant use). Products include:
Nembutal Sodium Solution 485

Phenobarbital (Potential for reduced efficacy and increased incidence of breakthrough bleeding and menstrual irregularities with concomitant use). Products include:
Arco-Lase Plus Tablets 592
Donnatal 2929
Donnatal Extentabs 2930

Phenylbutazone (Potential for reduced efficacy and increased incidence of breakthrough bleeding and menstrual irregularities with concomitant use).
No products indexed under this heading.

Phenytoin (Potential for reduced efficacy and increased incidence of breakthrough bleeding and menstrual irregularities with concomitant use). Products include:
Dilantin Infatabs 2624
Dilantin-125 Oral Suspension 2625

Phenytoin Sodium (Potential for reduced efficacy and increased incidence of breakthrough bleeding and menstrual irregularities with concomitant use). Products include:
Dilantin Kapseals 2622

Rifampin (Co-administration has been associated with reduced efficacy and increased incidence of breakthrough bleeding and menstrual irregularities). Products include:
Rifadin 765
Rifamate Capsules 767
Rifater Tablets 769

Secobarbital Sodium (Potential for reduced efficacy and increased incidence of breakthrough bleeding and menstrual irregularities with concomitant use).
No products indexed under this heading.

Tetracycline Hydrochloride (Potential for reduced efficacy and increased incidence of breakthrough bleeding and menstrual irregularities with concomitant use).
No products indexed under this heading.

Thiamylal Sodium (Potential for reduced efficacy and increased incidence of breakthrough bleeding and menstrual irregularities with concomitant use).
No products indexed under this heading.

Troleandomycin (May increase the risk of intrahepatic cholestasis). Products include:
Tao Capsules 2716

ALESSE-28 TABLETS

(Ethinyl Estradiol, Levonorgestrel) 3473
See Alesse-21 Tablets

ALEVE TABLETS, CAPLETS AND GELCAPS

(Naproxen Sodium) .... ■602
May interact with:

Acetaminophen (Concurrent administration with other pain relievers/fever reducers is not recommended unless advised by a physician). Products include:
Actifed Cold & Sinus Caplets and Tablets .... ■688
Alka-Seltzer Plus Liqui-Gels .... ■604
Alka-Seltzer Plus Cold & Flu Medicine Liqui-Gels .... ■604
Alka-Seltzer Plus Cold & Sinus Medicine Liqui-Gels .... ■604
Benadryl Allergy/Cold Tablets .... ■691
Benadryl Allergy Sinus Headache Caplets & Gelcaps .... ■693
Benadryl Severe Allergy & Sinus Headache Caplets .... ■694
Children's Cēpacol Sore Throat .... ■788
Comtrex Acute Head Cold & Sinus Pressure Relief Tablets .... ■627
Comtrex Deep Chest Cold & Congestion Relief Softgels .... ■627
Comtrex Flu Therapy & Fever Relief Daytime Caplets .... ■628
Comtrex Flu Therapy & Fever Relief Nighttime Tablets .... ■628
Comtrex Maximum Strength Multi-Symptom Cold & Cough Relief Tablets and Caplets .... ■626
Contac Severe Cold and Flu Caplets Maximum Strength .... ■746
Contac Severe Cold and Flu Caplets Non-Drowsy .... ■746
Coricidin 'D' Cold, Flu & Sinus Tablets .... ■737
Coricidin HBP Cold & Flu Tablets ... ■738
Coricidin HBP Maximum Strength Flu Tablets .... ■738
Coricidin HBP Night-Time Cold & Flu Tablets .... ■738
Darvon-N/Darvocet-N 1907
Dimetapp Cold and Fever Suspension .... ■775
Dimetapp Nighttime Flu Liquid .... ■776
Dimetapp Non-Drowsy Flu Syrup ... ■777
Drixoral Allergy/Sinus Extended-Release Tablets .... ■741
Drixoral Cold & Flu Extended-Release Tablets .... ■740
Aspirin Free Excedrin Caplets and Geltabs .... ■628
Excedrin Extra-Strength Tablets, Caplets, and Geltabs .... ■629
Excedrin Migraine 1070
Excedrin PM Tablets, Caplets, and Geltabs .... ■631
Goody's Body Pain Formula Powder .... ■620
Goody's Extra Strength Headache Powder .... ■620
Goody's Extra Strength Pain Relief Tablets .... ■620
Goody's PM Powder .... ■621
Hycomine Compound Tablets 1317
Lortab 3319
Lortab Elixir 3317
Maxidone Tablets CIII 3399
Maximum Strength Midol Menstrual Caplets and Gelcaps ... ■612
Maximum Strength Midol PMS Caplets and Gelcaps .... ■613
Maximum Strength Midol Teen Caplets .... ■612
Midrin Capsules 3464
Norco 5/325 Tablets CIII 3424
Norco 7.5/325 Tablets CIII 3425
Norco 10/325 Tablets CIII 3427
Norco 10/325 Tablets CIII 3425
Percocet Tablets 1326
Percogesic Aspirin-Free Coated Tablets .... ■667
Extra Strength Percogesic Aspirin-Free Coated Caplets .... ■665
Phrenilin 578
Robitussin Cold Caplets Multi-Symptom Cold & Flu .... ■781
Robitussin Cold Softgels Multi-Symptom Cold & Flu .... ■781
Robitussin Multi Symptom Honey Flu Liquid .... ■785
Robitussin Nighttime Honey Flu Liquid .... ■786
Sedapap Tablets 50 mg/650 mg ... 2225
Singlet Caplets .... ■761
Sinutab Sinus Allergy Medication, Maximum Strength Formula, Tablets & Caplets .... ■707
Sinutab Sinus Medication, Maximum Strength Without Drowsiness Formula, Tablets & Caplets .... ■707
Sudafed Cold & Cough Liquid Caps .... ■709
Sudafed Cold & Sinus Liquid Caps .... ■710
Sudafed Severe Cold .... ■711
Sudafed Sinus Headache Caplets ... ■712
Sudafed Sinus Headache Tablets ... ■712
Tavist Sinus Non-Drowsy Coated Caplets .... ■676
TheraFlu Regular Strength Cold & Cough Night Time Hot Liquid .... ■676
TheraFlu Regular Strength Cold & Sore Throat Night Time Hot Liquid .... ■676
TheraFlu Maximum Strength Flu & Congestion Non-Drowsy Hot Liquid .... ■677
TheraFlu Maximum Strength Flu & Cough Night Time Hot Liquid ... ■678
TheraFlu Maximum Strength Flu & Sore Throat Night Time Hot Liquid .... ■677
TheraFlu Maximum Strength Severe Cold & Congestion Night Time Caplets .... ■678
TheraFlu Maximum Strength Severe Cold & Congestion Night Time Hot Liquid .... ■678

TheraFlu Maximum Strength Severe Cold & Congestion Non-Drowsy ▣679
Triaminic Cold, Cough & Fever Liquid ▣681
Triaminic Cough & Sore Throat Liquid ▣682
Triaminic Cough & Sore Throat Softchews ▣684
Tylenol, Children's 2014
Children's Tylenol Allergy-D Liquid 2014
Children's Tylenol Cold Suspension Liquid and Chewable Tablets 2015
Children's Tylenol Cold Plus Cough Suspension Liquid and Chewable Tablets 2015
Children's Tylenol Flu Suspension Liquid 2015
Children's Tylenol Sinus Suspension Liquid 2017
Infants' Tylenol Cold Decongestant and Fever Reducer Concentrated Drops 2015
Infants' Tylenol Cold Decongestant and Fever Reducer Concentrated Drops Plus Cough 2015
Junior Strength Tylenol Soft Chews Chewable Tablets 2014
Tylenol 2009
Tylenol Allergy Sinus 2010
Tylenol Severe Allergy Caplets 2010
Multi-Symptom Tylenol Cold Complete Formula Caplets 2010
Multi-Symptom Tylenol Cold Non-Drowsy Caplets and Gelcaps 2010
Multi-Symptom Tylenol Cold Severe Congestion Non-Drowsy Caplets 2011
Maximum Strength Tylenol Flu NightTime Gelcaps 2011
Maximum Strength Tylenol Flu NightTime Liquid 2011
Maximum Strength Tylenol Flu Non-Drowsy Gelcaps 2011
Extra Strength Tylenol PM Caplets, Geltabs, and Gelcaps 2012
Maximum Strength Tylenol Sinus NightTime Caplets 2012
Maximum Strength Tylenol Sinus Non-Drowsy Geltabs, Gelcaps, Caplets, and Tablets 2012
Maximum Strength Tylenol Sore Throat Adult Liquid 2013
Tylenol with Codeine 2595
Women's Tylenol Menstrual Relief Caplets 2013
Tylox Capsules 2597
Ultracet Tablets 2597
Vanquish Caplets ▣617
Vicks 44M Cough, Cold & Flu Relief Liquid ▣725
Vicks DayQuil LiquiCaps/Liquid Multi-Symptom Cold/Flu Relief ▣727
Vicks NyQuil LiquiCaps/Liquid Multi-Symptom Cold/Flu Relief, Original and Cherry Flavors ▣727
Vicodin Tablets 516
Vicodin ES Tablets 517
Vicodin HP Tablets 518
Zydone Tablets 1330

Aspirin (Concurrent administration with other pain relievers/fever reducers is not recommended unless advised by a physician). Products include:
Aggrenox Capsules 1026
Alka-Seltzer ▣603
Alka-Seltzer Lemon Lime Antacid and Pain Reliever Effervescent Tablets ▣603
Alka-Seltzer Extra Strength Antacid and Pain Reliever Effervescent Tablets ▣603
Alka-Seltzer PM Effervescent Tablets ▣605
Genuine Bayer Tablets, Caplets and Gelcaps ▣606
Extra Strength Bayer Caplets and Gelcaps ▣610
Aspirin Regimen Bayer Children's Chewable Tablets (Orange or Cherry Flavored) ▣607
Bayer, Aspirin Regimen ▣606
Aspirin Regimen Bayer 81 mg Caplets with Calcium ▣607
Genuine Bayer Professional Labeling (Aspirin Regimen Bayer) ▣608
Extra Strength Bayer Arthritis Caplets ▣610
Extra Strength Bayer Plus Caplets ▣610
Extra Strength Bayer PM Caplets ▣611
BC Powder ▣619
BC Allergy Sinus Cold Powder ▣619
Arthritis Strength BC Powder ▣619
BC Sinus Cold Powder ▣619
Darvon Compound-65 Pulvules 1910
Ecotrin Enteric Coated Aspirin Low, Regular and Maximum Strength Tablets 1715
Excedrin Extra-Strength Tablets, Caplets, and Geltabs ▣629
Excedrin Migraine 1070
Goody's Body Pain Formula Powder ▣620
Goody's Extra Strength Headache Powder ▣620
Goody's Extra Strength Pain Relief Tablets ▣620
Percodan Tablets 1327
Robaxisal Tablets 2939
Soma Compound Tablets 3354
Soma Compound w/Codeine Tablets 3355
Vanquish Caplets ▣617

Ibuprofen (Concurrent administration with other pain relievers/fever reducers is not recommended unless advised by a physician). Products include:
Advil ▣771
Children's Advil Oral Suspension ▣773
Children's Advil Chewable Tablets ▣773
Advil Cold and Sinus Caplets ▣771
Advil Cold and Sinus Tablets ▣771
Advil Flu & Body Ache Caplets ▣772
Infants' Advil Drops ▣773
Junior Strength Advil Tablets ▣773
Junior Strength Advil Chewable Tablets ▣773
Advil Migraine Liquigels ▣772
Children's Motrin Oral Suspension and Chewable Tablets 2006
Children's Motrin Cold Oral Suspension 2007
Children's Motrin Oral Suspension ▣643
Motrin Suspension, Oral Drops, Chewable Tablets, and Caplets 2002
Infants' Motrin Concentrated Drops 2006
Junior Strength Motrin Caplets and Chewable Tablets 2006
Motrin IB Tablets, Caplets, and Gelcaps 2002
Motrin Migraine Pain Caplets 2005
Motrin Sinus Headache Caplets 2005
Vicoprofen Tablets 520

Naproxen (Concurrent administration with other pain relievers/fever reducers is not recommended unless advised by a physician). Products include:
EC-Naprosyn Delayed-Release Tablets 2967
Naprosyn Suspension 2967
Naprosyn Tablets 2967

Food Interactions

Alcohol (Individuals consuming 3 or more alcohol-containing drinks per day should consult their physicians for advice on when and how they should take this product).

ALEVE COLD & SINUS CAPLETS

(Naproxen Sodium, Pseudoephedrine Hydrochloride) ▣603
May interact with monoamine oxidase inhibitors and certain other agents. Compounds in these categories include:

Isocarboxazid (Concurrent and/or sequential use with MAO inhibitors is not recommended).
No products indexed under this heading.

Moclobemide (Concurrent and/or sequential use with MAO inhibitors is not recommended).
No products indexed under this heading.

Pargyline Hydrochloride (Concurrent and/or sequential use with MAO inhibitors is not recommended).
No products indexed under this heading.

Phenelzine Sulfate (Concurrent and/or sequential use with MAO inhibitors is not recommended). Products include:
Nardil Tablets 2653

Procarbazine Hydrochloride (Concurrent and/or sequential use with MAO inhibitors is not recommended). Products include:
Matulane Capsules 3246

Selegiline Hydrochloride (Concurrent and/or sequential use with MAO inhibitors is not recommended). Products include:
Eldepryl Capsules 3266

Tranylcypromine Sulfate (Concurrent and/or sequential use with MAO inhibitors is not recommended). Products include:
Parnate Tablets 1607

Food Interactions

Alcohol (Chronic heavy alcohol users, 3 or more drinks per day, should consult their physician for advice on when and how they should take pain relievers/fever reducers including naproxen).

ALFERON N INJECTION

(Interferon alfa-N3 (Human Leukocyte Derived)) 1770
None cited in PDR database.

ALKA-SELTZER ORIGINAL ANTACID AND PAIN RELIEVER EFFERVESCENT TABLETS

(Aspirin, Citric Acid, Sodium Bicarbonate) ▣603
May interact with oral anticoagulants, oral hypoglycemic agents, and certain other agents. Compounds in these categories include:

Acarbose (Concurrent use should be avoided unless directed by a doctor). Products include:
Precose Tablets 906

Antiarthritic Drugs, unspecified (Concurrent use should be avoided unless directed by a doctor).

Chlorpropamide (Concurrent use should be avoided unless directed by a doctor). Products include:
Diabinese Tablets 2680

Dicumarol (Concurrent use should be avoided unless directed by a doctor).
No products indexed under this heading.

Glimepiride (Concurrent use should be avoided unless directed by a doctor). Products include:
Amaryl Tablets 717

Glipizide (Concurrent use should be avoided unless directed by a doctor). Products include:
Glucotrol Tablets 2692
Glucotrol XL Extended Release Tablets 2693

Glyburide (Concurrent use should be avoided unless directed by a doctor). Products include:
DiaBeta Tablets 741
Glucovance Tablets 1086

Metformin Hydrochloride (Concurrent use should be avoided unless directed by a doctor). Products include:
Glucophage Tablets 1080
Glucophage XR Tablets 1080
Glucovance Tablets 1086

Miglitol (Concurrent use should be avoided unless directed by a doctor). Products include:
Glyset Tablets 2821

Pioglitazone Hydrochloride (Concurrent use should be avoided unless directed by a doctor). Products include:
Actos Tablets 3275

Prescription Drugs, unspecified (Antacids may interact with certain prescription drugs, consult a health-care professional).

Probenecid (Concurrent use with gout medications should be avoided unless directed by a doctor).
No products indexed under this heading.

Repaglinide (Concurrent use should be avoided unless directed by a doctor). Products include:
Prandin Tablets (0.5, 1, and 2 mg) 2432

Rosiglitazone Maleate (Concurrent use should be avoided unless directed by a doctor). Products include:
Avandia Tablets 1490

Sulfinpyrazone (Concurrent use with gout medications should be avoided unless directed by a doctor).
No products indexed under this heading.

Tolazamide (Concurrent use should be avoided unless directed by a doctor).
No products indexed under this heading.

Tolbutamide (Concurrent use should be avoided unless directed by a doctor).
No products indexed under this heading.

Troglitazone (Concurrent use should be avoided unless directed by a doctor).
No products indexed under this heading.

Warfarin Sodium (Concurrent use should be avoided unless directed by a doctor). Products include:
Coumadin for Injection 1243
Coumadin Tablets 1243
Warfarin Sodium Tablets, USP 3302

Food Interactions

Alcohol (Chronic heavy alcohol users, 3 or more drinks per day, should consult their physicians for advice on when and how they should take pain relievers/fever reducers including aspirin).

ALKA-SELTZER CHERRY ANTACID AND PAIN RELIEVER EFFERVESCENT TABLETS

(Aspirin, Citric Acid, Sodium Bicarbonate) ▣603
See Alka-Seltzer Original Antacid and Pain Reliever Effervescent Tablets

ALKA-SELTZER LEMON LIME ANTACID AND PAIN RELIEVER EFFERVESCENT TABLETS

(Aspirin, Citric Acid, Sodium Bicarbonate) ▣603
See Alka-Seltzer Original Antacid and Pain Reliever Effervescent Tablets

ALKA-SELTZER EXTRA STRENGTH ANTACID AND PAIN RELIEVER EFFERVESCENT TABLETS

(Aspirin, Citric Acid, Sodium Bicarbonate) ▣603
See Alka-Seltzer Original Antacid and Pain Reliever Effervescent Tablets

ALKA-SELTZER PLUS COLD MEDICINE LIQUI-GELS

(Acetaminophen, Chlorpheniramine Maleate, Pseudoephedrine Hydrochloride) ▣604
See Alka-Seltzer Plus Night-Time Cold Medicine Liqui-Gels

ALKA-SELTZER PLUS NIGHT-TIME COLD MEDICINE LIQUI-GELS

(Acetaminophen, Dextromethorphan Hydrobromide, Doxylamine Succinate, Pseudoephedrine Hydrochloride) ▣604
May interact with antihypertensives, hypnotics and sedatives, monoamine oxidase inhibitors, tranquilizers, and certain other agents. Compounds in these categories include:

Acebutolol Hydrochloride (Concurrent use with drugs for blood pressure is not recommended). Products include:

Sectral Capsules 3589

Alprazolam (May increase drowsiness effect). Products include:
Xanax Tablets 2865

Amlodipine Besylate (Concurrent use with drugs for blood pressure is not recommended). Products include:
Lotrel Capsules 2370
Norvasc Tablets 2704

Atenolol (Concurrent use with drugs for blood pressure is not recommended). Products include:
Tenoretic Tablets 690
Tenormin I.V. Injection 692

Benazepril Hydrochloride (Concurrent use with drugs for blood pressure is not recommended). Products include:
Lotensin Tablets 2365
Lotensin HCT Tablets 2367
Lotrel Capsules 2370

Bendroflumethiazide (Concurrent use with drugs for blood pressure is not recommended). Products include:
Corzide 40/5 Tablets 2247
Corzide 80/5 Tablets 2247

Betaxolol Hydrochloride (Concurrent use with drugs for blood pressure is not recommended). Products include:
Betoptic S Ophthalmic Suspension 537

Bisoprolol Fumarate (Concurrent use with drugs for blood pressure is not recommended). Products include:
Zebeta Tablets 1885
Ziac Tablets 1887

Buspirone Hydrochloride (May increase drowsiness effect).
No products indexed under this heading.

Candesartan Cilexetil (Concurrent use with drugs for blood pressure is not recommended). Products include:
Atacand Tablets 595
Atacand HCT Tablets 597

Captopril (Concurrent use with drugs for blood pressure is not recommended). Products include:
Captopril Tablets 2281

Carteolol Hydrochloride (Concurrent use with drugs for blood pressure is not recommended). Products include:
Carteolol Hydrochloride Ophthalmic Solution USP, 1% .... ⊙ 258
Ocupress Ophthalmic Solution, 1% Sterile .... ⊙ 303

Chlordiazepoxide (May increase drowsiness effect). Products include:
Limbitrol 1738

Chlordiazepoxide Hydrochloride (May increase drowsiness effect). Products include:
Librium Capsules 1736
Librium for Injection 1737

Chlorothiazide (Concurrent use with drugs for blood pressure is not recommended). Products include:
Aldoclor Tablets 2035
Diuril Oral 2087

Chlorothiazide Sodium (Concurrent use with drugs for blood pressure is not recommended). Products include:
Diuril Sodium Intravenous 2086

Chlorpromazine (May increase drowsiness effect). Products include:
Thorazine Suppositories 1656

Chlorpromazine Hydrochloride (May increase drowsiness effect). Products include:
Thorazine 1656

Chlorprothixene (May increase drowsiness effect).
No products indexed under this heading.

Chlorprothixene Hydrochloride (May increase drowsiness effect).
No products indexed under this heading.

Chlorthalidone (Concurrent use with drugs for blood pressure is not recommended). Products include:
Clorpres Tablets 1002
Combipres Tablets 1040
Tenoretic Tablets 690

Clonidine (Concurrent use with drugs for blood pressure is not recommended). Products include:
Catapres-TTS 1038

Clonidine Hydrochloride (Concurrent use with drugs for blood pressure is not recommended). Products include:
Catapres Tablets 1037
Clorpres Tablets 1002
Combipres Tablets 1040
Duraclon Injection 3057

Clorazepate Dipotassium (May increase drowsiness effect). Products include:
Tranxene 511

Deserpidine (Concurrent use with drugs for blood pressure is not recommended).
No products indexed under this heading.

Diazepam (May increase drowsiness effect). Products include:
Valium Injectable 3026
Valium Tablets 3047

Diazoxide (Concurrent use with drugs for blood pressure is not recommended).
No products indexed under this heading.

Diltiazem Hydrochloride (Concurrent use with drugs for blood pressure is not recommended). Products include:
Cardizem Injectable 1018
Cardizem Lyo-Ject Syringe 1018
Cardizem Monovial 1018
Cardizem CD Capsules 1016
Tiazac Capsules 1378

Doxazosin Mesylate (Concurrent use with drugs for blood pressure is not recommended). Products include:
Cardura Tablets 2668

Droperidol (May increase drowsiness effect).
No products indexed under this heading.

Enalapril Maleate (Concurrent use with drugs for blood pressure is not recommended). Products include:
Lexxel Tablets 608
Vaseretic Tablets 2204
Vasotec Tablets 2210

Enalaprilat (Concurrent use with drugs for blood pressure is not recommended). Products include:
Enalaprilat Injection 863
Vasotec I.V. Injection 2207

Eprosartan Mesylate (Concurrent use with drugs for blood pressure is not recommended). Products include:
Teveten Tablets 3327

Esmolol Hydrochloride (Concurrent use with drugs for blood pressure is not recommended). Products include:
Brevibloc Injection 858

Estazolam (May increase drowsiness effect). Products include:
ProSom Tablets 500

Ethchlorvynol (May increase drowsiness effect).
No products indexed under this heading.

Ethinamate (May increase drowsiness effect).
No products indexed under this heading.

Felodipine (Concurrent use with drugs for blood pressure is not recommended). Products include:
Lexxel Tablets 608
Plendil Extended-Release Tablets 623

Fluphenazine Decanoate (May increase drowsiness effect).
No products indexed under this heading.

Fluphenazine Enanthate (May increase drowsiness effect).
No products indexed under this heading.

Fluphenazine Hydrochloride (May increase drowsiness effect).
No products indexed under this heading.

Flurazepam Hydrochloride (May increase drowsiness effect).
No products indexed under this heading.

Fosinopril Sodium (Concurrent use with drugs for blood pressure is not recommended). Products include:
Monopril Tablets 1091
Monopril HCT 1094

Furosemide (Concurrent use with drugs for blood pressure is not recommended). Products include:
Furosemide Tablets 2284

Glutethimide (May increase drowsiness effect).
No products indexed under this heading.

Guanabenz Acetate (Concurrent use with drugs for blood pressure is not recommended).
No products indexed under this heading.

Guanethidine Monosulfate (Concurrent use with drugs for blood pressure is not recommended).
No products indexed under this heading.

Haloperidol (May increase drowsiness effect). Products include:
Haldol Injection, Tablets and Concentrate 2533

Haloperidol Decanoate (May increase drowsiness effect). Products include:
Haldol Decanoate 2535

Hydralazine Hydrochloride (Concurrent use with drugs for blood pressure is not recommended).
No products indexed under this heading.

Hydrochlorothiazide (Concurrent use with drugs for blood pressure is not recommended). Products include:
Accuretic Tablets 2614
Aldoril Tablets 2039
Atacand HCT Tablets 597
Avalide Tablets 1070
Diovan HCT Tablets 2338
Dyazide Capsules 1515
HydroDIURIL Tablets 2108
Hyzaar 2109
Inderide Tablets 3517
Inderide LA Long-Acting Capsules .. 3519
Lotensin HCT Tablets 2367
Maxzide 1008
Micardis HCT Tablets 1051
Microzide Capsules 3414
Moduretic Tablets 2138
Monopril HCT 1094
Prinzide Tablets 2168
Timolide Tablets 2187
Uniretic Tablets 3178
Vaseretic Tablets 2204
Zestoretic Tablets 695
Ziac Tablets 1887

Hydroflumethiazide (Concurrent use with drugs for blood pressure is not recommended). Products include:
Diucardin Tablets 3494

Hydroxyzine Hydrochloride (May increase drowsiness effect). Products include:
Atarax Tablets & Syrup 2667
Vistaril Intramuscular Solution 2738

Indapamide (Concurrent use with drugs for blood pressure is not recommended). Products include:
Indapamide Tablets 2286

Irbesartan (Concurrent use with drugs for blood pressure is not recommended). Products include:
Avalide Tablets 1070
Avapro Tablets 1074
Avapro Tablets 3076

Isocarboxazid (Concurrent and/or sequential use with MAO inhibitors is not recommended).
No products indexed under this heading.

Isradipine (Concurrent use with drugs for blood pressure is not recommended). Products include:
DynaCirc Capsules 2921
DynaCirc CR Tablets 2923

Labetalol Hydrochloride (Concurrent use with drugs for blood pressure is not recommended). Products include:
Normodyne Injection 3135
Normodyne Tablets 3137

Lisinopril (Concurrent use with drugs for blood pressure is not recommended). Products include:
Prinivil Tablets 2164
Prinzide Tablets 2168
Zestoretic Tablets 695
Zestril Tablets 698

Lorazepam (May increase drowsiness effect). Products include:
Ativan Injection 3478
Ativan Tablets 3482

Losartan Potassium (Concurrent use with drugs for blood pressure is not recommended). Products include:
Cozaar Tablets 2067
Hyzaar 2109

Loxapine Hydrochloride (May increase drowsiness effect).
No products indexed under this heading.

Loxapine Succinate (May increase drowsiness effect). Products include:
Loxitane Capsules 3398

Mecamylamine Hydrochloride (Concurrent use with drugs for blood pressure is not recommended). Products include:
Inversine Tablets 1850

Meprobamate (May increase drowsiness effect). Products include:
Miltown Tablets 3349

Mesoridazine Besylate (May increase drowsiness effect). Products include:
Serentil 1057

Methyclothiazide (Concurrent use with drugs for blood pressure is not recommended).
No products indexed under this heading.

Methyldopa (Concurrent use with drugs for blood pressure is not recommended). Products include:
Aldoclor Tablets 2035
Aldomet Tablets 2037
Aldoril Tablets 2039

Methyldopate Hydrochloride (Concurrent use with drugs for blood pressure is not recommended).
No products indexed under this heading.

Metolazone (Concurrent use with drugs for blood pressure is not recommended). Products include:
Mykrox Tablets 1168
Zaroxolyn Tablets 1177

Metoprolol Succinate (Concurrent use with drugs for blood pressure is not recommended). Products include:
Toprol-XL Tablets 651

Metoprolol Tartrate (Concurrent use with drugs for blood pressure is not recommended).
No products indexed under this heading.

Metyrosine (Concurrent use with drugs for blood pressure is not recommended). Products include:
Demser Capsules 2085

Mibefradil Dihydrochloride (Concurrent use with drugs for blood pressure is not recommended).
No products indexed under this heading.

Midazolam Hydrochloride (May increase drowsiness effect). Products include:
Versed Injection 3027

IMPORTANT NOTE: Always consult each drug listing in the patient's regimen for possible interactions.

Versed Syrup 3033

Minoxidil (Concurrent use with drugs for blood pressure is not recommended). Products include:
Rogaine Extra Strength for Men Topical Solution .... ▣721
Rogaine for Women Topical Solution .... ▣721

Moclobemide (Concurrent and/or sequential use with MAO inhibitors is not recommended).
No products indexed under this heading.

Moexipril Hydrochloride (Concurrent use with drugs for blood pressure is not recommended). Products include:
Uniretic Tablets 3178
Univasc Tablets 3181

Molindone Hydrochloride (May increase drowsiness effect). Products include:
Moban 1320

Nadolol (Concurrent use with drugs for blood pressure is not recommended). Products include:
Corgard Tablets 2245
Corzide 40/5 Tablets 2247
Corzide 80/5 Tablets 2247
Nadolol Tablets 2288

Nicardipine Hydrochloride (Concurrent use with drugs for blood pressure is not recommended). Products include:
Cardene I.V. 3485

Nifedipine (Concurrent use with drugs for blood pressure is not recommended). Products include:
Adalat CC Tablets 877
Procardia Capsules 2708
Procardia XL Extended Release Tablets 2710

Nisoldipine (Concurrent use with drugs for blood pressure is not recommended). Products include:
Sular Tablets 688

Nitroglycerin (Concurrent use with drugs for blood pressure is not recommended). Products include:
Nitro-Dur Transdermal Infusion System 3134
Nitro-Dur Transdermal Infusion System 1834
Nitrolingual Pumpspray 1355
Nitrostat Tablets 2658

Oxazepam (May increase drowsiness effect).
No products indexed under this heading.

Pargyline Hydrochloride (Concurrent and/or sequential use with MAO inhibitors is not recommended).
No products indexed under this heading.

Penbutolol Sulfate (Concurrent use with drugs for blood pressure is not recommended).
No products indexed under this heading.

Perindopril Erbumine (Concurrent use with drugs for blood pressure is not recommended). Products include:
Aceon Tablets (2 mg, 4 mg, 8 mg) 3249

Perphenazine (May increase drowsiness effect). Products include:
Etrafon 3115
Trilafon 3160

Phenelzine Sulfate (Concurrent and/or sequential use with MAO inhibitors is not recommended). Products include:
Nardil Tablets 2653

Phenoxybenzamine Hydrochloride (Concurrent use with drugs for blood pressure is not recommended). Products include:
Dibenzyline Capsules 3457

Phentolamine Mesylate (Concurrent use with drugs for blood pressure is not recommended).
No products indexed under this heading.

Pindolol (Concurrent use with drugs for blood pressure is not recommended).
No products indexed under this heading.

Polythiazide (Concurrent use with drugs for blood pressure is not recommended). Products include:
Minizide Capsules 2700
Renese Tablets 2712

Prazepam (May increase drowsiness effect).
No products indexed under this heading.

Prazosin Hydrochloride (Concurrent use with drugs for blood pressure is not recommended). Products include:
Minipress Capsules 2699
Minizide Capsules 2700

Procarbazine Hydrochloride (Concurrent and/or sequential use with MAO inhibitors is not recommended). Products include:
Matulane Capsules 3246

Prochlorperazine (May increase drowsiness effect). Products include:
Compazine 1505

Promethazine Hydrochloride (May increase drowsiness effect). Products include:
Mepergan Injection 3539
Phenergan Injection 3553
Phenergan 3556
Phenergan Syrup 3554
Phenergan with Codeine Syrup 3557
Phenergan with Dextromethorphan Syrup 3559
Phenergan VC Syrup 3560
Phenergan VC with Codeine Syrup 3561

Propofol (May increase drowsiness effect). Products include:
Diprivan Injectable Emulsion 667

Propranolol Hydrochloride (Concurrent use with drugs for blood pressure is not recommended). Products include:
Inderal 3513
Inderal LA Long-Acting Capsules 3516
Inderide Tablets 3517
Inderide LA Long-Acting Capsules 3519

Quazepam (May increase drowsiness effect).
No products indexed under this heading.

Quinapril Hydrochloride (Concurrent use with drugs for blood pressure is not recommended). Products include:
Accupril Tablets 2611
Accuretic Tablets 2614

Ramipril (Concurrent use with drugs for blood pressure is not recommended). Products include:
Altace Capsules 2233

Rauwolfia serpentina (Concurrent use with drugs for blood pressure is not recommended).
No products indexed under this heading.

Rescinnamine (Concurrent use with drugs for blood pressure is not recommended).
No products indexed under this heading.

Reserpine (Concurrent use with drugs for blood pressure is not recommended).
No products indexed under this heading.

Secobarbital Sodium (May increase drowsiness effect).
No products indexed under this heading.

Selegiline Hydrochloride (Concurrent and/or sequential use with MAO inhibitors is not recommended). Products include:
Eldepryl Capsules 3266

Sodium Nitroprusside (Concurrent use with drugs for blood pressure is not recommended).
No products indexed under this heading.

Sotalol Hydrochloride (Concurrent use with drugs for blood pressure is not recommended). Products include:
Betapace Tablets 950
Betapace AF Tablets 954

Spirapril Hydrochloride (Concurrent use with drugs for blood pressure is not recommended).
No products indexed under this heading.

Telmisartan (Concurrent use with drugs for blood pressure is not recommended). Products include:
Micardis Tablets 1049
Micardis HCT Tablets 1051

Temazepam (May increase drowsiness effect).
No products indexed under this heading.

Terazosin Hydrochloride (Concurrent use with drugs for blood pressure is not recommended). Products include:
Hytrin Capsules 464

Thioridazine Hydrochloride (May increase drowsiness effect). Products include:
Thioridazine Hydrochloride Tablets 2289

Thiothixene (May increase drowsiness effect). Products include:
Navane Capsules 2701
Thiothixene Capsules 2290

Timolol Maleate (Concurrent use with drugs for blood pressure is not recommended). Products include:
Blocadren Tablets 2046
Cosopt Sterile Ophthalmic Solution 2065
Timolide Tablets 2187
Timolol GFS .... ⊙266
Timoptic in Ocudose 2192
Timoptic Sterile Ophthalmic Solution 2190
Timoptic-XE Sterile Ophthalmic Gel Forming Solution 2194

Torsemide (Concurrent use with drugs for blood pressure is not recommended). Products include:
Demadex Tablets and Injection 2965

Trandolapril (Concurrent use with drugs for blood pressure is not recommended). Products include:
Mavik Tablets 478
Tarka Tablets 508

Tranylcypromine Sulfate (Concurrent and/or sequential use with MAO inhibitors is not recommended). Products include:
Parnate Tablets 1607

Triazolam (May increase drowsiness effect). Products include:
Halcion Tablets 2823

Trifluoperazine Hydrochloride (May increase drowsiness effect). Products include:
Stelazine 1640

Trimethaphan Camsylate (Concurrent use with drugs for blood pressure is not recommended).
No products indexed under this heading.

Valsartan (Concurrent use with drugs for blood pressure is not recommended). Products include:
Diovan Capsules 2337
Diovan HCT Tablets 2338

Verapamil Hydrochloride (Concurrent use with drugs for blood pressure is not recommended). Products include:
Covera-HS Tablets 3199
Isoptin SR Tablets 467
Tarka Tablets 508
Verelan Capsules 3184
Verelan PM Capsules 3186

Zaleplon (May increase drowsiness effect). Products include:
Sonata Capsules 3591

Zolpidem Tartrate (May increase drowsiness effect). Products include:
Ambien Tablets 3191

Food Interactions

Alcohol (Chronic heavy alcohol users, 3 or more drinks per day, should consult their physicians for advice on when and how they should take pain relievers/fever reducers including acetaminophen; increases drowsiness effect).

ALKA-SELTZER PLUS COLD & COUGH MEDICINE LIQUI-GELS

(Acetaminophen, Chlorpheniramine Maleate, Dextromethorphan Hydrobromide, Pseudoephedrine Hydrochloride) .... ▣604
See Alka-Seltzer Plus Night-Time Cold Medicine Liqui-Gels

ALKA-SELTZER PLUS COLD & FLU MEDICINE LIQUI-GELS

(Acetaminophen, Dextromethorphan Hydrobromide, Pseudoephedrine Hydrochloride) .... ▣604
See Alka-Seltzer Plus Night-Time Cold Medicine Liqui-Gels

ALKA-SELTZER PLUS COLD & SINUS MEDICINE LIQUI-GELS

(Acetaminophen, Pseudoephedrine Hydrochloride) .... ▣604
See Alka-Seltzer Plus Night-Time Cold Medicine Liqui-Gels

ALKA-SELTZER HEARTBURN RELIEF TABLETS

(Citric Acid, Sodium Bicarbonate) .... ▣604
May interact with:

Prescription Drugs, unspecified (Antacids may interact with certain unspecified prescription drugs).

ALKA-SELTZER PM EFFERVESCENT TABLETS

(Aspirin, Diphenhydramine Citrate) .... ▣605
May interact with oral anticoagulants, oral hypoglycemic agents, hypnotics and sedatives, tranquilizers, and certain other agents. Compounds in these categories include:

Acarbose (Concurrent use with antidiabetics should be avoided unless directed by a doctor). Products include:
Precose Tablets 906

Alprazolam (Concurrent use should be avoided). Products include:
Xanax Tablets 2865

Antiarthritic Drugs, unspecified (Concurrent use with drugs for arthritis should be avoided unless directed by a doctor).

Buspirone Hydrochloride (Concurrent use should be avoided).
No products indexed under this heading.

Chlordiazepoxide (Concurrent use should be avoided). Products include:
Limbitrol 1738

Chlordiazepoxide Hydrochloride (Concurrent use should be avoided). Products include:
Librium Capsules 1736
Librium for Injection 1737

Chlorpromazine (Concurrent use should be avoided). Products include:
Thorazine Suppositories 1656

Chlorpromazine Hydrochloride (Concurrent use should be avoided). Products include:
Thorazine 1656

Chlorpropamide (Concurrent use with antidiabetics should be avoided unless directed by a doctor). Products include:
- Diabinese Tablets 2680

Chlorprothixene (Concurrent use should be avoided).
- No products indexed under this heading.

Chlorprothixene Hydrochloride (Concurrent use should be avoided).
- No products indexed under this heading.

Clorazepate Dipotassium (Concurrent use should be avoided). Products include:
- Tranxene 511

Diazepam (Concurrent use should be avoided). Products include:
- Valium Injectable 3026
- Valium Tablets 3047

Dicumarol (Concurrent use with anticoagulants should be avoided unless directed by a doctor).
- No products indexed under this heading.

Droperidol (Concurrent use should be avoided).
- No products indexed under this heading.

Estazolam (Concurrent use should be avoided). Products include:
- ProSom Tablets 500

Ethchlorvynol (Concurrent use should be avoided).
- No products indexed under this heading.

Ethinamate (Concurrent use should be avoided).
- No products indexed under this heading.

Fluphenazine Decanoate (Concurrent use should be avoided).
- No products indexed under this heading.

Fluphenazine Enanthate (Concurrent use should be avoided).
- No products indexed under this heading.

Fluphenazine Hydrochloride (Concurrent use should be avoided).
- No products indexed under this heading.

Flurazepam Hydrochloride (Concurrent use should be avoided).
- No products indexed under this heading.

Glimepiride (Concurrent use with antidiabetics should be avoided unless directed by a doctor). Products include:
- Amaryl Tablets 717

Glipizide (Concurrent use with antidiabetics should be avoided unless directed by a doctor). Products include:
- Glucotrol Tablets 2692
- Glucotrol XL Extended Release Tablets 2693

Glutethimide (Concurrent use should be avoided).
- No products indexed under this heading.

Glyburide (Concurrent use with antidiabetics should be avoided unless directed by a doctor). Products include:
- DiaBeta Tablets 741
- Glucovance Tablets 1086

Haloperidol (Concurrent use should be avoided). Products include:
- Haldol Injection, Tablets and Concentrate 2533

Haloperidol Decanoate (Concurrent use should be avoided). Products include:
- Haldol Decanoate 2535

Hydroxyzine Hydrochloride (Concurrent use should be avoided). Products include:
- Atarax Tablets & Syrup 2667
- Vistaril Intramuscular Solution 2738

Lorazepam (Concurrent use should be avoided). Products include:
- Ativan Injection 3478
- Ativan Tablets 3482

Loxapine Hydrochloride (Concurrent use should be avoided).
- No products indexed under this heading.

Loxapine Succinate (Concurrent use should be avoided). Products include:
- Loxitane Capsules 3398

Meprobamate (Concurrent use should be avoided). Products include:
- Miltown Tablets 3349

Mesoridazine Besylate (Concurrent use should be avoided). Products include:
- Serentil 1057

Metformin Hydrochloride (Concurrent use with antidiabetics should be avoided unless directed by a doctor). Products include:
- Glucophage Tablets 1080
- Glucophage XR Tablets 1080
- Glucovance Tablets 1086

Midazolam Hydrochloride (Concurrent use should be avoided). Products include:
- Versed Injection 3027
- Versed Syrup 3033

Miglitol (Concurrent use with antidiabetics should be avoided unless directed by a doctor). Products include:
- Glyset Tablets 2821

Molindone Hydrochloride (Concurrent use should be avoided). Products include:
- Moban 1320

Oxazepam (Concurrent use should be avoided).
- No products indexed under this heading.

Perphenazine (Concurrent use should be avoided). Products include:
- Etrafon 3115
- Trilafon 3160

Pioglitazone Hydrochloride (Concurrent use with antidiabetics should be avoided unless directed by a doctor). Products include:
- Actos Tablets 3275

Prazepam (Concurrent use should be avoided).
- No products indexed under this heading.

Prochlorperazine (Concurrent use should be avoided). Products include:
- Compazine 1505

Promethazine Hydrochloride (Concurrent use should be avoided). Products include:
- Mepergan Injection 3539
- Phenergan Injection 3553
- Phenergan 3556
- Phenergan Syrup 3554
- Phenergan with Codeine Syrup 3557
- Phenergan with Dextromethorphan Syrup 3559
- Phenergan VC Syrup 3560
- Phenergan VC with Codeine Syrup 3561

Propofol (Concurrent use should be avoided). Products include:
- Diprivan Injectable Emulsion 667

Quazepam (Concurrent use should be avoided).
- No products indexed under this heading.

Repaglinide (Concurrent use with antidiabetics should be avoided unless directed by a doctor). Products include:
- Prandin Tablets (0.5, 1, and 2 mg) 2432

Rosiglitazone Maleate (Concurrent use with antidiabetics should be avoided unless directed by a doctor). Products include:
- Avandia Tablets 1490

Secobarbital Sodium (Concurrent use should be avoided).
- No products indexed under this heading.

Sulfinpyrazone (Concurrent use with gout medications should be avoided unless directed by a doctor).
- No products indexed under this heading.

Temazepam (Concurrent use should be avoided).
- No products indexed under this heading.

Thioridazine Hydrochloride (Concurrent use should be avoided). Products include:
- Thioridazine Hydrochloride Tablets 2289

Thiothixene (Concurrent use should be avoided). Products include:
- Navane Capsules 2701
- Thiothixene Capsules 2290

Tolazamide (Concurrent use with antidiabetics should be avoided unless directed by a doctor).
- No products indexed under this heading.

Tolbutamide (Concurrent use with antidiabetics should be avoided unless directed by a doctor).
- No products indexed under this heading.

Triazolam (Concurrent use should be avoided). Products include:
- Halcion Tablets 2823

Trifluoperazine Hydrochloride (Concurrent use should be avoided). Products include:
- Stelazine 1640

Troglitazone (Concurrent use with antidiabetics should be avoided unless directed by a doctor).
- No products indexed under this heading.

Warfarin Sodium (Concurrent use with anticoagulants should be avoided unless directed by a doctor). Products include:
- Coumadin for Injection 1243
- Coumadin Tablets 1243
- Warfarin Sodium Tablets, USP 3302

Zaleplon (Concurrent use should be avoided). Products include:
- Sonata Capsules 3591

Zolpidem Tartrate (Concurrent use should be avoided). Products include:
- Ambien Tablets 3191

Food Interactions

Alcohol (Chronic heavy alcohol users, 3 or more drinks per day, should consult their physicians for advice on when and how they should take pain relievers/fever reducers including aspirin; diphenhydramine is an antihistamine, therefore, concurrent use with alcoholic beverages should be avoided).

ALKERAN FOR INJECTION

(Melphalan Hydrochloride) 1465
May interact with:

Carmustine (BCNU) (Reduced threshold for BCNU lung toxicity). Products include:
- Gliadel Wafer 1723

Cisplatin (Affects melphalan kinetics by inducing renal dysfunction and subsequently altering melphalan clearance).
- No products indexed under this heading.

Cyclosporine (Potential for severe renal failure). Products include:
- Gengraf Capsules 457
- Neoral Soft Gelatin Capsules 2380
- Neoral Oral Solution 2380
- Sandimmune 2388

Nalidixic Acid (Increased incidence of severe hemorrhagic necrotic enterocolitis).
- No products indexed under this heading.

ALKERAN TABLETS

(Melphalan) 1466
None cited in PDR database.

ALL CLEAR EYE DROPS

(Naphazoline Hydrochloride, Polyethylene Glycol) .... ⊙ 252
None cited in PDR database.

ALL CLEAR AR EYE DROPS

(Hydroxypropyl Methylcellulose, Naphazoline Hydrochloride) .... ⊙ 252
None cited in PDR database.

ALL-BASIC CAPSULES

(Amino Acid Preparations) 2268
None cited in PDR database.

ALLEGRA CAPSULES

(Fexofenadine Hydrochloride) 712
May interact with erythromycin and certain other agents. Compounds in these categories include:

Aluminum Hydroxide (Administration of fexofenadine within 15 minutes of an aluminum and magnesium containing antacid decreased fexofenadine AUC by 41% and Cmax by 43%; Allegra should not be taken closely in time with aluminum and magnesium containing antacids). Products include:
- Amphojel Suspension (Mint Flavor) .... ■ 789
- Gaviscon Extra Strength Liquid .... ■ 751
- Gaviscon Extra Strength Tablets .... ■ 751
- Gaviscon Regular Strength Liquid .... ■ 751
- Gaviscon Regular Strength Tablets .... ■ 750
- Maalox Antacid/Anti-Gas Oral Suspension .... ■ 673
- Maalox Max Maximum Strength Antacid/Anti-Gas Liquid 2300
- Maalox Regular Strength Antacid/Antigas Liquid 2300
- Mylanta 1813
- Vanquish Caplets .... ■ 617

Erythromycin (Co-administration with erythromycin enhances fexofenadine gastrointestinal absorption thereby increasing plasma levels of fexofenadine; in vivo animal studies suggest that erythromycin may also decrease biliary excretion). Products include:
- Emgel 2% Topical Gel 1285
- Ery-Tab Tablets 448
- Erythromycin Base Filmtab Tablets 454
- Erythromycin Delayed-Release Capsules, USP 455
- PCE Dispertab Tablets 498

Erythromycin Estolate (Co-administration with erythromycin enhances fexofenadine gastrointestinal absorption thereby increasing plasma levels of fexofenadine; in vivo animal studies suggest that erythromycin may also decrease biliary excretion).
- No products indexed under this heading.

Erythromycin Ethylsuccinate (Co-administration with erythromycin enhances fexofenadine gastrointestinal absorption thereby increasing plasma levels of fexofenadine; in vivo animal studies suggest that erythromycin may also decrease biliary excretion). Products include:
- E.E.S. 450
- EryPed 446
- Pediazole Suspension 3050

Erythromycin Gluceptate (Co-administration with erythromycin enhances fexofenadine gastrointestinal absorption thereby increasing plasma levels of fexofenadine; in vivo animal studies suggest that erythromycin may also decrease biliary excretion).
- No products indexed under this heading.

Erythromycin Stearate (Co-administration with erythromycin enhances fexofenadine gastrointestinal absorption thereby increasing plasma levels of fexofenadine; in vivo animal studies suggest that erythromycin may also decrease biliary excretion). Products include:
- Erythrocin Stearate Filmtab Tablets 452

Ketoconazole (Co-administration with ketoconazole enhances fexofenadine gastrointestinal absorption thereby increasing plasma levels of fexofenadine; in vivo animal studies suggest that ketoconazole may also decrease fexofenadine gastrointestinal secretion). Products include:
- Nizoral 2% Cream 3620
- Nizoral A-D Shampoo 2008
- Nizoral 2% Shampoo 2007
- Nizoral Tablets 1791

Magnesium Hydroxide (Administration of fexofenadine within 15 minutes of an aluminum and magnesium containing antacid decreased fexofenadine AUC by 41% and Cmax by 43%; Allegra should not be taken closely in time with aluminum and magnesium containing antacids). Products include:
- Ex•Lax Milk of Magnesia Liquid .... ■670
- Maalox Antacid/Anti-Gas Oral Suspension .... ■673
- Maalox Max Maximum Strength Antacid/Anti-Gas Liquid 2300
- Maalox Regular Strength Antacid/Antigas Liquid 2300
- Mylanta Fast-Acting 1813
- Mylanta 1813
- Pepcid Complete Chewable Tablets 1815
- Phillips' Chewable Tablets .... ■615
- Phillips' Milk of Magnesia Liquid (Original, Cherry, & Mint) .... ■616
- Rolaids Tablets .... ■706
- Extra Strength Rolaids Tablets .... ■706
- Vanquish Caplets .... ■617

ALLEGRA TABLETS
(Fexofenadine Hydrochloride) 712
See Allegra Capsules

ALLEGRA-D EXTENDED-RELEASE TABLETS
(Fexofenadine Hydrochloride, Pseudoephedrine Hydrochloride) 714
May interact with erythromycin, cardiac glycosides, monoamine oxidase inhibitors, sympathomimetics, and certain other agents. Compounds in these categories include:

Albuterol (Combined effects of pseudoephedrine with other sympathomimetics on cardiovascular system may be harmful to the patient). Products include:
- Proventil Inhalation Aerosol 3142
- Ventolin Inhalation Aerosol and Refill 1679

Albuterol Sulfate (Combined effects of pseudoephedrine with other sympathomimetics on cardiovascular system may be harmful to the patient). Products include:
- AccuNeb Inhalation Solution 1230
- Combivent Inhalation Aerosol 1041
- DuoNeb Inhalation Solution 1233
- Proventil Inhalation Solution 0.083% 3146
- Proventil Repetabs Tablets 3148
- Proventil Solution for Inhalation 0.5% 3144
- Proventil HFA Inhalation Aerosol 3150
- Ventolin HFA Inhalation Aerosol 3618
- Volmax Extended-Release Tablets 2276

Deslanoside (Increased ectopic pacemaker activity can occur when pseudoephedrine is used concomitantly with digitalis).
No products indexed under this heading.

Digitoxin (Increased ectopic pacemaker activity can occur when pseudoephedrine is used concomitantly with digitalis).
No products indexed under this heading.

Digoxin (Increased ectopic pacemaker activity can occur when pseudoephedrine is used concomitantly with digitalis). Products include:
- Digitek Tablets 1003
- Lanoxicaps Capsules 1574
- Lanoxin Injection 1581
- Lanoxin Tablets 1587
- Lanoxin Elixir Pediatric 1578
- Lanoxin Injection Pediatric 1584

Dobutamine Hydrochloride (Combined effects of pseudoephedrine with other sympathomimetics on cardiovascular system may be harmful to the patient). Products include:
- Dobutrex Solution Vials 1914

Dopamine Hydrochloride (Combined effects of pseudoephedrine with other sympathomimetics on cardiovascular system may be harmful to the patient).
No products indexed under this heading.

Ephedrine Hydrochloride (Combined effects of pseudoephedrine with other sympathomimetics on cardiovascular system may be harmful to the patient). Products include:
- Primatene Tablets .... ■780

Ephedrine Sulfate (Combined effects of pseudoephedrine with other sympathomimetics on cardiovascular system may be harmful to the patient).
No products indexed under this heading.

Ephedrine Tannate (Combined effects of pseudoephedrine with other sympathomimetics on cardiovascular system may be harmful to the patient). Products include:
- Rynatuss Pediatric Suspension 3353
- Rynatuss Tablets 3353

Epinephrine (Combined effects of pseudoephedrine with other sympathomimetics on cardiovascular system may be harmful to the patient). Products include:
- Epifrin Sterile Ophthalmic Solution .... ⊙235
- EpiPen 1236
- Primatene Mist .... ■779
- Xylocaine with Epinephrine Injection 653

Epinephrine Bitartrate (Combined effects of pseudoephedrine with other sympathomimetics on cardiovascular system may be harmful to the patient). Products include:
- Sensorcaine 643

Epinephrine Hydrochloride (Combined effects of pseudoephedrine with other sympathomimetics on cardiovascular system may be harmful to the patient).
No products indexed under this heading.

Erythromycin (Co-administration with erythromycin enhances fexofenadine gastrointestinal absorption thereby increasing plasma levels of fexofenadine; in vivo animal studies suggest that erythromycin may also decrease biliary excretion). Products include:
- Emgel 2% Topical Gel 1285
- Ery-Tab Tablets 448
- Erythromycin Base Filmtab Tablets 454
- Erythromycin Delayed-Release Capsules, USP 455
- PCE Dispertab Tablets 498

Erythromycin Estolate (Co-administration with erythromycin enhances fexofenadine gastrointestinal absorption thereby increasing plasma levels of fexofenadine; in vivo animal studies suggest that erythromycin may also decrease biliary excretion).
No products indexed under this heading.

Erythromycin Ethylsuccinate (Co-administration with erythromycin enhances fexofenadine gastrointestinal absorption thereby increasing plasma levels of fexofenadine; in vivo animal studies suggest that erythromycin may also decrease biliary excretion). Products include:
- E.E.S. 450
- EryPed 446
- Pediazole Suspension 3050

Erythromycin Gluceptate (Co-administration with erythromycin enhances fexofenadine gastrointestinal absorption thereby increasing plasma levels of fexofenadine; in vivo animal studies suggest that erythromycin may also decrease biliary excretion).
No products indexed under this heading.

Erythromycin Stearate (Co-administration with erythromycin enhances fexofenadine gastrointestinal absorption thereby increasing plasma levels of fexofenadine; in vivo animal studies suggest that erythromycin may also decrease biliary excretion). Products include:
- Erythrocin Stearate Filmtab Tablets 452

Isocarboxazid (Concurrent and/or sequential use with MAO inhibitors is contraindicated).
No products indexed under this heading.

Isoproterenol Hydrochloride (Combined effects of pseudoephedrine with other sympathomimetics on cardiovascular system may be harmful to the patient).
No products indexed under this heading.

Isoproterenol Sulfate (Combined effects of pseudoephedrine with other sympathomimetics on cardiovascular system may be harmful to the patient).
No products indexed under this heading.

Ketoconazole (Co-administration with ketoconazole enhances fexofenadine gastrointestinal absorption thereby increasing plasma levels of fexofenadine; in vivo animal studies suggest that ketoconazole may also decrease fexofenadine gastrointestinal secretion). Products include:
- Nizoral 2% Cream 3620
- Nizoral A-D Shampoo 2008
- Nizoral 2% Shampoo 2007
- Nizoral Tablets 1791

Levalbuterol Hydrochloride (Combined effects of pseudoephedrine with other sympathomimetics on cardiovascular system may be harmful to the patient). Products include:
- Xopenex Inhalation Solution 3207

Mecamylamine Hydrochloride (Reduced antihypertensive effects). Products include:
- Inversine Tablets 1850

Metaproterenol Sulfate (Combined effects of pseudoephedrine with other sympathomimetics on cardiovascular system may be harmful to the patient). Products include:
- Alupent 1029

Metaraminol Bitartrate (Combined effects of pseudoephedrine with other sympathomimetics on cardiovascular system may be harmful to the patient). Products include:
- Aramine Injection 2043

Methoxamine Hydrochloride (Combined effects of pseudoephedrine with other sympathomimetics on cardiovascular system may be harmful to the patient).
No products indexed under this heading.

Methyldopa (Reduced antihypertensive effects). Products include:
- Aldoclor Tablets 2035
- Aldomet Tablets 2037
- Aldoril Tablets 2039

Methyldopate Hydrochloride (Reduced antihypertensive effects).
No products indexed under this heading.

Moclobemide (Concurrent and/or sequential use with MAO inhibitors is contraindicated).
No products indexed under this heading.

Norepinephrine Bitartrate (Combined effects of pseudoephedrine with other sympathomimetics on cardiovascular system may be harmful to the patient).
No products indexed under this heading.

Pargyline Hydrochloride (Concurrent and/or sequential use with MAO inhibitors is contraindicated).
No products indexed under this heading.

Phenelzine Sulfate (Concurrent and/or sequential use with MAO inhibitors is contraindicated). Products include:
- Nardil Tablets 2653

Phenylephrine Bitartrate (Combined effects of pseudoephedrine with other sympathomimetics on cardiovascular system may be harmful to the patient).
No products indexed under this heading.

Phenylephrine Hydrochloride (Combined effects of pseudoephedrine with other sympathomimetics on cardiovascular system may be harmful to the patient). Products include:
- Afrin Nasal Decongestant Children's Pump Mist .... ■734
- Extendryl 1361
- Hycomine Compound Tablets 1317
- Neo-Synephrine .... ■614
- Phenergan VC Syrup 3560
- Phenergan VC with Codeine Syrup 3561
- Preparation H Cream .... ■778
- Preparation H Cooling Gel .... ■778
- Preparation H .... ■778
- Vicks Sinex Nasal Spray and Ultra Fine Mist .... ■729

Phenylephrine Tannate (Combined effects of pseudoephedrine with other sympathomimetics on cardiovascular system may be harmful to the patient). Products include:
- Ryna-12 S Suspension 3351
- Reformulated Rynatan Pediatric Suspension 3352
- Rynatuss Pediatric Suspension 3353
- Rynatuss Tablets 3353

Phenylpropanolamine Hydrochloride (Combined effects of pseudoephedrine with other sympathomimetics on cardiovascular system may be harmful to the patient).
No products indexed under this heading.

Pirbuterol Acetate (Combined effects of pseudoephedrine with other sympathomimetics on cardiovascular system may be harmful to the patient). Products include:
- Maxair Autohaler 1981
- Maxair Inhaler 1984

Procarbazine Hydrochloride (Concurrent and/or sequential use with MAO inhibitors is contraindicated). Products include:
- Matulane Capsules 3246

Pseudoephedrine Sulfate (Combined effects of pseudoephedrine with other sympathomimetics on cardiovascular system may be harmful to the patient). Products include:
- Chlor-Trimeton Allergy/Decongestant Tablets .... ■736
- Claritin-D 12 Hour Extended Release Tablets 3102
- Claritin-D 24 Hour Extended Release Tablets 3104
- Coricidin 'D' Cold, Flu & Sinus Tablets .... ■737
- Drixoral Allergy/Sinus Extended-Release Tablets .... ■741
- Drixoral Cold & Allergy Sustained-Action Tablets .... ■740

Drixoral Cold & Flu Extended-Release Tablets 740
Drixoral Nasal Decongestant Long-Acting Non-Drowsy Tablets 740
Rynatan Tablets 3351

Reserpine (Reduced antihypertensive effects).
No products indexed under this heading.

Salmeterol Xinafoate (Combined effects of pseudoephedrine with other sympathomimetics on cardiovascular system may be harmful to the patient). Products include:
Advair Diskus 100/50 1448
Advair Diskus 250/50 1448
Advair Diskus 500/50 1448
Serevent Diskus 1637
Serevent Inhalation Aerosol 1633

Selegiline Hydrochloride (Concurrent and/or sequential use with MAO inhibitors is contraindicated). Products include:
Eldepryl Capsules 3266

Terbutaline Sulfate (Combined effects of pseudoephedrine with other sympathomimetics on cardiovascular system may be harmful to the patient). Products include:
Brethine Ampuls 2314
Brethine Tablets 2313

Tranylcypromine Sulfate (Concurrent and/or sequential use with MAO inhibitors is contraindicated). Products include:
Parnate Tablets 1607

Food Interactions

Diet, high-lipid (Co-administration with a high-fat meal decreased fexofenadine plasma concentrations Cmax and AUC and Tmax was delayed by 50%; the rate of extent of pseudoephedrine absorption was not affected by food; administration of Allegra-D with food should be avoided).

ALLUNA SLEEP TABLETS
(Valeriana officinalis) 837
None cited in PDR database.

ALOCRIL OPHTHALMIC SOLUTION
(Nedocromil Sodium) 545
None cited in PDR database.

ALOMIDE OPHTHALMIC SOLUTION
(Lodoxamide Tromethamine) .... ⊙204
None cited in PDR database.

ALOPRIM FOR INJECTION
(Allopurinol Sodium) 2292
May interact with cytotoxic drugs, thiazides, and certain other agents. Compounds in these categories include:

Amoxicillin Trihydrate (Co-administration of amoxicillin with allopurinol increases the frequency of rash).
No products indexed under this heading.

Ampicillin (Co-administration of ampicillin with allopurinol increases the frequency of rash).
No products indexed under this heading.

Ampicillin Sodium (Co-administration of ampicillin with allopurinol increases the frequency of rash). Products include:
Unasyn for Injection 2728

Azathioprine (Allopurinol inhibits the enzymatic oxidation of azathioprine to 6-thiouric acid; this interaction has been observed with oral allopurinol, usually with longer term therapy, reduction in oral dose of allopurinol has been suggested).
No products indexed under this heading.

Bendroflumethiazide (Co-administration of allopurinol and thiazide diuretics contribute to increased allopurinol toxicity). Products include:
Corzide 40/5 Tablets 2247
Corzide 80/5 Tablets 2247

Bleomycin Sulfate (Co-administration of allopurinol with cytotoxic agents including cyclophosphamide in patients with neoplastic disease, except leukemia, enhances the bone marrow suppression).
No products indexed under this heading.

Chlorothiazide (Co-administration of allopurinol and thiazide diuretics contribute to increased allopurinol toxicity). Products include:
Aldoclor Tablets 2035
Diuril Oral 2087

Chlorothiazide Sodium (Co-administration of allopurinol and thiazide diuretics contribute to increased allopurinol toxicity). Products include:
Diuril Sodium Intravenous 2086

Chlorpropamide (The half-life of chlorpropamide in the plasma may be prolonged by allopurinol, since allopurinol and chlorpropamide may compete for excretion in the renal tubule; the risk of hypoglycemia secondary to this interaction may be increased if used concurrently). Products include:
Diabinese Tablets 2680

Cyclophosphamide (Co-administration of allopurinol with cyclophosphamide in patients with neoplastic disease, except leukemia, enhances the bone marrow suppression).
No products indexed under this heading.

Cyclosporine (Co-administration may result in increased cyclosporine levels). Products include:
Gengraf Capsules 457
Neoral Soft Gelatin Capsules 2380
Neoral Oral Solution 2380
Sandimmune 2388

Daunorubicin Hydrochloride (Co-administration of allopurinol with cytotoxic agents including cyclophosphamide in patients with neoplastic disease, except leukemia, enhances the bone marrow suppression). Products include:
Cerubidine for Injection 947

Dicumarol (Allopurinol prolongs the half-life of dicumarol).
No products indexed under this heading.

Doxorubicin Hydrochloride (Co-administration of allopurinol with cytotoxic agents including cyclophosphamide in patients with neoplastic disease, except leukemia, enhances the bone marrow suppression). Products include:
Adriamycin PFS/RDF Injection 2767
Doxil Injection 566

Epirubicin Hydrochloride (Co-administration of allopurinol with cytotoxic agents including cyclophosphamide in patients with neoplastic disease, except leukemia, enhances the bone marrow suppression). Products include:
Ellence Injection 2806

Fluorouracil (Co-administration of allopurinol with cytotoxic agents including cyclophosphamide in patients with neoplastic disease, except leukemia, enhances the bone marrow suppression). Products include:
Carac Cream 1222
Efudex 1733
Fluoroplex 552

Hydrochlorothiazide (Co-administration of allopurinol and thiazide diuretics contribute to increased allopurinol toxicity). Products include:
Accuretic Tablets 2614
Aldoril Tablets 2039
Atacand HCT Tablets 597
Avalide Tablets 1070
Diovan HCT Tablets 2338
Dyazide Capsules 1515
HydroDIURIL Tablets 2108
Hyzaar 2109
Inderide Tablets 3517
Inderide LA Long-Acting Capsules .. 3519
Lotensin HCT Tablets 2367
Maxzide 1008
Micardis HCT Tablets 1051
Microzide Capsules 3414
Moduretic Tablets 2138
Monopril HCT 1094
Prinzide Tablets 2168
Timolide Tablets 2187
Uniretic Tablets 3178
Vaseretic Tablets 2204
Zestoretic Tablets 695
Ziac Tablets 1887

Hydroflumethiazide (Co-administration of allopurinol and thiazide diuretics contribute to increased allopurinol toxicity). Products include:
Diucardin Tablets 3494

Hydroxyurea (Co-administration of allopurinol with cytotoxic agents including cyclophosphamide in patients with neoplastic disease, except leukemia, enhances the bone marrow suppression). Products include:
Mylocel Tablets 2227

Mercaptopurine (Allopurinol inhibits the enzymatic oxidation of mercaptopurine to 6-thiouric acid; this interaction has been observed with oral allopurinol, usually with longer term therapy, reduction in oral dose of allopurinol has been suggested). Products include:
Purinethol Tablets 1615

Methotrexate Sodium (Co-administration of allopurinol with cytotoxic agents including cyclophosphamide in patients with neoplastic disease, except leukemia, enhances the bone marrow suppression).
No products indexed under this heading.

Methyclothiazide (Co-administration of allopurinol and thiazide diuretics contribute to increased allopurinol toxicity).
No products indexed under this heading.

Mitotane (Co-administration of allopurinol with cytotoxic agents including cyclophosphamide in patients with neoplastic disease, except leukemia, enhances the bone marrow suppression).
No products indexed under this heading.

Mitoxantrone Hydrochloride (Co-administration of allopurinol with cytotoxic agents including cyclophosphamide in patients with neoplastic disease, except leukemia, enhances the bone marrow suppression). Products include:
Novantrone for Injection 1760

Polythiazide (Co-administration of allopurinol and thiazide diuretics contribute to increased allopurinol toxicity). Products include:
Minizide Capsules 2700
Renese Tablets 2712

Probenecid (Co-administration of uricosuric agents decreases the inhibition of xanthine by oxypurinol and increases the urinary excretion of uric acid).
No products indexed under this heading.

Procarbazine Hydrochloride (Co-administration of allopurinol with cytotoxic agents including cyclophosphamide in patients with neoplastic disease, except leukemia, enhances the bone marrow suppression). Products include:
Matulane Capsules 3246

Sulfinpyrazone (Co-administration of uricosuric agents decreases the inhibition of xanthine by oxypurinol and increases the urinary excretion of uric acid).
No products indexed under this heading.

Tamoxifen Citrate (Co-administration of allopurinol with cytotoxic agents including cyclophosphamide in patients with neoplastic disease, except leukemia, enhances the bone marrow suppression). Products include:
Nolvadex Tablets 678

Vincristine Sulfate (Co-administration of allopurinol with cytotoxic agents including cyclophosphamide in patients with neoplastic disease, except leukemia, enhances the bone marrow suppression).
No products indexed under this heading.

ALORA TRANSDERMAL SYSTEM
(Estradiol) 3372
May interact with:

Medroxyprogesterone Acetate (Addition of progestin to estrogen replacement therapy may result in possible adverse effects on lipid and carbohydrate metabolism). Products include:
Depo-Provera Contraceptive Injection 2798
Lunelle Monthly Injection 2827
Premphase Tablets 3572
Prempro Tablets 3572
Provera Tablets 2853

ALPHAGAN OPHTHALMIC SOLUTION
(Brimonidine Tartrate) 545
May interact with anesthetics, antihypertensives, barbiturates, beta blockers, central nervous system depressants, cardiac glycosides, hypnotics and sedatives, monoamine oxidase inhibitors, narcotic analgesics, tricyclic antidepressants, and certain other agents. Compounds in these categories include:

Acebutolol Hydrochloride (Concurrent use of brimonidine, an alpha adrenergic agonist, with beta blockers (ophthalmic and systemic) may reduce pulse and blood pressure, however, in clinical trials brimonidine did not have any significant effects on pulse and blood pressure). Products include:
Sectral Capsules 3589

Alfentanil Hydrochloride (Possible additive or potentiating effect with CNS depressants).
No products indexed under this heading.

Alprazolam (Possible additive or potentiating effect with CNS depressants). Products include:
Xanax Tablets 2865

Amitriptyline Hydrochloride (Tricyclic antidepressants have been reported to blunt the hypotensive effect of systemic clonidine, an alpha adrenergic agonist; it is not known whether the concurrent use of these agents with brimonidine can lead to interference in IOP-lowering effect; caution is advised). Products include:
Etrafon 3115
Limbitrol 1738

Amlodipine Besylate (Concurrent use of brimonidine, an alpha adrenergic agonist, with antihypertensives may reduce pulse and blood pressure, however, in clinical trials brimonidine did not have any significant effects on pulse and blood pressure). Products include:

Lotrel Capsules 2370
Norvasc Tablets 2704

Amoxapine (Tricyclic antidepressants have been reported to blunt the hypotensive effect of systemic clonidine, an alpha adrenergic agonist; it is not known whether the concurrent use of these agents with brimonidine can lead to interference in IOP-lowering effect; caution is advised).
No products indexed under this heading.

Aprobarbital (Possible additive or potentiating effect with CNS depressants).
No products indexed under this heading.

Atenolol (Concurrent use of brimonidine, an alpha adrenergic agonist, with beta blockers (ophthalmic and systemic) may reduce pulse and blood pressure, however, in clinical trials brimonidine did not have any significant effects on pulse and blood pressure). Products include:
Tenoretic Tablets 690
Tenormin I.V. Injection 692

Benazepril Hydrochloride (Concurrent use of brimonidine, an alpha adrenergic agonist, with antihypertensives may reduce pulse and blood pressure, however, in clinical trials brimonidine did not have any significant effects on pulse and blood pressure). Products include:
Lotensin Tablets 2365
Lotensin HCT Tablets 2367
Lotrel Capsules 2370

Bendroflumethiazide (Concurrent use of brimonidine, an alpha adrenergic agonist, with antihypertensives may reduce pulse and blood pressure, however, in clinical trials brimonidine did not have any significant effects on pulse and blood pressure). Products include:
Corzide 40/5 Tablets 2247
Corzide 80/5 Tablets 2247

Betaxolol Hydrochloride (Concurrent use of brimonidine, an alpha adrenergic agonist, with beta blockers (ophthalmic and systemic) may reduce pulse and blood pressure, however, in clinical trials brimonidine did not have any significant effects on pulse and blood pressure). Products include:
Betoptic S Ophthalmic Suspension 537

Bisoprolol Fumarate (Concurrent use of brimonidine, an alpha adrenergic agonist, with beta blockers (ophthalmic and systemic) may reduce pulse and blood pressure, however, in clinical trials brimonidine did not have any significant effects on pulse and blood pressure). Products include:
Zebeta Tablets 1885
Ziac Tablets 1887

Buprenorphine Hydrochloride (Possible additive or potentiating effect with CNS depressants). Products include:
Buprenex Injectable 2918

Buspirone Hydrochloride (Possible additive or potentiating effect with CNS depressants).
No products indexed under this heading.

Butabarbital (Possible additive or potentiating effect with CNS depressants).
No products indexed under this heading.

Butalbital (Possible additive or potentiating effect with CNS depressants). Products include:
Phrenilin 578
Sedapap Tablets 50 mg/650 mg 2225

Candesartan Cilexetil (Concurrent use of brimonidine, an alpha adrenergic agonist, with antihypertensives may reduce pulse and blood pressure, however, in clinical trials brimonidine did not have any significant effects on pulse and blood pressure). Products include:
Atacand Tablets 595
Atacand HCT Tablets 597

Captopril (Concurrent use of brimonidine, an alpha adrenergic agonist, with antihypertensives may reduce pulse and blood pressure, however, in clinical trials brimonidine did not have any significant effects on pulse and blood pressure). Products include:
Captopril Tablets 2281

Carteolol Hydrochloride (Concurrent use of brimonidine, an alpha adrenergic agonist, with beta blockers (ophthalmic and systemic) may reduce pulse and blood pressure, however, in clinical trials brimonidine did not have any significant effects on pulse and blood pressure). Products include:
Carteolol Hydrochloride Ophthalmic Solution USP, 1% .... ⊙258
Ocupress Ophthalmic Solution, 1% Sterile .... ⊙303

Chlordiazepoxide (Possible additive or potentiating effect with CNS depressants). Products include:
Limbitrol 1738

Chlordiazepoxide Hydrochloride (Possible additive or potentiating effect with CNS depressants). Products include:
Librium Capsules 1736
Librium for Injection 1737

Chlorothiazide (Concurrent use of brimonidine, an alpha adrenergic agonist, with antihypertensives may reduce pulse and blood pressure, however, in clinical trials brimonidine did not have any significant effects on pulse and blood pressure). Products include:
Aldoclor Tablets 2035
Diuril Oral 2087

Chlorothiazide Sodium (Concurrent use of brimonidine, an alpha adrenergic agonist, with antihypertensives may reduce pulse and blood pressure, however, in clinical trials brimonidine did not have any significant effects on pulse and blood pressure). Products include:
Diuril Sodium Intravenous 2086

Chlorpromazine (Possible additive or potentiating effect with CNS depressants). Products include:
Thorazine Suppositories 1656

Chlorpromazine Hydrochloride (Possible additive or potentiating effect with CNS depressants). Products include:
Thorazine 1656

Chlorprothixene (Possible additive or potentiating effect with CNS depressants).
No products indexed under this heading.

Chlorprothixene Hydrochloride (Possible additive or potentiating effect with CNS depressants).
No products indexed under this heading.

Chlorprothixene Lactate (Possible additive or potentiating effect with CNS depressants).
No products indexed under this heading.

Chlorthalidone (Concurrent use of brimonidine, an alpha adrenergic agonist, with antihypertensives may reduce pulse and blood pressure, however, in clinical trials brimonidine did not have any significant effects on pulse and blood pressure). Products include:
Clorpres Tablets 1002
Combipres Tablets 1040
Tenoretic Tablets 690

Clomipramine Hydrochloride (Tricyclic antidepressants have been reported to blunt the hypotensive effect of systemic clonidine, an alpha adrenergic agonist; it is not known whether the concurrent use of these agents with brimonidine can lead to interference in IOP-lowering effect; caution is advised).
No products indexed under this heading.

Clonidine (Concurrent use of brimonidine, an alpha adrenergic agonist, with antihypertensives may reduce pulse and blood pressure, however, in clinical trials brimonidine did not have any significant effects on pulse and blood pressure). Products include:
Catapres-TTS 1038

Clonidine Hydrochloride (Concurrent use of brimonidine, an alpha adrenergic agonist, with antihypertensives may reduce pulse and blood pressure, however, in clinical trials brimonidine did not have any significant effects on pulse and blood pressure). Products include:
Catapres Tablets 1037
Clorpres Tablets 1002
Combipres Tablets 1040
Duraclon Injection 3057

Clorazepate Dipotassium (Possible additive or potentiating effect with CNS depressants). Products include:
Tranxene 511

Clozapine (Possible additive or potentiating effect with CNS depressants). Products include:
Clozaril Tablets 2319

Codeine Phosphate (Possible additive or potentiating effect with CNS depressants). Products include:
Phenergan with Codeine Syrup 3557
Phenergan VC with Codeine Syrup 3561
Robitussin A-C Syrup 2942
Robitussin-DAC Syrup 2942
Ryna-C Liquid .... ▣768
Soma Compound w/Codeine Tablets 3355
Tussi-Organidin NR Liquid 3350
Tussi-Organidin-S NR Liquid 3350
Tylenol with Codeine 2595

Deserpidine (Concurrent use of brimonidine, an alpha adrenergic agonist, with antihypertensives may reduce pulse and blood pressure, however, in clinical trials brimonidine did not have any significant effects on pulse and blood pressure).
No products indexed under this heading.

Desflurane (Possible additive or potentiating effect with CNS depressants). Products include:
Suprane Liquid for Inhalation 874

Desipramine Hydrochloride (Tricyclic antidepressants have been reported to blunt the hypotensive effect of systemic clonidine, an alpha adrenergic agonist; it is not known whether the concurrent use of these agents with brimonidine can lead to interference in IOP-lowering effect; caution is advised). Products include:
Norpramin Tablets 755

Deslanoside (Concurrent use of brimonidine, an alpha adrenergic agonist, with cardiac glycosides may reduce pulse and blood pressure, however, in clinical trials brimonidine did not have any significant effects on pulse and blood pressure).
No products indexed under this heading.

Dezocine (Possible additive or potentiating effect with CNS depressants).
No products indexed under this heading.

Diazepam (Possible additive or potentiating effect with CNS depressants). Products include:
Valium Injectable 3026
Valium Tablets 3047

Diazoxide (Concurrent use of brimonidine, an alpha adrenergic agonist, with antihypertensives may reduce pulse and blood pressure, however, in clinical trials brimonidine did not have any significant effects on pulse and blood pressure).
No products indexed under this heading.

Digitoxin (Concurrent use of brimonidine, an alpha adrenergic agonist, with cardiac glycosides may reduce pulse and blood pressure, however, in clinical trials brimonidine did not have any significant effects on pulse and blood pressure).
No products indexed under this heading.

Digoxin (Concurrent use of brimonidine, an alpha adrenergic agonist, with cardiac glycosides may reduce pulse and blood pressure, however, in clinical trials brimonidine did not have any significant effects on pulse and blood pressure). Products include:
Digitek Tablets 1003
Lanoxicaps Capsules 1574
Lanoxin Injection 1581
Lanoxin Tablets 1587
Lanoxin Elixir Pediatric 1578
Lanoxin Injection Pediatric 1584

Diltiazem Hydrochloride (Concurrent use of brimonidine, an alpha adrenergic agonist, with antihypertensives may reduce pulse and blood pressure, however, in clinical trials brimonidine did not have any significant effects on pulse and blood pressure). Products include:
Cardizem Injectable 1018
Cardizem Lyo-Ject Syringe 1018
Cardizem Monovial 1018
Cardizem CD Capsules 1016
Tiazac Capsules 1378

Doxazosin Mesylate (Concurrent use of brimonidine, an alpha adrenergic agonist, with antihypertensives may reduce pulse and blood pressure, however, in clinical trials brimonidine did not have any significant effects on pulse and blood pressure). Products include:
Cardura Tablets 2668

Doxepin Hydrochloride (Tricyclic antidepressants have been reported to blunt the hypotensive effect of systemic clonidine, an alpha adrenergic agonist; it is not known whether the concurrent use of these agents with brimonidine can lead to interference in IOP-lowering effect; caution is advised). Products include:
Sinequan 2713

Droperidol (Possible additive or potentiating effect with CNS depressants).
No products indexed under this heading.

Enalapril Maleate (Concurrent use of brimonidine, an alpha adrenergic agonist, with antihypertensives may reduce pulse and blood pressure, however, in clinical trials brimonidine did not have any significant effects on pulse and blood pressure). Products include:
Lexxel Tablets 608
Vaseretic Tablets 2204
Vasotec Tablets 2210

Enalaprilat (Concurrent use of brimonidine, an alpha adrenergic agonist, with antihypertensives may reduce pulse and blood pressure, however, in clinical trials brimonidine did not have any significant effects on pulse and blood pressure). Products include:
Enalaprilat Injection 863
Vasotec I.V. Injection 2207

Enflurane (Possible additive or potentiating effect with CNS depressants).
No products indexed under this heading.

Eprosartan Mesylate (Concurrent use of brimonidine, an alpha adrenergic agonist, with antihypertensives

may reduce pulse and blood pressure, however, in clinical trials brimonidine did not have any significant effects on pulse and blood pressure). Products include:
Teveten Tablets 3327

Esmolol Hydrochloride (Concurrent use of brimonidine, an alpha adrenergic agonist, with beta blockers (ophthalmic and systemic) may reduce pulse and blood pressure, however, in clinical trials brimonidine did not have any significant effects on pulse and blood pressure). Products include:
Brevibloc Injection 858

Estazolam (Possible additive or potentiating effect with CNS depressants). Products include:
ProSom Tablets 500

Ethchlorvynol (Possible additive or potentiating effect with CNS depressants).
No products indexed under this heading.

Ethinamate (Possible additive or potentiating effect with CNS depressants).
No products indexed under this heading.

Felodipine (Concurrent use of brimonidine, an alpha adrenergic agonist, with antihypertensives may reduce pulse and blood pressure, however, in clinical trials brimonidine did not have any significant effects on pulse and blood pressure).
Products include:
Lexxel Tablets 608
Plendil Extended-Release Tablets 623

Fentanyl (Possible additive or potentiating effect with CNS depressants). Products include:
Duragesic Transdermal System 1786

Fentanyl Citrate (Possible additive or potentiating effect with CNS depressants). Products include:
Actiq 1184

Fluphenazine Decanoate (Possible additive or potentiating effect with CNS depressants).
No products indexed under this heading.

Fluphenazine Enanthate (Possible additive or potentiating effect with CNS depressants).
No products indexed under this heading.

Fluphenazine Hydrochloride (Possible additive or potentiating effect with CNS depressants).
No products indexed under this heading.

Flurazepam Hydrochloride (Possible additive or potentiating effect with CNS depressants).
No products indexed under this heading.

Fosinopril Sodium (Concurrent use of brimonidine, an alpha adrenergic agonist, with antihypertensives may reduce pulse and blood pressure, however, in clinical trials brimonidine did not have any significant effects on pulse and blood pressure).
Products include:
Monopril Tablets 1091
Monopril HCT 1094

Furosemide (Concurrent use of brimonidine, an alpha adrenergic agonist, with antihypertensives may reduce pulse and blood pressure, however, in clinical trials brimonidine did not have any significant effects on pulse and blood pressure).
Products include:
Furosemide Tablets 2284

Glutethimide (Possible additive or potentiating effect with CNS depressants).
No products indexed under this heading.

Guanabenz Acetate (Concurrent use of brimonidine, an alpha adrenergic agonist, with antihypertensives may reduce pulse and blood pressure, however, in clinical trials brimonidine did not have any significant effects on pulse and blood pressure).
No products indexed under this heading.

Guanethidine Monosulfate (Concurrent use of brimonidine, an alpha adrenergic agonist, with antihypertensives may reduce pulse and blood pressure, however, in clinical trials brimonidine did not have any significant effects on pulse and blood pressure).
No products indexed under this heading.

Haloperidol (Possible additive or potentiating effect with CNS depressants). Products include:
Haldol Injection, Tablets and Concentrate 2533

Haloperidol Decanoate (Possible additive or potentiating effect with CNS depressants). Products include:
Haldol Decanoate 2535

Halothane (Possible additive or potentiating effect with CNS depressants). Products include:
Fluothane Inhalation 3508

Hydralazine Hydrochloride (Concurrent use of brimonidine, an alpha adrenergic agonist, with antihypertensives may reduce pulse and blood pressure, however, in clinical trials brimonidine did not have any significant effects on pulse and blood pressure).
No products indexed under this heading.

Hydrochlorothiazide (Concurrent use of brimonidine, an alpha adrenergic agonist, with antihypertensives may reduce pulse and blood pressure, however, in clinical trials brimonidine did not have any significant effects on pulse and blood pressure). Products include:
Accuretic Tablets 2614
Aldoril Tablets 2039
Atacand HCT Tablets 597
Avalide Tablets 1070
Diovan HCT Tablets 2338
Dyazide Capsules 1515
HydroDIURIL Tablets 2108
Hyzaar 2109
Inderide Tablets 3517
Inderide LA Long-Acting Capsules 3519
Lotensin HCT Tablets 2367
Maxzide 1008
Micardis HCT Tablets 1051
Microzide Capsules 3414
Moduretic Tablets 2138
Monopril HCT 1094
Prinzide Tablets 2168
Timolide Tablets 2187
Uniretic Tablets 3178
Vaseretic Tablets 2204
Zestoretic Tablets 695
Ziac Tablets 1887

Hydrocodone Bitartrate (Possible additive or potentiating effect with CNS depressants). Products include:
Hycodan 1316
Hycomine Compound Tablets 1317
Hycotuss Expectorant Syrup 1318
Lortab 3319
Lortab Elixir 3317
Maxidone Tablets CIII 3399
Norco 5/325 Tablets CIII 3424
Norco 7.5/325 Tablets CIII 3425
Norco 10/325 Tablets CIII 3427
Norco 10/325 Tablets CIII 3425
Vicodin Tablets 516
Vicodin ES Tablets 517
Vicodin HP Tablets 518
Vicodin Tuss Expectorant 519
Vicoprofen Tablets 520
Zydone Tablets 1330

Hydrocodone Polistirex (Possible additive or potentiating effect with CNS depressants). Products include:
Tussionex Pennkinetic Extended-Release Suspension 1174

Hydroflumethiazide (Concurrent use of brimonidine, an alpha adrenergic agonist, with antihypertensives may reduce pulse and blood pressure, however, in clinical trials brimonidine did not have any significant effects on pulse and blood pressure). Products include:
Diucardin Tablets 3494

Hydromorphone Hydrochloride (Possible additive or potentiating effect with CNS depressants).
Products include:
Dilaudid 441
Dilaudid Oral Liquid 445
Dilaudid Powder 441
Dilaudid Rectal Suppositories 441
Dilaudid Tablets 441
Dilaudid Tablets - 8 mg 445
Dilaudid-HP 443

Hydroxyzine Hydrochloride (Possible additive or potentiating effect with CNS depressants). Products include:
Atarax Tablets & Syrup 2667
Vistaril Intramuscular Solution 2738

Imipramine Hydrochloride (Tricyclic antidepressants have been reported to blunt the hypotensive effect of systemic clonidine, an alpha adrenergic agonist; it is not known whether the concurrent use of these agents with brimonidine can lead to interference in IOP-lowering effect; caution is advised).
No products indexed under this heading.

Imipramine Pamoate (Tricyclic antidepressants have been reported to blunt the hypotensive effect of systemic clonidine, an alpha adrenergic agonist; it is not known whether the concurrent use of these agents with brimonidine can lead to interference in IOP-lowering effect; caution is advised).
No products indexed under this heading.

Indapamide (Concurrent use of brimonidine, an alpha adrenergic agonist, with antihypertensives may reduce pulse and blood pressure, however, in clinical trials brimonidine did not have any significant effects on pulse and blood pressure).
Products include:
Indapamide Tablets 2286

Irbesartan (Concurrent use of brimonidine, an alpha adrenergic agonist, with antihypertensives may reduce pulse and blood pressure, however, in clinical trials brimonidine did not have any significant effects on pulse and blood pressure).
Products include:
Avalide Tablets 1070
Avapro Tablets 1074
Avapro Tablets 3076

Isocarboxazid (Concurrent use of brimonidine, an alpha adrenergic agonist, and MAO inhibitor is contraindicated).
No products indexed under this heading.

Isoflurane (Possible additive or potentiating effect with CNS depressants).
No products indexed under this heading.

Isradipine (Concurrent use of brimonidine, an alpha adrenergic agonist, with antihypertensives may reduce pulse and blood pressure, however, in clinical trials brimonidine did not have any significant effects on pulse and blood pressure).
Products include:
DynaCirc Capsules 2921
DynaCirc CR Tablets 2923

Ketamine Hydrochloride (Possible additive or potentiating effect with CNS depressants).
No products indexed under this heading.

Labetalol Hydrochloride (Concurrent use of brimonidine, an alpha adrenergic agonist, with beta blockers (ophthalmic and systemic) may reduce pulse and blood pressure, however, in clinical trials brimonidine did not have any significant effects on pulse and blood pressure).
Products include:
Normodyne Injection 3135
Normodyne Tablets 3137

Levobunolol Hydrochloride (Concurrent use of brimonidine, an alpha adrenergic agonist, with beta blockers (ophthalmic and systemic) may reduce pulse and blood pressure, however, in clinical trials brimonidine did not have any significant effects on pulse and blood pressure).
Products include:
Betagan ⊙ 228

Levomethadyl Acetate Hydrochloride (Possible additive or potentiating effect with CNS depressants).
No products indexed under this heading.

Levorphanol Tartrate (Possible additive or potentiating effect with CNS depressants). Products include:
Levo-Dromoran 1734
Levorphanol Tartrate Tablets 3059

Lisinopril (Concurrent use of brimonidine, an alpha adrenergic agonist, with antihypertensives may reduce pulse and blood pressure, however, in clinical trials brimonidine did not have any significant effects on pulse and blood pressure).
Products include:
Prinivil Tablets 2164
Prinzide Tablets 2168
Zestoretic Tablets 695
Zestril Tablets 698

Lorazepam (Possible additive or potentiating effect with CNS depressants). Products include:
Ativan Injection 3478
Ativan Tablets 3482

Losartan Potassium (Concurrent use of brimonidine, an alpha adrenergic agonist, with antihypertensives may reduce pulse and blood pressure, however, in clinical trials brimonidine did not have any significant effects on pulse and blood pressure). Products include:
Cozaar Tablets 2067
Hyzaar 2109

Loxapine Hydrochloride (Possible additive or potentiating effect with CNS depressants).
No products indexed under this heading.

Loxapine Succinate (Possible additive or potentiating effect with CNS depressants). Products include:
Loxitane Capsules 3398

Maprotiline Hydrochloride (Tricyclic antidepressants have been reported to blunt the hypotensive effect of systemic clonidine, an alpha adrenergic agonist; it is not known whether the concurrent use of these agents with brimonidine can lead to interference in IOP-lowering effect; caution is advised).
No products indexed under this heading.

Mecamylamine Hydrochloride (Concurrent use of brimonidine, an alpha adrenergic agonist, with antihypertensives may reduce pulse and blood pressure, however, in clinical trials brimonidine did not have any significant effects on pulse and blood pressure). Products include:
Inversine Tablets 1850

Meperidine Hydrochloride (Possible additive or potentiating effect with CNS depressants). Products include:
Demerol 3079
Mepergan Injection 3539

Mephobarbital (Possible additive or potentiating effect with CNS depressants).
No products indexed under this heading.

Meprobamate (Possible additive or potentiating effect with CNS depressants). Products include:
Miltown Tablets ... 3349

Mesoridazine Besylate (Possible additive or potentiating effect with CNS depressants). Products include:
Serentil ... 1057

Methadone Hydrochloride (Possible additive or potentiating effect with CNS depressants). Products include:
Dolophine Hydrochloride Tablets ... 3056

Methohexital Sodium (Possible additive or potentiating effect with CNS depressants). Products include:
Brevital Sodium for Injection, USP .. 1815

Methotrimeprazine (Possible additive or potentiating effect with CNS depressants).
No products indexed under this heading.

Methoxyflurane (Possible additive or potentiating effect with CNS depressants).
No products indexed under this heading.

Methyclothiazide (Concurrent use of brimonidine, an alpha adrenergic agonist, with antihypertensives may reduce pulse and blood pressure, however, in clinical trials brimonidine did not have any significant effects on pulse and blood pressure).
No products indexed under this heading.

Methyldopa (Concurrent use of brimonidine, an alpha adrenergic agonist, with antihypertensives may reduce pulse and blood pressure, however, in clinical trials brimonidine did not have any significant effects on pulse and blood pressure).
Products include:
Aldoclor Tablets ... 2035
Aldomet Tablets ... 2037
Aldoril Tablets ... 2039

Methyldopate Hydrochloride (Concurrent use of brimonidine, an alpha adrenergic agonist, with antihypertensives may reduce pulse and blood pressure, however, in clinical trials brimonidine did not have any significant effects on pulse and blood pressure).
No products indexed under this heading.

Metipranolol Hydrochloride (Concurrent use of brimonidine, an alpha adrenergic agonist, with beta blockers (ophthalmic and systemic) may reduce pulse and blood pressure, however, in clinical trials brimonidine did not have any significant effects on pulse and blood pressure).
No products indexed under this heading.

Metolazone (Concurrent use of brimonidine, an alpha adrenergic agonist, with antihypertensives may reduce pulse and blood pressure, however, in clinical trials brimonidine did not have any significant effects on pulse and blood pressure).
Products include:
Mykrox Tablets ... 1168
Zaroxolyn Tablets ... 1177

Metoprolol Succinate (Concurrent use of brimonidine, an alpha adrenergic agonist, with beta blockers (ophthalmic and systemic) may reduce pulse and blood pressure, however, in clinical trials brimonidine did not have any significant effects on pulse and blood pressure). Products include:
Toprol-XL Tablets ... 651

Metoprolol Tartrate (Concurrent use of brimonidine, an alpha adrenergic agonist, with beta blockers (ophthalmic and systemic) may reduce pulse and blood pressure, however, in clinical trials brimonidine did not have any significant effects on pulse and blood pressure).
No products indexed under this heading.

Metyrosine (Concurrent use of brimonidine, an alpha adrenergic agonist, with antihypertensives may reduce pulse and blood pressure, however, in clinical trials brimonidine did not have any significant effects on pulse and blood pressure).
Products include:
Demser Capsules ... 2085

Mibefradil Dihydrochloride (Concurrent use of brimonidine, an alpha adrenergic agonist, with antihypertensives may reduce pulse and blood pressure, however, in clinical trials brimonidine did not have any significant effects on pulse and blood pressure).
No products indexed under this heading.

Midazolam Hydrochloride (Possible additive or potentiating effect with CNS depressants). Products include:
Versed Injection ... 3027
Versed Syrup ... 3033

Minoxidil (Concurrent use of brimonidine, an alpha adrenergic agonist, with antihypertensives may reduce pulse and blood pressure, however, in clinical trials brimonidine did not have any significant effects on pulse and blood pressure).
Products include:
Rogaine Extra Strength for Men Topical Solution ... ▣721
Rogaine for Women Topical Solution ... ▣721

Moclobemide (Concurrent use of brimonidine, an alpha adrenergic agonist, and MAO inhibitor is contraindicated).
No products indexed under this heading.

Moexipril Hydrochloride (Concurrent use of brimonidine, an alpha adrenergic agonist, with antihypertensives may reduce pulse and blood pressure, however, in clinical trials brimonidine did not have any significant effects on pulse and blood pressure). Products include:
Uniretic Tablets ... 3178
Univasc Tablets ... 3181

Molindone Hydrochloride (Possible additive or potentiating effect with CNS depressants). Products include:
Moban ... 1320

Morphine Sulfate (Possible additive or potentiating effect with CNS depressants). Products include:
Astramorph/PF Injection, USP (Preservative-Free) ... 594
Duramorph Injection ... 1312
Infumorph 200 and Infumorph 500 Sterile Solutions ... 1314
Kadian Capsules ... 1335
MS Contin Tablets ... 2896
MSIR ... 2898
Oramorph SR Tablets ... 3062
Roxanol ... 3066

Nadolol (Concurrent use of brimonidine, an alpha adrenergic agonist, with beta blockers (ophthalmic and systemic) may reduce pulse and blood pressure, however, in clinical trials brimonidine did not have any significant effects on pulse and blood pressure). Products include:
Corgard Tablets ... 2245
Corzide 40/5 Tablets ... 2247
Corzide 80/5 Tablets ... 2247
Nadolol Tablets ... 2288

Nicardipine Hydrochloride (Concurrent use of brimonidine, an alpha adrenergic agonist, with antihypertensives may reduce pulse and blood pressure, however, in clinical trials brimonidine did not have any significant effects on pulse and blood pressure). Products include:
Cardene I.V. ... 3485

Nifedipine (Concurrent use of brimonidine, an alpha adrenergic agonist, with antihypertensives may reduce pulse and blood pressure, however, in clinical trials brimonidine did not have any significant effects on pulse and blood pressure).
Products include:
Adalat CC Tablets ... 877
Procardia Capsules ... 2708
Procardia XL Extended Release Tablets ... 2710

Nisoldipine (Concurrent use of brimonidine, an alpha adrenergic agonist, with antihypertensives may reduce pulse and blood pressure, however, in clinical trials brimonidine did not have any significant effects on pulse and blood pressure).
Products include:
Sular Tablets ... 688

Nitroglycerin (Concurrent use of brimonidine, an alpha adrenergic agonist, with antihypertensives may reduce pulse and blood pressure, however, in clinical trials brimonidine did not have any significant effects on pulse and blood pressure).
Products include:
Nitro-Dur Transdermal Infusion System ... 3134
Nitro-Dur Transdermal Infusion System ... 1834
Nitrolingual Pumpspray ... 1355
Nitrostat Tablets ... 2658

Nortriptyline Hydrochloride (Tricyclic antidepressants have been reported to blunt the hypotensive effect of systemic clonidine, an alpha adrenergic agonist; it is not known whether the concurrent use of these agents with brimonidine can lead to interference in IOP-lowering effect; caution is advised).
No products indexed under this heading.

Olanzapine (Possible additive or potentiating effect with CNS depressants). Products include:
Zyprexa Tablets ... 1973
Zyprexa ZYDIS Orally Disintegrating Tablets ... 1973

Oxazepam (Possible additive or potentiating effect with CNS depressants).
No products indexed under this heading.

Oxycodone Hydrochloride (Possible additive or potentiating effect with CNS depressants). Products include:
OxyContin Tablets ... 2912
OxyFast Oral Concentrate Solution . 2916
OxyIR Capsules ... 2916
Percocet Tablets ... 1326
Percodan Tablets ... 1327
Percolone Tablets ... 1327
Roxicodone ... 3067
Tylox Capsules ... 2597

Pargyline Hydrochloride (Concurrent use of brimonidine, an alpha adrenergic agonist, and MAO inhibitor is contraindicated).
No products indexed under this heading.

Penbutolol Sulfate (Concurrent use of brimonidine, an alpha adrenergic agonist, with beta blockers (ophthalmic and systemic) may reduce pulse and blood pressure, however, in clinical trials brimonidine did not have any significant effects on pulse and blood pressure).
No products indexed under this heading.

Pentobarbital Sodium (Possible additive or potentiating effect with CNS depressants). Products include:
Nembutal Sodium Solution ... 485

Perindopril Erbumine (Concurrent use of brimonidine, an alpha adrenergic agonist, with antihypertensives may reduce pulse and blood pressure, however, in clinical trials brimonidine did not have any significant effects on pulse and blood pressure). Products include:
Aceon Tablets (2 mg, 4 mg, 8 mg) ... 3249

Perphenazine (Possible additive or potentiating effect with CNS depressants). Products include:
Etrafon ... 3115
Trilafon ... 3160

Phenelzine Sulfate (Concurrent use of brimonidine, an alpha adrenergic agonist, and MAO inhibitor is contraindicated). Products include:
Nardil Tablets ... 2653

Phenobarbital (Possible additive or potentiating effect with CNS depressants). Products include:
Arco-Lase Plus Tablets ... 592
Donnatal ... 2929
Donnatal Extentabs ... 2930

Phenoxybenzamine Hydrochloride (Concurrent use of brimonidine, an alpha adrenergic agonist, with antihypertensives may reduce pulse and blood pressure, however, in clinical trials brimonidine did not have any significant effects on pulse and blood pressure). Products include:
Dibenzyline Capsules ... 3457

Phentolamine Mesylate (Concurrent use of brimonidine, an alpha adrenergic agonist, with antihypertensives may reduce pulse and blood pressure, however, in clinical trials brimonidine did not have any significant effects on pulse and blood pressure).
No products indexed under this heading.

Pindolol (Concurrent use of brimonidine, an alpha adrenergic agonist, with beta blockers (ophthalmic and systemic) may reduce pulse and blood pressure, however, in clinical trials brimonidine did not have any significant effects on pulse and blood pressure).
No products indexed under this heading.

Polythiazide (Concurrent use of brimonidine, an alpha adrenergic agonist, with antihypertensives may reduce pulse and blood pressure, however, in clinical trials brimonidine did not have any significant effects on pulse and blood pressure).
Products include:
Minizide Capsules ... 2700
Renese Tablets ... 2712

Prazepam (Possible additive or potentiating effect with CNS depressants).
No products indexed under this heading.

Prazosin Hydrochloride (Concurrent use of brimonidine, an alpha adrenergic agonist, with antihypertensives may reduce pulse and blood pressure, however, in clinical trials brimonidine did not have any significant effects on pulse and blood pressure). Products include:
Minipress Capsules ... 2699
Minizide Capsules ... 2700

Procarbazine Hydrochloride (Concurrent use of brimonidine, an alpha adrenergic agonist, and MAO inhibitor is contraindicated).
Products include:
Matulane Capsules ... 3246

Prochlorperazine (Possible additive or potentiating effect with CNS depressants). Products include:
Compazine ... 1505

Promethazine Hydrochloride (Possible additive or potentiating effect with CNS depressants).
Products include:
Mepergan Injection ... 3539
Phenergan Injection ... 3553
Phenergan ... 3556
Phenergan Syrup ... 3554
Phenergan with Codeine Syrup ... 3557
Phenergan with Dextromethorphan Syrup ... 3559
Phenergan VC Syrup ... 3560
Phenergan VC with Codeine Syrup .. 3561

Propofol (Possible additive or potentiating effect with CNS depressants). Products include:
Diprivan Injectable Emulsion 667

Propoxyphene Hydrochloride (Possible additive or potentiating effect with CNS depressants). Products include:
Darvon Pulvules 1909
Darvon Compound-65 Pulvules 1910

Propoxyphene Napsylate (Possible additive or potentiating effect with CNS depressants). Products include:
Darvon-N/Darvocet-N 1907
Darvon-N Tablets 1912

Propranolol Hydrochloride (Concurrent use of brimonidine, an alpha adrenergic agonist, with beta blockers (ophthalmic and systemic) may reduce pulse and blood pressure, however, in clinical trials brimonidine did not have any significant effects on pulse and blood pressure). Products include:
Inderal 3513
Inderal LA Long-Acting Capsules 3516
Inderide Tablets 3517
Inderide LA Long-Acting Capsules .. 3519

Protriptyline Hydrochloride (Tricyclic antidepressants have been reported to blunt the hypotensive effect of systemic clonidine, an alpha adrenergic agonist; it is not known whether the concurrent use of these agents with brimonidine can lead to interference in IOP-lowering effect; caution is advised). Products include:
Vivactil Tablets 2446
Vivactil Tablets 2217

Quazepam (Possible additive or potentiating effect with CNS depressants).
No products indexed under this heading.

Quetiapine Fumarate (Possible additive or potentiating effect with CNS depressants). Products include:
Seroquel Tablets 684

Quinapril Hydrochloride (Concurrent use of brimonidine, an alpha adrenergic agonist, with antihypertensives may reduce pulse and blood pressure, however, in clinical trials brimonidine did not have any significant effects on pulse and blood pressure). Products include:
Accupril Tablets 2611
Accuretic Tablets 2614

Ramipril (Concurrent use of brimonidine, an alpha adrenergic agonist, with antihypertensives may reduce pulse and blood pressure, however, in clinical trials brimonidine did not have any significant effects on pulse and blood pressure). Products include:
Altace Capsules 2233

Rauwolfia serpentina (Concurrent use of brimonidine, an alpha adrenergic agonist, with antihypertensives may reduce pulse and blood pressure, however, in clinical trials brimonidine did not have any significant effects on pulse and blood pressure).
No products indexed under this heading.

Remifentanil Hydrochloride (Possible additive or potentiating effect with CNS depressants).
No products indexed under this heading.

Rescinnamine (Concurrent use of brimonidine, an alpha adrenergic agonist, with antihypertensives may reduce pulse and blood pressure, however, in clinical trials brimonidine did not have any significant effects on pulse and blood pressure).
No products indexed under this heading.

Reserpine (Concurrent use of brimonidine, an alpha adrenergic agonist, with antihypertensives may reduce pulse and blood pressure, however, in clinical trials brimonidine did not have any significant effects on pulse and blood pressure).
No products indexed under this heading.

Risperidone (Possible additive or potentiating effect with CNS depressants). Products include:
Risperdal 1796

Secobarbital Sodium (Possible additive or potentiating effect with CNS depressants).
No products indexed under this heading.

Selegiline Hydrochloride (Concurrent use of brimonidine, an alpha adrenergic agonist, and MAO inhibitor is contraindicated). Products include:
Eldepryl Capsules 3266

Sevoflurane (Possible additive or potentiating effect with CNS depressants).
No products indexed under this heading.

Sodium Nitroprusside (Concurrent use of brimonidine, an alpha adrenergic agonist, with antihypertensives may reduce pulse and blood pressure, however, in clinical trials brimonidine did not have any significant effects on pulse and blood pressure).
No products indexed under this heading.

Sotalol Hydrochloride (Concurrent use of brimonidine, an alpha adrenergic agonist, with beta blockers (ophthalmic and systemic) may reduce pulse and blood pressure, however, in clinical trials brimonidine did not have any significant effects on pulse and blood pressure). Products include:
Betapace Tablets 950
Betapace AF Tablets 954

Spirapril Hydrochloride (Concurrent use of brimonidine, an alpha adrenergic agonist, with antihypertensives may reduce pulse and blood pressure, however, in clinical trials brimonidine did not have any significant effects on pulse and blood pressure).
No products indexed under this heading.

Sufentanil Citrate (Possible additive or potentiating effect with CNS depressants).
No products indexed under this heading.

Telmisartan (Concurrent use of brimonidine, an alpha adrenergic agonist, with antihypertensives may reduce pulse and blood pressure, however, in clinical trials brimonidine did not have any significant effects on pulse and blood pressure). Products include:
Micardis Tablets 1049
Micardis HCT Tablets 1051

Temazepam (Possible additive or potentiating effect with CNS depressants).
No products indexed under this heading.

Terazosin Hydrochloride (Concurrent use of brimonidine, an alpha adrenergic agonist, with antihypertensives may reduce pulse and blood pressure, however, in clinical trials brimonidine did not have any significant effects on pulse and blood pressure). Products include:
Hytrin Capsules 464

Thiamylal Sodium (Possible additive or potentiating effect with CNS depressants).
No products indexed under this heading.

Thioridazine Hydrochloride (Possible additive or potentiating effect with CNS depressants). Products include:
Thioridazine Hydrochloride Tablets 2289

Thiothixene (Possible additive or potentiating effect with CNS depressants). Products include:
Navane Capsules 2701
Thiothixene Capsules 2290

Timolol Hemihydrate (Concurrent use of brimonidine, an alpha adrenergic agonist, with beta blockers (ophthalmic and systemic) may reduce pulse and blood pressure, however, in clinical trials brimonidine did not have any significant effects on pulse and blood pressure). Products include:
Betimol Ophthalmic Solution .... ⊙324

Timolol Maleate (Concurrent use of brimonidine, an alpha adrenergic agonist, with beta blockers (ophthalmic and systemic) may reduce pulse and blood pressure, however, in clinical trials brimonidine did not have any significant effects on pulse and blood pressure). Products include:
Blocadren Tablets 2046
Cosopt Sterile Ophthalmic Solution 2065
Timolide Tablets 2187
Timolol GFS .... ⊙266
Timoptic in Ocudose 2192
Timoptic Sterile Ophthalmic Solution 2190
Timoptic-XE Sterile Ophthalmic Gel Forming Solution 2194

Torsemide (Concurrent use of brimonidine, an alpha adrenergic agonist, with antihypertensives may reduce pulse and blood pressure, however, in clinical trials brimonidine did not have any significant effects on pulse and blood pressure). Products include:
Demadex Tablets and Injection 2965

Trandolapril (Concurrent use of brimonidine, an alpha adrenergic agonist, with antihypertensives may reduce pulse and blood pressure, however, in clinical trials brimonidine did not have any significant effects on pulse and blood pressure). Products include:
Mavik Tablets 478
Tarka Tablets 508

Tranylcypromine Sulfate (Concurrent use of brimonidine, an alpha adrenergic agonist, and MAO inhibitor is contraindicated). Products include:
Parnate Tablets 1607

Triazolam (Possible additive or potentiating effect with CNS depressants). Products include:
Halcion Tablets 2823

Trifluoperazine Hydrochloride (Possible additive or potentiating effect with CNS depressants). Products include:
Stelazine 1640

Trimethaphan Camsylate (Concurrent use of brimonidine, an alpha adrenergic agonist, with antihypertensives may reduce pulse and blood pressure, however, in clinical trials brimonidine did not have any significant effects on pulse and blood pressure).
No products indexed under this heading.

Trimipramine Maleate (Tricyclic antidepressants have been reported to blunt the hypotensive effect of systemic clonidine, an alpha adrenergic agonist; it is not known whether the concurrent use of these agents with brimonidine can lead to interference in IOP-lowering effect; caution is advised). Products include:
Surmontil Capsules 3595

Valsartan (Concurrent use of brimonidine, an alpha adrenergic agonist, with antihypertensives may reduce pulse and blood pressure, however, in clinical trials brimonidine did not have any significant effects on pulse and blood pressure). Products include:
Diovan Capsules 2337
Diovan HCT Tablets 2338

Verapamil Hydrochloride (Concurrent use of brimonidine, an alpha adrenergic agonist, with antihypertensives may reduce pulse and blood pressure, however, in clinical trials brimonidine did not have any significant effects on pulse and blood pressure). Products include:
Covera-HS Tablets 3199
Isoptin SR Tablets 467
Tarka Tablets 508
Verelan Capsules 3184
Verelan PM Capsules 3186

Zaleplon (Possible additive or potentiating effect with CNS depressants). Products include:
Sonata Capsules 3591

Ziprasidone Hydrochloride (Possible additive or potentiating effect with CNS depressants). Products include:
Geodon Capsules 2688

Zolpidem Tartrate (Possible additive or potentiating effect with CNS depressants). Products include:
Ambien Tablets 3191

Food Interactions

Alcohol (Possible additive or potentiating effect with CNS depressants).

ALPHAGAN P OPHTHALMIC SOLUTION

(Brimonidine Tartrate) 546
See Alphagan Ophthalmic Solution

ALREX STERILE OPHTHALMIC SUSPENSION 0.2%

(Loteprednol Etabonate) .... ⊙256
None cited in PDR database.

ALTACE CAPSULES

(Ramipril) 2233

May interact with diuretics, lithium preparations, non-steroidal anti-inflammatory agents, potassium preparations, potassium sparing diuretics, and certain other agents. Compounds in these categories include:

Amiloride Hydrochloride (May result in excessive reduction of blood pressure after initiation of therapy; increased risk of hyperkalemia). Products include:
Midamor Tablets 2136
Moduretic Tablets 2138

Bendroflumethiazide (May result in excessive reduction of blood pressure after initiation of therapy). Products include:
Corzide 40/5 Tablets 2247
Corzide 80/5 Tablets 2247

Bumetanide (May result in excessive reduction of blood pressure after initiation of therapy).
No products indexed under this heading.

Celecoxib (Co-administration of ACE inhibitors with NSAID have been associated with worsening of renal failure and hyperkalemia). Products include:
Celebrex Capsules 2676
Celebrex Capsules 2780

Chlorothiazide (May result in excessive reduction of blood pressure after initiation of therapy). Products include:
Aldoclor Tablets 2035
Diuril Oral 2087

Chlorothiazide Sodium (May result in excessive reduction of blood pressure after initiation of therapy). Products include:
Diuril Sodium Intravenous 2086

Chlorthalidone (May result in excessive reduction of blood pressure after initiation of therapy). Products include:
- Clorpres Tablets ... 1002
- Combipres Tablets ... 1040
- Tenoretic Tablets ... 690

Diclofenac Potassium (Co-administration of ACE inhibitors with NSAID have been associated with worsening of renal failure and hyperkalemia). Products include:
- Cataflam Tablets ... 2315

Diclofenac Sodium (Co-administration of ACE inhibitors with NSAID have been associated with worsening of renal failure and hyperkalemia). Products include:
- Arthrotec Tablets ... 3195
- Voltaren Ophthalmic Sterile Ophthalmic Solution ... ⊙312
- Voltaren Tablets ... 2315
- Voltaren-XR Tablets ... 2315

Ethacrynic Acid (May result in excessive reduction of blood pressure after initiation of therapy). Products include:
- Edecrin Tablets ... 2091

Etodolac (Co-administration of ACE inhibitors with NSAID have been associated with worsening of renal failure and hyperkalemia). Products include:
- Lodine ... 3528
- Lodine XL Extended-Release Tablets ... 3530

Fenoprofen Calcium (Co-administration of ACE inhibitors with NSAID have been associated with worsening of renal failure and hyperkalemia).
- No products indexed under this heading.

Flurbiprofen (Co-administration of ACE inhibitors with NSAID have been associated with worsening of renal failure and hyperkalemia).
- No products indexed under this heading.

Furosemide (May result in excessive reduction of blood pressure after initiation of therapy). Products include:
- Furosemide Tablets ... 2284

Hydrochlorothiazide (May result in excessive reduction of blood pressure after initiation of therapy). Products include:
- Accuretic Tablets ... 2614
- Aldoril Tablets ... 2039
- Atacand HCT Tablets ... 597
- Avalide Tablets ... 1070
- Diovan HCT Tablets ... 2338
- Dyazide Capsules ... 1515
- HydroDIURIL Tablets ... 2108
- Hyzaar ... 2109
- Inderide Tablets ... 3517
- Inderide LA Long-Acting Capsules ... 3519
- Lotensin HCT Tablets ... 2367
- Maxzide ... 1008
- Micardis HCT Tablets ... 1051
- Microzide Capsules ... 3414
- Moduretic Tablets ... 2138
- Monopril HCT ... 1094
- Prinzide Tablets ... 2168
- Timolide Tablets ... 2187
- Uniretic Tablets ... 3178
- Vaseretic Tablets ... 2204
- Zestoretic Tablets ... 695
- Ziac Tablets ... 1887

Hydroflumethiazide (May result in excessive reduction of blood pressure after initiation of therapy). Products include:
- Diucardin Tablets ... 3494

Ibuprofen (Co-administration of ACE inhibitors with NSAID have been associated with worsening of renal failure and hyperkalemia). Products include:
- Advil ... ■771
- Children's Advil Oral Suspension ... ■773
- Children's Advil Chewable Tablets ... ■773
- Advil Cold and Sinus Caplets ... ■771
- Advil Cold and Sinus Tablets ... ■771
- Advil Flu & Body Ache Caplets ... ■772
- Infants' Advil Drops ... ■773
- Junior Strength Advil Tablets ... ■773
- Junior Strength Advil Chewable Tablets ... ■773
- Advil Migraine Liquigels ... ■772
- Children's Motrin Oral Suspension and Chewable Tablets ... 2006
- Children's Motrin Cold Oral Suspension ... 2007
- Children's Motrin Oral Suspension ... ■643
- Motrin Suspension, Oral Drops, Chewable Tablets, and Caplets ... 2002
- Infants' Motrin Concentrated Drops ... 2006
- Junior Strength Motrin Caplets and Chewable Tablets ... 2006
- Motrin IB Tablets, Caplets, and Gelcaps ... 2002
- Motrin Migraine Pain Caplets ... 2005
- Motrin Sinus Headache Caplets ... 2005
- Vicoprofen Tablets ... 520

Indapamide (May result in excessive reduction of blood pressure after initiation of therapy). Products include:
- Indapamide Tablets ... 2286

Indomethacin (Co-administration of ACE inhibitors with NSAID have been associated with worsening of renal failure and hyperkalemia). Products include:
- Indocin ... 2112

Indomethacin Sodium Trihydrate (Co-administration of ACE inhibitors with NSAID have been associated with worsening of renal failure and hyperkalemia). Products include:
- Indocin I.V. ... 2115

Ketoprofen (Co-administration of ACE inhibitors with NSAID have been associated with worsening of renal failure and hyperkalemia). Products include:
- Orudis Capsules ... 3548
- Orudis KT Tablets ... ■778
- Oruvail Capsules ... 3548

Ketorolac Tromethamine (Co-administration of ACE inhibitors with NSAID have been associated with worsening of renal failure and hyperkalemia). Products include:
- Acular Ophthalmic Solution ... 544
- Acular PF Ophthalmic Solution ... 544
- Toradol ... 3018

Lithium Carbonate (Increased serum lithium levels and symptoms of lithium toxicity). Products include:
- Eskalith ... 1527
- Lithium Carbonate ... 3061
- Lithobid Slow-Release Tablets ... 3255

Lithium Citrate (Increased serum lithium levels and symptoms of lithium toxicity). Products include:
- Lithium Citrate Syrup ... 3061

Meclofenamate Sodium (Co-administration of ACE inhibitors with NSAID have been associated with worsening of renal failure and hyperkalemia).
- No products indexed under this heading.

Mefenamic Acid (Co-administration of ACE inhibitors with NSAID have been associated with worsening of renal failure and hyperkalemia). Products include:
- Ponstel Capsules ... 1356

Meloxicam (Co-administration of ACE inhibitors with NSAID have been associated with worsening of renal failure and hyperkalemia). Products include:
- Mobic Tablets ... 1054

Methyclothiazide (May result in excessive reduction of blood pressure after initiation of therapy).
- No products indexed under this heading.

Metolazone (May result in excessive reduction of blood pressure after initiation of therapy). Products include:
- Mykrox Tablets ... 1168
- Zaroxolyn Tablets ... 1177

Nabumetone (Co-administration of ACE inhibitors with NSAID have been associated with worsening of renal failure and hyperkalemia). Products include:
- Relafen Tablets ... 1617

Naproxen (Co-administration of ACE inhibitors with NSAID have been associated with worsening of renal failure and hyperkalemia). Products include:
- EC-Naprosyn Delayed-Release Tablets ... 2967
- Naprosyn Suspension ... 2967
- Naprosyn Tablets ... 2967

Naproxen Sodium (Co-administration of ACE inhibitors with NSAID have been associated with worsening of renal failure and hyperkalemia). Products include:
- Aleve Tablets, Caplets and Gelcaps ... ■602
- Aleve Cold & Sinus Caplets ... ■603
- Anaprox Tablets ... 2967
- Anaprox DS Tablets ... 2967
- Naprelan Tablets ... 1293

Oxaprozin (Co-administration of ACE inhibitors with NSAID have been associated with worsening of renal failure and hyperkalemia).
- No products indexed under this heading.

Phenylbutazone (Co-administration of ACE inhibitors with NSAID have been associated with worsening of renal failure and hyperkalemia).
- No products indexed under this heading.

Piroxicam (Co-administration of ACE inhibitors with NSAID have been associated with worsening of renal failure and hyperkalemia). Products include:
- Feldene Capsules ... 2685

Polythiazide (May result in excessive reduction of blood pressure after initiation of therapy). Products include:
- Minizide Capsules ... 2700
- Renese Tablets ... 2712

Potassium Acid Phosphate (Increased risk of hyperkalemia). Products include:
- K-Phos Original (Sodium Free) Tablets ... 947

Potassium Bicarbonate (Increased risk of hyperkalemia).
- No products indexed under this heading.

Potassium Chloride (Increased risk of hyperkalemia). Products include:
- Chlor-3 ... 1361
- Colyte with Flavor Packs for Oral Solution ... 3170
- GoLYTELY and Pineapple Flavor GoLYTELY for Oral Solution ... 1068
- K-Dur Microburst Release System ER Tablets ... 1832
- Klor-Con M20/Klor-Con M10 Tablets ... 3329
- K-Lor Powder Packets ... 469
- K-Tab Filmtab Tablets ... 470
- Micro-K ... 3311
- NuLYTELY, Cherry Flavor, Lemon-Lime Flavor, and Orange Flavor NuLYTELY for Oral Solution ... 1068
- Rum-K ... 1363

Potassium Citrate (Increased risk of hyperkalemia). Products include:
- Urocit-K Tablets ... 2232

Potassium Gluconate (Increased risk of hyperkalemia).
- No products indexed under this heading.

Potassium Phosphate (Increased risk of hyperkalemia). Products include:
- K-Phos Neutral Tablets ... 946

Rofecoxib (Co-administration of ACE inhibitors with NSAID have been associated with worsening of renal failure and hyperkalemia). Products include:
- Vioxx ... 2213

Spironolactone (May result in excessive reduction of blood pressure after initiation of therapy; increased risk of hyperkalemia).
- No products indexed under this heading.

Sulindac (Co-administration of ACE inhibitors with NSAID have been associated with worsening of renal failure and hyperkalemia). Products include:
- Clinoril Tablets ... 2053

Tolmetin Sodium (Co-administration of ACE inhibitors with NSAID have been associated with worsening of renal failure and hyperkalemia). Products include:
- Tolectin ... 2589

Torsemide (May result in excessive reduction of blood pressure after initiation of therapy). Products include:
- Demadex Tablets and Injection ... 2965

Triamterene (May result in excessive reduction of blood pressure after initiation of therapy; increased risk of hyperkalemia). Products include:
- Dyazide Capsules ... 1515
- Dyrenium Capsules ... 3458
- Maxzide ... 1008

Food Interactions

Food, unspecified (The rate of absorption is reduced, not the extent of absorption).

Salt Substitutes, Potassium-Containing (Increases risk of hyperkalemia).

ALUPENT INHALATION AEROSOL

(Metaproterenol Sulfate) ... 1029

See Alupent Inhalation Solution

ALUPENT INHALATION SOLUTION

(Metaproterenol Sulfate) ... 1029

May interact with monoamine oxidase inhibitors, sympathomimetic aerosol bronchodilators, and tricyclic antidepressants. Compounds in these categories include:

Albuterol (Possible potentiation of adrenergic effects with beta adrenergic aerosol bronchodilators). Products include:
- Proventil Inhalation Aerosol ... 3142
- Ventolin Inhalation Aerosol and Refill ... 1679

Amitriptyline Hydrochloride (The action of beta adrenergic agonists on the vascular system may be potentiated). Products include:
- Etrafon ... 3115
- Limbitrol ... 1738

Amoxapine (The action of beta adrenergic agonists on the vascular system may be potentiated).
- No products indexed under this heading.

Bitolterol Mesylate (Possible potentiation of adrenergic effects with beta adrenergic aerosol bronchodilators).
- No products indexed under this heading.

Clomipramine Hydrochloride (The action of beta adrenergic agonists on the vascular system may be potentiated).
- No products indexed under this heading.

Desipramine Hydrochloride (The action of beta adrenergic agonists on the vascular system may be potentiated). Products include:
- Norpramin Tablets ... 755

Doxepin Hydrochloride (The action of beta adrenergic agonists on the vascular system may be potentiated). Products include:
- Sinequan ... 2713

Imipramine Hydrochloride (The action of beta adrenergic agonists on the vascular system may be

potentiated).
No products indexed under this heading.

Imipramine Pamoate (The action of beta adrenergic agonists on the vascular system may be potentiated).
No products indexed under this heading.

Isocarboxazid (The action of beta adrenergic agonists on the vascular system may be potentiated).
No products indexed under this heading.

Isoetharine (Possible potentiation of adrenergic effects with beta adrenergic aerosol bronchodilators).
No products indexed under this heading.

Isoproterenol Hydrochloride (Possible potentiation of adrenergic effects with beta adrenergic aerosol bronchodilators).
No products indexed under this heading.

Levalbuterol Hydrochloride (Possible potentiation of adrenergic effects with beta adrenergic aerosol bronchodilators). Products include:
Xopenex Inhalation Solution 3207

Maprotiline Hydrochloride (The action of beta adrenergic agonists on the vascular system may be potentiated).
No products indexed under this heading.

Moclobemide (The action of beta adrenergic agonists on the vascular system may be potentiated).
No products indexed under this heading.

Nortriptyline Hydrochloride (The action of beta adrenergic agonists on the vascular system may be potentiated).
No products indexed under this heading.

Pargyline Hydrochloride (The action of beta adrenergic agonists on the vascular system may be potentiated).
No products indexed under this heading.

Phenelzine Sulfate (The action of beta adrenergic agonists on the vascular system may be potentiated). Products include:
Nardil Tablets 2653

Pirbuterol Acetate (Possible potentiation of adrenergic effects with beta adrenergic aerosol bronchodilators). Products include:
Maxair Autohaler 1981
Maxair Inhaler 1984

Procarbazine Hydrochloride (The action of beta adrenergic agonists on the vascular system may be potentiated). Products include:
Matulane Capsules 3246

Protriptyline Hydrochloride (The action of beta adrenergic agonists on the vascular system may be potentiated). Products include:
Vivactil Tablets 2446
Vivactil Tablets 2217

Salmeterol Xinafoate (Possible potentiation of adrenergic effects with beta adrenergic aerosol bronchodilators). Products include:
Advair Diskus 100/50 1448
Advair Diskus 250/50 1448
Advair Diskus 500/50 1448
Serevent Diskus 1637
Serevent Inhalation Aerosol 1633

Selegiline Hydrochloride (The action of beta adrenergic agonists on the vascular system may be potentiated). Products include:
Eldepryl Capsules 3266

Terbutaline Sulfate (Possible potentiation of adrenergic effects with beta adrenergic aerosol bronchodilators). Products include:
Brethine Ampuls 2314
Brethine Tablets 2313

Tranylcypromine Sulfate (The action of beta adrenergic agonists on the vascular system may be potentiated). Products include:
Parnate Tablets 1607

Trimipramine Maleate (The action of beta adrenergic agonists on the vascular system may be potentiated). Products include:
Surmontil Capsules 3595

ALUSTRA CREAM
(Hydroquinone) 2018
None cited in PDR database.

AMARYL TABLETS
(Glimepiride) 717
May interact with beta blockers, corticosteroids, oral anticoagulants, diuretics, estrogens, insulin, monoamine oxidase inhibitors, non-steroidal anti-inflammatory agents, oral contraceptives, phenothiazines, salicylates, sulfonamides, sympathomimetics, thiazides, thyroid preparations, and certain other agents. Compounds in these categories include:

Acebutolol Hydrochloride (May potentiate hypoglycemic action). Products include:
Sectral Capsules 3589

Albuterol (Sympathomimetics tend to produce hyperglycemia and concurrent use may lead to loss of control). Products include:
Proventil Inhalation Aerosol 3142
Ventolin Inhalation Aerosol and Refill 1679

Albuterol Sulfate (Sympathomimetics tend to produce hyperglycemia and concurrent use may lead to loss of control). Products include:
AccuNeb Inhalation Solution 1230
Combivent Inhalation Aerosol 1041
DuoNeb Inhalation Solution 1233
Proventil Inhalation Solution 0.083% 3146
Proventil Repetabs Tablets 3148
Proventil Solution for Inhalation 0.5% 3144
Proventil HFA Inhalation Aerosol 3150
Ventolin HFA Inhalation Aerosol 3618
Volmax Extended-Release Tablets .. 2276

Amiloride Hydrochloride (Diuretics tend to produce hyperglycemia and concurrent use may lead to loss of control). Products include:
Midamor Tablets 2136
Moduretic Tablets 2138

Aspirin (Co-administration of aspirin (1 g tid) led to a 34% decrease in the mean glimepiride AUC and, therefore, a 34% increase in the mean CL/f; no hypoglycemic symptoms were reported). Products include:
Aggrenox Capsules 1026
Alka-Seltzer .... ▣603
Alka-Seltzer Lemon Lime Antacid and Pain Reliever Effervescent Tablets .... ▣603
Alka-Seltzer Extra Strength Antacid and Pain Reliever Effervescent Tablets .... ▣603
Alka-Seltzer PM Effervescent Tablets .... ▣605
Genuine Bayer Tablets, Caplets and Gelcaps .... ▣606
Extra Strength Bayer Caplets and Gelcaps .... ▣610
Aspirin Regimen Bayer Children's Chewable Tablets (Orange or Cherry Flavored) .... ▣607
Bayer, Aspirin Regimen .... ▣606
Aspirin Regimen Bayer 81 mg Caplets with Calcium .... ▣607
Genuine Bayer Professional Labeling (Aspirin Regimen Bayer) .... ▣608
Extra Strength Bayer Arthritis Caplets .... ▣610
Extra Strength Bayer Plus Caplets .... ▣610
Extra Strength Bayer PM Caplets .. ▣611
BC Powder .... ▣619
BC Allergy Sinus Cold Powder ...... ▣619
Arthritis Strength BC Powder .... ▣619
BC Sinus Cold Powder .... ▣619
Darvon Compound-65 Pulvules 1910
Ecotrin Enteric Coated Aspirin Low, Regular and Maximum Strength Tablets 1715
Excedrin Extra-Strength Tablets, Caplets, and Geltabs .... ▣629
Excedrin Migraine 1070
Goody's Body Pain Formula Powder .... ▣620
Goody's Extra Strength Headache Powder .... ▣620
Goody's Extra Strength Pain Relief Tablets .... ▣620
Percodan Tablets 1327
Robaxisal Tablets 2939
Soma Compound Tablets 3354
Soma Compound w/Codeine Tablets 3355
Vanquish Caplets .... ▣617

Atenolol (May potentiate hypoglycemic action). Products include:
Tenoretic Tablets 690
Tenormin I.V. Injection 692

Bendroflumethiazide (Diuretics tend to produce hyperglycemia and concurrent use may lead to loss of control). Products include:
Corzide 40/5 Tablets 2247
Corzide 80/5 Tablets 2247

Betamethasone Acetate (Corticosteroids tend to produce hyperglycemia and concurrent use may lead to loss of control). Products include:
Celestone Soluspan Injectable Suspension 3097

Betamethasone Sodium Phosphate (Corticosteroids tend to produce hyperglycemia and concurrent use may lead to loss of control). Products include:
Celestone Soluspan Injectable Suspension 3097

Betaxolol Hydrochloride (May potentiate hypoglycemic action). Products include:
Betoptic S Ophthalmic Suspension 537

Bisoprolol Fumarate (May potentiate hypoglycemic action). Products include:
Zebeta Tablets 1885
Ziac Tablets 1887

Bumetanide (Diuretics tend to produce hyperglycemia and concurrent use may lead to loss of control).
No products indexed under this heading.

Carteolol Hydrochloride (May potentiate hypoglycemic action). Products include:
Carteolol Hydrochloride Ophthalmic Solution USP, 1% ...... ⊙258
Ocupress Ophthalmic Solution, 1% Sterile .... ⊙303

Celecoxib (May potentiate hypoglycemic action). Products include:
Celebrex Capsules 2676
Celebrex Capsules 2780

Chloramphenicol (May potentiate hypoglycemic action). Products include:
Chloromycetin Ophthalmic Ointment, 1% .... ⊙296
Chloromycetin Ophthalmic Solution .... ⊙297
Chloroptic Sterile Ophthalmic Ointment .... ⊙234
Chloroptic Sterile Ophthalmic Solution .... ⊙235

Chloramphenicol Palmitate (May potentiate hypoglycemic action).
No products indexed under this heading.

Chloramphenicol Sodium Succinate (May potentiate hypoglycemic action).
No products indexed under this heading.

Chlorothiazide (Diuretics tend to produce hyperglycemia and concurrent use may lead to loss of control). Products include:
Aldoclor Tablets 2035
Diuril Oral 2087

Chlorothiazide Sodium (Diuretics tend to produce hyperglycemia and concurrent use may lead to loss of control). Products include:
Diuril Sodium Intravenous 2086

Chlorotrianisene (Estrogens tend to produce hyperglycemia and concurrent use may lead to loss of control).
No products indexed under this heading.

Chlorpromazine (Phenothiazines tend to produce hyperglycemia and concurrent use may lead to loss of control). Products include:
Thorazine Suppositories 1656

Chlorpromazine Hydrochloride (Phenothiazines tend to produce hyperglycemia and concurrent use may lead to loss of control). Products include:
Thorazine 1656

Chlorpropamide (May potentiate hypoglycemic action). Products include:
Diabinese Tablets 2680

Chlorthalidone (Diuretics tend to produce hyperglycemia and concurrent use may lead to loss of control). Products include:
Clorpres Tablets 1002
Combipres Tablets 1040
Tenoretic Tablets 690

Choline Magnesium Trisalicylate (May potentiate hypoglycemic action; clinical trials data indicate no evidence of significant adverse interaction with concurrent use). Products include:
Trilisate 2901

Cortisone Acetate (Corticosteroids tend to produce hyperglycemia and concurrent use may lead to loss of control). Products include:
Cortone Acetate Injectable Suspension 2059
Cortone Acetate Tablets 2061

Desogestrel (Oral contraceptives tend to produce hyperglycemia and concurrent use may lead to loss of control). Products include:
Cyclessa Tablets 2450
Desogen Tablets 2458
Mircette Tablets 2470
Ortho-Cept 21 Tablets 2546
Ortho-Cept 28 Tablets 2546

Dexamethasone (Corticosteroids tend to produce hyperglycemia and concurrent use may lead to loss of control). Products include:
Decadron Elixir 2078
Decadron Tablets 2079
TobraDex Ophthalmic Ointment 542
TobraDex Ophthalmic Suspension .. 541

Dexamethasone Acetate (Corticosteroids tend to produce hyperglycemia and concurrent use may lead to loss of control).
No products indexed under this heading.

Dexamethasone Sodium Phosphate (Corticosteroids tend to produce hyperglycemia and concurrent use may lead to loss of control). Products include:
Decadron Phosphate Injection 2081
Decadron Phosphate Sterile Ophthalmic Ointment 2083
Decadron Phosphate Sterile Ophthalmic Solution 2084
NeoDecadron Sterile Ophthalmic Solution 2144

Diclofenac Potassium (May potentiate hypoglycemic action). Products include:
Cataflam Tablets 2315

Diclofenac Sodium (May potentiate hypoglycemic action). Products include:
Arthrotec Tablets 3195
Voltaren Ophthalmic Sterile Ophthalmic Solution .... ⊙312
Voltaren Tablets 2315
Voltaren-XR Tablets 2315

Dicumarol (May potentiate hypoglycemic action).
No products indexed under this heading.

Dienestrol (Estrogens tend to produce hyperglycemia and concurrent use may lead to loss of control). Products include:
Ortho Dienestrol Cream 2554

Diethylstilbestrol (Estrogens tend to produce hyperglycemia and concurrent use may lead to loss of control).
No products indexed under this heading.

Diflunisal (May potentiate hypoglycemic action; clinical trials data indicate no evidence of significant adverse interaction with concurrent use). Products include:
Dolobid Tablets 2088

Dobutamine Hydrochloride (Sympathomimetics tend to produce hyperglycemia and concurrent use may lead to loss of control). Products include:
Dobutrex Solution Vials 1914

Dopamine Hydrochloride (Sympathomimetics tend to produce hyperglycemia and concurrent use may lead to loss of control).
No products indexed under this heading.

Ephedrine Hydrochloride (Sympathomimetics tend to produce hyperglycemia and concurrent use may lead to loss of control). Products include:
Primatene Tablets .... ■780

Ephedrine Sulfate (Sympathomimetics tend to produce hyperglycemia and concurrent use may lead to loss of control).
No products indexed under this heading.

Ephedrine Tannate (Sympathomimetics tend to produce hyperglycemia and concurrent use may lead to loss of control). Products include:
Rynatuss Pediatric Suspension 3353
Rynatuss Tablets 3353

Epinephrine (Sympathomimetics tend to produce hyperglycemia and concurrent use may lead to loss of control). Products include:
Epifrin Sterile Ophthalmic Solution .... ⊙235
EpiPen 1236
Primatene Mist .... ■779
Xylocaine with Epinephrine Injection 653

Epinephrine Bitartrate (Sympathomimetics tend to produce hyperglycemia and concurrent use may lead to loss of control). Products include:
Sensorcaine 643

Epinephrine Hydrochloride (Sympathomimetics tend to produce hyperglycemia and concurrent use may lead to loss of control).
No products indexed under this heading.

Esmolol Hydrochloride (May potentiate hypoglycemic action). Products include:
Brevibloc Injection 858

Estradiol (Estrogens tend to produce hyperglycemia and concurrent use may lead to loss of control). Products include:
Activella Tablets 2764
Alora Transdermal System 3372
Climara Transdermal System 958
CombiPatch Transdermal System .. 2323
Esclim Transdermal System 3460
Estrace Vaginal Cream 3358
Estrace Tablets 3361
Estring Vaginal Ring 2811
Ortho-Prefest Tablets 2570
Vagifem Tablets 2857
Vivelle Transdermal System 2412
Vivelle-Dot Transdermal System 2416

Estrogens, Conjugated (Estrogens tend to produce hyperglycemia and concurrent use may lead to loss of control). Products include:
Premarin Intravenous 3563
Premarin Tablets 3566
Premarin Vaginal Cream 3570
Premphase Tablets 3572
Prempro Tablets 3572

Estrogens, Esterified (Estrogens tend to produce hyperglycemia and concurrent use may lead to loss of control). Products include:
Estratest 3252
Menest Tablets 2254

Estropipate (Estrogens tend to produce hyperglycemia and concurrent use may lead to loss of control). Products include:
Ogen Tablets 2846
Ortho-Est Tablets 3464

Ethacrynic Acid (Diuretics tend to produce hyperglycemia and concurrent use may lead to loss of control). Products include:
Edecrin Tablets 2091

Ethinyl Estradiol (Estrogens tend to produce hyperglycemia and concurrent use may lead to loss of control). Products include:
Alesse-21 Tablets 3468
Alesse-28 Tablets 3473
Brevicon 28-Day Tablets 3380
Cyclessa Tablets 2450
Desogen Tablets 2458
Estinyl Tablets 3112
Estrostep 2627
femhrt Tablets 2635
Levlen 962
Levlite 21 Tablets 962
Levlite 28 Tablets 962
Levora Tablets 3389
Loestrin 21 Tablets 2642
Loestrin Fe Tablets 2642
Lo/Ovral Tablets 3532
Lo/Ovral-28 Tablets 3538
Low-Ogestrel-28 Tablets 3392
Microgestin Fe 1.5/30 Tablets 3407
Microgestin Fe 1/20 Tablets 3400
Mircette Tablets 2470
Modicon 2563
Necon 3415
Nordette-28 Tablets 2257
Norinyl 1 +35 28-Day Tablets 3380
Ogestrel 0.5/50-28 Tablets 3428
Ortho-Cept 21 Tablets 2546
Ortho-Cept 28 Tablets 2546
Ortho-Cyclen/Ortho Tri-Cyclen 2573
Ortho-Novum 2563
Ovcon 3364
Ovral Tablets 3551
Ovral-28 Tablets 3552
Tri-Levlen 962
Tri-Norinyl-28 Tablets 3433
Triphasil-21 Tablets 3600
Triphasil-28 Tablets 3605
Trivora Tablets 3439
Yasmin 28 Tablets 980
Zovia 3449

Ethynodiol Diacetate (Oral contraceptives tend to produce hyperglycemia and concurrent use may lead to loss of control). Products include:
Zovia 3449

Etodolac (May potentiate hypoglycemic action). Products include:
Lodine 3528
Lodine XL Extended-Release Tablets 3530

Fenoprofen Calcium (May potentiate hypoglycemic action).
No products indexed under this heading.

Fludrocortisone Acetate (Corticosteroids tend to produce hyperglycemia and concurrent use may lead to loss of control). Products include:
Florinef Acetate Tablets 2250

Fluphenazine Decanoate (Phenothiazines tend to produce hyperglycemia and concurrent use may lead to loss of control).
No products indexed under this heading.

Fluphenazine Enanthate (Phenothiazines tend to produce hyperglycemia and concurrent use may lead to loss of control).
No products indexed under this heading.

Fluphenazine Hydrochloride (Phenothiazines tend to produce hyperglycemia and concurrent use may lead to loss of control).
No products indexed under this heading.

Flurbiprofen (May potentiate hypoglycemic action).
No products indexed under this heading.

Furosemide (Diuretics tend to produce hyperglycemia and concurrent use may lead to loss of control). Products include:
Furosemide Tablets 2284

Glipizide (May potentiate hypoglycemic action). Products include:
Glucotrol Tablets 2692
Glucotrol XL Extended Release Tablets 2693

Glyburide (May potentiate hypoglycemic action). Products include:
DiaBeta Tablets 741
Glucovance Tablets 1086

Hydrochlorothiazide (Diuretics tend to produce hyperglycemia and concurrent use may lead to loss of control). Products include:
Accuretic Tablets 2614
Aldoril Tablets 2039
Atacand HCT Tablets 597
Avalide Tablets 1070
Diovan HCT Tablets 2338
Dyazide Capsules 1515
HydroDIURIL Tablets 2108
Hyzaar 2109
Inderide Tablets 3517
Inderide LA Long-Acting Capsules .. 3519
Lotensin HCT Tablets 2367
Maxzide 1008
Micardis HCT Tablets 1051
Microzide Capsules 3414
Moduretic Tablets 2138
Monopril HCT 1094
Prinzide Tablets 2168
Timolide Tablets 2187
Uniretic Tablets 3178
Vaseretic Tablets 2204
Zestoretic Tablets 695
Ziac Tablets 1887

Hydrocortisone (Corticosteroids tend to produce hyperglycemia and concurrent use may lead to loss of control). Products include:
Anusol-HC Cream 2.5% 2237
Cipro HC Otic Suspension 540
Cortaid Intensive Therapy Cream . ■717
Cortaid Maximum Strength Cream .... ■717
Cortisporin Ophthalmic Suspension Sterile .... ⊙297
Cortizone•5 .... ■699
Cortizone•10 .... ■699
Cortizone•10 Plus Creme .... ■700
Cortizone for Kids Creme .... ■699
Hydrocortone Tablets 2106
Massengill Medicated Soft Cloth Towelette .... ■753
VōSoL HC Otic Solution 3356

Hydrocortisone Acetate (Corticosteroids tend to produce hyperglycemia and concurrent use may lead to loss of control). Products include:
Analpram-HC 1338
Anusol HC-1 Hydrocortisone Anti-Itch Cream .... ■689
Anusol-HC Suppositories 2238
Cortaid .... ■717
Cortifoam Rectal Foam 3170
Cortisporin-TC Otic Suspension 2246
Hydrocortone Acetate Injectable Suspension 2103
Pramosone 1343
Proctocort Suppositories 2264
ProctoFoam-HC 3177
Terra-Cortril Ophthalmic Suspension 2716

Hydrocortisone Sodium Phosphate (Corticosteroids tend to produce hyperglycemia and concurrent use may lead to loss of control). Products include:
Hydrocortone Phosphate Injection, Sterile 2105

Hydrocortisone Sodium Succinate (Corticosteroids tend to produce hyperglycemia and concurrent use may lead to loss of control).
No products indexed under this heading.

Hydroflumethiazide (Diuretics tend to produce hyperglycemia and concurrent use may lead to loss of control). Products include:
Diucardin Tablets 3494

Ibuprofen (May potentiate hypoglycemic action). Products include:
Advil .... ■771
Children's Advil Oral Suspension ... ■773
Children's Advil Chewable Tablets . ■773
Advil Cold and Sinus Caplets .... ■771
Advil Cold and Sinus Tablets .... ■771
Advil Flu & Body Ache Caplets ...... ■772
Infants' Advil Drops .... ■773
Junior Strength Advil Tablets .... ■773
Junior Strength Advil Chewable Tablets .... ■773
Advil Migraine Liquigels .... ■772
Children's Motrin Oral Suspension and Chewable Tablets 2006
Children's Motrin Cold Oral Suspension 2007
Children's Motrin Oral Suspension .... ■643
Motrin Suspension, Oral Drops, Chewable Tablets, and Caplets 2002
Infants' Motrin Concentrated Drops 2006
Junior Strength Motrin Caplets and Chewable Tablets 2006
Motrin IB Tablets, Caplets, and Gelcaps 2002
Motrin Migraine Pain Caplets 2005
Motrin Sinus Headache Caplets 2005
Vicoprofen Tablets 520

Indapamide (Diuretics tend to produce hyperglycemia and concurrent use may lead to loss of control). Products include:
Indapamide Tablets 2286

Indomethacin (May potentiate hypoglycemic action). Products include:
Indocin 2112

Indomethacin Sodium Trihydrate (May potentiate hypoglycemic action). Products include:
Indocin I.V. 2115

Insulin, Human, Zinc Suspension (Co-administration of glimepiride with insulin may increase the potential for hypoglycemia). Products include:
Humulin L, 100 Units 1937
Humulin U, 100 Units 1943
Novolin L Human Insulin 10 ml Vials 2422

Insulin, Human NPH (Co-administration of glimepiride with insulin may increase the potential for hypoglycemia). Products include:
Humulin N, 100 Units 1939
Humulin N NPH Pen 1940
Novolin N Human Insulin 10 ml Vials 2422
Novolin N PenFill 2423
Novolin N Prefilled Syringe Disposable Insulin Delivery System 2425

Insulin, Human Regular (Co-administration of glimepiride with insulin may increase the potential for hypoglycemia). Products include:
Humulin R Regular (U 500) 1943
Humulin R, 100 Units 1941
Novolin R Human Insulin 10 ml Vials 2423
Novolin R PenFill 2423
Novolin R Prefilled Syringe Disposable Insulin Delivery System 2425
Velosulin BR Human Insulin 10 ml Vials 2435

Insulin, Human Regular and Human NPH Mixture (Co-administration of glimepiride with insulin may increase the potential for hypoglycemia). Products include:
Humulin 50/50, 100 Units 1934
Humulin 70/30, 100 Units 1935
Humulin 70/30 Pen 1936
Novolin 70/30 Human Insulin 10 ml Vials 2421
Novolin 70/30 PenFill 2423
Novolin 70/30 Prefilled Disposable Insulin Delivery System 2425

Insulin, NPH (Co-administration of glimepiride with insulin may increase the potential for hypoglycemia). Products include:

Iletin II, NPH (Pork), 100 Units 1946

Insulin, Regular (Co-administration of glimepiride with insulin may increase the potential for hypoglycemia). Products include:
Iletin II, Regular (Pork), 100 Units ... 1947

Insulin, Zinc Crystals (Co-administration of glimepiride with insulin may increase the potential for hypoglycemia).
No products indexed under this heading.

Insulin, Zinc Suspension (Co-administration of glimepiride with insulin may increase the potential for hypoglycemia). Products include:
Iletin II, Lente (Pork), 100 Units 1945

Insulin Aspart, Human Regular (Co-administration of glimepiride with insulin may increase the potential for hypoglycemia).
No products indexed under this heading.

Insulin glargine (Co-administration of glimepiride with insulin may increase the potential for hypoglycemia). Products include:
Lantus Injection 742

Insulin Lispro, Human (Co-administration of glimepiride with insulin may increase the potential for hypoglycemia). Products include:
Humalog 1926
Humalog Mix 75/25 Pen 1928

Insulin Lispro Protamine, Human (Co-administration of glimepiride with insulin may increase the potential for hypoglycemia). Products include:
Humalog Mix 75/25 Pen 1928

Isocarboxazid (May potentiate hypoglycemic action).
No products indexed under this heading.

Isoniazid (Isoniazid tends to produce hyperglycemia and concurrent use may lead to loss of control). Products include:
Rifamate Capsules 767
Rifater Tablets 769

Isoproterenol Hydrochloride (Sympathomimetics tend to produce hyperglycemia and concurrent use may lead to loss of control).
No products indexed under this heading.

Isoproterenol Sulfate (Sympathomimetics tend to produce hyperglycemia and concurrent use may lead to loss of control).
No products indexed under this heading.

Ketoprofen (May potentiate hypoglycemic action). Products include:
Orudis Capsules 3548
Orudis KT Tablets .... ▣778
Oruvail Capsules 3548

Ketorolac Tromethamine (May potentiate hypoglycemic action). Products include:
Acular Ophthalmic Solution 544
Acular PF Ophthalmic Solution 544
Toradol 3018

Labetalol Hydrochloride (May potentiate hypoglycemic action). Products include:
Normodyne Injection 3135
Normodyne Tablets 3137

Levalbuterol Hydrochloride (Sympathomimetics tend to produce hyperglycemia and concurrent use may lead to loss of control). Products include:
Xopenex Inhalation Solution 3207

Levobunolol Hydrochloride (May potentiate hypoglycemic action). Products include:
Betagan .... ⊙228

Levonorgestrel (Oral contraceptives tend to produce hyperglycemia and concurrent use may lead to loss of control). Products include:
Alesse-21 Tablets 3468
Alesse-28 Tablets 3473
Levlen 962
Levlite 21 Tablets 962
Levlite 28 Tablets 962
Levora Tablets 3389
Mirena Intrauterine System 974
Nordette-28 Tablets 2257
Norplant System 3543
Tri-Levlen 962
Triphasil-21 Tablets 3600
Triphasil-28 Tablets 3605
Trivora Tablets 3439

Levothyroxine Sodium (Thyroid products tend to produce hyperglycemia and concurrent use may lead to loss of control). Products include:
Levothroid Tablets 1373
Levoxyl Tablets 1819
Synthroid 505
Unithroid Tablets 3445

Liothyronine Sodium (Thyroid products tend to produce hyperglycemia and concurrent use may lead to loss of control). Products include:
Cytomel Tablets 1817
Triostat Injection 1825

Liotrix (Thyroid products tend to produce hyperglycemia and concurrent use may lead to loss of control).
No products indexed under this heading.

Magnesium Salicylate (May potentiate hypoglycemic action; clinical trials data indicate no evidence of significant adverse interaction with concurrent use). Products include:
Momentum Backache Relief Extra Strength Caplets .... ▣666

Meclofenamate Sodium (May potentiate hypoglycemic action).
No products indexed under this heading.

Mefenamic Acid (May potentiate hypoglycemic action). Products include:
Ponstel Capsules 1356

Meloxicam (May potentiate hypoglycemic action). Products include:
Mobic Tablets 1054

Mesoridazine Besylate (Phenothiazines tend to produce hyperglycemia and concurrent use may lead to loss of control). Products include:
Serentil 1057

Mestranol (Oral contraceptives tend to produce hyperglycemia and concurrent use may lead to loss of control). Products include:
Necon 1/50 Tablets 3415
Norinyl 1 + 50 28-Day Tablets 3380
Ortho-Novum 1/50▫28 Tablets 2556

Metaproterenol Sulfate (Sympathomimetics tend to produce hyperglycemia and concurrent use may lead to loss of control). Products include:
Alupent 1029

Metaraminol Bitartrate (Sympathomimetics tend to produce hyperglycemia and concurrent use may lead to loss of control). Products include:
Aramine Injection 2043

Metformin Hydrochloride (Co-administration of glimepiride with metformin may increase the potential for hypoglycemia). Products include:
Glucophage Tablets 1080
Glucophage XR Tablets 1080
Glucovance Tablets 1086

Methotrimeprazine (Phenothiazines tend to produce hyperglycemia and concurrent use may lead to loss of control).
No products indexed under this heading.

Methoxamine Hydrochloride (Sympathomimetics tend to produce hyperglycemia and concurrent use may lead to loss of control).
No products indexed under this heading.

Methyclothiazide (Diuretics tend to produce hyperglycemia and concurrent use may lead to loss of control).
No products indexed under this heading.

Methylprednisolone Acetate (Corticosteroids tend to produce hyperglycemia and concurrent use may lead to loss of control). Products include:
Depo-Medrol Injectable Suspension 2795

Methylprednisolone Sodium Succinate (Corticosteroids tend to produce hyperglycemia and concurrent use may lead to loss of control). Products include:
Solu-Medrol Sterile Powder 2855

Metipranolol Hydrochloride (May potentiate hypoglycemic action).
No products indexed under this heading.

Metolazone (Diuretics tend to produce hyperglycemia and concurrent use may lead to loss of control). Products include:
Mykrox Tablets 1168
Zaroxolyn Tablets 1177

Metoprolol Succinate (May potentiate hypoglycemic action). Products include:
Toprol-XL Tablets 651

Metoprolol Tartrate (May potentiate hypoglycemic action).
No products indexed under this heading.

Miconazole (A potential interaction between oral miconazole and oral hypoglycemic agents leading to severe hypoglycemia has been reported).
No products indexed under this heading.

Moclobemide (May potentiate hypoglycemic action).
No products indexed under this heading.

Nabumetone (May potentiate hypoglycemic action). Products include:
Relafen Tablets 1617

Nadolol (May potentiate hypoglycemic action). Products include:
Corgard Tablets 2245
Corzide 40/5 Tablets 2247
Corzide 80/5 Tablets 2247
Nadolol Tablets 2288

Naproxen (May potentiate hypoglycemic action). Products include:
EC-Naprosyn Delayed-Release Tablets 2967
Naprosyn Suspension 2967
Naprosyn Tablets 2967

Naproxen Sodium (May potentiate hypoglycemic action). Products include:
Aleve Tablets, Caplets and Gelcaps .... ▣602
Aleve Cold & Sinus Caplets .... ▣603
Anaprox Tablets 2967
Anaprox DS Tablets 2967
Naprelan Tablets 1293

Nicotinic Acid (Nicotinic acid tends to produce hyperglycemia and concurrent use may lead to loss of control).
No products indexed under this heading.

Norepinephrine Bitartrate (Sympathomimetics tend to produce hyperglycemia and concurrent use may lead to loss of control).
No products indexed under this heading.

Norethindrone (Oral contraceptives tend to produce hyperglycemia and concurrent use may lead to loss of control). Products include:
Brevicon 28-Day Tablets 3380
Micronor Tablets 2543
Modicon 2563
Necon 3415
Norinyl 1 +35 28-Day Tablets 3380
Norinyl 1 + 50 28-Day Tablets 3380
Nor-QD Tablets 3423
Ortho-Novum 2563
Ortho-Novum 1/50▫28 Tablets 2556
Ovcon 3364
Tri-Norinyl-28 Tablets 3433

Norethynodrel (Oral contraceptives tend to produce hyperglycemia and concurrent use may lead to loss of control).
No products indexed under this heading.

Norgestimate (Oral contraceptives tend to produce hyperglycemia and concurrent use may lead to loss of control). Products include:
Ortho-Cyclen/Ortho Tri-Cyclen 2573
Ortho-Prefest Tablets 2570

Norgestrel (Oral contraceptives tend to produce hyperglycemia and concurrent use may lead to loss of control). Products include:
Lo/Ovral Tablets 3532
Lo/Ovral-28 Tablets 3538
Low-Ogestrel-28 Tablets 3392
Ogestrel 0.5/50-28 Tablets 3428
Ovral Tablets 3551
Ovral-28 Tablets 3552
Ovrette Tablets 3552

Oxaprozin (May potentiate hypoglycemic action).
No products indexed under this heading.

Pargyline Hydrochloride (May potentiate hypoglycemic action).
No products indexed under this heading.

Penbutolol Sulfate (May potentiate hypoglycemic action).
No products indexed under this heading.

Perphenazine (Phenothiazines tend to produce hyperglycemia and concurrent use may lead to loss of control). Products include:
Etrafon 3115
Trilafon 3160

Phenelzine Sulfate (May potentiate hypoglycemic action). Products include:
Nardil Tablets 2653

Phenylbutazone (May potentiate hypoglycemic action).
No products indexed under this heading.

Phenylephrine Bitartrate (Sympathomimetics tend to produce hyperglycemia and concurrent use may lead to loss of control).
No products indexed under this heading.

Phenylephrine Hydrochloride (Sympathomimetics tend to produce hyperglycemia and concurrent use may lead to loss of control). Products include:
Afrin Nasal Decongestant Children's Pump Mist .... ▣734
Extendryl 1361
Hycomine Compound Tablets 1317
Neo-Synephrine .... ▣614
Phenergan VC Syrup 3560
Phenergan VC with Codeine Syrup . 3561
Preparation H Cream .... ▣778
Preparation H Cooling Gel .... ▣778
Preparation H .... ▣778
Vicks Sinex Nasal Spray and Ultra Fine Mist .... ▣729

Phenylephrine Tannate (Sympathomimetics tend to produce hyperglycemia and concurrent use may lead to loss of control). Products include:
Ryna-12 S Suspension 3351
Reformulated Rynatan Pediatric Suspension 3352
Rynatuss Pediatric Suspension 3353
Rynatuss Tablets 3353

Phenylpropanolamine Hydrochloride (Sympathomimetics tend to produce hyperglycemia and concurrent use may lead to loss of control).
No products indexed under this heading.

Phenytoin (Phenytoin tends to produce hyperglycemia and concurrent use may lead to loss of control). Products include:
Dilantin Infatabs 2624
Dilantin-125 Oral Suspension 2625

Phenytoin Sodium (Phenytoin tends to produce hyperglycemia and concurrent use may lead to loss of control). Products include:
- Dilantin Kapseals 2622

Pindolol (May potentiate hypoglycemic action).
- No products indexed under this heading.

Pirbuterol Acetate (Sympathomimetics tend to produce hyperglycemia and concurrent use may lead to loss of control). Products include:
- Maxair Autohaler 1981
- Maxair Inhaler 1984

Piroxicam (May potentiate hypoglycemic action). Products include:
- Feldene Capsules 2685

Polyestradiol Phosphate (Estrogens tend to produce hyperglycemia and concurrent use may lead to loss of control).
- No products indexed under this heading.

Polythiazide (Diuretics tend to produce hyperglycemia and concurrent use may lead to loss of control). Products include:
- Minizide Capsules 2700
- Renese Tablets 2712

Prednisolone Acetate (Corticosteroids tend to produce hyperglycemia and concurrent use may lead to loss of control). Products include:
- Blephamide Ophthalmic Ointment .. 547
- Blephamide Ophthalmic Suspension 548
- Poly-Pred Liquifilm Ophthalmic Suspension .... ⊙245
- Pred Forte Ophthalmic Suspension .... ⊙246
- Pred Mild Sterile Ophthalmic Suspension .... ⊙249
- Pred-G Ophthalmic Suspension ..... ⊙247
- Pred-G Sterile Ophthalmic Ointment .... ⊙248

Prednisolone Sodium Phosphate (Corticosteroids tend to produce hyperglycemia and concurrent use may lead to loss of control). Products include:
- Pediapred Oral Solution 1170

Prednisolone Tebutate (Corticosteroids tend to produce hyperglycemia and concurrent use may lead to loss of control).
- No products indexed under this heading.

Prednisone (Corticosteroids tend to produce hyperglycemia and concurrent use may lead to loss of control). Products include:
- Prednisone 3064

Probenecid (May potentiate hypoglycemic action).
- No products indexed under this heading.

Procarbazine Hydrochloride (May potentiate hypoglycemic action). Products include:
- Matulane Capsules 3246

Prochlorperazine (Phenothiazines tend to produce hyperglycemia and concurrent use may lead to loss of control). Products include:
- Compazine 1505

Promethazine Hydrochloride (Phenothiazines tend to produce hyperglycemia and concurrent use may lead to loss of control). Products include:
- Mepergan Injection 3539
- Phenergan Injection 3553
- Phenergan 3556
- Phenergan Syrup 3554
- Phenergan with Codeine Syrup 3557
- Phenergan with Dextromethorphan Syrup 3559
- Phenergan VC Syrup 3560
- Phenergan VC with Codeine Syrup . 3561

Propranolol Hydrochloride (Coadministration increases Cmax AUC, and T1/2 of glimepiride by 23%, 22% and 15% respectively and it decreased CL/f by 18%; no evidence of clinically significant adverse interactions). Products include:
- Inderal 3513
- Inderal LA Long-Acting Capsules 3516
- Inderide Tablets 3517
- Inderide LA Long-Acting Capsules .. 3519

Pseudoephedrine Hydrochloride (Sympathomimetics tend to produce hyperglycemia and concurrent use may lead to loss of control). Products include:
- Actifed Cold & Allergy Tablets .... ▣688
- Actifed Cold & Sinus Caplets and Tablets .... ▣688
- Advil Cold and Sinus Caplets .... ▣771
- Advil Cold and Sinus Tablets .... ▣771
- Advil Flu & Body Ache Caplets .... ▣772
- Aleve Cold & Sinus Caplets .... ▣603
- Alka-Seltzer Plus Liqui-Gels .... ▣604
- Alka-Seltzer Plus Cold & Flu Medicine Liqui-Gels .... ▣604
- Alka-Seltzer Plus Cold & Sinus Medicine Liqui-Gels .... ▣604
- Allegra-D Extended-Release Tablets 714
- BC Cold Powder .... ▣619
- Benadryl Allergy/Cold Tablets .... ▣691
- Benadryl Allergy/Congestion Tablets .... ▣692
- Benadryl Allergy & Sinus Liquid .... ▣693
- Benadryl Allergy & Sinus Fastmelt Tablets .... ▣693
- Benadryl Allergy Sinus Headache Caplets & Gelcaps .... ▣693
- Benadryl Severe Allergy & Sinus Headache Caplets .... ▣694
- Benadryl Children's Allergy/Cold Fastmelt Tablets .... ▣692
- Benylin Multi-Symptom Liquid .... ▣697
- Bromfed Capsules (Extended-Release) 2269
- Bromfed-PD Capsules (Extended-Release) 2269
- Children's Cēpacol Sore Throat .... ▣788
- Comtrex Acute Head Cold & Sinus Pressure Relief Tablets .... ▣627
- Comtrex Deep Chest Cold & Congestion Relief Softgels .... ▣627
- Comtrex Flu Therapy & Fever Relief Daytime Caplets .... ▣628
- Comtrex Flu Therapy & Fever Relief Nighttime Tablets .... ▣628
- Comtrex Maximum Strength Multi-Symptom Cold & Cough Relief Tablets and Caplets .... ▣626
- Contac Non-Drowsy 12 Hour Cold Caplets .... ▣745
- Contac Non-Drowsy Timed Release 12 Hour Cold Caplets .... ▣746
- Contac Severe Cold and Flu Caplets Maximum Strength .... ▣746
- Contac Severe Cold and Flu Caplets Non-Drowsy .... ▣746
- Dimetapp Elixir .... ▣777
- Dimetapp Cold and Fever Suspension .... ▣775
- Dimetapp DM Cold & Cough Elixir .... ▣775
- Dimetapp Nighttime Flu Liquid .... ▣776
- Dimetapp Non-Drowsy Flu Syrup .. ▣777
- Dimetapp Infant Drops Decongestant .... ▣775
- Dimetapp Infant Drops Decongestant Plus Cough .... ▣776
- Guaifed 2272
- Kronofed-A 1341
- Children's Motrin Cold Oral Suspension 2007
- Motrin Sinus Headache Caplets 2005
- PediaCare Cough-Cold Liquid .... ▣719
- PediaCare Infants' Drops Decongestant .... ▣719
- PediaCare Infants' Drops Decongestant Plus Cough .... ▣719
- PediaCare NightRest Cough-Cold Liquid .... ▣719
- Robitussin Cold Caplets Cold & Congestion .... ▣780
- Robitussin Cold Softgels Cold & Congestion .... ▣780
- Robitussin Cold Caplets Multi-Symptom Cold & Flu .... ▣781
- Robitussin Cold Softgels Multi-Symptom Cold & Flu .... ▣781
- Robitussin Cold Softgels Severe Congestion .... ▣782
- Robitussin Cough & Cold Infant Drops .... ▣782
- Robitussin Maximum Strength Cough & Cold Liquid .... ▣785
- Robitussin Pediatric Cough & Cold Formula Liquid .... ▣785
- Robitussin Multi Symptom Honey Flu Liquid .... ▣785
- Robitussin Nighttime Honey Flu Liquid .... ▣786
- Robitussin-CF Liquid .... ▣783
- Robitussin-DAC Syrup 2942
- Robitussin-PE Liquid .... ▣782
- Ryna .... ▣768
- Semprex-D Capsules 1172
- Singlet Caplets .... ▣761
- Sinutab Non-Drying Liquid Caps .... ▣706
- Sinutab Sinus Allergy Medication, Maximum Strength Formula, Tablets & Caplets .... ▣707
- Sinutab Sinus Medication, Maximum Strength Without Drowsiness Formula, Tablets & Caplets .... ▣707
- Sudafed 12 Hour Tablets .... ▣708
- Sudafed 24 Hour Tablets .... ▣708
- Children's Sudafed Cold & Cough Liquid .... ▣709
- Children's Sudafed Nasal Decongestant Chewables .... ▣711
- Children's Sudafed Nasal Decongestant Liquid Medication .... ▣711
- Sudafed Cold & Allergy Tablets .... ▣708
- Sudafed Cold & Cough Liquid Caps .... ▣709
- Sudafed Cold & Sinus Liquid Caps .... ▣710
- Sudafed Nasal Decongestant Tablets .... ▣710
- Sudafed Non-Drying Sinus Liquid Caps .... ▣712
- Sudafed Severe Cold .... ▣711
- Sudafed Sinus Headache Caplets .... ▣712
- Sudafed Sinus Headache Tablets . ▣712
- Tavist Sinus Non-Drowsy Coated Caplets .... ▣676
- TheraFlu Regular Strength Cold & Cough Night Time Hot Liquid .... ▣676
- TheraFlu Regular Strength Cold & Sore Throat Night Time Hot Liquid .... ▣676
- TheraFlu Maximum Strength Flu & Congestion Non-Drowsy Hot Liquid .... ▣677
- TheraFlu Maximum Strength Flu & Cough Night Time Hot Liquid .. ▣678
- TheraFlu Maximum Strength Flu & Sore Throat Night Time Hot Liquid .... ▣677
- TheraFlu Maximum Strength Severe Cold & Congestion Night Time Caplets .... ▣678
- TheraFlu Maximum Strength Severe Cold & Congestion Night Time Hot Liquid .... ▣678
- TheraFlu Maximum Strength Severe Cold & Congestion Non-Drowsy .... ▣679
- Triaminic Allergy Congestion Liquid .... ▣680
- Triaminic Chest Congestion Liquid .... ▣680
- Triaminic Cold & Allergy Liquid .... ▣681
- Triaminic Cold & Allergy Softchews .... ▣683
- Triaminic Cold & Cough Liquid .... ▣681
- Triaminic Cold & Cough Softchews .... ▣683
- Triaminic Cold & Night Time Cough Liquid .... ▣681
- Triaminic Cold, Cough & Fever Liquid .... ▣681
- Triaminic Cough Liquid .... ▣682
- Triaminic Cough & Congestion Liquid .... ▣682
- Triaminic Cough & Sore Throat Liquid .... ▣682
- Triaminic Cough & Sore Throat Softchews .... ▣684
- Children's Tylenol Allergy-D Liquid ... 2014
- Children's Tylenol Cold Suspension Liquid and Chewable Tablets 2015
- Children's Tylenol Cold Plus Cough Suspension Liquid and Chewable Tablets 2015
- Children's Tylenol Flu Suspension Liquid 2015
- Children's Tylenol Sinus Suspension Liquid 2017
- Infants' Tylenol Cold Decongestant and Fever Reducer Concentrated Drops 2015
- Infants' Tylenol Cold Decongestant and Fever Reducer Concentrated Drops Plus Cough .. 2015
- Tylenol Allergy Sinus 2010
- Multi-Symptom Tylenol Cold Complete Formula Caplets 2010
- Multi-Symptom Tylenol Cold Non-Drowsy Caplets and Gelcaps 2010
- Multi-Symptom Tylenol Cold Severe Congestion Non-Drowsy Caplets 2011
- Maximum Strength Tylenol Flu NightTime Gelcaps 2011
- Maximum Strength Tylenol Flu NightTime Liquid 2011
- Maximum Strength Tylenol Flu Non-Drowsy Gelcaps 2011
- Maximum Strength Tylenol Sinus NightTime Caplets 2012
- Maximum Strength Tylenol Sinus Non-Drowsy Geltabs, Gelcaps, Caplets, and Tablets 2012
- Vicks 44D Cough & Head Congestion Relief Liquid .... ▣724
- Vicks 44M Cough, Cold & Flu Relief Liquid .... ▣725
- Pediatric Vicks 44m Cough & Cold Relief .... ▣728
- Vicks DayQuil LiquiCaps/Liquid Multi-Symptom Cold/Flu Relief ... ▣727
- Children's Vicks NyQuil Cold/Cough Relief .... ▣726
- Vicks NyQuil LiquiCaps/Liquid Multi-Symptom Cold/Flu Relief, Original and Cherry Flavors .... ▣727
- Zephrex Tablets 3091
- Zephrex LA Tablets 3092
- Zyrtec-D 12 Hour Extended Relief Tablets 2758

Pseudoephedrine Sulfate (Sympathomimetics tend to produce hyperglycemia and concurrent use may lead to loss of control). Products include:
- Chlor-Trimeton Allergy/Decongestant Tablets .... ▣736
- Claritin-D 12 Hour Extended Release Tablets 3102
- Claritin-D 24 Hour Extended Release Tablets 3104
- Coricidin 'D' Cold, Flu & Sinus Tablets .... ▣737
- Drixoral Allergy/Sinus Extended-Release Tablets .... ▣741
- Drixoral Cold & Allergy Sustained-Action Tablets .... ▣740
- Drixoral Cold & Flu Extended-Release Tablets .... ▣740
- Drixoral Nasal Decongestant Long-Acting Non-Drowsy Tablets .... ▣740
- Rynatan Tablets 3351

Quinestrol (Estrogens tend to produce hyperglycemia and concurrent use may lead to loss of control).
- No products indexed under this heading.

Rofecoxib (May potentiate hypoglycemic action). Products include:
- Vioxx 2213

Salmeterol Xinafoate (Sympathomimetics tend to produce hyperglycemia and concurrent use may lead to loss of control). Products include:
- Advair Diskus 100/50 1448
- Advair Diskus 250/50 1448
- Advair Diskus 500/50 1448
- Serevent Diskus 1637
- Serevent Inhalation Aerosol 1633

Salsalate (May potentiate hypoglycemic action; clinical trials data indicate no evidence of significant adverse interaction with concurrent use).
- No products indexed under this heading.

Selegiline Hydrochloride (May potentiate hypoglycemic action). Products include:
- Eldepryl Capsules 3266

Sotalol Hydrochloride (May potentiate hypoglycemic action). Products include:
- Betapace Tablets 950
- Betapace AF Tablets 954

Spironolactone (Diuretics tend to produce hyperglycemia and concurrent use may lead to loss of control).
- No products indexed under this heading.

Sulfacytine (May potentiate hypoglycemic action).
- No products indexed under this heading.

Sulfamethizole (May potentiate hypoglycemic action). Products include:
- Urobiotic-250 Capsules 2731

Sulfamethoxazole (May potentiate hypoglycemic action). Products include:
- Bactrim 2949
- Septra Suspension 2265
- Septra Tablets 2265
- Septra DS Tablets 2265

Sulfasalazine (May potentiate hypoglycemic action). Products include:
- Azulfidine EN-tabs Tablets 2775

Sulfinpyrazone (May potentiate hypoglycemic action).
No products indexed under this heading.

Sulfisoxazole (May potentiate hypoglycemic action).
No products indexed under this heading.

Sulfisoxazole Acetyl (May potentiate hypoglycemic action). Products include:
- Pediazole Suspension 3050

Sulfisoxazole Diolamine (May potentiate hypoglycemic action).
No products indexed under this heading.

Sulindac (May potentiate hypoglycemic action). Products include:
- Clinoril Tablets 2053

Terbutaline Sulfate (Sympathomimetics tend to produce hyperglycemia and concurrent use may lead to loss of control). Products include:
- Brethine Ampuls 2314
- Brethine Tablets 2313

Thioridazine Hydrochloride (Phenothiazines tend to produce hyperglycemia and concurrent use may lead to loss of control). Products include:
- Thioridazine Hydrochloride Tablets 2289

Thyroglobulin (Thyroid products tend to produce hyperglycemia and concurrent use may lead to loss of control).
No products indexed under this heading.

Thyroid (Thyroid products tend to produce hyperglycemia and concurrent use may lead to loss of control).
No products indexed under this heading.

Thyroxine (Thyroid products tend to produce hyperglycemia and concurrent use may lead to loss of control).
No products indexed under this heading.

Thyroxine Sodium (Thyroid products tend to produce hyperglycemia and concurrent use may lead to loss of control).
No products indexed under this heading.

Timolol Hemihydrate (May potentiate hypoglycemic action). Products include:
- Betimol Ophthalmic Solution .... ⊙ 324

Timolol Maleate (May potentiate hypoglycemic action). Products include:
- Blocadren Tablets 2046
- Cosopt Sterile Ophthalmic Solution 2065
- Timolide Tablets 2187
- Timolol GFS .... ⊙ 266
- Timoptic in Ocudose 2192
- Timoptic Sterile Ophthalmic Solution 2190
- Timoptic-XE Sterile Ophthalmic Gel Forming Solution 2194

Tolazamide (May potentiate hypoglycemic action).
No products indexed under this heading.

Tolbutamide (May potentiate hypoglycemic action).
No products indexed under this heading.

Tolmetin Sodium (May potentiate hypoglycemic action). Products include:
- Tolectin 2589

Torsemide (Diuretics tend to produce hyperglycemia and concurrent use may lead to loss of control). Products include:
- Demadex Tablets and Injection 2965

Tranylcypromine Sulfate (May potentiate hypoglycemic action). Products include:
- Parnate Tablets 1607

Triamcinolone (Corticosteroids tend to produce hyperglycemia and concurrent use may lead to loss of control).
No products indexed under this heading.

Triamcinolone Acetonide (Corticosteroids tend to produce hyperglycemia and concurrent use may lead to loss of control). Products include:
- Azmacort Inhalation Aerosol 728
- Nasacort Nasal Inhaler 750
- Nasacort AQ Nasal Spray 752
- Tri-Nasal Spray 2274

Triamcinolone Diacetate (Corticosteroids tend to produce hyperglycemia and concurrent use may lead to loss of control).
No products indexed under this heading.

Triamcinolone Hexacetonide (Corticosteroids tend to produce hyperglycemia and concurrent use may lead to loss of control).
No products indexed under this heading.

Triamterene (Diuretics tend to produce hyperglycemia and concurrent use may lead to loss of control). Products include:
- Dyazide Capsules 1515
- Dyrenium Capsules 3458
- Maxzide 1008

Trifluoperazine Hydrochloride (Phenothiazines tend to produce hyperglycemia and concurrent use may lead to loss of control). Products include:
- Stelazine 1640

Warfarin Sodium (May potentiate hypoglycemic action). Products include:
- Coumadin for Injection 1243
- Coumadin Tablets 1243
- Warfarin Sodium Tablets, USP 3302

Food Interactions

Meal, unspecified (When glimepiride is given with meals the mean Tmax is slightly increased (12%) and mean Cmax and AUC are slightly decreased).

AMBIEN TABLETS

(Zolpidem Tartrate) 3191

May interact with central nervous system depressants and certain other agents. Compounds in these categories include:

Alfentanil Hydrochloride (Potential for enhanced CNS depressant effects of zolpidem).
No products indexed under this heading.

Alprazolam (Potential for enhanced CNS depressant effects of zolpidem). Products include:
- Xanax Tablets 2865

Aprobarbital (Potential for enhanced CNS depressant effects of zolpidem).
No products indexed under this heading.

Buprenorphine Hydrochloride (Potential for enhanced CNS depressant effects of zolpidem). Products include:
- Buprenex Injectable 2918

Buspirone Hydrochloride (Potential for enhanced CNS depressant effects of zolpidem).
No products indexed under this heading.

Butabarbital (Potential for enhanced CNS depressant effects of zolpidem).
No products indexed under this heading.

Butalbital (Potential for enhanced CNS depressant effects of zolpidem). Products include:
- Phrenilin 578
- Sedapap Tablets 50 mg/650 mg 2225

Chlordiazepoxide (Potential for enhanced CNS depressant effects of zolpidem). Products include:
- Limbitrol 1738

Chlordiazepoxide Hydrochloride (Potential for enhanced CNS depressant effects of zolpidem). Products include:
- Librium Capsules 1736
- Librium for Injection 1737

Chlorpromazine (Additive effect of decreased alertness and psychomotor performance; potential for enhanced CNS depressant effects of zolpidem). Products include:
- Thorazine Suppositories 1656

Chlorpromazine Hydrochloride (Additive effect of decreased alertness and psychomotor performance; potential for enhanced CNS depressant effects of zolpidem). Products include:
- Thorazine 1656

Chlorprothixene (Potential for enhanced CNS depressant effects of zolpidem).
No products indexed under this heading.

Chlorprothixene Hydrochloride (Potential for enhanced CNS depressant effects of zolpidem).
No products indexed under this heading.

Chlorprothixene Lactate (Potential for enhanced CNS depressant effects of zolpidem).
No products indexed under this heading.

Clorazepate Dipotassium (Potential for enhanced CNS depressant effects of zolpidem). Products include:
- Tranxene 511

Clozapine (Potential for enhanced CNS depressant effects of zolpidem). Products include:
- Clozaril Tablets 2319

Codeine Phosphate (Potential for enhanced CNS depressant effects of zolpidem). Products include:
- Phenergan with Codeine Syrup 3557
- Phenergan VC with Codeine Syrup 3561
- Robitussin A-C Syrup 2942
- Robitussin-DAC Syrup 2942
- Ryna-C Liquid .... ▣ 768
- Soma Compound w/Codeine Tablets 3355
- Tussi-Organidin NR Liquid 3350
- Tussi-Organidin-S NR Liquid 3350
- Tylenol with Codeine 2595

Desflurane (Potential for enhanced CNS depressant effects of zolpidem). Products include:
- Suprane Liquid for Inhalation 874

Dezocine (Potential for enhanced CNS depressant effects of zolpidem).
No products indexed under this heading.

Diazepam (Potential for enhanced CNS depressant effects of zolpidem). Products include:
- Valium Injectable 3026
- Valium Tablets 3047

Droperidol (Potential for enhanced CNS depressant effects of zolpidem).
No products indexed under this heading.

Enflurane (Potential for enhanced CNS depressant effects of zolpidem).
No products indexed under this heading.

Estazolam (Potential for enhanced CNS depressant effects of zolpidem). Products include:
- ProSom Tablets 500

Ethchlorvynol (Potential for enhanced CNS depressant effects of zolpidem).
No products indexed under this heading.

Ethinamate (Potential for enhanced CNS depressant effects of zolpidem).
No products indexed under this heading.

Fentanyl (Potential for enhanced CNS depressant effects of zolpidem). Products include:
- Duragesic Transdermal System 1786

Fentanyl Citrate (Potential for enhanced CNS depressant effects of zolpidem). Products include:
- Actiq 1184

Flumazenil (Zolpidem's sedative/hypnotic effect was reversed by flumazenil; however, no significant alterations in zolpidem pharmacokinetics was found). Products include:
- Romazicon Injection 3000

Fluoxetine Hydrochloride (Co-administration during multiple doses of both drugs at steady-state concentrations has resulted in a 17% increase in the zolpidem half-life; there was no evidence of an additive effect in psychomotor performance). Products include:
- Prozac Pulvules, Liquid, and Weekly Capsules 1238
- Sarafem Pulvules 1962

Fluphenazine Decanoate (Potential for enhanced CNS depressant effects of zolpidem).
No products indexed under this heading.

Fluphenazine Enanthate (Potential for enhanced CNS depressant effects of zolpidem).
No products indexed under this heading.

Fluphenazine Hydrochloride (Potential for enhanced CNS depressant effects of zolpidem).
No products indexed under this heading.

Flurazepam Hydrochloride (Potential for enhanced CNS depressant effects of zolpidem).
No products indexed under this heading.

Glutethimide (Potential for enhanced CNS depressant effects of zolpidem).
No products indexed under this heading.

Haloperidol (Co-administration in a single study revealed no effect on the pharmacokinetics or pharmacodynamics of zolpidem; however, there is a potential for enhanced CNS depressant effect of zolpidem). Products include:
- Haldol Injection, Tablets and Concentrate 2533

Haloperidol Decanoate (Co-administration in a single study revealed no effect on the pharmacokinetics or pharmacodynamics of zolpidem; however, there is a potential for enhanced CNS depressant effect of zolpidem). Products include:
- Haldol Decanoate 2535

Hydrocodone Bitartrate (Potential for enhanced CNS depressant effects of zolpidem). Products include:
- Hycodan 1316
- Hycomine Compound Tablets 1317
- Hycotuss Expectorant Syrup 1318
- Lortab 3319
- Lortab Elixir 3317
- Maxidone Tablets CIII 3399
- Norco 5/325 Tablets CIII 3424
- Norco 7.5/325 Tablets CIII 3425
- Norco 10/325 Tablets CIII 3427

Norco 10/325 Tablets CIII 3425
Vicodin Tablets 516
Vicodin ES Tablets 517
Vicodin HP Tablets 518
Vicodin Tuss Expectorant 519
Vicoprofen Tablets 520
Zydone Tablets 1330

Hydrocodone Polistirex (Potential for enhanced CNS depressant effects of zolpidem). Products include:
Tussionex Pennkinetic Extended-Release Suspension 1174

Hydromorphone Hydrochloride (Potential for enhanced CNS depressant effects of zolpidem). Products include:
Dilaudid 441
Dilaudid Oral Liquid 445
Dilaudid Powder 441
Dilaudid Rectal Suppositories 441
Dilaudid Tablets 441
Dilaudid Tablets - 8 mg 445
Dilaudid-HP 443

Hydroxyzine Hydrochloride (Potential for enhanced CNS depressant effects of zolpidem). Products include:
Atarax Tablets & Syrup 2667
Vistaril Intramuscular Solution 2738

Imipramine Hydrochloride (Co-administration produces 20% decrease in peak levels of imipramine with an additive effect of decreased alertness).
No products indexed under this heading.

Imipramine Pamoate (Co-administration produces 20% decrease in peak levels of imipramine with an additive effect of decreased alertness).
No products indexed under this heading.

Isoflurane (Potential for enhanced CNS depressant effects of zolpidem).
No products indexed under this heading.

Itraconazole (Co-administration has resulted in a 34% increse in AUC$_{0-\infty}$ of zolpidem; there was no significant pharmacodynamic effects of zolpidem on subjective drowsiness, postural sway, or pychomotor performance). Products include:
Sporanox Capsules 1800
Sporanox Injection 1804
Sporanox Injection 2509
Sporanox Oral Solution 1808
Sporanox Oral Solution 2512

Ketamine Hydrochloride (Potential for enhanced CNS depressant effects of zolpidem).
No products indexed under this heading.

Levomethadyl Acetate Hydrochloride (Potential for enhanced CNS depressant effects of zolpidem).
No products indexed under this heading.

Levorphanol Tartrate (Potential for enhanced CNS depressant effects of zolpidem). Products include:
Levo-Dromoran 1734
Levorphanol Tartrate Tablets 3059

Lorazepam (Potential for enhanced CNS depressant effects of zolpidem). Products include:
Ativan Injection 3478
Ativan Tablets 3482

Loxapine Hydrochloride (Potential for enhanced CNS depressant effects of zolpidem).
No products indexed under this heading.

Loxapine Succinate (Potential for enhanced CNS depressant effects of zolpidem). Products include:
Loxitane Capsules 3398

Meperidine Hydrochloride (Potential for enhanced CNS depressant effects of zolpidem). Products include:
Demerol 3079
Mepergan Injection 3539

Mephobarbital (Potential for enhanced CNS depressant effects of zolpidem).
No products indexed under this heading.

Meprobamate (Potential for enhanced CNS depressant effects of zolpidem). Products include:
Miltown Tablets 3349

Mesoridazine Besylate (Potential for enhanced CNS depressant effects of zolpidem). Products include:
Serentil 1057

Methadone Hydrochloride (Potential for enhanced CNS depressant effects of zolpidem). Products include:
Dolophine Hydrochloride Tablets 3056

Methohexital Sodium (Potential for enhanced CNS depressant effects of zolpidem). Products include:
Brevital Sodium for Injection, USP .. 1815

Methotrimeprazine (Potential for enhanced CNS depressant effects of zolpidem).
No products indexed under this heading.

Methoxyflurane (Potential for enhanced CNS depressant effects of zolpidem).
No products indexed under this heading.

Midazolam Hydrochloride (Potential for enhanced CNS depressant effects of zolpidem). Products include:
Versed Injection 3027
Versed Syrup 3033

Molindone Hydrochloride (Potential for enhanced CNS depressant effects of zolpidem). Products include:
Moban 1320

Morphine Sulfate (Potential for enhanced CNS depressant effects of zolpidem). Products include:
Astramorph/PF Injection, USP (Preservative-Free) 594
Duramorph Injection 1312
Infumorph 200 and Infumorph 500 Sterile Solutions 1314
Kadian Capsules 1335
MS Contin Tablets 2896
MSIR 2898
Oramorph SR Tablets 3062
Roxanol 3066

Olanzapine (Potential for enhanced CNS depressant effects of zolpidem). Products include:
Zyprexa Tablets 1973
Zyprexa ZYDIS Orally Disintegrating Tablets 1973

Oxazepam (Potential for enhanced CNS depressant effects of zolpidem).
No products indexed under this heading.

Oxycodone Hydrochloride (Potential for enhanced CNS depressant effects of zolpidem). Products include:
OxyContin Tablets 2912
OxyFast Oral Concentrate Solution . 2916
OxyIR Capsules 2916
Percocet Tablets 1326
Percodan Tablets 1327
Percolone Tablets 1327
Roxicodone 3067
Tylox Capsules 2597

Pentobarbital Sodium (Potential for enhanced CNS depressant effects of zolpidem). Products include:
Nembutal Sodium Solution 485

Perphenazine (Potential for enhanced CNS depressant effects of zolpidem). Products include:
Etrafon 3115
Trilafon 3160

Phenobarbital (Potential for enhanced CNS depressant effects of zolpidem). Products include:
Arco-Lase Plus Tablets 592
Donnatal 2929
Donnatal Extentabs 2930

Prazepam (Potential for enhanced CNS depressant effects of zolpidem).
No products indexed under this heading.

Prochlorperazine (Potential for enhanced CNS depressant effects of zolpidem). Products include:
Compazine 1505

Promethazine Hydrochloride (Potential for enhanced CNS depressant effects of zolpidem). Products include:
Mepergan Injection 3539
Phenergan Injection 3553
Phenergan 3556
Phenergan Syrup 3554
Phenergan with Codeine Syrup 3557
Phenergan with Dextromethorphan Syrup 3559
Phenergan VC Syrup 3560
Phenergan VC with Codeine Syrup .. 3561

Propofol (Potential for enhanced CNS depressant effects of zolpidem). Products include:
Diprivan Injectable Emulsion 667

Propoxyphene Hydrochloride (Potential for enhanced CNS depressant effects of zolpidem). Products include:
Darvon Pulvules 1909
Darvon Compound-65 Pulvules 1910

Propoxyphene Napsylate (Potential for enhanced CNS depressant effects of zolpidem). Products include:
Darvon-N/Darvocet-N 1907
Darvon-N Tablets 1912

Quazepam (Potential for enhanced CNS depressant effects of zolpidem).
No products indexed under this heading.

Quetiapine Fumarate (Potential for enhanced CNS depressant effects of zolpidem). Products include:
Seroquel Tablets 684

Remifentanil Hydrochloride (Potential for enhanced CNS depressant effects of zolpidem).
No products indexed under this heading.

Rifampin (Co-administration has resulted in significant reductions of the AUC, Cmax, and T½ of zolpidem together with significant reductions in the pharmacodynamic effects of zolpidem). Products include:
Rifadin 765
Rifamate Capsules 767
Rifater Tablets 769

Risperidone (Potential for enhanced CNS depressant effects of zolpidem). Products include:
Risperdal 1796

Secobarbital Sodium (Potential for enhanced CNS depressant effects of zolpidem).
No products indexed under this heading.

Sertraline Hydrochloride (Co-administration following consecutive nightly doses has resulted in significantly higher (43%) Cmax and significantly lower Tmax (53%) of zolpidem). Products include:
Zoloft 2751

Sevoflurane (Potential for enhanced CNS depressant effects of zolpidem).
No products indexed under this heading.

Sufentanil Citrate (Potential for enhanced CNS depressant effects of zolpidem).
No products indexed under this heading.

Temazepam (Potential for enhanced CNS depressant effects of zolpidem).
No products indexed under this heading.

Thiamylal Sodium (Potential for enhanced CNS depressant effects of zolpidem).
No products indexed under this heading.

Thioridazine Hydrochloride (Potential for enhanced CNS depressant effects of zolpidem). Products include:
Thioridazine Hydrochloride Tablets 2289

Thiothixene (Potential for enhanced CNS depressant effects of zolpidem). Products include:
Navane Capsules 2701
Thiothixene Capsules 2290

Triazolam (Potential for enhanced CNS depressant effects of zolpidem). Products include:
Halcion Tablets 2823

Trifluoperazine Hydrochloride (Potential for enhanced CNS depressant effects of zolpidem). Products include:
Stelazine 1640

Zaleplon (Potential for enhanced CNS depressant effects of zolpidem). Products include:
Sonata Capsules 3591

Ziprasidone Hydrochloride (Potential for enhanced CNS depressant effects of zolpidem). Products include:
Geodon Capsules 2688

Food Interactions

Alcohol (Co-administration produces additive effects on psychomotor performance).

Meal, unspecified (Mean AUC and Cmax decreased by 15% and 25% respectively, while Tmax was prolonged by 60%; for faster sleep onset, Ambien should not be administered with or immediately after meal).

AMBISOME FOR INJECTION

(Amphotericin B) 1383
May interact with aminoglycosides, antineoplastics, corticosteroids, curariform skeletal muscle relaxants, cardiac glycosides, imidazoles, and certain other agents. Compounds in these categories include:

ACTH (Concurrent use of ACTH and amphotericin B may potentiate hypokalemia which could predispose the patient to cardiac dysfunction).
No products indexed under this heading.

Altretamine (Concurrent use of antineoplastic agents and amphotericin B may enhance the potential for renal toxicity, bronchospasm, and hypotension). Products include:
Hexalen Capsules 2226

Amikacin Sulfate (Concurrent use of amphotericin B and other nephrotoxic agents, such as aminoglycosides, may enhance the potential for drug-induced renal toxicity).
No products indexed under this heading.

Anastrozole (Concurrent use of antineoplastic agents and amphotericin B may enhance the potential for renal toxicity, bronchospasm, and hypotension). Products include:
Arimidex Tablets 659

Asparaginase (Concurrent use of antineoplastic agents and amphotericin B may enhance the potential for renal toxicity, bronchospasm, and hypotension). Products include:
Elspar for Injection 2092

Atracurium Besylate (Amphotericin B-induced hypokalemia may enhance the curariform effect of

skeletal relaxants).
No products indexed under this heading.

Betamethasone Acetate (Concurrent use of corticosteroids and amphotericin B may potentiate hypokalemia which could predispose the patient to cardiac dysfunction). Products include:
Celestone Soluspan Injectable Suspension 3097

Betamethasone Sodium Phosphate (Concurrent use of corticosteroids and amphotericin B may potentiate hypokalemia which could predispose the patient to cardiac dysfunction). Products include:
Celestone Soluspan Injectable Suspension 3097

Bicalutamide (Concurrent use of antineoplastic agents and amphotericin B may enhance the potential for renal toxicity, bronchospasm, and hypotension). Products include:
Casodex Tablets 662

Bleomycin Sulfate (Concurrent use of antineoplastic agents and amphotericin B may enhance the potential for renal toxicity, bronchospasm, and hypotension).
No products indexed under this heading.

Busulfan (Concurrent use of antineoplastic agents and amphotericin B may enhance the potential for renal toxicity, bronchospasm, and hypotension). Products include:
Myleran Tablets 1603

Carboplatin (Concurrent use of antineoplastic agents and amphotericin B may enhance the potential for renal toxicity, bronchospasm, and hypotension). Products include:
Paraplatin for Injection 1126

Carmustine (BCNU) (Concurrent use of antineoplastic agents and amphotericin B may enhance the potential for renal toxicity, bronchospasm, and hypotension). Products include:
Gliadel Wafer 1723

Chlorambucil (Concurrent use of antineoplastic agents and amphotericin B may enhance the potential for renal toxicity, bronchospasm, and hypotension). Products include:
Leukeran Tablets 1591

Cisplatin (Concurrent use of antineoplastic agents and amphotericin B may enhance the potential for renal toxicity, bronchospasm, and hypotension).
No products indexed under this heading.

Clotrimazole (Imidazoles may induce fungal resistance to amphotericin B; combination therapy should be administered with caution, especially in immunocompromised patients). Products include:
Gyne-Lotrimin 3, 3-Day Cream .... ▣741
Lotrimin AF Cream, Lotion, Solution, and Jock Itch Cream .... ▣742
Lotrimin 3128
Lotrisone 3129
Mycelex Troche 573
Mycelex-7 Combination-Pack Vaginal Inserts & External Vulvar Cream .... ▣614
Mycelex-7 Vaginal Cream .... ▣614
Mycelex-7 Vaginal Cream with 7 Disposable Applicators .... ▣614

Cortisone Acetate (Concurrent use of corticosteroids and amphotericin B may potentiate hypokalemia which could predispose the patient to cardiac dysfunction). Products include:
Cortone Acetate Injectable Suspension 2059
Cortone Acetate Tablets 2061

Cyclophosphamide (Concurrent use of antineoplastic agents and amphotericin B may enhance the potential for renal toxicity, bronchospasm, and hypotension).
No products indexed under this heading.

Cyclosporine (Concurrent use of amphotericin B and other nephrotoxic agents, such as cyclosporine, may enhance the potential for drug-induced renal toxicity). Products include:
Gengraf Capsules 457
Neoral Soft Gelatin Capsules 2380
Neoral Oral Solution 2380
Sandimmune 2388

Dacarbazine (Concurrent use of antineoplastic agents and amphotericin B may enhance the potential for renal toxicity, bronchospasm, and hypotension). Products include:
DTIC-Dome 902

Daunorubicin Citrate (Concurrent use of antineoplastic agents and amphotericin B may enhance the potential for renal toxicity, bronchospasm, and hypotension). Products include:
DaunoXome Injection 1442

Daunorubicin Hydrochloride (Concurrent use of antineoplastic agents and amphotericin B may enhance the potential for renal toxicity, bronchospasm, and hypotension). Products include:
Cerubidine for Injection 947

Denileukin Diftitox (Concurrent use of antineoplastic agents and amphotericin B may enhance the potential for renal toxicity, bronchospasm, and hypotension).
No products indexed under this heading.

Deslanoside (Concurrent use of digitalis and amphotericin B may induce hypokalemia and may potentiate digitalis toxicity).
No products indexed under this heading.

Dexamethasone (Concurrent use of corticosteroids and amphotericin B may potentiate hypokalemia which could predispose the patient to cardiac dysfunction). Products include:
Decadron Elixir 2078
Decadron Tablets 2079
TobraDex Ophthalmic Ointment 542
TobraDex Ophthalmic Suspension 541

Dexamethasone Acetate (Concurrent use of corticosteroids and amphotericin B may potentiate hypokalemia which could predispose the patient to cardiac dysfunction).
No products indexed under this heading.

Dexamethasone Sodium Phosphate (Concurrent use of corticosteroids and amphotericin B may potentiate hypokalemia which could predispose the patient to cardiac dysfunction). Products include:
Decadron Phosphate Injection 2081
Decadron Phosphate Sterile Ophthalmic Ointment 2083
Decadron Phosphate Sterile Ophthalmic Solution 2084
NeoDecadron Sterile Ophthalmic Solution 2144

Digitoxin (Concurrent use of digitalis and amphotericin B may induce hypokalemia and may potentiate digitalis toxicity).
No products indexed under this heading.

Digoxin (Concurrent use of digitalis and amphotericin B may induce hypokalemia and may potentiate digitalis toxicity). Products include:
Digitek Tablets 1003
Lanoxicaps Capsules 1574
Lanoxin Injection 1581
Lanoxin Tablets 1587
Lanoxin Elixir Pediatric 1578
Lanoxin Injection Pediatric 1584

Docetaxel (Concurrent use of antineoplastic agents and amphotericin B may enhance the potential for renal toxicity, bronchospasm, and hypotension). Products include:
Taxotere for Injection Concentrate 778

Doxorubicin Hydrochloride (Concurrent use of antineoplastic agents and amphotericin B may enhance the potential for renal toxicity, bronchospasm, and hypotension). Products include:
Adriamycin PFS/RDF Injection 2767
Doxil Injection 566

Epirubicin Hydrochloride (Concurrent use of antineoplastic agents and amphotericin B may enhance the potential for renal toxicity, bronchospasm, and hypotension). Products include:
Ellence Injection 2806

Estramustine Phosphate Sodium (Concurrent use of antineoplastic agents and amphotericin B may enhance the potential for renal toxicity, bronchospasm, and hypotension). Products include:
Emcyt Capsules 2810

Etoposide (Concurrent use of antineoplastic agents and amphotericin B may enhance the potential for renal toxicity, bronchospasm, and hypotension).
No products indexed under this heading.

Exemestane (Concurrent use of antineoplastic agents and amphotericin B may enhance the potential for renal toxicity, bronchospasm, and hypotension). Products include:
Aromasin Tablets 2769

Floxuridine (Concurrent use of antineoplastic agents and amphotericin B may enhance the potential for renal toxicity, bronchospasm, and hypotension). Products include:
Sterile FUDR 2974

Fluconazole (Imidazoles may induce fungal resistance to amphotericin B; combination therapy should be administered with caution, especially in immunocompromised patients). Products include:
Diflucan Tablets, Injection, and Oral Suspension 2681

Flucytosine (Concurrent use may increase the toxicity of flucytosine by possibly increasing its cellular uptake and/or impairing its renal excretion). Products include:
Ancobon Capsules 1730

Fludrocortisone Acetate (Concurrent use of corticosteroids and amphotericin B may potentiate hypokalemia which could predispose the patient to cardiac dysfunction). Products include:
Florinef Acetate Tablets 2250

Fluorouracil (Concurrent use of antineoplastic agents and amphotericin B may enhance the potential for renal toxicity, bronchospasm, and hypotension). Products include:
Carac Cream 1222
Efudex 1733
Fluoroplex 552

Flutamide (Concurrent use of antineoplastic agents and amphotericin B may enhance the potential for renal toxicity, bronchospasm, and hypotension). Products include:
Eulexin Capsules 3118

Gemcitabine Hydrochloride (Concurrent use of antineoplastic agents and amphotericin B may enhance the potential for renal toxicity, bronchospasm, and hypotension). Products include:
Gemzar for Injection 1919

Gentamicin Sulfate (Concurrent use of amphotericin B and other nephrotoxic agents, such as aminoglycosides, may enhance the potential for drug-induced renal toxicity). Products include:
Genoptic Ophthalmic Ointment .... ⊙239
Genoptic Sterile Ophthalmic Solution .... ⊙239
Pred-G Ophthalmic Suspension .... ⊙247
Pred-G Sterile Ophthalmic Ointment .... ⊙248

Hydrocortisone (Concurrent use of corticosteroids and amphotericin B may potentiate hypokalemia which could predispose the patient to cardiac dysfunction). Products include:
Anusol-HC Cream 2.5% 2237
Cipro HC Otic Suspension 540
Cortaid Intensive Therapy Cream .... ▣717
Cortaid Maximum Strength Cream .... ▣717
Cortisporin Ophthalmic Suspension Sterile .... ⊙297
Cortizone•5 .... ▣699
Cortizone•10 .... ▣699
Cortizone•10 Plus Creme .... ▣700
Cortizone for Kids Creme .... ▣699
Hydrocortone Tablets 2106
Massengill Medicated Soft Cloth Towelette .... ▣753
VōSoL HC Otic Solution 3356

Hydrocortisone Acetate (Concurrent use of corticosteroids and amphotericin B may potentiate hypokalemia which could predispose the patient to cardiac dysfunction). Products include:
Analpram-HC 1338
Anusol HC-1 Hydrocortisone Anti-Itch Cream .... ▣689
Anusol-HC Suppositories 2238
Cortaid .... ▣717
Cortifoam Rectal Foam 3170
Cortisporin-TC Otic Suspension 2246
Hydrocortone Acetate Injectable Suspension 2103
Pramosone 1343
Proctocort Suppositories 2264
ProctoFoam-HC 3177
Terra-Cortril Ophthalmic Suspension 2716

Hydrocortisone Sodium Phosphate (Concurrent use of corticosteroids and amphotericin B may potentiate hypokalemia which could predispose the patient to cardiac dysfunction). Products include:
Hydrocortone Phosphate Injection, Sterile 2105

Hydrocortisone Sodium Succinate (Concurrent use of corticosteroids and amphotericin B may potentiate hypokalemia which could predispose the patient to cardiac dysfunction).
No products indexed under this heading.

Hydroxyurea (Concurrent use of antineoplastic agents and amphotericin B may enhance the potential for renal toxicity, bronchospasm, and hypotension). Products include:
Mylocel Tablets 2227

Idarubicin Hydrochloride (Concurrent use of antineoplastic agents and amphotericin B may enhance the potential for renal toxicity, bronchospasm, and hypotension). Products include:
Idamycin PFS Injection 2825

Ifosfamide (Concurrent use of antineoplastic agents and amphotericin B may enhance the potential for renal toxicity, bronchospasm, and hypotension). Products include:
Ifex for Injection 1123

Interferon alfa-2A, Recombinant (Concurrent use of antineoplastic agents and amphotericin B may enhance the potential for renal toxicity, bronchospasm, and hypotension). Products include:
Roferon-A Injection 2996

Interferon alfa-2B, Recombinant (Concurrent use of antineoplastic agents and amphotericin B may enhance the potential for renal toxicity, bronchospasm, and hypotension). Products include:
Intron A for Injection 3120
Rebetron Combination Therapy 3153

Irinotecan Hydrochloride (Concurrent use of antineoplastic agents and amphotericin B may enhance the potential for renal toxicity, broncho-

spasm, and hypotension).
No products indexed under this heading.

Kanamycin Sulfate (Concurrent use of amphotericin B and other nephrotoxic agents, such as aminoglycosides, may enhance the potential for drug-induced renal toxicity).
No products indexed under this heading.

Ketoconazole (Imidazoles may induce fungal resistance to amphotericin B; combination therapy should be administered with caution, especially in immunocompromised patients). Products include:
Nizoral 2% Cream 3620
Nizoral A-D Shampoo 2008
Nizoral 2% Shampoo 2007
Nizoral Tablets 1791

Levamisole Hydrochloride (Concurrent use of antineoplastic agents and amphotericin B may enhance the potential for renal toxicity, bronchospasm, and hypotension). Products include:
Ergamisol Tablets 1789

Lomustine (CCNU) (Concurrent use of antineoplastic agents and amphotericin B may enhance the potential for renal toxicity, bronchospasm, and hypotension).
No products indexed under this heading.

Mechlorethamine Hydrochloride (Concurrent use of antineoplastic agents and amphotericin B may enhance the potential for renal toxicity, bronchospasm, and hypotension). Products include:
Mustargen for Injection 2142

Megestrol Acetate (Concurrent use of antineoplastic agents and amphotericin B may enhance the potential for renal toxicity, bronchospasm, and hypotension). Products include:
Megace Oral Suspension 1124

Melphalan (Concurrent use of antineoplastic agents and amphotericin B may enhance the potential for renal toxicity, bronchospasm, and hypotension). Products include:
Alkeran Tablets 1466

Mercaptopurine (Concurrent use of antineoplastic agents and amphotericin B may enhance the potential for renal toxicity, bronchospasm, and hypotension). Products include:
Purinethol Tablets 1615

Methotrexate Sodium (Concurrent use of antineoplastic agents and amphotericin B may enhance the potential for renal toxicity, bronchospasm, and hypotension).
No products indexed under this heading.

Methylprednisolone Acetate (Concurrent use of corticosteroids and amphotericin B may potentiate hypokalemia which could predispose the patient to cardiac dysfunction). Products include:
Depo-Medrol Injectable Suspension 2795

Methylprednisolone Sodium Succinate (Concurrent use of corticosteroids and amphotericin B may potentiate hypokalemia which could predispose the patient to cardiac dysfunction). Products include:
Solu-Medrol Sterile Powder 2855

Miconazole (Imidazoles may induce fungal resistance to amphotericin B; combination therapy should be administered with caution, especially in immunocompromised patients).
No products indexed under this heading.

Miconazole Nitrate (Imidazoles may induce fungal resistance to amphotericin B; combination therapy should be administered with caution, especially in immunocompromised patients). Products include:
Desenex .... ▣668
Desenex Jock Itch Spray Powder .. ▣668
Lotrimin AF Spray Powder, Spray Liquid, Spray Deodorant Powder, Shaker Powder and Jock Itch Spray Powder .... ▣742

Mitomycin (Mitomycin-C) (Concurrent use of antineoplastic agents and amphotericin B may enhance the potential for renal toxicity, bronchospasm, and hypotension).
No products indexed under this heading.

Mitotane (Concurrent use of antineoplastic agents and amphotericin B may enhance the potential for renal toxicity, bronchospasm, and hypotension).
No products indexed under this heading.

Mitoxantrone Hydrochloride (Concurrent use of antineoplastic agents and amphotericin B may enhance the potential for renal toxicity, bronchospasm, and hypotension). Products include:
Novantrone for Injection 1760

Mivacurium Chloride (Amphotericin B-induced hypokalemia may enhance the curariform effect of skeletal relaxants).
No products indexed under this heading.

Paclitaxel (Concurrent use of antineoplastic agents and amphotericin B may enhance the potential for renal toxicity, bronchospasm, and hypotension). Products include:
Taxol Injection 1129

Pancuronium Bromide (Amphotericin B-induced hypokalemia may enhance the curariform effect of skeletal relaxants).
No products indexed under this heading.

Pentamidine Isethionate (Concurrent use of amphotericin B and other nephrotoxic agents, such as pentamidine, may enhance the potential for drug-induced renal toxicity).
No products indexed under this heading.

Prednisolone Acetate (Concurrent use of corticosteroids and amphotericin B may potentiate hypokalemia which could predispose the patient to cardiac dysfunction). Products include:
Blephamide Ophthalmic Ointment .. 547
Blephamide Ophthalmic Suspension 548
Poly-Pred Liquifilm Ophthalmic Suspension .... ⊙245
Pred Forte Ophthalmic Suspension .... ⊙246
Pred Mild Sterile Ophthalmic Suspension .... ⊙249
Pred-G Ophthalmic Suspension .... ⊙247
Pred-G Sterile Ophthalmic Ointment .... ⊙248

Prednisolone Sodium Phosphate (Concurrent use of corticosteroids and amphotericin B may potentiate hypokalemia which could predispose the patient to cardiac dysfunction). Products include:
Pediapred Oral Solution 1170

Prednisolone Tebutate (Concurrent use of corticosteroids and amphotericin B may potentiate hypokalemia which could predispose the patient to cardiac dysfunction).
No products indexed under this heading.

Prednisone (Concurrent use of corticosteroids and amphotericin B may potentiate hypokalemia which could predispose the patient to cardiac dysfunction). Products include:
Prednisone 3064

Procarbazine Hydrochloride (Concurrent use of antineoplastic agents and amphotericin B may enhance the potential for renal toxicity, bronchospasm, and hypotension). Products include:
Matulane Capsules 3246

Rapacuronium Bromide (Amphotericin B-induced hypokalemia may enhance the curariform effect of skeletal relaxants).
No products indexed under this heading.

Rocuronium Bromide (Amphotericin B-induced hypokalemia may enhance the curariform effect of skeletal relaxants). Products include:
Zemuron Injection 2491

Streptomycin Sulfate (Concurrent use of amphotericin B and other nephrotoxic agents, such as aminoglycosides, may enhance the potential for drug-induced renal toxicity). Products include:
Streptomycin Sulfate Injection 2714

Streptozocin (Concurrent use of antineoplastic agents and amphotericin B may enhance the potential for renal toxicity, bronchospasm, and hypotension).
No products indexed under this heading.

Tamoxifen Citrate (Concurrent use of antineoplastic agents and amphotericin B may enhance the potential for renal toxicity, bronchospasm, and hypotension). Products include:
Nolvadex Tablets 678

Teniposide (Concurrent use of antineoplastic agents and amphotericin B may enhance the potential for renal toxicity, bronchospasm, and hypotension).
No products indexed under this heading.

Thioguanine (Concurrent use of antineoplastic agents and amphotericin B may enhance the potential for renal toxicity, bronchospasm, and hypotension). Products include:
Tabloid Tablets 1642

Thiotepa (Concurrent use of antineoplastic agents and amphotericin B may enhance the potential for renal toxicity, bronchospasm, and hypotension). Products include:
Thioplex for Injection 1765

Tobramycin (Concurrent use of amphotericin B and other nephrotoxic agents, such as aminoglycosides, may enhance the potential for drug-induced renal toxicity). Products include:
TOBI Solution for Inhalation 1206
TobraDex Ophthalmic Ointment 542
TobraDex Ophthalmic Suspension .. 541
Tobrex Ophthalmic Ointment .... ⊙220
Tobrex Ophthalmic Solution .... ⊙221

Tobramycin Sulfate (Concurrent use of amphotericin B and other nephrotoxic agents, such as aminoglycosides, may enhance the potential for drug-induced renal toxicity). Products include:
Nebcin Vials, Hyporets & ADD-Vantage 1955

Topotecan Hydrochloride (Concurrent use of antineoplastic agents and amphotericin B may enhance the potential for renal toxicity, bronchospasm, and hypotension). Products include:
Hycamtin for Injection 1546

Toremifene Citrate (Concurrent use of antineoplastic agents and amphotericin B may enhance the potential for renal toxicity, bronchospasm, and hypotension). Products include:
Fareston Tablets 3237

Triamcinolone (Concurrent use of corticosteroids and amphotericin B may potentiate hypokalemia which could predispose the patient to cardiac dysfunction).
No products indexed under this heading.

Triamcinolone Acetonide (Concurrent use of corticosteroids and amphotericin B may potentiate hypokalemia which could predispose the patient to cardiac dysfunction). Products include:
Azmacort Inhalation Aerosol 728
Nasacort Nasal Inhaler 750
Nasacort AQ Nasal Spray 752
Tri-Nasal Spray 2274

Triamcinolone Diacetate (Concurrent use of corticosteroids and amphotericin B may potentiate hypokalemia which could predispose the patient to cardiac dysfunction).
No products indexed under this heading.

Triamcinolone Hexacetonide (Concurrent use of corticosteroids and amphotericin B may potentiate hypokalemia which could predispose the patient to cardiac dysfunction).
No products indexed under this heading.

Tubocurarine Chloride (Amphotericin B-induced hypokalemia may enhance the curariform effect of skeletal relaxants).
No products indexed under this heading.

Valrubicin (Concurrent use of antineoplastic agents and amphotericin B may enhance the potential for renal toxicity, bronchospasm, and hypotension). Products include:
Valstar Sterile Solution for Intravesical Instillation 1175

Vecuronium Bromide (Amphotericin B-induced hypokalemia may enhance the curariform effect of skeletal relaxants). Products include:
Norcuron for Injection 2478

Vincristine Sulfate (Concurrent use of antineoplastic agents and amphotericin B may enhance the potential for renal toxicity, bronchospasm, and hypotension).
No products indexed under this heading.

Vinorelbine Tartrate (Concurrent use of antineoplastic agents and amphotericin B may enhance the potential for renal toxicity, bronchospasm, and hypotension). Products include:
Navelbine Injection 1604

AMBROTOSE POWDER

(Glucosamine Hydrochloride) .... ▣819
None cited in PDR database.

AMBROTOSE WITH LECITHIN CAPSULES

(Lecithin) .... ▣819
None cited in PDR database.

AMERGE TABLETS

(Naratriptan Hydrochloride) 1467
May interact with 5HT1-receptor agonists, ergot-containing drugs, oral contraceptives, and selective serotonin reuptake inhibitors. Compounds in these categories include:

Citalopram Hydrobromide (Co-administration of 5-HT_1 agonists with selective serotonin reuptake inhibitors (SSRIs) has resulted, rarely, in hyperreflexia, weakness, and incoordination). Products include:
Celexa 1365

Desogestrel (Co-administration with oral contraceptives has resulted in reduced clearance by 32% and volume of distribution by 22%, producing slightly higher concentrations of naratriptan). Products include:
Cyclessa Tablets 2450
Desogen Tablets 2458
Mircette Tablets 2470
Ortho-Cept 21 Tablets 2546
Ortho-Cept 28 Tablets 2546

Dihydroergotamine Mesylate (Ergot-containing drugs have been reported to cause prolonged vaso-

spastic reactions; because there is a theoretical basis that these effects may be additive, use of ergot-type agents and naratriptan within 24 hours is contraindicated). Products include:

D.H.E. 45 Injection 2334
Migranal Nasal Spray 2376

Ergonovine Maleate (Ergot-containing drugs have been reported to cause prolonged vasospastic reactions; because there is a theoretical basis that these effects may be additive, use of ergot-type agents and naratriptan within 24 hours is contraindicated).

No products indexed under this heading.

Ergotamine Tartrate (Ergot-containing drugs have been reported to cause prolonged vasospastic reactions; because there is a theoretical basis that these effects may be additive, use of ergot-type agents and naratriptan within 24 hours is contraindicated).

No products indexed under this heading.

Ethinyl Estradiol (Co-administration with oral contraceptives has resulted in reduced clearance by 32% and volume of distribution by 22%, producing slightly higher concentrations of naratriptan). Products include:

Alesse-21 Tablets 3468
Alesse-28 Tablets 3473
Brevicon 28-Day Tablets 3380
Cyclessa Tablets 2450
Desogen Tablets 2458
Estinyl Tablets 3112
Estrostep 2627
femhrt Tablets 2635
Levlen 962
Levlite 21 Tablets 962
Levlite 28 Tablets 962
Levora Tablets 3389
Loestrin 21 Tablets 2642
Loestrin Fe Tablets 2642
Lo/Ovral Tablets 3532
Lo/Ovral-28 Tablets 3538
Low-Ogestrel-28 Tablets 3392
Microgestin Fe 1.5/30 Tablets 3407
Microgestin Fe 1/20 Tablets 3400
Mircette Tablets 2470
Modicon 2563
Necon 3415
Nordette-28 Tablets 2257
Norinyl 1 +35 28-Day Tablets 3380
Ogestrel 0.5/50-28 Tablets 3428
Ortho-Cept 21 Tablets 2546
Ortho-Cept 28 Tablets 2546
Ortho-Cyclen/Ortho Tri-Cyclen 2573
Ortho-Novum 2563
Ovcon 3364
Ovral Tablets 3551
Ovral-28 Tablets 3552
Tri-Levlen 962
Tri-Norinyl-28 Tablets 3433
Triphasil-21 Tablets 3600
Triphasil-28 Tablets 3605
Trivora Tablets 3439
Yasmin 28 Tablets 980
Zovia 3449

Ethynodiol Diacetate (Co-administration with oral contraceptives has resulted in reduced clearance by 32% and volume of distribution by 22%, producing slightly higher concentrations of naratriptan). Products include:

Zovia 3449

Fluoxetine Hydrochloride (Co-administration of 5-HT_1 agonists with selective serotonin reuptake inhibitors (SSRIs) has resulted, rarely, in hyperreflexia, weakness, and incoordination). Products include:

Prozac Pulvules, Liquid, and Weekly Capsules 1238
Sarafem Pulvules 1962

Fluvoxamine Maleate (Co-administration of 5-HT_1 agonists with selective serotonin reuptake inhibitors (SSRIs) has resulted, rarely, in hyperreflexia, weakness, and incoordination). Products include:

Luvox Tablets (25, 50, 100 mg) 3256

Levonorgestrel (Co-administration with oral contraceptives has resulted in reduced clearance by 32% and volume of distribution by 22%, producing slightly higher concentrations of naratriptan). Products include:

Alesse-21 Tablets 3468
Alesse-28 Tablets 3473
Levlen 962
Levlite 21 Tablets 962
Levlite 28 Tablets 962
Levora Tablets 3389
Mirena Intrauterine System 974
Nordette-28 Tablets 2257
Norplant System 3543
Tri-Levlen 962
Triphasil-21 Tablets 3600
Triphasil-28 Tablets 3605
Trivora Tablets 3439

Mestranol (Co-administration with oral contraceptives has resulted in reduced clearance by 32% and volume of distribution by 22%, producing slightly higher concentrations of naratriptan). Products include:

Necon 1/50 Tablets 3415
Norinyl 1 + 50 28-Day Tablets 3380
Ortho-Novum 1/50□28 Tablets 2556

Methylergonovine Maleate (Ergot-containing drugs have been reported to cause prolonged vasospastic reactions; because there is a theoretical basis that these effects may be additive, use of ergot-type agents and naratriptan within 24 hours is contraindicated).

No products indexed under this heading.

Methysergide Maleate (Ergot-containing drugs have been reported to cause prolonged vasospastic reactions; because there is a theoretical basis that these effects may be additive, use of ergot-type agents and naratriptan within 24 hours is contraindicated).

No products indexed under this heading.

Norethindrone (Co-administration with oral contraceptives has resulted in reduced clearance by 32% and volume of distribution by 22%, producing slightly higher concentrations of naratriptan). Products include:

Brevicon 28-Day Tablets 3380
Micronor Tablets 2543
Modicon 2563
Necon 3415
Norinyl 1 +35 28-Day Tablets 3380
Norinyl 1 + 50 28-Day Tablets 3380
Nor-QD Tablets 3423
Ortho-Novum 2563
Ortho-Novum 1/50□28 Tablets 2556
Ovcon 3364
Tri-Norinyl-28 Tablets 3433

Norethynodrel (Co-administration with oral contraceptives has resulted in reduced clearance by 32% and volume of distribution by 22%, producing slightly higher concentrations of naratriptan).

No products indexed under this heading.

Norgestimate (Co-administration with oral contraceptives has resulted in reduced clearance by 32% and volume of distribution by 22%, producing slightly higher concentrations of naratriptan). Products include:

Ortho-Cyclen/Ortho Tri-Cyclen 2573
Ortho-Prefest Tablets 2570

Norgestrel (Co-administration with oral contraceptives has resulted in reduced clearance by 32% and volume of distribution by 22%, producing slightly higher concentrations of naratriptan). Products include:

Lo/Ovral Tablets 3532
Lo/Ovral-28 Tablets 3538
Low-Ogestrel-28 Tablets 3392
Ogestrel 0.5/50-28 Tablets 3428
Ovral Tablets 3551
Ovral-28 Tablets 3552
Ovrette Tablets 3552

Paroxetine Hydrochloride (Co-administration of 5-HT_1 agonists with selective serotonin reuptake inhibitors (SSRIs) has resulted, rarely, in hyperreflexia, weakness, and incoordination). Products include:

Paxil 1609

Rizatriptan Benzoate (Co-administration with other 5-HT_1 agonists within 24 hours of each other is contraindicated because of the vasospastic effects may be additive). Products include:

Maxalt Tablets 2120
Maxalt-MLT Orally Disintegrating Tablets 2120

Sertraline Hydrochloride (Co-administration of 5-HT_1 agonists with selective serotonin reuptake inhibitors (SSRIs) has resulted, rarely, in hyperreflexia, weakness, and incoordination). Products include:

Zoloft 2751

Sumatriptan (Co-administration with other 5-HT1 agonists within 24 hours of each other is contraindicated because of the vasospastic effects may be additive). Products include:

Imitrex Nasal Spray 1554

Sumatriptan Succinate (Co-administration with other 5-HT1 agonists within 24 hours of each other is contraindicated because of the vasospastic effects may be additive). Products include:

Imitrex Injection 1549
Imitrex Tablets 1558

Zolmitriptan (Co-administration with other 5-HT1 agonists within 24 hours of each other is contraindicated because of the vasospastic effects may be additive). Products include:

Zomig Tablets 708
Zomig-ZMT Tablets 708

AMERICAINE ANESTHETIC LUBRICANT

(Benzocaine) 1162
None cited in PDR database.

AMERICAINE OTIC TOPICAL ANESTHETIC EAR DROPS

(Benzocaine) 1162
None cited in PDR database.

AMICAR INJECTION

(Aminocaproic Acid) 3608
None cited in PDR database.

AMICAR SYRUP

(Aminocaproic Acid) 3608
None cited in PDR database.

AMICAR TABLETS

(Aminocaproic Acid) 3608
None cited in PDR database.

AMINO-CERV CREME

(L-Cystine, Inositol, Methionine, Sodium Propionate, Urea) 2231
None cited in PDR database.

AMINOHIPPURATE SODIUM PAH INJECTION

(Aminohippurate Sodium) 2041
May interact with sulfonamides and certain other agents. Compounds in these categories include:

Bendroflumethiazide (Co-administration with sulfonamides interfere with chemical color development essential to the analytical procedures). Products include:

Corzide 40/5 Tablets 2247
Corzide 80/5 Tablets 2247

Chlorothiazide (Co-administration with sulfonamides interfere with chemical color development essential to the analytical procedures). Products include:

Aldoclor Tablets 2035
Diuril Oral 2087

Chlorothiazide Sodium (Co-administration with sulfonamides interfere with chemical color development essential to the analytical procedures). Products include:

Diuril Sodium Intravenous 2086

Chlorpropamide (Co-administration with sulfonamides interfere with chemical color development essential to the analytical procedures). Products include:

Diabinese Tablets 2680

Glipizide (Co-administration with sulfonamides interfere with chemical color development essential to the analytical procedures). Products include:

Glucotrol Tablets 2692
Glucotrol XL Extended Release Tablets 2693

Glyburide (Co-administration with sulfonamides interfere with chemical color development essential to the analytical procedures). Products include:

DiaBeta Tablets 741
Glucovance Tablets 1086

Hydrochlorothiazide (Co-administration with sulfonamides interfere with chemical color development essential to the analytical procedures). Products include:

Accuretic Tablets 2614
Aldoril Tablets 2039
Atacand HCT Tablets 597
Avalide Tablets 1070
Diovan HCT Tablets 2338
Dyazide Capsules 1515
HydroDIURIL Tablets 2108
Hyzaar 2109
Inderide Tablets 3517
Inderide LA Long-Acting Capsules 3519
Lotensin HCT Tablets 2367
Maxzide 1008
Micardis HCT Tablets 1051
Microzide Capsules 3414
Moduretic Tablets 2138
Monopril HCT 1094
Prinzide Tablets 2168
Timolide Tablets 2187
Uniretic Tablets 3178
Vaseretic Tablets 2204
Zestoretic Tablets 695
Ziac Tablets 1887

Hydroflumethiazide (Co-administration with sulfonamides interfere with chemical color development essential to the analytical procedures). Products include:

Diucardin Tablets 3494

Methyclothiazide (Co-administration with sulfonamides interfere with chemical color development essential to the analytical procedures).

No products indexed under this heading.

Polythiazide (Co-administration with sulfonamides interfere with chemical color development essential to the analytical procedures). Products include:

Minizide Capsules 2700
Renese Tablets 2712

Probenecid (Tubular secretion of PAH depressed).

No products indexed under this heading.

Procaine Hydrochloride (Renal clearance measurements impaired).

No products indexed under this heading.

Sulfacytine (Co-administration with sulfonamides interfere with chemical color development essential to the analytical procedures).

No products indexed under this heading.

Sulfamethizole (Co-administration with sulfonamides interfere with chemical color development essential to the analytical procedures). Products include:

Urobiotic-250 Capsules 2731

Sulfamethoxazole (Co-administration with sulfonamides interfere with chemical color development essential to the analytical procedures). Products include:

Bactrim 2949

Septra Suspension 2265
Septra Tablets 2265
Septra DS Tablets 2265

Sulfasalazine (Co-administration with sulfonamides interfere with chemical color development essential to the analytical procedures). Products include:
Azulfidine EN-tabs Tablets 2775

Sulfinpyrazone (Co-administration with sulfonamides interfere with chemical color development essential to the analytical procedures).
No products indexed under this heading.

Sulfisoxazole (Co-administration with sulfonamides interfere with chemical color development essential to the analytical procedures).
No products indexed under this heading.

Sulfisoxazole Acetyl (Co-administration with sulfonamides interfere with chemical color development essential to the analytical procedures). Products include:
Pediazole Suspension 3050

Sulfisoxazole Diolamine (Co-administration with sulfonamides interfere with chemical color development essential to the analytical procedures).
No products indexed under this heading.

Tolazamide (Co-administration with sulfonamides interfere with chemical color development essential to the analytical procedures).
No products indexed under this heading.

Tolbutamide (Co-administration with sulfonamides interfere with chemical color development essential to the analytical procedures).
No products indexed under this heading.

AMOXIL CHEWABLE TABLETS

(Amoxicillin) 1471
See Amoxil Tablets

AMOXIL FOR ORAL SUSPENSION

(Amoxicillin) 1471
See Amoxil Tablets

AMOXIL PEDIATRIC DROPS FOR ORAL SUSPENSION

(Amoxicillin) 1471
See Amoxil Tablets

AMOXIL TABLETS

(Amoxicillin) 1471
May interact with macrolide antibiotics, tetracyclines, and certain other agents. Compounds in these categories include:

Azithromycin Dihydrate (May interfere with bactericidal effects of penicillin; this has been demonstrated in vitro, however, the clinical significance of the interaction is not well documented). Products include:
Zithromax 2743
Zithromax for IV Infusion 2748
Zithromax for Oral Suspension, 300 mg, 600 mg, 900 mg, 1200 mg 2739
Zithromax Tablets, 250 mg 2739

Chloramphenicol Sodium Succinate (May interfere with bactericidal effects of penicillin; this has been demonstrated in vitro, however, the clinical significance of the interaction is not well documented).
No products indexed under this heading.

Clarithromycin (May interfere with bactericidal effects of penicillin; this has been demonstrated in vitro, however, the clinical significance of the interaction is not well documented). Products include:
Biaxin/Biaxin XL 403
PREVPAC 3298

Demeclocycline Hydrochloride (May interfere with bactericidal effects of penicillin; this has been demonstrated in vitro, however, the clinical significance of the interaction is not well documented). Products include:
Declomycin Tablets 1855

Dirithromycin (May interfere with bactericidal effects of penicillin; this has been demonstrated in vitro, however, the clinical significance of the interaction is not well documented). Products include:
Dynabac Tablets 2269

Doxycycline Calcium (May interfere with bactericidal effects of penicillin; this has been demonstrated in vitro, however, the clinical significance of the interaction is not well documented). Products include:
Vibramycin Calcium Oral Suspension Syrup 2735

Doxycycline Hyclate (May interfere with bactericidal effects of penicillin; this has been demonstrated in vitro, however, the clinical significance of the interaction is not well documented). Products include:
Doryx Coated Pellet Filled Capsules 3357
Periostat Tablets 1208
Vibramycin Hyclate Capsules 2735
Vibramycin Hyclate Intravenous 2737
Vibra-Tabs Film Coated Tablets 2735

Doxycycline Monohydrate (May interfere with bactericidal effects of penicillin; this has been demonstrated in vitro, however, the clinical significance of the interaction is not well documented). Products include:
Monodox Capsules 2442
Vibramycin Monohydrate for Oral Suspension 2735

Erythromycin (May interfere with bactericidal effects of penicillin; this has been demonstrated in vitro, however, the clinical significance of the interaction is not well documented). Products include:
Emgel 2% Topical Gel 1285
Ery-Tab Tablets 448
Erythromycin Base Filmtab Tablets . 454
Erythromycin Delayed-Release Capsules, USP 455
PCE Dispertab Tablets 498

Erythromycin Estolate (May interfere with bactericidal effects of penicillin; this has been demonstrated in vitro, however, the clinical significance of the interaction is not well documented).
No products indexed under this heading.

Erythromycin Ethylsuccinate (May interfere with bactericidal effects of penicillin; this has been demonstrated in vitro, however, the clinical significance of the interaction is not well documented). Products include:
E.E.S. 450
EryPed 446
Pediazole Suspension 3050

Erythromycin Gluceptate (May interfere with bactericidal effects of penicillin; this has been demonstrated in vitro, however, the clinical significance of the interaction is not well documented).
No products indexed under this heading.

Erythromycin Stearate (May interfere with bactericidal effects of penicillin; this has been demonstrated in vitro, however, the clinical significance of the interaction is not well documented). Products include:
Erythrocin Stearate Filmtab Tablets 452

Methacycline Hydrochloride (May interfere with bactericidal effects of penicillin; this has been demonstrated in vitro, however, the clinical significance of the interaction is not well documented).
No products indexed under this heading.

Minocycline Hydrochloride (May interfere with bactericidal effects of penicillin; this has been demonstrated in vitro, however, the clinical significance of the interaction is not well documented). Products include:
Dynacin Capsules 2019
Minocin Intravenous 1862
Minocin Oral Suspension 1865
Minocin Pellet-Filled Capsules 1863

Oxytetracycline Hydrochloride (May interfere with bactericidal effects of penicillin; this has been demonstrated in vitro, however, the clinical significance of the interaction is not well documented). Products include:
Terra-Cortril Ophthalmic Suspension 2716
Urobiotic-250 Capsules 2731

Probenecid (Decreases the renal tubular secretion of amoxicillin; concurrent use may result in increased and prolonged blood levels).
No products indexed under this heading.

Sulfamethoxazole (May interfere with bactericidal effects of penicillin; this has been demonstrated in vitro, however, the clinical significance of the interaction is not well documented). Products include:
Bactrim 2949
Septra Suspension 2265
Septra Tablets 2265
Septra DS Tablets 2265

Sulfisoxazole Acetyl (May interfere with bactericidal effects of penicillin; this has been demonstrated in vitro, however, the clinical significance of the interaction is not well documented). Products include:
Pediazole Suspension 3050

Tetracycline Hydrochloride (May interfere with bactericidal effects of penicillin; this has been demonstrated in vitro, however, the clinical significance of the interaction is not well documented).
No products indexed under this heading.

Troleandomycin (May interfere with bactericidal effects of penicillin; this has been demonstrated in vitro, however, the clinical significance of the interaction is not well documented). Products include:
Tao Capsules 2716

AMPHOJEL SUSPENSION (MINT FLAVOR)

(Aluminum Hydroxide) ....▣ 789
May interact with tetracyclines. Compounds in these categories include:

Demeclocycline Hydrochloride (Concurrent administration should be avoided). Products include:
Declomycin Tablets 1855

Doxycycline Calcium (Concurrent administration should be avoided). Products include:
Vibramycin Calcium Oral Suspension Syrup 2735

Doxycycline Hyclate (Concurrent administration should be avoided). Products include:
Doryx Coated Pellet Filled Capsules 3357
Periostat Tablets 1208
Vibramycin Hyclate Capsules 2735
Vibramycin Hyclate Intravenous 2737
Vibra-Tabs Film Coated Tablets 2735

Doxycycline Monohydrate (Concurrent administration should be avoided). Products include:
Monodox Capsules 2442
Vibramycin Monohydrate for Oral Suspension 2735

Methacycline Hydrochloride (Concurrent administration should be avoided).
No products indexed under this heading.

Minocycline Hydrochloride (Concurrent administration should be avoided). Products include:
Dynacin Capsules 2019
Minocin Intravenous 1862
Minocin Oral Suspension 1865
Minocin Pellet-Filled Capsules 1863

Oxytetracycline (Concurrent administration should be avoided).
No products indexed under this heading.

Oxytetracycline Hydrochloride (Concurrent administration should be avoided). Products include:
Terra-Cortril Ophthalmic Suspension 2716
Urobiotic-250 Capsules 2731

Prescription Drugs, unspecified (Effect resulting from coadministration not specified).

Tetracycline Hydrochloride (Concurrent administration should be avoided).
No products indexed under this heading.

AMPHOTEC

(Amphotericin B, Cholesteryl Sulfate Complex) 1774
May interact with aminoglycosides, antineoplastics, corticosteroids, curariform skeletal muscle relaxants, cardiac glycosides, imidazoles, and certain other agents. Compounds in these categories include:

ACTH (Concurrent use with ACTH may potentiate hypokalemia, which could predispose the patient to cardiac dysfunction).
No products indexed under this heading.

Altretamine (Concurrent use with antineoplastic agents may enhance the potential for renal toxicity, bronchospasm, and hypotension). Products include:
Hexalen Capsules 2226

Amikacin Sulfate (Concurrent use may enhance the potential for drug-induced renal toxicity).
No products indexed under this heading.

Anastrozole (Concurrent use with antineoplastic agents may enhance the potential for renal toxicity, bronchospasm, and hypotension). Products include:
Arimidex Tablets 659

Asparaginase (Concurrent use with antineoplastic agents may enhance the potential for renal toxicity, bronchospasm, and hypotension). Products include:
Elspar for Injection 2092

Atracurium Besylate (Amphotericin B-induced hypokalemia may enhance the curariform effect of skeletal relaxants).
No products indexed under this heading.

Betamethasone Acetate (Concurrent use with corticosteroids may potentiate hypokalemia, which could predispose the patient to cardiac dysfunction). Products include:
Celestone Soluspan Injectable Suspension 3097

Betamethasone Sodium Phosphate (Concurrent use with corticosteroids may potentiate hypokalemia, which could predispose the patient to cardiac dysfunction). Products include:
Celestone Soluspan Injectable Suspension 3097

Bicalutamide (Concurrent use with antineoplastic agents may enhance

the potential for renal toxicity, bronchospasm, and hypotension). Products include:

Casodex Tablets 662

Bleomycin Sulfate (Concurrent use with antineoplastic agents may enhance the potential for renal toxicity, bronchospasm, and hypotension).

No products indexed under this heading.

Busulfan (Concurrent use with antineoplastic agents may enhance the potential for renal toxicity, bronchospasm, and hypotension). Products include:

Myleran Tablets 1603

Carboplatin (Concurrent use with antineoplastic agents may enhance the potential for renal toxicity, bronchospasm, and hypotension). Products include:

Paraplatin for Injection 1126

Carmustine (BCNU) (Concurrent use with antineoplastic agents may enhance the potential for renal toxicity, bronchospasm, and hypotension). Products include:

Gliadel Wafer 1723

Chlorambucil (Concurrent use with antineoplastic agents may enhance the potential for renal toxicity, bronchospasm, and hypotension). Products include:

Leukeran Tablets 1591

Cisplatin (Concurrent use with antineoplastic agents may enhance the potential for renal toxicity, bronchospasm, and hypotension).

No products indexed under this heading.

Clotrimazole (Antagonism between amphotericin B and imidazole derivatives which inhibit ergosterol synthesis, has been reported; clinical significance of this finding has not been determined). Products include:

Gyne-Lotrimin 3, 3-Day Cream ......▣741
Lotrimin AF Cream, Lotion, Solution, and Jock Itch Cream ....▣742
Lotrimin 3128
Lotrisone 3129
Mycelex Troche 573
Mycelex-7 Combination-Pack Vaginal Inserts & External Vulvar Cream ....▣614
Mycelex-7 Vaginal Cream ....▣614
Mycelex-7 Vaginal Cream with 7 Disposable Applicators ....▣614

Cortisone Acetate (Concurrent use with corticosteroids may potentiate hypokalemia, which could predispose the patient to cardiac dysfunction). Products include:

Cortone Acetate Injectable Suspension 2059
Cortone Acetate Tablets 2061

Cyclophosphamide (Concurrent use with antineoplastic agents may enhance the potential for renal toxicity, bronchospasm, and hypotension).

No products indexed under this heading.

Cyclosporine (Concurrent use may result in increased potential for renal toxicity, however, the renal toxicity in amphotericin B-deoxycholate treated patients had a significantly higher toxicity than Amphotec). Products include:

Gengraf Capsules 457
Neoral Soft Gelatin Capsules 2380
Neoral Oral Solution 2380
Sandimmune 2388

Dacarbazine (Concurrent use with antineoplastic agents may enhance the potential for renal toxicity, bronchospasm, and hypotension). Products include:

DTIC-Dome 902

Daunorubicin Citrate (Concurrent use with antineoplastic agents may enhance the potential for renal toxicity, bronchospasm, and hypotension). Products include:

DaunoXome Injection 1442

Daunorubicin Hydrochloride (Concurrent use with antineoplastic agents may enhance the potential for renal toxicity, bronchospasm, and hypotension). Products include:

Cerubidine for Injection 947

Denileukin Diftitox (Concurrent use with antineoplastic agents may enhance the potential for renal toxicity, bronchospasm, and hypotension).

No products indexed under this heading.

Deslanoside (Concurrent use may induce hypokalemia and may potentiate digitalis toxicity).

No products indexed under this heading.

Dexamethasone (Concurrent use with corticosteroids may potentiate hypokalemia, which could predispose the patient to cardiac dysfunction). Products include:

Decadron Elixir 2078
Decadron Tablets 2079
TobraDex Ophthalmic Ointment 542
TobraDex Ophthalmic Suspension .. 541

Dexamethasone Acetate (Concurrent use with corticosteroids may potentiate hypokalemia, which could predispose the patient to cardiac dysfunction).

No products indexed under this heading.

Dexamethasone Sodium Phosphate (Concurrent use with corticosteroids may potentiate hypokalemia, which could predispose the patient to cardiac dysfunction). Products include:

Decadron Phosphate Injection 2081
Decadron Phosphate Sterile Ophthalmic Ointment 2083
Decadron Phosphate Sterile Ophthalmic Solution 2084
NeoDecadron Sterile Ophthalmic Solution 2144

Digitoxin (Concurrent use may induce hypokalemia and may potentiate digitalis toxicity).

No products indexed under this heading.

Digoxin (Concurrent use may induce hypokalemia and may potentiate digitalis toxicity). Products include:

Digitek Tablets 1003
Lanoxicaps Capsules 1574
Lanoxin Injection 1581
Lanoxin Tablets 1587
Lanoxin Elixir Pediatric 1578
Lanoxin Injection Pediatric 1584

Docetaxel (Concurrent use with antineoplastic agents may enhance the potential for renal toxicity, bronchospasm, and hypotension). Products include:

Taxotere for Injection Concentrate 778

Doxorubicin Hydrochloride (Concurrent use with antineoplastic agents may enhance the potential for renal toxicity, bronchospasm, and hypotension). Products include:

Adriamycin PFS/RDF Injection 2767
Doxil Injection 566

Epirubicin Hydrochloride (Concurrent use with antineoplastic agents may enhance the potential for renal toxicity, bronchospasm, and hypotension). Products include:

Ellence Injection 2806

Estramustine Phosphate Sodium (Concurrent use with antineoplastic agents may enhance the potential for renal toxicity, bronchospasm, and hypotension). Products include:

Emcyt Capsules 2810

Etoposide (Concurrent use with antineoplastic agents may enhance the potential for renal toxicity, bronchospasm, and hypotension).

No products indexed under this heading.

Exemestane (Concurrent use with antineoplastic agents may enhance the potential for renal toxicity, bronchospasm, and hypotension). Products include:

Aromasin Tablets 2769

Floxuridine (Concurrent use with antineoplastic agents may enhance the potential for renal toxicity, bronchospasm, and hypotension). Products include:

Sterile FUDR 2974

Fluconazole (Antagonism between amphotericin B and imidazole derivatives which inhibit ergosterol synthesis, has been reported; clinical significance of this finding has not been determined). Products include:

Diflucan Tablets, Injection, and Oral Suspension 2681

Flucytosine (Concurrent use may increase the toxicity of flucytosine by possibly increasing its cellular uptake and/or impairing its renal excretion). Products include:

Ancobon Capsules 1730

Fludrocortisone Acetate (Concurrent use with corticosteroids may potentiate hypokalemia, which could predispose the patient to cardiac dysfunction). Products include:

Florinef Acetate Tablets 2250

Fluorouracil (Concurrent use with antineoplastic agents may enhance the potential for renal toxicity, bronchospasm, and hypotension). Products include:

Carac Cream 1222
Efudex 1733
Fluoroplex 552

Flutamide (Concurrent use with antineoplastic agents may enhance the potential for renal toxicity, bronchospasm, and hypotension). Products include:

Eulexin Capsules 3118

Gemcitabine Hydrochloride (Concurrent use with antineoplastic agents may enhance the potential for renal toxicity, bronchospasm, and hypotension). Products include:

Gemzar for Injection 1919

Gentamicin Sulfate (Concurrent use may enhance the potential for drug-induced renal toxicity). Products include:

Genoptic Ophthalmic Ointment ..... ⊙239
Genoptic Sterile Ophthalmic Solution .... ⊙239
Pred-G Ophthalmic Suspension ..... ⊙247
Pred-G Sterile Ophthalmic Ointment .... ⊙248

Hydrocortisone (Concurrent use with corticosteroids may potentiate hypokalemia, which could predispose the patient to cardiac dysfunction). Products include:

Anusol-HC Cream 2.5% 2237
Cipro HC Otic Suspension 540
Cortaid Intensive Therapy Cream . ▣717
Cortaid Maximum Strength Cream .... ▣717
Cortisporin Ophthalmic Suspension Sterile .... ⊙297
Cortizone•5 .... ▣699
Cortizone•10 .... ▣699
Cortizone•10 Plus Creme .... ▣700
Cortizone for Kids Creme .... ▣699
Hydrocortone Tablets 2106
Massengill Medicated Soft Cloth Towelette .... ▣753
VōSoL HC Otic Solution 3356

Hydrocortisone Acetate (Concurrent use with corticosteroids may potentiate hypokalemia, which could predispose the patient to cardiac dysfunction). Products include:

Analpram-HC 1338
Anusol HC-1 Hydrocortisone Anti-Itch Cream .... ▣689
Anusol-HC Suppositories 2238
Cortaid .... ▣717
Cortifoam Rectal Foam 3170
Cortisporin-TC Otic Suspension 2246
Hydrocortone Acetate Injectable Suspension 2103
Pramosone 1343
Proctocort Suppositories 2264
ProctoFoam-HC 3177
Terra-Cortril Ophthalmic Suspension 2716

Hydrocortisone Sodium Phosphate (Concurrent use with corticosteroids may potentiate hypokalemia, which could predispose the patient to cardiac dysfunction). Products include:

Hydrocortone Phosphate Injection, Sterile 2105

Hydrocortisone Sodium Succinate (Concurrent use with corticosteroids may potentiate hypokalemia, which could predispose the patient to cardiac dysfunction).

No products indexed under this heading.

Hydroxyurea (Concurrent use with antineoplastic agents may enhance the potential for renal toxicity, bronchospasm, and hypotension). Products include:

Mylocel Tablets 2227

Idarubicin Hydrochloride (Concurrent use with antineoplastic agents may enhance the potential for renal toxicity, bronchospasm, and hypotension). Products include:

Idamycin PFS Injection 2825

Ifosfamide (Concurrent use with antineoplastic agents may enhance the potential for renal toxicity, bronchospasm, and hypotension). Products include:

Ifex for Injection 1123

Interferon alfa-2A, Recombinant (Concurrent use with antineoplastic agents may enhance the potential for renal toxicity, bronchospasm, and hypotension). Products include:

Roferon-A Injection 2996

Interferon alfa-2B, Recombinant (Concurrent use with antineoplastic agents may enhance the potential for renal toxicity, bronchospasm, and hypotension). Products include:

Intron A for Injection 3120
Rebetron Combination Therapy 3153

Irinotecan Hydrochloride (Concurrent use with antineoplastic agents may enhance the potential for renal toxicity, bronchospasm, and hypotension).

No products indexed under this heading.

Kanamycin Sulfate (Concurrent use may enhance the potential for drug-induced renal toxicity).

No products indexed under this heading.

Ketoconazole (Antagonism between amphotericin B and imidazole derivatives which inhibit ergosterol synthesis, has been reported; clinical significance of this finding has not been determined). Products include:

Nizoral 2% Cream 3620
Nizoral A-D Shampoo 2008
Nizoral 2% Shampoo 2007
Nizoral Tablets 1791

Levamisole Hydrochloride (Concurrent use with antineoplastic agents may enhance the potential for renal toxicity, bronchospasm, and hypotension). Products include:

Ergamisol Tablets 1789

Lomustine (CCNU) (Concurrent use with antineoplastic agents may enhance the potential for renal toxicity, bronchospasm, and hypotension).

No products indexed under this heading.

Mechlorethamine Hydrochloride (Concurrent use with antineoplastic agents may enhance the potential for renal toxicity, bronchospasm, and hypotension). Products include:

Mustargen for Injection 2142

Megestrol Acetate (Concurrent use with antineoplastic agents may enhance the potential for renal toxicity, bronchospasm, and hypotension). Products include:

Megace Oral Suspension 1124

Melphalan (Concurrent use with antineoplastic agents may enhance the potential for renal toxicity, bronchospasm, and hypotension). Products include:
Alkeran Tablets 1466

Mercaptopurine (Concurrent use with antineoplastic agents may enhance the potential for renal toxicity, bronchospasm, and hypotension). Products include:
Purinethol Tablets 1615

Methotrexate Sodium (Concurrent use with antineoplastic agents may enhance the potential for renal toxicity, bronchospasm, and hypotension).
No products indexed under this heading.

Methylprednisolone Acetate (Concurrent use with corticosteroids may potentiate hypokalemia, which could predispose the patient to cardiac dysfunction). Products include:
Depo-Medrol Injectable Suspension 2795

Methylprednisolone Sodium Succinate (Concurrent use with corticosteroids may potentiate hypokalemia, which could predispose the patient to cardiac dysfunction). Products include:
Solu-Medrol Sterile Powder 2855

Miconazole (Antagonism between amphotericin B and imidazole derivatives which inhibit ergosterol synthesis, has been reported; clinical significance of this finding has not been determined).
No products indexed under this heading.

Miconazole Nitrate (Antagonism between amphotericin B and imidazole derivatives which inhibit ergosterol synthesis, has been reported; clinical significance of this finding has not been determined). Products include:
Desenex .... ⊡668
Desenex Jock Itch Spray Powder . ⊡668
Lotrimin AF Spray Powder, Spray Liquid, Spray Deodorant Powder, Shaker Powder and Jock Itch Spray Powder .... ⊡742

Mitomycin (Mitomycin-C) (Concurrent use with antineoplastic agents may enhance the potential for renal toxicity, bronchospasm, and hypotension).
No products indexed under this heading.

Mitotane (Concurrent use with antineoplastic agents may enhance the potential for renal toxicity, bronchospasm, and hypotension).
No products indexed under this heading.

Mitoxantrone Hydrochloride (Concurrent use with antineoplastic agents may enhance the potential for renal toxicity, bronchospasm, and hypotension). Products include:
Novantrone for Injection 1760

Mivacurium Chloride (Amphotericin B-induced hypokalemia may enhance the curariform effect of skeletal relaxants).
No products indexed under this heading.

Paclitaxel (Concurrent use with antineoplastic agents may enhance the potential for renal toxicity, bronchospasm, and hypotension). Products include:
Taxol Injection 1129

Pancuronium Bromide (Amphotericin B-induced hypokalemia may enhance the curariform effect of skeletal relaxants).
No products indexed under this heading.

Pentamidine Isethionate (Concurrent use may enhance the potential for drug-induced renal toxicity).
No products indexed under this heading.

Prednisolone Acetate (Concurrent use with corticosteroids may potentiate hypokalemia, which could predispose the patient to cardiac dysfunction). Products include:
Blephamide Ophthalmic Ointment ... 547
Blephamide Ophthalmic Suspension 548
Poly-Pred Liquifilm Ophthalmic Suspension .... ⊙245
Pred Forte Ophthalmic Suspension .... ⊙246
Pred Mild Sterile Ophthalmic Suspension .... ⊙249
Pred-G Ophthalmic Suspension ..... ⊙247
Pred-G Sterile Ophthalmic Ointment .... ⊙248

Prednisolone Sodium Phosphate (Concurrent use with corticosteroids may potentiate hypokalemia, which could predispose the patient to cardiac dysfunction). Products include:
Pediapred Oral Solution 1170

Prednisolone Tebutate (Concurrent use with corticosteroids may potentiate hypokalemia, which could predispose the patient to cardiac dysfunction).
No products indexed under this heading.

Prednisone (Concurrent use with corticosteroids may potentiate hypokalemia, which could predispose the patient to cardiac dysfunction). Products include:
Prednisone 3064

Procarbazine Hydrochloride (Concurrent use with antineoplastic agents may enhance the potential for renal toxicity, bronchospasm, and hypotension). Products include:
Matulane Capsules 3246

Rapacuronium Bromide (Amphotericin B-induced hypokalemia may enhance the curariform effect of skeletal relaxants).
No products indexed under this heading.

Rocuronium Bromide (Amphotericin B-induced hypokalemia may enhance the curariform effect of skeletal relaxants). Products include:
Zemuron Injection 2491

Streptomycin Sulfate (Concurrent use may enhance the potential for drug-induced renal toxicity). Products include:
Streptomycin Sulfate Injection 2714

Streptozocin (Concurrent use with antineoplastic agents may enhance the potential for renal toxicity, bronchospasm, and hypotension).
No products indexed under this heading.

Tacrolimus (Concurrent use may result in increased potential for renal toxicity, however, the renal toxicity in amphotericin B-deoxycholate treated patients had a significantly higher toxicity than Amphotec). Products include:
Prograf 1393
Protopic Ointment 1397

Tamoxifen Citrate (Concurrent use with antineoplastic agents may enhance the potential for renal toxicity, bronchospasm, and hypotension). Products include:
Nolvadex Tablets 678

Teniposide (Concurrent use with antineoplastic agents may enhance the potential for renal toxicity, bronchospasm, and hypotension).
No products indexed under this heading.

Thioguanine (Concurrent use with antineoplastic agents may enhance the potential for renal toxicity, bronchospasm, and hypotension). Products include:
Tabloid Tablets 1642

Thiotepa (Concurrent use with antineoplastic agents may enhance the potential for renal toxicity, bronchospasm, and hypotension). Products include:
Thioplex for Injection 1765

Tobramycin (Concurrent use may enhance the potential for drug-induced renal toxicity). Products include:
TOBI Solution for Inhalation 1206
TobraDex Ophthalmic Ointment 542
TobraDex Ophthalmic Suspension .. 541
Tobrex Ophthalmic Ointment .... ⊙220
Tobrex Ophthalmic Solution .... ⊙221

Tobramycin Sulfate (Concurrent use may enhance the potential for drug-induced renal toxicity). Products include:
Nebcin Vials, Hyporets & ADD-Vantage 1955

Topotecan Hydrochloride (Concurrent use with antineoplastic agents may enhance the potential for renal toxicity, bronchospasm, and hypotension). Products include:
Hycamtin for Injection 1546

Toremifene Citrate (Concurrent use with antineoplastic agents may enhance the potential for renal toxicity, bronchospasm, and hypotension). Products include:
Fareston Tablets 3237

Triamcinolone (Concurrent use with corticosteroids may potentiate hypokalemia, which could predispose the patient to cardiac dysfunction).
No products indexed under this heading.

Triamcinolone Acetonide (Concurrent use with corticosteroids may potentiate hypokalemia, which could predispose the patient to cardiac dysfunction). Products include:
Azmacort Inhalation Aerosol 728
Nasacort Nasal Inhaler 750
Nasacort AQ Nasal Spray 752
Tri-Nasal Spray 2274

Triamcinolone Diacetate (Concurrent use with corticosteroids may potentiate hypokalemia, which could predispose the patient to cardiac dysfunction).
No products indexed under this heading.

Triamcinolone Hexacetonide (Concurrent use with corticosteroids may potentiate hypokalemia, which could predispose the patient to cardiac dysfunction).
No products indexed under this heading.

Tubocurarine Chloride (Amphotericin B-induced hypokalemia may enhance the curariform effect of skeletal relaxants).
No products indexed under this heading.

Valrubicin (Concurrent use with antineoplastic agents may enhance the potential for renal toxicity, bronchospasm, and hypotension). Products include:
Valstar Sterile Solution for Intravesical Instillation 1175

Vecuronium Bromide (Amphotericin B-induced hypokalemia may enhance the curariform effect of skeletal relaxants). Products include:
Norcuron for Injection 2478

Vincristine Sulfate (Concurrent use with antineoplastic agents may enhance the potential for renal toxicity, bronchospasm, and hypotension).
No products indexed under this heading.

Vinorelbine Tartrate (Concurrent use with antineoplastic agents may enhance the potential for renal toxicity, bronchospasm, and hypotension). Products include:
Navelbine Injection 1604

AMVISC PLUS
(Sodium Hyaluronate) .... ⊙329
None cited in PDR database.

ANADROL-50 TABLETS
(Oxymetholone) 3321
May interact with oral anticoagulants, oral hypoglycemic agents, and insulin. Compounds in these categories include:

Acarbose (Anabolic steroids tend to decrease glucose tolerance; oral hypoglycemic dosage may need to be adjusted in diabetic patients). Products include:
Precose Tablets 906

Chlorpropamide (Anabolic steroids tend to decrease glucose tolerance; oral hypoglycemic dosage may need to be adjusted in diabetic patients). Products include:
Diabinese Tablets 2680

Dicumarol (Anabolic steroids may cause suppression of clotting factors II, V, VII, and X, an increase in prothrombin time, and increased sensitivity to anticoagulants; dosage of anticoagulants may need to be adjusted).
No products indexed under this heading.

Glimepiride (Anabolic steroids tend to decrease glucose tolerance; oral hypoglycemic dosage may need to be adjusted in diabetic patients). Products include:
Amaryl Tablets 717

Glipizide (Anabolic steroids tend to decrease glucose tolerance; oral hypoglycemic dosage may need to be adjusted in diabetic patients). Products include:
Glucotrol Tablets 2692
Glucotrol XL Extended Release Tablets 2693

Glyburide (Anabolic steroids tend to decrease glucose tolerance; oral hypoglycemic dosage may need to be adjusted in diabetic patients). Products include:
DiaBeta Tablets 741
Glucovance Tablets 1086

Insulin, Human, Zinc Suspension (Anabolic steroids tend to decrease glucose tolerance; insulin dosage may need to be adjusted in diabetic patients). Products include:
Humulin L, 100 Units 1937
Humulin U, 100 Units 1943
Novolin L Human Insulin 10 ml Vials 2422

Insulin, Human NPH (Anabolic steroids tend to decrease glucose tolerance; insulin dosage may need to be adjusted in diabetic patients). Products include:
Humulin N, 100 Units 1939
Humulin N NPH Pen 1940
Novolin N Human Insulin 10 ml Vials 2422
Novolin N PenFill 2423
Novolin N Prefilled Syringe Disposable Insulin Delivery System 2425

Insulin, Human Regular (Anabolic steroids tend to decrease glucose tolerance; insulin dosage may need to be adjusted in diabetic patients). Products include:
Humulin R Regular (U-500) 1943
Humulin R, 100 Units 1941
Novolin R Human Insulin 10 ml Vials 2423
Novolin R PenFill 2423
Novolin R Prefilled Syringe Disposable Insulin Delivery System 2425
Velosulin BR Human Insulin 10 ml Vials 2435

Insulin, Human Regular and Human NPH Mixture (Anabolic steroids tend to decrease glucose tolerance; insulin dosage may need to be adjusted in diabetic patients). Products include:
Humulin 50/50, 100 Units 1934
Humulin 70/30, 100 Units 1935
Humulin 70/30 Pen 1936
Novolin 70/30 Human Insulin 10 ml Vials 2421
Novolin 70/30 PenFill 2423

Novolin 70/30 Prefilled Disposable Insulin Delivery System 2425

Insulin, NPH (Anabolic steroids tend to decrease glucose tolerance; insulin dosage may need to be adjusted in diabetic patients). Products include:
Iletin II, NPH (Pork), 100 Units 1946

Insulin, Regular (Anabolic steroids tend to decrease glucose tolerance; insulin dosage may need to be adjusted in diabetic patients). Products include:
Iletin II, Regular (Pork), 100 Units ... 1947

Insulin, Zinc Crystals (Anabolic steroids tend to decrease glucose tolerance; insulin dosage may need to be adjusted in diabetic patients).
No products indexed under this heading.

Insulin, Zinc Suspension (Anabolic steroids tend to decrease glucose tolerance; insulin dosage may need to be adjusted in diabetic patients). Products include:
Iletin II, Lente (Pork), 100 Units 1945

Insulin Aspart, Human Regular (Anabolic steroids tend to decrease glucose tolerance; insulin dosage may need to be adjusted in diabetic patients).
No products indexed under this heading.

Insulin glargine (Anabolic steroids tend to decrease glucose tolerance; insulin dosage may need to be adjusted in diabetic patients). Products include:
Lantus Injection 742

Insulin Lispro, Human (Anabolic steroids tend to decrease glucose tolerance; insulin dosage may need to be adjusted in diabetic patients). Products include:
Humalog 1926
Humalog Mix 75/25 Pen 1928

Insulin Lispro Protamine, Human (Anabolic steroids tend to decrease glucose tolerance; insulin dosage may need to be adjusted in diabetic patients). Products include:
Humalog Mix 75/25 Pen 1928

Metformin Hydrochloride (Anabolic steroids tend to decrease glucose tolerance; oral hypoglycemic dosage may need to be adjusted in diabetic patients). Products include:
Glucophage Tablets 1080
Glucophage XR Tablets 1080
Glucovance Tablets 1086

Miglitol (Anabolic steroids tend to decrease glucose tolerance; oral hypoglycemic dosage may need to be adjusted in diabetic patients). Products include:
Glyset Tablets 2821

Pioglitazone Hydrochloride (Anabolic steroids tend to decrease glucose tolerance; oral hypoglycemic dosage may need to be adjusted in diabetic patients). Products include:
Actos Tablets 3275

Repaglinide (Anabolic steroids tend to decrease glucose tolerance; oral hypoglycemic dosage may need to be adjusted in diabetic patients). Products include:
Prandin Tablets (0.5, 1, and 2 mg) 2432

Rosiglitazone Maleate (Anabolic steroids tend to decrease glucose tolerance; oral hypoglycemic dosage may need to be adjusted in diabetic patients). Products include:
Avandia Tablets 1490

Tolazamide (Anabolic steroids tend to decrease glucose tolerance; oral hypoglycemic dosage may need to be adjusted in diabetic patients).
No products indexed under this heading.

Tolbutamide (Anabolic steroids tend to decrease glucose tolerance; oral hypoglycemic dosage may need to be adjusted in diabetic patients).
No products indexed under this heading.

Troglitazone (Anabolic steroids tend to decrease glucose tolerance; oral hypoglycemic dosage may need to be adjusted in diabetic patients).
No products indexed under this heading.

Warfarin Sodium (Anabolic steroids may cause suppression of clotting factors II, V, VII, and X, an increase in prothrombin time, and increased sensitivity to anticoagulants; dosage of anticoagulants may need to be adjusted). Products include:
Coumadin for Injection 1243
Coumadin Tablets 1243
Warfarin Sodium Tablets, USP 3302

ANALPRAM HC LOTION 2.5%

(Hydrocortisone Acetate, Pramoxine Hydrochloride) 1338
None cited in PDR database.

ANALPRAM-HC RECTAL CREAM 1% AND 2.5%

(Hydrocortisone Acetate, Pramoxine Hydrochloride) 1338
None cited in PDR database.

ANAPROX TABLETS

(Naproxen Sodium) 2967
See EC-Naprosyn Delayed-Release Tablets

ANAPROX DS TABLETS

(Naproxen Sodium) 2967
See EC-Naprosyn Delayed-Release Tablets

BABY ANBESOL GEL

(Benzocaine) 774
None cited in PDR database.

JUNIOR ANBESOL GEL

(Benzocaine) 774
None cited in PDR database.

MAXIMUM STRENGTH ANBESOL GEL

(Benzocaine) 774
None cited in PDR database.

MAXIMUM STRENGTH ANBESOL LIQUID

(Benzocaine) 774
None cited in PDR database.

ANCEF FOR INJECTION

(Cefazolin Sodium) 1474
May interact with:

Probenecid (Increased and prolonged cephalosporin blood levels).
No products indexed under this heading.

ANCEF INJECTION

(Cefazolin Sodium) 1474
See Ancef for Injection

ANCOBON CAPSULES

(Flucytosine) 1730
May interact with:

Amphotericin B (Antifungal synergism between flucytosine and amphotericin B has been reported). Products include:
Abelcet Injection 1273
AmBisome for Injection 1383
Amphotec 1774

Cytarabine Liposome (Cytosine arabinoside has been reported to inactivate the antifungal activity of flucytosine by competitive inhibition). Products include:
DepoCyt Injection 1197

Cytosine Arabinoside (Inactivation of Ancobon's antifungal activity).
No products indexed under this heading.

Drugs that Impair Glomerular Filtration (Biological half-life of Ancobon may be prolonged).
No products indexed under this heading.

ANDRODERM TRANSDERMAL SYSTEM CIII

(Testosterone) 3377
May interact with oral anticoagulants, insulin, and certain other agents. Compounds in these categories include:

Dicumarol (Potential for decreased requirements of oral anticoagulants).
No products indexed under this heading.

Insulin, Human, Zinc Suspension (In diabetic patients androgens may decrease blood glucose and, therefore, insulin requirements). Products include:
Humulin L, 100 Units 1937
Humulin U, 100 Units 1943
Novolin L Human Insulin 10 ml Vials 2422

Insulin, Human NPH (In diabetic patients androgens may decrease blood glucose and, therefore, insulin requirements). Products include:
Humulin N, 100 Units 1939
Humulin N NPH Pen 1940
Novolin N Human Insulin 10 ml Vials 2422
Novolin N PenFill 2423
Novolin N Prefilled Syringe Disposable Insulin Delivery System 2425

Insulin, Human Regular (In diabetic patients androgens may decrease blood glucose and, therefore, insulin requirements). Products include:
Humulin R Regular (U-500) 1943
Humulin R, 100 Units 1941
Novolin R Human Insulin 10 ml Vials 2423
Novolin R PenFill 2423
Novolin R Prefilled Syringe Disposable Insulin Delivery System 2425
Velosulin BR Human Insulin 10 ml Vials 2435

Insulin, Human Regular and Human NPH Mixture (In diabetic patients androgens may decrease blood glucose and, therefore, insulin requirements). Products include:
Humulin 50/50, 100 Units 1934
Humulin 70/30, 100 Units 1935
Humulin 70/30 Pen 1936
Novolin 70/30 Human Insulin 10 ml Vials 2421
Novolin 70/30 PenFill 2423
Novolin 70/30 Prefilled Disposable Insulin Delivery System 2425

Insulin, NPH (In diabetic patients androgens may decrease blood glucose and, therefore, insulin requirements). Products include:
Iletin II, NPH (Pork), 100 Units 1946

Insulin, Regular (In diabetic patients androgens may decrease blood glucose and, therefore, insulin requirements). Products include:
Iletin II, Regular (Pork), 100 Units ... 1947

Insulin, Zinc Crystals (In diabetic patients androgens may decrease blood glucose and, therefore, insulin requirements).
No products indexed under this heading.

Insulin, Zinc Suspension (In diabetic patients androgens may decrease blood glucose and, therefore, insulin requirements). Products include:
Iletin II, Lente (Pork), 100 Units 1945

Insulin Aspart, Human Regular (In diabetic patients androgens may decrease blood glucose and, therefore, insulin requirements).
No products indexed under this heading.

Insulin glargine (In diabetic patients androgens may decrease blood glucose and, therefore, insulin requirements). Products include:
Lantus Injection 742

Insulin Lispro, Human (In diabetic patients androgens may decrease blood glucose and, therefore, insulin requirements). Products include:
Humalog 1926
Humalog Mix 75/25 Pen 1928

Insulin Lispro Protamine, Human (In diabetic patients androgens may decrease blood glucose and, therefore, insulin requirements). Products include:
Humalog Mix 75/25 Pen 1928

Oxyphenbutazone (Concurrent administration may result in elevated serum levels of oxyphenbutazone).
No products indexed under this heading.

Warfarin Sodium (Potential for decreased requirements of oral anticoagulants). Products include:
Coumadin for Injection 1243
Coumadin Tablets 1243
Warfarin Sodium Tablets, USP 3302

ANDROGEL

(Testosterone) 3322
May interact with corticosteroids, insulin, and certain other agents. Compounds in these categories include:

ACTH (Co-administration of testosterone with ACTH may enhance edema formation).
No products indexed under this heading.

Betamethasone Acetate (Co-administration of testosterone with corticosteroids may enhance edema formation). Products include:
Celestone Soluspan Injectable Suspension 3097

Betamethasone Sodium Phosphate (Co-administration of testosterone with corticosteroids may enhance edema formation). Products include:
Celestone Soluspan Injectable Suspension 3097

Cortisone Acetate (Co-administration of testosterone with corticosteroids may enhance edema formation). Products include:
Cortone Acetate Injectable Suspension 2059
Cortone Acetate Tablets 2061

Dexamethasone (Co-administration of testosterone with corticosteroids may enhance edema formation). Products include:
Decadron Elixir 2078
Decadron Tablets 2079
TobraDex Ophthalmic Ointment 542
TobraDex Ophthalmic Suspension .. 541

Dexamethasone Acetate (Co-administration of testosterone with corticosteroids may enhance edema formation).
No products indexed under this heading.

Dexamethasone Sodium Phosphate (Co-administration of testosterone with corticosteroids may enhance edema formation). Products include:
Decadron Phosphate Injection 2081
Decadron Phosphate Sterile Ophthalmic Ointment 2083
Decadron Phosphate Sterile Ophthalmic Solution 2084
NeoDecadron Sterile Ophthalmic Solution 2144

Fludrocortisone Acetate (Co-administration of testosterone with corticosteroids may enhance edema formation). Products include:
Florinef Acetate Tablets 2250

Hydrocortisone (Co-administration of testosterone with corticosteroids may enhance edema formation). Products include:
Anusol-HC Cream 2.5% 2237
Cipro HC Otic Suspension 540
Cortaid Intensive Therapy Cream .. 717
Cortaid Maximum Strength Cream 717

IMPORTANT NOTE: Always consult each drug listing in the patient's regimen for possible interactions.

Cortisporin Ophthalmic Suspension Sterile ⊙297
Cortizone•5 ▣699
Cortizone•10 ▣699
Cortizone•10 Plus Creme ▣700
Cortizone for Kids Creme ▣699
Hydrocortone Tablets 2106
Massengill Medicated Soft Cloth Towelette ▣753
VōSoL HC Otic Solution 3356

Hydrocortisone Acetate (Co-administration of testosterone with corticosteroids may enhance edema formation). Products include:
Analpram-HC 1338
Anusol HC-1 Hydrocortisone Anti-Itch Cream ▣689
Anusol-HC Suppositories 2238
Cortaid ▣717
Cortifoam Rectal Foam 3170
Cortisporin-TC Otic Suspension 2246
Hydrocortone Acetate Injectable Suspension 2103
Pramosone 1343
Proctocort Suppositories 2264
ProctoFoam-HC 3177
Terra-Cortril Ophthalmic Suspension 2716

Hydrocortisone Sodium Phosphate (Co-administration of testosterone with corticosteroids may enhance edema formation). Products include:
Hydrocortone Phosphate Injection, Sterile 2105

Hydrocortisone Sodium Succinate (Co-administration of testosterone with corticosteroids may enhance edema formation).
No products indexed under this heading.

Insulin, Human, Zinc Suspension (In diabetic patients, the metabolic effects of androgens may decrease blood glucose and, therefore, insulin requirements). Products include:
Humulin L, 100 Units 1937
Humulin U, 100 Units 1943
Novolin L Human Insulin 10 ml Vials 2422

Insulin, Human NPH (In diabetic patients, the metabolic effects of androgens may decrease blood glucose and, therefore, insulin requirements). Products include:
Humulin N, 100 Units 1939
Humulin N NPH Pen 1940
Novolin N Human Insulin 10 ml Vials 2422
Novolin N PenFill 2423
Novolin N Prefilled Syringe Disposable Insulin Delivery System 2425

Insulin, Human Regular (In diabetic patients, the metabolic effects of androgens may decrease blood glucose and, therefore, insulin requirements). Products include:
Humulin R Regular (U-500) 1943
Humulin R, 100 Units 1941
Novolin R Human Insulin 10 ml Vials 2423
Novolin R PenFill 2423
Novolin R Prefilled Syringe Disposable Insulin Delivery System 2425
Velosulin BR Human Insulin 10 ml Vials 2435

Insulin, Human Regular and Human NPH Mixture (In diabetic patients, the metabolic effects of androgens may decrease blood glucose and, therefore, insulin requirements). Products include:
Humulin 50/50, 100 Units 1934
Humulin 70/30, 100 Units 1935
Humulin 70/30 Pen 1936
Novolin 70/30 Human Insulin 10 ml Vials 2421
Novolin 70/30 PenFill 2423
Novolin 70/30 Prefilled Disposable Insulin Delivery System 2425

Insulin, NPH (In diabetic patients, the metabolic effects of androgens may decrease blood glucose and, therefore, insulin requirements). Products include:
Iletin II, NPH (Pork), 100 Units 1946

Insulin, Regular (In diabetic patients, the metabolic effects of androgens may decrease blood glucose and, therefore, insulin requirements). Products include:
Iletin II, Regular (Pork), 100 Units 1947

Insulin, Zinc Crystals (In diabetic patients, the metabolic effects of androgens may decrease blood glucose and, therefore, insulin requirements).
No products indexed under this heading.

Insulin, Zinc Suspension (In diabetic patients, the metabolic effects of androgens may decrease blood glucose and, therefore, insulin requirements). Products include:
Iletin II, Lente (Pork), 100 Units 1945

Insulin Aspart, Human Regular (In diabetic patients, the metabolic effects of androgens may decrease blood glucose and, therefore, insulin requirements).
No products indexed under this heading.

Insulin glargine (In diabetic patients, the metabolic effects of androgens may decrease blood glucose and, therefore, insulin requirements). Products include:
Lantus Injection 742

Insulin Lispro, Human (In diabetic patients, the metabolic effects of androgens may decrease blood glucose and, therefore, insulin requirements). Products include:
Humalog 1926
Humalog Mix 75/25 Pen 1928

Insulin Lispro Protamine, Human (In diabetic patients, the metabolic effects of androgens may decrease blood glucose and, therefore, insulin requirements). Products include:
Humalog Mix 75/25 Pen 1928

Methylprednisolone Acetate (Co-administration of testosterone with corticosteroids may enhance edema formation). Products include:
Depo-Medrol Injectable Suspension 2795

Methylprednisolone Sodium Succinate (Co-administration of testosterone with corticosteroids may enhance edema formation). Products include:
Solu-Medrol Sterile Powder 2855

Oxyphenbutazone (Co-administration of androgens and oxyphenbutazone may result in elevated serum levels of oxyphenbutazone).
No products indexed under this heading.

Prednisolone Acetate (Co-administration of testosterone with corticosteroids may enhance edema formation). Products include:
Blephamide Ophthalmic Ointment 547
Blephamide Ophthalmic Suspension 548
Poly-Pred Liquifilm Ophthalmic Suspension ⊙245
Pred Forte Ophthalmic Suspension ⊙246
Pred Mild Sterile Ophthalmic Suspension ⊙249
Pred-G Ophthalmic Suspension ⊙247
Pred-G Sterile Ophthalmic Ointment ⊙248

Prednisolone Sodium Phosphate (Co-administration of testosterone with corticosteroids may enhance edema formation). Products include:
Pediapred Oral Solution 1170

Prednisolone Tebutate (Co-administration of testosterone with corticosteroids may enhance edema formation).
No products indexed under this heading.

Prednisone (Co-administration of testosterone with corticosteroids may enhance edema formation). Products include:
Prednisone 3064

Propranolol Hydrochloride (Co-administration of injectable testosterone cypionate has resulted in an increased clearance of propranolol). Products include:
Inderal 3513
Inderal LA Long-Acting Capsules 3516
Inderide Tablets 3517
Inderide LA Long-Acting Capsules 3519

Triamcinolone (Co-administration of testosterone with corticosteroids may enhance edema formation).
No products indexed under this heading.

Triamcinolone Acetonide (Co-administration of testosterone with corticosteroids may enhance edema formation). Products include:
Azmacort Inhalation Aerosol 728
Nasacort Nasal Inhaler 750
Nasacort AQ Nasal Spray 752
Tri-Nasal Spray 2274

Triamcinolone Diacetate (Co-administration of testosterone with corticosteroids may enhance edema formation).
No products indexed under this heading.

Triamcinolone Hexacetonide (Co-administration of testosterone with corticosteroids may enhance edema formation).
No products indexed under this heading.

ANDROID CAPSULES, 10 MG

(Methyltestosterone) 1731
May interact with oral anticoagulants, insulin, and certain other agents. Compounds in these categories include:

Dicumarol (Decreased anticoagulant requirements).
No products indexed under this heading.

Insulin, Human, Zinc Suspension (In diabetic patients the metabolic effects of androgens may decrease blood glucose and insulin requirements). Products include:
Humulin L, 100 Units 1937
Humulin U, 100 Units 1943
Novolin L Human Insulin 10 ml Vials 2422

Insulin, Human NPH (In diabetic patients the metabolic effects of androgens may decrease blood glucose and insulin requirements). Products include:
Humulin N, 100 Units 1939
Humulin N NPH Pen 1940
Novolin N Human Insulin 10 ml Vials 2422
Novolin N PenFill 2423
Novolin N Prefilled Syringe Disposable Insulin Delivery System 2425

Insulin, Human Regular (In diabetic patients the metabolic effects of androgens may decrease blood glucose and insulin requirements). Products include:
Humulin R Regular (U-500) 1943
Humulin R, 100 Units 1941
Novolin R Human Insulin 10 ml Vials 2423
Novolin R PenFill 2423
Novolin R Prefilled Syringe Disposable Insulin Delivery System 2425
Velosulin BR Human Insulin 10 ml Vials 2435

Insulin, Human Regular and Human NPH Mixture (In diabetic patients the metabolic effects of androgens may decrease blood glucose and insulin requirements). Products include:
Humulin 50/50, 100 Units 1934
Humulin 70/30, 100 Units 1935
Humulin 70/30 Pen 1936
Novolin 70/30 Human Insulin 10 ml Vials 2421
Novolin 70/30 PenFill 2423
Novolin 70/30 Prefilled Disposable Insulin Delivery System 2425

Insulin, NPH (In diabetic patients the metabolic effects of androgens may decrease blood glucose and insulin requirements). Products include:
Iletin II, NPH (Pork), 100 Units 1946

Insulin, Regular (In diabetic patients the metabolic effects of androgens may decrease blood glucose and insulin requirements). Products include:
Iletin II, Regular (Pork), 100 Units 1947

Insulin, Zinc Crystals (In diabetic patients the metabolic effects of androgens may decrease blood glucose and insulin requirements).
No products indexed under this heading.

Insulin, Zinc Suspension (In diabetic patients the metabolic effects of androgens may decrease blood glucose and insulin requirements). Products include:
Iletin II, Lente (Pork), 100 Units 1945

Insulin Aspart, Human Regular (In diabetic patients the metabolic effects of androgens may decrease blood glucose and insulin requirements).
No products indexed under this heading.

Insulin glargine (In diabetic patients the metabolic effects of androgens may decrease blood glucose and insulin requirements). Products include:
Lantus Injection 742

Insulin Lispro, Human (In diabetic patients the metabolic effects of androgens may decrease blood glucose and insulin requirements). Products include:
Humalog 1926
Humalog Mix 75/25 Pen 1928

Insulin Lispro Protamine, Human (In diabetic patients the metabolic effects of androgens may decrease blood glucose and insulin requirements). Products include:
Humalog Mix 75/25 Pen 1928

Oxyphenbutazone (Concurrent use may result in elevated serum levels of oxyphenbutazone).
No products indexed under this heading.

Warfarin Sodium (Decreased anticoagulant requirements). Products include:
Coumadin for Injection 1243
Coumadin Tablets 1243
Warfarin Sodium Tablets, USP 3302

ANECTINE INJECTION

(Succinylcholine Chloride) 1476
May interact with beta blockers, glucocorticoids, monoamine oxidase inhibitors, neuromuscular blocking agents, oral contraceptives, and certain other agents. Compounds in these categories include:

Acebutolol Hydrochloride (Enhances neuromuscular blocking action). Products include:
Sectral Capsules 3589

Antibiotics, non-penicillin, unspecified (Enhances neuromuscular blocking action).

Anticancer Drugs, unspecified (Prolong respiratory depression).

Aprotinin (Enhances neuromuscular blocking action). Products include:
Trasylol Injection 909

Atenolol (Enhances neuromuscular blocking action). Products include:
Tenoretic Tablets 690
Tenormin I.V. Injection 692

Atracurium Besylate (Possible synergistic or antagonistic effect if co-administered during the same

procedure).
No products indexed under this heading.

Betamethasone Acetate (Chronic use of glucocorticoids enhances neuromuscular blocking effect by reducing plasma cholinesterase activity). Products include:
Celestone Soluspan Injectable Suspension 3097

Betamethasone Sodium Phosphate (Chronic use of glucocorticoids enhances neuromuscular blocking effect by reducing plasma cholinesterase activity). Products include:
Celestone Soluspan Injectable Suspension 3097

Betaxolol Hydrochloride (Enhances neuromuscular blocking action). Products include:
Betoptic S Ophthalmic Suspension 537

Bisoprolol Fumarate (Enhances neuromuscular blocking action). Products include:
Zebeta Tablets 1885
Ziac Tablets 1887

Carteolol Hydrochloride (Enhances neuromuscular blocking action). Products include:
Carteolol Hydrochloride Ophthalmic Solution USP, 1% .... ⊙258
Ocupress Ophthalmic Solution, 1% Sterile .... ⊙303

Chloroquine Hydrochloride (Enhances neuromuscular blocking action).
No products indexed under this heading.

Chloroquine Phosphate (Enhances neuromuscular blocking action). Products include:
Aralen Tablets 3075

Cisatracurium Besylate (Possible synergistic or antagonistic effect if co-administered during the same procedure).
No products indexed under this heading.

Cortisone Acetate (Chronic use of glucocorticoids enhances neuromuscular blocking effect by reducing plasma cholinesterase activity). Products include:
Cortone Acetate Injectable Suspension 2059
Cortone Acetate Tablets 2061

Desflurane (Enhances neuromuscular blocking action). Products include:
Suprane Liquid for Inhalation 874

Desogestrel (Chronic use of oral contraceptives enhances neuromuscular blocking effect by reducing plasma cholinesterase activity). Products include:
Cyclessa Tablets 2450
Desogen Tablets 2458
Mircette Tablets 2470
Ortho-Cept 21 Tablets 2546
Ortho-Cept 28 Tablets 2546

Dexamethasone (Chronic use of glucocorticoids enhances neuromuscular blocking effect by reducing plasma cholinesterase activity). Products include:
Decadron Elixir 2078
Decadron Tablets 2079
TobraDex Ophthalmic Ointment 542
TobraDex Ophthalmic Suspension 541

Dexamethasone Acetate (Chronic use of glucocorticoids enhances neuromuscular blocking effect by reducing plasma cholinesterase activity).
No products indexed under this heading.

Dexamethasone Sodium Phosphate (Chronic use of glucocorticoids enhances neuromuscular blocking effect by reducing plasma cholinesterase activity). Products include:
Decadron Phosphate Injection 2081
Decadron Phosphate Sterile Ophthalmic Ointment 2083
Decadron Phosphate Sterile Ophthalmic Solution 2084
NeoDecadron Sterile Ophthalmic Solution 2144

Diethyl Ether (Enhances neuromuscular blocking action).
No products indexed under this heading.

Doxacurium Chloride (Possible synergistic or antagonistic effect if co-administered during the same procedure).
No products indexed under this heading.

Echothiophate Iodide (Prolongs respiratory depression).
No products indexed under this heading.

Esmolol Hydrochloride (Enhances neuromuscular blocking action). Products include:
Brevibloc Injection 858

Ethinyl Estradiol (Chronic use of oral contraceptives enhances neuromuscular blocking effect by reducing plasma cholinesterase activity). Products include:
Alesse-21 Tablets 3468
Alesse-28 Tablets 3473
Brevicon 28-Day Tablets 3380
Cyclessa Tablets 2450
Desogen Tablets 2458
Estinyl Tablets 3112
Estrostep 2627
femhrt Tablets 2635
Levlen 962
Levlite 21 Tablets 962
Levlite 28 Tablets 962
Levora Tablets 3389
Loestrin 21 Tablets 2642
Loestrin Fe Tablets 2642
Lo/Ovral Tablets 3532
Lo/Ovral-28 Tablets 3538
Low-Ogestrel-28 Tablets 3392
Microgestin Fe 1.5/30 Tablets 3407
Microgestin Fe 1/20 Tablets 3400
Mircette Tablets 2470
Modicon 2563
Necon 3415
Nordette-28 Tablets 2257
Norinyl 1 +35 28-Day Tablets 3380
Ogestrel 0.5/50-28 Tablets 3428
Ortho-Cept 21 Tablets 2546
Ortho-Cept 28 Tablets 2546
Ortho-Cyclen/Ortho Tri-Cyclen 2573
Ortho-Novum 2563
Ovcon 3364
Ovral Tablets 3551
Ovral-28 Tablets 3552
Tri-Levlen 962
Tri-Norinyl-28 Tablets 3433
Triphasil-21 Tablets 3600
Triphasil-28 Tablets 3605
Trivora Tablets 3439
Yasmin 28 Tablets 980
Zovia 3449

Ethynodiol Diacetate (Chronic use of oral contraceptives enhances neuromuscular blocking effect by reducing plasma cholinesterase activity). Products include:
Zovia 3449

Fludrocortisone Acetate (Chronic use of glucocorticoids enhances neuromuscular blocking effect by reducing plasma cholinesterase activity). Products include:
Florinef Acetate Tablets 2250

Hydrocortisone (Chronic use of glucocorticoids enhances neuromuscular blocking effect by reducing plasma cholinesterase activity). Products include:
Anusol-HC Cream 2.5% 2237
Cipro HC Otic Suspension 540
Cortaid Intensive Therapy Cream .... ▣717
Cortaid Maximum Strength Cream .... ▣717
Cortisporin Ophthalmic Suspension Sterile .... ⊙297
Cortizone•5 .... ▣699
Cortizone•10 .... ▣699
Cortizone•10 Plus Creme .... ▣700
Cortizone for Kids Creme .... ▣699
Hydrocortone Tablets 2106
Massengill Medicated Soft Cloth Towelette .... ▣753
VōSoL HC Otic Solution 3356

Hydrocortisone Acetate (Chronic use of glucocorticoids enhances neuromuscular blocking effect by reducing plasma cholinesterase activity). Products include:
Analpram-HC 1338
Anusol HC-1 Hydrocortisone Anti-Itch Cream .... ▣689
Anusol-HC Suppositories 2238
Cortaid .... ▣717
Cortifoam Rectal Foam 3170
Cortisporin-TC Otic Suspension 2246
Hydrocortone Acetate Injectable Suspension 2103
Pramosone 1343
Proctocort Suppositories 2264
ProctoFoam-HC 3177
Terra-Cortril Ophthalmic Suspension 2716

Hydrocortisone Sodium Phosphate (Chronic use of glucocorticoids enhances neuromuscular blocking effect by reducing plasma cholinesterase activity). Products include:
Hydrocortone Phosphate Injection, Sterile 2105

Hydrocortisone Sodium Succinate (Chronic use of glucocorticoids enhances neuromuscular blocking effect by reducing plasma cholinesterase activity).
No products indexed under this heading.

Isocarboxazid (Chronic use of certain unspecified MAO inhibitors enhances neuromuscular blocking effect by reducing plasma cholinesterase activity).
No products indexed under this heading.

Isoflurane (Enhances neuromuscular blocking action).
No products indexed under this heading.

Labetalol Hydrochloride (Enhances neuromuscular blocking action). Products include:
Normodyne Injection 3135
Normodyne Tablets 3137

Levobunolol Hydrochloride (Enhances neuromuscular blocking action). Products include:
Betagan .... ⊙228

Levonorgestrel (Chronic use of oral contraceptives enhances neuromuscular blocking effect by reducing plasma cholinesterase activity). Products include:
Alesse-21 Tablets 3468
Alesse-28 Tablets 3473
Levlen 962
Levlite 21 Tablets 962
Levlite 28 Tablets 962
Levora Tablets 3389
Mirena Intrauterine System 974
Nordette-28 Tablets 2257
Norplant System 3543
Tri-Levlen 962
Triphasil-21 Tablets 3600
Triphasil-28 Tablets 3605
Trivora Tablets 3439

Lidocaine Hydrochloride (Enhances neuromuscular blocking action). Products include:
Bactine First Aid Liquid .... ▣611
Xylocaine Injections 653

Lithium Carbonate (Enhances neuromuscular blocking action). Products include:
Eskalith 1527
Lithium Carbonate 3061
Lithobid Slow-Release Tablets 3255

Magnesium Sulfate Injection (Enhances neuromuscular blocking action).
No products indexed under this heading.

Mestranol (Chronic use of oral contraceptives enhances neuromuscular blocking effect by reducing plasma cholinesterase activity). Products include:
Necon 1/50 Tablets 3415
Norinyl 1 + 50 28-Day Tablets 3380
Ortho-Novum 1/50□28 Tablets 2556

Methylprednisolone Acetate (Chronic use of glucocorticoids enhances neuromuscular blocking effect by reducing plasma cholinesterase activity). Products include:
Depo-Medrol Injectable Suspension 2795

Methylprednisolone Sodium Succinate (Chronic use of glucocorticoids enhances neuromuscular blocking effect by reducing plasma cholinesterase activity). Products include:
Solu-Medrol Sterile Powder 2855

Metipranolol Hydrochloride (Enhances neuromuscular blocking action).
No products indexed under this heading.

Metoclopramide Hydrochloride (Enhances neuromuscular blocking action). Products include:
Reglan 2935

Metocurine Iodide (Possible synergistic or antagonistic effect if co-administered during the same procedure).
No products indexed under this heading.

Metoprolol Succinate (Enhances neuromuscular blocking action). Products include:
Toprol-XL Tablets 651

Metoprolol Tartrate (Enhances neuromuscular blocking action).
No products indexed under this heading.

Mivacurium Chloride (Possible synergistic or antagonistic effect if co-administered during the same procedure).
No products indexed under this heading.

Moclobemide (Chronic use of certain unspecified MAO inhibitors enhances neuromuscular blocking effect by reducing plasma cholinesterase activity).
No products indexed under this heading.

Nadolol (Enhances neuromuscular blocking action). Products include:
Corgard Tablets 2245
Corzide 40/5 Tablets 2247
Corzide 80/5 Tablets 2247
Nadolol Tablets 2288

Norethindrone (Chronic use of oral contraceptives enhances neuromuscular blocking effect by reducing plasma cholinesterase activity). Products include:
Brevicon 28-Day Tablets 3380
Micronor Tablets 2543
Modicon 2563
Necon 3415
Norinyl 1 +35 28-Day Tablets 3380
Norinyl 1 + 50 28-Day Tablets 3380
Nor-QD Tablets 3423
Ortho-Novum 2563
Ortho-Novum 1/50□28 Tablets 2556
Ovcon 3364
Tri-Norinyl-28 Tablets 3433

Norethynodrel (Chronic use of oral contraceptives enhances neuromuscular blocking effect by reducing plasma cholinesterase activity).
No products indexed under this heading.

Norgestimate (Chronic use of oral contraceptives enhances neuromuscular blocking effect by reducing plasma cholinesterase activity). Products include:
Ortho-Cyclen/Ortho Tri-Cyclen 2573
Ortho-Prefest Tablets 2570

Norgestrel (Chronic use of oral contraceptives enhances neuromuscular blocking effect by reducing plasma cholinesterase activity). Products include:
Lo/Ovral Tablets 3532
Lo/Ovral-28 Tablets 3538
Low-Ogestrel-28 Tablets 3392
Ogestrel 0.5/50-28 Tablets 3428
Ovral Tablets 3551
Ovral-28 Tablets 3552
Ovrette Tablets 3552

Oxytocin (Enhances neuromuscular blocking action).
No products indexed under this heading.

Oxytocin (Nasal Spray) (Enhances neuromuscular blocking action).
No products indexed under this heading.

Pancuronium Bromide (Possible synergistic or antagonistic effect if co-administered during the same procedure).
No products indexed under this heading.

Pargyline Hydrochloride (Chronic use of certain unspecified MAO inhibitors enhances neuromuscular blocking effect by reducing plasma cholinesterase activity).
No products indexed under this heading.

Penbutolol Sulfate (Enhances neuromuscular blocking action).
No products indexed under this heading.

Phenelzine Sulfate (Chronic use of certain unspecified MAO inhibitors enhances neuromuscular blocking effect by reducing plasma cholinesterase activity). Products include:
Nardil Tablets 2653

Pindolol (Enhances neuromuscular blocking action).
No products indexed under this heading.

Prednisolone Acetate (Chronic use of glucocorticoids enhances neuromuscular blocking effect by reducing plasma cholinesterase activity). Products include:
Blephamide Ophthalmic Ointment ... 547
Blephamide Ophthalmic Suspension 548
Poly-Pred Liquifilm Ophthalmic Suspension .... ⊙245
Pred Forte Ophthalmic Suspension .... ⊙246
Pred Mild Sterile Ophthalmic Suspension .... ⊙249
Pred-G Ophthalmic Suspension ..... ⊙247
Pred-G Sterile Ophthalmic Ointment .... ⊙248

Prednisolone Sodium Phosphate (Chronic use of glucocorticoids enhances neuromuscular blocking effect by reducing plasma cholinesterase activity). Products include:
Pediapred Oral Solution 1170

Prednisolone Tebutate (Chronic use of glucocorticoids enhances neuromuscular blocking effect by reducing plasma cholinesterase activity).
No products indexed under this heading.

Prednisone (Chronic use of glucocorticoids enhances neuromuscular blocking effect by reducing plasma cholinesterase activity). Products include:
Prednisone 3064

Procainamide Hydrochloride (Enhances neuromuscular blocking action). Products include:
Procanbid Extended-Release Tablets 2262

Procarbazine Hydrochloride (Chronic use of certain unspecified MAO inhibitors enhances neuromuscular blocking effect by reducing plasma cholinesterase activity). Products include:
Matulane Capsules 3246

Promazine Hydrochloride (Enhances neuromuscular blocking action).
No products indexed under this heading.

Propranolol Hydrochloride (Enhances neuromuscular blocking action). Products include:
Inderal 3513
Inderal LA Long-Acting Capsules 3516
Inderide Tablets 3517
Inderide LA Long-Acting Capsules .. 3519

Quinidine Gluconate (Enhances neuromuscular blocking action). Products include:
Quinaglute Dura-Tabs Tablets 978

Quinidine Polygalacturonate (Enhances neuromuscular blocking action).
No products indexed under this heading.

Quinidine Sulfate (Enhances neuromuscular blocking action). Products include:
Quinidex Extentabs 2933

Quinine (Enhances neuromuscular blocking action).
No products indexed under this heading.

Rapacuronium Bromide (Possible synergistic or antagonistic effect if co-administered during the same procedure).
No products indexed under this heading.

Rocuronium Bromide (Possible synergistic or antagonistic effect if co-administered during the same procedure). Products include:
Zemuron Injection 2491

Selegiline Hydrochloride (Chronic use of certain unspecified MAO inhibitors enhances neuromuscular blocking effect by reducing plasma cholinesterase activity). Products include:
Eldepryl Capsules 3266

Sotalol Hydrochloride (Enhances neuromuscular blocking action). Products include:
Betapace Tablets 950
Betapace AF Tablets 954

Terbutaline Sulfate (Enhances neuromuscular blocking action). Products include:
Brethine Ampuls 2314
Brethine Tablets 2313

Timolol Hemihydrate (Enhances neuromuscular blocking action). Products include:
Betimol Ophthalmic Solution .... ⊙324

Timolol Maleate (Enhances neuromuscular blocking action). Products include:
Blocadren Tablets 2046
Cosopt Sterile Ophthalmic Solution 2065
Timolide Tablets 2187
Timolol GFS .... ⊙266
Timoptic in Ocudose 2192
Timoptic Sterile Ophthalmic Solution 2190
Timoptic-XE Sterile Ophthalmic Gel Forming Solution 2194

Tranylcypromine Sulfate (Chronic use of certain unspecified MAO inhibitors enhances neuromuscular blocking effect by reducing plasma cholinesterase activity). Products include:
Parnate Tablets 1607

Triamcinolone (Chronic use of glucocorticoids enhances neuromuscular blocking effect by reducing plasma cholinesterase activity).
No products indexed under this heading.

Triamcinolone Acetonide (Chronic use of glucocorticoids enhances neuromuscular blocking effect by reducing plasma cholinesterase activity). Products include:
Azmacort Inhalation Aerosol 728
Nasacort Nasal Inhaler 750
Nasacort AQ Nasal Spray 752
Tri-Nasal Spray 2274

Triamcinolone Diacetate (Chronic use of glucocorticoids enhances neuromuscular blocking effect by reducing plasma cholinesterase activity).
No products indexed under this heading.

Triamcinolone Hexacetonide (Chronic use of glucocorticoids enhances neuromuscular blocking effect by reducing plasma cholinesterase activity).
No products indexed under this heading.

Trimethaphan Camsylate (Enhances neuromuscular blocking action).
No products indexed under this heading.

Vecuronium Bromide (Possible synergistic or antagonistic effect if co-administered during the same procedure). Products include:
Norcuron for Injection 2478

ANTABUSE TABLETS
(Disulfiram) 3474
May interact with oral anticoagulants, phenytoin, and certain other agents. Compounds in these categories include:

Dicumarol (Disulfiram may prolong prothrombin time; it may be necessary to adjust the dosage of oral anticoagulants).
No products indexed under this heading.

Fosphenytoin Sodium (Co-administration with disulfiram and phenytoin can lead to an increase in phenytoin levels resulting in phenytoin intoxication; baseline phenytoin serum level should be obtained prior to initiation of disulfiram therapy; subsequently phenytoin levels should be determined on different days for evidence of an increase or continuous rise in its levels and dosage adjusted accordingly). Products include:
Cerebyx Injection 2619

Isoniazid (Co-administration can result in unsteady gait or marked changes in mental status; the disulfiram should be discontinued if such signs appear). Products include:
Rifamate Capsules 767
Rifater Tablets 769

Metronidazole (Co-administration has resulted in psychotic reactions; patients who are receiving or have recently received metronidazole should not be given Antabuse). Products include:
MetroCream 1404
MetroGel 1405
MetroGel-Vaginal Gel 1986
MetroLotion 1405
Noritate Cream 1224

Metronidazole Hydrochloride (Co-administration has resulted in psychotic reactions; patients who are receiving or have recently received metronidazole should not be given Antabuse).
No products indexed under this heading.

Paraldehyde (Patients who are receiving or have recently received paraldehyde should not be given Antabuse).
No products indexed under this heading.

Phenytoin (Co-administration with disulfiram and phenytoin can lead to an increase in phenytoin levels resulting in phenytoin intoxication; baseline phenytoin serum level should be obtained prior to initiation of disulfiram therapy; subsequently phenytoin levels should be determined on different days for evidence of an increase or continuous rise in its levels and dosage adjusted accordingly). Products include:
Dilantin Infatabs 2624
Dilantin-125 Oral Suspension 2625

Phenytoin Sodium (Co-administration with disulfiram and phenytoin can lead to an increase in phenytoin levels resulting in phenytoin intoxication; baseline phenytoin serum level should be obtained prior to initiation of disulfiram therapy; subsequently phenytoin levels should be determined on different days for evidence of an increase or continuous rise in its levels and dosage adjusted accordingly). Products include:
Dilantin Kapseals 2622

Warfarin Sodium (Disulfiram may prolong prothrombin time; it may be necessary to adjust the dosage of oral anticoagulants). Products include:
Coumadin for Injection 1243
Coumadin Tablets 1243
Warfarin Sodium Tablets, USP 3302

Food Interactions

Alcohol (Antabuse plus alcohol, even small amounts, produces flushing, throbbing in head and neck, throbbing headache, respiratory difficulty, nausea, copious vomiting, thirst, dyspnea, chest pain, palpitations, and other serious cardiovascular and respiratory reactions resulting in possible fatality; concurrent use with alcohol or alcohol containing preparations, such as cough syrups, tonics, sauces, and even after shave lotions and back rubs is contraindicated).

ANTABUSE TABLETS
(Disulfiram) 2444
May interact with oral anticoagulants and phenytoin. Compounds in these categories include:

Dicumarol (Disulfiram may prolong prothrombin time).
No products indexed under this heading.

Fosphenytoin Sodium (Co-administration can result in an increase in phenytoin levels leading to phenytoin intoxication). Products include:
Cerebyx Injection 2619

Isoniazid (Co-administration may lead to unsteady gait or mixed changes in mental status). Products include:
Rifamate Capsules 767
Rifater Tablets 769

Metronidazole (Co-administration has resulted in psychotic reactions; concurrent use is contraindicated). Products include:
MetroCream 1404
MetroGel 1405
MetroGel-Vaginal Gel 1986
MetroLotion 1405
Noritate Cream 1224

Metronidazole Hydrochloride (Co-administration has resulted in psychotic reactions; concurrent use is contraindicated).
No products indexed under this heading.

Paraldehyde (Concurrent use is contraindicated due to possibility of disulfiram-alcohol reactions).
No products indexed under this heading.

Phenytoin (Co-administration can result in an increase in phenytoin levels leading to phenytoin intoxication). Products include:
Dilantin Infatabs 2624
Dilantin-125 Oral Suspension 2625

Phenytoin Sodium (Co-administration can result in an increase in phenytoin levels leading to phenytoin intoxication). Products include:
Dilantin Kapseals 2622

Warfarin Sodium (Disulfiram may prolong prothrombin time). Products include:
Coumadin for Injection 1243
Coumadin Tablets 1243
Warfarin Sodium Tablets, USP 3302

Food Interactions

Alcohol (Disulfiram plus alcohol, even small amounts, produce flushing, throbbing in head and neck, throbbing headache, respiratory difficulty, nausea, vomiting, and confusion; concurrent use with alcohol-containing preparations, such as cough syrups, tonics, sauces, vinegars,

and even aftershave lotion and back rubs should be avoided).

ANTAGON INJECTION
(Ganirelix acetate) 2447
None cited in PDR database.

ANTIOXIDANT BOOSTER CAPLETS
(Herbals with Vitamins & Minerals)...................................... ⊞794
None cited in PDR database.

ANTIVENIN (BLACK WIDOW SPIDER ANTIVENIN)
(Black Widow Spider Antivenin (Equine)).. 2042
None cited in PDR database.

ANTIVENIN (MICRURUS FULVIUS)
(Antivenin (Micrurus Fulvius)) 3477
May interact with beta blockers and narcotic analgesics. Compounds in these categories include:

Acebutolol Hydrochloride (Co-administration with beta-adrenergic blockers has been associated with an increased severity of acute anaphylaxis; anaphylaxis may be resistant and prolonged; altered or larger than usual doses of epinephrine may be required to treat anaphylaxis). Products include:
Sectral Capsules 3589

Alfentanil Hydrochloride (Co-administration with drugs that depress respiration, such as narcotic analgesics, are contraindicated).
No products indexed under this heading.

Atenolol (Co-administration with beta-adrenergic blockers has been associated with an increased severity of acute anaphylaxis; anaphylaxis may be resistant and prolonged; altered or larger than usual doses of epinephrine may be required to treat anaphylaxis). Products include:
Tenoretic Tablets 690
Tenormin I.V. Injection 692

Betaxolol Hydrochloride (Co-administration with beta-adrenergic blockers has been associated with an increased severity of acute anaphylaxis; anaphylaxis may be resistant and prolonged; altered or larger than usual doses of epinephrine may be required to treat anaphylaxis). Products include:
Betoptic S Ophthalmic Suspension 537

Bisoprolol Fumarate (Co-administration with beta-adrenergic blockers has been associated with an increased severity of acute anaphylaxis; anaphylaxis may be resistant and prolonged; altered or larger than usual doses of epinephrine may be required to treat anaphylaxis). Products include:
Zebeta Tablets 1885
Ziac Tablets 1887

Buprenorphine Hydrochloride (Co-administration with drugs that depress respiration, such as narcotic analgesics, are contraindicated). Products include:
Buprenex Injectable 2918

Carteolol Hydrochloride (Co-administration with beta-adrenergic blockers has been associated with an increased severity of acute anaphylaxis; anaphylaxis may be resistant and prolonged; altered or larger than usual doses of epinephrine may be required to treat anaphylaxis). Products include:
Carteolol Hydrochloride Ophthalmic Solution USP, 1% ..... ⊙258
Ocupress Ophthalmic Solution, 1% Sterile .... ⊙303

Codeine Phosphate (Co-administration with drugs that depress respiration, such as narcotic analgesics, are contraindicated). Products include:
Phenergan with Codeine Syrup 3557
Phenergan VC with Codeine Syrup .. 3561
Robitussin A-C Syrup 2942
Robitussin-DAC Syrup 2942
Ryna-C Liquid .... ⊞768
Soma Compound w/Codeine Tablets 3355
Tussi-Organidin NR Liquid 3350
Tussi-Organidin-S NR Liquid 3350
Tylenol with Codeine 2595

Dezocine (Co-administration with drugs that depress respiration, such as narcotic analgesics, are contraindicated).
No products indexed under this heading.

Esmolol Hydrochloride (Co-administration with beta-adrenergic blockers has been associated with an increased severity of acute anaphylaxis; anaphylaxis may be resistant and prolonged; altered or larger than usual doses of epinephrine may be required to treat anaphylaxis). Products include:
Brevibloc Injection 858

Fentanyl (Co-administration with drugs that depress respiration, such as narcotic analgesics, are contraindicated). Products include:
Duragesic Transdermal System 1786

Fentanyl Citrate (Co-administration with drugs that depress respiration, such as narcotic analgesics, are contraindicated). Products include:
Actiq 1184

Hydrocodone Bitartrate (Co-administration with drugs that depress respiration, such as narcotic analgesics, are contraindicated). Products include:
Hycodan 1316
Hycomine Compound Tablets 1317
Hycotuss Expectorant Syrup 1318
Lortab 3319
Lortab Elixir 3317
Maxidone Tablets CIII 3399
Norco 5/325 Tablets CIII 3424
Norco 7.5/325 Tablets CIII 3425
Norco 10/325 Tablets CIII 3427
Norco 10/325 Tablets CIII 3425
Vicodin Tablets 516
Vicodin ES Tablets 517
Vicodin HP Tablets 518
Vicodin Tuss Expectorant 519
Vicoprofen Tablets 520
Zydone Tablets 1330

Hydrocodone Polistirex (Co-administration with drugs that depress respiration, such as narcotic analgesics, are contraindicated). Products include:
Tussionex Pennkinetic Extended-Release Suspension 1174

Hydromorphone Hydrochloride (Co-administration with drugs that depress respiration, such as narcotic analgesics, are contraindicated). Products include:
Dilaudid 441
Dilaudid Oral Liquid 445
Dilaudid Powder 441
Dilaudid Rectal Suppositories 441
Dilaudid Tablets 441
Dilaudid Tablets - 8 mg 445
Dilaudid-HP 443

Labetalol Hydrochloride (Co-administration with beta-adrenergic blockers has been associated with an increased severity of acute anaphylaxis; anaphylaxis may be resistant and prolonged; altered or larger than usual doses of epinephrine may be required to treat anaphylaxis). Products include:
Normodyne Injection 3135
Normodyne Tablets 3137

Levobunolol Hydrochloride (Co-administration with beta-adrenergic blockers has been associated with an increased severity of acute anaphylaxis; anaphylaxis may be resistant and prolonged; altered or larger than usual doses of epinephrine may be required to treat anaphylaxis). Products include:
Betagan .... ⊙228

Levorphanol Tartrate (Co-administration with drugs that depress respiration, such as narcotic analgesics, are contraindicated). Products include:
Levo-Dromoran 1734
Levorphanol Tartrate Tablets 3059

Meperidine Hydrochloride (Co-administration with drugs that depress respiration, such as narcotic analgesics, are contraindicated). Products include:
Demerol 3079
Mepergan Injection 3539

Methadone Hydrochloride (Co-administration with drugs that depress respiration, such as narcotic analgesics, are contraindicated). Products include:
Dolophine Hydrochloride Tablets 3056

Metipranolol Hydrochloride (Co-administration with beta-adrenergic blockers has been associated with an increased severity of acute anaphylaxis; anaphylaxis may be resistant and prolonged; altered or larger than usual doses of epinephrine may be required to treat anaphylaxis).
No products indexed under this heading.

Metoprolol Succinate (Co-administration with beta-adrenergic blockers has been associated with an increased severity of acute anaphylaxis; anaphylaxis may be resistant and prolonged; altered or larger than usual doses of epinephrine may be required to treat anaphylaxis). Products include:
Toprol-XL Tablets 651

Metoprolol Tartrate (Co-administration with beta-adrenergic blockers has been associated with an increased severity of acute anaphylaxis; anaphylaxis may be resistant and prolonged; altered or larger than usual doses of epinephrine may be required to treat anaphylaxis).
No products indexed under this heading.

Morphine Sulfate (Co-administration with drugs that depress respiration, such as narcotic analgesics, are contraindicated). Products include:
Astramorph/PF Injection, USP (Preservative-Free) 594
Duramorph Injection 1312
Infumorph 200 and Infumorph 500 Sterile Solutions 1314
Kadian Capsules 1335
MS Contin Tablets 2896
MSIR 2898
Oramorph SR Tablets 3062
Roxanol 3066

Nadolol (Co-administration with beta-adrenergic blockers has been associated with an increased severity of acute anaphylaxis; anaphylaxis may be resistant and prolonged; altered or larger than usual doses of epinephrine may be required to treat anaphylaxis). Products include:
Corgard Tablets 2245
Corzide 40/5 Tablets 2247
Corzide 80/5 Tablets 2247
Nadolol Tablets 2288

Oxycodone Hydrochloride (Co-administration with drugs that depress respiration, such as narcotic analgesics, are contraindicated). Products include:
OxyContin Tablets 2912
OxyFast Oral Concentrate Solution . 2916
OxyIR Capsules 2916
Percocet Tablets 1326
Percodan Tablets 1327
Percolone Tablets 1327
Roxicodone 3067
Tylox Capsules 2597

Penbutolol Sulfate (Co-administration with beta-adrenergic blockers has been associated with an increased severity of acute anaphylaxis; anaphylaxis may be resistant and prolonged; altered or larger than usual doses of epinephrine may be required to treat anaphylaxis).
No products indexed under this heading.

Pindolol (Co-administration with beta-adrenergic blockers has been associated with an increased severity of acute anaphylaxis; anaphylaxis may be resistant and prolonged; altered or larger than usual doses of epinephrine may be required to treat anaphylaxis).
No products indexed under this heading.

Propoxyphene Hydrochloride (Co-administration with drugs that depress respiration, such as narcotic analgesics, are contraindicated). Products include:
Darvon Pulvules 1909
Darvon Compound-65 Pulvules 1910

Propoxyphene Napsylate (Co-administration with drugs that depress respiration, such as narcotic analgesics, are contraindicated). Products include:
Darvon-N/Darvocet-N 1907
Darvon-N Tablets 1912

Propranolol Hydrochloride (Co-administration with beta-adrenergic blockers has been associated with an increased severity of acute anaphylaxis; anaphylaxis may be resistant and prolonged; altered or larger than usual doses of epinephrine may be required to treat anaphylaxis). Products include:
Inderal 3513
Inderal LA Long-Acting Capsules 3516
Inderide Tablets 3517
Inderide LA Long-Acting Capsules .. 3519

Remifentanil Hydrochloride (Co-administration with drugs that depress respiration, such as narcotic analgesics, are contraindicated).
No products indexed under this heading.

Sotalol Hydrochloride (Co-administration with beta-adrenergic blockers has been associated with an increased severity of acute anaphylaxis; anaphylaxis may be resistant and prolonged; altered or larger than usual doses of epinephrine may be required to treat anaphylaxis). Products include:
Betapace Tablets 950
Betapace AF Tablets 954

Sufentanil Citrate (Co-administration with drugs that depress respiration, such as narcotic analgesics, are contraindicated).
No products indexed under this heading.

Timolol Hemihydrate (Co-administration with beta-adrenergic blockers has been associated with an increased severity of acute anaphylaxis; anaphylaxis may be resistant and prolonged; altered or larger than usual doses of epinephrine may be required to treat anaphylaxis). Products include:
Betimol Ophthalmic Solution .... ⊙324

Timolol Maleate (Co-administration with beta-adrenergic blockers has been associated with an increased severity of acute anaphylaxis; anaphylaxis may be resistant and prolonged; altered or larger than usual doses of epinephrine may be required to treat anaphylaxis). Products include:
Blocadren Tablets 2046
Cosopt Sterile Ophthalmic Solution 2065
Timolide Tablets 2187
Timolol GFS .... ⊙266
Timoptic in Ocudose 2192
Timoptic Sterile Ophthalmic Solution 2190

IMPORTANT NOTE: Always consult each drug listing in the patient's regimen for possible interactions.

Timoptic-XE Sterile Ophthalmic Gel Forming Solution 2194

ANTIVENIN POLYVALENT

(Antivenin (Crotalidae) Polyvalent) 3475

May interact with beta blockers. Compounds in these categories include:

Acebutolol Hydrochloride (Co-administration with beta-adrenergic blockers has been associated with an increased severity of acute anaphylaxis; anaphylaxis may be resistant and prolonged; altered or larger than usual doses of epinephrine may be required to treat anaphylaxis). Products include:

- Sectral Capsules 3589

Atenolol (Co-administration with beta-adrenergic blockers has been associated with an increased severity of acute anaphylaxis; anaphylaxis may be resistant and prolonged; altered or larger than usual doses of epinephrine may be required to treat anaphylaxis). Products include:

- Tenoretic Tablets 690
- Tenormin I.V. Injection 692

Betaxolol Hydrochloride (Co-administration with beta-adrenergic blockers has been associated with an increased severity of acute anaphylaxis; anaphylaxis may be resistant and prolonged; altered or larger than usual doses of epinephrine may be required to treat anaphylaxis). Products include:

- Betoptic S Ophthalmic Suspension 537

Bisoprolol Fumarate (Co-administration with beta-adrenergic blockers has been associated with an increased severity of acute anaphylaxis; anaphylaxis may be resistant and prolonged; altered or larger than usual doses of epinephrine may be required to treat anaphylaxis). Products include:

- Zebeta Tablets 1885
- Ziac Tablets 1887

Carteolol Hydrochloride (Co-administration with beta-adrenergic blockers has been associated with an increased severity of acute anaphylaxis; anaphylaxis may be resistant and prolonged; altered or larger than usual doses of epinephrine may be required to treat anaphylaxis). Products include:

- Carteolol Hydrochloride Ophthalmic Solution USP, 1% ..... ⊙ 258
- Ocupress Ophthalmic Solution, 1% Sterile .... ⊙ 303

Esmolol Hydrochloride (Co-administration with beta-adrenergic blockers has been associated with an increased severity of acute anaphylaxis; anaphylaxis may be resistant and prolonged; altered or larger than usual doses of epinephrine may be required to treat anaphylaxis). Products include:

- Brevibloc Injection 858

Labetalol Hydrochloride (Co-administration with beta-adrenergic blockers has been associated with an increased severity of acute anaphylaxis; anaphylaxis may be resistant and prolonged; altered or larger than usual doses of epinephrine may be required to treat anaphylaxis). Products include:

- Normodyne Injection 3135
- Normodyne Tablets 3137

Levobunolol Hydrochloride (Co-administration with beta-adrenergic blockers has been associated with an increased severity of acute anaphylaxis; anaphylaxis may be resistant and prolonged; altered or larger than usual doses of epinephrine may be required to treat anaphylaxis). Products include:

- Betagan .... ⊙ 228

Metipranolol Hydrochloride (Co-administration with beta-adrenergic blockers has been associated with an increased severity of acute anaphylaxis; anaphylaxis may be resistant and prolonged; altered or larger than usual doses of epinephrine may be required to treat anaphylaxis).

No products indexed under this heading.

Metoprolol Succinate (Co-administration with beta-adrenergic blockers has been associated with an increased severity of acute anaphylaxis; anaphylaxis may be resistant and prolonged; altered or larger than usual doses of epinephrine may be required to treat anaphylaxis). Products include:

- Toprol-XL Tablets 651

Metoprolol Tartrate (Co-administration with beta-adrenergic blockers has been associated with an increased severity of acute anaphylaxis; anaphylaxis may be resistant and prolonged; altered or larger than usual doses of epinephrine may be required to treat anaphylaxis).

No products indexed under this heading.

Nadolol (Co-administration with beta-adrenergic blockers has been associated with an increased severity of acute anaphylaxis; anaphylaxis may be resistant and prolonged; altered or larger than usual doses of epinephrine may be required to treat anaphylaxis). Products include:

- Corgard Tablets 2245
- Corzide 40/5 Tablets 2247
- Corzide 80/5 Tablets 2247
- Nadolol Tablets 2288

Penbutolol Sulfate (Co-administration with beta-adrenergic blockers has been associated with an increased severity of acute anaphylaxis; anaphylaxis may be resistant and prolonged; altered or larger than usual doses of epinephrine may be required to treat anaphylaxis).

No products indexed under this heading.

Pindolol (Co-administration with beta-adrenergic blockers has been associated with an increased severity of acute anaphylaxis; anaphylaxis may be resistant and prolonged; altered or larger than usual doses of epinephrine may be required to treat anaphylaxis).

No products indexed under this heading.

Propranolol Hydrochloride (Co-administration with beta-adrenergic blockers has been associated with an increased severity of acute anaphylaxis; anaphylaxis may be resistant and prolonged; altered or larger than usual doses of epinephrine may be required to treat anaphylaxis). Products include:

- Inderal 3513
- Inderal LA Long-Acting Capsules 3516
- Inderide Tablets 3517
- Inderide LA Long-Acting Capsules .. 3519

Sotalol Hydrochloride (Co-administration with beta-adrenergic blockers has been associated with an increased severity of acute anaphylaxis; anaphylaxis may be resistant and prolonged; altered or larger than usual doses of epinephrine may be required to treat anaphylaxis). Products include:

- Betapace Tablets 950
- Betapace AF Tablets 954

Timolol Hemihydrate (Co-administration with beta-adrenergic blockers has been associated with an increased severity of acute anaphylaxis; anaphylaxis may be resistant and prolonged; altered or larger than usual doses of epinephrine may be required to treat anaphylaxis). Products include:

- Betimol Ophthalmic Solution .... ⊙ 324

Timolol Maleate (Co-administration with beta-adrenergic blockers has been associated with an increased severity of acute anaphylaxis; anaphylaxis may be resistant and prolonged; altered or larger than usual doses of epinephrine may be required to treat anaphylaxis). Products include:

- Blocadren Tablets 2046
- Cosopt Sterile Ophthalmic Solution 2065
- Timolide Tablets 2187
- Timolol GFS .... ⊙ 266
- Timoptic in Ocudose 2192
- Timoptic Sterile Ophthalmic Solution 2190
- Timoptic-XE Sterile Ophthalmic Gel Forming Solution 2194

ANTIVERT, ANTIVERT/25, & ANTIVERT/50 TABLETS

(Meclizine Hydrochloride) 2664

Food Interactions

Alcohol (Concurrent use should be avoided).

ANUSOL HC-1 HYDROCORTISONE ANTI-ITCH CREAM

(Hydrocortisone Acetate) .... ▣ 689

None cited in PDR database.

ANUSOL OINTMENT

(Mineral Oil, Pramoxine Hydrochloride, Zinc Oxide) .... ▣ 688

None cited in PDR database.

ANUSOL SUPPOSITORIES

(Starch) .... ▣ 689

None cited in PDR database.

ANUSOL-HC CREAM 2.5%

(Hydrocortisone) 2237

None cited in PDR database.

ANUSOL-HC SUPPOSITORIES

(Hydrocortisone Acetate) 2238

None cited in PDR database.

ANZEMET INJECTION

(Dolasetron Mesylate) 719

See Anzemet Tablets

ANZEMET TABLETS

(Dolasetron Mesylate) 722

May interact with:

Atenolol (Decreases hydrodolasetron clearance by 27%). Products include:

- Tenoretic Tablets 690
- Tenormin I.V. Injection 692

Cimetidine (Co-administration of dolasetron with cimetidine, a nonselective inhibitor of CYP450, has resulted in increased blood levels of dolasetron by 24%). Products include:

- Tagamet HB 200 Suspension .... ▣ 762
- Tagamet HB 200 Tablets .... ▣ 761
- Tagamet Tablets 1644

Cimetidine Hydrochloride (Co-administration of dolasetron with cimetidine, a nonselective inhibitor of CYP450, has resulted in increased blood levels of dolasetron by 24%). Products include:

- Tagamet 1644

Rifampin (Co-administration of dolasetron with rifampin, a potent inducer of CYP450, has resulted in decreased blood levels of dolasetron by 28%). Products include:

- Rifadin 765
- Rifamate Capsules 767
- Rifater Tablets 769

APHTHASOL ORAL PASTE

(Amlexanox) 1025

None cited in PDR database.

APLIGRAF

(Graftskin) 2305

May interact with cytotoxic drugs and certain other agents. Compounds in these categories include:

Bleomycin Sulfate (In *in vitro* and *in vivo* histology studies, exposure to cytotoxic agents degraded Apligraf; concurrent use should be avoided).

No products indexed under this heading.

Chlorhexidine Gluconate (In *in vitro* and *in vivo* histology studies, exposure to chlorhexidine degraded Apligraf; concurrent use should be avoided). Products include:

- Betasept Surgical Scrub 2895

Cyclophosphamide (In *in vitro* and *in vivo* histology studies, exposure to cytotoxic agents degraded Apligraf; concurrent use should be avoided).

No products indexed under this heading.

Dakin's solution (In *in vitro* and *in vivo* histology studies, exposure to Dakin's solution degraded Apligraf; reduces Apligraf cell viability; concurrent use should be avoided).

No products indexed under this heading.

Daunorubicin Hydrochloride (In *in vitro* and *in vivo* histology studies, exposure to cytotoxic agents degraded Apligraf; concurrent use should be avoided). Products include:

- Cerubidine for Injection 947

Doxorubicin Hydrochloride (In *in vitro* and *in vivo* histology studies, exposure to cytotoxic agents degraded Apligraf; concurrent use should be avoided). Products include:

- Adriamycin PFS/RDF Injection 2767
- Doxil Injection 566

Epirubicin Hydrochloride (In *in vitro* and *in vivo* histology studies, exposure to cytotoxic agents degraded Apligraf; concurrent use should be avoided). Products include:

- Ellence Injection 2806

Fluorouracil (In *in vitro* and *in vivo* histology studies, exposure to cytotoxic agents degraded Apligraf; concurrent use should be avoided). Products include:

- Carac Cream 1222
- Efudex 1733
- Fluoroplex 552

Hydroxyurea (In *in vitro* and *in vivo* histology studies, exposure to cytotoxic agents degraded Apligraf; concurrent use should be avoided). Products include:

- Mylocel Tablets 2227

Mafenide Acetate (In *in vitro* and *in vivo* histology studies, exposure to mafenide acetate degraded Apligraf; reduces Apligraf cell viability; concurrent use should be avoided). Products include:

- Sulfamylon Cream 1011
- Sulfamylon Topical Solution 1011

Methotrexate Sodium (In *in vitro* and *in vivo* histology studies, exposure to cytotoxic agents degraded Apligraf; concurrent use should be avoided).

No products indexed under this heading.

Mitotane (In *in vitro* and *in vivo* histology studies, exposure to cytotoxic agents degraded Apligraf; concurrent use should be avoided).

No products indexed under this heading.

Mitoxantrone Hydrochloride (In *in vitro* and *in vivo* histology studies, exposure to cytotoxic agents degraded Apligraf; concurrent use should be avoided). Products include:

- Novantrone for Injection 1760

Nystatin (Reduces Apligraf cell viability). Products include:

- Nystatin Vaginal Tablets, USP 2445
- Nystop Topical Powder USP 2608

Polymyxin B Sulfate (Reduces Apligraf cell viability). Products include:

Betadine Brand First Aid Antibiotics & Moisturizer Ointment 2894
Betadine Brand Plus First Aid Antibiotics & Pain Reliever Ointment 2894
Cortisporin Ophthalmic Suspension Sterile .... ⊙297
Neosporin G.U. Irrigant Sterile 2256
Neosporin Ointment .... ▣704
Neosporin Ophthalmic Ointment Sterile .... ⊙299
Neosporin Ophthalmic Solution Sterile .... ⊙300
Neosporin + Pain Relief Maximum Strength Cream .... ▣704
Neosporin + Pain Relief Maximum Strength Ointment .... ▣704
Poly-Pred Liquifilm Ophthalmic Suspension .... ⊙245
Polysporin Ointment .... ▣706
Polysporin Ophthalmic Ointment Sterile .... ⊙301
Polysporin Powder .... ▣706
Polytrim Ophthalmic Solution 556

Povidone Iodine (In *in vitro* and *in vivo* histology studies, exposure to povidone iodine solution degraded Apligraf; concurrent use should be avoided). Products include:
Betadine Medicated Douche 2894
Betadine Ointment 2894
Betadine PrepStick Applicator 2894
Betadine PrepStick Plus Applicator 2894
Betadine Skin Cleanser 2895
Betadine Solution 2895
Betadine Surgical Scrub 2895
Massengill Medicated Disposable Douche .... ▣753

Procarbazine Hydrochloride (In *in vitro* and *in vivo* histology studies, exposure to cytotoxic agents degraded Apligraf; concurrent use should be avoided). Products include:
Matulane Capsules 3246

Scarlet Red Dressing (In *in vitro* and *in vivo* histology studies, exposure to Scarlet Red Dressing degraded Apligraf; concurrent use should be avoided).
No products indexed under this heading.

Tamoxifen Citrate (In *in vitro* and *in vivo* histology studies, exposure to cytotoxic agents degraded Apligraf; concurrent use should be avoided). Products include:
Nolvadex Tablets 678

Tincoban (In *in vitro* and *in vivo* histology studies, exposure to tincoban agents degraded Apligraf; concurrent use should be avoided).
No products indexed under this heading.

Vincristine Sulfate (In *in vitro* and *in vivo* histology studies, exposure to cytotoxic agents degraded Apligraf; concurrent use should be avoided).
No products indexed under this heading.

Zinc Sulfate (In *in vitro* and *in vivo* histology studies, exposure to zinc sulfate agents degraded Apligraf; concurrent use should be avoided). Products include:
Clear Eyes ACR Astringent/Lubricant Eye Redness Reliever .... ⊙322
Visine A.C. Seasonal Relief From Pollen & Dust Eye Drops .... ⊙314

APLISOL INJECTION

(Tuberculin, Purified Protein Derivative, Diluted) 2609

May interact with corticosteroids, immunosuppressive agents, and certain other agents. Compounds in these categories include:

Azathioprine (In patients receiving immunosuppressive agents, reactivity to the test may be depressed or suppressed).
No products indexed under this heading.

Basiliximab (In patients receiving immunosuppressive agents, reactivity to the test may be depressed or suppressed). Products include:
Simulect for Injection 2399

Betamethasone Acetate (In patients receiving corticosteroids, reactivity to the test may be depressed or suppressed). Products include:
Celestone Soluspan Injectable Suspension 3097

Betamethasone Sodium Phosphate (In patients receiving corticosteroids, reactivity to the test may be depressed or suppressed). Products include:
Celestone Soluspan Injectable Suspension 3097

Cortisone Acetate (In patients receiving corticosteroids, reactivity to the test may be depressed or suppressed). Products include:
Cortone Acetate Injectable Suspension 2059
Cortone Acetate Tablets 2061

Cyclosporine (In patients receiving immunosuppressive agents, reactivity to the test may be depressed or suppressed). Products include:
Gengraf Capsules 457
Neoral Soft Gelatin Capsules 2380
Neoral Oral Solution 2380
Sandimmune 2388

Dexamethasone (In patients receiving corticosteroids, reactivity to the test may be depressed or suppressed). Products include:
Decadron Elixir 2078
Decadron Tablets 2079
TobraDex Ophthalmic Ointment 542
TobraDex Ophthalmic Suspension 541

Dexamethasone Acetate (In patients receiving corticosteroids, reactivity to the test may be depressed or suppressed).
No products indexed under this heading.

Dexamethasone Sodium Phosphate (In patients receiving corticosteroids, reactivity to the test may be depressed or suppressed). Products include:
Decadron Phosphate Injection 2081
Decadron Phosphate Sterile Ophthalmic Ointment 2083
Decadron Phosphate Sterile Ophthalmic Solution 2084
NeoDecadron Sterile Ophthalmic Solution 2144

Fludrocortisone Acetate (In patients receiving corticosteroids, reactivity to the test may be depressed or suppressed). Products include:
Florinef Acetate Tablets 2250

Hydrocortisone (In patients receiving corticosteroids, reactivity to the test may be depressed or suppressed). Products include:
Anusol-HC Cream 2.5% 2237
Cipro HC Otic Suspension 540
Cortaid Intensive Therapy Cream .... ▣717
Cortaid Maximum Strength Cream .... ▣717
Cortisporin Ophthalmic Suspension Sterile .... ⊙297
Cortizone•5 .... ▣699
Cortizone•10 .... ▣699
Cortizone•10 Plus Creme .... ▣700
Cortizone for Kids Creme .... ▣699
Hydrocortone Tablets 2106
Massengill Medicated Soft Cloth Towelette .... ▣753
VōSoL HC Otic Solution 3356

Hydrocortisone Acetate (In patients receiving corticosteroids, reactivity to the test may be depressed or suppressed). Products include:
Analpram-HC 1338
Anusol HC-1 Hydrocortisone Anti-Itch Cream .... ▣689
Anusol-HC Suppositories 2238
Cortaid .... ▣717
Cortifoam Rectal Foam 3170
Cortisporin-TC Otic Suspension 2246
Hydrocortone Acetate Injectable Suspension 2103
Pramosone 1343
Proctocort Suppositories 2264
ProctoFoam-HC 3177
Terra-Cortril Ophthalmic Suspension 2716

Hydrocortisone Sodium Phosphate (In patients receiving corticosteroids, reactivity to the test may be depressed or suppressed). Products include:
Hydrocortone Phosphate Injection, Sterile 2105

Hydrocortisone Sodium Succinate (In patients receiving corticosteroids, reactivity to the test may be depressed or suppressed).
No products indexed under this heading.

Live Virus Vaccines (The reactivity to PPD may be temporarily depressed by certain live virus vaccines).
No products indexed under this heading.

Methylprednisolone Acetate (In patients receiving corticosteroids, reactivity to the test may be depressed or suppressed). Products include:
Depo-Medrol Injectable Suspension 2795

Methylprednisolone Sodium Succinate (In patients receiving corticosteroids, reactivity to the test may be depressed or suppressed). Products include:
Solu-Medrol Sterile Powder 2855

Muromonab-CD3 (In patients receiving immunosuppressive agents, reactivity to the test may be depressed or suppressed). Products include:
Orthoclone OKT3 Sterile Solution 2498

Mycophenolate Mofetil (In patients receiving immunosuppressive agents, reactivity to the test may be depressed or suppressed). Products include:
CellCept Capsules 2951
CellCept Oral Suspension 2951
CellCept Tablets 2951

Prednisolone Acetate (In patients receiving corticosteroids, reactivity to the test may be depressed or suppressed). Products include:
Blephamide Ophthalmic Ointment 547
Blephamide Ophthalmic Suspension 548
Poly-Pred Liquifilm Ophthalmic Suspension .... ⊙245
Pred Forte Ophthalmic Suspension .... ⊙246
Pred Mild Sterile Ophthalmic Suspension .... ⊙249
Pred-G Ophthalmic Suspension .... ⊙247
Pred-G Sterile Ophthalmic Ointment .... ⊙248

Prednisolone Sodium Phosphate (In patients receiving corticosteroids, reactivity to the test may be depressed or suppressed). Products include:
Pediapred Oral Solution 1170

Prednisolone Tebutate (In patients receiving corticosteroids, reactivity to the test may be depressed or suppressed).
No products indexed under this heading.

Prednisone (In patients receiving corticosteroids, reactivity to the test may be depressed or suppressed). Products include:
Prednisone 3064

Sirolimus (In patients receiving immunosuppressive agents, reactivity to the test may be depressed or suppressed). Products include:
Rapamune Oral Solution and Tablets 3584

Tacrolimus (In patients receiving immunosuppressive agents, reactivity to the test may be depressed or suppressed). Products include:
Prograf 1393
Protopic Ointment 1397

Triamcinolone (In patients receiving corticosteroids, reactivity to the test may be depressed or suppressed).
No products indexed under this heading.

Triamcinolone Acetonide (In patients receiving corticosteroids, reactivity to the test may be depressed or suppressed). Products include:
Azmacort Inhalation Aerosol 728
Nasacort Nasal Inhaler 750
Nasacort AQ Nasal Spray 752
Tri-Nasal Spray 2274

Triamcinolone Diacetate (In patients receiving corticosteroids, reactivity to the test may be depressed or suppressed).
No products indexed under this heading.

Triamcinolone Hexacetonide (In patients receiving corticosteroids, reactivity to the test may be depressed or suppressed).
No products indexed under this heading.

AQUAMEPHYTON INJECTION

(Vitamin K_1) 2042

May interact with oral anticoagulants. Compounds in these categories include:

Dicumarol (Temporary resistance to anticoagulants).
No products indexed under this heading.

Warfarin Sodium (Temporary resistance to anticoagulants). Products include:
Coumadin for Injection 1243
Coumadin Tablets 1243
Warfarin Sodium Tablets, USP 3302

AQUASOL A PARENTERAL

(Vitamin A) 593

May interact with oral contraceptives. Compounds in these categories include:

Desogestrel (Potential for a significant increase in plasma vitamin A levels). Products include:
Cyclessa Tablets 2450
Desogen Tablets 2458
Mircette Tablets 2470
Ortho-Cept 21 Tablets 2546
Ortho-Cept 28 Tablets 2546

Ethinyl Estradiol (Potential for a significant increase in plasma vitamin A levels). Products include:
Alesse-21 Tablets 3468
Alesse-28 Tablets 3473
Brevicon 28-Day Tablets 3380
Cyclessa Tablets 2450
Desogen Tablets 2458
Estinyl Tablets 3112
Estrostep 2627
femhrt Tablets 2635
Levlen 962
Levlite 21 Tablets 962
Levlite 28 Tablets 962
Levora Tablets 3389
Loestrin 21 Tablets 2642
Loestrin Fe Tablets 2642
Lo/Ovral Tablets 3532
Lo/Ovral-28 Tablets 3538
Low-Ogestrel-28 Tablets 3392
Microgestin Fe 1.5/30 Tablets 3407
Microgestin Fe 1/20 Tablets 3400
Mircette Tablets 2470
Modicon 2563
Necon 3415
Nordette-28 Tablets 2257
Norinyl 1 +35 28-Day Tablets 3380
Ogestrel 0.5/50-28 Tablets 3428
Ortho-Cept 21 Tablets 2546
Ortho-Cept 28 Tablets 2546
Ortho-Cyclen/Ortho Tri-Cyclen 2573
Ortho-Novum 2563
Ovcon 3364
Ovral Tablets 3551
Ovral-28 Tablets 3552
Tri-Levlen 962
Tri-Norinyl-28 Tablets 3433
Triphasil-21 Tablets 3600
Triphasil-28 Tablets 3605

Trivora Tablets 3439
Yasmin 28 Tablets 980
Zovia 3449

Ethynodiol Diacetate (Potential for a significant increase in plasma vitamin A levels). Products include:
Zovia 3449

Levonorgestrel (Potential for a significant increase in plasma vitamin A levels). Products include:
Alesse-21 Tablets 3468
Alesse-28 Tablets 3473
Levlen 962
Levlite 21 Tablets 962
Levlite 28 Tablets 962
Levora Tablets 3389
Mirena Intrauterine System 974
Nordette-28 Tablets 2257
Norplant System 3543
Tri-Levlen 962
Triphasil-21 Tablets 3600
Triphasil-28 Tablets 3605
Trivora Tablets 3439

Mestranol (Potential for a significant increase in plasma vitamin A levels). Products include:
Necon 1/50 Tablets 3415
Norinyl 1 + 50 28-Day Tablets 3380
Ortho-Novum 1/50□28 Tablets 2556

Norethindrone (Potential for a significant increase in plasma vitamin A levels). Products include:
Brevicon 28-Day Tablets 3380
Micronor Tablets 2543
Modicon 2563
Necon 3415
Norinyl 1 +35 28-Day Tablets 3380
Norinyl 1 + 50 28-Day Tablets 3380
Nor-QD Tablets 3423
Ortho-Novum 2563
Ortho-Novum 1/50□28 Tablets 2556
Ovcon 3364
Tri-Norinyl-28 Tablets 3433

Norethynodrel (Potential for a significant increase in plasma vitamin A levels).
No products indexed under this heading.

Norgestimate (Potential for a significant increase in plasma vitamin A levels). Products include:
Ortho-Cyclen/Ortho Tri-Cyclen 2573
Ortho-Prefest Tablets 2570

Norgestrel (Potential for a significant increase in plasma vitamin A levels). Products include:
Lo/Ovral Tablets 3532
Lo/Ovral-28 Tablets 3538
Low-Ogestrel-28 Tablets 3392
Ogestrel 0.5/50-28 Tablets 3428
Ovral Tablets 3551
Ovral-28 Tablets 3552
Ovrette Tablets 3552

ARALEN TABLETS

(Chloroquine Phosphate) 3075
May interact with:

Hepatotoxic Drugs, unspecified (Caution should be exercised when used in conjunction with known hepatotoxic drugs).

ARAMINE INJECTION

(Metaraminol Bitartrate) 2043
May interact with cardiac glycosides, monoamine oxidase inhibitors, tricyclic antidepressants, and certain other agents. Compounds in these categories include:

Amitriptyline Hydrochloride (Potentiates pressor effect). Products include:
Etrafon 3115
Limbitrol 1738

Amoxapine (Potentiates pressor effect).
No products indexed under this heading.

Clomipramine Hydrochloride (Potentiates pressor effect).
No products indexed under this heading.

Desipramine Hydrochloride (Potentiates pressor effect). Products include:
Norpramin Tablets 755

Deslanoside (May cause ectopic arrhythmic reaction).
No products indexed under this heading.

Digitoxin (May cause ectopic arrhythmic reaction).
No products indexed under this heading.

Digoxin (May cause ectopic arrhythmic reaction). Products include:
Digitek Tablets 1003
Lanoxicaps Capsules 1574
Lanoxin Injection 1581
Lanoxin Tablets 1587
Lanoxin Elixir Pediatric 1578
Lanoxin Injection Pediatric 1584

Doxepin Hydrochloride (Potentiates pressor effect). Products include:
Sinequan 2713

Halothane (Concurrent use should be avoided). Products include:
Fluothane Inhalation 3508

Imipramine Hydrochloride (Potentiates pressor effect).
No products indexed under this heading.

Imipramine Pamoate (Potentiates pressor effect).
No products indexed under this heading.

Isocarboxazid (Potentiates pressor effect).
No products indexed under this heading.

Maprotiline Hydrochloride (Potentiates pressor effect).
No products indexed under this heading.

Moclobemide (Potentiates pressor effect).
No products indexed under this heading.

Nortriptyline Hydrochloride (Potentiates pressor effect).
No products indexed under this heading.

Pargyline Hydrochloride (Potentiates pressor effect).
No products indexed under this heading.

Phenelzine Sulfate (Potentiates pressor effect). Products include:
Nardil Tablets 2653

Procarbazine Hydrochloride (Potentiates pressor effect). Products include:
Matulane Capsules 3246

Protriptyline Hydrochloride (Potentiates pressor effect). Products include:
Vivactil Tablets 2446
Vivactil Tablets 2217

Selegiline Hydrochloride (Potentiates pressor effect). Products include:
Eldepryl Capsules 3266

Tranylcypromine Sulfate (Potentiates pressor effect). Products include:
Parnate Tablets 1607

Trimipramine Maleate (Potentiates pressor effect). Products include:
Surmontil Capsules 3595

ARAVA TABLETS

(Leflunomide) 724
May interact with:

Charcoal, Activated (Co-administration has resulted in a rapid and significant decrease in plasma M1 (the active metabolite of leflunomide) concentration).
No products indexed under this heading.

Cholestyramine (Co-administration has resulted in a rapid and significant decrease in plasma M1 (the active metabolite of leflunomide) concentration).
No products indexed under this heading.

Diclofenac Potassium (*In-vitro* co-administration has resulted in increased in free fraction of diclofenac; the clinical significance is unknown). Products include:
Cataflam Tablets 2315

Diclofenac Sodium (*In-vitro* co-administration has resulted in increased in free fraction of diclofenac; the clinical significance is unknown). Products include:
Arthrotec Tablets 3195
Voltaren Ophthalmic Sterile Ophthalmic Solution .... ⊙312
Voltaren Tablets 2315
Voltaren-XR Tablets 2315

Hepatotoxic Drugs, unspecified (Leflunomide treatment is associated with elevations of liver enzymes; co-adminstration may increase the risk of hepatotoxicity).

Ibuprofen (*In-vitro* co-administration has resulted in increased in free fraction of ibuprofen; the clinical significance is unknown). Products include:
Advil .... ▣771
Children's Advil Oral Suspension .... ▣773
Children's Advil Chewable Tablets .... ▣773
Advil Cold and Sinus Caplets .... ▣771
Advil Cold and Sinus Tablets .... ▣771
Advil Flu & Body Ache Caplets .... ▣772
Infants' Advil Drops .... ▣773
Junior Strength Advil Tablets .... ▣773
Junior Strength Advil Chewable Tablets .... ▣773
Advil Migraine Liquigels .... ▣772
Children's Motrin Oral Suspension and Chewable Tablets 2006
Children's Motrin Cold Oral Suspension 2007
Children's Motrin Oral Suspension .... ▣643
Motrin Suspension, Oral Drops, Chewable Tablets, and Caplets 2002
Infants' Motrin Concentrated Drops 2006
Junior Strength Motrin Caplets and Chewable Tablets 2006
Motrin IB Tablets, Caplets, and Gelcaps 2002
Motrin Migraine Pain Caplets 2005
Motrin Sinus Headache Caplets 2005
Vicoprofen Tablets 520

Methotrexate Sodium (Co-administration increases the risk of hepatotoxicity; concurrent use has not demonstrated any pharmacokinetic interaction).
No products indexed under this heading.

Rifampin (Co-administration has resulted in increased M1 peak levels). Products include:
Rifadin 765
Rifamate Capsules 767
Rifater Tablets 769

Tolbutamide (*In-vitro* co-administration has resulted in increased in free fraction of tolbutamide).
No products indexed under this heading.

ARCO-LASE TABLETS

(Amylase, Cellulase, Lipase, Protease) 592
None cited in PDR database.

ARCO-LASE PLUS TABLETS

(Amylase, Cellulase, Hyoscyamine Sulfate, Lipase, Phenobarbital, Protease) 592
None cited in PDR database.

AREDIA FOR INJECTION

(Pamidronate Disodium) 2309
None cited in PDR database.

ARGATROBAN INJECTION

(Argatroban) 1478
May interact with anticoagulants, thrombolytics, and certain other agents. Compounds in these categories include:

Alteplase, Recombinant (Co-administration with thrombolytic agents may increase the risk of bleeding). Products include:
Activase I.V. 1410
Cathflo Activase 3611

Anistreplase (Co-administration with thrombolytic agents may increase the risk of bleeding).
No products indexed under this heading.

Ardeparin Sodium (Co-administration with other anticoagulants may increase the risk of bleeding).
No products indexed under this heading.

Aspirin (Co-administration with antiplatelet agents, such as aspirin, may increase the risk of bleeding). Products include:
Aggrenox Capsules 1026
Alka-Seltzer .... ▣603
Alka-Seltzer Lemon Lime Antacid and Pain Reliever Effervescent Tablets .... ▣603
Alka-Seltzer Extra Strength Antacid and Pain Reliever Effervescent Tablets .... ▣603
Alka-Seltzer PM Effervescent Tablets .... ▣605
Genuine Bayer Tablets, Caplets and Gelcaps .... ▣606
Extra Strength Bayer Caplets and Gelcaps .... ▣610
Aspirin Regimen Bayer Children's Chewable Tablets (Orange or Cherry Flavored) .... ▣607
Bayer, Aspirin Regimen .... ▣606
Aspirin Regimen Bayer 81 mg Caplets with Calcium .... ▣607
Genuine Bayer Professional Labeling (Aspirin Regimen Bayer) .... ▣608
Extra Strength Bayer Arthritis Caplets .... ▣610
Extra Strength Bayer Plus Caplets .... ▣610
Extra Strength Bayer PM Caplets .... ▣611
BC Powder .... ▣619
BC Allergy Sinus Cold Powder .... ▣619
Arthritis Strength BC Powder .... ▣619
BC Sinus Cold Powder .... ▣619
Darvon Compound-65 Pulvules 1910
Ecotrin Enteric Coated Aspirin Low, Regular and Maximum Strength Tablets 1715
Excedrin Extra-Strength Tablets, Caplets, and Geltabs .... ▣629
Excedrin Migraine 1070
Goody's Body Pain Formula Powder .... ▣620
Goody's Extra Strength Headache Powder .... ▣620
Goody's Extra Strength Pain Relief Tablets .... ▣620
Percodan Tablets 1327
Robaxisal Tablets 2939
Soma Compound Tablets 3354
Soma Compound w/Codeine Tablets 3355
Vanquish Caplets .... ▣617

Clopidogrel Bisulfate (Co-administration with antiplatelet agents may increase the risk of bleeding). Products include:
Plavix Tablets 1097
Plavix Tablets 3084

Dalteparin Sodium (Co-administration with other anticoagulants may increase the risk of bleeding). Products include:
Fragmin Injection 2814

Danaparoid Sodium (Co-administration with other anticoagulants may increase the risk of bleeding). Products include:
Orgaran Injection 2480

Dicumarol (Co-administration with other anticoagulants may increase the risk of bleeding).
No products indexed under this heading.

Dipyridamole (Co-administration with antiplatelet agents may increase the risk of bleeding). Products include:

Aggrenox Capsules 1026
Persantine Tablets 1057

Enoxaparin (Co-administration with other anticoagulants may increase the risk of bleeding). Products include:

Lovenox Injection 746

Heparin Sodium (Co-administration with other anticoagulants may increase the risk of bleeding). Products include:

Heparin Lock Flush Solution 3509
Heparin Sodium Injection 3511

Reteplase (Co-administration with thrombolytic agents may increase the risk of bleeding). Products include:

Retavase Vials 1182

Streptokinase (Co-administration with thrombolytic agents may increase the risk of bleeding). Products include:

Streptase for Infusion 647

Tinzaparin sodium (Co-administration with other anticoagulants may increase the risk of bleeding). Products include:

Innohep Injection 1248

Urokinase (Co-administration with thrombolytic agents may increase the risk of bleeding).

No products indexed under this heading.

Warfarin Sodium (Co-administration with other anticoagulants may increase the risk of bleeding). Products include:

Coumadin for Injection 1243
Coumadin Tablets 1243
Warfarin Sodium Tablets, USP 3302

ARICEPT TABLETS

(Donepezil Hydrochloride) 2665

May interact with anticholinergics, dexamethasone, non-steroidal anti-inflammatory agents, phenytoin, quinidine, and certain other agents. Compounds in these categories include:

Atropine Sulfate (Donepezil, a cholinesterase inhibitor, has the potential to interfere with the activity of anticholinergic medications). Products include:

Donnatal 2929
Donnatal Extentabs 2930
Motofen Tablets 577
Prosed/DS Tablets 3268
Urised Tablets 2876

Belladonna Alkaloids (Donepezil, a cholinesterase inhibitor, has the potential to interfere with the activity of anticholinergic medications). Products include:

Hyland's Teething Tablets .... ▣766
Urimax Tablets 1769

Benztropine Mesylate (Donepezil, a cholinesterase inhibitor, has the potential to interfere with the activity of anticholinergic medications). Products include:

Cogentin 2055

Bethanechol Chloride (Potential for synergistic effect). Products include:

Urecholine 2198
Urecholine Tablets 2445

Biperiden Hydrochloride (Donepezil, a cholinesterase inhibitor, has the potential to interfere with the activity of anticholinergic medications). Products include:

Akineton 402

Carbamazepine (Inducers of CYP2D6 and CYP3A4, such as carbamazepine, could increase the rate of elimination of donepezil). Products include:

Carbatrol Capsules 3234
Tegretol/Tegretol-XR 2404

Celecoxib (Cholinesterase inhibitors, such as donepezil, may be expected to increase gastric acid secretion due to increased cholinergic activity, therefore, patients on concurrent NSAID therapy should be monitored closely for increased risk of developing ulcers or symptoms of active or occult gastrointestinal bleeding). Products include:

Celebrex Capsules 2676
Celebrex Capsules 2780

Clidinium Bromide (Donepezil, a cholinesterase inhibitor, has the potential to interfere with the activity of anticholinergic medications).

No products indexed under this heading.

Dexamethasone (Inducers of CYP2D6 and CYP3A4, such as dexamethasone, could increase the rate of elimination of donepezil). Products include:

Decadron Elixir 2078
Decadron Tablets 2079
TobraDex Ophthalmic Ointment 542
TobraDex Ophthalmic Suspension 541

Dexamethasone Acetate (Inducers of CYP2D6 and CYP3A4, such as dexamethasone, could increase the rate of elimination of donepezil).

No products indexed under this heading.

Dexamethasone Sodium Phosphate (Inducers of CYP2D6 and CYP3A4, such as dexamethasone, could increase the rate of elimination of donepezil). Products include:

Decadron Phosphate Injection 2081
Decadron Phosphate Sterile Ophthalmic Ointment 2083
Decadron Phosphate Sterile Ophthalmic Solution 2084
NeoDecadron Sterile Ophthalmic Solution 2144

Diclofenac Potassium (Cholinesterase inhibitors, such as donepezil, may be expected to increase gastric acid secretion due to increased cholinergic activity, therefore, patients on concurrent NSAID therapy should be monitored closely for increased risk of developing ulcers or symptoms of active or occult gastrointestinal bleeding). Products include:

Cataflam Tablets 2315

Diclofenac Sodium (Cholinesterase inhibitors, such as donepezil, may be expected to increase gastric acid secretion due to increased cholinergic activity, therefore, patients on concurrent NSAID therapy should be monitored closely for increased risk of developing ulcers or symptoms of active or occult gastrointestinal bleeding). Products include:

Arthrotec Tablets 3195
Voltaren Ophthalmic Sterile Ophthalmic Solution .... ⊙312
Voltaren Tablets 2315
Voltaren-XR Tablets 2315

Dicyclomine Hydrochloride (Donepezil, a cholinesterase inhibitor, has the potential to interfere with the activity of anticholinergic medications).

No products indexed under this heading.

Etodolac (Cholinesterase inhibitors, such as donepezil, may be expected to increase gastric acid secretion due to increased cholinergic activity, therefore, patients on concurrent NSAID therapy should be monitored closely for increased risk of developing ulcers or symptoms of active or occult gastrointestinal bleeding). Products include:

Lodine 3528
Lodine XL Extended-Release Tablets 3530

Fenoprofen Calcium (Cholinesterase inhibitors, such as donepezil, may be expected to increase gastric acid secretion due to increased cholinergic activity, therefore, patients on concurrent NSAID therapy should be monitored closely for increased risk of developing ulcers or symptoms of active or occult gastrointestinal bleeding).

No products indexed under this heading.

Flurbiprofen (Cholinesterase inhibitors, such as donepezil, may be expected to increase gastric acid secretion due to increased cholinergic activity, therefore, patients on concurrent NSAID therapy should be monitored closely for increased risk of developing ulcers or symptoms of active or occult gastrointestinal bleeding).

No products indexed under this heading.

Fosphenytoin Sodium (Inducers of CYP2D6 and CYP3A4, such as phenytoin, could increase the rate of elimination of donepezil). Products include:

Cerebyx Injection 2619

Glycopyrrolate (Donepezil, a cholinesterase inhibitor, has the potential to interfere with the activity of anticholinergic medications). Products include:

Robinul Forte Tablets 1358
Robinul Injectable 2940
Robinul Tablets 1358

Hyoscyamine (Donepezil, a cholinesterase inhibitor, has the potential to interfere with the activity of anticholinergic medications). Products include:

Urised Tablets 2876

Hyoscyamine Sulfate (Donepezil, a cholinesterase inhibitor, has the potential to interfere with the activity of anticholinergic medications). Products include:

Arco-Lase Plus Tablets 592
Donnatal 2929
Donnatal Extentabs 2930
Levsin/Levsinex/Levbid 3172
NuLev Orally Disintegrating Tablets 3176
Prosed/DS Tablets 3268
Urimax Tablets 1769

Ibuprofen (Cholinesterase inhibitors, such as donepezil, may be expected to increase gastric acid secretion due to increased cholinergic activity, therefore, patients on concurrent NSAID therapy should be monitored closely for increased risk of developing ulcers or symptoms of active or occult gastrointestinal bleeding). Products include:

Advil .... ▣771
Children's Advil Oral Suspension .... ▣773
Children's Advil Chewable Tablets .... ▣773
Advil Cold and Sinus Caplets .... ▣771
Advil Cold and Sinus Tablets .... ▣771
Advil Flu & Body Ache Caplets .... ▣772
Infants' Advil Drops .... ▣773
Junior Strength Advil Tablets .... ▣773
Junior Strength Advil Chewable Tablets .... ▣773
Advil Migraine Liquigels .... ▣772
Children's Motrin Oral Suspension and Chewable Tablets 2006
Children's Motrin Cold Oral Suspension 2007
Children's Motrin Oral Suspension .... ▣643
Motrin Suspension, Oral Drops, Chewable Tablets, and Caplets 2002
Infants' Motrin Concentrated Drops 2006
Junior Strength Motrin Caplets and Chewable Tablets 2006
Motrin IB Tablets, Caplets, and Gelcaps 2002
Motrin Migraine Pain Caplets 2005
Motrin Sinus Headache Caplets 2005
Vicoprofen Tablets 520

Indomethacin (Cholinesterase inhibitors, such as donepezil, may be expected to increase gastric acid secretion due to increased cholinergic activity, therefore, patients on concurrent NSAID therapy should be monitored closely for increased risk of developing ulcers or symptoms of active or occult gastrointestinal bleeding). Products include:

Indocin 2112

Indomethacin Sodium Trihydrate (Cholinesterase inhibitors, such as donepezil, may be expected to increase gastric acid secretion due to increased cholinergic activity, therefore, patients on concurrent NSAID therapy should be monitored closely for increased risk of developing ulcers or symptoms of active or occult gastrointestinal bleeding). Products include:

Indocin I.V. 2115

Ipratropium Bromide (Donepezil, a cholinesterase inhibitor, has the potential to interfere with the activity of anticholinergic medications). Products include:

Atrovent Inhalation Aerosol 1030
Atrovent Inhalation Solution 1031
Atrovent Nasal Spray 0.03% 1032
Atrovent Nasal Spray 0.06% 1033
Combivent Inhalation Aerosol 1041
DuoNeb Inhalation Solution 1233

Ketoconazole (Inhibitors of CYP450, 2D6 and 3A4, such as ketoconazole, inhibit donepezil metabolism in vitro). Products include:

Nizoral 2% Cream 3620
Nizoral A-D Shampoo 2008
Nizoral 2% Shampoo 2007
Nizoral Tablets 1791

Ketoprofen (Cholinesterase inhibitors, such as donepezil, may be expected to increase gastric acid secretion due to increased cholinergic activity, therefore, patients on concurrent NSAID therapy should be monitored closely for increased risk of developing ulcers or symptoms of active or occult gastrointestinal bleeding). Products include:

Orudis Capsules 3548
Orudis KT Tablets .... ▣778
Oruvail Capsules 3548

Ketorolac Tromethamine (Cholinesterase inhibitors, such as donepezil, may be expected to increase gastric acid secretion due to increased cholinergic activity, therefore, patients on concurrent NSAID therapy should be monitored closely for increased risk of developing ulcers or symptoms of active or occult gastrointestinal bleeding). Products include:

Acular Ophthalmic Solution 544
Acular PF Ophthalmic Solution 544
Toradol 3018

Meclofenamate Sodium (Cholinesterase inhibitors, such as donepezil, may be expected to increase gastric acid secretion due to increased cholinergic activity, therefore, patients on concurrent NSAID therapy should be monitored closely for increased risk of developing ulcers or symptoms of active or occult gastrointestinal bleeding).

No products indexed under this heading.

Mefenamic Acid (Cholinesterase inhibitors, such as donepezil, may be expected to increase gastric acid secretion due to increased cholinergic activity, therefore, patients on concurrent NSAID therapy should be monitored closely for increased risk of developing ulcers or symptoms of active or occult gastrointestinal bleeding). Products include:

Ponstel Capsules 1356

Meloxicam (Cholinesterase inhibitors, such as donepezil, may be expected to increase gastric acid secretion due to increased cholinergic activity, therefore, patients on concurrent NSAID therapy should be monitored closely for increased risk of developing ulcers or symptoms of active or occult gastrointestinal bleeding). Products include:

Mobic Tablets 1054

Mepenzolate Bromide (Donepezil, a cholinesterase inhibitor, has the

potential to interfere with the activity of anticholinergic medications).

No products indexed under this heading.

Nabumetone (Cholinesterase inhibitors, such as donepezil, may be expected to increase gastric acid secretion due to increased cholinergic activity, therefore, patients on concurrent NSAID therapy should be monitored closely for increased risk of developing ulcers or symptoms of active or occult gastrointestinal bleeding). Products include:

Relafen Tablets 1617

Naproxen (Cholinesterase inhibitors, such as donepezil, may be expected to increase gastric acid secretion due to increased cholinergic activity, therefore, patients on concurrent NSAID therapy should be monitored closely for increased risk of developing ulcers or symptoms of active or occult gastrointestinal bleeding). Products include:

EC-Naprosyn Delayed-Release Tablets........ 2967
Naprosyn Suspension 2967
Naprosyn Tablets 2967

Naproxen Sodium (Cholinesterase inhibitors, such as donepezil, may be expected to increase gastric acid secretion due to increased cholinergic activity, therefore, patients on concurrent NSAID therapy should be monitored closely for increased risk of developing ulcers or symptoms of active or occult gastrointestinal bleeding). Products include:

Aleve Tablets, Caplets and Gelcaps........ ▣602
Aleve Cold & Sinus Caplets .... ▣603
Anaprox Tablets 2967
Anaprox DS Tablets 2967
Naprelan Tablets 1293

Oxaprozin (Cholinesterase inhibitors, such as donepezil, may be expected to increase gastric acid secretion due to increased cholinergic activity, therefore, patients on concurrent NSAID therapy should be monitored closely for increased risk of developing ulcers or symptoms of active or occult gastrointestinal bleeding).

No products indexed under this heading.

Oxybutynin Chloride (Donepezil, a cholinesterase inhibitor, has the potential to interfere with the activity of anticholinergic medications). Products include:

Ditropan XL Extended Release Tablets........ 564

Phenobarbital (Inducers of CYP2D6 and CYP3A4, such as phenobarbital, could increase the rate of elimination of donepezil). Products include:

Arco-Lase Plus Tablets 592
Donnatal 2929
Donnatal Extentabs 2930

Phenylbutazone (Cholinesterase inhibitors, such as donepezil, may be expected to increase gastric acid secretion due to increased cholinergic activity, therefore, patients on concurrent NSAID therapy should be monitored closely for increased risk of developing ulcers or symptoms of active or occult gastrointestinal bleeding).

No products indexed under this heading.

Phenytoin (Inducers of CYP2D6 and CYP3A4, such as phenytoin, could increase the rate of elimination of donepezil). Products include:

Dilantin Infatabs 2624
Dilantin-125 Oral Suspension 2625

Phenytoin Sodium (Inducers of CYP2D6 and CYP3A4, such as phenytoin, could increase the rate of elimination of donepezil). Products include:

Dilantin Kapseals 2622

Piroxicam (Cholinesterase inhibitors, such as donepezil, may be expected to increase gastric acid secretion due to increased cholinergic activity, therefore, patients on concurrent NSAID therapy should be monitored closely for increased risk of developing ulcers or symptoms of active or occult gastrointestinal bleeding). Products include:

Feldene Capsules 2685

Procyclidine Hydrochloride (Donepezil, a cholinesterase inhibitor, has the potential to interfere with the activity of anticholinergic medications).

No products indexed under this heading.

Propantheline Bromide (Donepezil, a cholinesterase inhibitor, has the potential to interfere with the activity of anticholinergic medications).

No products indexed under this heading.

Quinidine Gluconate (Inhibitors of CYP450, 2D6 and 3A4, such as quinidine, inhibit donepezil metabolism in vitro). Products include:

Quinaglute Dura-Tabs Tablets 978

Quinidine Polygalacturonate (Inhibitors of CYP450, 2D6 and 3A4, such as quinidine, inhibit donepezil metabolism in vitro).

No products indexed under this heading.

Quinidine Sulfate (Inhibitors of CYP450, 2D6 and 3A4, such as quinidine, inhibit donepezil metabolism in vitro). Products include:

Quinidex Extentabs 2933

Rifampin (Inducers of CYP2D6 and CYP3A4, such as rifampin, could increase the rate of elimination of donepezil). Products include:

Rifadin 765
Rifamate Capsules 767
Rifater Tablets 769

Rofecoxib (Cholinesterase inhibitors, such as donepezil, may be expected to increase gastric acid secretion due to increased cholinergic activity, therefore, patients on concurrent NSAID therapy should be monitored closely for increased risk of developing ulcers or symptoms of active or occult gastrointestinal bleeding). Products include:

Vioxx 2213

Scopolamine (Donepezil, a cholinesterase inhibitor, has the potential to interfere with the activity of anticholinergic medications). Products include:

Transderm Scōp Transdermal Therapeutic System........ 2302

Scopolamine Hydrobromide (Donepezil, a cholinesterase inhibitor, has the potential to interfere with the activity of anticholinergic medications). Products include:

Donnatal 2929
Donnatal Extentabs 2930

Succinylcholine Chloride (Potential for synergistic effect). Products include:

Anectine Injection 1476

Sulindac (Cholinesterase inhibitors, such as donepezil, may be expected to increase gastric acid secretion due to increased cholinergic activity, therefore, patients on concurrent NSAID therapy should be monitored closely for increased risk of developing ulcers or symptoms of active or occult gastrointestinal bleeding). Products include:

Clinoril Tablets 2053

Tolmetin Sodium (Cholinesterase inhibitors, such as donepezil, may be expected to increase gastric acid secretion due to increased cholinergic activity, therefore, patients on concurrent NSAID therapy should be monitored closely for increased risk of developing ulcers or symptoms of active or occult gastrointestinal bleeding). Products include:

Tolectin 2589

Tolterodine Tartrate (Donepezil, a cholinesterase inhibitor, has the potential to interfere with the activity of anticholinergic medications). Products include:

Detrol Tablets 3623
Detrol LA Capsules 2801

Tridihexethyl Chloride (Donepezil, a cholinesterase inhibitor, has the potential to interfere with the activity of anticholinergic medications).

No products indexed under this heading.

Trihexyphenidyl Hydrochloride (Donepezil, a cholinesterase inhibitor, has the potential to interfere with the activity of anticholinergic medications). Products include:

Artane 1855

ARICEPT TABLETS

(Donepezil Hydrochloride) 1270

May interact with anticholinergics, dexamethasone, non-steroidal anti-inflammatory agents, phenytoin, quinidine, and certain other agents. Compounds in these categories include:

Atropine Sulfate (Donepezil, a cholinesterase inhibitor, has the potential to interfere with the activity of anticholinergic medications). Products include:

Donnatal 2929
Donnatal Extentabs 2930
Motofen Tablets 577
Prosed/DS Tablets 3268
Urised Tablets 2876

Belladonna Alkaloids (Donepezil, a cholinesterase inhibitor, has the potential to interfere with the activity of anticholinergic medications). Products include:

Hyland's Teething Tablets .... ▣766
Urimax Tablets 1769

Benztropine Mesylate (Donepezil, a cholinesterase inhibitor, has the potential to interfere with the activity of anticholinergic medications). Products include:

Cogentin 2055

Bethanechol Chloride (Potential for synergistic effect). Products include:

Urecholine 2198
Urecholine Tablets 2445

Biperiden Hydrochloride (Donepezil, a cholinesterase inhibitor, has the potential to interfere with the activity of anticholinergic medications). Products include:

Akineton 402

Carbamazepine (Inducers of CYP2D6 and CYP3A4, such as carbamazepine, could increase the rate of elimination of donepezil). Products include:

Carbatrol Capsules 3234
Tegretol/Tegretol-XR 2404

Celecoxib (Cholinesterase inhibitors, such as donepezil, may be expected to increase gastric acid secretion due to increased cholinergic activity, therefore, patients on concurrent NSAID therapy should be monitored closely for increased risk of developing ulcers or symptoms of active or occult gastrointestinal bleeding). Products include:

Celebrex Capsules 2676
Celebrex Capsules 2780

Clidinium Bromide (Donepezil, a cholinesterase inhibitor, has the potential to interfere with the activity of anticholinergic medications).

No products indexed under this heading.

Dexamethasone (Inducers of CYP2D6 and CYP3A4, such as dexamethasone, could increase the rate of elimination of donepezil). Products include:

Decadron Elixir 2078
Decadron Tablets 2079
TobraDex Ophthalmic Ointment 542
TobraDex Ophthalmic Suspension 541

Dexamethasone Acetate (Inducers of CYP2D6 and CYP3A4, such as dexamethasone, could increase the rate of elimination of donepezil).

No products indexed under this heading.

Dexamethasone Sodium Phosphate (Inducers of CYP2D6 and CYP3A4, such as dexamethasone, could increase the rate of elimination of donepezil). Products include:

Decadron Phosphate Injection 2081
Decadron Phosphate Sterile Ophthalmic Ointment........ 2083
Decadron Phosphate Sterile Ophthalmic Solution 2084
NeoDecadron Sterile Ophthalmic Solution........ 2144

Diclofenac Potassium (Cholinesterase inhibitors, such as donepezil, may be expected to increase gastric acid secretion due to increased cholinergic activity, therefore, patients on concurrent NSAID therapy should be monitored closely for increased risk of developing ulcers or symptoms of active or occult gastrointestinal bleeding). Products include:

Cataflam Tablets 2315

Diclofenac Sodium (Cholinesterase inhibitors, such as donepezil, may be expected to increase gastric acid secretion due to increased cholinergic activity, therefore, patients on concurrent NSAID therapy should be monitored closely for increased risk of developing ulcers or symptoms of active or occult gastrointestinal bleeding). Products include:

Arthrotec Tablets 3195
Voltaren Ophthalmic Sterile Ophthalmic Solution........ ⊙312
Voltaren Tablets 2315
Voltaren-XR Tablets 2315

Dicyclomine Hydrochloride (Donepezil, a cholinesterase inhibitor, has the potential to interfere with the activity of anticholinergic medications).

No products indexed under this heading.

Etodolac (Cholinesterase inhibitors, such as donepezil, may be expected to increase gastric acid secretion due to increased cholinergic activity, therefore, patients on concurrent NSAID therapy should be monitored closely for increased risk of developing ulcers or symptoms of active or occult gastrointestinal bleeding). Products include:

Lodine 3528
Lodine XL Extended-Release Tablets........ 3530

Fenoprofen Calcium (Cholinesterase inhibitors, such as donepezil, may be expected to increase gastric acid secretion due to increased cholinergic activity, therefore, patients on concurrent NSAID therapy should be monitored closely for increased risk of developing ulcers or symptoms of active or occult gastrointestinal bleeding).

No products indexed under this heading.

Flurbiprofen (Cholinesterase inhibitors, such as donepezil, may be expected to increase gastric acid secretion due to increased cholinergic activity, therefore, patients on concurrent NSAID therapy should be monitored closely for increased risk of developing ulcers or symptoms of active or occult gastrointestinal bleeding).

No products indexed under this heading.

Fosphenytoin Sodium (Inducers of CYP2D6 and CYP3A4, such as phenytoin, could increase the rate of elimination of donepezil). Products include:

Cerebyx Injection 2619

Glycopyrrolate (Donepezil, a cholinesterase inhibitor, has the potential to interfere with the activity of anticholinergic medications). Products include:

Robinul Forte Tablets 1358
Robinul Injectable 2940
Robinul Tablets 1358

Hyoscyamine (Donepezil, a cholinesterase inhibitor, has the potential to interfere with the activity of anticholinergic medications). Products include:

Urised Tablets 2876

Hyoscyamine Sulfate (Donepezil, a cholinesterase inhibitor, has the potential to interfere with the activity of anticholinergic medications). Products include:

Arco-Lase Plus Tablets 592
Donnatal 2929
Donnatal Extentabs 2930
Levsin/Levsinex/Levbid 3172
NuLev Orally Disintegrating Tablets 3176
Prosed/DS Tablets 3268
Urimax Tablets 1769

Ibuprofen (Cholinesterase inhibitors, such as donepezil, may be expected to increase gastric acid secretion due to increased cholinergic activity, therefore, patients on concurrent NSAID therapy should be monitored closely for increased risk of developing ulcers or symptoms of active or occult gastrointestinal bleeding). Products include:

Advil 771
Children's Advil Oral Suspension 773
Children's Advil Chewable Tablets 773
Advil Cold and Sinus Caplets 771
Advil Cold and Sinus Tablets 771
Advil Flu & Body Ache Caplets 772
Infants' Advil Drops 773
Junior Strength Advil Tablets 773
Junior Strength Advil Chewable Tablets 773
Advil Migraine Liquigels 772
Children's Motrin Oral Suspension and Chewable Tablets 2006
Children's Motrin Cold Oral Suspension 2007
Children's Motrin Oral Suspension 643
Motrin Suspension, Oral Drops, Chewable Tablets, and Caplets 2002
Infants' Motrin Concentrated Drops 2006
Junior Strength Motrin Caplets and Chewable Tablets 2006
Motrin IB Tablets, Caplets, and Gelcaps 2002
Motrin Migraine Pain Caplets 2005
Motrin Sinus Headache Caplets 2005
Vicoprofen Tablets 520

Indomethacin (Cholinesterase inhibitors, such as donepezil, may be expected to increase gastric acid secretion due to increased cholinergic activity, therefore, patients on concurrent NSAID therapy should be monitored closely for increased risk of developing ulcers or symptoms of active or occult gastrointestinal bleeding). Products include:

Indocin 2112

Indomethacin Sodium Trihydrate (Cholinesterase inhibitors, such as donepezil, may be expected to increase gastric acid secretion due to increased cholinergic activity, therefore, patients on concurrent NSAID therapy should be monitored closely for increased risk of developing ulcers or symptoms of active or occult gastrointestinal bleeding). Products include:

Indocin I.V. 2115

Ipratropium Bromide (Donepezil, a cholinesterase inhibitor, has the potential to interfere with the activity of anticholinergic medications). Products include:

Atrovent Inhalation Aerosol 1030
Atrovent Inhalation Solution 1031
Atrovent Nasal Spray 0.03% 1032
Atrovent Nasal Spray 0.06% 1033
Combivent Inhalation Aerosol 1041
DuoNeb Inhalation Solution 1233

Ketoconazole (Inhibitors of CYP450, 2D6 and 3A4, such as ketoconazole, inhibit donepezil metabolism in vitro). Products include:

Nizoral 2% Cream 3620
Nizoral A-D Shampoo 2008
Nizoral 2% Shampoo 2007
Nizoral Tablets 1791

Ketoprofen (Cholinesterase inhibitors, such as donepezil, may be expected to increase gastric acid secretion due to increased cholinergic activity, therefore, patients on concurrent NSAID therapy should be monitored closely for increased risk of developing ulcers or symptoms of active or occult gastrointestinal bleeding). Products include:

Orudis Capsules 3548
Orudis KT Tablets 778
Oruvail Capsules 3548

Ketorolac Tromethamine (Cholinesterase inhibitors, such as donepezil, may be expected to increase gastric acid secretion due to increased cholinergic activity, therefore, patients on concurrent NSAID therapy should be monitored closely for increased risk of developing ulcers or symptoms of active or occult gastrointestinal bleeding). Products include:

Acular Ophthalmic Solution 544
Acular PF Ophthalmic Solution 544
Toradol 3018

Meclofenamate Sodium (Cholinesterase inhibitors, such as donepezil, may be expected to increase gastric acid secretion due to increased cholinergic activity, therefore, patients on concurrent NSAID therapy should be monitored closely for increased risk of developing ulcers or symptoms of active or occult gastrointestinal bleeding).

No products indexed under this heading.

Mefenamic Acid (Cholinesterase inhibitors, such as donepezil, may be expected to increase gastric acid secretion due to increased cholinergic activity, therefore, patients on concurrent NSAID therapy should be monitored closely for increased risk of developing ulcers or symptoms of active or occult gastrointestinal bleeding). Products include:

Ponstel Capsules 1356

Meloxicam (Cholinesterase inhibitors, such as donepezil, may be expected to increase gastric acid secretion due to increased cholinergic activity, therefore, patients on concurrent NSAID therapy should be monitored closely for increased risk of developing ulcers or symptoms of active or occult gastrointestinal bleeding). Products include:

Mobic Tablets 1054

Mepenzolate Bromide (Donepezil, a cholinesterase inhibitor, has the potential to interfere with the activity of anticholinergic medications).

No products indexed under this heading.

Nabumetone (Cholinesterase inhibitors, such as donepezil, may be expected to increase gastric acid secretion due to increased cholinergic activity, therefore, patients on concurrent NSAID therapy should be monitored closely for increased risk of developing ulcers or symptoms of active or occult gastrointestinal bleeding). Products include:

Relafen Tablets 1617

Naproxen (Cholinesterase inhibitors, such as donepezil, may be expected to increase gastric acid secretion due to increased cholinergic activity, therefore, patients on concurrent NSAID therapy should be monitored closely for increased risk of developing ulcers or symptoms of active or occult gastrointestinal bleeding). Products include:

EC-Naprosyn Delayed-Release Tablets 2967
Naprosyn Suspension 2967
Naprosyn Tablets 2967

Naproxen Sodium (Cholinesterase inhibitors, such as donepezil, may be expected to increase gastric acid secretion due to increased cholinergic activity, therefore, patients on concurrent NSAID therapy should be monitored closely for increased risk of developing ulcers or symptoms of active or occult gastrointestinal bleeding). Products include:

Aleve Tablets, Caplets and Gelcaps 602
Aleve Cold & Sinus Caplets 603
Anaprox Tablets 2967
Anaprox DS Tablets 2967
Naprelan Tablets 1293

Oxaprozin (Cholinesterase inhibitors, such as donepezil, may be expected to increase gastric acid secretion due to increased cholinergic activity, therefore, patients on concurrent NSAID therapy should be monitored closely for increased risk of developing ulcers or symptoms of active or occult gastrointestinal bleeding).

No products indexed under this heading.

Oxybutynin Chloride (Donepezil, a cholinesterase inhibitor, has the potential to interfere with the activity of anticholinergic medications). Products include:

Ditropan XL Extended Release Tablets 564

Phenobarbital (Inducers of CYP2D6 and CYP3A4, such as phenobarbital, could increase the rate of elimination of donepezil). Products include:

Arco-Lase Plus Tablets 592
Donnatal 2929
Donnatal Extentabs 2930

Phenylbutazone (Cholinesterase inhibitors, such as donepezil, may be expected to increase gastric acid secretion due to increased cholinergic activity, therefore, patients on concurrent NSAID therapy should be monitored closely for increased risk of developing ulcers or symptoms of active or occult gastrointestinal bleeding).

No products indexed under this heading.

Phenytoin (Inducers of CYP2D6 and CYP3A4, such as phenytoin, could increase the rate of elimination of donepezil). Products include:

Dilantin Infatabs 2624
Dilantin-125 Oral Suspension 2625

Phenytoin Sodium (Inducers of CYP2D6 and CYP3A4, such as phenytoin, could increase the rate of elimination of donepezil). Products include:

Dilantin Kapseals 2622

Piroxicam (Cholinesterase inhibitors, such as donepezil, may be expected to increase gastric acid secretion due to increased cholinergic activity, therefore, patients on concurrent NSAID therapy should be monitored closely for increased risk of developing ulcers or symptoms of active or occult gastrointestinal bleeding). Products include:

Feldene Capsules 2685

Procyclidine Hydrochloride (Donepezil, a cholinesterase inhibitor, has the potential to interfere with the activity of anticholinergic medications).

No products indexed under this heading.

Propantheline Bromide (Donepezil, a cholinesterase inhibitor, has the potential to interfere with the activity of anticholinergic medications).

No products indexed under this heading.

Quinidine Gluconate (Inhibitors of CYP450, 2D6 and 3A4, such as quinidine, inhibit donepezil metabolism in vitro). Products include:

Quinaglute Dura-Tabs Tablets 978

Quinidine Polygalacturonate (Inhibitors of CYP450, 2D6 and 3A4, such as quinidine, inhibit donepezil metabolism in vitro).

No products indexed under this heading.

Quinidine Sulfate (Inhibitors of CYP450, 2D6 and 3A4, such as quinidine, inhibit donepezil metabolism in vitro). Products include:

Quinidex Extentabs 2933

Rifampin (Inducers of CYP2D6 and CYP3A4, such as rifampin, could increase the rate of elimination of donepezil). Products include:

Rifadin 765
Rifamate Capsules 767
Rifater Tablets 769

Rofecoxib (Cholinesterase inhibitors, such as donepezil, may be expected to increase gastric acid secretion due to increased cholinergic activity, therefore, patients on concurrent NSAID therapy should be monitored closely for increased risk of developing ulcers or symptoms of active or occult gastrointestinal bleeding). Products include:

Vioxx 2213

Scopolamine (Donepezil, a cholinesterase inhibitor, has the potential to interfere with the activity of anticholinergic medications). Products include:

Transderm Scōp Transdermal Therapeutic System 2302

Scopolamine Hydrobromide (Donepezil, a cholinesterase inhibitor, has the potential to interfere with the activity of anticholinergic medications). Products include:

Donnatal 2929
Donnatal Extentabs 2930

Succinylcholine Chloride (Potential for synergistic effect). Products include:

Anectine Injection 1476

Sulindac (Cholinesterase inhibitors, such as donepezil, may be expected to increase gastric acid secretion due to increased cholinergic activity, therefore, patients on concurrent NSAID therapy should be monitored closely for increased risk of developing ulcers or symptoms of active or occult gastrointestinal bleeding). Products include:

Clinoril Tablets 2053

Tolmetin Sodium (Cholinesterase inhibitors, such as donepezil, may be expected to increase gastric acid secretion due to increased cholinergic activity, therefore, patients on concurrent NSAID therapy should be monitored closely for increased risk of developing ulcers or symptoms of active or occult gastrointestinal bleeding). Products include:

Tolectin 2589

Tolterodine Tartrate (Donepezil, a cholinesterase inhibitor, has the potential to interfere with the activity of anticholinergic medications). Products include:

Detrol Tablets 3623
Detrol LA Capsules 2801

Tridihexethyl Chloride (Donepezil, a cholinesterase inhibitor, has the potential to interfere with the activity of anticholinergic medications).

No products indexed under this heading.

Trihexyphenidyl Hydrochloride (Donepezil, a cholinesterase inhibitor, has the potential to interfere with the activity of anticholinergic medications). Products include:

Artane 1855

ARIMIDEX TABLETS

(Anastrozole) 659
None cited in PDR database.

AROMASIN TABLETS

(Exemestane) 2769
May interact with phenytoin and certain other agents. Compounds in these categories include:

Carbamazepine (Exemestane is metabolized by CYP3A4; co-administration with known inducers of CYP3A4, such as carbamazepine, may result in possible decrease of exemestane plasma levels). Products include:
- Carbatrol Capsules 3234
- Tegretol/Tegretol-XR 2404

Fosphenytoin Sodium (Exemestane is metabolized by CYP3A4; co-administration with known inducers of CYP3A4, such as phenytoin, may result in possible decrease of exemestane plasma levels). Products include:
- Cerebyx Injection 2619

Phenobarbital (Exemestane is metabolized by CYP3A4; co-administration with known inducers of CYP3A4, such as phenobarbital, may result in possible decrease of exemestane plasma levels). Products include:
- Arco-Lase Plus Tablets 592
- Donnatal 2929
- Donnatal Extentabs 2930

Phenytoin (Exemestane is metabolized by CYP3A4; co-administration with known inducers of CYP3A4, such as phenytoin, may result in possible decrease of exemestane plasma levels). Products include:
- Dilantin Infatabs 2624
- Dilantin-125 Oral Suspension 2625

Phenytoin Sodium (Exemestane is metabolized by CYP3A4; co-administration with known inducers of CYP3A4, such as phenytoin, may result in possible decrease of exemestane plasma levels). Products include:
- Dilantin Kapseals 2622

Rifampin (Exemestane is metabolized by CYP3A4; co-administration with known inducers of CYP3A4, such as rifampin, may result in possible decrease of exemestane plasma levels). Products include:
- Rifadin 765
- Rifamate Capsules 767
- Rifater Tablets 769

Food Interactions

Food, unspecified (Exemestane plasma levels increased approximately 40% after high-fat breakfast).

ARTANE ELIXIR

(Trihexyphenidyl Hydrochloride) 1855
May interact with:

Levodopa (The usual dose of each may need to be reduced when used concomitantly). Products include:
- Sinemet Tablets 1253
- Sinemet CR Tablets 1255

ARTANE TABLETS

(Trihexyphenidyl Hydrochloride) 1855
See Artane Elixir

ARTHROTEC TABLETS

(Diclofenac Sodium, Misoprostol) 3195
May interact with antacids, antihypertensives, diuretics, oral hypoglycemic agents, insulin, lithium preparations, potassium sparing diuretics, and certain other agents. Compounds in these categories include:

Acarbose (Diclofenac may alter a diabetic patient's response to oral hypoglycemic agents; both hypo- and hyperglycemic effects have been reported). Products include:
- Precose Tablets 906

Acebutolol Hydrochloride (NSAIDs can inhibit the activity of antihypertensives). Products include:
- Sectral Capsules 3589

Aluminum Carbonate (Antacids reduce the bioavailability of misoprostol acid and may delay absorption of diclofenac).
No products indexed under this heading.

Aluminum Hydroxide (Antacids reduce the bioavailability of misoprostol acid and may delay absorption of diclofenac). Products include:
- Amphojel Suspension (Mint Flavor) .... ▣789
- Gaviscon Extra Strength Liquid .... ▣751
- Gaviscon Extra Strength Tablets .... ▣751
- Gaviscon Regular Strength Liquid .... ▣751
- Gaviscon Regular Strength Tablets .... ▣750
- Maalox Antacid/Anti-Gas Oral Suspension .... ▣673
- Maalox Max Maximum Strength Antacid/Anti-Gas Liquid 2300
- Maalox Regular Strength Antacid/Antigas Liquid 2300
- Mylanta 1813
- Vanquish Caplets .... ▣617

Amiloride Hydrochloride (Co-administration with potassium-sparing diuretics may be associated with increased serum potassium levels). Products include:
- Midamor Tablets 2136
- Moduretic Tablets 2138

Amlodipine Besylate (NSAIDs can inhibit the activity of antihypertensives). Products include:
- Lotrel Capsules 2370
- Norvasc Tablets 2704

Aspirin (Co-administration is not recommended because diclofenac sodium is displaced from its binding sites by aspirin resulting in lower plasma concentrations, peak plasma levels and AUC values). Products include:
- Aggrenox Capsules 1026
- Alka-Seltzer .... ▣603
- Alka-Seltzer Lemon Lime Antacid and Pain Reliever Effervescent Tablets .... ▣603
- Alka-Seltzer Extra Strength Antacid and Pain Reliever Effervescent Tablets .... ▣603
- Alka-Seltzer PM Effervescent Tablets .... ▣605
- Genuine Bayer Tablets, Caplets and Gelcaps .... ▣606
- Extra Strength Bayer Caplets and Gelcaps .... ▣610
- Aspirin Regimen Bayer Children's Chewable Tablets (Orange or Cherry Flavored) .... ▣607
- Bayer, Aspirin Regimen .... ▣606
- Aspirin Regimen Bayer 81 mg Caplets with Calcium .... ▣607
- Genuine Bayer Professional Labeling (Aspirin Regimen Bayer) .... ▣608
- Extra Strength Bayer Arthritis Caplets .... ▣610
- Extra Strength Bayer Plus Caplets .... ▣610
- Extra Strength Bayer PM Caplets .... ▣611
- BC Powder .... ▣619
- BC Allergy Sinus Cold Powder .... ▣619
- Arthritis Strength BC Powder .... ▣619
- BC Sinus Cold Powder .... ▣619
- Darvon Compound-65 Pulvules 1910
- Ecotrin Enteric Coated Aspirin Low, Regular and Maximum Strength Tablets 1715
- Excedrin Extra-Strength Tablets, Caplets, and Geltabs .... ▣629
- Excedrin Migraine 1070
- Goody's Body Pain Formula Powder .... ▣620
- Goody's Extra Strength Headache Powder .... ▣620
- Goody's Extra Strength Pain Relief Tablets .... ▣620
- Percodan Tablets 1327
- Robaxisal Tablets 2939
- Soma Compound Tablets 3354
- Soma Compound w/Codeine Tablets 3355
- Vanquish Caplets .... ▣617

Atenolol (NSAIDs can inhibit the activity of antihypertensives). Products include:
- Tenoretic Tablets 690
- Tenormin I.V. Injection 692

Benazepril Hydrochloride (NSAIDs can inhibit the activity of antihypertensives). Products include:
- Lotensin Tablets 2365
- Lotensin HCT Tablets 2367
- Lotrel Capsules 2370

Bendroflumethiazide (NSAIDs can inhibit the activity of diuretics). Products include:
- Corzide 40/5 Tablets 2247
- Corzide 80/5 Tablets 2247

Betaxolol Hydrochloride (NSAIDs can inhibit the activity of antihypertensives). Products include:
- Betoptic S Ophthalmic Suspension 537

Bisoprolol Fumarate (NSAIDs can inhibit the activity of antihypertensives). Products include:
- Zebeta Tablets 1885
- Ziac Tablets 1887

Bumetanide (NSAIDs can inhibit the activity of diuretics).
No products indexed under this heading.

Candesartan Cilexetil (NSAIDs can inhibit the activity of antihypertensives). Products include:
- Atacand Tablets 595
- Atacand HCT Tablets 597

Captopril (NSAIDs can inhibit the activity of antihypertensives). Products include:
- Captopril Tablets 2281

Carteolol Hydrochloride (NSAIDs can inhibit the activity of antihypertensives). Products include:
- Carteolol Hydrochloride Ophthalmic Solution USP, 1% .... ⊙258
- Ocupress Ophthalmic Solution, 1% Sterile .... ⊙303

Chlorothiazide (NSAIDs can inhibit the activity of diuretics). Products include:
- Aldoclor Tablets 2035
- Diuril Oral 2087

Chlorothiazide Sodium (NSAIDs can inhibit the activity of diuretics). Products include:
- Diuril Sodium Intravenous 2086

Chlorpropamide (Diclofenac may alter a diabetic patient's response to oral hypoglycemic agents; both hypo- and hyperglycemic effects have been reported). Products include:
- Diabinese Tablets 2680

Chlorthalidone (NSAIDs can inhibit the activity of diuretics). Products include:
- Clorpres Tablets 1002
- Combipres Tablets 1040
- Tenoretic Tablets 690

Clonidine (NSAIDs can inhibit the activity of antihypertensives). Products include:
- Catapres-TTS 1038

Clonidine Hydrochloride (NSAIDs can inhibit the activity of antihypertensives). Products include:
- Catapres Tablets 1037
- Clorpres Tablets 1002
- Combipres Tablets 1040
- Duraclon Injection 3057

Cyclosporine (NSAIDs may affect renal prostaglandins and increase the toxicity of certain drugs, including cyclosporine; potential for increased cyclosporine-induced nephrotoxicity). Products include:
- Gengraf Capsules 457
- Neoral Soft Gelatin Capsules 2380
- Neoral Oral Solution 2380
- Sandimmune 2388

Deserpidine (NSAIDs can inhibit the activity of antihypertensives).
No products indexed under this heading.

Diazoxide (NSAIDs can inhibit the activity of antihypertensives).
No products indexed under this heading.

Digoxin (Co-administration of digoxin with diclofenac has resulted in elevated digoxin levels). Products include:
- Digitek Tablets 1003
- Lanoxicaps Capsules 1574
- Lanoxin Injection 1581
- Lanoxin Tablets 1587
- Lanoxin Elixir Pediatric 1578
- Lanoxin Injection Pediatric 1584

Diltiazem Hydrochloride (NSAIDs can inhibit the activity of antihypertensives). Products include:
- Cardizem Injectable 1018
- Cardizem Lyo-Ject Syringe 1018
- Cardizem Monovial 1018
- Cardizem CD Capsules 1016
- Tiazac Capsules 1378

Doxazosin Mesylate (NSAIDs can inhibit the activity of antihypertensives). Products include:
- Cardura Tablets 2668

Enalapril Maleate (NSAIDs can inhibit the activity of antihypertensives). Products include:
- Lexxel Tablets 608
- Vaseretic Tablets 2204
- Vasotec Tablets 2210

Enalaprilat (NSAIDs can inhibit the activity of antihypertensives). Products include:
- Enalaprilat Injection 863
- Vasotec I.V. Injection 2207

Eprosartan Mesylate (NSAIDs can inhibit the activity of antihypertensives). Products include:
- Teveten Tablets 3327

Esmolol Hydrochloride (NSAIDs can inhibit the activity of antihypertensives). Products include:
- Brevibloc Injection 858

Ethacrynic Acid (NSAIDs can inhibit the activity of diuretics). Products include:
- Edecrin Tablets 2091

Felodipine (NSAIDs can inhibit the activity of antihypertensives). Products include:
- Lexxel Tablets 608
- Plendil Extended-Release Tablets 623

Fosinopril Sodium (NSAIDs can inhibit the activity of antihypertensives). Products include:
- Monopril Tablets 1091
- Monopril HCT 1094

Furosemide (NSAIDs can inhibit the activity of diuretics). Products include:
- Furosemide Tablets 2284

Glimepiride (Diclofenac may alter a diabetic patient's response to oral hypoglycemic agents; both hypo- and hyperglycemic effects have been reported). Products include:
- Amaryl Tablets 717

Glipizide (Diclofenac may alter a diabetic patient's response to oral hypoglycemic agents; both hypo- and hyperglycemic effects have been reported). Products include:
- Glucotrol Tablets 2692
- Glucotrol XL Extended Release Tablets 2693

Glyburide (Diclofenac may alter a diabetic patient's response to oral hypoglycemic agents; both hypo- and hyperglycemic effects have been reported). Products include:
- DiaBeta Tablets 741
- Glucovance Tablets 1086

Guanabenz Acetate (NSAIDs can inhibit the activity of antihypertensives).
No products indexed under this heading.

Guanethidine Monosulfate (NSAIDs can inhibit the activity of antihypertensives).
No products indexed under this heading.

Hydralazine Hydrochloride (NSAIDs can inhibit the activity of antihypertensives).
No products indexed under this heading.

Hydrochlorothiazide (NSAIDs can inhibit the activity of diuretics). Products include:
- Accuretic Tablets ... 2614
- Aldoril Tablets ... 2039
- Atacand HCT Tablets ... 597
- Avalide Tablets ... 1070
- Diovan HCT Tablets ... 2338
- Dyazide Capsules ... 1515
- HydroDIURIL Tablets ... 2108
- Hyzaar ... 2109
- Inderide Tablets ... 3517
- Inderide LA Long-Acting Capsules .. 3519
- Lotensin HCT Tablets ... 2367
- Maxzide ... 1008
- Micardis HCT Tablets ... 1051
- Microzide Capsules ... 3414
- Moduretic Tablets ... 2138
- Monopril HCT ... 1094
- Prinzide Tablets ... 2168
- Timolide Tablets ... 2187
- Uniretic Tablets ... 3178
- Vaseretic Tablets ... 2204
- Zestoretic Tablets ... 695
- Ziac Tablets ... 1887

Hydroflumethiazide (NSAIDs can inhibit the activity of diuretics). Products include:
- Diucardin Tablets ... 3494

Indapamide (NSAIDs can inhibit the activity of diuretics). Products include:
- Indapamide Tablets ... 2286

Insulin, Human, Zinc Suspension (Diclofenac may alter a diabetic patient's response to insulin; both hypo- and hyperglycemic effects have been reported). Products include:
- Humulin L, 100 Units ... 1937
- Humulin U, 100 Units ... 1943
- Novolin L Human Insulin 10 ml Vials ... 2422

Insulin, Human NPH (Diclofenac may alter a diabetic patient's response to insulin; both hypo- and hyperglycemic effects have been reported). Products include:
- Humulin N, 100 Units ... 1939
- Humulin N NPH Pen ... 1940
- Novolin N Human Insulin 10 ml Vials ... 2422
- Novolin N PenFill ... 2423
- Novolin N Prefilled Syringe Disposable Insulin Delivery System ... 2425

Insulin, Human Regular (Diclofenac may alter a diabetic patient's response to insulin; both hypo- and hyperglycemic effects have been reported). Products include:
- Humulin R Regular (U-500) ... 1943
- Humulin R, 100 Units ... 1941
- Novolin R Human Insulin 10 ml Vials ... 2423
- Novolin R PenFill ... 2423
- Novolin R Prefilled Syringe Disposable Insulin Delivery System ... 2425
- Velosulin BR Human Insulin 10 ml Vials ... 2435

Insulin, Human Regular and Human NPH Mixture (Diclofenac may alter a diabetic patient's response to insulin; both hypo- and hyperglycemic effects have been reported). Products include:
- Humulin 50/50, 100 Units ... 1934
- Humulin 70/30, 100 Units ... 1935
- Humulin 70/30 Pen ... 1936
- Novolin 70/30 Human Insulin 10 ml Vials ... 2421
- Novolin 70/30 PenFill ... 2423
- Novolin 70/30 Prefilled Disposable Insulin Delivery System ... 2425

Insulin, NPH (Diclofenac may alter a diabetic patient's response to insulin; both hypo- and hyperglycemic effects have been reported). Products include:
- Iletin II, NPH (Pork), 100 Units ... 1946

Insulin, Regular (Diclofenac may alter a diabetic patient's response to insulin; both hypo- and hyperglycemic effects have been reported). Products include:
- Iletin II, Regular (Pork), 100 Units ... 1947

Insulin, Zinc Crystals (Diclofenac may alter a diabetic patient's response to insulin; both hypo- and hyperglycemic effects have been reported).
No products indexed under this heading.

Insulin, Zinc Suspension (Diclofenac may alter a diabetic patient's response to insulin; both hypo- and hyperglycemic effects have been reported). Products include:
- Iletin II, Lente (Pork), 100 Units ... 1945

Insulin Aspart, Human Regular (Diclofenac may alter a diabetic patient's response to insulin; both hypo- and hyperglycemic effects have been reported).
No products indexed under this heading.

Insulin glargine (Diclofenac may alter a diabetic patient's response to insulin; both hypo- and hyperglycemic effects have been reported). Products include:
- Lantus Injection ... 742

Insulin Lispro, Human (Diclofenac may alter a diabetic patient's response to insulin; both hypo- and hyperglycemic effects have been reported). Products include:
- Humalog ... 1926
- Humalog Mix 75/25 Pen ... 1928

Insulin Lispro Protamine, Human (Diclofenac may alter a diabetic patient's response to insulin; both hypo- and hyperglycemic effects have been reported). Products include:
- Humalog Mix 75/25 Pen ... 1928

Irbesartan (NSAIDs can inhibit the activity of antihypertensives). Products include:
- Avalide Tablets ... 1070
- Avapro Tablets ... 1074
- Avapro Tablets ... 3076

Isradipine (NSAIDs can inhibit the activity of antihypertensives). Products include:
- DynaCirc Capsules ... 2921
- DynaCirc CR Tablets ... 2923

Labetalol Hydrochloride (NSAIDs can inhibit the activity of antihypertensives). Products include:
- Normodyne Injection ... 3135
- Normodyne Tablets ... 3137

Lisinopril (NSAIDs can inhibit the activity of antihypertensives). Products include:
- Prinivil Tablets ... 2164
- Prinzide Tablets ... 2168
- Zestoretic Tablets ... 695
- Zestril Tablets ... 698

Lithium Carbonate (NSAIDs have produced an elevation of plasma lithium levels and a reduction in renal lithium clearance). Products include:
- Eskalith ... 1527
- Lithium Carbonate ... 3061
- Lithobid Slow-Release Tablets ... 3255

Lithium Citrate (NSAIDs have produced an elevation of plasma lithium levels and a reduction in renal lithium clearance). Products include:
- Lithium Citrate Syrup ... 3061

Losartan Potassium (NSAIDs can inhibit the activity of antihypertensives). Products include:
- Cozaar Tablets ... 2067
- Hyzaar ... 2109

Magaldrate (Antacids reduce the bioavailability of misoprostol acid and may delay absorption of diclofenac).
No products indexed under this heading.

Magnesium Hydroxide (Antacids reduce the bioavailability of misoprostol acid and may delay absorption of diclofenac; magnesium-containing antacids exacerbate misoprostol-associated diarrhea). Products include:
- Ex•Lax Milk of Magnesia Liquid ... ▣670
- Maalox Antacid/Anti-Gas Oral Suspension ... ▣673
- Maalox Max Maximum Strength Antacid/Anti-Gas Liquid ... 2300
- Maalox Regular Strength Antacid/Antigas Liquid ... 2300
- Mylanta Fast-Acting ... 1813
- Mylanta ... 1813
- Pepcid Complete Chewable Tablets ... 1815
- Phillips' Chewable Tablets ... ▣615
- Phillips' Milk of Magnesia Liquid (Original, Cherry, & Mint) ... ▣616
- Rolaids Tablets ... ▣706
- Extra Strength Rolaids Tablets ... ▣706
- Vanquish Caplets ... ▣617

Magnesium Oxide (Antacids reduce the bioavailability of misoprostol acid and may delay absorption of diclofenac; magnesium-containing antacids exacerbate misoprostol-associated diarrhea). Products include:
- Beelith Tablets ... 946
- Mag-Ox 400 Tablets ... 1024
- Uro-Mag Capsules ... 1024

Mecamylamine Hydrochloride (NSAIDs can inhibit the activity of antihypertensives). Products include:
- Inversine Tablets ... 1850

Metformin Hydrochloride (Diclofenac may alter a diabetic patient's response to oral hypoglycemic agents; both hypo- and hyperglycemic effects have been reported). Products include:
- Glucophage Tablets ... 1080
- Glucophage XR Tablets ... 1080
- Glucovance Tablets ... 1086

Methotrexate Sodium (NSAIDs may affect renal prostaglandins and increase the toxicity of certain drugs, including methotrexate; potential for increased serum methotrexate concentrations).
No products indexed under this heading.

Methyclothiazide (NSAIDs can inhibit the activity of diuretics).
No products indexed under this heading.

Methyldopa (NSAIDs can inhibit the activity of antihypertensives). Products include:
- Aldoclor Tablets ... 2035
- Aldomet Tablets ... 2037
- Aldoril Tablets ... 2039

Methyldopate Hydrochloride (NSAIDs can inhibit the activity of antihypertensives).
No products indexed under this heading.

Metolazone (NSAIDs can inhibit the activity of diuretics). Products include:
- Mykrox Tablets ... 1168
- Zaroxolyn Tablets ... 1177

Metoprolol Succinate (NSAIDs can inhibit the activity of antihypertensives). Products include:
- Toprol-XL Tablets ... 651

Metoprolol Tartrate (NSAIDs can inhibit the activity of antihypertensives).
No products indexed under this heading.

Metyrosine (NSAIDs can inhibit the activity of antihypertensives). Products include:
- Demser Capsules ... 2085

Mibefradil Dihydrochloride (NSAIDs can inhibit the activity of antihypertensives).
No products indexed under this heading.

Miglitol (Diclofenac may alter a diabetic patient's response to oral hypoglycemic agents; both hypo- and hyperglycemic effects have been reported). Products include:
- Glyset Tablets ... 2821

Minoxidil (NSAIDs can inhibit the activity of antihypertensives). Products include:
- Rogaine Extra Strength for Men Topical Solution ... ▣721
- Rogaine for Women Topical Solution ... ▣721

Moexipril Hydrochloride (NSAIDs can inhibit the activity of antihypertensives). Products include:
- Uniretic Tablets ... 3178
- Univasc Tablets ... 3181

Nadolol (NSAIDs can inhibit the activity of antihypertensives). Products include:
- Corgard Tablets ... 2245
- Corzide 40/5 Tablets ... 2247
- Corzide 80/5 Tablets ... 2247
- Nadolol Tablets ... 2288

Nicardipine Hydrochloride (NSAIDs can inhibit the activity of antihypertensives). Products include:
- Cardene I.V. ... 3485

Nifedipine (NSAIDs can inhibit the activity of antihypertensives). Products include:
- Adalat CC Tablets ... 877
- Procardia Capsules ... 2708
- Procardia XL Extended Release Tablets ... 2710

Nisoldipine (NSAIDs can inhibit the activity of antihypertensives). Products include:
- Sular Tablets ... 688

Nitroglycerin (NSAIDs can inhibit the activity of antihypertensives). Products include:
- Nitro-Dur Transdermal Infusion System ... 3134
- Nitro-Dur Transdermal Infusion System ... 1834
- Nitrolingual Pumpspray ... 1355
- Nitrostat Tablets ... 2658

Penbutolol Sulfate (NSAIDs can inhibit the activity of antihypertensives).
No products indexed under this heading.

Perindopril Erbumine (NSAIDs can inhibit the activity of antihypertensives). Products include:
- Aceon Tablets (2 mg, 4 mg, 8 mg) ... 3249

Phenobarbital (Co-administration in patients on chronic phenobarbital therapy has resulted in phenobarbital toxicity). Products include:
- Arco-Lase Plus Tablets ... 592
- Donnatal ... 2929
- Donnatal Extentabs ... 2930

Phenoxybenzamine Hydrochloride (NSAIDs can inhibit the activity of antihypertensives). Products include:
- Dibenzyline Capsules ... 3457

Phentolamine Mesylate (NSAIDs can inhibit the activity of antihypertensives).
No products indexed under this heading.

Pindolol (NSAIDs can inhibit the activity of antihypertensives).
No products indexed under this heading.

Pioglitazone Hydrochloride (Diclofenac may alter a diabetic patient's response to oral hypoglycemic agents; both hypo- and hyperglycemic effects have been reported). Products include:
- Actos Tablets ... 3275

Polythiazide (NSAIDs can inhibit the activity of diuretics). Products include:
- Minizide Capsules ... 2700
- Renese Tablets ... 2712

Prazosin Hydrochloride (NSAIDs can inhibit the activity of antihypertensives). Products include:
- Minipress Capsules ... 2699
- Minizide Capsules ... 2700

Propranolol Hydrochloride (NSAIDs can inhibit the activity of antihypertensives). Products include:

Inderal 3513
Inderal LA Long-Acting Capsules 3516
Inderide Tablets 3517
Inderide LA Long-Acting Capsules .. 3519

Quinapril Hydrochloride (NSAIDs can inhibit the activity of antihypertensives). Products include:
Accupril Tablets 2611
Accuretic Tablets 2614

Ramipril (NSAIDs can inhibit the activity of antihypertensives). Products include:
Altace Capsules 2233

Rauwolfia serpentina (NSAIDs can inhibit the activity of antihypertensives).
No products indexed under this heading.

Repaglinide (Diclofenac may alter a diabetic patient's response to oral hypoglycemic agents; both hypo- and hyperglycemic effects have been reported). Products include:
Prandin Tablets (0.5, 1, and 2 mg) 2432

Rescinnamine (NSAIDs can inhibit the activity of antihypertensives).
No products indexed under this heading.

Reserpine (NSAIDs can inhibit the activity of antihypertensives).
No products indexed under this heading.

Rosiglitazone Maleate (Diclofenac may alter a diabetic patient's response to oral hypoglycemic agents; both hypo- and hyperglycemic effects have been reported). Products include:
Avandia Tablets 1490

Sodium Bicarbonate (Antacids reduce the bioavailability of misoprostol acid and may delay absorption of diclofenac). Products include:
Alka-Seltzer .... ◘603
Alka-Seltzer Lemon Lime Antacid and Pain Reliever Effervescent Tablets .... ◘603
Alka-Seltzer Extra Strength Antacid and Pain Reliever Effervescent Tablets .... ◘603
Alka-Seltzer Heartburn Relief Tablets .... ◘604
Ceo-Two Evacuant Suppository .... ◘618
Colyte with Flavor Packs for Oral Solution 3170
GoLYTELY and Pineapple Flavor GoLYTELY for Oral Solution 1068
NuLYTELY, Cherry Flavor, Lemon-Lime Flavor, and Orange Flavor NuLYTELY for Oral Solution 1068

Sodium Nitroprusside (NSAIDs can inhibit the activity of antihypertensives).
No products indexed under this heading.

Sotalol Hydrochloride (NSAIDs can inhibit the activity of antihypertensives). Products include:
Betapace Tablets 950
Betapace AF Tablets 954

Spirapril Hydrochloride (NSAIDs can inhibit the activity of antihypertensives).
No products indexed under this heading.

Spironolactone (Co-administration with potassium-sparing diuretics may be associated with increased serum potassium levels).
No products indexed under this heading.

Telmisartan (NSAIDs can inhibit the activity of antihypertensives). Products include:
Micardis Tablets 1049
Micardis HCT Tablets 1051

Terazosin Hydrochloride (NSAIDs can inhibit the activity of antihypertensives). Products include:
Hytrin Capsules 464

Timolol Maleate (NSAIDs can inhibit the activity of antihypertensives). Products include:
Blocadren Tablets 2046
Cosopt Sterile Ophthalmic Solution 2065
Timolide Tablets 2187
Timolol GFS .... ⊙266
Timoptic in Ocudose 2192
Timoptic Sterile Ophthalmic Solution 2190
Timoptic-XE Sterile Ophthalmic Gel Forming Solution 2194

Tolazamide (Diclofenac may alter a diabetic patient's response to oral hypoglycemic agents; both hypo- and hyperglycemic effects have been reported).
No products indexed under this heading.

Tolbutamide (Diclofenac may alter a diabetic patient's response to oral hypoglycemic agents; both hypo- and hyperglycemic effects have been reported).
No products indexed under this heading.

Torsemide (NSAIDs can inhibit the activity of diuretics). Products include:
Demadex Tablets and Injection 2965

Trandolapril (NSAIDs can inhibit the activity of antihypertensives). Products include:
Mavik Tablets 478
Tarka Tablets 508

Triamterene (Co-administration with potassium-sparing diuretics may be associated with increased serum potassium levels). Products include:
Dyazide Capsules 1515
Dyrenium Capsules 3458
Maxzide 1008

Trimethaphan Camsylate (NSAIDs can inhibit the activity of antihypertensives).
No products indexed under this heading.

Troglitazone (Diclofenac may alter a diabetic patient's response to oral hypoglycemic agents; both hypo- and hyperglycemic effects have been reported).
No products indexed under this heading.

Valsartan (NSAIDs can inhibit the activity of antihypertensives). Products include:
Diovan Capsules 2337
Diovan HCT Tablets 2338

Verapamil Hydrochloride (NSAIDs can inhibit the activity of antihypertensives). Products include:
Covera-HS Tablets 3199
Isoptin SR Tablets 467
Tarka Tablets 508
Verelan Capsules 3184
Verelan PM Capsules 3186

Warfarin Sodium (The effects of warfarin and NSAIDs on GI bleeding are synergistic, such that users of both drugs together have a risk of serious bleeding greater than users of either drug alone). Products include:
Coumadin for Injection 1243
Coumadin Tablets 1243
Warfarin Sodium Tablets, USP 3302

ASACOL DELAYED-RELEASE TABLETS

(Mesalamine) 2884
None cited in PDR database.

ASTELIN NASAL SPRAY

(Azelastine Hydrochloride) 3339
May interact with antihistamines, central nervous system depressants, and certain other agents. Compounds in these categories include:

Acrivastine (Co-administration may result in additional reduction in alertness and impairment of CNS performance; concurrent use with other antihistamines should be avoided). Products include:
Semprex-D Capsules 1172

Alfentanil Hydrochloride (Co-administration may result in additional reduction in alertness and impairment of CNS performance).
No products indexed under this heading.

Alprazolam (Co-administration may result in additional reduction in alertness and impairment of CNS performance). Products include:
Xanax Tablets 2865

Aprobarbital (Co-administration may result in additional reduction in alertness and impairment of CNS performance).
No products indexed under this heading.

Astemizole (Co-administration may result in additional reduction in alertness and impairment of CNS performance; concurrent use with other antihistamines should be avoided).
No products indexed under this heading.

Azatadine Maleate (Co-administration may result in additional reduction in alertness and impairment of CNS performance; concurrent use with other antihistamines should be avoided). Products include:
Rynatan Tablets 3351

Bromodiphenhydramine Hydrochloride (Co-administration may result in additional reduction in alertness and impairment of CNS performance; concurrent use with other antihistamines should be avoided).
No products indexed under this heading.

Brompheniramine Maleate (Co-administration may result in additional reduction in alertness and impairment of CNS performance; concurrent use with other antihistamines should be avoided). Products include:
Bromfed Capsules (Extended-Release) 2269
Bromfed-PD Capsules (Extended-Release) 2269
Comtrex Acute Head Cold & Sinus Pressure Relief Tablets .... ◘627
Dimetapp Elixir .... ◘777
Dimetapp Cold and Fever Suspension .... ◘775
Dimetapp DM Cold & Cough Elixir . ◘775
Dimetapp Nighttime Flu Liquid .... ◘776

Buprenorphine Hydrochloride (Co-administration may result in additional reduction in alertness and impairment of CNS performance). Products include:
Buprenex Injectable 2918

Buspirone Hydrochloride (Co-administration may result in additional reduction in alertness and impairment of CNS performance).
No products indexed under this heading.

Butabarbital (Co-administration may result in additional reduction in alertness and impairment of CNS performance).
No products indexed under this heading.

Butalbital (Co-administration may result in additional reduction in alertness and impairment of CNS performance). Products include:
Phrenilin 578
Sedapap Tablets 50 mg/650 mg ... 2225

Cetirizine Hydrochloride (Co-administration may result in additional reduction in alertness and impairment of CNS performance; concurrent use with other antihistamines should be avoided). Products include:
Zyrtec 2756
Zyrtec-D 12 Hour Extended Relief Tablets 2758

Chlordiazepoxide (Co-administration may result in additional reduction in alertness and impairment of CNS performance). Products include:
Limbitrol 1738

Chlordiazepoxide Hydrochloride (Co-administration may result in additional reduction in alertness and impairment of CNS performance). Products include:
Librium Capsules 1736
Librium for Injection 1737

Chlorpheniramine Maleate (Co-administration may result in additional reduction in alertness and impairment of CNS performance; concurrent use with other antihistamines should be avoided). Products include:
Actifed Cold & Sinus Caplets and Tablets .... ◘688
Alka-Seltzer Plus Liqui-Gels .... ◘604
BC Allergy Sinus Cold Powder .... ◘619
Chlor-Trimeton Allergy Tablets .... ◘735
Chlor-Trimeton Allergy/Decongestant Tablets .... ◘736
Comtrex Flu Therapy & Fever Relief Nighttime Tablets .... ◘628
Comtrex Maximum Strength Multi-Symptom Cold & Cough Relief Tablets and Caplets .... ◘626
Contac Severe Cold and Flu Caplets Maximum Strength .... ◘746
Coricidin 'D' Cold, Flu & Sinus Tablets .... ◘737
Coricidin/Coricidin D .... ◘738
Coricidin HBP Maximum Strength Flu Tablets .... ◘738
Extendryl 1361
Hycomine Compound Tablets 1317
Kronofed-A 1341
PediaCare Cough-Cold Liquid .... ◘719
PediaCare NightRest Cough-Cold Liquid .... ◘719
Robitussin Nighttime Honey Flu Liquid .... ◘786
Ryna .... ◘768
Singlet Caplets .... ◘761
Sinutab Sinus Allergy Medication, Maximum Strength Formula, Tablets & Caplets .... ◘707
Sudafed Cold & Allergy Tablets .... ◘708
TheraFlu Regular Strength Cold & Cough Night Time Hot Liquid .... ◘676
TheraFlu Regular Strength Cold & Sore Throat Night Time Hot Liquid .... ◘676
TheraFlu Maximum Strength Flu & Cough Night Time Hot Liquid .. ◘678
TheraFlu Maximum Strength Flu & Sore Throat Night Time Hot Liquid .... ◘677
TheraFlu Maximum Strength Severe Cold & Congestion Night Time Caplets .... ◘678
TheraFlu Maximum Strength Severe Cold & Congestion Night Time Hot Liquid .... ◘678
Triaminic Cold & Allergy Liquid .... ◘681
Triaminic Cold & Allergy Softchews .... ◘683
Triaminic Cold & Cough Liquid .... ◘681
Triaminic Cold & Cough Softchews .... ◘683
Triaminic Cold & Night Time Cough Liquid .... ◘681
Triaminic Cold, Cough & Fever Liquid .... ◘681
Children's Tylenol Cold Suspension Liquid and Chewable Tablets 2015
Children's Tylenol Cold Plus Cough Suspension Liquid and Chewable Tablets 2015
Children's Tylenol Flu Suspension Liquid 2015
Maximum Strength Tylenol Allergy Sinus Caplets, Gelcaps, and Geltabs 2010
Multi-Symptom Tylenol Cold Complete Formula Caplets 2010
Vicks 44M Cough, Cold & Flu Relief Liquid .... ◘725
Pediatric Vicks 44m Cough & Cold Relief .... ◘728
Children's Vicks NyQuil Cold/Cough Relief .... ◘726

Chlorpheniramine Polistirex (Co-administration may result in additional reduction in alertness and impairment of CNS performance; concurrent use with other antihistamines should be avoided). Products include:
Tussionex Pennkinetic Extended-Release Suspension 1174

Chlorpheniramine Tannate (Co-administration may result in additional reduction in alertness and impairment-

ment of CNS performance; concurrent use with other antihistamines should be avoided). Products include:
- Reformulated Rynatan Pediatric Suspension 3352
- Rynatuss Pediatric Suspension 3353
- Rynatuss Tablets 3353
- Tussi-12 S Suspension 3356
- Tussi-12 Tablets 3356

Chlorpromazine (Co-administration may result in additional reduction in alertness and impairment of CNS performance). Products include:
- Thorazine Suppositories 1656

Chlorpromazine Hydrochloride (Co-administration may result in additional reduction in alertness and impairment of CNS performance). Products include:
- Thorazine 1656

Chlorprothixene (Co-administration may result in additional reduction in alertness and impairment of CNS performance).
No products indexed under this heading.

Chlorprothixene Hydrochloride (Co-administration may result in additional reduction in alertness and impairment of CNS performance).
No products indexed under this heading.

Chlorprothixene Lactate (Co-administration may result in additional reduction in alertness and impairment of CNS performance).
No products indexed under this heading.

Cimetidine (Increases the mean Cmax and AUC of orally administered azelastine by approximately 65%). Products include:
- Tagamet HB 200 Suspension 762
- Tagamet HB 200 Tablets 761
- Tagamet Tablets 1644

Cimetidine Hydrochloride (Co-administration of oral azelastine and cimetidine has resulted in increased mean Cmax and AUC of azelastine). Products include:
- Tagamet 1644

Clemastine Fumarate (Co-administration may result in additional reduction in alertness and impairment of CNS performance; concurrent use with other antihistamines should be avoided). Products include:
- Tavist 12 Hour Allergy Tablets 676

Clorazepate Dipotassium (Co-administration may result in additional reduction in alertness and impairment of CNS performance). Products include:
- Tranxene 511

Clozapine (Co-administration may result in additional reduction in alertness and impairment of CNS performance). Products include:
- Clozaril Tablets 2319

Codeine Phosphate (Co-administration may result in additional reduction in alertness and impairment of CNS performance). Products include:
- Phenergan with Codeine Syrup 3557
- Phenergan VC with Codeine Syrup .. 3561
- Robitussin A-C Syrup 2942
- Robitussin-DAC Syrup 2942
- Ryna-C Liquid 768
- Soma Compound w/Codeine Tablets 3355
- Tussi-Organidin NR Liquid 3350
- Tussi-Organidin-S NR Liquid 3350
- Tylenol with Codeine 2595

Cyproheptadine Hydrochloride (Co-administration may result in additional reduction in alertness and impairment of CNS performance; concurrent use with other antihistamines should be avoided). Products include:
- Periactin Tablets 2155

Desflurane (Co-administration may result in additional reduction in alertness and impairment of CNS performance). Products include:
- Suprane Liquid for Inhalation 874

Dexchlorpheniramine Maleate (Co-administration may result in additional reduction in alertness and impairment of CNS performance; concurrent use with other antihistamines should be avoided).
No products indexed under this heading.

Dezocine (Co-administration may result in additional reduction in alertness and impairment of CNS performance).
No products indexed under this heading.

Diazepam (Co-administration may result in additional reduction in alertness and impairment of CNS performance). Products include:
- Valium Injectable 3026
- Valium Tablets 3047

Diphenhydramine Citrate (Co-administration may result in additional reduction in alertness and impairment of CNS performance; concurrent use with other antihistamines should be avoided). Products include:
- Alka-Seltzer PM Effervescent Tablets 605
- Benadryl Allergy & Sinus Fastmelt Tablets 693
- Benadryl Children's Allergy/Cold Fastmelt Tablets 692
- Excedrin PM Tablets, Caplets, and Geltabs 631
- Goody's PM Powder 621

Diphenhydramine Hydrochloride (Co-administration may result in additional reduction in alertness and impairment of CNS performance; concurrent use with other antihistamines should be avoided). Products include:
- Extra Strength Bayer PM Caplets 611
- Benadryl Allergy Chewables 689
- Benadryl Allergy 691
- Benadryl Allergy Liquid 690
- Benadryl Allergy/Cold Tablets 691
- Benadryl Allergy/Congestion Tablets 692
- Benadryl Allergy & Sinus Liquid 693
- Benadryl Allergy Sinus Headache Caplets & Gelcaps 693
- Benadryl Severe Allergy & Sinus Headache Caplets 694
- Benadryl Dye-Free Allergy Liquid ... 690
- Benadryl Dye-Free Allergy Liqui-Gels Softgels 690
- Benadryl Itch Relief Stick Extra Strength 695
- Benadryl Cream 695
- Benadryl Gel 695
- Benadryl Spray 696
- Benadryl Parenteral 2617
- Coricidin HBP Night-Time Cold & Flu Tablets 738
- Nytol QuickCaps Caplets 622
- Maximum Strength Nytol QuickGels Softgels 621
- Extra Strength Percogesic Aspirin-Free Coated Caplets 665
- Simply Sleep Caplets 2008
- Sominex Original Formula Tablets . 761
- Children's Tylenol Allergy-D Liquid ... 2014
- Maximum Strength Tylenol Allergy Sinus NightTime Caplets 2010
- Tylenol Severe Allergy Caplets 2010
- Maximum Strength Tylenol Flu NightTime Gelcaps 2011
- Extra Strength Tylenol PM Caplets, Geltabs, and Gelcaps 2012
- Unisom Maximum Strength SleepGels 713

Diphenylpyraline Hydrochloride (Co-administration may result in additional reduction in alertness and impairment of CNS performance; concurrent use with other antihistamines should be avoided).
No products indexed under this heading.

Droperidol (Co-administration may result in additional reduction in alertness and impairment of CNS performance).
No products indexed under this heading.

Enflurane (Co-administration may result in additional reduction in alertness and impairment of CNS performance).
No products indexed under this heading.

Estazolam (Co-administration may result in additional reduction in alertness and impairment of CNS performance). Products include:
- ProSom Tablets 500

Ethchlorvynol (Co-administration may result in additional reduction in alertness and impairment of CNS performance).
No products indexed under this heading.

Ethinamate (Co-administration may result in additional reduction in alertness and impairment of CNS performance).
No products indexed under this heading.

Fentanyl (Co-administration may result in additional reduction in alertness and impairment of CNS performance). Products include:
- Duragesic Transdermal System 1786

Fentanyl Citrate (Co-administration may result in additional reduction in alertness and impairment of CNS performance). Products include:
- Actiq 1184

Fexofenadine Hydrochloride (Co-administration may result in additional reduction in alertness and impairment of CNS performance; concurrent use with other antihistamines should be avoided). Products include:
- Allegra 712
- Allegra-D Extended-Release Tablets 714

Fluphenazine Decanoate (Co-administration may result in additional reduction in alertness and impairment of CNS performance).
No products indexed under this heading.

Fluphenazine Enanthate (Co-administration may result in additional reduction in alertness and impairment of CNS performance).
No products indexed under this heading.

Fluphenazine Hydrochloride (Co-administration may result in additional reduction in alertness and impairment of CNS performance).
No products indexed under this heading.

Flurazepam Hydrochloride (Co-administration may result in additional reduction in alertness and impairment of CNS performance).
No products indexed under this heading.

Glutethimide (Co-administration may result in additional reduction in alertness and impairment of CNS performance).
No products indexed under this heading.

Haloperidol (Co-administration may result in additional reduction in alertness and impairment of CNS performance). Products include:
- Haldol Injection, Tablets and Concentrate 2533

Haloperidol Decanoate (Co-administration may result in additional reduction in alertness and impairment of CNS performance). Products include:
- Haldol Decanoate 2535

Hydrocodone Bitartrate (Co-administration may result in additional reduction in alertness and impairment of CNS performance). Products include:
- Hycodan 1316
- Hycomine Compound Tablets 1317
- Hycotuss Expectorant Syrup 1318
- Lortab 3319
- Lortab Elixir 3317
- Maxidone Tablets CIII 3399
- Norco 5/325 Tablets CIII 3424
- Norco 7.5/325 Tablets CIII 3425
- Norco 10/325 Tablets CIII 3427
- Norco 10/325 Tablets CIII 3425
- Vicodin Tablets 516
- Vicodin ES Tablets 517
- Vicodin HP Tablets 518
- Vicodin Tuss Expectorant 519
- Vicoprofen Tablets 520
- Zydone Tablets 1330

Hydrocodone Polistirex (Co-administration may result in additional reduction in alertness and impairment of CNS performance). Products include:
- Tussionex Pennkinetic Extended-Release Suspension 1174

Hydromorphone Hydrochloride (Co-administration may result in additional reduction in alertness and impairment of CNS performance). Products include:
- Dilaudid 441
- Dilaudid Oral Liquid 445
- Dilaudid Powder 441
- Dilaudid Rectal Suppositories 441
- Dilaudid Tablets 441
- Dilaudid Tablets - 8 mg 445
- Dilaudid-HP 443

Hydroxyzine Hydrochloride (Co-administration may result in additional reduction in alertness and impairment of CNS performance). Products include:
- Atarax Tablets & Syrup 2667
- Vistaril Intramuscular Solution 2738

Isoflurane (Co-administration may result in additional reduction in alertness and impairment of CNS performance).
No products indexed under this heading.

Ketamine Hydrochloride (Co-administration may result in additional reduction in alertness and impairment of CNS performance).
No products indexed under this heading.

Ketoconazole (Co-administration of oral azelastine and ketoconazole interfere with the measurement of azelastine plasma concentrations, however, no effects on QTc have been observed). Products include:
- Nizoral 2% Cream 3620
- Nizoral A-D Shampoo 2008
- Nizoral 2% Shampoo 2007
- Nizoral Tablets 1791

Levomethadyl Acetate Hydrochloride (Co-administration may result in additional reduction in alertness and impairment of CNS performance).
No products indexed under this heading.

Levorphanol Tartrate (Co-administration may result in additional reduction in alertness and impairment of CNS performance). Products include:
- Levo-Dromoran 1734
- Levorphanol Tartrate Tablets 3059

Loratadine (Co-administration may result in additional reduction in alertness and impairment of CNS performance; concurrent use with other antihistamines should be avoided). Products include:
- Claritin 3100
- Claritin-D 12 Hour Extended Release Tablets 3102
- Claritin-D 24 Hour Extended Release Tablets 3104

Lorazepam (Co-administration may result in additional reduction in alertness and impairment of CNS performance). Products include:
- Ativan Injection 3478
- Ativan Tablets 3482

Loxapine Hydrochloride (Co-administration may result in additional reduction in alertness and impair-

ment of CNS performance).
No products indexed under this heading.

Loxapine Succinate (Co-administration may result in additional reduction in alertness and impairment of CNS performance). Products include:
Loxitane Capsules 3398

Meperidine Hydrochloride (Co-administration may result in additional reduction in alertness and impairment of CNS performance). Products include:
Demerol 3079
Mepergan Injection 3539

Mephobarbital (Co-administration may result in additional reduction in alertness and impairment of CNS performance).
No products indexed under this heading.

Meprobamate (Co-administration may result in additional reduction in alertness and impairment of CNS performance). Products include:
Miltown Tablets 3349

Mesoridazine Besylate (Co-administration may result in additional reduction in alertness and impairment of CNS performance). Products include:
Serentil 1057

Methadone Hydrochloride (Co-administration may result in additional reduction in alertness and impairment of CNS performance). Products include:
Dolophine Hydrochloride Tablets 3056

Methdilazine Hydrochloride (Co-administration may result in additional reduction in alertness and impairment of CNS performance; concurrent use with other antihistamines should be avoided).
No products indexed under this heading.

Methohexital Sodium (Co-administration may result in additional reduction in alertness and impairment of CNS performance). Products include:
Brevital Sodium for Injection, USP .. 1815

Methotrimeprazine (Co-administration may result in additional reduction in alertness and impairment of CNS performance).
No products indexed under this heading.

Methoxyflurane (Co-administration may result in additional reduction in alertness and impairment of CNS performance).
No products indexed under this heading.

Midazolam Hydrochloride (Co-administration may result in additional reduction in alertness and impairment of CNS performance). Products include:
Versed Injection 3027
Versed Syrup 3033

Molindone Hydrochloride (Co-administration may result in additional reduction in alertness and impairment of CNS performance). Products include:
Moban 1320

Morphine Sulfate (Co-administration may result in additional reduction in alertness and impairment of CNS performance). Products include:
Astramorph/PF Injection, USP (Preservative-Free) 594
Duramorph Injection 1312
Infumorph 200 and Infumorph 500 Sterile Solutions 1314
Kadian Capsules 1335
MS Contin Tablets 2896
MSIR 2898
Oramorph SR Tablets 3062
Roxanol 3066

Olanzapine (Co-administration may result in additional reduction in alertness and impairment of CNS performance). Products include:
Zyprexa Tablets 1973
Zyprexa ZYDIS Orally Disintegrating Tablets 1973

Oxazepam (Co-administration may result in additional reduction in alertness and impairment of CNS performance).
No products indexed under this heading.

Oxycodone Hydrochloride (Co-administration may result in additional reduction in alertness and impairment of CNS performance). Products include:
OxyContin Tablets 2912
OxyFast Oral Concentrate Solution . 2916
OxyIR Capsules 2916
Percocet Tablets 1326
Percodan Tablets 1327
Percolone Tablets 1327
Roxicodone 3067
Tylox Capsules 2597

Pentobarbital Sodium (Co-administration may result in additional reduction in alertness and impairment of CNS performance). Products include:
Nembutal Sodium Solution 485

Perphenazine (Co-administration may result in additional reduction in alertness and impairment of CNS performance). Products include:
Etrafon 3115
Trilafon 3160

Phenobarbital (Co-administration may result in additional reduction in alertness and impairment of CNS performance). Products include:
Arco-Lase Plus Tablets 592
Donnatal 2929
Donnatal Extentabs 2930

Prazepam (Co-administration may result in additional reduction in alertness and impairment of CNS performance).
No products indexed under this heading.

Prochlorperazine (Co-administration may result in additional reduction in alertness and impairment of CNS performance). Products include:
Compazine 1505

Promethazine Hydrochloride (Co-administration may result in additional reduction in alertness and impairment of CNS performance; concurrent use with other antihistamines should be avoided). Products include:
Mepergan Injection 3539
Phenergan Injection 3553
Phenergan 3556
Phenergan Syrup 3554
Phenergan with Codeine Syrup 3557
Phenergan with Dextromethorphan Syrup 3559
Phenergan VC Syrup 3560
Phenergan VC with Codeine Syrup .. 3561

Propofol (Co-administration may result in additional reduction in alertness and impairment of CNS performance). Products include:
Diprivan Injectable Emulsion 667

Propoxyphene Hydrochloride (Co-administration may result in additional reduction in alertness and impairment of CNS performance). Products include:
Darvon Pulvules 1909
Darvon Compound-65 Pulvules 1910

Propoxyphene Napsylate (Co-administration may result in additional reduction in alertness and impairment of CNS performance). Products include:
Darvon-N/Darvocet-N 1907
Darvon-N Tablets 1912

Pyrilamine Maleate (Co-administration may result in additional reduction in alertness and impairment of CNS performance; concurrent use with other antihistamines should be avoided). Products include:
Maximum Strength Midol Menstrual Caplets and Gelcaps .... ■612
Maximum Strength Midol PMS Caplets and Gelcaps .... ■613

Pyrilamine Tannate (Co-administration may result in additional reduction in alertness and impairment of CNS performance; concurrent use with other antihistamines should be avoided). Products include:
Ryna-12 S Suspension 3351

Quazepam (Co-administration may result in additional reduction in alertness and impairment of CNS performance).
No products indexed under this heading.

Quetiapine Fumarate (Co-administration may result in additional reduction in alertness and impairment of CNS performance). Products include:
Seroquel Tablets 684

Remifentanil Hydrochloride (Co-administration may result in additional reduction in alertness and impairment of CNS performance).
No products indexed under this heading.

Risperidone (Co-administration may result in additional reduction in alertness and impairment of CNS performance). Products include:
Risperdal 1796

Secobarbital Sodium (Co-administration may result in additional reduction in alertness and impairment of CNS performance).
No products indexed under this heading.

Sevoflurane (Co-administration may result in additional reduction in alertness and impairment of CNS performance).
No products indexed under this heading.

Sufentanil Citrate (Co-administration may result in additional reduction in alertness and impairment of CNS performance).
No products indexed under this heading.

Temazepam (Co-administration may result in additional reduction in alertness and impairment of CNS performance).
No products indexed under this heading.

Terfenadine (Co-administration may result in additional reduction in alertness and impairment of CNS performance; concurrent use with other antihistamines should be avoided).
No products indexed under this heading.

Thiamylal Sodium (Co-administration may result in additional reduction in alertness and impairment of CNS performance).
No products indexed under this heading.

Thioridazine Hydrochloride (Co-administration may result in additional reduction in alertness and impairment of CNS performance). Products include:
Thioridazine Hydrochloride Tablets 2289

Thiothixene (Co-administration may result in additional reduction in alertness and impairment of CNS performance). Products include:
Navane Capsules 2701
Thiothixene Capsules 2290

Triazolam (Co-administration may result in additional reduction in alertness and impairment of CNS performance). Products include:
Halcion Tablets 2823

Trifluoperazine Hydrochloride (Co-administration may result in additional reduction in alertness and impairment of CNS performance). Products include:
Stelazine 1640

Trimeprazine Tartrate (Co-administration may result in additional reduction in alertness and impairment of CNS performance; concurrent use with other antihistamines should be avoided).
No products indexed under this heading.

Tripelennamine Hydrochloride (Co-administration may result in additional reduction in alertness and impairment of CNS performance; concurrent use with other antihistamines should be avoided).
No products indexed under this heading.

Triprolidine Hydrochloride (Co-administration may result in additional reduction in alertness and impairment of CNS performance; concurrent use with other antihistamines should be avoided). Products include:
Actifed Cold & Allergy Tablets .... ■688

Zaleplon (Co-administration may result in additional reduction in alertness and impairment of CNS performance). Products include:
Sonata Capsules 3591

Ziprasidone Hydrochloride (Co-administration may result in additional reduction in alertness and impairment of CNS performance). Products include:
Geodon Capsules 2688

Zolpidem Tartrate (Co-administration may result in additional reduction in alertness and impairment of CNS performance). Products include:
Ambien Tablets 3191

Food Interactions

Alcohol (Concurrent use may result in additional reduction in alertness and impairment of CNS performance; alcohol intake should be avoided).

ASTRAMORPH/PF INJECTION, USP (PRESERVATIVE-FREE)

(Morphine Sulfate) 594
May interact with antihistamines, butyrophenones, central nervous system depressants, anticoagulants, parenterally administered corticosteroids, hypnotics and sedatives, monoamine oxidase inhibitors, antipsychotic agents, phenothiazines, psychotropics, tricyclic antidepressants, and certain other agents. Compounds in these categories include:

Acrivastine (Potentiation of depressant effects of morphine). Products include:
Semprex-D Capsules 1172

Alfentanil Hydrochloride (Potentiation of depressant effects of morphine).
No products indexed under this heading.

Alprazolam (Potentiation of depressant effects of morphine). Products include:
Xanax Tablets 2865

Amitriptyline Hydrochloride (Potentiation of depressant effects of morphine). Products include:
Etrafon 3115
Limbitrol 1738

Amoxapine (Potentiation of depressant effects of morphine).
No products indexed under this heading.

Aprobarbital (Potentiation of depressant effects of morphine).
No products indexed under this heading.

Ardeparin Sodium (Administration of morphine by epidural or intrathecal route is contraindicated in presence of concomitant anticoagulant therapy).
No products indexed under this heading.

Astemizole (Potentiation of depressant effects of morphine).
No products indexed under this heading.

Azatadine Maleate (Potentiation of depressant effects of morphine). Products include:
Rynatan Tablets ... 3351

Bromodiphenhydramine Hydrochloride (Potentiation of depressant effects of morphine).
No products indexed under this heading.

Brompheniramine Maleate (Potentiation of depressant effects of morphine). Products include:
Bromfed Capsules (Extended-Release) ... 2269
Bromfed-PD Capsules (Extended-Release) ... 2269
Comtrex Acute Head Cold & Sinus Pressure Relief Tablets ... ■627
Dimetapp Elixir ... ■777
Dimetapp Cold and Fever Suspension ... ■775
Dimetapp DM Cold & Cough Elixir ... ■775
Dimetapp Nighttime Flu Liquid ... ■776

Buprenorphine Hydrochloride (Potentiation of depressant effects of morphine). Products include:
Buprenex Injectable ... 2918

Buspirone Hydrochloride (Potentiation of depressant effects of morphine).
No products indexed under this heading.

Butabarbital (Potentiation of depressant effects of morphine).
No products indexed under this heading.

Butalbital (Potentiation of depressant effects of morphine). Products include:
Phrenilin ... 578
Sedapap Tablets 50 mg/650 mg ... 2225

Cetirizine Hydrochloride (Potentiation of depressant effects of morphine). Products include:
Zyrtec ... 2756
Zyrtec-D 12 Hour Extended Relief Tablets ... 2758

Chlordiazepoxide (Potentiation of depressant effects of morphine). Products include:
Limbitrol ... 1738

Chlordiazepoxide Hydrochloride (Potentiation of depressant effects of morphine). Products include:
Librium Capsules ... 1736
Librium for Injection ... 1737

Chlorpheniramine Maleate (Potentiation of depressant effects of morphine). Products include:
Actifed Cold & Sinus Caplets and Tablets ... ■688
Alka-Seltzer Plus Liqui-Gels ... ■604
BC Allergy Sinus Cold Powder ... ■619
Chlor-Trimeton Allergy Tablets ... ■735
Chlor-Trimeton Allergy/Decongestant Tablets ... ■736
Comtrex Flu Therapy & Fever Relief Nighttime Tablets ... ■628
Comtrex Maximum Strength Multi-Symptom Cold & Cough Relief Tablets and Caplets ... ■626
Contac Severe Cold and Flu Caplets Maximum Strength ... ■746
Coricidin 'D' Cold, Flu & Sinus Tablets ... ■737
Coricidin/Coricidin D ... ■738
Coricidin HBP Maximum Strength Flu Tablets ... ■738
Extendryl ... 1361
Hycomine Compound Tablets ... 1317
Kronofed-A ... 1341
PediaCare Cough-Cold Liquid ... ■719
PediaCare NightRest Cough-Cold Liquid ... ■719
Robitussin Nighttime Honey Flu Liquid ... ■786
Ryna ... ■768
Singlet Caplets ... ■761
Sinutab Sinus Allergy Medication, Maximum Strength Formula, Tablets & Caplets ... ■707
Sudafed Cold & Allergy Tablets ... ■708
TheraFlu Regular Strength Cold & Cough Night Time Hot Liquid ... ■676
TheraFlu Regular Strength Cold & Sore Throat Night Time Hot Liquid ... ■676
TheraFlu Maximum Strength Flu & Cough Night Time Hot Liquid ... ■678
TheraFlu Maximum Strength Flu & Sore Throat Night Time Hot Liquid ... ■677
TheraFlu Maximum Strength Severe Cold & Congestion Night Time Caplets ... ■678
TheraFlu Maximum Strength Severe Cold & Congestion Night Time Hot Liquid ... ■678
Triaminic Cold & Allergy Liquid ... ■681
Triaminic Cold & Allergy Softchews ... ■683
Triaminic Cold & Cough Liquid ... ■681
Triaminic Cold & Cough Softchews ... ■683
Triaminic Cold & Night Time Cough Liquid ... ■681
Triaminic Cold, Cough & Fever Liquid ... ■681
Children's Tylenol Cold Suspension Liquid and Chewable Tablets ... 2015
Children's Tylenol Cold Plus Cough Suspension Liquid and Chewable Tablets ... 2015
Children's Tylenol Flu Suspension Liquid ... 2015
Maximum Strength Tylenol Allergy Sinus Caplets, Gelcaps, and Geltabs ... 2010
Multi-Symptom Tylenol Cold Complete Formula Caplets ... 2010
Vicks 44M Cough, Cold & Flu Relief Liquid ... ■725
Pediatric Vicks 44m Cough & Cold Relief ... ■728
Children's Vicks NyQuil Cold/Cough Relief ... ■726

Chlorpheniramine Polistirex (Potentiation of depressant effects of morphine). Products include:
Tussionex Pennkinetic Extended-Release Suspension ... 1174

Chlorpheniramine Tannate (Potentiation of depressant effects of morphine). Products include:
Reformulated Rynatan Pediatric Suspension ... 3352
Rynatuss Pediatric Suspension ... 3353
Rynatuss Tablets ... 3353
Tussi-12 S Suspension ... 3356
Tussi-12 Tablets ... 3356

Chlorpromazine (Potentiation of depressant effects of morphine; increased risk of respiratory depression). Products include:
Thorazine Suppositories ... 1656

Chlorpromazine Hydrochloride (Potentiation of depressant effects of morphine; increased risk of respiratory depression). Products include:
Thorazine ... 1656

Chlorprothixene (Potentiation of depressant effects of morphine; increased risk of respiratory depression).
No products indexed under this heading.

Chlorprothixene Hydrochloride (Potentiation of depressant effects of morphine; increased risk of respiratory depression).
No products indexed under this heading.

Chlorprothixene Lactate (Potentiation of depressant effects of morphine; increased risk of respiratory depression).
No products indexed under this heading.

Clemastine Fumarate (Potentiation of depressant effects of morphine). Products include:
Tavist 12 Hour Allergy Tablets ... ■676

Clomipramine Hydrochloride (Potentiation of depressant effects of morphine).
No products indexed under this heading.

Clorazepate Dipotassium (Potentiation of depressant effects of morphine). Products include:
Tranxene ... 511

Clozapine (Potentiation of depressant effects of morphine; increased risk of respiratory depression). Products include:
Clozaril Tablets ... 2319

Codeine Phosphate (Potentiation of depressant effects of morphine). Products include:
Phenergan with Codeine Syrup ... 3557
Phenergan VC with Codeine Syrup ... 3561
Robitussin A-C Syrup ... 2942
Robitussin-DAC Syrup ... 2942
Ryna-C Liquid ... ■768
Soma Compound w/Codeine Tablets ... 3355
Tussi-Organidin NR Liquid ... 3350
Tussi-Organidin-S NR Liquid ... 3350
Tylenol with Codeine ... 2595

Cyproheptadine Hydrochloride (Potentiation of depressant effects of morphine). Products include:
Periactin Tablets ... 2155

Dalteparin Sodium (Administration of morphine by epidural or intrathecal route is contraindicated in presence of concomitant anticoagulant therapy). Products include:
Fragmin Injection ... 2814

Danaparoid Sodium (Administration of morphine by epidural or intrathecal route is contraindicated in presence of concomitant anticoagulant therapy). Products include:
Orgaran Injection ... 2480

Desflurane (Potentiation of depressant effects of morphine). Products include:
Suprane Liquid for Inhalation ... 874

Desipramine Hydrochloride (Potentiation of depressant effects of morphine). Products include:
Norpramin Tablets ... 755

Dexamethasone Acetate (Administration of morphine by epidural or intrathecal route is contraindicated in presence of concomitantly administered parenteral corticosteroids within 2 weeks).
No products indexed under this heading.

Dexamethasone Sodium Phosphate (Administration of morphine by epidural or intrathecal route is contraindicated in presence of concomitantly administered parenteral corticosteroids within 2 weeks). Products include:
Decadron Phosphate Injection ... 2081
Decadron Phosphate Sterile Ophthalmic Ointment ... 2083
Decadron Phosphate Sterile Ophthalmic Solution ... 2084
NeoDecadron Sterile Ophthalmic Solution ... 2144

Dexchlorpheniramine Maleate (Potentiation of depressant effects of morphine).
No products indexed under this heading.

Dezocine (Potentiation of depressant effects of morphine).
No products indexed under this heading.

Diazepam (Potentiation of depressant effects of morphine). Products include:
Valium Injectable ... 3026
Valium Tablets ... 3047

Dicumarol (Administration of morphine by epidural or intrathecal route is contraindicated in presence of concomitant anticoagulant therapy).
No products indexed under this heading.

Diphenhydramine Citrate (Potentiation of depressant effects of morphine). Products include:
Alka-Seltzer PM Effervescent Tablets ... ■605
Benadryl Allergy & Sinus Fastmelt Tablets ... ■693
Benadryl Children's Allergy/Cold Fastmelt Tablets ... ■692
Excedrin PM Tablets, Caplets, and Geltabs ... ■631
Goody's PM Powder ... ■621

Diphenhydramine Hydrochloride (Potentiation of depressant effects of morphine). Products include:
Extra Strength Bayer PM Caplets ... ■611
Benadryl Allergy Chewables ... ■689
Benadryl Allergy ... ■691
Benadryl Allergy Liquid ... ■690
Benadryl Allergy/Cold Tablets ... ■691
Benadryl Allergy/Congestion Tablets ... ■692
Benadryl Allergy & Sinus Liquid ... ■693
Benadryl Allergy Sinus Headache Caplets & Gelcaps ... ■693
Benadryl Severe Allergy & Sinus Headache Caplets ... ■694
Benadryl Dye-Free Allergy Liquid ... ■690
Benadryl Dye-Free Allergy Liqui-Gels Softgels ... ■690
Benadryl Itch Relief Stick Extra Strength ... ■695
Benadryl Cream ... ■695
Benadryl Gel ... ■695
Benadryl Spray ... ■696
Benadryl Parenteral ... 2617
Coricidin HBP Night-Time Cold & Flu Tablets ... ■738
Nytol QuickCaps Caplets ... ■622
Maximum Strength Nytol QuickGels Softgels ... ■621
Extra Strength Percogesic Aspirin-Free Coated Caplets ... ■665
Simply Sleep Caplets ... 2008
Sominex Original Formula Tablets ... ■761
Children's Tylenol Allergy-D Liquid ... 2014
Maximum Strength Tylenol Allergy Sinus NightTime Caplets ... 2010
Tylenol Severe Allergy Caplets ... 2010
Maximum Strength Tylenol Flu NightTime Gelcaps ... 2011
Extra Strength Tylenol PM Caplets, Geltabs, and Gelcaps ... 2012
Unisom Maximum Strength SleepGels ... ■713

Diphenylpyraline Hydrochloride (Potentiation of depressant effects of morphine).
No products indexed under this heading.

Doxepin Hydrochloride (Potentiation of depressant effects of morphine). Products include:
Sinequan ... 2713

Droperidol (Potentiation of depressant effects of morphine).
No products indexed under this heading.

Enflurane (Potentiation of depressant effects of morphine).
No products indexed under this heading.

Enoxaparin (Administration of morphine by epidural or intrathecal route is contraindicated in presence of concomitant anticoagulant therapy). Products include:
Lovenox Injection ... 746

Estazolam (Potentiation of depressant effects of morphine). Products include:
ProSom Tablets ... 500

Ethchlorvynol (Potentiation of depressant effects of morphine).
No products indexed under this heading.

Ethinamate (Potentiation of depressant effects of morphine).
No products indexed under this heading.

Fentanyl (Potentiation of depressant effects of morphine). Products include:
Duragesic Transdermal System ... 1786

Fentanyl Citrate (Potentiation of depressant effects of morphine). Products include:
Actiq ... 1184

Fexofenadine Hydrochloride (Potentiation of depressant effects of morphine). Products include:
Allegra ... 712
Allegra-D Extended-Release Tablets ... 714

IMPORTANT NOTE: Always consult each drug listing in the patient's regimen for possible interactions.

Fluphenazine Decanoate (Potentiation of depressant effects of morphine; increased risk of respiratory depression).
No products indexed under this heading.

Fluphenazine Enanthate (Potentiation of depressant effects of morphine; increased risk of respiratory depression).
No products indexed under this heading.

Fluphenazine Hydrochloride (Potentiation of depressant effects of morphine; increased risk of respiratory depression).
No products indexed under this heading.

Flurazepam Hydrochloride (Potentiation of depressant effects of morphine).
No products indexed under this heading.

Glutethimide (Potentiation of depressant effects of morphine).
No products indexed under this heading.

Haloperidol (Potentiation of depressant effects of morphine). Products include:
- Haldol Injection, Tablets and Concentrate 2533

Haloperidol Decanoate (Potentiation of depressant effects of morphine; increased risk of respiratory depression). Products include:
- Haldol Decanoate 2535

Heparin Sodium (Administration of morphine by epidural or intrathecal route is contraindicated in presence of concomitant anticoagulant therapy). Products include:
- Heparin Lock Flush Solution 3509
- Heparin Sodium Injection 3511

Hydrocodone Bitartrate (Potentiation of depressant effects of morphine). Products include:
- Hycodan 1316
- Hycomine Compound Tablets 1317
- Hycotuss Expectorant Syrup 1318
- Lortab 3319
- Lortab Elixir 3317
- Maxidone Tablets CIII 3399
- Norco 5/325 Tablets CIII 3424
- Norco 7.5/325 Tablets CIII 3425
- Norco 10/325 Tablets CIII 3427
- Norco 10/325 Tablets CIII 3425
- Vicodin Tablets 516
- Vicodin ES Tablets 517
- Vicodin HP Tablets 518
- Vicodin Tuss Expectorant 519
- Vicoprofen Tablets 520
- Zydone Tablets 1330

Hydrocodone Polistirex (Potentiation of depressant effects of morphine). Products include:
- Tussionex Pennkinetic Extended-Release Suspension 1174

Hydrocortisone Acetate (Administration of morphine by epidural or intrathecal route is contraindicated in presence of concomitantly administered parenteral corticosteroids within 2 weeks). Products include:
- Analpram-HC 1338
- Anusol HC-1 Hydrocortisone Anti-Itch Cream .... ▣689
- Anusol-HC Suppositories 2238
- Cortaid .... ▣717
- Cortifoam Rectal Foam 3170
- Cortisporin-TC Otic Suspension 2246
- Hydrocortone Acetate Injectable Suspension 2103
- Pramosone 1343
- Proctocort Suppositories 2264
- ProctoFoam-HC 3177
- Terra-Cortril Ophthalmic Suspension 2716

Hydrocortisone Sodium Phosphate (Administration of morphine by epidural or intrathecal route is contraindicated in presence of concomitantly administered parenteral corticosteroids within 2 weeks). Products include:
- Hydrocortone Phosphate Injection, Sterile 2105

Hydrocortisone Sodium Succinate (Administration of morphine by epidural or intrathecal route is contraindicated in presence of concomitantly administered parenteral corticosteroids within 2 weeks).
No products indexed under this heading.

Hydromorphone Hydrochloride (Potentiation of depressant effects of morphine). Products include:
- Dilaudid 441
- Dilaudid Oral Liquid 445
- Dilaudid Powder 441
- Dilaudid Rectal Suppositories 441
- Dilaudid Tablets 441
- Dilaudid Tablets - 8 mg 445
- Dilaudid-HP 443

Hydroxyzine Hydrochloride (Potentiation of depressant effects of morphine). Products include:
- Atarax Tablets & Syrup 2667
- Vistaril Intramuscular Solution 2738

Imipramine Hydrochloride (Potentiation of depressant effects of morphine).
No products indexed under this heading.

Imipramine Pamoate (Potentiation of depressant effects of morphine).
No products indexed under this heading.

Isocarboxazid (Concomitant use potentiates depressant effects of morphine).
No products indexed under this heading.

Isoflurane (Potentiation of depressant effects of morphine).
No products indexed under this heading.

Ketamine Hydrochloride (Potentiation of depressant effects of morphine).
No products indexed under this heading.

Levomethadyl Acetate Hydrochloride (Potentiation of depressant effects of morphine).
No products indexed under this heading.

Levorphanol Tartrate (Potentiation of depressant effects of morphine). Products include:
- Levo-Dromoran 1734
- Levorphanol Tartrate Tablets 3059

Lithium Carbonate (Potentiation of depressant effects of morphine; increased risk of respiratory depression). Products include:
- Eskalith 1527
- Lithium Carbonate 3061
- Lithobid Slow-Release Tablets 3255

Lithium Citrate (Potentiation of depressant effects of morphine; increased risk of respiratory depression). Products include:
- Lithium Citrate Syrup 3061

Loratadine (Potentiation of depressant effects of morphine). Products include:
- Claritin 3100
- Claritin-D 12 Hour Extended Release Tablets 3102
- Claritin-D 24 Hour Extended Release Tablets 3104

Lorazepam (Potentiation of depressant effects of morphine). Products include:
- Ativan Injection 3478
- Ativan Tablets 3482

Loxapine Hydrochloride (Potentiation of depressant effects of morphine; increased risk of respiratory depression).
No products indexed under this heading.

Loxapine Succinate (Potentiation of depressant effects of morphine). Products include:
- Loxitane Capsules 3398

Maprotiline Hydrochloride (Potentiation of depressant effects of morphine).
No products indexed under this heading.

Meperidine Hydrochloride (Potentiation of depressant effects of morphine). Products include:
- Demerol 3079
- Mepergan Injection 3539

Mephobarbital (Potentiation of depressant effects of morphine).
No products indexed under this heading.

Meprobamate (Potentiation of depressant effects of morphine). Products include:
- Miltown Tablets 3349

Mesoridazine Besylate (Potentiation of depressant effects of morphine; increased risk of respiratory depression). Products include:
- Serentil 1057

Methadone Hydrochloride (Potentiation of depressant effects of morphine). Products include:
- Dolophine Hydrochloride Tablets 3056

Methdilazine Hydrochloride (Potentiation of depressant effects of morphine).
No products indexed under this heading.

Methohexital Sodium (Potentiation of depressant effects of morphine). Products include:
- Brevital Sodium for Injection, USP 1815

Methotrimeprazine (Potentiation of depressant effects of morphine).
No products indexed under this heading.

Methoxyflurane (Potentiation of depressant effects of morphine).
No products indexed under this heading.

Methylprednisolone Acetate (Administration of morphine by epidural or intrathecal route is contraindicated in presence of concomitantly administered parenteral corticosteroids within 2 weeks). Products include:
- Depo-Medrol Injectable Suspension 2795

Methylprednisolone Sodium Succinate (Administration of morphine by epidural or intrathecal route is contraindicated in presence of concomitantly administered parenteral corticosteroids within 2 weeks). Products include:
- Solu-Medrol Sterile Powder 2855

Midazolam Hydrochloride (Potentiation of depressant effects of morphine). Products include:
- Versed Injection 3027
- Versed Syrup 3033

Moclobemide (Concomitant use potentiates depressant effects of morphine).
No products indexed under this heading.

Molindone Hydrochloride (Potentiation of depressant effects of morphine; increased risk of respiratory depression with neuroleptics). Products include:
- Moban 1320

Nortriptyline Hydrochloride (Potentiation of depressant effects of morphine).
No products indexed under this heading.

Olanzapine (Potentiation of depressant effects of morphine). Products include:
- Zyprexa Tablets 1973
- Zyprexa ZYDIS Orally Disintegrating Tablets 1973

Oxazepam (Potentiation of depressant effects of morphine).
No products indexed under this heading.

Oxycodone Hydrochloride (Potentiation of depressant effects of morphine). Products include:
- OxyContin Tablets 2912
- OxyFast Oral Concentrate Solution 2916
- OxyIR Capsules 2916
- Percocet Tablets 1326
- Percodan Tablets 1327
- Percolone Tablets 1327
- Roxicodone 3067
- Tylox Capsules 2597

Pargyline Hydrochloride (Concomitant use potentiates depressant effects of morphine).
No products indexed under this heading.

Pentobarbital Sodium (Potentiation of depressant effects of morphine). Products include:
- Nembutal Sodium Solution 485

Perphenazine (Potentiation of depressant effects of morphine). Products include:
- Etrafon 3115
- Trilafon 3160

Phenelzine Sulfate (Concomitant use potentiates depressant effects of morphine). Products include:
- Nardil Tablets 2653

Phenobarbital (Potentiation of depressant effects of morphine). Products include:
- Arco-Lase Plus Tablets 592
- Donnatal 2929
- Donnatal Extentabs 2930

Pimozide (Potentiation of depressant effects of morphine; increased risk of respiratory depression). Products include:
- Orap Tablets 1407

Prazepam (Potentiation of depressant effects of morphine).
No products indexed under this heading.

Prednisolone Acetate (Administration of morphine by epidural or intrathecal route is contraindicated in presence of concomitantly administered parenteral corticosteroids within 2 weeks). Products include:
- Blephamide Ophthalmic Ointment 547
- Blephamide Ophthalmic Suspension 548
- Poly-Pred Liquifilm Ophthalmic Suspension .... ⊙245
- Pred Forte Ophthalmic Suspension .... ⊙246
- Pred Mild Sterile Ophthalmic Suspension .... ⊙249
- Pred-G Ophthalmic Suspension .... ⊙247
- Pred-G Sterile Ophthalmic Ointment .... ⊙248

Prednisolone Sodium Phosphate (Administration of morphine by epidural or intrathecal route is contraindicated in presence of concomitantly administered parenteral corticosteroids within 2 weeks). Products include:
- Pediapred Oral Solution 1170

Prednisolone Tebutate (Administration of morphine by epidural or intrathecal route is contraindicated in presence of concomitantly administered parenteral corticosteroids within 2 weeks).
No products indexed under this heading.

Procarbazine Hydrochloride (Concomitant use potentiates depressant effects of morphine). Products include:
- Matulane Capsules 3246

Prochlorperazine (Potentiation of depressant effects of morphine; increased risk of respiratory depression). Products include:
- Compazine 1505

Promethazine Hydrochloride (Potentiation of depressant effects of morphine; increased risk of respiratory depression). Products include:
- Mepergan Injection 3539
- Phenergan Injection 3553
- Phenergan 3556
- Phenergan Syrup 3554
- Phenergan with Codeine Syrup 3557
- Phenergan with Dextromethorphan Syrup 3559
- Phenergan VC Syrup 3560
- Phenergan VC with Codeine Syrup 3561

Propofol (Potentiation of depressant effects of morphine). Products include:
Diprivan Injectable Emulsion 667

Propoxyphene Hydrochloride (Potentiation of depressant effects of morphine). Products include:
Darvon Pulvules 1909
Darvon Compound-65 Pulvules 1910

Propoxyphene Napsylate (Potentiation of depressant effects of morphine). Products include:
Darvon-N/Darvocet-N 1907
Darvon-N Tablets 1912

Protriptyline Hydrochloride (Potentiation of depressant effects of morphine). Products include:
Vivactil Tablets 2446
Vivactil Tablets 2217

Pyrilamine Maleate (Potentiation of depressant effects of morphine). Products include:
Maximum Strength Midol Menstrual Caplets and Gelcaps 612
Maximum Strength Midol PMS Caplets and Gelcaps 613

Pyrilamine Tannate (Potentiation of depressant effects of morphine). Products include:
Ryna-12 S Suspension 3351

Quazepam (Potentiation of depressant effects of morphine).
No products indexed under this heading.

Quetiapine Fumarate (Potentiation of depressant effects of morphine). Products include:
Seroquel Tablets 684

Remifentanil Hydrochloride (Potentiation of depressant effects of morphine).
No products indexed under this heading.

Risperidone (Potentiation of depressant effects of morphine). Products include:
Risperdal 1796

Secobarbital Sodium (Potentiation of depressant effects of morphine).
No products indexed under this heading.

Selegiline Hydrochloride (Concomitant use potentiates depressant effects of morphine). Products include:
Eldepryl Capsules 3266

Sevoflurane (Potentiation of depressant effects of morphine).
No products indexed under this heading.

Sufentanil Citrate (Potentiation of depressant effects of morphine).
No products indexed under this heading.

Temazepam (Potentiation of depressant effects of morphine).
No products indexed under this heading.

Terfenadine (Potentiation of depressant effects of morphine).
No products indexed under this heading.

Thiamylal Sodium (Potentiation of depressant effects of morphine).
No products indexed under this heading.

Thioridazine Hydrochloride (Potentiation of depressant effects of morphine; increased risk of respiratory depression). Products include:
Thioridazine Hydrochloride Tablets 2289

Thiothixene (Potentiation of depressant effects of morphine; increased risk of respiratory depression). Products include:
Navane Capsules 2701
Thiothixene Capsules 2290

Tinzaparin sodium (Administration of morphine by epidural or intrathecal route is contraindicated in presence of concomitant anticoagulant therapy). Products include:
Innohep Injection 1248

Tranylcypromine Sulfate (Concomitant use potentiates depressant effects of morphine). Products include:
Parnate Tablets 1607

Triamcinolone Acetonide (Administration of morphine by epidural or intrathecal route is contraindicated in presence of concomitantly administered parenteral corticosteroids within 2 weeks). Products include:
Azmacort Inhalation Aerosol 728
Nasacort Nasal Inhaler 750
Nasacort AQ Nasal Spray 752
Tri-Nasal Spray 2274

Triamcinolone Diacetate (Administration of morphine by epidural or intrathecal route is contraindicated in presence of concomitantly administered parenteral corticosteroids within 2 weeks).
No products indexed under this heading.

Triamcinolone Hexacetonide (Administration of morphine by epidural or intrathecal route is contraindicated in presence of concomitantly administered parenteral corticosteroids within 2 weeks).
No products indexed under this heading.

Triazolam (Potentiation of depressant effects of morphine). Products include:
Halcion Tablets 2823

Trifluoperazine Hydrochloride (Potentiation of depressant effects of morphine; increased risk of respiratory depression). Products include:
Stelazine 1640

Trimeprazine Tartrate (Potentiation of depressant effects of morphine).
No products indexed under this heading.

Trimipramine Maleate (Potentiation of depressant effects of morphine). Products include:
Surmontil Capsules 3595

Tripelennamine Hydrochloride (Potentiation of depressant effects of morphine).
No products indexed under this heading.

Triprolidine Hydrochloride (Potentiation of depressant effects of morphine). Products include:
Actifed Cold & Allergy Tablets 688

Warfarin Sodium (Administration of morphine by epidural or intrathecal route is contraindicated in presence of concomitant anticoagulant therapy). Products include:
Coumadin for Injection 1243
Coumadin Tablets 1243
Warfarin Sodium Tablets, USP 3302

Zaleplon (Potentiation of depressant effects of morphine). Products include:
Sonata Capsules 3591

Ziprasidone Hydrochloride (Potentiation of depressant effects of morphine). Products include:
Geodon Capsules 2688

Zolpidem Tartrate (Potentiation of depressant effects of morphine). Products include:
Ambien Tablets 3191

Food Interactions

Alcohol (Potentiation of depressant effects of morphine).

ATACAND TABLETS

(Candesartan Cilexetil) 595
None cited in PDR database.

ATACAND HCT TABLETS

(Candesartan Cilexetil, Hydrochlorothiazide) 597
May interact with:

Acarbose (Hyperglycemia may occur with thiazide diuretics; dosage adjustment of the antidiabetic drugs may be required). Products include:
Precose Tablets 906

Acebutolol Hydrochloride (Co-administration with other antihypertensive drugs may result in additive effect or potentiation of the antihypertensive effects with a potential for aggravation of orthostatic hypotension). Products include:
Sectral Capsules 3589

ACTH (Co-administration with ACTH intensifies the electrolyte depletion, particularly hypokalemia).
No products indexed under this heading.

Alfentanil Hydrochloride (Narcotics may aggravate orthostatic hypotension produced by hydrochlorothiazide).
No products indexed under this heading.

Amlodipine Besylate (Co-administration with other antihypertensive drugs may result in additive effect or potentiation of the antihypertensive effects with a potential for aggravation of orthostatic hypotension). Products include:
Lotrel Capsules 2370
Norvasc Tablets 2704

Aprobarbital (Barbiturates may aggravate orthostatic hypotension produced by hydrochlorothiazide).
No products indexed under this heading.

Atenolol (Co-administration with other antihypertensive drugs may result in additive effect or potentiation of the antihypertensive effects with a potential for aggravation of orthostatic hypotension). Products include:
Tenoretic Tablets 690
Tenormin I.V. Injection 692

Atracurium Besylate (Possible increased responsiveness to the muscle relaxant).
No products indexed under this heading.

Benazepril Hydrochloride (Co-administration with other antihypertensive drugs may result in additive effect or potentiation of the antihypertensive effects with a potential for aggravation of orthostatic hypotension). Products include:
Lotensin Tablets 2365
Lotensin HCT Tablets 2367
Lotrel Capsules 2370

Bendroflumethiazide (Co-administration with other antihypertensive drugs may result in additive effect or potentiation of the antihypertensive effects with a potential for aggravation of orthostatic hypotension). Products include:
Corzide 40/5 Tablets 2247
Corzide 80/5 Tablets 2247

Betamethasone Acetate (Co-administration with corticosteroids intensifies the electrolyte depletion, particularly hypokalemia). Products include:
Celestone Soluspan Injectable Suspension 3097

Betamethasone Sodium Phosphate (Co-administration with corticosteroids intensifies the electrolyte depletion, particularly hypokalemia). Products include:
Celestone Soluspan Injectable Suspension 3097

Betaxolol Hydrochloride (Co-administration with other antihypertensive drugs may result in additive effect or potentiation of the antihypertensive effects with a potential for aggravation of orthostatic hypotension). Products include:
Betoptic S Ophthalmic Suspension 537

Bisoprolol Fumarate (Co-administration with other antihypertensive drugs may result in additive effect or potentiation of the antihypertensive effects with a potential for aggravation of orthostatic hypotension). Products include:
Zebeta Tablets 1885
Ziac Tablets 1887

Buprenorphine Hydrochloride (Narcotics may aggravate orthostatic hypotension produced by hydrochlorothiazide). Products include:
Buprenex Injectable 2918

Butabarbital (Barbiturates may aggravate orthostatic hypotension produced by hydrochlorothiazide).
No products indexed under this heading.

Butalbital (Barbiturates may aggravate orthostatic hypotension produced by hydrochlorothiazide). Products include:
Phrenilin 578
Sedapap Tablets 50 mg/650 mg 2225

Captopril (Co-administration with other antihypertensive drugs may result in additive effect or potentiation of the antihypertensive effects with a potential for aggravation of orthostatic hypotension). Products include:
Captopril Tablets 2281

Carteolol Hydrochloride (Co-administration with other antihypertensive drugs may result in additive effect or potentiation of the antihypertensive effects with a potential for aggravation of orthostatic hypotension). Products include:
Carteolol Hydrochloride Ophthalmic Solution USP, 1% .... ⊙258
Ocupress Ophthalmic Solution, 1% Sterile .... ⊙303

Celecoxib (Co-administration of non-steroidal anti-inflammatory agents can reduce the diuretic, natriuretic, and antihypertensive effects of thiazide diuretics). Products include:
Celebrex Capsules 2676
Celebrex Capsules 2780

Chlorothiazide (Co-administration with other antihypertensive drugs may result in additive effect or potentiation of the antihypertensive effects with a potential for aggravation of orthostatic hypotension). Products include:
Aldoclor Tablets 2035
Diuril Oral 2087

Chlorothiazide Sodium (Co-administration with other antihypertensive drugs may result in additive effect or potentiation of the antihypertensive effects with a potential for aggravation of orthostatic hypotension). Products include:
Diuril Sodium Intravenous 2086

Chlorpropamide (Hyperglycemia may occur with thiazide diuretics; dosage adjustment of the antidiabetic drugs may be required). Products include:
Diabinese Tablets 2680

Chlorthalidone (Co-administration with other antihypertensive drugs may result in additive effect or potentiation of the antihypertensive effects with a potential for aggravation of orthostatic hypotension). Products include:
Clorpres Tablets 1002
Combipres Tablets 1040
Tenoretic Tablets 690

Cholestyramine (Co-administration with anionic exchange resins, such as cholestyramine, binds the hydrochlorothiazide and reduces its absorption by up to 85 percent).
No products indexed under this heading.

Cisatracurium Besylate (Possible increased responsiveness to the muscle relaxant).
No products indexed under this heading.

Clonidine (Co-administration with other antihypertensive drugs may result in additive effect or potentiation of the antihypertensive effects with a potential for aggravation of orthostatic hypotension). Products include:

Catapres-TTS 1038

Clonidine Hydrochloride (Co-administration with other antihypertensive drugs may result in additive effect or potentiation of the antihypertensive effects with a potential for aggravation of orthostatic hypotension). Products include:

Catapres Tablets 1037
Clorpres Tablets 1002
Combipres Tablets 1040
Duraclon Injection 3057

Codeine Phosphate (Narcotics may aggravate orthostatic hypotension produced by hydrochlorothiazide). Products include:

Phenergan with Codeine Syrup 3557
Phenergan VC with Codeine Syrup . 3561
Robitussin A-C Syrup 2942
Robitussin-DAC Syrup 2942
Ryna-C Liquid .... ▣768
Soma Compound w/Codeine Tablets 3355
Tussi-Organidin NR Liquid 3350
Tussi-Organidin-S NR Liquid 3350
Tylenol with Codeine 2595

Colestipol Hydrochloride (Co-administration with anionic exchange resins, such as colestipol, binds the hydrochlorothiazide and reduces its absorption by up to 43 percent). Products include:

Colestid Tablets 2791

Cortisone Acetate (Co-administration with corticosteroids intensifies the electrolyte depletion, particularly hypokalemia). Products include:

Cortone Acetate Injectable Suspension 2059
Cortone Acetate Tablets 2061

Deserpidine (Co-administration with other antihypertensive drugs may result in additive effect or potentiation of the antihypertensive effects with a potential for aggravation of orthostatic hypotension).

No products indexed under this heading.

Dexamethasone (Co-administration with corticosteroids intensifies the electrolyte depletion, particularly hypokalemia). Products include:

Decadron Elixir 2078
Decadron Tablets 2079
TobraDex Ophthalmic Ointment 542
TobraDex Ophthalmic Suspension .. 541

Dexamethasone Acetate (Co-administration with corticosteroids intensifies the electrolyte depletion, particularly hypokalemia).

No products indexed under this heading.

Dexamethasone Sodium Phosphate (Co-administration with corticosteroids intensifies the electrolyte depletion, particularly hypokalemia). Products include:

Decadron Phosphate Injection 2081
Decadron Phosphate Sterile Ophthalmic Ointment 2083
Decadron Phosphate Sterile Ophthalmic Solution 2084
NeoDecadron Sterile Ophthalmic Solution 2144

Dezocine (Narcotics may aggravate orthostatic hypotension produced by hydrochlorothiazide).

No products indexed under this heading.

Diazoxide (Co-administration with other antihypertensive drugs may result in additive effect or potentiation of the antihypertensive effects with a potential for aggravation of orthostatic hypotension).

No products indexed under this heading.

Diclofenac Potassium (Co-administration of non-steroidal anti-inflammatory agents can reduce the diuretic, natriuretic, and antihypertensive effects of thiazide diuretics). Products include:

Cataflam Tablets 2315

Diclofenac Sodium (Co-administration of non-steroidal anti-inflammatory agents can reduce the diuretic, natriuretic, and antihypertensive effects of thiazide diuretics). Products include:

Arthrotec Tablets 3195
Voltaren Ophthalmic Sterile Ophthalmic Solution .... ⊙312
Voltaren Tablets 2315
Voltaren-XR Tablets 2315

Diltiazem Hydrochloride (Co-administration with other antihypertensive drugs may result in additive effect or potentiation of the antihypertensive effects with a potential for aggravation of orthostatic hypotension). Products include:

Cardizem Injectable 1018
Cardizem Lyo-Ject Syringe 1018
Cardizem Monovial 1018
Cardizem CD Capsules 1016
Tiazac Capsules 1378

Doxazosin Mesylate (Co-administration with other antihypertensive drugs may result in additive effect or potentiation of the antihypertensive effects with a potential for aggravation of orthostatic hypotension). Products include:

Cardura Tablets 2668

Enalapril Maleate (Co-administration with other antihypertensive drugs may result in additive effect or potentiation of the antihypertensive effects with a potential for aggravation of orthostatic hypotension). Products include:

Lexxel Tablets 608
Vaseretic Tablets 2204
Vasotec Tablets 2210

Enalaprilat (Co-administration with other antihypertensive drugs may result in additive effect or potentiation of the antihypertensive effects with a potential for aggravation of orthostatic hypotension). Products include:

Enalaprilat injection 863
Vasotec I.V. Injection 2207

Eprosartan Mesylate (Co-administration with other antihypertensive drugs may result in additive effect or potentiation of the antihypertensive effects with a potential for aggravation of orthostatic hypotension). Products include:

Teveten Tablets 3327

Esmolol Hydrochloride (Co-administration with other antihypertensive drugs may result in additive effect or potentiation of the antihypertensive effects with a potential for aggravation of orthostatic hypotension). Products include:

Brevibloc Injection 858

Etodolac (Co-administration of non-steroidal anti-inflammatory agents can reduce the diuretic, natriuretic, and antihypertensive effects of thiazide diuretics). Products include:

Lodine 3528
Lodine XL Extended-Release Tablets 3530

Felodipine (Co-administration with other antihypertensive drugs may result in additive effect or potentiation of the antihypertensive effects with a potential for aggravation of orthostatic hypotension). Products include:

Lexxel Tablets 608
Plendil Extended-Release Tablets ... 623

Fenoprofen Calcium (Co-administration of non-steroidal anti-inflammatory agents can reduce the diuretic, natriuretic, and antihypertensive effects of thiazide diuretics).

No products indexed under this heading.

Fentanyl (Narcotics may aggravate orthostatic hypotension produced by hydrochlorothiazide). Products include:

Duragesic Transdermal System 1786

Fentanyl Citrate (Narcotics may aggravate orthostatic hypotension produced by hydrochlorothiazide). Products include:

Actiq 1184

Fludrocortisone Acetate (Co-administration with corticosteroids intensifies the electrolyte depletion, particularly hypokalemia). Products include:

Florinef Acetate Tablets 2250

Flurbiprofen (Co-administration of non-steroidal anti-inflammatory agents can reduce the diuretic, natriuretic, and antihypertensive effects of thiazide diuretics).

No products indexed under this heading.

Fosinopril Sodium (Co-administration with other antihypertensive drugs may result in additive effect or potentiation of the antihypertensive effects with a potential for aggravation of orthostatic hypotension). Products include:

Monopril Tablets 1091
Monopril HCT 1094

Furosemide (Co-administration with other antihypertensive drugs may result in additive effect or potentiation of the antihypertensive effects with a potential for aggravation of orthostatic hypotension). Products include:

Furosemide Tablets 2284

Glimepiride (Hyperglycemia may occur with thiazide diuretics; dosage adjustment of the antidiabetic drugs may be required). Products include:

Amaryl Tablets 717

Glipizide (Hyperglycemia may occur with thiazide diuretics; dosage adjustment of the antidiabetic drugs may be required). Products include:

Glucotrol Tablets 2692
Glucotrol XL Extended Release Tablets 2693

Glyburide (Hyperglycemia may occur with thiazide diuretics; dosage adjustment of the antidiabetic drugs may be required). Products include:

DiaBeta Tablets 741
Glucovance Tablets 1086

Guanabenz Acetate (Co-administration with other antihypertensive drugs may result in additive effect or potentiation of the antihypertensive effects with a potential for aggravation of orthostatic hypotension).

No products indexed under this heading.

Guanethidine Monosulfate (Co-administration with other antihypertensive drugs may result in additive effect or potentiation of the antihypertensive effects with a potential for aggravation of orthostatic hypotension).

No products indexed under this heading.

Hydralazine Hydrochloride (Co-administration with other antihypertensive drugs may result in additive effect or potentiation of the antihypertensive effects with a potential for aggravation of orthostatic hypotension).

No products indexed under this heading.

Hydrocodone Bitartrate (Narcotics may aggravate orthostatic hypotension produced by hydrochlorothiazide). Products include:

Hycodan 1316
Hycomine Compound Tablets 1317
Hycotuss Expectorant Syrup 1318
Lortab 3319
Lortab Elixir 3317
Maxidone Tablets CIII 3399
Norco 5/325 Tablets CIII 3424
Norco 7.5/325 Tablets CIII 3425
Norco 10/325 Tablets CIII 3427
Norco 10/325 Tablets CIII 3425
Vicodin Tablets 516
Vicodin ES Tablets 517
Vicodin HP Tablets 518
Vicodin Tuss Expectorant 519
Vicoprofen Tablets 520
Zydone Tablets 1330

Hydrocodone Polistirex (Narcotics may aggravate orthostatic hypotension produced by hydrochlorothiazide). Products include:

Tussionex Pennkinetic Extended-Release Suspension 1174

Hydrocortisone (Co-administration with corticosteroids intensifies the electrolyte depletion, particularly hypokalemia). Products include:

Anusol-HC Cream 2.5% 2237
Cipro HC Otic Suspension 540
Cortaid Intensive Therapy Cream . ▣717
Cortaid Maximum Strength Cream .... ▣717
Cortisporin Ophthalmic Suspension Sterile .... ⊙297
Cortizone•5 .... ▣699
Cortizone•10 .... ▣699
Cortizone•10 Plus Creme .... ▣700
Cortizone for Kids Creme .... ▣699
Hydrocortone Tablets 2106
Massengill Medicated Soft Cloth Towelette .... ▣753
VōSoL HC Otic Solution 3356

Hydrocortisone Acetate (Co-administration with corticosteroids intensifies the electrolyte depletion, particularly hypokalemia). Products include:

Analpram-HC 1338
Anusol HC-1 Hydrocortisone Anti-Itch Cream .... ▣689
Anusol-HC Suppositories 2238
Cortaid .... ▣717
Cortifoam Rectal Foam 3170
Cortisporin-TC Otic Suspension 2246
Hydrocortone Acetate Injectable Suspension 2103
Pramosone 1343
Proctocort Suppositories 2264
ProctoFoam-HC 3177
Terra-Cortril Ophthalmic Suspension 2716

Hydrocortisone Sodium Phosphate (Co-administration with corticosteroids intensifies the electrolyte depletion, particularly hypokalemia). Products include:

Hydrocortone Phosphate Injection, Sterile 2105

Hydrocortisone Sodium Succinate (Co-administration with corticosteroids intensifies the electrolyte depletion, particularly hypokalemia).

No products indexed under this heading.

Hydroflumethiazide (Co-administration with other antihypertensive drugs may result in additive effect or potentiation of the antihypertensive effects with a potential for aggravation of orthostatic hypotension). Products include:

Diucardin Tablets 3494

Hydromorphone Hydrochloride (Narcotics may aggravate orthostatic hypotension produced by hydrochlorothiazide). Products include:

Dilaudid 441
Dilaudid Oral Liquid 445
Dilaudid Powder 441
Dilaudid Rectal Suppositories 441
Dilaudid Tablets 441
Dilaudid Tablets - 8 mg 445
Dilaudid-HP 443

Ibuprofen (Co-administration of non-steroidal anti-inflammatory agents can reduce the diuretic, natriuretic, and antihypertensive effects of thiazide diuretics). Products include:

Advil .... ▣771
Children's Advil Oral Suspension ... ▣773
Children's Advil Chewable Tablets . ▣773
Advil Cold and Sinus Caplets .... ▣771

Advil Cold and Sinus Tablets .... ■771
Advil Flu & Body Ache Caplets ...... ■772
Infants' Advil Drops .... ■773
Junior Strength Advil Tablets .... ■773
Junior Strength Advil Chewable Tablets .... ■773
Advil Migraine Liquigels .... ■772
Children's Motrin Oral Suspension and Chewable Tablets.................. 2006
Children's Motrin Cold Oral Suspension.................................... 2007
Children's Motrin Oral Suspension.............................. ■643
Motrin Suspension, Oral Drops, Chewable Tablets, and Caplets.... 2002
Infants' Motrin Concentrated Drops.. 2006
Junior Strength Motrin Caplets and Chewable Tablets........................ 2006
Motrin IB Tablets, Caplets, and Gelcaps.................................... 2002
Motrin Migraine Pain Caplets 2005
Motrin Sinus Headache Caplets 2005
Vicoprofen Tablets 520

Indapamide (Co-administration with other antihypertensive drugs may result in additive effect or potentiation of the antihypertensive effects with a potential for aggravation of orthostatic hypotension). Products include:
Indapamide Tablets 2286

Indomethacin (Co-administration of non-steroidal anti-inflammatory agents can reduce the diuretic, natriuretic, and antihypertensive effects of thiazide diuretics). Products include:
Indocin 2112

Indomethacin Sodium Trihydrate (Co-administration of non-steroidal anti-inflammatory agents can reduce the diuretic, natriuretic, and antihypertensive effects of thiazide diuretics). Products include:
Indocin I.V. 2115

Insulin, Human, Zinc Suspension (Hyperglycemia may occur with thiazide diuretics; dosage adjustment of the insulin may be required). Products include:
Humulin L, 100 Units 1937
Humulin U, 100 Units 1943
Novolin L Human Insulin 10 ml Vials 2422

Insulin, Human NPH (Hyperglycemia may occur with thiazide diuretics; dosage adjustment of the insulin may be required). Products include:
Humulin N, 100 Units 1939
Humulin N NPH Pen 1940
Novolin N Human Insulin 10 ml Vials 2422
Novolin N PenFill 2423
Novolin N Prefilled Syringe Disposable Insulin Delivery System 2425

Insulin, Human Regular (Hyperglycemia may occur with thiazide diuretics; dosage adjustment of the insulin may be required). Products include:
Humulin R Regular (U-500) 1943
Humulin R, 100 Units 1941
Novolin R Human Insulin 10 ml Vials 2423
Novolin R PenFill 2423
Novolin R Prefilled Syringe Disposable Insulin Delivery System 2425
Velosulin BR Human Insulin 10 ml Vials 2435

Insulin, Human Regular and Human NPH Mixture (Hyperglycemia may occur with thiazide diuretics; dosage adjustment of the insulin may be required). Products include:
Humulin 50/50, 100 Units 1934
Humulin 70/30, 100 Units 1935
Humulin 70/30 Pen 1936
Novolin 70/30 Human Insulin 10 ml Vials 2421
Novolin 70/30 PenFill 2423
Novolin 70/30 Prefilled Disposable Insulin Delivery System 2425

Insulin, NPH (Hyperglycemia may occur with thiazide diuretics; dosage adjustment of the insulin may be required). Products include:
Iletin II, NPH (Pork), 100 Units 1946

Insulin, Regular (Hyperglycemia may occur with thiazide diuretics; dosage adjustment of the insulin may be required). Products include:
Iletin II, Regular (Pork), 100 Units ... 1947

Insulin, Zinc Crystals (Hyperglycemia may occur with thiazide diuretics; dosage adjustment of the insulin may be required).
No products indexed under this heading.

Insulin, Zinc Suspension (Hyperglycemia may occur with thiazide diuretics; dosage adjustment of the insulin may be required). Products include:
Iletin II, Lente (Pork), 100 Units 1945

Insulin Aspart, Human Regular (Hyperglycemia may occur with thiazide diuretics; dosage adjustment of the insulin may be required).
No products indexed under this heading.

Insulin glargine (Hyperglycemia may occur with thiazide diuretics; dosage adjustment of the insulin may be required). Products include:
Lantus Injection 742

Insulin Lispro, Human (Hyperglycemia may occur with thiazide diuretics; dosage adjustment of the insulin may be required). Products include:
Humalog 1926
Humalog Mix 75/25 Pen 1928

Insulin Lispro Protamine, Human (Hyperglycemia may occur with thiazide diuretics; dosage adjustment of the insulin may be required). Products include:
Humalog Mix 75/25 Pen 1928

Irbesartan (Co-administration with other antihypertensive drugs may result in additive effect or potentiation of the antihypertensive effects with a potential for aggravation of orthostatic hypotension). Products include:
Avalide Tablets 1070
Avapro Tablets 1074
Avapro Tablets 3076

Isradipine (Co-administration with other antihypertensive drugs may result in additive effect or potentiation of the antihypertensive effects with a potential for aggravation of orthostatic hypotension). Products include:
DynaCirc Capsules 2921
DynaCirc CR Tablets 2923

Ketoprofen (Co-administration of non-steroidal anti-inflammatory agents can reduce the diuretic, natriuretic, and antihypertensive effects of thiazide diuretics). Products include:
Orudis Capsules 3548
Orudis KT Tablets .... ■778
Oruvail Capsules 3548

Ketorolac Tromethamine (Co-administration of non-steroidal anti-inflammatory agents can reduce the diuretic, natriuretic, and antihypertensive effects of thiazide diuretics). Products include:
Acular Ophthalmic Solution 544
Acular PF Ophthalmic Solution 544
Toradol 3018

Labetalol Hydrochloride (Co-administration with other antihypertensive drugs may result in additive effect or potentiation of the antihypertensive effects with a potential for aggravation of orthostatic hypotension). Products include:
Normodyne Injection 3135
Normodyne Tablets 3137

Levorphanol Tartrate (Narcotics may aggravate orthostatic hypotension produced by hydrochlorothiazide). Products include:
Levo-Dromoran 1734
Levorphanol Tartrate Tablets 3059

Lisinopril (Co-administration with other antihypertensive drugs may result in additive effect or potentiation of the antihypertensive effects with a potential for aggravation of orthostatic hypotension). Products include:
Prinivil Tablets 2164
Prinzide Tablets 2168
Zestoretic Tablets 695
Zestril Tablets 698

Lithium Carbonate (Diuretic agents reduce the renal clearance of lithium and can cause a high risk of lithium toxicity; in general, lithium should not be given with diuretics). Products include:
Eskalith 1527
Lithium Carbonate 3061
Lithobid Slow-Release Tablets 3255

Lithium Citrate (Diuretic agents reduce the renal clearance of lithium and can cause a high risk of lithium toxicity; in general, lithium should not be given with diuretics). Products include:
Lithium Citrate Syrup 3061

Losartan Potassium (Co-administration with other antihypertensive drugs may result in additive effect or potentiation of the antihypertensive effects with a potential for aggravation of orthostatic hypotension). Products include:
Cozaar Tablets 2067
Hyzaar 2109

Mecamylamine Hydrochloride (Co-administration with other antihypertensive drugs may result in additive effect or potentiation of the antihypertensive effects with a potential for aggravation of orthostatic hypotension). Products include:
Inversine Tablets 1850

Meclofenamate Sodium (Co-administration of non-steroidal anti-inflammatory agents can reduce the diuretic, natriuretic, and antihypertensive effects of thiazide diuretics).
No products indexed under this heading.

Mefenamic Acid (Co-administration of non-steroidal anti-inflammatory agents can reduce the diuretic, natriuretic, and antihypertensive effects of thiazide diuretics). Products include:
Ponstel Capsules 1356

Meloxicam (Co-administration of non-steroidal anti-inflammatory agents can reduce the diuretic, natriuretic, and antihypertensive effects of thiazide diuretics). Products include:
Mobic Tablets 1054

Meperidine Hydrochloride (Narcotics may aggravate orthostatic hypotension produced by hydrochlorothiazide). Products include:
Demerol 3079
Mepergan Injection 3539

Mephobarbital (Barbiturates may aggravate orthostatic hypotension produced by hydrochlorothiazide).
No products indexed under this heading.

Metformin Hydrochloride (Hyperglycemia may occur with thiazide diuretics; dosage adjustment of the antidiabetic drugs may be required). Products include:
Glucophage Tablets 1080
Glucophage XR Tablets 1080
Glucovance Tablets 1086

Methadone Hydrochloride (Narcotics may aggravate orthostatic hypotension produced by hydrochlorothiazide). Products include:
Dolophine Hydrochloride Tablets 3056

Methyclothiazide (Co-administration with other antihypertensive drugs may result in additive effect or potentiation of the antihypertensive effects with a potential for aggravation of orthostatic hypotension).
No products indexed under this heading.

Methyldopa (Co-administration with other antihypertensive drugs may result in additive effect or potentiation of the antihypertensive effects with a potential for aggravation of orthostatic hypotension). Products include:
Aldoclor Tablets 2035
Aldomet Tablets 2037
Aldoril Tablets 2039

Methyldopate Hydrochloride (Co-administration with other antihypertensive drugs may result in additive effect or potentiation of the antihypertensive effects with a potential for aggravation of orthostatic hypotension).
No products indexed under this heading.

Methylprednisolone Acetate (Co-administration with corticosteroids intensifies the electrolyte depletion, particularly hypokalemia). Products include:
Depo-Medrol Injectable Suspension 2795

Methylprednisolone Sodium Succinate (Co-administration with corticosteroids intensifies the electrolyte depletion, particularly hypokalemia). Products include:
Solu-Medrol Sterile Powder 2855

Metocurine Iodide (Possible increased responsiveness to the muscle relaxant).
No products indexed under this heading.

Metolazone (Co-administration with other antihypertensive drugs may result in additive effect or potentiation of the antihypertensive effects with a potential for aggravation of orthostatic hypotension). Products include:
Mykrox Tablets 1168
Zaroxolyn Tablets 1177

Metoprolol Succinate (Co-administration with other antihypertensive drugs may result in additive effect or potentiation of the antihypertensive effects with a potential for aggravation of orthostatic hypotension). Products include:
Toprol-XL Tablets 651

Metoprolol Tartrate (Co-administration with other antihypertensive drugs may result in additive effect or potentiation of the antihypertensive effects with a potential for aggravation of orthostatic hypotension).
No products indexed under this heading.

Metyrosine (Co-administration with other antihypertensive drugs may result in additive effect or potentiation of the antihypertensive effects with a potential for aggravation of orthostatic hypotension). Products include:
Demser Capsules 2085

Mibefradil Dihydrochloride (Co-administration with other antihypertensive drugs may result in additive effect or potentiation of the antihypertensive effects with a potential for aggravation of orthostatic hypotension).
No products indexed under this heading.

Miglitol (Hyperglycemia may occur with thiazide diuretics; dosage adjustment of the antidiabetic drugs may be required). Products include:
Glyset Tablets 2821

Minoxidil (Co-administration with other antihypertensive drugs may result in additive effect or potentiation of the antihypertensive effects with a potential for aggravation of orthostatic hypotension). Products include:
Rogaine Extra Strength for Men Topical Solution .... ■721

Rogaine for Women Topical Solution ▣ 721

Mivacurium Chloride (Possible increased responsiveness to the muscle relaxant).
No products indexed under this heading.

Moexipril Hydrochloride (Co-administration with other antihypertensive drugs may result in additive effect or potentiation of the antihypertensive effects with a potential for aggravation of orthostatic hypotension). Products include:
- Uniretic Tablets ... 3178
- Univasc Tablets ... 3181

Morphine Sulfate (Narcotics may aggravate orthostatic hypotension produced by hydrochlorothiazide). Products include:
- Astramorph/PF Injection, USP (Preservative-Free) ... 594
- Duramorph Injection ... 1312
- Infumorph 200 and Infumorph 500 Sterile Solutions ... 1314
- Kadian Capsules ... 1335
- MS Contin Tablets ... 2896
- MSIR ... 2898
- Oramorph SR Tablets ... 3062
- Roxanol ... 3066

Nabumetone (Co-administration of non-steroidal anti-inflammatory agents can reduce the diuretic, natriuretic, and antihypertensive effects of thiazide diuretics). Products include:
- Relafen Tablets ... 1617

Nadolol (Co-administration with other antihypertensive drugs may result in additive effect or potentiation of the antihypertensive effects with a potential for aggravation of orthostatic hypotension). Products include:
- Corgard Tablets ... 2245
- Corzide 40/5 Tablets ... 2247
- Corzide 80/5 Tablets ... 2247
- Nadolol Tablets ... 2288

Naproxen (Co-administration of non-steroidal anti-inflammatory agents can reduce the diuretic, natriuretic, and antihypertensive effects of thiazide diuretics). Products include:
- EC-Naprosyn Delayed-Release Tablets ... 2967
- Naprosyn Suspension ... 2967
- Naprosyn Tablets ... 2967

Naproxen Sodium (Co-administration of non-steroidal anti-inflammatory agents can reduce the diuretic, natriuretic, and antihypertensive effects of thiazide diuretics). Products include:
- Aleve Tablets, Caplets and Gelcaps ▣ 602
- Aleve Cold & Sinus Caplets ▣ 603
- Anaprox Tablets ... 2967
- Anaprox DS Tablets ... 2967
- Naprelan Tablets ... 1293

Nicardipine Hydrochloride (Co-administration with other antihypertensive drugs may result in additive effect or potentiation of the antihypertensive effects with a potential for aggravation of orthostatic hypotension). Products include:
- Cardene I.V. ... 3485

Nifedipine (Co-administration with other antihypertensive drugs may result in additive effect or potentiation of the antihypertensive effects with a potential for aggravation of orthostatic hypotension). Products include:
- Adalat CC Tablets ... 877
- Procardia Capsules ... 2708
- Procardia XL Extended Release Tablets ... 2710

Nisoldipine (Co-administration with other antihypertensive drugs may result in additive effect or potentiation of the antihypertensive effects with a potential for aggravation of orthostatic hypotension). Products include:
- Sular Tablets ... 688

Nitroglycerin (Co-administration with other antihypertensive drugs may result in additive effect or potentiation of the antihypertensive effects with a potential for aggravation of orthostatic hypotension). Products include:
- Nitro-Dur Transdermal Infusion System ... 3134
- Nitro-Dur Transdermal Infusion System ... 1834
- Nitrolingual Pumpspray ... 1355
- Nitrostat Tablets ... 2658

Norepinephrine Bitartrate (Possible decreased response to pressor amines).
No products indexed under this heading.

Oxaprozin (Co-administration of non-steroidal anti-inflammatory agents can reduce the diuretic, natriuretic, and antihypertensive effects of thiazide diuretics).
No products indexed under this heading.

Oxycodone Hydrochloride (Narcotics may aggravate orthostatic hypotension produced by hydrochlorothiazide). Products include:
- OxyContin Tablets ... 2912
- OxyFast Oral Concentrate Solution ... 2916
- OxyIR Capsules ... 2916
- Percocet Tablets ... 1326
- Percodan Tablets ... 1327
- Percolone Tablets ... 1327
- Roxicodone ... 3067
- Tylox Capsules ... 2597

Pancuronium Bromide (Possible increased responsiveness to the muscle relaxant).
No products indexed under this heading.

Penbutolol Sulfate (Co-administration with other antihypertensive drugs may result in additive effect or potentiation of the antihypertensive effects with a potential for aggravation of orthostatic hypotension).
No products indexed under this heading.

Pentobarbital Sodium (Barbiturates may aggravate orthostatic hypotension produced by hydrochlorothiazide). Products include:
- Nembutal Sodium Solution ... 485

Perindopril Erbumine (Co-administration with other antihypertensive drugs may result in additive effect or potentiation of the antihypertensive effects with a potential for aggravation of orthostatic hypotension). Products include:
- Aceon Tablets (2 mg, 4 mg, 8 mg) ... 3249

Phenobarbital (Barbiturates may aggravate orthostatic hypotension produced by hydrochlorothiazide). Products include:
- Arco-Lase Plus Tablets ... 592
- Donnatal ... 2929
- Donnatal Extentabs ... 2930

Phenoxybenzamine Hydrochloride (Co-administration with other antihypertensive drugs may result in additive effect or potentiation of the antihypertensive effects with a potential for aggravation of orthostatic hypotension). Products include:
- Dibenzyline Capsules ... 3457

Phentolamine Mesylate (Co-administration with other antihypertensive drugs may result in additive effect or potentiation of the antihypertensive effects with a potential for aggravation of orthostatic hypotension).
No products indexed under this heading.

Phenylbutazone (Co-administration of non-steroidal anti-inflammatory agents can reduce the diuretic, natriuretic, and antihypertensive effects of thiazide diuretics).
No products indexed under this heading.

Pindolol (Co-administration with other antihypertensive drugs may result in additive effect or potentiation of the antihypertensive effects with a potential for aggravation of orthostatic hypotension).
No products indexed under this heading.

Pioglitazone Hydrochloride (Hyperglycemia may occur with thiazide diuretics; dosage adjustment of the antidiabetic drugs may be required). Products include:
- Actos Tablets ... 3275

Piroxicam (Co-administration of non-steroidal anti-inflammatory agents can reduce the diuretic, natriuretic, and antihypertensive effects of thiazide diuretics). Products include:
- Feldene Capsules ... 2685

Polythiazide (Co-administration with other antihypertensive drugs may result in additive effect or potentiation of the antihypertensive effects with a potential for aggravation of orthostatic hypotension). Products include:
- Minizide Capsules ... 2700
- Renese Tablets ... 2712

Prazosin Hydrochloride (Co-administration with other antihypertensive drugs may result in additive effect or potentiation of the antihypertensive effects with a potential for aggravation of orthostatic hypotension). Products include:
- Minipress Capsules ... 2699
- Minizide Capsules ... 2700

Prednisolone Acetate (Co-administration with corticosteroids intensifies the electrolyte depletion, particularly hypokalemia). Products include:
- Blephamide Ophthalmic Ointment ... 547
- Blephamide Ophthalmic Suspension ... 548
- Poly-Pred Liquifilm Ophthalmic Suspension ⊙ 245
- Pred Forte Ophthalmic Suspension ⊙ 246
- Pred Mild Sterile Ophthalmic Suspension ⊙ 249
- Pred-G Ophthalmic Suspension ⊙ 247
- Pred-G Sterile Ophthalmic Ointment ⊙ 248

Prednisolone Sodium Phosphate (Co-administration with corticosteroids intensifies the electrolyte depletion, particularly hypokalemia). Products include:
- Pediapred Oral Solution ... 1170

Prednisolone Tebutate (Co-administration with corticosteroids intensifies the electrolyte depletion, particularly hypokalemia).
No products indexed under this heading.

Prednisone (Co-administration with corticosteroids intensifies the electrolyte depletion, particularly hypokalemia). Products include:
- Prednisone ... 3064

Propoxyphene Hydrochloride (Narcotics may aggravate orthostatic hypotension produced by hydrochlorothiazide). Products include:
- Darvon Pulvules ... 1909
- Darvon Compound-65 Pulvules ... 1910

Propoxyphene Napsylate (Narcotics may aggravate orthostatic hypotension produced by hydrochlorothiazide). Products include:
- Darvon-N/Darvocet-N ... 1907
- Darvon-N Tablets ... 1912

Propranolol Hydrochloride (Co-administration with other antihypertensive drugs may result in additive effect or potentiation of the antihypertensive effects with a potential for aggravation of orthostatic hypotension). Products include:
- Inderal ... 3513
- Inderal LA Long-Acting Capsules ... 3516
- Inderide Tablets ... 3517
- Inderide LA Long-Acting Capsules ... 3519

Quinapril Hydrochloride (Co-administration with other antihypertensive drugs may result in additive effect or potentiation of the antihypertensive effects with a potential for aggravation of orthostatic hypotension). Products include:
- Accupril Tablets ... 2611
- Accuretic Tablets ... 2614

Ramipril (Co-administration with other antihypertensive drugs may result in additive effect or potentiation of the antihypertensive effects with a potential for aggravation of orthostatic hypotension). Products include:
- Altace Capsules ... 2233

Rapacuronium Bromide (Possible increased responsiveness to the muscle relaxant).
No products indexed under this heading.

Rauwolfia serpentina (Co-administration with other antihypertensive drugs may result in additive effect or potentiation of the antihypertensive effects with a potential for aggravation of orthostatic hypotension).
No products indexed under this heading.

Remifentanil Hydrochloride (Narcotics may aggravate orthostatic hypotension produced by hydrochlorothiazide).
No products indexed under this heading.

Repaglinide (Hyperglycemia may occur with thiazide diuretics; dosage adjustment of the antidiabetic drugs may be required). Products include:
- Prandin Tablets (0.5, 1, and 2 mg) ... 2432

Rescinnamine (Co-administration with other antihypertensive drugs may result in additive effect or potentiation of the antihypertensive effects with a potential for aggravation of orthostatic hypotension).
No products indexed under this heading.

Reserpine (Co-administration with other antihypertensive drugs may result in additive effect or potentiation of the antihypertensive effects with a potential for aggravation of orthostatic hypotension).
No products indexed under this heading.

Rocuronium Bromide (Possible increased responsiveness to the muscle relaxant). Products include:
- Zemuron Injection ... 2491

Rofecoxib (Co-administration of non-steroidal anti-inflammatory agents can reduce the diuretic, natriuretic, and antihypertensive effects of thiazide diuretics). Products include:
- Vioxx ... 2213

Rosiglitazone Maleate (Hyperglycemia may occur with thiazide diuretics; dosage adjustment of the antidiabetic drugs may be required). Products include:
- Avandia Tablets ... 1490

Secobarbital Sodium (Barbiturates may aggravate orthostatic hypotension produced by hydrochlorothiazide).
No products indexed under this heading.

Sodium Nitroprusside (Co-administration with other antihypertensive drugs may result in additive effect or potentiation of the antihypertensive effects with a potential for aggravation of orthostatic hypotension).
No products indexed under this heading.

Sotalol Hydrochloride (Co-administration with other antihypertensive drugs may result in additive effect or potentiation of the antihypertensive effects with a potential for aggravation of orthostatic hypotension). Products include:
- Betapace Tablets 950
- Betapace AF Tablets 954

Spirapril Hydrochloride (Co-administration with other antihypertensive drugs may result in additive effect or potentiation of the antihypertensive effects with a potential for aggravation of orthostatic hypotension).
No products indexed under this heading.

Sufentanil Citrate (Narcotics may aggravate orthostatic hypotension produced by hydrochlorothiazide).
No products indexed under this heading.

Sulindac (Co-administration of non-steroidal anti-inflammatory agents can reduce the diuretic, natriuretic, and antihypertensive effects of thiazide diuretics). Products include:
- Clinoril Tablets 2053

Telmisartan (Co-administration with other antihypertensive drugs may result in additive effect or potentiation of the antihypertensive effects with a potential for aggravation of orthostatic hypotension). Products include:
- Micardis Tablets 1049
- Micardis HCT Tablets 1051

Terazosin Hydrochloride (Co-administration with other antihypertensive drugs may result in additive effect or potentiation of the antihypertensive effects with a potential for aggravation of orthostatic hypotension). Products include:
- Hytrin Capsules 464

Thiamylal Sodium (Barbiturates may aggravate orthostatic hypotension produced by hydrochlorothiazide).
No products indexed under this heading.

Timolol Maleate (Co-administration with other antihypertensive drugs may result in additive effect or potentiation of the antihypertensive effects with a potential for aggravation of orthostatic hypotension).
Products include:
- Blocadren Tablets 2046
- Cosopt Sterile Ophthalmic Solution 2065
- Timolide Tablets 2187
- Timolol GFS .... ⊙266
- Timoptic in Ocudose 2192
- Timoptic Sterile Ophthalmic Solution 2190
- Timoptic-XE Sterile Ophthalmic Gel Forming Solution 2194

Tolazamide (Hyperglycemia may occur with thiazide diuretics; dosage adjustment of the antidiabetic drugs may be required).
No products indexed under this heading.

Tolbutamide (Hyperglycemia may occur with thiazide diuretics; dosage adjustment of the antidiabetic drugs may be required).
No products indexed under this heading.

Tolmetin Sodium (Co-administration of non-steroidal anti-inflammatory agents can reduce the diuretic, natriuretic, and antihypertensive effects of thiazide diuretics).
Products include:
- Tolectin 2589

Torsemide (Co-administration with other antihypertensive drugs may result in additive effect or potentiation of the antihypertensive effects with a potential for aggravation of orthostatic hypotension). Products include:
- Demadex Tablets and Injection 2965

Trandolapril (Co-administration with other antihypertensive drugs may result in additive effect or potentiation of the antihypertensive effects with a potential for aggravation of orthostatic hypotension). Products include:
- Mavik Tablets 478
- Tarka Tablets 508

Triamcinolone (Co-administration with corticosteroids intensifies the electrolyte depletion, particularly hypokalemia).
No products indexed under this heading.

Triamcinolone Acetonide (Co-administration with corticosteroids intensifies the electrolyte depletion, particularly hypokalemia). Products include:
- Azmacort Inhalation Aerosol 728
- Nasacort Nasal Inhaler 750
- Nasacort AQ Nasal Spray 752
- Tri-Nasal Spray 2274

Triamcinolone Diacetate (Co-administration with corticosteroids intensifies the electrolyte depletion, particularly hypokalemia).
No products indexed under this heading.

Triamcinolone Hexacetonide (Co-administration with corticosteroids intensifies the electrolyte depletion, particularly hypokalemia).
No products indexed under this heading.

Trimethaphan Camsylate (Co-administration with other antihypertensive drugs may result in additive effect or potentiation of the antihypertensive effects with a potential for aggravation of orthostatic hypotension).
No products indexed under this heading.

Troglitazone (Hyperglycemia may occur with thiazide diuretics; dosage adjustment of the antidiabetic drugs may be required).
No products indexed under this heading.

Tubocurarine Chloride (Possible increased responsiveness to the muscle relaxant).
No products indexed under this heading.

Valsartan (Co-administration with other antihypertensive drugs may result in additive effect or potentiation of the antihypertensive effects with a potential for aggravation of orthostatic hypotension). Products include:
- Diovan Capsules 2337
- Diovan HCT Tablets 2338

Vecuronium Bromide (Possible increased responsiveness to the muscle relaxant). Products include:
- Norcuron for Injection 2478

Verapamil Hydrochloride (Co-administration with other antihypertensive drugs may result in additive effect or potentiation of the antihypertensive effects with a potential for aggravation of orthostatic hypotension). Products include:
- Covera-HS Tablets 3199
- Isoptin SR Tablets 467
- Tarka Tablets 508
- Verelan Capsules 3184
- Verelan PM Capsules 3186

Food Interactions

Alcohol (May aggravate orthostatic hypotension produced by hydrochlorothiazide).

ATARAX TABLETS & SYRUP

(Hydroxyzine Hydrochloride) 2667
May interact with barbiturates, central nervous system depressants, narcotic analgesics, and certain other agents. Compounds in these categories include:

Alfentanil Hydrochloride (The potentiating action of hydroxyzine must be considered when it is used concurrently).
No products indexed under this heading.

Alprazolam (The potentiating action of hydroxyzine must be considered when it is used concurrently). Products include:
- Xanax Tablets 2865

Aprobarbital (The potentiating action of hydroxyzine must be considered when it is used concurrently).
No products indexed under this heading.

Buprenorphine Hydrochloride (The potentiating action of hydroxyzine must be considered when it is used concurrently). Products include:
- Buprenex Injectable 2918

Buspirone Hydrochloride (The potentiating action of hydroxyzine must be considered when it is used concurrently).
No products indexed under this heading.

Butabarbital (The potentiating action of hydroxyzine must be considered when it is used concurrently).
No products indexed under this heading.

Butalbital (The potentiating action of hydroxyzine must be considered when it is used concurrently).
Products include:
- Phrenilin 578
- Sedapap Tablets 50 mg/650 mg 2225

Chlordiazepoxide (The potentiating action of hydroxyzine must be considered when it is used concurrently). Products include:
- Limbitrol 1738

Chlordiazepoxide Hydrochloride (The potentiating action of hydroxyzine must be considered when it is used concurrently). Products include:
- Librium Capsules 1736
- Librium for Injection 1737

Chlorpromazine (The potentiating action of hydroxyzine must be considered when it is used concurrently). Products include:
- Thorazine Suppositories 1656

Chlorpromazine Hydrochloride (The potentiating action of hydroxyzine must be considered when it is used concurrently). Products include:
- Thorazine 1656

Chlorprothixene (The potentiating action of hydroxyzine must be considered when it is used concurrently).
No products indexed under this heading.

Chlorprothixene Hydrochloride (The potentiating action of hydroxyzine must be considered when it is used concurrently).
No products indexed under this heading.

Chlorprothixene Lactate (The potentiating action of hydroxyzine must be considered when it is used concurrently).
No products indexed under this heading.

Clorazepate Dipotassium (The potentiating action of hydroxyzine must be considered when it is used concurrently). Products include:
- Tranxene 511

Clozapine (The potentiating action of hydroxyzine must be considered when it is used concurrently).
Products include:
- Clozaril Tablets 2319

Codeine Phosphate (The potentiating action of hydroxyzine must be considered when it is used concurrently). Products include:
- Phenergan with Codeine Syrup 3557
- Phenergan VC with Codeine Syrup 3561
- Robitussin A-C Syrup 2942
- Robitussin-DAC Syrup 2942
- Ryna-C Liquid .... ▣768
- Soma Compound w/Codeine Tablets 3355
- Tussi-Organidin NR Liquid 3350
- Tussi-Organidin-S NR Liquid 3350
- Tylenol with Codeine 2595

Desflurane (The potentiating action of hydroxyzine must be considered when it is used concurrently).
Products include:
- Suprane Liquid for Inhalation 874

Dezocine (The potentiating action of hydroxyzine must be considered when it is used concurrently).
No products indexed under this heading.

Diazepam (The potentiating action of hydroxyzine must be considered when it is used concurrently).
Products include:
- Valium Injectable 3026
- Valium Tablets 3047

Droperidol (The potentiating action of hydroxyzine must be considered when it is used concurrently).
No products indexed under this heading.

Enflurane (The potentiating action of hydroxyzine must be considered when it is used concurrently).
No products indexed under this heading.

Estazolam (The potentiating action of hydroxyzine must be considered when it is used concurrently).
Products include:
- ProSom Tablets 500

Ethchlorvynol (The potentiating action of hydroxyzine must be considered when it is used concurrently).
No products indexed under this heading.

Ethinamate (The potentiating action of hydroxyzine must be considered when it is used concurrently).
No products indexed under this heading.

Fentanyl (The potentiating action of hydroxyzine must be considered when it is used concurrently).
Products include:
- Duragesic Transdermal System 1786

Fentanyl Citrate (The potentiating action of hydroxyzine must be considered when it is used concurrently). Products include:
- Actiq 1184

Fluphenazine Decanoate (The potentiating action of hydroxyzine must be considered when it is used concurrently).
No products indexed under this heading.

Fluphenazine Enanthate (The potentiating action of hydroxyzine must be considered when it is used concurrently).
No products indexed under this heading.

Fluphenazine Hydrochloride (The potentiating action of hydroxyzine must be considered when it is used concurrently).
No products indexed under this heading.

Flurazepam Hydrochloride (The potentiating action of hydroxyzine must be considered when it is used concurrently).
No products indexed under this heading.

Glutethimide (The potentiating action of hydroxyzine must be considered when it is used concurrently).
No products indexed under this heading.

Haloperidol (The potentiating action of hydroxyzine must be considered when it is used concurrently). Products include:
Haldol Injection, Tablets and Concentrate 2533

Haloperidol Decanoate (The potentiating action of hydroxyzine must be considered when it is used concurrently). Products include:
Haldol Decanoate 2535

Hydrocodone Bitartrate (The potentiating action of hydroxyzine must be considered when it is used concurrently). Products include:
Hycodan 1316
Hycomine Compound Tablets 1317
Hycotuss Expectorant Syrup 1318
Lortab 3319
Lortab Elixir 3317
Maxidone Tablets CIII 3399
Norco 5/325 Tablets CIII 3424
Norco 7.5/325 Tablets CIII 3425
Norco 10/325 Tablets CIII 3427
Norco 10/325 Tablets CIII 3425
Vicodin Tablets 516
Vicodin ES Tablets 517
Vicodin HP Tablets 518
Vicodin Tuss Expectorant 519
Vicoprofen Tablets 520
Zydone Tablets 1330

Hydrocodone Polistirex (The potentiating action of hydroxyzine must be considered when it is used concurrently). Products include:
Tussionex Pennkinetic Extended-Release Suspension 1174

Hydromorphone Hydrochloride (The potentiating action of hydroxyzine must be considered when it is used concurrently). Products include:
Dilaudid 441
Dilaudid Oral Liquid 445
Dilaudid Powder 441
Dilaudid Rectal Suppositories 441
Dilaudid Tablets 441
Dilaudid Tablets - 8 mg 445
Dilaudid-HP 443

Isoflurane (The potentiating action of hydroxyzine must be considered when it is used concurrently).
No products indexed under this heading.

Ketamine Hydrochloride (The potentiating action of hydroxyzine must be considered when it is used concurrently).
No products indexed under this heading.

Levomethadyl Acetate Hydrochloride (The potentiating action of hydroxyzine must be considered when it is used concurrently).
No products indexed under this heading.

Levorphanol Tartrate (The potentiating action of hydroxyzine must be considered when it is used concurrently). Products include:
Levo-Dromoran 1734
Levorphanol Tartrate Tablets 3059

Lorazepam (The potentiating action of hydroxyzine must be considered when it is used concurrently). Products include:
Ativan Injection 3478
Ativan Tablets 3482

Loxapine Hydrochloride (The potentiating action of hydroxyzine must be considered when it is used concurrently).
No products indexed under this heading.

Loxapine Succinate (The potentiating action of hydroxyzine must be considered when it is used concurrently). Products include:
Loxitane Capsules 3398

Meperidine Hydrochloride (The potentiating action of hydroxyzine must be considered when it is used concurrently). Products include:
Demerol 3079
Mepergan Injection 3539

Mephobarbital (The potentiating action of hydroxyzine must be considered when it is used concurrently).
No products indexed under this heading.

Meprobamate (The potentiating action of hydroxyzine must be considered when it is used concurrently). Products include:
Miltown Tablets 3349

Mesoridazine Besylate (The potentiating action of hydroxyzine must be considered when it is used concurrently). Products include:
Serentil 1057

Methadone Hydrochloride (The potentiating action of hydroxyzine must be considered when it is used concurrently). Products include:
Dolophine Hydrochloride Tablets 3056

Methohexital Sodium (The potentiating action of hydroxyzine must be considered when it is used concurrently). Products include:
Brevital Sodium for Injection, USP 1815

Methotrimeprazine (The potentiating action of hydroxyzine must be considered when it is used concurrently).
No products indexed under this heading.

Methoxyflurane (The potentiating action of hydroxyzine must be considered when it is used concurrently).
No products indexed under this heading.

Midazolam Hydrochloride (The potentiating action of hydroxyzine must be considered when it is used concurrently). Products include:
Versed Injection 3027
Versed Syrup 3033

Molindone Hydrochloride (The potentiating action of hydroxyzine must be considered when it is used concurrently). Products include:
Moban 1320

Morphine Sulfate (The potentiating action of hydroxyzine must be considered when it is used concurrently). Products include:
Astramorph/PF Injection, USP (Preservative-Free) 594
Duramorph Injection 1312
Infumorph 200 and Infumorph 500 Sterile Solutions 1314
Kadian Capsules 1335
MS Contin Tablets 2896
MSIR 2898
Oramorph SR Tablets 3062
Roxanol 3066

Non-narcotic Analgesics, unspecified (Potentiated action of non-narcotic analgesics).

Olanzapine (The potentiating action of hydroxyzine must be considered when it is used concurrently). Products include:
Zyprexa Tablets 1973
Zyprexa ZYDIS Orally Disintegrating Tablets 1973

Oxazepam (The potentiating action of hydroxyzine must be considered when it is used concurrently).
No products indexed under this heading.

Oxycodone Hydrochloride (The potentiating action of hydroxyzine must be considered when it is used concurrently). Products include:
OxyContin Tablets 2912
OxyFast Oral Concentrate Solution 2916
OxyIR Capsules 2916
Percocet Tablets 1326
Percodan Tablets 1327
Percolone Tablets 1327
Roxicodone 3067
Tylox Capsules 2597

Pentobarbital Sodium (The potentiating action of hydroxyzine must be considered when it is used concurrently). Products include:
Nembutal Sodium Solution 485

Perphenazine (The potentiating action of hydroxyzine must be considered when it is used concurrently). Products include:
Etrafon 3115
Trilafon 3160

Phenobarbital (The potentiating action of hydroxyzine must be considered when it is used concurrently). Products include:
Arco-Lase Plus Tablets 592
Donnatal 2929
Donnatal Extentabs 2930

Prazepam (The potentiating action of hydroxyzine must be considered when it is used concurrently).
No products indexed under this heading.

Prochlorperazine (The potentiating action of hydroxyzine must be considered when it is used concurrently). Products include:
Compazine 1505

Promethazine Hydrochloride (The potentiating action of hydroxyzine must be considered when it is used concurrently). Products include:
Mepergan Injection 3539
Phenergan Injection 3553
Phenergan 3556
Phenergan Syrup 3554
Phenergan with Codeine Syrup 3557
Phenergan with Dextromethorphan Syrup 3559
Phenergan VC Syrup 3560
Phenergan VC with Codeine Syrup 3561

Propofol (The potentiating action of hydroxyzine must be considered when it is used concurrently). Products include:
Diprivan Injectable Emulsion 667

Propoxyphene Hydrochloride (The potentiating action of hydroxyzine must be considered when it is used concurrently). Products include:
Darvon Pulvules 1909
Darvon Compound-65 Pulvules 1910

Propoxyphene Napsylate (The potentiating action of hydroxyzine must be considered when it is used concurrently). Products include:
Darvon-N/Darvocet-N 1907
Darvon-N Tablets 1912

Quazepam (The potentiating action of hydroxyzine must be considered when it is used concurrently).
No products indexed under this heading.

Quetiapine Fumarate (The potentiating action of hydroxyzine must be considered when it is used concurrently). Products include:
Seroquel Tablets 684

Remifentanil Hydrochloride (The potentiating action of hydroxyzine must be considered when it is used concurrently).
No products indexed under this heading.

Risperidone (The potentiating action of hydroxyzine must be considered when it is used concurrently). Products include:
Risperdal 1796

Secobarbital Sodium (The potentiating action of hydroxyzine must be considered when it is used concurrently).
No products indexed under this heading.

Sevoflurane (The potentiating action of hydroxyzine must be considered when it is used concurrently).
No products indexed under this heading.

Sufentanil Citrate (The potentiating action of hydroxyzine must be considered when it is used concurrently).
No products indexed under this heading.

Temazepam (The potentiating action of hydroxyzine must be considered when it is used concurrently).
No products indexed under this heading.

Thiamylal Sodium (The potentiating action of hydroxyzine must be considered when it is used concurrently).
No products indexed under this heading.

Thioridazine Hydrochloride (The potentiating action of hydroxyzine must be considered when it is used concurrently). Products include:
Thioridazine Hydrochloride Tablets 2289

Thiothixene (The potentiating action of hydroxyzine must be considered when it is used concurrently). Products include:
Navane Capsules 2701
Thiothixene Capsules 2290

Triazolam (The potentiating action of hydroxyzine must be considered when it is used concurrently). Products include:
Halcion Tablets 2823

Trifluoperazine Hydrochloride (The potentiating action of hydroxyzine must be considered when it is used concurrently). Products include:
Stelazine 1640

Zaleplon (The potentiating action of hydroxyzine must be considered when it is used concurrently). Products include:
Sonata Capsules 3591

Ziprasidone Hydrochloride (The potentiating action of hydroxyzine must be considered when it is used concurrently). Products include:
Geodon Capsules 2688

Zolpidem Tartrate (The potentiating action of hydroxyzine must be considered when it is used concurrently). Products include:
Ambien Tablets 3191

Food Interactions

Alcohol (Increased effect of alcohol).

ATIVAN INJECTION

(Lorazepam) 3478
May interact with barbiturates, central nervous system depressants, antidepressant drugs, monoamine oxidase inhibitors, phenothiazines, valproate, and certain other agents. Compounds in these categories include:

Alfentanil Hydrochloride (Co-administration results in additive CNS depression of the central nervous system).
No products indexed under this heading.

Alprazolam (Co-administration results in additive CNS depression of the central nervous system). Products include:
Xanax Tablets 2865

Amitriptyline Hydrochloride (Co-administration results in additive CNS depression of the central nervous system). Products include:
Etrafon 3115
Limbitrol 1738

Amoxapine (Co-administration results in additive CNS depression of the central nervous system).
No products indexed under this heading.

Aprobarbital (Co-administration results in additive CNS depression of the central nervous system).
No products indexed under this heading.

Buprenorphine Hydrochloride (Co-administration results in additive CNS depression of the central nervous system). Products include:

- Buprenex Injectable 2918

Bupropion Hydrochloride (Co-administration results in additive CNS depression of the central nervous system). Products include:
- Wellbutrin Tablets 1680
- Wellbutrin SR Sustained-Release Tablets 1684
- Zyban Sustained-Release Tablets 1710

Buspirone Hydrochloride (Co-administration results in additive CNS depression of the central nervous system).
No products indexed under this heading.

Butabarbital (Co-administration results in additive CNS depression of the central nervous system).
No products indexed under this heading.

Butalbital (Co-administration results in additive CNS depression of the central nervous system). Products include:
- Phrenilin 578
- Sedapap Tablets 50 mg/650 mg 2225

Chlordiazepoxide (Co-administration results in additive CNS depression of the central nervous system). Products include:
- Limbitrol 1738

Chlordiazepoxide Hydrochloride (Co-administration results in additive CNS depression of the central nervous system). Products include:
- Librium Capsules 1736
- Librium for Injection 1737

Chlorpromazine (Co-administration results in additive CNS depression of the central nervous system). Products include:
- Thorazine Suppositories 1656

Chlorpromazine Hydrochloride (Co-administration results in additive CNS depression of the central nervous system). Products include:
- Thorazine 1656

Chlorprothixene (Co-administration results in additive CNS depression of the central nervous system).
No products indexed under this heading.

Chlorprothixene Hydrochloride (Co-administration results in additive CNS depression of the central nervous system).
No products indexed under this heading.

Chlorprothixene Lactate (Co-administration results in additive CNS depression of the central nervous system).
No products indexed under this heading.

Citalopram Hydrobromide (Co-administration results in additive CNS depression of the central nervous system). Products include:
- Celexa 1365

Clorazepate Dipotassium (Co-administration results in additive CNS depression of the central nervous system). Products include:
- Tranxene 511

Clozapine (Co-administration has resulted in marked sedation, excessive salivation, ataxia, and rarely, death). Products include:
- Clozaril Tablets 2319

Codeine Phosphate (Co-administration results in additive CNS depression of the central nervous system). Products include:
- Phenergan with Codeine Syrup 3557
- Phenergan VC with Codeine Syrup 3561
- Robitussin A-C Syrup 2942
- Robitussin-DAC Syrup 2942
- Ryna-C Liquid 768
- Soma Compound w/Codeine Tablets 3355
- Tussi-Organidin NR Liquid 3350
- Tussi-Organidin-S NR Liquid 3350
- Tylenol with Codeine 2595

Desflurane (Co-administration results in additive CNS depression of the central nervous system). Products include:
- Suprane Liquid for Inhalation 874

Desipramine Hydrochloride (Co-administration results in additive CNS depression of the central nervous system). Products include:
- Norpramin Tablets 755

Dezocine (Co-administration results in additive CNS depression of the central nervous system).
No products indexed under this heading.

Diazepam (Co-administration results in additive CNS depression of the central nervous system). Products include:
- Valium Injectable 3026
- Valium Tablets 3047

Divalproex Sodium (Co-administration of injectable lorazepam and valproate has resulted in decreased total clearance of lorazepam by 40% and decreased formation rate of lorazepam glucuronide by 55%). Products include:
- Depakote Sprinkle Capsules 426
- Depakote Tablets 430
- Depakote ER Tablets 436

Doxepin Hydrochloride (Co-administration results in additive CNS depression of the central nervous system). Products include:
- Sinequan 2713

Droperidol (Co-administration results in additive CNS depression of the central nervous system).
No products indexed under this heading.

Enflurane (Co-administration results in additive CNS depression of the central nervous system).
No products indexed under this heading.

Estazolam (Co-administration results in additive CNS depression of the central nervous system). Products include:
- ProSom Tablets 500

Ethchlorvynol (Co-administration results in additive CNS depression of the central nervous system).
No products indexed under this heading.

Ethinamate (Co-administration results in additive CNS depression of the central nervous system).
No products indexed under this heading.

Ethinyl Estradiol (Co-administration with injectable lorazepam and norethindrone acetate/ethinyl estradiol containing oral contraceptives was associated with a 55% decrease in half-life, a 50% increase in the volume of distribution, thereby resulting in an almost 3.7-fold increase in total clearance of lorazepam). Products include:
- Alesse-21 Tablets 3468
- Alesse-28 Tablets 3473
- Brevicon 28-Day Tablets 3380
- Cyclessa Tablets 2450
- Desogen Tablets 2458
- Estinyl Tablets 3112
- Estrostep 2627
- femhrt Tablets 2635
- Levlen 962
- Levlite 21 Tablets 962
- Levlite 28 Tablets 962
- Levora Tablets 3389
- Loestrin 21 Tablets 2642
- Loestrin Fe Tablets 2642
- Lo/Ovral Tablets 3532
- Lo/Ovral-28 Tablets 3538
- Low-Ogestrel-28 Tablets 3392
- Microgestin Fe 1.5/30 Tablets 3407
- Microgestin Fe 1/20 Tablets 3400
- Mircette Tablets 2470
- Modicon 2563
- Necon 3415
- Nordette-28 Tablets 2257
- Norinyl 1 + 35 28-Day Tablets 3380
- Ogestrel 0.5/50-28 Tablets 3428
- Ortho-Cept 21 Tablets 2546
- Ortho-Cept 28 Tablets 2546
- Ortho-Cyclen/Ortho Tri-Cyclen 2573
- Ortho-Novum 2563
- Ovcon 3364
- Ovral Tablets 3551
- Ovral-28 Tablets 3552
- Tri-Levlen 962
- Tri-Norinyl-28 Tablets 3433
- Triphasil-21 Tablets 3600
- Triphasil-28 Tablets 3605
- Trivora Tablets 3439
- Yasmin 28 Tablets 980
- Zovia 3449

Fentanyl (Co-administration results in additive CNS depression of the central nervous system). Products include:
- Duragesic Transdermal System 1786

Fentanyl Citrate (Co-administration results in additive CNS depression of the central nervous system). Products include:
- Actiq 1184

Fluoxetine Hydrochloride (Co-administration results in additive CNS depression of the central nervous system). Products include:
- Prozac Pulvules, Liquid, and Weekly Capsules 1238
- Sarafem Pulvules 1962

Fluphenazine Decanoate (Co-administration results in additive CNS depression of the central nervous system).
No products indexed under this heading.

Fluphenazine Enanthate (Co-administration results in additive CNS depression of the central nervous system).
No products indexed under this heading.

Fluphenazine Hydrochloride (Co-administration results in additive CNS depression of the central nervous system).
No products indexed under this heading.

Flurazepam Hydrochloride (Co-administration results in additive CNS depression of the central nervous system).
No products indexed under this heading.

Glutethimide (Co-administration results in additive CNS depression of the central nervous system).
No products indexed under this heading.

Haloperidol (Co-administration has resulted in apnea, coma, bradycardia, arrhythmia, heart arrest, and death). Products include:
- Haldol Injection, Tablets and Concentrate 2533

Haloperidol Decanoate (Co-administration has resulted in apnea, coma, bradycardia, arrhythmia, heart arrest, and death). Products include:
- Haldol Decanoate 2535

Hydrocodone Bitartrate (Co-administration results in additive CNS depression of the central nervous system). Products include:
- Hycodan 1316
- Hycomine Compound Tablets 1317
- Hycotuss Expectorant Syrup 1318
- Lortab 3319
- Lortab Elixir 3317
- Maxidone Tablets CIII 3399
- Norco 5/325 Tablets CIII 3424
- Norco 7.5/325 Tablets CIII 3425
- Norco 10/325 Tablets CIII 3427
- Norco 10/325 Tablets CIII 3425
- Vicodin Tablets 516
- Vicodin ES Tablets 517
- Vicodin HP Tablets 518
- Vicodin Tuss Expectorant 519
- Vicoprofen Tablets 520
- Zydone Tablets 1330

Hydrocodone Polistirex (Co-administration results in additive CNS depression of the central nervous system). Products include:
- Tussionex Pennkinetic Extended-Release Suspension 1174

Hydromorphone Hydrochloride (Co-administration results in additive CNS depression of the central nervous system). Products include:
- Dilaudid 441
- Dilaudid Oral Liquid 445
- Dilaudid Powder 441
- Dilaudid Rectal Suppositories 441
- Dilaudid Tablets 441
- Dilaudid Tablets - 8 mg 445
- Dilaudid-HP 443

Hydroxyzine Hydrochloride (Co-administration results in additive CNS depression of the central nervous system). Products include:
- Atarax Tablets & Syrup 2667
- Vistaril Intramuscular Solution 2738

Imipramine Hydrochloride (Co-administration results in additive CNS depression of the central nervous system).
No products indexed under this heading.

Imipramine Pamoate (Co-administration results in additive CNS depression of the central nervous system).
No products indexed under this heading.

Isocarboxazid (Co-administration results in additive CNS depression of the central nervous system).
No products indexed under this heading.

Isoflurane (Co-administration results in additive CNS depression of the central nervous system).
No products indexed under this heading.

Ketamine Hydrochloride (Co-administration results in additive CNS depression of the central nervous system).
No products indexed under this heading.

Levomethadyl Acetate Hydrochloride (Co-administration results in additive CNS depression of the central nervous system).
No products indexed under this heading.

Levorphanol Tartrate (Co-administration results in additive CNS depression of the central nervous system). Products include:
- Levo-Dromoran 1734
- Levorphanol Tartrate Tablets 3059

Loxapine Hydrochloride (Co-administration has resulted in rare reports of significant respiratory depression, stupor, and/or hypotension).
No products indexed under this heading.

Loxapine Succinate (Co-administration has resulted in rare reports of significant respiratory depression, stupor, and/or hypotension). Products include:
- Loxitane Capsules 3398

Maprotiline Hydrochloride (Co-administration results in additive CNS depression of the central nervous system).
No products indexed under this heading.

Meperidine Hydrochloride (Co-administration results in additive CNS depression of the central nervous system). Products include:
- Demerol 3079
- Mepergan Injection 3539

Mephobarbital (Co-administration results in additive CNS depression of the central nervous system).
No products indexed under this heading.

Meprobamate (Co-administration results in additive CNS depression of the central nervous system). Products include:
- Miltown Tablets 3349

IMPORTANT NOTE: Always consult each drug listing in the patient's regimen for possible interactions.

Mesoridazine Besylate (Co-administration results in additive CNS depression of the central nervous system). Products include:
Serentil 1057

Methadone Hydrochloride (Co-administration results in additive CNS depression of the central nervous system). Products include:
Dolophine Hydrochloride Tablets 3056

Methohexital Sodium (Co-administration results in additive CNS depression of the central nervous system). Products include:
Brevital Sodium for Injection, USP .. 1815

Methotrimeprazine (Co-administration results in additive CNS depression of the central nervous system).
No products indexed under this heading.

Methoxyflurane (Co-administration results in additive CNS depression of the central nervous system).
No products indexed under this heading.

Midazolam Hydrochloride (Co-administration results in additive CNS depression of the central nervous system). Products include:
Versed Injection 3027
Versed Syrup 3033

Mirtazapine (Co-administration results in additive CNS depression of the central nervous system). Products include:
Remeron Tablets 2483
Remeron SolTab Tablets 2486

Moclobemide (Co-administration results in additive CNS depression of the central nervous system).
No products indexed under this heading.

Molindone Hydrochloride (Co-administration results in additive CNS depression of the central nervous system). Products include:
Moban 1320

Morphine Sulfate (Co-administration results in additive CNS depression of the central nervous system). Products include:
Astramorph/PF Injection, USP (Preservative-Free) 594
Duramorph Injection 1312
Infumorph 200 and Infumorph 500 Sterile Solutions 1314
Kadian Capsules 1335
MS Contin Tablets 2896
MSIR 2898
Oramorph SR Tablets 3062
Roxanol 3066

Nefazodone Hydrochloride (Co-administration results in additive CNS depression of the central nervous system). Products include:
Serzone Tablets 1104

Norethindrone (Co-administration with injectable lorazepam and norethindrone acetate/ethinyl estradiol containing oral contraceptives was associated with a 55% decrease in half-life, a 50% increase in the volume of distribution, thereby resulting in an almost 3.7-fold increase in total clearance of lorazepam). Products include:
Brevicon 28-Day Tablets 3380
Micronor Tablets 2543
Modicon 2563
Necon 3415
Norinyl 1 +35 28-Day Tablets 3380
Norinyl 1 + 50 28-Day Tablets 3380
Nor-QD Tablets 3423
Ortho-Novum 2563
Ortho-Novum 1/50□28 Tablets 2556
Ovcon 3364
Tri-Norinyl-28 Tablets 3433

Norethindrone Acetate (Co-administration with injectable lorazepam and norethindrone acetate/ethinyl estradiol containing oral contraceptives was associated with a 55% decrease in half-life, a 50% increase in the volume of distribution, thereby resulting in an almost 3.7-fold increase in total clearance of lorazepam). Products include:
Activella Tablets 2764
Aygestin Tablets 1333
CombiPatch Transdermal System .. 2323
Estrostep 2627
femhrt Tablets 2635
Loestrin 21 Tablets 2642
Loestrin Fe Tablets 2642
Microgestin Fe 1.5/30 Tablets 3407
Microgestin Fe 1/20 Tablets 3400

Nortriptyline Hydrochloride (Co-administration results in additive CNS depression of the central nervous system).
No products indexed under this heading.

Olanzapine (Co-administration results in additive CNS depression of the central nervous system). Products include:
Zyprexa Tablets 1973
Zyprexa ZYDIS Orally Disintegrating Tablets 1973

Oxazepam (Co-administration results in additive CNS depression of the central nervous system).
No products indexed under this heading.

Oxycodone Hydrochloride (Co-administration results in additive CNS depression of the central nervous system). Products include:
OxyContin Tablets 2912
OxyFast Oral Concentrate Solution . 2916
OxyIR Capsules 2916
Percocet Tablets 1326
Percodan Tablets 1327
Percolone Tablets 1327
Roxicodone 3067
Tylox Capsules 2597

Pargyline Hydrochloride (Co-administration results in additive CNS depression of the central nervous system).
No products indexed under this heading.

Paroxetine Hydrochloride (Co-administration results in additive CNS depression of the central nervous system). Products include:
Paxil 1609

Pentobarbital Sodium (Co-administration results in additive CNS depression of the central nervous system). Products include:
Nembutal Sodium Solution 485

Perphenazine (Co-administration results in additive CNS depression of the central nervous system). Products include:
Etrafon 3115
Trilafon 3160

Phenelzine Sulfate (Co-administration results in additive CNS depression of the central nervous system). Products include:
Nardil Tablets 2653

Phenobarbital (Co-administration results in additive CNS depression of the central nervous system). Products include:
Arco-Lase Plus Tablets 592
Donnatal 2929
Donnatal Extentabs 2930

Prazepam (Co-administration results in additive CNS depression of the central nervous system).
No products indexed under this heading.

Probenecid (Co-administration of injectable lorazepam with probenecid has resulted in a prolongation of lorazepam half-life by 130% and a decrease in its clearance by 45%).
No products indexed under this heading.

Procarbazine Hydrochloride (Co-administration results in additive CNS depression of the central nervous system). Products include:
Matulane Capsules 3246

Prochlorperazine (Co-administration results in additive CNS depression of the central nervous system). Products include:
Compazine 1505

Promethazine Hydrochloride (Co-administration results in additive CNS depression of the central nervous system). Products include:
Mepergan Injection 3539
Phenergan Injection 3553
Phenergan 3556
Phenergan Syrup 3554
Phenergan with Codeine Syrup 3557
Phenergan with Dextromethorphan Syrup 3559
Phenergan VC Syrup 3560
Phenergan VC with Codeine Syrup .. 3561

Propofol (Co-administration results in additive CNS depression of the central nervous system). Products include:
Diprivan Injectable Emulsion 667

Propoxyphene Hydrochloride (Co-administration results in additive CNS depression of the central nervous system). Products include:
Darvon Pulvules 1909
Darvon Compound-65 Pulvules 1910

Propoxyphene Napsylate (Co-administration results in additive CNS depression of the central nervous system). Products include:
Darvon-N/Darvocet-N 1907
Darvon-N Tablets 1912

Protriptyline Hydrochloride (Co-administration results in additive CNS depression of the central nervous system). Products include:
Vivactil Tablets 2446
Vivactil Tablets 2217

Quazepam (Co-administration results in additive CNS depression of the central nervous system).
No products indexed under this heading.

Quetiapine Fumarate (Co-administration results in additive CNS depression of the central nervous system). Products include:
Seroquel Tablets 684

Remifentanil Hydrochloride (Co-administration results in additive CNS depression of the central nervous system).
No products indexed under this heading.

Risperidone (Co-administration results in additive CNS depression of the central nervous system). Products include:
Risperdal 1796

Scopolamine (Co-administration of scopolamine with injectible lorazepam has resulted in increased incidence of sedation, hallucinations, and irrational behavior). Products include:
Transderm Scōp Transdermal Therapeutic System 2302

Scopolamine Hydrobromide (Co-administration of scopolamine with injectible lorazepam has resulted in increased incidence of sedation, hallucinations, and irrational behavior). Products include:
Donnatal 2929
Donnatal Extentabs 2930

Secobarbital Sodium (Co-administration results in additive CNS depression of the central nervous system).
No products indexed under this heading.

Selegiline Hydrochloride (Co-administration results in additive CNS depression of the central nervous system). Products include:
Eldepryl Capsules 3266

Sertraline Hydrochloride (Co-administration results in additive CNS depression of the central nervous system). Products include:
Zoloft 2751

Sevoflurane (Co-administration results in additive CNS depression of the central nervous system).
No products indexed under this heading.

Sufentanil Citrate (Co-administration results in additive CNS depression of the central nervous system).
No products indexed under this heading.

Temazepam (Co-administration results in additive CNS depression of the central nervous system).
No products indexed under this heading.

Thiamylal Sodium (Co-administration results in additive CNS depression of the central nervous system).
No products indexed under this heading.

Thioridazine Hydrochloride (Co-administration results in additive CNS depression of the central nervous system). Products include:
Thioridazine Hydrochloride Tablets 2289

Thiothixene (Co-administration results in additive CNS depression of the central nervous system). Products include:
Navane Capsules 2701
Thiothixene Capsules 2290

Tranylcypromine Sulfate (Co-administration results in additive CNS depression of the central nervous system). Products include:
Parnate Tablets 1607

Trazodone Hydrochloride (Co-administration results in additive CNS depression of the central nervous system).
No products indexed under this heading.

Triazolam (Co-administration results in additive CNS depression of the central nervous system). Products include:
Halcion Tablets 2823

Trifluoperazine Hydrochloride (Co-administration results in additive CNS depression of the central nervous system). Products include:
Stelazine 1640

Trimipramine Maleate (Co-administration results in additive CNS depression of the central nervous system). Products include:
Surmontil Capsules 3595

Valproate Sodium (Co-administration of injectable lorazepam and valproate has resulted in decreased total clearance of lorazepam by 40% and decreased formation rate of lorazepam glucuronide by 55%). Products include:
Depacon Injection 416

Valproic Acid (Co-administration of injectable lorazepam and valproate has resulted in decreased total clearance of lorazepam by 40% and decreased formation rate of lorazepam glucuronide by 55%). Products include:
Depakene 421

Venlafaxine Hydrochloride (Co-administration results in additive CNS depression of the central nervous system). Products include:
Effexor Tablets 3495
Effexor XR Capsules 3499

Zaleplon (Co-administration results in additive CNS depression of the central nervous system). Products include:
Sonata Capsules 3591

Ziprasidone Hydrochloride (Co-administration results in additive CNS depression of the central nervous system). Products include:
Geodon Capsules 2688

Zolpidem Tartrate (Co-administration results in additive CNS depression of the central nervous system). Products include:
Ambien Tablets 3191

Food Interactions

Alcohol (Concurrent use results in additive CNS depression of the central nervous system).

ATIVAN TABLETS

(Lorazepam) 3482
See Ativan Injection

ATROMID-S CAPSULES

(Clofibrate) 3483
May interact with anticoagulants and certain other agents. Compounds in these categories include:

Ardeparin Sodium (To prevent bleeding complications, anticoagulant dosage should be reduced generally by one-half).
No products indexed under this heading.

Dalteparin Sodium (To prevent bleeding complications, anticoagulant dosage should be reduced generally by one-half). Products include:
Fragmin Injection 2814

Danaparoid Sodium (To prevent bleeding complications, anticoagulant dosage should be reduced generally by one-half). Products include:
Orgaran Injection 2480

Dicumarol (To prevent bleeding complications, anticoagulant dosage should be reduced generally by one-half).
No products indexed under this heading.

Enoxaparin (To prevent bleeding complications, anticoagulant dosage should be reduced generally by one-half). Products include:
Lovenox Injection 746

Heparin Sodium (To prevent bleeding complications, anticoagulant dosage should be reduced generally by one-half). Products include:
Heparin Lock Flush Solution 3509
Heparin Sodium Injection 3511

Lovastatin (Potential for fulminant rhabdomyolysis, myopathy, and acute renal failure). Products include:
Mevacor Tablets 2132

Phenytoin (Atromid-S may displace phenytoin from its binding site). Products include:
Dilantin Infatabs 2624
Dilantin-125 Oral Suspension 2625

Phenytoin Sodium (Atromid-S may displace phenytoin from its binding site). Products include:
Dilantin Kapseals 2622

Tinzaparin sodium (To prevent bleeding complications, anticoagulant dosage should be reduced generally by one-half). Products include:
Innohep Injection 1248

Tolbutamide (Increased hypoglycemic effect; Atromid-S may displace tolbutamide from its binding site).
No products indexed under this heading.

Warfarin Sodium (To prevent bleeding complications, anticoagulant dosage should be reduced generally by one-half). Products include:
Coumadin for Injection 1243
Coumadin Tablets 1243
Warfarin Sodium Tablets, USP 3302

ATROVENT INHALATION AEROSOL

(Ipratropium Bromide) 1030
None cited in PDR database.

ATROVENT INHALATION SOLUTION

(Ipratropium Bromide) 1031
None cited in PDR database.

ATROVENT NASAL SPRAY 0.03%

(Ipratropium Bromide) 1032
May interact with anticholinergics. Compounds in these categories include:

Atropine Sulfate (Some potential for an additive interaction with other concomitantly administered anticholinergic drugs). Products include:
Donnatal 2929
Donnatal Extentabs 2930
Motofen Tablets 577
Prosed/DS Tablets 3268
Urised Tablets 2876

Belladonna Alkaloids (Some potential for an additive interaction with other concomitantly administered anticholinergic drugs). Products include:
Hyland's Teething Tablets 766
Urimax Tablets 1769

Benztropine Mesylate (Some potential for an additive interaction with other concomitantly administered anticholinergic drugs). Products include:
Cogentin 2055

Biperiden Hydrochloride (Some potential for an additive interaction with other concomitantly administered anticholinergic drugs). Products include:
Akineton 402

Clidinium Bromide (Some potential for an additive interaction with other concomitantly administered anticholinergic drugs).
No products indexed under this heading.

Dicyclomine Hydrochloride (Some potential for an additive interaction with other concomitantly administered anticholinergic drugs).
No products indexed under this heading.

Glycopyrrolate (Some potential for an additive interaction with other concomitantly administered anticholinergic drugs). Products include:
Robinul Forte Tablets 1358
Robinul Injectable 2940
Robinul Tablets 1358

Hyoscyamine (Some potential for an additive interaction with other concomitantly administered anticholinergic drugs). Products include:
Urised Tablets 2876

Hyoscyamine Sulfate (Some potential for an additive interaction with other concomitantly administered anticholinergic drugs). Products include:
Arco-Lase Plus Tablets 592
Donnatal 2929
Donnatal Extentabs 2930
Levsin/Levsinex/Levbid 3172
NuLev Orally Disintegrating Tablets 3176
Prosed/DS Tablets 3268
Urimax Tablets 1769

Mepenzolate Bromide (Some potential for an additive interaction with other concomitantly administered anticholinergic drugs).
No products indexed under this heading.

Oxybutynin Chloride (Some potential for an additive interaction with other concomitantly administered anticholinergic drugs). Products include:
Ditropan XL Extended Release Tablets 564

Procyclidine Hydrochloride (Some potential for an additive interaction with other concomitantly administered anticholinergic drugs).
No products indexed under this heading.

Propantheline Bromide (Some potential for an additive interaction with other concomitantly administered anticholinergic drugs).
No products indexed under this heading.

Scopolamine (Some potential for an additive interaction with other concomitantly administered anticholinergic drugs). Products include:
Transderm Scōp Transdermal Therapeutic System 2302

Scopolamine Hydrobromide (Some potential for an additive interaction with other concomitantly administered anticholinergic drugs). Products include:
Donnatal 2929
Donnatal Extentabs 2930

Tolterodine Tartrate (Some potential for an additive interaction with other concomitantly administered anticholinergic drugs). Products include:
Detrol Tablets 3623
Detrol LA Capsules 2801

Tridihexethyl Chloride (Some potential for an additive interaction with other concomitantly administered anticholinergic drugs).
No products indexed under this heading.

Trihexyphenidyl Hydrochloride (Some potential for an additive interaction with other concomitantly administered anticholinergic drugs). Products include:
Artane 1855

ATROVENT NASAL SPRAY 0.06%

(Ipratropium Bromide) 1033
May interact with anticholinergics. Compounds in these categories include:

Atropine Sulfate (Some potential for an additive interaction with other concomitantly administered anticholinergic drugs). Products include:
Donnatal 2929
Donnatal Extentabs 2930
Motofen Tablets 577
Prosed/DS Tablets 3268
Urised Tablets 2876

Belladonna Alkaloids (Some potential for an additive interaction with other concomitantly administered anticholinergic drugs). Products include:
Hyland's Teething Tablets 766
Urimax Tablets 1769

Benztropine Mesylate (Some potential for an additive interaction with other concomitantly administered anticholinergic drugs). Products include:
Cogentin 2055

Biperiden Hydrochloride (Some potential for an additive interaction with other concomitantly administered anticholinergic drugs). Products include:
Akineton 402

Clidinium Bromide (Some potential for an additive interaction with other concomitantly administered anticholinergic drugs).
No products indexed under this heading.

Dicyclomine Hydrochloride (Some potential for an additive interaction with other concomitantly administered anticholinergic drugs).
No products indexed under this heading.

Glycopyrrolate (Some potential for an additive interaction with other concomitantly administered anticholinergic drugs). Products include:
Robinul Forte Tablets 1358
Robinul Injectable 2940
Robinul Tablets 1358

Hyoscyamine (Some potential for an additive interaction with other concomitantly administered anticholinergic drugs). Products include:
Urised Tablets 2876

Hyoscyamine Sulfate (Some potential for an additive interaction with other concomitantly administered anticholinergic drugs). Products include:
Arco-Lase Plus Tablets 592
Donnatal 2929
Donnatal Extentabs 2930
Levsin/Levsinex/Levbid 3172
NuLev Orally Disintegrating Tablets 3176
Prosed/DS Tablets 3268
Urimax Tablets 1769

Mepenzolate Bromide (Some potential for an additive interaction with other concomitantly administered anticholinergic drugs).
No products indexed under this heading.

Oxybutynin Chloride (Some potential for an additive interaction with other concomitantly administered anticholinergic drugs). Products include:
Ditropan XL Extended Release Tablets 564

Procyclidine Hydrochloride (Some potential for an additive interaction with other concomitantly administered anticholinergic drugs).
No products indexed under this heading.

Propantheline Bromide (Some potential for an additive interaction with other concomitantly administered anticholinergic drugs).
No products indexed under this heading.

Scopolamine (Some potential for an additive interaction with other concomitantly administered anticholinergic drugs). Products include:
Transderm Scōp Transdermal Therapeutic System 2302

Scopolamine Hydrobromide (Some potential for an additive interaction with other concomitantly administered anticholinergic drugs). Products include:
Donnatal 2929
Donnatal Extentabs 2930

Tolterodine Tartrate (Some potential for an additive interaction with other concomitantly administered anticholinergic drugs). Products include:
Detrol Tablets 3623
Detrol LA Capsules 2801

Tridihexethyl Chloride (Some potential for an additive interaction with other concomitantly administered anticholinergic drugs).
No products indexed under this heading.

Trihexyphenidyl Hydrochloride (Some potential for an additive interaction with other concomitantly administered anticholinergic drugs). Products include:
Artane 1855

ATTENUVAX

(Measles Virus Vaccine Live) 2044
May interact with immunosuppressive agents. Compounds in these categories include:

Azathioprine (Concurrent use in individuals on immunosuppressive therapy is contraindicated).
No products indexed under this heading.

Basiliximab (Concurrent use in individuals on immunosuppressive therapy is contraindicated). Products include:
Simulect for Injection 2399

Cyclosporine (Concurrent use in individuals on immunosuppressive therapy is contraindicated). Products include:
Gengraf Capsules 457
Neoral Soft Gelatin Capsules 2380
Neoral Oral Solution 2380
Sandimmune 2388

Muromonab-CD3 (Concurrent use in individuals on immunosuppressive therapy is contraindicated). Products include:
- Orthoclone OKT3 Sterile Solution ... 2498

Mycophenolate Mofetil (Concurrent use in individuals on immunosuppressive therapy is contraindicated). Products include:
- CellCept Capsules ... 2951
- CellCept Oral Suspension ... 2951
- CellCept Tablets ... 2951

Sirolimus (Concurrent use in individuals on immunosuppressive therapy is contraindicated). Products include:
- Rapamune Oral Solution and Tablets ... 3584

Tacrolimus (Concurrent use in individuals on immunosuppressive therapy is contraindicated). Products include:
- Prograf ... 1393
- Protopic Ointment ... 1397

AUGMENTIN CHEWABLE TABLETS
(Amoxicillin, Clavulanate Potassium) ... 1482
See Augmentin ES-600 Powder for Oral Suspension

AUGMENTIN POWDER FOR ORAL SUSPENSION
(Amoxicillin, Clavulanate Potassium) ... 1482
See Augmentin ES-600 Powder for Oral Suspension

AUGMENTIN TABLETS
(Amoxicillin, Clavulanate Potassium) ... 1485
See Augmentin ES-600 Powder for Oral Suspension

AUGMENTIN ES-600 POWDER FOR ORAL SUSPENSION
(Amoxicillin, Clavulanate Potassium) ... 1487
May interact with oral contraceptives and certain other agents. Compounds in these categories include:

Allopurinol (Co-administration of ampicillin with allopurinol substantially increases the incidence of rashes; there are no data with Augmentin and allopurinol administered concurrently).
No products indexed under this heading.

Desogestrel (Potential for reduced efficacy of oral contraceptives). Products include:
- Cyclessa Tablets ... 2450
- Desogen Tablets ... 2458
- Mircette Tablets ... 2470
- Ortho-Cept 21 Tablets ... 2546
- Ortho-Cept 28 Tablets ... 2546

Ethinyl Estradiol (Potential for reduced efficacy of oral contraceptives). Products include:
- Alesse-21 Tablets ... 3468
- Alesse-28 Tablets ... 3473
- Brevicon 28-Day Tablets ... 3380
- Cyclessa Tablets ... 2450
- Desogen Tablets ... 2458
- Estinyl Tablets ... 3112
- Estrostep ... 2627
- femhrt Tablets ... 2635
- Levlen ... 962
- Levlite 21 Tablets ... 962
- Levlite 28 Tablets ... 962
- Levora Tablets ... 3389
- Loestrin 21 Tablets ... 2642
- Loestrin Fe Tablets ... 2642
- Lo/Ovral Tablets ... 3532
- Lo/Ovral-28 Tablets ... 3538
- Low-Ogestrel-28 Tablets ... 3392
- Microgestin Fe 1.5/30 Tablets ... 3407
- Microgestin Fe 1/20 Tablets ... 3400
- Mircette Tablets ... 2470
- Modicon ... 2563
- Necon ... 3415
- Nordette-28 Tablets ... 2257
- Norinyl 1 +35 28-Day Tablets ... 3380
- Ogestrel 0.5/50-28 Tablets ... 3428
- Ortho-Cept 21 Tablets ... 2546
- Ortho-Cept 28 Tablets ... 2546
- Ortho-Cyclen/Ortho Tri-Cyclen ... 2573
- Ortho-Novum ... 2563
- Ovcon ... 3364
- Ovral Tablets ... 3551
- Ovral-28 Tablets ... 3552
- Tri-Levlen ... 962
- Tri-Norinyl-28 Tablets ... 3433
- Triphasil-21 Tablets ... 3600
- Triphasil-28 Tablets ... 3605
- Trivora Tablets ... 3439
- Yasmin 28 Tablets ... 980
- Zovia ... 3449

Ethynodiol Diacetate (Potential for reduced efficacy of oral contraceptives). Products include:
- Zovia ... 3449

Levonorgestrel (Potential for reduced efficacy of oral contraceptives). Products include:
- Alesse-21 Tablets ... 3468
- Alesse-28 Tablets ... 3473
- Levlen ... 962
- Levlite 21 Tablets ... 962
- Levlite 28 Tablets ... 962
- Levora Tablets ... 3389
- Mirena Intrauterine System ... 974
- Nordette-28 Tablets ... 2257
- Norplant System ... 3543
- Tri-Levlen ... 962
- Triphasil-21 Tablets ... 3600
- Triphasil-28 Tablets ... 3605
- Trivora Tablets ... 3439

Mestranol (Potential for reduced efficacy of oral contraceptives). Products include:
- Necon 1/50 Tablets ... 3415
- Norinyl 1 + 50 28-Day Tablets ... 3380
- Ortho-Novum 1/50▫28 Tablets ... 2556

Norethindrone (Potential for reduced efficacy of oral contraceptives). Products include:
- Brevicon 28-Day Tablets ... 3380
- Micronor Tablets ... 2543
- Modicon ... 2563
- Necon ... 3415
- Norinyl 1 +35 28-Day Tablets ... 3380
- Norinyl 1 + 50 28-Day Tablets ... 3380
- Nor-QD Tablets ... 3423
- Ortho-Novum ... 2563
- Ortho-Novum 1/50▫28 Tablets ... 2556
- Ovcon ... 3364
- Tri-Norinyl-28 Tablets ... 3433

Norethynodrel (Potential for reduced efficacy of oral contraceptives).
No products indexed under this heading.

Norgestimate (Potential for reduced efficacy of oral contraceptives). Products include:
- Ortho-Cyclen/Ortho Tri-Cyclen ... 2573
- Ortho-Prefest Tablets ... 2570

Norgestrel (Potential for reduced efficacy of oral contraceptives). Products include:
- Lo/Ovral Tablets ... 3532
- Lo/Ovral-28 Tablets ... 3538
- Low-Ogestrel-28 Tablets ... 3392
- Ogestrel 0.5/50-28 Tablets ... 3428
- Ovral Tablets ... 3551
- Ovral-28 Tablets ... 3552
- Ovrette Tablets ... 3552

Probenecid (Decreases the renal tubular secretion of amoxicillin; concurrent use may result in increased and prolonged blood levels of amoxicillin, therefore concomitant use is not recommended).
No products indexed under this heading.

AURALGAN OTIC SOLUTION
(Antipyrine, Benzocaine, Glycerin) ... 3485
None cited in PDR database.

AUTOPLEX T
(Anti-Inhibitor Coagulant Complex) ... 2294
May interact with:

Aminocaproic Acid (Concomitant use with antifibrinolytic agents should be avoided). Products include:
- Amicar Injection ... 3608
- Amicar Syrup ... 3608
- Amicar Tablets ... 3608

Tranexamic Acid (Concomitant use with antifibrinolytic agents should be avoided).
No products indexed under this heading.

AVALIDE TABLETS
(Hydrochlorothiazide, Irbesartan) ... 1070
May interact with antihypertensives, barbiturates, corticosteroids, cardiac glycosides, oral hypoglycemic agents, insulin, lithium preparations, narcotic analgesics, nondepolarizing neuromuscular blocking agents, nonsteroidal anti-inflammatory agents, and certain other agents. Compounds in these categories include:

Acarbose (Hydrochlorothiazide may cause hyperglycemia, therefore, dosage adjustment of oral hypoglycemic agent may be required). Products include:
- Precose Tablets ... 906

Acebutolol Hydrochloride (Hydrochlorothiazide may add to or potentiate the therapeutic effect of other antihypertensive drugs). Products include:
- Sectral Capsules ... 3589

ACTH (Co-administration with ACTH intensifies electrolyte depletion particularly hypokalemia).
No products indexed under this heading.

Alfentanil Hydrochloride (Potentiation of orthostatic hypotension).
No products indexed under this heading.

Amlodipine Besylate (Hydrochlorothiazide may add to or potentiate the therapeutic effect of other antihypertensive drugs). Products include:
- Lotrel Capsules ... 2370
- Norvasc Tablets ... 2704

Aprobarbital (Potentiation of orthostatic hypotension).
No products indexed under this heading.

Atenolol (Hydrochlorothiazide may add to or potentiate the therapeutic effect of other antihypertensive drugs). Products include:
- Tenoretic Tablets ... 690
- Tenormin I.V. Injection ... 692

Atracurium Besylate (Possible increased responsiveness to the muscle relaxants).
No products indexed under this heading.

Benazepril Hydrochloride (Hydrochlorothiazide may add to or potentiate the therapeutic effect of other antihypertensive drugs). Products include:
- Lotensin Tablets ... 2365
- Lotensin HCT Tablets ... 2367
- Lotrel Capsules ... 2370

Bendroflumethiazide (Hydrochlorothiazide may add to or potentiate the therapeutic effect of other antihypertensive drugs). Products include:
- Corzide 40/5 Tablets ... 2247
- Corzide 80/5 Tablets ... 2247

Betamethasone Acetate (Co-administration with corticosteroids intensifies electrolyte depletion particularly hypokalemia). Products include:
- Celestone Soluspan Injectable Suspension ... 3097

Betamethasone Sodium Phosphate (Co-administration with corticosteroids intensifies electrolyte depletion particularly hypokalemia). Products include:
- Celestone Soluspan Injectable Suspension ... 3097

Betaxolol Hydrochloride (Hydrochlorothiazide may add to or potentiate the therapeutic effect of other antihypertensive drugs). Products include:
- Betoptic S Ophthalmic Suspension ... 537

Bisoprolol Fumarate (Hydrochlorothiazide may add to or potentiate the therapeutic effect of other antihypertensive drugs). Products include:
- Zebeta Tablets ... 1885
- Ziac Tablets ... 1887

Buprenorphine Hydrochloride (Potentiation of orthostatic hypotension). Products include:
- Buprenex Injectable ... 2918

Butabarbital (Potentiation of orthostatic hypotension).
No products indexed under this heading.

Butalbital (Potentiation of orthostatic hypotension). Products include:
- Phrenilin ... 578
- Sedapap Tablets 50 mg/650 mg ... 2225

Candesartan Cilexetil (Hydrochlorothiazide may add to or potentiate the therapeutic effect of other antihypertensive drugs). Products include:
- Atacand Tablets ... 595
- Atacand HCT Tablets ... 597

Captopril (Hydrochlorothiazide may add to or potentiate the therapeutic effect of other antihypertensive drugs). Products include:
- Captopril Tablets ... 2281

Carteolol Hydrochloride (Hydrochlorothiazide may add to or potentiate the therapeutic effect of other antihypertensive drugs). Products include:
- Carteolol Hydrochloride Ophthalmic Solution USP, 1% ... ⊙258
- Ocupress Ophthalmic Solution, 1% Sterile ... ⊙303

Celecoxib (Co-administration with non-steroidal anti-inflammatory agents may reduce the natriuretic and antihypertensive effects of thiazides). Products include:
- Celebrex Capsules ... 2676
- Celebrex Capsules ... 2780

Chlorothiazide (Hydrochlorothiazide may add to or potentiate the therapeutic effect of other antihypertensive drugs). Products include:
- Aldoclor Tablets ... 2035
- Diuril Oral ... 2087

Chlorothiazide Sodium (Hydrochlorothiazide may add to or potentiate the therapeutic effect of other antihypertensive drugs). Products include:
- Diuril Sodium Intravenous ... 2086

Chlorpropamide (Hydrochlorothiazide may cause hyperglycemia, therefore, dosage adjustment of oral hypoglycemic agent may be required). Products include:
- Diabinese Tablets ... 2680

Chlorthalidone (Hydrochlorothiazide may add to or potentiate the therapeutic effect of other antihypertensive drugs). Products include:
- Clorpres Tablets ... 1002
- Combipres Tablets ... 1040
- Tenoretic Tablets ... 690

Cholestyramine (Absorption of hydrochlorothiazide is impaired in the presence of anionic exchange resins; single dose of cholestyramine binds the hydrochlorothiazide and reduces its absorption from GI tract by 85%).
No products indexed under this heading.

Cisatracurium Besylate (Possible increased responsiveness to the muscle relaxants).
No products indexed under this heading.

Clonidine (Hydrochlorothiazide may add to or potentiate the therapeutic effect of other antihypertensive drugs). Products include:
- Catapres-TTS ... 1038

Clonidine Hydrochloride (Hydrochlorothiazide may add to or potenti-

ate the therapeutic effect of other antihypertensive drugs). Products include:

- Catapres Tablets 1037
- Clorpres Tablets 1002
- Combipres Tablets 1040
- Duraclon Injection 3057

Codeine Phosphate (Potentiation of orthostatic hypotension). Products include:

- Phenergan with Codeine Syrup 3557
- Phenergan VC with Codeine Syrup .. 3561
- Robitussin A-C Syrup 2942
- Robitussin-DAC Syrup 2942
- Ryna-C Liquid .... ▣768
- Soma Compound w/Codeine Tablets 3355
- Tussi-Organidin NR Liquid 3350
- Tussi-Organidin-S NR Liquid 3350
- Tylenol with Codeine 2595

Colestipol Hydrochloride (Absorption of hydrochlorothiazide is impaired in the presence of anionic exchange resins; single dose of colestipol binds the hydrochlorothiazide and reduces its absorption from GI tract by 43%). Products include:

- Colestid Tablets 2791

Cortisone Acetate (Co-administration with corticosteroids intensifies electrolyte depletion particularly hypokalemia). Products include:

- Cortone Acetate Injectable Suspension 2059
- Cortone Acetate Tablets 2061

Deserpidine (Hydrochlorothiazide may add to or potentiate the therapeutic effect of other antihypertensive drugs).

No products indexed under this heading.

Deslanoside (Concurrent digitalis therapy may exaggerate metabolic effects of hypokalemia, especially myocardial effects, e.g., increased ventricular irritability).

No products indexed under this heading.

Dexamethasone (Co-administration with corticosteroids intensifies electrolyte depletion particularly hypokalemia). Products include:

- Decadron Elixir 2078
- Decadron Tablets 2079
- TobraDex Ophthalmic Ointment 542
- TobraDex Ophthalmic Suspension .. 541

Dexamethasone Acetate (Co-administration with corticosteroids intensifies electrolyte depletion particularly hypokalemia).

No products indexed under this heading.

Dexamethasone Sodium Phosphate (Co-administration with corticosteroids intensifies electrolyte depletion particularly hypokalemia). Products include:

- Decadron Phosphate Injection 2081
- Decadron Phosphate Sterile Ophthalmic Ointment 2083
- Decadron Phosphate Sterile Ophthalmic Solution 2084
- NeoDecadron Sterile Ophthalmic Solution 2144

Dezocine (Potentiation of orthostatic hypotension).

No products indexed under this heading.

Diazoxide (Hydrochlorothiazide may add to or potentiate the therapeutic effect of other antihypertensive drugs).

No products indexed under this heading.

Diclofenac Potassium (Co-administration with non-steroidal anti-inflammatory agents may reduce the natriuretic and antihypertensive effects of thiazides). Products include:

- Cataflam Tablets 2315

Diclofenac Sodium (Co-administration with non-steroidal anti-inflammatory agents may reduce the natriuretic and antihypertensive effects of thiazides). Products include:

- Arthrotec Tablets 3195
- Voltaren Ophthalmic Sterile Ophthalmic Solution .... ⊙312
- Voltaren Tablets 2315
- Voltaren-XR Tablets 2315

Digitoxin (Concurrent digitalis therapy may exaggerate metabolic effects of hypokalemia, especially myocardial effects, e.g., increased ventricular irritability).

No products indexed under this heading.

Digoxin (Concurrent digitalis therapy may exaggerate metabolic effects of hypokalemia, especially myocardial effects, e.g., increased ventricular irritability). Products include:

- Digitek Tablets 1003
- Lanoxicaps Capsules 1574
- Lanoxin Injection 1581
- Lanoxin Tablets 1587
- Lanoxin Elixir Pediatric 1578
- Lanoxin Injection Pediatric 1584

Diltiazem Hydrochloride (Hydrochlorothiazide may add to or potentiate the therapeutic effect of other antihypertensive drugs). Products include:

- Cardizem Injectable 1018
- Cardizem Lyo-Ject Syringe 1018
- Cardizem Monovial 1018
- Cardizem CD Capsules 1016
- Tiazac Capsules 1378

Doxazosin Mesylate (Hydrochlorothiazide may add to or potentiate the therapeutic effect of other antihypertensive drugs). Products include:

- Cardura Tablets 2668

Enalapril Maleate (Hydrochlorothiazide may add to or potentiate the therapeutic effect of other antihypertensive drugs). Products include:

- Lexxel Tablets 608
- Vaseretic Tablets 2204
- Vasotec Tablets 2210

Enalaprilat (Hydrochlorothiazide may add to or potentiate the therapeutic effect of other antihypertensive drugs). Products include:

- Enalaprilat Injection 863
- Vasotec I.V. Injection 2207

Eprosartan Mesylate (Hydrochlorothiazide may add to or potentiate the therapeutic effect of other antihypertensive drugs). Products include:

- Teveten Tablets 3327

Esmolol Hydrochloride (Hydrochlorothiazide may add to or potentiate the therapeutic effect of other antihypertensive drugs). Products include:

- Brevibloc Injection 858

Etodolac (Co-administration with non-steroidal anti-inflammatory agents may reduce the natriuretic and antihypertensive effects of thiazides). Products include:

- Lodine 3528
- Lodine XL Extended-Release Tablets 3530

Felodipine (Hydrochlorothiazide may add to or potentiate the therapeutic effect of other antihypertensive drugs). Products include:

- Lexxel Tablets 608
- Plendil Extended-Release Tablets 623

Fenoprofen Calcium (Co-administration with non-steroidal anti-inflammatory agents may reduce the natriuretic and antihypertensive effects of thiazides).

No products indexed under this heading.

Fentanyl (Potentiation of orthostatic hypotension). Products include:

- Duragesic Transdermal System 1786

Fentanyl Citrate (Potentiation of orthostatic hypotension). Products include:

- Actiq 1184

Fludrocortisone Acetate (Co-administration with corticosteroids intensifies electrolyte depletion particularly hypokalemia). Products include:

- Florinef Acetate Tablets 2250

Flurbiprofen (Co-administration with non-steroidal anti-inflammatory agents may reduce the natriuretic and antihypertensive effects of thiazides).

No products indexed under this heading.

Fosinopril Sodium (Hydrochlorothiazide may add to or potentiate the therapeutic effect of other antihypertensive drugs). Products include:

- Monopril Tablets 1091
- Monopril HCT 1094

Furosemide (Hydrochlorothiazide may add to or potentiate the therapeutic effect of other antihypertensive drugs). Products include:

- Furosemide Tablets 2284

Glimepiride (Hydrochlorothiazide may cause hyperglycemia, therefore, dosage adjustment of oral hypoglycemic agent may be required). Products include:

- Amaryl Tablets 717

Glipizide (Hydrochlorothiazide may cause hyperglycemia, therefore, dosage adjustment of oral hypoglycemic agent may be required). Products include:

- Glucotrol Tablets 2692
- Glucotrol XL Extended Release Tablets 2693

Glyburide (Hydrochlorothiazide may cause hyperglycemia, therefore, dosage adjustment of oral hypoglycemic agent may be required). Products include:

- DiaBeta Tablets 741
- Glucovance Tablets 1086

Guanabenz Acetate (Hydrochlorothiazide may add to or potentiate the therapeutic effect of other antihypertensive drugs).

No products indexed under this heading.

Guanethidine Monosulfate (Hydrochlorothiazide may add to or potentiate the therapeutic effect of other antihypertensive drugs).

No products indexed under this heading.

Hydralazine Hydrochloride (Hydrochlorothiazide may add to or potentiate the therapeutic effect of other antihypertensive drugs).

No products indexed under this heading.

Hydrocodone Bitartrate (Potentiation of orthostatic hypotension). Products include:

- Hycodan 1316
- Hycomine Compound Tablets 1317
- Hycotuss Expectorant Syrup 1318
- Lortab 3319
- Lortab Elixir 3317
- Maxidone Tablets CIII 3399
- Norco 5/325 Tablets CIII 3424
- Norco 7.5/325 Tablets CIII 3425
- Norco 10/325 Tablets CIII 3427
- Norco 10/325 Tablets CIII 3425
- Vicodin Tablets 516
- Vicodin ES Tablets 517
- Vicodin HP Tablets 518
- Vicodin Tuss Expectorant 519
- Vicoprofen Tablets 520
- Zydone Tablets 1330

Hydrocodone Polistirex (Potentiation of orthostatic hypotension). Products include:

- Tussionex Pennkinetic Extended-Release Suspension 1174

Hydrocortisone (Co-administration with corticosteroids intensifies electrolyte depletion particularly hypokalemia). Products include:

- Anusol-HC Cream 2.5% 2237
- Cipro HC Otic Suspension 540
- Cortaid Intensive Therapy Cream .. ▣717
- Cortaid Maximum Strength Cream .... ▣717
- Cortisporin Ophthalmic Suspension Sterile .... ⊙297
- Cortizone•5 .... ▣699
- Cortizone•10 .... ▣699
- Cortizone•10 Plus Creme .... ▣700
- Cortizone for Kids Creme .... ▣699
- Hydrocortone Tablets 2106
- Massengill Medicated Soft Cloth Towelette .... ▣753
- VōSoL HC Otic Solution 3356

Hydrocortisone Acetate (Co-administration with corticosteroids intensifies electrolyte depletion particularly hypokalemia). Products include:

- Analpram-HC 1338
- Anusol HC-1 Hydrocortisone Anti-Itch Cream .... ▣689
- Anusol-HC Suppositories 2238
- Cortaid .... ▣717
- Cortifoam Rectal Foam 3170
- Cortisporin-TC Otic Suspension 2246
- Hydrocortone Acetate Injectable Suspension 2103
- Pramosone 1343
- Proctocort Suppositories 2264
- ProctoFoam-HC 3177
- Terra-Cortril Ophthalmic Suspension 2716

Hydrocortisone Sodium Phosphate (Co-administration with corticosteroids intensifies electrolyte depletion particularly hypokalemia). Products include:

- Hydrocortone Phosphate Injection, Sterile 2105

Hydrocortisone Sodium Succinate (Co-administration with corticosteroids intensifies electrolyte depletion particularly hypokalemia).

No products indexed under this heading.

Hydroflumethiazide (Hydrochlorothiazide may add to or potentiate the therapeutic effect of other antihypertensive drugs). Products include:

- Diucardin Tablets 3494

Hydromorphone Hydrochloride (Potentiation of orthostatic hypotension). Products include:

- Dilaudid 441
- Dilaudid Oral Liquid 445
- Dilaudid Powder 441
- Dilaudid Rectal Suppositories 441
- Dilaudid Tablets 441
- Dilaudid Tablets - 8 mg 445
- Dilaudid-HP 443

Ibuprofen (Co-administration with non-steroidal anti-inflammatory agents may reduce the natriuretic and antihypertensive effects of thiazides). Products include:

- Advil .... ▣771
- Children's Advil Oral Suspension .... ▣773
- Children's Advil Chewable Tablets .. ▣773
- Advil Cold and Sinus Caplets .... ▣771
- Advil Cold and Sinus Tablets .... ▣771
- Advil Flu & Body Ache Caplets .... ▣772
- Infants' Advil Drops .... ▣773
- Junior Strength Advil Tablets .... ▣773
- Junior Strength Advil Chewable Tablets .... ▣773
- Advil Migraine Liquigels .... ▣772
- Children's Motrin Oral Suspension and Chewable Tablets 2006
- Children's Motrin Cold Oral Suspension 2007
- Children's Motrin Oral Suspension .... ▣643
- Motrin Suspension, Oral Drops, Chewable Tablets, and Caplets 2002
- Infants' Motrin Concentrated Drops 2006
- Junior Strength Motrin Caplets and Chewable Tablets 2006
- Motrin IB Tablets, Caplets, and Gelcaps 2002
- Motrin Migraine Pain Caplets 2005
- Motrin Sinus Headache Caplets 2005
- Vicoprofen Tablets 520

Indapamide (Hydrochlorothiazide may add to or potentiate the therapeutic effect of other antihypertensive drugs). Products include:

- Indapamide Tablets 2286

Indomethacin (Co-administration with non-steroidal anti-inflammatory agents may reduce the natriuretic and antihypertensive effects of thiazides). Products include:

- Indocin 2112

Indomethacin Sodium Trihydrate (Co-administration with non-

steroidal anti-inflammatory agents may reduce the natriuretic and antihypertensive effects of thiazides). Products include:
- Indocin I.V. 2115

Insulin, Human, Zinc Suspension (Hydrochlorothiazide may cause hyperglycemia, therefore, dosage adjustment of insulin may be required). Products include:
- Humulin L, 100 Units 1937
- Humulin U, 100 Units 1943
- Novolin L Human Insulin 10 ml Vials 2422

Insulin, Human NPH (Hydrochlorothiazide may cause hyperglycemia, therefore, dosage adjustment of insulin may be required). Products include:
- Humulin N, 100 Units 1939
- Humulin N NPH Pen 1940
- Novolin N Human Insulin 10 ml Vials 2422
- Novolin N PenFill 2423
- Novolin N Prefilled Syringe Disposable Insulin Delivery System 2425

Insulin, Human Regular (Hydrochlorothiazide may cause hyperglycemia, therefore, dosage adjustment of insulin may be required). Products include:
- Humulin R Regular (U-500) 1943
- Humulin R, 100 Units 1941
- Novolin R Human Insulin 10 ml Vials 2423
- Novolin R PenFill 2423
- Novolin R Prefilled Syringe Disposable Insulin Delivery System 2425
- Velosulin BR Human Insulin 10 ml Vials 2435

Insulin, Human Regular and Human NPH Mixture (Hydrochlorothiazide may cause hyperglycemia, therefore, dosage adjustment of insulin may be required). Products include:
- Humulin 50/50, 100 Units 1934
- Humulin 70/30, 100 Units 1935
- Humulin 70/30 Pen 1936
- Novolin 70/30 Human Insulin 10 ml Vials 2421
- Novolin 70/30 PenFill 2423
- Novolin 70/30 Prefilled Disposable Insulin Delivery System 2425

Insulin, NPH (Hydrochlorothiazide may cause hyperglycemia, therefore, dosage adjustment of insulin may be required). Products include:
- Iletin II, NPH (Pork), 100 Units 1946

Insulin, Regular (Hydrochlorothiazide may cause hyperglycemia, therefore, dosage adjustment of insulin may be required). Products include:
- Iletin II, Regular (Pork), 100 Units 1947

Insulin, Zinc Crystals (Hydrochlorothiazide may cause hyperglycemia, therefore, dosage adjustment of insulin may be required).
- No products indexed under this heading.

Insulin, Zinc Suspension (Hydrochlorothiazide may cause hyperglycemia, therefore, dosage adjustment of insulin may be required). Products include:
- Iletin II, Lente (Pork), 100 Units 1945

Insulin Aspart, Human Regular (Hydrochlorothiazide may cause hyperglycemia, therefore, dosage adjustment of insulin may be required).
- No products indexed under this heading.

Insulin glargine (Hydrochlorothiazide may cause hyperglycemia, therefore, dosage adjustment of insulin may be required). Products include:
- Lantus Injection 742

Insulin Lispro, Human (Hydrochlorothiazide may cause hyperglycemia, therefore, dosage adjustment of insulin may be required). Products include:
- Humalog 1926
- Humalog Mix 75/25 Pen 1928

Insulin Lispro Protamine, Human (Hydrochlorothiazide may cause hyperglycemia, therefore, dosage adjustment of insulin may be required). Products include:
- Humalog Mix 75/25 Pen 1928

Isradipine (Hydrochlorothiazide may add to or potentiate the therapeutic effect of other antihypertensive drugs). Products include:
- DynaCirc Capsules 2921
- DynaCirc CR Tablets 2923

Ketoprofen (Co-administration with non-steroidal anti-inflammatory agents may reduce the natriuretic and antihypertensive effects of thiazides). Products include:
- Orudis Capsules 3548
- Orudis KT Tablets .... ▣778
- Oruvail Capsules 3548

Ketorolac Tromethamine (Co-administration with non-steroidal anti-inflammatory agents may reduce the natriuretic and antihypertensive effects of thiazides). Products include:
- Acular Ophthalmic Solution 544
- Acular PF Ophthalmic Solution 544
- Toradol 3018

Labetalol Hydrochloride (Hydrochlorothiazide may add to or potentiate the therapeutic effect of other antihypertensive drugs). Products include:
- Normodyne Injection 3135
- Normodyne Tablets 3137

Levorphanol Tartrate (Potentiation of orthostatic hypotension). Products include:
- Levo-Dromoran 1734
- Levorphanol Tartrate Tablets 3059

Lisinopril (Hydrochlorothiazide may add to or potentiate the therapeutic effect of other antihypertensive drugs). Products include:
- Prinivil Tablets 2164
- Prinzide Tablets 2168
- Zestoretic Tablets 695
- Zestril Tablets 698

Lithium Carbonate (Diuretics reduce lithium's renal clearance and add a high risk of lithium toxicity). Products include:
- Eskalith 1527
- Lithium Carbonate 3061
- Lithobid Slow-Release Tablets 3255

Lithium Citrate (Diuretics reduce lithium's renal clearance and add a high risk of lithium toxicity). Products include:
- Lithium Citrate Syrup 3061

Losartan Potassium (Hydrochlorothiazide may add to or potentiate the therapeutic effect of other antihypertensive drugs). Products include:
- Cozaar Tablets 2067
- Hyzaar 2109

Mecamylamine Hydrochloride (Hydrochlorothiazide may add to or potentiate the therapeutic effect of other antihypertensive drugs). Products include:
- Inversine Tablets 1850

Meclofenamate Sodium (Co-administration with non-steroidal anti-inflammatory agents may reduce the natriuretic and antihypertensive effects of thiazides).
- No products indexed under this heading.

Mefenamic Acid (Co-administration with non-steroidal anti-inflammatory agents may reduce the natriuretic and antihypertensive effects of thiazides). Products include:
- Ponstel Capsules 1356

Meloxicam (Co-administration with non-steroidal anti-inflammatory agents may reduce the natriuretic and antihypertensive effects of thiazides). Products include:
- Mobic Tablets 1054

Meperidine Hydrochloride (Potentiation of orthostatic hypotension). Products include:
- Demerol 3079
- Mepergan Injection 3539

Mephobarbital (Potentiation of orthostatic hypotension).
- No products indexed under this heading.

Metformin Hydrochloride (Hydrochlorothiazide may cause hyperglycemia, therefore, dosage adjustment of oral hypoglycemic agent may be required). Products include:
- Glucophage Tablets 1080
- Glucophage XR Tablets 1080
- Glucovance Tablets 1086

Methadone Hydrochloride (Potentiation of orthostatic hypotension). Products include:
- Dolophine Hydrochloride Tablets 3056

Methyclothiazide (Hydrochlorothiazide may add to or potentiate the therapeutic effect of other antihypertensive drugs).
- No products indexed under this heading.

Methyldopa (Hydrochlorothiazide may add to or potentiate the therapeutic effect of other antihypertensive drugs). Products include:
- Aldoclor Tablets 2035
- Aldomet Tablets 2037
- Aldoril Tablets 2039

Methyldopate Hydrochloride (Hydrochlorothiazide may add to or potentiate the therapeutic effect of other antihypertensive drugs).
- No products indexed under this heading.

Methylprednisolone Acetate (Co-administration with corticosteroids intensifies electrolyte depletion particularly hypokalemia). Products include:
- Depo-Medrol Injectable Suspension 2795

Methylprednisolone Sodium Succinate (Co-administration with corticosteroids intensifies electrolyte depletion particularly hypokalemia). Products include:
- Solu-Medrol Sterile Powder 2855

Metocurine Iodide (Possible increased responsiveness to the muscle relaxants).
- No products indexed under this heading.

Metolazone (Hydrochlorothiazide may add to or potentiate the therapeutic effect of other antihypertensive drugs). Products include:
- Mykrox Tablets 1168
- Zaroxolyn Tablets 1177

Metoprolol Succinate (Hydrochlorothiazide may add to or potentiate the therapeutic effect of other antihypertensive drugs). Products include:
- Toprol-XL Tablets 651

Metoprolol Tartrate (Hydrochlorothiazide may add to or potentiate the therapeutic effect of other antihypertensive drugs).
- No products indexed under this heading.

Metyrosine (Hydrochlorothiazide may add to or potentiate the therapeutic effect of other antihypertensive drugs). Products include:
- Demser Capsules 2085

Mibefradil Dihydrochloride (Hydrochlorothiazide may add to or potentiate the therapeutic effect of other antihypertensive drugs).
- No products indexed under this heading.

Miglitol (Hydrochlorothiazide may cause hyperglycemia, therefore, dosage adjustment of oral hypoglycemic agent may be required). Products include:
- Glyset Tablets 2821

Minoxidil (Hydrochlorothiazide may add to or potentiate the therapeutic effect of other antihypertensive drugs). Products include:
- Rogaine Extra Strength for Men Topical Solution .... ▣721
- Rogaine for Women Topical Solution .... ▣721

Mivacurium Chloride (Possible increased responsiveness to the muscle relaxants).
- No products indexed under this heading.

Moexipril Hydrochloride (Hydrochlorothiazide may add to or potentiate the therapeutic effect of other antihypertensive drugs). Products include:
- Uniretic Tablets 3178
- Univasc Tablets 3181

Morphine Sulfate (Potentiation of orthostatic hypotension). Products include:
- Astramorph/PF Injection, USP (Preservative-Free) 594
- Duramorph Injection 1312
- Infumorph 200 and Infumorph 500 Sterile Solutions 1314
- Kadian Capsules 1335
- MS Contin Tablets 2896
- MSIR 2898
- Oramorph SR Tablets 3062
- Roxanol 3066

Nabumetone (Co-administration with non-steroidal anti-inflammatory agents may reduce the natriuretic and antihypertensive effects of thiazides). Products include:
- Relafen Tablets 1617

Nadolol (Hydrochlorothiazide may add to or potentiate the therapeutic effect of other antihypertensive drugs). Products include:
- Corgard Tablets 2245
- Corzide 40/5 Tablets 2247
- Corzide 80/5 Tablets 2247
- Nadolol Tablets 2288

Naproxen (Co-administration with non-steroidal anti-inflammatory agents may reduce the natriuretic and antihypertensive effects of thiazides). Products include:
- EC-Naprosyn Delayed-Release Tablets 2967
- Naprosyn Suspension 2967
- Naprosyn Tablets 2967

Naproxen Sodium (Co-administration with non-steroidal anti-inflammatory agents may reduce the natriuretic and antihypertensive effects of thiazides). Products include:
- Aleve Tablets, Caplets and Gelcaps .... ▣602
- Aleve Cold & Sinus Caplets .... ▣603
- Anaprox Tablets 2967
- Anaprox DS Tablets 2967
- Naprelan Tablets 1293

Nicardipine Hydrochloride (Hydrochlorothiazide may add to or potentiate the therapeutic effect of other antihypertensive drugs). Products include:
- Cardene I.V. 3485

Nifedipine (In vitro studies show significant inhibition of the formation of oxidized irbesartan metabolites with the known cytochrome CYP 2C9 substrate/inhibitor, nifedipine; the pharmacokinetics of irbesartan were not affected by co-administration of nifedipine; hydrochlorothiazide may add to or potentiate the therapeutic effect of other antihypertensive drugs). Products include:
- Adalat CC Tablets 877
- Procardia Capsules 2708
- Procardia XL Extended Release Tablets 2710

Nisoldipine (Hydrochlorothiazide may add to or potentiate the therapeutic effect of other antihypertensive drugs). Products include:
- Sular Tablets 688

Nitroglycerin (Hydrochlorothiazide may add to or potentiate the therapeutic effect of other antihypertensive drugs). Products include:
- Nitro-Dur Transdermal Infusion System 3134
- Nitro-Dur Transdermal Infusion System 1834
- Nitrolingual Pumpspray 1355
- Nitrostat Tablets 2658

Norepinephrine Bitartrate (Thiazides may decrease arterial responsiveness to norepinephrine).
- No products indexed under this heading.

Oxaprozin (Co-administration with non-steroidal anti-inflammatory agents may reduce the natriuretic and antihypertensive effects of thiazides).
- No products indexed under this heading.

Oxycodone Hydrochloride (Potentiation of orthostatic hypotension). Products include:
- OxyContin Tablets 2912
- OxyFast Oral Concentrate Solution .. 2916
- OxyIR Capsules 2916
- Percocet Tablets 1326
- Percodan Tablets 1327
- Percolone Tablets 1327
- Roxicodone 3067
- Tylox Capsules 2597

Pancuronium Bromide (Possible increased responsiveness to the muscle relaxants).
- No products indexed under this heading.

Penbutolol Sulfate (Hydrochlorothiazide may add to or potentiate the therapeutic effect of other antihypertensive drugs).
- No products indexed under this heading.

Pentobarbital Sodium (Potentiation of orthostatic hypotension). Products include:
- Nembutal Sodium Solution 485

Perindopril Erbumine (Hydrochlorothiazide may add to or potentiate the therapeutic effect of other antihypertensive drugs). Products include:
- Aceon Tablets (2 mg, 4 mg, 8 mg) 3249

Phenobarbital (Potentiation of orthostatic hypotension). Products include:
- Arco-Lase Plus Tablets 592
- Donnatal 2929
- Donnatal Extentabs 2930

Phenoxybenzamine Hydrochloride (Hydrochlorothiazide may add to or potentiate the therapeutic effect of other antihypertensive drugs). Products include:
- Dibenzyline Capsules 3457

Phentolamine Mesylate (Hydrochlorothiazide may add to or potentiate the therapeutic effect of other antihypertensive drugs).
- No products indexed under this heading.

Phenylbutazone (Co-administration with non-steroidal anti-inflammatory agents may reduce the natriuretic and antihypertensive effects of thiazides).
- No products indexed under this heading.

Pindolol (Hydrochlorothiazide may add to or potentiate the therapeutic effect of other antihypertensive drugs).
- No products indexed under this heading.

Pioglitazone Hydrochloride (Hydrochlorothiazide may cause hyperglycemia, therefore, dosage adjustment of oral hypoglycemic agent may be required). Products include:
- Actos Tablets 3275

Piroxicam (Co-administration with non-steroidal anti-inflammatory agents may reduce the natriuretic and antihypertensive effects of thiazides). Products include:
- Feldene Capsules 2685

Polythiazide (Hydrochlorothiazide may add to or potentiate the therapeutic effect of other antihypertensive drugs). Products include:
- Minizide Capsules 2700
- Renese Tablets 2712

Prazosin Hydrochloride (Hydrochlorothiazide may add to or potentiate the therapeutic effect of other antihypertensive drugs). Products include:
- Minipress Capsules 2699
- Minizide Capsules 2700

Prednisolone Acetate (Co-administration with corticosteroids intensifies electrolyte depletion particularly hypokalemia). Products include:
- Blephamide Ophthalmic Ointment .. 547
- Blephamide Ophthalmic Suspension 548
- Poly-Pred Liquifilm Ophthalmic Suspension .... ⊙245
- Pred Forte Ophthalmic Suspension .... ⊙246
- Pred Mild Sterile Ophthalmic Suspension .... ⊙249
- Pred-G Ophthalmic Suspension .... ⊙247
- Pred-G Sterile Ophthalmic Ointment .... ⊙248

Prednisolone Sodium Phosphate (Co-administration with corticosteroids intensifies electrolyte depletion particularly hypokalemia). Products include:
- Pediapred Oral Solution 1170

Prednisolone Tebutate (Co-administration with corticosteroids intensifies electrolyte depletion particularly hypokalemia).
- No products indexed under this heading.

Prednisone (Co-administration with corticosteroids intensifies electrolyte depletion particularly hypokalemia). Products include:
- Prednisone 3064

Propoxyphene Hydrochloride (Potentiation of orthostatic hypotension). Products include:
- Darvon Pulvules 1909
- Darvon Compound-65 Pulvules 1910

Propoxyphene Napsylate (Potentiation of orthostatic hypotension). Products include:
- Darvon-N/Darvocet-N 1907
- Darvon-N Tablets 1912

Propranolol Hydrochloride (Hydrochlorothiazide may add to or potentiate the therapeutic effect of other antihypertensive drugs). Products include:
- Inderal 3513
- Inderal LA Long-Acting Capsules 3516
- Inderide Tablets 3517
- Inderide LA Long-Acting Capsules .. 3519

Quinapril Hydrochloride (Hydrochlorothiazide may add to or potentiate the therapeutic effect of other antihypertensive drugs). Products include:
- Accupril Tablets 2611
- Accuretic Tablets 2614

Ramipril (Hydrochlorothiazide may add to or potentiate the therapeutic effect of other antihypertensive drugs). Products include:
- Altace Capsules 2233

Rapacuronium Bromide (Possible increased responsiveness to the muscle relaxants).
- No products indexed under this heading.

Rauwolfia serpentina (Hydrochlorothiazide may add to or potentiate the therapeutic effect of other antihypertensive drugs).
- No products indexed under this heading.

Remifentanil Hydrochloride (Potentiation of orthostatic hypotension).
- No products indexed under this heading.

Repaglinide (Hydrochlorothiazide may cause hyperglycemia, therefore, dosage adjustment of oral hypoglycemic agent may be required). Products include:
- Prandin Tablets (0.5, 1, and 2 mg) 2432

Rescinnamine (Hydrochlorothiazide may add to or potentiate the therapeutic effect of other antihypertensive drugs).
- No products indexed under this heading.

Reserpine (Hydrochlorothiazide may add to or potentiate the therapeutic effect of other antihypertensive drugs).
- No products indexed under this heading.

Rocuronium Bromide (Possible increased responsiveness to the muscle relaxants). Products include:
- Zemuron Injection 2491

Rofecoxib (Co-administration with non-steroidal anti-inflammatory agents may reduce the natriuretic and antihypertensive effects of thiazides). Products include:
- Vioxx 2213

Rosiglitazone Maleate (Hydrochlorothiazide may cause hyperglycemia, therefore, dosage adjustment of oral hypoglycemic agent may be required). Products include:
- Avandia Tablets 1490

Secobarbital Sodium (Potentiation of orthostatic hypotension).
- No products indexed under this heading.

Sodium Nitroprusside (Hydrochlorothiazide may add to or potentiate the therapeutic effect of other antihypertensive drugs).
- No products indexed under this heading.

Sotalol Hydrochloride (Hydrochlorothiazide may add to or potentiate the therapeutic effect of other antihypertensive drugs). Products include:
- Betapace Tablets 950
- Betapace AF Tablets 954

Spirapril Hydrochloride (Hydrochlorothiazide may add to or potentiate the therapeutic effect of other antihypertensive drugs).
- No products indexed under this heading.

Sufentanil Citrate (Potentiation of orthostatic hypotension).
- No products indexed under this heading.

Sulindac (Co-administration with non-steroidal anti-inflammatory agents may reduce the natriuretic and antihypertensive effects of thiazides). Products include:
- Clinoril Tablets 2053

Telmisartan (Hydrochlorothiazide may add to or potentiate the therapeutic effect of other antihypertensive drugs). Products include:
- Micardis Tablets 1049
- Micardis HCT Tablets 1051

Terazosin Hydrochloride (Hydrochlorothiazide may add to or potentiate the therapeutic effect of other antihypertensive drugs). Products include:
- Hytrin Capsules 464

Thiamylal Sodium (Potentiation of orthostatic hypotension).
- No products indexed under this heading.

Timolol Maleate (Hydrochlorothiazide may add to or potentiate the therapeutic effect of other antihypertensive drugs). Products include:
- Blocadren Tablets 2046
- Cosopt Sterile Ophthalmic Solution 2065
- Timolide Tablets 2187
- Timolol GFS .... ⊙266
- Timoptic in Ocudose 2192
- Timoptic Sterile Ophthalmic Solution 2190
- Timoptic-XE Sterile Ophthalmic Gel Forming Solution 2194

Tolazamide (Hydrochlorothiazide may cause hyperglycemia, therefore, dosage adjustment of oral hypoglycemic agent may be required).
- No products indexed under this heading.

Tolbutamide (In vitro studies show significant inhibition of the formation of oxidized irbesartan metabolites with the known cytochrome CYP 2C9 substrate/inhibitor, tolbutamide; hydrochlorothiazide may cause hyperglycemia, therefore dosage adjustment of oral hypoglycemic agent may be required).
- No products indexed under this heading.

Tolmetin Sodium (Co-administration with non-steroidal anti-inflammatory agents may reduce the natriuretic and antihypertensive effects of thiazides). Products include:
- Tolectin 2589

Torsemide (Hydrochlorothiazide may add to or potentiate the therapeutic effect of other antihypertensive drugs). Products include:
- Demadex Tablets and Injection 2965

Trandolapril (Hydrochlorothiazide may add to or potentiate the therapeutic effect of other antihypertensive drugs). Products include:
- Mavik Tablets 478
- Tarka Tablets 508

Triamcinolone (Co-administration with corticosteroids intensifies electrolyte depletion particularly hypokalemia).
- No products indexed under this heading.

Triamcinolone Acetonide (Co-administration with corticosteroids intensifies electrolyte depletion particularly hypokalemia). Products include:
- Azmacort Inhalation Aerosol 728
- Nasacort Nasal Inhaler 750
- Nasacort AQ Nasal Spray 752
- Tri-Nasal Spray 2274

Triamcinolone Diacetate (Co-administration with corticosteroids intensifies electrolyte depletion particularly hypokalemia).
- No products indexed under this heading.

Triamcinolone Hexacetonide (Co-administration with corticosteroids intensifies electrolyte depletion particularly hypokalemia).
- No products indexed under this heading.

Trimethaphan Camsylate (Hydrochlorothiazide may add to or potentiate the therapeutic effect of other antihypertensive drugs).
- No products indexed under this heading.

Troglitazone (Hydrochlorothiazide may cause hyperglycemia, therefore, dosage adjustment of oral hypoglycemic agent may be required).
- No products indexed under this heading.

Tubocurarine Chloride (Possible increased responsiveness to the muscle relaxants).
- No products indexed under this heading.

Valsartan (Hydrochlorothiazide may add to or potentiate the therapeutic effect of other antihypertensive drugs). Products include:
- Diovan Capsules 2337
- Diovan HCT Tablets 2338

Vecuronium Bromide (Possible increased responsiveness to the muscle relaxants). Products include:
- Norcuron for Injection 2478

Verapamil Hydrochloride (Hydrochlorothiazide may add to or potentiate the therapeutic effect of other antihypertensive drugs). Products include:
- Covera-HS Tablets 3199
- Isoptin SR Tablets 467
- Tarka Tablets 508
- Verelan Capsules 3184
- Verelan PM Capsules 3186

Food Interactions

Alcohol (Potentiation of orthostatic hypotension).

AVANDIA TABLETS

(Rosiglitazone Maleate) 1490

May interact with insulin. Compounds in these categories include:

Insulin, Human, Zinc Suspension (Co-administration of rosiglitazone with insulin has resulted in increased incidence of cardiac failure and other cardiovascular adverse events). Products include:
- Humulin L, 100 Units 1937
- Humulin U, 100 Units 1943
- Novolin L Human Insulin 10 ml Vials 2422

Insulin, Human NPH (Co-administration of rosiglitazone with insulin has resulted in increased incidence of cardiac failure and other cardiovascular adverse events). Products include:
- Humulin N, 100 Units 1939
- Humulin N NPH Pen 1940
- Novolin N Human Insulin 10 ml Vials 2422
- Novolin N PenFill 2423
- Novolin N Prefilled Syringe Disposable Insulin Delivery System 2425

Insulin, Human Regular (Co-administration of rosiglitazone with insulin has resulted in increased incidence of cardiac failure and other cardiovascular adverse events). Products include:
- Humulin R Regular (U-500) 1943
- Humulin R, 100 Units 1941
- Novolin R Human Insulin 10 ml Vials 2423
- Novolin R PenFill 2423
- Novolin R Prefilled Syringe Disposable Insulin Delivery System 2425
- Velosulin BR Human Insulin 10 ml Vials 2435

Insulin, Human Regular and Human NPH Mixture (Co-administration of rosiglitazone with insulin has resulted in increased incidence of cardiac failure and other cardiovascular adverse events). Products include:
- Humulin 50/50, 100 Units 1934
- Humulin 70/30, 100 Units 1935
- Humulin 70/30 Pen 1936
- Novolin 70/30 Human Insulin 10 ml Vials 2421
- Novolin 70/30 PenFill 2423
- Novolin 70/30 Prefilled Disposable Insulin Delivery System 2425

Insulin, NPH (Co-administration of rosiglitazone with insulin has resulted in increased incidence of cardiac failure and other cardiovascular adverse events). Products include:
- Iletin II, NPH (Pork), 100 Units 1946

Insulin, Regular (Co-administration of rosiglitazone with insulin has resulted in increased incidence of cardiac failure and other cardiovascular adverse events). Products include:
- Iletin II, Regular (Pork), 100 Units 1947

Insulin, Zinc Crystals (Co-administration of rosiglitazone with insulin has resulted in increased incidence of cardiac failure and other cardiovascular adverse events).

No products indexed under this heading.

Insulin, Zinc Suspension (Co-administration of rosiglitazone with insulin has resulted in increased incidence of cardiac failure and other cardiovascular adverse events). Products include:
- Iletin II, Lente (Pork), 100 Units 1945

Insulin Aspart, Human Regular (Co-administration of rosiglitazone with insulin has resulted in increased incidence of cardiac failure and other cardiovascular adverse events).

No products indexed under this heading.

Insulin glargine (Co-administration of rosiglitazone with insulin has resulted in increased incidence of cardiac failure and other cardiovascular adverse events). Products include:
- Lantus Injection 742

Insulin Lispro, Human (Co-administration of rosiglitazone with insulin has resulted in increased incidence of cardiac failure and other cardiovascular adverse events). Products include:
- Humalog 1926
- Humalog Mix 75/25 Pen 1928

Insulin Lispro Protamine, Human (Co-administration of rosiglitazone with insulin has resulted in increased incidence of cardiac failure and other cardiovascular adverse events). Products include:
- Humalog Mix 75/25 Pen 1928

AVAPRO TABLETS

(Irbesartan) 1074

None cited in PDR database.

AVAPRO TABLETS

(Irbesartan) 3076

None cited in PDR database.

AVC CREAM

(Sulfanilamide) 1350

None cited in PDR database.

AVC SUPPOSITORIES

(Sulfanilamide) 1350

None cited in PDR database.

AVELOX TABLETS

(Moxifloxacin Hydrochloride) 879

May interact with antacids containing aluminum, calcium and magnesium, erythromycin, iron containing oral preparations, non-steroidal anti-inflammatory agents, phenothiazines, quinidine, tricyclic antidepressants, and certain other agents. Compounds in these categories include:

Aluminum Carbonate (Co-administration of quinolones, such as moxifloxacin, with antacids containing magnesium, calcium, or aluminum may substantially interfere with the absorption of quinolones; moxifloxacin should be taken at least 4 hours before or 8 hours after ingestionof antacids).

No products indexed under this heading.

Aluminum Hydroxide (Co-administration of quinolones, such as moxifloxacin, with antacids containing magnesium, calcium, or aluminum may substantially interfere with the absorption of quinolones; moxifloxacin should be taken at least 4 hours before or 8 hours after ingestionof antacids). Products include:
- Amphojel Suspension (Mint Flavor) .... ■ 789
- Gaviscon Extra Strength Liquid .... ■ 751
- Gaviscon Extra Strength Tablets .... ■ 751
- Gaviscon Regular Strength Liquid . ■ 751
- Gaviscon Regular Strength Tablets .... ■ 750
- Maalox Antacid/Anti-Gas Oral Suspension .... ■ 673
- Maalox Max Maximum Strength Antacid/Anti-Gas Liquid 2300
- Maalox Regular Strength Antacid/Antigas Liquid 2300
- Mylanta 1813
- Vanquish Caplets .... ■ 617

Amiodarone Hydrochloride (Moxifloxacin has been shown to prolong the QT interval; concurrent use with class 1A antiarrhythmic agents, such as amiodarone, should be avoided). Products include:
- Cordarone Intravenous 3491
- Cordarone Tablets 3487
- Pacerone Tablets 3331

Amitriptyline Hydrochloride (Moxifloxacin has been shown to prolong the QT interval; an additive effect with co-administration cannot be excluded). Products include:
- Etrafon 3115
- Limbitrol 1738

Amoxapine (Moxifloxacin has been shown to prolong the QT interval; an additive effect with co-administration cannot be excluded).

No products indexed under this heading.

Calcium Carbonate (Co-administration of quinolones, such as moxifloxacin, with antacids containing magnesium, calcium or aluminum may substantially interfere with the absorption of quinolones; moxifloxacin should be taken at least 4 hours before or 8 hours after ingestion of antacids). Products include:
- Aspirin Regimen Bayer 81 mg Caplets with Calcium .... ■ 607
- Extra Strength Bayer Plus Caplets .... ■ 610
- Caltrate 600 Tablets .... ■ 814
- Caltrate 600 PLUS .... ■ 815
- Caltrate 600 + D Tablets .... ■ 814
- Caltrate 600 + Soy Tablets .... ■ 814
- D-Cal Chewable Caplets .... ■ 794
- Florical Capsules and Tablets 2223
- Quick Dissolve Maalox Max Maximum Strength Antacid/Antigas Tablets 2301
- Quick Dissolve Maalox Regular Strength Antacid Tablets 2301
- Marblen Suspension .... ■ 633
- Monocal Tablets 2223
- Mylanta Fast-Acting 1813
- Mylanta Calci Tabs .... ■ 636
- One-A-Day Bedtime & Rest Tablets .... ■ 805
- One-A-Day Calcium Plus Chewable Tablets .... ■ 805
- Os-Cal Chewable Tablets .... ■ 838
- Pepcid Complete Chewable Tablets 1815
- ReSource Wellness CalciWise Soft Chews .... ■ 824
- Rolaids Tablets .... ■ 706
- Extra Strength Rolaids Tablets .... ■ 706
- Slow-Mag Tablets .... ■ 835
- Titralac .... ■ 640
- 3M Titralac Plus Antacid Tablets .... ■ 640
- Tums .... ■ 763

Celecoxib (Co-administration of a non-steroidal anti-inflammatory agent with a quinolone may increase the risks of CNS stimulation and convulsions; this interaction has not been observed with moxifloxacin clinical and preclinical trials). Products include:
- Celebrex Capsules 2676
- Celebrex Capsules 2780

Chlorpromazine (Moxifloxacin has been shown to prolong the QT interval; co-administration with antipsychotic phenothiazines cannot be excluded). Products include:
- Thorazine Suppositories 1656

Chlorpromazine Hydrochloride (Moxifloxacin has been shown to prolong the QT interval; co-administration with antipsychotic phenothiazines cannot be excluded). Products include:
- Thorazine 1656

Cisapride (Moxifloxacin has been shown to prolong the QT interval; an additive effect with co-administration cannot be excluded).

No products indexed under this heading.

Clomipramine Hydrochloride (Moxifloxacin has been shown to prolong the QT interval; an additive effect with co-administration cannot be excluded).

No products indexed under this heading.

Desipramine Hydrochloride (Moxifloxacin has been shown to prolong the QT interval; an additive effect with co-administration cannot be excluded). Products include:
- Norpramin Tablets 755

Diclofenac Potassium (Co-administration of a non-steroidal anti-inflammatory agent with a quinolone may increase the risks of CNS stimulation and convulsions; this interaction has not been observed with moxifloxacin clinical and preclinical trials). Products include:
- Cataflam Tablets 2315

Diclofenac Sodium (Co-administration of a non-steroidal anti-inflammatory agent with a quinolone may increase the risks of CNS stimulation and convulsions; this interaction has not been observed with moxifloxacin clinical and preclinical trials). Products include:
- Arthrotec Tablets 3195
- Voltaren Ophthalmic Sterile Ophthalmic Solution .... ⊙ 312
- Voltaren Tablets 2315
- Voltaren-XR Tablets 2315

Didanosine (Co-administration of quinolones, such as moxifloxacin, with antacids contained in Videx chewable/buffered tablets or the pediatric powder for oral solution may substantially interfere with the absorption of quinolones; moxifloxacin should be taken at least 4 hours before or 8 hours after ingestion of Videx). Products include:
- Videx 1138
- Videx EC Capsules 1143

Digoxin (Co-administration in healthy individuals has resulted in the increase in mean digoxin Cmax by about 50% during the distribution phase of digoxin; this transient increase in digoxin Cmax is not viewed to be clinically significant). Products include:
- Digitek Tablets 1003
- Lanoxicaps Capsules 1574
- Lanoxin Injection 1581
- Lanoxin Tablets 1587
- Lanoxin Elixir Pediatric 1578
- Lanoxin Injection Pediatric 1584

Doxepin Hydrochloride (Moxifloxacin has been shown to prolong the QT interval; an additive effect with co-administration cannot be excluded). Products include:
- Sinequan 2713

Erythromycin (Moxifloxacin has been shown to prolong the QT interval; an additive effect with co-administration cannot be excluded). Products include:
- Emgel 2% Topical Gel 1285
- Ery-Tab Tablets 448
- Erythromycin Base Filmtab Tablets . 454
- Erythromycin Delayed-Release Capsules, USP 455
- PCE Dispertab Tablets 498

Erythromycin Estolate (Moxifloxacin has been shown to prolong the QT interval; an additive effect with co-administration cannot be excluded).

No products indexed under this heading.

Erythromycin Ethylsuccinate (Moxifloxacin has been shown to prolong the QT interval; an additive effect with co-administration cannot be excluded). Products include:
- E.E.S. 450

(■ Described in PDR For Nonprescription Drugs) (⊙ Described in PDR For Ophthalmic Medicines™)

EryPed 446
Pediazole Suspension 3050

Erythromycin Gluceptate (Moxifloxacin has been shown to prolong the QT interval; an additive effect with co-administration cannot be excluded).
No products indexed under this heading.

Erythromycin Stearate (Moxifloxacin has been shown to prolong the QT interval; an additive effect with co-administration cannot be excluded). Products include:
Erythrocin Stearate Filmtab Tablets 452

Etodolac (Co-administration of a non-steroidal anti-inflammatory agent with a quinolone may increase the risks of CNS stimulation and convulsions; this interaction has not been observed with moxifloxacin clinical and preclinical trials). Products include:
Lodine 3528
Lodine XL Extended-Release Tablets 3530

Fenoprofen Calcium (Co-administration of a non-steroidal anti-inflammatory agent with a quinolone may increase the risks of CNS stimulation and convulsions; this interaction has not been observed with moxifloxacin clinical and preclinical trials).
No products indexed under this heading.

Ferrous Fumarate (Co-administration of quinolones, such as moxifloxacin, with iron-containing products may substantially interfere with the absorption of quinolones; moxifloxacin should be taken at least 4 hours before or 8 hours after ingestion of iron-containing products). Products include:
New Formulation Chromagen OB Capsules 3094
Loestrin Fe Tablets 2642
NataChew Tablets 3364

Ferrous Gluconate (Co-administration of quinolones, such as moxifloxacin, with iron-containing products may substantially interfere with the absorption of quinolones; moxifloxacin should be taken at least 4 hours before or 8 hours after ingestion of iron-containing products). Products include:
Fergon Iron Tablets .... ▣802

Ferrous Sulfate (Co-administration of moxifloxacin with ferrous sulfate has resulted in reduced mean AUC (39%) and Cmax (59%) of moxifloxacin; moxifloxacin should be taken at least 4 hours before or 8 hours after ingestion of ferrous sulfate). Products include:
Feosol Tablets 1717
Slow Fe Tablets .... ▣827
Slow Fe with Folic Acid Tablets ..... ▣828

Fluphenazine Decanoate (Moxifloxacin has been shown to prolong the QT interval; co-administration with antipsychotic phenothiazines cannot be excluded).
No products indexed under this heading.

Fluphenazine Enanthate (Moxifloxacin has been shown to prolong the QT interval; co-administration with antipsychotic phenothiazines cannot be excluded).
No products indexed under this heading.

Fluphenazine Hydrochloride (Moxifloxacin has been shown to prolong the QT interval; co-administration with antipsychotic phenothiazines cannot be excluded).
No products indexed under this heading.

Flurbiprofen (Co-administration of a non-steroidal anti-inflammatory agent with a quinolone may increase the risks of CNS stimulation and convulsions; this interaction has not been observed with moxifloxacin clinical and preclinical trials).
No products indexed under this heading.

Glyburide (Co-administration has resulted in reduced mean AUC and Cmax by 12% and 21% respectively; blood glucose levels were decreased slightly in patients on concurrent therapy; these interaction results are not viewed as clinically significant). Products include:
DiaBeta Tablets 741
Glucovance Tablets 1086

Ibuprofen (Co-administration of a non-steroidal anti-inflammatory agent with a quinolone may increase the risks of CNS stimulation and convulsions; this interaction has not been observed with moxifloxacin clinical and preclinical trials). Products include:
Advil .... ▣771
Children's Advil Oral Suspension ... ▣773
Children's Advil Chewable Tablets . ▣773
Advil Cold and Sinus Caplets .... ▣771
Advil Cold and Sinus Tablets .... ▣771
Advil Flu & Body Ache Caplets .... ▣772
Infants' Advil Drops .... ▣773
Junior Strength Advil Tablets .... ▣773
Junior Strength Advil Chewable Tablets .... ▣773
Advil Migraine Liquigels .... ▣772
Children's Motrin Oral Suspension and Chewable Tablets 2006
Children's Motrin Cold Oral Suspension 2007
Children's Motrin Oral Suspension .... ▣643
Motrin Suspension, Oral Drops, Chewable Tablets, and Caplets 2002
Infants' Motrin Concentrated Drops 2006
Junior Strength Motrin Caplets and Chewable Tablets 2006
Motrin IB Tablets, Caplets, and Gelcaps 2002
Motrin Migraine Pain Caplets 2005
Motrin Sinus Headache Caplets 2005
Vicoprofen Tablets 520

Imipramine Hydrochloride (Moxifloxacin has been shown to prolong the QT interval; an additive effect with co-administration cannot be excluded).
No products indexed under this heading.

Imipramine Pamoate (Moxifloxacin has been shown to prolong the QT interval; an additive effect with co-administration cannot be excluded).
No products indexed under this heading.

Indomethacin (Co-administration of a non-steroidal anti-inflammatory agent with a quinolone may increase the risks of CNS stimulation and convulsions; this interaction has not been observed with moxifloxacin clinical and preclinical trials). Products include:
Indocin 2112

Indomethacin Sodium Trihydrate (Co-administration of a non-steroidal anti-inflammatory agent with a quinolone may increase the risks of CNS stimulation and convulsions; this interaction has not been observed with moxifloxacin clinical and preclinical trials). Products include:
Indocin I.V. 2115

Iron (Co-administration of quinolones, such as moxifloxacin, with iron-containing products may substantially interfere with the absorption of quinolones; moxifloxacin should be taken at least 4 hours before or 8 hours after ingestion of iron-containing products).
No products indexed under this heading.

Ketoprofen (Co-administration of a non-steroidal anti-inflammatory agent with a quinolone may increase the risks of CNS stimulation and convulsions; this interaction has not been observed with moxifloxacin clinical and preclinical trials). Products include:
Orudis Capsules 3548
Orudis KT Tablets .... ▣778
Oruvail Capsules 3548

Ketorolac Tromethamine (Co-administration of a non-steroidal anti-inflammatory agent with a quinolone may increase the risks of CNS stimulation and convulsions; this interaction has not been observed with moxifloxacin clinical and preclinical trials). Products include:
Acular Ophthalmic Solution 544
Acular PF Ophthalmic Solution 544
Toradol 3018

Magaldrate (Co-administration of quinolones, such as moxifloxacin, with antacids containing magnesium, calcium, or aluminum may substantially interfere with the absorption of quinolones; moxifloxacin should be taken at least 4 hours before or 8 hours after ingestionof antacids).
No products indexed under this heading.

Magnesium Hydroxide (Co-administration of quinolones, such as moxifloxacin, with antacids containing magnesium, calcium, or aluminum may substantially interfere with the absorption of quinolones; moxifloxacin should be taken at least 4 hours before or 8 hours after ingestionof antacids). Products include:
Ex•Lax Milk of Magnesia Liquid .... ▣670
Maalox Antacid/Anti-Gas Oral Suspension .... ▣673
Maalox Max Maximum Strength Antacid/Anti-Gas Liquid 2300
Maalox Regular Strength Antacid/Antigas Liquid 2300
Mylanta Fast-Acting 1813
Mylanta 1813
Pepcid Complete Chewable Tablets 1815
Phillips' Chewable Tablets .... ▣615
Phillips' Milk of Magnesia Liquid (Original, Cherry, & Mint) .... ▣616
Rolaids Tablets .... ▣706
Extra Strength Rolaids Tablets ...... ▣706
Vanquish Caplets .... ▣617

Magnesium Oxide (Co-administration of quinolones, such as moxifloxacin, with antacids containing magnesium, calcium, or aluminum may substantially interfere with the absorption of quinolones; moxifloxacin should be taken at least 4 hours before or 8 hours after ingestionof antacids). Products include:
Beelith Tablets 946
Mag-Ox 400 Tablets 1024
Uro-Mag Capsules 1024

Maprotiline Hydrochloride (Moxifloxacin has been shown to prolong the QT interval; an additive effect with co-administration cannot be excluded).
No products indexed under this heading.

Meclofenamate Sodium (Co-administration of a non-steroidal anti-inflammatory agent with a quinolone may increase the risks of CNS stimulation and convulsions; this interaction has not been observed with moxifloxacin clinical and preclinical trials).
No products indexed under this heading.

Mefenamic Acid (Co-administration of a non-steroidal anti-inflammatory agent with a quinolone may increase the risks of CNS stimulation and convulsions; this interaction has not been observed with moxifloxacin clinical and preclinical trials). Products include:
Ponstel Capsules 1356

Meloxicam (Co-administration of a non-steroidal anti-inflammatory agent with a quinolone may increase the risks of CNS stimulation and convulsions; this interaction has not been observed with moxifloxacin clinical and preclinical trials). Products include:
Mobic Tablets 1054

Mesoridazine Besylate (Moxifloxacin has been shown to prolong the QT interval; co-administration with antipsychotic phenothiazines cannot be excluded). Products include:
Serentil 1057

Methotrimeprazine (Moxifloxacin has been shown to prolong the QT interval; co-administration with antipsychotic phenothiazines cannot be excluded).
No products indexed under this heading.

Nabumetone (Co-administration of a non-steroidal anti-inflammatory agent with a quinolone may increase the risks of CNS stimulation and convulsions; this interaction has not been observed with moxifloxacin clinical and preclinical trials). Products include:
Relafen Tablets 1617

Naproxen (Co-administration of a non-steroidal anti-inflammatory agent with a quinolone may increase the risks of CNS stimulation and convulsions; this interaction has not been observed with moxifloxacin clinical and preclinical trials). Products include:
EC-Naprosyn Delayed-Release Tablets 2967
Naprosyn Suspension 2967
Naprosyn Tablets 2967

Naproxen Sodium (Co-administration of a non-steroidal anti-inflammatory agent with a quinolone may increase the risks of CNS stimulation and convulsions; this interaction has not been observed with moxifloxacin clinical and preclinical trials). Products include:
Aleve Tablets, Caplets and Gelcaps .... ▣602
Aleve Cold & Sinus Caplets .... ▣603
Anaprox Tablets 2967
Anaprox DS Tablets 2967
Naprelan Tablets 1293

Nortriptyline Hydrochloride (Moxifloxacin has been shown to prolong the QT interval; an additive effect with co-administration cannot be excluded).
No products indexed under this heading.

Oxaprozin (Co-administration of a non-steroidal anti-inflammatory agent with a quinolone may increase the risks of CNS stimulation and convulsions; this interaction has not been observed with moxifloxacin clinical and preclinical trials).
No products indexed under this heading.

Perphenazine (Moxifloxacin has been shown to prolong the QT interval; co-administration with antipsychotic phenothiazines cannot be excluded). Products include:
Etrafon 3115
Trilafon 3160

Phenylbutazone (Co-administration of a non-steroidal anti-inflammatory agent with a quinolone may increase the risks of CNS stimulation and convulsions; this interaction has not been observed with moxifloxacin clinical and preclinical trials).
No products indexed under this heading.

Piroxicam (Co-administration of a non-steroidal anti-inflammatory agent with a quinolone may increase the risks of CNS stimulation and convul-

sions; this interaction has not been observed with moxifloxacin clinical and preclinical trials). Products include:

Feldene Capsules 2685

Polysaccharide-Iron Complex (Co-administration of quinolones, such as moxifloxacin, with iron-containing products may substantially interfere with the absorption of quinolones; moxifloxacin should be taken at least 4 hours before or 8 hours after ingestion of iron-containing products). Products include:

Niferex 3176
Niferex-150 Capsules 3176
Nu-Iron 150 Capsules 2224

Procainamide Hydrochloride (Moxifloxacin has been shown to prolong the QT interval; concurrent use with class 1A antiarrhythmic agents, such as procainamide, should be avoided). Products include:

Procanbid Extended-Release Tablets 2262

Prochlorperazine (Moxifloxacin has been shown to prolong the QT interval; co-administration with antipsychotic phenothiazines cannot be excluded). Products include:

Compazine 1505

Promethazine Hydrochloride (Moxifloxacin has been shown to prolong the QT interval; co-administration with antipsychotic phenothiazines cannot be excluded). Products include:

Mepergan Injection 3539
Phenergan Injection 3553
Phenergan 3556
Phenergan Syrup 3554
Phenergan with Codeine Syrup 3557
Phenergan with Dextromethorphan Syrup 3559
Phenergan VC Syrup 3560
Phenergan VC with Codeine Syrup 3561

Protriptyline Hydrochloride (Moxifloxacin has been shown to prolong the QT interval; an additive effect with co-administration cannot be excluded). Products include:

Vivactil Tablets 2446
Vivactil Tablets 2217

Quinidine Gluconate (Moxifloxacin has been shown to prolong the QT interval; concurrent use with class 1A antiarrhythmic agents, such as quinidine, should be avoided). Products include:

Quinaglute Dura-Tabs Tablets 978

Quinidine Polygalacturonate (Moxifloxacin has been shown to prolong the QT interval; concurrent use with class 1A antiarrhythmic agents, such as quinidine, should be avoided).

No products indexed under this heading.

Quinidine Sulfate (Moxifloxacin has been shown to prolong the QT interval; concurrent use with class 1A antiarrhythmic agents, such as quinidine, should be avoided). Products include:

Quinidex Extentabs 2933

Rofecoxib (Co-administration of a non-steroidal anti-inflammatory agent with a quinolone may increase the risks of CNS stimulation and convulsions; this interaction has not been observed with moxifloxacin clinical and preclinical trials). Products include:

Vioxx 2213

Sotalol Hydrochloride (Moxifloxacin has been shown to prolong the QT interval; concurrent use with class III antiarrhythmic agents, such as sotalol, should be avoided). Products include:

Betapace Tablets 950
Betapace AF Tablets 954

Sucralfate (Co-administration of quinolones, such as moxifloxacin, with sucralfate may substantially interfere with the absorption of quinolones; moxifloxacin should be taken at least 4 hours before or 8 hours after ingestion of sucralfate). Products include:

Carafate Suspension 731
Carafate Tablets 730

Sulindac (Co-administration of a non-steroidal anti-inflammatory agent with a quinolone may increase the risks of CNS stimulation and convulsions; this interaction has not been observed with moxifloxacin clinical and preclinical trials). Products include:

Clinoril Tablets 2053

Thioridazine Hydrochloride (Moxifloxacin has been shown to prolong the QT interval; co-administration with antipsychotic phenothiazines cannot be excluded). Products include:

Thioridazine Hydrochloride Tablets 2289

Tolmetin Sodium (Co-administration of a non-steroidal anti-inflammatory agent with a quinolone may increase the risks of CNS stimulation and convulsions; this interaction has not been observed with moxifloxacin clinical and preclinical trials). Products include:

Tolectin 2589

Trifluoperazine Hydrochloride (Moxifloxacin has been shown to prolong the QT interval; co-administration with antipsychotic phenothiazines cannot be excluded). Products include:

Stelazine 1640

Trimipramine Maleate (Moxifloxacin has been shown to prolong the QT interval; an additive effect with co-administration cannot be excluded). Products include:

Surmontil Capsules 3595

Zinc Sulfate (Co-administration of quinolones, such as moxifloxacin, with zinc-containing products may substantially interfere with the absorption of quinolones; moxifloxacin should be taken at least 4 hours before or 8 hours after ingestion of zinc-containing products). Products include:

Clear Eyes ACR Astringent/Lubricant Eye Redness Reliever .... ⊙ 322
Visine A.C. Seasonal Relief From Pollen & Dust Eye Drops .... ⊙ 314

AVITA CREAM

(Tretinoin) 999
May interact with:

Concomitant Topical Acne Therapy (Effect not specified).

No products indexed under this heading.

Resorcinol (Caution should be exercised).

No products indexed under this heading.

Salicylic Acid (Caution should be exercised). Products include:

Clear Away Gel with Aloe Wart Remover System .... ▣ 736
Clear Away Liquid Wart Remover System .... ▣ 736
Clear Away One Step Wart Remover .... ▣ 737
Clear Away One Step Wart Remover for Kids .... ▣ 737
Clear Away One Step Plantar Wart Remover .... ▣ 737
Compound W One Step Pads for Kids .... ▣ 664
Compound W One Step Plantar Pads .... ▣ 664
Compound W One Step Wart Remover Pads .... ▣ 664
Compound W Wart Remover Gel .... ▣ 665
Compound W Wart Remover Liquid .... ▣ 665
Wart-Off Liquid .... ▣ 716

Sulfur (Caution should be exercised). Products include:

Plexion 2024

Topical Medications (Effect not specified).

No products indexed under this heading.

AVITA GEL

(Tretinoin) 1000
See Avita Cream

AVONEX

(Interferon Beta-1a) 1013
May interact with:

Bone Marrow Depressants, unspecified (Co-administration with myelosuppressive agents requires careful patient monitoring).

AXERT TABLETS

(Almotriptan Malate) 2772
May interact with 5HT1-receptor agonists, ergot-containing drugs, erythromycin, selective serotonin reuptake inhibitors, and certain other agents. Compounds in these categories include:

Citalopram Hydrobromide (Co-administration of SSRI and 5HT1 agonist have been rarely reported to cause weakness, hyperreflexia, and incoordination). Products include:

Celexa 1365

Dihydroergotamine Mesylate (Ergot-containing drugs have been reported to cause prolonged vasospastic reactions; because there is a theoretical basis that these effects may be additive, use of ergot-type agents and almotriptan within 24 hours is contraindicated). Products include:

D.H.E. 45 Injection 2334
Migranal Nasal Spray 2376

Ergonovine Maleate (Ergot-containing drugs have been reported to cause prolonged vasospastic reactions; because there is a theoretical basis that these effects may be additive, use of ergot-type agents and almotriptan within 24 hours is contraindicated).

No products indexed under this heading.

Ergotamine Tartrate (Ergot-containing drugs have been reported to cause prolonged vasospastic reactions; because there is a theoretical basis that these effects may be additive, use of ergot-type agents and almotriptan within 24 hours is contraindicated).

No products indexed under this heading.

Erythromycin (Co-administration with other potent inhibitors of CYP3A4 inhibitors, such as erythromycin, may result in increased exposures to almotriptan). Products include:

Emgel 2% Topical Gel 1285
Ery-Tab Tablets 448
Erythromycin Base Filmtab Tablets 454
Erythromycin Delayed-Release Capsules, USP 455
PCE Dispertab Tablets 498

Erythromycin Estolate (Co-administration with other potent inhibitors of CYP3A4 inhibitors, such as erythromycin, may result in increased exposures to almotriptan).

No products indexed under this heading.

Erythromycin Ethylsuccinate (Co-administration with other potent inhibitors of CYP3A4 inhibitors, such as erythromycin, may result in increased exposures to almotriptan). Products include:

E.E.S. 450
EryPed 446
Pediazole Suspension 3050

Erythromycin Gluceptate (Co-administration with other potent inhibitors of CYP3A4 inhibitors, such as erythromycin, may result in increased exposures to almotriptan).

No products indexed under this heading.

Erythromycin Stearate (Co-administration with other potent inhibitors of CYP3A4 inhibitors, such as erythromycin, may result in increased exposures to almotriptan). Products include:

Erythrocin Stearate Filmtab Tablets 452

Fluoxetine Hydrochloride (Co-administration has resulted in an increase in maximal concentrations of almotriptan by 18%; this difference is not clinically significant; co-administration of SSRI and 5HT1 agonist have been rarely reported to cause weakness, hyperreflexia, and incoordination). Products include:

Prozac Pulvules, Liquid, and Weekly Capsules 1238
Sarafem Pulvules 1962

Fluvoxamine Maleate (Co-administration of SSRI and 5HT1 agonist have been rarely reported to cause weakness, hyperreflexia, and incoordination). Products include:

Luvox Tablets (25, 50, 100 mg) 3256

Itraconazole (Co-administration with other potent inhibitors of CYP3A4 inhibitors, such as itraconazole, may result in increased exposures to almotriptan). Products include:

Sporanox Capsules 1800
Sporanox Injection 1804
Sporanox Injection 2509
Sporanox Oral Solution 1808
Sporanox Oral Solution 2512

Ketoconazole (Co-administration has resulted in an approximately 60% increase in the AUC and maximal plasma concentrations of almotriptan). Products include:

Nizoral 2% Cream 3620
Nizoral A-D Shampoo 2008
Nizoral 2% Shampoo 2007
Nizoral Tablets 1791

Methylergonovine Maleate (Ergot-containing drugs have been reported to cause prolonged vasospastic reactions; because there is a theoretical basis that these effects may be additive, use of ergot-type agents and almotriptan within 24 hours is contraindicated).

No products indexed under this heading.

Methysergide Maleate (Ergot-containing drugs have been reported to cause prolonged vasospastic reactions; because there is a theoretical basis that these effects may be additive, use of ergot-type agents and almotriptan within 24 hours is contraindicated).

No products indexed under this heading.

Moclobemide (Co-administration has resulted in a 27% decrease in almotriptan clearance).

No products indexed under this heading.

Naratriptan Hydrochloride (Co-administration with other 5HT1 agonists within 24 hours of treatment with almotriptan is contraindicated). Products include:

Amerge Tablets 1467

Paroxetine Hydrochloride (Co-administration of SSRI and 5HT1 agonist have been rarely reported to cause weakness, hyperreflexia, and incoordination). Products include:

Paxil 1609

Ritonavir (Co-administration with other potent inhibitors of CYP3A4 inhibitors, such as ritonavir, may result in increased exposures to almotriptan). Products include:

Kaletra Capsules 471
Kaletra Oral Solution 471
Norvir Capsules 487
Norvir Oral Solution 487

Rizatriptan Benzoate (Co-administration with other 5HT1 agonists within 24 hours of treatment with almotriptan is contraindicated). Products include:
Maxalt Tablets 2120
Maxalt-MLT Orally Disintegrating Tablets 2120

Sertraline Hydrochloride (Co-administration of SSRI and 5HT1 agonist have been rarely reported to cause weakness, hyperreflexia, and incoordination). Products include:
Zoloft 2751

Sumatriptan (Co-administration with other 5HT1 agonists within 24 hours of treatment with almotriptan is contraindicated). Products include:
Imitrex Nasal Spray 1554

Sumatriptan Succinate (Co-administration with other 5HT1 agonists within 24 hours of treatment with almotriptan is contraindicated). Products include:
Imitrex Injection 1549
Imitrex Tablets 1558

Verapamil Hydrochloride (Co-administration has resulted in a 20% increase in AUC and a 24% increase in maximal plasma concentrations of almotriptan; neither of these changes is clinically significant). Products include:
Covera-HS Tablets 3199
Isoptin SR Tablets 467
Tarka Tablets 508
Verelan Capsules 3184
Verelan PM Capsules 3186

Zolmitriptan (Co-administration with other 5HT1 agonists within 24 hours of treatment with almotriptan is contraindicated). Products include:
Zomig Tablets 708
Zomig-ZMT Tablets 708

AXID PULVULES

(Nizatidine) 2919
May interact with:

Aspirin (Increased serum salicylate levels when nizatidine is given concurrently with very high doses (3,900 mg) of aspirin). Products include:
Aggrenox Capsules 1026
Alka-Seltzer ▣603
Alka-Seltzer Lemon Lime Antacid and Pain Reliever Effervescent Tablets ▣603
Alka-Seltzer Extra Strength Antacid and Pain Reliever Effervescent Tablets ▣603
Alka-Seltzer PM Effervescent Tablets ▣605
Genuine Bayer Tablets, Caplets and Gelcaps ▣606
Extra Strength Bayer Caplets and Gelcaps ▣610
Aspirin Regimen Bayer Children's Chewable Tablets (Orange or Cherry Flavored) ▣607
Bayer, Aspirin Regimen ▣606
Aspirin Regimen Bayer 81 mg Caplets with Calcium ▣607
Genuine Bayer Professional Labeling (Aspirin Regimen Bayer) ▣608
Extra Strength Bayer Arthritis Caplets ▣610
Extra Strength Bayer Plus Caplets ▣610
Extra Strength Bayer PM Caplets ▣611
BC Powder ▣619
BC Allergy Sinus Cold Powder ▣619
Arthritis Strength BC Powder ▣619
BC Sinus Cold Powder ▣619
Darvon Compound-65 Pulvules 1910
Ecotrin Enteric Coated Aspirin Low, Regular and Maximum Strength Tablets 1715
Excedrin Extra-Strength Tablets, Caplets, and Geltabs ▣629
Excedrin Migraine 1070
Goody's Body Pain Formula Powder ▣620
Goody's Extra Strength Headache Powder ▣620
Goody's Extra Strength Pain Relief Tablets ▣620
Percodan Tablets 1327
Robaxisal Tablets 2939
Soma Compound Tablets 3354
Soma Compound w/Codeine Tablets 3355
Vanquish Caplets ▣617

AXID PULVULES

(Nizatidine) 1903
May interact with:

Aspirin (Increased serum salicylate levels when nizatidine is given concurrently with very high doses (3,900 mg) of aspirin). Products include:
Aggrenox Capsules 1026
Alka-Seltzer ▣603
Alka-Seltzer Lemon Lime Antacid and Pain Reliever Effervescent Tablets ▣603
Alka-Seltzer Extra Strength Antacid and Pain Reliever Effervescent Tablets ▣603
Alka-Seltzer PM Effervescent Tablets ▣605
Genuine Bayer Tablets, Caplets and Gelcaps ▣606
Extra Strength Bayer Caplets and Gelcaps ▣610
Aspirin Regimen Bayer Children's Chewable Tablets (Orange or Cherry Flavored) ▣607
Bayer, Aspirin Regimen ▣606
Aspirin Regimen Bayer 81 mg Caplets with Calcium ▣607
Genuine Bayer Professional Labeling (Aspirin Regimen Bayer) ▣608
Extra Strength Bayer Arthritis Caplets ▣610
Extra Strength Bayer Plus Caplets ▣610
Extra Strength Bayer PM Caplets ▣611
BC Powder ▣619
BC Allergy Sinus Cold Powder ▣619
Arthritis Strength BC Powder ▣619
BC Sinus Cold Powder ▣619
Darvon Compound-65 Pulvules 1910
Ecotrin Enteric Coated Aspirin Low, Regular and Maximum Strength Tablets 1715
Excedrin Extra-Strength Tablets, Caplets, and Geltabs ▣629
Excedrin Migraine 1070
Goody's Body Pain Formula Powder ▣620
Goody's Extra Strength Headache Powder ▣620
Goody's Extra Strength Pain Relief Tablets ▣620
Percodan Tablets 1327
Robaxisal Tablets 2939
Soma Compound Tablets 3354
Soma Compound w/Codeine Tablets 3355
Vanquish Caplets ▣617

AYGESTIN TABLETS

(Norethindrone Acetate) 1333
None cited in PDR database.

AZACTAM FOR INJECTION

(Aztreonam) 1276
May interact with aminoglycosides and certain other agents. Compounds in these categories include:

Amikacin Sulfate (Renal function should be monitored if used concurrently or if higher dosages of aminoglycosides are used because of the potential nephrotoxicity and ototoxicity of aminoglycoside antibiotics).
No products indexed under this heading.

Cefoxitin Sodium (May induce high levels of beta-lacatamase in vitro in some gram-negative aerobes; may antagonize aztreonam). Products include:
Mefoxin for Injection 2124
Mefoxin Premixed Intravenous Solution 2127

Gentamicin Sulfate (Renal function should be monitored if used concurrently or if higher dosages of aminoglycosides are used because of the potential nephrotoxicity and ototoxicity of aminoglycoside antibiotics). Products include:
Genoptic Ophthalmic Ointment ⊙239
Genoptic Sterile Ophthalmic Solution ⊙239
Pred-G Ophthalmic Suspension ⊙247
Pred-G Sterile Ophthalmic Ointment ⊙248

Imipenem (May induce high levels of beta-lacatamase in vitro in some gram-negative aerobes; may antagonize aztreonam). Products include:
Primaxin I.M. 2158
Primaxin I.V. 2160

Kanamycin Sulfate (Renal function should be monitored if used concurrently or if higher dosages of aminoglycosides are used because of the potential nephrotoxicity and ototoxicity of aminoglycoside antibiotics).
No products indexed under this heading.

Streptomycin Sulfate (Renal function should be monitored if used concurrently or if higher dosages of aminoglycosides are used because of the potential nephrotoxicity and ototoxicity of aminoglycoside antibiotics). Products include:
Streptomycin Sulfate Injection 2714

Tobramycin (Renal function should be monitored if used concurrently or if higher dosages of aminoglycosides are used because of the potential nephrotoxicity and ototoxicity of aminoglycoside antibiotics). Products include:
TOBI Solution for Inhalation 1206
TobraDex Ophthalmic Ointment 542
TobraDex Ophthalmic Suspension 541
Tobrex Ophthalmic Ointment ⊙220
Tobrex Ophthalmic Solution ⊙221

Tobramycin Sulfate (Renal function should be monitored if used concurrently or if higher dosages of aminoglycosides are used because of the potential nephrotoxicity and ototoxicity of aminoglycoside antibiotics). Products include:
Nebcin Vials, Hyporets & ADD-Vantage 1955

AZELEX CREAM

(Azelaic Acid) 547
None cited in PDR database.

AZMACORT INHALATION AEROSOL

(Triamcinolone Acetonide) 728
May interact with:

Prednisone (Potential for increased likelihood of HPA suppression). Products include:
Prednisone 3064

AZOPT OPHTHALMIC SUSPENSION

(Brinzolamide) 536
May interact with carbonic anhydrase inhibitors and salicylates. Compounds in these categories include:

Acetazolamide (There is a potential for an additive effect on the known systemic effects of carbonic anhydrase inhibition in patients receiving an oral carbonic anhydrase inhibitor and brinzolamide; co-administration is not recommended). Products include:
Diamox Sequels Sustained Release Capsules ⊙270
Diamox Tablets ⊙269

Aspirin (Co-administration with high dose salicylate and oral carbonic anhydrase inhibitor has resulted in rare instances of drug interactions). Products include:
Aggrenox Capsules 1026
Alka-Seltzer ▣603
Alka-Seltzer Lemon Lime Antacid and Pain Reliever Effervescent Tablets ▣603
Alka-Seltzer Extra Strength Antacid and Pain Reliever Effervescent Tablets ▣603
Alka-Seltzer PM Effervescent Tablets ▣605
Genuine Bayer Tablets, Caplets and Gelcaps ▣606
Extra Strength Bayer Caplets and Gelcaps ▣610
Aspirin Regimen Bayer Children's Chewable Tablets (Orange or Cherry Flavored) ▣607
Bayer, Aspirin Regimen ▣606
Aspirin Regimen Bayer 81 mg Caplets with Calcium ▣607
Genuine Bayer Professional Labeling (Aspirin Regimen Bayer) ▣608
Extra Strength Bayer Arthritis Caplets ▣610
Extra Strength Bayer Plus Caplets ▣610
Extra Strength Bayer PM Caplets ▣611
BC Powder ▣619
BC Allergy Sinus Cold Powder ▣619
Arthritis Strength BC Powder ▣619
BC Sinus Cold Powder ▣619
Darvon Compound-65 Pulvules 1910
Ecotrin Enteric Coated Aspirin Low, Regular and Maximum Strength Tablets 1715
Excedrin Extra-Strength Tablets, Caplets, and Geltabs ▣629
Excedrin Migraine 1070
Goody's Body Pain Formula Powder ▣620
Goody's Extra Strength Headache Powder ▣620
Goody's Extra Strength Pain Relief Tablets ▣620
Percodan Tablets 1327
Robaxisal Tablets 2939
Soma Compound Tablets 3354
Soma Compound w/Codeine Tablets 3355
Vanquish Caplets ▣617

Choline Magnesium Trisalicylate (Co-administration with high dose salicylate and oral carbonic anhydrase inhibitor has resulted in rare instances of drug interactions). Products include:
Trilisate 2901

Dichlorphenamide (There is a potential for an additive effect on the known systemic effects of carbonic anhydrase inhibition in patients receiving an oral carbonic anhydrase inhibitor and brinzolamide; co-administration is not recommended). Products include:
Daranide Tablets 2077

Diflunisal (Co-administration with high dose salicylate and oral carbonic anhydrase inhibitor has resulted in rare instances of drug interactions). Products include:
Dolobid Tablets 2088

Dorzolamide Hydrochloride (There is a potential for an additive effect on the known systemic effects of carbonic anhydrase inhibition in patients receiving an oral carbonic anhydrase inhibitor and brinzolamide; co-administration is not recommended). Products include:
Cosopt Sterile Ophthalmic Solution 2065
Trusopt Sterile Ophthalmic Solution 2196

Magnesium Salicylate (Co-administration with high dose salicylate and oral carbonic anhydrase inhibitor has resulted in rare instances of drug interactions). Products include:
Momentum Backache Relief Extra Strength Caplets ▣666

Methazolamide (There is a potential for an additive effect on the known systemic effects of carbonic anhydrase inhibition in patients receiving an oral carbonic anhydrase inhibitor and brinzolamide; co-administration is not recommended). Products include:
Neptazane Tablets ⊙271

Salsalate (Co-administration with high dose salicylate and oral carbonic anhydrase inhibitor has resulted in rare instances of drug interactions).
No products indexed under this heading.

AZULFIDINE EN-TABS TABLETS
(Sulfasalazine) 2775
May interact with:

Digoxin (Reduced absorption of digoxin). Products include:
- Digitek Tablets 1003
- Lanoxicaps Capsules 1574
- Lanoxin Injection 1581
- Lanoxin Tablets 1587
- Lanoxin Elixir Pediatric 1578
- Lanoxin Injection Pediatric 1584

Folic Acid (Reduced absorption of folic acid). Products include:
- Bevitamel Tablets 3459
- Nicomide Tablets 3247
- Slow Fe with Folic Acid Tablets ....◘ 828

BACTINE FIRST AID LIQUID
(Benzalkonium Chloride, Lidocaine Hydrochloride) .... ◘ 611
None cited in PDR database.

BACTRIM PEDIATRIC SUSPENSION
(Sulfamethoxazole, Trimethoprim) 2949
See Bactrim DS Tablets

BACTRIM TABLETS
(Sulfamethoxazole, Trimethoprim) 2949
See Bactrim DS Tablets

BACTRIM DS TABLETS
(Sulfamethoxazole, Trimethoprim) 2949
May interact with oral hypoglycemic agents, phenytoin, thiazides, tricyclic antidepressants, and certain other agents. Compounds in these categories include:

Acarbose (Sulfonamides potentiate the effect of oral hypoglycemic agents). Products include:
- Precose Tablets 906

Amantadine Hydrochloride (Co-adminstration has resulted in a single case of toxic delirium). Products include:
- Symmetrel 1328

Amitriptyline Hydrochloride (The efficacy of tricyclic antidepressants can decrease when co-administered with Bactrim). Products include:
- Etrafon 3115
- Limbitrol 1738

Amoxapine (The efficacy of tricyclic antidepressants can decrease when co-administered with Bactrim).
No products indexed under this heading.

Bendroflumethiazide (Co-administration of thiazide diuretics with Bactrim, especially in elderly patients, can result in an increased incidence of thrombocytopenia with purpura). Products include:
- Corzide 40/5 Tablets 2247
- Corzide 80/5 Tablets 2247

Chlorothiazide (Co-administration of thiazide diuretics with Bactrim, especially in elderly patients, can result in an increased incidence of thrombocytopenia with purpura). Products include:
- Aldoclor Tablets 2035
- Diuril Oral 2087

Chlorothiazide Sodium (Co-administration of thiazide diuretics with Bactrim, especially in elderly patients, can result in an increased incidence of thrombocytopenia with purpura). Products include:
- Diuril Sodium Intravenous 2086

Chlorpropamide (Sulfonamides potentiate the effect of oral hypoglycemic agents). Products include:
- Diabinese Tablets 2680

Clomipramine Hydrochloride (The efficacy of tricyclic antidepressants can decrease when co-administered with Bactrim).
No products indexed under this heading.

Cyclosporine (Co-administration in renal transplant recipients has resulted in marked but reversible nephrotoxicity). Products include:
- Gengraf Capsules 457
- Neoral Soft Gelatin Capsules 2380
- Neoral Oral Solution 2380
- Sandimmune 2388

Desipramine Hydrochloride (The efficacy of tricyclic antidepressants can decrease when co-administered with Bactrim). Products include:
- Norpramin Tablets 755

Digoxin (Co-administration of digoxin with Bactrim, especially in elderly patients, can result in increased digoxin blood levels). Products include:
- Digitek Tablets 1003
- Lanoxicaps Capsules 1574
- Lanoxin Injection 1581
- Lanoxin Tablets 1587
- Lanoxin Elixir Pediatric 1578
- Lanoxin Injection Pediatric 1584

Doxepin Hydrochloride (The efficacy of tricyclic antidepressants can decrease when co-administered with Bactrim). Products include:
- Sinequan 2713

Fosphenytoin Sodium (Bactrim may inhibit hepatic metabolism of phenytoin; Bactrim, given at a common clinical dosage, increased the phenytoin half-life by 39% and decreased the phenytoin metabolic clearance rate by 27%). Products include:
- Cerebyx Injection 2619

Glimepiride (Sulfonamides potentiate the effect of oral hypoglycemic agents). Products include:
- Amaryl Tablets 717

Glipizide (Sulfonamides potentiate the effect of oral hypoglycemic agents). Products include:
- Glucotrol Tablets 2692
- Glucotrol XL Extended Release Tablets 2693

Glyburide (Sulfonamides potentiate the effect of oral hypoglycemic agents). Products include:
- DiaBeta Tablets 741
- Glucovance Tablets 1086

Hydrochlorothiazide (Co-administration of thiazide diuretics with Bactrim, especially in elderly patients, can result in an increased incidence of thrombocytopenia with purpura). Products include:
- Accuretic Tablets 2614
- Aldoril Tablets 2039
- Atacand HCT Tablets 597
- Avalide Tablets 1070
- Diovan HCT Tablets 2338
- Dyazide Capsules 1515
- HydroDIURIL Tablets 2108
- Hyzaar 2109
- Inderide Tablets 3517
- Inderide LA Long-Acting Capsules .. 3519
- Lotensin HCT Tablets 2367
- Maxzide 1008
- Micardis HCT Tablets 1051
- Microzide Capsules 3414
- Moduretic Tablets 2138
- Monopril HCT 1094
- Prinzide Tablets 2168
- Timolide Tablets 2187
- Uniretic Tablets 3178
- Vaseretic Tablets 2204
- Zestoretic Tablets 695
- Ziac Tablets 1887

Hydroflumethiazide (Co-administration of thiazide diuretics with Bactrim, especially in elderly patients, can result in an increased incidence of thrombocytopenia with purpura). Products include:
- Diucardin Tablets 3494

Imipramine Hydrochloride (The efficacy of tricyclic antidepressants can decrease when co-administered with Bactrim).
No products indexed under this heading.

Imipramine Pamoate (The efficacy of tricyclic antidepressants can decrease when co-administered with Bactrim).
No products indexed under this heading.

Indomethacin (Increases sulfamethoxazole blood levels). Products include:
- Indocin 2112

Maprotiline Hydrochloride (The efficacy of tricyclic antidepressants can decrease when co-administered with Bactrim).
No products indexed under this heading.

Metformin Hydrochloride (Sulfonamides potentiate the effect of oral hypoglycemic agents). Products include:
- Glucophage Tablets 1080
- Glucophage XR Tablets 1080
- Glucovance Tablets 1086

Methotrexate Sodium (Sulfonamides can displace methotrexate from protein binding sites and can compete with the renal transport of methotrexate, thus increasing free methotrexate concentrations).
No products indexed under this heading.

Methyclothiazide (Co-administration of thiazide diuretics with Bactrim, especially in elderly patients, can result in an increased incidence of thrombocytopenia with purpura).
No products indexed under this heading.

Miglitol (Sulfonamides potentiate the effect of oral hypoglycemic agents). Products include:
- Glyset Tablets 2821

Nortriptyline Hydrochloride (The efficacy of tricyclic antidepressants can decrease when co-administered with Bactrim).
No products indexed under this heading.

Phenytoin (Bactrim may inhibit hepatic metabolism of phenytoin; Bactrim, given at a common clinical dosage, increased the phenytoin half-life by 39% and decreased the phenytoin metabolic clearance rate by 27%). Products include:
- Dilantin Infatabs 2624
- Dilantin-125 Oral Suspension 2625

Phenytoin Sodium (Bactrim may inhibit hepatic metabolism of phenytoin; Bactrim, given at a common clinical dosage, increased the phenytoin half-life by 39% and decreased the phenytoin metabolic clearance rate by 27%). Products include:
- Dilantin Kapseals 2622

Pioglitazone Hydrochloride (Sulfonamides potentiate the effect of oral hypoglycemic agents). Products include:
- Actos Tablets 3275

Polythiazide (Co-administration of thiazide diuretics with Bactrim, especially in elderly patients, can result in an increased incidence of thrombocytopenia with purpura). Products include:
- Minizide Capsules 2700
- Renese Tablets 2712

Protriptyline Hydrochloride (The efficacy of tricyclic antidepressants can decrease when co-administered with Bactrim). Products include:
- Vivactil Tablets 2446
- Vivactil Tablets 2217

Pyrimethamine (Potential for megaloblastic anemia with concurrent use). Products include:
- Daraprim Tablets 1511

Repaglinide (Sulfonamides potentiate the effect of oral hypoglycemic agents). Products include:
- Prandin Tablets (0.5, 1, and 2 mg) 2432

Rosiglitazone Maleate (Sulfonamides potentiate the effect of oral hypoglycemic agents). Products include:
- Avandia Tablets 1490

Tolazamide (Sulfonamides potentiate the effect of oral hypoglycemic agents).
No products indexed under this heading.

Tolbutamide (Sulfonamides potentiate the effect of oral hypoglycemic agents).
No products indexed under this heading.

Trimipramine Maleate (The efficacy of tricyclic antidepressants can decrease when co-administered with Bactrim). Products include:
- Surmontil Capsules 3595

Troglitazone (Sulfonamides potentiate the effect of oral hypoglycemic agents).
No products indexed under this heading.

Warfarin Sodium (Bactrim may prolong the prothrombin time in patients receiving warfarin). Products include:
- Coumadin for Injection 1243
- Coumadin Tablets 1243
- Warfarin Sodium Tablets, USP 3302

BACTROBAN CREAM
(Mupirocin Calcium) 1494
None cited in PDR database.

BACTROBAN NASAL
(Mupirocin Calcium) 1495
None cited in PDR database.

BACTROBAN OINTMENT
(Mupirocin) 1496
None cited in PDR database.

BALMEX DIAPER RASH OINTMENT
(Zinc Oxide) .... ◘ 619
None cited in PDR database.

BALMEX MEDICATED PLUS BABY POWDER
(Corn Starch, Zinc Oxide) .... ◘ 619
None cited in PDR database.

BAYCOL TABLETS
(Cerivastatin Sodium) 883
May interact with erythromycin, fibrates, and certain other agents. Compounds in these categories include:

Cholestyramine (Co-administration has resulted in decrease of more than 22% for AUC and 40% for Cmax when compared to dosing cerivastatin alone; a dosing schedule of cerivastatin given at bedtime and cholestyramine given before the evening meal would not result in a significant decrease in clinical effect of cerivastatin).
No products indexed under this heading.

Clofibrate (The risk of myopathy during treatment with other HMG-CoA reductase inhibitor has increased with concurrent use of fibric acid derivatives; combined therapy should be avoided). Products include:
- Atromid-S Capsules 3483

Cyclosporine (The risk of myopathy during treatment with other HMG-CoA reductase inhibitor has increased with concurrent use of cyclosporine). Products include:
- Gengraf Capsules 457
- Neoral Soft Gelatin Capsules 2380
- Neoral Oral Solution 2380
- Sandimmune 2388

Erythromycin (Co-administration has resulted in increased steady-state cerivastatin AUC (50%) and Cmax (24%); the risk of myopathy during treatment with other HMG-CoA reductase inhibitor has increased with concurrent use of erythromycin). Products include:

Emgel 2% Topical Gel 1285
Ery-Tab Tablets 448
Erythromycin Base Filmtab Tablets . 454
Erythromycin Delayed-Release Capsules, USP 455
PCE Dispertab Tablets 498

Erythromycin Estolate (Co-administration has resulted in increased steady-state cerivastatin AUC (50%) and Cmax (24%); the risk of myopathy during treatment with other HMG-CoA reductase inhibitor has increased with concurrent use of erythromycin).
No products indexed under this heading.

Erythromycin Ethylsuccinate (Co-administration has resulted in increased steady-state cerivastatin AUC (50%) and Cmax (24%); the risk of myopathy during treatment with other HMG-CoA reductase inhibitor has increased with concurrent use of erythromycin). Products include:
E.E.S. 450
EryPed 446
Pediazole Suspension 3050

Erythromycin Gluceptate (Co-administration has resulted in increased steady-state cerivastatin AUC (50%) and Cmax (24%); the risk of myopathy during treatment with other HMG-CoA reductase inhibitor has increased with concurrent use of erythromycin).
No products indexed under this heading.

Erythromycin Stearate (Co-administration has resulted in increased steady-state cerivastatin AUC (50%) and Cmax (24%); the risk of myopathy during treatment with other HMG-CoA reductase inhibitor has increased with concurrent use of erythromycin). Products include:
Erythrocin Stearate Filmtab Tablets 452

Fenofibrate (The risk of myopathy during treatment with other HMG-CoA reductase inhibitor has increased with concurrent use of fibric acid derivatives; combined therapy should be avoided). Products include:
Tricor Capsules, Micronized 513

Gemfibrozil (Co-administration has resulted in rhabdomyolysis and associated renal failure; concurrent use is contraindicated). Products include:
Lopid Tablets 2650

Itraconazole (The risk of myopathy during treatment with other HMG-CoA reductase inhibitor has increased with concurrent use of itraconazole). Products include:
Sporanox Capsules 1800
Sporanox Injection 1804
Sporanox Injection 2509
Sporanox Oral Solution 1808
Sporanox Oral Solution 2512

Niacin (The risk of myopathy during treatment with other HMG-CoA reductase inhibitor has increased with concurrent use of lipid-lowering dose of niacin). Products include:
Niaspan Extended-Release Tablets 1846
Nicotinex Elixir .... ■633

GENUINE BAYER TABLETS, CAPLETS AND GELCAPS
(Aspirin) .... ■606
See Extra Strength Bayer Plus Caplets

EXTRA STRENGTH BAYER CAPLETS AND GELCAPS
(Aspirin) .... ■610
See Extra Strength Bayer Plus Caplets

ASPIRIN REGIMEN BAYER CHILDREN'S CHEWABLE TABLETS (ORANGE OR CHERRY FLAVORED)
(Aspirin) .... ■607
See Extra Strength Bayer Plus Caplets

ASPIRIN REGIMEN BAYER ADULT LOW STRENGTH 81 MG TABLETS
(Aspirin) .... ■606
See Extra Strength Bayer Plus Caplets

ASPIRIN REGIMEN BAYER 81 MG CAPLETS WITH CALCIUM
(Aspirin, Calcium Carbonate) .... ■607
See Extra Strength Bayer Plus Caplets

ASPIRIN REGIMEN BAYER REGULAR STRENGTH 325 MG CAPLETS
(Aspirin) .... ■606
See Extra Strength Bayer Plus Caplets

GENUINE BAYER PROFESSIONAL LABELING (ASPIRIN REGIMEN BAYER)
(Aspirin) .... ■608
May interact with oral anticoagulants, oral hypoglycemic agents, and certain other agents. Compounds in these categories include:

Acarbose (Concurrent use should be avoided unless directed by a doctor). Products include:
Precose Tablets 906

Aluminum Carbonate (Co-administration of nonabsorbable antacids may alter the rate of absorption of aspirin, thereby resulting in a decreased acetylsalicylic acid/salicylate ratio in plasma; clinical significance of this interaction is unknown).
No products indexed under this heading.

Aluminum Hydroxide (Co-administration of nonabsorbable antacids may alter the rate of absorption of aspirin, thereby resulting in a decreased acetylsalicylic acid/salicylate ratio in plasma; clinical significance of this interaction is unknown). Products include:
Amphojel Suspension (Mint Flavor) .... ■789
Gaviscon Extra Strength Liquid .... ■751
Gaviscon Extra Strength Tablets .... ■751
Gaviscon Regular Strength Liquid .... ■751
Gaviscon Regular Strength Tablets .... ■750
Maalox Antacid/Anti-Gas Oral Suspension .... ■673
Maalox Max Maximum Strength Antacid/Anti-Gas Liquid 2300
Maalox Regular Strength Antacid/Antigas Liquid 2300
Mylanta 1813
Vanquish Caplets .... ■617

Antiarthritic Drugs, unspecified (Concurrent use should be avoided unless directed by a doctor).

Chlorpropamide (Concurrent use should be avoided unless directed by a doctor). Products include:
Diabinese Tablets 2680

Dicumarol (Concurrent use should be avoided unless directed by a doctor).
No products indexed under this heading.

Glimepiride (Concurrent use should be avoided unless directed by a doctor). Products include:
Amaryl Tablets 717

Glipizide (Concurrent use should be avoided unless directed by a doctor). Products include:
Glucotrol Tablets 2692
Glucotrol XL Extended Release Tablets 2693

Glyburide (Concurrent use should be avoided unless directed by a doctor). Products include:
DiaBeta Tablets 741
Glucovance Tablets 1086

Magnesium Hydroxide (Co-administration of nonabsorbable antacids may alter the rate of absorption of aspirin, thereby resulting in a decreased acetylsalicylic acid/salicylate ratio in plasma; clinical significance of this interaction is unknown). Products include:
Ex•Lax Milk of Magnesia Liquid .... ■670
Maalox Antacid/Anti-Gas Oral Suspension .... ■673
Maalox Max Maximum Strength Antacid/Anti-Gas Liquid 2300
Maalox Regular Strength Antacid/Antigas Liquid 2300
Mylanta Fast-Acting 1813
Mylanta 1813
Pepcid Complete Chewable Tablets 1815
Phillips' Chewable Tablets .... ■615
Phillips' Milk of Magnesia Liquid (Original, Cherry, & Mint) .... ■616
Rolaids Tablets .... ■706
Extra Strength Rolaids Tablets .... ■706
Vanquish Caplets .... ■617

Magnesium Oxide (Co-administration of nonabsorbable antacids may alter the rate of absorption of aspirin, thereby resulting in a decreased acetylsalicylic acid/salicylate ratio in plasma; clinical significance of this interaction is unknown). Products include:
Beelith Tablets 946
Mag-Ox 400 Tablets 1024
Uro-Mag Capsules 1024

Metformin Hydrochloride (Concurrent use should be avoided unless directed by a doctor). Products include:
Glucophage Tablets 1080
Glucophage XR Tablets 1080
Glucovance Tablets 1086

Miglitol (Concurrent use should be avoided unless directed by a doctor). Products include:
Glyset Tablets 2821

Pioglitazone Hydrochloride (Concurrent use should be avoided unless directed by a doctor). Products include:
Actos Tablets 3275

Probenecid (Concurrent use with gout medications should be avoided unless directed by a doctor).
No products indexed under this heading.

Repaglinide (Concurrent use should be avoided unless directed by a doctor). Products include:
Prandin Tablets (0.5, 1, and 2 mg) 2432

Rosiglitazone Maleate (Concurrent use should be avoided unless directed by a doctor). Products include:
Avandia Tablets 1490

Sodium Bicarbonate (Co-administration of absorbable antacids at therapeutic doses may increase the clearance of salicylates in some individuals; clinical significance of this interaction is unknown). Products include:
Alka-Seltzer .... ■603
Alka-Seltzer Lemon Lime Antacid and Pain Reliever Effervescent Tablets .... ■603
Alka-Seltzer Extra Strength Antacid and Pain Reliever Effervescent Tablets .... ■603
Alka-Seltzer Heartburn Relief Tablets .... ■604
Ceo-Two Evacuant Suppository .... ■618
Colyte with Flavor Packs for Oral Solution 3170
GoLYTELY and Pineapple Flavor GoLYTELY for Oral Solution 1068
NuLYTELY, Cherry Flavor, Lemon-Lime Flavor, and Orange Flavor NuLYTELY for Oral Solution 1068

Sulfinpyrazone (Concurrent use with gout medications should be avoided unless directed by a doctor).
No products indexed under this heading.

Tolazamide (Concurrent use should be avoided unless directed by a doctor).
No products indexed under this heading.

Tolbutamide (Concurrent use should be avoided unless directed by a doctor).
No products indexed under this heading.

Troglitazone (Concurrent use should be avoided unless directed by a doctor).
No products indexed under this heading.

Warfarin Sodium (Concurrent use should be avoided unless directed by a doctor). Products include:
Coumadin for Injection 1243
Coumadin Tablets 1243
Warfarin Sodium Tablets, USP 3302

EXTRA STRENGTH BAYER ARTHRITIS CAPLETS
(Aspirin) .... ■610
See Extra Strength Bayer Plus Caplets

EXTRA STRENGTH BAYER PLUS CAPLETS
(Aspirin, Calcium Carbonate) .... ■610
May interact with oral anticoagulants, oral hypoglycemic agents, and certain other agents. Compounds in these categories include:

Acarbose (Concurrent use should be avoided unless directed by a doctor). Products include:
Precose Tablets 906

Antiarthritic Drugs, unspecified (Concurrent use should be avoided unless directed by a doctor).

Chlorpropamide (Concurrent use should be avoided unless directed by a doctor). Products include:
Diabinese Tablets 2680

Dicumarol (Concurrent use should be avoided unless directed by a doctor).
No products indexed under this heading.

Glimepiride (Concurrent use should be avoided unless directed by a doctor). Products include:
Amaryl Tablets 717

Glipizide (Concurrent use should be avoided unless directed by a doctor). Products include:
Glucotrol Tablets 2692
Glucotrol XL Extended Release Tablets 2693

Glyburide (Concurrent use should be avoided unless directed by a doctor). Products include:
DiaBeta Tablets 741
Glucovance Tablets 1086

Metformin Hydrochloride (Concurrent use should be avoided unless directed by a doctor). Products include:
Glucophage Tablets 1080
Glucophage XR Tablets 1080
Glucovance Tablets 1086

Miglitol (Concurrent use should be avoided unless directed by a doctor). Products include:
Glyset Tablets 2821

Pioglitazone Hydrochloride (Concurrent use should be avoided unless directed by a doctor). Products include:
Actos Tablets 3275

Probenecid (Concurrent use with gout medications should be avoided unless directed by a doctor).
No products indexed under this heading.

Repaglinide (Concurrent use should be avoided unless directed by a doctor). Products include:
Prandin Tablets (0.5, 1, and 2 mg) 2432

Rosiglitazone Maleate (Concurrent use should be avoided unless directed by a doctor). Products include:

Avandia Tablets 1490

Sulfinpyrazone (Concurrent use with gout medications should be avoided unless directed by a doctor).
No products indexed under this heading.

Tolazamide (Concurrent use should be avoided unless directed by a doctor).
No products indexed under this heading.

Tolbutamide (Concurrent use should be avoided unless directed by a doctor).
No products indexed under this heading.

Troglitazone (Concurrent use should be avoided unless directed by a doctor).
No products indexed under this heading.

Warfarin Sodium (Concurrent use should be avoided unless directed by a doctor). Products include:
Coumadin for Injection 1243
Coumadin Tablets 1243
Warfarin Sodium Tablets, USP 3302

Food Interactions

Alcohol (Chronic heavy alcohol users, 3 or more drinks per day, should consult their physicians for advice on when and how they should take pain relievers/ fever reducers including aspirin).

EXTRA STRENGTH BAYER PM CAPLETS

(Aspirin, Diphenhydramine Hydrochloride) .... ■ 611

May interact with oral anticoagulants, oral hypoglycemic agents, hypnotics and sedatives, tranquilizers, and certain other agents. Compounds in these categories include:

Acarbose (Concurrent use should be avoided unless directed by a doctor). Products include:
Precose Tablets 906

Alprazolam (Concurrent use not recommended). Products include:
Xanax Tablets 2865

Antiarthritic Drugs, unspecified (Concurrent use with arthritis medications should be avoided unless directed by a doctor).

Buspirone Hydrochloride (Concurrent use not recommended).
No products indexed under this heading.

Chlordiazepoxide (Concurrent use not recommended). Products include:
Limbitrol 1738

Chlordiazepoxide Hydrochloride (Concurrent use not recommended). Products include:
Librium Capsules 1736
Librium for Injection 1737

Chlorpromazine (Concurrent use not recommended). Products include:
Thorazine Suppositories 1656

Chlorpromazine Hydrochloride (Concurrent use not recommended). Products include:
Thorazine 1656

Chlorpropamide (Concurrent use should be avoided unless directed by a doctor). Products include:
Diabinese Tablets 2680

Chlorprothixene (Concurrent use not recommended).
No products indexed under this heading.

Chlorprothixene Hydrochloride (Concurrent use not recommended).
No products indexed under this heading.

Clorazepate Dipotassium (Concurrent use not recommended). Products include:
Tranxene 511

Diazepam (Concurrent use not recommended). Products include:
Valium Injectable 3026
Valium Tablets 3047

Dicumarol (Concurrent use should be avoided unless directed by a doctor).
No products indexed under this heading.

Droperidol (Concurrent use not recommended).
No products indexed under this heading.

Estazolam (Concurrent use not recommended). Products include:
ProSom Tablets 500

Ethchlorvynol (Concurrent use not recommended).
No products indexed under this heading.

Ethinamate (Concurrent use not recommended).
No products indexed under this heading.

Fluphenazine Decanoate (Concurrent use not recommended).
No products indexed under this heading.

Fluphenazine Enanthate (Concurrent use not recommended).
No products indexed under this heading.

Fluphenazine Hydrochloride (Concurrent use not recommended).
No products indexed under this heading.

Flurazepam Hydrochloride (Concurrent use not recommended).
No products indexed under this heading.

Glimepiride (Concurrent use should be avoided unless directed by a doctor). Products include:
Amaryl Tablets 717

Glipizide (Concurrent use should be avoided unless directed by a doctor). Products include:
Glucotrol Tablets 2692
Glucotrol XL Extended Release Tablets 2693

Glutethimide (Concurrent use not recommended).
No products indexed under this heading.

Glyburide (Concurrent use should be avoided unless directed by a doctor). Products include:
DiaBeta Tablets 741
Glucovance Tablets 1086

Haloperidol (Concurrent use not recommended). Products include:
Haldol Injection, Tablets and Concentrate 2533

Haloperidol Decanoate (Concurrent use not recommended). Products include:
Haldol Decanoate 2535

Hydroxyzine Hydrochloride (Concurrent use not recommended). Products include:
Atarax Tablets & Syrup 2667
Vistaril Intramuscular Solution 2738

Lorazepam (Concurrent use not recommended). Products include:
Ativan Injection 3478
Ativan Tablets 3482

Loxapine Hydrochloride (Concurrent use not recommended).
No products indexed under this heading.

Loxapine Succinate (Concurrent use not recommended). Products include:
Loxitane Capsules 3398

Meprobamate (Concurrent use not recommended). Products include:
Miltown Tablets 3349

Mesoridazine Besylate (Concurrent use not recommended). Products include:
Serentil 1057

Metformin Hydrochloride (Concurrent use should be avoided unless directed by a doctor). Products include:
Glucophage Tablets 1080
Glucophage XR Tablets 1080
Glucovance Tablets 1086

Midazolam Hydrochloride (Concurrent use not recommended). Products include:
Versed Injection 3027
Versed Syrup 3033

Miglitol (Concurrent use should be avoided unless directed by a doctor). Products include:
Glyset Tablets 2821

Molindone Hydrochloride (Concurrent use not recommended). Products include:
Moban 1320

Oxazepam (Concurrent use not recommended).
No products indexed under this heading.

Perphenazine (Concurrent use not recommended). Products include:
Etrafon 3115
Trilafon 3160

Pioglitazone Hydrochloride (Concurrent use should be avoided unless directed by a doctor). Products include:
Actos Tablets 3275

Prazepam (Concurrent use not recommended).
No products indexed under this heading.

Probenecid (Concurrent use with gout medications should be avoided unless directed by a doctor).
No products indexed under this heading.

Prochlorperazine (Concurrent use not recommended). Products include:
Compazine 1505

Promethazine Hydrochloride (Concurrent use not recommended). Products include:
Mepergan Injection 3539
Phenergan Injection 3553
Phenergan 3556
Phenergan Syrup 3554
Phenergan with Codeine Syrup 3557
Phenergan with Dextromethorphan Syrup 3559
Phenergan VC Syrup 3560
Phenergan VC with Codeine Syrup . 3561

Propofol (Concurrent use not recommended). Products include:
Diprivan Injectable Emulsion 667

Quazepam (Concurrent use not recommended).
No products indexed under this heading.

Repaglinide (Concurrent use should be avoided unless directed by a doctor). Products include:
Prandin Tablets (0.5, 1, and 2 mg) 2432

Rosiglitazone Maleate (Concurrent use should be avoided unless directed by a doctor). Products include:
Avandia Tablets 1490

Secobarbital Sodium (Concurrent use not recommended).
No products indexed under this heading.

Sulfinpyrazone (Concurrent use with gout medications should be avoided unless directed by a doctor).
No products indexed under this heading.

Temazepam (Concurrent use not recommended).
No products indexed under this heading.

Thioridazine Hydrochloride (Concurrent use not recommended). Products include:
Thioridazine Hydrochloride Tablets 2289

Thiothixene (Concurrent use not recommended). Products include:
Navane Capsules 2701
Thiothixene Capsules 2290

Tolazamide (Concurrent use should be avoided unless directed by a doctor).
No products indexed under this heading.

Tolbutamide (Concurrent use should be avoided unless directed by a doctor).
No products indexed under this heading.

Triazolam (Concurrent use not recommended). Products include:
Halcion Tablets 2823

Trifluoperazine Hydrochloride (Concurrent use not recommended). Products include:
Stelazine 1640

Troglitazone (Concurrent use should be avoided unless directed by a doctor).
No products indexed under this heading.

Warfarin Sodium (Concurrent use should be avoided unless directed by a doctor). Products include:
Coumadin for Injection 1243
Coumadin Tablets 1243
Warfarin Sodium Tablets, USP 3302

Zaleplon (Concurrent use not recommended). Products include:
Sonata Capsules 3591

Zolpidem Tartrate (Concurrent use not recommended). Products include:
Ambien Tablets 3191

Food Interactions

Alcohol (Chronic heavy alcohol users, 3 or more drinks per day, should consult their physicians for advice on when and how they should take pain relievers/ fever reducers including aspirin).

BAYGAM

(Globulin, Immune (Human)) 914
None cited in PDR database.

BAYHEP B

(Hepatitis B Immune Globulin (Human)) 915
May interact with:

Vaccines (Live) (May interfere with response. Use should be deferred for 3 months after administration of HyperHep).
No products indexed under this heading.

BAYRAB

(Rabies Immune Globulin (Human)) 917
May interact with:

Measles, Mumps & Rubella Virus Vaccine, Live (Interference with the response to live viral vaccines). Products include:
M-M-R II 2118

Measles & Rubella Virus Vaccine Live (Interference with the response to live viral vaccines).
No products indexed under this heading.

Measles Virus Vaccine Live (Interference with the response to live viral vaccines). Products include:
Attenuvax 2044

Mumps Virus Vaccine, Live (Interference with the response to live viral vaccines). Products include:
Mumpsvax 2141

Poliovirus Vaccine, Live, Oral, Trivalent, Types 1,2,3 (Sabin) (Interference with the response to live viral vaccines).
No products indexed under this heading.

Rubella & Mumps Virus Vaccine Live (Interference with the response to live viral vaccines).
No products indexed under this heading.

Rubella Virus Vaccine Live (Interference with the response to live viral vaccines). Products include:
Meruvax II 2130

BAYRHO-D FULL DOSE
(Rh_o (D) Immune Globulin (Human)) ... 921
May interact with:

Measles, Mumps & Rubella Virus Vaccine, Live (Interference with response to live vaccines). Products include:
M-M-R II 2118

Measles & Rubella Virus Vaccine Live (Interference with response to live vaccines).
No products indexed under this heading.

Measles Virus Vaccine Live (Interference with response to live vaccines). Products include:
Attenuvax 2044

Rubella & Mumps Virus Vaccine Live (Interference with response to live vaccines).
No products indexed under this heading.

Rubella Virus Vaccine Live (Interference with response to live vaccines). Products include:
Meruvax II 2130

BAYRHO-D MINI-DOSE
(Rh_o (D) Immune Globulin (Human)) ... 919
See BayRho-D Full Dose

BAYTET
(Tetanus Immune Globulin (Human)) 923
May interact with:

Vaccines (Live) (May interfere with response. Use should be deferred for 3 months).
No products indexed under this heading.

BC POWDER
(Aspirin, Caffeine, Salicylamide) ...... ▣619
See BC Allergy Sinus Cold Powder

BC ALLERGY SINUS COLD POWDER
(Aspirin, Chlorpheniramine Maleate, Pseudoephedrine Hydrochloride).............................. ▣619
May interact with monoamine oxidase inhibitors and certain other agents. Compounds in these categories include:

Isocarboxazid (Concurrent use with MAO inhibitors is not recommended; consult your doctor).
No products indexed under this heading.

Moclobemide (Concurrent use with MAO inhibitors is not recommended; consult your doctor).
No products indexed under this heading.

Pargyline Hydrochloride (Concurrent use with MAO inhibitors is not recommended; consult your doctor).
No products indexed under this heading.

Phenelzine Sulfate (Concurrent use with MAO inhibitors is not recommended; consult your doctor). Products include:
Nardil Tablets 2653

Procarbazine Hydrochloride (Concurrent use with MAO inhibitors is not recommended; consult your doctor). Products include:
Matulane Capsules 3246

Selegiline Hydrochloride (Concurrent use with MAO inhibitors is not recommended; consult your doctor). Products include:
Eldepryl Capsules 3266

Tranylcypromine Sulfate (Concurrent use with MAO inhibitors is not recommended; consult your doctor). Products include:
Parnate Tablets 1607

Food Interactions

Alcohol (Individuals consuming 3 or more alcohol-containing drinks per day should consult their physician for advice on when and how they should take this product; increases drowsiness; avoid concurrent use).

ARTHRITIS STRENGTH BC POWDER
(Aspirin, Caffeine, Salicylamide) ...... ▣619
See BC Allergy Sinus Cold Powder

BC SINUS COLD POWDER
(Aspirin, Pseudoephedrine Hydrochloride).............................. ▣619
See BC Allergy Sinus Cold Powder

BEANO LIQUID
(Alpha Galactosidase Enzyme) .... ▣809
None cited in PDR database.

BEANO TABLETS
(Alpha Galactosidase Enzyme) .... ▣809
None cited in PDR database.

BEBULIN VH
(Factor IX Complex) 840
None cited in PDR database.

BECONASE INHALATION AEROSOL
(Beclomethasone Dipropionate) 1497
None cited in PDR database.

BECONASE AQ NASAL SPRAY
(Beclomethasone Dipropionate Monohydrate) 1498
None cited in PDR database.

BEELITH TABLETS
(Magnesium Oxide, Vitamin B_6) 946
May interact with:

Prescription Drugs, unspecified (Concurrent use should be avoided).

BENADRYL ALLERGY CHEWABLES
(Diphenhydramine Hydrochloride) .... ▣689
See Benadryl Allergy Kapseal Capsules

BENADRYL ALLERGY KAPSEAL CAPSULES
(Diphenhydramine Hydrochloride) .... ▣691
May interact with hypnotics and sedatives, tranquilizers, and certain other agents. Compounds in these categories include:

Alprazolam (May increase drowsiness effect). Products include:
Xanax Tablets 2865

Buspirone Hydrochloride (May increase drowsiness effect).
No products indexed under this heading.

Chlordiazepoxide (May increase drowsiness effect). Products include:
Limbitrol 1738

Chlordiazepoxide Hydrochloride (May increase drowsiness effect). Products include:
Librium Capsules 1736
Librium for Injection 1737

Chlorpromazine (May increase drowsiness effect). Products include:
Thorazine Suppositories 1656

Chlorpromazine Hydrochloride (May increase drowsiness effect). Products include:
Thorazine 1656

Chlorprothixene (May increase drowsiness effect).
No products indexed under this heading.

Chlorprothixene Hydrochloride (May increase drowsiness effect).
No products indexed under this heading.

Clorazepate Dipotassium (May increase drowsiness effect). Products include:
Tranxene 511

Diazepam (May increase drowsiness effect). Products include:
Valium Injectable 3026
Valium Tablets 3047

Droperidol (May increase drowsiness effect).
No products indexed under this heading.

Estazolam (May increase drowsiness effect). Products include:
ProSom Tablets 500

Ethchlorvynol (May increase drowsiness effect).
No products indexed under this heading.

Ethinamate (May increase drowsiness effect).
No products indexed under this heading.

Fluphenazine Decanoate (May increase drowsiness effect).
No products indexed under this heading.

Fluphenazine Enanthate (May increase drowsiness effect).
No products indexed under this heading.

Fluphenazine Hydrochloride (May increase drowsiness effect).
No products indexed under this heading.

Flurazepam Hydrochloride (May increase drowsiness effect).
No products indexed under this heading.

Glutethimide (May increase drowsiness effect).
No products indexed under this heading.

Haloperidol (May increase drowsiness effect). Products include:
Haldol Injection, Tablets and Concentrate 2533

Haloperidol Decanoate (May increase drowsiness effect). Products include:
Haldol Decanoate 2535

Hydroxyzine Hydrochloride (May increase drowsiness effect). Products include:
Atarax Tablets & Syrup 2667
Vistaril Intramuscular Solution 2738

Lorazepam (May increase drowsiness effect). Products include:
Ativan Injection 3478
Ativan Tablets 3482

Loxapine Hydrochloride (May increase drowsiness effect).
No products indexed under this heading.

Loxapine Succinate (May increase drowsiness effect). Products include:
Loxitane Capsules 3398

Meprobamate (May increase drowsiness effect). Products include:
Miltown Tablets 3349

Mesoridazine Besylate (May increase drowsiness effect). Products include:
Serentil 1057

Midazolam Hydrochloride (May increase drowsiness effect). Products include:
Versed Injection 3027
Versed Syrup 3033

Molindone Hydrochloride (May increase drowsiness effect). Products include:
Moban 1320

Oxazepam (May increase drowsiness effect).
No products indexed under this heading.

Perphenazine (May increase drowsiness effect). Products include:
Etrafon 3115
Trilafon 3160

Prazepam (May increase drowsiness effect).
No products indexed under this heading.

Prochlorperazine (May increase drowsiness effect). Products include:
Compazine 1505

Promethazine Hydrochloride (May increase drowsiness effect). Products include:
Mepergan Injection 3539
Phenergan Injection 3553
Phenergan 3556
Phenergan Syrup 3554
Phenergan with Codeine Syrup 3557
Phenergan with Dextromethorphan Syrup 3559
Phenergan VC Syrup 3560
Phenergan VC with Codeine Syrup . 3561

Propofol (May increase drowsiness effect). Products include:
Diprivan Injectable Emulsion 667

Quazepam (May increase drowsiness effect).
No products indexed under this heading.

Secobarbital Sodium (May increase drowsiness effect).
No products indexed under this heading.

Temazepam (May increase drowsiness effect).
No products indexed under this heading.

Thioridazine Hydrochloride (May increase drowsiness effect). Products include:
Thioridazine Hydrochloride Tablets 2289

Thiothixene (May increase drowsiness effect). Products include:
Navane Capsules 2701
Thiothixene Capsules 2290

Triazolam (May increase drowsiness effect). Products include:
Halcion Tablets 2823

Trifluoperazine Hydrochloride (May increase drowsiness effect). Products include:
Stelazine 1640

Zaleplon (May increase drowsiness effect). Products include:
Sonata Capsules 3591

Zolpidem Tartrate (May increase drowsiness effect). Products include:
Ambien Tablets 3191

Food Interactions

Alcohol (May increase drowsiness effect).

BENADRYL ALLERGY LIQUID
(Diphenhydramine Hydrochloride) .... ▣690
See Benadryl Allergy Kapseal Capsules

BENADRYL ALLERGY ULTRATAB TABLETS
(Diphenhydramine Hydrochloride) .... ▣691
See Benadryl Allergy Kapseal Capsules

BENADRYL ALLERGY/ COLD TABLETS
(Acetaminophen, Diphenhydramine Hydrochloride, Pseudoephedrine Hydrochloride) ...... ▣691
May interact with hypnotics and sedatives, monoamine oxidase inhibitors, tranquilizers, and certain other agents. Compounds in these categories include:

Alprazolam (May increase drowsiness effect). Products include:
Xanax Tablets 2865

Buspirone Hydrochloride (May increase drowsiness effect).
No products indexed under this heading.

IMPORTANT NOTE: Always consult each drug listing in the patient's regimen for possible interactions.

Chlordiazepoxide (May increase drowsiness effect). Products include:
Limbitrol 1738

Chlordiazepoxide Hydrochloride (May increase drowsiness effect). Products include:
Librium Capsules 1736
Librium for Injection 1737

Chlorpromazine (May increase drowsiness effect). Products include:
Thorazine Suppositories 1656

Chlorpromazine Hydrochloride (May increase drowsiness effect). Products include:
Thorazine 1656

Chlorprothixene (May increase drowsiness effect).
No products indexed under this heading.

Chlorprothixene Hydrochloride (May increase drowsiness effect).
No products indexed under this heading.

Clorazepate Dipotassium (May increase drowsiness effect). Products include:
Tranxene 511

Diazepam (May increase drowsiness effect). Products include:
Valium Injectable 3026
Valium Tablets 3047

Droperidol (May increase drowsiness effect).
No products indexed under this heading.

Estazolam (May increase drowsiness effect). Products include:
ProSom Tablets 500

Ethchlorvynol (May increase drowsiness effect).
No products indexed under this heading.

Ethinamate (May increase drowsiness effect).
No products indexed under this heading.

Fluphenazine Decanoate (May increase drowsiness effect).
No products indexed under this heading.

Fluphenazine Enanthate (May increase drowsiness effect).
No products indexed under this heading.

Fluphenazine Hydrochloride (May increase drowsiness effect).
No products indexed under this heading.

Flurazepam Hydrochloride (May increase drowsiness effect).
No products indexed under this heading.

Glutethimide (May increase drowsiness effect).
No products indexed under this heading.

Haloperidol (May increase drowsiness effect). Products include:
Haldol Injection, Tablets and Concentrate 2533

Haloperidol Decanoate (May increase drowsiness effect). Products include:
Haldol Decanoate 2535

Hydroxyzine Hydrochloride (May increase drowsiness effect). Products include:
Atarax Tablets & Syrup 2667
Vistaril Intramuscular Solution 2738

Isocarboxazid (Concurrent and/or sequential use is not recommended).
No products indexed under this heading.

Lorazepam (May increase drowsiness effect). Products include:
Ativan Injection 3478
Ativan Tablets 3482

Loxapine Hydrochloride (May increase drowsiness effect).
No products indexed under this heading.

Loxapine Succinate (May increase drowsiness effect). Products include:
Loxitane Capsules 3398

Meprobamate (May increase drowsiness effect). Products include:
Miltown Tablets 3349

Mesoridazine Besylate (May increase drowsiness effect). Products include:
Serentil 1057

Midazolam Hydrochloride (May increase drowsiness effect). Products include:
Versed Injection 3027
Versed Syrup 3033

Moclobemide (Concurrent and/or sequential use is not recommended).
No products indexed under this heading.

Molindone Hydrochloride (May increase drowsiness effect). Products include:
Moban 1320

Oxazepam (May increase drowsiness effect).
No products indexed under this heading.

Pargyline Hydrochloride (Concurrent and/or sequential use is not recommended).
No products indexed under this heading.

Perphenazine (May increase drowsiness effect). Products include:
Etrafon 3115
Trilafon 3160

Phenelzine Sulfate (Concurrent and/or sequential use is not recommended). Products include:
Nardil Tablets 2653

Prazepam (May increase drowsiness effect).
No products indexed under this heading.

Procarbazine Hydrochloride (Concurrent and/or sequential use is not recommended). Products include:
Matulane Capsules 3246

Prochlorperazine (May increase drowsiness effect). Products include:
Compazine 1505

Promethazine Hydrochloride (May increase drowsiness effect). Products include:
Mepergan Injection 3539
Phenergan Injection 3553
Phenergan 3556
Phenergan Syrup 3554
Phenergan with Codeine Syrup 3557
Phenergan with Dextromethorphan Syrup 3559
Phenergan VC Syrup 3560
Phenergan VC with Codeine Syrup 3561

Propofol (May increase drowsiness effect). Products include:
Diprivan Injectable Emulsion 667

Quazepam (May increase drowsiness effect).
No products indexed under this heading.

Secobarbital Sodium (May increase drowsiness effect).
No products indexed under this heading.

Selegiline Hydrochloride (Concurrent and/or sequential use is not recommended). Products include:
Eldepryl Capsules 3266

Temazepam (May increase drowsiness effect).
No products indexed under this heading.

Thioridazine Hydrochloride (May increase drowsiness effect). Products include:
Thioridazine Hydrochloride Tablets 2289

Thiothixene (May increase drowsiness effect). Products include:
Navane Capsules 2701
Thiothixene Capsules 2290

Tranylcypromine Sulfate (Concurrent and/or sequential use is not recommended). Products include:
Parnate Tablets 1607

Triazolam (May increase drowsiness effect). Products include:
Halcion Tablets 2823

Trifluoperazine Hydrochloride (May increase drowsiness effect). Products include:
Stelazine 1640

Zaleplon (May increase drowsiness effect). Products include:
Sonata Capsules 3591

Zolpidem Tartrate (May increase drowsiness effect). Products include:
Ambien Tablets 3191

Food Interactions

Alcohol (May increase drowsiness effect).

BENADRYL ALLERGY/CONGESTION TABLETS
(Diphenhydramine Hydrochloride, Pseudoephedrine Hydrochloride) .... ▣692
May interact with hypnotics and sedatives, monoamine oxidase inhibitors, tranquilizers, and certain other agents. Compounds in these categories include:

Alprazolam (May increase the drowsiness effect). Products include:
Xanax Tablets 2865

Buspirone Hydrochloride (May increase the drowsiness effect).
No products indexed under this heading.

Chlordiazepoxide (May increase the drowsiness effect). Products include:
Limbitrol 1738

Chlordiazepoxide Hydrochloride (May increase the drowsiness effect). Products include:
Librium Capsules 1736
Librium for Injection 1737

Chlorpromazine (May increase the drowsiness effect). Products include:
Thorazine Suppositories 1656

Chlorpromazine Hydrochloride (May increase the drowsiness effect). Products include:
Thorazine 1656

Chlorprothixene (May increase the drowsiness effect).
No products indexed under this heading.

Chlorprothixene Hydrochloride (May increase the drowsiness effect).
No products indexed under this heading.

Clorazepate Dipotassium (May increase the drowsiness effect). Products include:
Tranxene 511

Diazepam (May increase the drowsiness effect). Products include:
Valium Injectable 3026
Valium Tablets 3047

Droperidol (May increase the drowsiness effect).
No products indexed under this heading.

Estazolam (May increase the drowsiness effect). Products include:
ProSom Tablets 500

Ethchlorvynol (May increase the drowsiness effect).
No products indexed under this heading.

Ethinamate (May increase the drowsiness effect).
No products indexed under this heading.

Fluphenazine Decanoate (May increase the drowsiness effect).
No products indexed under this heading.

Fluphenazine Enanthate (May increase the drowsiness effect).
No products indexed under this heading.

Fluphenazine Hydrochloride (May increase the drowsiness effect).
No products indexed under this heading.

Flurazepam Hydrochloride (May increase the drowsiness effect).
No products indexed under this heading.

Glutethimide (May increase the drowsiness effect).
No products indexed under this heading.

Haloperidol (May increase the drowsiness effect). Products include:
Haldol Injection, Tablets and Concentrate 2533

Haloperidol Decanoate (May increase the drowsiness effect). Products include:
Haldol Decanoate 2535

Hydroxyzine Hydrochloride (May increase the drowsiness effect). Products include:
Atarax Tablets & Syrup 2667
Vistaril Intramuscular Solution 2738

Isocarboxazid (Concurrent and/or sequential use is not recommended).
No products indexed under this heading.

Lorazepam (May increase the drowsiness effect). Products include:
Ativan Injection 3478
Ativan Tablets 3482

Loxapine Hydrochloride (May increase the drowsiness effect).
No products indexed under this heading.

Loxapine Succinate (May increase the drowsiness effect). Products include:
Loxitane Capsules 3398

Meprobamate (May increase the drowsiness effect). Products include:
Miltown Tablets 3349

Mesoridazine Besylate (May increase the drowsiness effect). Products include:
Serentil 1057

Midazolam Hydrochloride (May increase the drowsiness effect). Products include:
Versed Injection 3027
Versed Syrup 3033

Moclobemide (Concurrent and/or sequential use is not recommended).
No products indexed under this heading.

Molindone Hydrochloride (May increase the drowsiness effect). Products include:
Moban 1320

Oxazepam (May increase the drowsiness effect).
No products indexed under this heading.

Pargyline Hydrochloride (Concurrent and/or sequential use is not recommended).
No products indexed under this heading.

Perphenazine (May increase the drowsiness effect). Products include:
Etrafon 3115
Trilafon 3160

Phenelzine Sulfate (Concurrent and/or sequential use is not recommended). Products include:
Nardil Tablets 2653

Prazepam (May increase the drowsiness effect).
No products indexed under this heading.

Procarbazine Hydrochloride (Concurrent and/or sequential use is not recommended). Products include:
Matulane Capsules 3246

Prochlorperazine (May increase the drowsiness effect). Products include:
Compazine 1505

Promethazine Hydrochloride (May increase the drowsiness effect). Products include:
Mepergan Injection 3539
Phenergan Injection 3553
Phenergan 3556
Phenergan Syrup 3554
Phenergan with Codeine Syrup 3557
Phenergan with Dextromethorphan Syrup 3559
Phenergan VC Syrup 3560
Phenergan VC with Codeine Syrup .. 3561

Propofol (May increase the drowsiness effect). Products include:
Diprivan Injectable Emulsion 667

Quazepam (May increase the drowsiness effect).
No products indexed under this heading.

Secobarbital Sodium (May increase the drowsiness effect).
No products indexed under this heading.

Selegiline Hydrochloride (Concurrent and/or sequential use is not recommended). Products include:
Eldepryl Capsules 3266

Temazepam (May increase the drowsiness effect).
No products indexed under this heading.

Thioridazine Hydrochloride (May increase the drowsiness effect). Products include:
Thioridazine Hydrochloride Tablets 2289

Thiothixene (May increase the drowsiness effect). Products include:
Navane Capsules 2701
Thiothixene Capsules 2290

Tranylcypromine Sulfate (Concurrent and/or sequential use is not recommended). Products include:
Parnate Tablets 1607

Triazolam (May increase the drowsiness effect). Products include:
Halcion Tablets 2823

Trifluoperazine Hydrochloride (May increase the drowsiness effect). Products include:
Stelazine 1640

Zaleplon (May increase the drowsiness effect). Products include:
Sonata Capsules 3591

Zolpidem Tartrate (May increase the drowsiness effect). Products include:
Ambien Tablets 3191

Food Interactions

Alcohol (Increases the drowsiness effect; avoid concomitant use).

BENADRYL ALLERGY & SINUS LIQUID

(Diphenhydramine Hydrochloride, Pseudoephedrine Hydrochloride) 693
May interact with hypnotics and sedatives, monoamine oxidase inhibitors, tranquilizers, and certain other agents. Compounds in these categories include:

Alprazolam (May increase drowsiness effect; consult your physician). Products include:
Xanax Tablets 2865

Buspirone Hydrochloride (May increase drowsiness effect; consult your physician).
No products indexed under this heading.

Chlordiazepoxide (May increase drowsiness effect; consult your physician). Products include:
Limbitrol 1738

Chlordiazepoxide Hydrochloride (May increase drowsiness effect; consult your physician). Products include:
Librium Capsules 1736
Librium for Injection 1737

Chlorpromazine (May increase drowsiness effect; consult your physician). Products include:
Thorazine Suppositories 1656

Chlorpromazine Hydrochloride (May increase drowsiness effect; consult your physician). Products include:
Thorazine 1656

Chlorprothixene (May increase drowsiness effect; consult your physician).
No products indexed under this heading.

Chlorprothixene Hydrochloride (May increase drowsiness effect; consult your physician).
No products indexed under this heading.

Clorazepate Dipotassium (May increase drowsiness effect; consult your physician). Products include:
Tranxene 511

Diazepam (May increase drowsiness effect; consult your physician). Products include:
Valium Injectable 3026
Valium Tablets 3047

Droperidol (May increase drowsiness effect; consult your physician).
No products indexed under this heading.

Estazolam (May increase drowsiness effect; consult your physician). Products include:
ProSom Tablets 500

Ethchlorvynol (May increase drowsiness effect; consult your physician).
No products indexed under this heading.

Ethinamate (May increase drowsiness effect; consult your physician).
No products indexed under this heading.

Fluphenazine Decanoate (May increase drowsiness effect; consult your physician).
No products indexed under this heading.

Fluphenazine Enanthate (May increase drowsiness effect; consult your physician).
No products indexed under this heading.

Fluphenazine Hydrochloride (May increase drowsiness effect; consult your physician).
No products indexed under this heading.

Flurazepam Hydrochloride (May increase drowsiness effect; consult your physician).
No products indexed under this heading.

Glutethimide (May increase drowsiness effect; consult your physician).
No products indexed under this heading.

Haloperidol (May increase drowsiness effect; consult your physician). Products include:
Haldol Injection, Tablets and Concentrate 2533

Haloperidol Decanoate (May increase drowsiness effect; consult your physician). Products include:
Haldol Decanoate 2535

Hydroxyzine Hydrochloride (May increase drowsiness effect; consult your physician). Products include:
Atarax Tablets & Syrup 2667
Vistaril Intramuscular Solution 2738

Isocarboxazid (Concurrent and/or sequential use is not recommended).
No products indexed under this heading.

Lorazepam (May increase drowsiness effect; consult your physician). Products include:
Ativan Injection 3478
Ativan Tablets 3482

Loxapine Hydrochloride (May increase drowsiness effect; consult your physician).
No products indexed under this heading.

Loxapine Succinate (May increase drowsiness effect; consult your physician). Products include:
Loxitane Capsules 3398

Meprobamate (May increase drowsiness effect; consult your physician). Products include:
Miltown Tablets 3349

Mesoridazine Besylate (May increase drowsiness effect; consult your physician). Products include:
Serentil 1057

Midazolam Hydrochloride (May increase drowsiness effect; consult your physician). Products include:
Versed Injection 3027
Versed Syrup 3033

Moclobemide (Concurrent and/or sequential use is not recomended).
No products indexed under this heading.

Molindone Hydrochloride (May increase drowsiness effect; consult your physician). Products include:
Moban 1320

Oxazepam (May increase drowsiness effect; consult your physician).
No products indexed under this heading.

Pargyline Hydrochloride (Concurrent and/or sequential use is not recommended).
No products indexed under this heading.

Perphenazine (May increase drowsiness effect; consult your physician). Products include:
Etrafon 3115
Trilafon 3160

Phenelzine Sulfate (Concurrent and/or sequential use is not recommended). Products include:
Nardil Tablets 2653

Prazepam (May increase drowsiness effect; consult your physician).
No products indexed under this heading.

Procarbazine Hydrochloride (Concurrent and/or sequential use is not recommended). Products include:
Matulane Capsules 3246

Prochlorperazine (May increase drowsiness effect; consult your physician). Products include:
Compazine 1505

Promethazine Hydrochloride (May increase drowsiness effect; consult your physician). Products include:
Mepergan Injection 3539
Phenergan Injection 3553
Phenergan 3556
Phenergan Syrup 3554
Phenergan with Codeine Syrup 3557
Phenergan with Dextromethorphan Syrup 3559
Phenergan VC Syrup 3560
Phenergan VC with Codeine Syrup . 3561

Propofol (May increase drowsiness effect; consult your physician). Products include:
Diprivan Injectable Emulsion 667

Quazepam (May increase drowsiness effect; consult your physician).
No products indexed under this heading.

Secobarbital Sodium (May increase drowsiness effect; consult your physician).
No products indexed under this heading.

Selegiline Hydrochloride (Concurrent and/or sequential use is not recommended). Products include:
Eldepryl Capsules 3266

Temazepam (May increase drowsiness effect; consult your physician).
No products indexed under this heading.

Thioridazine Hydrochloride (May increase drowsiness effect; consult your physician). Products include:
Thioridazine Hydrochloride Tablets 2289

Thiothixene (May increase drowsiness effect; consult your physician). Products include:
Navane Capsules 2701
Thiothixene Capsules 2290

Tranylcypromine Sulfate (Concurrent and/or sequential use is not recommended). Products include:
Parnate Tablets 1607

Triazolam (May increase drowsiness effect; consult your physician). Products include:
Halcion Tablets 2823

Trifluoperazine Hydrochloride (May increase drowsiness effect; consult your physician). Products include:
Stelazine 1640

Zaleplon (May increase drowsiness effect; consult your physician). Products include:
Sonata Capsules 3591

Zolpidem Tartrate (May increase drowsiness effect; consult your physician). Products include:
Ambien Tablets 3191

Food Interactions

Alcohol (May increase drowsiness effect; avoid concurrent use).

BENADRYL ALLERGY & SINUS FASTMELT TABLETS

(Diphenhydramine Citrate, Pseudoephedrine Hydrochloride) 693
See Benadryl Children's Allergy/Cold Fastmelt Tablets

BENADRYL ALLERGY SINUS HEADACHE CAPLETS & GELCAPS

(Acetaminophen, Diphenhydramine Hydrochloride, Pseudoephedrine Hydrochloride) 693
May interact with hypnotics and sedatives, monoamine oxidase inhibitors, tranquilizers, and certain other agents. Compounds in these categories include:

Alprazolam (May increase drowsiness effect). Products include:
Xanax Tablets 2865

Buspirone Hydrochloride (May increase drowsiness effect).
No products indexed under this heading.

Chlordiazepoxide (May increase drowsiness effect). Products include:
Limbitrol 1738

Chlordiazepoxide Hydrochloride (May increase drowsiness effect). Products include:
Librium Capsules 1736
Librium for Injection 1737

Chlorpromazine (May increase drowsiness effect). Products include:
Thorazine Suppositories 1656

Chlorpromazine Hydrochloride (May increase drowsiness effect). Products include:
Thorazine 1656

Chlorprothixene (May increase drowsiness effect).
No products indexed under this heading.

Chlorprothixene Hydrochloride (May increase drowsiness effect).
No products indexed under this heading.

Clorazepate Dipotassium (May increase drowsiness effect). Products include:
Tranxene 511

Diazepam (May increase drowsiness effect). Products include:
Valium Injectable 3026
Valium Tablets 3047

Droperidol (May increase drowsiness effect).
No products indexed under this heading.

Estazolam (May increase drowsiness effect). Products include:
ProSom Tablets 500

Ethchlorvynol (May increase drowsiness effect).
No products indexed under this heading.

Ethinamate (May increase drowsiness effect).
No products indexed under this heading.

Fluphenazine Decanoate (May increase drowsiness effect).
No products indexed under this heading.

Fluphenazine Enanthate (May increase drowsiness effect).
No products indexed under this heading.

Fluphenazine Hydrochloride (May increase drowsiness effect).
No products indexed under this heading.

Flurazepam Hydrochloride (May increase drowsiness effect).
No products indexed under this heading.

Glutethimide (May increase drowsiness effect).
No products indexed under this heading.

Haloperidol (May increase drowsiness effect). Products include:
Haldol Injection, Tablets and Concentrate 2533

Haloperidol Decanoate (May increase drowsiness effect). Products include:
Haldol Decanoate 2535

Hydroxyzine Hydrochloride (May increase drowsiness effect). Products include:
Atarax Tablets & Syrup 2667
Vistaril Intramuscular Solution 2738

Isocarboxazid (Concurrent and/or sequential use is not recommended).
No products indexed under this heading.

Lorazepam (May increase drowsiness effect). Products include:
Ativan Injection 3478
Ativan Tablets 3482

Loxapine Hydrochloride (May increase drowsiness effect).
No products indexed under this heading.

Loxapine Succinate (May increase drowsiness effect). Products include:
Loxitane Capsules 3398

Meprobamate (May increase drowsiness effect). Products include:
Miltown Tablets 3349

Mesoridazine Besylate (May increase drowsiness effect). Products include:
Serentil 1057

Midazolam Hydrochloride (May increase drowsiness effect). Products include:
Versed Injection 3027
Versed Syrup 3033

Moclobemide (Concurrent and/or sequential use is not recommended).
No products indexed under this heading.

Molindone Hydrochloride (May increase drowsiness effect). Products include:
Moban 1320

Oxazepam (May increase drowsiness effect).
No products indexed under this heading.

Pargyline Hydrochloride (Concurrent and/or sequential use is not recommended).
No products indexed under this heading.

Perphenazine (May increase drowsiness effect). Products include:
Etrafon 3115
Trilafon 3160

Phenelzine Sulfate (Concurrent and/or sequential use is not recommended). Products include:
Nardil Tablets 2653

Prazepam (May increase drowsiness effect).
No products indexed under this heading.

Procarbazine Hydrochloride (Concurrent and/or sequential use is not recommended). Products include:
Matulane Capsules 3246

Prochlorperazine (May increase drowsiness effect). Products include:
Compazine 1505

Promethazine Hydrochloride (May increase drowsiness effect). Products include:
Mepergan Injection 3539
Phenergan Injection 3553
Phenergan 3556
Phenergan Syrup 3554
Phenergan with Codeine Syrup 3557
Phenergan with Dextromethorphan Syrup 3559
Phenergan VC Syrup 3560
Phenergan VC with Codeine Syrup 3561

Propofol (May increase drowsiness effect). Products include:
Diprivan Injectable Emulsion 667

Quazepam (May increase drowsiness effect).
No products indexed under this heading.

Secobarbital Sodium (May increase drowsiness effect).
No products indexed under this heading.

Selegiline Hydrochloride (Concurrent and/or sequential use is not recommended). Products include:
Eldepryl Capsules 3266

Temazepam (May increase drowsiness effect).
No products indexed under this heading.

Thioridazine Hydrochloride (May increase drowsiness effect). Products include:
Thioridazine Hydrochloride Tablets 2289

Thiothixene (May increase drowsiness effect). Products include:
Navane Capsules 2701
Thiothixene Capsules 2290

Tranylcypromine Sulfate (Concurrent and/or sequential use is not recommended). Products include:
Parnate Tablets 1607

Triazolam (May increase drowsiness effect). Products include:
Halcion Tablets 2823

Trifluoperazine Hydrochloride (May increase drowsiness effect). Products include:
Stelazine 1640

Zaleplon (May increase drowsiness effect). Products include:
Sonata Capsules 3591

Zolpidem Tartrate (May increase drowsiness effect). Products include:
Ambien Tablets 3191

Food Interactions

Alcohol (May increase drowsiness effect).

BENADRYL SEVERE ALLERGY & SINUS HEADACHE CAPLETS

(Acetaminophen, Diphenhydramine Hydrochloride, Pseudoephedrine Hydrochloride) .... ■694
May interact with hypnotics and sedatives, monoamine oxidase inhibitors, tranquilizers, and certain other agents. Compounds in these categories include:

Alprazolam (May increase drowsiness). Products include:
Xanax Tablets 2865

Buspirone Hydrochloride (May increase drowsiness).
No products indexed under this heading.

Chlordiazepoxide (May increase drowsiness). Products include:
Limbitrol 1738

Chlordiazepoxide Hydrochloride (May increase drowsiness). Products include:
Librium Capsules 1736
Librium for Injection 1737

Chlorpromazine (May increase drowsiness). Products include:
Thorazine Suppositories 1656

Chlorpromazine Hydrochloride (May increase drowsiness). Products include:
Thorazine 1656

Chlorprothixene (May increase drowsiness).
No products indexed under this heading.

Chlorprothixene Hydrochloride (May increase drowsiness).
No products indexed under this heading.

Clorazepate Dipotassium (May increase drowsiness). Products include:
Tranxene 511

Diazepam (May increase drowsiness). Products include:
Valium Injectable 3026
Valium Tablets 3047

Droperidol (May increase drowsiness).
No products indexed under this heading.

Estazolam (May increase drowsiness). Products include:
ProSom Tablets 500

Ethchlorvynol (May increase drowsiness).
No products indexed under this heading.

Ethinamate (May increase drowsiness).
No products indexed under this heading.

Fluphenazine Decanoate (May increase drowsiness).
No products indexed under this heading.

Fluphenazine Enanthate (May increase drowsiness).
No products indexed under this heading.

Fluphenazine Hydrochloride (May increase drowsiness).
No products indexed under this heading.

Flurazepam Hydrochloride (May increase drowsiness).
No products indexed under this heading.

Glutethimide (May increase drowsiness).
No products indexed under this heading.

Haloperidol (May increase drowsiness). Products include:
Haldol Injection, Tablets and Concentrate 2533

Haloperidol Decanoate (May increase drowsiness). Products include:
Haldol Decanoate 2535

Hydroxyzine Hydrochloride (May increase drowsiness). Products include:
Atarax Tablets & Syrup 2667
Vistaril Intramuscular Solution 2738

Isocarboxazid (Concurrent and/or sequential use with MAO inhibitors is not recommended).
No products indexed under this heading.

Lorazepam (May increase drowsiness). Products include:
Ativan Injection 3478
Ativan Tablets 3482

Loxapine Hydrochloride (May increase drowsiness).
No products indexed under this heading.

Loxapine Succinate (May increase drowsiness). Products include:
Loxitane Capsules 3398

Meprobamate (May increase drowsiness). Products include:
Miltown Tablets 3349

Mesoridazine Besylate (May increase drowsiness). Products include:
Serentil 1057

Midazolam Hydrochloride (May increase drowsiness). Products include:
Versed Injection 3027
Versed Syrup 3033

Moclobemide (Concurrent and/or sequential use with MAO inhibitors is not recommended).
No products indexed under this heading.

Molindone Hydrochloride (May increase drowsiness). Products include:
Moban 1320

Oxazepam (May increase drowsiness).
No products indexed under this heading.

Pargyline Hydrochloride (Concurrent and/or sequential use with MAO inhibitors is not recommended).
No products indexed under this heading.

Perphenazine (May increase drowsiness). Products include:
Etrafon 3115
Trilafon 3160

Phenelzine Sulfate (Concurrent and/or sequential use with MAO inhibitors is not recommended). Products include:
Nardil Tablets 2653

Prazepam (May increase drowsiness).
No products indexed under this heading.

Procarbazine Hydrochloride (Concurrent and/or sequential use with MAO inhibitors is not recommended). Products include:
Matulane Capsules 3246

Prochlorperazine (May increase drowsiness). Products include:
Compazine 1505

Promethazine Hydrochloride (May increase drowsiness). Products include:
Mepergan Injection 3539
Phenergan Injection 3553
Phenergan 3556
Phenergan Syrup 3554
Phenergan with Codeine Syrup 3557
Phenergan with Dextromethorphan Syrup 3559
Phenergan VC Syrup 3560
Phenergan VC with Codeine Syrup 3561

Propofol (May increase drowsiness). Products include:
Diprivan Injectable Emulsion 667

Quazepam (May increase drowsiness).
No products indexed under this heading.

Secobarbital Sodium (May increase drowsiness).
No products indexed under this heading.

Selegiline Hydrochloride (Concurrent and/or sequential use with MAO inhibitors is not recommended). Products include:
Eldepryl Capsules 3266

Temazepam (May increase drowsiness).
No products indexed under this heading.

Thioridazine Hydrochloride (May increase drowsiness). Products include:
Thioridazine Hydrochloride Tablets........ 2289

Thiothixene (May increase drowsiness). Products include:
Navane Capsules 2701
Thiothixene Capsules 2290

Tranylcypromine Sulfate (Concurrent and/or sequential use with MAO inhibitors is not recommended). Products include:
Parnate Tablets 1607

Triazolam (May increase drowsiness). Products include:
Halcion Tablets 2823

Trifluoperazine Hydrochloride (May increase drowsiness). Products include:
Stelazine 1640

Zaleplon (May increase drowsiness). Products include:
Sonata Capsules 3591

Zolpidem Tartrate (May increase drowsiness). Products include:
Ambien Tablets 3191

Food Interactions

Alcohol (Chronic heavy alcohol users, 3 or more drinks per day, should consult their physician for advice on when and how they should take pain relievers/fever reducers including acetaminophen; increases drowsiness effect).

BENADRYL CHILDREN'S ALLERGY/COLD FASTMELT TABLETS

(Diphenhydramine Citrate, Pseudoephedrine Hydrochloride) ....▣692
May interact with hypnotics and sedatives, monoamine oxidase inhibitors, tranquilizers, and certain other agents. Compounds in these categories include:

Alprazolam (May increase drowsiness). Products include:
Xanax Tablets 2865

Buspirone Hydrochloride (May increase drowsiness).
No products indexed under this heading.

Chlordiazepoxide (May increase drowsiness). Products include:
Limbitrol 1738

Chlordiazepoxide Hydrochloride (May increase drowsiness). Products include:
Librium Capsules 1736
Librium for Injection 1737

Chlorpromazine (May increase drowsiness). Products include:
Thorazine Suppositories 1656

Chlorpromazine Hydrochloride (May increase drowsiness). Products include:
Thorazine 1656

Chlorprothixene (May increase drowsiness).
No products indexed under this heading.

Chlorprothixene Hydrochloride (May increase drowsiness).
No products indexed under this heading.

Clorazepate Dipotassium (May increase drowsiness). Products include:
Tranxene 511

Diazepam (May increase drowsiness). Products include:
Valium Injectable 3026
Valium Tablets 3047

Droperidol (May increase drowsiness).
No products indexed under this heading.

Estazolam (May increase drowsiness). Products include:
ProSom Tablets 500

Ethchlorvynol (May increase drowsiness).
No products indexed under this heading.

Ethinamate (May increase drowsiness).
No products indexed under this heading.

Fluphenazine Decanoate (May increase drowsiness).
No products indexed under this heading.

Fluphenazine Enanthate (May increase drowsiness).
No products indexed under this heading.

Fluphenazine Hydrochloride (May increase drowsiness).
No products indexed under this heading.

Flurazepam Hydrochloride (May increase drowsiness).
No products indexed under this heading.

Glutethimide (May increase drowsiness).
No products indexed under this heading.

Haloperidol (May increase drowsiness). Products include:
Haldol Injection, Tablets and Concentrate 2533

Haloperidol Decanoate (May increase drowsiness). Products include:
Haldol Decanoate 2535

Hydroxyzine Hydrochloride (May increase drowsiness). Products include:
Atarax Tablets & Syrup 2667
Vistaril Intramuscular Solution 2738

Isocarboxazid (Concurrent and/or sequential use with MAO inhibitors is not recommended).
No products indexed under this heading.

Lorazepam (May increase drowsiness). Products include:
Ativan Injection 3478
Ativan Tablets 3482

Loxapine Hydrochloride (May increase drowsiness).
No products indexed under this heading.

Loxapine Succinate (May increase drowsiness). Products include:
Loxitane Capsules 3398

Meprobamate (May increase drowsiness). Products include:
Miltown Tablets 3349

Mesoridazine Besylate (May increase drowsiness). Products include:
Serentil 1057

Midazolam Hydrochloride (May increase drowsiness). Products include:
Versed Injection 3027
Versed Syrup 3033

Moclobemide (Concurrent and/or sequential use with MAO inhibitors is not recommended).
No products indexed under this heading.

Molindone Hydrochloride (May increase drowsiness). Products include:
Moban 1320

Oxazepam (May increase drowsiness).
No products indexed under this heading.

Pargyline Hydrochloride (Concurrent and/or sequential use with MAO inhibitors is not recommended).
No products indexed under this heading.

Perphenazine (May increase drowsiness). Products include:
Etrafon 3115
Trilafon 3160

Phenelzine Sulfate (Concurrent and/or sequential use with MAO inhibitors is not recommended). Products include:
Nardil Tablets 2653

Prazepam (May increase drowsiness).
No products indexed under this heading.

Procarbazine Hydrochloride (Concurrent and/or sequential use with MAO inhibitors is not recommended). Products include:
Matulane Capsules 3246

Prochlorperazine (May increase drowsiness). Products include:
Compazine 1505

Promethazine Hydrochloride (May increase drowsiness). Products include:
Mepergan Injection 3539
Phenergan Injection 3553
Phenergan 3556
Phenergan Syrup 3554
Phenergan with Codeine Syrup 3557
Phenergan with Dextromethorphan Syrup 3559
Phenergan VC Syrup 3560
Phenergan VC with Codeine Syrup 3561

Propofol (May increase drowsiness). Products include:
Diprivan Injectable Emulsion 667

Quazepam (May increase drowsiness).
No products indexed under this heading.

Secobarbital Sodium (May increase drowsiness).
No products indexed under this heading.

Selegiline Hydrochloride (Concurrent and/or sequential use with MAO inhibitors is not recommended). Products include:
Eldepryl Capsules 3266

Temazepam (May increase drowsiness).
No products indexed under this heading.

Thioridazine Hydrochloride (May increase drowsiness). Products include:
Thioridazine Hydrochloride Tablets 2289

Thiothixene (May increase drowsiness). Products include:
Navane Capsules 2701
Thiothixene Capsules 2290

Tranylcypromine Sulfate (Concurrent and/or sequential use with MAO inhibitors is not recommended). Products include:
Parnate Tablets 1607

Triazolam (May increase drowsiness). Products include:
Halcion Tablets 2823

Trifluoperazine Hydrochloride (May increase drowsiness). Products include:
Stelazine 1640

Zaleplon (May increase drowsiness). Products include:
Sonata Capsules 3591

Zolpidem Tartrate (May increase drowsiness). Products include:
Ambien Tablets 3191

Food Interactions

Alcohol (May increase drowsiness).

BENADRYL DYE-FREE ALLERGY LIQUID

(Diphenhydramine Hydrochloride)........ ▣690
May interact with hypnotics and sedatives, tranquilizers, and certain other agents. Compounds in these categories include:

Alprazolam (May increase the drowsiness effect). Products include:
Xanax Tablets 2865

Buspirone Hydrochloride (May increase the drowsiness effect).
No products indexed under this heading.

Chlordiazepoxide (May increase the drowsiness effect). Products include:
Limbitrol 1738

Chlordiazepoxide Hydrochloride (May increase the drowsiness effect). Products include:
Librium Capsules 1736
Librium for Injection 1737

Chlorpromazine (May increase the drowsiness effect). Products include:
Thorazine Suppositories 1656

Chlorpromazine Hydrochloride (May increase the drowsiness effect). Products include:
Thorazine 1656

Chlorprothixene (May increase the drowsiness effect).
No products indexed under this heading.

Chlorprothixene Hydrochloride (May increase the drowsiness effect).
No products indexed under this heading.

Clorazepate Dipotassium (May increase the drowsiness effect). Products include:
Tranxene 511

Diazepam (May increase the drowsiness effect). Products include:
Valium Injectable 3026
Valium Tablets 3047

Droperidol (May increase the drowsiness effect).
No products indexed under this heading.

Estazolam (May increase the drowsiness effect). Products include:
ProSom Tablets 500

Ethchlorvynol (May increase the drowsiness effect).
No products indexed under this heading.

Ethinamate (May increase the drowsiness effect).
No products indexed under this heading.

Fluphenazine Decanoate (May increase the drowsiness effect).
No products indexed under this heading.

Fluphenazine Enanthate (May increase the drowsiness effect).
No products indexed under this heading.

Fluphenazine Hydrochloride (May increase the drowsiness effect).
No products indexed under this heading.

Flurazepam Hydrochloride (May increase the drowsiness effect).
No products indexed under this heading.

Glutethimide (May increase the drowsiness effect).
No products indexed under this heading.

Haloperidol (May increase the drowsiness effect). Products include:
Haldol Injection, Tablets and Concentrate 2533

Haloperidol Decanoate (May increase the drowsiness effect). Products include:
Haldol Decanoate 2535

Hydroxyzine Hydrochloride (May increase the drowsiness effect). Products include:
- Atarax Tablets & Syrup 2667
- Vistaril Intramuscular Solution 2738

Lorazepam (May increase the drowsiness effect). Products include:
- Ativan Injection 3478
- Ativan Tablets 3482

Loxapine Hydrochloride (May increase the drowsiness effect).
- No products indexed under this heading.

Loxapine Succinate (May increase the drowsiness effect). Products include:
- Loxitane Capsules 3398

Meprobamate (May increase the drowsiness effect). Products include:
- Miltown Tablets 3349

Mesoridazine Besylate (May increase the drowsiness effect). Products include:
- Serentil 1057

Midazolam Hydrochloride (May increase the drowsiness effect). Products include:
- Versed Injection 3027
- Versed Syrup 3033

Molindone Hydrochloride (May increase the drowsiness effect). Products include:
- Moban 1320

Oxazepam (May increase the drowsiness effect).
- No products indexed under this heading.

Perphenazine (May increase the drowsiness effect). Products include:
- Etrafon 3115
- Trilafon 3160

Prazepam (May increase the drowsiness effect).
- No products indexed under this heading.

Prochlorperazine (May increase the drowsiness effect). Products include:
- Compazine 1505

Promethazine Hydrochloride (May increase the drowsiness effect). Products include:
- Mepergan Injection 3539
- Phenergan Injection 3553
- Phenergan 3556
- Phenergan Syrup 3554
- Phenergan with Codeine Syrup 3557
- Phenergan with Dextromethorphan Syrup 3559
- Phenergan VC Syrup 3560
- Phenergan VC with Codeine Syrup . 3561

Propofol (May increase the drowsiness effect). Products include:
- Diprivan Injectable Emulsion 667

Quazepam (May increase the drowsiness effect).
- No products indexed under this heading.

Secobarbital Sodium (May increase the drowsiness effect).
- No products indexed under this heading.

Temazepam (May increase the drowsiness effect).
- No products indexed under this heading.

Thioridazine Hydrochloride (May increase the drowsiness effect). Products include:
- Thioridazine Hydrochloride Tablets 2289

Thiothixene (May increase the drowsiness effect). Products include:
- Navane Capsules 2701
- Thiothixene Capsules 2290

Triazolam (May increase the drowsiness effect). Products include:
- Halcion Tablets 2823

Trifluoperazine Hydrochloride (May increase the drowsiness effect). Products include:
- Stelazine 1640

Zaleplon (May increase the drowsiness effect). Products include:
- Sonata Capsules 3591

Zolpidem Tartrate (May increase the drowsiness effect). Products include:
- Ambien Tablets 3191

Food Interactions

Alcohol (May increase the drowsiness effect).

BENADRYL DYE-FREE ALLERGY LIQUI-GELS SOFTGELS

(Diphenhydramine Hydrochloride)................................ ■690

May interact with hypnotics and sedatives, tranquilizers, and certain other agents. Compounds in these categories include:

Alprazolam (May increase the drowsiness effect). Products include:
- Xanax Tablets 2865

Buspirone Hydrochloride (May increase the drowsiness effect).
- No products indexed under this heading.

Chlordiazepoxide (May increase the drowsiness effect). Products include:
- Limbitrol 1738

Chlordiazepoxide Hydrochloride (May increase the drowsiness effect). Products include:
- Librium Capsules 1736
- Librium for Injection 1737

Chlorpromazine (May increase the drowsiness effect). Products include:
- Thorazine Suppositories 1656

Chlorpromazine Hydrochloride (May increase the drowsiness effect). Products include:
- Thorazine 1656

Chlorprothixene (May increase the drowsiness effect).
- No products indexed under this heading.

Chlorprothixene Hydrochloride (May increase the drowsiness effect).
- No products indexed under this heading.

Clorazepate Dipotassium (May increase the drowsiness effect). Products include:
- Tranxene 511

Diazepam (May increase the drowsiness effect). Products include:
- Valium Injectable 3026
- Valium Tablets 3047

Droperidol (May increase the drowsiness effect).
- No products indexed under this heading.

Estazolam (May increase the drowsiness effect). Products include:
- ProSom Tablets 500

Ethchlorvynol (May increase the drowsiness effect).
- No products indexed under this heading.

Ethinamate (May increase the drowsiness effect).
- No products indexed under this heading.

Fluphenazine Decanoate (May increase the drowsiness effect).
- No products indexed under this heading.

Fluphenazine Enanthate (May increase the drowsiness effect).
- No products indexed under this heading.

Fluphenazine Hydrochloride (May increase the drowsiness effect).
- No products indexed under this heading.

Flurazepam Hydrochloride (May increase the drowsiness effect).
- No products indexed under this heading.

Glutethimide (May increase the drowsiness effect).
- No products indexed under this heading.

Haloperidol (May increase the drowsiness effect). Products include:
- Haldol Injection, Tablets and Concentrate 2533

Haloperidol Decanoate (May increase the drowsiness effect). Products include:
- Haldol Decanoate 2535

Hydroxyzine Hydrochloride (May increase the drowsiness effect). Products include:
- Atarax Tablets & Syrup 2667
- Vistaril Intramuscular Solution 2738

Lorazepam (May increase the drowsiness effect). Products include:
- Ativan Injection 3478
- Ativan Tablets 3482

Loxapine Hydrochloride (May increase the drowsiness effect).
- No products indexed under this heading.

Loxapine Succinate (May increase the drowsiness effect). Products include:
- Loxitane Capsules 3398

Meprobamate (May increase the drowsiness effect). Products include:
- Miltown Tablets 3349

Mesoridazine Besylate (May increase the drowsiness effect). Products include:
- Serentil 1057

Midazolam Hydrochloride (May increase the drowsiness effect). Products include:
- Versed Injection 3027
- Versed Syrup 3033

Molindone Hydrochloride (May increase the drowsiness effect). Products include:
- Moban 1320

Oxazepam (May increase the drowsiness effect).
- No products indexed under this heading.

Perphenazine (May increase the drowsiness effect). Products include:
- Etrafon 3115
- Trilafon 3160

Prazepam (May increase the drowsiness effect).
- No products indexed under this heading.

Prochlorperazine (May increase the drowsiness effect). Products include:
- Compazine 1505

Promethazine Hydrochloride (May increase the drowsiness effect). Products include:
- Mepergan Injection 3539
- Phenergan Injection 3553
- Phenergan 3556
- Phenergan Syrup 3554
- Phenergan with Codeine Syrup 3557
- Phenergan with Dextromethorphan Syrup 3559
- Phenergan VC Syrup 3560
- Phenergan VC with Codeine Syrup . 3561

Propofol (May increase the drowsiness effect). Products include:
- Diprivan Injectable Emulsion 667

Quazepam (May increase the drowsiness effect).
- No products indexed under this heading.

Secobarbital Sodium (May increase the drowsiness effect).
- No products indexed under this heading.

Temazepam (May increase the drowsiness effect).
- No products indexed under this heading.

Thioridazine Hydrochloride (May increase the drowsiness effect). Products include:
- Thioridazine Hydrochloride Tablets 2289

Thiothixene (May increase the drowsiness effect). Products include:
- Navane Capsules 2701
- Thiothixene Capsules 2290

Triazolam (May increase the drowsiness effect). Products include:
- Halcion Tablets 2823

Trifluoperazine Hydrochloride (May increase the drowsiness effect). Products include:
- Stelazine 1640

Zaleplon (May increase the drowsiness effect). Products include:
- Sonata Capsules 3591

Zolpidem Tartrate (May increase the drowsiness effect). Products include:
- Ambien Tablets 3191

Food Interactions

Alcohol (May increase the drowsiness effect).

BENADRYL ITCH RELIEF STICK EXTRA STRENGTH

(Diphenhydramine Hydrochloride, Zinc Acetate)............ ■695

None cited in PDR database.

BENADRYL ITCH STOPPING CREAM ORIGINAL STRENGTH

(Diphenhydramine Hydrochloride, Zinc Acetate)............ ■695

May interact with:

Diphenhydramine (Concurrent use with other diphenhydramine-containing product is not recommended).
- No products indexed under this heading.

BENADRYL ITCH STOPPING CREAM EXTRA STRENGTH

(Diphenhydramine Hydrochloride, Zinc Acetate)............ ■695

See Benadryl Itch Stopping Cream Original Strength

BENADRYL ITCH STOPPING GEL ORIGINAL STRENGTH

(Diphenhydramine Hydrochloride)................................ ■695

May interact with:

Diphenhydramine (Concurrent use with other diphenhydramine-containing product is not recommended).
- No products indexed under this heading.

BENADRYL ITCH STOPPING GEL EXTRA STRENGTH

(Diphenhydramine Hydrochloride)................................ ■695

See Benadryl Itch Stopping Gel Original Strength

BENADRYL ITCH STOPPING SPRAY ORIGINAL STRENGTH

(Diphenhydramine Hydrochloride, Zinc Acetate)............ ■696

None cited in PDR database.

BENADRYL ITCH STOPPING SPRAY EXTRA STRENGTH

(Diphenhydramine Hydrochloride, Zinc Acetate)............ ■696

See Benadryl Itch Stopping Spray Original Strength

BENADRYL PARENTERAL

(Diphenhydramine Hydrochloride) 2617

May interact with central nervous system depressants, monoamine oxidase inhibitors, and certain other agents. Compounds in these categories include:

Alfentanil Hydrochloride (Additive effects).
No products indexed under this heading.

Alprazolam (Additive effects). Products include:
Xanax Tablets 2865

Aprobarbital (Additive effects).
No products indexed under this heading.

Buprenorphine Hydrochloride (Additive effects). Products include:
Buprenex Injectable 2918

Buspirone Hydrochloride (Additive effects).
No products indexed under this heading.

Butabarbital (Additive effects).
No products indexed under this heading.

Butalbital (Additive effects). Products include:
Phrenilin 578
Sedapap Tablets 50 mg/650 mg 2225

Chlordiazepoxide (Additive effects). Products include:
Limbitrol 1738

Chlordiazepoxide Hydrochloride (Additive effects). Products include:
Librium Capsules 1736
Librium for Injection 1737

Chlorpromazine (Additive effects). Products include:
Thorazine Suppositories 1656

Chlorpromazine Hydrochloride (Additive effects). Products include:
Thorazine 1656

Chlorprothixene (Additive effects).
No products indexed under this heading.

Chlorprothixene Hydrochloride (Additive effects).
No products indexed under this heading.

Chlorprothixene Lactate (Additive effects).
No products indexed under this heading.

Clorazepate Dipotassium (Additive effects). Products include:
Tranxene 511

Clozapine (Additive effects). Products include:
Clozaril Tablets 2319

Codeine Phosphate (Additive effects). Products include:
Phenergan with Codeine Syrup 3557
Phenergan VC with Codeine Syrup 3561
Robitussin A-C Syrup 2942
Robitussin-DAC Syrup 2942
Ryna-C Liquid 768
Soma Compound w/Codeine Tablets 3355
Tussi-Organidin NR Liquid 3350
Tussi-Organidin-S NR Liquid 3350
Tylenol with Codeine 2595

Desflurane (Additive effects). Products include:
Suprane Liquid for Inhalation 874

Dezocine (Additive effects).
No products indexed under this heading.

Diazepam (Additive effects). Products include:
Valium Injectable 3026
Valium Tablets 3047

Droperidol (Additive effects).
No products indexed under this heading.

Enflurane (Additive effects).
No products indexed under this heading.

Estazolam (Additive effects). Products include:
ProSom Tablets 500

Ethchlorvynol (Additive effects).
No products indexed under this heading.

Ethinamate (Additive effects).
No products indexed under this heading.

Fentanyl (Additive effects). Products include:
Duragesic Transdermal System 1786

Fentanyl Citrate (Additive effects). Products include:
Actiq 1184

Fluphenazine Decanoate (Additive effects).
No products indexed under this heading.

Fluphenazine Enanthate (Additive effects).
No products indexed under this heading.

Fluphenazine Hydrochloride (Additive effects).
No products indexed under this heading.

Flurazepam Hydrochloride (Additive effects).
No products indexed under this heading.

Glutethimide (Additive effects).
No products indexed under this heading.

Haloperidol (Additive effects). Products include:
Haldol Injection, Tablets and Concentrate 2533

Haloperidol Decanoate (Additive effects). Products include:
Haldol Decanoate 2535

Hydrocodone Bitartrate (Additive effects). Products include:
Hycodan 1316
Hycomine Compound Tablets 1317
Hycotuss Expectorant Syrup 1318
Lortab 3319
Lortab Elixir 3317
Maxidone Tablets CIII 3399
Norco 5/325 Tablets CIII 3424
Norco 7.5/325 Tablets CIII 3425
Norco 10/325 Tablets CIII 3427
Norco 10/325 Tablets CIII 3425
Vicodin Tablets 516
Vicodin ES Tablets 517
Vicodin HP Tablets 518
Vicodin Tuss Expectorant 519
Vicoprofen Tablets 520
Zydone Tablets 1330

Hydrocodone Polistirex (Additive effects). Products include:
Tussionex Pennkinetic Extended-Release Suspension 1174

Hydromorphone Hydrochloride (Additive effects). Products include:
Dilaudid 441
Dilaudid Oral Liquid 445
Dilaudid Powder 441
Dilaudid Rectal Suppositories 441
Dilaudid Tablets 441
Dilaudid Tablets - 8 mg 445
Dilaudid-HP 443

Hydroxyzine Hydrochloride (Additive effects). Products include:
Atarax Tablets & Syrup 2667
Vistaril Intramuscular Solution 2738

Isocarboxazid (MAO inhibitors prolong and intensify the anticholinergic effects of antihistamines).
No products indexed under this heading.

Isoflurane (Additive effects).
No products indexed under this heading.

Ketamine Hydrochloride (Additive effects).
No products indexed under this heading.

Levomethadyl Acetate Hydrochloride (Additive effects).
No products indexed under this heading.

Levorphanol Tartrate (Additive effects). Products include:
Levo-Dromoran 1734
Levorphanol Tartrate Tablets 3059

Lorazepam (Additive effects). Products include:
Ativan Injection 3478
Ativan Tablets 3482

Loxapine Hydrochloride (Additive effects).
No products indexed under this heading.

Loxapine Succinate (Additive effects). Products include:
Loxitane Capsules 3398

Meperidine Hydrochloride (Additive effects). Products include:
Demerol 3079
Mepergan Injection 3539

Mephobarbital (Additive effects).
No products indexed under this heading.

Meprobamate (Additive effects). Products include:
Miltown Tablets 3349

Mesoridazine Besylate (Additive effects). Products include:
Serentil 1057

Methadone Hydrochloride (Additive effects). Products include:
Dolophine Hydrochloride Tablets 3056

Methohexital Sodium (Additive effects). Products include:
Brevital Sodium for Injection, USP 1815

Methotrimeprazine (Additive effects).
No products indexed under this heading.

Methoxyflurane (Additive effects).
No products indexed under this heading.

Midazolam Hydrochloride (Additive effects). Products include:
Versed Injection 3027
Versed Syrup 3033

Moclobemide (MAO inhibitors prolong and intensify the anticholinergic effects of antihistamines).
No products indexed under this heading.

Molindone Hydrochloride (Additive effects). Products include:
Moban 1320

Morphine Sulfate (Additive effects). Products include:
Astramorph/PF Injection, USP (Preservative-Free) 594
Duramorph Injection 1312
Infumorph 200 and Infumorph 500 Sterile Solutions 1314
Kadian Capsules 1335
MS Contin Tablets 2896
MSIR 2898
Oramorph SR Tablets 3062
Roxanol 3066

Olanzapine (Additive effects). Products include:
Zyprexa Tablets 1973
Zyprexa ZYDIS Orally Disintegrating Tablets 1973

Oxazepam (Additive effects).
No products indexed under this heading.

Oxycodone Hydrochloride (Additive effects). Products include:
OxyContin Tablets 2912
OxyFast Oral Concentrate Solution 2916
OxyIR Capsules 2916
Percocet Tablets 1326
Percodan Tablets 1327
Percolone Tablets 1327
Roxicodone 3067
Tylox Capsules 2597

Pargyline Hydrochloride (MAO inhibitors prolong and intensify the anticholinergic effects of antihistamines).
No products indexed under this heading.

Pentobarbital Sodium (Additive effects). Products include:
Nembutal Sodium Solution 485

Perphenazine (Additive effects). Products include:
Etrafon 3115
Trilafon 3160

Phenelzine Sulfate (MAO inhibitors prolong and intensify the anticholinergic effects of antihistamines). Products include:
Nardil Tablets 2653

Phenobarbital (Additive effects). Products include:
Arco-Lase Plus Tablets 592
Donnatal 2929
Donnatal Extentabs 2930

Prazepam (Additive effects).
No products indexed under this heading.

Procarbazine Hydrochloride (MAO inhibitors prolong and intensify the anticholinergic effects of antihistamines). Products include:
Matulane Capsules 3246

Prochlorperazine (Additive effects). Products include:
Compazine 1505

Promethazine Hydrochloride (Additive effects). Products include:
Mepergan Injection 3539
Phenergan Injection 3553
Phenergan 3556
Phenergan Syrup 3554
Phenergan with Codeine Syrup 3557
Phenergan with Dextromethorphan Syrup 3559
Phenergan VC Syrup 3560
Phenergan VC with Codeine Syrup 3561

Propofol (Additive effects). Products include:
Diprivan Injectable Emulsion 667

Propoxyphene Hydrochloride (Additive effects). Products include:
Darvon Pulvules 1909
Darvon Compound-65 Pulvules 1910

Propoxyphene Napsylate (Additive effects). Products include:
Darvon-N/Darvocet-N 1907
Darvon-N Tablets 1912

Quazepam (Additive effects).
No products indexed under this heading.

Quetiapine Fumarate (Additive effects). Products include:
Seroquel Tablets 684

Remifentanil Hydrochloride (Additive effects).
No products indexed under this heading.

Risperidone (Additive effects). Products include:
Risperdal 1796

Secobarbital Sodium (Additive effects).
No products indexed under this heading.

Selegiline Hydrochloride (MAO inhibitors prolong and intensify the anticholinergic effects of antihistamines). Products include:
Eldepryl Capsules 3266

Sevoflurane (Additive effects).
No products indexed under this heading.

Sufentanil Citrate (Additive effects).
No products indexed under this heading.

Temazepam (Additive effects).
No products indexed under this heading.

Thiamylal Sodium (Additive effects).
No products indexed under this heading.

Thioridazine Hydrochloride (Additive effects). Products include:
Thioridazine Hydrochloride Tablets 2289

Thiothixene (Additive effects). Products include:
Navane Capsules 2701
Thiothixene Capsules 2290

Tranylcypromine Sulfate (MAO inhibitors prolong and intensify the anticholinergic effects of antihistamines). Products include:
Parnate Tablets 1607

Triazolam (Additive effects). Products include:
Halcion Tablets 2823

Trifluoperazine Hydrochloride (Additive effects). Products include:
Stelazine 1640

Zaleplon (Additive effects). Products include:
Sonata Capsules 3591

Ziprasidone Hydrochloride (Additive effects). Products include:
Geodon Capsules 2688

Zolpidem Tartrate (Additive effects). Products include:

IMPORTANT NOTE: Always consult each drug listing in the patient's regimen for possible interactions.

Ambien Tablets 3191

Food Interactions

Alcohol (Additive effects).

BENEFIX FOR INJECTION
(Antihemophilic Factor (Recombinant)) 1432
None cited in PDR database.

BENGAY EXTERNAL ANALGESIC PRODUCTS
(Menthol, Methyl Salicylate) .... ▣696
None cited in PDR database.

BENOQUIN CREAM 20%
(Monobenzone) 1732
None cited in PDR database.

BENYLIN ADULT FORMULA COUGH SUPPRESSANT LIQUID
(Dextromethorphan Hydrobromide) .... ▣696
May interact with monoamine oxidase inhibitors. Compounds in these categories include:

Isocarboxazid (Concurrent and/or sequential use should be avoided).
No products indexed under this heading.

Moclobemide (Concurrent and/or sequential use should be avoided).
No products indexed under this heading.

Pargyline Hydrochloride (Concurrent and/or sequential use should be avoided).
No products indexed under this heading.

Phenelzine Sulfate (Concurrent and/or sequential use should be avoided). Products include:
Nardil Tablets 2653

Procarbazine Hydrochloride (Concurrent and/or sequential use should be avoided). Products include:
Matulane Capsules 3246

Selegiline Hydrochloride (Concurrent and/or sequential use should be avoided). Products include:
Eldepryl Capsules 3266

Tranylcypromine Sulfate (Concurrent and/or sequential use should be avoided). Products include:
Parnate Tablets 1607

BENYLIN COUGH SUPPRESSANT/ EXPECTORANT LIQUID
(Dextromethorphan Hydrobromide, Guaifenesin) .... ▣697
May interact with monoamine oxidase inhibitors. Compounds in these categories include:

Isocarboxazid (Concurrent and/or sequential use is not recommended).
No products indexed under this heading.

Moclobemide (Concurrent and/or sequential use is not recommended).
No products indexed under this heading.

Pargyline Hydrochloride (Concurrent and/or sequential use is not recommended).
No products indexed under this heading.

Phenelzine Sulfate (Concurrent and/or sequential use is not recommended). Products include:
Nardil Tablets 2653

Procarbazine Hydrochloride (Concurrent and/or sequential use is not recommended). Products include:
Matulane Capsules 3246

Selegiline Hydrochloride (Concurrent and/or sequential use is not recommended). Products include:
Eldepryl Capsules 3266

Tranylcypromine Sulfate (Concurrent and/or sequential use is not recommended). Products include:
Parnate Tablets 1607

BENYLIN MULTI-SYMPTOM LIQUID
(Dextromethorphan Hydrobromide, Guaifenesin, Pseudoephedrine Hydrochloride) .... ▣697
May interact with monoamine oxidase inhibitors. Compounds in these categories include:

Isocarboxazid (Concurrent and/or sequential use is not recommended).
No products indexed under this heading.

Moclobemide (Concurrent and/or sequential use is not recommended).
No products indexed under this heading.

Pargyline Hydrochloride (Concurrent and/or sequential use is not recommended).
No products indexed under this heading.

Phenelzine Sulfate (Concurrent and/or sequential use is not recommended). Products include:
Nardil Tablets 2653

Procarbazine Hydrochloride (Concurrent and/or sequential use is not recommended). Products include:
Matulane Capsules 3246

Selegiline Hydrochloride (Concurrent and/or sequential use is not recommended). Products include:
Eldepryl Capsules 3266

Tranylcypromine Sulfate (Concurrent and/or sequential use is not recommended). Products include:
Parnate Tablets 1607

BENYLIN PEDIATRIC COUGH SUPPRESSANT LIQUID
(Dextromethorphan Hydrobromide) .... ▣698
May interact with monoamine oxidase inhibitors. Compounds in these categories include:

Isocarboxazid (Concurrent and/or sequential use should be avoided).
No products indexed under this heading.

Moclobemide (Concurrent and/or sequential use should be avoided).
No products indexed under this heading.

Pargyline Hydrochloride (Concurrent and/or sequential use should be avoided).
No products indexed under this heading.

Phenelzine Sulfate (Concurrent and/or sequential use should be avoided). Products include:
Nardil Tablets 2653

Procarbazine Hydrochloride (Concurrent and/or sequential use should be avoided). Products include:
Matulane Capsules 3246

Selegiline Hydrochloride (Concurrent and/or sequential use should be avoided). Products include:
Eldepryl Capsules 3266

Tranylcypromine Sulfate (Concurrent and/or sequential use should be avoided). Products include:
Parnate Tablets 1607

BENZACLIN TOPICAL GEL
(Benzoyl Peroxide, Clindamycin Phosphate) 1220
May interact with:

Concomitant Topical Acne Therapy (Possible cumulative irritancy effect may occur, especially with the use of peeling, desquamating, or abrasive agents).
No products indexed under this heading.

BETA-C TABLETS
(Allium sativum, Bioflavonoids, Hesperidin Complex, Vitamin A, Vitamin C) .... ▣811
None cited in PDR database.

BETADINE BRAND FIRST AID ANTIBIOTICS & MOISTURIZER OINTMENT
(Bacitracin Zinc, Polymyxin B Sulfate) 2894
None cited in PDR database.

BETADINE BRAND PLUS FIRST AID ANTIBIOTICS & PAIN RELIEVER OINTMENT
(Bacitracin Zinc, Polymyxin B Sulfate, Pramoxine Hydrochloride) 2894
None cited in PDR database.

BETADINE MEDICATED DOUCHE
(Povidone Iodine) 2894
None cited in PDR database.

BETADINE OINTMENT
(Povidone Iodine) 2894
None cited in PDR database.

BETADINE PREPSTICK APPLICATOR
(Povidone Iodine) 2894
None cited in PDR database.

BETADINE PREPSTICK PLUS APPLICATOR
(Povidone Iodine) 2894
None cited in PDR database.

BETADINE SKIN CLEANSER
(Povidone Iodine) 2895
None cited in PDR database.

BETADINE SOLUTION
(Povidone Iodine) 2895
None cited in PDR database.

BETADINE SURGICAL SCRUB
(Povidone Iodine) 2895
None cited in PDR database.

BETAGAN LIQUIFILM
(Levobunolol Hydrochloride) .... ⊙228
See Betagan Liquifilm with C CAP Compliance Cap

BETAGAN LIQUIFILM WITH C CAP COMPLIANCE CAP
(Levobunolol Hydrochloride) .... ⊙228
May interact with beta blockers, cardiac glycosides, phenothiazines, and certain other agents. Compounds in these categories include:

Acebutolol Hydrochloride (Co-administration with oral beta blockers may result in additive effect either on intraocular pressure or on the known systemic effects of beta blockade). Products include:
Sectral Capsules 3589

Atenolol (Co-administration with oral beta blockers may result in additive effect either on intraocular pressure or on the known systemic effects of beta blockade). Products include:
Tenoretic Tablets 690
Tenormin I.V. Injection 692

Betaxolol Hydrochloride (Co-administration with oral beta blockers may result in additive effect either on intraocular pressure or on the known systemic effects of beta blockade). Products include:
Betoptic S Ophthalmic Suspension 537

Bisoprolol Fumarate (Co-administration with oral beta blockers may result in additive effect either on intraocular pressure or on the known systemic effects of beta blockade). Products include:
Zebeta Tablets 1885
Ziac Tablets 1887

Carteolol Hydrochloride (Co-administration with oral beta blockers may result in additive effect either on intraocular pressure or on the known systemic effects of beta blockade). Products include:
Carteolol Hydrochloride Ophthalmic Solution USP, 1% .... ⊙258
Ocupress Ophthalmic Solution, 1% Sterile .... ⊙303

Chlorpromazine (Co-administration with phenothiazine-related compounds may have an additive hypotensive effect due to inhibition of each other's metabolism). Products include:
Thorazine Suppositories 1656

Chlorpromazine Hydrochloride (Co-administration with phenothiazine-related compounds may have an additive hypotensive effect due to inhibition of each other's metabolism). Products include:
Thorazine 1656

Deserpidine (Possible additive effects and production of hypotension and/or bradycardia when beta blocker is concurrently used with catecholamine-depleting drugs).
No products indexed under this heading.

Deslanoside (Co-administration with digitalis and calcium channel blockers may have an additive effect on prolonging atrioventricular conduction time).
No products indexed under this heading.

Digitoxin (Co-administration with digitalis and calcium channel blockers may have an additive effect on prolonging atrioventricular conduction time).
No products indexed under this heading.

Digoxin (Co-administration with digitalis and calcium channel blockers may have an additive effect on prolonging atrioventricular conduction time). Products include:
Digitek Tablets 1003
Lanoxicaps Capsules 1574
Lanoxin Injection 1581
Lanoxin Tablets 1587
Lanoxin Elixir Pediatric 1578
Lanoxin Injection Pediatric 1584

Epinephrine (Concurrent use in patients with history of atopy or severe anaphylactic reaction to allergens may be unresponsive to the usual doses of epinephrine used to treat anaphylactic reaction; mydriasis may result with concomitant epinephrine). Products include:
Epifrin Sterile Ophthalmic Solution .... ⊙235
EpiPen 1236
Primatene Mist .... ▣779
Xylocaine with Epinephrine Injection 653

Epinephrine Hydrochloride (Concurrent use in patients with history of atopy or severe anaphylactic reaction to allergens may be unresponsive to the usual doses of epinephrine used to treat anaphylactic reaction; mydriasis may result with concomitant epinephrine).
No products indexed under this heading.

Esmolol Hydrochloride (Co-administration with oral beta blockers may result in additive effect either on intraocular pressure or on the known systemic effects of beta blockade). Products include:

Brevibloc Injection........................... 858

Fluphenazine Decanoate (Co-administration with phenothiazine-related compounds may have an additive hypotensive effect due to inhibition of each other's metabolism).
No products indexed under this heading.

Fluphenazine Enanthate (Co-administration with phenothiazine-related compounds may have an additive hypotensive effect due to inhibition of each other's metabolism).
No products indexed under this heading.

Fluphenazine Hydrochloride (Co-administration with phenothiazine-related compounds may have an additive hypotensive effect due to inhibition of each other's metabolism).
No products indexed under this heading.

Labetalol Hydrochloride (Co-administration with oral beta blockers may result in additive effect either on intraocular pressure or on the known systemic effects of beta blockade). Products include:
Normodyne Injection 3135
Normodyne Tablets 3137

Mesoridazine Besylate (Co-administration with phenothiazine-related compounds may have an additive hypotensive effect due to inhibition of each other's metabolism). Products include:
Serentil 1057

Methotrimeprazine (Co-administration with phenothiazine-related compounds may have an additive hypotensive effect due to inhibition of each other's metabolism).
No products indexed under this heading.

Metipranolol Hydrochloride (Co-administration with oral beta blockers may result in additive effect either on intraocular pressure or on the known systemic effects of beta blockade).
No products indexed under this heading.

Metoprolol Succinate (Co-administration with oral beta blockers may result in additive effect either on intraocular pressure or on the known systemic effects of beta blockade). Products include:
Toprol-XL Tablets 651

Metoprolol Tartrate (Co-administration with oral beta blockers may result in additive effect either on intraocular pressure or on the known systemic effects of beta blockade).
No products indexed under this heading.

Nadolol (Co-administration with oral beta blockers may result in additive effect either on intraocular pressure or on the known systemic effects of beta blockade). Products include:
Corgard Tablets 2245
Corzide 40/5 Tablets 2247
Corzide 80/5 Tablets 2247
Nadolol Tablets 2288

Penbutolol Sulfate (Co-administration with oral beta blockers may result in additive effect either on intraocular pressure or on the known systemic effects of beta blockade).
No products indexed under this heading.

Perphenazine (Co-administration with phenothiazine-related compounds may have an additive hypotensive effect due to inhibition of each other's metabolism). Products include:
Etrafon 3115

Trilafon 3160

Pindolol (Co-administration with oral beta blockers may result in additive effect either on intraocular pressure or on the known systemic effects of beta blockade).
No products indexed under this heading.

Prochlorperazine (Co-administration with phenothiazine-related compounds may have an additive hypotensive effect due to inhibition of each other's metabolism). Products include:
Compazine 1505

Promethazine Hydrochloride (Co-administration with phenothiazine-related compounds may have an additive hypotensive effect due to inhibition of each other's metabolism). Products include:
Mepergan Injection 3539
Phenergan Injection 3553
Phenergan 3556
Phenergan Syrup 3554
Phenergan with Codeine Syrup 3557
Phenergan with Dextromethorphan Syrup 3559
Phenergan VC Syrup 3560
Phenergan VC with Codeine Syrup .3561

Propranolol Hydrochloride (Co-administration with oral beta blockers may result in additive effect either on intraocular pressure or on the known systemic effects of beta blockade). Products include:
Inderal 3513
Inderal LA Long-Acting Capsules 3516
Inderide Tablets 3517
Inderide LA Long-Acting Capsules ..3519

Rauwolfia serpentina (Possible additive effects and production of hypotension and/or bradycardia when beta blocker is concurrently used with catecholamine-depleting drugs).
No products indexed under this heading.

Rescinnamine (Possible additive effects and production of hypotension and/or bradycardia when beta blocker is concurrently used with catecholamine-depleting drugs).
No products indexed under this heading.

Reserpine (Possible additive effects and production of hypotension and/or bradycardia when beta blocker is concurrently used with catecholamine-depleting drugs).
No products indexed under this heading.

Sotalol Hydrochloride (Co-administration with oral beta blockers may result in additive effect either on intraocular pressure or on the known systemic effects of beta blockade). Products include:
Betapace Tablets 950
Betapace AF Tablets 954

Thioridazine Hydrochloride (Co-administration with phenothiazine-related compounds may have an additive hypotensive effect due to inhibition of each other's metabolism). Products include:
Thioridazine Hydrochloride Tablets 2289

Timolol Hemihydrate (Co-administration with oral beta blockers may result in additive effect either on intraocular pressure or on the known systemic effects of beta blockade). Products include:
Betimol Ophthalmic Solution ....⊙324

Timolol Maleate (Co-administration with oral beta blockers may result in additive effect either on intraocular pressure or on the known systemic effects of beta blockade). Products include:
Blocadren Tablets 2046
Cosopt Sterile Ophthalmic Solution 2065
Timolide Tablets 2187
Timolol GFS ....⊙266
Timoptic in Ocudose 2192
Timoptic Sterile Ophthalmic Solution..2190
Timoptic-XE Sterile Ophthalmic Gel Forming Solution 2194

Trifluoperazine Hydrochloride (Co-administration with phenothiazine-related compounds may have an additive hypotensive effect due to inhibition of each other's metabolism). Products include:
Stelazine 1640

BETAPACE TABLETS

(Sotalol Hydrochloride) 950
See Betapace AF Tablets

BETAPACE AF TABLETS

(Sotalol Hydrochloride) 954
May interact with antacids containing aluminum, calcium and magnesium, beta$_2$ agonists, calcium channel blockers, oral hypoglycemic agents, insulin, macrolide antibiotics, phenothiazines, quinidine, tricyclic antidepressants, and certain other agents. Compounds in these categories include:

Acarbose (Hyperglycemia may occur, and the dosage of oral hypoglycemic agents may require adjustment; beta blocker may mask the symptoms of hypoglycemia). Products include:
Precose Tablets 906

Albuterol (Beta-agonists may have to be administered in increased dosages when used concomitantly with sotalol). Products include:
Proventil Inhalation Aerosol 3142
Ventolin Inhalation Aerosol and Refill 1679

Albuterol Sulfate (Beta-agonists may have to be administered in increased dosages when used concomitantly with sotalol). Products include:
AccuNeb Inhalation Solution 1230
Combivent Inhalation Aerosol 1041
DuoNeb Inhalation Solution 1233
Proventil Inhalation Solution 0.083% 3146
Proventil Repetabs Tablets 3148
Proventil Solution for Inhalation 0.5% 3144
Proventil HFA Inhalation Aerosol 3150
Ventolin HFA Inhalation Aerosol 3618
Volmax Extended-Release Tablets ..2276

Aluminum Carbonate (Co-administration within 2 hours of antacids containing aluminum oxide and magnesium hydroxide should be avoided because it may result in a reduction in Cmax and AUC of 26% and 20% respectively and consequently in a 20% reduction in the bradycardic effect at rest).
No products indexed under this heading.

Aluminum Hydroxide (Co-administration within 2 hours of antacids containing aluminum oxide and magnesium hydroxide should be avoided because it may result in a reduction in Cmax and AUC of 26% and 20% respectively and consequently in a 20% reduction in the bradycardic effect at rest). Products include:
Amphojel Suspension (Mint Flavor) ....▣789
Gaviscon Extra Strength Liquid .....▣751
Gaviscon Extra Strength Tablets .....▣751
Gaviscon Regular Strength Liquid .▣751
Gaviscon Regular Strength Tablets ....▣750
Maalox Antacid/Anti-Gas Oral Suspension ....▣673
Maalox Max Maximum Strength Antacid/Anti-Gas Liquid 2300
Maalox Regular Strength Antacid/Antigas Liquid 2300
Mylanta 1813
Vanquish Caplets ....▣617

Amiodarone Hydrochloride (Co-administration with class III antiarrhythmics, such as amiodarone, is not recommended because of their potential to prolong refractoriness; in clinical trials, Betapace AF was not administered to patients previously treated with oral amiodarone for >1 month in the previous 3 months). Products include:
Cordarone Intravenous 3491
Cordarone Tablets 3487
Pacerone Tablets 3331

Amitriptyline Hydrochloride (Co-administration with other drugs that prolong the QT interval, such as tricyclic antidepressants, has not been studied and is not recommended). Products include:
Etrafon 3115
Limbitrol 1738

Amlodipine Besylate (Co-administration with calcium channel blocking drugs can result in possible additive effects on A-V conduction or ventricular function; potential for additive effects on blood pressure, possibly leading to hypotension). Products include:
Lotrel Capsules 2370
Norvasc Tablets 2704

Amoxapine (Co-administration with other drugs that prolong the QT interval, such as tricyclic antidepressants, has not been studied and is not recommended).
No products indexed under this heading.

Astemizole (Co-administration with other drugs known to prolong the QT interval, such as astemizole, has not been studied; concurrent use requires caution).
No products indexed under this heading.

Azithromycin Dihydrate (Co-administration with other drugs that prolong the QT interval, such as certain oral macrolides, has not been studied and is not recommended). Products include:
Zithromax 2743
Zithromax for IV Infusion 2748
Zithromax for Oral Suspension, 300 mg, 600 mg, 900 mg, 1200 mg 2739
Zithromax Tablets, 250 mg 2739

Bepridil Hydrochloride (Co-administration with other drugs that prolong the QT interval, such as bepridil, has not been studied and is not recommended; concurrent use with calcium channel blocking drugs can result in possible additive effects on A-V conduction or ventricular function; potential for additive effects on blood pressure, possibly leading to hypotension). Products include:
Vascor Tablets 2602

Bitolterol Mesylate (Beta-agonists may have to be administered in increased dosages when used concomitantly with sotalol).
No products indexed under this heading.

Chlorpromazine (Co-administration with other drugs that prolong the QT interval, such as some phenothiazines, has not been studied and is not recommended). Products include:
Thorazine Suppositories 1656

Chlorpromazine Hydrochloride (Co-administration with other drugs that prolong the QT interval, such as some phenothiazines, has not been studied and is not recommended). Products include:
Thorazine 1656

Chlorpropamide (Hyperglycemia may occur, and the dosage of oral hypoglycemic agents may require adjustment; beta blocker may mask the symptoms of hypoglycemia). Products include:
Diabinese Tablets 2680

Cisapride (Co-administration with other drugs that prolong the QT

interval, such as cisapride, has not been studied and is not recommended).
No products indexed under this heading.

Clarithromycin (Co-administration with other drugs that prolong the QT interval, such as certain oral macrolides, has not been studied and is not recommended). Products include:
Biaxin/Biaxin XL ... 403
PREVPAC ... 3298

Clomipramine Hydrochloride (Co-administration with other drugs that prolong the QT interval, such as tricyclic antidepressants, has not been studied and is not recommended).
No products indexed under this heading.

Clonidine (Beta-blocking drugs may potentiate the rebound hypertension sometimes observed after discontinuation of clonidine). Products include:
Catapres-TTS ... 1038

Clonidine Hydrochloride (Beta-blocking drugs may potentiate the rebound hypertension sometimes observed after discontinuation of clonidine). Products include:
Catapres Tablets ... 1037
Clorpres Tablets ... 1002
Combipres Tablets ... 1040
Duraclon Injection ... 3057

Desipramine Hydrochloride (Co-administration with other drugs that prolong the QT interval, such as tricyclic antidepressants, has not been studied and is not recommended). Products include:
Norpramin Tablets ... 755

Digoxin (Proarrhythmic events were more common in sotalol treated patients also receiving digoxin). Products include:
Digitek Tablets ... 1003
Lanoxicaps Capsules ... 1574
Lanoxin Injection ... 1581
Lanoxin Tablets ... 1587
Lanoxin Elixir Pediatric ... 1578
Lanoxin Injection Pediatric ... 1584

Diltiazem Hydrochloride (Co-administration with calcium channel blocking drugs can result in possible additive effects on A-V conduction or ventricular function; potential for additive effects on blood pressure, possibly leading to hypotension). Products include:
Cardizem Injectable ... 1018
Cardizem Lyo-Ject Syringe ... 1018
Cardizem Monovial ... 1018
Cardizem CD Capsules ... 1016
Tiazac Capsules ... 1378

Dirithromycin (Co-administration with other drugs that prolong the QT interval, such as certain oral macrolides, has not been studied and is not recommended). Products include:
Dynabac Tablets ... 2269

Disopyramide Phosphate (Co-administration with class I antiarrhythmics, such as disopyramide, is not recommended because of their potential to prolong refractoriness).
No products indexed under this heading.

Doxepin Hydrochloride (Co-administration with other drugs that prolong the QT interval, such as tricyclic antidepressants, has not been studied and is not recommended). Products include:
Sinequan ... 2713

Ephedrine Hydrochloride (Beta-agonists may have to be administered in increased dosages when used concomitantly with sotalol). Products include:
Primatene Tablets ... ▣780

Ephedrine Sulfate (Beta-agonists may have to be administered in increased dosages when used concomitantly with sotalol).
No products indexed under this heading.

Ephedrine Tannate (Beta-agonists may have to be administered in increased dosages when used concomitantly with sotalol). Products include:
Rynatuss Pediatric Suspension ... 3353
Rynatuss Tablets ... 3353

Epinephrine (Beta-agonists may have to be administered in increased dosages when used concomitantly with sotalol). Products include:
Epifrin Sterile Ophthalmic Solution ... ⊙235
EpiPen ... 1236
Primatene Mist ... ▣779
Xylocaine with Epinephrine Injection ... 653

Epinephrine Hydrochloride (Beta-agonists may have to be administered in increased dosages when used concomitantly with sotalol).
No products indexed under this heading.

Erythromycin (Co-administration with other drugs that prolong the QT interval, such as certain oral macrolides, has not been studied and is not recommended). Products include:
Emgel 2% Topical Gel ... 1285
Ery-Tab Tablets ... 448
Erythromycin Base Filmtab Tablets . 454
Erythromycin Delayed-Release Capsules, USP ... 455
PCE Dispertab Tablets ... 498

Erythromycin Estolate (Co-administration with other drugs that prolong the QT interval, such as certain oral macrolides, has not been studied and is not recommended).
No products indexed under this heading.

Erythromycin Ethylsuccinate (Co-administration with other drugs that prolong the QT interval, such as certain oral macrolides, has not been studied and is not recommended). Products include:
E.E.S. ... 450
EryPed ... 446
Pediazole Suspension ... 3050

Erythromycin Gluceptate (Co-administration with other drugs that prolong the QT interval, such as certain oral macrolides, has not been studied and is not recommended).
No products indexed under this heading.

Erythromycin Stearate (Co-administration with other drugs that prolong the QT interval, such as certain oral macrolides, has not been studied and is not recommended). Products include:
Erythrocin Stearate Filmtab Tablets ... 452

Felodipine (Co-administration with calcium channel blocking drugs can result in possible additive effects on A-V conduction or ventricular function; potential for additive effects on blood pressure, possibly leading to hypotension). Products include:
Lexxel Tablets ... 608
Plendil Extended-Release Tablets ... 623

Fluphenazine Decanoate (Co-administration with other drugs that prolong the QT interval, such as some phenothiazines, has not been studied and is not recommended).
No products indexed under this heading.

Fluphenazine Enanthate (Co-administration with other drugs that prolong the QT interval, such as some phenothiazines, has not been studied and is not recommended).
No products indexed under this heading.

Fluphenazine Hydrochloride (Co-administration with other drugs that prolong the QT interval, such as some phenothiazines, has not been studied and is not recommended).
No products indexed under this heading.

Glimepiride (Hyperglycemia may occur, and the dosage of oral hypoglycemic agents may require adjustment; beta blocker may mask the symptoms of hypoglycemia). Products include:
Amaryl Tablets ... 717

Glipizide (Hyperglycemia may occur, and the dosage of oral hypoglycemic agents may require adjustment; beta blocker may mask the symptoms of hypoglycemia). Products include:
Glucotrol Tablets ... 2692
Glucotrol XL Extended Release Tablets ... 2693

Glyburide (Hyperglycemia may occur, and the dosage of oral hypoglycemic agents may require adjustment; beta blocker may mask the symptoms of hypoglycemia). Products include:
DiaBeta Tablets ... 741
Glucovance Tablets ... 1086

Guanethidine Monosulfate (Co-administration of beta blocker with catecholamine-depleting drugs, such as guanethidine, may produce an excessive reduction of resting sympathetic nervous tone; patients should be closely monitored for evidence of hypotension and/or marked bradycardiawhich may produce syncope).
No products indexed under this heading.

Imipramine Hydrochloride (Co-administration with other drugs that prolong the QT interval, such as tricyclic antidepressants, has not been studied and is not recommended).
No products indexed under this heading.

Imipramine Pamoate (Co-administration with other drugs that prolong the QT interval, such as tricyclic antidepressants, has not been studied and is not recommended).
No products indexed under this heading.

Insulin, Human, Zinc Suspension (Hyperglycemia may occur, and the dosage of insulin may require adjustment; beta blocker may mask the symptoms of hypoglycemia). Products include:
Humulin L, 100 Units ... 1937
Humulin U, 100 Units ... 1943
Novolin L Human Insulin 10 ml Vials ... 2422

Insulin, Human NPH (Hyperglycemia may occur, and the dosage of insulin may require adjustment; beta blocker may mask the symptoms of hypoglycemia). Products include:
Humulin N, 100 Units ... 1939
Humulin N NPH Pen ... 1940
Novolin N Human Insulin 10 ml Vials ... 2422
Novolin N PenFill ... 2423
Novolin N Prefilled Syringe Disposable Insulin Delivery System ... 2425

Insulin, Human Regular (Hyperglycemia may occur, and the dosage of insulin may require adjustment; beta blocker may mask the symptoms of hypoglycemia). Products include:
Humulin R Regular (U-500) ... 1943
Humulin R, 100 Units ... 1941
Novolin R Human Insulin 10 ml Vials ... 2423
Novolin R PenFill ... 2423
Novolin R Prefilled Syringe Disposable Insulin Delivery System ... 2425
Velosulin BR Human Insulin 10 ml Vials ... 2435

Insulin, Human Regular and Human NPH Mixture (Hyperglycemia may occur, and the dosage of insulin may require adjustment; beta blocker may mask the symptoms of hypoglycemia). Products include:
Humulin 50/50, 100 Units ... 1934
Humulin 70/30, 100 Units ... 1935
Humulin 70/30 Pen ... 1936
Novolin 70/30 Human Insulin 10 ml Vials ... 2421
Novolin 70/30 PenFill ... 2423
Novolin 70/30 Prefilled Disposable Insulin Delivery System ... 2425

Insulin, NPH (Hyperglycemia may occur, and the dosage of insulin may require adjustment; beta blocker may mask the symptoms of hypoglycemia). Products include:
Iletin II, NPH (Pork), 100 Units ... 1946

Insulin, Regular (Hyperglycemia may occur, and the dosage of insulin may require adjustment; beta blocker may mask the symptoms of hypoglycemia). Products include:
Iletin II, Regular (Pork), 100 Units ... 1947

Insulin, Zinc Crystals (Hyperglycemia may occur, and the dosage of insulin may require adjustment; beta blocker may mask the symptoms of hypoglycemia).
No products indexed under this heading.

Insulin, Zinc Suspension (Hyperglycemia may occur, and the dosage of insulin may require adjustment; beta blocker may mask the symptoms of hypoglycemia). Products include:
Iletin II, Lente (Pork), 100 Units ... 1945

Insulin Aspart, Human Regular (Hyperglycemia may occur, and the dosage of insulin may require adjustment; beta blocker may mask the symptoms of hypoglycemia).
No products indexed under this heading.

Insulin glargine (Hyperglycemia may occur, and the dosage of insulin may require adjustment; beta blocker may mask the symptoms of hypoglycemia). Products include:
Lantus Injection ... 742

Insulin Lispro, Human (Hyperglycemia may occur, and the dosage of insulin may require adjustment; beta blocker may mask the symptoms of hypoglycemia). Products include:
Humalog ... 1926
Humalog Mix 75/25 Pen ... 1928

Insulin Lispro Protamine, Human (Hyperglycemia may occur, and the dosage of insulin may require adjustment; beta blocker may mask the symptoms of hypoglycemia). Products include:
Humalog Mix 75/25 Pen ... 1928

Isoetharine (Beta-agonists may have to be administered in increased dosages when used concomitantly with sotalol).
No products indexed under this heading.

Isoproterenol Hydrochloride (Beta-agonists may have to be administered in increased dosages when used concomitantly with sotalol).
No products indexed under this heading.

Isoproterenol Sulfate (Beta-agonists may have to be administered in increased dosages when used concomitantly with sotalol).
No products indexed under this heading.

Isradipine (Co-administration with calcium channel blocking drugs can result in possible additive effects on A-V conduction or ventricular function; potential for additive effects on blood pressure, possibly leading to hypotension). Products include:
DynaCirc Capsules ... 2921
DynaCirc CR Tablets ... 2923

Levalbuterol Hydrochloride (Beta-agonists may have to be

administered in increased dosages when used concomitantly with sotalol). Products include:

Xopenex Inhalation Solution 3207

Magaldrate (Co-administration within 2 hours of antacids containing aluminum oxide and magnesium hydroxide should be avoided because it may result in a reduction in Cmax and AUC of 26% and 20% respectively and consequently in a 20% reduction in the bradycardic effect at rest).

No products indexed under this heading.

Magnesium Hydroxide (Co-administration within 2 hours of antacids containing aluminum oxide and magnesium hydroxide should be avoided because it may result in a reduction in Cmax and AUC of 26% and 20% respectively and consequently in a 20% reduction in the bradycardic effect at rest). Products include:

Ex•Lax Milk of Magnesia Liquid 670
Maalox Antacid/Anti-Gas Oral Suspension 673
Maalox Max Maximum Strength Antacid/Anti-Gas Liquid 2300
Maalox Regular Strength Antacid/Antigas Liquid 2300
Mylanta Fast-Acting 1813
Mylanta 1813
Pepcid Complete Chewable Tablets 1815
Phillips' Chewable Tablets 615
Phillips' Milk of Magnesia Liquid (Original, Cherry, & Mint) 616
Rolaids Tablets 706
Extra Strength Rolaids Tablets 706
Vanquish Caplets 617

Magnesium Oxide (Co-administration within 2 hours of antacids containing aluminum oxide and magnesium hydroxide should be avoided because it may result in a reduction in Cmax and AUC of 26% and 20% respectively and consequently in a 20% reduction in the bradycardic effect at rest). Products include:

Beelith Tablets 946
Mag-Ox 400 Tablets 1024
Uro-Mag Capsules 1024

Maprotiline Hydrochloride (Co-administration with other drugs that prolong the QT interval, such as tricyclic antidepressants, has not been studied and is not recommended).

No products indexed under this heading.

Mesoridazine Besylate (Co-administration with other drugs that prolong the QT interval, such as some phenothiazines, has not been studied and is not recommended). Products include:

Serentil 1057

Metaproterenol Sulfate (Beta-agonists may have to be administered in increased dosages when used concomitantly with sotalol). Products include:

Alupent 1029

Metformin Hydrochloride (Hyperglycemia may occur, and the dosage of oral hypoglycemic agents may require adjustment; beta blocker may mask the symptoms of hypoglycemia). Products include:

Glucophage Tablets 1080
Glucophage XR Tablets 1080
Glucovance Tablets 1086

Methotrimeprazine (Co-administration with other drugs that prolong the QT interval, such as some phenothiazines, has not been studied and is not recommended).

No products indexed under this heading.

Mibefradil Dihydrochloride (Co-administration with calcium channel blocking drugs can result in possible additive effects on A-V conduction or ventricular function; potential for additive effects on blood pressure, possibly leading to hypotension).

No products indexed under this heading.

Miglitol (Hyperglycemia may occur, and the dosage of oral hypoglycemic agents may require adjustment; beta blocker may mask the symptoms of hypoglycemia). Products include:

Glyset Tablets 2821

Nicardipine Hydrochloride (Co-administration with calcium channel blocking drugs can result in possible additive effects on A-V conduction or ventricular function; potential for additive effects on blood pressure, possibly leading to hypotension). Products include:

Cardene I.V. 3485

Nifedipine (Co-administration with calcium channel blocking drugs can result in possible additive effects on A-V conduction or ventricular function; potential for additive effects on blood pressure, possibly leading to hypotension). Products include:

Adalat CC Tablets 877
Procardia Capsules 2708
Procardia XL Extended Release Tablets 2710

Nimodipine (Co-administration with calcium channel blocking drugs can result in possible additive effects on A-V conduction or ventricular function; potential for additive effects on blood pressure, possibly leading to hypotension). Products include:

Nimotop Capsules 904

Nisoldipine (Co-administration with calcium channel blocking drugs can result in possible additive effects on A-V conduction or ventricular function; potential for additive effects on blood pressure, possibly leading to hypotension). Products include:

Sular Tablets 688

Nortriptyline Hydrochloride (Co-administration with other drugs that prolong the QT interval, such as tricyclic antidepressants, has not been studied and is not recommended).

No products indexed under this heading.

Perphenazine (Co-administration with other drugs that prolong the QT interval, such as some phenothiazines, has not been studied and is not recommended). Products include:

Etrafon 3115
Trilafon 3160

Pioglitazone Hydrochloride (Hyperglycemia may occur, and the dosage of oral hypoglycemic agents may require adjustment; beta blocker may mask the symptoms of hypoglycemia). Products include:

Actos Tablets 3275

Pirbuterol Acetate (Beta-agonists may have to be administered in increased dosages when used concomitantly with sotalol). Products include:

Maxair Autohaler 1981
Maxair Inhaler 1984

Procainamide Hydrochloride (Co-administration with class I antiarrhythmics, such as procainamide, is not recommended because of their potential to prolong refractoriness). Products include:

Procanbid Extended-Release Tablets 2262

Prochlorperazine (Co-administration with other drugs that prolong the QT interval, such as some phenothiazines, has not been studied and is not recommended). Products include:

Compazine 1505

Promethazine Hydrochloride (Co-administration with other drugs that prolong the QT interval, such as some phenothiazines, has not been studied and is not recommended). Products include:

Mepergan Injection 3539
Phenergan Injection 3553
Phenergan 3556
Phenergan Syrup 3554
Phenergan with Codeine Syrup 3557
Phenergan with Dextromethorphan Syrup 3559
Phenergan VC Syrup 3560
Phenergan VC with Codeine Syrup .. 3561

Protriptyline Hydrochloride (Co-administration with other drugs that prolong the QT interval, such as tricyclic antidepressants, has not been studied and is not recommended). Products include:

Vivactil Tablets 2446
Vivactil Tablets 2217

Quinidine Gluconate (Co-administration with class I antiarrhythmics, such as quinidine, is not recommended because of their potential to prolong refractoriness). Products include:

Quinaglute Dura-Tabs Tablets 978

Quinidine Polygalacturonate (Co-administration with class I antiarrhythmics, such as quinidine, is not recommended because of their potential to prolong refractoriness).

No products indexed under this heading.

Quinidine Sulfate (Co-administration with class I antiarrhythmics, such as quinidine, is not recommended because of their potential to prolong refractoriness). Products include:

Quinidex Extentabs 2933

Repaglinide (Hyperglycemia may occur, and the dosage of oral hypoglycemic agents may require adjustment; beta blocker may mask the symptoms of hypoglycemia). Products include:

Prandin Tablets (0.5, 1, and 2 mg) 2432

Reserpine (Co-administration of beta blocker with catecholamine-depleting drugs, such as reserpine, may produce an excessive reduction of resting sympathetic nervous tone; patients should be closely monitored for evidence of hypotension and/or marked bradycardia which may produce syncope).

No products indexed under this heading.

Rosiglitazone Maleate (Hyperglycemia may occur, and the dosage of oral hypoglycemic agents may require adjustment; beta blocker may mask the symptoms of hypoglycemia). Products include:

Avandia Tablets 1490

Salmeterol Xinafoate (Beta-agonists may have to be administered in increased dosages when used concomitantly with sotalol). Products include:

Advair Diskus 100/50 1448
Advair Diskus 250/50 1448
Advair Diskus 500/50 1448
Serevent Diskus 1637
Serevent Inhalation Aerosol 1633

Terbutaline Sulfate (Beta-agonists may have to be administered in increased dosages when used concomitantly with sotalol). Products include:

Brethine Ampuls 2314
Brethine Tablets 2313

Thioridazine Hydrochloride (Co-administration with other drugs that prolong the QT interval, such as some phenothiazines, has not been studied and is not recommended). Products include:

Thioridazine Hydrochloride Tablets 2289

Tolazamide (Hyperglycemia may occur, and the dosage of oral hypoglycemic agents may require adjustment; beta blocker may mask the symptoms of hypoglycemia).

No products indexed under this heading.

Tolbutamide (Hyperglycemia may occur, and the dosage of oral hypoglycemic agents may require adjustment; beta blocker may mask the symptoms of hypoglycemia).

No products indexed under this heading.

Trifluoperazine Hydrochloride (Co-administration with other drugs that prolong the QT interval, such as some phenothiazines, has not been studied and is not recommended). Products include:

Stelazine 1640

Trimipramine Maleate (Co-administration with other drugs that prolong the QT interval, such as tricyclic antidepressants, has not been studied and is not recommended). Products include:

Surmontil Capsules 3595

Troglitazone (Hyperglycemia may occur, and the dosage of oral hypoglycemic agents may require adjustment; beta blocker may mask the symptoms of hypoglycemia).

No products indexed under this heading.

Troleandomycin (Co-administration with other drugs that prolong the QT interval, such as certain oral macrolides, has not been studied and is not recommended). Products include:

Tao Capsules 2716

Verapamil Hydrochloride (Co-administration with calcium channel blocking drugs can result in possible additive effects on A-V conduction or ventricular function; potential for additive effects on blood pressure, possibly leading to hypotension). Products include:

Covera-HS Tablets 3199
Isoptin SR Tablets 467
Tarka Tablets 508
Verelan Capsules 3184
Verelan PM Capsules 3186

BETASEPT SURGICAL SCRUB

(Chlorhexidine Gluconate) 2895
None cited in PDR database.

BETASERON FOR SC INJECTION

(Interferon Beta-1b) 988
None cited in PDR database.

BETAXON OPHTHALMIC SUSPENSION

(Levobetaxolol Hydrochloride) 537
May interact with adrenergic augmenting psychotropics, beta blockers, and certain other agents. Compounds in these categories include:

Acebutolol Hydrochloride (Co-administration with oral beta-adrenergic blocking agents may result in potential additive effects on systemic beta-blockade). Products include:

Sectral Capsules 3589

Atenolol (Co-administration with oral beta-adrenergic blocking agents may result in potential additive effects on systemic beta-blockade). Products include:

Tenoretic Tablets 690
Tenormin I.V. Injection 692

Betaxolol Hydrochloride (Co-administration with oral beta-adrenergic blocking agents may result in potential additive effects on systemic beta-blockade). Products include:

Betoptic S Ophthalmic Suspension 537

Bisoprolol Fumarate (Co-administration with oral beta-adrenergic blocking agents may result in potential additive effects on systemic beta-blockade). Products include:

Zebeta Tablets 1885
Ziac Tablets 1887

Carteolol Hydrochloride (Co-administration with oral beta-adrener-

gic blocking agents may result in potential additive effects on systemic beta-blockade). Products include:
- Carteolol Hydrochloride Ophthalmic Solution USP, 1% ..... ⊙ 258
- Ocupress Ophthalmic Solution, 1% Sterile ..... ⊙ 303

Epinephrine (Concurrent use in patients with history of atopy or severe anaphylactic reaction to allergens may be unresponsive to the usual doses of epinephrine used to treat anaphylactic reaction). Products include:
- Epifrin Sterile Ophthalmic Solution ..... ⊙ 235
- EpiPen 1236
- Primatene Mist ..... ▣ 779
- Xylocaine with Epinephrine Injection 653

Epinephrine Hydrochloride (Concurrent use in patients with history of atopy or severe anaphylactic reaction to allergens may be unresponsive to the usual doses of epinephrine used to treat anaphylactic reaction).
No products indexed under this heading.

Esmolol Hydrochloride (Co-administration with oral beta-adrenergic blocking agents may result in potential additive effects on systemic beta-blockade). Products include:
- Brevibloc Injection 858

Guanethidine Monosulfate (Co-administration with catecholamine-depleting drugs, such as guanethidine, may result in possible additive effects and production of hypotension and/or bradycardia).
No products indexed under this heading.

Isocarboxazid (Levobetaxolol is an adrenergic blocking agent; therefore, caution should be exercised in patients using concomitant adrenergic psychotropic drugs).
No products indexed under this heading.

Labetalol Hydrochloride (Co-administration with oral beta-adrenergic blocking agents may result in potential additive effects on systemic beta-blockade). Products include:
- Normodyne Injection 3135
- Normodyne Tablets 3137

Levobunolol Hydrochloride (Co-administration with oral beta-adrenergic blocking agents may result in potential additive effects on systemic beta-blockade). Products include:
- Betagan ..... ⊙ 228

Metipranolol Hydrochloride (Co-administration with oral beta-adrenergic blocking agents may result in potential additive effects on systemic beta-blockade).
No products indexed under this heading.

Metoprolol Succinate (Co-administration with oral beta-adrenergic blocking agents may result in potential additive effects on systemic beta-blockade). Products include:
- Toprol-XL Tablets 651

Metoprolol Tartrate (Co-administration with oral beta-adrenergic blocking agents may result in potential additive effects on systemic beta-blockade).
No products indexed under this heading.

Nadolol (Co-administration with oral beta-adrenergic blocking agents may result in potential additive effects on systemic beta-blockade). Products include:
- Corgard Tablets 2245
- Corzide 40/5 Tablets 2247
- Corzide 80/5 Tablets 2247
- Nadolol Tablets 2288

Pargyline Hydrochloride (Levobetaxolol is an adrenergic blocking agent; therefore, caution should be exercised in patients using concomitant adrenergic psychotropic drugs).
No products indexed under this heading.

Penbutolol Sulfate (Co-administration with oral beta-adrenergic blocking agents may result in potential additive effects on systemic beta-blockade).
No products indexed under this heading.

Phenelzine Sulfate (Levobetaxolol is an adrenergic blocking agent; therefore, caution should be exercised in patients using concomitant adrenergic psychotropic drugs). Products include:
- Nardil Tablets 2653

Pindolol (Co-administration with oral beta-adrenergic blocking agents may result in potential additive effects on systemic beta-blockade).
No products indexed under this heading.

Propranolol Hydrochloride (Co-administration with oral beta-adrenergic blocking agents may result in potential additive effects on systemic beta-blockade). Products include:
- Inderal 3513
- Inderal LA Long-Acting Capsules 3516
- Inderide Tablets 3517
- Inderide LA Long-Acting Capsules 3519

Reserpine (Co-administration with catecholamine-depleting drugs, such as reserpine, may result in possible additive effects and production of hypotension and/or bradycardia).
No products indexed under this heading.

Sotalol Hydrochloride (Co-administration with oral beta-adrenergic blocking agents may result in potential additive effects on systemic beta-blockade). Products include:
- Betapace Tablets 950
- Betapace AF Tablets 954

Timolol Hemihydrate (Co-administration with oral beta-adrenergic blocking agents may result in potential additive effects on systemic beta-blockade). Products include:
- Betimol Ophthalmic Solution ..... ⊙ 324

Timolol Maleate (Co-administration with oral beta-adrenergic blocking agents may result in potential additive effects on systemic beta-blockade). Products include:
- Blocadren Tablets 2046
- Cosopt Sterile Ophthalmic Solution 2065
- Timolide Tablets 2187
- Timolol GFS ..... ⊙ 266
- Timoptic in Ocudose 2192
- Timoptic Sterile Ophthalmic Solution 2190
- Timoptic-XE Sterile Ophthalmic Gel Forming Solution 2194

Tranylcypromine Sulfate (Levobetaxolol is an adrenergic blocking agent; therefore, caution should be exercised in patients using concomitant adrenergic psychotropic drugs). Products include:
- Parnate Tablets 1607

BETIMOL OPHTHALMIC SOLUTION

(Timolol Hemihydrate) ..... ⊙ 324
May interact with beta blockers, calcium channel blockers, cardiac glycosides, and certain other agents. Compounds in these categories include:

Acebutolol Hydrochloride (Concurrent use with systemic beta blockers may result in additive effect either on the intraocular pressure or the known systemic effect of beta blockade). Products include:
- Sectral Capsules 3589

Amlodipine Besylate (Possible atrioventricular conduction disturbances, left ventricular failure, and hypotension). Products include:
- Lotrel Capsules 2370
- Norvasc Tablets 2704

Atenolol (Concurrent use with systemic beta blockers may result in additive effect either on the intraocular pressure or the known systemic effect of beta blockade). Products include:
- Tenoretic Tablets 690
- Tenormin I.V. Injection 692

Bepridil Hydrochloride (Possible atrioventricular conduction disturbances, left ventricular failure, and hypotension). Products include:
- Vascor Tablets 2602

Betaxolol Hydrochloride (Concurrent use with systemic beta blockers may result in additive effect either on the intraocular pressure or the known systemic effect of beta blockade). Products include:
- Betoptic S Ophthalmic Suspension 537

Bisoprolol Fumarate (Concurrent use with systemic beta blockers may result in additive effect either on the intraocular pressure or the known systemic effect of beta blockade). Products include:
- Zebeta Tablets 1885
- Ziac Tablets 1887

Carteolol Hydrochloride (Concurrent use with systemic beta blockers may result in additive effect either on the intraocular pressure or the known systemic effect of beta blockade). Products include:
- Carteolol Hydrochloride Ophthalmic Solution USP, 1% ..... ⊙ 258
- Ocupress Ophthalmic Solution, 1% Sterile ..... ⊙ 303

Deslanoside (Concomitant use of beta blockers with digitalis and calcium antagonists may have additive effects in prolonging atrioventricular conduction time).
No products indexed under this heading.

Digitoxin (Concomitant use of beta blockers with digitalis and calcium antagonists may have additive effects in prolonging atrioventricular conduction time).
No products indexed under this heading.

Digoxin (Concomitant use of beta blockers with digitalis and calcium antagonists may have additive effects in prolonging atrioventricular conduction time). Products include:
- Digitek Tablets 1003
- Lanoxicaps Capsules 1574
- Lanoxin Injection 1581
- Lanoxin Tablets 1587
- Lanoxin Elixir Pediatric 1578
- Lanoxin Injection Pediatric 1584

Diltiazem Hydrochloride (Possible atrioventricular conduction disturbances, left ventricular failure, and hypotension). Products include:
- Cardizem Injectable 1018
- Cardizem Lyo-Ject Syringe 1018
- Cardizem Monovial 1018
- Cardizem CD Capsules 1016
- Tiazac Capsules 1378

Epinephrine (Patients with a history of atopy or anaphylactic reactions to a variety of allergens may be unresponsive to the usual dose of injectable epinephrine used to treat allergic reactions). Products include:
- Epifrin Sterile Ophthalmic Solution ..... ⊙ 235
- EpiPen 1236
- Primatene Mist ..... ▣ 779
- Xylocaine with Epinephrine Injection 653

Epinephrine Bitartrate (Patients with a history of atopy or anaphylactic reactions to a variety of allergens may be unresponsive to the usual dose of injectable epinephrine used to treat allergic reactions). Products include:
- Sensorcaine 643

Esmolol Hydrochloride (Concurrent use with systemic beta blockers may result in additive effect either on the intraocular pressure or the known systemic effect of beta blockade). Products include:
- Brevibloc Injection 858

Felodipine (Possible atrioventricular conduction disturbances, left ventricular failure, and hypotension). Products include:
- Lexxel Tablets 608
- Plendil Extended-Release Tablets 623

Isradipine (Possible atrioventricular conduction disturbances, left ventricular failure, and hypotension). Products include:
- DynaCirc Capsules 2921
- DynaCirc CR Tablets 2923

Labetalol Hydrochloride (Concurrent use with systemic beta blockers may result in additive effect either on the intraocular pressure or the known systemic effect of beta blockade). Products include:
- Normodyne Injection 3135
- Normodyne Tablets 3137

Levobunolol Hydrochloride (Concurrent use with systemic beta blockers may result in additive effect either on the intraocular pressure or the known systemic effect of beta blockade). Products include:
- Betagan ..... ⊙ 228

Metipranolol Hydrochloride (Concurrent use with systemic beta blockers may result in additive effect either on the intraocular pressure or the known systemic effect of beta blockade).
No products indexed under this heading.

Metoprolol Succinate (Concurrent use with systemic beta blockers may result in additive effect either on the intraocular pressure or the known systemic effect of beta blockade). Products include:
- Toprol-XL Tablets 651

Metoprolol Tartrate (Concurrent use with systemic beta blockers may result in additive effect either on the intraocular pressure or the known systemic effect of beta blockade).
No products indexed under this heading.

Mibefradil Dihydrochloride (Possible atrioventricular conduction disturbances, left ventricular failure, and hypotension).
No products indexed under this heading.

Nadolol (Concurrent use with systemic beta blockers may result in additive effect either on the intraocular pressure or the known systemic effect of beta blockade). Products include:
- Corgard Tablets 2245
- Corzide 40/5 Tablets 2247
- Corzide 80/5 Tablets 2247
- Nadolol Tablets 2288

Nicardipine Hydrochloride (Possible atrioventricular conduction disturbances, left ventricular failure, and hypotension). Products include:
- Cardene I.V. 3485

Nifedipine (Possible atrioventricular conduction disturbances, left ventricular failure, and hypotension). Products include:
- Adalat CC Tablets 877
- Procardia Capsules 2708
- Procardia XL Extended Release Tablets 2710

Nimodipine (Possible atrioventricular conduction disturbances, left ventricular failure, and hypotension). Products include:
- Nimotop Capsules 904

Nisoldipine (Possible atrioventricular conduction disturbances, left ventricular failure, and hypotension). Products include:
- Sular Tablets 688

Penbutolol Sulfate (Concurrent use with systemic beta blockers may

result in additive effect either on the intraocular pressure or the known systemic effect of beta blockade).
No products indexed under this heading.

Pindolol (Concurrent use with systemic beta blockers may result in additive effect either on the intraocular pressure or the known systemic effect of beta blockade).
No products indexed under this heading.

Propranolol Hydrochloride (Concurrent use with systemic beta blockers may result in additive effect either on the intraocular pressure or the known systemic effect of beta blockade). Products include:
Inderal 3513
Inderal LA Long-Acting Capsules 3516
Inderide Tablets 3517
Inderide LA Long-Acting Capsules .. 3519

Sotalol Hydrochloride (Concurrent use with systemic beta blockers may result in additive effect either on the intraocular pressure or the known systemic effect of beta blockade). Products include:
Betapace Tablets 950
Betapace AF Tablets 954

Timolol Maleate (Concurrent use with systemic beta blockers may result in additive effect either on the intraocular pressure or the known systemic effect of beta blockade). Products include:
Blocadren Tablets 2046
Cosopt Sterile Ophthalmic Solution 2065
Timolide Tablets 2187
Timolol GFS .... ⊙266
Timoptic in Ocudose 2192
Timoptic Sterile Ophthalmic Solution 2190
Timoptic-XE Sterile Ophthalmic Gel Forming Solution 2194

Verapamil Hydrochloride (Possible atrioventricular conduction disturbances, left ventricular failure, and hypotension). Products include:
Covera-HS Tablets 3199
Isoptin SR Tablets 467
Tarka Tablets 508
Verelan Capsules 3184
Verelan PM Capsules 3186

BETOPTIC S OPHTHALMIC SUSPENSION

(Betaxolol Hydrochloride) 537
May interact with adrenergic augmenting psychotropics, beta blockers, and certain other agents. Compounds in these categories include:

Acebutolol Hydrochloride (Co-administration with oral beta blockers may result in additive effects either on intraocular pressure or on the known systemic effects of beta blockade). Products include:
Sectral Capsules 3589

Atenolol (Co-administration with oral beta blockers may result in additive effects either on intraocular pressure or on the known systemic effects of beta blockade). Products include:
Tenoretic Tablets 690
Tenormin I.V. Injection 692

Bisoprolol Fumarate (Co-administration with oral beta blockers may result in additive effects either on intraocular pressure or on the known systemic effects of beta blockade). Products include:
Zebeta Tablets 1885
Ziac Tablets 1887

Carteolol Hydrochloride (Co-administration with oral beta blockers may result in additive effects either on intraocular pressure or on the known systemic effects of beta blockade). Products include:
Carteolol Hydrochloride Ophthalmic Solution USP, 1% .... ⊙258
Ocupress Ophthalmic Solution, 1% Sterile .... ⊙303

Deserpidine (Possible additive effects and production of hypotension and/or bradycardia when beta blocker is concurrently used with catecholamine depleting drugs).
No products indexed under this heading.

Epinephrine (Concurrent use in patients with history of atopy or severe anaphylactic reaction to allergens may be unresponsive to the usual doses of epinephrine used to treat anaphylactic reaction). Products include:
Epifrin Sterile Ophthalmic Solution .... ⊙235
EpiPen 1236
Primatene Mist 779
Xylocaine with Epinephrine Injection 653

Epinephrine Hydrochloride (Concurrent use in patients with history of atopy or severe anaphylactic reaction to allergens may be unresponsive to the usual doses of epinephrine used to treat anaphylactic reaction).
No products indexed under this heading.

Esmolol Hydrochloride (Co-administration with oral beta blockers may result in additive effects either on intraocular pressure or on the known systemic effects of beta blockade). Products include:
Brevibloc Injection 858

Isocarboxazid (Exercise caution when used concurrently with adrenergic psychotropic drugs).
No products indexed under this heading.

Labetalol Hydrochloride (Co-administration with oral beta blockers may result in additive effects either on intraocular pressure or on the known systemic effects of beta blockade). Products include:
Normodyne Injection 3135
Normodyne Tablets 3137

Levobunolol Hydrochloride (Co-administration with oral beta blockers may result in additive effects either on intraocular pressure or on the known systemic effects of beta blockade). Products include:
Betagan .... ⊙228

Metipranolol Hydrochloride (Co-administration with oral beta blockers may result in additive effects either on intraocular pressure or on the known systemic effects of beta blockade).
No products indexed under this heading.

Metoprolol Succinate (Co-administration with oral beta blockers may result in additive effects either on intraocular pressure or on the known systemic effects of beta blockade). Products include:
Toprol-XL Tablets 651

Metoprolol Tartrate (Co-administration with oral beta blockers may result in additive effects either on intraocular pressure or on the known systemic effects of beta blockade).
No products indexed under this heading.

Nadolol (Co-administration with oral beta blockers may result in additive effects either on intraocular pressure or on the known systemic effects of beta blockade). Products include:
Corgard Tablets 2245
Corzide 40/5 Tablets 2247
Corzide 80/5 Tablets 2247
Nadolol Tablets 2288

Pargyline Hydrochloride (Exercise caution when used concurrently with adrenergic psychotropic drugs).
No products indexed under this heading.

Penbutolol Sulfate (Co-administration with oral beta blockers may result in additive effects either on intraocular pressure or on the known systemic effects of beta blockade).
No products indexed under this heading.

Phenelzine Sulfate (Exercise caution when used concurrently with adrenergic psychotropic drugs). Products include:
Nardil Tablets 2653

Pindolol (Co-administration with oral beta blockers may result in additive effects either on intraocular pressure or on the known systemic effects of beta blockade).
No products indexed under this heading.

Propranolol Hydrochloride (Co-administration with oral beta blockers may result in additive effects either on intraocular pressure or on the known systemic effects of beta blockade). Products include:
Inderal 3513
Inderal LA Long-Acting Capsules 3516
Inderide Tablets 3517
Inderide LA Long-Acting Capsules .. 3519

Rauwolfia serpentina (Possible additive effects and production of hypotension and/or bradycardia when beta blocker is concurrently used with catecholamine depleting drugs).
No products indexed under this heading.

Rescinnamine (Possible additive effects and production of hypotension and/or bradycardia when beta blocker is concurrently used with catecholamine depleting drugs).
No products indexed under this heading.

Reserpine (Possible additive effects and production of hypotension and/or bradycardia when beta blocker is concurrently used with catecholamine depleting drugs).
No products indexed under this heading.

Sotalol Hydrochloride (Co-administration with oral beta blockers may result in additive effects either on intraocular pressure or on the known systemic effects of beta blockade). Products include:
Betapace Tablets 950
Betapace AF Tablets 954

Timolol Hemihydrate (Co-administration with oral beta blockers may result in additive effects either on intraocular pressure or on the known systemic effects of beta blockade). Products include:
Betimol Ophthalmic Solution .... ⊙324

Timolol Maleate (Co-administration with oral beta blockers may result in additive effects either on intraocular pressure or on the known systemic effects of beta blockade). Products include:
Blocadren Tablets 2046
Cosopt Sterile Ophthalmic Solution 2065
Timolide Tablets 2187
Timolol GFS .... ⊙266
Timoptic in Ocudose 2192
Timoptic Sterile Ophthalmic Solution 2190
Timoptic-XE Sterile Ophthalmic Gel Forming Solution 2194

Tranylcypromine Sulfate (Exercise caution when used concurrently with adrenergic psychotropic drugs). Products include:
Parnate Tablets 1607

BEVITAMEL TABLETS

(Folic Acid, Melatonin, Vitamin B_{12}) 3459
None cited in PDR database.

BIAXIN FILMTAB TABLETS

(Clarithromycin) 403
May interact with oral anticoagulants, oral hypoglycemic agents, insulin, phenytoin, valproate, theophylline, and certain other agents. Compounds in these categories include:

Acarbose (Clarithromycin, in rare cases, causes hypoglycemia, some of which have occurred in patients taking oral hypoglycemic agents). Products include:
Precose Tablets 906

Alfentanil Hydrochloride (Concurrent use of erythromycin and/or clarithromycin in patients receiving drugs metabolized by the cytochrome P450 system may be associated with elevation in serum levels of alfentanil).
No products indexed under this heading.

Aminophylline (Co-administration in patients who are receiving high doses of theophylline may be associated with an increase in serum theophylline levels and potential theophylline toxicity).
No products indexed under this heading.

Astemizole (Concurrent use of erythromycin in patients receiving astemizole has resulted in prolonged QT interval and torsade de pointes; because clarithromycin is metabolized by P450, co-administration is not recommended).
No products indexed under this heading.

Bromocriptine Mesylate (Concurrent use of erythromycin and/or clarithromycin in patients receiving drugs metabolized by the cytochrome P450 system may be associated with elevation in serum levels of bromocriptine).
No products indexed under this heading.

Carbamazepine (Potential for increased serum concentration of carbamazepine). Products include:
Carbatrol Capsules 3234
Tegretol/Tegretol-XR 2404

Chlorpropamide (Clarithromycin, in rare cases, causes hypoglycemia, some of which have occurred in patients taking oral hypoglycemic agents). Products include:
Diabinese Tablets 2680

Cisapride (Concurrent use of erythromycin and/or clarithromycin in patients receiving cisapride has been reported to result in rare cases of cardiovascular adverse events including prolonged QT interval, ventricular tachycardia, ventricular fibrillation, and torsade de pointes, and death have been reported; co-administration is contraindicated).
No products indexed under this heading.

Cyclosporine (Concurrent use of erythromycin and/or clarithromycin in patients receiving drugs metabolized by the cytochrome P450 system may be associated with elevation in serum levels of cyclosporine). Products include:
Gengraf Capsules 457
Neoral Soft Gelatin Capsules 2380
Neoral Oral Solution 2380
Sandimmune 2388

Dicumarol (Co-administration may result in the potentiation of oral anticoagulant effects).
No products indexed under this heading.

Digoxin (Concomitant use has resulted in elevated digoxin serum concentrations and some patients have shown signs of digoxin toxicity, including arrhythmias). Products include:
Digitek Tablets 1003
Lanoxicaps Capsules 1574

Lanoxin Injection 1581
Lanoxin Tablets 1587
Lanoxin Elixir Pediatric 1578
Lanoxin Injection Pediatric 1584

Dihydroergotamine Mesylate (Co-administration has been associated in some patients with acute ergot toxicity characterized by severe peripheral vasospasm and dysesthesia). Products include:
D.H.E. 45 Injection 2334
Migranal Nasal Spray 2376

Disopyramide Phosphate (Concurrent use of erythromycin and/or clarithromycin in patients receiving drugs metabolized by the cytochrome P450 system may be associated with elevation in serum levels of disopyramide).
No products indexed under this heading.

Divalproex Sodium (Concurrent use of erythromycin and/or clarithromycin in patients receiving drugs metabolized by the cytochrome P450 system may be associated with elevation in serum levels of valproate). Products include:
Depakote Sprinkle Capsules 426
Depakote Tablets 430
Depakote ER Tablets 436

Dyphylline (Co-administration in patients who are receiving high doses of theophylline may be associated with an increase in serum theophylline levels and potential theophylline toxicity). Products include:
Lufyllin Tablets 3347
Lufyllin-400 Tablets 3347
Lufyllin-GG Elixir 3348
Lufyllin-GG Tablets 3348

Ergotamine Tartrate (Co-administration has been associated in some patients with acute ergot toxicity characterized by severe peripheral vasospasm and dysesthesia).
No products indexed under this heading.

Fluconazole (Co-administration has resulted in increases in the mean steady-state clarithromycin Cmin and AUC). Products include:
Diflucan Tablets, Injection, and Oral Suspension 2681

Fosphenytoin Sodium (Concurrent use of erythromycin and/or clarithromycin in patients receiving drugs metabolized by the cytochrome P450 system may be associated with elevation in serum levels of phenytoin). Products include:
Cerebyx Injection 2619

Glimepiride (Clarithromycin, in rare cases, causes hypoglycemia, some of which have occurred in patients taking oral hypoglycemic agents). Products include:
Amaryl Tablets 717

Glipizide (Clarithromycin, in rare cases, causes hypoglycemia, some of which have occurred in patients taking oral hypoglycemic agents). Products include:
Glucotrol Tablets 2692
Glucotrol XL Extended Release Tablets 2693

Glyburide (Clarithromycin, in rare cases, causes hypoglycemia, some of which have occurred in patients taking oral hypoglycemic agents). Products include:
DiaBeta Tablets 741
Glucovance Tablets 1086

Hexobarbital (Concurrent use of erythromycin and/or clarithromycin in patients receiving drugs metabolized by the cytochrome P450 system may be associated with elevation in serum levels of hexobarbital).

Insulin, Human, Zinc Suspension (Clarithromycin, in rare cases, causes hypoglycemia, some of which have occurred in patients taking insulin). Products include:
Humulin L, 100 Units 1937
Humulin U, 100 Units 1943
Novolin L Human Insulin 10 ml Vials 2422

Insulin, Human NPH (Clarithromycin, in rare cases, causes hypoglycemia, some of which have occurred in patients taking insulin). Products include:
Humulin N, 100 Units 1939
Humulin N NPH Pen 1940
Novolin N Human Insulin 10 ml Vials 2422
Novolin N PenFill 2423
Novolin N Prefilled Syringe Disposable Insulin Delivery System 2425

Insulin, Human Regular (Clarithromycin, in rare cases, causes hypoglycemia, some of which have occurred in patients taking insulin). Products include:
Humulin R Regular (U-500) 1943
Humulin R, 100 Units 1941
Novolin R Human Insulin 10 ml Vials 2423
Novolin R PenFill 2423
Novolin R Prefilled Syringe Disposable Insulin Delivery System 2425
Velosulin BR Human Insulin 10 ml Vials 2435

Insulin, Human Regular and Human NPH Mixture (Clarithromycin, in rare cases, causes hypoglycemia, some of which have occurred in patients taking insulin). Products include:
Humulin 50/50, 100 Units 1934
Humulin 70/30, 100 Units 1935
Humulin 70/30 Pen 1936
Novolin 70/30 Human Insulin 10 ml Vials 2421
Novolin 70/30 PenFill 2423
Novolin 70/30 Prefilled Disposable Insulin Delivery System 2425

Insulin, NPH (Clarithromycin, in rare cases, causes hypoglycemia, some of which have occurred in patients taking insulin). Products include:
Iletin II, NPH (Pork), 100 Units 1946

Insulin, Regular (Clarithromycin, in rare cases, causes hypoglycemia, some of which have occurred in patients taking insulin). Products include:
Iletin II, Regular (Pork), 100 Units ... 1947

Insulin, Zinc Crystals (Clarithromycin, in rare cases, causes hypoglycemia, some of which have occurred in patients taking insulin).
No products indexed under this heading.

Insulin, Zinc Suspension (Clarithromycin, in rare cases, causes hypoglycemia, some of which have occurred in patients taking insulin). Products include:
Iletin II, Lente (Pork), 100 Units 1945

Insulin Aspart, Human Regular (Clarithromycin, in rare cases, causes hypoglycemia, some of which have occurred in patients taking insulin).
No products indexed under this heading.

Insulin glargine (Clarithromycin, in rare cases, causes hypoglycemia, some of which have occurred in patients taking insulin). Products include:
Lantus Injection 742

Insulin Lispro, Human (Clarithromycin, in rare cases, causes hypoglycemia, some of which have occurred in patients taking insulin). Products include:
Humalog 1926
Humalog Mix 75/25 Pen 1928

Insulin Lispro Protamine, Human (Clarithromycin, in rare cases, causes hypoglycemia, some of which have occurred in patients taking insulin). Products include:
Humalog Mix 75/25 Pen 1928

Lovastatin (As with other macrolides, clarithromycin has been reported to increase concentrations of HMG-CoA reductase inhibitors, such as lovastatin, through inhibition of CYP450 metabolism of simvastatin; rare reports of rhabdomyolysis have been reported). Products include:
Mevacor Tablets 2132

Metformin Hydrochloride (Clarithromycin, in rare cases, causes hypoglycemia, some of which have occurred in patients taking oral hypoglycemic agents). Products include:
Glucophage Tablets 1080
Glucophage XR Tablets 1080
Glucovance Tablets 1086

Miglitol (Clarithromycin, in rare cases, causes hypoglycemia, some of which have occurred in patients taking oral hypoglycemic agents). Products include:
Glyset Tablets 2821

Omeprazole (Co-administration increases the steady-state plasma concentrations, Cmax, AUC 0-24, and T 1/2 of omeprazole). Products include:
Prilosec Delayed-Release Capsules 628

Phenytoin (Concurrent use of erythromycin and/or clarithromycin in patients receiving drugs metabolized by the cytochrome P450 system may be associated with elevation in serum levels of phenytoin). Products include:
Dilantin Infatabs 2624
Dilantin-125 Oral Suspension 2625

Phenytoin Sodium (Concurrent use of erythromycin and/or clarithromycin in patients receiving drugs metabolized by the cytochrome P450 system may be associated with elevation in serum levels of phenytoin). Products include:
Dilantin Kapseals 2622

Pimozide (Concurrent use of erythromycin and/or clarithromycin in patients receiving pimozide has been reported to result in rare cases of cardiovascular adverse events including prolonged QT interval, ventricular tachycardia, ventricular fibrillation, and torsade de pointes, and death have been reported; co-administration is contraindicated). Products include:
Orap Tablets 1407

Pioglitazone Hydrochloride (Clarithromycin, in rare cases, causes hypoglycemia, some of which have occurred in patients taking oral hypoglycemic agents). Products include:
Actos Tablets 3275

Ranitidine Bismuth Citrate (Co-administration has resulted in increased plasma ranitidine concentrations (57%), increased plasma bismuth trough concentrations (48%), and increased 14-hydroxy-clarithromycin plasma concentrations (31%); these effects are clinically insignificant).
No products indexed under this heading.

Repaglinide (Clarithromycin, in rare cases, causes hypoglycemia, some of which have occurred in patients taking oral hypoglycemic agents). Products include:
Prandin Tablets (0.5, 1, and 2 mg) 2432

Ritonavir (Co-administration has resulted in a 77% increase in clarithromycin AUC and a 100% decrease in the AUC of 14-OH clarithromycin; dosage adjustments may be needed if clarithromycin is administered to patients with renal impairment). Products include:
Kaletra Capsules 471
Kaletra Oral Solution 471
Norvir Capsules 487
Norvir Oral Solution 487

Rosiglitazone Maleate (Clarithromycin, in rare cases, causes hypoglycemia, some of which have occurred in patients taking oral hypoglycemic agents). Products include:
Avandia Tablets 1490

Simvastatin (As with other macrolides, clarithromycin has been reported to increase concentrations of HMG-CoA reductase inhibitors, such as simvastatin, through inhibition of CYP450 metabolism of simvastatin; rare reports of rhabdomyolysis have been reported). Products include:
Zocor Tablets 2219

Tacrolimus (Concurrent use of erythromycin and/or clarithromycin in patients receiving drugs metabolized by the cytochrome P450 system may be associated with elevation in serum levels of tacrolimus). Products include:
Prograf 1393
Protopic Ointment 1397

Terfenadine (Co-administration has resulted in increase in active metabolite of terfenadine by 3-fold; rare cases of cardiovascular adverse events including prolonged QT interval, ventricular tachycardia, ventricular fibrillation, and torsade de pointes, and death have been reported; co-administration is contraindicated).
No products indexed under this heading.

Theophylline (Co-administration in patients who are receiving high doses of theophylline may be associated with an increase in serum theophylline levels and potential theophylline toxicity). Products include:
Aerolate 1361
Theo-Dur Extended-Release Tablets 1835
Uni-Dur Extended-Release Tablets .. 1841
Uniphyl 400 mg and 600 mg Tablets 2903

Theophylline Calcium Salicylate (Co-administration in patients who are receiving high doses of theophylline may be associated with an increase in serum theophylline levels and potential theophylline toxicity).
No products indexed under this heading.

Theophylline Sodium Glycinate (Co-administration in patients who are receiving high doses of theophylline may be associated with an increase in serum theophylline levels and potential theophylline toxicity).
No products indexed under this heading.

Tolazamide (Clarithromycin, in rare cases, causes hypoglycemia, some of which have occurred in patients taking oral hypoglycemic agents).
No products indexed under this heading.

Tolbutamide (Clarithromycin, in rare cases, causes hypoglycemia, some of which have occurred in patients taking oral hypoglycemic agents).
No products indexed under this heading.

Triazolam (Erythromycin, another macrolide antibiotic, has been reported to decrease the clearance of triazolam and, thus, may increase the pharmacologic effect of the triazolam; concomitant use has resulted in somnolence and confusion). Products include:
Halcion Tablets 2823

Troglitazone (Clarithromycin, in rare cases, causes hypoglycemia, some of which have occurred in patients taking oral hypoglycemic

agents).

No products indexed under this heading.

Valproate Sodium (Concurrent use of erythromycin and/or clarithromycin in patients receiving drugs metabolized by the cytochrome P450 system may be associated with elevation in serum levels of valproate). Products include:

- Depacon Injection 416

Valproic Acid (Concurrent use of erythromycin and/or clarithromycin in patients receiving drugs metabolized by the cytochrome P450 system may be associated with elevation in serum levels of valproate). Products include:

- Depakene 421

Warfarin Sodium (Coadministration may result in the potentiation of oral anticoagulant effects). Products include:

- Coumadin for Injection 1243
- Coumadin Tablets 1243
- Warfarin Sodium Tablets, USP 3302

Zidovudine (Potential for decreased steady-state zidovudine concentration). Products include:

- Combivir Tablets 1502
- Retrovir 1625
- Retrovir IV Infusion 1629
- Trizivir Tablets 1669

Food Interactions

Food, unspecified (Food slightly delays both the onset of absorption and the formation of the active metabolite, but does not affect the extent of bioavailability; Biaxin may be administered without regard to food).

BIAXIN FOR ORAL SUSPENSION
(Clarithromycin) 403
See Biaxin Filmtab Tablets

BIAXIN XL FILMTAB TABLETS
(Clarithromycin) 403
See Biaxin Filmtab Tablets

BICILLIN C-R 900/300 INJECTION
(Penicillin G Benzathine, Penicillin G Procaine) 2240
May interact with tetracyclines and certain other agents. Compounds in these categories include:

Demeclocycline Hydrochloride (May antagonize the bactericidal effect of penicillin). Products include:

- Declomycin Tablets 1855

Doxycycline Calcium (May antagonize the bactericidal effect of penicillin). Products include:

- Vibramycin Calcium Oral Suspension Syrup 2735

Doxycycline Hyclate (May antagonize the bactericidal effect of penicillin). Products include:

- Doryx Coated Pellet Filled Capsules 3357
- Periostat Tablets 1208
- Vibramycin Hyclate Capsules 2735
- Vibramycin Hyclate Intravenous 2737
- Vibra-Tabs Film Coated Tablets 2735

Doxycycline Monohydrate (May antagonize the bactericidal effect of penicillin). Products include:

- Monodox Capsules 2442
- Vibramycin Monohydrate for Oral Suspension 2735

Methacycline Hydrochloride (May antagonize the bactericidal effect of penicillin).

No products indexed under this heading.

Minocycline Hydrochloride (May antagonize the bactericidal effect of penicillin). Products include:

- Dynacin Capsules 2019
- Minocin Intravenous 1862
- Minocin Oral Suspension 1865
- Minocin Pellet-Filled Capsules 1863

Oxytetracycline Hydrochloride (May antagonize the bactericidal effect of penicillin). Products include:

- Terra-Cortril Ophthalmic Suspension 2716
- Urobiotic-250 Capsules 2731

Probenecid (Concurrent administration increases and prolongs serum penicillin levels).

No products indexed under this heading.

Tetracycline Hydrochloride (May antagonize the bactericidal effect of penicillin).

No products indexed under this heading.

BICILLIN C-R INJECTION
(Penicillin G Benzathine, Penicillin G Procaine) 2238
See Bicillin C-R 900/300 Injection

BICILLIN L-A INJECTION
(Penicillin G Benzathine) 2242
May interact with tetracyclines and certain other agents. Compounds in these categories include:

Demeclocycline Hydrochloride (May antagonize the bactericidal effect of penicillin). Products include:

- Declomycin Tablets 1855

Doxycycline Calcium (May antagonize the bactericidal effect of penicillin). Products include:

- Vibramycin Calcium Oral Suspension Syrup 2735

Doxycycline Hyclate (May antagonize the bactericidal effect of penicillin). Products include:

- Doryx Coated Pellet Filled Capsules 3357
- Periostat Tablets 1208
- Vibramycin Hyclate Capsules 2735
- Vibramycin Hyclate Intravenous 2737
- Vibra-Tabs Film Coated Tablets 2735

Doxycycline Monohydrate (May antagonize the bactericidal effect of penicillin). Products include:

- Monodox Capsules 2442
- Vibramycin Monohydrate for Oral Suspension 2735

Methacycline Hydrochloride (May antagonize the bactericidal effect of penicillin).

No products indexed under this heading.

Minocycline Hydrochloride (May antagonize the bactericidal effect of penicillin). Products include:

- Dynacin Capsules 2019
- Minocin Intravenous 1862
- Minocin Oral Suspension 1865
- Minocin Pellet-Filled Capsules 1863

Oxytetracycline Hydrochloride (May antagonize the bactericidal effect of penicillin). Products include:

- Terra-Cortril Ophthalmic Suspension 2716
- Urobiotic-250 Capsules 2731

Probenecid (Increases serum penicillin levels).

No products indexed under this heading.

Tetracycline Hydrochloride (May antagonize the bactericidal effect of penicillin).

No products indexed under this heading.

BILTRICIDE TABLETS
(Praziquantel) 887
None cited in PDR database.

BIOCHOICE IMMUNE[26] POWDER AND CAPSULES
(Egg Product) 818
None cited in PDR database.

BIOCHOICE IMMUNE SUPPORT POWDER
(Egg Product, Vitamins with Minerals) 818
None cited in PDR database.

BIO-COMPLEX 5000 GENTLE FOAMING CLEANSER
(Aloe vera) 769
None cited in PDR database.

BIO-COMPLEX 5000 REVITALIZING CONDITIONER
(Octyl Methoxycinnamate) 769
None cited in PDR database.

BIO-COMPLEX 5000 REVITALIZING SHAMPOO
(Octyl Methoxycinnamate) 770
None cited in PDR database.

BIOLEAN CAPSULES AND TABLETS
(Amino Acid Preparations, Ephedra, Herbals, Multiple) 842
May interact with monoamine oxidase inhibitors and certain other agents. Compounds in these categories include:

Caffeine (Caffeine intake should be minimized while consuming this product; simultaneous or same day consumption should be avoided). Products include:

- BC Powder 619
- Arthritis Strength BC Powder 619
- Darvon Compound-65 Pulvules 1910
- Aspirin Free Excedrin Caplets and Geltabs 628
- Excedrin Extra-Strength Tablets, Caplets, and Geltabs 629
- Excedrin Migraine 1070
- Goody's Extra Strength Headache Powder 620
- Goody's Extra Strength Pain Relief Tablets 620
- Hycomine Compound Tablets 1317
- Maximum Strength Midol Menstrual Caplets and Gelcaps 612
- Vanquish Caplets 617
- Vivarin 763

Isocarboxazid (Concurrent use with MAO inhibitors should be undertaken with healthcare professional's supervision).

No products indexed under this heading.

Moclobemide (Concurrent use with MAO inhibitors should be undertaken with healthcare professional's supervision).

No products indexed under this heading.

Pargyline Hydrochloride (Concurrent use with MAO inhibitors should be undertaken with healthcare professional's supervision).

No products indexed under this heading.

Phenelzine Sulfate (Concurrent use with MAO inhibitors should be undertaken with healthcare professional's supervision). Products include:

- Nardil Tablets 2653

Phenylpropanolamine Hydrochloride (Concurrent use should be undertaken with healthcare professional's supervision).

No products indexed under this heading.

Procarbazine Hydrochloride (Concurrent use with MAO inhibitors should be undertaken with healthcare professional's supervision). Products include:

- Matulane Capsules 3246

Pseudoephedrine Hydrochloride (Concurrent use should be undertaken with healthcare professional's supervision). Products include:

- Actifed Cold & Allergy Tablets 688
- Actifed Cold & Sinus Caplets and Tablets 688
- Advil Cold and Sinus Caplets 771
- Advil Cold and Sinus Tablets 771
- Advil Flu & Body Ache Caplets 772
- Aleve Cold & Sinus Caplets 603
- Alka-Seltzer Plus Liqui-Gels 604
- Alka-Seltzer Plus Cold & Flu Medicine Liqui-Gels 604
- Alka-Seltzer Plus Cold & Sinus Medicine Liqui-Gels 604
- Allegra-D Extended-Release Tablets 714
- BC Cold Powder 619
- Benadryl Allergy/Cold Tablets 691
- Benadryl Allergy/Congestion Tablets 692
- Benadryl Allergy & Sinus Liquid 693
- Benadryl Allergy & Sinus Fastmelt Tablets 693
- Benadryl Allergy Sinus Headache Caplets & Gelcaps 693
- Benadryl Severe Allergy & Sinus Headache Caplets 694
- Benadryl Children's Allergy/Cold Fastmelt Tablets 692
- Benylin Multi-Symptom Liquid 697
- Bromfed Capsules (Extended-Release) 2269
- Bromfed-PD Capsules (Extended-Release) 2269
- Children's Cēpacol Sore Throat 788
- Comtrex Acute Head Cold & Sinus Pressure Relief Tablets 627
- Comtrex Deep Chest Cold & Congestion Relief Softgels 627
- Comtrex Flu Therapy & Fever Relief Daytime Caplets 628
- Comtrex Flu Therapy & Fever Relief Nighttime Tablets 628
- Comtrex Maximum Strength Multi-Symptom Cold & Cough Relief Tablets and Caplets 626
- Contac Non-Drowsy 12 Hour Cold Caplets 745
- Contac Non-Drowsy Timed Release 12 Hour Cold Caplets 746
- Contac Severe Cold and Flu Caplets Maximum Strength 746
- Contac Severe Cold and Flu Caplets Non-Drowsy 746
- Dimetapp Elixir 777
- Dimetapp Cold and Fever Suspension 775
- Dimetapp DM Cold & Cough Elixir 775
- Dimetapp Nighttime Flu Liquid 776
- Dimetapp Non-Drowsy Flu Syrup 777
- Dimetapp Infant Drops Decongestant 775
- Dimetapp Infant Drops Decongestant Plus Cough 776
- Guaifed 2272
- Kronofed-A 1341
- Children's Motrin Cold Oral Suspension 2007
- Motrin Sinus Headache Caplets 2005
- PediaCare Cough-Cold Liquid 719
- PediaCare Infants' Drops Decongestant 719
- PediaCare Infants' Drops Decongestant Plus Cough 719
- PediaCare NightRest Cough-Cold Liquid 719
- Robitussin Cold Caplets Cold & Congestion 780
- Robitussin Cold Softgels Cold & Congestion 780
- Robitussin Cold Caplets Multi-Symptom Cold & Flu 781
- Robitussin Cold Softgels Multi-Symptom Cold & Flu 781
- Robitussin Cold Softgels Severe Congestion 782
- Robitussin Cough & Cold Infant Drops 782
- Robitussin Maximum Strength Cough & Cold Liquid 785
- Robitussin Pediatric Cough & Cold Formula Liquid 785
- Robitussin Multi Symptom Honey Flu Liquid 785
- Robitussin Nighttime Honey Flu Liquid 786
- Robitussin-CF Liquid 783
- Robitussin-DAC Syrup 2942
- Robitussin-PE Liquid 782
- Ryna 768
- Semprex-D Capsules 1172
- Singlet Caplets 761
- Sinutab Non-Drying Liquid Caps 706
- Sinutab Sinus Allergy Medication, Maximum Strength Formula, Tablets & Caplets 707
- Sinutab Sinus Medication, Maximum Strength Without Drowsiness Formula, Tablets & Caplets 707
- Sudafed 12 Hour Tablets 708
- Sudafed 24 Hour Tablets 708
- Children's Sudafed Cold & Cough Liquid 709
- Children's Sudafed Nasal Decongestant Chewables 711

Children's Sudafed Nasal Decongestant Liquid Medication ▣711
Sudafed Cold & Allergy Tablets ▣708
Sudafed Cold & Cough Liquid Caps ▣709
Sudafed Cold & Sinus Liquid Caps ▣710
Sudafed Nasal Decongestant Tablets ▣710
Sudafed Non-Drying Sinus Liquid Caps ▣712
Sudafed Severe Cold ▣711
Sudafed Sinus Headache Caplets ▣712
Sudafed Sinus Headache Tablets ▣712
Tavist Sinus Non-Drowsy Coated Caplets ▣676
TheraFlu Regular Strength Cold & Cough Night Time Hot Liquid ▣676
TheraFlu Regular Strength Cold & Sore Throat Night Time Hot Liquid ▣676
TheraFlu Maximum Strength Flu & Congestion Non-Drowsy Hot Liquid ▣677
TheraFlu Maximum Strength Flu & Cough Night Time Hot Liquid ▣678
TheraFlu Maximum Strength Flu & Sore Throat Night Time Hot Liquid ▣677
TheraFlu Maximum Strength Severe Cold & Congestion Night Time Caplets ▣678
TheraFlu Maximum Strength Severe Cold & Congestion Night Time Hot Liquid ▣678
TheraFlu Maximum Strength Severe Cold & Congestion Non-Drowsy ▣679
Triaminic Allergy Congestion Liquid ▣680
Triaminic Chest Congestion Liquid ▣680
Triaminic Cold & Allergy Liquid ▣681
Triaminic Cold & Allergy Softchews ▣683
Triaminic Cold & Cough Liquid ▣681
Triaminic Cold & Cough Softchews ▣683
Triaminic Cold & Night Time Cough Liquid ▣681
Triaminic Cold, Cough & Fever Liquid ▣681
Triaminic Cough Liquid ▣682
Triaminic Cough & Congestion Liquid ▣682
Triaminic Cough & Sore Throat Liquid ▣682
Triaminic Cough & Sore Throat Softchews ▣684
Children's Tylenol Allergy-D Liquid 2014
Children's Tylenol Cold Suspension Liquid and Chewable Tablets 2015
Children's Tylenol Cold Plus Cough Suspension Liquid and Chewable Tablets 2015
Children's Tylenol Flu Suspension Liquid 2015
Children's Tylenol Sinus Suspension Liquid 2017
Infants' Tylenol Cold Decongestant and Fever Reducer Concentrated Drops 2015
Infants' Tylenol Cold Decongestant and Fever Reducer Concentrated Drops Plus Cough 2015
Tylenol Allergy Sinus 2010
Multi-Symptom Tylenol Cold Complete Formula Caplets 2010
Multi-Symptom Tylenol Cold Non-Drowsy Caplets and Gelcaps 2010
Multi-Symptom Tylenol Cold Severe Congestion Non-Drowsy Caplets 2011
Maximum Strength Tylenol Flu NightTime Gelcaps 2011
Maximum Strength Tylenol Flu NightTime Liquid 2011
Maximum Strength Tylenol Flu Non-Drowsy Gelcaps 2011
Maximum Strength Tylenol Sinus NightTime Caplets 2012
Maximum Strength Tylenol Sinus Non-Drowsy Geltabs, Gelcaps, Caplets, and Tablets 2012
Vicks 44D Cough & Head Congestion Relief Liquid ▣724
Vicks 44M Cough, Cold & Flu Relief Liquid ▣725
Pediatric Vicks 44m Cough & Cold Relief ▣728
Vicks DayQuil LiquiCaps/Liquid Multi-Symptom Cold/Flu Relief ▣727
Children's Vicks NyQuil Cold/Cough Relief ▣726
Vicks NyQuil LiquiCaps/Liquid Multi-Symptom Cold/Flu Relief, Original and Cherry Flavors ▣727
Zephrex Tablets 3091
Zephrex LA Tablets 3092
Zyrtec-D 12 Hour Extended Relief Tablets 2758

Selegiline Hydrochloride (Concurrent use with MAO inhibitors should be undertaken with healthcare professional's supervision). Products include:
Eldepryl Capsules 3266

Tranylcypromine Sulfate (Concurrent use with MAO inhibitors should be undertaken with healthcare professional's supervision). Products include:
Parnate Tablets 1607

BIOLEAN ACCELERATOR TABLETS

(Amino Acid Preparations, Herbals, Multiple) ▣842
May interact with anorexiants and antidepressant drugs. Compounds in these categories include:

Amitriptyline Hydrochloride (Effect of concurrent use is not specified). Products include:
Etrafon 3115
Limbitrol 1738

Amoxapine (Effect of concurrent use is not specified).
No products indexed under this heading.

Amphetamine Resins (Effect of concurrent use is not specified).
No products indexed under this heading.

Benzphetamine Hydrochloride (Effect of concurrent use is not specified).
No products indexed under this heading.

Bupropion Hydrochloride (Effect of concurrent use is not specified). Products include:
Wellbutrin Tablets 1680
Wellbutrin SR Sustained-Release Tablets 1684
Zyban Sustained-Release Tablets 1710

Citalopram Hydrobromide (Effect of concurrent use is not specified). Products include:
Celexa 1365

Desipramine Hydrochloride (Effect of concurrent use is not specified). Products include:
Norpramin Tablets 755

Dextroamphetamine Sulfate (Effect of concurrent use is not specified). Products include:
Adderall Tablets 3231
Adderall XR Capsules
Dexedrine 1512
DextroStat Tablets 3236

Diethylpropion Hydrochloride (Effect of concurrent use is not specified).
No products indexed under this heading.

Doxepin Hydrochloride (Effect of concurrent use is not specified). Products include:
Sinequan 2713

Fenfluramine Hydrochloride (Effect of concurrent use is not specified).
No products indexed under this heading.

Fluoxetine Hydrochloride (Effect of concurrent use is not specified). Products include:
Prozac Pulvules, Liquid, and Weekly Capsules 1238
Sarafem Pulvules 1962

Imipramine Hydrochloride (Effect of concurrent use is not specified).
No products indexed under this heading.

Imipramine Pamoate (Effect of concurrent use is not specified).
No products indexed under this heading.

Isocarboxazid (Effect of concurrent use is not specified).
No products indexed under this heading.

Maprotiline Hydrochloride (Effect of concurrent use is not specified).
No products indexed under this heading.

Mazindol (Effect of concurrent use is not specified).
No products indexed under this heading.

Methamphetamine Hydrochloride (Effect of concurrent use is not specified). Products include:
Desoxyn Tablets 440

Mirtazapine (Effect of concurrent use is not specified). Products include:
Remeron Tablets 2483
Remeron SolTab Tablets 2486

Nefazodone Hydrochloride (Effect of concurrent use is not specified). Products include:
Serzone Tablets 1104

Nortriptyline Hydrochloride (Effect of concurrent use is not specified).
No products indexed under this heading.

Paroxetine Hydrochloride (Effect of concurrent use is not specified). Products include:
Paxil 1609

Phendimetrazine Tartrate (Effect of concurrent use is not specified). Products include:
Bontril Slow-Release Capsules 576

Phenelzine Sulfate (Effect of concurrent use is not specified). Products include:
Nardil Tablets 2653

Phenmetrazine Hydrochloride (Effect of concurrent use is not specified).
No products indexed under this heading.

Protriptyline Hydrochloride (Effect of concurrent use is not specified). Products include:
Vivactil Tablets 2446
Vivactil Tablets 2217

Sertraline Hydrochloride (Effect of concurrent use is not specified). Products include:
Zoloft 2751

Sibutramine Hydrochloride Monohydrate (Effect of concurrent use is not specified). Products include:
Meridia Capsules 481

Tranylcypromine Sulfate (Effect of concurrent use is not specified). Products include:
Parnate Tablets 1607

Trazodone Hydrochloride (Effect of concurrent use is not specified).
No products indexed under this heading.

Trimipramine Maleate (Effect of concurrent use is not specified). Products include:
Surmontil Capsules 3595

Venlafaxine Hydrochloride (Effect of concurrent use is not specified). Products include:
Effexor Tablets 3495
Effexor XR Capsules 3499

BIOLEAN FREE TABLETS

(Amino Acid Preparations, Ginkgo biloba, Ginseng) ▣843
May interact with anorexiants, monoamine oxidase inhibitors, and certain other agents. Compounds in these categories include:

Amphetamine Resins (Concurrent use with appetite suppressants is not recommended).
No products indexed under this heading.

Benzphetamine Hydrochloride (Concurrent use with appetite suppressants is not recommended).
No products indexed under this heading.

Caffeine-containing medications (Concurrent caffeine intake should be minimized).

Dextroamphetamine Sulfate (Concurrent use with appetite suppressants is not recommended). Products include:
Adderall Tablets 3231
Adderall XR Capsules
Dexedrine 1512
DextroStat Tablets 3236

Diethylpropion Hydrochloride (Concurrent use with appetite suppressants is not recommended).
No products indexed under this heading.

Fenfluramine Hydrochloride (Concurrent use with appetite suppressants is not recommended).
No products indexed under this heading.

Isocarboxazid (Concurrent use with MAO inhibitors is not recommended).
No products indexed under this heading.

Mazindol (Concurrent use with appetite suppressants is not recommended).
No products indexed under this heading.

Methamphetamine Hydrochloride (Concurrent use with appetite suppressants is not recommended). Products include:
Desoxyn Tablets 440

Moclobemide (Concurrent use with MAO inhibitors is not recommended).
No products indexed under this heading.

Pargyline Hydrochloride (Concurrent use with MAO inhibitors is not recommended).
No products indexed under this heading.

Phendimetrazine Tartrate (Concurrent use with appetite suppressants is not recommended). Products include:
Bontril Slow-Release Capsules 576

Phenelzine Sulfate (Concurrent use with MAO inhibitors is not recommended). Products include:
Nardil Tablets 2653

Phenmetrazine Hydrochloride (Concurrent use with appetite suppressants is not recommended).
No products indexed under this heading.

Procarbazine Hydrochloride (Concurrent use with MAO inhibitors is not recommended). Products include:
Matulane Capsules 3246

Selegiline Hydrochloride (Concurrent use with MAO inhibitors is not recommended). Products include:
Eldepryl Capsules 3266

Sibutramine Hydrochloride Monohydrate (Concurrent use with appetite suppressants is not recommended). Products include:
Meridia Capsules 481

Tranylcypromine Sulfate (Concurrent use with MAO inhibitors is not recommended). Products include:
Parnate Tablets 1607

Food Interactions

Beverages, caffeine-containing (Concurrent caffeine intake should be minimized).

BIOLEAN LIPOTRIM CAPSULES

(Herbals with Minerals) ▣843
None cited in PDR database.

BIOMUNE OSF EXPRESS SPRAY

(Homeopathic Formulations) ▣640
None cited in PDR database.

BIOMUNE OSF PLUS CAPSULES
(Astragalus, Colostrum, Whey) .... ▣820
None cited in PDR database.

BION TEARS LUBRICANT EYE DROPS
(Dextran 70, Hydroxypropyl Methylcellulose)............................ 538
None cited in PDR database.

BIOS LIFE 2 DRINK MIX
(Fiber, Vitamins with Minerals) 3321
None cited in PDR database.

BIOTIN CAPSULES
(Biotin) 2223
None cited in PDR database.

BLEPH-10 OPHTHALMIC OINTMENT 10%
(Sulfacetamide Sodium) .... ⊙230
May interact with silver preparations. Compounds in these categories include:

Silver Nitrate (Incompatible).
No products indexed under this heading.

BLEPH-10 OPHTHALMIC SOLUTION 10%
(Sulfacetamide Sodium) .... ⊙230
See Bleph-10 Ophthalmic Ointment 10%

BLEPHAMIDE OPHTHALMIC OINTMENT
(Prednisolone Acetate, Sulfacetamide Sodium) 547
May interact with para-aminobenzoic acid based local anesthetics and silver preparations. Compounds in these categories include:

Procaine Hydrochloride (May antagonize the action of sulfonamide).
No products indexed under this heading.

Silver Nitrate (Blephamide ointment is incompatible with silver preparations).
No products indexed under this heading.

Tetracaine Hydrochloride (May antagonize the action of sulfonamide). Products include:
Cēpacol Viractin Cold Sore and Fever Blister Treatment, Gel ....▣788
Cetacaine Topical Anesthetic 1196

BLEPHAMIDE OPHTHALMIC SUSPENSION
(Prednisolone Acetate, Sulfacetamide Sodium) 548
May interact with para-aminobenzoic acid based local anesthetics and certain other agents. Compounds in these categories include:

Procaine Hydrochloride (Local anesthetics related to p-amino benzoic acid may antagonize the action of the sulfonamides).
No products indexed under this heading.

Silver Nitrate (Blephamide ophthalmic suspension is incompatible with silver preparations).
No products indexed under this heading.

Tetracaine Hydrochloride (Local anesthetics related to p-amino benzoic acid may antagonize the action of the sulfonamides). Products include:
Cēpacol Viractin Cold Sore and Fever Blister Treatment, Gel ....▣788
Cetacaine Topical Anesthetic 1196

BLOCADREN TABLETS
(Timolol Maleate) 2046
May interact with catecholamine depleting drugs, calcium channel blockers, cardiac glycosides, oral hypoglycemic agents, insulin, nonsteroidal anti-inflammatory agents, quinidine, and certain other agents. Compounds in these categories include:

Acarbose (Beta blockers may mask the signs and symptoms of acute hypoglycemia). Products include:
Precose Tablets 906

Amlodipine Besylate (AV conduction disturbances; left ventricular failure). Products include:
Lotrel Capsules 2370
Norvasc Tablets 2704

Bepridil Hydrochloride (AV conduction disturbances; left ventricular failure). Products include:
Vascor Tablets 2602

Celecoxib (Blunting of the antihypertensive effect). Products include:
Celebrex Capsules 2676
Celebrex Capsules 2780

Chlorpropamide (Beta blockers may mask the signs and symptoms of acute hypoglycemia). Products include:
Diabinese Tablets 2680

Clonidine (Beta adrenergic blocking agents may exacerbate the rebound hypertension). Products include:
Catapres-TTS 1038

Clonidine Hydrochloride (Beta adrenergic blocking agents may exacerbate the rebound hypertension). Products include:
Catapres Tablets 1037
Clorpres Tablets 1002
Combipres Tablets 1040
Duraclon Injection 3057

Deserpidine (Additive effects; hypotension and/or bradycardia).
No products indexed under this heading.

Deslanoside (Additive effects in prolonging AV conduction time).
No products indexed under this heading.

Diclofenac Potassium (Blunting of the antihypertensive effect). Products include:
Cataflam Tablets 2315

Diclofenac Sodium (Blunting of the antihypertensive effect). Products include:
Arthrotec Tablets 3195
Voltaren Ophthalmic Sterile Ophthalmic Solution .... ⊙312
Voltaren Tablets 2315
Voltaren-XR Tablets 2315

Digitoxin (Additive effects in prolonging AV conduction time).
No products indexed under this heading.

Digoxin (Additive effects in prolonging AV conduction time). Products include:
Digitek Tablets 1003
Lanoxicaps Capsules 1574
Lanoxin Injection 1581
Lanoxin Tablets 1587
Lanoxin Elixir Pediatric 1578
Lanoxin Injection Pediatric 1584

Diltiazem Hydrochloride (AV conduction disturbances; left ventricular failure). Products include:
Cardizem Injectable 1018
Cardizem Lyo-Ject Syringe 1018
Cardizem Monovial 1018
Cardizem CD Capsules 1016
Tiazac Capsules 1378

Epinephrine (Patients with a history of atopy or severe anaphylactic reaction to variety of allergens may be unresponsive to the usual dose of epinephrine to treat anaphylactic reactions). Products include:
Epifrin Sterile Ophthalmic Solution .... ⊙235
EpiPen 1236
Primatene Mist ....▣779
Xylocaine with Epinephrine Injection 653

Epinephrine Hydrochloride (Patients with a history of atopy or severe anaphylactic reaction to variety of allergens may be unresponsive to the usual dose of epinephrine to treat anaphylactic reactions).
No products indexed under this heading.

Etodolac (Blunting of the antihypertensive effect). Products include:
Lodine 3528
Lodine XL Extended-Release Tablets 3530

Felodipine (AV conduction disturbances; left ventricular failure). Products include:
Lexxel Tablets 608
Plendil Extended-Release Tablets ... 623

Fenoprofen Calcium (Blunting of the antihypertensive effect).
No products indexed under this heading.

Flurbiprofen (Blunting of the antihypertensive effect).
No products indexed under this heading.

Glimepiride (Beta blockers may mask the signs and symptoms of acute hypoglycemia). Products include:
Amaryl Tablets 717

Glipizide (Beta blockers may mask the signs and symptoms of acute hypoglycemia). Products include:
Glucotrol Tablets 2692
Glucotrol XL Extended Release Tablets 2693

Glyburide (Beta blockers may mask the signs and symptoms of acute hypoglycemia). Products include:
DiaBeta Tablets 741
Glucovance Tablets 1086

Guanethidine Monosulfate (Additive effects; hypotension and/or bradycardia).
No products indexed under this heading.

Ibuprofen (Blunting of the antihypertensive effect). Products include:
Advil ....▣771
Children's Advil Oral Suspension ...▣773
Children's Advil Chewable Tablets .▣773
Advil Cold and Sinus Caplets ....▣771
Advil Cold and Sinus Tablets ....▣771
Advil Flu & Body Ache Caplets ......▣772
Infants' Advil Drops ....▣773
Junior Strength Advil Tablets ....▣773
Junior Strength Advil Chewable Tablets ....▣773
Advil Migraine Liquigels ....▣772
Children's Motrin Oral Suspension and Chewable Tablets 2006
Children's Motrin Cold Oral Suspension 2007
Children's Motrin Oral Suspension ....▣643
Motrin Suspension, Oral Drops, Chewable Tablets, and Caplets 2002
Infants' Motrin Concentrated Drops 2006
Junior Strength Motrin Caplets and Chewable Tablets 2006
Motrin IB Tablets, Caplets, and Gelcaps 2002
Motrin Migraine Pain Caplets 2005
Motrin Sinus Headache Caplets 2005
Vicoprofen Tablets 520

Indomethacin (Blunting of the antihypertensive effect). Products include:
Indocin 2112

Indomethacin Sodium Trihydrate (Blunting of the antihypertensive effect). Products include:
Indocin I.V. 2115

Insulin, Human, Zinc Suspension (Beta blockers may mask the signs and symptoms of acute hypoglycemia). Products include:
Humulin L, 100 Units 1937
Humulin U, 100 Units 1943
Novolin L Human Insulin 10 ml Vials 2422

Insulin, Human NPH (Beta blockers may mask the signs and symptoms of acute hypoglycemia). Products include:
Humulin N, 100 Units 1939
Humulin N NPH Pen 1940
Novolin N Human Insulin 10 ml Vials 2422
Novolin N PenFill 2423
Novolin N Prefilled Syringe Disposable Insulin Delivery System 2425

Insulin, Human Regular (Beta blockers may mask the signs and symptoms of acute hypoglycemia). Products include:
Humulin R Regular (U-500) 1943
Humulin R, 100 Units 1941
Novolin R Human Insulin 10 ml Vials 2423
Novolin R PenFill 2423
Novolin R Prefilled Syringe Disposable Insulin Delivery System 2425
Velosulin BR Human Insulin 10 ml Vials 2435

Insulin, Human Regular and Human NPH Mixture (Beta blockers may mask the signs and symptoms of acute hypoglycemia). Products include:
Humulin 50/50, 100 Units 1934
Humulin 70/30, 100 Units 1935
Humulin 70/30 Pen 1936
Novolin 70/30 Human Insulin 10 ml Vials 2421
Novolin 70/30 PenFill 2423
Novolin 70/30 Prefilled Disposable Insulin Delivery System 2425

Insulin, NPH (Beta blockers may mask the signs and symptoms of acute hypoglycemia). Products include:
Iletin II, NPH (Pork), 100 Units 1946

Insulin, Regular (Beta blockers may mask the signs and symptoms of acute hypoglycemia). Products include:
Iletin II, Regular (Pork), 100 Units ... 1947

Insulin, Zinc Crystals (Beta blockers may mask the signs and symptoms of acute hypoglycemia).
No products indexed under this heading.

Insulin, Zinc Suspension (Beta blockers may mask the signs and symptoms of acute hypoglycemia). Products include:
Iletin II, Lente (Pork), 100 Units 1945

Insulin Aspart, Human Regular (Beta blockers may mask the signs and symptoms of acute hypoglycemia).
No products indexed under this heading.

Insulin glargine (Beta blockers may mask the signs and symptoms of acute hypoglycemia). Products include:
Lantus Injection 742

Insulin Lispro, Human (Beta blockers may mask the signs and symptoms of acute hypoglycemia). Products include:
Humalog 1926
Humalog Mix 75/25 Pen 1928

Insulin Lispro Protamine, Human (Beta blockers may mask the signs and symptoms of acute hypoglycemia). Products include:
Humalog Mix 75/25 Pen 1928

Isradipine (AV conduction disturbances; left ventricular failure). Products include:
DynaCirc Capsules 2921
DynaCirc CR Tablets 2923

Ketoprofen (Blunting of the antihypertensive effect). Products include:
Orudis Capsules 3548
Orudis KT Tablets ....▣778
Oruvail Capsules 3548

Ketorolac Tromethamine (Blunting of the antihypertensive effect). Products include:
Acular Ophthalmic Solution 544
Acular PF Ophthalmic Solution 544

IMPORTANT NOTE: Always consult each drug listing in the patient's regimen for possible interactions.

Toradol 3018

Meclofenamate Sodium (Blunting of the antihypertensive effect).
No products indexed under this heading.

Mefenamic Acid (Blunting of the antihypertensive effect). Products include:
Ponstel Capsules 1356

Meloxicam (Blunting of the antihypertensive effect). Products include:
Mobic Tablets 1054

Metformin Hydrochloride (Beta blockers may mask the signs and symptoms of acute hypoglycemia). Products include:
Glucophage Tablets 1080
Glucophage XR Tablets 1080
Glucovance Tablets 1086

Mibefradil Dihydrochloride (AV conduction disturbances; left ventricular failure).
No products indexed under this heading.

Miglitol (Beta blockers may mask the signs and symptoms of acute hypoglycemia). Products include:
Glyset Tablets 2821

Nabumetone (Blunting of the antihypertensive effect). Products include:
Relafen Tablets 1617

Naproxen (Blunting of the antihypertensive effect). Products include:
EC-Naprosyn Delayed-Release Tablets 2967
Naprosyn Suspension 2967
Naprosyn Tablets 2967

Naproxen Sodium (Blunting of the antihypertensive effect). Products include:
Aleve Tablets, Caplets and Gelcaps .... ■602
Aleve Cold & Sinus Caplets .... ■603
Anaprox Tablets 2967
Anaprox DS Tablets 2967
Naprelan Tablets 1293

Nicardipine Hydrochloride (AV conduction disturbances; left ventricular failure). Products include:
Cardene I.V. 3485

Nifedipine (Hypotension). Products include:
Adalat CC Tablets 877
Procardia Capsules 2708
Procardia XL Extended Release Tablets 2710

Nimodipine (AV conduction disturbances; left ventricular failure). Products include:
Nimotop Capsules 904

Nisoldipine (AV conduction disturbances; left ventricular failure). Products include:
Sular Tablets 688

Oxaprozin (Blunting of the antihypertensive effect).
No products indexed under this heading.

Phenylbutazone (Blunting of the antihypertensive effect).
No products indexed under this heading.

Pioglitazone Hydrochloride (Beta blockers may mask the signs and symptoms of acute hypoglycemia). Products include:
Actos Tablets 3275

Piroxicam (Blunting of the antihypertensive effect). Products include:
Feldene Capsules 2685

Quinidine Gluconate (Co-administration has resulted in potentiated systemic beta-blockade, such as decreased heart rate). Products include:
Quinaglute Dura-Tabs Tablets 978

Quinidine Polygalacturonate (Co-administration has resulted in potentiated systemic beta-blockade, such as decreased heart rate).
No products indexed under this heading.

Quinidine Sulfate (Co-administration has resulted in potentiated systemic beta-blockade, such as decreased heart rate). Products include:
Quinidex Extentabs 2933

Rauwolfia serpentina (Additive effects; hypotension and/or bradycardia).
No products indexed under this heading.

Repaglinide (Beta blockers may mask the signs and symptoms of acute hypoglycemia). Products include:
Prandin Tablets (0.5, 1, and 2 mg) 2432

Rescinnamine (Additive effects; hypotension and/or bradycardia).
No products indexed under this heading.

Reserpine (Additive effects; hypotension and/or bradycardia).
No products indexed under this heading.

Rofecoxib (Blunting of the antihypertensive effect). Products include:
Vioxx 2213

Rosiglitazone Maleate (Beta blockers may mask the signs and symptoms of acute hypoglycemia). Products include:
Avandia Tablets 1490

Sulindac (Blunting of the antihypertensive effect). Products include:
Clinoril Tablets 2053

Tolazamide (Beta blockers may mask the signs and symptoms of acute hypoglycemia).
No products indexed under this heading.

Tolbutamide (Beta blockers may mask the signs and symptoms of acute hypoglycemia).
No products indexed under this heading.

Tolmetin Sodium (Blunting of the antihypertensive effect). Products include:
Tolectin 2589

Troglitazone (Beta blockers may mask the signs and symptoms of acute hypoglycemia).
No products indexed under this heading.

Verapamil Hydrochloride (AV conduction disturbances; left ventricular failure). Products include:
Covera-HS Tablets 3199
Isoptin SR Tablets 467
Tarka Tablets 508
Verelan Capsules 3184
Verelan PM Capsules 3186

BODYLEAN POWDER
(Amino Acid Preparations, Vitamins with Minerals) .... ■795
None cited in PDR database.

BONTRIL SLOW-RELEASE CAPSULES
(Phendimetrazine Tartrate) 576
May interact with insulin, monoamine oxidase inhibitors, and certain other agents. Compounds in these categories include:

Guanethidine Monosulfate (Hypotensive effect of guanethidine may be decreased).
No products indexed under this heading.

Insulin, Human, Zinc Suspension (Insulin requirement may be altered). Products include:
Humulin L, 100 Units 1937
Humulin U, 100 Units 1943
Novolin L Human Insulin 10 ml Vials 2422

Insulin, Human NPH (Insulin requirement may be altered). Products include:
Humulin N, 100 Units 1939
Humulin N NPH Pen 1940
Novolin N Human Insulin 10 ml Vials 2422
Novolin N PenFill 2423
Novolin N Prefilled Syringe Disposable Insulin Delivery System 2425

Insulin, Human Regular (Insulin requirement may be altered). Products include:
Humulin R Regular (U-500) 1943
Humulin R, 100 Units 1941
Novolin R Human Insulin 10 ml Vials 2423
Novolin R PenFill 2423
Novolin R Prefilled Syringe Disposable Insulin Delivery System 2425
Velosulin BR Human Insulin 10 ml Vials 2435

Insulin, Human Regular and Human NPH Mixture (Insulin requirement may be altered). Products include:
Humulin 50/50, 100 Units 1934
Humulin 70/30, 100 Units 1935
Humulin 70/30 Pen 1936
Novolin 70/30 Human Insulin 10 ml Vials 2421
Novolin 70/30 PenFill 2423
Novolin 70/30 Prefilled Disposable Insulin Delivery System 2425

Insulin, NPH (Insulin requirement may be altered). Products include:
Iletin II, NPH (Pork), 100 Units 1946

Insulin, Regular (Insulin requirement may be altered). Products include:
Iletin II, Regular (Pork), 100 Units ... 1947

Insulin, Zinc Crystals (Insulin requirement may be altered).
No products indexed under this heading.

Insulin, Zinc Suspension (Insulin requirement may be altered). Products include:
Iletin II, Lente (Pork), 100 Units 1945

Insulin Aspart, Human Regular (Insulin requirement may be altered).
No products indexed under this heading.

Insulin glargine (Insulin requirement may be altered). Products include:
Lantus Injection 742

Insulin Lispro, Human (Insulin requirement may be altered). Products include:
Humalog 1926
Humalog Mix 75/25 Pen 1928

Insulin Lispro Protamine, Human (Insulin requirement may be altered). Products include:
Humalog Mix 75/25 Pen 1928

Isocarboxazid (Potential for hypertensive crisis).
No products indexed under this heading.

Moclobemide (Potential for hypertensive crisis).
No products indexed under this heading.

Pargyline Hydrochloride (Potential for hypertensive crisis).
No products indexed under this heading.

Phenelzine Sulfate (Potential for hypertensive crisis). Products include:
Nardil Tablets 2653

Procarbazine Hydrochloride (Potential for hypertensive crisis). Products include:
Matulane Capsules 3246

Selegiline Hydrochloride (Potential for hypertensive crisis). Products include:
Eldepryl Capsules 3266

Tranylcypromine Sulfate (Potential for hypertensive crisis). Products include:
Parnate Tablets 1607

BOTOX PURIFIED NEUROTOXIN COMPLEX
(Botulinum Toxin Type A) 549
None cited in PDR database.

BRETHINE AMPULS
(Terbutaline Sulfate) 2314
See Brethine Tablets

BRETHINE TABLETS
(Terbutaline Sulfate) 2313
May interact with beta blockers, monoamine oxidase inhibitors, potassium-depleting diuretics, sympathomimetics, and tricyclic antidepressants. Compounds in these categories include:

Acebutolol Hydrochloride (Beta-adrenergic blocking agents not only block the pulmonary effect of beta-agonists but may produce severe bronchospasm in asthmatic patients). Products include:
Sectral Capsules 3589

Albuterol (Co-administration of terbutaline with other sympathomimetic agents is not recommended, since the combined effect on the cardiovascular system may be deleterious to the patient; however, this does not preclude the use of an aerosol beta agonist for the relief of an acute bronchospasm in patients receiving chronic oral therapy with terbutaline). Products include:
Proventil Inhalation Aerosol 3142
Ventolin Inhalation Aerosol and Refill 1679

Albuterol Sulfate (Co-administration of terbutaline with other sympathomimetic agents is not recommended, since the combined effect on the cardiovascular system may be deleterious to the patient; however, this does not preclude the use of an aerosol beta agonist for the relief of an acute bronchospasm in patients receiving chronic oral therapy with terbutaline). Products include:
AccuNeb Inhalation Solution 1230
Combivent Inhalation Aerosol 1041
DuoNeb Inhalation Solution 1233
Proventil Inhalation Solution 0.083% 3146
Proventil Repetabs Tablets 3148
Proventil Solution for Inhalation 0.5% 3144
Proventil HFA Inhalation Aerosol 3150
Ventolin HFA Inhalation Aerosol 3618
Volmax Extended-Release Tablets .. 2276

Amitriptyline Hydrochloride (The action of terbutaline on the vascular system may be potentiated; concurrent and/or sequential use should be undertaken with extreme caution). Products include:
Etrafon 3115
Limbitrol 1738

Amoxapine (The action of terbutaline on the vascular system may be potentiated; concurrent and/or sequential use should be undertaken with extreme caution).
No products indexed under this heading.

Atenolol (Beta-adrenergic blocking agents not only block the pulmonary effect of beta-agonists but may produce severe bronchospasm in asthmatic patients). Products include:
Tenoretic Tablets 690
Tenormin I.V. Injection 692

Bendroflumethiazide (The ECG changes and/or hypokalemia that may result from the administration of non-potassium sparing diuretics can be acutely worsened by beta-agonists, especially when the recommended dose of beta-agonist is exceeded). Products include:
Corzide 40/5 Tablets 2247
Corzide 80/5 Tablets 2247

Betaxolol Hydrochloride (Beta-adrenergic blocking agents not only block the pulmonary effect of beta-agonists but may produce severe bronchospasm in asthmatic patients). Products include:
Betoptic S Ophthalmic Suspension 537

Bisoprolol Fumarate (Beta-adrenergic blocking agents not only block the pulmonary effect of beta-agonists but may produce severe bronchospasm in asthmatic patients). Products include:
Zebeta Tablets 1885
Ziac Tablets 1887

Bumetanide (The ECG changes and/or hypokalemia that may result from the administration of non-potassium sparing diuretics can be acutely worsened by beta-agonists, especially when the recommended dose of beta-agonist is exceeded).
No products indexed under this heading.

Carteolol Hydrochloride (Beta-adrenergic blocking agents not only block the pulmonary effect of beta-agonists but may produce severe bronchospasm in asthmatic patients). Products include:
Carteolol Hydrochloride Ophthalmic Solution USP, 1% .... ⊙ 258
Ocupress Ophthalmic Solution, 1% Sterile .... ⊙ 303

Chlorothiazide (The ECG changes and/or hypokalemia that may result from the administration of non-potassium sparing diuretics can be acutely worsened by beta-agonists, especially when the recommended dose of beta-agonist is exceeded). Products include:
Aldoclor Tablets 2035
Diuril Oral 2087

Chlorothiazide Sodium (The ECG changes and/or hypokalemia that may result from the administration of non-potassium sparing diuretics can be acutely worsened by beta-agonists, especially when the recommended dose of beta-agonist is exceeded). Products include:
Diuril Sodium Intravenous 2086

Clomipramine Hydrochloride (The action of terbutaline on the vascular system may be potentiated; concurrent and/or sequential use should be undertaken with extreme caution).
No products indexed under this heading.

Desipramine Hydrochloride (The action of terbutaline on the vascular system may be potentiated; concurrent and/or sequential use should be undertaken with extreme caution). Products include:
Norpramin Tablets 755

Dobutamine Hydrochloride (Co-administration of terbutaline with other sympathomimetic agents is not recommended, since the combined effect on the cardiovascular system may be deleterious to the patient; however, this does not preclude the use of an aerosol beta agonist for the relief of an acute bronchospasm in patients receiving chronic oral therapy with terbutaline). Products include:
Dobutrex Solution Vials 1914

Dopamine Hydrochloride (Co-administration of terbutaline with other sympathomimetic agents is not recommended, since the combined effect on the cardiovascular system may be deleterious to the patient; however, this does not preclude the use of an aerosol beta agonist for the relief of an acute bronchospasm in patients receiving chronic oral therapy with terbutaline).
No products indexed under this heading.

Doxepin Hydrochloride (The action of terbutaline on the vascular system may be potentiated; concurrent and/or sequential use should be undertaken with extreme caution). Products include:
Sinequan 2713

Ephedrine Hydrochloride (Co-administration of terbutaline with other sympathomimetic agents is not recommended, since the combined effect on the cardiovascular system may be deleterious to the patient; however, this does not preclude the use of an aerosol beta agonist for the relief of an acute bronchospasm in patients receiving chronic oral therapy with terbutaline). Products include:
Primatene Tablets .... ▣ 780

Ephedrine Sulfate (Co-administration of terbutaline with other sympathomimetic agents is not recommended, since the combined effect on the cardiovascular system may be deleterious to the patient; however, this does not preclude the use of an aerosol beta agonist for the relief of an acute bronchospasm in patients receiving chronic oral therapy with terbutaline).
No products indexed under this heading.

Ephedrine Tannate (Co-administration of terbutaline with other sympathomimetic agents is not recommended, since the combined effect on the cardiovascular system may be deleterious to the patient; however, this does not preclude the use of an aerosol beta agonist for the relief of an acute bronchospasm in patients receiving chronic oral therapy with terbutaline). Products include:
Rynatuss Pediatric Suspension 3353
Rynatuss Tablets 3353

Epinephrine (Co-administration of terbutaline with other sympathomimetic agents is not recommended, since the combined effect on the cardiovascular system may be deleterious to the patient; however, this does not preclude the use of an aerosol beta agonist for the relief of an acute bronchospasm in patients receiving chronic oral therapy with terbutaline). Products include:
Epifrin Sterile Ophthalmic Solution .... ⊙ 235
EpiPen 1236
Primatene Mist .... ▣ 779
Xylocaine with Epinephrine Injection 653

Epinephrine Bitartrate (Co-administration of terbutaline with other sympathomimetic agents is not recommended, since the combined effect on the cardiovascular system may be deleterious to the patient; however, this does not preclude the use of an aerosol beta agonist for the relief of an acute bronchospasm in patients receiving chronic oral therapy with terbutaline). Products include:
Sensorcaine 643

Epinephrine Hydrochloride (Co-administration of terbutaline with other sympathomimetic agents is not recommended, since the combined effect on the cardiovascular system may be deleterious to the patient; however, this does not preclude the use of an aerosol beta agonist for the relief of an acute bronchospasm in patients receiving chronic oral therapy with terbutaline).
No products indexed under this heading.

Esmolol Hydrochloride (Beta-adrenergic blocking agents not only block the pulmonary effect of beta-agonists but may produce severe bronchospasm in asthmatic patients). Products include:
Brevibloc Injection 858

Ethacrynic Acid (The ECG changes and/or hypokalemia that may result from the administration of non-potassium sparing diuretics can be acutely worsened by beta-agonists, especially when the recommended dose of beta-agonist is exceeded). Products include:
Edecrin Tablets 2091

Furosemide (The ECG changes and/or hypokalemia that may result from the administration of non-potassium sparing diuretics can be acutely worsened by beta-agonists, especially when the recommended dose of beta-agonist is exceeded). Products include:
Furosemide Tablets 2284

Hydrochlorothiazide (The ECG changes and/or hypokalemia that may result from the administration of non-potassium sparing diuretics can be acutely worsened by beta-agonists, especially when the recommended dose of beta-agonist is exceeded). Products include:
Accuretic Tablets 2614
Aldoril Tablets 2039
Atacand HCT Tablets 597
Avalide Tablets 1070
Diovan HCT Tablets 2338
Dyazide Capsules 1515
HydroDIURIL Tablets 2108
Hyzaar 2109
Inderide Tablets 3517
Inderide LA Long-Acting Capsules .. 3519
Lotensin HCT Tablets 2367
Maxzide 1008
Micardis HCT Tablets 1051
Microzide Capsules 3414
Moduretic Tablets 2138
Monopril HCT 1094
Prinzide Tablets 2168
Timolide Tablets 2187
Uniretic Tablets 3178
Vaseretic Tablets 2204
Zestoretic Tablets 695
Ziac Tablets 1887

Hydroflumethiazide (The ECG changes and/or hypokalemia that may result from the administration of non-potassium sparing diuretics can be acutely worsened by beta-agonists, especially when the recommended dose of beta-agonist is exceeded). Products include:
Diucardin Tablets 3494

Imipramine Hydrochloride (The action of terbutaline on the vascular system may be potentiated; concurrent and/or sequential use should be undertaken with extreme caution).
No products indexed under this heading.

Imipramine Pamoate (The action of terbutaline on the vascular system may be potentiated; concurrent and/or sequential use should be undertaken with extreme caution).
No products indexed under this heading.

Isocarboxazid (The action of terbutaline on the vascular system may be potentiated; concurrent and/or sequential use should be undertaken with extreme caution).
No products indexed under this heading.

Isoproterenol Hydrochloride (Co-administration of terbutaline with other sympathomimetic agents is not recommended, since the combined effect on the cardiovascular system may be deleterious to the patient; however, this does not preclude the use of an aerosol beta agonist for the relief of an acute bronchospasm in patients receiving chronic oral therapy with terbutaline).
No products indexed under this heading.

Isoproterenol Sulfate (Co-administration of terbutaline with other sympathomimetic agents is not recommended, since the combined effect on the cardiovascular system may be deleterious to the patient; however, this does not preclude the use of an aerosol beta agonist for the relief of an acute bronchospasm in patients receiving chronic oral therapy with terbutaline).
No products indexed under this heading.

Labetalol Hydrochloride (Beta-adrenergic blocking agents not only block the pulmonary effect of beta-agonists but may produce severe bronchospasm in asthmatic patients). Products include:
Normodyne Injection 3135
Normodyne Tablets 3137

Levalbuterol Hydrochloride (Co-administration of terbutaline with other sympathomimetic agents is not recommended, since the combined effect on the cardiovascular system may be deleterious to the patient; however, this does not preclude the use of an aerosol beta agonist for the relief of an acute bronchospasm in patients receiving chronic oral therapy with terbutaline). Products include:
Xopenex Inhalation Solution 3207

Levobunolol Hydrochloride (Beta-adrenergic blocking agents not only block the pulmonary effect of beta-agonists but may produce severe bronchospasm in asthmatic patients). Products include:
Betagan .... ⊙ 228

Maprotiline Hydrochloride (The action of terbutaline on the vascular system may be potentiated; concurrent and/or sequential use should be undertaken with extreme caution).
No products indexed under this heading.

Metaproterenol Sulfate (Co-administration of terbutaline with other sympathomimetic agents is not recommended, since the combined effect on the cardiovascular system may be deleterious to the patient; however, this does not preclude the use of an aerosol beta agonist for the relief of an acute bronchospasm in patients receiving chronic oral therapy with terbutaline). Products include:
Alupent 1029

Metaraminol Bitartrate (Co-administration of terbutaline with other sympathomimetic agents is not recommended, since the combined effect on the cardiovascular system may be deleterious to the patient; however, this does not preclude the use of an aerosol beta agonist for the relief of an acute bronchospasm in patients receiving chronic oral therapy with terbutaline). Products include:
Aramine Injection 2043

Methoxamine Hydrochloride (Co-administration of terbutaline with other sympathomimetic agents is not recommended, since the combined effect on the cardiovascular system may be deleterious to the patient; however, this does not preclude the use of an aerosol beta agonist for the relief of an acute bronchospasm in patients receiving chronic oral therapy with terbutaline).
No products indexed under this heading.

Methyclothiazide (The ECG changes and/or hypokalemia that may result from the administration of non-potassium sparing diuretics can be acutely worsened by beta-agonists, especially when the recommended dose of beta-agonist is exceeded).
No products indexed under this heading.

Metipranolol Hydrochloride (Beta-adrenergic blocking agents not only block the pulmonary effect of beta-agonists but may produce severe bronchospasm in asthmatic

patients).
No products indexed under this heading.

Metoprolol Succinate (Beta-adrenergic blocking agents not only block the pulmonary effect of beta-agonists but may produce severe bronchospasm in asthmatic patients). Products include:
- Toprol-XL Tablets 651

Metoprolol Tartrate (Beta-adrenergic blocking agents not only block the pulmonary effect of beta-agonists but may produce severe bronchospasm in asthmatic patients).
No products indexed under this heading.

Moclobemide (The action of terbutaline on the vascular system may be potentiated; concurrent and/or sequential use should be undertaken with extreme caution).
No products indexed under this heading.

Nadolol (Beta-adrenergic blocking agents not only block the pulmonary effect of beta-agonists but may produce severe bronchospasm in asthmatic patients). Products include:
- Corgard Tablets 2245
- Corzide 40/5 Tablets 2247
- Corzide 80/5 Tablets 2247
- Nadolol Tablets 2288

Norepinephrine Bitartrate (Co-administration of terbutaline with other sympathomimetic agents is not recommended, since the combined effect on the cardiovascular system may be deleterious to the patient; however, this does not preclude the use of an aerosol beta agonist for the relief of an acute bronchospasm in patients receiving chronic oral therapy with terbutaline).
No products indexed under this heading.

Nortriptyline Hydrochloride (The action of terbutaline on the vascular system may be potentiated; concurrent and/or sequential use should be undertaken with extreme caution).
No products indexed under this heading.

Pargyline Hydrochloride (The action of terbutaline on the vascular system may be potentiated; concurrent and/or sequential use should be undertaken with extreme caution).
No products indexed under this heading.

Penbutolol Sulfate (Beta-adrenergic blocking agents not only block the pulmonary effect of beta-agonists but may produce severe bronchospasm in asthmatic patients).
No products indexed under this heading.

Phenelzine Sulfate (The action of terbutaline on the vascular system may be potentiated; concurrent and/or sequential use should be undertaken with extreme caution). Products include:
- Nardil Tablets 2653

Phenylephrine Bitartrate (Co-administration of terbutaline with other sympathomimetic agents is not recommended, since the combined effect on the cardiovascular system may be deleterious to the patient; however, this does not preclude the use of an aerosol beta agonist for the relief of an acute bronchospasm in patients receiving chronic oral therapy with terbutaline).
No products indexed under this heading.

Phenylephrine Hydrochloride (Co-administration of terbutaline with other sympathomimetic agents is not recommended, since the combined effect on the cardiovascular system may be deleterious to the patient; however, this does not preclude the use of an aerosol beta agonist for the relief of an acute bronchospasm in patients receiving chronic oral therapy with terbutaline). Products include:
- Afrin Nasal Decongestant Children's Pump Mist .... ■734
- Extendryl 1361
- Hycomine Compound Tablets 1317
- Neo-Synephrine .... ■614
- Phenergan VC Syrup 3560
- Phenergan VC with Codeine Syrup 3561
- Preparation H Cream .... ■778
- Preparation H Cooling Gel .... ■778
- Preparation H .... ■778
- Vicks Sinex Nasal Spray and Ultra Fine Mist .... ■729

Phenylephrine Tannate (Co-administration of terbutaline with other sympathomimetic agents is not recommended, since the combined effect on the cardiovascular system may be deleterious to the patient; however, this does not preclude the use of an aerosol beta agonist for the relief of an acute bronchospasm in patients receiving chronic oral therapy with terbutaline). Products include:
- Ryna-12 S Suspension 3351
- Reformulated Rynatan Pediatric Suspension 3352
- Rynatuss Pediatric Suspension 3353
- Rynatuss Tablets 3353

Phenylpropanolamine Hydrochloride (Co-administration of terbutaline with other sympathomimetic agents is not recommended, since the combined effect on the cardiovascular system may be deleterious to the patient; however, this does not preclude the use of an aerosol beta agonist for the relief of an acute bronchospasm in patients receiving chronic oral therapy with terbutaline).
No products indexed under this heading.

Pindolol (Beta-adrenergic blocking agents not only block the pulmonary effect of beta-agonists but may produce severe bronchospasm in asthmatic patients).
No products indexed under this heading.

Pirbuterol Acetate (Co-administration of terbutaline with other sympathomimetic agents is not recommended, since the combined effect on the cardiovascular system may be deleterious to the patient; however, this does not preclude the use of an aerosol beta agonist for the relief of an acute bronchospasm in patients receiving chronic oral therapy with terbutaline). Products include:
- Maxair Autohaler 1981
- Maxair Inhaler 1984

Polythiazide (The ECG changes and/or hypokalemia that may result from the administration of non-potassium sparing diuretics can be acutely worsened by beta-agonists, especially when the recommended dose of beta-agonist is exceeded). Products include:
- Minizide Capsules 2700
- Renese Tablets 2712

Procarbazine Hydrochloride (The action of terbutaline on the vascular system may be potentiated; concurrent and/or sequential use should be undertaken with extreme caution). Products include:
- Matulane Capsules 3246

Propranolol Hydrochloride (Beta-adrenergic blocking agents not only block the pulmonary effect of beta-agonists but may produce severe bronchospasm in asthmatic patients). Products include:
- Inderal 3513
- Inderal LA Long-Acting Capsules 3516
- Inderide Tablets 3517
- Inderide LA Long-Acting Capsules 3519

Protriptyline Hydrochloride (The action of terbutaline on the vascular system may be potentiated; concurrent and/or sequential use should be undertaken with extreme caution). Products include:
- Vivactil Tablets 2446
- Vivactil Tablets 2217

Pseudoephedrine Hydrochloride (Co-administration of terbutaline with other sympathomimetic agents is not recommended, since the combined effect on the cardiovascular system may be deleterious to the patient; however, this does not preclude the use of an aerosol beta agonist for the relief of an acute bronchospasm in patients receiving chronic oral therapy with terbutaline). Products include:
- Actifed Cold & Allergy Tablets .... ■688
- Actifed Cold & Sinus Caplets and Tablets .... ■688
- Advil Cold and Sinus Caplets .... ■771
- Advil Cold and Sinus Tablets .... ■771
- Advil Flu & Body Ache Caplets .... ■772
- Aleve Cold & Sinus Caplets .... ■603
- Alka-Seltzer Plus Liqui-Gels .... ■604
- Alka-Seltzer Plus Cold & Flu Medicine Liqui-Gels .... ■604
- Alka-Seltzer Plus Cold & Sinus Medicine Liqui-Gels .... ■604
- Allegra-D Extended-Release Tablets 714
- BC Cold Powder .... ■619
- Benadryl Allergy/Cold Tablets .... ■691
- Benadryl Allergy/Congestion Tablets .... ■692
- Benadryl Allergy & Sinus Liquid .... ■693
- Benadryl Allergy & Sinus Fastmelt Tablets .... ■693
- Benadryl Allergy Sinus Headache Caplets & Gelcaps .... ■693
- Benadryl Severe Allergy & Sinus Headache Caplets .... ■694
- Benadryl Children's Allergy/Cold Fastmelt Tablets .... ■692
- Benylin Multi-Symptom Liquid .... ■697
- Bromfed Capsules (Extended-Release) 2269
- Bromfed-PD Capsules (Extended-Release) 2269
- Children's Cēpacol Sore Throat .... ■788
- Comtrex Acute Head Cold & Sinus Pressure Relief Tablets .... ■627
- Comtrex Deep Chest Cold & Congestion Relief Softgels .... ■627
- Comtrex Flu Therapy & Fever Relief Daytime Caplets .... ■628
- Comtrex Flu Therapy & Fever Relief Nighttime Tablets .... ■628
- Comtrex Maximum Strength Multi-Symptom Cold & Cough Relief Tablets and Caplets .... ■626
- Contac Non-Drowsy 12 Hour Cold Caplets .... ■745
- Contac Non-Drowsy Timed Release 12 Hour Cold Caplets .... ■746
- Contac Severe Cold and Flu Caplets Maximum Strength .... ■746
- Contac Severe Cold and Flu Caplets Non-Drowsy .... ■746
- Dimetapp Elixir .... ■777
- Dimetapp Cold and Fever Suspension .... ■775
- Dimetapp DM Cold & Cough Elixir .... ■775
- Dimetapp Nighttime Flu Liquid .... ■776
- Dimetapp Non-Drowsy Flu Syrup .... ■777
- Dimetapp Infant Drops Decongestant .... ■775
- Dimetapp Infant Drops Decongestant Plus Cough .... ■776
- Guaifed 2272
- Kronofed-A 1341
- Children's Motrin Cold Oral Suspension 2007
- Motrin Sinus Headache Caplets 2005
- PediaCare Cough-Cold Liquid .... ■719
- PediaCare Infants' Drops Decongestant .... ■719
- PediaCare Infants' Drops Decongestant Plus Cough .... ■719
- PediaCare NightRest Cough-Cold Liquid .... ■719
- Robitussin Cold Caplets Cold & Congestion .... ■780
- Robitussin Cold Softgels Cold & Congestion .... ■780
- Robitussin Cold Caplets Multi-Symptom Cold & Flu .... ■781
- Robitussin Cold Softgels Multi-Symptom Cold & Flu .... ■781
- Robitussin Cold Softgels Severe Congestion .... ■782
- Robitussin Cough & Cold Infant Drops .... ■782
- Robitussin Maximum Strength Cough & Cold Liquid .... ■785
- Robitussin Pediatric Cough & Cold Formula Liquid .... ■785
- Robitussin Multi Symptom Honey Flu Liquid .... ■785
- Robitussin Nighttime Honey Flu Liquid .... ■786
- Robitussin-CF Liquid .... ■783
- Robitussin-DAC Syrup 2942
- Robitussin-PE Liquid .... ■782
- Ryna .... ■768
- Semprex-D Capsules 1172
- Singlet Caplets .... ■761
- Sinutab Non-Drying Liquid Caps .... ■706
- Sinutab Sinus Allergy Medication, Maximum Strength Formula, Tablets & Caplets .... ■707
- Sinutab Sinus Medication, Maximum Strength Without Drowsiness Formula, Tablets & Caplets .... ■707
- Sudafed 12 Hour Tablets .... ■708
- Sudafed 24 Hour Tablets .... ■708
- Children's Sudafed Cold & Cough Liquid .... ■709
- Children's Sudafed Nasal Decongestant Chewables .... ■711
- Children's Sudafed Nasal Decongestant Liquid Medication .... ■711
- Sudafed Cold & Allergy Tablets .... ■708
- Sudafed Cold & Cough Liquid Caps .... ■709
- Sudafed Cold & Sinus Liquid Caps .... ■710
- Sudafed Nasal Decongestant Tablets .... ■710
- Sudafed Non-Drying Sinus Liquid Caps .... ■712
- Sudafed Severe Cold .... ■711
- Sudafed Sinus Headache Caplets .... ■712
- Sudafed Sinus Headache Tablets .... ■712
- Tavist Sinus Non-Drowsy Coated Caplets .... ■676
- TheraFlu Regular Strength Cold & Cough Night Time Hot Liquid .... ■676
- TheraFlu Regular Strength Cold & Sore Throat Night Time Hot Liquid .... ■676
- TheraFlu Maximum Strength Flu & Congestion Non-Drowsy Hot Liquid .... ■677
- TheraFlu Maximum Strength Flu & Cough Night Time Hot Liquid .... ■678
- TheraFlu Maximum Strength Flu & Sore Throat Night Time Hot Liquid .... ■677
- TheraFlu Maximum Strength Severe Cold & Congestion Night Time Caplets .... ■678
- TheraFlu Maximum Strength Severe Cold & Congestion Night Time Hot Liquid .... ■678
- TheraFlu Maximum Strength Severe Cold & Congestion Non-Drowsy .... ■679
- Triaminic Allergy Congestion Liquid .... ■680
- Triaminic Chest Congestion Liquid .... ■680
- Triaminic Cold & Allergy Liquid .... ■681
- Triaminic Cold & Allergy Softchews .... ■683
- Triaminic Cold & Cough Liquid .... ■681
- Triaminic Cold & Cough Softchews .... ■683
- Triaminic Cold & Night Time Cough Liquid .... ■681
- Triaminic Cold, Cough & Fever Liquid .... ■681
- Triaminic Cough Liquid .... ■682
- Triaminic Cough & Congestion Liquid .... ■682
- Triaminic Cough & Sore Throat Liquid .... ■682
- Triaminic Cough & Sore Throat Softchews .... ■684
- Children's Tylenol Allergy-D Liquid 2014
- Children's Tylenol Cold Suspension Liquid and Chewable Tablets 2015
- Children's Tylenol Cold Plus Cough Suspension Liquid and Chewable Tablets 2015
- Children's Tylenol Flu Suspension Liquid 2015
- Children's Tylenol Sinus Suspension Liquid 2017
- Infants' Tylenol Cold Decongestant and Fever Reducer Concentrated Drops 2015

Infants' Tylenol Cold Decongestant and Fever Reducer Concentrated Drops Plus Cough.. 2015
Tylenol Allergy Sinus ... 2010
Multi-Symptom Tylenol Cold Complete Formula Caplets ... 2010
Multi-Symptom Tylenol Cold Non-Drowsy Caplets and Gelcaps ... 2010
Multi-Symptom Tylenol Cold Severe Congestion Non-Drowsy Caplets ... 2011
Maximum Strength Tylenol Flu NightTime Gelcaps ... 2011
Maximum Strength Tylenol Flu NightTime Liquid ... 2011
Maximum Strength Tylenol Flu Non-Drowsy Gelcaps ... 2011
Maximum Strength Tylenol Sinus NightTime Caplets ... 2012
Maximum Strength Tylenol Sinus Non-Drowsy Geltabs, Gelcaps, Caplets, and Tablets ... 2012
Vicks 44D Cough & Head Congestion Relief Liquid ... ▣724
Vicks 44M Cough, Cold & Flu Relief Liquid ... ▣725
Pediatric Vicks 44m Cough & Cold Relief ... ▣728
Vicks DayQuil LiquiCaps/Liquid Multi-Symptom Cold/Flu Relief ... ▣727
Children's Vicks NyQuil Cold/Cough Relief ... ▣726
Vicks NyQuil LiquiCaps/Liquid Multi-Symptom Cold/Flu Relief, Original and Cherry Flavors ... ▣727
Zephrex Tablets ... 3091
Zephrex LA Tablets ... 3092
Zyrtec-D 12 Hour Extended Relief Tablets ... 2758

Pseudoephedrine Sulfate (Co-administration of terbutaline with other sympathomimetic agents is not recommended, since the combined effect on the cardiovascular system may be deleterious to the patient; however, this does not preclude the use of an aerosol beta agonist for the relief of an acute bronchospasm in patients receiving chronic oral therapy with terbutaline). Products include:
Chlor-Trimeton Allergy/Decongestant Tablets ... ▣736
Claritin-D 12 Hour Extended Release Tablets ... 3102
Claritin-D 24 Hour Extended Release Tablets ... 3104
Coricidin 'D' Cold, Flu & Sinus Tablets ... ▣737
Drixoral Allergy/Sinus Extended-Release Tablets ... ▣741
Drixoral Cold & Allergy Sustained-Action Tablets ... ▣740
Drixoral Cold & Flu Extended-Release Tablets ... ▣740
Drixoral Nasal Decongestant Long-Acting Non-Drowsy Tablets ... ▣740
Rynatan Tablets ... 3351

Salmeterol Xinafoate (Co-administration of terbutaline with other sympathomimetic agents is not recommended, since the combined effect on the cardiovascular system may be deleterious to the patient; however, this does not preclude the use of an aerosol beta agonist for the relief of an acute bronchospasm in patients receiving chronic oral therapy with terbutaline). Products include:
Advair Diskus 100/50 ... 1448
Advair Diskus 250/50 ... 1448
Advair Diskus 500/50 ... 1448
Serevent Diskus ... 1637
Serevent Inhalation Aerosol ... 1633

Selegiline Hydrochloride (The action of terbutaline on the vascular system may be potentiated; concurrent and/or sequential use should be undertaken with extreme caution). Products include:
Eldepryl Capsules ... 3266

Sotalol Hydrochloride (Beta-adrenergic blocking agents not only block the pulmonary effect of beta-agonists but may produce severe bronchospasm in asthmatic patients). Products include:
Betapace Tablets ... 950
Betapace AF Tablets ... 954

Timolol Hemihydrate (Beta-adrenergic blocking agents not only block the pulmonary effect of beta-agonists but may produce severe bronchospasm in asthmatic patients). Products include:
Betimol Ophthalmic Solution ... ⊙324

Timolol Maleate (Beta-adrenergic blocking agents not only block the pulmonary effect of beta-agonists but may produce severe bronchospasm in asthmatic patients). Products include:
Blocadren Tablets ... 2046
Cosopt Sterile Ophthalmic Solution ... 2065
Timolide Tablets ... 2187
Timolol GFS ... ⊙266
Timoptic in Ocudose ... 2192
Timoptic Sterile Ophthalmic Solution ... 2190
Timoptic-XE Sterile Ophthalmic Gel Forming Solution ... 2194

Torsemide (The ECG changes and/or hypokalemia that may result from the administration of non-potassium sparing diuretics can be acutely worsened by beta-agonists, especially when the recommended dose of beta-agonist is exceeded). Products include:
Demadex Tablets and Injection ... 2965

Tranylcypromine Sulfate (The action of terbutaline on the vascular system may be potentiated; concurrent and/or sequential use should be undertaken with extreme caution). Products include:
Parnate Tablets ... 1607

Trimipramine Maleate (The action of terbutaline on the vascular system may be potentiated; concurrent and/or sequential use should be undertaken with extreme caution). Products include:
Surmontil Capsules ... 3595

BREVIBLOC INJECTION

(Esmolol Hydrochloride) ... 858
May interact with oral hypoglycemic agents, insulin, and certain other agents. Compounds in these categories include:

Acarbose (Beta blockers may mask tachycardia occurring with hypoglycemia). Products include:
Precose Tablets ... 906

Chlorpropamide (Beta blockers may mask tachycardia occurring with hypoglycemia). Products include:
Diabinese Tablets ... 2680

Digoxin (Increased digoxin levels by 10-20% when concomitantly administered by intravenous route). Products include:
Digitek Tablets ... 1003
Lanoxicaps Capsules ... 1574
Lanoxin Injection ... 1581
Lanoxin Tablets ... 1587
Lanoxin Elixir Pediatric ... 1578
Lanoxin Injection Pediatric ... 1584

Dopamine Hydrochloride (Concurrent use is not recommended to control supraventricular tachycardia because of the danger of blocking cardiac contractility when systemic vascular resistance is high).
No products indexed under this heading.

Epinephrine Hydrochloride (Concurrent use is not recommended to control supraventricular tachycardia because of the danger of blocking cardiac contractility when systemic vascular resistance is high; potential for unresponsiveness to the usual dose of epinephrine to treat allergic reaction).
No products indexed under this heading.

Glimepiride (Beta blockers may mask tachycardia occurring with hypoglycemia). Products include:
Amaryl Tablets ... 717

Glipizide (Beta blockers may mask tachycardia occurring with hypoglycemia). Products include:
Glucotrol Tablets ... 2692
Glucotrol XL Extended Release Tablets ... 2693

Glyburide (Beta blockers may mask tachycardia occurring with hypoglycemia). Products include:
DiaBeta Tablets ... 741
Glucovance Tablets ... 1086

Insulin, Human, Zinc Suspension (Beta blockers may mask tachycardia occurring with hypoglycemia). Products include:
Humulin L, 100 Units ... 1937
Humulin U, 100 Units ... 1943
Novolin L Human Insulin 10 ml Vials ... 2422

Insulin, Human NPH (Beta blockers may mask tachycardia occurring with hypoglycemia). Products include:
Humulin N, 100 Units ... 1939
Humulin N NPH Pen ... 1940
Novolin N Human Insulin 10 ml Vials ... 2422
Novolin N PenFill ... 2423
Novolin N Prefilled Syringe Disposable Insulin Delivery System ... 2425

Insulin, Human Regular (Beta blockers may mask tachycardia occurring with hypoglycemia). Products include:
Humulin R Regular (U-500) ... 1943
Humulin R, 100 Units ... 1941
Novolin R Human Insulin 10 ml Vials ... 2423
Novolin R PenFill ... 2423
Novolin R Prefilled Syringe Disposable Insulin Delivery System ... 2425
Velosulin BR Human Insulin 10 ml Vials ... 2435

Insulin, Human Regular and Human NPH Mixture (Beta blockers may mask tachycardia occurring with hypoglycemia). Products include:
Humulin 50/50, 100 Units ... 1934
Humulin 70/30, 100 Units ... 1935
Humulin 70/30 Pen ... 1936
Novolin 70/30 Human Insulin 10 ml Vials ... 2421
Novolin 70/30 PenFill ... 2423
Novolin 70/30 Prefilled Disposable Insulin Delivery System ... 2425

Insulin, NPH (Beta blockers may mask tachycardia occurring with hypoglycemia). Products include:
Iletin II, NPH (Pork), 100 Units ... 1946

Insulin, Regular (Beta blockers may mask tachycardia occurring with hypoglycemia). Products include:
Iletin II, Regular (Pork), 100 Units ... 1947

Insulin, Zinc Crystals (Beta blockers may mask tachycardia occurring with hypoglycemia).
No products indexed under this heading.

Insulin, Zinc Suspension (Beta blockers may mask tachycardia occurring with hypoglycemia). Products include:
Iletin II, Lente (Pork), 100 Units ... 1945

Insulin Aspart, Human Regular (Beta blockers may mask tachycardia occurring with hypoglycemia).
No products indexed under this heading.

Insulin glargine (Beta blockers may mask tachycardia occurring with hypoglycemia). Products include:
Lantus Injection ... 742

Insulin Lispro, Human (Beta blockers may mask tachycardia occurring with hypoglycemia). Products include:
Humalog ... 1926
Humalog Mix 75/25 Pen ... 1928

Insulin Lispro Protamine, Human (Beta blockers may mask tachycardia occurring with hypoglycemia). Products include:
Humalog Mix 75/25 Pen ... 1928

Metformin Hydrochloride (Beta blockers may mask tachycardia occurring with hypoglycemia). Products include:
Glucophage Tablets ... 1080
Glucophage XR Tablets ... 1080
Glucovance Tablets ... 1086

Miglitol (Beta blockers may mask tachycardia occurring with hypoglycemia). Products include:
Glyset Tablets ... 2821

Morphine Sulfate (Intravenous morphine increases Brevibloc steady-state blood levels by 46%). Products include:
Astramorph/PF Injection, USP (Preservative-Free) ... 594
Duramorph Injection ... 1312
Infumorph 200 and Infumorph 500 Sterile Solutions ... 1314
Kadian Capsules ... 1335
MS Contin Tablets ... 2896
MSIR ... 2898
Oramorph SR Tablets ... 3062
Roxanol ... 3066

Norepinephrine Hydrochloride (Concurrent use is not recommended to control supraventricular tachycardia because of the danger of blocking cardiac contractility when systemic vascular resistance is high).
No products indexed under this heading.

Pioglitazone Hydrochloride (Beta blockers may mask tachycardia occurring with hypoglycemia). Products include:
Actos Tablets ... 3275

Repaglinide (Beta blockers may mask tachycardia occurring with hypoglycemia). Products include:
Prandin Tablets (0.5, 1, and 2 mg) ... 2432

Reserpine (Potential for additive effect; hypotension or marked bradycardia which may result in vertigo, syncope, or postural hypotension).
No products indexed under this heading.

Rosiglitazone Maleate (Beta blockers may mask tachycardia occurring with hypoglycemia). Products include:
Avandia Tablets ... 1490

Succinylcholine Chloride (Prolonged neuromuscular blockade from five minutes to eight minutes). Products include:
Anectine Injection ... 1476

Tolazamide (Beta blockers may mask tachycardia occurring with hypoglycemia).
No products indexed under this heading.

Tolbutamide (Beta blockers may mask tachycardia occurring with hypoglycemia).
No products indexed under this heading.

Troglitazone (Beta blockers may mask tachycardia occurring with hypoglycemia).
No products indexed under this heading.

Verapamil Hydrochloride (Potential for fatal cardiac arrests in patients with depressed myocardial function). Products include:
Covera-HS Tablets ... 3199
Isoptin SR Tablets ... 467
Tarka Tablets ... 508
Verelan Capsules ... 3184
Verelan PM Capsules ... 3186

Warfarin Sodium (Brevibloc concentrations were equivocally higher when given with Warfarin). Products include:
Coumadin for Injection ... 1243
Coumadin Tablets ... 1243
Warfarin Sodium Tablets, USP ... 3302

BREVICON 28-DAY TABLETS

(Ethinyl Estradiol, Norethindrone) 3380
May interact with barbiturates, phenytoin, tetracyclines, and certain other agents. Compounds in these categories include:

Ampicillin (Potential for reduced efficacy and increased incidence of breakthrough bleeding and menstrual irregularities with concomitant use).
No products indexed under this heading.

Ampicillin Sodium (Potential for reduced efficacy and increased incidence of breakthrough bleeding and menstrual irregularities with concomitant use). Products include:
Unasyn for Injection 2728

Aprobarbital (Potential for reduced efficacy and increased incidence of breakthrough bleeding and menstrual irregularities with concomitant use).
No products indexed under this heading.

Butabarbital (Potential for reduced efficacy and increased incidence of breakthrough bleeding and menstrual irregularities with concomitant use).
No products indexed under this heading.

Butalbital (Potential for reduced efficacy and increased incidence of breakthrough bleeding and menstrual irregularities with concomitant use). Products include:
Phrenilin 578
Sedapap Tablets 50 mg/650 mg ... 2225

Demeclocycline Hydrochloride (Potential for reduced efficacy and increased incidence of breakthrough bleeding and menstrual irregularities with concomitant use). Products include:
Declomycin Tablets 1855

Doxycycline Calcium (Potential for reduced efficacy and increased incidence of breakthrough bleeding and menstrual irregularities with concomitant use). Products include:
Vibramycin Calcium Oral Suspension Syrup 2735

Doxycycline Hyclate (Potential for reduced efficacy and increased incidence of breakthrough bleeding and menstrual irregularities with concomitant use). Products include:
Doryx Coated Pellet Filled Capsules 3357
Periostat Tablets 1208
Vibramycin Hyclate Capsules 2735
Vibramycin Hyclate Intravenous 2737
Vibra-Tabs Film Coated Tablets 2735

Doxycycline Monohydrate (Potential for reduced efficacy and increased incidence of breakthrough bleeding and menstrual irregularities with concomitant use). Products include:
Monodox Capsules 2442
Vibramycin Monohydrate for Oral Suspension 2735

Fosphenytoin Sodium (Potential for reduced efficacy and increased incidence of breakthrough bleeding and menstrual irregularities with concomitant use). Products include:
Cerebyx Injection 2619

Griseofulvin (Potential for reduced efficacy and increased incidence of breakthrough bleeding and menstrual irregularities with concomitant use). Products include:
Grifulvin V Tablets Microsize and Oral Suspension Microsize 2518
Gris-PEG Tablets 2661

Mephobarbital (Potential for reduced efficacy and increased incidence of breakthrough bleeding and menstrual irregularities with concomitant use).
No products indexed under this heading.

Methacycline Hydrochloride (Potential for reduced efficacy and increased incidence of breakthrough bleeding and menstrual irregularities with concomitant use).
No products indexed under this heading.

Minocycline Hydrochloride (Potential for reduced efficacy and increased incidence of breakthrough bleeding and menstrual irregularities with concomitant use). Products include:
Dynacin Capsules 2019
Minocin Intravenous 1862
Minocin Oral Suspension 1865
Minocin Pellet-Filled Capsules 1863

Oxytetracycline Hydrochloride (Potential for reduced efficacy and increased incidence of breakthrough bleeding and menstrual irregularities with concomitant use). Products include:
Terra-Cortril Ophthalmic Suspension 2716
Urobiotic-250 Capsules 2731

Pentobarbital Sodium (Potential for reduced efficacy and increased incidence of breakthrough bleeding and menstrual irregularities with concomitant use). Products include:
Nembutal Sodium Solution 485

Phenobarbital (Potential for reduced efficacy and increased incidence of breakthrough bleeding and menstrual irregularities with concomitant use). Products include:
Arco-Lase Plus Tablets 592
Donnatal 2929
Donnatal Extentabs 2930

Phenylbutazone (Potential for reduced efficacy and increased incidence of breakthrough bleeding and menstrual irregularities with concomitant use).
No products indexed under this heading.

Phenytoin (Potential for reduced efficacy and increased incidence of breakthrough bleeding and menstrual irregularities with concomitant use). Products include:
Dilantin Infatabs 2624
Dilantin-125 Oral Suspension 2625

Phenytoin Sodium (Potential for reduced efficacy and increased incidence of breakthrough bleeding and menstrual irregularities with concomitant use). Products include:
Dilantin Kapseals 2622

Rifampin (Co-administration has been associated with reduced efficacy and increased incidence of breakthrough bleeding and menstrual irregularities). Products include:
Rifadin 765
Rifamate Capsules 767
Rifater Tablets 769

Secobarbital Sodium (Potential for reduced efficacy and increased incidence of breakthrough bleeding and menstrual irregularities with concomitant use).
No products indexed under this heading.

Tetracycline Hydrochloride (Potential for reduced efficacy and increased incidence of breakthrough bleeding and menstrual irregularities with concomitant use).
No products indexed under this heading.

Thiamylal Sodium (Potential for reduced efficacy and increased incidence of breakthrough bleeding and menstrual irregularities with concomitant use).
No products indexed under this heading.

BREVITAL SODIUM FOR INJECTION, USP

(Methohexital Sodium) 1815
May interact with barbiturates, corticosteroids, oral anticoagulants, phenytoin, and certain other agents. Compounds in these categories include:

Aprobarbital (Prior chronic administration of barbiturates appears to reduce the effectiveness of methohexital sodium).
No products indexed under this heading.

Betamethasone Acetate (Barbiturates may influence the absorption and elimination of other concomitantly used drugs, such as corticosteroids). Products include:
Celestone Soluspan Injectable Suspension 3097

Betamethasone Sodium Phosphate (Barbiturates may influence the absorption and elimination of other concomitantly used drugs, such as corticosteroids). Products include:
Celestone Soluspan Injectable Suspension 3097

Butabarbital (Prior chronic administration of barbiturates appears to reduce the effectiveness of methohexital sodium).
No products indexed under this heading.

Butalbital (Prior chronic administration of barbiturates appears to reduce the effectiveness of methohexital sodium). Products include:
Phrenilin 578
Sedapap Tablets 50 mg/650 mg ... 2225

Cortisone Acetate (Barbiturates may influence the absorption and elimination of other concomitantly used drugs, such as corticosteroids). Products include:
Cortone Acetate Injectable Suspension 2059
Cortone Acetate Tablets 2061

Dexamethasone (Barbiturates may influence the absorption and elimination of other concomitantly used drugs, such as corticosteroids). Products include:
Decadron Elixir 2078
Decadron Tablets 2079
TobraDex Ophthalmic Ointment 542
TobraDex Ophthalmic Suspension .. 541

Dexamethasone Acetate (Barbiturates may influence the absorption and elimination of other concomitantly used drugs, such as corticosteroids).
No products indexed under this heading.

Dexamethasone Sodium Phosphate (Barbiturates may influence the absorption and elimination of other concomitantly used drugs, such as corticosteroids). Products include:
Decadron Phosphate Injection 2081
Decadron Phosphate Sterile Ophthalmic Ointment 2083
Decadron Phosphate Sterile Ophthalmic Solution 2084
NeoDecadron Sterile Ophthalmic Solution 2144

Dicumarol (Barbiturates may influence the absorption and elimination of other concomitantly used drugs, such as anticoagulants).
No products indexed under this heading.

Fludrocortisone Acetate (Barbiturates may influence the absorption and elimination of other concomitantly used drugs, such as corticosteroids). Products include:
Florinef Acetate Tablets 2250

Fosphenytoin Sodium (Prior chronic administration of phenytoin appears to reduce the effectiveness of methohexital sodium; barbiturates may influence the absorption and elimination of other concomitantly used drugs, such as phenytoin). Products include:
Cerebyx Injection 2619

Halothane (Barbiturates may influence the absorption and elimination of other concomitantly used drugs, such as halothane). Products include:
Fluothane Inhalation 3508

Hydrocortisone (Barbiturates may influence the absorption and elimination of other concomitantly used drugs, such as corticosteroids). Products include:
Anusol-HC Cream 2.5% 2237
Cipro HC Otic Suspension 540
Cortaid Intensive Therapy Cream .. ■717
Cortaid Maximum Strength Cream .... ■717
Cortisporin Ophthalmic Suspension Sterile .... ⊙297
Cortizone•5 .... ■699
Cortizone•10 .... ■699
Cortizone•10 Plus Creme .... ■700
Cortizone for Kids Creme .... ■699
Hydrocortone Tablets 2106
Massengill Medicated Soft Cloth Towelette .... ■753
VōSoL HC Otic Solution 3356

Hydrocortisone Acetate (Barbiturates may influence the absorption and elimination of other concomitantly used drugs, such as corticosteroids). Products include:
Analpram-HC 1338
Anusol HC-1 Hydrocortisone Anti-Itch Cream .... ■689
Anusol-HC Suppositories 2238
Cortaid .... ■717
Cortifoam Rectal Foam 3170
Cortisporin-TC Otic Suspension 2246
Hydrocortone Acetate Injectable Suspension 2103
Pramosone 1343
Proctocort Suppositories 2264
ProctoFoam-HC 3177
Terra-Cortril Ophthalmic Suspension 2716

Hydrocortisone Sodium Phosphate (Barbiturates may influence the absorption and elimination of other concomitantly used drugs, such as corticosteroids). Products include:
Hydrocortone Phosphate Injection, Sterile 2105

Hydrocortisone Sodium Succinate (Barbiturates may influence the absorption and elimination of other concomitantly used drugs, such as corticosteroids).
No products indexed under this heading.

Mephobarbital (Prior chronic administration of barbiturates appears to reduce the effectiveness of methohexital sodium).
No products indexed under this heading.

Methylprednisolone Acetate (Barbiturates may influence the absorption and elimination of other concomitantly used drugs, such as corticosteroids). Products include:
Depo-Medrol Injectable Suspension 2795

Methylprednisolone Sodium Succinate (Barbiturates may influence the absorption and elimination of other concomitantly used drugs, such as corticosteroids). Products include:
Solu-Medrol Sterile Powder 2855

Pentobarbital Sodium (Prior chronic administration of barbiturates appears to reduce the effectiveness of methohexital sodium). Products include:
Nembutal Sodium Solution 485

Phenobarbital (Prior chronic administration of barbiturates appears to reduce the effectiveness of methohexital sodium). Products include:
Arco-Lase Plus Tablets 592
Donnatal 2929
Donnatal Extentabs 2930

Phenytoin (Prior chronic administration of phenytoin appears to reduce the effectiveness of methohexital sodium; barbiturates may influence the absorption and elimination of other concomitantly used drugs, such as phenytoin). Products include:
- Dilantin Infatabs ... 2624
- Dilantin-125 Oral Suspension ... 2625

Phenytoin Sodium (Prior chronic administration of phenytoin appears to reduce the effectiveness of methohexital sodium; barbiturates may influence the absorption and elimination of other concomitantly used drugs, such as phenytoin). Products include:
- Dilantin Kapseals ... 2622

Prednisolone Acetate (Barbiturates may influence the absorption and elimination of other concomitantly used drugs, such as corticosteroids). Products include:
- Blephamide Ophthalmic Ointment ... 547
- Blephamide Ophthalmic Suspension ... 548
- Poly-Pred Liquifilm Ophthalmic Suspension ... ⊙245
- Pred Forte Ophthalmic Suspension ... ⊙246
- Pred Mild Sterile Ophthalmic Suspension ... ⊙249
- Pred-G Ophthalmic Suspension ... ⊙247
- Pred-G Sterile Ophthalmic Ointment ... ⊙248

Prednisolone Sodium Phosphate (Barbiturates may influence the absorption and elimination of other concomitantly used drugs, such as corticosteroids). Products include:
- Pediapred Oral Solution ... 1170

Prednisolone Tebutate (Barbiturates may influence the absorption and elimination of other concomitantly used drugs, such as corticosteroids).
- No products indexed under this heading.

Prednisone (Barbiturates may influence the absorption and elimination of other concomitantly used drugs, such as corticosteroids). Products include:
- Prednisone ... 3064

Propylene Glycol (Barbiturates may influence the absorption and elimination of other concomitantly used drugs, such as propylene glycol-containing solutions). Products include:
- Moisture Eyes Eye Drops ... ⊙252
- Moisture Eyes Preservative Free Eye Drops ... ⊙253

Secobarbital Sodium (Prior chronic administration of barbiturates appears to reduce the effectiveness of methohexital sodium).
- No products indexed under this heading.

Thiamylal Sodium (Prior chronic administration of barbiturates appears to reduce the effectiveness of methohexital sodium).
- No products indexed under this heading.

Triamcinolone (Barbiturates may influence the absorption and elimination of other concomitantly used drugs, such as corticosteroids).
- No products indexed under this heading.

Triamcinolone Acetonide (Barbiturates may influence the absorption and elimination of other concomitantly used drugs, such as corticosteroids). Products include:
- Azmacort Inhalation Aerosol ... 728
- Nasacort Nasal Inhaler ... 750
- Nasacort AQ Nasal Spray ... 752
- Tri-Nasal Spray ... 2274

Triamcinolone Diacetate (Barbiturates may influence the absorption and elimination of other concomitantly used drugs, such as corticosteroids).
- No products indexed under this heading.

Triamcinolone Hexacetonide (Barbiturates may influence the absorption and elimination of other concomitantly used drugs, such as corticosteroids).
- No products indexed under this heading.

Warfarin Sodium (Barbiturates may influence the absorption and elimination of other concomitantly used drugs, such as anticoagulants). Products include:
- Coumadin for Injection ... 1243
- Coumadin Tablets ... 1243
- Warfarin Sodium Tablets, USP ... 3302

Food Interactions

Alcohol (Barbiturates may influence the absorption and elimination of other concomitantly used drugs, such as ethyl alcohol).

BREVOXYL-4 CLEANSING LOTION
(Benzoyl Peroxide) ... 3269
None cited in PDR database.

BREVOXYL-4 CREAMY WASH
(Benzoyl Peroxide) ... 3270
None cited in PDR database.

BREVOXYL-4 GEL
(Benzoyl Peroxide) ... 3269
None cited in PDR database.

BREVOXYL-8 CLEANSING LOTION
(Benzoyl Peroxide) ... 3269
None cited in PDR database.

BREVOXYL-8 CREAMY WASH
(Benzoyl Peroxide) ... 3270
None cited in PDR database.

BREVOXYL-8 GEL
(Benzoyl Peroxide) ... 3269
None cited in PDR database.

BRITE-LIFE CAPLETS
(Hypericum, Vitamin B_6) ... ■795
None cited in PDR database.

BROMFED CAPSULES (EXTENDED-RELEASE)
(Brompheniramine Maleate, Pseudoephedrine Hydrochloride) ... 2269
May interact with beta blockers, central nervous system depressants, monoamine oxidase inhibitors, veratrum alkaloids, and certain other agents. Compounds in these categories include:

Acebutolol Hydrochloride (Co-administration with beta adrenergic blockers increases the effects of sympathomimetics). Products include:
- Sectral Capsules ... 3589

Alfentanil Hydrochloride (Co-administration may have an additive effect).
- No products indexed under this heading.

Alprazolam (Co-administration may have an additive effect). Products include:
- Xanax Tablets ... 2865

Aprobarbital (Co-administration may have an additive effect).
- No products indexed under this heading.

Atenolol (Co-administration with beta adrenergic blockers increases the effects of sympathomimetics). Products include:
- Tenoretic Tablets ... 690
- Tenormin I.V. Injection ... 692

Betaxolol Hydrochloride (Co-administration with beta adrenergic blockers increases the effects of sympathomimetics). Products include:
- Betoptic S Ophthalmic Suspension ... 537

Bisoprolol Fumarate (Co-administration with beta adrenergic blockers increases the effects of sympathomimetics). Products include:
- Zebeta Tablets ... 1885
- Ziac Tablets ... 1887

Buprenorphine Hydrochloride (Co-administration may have an additive effect). Products include:
- Buprenex Injectable ... 2918

Buspirone Hydrochloride (Co-administration may have an additive effect).
- No products indexed under this heading.

Butabarbital (Co-administration may have an additive effect).
- No products indexed under this heading.

Butalbital (Co-administration may have an additive effect). Products include:
- Phrenilin ... 578
- Sedapap Tablets 50 mg/650 mg ... 2225

Carteolol Hydrochloride (Co-administration with beta adrenergic blockers increases the effects of sympathomimetics). Products include:
- Carteolol Hydrochloride Ophthalmic Solution USP, 1% ... ⊙258
- Ocupress Ophthalmic Solution, 1% Sterile ... ⊙303

Chlordiazepoxide (Co-administration may have an additive effect). Products include:
- Limbitrol ... 1738

Chlordiazepoxide Hydrochloride (Co-administration may have an additive effect). Products include:
- Librium Capsules ... 1736
- Librium for Injection ... 1737

Chlorpromazine (Co-administration may have an additive effect). Products include:
- Thorazine Suppositories ... 1656

Chlorpromazine Hydrochloride (Co-administration may have an additive effect). Products include:
- Thorazine ... 1656

Chlorprothixene (Co-administration may have an additive effect).
- No products indexed under this heading.

Chlorprothixene Hydrochloride (Co-administration may have an additive effect).
- No products indexed under this heading.

Chlorprothixene Lactate (Co-administration may have an additive effect).
- No products indexed under this heading.

Clorazepate Dipotassium (Co-administration may have an additive effect). Products include:
- Tranxene ... 511

Clozapine (Co-administration may have an additive effect). Products include:
- Clozaril Tablets ... 2319

Codeine Phosphate (Co-administration may have an additive effect). Products include:
- Phenergan with Codeine Syrup ... 3557
- Phenergan VC with Codeine Syrup ... 3561
- Robitussin A-C Syrup ... 2942
- Robitussin-DAC Syrup ... 2942
- Ryna-C Liquid ... ■768
- Soma Compound w/Codeine Tablets ... 3355
- Tussi-Organidin NR Liquid ... 3350
- Tussi-Organidin-S NR Liquid ... 3350
- Tylenol with Codeine ... 2595

Cryptenamine Preparations (Reduced antihypertensive effects).
- No products indexed under this heading.

Desflurane (Co-administration may have an additive effect). Products include:
- Suprane Liquid for Inhalation ... 874

Dezocine (Co-administration may have an additive effect).
- No products indexed under this heading.

Diazepam (Co-administration may have an additive effect). Products include:
- Valium Injectable ... 3026
- Valium Tablets ... 3047

Droperidol (Co-administration may have an additive effect).
- No products indexed under this heading.

Enflurane (Co-administration may have an additive effect).
- No products indexed under this heading.

Esmolol Hydrochloride (Co-administration with beta adrenergic blockers increases the effects of sympathomimetics). Products include:
- Brevibloc Injection ... 858

Estazolam (Co-administration may have an additive effect). Products include:
- ProSom Tablets ... 500

Ethchlorvynol (Co-administration may have an additive effect).
- No products indexed under this heading.

Ethinamate (Co-administration may have an additive effect).
- No products indexed under this heading.

Fentanyl (Co-administration may have an additive effect). Products include:
- Duragesic Transdermal System ... 1786

Fentanyl Citrate (Co-administration may have an additive effect). Products include:
- Actiq ... 1184

Fluphenazine Decanoate (Co-administration may have an additive effect).
- No products indexed under this heading.

Fluphenazine Enanthate (Co-administration may have an additive effect).
- No products indexed under this heading.

Fluphenazine Hydrochloride (Co-administration may have an additive effect).
- No products indexed under this heading.

Flurazepam Hydrochloride (Co-administration may have an additive effect).
- No products indexed under this heading.

Glutethimide (Co-administration may have an additive effect).
- No products indexed under this heading.

Haloperidol (Co-administration may have an additive effect). Products include:
- Haldol Injection, Tablets and Concentrate ... 2533

Haloperidol Decanoate (Co-administration may have an additive effect). Products include:
- Haldol Decanoate ... 2535

Hydrocodone Bitartrate (Co-administration may have an additive effect). Products include:
- Hycodan ... 1316
- Hycomine Compound Tablets ... 1317
- Hycotuss Expectorant Syrup ... 1318
- Lortab ... 3319
- Lortab Elixir ... 3317
- Maxidone Tablets CIII ... 3399
- Norco 5/325 Tablets CIII ... 3424
- Norco 7.5/325 Tablets CIII ... 3425
- Norco 10/325 Tablets CIII ... 3427
- Norco 10/325 Tablets CIII ... 3425
- Vicodin Tablets ... 516

Vicodin ES Tablets 517
Vicodin HP Tablets 518
Vicodin Tuss Expectorant 519
Vicoprofen Tablets 520
Zydone Tablets 1330

Hydrocodone Polistirex (Co-administration may have an additive effect). Products include:
Tussionex Pennkinetic Extended-Release Suspension 1174

Hydromorphone Hydrochloride (Co-administration may have an additive effect). Products include:
Dilaudid 441
Dilaudid Oral Liquid 445
Dilaudid Powder 441
Dilaudid Rectal Suppositories 441
Dilaudid Tablets 441
Dilaudid Tablets - 8 mg 445
Dilaudid-HP 443

Hydroxyzine Hydrochloride (Co-administration may have an additive effect). Products include:
Atarax Tablets & Syrup 2667
Vistaril Intramuscular Solution 2738

Isocarboxazid (Co-administration with monoamine oxidase inhibitors increases the effects of sympathomimetics; concurrent use is contraindicated).
No products indexed under this heading.

Isoflurane (Co-administration may have an additive effect).
No products indexed under this heading.

Ketamine Hydrochloride (Co-administration may have an additive effect).
No products indexed under this heading.

Labetalol Hydrochloride (Co-administration with beta adrenergic blockers increases the effects of sympathomimetics). Products include:
Normodyne Injection 3135
Normodyne Tablets 3137

Levobunolol Hydrochloride (Co-administration with beta adrenergic blockers increases the effects of sympathomimetics). Products include:
Betagan .... ⊙228

Levomethadyl Acetate Hydrochloride (Co-administration may have an additive effect).
No products indexed under this heading.

Levorphanol Tartrate (Co-administration may have an additive effect). Products include:
Levo-Dromoran 1734
Levorphanol Tartrate Tablets 3059

Lorazepam (Co-administration may have an additive effect). Products include:
Ativan Injection 3478
Ativan Tablets 3482

Loxapine Hydrochloride (Co-administration may have an additive effect).
No products indexed under this heading.

Loxapine Succinate (Co-administration may have an additive effect). Products include:
Loxitane Capsules 3398

Mecamylamine Hydrochloride (Reduced antihypertensive effects). Products include:
Inversine Tablets 1850

Meperidine Hydrochloride (Co-administration may have an additive effect). Products include:
Demerol 3079
Mepergan Injection 3539

Mephobarbital (Co-administration may have an additive effect).
No products indexed under this heading.

Meprobamate (Co-administration may have an additive effect). Products include:
Miltown Tablets 3349

Mesoridazine Besylate (Co-administration may have an additive effect). Products include:
Serentil 1057

Methadone Hydrochloride (Co-administration may have an additive effect). Products include:
Dolophine Hydrochloride Tablets 3056

Methohexital Sodium (Co-administration may have an additive effect). Products include:
Brevital Sodium for Injection, USP 1815

Methotrimeprazine (Co-administration may have an additive effect).
No products indexed under this heading.

Methoxyflurane (Co-administration may have an additive effect).
No products indexed under this heading.

Methyldopa (Reduced antihypertensive effects). Products include:
Aldoclor Tablets 2035
Aldomet Tablets 2037
Aldoril Tablets 2039

Methyldopate Hydrochloride (Reduced antihypertensive effects).
No products indexed under this heading.

Metipranolol Hydrochloride (Co-administration with beta adrenergic blockers increases the effects of sympathomimetics).
No products indexed under this heading.

Metoprolol Succinate (Co-administration with beta adrenergic blockers increases the effects of sympathomimetics). Products include:
Toprol-XL Tablets 651

Metoprolol Tartrate (Co-administration with beta adrenergic blockers increases the effects of sympathomimetics).
No products indexed under this heading.

Midazolam Hydrochloride (Co-administration may have an additive effect). Products include:
Versed Injection 3027
Versed Syrup 3033

Moclobemide (Co-administration with monoamine oxidase inhibitors increases the effects of sympathomimetics; concurrent use is contraindicated).
No products indexed under this heading.

Molindone Hydrochloride (Co-administration may have an additive effect). Products include:
Moban 1320

Morphine Sulfate (Co-administration may have an additive effect). Products include:
Astramorph/PF Injection, USP (Preservative-Free) 594
Duramorph Injection 1312
Infumorph 200 and Infumorph 500 Sterile Solutions 1314
Kadian Capsules 1335
MS Contin Tablets 2896
MSIR 2898
Oramorph SR Tablets 3062
Roxanol 3066

Nadolol (Co-administration with beta adrenergic blockers increases the effects of sympathomimetics). Products include:
Corgard Tablets 2245
Corzide 40/5 Tablets 2247
Corzide 80/5 Tablets 2247
Nadolol Tablets 2288

Olanzapine (Co-administration may have an additive effect). Products include:
Zyprexa Tablets 1973
Zyprexa ZYDIS Orally Disintegrating Tablets 1973

Oxazepam (Co-administration may have an additive effect).
No products indexed under this heading.

Oxycodone Hydrochloride (Co-administration may have an additive effect). Products include:
OxyContin Tablets 2912
OxyFast Oral Concentrate Solution 2916
OxyIR Capsules 2916
Percocet Tablets 1326
Percodan Tablets 1327
Percolone Tablets 1327
Roxicodone 3067
Tylox Capsules 2597

Pargyline Hydrochloride (Co-administration with monoamine oxidase inhibitors increases the effects of sympathomimetics; concurrent use is contraindicated).
No products indexed under this heading.

Penbutolol Sulfate (Co-administration with beta adrenergic blockers increases the effects of sympathomimetics).
No products indexed under this heading.

Pentobarbital Sodium (Co-administration may have an additive effect). Products include:
Nembutal Sodium Solution 485

Perphenazine (Co-administration may have an additive effect). Products include:
Etrafon 3115
Trilafon 3160

Phenelzine Sulfate (Co-administration with monoamine oxidase inhibitors increases the effects of sympathomimetics; concurrent use is contraindicated). Products include:
Nardil Tablets 2653

Phenobarbital (Co-administration may have an additive effect). Products include:
Arco-Lase Plus Tablets 592
Donnatal 2929
Donnatal Extentabs 2930

Pindolol (Co-administration with beta adrenergic blockers increases the effects of sympathomimetics).
No products indexed under this heading.

Prazepam (Co-administration may have an additive effect).
No products indexed under this heading.

Procarbazine Hydrochloride (Co-administration with monoamine oxidase inhibitors increases the effects of sympathomimetics; concurrent use is contraindicated). Products include:
Matulane Capsules 3246

Prochlorperazine (Co-administration may have an additive effect). Products include:
Compazine 1505

Promethazine Hydrochloride (Co-administration may have an additive effect). Products include:
Mepergan Injection 3539
Phenergan Injection 3553
Phenergan 3556
Phenergan Syrup 3554
Phenergan with Codeine Syrup 3557
Phenergan with Dextromethorphan Syrup 3559
Phenergan VC Syrup 3560
Phenergan VC with Codeine Syrup 3561

Propofol (Co-administration may have an additive effect). Products include:
Diprivan Injectable Emulsion 667

Propoxyphene Hydrochloride (Co-administration may have an additive effect). Products include:
Darvon Pulvules 1909
Darvon Compound-65 Pulvules 1910

Propoxyphene Napsylate (Co-administration may have an additive effect). Products include:
Darvon-N/Darvocet-N 1907
Darvon-N Tablets 1912

Propranolol Hydrochloride (Co-administration with beta adrenergic blockers increases the effects of sympathomimetics). Products include:
Inderal 3513
Inderal LA Long-Acting Capsules 3516
Inderide Tablets 3517
Inderide LA Long-Acting Capsules 3519

Quazepam (Co-administration may have an additive effect).
No products indexed under this heading.

Quetiapine Fumarate (Co-administration may have an additive effect). Products include:
Seroquel Tablets 684

Remifentanil Hydrochloride (Co-administration may have an additive effect).
No products indexed under this heading.

Reserpine (Reduced antihypertensive effects).
No products indexed under this heading.

Risperidone (Co-administration may have an additive effect). Products include:
Risperdal 1796

Secobarbital Sodium (Co-administration may have an additive effect).
No products indexed under this heading.

Selegiline Hydrochloride (Co-administration with monoamine oxidase inhibitors increases the effects of sympathomimetics; concurrent use is contraindicated). Products include:
Eldepryl Capsules 3266

Sevoflurane (Co-administration may have an additive effect).
No products indexed under this heading.

Sotalol Hydrochloride (Co-administration with beta adrenergic blockers increases the effects of sympathomimetics). Products include:
Betapace Tablets 950
Betapace AF Tablets 954

Sufentanil Citrate (Co-administration may have an additive effect).
No products indexed under this heading.

Temazepam (Co-administration may have an additive effect).
No products indexed under this heading.

Thiamylal Sodium (Co-administration may have an additive effect).
No products indexed under this heading.

Thioridazine Hydrochloride (Co-administration may have an additive effect). Products include:
Thioridazine Hydrochloride Tablets 2289

Thiothixene (Co-administration may have an additive effect). Products include:
Navane Capsules 2701
Thiothixene Capsules 2290

Timolol Hemihydrate (Co-administration with beta adrenergic blockers increases the effects of sympathomimetics). Products include:
Betimol Ophthalmic Solution .... ⊙324

Timolol Maleate (Co-administration with beta adrenergic blockers increases the effects of sympathomimetics). Products include:
Blocadren Tablets 2046
Cosopt Sterile Ophthalmic Solution 2065
Timolide Tablets 2187
Timolol GFS .... ⊙266
Timoptic in Ocudose 2192
Timoptic Sterile Ophthalmic Solution 2190
Timoptic-XE Sterile Ophthalmic Gel Forming Solution 2194

Tranylcypromine Sulfate (Co-administration with monoamine oxidase inhibitors increases the effects of sympathomimetics; concurrent use is contraindicated). Products include:
Parnate Tablets 1607

Triazolam (Co-administration may have an additive effect). Products include:
Halcion Tablets 2823

Trifluoperazine Hydrochloride (Co-administration may have an additive effect). Products include:
Stelazine 1640

Zaleplon (Co-administration may have an additive effect). Products include:
Sonata Capsules 3591

Ziprasidone Hydrochloride (Co-administration may have an additive effect). Products include:
Geodon Capsules 2688

Zolpidem Tartrate (Co-administration may have an additive effect). Products include:
Ambien Tablets 3191

Food Interactions

Alcohol (Co-administration may have an additive effect).

BROMFED-PD CAPSULES (EXTENDED-RELEASE)

(Brompheniramine Maleate, Pseudoephedrine Hydrochloride)....... 2269
See Bromfed Capsules (Extended-Release)

BUGS BUNNY CHILDREN'S MULTIVITAMIN PLUS EXTRA C CHEWABLE TABLETS (SUGAR FREE)

(Vitamins with Minerals) 804
None cited in PDR database.

BUGS BUNNY CHILDREN'S MULTIVITAMIN PLUS IRON CHEWABLE TABLETS

(Vitamins with Iron) 802
None cited in PDR database.

BUGS BUNNY COMPLETE CHILDREN'S MULTIVITAMIN/ MULTIMINERAL CHEWABLE TABLETS (SUGAR FREE)

(Vitamins with Minerals) 803
None cited in PDR database.

BUMINATE 5% SOLUTION, USP

(Albumin (human)) 841
None cited in PDR database.

BUMINATE 25% SOLUTION, USP

(Albumin (human)) 842
None cited in PDR database.

BUPRENEX INJECTABLE

(Buprenorphine Hydrochloride) 2918
May interact with antihistamines, benzodiazepines, central nervous system depressants, erythromycin, general anesthetics, hypnotics and sedatives, monoamine oxidase inhibitors, narcotic analgesics, phenothiazines, phenytoin, tranquilizers, and certain other agents. Compounds in these categories include:

Acrivastine (Increased CNS depression). Products include:
Semprex-D Capsules 1172

Alfentanil Hydrochloride (Increased CNS depression).
No products indexed under this heading.

Alprazolam (Increased CNS depression). Products include:
Xanax Tablets 2865

Aprobarbital (Increased CNS depression).
No products indexed under this heading.

Astemizole (Increased CNS depression).
No products indexed under this heading.

Azatadine Maleate (Increased CNS depression). Products include:
Rynatan Tablets 3351

Bromodiphenhydramine Hydrochloride (Increased CNS depression).
No products indexed under this heading.

Brompheniramine Maleate (Increased CNS depression).
Products include:
Bromfed Capsules (Extended-Release)........................ 2269
Bromfed-PD Capsules (Extended-Release)........................ 2269
Comtrex Acute Head Cold & Sinus Pressure Relief Tablets...... 627
Dimetapp Elixir 777
Dimetapp Cold and Fever Suspension........................ 775
Dimetapp DM Cold & Cough Elixir . 775
Dimetapp Nighttime Flu Liquid 776

Buspirone Hydrochloride (Increased CNS depression).
No products indexed under this heading.

Butabarbital (Increased CNS depression).
No products indexed under this heading.

Butalbital (Increased CNS depression). Products include:
Phrenilin 578
Sedapap Tablets 50 mg/650 mg 2225

Carbamazepine (Buprenorphine is metabolized by the CYP3A4 isoenzyme; co-administration with inducers of CYP3A4, such as carbamazepine, may cause increase in clearance of buprenorphine).
Products include:
Carbatrol Capsules 3234
Tegretol/Tegretol-XR 2404

Cetirizine Hydrochloride (Increased CNS depression).
Products include:
Zyrtec 2756
Zyrtec-D 12 Hour Extended Relief Tablets........................ 2758

Chlordiazepoxide (Increased CNS depression). Products include:
Limbitrol 1738

Chlordiazepoxide Hydrochloride (Increased CNS depression).
Products include:
Librium Capsules 1736
Librium for Injection 1737

Chlorpheniramine Maleate (Increased CNS depression).
Products include:
Actifed Cold & Sinus Caplets and Tablets........................ 688
Alka-Seltzer Plus Liqui-Gels 604
BC Allergy Sinus Cold Powder 619
Chlor-Trimeton Allergy Tablets 735
Chlor-Trimeton Allergy/Decongestant Tablets...... 736
Comtrex Flu Therapy & Fever Relief Nighttime Tablets 628
Comtrex Maximum Strength Multi-Symptom Cold & Cough Relief Tablets and Caplets........... 626
Contac Severe Cold and Flu Caplets Maximum Strength......... 746
Coricidin 'D' Cold, Flu & Sinus Tablets........................ 737
Coricidin/Coricidin D 738
Coricidin HBP Maximum Strength Flu Tablets........................ 738
Extendryl 1361
Hycomine Compound Tablets 1317
Kronofed-A 1341
PediaCare Cough-Cold Liquid 719
PediaCare NightRest Cough-Cold Liquid........................ 719
Robitussin Nighttime Honey Flu Liquid........................ 786
Ryna 768
Singlet Caplets 761
Sinutab Sinus Allergy Medication, Maximum Strength Formula, Tablets & Caplets........................ 707
Sudafed Cold & Allergy Tablets 708
TheraFlu Regular Strength Cold & Cough Night Time Hot Liquid........ 676
TheraFlu Regular Strength Cold & Sore Throat Night Time Hot Liquid........................ 676
TheraFlu Maximum Strength Flu & Cough Night Time Hot Liquid .. 678
TheraFlu Maximum Strength Flu & Sore Throat Night Time Hot Liquid........................ 677
TheraFlu Maximum Strength Severe Cold & Congestion Night Time Caplets........................ 678
TheraFlu Maximum Strength Severe Cold & Congestion Night Time Hot Liquid........................ 678
Triaminic Cold & Allergy Liquid 681
Triaminic Cold & Allergy Softchews........................ 683
Triaminic Cold & Cough Liquid 681
Triaminic Cold & Cough Softchews........................ 683
Triaminic Cold & Night Time Cough Liquid........................ 681
Triaminic Cold, Cough & Fever Liquid........................ 681
Children's Tylenol Cold Suspension Liquid and Chewable Tablets........................ 2015
Children's Tylenol Cold Plus Cough Suspension Liquid and Chewable Tablets........................ 2015
Children's Tylenol Flu Suspension Liquid........................ 2015
Maximum Strength Tylenol Allergy Sinus Caplets, Gelcaps, and Geltabs........................ 2010
Multi-Symptom Tylenol Cold Complete Formula Caplets........... 2010
Vicks 44M Cough, Cold & Flu Relief Liquid........................ 725
Pediatric Vicks 44m Cough & Cold Relief........................ 728
Children's Vicks NyQuil Cold/Cough Relief........................ 726

Chlorpheniramine Polistirex (Increased CNS depression).
Products include:
Tussionex Pennkinetic Extended-Release Suspension....... 1174

Chlorpheniramine Tannate (Increased CNS depression).
Products include:
Reformulated Rynatan Pediatric Suspension........................ 3352
Rynatuss Pediatric Suspension 3353
Rynatuss Tablets 3353
Tussi-12 S Suspension 3356
Tussi-12 Tablets 3356

Chlorpromazine (Increased CNS depression). Products include:
Thorazine Suppositories 1656

Chlorpromazine Hydrochloride (Increased CNS depression).
Products include:
Thorazine 1656

Chlorprothixene (Increased CNS depression).
No products indexed under this heading.

Chlorprothixene Hydrochloride (Increased CNS depression).
No products indexed under this heading.

Chlorprothixene Lactate (Increased CNS depression).
No products indexed under this heading.

Clemastine Fumarate (Increased CNS depression). Products include:
Tavist 12 Hour Allergy Tablets 676

Clorazepate Dipotassium (Increased CNS depression).
Products include:
Tranxene 511

Clozapine (Increased CNS depression). Products include:
Clozaril Tablets 2319

Codeine Phosphate (Increased CNS depression). Products include:
Phenergan with Codeine Syrup 3557
Phenergan VC with Codeine Syrup .. 3561
Robitussin A-C Syrup 2942
Robitussin-DAC Syrup 2942
Ryna-C Liquid 768
Soma Compound w/Codeine Tablets........................ 3355
Tussi-Organidin NR Liquid 3350
Tussi-Organidin-S NR Liquid 3350
Tylenol with Codeine 2595

Cyproheptadine Hydrochloride (Increased CNS depression).
Products include:
Periactin Tablets 2155

Desflurane (Increased CNS depression). Products include:
Suprane Liquid for Inhalation 874

Dexchlorpheniramine Maleate (Increased CNS depression).
No products indexed under this heading.

Dezocine (Increased CNS depression).
No products indexed under this heading.

Diazepam (Concurrent use has resulted in respiratory and cardiovascular collapse; increased CNS depression). Products include:
Valium Injectable 3026
Valium Tablets 3047

Diphenhydramine Citrate (Increased CNS depression).
Products include:
Alka-Seltzer PM Effervescent Tablets........................ 605
Benadryl Allergy & Sinus Fastmelt Tablets........................ 693
Benadryl Children's Allergy/Cold Fastmelt Tablets........................ 692
Excedrin PM Tablets, Caplets, and Geltabs........................ 631
Goody's PM Powder 621

Diphenhydramine Hydrochloride (Increased CNS depression).
Products include:
Extra Strength Bayer PM Caplets........................ 611
Benadryl Allergy Chewables 689
Benadryl Allergy 691
Benadryl Allergy Liquid 690
Benadryl Allergy/Cold Tablets 691
Benadryl Allergy/Congestion Tablets........................ 692
Benadryl Allergy & Sinus Liquid 693
Benadryl Allergy Sinus Headache Caplets & Gelcaps........................ 693
Benadryl Severe Allergy & Sinus Headache Caplets........................ 694
Benadryl Dye-Free Allergy Liquid 690
Benadryl Dye-Free Allergy Liqui-Gels Softgels........................ 690
Benadryl Itch Relief Stick Extra Strength........................ 695
Benadryl Cream 695
Benadryl Gel 695
Benadryl Spray 696
Benadryl Parenteral 2617
Coricidin HBP Night-Time Cold & Flu Tablets........................ 738
Nytol QuickCaps Caplets 622
Maximum Strength Nytol QuickGels Softgels........................ 621
Extra Strength Percogesic Aspirin-Free Coated Caplets........ 665
Simply Sleep Caplets 2008
Sominex Original Formula Tablets . 761
Children's Tylenol Allergy-D Liquid ... 2014
Maximum Strength Tylenol Allergy Sinus NightTime Caplets........................ 2010
Tylenol Severe Allergy Caplets 2010
Maximum Strength Tylenol Flu NightTime Gelcaps........................ 2011
Extra Strength Tylenol PM Caplets, Geltabs, and Gelcaps........................ 2012
Unisom Maximum Strength SleepGels........................ 713

Diphenylpyraline Hydrochloride (Increased CNS depression).
No products indexed under this heading.

Droperidol (Increased CNS depression).
No products indexed under this heading.

Enflurane (Increased CNS depression).
No products indexed under this heading.

Erythromycin (Buprenorphine is metabolized by the CYP3A4 isoenzyme; co-administration with inhibitors of CYP3A4, such as erythromy-

IMPORTANT NOTE: Always consult each drug listing in the patient's regimen for possible interactions.

cin, may cause decrease in clearance of buprenorphine). Products include:
- Emgel 2% Topical Gel ... 1285
- Ery-Tab Tablets ... 448
- Erythromycin Base Filmtab Tablets ... 454
- Erythromycin Delayed-Release Capsules, USP ... 455
- PCE Dispertab Tablets ... 498

Erythromycin Estolate (Buprenorphine is metabolized by the CYP3A4 isoenzyme; co-administration with inhibitors of CYP3A4, such as erythromycin, may cause decrease in clearance of buprenorphine).
No products indexed under this heading.

Erythromycin Ethylsuccinate (Buprenorphine is metabolized by the CYP3A4 isoenzyme; co-administration with inhibitors of CYP3A4, such as erythromycin, may cause decrease in clearance of buprenorphine). Products include:
- E.E.S. ... 450
- EryPed ... 446
- Pediazole Suspension ... 3050

Erythromycin Gluceptate (Buprenorphine is metabolized by the CYP3A4 isoenzyme; co-administration with inhibitors of CYP3A4, such as erythromycin, may cause decrease in clearance of buprenorphine).
No products indexed under this heading.

Erythromycin Stearate (Buprenorphine is metabolized by the CYP3A4 isoenzyme; co-administration with inhibitors of CYP3A4, such as erythromycin, may cause decrease in clearance of buprenorphine). Products include:
- Erythrocin Stearate Filmtab Tablets ... 452

Estazolam (Increased CNS depression). Products include:
- ProSom Tablets ... 500

Ethchlorvynol (Increased CNS depression).
No products indexed under this heading.

Ethinamate (Increased CNS depression).
No products indexed under this heading.

Fentanyl (Increased CNS depression). Products include:
- Duragesic Transdermal System ... 1786

Fentanyl Citrate (Increased CNS depression). Products include:
- Actiq ... 1184

Fexofenadine Hydrochloride (Increased CNS depression). Products include:
- Allegra ... 712
- Allegra-D Extended-Release Tablets ... 714

Fluphenazine Decanoate (Increased CNS depression).
No products indexed under this heading.

Fluphenazine Enanthate (Increased CNS depression).
No products indexed under this heading.

Fluphenazine Hydrochloride (Increased CNS depression).
No products indexed under this heading.

Flurazepam Hydrochloride (Increased CNS depression).
No products indexed under this heading.

Fosphenytoin Sodium (Buprenorphine is metabolized by the CYP3A4 isoenzyme; co-administration with inducers of CYP3A4, such as phenytoin, may cause increase in clearance of buprenorphine). Products include:
- Cerebyx Injection ... 2619

Glutethimide (Increased CNS depression).
No products indexed under this heading.

Halazepam (Increased CNS depression).
No products indexed under this heading.

Haloperidol (Increased CNS depression). Products include:
- Haldol Injection, Tablets and Concentrate ... 2533

Haloperidol Decanoate (Increased CNS depression). Products include:
- Haldol Decanoate ... 2535

Hydrocodone Bitartrate (Increased CNS depression). Products include:
- Hycodan ... 1316
- Hycomine Compound Tablets ... 1317
- Hycotuss Expectorant Syrup ... 1318
- Lortab ... 3319
- Lortab Elixir ... 3317
- Maxidone Tablets CIII ... 3399
- Norco 5/325 Tablets CIII ... 3424
- Norco 7.5/325 Tablets CIII ... 3425
- Norco 10/325 Tablets CIII ... 3427
- Norco 10/325 Tablets CIII ... 3425
- Vicodin Tablets ... 516
- Vicodin ES Tablets ... 517
- Vicodin HP Tablets ... 518
- Vicodin Tuss Expectorant ... 519
- Vicoprofen Tablets ... 520
- Zydone Tablets ... 1330

Hydrocodone Polistirex (Increased CNS depression). Products include:
- Tussionex Pennkinetic Extended-Release Suspension ... 1174

Hydromorphone Hydrochloride (Increased CNS depression). Products include:
- Dilaudid ... 441
- Dilaudid Oral Liquid ... 445
- Dilaudid Powder ... 441
- Dilaudid Rectal Suppositories ... 441
- Dilaudid Tablets ... 441
- Dilaudid Tablets - 8 mg ... 445
- Dilaudid-HP ... 443

Hydroxyzine Hydrochloride (Increased CNS depression). Products include:
- Atarax Tablets & Syrup ... 2667
- Vistaril Intramuscular Solution ... 2738

Isocarboxazid (Effect unspecified; caution should be exercised).
No products indexed under this heading.

Isoflurane (Increased CNS depression).
No products indexed under this heading.

Ketamine Hydrochloride (Increased CNS depression).
No products indexed under this heading.

Ketoconazole (Buprenorphine is matabolized by the CYP3A4 isoenzyme; co-administration with inhibitors of CYP3A4, such as ketoconazole, may cause decrease in clearance of buprenorphine). Products include:
- Nizoral 2% Cream ... 3620
- Nizoral A-D Shampoo ... 2008
- Nizoral 2% Shampoo ... 2007
- Nizoral Tablets ... 1791

Levomethadyl Acetate Hydrochloride (Increased CNS depression).
No products indexed under this heading.

Levorphanol Tartrate (Increased CNS depression). Products include:
- Levo-Dromoran ... 1734
- Levorphanol Tartrate Tablets ... 3059

Loratadine (Increased CNS depression). Products include:
- Claritin ... 3100
- Claritin-D 12 Hour Extended Release Tablets ... 3102
- Claritin-D 24 Hour Extended Release Tablets ... 3104

Lorazepam (Increased CNS depression). Products include:
- Ativan Injection ... 3478
- Ativan Tablets ... 3482

Loxapine Hydrochloride (Increased CNS depression).
No products indexed under this heading.

Loxapine Succinate (Increased CNS depression). Products include:
- Loxitane Capsules ... 3398

Meperidine Hydrochloride (Increased CNS depression). Products include:
- Demerol ... 3079
- Mepergan Injection ... 3539

Mephobarbital (Increased CNS depression).
No products indexed under this heading.

Meprobamate (Increased CNS depression). Products include:
- Miltown Tablets ... 3349

Mesoridazine Besylate (Increased CNS depression). Products include:
- Serentil ... 1057

Methadone Hydrochloride (Increased CNS depression). Products include:
- Dolophine Hydrochloride Tablets ... 3056

Methdilazine Hydrochloride (Increased CNS depression).
No products indexed under this heading.

Methohexital Sodium (Increased CNS depression). Products include:
- Brevital Sodium for Injection, USP ... 1815

Methotrimeprazine (Increased CNS depression).
No products indexed under this heading.

Methoxyflurane (Increased CNS depression).
No products indexed under this heading.

Midazolam Hydrochloride (Increased CNS depression). Products include:
- Versed Injection ... 3027
- Versed Syrup ... 3033

Moclobemide (Effect unspecified; caution should be exercised).
No products indexed under this heading.

Molindone Hydrochloride (Increased CNS depression). Products include:
- Moban ... 1320

Morphine Sulfate (Increased CNS depression). Products include:
- Astramorph/PF Injection, USP (Preservative-Free) ... 594
- Duramorph Injection ... 1312
- Infumorph 200 and Infumorph 500 Sterile Solutions ... 1314
- Kadian Capsules ... 1335
- MS Contin Tablets ... 2896
- MSIR ... 2898
- Oramorph SR Tablets ... 3062
- Roxanol ... 3066

Olanzapine (Increased CNS depression). Products include:
- Zyprexa Tablets ... 1973
- Zyprexa ZYDIS Orally Disintegrating Tablets ... 1973

Oxazepam (Increased CNS depression).
No products indexed under this heading.

Oxycodone Hydrochloride (Increased CNS depression). Products include:
- OxyContin Tablets ... 2912
- OxyFast Oral Concentrate Solution ... 2916
- OxyIR Capsules ... 2916
- Percocet Tablets ... 1326
- Percodan Tablets ... 1327
- Percolone Tablets ... 1327
- Roxicodone ... 3067
- Tylox Capsules ... 2597

Pargyline Hydrochloride (Effect unspecified; caution should be exercised).
No products indexed under this heading.

Pentobarbital Sodium (Increased CNS depression). Products include:
- Nembutal Sodium Solution ... 485

Perphenazine (Increased CNS depression). Products include:
- Etrafon ... 3115
- Trilafon ... 3160

Phenelzine Sulfate (Effect unspecified; caution should be exercised). Products include:
- Nardil Tablets ... 2653

Phenobarbital (Increased CNS depression). Products include:
- Arco-Lase Plus Tablets ... 592
- Donnatal ... 2929
- Donnatal Extentabs ... 2930

Phenprocoumon (Potential for purpura).
No products indexed under this heading.

Phenytoin (Buprenorphine is metabolized by the CYP3A4 isoenzyme; co-administration with inducers of CYP3A4, such as phenytoin, may cause increase in clearance of buprenorphine). Products include:
- Dilantin Infatabs ... 2624
- Dilantin-125 Oral Suspension ... 2625

Phenytoin Sodium (Buprenorphine is metabolized by the CYP3A4 isoenzyme; co-administration with inducers of CYP3A4, such as phenytoin, may cause increase in clearance of buprenorphine). Products include:
- Dilantin Kapseals ... 2622

Prazepam (Increased CNS depression).
No products indexed under this heading.

Procarbazine Hydrochloride (Effect unspecified; caution should be exercised). Products include:
- Matulane Capsules ... 3246

Prochlorperazine (Increased CNS depression). Products include:
- Compazine ... 1505

Promethazine Hydrochloride (Increased CNS depression). Products include:
- Mepergan Injection ... 3539
- Phenergan Injection ... 3553
- Phenergan ... 3556
- Phenergan Syrup ... 3554
- Phenergan with Codeine Syrup ... 3557
- Phenergan with Dextromethorphan Syrup ... 3559
- Phenergan VC Syrup ... 3560
- Phenergan VC with Codeine Syrup ... 3561

Propofol (Increased CNS depression). Products include:
- Diprivan Injectable Emulsion ... 667

Propoxyphene Hydrochloride (Increased CNS depression). Products include:
- Darvon Pulvules ... 1909
- Darvon Compound-65 Pulvules ... 1910

Propoxyphene Napsylate (Increased CNS depression). Products include:
- Darvon-N/Darvocet-N ... 1907
- Darvon-N Tablets ... 1912

Pyrilamine Maleate (Increased CNS depression). Products include:
- Maximum Strength Midol Menstrual Caplets and Gelcaps ... ▣612
- Maximum Strength Midol PMS Caplets and Gelcaps ... ▣613

Pyrilamine Tannate (Increased CNS depression). Products include:
- Ryna-12 S Suspension ... 3351

Quazepam (Increased CNS depression).
No products indexed under this heading.

Quetiapine Fumarate (Increased CNS depression). Products include:
- Seroquel Tablets ... 684

Remifentanil Hydrochloride (Increased CNS depression).
No products indexed under this heading.

Rifampin (Buprenorphine is metabolized by the CYP3A4 isoenzyme; co-administration with inducers of CYP3A4, such as rifampin, may cause increase in clearance of buprenorphine). Products include:
- Rifadin ... 765

Rifamate Capsules 767
Rifater Tablets 769

Risperidone (Increased CNS depression). Products include:
Risperdal 1796

Ritonavir (Buprenorphine is metabolized by the CYP3A4 isoenzyme; co-administration with inhibitors of CYP3A4, such as ritonavir, may cause decrease in clearance of buprenorphine). Products include:
Kaletra Capsules 471
Kaletra Oral Solution 471
Norvir Capsules 487
Norvir Oral Solution 487

Secobarbital Sodium (Increased CNS depression).
No products indexed under this heading.

Selegiline Hydrochloride (Effect unspecified; caution should be exercised). Products include:
Eldepryl Capsules 3266

Sevoflurane (Increased CNS depression).
No products indexed under this heading.

Sufentanil Citrate (Increased CNS depression).
No products indexed under this heading.

Temazepam (Increased CNS depression).
No products indexed under this heading.

Terfenadine (Increased CNS depression).
No products indexed under this heading.

Thiamylal Sodium (Increased CNS depression).
No products indexed under this heading.

Thioridazine Hydrochloride (Increased CNS depression). Products include:
Thioridazine Hydrochloride Tablets 2289

Thiothixene (Increased CNS depression). Products include:
Navane Capsules 2701
Thiothixene Capsules 2290

Tranylcypromine Sulfate (Effect unspecified; caution should be exercised). Products include:
Parnate Tablets 1607

Triazolam (Increased CNS depression). Products include:
Halcion Tablets 2823

Trifluoperazine Hydrochloride (Increased CNS depression). Products include:
Stelazine 1640

Trimeprazine Tartrate (Increased CNS depression).
No products indexed under this heading.

Tripelennamine Hydrochloride (Increased CNS depression).
No products indexed under this heading.

Triprolidine Hydrochloride (Increased CNS depression). Products include:
Actifed Cold & Allergy Tablets .... ■688

Zaleplon (Increased CNS depression). Products include:
Sonata Capsules 3591

Ziprasidone Hydrochloride (Increased CNS depression). Products include:
Geodon Capsules 2688

Zolpidem Tartrate (Increased CNS depression). Products include:
Ambien Tablets 3191

Food Interactions

Alcohol (Increased CNS depression).

CAFCIT INJECTION
(Caffeine Citrate) 1035
See Cafcit Oral Solution

CAFCIT ORAL SOLUTION
(Caffeine Citrate) 1035
May interact with phenytoin, theophylline, and certain other agents. Compounds in these categories include:

Aminophylline (Interconversion between caffeine and theophylline has been reported in preterm neonates; the concurrent use of these drugs is not recommended).
No products indexed under this heading.

Cimetidine (Co-administration of caffeine with cimetidine may result in reduced caffeine elimination; lower doses of caffeine may be needed). Products include:
Tagamet HB 200 Suspension .... ■762
Tagamet HB 200 Tablets .... ■761
Tagamet Tablets 1644

Cimetidine Hydrochloride (Co-administration of caffeine with cimetidine may result in reduced caffeine elimination; lower doses of caffeine may be needed). Products include:
Tagamet 1644

Dyphylline (Interconversion between caffeine and theophylline has been reported in preterm neonates; the concurrent use of these drugs is not recommended). Products include:
Lufyllin Tablets 3347
Lufyllin-400 Tablets 3347
Lufyllin-GG Elixir 3348
Lufyllin-GG Tablets 3348

Fosphenytoin Sodium (Co-administration of caffeine with phenytoin may result in increased caffeine elimination; higher doses of caffeine may be needed). Products include:
Cerebyx Injection 2619

Ketoconazole (Co-administration of caffeine with ketoconazole may result in reduced caffeine elimination; lower doses of caffeine may be needed). Products include:
Nizoral 2% Cream 3620
Nizoral A-D Shampoo 2008
Nizoral 2% Shampoo 2007
Nizoral Tablets 1791

Ketoprofen (Co-administration results in reduced urine volume in healthy volunteers). Products include:
Orudis Capsules 3548
Orudis KT Tablets .... ■778
Oruvail Capsules 3548

Phenobarbital (Co-administration of caffeine with phenobarbital may result in increased caffeine elimination; higher doses of caffeine may be needed). Products include:
Arco-Lase Plus Tablets 592
Donnatal 2929
Donnatal Extentabs 2930

Phenytoin (Co-administration of caffeine with phenytoin may result in increased caffeine elimination; higher doses of caffeine may be needed). Products include:
Dilantin Infatabs 2624
Dilantin-125 Oral Suspension 2625

Phenytoin Sodium (Co-administration of caffeine with phenytoin may result in increased caffeine elimination; higher doses of caffeine may be needed). Products include:
Dilantin Kapseals 2622

Theophylline (Interconversion between caffeine and theophylline has been reported in preterm neonates; the concurrent use of these drugs is not recommended). Products include:
Aerolate 1361
Theo-Dur Extended-Release Tablets 1835
Uni-Dur Extended-Release Tablets .. 1841
Uniphyl 400 mg and 600 mg Tablets 2903

Theophylline Calcium Salicylate (Interconversion between caffeine and theophylline has been reported in preterm neonates; the concurrent use of these drugs is not recommended).
No products indexed under this heading.

Theophylline Sodium Glycinate (Interconversion between caffeine and theophylline has been reported in preterm neonates; the concurrent use of these drugs is not recommended).
No products indexed under this heading.

CALADRYL LOTION
(Calamine, Pramoxine Hydrochloride) .... ■698
None cited in PDR database.

CALADRYL CLEAR LOTION
(Pramoxine Hydrochloride, Zinc Acetate) .... ■698
None cited in PDR database.

CALCIJEX INJECTION
(Calcitriol) 411
May interact with:

Magnesium Carbonate (Co-administration with magnesium-containing antacids may lead to the development of hypermagnesemia; concurrent use should be avoided). Products include:
Gaviscon Extra Strength Liquid ..... ■751
Gaviscon Extra Strength Tablets .... ■751
Gaviscon Regular Strength Liquid . ■751
Marblen Suspension .... ■633
One-A-Day Calcium Plus Chewable Tablets .... ■805

Magnesium Hydroxide (Co-administration with magnesium-containing antacids may lead to the development of hypermagnesemia; concurrent use should be avoided). Products include:
Ex•Lax Milk of Magnesia Liquid ..... ■670
Maalox Antacid/Anti-Gas Oral Suspension .... ■673
Maalox Max Maximum Strength Antacid/Anti-Gas Liquid 2300
Maalox Regular Strength Antacid/Antigas Liquid 2300
Mylanta Fast-Acting 1813
Mylanta 1813
Pepcid Complete Chewable Tablets 1815
Phillips' Chewable Tablets .... ■615
Phillips' Milk of Magnesia Liquid (Original, Cherry, & Mint) .... ■616
Rolaids Tablets .... ■706
Extra Strength Rolaids Tablets .... ■706
Vanquish Caplets .... ■617

Vitamin D (Since calcitriol is the most potent metabolite of vitamin D available, vitamin D and its derivatives should be withheld during treatment). Products include:
Active Calcium Tablets 3335
Caltrate 600 PLUS .... ■815
Caltrate 600 + D Tablets .... ■814
Centrum Focused Formulas Bone Health Tablets .... ■815
Citracal Caplets + D .... ■823
D-Cal Chewable Caplets .... ■794
One-A-Day Calcium Plus Chewable Tablets .... ■805
Os-Cal 250 + D Tablets .... ■838
Os-Cal 500 + D Tablets .... ■839

CALCIUM DISODIUM VERSENATE INJECTION
(Calcium Disodium Edetate) 1980
May interact with:

Insulin, Human, Zinc Suspension (Interference with the action of zinc insulin by chelating the zinc). Products include:
Humulin L, 100 Units 1937
Humulin U, 100 Units 1943
Novolin L Human Insulin 10 ml Vials 2422

Insulin, Zinc Crystals (Interference with the action of zinc insulin by chelating the zinc).
No products indexed under this heading.

Insulin, Zinc Suspension (Interference with the action of zinc insulin by chelating the zinc). Products include:
Iletin II, Lente (Pork), 100 Units 1945

Steroids, unspecified (Enhances renal toxicity of edetate calcium disodium in animals).
No products indexed under this heading.

CALTRATE 600 TABLETS
(Calcium Carbonate) .... ■814
None cited in PDR database.

CALTRATE 600 + CHEWABLES
(Calcium Carbonate, Vitamin D, Vitamins with Minerals) .... ■815
None cited in PDR database.

CALTRATE 600 + TABLETS
(Calcium Carbonate, Minerals, Multiple, Vitamin D) .... ■815
None cited in PDR database.

CALTRATE 600 + D TABLETS
(Calcium Carbonate, Vitamin D) ...... ■814
None cited in PDR database.

CALTRATE 600 + SOY TABLETS
(Calcium Carbonate) .... ■814
None cited in PDR database.

CAMPATH AMPULES
(Alemtuzumab) 992
May interact with:

Live Virus Vaccines (Patients who have recently received Campath, should not be immunized with live viral vaccines due to their immunosuppression).
No products indexed under this heading.

CANASA RECTAL SUPPOSITORIES
(Mesalamine) 829
May interact with:

Sulfasalazine (Patients on concurrent oral products that contain or release mesalamine should be carefully monitored with urinalysis, BUN and creatinine testing). Products include:
Azulfidine EN-tabs Tablets 2775

CANCIDAS FOR INJECTION
(Caspofungin acetate) 2048
May interact with dexamethasone, phenytoin, and certain other agents. Compounds in these categories include:

Carbamazepine (The results from regression analyses of patient pharmacokinetic data suggest that co-administration of inducers of drug clearance and/or mixed inducer/inhibitors with caspofungin may result in clinically meaningful reductions in caspofungin concentrations; an increase in the daily dose of caspofungin to 70 mg, following the usual 70-mg loading dose, should be considered in patients who are not clinically responding during concomitant therapy). Products include:
Carbatrol Capsules 3234
Tegretol/Tegretol-XR 2404

Cyclosporine (Co-administration with cyclosporine results in increased AUC of caspofungin by approximately 35%; there were transient increases in liver ALT and AST during co-administration; concomitant use is not recommended unless the potential benefit outweighs the potential risk to the patient). Products include:
Gengraf Capsules 457
Neoral Soft Gelatin Capsules 2380
Neoral Oral Solution 2380

Sandimmune 2388

Dexamethasone (The results from regression analyses of patient pharmacokinetic data suggest that co-administration of inducers of drug clearance and/or mixed inducer/inhibitors with caspofungin may result in clinically meaningful reductions in caspofungin concentrations; an increase in the daily dose of caspofungin to 70 mg, following the usual 70-mg loading dose, should be considered in patients who are not clinically responding during concomitant therapy). Products include:

Decadron Elixir 2078
Decadron Tablets 2079
TobraDex Ophthalmic Ointment 542
TobraDex Ophthalmic Suspension .. 541

Dexamethasone Acetate (The results from regression analyses of patient pharmacokinetic data suggest that co-administration of inducers of drug clearance and/or mixed inducer/inhibitors with caspofungin may result in clinically meaningful reductions in caspofungin concentrations; an increase in the daily dose of caspofungin to 70 mg, following the usual 70-mg loading dose, should be considered in patients who are not clinically responding during concomitant therapy).

No products indexed under this heading.

Dexamethasone Sodium Phosphate (The results from regression analyses of patient pharmacokinetic data suggest that co-administration of inducers of drug clearance and/or mixed inducer/inhibitors with caspofungin may result in clinically meaningful reductions in caspofungin concentrations; an increase in the daily dose of caspofungin to 70 mg, following the usual 70-mg loading dose, should be considered in patients who are not clinically responding during concomitant therapy). Products include:

Decadron Phosphate Injection 2081
Decadron Phosphate Sterile Ophthalmic Ointment 2083
Decadron Phosphate Sterile Ophthalmic Solution 2084
NeoDecadron Sterile Ophthalmic Solution 2144

Efavirenz (The results from regression analyses of patient pharmacokinetic data suggest that co-administration of inducers of drug clearance and/or mixed inducer/inhibitors with caspofungin may result in clinically meaningful reductions in caspofungin concentrations; an increase in the daily dose of caspofungin to 70 mg, following the usual 70-mg loading dose, should be considered in patients who are not clinically responding during concomitant therapy). Products include:

Sustiva Capsules 1258

Fosphenytoin Sodium (The results from regression analyses of patient pharmacokinetic data suggest that co-administration of inducers of drug clearance and/or mixed inducer/inhibitors with caspofungin may result in clinically meaningful reductions in caspofungin concentrations; an increase in the daily dose of caspofungin to 70 mg, following the usual 70-mg loading dose, should be considered in patients who are not clinically responding during concomitant therapy). Products include:

Cerebyx Injection 2619

Nelfinavir Mesylate (The results from regression analyses of patient pharmacokinetic data suggest that co-administration of inducers of drug clearance and/or mixed inducer/inhibitors with caspofungin may result in clinically meaningful reductions in caspofungin concentrations; an increase in the daily dose of caspofungin to 70 mg, following the usual 70-mg loading dose, should be considered in patients who are not clinically responding during concomitant therapy). Products include:

Viracept 532

Nevirapine (The results from regression analyses of patient pharmacokinetic data suggest that co-administration of inducers of drug clearance and/or mixed inducer/inhibitors with caspofungin may result in clinically meaningful reductions in caspofungin concentrations; an increase in the daily dose of caspofungin to 70 mg, following the usual 70-mg loading dose, should be considered in patients who are not clinically responding during concomitant therapy). Products include:

Viramune Oral Suspension 1060
Viramune Tablets 1060

Phenytoin (The results from regression analyses of patient pharmacokinetic data suggest that co-administration of inducers of drug clearance and/or mixed inducer/inhibitors with caspofungin may result in clinically meaningful reductions in caspofungin concentrations; an increase in the daily dose of caspofungin to 70 mg, following the usual 70-mg loading dose, should be considered in patients who are not clinically responding during concomitant therapy). Products include:

Dilantin Infatabs 2624
Dilantin-125 Oral Suspension 2625

Phenytoin Sodium (The results from regression analyses of patient pharmacokinetic data suggest that co-administration of inducers of drug clearance and/or mixed inducer/inhibitors with caspofungin may result in clinically meaningful reductions in caspofungin concentrations; an increase in the daily dose of caspofungin to 70 mg, following the usual 70-mg loading dose, should be considered in patients who are not clinically responding during concomitant therapy). Products include:

Dilantin Kapseals 2622

Rifampin (The results from regression analyses of patient pharmacokinetic data suggest that co-administration of inducers of drug clearance and/or mixed inducer/inhibitors with caspofungin may result in clinically meaningful reductions in caspofungin concentrations; an increase in the daily dose of caspofungin to 70 mg, following the usual 70-mg loading dose, should be considered in patients who are not clinically responding during concomitant therapy). Products include:

Rifadin 765
Rifamate Capsules 767
Rifater Tablets 769

Tacrolimus (Co-administration with tacrolimus reduces the AUC of tacrolimus by approximately 20%, peak blood concentration by 16% and 12-hour blood concentration by 26%; standard monitoring of tacrolimus blood concentrations and appropriate tacrolimus dosage adjustments are recommended). Products include:

Prograf 1393
Protopic Ointment 1397

CAPEX SHAMPOO

(Fluocinolone Acetonide) 1400
None cited in PDR database.

CAPTOPRIL TABLETS

(Captopril) 2281
May interact with beta blockers, diuretics, ganglionic blocking agents, lithium preparations, nitrates and nitrites, non-steroidal anti-inflammatory agents, peripheral adrenergic blockers, potassium preparations, inhibitors of endogenous prostaglandin synthesis, potassium sparing diuretics, agents causing renin release, thiazides, vasodilators, and certain other agents. Compounds in these categories include:

Acebutolol Hydrochloride (Less than additive antihypertensive effect). Products include:

Sectral Capsules 3589

Amiloride Hydrochloride (Hypotension; increased serum potassium). Products include:

Midamor Tablets 2136
Moduretic Tablets 2138

Amyl Nitrite (Discontinue before starting captopril; if resumed administer at lower dosage).

No products indexed under this heading.

Aspirin (Antihypertensive effects of captopril reduced). Products include:

Aggrenox Capsules 1026
Alka-Seltzer .... ▣603
Alka-Seltzer Lemon Lime Antacid and Pain Reliever Effervescent Tablets .... ▣603
Alka-Seltzer Extra Strength Antacid and Pain Reliever Effervescent Tablets .... ▣603
Alka-Seltzer PM Effervescent Tablets .... ▣605
Genuine Bayer Tablets, Caplets and Gelcaps .... ▣606
Extra Strength Bayer Caplets and Gelcaps .... ▣610
Aspirin Regimen Bayer Children's Chewable Tablets (Orange or Cherry Flavored) .... ▣607
Bayer, Aspirin Regimen .... ▣606
Aspirin Regimen Bayer 81 mg Caplets with Calcium .... ▣607
Genuine Bayer Professional Labeling (Aspirin Regimen Bayer) .... ▣608
Extra Strength Bayer Arthritis Caplets .... ▣610
Extra Strength Bayer Plus Caplets .... ▣610
Extra Strength Bayer PM Caplets .. ▣611
BC Powder .... ▣619
BC Allergy Sinus Cold Powder ...... ▣619
Arthritis Strength BC Powder .... ▣619
BC Sinus Cold Powder .... ▣619
Darvon Compound-65 Pulvules 1910
Ecotrin Enteric Coated Aspirin Low, Regular and Maximum Strength Tablets 1715
Excedrin Extra-Strength Tablets, Caplets, and Geltabs .... ▣629
Excedrin Migraine 1070
Goody's Body Pain Formula Powder .... ▣620
Goody's Extra Strength Headache Powder .... ▣620
Goody's Extra Strength Pain Relief Tablets .... ▣620
Percodan Tablets 1327
Robaxisal Tablets 2939
Soma Compound Tablets 3354
Soma Compound w/Codeine Tablets 3355
Vanquish Caplets .... ▣617

Atenolol (Less than additive antihypertensive effect). Products include:

Tenoretic Tablets 690
Tenormin I.V. Injection 692

Bendroflumethiazide (Captopril's effect will be augmented). Products include:

Corzide 40/5 Tablets 2247
Corzide 80/5 Tablets 2247

Betaxolol Hydrochloride (Less than additive antihypertensive effect). Products include:

Betoptic S Ophthalmic Suspension 537

Bisoprolol Fumarate (Less than additive antihypertensive effect). Products include:

Zebeta Tablets 1885
Ziac Tablets 1887

Bumetanide (Captopril's effect will be augmented; hypotension).

No products indexed under this heading.

Carteolol Hydrochloride (Less than additive antihypertensive effect). Products include:

Carteolol Hydrochloride Ophthalmic Solution USP, 1% ..... ⊙258
Ocupress Ophthalmic Solution, 1% Sterile .... ⊙303

Celecoxib (Antihypertensive effects of captopril reduced). Products include:

Celebrex Capsules 2676
Celebrex Capsules 2780

Chlorothiazide (Captopril's effect will be augmented). Products include:

Aldoclor Tablets 2035
Diuril Oral 2087

Chlorothiazide Sodium (Captopril's effect will be augmented). Products include:

Diuril Sodium Intravenous 2086

Chlorthalidone (Captopril's effect will be augmented; hypotension; increased serum potassium). Products include:

Clorpres Tablets 1002
Combipres Tablets 1040
Tenoretic Tablets 690

Deserpidine (Use with caution).

No products indexed under this heading.

Diazoxide (Drugs having vasodilator activity should, if possible, be discontinued before starting captopril).

No products indexed under this heading.

Diclofenac Potassium (Antihypertensive effects of captopril reduced). Products include:

Cataflam Tablets 2315

Diclofenac Sodium (Antihypertensive effects of captopril reduced). Products include:

Arthrotec Tablets 3195
Voltaren Ophthalmic Sterile Ophthalmic Solution .... ⊙312
Voltaren Tablets 2315
Voltaren-XR Tablets 2315

Epoprostenol Sodium (Drugs having vasodilator activity should, if possible, be discontinued before starting captopril). Products include:

Flolan for Injection 1528

Erythrityl Tetranitrate (Discontinue before starting captopril; if resumed administer at lower dosage).

No products indexed under this heading.

Esmolol Hydrochloride (Less than additive antihypertensive effect). Products include:

Brevibloc Injection 858

Ethacrynic Acid (Captopril's effect will be augmented; hypotension). Products include:

Edecrin Tablets 2091

Etodolac (Antihypertensive effects of captopril reduced). Products include:

Lodine 3528
Lodine XL Extended-Release Tablets 3530

Fenoprofen Calcium (Antihypertensive effects of captopril reduced).

No products indexed under this heading.

Flurbiprofen (Antihypertensive effects of captopril reduced).

No products indexed under this heading.

Furosemide (Captopril's effect will be augmented; hypotension). Products include:

Furosemide Tablets 2284

Guanethidine Monosulfate (Use with caution).

No products indexed under this heading.

Hydralazine Hydrochloride (Drugs having vasodilator activity should, if possible, be discontinued before starting captopril).

No products indexed under this heading.

Hydrochlorothiazide (Captopril's effect will be augmented). Products include:

Accuretic Tablets 2614
Aldoril Tablets 2039
Atacand HCT Tablets 597
Avalide Tablets 1070
Diovan HCT Tablets 2338
Dyazide Capsules 1515
HydroDIURIL Tablets 2108
Hyzaar 2109

Inderide Tablets ... 3517
Inderide LA Long-Acting Capsules .. 3519
Lotensin HCT Tablets ... 2367
Maxzide ... 1008
Micardis HCT Tablets ... 1051
Microzide Capsules ... 3414
Moduretic Tablets ... 2138
Monopril HCT ... 1094
Prinzide Tablets ... 2168
Timolide Tablets ... 2187
Uniretic Tablets ... 3178
Vaseretic Tablets ... 2204
Zestoretic Tablets ... 695
Ziac Tablets ... 1887

Hydroflumethiazide (Captopril's effect will be augmented). Products include:
Diucardin Tablets ... 3494

Ibuprofen (Antihypertensive effects of captopril reduced). Products include:
Advil ... ■771
Children's Advil Oral Suspension ... ■773
Children's Advil Chewable Tablets ... ■773
Advil Cold and Sinus Caplets ... ■771
Advil Cold and Sinus Tablets ... ■771
Advil Flu & Body Ache Caplets ... ■772
Infants' Advil Drops ... ■773
Junior Strength Advil Tablets ... ■773
Junior Strength Advil Chewable Tablets ... ■773
Advil Migraine Liquigels ... ■772
Children's Motrin Oral Suspension and Chewable Tablets ... 2006
Children's Motrin Cold Oral Suspension ... 2007
Children's Motrin Oral Suspension ... ■643
Motrin Suspension, Oral Drops, Chewable Tablets, and Caplets ... 2002
Infants' Motrin Concentrated Drops ... 2006
Junior Strength Motrin Caplets and Chewable Tablets ... 2006
Motrin IB Tablets, Caplets, and Gelcaps ... 2002
Motrin Migraine Pain Caplets ... 2005
Motrin Sinus Headache Caplets ... 2005
Vicoprofen Tablets ... 520

Indapamide (Captopril's effect will be augmented; hypotension). Products include:
Indapamide Tablets ... 2286

Indomethacin (Antihypertensive effects of captopril reduced). Products include:
Indocin ... 2112

Indomethacin Sodium Trihydrate (Antihypertensive effects of captopril reduced). Products include:
Indocin I.V. ... 2115

Isosorbide Dinitrate (Discontinue before starting captopril; if resumed administer at lower dosage). Products include:
Isordil Sublingual Tablets ... 3525
Isordil Titradose Tablets ... 3526

Isosorbide Mononitrate (Discontinue before starting captopril; if resumed administer at lower dosage). Products include:
Imdur Tablets ... 1826
Ismo Tablets ... 3524

Ketoprofen (Antihypertensive effects of captopril reduced). Products include:
Orudis Capsules ... 3548
Orudis KT Tablets ... ■778
Oruvail Capsules ... 3548

Ketorolac Tromethamine (Antihypertensive effects of captopril reduced). Products include:
Acular Ophthalmic Solution ... 544
Acular PF Ophthalmic Solution ... 544
Toradol ... 3018

Labetalol Hydrochloride (Less than additive antihypertensive effect). Products include:
Normodyne Injection ... 3135
Normodyne Tablets ... 3137

Levobunolol Hydrochloride (Less than additive antihypertensive effect). Products include:
Betagan ... ⊙228

Lithium Carbonate (Increased serum lithium levels and symptoms of lithium toxicity). Products include:
Eskalith ... 1527
Lithium Carbonate ... 3061
Lithobid Slow-Release Tablets ... 3255

Lithium Citrate (Increased serum lithium levels and symptoms of lithium toxicity). Products include:
Lithium Citrate Syrup ... 3061

Mecamylamine Hydrochloride (Use with caution). Products include:
Inversine Tablets ... 1850

Meclofenamate Sodium (Antihypertensive effects of captopril reduced).
No products indexed under this heading.

Mefenamic Acid (Antihypertensive effects of captopril reduced). Products include:
Ponstel Capsules ... 1356

Meloxicam (Antihypertensive effects of captopril reduced). Products include:
Mobic Tablets ... 1054

Methyclothiazide (Captopril's effect will be augmented).
No products indexed under this heading.

Metipranolol Hydrochloride (Less than additive antihypertensive effect).
No products indexed under this heading.

Metolazone (Captopril's effect will be augmented; hypotension). Products include:
Mykrox Tablets ... 1168
Zaroxolyn Tablets ... 1177

Metoprolol Succinate (Less than additive antihypertensive effect). Products include:
Toprol-XL Tablets ... 651

Metoprolol Tartrate (Less than additive antihypertensive effect).
No products indexed under this heading.

Minoxidil (Drugs having vasodilator activity should, if possible, be discontinued before starting captopril). Products include:
Rogaine Extra Strength for Men Topical Solution ... ■721
Rogaine for Women Topical Solution ... ■721

Nabumetone (Antihypertensive effects of captopril reduced). Products include:
Relafen Tablets ... 1617

Nadolol (Less than additive antihypertensive effect). Products include:
Corgard Tablets ... 2245
Corzide 40/5 Tablets ... 2247
Corzide 80/5 Tablets ... 2247
Nadolol Tablets ... 2288

Naproxen (Antihypertensive effects of captopril reduced). Products include:
EC-Naprosyn Delayed-Release Tablets ... 2967
Naprosyn Suspension ... 2967
Naprosyn Tablets ... 2967

Naproxen Sodium (Antihypertensive effects of captopril reduced). Products include:
Aleve Tablets, Caplets and Gelcaps ... ■602
Aleve Cold & Sinus Caplets ... ■603
Anaprox Tablets ... 2967
Anaprox DS Tablets ... 2967
Naprelan Tablets ... 1293

Nitroglycerin (Discontinue before starting captopril; if resumed administer at lower dosage). Products include:
Nitro-Dur Transdermal Infusion System ... 3134
Nitro-Dur Transdermal Infusion System ... 1834
Nitrolingual Pumpspray ... 1355
Nitrostat Tablets ... 2658

Oxaprozin (Antihypertensive effects of captopril reduced).
No products indexed under this heading.

Penbutolol Sulfate (Less than additive antihypertensive effect).
No products indexed under this heading.

Pentaerythritol Tetranitrate (Discontinue before starting captopril; if resumed administer at lower dosage).
No products indexed under this heading.

Phenylbutazone (Antihypertensive effects of captopril reduced).
No products indexed under this heading.

Pindolol (Less than additive antihypertensive effect).
No products indexed under this heading.

Piroxicam (Antihypertensive effects of captopril reduced). Products include:
Feldene Capsules ... 2685

Polythiazide (Captopril's effect will be augmented). Products include:
Minizide Capsules ... 2700
Renese Tablets ... 2712

Potassium Acid Phosphate (Potential for significant increase in serum potassium). Products include:
K-Phos Original (Sodium Free) Tablets ... 947

Potassium Bicarbonate (Potential for significant increase in serum potassium).
No products indexed under this heading.

Potassium Chloride (Potential for significant increase in serum potassium). Products include:
Chlor-3 ... 1361
Colyte with Flavor Packs for Oral Solution ... 3170
GoLYTELY and Pineapple Flavor GoLYTELY for Oral Solution ... 1068
K-Dur Microburst Release System ER Tablets ... 1832
Klor-Con M20/Klor-Con M10 Tablets ... 3329
K-Lor Powder Packets ... 469
K-Tab Filmtab Tablets ... 470
Micro-K ... 3311
NuLYTELY, Cherry Flavor, Lemon-Lime Flavor, and Orange Flavor NuLYTELY for Oral Solution ... 1068
Rum-K ... 1363

Potassium Citrate (Potential for significant increase in serum potassium). Products include:
Urocit-K Tablets ... 2232

Potassium Gluconate (Potential for significant increase in serum potassium).
No products indexed under this heading.

Potassium Phosphate (Potential for significant increase in serum potassium). Products include:
K-Phos Neutral Tablets ... 946

Prazosin Hydrochloride (Use with caution). Products include:
Minipress Capsules ... 2699
Minizide Capsules ... 2700

Propranolol Hydrochloride (Less than additive antihypertensive effect). Products include:
Inderal ... 3513
Inderal LA Long-Acting Capsules ... 3516
Inderide Tablets ... 3517
Inderide LA Long-Acting Capsules .. 3519

Rauwolfia serpentina (Use with caution).
No products indexed under this heading.

Rescinnamine (Use with caution).
No products indexed under this heading.

Reserpine (Use with caution).
No products indexed under this heading.

Rofecoxib (Antihypertensive effects of captopril reduced). Products include:
Vioxx ... 2213

Sotalol Hydrochloride (Less than additive antihypertensive effect). Products include:
Betapace Tablets ... 950
Betapace AF Tablets ... 954

Spironolactone (Captopril's effect will be augmented; hypotension; increased serum potassium).
No products indexed under this heading.

Sulindac (Antihypertensive effects of captopril reduced). Products include:
Clinoril Tablets ... 2053

Terazosin Hydrochloride (Use with caution). Products include:
Hytrin Capsules ... 464

Timolol Hemihydrate (Less than additive antihypertensive effect). Products include:
Betimol Ophthalmic Solution ... ⊙324

Timolol Maleate (Less than additive antihypertensive effect). Products include:
Blocadren Tablets ... 2046
Cosopt Sterile Ophthalmic Solution ... 2065
Timolide Tablets ... 2187
Timolol GFS ... ⊙266
Timoptic in Ocudose ... 2192
Timoptic Sterile Ophthalmic Solution ... 2190
Timoptic-XE Sterile Ophthalmic Gel Forming Solution ... 2194

Tolmetin Sodium (Antihypertensive effects of captopril reduced). Products include:
Tolectin ... 2589

Torsemide (Captopril's effect will be augmented; hypotension). Products include:
Demadex Tablets and Injection ... 2965

Triamterene (Captopril's effect will be augmented; hypotension; increased serum potassium). Products include:
Dyazide Capsules ... 1515
Dyrenium Capsules ... 3458
Maxzide ... 1008

Trimethaphan Camsylate (Use with caution).
No products indexed under this heading.

Food Interactions

Food, unspecified (Reduces absorption by about 30% to 40%; should be given one hour before meals).

CARAC CREAM
(Fluorouracil) ... 1222
None cited in PDR database.

CARAFATE SUSPENSION
(Sucralfate) ... 731
May interact with fluoroquinolone antibiotics, quinidine, theophylline, and certain other agents. Compounds in these categories include:

Alatrofloxacin Mesylate (Potential for reduced extent of absorption (bioavailability) with concomitant oral administration; dosing the concomitant medication 2 hours before sucralfate eliminates the interaction). Products include:
Trovan I.V. ... 2722

Aluminum Carbonate (Simultaneous administration within one-half hour before or after sucralfate should be avoided; may increase the total body burden of aluminum).
No products indexed under this heading.

Aluminum Hydroxide (Simultaneous administration within one-half hour before or after sucralfate should be avoided; may increase the total body burden of aluminum). Products include:
Amphojel Suspension (Mint Flavor) ... ■789
Gaviscon Extra Strength Liquid ... ■751
Gaviscon Extra Strength Tablets ... ■751
Gaviscon Regular Strength Liquid ... ■751

Gaviscon Regular Strength Tablets ▣750
Maalox Antacid/Anti-Gas Oral Suspension ▣673
Maalox Max Maximum Strength Antacid/Anti-Gas Liquid 2300
Maalox Regular Strength Antacid/Antigas Liquid 2300
Mylanta 1813
Vanquish Caplets ▣617

Aminophylline (Simultaneous administration results in reduced oral absorption of theophylline).
No products indexed under this heading.

Cimetidine (Simultaneous administration results in reduced oral absorption of oral cimetidine; dosing the concomitant medication 2 hours before sucralfate eliminates the interaction). Products include:
Tagamet HB 200 Suspension ▣762
Tagamet HB 200 Tablets ▣761
Tagamet Tablets 1644

Cimetidine Hydrochloride (Simultaneous administration results in reduced oral absorption of oral cimetidine; dosing the concomitant medication 2 hours before sucralfate eliminates the interaction). Products include:
Tagamet 1644

Ciprofloxacin (Potential for reduced extent of absorption (bioavailability) with concomitant oral administration; dosing the concomitant medication 2 hours before sucralfate eliminates the interaction). Products include:
Cipro I.V. 893
Cipro I.V. Pharmacy Bulk Package 897
Cipro Oral Suspension 887

Ciprofloxacin Hydrochloride (Potential for reduced extent of absorption (bioavailability) with concomitant oral administration; dosing the concomitant medication 2 hours before sucralfate eliminates the interaction). Products include:
Ciloxan 538
Cipro HC Otic Suspension 540
Cipro Tablets 887

Digoxin (Simultaneous administration results in reduced oral absorption of oral digoxin; dosing the concomitant medication 2 hours before sucralfate eliminates the interaction). Products include:
Digitek Tablets 1003
Lanoxicaps Capsules 1574
Lanoxin Injection 1581
Lanoxin Tablets 1587
Lanoxin Elixir Pediatric 1578
Lanoxin Injection Pediatric 1584

Dyphylline (Simultaneous administration results in reduced oral absorption of theophylline). Products include:
Lufyllin Tablets 3347
Lufyllin-400 Tablets 3347
Lufyllin-GG Elixir 3348
Lufyllin-GG Tablets 3348

Enoxacin (Potential for reduced extent of absorption (bioavailability) with concomitant oral administration; dosing the concomitant medication 2 hours before sucralfate eliminates the interaction).
No products indexed under this heading.

Grepafloxacin Hydrochloride (Potential for reduced extent of absorption (bioavailability) with concomitant oral administration; dosing the concomitant medication 2 hours before sucralfate eliminates the interaction).
No products indexed under this heading.

Ketoconazole (Simultaneous administration results in reduced oral absorption of oral ketoconazole). Products include:
Nizoral 2% Cream 3620
Nizoral A-D Shampoo 2008
Nizoral 2% Shampoo 2007
Nizoral Tablets 1791

Levothyroxine Sodium (Potential for reduced extent of absorption (bioavailability) with concomitant oral administration). Products include:
Levothroid Tablets 1373
Levoxyl Tablets 1819
Synthroid 505
Unithroid Tablets 3445

Lomefloxacin Hydrochloride (Potential for reduced extent of absorption (bioavailability) with concomitant oral administration; dosing the concomitant medication 2 hours before sucralfate eliminates the interaction).
No products indexed under this heading.

Magnesium Hydroxide (Simultaneous administration within one-half hour before or after sucralfate should be avoided; may increase the total body burden of aluminum). Products include:
Ex•Lax Milk of Magnesia Liquid ▣670
Maalox Antacid/Anti-Gas Oral Suspension ▣673
Maalox Max Maximum Strength Antacid/Anti-Gas Liquid 2300
Maalox Regular Strength Antacid/Antigas Liquid 2300
Mylanta Fast-Acting 1813
Mylanta 1813
Pepcid Complete Chewable Tablets 1815
Phillips' Chewable Tablets ▣615
Phillips' Milk of Magnesia Liquid (Original, Cherry, & Mint) ▣616
Rolaids Tablets ▣706
Extra Strength Rolaids Tablets ▣706
Vanquish Caplets ▣617

Magnesium Oxide (Simultaneous administration within one-half hour before or after sucralfate should be avoided; may increase the total body burden of aluminum). Products include:
Beelith Tablets 946
Mag-Ox 400 Tablets 1024
Uro-Mag Capsules 1024

Moxifloxacin Hydrochloride (Potential for reduced extent of absorption (bioavailability) with concomitant oral administration; dosing the concomitant medication 2 hours before sucralfate eliminates the interaction). Products include:
Avelox Tablets 879

Norfloxacin (Potential for reduced extent of absorption (bioavailability) with concomitant oral administration; dosing the concomitant medication 2 hours before sucralfate eliminates the interaction). Products include:
Chibroxin Sterile Ophthalmic Solution 2051
Noroxin Tablets 2145

Ofloxacin (Potential for reduced extent of absorption (bioavailability) with concomitant oral administration; dosing the concomitant medication 2 hours before sucralfate eliminates the interaction). Products include:
Floxin I.V. 2526
Floxin Otic Solution 1219
Floxin Tablets 2529
Ocuflox Ophthalmic Solution 554

Phenytoin (Simultaneous administration results in reduced oral absorption of oral phenytoin). Products include:
Dilantin Infatabs 2624
Dilantin-125 Oral Suspension 2625

Phenytoin Sodium (Simultaneous administration results in reduced oral absorption of oral phenytoin). Products include:
Dilantin Kapseals 2622

Quinidine Gluconate (Potential for reduced extent of absorption (bioavailability) with concomitant oral administration). Products include:
Quinaglute Dura-Tabs Tablets 978

Quinidine Polygalacturonate (Potential for reduced extent of absorption (bioavailability) with concomitant oral administration).
No products indexed under this heading.

Quinidine Sulfate (Potential for reduced extent of absorption (bioavailability) with concomitant oral administration). Products include:
Quinidex Extentabs 2933

Ranitidine Hydrochloride (Simultaneous administration results in reduced oral absorption of oral ranitidine; dosing the concomitant medication 2 hours before sucralfate eliminates the interaction). Products include:
Zantac 1690
Zantac Injection 1688
Zantac 75 Tablets ▣717

Tetracycline Hydrochloride (Simultaneous administration results in reduced oral absorption of oral tetracycline).
No products indexed under this heading.

Theophylline (Simultaneous administration results in reduced oral absorption of theophylline). Products include:
Aerolate 1361
Theo-Dur Extended-Release Tablets 1835
Uni-Dur Extended-Release Tablets 1841
Uniphyl 400 mg and 600 mg Tablets 2903

Theophylline Calcium Salicylate (Simultaneous administration results in reduced oral absorption of theophylline).
No products indexed under this heading.

Theophylline Sodium Glycinate (Simultaneous administration results in reduced oral absorption of theophylline).
No products indexed under this heading.

Trovafloxacin Mesylate (Potential for reduced extent of absorption (bioavailability) with concomitant oral administration; dosing the concomitant medication 2 hours before sucralfate eliminates the interaction). Products include:
Trovan Tablets 2722

Warfarin Sodium (Subtherapeutic prothrombin times with concomitant warfarin and sucralfate have been reported in spontaneous and published reports; clinical studies have demonstrated no changes in the prothrombin time with the addition of sucralfate to chronic warfarin therapy). Products include:
Coumadin for Injection 1243
Coumadin Tablets 1243
Warfarin Sodium Tablets, USP 3302

CARAFATE TABLETS
(Sucralfate) 730
May interact with fluoroquinolone antibiotics, quinidine, theophylline, and certain other agents. Compounds in these categories include:

Alatrofloxacin Mesylate (Potential for reduced extent of absorption (bioavailability) with concomitant oral administration; dosing the concomitant medication 2 hours before sucralfate eliminates the interaction). Products include:
Trovan I.V. 2722

Aluminum Carbonate (Simultaneous administration within one-half hour before or after sucralfate should be avoided; may increase the total body burden of aluminum).
No products indexed under this heading.

Aluminum Hydroxide (Simultaneous administration within one-half hour before or after sucralfate should be avoided; may increase the total body burden of aluminum). Products include:
Amphojel Suspension (Mint Flavor) ▣789
Gaviscon Extra Strength Liquid ▣751
Gaviscon Extra Strength Tablets ▣751
Gaviscon Regular Strength Liquid ▣751
Gaviscon Regular Strength Tablets ▣750
Maalox Antacid/Anti-Gas Oral Suspension ▣673
Maalox Max Maximum Strength Antacid/Anti-Gas Liquid 2300
Maalox Regular Strength Antacid/Antigas Liquid 2300
Mylanta 1813
Vanquish Caplets ▣617

Aminophylline (Simultaneous administration results in reduced oral absorption of theophylline).
No products indexed under this heading.

Cimetidine (Simultaneous administration results in reduced oral absorption of oral cimetidine; dosing the concomitant medication 2 hours before sucralfate eliminates the interaction). Products include:
Tagamet HB 200 Suspension ▣762
Tagamet HB 200 Tablets ▣761
Tagamet Tablets 1644

Cimetidine Hydrochloride (Simultaneous administration results in reduced oral absorption of oral cimetidine; dosing the concomitant medication 2 hours before sucralfate eliminates the interaction). Products include:
Tagamet 1644

Ciprofloxacin (Potential for reduced extent of absorption (bioavailability) with concomitant oral administration; dosing the concomitant medication 2 hours before sucralfate eliminates the interaction). Products include:
Cipro I.V. 893
Cipro I.V. Pharmacy Bulk Package 897
Cipro Oral Suspension 887

Ciprofloxacin Hydrochloride (Potential for reduced extent of absorption (bioavailability) with concomitant oral administration; dosing the concomitant medication 2 hours before sucralfate eliminates the interaction). Products include:
Ciloxan 538
Cipro HC Otic Suspension 540
Cipro Tablets 887

Digoxin (Simultaneous administration results in reduced oral absorption of oral digoxin; dosing the concomitant medication 2 hours before sucralfate eliminates the interaction). Products include:
Digitek Tablets 1003
Lanoxicaps Capsules 1574
Lanoxin Injection 1581
Lanoxin Tablets 1587
Lanoxin Elixir Pediatric 1578
Lanoxin Injection Pediatric 1584

Dyphylline (Simultaneous administration results in reduced oral absorption of theophylline). Products include:
Lufyllin Tablets 3347
Lufyllin-400 Tablets 3347
Lufyllin-GG Elixir 3348
Lufyllin-GG Tablets 3348

Enoxacin (Potential for reduced extent of absorption (bioavailability) with concomitant oral administration; dosing the concomitant medication 2 hours before sucralfate eliminates the interaction).
No products indexed under this heading.

Grepafloxacin Hydrochloride (Potential for reduced extent of absorption (bioavailability) with concomitant oral administration; dosing the concomitant medication 2 hours before sucralfate eliminates the interaction).
No products indexed under this heading.

Ketoconazole (Simultaneous administration results in reduced oral absorption of oral ketoconazole). Products include:

Nizoral 2% Cream 3620
Nizoral A-D Shampoo 2008
Nizoral 2% Shampoo 2007
Nizoral Tablets 1791

Levothyroxine Sodium (Potential for reduced extent of absorption (bioavailability) with concomitant oral administration). Products include:
Levothroid Tablets 1373
Levoxyl Tablets 1819
Synthroid 505
Unithroid Tablets 3445

Lomefloxacin Hydrochloride (Potential for reduced extent of absorption (bioavailability) with concomitant oral administration; dosing the concomitant medication 2 hours before sucralfate eliminates the interaction).
No products indexed under this heading.

Magnesium Hydroxide (Simultaneous administration within one-half hour before or after sucralfate should be avoided; may increase the total body burden of aluminum). Products include:
Ex•Lax Milk of Magnesia Liquid .... ▣670
Maalox Antacid/Anti-Gas Oral Suspension.................... ▣673
Maalox Max Maximum Strength Antacid/Anti-Gas Liquid 2300
Maalox Regular Strength Antacid/Antigas Liquid 2300
Mylanta Fast-Acting 1813
Mylanta 1813
Pepcid Complete Chewable Tablets.................... 1815
Phillips' Chewable Tablets .... ▣615
Phillips' Milk of Magnesia Liquid (Original, Cherry, & Mint).................... ▣616
Rolaids Tablets .... ▣706
Extra Strength Rolaids Tablets ...... ▣706
Vanquish Caplets .... ▣617

Magnesium Oxide (Simultaneous administration within one-half hour before or after sucralfate should be avoided; may increase the total body burden of aluminum). Products include:
Beelith Tablets 946
Mag-Ox 400 Tablets 1024
Uro-Mag Capsules 1024

Moxifloxacin Hydrochloride (Potential for reduced extent of absorption (bioavailability) with concomitant oral administration; dosing the concomitant medication 2 hours before sucralfate eliminates the interaction). Products include:
Avelox Tablets 879

Norfloxacin (Potential for reduced extent of absorption (bioavailability) with concomitant oral administration; dosing the concomitant medication 2 hours before sucralfate eliminates the interaction). Products include:
Chibroxin Sterile Ophthalmic Solution.................... 2051
Noroxin Tablets 2145

Ofloxacin (Potential for reduced extent of absorption (bioavailability) with concomitant oral administration; dosing the concomitant medication 2 hours before sucralfate eliminates the interaction). Products include:
Floxin I.V. 2526
Floxin Otic Solution 1219
Floxin Tablets 2529
Ocuflox Ophthalmic Solution 554

Phenytoin (Simultaneous administration results in reduced oral absorption of oral phenytoin). Products include:
Dilantin Infatabs 2624
Dilantin-125 Oral Suspension 2625

Phenytoin Sodium (Simultaneous administration results in reduced oral absorption of oral phenytoin). Products include:
Dilantin Kapseals 2622

Quinidine Gluconate (Potential for reduced extent of absorption (bioavailability) with concomitant oral administration). Products include:
Quinaglute Dura-Tabs Tablets 978

Quinidine Polygalacturonate (Potential for reduced extent of absorption (bioavailability) with concomitant oral administration).
No products indexed under this heading.

Quinidine Sulfate (Potential for reduced extent of absorption (bioavailability) with concomitant oral administration). Products include:
Quinidex Extentabs 2933

Ranitidine Hydrochloride (Simultaneous administration results in reduced oral absorption of oral ranitidine; dosing the concomitant medication 2 hours before sucralfate eliminates the interaction). Products include:
Zantac 1690
Zantac Injection 1688
Zantac 75 Tablets .... ▣717

Tetracycline Hydrochloride (Simultaneous administration results in reduced oral absorption of oral tetracycline).
No products indexed under this heading.

Theophylline (Simultaneous administration results in reduced oral absorption of theophylline). Products include:
Aerolate 1361
Theo-Dur Extended-Release Tablets 1835
Uni-Dur Extended-Release Tablets .. 1841
Uniphyl 400 mg and 600 mg Tablets 2903

Theophylline Calcium Salicylate (Simultaneous administration results in reduced oral absorption of theophylline).
No products indexed under this heading.

Theophylline Sodium Glycinate (Simultaneous administration results in reduced oral absorption of theophylline).
No products indexed under this heading.

Trovafloxacin Mesylate (Potential for reduced extent of absorption (bioavailability) with concomitant oral administration; dosing the concomitant medication 2 hours before sucralfate eliminates the interaction). Products include:
Trovan Tablets 2722

Warfarin Sodium (Subtherapeutic prothrombin times with concomitant warfarin and sucralfate have been reported in spontaneous and published reports; clinical studies have demonstrated no changes in the prothrombin time with the addition of sucralfate to chronic warfarin therapy). Products include:
Coumadin for Injection 1243
Coumadin Tablets 1243
Warfarin Sodium Tablets, USP 3302

CARBATROL CAPSULES

(Carbamazepine) 3234

May interact with doxycycline, anticonvulsants, erythromycin, lithium preparations, macrolide antibiotics, monoamine oxidase inhibitors, antipsychotic agents, oral contraceptives, phenytoin, valproate, theophylline, and certain other agents. Compounds in these categories include:

Acetaminophen (Carbamazepine induces hepatic CYP activity and causes or would be expected to decrease plasma levels of acetaminophen). Products include:
Actifed Cold & Sinus Caplets and Tablets.................... ▣688
Alka-Seltzer Plus Liqui-Gels .... ▣604
Alka-Seltzer Plus Cold & Flu Medicine Liqui-Gels.................... ▣604
Alka-Seltzer Plus Cold & Sinus Medicine Liqui-Gels.................... ▣604
Benadryl Allergy/Cold Tablets .... ▣691
Benadryl Allergy Sinus Headache Caplets & Gelcaps.................... ▣693
Benadryl Severe Allergy & Sinus Headache Caplets.................... ▣694
Children's Cēpacol Sore Throat .... ▣788
Comtrex Acute Head Cold & Sinus Pressure Relief Tablets ..... ▣627
Comtrex Deep Chest Cold & Congestion Relief Softgels......... ▣627
Comtrex Flu Therapy & Fever Relief Daytime Caplets .... ▣628
Comtrex Flu Therapy & Fever Relief Nighttime Tablets .... ▣628
Comtrex Maximum Strength Multi-Symptom Cold & Cough Relief Tablets and Caplets.......... ▣626
Contac Severe Cold and Flu Caplets Maximum Strength.......... ▣746
Contac Severe Cold and Flu Caplets Non-Drowsy .... ▣746
Coricidin 'D' Cold, Flu & Sinus Tablets.................... ▣737
Coricidin HBP Cold & Flu Tablets ... ▣738
Coricidin HBP Maximum Strength Flu Tablets.................... ▣738
Coricidin HBP Night-Time Cold & Flu Tablets.................... ▣738
Darvon-N/Darvocet-N 1907
Dimetapp Cold and Fever Suspension.................... ▣775
Dimetapp Nighttime Flu Liquid .... ▣776
Dimetapp Non-Drowsy Flu Syrup .... ▣777
Drixoral Allergy/Sinus Extended-Release Tablets .... ▣741
Drixoral Cold & Flu Extended-Release Tablets.......... ▣740
Aspirin Free Excedrin Caplets and Geltabs.................... ▣628
Excedrin Extra-Strength Tablets, Caplets, and Geltabs .... ▣629
Excedrin Migraine 1070
Excedrin PM Tablets, Caplets, and Geltabs .... ▣631
Goody's Body Pain Formula Powder.................... ▣620
Goody's Extra Strength Headache Powder.................... ▣620
Goody's Extra Strength Pain Relief Tablets.................... ▣620
Goody's PM Powder .... ▣621
Hycomine Compound Tablets 1317
Lortab 3319
Lortab Elixir 3317
Maxidone Tablets CIII 3399
Maximum Strength Midol Menstrual Caplets and Gelcaps.. ▣612
Maximum Strength Midol PMS Caplets and Gelcaps.................... ▣613
Maximum Strength Midol Teen Caplets.................... ▣612
Midrin Capsules 3464
Norco 5/325 Tablets CIII 3424
Norco 7.5/325 Tablets CIII 3425
Norco 10/325 Tablets CIII 3427
Norco 10/325 Tablets CIII 3425
Percocet Tablets 1326
Percogesic Aspirin-Free Coated Tablets.................... ▣667
Extra Strength Percogesic Aspirin-Free Coated Caplets.......... ▣665
Phrenilin 578
Robitussin Cold Caplets Multi-Symptom Cold & Flu.......... ▣781
Robitussin Cold Softgels Multi-Symptom Cold & Flu.......... ▣781
Robitussin Multi Symptom Honey Flu Liquid.................... ▣785
Robitussin Nighttime Honey Flu Liquid.................... ▣786
Sedapap Tablets 50 mg/650 mg 2225
Singlet Caplets .... ▣761
Sinutab Sinus Allergy Medication, Maximum Strength Formula, Tablets & Caplets.................... ▣707
Sinutab Sinus Medication, Maximum Strength Without Drowsiness Formula, Tablets & Caplets.................... ▣707
Sudafed Cold & Cough Liquid Caps .... ▣709
Sudafed Cold & Sinus Liquid Caps .... ▣710
Sudafed Severe Cold .... ▣711
Sudafed Sinus Headache Caplets . ▣712
Sudafed Sinus Headache Tablets .. ▣712
Tavist Sinus Non-Drowsy Coated Caplets.................... ▣676
TheraFlu Regular Strength Cold & Cough Night Time Hot Liquid........ ▣676
TheraFlu Regular Strength Cold & Sore Throat Night Time Hot Liquid.................... ▣676
TheraFlu Maximum Strength Flu & Congestion Non-Drowsy Hot Liquid.................... ▣677
TheraFlu Maximum Strength Flu & Cough Night Time Hot Liquid.. ▣678
TheraFlu Maximum Strength Flu & Sore Throat Night Time Hot Liquid.................... ▣677
TheraFlu Maximum Strength Severe Cold & Congestion Night Time Caplets.................... ▣678
TheraFlu Maximum Strength Severe Cold & Congestion Night Time Hot Liquid.......... ▣678
TheraFlu Maximum Strength Severe Cold & Congestion Non-Drowsy.................... ▣679
Triaminic Cold, Cough & Fever Liquid.................... ▣681
Triaminic Cough & Sore Throat Liquid.................... ▣682
Triaminic Cough & Sore Throat Softchews.................... ▣684
Tylenol, Children's 2014
Children's Tylenol Allergy-D Liquid ... 2014
Children's Tylenol Cold Suspension Liquid and Chewable Tablets.................... 2015
Children's Tylenol Cold Plus Cough Suspension Liquid and Chewable Tablets.................... 2015
Children's Tylenol Flu Suspension Liquid.................... 2015
Children's Tylenol Sinus Suspension Liquid.................... 2017
Infants' Tylenol Cold Decongestant and Fever Reducer Concentrated Drops.................... 2015
Infants' Tylenol Cold Decongestant and Fever Reducer Concentrated Drops Plus Cough.. 2015
Junior Strength Tylenol Soft Chews Chewable Tablets.................... 2014
Tylenol 2009
Tylenol Allergy Sinus 2010
Tylenol Severe Allergy Caplets 2010
Multi-Symptom Tylenol Cold Complete Formula Caplets.......... 2010
Multi-Symptom Tylenol Cold Non-Drowsy Caplets and Gelcaps.................... 2010
Multi-Symptom Tylenol Cold Severe Congestion Non-Drowsy Caplets 2011
Maximum Strength Tylenol Flu NightTime Gelcaps.................... 2011
Maximum Strength Tylenol Flu NightTime Liquid.................... 2011
Maximum Strength Tylenol Flu Non-Drowsy Gelcaps.................... 2011
Extra Strength Tylenol PM Caplets, Geltabs, and Gelcaps.................... 2012
Maximum Strength Tylenol Sinus NightTime Caplets.................... 2012
Maximum Strength Tylenol Sinus Non-Drowsy Geltabs, Gelcaps, Caplets, and Tablets.................... 2012
Maximum Strength Tylenol Sore Throat Adult Liquid.................... 2013
Tylenol with Codeine 2595
Women's Tylenol Menstrual Relief Caplets 2013
Tylox Capsules 2597
Ultracet Tablets 2597
Vanquish Caplets .... ▣617
Vicks 44M Cough, Cold & Flu Relief Liquid.................... ▣725
Vicks DayQuil LiquiCaps/Liquid Multi-Symptom Cold/Flu Relief... ▣727
Vicks NyQuil LiquiCaps/Liquid Multi-Symptom Cold/Flu Relief, Original and Cherry Flavors.......... ▣727
Vicodin Tablets 516
Vicodin ES Tablets 517
Vicodin HP Tablets 518
Zydone Tablets 1330

Alprazolam (Carbamazepine induces hepatic CYP activity and causes or would be expected to decrease plasma levels of alprazolam). Products include:
Xanax Tablets 2865

Aminophylline (Inducers of CYP3A4, such as theophylline, can increase the rate of carbamazepine metabolism and can thus decrease plasma carbamazepine levels; carbamazepine induces hepatic CYP activity and causes or would be expected to decrease plasma levels of theophylline).
No products indexed under this heading.

Azithromycin Dihydrate (Inhibitors of CYP3A4, such as macrolides, inhibit carbamazepine metabolism and thus increase plasma carbamazepine levels). Products include:
Zithromax 2743
Zithromax for IV Infusion 2748

IMPORTANT NOTE: Always consult each drug listing in the patient's regimen for possible interactions.

Zithromax for Oral Suspension, 300 mg, 600 mg, 900 mg, 1200 mg 2739
Zithromax Tablets, 250 mg 2739

Chlorpromazine (Co-administration with psychotropic agents has resulted in isolated cases of neuroleptic malignant syndrome). Products include:
Thorazine Suppositories 1656

Chlorpromazine Hydrochloride (Co-administration with psychotropic agents has resulted in isolated cases of neuroleptic malignant syndrome). Products include:
Thorazine 1656

Chlorprothixene (Co-administration with psychotropic agents has resulted in isolated cases of neuroleptic malignant syndrome).
No products indexed under this heading.

Chlorprothixene Hydrochloride (Co-administration with psychotropic agents has resulted in isolated cases of neuroleptic malignant syndrome).
No products indexed under this heading.

Cimetidine (Inhibitors of CYP3A4, such as cimetidine, inhibit carbamazepine metabolism and thus increase plasma carbamazepine levels). Products include:
Tagamet HB 200 Suspension .... ▣ 762
Tagamet HB 200 Tablets .... ▣ 761
Tagamet Tablets 1644

Cimetidine Hydrochloride (Inhibitors of CYP3A4, such as cimetidine, inhibit carbamazepine metabolism and thus increase plasma carbamazepine levels). Products include:
Tagamet 1644

Cisplatin (Inducers of CYP3A4, such as cisplatin, can increase the rate of carbamazepine metabolism and can thus decrease plasma carbamazepine levels).
No products indexed under this heading.

Clarithromycin (Inhibitors of CYP3A4, such as clarithromycin, inhibit carbamazepine metabolism and thus increase plasma carbamazepine levels). Products include:
Biaxin/Biaxin XL 403
PREVPAC 3298

Clomipramine Hydrochloride (Carbamazepine can increase plasma levels of clomipramine).
No products indexed under this heading.

Clonazepam (Carbamazepine induces hepatic CYP activity and causes or would be expected to decrease plasma levels of clonazepine; alterations of thyroid function have been reported in combination therapy with other anticonvulsants). Products include:
Klonopin Tablets 2983

Clozapine (Carbamazepine induces hepatic CYP activity and causes or would be expected to decrease plasma levels of clozapine). Products include:
Clozaril Tablets 2319

Danazol (Inhibitors of CYP3A4, such as danazol, inhibit carbamazepine metabolism and thus increase plasma carbamazepine levels).
No products indexed under this heading.

Desogestrel (Carbamazepine induces hepatic CYP activity and causes or would be expected to decrease plasma levels of oral contraceptives; breakthrough bleeding has been reported among patients receiving concomitant oral contraceptives and their reliability may be adversely affected). Products include:
Cyclessa Tablets 2450
Desogen Tablets 2458
Mircette Tablets 2470
Ortho-Cept 21 Tablets 2546
Ortho-Cept 28 Tablets 2546

Dicumarol (Carbamazepine induces hepatic CYP activity and causes or would be expected to decrease plasma levels of dicumarol).
No products indexed under this heading.

Diltiazem Hydrochloride (Inhibitors of CYP3A4, such as diltiazem, inhibit carbamazepine metabolism and thus increase plasma carbamazepine levels). Products include:
Cardizem Injectable 1018
Cardizem Lyo-Ject Syringe 1018
Cardizem Monovial 1018
Cardizem CD Capsules 1016
Tiazac Capsules 1378

Dirithromycin (Inhibitors of CYP3A4, such as macrolides, inhibit carbamazepine metabolism and thus increase plasma carbamazepine levels). Products include:
Dynabac Tablets 2269

Divalproex Sodium (Alterations of thyroid function have been reported in combination therapy with other anticonvulsants). Products include:
Depakote Sprinkle Capsules 426
Depakote Tablets 430
Depakote ER Tablets 436

Doxorubicin Hydrochloride (Inducers of CYP3A4, such as doxorubicin, can increase the rate of carbamazepine metabolism and can thus decrease plasma carbamazepine levels). Products include:
Adriamycin PFS/RDF Injection 2767
Doxil Injection 566

Doxycycline Calcium (Carbamazepine induces hepatic CYP activity and causes or would be expected to decrease plasma levels of doxycycline). Products include:
Vibramycin Calcium Oral Suspension Syrup 2735

Doxycycline Hyclate (Carbamazepine induces hepatic CYP activity and causes or would be expected to decrease plasma levels of doxycycline). Products include:
Doryx Coated Pellet Filled Capsules 3357
Periostat Tablets 1208
Vibramycin Hyclate Capsules 2735
Vibramycin Hyclate Intravenous 2737
Vibra-Tabs Film Coated Tablets 2735

Doxycycline Monohydrate (Carbamazepine induces hepatic CYP activity and causes or would be expected to decrease plasma levels of doxycycline). Products include:
Monodox Capsules 2442
Vibramycin Monohydrate for Oral Suspension 2735

Dyphylline (Inducers of CYP3A4, such as theophylline, can increase the rate of carbamazepine metabolism and can thus decrease plasma carbamazepine levels; carbamazepine induces hepatic CYP activity and causes or would be expected to decrease plasma levels of theophylline). Products include:
Lufyllin Tablets 3347
Lufyllin-400 Tablets 3347
Lufyllin-GG Elixir 3348
Lufyllin-GG Tablets 3348

Erythromycin (Inhibitors of CYP3A4, such as erythromycin, inhibit carbamazepine metabolism and thus increase plasma carbamazepine levels). Products include:
Emgel 2% Topical Gel 1285
Ery-Tab Tablets 448
Erythromycin Base Filmtab Tablets 454
Erythromycin Delayed-Release Capsules, USP 455
PCE Dispertab Tablets 498

Erythromycin Estolate (Inhibitors of CYP3A4, such as erythromycin, inhibit carbamazepine metabolism and thus increase plasma carbamazepine levels).
No products indexed under this heading.

Erythromycin Ethylsuccinate (Inhibitors of CYP3A4, such as erythromycin, inhibit carbamazepine metabolism and thus increase plasma carbamazepine levels). Products include:
E.E.S. 450
EryPed 446
Pediazole Suspension 3050

Erythromycin Gluceptate (Inhibitors of CYP3A4, such as erythromycin, inhibit carbamazepine metabolism and thus increase plasma carbamazepine levels).
No products indexed under this heading.

Erythromycin Stearate (Inhibitors of CYP3A4, such as erythromycin, inhibit carbamazepine metabolism and thus increase plasma carbamazepine levels). Products include:
Erythrocin Stearate Filmtab Tablets 452

Ethinyl Estradiol (Carbamazepine induces hepatic CYP activity and causes or would be expected to decrease plasma levels of oral contraceptives; breakthrough bleeding has been reported among patients receiving concomitant oral contraceptives and their reliability may be adversely affected). Products include:
Alesse-21 Tablets 3468
Alesse-28 Tablets 3473
Brevicon 28-Day Tablets 3380
Cyclessa Tablets 2450
Desogen Tablets 2458
Estinyl Tablets 3112
Estrostep 2627
femhrt Tablets 2635
Levlen 962
Levlite 21 Tablets 962
Levlite 28 Tablets 962
Levora Tablets 3389
Loestrin 21 Tablets 2642
Loestrin Fe Tablets 2642
Lo/Ovral Tablets 3532
Lo/Ovral-28 Tablets 3538
Low-Ogestrel-28 Tablets 3392
Microgestin Fe 1.5/30 Tablets 3407
Microgestin Fe 1/20 Tablets 3400
Mircette Tablets 2470
Modicon 2563
Necon 3415
Nordette-28 Tablets 2257
Norinyl 1 +35 28-Day Tablets 3380
Ogestrel 0.5/50-28 Tablets 3428
Ortho-Cept 21 Tablets 2546
Ortho-Cept 28 Tablets 2546
Ortho-Cyclen/Ortho Tri-Cyclen 2573
Ortho-Novum 2563
Ovcon 3364
Ovral Tablets 3551
Ovral-28 Tablets 3552
Tri-Levlen 962
Tri-Norinyl-28 Tablets 3433
Triphasil-21 Tablets 3600
Triphasil-28 Tablets 3605
Trivora Tablets 3439
Yasmin 28 Tablets 980
Zovia 3449

Ethosuximide (Carbamazepine induces hepatic CYP activity and causes or would be expected to decrease plasma levels of ethosuximide; alterations of thyroid function have been reported in combination therapy with other anticonvulsants). Products include:
Zarontin Capsules 2659
Zarontin Syrup 2660

Ethotoin (Alterations of thyroid function have been reported in combination therapy with other anticonvulsants).
No products indexed under this heading.

Ethynodiol Diacetate (Carbamazepine induces hepatic CYP activity and causes or would be expected to decrease plasma levels of oral contraceptives; breakthrough bleeding has been reported among patients receiving concomitant oral contraceptives and their reliability may be adversely affected). Products include:
Zovia 3449

Felbamate (Inducers of CYP3A4, such as felbamate, can increase the rate of carbamazepine metabolism and can thus decrease plasma carbamazepine levels; alterations of thyroid function have been reported in combination therapy with other anticonvulsants). Products include:
Felbatol 3343

Fluoxetine Hydrochloride (Inhibitors of CYP3A4, such as fluoxetine, inhibit carbamazepine metabolism and thus increase plasma carbamazepine levels). Products include:
Prozac Pulvules, Liquid, and Weekly Capsules 1238
Sarafem Pulvules 1962

Fluphenazine Decanoate (Co-administration with psychotropic agents has resulted in isolated cases of neuroleptic malignant syndrome).
No products indexed under this heading.

Fluphenazine Enanthate (Co-administration with psychotropic agents has resulted in isolated cases of neuroleptic malignant syndrome).
No products indexed under this heading.

Fluphenazine Hydrochloride (Co-administration with psychotropic agents has resulted in isolated cases of neuroleptic malignant syndrome).
No products indexed under this heading.

Fosphenytoin Sodium (Alterations of thyroid function have been reported in combination therapy with other anticonvulsants). Products include:
Cerebyx Injection 2619

Haloperidol (Carbamazepine induces hepatic CYP activity and causes or would be expected to decrease plasma levels of haloperidol). Products include:
Haldol Injection, Tablets and Concentrate 2533

Haloperidol Decanoate (Carbamazepine induces hepatic CYP activity and causes or would be expected to decrease plasma levels of haloperidol). Products include:
Haldol Decanoate 2535

Isocarboxazid (Because of the relationship of carbamazepine to other tricyclic compounds, on theoretical grounds, co-administration with MAO inhibitors is contraindicated).
No products indexed under this heading.

Isoniazid (Inhibitors of CYP3A4, such as isoniazid, inhibit carbamazepine metabolism and thus increase plasma carbamazepine levels). Products include:
Rifamate Capsules 767
Rifater Tablets 769

Itraconazole (Inhibitors of CYP3A4, such as itraconazole, inhibit carbamazepine metabolism and thus increase plasma carbamazepine levels). Products include:
Sporanox Capsules 1800
Sporanox Injection 1804
Sporanox Injection 2509
Sporanox Oral Solution 1808
Sporanox Oral Solution 2512

Ketoconazole (Inhibitors of CYP3A4, such as ketoconazole, inhibit carbamazepine metabolism and thus increase plasma carbamazepine levels). Products include:
Nizoral 2% Cream 3620
Nizoral A-D Shampoo 2008
Nizoral 2% Shampoo 2007
Nizoral Tablets 1791

Lamotrigine (Alterations of thyroid function have been reported in combination therapy with other anticonvulsants). Products include:

Lamictal 1567

Levetiracetam (Alterations of thyroid function have been reported in combination therapy with other anticonvulsants). Products include:

Keppra Tablets 3314

Levonorgestrel (Carbamazepine induces hepatic CYP activity and causes or would be expected to decrease plasma levels of oral contraceptives; breakthrough bleeding has been reported among patients receiving concomitant oral contraceptives and their reliability may be adversely affected). Products include:

Alesse-21 Tablets 3468
Alesse-28 Tablets 3473
Levlen 962
Levlite 21 Tablets 962
Levlite 28 Tablets 962
Levora Tablets 3389
Mirena Intrauterine System 974
Nordette-28 Tablets 2257
Norplant System 3543
Tri-Levlen 962
Triphasil-21 Tablets 3600
Triphasil-28 Tablets 3605
Trivora Tablets 3439

Lithium Carbonate (Co-administration with psychotropic agents has resulted in isolated cases of neuroleptic malignant syndrome). Products include:

Eskalith 1527
Lithium Carbonate 3061
Lithobid Slow-Release Tablets 3255

Lithium Citrate (Co-administration with psychotropic agents has resulted in isolated cases of neuroleptic malignant syndrome). Products include:

Lithium Citrate Syrup 3061

Loratadine (Inhibitors of CYP3A4, such as loratadine, inhibit carbamazepine metabolism and thus increase plasma carbamazepine levels). Products include:

Claritin 3100
Claritin-D 12 Hour Extended Release Tablets 3102
Claritin-D 24 Hour Extended Release Tablets 3104

Loxapine Hydrochloride (Co-administration with psychotropic agents has resulted in isolated cases of neuroleptic malignant syndrome).

No products indexed under this heading.

Loxapine Succinate (Co-administration with psychotropic agents has resulted in isolated cases of neuroleptic malignant syndrome). Products include:

Loxitane Capsules 3398

Mephenytoin (Alterations of thyroid function have been reported in combination therapy with other anticonvulsants).

No products indexed under this heading.

Mesoridazine Besylate (Co-administration with psychotropic agents has resulted in isolated cases of neuroleptic malignant syndrome). Products include:

Serentil 1057

Mestranol (Carbamazepine induces hepatic CYP activity and causes or would be expected to decrease plasma levels of oral contraceptives; breakthrough bleeding has been reported among patients receiving concomitant oral contraceptives and their reliability may be adversely affected). Products include:

Necon 1/50 Tablets 3415
Norinyl 1 + 50 28-Day Tablets 3380
Ortho-Novum 1/50□28 Tablets 2556

Methotrimeprazine (Co-administration with psychotropic agents has resulted in isolated cases of neuroleptic malignant syndrome).

No products indexed under this heading.

Methsuximide (Carbamezapine induces hepatic CYP activity and causes or would be expected to decrease plasma levels of methsuximide; alterations of thyroid function have been reported in combination therapy with other anticonvulsants). Products include:

Celontin Capsules 2618

Moclobemide (Because of the relationship of carbamazepine to other tricyclic compounds, on theoretical grounds, co-administration with MAO inhibitors is contraindicated).

No products indexed under this heading.

Molindone Hydrochloride (Co-administration with psychotropic agents has resulted in isolated cases of neuroleptic malignant syndrome). Products include:

Moban 1320

Niacinamide (Inhibitors of CYP3A4, such as niacinamide, inhibit carbamazepine metabolism and thus increase plasma carbamazepine levels).

No products indexed under this heading.

Nicotinamide (Inhibitors of CYP3A4, such as nicotinamide, inhibit carbamazepine metabolism and thus increase plasma carbamazepine levels). Products include:

Nicomide Tablets 3247

Norethindrone (Carbamazepine induces hepatic CYP activity and causes or would be expected to decrease plasma levels of oral contraceptives; breakthrough bleeding has been reported among patients receiving concomitant oral contraceptives and their reliability may be adversely affected). Products include:

Brevicon 28-Day Tablets 3380
Micronor Tablets 2543
Modicon 2563
Necon 3415
Norinyl 1 +35 28-Day Tablets 3380
Norinyl 1 + 50 28-Day Tablets 3380
Nor-QD Tablets 3423
Ortho-Novum 2563
Ortho-Novum 1/50□28 Tablets 2556
Ovcon 3364
Tri-Norinyl-28 Tablets 3433

Norethynodrel (Carbamazepine induces hepatic CYP activity and causes or would be expected to decrease plasma levels of oral contraceptives; breakthrough bleeding has been reported among patients receiving concomitant oral contraceptives and their reliability may be adversely affected).

No products indexed under this heading.

Norgestimate (Carbamazepine induces hepatic CYP activity and causes or would be expected to decrease plasma levels of oral contraceptives; breakthrough bleeding has been reported among patients receiving concomitant oral contraceptives and their reliability may be adversely affected). Products include:

Ortho-Cyclen/Ortho Tri-Cyclen 2573
Ortho-Prefest Tablets 2570

Norgestrel (Carbamazepine induces hepatic CYP activity and causes or would be expected to decrease plasma levels of oral contraceptives; breakthrough bleeding has been reported among patients receiving concomitant oral contraceptives and their reliability may be adversely affected). Products include:

Lo/Ovral Tablets 3532
Lo/Ovral-28 Tablets 3538
Low-Ogestrel-28 Tablets 3392
Ogestrel 0.5/50-28 Tablets 3428
Ovral Tablets 3551
Ovral-28 Tablets 3552
Ovrette Tablets 3552

Olanzapine (Co-administration with psychotropic agents has resulted in isolated cases of neuroleptic malignant syndrome). Products include:

Zyprexa Tablets 1973
Zyprexa ZYDIS Orally Disintegrating Tablets 1973

Oxcarbazepine (Alterations of thyroid function have been reported in combination therapy with other anticonvulsants). Products include:

Trileptal Oral Suspension 2407
Trileptal Tablets 2407

Paramethadione (Alterations of thyroid function have been reported in combination therapy with other anticonvulsants).

No products indexed under this heading.

Pargyline Hydrochloride (Because of the relationship of carbamazepine to other tricyclic compounds, on theoretical grounds, co-administration with MAO inhibitors is contraindicated).

No products indexed under this heading.

Perphenazine (Co-administration with psychotropic agents has resulted in isolated cases of neuroleptic malignant syndrome). Products include:

Etrafon 3115
Trilafon 3160

Phenacemide (Alterations of thyroid function have been reported in combination therapy with other anticonvulsants).

No products indexed under this heading.

Phenelzine Sulfate (Because of the relationship of carbamazepine to other tricyclic compounds, on theoretical grounds, co-administration with MAO inhibitors is contraindicated). Products include:

Nardil Tablets 2653

Phenobarbital (Inducers of CYP3A4, such as phenobarbital, can increase the rate of carbamazepine metabolism and can thus decrease plasma carbamazepine levels; alterations of thyroid function have been reported in combination therapy with other anticonvulsants). Products include:

Arco-Lase Plus Tablets 592
Donnatal 2929
Donnatal Extentabs 2930

Phensuximide (Carbamezapine induces hepatic CYP activity and causes or would be expected to decrease plasma levels of phensuximide; alterations of thyroid function have been reported in combination therapy with other anticonvulsants).

No products indexed under this heading.

Phenytoin (Alterations of thyroid function have been reported in combination therapy with other anticonvulsants). Products include:

Dilantin Infatabs 2624
Dilantin-125 Oral Suspension 2625

Phenytoin Sodium (Alterations of thyroid function have been reported in combination therapy with other anticonvulsants). Products include:

Dilantin Kapseals 2622

Pimozide (Co-administration with psychotropic agents has resulted in isolated cases of neuroleptic malignant syndrome). Products include:

Orap Tablets 1407

Primidone (Inducers of CYP3A4, such as primidone, can increase the rate of carbamazepine metabolism and can thus decrease plasma carbamazepine levels; carbamazepine increases levels of primidone; alterations of thyroid function have been reported in combination therapy with other anticonvulsants).

No products indexed under this heading.

Procarbazine Hydrochloride (Because of the relationship of carbamazepine to other tricyclic compounds, on theoretical grounds, co-administration with MAO inhibitors is contraindicated). Products include:

Matulane Capsules 3246

Prochlorperazine (Co-administration with psychotropic agents has resulted in isolated cases of neuroleptic malignant syndrome). Products include:

Compazine 1505

Promethazine Hydrochloride (Co-administration with psychotropic agents has resulted in isolated cases of neuroleptic malignant syndrome). Products include:

Mepergan Injection 3539
Phenergan Injection 3553
Phenergan 3556
Phenergan Syrup 3554
Phenergan with Codeine Syrup 3557
Phenergan with Dextromethorphan Syrup 3559
Phenergan VC Syrup 3560
Phenergan VC with Codeine Syrup .. 3561

Propoxyphene Hydrochloride (Inhibitors of CYP3A4, such as propoxyphene, inhibit carbamazepine metabolism and thus increase plasma carbamazepine levels). Products include:

Darvon Pulvules 1909
Darvon Compound-65 Pulvules 1910

Propoxyphene Napsylate (Inhibitors of CYP3A4, such as propoxyphene, inhibit carbamazepine metabolism and thus increase plasma carbamazepine levels). Products include:

Darvon-N/Darvocet-N 1907
Darvon-N Tablets 1912

Quetiapine Fumarate (Co-administration with psychotropic agents has resulted in isolated cases of neuroleptic malignant syndrome). Products include:

Seroquel Tablets 684

Rifampin (Inducers of CYP3A4, such as rifampin, can increase the rate of carbamazepine metabolism and can thus decrease plasma carbamazepine levels). Products include:

Rifadin 765
Rifamate Capsules 767
Rifater Tablets 769

Risperidone (Co-administration with psychotropic agents has resulted in isolated cases of neuroleptic malignant syndrome). Products include:

Risperdal 1796

Selegiline Hydrochloride (Because of the relationship of carbamazepine to other tricyclic compounds, on theoretical grounds, co-administration with MAO inhibitors is contraindicated). Products include:

Eldepryl Capsules 3266

Terfenadine (Inhibitors of CYP3A4, such as terfenadine, inhibit carbamazepine metabolism and thus increase plasma carbamazepine levels).

No products indexed under this heading.

Theophylline (Inducers of CYP3A4, such as theophylline, can increase the rate of carbamazepine metabolism and can thus decrease plasma carbamazepine levels; carbamazepine induces hepatic CYP activity and causes or would be expected to decrease plasma levels of theophylline). Products include:

Aerolate 1361
Theo-Dur Extended-Release Tablets 1835
Uni-Dur Extended-Release Tablets .. 1841

Uniphyl 400 mg and 600 mg Tablets 2903

Theophylline Calcium Salicylate (Inducers of CYP3A4, such as theophylline, can increase the rate of carbamazepine metabolism and can thus decrease plasma carbamazepine levels; carbamazepine induces hepatic CYP activity and causes or would be expected to decrease plasma levels of theophylline).
No products indexed under this heading.

Theophylline Sodium Glycinate (Inducers of CYP3A4, such as theophylline, can increase the rate of carbamazepine metabolism and can thus decrease plasma carbamazepine levels; carbamazepine induces hepatic CYP activity and causes or would be expected to decrease plasma levels of theophylline).
No products indexed under this heading.

Thioridazine Hydrochloride (Co-administration with psychotropic agents has resulted in isolated cases of neuroleptic malignant syndrome). Products include:
Thioridazine Hydrochloride Tablets 2289

Thiothixene (Co-administration with psychotropic agents has resulted in isolated cases of neuroleptic malignant syndrome). Products include:
Navane Capsules 2701
Thiothixene Capsules 2290

Tiagabine Hydrochloride (Alterations of thyroid function have been reported in combination therapy with other anticonvulsants). Products include:
Gabitril Tablets 1189

Topiramate (Alterations of thyroid function have been reported in combination therapy with other anticonvulsants). Products include:
Topamax Sprinkle Capsules 2590
Topamax Tablets 2590

Tranylcypromine Sulfate (Because of the relationship of carbamazepine to other tricyclic compounds, on theoretical grounds, co-administration with MAO inhibitors is contraindicated). Products include:
Parnate Tablets 1607

Trifluoperazine Hydrochloride (Co-administration with psychotropic agents has resulted in isolated cases of neuroleptic malignant syndrome). Products include:
Stelazine 1640

Trimethadione (Alterations of thyroid function have been reported in combination therapy with other anticonvulsants).
No products indexed under this heading.

Troleandomycin (Inhibitors of CYP3A4, such as troleandomycin, inhibit carbamazepine metabolism and thus increase plasma carbamazepine levels). Products include:
Tao Capsules 2716

Valproate Sodium (Alterations of thyroid function have been reported in combination therapy with other anticonvulsants). Products include:
Depacon Injection 416

Valproic Acid (Alterations of thyroid function have been reported in combination therapy with other anticonvulsants). Products include:
Depakene 421

Verapamil Hydrochloride (Inhibitors of CYP3A4, such as verapamil, inhibit carbamazepine metabolism and thus increase plasma carbamazepine levels). Products include:
Covera-HS Tablets 3199
Isoptin SR Tablets 467
Tarka Tablets 508
Verelan Capsules 3184
Verelan PM Capsules 3186

Warfarin Sodium (Carbamezepine induces hepatic CYP activity and causes or would be expected to decrease plasma levels of warfarin). Products include:
Coumadin for Injection 1243
Coumadin Tablets 1243
Warfarin Sodium Tablets, USP 3302

Ziprasidone Hydrochloride (Co-administration with psychotropic agents has resulted in isolated cases of neuroleptic malignant syndrome). Products include:
Geodon Capsules 2688

Zonisamide (Alterations of thyroid function have been reported in combination therapy with other anticonvulsants). Products include:
Zonegran Capsules 1307

Food Interactions

Food, unspecified (A high fat meal increased the rat of absorption of a single 400 mg dose but not the AUC; elimination half-life remains unchanged between fasting and fed states).

CARDENE I.V.

(Nicardipine Hydrochloride) 3485
May interact with beta blockers and certain other agents. Compounds in these categories include:

Acebutolol Hydrochloride (In vitro and in some patients a negative inotropic effect has been observed with Cardene I.V., therefore, caution should be exercised when co-administered with beta blocker in patients with CHF or significant left ventricular dysfunction). Products include:
Sectral Capsules 3589

Atenolol (In vitro and in some patients a negative inotropic effect has been observed with Cardene I.V., therefore, caution should be exercised when co-administered with beta blocker in patients with CHF or significant left ventricular dysfunction). Products include:
Tenoretic Tablets 690
Tenormin I.V. Injection 692

Betaxolol Hydrochloride (In vitro and in some patients a negative inotropic effect has been observed with Cardene I.V., therefore, caution should be exercised when co-administered with beta blocker in patients with CHF or significant left ventricular dysfunction). Products include:
Betoptic S Ophthalmic Suspension 537

Bisoprolol Fumarate (In vitro and in some patients a negative inotropic effect has been observed with Cardene I.V., therefore, caution should be exercised when co-administered with beta blocker in patients with CHF or significant left ventricular dysfunction). Products include:
Zebeta Tablets 1885
Ziac Tablets 1887

Carteolol Hydrochloride (In vitro and in some patients a negative inotropic effect has been observed with Cardene I.V., therefore, caution should be exercised when co-administered with beta blocker in patients with CHF or significant left ventricular dysfunction). Products include:
Carteolol Hydrochloride Ophthalmic Solution USP, 1% .... ⊙258
Ocupress Ophthalmic Solution, 1% Sterile .... ⊙303

Cimetidine (Co-administration of cimetidine with Cardene Capsules increases nicardipine plasma concentration). Products include:
Tagamet HB 200 Suspension .... ▣762
Tagamet HB 200 Tablets .... ▣761
Tagamet Tablets 1644

Cimetidine Hydrochloride (Co-administration of cimetidine with Cardene Capsules increases nicardipine plasma concentration). Products include:
Tagamet 1644

Cyclosporine (Co-administration of Cardene Capsules and cyclosporine results in elevated plasma cyclosporine levels). Products include:
Gengraf Capsules 457
Neoral Soft Gelatin Capsules 2380
Neoral Oral Solution 2380
Sandimmune 2388

Digoxin (No alteration in digoxin plasma levels, however, as a precaution, digoxin levels should be evaluated when concomitant therapy is initiated). Products include:
Digitek Tablets 1003
Lanoxicaps Capsules 1574
Lanoxin Injection 1581
Lanoxin Tablets 1587
Lanoxin Elixir Pediatric 1578
Lanoxin Injection Pediatric 1584

Esmolol Hydrochloride (In vitro and in some patients a negative inotropic effect has been observed with Cardene I.V., therefore, caution should be exercised when co-administered with beta blocker in patients with CHF or significant left ventricular dysfunction). Products include:
Brevibloc Injection 858

Fentanyl (Potential for hypotension with fentanyl anesthesia when used with calcium channel blocker and beta blocker; such reaction has not been observed with Cardene I.V. during clinical trials). Products include:
Duragesic Transdermal System 1786

Fentanyl Citrate (Potential for hypotension with fentanyl anesthesia when used with calcium channel blocker and beta blocker; such reaction has not been observed with Cardene I.V. during clinical trials). Products include:
Actiq 1184

Labetalol Hydrochloride (In vitro and in some patients a negative inotropic effect has been observed with Cardene I.V., therefore, caution should be exercised when co-administered with beta blocker in patients with CHF or significant left ventricular dysfunction). Products include:
Normodyne Injection 3135
Normodyne Tablets 3137

Levobunolol Hydrochloride (In vitro and in some patients a negative inotropic effect has been observed with Cardene I.V., therefore, caution should be exercised when co-administered with beta blocker in patients with CHF or significant left ventricular dysfunction). Products include:
Betagan .... ⊙228

Metipranolol Hydrochloride (In vitro and in some patients a negative inotropic effect has been observed with Cardene I.V., therefore, caution should be exercised when co-administered with beta blocker in patients with CHF or significant left ventricular dysfunction).
No products indexed under this heading.

Metoprolol Succinate (In vitro and in some patients a negative inotropic effect has been observed with Cardene I.V., therefore, caution should be exercised when co-administered with beta blocker in patients with CHF or significant left ventricular dysfunction). Products include:
Toprol-XL Tablets 651

Metoprolol Tartrate (In vitro and in some patients a negative inotropic effect has been observed with Cardene I.V., therefore, caution should be exercised when co-administered with beta blocker in patients with CHF or significant left ventricular dysfunction).
No products indexed under this heading.

Nadolol (In vitro and in some patients a negative inotropic effect has been observed with Cardene I.V., therefore, caution should be exercised when co-administered with beta blocker in patients with CHF or significant left ventricular dysfunction). Products include:
Corgard Tablets 2245
Corzide 40/5 Tablets 2247
Corzide 80/5 Tablets 2247
Nadolol Tablets 2288

Penbutolol Sulfate (In vitro and in some patients a negative inotropic effect has been observed with Cardene I.V., therefore, caution should be exercised when co-administered with beta blocker in patients with CHF or significant left ventricular dysfunction).
No products indexed under this heading.

Pindolol (In vitro and in some patients a negative inotropic effect has been observed with Cardene I.V., therefore, caution should be exercised when co-administered with beta blocker in patients with CHF or significant left ventricular dysfunction).
No products indexed under this heading.

Propranolol Hydrochloride (In vitro and in some patients a negative inotropic effect has been observed with Cardene I.V., therefore, caution should be exercised when co-administered with beta blocker in patients with CHF or significant left ventricular dysfunction). Products include:
Inderal 3513
Inderal LA Long-Acting Capsules 3516
Inderide Tablets 3517
Inderide LA Long-Acting Capsules 3519

Sotalol Hydrochloride (In vitro and in some patients a negative inotropic effect has been observed with Cardene I.V., therefore, caution should be exercised when co-administered with beta blocker in patients with CHF or significant left ventricular dysfunction). Products include:
Betapace Tablets 950
Betapace AF Tablets 954

Timolol Hemihydrate (In vitro and in some patients a negative inotropic effect has been observed with Cardene I.V., therefore, caution should be exercised when co-administered with beta blocker in patients with CHF or significant left ventricular dysfunction). Products include:
Betimol Ophthalmic Solution .... ⊙324

Timolol Maleate (In vitro and in some patients a negative inotropic effect has been observed with Cardene I.V., therefore, caution should be exercised when co-administered with beta blocker in patients with CHF or significant left ventricular dysfunction). Products include:
Blocadren Tablets 2046
Cosopt Sterile Ophthalmic Solution 2065
Timolide Tablets 2187
Timolol GFS .... ⊙266
Timoptic in Ocudose 2192
Timoptic Sterile Ophthalmic Solution 2190
Timoptic-XE Sterile Ophthalmic Gel Forming Solution 2194

CARDIO ESSENTIALS CAPSULES

(Coenzyme Q-10) 3321
None cited in PDR database.

CARDIOPTIMA DRINK MIX PACKETS

(Amino Acid Preparations, Herbals with Vitamins & Minerals) .... ▣795
None cited in PDR database.

CARDIZEM INJECTABLE
(Diltiazem Hydrochloride) 1018
See Cardizem CD Capsules

CARDIZEM LYO-JECT SYRINGE
(Diltiazem Hydrochloride) 1018
See Cardizem CD Capsules

CARDIZEM MONOVIAL
(Diltiazem Hydrochloride) 1018
See Cardizem CD Capsules

CARDIZEM CD CAPSULES
(Diltiazem Hydrochloride) 1016
May interact with anesthetics, beta blockers, cardiac glycosides, and certain other agents. Compounds in these categories include:

Acebutolol Hydrochloride (Concomitant use of diltiazem with beta blockers may result in additive effect on cardiac conduction; intravenous diltiazem and intravenous beta-blockers should not be administered together or in close proximity). Products include:
Sectral Capsules 3589

Alfentanil Hydrochloride (Calcium channel blockers potentiate the depression of cardiac contractility, conductivity, and automaticity as well as vascular dilation associated with anesthetics).
No products indexed under this heading.

Amiodarone Hydrochloride (Agents known to affect cardiac contractility, such as amiodarone, may produce additive inhibition of cardiac conduction leading to increased risk of AV block). Products include:
Cordarone Intravenous 3491
Cordarone Tablets 3487
Pacerone Tablets 3331

Atenolol (Concomitant use of diltiazem with beta blockers may result in additive effect on cardiac conduction; intravenous diltiazem and intravenous beta-blockers should not be administered together or in close proximity). Products include:
Tenoretic Tablets 690
Tenormin I.V. Injection 692

Betaxolol Hydrochloride (Concomitant use of diltiazem with beta blockers may result in additive effect on cardiac conduction; intravenous diltiazem and intravenous beta-blockers should not be administered together or in close proximity). Products include:
Betoptic S Ophthalmic Suspension 537

Bisoprolol Fumarate (Concomitant use of diltiazem with beta blockers may result in additive effect on cardiac conduction; intravenous diltiazem and intravenous beta-blockers should not be administered together or in close proximity). Products include:
Zebeta Tablets 1885
Ziac Tablets 1887

Carbamazepine (Co-administration has resulted in increased serum levels of carbamazepine resulting in toxicity in some patients). Products include:
Carbatrol Capsules 3234
Tegretol/Tegretol-XR 2404

Carteolol Hydrochloride (Concomitant use of diltiazem with beta blockers may result in additive effect on cardiac conduction; intravenous diltiazem and intravenous beta-blockers should not be administered together or in close proximity). Products include:
Carteolol Hydrochloride Ophthalmic Solution USP, 1% ..... ⊙258
Ocupress Ophthalmic Solution, 1% Sterile .... ⊙303

Cimetidine (Co-administration has resulted in inhibition of hepatic cytochrome P450 by cimetidine producing significant increase in peak diltiazem plasma levels and AUC; an adjustment in diltiazem dosage may be warranted). Products include:
Tagamet HB 200 Suspension 762
Tagamet HB 200 Tablets 761
Tagamet Tablets 1644

Cimetidine Hydrochloride (Co-administration has resulted in inhibition of hepatic cytochrome P450 by cimetidine producing significant increase in peak diltiazem plasma levels and AUC; an adjustment in diltiazem dosage may be warranted). Products include:
Tagamet 1644

Cyclosporine (Diltiazem inhibits cytochrome P450 3A enzyme and co-administration may result in increased cyclosporine concentrations; a reduction in cyclosporine dose may be required, especially in renal and cardiac transplant recipients). Products include:
Gengraf Capsules 457
Neoral Soft Gelatin Capsules 2380
Neoral Oral Solution 2380
Sandimmune 2388

Deslanoside (Concomitant use of diltiazem with digitalis may result in additive effects on cardiac conduction).
No products indexed under this heading.

Digitoxin (Concomitant use of diltiazem with digitalis may result in additive effects on cardiac conduction).
No products indexed under this heading.

Digoxin (Co-administration has resulted in increased plasma digoxin concentrations in some patients; concomitant use of diltiazem with digitalis may result in additive effects on cardiac conduction). Products include:
Digitek Tablets 1003
Lanoxicaps Capsules 1574
Lanoxin Injection 1581
Lanoxin Tablets 1587
Lanoxin Elixir Pediatric 1578
Lanoxin Injection Pediatric 1584

Enflurane (Calcium channel blockers potentiate the depression of cardiac contractility, conductivity, and automaticity as well as vascular dilation associated with anesthetics).
No products indexed under this heading.

Esmolol Hydrochloride (Concomitant use of diltiazem with beta blockers may result in additive effect on cardiac conduction; intravenous diltiazem and intravenous beta-blockers should not be administered together or in close proximity). Products include:
Brevibloc Injection 858

Fentanyl Citrate (Calcium channel blockers potentiate the depression of cardiac contractility, conductivity, and automaticity as well as vascular dilation associated with anesthetics). Products include:
Actiq 1184

Fluoxetine Hydrochloride (Diltiazem undergoes biotransformation by cytochrome P450 mixed function oxidase; co-administration may result in increased serum concentrations of diltiazem, probably due to inhibited oxidative metabolism of diltiazem by fluoxetine). Products include:
Prozac Pulvules, Liquid, and Weekly Capsules 1238
Sarafem Pulvules 1962

Fluvoxamine Maleate (Diltiazem undergoes biotransformation by cytochrome P450 mixed function oxidase; co-administration may result in increased serum concentrations of diltiazem, probably due to inhibited oxidative metabolism of diltiazem by fluvoxamine). Products include:
Luvox Tablets (25, 50, 100 mg) 3256

Halothane (Calcium channel blockers potentiate the depression of cardiac contractility, conductivity, and automaticity as well as vascular dilation associated with anesthetics). Products include:
Fluothane Inhalation 3508

Isoflurane (Calcium channel blockers potentiate the depression of cardiac contractility, conductivity, and automaticity as well as vascular dilation associated with anesthetics).
No products indexed under this heading.

Ketamine Hydrochloride (Calcium channel blockers potentiate the depression of cardiac contractility, conductivity, and automaticity as well as vascular dilation associated with anesthetics).
No products indexed under this heading.

Labetalol Hydrochloride (Concomitant use of diltiazem with beta blockers may result in additive effect on cardiac conduction; intravenous diltiazem and intravenous beta-blockers should not be administered together or in close proximity). Products include:
Normodyne Injection 3135
Normodyne Tablets 3137

Levobunolol Hydrochloride (Concomitant use of diltiazem with beta blockers may result in additive effect on cardiac conduction; intravenous diltiazem and intravenous beta-blockers should not be administered together or in close proximity). Products include:
Betagan .... ⊙228

Methohexital Sodium (Calcium channel blockers potentiate the depression of cardiac contractility, conductivity, and automaticity as well as vascular dilation associated with anesthetics). Products include:
Brevital Sodium for Injection, USP .. 1815

Metipranolol Hydrochloride (Concomitant use of diltiazem with beta blockers may result in additive effect on cardiac conduction; intravenous diltiazem and intravenous beta-blockers should not be administered together or in close proximity).
No products indexed under this heading.

Metoprolol Succinate (Concomitant use of diltiazem with beta blockers may result in additive effect on cardiac conduction; intravenous diltiazem and intravenous beta-blockers should not be administered together or in close proximity). Products include:
Toprol-XL Tablets 651

Metoprolol Tartrate (Concomitant use of diltiazem with beta blockers may result in additive effect on cardiac conduction; intravenous diltiazem and intravenous beta-blockers should not be administered together or in close proximity).
No products indexed under this heading.

Midazolam Hydrochloride (Calcium channel blockers potentiate the depression of cardiac contractility, conductivity, and automaticity as well as vascular dilation associated with anesthetics). Products include:
Versed Injection 3027
Versed Syrup 3033

Nadolol (Concomitant use of diltiazem with beta blockers may result in additive effect on cardiac conduction; intravenous diltiazem and intravenous beta-blockers should not be administered together or in close proximity). Products include:
Corgard Tablets 2245
Corzide 40/5 Tablets 2247
Corzide 80/5 Tablets 2247
Nadolol Tablets 2288

Penbutolol Sulfate (Concomitant use of diltiazem with beta blockers may result in additive effect on cardiac conduction; intravenous diltiazem and intravenous beta-blockers should not be administered together or in close proximity).
No products indexed under this heading.

Pindolol (Concomitant use of diltiazem with beta blockers may result in additive effect on cardiac conduction; intravenous diltiazem and intravenous beta-blockers should not be administered together or in close proximity).
No products indexed under this heading.

Propofol (Calcium channel blockers potentiate the depression of cardiac contractility, conductivity, and automaticity as well as vascular dilation associated with anesthetics). Products include:
Diprivan Injectable Emulsion 667

Propranolol Hydrochloride (Co-administration has resulted in increased propranolol levels and bioavailability of propranolol was increased approximately 50%; concomitant use of diltiazem with beta blockers may result in additive effect on cardiac conduction; intravenous diltiazem and intravenous beta-blockers should not be administered together or in close proximity). Products include:
Inderal 3513
Inderal LA Long-Acting Capsules 3516
Inderide Tablets 3517
Inderide LA Long-Acting Capsules .. 3519

Ranitidine Hydrochloride (Co-administration produces smaller, nonsignificant increase in diltiazem plasma levels). Products include:
Zantac 1690
Zantac Injection 1688
Zantac 75 Tablets 717

Remifentanil Hydrochloride (Calcium channel blockers potentiate the depression of cardiac contractility, conductivity, and automaticity as well as vascular dilation associated with anesthetics).
No products indexed under this heading.

Ritonavir (Diltiazem undergoes biotransformation by cytochrome P450 mixed function oxidase; co-administration may result in increased serum concentrations of diltiazem, probably due to decreased diltiazem metabolism). Products include:
Kaletra Capsules 471
Kaletra Oral Solution 471
Norvir Capsules 487
Norvir Oral Solution 487

Sotalol Hydrochloride (Concomitant use of diltiazem with beta blockers may result in additive effect on cardiac conduction; intravenous diltiazem and intravenous beta-blockers should not be administered together or in close proximity). Products include:
Betapace Tablets 950
Betapace AF Tablets 954

Sufentanil Citrate (Calcium channel blockers potentiate the depression of cardiac contractility, conductivity, and automaticity as well as vascular dilation associated with anesthetics).
No products indexed under this heading.

Thiamylal Sodium (Calcium channel blockers potentiate the depression of cardiac contractility, conductivity, and automaticity as well as vascular dilation associated with

anesthetics).
No products indexed under this heading.

Timolol Hemihydrate (Concomitant use of diltiazem with beta blockers may result in additive effect on cardiac conduction; intravenous diltiazem and intravenous beta-blockers should not be administered together or in close proximity). Products include:
Betimol Ophthalmic Solution .... ⊙ 324

Timolol Maleate (Concomitant use of diltiazem with beta blockers may result in additive effect on cardiac conduction; intravenous diltiazem and intravenous beta-blockers should not be administered together or in close proximity). Products include:
Blocadren Tablets 2046
Cosopt Sterile Ophthalmic Solution.. 2065
Timolide Tablets 2187
Timolol GFS .... ⊙ 266
Timoptic in Ocudose 2192
Timoptic Sterile Ophthalmic Solution 2190
Timoptic-XE Sterile Ophthalmic Gel Forming Solution 2194

CARDURA TABLETS
(Doxazosin Mesylate) 2668
May interact with:

Cimetidine (Co-administration with oral cimetidine has resulted in a 10% increase in mean AUC of doxazosin and a slight but statistically insignificant increase in mean Cmax and mean half-life of doxazosin). Products include:
Tagamet HB 200 Suspension ....▣ 762
Tagamet HB 200 Tablets ....▣ 761
Tagamet Tablets 1644

Cimetidine Hydrochloride (Co-administration with oral cimetidine has resulted in a 10% increase in mean AUC of doxazosin and a slight but statistically insignificant increase in mean Cmax and mean half-life of doxazosin). Products include:
Tagamet 1644

CARNITOR INJECTION
(Levocarnitine) 3242
None cited in PDR database.

CARNITOR TABLETS AND ORAL SOLUTION
(Levocarnitine) 3245
None cited in PDR database.

CARTEOLOL HYDROCHLORIDE OPHTHALMIC SOLUTION USP, 1%
(Carteolol Hydrochloride) .... ⊙ 258
May interact with beta blockers and certain other agents. Compounds in these categories include:

Acebutolol Hydrochloride (Co-administration with oral beta-adrenergic blocking agents may result in potential additive effects on systemic beta-blockade). Products include:
Sectral Capsules 3589

Atenolol (Co-administration with oral beta-adrenergic blocking agents may result in potential additive effects on systemic beta-blockade). Products include:
Tenoretic Tablets 690
Tenormin I.V. Injection 692

Betaxolol Hydrochloride (Co-administration with oral beta-adrenergic blocking agents may result in potential additive effects on systemic beta-blockade). Products include:
Betoptic S Ophthalmic Suspension 537

Bisoprolol Fumarate (Co-administration with oral beta-adrenergic blocking agents may result in potential additive effects on systemic beta-blockade). Products include:
Zebeta Tablets 1885
Ziac Tablets 1887

Esmolol Hydrochloride (Co-administration with oral beta-adrenergic blocking agents may result in potential additive effects on systemic beta-blockade). Products include:
Brevibloc Injection 858

Guanethidine Monosulfate (Co-administration with catecholamine-depleting drugs, such as guanethidine, may result in possible additive effects and production of hypotension and/or marked bradycardia, which may produce vertigo, syncope, or postural hypertension).
No products indexed under this heading.

Labetalol Hydrochloride (Co-administration with oral beta-adrenergic blocking agents may result in potential additive effects on systemic beta-blockade). Products include:
Normodyne Injection 3135
Normodyne Tablets 3137

Levobunolol Hydrochloride (Co-administration with oral beta-adrenergic blocking agents may result in potential additive effects on systemic beta-blockade). Products include:
Betagan .... ⊙ 228

Metipranolol Hydrochloride (Co-administration with oral beta-adrenergic blocking agents may result in potential additive effects on systemic beta-blockade).
No products indexed under this heading.

Metoprolol Succinate (Co-administration with oral beta-adrenergic blocking agents may result in potential additive effects on systemic beta-blockade). Products include:
Toprol-XL Tablets 651

Metoprolol Tartrate (Co-administration with oral beta-adrenergic blocking agents may result in potential additive effects on systemic beta-blockade).
No products indexed under this heading.

Nadolol (Co-administration with oral beta-adrenergic blocking agents may result in potential additive effects on systemic beta-blockade). Products include:
Corgard Tablets 2245
Corzide 40/5 Tablets 2247
Corzide 80/5 Tablets 2247
Nadolol Tablets 2288

Penbutolol Sulfate (Co-administration with oral beta-adrenergic blocking agents may result in potential additive effects on systemic beta-blockade).
No products indexed under this heading.

Pindolol (Co-administration with oral beta-adrenergic blocking agents may result in potential additive effects on systemic beta-blockade).
No products indexed under this heading.

Propranolol Hydrochloride (Co-administration with oral beta-adrenergic blocking agents may result in potential additive effects on systemic beta-blockade). Products include:
Inderal 3513
Inderal LA Long-Acting Capsules 3516
Inderide Tablets 3517
Inderide LA Long-Acting Capsules .. 3519

Reserpine (Co-administration with catecholamine-depleting drugs, such as reserpine, may result in possible additive effects and production of hypotension and/or marked bradycardia, which may produce vertigo, syncope, or postural hypertension).
No products indexed under this heading.

Sotalol Hydrochloride (Co-administration with oral beta-adrenergic blocking agents may result in potential additive effects on systemic beta-blockade). Products include:
Betapace Tablets 950
Betapace AF Tablets 954

Timolol Hemihydrate (Co-administration with oral beta-adrenergic blocking agents may result in potential additive effects on systemic beta-blockade). Products include:
Betimol Ophthalmic Solution .... ⊙ 324

Timolol Maleate (Co-administration with oral beta-adrenergic blocking agents may result in potential additive effects on systemic beta-blockade). Products include:
Blocadren Tablets 2046
Cosopt Sterile Ophthalmic Solution 2065
Timolide Tablets 2187
Timolol GFS .... ⊙ 266
Timoptic in Ocudose 2192
Timoptic Sterile Ophthalmic Solution 2190
Timoptic-XE Sterile Ophthalmic Gel Forming Solution 2194

CASODEX TABLETS
(Bicalutamide) 662
May interact with oral anticoagulants. Compounds in these categories include:

Dicumarol (Bicalutamide can displace coumarin anticoagulant from their protein-binding sites as shown in *in vitro* studies; close monitoring of prothrombin time is advised).
No products indexed under this heading.

Warfarin Sodium (Bicalutamide can displace coumarin anticoagulant from their protein-binding sites as shown in *in vitro* studies; close monitoring of prothrombin time is advised). Products include:
Coumadin for Injection 1243
Coumadin Tablets 1243
Warfarin Sodium Tablets, USP 3302

CATAFLAM TABLETS
(Diclofenac Potassium) 2315
See Voltaren Tablets

CATALYST CAPSULES
(Amino Acid Preparations) .... ▣ 796
None cited in PDR database.

CATAPRES TABLETS
(Clonidine Hydrochloride) 1037
May interact with barbiturates, beta blockers, calcium channel blockers, cardiac glycosides, hypnotics and sedatives, tricyclic antidepressants, and certain other agents. Compounds in these categories include:

Acebutolol Hydrochloride (Co-administration with agents known to affect sinus node function or AV nodal conduction, such as beta blockers, may result in additive effects such as bradycardia and AV block). Products include:
Sectral Capsules 3589

Amitriptyline Hydrochloride (Co-administration may reduce the hypotensive effects; dosage adjustment may be necessary; concurrent use has resulted in corneal lesions in rats within 5 days). Products include:
Etrafon 3115
Limbitrol 1738

Amlodipine Besylate (Co-administration with agents known to affect sinus node function or AV nodal conduction, such as calcium channel blockers, may result in additive effects such as bradycardia and AV block). Products include:
Lotrel Capsules 2370
Norvasc Tablets 2704

Amoxapine (Co-administration may reduce the hypotensive effects; dosage adjustment may be necessary).
No products indexed under this heading.

Aprobarbital (Clonidine may potentiate the CNS-depressive effects).
No products indexed under this heading.

Atenolol (Co-administration with agents known to affect sinus node function or AV nodal conduction, such as beta blockers, may result in additive effects such as bradycardia and AV block). Products include:
Tenoretic Tablets 690
Tenormin I.V. Injection 692

Bepridil Hydrochloride (Co-administration with agents known to affect sinus node function or AV nodal conduction, such as calcium channel blockers, may result in additive effects such as bradycardia and AV block). Products include:
Vascor Tablets 2602

Betaxolol Hydrochloride (Co-administration with agents known to affect sinus node function or AV nodal conduction, such as beta blockers, may result in additive effects such as bradycardia and AV block). Products include:
Betoptic S Ophthalmic Suspension 537

Bisoprolol Fumarate (Co-administration with agents known to affect sinus node function or AV nodal conduction, such as beta blockers, may result in additive effects such as bradycardia and AV block). Products include:
Zebeta Tablets 1885
Ziac Tablets 1887

Butabarbital (Clonidine may potentiate the CNS-depressive effects).
No products indexed under this heading.

Butalbital (Clonidine may potentiate the CNS-depressive effects). Products include:
Phrenilin 578
Sedapap Tablets 50 mg/650 mg ... 2225

Carteolol Hydrochloride (Co-administration with agents known to affect sinus node function or AV nodal conduction, such as beta blockers, may result in additive effects such as bradycardia and AV block). Products include:
Carteolol Hydrochloride Ophthalmic Solution USP, 1% ..... ⊙ 258
Ocupress Ophthalmic Solution, 1% Sterile .... ⊙ 303

Clomipramine Hydrochloride (Co-administration may reduce the hypotensive effects; dosage adjustment may be necessary).
No products indexed under this heading.

Desipramine Hydrochloride (Co-administration may reduce the hypotensive effects; dosage adjustment may be necessary). Products include:
Norpramin Tablets 755

Deslanoside (Co-administration with agents known to affect sinus node function or AV nodal conduction, such as digitalis, may result in additive effects such as bradycardia and AV block).
No products indexed under this heading.

Digitoxin (Co-administration with agents known to affect sinus node function or AV nodal conduction, such as digitalis, may result in additive effects such as bradycardia and AV block).
No products indexed under this heading.

Digoxin (Co-administration with agents known to affect sinus node function or AV nodal conduction, such as digitalis, may result in additive effects such as bradycardia and AV block). Products include:
Digitek Tablets 1003
Lanoxicaps Capsules 1574
Lanoxin Injection 1581

Lanoxin Tablets 1587
Lanoxin Elixir Pediatric 1578
Lanoxin Injection Pediatric 1584

Diltiazem Hydrochloride (Co-administration with agents known to affect sinus node function or AV nodal conduction, such as calcium channel blockers, may result in additive effects such as bradycardia and AV block). Products include:
Cardizem Injectable 1018
Cardizem Lyo-Ject Syringe 1018
Cardizem Monovial 1018
Cardizem CD Capsules 1016
Tiazac Capsules 1378

Doxepin Hydrochloride (Co-administration may reduce the hypotensive effects; dosage adjustment may be necessary). Products include:
Sinequan 2713

Esmolol Hydrochloride (Co-administration with agents known to affect sinus node function or AV nodal conduction, such as beta blockers, may result in additive effects such as bradycardia and AV block). Products include:
Brevibloc Injection 858

Estazolam (Clonidine may potentiate the CNS-depressive effects). Products include:
ProSom Tablets 500

Ethchlorvynol (Clonidine may potentiate the CNS-depressive effects).
No products indexed under this heading.

Ethinamate (Clonidine may potentiate the CNS-depressive effects).
No products indexed under this heading.

Felodipine (Co-administration with agents known to affect sinus node function or AV nodal conduction, such as calcium channel blockers, may result in additive effects such as bradycardia and AV block). Products include:
Lexxel Tablets 608
Plendil Extended-Release Tablets 623

Flurazepam Hydrochloride (Clonidine may potentiate the CNS-depressive effects).
No products indexed under this heading.

Glutethimide (Clonidine may potentiate the CNS-depressive effects).
No products indexed under this heading.

Imipramine Hydrochloride (Co-administration may reduce the hypotensive effects; dosage adjustment may be necessary).
No products indexed under this heading.

Imipramine Pamoate (Co-administration may reduce the hypotensive effects; dosage adjustment may be necessary).
No products indexed under this heading.

Isradipine (Co-administration with agents known to affect sinus node function or AV nodal conduction, such as calcium channel blockers, may result in additive effects such as bradycardia and AV block). Products include:
DynaCirc Capsules 2921
DynaCirc CR Tablets 2923

Labetalol Hydrochloride (Co-administration with agents known to affect sinus node function or AV nodal conduction, such as beta blockers, may result in additive effects such as bradycardia and AV block). Products include:
Normodyne Injection 3135
Normodyne Tablets 3137

Levobunolol Hydrochloride (Co-administration with agents known to affect sinus node function or AV nodal conduction, such as beta blockers, may result in additive effects such as bradycardia and AV block). Products include:
Betagan .... ⊙228

Lorazepam (Clonidine may potentiate the CNS-depressive effects). Products include:
Ativan Injection 3478
Ativan Tablets 3482

Maprotiline Hydrochloride (Co-administration may reduce the hypotensive effects; dosage adjustment may be necessary).
No products indexed under this heading.

Mephobarbital (Clonidine may potentiate the CNS-depressive effects).
No products indexed under this heading.

Metipranolol Hydrochloride (Co-administration with agents known to affect sinus node function or AV nodal conduction, such as beta blockers, may result in additive effects such as bradycardia and AV block).
No products indexed under this heading.

Metoprolol Succinate (Co-administration with agents known to affect sinus node function or AV nodal conduction, such as beta blockers, may result in additive effects such as bradycardia and AV block). Products include:
Toprol-XL Tablets 651

Metoprolol Tartrate (Co-administration with agents known to affect sinus node function or AV nodal conduction, such as beta blockers, may result in additive effects such as bradycardia and AV block).
No products indexed under this heading.

Mibefradil Dihydrochloride (Co-administration with agents known to affect sinus node function or AV nodal conduction, such as calcium channel blockers, may result in additive effects such as bradycardia and AV block).
No products indexed under this heading.

Midazolam Hydrochloride (Clonidine may potentiate the CNS-depressive effects). Products include:
Versed Injection 3027
Versed Syrup 3033

Nadolol (Co-administration with agents known to affect sinus node function or AV nodal conduction, such as beta blockers, may result in additive effects such as bradycardia and AV block). Products include:
Corgard Tablets 2245
Corzide 40/5 Tablets 2247
Corzide 80/5 Tablets 2247
Nadolol Tablets 2288

Nicardipine Hydrochloride (Co-administration with agents known to affect sinus node function or AV nodal conduction, such as calcium channel blockers, may result in additive effects such as bradycardia and AV block). Products include:
Cardene I.V. 3485

Nifedipine (Co-administration with agents known to affect sinus node function or AV nodal conduction, such as calcium channel blockers, may result in additive effects such as bradycardia and AV block). Products include:
Adalat CC Tablets 877
Procardia Capsules 2708
Procardia XL Extended Release Tablets 2710

Nimodipine (Co-administration with agents known to affect sinus node function or AV nodal conduction, such as calcium channel blockers, may result in additive effects such as bradycardia and AV block). Products include:
Nimotop Capsules 904

Nisoldipine (Co-administration with agents known to affect sinus node function or AV nodal conduction, such as calcium channel blockers, may result in additive effects such as bradycardia and AV block). Products include:
Sular Tablets 688

Nortriptyline Hydrochloride (Co-administration may reduce the hypotensive effects; dosage adjustment may be necessary).
No products indexed under this heading.

Penbutolol Sulfate (Co-administration with agents known to affect sinus node function or AV nodal conduction, such as beta blockers, may result in additive effects such as bradycardia and AV block).
No products indexed under this heading.

Pentobarbital Sodium (Clonidine may potentiate the CNS-depressive effects). Products include:
Nembutal Sodium Solution 485

Phenobarbital (Clonidine may potentiate the CNS-depressive effects). Products include:
Arco-Lase Plus Tablets 592
Donnatal 2929
Donnatal Extentabs 2930

Pindolol (Co-administration with agents known to affect sinus node function or AV nodal conduction, such as beta blockers, may result in additive effects such as bradycardia and AV block).
No products indexed under this heading.

Propofol (Clonidine may potentiate the CNS-depressive effects). Products include:
Diprivan Injectable Emulsion 667

Propranolol Hydrochloride (Co-administration with agents known to affect sinus node function or AV nodal conduction, such as beta blockers, may result in additive effects such as bradycardia and AV block). Products include:
Inderal 3513
Inderal LA Long-Acting Capsules 3516
Inderide Tablets 3517
Inderide LA Long-Acting Capsules 3519

Protriptyline Hydrochloride (Co-administration may reduce the hypotensive effects; dosage adjustment may be necessary). Products include:
Vivactil Tablets 2446
Vivactil Tablets 2217

Quazepam (Clonidine may potentiate the CNS-depressive effects).
No products indexed under this heading.

Secobarbital Sodium (Clonidine may potentiate the CNS-depressive effects).
No products indexed under this heading.

Sotalol Hydrochloride (Co-administration with agents known to affect sinus node function or AV nodal conduction, such as beta blockers, may result in additive effects such as bradycardia and AV block). Products include:
Betapace Tablets 950
Betapace AF Tablets 954

Temazepam (Clonidine may potentiate the CNS-depressive effects).
No products indexed under this heading.

Thiamylal Sodium (Clonidine may potentiate the CNS-depressive effects).
No products indexed under this heading.

Timolol Hemihydrate (Co-administration with agents known to affect sinus node function or AV nodal conduction, such as beta blockers, may result in additive effects such as bradycardia and AV block). Products include:
Betimol Ophthalmic Solution .... ⊙324

Timolol Maleate (Co-administration with agents known to affect sinus node function or AV nodal conduction, such as beta blockers, may result in additive effects such as bradycardia and AV block). Products include:
Blocadren Tablets 2046
Cosopt Sterile Ophthalmic Solution 2065
Timolide Tablets 2187
Timolol GFS .... ⊙266
Timoptic in Ocudose 2192
Timoptic Sterile Ophthalmic Solution 2190
Timoptic-XE Sterile Ophthalmic Gel Forming Solution 2194

Triazolam (Clonidine may potentiate the CNS-depressive effects). Products include:
Halcion Tablets 2823

Trimipramine Maleate (Co-administration may reduce the hypotensive effects; dosage adjustment may be necessary). Products include:
Surmontil Capsules 3595

Verapamil Hydrochloride (Co-administration with agents known to affect sinus node function or AV nodal conduction, such as calcium channel blockers, may result in additive effects such as bradycardia and AV block). Products include:
Covera-HS Tablets 3199
Isoptin SR Tablets 467
Tarka Tablets 508
Verelan Capsules 3184
Verelan PM Capsules 3186

Zaleplon (Clonidine may potentiate the CNS-depressive effects). Products include:
Sonata Capsules 3591

Zolpidem Tartrate (Clonidine may potentiate the CNS-depressive effects). Products include:
Ambien Tablets 3191

Food Interactions

Alcohol (Clonidine may potentiate the CNS-depressive effects).

CATAPRES-TTS

(Clonidine) 1038

May interact with barbiturates, beta blockers, calcium channel blockers, cardiac glycosides, hypnotics and sedatives, tricyclic antidepressants, and certain other agents. Compounds in these categories include:

Acebutolol Hydrochloride (Co-administration with agents known to affect sinus node function or AV nodal conduction, such as beta blockers, may result in additive effects such as bradycardia and AV block). Products include:
Sectral Capsules 3589

Amitriptyline Hydrochloride (Co-administration may reduce the hypotensive effects; dosage adjustment may be necessary; concurrent use has resulted in corneal lesions in rats within 5 days). Products include:
Etrafon 3115
Limbitrol 1738

Amlodipine Besylate (Co-administration with agents known to affect sinus node function or AV nodal conduction, such as calcium channel blockers, may result in additive effects such as bradycardia and AV block). Products include:
Lotrel Capsules 2370
Norvasc Tablets 2704

Amoxapine (Co-administration may reduce the hypotensive effects; dos-

age adjustment may be necessary).
No products indexed under this heading.

Aprobarbital (Clonidine may potentiate the CNS-depressive effects).
No products indexed under this heading.

Atenolol (Co-administration with agents known to affect sinus node function or AV nodal conduction, such as beta blockers, may result in additive effects such as bradycardia and AV block). Products include:
Tenoretic Tablets 690
Tenormin I.V. Injection 692

Bepridil Hydrochloride (Co-administration with agents known to affect sinus node function or AV nodal conduction, such as calcium channel blockers, may result in additive effects such as bradycardia and AV block). Products include:
Vascor Tablets 2602

Betaxolol Hydrochloride (Co-administration with agents known to affect sinus node function or AV nodal conduction, such as beta blockers, may result in additive effects such as bradycardia and AV block). Products include:
Betoptic S Ophthalmic Suspension 537

Bisoprolol Fumarate (Co-administration with agents known to affect sinus node function or AV nodal conduction, such as beta blockers, may result in additive effects such as bradycardia and AV block). Products include:
Zebeta Tablets 1885
Ziac Tablets 1887

Butabarbital (Clonidine may potentiate the CNS-depressive effects).
No products indexed under this heading.

Butalbital (Clonidine may potentiate the CNS-depressive effects).
Products include:
Phrenilin 578
Sedapap Tablets 50 mg/650 mg 2225

Carteolol Hydrochloride (Co-administration with agents known to affect sinus node function or AV nodal conduction, such as beta blockers, may result in additive effects such as bradycardia and AV block). Products include:
Carteolol Hydrochloride Ophthalmic Solution USP, 1% .... ⊙ 258
Ocupress Ophthalmic Solution, 1% Sterile .... ⊙ 303

Clomipramine Hydrochloride (Co-administration may reduce the hypotensive effects; dosage adjustment may be necessary).
No products indexed under this heading.

Desipramine Hydrochloride (Co-administration may reduce the hypotensive effects; dosage adjustment may be necessary). Products include:
Norpramin Tablets 755

Deslanoside (Co-administration with agents known to affect sinus node function or AV nodal conduction, such as digitalis, may result in additive effects such as bradycardia and AV block).
No products indexed under this heading.

Digitoxin (Co-administration with agents known to affect sinus node function or AV nodal conduction, such as digitalis, may result in additive effects such as bradycardia and AV block).
No products indexed under this heading.

Digoxin (Co-administration with agents known to affect sinus node function or AV nodal conduction, such as digitalis, may result in additive effects such as bradycardia and AV block). Products include:
Digitek Tablets 1003
Lanoxicaps Capsules 1574
Lanoxin Injection 1581
Lanoxin Tablets 1587
Lanoxin Elixir Pediatric 1578
Lanoxin Injection Pediatric 1584

Diltiazem Hydrochloride (Co-administration with agents known to affect sinus node function or AV nodal conduction, such as calcium channel blockers, may result in additive effects such as bradycardia and AV block). Products include:
Cardizem Injectable 1018
Cardizem Lyo-Ject Syringe 1018
Cardizem Monovial 1018
Cardizem CD Capsules 1016
Tiazac Capsules 1378

Doxepin Hydrochloride (Co-administration may reduce the hypotensive effects; dosage adjustment may be necessary). Products include:
Sinequan 2713

Esmolol Hydrochloride (Co-administration with agents known to affect sinus node function or AV nodal conduction, such as beta blockers, may result in additive effects such as bradycardia and AV block). Products include:
Brevibloc Injection 858

Estazolam (Clonidine may potentiate the CNS-depressive effects).
Products include:
ProSom Tablets 500

Ethchlorvynol (Clonidine may potentiate the CNS-depressive effects).
No products indexed under this heading.

Ethinamate (Clonidine may potentiate the CNS-depressive effects).
No products indexed under this heading.

Felodipine (Co-administration with agents known to affect sinus node function or AV nodal conduction, such as calcium channel blockers, may result in additive effects such as bradycardia and AV block).
Products include:
Lexxel Tablets 608
Plendil Extended-Release Tablets 623

Flurazepam Hydrochloride (Clonidine may potentiate the CNS-depressive effects).
No products indexed under this heading.

Glutethimide (Clonidine may potentiate the CNS-depressive effects).
No products indexed under this heading.

Imipramine Hydrochloride (Co-administration may reduce the hypotensive effects; dosage adjustment may be necessary).
No products indexed under this heading.

Imipramine Pamoate (Co-administration may reduce the hypotensive effects; dosage adjustment may be necessary).
No products indexed under this heading.

Isradipine (Co-administration with agents known to affect sinus node function or AV nodal conduction, such as calcium channel blockers, may result in additive effects such as bradycardia and AV block).
Products include:
DynaCirc Capsules 2921
DynaCirc CR Tablets 2923

Labetalol Hydrochloride (Co-administration with agents known to affect sinus node function or AV nodal conduction, such as beta blockers, may result in additive effects such as bradycardia and AV block). Products include:
Normodyne Injection 3135
Normodyne Tablets 3137

Levobunolol Hydrochloride (Co-administration with agents known to affect sinus node function or AV nodal conduction, such as beta blockers, may result in additive effects such as bradycardia and AV block). Products include:
Betagan .... ⊙ 228

Lorazepam (Clonidine may potentiate the CNS-depressive effects).
Products include:
Ativan Injection 3478
Ativan Tablets 3482

Maprotiline Hydrochloride (Co-administration may reduce the hypotensive effects; dosage adjustment may be necessary).
No products indexed under this heading.

Mephobarbital (Clonidine may potentiate the CNS-depressive effects).
No products indexed under this heading.

Metipranolol Hydrochloride (Co-administration with agents known to affect sinus node function or AV nodal conduction, such as beta blockers, may result in additive effects such as bradycardia and AV block).
No products indexed under this heading.

Metoprolol Succinate (Co-administration with agents known to affect sinus node function or AV nodal conduction, such as beta blockers, may result in additive effects such as bradycardia and AV block). Products include:
Toprol-XL Tablets 651

Metoprolol Tartrate (Co-administration with agents known to affect sinus node function or AV nodal conduction, such as beta blockers, may result in additive effects such as bradycardia and AV block).
No products indexed under this heading.

Mibefradil Dihydrochloride (Co-administration with agents known to affect sinus node function or AV nodal conduction, such as calcium channel blockers, may result in additive effects such as bradycardia and AV block).
No products indexed under this heading.

Midazolam Hydrochloride (Clonidine may potentiate the CNS-depressive effects). Products include:
Versed Injection 3027
Versed Syrup 3033

Nadolol (Co-administration with agents known to affect sinus node function or AV nodal conduction, such as beta blockers, may result in additive effects such as bradycardia and AV block). Products include:
Corgard Tablets 2245
Corzide 40/5 Tablets 2247
Corzide 80/5 Tablets 2247
Nadolol Tablets 2288

Nicardipine Hydrochloride (Co-administration with agents known to affect sinus node function or AV nodal conduction, such as calcium channel blockers, may result in additive effects such as bradycardia and AV block). Products include:
Cardene I.V. 3485

Nifedipine (Co-administration with agents known to affect sinus node function or AV nodal conduction, such as calcium channel blockers, may result in additive effects such as bradycardia and AV block).
Products include:
Adalat CC Tablets 877
Procardia Capsules 2708
Procardia XL Extended Release Tablets 2710

Nimodipine (Co-administration with agents known to affect sinus node function or AV nodal conduction, such as calcium channel blockers, may result in additive effects such as bradycardia and AV block).
Products include:
Nimotop Capsules 904

Nisoldipine (Co-administration with agents known to affect sinus node function or AV nodal conduction, such as calcium channel blockers, may result in additive effects such as bradycardia and AV block).
Products include:
Sular Tablets 688

Nortriptyline Hydrochloride (Co-administration may reduce the hypotensive effects; dosage adjustment may be necessary).
No products indexed under this heading.

Penbutolol Sulfate (Co-administration with agents known to affect sinus node function or AV nodal conduction, such as beta blockers, may result in additive effects such as bradycardia and AV block).
No products indexed under this heading.

Pentobarbital Sodium (Clonidine may potentiate the CNS-depressive effects). Products include:
Nembutal Sodium Solution 485

Phenobarbital (Clonidine may potentiate the CNS-depressive effects). Products include:
Arco-Lase Plus Tablets 592
Donnatal 2929
Donnatal Extentabs 2930

Pindolol (Co-administration with agents known to affect sinus node function or AV nodal conduction, such as beta blockers, may result in additive effects such as bradycardia and AV block).
No products indexed under this heading.

Propofol (Clonidine may potentiate the CNS-depressive effects).
Products include:
Diprivan Injectable Emulsion 667

Propranolol Hydrochloride (Co-administration with agents known to affect sinus node function or AV nodal conduction, such as beta blockers, may result in additive effects such as bradycardia and AV block). Products include:
Inderal 3513
Inderal LA Long-Acting Capsules 3516
Inderide Tablets 3517
Inderide LA Long-Acting Capsules 3519

Protriptyline Hydrochloride (Co-administration may reduce the hypotensive effects; dosage adjustment may be necessary). Products include:
Vivactil Tablets 2446
Vivactil Tablets 2217

Quazepam (Clonidine may potentiate the CNS-depressive effects).
No products indexed under this heading.

Secobarbital Sodium (Clonidine may potentiate the CNS-depressive effects).
No products indexed under this heading.

Sotalol Hydrochloride (Co-administration with agents known to affect sinus node function or AV nodal conduction, such as beta blockers, may result in additive effects such as bradycardia and AV block). Products include:
Betapace Tablets 950
Betapace AF Tablets 954

Temazepam (Clonidine may potentiate the CNS-depressive effects).
No products indexed under this heading.

Thiamylal Sodium (Clonidine may potentiate the CNS-depressive

effects).
No products indexed under this heading.

Timolol Hemihydrate (Co-administration with agents known to affect sinus node function or AV nodal conduction, such as beta blockers, may result in additive effects such as bradycardia and AV block). Products include:
Betimol Ophthalmic Solution .... ⊙324

Timolol Maleate (Co-administration with agents known to affect sinus node function or AV nodal conduction, such as beta blockers, may result in additive effects such as bradycardia and AV block). Products include:
Blocadren Tablets 2046
Cosopt Sterile Ophthalmic Solution 2065
Timolide Tablets 2187
Timolol GFS .... ⊙266
Timoptic in Ocudose 2192
Timoptic Sterile Ophthalmic Solution 2190
Timoptic-XE Sterile Ophthalmic Gel Forming Solution 2194

Triazolam (Clonidine may potentiate the CNS-depressive effects). Products include:
Halcion Tablets 2823

Trimipramine Maleate (Co-administration may reduce the hypotensive effects; dosage adjustment may be necessary). Products include:
Surmontil Capsules 3595

Verapamil Hydrochloride (Co-administration with agents known to affect sinus node function or AV nodal conduction, such as calcium channel blockers, may result in additive effects such as bradycardia and AV block). Products include:
Covera-HS Tablets 3199
Isoptin SR Tablets 467
Tarka Tablets 508
Verelan Capsules 3184
Verelan PM Capsules 3186

Zaleplon (Clonidine may potentiate the CNS-depressive effects). Products include:
Sonata Capsules 3591

Zolpidem Tartrate (Clonidine may potentiate the CNS-depressive effects). Products include:
Ambien Tablets 3191

Food Interactions

Alcohol (Clonidine may potentiate the CNS-depressive effects).

CATHFLO ACTIVASE
(Alteplase, Recombinant) 3611
See Activase I.V.

CAVERJECT STERILE POWDER
(Alprostadil) 2777
May interact with:

Heparin Sodium (Patients on anticoagulants, such as heparin, may have increased propensity for bleeding after intracavernosal injection). Products include:
Heparin Lock Flush Solution 3509
Heparin Sodium Injection 3511

Sildenafil Citrate (The safety and efficacy of combination therapy with other vasoactive agents, such as sildenafil, have not been studied; therefore, such combinations are not recommended). Products include:
Viagra Tablets 2732

Warfarin Sodium (Patients on anticoagulants, such as warfarin, may have increased propensity for bleeding after intracavernosal injection). Products include:
Coumadin for Injection 1243
Coumadin Tablets 1243
Warfarin Sodium Tablets, USP 3302

CECLOR CD TABLETS
(Cefaclor) 1279
May interact with:

Aluminum Hydroxide (Co-administration with magnesium or aluminum hydroxide-containing antacids, when taken within 1 hour of administration, results in diminished extent of absorption). Products include:
Amphojel Suspension (Mint Flavor) .... ▣789
Gaviscon Extra Strength Liquid .... ▣751
Gaviscon Extra Strength Tablets .... ▣751
Gaviscon Regular Strength Liquid .... ▣751
Gaviscon Regular Strength Tablets .... ▣750
Maalox Antacid/Anti-Gas Oral Suspension .... ▣673
Maalox Max Maximum Strength Antacid/Anti-Gas Liquid 2300
Maalox Regular Strength Antacid/Antigas Liquid 2300
Mylanta 1813
Vanquish Caplets .... ▣617

Magnesium Hydroxide (Co-administration with magnesium or aluminum hydroxide-containing antacids, when taken within 1 hour of administration, results in diminished extent of absorption). Products include:
Ex•Lax Milk of Magnesia Liquid .... ▣670
Maalox Antacid/Anti-Gas Oral Suspension .... ▣673
Maalox Max Maximum Strength Antacid/Anti-Gas Liquid 2300
Maalox Regular Strength Antacid/Antigas Liquid 2300
Mylanta Fast-Acting 1813
Mylanta 1813
Pepcid Complete Chewable Tablets 1815
Phillips' Chewable Tablets .... ▣615
Phillips' Milk of Magnesia Liquid (Original, Cherry, & Mint) .... ▣616
Rolaids Tablets .... ▣706
Extra Strength Rolaids Tablets .... ▣706
Vanquish Caplets .... ▣617

Probenecid (Inhibits the renal excretion of cefaclor).
No products indexed under this heading.

Warfarin Sodium (Co-administration has resulted in rare reports of increased prothrombin time with or without clinical bleeding). Products include:
Coumadin for Injection 1243
Coumadin Tablets 1243
Warfarin Sodium Tablets, USP 3302

Food Interactions

Food, unspecified (The extent of absorption (AUC) and the maximum plasma concentration (Cmax) of cefaclor from Ceclor CD are greater when it is taken with food).

CECLOR PULVULES
(Cefaclor) 1905
May interact with oral anticoagulants and certain other agents. Compounds in these categories include:

Dicumarol (Co-administration has resulted in increased anticoagulant effect).
No products indexed under this heading.

Probenecid (Inhibits renal excretion of cefaclor).
No products indexed under this heading.

Warfarin Sodium (Co-administration has resulted in increased anticoagulant effect). Products include:
Coumadin for Injection 1243
Coumadin Tablets 1243
Warfarin Sodium Tablets, USP 3302

CECLOR SUSPENSION
(Cefaclor) 1905
See Ceclor Pulvules

CEDAX CAPSULES
(Ceftibuten Dihydrate) 1021
May interact with:

Ranitidine Hydrochloride (Ranitidine increases the ceftibuten Cmax by 23% and AUC by 16%; clinical relevance in this interaction is not known). Products include:
Zantac 1690
Zantac Injection 1688
Zantac 75 Tablets .... ▣717

Food Interactions

Food, unspecified (Food delays the time of Cmax, decreases the Cmax, and the extent of absorption (AUC); ceftibuten oral suspension should be taken at least 2 hours before meal or at least 1 hour after meal).

CEDAX ORAL SUSPENSION
(Ceftibuten Dihydrate) 1021
See Cedax Capsules

CEFIZOX FOR INTRAMUSCULAR OR INTRAVENOUS USE
(Ceftizoxime Sodium) 1390
May interact with aminoglycosides. Compounds in these categories include:

Amikacin Sulfate (Co-administration of other cephalosporins with aminoglycosides has resulted in nephrotoxicity).
No products indexed under this heading.

Gentamicin Sulfate (Co-administration of other cephalosporins with aminoglycosides has resulted in nephrotoxicity). Products include:
Genoptic Ophthalmic Ointment .... ⊙239
Genoptic Sterile Ophthalmic Solution .... ⊙239
Pred-G Ophthalmic Suspension .... ⊙247
Pred-G Sterile Ophthalmic Ointment .... ⊙248

Kanamycin Sulfate (Co-administration of other cephalosporins with aminoglycosides has resulted in nephrotoxicity).
No products indexed under this heading.

Streptomycin Sulfate (Co-administration of other cephalosporins with aminoglycosides has resulted in nephrotoxicity). Products include:
Streptomycin Sulfate Injection 2714

Tobramycin (Co-administration of other cephalosporins with aminoglycosides has resulted in nephrotoxicity). Products include:
TOBI Solution for Inhalation 1206
TobraDex Ophthalmic Ointment 542
TobraDex Ophthalmic Suspension 541
Tobrex Ophthalmic Ointment .... ⊙220
Tobrex Ophthalmic Solution .... ⊙221

Tobramycin Sulfate (Co-administration of other cephalosporins with aminoglycosides has resulted in nephrotoxicity). Products include:
Nebcin Vials, Hyporets & ADD-Vantage 1955

CEFOBID INTRAVENOUS/ INTRAMUSCULAR
(Cefoperazone) 2671
See Cefobid Pharmacy Bulk Package - Not for Direct Infusion

CEFOBID PHARMACY BULK PACKAGE - NOT FOR DIRECT INFUSION
(Cefoperazone Sodium) 2673
May interact with aminoglycosides and certain other agents. Compounds in these categories include:

Amikacin Sulfate (Potential for nephrotoxicity).
No products indexed under this heading.

Gentamicin Sulfate (Potential for nephrotoxicity). Products include:
Genoptic Ophthalmic Ointment .... ⊙239
Genoptic Sterile Ophthalmic Solution .... ⊙239
Pred-G Ophthalmic Suspension .... ⊙247
Pred-G Sterile Ophthalmic Ointment .... ⊙248

Kanamycin Sulfate (Potential for nephrotoxicity).
No products indexed under this heading.

Streptomycin Sulfate (Potential for nephrotoxicity). Products include:
Streptomycin Sulfate Injection 2714

Tobramycin (Potential for nephrotoxicity). Products include:
TOBI Solution for Inhalation 1206
TobraDex Ophthalmic Ointment 542
TobraDex Ophthalmic Suspension 541
Tobrex Ophthalmic Ointment .... ⊙220
Tobrex Ophthalmic Solution .... ⊙221

Tobramycin Sulfate (Potential for nephrotoxicity). Products include:
Nebcin Vials, Hyporets & ADD-Vantage 1955

Food Interactions

Alcohol (A disulfiram-like reaction characterized by flushing, sweating, headache, and tachycardia has been reported when alcohol was ingested within 72 hours after Cefobid administration).

CEFOTAN FOR INJECTION
(Cefotetan) 664
May interact with aminoglycosides and certain other agents. Compounds in these categories include:

Amikacin Sulfate (Cefotetan increases serum creatinine; concurrent use may lead to potentiation of nephrotoxicity).
No products indexed under this heading.

Gentamicin Sulfate (Cefotetan increases serum creatinine; concurrent use may lead to potentiation of nephrotoxicity). Products include:
Genoptic Ophthalmic Ointment .... ⊙239
Genoptic Sterile Ophthalmic Solution .... ⊙239
Pred-G Ophthalmic Suspension .... ⊙247
Pred-G Sterile Ophthalmic Ointment .... ⊙248

Kanamycin Sulfate (Cefotetan increases serum creatinine; concurrent use may lead to potentiation of nephrotoxicity).
No products indexed under this heading.

Streptomycin Sulfate (Cefotetan increases serum creatinine; concurrent use may lead to potentiation of nephrotoxicity). Products include:
Streptomycin Sulfate Injection 2714

Tobramycin (Cefotetan increases serum creatinine; concurrent use may lead to potentiation of nephrotoxicity). Products include:
TOBI Solution for Inhalation 1206
TobraDex Ophthalmic Ointment 542
TobraDex Ophthalmic Suspension 541
Tobrex Ophthalmic Ointment .... ⊙220
Tobrex Ophthalmic Solution .... ⊙221

Tobramycin Sulfate (Cefotetan increases serum creatinine; concurrent use may lead to potentiation of nephrotoxicity). Products include:
Nebcin Vials, Hyporets & ADD-Vantage 1955

Food Interactions

Alcohol (When ingested within 72 hours after Cefotan administration may cause disulfiram-like reactions, including flushing, headache, sweating and tachycardia).

CEFOTAN INJECTION
(Cefotetan) 664
See Cefotan for Injection

CEFTIN FOR ORAL SUSPENSION
(Cefuroxime Axetil) 1898
See Ceftin Tablets

CEFTIN TABLETS

(Cefuroxime Axetil) ... 1898

May interact with drugs that reduce gastric acidity and certain other agents. Compounds in these categories include:

Aluminum Carbonate (Drugs that reduce gastric acidity may result in a lower bioavailability of Ceftin compared with that of fasting state and tend to cancel the effect of postprandial absorption).

No products indexed under this heading.

Aluminum Hydroxide (Drugs that reduce gastric acidity may result in a lower bioavailability of Ceftin compared with that of fasting state and tend to cancel the effect of postprandial absorption). Products include:

Amphojel Suspension (Mint Flavor) ... ▣789
Gaviscon Extra Strength Liquid ... ▣751
Gaviscon Extra Strength Tablets ... ▣751
Gaviscon Regular Strength Liquid ... ▣751
Gaviscon Regular Strength Tablets ... ▣750
Maalox Antacid/Anti-Gas Oral Suspension ... ▣673
Maalox Max Maximum Strength Antacid/Anti-Gas Liquid ... 2300
Maalox Regular Strength Antacid/Antigas Liquid ... 2300
Mylanta ... 1813
Vanquish Caplets ... ▣617

Cimetidine (Drugs that reduce gastric acidity may result in a lower bioavailability of Ceftin compared with that of fasting state and tend to cancel the effect of postprandial absorption). Products include:

Tagamet HB 200 Suspension ... ▣762
Tagamet HB 200 Tablets ... ▣761
Tagamet Tablets ... 1644

Cimetidine Hydrochloride (Drugs that reduce gastric acidity may result in a lower bioavailability of Ceftin compared with that of fasting state and tend to cancel the effect of postprandial absorption). Products include:

Tagamet ... 1644

Esomeprazole Magnesium (Drugs that reduce gastric acidity may result in a lower bioavailability of Ceftin compared with that of fasting state and tend to cancel the effect of postprandial absorption). Products include:

Nexium Delayed-Release Capsules ... 619

Famotidine (Drugs that reduce gastric acidity may result in a lower bioavailability of Ceftin compared with that of fasting state and tend to cancel the effect of postprandial absorption). Products include:

Famotidine Injection ... 866
Pepcid AC ... 1814
Pepcid Complete Chewable Tablets ... 1815
Pepcid Injection ... 2153
Pepcid for Oral Suspension ... 2150
Pepcid RPD Orally Disintegrating Tablets ... 2150
Pepcid Tablets ... 2150

Lansoprazole (Drugs that reduce gastric acidity may result in a lower bioavailability of Ceftin compared with that of fasting state and tend to cancel the effect of postprandial absorption). Products include:

Prevacid Delayed-Release Capsules ... 3292
PREVPAC ... 3298

Magnesium Hydroxide (Drugs that reduce gastric acidity may result in a lower bioavailability of Ceftin compared with that of fasting state and tend to cancel the effect of postprandial absorption). Products include:

Ex•Lax Milk of Magnesia Liquid ... ▣670
Maalox Antacid/Anti-Gas Oral Suspension ... ▣673
Maalox Max Maximum Strength Antacid/Anti-Gas Liquid ... 2300
Maalox Regular Strength Antacid/Antigas Liquid ... 2300
Mylanta Fast-Acting ... 1813
Mylanta ... 1813
Pepcid Complete Chewable Tablets ... 1815
Phillips' Chewable Tablets ... ▣615
Phillips' Milk of Magnesia Liquid (Original, Cherry, & Mint) ... ▣616
Rolaids Tablets ... ▣706
Extra Strength Rolaids Tablets ... ▣706
Vanquish Caplets ... ▣617

Nizatidine (Drugs that reduce gastric acidity may result in a lower bioavailability of Ceftin compared with that of fasting state and tend to cancel the effect of postprandial absorption). Products include:

Axid Pulvules ... 1903
Axid Pulvules ... 2919

Omeprazole (Drugs that reduce gastric acidity may result in a lower bioavailability of Ceftin compared with that of fasting state and tend to cancel the effect of postprandial absorption). Products include:

Prilosec Delayed-Release Capsules ... 628

Probenecid (Increases serum concentration of cefuroxime).

No products indexed under this heading.

Rabeprazole Sodium (Drugs that reduce gastric acidity may result in a lower bioavailability of Ceftin compared with that of fasting state and tend to cancel the effect of postprandial absorption). Products include:

Aciphex Tablets ... 1267
Aciphex Tablets ... 1783

Ranitidine Hydrochloride (Drugs that reduce gastric acidity may result in a lower bioavailability of Ceftin compared with that of fasting state and tend to cancel the effect of postprandial absorption). Products include:

Zantac ... 1690
Zantac Injection ... 1688
Zantac 75 Tablets ... ▣717

Food Interactions

Food, unspecified (Absorption is greater when taken after food).

CEFZIL FOR ORAL SUSPENSION

(Cefprozil) ... 1076

See Cefzil Tablets

CEFZIL TABLETS

(Cefprozil) ... 1076

May interact with aminoglycosides and certain other agents. Compounds in these categories include:

Amikacin Sulfate (Potential for nephrotoxicity).

No products indexed under this heading.

Gentamicin Sulfate (Potential for nephrotoxicity). Products include:

Genoptic Ophthalmic Ointment ... ⊙239
Genoptic Sterile Ophthalmic Solution ... ⊙239
Pred-G Ophthalmic Suspension ... ⊙247
Pred-G Sterile Ophthalmic Ointment ... ⊙248

Kanamycin Sulfate (Potential for nephrotoxicity).

No products indexed under this heading.

Probenecid (Doubles the AUC for cefprozil).

No products indexed under this heading.

Streptomycin Sulfate (Potential for nephrotoxicity). Products include:

Streptomycin Sulfate Injection ... 2714

Tobramycin (Potential for nephrotoxicity). Products include:

TOBI Solution for Inhalation ... 1206
TobraDex Ophthalmic Ointment ... 542
TobraDex Ophthalmic Suspension ... 541
Tobrex Ophthalmic Ointment ... ⊙220
Tobrex Ophthalmic Solution ... ⊙221

Tobramycin Sulfate (Potential for nephrotoxicity). Products include:

Nebcin Vials, Hyporets & ADD-Vantage ... 1955

CELEBREX CAPSULES

(Celecoxib) ... 2780

May interact with ACE inhibitors, antacids containing aluminum, calcium and magnesium, lithium preparations, thiazides, and certain other agents. Compounds in these categories include:

Aluminum Carbonate (Co-administration with an aluminum-and-magnesium-containing antacid resulted in a reduction in plasma celecoxib concentration with a decrease of 37% in C_{max} and 10% in AUC).

No products indexed under this heading.

Aluminum Hydroxide (Co-administration with an aluminum-and-magnesium-containing antacid resulted in a reduction in plasma celecoxib concentration with a decrease of 37% in C_{max} and 10% in AUC). Products include:

Amphojel Suspension (Mint Flavor) ... ▣789
Gaviscon Extra Strength Liquid ... ▣751
Gaviscon Extra Strength Tablets ... ▣751
Gaviscon Regular Strength Liquid ... ▣751
Gaviscon Regular Strength Tablets ... ▣750
Maalox Antacid/Anti-Gas Oral Suspension ... ▣673
Maalox Max Maximum Strength Antacid/Anti-Gas Liquid ... 2300
Maalox Regular Strength Antacid/Antigas Liquid ... 2300
Mylanta ... 1813
Vanquish Caplets ... ▣617

Amiodarone Hydrochloride (Co-administration of celecoxib with drugs known to inhibit CYP4502C9, such as amiodarone, may result in increased plasma concentration; caution should be exercised if used concurrently). Products include:

Cordarone Intravenous ... 3491
Cordarone Tablets ... 3487
Pacerone Tablets ... 3331

Aspirin (Co-administration may result in an increased rate of GI ulceration or other complications; low dose of aspirin can be used with celecoxib). Products include:

Aggrenox Capsules ... 1026
Alka-Seltzer ... ▣603
Alka-Seltzer Lemon Lime Antacid and Pain Reliever Effervescent Tablets ... ▣603
Alka-Seltzer Extra Strength Antacid and Pain Reliever Effervescent Tablets ... ▣603
Alka-Seltzer PM Effervescent Tablets ... ▣605
Genuine Bayer Tablets, Caplets and Gelcaps ... ▣606
Extra Strength Bayer Caplets and Gelcaps ... ▣610
Aspirin Regimen Bayer Children's Chewable Tablets (Orange or Cherry Flavored) ... ▣607
Bayer, Aspirin Regimen ... ▣606
Aspirin Regimen Bayer 81 mg Caplets with Calcium ... ▣607
Genuine Bayer Professional Labeling (Aspirin Regimen Bayer) ... ▣608
Extra Strength Bayer Arthritis Caplets ... ▣610
Extra Strength Bayer Plus Caplets ... ▣610
Extra Strength Bayer PM Caplets ... ▣611
BC Powder ... ▣619
BC Allergy Sinus Cold Powder ... ▣619
Arthritis Strength BC Powder ... ▣619
BC Sinus Cold Powder ... ▣619
Darvon Compound-65 Pulvules ... 1910
Ecotrin Enteric Coated Aspirin Low, Regular and Maximum Strength Tablets ... 1715
Excedrin Extra-Strength Tablets, Caplets, and Geltabs ... ▣629
Excedrin Migraine ... 1070
Goody's Body Pain Formula Powder ... ▣620
Goody's Extra Strength Headache Powder ... ▣620
Goody's Extra Strength Pain Relief Tablets ... ▣620
Percodan Tablets ... 1327
Robaxisal Tablets ... 2939
Soma Compound Tablets ... 3354
Soma Compound w/Codeine Tablets ... 3355
Vanquish Caplets ... ▣617

Benazepril Hydrochloride (Co-administration of NSAID with ACE inhibitors may result in diminished antihypertensive effect of ACE inhibitors). Products include:

Lotensin Tablets ... 2365
Lotensin HCT Tablets ... 2367
Lotrel Capsules ... 2370

Bendroflumethiazide (Co-administration of NSAID with thiazides may result in reduced natriuretic effect of thiazide diuretics). Products include:

Corzide 40/5 Tablets ... 2247
Corzide 80/5 Tablets ... 2247

Captopril (Co-administration of NSAID with ACE inhibitors may result in diminished antihypertensive effect of ACE inhibitors). Products include:

Captopril Tablets ... 2281

Chlorothiazide (Co-administration of NSAID with thiazides may result in reduced natriuretic effect of thiazide diuretics). Products include:

Aldoclor Tablets ... 2035
Diuril Oral ... 2087

Chlorothiazide Sodium (Co-administration of NSAID with thiazides may result in reduced natriuretic effect of thiazide diuretics). Products include:

Diuril Sodium Intravenous ... 2086

Enalapril Maleate (Co-administration of NSAID with ACE inhibitors may result in diminished antihypertensive effect of ACE inhibitors). Products include:

Lexxel Tablets ... 608
Vaseretic Tablets ... 2204
Vasotec Tablets ... 2210

Enalaprilat (Co-administration of NSAID with ACE inhibitors may result in diminished antihypertensive effect of ACE inhibitors). Products include:

Enalaprilat Injection ... 863
Vasotec I.V. Injection ... 2207

Fluconazole (Co-administration has resulted in a two-fold increase in celecoxib plasma concentration due to inhibition of celecoxib metabolism via P4502C9). Products include:

Diflucan Tablets, Injection, and Oral Suspension ... 2681

Fosinopril Sodium (Co-administration of NSAID with ACE inhibitors may result in diminished antihypertensive effect of ACE inhibitors). Products include:

Monopril Tablets ... 1091
Monopril HCT ... 1094

Furosemide (Co-administration of NSAID with thiazides may result in reduced natriuretic effect of furosemide). Products include:

Furosemide Tablets ... 2284

Hydrochlorothiazide (Co-administration of NSAID with thiazides may result in reduced natriuretic effect of thiazide diuretics). Products include:

Accuretic Tablets ... 2614
Aldoril Tablets ... 2039
Atacand HCT Tablets ... 597
Avalide Tablets ... 1070
Diovan HCT Tablets ... 2338
Dyazide Capsules ... 1515
HydroDIURIL Tablets ... 2108
Hyzaar ... 2109
Inderide Tablets ... 3517
Inderide LA Long-Acting Capsules ... 3519
Lotensin HCT Tablets ... 2367
Maxzide ... 1008
Micardis HCT Tablets ... 1051
Microzide Capsules ... 3414
Moduretic Tablets ... 2138
Monopril HCT ... 1094
Prinzide Tablets ... 2168
Timolide Tablets ... 2187
Uniretic Tablets ... 3178

Vaseretic Tablets 2204
Zestoretic Tablets 695
Ziac Tablets 1887

Hydroflumethiazide (Co-administration of NSAID with thiazides may result in reduced natriuretic effect of thiazide diuretics). Products include:

Diucardin Tablets 3494

Itraconazole (Co-administration of celecoxib with drugs known to inhibit CYP4502C9, such as itraconazole, may result in increased plasma concentration; caution should be exercised if used concurrently). Products include:

Sporanox Capsules 1800
Sporanox Injection 1804
Sporanox Injection 2509
Sporanox Oral Solution 1808
Sporanox Oral Solution 2512

Ketoconazole (Co-administration of celecoxib with drugs known to inhibit CYP4502C9, such as ketoconazole, may result in increased plasma concentration; caution should be exercised if used concurrently). Products include:

Nizoral 2% Cream 3620
Nizoral A-D Shampoo 2008
Nizoral 2% Shampoo 2007
Nizoral Tablets 1791

Lisinopril (Co-administration of NSAID with ACE inhibitors may result in diminished antihypertensive effect of ACE inhibitors). Products include:

Prinivil Tablets 2164
Prinzide Tablets 2168
Zestoretic Tablets 695
Zestril Tablets 698

Lithium Carbonate (Co-administration has resulted in increased steady-state lithium plasma levels). Products include:

Eskalith 1527
Lithium Carbonate 3061
Lithobid Slow-Release Tablets 3255

Lithium Citrate (Co-administration has resulted in increased steady-state lithium plasma levels). Products include:

Lithium Citrate Syrup 3061

Magaldrate (Co-administration with an aluminum-and-magnesium-containing antacid resulted in a reduction in plasma celecoxib concentration with a decrease of 37% in Cmax and 10% in AUC).

No products indexed under this heading.

Magnesium Hydroxide (Co-administration with an aluminum-and-magnesium-containing antacid resulted in a reduction in plasma celecoxib concentration with a decrease of 37% in Cmax and 10% in AUC). Products include:

Ex•Lax Milk of Magnesia Liquid 670
Maalox Antacid/Anti-Gas Oral Suspension 673
Maalox Max Maximum Strength Antacid/Anti-Gas Liquid 2300
Maalox Regular Strength Antacid/Antigas Liquid 2300
Mylanta Fast-Acting 1813
Mylanta 1813
Pepcid Complete Chewable Tablets 1815
Phillips' Chewable Tablets 615
Phillips' Milk of Magnesia Liquid (Original, Cherry, & Mint) 616
Rolaids Tablets 706
Extra Strength Rolaids Tablets 706
Vanquish Caplets 617

Magnesium Oxide (Co-administration with an aluminum-and-magnesium-containing antacid resulted in a reduction in plasma celecoxib concentration with a decrease of 37% in Cmax and 10% in AUC). Products include:

Beelith Tablets 946
Mag-Ox 400 Tablets 1024
Uro-Mag Capsules 1024

Methyclothiazide (Co-administration of NSAID with thiazides may result in reduced natriuretic effect of thiazide diuretics).

No products indexed under this heading.

Moexipril Hydrochloride (Co-administration of NSAID with ACE inhibitors may result in diminished antihypertensive effect of ACE inhibitors). Products include:

Uniretic Tablets 3178
Univasc Tablets 3181

Perindopril Erbumine (Co-administration of NSAID with ACE inhibitors may result in diminished antihypertensive effect of ACE inhibitors). Products include:

Aceon Tablets (2 mg, 4 mg, 8 mg) 3249

Polythiazide (Co-administration of NSAID with thiazides may result in reduced natriuretic effect of thiazide diuretics). Products include:

Minizide Capsules 2700
Renese Tablets 2712

Quinapril Hydrochloride (Co-administration of NSAID with ACE inhibitors may result in diminished antihypertensive effect of ACE inhibitors). Products include:

Accupril Tablets 2611
Accuretic Tablets 2614

Ramipril (Co-administration of NSAID with ACE inhibitors may result in diminished antihypertensive effect of ACE inhibitors). Products include:

Altace Capsules 2233

Spirapril Hydrochloride (Co-administration of NSAID with ACE inhibitors may result in diminished antihypertensive effect of ACE inhibitors).

No products indexed under this heading.

Trandolapril (Co-administration of NSAID with ACE inhibitors may result in diminished antihypertensive effect of ACE inhibitors). Products include:

Mavik Tablets 478
Tarka Tablets 508

Warfarin Sodium (Co-administration in the predominantly elderly patients has resulted in increases in prothrombin time and bleeding). Products include:

Coumadin for Injection 1243
Coumadin Tablets 1243
Warfarin Sodium Tablets, USP 3302

Food Interactions

Food, unspecified (Co-administration with a high-fat meal delayed peak plasma levels for about 1 to 2 hours with an increase in total absorption (AUC) of 10% to 20%; Celebrex can be administered without regard to the timing of meals).

CELEBREX CAPSULES

(Celecoxib) 2676

May interact with ACE inhibitors, antacids containing aluminum, calcium and magnesium, lithium preparations, thiazides, and certain other agents. Compounds in these categories include:

Aluminum Carbonate (Co-administration with an aluminum-and-magnesium-containing antacid resulted in a reduction in plasma celecoxib concentration with a decrease of 37% in Cmax and 10% in AUC).

No products indexed under this heading.

Aluminum Hydroxide (Co-administration with an aluminum-and-magnesium-containing antacid resulted in a reduction in plasma celecoxib concentration with a decrease of 37% in Cmax and 10% in AUC). Products include:

Amphojel Suspension (Mint Flavor) 789
Gaviscon Extra Strength Liquid 751
Gaviscon Extra Strength Tablets 751
Gaviscon Regular Strength Liquid 751
Gaviscon Regular Strength Tablets 750
Maalox Antacid/Anti-Gas Oral Suspension 673
Maalox Max Maximum Strength Antacid/Anti-Gas Liquid 2300
Maalox Regular Strength Antacid/Antigas Liquid 2300
Mylanta 1813
Vanquish Caplets 617

Amiodarone Hydrochloride (Co-administration of celecoxib with drugs known to inhibit CYP4502C9, such as amiodarone, may result in increased plasma concentration; caution should be exercised if used concurrently). Products include:

Cordarone Intravenous 3491
Cordarone Tablets 3487
Pacerone Tablets 3331

Aspirin (Co-administration may result in an increased rate of GI ulceration or other complications; low dose of aspirin can be used with celecoxib). Products include:

Aggrenox Capsules 1026
Alka-Seltzer 603
Alka-Seltzer Lemon Lime Antacid and Pain Reliever Effervescent Tablets 603
Alka-Seltzer Extra Strength Antacid and Pain Reliever Effervescent Tablets 603
Alka-Seltzer PM Effervescent Tablets 605
Genuine Bayer Tablets, Caplets and Gelcaps 606
Extra Strength Bayer Caplets and Gelcaps 610
Aspirin Regimen Bayer Children's Chewable Tablets (Orange or Cherry Flavored) 607
Bayer, Aspirin Regimen 606
Aspirin Regimen Bayer 81 mg Caplets with Calcium 607
Genuine Bayer Professional Labeling (Aspirin Regimen Bayer) 608
Extra Strength Bayer Arthritis Caplets 610
Extra Strength Bayer Plus Caplets 610
Extra Strength Bayer PM Caplets 611
BC Powder 619
BC Allergy Sinus Cold Powder 619
Arthritis Strength BC Powder 619
BC Sinus Cold Powder 619
Darvon Compound-65 Pulvules 1910
Ecotrin Enteric Coated Aspirin Low, Regular and Maximum Strength Tablets 1715
Excedrin Extra-Strength Tablets, Caplets, and Geltabs 629
Excedrin Migraine 1070
Goody's Body Pain Formula Powder 620
Goody's Extra Strength Headache Powder 620
Goody's Extra Strength Pain Relief Tablets 620
Percodan Tablets 1327
Robaxisal Tablets 2939
Soma Compound Tablets 3354
Soma Compound w/Codeine Tablets 3355
Vanquish Caplets 617

Benazepril Hydrochloride (Co-administration of NSAID with ACE inhibitors may result in diminished antihypertensive effect of ACE inhibitors). Products include:

Lotensin Tablets 2365
Lotensin HCT Tablets 2367
Lotrel Capsules 2370

Bendroflumethiazide (Co-administration of NSAID with thiazides may result in reduced natriuretic effect of thiazide diuretics). Products include:

Corzide 40/5 Tablets 2247
Corzide 80/5 Tablets 2247

Captopril (Co-administration of NSAID with ACE inhibitors may result in diminished antihypertensive effect of ACE inhibitors). Products include:

Captopril Tablets 2281

Chlorothiazide (Co-administration of NSAID with thiazides may result in reduced natriuretic effect of thiazide diuretics). Products include:

Aldoclor Tablets 2035
Diuril Oral 2087

Chlorothiazide Sodium (Co-administration of NSAID with thiazides may result in reduced natriuretic effect of thiazide diuretics). Products include:

Diuril Sodium Intravenous 2086

Enalapril Maleate (Co-administration of NSAID with ACE inhibitors may result in diminished antihypertensive effect of ACE inhibitors). Products include:

Lexxel Tablets 608
Vaseretic Tablets 2204
Vasotec Tablets 2210

Enalaprilat (Co-administration of NSAID with ACE inhibitors may result in diminished antihypertensive effect of ACE inhibitors). Products include:

Enalaprilat Injection 863
Vasotec I.V. Injection 2207

Fluconazole (Co-administration has resulted in a two-fold increase in celecoxib plasma concentration due to inhibition of celecoxib metabolism via P4502C9). Products include:

Diflucan Tablets, Injection, and Oral Suspension 2681

Fosinopril Sodium (Co-administration of NSAID with ACE inhibitors may result in diminished antihypertensive effect of ACE inhibitors). Products include:

Monopril Tablets 1091
Monopril HCT 1094

Furosemide (Co-administration of NSAID with thiazides may result in reduced natriuretic effect of furosemide). Products include:

Furosemide Tablets 2284

Hydrochlorothiazide (Co-administration of NSAID with thiazides may result in reduced natriuretic effect of thiazide diuretics). Products include:

Accuretic Tablets 2614
Aldoril Tablets 2039
Atacand HCT Tablets 597
Avalide Tablets 1070
Diovan HCT Tablets 2338
Dyazide Capsules 1515
HydroDIURIL Tablets 2108
Hyzaar 2109
Inderide Tablets 3517
Inderide LA Long-Acting Capsules 3519
Lotensin HCT Tablets 2367
Maxzide 1008
Micardis HCT Tablets 1051
Microzide Capsules 3414
Moduretic Tablets 2138
Monopril HCT 1094
Prinzide Tablets 2168
Timolide Tablets 2187
Uniretic Tablets 3178
Vaseretic Tablets 2204
Zestoretic Tablets 695
Ziac Tablets 1887

Hydroflumethiazide (Co-administration of NSAID with thiazides may result in reduced natriuretic effect of thiazide diuretics). Products include:

Diucardin Tablets 3494

Itraconazole (Co-administration of celecoxib with drugs known to inhibit CYP4502C9, such as itraconazole, may result in increased plasma concentration; caution should be exercised if used concurrently). Products include:

Sporanox Capsules 1800
Sporanox Injection 1804
Sporanox Injection 2509
Sporanox Oral Solution 1808
Sporanox Oral Solution 2512

Ketoconazole (Co-administration of celecoxib with drugs known to inhibit CYP4502C9, such as ketoconazole, may result in increased plasma concentration; caution should be exercised if used concurrently). Products include:

Nizoral 2% Cream 3620
Nizoral A-D Shampoo 2008
Nizoral 2% Shampoo 2007
Nizoral Tablets 1791

Lisinopril (Co-administration of NSAID with ACE inhibitors may result

in diminished antihypertensive effect of ACE inhibitors). Products include:
- Prinivil Tablets 2164
- Prinzide Tablets 2168
- Zestoretic Tablets 695
- Zestril Tablets 698

Lithium Carbonate (Co-administration has resulted in increased steady-state lithium plasma levels). Products include:
- Eskalith 1527
- Lithium Carbonate 3061
- Lithobid Slow-Release Tablets 3255

Lithium Citrate (Co-administration has resulted in increased steady-state lithium plasma levels). Products include:
- Lithium Citrate Syrup 3061

Magaldrate (Co-administration with an aluminum-and-magnesium-containing antacid resulted in a reduction in plasma celecoxib concentration with a decrease of 37% in Cmax and 10% in AUC).
No products indexed under this heading.

Magnesium Hydroxide (Co-administration with an aluminum-and-magnesium-containing antacid resulted in a reduction in plasma celecoxib concentration with a decrease of 37% in Cmax and 10% in AUC). Products include:
- Ex•Lax Milk of Magnesia Liquid .... ■670
- Maalox Antacid/Anti-Gas Oral Suspension .... ■673
- Maalox Max Maximum Strength Antacid/Anti-Gas Liquid 2300
- Maalox Regular Strength Antacid/Antigas Liquid 2300
- Mylanta Fast-Acting 1813
- Mylanta 1813
- Pepcid Complete Chewable Tablets 1815
- Phillips' Chewable Tablets .... ■615
- Phillips' Milk of Magnesia Liquid (Original, Cherry, & Mint) .... ■616
- Rolaids Tablets .... ■706
- Extra Strength Rolaids Tablets .... ■706
- Vanquish Caplets .... ■617

Magnesium Oxide (Co-administration with an aluminum-and-magnesium-containing antacid resulted in a reduction in plasma celecoxib concentration with a decrease of 37% in Cmax and 10% in AUC). Products include:
- Beelith Tablets 946
- Mag-Ox 400 Tablets 1024
- Uro-Mag Capsules 1024

Methyclothiazide (Co-administration of NSAID with thiazides may result in reduced natriuretic effect of thiazide diuretics).
No products indexed under this heading.

Moexipril Hydrochloride (Co-administration of NSAID with ACE inhibitors may result in diminished antihypertensive effect of ACE inhibitors). Products include:
- Uniretic Tablets 3178
- Univasc Tablets 3181

Perindopril Erbumine (Co-administration of NSAID with ACE inhibitors may result in diminished antihypertensive effect of ACE inhibitors). Products include:
- Aceon Tablets (2 mg, 4 mg, 8 mg) 3249

Polythiazide (Co-administration of NSAID with thiazides may result in reduced natriuretic effect of thiazide diuretics). Products include:
- Minizide Capsules 2700
- Renese Tablets 2712

Quinapril Hydrochloride (Co-administration of NSAID with ACE inhibitors may result in diminished antihypertensive effect of ACE inhibitors). Products include:
- Accupril Tablets 2611
- Accuretic Tablets 2614

Ramipril (Co-administration of NSAID with ACE inhibitors may result in diminished antihypertensive effect of ACE inhibitors). Products include:
- Altace Capsules 2233

Spirapril Hydrochloride (Co-administration of NSAID with ACE inhibitors may result in diminished antihypertensive effect of ACE inhibitors).
No products indexed under this heading.

Trandolapril (Co-administration of NSAID with ACE inhibitors may result in diminished antihypertensive effect of ACE inhibitors). Products include:
- Mavik Tablets 478
- Tarka Tablets 508

Warfarin Sodium (Co-administration in the predominantly elderly patients has resulted in increases in prothrombin time and bleeding). Products include:
- Coumadin for Injection 1243
- Coumadin Tablets 1243
- Warfarin Sodium Tablets, USP 3302

Food Interactions

Food, unspecified (Co-administration with a high-fat meal delayed peak plasma levels for about 1 to 2 hours with an increase in total absorption (AUC) of 10% to 20%; Celebrex can be administered without regard to the timing of meals).

CELESTIAL SEASONINGS SOOTHERS THROAT DROPS

(Menthol, Pectin) .... ■685
None cited in PDR database.

CELESTONE SOLUSPAN INJECTABLE SUSPENSION

(Betamethasone Acetate, Betamethasone Sodium Phosphate) 3097
May interact with oral hypoglycemic agents and insulin. Compounds in these categories include:

Acarbose (Increased requirements for oral hypoglycemic agents in diabetes). Products include:
- Precose Tablets 906

Aspirin (Concurrent use in hypoprothrombinemia may be undertaken with caution). Products include:
- Aggrenox Capsules 1026
- Alka-Seltzer .... ■603
- Alka-Seltzer Lemon Lime Antacid and Pain Reliever Effervescent Tablets .... ■603
- Alka-Seltzer Extra Strength Antacid and Pain Reliever Effervescent Tablets .... ■603
- Alka-Seltzer PM Effervescent Tablets .... ■605
- Genuine Bayer Tablets, Caplets and Gelcaps .... ■606
- Extra Strength Bayer Caplets and Gelcaps .... ■610
- Aspirin Regimen Bayer Children's Chewable Tablets (Orange or Cherry Flavored) .... ■607
- Bayer, Aspirin Regimen .... ■606
- Aspirin Regimen Bayer 81 mg Caplets with Calcium .... ■607
- Genuine Bayer Professional Labeling (Aspirin Regimen Bayer) .... ■608
- Extra Strength Bayer Arthritis Caplets .... ■610
- Extra Strength Bayer Plus Caplets .... ■610
- Extra Strength Bayer PM Caplets .... ■611
- BC Powder .... ■619
- BC Allergy Sinus Cold Powder .... ■619
- Arthritis Strength BC Powder .... ■619
- BC Sinus Cold Powder .... ■619
- Darvon Compound-65 Pulvules 1910
- Ecotrin Enteric Coated Aspirin Low, Regular and Maximum Strength Tablets 1715
- Excedrin Extra-Strength Tablets, Caplets, and Geltabs .... ■629
- Excedrin Migraine 1070
- Goody's Body Pain Formula Powder .... ■620
- Goody's Extra Strength Headache Powder .... ■620
- Goody's Extra Strength Pain Relief Tablets .... ■620
- Percodan Tablets 1327
- Robaxisal Tablets 2939
- Soma Compound Tablets 3354
- Soma Compound w/Codeine Tablets 3355
- Vanquish Caplets .... ■617

Chlorpropamide (Increased requirements for oral hypoglycemic agents in diabetes). Products include:
- Diabinese Tablets 2680

Glimepiride (Increased requirements for oral hypoglycemic agents in diabetes). Products include:
- Amaryl Tablets 717

Glipizide (Increased requirements for oral hypoglycemic agents in diabetes). Products include:
- Glucotrol Tablets 2692
- Glucotrol XL Extended Release Tablets 2693

Glyburide (Increased requirements for oral hypoglycemic agents in diabetes). Products include:
- DiaBeta Tablets 741
- Glucovance Tablets 1086

Immunization (Neurological complications).
No products indexed under this heading.

Insulin, Human, Zinc Suspension (Increased requirements for insulin in diabetes). Products include:
- Humulin L, 100 Units 1937
- Humulin U, 100 Units 1943
- Novolin L Human Insulin 10 ml Vials 2422

Insulin, Human NPH (Increased requirements for insulin in diabetes). Products include:
- Humulin N, 100 Units 1939
- Humulin N NPH Pen 1940
- Novolin N Human Insulin 10 ml Vials 2422
- Novolin N PenFill 2423
- Novolin N Prefilled Syringe Disposable Insulin Delivery System 2425

Insulin, Human Regular (Increased requirements for insulin in diabetes). Products include:
- Humulin R Regular (U-500) 1943
- Humulin R, 100 Units 1941
- Novolin R Human Insulin 10 ml Vials 2423
- Novolin R PenFill 2423
- Novolin R Prefilled Syringe Disposable Insulin Delivery System 2425
- Velosulin BR Human Insulin 10 ml Vials 2435

Insulin, Human Regular and Human NPH Mixture (Increased requirements for insulin in diabetes). Products include:
- Humulin 50/50, 100 Units 1934
- Humulin 70/30, 100 Units 1935
- Humulin 70/30 Pen 1936
- Novolin 70/30 Human Insulin 10 ml Vials 2421
- Novolin 70/30 PenFill 2423
- Novolin 70/30 Prefilled Disposable Insulin Delivery System 2425

Insulin, NPH (Increased requirements for insulin in diabetes). Products include:
- Iletin II, NPH (Pork), 100 Units 1946

Insulin, Regular (Increased requirements for insulin in diabetes). Products include:
- Iletin II, Regular (Pork), 100 Units 1947

Insulin, Zinc Crystals (Increased requirements for insulin in diabetes).
No products indexed under this heading.

Insulin, Zinc Suspension (Increased requirements for insulin in diabetes). Products include:
- Iletin II, Lente (Pork), 100 Units 1945

Insulin Aspart, Human Regular (Increased requirements for insulin in diabetes).
No products indexed under this heading.

Insulin glargine (Increased requirements for insulin in diabetes). Products include:
- Lantus Injection 742

Insulin Lispro, Human (Increased requirements for insulin in diabetes). Products include:
- Humalog 1926
- Humalog Mix 75/25 Pen 1928

Insulin Lispro Protamine, Human (Increased requirements for insulin in diabetes). Products include:
- Humalog Mix 75/25 Pen 1928

Metformin Hydrochloride (Increased requirements for oral hypoglycemic agents in diabetes). Products include:
- Glucophage Tablets 1080
- Glucophage XR Tablets 1080
- Glucovance Tablets 1086

Miglitol (Increased requirements for oral hypoglycemic agents in diabetes). Products include:
- Glyset Tablets 2821

Pioglitazone Hydrochloride (Increased requirements for oral hypoglycemic agents in diabetes). Products include:
- Actos Tablets 3275

Repaglinide (Increased requirements for oral hypoglycemic agents in diabetes). Products include:
- Prandin Tablets (0.5, 1, and 2 mg) 2432

Rosiglitazone Maleate (Increased requirements for oral hypoglycemic agents in diabetes). Products include:
- Avandia Tablets 1490

Tolazamide (Increased requirements for oral hypoglycemic agents in diabetes).
No products indexed under this heading.

Tolbutamide (Increased requirements for oral hypoglycemic agents in diabetes).
No products indexed under this heading.

Troglitazone (Increased requirements for oral hypoglycemic agents in diabetes).
No products indexed under this heading.

CELESTONE SYRUP

(Betamethasone) 3099
See Celestone Soluspan Injectable Suspension

CELEXA ORAL SOLUTION

(Citalopram Hydrobromide) 1365
See Celexa Tablets

CELEXA TABLETS

(Citalopram Hydrobromide) 1365
May interact with erythromycin, lithium preparations, macrolide antibiotics, monoamine oxidase inhibitors, tricyclic antidepressants, and certain other agents. Compounds in these categories include:

Amitriptyline Hydrochloride (Co-administration of imipramine with citalopram has resulted in a 50% increase in active metabolite, desipramine concentration; the clinical significance of these findings is unknown; caution is indicated if tricyclic antidepressants are co-administered with citalopram, a relatively weak inhibitor of CYP2D6). Products include:
- Etrafon 3115
- Limbitrol 1738

Amoxapine (Co-administration of imipramine with citalopram has resulted in a 50% increase in active metabolite, desipramine concentration; the clinical significance of these findings is unknown; caution is indicated if tricyclic antidepressants are co-administered with citalopram, a relatively weak inhibitor of CYP2D6).
No products indexed under this heading.

Azithromycin Dihydrate (Co-administration with potent inhibitors

of CYP3A4, such as macrolide antibiotics, may decrease the clearance of citalopram). Products include:
Zithromax 2743
Zithromax for IV Infusion 2748
Zithromax for Oral Suspension, 300 mg, 600 mg, 900 mg, 1200 mg.................................... 2739
Zithromax Tablets, 250 mg 2739

Carbamazepine (Given the enzyme inducing properties of carbamazepine, the possibility that carbamazepine might increase the clearance of citalopram should be considered if the two drugs are co-administered; during pharmacokinetic studies, the citalopram levels were unaffected with concurrent use). Products include:
Carbatrol Capsules 3234
Tegretol/Tegretol-XR 2404

Cimetidine (Co-administration has resulted in an increase in citalopram AUC and Cmax by 43% and 39% respectively; the clinical significance of these findings is unknown). Products include:
Tagamet HB 200 Suspension 762
Tagamet HB 200 Tablets 761
Tagamet Tablets 1644

Cimetidine Hydrochloride (Co-administration has resulted in an increase in citalopram AUC and Cmax by 43% and 39% respectively; the clinical significance of these findings is unknown). Products include:
Tagamet 1644

Clarithromycin (Co-administration with potent inhibitors of CYP3A4, such as macrolide antibiotics, may decrease the clearance of citalopram). Products include:
Biaxin/Biaxin XL 403
PREVPAC 3298

Clomipramine Hydrochloride (Co-administration of imipramine with citalopram has resulted in a 50% increase in active metabolite, desipramine concentration; the clinical significance of these findings is unknown; caution is indicated if tricyclic antidepressants are co-administered with citalopram, a relatively weak inhibitor of CYP2D6).
No products indexed under this heading.

Desipramine Hydrochloride (Co-administration of imipramine with citalopram has resulted in a 50% increase in active metabolite, desipramine concentration; the clinical significance of these findings is unknown; caution is indicated if tricyclic antidepressants are co-administered with citalopram, a relatively weak inhibitor of CYP2D6). Products include:
Norpramin Tablets 755

Dirithromycin (Co-administration with potent inhibitors of CYP3A4, such as macrolide antibiotics, may decrease the clearance of citalopram). Products include:
Dynabac Tablets 2269

Doxepin Hydrochloride (Co-administration of imipramine with citalopram has resulted in a 50% increase in active metabolite, desipramine concentration; the clinical significance of these findings is unknown; caution is indicated if tricyclic antidepressants are co-administered with citalopram, a relatively weak inhibitor of CYP2D6). Products include:
Sinequan 2713

Erythromycin (Co-administration with potent inhibitors of CYP3A4, such as erythromycin, may decrease the clearance of citalopram). Products include:
Emgel 2% Topical Gel 1285
Ery-Tab Tablets 448
Erythromycin Base Filmtab Tablets . 454
Erythromycin Delayed-Release Capsules, USP 455
PCE Dispertab Tablets 498

Erythromycin Estolate (Co-administration with potent inhibitors of CYP3A4, such as erythromycin, may decrease the clearance of citalopram).
No products indexed under this heading.

Erythromycin Ethylsuccinate (Co-administration with potent inhibitors of CYP3A4, such as erythromycin, may decrease the clearance of citalopram). Products include:
E.E.S. 450
EryPed 446
Pediazole Suspension 3050

Erythromycin Gluceptate (Co-administration with potent inhibitors of CYP3A4, such as erythromycin, may decrease the clearance of citalopram).
No products indexed under this heading.

Erythromycin Stearate (Co-administration with potent inhibitors of CYP3A4, such as erythromycin, may decrease the clearance of citalopram). Products include:
Erythrocin Stearate Filmtab Tablets 452

Fluconazole (Co-administration with potent inhibitors of CYP3A4, such as fluconazole, may decrease the clearance of citalopram). Products include:
Diflucan Tablets, Injection, and Oral Suspension 2681

Imipramine Hydrochloride (Co-administration of imipramine with citalopram has resulted in a 50% increase in active metabolite, desipramine concentration; the clinical significance of these findings is unknown; caution is indicated if tricyclic antidepressants are co-administered with citalopram, a relatively weak inhibitor of CYP2D6).
No products indexed under this heading.

Imipramine Pamoate (Co-administration of imipramine with citalopram has resulted in a 50% increase in active metabolite, desipramine concentration; the clinical significance of these findings is unknown; caution is indicated if tricyclic antidepressants are co-administered with citalopram, a relatively weak inhibitor of CYP2D6).
No products indexed under this heading.

Isocarboxazid (Co-administration of serotonin reuptake inhibitors and MAO inhibitors has resulted in serious, sometimes fatal, reactions including hyperthermia, rigidity, myoclonus, and other potentially serious adverse reactions; concurrent and/or sequential use is contraindicated).
No products indexed under this heading.

Itraconazole (Co-administration with potent inhibitors of CYP3A4, such as itraconazole, may decrease the clearance of citalopram). Products include:
Sporanox Capsules 1800
Sporanox Injection 1804
Sporanox Injection 2509
Sporanox Oral Solution 1808
Sporanox Oral Solution 2512

Ketoconazole (Co-administration with potent inhibitors of CYP3A4, such as ketoconazole, may decrease the clearance of citalopram). Products include:
Nizoral 2% Cream 3620
Nizoral A-D Shampoo 2008
Nizoral 2% Shampoo 2007
Nizoral Tablets 1791

Lithium Carbonate (Plasma lithium levels should be monitored, if used concurrently, lithium may enhance the serotonergic effects of citalopram; co-administration during clinical trials had no significant effect on the pharmacokinetics of either drug). Products include:
Eskalith 1527
Lithium Carbonate 3061
Lithobid Slow-Release Tablets 3255

Lithium Citrate (Plasma lithium levels should be monitored, if used concurrently, lithium may enhance the serotonergic effects of citalopram; co-administration during clinical trials had no significant effect on the pharmacokinetics of either drug). Products include:
Lithium Citrate Syrup 3061

Maprotiline Hydrochloride (Co-administration of imipramine with citalopram has resulted in a 50% increase in active metabolite, desipramine concentration; the clinical significance of these findings is unknown; caution is indicated if tricyclic antidepressants are co-administered with citalopram, a relatively weak inhibitor of CYP2D6).
No products indexed under this heading.

Metoprolol Succinate (Co-administration has resulted in a two-fold increase in the plasma levels of metoprolol; increased plasma levels of metoprolol have been associated with decreased cardioselectivity; no clinically significant effects on the blood pressure or heart rate has been reported with concurrent use). Products include:
Toprol-XL Tablets 651

Metoprolol Tartrate (Co-administration has resulted in a two-fold increase in the plasma levels of metoprolol; increased plasma levels of metoprolol have been associated with decreased cardioselectivity; no clinically significant effects on the blood pressure or heart rate has been reported with concurrent use).
No products indexed under this heading.

Moclobemide (Co-administration of serotonin reuptake inhibitors and MAO inhibitors has resulted in serious, sometimes fatal, reactions including hyperthermia, rigidity, myoclonus, and other potentially serious adverse reactions; concurrent and/or sequential use is contraindicated).
No products indexed under this heading.

Nortriptyline Hydrochloride (Co-administration of imipramine with citalopram has resulted in a 50% increase in active metabolite, desipramine concentration; the clinical significance of these findings is unknown; caution is indicated if tricyclic antidepressants are co-administered with citalopram, a relatively weak inhibitor of CYP2D6).
No products indexed under this heading.

Omeprazole (Co-administration with potent inhibitors of CYP2C19, such as omeprazole, may decrease the clearance of citalopram). Products include:
Prilosec Delayed-Release Capsules 628

Pargyline Hydrochloride (Co-administration of serotonin reuptake inhibitors and MAO inhibitors has resulted in serious, sometimes fatal, reactions including hyperthermia, rigidity, myoclonus, and other potentially serious adverse reactions; concurrent and/or sequential use is contraindicated).
No products indexed under this heading.

Phenelzine Sulfate (Co-administration of serotonin reuptake inhibitors and MAO inhibitors has resulted in serious, sometimes fatal, reactions including hyperthermia, rigidity, myoclonus, and other potentially serious adverse reactions; concurrent and/or sequential use is contraindicated). Products include:
Nardil Tablets 2653

Procarbazine Hydrochloride (Co-administration of serotonin reuptake inhibitors and MAO inhibitors has resulted in serious, sometimes fatal, reactions including hyperthermia, rigidity, myoclonus, and other potentially serious adverse reactions; concurrent and/or sequential use is contraindicated). Products include:
Matulane Capsules 3246

Protriptyline Hydrochloride (Co-administration of imipramine with citalopram has resulted in a 50% increase in active metabolite, desipramine concentration; the clinical significance of these findings is unknown; caution is indicated if tricyclic antidepressants are co-administered with citalopram, a relatively weak inhibitor of CYP2D6). Products include:
Vivactil Tablets 2446
Vivactil Tablets 2217

Selegiline Hydrochloride (Co-administration of serotonin reuptake inhibitors and MAO inhibitors has resulted in serious, sometimes fatal, reactions including hyperthermia, rigidity, myoclonus, and other potentially serious adverse reactions; concurrent and/or sequential use is contraindicated). Products include:
Eldepryl Capsules 3266

Tranylcypromine Sulfate (Co-administration of serotonin reuptake inhibitors and MAO inhibitors has resulted in serious, sometimes fatal, reactions including hyperthermia, rigidity, myoclonus, and other potentially serious adverse reactions; concurrent and/or sequential use is contraindicated). Products include:
Parnate Tablets 1607

Trimipramine Maleate (Co-administration of imipramine with citalopram has resulted in a 50% increase in active metabolite, desipramine concentration; the clinical significance of these findings is unknown; caution is indicated if tricyclic antidepressants are co-administered with citalopram, a relatively weak inhibitor of CYP2D6). Products include:
Surmontil Capsules 3595

Troleandomycin (Co-administration with potent inhibitors of CYP3A4, such as macrolide antibiotics, may decrease the clearance of citalopram). Products include:
Tao Capsules 2716

Warfarin Sodium (Co-administration has resulted in increased prothrombin time by 5%, the clinical significance of which is unknown). Products include:
Coumadin for Injection 1243
Coumadin Tablets 1243
Warfarin Sodium Tablets, USP 3302

Food Interactions

Alcohol (Concurrent use is not recommended; although, citalopram did not potentiate cognitive and motor effects of alcohol).

CELLCEPT CAPSULES

(Mycophenolate Mofetil) 2951
May interact with:

Acyclovir (Potential for these two drugs to compete for tubular secretion further increasing the concentrations of both drugs; AUCs were increased 10.6% for phenolic glucuronide of mycophenolate mofetil and 21.9% for acyclovir). Products include:
Zovirax 1706
Zovirax Ointment 1707

Acyclovir Sodium (Potential for these two drugs to compete for tubular secretion further increasing the concentrations of both drugs; AUCs were increased 10.6% for phenolic glucuronide of mycophenolate mofetil and 21.9% for acyclovir). Products include:
- Zovirax for Injection 1708

Aluminum Hydroxide (Potential for decreased absorption when CellCept is administered with the antacids containing aluminum and magnesium hydroxide; avoid simultaneous administration). Products include:
- Amphojel Suspension (Mint Flavor) .... ▣789
- Gaviscon Extra Strength Liquid .... ▣751
- Gaviscon Extra Strength Tablets .... ▣751
- Gaviscon Regular Strength Liquid .... ▣751
- Gaviscon Regular Strength Tablets .... ▣750
- Maalox Antacid/Anti-Gas Oral Suspension .... ▣673
- Maalox Max Maximum Strength Antacid/Anti-Gas Liquid 2300
- Maalox Regular Strength Antacid/Antigas Liquid 2300
- Mylanta 1813
- Vanquish Caplets .... ▣617

Antibiotics, unspecified (Drugs that alter gastrointestinal flora may interact with mycophenolate mofetil by disrupting enterohepatic recirculation).

Azathioprine (Concomitant administration is not recommended because such co-administration has not been studied clinically).
- No products indexed under this heading.

Azathioprine Sodium (Concomitant administration is not recommended because such co-administration has not been studied clinically).
- No products indexed under this heading.

Cholestyramine (Decreased AUC of mycophenolate mofetil by approximately 40%; concomitant use with agents that may interfere with enterohepatic circulation should be avoided).
- No products indexed under this heading.

Ethinyl Estradiol (Possiblity of changes in the pharmacokinetics of the oral contraceptives under long term dosing conditions with CellCept which might adversely affect the efficacy of the oral contraceptive). Products include:
- Alesse-21 Tablets 3468
- Alesse-28 Tablets 3473
- Brevicon 28-Day Tablets 3380
- Cyclessa Tablets 2450
- Desogen Tablets 2458
- Estinyl Tablets 3112
- Estrostep 2627
- femhrt Tablets 2635
- Levlen 962
- Levlite 21 Tablets 962
- Levlite 28 Tablets 962
- Levora Tablets 3389
- Loestrin 21 Tablets 2642
- Loestrin Fe Tablets 2642
- Lo/Ovral Tablets 3532
- Lo/Ovral-28 Tablets 3538
- Low-Ogestrel-28 Tablets 3392
- Microgestin Fe 1.5/30 Tablets 3407
- Microgestin Fe 1/20 Tablets 3400
- Mircette Tablets 2470
- Modicon 2563
- Necon 3415
- Nordette-28 Tablets 2257
- Norinyl 1 +35 28-Day Tablets 3380
- Ogestrel 0.5/50-28 Tablets 3428
- Ortho-Cept 21 Tablets 2546
- Ortho-Cept 28 Tablets 2546
- Ortho-Cyclen/Ortho Tri-Cyclen 2573
- Ortho-Novum 2563
- Ovcon 3364
- Ovral Tablets 3551
- Ovral-28 Tablets 3552
- Tri-Levlen 962
- Tri-Norinyl-28 Tablets 3433
- Triphasil-21 Tablets 3600
- Triphasil-28 Tablets 3605
- Trivora Tablets 3439
- Yasmin 28 Tablets 980
- Zovia 3449

Ganciclovir Sodium (Potential for these two drugs to compete for tubular secretion further increasing the concentrations of both drugs). Products include:
- Cytovene-IV 2959

Magnesium Hydroxide (Potential for decreased absorption when CellCept is administered with the antacids containing aluminum and magnesium hydroxide; avoid simultaneous administration). Products include:
- Ex•Lax Milk of Magnesia Liquid .... ▣670
- Maalox Antacid/Anti-Gas Oral Suspension .... ▣673
- Maalox Max Maximum Strength Antacid/Anti-Gas Liquid 2300
- Maalox Regular Strength Antacid/Antigas Liquid 2300
- Mylanta Fast-Acting 1813
- Mylanta 1813
- Pepcid Complete Chewable Tablets 1815
- Phillips' Chewable Tablets .... ▣615
- Phillips' Milk of Magnesia Liquid (Original, Cherry, & Mint) .... ▣616
- Rolaids Tablets .... ▣706
- Extra Strength Rolaids Tablets .... ▣706
- Vanquish Caplets .... ▣617

Norethindrone (Possiblity of changes in the pharmacokinetics of the oral contraceptives under long term dosing conditions with CellCept which might adversely affect the efficacy of the oral contraceptive). Products include:
- Brevicon 28-Day Tablets 3380
- Micronor Tablets 2543
- Modicon 2563
- Necon 3415
- Norinyl 1 +35 28-Day Tablets 3380
- Norinyl 1 + 50 28-Day Tablets 3380
- Nor-QD Tablets 3423
- Ortho-Novum 2563
- Ortho-Novum 1/50□28 Tablets 2556
- Ovcon 3364
- Tri-Norinyl-28 Tablets 3433

Probenecid (Potential for increased plasma concentration of MPA).
- No products indexed under this heading.

Food Interactions

Food, unspecified (Food has no effect on MPA AUC, but has been shown to decrease MPA Cmax by 40%; it is recommended that CellCept be administered on an empty stomach).

CELLCEPT INTRAVENOUS

(Mycophenolate Mofetil Hydrochloride) 2951
See CellCept Capsules

CELLCEPT ORAL SUSPENSION

(Mycophenolate Mofetil) 2951
See CellCept Capsules

CELLCEPT TABLETS

(Mycophenolate Mofetil) 2951
See CellCept Capsules

CELLUVISC LUBRICANT EYE DROPS

(Carboxymethylcellulose Sodium) .... ⊙234
None cited in PDR database.

CELONTIN CAPSULES

(Methsuximide) 2618
May interact with anticonvulsants. Compounds in these categories include:

Carbamazepine (Effect not specified; periodic serum level determination may be necessary). Products include:
- Carbatrol Capsules 3234
- Tegretol/Tegretol-XR 2404

Divalproex Sodium (Effect not specified; periodic serum level determination may be necessary). Products include:
- Depakote Sprinkle Capsules 426
- Depakote Tablets 430
- Depakote ER Tablets 436

Ethosuximide (Effect not specified; periodic serum level determination may be necessary). Products include:
- Zarontin Capsules 2659
- Zarontin Syrup 2660

Ethotoin (Effect not specified; periodic serum level determination may be necessary).
- No products indexed under this heading.

Felbamate (Effect not specified; periodic serum level determination may be necessary). Products include:
- Felbatol 3343

Fosphenytoin Sodium (Effect not specified; periodic serum level determination may be necessary). Products include:
- Cerebyx Injection 2619

Lamotrigine (Effect not specified; periodic serum level determination may be necessary). Products include:
- Lamictal 1567

Levetiracetam (Effect not specified; periodic serum level determination may be necessary). Products include:
- Keppra Tablets 3314

Mephenytoin (Effect not specified; periodic serum level determination may be necessary).
- No products indexed under this heading.

Oxcarbazepine (Effect not specified; periodic serum level determination may be necessary). Products include:
- Trileptal Oral Suspension 2407
- Trileptal Tablets 2407

Paramethadione (Effect not specified; periodic serum level determination may be necessary).
- No products indexed under this heading.

Phenacemide (Effect not specified; periodic serum level determination may be necessary).
- No products indexed under this heading.

Phenobarbital (Increased plasma concentration of phenobarbital). Products include:
- Arco-Lase Plus Tablets 592
- Donnatal 2929
- Donnatal Extentabs 2930

Phensuximide (Effect not specified; periodic serum level determination may be necessary).
- No products indexed under this heading.

Phenytoin (Increased plasma concentration of phenytoin). Products include:
- Dilantin Infatabs 2624
- Dilantin-125 Oral Suspension 2625

Phenytoin Sodium (Increased plasma concentration of phenytoin). Products include:
- Dilantin Kapseals 2622

Primidone (Effect not specified; periodic serum level determination may be necessary).
- No products indexed under this heading.

Tiagabine Hydrochloride (Effect not specified; periodic serum level determination may be necessary). Products include:
- Gabitril Tablets 1189

Topiramate (Effect not specified; periodic serum level determination may be necessary). Products include:
- Topamax Sprinkle Capsules 2590
- Topamax Tablets 2590

Trimethadione (Effect not specified; periodic serum level determination may be necessary).
- No products indexed under this heading.

Valproate Sodium (Effect not specified; periodic serum level determination may be necessary). Products include:
- Depacon Injection 416

Valproic Acid (Effect not specified; periodic serum level determination may be necessary). Products include:
- Depakene 421

Zonisamide (Effect not specified; periodic serum level determination may be necessary). Products include:
- Zonegran Capsules 1307

CENESTIN TABLETS

(Estrogens, Conjugated, Synthetic A) 1263
None cited in PDR database.

CENTRUM ECHINACEA SOFTGELS

(Echinacea angustifolia) .... ▣852
None cited in PDR database.

CENTRUM FOCUSED FORMULAS BONE HEALTH TABLETS

(Minerals, Multiple, Vitamin D) .... ▣815
None cited in PDR database.

CENTRUM FOCUSED FORMULAS ENERGY TABLETS

(Ginseng, Vitamin B Complex) .... ▣816
None cited in PDR database.

CENTRUM FOCUSED FORMULAS HEART TABLETS

(Allium sativum, Coenzyme Q-10, Vitamins with Minerals) .... ▣816
None cited in PDR database.

CENTRUM FOCUSED FORMULAS MENTAL CLARITY TABLETS

(Ginkgo biloba, Vitamins with Minerals) .... ▣816
None cited in PDR database.

CENTRUM FOCUSED FORMULAS PROSTATE SOFTGELS

(Serenoa repens, Vitamin A) .... ▣816
None cited in PDR database.

CENTRUM GINKGO BILOBA SOFTGELS

(Ginkgo biloba) .... ▣852
None cited in PDR database.

CENTRUM GINSENG SOFTGELS

(Ginseng) .... ▣853
None cited in PDR database.

CENTRUM KIDS COMPLETE CHILDREN'S CHEWABLES

(Vitamins with Minerals) .... ▣817
None cited in PDR database.

CENTRUM PERFORMANCE MULTIVITAMIN-MULTIMINERAL TABLETS

(Vitamins with Minerals) .... ▣817
None cited in PDR database.

CENTRUM SAW PALMETTO SOFTGELS

(Serenoa repens) .... ▣853
None cited in PDR database.

CENTRUM ST. JOHN'S WORT SOFTGELS

(Hypericum) .... ▣853
None cited in PDR database.

CENTRUM TABLETS
(Vitamins with Minerals) ■ 815
None cited in PDR database.

CENTRUM SILVER TABLETS
(Vitamins with Minerals) ■ 818
None cited in PDR database.

CEO-TWO EVACUANT SUPPOSITORY
(Potassium Bitartrate, Sodium Bicarbonate) ■ 618
None cited in PDR database.

CĒPACOL ANTISEPTIC MOUTHWASH/GARGLE, ORIGINAL
(Cetylpyridinium Chloride) ■ 786
None cited in PDR database.

CĒPACOL ANTISEPTIC MOUTHWASH/GARGLE, MINT
(Cetylpyridinium Chloride) ■ 786
None cited in PDR database.

CHILDREN'S CĒPACOL SORE THROAT FORMULA, CHERRY FLAVOR LIQUID
(Acetaminophen, Pseudoephedrine Hydrochloride) ■ 788
May interact with monoamine oxidase inhibitors. Compounds in these categories include:

Isocarboxazid (Concurrent and/or sequential use with MAO inhibitors is not recommended).
No products indexed under this heading.

Moclobemide (Concurrent and/or sequential use with MAO inhibitors is not recommended).
No products indexed under this heading.

Pargyline Hydrochloride (Concurrent and/or sequential use with MAO inhibitors is not recommended).
No products indexed under this heading.

Phenelzine Sulfate (Concurrent and/or sequential use with MAO inhibitors is not recommended). Products include:
Nardil Tablets 2653

Procarbazine Hydrochloride (Concurrent and/or sequential use with MAO inhibitors is not recommended). Products include:
Matulane Capsules 3246

Selegiline Hydrochloride (Concurrent and/or sequential use with MAO inhibitors is not recommended). Products include:
Eldepryl Capsules 3266

Tranylcypromine Sulfate (Concurrent and/or sequential use with MAO inhibitors is not recommended). Products include:
Parnate Tablets 1607

CHILDREN'S CĒPACOL SORE THROAT FORMULA, GRAPE FLAVOR LIQUID
(Acetaminophen, Pseudoephedrine Hydrochloride) ■ 788
See Children's Cēpacol Sore Throat Formula, Cherry Flavor Liquid

CĒPACOL MAXIMUM STRENGTH SUGAR FREE SORE THROAT LOZENGES, CHERRY FLAVOR
(Benzocaine, Menthol) ■ 787
None cited in PDR database.

CĒPACOL MAXIMUM STRENGTH SUGAR FREE SORE THROAT LOZENGES, COOL MINT FLAVOR
(Benzocaine, Menthol) ■ 787
None cited in PDR database.

CĒPACOL MAXIMUM STRENGTH SORE THROAT LOZENGES, CHERRY FLAVOR
(Benzocaine, Menthol) ■ 787
None cited in PDR database.

CĒPACOL MAXIMUM STRENGTH SORE THROAT LOZENGES, MINT FLAVOR
(Benzocaine, Menthol) ■ 787
None cited in PDR database.

CĒPACOL REGULAR STRENGTH SORE THROAT LOZENGES, CHERRY FLAVOR
(Menthol) ■ 787
None cited in PDR database.

CĒPACOL REGULAR STRENGTH SORE THROAT LOZENGES, ORIGINAL MINT FLAVOR
(Menthol) ■ 787
None cited in PDR database.

CĒPACOL MAXIMUM STRENGTH SORE THROAT SPRAY, CHERRY FLAVOR
(Dyclonine Hydrochloride) ■ 787
None cited in PDR database.

CĒPACOL MAXIMUM STRENGTH SORE THROAT SPRAY, COOL MENTHOL FLAVOR
(Dyclonine Hydrochloride) ■ 787
None cited in PDR database.

CĒPACOL VIRACTIN COLD SORE AND FEVER BLISTER TREATMENT, CREAM
(Tetracaine) ■ 788
None cited in PDR database.

CĒPACOL VIRACTIN COLD SORE AND FEVER BLISTER TREATMENT, GEL
(Tetracaine Hydrochloride) ■ 788
None cited in PDR database.

CEPTAZ FOR INJECTION
(Ceftazidime) 1499
May interact with aminoglycosides and certain other agents. Compounds in these categories include:

Amikacin Sulfate (Potential for nephrotoxicity following concomitant administration).
No products indexed under this heading.

Chloramphenicol (Possible antagonism in vivo). Products include:
Chloromycetin Ophthalmic Ointment, 1% ⊙ 296
Chloromycetin Ophthalmic Solution ⊙ 297
Chloroptic Sterile Ophthalmic Ointment ⊙ 234
Chloroptic Sterile Ophthalmic Solution ⊙ 235

Chloramphenicol Palmitate (Possible antagonism in vivo).
No products indexed under this heading.

Chloramphenicol Sodium Succinate (Possible antagonism in vivo).
No products indexed under this heading.

Furosemide (Potential for nephrotoxicity following concomitant administration). Products include:
Furosemide Tablets 2284

Gentamicin Sulfate (Potential for nephrotoxicity following concomitant administration). Products include:
Genoptic Ophthalmic Ointment ⊙ 239
Genoptic Sterile Ophthalmic Solution ⊙ 239
Pred-G Ophthalmic Suspension ⊙ 247
Pred-G Sterile Ophthalmic Ointment ⊙ 248

Kanamycin Sulfate (Potential for nephrotoxicity following concomitant administration).
No products indexed under this heading.

Streptomycin Sulfate (Potential for nephrotoxicity following concomitant administration). Products include:
Streptomycin Sulfate Injection 2714

Tobramycin (Potential for nephrotoxicity following concomitant administration). Products include:
TOBI Solution for Inhalation 1206
TobraDex Ophthalmic Ointment 542
TobraDex Ophthalmic Suspension 541
Tobrex Ophthalmic Ointment ⊙ 220
Tobrex Ophthalmic Solution ⊙ 221

Tobramycin Sulfate (Potential for nephrotoxicity following concomitant administration). Products include:
Nebcin Vials, Hyporets & ADD-Vantage 1955

CEREBYX INJECTION
(Fosphenytoin Sodium) 2619
May interact with corticosteroids, oral anticoagulants, estrogens, histamine H_2-receptor antagonists, oral contraceptives, phenothiazines, quinidine, salicylates, succinimides, sulfonamides, tricyclic antidepressants, theophylline, and certain other agents. Compounds in these categories include:

Aminophylline (Efficacy of theophylline is impaired by phenytoin).
No products indexed under this heading.

Amiodarone Hydrochloride (Co-administration may increase plasma phenytoin concentration). Products include:
Cordarone Intravenous 3491
Cordarone Tablets 3487
Pacerone Tablets 3331

Amitriptyline Hydrochloride (Tricyclic antidepressants may precipitate seizures in susceptible patients; Cerebyx dosage may need to be adjusted). Products include:
Etrafon 3115
Limbitrol 1738

Amoxapine (Tricyclic antidepressants may precipitate seizures in susceptible patients; Cerebyx dosage may need to be adjusted).
No products indexed under this heading.

Aspirin (Co-administration may increase plasma phenytoin concentration). Products include:
Aggrenox Capsules 1026
Alka-Seltzer ■ 603
Alka-Seltzer Lemon Lime Antacid and Pain Reliever Effervescent Tablets ■ 603
Alka-Seltzer Extra Strength Antacid and Pain Reliever Effervescent Tablets ■ 603
Alka-Seltzer PM Effervescent Tablets ■ 605
Genuine Bayer Tablets, Caplets and Gelcaps ■ 606
Extra Strength Bayer Caplets and Gelcaps ■ 610
Aspirin Regimen Bayer Children's Chewable Tablets (Orange or Cherry Flavored) ■ 607
Bayer, Aspirin Regimen ■ 606
Aspirin Regimen Bayer 81 mg Caplets with Calcium ■ 607
Genuine Bayer Professional Labeling (Aspirin Regimen Bayer) ■ 608
Extra Strength Bayer Arthritis Caplets ■ 610
Extra Strength Bayer Plus Caplets ■ 610
Extra Strength Bayer PM Caplets ■ 611
BC Powder ■ 619
BC Allergy Sinus Cold Powder ■ 619
Arthritis Strength BC Powder ■ 619
BC Sinus Cold Powder ■ 619
Darvon Compound-65 Pulvules 1910
Ecotrin Enteric Coated Aspirin Low, Regular and Maximum Strength Tablets 1715
Excedrin Extra-Strength Tablets, Caplets, and Geltabs ■ 629
Excedrin Migraine 1070
Goody's Body Pain Formula Powder ■ 620
Goody's Extra Strength Headache Powder ■ 620
Goody's Extra Strength Pain Relief Tablets ■ 620
Percodan Tablets 1327
Robaxisal Tablets 2939
Soma Compound Tablets 3354
Soma Compound w/Codeine Tablets 3355
Vanquish Caplets ■ 617

Bendroflumethiazide (Co-administration with sulfonamides may increase plasma phenytoin concentration). Products include:
Corzide 40/5 Tablets 2247
Corzide 80/5 Tablets 2247

Betamethasone Acetate (Efficacy of corticosteroids is impaired by phenytoin). Products include:
Celestone Soluspan Injectable Suspension 3097

Betamethasone Sodium Phosphate (Efficacy of corticosteroids is impaired by phenytoin). Products include:
Celestone Soluspan Injectable Suspension 3097

Carbamazepine (Co-administration may decrease plasma phenytoin concentration). Products include:
Carbatrol Capsules 3234
Tegretol/Tegretol-XR 2404

Chloramphenicol (Co-administration may increase plasma phenytoin concentration). Products include:
Chloromycetin Ophthalmic Ointment, 1% ⊙ 296
Chloromycetin Ophthalmic Solution ⊙ 297
Chloroptic Sterile Ophthalmic Ointment ⊙ 234
Chloroptic Sterile Ophthalmic Solution ⊙ 235

Chloramphenicol Palmitate (Co-administration may increase plasma phenytoin concentration).
No products indexed under this heading.

Chloramphenicol Sodium Succinate (Co-administration may increase plasma phenytoin concentration).
No products indexed under this heading.

Chlordiazepoxide (Co-administration may increase plasma phenytoin concentration). Products include:
Limbitrol 1738

Chlordiazepoxide Hydrochloride (Co-administration may increase plasma phenytoin concentration). Products include:
Librium Capsules 1736
Librium for Injection 1737

Chlorothiazide (Co-administration with sulfonamides may increase plasma phenytoin concentration). Products include:
Aldoclor Tablets 2035
Diuril Oral 2087

Chlorothiazide Sodium (Co-administration with sulfonamides may increase plasma phenytoin concentration). Products include:
Diuril Sodium Intravenous 2086

Chlorotrianisene (Co-administration with estrogens may increase plasma phenytoin concentration; efficacy of estrogens is impaired by phenytoin).
No products indexed under this heading.

Chlorpromazine (Co-administration with phenothiazines may increase plasma phenytoin concentration). Products include:

Thorazine Suppositories 1656

Chlorpromazine Hydrochloride (Co-administration with phenothiazines may increase plasma phenytoin concentration). Products include:
Thorazine 1656

Chlorpropamide (Co-administration with sulfonamides may increase plasma phenytoin concentration). Products include:
Diabinese Tablets 2680

Choline Magnesium Trisalicylate (Co-administration may increase plasma phenytoin concentration). Products include:
Trilisate 2901

Cimetidine (Co-administration may increase plasma phenytoin concentration). Products include:
Tagamet HB 200 Suspension .... ■ 762
Tagamet HB 200 Tablets .... ■ 761
Tagamet Tablets 1644

Cimetidine Hydrochloride (Co-administration may increase plasma phenytoin concentration). Products include:
Tagamet 1644

Clomipramine Hydrochloride (Tricyclic antidepressants may precipitate seizures in susceptible patients; Cerebyx dosage may need to be adjusted).
No products indexed under this heading.

Cortisone Acetate (Efficacy of corticosteroids is impaired by phenytoin). Products include:
Cortone Acetate Injectable Suspension 2059
Cortone Acetate Tablets 2061

Desipramine Hydrochloride (Tricyclic antidepressants may precipitate seizures in susceptible patients; Cerebyx dosage may need to be adjusted). Products include:
Norpramin Tablets 755

Desogestrel (Efficacy of oral contraceptives impaired by phenytoin). Products include:
Cyclessa Tablets 2450
Desogen Tablets 2458
Mircette Tablets 2470
Ortho-Cept 21 Tablets 2546
Ortho-Cept 28 Tablets 2546

Dexamethasone (Efficacy of corticosteroids is impaired by phenytoin). Products include:
Decadron Elixir 2078
Decadron Tablets 2079
TobraDex Ophthalmic Ointment 542
TobraDex Ophthalmic Suspension 541

Dexamethasone Acetate (Efficacy of corticosteroids is impaired by phenytoin).
No products indexed under this heading.

Dexamethasone Sodium Phosphate (Efficacy of corticosteroids is impaired by phenytoin). Products include:
Decadron Phosphate Injection 2081
Decadron Phosphate Sterile Ophthalmic Ointment 2083
Decadron Phosphate Sterile Ophthalmic Solution 2084
NeoDecadron Sterile Ophthalmic Solution 2144

Diazepam (Co-administration may increase plasma phenytoin concentration). Products include:
Valium Injectable 3026
Valium Tablets 3047

Dicumarol (Co-administration may increase plasma phenytoin concentration; efficacy of coumarin is impaired by phenytoin).
No products indexed under this heading.

Dienestrol (Co-administration with estrogens may increase plasma phenytoin concentration; efficacy of estrogens is impaired by phenytoin). Products include:
Ortho Dienestrol Cream 2554

Diethylstilbestrol (Co-administration with estrogens may increase plasma phenytoin concentration; efficacy of estrogens is impaired by phenytoin).
No products indexed under this heading.

Diflunisal (Co-administration may increase plasma phenytoin concentration). Products include:
Dolobid Tablets 2088

Digitoxin (Efficacy of digitoxin is impaired by phenytoin).
No products indexed under this heading.

Disulfiram (Co-administration may increase plasma phenytoin concentration). Products include:
Antabuse Tablets 2444
Antabuse Tablets 3474

Divalproex Sodium (Co-administration may result in either decrease or increase in plasma phenytoin concentrations; unpredictable effect of phenytoin on valproate plasma concentrations). Products include:
Depakote Sprinkle Capsules 426
Depakote Tablets 430
Depakote ER Tablets 436

Doxepin Hydrochloride (Tricyclic antidepressants may precipitate seizures in susceptible patients; Cerebyx dosage may need to be adjusted). Products include:
Sinequan 2713

Doxycycline Calcium (Efficacy of doxycycline is impaired by phenytoin). Products include:
Vibramycin Calcium Oral Suspension Syrup 2735

Doxycycline Hyclate (Efficacy of doxycycline is impaired by phenytoin). Products include:
Doryx Coated Pellet Filled Capsules 3357
Periostat Tablets 1208
Vibramycin Hyclate Capsules 2735
Vibramycin Hyclate Intravenous 2737
Vibra-Tabs Film Coated Tablets 2735

Doxycycline Monohydrate (Efficacy of doxycycline is impaired by phenytoin). Products include:
Monodox Capsules 2442
Vibramycin Monohydrate for Oral Suspension 2735

Dyphylline (Efficacy of theophylline is impaired by phenytoin). Products include:
Lufyllin Tablets 3347
Lufyllin-400 Tablets 3347
Lufyllin-GG Elixir 3348
Lufyllin-GG Tablets 3348

Estradiol (Co-administration with estrogens may increase plasma phenytoin concentration; efficacy of estrogens is impaired by phenytoin). Products include:
Activella Tablets 2764
Alora Transdermal System 3372
Climara Transdermal System 958
CombiPatch Transdermal System .. 2323
Esclim Transdermal System 3460
Estrace Vaginal Cream 3358
Estrace Tablets 3361
Estring Vaginal Ring 2811
Ortho-Prefest Tablets 2570
Vagifem Tablets 2857
Vivelle Transdermal System 2412
Vivelle-Dot Transdermal System 2416

Estrogens, Conjugated (Co-administration with estrogens may increase plasma phenytoin concentration; efficacy of estrogens is impaired by phenytoin). Products include:
Premarin Intravenous 3563
Premarin Tablets 3566
Premarin Vaginal Cream 3570
Premphase Tablets 3572
Prempro Tablets 3572

Estrogens, Esterified (Co-administration with estrogens may increase plasma phenytoin concentration; efficacy of estrogens is impaired by phenytoin). Products include:
Estratest 3252
Menest Tablets 2254

Estropipate (Co-administration with estrogens may increase plasma phenytoin concentration; efficacy of estrogens is impaired by phenytoin). Products include:
Ogen Tablets 2846
Ortho-Est Tablets 3464

Ethinyl Estradiol (Co-administration with estrogens may increase plasma phenytoin concentration; efficacy of estrogens is impaired by phenytoin). Products include:
Alesse-21 Tablets 3468
Alesse-28 Tablets 3473
Brevicon 28-Day Tablets 3380
Cyclessa Tablets 2450
Desogen Tablets 2458
Estinyl Tablets 3112
Estrostep 2627
femhrt Tablets 2635
Levlen 962
Levlite 21 Tablets 962
Levlite 28 Tablets 962
Levora Tablets 3389
Loestrin 21 Tablets 2642
Loestrin Fe Tablets 2642
Lo/Ovral Tablets 3532
Lo/Ovral-28 Tablets 3538
Low-Ogestrel-28 Tablets 3392
Microgestin Fe 1.5/30 Tablets 3407
Microgestin Fe 1/20 Tablets 3400
Mircette Tablets 2470
Modicon 2563
Necon 3415
Nordette-28 Tablets 2257
Norinyl 1 +35 28-Day Tablets 3380
Ogestrel 0.5/50-28 Tablets 3428
Ortho-Cept 21 Tablets 2546
Ortho-Cept 28 Tablets 2546
Ortho-Cyclen/Ortho Tri-Cyclen 2573
Ortho-Novum 2563
Ovcon 3364
Ovral Tablets 3551
Ovral-28 Tablets 3552
Tri-Levlen 962
Tri-Norinyl-28 Tablets 3433
Triphasil-21 Tablets 3600
Triphasil-28 Tablets 3605
Trivora Tablets 3439
Yasmin 28 Tablets 980
Zovia 3449

Ethosuximide (Co-administration may increase plasma phenytoin concentration). Products include:
Zarontin Capsules 2659
Zarontin Syrup 2660

Ethynodiol Diacetate (Efficacy of oral contraceptives impaired by phenytoin). Products include:
Zovia 3449

Famotidine (Co-administration may increase plasma phenytoin concentration). Products include:
Famotidine Injection 866
Pepcid AC 1814
Pepcid Complete Chewable Tablets 1815
Pepcid Injection 2153
Pepcid for Oral Suspension 2150
Pepcid RPD Orally Disintegrating Tablets 2150
Pepcid Tablets 2150

Fludrocortisone Acetate (Efficacy of corticosteroids is impaired by phenytoin). Products include:
Florinef Acetate Tablets 2250

Fluoxetine Hydrochloride (Co-administration may increase plasma phenytoin concentration). Products include:
Prozac Pulvules, Liquid, and Weekly Capsules 1238
Sarafem Pulvules 1962

Fluphenazine Decanoate (Co-administration with phenothiazines may increase plasma phenytoin concentration).
No products indexed under this heading.

Fluphenazine Enanthate (Co-administration with phenothiazines may increase plasma phenytoin concentration).
No products indexed under this heading.

Fluphenazine Hydrochloride (Co-administration with phenothiazines may increase plasma phenytoin concentration).
No products indexed under this heading.

Furosemide (Efficacy of furosemide is impaired by phenytoin). Products include:
Furosemide Tablets 2284

Glipizide (Co-administration with sulfonamides may increase plasma phenytoin concentration). Products include:
Glucotrol Tablets 2692
Glucotrol XL Extended Release Tablets 2693

Glyburide (Co-administration with sulfonamides may increase plasma phenytoin concentration). Products include:
DiaBeta Tablets 741
Glucovance Tablets 1086

Halothane (Co-administration may increase plasma phenytoin concentration). Products include:
Fluothane Inhalation 3508

Hydrochlorothiazide (Co-administration with sulfonamides may increase plasma phenytoin concentration). Products include:
Accuretic Tablets 2614
Aldoril Tablets 2039
Atacand HCT Tablets 597
Avalide Tablets 1070
Diovan HCT Tablets 2338
Dyazide Capsules 1515
HydroDIURIL Tablets 2108
Hyzaar 2109
Inderide Tablets 3517
Inderide LA Long-Acting Capsules .. 3519
Lotensin HCT Tablets 2367
Maxzide 1008
Micardis HCT Tablets 1051
Microzide Capsules 3414
Moduretic Tablets 2138
Monopril HCT 1094
Prinzide Tablets 2168
Timolide Tablets 2187
Uniretic Tablets 3178
Vaseretic Tablets 2204
Zestoretic Tablets 695
Ziac Tablets 1887

Hydrocortisone (Efficacy of corticosteroids is impaired by phenytoin). Products include:
Anusol-HC Cream 2.5% 2237
Cipro HC Otic Suspension 540
Cortaid Intensive Therapy Cream . ■ 717
Cortaid Maximum Strength Cream .... ■ 717
Cortisporin Ophthalmic Suspension Sterile .... ⊙ 297
Cortizone•5 .... ■ 699
Cortizone•10 .... ■ 699
Cortizone•10 Plus Creme .... ■ 700
Cortizone for Kids Creme .... ■ 699
Hydrocortone Tablets 2106
Massengill Medicated Soft Cloth Towelette .... ■ 753
VōSoL HC Otic Solution 3356

Hydrocortisone Acetate (Efficacy of corticosteroids is impaired by phenytoin). Products include:
Analpram-HC 1338
Anusol HC-1 Hydrocortisone Anti-Itch Cream .... ■ 689
Anusol-HC Suppositories 2238
Cortaid .... ■ 717
Cortifoam Rectal Foam 3170
Cortisporin-TC Otic Suspension 2246
Hydrocortone Acetate Injectable Suspension 2103
Pramosone 1343
Proctocort Suppositories 2264
ProctoFoam-HC 3177
Terra-Cortril Ophthalmic Suspension 2716

Hydrocortisone Sodium Phosphate (Efficacy of corticosteroids is impaired by phenytoin). Products include:
Hydrocortone Phosphate Injection, Sterile 2105

Hydrocortisone Sodium Succinate (Efficacy of corticosteroids is impaired by phenytoin).
No products indexed under this heading.

Hydroflumethiazide (Co-administration with sulfonamides may increase plasma phenytoin concentration). Products include:
Diucardin Tablets 3494

Imipramine Hydrochloride (Tricyclic antidepressants may precipitate seizures in susceptible patients; Cerebyx dosage may need to be adjusted).
No products indexed under this heading.

Imipramine Pamoate (Tricyclic antidepressants may precipitate seizures in susceptible patients; Cerebyx dosage may need to be adjusted).
No products indexed under this heading.

Isoniazid (Co-administration may increase plasma phenytoin concentration). Products include:
Rifamate Capsules 767
Rifater Tablets 769

Levonorgestrel (Efficacy of oral contraceptives impaired by phenytoin). Products include:
Alesse-21 Tablets 3468
Alesse-28 Tablets 3473
Levlen 962
Levlite 21 Tablets 962
Levlite 28 Tablets 962
Levora Tablets 3389
Mirena Intrauterine System 974
Nordette-28 Tablets 2257
Norplant System 3543
Tri-Levlen 962
Triphasil-21 Tablets 3600
Triphasil-28 Tablets 3605
Trivora Tablets 3439

Magnesium Salicylate (Co-administration may increase plasma phenytoin concentration). Products include:
Momentum Backache Relief Extra Strength Caplets .... ▣666

Maprotiline Hydrochloride (Tricyclic antidepressants may precipitate seizures in susceptible patients; Cerebyx dosage may need to be adjusted).
No products indexed under this heading.

Mesoridazine Besylate (Co-administration with phenothiazines may increase plasma phenytoin concentration). Products include:
Serentil 1057

Mestranol (Efficacy of oral contraceptives impaired by phenytoin). Products include:
Necon 1/50 Tablets 3415
Norinyl 1 + 50 28-Day Tablets 3380
Ortho-Novum 1/50▫28 Tablets 2556

Methotrimeprazine (Co-administration with phenothiazines may increase plasma phenytoin concentration).
No products indexed under this heading.

Methsuximide (Co-administration may increase plasma phenytoin concentration). Products include:
Celontin Capsules 2618

Methyclothiazide (Co-administration with sulfonamides may increase plasma phenytoin concentration).
No products indexed under this heading.

Methylphenidate Hydrochloride (Co-administration may increase plasma phenytoin concentration). Products include:
Concerta Extended-Release Tablets 1998
Concerta Tablets 561
Metadate CD Capsules 1164
Metadate ER Tablets 1167
Methylin Tablets 1995
Methylin ER Tablets 1995
Ritalin 2387

Methylprednisolone Acetate (Efficacy of corticosteroids is impaired by phenytoin). Products include:
Depo-Medrol Injectable Suspension 2795

Methylprednisolone Sodium Succinate (Efficacy of corticosteroids is impaired by phenytoin). Products include:
Solu-Medrol Sterile Powder 2855

Nizatidine (Co-administration may increase plasma phenytoin concentration). Products include:
Axid Pulvules 1903
Axid Pulvules 2919

Norethindrone (Efficacy of oral contraceptives impaired by phenytoin). Products include:
Brevicon 28-Day Tablets 3380
Micronor Tablets 2543
Modicon 2563
Necon 3415
Norinyl 1 +35 28-Day Tablets 3380
Norinyl 1 + 50 28-Day Tablets 3380
Nor-QD Tablets 3423
Ortho-Novum 2563
Ortho-Novum 1/50▫28 Tablets 2556
Ovcon 3364
Tri-Norinyl-28 Tablets 3433

Norethynodrel (Efficacy of oral contraceptives impaired by phenytoin).
No products indexed under this heading.

Norgestimate (Efficacy of oral contraceptives impaired by phenytoin). Products include:
Ortho-Cyclen/Ortho Tri-Cyclen 2573
Ortho-Prefest Tablets 2570

Norgestrel (Efficacy of oral contraceptives impaired by phenytoin). Products include:
Lo/Ovral Tablets 3532
Lo/Ovral-28 Tablets 3538
Low-Ogestrel-28 Tablets 3392
Ogestrel 0.5/50-28 Tablets 3428
Ovral Tablets 3551
Ovral-28 Tablets 3552
Ovrette Tablets 3552

Nortriptyline Hydrochloride (Tricyclic antidepressants may precipitate seizures in susceptible patients; Cerebyx dosage may need to be adjusted).
No products indexed under this heading.

Perphenazine (Co-administration with phenothiazines may increase plasma phenytoin concentration). Products include:
Etrafon 3115
Trilafon 3160

Phenobarbital (Co-administration may result in either decrease or increase in plasma phenytoin concentrations; unpredictable effect of phenytoin on phenobarbital plasma concentrations). Products include:
Arco-Lase Plus Tablets 592
Donnatal 2929
Donnatal Extentabs 2930

Phensuximide (Co-administration may increase plasma phenytoin concentration).
No products indexed under this heading.

Phenylbutazone (Co-administration may increase plasma phenytoin concentration).
No products indexed under this heading.

Polyestradiol Phosphate (Co-administration with estrogens may increase plasma phenytoin concentration; efficacy of estrogens is impaired by phenytoin).
No products indexed under this heading.

Polythiazide (Co-administration with sulfonamides may increase plasma phenytoin concentration). Products include:
Minizide Capsules 2700
Renese Tablets 2712

Prednisolone Acetate (Efficacy of corticosteroids is impaired by phenytoin). Products include:
Blephamide Ophthalmic Ointment 547
Blephamide Ophthalmic Suspension 548
Poly-Pred Liquifilm Ophthalmic Suspension .... ⊙245
Pred Forte Ophthalmic Suspension .... ⊙246
Pred Mild Sterile Ophthalmic Suspension .... ⊙249
Pred-G Ophthalmic Suspension .... ⊙247
Pred-G Sterile Ophthalmic Ointment .... ⊙248

Prednisolone Sodium Phosphate (Efficacy of corticosteroids is impaired by phenytoin). Products include:
Pediapred Oral Solution 1170

Prednisolone Tebutate (Efficacy of corticosteroids is impaired by phenytoin).
No products indexed under this heading.

Prednisone (Efficacy of corticosteroids is impaired by phenytoin). Products include:
Prednisone 3064

Prochlorperazine (Co-administration with phenothiazines may increase plasma phenytoin concentration). Products include:
Compazine 1505

Promethazine Hydrochloride (Co-administration with phenothiazines may increase plasma phenytoin concentration). Products include:
Mepergan Injection 3539
Phenergan Injection 3553
Phenergan 3556
Phenergan Syrup 3554
Phenergan with Codeine Syrup 3557
Phenergan with Dextromethorphan Syrup 3559
Phenergan VC Syrup 3560
Phenergan VC with Codeine Syrup 3561

Protriptyline Hydrochloride (Tricyclic antidepressants may precipitate seizures in susceptible patients; Cerebyx dosage may need to be adjusted). Products include:
Vivactil Tablets 2446
Vivactil Tablets 2217

Quinestrol (Co-administration with estrogens may increase plasma phenytoin concentration; efficacy of estrogens is impaired by phenytoin).
No products indexed under this heading.

Quinidine Gluconate (Efficacy of quinidine is impaired by phenytoin). Products include:
Quinaglute Dura-Tabs Tablets 978

Quinidine Polygalacturonate (Efficacy of quinidine is impaired by phenytoin).
No products indexed under this heading.

Quinidine Sulfate (Efficacy of quinidine is impaired by phenytoin). Products include:
Quinidex Extentabs 2933

Ranitidine Bismuth Citrate (Co-administration may increase plasma phenytoin concentration).
No products indexed under this heading.

Ranitidine Hydrochloride (Co-administration may increase plasma phenytoin concentration). Products include:
Zantac 1690
Zantac Injection 1688
Zantac 75 Tablets .... ▣717

Reserpine (Co-administration may decrease plasma phenytoin concentration).
No products indexed under this heading.

Rifampin (Efficacy of rifampin is impaired by phenytoin). Products include:
Rifadin 765
Rifamate Capsules 767
Rifater Tablets 769

Salsalate (Co-administration may increase plasma phenytoin concentration).
No products indexed under this heading.

Sulfacytine (Co-administration with sulfonamides may increase plasma phenytoin concentration).

Sulfamethizole (Co-administration with sulfonamides may increase plasma phenytoin concentration). Products include:
Urobiotic-250 Capsules 2731

Sulfamethoxazole (Co-administration with sulfonamides may increase plasma phenytoin concentration). Products include:
Bactrim 2949
Septra Suspension 2265
Septra Tablets 2265
Septra DS Tablets 2265

Sulfasalazine (Co-administration with sulfonamides may increase plasma phenytoin concentration). Products include:
Azulfidine EN-tabs Tablets 2775

Sulfinpyrazone (Co-administration with sulfonamides may increase plasma phenytoin concentration).
No products indexed under this heading.

Sulfisoxazole (Co-administration with sulfonamides may increase plasma phenytoin concentration).
No products indexed under this heading.

Sulfisoxazole Acetyl (Co-administration with sulfonamides may increase plasma phenytoin concentration). Products include:
Pediazole Suspension 3050

Sulfisoxazole Diolamine (Co-administration with sulfonamides may increase plasma phenytoin concentration).
No products indexed under this heading.

Theophylline (Efficacy of theophylline is impaired by phenytoin). Products include:
Aerolate 1361
Theo-Dur Extended-Release Tablets 1835
Uni-Dur Extended-Release Tablets 1841
Uniphyl 400 mg and 600 mg Tablets 2903

Theophylline Calcium Salicylate (Efficacy of theophylline is impaired by phenytoin).
No products indexed under this heading.

Theophylline Sodium Glycinate (Efficacy of theophylline is impaired by phenytoin).
No products indexed under this heading.

Thioridazine Hydrochloride (Co-administration with phenothiazines may increase plasma phenytoin concentration). Products include:
Thioridazine Hydrochloride Tablets 2289

Tolazamide (Co-administration with sulfonamides may increase plasma phenytoin concentration).
No products indexed under this heading.

Tolbutamide (Co-administration may increase plasma phenytoin concentration).
No products indexed under this heading.

Trazodone Hydrochloride (Co-administration may increase plasma phenytoin concentration).
No products indexed under this heading.

Triamcinolone (Efficacy of corticosteroids is impaired by phenytoin).
No products indexed under this heading.

Triamcinolone Acetonide (Efficacy of corticosteroids is impaired by phenytoin). Products include:
Azmacort Inhalation Aerosol 728
Nasacort Nasal Inhaler 750

IMPORTANT NOTE: Always consult each drug listing in the patient's regimen for possible interactions.

Nasacort AQ Nasal Spray 752
Tri-Nasal Spray 2274

Triamcinolone Diacetate (Efficacy of corticosteroids is impaired by phenytoin).
No products indexed under this heading.

Triamcinolone Hexacetonide (Efficacy of corticosteroids is impaired by phenytoin).
No products indexed under this heading.

Trifluoperazine Hydrochloride (Co-administration with phenothiazines may increase plasma phenytoin concentration). Products include:
Stelazine 1640

Trimipramine Maleate (Tricyclic antidepressants may precipitate seizures in susceptible patients; Cerebyx dosage may need to be adjusted). Products include:
Surmontil Capsules 3595

Valproic Acid (Co-administration may result in either decrease or increase in plasma phenytoin concentrations; unpredictable effect of phenytoin on valproic acid plasma concentrations). Products include:
Depakene 421

Vitamin D (Efficacy of vitamin D is impaired by phenytoin). Products include:
Active Calcium Tablets 3335
Caltrate 600 PLUS .... ■815
Caltrate 600 + D Tablets .... ■814
Centrum Focused Formulas Bone Health Tablets .... ■815
Citracal Caplets + D .... ■823
D-Cal Chewable Caplets .... ■794
One-A-Day Calcium Plus Chewable Tablets .... ■805
Os-Cal 250 + D Tablets .... ■838
Os-Cal 500 + D Tablets .... ■839

Warfarin Sodium (Efficacy of coumarin is impaired by phenytoin). Products include:
Coumadin for Injection 1243
Coumadin Tablets 1243
Warfarin Sodium Tablets, USP 3302

Food Interactions

Alcohol (Acute alcohol intake may increase plasma phenytoin concentration; chronic alcohol abuse may decrease plasma phenytoin concentration).

CEREZYME FOR INJECTION

(Imiglucerase) 1438
None cited in PDR database.

CERTS COOL MINT DROPS

(Breath Freshener) .... ■685
None cited in PDR database.

CERTS POWERFUL MINTS

(Breath Freshener) .... ■686
None cited in PDR database.

CERUBIDINE FOR INJECTION

(Daunorubicin Hydrochloride) 947
May interact with:

Bone Marrow Depressants, unspecified (Therapy with Cerubidine should not be started in patients with pre-existing drug-induced myelosuppression).

Cyclophosphamide (Co-administration increases the risk of cardiotoxicity).
No products indexed under this heading.

Doxorubicin Hydrochloride (Use of daunorubicin in a patient who has previously received doxorubicin increases the risk of cardiotoxicity; daunorubicin should not be used in patients who have previously received the recommended maximum cumulative doses of doxorubicin or daunorubicin). Products include:
Adriamycin PFS/RDF Injection 2767
Doxil Injection 566

Methotrexate Sodium (Co-administration with hepatotoxic drugs, such as methotrexate, may impair liver function and increase the risk of toxicity).
No products indexed under this heading.

CERUMENEX EARDROPS

(Triethanolamine Polypeptide Oleate-Condensate) 2895
None cited in PDR database.

CERVIDIL VAGINAL INSERT

(Dinoprostone) 1369
May interact with oxytocic drugs. Compounds in these categories include:

Ergonovine Maleate (Dinoprostone may augment the activity of oxytocic agents and concomitant use is not recommended; a dosing interval of at least 30 minutes is recommended for sequential use).
No products indexed under this heading.

Methylergonovine Maleate (Dinoprostone may augment the activity of oxytocic agents and concomitant use is not recommended; a dosing interval of at least 30 minutes is recommended for sequential use).
No products indexed under this heading.

Oxytocin (Dinoprostone may augment the activity of oxytocic agents and concomitant use is not recommended; a dosing interval of at least 30 minutes is recommended for sequential use).
No products indexed under this heading.

CETACAINE TOPICAL ANESTHETIC

(Benzocaine, Butyl Aminobenzoate, Tetracaine Hydrochloride) 1196
None cited in PDR database.

CETROTIDE FOR INJECTION

(Cetrorelix Acetate) 3209
None cited in PDR database.

C-GRAMS CAPLETS

(Vitamin C) .... ■795
None cited in PDR database.

CHELATED MINERAL TABLETS

(Minerals, Multiple) 3335
None cited in PDR database.

CHEMET CAPSULES

(Succimer) 3078
May interact with:

Calcium Disodium Edetate (Concomitant administration is not recommended). Products include:
Calcium Disodium Versenate Injection 1980

CHIBROXIN STERILE OPHTHALMIC SOLUTION

(Norfloxacin) 2051
May interact with oral anticoagulants, theophylline, and certain other agents. Compounds in these categories include:

Aminophylline (Potential elevation of serum theophylline concentrations).
No products indexed under this heading.

Caffeine (Interferes with the metabolism of caffeine). Products include:
BC Powder .... ■619
Arthritis Strength BC Powder .... ■619
Darvon Compound-65 Pulvules 1910
Aspirin Free Excedrin Caplets and Geltabs .... ■628
Excedrin Extra-Strength Tablets, Caplets, and Geltabs .... ■629
Excedrin Migraine 1070
Goody's Extra Strength Headache Powder .... ■620
Goody's Extra Strength Pain Relief Tablets .... ■620
Hycomine Compound Tablets 1317
Maximum Strength Midol Menstrual Caplets and Gelcaps .... ■612
Vanquish Caplets .... ■617
Vivarin .... ■763

Cyclosporine (Elevated serum levels of cyclosporine). Products include:
Gengraf Capsules 457
Neoral Soft Gelatin Capsules 2380
Neoral Oral Solution 2380
Sandimmune 2388

Dicumarol (Enhanced effects of anticoagulant).
No products indexed under this heading.

Dyphylline (Potential elevation of serum theophylline concentrations). Products include:
Lufyllin Tablets 3347
Lufyllin-400 Tablets 3347
Lufyllin-GG Elixir 3348
Lufyllin-GG Tablets 3348

Theophylline (Potential elevation of serum theophylline concentrations). Products include:
Aerolate 1361
Theo-Dur Extended-Release Tablets 1835
Uni-Dur Extended-Release Tablets 1841
Uniphyl 400 mg and 600 mg Tablets 2903

Theophylline Calcium Salicylate (Potential elevation of serum theophylline concentrations).
No products indexed under this heading.

Theophylline Sodium Glycinate (Potential elevation of serum theophylline concentrations).
No products indexed under this heading.

Warfarin Sodium (Enhanced effects of anticoagulant). Products include:
Coumadin for Injection 1243
Coumadin Tablets 1243
Warfarin Sodium Tablets, USP 3302

CHIROCAINE INJECTION

(Levobupivacaine Hydrochloride) 2909
May interact with erythromycin, local anesthetics, phenytoin, and certain other agents. Compounds in these categories include:

Bupivacaine Hydrochloride (Co-administration with other local anesthetics may produce additive toxic effects). Products include:
Sensorcaine 643
Sensorcaine-MPF Injection 643

Chloroprocaine Hydrochloride (Co-administration with other local anesthetics may produce additive toxic effects). Products include:
Nesacaine/Nesacaine MPF 617

Clarithromycin (In vitro studies indicate CYP3A4 and CYP1A2 mediate the metabolism of levobupivacaine; it is likely that the metabolism of levobupivacaine may be affected by the known CYP1A2 inhibitors, such as clarithromycin). Products include:
Biaxin/Biaxin XL 403
PREVPAC 3298

Erythromycin (In vitro studies indicate CYP3A4 and CYP1A2 mediate the metabolism of levobupivacaine; it is likely that the metabolism of levobupivacaine may be affected by the known CYP3A4 inhibitors, such as erythromycin). Products include:
Emgel 2% Topical Gel 1285
Ery-Tab Tablets 448
Erythromycin Base Filmtab Tablets 454
Erythromycin Delayed-Release Capsules, USP 455
PCE Dispertab Tablets 498

Erythromycin Estolate (In vitro studies indicate CYP3A4 and CYP1A2 mediate the metabolism of levobupivacaine; it is likely that the metabolism of levobupivacaine may be affected by the known CYP3A4 inhibitors, such as erythromycin).
No products indexed under this heading.

Erythromycin Ethylsuccinate (In vitro studies indicate CYP3A4 and CYP1A2 mediate the metabolism of levobupivacaine; it is likely that the metabolism of levobupivacaine may be affected by the known CYP3A4 inhibitors, such as erythromycin). Products include:
E.E.S. 450
EryPed 446
Pediazole Suspension 3050

Erythromycin Gluceptate (In vitro studies indicate CYP3A4 and CYP1A2 mediate the metabolism of levobupivacaine; it is likely that the metabolism of levobupivacaine may be affected by the known CYP3A4 inhibitors, such as erythromycin).
No products indexed under this heading.

Erythromycin Stearate (In vitro studies indicate CYP3A4 and CYP1A2 mediate the metabolism of levobupivacaine; it is likely that the metabolism of levobupivacaine may be affected by the known CYP3A4 inhibitors, such as erythromycin). Products include:
Erythrocin Stearate Filmtab Tablets 452

Etidocaine Hydrochloride (Co-administration with other local anesthetics may produce additive toxic effects). Products include:
Duranest Injections 600

Fosphenytoin Sodium (In vitro studies indicate CYP3A4 and CYP1A2 mediate the metabolism of levobupivacaine; it is likely that the metabolism of levobupivacaine may be affected by the known CYP3A4 inducers, such as phenytoin). Products include:
Cerebyx Injection 2619

Furafylline (In vitro studies indicate CYP3A4 and CYP1A2 mediate the metabolism of levobupivacaine; it is likely that the metabolism of levobupivacaine may be affected by the known CYP1A2 inhibitors, such as furafylline).
No products indexed under this heading.

Ketoconazole (In vitro studies indicate CYP3A4 and CYP1A2 mediate the metabolism of levobupivacaine; it is likely that the metabolism of levobupivacaine may be affected by the known CYP3A4 inhibitors, such as azole antimycotics ketoconazole). Products include:
Nizoral 2% Cream 3620
Nizoral A-D Shampoo 2008
Nizoral 2% Shampoo 2007
Nizoral Tablets 1791

Lidocaine Hydrochloride (Co-administration with other local anesthetics may produce additive toxic effects). Products include:
Bactine First Aid Liquid .... ■611
Xylocaine Injections 653

Mepivacaine Hydrochloride (Co-administration with other local anesthetics may produce additive toxic effects). Products include:
Polocaine Injection, USP 625
Polocaine-MPF Injection, USP 625

Omeprazole (In vitro studies indicate CYP3A4 and CYP1A2 mediate the metabolism of levobupivacaine; it is likely that the metabolism of

levobupivacaine may be affected by the known CYP1A2 inducers, such as omeprazole). Products include:
- Prilosec Delayed-Release Capsules 628

Phenobarbital (In vitro studies indicate CYP3A4 and CYP1A2 mediate the metabolism of levobupivacaine; it is likely that the metabolism of levobupivacaine may be affected by the known CYP3A4 inducers, such as phenobarbital). Products include:
- Arco-Lase Plus Tablets 592
- Donnatal 2929
- Donnatal Extentabs 2930

Phenytoin (In vitro studies indicate CYP3A4 and CYP1A2 mediate the metabolism of levobupivacaine; it is likely that the metabolism of levobupivacaine may be affected by the known CYP3A4 inducers, such as phenytoin). Products include:
- Dilantin Infatabs 2624
- Dilantin-125 Oral Suspension 2625

Phenytoin Sodium (In vitro studies indicate CYP3A4 and CYP1A2 mediate the metabolism of levobupivacaine; it is likely that the metabolism of levobupivacaine may be affected by the known CYP3A4 inducers, such as phenytoin). Products include:
- Dilantin Kapseals 2622

Procaine Hydrochloride (Co-administration with other local anesthetics may produce additive toxic effects).
- No products indexed under this heading.

Rifampin (In vitro studies indicate CYP3A4 and CYP1A2 mediate the metabolism of levobupivacaine; it is likely that the metabolism of levobupivacaine may be affected by the known CYP3A4 inducers, such as rifampin). Products include:
- Rifadin 765
- Rifamate Capsules 767
- Rifater Tablets 769

Ritonavir (In vitro studies indicate CYP3A4 and CYP1A2 mediate the metabolism of levobupivacaine; it is likely that the metabolism of levobupivacaine may be affected by the known CYP3A4 inhibitors, such as protease inhibitor ritonavir). Products include:
- Kaletra Capsules 471
- Kaletra Oral Solution 471
- Norvir Capsules 487
- Norvir Oral Solution 487

Tetracaine Hydrochloride (Co-administration with other local anesthetics may produce additive toxic effects). Products include:
- Cēpacol Viractin Cold Sore and Fever Blister Treatment, Gel .... ▣788
- Cetacaine Topical Anesthetic 1196

Verapamil Hydrochloride (In vitro studies indicate CYP3A4 and CYP1A2 mediate the metabolism of levobupivacaine; it is likely that the metabolism of levobupivacaine may be affected by the known CYP3A4 inhibitors, such as verapamil). Products include:
- Covera-HS Tablets 3199
- Isoptin SR Tablets 467
- Tarka Tablets 508
- Verelan Capsules 3184
- Verelan PM Capsules 3186

CHLOR-3
(Potassium Chloride) 1361
None cited in PDR database.

CHLOROMYCETIN OPHTHALMIC OINTMENT, 1%
(Chloramphenicol) .... ⊙296
None cited in PDR database.

CHLOROMYCETIN OPHTHALMIC SOLUTION
(Chloramphenicol) .... ⊙297
None cited in PDR database.

CHLOROPTIC STERILE OPHTHALMIC OINTMENT
(Chloramphenicol) .... ⊙234
None cited in PDR database.

CHLOROPTIC STERILE OPHTHALMIC SOLUTION
(Chloramphenicol) .... ⊙235
None cited in PDR database.

CHLOR-TRIMETON ALLERGY TABLETS
(Chlorpheniramine Maleate) .... ▣735
May interact with hypnotics and sedatives, tranquilizers, and certain other agents. Compounds in these categories include:

Alprazolam (May increase drowsiness effect). Products include:
- Xanax Tablets 2865

Buspirone Hydrochloride (May increase drowsiness effect).
- No products indexed under this heading.

Chlordiazepoxide (May increase drowsiness effect). Products include:
- Limbitrol 1738

Chlordiazepoxide Hydrochloride (May increase drowsiness effect). Products include:
- Librium Capsules 1736
- Librium for Injection 1737

Chlorpromazine (May increase drowsiness effect). Products include:
- Thorazine Suppositories 1656

Chlorpromazine Hydrochloride (May increase drowsiness effect). Products include:
- Thorazine 1656

Chlorprothixene (May increase drowsiness effect).
- No products indexed under this heading.

Chlorprothixene Hydrochloride (May increase drowsiness effect).
- No products indexed under this heading.

Clorazepate Dipotassium (May increase drowsiness effect). Products include:
- Tranxene 511

Diazepam (May increase drowsiness effect). Products include:
- Valium Injectable 3026
- Valium Tablets 3047

Droperidol (May increase drowsiness effect).
- No products indexed under this heading.

Estazolam (May increase drowsiness effect). Products include:
- ProSom Tablets 500

Ethchlorvynol (May increase drowsiness effect).
- No products indexed under this heading.

Ethinamate (May increase drowsiness effect).
- No products indexed under this heading.

Fluphenazine Decanoate (May increase drowsiness effect).
- No products indexed under this heading.

Fluphenazine Enanthate (May increase drowsiness effect).
- No products indexed under this heading.

Fluphenazine Hydrochloride (May increase drowsiness effect).
- No products indexed under this heading.

Flurazepam Hydrochloride (May increase drowsiness effect).
- No products indexed under this heading.

Glutethimide (May increase drowsiness effect).
- No products indexed under this heading.

Haloperidol (May increase drowsiness effect). Products include:
- Haldol Injection, Tablets and Concentrate 2533

Haloperidol Decanoate (May increase drowsiness effect). Products include:
- Haldol Decanoate 2535

Hydroxyzine Hydrochloride (May increase drowsiness effect). Products include:
- Atarax Tablets & Syrup 2667
- Vistaril Intramuscular Solution 2738

Lorazepam (May increase drowsiness effect). Products include:
- Ativan Injection 3478
- Ativan Tablets 3482

Loxapine Hydrochloride (May increase drowsiness effect).
- No products indexed under this heading.

Loxapine Succinate (May increase drowsiness effect). Products include:
- Loxitane Capsules 3398

Meprobamate (May increase drowsiness effect). Products include:
- Miltown Tablets 3349

Mesoridazine Besylate (May increase drowsiness effect). Products include:
- Serentil 1057

Midazolam Hydrochloride (May increase drowsiness effect). Products include:
- Versed Injection 3027
- Versed Syrup 3033

Molindone Hydrochloride (May increase drowsiness effect). Products include:
- Moban 1320

Oxazepam (May increase drowsiness effect).
- No products indexed under this heading.

Perphenazine (May increase drowsiness effect). Products include:
- Etrafon 3115
- Trilafon 3160

Prazepam (May increase drowsiness effect).
- No products indexed under this heading.

Prochlorperazine (May increase drowsiness effect). Products include:
- Compazine 1505

Promethazine Hydrochloride (May increase drowsiness effect). Products include:
- Mepergan Injection 3539
- Phenergan Injection 3553
- Phenergan 3556
- Phenergan Syrup 3554
- Phenergan with Codeine Syrup 3557
- Phenergan with Dextromethorphan Syrup 3559
- Phenergan VC Syrup 3560
- Phenergan VC with Codeine Syrup 3561

Propofol (May increase drowsiness effect). Products include:
- Diprivan Injectable Emulsion 667

Quazepam (May increase drowsiness effect).
- No products indexed under this heading.

Secobarbital Sodium (May increase drowsiness effect).
- No products indexed under this heading.

Temazepam (May increase drowsiness effect).
- No products indexed under this heading.

Thioridazine Hydrochloride (May increase drowsiness effect). Products include:
- Thioridazine Hydrochloride Tablets 2289

Thiothixene (May increase drowsiness effect). Products include:
- Navane Capsules 2701
- Thiothixene Capsules 2290

Triazolam (May increase drowsiness effect). Products include:
- Halcion Tablets 2823

Trifluoperazine Hydrochloride (May increase drowsiness effect). Products include:
- Stelazine 1640

Zaleplon (May increase drowsiness effect). Products include:
- Sonata Capsules 3591

Zolpidem Tartrate (May increase drowsiness effect). Products include:
- Ambien Tablets 3191

Food Interactions

Alcohol (May increase drowsiness effect, avoid alcoholic beverages).

CHLOR-TRIMETON ALLERGY/ DECONGESTANT TABLETS
(Chlorpheniramine Maleate, Pseudoephedrine Sulfate) .... ▣736
May interact with hypnotics and sedatives, monoamine oxidase inhibitors, tranquilizers, and certain other agents. Compounds in these categories include:

Alprazolam (May increase drowsiness effect). Products include:
- Xanax Tablets 2865

Buspirone Hydrochloride (May increase drowsiness effect).
- No products indexed under this heading.

Chlordiazepoxide (May increase drowsiness effect). Products include:
- Limbitrol 1738

Chlordiazepoxide Hydrochloride (May increase drowsiness effect). Products include:
- Librium Capsules 1736
- Librium for Injection 1737

Chlorpromazine (May increase drowsiness effect). Products include:
- Thorazine Suppositories 1656

Chlorpromazine Hydrochloride (May increase drowsiness effect). Products include:
- Thorazine 1656

Chlorprothixene (May increase drowsiness effect).
- No products indexed under this heading.

Chlorprothixene Hydrochloride (May increase drowsiness effect).
- No products indexed under this heading.

Clorazepate Dipotassium (May increase drowsiness effect). Products include:
- Tranxene 511

Diazepam (May increase drowsiness effect). Products include:
- Valium Injectable 3026
- Valium Tablets 3047

Droperidol (May increase drowsiness effect).
- No products indexed under this heading.

Estazolam (May increase drowsiness effect). Products include:
- ProSom Tablets 500

Ethchlorvynol (May increase drowsiness effect).
- No products indexed under this heading.

Ethinamate (May increase drowsiness effect).
- No products indexed under this heading.

Fluphenazine Decanoate (May increase drowsiness effect).
- No products indexed under this heading.

Fluphenazine Enanthate (May increase drowsiness effect).
- No products indexed under this heading.

Fluphenazine Hydrochloride (May increase drowsiness effect).
- No products indexed under this heading.

Flurazepam Hydrochloride (May increase drowsiness effect).
No products indexed under this heading.

Glutethimide (May increase drowsiness effect).
No products indexed under this heading.

Haloperidol (May increase drowsiness effect). Products include:
- Haldol Injection, Tablets and Concentrate ... 2533

Haloperidol Decanoate (May increase drowsiness effect). Products include:
- Haldol Decanoate ... 2535

Hydroxyzine Hydrochloride (May increase drowsiness effect). Products include:
- Atarax Tablets & Syrup ... 2667
- Vistaril Intramuscular Solution ... 2738

Isocarboxazid (Concurrent and/or sequential use is not recommended).
No products indexed under this heading.

Lorazepam (May increase drowsiness effect). Products include:
- Ativan Injection ... 3478
- Ativan Tablets ... 3482

Loxapine Hydrochloride (May increase drowsiness effect).
No products indexed under this heading.

Loxapine Succinate (May increase drowsiness effect). Products include:
- Loxitane Capsules ... 3398

Meprobamate (May increase drowsiness effect). Products include:
- Miltown Tablets ... 3349

Mesoridazine Besylate (May increase drowsiness effect). Products include:
- Serentil ... 1057

Midazolam Hydrochloride (May increase drowsiness effect). Products include:
- Versed Injection ... 3027
- Versed Syrup ... 3033

Moclobemide (Concurrent and/or sequential use is not recommended).
No products indexed under this heading.

Molindone Hydrochloride (May increase drowsiness effect). Products include:
- Moban ... 1320

Oxazepam (May increase drowsiness effect).
No products indexed under this heading.

Pargyline Hydrochloride (Concurrent and/or sequential use is not recommended).
No products indexed under this heading.

Perphenazine (May increase drowsiness effect). Products include:
- Etrafon ... 3115
- Trilafon ... 3160

Phenelzine Sulfate (Concurrent and/or sequential use is not recommended). Products include:
- Nardil Tablets ... 2653

Prazepam (May increase drowsiness effect).
No products indexed under this heading.

Procarbazine Hydrochloride (Concurrent and/or sequential use is not recommended). Products include:
- Matulane Capsules ... 3246

Prochlorperazine (May increase drowsiness effect). Products include:
- Compazine ... 1505

Promethazine Hydrochloride (May increase drowsiness effect). Products include:
- Mepergan Injection ... 3539
- Phenergan Injection ... 3553
- Phenergan ... 3556
- Phenergan Syrup ... 3554
- Phenergan with Codeine Syrup ... 3557
- Phenergan with Dextromethorphan Syrup ... 3559
- Phenergan VC Syrup ... 3560
- Phenergan VC with Codeine Syrup ... 3561

Propofol (May increase drowsiness effect). Products include:
- Diprivan Injectable Emulsion ... 667

Quazepam (May increase drowsiness effect).
No products indexed under this heading.

Secobarbital Sodium (May increase drowsiness effect).
No products indexed under this heading.

Selegiline Hydrochloride (Concurrent and/or sequential use is not recommended). Products include:
- Eldepryl Capsules ... 3266

Temazepam (May increase drowsiness effect).
No products indexed under this heading.

Thioridazine Hydrochloride (May increase drowsiness effect). Products include:
- Thioridazine Hydrochloride Tablets ... 2289

Thiothixene (May increase drowsiness effect). Products include:
- Navane Capsules ... 2701
- Thiothixene Capsules ... 2290

Tranylcypromine Sulfate (Concurrent and/or sequential use is not recommended). Products include:
- Parnate Tablets ... 1607

Triazolam (May increase drowsiness effect). Products include:
- Halcion Tablets ... 2823

Trifluoperazine Hydrochloride (May increase drowsiness effect). Products include:
- Stelazine ... 1640

Zaleplon (May increase drowsiness effect). Products include:
- Sonata Capsules ... 3591

Zolpidem Tartrate (May increase drowsiness effect). Products include:
- Ambien Tablets ... 3191

Food Interactions

Alcohol (May increase drowsiness effect).

NEW FORMULATION CHROMAGEN OB CAPSULES

(Ferrous Fumarate, Vitamins, Prenatal, Vitamins with Minerals) ... 3094
None cited in PDR database.

CILOXAN OPHTHALMIC OINTMENT

(Ciprofloxacin Hydrochloride) ... 538
See Ciloxan Ophthalmic Solution

CILOXAN OPHTHALMIC SOLUTION

(Ciprofloxacin Hydrochloride) ... 538
May interact with oral anticoagulants, theophylline, and certain other agents. Compounds in these categories include:

Aminophylline (Systemic administration of quinolones elevates plasma concentrations of theophylline).
No products indexed under this heading.

Caffeine-containing medications (Interference with caffeine metabolism with systemic quinolones).
No products indexed under this heading.

Cyclosporine (Concomitant administration with systemic quinolones may result in transient elevations in serum creatinine). Products include:
- Gengraf Capsules ... 457
- Neoral Soft Gelatin Capsules ... 2380
- Neoral Oral Solution ... 2380
- Sandimmune ... 2388

Dicumarol (Enhanced anticoagulant effect with systemic quinolones).
No products indexed under this heading.

Dyphylline (Systemic administration of quinolones elevates plasma concentrations of theophylline). Products include:
- Lufyllin Tablets ... 3347
- Lufyllin-400 Tablets ... 3347
- Lufyllin-GG Elixir ... 3348
- Lufyllin-GG Tablets ... 3348

Theophylline (Systemic administration of quinolones elevates plasma concentrations of theophylline). Products include:
- Aerolate ... 1361
- Theo-Dur Extended-Release Tablets ... 1835
- Uni-Dur Extended-Release Tablets ... 1841
- Uniphyl 400 mg and 600 mg Tablets ... 2903

Theophylline Calcium Salicylate (Systemic administration of quinolones elevates plasma concentrations of theophylline).
No products indexed under this heading.

Theophylline Sodium Glycinate (Systemic administration of quinolones elevates plasma concentrations of theophylline).
No products indexed under this heading.

Warfarin Sodium (Enhanced anticoagulant effect with systemic quinolones). Products include:
- Coumadin for Injection ... 1243
- Coumadin Tablets ... 1243
- Warfarin Sodium Tablets, USP ... 3302

CIPRO HC OTIC SUSPENSION

(Ciprofloxacin Hydrochloride, Hydrocortisone) ... 540
None cited in PDR database.

CIPRO I.V.

(Ciprofloxacin) ... 893
See Cipro Tablets

CIPRO I.V. PHARMACY BULK PACKAGE

(Ciprofloxacin) ... 897
See Cipro Tablets

CIPRO ORAL SUSPENSION

(Ciprofloxacin) ... 887
See Cipro Tablets

CIPRO TABLETS

(Ciprofloxacin Hydrochloride) ... 887
May interact with antacids containing aluminum, calcium and magnesium, calcium preparations, oral anticoagulants, iron containing oral preparations, phenytoin, theophylline, and certain other agents. Compounds in these categories include:

Aluminum Carbonate (Concurrent administration of these antacids may substantially interfere with the oral absorption of ciprofloxacin; antacids may be administered either 2 hours after or 6 hours before ciprofloxacin dosing without a significant decrease in bioavailability).
No products indexed under this heading.

Aluminum Hydroxide (Concurrent administration of these antacids may substantially interfere with the oral absorption of ciprofloxacin; antacids may be administered either 2 hours after or 6 hours before ciprofloxacin dosing without a significant decrease in bioavailability). Products include:
- Amphojel Suspension (Mint Flavor) ... ▣789
- Gaviscon Extra Strength Liquid ... ▣751
- Gaviscon Extra Strength Tablets ... ▣751
- Gaviscon Regular Strength Liquid ... ▣751
- Gaviscon Regular Strength Tablets ... ▣750
- Maalox Antacid/Anti-Gas Oral Suspension ... ▣673
- Maalox Max Maximum Strength Antacid/Anti-Gas Liquid ... 2300
- Maalox Regular Strength Antacid/Antigas Liquid ... 2300
- Mylanta ... 1813
- Vanquish Caplets ... ▣617

Aminophylline (Potential for severe and fatal reactions including cardiac arrest, seizures, respiratory failure and status epilepticus; concurrent use should be avoided or serum levels of theophylline should be monitored carefully).
No products indexed under this heading.

Caffeine (Reduced clearance of caffeine and a prolongation of its serum half-life). Products include:
- BC Powder ... ▣619
- Arthritis Strength BC Powder ... ▣619
- Darvon Compound-65 Pulvules ... 1910
- Aspirin Free Excedrin Caplets and Geltabs ... ▣628
- Excedrin Extra-Strength Tablets, Caplets, and Geltabs ... ▣629
- Excedrin Migraine ... 1070
- Goody's Extra Strength Headache Powder ... ▣620
- Goody's Extra Strength Pain Relief Tablets ... ▣620
- Hycomine Compound Tablets ... 1317
- Maximum Strength Midol Menstrual Caplets and Gelcaps ... ▣612
- Vanquish Caplets ... ▣617
- Vivarin ... ▣763

Calcium Carbonate (Co-administration with calcium-containing products may substantially interfere with the oral absorption of quinolones; these preparations may be taken six hours before or two hours after taking ciprofloxacin). Products include:
- Aspirin Regimen Bayer 81 mg Caplets with Calcium ... ▣607
- Extra Strength Bayer Plus Caplets ... ▣610
- Caltrate 600 Tablets ... ▣814
- Caltrate 600 PLUS ... ▣815
- Caltrate 600 + D Tablets ... ▣814
- Caltrate 600 + Soy Tablets ... ▣814
- D-Cal Chewable Caplets ... ▣794
- Florical Capsules and Tablets ... 2223
- Quick Dissolve Maalox Max Maximum Strength Antacid/Antigas Tablets ... 2301
- Quick Dissolve Maalox Regular Strength Antacid Tablets ... 2301
- Marblen Suspension ... ▣633
- Monocal Tablets ... 2223
- Mylanta Fast-Acting ... 1813
- Mylanta Calci Tabs ... ▣636
- One-A-Day Bedtime & Rest Tablets ... ▣805
- One-A-Day Calcium Plus Chewable Tablets ... ▣805
- Os-Cal Chewable Tablets ... ▣838
- Pepcid Complete Chewable Tablets ... 1815
- ReSource Wellness CalciWise Soft Chews ... ▣824
- Rolaids Tablets ... ▣706
- Extra Strength Rolaids Tablets ... ▣706
- Slow-Mag Tablets ... ▣835
- Titralac ... ▣640
- 3M Titralac Plus Antacid Tablets ... ▣640
- Tums ... ▣763

Calcium Chloride (Co-administration with calcium-containing products may substantially interfere with the oral absorption of quinolones; these preparations may be taken six hours before or two hours after taking ciprofloxacin).
No products indexed under this heading.

Calcium Citrate (Co-administration with calcium-containing products may substantially interfere with the oral absorption of quinolones; these preparations may be taken six hours before or two hours after taking ciprofloxacin). Products include:
- Active Calcium Tablets ... 3335
- Citracal Liquitab Tablets ... ▣823
- Citracal Tablets ... 2231
- Citracal Caplets + D ... ▣823

Calcium Glubionate (Co-administration with calcium-containing products may substantially interfere with the oral absorption of quinolones; these preparations

may be taken six hours before or two hours after taking ciprofloxacin).
No products indexed under this heading.

Cyclosporine (Transient elevations in serum creatinine). Products include:
Gengraf Capsules 457
Neoral Soft Gelatin Capsules 2380
Neoral Oral Solution 2380
Sandimmune 2388

Dicumarol (Enhanced effects of anticoagulant).
No products indexed under this heading.

Didanosine (Didanosine (Videx) chewable tablets or pediatric powder for oral solution contains aluminum-magnesium-based antacid; co-administration may interfere with Cipro oral aborption; these preparations may be taken six hours before or two hours after taking ciprofloxacin). Products include:
Videx 1138
Videx EC Capsules 1143

Dyphylline (Potential for severe and fatal reactions including cardiac arrest, seizures, respiratory failure and status epilepticus; concurrent use should be avoided or serum levels of theophylline should be monitored carefully). Products include:
Lufyllin Tablets 3347
Lufyllin-400 Tablets 3347
Lufyllin-GG Elixir 3348
Lufyllin-GG Tablets 3348

Ferrous Fumarate (Co-administration with iron-containing products may substantially interfere with the oral absorption of quinolones; these preparations may be taken six hours before or two hours after taking ciprofloxacin). Products include:
New Formulation Chromagen OB Capsules 3094
Loestrin Fe Tablets 2642
NataChew Tablets 3364

Ferrous Gluconate (Co-administration with iron-containing products may substantially interfere with the oral absorption of quinolones; these preparations may be taken six hours before or two hours after taking ciprofloxacin). Products include:
Fergon Iron Tablets .... ◙802

Ferrous Sulfate (Co-administration with iron-containing products may substantially interfere with the oral absorption of quinolones; these preparations may be taken six hours before or two hours after taking ciprofloxacin). Products include:
Feosol Tablets 1717
Slow Fe Tablets .... ◙827
Slow Fe with Folic Acid Tablets ...... ◙828

Fosphenytoin Sodium (Potential for change in serum phenytoin levels). Products include:
Cerebyx Injection 2619

Glyburide (Co-administration, on rare occasions, has resulted in severe hypoglycemia). Products include:
DiaBeta Tablets 741
Glucovance Tablets 1086

Iron (Co-administration with iron-containing products may substantially interfere with the oral absorption of quinolones; these preparations may be taken six hours before or two hours after taking ciprofloxacin).
No products indexed under this heading.

Magaldrate (Concurrent administration of these antacids may substantially interfere with the oral absorption of ciprofloxacin; antacids may be administered either 2 hours after or 6 hours before ciprofloxacin dosing without a significant decrease in bioavailability).
No products indexed under this heading.

Magnesium Hydroxide (Concurrent administration of these antacids may substantially interfere with the oral absorption of ciprofloxacin; antacids may be administered either 2 hours after or 6 hours before ciprofloxacin dosing without a significant decrease in bioavailability). Products include:
Ex•Lax Milk of Magnesia Liquid .... ◙670
Maalox Antacid/Anti-Gas Oral Suspension.. ◙673
Maalox Max Maximum Strength Antacid/Anti-Gas Liquid 2300
Maalox Regular Strength Antacid/Antigas Liquid 2300
Mylanta Fast-Acting 1813
Mylanta 1813
Pepcid Complete Chewable Tablets... 1815
Phillips' Chewable Tablets .... ◙615
Phillips' Milk of Magnesia Liquid (Original, Cherry, & Mint) .... ◙616
Rolaids Tablets .... ◙706
Extra Strength Rolaids Tablets ...... ◙706
Vanquish Caplets .... ◙617

Magnesium Oxide (Concurrent administration of these antacids may substantially interfere with the oral absorption of ciprofloxacin; antacids may be administered either 2 hours after or 6 hours before ciprofloxacin dosing without a significant decrease in bioavailability). Products include:
Beelith Tablets 946
Mag-Ox 400 Tablets 1024
Uro-Mag Capsules 1024

Phenytoin (Potential for change in serum phenytoin levels). Products include:
Dilantin Infatabs 2624
Dilantin-125 Oral Suspension 2625

Phenytoin Sodium (Potential for change in serum phenytoin levels). Products include:
Dilantin Kapseals 2622

Polysaccharide-Iron Complex (Co-administration with iron-containing products may substantially interfere with the oral absorption of quinolones; these preparations may be taken six hours before or two hours after taking ciprofloxacin). Products include:
Niferex 3176
Niferex-150 Capsules 3176
Nu-Iron 150 Capsules 2224

Probenecid (Interferes with renal tubular secretion of ciprofloxacin).
No products indexed under this heading.

Sucralfate (Co-administration with sucralfate may substantially interfere with the oral aborption of quinolones; these preparations may be taken six hours before or two hours after taking ciprofloxacin). Products include:
Carafate Suspension 731
Carafate Tablets 730

Theophylline (Potential for severe and fatal reactions including cardiac arrest, seizures, respiratory failure and status epilepticus; concurrent use should be avoided or serum levels of theophylline should be monitored carefully). Products include:
Aerolate 1361
Theo-Dur Extended-Release Tablets 1835
Uni-Dur Extended-Release Tablets .. 1841
Uniphyl 400 mg and 600 mg Tablets 2903

Theophylline Calcium Salicylate (Potential for severe and fatal reactions including cardiac arrest, seizures, respiratory failure and status epilepticus; concurrent use should be avoided or serum levels of theophylline should be monitored carefully).
No products indexed under this heading.

Theophylline Sodium Glycinate (Potential for severe and fatal reactions including cardiac arrest, seizures, respiratory failure and status epilepticus; concurrent use should be avoided or serum levels of theophylline should be monitored carefully).
No products indexed under this heading.

Warfarin Sodium (Enhanced effects of anticoagulant). Products include:
Coumadin for Injection 1243
Coumadin Tablets 1243
Warfarin Sodium Tablets, USP 3302

Zinc Sulfate (Co-administration with zinc-containing products may substantially interfere with the oral absorption of quinolones; these preparations may be taken six hours before or two hours after taking ciprofloxacin). Products include:
Clear Eyes ACR Astringent/Lubricant Eye Redness Reliever .... ⊙322
Visine A.C. Seasonal Relief From Pollen & Dust Eye Drops .... ⊙314

Food Interactions

Dairy products (Oral ciprofloxacin should not be taken concurrently with milk or yogurt alone, since absorption of ciprofloxacin may be significantly reduced; dietary calcium as part of a meal, however, does not significantly affect ciprofloxacin absorption).

Food, unspecified (Delays the oral absorption of the drug resulting in peak concentrations that are closer to 2 hours after dosing).

CITRACAL LIQUITAB TABLETS
(Calcium Citrate) .... ◙823
None cited in PDR database.

CITRACAL PRENATAL RX TABLETS
(Vitamins, Prenatal) 2231
None cited in PDR database.

CITRACAL TABLETS
(Calcium Citrate) 2231
None cited in PDR database.

CITRACAL CAPLETS + D
(Calcium Citrate, Vitamin D) .... ◙823
None cited in PDR database.

CITRUCEL CAPLETS
(Methylcellulose) .... ◙745
None cited in PDR database.

CITRUCEL ORANGE FLAVOR POWDER
(Methylcellulose) .... ◙744
None cited in PDR database.

CITRUCEL SUGAR FREE ORANGE FLAVOR POWDER
(Methylcellulose) .... ◙745
None cited in PDR database.

CLAFORAN INJECTION
(Cefotaxime Sodium) 732
May interact with aminoglycosides. Compounds in these categories include:

Amikacin Sulfate (Increased nephrotoxicity).
No products indexed under this heading.

Gentamicin Sulfate (Increased nephrotoxicity). Products include:
Genoptic Ophthalmic Ointment ..... ⊙239
Genoptic Sterile Ophthalmic Solution .... ⊙239
Pred-G Ophthalmic Suspension ..... ⊙247
Pred-G Sterile Ophthalmic Ointment .... ⊙248

Kanamycin Sulfate (Increased nephrotoxicity).
No products indexed under this heading.

Streptomycin Sulfate (Increased nephrotoxicity). Products include:
Streptomycin Sulfate Injection 2714

Tobramycin (Increased nephrotoxicity). Products include:
TOBI Solution for Inhalation 1206
TobraDex Ophthalmic Ointment 542
TobraDex Ophthalmic Suspension .. 541
Tobrex Ophthalmic Ointment .... ⊙220
Tobrex Ophthalmic Solution .... ⊙221

Tobramycin Sulfate (Increased nephrotoxicity). Products include:
Nebcin Vials, Hyporets & ADD-Vantage 1955

CLARITIN REDITABS
(Loratadine) 3100
See Claritin Tablets

CLARITIN SYRUP
(Loratadine) 3100
See Claritin Tablets

CLARITIN TABLETS
(Loratadine) 3100
May interact with erythromycin and certain other agents. Compounds in these categories include:

Cimetidine (Increased plasma concentrations (AUC 0-24 hours) of loratadine and/or decarboethoxyloratadine have been reported following co-administration; no clinically relevant changes in the safety profile of loratadine have been observed). Products include:
Tagamet HB 200 Suspension .... ◙762
Tagamet HB 200 Tablets .... ◙761
Tagamet Tablets 1644

Cimetidine Hydrochloride (Increased plasma concentrations (AUC 0-24 hours) of loratadine and/or decarboethoxyloratadine have been reported following co-administration; no clinically relevant changes in the safety profile of loratadine have been observed). Products include:
Tagamet 1644

Erythromycin (Increased plasma concentrations (AUC 0-24 hours) of loratadine and/or decarboethoxyloratadine have been reported following co-administration; no clinically relevant changes in the safety profile of loratadine have been observed). Products include:
Emgel 2% Topical Gel 1285
Ery-Tab Tablets 448
Erythromycin Base Filmtab Tablets . 454
Erythromycin Delayed-Release Capsules, USP 455
PCE Dispertab Tablets 498

Erythromycin Estolate (Increased plasma concentrations (AUC 0-24 hours) of loratadine and/or decarboethoxyloratadine have been reported following co-administration; no clinically relevant changes in the safety profile of loratadine have been observed).
No products indexed under this heading.

Erythromycin Ethylsuccinate (Increased plasma concentrations (AUC 0-24 hours) of loratadine and/or decarboethoxyloratadine have been reported following co-administration; no clinically relevant changes in the safety profile of loratadine have been observed). Products include:
E.E.S. 450
EryPed 446
Pediazole Suspension 3050

Erythromycin Gluceptate (Increased plasma concentrations (AUC 0-24 hours) of loratadine and/or decarboethoxyloratadine have been reported following co-administration; no clinically relevant changes in the safety profile of loratadine have been observed).
No products indexed under this heading.

Erythromycin Stearate (Increased plasma concentrations (AUC 0-24 hours) of loratadine and/or decarboethoxyloratadine have been reported following co-administration; no clinically relevant changes in the safety profile of loratadine have been observed). Products include:
- Erythrocin Stearate Filmtab Tablets 452

Ketoconazole (Increased plasma concentrations (AUC 0-24 hours) of loratadine and/or decarboethoxyloratadine have been reported following co-administration; no clinically relevant changes in the safety profile of loratadine have been observed). Products include:
- Nizoral 2% Cream 3620
- Nizoral A-D Shampoo 2008
- Nizoral 2% Shampoo 2007
- Nizoral Tablets 1791

Food Interactions

Meal, unspecified (Food increases the AUC by approximately 73%, the time to peak plasma concentration is delayed by one-hour).

CLARITIN-D 12 HOUR EXTENDED RELEASE TABLETS

(Loratadine, Pseudoephedrine Sulfate) 3102

See Claritin-D 24 Hour Extended Release Tablets

CLARITIN-D 24 HOUR EXTENDED RELEASE TABLETS

(Loratadine, Pseudoephedrine Sulfate) 3104

May interact with beta blockers, erythromycin, cardiac glycosides, monoamine oxidase inhibitors, veratrum alkaloids, and certain other agents. Compounds in these categories include:

Acebutolol Hydrochloride (Sympathomimetics may reduce the antihypertensive effects of beta-adrenergic blocking agents). Products include:
- Sectral Capsules 3589

Atenolol (Sympathomimetics may reduce the antihypertensive effects of beta-adrenergic blocking agents). Products include:
- Tenoretic Tablets 690
- Tenormin I.V. Injection 692

Betaxolol Hydrochloride (Sympathomimetics may reduce the antihypertensive effects of beta-adrenergic blocking agents). Products include:
- Betoptic S Ophthalmic Suspension 537

Bisoprolol Fumarate (Sympathomimetics may reduce the antihypertensive effects of beta-adrenergic blocking agents). Products include:
- Zebeta Tablets 1885
- Ziac Tablets 1887

Carteolol Hydrochloride (Sympathomimetics may reduce the antihypertensive effects of beta-adrenergic blocking agents). Products include:
- Carteolol Hydrochloride Ophthalmic Solution USP, 1% .... ⊙258
- Ocupress Ophthalmic Solution, 1% Sterile .... ⊙303

Cimetidine (Increased plasma concentrations (AUC 0-24 hours) or loratadine and/or descarboethoxyloratadine have been reported following co-administration; no clinically relevant changes in the safety profile of loratadine have been observed). Products include:
- Tagamet HB 200 Suspension .... ▣762
- Tagamet HB 200 Tablets .... ▣761
- Tagamet Tablets 1644

Cimetidine Hydrochloride (Increased plasma concentrations (AUC 0-24 hours) or loratadine and/or descarboethoxyloratadine have been reported following co-administration; no clinically relevant changes in the safety profile of loratadine have been observed). Products include:
- Tagamet 1644

Cryptenamine Preparations (Sympathomimetics may reduce the antihypertensive effects of veratrum alkaloids).
- No products indexed under this heading.

Deslanoside (Increased ectopic pacemaker activity can occur when pseudoephedrine is used concomitantly with digitalis).
- No products indexed under this heading.

Digitoxin (Increased ectopic pacemaker activity can occur when pseudoephedrine is used concomitantly with digitalis).
- No products indexed under this heading.

Digoxin (Increased ectopic pacemaker activity can occur when pseudoephedrine is used concomitantly with digitalis). Products include:
- Digitek Tablets 1003
- Lanoxicaps Capsules 1574
- Lanoxin Injection 1581
- Lanoxin Tablets 1587
- Lanoxin Elixir Pediatric 1578
- Lanoxin Injection Pediatric 1584

Erythromycin (Increased plasma concentrations (AUC 0-24 hours) or loratadine and/or descarboethoxyloratadine have been reported following co-administration; no clinically relevant changes in the safety profile of loratadine have been observed; plasma concentrations (AUC 0-24 hours) of erythromycin decreased 15% with co-administration; the clinical significance is unknown). Products include:
- Emgel 2% Topical Gel 1285
- Ery-Tab Tablets 448
- Erythromycin Base Filmtab Tablets 454
- Erythromycin Delayed-Release Capsules, USP 455
- PCE Dispertab Tablets 498

Erythromycin Estolate (Increased plasma concentrations (AUC 0-24 hours) or loratadine and/or descarboethoxyloratadine have been reported following co-administration; no clinically relevant changes in the safety profile of loratadine have been observed; plasma concentrations (AUC 0-24 hours) of erythromycin decreased 15% with co-administration; the clinical significance is unknown).
- No products indexed under this heading.

Erythromycin Ethylsuccinate (Increased plasma concentrations (AUC 0-24 hours) or loratadine and/or descarboethoxyloratadine have been reported following co-administration; no clinically relevant changes in the safety profile of loratadine have been observed; plasma concentrations (AUC 0-24 hours) of erythromycin decreased 15% with co-administration; the clinical significance is unknown). Products include:
- E.E.S. 450
- EryPed 446
- Pediazole Suspension 3050

Erythromycin Gluceptate (Increased plasma concentrations (AUC 0-24 hours) or loratadine and/or descarboethoxyloratadine have been reported following co-administration; no clinically relevant changes in the safety profile of loratadine have been observed; plasma concentrations (AUC 0-24 hours) of erythromycin decreased 15% with co-administration; the clinical significance is unknown).
- No products indexed under this heading.

Erythromycin Stearate (Increased plasma concentrations (AUC 0-24 hours) or loratadine and/or descarboethoxyloratadine have been reported following co-administration; no clinically relevant changes in the safety profile of loratadine have been observed; plasma concentrations (AUC 0-24 hours) of erythromycin decreased 15% with co-administration; the clinical significance is unknown). Products include:
- Erythrocin Stearate Filmtab Tablets 452

Esmolol Hydrochloride (Sympathomimetics may reduce the antihypertensive effects of beta-adrenergic blocking agents). Products include:
- Brevibloc Injection 858

Isocarboxazid (Concurrent and/or sequential use with MAO inhibitors is contraindicated).
- No products indexed under this heading.

Ketoconazole (Increased plasma concentrations (AUC 0-24 hours) or loratadine and/or descarboethoxyloratadine have been reported following co-administration; no clinically relevant changes in the safety profile of loratadine have been observed). Products include:
- Nizoral 2% Cream 3620
- Nizoral A-D Shampoo 2008
- Nizoral 2% Shampoo 2007
- Nizoral Tablets 1791

Labetalol Hydrochloride (Sympathomimetics may reduce the antihypertensive effects of beta-adrenergic blocking agents). Products include:
- Normodyne Injection 3135
- Normodyne Tablets 3137

Levobunolol Hydrochloride (Sympathomimetics may reduce the antihypertensive effects of beta-adrenergic blocking agents). Products include:
- Betagan .... ⊙228

Mecamylamine Hydrochloride (Sympathomimetics may reduce the antihypertensive effects of mecamylamine). Products include:
- Inversine Tablets 1850

Methyldopa (Sympathomimetics may reduce the antihypertensive effects of methyldopa). Products include:
- Aldoclor Tablets 2035
- Aldomet Tablets 2037
- Aldoril Tablets 2039

Methyldopate Hydrochloride (Sympathomimetics may reduce the antihypertensive effects of methyldopa).
- No products indexed under this heading.

Metipranolol Hydrochloride (Sympathomimetics may reduce the antihypertensive effects of beta-adrenergic blocking agents).
- No products indexed under this heading.

Metoprolol Succinate (Sympathomimetics may reduce the antihypertensive effects of beta-adrenergic blocking agents). Products include:
- Toprol-XL Tablets 651

Metoprolol Tartrate (Sympathomimetics may reduce the antihypertensive effects of beta-adrenergic blocking agents).
- No products indexed under this heading.

Moclobemide (Concurrent and/or sequential use with MAO inhibitors is contraindicated).
- No products indexed under this heading.

Nadolol (Sympathomimetics may reduce the antihypertensive effects of beta-adrenergic blocking agents). Products include:
- Corgard Tablets 2245
- Corzide 40/5 Tablets 2247
- Corzide 80/5 Tablets 2247
- Nadolol Tablets 2288

Pargyline Hydrochloride (Concurrent and/or sequential use with MAO inhibitors is contraindicated).
- No products indexed under this heading.

Penbutolol Sulfate (Sympathomimetics may reduce the antihypertensive effects of beta-adrenergic blocking agents).
- No products indexed under this heading.

Phenelzine Sulfate (Concurrent and/or sequential use with MAO inhibitors is contraindicated). Products include:
- Nardil Tablets 2653

Pindolol (Sympathomimetics may reduce the antihypertensive effects of beta-adrenergic blocking agents).
- No products indexed under this heading.

Procarbazine Hydrochloride (Concurrent and/or sequential use with MAO inhibitors is contraindicated). Products include:
- Matulane Capsules 3246

Propranolol Hydrochloride (Sympathomimetics may reduce the antihypertensive effects of beta-adrenergic blocking agents). Products include:
- Inderal 3513
- Inderal LA Long-Acting Capsules 3516
- Inderide Tablets 3517
- Inderide LA Long-Acting Capsules 3519

Reserpine (Sympathomimetics may reduce the antihypertensive effects of reserpine).
- No products indexed under this heading.

Selegiline Hydrochloride (Concurrent and/or sequential use with MAO inhibitors is contraindicated). Products include:
- Eldepryl Capsules 3266

Sotalol Hydrochloride (Sympathomimetics may reduce the antihypertensive effects of beta-adrenergic blocking agents). Products include:
- Betapace Tablets 950
- Betapace AF Tablets 954

Timolol Hemihydrate (Sympathomimetics may reduce the antihypertensive effects of beta-adrenergic blocking agents). Products include:
- Betimol Ophthalmic Solution .... ⊙324

Timolol Maleate (Sympathomimetics may reduce the antihypertensive effects of beta-adrenergic blocking agents). Products include:
- Blocadren Tablets 2046
- Cosopt Sterile Ophthalmic Solution 2065
- Timolide Tablets 2187
- Timolol GFS .... ⊙266
- Timoptic in Ocudose 2192
- Timoptic Sterile Ophthalmic Solution 2190
- Timoptic-XE Sterile Ophthalmic Gel Forming Solution 2194

Tranylcypromine Sulfate (Concurrent and/or sequential use with MAO inhibitors is contraindicated). Products include:
- Parnate Tablets 1607

Food Interactions

Food, unspecified (Increases the AUC of loratadine by approximately 125% and Cmax by approximately 80%, however, food did not significantly affect the pharmacokinetics of pseudoephedrine or descarboethoxyloratadine).

CLEAR AWAY GEL WITH ALOE WART REMOVER SYSTEM

(Salicylic Acid) .... ▣736

None cited in PDR database.

CLEAR AWAY LIQUID WART REMOVER SYSTEM

(Salicylic Acid) .... ▣736

None cited in PDR database.

CLEAR AWAY ONE STEP WART REMOVER
(Salicylic Acid) 737
None cited in PDR database.

CLEAR AWAY ONE STEP WART REMOVER FOR KIDS
(Salicylic Acid) 737
None cited in PDR database.

CLEAR AWAY ONE STEP PLANTAR WART REMOVER
(Salicylic Acid) 737
None cited in PDR database.

CLEAR EYES ACR ASTRINGENT/LUBRICANT EYE REDNESS RELIEVER
(Glycerin, Naphazoline Hydrochloride, Zinc Sulfate)............ ⊙ 322
None cited in PDR database.

CLEAR EYES CLR SOOTHING DROPS
(Glycerin, Hydroxypropyl Methylcellulose, Sodium Chloride) .... ⊙ 322
None cited in PDR database.

CLEAR EYES LUBRICANT EYE REDNESS RELIEVER
(Glycerin, Naphazoline Hydrochloride) .... ⊙ 322
None cited in PDR database.

CLEOCIN HCL CAPSULES
(Clindamycin Hydrochloride) 2784
See Cleocin Phosphate Sterile Solution

CLEOCIN PHOSPHATE STERILE SOLUTION
(Clindamycin Phosphate) 2785
May interact with erythromycin, neuromuscular blocking agents, and certain other agents. Compounds in these categories include:

Atracurium Besylate (Clindamycin has been shown to have neuromuscular blocking properties that may enhance the action of other neuromuscular blocking agents).
No products indexed under this heading.

Cisatracurium Besylate (Clindamycin has been shown to have neuromuscular blocking properties that may enhance the action of other neuromuscular blocking agents).
No products indexed under this heading.

Diphenoxylate Hydrochloride (May prolong and/or worsen colitis).
No products indexed under this heading.

Doxacurium Chloride (Clindamycin has been shown to have neuromuscular blocking properties that may enhance the action of other neuromuscular blocking agents).
No products indexed under this heading.

Erythromycin (Antagonism has been demonstrated between clindamycin and erythromycin *in vitro* because of possible clinical significance, these two drugs should not be administered concurrently). Products include:
- Emgel 2% Topical Gel 1285
- Ery-Tab Tablets 448
- Erythromycin Base Filmtab Tablets . 454
- Erythromycin Delayed-Release Capsules, USP 455
- PCE Dispertab Tablets 498

Erythromycin Estolate (Antagonism has been demonstrated between clindamycin and erythromycin *in vitro* because of possible clinical significance, these two drugs should not be administered concurrently).
No products indexed under this heading.

Erythromycin Ethylsuccinate (Antagonism has been demonstrated between clindamycin and erythromycin *in vitro* because of possible clinical significance, these two drugs should not be administered concurrently). Products include:
- E.E.S. 450
- EryPed 446
- Pediazole Suspension 3050

Erythromycin Gluceptate (Antagonism has been demonstrated between clindamycin and erythromycin *in vitro* because of possible clinical significance, these two drugs should not be administered concurrently).
No products indexed under this heading.

Erythromycin Stearate (Antagonism has been demonstrated between clindamycin and erythromycin in vitro because of possible clinical significance, these two drugs should not be administered concurrently). Products include:
- Erythrocin Stearate Filmtab Tablets 452

Metocurine Iodide (Clindamycin has been shown to have neuromuscular blocking properties that may enhance the action of other neuromuscular blocking agents).
No products indexed under this heading.

Mivacurium Chloride (Clindamycin has been shown to have neuromuscular blocking properties that may enhance the action of other neuromuscular blocking agents).
No products indexed under this heading.

Pancuronium Bromide (Clindamycin has been shown to have neuromuscular blocking properties that may enhance the action of other neuromuscular blocking agents).
No products indexed under this heading.

Rapacuronium Bromide (Clindamycin has been shown to have neuromuscular blocking properties that may enhance the action of other neuromuscular blocking agents).
No products indexed under this heading.

Rocuronium Bromide (Clindamycin has been shown to have neuromuscular blocking properties that may enhance the action of other neuromuscular blocking agents). Products include:
- Zemuron Injection 2491

Succinylcholine Chloride (Clindamycin has been shown to have neuromuscular blocking properties that may enhance the action of other neuromuscular blocking agents). Products include:
- Anectine Injection 1476

Vecuronium Bromide (Clindamycin has been shown to have neuromuscular blocking properties that may enhance the action of other neuromuscular blocking agents). Products include:
- Norcuron for Injection 2478

CLEOCIN T TOPICAL GEL
(Clindamycin Phosphate) 2790
May interact with neuromuscular blocking agents. Compounds in these categories include:

Atracurium Besylate (Clindamycin has neuromuscular blocking properties that may enhance the action of other neuromuscular blocking agents).
No products indexed under this heading.

Cisatracurium Besylate (Clindamycin has neuromuscular blocking properties that may enhance the action of other neuromuscular blocking agents).
No products indexed under this heading.

Doxacurium Chloride (Clindamycin has neuromuscular blocking properties that may enhance the action of other neuromuscular blocking agents).
No products indexed under this heading.

Metocurine Iodide (Clindamycin has neuromuscular blocking properties that may enhance the action of other neuromuscular blocking agents).
No products indexed under this heading.

Mivacurium Chloride (Clindamycin has neuromuscular blocking properties that may enhance the action of other neuromuscular blocking agents).
No products indexed under this heading.

Pancuronium Bromide (Clindamycin has neuromuscular blocking properties that may enhance the action of other neuromuscular blocking agents).
No products indexed under this heading.

Rapacuronium Bromide (Clindamycin has neuromuscular blocking properties that may enhance the action of other neuromuscular blocking agents).
No products indexed under this heading.

Rocuronium Bromide (Clindamycin has neuromuscular blocking properties that may enhance the action of other neuromuscular blocking agents). Products include:
- Zemuron Injection 2491

Succinylcholine Chloride (Clindamycin has neuromuscular blocking properties that may enhance the action of other neuromuscular blocking agents). Products include:
- Anectine Injection 1476

Vecuronium Bromide (Clindamycin has neuromuscular blocking properties that may enhance the action of other neuromuscular blocking agents). Products include:
- Norcuron for Injection 2478

CLEOCIN T TOPICAL LOTION
(Clindamycin Phosphate) 2790
See Cleocin T Topical Gel

CLEOCIN T TOPICAL SOLUTION
(Clindamycin Phosphate) 2790
See Cleocin T Topical Gel

CLEOCIN VAGINAL CREAM
(Clindamycin Phosphate) 2788
See Cleocin Vaginal Ovules

CLEOCIN VAGINAL OVULES
(Clindamycin Phosphate) 2789
May interact with neuromuscular blocking agents. Compounds in these categories include:

Atracurium Besylate (Clindamycin has been shown to have neuromuscular blocking properties; coadministration of clindamycin with neuromuscular blocking agents may enhance action of these neuromuscular blocking agents).
No products indexed under this heading.

Cisatracurium Besylate (Clindamycin has been shown to have neuromuscular blocking properties; coadministration of clindamycin with neuromuscular blocking agents may enhance action of these neuromuscular blocking agents).
No products indexed under this heading.

Doxacurium Chloride (Clindamycin has been shown to have neuromuscular blocking properties; coadministration of clindamycin with neuromuscular blocking agents may enhance action of these neuromuscular blocking agents).
No products indexed under this heading.

Metocurine Iodide (Clindamycin has been shown to have neuromuscular blocking properties; coadministration of clindamycin with neuromuscular blocking agents may enhance action of these neuromuscular blocking agents).
No products indexed under this heading.

Mivacurium Chloride (Clindamycin has been shown to have neuromuscular blocking properties; coadministration of clindamycin with neuromuscular blocking agents may enhance action of these neuromuscular blocking agents).
No products indexed under this heading.

Pancuronium Bromide (Clindamycin has been shown to have neuromuscular blocking properties; coadministration of clindamycin with neuromuscular blocking agents may enhance action of these neuromuscular blocking agents).
No products indexed under this heading.

Rapacuronium Bromide (Clindamycin has been shown to have neuromuscular blocking properties; coadministration of clindamycin with neuromuscular blocking agents may enhance action of these neuromuscular blocking agents).
No products indexed under this heading.

Rocuronium Bromide (Clindamycin has been shown to have neuromuscular blocking properties; coadministration of clindamycin with neuromuscular blocking agents may enhance action of these neuromuscular blocking agents). Products include:
- Zemuron Injection 2491

Succinylcholine Chloride (Clindamycin has been shown to have neuromuscular blocking properties; coadministration of clindamycin with neuromuscular blocking agents may enhance action of these neuromuscular blocking agents). Products include:
- Anectine Injection 1476

Vecuronium Bromide (Clindamycin has been shown to have neuromuscular blocking properties; coadministration of clindamycin with neuromuscular blocking agents may enhance action of these neuromuscular blocking agents). Products include:
- Norcuron for Injection 2478

CLIMARA TRANSDERMAL SYSTEM
(Estradiol) 958
May interact with:

Medroxyprogesterone Acetate (Potential for adverse effects on carbohydrate and lipid metabolism). Products include:
- Depo-Provera Contraceptive Injection 2798
- Lunelle Monthly Injection 2827
- Premphase Tablets 3572
- Prempro Tablets 3572
- Provera Tablets 2853

CLINAC BPO GEL USP
(Benzoyl Peroxide) 1339
None cited in PDR database.

CLINDAGEL
(Clindamycin Phosphate) 1401
May interact with neuromuscular blocking agents. Compounds in these categories include:

Atracurium Besylate (Clindamycin has neuromuscular blocking properties that may enhance the action of other neuromuscular blocking agents).
No products indexed under this heading.

Cisatracurium Besylate (Clindamycin has neuromuscular blocking properties that may enhance the action of other neuromuscular blocking agents).
No products indexed under this heading.

Doxacurium Chloride (Clindamycin has neuromuscular blocking properties that may enhance the action of other neuromuscular blocking agents).
No products indexed under this heading.

Metocurine Iodide (Clindamycin has neuromuscular blocking properties that may enhance the action of other neuromuscular blocking agents).
No products indexed under this heading.

Mivacurium Chloride (Clindamycin has neuromuscular blocking properties that may enhance the action of other neuromuscular blocking agents).
No products indexed under this heading.

Pancuronium Bromide (Clindamycin has neuromuscular blocking properties that may enhance the action of other neuromuscular blocking agents).
No products indexed under this heading.

Rapacuronium Bromide (Clindamycin has neuromuscular blocking properties that may enhance the action of other neuromuscular blocking agents).
No products indexed under this heading.

Rocuronium Bromide (Clindamycin has neuromuscular blocking properties that may enhance the action of other neuromuscular blocking agents). Products include:
Zemuron Injection 2491

Succinylcholine Chloride (Clindamycin has neuromuscular blocking properties that may enhance the action of other neuromuscular blocking agents). Products include:
Anectine Injection 1476

Vecuronium Bromide (Clindamycin has neuromuscular blocking properties that may enhance the action of other neuromuscular blocking agents). Products include:
Norcuron for Injection 2478

CLINDETS PLEDGETS
(Clindamycin Phosphate) 3270
May interact with neuromuscular blocking agents. Compounds in these categories include:

Atracurium Besylate (Clindamycin has neuromuscular blocking properties and it may enhance the neuromuscular blocking agents).
No products indexed under this heading.

Cisatracurium Besylate (Clindamycin has neuromuscular blocking properties and it may enhance the neuromuscular blocking agents).
No products indexed under this heading.

Doxacurium Chloride (Clindamycin has neuromuscular blocking properties and it may enhance the neuromuscular blocking agents).
No products indexed under this heading.

Metocurine Iodide (Clindamycin has neuromuscular blocking properties and it may enhance the neuromuscular blocking agents).
No products indexed under this heading.

Mivacurium Chloride (Clindamycin has neuromuscular blocking properties and it may enhance the neuromuscular blocking agents).
No products indexed under this heading.

Pancuronium Bromide (Clindamycin has neuromuscular blocking properties and it may enhance the neuromuscular blocking agents).
No products indexed under this heading.

Rapacuronium Bromide (Clindamycin has neuromuscular blocking properties and it may enhance the neuromuscular blocking agents).
No products indexed under this heading.

Rocuronium Bromide (Clindamycin has neuromuscular blocking properties and it may enhance the neuromuscular blocking agents). Products include:
Zemuron Injection 2491

Succinylcholine Chloride (Clindamycin has neuromuscular blocking properties and it may enhance the neuromuscular blocking agents). Products include:
Anectine Injection 1476

Vecuronium Bromide (Clindamycin has neuromuscular blocking properties and it may enhance the neuromuscular blocking agents). Products include:
Norcuron for Injection 2478

CLINICAL CARE ANTIMICROBIAL WOUND CLEANSER
(Benzethonium Chloride) .... ■632
None cited in PDR database.

CLINORIL TABLETS
(Sulindac) 2053
May interact with oral anticoagulants, oral hypoglycemic agents, non-steroidal anti-inflammatory agents, and certain other agents. Compounds in these categories include:

Acarbose (Special attention should be paid to patients taking higher doses than those recommended and to patients with renal or metabolic impairment). Products include:
Precose Tablets 906

Aspirin (Increased gastrointestinal reactions). Products include:
Aggrenox Capsules 1026
Alka-Seltzer .... ■603
Alka-Seltzer Lemon Lime Antacid and Pain Reliever Effervescent Tablets .... ■603
Alka-Seltzer Extra Strength Antacid and Pain Reliever Effervescent Tablets .... ■603
Alka-Seltzer PM Effervescent Tablets .... ■605
Genuine Bayer Tablets, Caplets and Gelcaps .... ■606
Extra Strength Bayer Caplets and Gelcaps .... ■610
Aspirin Regimen Bayer Children's Chewable Tablets (Orange or Cherry Flavored) .... ■607
Bayer, Aspirin Regimen .... ■606
Aspirin Regimen Bayer 81 mg Caplets with Calcium .... ■607
Genuine Bayer Professional Labeling (Aspirin Regimen Bayer) .... ■608
Extra Strength Bayer Arthritis Caplets .... ■610
Extra Strength Bayer Plus Caplets .... ■610
Extra Strength Bayer PM Caplets .... ■611
BC Powder .... ■619
BC Allergy Sinus Cold Powder .... ■619
Arthritis Strength BC Powder .... ■619
BC Sinus Cold Powder .... ■619
Darvon Compound-65 Pulvules 1910
Ecotrin Enteric Coated Aspirin Low, Regular and Maximum Strength Tablets 1715
Excedrin Extra-Strength Tablets, Caplets, and Geltabs .... ■629
Excedrin Migraine 1070
Goody's Body Pain Formula Powder .... ■620
Goody's Extra Strength Headache Powder .... ■620
Goody's Extra Strength Pain Relief Tablets .... ■620
Percodan Tablets 1327
Robaxisal Tablets 2939
Soma Compound Tablets 3354
Soma Compound w/Codeine Tablets 3355
Vanquish Caplets .... ■617

Aspirin, Enteric Coated (Increased gastrointestinal reactions).
No products indexed under this heading.

Celecoxib (Concomitant use is not recommended due to the increased possibility of gastrointestinal toxicity, with little or no increase in efficacy). Products include:
Celebrex Capsules 2676
Celebrex Capsules 2780

Chlorpropamide (Special attention should be paid to patients taking higher doses than those recommended and to patients with renal or metabolic impairment). Products include:
Diabinese Tablets 2680

Cyclosporine (Increased cyclosporine-induced toxicity). Products include:
Gengraf Capsules 457
Neoral Soft Gelatin Capsules 2380
Neoral Oral Solution 2380
Sandimmune 2388

Diclofenac Potassium (Concomitant use is not recommended due to the increased possibility of gastrointestinal toxicity, with little or no increase in efficacy). Products include:
Cataflam Tablets 2315

Diclofenac Sodium (Concomitant use is not recommended due to the increased possibility of gastrointestinal toxicity, with little or no increase in efficacy). Products include:
Arthrotec Tablets 3195
Voltaren Ophthalmic Sterile Ophthalmic Solution .... ⊙312
Voltaren Tablets 2315
Voltaren-XR Tablets 2315

Dicumarol (Special attention should be paid to patients taking higher doses than those recommended and to patients with renal or metabolic impairment).
No products indexed under this heading.

Diflunisal (Decreased plasma levels of sulindac). Products include:
Dolobid Tablets 2088

DMSO (Reduced efficacy of sulindac; peripheral neuropathy).
No products indexed under this heading.

Etodolac (Concomitant use is not recommended due to the increased possibility of gastrointestinal toxicity, with little or no increase in efficacy). Products include:
Lodine 3528
Lodine XL Extended-Release Tablets 3530

Fenoprofen Calcium (Concomitant use is not recommended due to the increased possibility of gastrointestinal toxicity, with little or no increase in efficacy).
No products indexed under this heading.

Flurbiprofen (Concomitant use is not recommended due to the increased possibility of gastrointestinal toxicity, with little or no increase in efficacy).
No products indexed under this heading.

Furosemide (Clinoril may blunt the renal response to I.V. furosemide). Products include:
Furosemide Tablets 2284

Glimepiride (Special attention should be paid to patients taking higher doses than those recommended and to patients with renal or metabolic impairment). Products include:
Amaryl Tablets 717

Glipizide (Special attention should be paid to patients taking higher doses than those recommended and to patients with renal or metabolic impairment). Products include:
Glucotrol Tablets 2692
Glucotrol XL Extended Release Tablets 2693

Glyburide (Special attention should be paid to patients taking higher doses than those recommended and to patients with renal or metabolic impairment). Products include:
DiaBeta Tablets 741
Glucovance Tablets 1086

Ibuprofen (Concomitant use is not recommended due to the increased possibility of gastrointestinal toxicity, with little or no increase in efficacy). Products include:
Advil .... ■771
Children's Advil Oral Suspension .... ■773
Children's Advil Chewable Tablets .... ■773
Advil Cold and Sinus Caplets .... ■771
Advil Cold and Sinus Tablets .... ■771
Advil Flu & Body Ache Caplets .... ■772
Infants' Advil Drops .... ■773
Junior Strength Advil Tablets .... ■773
Junior Strength Advil Chewable Tablets .... ■773
Advil Migraine Liquigels .... ■772
Children's Motrin Oral Suspension and Chewable Tablets 2006
Children's Motrin Cold Oral Suspension 2007
Children's Motrin Oral Suspension .... ■643
Motrin Suspension, Oral Drops, Chewable Tablets, and Caplets 2002
Infants' Motrin Concentrated Drops 2006
Junior Strength Motrin Caplets and Chewable Tablets 2006
Motrin IB Tablets, Caplets, and Gelcaps 2002
Motrin Migraine Pain Caplets 2005
Motrin Sinus Headache Caplets 2005
Vicoprofen Tablets 520

Indomethacin (Concomitant use is not recommended due to the increased possibility of gastrointestinal toxicity, with little or no increase in efficacy). Products include:
Indocin 2112

Indomethacin Sodium Trihydrate (Concomitant use is not recommended due to the increased possibility of gastrointestinal toxicity, with little or no increase in efficacy). Products include:
Indocin I.V. 2115

Ketoprofen (Concomitant use is not recommended due to the increased possibility of gastrointestinal toxicity, with little or no increase in efficacy). Products include:
Orudis Capsules 3548
Orudis KT Tablets .... ■778
Oruvail Capsules 3548

Ketorolac Tromethamine (Concomitant use is not recommended due to the increased possibility of gastrointestinal toxicity, with little or no increase in efficacy). Products include:
Acular Ophthalmic Solution 544
Acular PF Ophthalmic Solution 544
Toradol 3018

Meclofenamate Sodium (Concomitant use is not recommended

due to the increased possibility of gastrointestinal toxicity, with little or no increase in efficacy).
No products indexed under this heading.

Mefenamic Acid (Concomitant use is not recommended due to the increased possibility of gastrointestinal toxicity, with little or no increase in efficacy). Products include:
Ponstel Capsules 1356

Meloxicam (Concomitant use is not recommended due to the increased possibility of gastrointestinal toxicity, with little or no increase in efficacy). Products include:
Mobic Tablets 1054

Metformin Hydrochloride (Special attention should be paid to patients taking higher doses than those recommended and to patients with renal or metabolic impairment). Products include:
Glucophage Tablets 1080
Glucophage XR Tablets 1080
Glucovance Tablets 1086

Methotrexate Sodium (Decreased tubular secretion of methotrexate and potentiation of its toxicity).
No products indexed under this heading.

Miglitol (Special attention should be paid to patients taking higher doses than those recommended and to patients with renal or metabolic impairment). Products include:
Glyset Tablets 2821

Nabumetone (Concomitant use is not recommended due to the increased possibility of gastrointestinal toxicity, with little or no increase in efficacy). Products include:
Relafen Tablets 1617

Naproxen (Concomitant use is not recommended due to the increased possibility of gastrointestinal toxicity, with little or no increase in efficacy). Products include:
EC-Naprosyn Delayed-Release Tablets 2967
Naprosyn Suspension 2967
Naprosyn Tablets 2967

Naproxen Sodium (Concomitant use is not recommended due to the increased possibility of gastrointestinal toxicity, with little or no increase in efficacy). Products include:
Aleve Tablets, Caplets and Gelcaps .... ▣602
Aleve Cold & Sinus Caplets .... ▣603
Anaprox Tablets 2967
Anaprox DS Tablets 2967
Naprelan Tablets 1293

Oxaprozin (Concomitant use is not recommended due to the increased possibility of gastrointestinal toxicity, with little or no increase in efficacy).
No products indexed under this heading.

Phenylbutazone (Concomitant use is not recommended due to the increased possibility of gastrointestinal toxicity, with little or no increase in efficacy).
No products indexed under this heading.

Pioglitazone Hydrochloride (Special attention should be paid to patients taking higher doses than those recommended and to patients with renal or metabolic impairment). Products include:
Actos Tablets 3275

Piroxicam (Concomitant use is not recommended due to the increased possibility of gastrointestinal toxicity, with little or no increase in efficacy). Products include:
Feldene Capsules 2685

Probenecid (Increased plasma levels of sulindac; modest reduction in uricosuric action of probenecid).
No products indexed under this heading.

Repaglinide (Special attention should be paid to patients taking higher doses than those recommended and to patients with renal or metabolic impairment). Products include:
Prandin Tablets (0.5, 1, and 2 mg) 2432

Rofecoxib (Concomitant use is not recommended due to the increased possibility of gastrointestinal toxicity, with little or no increase in efficacy). Products include:
Vioxx 2213

Rosiglitazone Maleate (Special attention should be paid to patients taking higher doses than those recommended and to patients with renal or metabolic impairment). Products include:
Avandia Tablets 1490

Tolazamide (Special attention should be paid to patients taking higher doses than those recommended and to patients with renal or metabolic impairment).
No products indexed under this heading.

Tolbutamide (Special attention should be paid to patients taking higher doses than those recommended and to patients with renal or metabolic impairment).
No products indexed under this heading.

Tolmetin Sodium (Concomitant use is not recommended due to the increased possibility of gastrointestinal toxicity, with little or no increase in efficacy). Products include:
Tolectin 2589

Troglitazone (Special attention should be paid to patients taking higher doses than those recommended and to patients with renal or metabolic impairment).
No products indexed under this heading.

Warfarin Sodium (Special attention should be paid to patients taking higher doses than those recommended and to patients with renal or metabolic impairment). Products include:
Coumadin for Injection 1243
Coumadin Tablets 1243
Warfarin Sodium Tablets, USP 3302

Food Interactions

Food, unspecified (The peak plasma concentrations of biologically active sulfide metabolite is delayed slightly in the presence of food).

CLOBEVATE GEL
(Clobetasol Propionate) 3271
None cited in PDR database.

CLOMID TABLETS
(Clomiphene Citrate) 735
None cited in PDR database.

CLORPACTIN WCS-90
(Sodium Oxychlorosene) 1723
None cited in PDR database.

CLORPRES TABLETS
(Chlorthalidone, Clonidine Hydrochloride) 1002
May interact with antihypertensives, barbiturates, beta blockers, cardiac glycosides, oral hypoglycemic agents, hypnotics and sedatives, insulin, lithium preparations, narcotic analgesics, tricyclic antidepressants, and certain other agents. Compounds in these categories include:

Acarbose (Chlorthalidone causes hyperglycemia; higher dosage of oral hypoglycemic agents may be required). Products include:
Precose Tablets 906

Acebutolol Hydrochloride (Chlorthalidone may add to or potentiate the action of other antihypertensives; if therapy is to be discontinued in patients receiving clonidine and beta blockers concurrently, beta blockers should be discontinued several days before the gradual withdrawal of clonidine). Products include:
Sectral Capsules 3589

Alfentanil Hydrochloride (Orthostatic hypotension may be aggravated by narcotics; orthostatic hypotension may be aggravated by barbiturates).
No products indexed under this heading.

Amitriptyline Hydrochloride (Co-administration of clonidine with tricyclic antidepressants may result in reduced effect of clonidine, necessitating an increase in dosage; concurrent use enhances the manifestation of corneal lesions in rats). Products include:
Etrafon 3115
Limbitrol 1738

Amlodipine Besylate (Chlorthalidone may add to or potentiate the action of other antihypertensives). Products include:
Lotrel Capsules 2370
Norvasc Tablets 2704

Amoxapine (Co-administration of clonidine with tricyclic antidepressants may result in reduced effect of clonidine, necessitating an increase in dosage).
No products indexed under this heading.

Aprobarbital (Clonidine may enhance the CNS-depressive effects of barbiturates; orthostatic hypotension may be aggravated by barbiturates).
No products indexed under this heading.

Atenolol (Chlorthalidone may add to or potentiate the action of other antihypertensives; if therapy is to be discontinued in patients receiving clonidine and beta blockers concurrently, beta blockers should be discontinued several days before the gradual withdrawal of clonidine). Products include:
Tenoretic Tablets 690
Tenormin I.V. Injection 692

Benazepril Hydrochloride (Chlorthalidone may add to or potentiate the action of other antihypertensives). Products include:
Lotensin Tablets 2365
Lotensin HCT Tablets 2367
Lotrel Capsules 2370

Bendroflumethiazide (Chlorthalidone may add to or potentiate the action of other antihypertensives). Products include:
Corzide 40/5 Tablets 2247
Corzide 80/5 Tablets 2247

Betaxolol Hydrochloride (Chlorthalidone may add to or potentiate the action of other antihypertensives; if therapy is to be discontinued in patients receiving clonidine and beta blockers concurrently, beta blockers should be discontinued several days before the gradual withdrawal of clonidine). Products include:
Betoptic S Ophthalmic Suspension 537

Bisoprolol Fumarate (Chlorthalidone may add to or potentiate the action of other antihypertensives; if therapy is to be discontinued in patients receiving clonidine and beta blockers concurrently, beta blockers should be discontinued several days before the gradual withdrawal of clonidine). Products include:
Zebeta Tablets 1885
Ziac Tablets 1887

Buprenorphine Hydrochloride (Orthostatic hypotension may be aggravated by narcotics; orthostatic hypotension may be aggravated by barbiturates). Products include:
Buprenex Injectable 2918

Butabarbital (Clonidine may enhance the CNS-depressive effects of barbiturates; orthostatic hypotension may be aggravated by barbiturates).
No products indexed under this heading.

Butalbital (Clonidine may enhance the CNS-depressive effects of barbiturates; orthostatic hypotension may be aggravated by barbiturates). Products include:
Phrenilin 578
Sedapap Tablets 50 mg/650 mg 2225

Candesartan Cilexetil (Chlorthalidone may add to or potentiate the action of other antihypertensives). Products include:
Atacand Tablets 595
Atacand HCT Tablets 597

Captopril (Chlorthalidone may add to or potentiate the action of other antihypertensives). Products include:
Captopril Tablets 2281

Carteolol Hydrochloride (Chlorthalidone may add to or potentiate the action of other antihypertensives; if therapy is to be discontinued in patients receiving clonidine and beta blockers concurrently, beta blockers should be discontinued several days before the gradual withdrawal of clonidine). Products include:
Carteolol Hydrochloride Ophthalmic Solution USP, 1% .... ⊙258
Ocupress Ophthalmic Solution, 1% Sterile .... ⊙303

Chlorothiazide (Chlorthalidone may add to or potentiate the action of other antihypertensives). Products include:
Aldoclor Tablets 2035
Diuril Oral 2087

Chlorothiazide Sodium (Chlorthalidone may add to or potentiate the action of other antihypertensives). Products include:
Diuril Sodium Intravenous 2086

Chlorpropamide (Chlorthalidone causes hyperglycemia; higher dosage of oral hypoglycemic agents may be required). Products include:
Diabinese Tablets 2680

Clomipramine Hydrochloride (Co-administration of clonidine with tricyclic antidepressants may result in reduced effect of clonidine, necessitating an increase in dosage).
No products indexed under this heading.

Clonidine (Chlorthalidone may add to or potentiate the action of other antihypertensives). Products include:
Catapres-TTS 1038

Codeine Phosphate (Orthostatic hypotension may be aggravated by narcotics; orthostatic hypotension may be aggravated by barbiturates). Products include:
Phenergan with Codeine Syrup 3557
Phenergan VC with Codeine Syrup 3561
Robitussin A-C Syrup 2942
Robitussin-DAC Syrup 2942
Ryna-C Liquid .... ▣768
Soma Compound w/Codeine Tablets 3355
Tussi-Organidin NR Liquid 3350
Tussi-Organidin-S NR Liquid 3350
Tylenol with Codeine 2595

Deserpidine (Chlorthalidone may add to or potentiate the action of other antihypertensives).
No products indexed under this heading.

Desipramine Hydrochloride (Co-administration of clonidine with tricyclic antidepressants may result in reduced effect of clonidine, necessitating an increase in dosage). Products include:
Norpramin Tablets 755

Deslanoside (Digitalis therapy may exaggerate the metabolic effects of hypokalemia especially with reference to myocardial activity).
No products indexed under this heading.

Dezocine (Orthostatic hypotension may be aggravated by narcotics; orthostatic hypotension may be aggravated by barbiturates).
No products indexed under this heading.

Diazoxide (Chlorthalidone may add to or potentiate the action of other antihypertensives).
No products indexed under this heading.

Digitoxin (Digitalis therapy may exaggerate the metabolic effects of hypokalemia especially with reference to myocardial activity).
No products indexed under this heading.

Digoxin (Digitalis therapy may exaggerate the metabolic effects of hypokalemia especially with reference to myocardial activity). Products include:
Digitek Tablets ... 1003
Lanoxicaps Capsules ... 1574
Lanoxin Injection ... 1581
Lanoxin Tablets ... 1587
Lanoxin Elixir Pediatric ... 1578
Lanoxin Injection Pediatric ... 1584

Diltiazem Hydrochloride (Chlorthalidone may add to or potentiate the action of other antihypertensives). Products include:
Cardizem Injectable ... 1018
Cardizem Lyo-Ject Syringe ... 1018
Cardizem Monovial ... 1018
Cardizem CD Capsules ... 1016
Tiazac Capsules ... 1378

Doxazosin Mesylate (Chlorthalidone may add to or potentiate the action of other antihypertensives). Products include:
Cardura Tablets ... 2668

Doxepin Hydrochloride (Co-administration of clonidine with tricyclic antidepressants may result in reduced effect of clonidine, necessitating an increase in dosage). Products include:
Sinequan ... 2713

Enalapril Maleate (Chlorthalidone may add to or potentiate the action of other antihypertensives). Products include:
Lexxel Tablets ... 608
Vaseretic Tablets ... 2204
Vasotec Tablets ... 2210

Enalaprilat (Chlorthalidone may add to or potentiate the action of other antihypertensives). Products include:
Enalaprilat Injection ... 863
Vasotec I.V. Injection ... 2207

Eprosartan Mesylate (Chlorthalidone may add to or potentiate the action of other antihypertensives). Products include:
Teveten Tablets ... 3327

Esmolol Hydrochloride (Chlorthalidone may add to or potentiate the action of other antihypertensives; if therapy is to be discontinued in patients receiving clonidine and beta blockers concurrently, beta blockers should be discontinued several days before the gradual withdrawal of clonidine). Products include:
Brevibloc Injection ... 858

Estazolam (Clonidine may enhance the CNS-depressive effects of other sedatives). Products include:
ProSom Tablets ... 500

Ethchlorvynol (Clonidine may enhance the CNS-depressive effects of other sedatives).
No products indexed under this heading.

Ethinamate (Clonidine may enhance the CNS-depressive effects of other sedatives).
No products indexed under this heading.

Felodipine (Chlorthalidone may add to or potentiate the action of other antihypertensives). Products include:
Lexxel Tablets ... 608
Plendil Extended-Release Tablets ... 623

Fentanyl (Orthostatic hypotension may be aggravated by narcotics; orthostatic hypotension may be aggravated by barbiturates). Products include:
Duragesic Transdermal System ... 1786

Fentanyl Citrate (Orthostatic hypotension may be aggravated by narcotics; orthostatic hypotension may be aggravated by barbiturates). Products include:
Actiq ... 1184

Flurazepam Hydrochloride (Clonidine may enhance the CNS-depressive effects of other sedatives).
No products indexed under this heading.

Fosinopril Sodium (Chlorthalidone may add to or potentiate the action of other antihypertensives). Products include:
Monopril Tablets ... 1091
Monopril HCT ... 1094

Furosemide (Chlorthalidone may add to or potentiate the action of other antihypertensives). Products include:
Furosemide Tablets ... 2284

Glimepiride (Chlorthalidone causes hyperglycemia; higher dosage of oral hypoglycemic agents may be required). Products include:
Amaryl Tablets ... 717

Glipizide (Chlorthalidone causes hyperglycemia; higher dosage of oral hypoglycemic agents may be required). Products include:
Glucotrol Tablets ... 2692
Glucotrol XL Extended Release Tablets ... 2693

Glutethimide (Clonidine may enhance the CNS-depressive effects of other sedatives).
No products indexed under this heading.

Glyburide (Chlorthalidone causes hyperglycemia; higher dosage of oral hypoglycemic agents may be required). Products include:
DiaBeta Tablets ... 741
Glucovance Tablets ... 1086

Guanabenz Acetate (Chlorthalidone may add to or potentiate the action of other antihypertensives).
No products indexed under this heading.

Guanethidine Monosulfate (Chlorthalidone may add to or potentiate the action of other antihypertensives).
No products indexed under this heading.

Hydralazine Hydrochloride (Chlorthalidone may add to or potentiate the action of other antihypertensives).
No products indexed under this heading.

Hydrochlorothiazide (Chlorthalidone may add to or potentiate the action of other antihypertensives). Products include:
Accuretic Tablets ... 2614
Aldoril Tablets ... 2039
Atacand HCT Tablets ... 597
Avalide Tablets ... 1070
Diovan HCT Tablets ... 2338
Dyazide Capsules ... 1515
HydroDIURIL Tablets ... 2108
Hyzaar ... 2109
Inderide Tablets ... 3517
Inderide LA Long-Acting Capsules ... 3519
Lotensin HCT Tablets ... 2367
Maxzide ... 1008
Micardis HCT Tablets ... 1051
Microzide Capsules ... 3414
Moduretic Tablets ... 2138
Monopril HCT ... 1094
Prinzide Tablets ... 2168
Timolide Tablets ... 2187
Uniretic Tablets ... 3178
Vaseretic Tablets ... 2204
Zestoretic Tablets ... 695
Ziac Tablets ... 1887

Hydrocodone Bitartrate (Orthostatic hypotension may be aggravated by narcotics; orthostatic hypotension may be aggravated by barbiturates). Products include:
Hycodan ... 1316
Hycomine Compound Tablets ... 1317
Hycotuss Expectorant Syrup ... 1318
Lortab ... 3319
Lortab Elixir ... 3317
Maxidone Tablets CIII ... 3399
Norco 5/325 Tablets CIII ... 3424
Norco 7.5/325 Tablets CIII ... 3425
Norco 10/325 Tablets CIII ... 3427
Norco 10/325 Tablets CIII ... 3425
Vicodin Tablets ... 516
Vicodin ES Tablets ... 517
Vicodin HP Tablets ... 518
Vicodin Tuss Expectorant ... 519
Vicoprofen Tablets ... 520
Zydone Tablets ... 1330

Hydrocodone Polistirex (Orthostatic hypotension may be aggravated by narcotics; orthostatic hypotension may be aggravated by barbiturates). Products include:
Tussionex Pennkinetic Extended-Release Suspension ... 1174

Hydroflumethiazide (Chlorthalidone may add to or potentiate the action of other antihypertensives). Products include:
Diucardin Tablets ... 3494

Hydromorphone Hydrochloride (Orthostatic hypotension may be aggravated by narcotics; orthostatic hypotension may be aggravated by barbiturates). Products include:
Dilaudid ... 441
Dilaudid Oral Liquid ... 445
Dilaudid Powder ... 441
Dilaudid Rectal Suppositories ... 441
Dilaudid Tablets ... 441
Dilaudid Tablets - 8 mg ... 445
Dilaudid-HP ... 443

Imipramine Hydrochloride (Co-administration of clonidine with tricyclic antidepressants may result in reduced effect of clonidine, necessitating an increase in dosage).
No products indexed under this heading.

Imipramine Pamoate (Co-administration of clonidine with tricyclic antidepressants may result in reduced effect of clonidine, necessitating an increase in dosage).
No products indexed under this heading.

Indapamide (Chlorthalidone may add to or potentiate the action of other antihypertensives). Products include:
Indapamide Tablets ... 2286

Insulin, Human, Zinc Suspension (Chlorthalidone causes hyperglycemia; insulin requirements may be increased, decreased, or unchanged). Products include:
Humulin L, 100 Units ... 1937
Humulin U, 100 Units ... 1943
Novolin L Human Insulin 10 ml Vials ... 2422

Insulin, Human NPH (Chlorthalidone causes hyperglycemia; insulin requirements may be increased, decreased, or unchanged). Products include:
Humulin N, 100 Units ... 1939
Humulin N NPH Pen ... 1940
Novolin N Human Insulin 10 ml Vials ... 2422
Novolin N PenFill ... 2423
Novolin N Prefilled Syringe Disposable Insulin Delivery System ... 2425

Insulin, Human Regular (Chlorthalidone causes hyperglycemia; insulin requirements may be increased, decreased, or unchanged). Products include:
Humulin R Regular (U-500) ... 1943
Humulin R, 100 Units ... 1941
Novolin R Human Insulin 10 ml Vials ... 2423
Novolin R PenFill ... 2423
Novolin R Prefilled Syringe Disposable Insulin Delivery System ... 2425
Velosulin BR Human Insulin 10 ml Vials ... 2435

Insulin, Human Regular and Human NPH Mixture (Chlorthalidone causes hyperglycemia; insulin requirements may be increased, decreased, or unchanged). Products include:
Humulin 50/50, 100 Units ... 1934
Humulin 70/30, 100 Units ... 1935
Humulin 70/30 Pen ... 1936
Novolin 70/30 Human Insulin 10 ml Vials ... 2421
Novolin 70/30 PenFill ... 2423
Novolin 70/30 Prefilled Disposable Insulin Delivery System ... 2425

Insulin, NPH (Chlorthalidone causes hyperglycemia; insulin requirements may be increased, decreased, or unchanged). Products include:
Iletin II, NPH (Pork), 100 Units ... 1946

Insulin, Regular (Chlorthalidone causes hyperglycemia; insulin requirements may be increased, decreased, or unchanged). Products include:
Iletin II, Regular (Pork), 100 Units ... 1947

Insulin, Zinc Crystals (Chlorthalidone causes hyperglycemia; insulin requirements may be increased, decreased, or unchanged).
No products indexed under this heading.

Insulin, Zinc Suspension (Chlorthalidone causes hyperglycemia; insulin requirements may be increased, decreased, or unchanged). Products include:
Iletin II, Lente (Pork), 100 Units ... 1945

Insulin Aspart, Human Regular (Chlorthalidone causes hyperglycemia; insulin requirements may be increased, decreased, or unchanged).
No products indexed under this heading.

Insulin glargine (Chlorthalidone causes hyperglycemia; insulin requirements may be increased, decreased, or unchanged). Products include:
Lantus Injection ... 742

Insulin Lispro, Human (Chlorthalidone causes hyperglycemia; insulin requirements may be increased, decreased, or unchanged). Products include:
Humalog ... 1926
Humalog Mix 75/25 Pen ... 1928

Insulin Lispro Protamine, Human (Chlorthalidone causes hyperglycemia; insulin requirements may be increased, decreased, or unchanged). Products include:
Humalog Mix 75/25 Pen ... 1928

Irbesartan (Chlorthalidone may add to or potentiate the action of other antihypertensives). Products include:
Avalide Tablets ... 1070
Avapro Tablets ... 1074
Avapro Tablets ... 3076

Isradipine (Chlorthalidone may add to or potentiate the action of other antihypertensives). Products include:
DynaCirc Capsules ... 2921
DynaCirc CR Tablets ... 2923

Labetalol Hydrochloride (Chlorthalidone may add to or potentiate the action of other antihypertensives; if therapy is to be discontinued in patients receiving clonidine and beta blockers concurrently, beta blockers should be discontinued

several days before the gradual withdrawal of clonidine). Products include:

Normodyne Injection 3135
Normodyne Tablets 3137

Levobunolol Hydrochloride (Chlorthalidone may add to or potentiate the action of other antihypertensives; if therapy is to be discontinued in patients receiving clonidine and beta blockers concurrently, beta blockers should be discontinued several days before the gradual withdrawal of clonidine). Products include:

Betagan .... ⊙228

Levorphanol Tartrate (Orthostatic hypotension may be aggravated by narcotics; orthostatic hypotension may be aggravated by barbiturates). Products include:

Levo-Dromoran 1734
Levorphanol Tartrate Tablets 3059

Lisinopril (Chlorthalidone may add to or potentiate the action of other antihypertensives). Products include:

Prinivil Tablets 2164
Prinzide Tablets 2168
Zestoretic Tablets 695
Zestril Tablets 698

Lithium Carbonate (Chlorthalidone reduces renal clearance of lithium, increasing the risk of lithium toxicity). Products include:

Eskalith 1527
Lithium Carbonate 3061
Lithobid Slow-Release Tablets 3255

Lithium Citrate (Chlorthalidone reduces renal clearance of lithium, increasing the risk of lithium toxicity). Products include:

Lithium Citrate Syrup 3061

Lorazepam (Clonidine may enhance the CNS-depressive effects of other sedatives). Products include:

Ativan Injection 3478
Ativan Tablets 3482

Losartan Potassium (Chlorthalidone may add to or potentiate the action of other antihypertensives). Products include:

Cozaar Tablets 2067
Hyzaar 2109

Maprotiline Hydrochloride (Co-administration of clonidine with tricyclic antidepressants may result in reduced effect of clonidine, necessitating an increase in dosage).

No products indexed under this heading.

Mecamylamine Hydrochloride (Chlorthalidone may add to or potentiate the action of other antihypertensives). Products include:

Inversine Tablets 1850

Meperidine Hydrochloride (Orthostatic hypotension may be aggravated by narcotics; orthostatic hypotension may be aggravated by barbiturates). Products include:

Demerol 3079
Mepergan Injection 3539

Mephobarbital (Clonidine may enhance the CNS-depressive effects of barbiturates; orthostatic hypotension may be aggravated by barbiturates).

No products indexed under this heading.

Metformin Hydrochloride (Chlorthalidone causes hyperglycemia; higher dosage of oral hypoglycemic agents may be required). Products include:

Glucophage Tablets 1080
Glucophage XR Tablets 1080
Glucovance Tablets 1086

Methadone Hydrochloride (Orthostatic hypotension may be aggravated by narcotics; orthostatic hypotension may be aggravated by barbiturates). Products include:

Dolophine Hydrochloride Tablets 3056

Methyclothiazide (Chlorthalidone may add to or potentiate the action of other antihypertensives).

No products indexed under this heading.

Methyldopa (Chlorthalidone may add to or potentiate the action of other antihypertensives). Products include:

Aldoclor Tablets 2035
Aldomet Tablets 2037
Aldoril Tablets 2039

Methyldopate Hydrochloride (Chlorthalidone may add to or potentiate the action of other antihypertensives).

No products indexed under this heading.

Metipranolol Hydrochloride (Chlorthalidone may add to or potentiate the action of other antihypertensives; if therapy is to be discontinued in patients receiving clonidine and beta blockers concurrently, beta blockers should be discontinued several days before the gradual withdrawal of clonidine).

No products indexed under this heading.

Metolazone (Chlorthalidone may add to or potentiate the action of other antihypertensives). Products include:

Mykrox Tablets 1168
Zaroxolyn Tablets 1177

Metoprolol Succinate (Chlorthalidone may add to or potentiate the action of other antihypertensives; if therapy is to be discontinued in patients receiving clonidine and beta blockers concurrently, beta blockers should be discontinued several days before the gradual withdrawal of clonidine). Products include:

Toprol-XL Tablets 651

Metoprolol Tartrate (Chlorthalidone may add to or potentiate the action of other antihypertensives; if therapy is to be discontinued in patients receiving clonidine and beta blockers concurrently, beta blockers should be discontinued several days before the gradual withdrawal of clonidine).

No products indexed under this heading.

Metyrosine (Chlorthalidone may add to or potentiate the action of other antihypertensives). Products include:

Demser Capsules 2085

Mibefradil Dihydrochloride (Chlorthalidone may add to or potentiate the action of other antihypertensives).

No products indexed under this heading.

Midazolam Hydrochloride (Clonidine may enhance the CNS-depressive effects of other sedatives). Products include:

Versed Injection 3027
Versed Syrup 3033

Miglitol (Chlorthalidone causes hyperglycemia; higher dosage of oral hypoglycemic agents may be required). Products include:

Glyset Tablets 2821

Minoxidil (Chlorthalidone may add to or potentiate the action of other antihypertensives). Products include:

Rogaine Extra Strength for Men Topical Solution .... ▣721
Rogaine for Women Topical Solution .... ▣721

Moexipril Hydrochloride (Chlorthalidone may add to or potentiate the action of other antihypertensives). Products include:

Uniretic Tablets 3178
Univasc Tablets 3181

Morphine Sulfate (Orthostatic hypotension may be aggravated by narcotics; orthostatic hypotension may be aggravated by barbiturates). Products include:

Astramorph/PF Injection, USP (Preservative-Free)..................... 594
Duramorph Injection 1312
Infumorph 200 and Infumorph 500 Sterile Solutions 1314
Kadian Capsules 1335
MS Contin Tablets 2896
MSIR 2898
Oramorph SR Tablets 3062
Roxanol 3066

Nadolol (Chlorthalidone may add to or potentiate the action of other antihypertensives; if therapy is to be discontinued in patients receiving clonidine and beta blockers concurrently, beta blockers should be discontinued several days before the gradual withdrawal of clonidine). Products include:

Corgard Tablets 2245
Corzide 40/5 Tablets 2247
Corzide 80/5 Tablets 2247
Nadolol Tablets 2288

Nicardipine Hydrochloride (Chlorthalidone may add to or potentiate the action of other antihypertensives). Products include:

Cardene I.V. 3485

Nifedipine (Chlorthalidone may add to or potentiate the action of other antihypertensives). Products include:

Adalat CC Tablets 877
Procardia Capsules 2708
Procardia XL Extended Release Tablets 2710

Nisoldipine (Chlorthalidone may add to or potentiate the action of other antihypertensives). Products include:

Sular Tablets 688

Nitroglycerin (Chlorthalidone may add to or potentiate the action of other antihypertensives). Products include:

Nitro-Dur Transdermal Infusion System 3134
Nitro-Dur Transdermal Infusion System 1834
Nitrolingual Pumpspray 1355
Nitrostat Tablets 2658

Norepinephrine Bitartrate (Chlorthalidone may decrease arterial responsiveness to norepinephrine).

No products indexed under this heading.

Nortriptyline Hydrochloride (Co-administration of clonidine with tricyclic antidepressants may result in reduced effect of clonidine, necessitating an increase in dosage).

No products indexed under this heading.

Oxycodone Hydrochloride (Orthostatic hypotension may be aggravated by narcotics; orthostatic hypotension may be aggravated by barbiturates). Products include:

OxyContin Tablets 2912
OxyFast Oral Concentrate Solution . 2916
OxyIR Capsules 2916
Percocet Tablets 1326
Percodan Tablets 1327
Percolone Tablets 1327
Roxicodone 3067
Tylox Capsules 2597

Penbutolol Sulfate (Chlorthalidone may add to or potentiate the action of other antihypertensives; if therapy is to be discontinued in patients receiving clonidine and beta blockers concurrently, beta blockers should be discontinued several days before the gradual withdrawal of clonidine).

No products indexed under this heading.

Pentobarbital Sodium (Clonidine may enhance the CNS-depressive effects of barbiturates; orthostatic hypotension may be aggravated by barbiturates). Products include:

Nembutal Sodium Solution 485

Perindopril Erbumine (Chlorthalidone may add to or potentiate the action of other antihypertensives). Products include:

Aceon Tablets (2 mg, 4 mg, 8 mg).. 3249

Phenobarbital (Clonidine may enhance the CNS-depressive effects of barbiturates; orthostatic hypotension may be aggravated by barbiturates). Products include:

Arco-Lase Plus Tablets 592
Donnatal 2929
Donnatal Extentabs 2930

Phenoxybenzamine Hydrochloride (Chlorthalidone may add to or potentiate the action of other antihypertensives). Products include:

Dibenzyline Capsules 3457

Phentolamine Mesylate (Chlorthalidone may add to or potentiate the action of other antihypertensives).

No products indexed under this heading.

Pindolol (Chlorthalidone may add to or potentiate the action of other antihypertensives; if therapy is to be discontinued in patients receiving clonidine and beta blockers concurrently, beta blockers should be discontinued several days before the gradual withdrawal of clonidine).

No products indexed under this heading.

Pioglitazone Hydrochloride (Chlorthalidone causes hyperglycemia; higher dosage of oral hypoglycemic agents may be required). Products include:

Actos Tablets 3275

Polythiazide (Chlorthalidone may add to or potentiate the action of other antihypertensives). Products include:

Minizide Capsules 2700
Renese Tablets 2712

Prazosin Hydrochloride (Chlorthalidone may add to or potentiate the action of other antihypertensives). Products include:

Minipress Capsules 2699
Minizide Capsules 2700

Propofol (Clonidine may enhance the CNS-depressive effects of other sedatives). Products include:

Diprivan Injectable Emulsion 667

Propoxyphene Hydrochloride (Orthostatic hypotension may be aggravated by narcotics; orthostatic hypotension may be aggravated by barbiturates). Products include:

Darvon Pulvules 1909
Darvon Compound-65 Pulvules 1910

Propoxyphene Napsylate (Orthostatic hypotension may be aggravated by narcotics; orthostatic hypotension may be aggravated by barbiturates). Products include:

Darvon-N/Darvocet-N 1907
Darvon-N Tablets 1912

Propranolol Hydrochloride (Chlorthalidone may add to or potentiate the action of other antihypertensives; if therapy is to be discontinued in patients receiving clonidine and beta blockers concurrently, beta blockers should be discontinued several days before the gradual withdrawal of clonidine). Products include:

Inderal 3513
Inderal LA Long-Acting Capsules 3516
Inderide Tablets 3517
Inderide LA Long-Acting Capsules .. 3519

Protriptyline Hydrochloride (Co-administration of clonidine with tricyclic antidepressants may result in reduced effect of clonidine, necessitating an increase in dosage). Products include:

Vivactil Tablets 2446
Vivactil Tablets 2217

Quazepam (Clonidine may enhance the CNS-depressive effects of other

sedatives).
No products indexed under this heading.

Quinapril Hydrochloride (Chlorthalidone may add to or potentiate the action of other antihypertensives). Products include:
Accupril Tablets 2611
Accuretic Tablets 2614

Ramipril (Chlorthalidone may add to or potentiate the action of other antihypertensives). Products include:
Altace Capsules 2233

Rauwolfia serpentina (Chlorthalidone may add to or potentiate the action of other antihypertensives).
No products indexed under this heading.

Remifentanil Hydrochloride (Orthostatic hypotension may be aggravated by narcotics; orthostatic hypotension may be aggravated by barbiturates).
No products indexed under this heading.

Repaglinide (Chlorthalidone causes hyperglycemia; higher dosage of oral hypoglycemic agents may be required). Products include:
Prandin Tablets (0.5, 1, and 2 mg).......... 2432

Rescinnamine (Chlorthalidone may add to or potentiate the action of other antihypertensives).
No products indexed under this heading.

Reserpine (Chlorthalidone may add to or potentiate the action of other antihypertensives).
No products indexed under this heading.

Rosiglitazone Maleate (Chlorthalidone causes hyperglycemia; higher dosage of oral hypoglycemic agents may be required). Products include:
Avandia Tablets 1490

Secobarbital Sodium (Clonidine may enhance the CNS-depressive effects of barbiturates; orthostatic hypotension may be aggravated by barbiturates).
No products indexed under this heading.

Sodium Nitroprusside (Chlorthalidone may add to or potentiate the action of other antihypertensives).
No products indexed under this heading.

Sotalol Hydrochloride (Chlorthalidone may add to or potentiate the action of other antihypertensives; if therapy is to be discontinued in patients receiving clonidine and beta blockers concurrently, beta blockers should be discontinued several days before the gradual withdrawal of clonidine). Products include:
Betapace Tablets 950
Betapace AF Tablets 954

Spirapril Hydrochloride (Chlorthalidone may add to or potentiate the action of other antihypertensives).
No products indexed under this heading.

Sufentanil Citrate (Orthostatic hypotension may be aggravated by narcotics; orthostatic hypotension may be aggravated by barbiturates).
No products indexed under this heading.

Telmisartan (Chlorthalidone may add to or potentiate the action of other antihypertensives). Products include:
Micardis Tablets 1049
Micardis HCT Tablets 1051

Temazepam (Clonidine may enhance the CNS-depressive effects of other sedatives).
No products indexed under this heading.

Terazosin Hydrochloride (Chlorthalidone may add to or potentiate the action of other antihypertensives). Products include:
Hytrin Capsules 464

Thiamylal Sodium (Clonidine may enhance the CNS-depressive effects of barbiturates; orthostatic hypotension may be aggravated by barbiturates).
No products indexed under this heading.

Timolol Hemihydrate (Chlorthalidone may add to or potentiate the action of other antihypertensives; if therapy is to be discontinued in patients receiving clonidine and beta blockers concurrently, beta blockers should be discontinued several days before the gradual withdrawal of clonidine). Products include:
Betimol Ophthalmic Solution .... ⊙324

Timolol Maleate (Chlorthalidone may add to or potentiate the action of other antihypertensives; if therapy is to be discontinued in patients receiving clonidine and beta blockers concurrently, beta blockers should be discontinued several days before the gradual withdrawal of clonidine). Products include:
Blocadren Tablets 2046
Cosopt Sterile Ophthalmic Solution.......... 2065
Timolide Tablets 2187
Timolol GFS .... ⊙266
Timoptic in Ocudose 2192
Timoptic Sterile Ophthalmic Solution.......... 2190
Timoptic-XE Sterile Ophthalmic Gel Forming Solution.......... 2194

Tolazamide (Chlorthalidone causes hyperglycemia; higher dosage of oral hypoglycemic agents may be required).
No products indexed under this heading.

Tolbutamide (Chlorthalidone causes hyperglycemia; higher dosage of oral hypoglycemic agents may be required).
No products indexed under this heading.

Torsemide (Chlorthalidone may add to or potentiate the action of other antihypertensives). Products include:
Demadex Tablets and Injection 2965

Trandolapril (Chlorthalidone may add to or potentiate the action of other antihypertensives). Products include:
Mavik Tablets 478
Tarka Tablets 508

Triazolam (Clonidine may enhance the CNS-depressive effects of other sedatives). Products include:
Halcion Tablets 2823

Trimethaphan Camsylate (Chlorthalidone may add to or potentiate the action of other antihypertensives).
No products indexed under this heading.

Trimipramine Maleate (Co-administration of clonidine with tricyclic antidepressants may result in reduced effect of clonidine, necessitating an increase in dosage). Products include:
Surmontil Capsules 3595

Troglitazone (Chlorthalidone causes hyperglycemia; higher dosage of oral hypoglycemic agents may be required).
No products indexed under this heading.

Tubocurarine Chloride (Chlorthalidone may increase responsiveness to tubocurarine).
No products indexed under this heading.

Valsartan (Chlorthalidone may add to or potentiate the action of other antihypertensives). Products include:
Diovan Capsules 2337
Diovan HCT Tablets 2338

Verapamil Hydrochloride (Chlorthalidone may add to or potentiate the action of other antihypertensives). Products include:
Covera-HS Tablets 3199
Isoptin SR Tablets 467
Tarka Tablets 508
Verelan Capsules 3184
Verelan PM Capsules 3186

Zaleplon (Clonidine may enhance the CNS-depressive effects of other sedatives). Products include:
Sonata Capsules 3591

Zolpidem Tartrate (Clonidine may enhance the CNS-depressive effects of other sedatives). Products include:
Ambien Tablets 3191

Food Interactions

Alcohol (Clonidine may enhance the CNS-depressive effects of alcohol; orthostatic hypotension may be aggravated by alcohol).

CLOZARIL TABLETS

(Clozapine) 2319
May interact with antihypertensives, belladona products, benzodiazepines, antidepressant drugs, erythromycin, phenytoin, psychotropics, quinidine, selective serotonin reuptake inhibitors, and certain other agents. Compounds in these categories include:

Acebutolol Hydrochloride (Hypotensive effects potentiated). Products include:
Sectral Capsules 3589

Alprazolam (Co-administration with benzodiazepines or other psychotropic agents may be accompanied by profound collapse and respiratory and/or cardiac arrest; caution is advised if used concurrently). Products include:
Xanax Tablets 2865

Amitriptyline Hydrochloride (Concomitant use of clozapine with other drugs metabolized by cytochrome P450IID6 may require lower than usual doses prescribed for either drug). Products include:
Etrafon 3115
Limbitrol 1738

Amlodipine Besylate (Hypotensive effects potentiated). Products include:
Lotrel Capsules 2370
Norvasc Tablets 2704

Amoxapine (Concomitant use of clozapine with other drugs metabolized by cytochrome P450IID6 may require lower than usual doses prescribed for either drug).
No products indexed under this heading.

Atenolol (Hypotensive effects potentiated). Products include:
Tenoretic Tablets 690
Tenormin I.V. Injection 692

Atropine Sulfate (Anticholinergic effects potentiated). Products include:
Donnatal 2929
Donnatal Extentabs 2930
Motofen Tablets 577
Prosed/DS Tablets 3268
Urised Tablets 2876

Belladonna Alkaloids (Anticholinergic effects potentiated). Products include:
Hyland's Teething Tablets .... ▣766
Urimax Tablets 1769

Benazepril Hydrochloride (Hypotensive effects potentiated). Products include:
Lotensin Tablets 2365
Lotensin HCT Tablets 2367
Lotrel Capsules 2370

Bendroflumethiazide (Hypotensive effects potentiated). Products include:
Corzide 40/5 Tablets 2247
Corzide 80/5 Tablets 2247

Betaxolol Hydrochloride (Hypotensive effects potentiated). Products include:
Betoptic S Ophthalmic Suspension 537

Bisoprolol Fumarate (Hypotensive effects potentiated). Products include:
Zebeta Tablets 1885
Ziac Tablets 1887

Bone Marrow Depressants, unspecified (Increases the risk and/or severity of bone marrow suppression).

Bupropion Hydrochloride (Concomitant use of clozapine with other drugs metabolized by cytochrome P450IID6 may require lower than usual doses prescribed for either drug). Products include:
Wellbutrin Tablets 1680
Wellbutrin SR Sustained-Release Tablets 1684
Zyban Sustained-Release Tablets 1710

Buspirone Hydrochloride (Co-administration with benzodiazepines or other psychotropic agents may be accompanied by profound collapse and respiratory and/or cardiac arrest; caution is advised if used concurrently).
No products indexed under this heading.

Candesartan Cilexetil (Hypotensive effects potentiated). Products include:
Atacand Tablets 595
Atacand HCT Tablets 597

Captopril (Hypotensive effects potentiated). Products include:
Captopril Tablets 2281

Carbamazepine (Concomitant use is not recommended; discontinuation of concomitant carbamazepine administration may result in increase in clozapine levels). Products include:
Carbatrol Capsules 3234
Tegretol/Tegretol-XR 2404

Carteolol Hydrochloride (Hypotensive effects potentiated). Products include:
Carteolol Hydrochloride Ophthalmic Solution USP, 1% .... ⊙258
Ocupress Ophthalmic Solution, 1% Sterile .... ⊙303

Chlordiazepoxide (Co-administration with benzodiazepines or other psychotropic agents may be accompanied by profound collapse and respiratory and/or cardiac arrest; caution is advised if used concurrently). Products include:
Limbitrol 1738

Chlordiazepoxide Hydrochloride (Co-administration with benzodiazepines or other psychotropic agents may be accompanied by profound collapse and respiratory and/or cardiac arrest; caution is advised if used concurrently). Products include:
Librium Capsules 1736
Librium for Injection 1737

Chlorothiazide (Hypotensive effects potentiated). Products include:
Aldoclor Tablets 2035
Diuril Oral 2087

Chlorothiazide Sodium (Hypotensive effects potentiated). Products include:
Diuril Sodium Intravenous 2086

Chlorpromazine (Co-administration with benzodiazepines or other psychotropic agents may be accompanied by profound collapse and respiratory and/or cardiac arrest; caution is advised if used concurrently). Products include:
Thorazine Suppositories 1656

Chlorpromazine Hydrochloride (Co-administration with benzodiazepines or other psychotropic agents may be accompanied by profound

collapse and respiratory and/or cardiac arrest; caution is advised if used concurrently). Products include:
Thorazine ... 1656

Chlorprothixene (Co-administration with benzodiazepines or other psychotropic agents may be accompanied by profound collapse and respiratory and/or cardiac arrest; caution is advised if used concurrently).
No products indexed under this heading.

Chlorprothixene Hydrochloride (Co-administration with benzodiazepines or other psychotropic agents may be accompanied by profound collapse and respiratory and/or cardiac arrest; caution is advised if used concurrently).
No products indexed under this heading.

Chlorthalidone (Hypotensive effects potentiated). Products include:
Clorpres Tablets ... 1002
Combipres Tablets ... 1040
Tenoretic Tablets ... 690

Cimetidine (May increase plasma levels of clozapine, potentially resulting in adverse effects). Products include:
Tagamet HB 200 Suspension ... 762
Tagamet HB 200 Tablets ... 761
Tagamet Tablets ... 1644

Cimetidine Hydrochloride (May increase levels of clozapine potentially resulting in adverse effects). Products include:
Tagamet ... 1644

Citalopram Hydrobromide (Elevated serum levels of clozapine have been observed when co-administered with selective serotonin reuptake inhibitors; a reduced clozapine dose should be considered). Products include:
Celexa ... 1365

Clonidine (Hypotensive effects potentiated). Products include:
Catapres-TTS ... 1038

Clonidine Hydrochloride (Hypotensive effects potentiated). Products include:
Catapres Tablets ... 1037
Clorpres Tablets ... 1002
Combipres Tablets ... 1040
Duraclon Injection ... 3057

Clorazepate Dipotassium (Co-administration with benzodiazepines or other psychotropic agents may be accompanied by profound collapse and respiratory and/or cardiac arrest; caution is advised if used concurrently). Products include:
Tranxene ... 511

CNS-Active Drugs, unspecified (Caution is advised).

Deserpidine (Hypotensive effects potentiated).
No products indexed under this heading.

Desipramine Hydrochloride (Concomitant use of clozapine with other drugs metabolized by cytochrome P450IID6 may require lower than usual doses prescribed for either drug). Products include:
Norpramin Tablets ... 755

Diazepam (Co-administration with benzodiazepines or other psychotropic agents may be accompanied by profound collapse and respiratory and/or cardiac arrest; caution is advised if used concurrently). Products include:
Valium Injectable ... 3026
Valium Tablets ... 3047

Diazoxide (Hypotensive effects potentiated).
No products indexed under this heading.

Digitoxin (Co-administration with other highly protein-bound drugs, such as digitoxin, may cause an increase in plasma concentrations of warfarin, potentially resulting in adverse effects).
No products indexed under this heading.

Digoxin (Increase in plasma concentrations resulting in adverse affects). Products include:
Digitek Tablets ... 1003
Lanoxicaps Capsules ... 1574
Lanoxin Injection ... 1581
Lanoxin Tablets ... 1587
Lanoxin Elixir Pediatric ... 1578
Lanoxin Injection Pediatric ... 1584

Diltiazem Hydrochloride (Hypotensive effects potentiated). Products include:
Cardizem Injectable ... 1018
Cardizem Lyo-Ject Syringe ... 1018
Cardizem Monovial ... 1018
Cardizem CD Capsules ... 1016
Tiazac Capsules ... 1378

Doxazosin Mesylate (Hypotensive effects potentiated). Products include:
Cardura Tablets ... 2668

Doxepin Hydrochloride (Concomitant use of clozapine with other drugs metabolized by cytochrome P450IID6 may require lower than usual doses prescribed for either drug). Products include:
Sinequan ... 2713

Droperidol (Co-administration with benzodiazepines or other psychotropic agents may be accompanied by profound collapse and respiratory and/or cardiac arrest; caution is advised if used concurrently).
No products indexed under this heading.

Enalapril Maleate (Hypotensive effects potentiated). Products include:
Lexxel Tablets ... 608
Vaseretic Tablets ... 2204
Vasotec Tablets ... 2210

Enalaprilat (Hypotensive effects potentiated). Products include:
Enalaprilat Injection ... 863
Vasotec I.V. Injection ... 2207

Encainide Hydrochloride (Concomitant use of clozapine with other drugs metabolized by cytochrome P450IID6 may require lower than usual doses).
No products indexed under this heading.

Epinephrine Hydrochloride (Possible reverse epinephrine effect).
No products indexed under this heading.

Eprosartan Mesylate (Hypotensive effects potentiated). Products include:
Teveten Tablets ... 3327

Erythromycin (May increase plasma levels of clozapine, potentially resulting in adverse effects). Products include:
Emgel 2% Topical Gel ... 1285
Ery-Tab Tablets ... 448
Erythromycin Base Filmtab Tablets ... 454
Erythromycin Delayed-Release Capsules, USP ... 455
PCE Dispertab Tablets ... 498

Erythromycin Estolate (May increase plasma levels of clozapine, potentially resulting in adverse effects).
No products indexed under this heading.

Erythromycin Ethylsuccinate (May increase plasma levels of clozapine, potentially resulting in adverse effects). Products include:
E.E.S. ... 450
EryPed ... 446
Pediazole Suspension ... 3050

Erythromycin Gluceptate (May increase plasma levels of clozapine, potentially resulting in adverse effects).
No products indexed under this heading.

Erythromycin Stearate (May increase plasma levels of clozapine, potentially resulting in adverse effects). Products include:
Erythrocin Stearate Filmtab Tablets ... 452

Esmolol Hydrochloride (Hypotensive effects potentiated). Products include:
Brevibloc Injection ... 858

Estazolam (Co-administration with benzodiazepines or other psychotropic agents may be accompanied by profound collapse and respiratory and/or cardiac arrest; caution is advised if used concurrently). Products include:
ProSom Tablets ... 500

Felodipine (Hypotensive effects potentiated). Products include:
Lexxel Tablets ... 608
Plendil Extended-Release Tablets ... 623

Flecainide Acetate (Concomitant use of clozapine with other drugs metabolized by cytochrome P450IID6 may require lower than usual doses prescribed for either drug). Products include:
Tambocor Tablets ... 1990

Fluoxetine Hydrochloride (Co-administration in schizophrenic patients has resulted in elevated mean trough concentrations of clozapine and its metabolites by less than two-fold compared to baseline concentrations; a reduced clozapine dose should be considered). Products include:
Prozac Pulvules, Liquid, and Weekly Capsules ... 1238
Sarafem Pulvules ... 1962

Fluphenazine Decanoate (Co-administration with benzodiazepines or other psychotropic agents may be accompanied by profound collapse and respiratory and/or cardiac arrest; caution is advised if used concurrently).
No products indexed under this heading.

Fluphenazine Enanthate (Co-administration with benzodiazepines or other psychotropic agents may be accompanied by profound collapse and respiratory and/or cardiac arrest; caution is advised if used concurrently).
No products indexed under this heading.

Fluphenazine Hydrochloride (Co-administration with benzodiazepines or other psychotropic agents may be accompanied by profound collapse and respiratory and/or cardiac arrest; caution is advised if used concurrently).
No products indexed under this heading.

Flurazepam Hydrochloride (Co-administration with benzodiazepines or other psychotropic agents may be accompanied by profound collapse and respiratory and/or cardiac arrest; caution is advised if used concurrently).
No products indexed under this heading.

Fluvoxamine Maleate (Co-administration in schizophrenic patients has resulted in elevated mean trough concentrations of clozapine and its metabolites by about three-fold compared to baseline concentrations; a reduced clozapine dose should be considered). Products include:
Luvox Tablets (25, 50, 100 mg) ... 3256

Fosinopril Sodium (Hypotensive effects potentiated). Products include:
Monopril Tablets ... 1091
Monopril HCT ... 1094

Fosphenytoin Sodium (May decrease clozapine plasma levels, a decrease in effectiveness of a previously effective clozapine dose). Products include:
Cerebyx Injection ... 2619

Furosemide (Hypotensive effects potentiated). Products include:
Furosemide Tablets ... 2284

Guanabenz Acetate (Hypotensive effects potentiated).
No products indexed under this heading.

Guanethidine Monosulfate (Hypotensive effects potentiated).
No products indexed under this heading.

Halazepam (Co-administration with benzodiazepines or other psychotropic agents may be accompanied by profound collapse and respiratory and/or cardiac arrest; caution is advised if used concurrently).
No products indexed under this heading.

Haloperidol (Co-administration with benzodiazepines or other psychotropic agents may be accompanied by profound collapse and respiratory and/or cardiac arrest; caution is advised if used concurrently). Products include:
Haldol Injection, Tablets and Concentrate ... 2533

Haloperidol Decanoate (Co-administration with benzodiazepines or other psychotropic agents may be accompanied by profound collapse and respiratory and/or cardiac arrest; caution is advised if used concurrently). Products include:
Haldol Decanoate ... 2535

Hydralazine Hydrochloride (Hypotensive effects potentiated).
No products indexed under this heading.

Hydrochlorothiazide (Hypotensive effects potentiated). Products include:
Accuretic Tablets ... 2614
Aldoril Tablets ... 2039
Atacand HCT Tablets ... 597
Avalide Tablets ... 1070
Diovan HCT Tablets ... 2338
Dyazide Capsules ... 1515
HydroDIURIL Tablets ... 2108
Hyzaar ... 2109
Inderide Tablets ... 3517
Inderide LA Long-Acting Capsules ... 3519
Lotensin HCT Tablets ... 2367
Maxzide ... 1008
Micardis HCT Tablets ... 1051
Microzide Capsules ... 3414
Moduretic Tablets ... 2138
Monopril HCT ... 1094
Prinzide Tablets ... 2168
Timolide Tablets ... 2187
Uniretic Tablets ... 3178
Vaseretic Tablets ... 2204
Zestoretic Tablets ... 695
Ziac Tablets ... 1887

Hydroflumethiazide (Hypotensive effects potentiated). Products include:
Diucardin Tablets ... 3494

Hydroxyzine Hydrochloride (Co-administration with benzodiazepines or other psychotropic agents may be accompanied by profound collapse and respiratory and/or cardiac arrest; caution is advised if used concurrently). Products include:
Atarax Tablets & Syrup ... 2667
Vistaril Intramuscular Solution ... 2738

Hyoscyamine (Anticholinergic effects potentiated). Products include:
Urised Tablets ... 2876

Hyoscyamine Sulfate (Anticholinergic effects potentiated). Products include:
Arco-Lase Plus Tablets ... 592
Donnatal ... 2929
Donnatal Extentabs ... 2930
Levsin/Levsinex/Levbid ... 3172

NuLev Orally Disintegrating Tablets ... 3176
Prosed/DS Tablets ... 3268
Urimax Tablets ... 1769

Imipramine Hydrochloride (Concomitant use of clozapine with other drugs metabolized by cytochrome P450IID6 may require lower than usual doses prescribed for either drug).
No products indexed under this heading.

Imipramine Pamoate (Concomitant use of clozapine with other drugs metabolized by cytochrome P450IID6 may require lower than usual doses prescribed for either drug).
No products indexed under this heading.

Indapamide (Hypotensive effects potentiated). Products include:
Indapamide Tablets ... 2286

Irbesartan (Hypotensive effects potentiated). Products include:
Avalide Tablets ... 1070
Avapro Tablets ... 1074
Avapro Tablets ... 3076

Isocarboxazid (Concomitant use of clozapine with other drugs metabolized by cytochrome P450IID6 may require lower than usual doses prescribed for either drug).
No products indexed under this heading.

Isradipine (Hypotensive effects potentiated). Products include:
DynaCirc Capsules ... 2921
DynaCirc CR Tablets ... 2923

Labetalol Hydrochloride (Hypotensive effects potentiated). Products include:
Normodyne Injection ... 3135
Normodyne Tablets ... 3137

Lisinopril (Hypotensive effects potentiated). Products include:
Prinivil Tablets ... 2164
Prinzide Tablets ... 2168
Zestoretic Tablets ... 695
Zestril Tablets ... 698

Lithium Carbonate (Co-administration with benzodiazepines or other psychotropic agents may be accompanied by profound collapse and respiratory and/or cardiac arrest; caution is advised if used concurrently). Products include:
Eskalith ... 1527
Lithium Carbonate ... 3061
Lithobid Slow-Release Tablets ... 3255

Lithium Citrate (Co-administration with benzodiazepines or other psychotropic agents may be accompanied by profound collapse and respiratory and/or cardiac arrest; caution is advised if used concurrently). Products include:
Lithium Citrate Syrup ... 3061

Lorazepam (Co-administration with benzodiazepines or other psychotropic agents may be accompanied by profound collapse and respiratory and/or cardiac arrest; caution is advised if used concurrently). Products include:
Ativan Injection ... 3478
Ativan Tablets ... 3482

Losartan Potassium (Hypotensive effects potentiated). Products include:
Cozaar Tablets ... 2067
Hyzaar ... 2109

Loxapine Hydrochloride (Co-administration with benzodiazepines or other psychotropic agents may be accompanied by profound collapse and respiratory and/or cardiac arrest; caution is advised if used concurrently).
No products indexed under this heading.

Loxapine Succinate (Co-administration with benzodiazepines or other psychotropic agents may be accompanied by profound collapse and respiratory and/or cardiac arrest; caution is advised if used concurrently). Products include:
Loxitane Capsules ... 3398

Maprotiline Hydrochloride (Concomitant use of clozapine with other drugs metabolized by cytochrome P450IID6 may require lower than usual doses prescribed for either drug).
No products indexed under this heading.

Mecamylamine Hydrochloride (Hypotensive effects potentiated). Products include:
Inversine Tablets ... 1850

Meprobamate (Co-administration with benzodiazepines or other psychotropic agents may be accompanied by profound collapse and respiratory and/or cardiac arrest; caution is advised if used concurrently). Products include:
Miltown Tablets ... 3349

Mesoridazine Besylate (Co-administration with benzodiazepines or other psychotropic agents may be accompanied by profound collapse and respiratory and/or cardiac arrest; caution is advised if used concurrently). Products include:
Serentil ... 1057

Methyclothiazide (Hypotensive effects potentiated).
No products indexed under this heading.

Methyldopa (Hypotensive effects potentiated). Products include:
Aldoclor Tablets ... 2035
Aldomet Tablets ... 2037
Aldoril Tablets ... 2039

Methyldopate Hydrochloride (Hypotensive effects potentiated).
No products indexed under this heading.

Metolazone (Hypotensive effects potentiated). Products include:
Mykrox Tablets ... 1168
Zaroxolyn Tablets ... 1177

Metoprolol Succinate (Hypotensive effects potentiated). Products include:
Toprol-XL Tablets ... 651

Metoprolol Tartrate (Hypotensive effects potentiated).
No products indexed under this heading.

Metyrosine (Hypotensive effects potentiated). Products include:
Demser Capsules ... 2085

Mibefradil Dihydrochloride (Hypotensive effects potentiated).
No products indexed under this heading.

Midazolam Hydrochloride (Co-administration with benzodiazepines or other psychotropic agents may be accompanied by profound collapse and respiratory and/or cardiac arrest; caution is advised if used concurrently). Products include:
Versed Injection ... 3027
Versed Syrup ... 3033

Minoxidil (Hypotensive effects potentiated). Products include:
Rogaine Extra Strength for Men Topical Solution ... ▣721
Rogaine for Women Topical Solution ... ▣721

Mirtazapine (Concomitant use of clozapine with other drugs metabolized by cytochrome P450IID6 may require lower than usual doses prescribed for either drug). Products include:
Remeron Tablets ... 2483
Remeron SolTab Tablets ... 2486

Moexipril Hydrochloride (Hypotensive effects potentiated). Products include:
Uniretic Tablets ... 3178
Univasc Tablets ... 3181

Molindone Hydrochloride (Co-administration with benzodiazepines or other psychotropic agents may be accompanied by profound collapse and respiratory and/or cardiac arrest; caution is advised if used concurrently). Products include:
Moban ... 1320

Nadolol (Hypotensive effects potentiated). Products include:
Corgard Tablets ... 2245
Corzide 40/5 Tablets ... 2247
Corzide 80/5 Tablets ... 2247
Nadolol Tablets ... 2288

Nefazodone Hydrochloride (Concomitant use of clozapine with other drugs metabolized by cytochrome P450IID6 may require lower than usual doses prescribed for either drug). Products include:
Serzone Tablets ... 1104

Nicardipine Hydrochloride (Hypotensive effects potentiated). Products include:
Cardene I.V. ... 3485

Nifedipine (Hypotensive effects potentiated). Products include:
Adalat CC Tablets ... 877
Procardia Capsules ... 2708
Procardia XL Extended Release Tablets ... 2710

Nisoldipine (Hypotensive effects potentiated). Products include:
Sular Tablets ... 688

Nitroglycerin (Hypotensive effects potentiated). Products include:
Nitro-Dur Transdermal Infusion System ... 3134
Nitro-Dur Transdermal Infusion System ... 1834
Nitrolingual Pumpspray ... 1355
Nitrostat Tablets ... 2658

Norepinephrine Bitartrate (Possible reverse epinephrine effect).
No products indexed under this heading.

Nortriptyline Hydrochloride (Concomitant use of clozapine with other drugs metabolized by cytochrome P450IID6 may require lower than usual doses prescribed for either drug).
No products indexed under this heading.

Olanzapine (Co-administration with benzodiazepines or other psychotropic agents may be accompanied by profound collapse and respiratory and/or cardiac arrest; caution is advised if used concurrently). Products include:
Zyprexa Tablets ... 1973
Zyprexa ZYDIS Orally Disintegrating Tablets ... 1973

Oxazepam (Co-administration with benzodiazepines or other psychotropic agents may be accompanied by profound collapse and respiratory and/or cardiac arrest; caution is advised if used concurrently).
No products indexed under this heading.

Paroxetine Hydrochloride (Co-administration in schizophrenic patients has resulted in elevated mean trough concentrations of clozapine and its metabolites by less than two-fold compared to baseline concentrations; a reduced clozapine dose should be considered). Products include:
Paxil ... 1609

Penbutolol Sulfate (Hypotensive effects potentiated).
No products indexed under this heading.

Perindopril Erbumine (Hypotensive effects potentiated). Products include:
Aceon Tablets (2 mg, 4 mg, 8 mg) ... 3249

Perphenazine (Co-administration with benzodiazepines or other psychotropic agents may be accompanied by profound collapse and respiratory and/or cardiac arrest; caution is advised if used concurrently). Products include:
Etrafon ... 3115
Trilafon ... 3160

Phenelzine Sulfate (Concomitant use of clozapine with other drugs metabolized by cytochrome P450IID6 may require lower than usual doses prescribed for either drug). Products include:
Nardil Tablets ... 2653

Phenoxybenzamine Hydrochloride (Hypotensive effects potentiated). Products include:
Dibenzyline Capsules ... 3457

Phentolamine Mesylate (Hypotensive effects potentiated).
No products indexed under this heading.

Phenytoin (May decrease clozapine plasma levels, a decrease in effectiveness of a previously effective clozapine dose). Products include:
Dilantin Infatabs ... 2624
Dilantin-125 Oral Suspension ... 2625

Phenytoin Sodium (May decrease clozapine plasma levels, a decrease in effectiveness of a previously effective clozapine dose). Products include:
Dilantin Kapseals ... 2622

Pindolol (Hypotensive effects potentiated).
No products indexed under this heading.

Polythiazide (Hypotensive effects potentiated). Products include:
Minizide Capsules ... 2700
Renese Tablets ... 2712

Prazepam (Co-administration with benzodiazepines or other psychotropic agents may be accompanied by profound collapse and respiratory and/or cardiac arrest; caution is advised if used concurrently).
No products indexed under this heading.

Prazosin Hydrochloride (Hypotensive effects potentiated). Products include:
Minipress Capsules ... 2699
Minizide Capsules ... 2700

Prochlorperazine (Co-administration with benzodiazepines or other psychotropic agents may be accompanied by profound collapse and respiratory and/or cardiac arrest; caution is advised if used concurrently). Products include:
Compazine ... 1505

Promethazine Hydrochloride (Co-administration with benzodiazepines or other psychotropic agents may be accompanied by profound collapse and respiratory and/or cardiac arrest; caution is advised if used concurrently). Products include:
Mepergan Injection ... 3539
Phenergan Injection ... 3553
Phenergan ... 3556
Phenergan Syrup ... 3554
Phenergan with Codeine Syrup ... 3557
Phenergan with Dextromethorphan Syrup ... 3559
Phenergan VC Syrup ... 3560
Phenergan VC with Codeine Syrup ... 3561

Propafenone Hydrochloride (Concomitant use of clozapine with other drugs metabolized by cytochrome P450IID6 may require lower than usual doses prescribed for either drug). Products include:
Rythmol Tablets – 150 mg, 225 mg, 300 mg ... 502

Propranolol Hydrochloride (Hypotensive effects potentiated). Products include:
Inderal ... 3513
Inderal LA Long-Acting Capsules ... 3516
Inderide Tablets ... 3517
Inderide LA Long-Acting Capsules ... 3519

Protriptyline Hydrochloride (Concomitant use of clozapine with other

drugs metabolized by cytochrome P450IID6 may require lower than usual doses prescribed for either drug). Products include:
- Vivactil Tablets ... 2446
- Vivactil Tablets ... 2217

Quazepam (Co-administration with benzodiazepines or other psychotropic agents may be accompanied by profound collapse and respiratory and/or cardiac arrest; caution is advised if used concurrently).
- No products indexed under this heading.

Quetiapine Fumarate (Co-administration with benzodiazepines or other psychotropic agents may be accompanied by profound collapse and respiratory and/or cardiac arrest; caution is advised if used concurrently). Products include:
- Seroquel Tablets ... 684

Quinapril Hydrochloride (Hypotensive effects potentiated). Products include:
- Accupril Tablets ... 2611
- Accuretic Tablets ... 2614

Quinidine Gluconate (Co-administration with drugs that inhibit CYP4502D6, such as quinidine, may require lower than usually prescribed doses for either clozapine or quinidine). Products include:
- Quinaglute Dura-Tabs Tablets ... 978

Quinidine Polygalacturonate (Co-administration with drugs that inhibit CYP4502D6, such as quinidine, may require lower than usually prescribed doses for either clozapine or quinidine).
- No products indexed under this heading.

Quinidine Sulfate (Co-administration with drugs that inhibit CYP4502D6, such as quinidine, may require lower than usually prescribed doses for either clozapine or quinidine). Products include:
- Quinidex Extentabs ... 2933

Ramipril (Hypotensive effects potentiated). Products include:
- Altace Capsules ... 2233

Rauwolfia serpentina (Hypotensive effects potentiated).
- No products indexed under this heading.

Rescinnamine (Hypotensive effects potentiated).
- No products indexed under this heading.

Reserpine (Hypotensive effects potentiated).
- No products indexed under this heading.

Risperidone (Co-administration with benzodiazepines or other psychotropic agents may be accompanied by profound collapse and respiratory and/or cardiac arrest; caution is advised if used concurrently). Products include:
- Risperdal ... 1796

Scopolamine (Anticholinergic effects potentiated). Products include:
- Transderm Scōp Transdermal Therapeutic System ... 2302

Scopolamine Hydrobromide (Anticholinergic effects potentiated). Products include:
- Donnatal ... 2929
- Donnatal Extentabs ... 2930

Sertraline Hydrochloride (Co-administration in schizophrenic patients has resulted in elevated mean trough concentrations of clozapine and its metabolites by less than two-fold compared to baseline concentrations; a reduced clozapine dose should be considered). Products include:
- Zoloft ... 2751

Sodium Nitroprusside (Hypotensive effects potentiated).
- No products indexed under this heading.

Sotalol Hydrochloride (Hypotensive effects potentiated). Products include:
- Betapace Tablets ... 950
- Betapace AF Tablets ... 954

Spirapril Hydrochloride (Hypotensive effects potentiated).
- No products indexed under this heading.

Telmisartan (Hypotensive effects potentiated). Products include:
- Micardis Tablets ... 1049
- Micardis HCT Tablets ... 1051

Temazepam (Co-administration with benzodiazepines or other psychotropic agents may be accompanied by profound collapse and respiratory and/or cardiac arrest; caution is advised if used concurrently).
- No products indexed under this heading.

Terazosin Hydrochloride (Hypotensive effects potentiated). Products include:
- Hytrin Capsules ... 464

Thioridazine Hydrochloride (Co-administration with benzodiazepines or other psychotropic agents may be accompanied by profound collapse and respiratory and/or cardiac arrest; caution is advised if used concurrently). Products include:
- Thioridazine Hydrochloride Tablets ... 2289

Thiothixene (Co-administration with benzodiazepines or other psychotropic agents may be accompanied by profound collapse and respiratory and/or cardiac arrest; caution is advised if used concurrently). Products include:
- Navane Capsules ... 2701
- Thiothixene Capsules ... 2290

Timolol Maleate (Hypotensive effects potentiated). Products include:
- Blocadren Tablets ... 2046
- Cosopt Sterile Ophthalmic Solution ... 2065
- Timolide Tablets ... 2187
- Timolol GFS ... ⊙ 266
- Timoptic in Ocudose ... 2192
- Timoptic Sterile Ophthalmic Solution ... 2190
- Timoptic-XE Sterile Ophthalmic Gel Forming Solution ... 2194

Torsemide (Hypotensive effects potentiated). Products include:
- Demadex Tablets and Injection ... 2965

Trandolapril (Hypotensive effects potentiated). Products include:
- Mavik Tablets ... 478
- Tarka Tablets ... 508

Tranylcypromine Sulfate (Concomitant use of clozapine with other drugs metabolized by cytochrome P450IID6 may require lower than usual doses prescribed for either drug). Products include:
- Parnate Tablets ... 1607

Trazodone Hydrochloride (Concomitant use of clozapine with other drugs metabolized by cytochrome P450IID6 may require lower than usual doses prescribed for either drug).
- No products indexed under this heading.

Triazolam (Co-administration with benzodiazepines or other psychotropic agents may be accompanied by profound collapse and respiratory and/or cardiac arrest; caution is advised if used concurrently). Products include:
- Halcion Tablets ... 2823

Trifluoperazine Hydrochloride (Co-administration with benzodiazepines or other psychotropic agents may be accompanied by profound collapse and respiratory and/or cardiac arrest; caution is advised if used concurrently). Products include:
- Stelazine ... 1640

Trimethaphan Camsylate (Hypotensive effects potentiated).
- No products indexed under this heading.

Trimipramine Maleate (Concomitant use of clozapine with other drugs metabolized by cytochrome P450IID6 may require lower than usual doses prescribed for either drug). Products include:
- Surmontil Capsules ... 3595

Valsartan (Hypotensive effects potentiated). Products include:
- Diovan Capsules ... 2337
- Diovan HCT Tablets ... 2338

Venlafaxine Hydrochloride (Concomitant use of clozapine with other drugs metabolized by cytochrome P450IID6 may require lower than usual doses prescribed for either drug). Products include:
- Effexor Tablets ... 3495
- Effexor XR Capsules ... 3499

Verapamil Hydrochloride (Hypotensive effects potentiated). Products include:
- Covera-HS Tablets ... 3199
- Isoptin SR Tablets ... 467
- Tarka Tablets ... 508
- Verelan Capsules ... 3184
- Verelan PM Capsules ... 3186

Warfarin Sodium (Co-administration with other highly protein-bound drugs, such as warfarin, may cause an increase in plasma concentrations of warfarin, potentially resulting in adverse effects). Products include:
- Coumadin for Injection ... 1243
- Coumadin Tablets ... 1243
- Warfarin Sodium Tablets, USP ... 3302

Ziprasidone Hydrochloride (Co-administration with benzodiazepines or other psychotropic agents may be accompanied by profound collapse and respiratory and/or cardiac arrest; caution is advised if used concurrently). Products include:
- Geodon Capsules ... 2688

Food Interactions

Alcohol (Caution is advised with concomitant use).

COGENTIN INJECTION

(Benztropine Mesylate) ... 2055

May interact with anticholinergics, dopamine antagonists, belladona products, butyrophenones, phenothiazines, and tricyclic antidepressants. Compounds in these categories include:

Amitriptyline Hydrochloride (Potential for paralytic ileus, hyperthermia and heat stroke). Products include:
- Etrafon ... 3115
- Limbitrol ... 1738

Amoxapine (Potential for paralytic ileus, hyperthermia and heat stroke).
- No products indexed under this heading.

Atropine Sulfate (Potential for paralytic ileus, hyperthermia and heat stroke). Products include:
- Donnatal ... 2929
- Donnatal Extentabs ... 2930
- Motofen Tablets ... 577
- Prosed/DS Tablets ... 3268
- Urised Tablets ... 2876

Belladonna Alkaloids (Potential for paralytic ileus, hyperthermia and heat stroke). Products include:
- Hyland's Teething Tablets ... 766
- Urimax Tablets ... 1769

Biperiden Hydrochloride (Potential for paralytic ileus, hyperthermia and heat stroke). Products include:
- Akineton ... 402

Chlorpromazine (Potential for paralytic ileus, hyperthermia and heat stroke). Products include:
- Thorazine Suppositories ... 1656

Chlorpromazine Hydrochloride (Potential for paralytic ileus, hyperthermia and heat stroke). Products include:
- Thorazine ... 1656

Clidinium Bromide (Potential for paralytic ileus, hyperthermia and heat stroke).
- No products indexed under this heading.

Clomipramine Hydrochloride (Potential for paralytic ileus, hyperthermia and heat stroke).
- No products indexed under this heading.

Clozapine (Potential for paralytic ileus, hyperthermia and heat stroke). Products include:
- Clozaril Tablets ... 2319

Desipramine Hydrochloride (Potential for paralytic ileus, hyperthermia and heat stroke). Products include:
- Norpramin Tablets ... 755

Dicyclomine Hydrochloride (Potential for paralytic ileus, hyperthermia and heat stroke).
- No products indexed under this heading.

Doxepin Hydrochloride (Potential for paralytic ileus, hyperthermia and heat stroke). Products include:
- Sinequan ... 2713

Fluphenazine Decanoate (Potential for paralytic ileus, hyperthermia and heat stroke).
- No products indexed under this heading.

Fluphenazine Enanthate (Potential for paralytic ileus, hyperthermia and heat stroke).
- No products indexed under this heading.

Fluphenazine Hydrochloride (Potential for paralytic ileus, hyperthermia and heat stroke).
- No products indexed under this heading.

Glycopyrrolate (Potential for paralytic ileus, hyperthermia and heat stroke). Products include:
- Robinul Forte Tablets ... 1358
- Robinul Injectable ... 2940
- Robinul Tablets ... 1358

Haloperidol (Potential for paralytic ileus, hyperthermia and heat stroke). Products include:
- Haldol Injection, Tablets and Concentrate ... 2533

Haloperidol Decanoate (Potential for paralytic ileus, hyperthermia and heat stroke). Products include:
- Haldol Decanoate ... 2535

Hyoscyamine (Potential for paralytic ileus, hyperthermia and heat stroke). Products include:
- Urised Tablets ... 2876

Hyoscyamine Sulfate (Potential for paralytic ileus, hyperthermia and heat stroke). Products include:
- Arco-Lase Plus Tablets ... 592
- Donnatal ... 2929
- Donnatal Extentabs ... 2930
- Levsin/Levsinex/Levbid ... 3172
- NuLev Orally Disintegrating Tablets ... 3176
- Prosed/DS Tablets ... 3268
- Urimax Tablets ... 1769

Imipramine Hydrochloride (Potential for paralytic ileus, hyperthermia and heat stroke).
- No products indexed under this heading.

Imipramine Pamoate (Potential for paralytic ileus, hyperthermia and heat stroke).
- No products indexed under this heading.

Ipratropium Bromide (Potential for paralytic ileus, hyperthermia and heat stroke). Products include:
- Atrovent Inhalation Aerosol ... 1030
- Atrovent Inhalation Solution ... 1031
- Atrovent Nasal Spray 0.03% ... 1032

Atrovent Nasal Spray 0.06% 1033
Combivent Inhalation Aerosol 1041
DuoNeb Inhalation Solution 1233

Maprotiline Hydrochloride (Potential for paralytic ileus, hyperthermia and heat stroke).
No products indexed under this heading.

Mepenzolate Bromide (Potential for paralytic ileus, hyperthermia and heat stroke).
No products indexed under this heading.

Mesoridazine Besylate (Potential for paralytic ileus, hyperthermia and heat stroke). Products include:
Serentil 1057

Methotrimeprazine (Potential for paralytic ileus, hyperthermia and heat stroke).
No products indexed under this heading.

Metoclopramide Hydrochloride (Potential for paralytic ileus, hyperthermia and heat stroke). Products include:
Reglan 2935

Nortriptyline Hydrochloride (Potential for paralytic ileus, hyperthermia and heat stroke).
No products indexed under this heading.

Olanzapine (Potential for paralytic ileus, hyperthermia and heat stroke). Products include:
Zyprexa Tablets 1973
Zyprexa ZYDIS Orally Disintegrating Tablets 1973

Oxybutynin Chloride (Potential for paralytic ileus, hyperthermia and heat stroke). Products include:
Ditropan XL Extended Release Tablets 564

Perphenazine (Potential for paralytic ileus, hyperthermia and heat stroke). Products include:
Etrafon 3115
Trilafon 3160

Pimozide (Potential for paralytic ileus, hyperthermia and heat stroke). Products include:
Orap Tablets 1407

Prochlorperazine (Potential for paralytic ileus, hyperthermia and heat stroke). Products include:
Compazine 1505

Procyclidine Hydrochloride (Potential for paralytic ileus, hyperthermia and heat stroke).
No products indexed under this heading.

Promethazine Hydrochloride (Potential for paralytic ileus, hyperthermia and heat stroke). Products include:
Mepergan Injection 3539
Phenergan Injection 3553
Phenergan 3556
Phenergan Syrup 3554
Phenergan with Codeine Syrup 3557
Phenergan with Dextromethorphan Syrup 3559
Phenergan VC Syrup 3560
Phenergan VC with Codeine Syrup . 3561

Propantheline Bromide (Potential for paralytic ileus, hyperthermia and heat stroke).
No products indexed under this heading.

Protriptyline Hydrochloride (Potential for paralytic ileus, hyperthermia and heat stroke). Products include:
Vivactil Tablets 2446
Vivactil Tablets 2217

Quetiapine Fumarate (Potential for paralytic ileus, hyperthermia and heat stroke). Products include:
Seroquel Tablets 684

Scopolamine (Potential for paralytic ileus, hyperthermia and heat stroke). Products include:
Transderm Scōp Transdermal Therapeutic System 2302

Scopolamine Hydrobromide (Potential for paralytic ileus, hyperthermia and heat stroke). Products include:
Donnatal 2929
Donnatal Extentabs 2930

Thioridazine Hydrochloride (Potential for paralytic ileus, hyperthermia and heat stroke). Products include:
Thioridazine Hydrochloride Tablets 2289

Tolterodine Tartrate (Potential for paralytic ileus, hyperthermia and heat stroke). Products include:
Detrol Tablets 3623
Detrol LA Capsules 2801

Tridihexethyl Chloride (Potential for paralytic ileus, hyperthermia and heat stroke).
No products indexed under this heading.

Trifluoperazine Hydrochloride (Potential for paralytic ileus, hyperthermia and heat stroke). Products include:
Stelazine 1640

Trihexyphenidyl Hydrochloride (Potential for paralytic ileus, hyperthermia and heat stroke). Products include:
Artane 1855

Trimipramine Maleate (Potential for paralytic ileus, hyperthermia and heat stroke). Products include:
Surmontil Capsules 3595

COGENTIN TABLETS

(Benztropine Mesylate) 2055
See Cogentin Injection

COGNEX CAPSULES

(Tacrine Hydrochloride) 1351
May interact with anticholinergics, cholinergic agents, non-steroidal anti-inflammatory agents, theophylline, and certain other agents. Compounds in these categories include:

Aminophylline (Co-administration increases theophylline elimination half-life and average plasma theophylline concentrations by approximately two-fold).
No products indexed under this heading.

Atropine Sulfate (Tacrine has potential to interfere with the activity of anticholinergic drugs). Products include:
Donnatal 2929
Donnatal Extentabs 2930
Motofen Tablets 577
Prosed/DS Tablets 3268
Urised Tablets 2876

Belladonna Alkaloids (Tacrine has potential to interfere with the activity of anticholinergic drugs). Products include:
Hyland's Teething Tablets .... ▣766
Urimax Tablets 1769

Benztropine Mesylate (Tacrine has potential to interfere with the activity of anticholinergic drugs). Products include:
Cogentin 2055

Bethanechol Chloride (Concurrent administration with cholinergic agonist may result in synergistic effect). Products include:
Urecholine 2198
Urecholine Tablets 2445

Biperiden Hydrochloride (Tacrine has potential to interfere with the activity of anticholinergic drugs). Products include:
Akineton 402

Celecoxib (Patients receiving concurrent NSAIDs are at increased risk of developing ulcers since tacrine may be expected to increase gastric acid secretion due to increased cholinergic activity; patients receiving combined therapy should be monitored closely for symptoms of active or occult gastrointestinal disease). Products include:
Celebrex Capsules 2676
Celebrex Capsules 2780

Cevimeline Hydrochloride (Concurrent administration may result in synergistic effect). Products include:
Evoxac Capsules 1217

Cimetidine (Increases Cmax and AUC of tacrine by approximately 54% and 64% respectively). Products include:
Tagamet HB 200 Suspension .... ▣762
Tagamet HB 200 Tablets .... ▣761
Tagamet Tablets 1644

Cimetidine Hydrochloride (Increases Cmax and AUC of tacrine by approximately 54% and 64% respectively). Products include:
Tagamet 1644

Clidinium Bromide (Tacrine has potential to interfere with the activity of anticholinergic drugs).
No products indexed under this heading.

Diclofenac Potassium (Patients receiving concurrent NSAIDs are at increased risk of developing ulcers since tacrine may be expected to increase gastric acid secretion due to increased cholinergic activity; patients receiving combined therapy should be monitored closely for symptoms of active or occult gastrointestinal disease). Products include:
Cataflam Tablets 2315

Diclofenac Sodium (Patients receiving concurrent NSAIDs are at increased risk of developing ulcers since tacrine may be expected to increase gastric acid secretion due to increased cholinergic activity; patients receiving combined therapy should be monitored closely for symptoms of active or occult gastrointestinal disease). Products include:
Arthrotec Tablets 3195
Voltaren Ophthalmic Sterile Ophthalmic Solution .... ⊙312
Voltaren Tablets 2315
Voltaren-XR Tablets 2315

Dicyclomine Hydrochloride (Tacrine has potential to interfere with the activity of anticholinergic drugs).
No products indexed under this heading.

Donepezil Hydrochloride (Concurrent administration may result in synergistic effect). Products include:
Aricept Tablets 1270
Aricept Tablets 2665

Dyphylline (Co-administration increases theophylline elimination half-life and average plasma theophylline concentrations by approximately two-fold). Products include:
Lufyllin Tablets 3347
Lufyllin-400 Tablets 3347
Lufyllin-GG Elixir 3348
Lufyllin-GG Tablets 3348

Edrophonium Chloride (Concurrent administration may result in synergistic effect). Products include:
Tensilon Injectable 1745

Etodolac (Patients receiving concurrent NSAIDs are at increased risk of developing ulcers since tacrine may be expected to increase gastric acid secretion due to increased cholinergic activity; patients receiving combined therapy should be monitored closely for symptoms of active or occult gastrointestinal disease). Products include:
Lodine 3528
Lodine XL Extended-Release Tablets 3530

Fenoprofen Calcium (Patients receiving concurrent NSAIDs are at increased risk of developing ulcers since tacrine may be expected to increase gastric acid secretion due to increased cholinergic activity; patients receiving combined therapy should be monitored closely for symptoms of active or occult gastrointestinal disease).
No products indexed under this heading.

Flurbiprofen (Patients receiving concurrent NSAIDs are at increased risk of developing ulcers since tacrine may be expected to increase gastric acid secretion due to increased cholinergic activity; patients receiving combined therapy should be monitored closely for symptoms of active or occult gastrointestinal disease).
No products indexed under this heading.

Fluvoxamine Maleate (Co-administration was associated with five- and eight-fold increases in tacrine Cmax and AUC, respectively, compared to the administration of tacrine alone; nausea, vomiting, sweating, and diarrhea have resulted following concurrent use). Products include:
Luvox Tablets (25, 50, 100 mg) 3256

Galantamine Hydrobromide (Concurrent administration may result in synergistic effect). Products include:
Reminyl Oral Solution 1792
Reminyl Tablets 1792

Glycopyrrolate (Tacrine has potential to interfere with the activity of anticholinergic drugs). Products include:
Robinul Forte Tablets 1358
Robinul Injectable 2940
Robinul Tablets 1358

Hyoscyamine (Tacrine has potential to interfere with the activity of anticholinergic drugs). Products include:
Urised Tablets 2876

Hyoscyamine Sulfate (Tacrine has potential to interfere with the activity of anticholinergic drugs). Products include:
Arco-Lase Plus Tablets 592
Donnatal 2929
Donnatal Extentabs 2930
Levsin/Levsinex/Levbid 3172
NuLev Orally Disintegrating Tablets 3176
Prosed/DS Tablets 3268
Urimax Tablets 1769

Ibuprofen (Patients receiving concurrent NSAIDs are at increased risk of developing ulcers since tacrine may be expected to increase gastric acid secretion due to increased cholinergic activity; patients receiving combined therapy should be monitored closely for symptoms of active or occult gastrointestinal disease). Products include:
Advil .... ▣771
Children's Advil Oral Suspension .... ▣773
Children's Advil Chewable Tablets .. ▣773
Advil Cold and Sinus Caplets .... ▣771
Advil Cold and Sinus Tablets .... ▣771
Advil Flu & Body Ache Caplets ...... ▣772
Infants' Advil Drops .... ▣773
Junior Strength Advil Tablets .... ▣773
Junior Strength Advil Chewable Tablets .... ▣773
Advil Migraine Liquigels .... ▣772
Children's Motrin Oral Suspension and Chewable Tablets 2006
Children's Motrin Cold Oral Suspension 2007
Children's Motrin Oral Suspension .... ▣643
Motrin Suspension, Oral Drops, Chewable Tablets, and Caplets 2002
Infants' Motrin Concentrated Drops 2006
Junior Strength Motrin Caplets and Chewable Tablets 2006
Motrin IB Tablets, Caplets, and Gelcaps 2002
Motrin Migraine Pain Caplets 2005
Motrin Sinus Headache Caplets 2005
Vicoprofen Tablets 520

Indomethacin (Patients receiving concurrent NSAIDs are at increased risk of developing ulcers since

tacrine may be expected to increase gastric acid secretion due to increased cholinergic activity; patients receiving combined therapy should be monitored closely for symptoms of active or occult gastrointestinal disease). Products include:

Indocin 2112

Indomethacin Sodium Trihydrate (Patients receiving concurrent NSAIDs are at increased risk of developing ulcers since tacrine may be expected to increase gastric acid secretion due to increased cholinergic activity; patients receiving combined therapy should be monitored closely for symptoms of active or occult gastrointestinal disease). Products include:

Indocin I.V. 2115

Ipratropium Bromide (Tacrine has potential to interfere with the activity of anticholinergic drugs). Products include:

Atrovent Inhalation Aerosol 1030
Atrovent Inhalation Solution 1031
Atrovent Nasal Spray 0.03% 1032
Atrovent Nasal Spray 0.06% 1033
Combivent Inhalation Aerosol 1041
DuoNeb Inhalation Solution 1233

Ketoprofen (Patients receiving concurrent NSAIDs are at increased risk of developing ulcers since tacrine may be expected to increase gastric acid secretion due to increased cholinergic activity; patients receiving combined therapy should be monitored closely for symptoms of active or occult gastrointestinal disease). Products include:

Orudis Capsules 3548
Orudis KT Tablets .... ▣778
Oruvail Capsules 3548

Ketorolac Tromethamine (Patients receiving concurrent NSAIDs are at increased risk of developing ulcers since tacrine may be expected to increase gastric acid secretion due to increased cholinergic activity; patients receiving combined therapy should be monitored closely for symptoms of active or occult gastrointestinal disease). Products include:

Acular Ophthalmic Solution 544
Acular PF Ophthalmic Solution 544
Toradol 3018

Meclofenamate Sodium (Patients receiving concurrent NSAIDs are at increased risk of developing ulcers since tacrine may be expected to increase gastric acid secretion due to increased cholinergic activity; patients receiving combined therapy should be monitored closely for symptoms of active or occult gastrointestinal disease).

No products indexed under this heading.

Mefenamic Acid (Patients receiving concurrent NSAIDs are at increased risk of developing ulcers since tacrine may be expected to increase gastric acid secretion due to increased cholinergic activity; patients receiving combined therapy should be monitored closely for symptoms of active or occult gastrointestinal disease). Products include:

Ponstel Capsules 1356

Meloxicam (Patients receiving concurrent NSAIDs are at increased risk of developing ulcers since tacrine may be expected to increase gastric acid secretion due to increased cholinergic activity; patients receiving combined therapy should be monitored closely for symptoms of active or occult gastrointestinal disease). Products include:

Mobic Tablets 1054

Mepenzolate Bromide (Tacrine has potential to interfere with the activity of anticholinergic drugs).

No products indexed under this heading.

Nabumetone (Patients receiving concurrent NSAIDs are at increased risk of developing ulcers since tacrine may be expected to increase gastric acid secretion due to increased cholinergic activity; patients receiving combined therapy should be monitored closely for symptoms of active or occult gastrointestinal disease). Products include:

Relafen Tablets 1617

Naproxen (Patients receiving concurrent NSAIDs are at increased risk of developing ulcers since tacrine may be expected to increase gastric acid secretion due to increased cholinergic activity; patients receiving combined therapy should be monitored closely for symptoms of active or occult gastrointestinal disease). Products include:

EC-Naprosyn Delayed-Release Tablets 2967
Naprosyn Suspension 2967
Naprosyn Tablets 2967

Naproxen Sodium (Patients receiving concurrent NSAIDs are at increased risk of developing ulcers since tacrine may be expected to increase gastric acid secretion due to increased cholinergic activity; patients receiving combined therapy should be monitored closely for symptoms of active or occult gastrointestinal disease). Products include:

Aleve Tablets, Caplets and Gelcaps .... ▣602
Aleve Cold & Sinus Caplets .... ▣603
Anaprox Tablets 2967
Anaprox DS Tablets 2967
Naprelan Tablets 1293

Neostigmine Bromide (Concurrent administration may result in synergistic effect). Products include:

Prostigmin Tablets 1744

Neostigmine Methylsulfate (Concurrent administration may result in synergistic effect). Products include:

Prostigmin Injectable 1744

Oxaprozin (Patients receiving concurrent NSAIDs are at increased risk of developing ulcers since tacrine may be expected to increase gastric acid secretion due to increased cholinergic activity; patients receiving combined therapy should be monitored closely for symptoms of active or occult gastrointestinal disease).

No products indexed under this heading.

Oxybutynin Chloride (Tacrine has potential to interfere with the activity of anticholinergic drugs). Products include:

Ditropan XL Extended Release Tablets 564

Phenylbutazone (Patients receiving concurrent NSAIDs are at increased risk of developing ulcers since tacrine may be expected to increase gastric acid secretion due to increased cholinergic activity; patients receiving combined therapy should be monitored closely for symptoms of active or occult gastrointestinal disease).

No products indexed under this heading.

Piroxicam (Patients receiving concurrent NSAIDs are at increased risk of developing ulcers since tacrine may be expected to increase gastric acid secretion due to increased cholinergic activity; patients receiving combined therapy should be monitored closely for symptoms of active or occult gastrointestinal disease). Products include:

Feldene Capsules 2685

Procyclidine Hydrochloride (Tacrine has potential to interfere with the activity of anticholinergic drugs).

No products indexed under this heading.

Propantheline Bromide (Tacrine has potential to interfere with the activity of anticholinergic drugs).

No products indexed under this heading.

Pyridostigmine Bromide (Concurrent administration may result in synergistic effect). Products include:

Mestinon 1740

Rivastigmine Tartrate (Concurrent administration may result in synergistic effect). Products include:

Exelon Capsules 2342
Exelon Oral Solution 2345

Rofecoxib (Patients receiving concurrent NSAIDs are at increased risk of developing ulcers since tacrine may be expected to increase gastric acid secretion due to increased cholinergic activity; patients receiving combined therapy should be monitored closely for symptoms of active or occult gastrointestinal disease). Products include:

Vioxx 2213

Scopolamine (Tacrine has potential to interfere with the activity of anticholinergic drugs). Products include:

Transderm Scōp Transdermal Therapeutic System 2302

Scopolamine Hydrobromide (Tacrine has potential to interfere with the activity of anticholinergic drugs). Products include:

Donnatal 2929
Donnatal Extentabs 2930

Succinylcholine Chloride (Tacrine, as a cholinesterase inhibitor, may exaggerate succinylcholine-type muscle relaxation during anesthesia). Products include:

Anectine Injection 1476

Sulindac (Patients receiving concurrent NSAIDs are at increased risk of developing ulcers since tacrine may be expected to increase gastric acid secretion due to increased cholinergic activity; patients receiving combined therapy should be monitored closely for symptoms of active or occult gastrointestinal disease). Products include:

Clinoril Tablets 2053

Theophylline (Co-administration increases theophylline elimination half-life and average plasma theophylline concentrations by approximately two-fold). Products include:

Aerolate 1361
Theo-Dur Extended-Release Tablets 1835
Uni-Dur Extended-Release Tablets 1841
Uniphyl 400 mg and 600 mg Tablets 2903

Theophylline Calcium Salicylate (Co-administration increases theophylline elimination half-life and average plasma theophylline concentrations by approximately two-fold).

No products indexed under this heading.

Theophylline Sodium Glycinate (Co-administration increases theophylline elimination half-life and average plasma theophylline concentrations by approximately two-fold).

No products indexed under this heading.

Tolmetin Sodium (Patients receiving concurrent NSAIDs are at increased risk of developing ulcers since tacrine may be expected to increase gastric acid secretion due to increased cholinergic activity; patients receiving combined therapy should be monitored closely for symptoms of active or occult gastrointestinal disease). Products include:

Tolectin 2589

Tolterodine Tartrate (Tacrine has potential to interfere with the activity of anticholinergic drugs). Products include:

Detrol Tablets 3623
Detrol LA Capsules 2801

Tridihexethyl Chloride (Tacrine has potential to interfere with the activity of anticholinergic drugs).

No products indexed under this heading.

Trihexyphenidyl Hydrochloride (Tacrine has potential to interfere with the activity of anticholinergic drugs). Products include:

Artane 1855

Food Interactions

Food, unspecified (Food reduces tacrine bioavailability by approximately 30% to 40%; no effect if tacrine is administered at least one hour before meals).

COLACE CAPSULES, SYRUP, LIQUID

(Docusate Sodium) 3236
None cited in PDR database.

COLAZAL CAPSULES

(Balsalazide Disodium) 3069
May interact with:

Antibiotics, unspecified (Use of orally administered antibiotics could, theoretically, interfere with the release of mesalamine in the colon).

COLD SEASON NUTRITION BOOSTER CAPSULES

(Astragalus, Echinacea, Herbals, Multiple) .... ▣796
None cited in PDR database.

COLESTID TABLETS

(Colestipol Hydrochloride) 2791
May interact with cardiac glycosides, tetracyclines, and certain other agents. Compounds in these categories include:

Chlorothiazide (The absorption of chlorothiazide as reflected in urinary excretion is markedly decreased even when administered one hour before colestipol). Products include:

Aldoclor Tablets 2035
Diuril Oral 2087

Demeclocycline Hydrochloride (Simultaneous administration results in decreased absorption of oral tetracyclines). Products include:

Declomycin Tablets 1855

Deslanoside (Potential for binding of digitalis glycosides).

No products indexed under this heading.

Digitoxin (Potential for binding of digitalis glycosides).

No products indexed under this heading.

Digoxin (Potential for binding of digitalis glycosides). Products include:

Digitek Tablets 1003
Lanoxicaps Capsules 1574
Lanoxin Injection 1581
Lanoxin Tablets 1587
Lanoxin Elixir Pediatric 1578
Lanoxin Injection Pediatric 1584

Doxycycline Calcium (Simultaneous administration results in decreased absorption of oral tetracyclines). Products include:

Vibramycin Calcium Oral Suspension Syrup 2735

Doxycycline Hyclate (Simultaneous administration results in decreased absorption of oral tetracyclines). Products include:

Doryx Coated Pellet Filled Capsules 3357
Periostat Tablets 1208
Vibramycin Hyclate Capsules 2735
Vibramycin Hyclate Intravenous 2737
Vibra-Tabs Film Coated Tablets 2735

Doxycycline Monohydrate (Simultaneous administration results in decreased absorption of oral tetracyclines). Products include:

Monodox Capsules 2442
Vibramycin Monohydrate for Oral Suspension 2735

Folic Acid (Colestipol may reduce absorption of oral folic acid). Products include:
Bevitamel Tablets 3459
Nicomide Tablets 3247
Slow Fe with Folic Acid Tablets ..... ◙ 828

Furosemide (Simultaneous administration results in decreased absorption of oral furosemide). Products include:
Furosemide Tablets 2284

Gemfibrozil (Simultaneous administration results in decreased absorption of gemfibrozil). Products include:
Lopid Tablets 2650

Hydrochlorothiazide (Simultaneous administration results in decreased absorption of hydrochlorothiazide). Products include:
Accuretic Tablets 2614
Aldoril Tablets 2039
Atacand HCT Tablets 597
Avalide Tablets 1070
Diovan HCT Tablets 2338
Dyazide Capsules 1515
HydroDIURIL Tablets 2108
Hyzaar 2109
Inderide Tablets 3517
Inderide LA Long-Acting Capsules .. 3519
Lotensin HCT Tablets 2367
Maxzide 1008
Micardis HCT Tablets 1051
Microzide Capsules 3414
Moduretic Tablets 2138
Monopril HCT 1094
Prinzide Tablets 2168
Timolide Tablets 2187
Uniretic Tablets 3178
Vaseretic Tablets 2204
Zestoretic Tablets 695
Ziac Tablets 1887

Hydrocortisone (Bile acid binding agents may interfere with the absorption of oral hydrocortisone). Products include:
Anusol-HC Cream 2.5% 2237
Cipro HC Otic Suspension 540
Cortaid Intensive Therapy Cream . ◙ 717
Cortaid Maximum Strength Cream .... ◙ 717
Cortisporin Ophthalmic Suspension Sterile .... ⊙ 297
Cortizone•5 .... ◙ 699
Cortizone•10 .... ◙ 699
Cortizone•10 Plus Creme .... ◙ 700
Cortizone for Kids Creme .... ◙ 699
Hydrocortone Tablets 2106
Massengill Medicated Soft Cloth Towelette .... ◙ 753
VōSoL HC Otic Solution 3356

Methacycline Hydrochloride (Simultaneous administration results in decreased absorption of oral tetracyclines).
No products indexed under this heading.

Minocycline Hydrochloride (Simultaneous administration results in decreased absorption of oral tetracyclines). Products include:
Dynacin Capsules 2019
Minocin Intravenous 1862
Minocin Oral Suspension 1865
Minocin Pellet-Filled Capsules 1863

Oxytetracycline Hydrochloride (Simultaneous administration results in decreased absorption of oral tetracyclines). Products include:
Terra-Cortril Ophthalmic Suspension 2716
Urobiotic-250 Capsules 2731

Penicillin G Potassium (Simultaneous administration results in decreased absorption of oral penicillin G). Products include:
Pfizerpen for Injection 2707

Phytonadione (Colestipol may reduce absorption of oral fat soluble vitamins).
No products indexed under this heading.

Potassium Phosphate (Bile acid binding agents may interfere with the absorption of oral phosphate supplements). Products include:
K-Phos Neutral Tablets 946

Propranolol Hydrochloride (Repeated doses of colestipol given prior to a single dose of propranolol has resulted in decreased propranolol absorption; statistically significant effect on the rate of absorption has been noted). Products include:
Inderal 3513
Inderal LA Long-Acting Capsules 3516
Inderide Tablets 3517
Inderide LA Long-Acting Capsules .. 3519

Tetracycline Hydrochloride (Simultaneous administration results in decreased absorption of oral tetracyclines).
No products indexed under this heading.

Vitamin A (Colestipol may reduce absorption of oral fat soluble vitamins). Products include:
Aquasol A Parenteral 593
Beta-C Tablets .... ◙ 811
Centrum Focused Formulas Prostate Softgels .... ◙ 816

Vitamin D (Colestipol may reduce absorption of oral fat soluble vitamins). Products include:
Active Calcium Tablets 3335
Caltrate 600 PLUS .... ◙ 815
Caltrate 600 + D Tablets .... ◙ 814
Centrum Focused Formulas Bone Health Tablets .... ◙ 815
Citracal Caplets + D .... ◙ 823
D-Cal Chewable Caplets .... ◙ 794
One-A-Day Calcium Plus Chewable Tablets .... ◙ 805
Os-Cal 250 + D Tablets .... ◙ 838
Os-Cal 500 + D Tablets .... ◙ 839

Vitamin K (Colestipol may reduce absorption of oral fat soluble vitamins).
No products indexed under this heading.

COLLAGENASE SANTYL OINTMENT

(Collagenase) 3248
May interact with:

Cortisone Acetate (Chronic concurrent use may result in systemic manifestations of hypersensitivity to collagenase). Products include:
Cortone Acetate Injectable Suspension 2059
Cortone Acetate Tablets 2061

COLLYRIUM EYE WASH

(Boric Acid, Sodium Borate) .... ⊙ 252
None cited in PDR database.

COLY-MYCIN M PARENTERAL

(Colistimethate Sodium) 2243
May interact with aminoglycosides and certain other agents. Compounds in these categories include:

Amikacin Sulfate (Certain antibiotics, such as aminoglycosides, have been reported to interfere with the nerve transmission at the neuromuscular junction; co-administration should be avoided except with the greatest caution).
No products indexed under this heading.

Cephalothin Sodium (May enhance the nephrotoxicity; co-administration should be avoided).

Decamethonium (May potentiate the neuromuscular blocking effect).

Gallamine (May potentiate the neuromuscular blocking effect).

Gentamicin Sulfate (Certain antibiotics, such as aminoglycosides, have been reported to interfere with the nerve transmission at the neuromuscular junction; co-administration should be avoided except with the greatest caution). Products include:
Genoptic Ophthalmic Ointment .... ⊙ 239
Genoptic Sterile Ophthalmic Solution .... ⊙ 239
Pred-G Ophthalmic Suspension .... ⊙ 247
Pred-G Sterile Ophthalmic Ointment .... ⊙ 248

Kanamycin Sulfate (Certain antibiotics, such as aminoglycosides, have been reported to interfere with the nerve transmission at the neuromuscular junction; co-administration should be avoided except with the greatest caution).
No products indexed under this heading.

Polymyxin (Certain antibiotics, such as polymyxin, have been reported to interfere with the nerve transmission at the neuromuscular junction; co-administration should be avoided except with the greatest caution).
No products indexed under this heading.

Sodium Citrate (May potentiate the neuromuscular blocking effect).
No products indexed under this heading.

Streptomycin Sulfate (Certain antibiotics, such as aminoglycosides, have been reported to interfere with the nerve transmission at the neuromuscular junction; co-administration should be avoided except with the greatest caution). Products include:
Streptomycin Sulfate Injection 2714

Succinylcholine Chloride (May potentiate the neuromuscular blocking effect). Products include:
Anectine Injection 1476

Tobramycin (Certain antibiotics, such as aminoglycosides, have been reported to interfere with the nerve transmission at the neuromuscular junction; co-administration should be avoided except with the greatest caution). Products include:
TOBI Solution for Inhalation 1206
TobraDex Ophthalmic Ointment 542
TobraDex Ophthalmic Suspension 541
Tobrex Ophthalmic Ointment .... ⊙ 220
Tobrex Ophthalmic Solution .... ⊙ 221

Tobramycin Sulfate (Certain antibiotics, such as aminoglycosides, have been reported to interfere with the nerve transmission at the neuromuscular junction; co-administration should be avoided except with the greatest caution). Products include:
Nebcin Vials, Hyporets & ADD-Vantage 1955

Tubocurarine Chloride (May potentiate the neuromuscular blocking effect).
No products indexed under this heading.

COLYTE WITH FLAVOR PACKS FOR ORAL SOLUTION

(Polyethylene Glycol, Potassium Chloride, Sodium Bicarbonate, Sodium Chloride, Sodium Sulfate) 3170
May interact with:

Oral Medications, unspecified (Those administered within one hour of Colyte usage may be flushed from the gastrointestinal tract and not absorbed).

COMBIPATCH TRANSDERMAL SYSTEM

(Estradiol, Norethindrone Acetate) 2323
None cited in PDR database.

COMBIPRES TABLETS

(Chlorthalidone, Clonidine Hydrochloride) 1040
May interact with antihypertensives, barbiturates, oral hypoglycemic agents, hypnotics and sedatives, insulin, lithium preparations, narcotic analgesics, tricyclic antidepressants, and certain other agents. Compounds in these categories include:

Acarbose (Higher dosage of oral hypoglycemic agents may be required). Products include:
Precose Tablets 906

Acebutolol Hydrochloride (Chlorthalidone may add to or potentiate the action of other antihypertensive drugs). Products include:
Sectral Capsules 3589

Alfentanil Hydrochloride (Orthostatic hypotension produced by chlorthalidone may be aggravated by narcotics).
No products indexed under this heading.

Amitriptyline Hydrochloride (Amitriptyline in combination with clonidine enhances the manifestation of corneal lesions in rats; co-administration therapy may result in reduced effect of clonidine, thus necessitating an increase in dosage). Products include:
Etrafon 3115
Limbitrol 1738

Amlodipine Besylate (Chlorthalidone may add to or potentiate the action of other antihypertensive drugs). Products include:
Lotrel Capsules 2370
Norvasc Tablets 2704

Amoxapine (Co-administration results in reduced effect of clonidine, thus necessitating an increase in dosage).
No products indexed under this heading.

Aprobarbital (Orthostatic hypotension produced by chlorthalidone may be aggravated by barbiturates; potential for enhanced CNS-depressive effects).
No products indexed under this heading.

Atenolol (Chlorthalidone may add to or potentiate the action of other antihypertensive drugs). Products include:
Tenoretic Tablets 690
Tenormin I.V. Injection 692

Benazepril Hydrochloride (Chlorthalidone may add to or potentiate the action of other antihypertensive drugs). Products include:
Lotensin Tablets 2365
Lotensin HCT Tablets 2367
Lotrel Capsules 2370

Bendroflumethiazide (Chlorthalidone may add to or potentiate the action of other antihypertensive drugs). Products include:
Corzide 40/5 Tablets 2247
Corzide 80/5 Tablets 2247

Betaxolol Hydrochloride (Chlorthalidone may add to or potentiate the action of other antihypertensive drugs). Products include:
Betoptic S Ophthalmic Suspension 537

Bisoprolol Fumarate (Chlorthalidone may add to or potentiate the action of other antihypertensive drugs). Products include:
Zebeta Tablets 1885
Ziac Tablets 1887

Buprenorphine Hydrochloride (Orthostatic hypotension produced by chlorthalidone may be aggravated by narcotics). Products include:
Buprenex Injectable 2918

Butabarbital (Orthostatic hypotension produced by chlorthalidone may be aggravated by barbiturates; potential for enhanced CNS-depressive effects).
No products indexed under this heading.

Butalbital (Orthostatic hypotension produced by chlorthalidone may be aggravated by barbiturates; potential for enhanced CNS-depressive effects). Products include:
Phrenilin 578
Sedapap Tablets 50 mg/650 mg ... 2225

Candesartan Cilexetil (Chlorthalidone may add to or potentiate the action of other antihypertensive drugs). Products include:

Atacand Tablets 595
Atacand HCT Tablets 597

Captopril (Chlorthalidone may add to or potentiate the action of other antihypertensive drugs). Products include:
Captopril Tablets 2281

Carteolol Hydrochloride (Chlorthalidone may add to or potentiate the action of other antihypertensive drugs). Products include:
Carteolol Hydrochloride Ophthalmic Solution USP, 1% ..... ⊙258
Ocupress Ophthalmic Solution, 1% Sterile ..... ⊙303

Chlorothiazide (Chlorthalidone may add to or potentiate the action of other antihypertensive drugs). Products include:
Aldoclor Tablets 2035
Diuril Oral 2087

Chlorothiazide Sodium (Chlorthalidone may add to or potentiate the action of other antihypertensive drugs). Products include:
Diuril Sodium Intravenous 2086

Chlorpropamide (Higher dosage of oral hypoglycemic agents may be required). Products include:
Diabinese Tablets 2680

Clomipramine Hydrochloride (Co-administration results in reduced effect of clonidine, thus necessitating an increase in dosage).
No products indexed under this heading.

Clonidine (Chlorthalidone may add to or potentiate the action of other antihypertensive drugs). Products include:
Catapres-TTS 1038

Codeine Phosphate (Orthostatic hypotension produced by chlorthalidone may be aggravated by narcotics). Products include:
Phenergan with Codeine Syrup 3557
Phenergan VC with Codeine Syrup 3561
Robitussin A-C Syrup 2942
Robitussin-DAC Syrup 2942
Ryna-C Liquid ..... ▣768
Soma Compound w/Codeine Tablets 3355
Tussi-Organidin NR Liquid 3350
Tussi-Organidin-S NR Liquid 3350
Tylenol with Codeine 2595

Deserpidine (Chlorthalidone may add to or potentiate the action of other antihypertensive drugs).
No products indexed under this heading.

Desipramine Hydrochloride (Co-administration results in reduced effect of clonidine, thus necessitating an increase in dosage). Products include:
Norpramin Tablets 755

Dezocine (Orthostatic hypotension produced by chlorthalidone may be aggravated by narcotics).
No products indexed under this heading.

Diazoxide (Chlorthalidone may add to or potentiate the action of other antihypertensive drugs).
No products indexed under this heading.

Diltiazem Hydrochloride (Chlorthalidone may add to or potentiate the action of other antihypertensive drugs). Products include:
Cardizem Injectable 1018
Cardizem Lyo-Ject Syringe 1018
Cardizem Monovial 1018
Cardizem CD Capsules 1016
Tiazac Capsules 1378

Doxazosin Mesylate (Chlorthalidone may add to or potentiate the action of other antihypertensive drugs). Products include:
Cardura Tablets 2668

Doxepin Hydrochloride (Co-administration results in reduced effect of clonidine, thus necessitating an increase in dosage). Products include:
Sinequan 2713

Enalapril Maleate (Chlorthalidone may add to or potentiate the action of other antihypertensive drugs). Products include:
Lexxel Tablets 608
Vaseretic Tablets 2204
Vasotec Tablets 2210

Enalaprilat (Chlorthalidone may add to or potentiate the action of other antihypertensive drugs). Products include:
Enalaprilat Injection 863
Vasotec I.V. Injection 2207

Eprosartan Mesylate (Chlorthalidone may add to or potentiate the action of other antihypertensive drugs). Products include:
Teveten Tablets 3327

Esmolol Hydrochloride (Chlorthalidone may add to or potentiate the action of other antihypertensive drugs). Products include:
Brevibloc Injection 858

Estazolam (Enhanced CNS-depressive effects). Products include:
ProSom Tablets 500

Ethchlorvynol (Enhanced CNS-depressive effects).
No products indexed under this heading.

Ethinamate (Enhanced CNS-depressive effects).
No products indexed under this heading.

Felodipine (Chlorthalidone may add to or potentiate the action of other antihypertensive drugs). Products include:
Lexxel Tablets 608
Plendil Extended-Release Tablets 623

Fentanyl (Orthostatic hypotension produced by chlorthalidone may be aggravated by narcotics). Products include:
Duragesic Transdermal System 1786

Fentanyl Citrate (Orthostatic hypotension produced by chlorthalidone may be aggravated by narcotics). Products include:
Actiq 1184

Flurazepam Hydrochloride (Enhanced CNS-depressive effects).
No products indexed under this heading.

Fosinopril Sodium (Chlorthalidone may add to or potentiate the action of other antihypertensive drugs). Products include:
Monopril Tablets 1091
Monopril HCT 1094

Furosemide (Chlorthalidone may add to or potentiate the action of other antihypertensive drugs). Products include:
Furosemide Tablets 2284

Glimepiride (Higher dosage of oral hypoglycemic agents may be required). Products include:
Amaryl Tablets 717

Glipizide (Higher dosage of oral hypoglycemic agents may be required). Products include:
Glucotrol Tablets 2692
Glucotrol XL Extended Release Tablets 2693

Glutethimide (Enhanced CNS-depressive effects).
No products indexed under this heading.

Glyburide (Higher dosage of oral hypoglycemic agents may be required). Products include:
DiaBeta Tablets 741
Glucovance Tablets 1086

Guanabenz Acetate (Chlorthalidone may add to or potentiate the action of other antihypertensive drugs).
No products indexed under this heading.

Guanethidine Monosulfate (Chlorthalidone may add to or potentiate the action of other antihypertensive drugs).
No products indexed under this heading.

Hydralazine Hydrochloride (Chlorthalidone may add to or potentiate the action of other antihypertensive drugs).
No products indexed under this heading.

Hydrochlorothiazide (Chlorthalidone may add to or potentiate the action of other antihypertensive drugs). Products include:
Accuretic Tablets 2614
Aldoril Tablets 2039
Atacand HCT Tablets 597
Avalide Tablets 1070
Diovan HCT Tablets 2338
Dyazide Capsules 1515
HydroDIURIL Tablets 2108
Hyzaar 2109
Inderide Tablets 3517
Inderide LA Long-Acting Capsules 3519
Lotensin HCT Tablets 2367
Maxzide 1008
Micardis HCT Tablets 1051
Microzide Capsules 3414
Moduretic Tablets 2138
Monopril HCT 1094
Prinzide Tablets 2168
Timolide Tablets 2187
Uniretic Tablets 3178
Vaseretic Tablets 2204
Zestoretic Tablets 695
Ziac Tablets 1887

Hydrocodone Bitartrate (Orthostatic hypotension produced by chlorthalidone may be aggravated by narcotics). Products include:
Hycodan 1316
Hycomine Compound Tablets 1317
Hycotuss Expectorant Syrup 1318
Lortab 3319
Lortab Elixir 3317
Maxidone Tablets CIII 3399
Norco 5/325 Tablets CIII 3424
Norco 7.5/325 Tablets CIII 3425
Norco 10/325 Tablets CIII 3427
Norco 10/325 Tablets CIII 3425
Vicodin Tablets 516
Vicodin ES Tablets 517
Vicodin HP Tablets 518
Vicodin Tuss Expectorant 519
Vicoprofen Tablets 520
Zydone Tablets 1330

Hydrocodone Polistirex (Orthostatic hypotension produced by chlorthalidone may be aggravated by narcotics). Products include:
Tussionex Pennkinetic Extended-Release Suspension 1174

Hydroflumethiazide (Chlorthalidone may add to or potentiate the action of other antihypertensive drugs). Products include:
Diucardin Tablets 3494

Hydromorphone Hydrochloride (Orthostatic hypotension produced by chlorthalidone may be aggravated by narcotics). Products include:
Dilaudid 441
Dilaudid Oral Liquid 445
Dilaudid Powder 441
Dilaudid Rectal Suppositories 441
Dilaudid Tablets 441
Dilaudid Tablets - 8 mg 445
Dilaudid-HP 443

Imipramine Hydrochloride (Co-administration results in reduced effect of clonidine, thus necessitating an increase in dosage).
No products indexed under this heading.

Imipramine Pamoate (Co-administration results in reduced effect of clonidine, thus necessitating an increase in dosage).
No products indexed under this heading.

Indapamide (Chlorthalidone may add to or potentiate the action of other antihypertensive drugs). Products include:
Indapamide Tablets 2286

Insulin, Human, Zinc Suspension (Insulin requirements in diabetic patients may be increased, decreased or unchanged). Products include:
Humulin L, 100 Units 1937
Humulin U, 100 Units 1943
Novolin L Human Insulin 10 ml Vials 2422

Insulin, Human NPH (Insulin requirements in diabetic patients may be increased, decreased or unchanged). Products include:
Humulin N, 100 Units 1939
Humulin N NPH Pen 1940
Novolin N Human Insulin 10 ml Vials 2422
Novolin N PenFill 2423
Novolin N Prefilled Syringe Disposable Insulin Delivery System 2425

Insulin, Human Regular (Insulin requirements in diabetic patients may be increased, decreased or unchanged). Products include:
Humulin R Regular (U-500) 1943
Humulin R, 100 Units 1941
Novolin R Human Insulin 10 ml Vials 2423
Novolin R PenFill 2423
Novolin R Prefilled Syringe Disposable Insulin Delivery System 2425
Velosulin BR Human Insulin 10 ml Vials 2435

Insulin, Human Regular and Human NPH Mixture (Insulin requirements in diabetic patients may be increased, decreased or unchanged). Products include:
Humulin 50/50, 100 Units 1934
Humulin 70/30, 100 Units 1935
Humulin 70/30 Pen 1936
Novolin 70/30 Human Insulin 10 ml Vials 2421
Novolin 70/30 PenFill 2423
Novolin 70/30 Prefilled Disposable Insulin Delivery System 2425

Insulin, NPH (Insulin requirements in diabetic patients may be increased, decreased or unchanged). Products include:
Iletin II, NPH (Pork), 100 Units 1946

Insulin, Regular (Insulin requirements in diabetic patients may be increased, decreased or unchanged). Products include:
Iletin II, Regular (Pork), 100 Units 1947

Insulin, Zinc Crystals (Insulin requirements in diabetic patients may be increased, decreased or unchanged).
No products indexed under this heading.

Insulin, Zinc Suspension (Insulin requirements in diabetic patients may be increased, decreased or unchanged). Products include:
Iletin II, Lente (Pork), 100 Units 1945

Insulin Aspart, Human Regular (Insulin requirements in diabetic patients may be increased, decreased or unchanged).
No products indexed under this heading.

Insulin glargine (Insulin requirements in diabetic patients may be increased, decreased or unchanged). Products include:
Lantus Injection 742

Insulin Lispro, Human (Insulin requirements in diabetic patients may be increased, decreased or unchanged). Products include:
Humalog 1926
Humalog Mix 75/25 Pen 1928

Insulin Lispro Protamine, Human (Insulin requirements in diabetic patients may be increased, decreased or unchanged). Products include:
Humalog Mix 75/25 Pen 1928

Irbesartan (Chlorthalidone may add to or potentiate the action of other antihypertensive drugs). Products include:
Avalide Tablets 1070
Avapro Tablets 1074

Avapro Tablets ... 3076

Isradipine (Chlorthalidone may add to or potentiate the action of other antihypertensive drugs). Products include:
DynaCirc Capsules ... 2921
DynaCirc CR Tablets ... 2923

Labetalol Hydrochloride (Chlorthalidone may add to or potentiate the action of other antihypertensive drugs). Products include:
Normodyne Injection ... 3135
Normodyne Tablets ... 3137

Levorphanol Tartrate (Orthostatic hypotension produced by chlorthalidone may be aggravated by narcotics). Products include:
Levo-Dromoran ... 1734
Levorphanol Tartrate Tablets ... 3059

Lisinopril (Chlorthalidone may add to or potentiate the action of other antihypertensive drugs). Products include:
Prinivil Tablets ... 2164
Prinzide Tablets ... 2168
Zestoretic Tablets ... 695
Zestril Tablets ... 698

Lithium Carbonate (Reduced renal lithium clearance and increased risk of lithium toxicity). Products include:
Eskalith ... 1527
Lithium Carbonate ... 3061
Lithobid Slow-Release Tablets ... 3255

Lithium Citrate (Reduced renal lithium clearance and increased risk of lithium toxicity). Products include:
Lithium Citrate Syrup ... 3061

Lorazepam (Enhanced CNS-depressive effects). Products include:
Ativan Injection ... 3478
Ativan Tablets ... 3482

Losartan Potassium (Chlorthalidone may add to or potentiate the action of other antihypertensive drugs). Products include:
Cozaar Tablets ... 2067
Hyzaar ... 2109

Maprotiline Hydrochloride (Co-administration results in reduced effect of clonidine, thus necessitating an increase in dosage).
No products indexed under this heading.

Mecamylamine Hydrochloride (Chlorthalidone may add to or potentiate the action of other antihypertensive drugs). Products include:
Inversine Tablets ... 1850

Meperidine Hydrochloride (Orthostatic hypotension produced by chlorthalidone may be aggravated by narcotics). Products include:
Demerol ... 3079
Mepergan Injection ... 3539

Mephobarbital (Orthostatic hypotension produced by chlorthalidone may be aggravated by barbiturates; potential for enhanced CNS-depressive effects).
No products indexed under this heading.

Metformin Hydrochloride (Higher dosage of oral hypoglycemic agents may be required). Products include:
Glucophage Tablets ... 1080
Glucophage XR Tablets ... 1080
Glucovance Tablets ... 1086

Methadone Hydrochloride (Orthostatic hypotension produced by chlorthalidone may be aggravated by narcotics). Products include:
Dolophine Hydrochloride Tablets ... 3056

Methyclothiazide (Chlorthalidone may add to or potentiate the action of other antihypertensive drugs).
No products indexed under this heading.

Methyldopa (Chlorthalidone may add to or potentiate the action of other antihypertensive drugs). Products include:
Aldoclor Tablets ... 2035
Aldomet Tablets ... 2037
Aldoril Tablets ... 2039

Methyldopate Hydrochloride (Chlorthalidone may add to or potentiate the action of other antihypertensive drugs).
No products indexed under this heading.

Metolazone (Chlorthalidone may add to or potentiate the action of other antihypertensive drugs). Products include:
Mykrox Tablets ... 1168
Zaroxolyn Tablets ... 1177

Metoprolol Succinate (Chlorthalidone may add to or potentiate the action of other antihypertensive drugs). Products include:
Toprol-XL Tablets ... 651

Metoprolol Tartrate (Chlorthalidone may add to or potentiate the action of other antihypertensive drugs).
No products indexed under this heading.

Metyrosine (Chlorthalidone may add to or potentiate the action of other antihypertensive drugs). Products include:
Demser Capsules ... 2085

Mibefradil Dihydrochloride (Chlorthalidone may add to or potentiate the action of other antihypertensive drugs).
No products indexed under this heading.

Midazolam Hydrochloride (Enhanced CNS-depressive effects). Products include:
Versed Injection ... 3027
Versed Syrup ... 3033

Miglitol (Higher dosage of oral hypoglycemic agents may be required). Products include:
Glyset Tablets ... 2821

Minoxidil (Chlorthalidone may add to or potentiate the action of other antihypertensive drugs). Products include:
Rogaine Extra Strength for Men Topical Solution ... ▣ 721
Rogaine for Women Topical Solution ... ▣ 721

Moexipril Hydrochloride (Chlorthalidone may add to or potentiate the action of other antihypertensive drugs). Products include:
Uniretic Tablets ... 3178
Univasc Tablets ... 3181

Morphine Sulfate (Orthostatic hypotension produced by chlorthalidone may be aggravated by narcotics). Products include:
Astramorph/PF Injection, USP (Preservative-Free) ... 594
Duramorph Injection ... 1312
Infumorph 200 and Infumorph 500 Sterile Solutions ... 1314
Kadian Capsules ... 1335
MS Contin Tablets ... 2896
MSIR ... 2898
Oramorph SR Tablets ... 3062
Roxanol ... 3066

Nadolol (Chlorthalidone may add to or potentiate the action of other antihypertensive drugs). Products include:
Corgard Tablets ... 2245
Corzide 40/5 Tablets ... 2247
Corzide 80/5 Tablets ... 2247
Nadolol Tablets ... 2288

Nicardipine Hydrochloride (Chlorthalidone may add to or potentiate the action of other antihypertensive drugs). Products include:
Cardene I.V. ... 3485

Nifedipine (Chlorthalidone may add to or potentiate the action of other antihypertensive drugs). Products include:
Adalat CC Tablets ... 877
Procardia Capsules ... 2708
Procardia XL Extended Release Tablets ... 2710

Nisoldipine (Chlorthalidone may add to or potentiate the action of other antihypertensive drugs). Products include:
Sular Tablets ... 688

Nitroglycerin (Chlorthalidone may add to or potentiate the action of other antihypertensive drugs). Products include:
Nitro-Dur Transdermal Infusion System ... 3134
Nitro-Dur Transdermal Infusion System ... 1834
Nitrolingual Pumpspray ... 1355
Nitrostat Tablets ... 2658

Norepinephrine Bitartrate (Decreased arterial responsiveness to norepinephrine).
No products indexed under this heading.

Nortriptyline Hydrochloride (Co-administration results in reduced effect of clonidine, thus necessitating an increase in dosage).
No products indexed under this heading.

Oxycodone Hydrochloride (Orthostatic hypotension produced by chlorthalidone may be aggravated by narcotics). Products include:
OxyContin Tablets ... 2912
OxyFast Oral Concentrate Solution ... 2916
OxyIR Capsules ... 2916
Percocet Tablets ... 1326
Percodan Tablets ... 1327
Percolone Tablets ... 1327
Roxicodone ... 3067
Tylox Capsules ... 2597

Papaverine (Drug-induced hepatitis (one case)).
No products indexed under this heading.

Penbutolol Sulfate (Chlorthalidone may add to or potentiate the action of other antihypertensive drugs).
No products indexed under this heading.

Pentobarbital Sodium (Orthostatic hypotension produced by chlorthalidone may be aggravated by barbiturates; potential for enhanced CNS-depressive effects). Products include:
Nembutal Sodium Solution ... 485

Perindopril Erbumine (Chlorthalidone may add to or potentiate the action of other antihypertensive drugs). Products include:
Aceon Tablets (2 mg, 4 mg, 8 mg) ... 3249

Phenobarbital (Orthostatic hypotension produced by chlorthalidone may be aggravated by barbiturates; potential for enhanced CNS-depressive effects). Products include:
Arco-Lase Plus Tablets ... 592
Donnatal ... 2929
Donnatal Extentabs ... 2930

Phenoxybenzamine Hydrochloride (Chlorthalidone may add to or potentiate the action of other antihypertensive drugs). Products include:
Dibenzyline Capsules ... 3457

Phentolamine Mesylate (Chlorthalidone may add to or potentiate the action of other antihypertensive drugs).
No products indexed under this heading.

Pindolol (Chlorthalidone may add to or potentiate the action of other antihypertensive drugs).
No products indexed under this heading.

Pioglitazone Hydrochloride (Higher dosage of oral hypoglycemic agents may be required). Products include:
Actos Tablets ... 3275

Polythiazide (Chlorthalidone may add to or potentiate the action of other antihypertensive drugs). Products include:
Minizide Capsules ... 2700
Renese Tablets ... 2712

Prazosin Hydrochloride (Chlorthalidone may add to or potentiate the action of other antihypertensive drugs). Products include:
Minipress Capsules ... 2699
Minizide Capsules ... 2700

Propofol (Enhanced CNS-depressive effects). Products include:
Diprivan Injectable Emulsion ... 667

Propoxyphene Hydrochloride (Orthostatic hypotension produced by chlorthalidone may be aggravated by narcotics). Products include:
Darvon Pulvules ... 1909
Darvon Compound-65 Pulvules ... 1910

Propoxyphene Napsylate (Orthostatic hypotension produced by chlorthalidone may be aggravated by narcotics). Products include:
Darvon-N/Darvocet-N ... 1907
Darvon-N Tablets ... 1912

Propranolol Hydrochloride (Chlorthalidone may add to or potentiate the action of other antihypertensive drugs). Products include:
Inderal ... 3513
Inderal LA Long-Acting Capsules ... 3516
Inderide Tablets ... 3517
Inderide LA Long-Acting Capsules ... 3519

Protriptyline Hydrochloride (Co-administration results in reduced effect of clonidine, thus necessitating an increase in dosage). Products include:
Vivactil Tablets ... 2446
Vivactil Tablets ... 2217

Quazepam (Enhanced CNS-depressive effects).
No products indexed under this heading.

Quinapril Hydrochloride (Chlorthalidone may add to or potentiate the action of other antihypertensive drugs). Products include:
Accupril Tablets ... 2611
Accuretic Tablets ... 2614

Ramipril (Chlorthalidone may add to or potentiate the action of other antihypertensive drugs). Products include:
Altace Capsules ... 2233

Rauwolfia serpentina (Chlorthalidone may add to or potentiate the action of other antihypertensive drugs).
No products indexed under this heading.

Remifentanil Hydrochloride (Orthostatic hypotension produced by chlorthalidone may be aggravated by narcotics).
No products indexed under this heading.

Repaglinide (Higher dosage of oral hypoglycemic agents may be required). Products include:
Prandin Tablets (0.5, 1, and 2 mg) ... 2432

Rescinnamine (Chlorthalidone may add to or potentiate the action of other antihypertensive drugs).
No products indexed under this heading.

Reserpine (Chlorthalidone may add to or potentiate the action of other antihypertensive drugs).
No products indexed under this heading.

Rosiglitazone Maleate (Higher dosage of oral hypoglycemic agents may be required). Products include:
Avandia Tablets ... 1490

Secobarbital Sodium (Orthostatic hypotension produced by chlorthalidone may be aggravated by barbiturates; potential for enhanced CNS-depressive effects).
No products indexed under this heading.

Sodium Nitroprusside (Chlorthalidone may add to or potentiate the action of other antihypertensive drugs).
No products indexed under this heading.

Sotalol Hydrochloride (Chlorthalidone may add to or potentiate the action of other antihypertensive drugs). Products include:

Betapace Tablets 950
Betapace AF Tablets 954

Spirapril Hydrochloride (Chlorthalidone may add to or potentiate the action of other antihypertensive drugs).

No products indexed under this heading.

Sufentanil Citrate (Orthostatic hypotension produced by chlorthalidone may be aggravated by narcotics).

No products indexed under this heading.

Telmisartan (Chlorthalidone may add to or potentiate the action of other antihypertensive drugs). Products include:

Micardis Tablets 1049
Micardis HCT Tablets 1051

Temazepam (Enhanced CNS-depressive effects).

No products indexed under this heading.

Terazosin Hydrochloride (Chlorthalidone may add to or potentiate the action of other antihypertensive drugs). Products include:

Hytrin Capsules 464

Thiamylal Sodium (Orthostatic hypotension produced by chlorthalidone may be aggravated by barbiturates; potential for enhanced CNS-depressive effects).

No products indexed under this heading.

Timolol Maleate (Chlorthalidone may add to or potentiate the action of other antihypertensive drugs). Products include:

Blocadren Tablets 2046
Cosopt Sterile Ophthalmic Solution 2065
Timolide Tablets 2187
Timolol GFS ⊙ 266
Timoptic in Ocudose 2192
Timoptic Sterile Ophthalmic Solution 2190
Timoptic-XE Sterile Ophthalmic Gel Forming Solution 2194

Tolazamide (Higher dosage of oral hypoglycemic agents may be required).

No products indexed under this heading.

Tolbutamide (Higher dosage of oral hypoglycemic agents may be required).

No products indexed under this heading.

Torsemide (Chlorthalidone may add to or potentiate the action of other antihypertensive drugs). Products include:

Demadex Tablets and Injection 2965

Trandolapril (Chlorthalidone may add to or potentiate the action of other antihypertensive drugs). Products include:

Mavik Tablets 478
Tarka Tablets 508

Triazolam (Enhanced CNS-depressive effects). Products include:

Halcion Tablets 2823

Trimethaphan Camsylate (Chlorthalidone may add to or potentiate the action of other antihypertensive drugs).

No products indexed under this heading.

Trimipramine Maleate (Co-administration results in reduced effect of clonidine, thus necessitating an increase in dosage). Products include:

Surmontil Capsules 3595

Troglitazone (Higher dosage of oral hypoglycemic agents may be required).

No products indexed under this heading.

Tubocurarine Chloride (Increased responsiveness to tubocurarine).

No products indexed under this heading.

Valsartan (Chlorthalidone may add to or potentiate the action of other antihypertensive drugs). Products include:

Diovan Capsules 2337
Diovan HCT Tablets 2338

Verapamil Hydrochloride (Chlorthalidone may add to or potentiate the action of other antihypertensive drugs). Products include:

Covera-HS Tablets 3199
Isoptin SR Tablets 467
Tarka Tablets 508
Verelan Capsules 3184
Verelan PM Capsules 3186

Zaleplon (Enhanced CNS-depressive effects). Products include:

Sonata Capsules 3591

Zolpidem Tartrate (Enhanced CNS-depressive effects). Products include:

Ambien Tablets 3191

Food Interactions

Alcohol (Orthostatic hypotension produced by chlorthalidone may be aggravated by alcohol; potential for enhanced CNS-depressive effects).

COMBIVENT INHALATION AEROSOL

(Albuterol Sulfate, Ipratropium Bromide) 1041

May interact with anticholinergics, beta blockers, monoamine oxidase inhibitors, potassium-depleting diuretics, sympathomimetics, and tricyclic antidepressants. Compounds in these categories include:

Acebutolol Hydrochloride (Co-administration with beta blockers inhibits the effects of each other). Products include:

Sectral Capsules 3589

Albuterol (Co-administration with other sympathomimetic agents increases the risk of adverse cardiovascular effects). Products include:

Proventil Inhalation Aerosol 3142
Ventolin Inhalation Aerosol and Refill 1679

Amitriptyline Hydrochloride (Co-administration with tricyclic antidepressant can potentiate the action of albuterol on the cardiovascular system). Products include:

Etrafon 3115
Limbitrol 1738

Amoxapine (Co-administration with tricyclic antidepressant can potentiate the action of albuterol on the cardiovascular system).

No products indexed under this heading.

Atenolol (Co-administration with beta blockers inhibits the effects of each other). Products include:

Tenoretic Tablets 690
Tenormin I.V. Injection 692

Atropine Sulfate (Co-administration has some potential for additive anticholinergic effects; caution is advised). Products include:

Donnatal 2929
Donnatal Extentabs 2930
Motofen Tablets 577
Prosed/DS Tablets 3268
Urised Tablets 2876

Belladonna Alkaloids (Co-administration has some potential for additive anticholinergic effects; caution is advised). Products include:

Hyland's Teething Tablets ▣ 766
Urimax Tablets 1769

Bendroflumethiazide (Co-administration with non-potassium-sparing diuretics can result in acute worsening of ECG changes and/or hypokalemia, especially when recommended dose of the beta agonist is exceeded; clinical significance of this interaction is unknown). Products include:

Corzide 40/5 Tablets 2247
Corzide 80/5 Tablets 2247

Benztropine Mesylate (Co-administration has some potential for additive anticholinergic effects; caution is advised). Products include:

Cogentin 2055

Betaxolol Hydrochloride (Co-administration with beta blockers inhibits the effects of each other). Products include:

Betoptic S Ophthalmic Suspension 537

Biperiden Hydrochloride (Co-administration has some potential for additive anticholinergic effects; caution is advised). Products include:

Akineton 402

Bisoprolol Fumarate (Co-administration with beta blockers inhibits the effects of each other). Products include:

Zebeta Tablets 1885
Ziac Tablets 1887

Bumetanide (Co-administration with non-potassium-sparing diuretics can result in acute worsening of ECG changes and/or hypokalemia, especially when recommended dose of the beta agonist is exceeded; clinical significance of this interaction is unknown).

No products indexed under this heading.

Carteolol Hydrochloride (Co-administration with beta blockers inhibits the effects of each other). Products include:

Carteolol Hydrochloride Ophthalmic Solution USP, 1% ⊙ 258
Ocupress Ophthalmic Solution, 1% Sterile ⊙ 303

Chlorothiazide (Co-administration with non-potassium-sparing diuretics can result in acute worsening of ECG changes and/or hypokalemia, especially when recommended dose of the beta agonist is exceeded; clinical significance of this interaction is unknown). Products include:

Aldoclor Tablets 2035
Diuril Oral 2087

Chlorothiazide Sodium (Co-administration with non-potassium-sparing diuretics can result in acute worsening of ECG changes and/or hypokalemia, especially when recommended dose of the beta agonist is exceeded; clinical significance of this interaction is unknown). Products include:

Diuril Sodium Intravenous 2086

Clidinium Bromide (Co-administration has some potential for additive anticholinergic effects; caution is advised).

No products indexed under this heading.

Clomipramine Hydrochloride (Co-administration with tricyclic antidepressant can potentiate the action of albuterol on the cardiovascular system).

No products indexed under this heading.

Desipramine Hydrochloride (Co-administration with tricyclic antidepressant can potentiate the action of albuterol on the cardiovascular system). Products include:

Norpramin Tablets 755

Dicyclomine Hydrochloride (Co-administration has some potential for additive anticholinergic effects; caution is advised).

No products indexed under this heading.

Dobutamine Hydrochloride (Co-administration with other sympathomimetic agents increases the risk of adverse cardiovascular effects). Products include:

Dobutrex Solution Vials 1914

Dopamine Hydrochloride (Co-administration with other sympathomimetic agents increases the risk of adverse cardiovascular effects).

No products indexed under this heading.

Doxepin Hydrochloride (Co-administration with tricyclic antidepressant can potentiate the action of albuterol on the cardiovascular system). Products include:

Sinequan 2713

Ephedrine Hydrochloride (Co-administration with other sympathomimetic agents increases the risk of adverse cardiovascular effects). Products include:

Primatene Tablets ▣ 780

Ephedrine Sulfate (Co-administration with other sympathomimetic agents increases the risk of adverse cardiovascular effects).

No products indexed under this heading.

Ephedrine Tannate (Co-administration with other sympathomimetic agents increases the risk of adverse cardiovascular effects). Products include:

Rynatuss Pediatric Suspension 3353
Rynatuss Tablets 3353

Epinephrine (Co-administration with other sympathomimetic agents increases the risk of adverse cardiovascular effects). Products include:

Epifrin Sterile Ophthalmic Solution ⊙ 235
EpiPen 1236
Primatene Mist ▣ 779
Xylocaine with Epinephrine Injection 653

Epinephrine Bitartrate (Co-administration with other sympathomimetic agents increases the risk of adverse cardiovascular effects). Products include:

Sensorcaine 643

Epinephrine Hydrochloride (Co-administration with other sympathomimetic agents increases the risk of adverse cardiovascular effects).

No products indexed under this heading.

Esmolol Hydrochloride (Co-administration with beta blockers inhibits the effects of each other). Products include:

Brevibloc Injection 858

Ethacrynic Acid (Co-administration with non-potassium-sparing diuretics can result in acute worsening of ECG changes and/or hypokalemia, especially when recommended dose of the beta agonist is exceeded; clinical significance of this interaction is unknown). Products include:

Edecrin Tablets 2091

Furosemide (Co-administration with non-potassium-sparing diuretics can result in acute worsening of ECG changes and/or hypokalemia, especially when recommended dose of the beta agonist is exceeded; clinical significance of this interaction is unknown). Products include:

Furosemide Tablets 2284

Glycopyrrolate (Co-administration has some potential for additive anticholinergic effects; caution is advised). Products include:

Robinul Forte Tablets 1358
Robinul Injectable 2940
Robinul Tablets 1358

Hydrochlorothiazide (Co-administration with non-potassium-sparing diuretics can result in acute

worsening of ECG changes and/or hypokalemia, especially when recommended dose of the beta agonist is exceeded; clinical significance of this interaction is unknown). Products include:

Accuretic Tablets 2614
Aldoril Tablets 2039
Atacand HCT Tablets 597
Avalide Tablets 1070
Diovan HCT Tablets 2338
Dyazide Capsules 1515
HydroDIURIL Tablets 2108
Hyzaar 2109
Inderide Tablets 3517
Inderide LA Long-Acting Capsules .. 3519
Lotensin HCT Tablets 2367
Maxzide 1008
Micardis HCT Tablets 1051
Microzide Capsules 3414
Moduretic Tablets 2138
Monopril HCT 1094
Prinzide Tablets 2168
Timolide Tablets 2187
Uniretic Tablets 3178
Vaseretic Tablets 2204
Zestoretic Tablets 695
Ziac Tablets 1887

Hydroflumethiazide (Co-administration with non-potassium-sparing diuretics can result in acute worsening of ECG changes and/or hypokalemia, especially when recommended dose of the beta agonist is exceeded; clinical significance of this interaction is unknown). Products include:

Diucardin Tablets 3494

Hyoscyamine (Co-administration has some potential for additive anticholinergic effects; caution is advised). Products include:

Urised Tablets 2876

Hyoscyamine Sulfate (Co-administration has some potential for additive anticholinergic effects; caution is advised). Products include:

Arco-Lase Plus Tablets 592
Donnatal 2929
Donnatal Extentabs 2930
Levsin/Levsinex/Levbid 3172
NuLev Orally Disintegrating Tablets 3176
Prosed/DS Tablets 3268
Urimax Tablets 1769

Imipramine Hydrochloride (Co-administration with tricyclic antidepressant can potentiate the action of albuterol on the cardiovascular system).

No products indexed under this heading.

Imipramine Pamoate (Co-administration with tricyclic antidepressant can potentiate the action of albuterol on the cardiovascular system).

No products indexed under this heading.

Isocarboxazid (Co-administration with MAO inhibitor can potentiate the action of albuterol on the cardiovascular system).

No products indexed under this heading.

Isoproterenol Hydrochloride (Co-administration with other sympathomimetic agents increases the risk of adverse cardiovascular effects).

No products indexed under this heading.

Isoproterenol Sulfate (Co-administration with other sympathomimetic agents increases the risk of adverse cardiovascular effects).

No products indexed under this heading.

Labetalol Hydrochloride (Co-administration with beta blockers inhibits the effects of each other). Products include:

Normodyne Injection 3135
Normodyne Tablets 3137

Levalbuterol Hydrochloride (Co-administration with other sympathomimetic agents increases the risk of adverse cardiovascular effects). Products include:

Xopenex Inhalation Solution 3207

Levobunolol Hydrochloride (Co-administration with beta blockers inhibits the effects of each other). Products include:

Betagan .... ⊙228

Maprotiline Hydrochloride (Co-administration with tricyclic antidepressant can potentiate the action of albuterol on the cardiovascular system).

No products indexed under this heading.

Mepenzolate Bromide (Co-administration has some potential for additive anticholinergic effects; caution is advised).

No products indexed under this heading.

Metaproterenol Sulfate (Co-administration with other sympathomimetic agents increases the risk of adverse cardiovascular effects). Products include:

Alupent 1029

Metaraminol Bitartrate (Co-administration with other sympathomimetic agents increases the risk of adverse cardiovascular effects). Products include:

Aramine Injection 2043

Methoxamine Hydrochloride (Co-administration with other sympathomimetic agents increases the risk of adverse cardiovascular effects).

No products indexed under this heading.

Methyclothiazide (Co-administration with non-potassium-sparing diuretics can result in acute worsening of ECG changes and/or hypokalemia, especially when recommended dose of the beta agonist is exceeded; clinical significance of this interaction is unknown).

No products indexed under this heading.

Metipranolol Hydrochloride (Co-administration with beta blockers inhibits the effects of each other).

No products indexed under this heading.

Metoprolol Succinate (Co-administration with beta blockers inhibits the effects of each other). Products include:

Toprol-XL Tablets 651

Metoprolol Tartrate (Co-administration with beta blockers inhibits the effects of each other).

No products indexed under this heading.

Moclobemide (Co-administration with MAO inhibitor can potentiate the action of albuterol on the cardiovascular system).

No products indexed under this heading.

Nadolol (Co-administration with beta blockers inhibits the effects of each other). Products include:

Corgard Tablets 2245
Corzide 40/5 Tablets 2247
Corzide 80/5 Tablets 2247
Nadolol Tablets 2288

Norepinephrine Bitartrate (Co-administration with other sympathomimetic agents increases the risk of adverse cardiovascular effects).

No products indexed under this heading.

Nortriptyline Hydrochloride (Co-administration with tricyclic antidepressant can potentiate the action of albuterol on the cardiovascular system).

No products indexed under this heading.

Oxybutynin Chloride (Co-administration has some potential for additive anticholinergic effects; caution is advised). Products include:

Ditropan XL Extended Release Tablets 564

Pargyline Hydrochloride (Co-administration with MAO inhibitor can potentiate the action of albuterol on the cardiovascular system).

No products indexed under this heading.

Penbutolol Sulfate (Co-administration with beta blockers inhibits the effects of each other).

No products indexed under this heading.

Phenelzine Sulfate (Co-administration with MAO inhibitor can potentiate the action of albuterol on the cardiovascular system). Products include:

Nardil Tablets 2653

Phenylephrine Bitartrate (Co-administration with other sympathomimetic agents increases the risk of adverse cardiovascular effects).

No products indexed under this heading.

Phenylephrine Hydrochloride (Co-administration with other sympathomimetic agents increases the risk of adverse cardiovascular effects). Products include:

Afrin Nasal Decongestant Children's Pump Mist .... ▣734
Extendryl 1361
Hycomine Compound Tablets 1317
Neo-Synephrine .... ▣614
Phenergan VC Syrup 3560
Phenergan VC with Codeine Syrup . 3561
Preparation H Cream .... ▣778
Preparation H Cooling Gel .... ▣778
Preparation H .... ▣778
Vicks Sinex Nasal Spray and Ultra Fine Mist .... ▣729

Phenylephrine Tannate (Co-administration with other sympathomimetic agents increases the risk of adverse cardiovascular effects). Products include:

Ryna-12 S Suspension 3351
Reformulated Rynatan Pediatric Suspension 3352
Rynatuss Pediatric Suspension 3353
Rynatuss Tablets 3353

Phenylpropanolamine Hydrochloride (Co-administration with other sympathomimetic agents increases the risk of adverse cardiovascular effects).

No products indexed under this heading.

Pindolol (Co-administration with beta blockers inhibits the effects of each other).

No products indexed under this heading.

Pirbuterol Acetate (Co-administration with other sympathomimetic agents increases the risk of adverse cardiovascular effects). Products include:

Maxair Autohaler 1981
Maxair Inhaler 1984

Polythiazide (Co-administration with non-potassium-sparing diuretics can result in acute worsening of ECG changes and/or hypokalemia, especially when recommended dose of the beta agonist is exceeded; clinical significance of this interaction is unknown). Products include:

Minizide Capsules 2700
Renese Tablets 2712

Procarbazine Hydrochloride (Co-administration with MAO inhibitor can potentiate the action of albuterol on the cardiovascular system). Products include:

Matulane Capsules 3246

Procyclidine Hydrochloride (Co-administration has some potential for additive anticholinergic effects; caution is advised).

No products indexed under this heading.

Propantheline Bromide (Co-administration has some potential for additive anticholinergic effects; caution is advised).

No products indexed under this heading.

Propranolol Hydrochloride (Co-administration with beta blockers inhibits the effects of each other). Products include:

Inderal 3513
Inderal LA Long-Acting Capsules 3516
Inderide Tablets 3517
Inderide LA Long-Acting Capsules .. 3519

Protriptyline Hydrochloride (Co-administration with tricyclic antidepressant can potentiate the action of albuterol on the cardiovascular system). Products include:

Vivactil Tablets 2446
Vivactil Tablets 2217

Pseudoephedrine Hydrochloride (Co-administration with other sympathomimetic agents increases the risk of adverse cardiovascular effects). Products include:

Actifed Cold & Allergy Tablets .... ▣688
Actifed Cold & Sinus Caplets and Tablets .... ▣688
Advil Cold and Sinus Caplets .... ▣771
Advil Cold and Sinus Tablets .... ▣771
Advil Flu & Body Ache Caplets .... ▣772
Aleve Cold & Sinus Caplets .... ▣603
Alka-Seltzer Plus Liqui-Gels .... ▣604
Alka-Seltzer Plus Cold & Flu Medicine Liqui-Gels .... ▣604
Alka-Seltzer Plus Cold & Sinus Medicine Liqui-Gels .... ▣604
Allegra-D Extended-Release Tablets 714
BC Cold Powder .... ▣619
Benadryl Allergy/Cold Tablets .... ▣691
Benadryl Allergy/Congestion Tablets .... ▣692
Benadryl Allergy & Sinus Liquid .... ▣693
Benadryl Allergy & Sinus Fastmelt Tablets .... ▣693
Benadryl Allergy Sinus Headache Caplets & Gelcaps .... ▣693
Benadryl Severe Allergy & Sinus Headache Caplets .... ▣694
Benadryl Children's Allergy/Cold Fastmelt Tablets .... ▣692
Benylin Multi-Symptom Liquid .... ▣697
Bromfed Capsules (Extended-Release) 2269
Bromfed-PD Capsules (Extended-Release) 2269
Children's Cēpacol Sore Throat .... ▣788
Comtrex Acute Head Cold & Sinus Pressure Relief Tablets .... ▣627
Comtrex Deep Chest Cold & Congestion Relief Softgels .... ▣627
Comtrex Flu Therapy & Fever Relief Daytime Caplets .... ▣628
Comtrex Flu Therapy & Fever Relief Nighttime Tablets .... ▣628
Comtrex Maximum Strength Multi-Symptom Cold & Cough Relief Tablets and Caplets .... ▣626
Contac Non-Drowsy 12 Hour Cold Caplets .... ▣745
Contac Non-Drowsy Timed Release 12 Hour Cold Caplets ... ▣746
Contac Severe Cold and Flu Caplets Maximum Strength .... ▣746
Contac Severe Cold and Flu Caplets Non-Drowsy .... ▣746
Dimetapp Elixir .... ▣777
Dimetapp Cold and Fever Suspension .... ▣775
Dimetapp DM Cold & Cough Elixir . ▣775
Dimetapp Nighttime Flu Liquid .... ▣776
Dimetapp Non-Drowsy Flu Syrup .. ▣777
Dimetapp Infant Drops Decongestant .... ▣775
Dimetapp Infant Drops Decongestant Plus Cough .... ▣776
Guaifed 2272
Kronofed-A 1341
Children's Motrin Cold Oral Suspension 2007
Motrin Sinus Headache Caplets 2005
PediaCare Cough-Cold Liquid .... ▣719
PediaCare Infants' Drops Decongestant .... ▣719
PediaCare Infants' Drops Decongestant Plus Cough .... ▣719
PediaCare NightRest Cough-Cold Liquid .... ▣719
Robitussin Cold Caplets Cold & Congestion .... ▣780

Robitussin Cold Softgels Cold & Congestion ▣780
Robitussin Cold Caplets Multi-Symptom Cold & Flu ▣781
Robitussin Cold Softgels Multi-Symptom Cold & Flu ▣781
Robitussin Cold Softgels Severe Congestion ▣782
Robitussin Cough & Cold Infant Drops ▣782
Robitussin Maximum Strength Cough & Cold Liquid ▣785
Robitussin Pediatric Cough & Cold Formula Liquid ▣785
Robitussin Multi Symptom Honey Flu Liquid ▣785
Robitussin Nighttime Honey Flu Liquid ▣786
Robitussin-CF Liquid ▣783
Robitussin-DAC Syrup 2942
Robitussin-PE Liquid ▣782
Ryna ▣768
Semprex-D Capsules 1172
Singlet Caplets ▣761
Sinutab Non-Drying Liquid Caps ▣706
Sinutab Sinus Allergy Medication, Maximum Strength Formula, Tablets & Caplets ▣707
Sinutab Sinus Medication, Maximum Strength Without Drowsiness Formula, Tablets & Caplets ▣707
Sudafed 12 Hour Tablets ▣708
Sudafed 24 Hour Tablets ▣708
Children's Sudafed Cold & Cough Liquid ▣709
Children's Sudafed Nasal Decongestant Chewables ▣711
Children's Sudafed Nasal Decongestant Liquid Medication ▣711
Sudafed Cold & Allergy Tablets ▣708
Sudafed Cold & Cough Liquid Caps ▣709
Sudafed Cold & Sinus Liquid Caps ▣710
Sudafed Nasal Decongestant Tablets ▣710
Sudafed Non-Drying Sinus Liquid Caps ▣712
Sudafed Severe Cold ▣711
Sudafed Sinus Headache Caplets ▣712
Sudafed Sinus Headache Tablets ▣712
Tavist Sinus Non-Drowsy Coated Caplets ▣676
TheraFlu Regular Strength Cold & Cough Night Time Hot Liquid ▣676
TheraFlu Regular Strength Cold & Sore Throat Night Time Hot Liquid ▣676
TheraFlu Maximum Strength Flu & Congestion Non-Drowsy Hot Liquid ▣677
TheraFlu Maximum Strength Flu & Cough Night Time Hot Liquid ▣678
TheraFlu Maximum Strength Flu & Sore Throat Night Time Hot Liquid ▣677
TheraFlu Maximum Strength Severe Cold & Congestion Night Time Caplets ▣678
TheraFlu Maximum Strength Severe Cold & Congestion Night Time Hot Liquid ▣678
TheraFlu Maximum Strength Severe Cold & Congestion Non-Drowsy ▣679
Triaminic Allergy Congestion Liquid ▣680
Triaminic Chest Congestion Liquid ▣680
Triaminic Cold & Allergy Liquid ▣681
Triaminic Cold & Allergy Softchews ▣683
Triaminic Cold & Cough Liquid ▣681
Triaminic Cold & Cough Softchews ▣683
Triaminic Cold & Night Time Cough Liquid ▣681
Triaminic Cold, Cough & Fever Liquid ▣681
Triaminic Cough Liquid ▣682
Triaminic Cough & Congestion Liquid ▣682
Triaminic Cough & Sore Throat Liquid ▣682
Triaminic Cough & Sore Throat Softchews ▣684
Children's Tylenol Allergy-D Liquid 2014
Children's Tylenol Cold Suspension Liquid and Chewable Tablets 2015
Children's Tylenol Cold Plus Cough Suspension Liquid and Chewable Tablets 2015
Children's Tylenol Flu Suspension Liquid 2015
Children's Tylenol Sinus Suspension Liquid 2017
Infants' Tylenol Cold Decongestant and Fever Reducer Concentrated Drops 2015
Infants' Tylenol Cold Decongestant and Fever Reducer Concentrated Drops Plus Cough 2015
Tylenol Allergy Sinus 2010
Multi-Symptom Tylenol Cold Complete Formula Caplets 2010
Multi-Symptom Tylenol Cold Non-Drowsy Caplets and Gelcaps 2010
Multi-Symptom Tylenol Cold Severe Congestion Non-Drowsy Caplets 2011
Maximum Strength Tylenol Flu NightTime Gelcaps 2011
Maximum Strength Tylenol Flu NightTime Liquid 2011
Maximum Strength Tylenol Flu Non-Drowsy Gelcaps 2011
Maximum Strength Tylenol Sinus NightTime Caplets 2012
Maximum Strength Tylenol Sinus Non-Drowsy Geltabs, Gelcaps, Caplets, and Tablets 2012
Vicks 44D Cough & Head Congestion Relief Liquid ▣724
Vicks 44M Cough, Cold & Flu Relief Liquid ▣725
Pediatric Vicks 44m Cough & Cold Relief ▣728
Vicks DayQuil LiquiCaps/Liquid Multi-Symptom Cold/Flu Relief ▣727
Children's Vicks NyQuil Cold/Cough Relief ▣726
Vicks NyQuil LiquiCaps/Liquid Multi-Symptom Cold/Flu Relief, Original and Cherry Flavors ▣727
Zephrex Tablets 3091
Zephrex LA Tablets 3092
Zyrtec-D 12 Hour Extended Relief Tablets 2758

Pseudoephedrine Sulfate (Co-administration with other sympathomimetic agents increases the risk of adverse cardiovascular effects). Products include:
Chlor-Trimeton Allergy/Decongestant Tablets ▣736
Claritin-D 12 Hour Extended Release Tablets 3102
Claritin-D 24 Hour Extended Release Tablets 3104
Coricidin 'D' Cold, Flu & Sinus Tablets ▣737
Drixoral Allergy/Sinus Extended-Release Tablets ▣741
Drixoral Cold & Allergy Sustained-Action Tablets ▣740
Drixoral Cold & Flu Extended-Release Tablets ▣740
Drixoral Nasal Decongestant Long-Acting Non-Drowsy Tablets ▣740
Rynatan Tablets 3351

Salmeterol Xinafoate (Co-administration with other sympathomimetic agents increases the risk of adverse cardiovascular effects). Products include:
Advair Diskus 100/50 1448
Advair Diskus 250/50 1448
Advair Diskus 500/50 1448
Serevent Diskus 1637
Serevent Inhalation Aerosol 1633

Scopolamine (Co-administration has some potential for additive anticholinergic effects; caution is advised). Products include:
Transderm Scōp Transdermal Therapeutic System 2302

Scopolamine Hydrobromide (Co-administration has some potential for additive anticholinergic effects; caution is advised). Products include:
Donnatal 2929
Donnatal Extentabs 2930

Selegiline Hydrochloride (Co-administration with MAO inhibitor can potentiate the action of albuterol on the cardiovascular system). Products include:
Eldepryl Capsules 3266

Sotalol Hydrochloride (Co-administration with beta blockers inhibits the effects of each other). Products include:
Betapace Tablets 950
Betapace AF Tablets 954

Terbutaline Sulfate (Co-administration with other sympathomimetic agents increases the risk of adverse cardiovascular effects). Products include:
Brethine Ampuls 2314
Brethine Tablets 2313

Timolol Hemihydrate (Co-administration with beta blockers inhibits the effects of each other). Products include:
Betimol Ophthalmic Solution ⊙324

Timolol Maleate (Co-administration with beta blockers inhibits the effects of each other). Products include:
Blocadren Tablets 2046
Cosopt Sterile Ophthalmic Solution 2065
Timolide Tablets 2187
Timolol GFS ⊙266
Timoptic in Ocudose 2192
Timoptic Sterile Ophthalmic Solution 2190
Timoptic-XE Sterile Ophthalmic Gel Forming Solution 2194

Tolterodine Tartrate (Co-administration has some potential for additive anticholinergic effects; caution is advised). Products include:
Detrol Tablets 3623
Detrol LA Capsules 2801

Torsemide (Co-administration with non-potassium-sparing diuretics can result in acute worsening of ECG changes and/or hypokalemia, especially when recommended dose of the beta agonist is exceeded; clinical significance of this interaction is unknown). Products include:
Demadex Tablets and Injection 2965

Tranylcypromine Sulfate (Co-administration with MAO inhibitor can potentiate the action of albuterol on the cardiovascular system). Products include:
Parnate Tablets 1607

Tridihexethyl Chloride (Co-administration has some potential for additive anticholinergic effects; caution is advised).
No products indexed under this heading.

Trihexyphenidyl Hydrochloride (Co-administration has some potential for additive anticholinergic effects; caution is advised). Products include:
Artane 1855

Trimipramine Maleate (Co-administration with tricyclic antidepressant can potentiate the action of albuterol on the cardiovascular system). Products include:
Surmontil Capsules 3595

COMBIVIR TABLETS

(Lamivudine, Zidovudine) 1502
May interact with cytotoxic drugs and certain other agents. Compounds in these categories include:

Bleomycin Sulfate (May increase the hematologic toxicity of zidovudine).
No products indexed under this heading.

Bone Marrow Depressants, unspecified (May increase the hematologic toxicity of zidovudine).

Cyclophosphamide (May increase the hematologic toxicity of zidovudine).
No products indexed under this heading.

Daunorubicin Hydrochloride (May increase the hematologic toxicity of zidovudine). Products include:
Cerubidine for Injection 947

Doxorubicin Hydrochloride (May increase the hematologic toxicity of zidovudine). Products include:
Adriamycin PFS/RDF Injection 2767
Doxil Injection 566

Epirubicin Hydrochloride (May increase the hematologic toxicity of zidovudine). Products include:
Ellence Injection 2806

Fluorouracil (May increase the hematologic toxicity of zidovudine). Products include:
Carac Cream 1222
Efudex 1733
Fluoroplex 552

Ganciclovir Sodium (May increase the hematologic toxicity of zidovudine). Products include:
Cytovene-IV 2959

Hydroxyurea (May increase the hematologic toxicity of zidovudine). Products include:
Mylocel Tablets 2227

Interferon alfa-2A, Recombinant (May increase the hematologic toxicity of zidovudine). Products include:
Roferon-A Injection 2996

Interferon alfa-2B, Recombinant (May increase the hematologic toxicity of zidovudine). Products include:
Intron A for Injection 3120
Rebetron Combination Therapy 3153

Methotrexate Sodium (May increase the hematologic toxicity of zidovudine).
No products indexed under this heading.

Mitotane (May increase the hematologic toxicity of zidovudine).
No products indexed under this heading.

Mitoxantrone Hydrochloride (May increase the hematologic toxicity of zidovudine). Products include:
Novantrone for Injection 1760

Procarbazine Hydrochloride (May increase the hematologic toxicity of zidovudine). Products include:
Matulane Capsules 3246

Tamoxifen Citrate (May increase the hematologic toxicity of zidovudine). Products include:
Nolvadex Tablets 678

Vincristine Sulfate (May increase the hematologic toxicity of zidovudine).
No products indexed under this heading.

COMPAZINE INJECTION

(Prochlorperazine) 1505
See Compazine Tablets

COMPAZINE SPANSULE CAPSULES

(Prochlorperazine) 1505
See Compazine Tablets

COMPAZINE SUPPOSITORIES

(Prochlorperazine) 1505
See Compazine Tablets

COMPAZINE SYRUP

(Prochlorperazine) 1505
See Compazine Tablets

COMPAZINE TABLETS

(Prochlorperazine) 1505
May interact with antihistamines, barbiturates, antineoplastics, central nervous system depressants, oral anticoagulants, anticonvulsants, general anesthetics, narcotic analgesics, thiazides, and certain other agents. Compounds in these categories include:

Acrivastine (Phenothiazines may intensify or prolong the action of other central nervous system depressants). Products include:
Semprex-D Capsules 1172

Alfentanil Hydrochloride (Phenothiazines may intensify or prolong the action of other central nervous system depressants).
No products indexed under this heading.

Alprazolam (Phenothiazines may intensify or prolong the action of other central nervous system depressants). Products include:
- Xanax Tablets ... 2865

Altretamine (Vomiting as a sign of toxicity of antineoplastic agents may be obscured by the antiemetic effect of Compazine). Products include:
- Hexalen Capsules ... 2226

Anastrozole (Vomiting as a sign of toxicity of antineoplastic agents may be obscured by the antiemetic effect of Compazine). Products include:
- Arimidex Tablets ... 659

Aprobarbital (Phenothiazines may intensify or prolong the action of other central nervous system depressants).
- No products indexed under this heading.

Asparaginase (Vomiting as a sign of toxicity of antineoplastic agents may be obscured by the antiemetic effect of Compazine). Products include:
- Elspar for Injection ... 2092

Astemizole (Phenothiazines may intensify or prolong the action of other central nervous system depressants).
- No products indexed under this heading.

Atropine Sulfate (Phenothiazines may intensify or prolong the action of atropine). Products include:
- Donnatal ... 2929
- Donnatal Extentabs ... 2930
- Motofen Tablets ... 577
- Prosed/DS Tablets ... 3268
- Urised Tablets ... 2876

Azatadine Maleate (Phenothiazines may intensify or prolong the action of other central nervous system depressants). Products include:
- Rynatan Tablets ... 3351

Bendroflumethiazide (Accentuates the orthostatic hypotension that may occur with phenothiazines). Products include:
- Corzide 40/5 Tablets ... 2247
- Corzide 80/5 Tablets ... 2247

Bicalutamide (Vomiting as a sign of toxicity of antineoplastic agents may be obscured by the antiemetic effect of Compazine). Products include:
- Casodex Tablets ... 662

Bleomycin Sulfate (Vomiting as a sign of toxicity of antineoplastic agents may be obscured by the antiemetic effect of Compazine).
- No products indexed under this heading.

Bromodiphenhydramine Hydrochloride (Phenothiazines may intensify or prolong the action of other central nervous system depressants).
- No products indexed under this heading.

Brompheniramine Maleate (Phenothiazines may intensify or prolong the action of other central nervous system depressants). Products include:
- Bromfed Capsules (Extended-Release) ... 2269
- Bromfed-PD Capsules (Extended-Release) ... 2269
- Comtrex Acute Head Cold & Sinus Pressure Relief Tablets ... ▣627
- Dimetapp Elixir ... ▣777
- Dimetapp Cold and Fever Suspension ... ▣775
- Dimetapp DM Cold & Cough Elixir ... ▣775
- Dimetapp Nighttime Flu Liquid ... ▣776

Buprenorphine Hydrochloride (Phenothiazines may intensify or prolong the action of other central nervous system depressants). Products include:
- Buprenex Injectable ... 2918

Buspirone Hydrochloride (Phenothiazines may intensify or prolong the action of other central nervous system depressants).
- No products indexed under this heading.

Busulfan (Vomiting as a sign of toxicity of antineoplastic agents may be obscured by the antiemetic effect of Compazine). Products include:
- Myleran Tablets ... 1603

Butabarbital (Phenothiazines may intensify or prolong the action of other central nervous system depressants).
- No products indexed under this heading.

Butalbital (Phenothiazines may intensify or prolong the action of other central nervous system depressants). Products include:
- Phrenilin ... 578
- Sedapap Tablets 50 mg/650 mg ... 2225

Carbamazepine (Phenothiazines may lower convulsive threshold; dosage adjustments of anticonvulsant may be necessary). Products include:
- Carbatrol Capsules ... 3234
- Tegretol/Tegretol-XR ... 2404

Carboplatin (Vomiting as a sign of toxicity of antineoplastic agents may be obscured by the antiemetic effect of Compazine). Products include:
- Paraplatin for Injection ... 1126

Carmustine (BCNU) (Vomiting as a sign of toxicity of antineoplastic agents may be obscured by the antiemetic effect of Compazine). Products include:
- Gliadel Wafer ... 1723

Cetirizine Hydrochloride (Phenothiazines may intensify or prolong the action of other central nervous system depressants). Products include:
- Zyrtec ... 2756
- Zyrtec-D 12 Hour Extended Relief Tablets ... 2758

Chlorambucil (Vomiting as a sign of toxicity of antineoplastic agents may be obscured by the antiemetic effect of Compazine). Products include:
- Leukeran Tablets ... 1591

Chlordiazepoxide (Phenothiazines may intensify or prolong the action of other central nervous system depressants). Products include:
- Limbitrol ... 1738

Chlordiazepoxide Hydrochloride (Phenothiazines may intensify or prolong the action of other central nervous system depressants). Products include:
- Librium Capsules ... 1736
- Librium for Injection ... 1737

Chlorothiazide (Accentuates the orthostatic hypotension that may occur with phenothiazines). Products include:
- Aldoclor Tablets ... 2035
- Diuril Oral ... 2087

Chlorothiazide Sodium (Accentuates the orthostatic hypotension that may occur with phenothiazines). Products include:
- Diuril Sodium Intravenous ... 2086

Chlorpheniramine Maleate (Phenothiazines may intensify or prolong the action of other central nervous system depressants). Products include:
- Actifed Cold & Sinus Caplets and Tablets ... ▣688
- Alka-Seltzer Plus Liqui-Gels ... ▣604
- BC Allergy Sinus Cold Powder ... ▣619
- Chlor-Trimeton Allergy Tablets ... ▣735
- Chlor-Trimeton Allergy/Decongestant Tablets ... ▣736
- Comtrex Flu Therapy & Fever Relief Nighttime Tablets ... ▣628
- Comtrex Maximum Strength Multi-Symptom Cold & Cough Relief Tablets and Caplets ... ▣626
- Contac Severe Cold and Flu Caplets Maximum Strength ... ▣746
- Coricidin 'D' Cold, Flu & Sinus Tablets ... ▣737
- Coricidin/Coricidin D ... ▣738
- Coricidin HBP Maximum Strength Flu Tablets ... ▣738
- Extendryl ... 1361
- Hycomine Compound Tablets ... 1317
- Kronofed-A ... 1341
- PediaCare Cough-Cold Liquid ... ▣719
- PediaCare NightRest Cough-Cold Liquid ... ▣719
- Robitussin Nighttime Honey Flu Liquid ... ▣786
- Ryna ... ▣768
- Singlet Caplets ... ▣761
- Sinutab Sinus Allergy Medication, Maximum Strength Formula, Tablets & Caplets ... ▣707
- Sudafed Cold & Allergy Tablets ... ▣708
- TheraFlu Regular Strength Cold & Cough Night Time Hot Liquid ... ▣676
- TheraFlu Regular Strength Cold & Sore Throat Night Time Hot Liquid ... ▣676
- TheraFlu Maximum Strength Flu & Cough Night Time Hot Liquid ... ▣678
- TheraFlu Maximum Strength Flu & Sore Throat Night Time Hot Liquid ... ▣677
- TheraFlu Maximum Strength Severe Cold & Congestion Night Time Caplets ... ▣678
- TheraFlu Maximum Strength Severe Cold & Congestion Night Time Hot Liquid ... ▣678
- Triaminic Cold & Allergy Liquid ... ▣681
- Triaminic Cold & Allergy Softchews ... ▣683
- Triaminic Cold & Cough Liquid ... ▣681
- Triaminic Cold & Cough Softchews ... ▣683
- Triaminic Cold & Night Time Cough Liquid ... ▣681
- Triaminic Cold, Cough & Fever Liquid ... ▣681
- Children's Tylenol Cold Suspension Liquid and Chewable Tablets ... 2015
- Children's Tylenol Cold Plus Cough Suspension Liquid and Chewable Tablets ... 2015
- Children's Tylenol Flu Suspension Liquid ... 2015
- Maximum Strength Tylenol Allergy Sinus Caplets, Gelcaps, and Geltabs ... 2010
- Multi-Symptom Tylenol Cold Complete Formula Caplets ... 2010
- Vicks 44M Cough, Cold & Flu Relief Liquid ... ▣725
- Pediatric Vicks 44m Cough & Cold Relief ... ▣728
- Children's Vicks NyQuil Cold/Cough Relief ... ▣726

Chlorpheniramine Polistirex (Phenothiazines may intensify or prolong the action of other central nervous system depressants). Products include:
- Tussionex Pennkinetic Extended-Release Suspension ... 1174

Chlorpheniramine Tannate (Phenothiazines may intensify or prolong the action of other central nervous system depressants). Products include:
- Reformulated Rynatan Pediatric Suspension ... 3352
- Rynatuss Pediatric Suspension ... 3353
- Rynatuss Tablets ... 3353
- Tussi-12 S Suspension ... 3356
- Tussi-12 Tablets ... 3356

Chlorpromazine (Phenothiazines may intensify or prolong the action of other central nervous system depressants). Products include:
- Thorazine Suppositories ... 1656

Chlorpromazine Hydrochloride (Phenothiazines may intensify or prolong the action of other central nervous system depressants). Products include:
- Thorazine ... 1656

Chlorprothixene (Phenothiazines may intensify or prolong the action of other central nervous system depressants).
- No products indexed under this heading.

Chlorprothixene Hydrochloride (Phenothiazines may intensify or prolong the action of other central nervous system depressants).
- No products indexed under this heading.

Chlorprothixene Lactate (Phenothiazines may intensify or prolong the action of other central nervous system depressants).
- No products indexed under this heading.

Cisplatin (Vomiting as a sign of toxicity of antineoplastic agents may be obscured by the antiemetic effect of Compazine).
- No products indexed under this heading.

Clemastine Fumarate (Phenothiazines may intensify or prolong the action of other central nervous system depressants). Products include:
- Tavist 12 Hour Allergy Tablets ... ▣676

Clorazepate Dipotassium (Phenothiazines may intensify or prolong the action of other central nervous system depressants). Products include:
- Tranxene ... 511

Clozapine (Phenothiazines may intensify or prolong the action of other central nervous system depressants). Products include:
- Clozaril Tablets ... 2319

Codeine Phosphate (Phenothiazines may intensify or prolong the action of other central nervous system depressants). Products include:
- Phenergan with Codeine Syrup ... 3557
- Phenergan VC with Codeine Syrup ... 3561
- Robitussin A-C Syrup ... 2942
- Robitussin-DAC Syrup ... 2942
- Ryna-C Liquid ... ▣768
- Soma Compound w/Codeine Tablets ... 3355
- Tussi-Organidin NR Liquid ... 3350
- Tussi-Organidin-S NR Liquid ... 3350
- Tylenol with Codeine ... 2595

Cyclophosphamide (Vomiting as a sign of toxicity of antineoplastic agents may be obscured by the antiemetic effect of Compazine).
- No products indexed under this heading.

Cyproheptadine Hydrochloride (Phenothiazines may intensify or prolong the action of other central nervous system depressants). Products include:
- Periactin Tablets ... 2155

Dacarbazine (Vomiting as a sign of toxicity of antineoplastic agents may be obscured by the antiemetic effect of Compazine). Products include:
- DTIC-Dome ... 902

Daunorubicin Citrate (Vomiting as a sign of toxicity of antineoplastic agents may be obscured by the antiemetic effect of Compazine). Products include:
- DaunoXome Injection ... 1442

Daunorubicin Hydrochloride (Vomiting as a sign of toxicity of antineoplastic agents may be obscured by the antiemetic effect of Compazine). Products include:
- Cerubidine for Injection ... 947

Denileukin Diftitox (Vomiting as a sign of toxicity of antineoplastic agents may be obscured by the antiemetic effect of Compazine).
- No products indexed under this heading.

Desflurane (Phenothiazines may intensify or prolong the action of other central nervous system depressants). Products include:
- Suprane Liquid for Inhalation ... 874

Dexchlorpheniramine Maleate (Phenothiazines may intensify or prolong the action of other central nervous system depressants).
- No products indexed under this heading.

Dezocine (Phenothiazines may intensify or prolong the action of other central nervous system

depressants).
No products indexed under this heading.

Diazepam (Phenothiazines may intensify or prolong the action of other central nervous system depressants). Products include:
Valium Injectable 3026
Valium Tablets 3047

Dicumarol (Diminished effect of oral anticoagulants).
No products indexed under this heading.

Diphenhydramine Citrate (Phenothiazines may intensify or prolong the action of other central nervous system depressants). Products include:
Alka-Seltzer PM Effervescent Tablets 605
Benadryl Allergy & Sinus Fastmelt Tablets 693
Benadryl Children's Allergy/Cold Fastmelt Tablets 692
Excedrin PM Tablets, Caplets, and Geltabs 631
Goody's PM Powder 621

Diphenhydramine Hydrochloride (Phenothiazines may intensify or prolong the action of other central nervous system depressants). Products include:
Extra Strength Bayer PM Caplets 611
Benadryl Allergy Chewables 689
Benadryl Allergy 691
Benadryl Allergy Liquid 690
Benadryl Allergy/Cold Tablets 691
Benadryl Allergy/Congestion Tablets 692
Benadryl Allergy & Sinus Liquid 693
Benadryl Allergy Sinus Headache Caplets & Gelcaps 693
Benadryl Severe Allergy & Sinus Headache Caplets 694
Benadryl Dye-Free Allergy Liquid 690
Benadryl Dye-Free Allergy Liqui-Gels Softgels 690
Benadryl Itch Relief Stick Extra Strength 695
Benadryl Cream 695
Benadryl Gel 695
Benadryl Spray 696
Benadryl Parenteral 2617
Coricidin HBP Night-Time Cold & Flu Tablets 738
Nytol QuickCaps Caplets 622
Maximum Strength Nytol QuickGels Softgels 621
Extra Strength Percogesic Aspirin-Free Coated Caplets 665
Simply Sleep Caplets 2008
Sominex Original Formula Tablets 761
Children's Tylenol Allergy-D Liquid 2014
Maximum Strength Tylenol Allergy Sinus NightTime Caplets 2010
Tylenol Severe Allergy Caplets 2010
Maximum Strength Tylenol Flu NightTime Gelcaps 2011
Extra Strength Tylenol PM Caplets, Geltabs, and Gelcaps 2012
Unisom Maximum Strength SleepGels 713

Diphenylpyraline Hydrochloride (Phenothiazines may intensify or prolong the action of other central nervous system depressants).
No products indexed under this heading.

Divalproex Sodium (Phenothiazines may lower convulsive threshold; dosage adjustments of anticonvulsant may be necessary). Products include:
Depakote Sprinkle Capsules 426
Depakote Tablets 430
Depakote ER Tablets 436

Docetaxel (Vomiting as a sign of toxicity of antineoplastic agents may be obscured by the antiemetic effect of Compazine). Products include:
Taxotere for Injection Concentrate 778

Doxorubicin Hydrochloride (Vomiting as a sign of toxicity of antineoplastic agents may be obscured by the antiemetic effect of Compazine). Products include:
Adriamycin PFS/RDF Injection 2767
Doxil Injection 566

Droperidol (Phenothiazines may intensify or prolong the action of other central nervous system depressants).
No products indexed under this heading.

Enflurane (Phenothiazines may intensify or prolong the action of other central nervous system depressants).
No products indexed under this heading.

Epinephrine (Potential for paradoxical lowering of blood pressure). Products include:
Epifrin Sterile Ophthalmic Solution .... ⊙235
EpiPen 1236
Primatene Mist 779
Xylocaine with Epinephrine Injection 653

Epinephrine Hydrochloride (Potential for paradoxical lowering of blood pressure).
No products indexed under this heading.

Epirubicin Hydrochloride (Vomiting as a sign of toxicity of antineoplastic agents may be obscured by the antiemetic effect of Compazine). Products include:
Ellence Injection 2806

Estazolam (Phenothiazines may intensify or prolong the action of other central nervous system depressants). Products include:
ProSom Tablets 500

Estramustine Phosphate Sodium (Vomiting as a sign of toxicity of antineoplastic agents may be obscured by the antiemetic effect of Compazine). Products include:
Emcyt Capsules 2810

Ethchlorvynol (Phenothiazines may intensify or prolong the action of other central nervous system depressants).
No products indexed under this heading.

Ethinamate (Phenothiazines may intensify or prolong the action of other central nervous system depressants).
No products indexed under this heading.

Ethosuximide (Phenothiazines may lower convulsive threshold; dosage adjustments of anticonvulsant may be necessary). Products include:
Zarontin Capsules 2659
Zarontin Syrup 2660

Ethotoin (Phenothiazines may lower convulsive threshold; dosage adjustments of anticonvulsant may be necessary).
No products indexed under this heading.

Etoposide (Vomiting as a sign of toxicity of antineoplastic agents may be obscured by the antiemetic effect of Compazine).
No products indexed under this heading.

Exemestane (Vomiting as a sign of toxicity of antineoplastic agents may be obscured by the antiemetic effect of Compazine). Products include:
Aromasin Tablets 2769

Felbamate (Phenothiazines may lower convulsive threshold; dosage adjustments of anticonvulsant may be necessary). Products include:
Felbatol 3343

Fentanyl (Phenothiazines may intensify or prolong the action of other central nervous system depressants). Products include:
Duragesic Transdermal System 1786

Fentanyl Citrate (Phenothiazines may intensify or prolong the action of other central nervous system depressants). Products include:
Actiq 1184

Fexofenadine Hydrochloride (Phenothiazines may intensify or prolong the action of other central nervous system depressants). Products include:
Allegra 712
Allegra-D Extended-Release Tablets 714

Floxuridine (Vomiting as a sign of toxicity of antineoplastic agents may be obscured by the antiemetic effect of Compazine). Products include:
Sterile FUDR 2974

Fluorouracil (Vomiting as a sign of toxicity of antineoplastic agents may be obscured by the antiemetic effect of Compazine). Products include:
Carac Cream 1222
Efudex 1733
Fluoroplex 552

Fluphenazine Decanoate (Phenothiazines may intensify or prolong the action of other central nervous system depressants).
No products indexed under this heading.

Fluphenazine Enanthate (Phenothiazines may intensify or prolong the action of other central nervous system depressants).
No products indexed under this heading.

Fluphenazine Hydrochloride (Phenothiazines may intensify or prolong the action of other central nervous system depressants).
No products indexed under this heading.

Flurazepam Hydrochloride (Phenothiazines may intensify or prolong the action of other central nervous system depressants).
No products indexed under this heading.

Flutamide (Vomiting as a sign of toxicity of antineoplastic agents may be obscured by the antiemetic effect of Compazine). Products include:
Eulexin Capsules 3118

Fosphenytoin Sodium (Phenothiazines may lower convulsive threshold; dosage adjustments of anticonvulsant may be necessary). Products include:
Cerebyx Injection 2619

Gemcitabine Hydrochloride (Vomiting as a sign of toxicity of antineoplastic agents may be obscured by the antiemetic effect of Compazine). Products include:
Gemzar for Injection 1919

Glutethimide (Phenothiazines may intensify or prolong the action of other central nervous system depressants).
No products indexed under this heading.

Guanadrel Sulfate (Coadministration may counteract antihypertensive effects of guanadrel).
No products indexed under this heading.

Guanethidine Monosulfate (Coadministration may counteract antihypertensive effects of guanethidine).
No products indexed under this heading.

Haloperidol (Phenothiazines may intensify or prolong the action of other central nervous system depressants). Products include:
Haldol Injection, Tablets and Concentrate 2533

Haloperidol Decanoate (Phenothiazines may intensify or prolong the action of other central nervous system depressants). Products include:
Haldol Decanoate 2535

Hydrochlorothiazide (Accentuates the orthostatic hypotension that may occur with phenothiazines). Products include:
Accuretic Tablets 2614
Aldoril Tablets 2039
Atacand HCT Tablets 597
Avalide Tablets 1070
Diovan HCT Tablets 2338
Dyazide Capsules 1515
HydroDIURIL Tablets 2108
Hyzaar 2109
Inderide Tablets 3517
Inderide LA Long-Acting Capsules 3519
Lotensin HCT Tablets 2367
Maxzide 1008
Micardis HCT Tablets 1051
Microzide Capsules 3414
Moduretic Tablets 2138
Monopril HCT 1094
Prinzide Tablets 2168
Timolide Tablets 2187
Uniretic Tablets 3178
Vaseretic Tablets 2204
Zestoretic Tablets 695
Ziac Tablets 1887

Hydrocodone Bitartrate (Phenothiazines may intensify or prolong the action of other central nervous system depressants). Products include:
Hycodan 1316
Hycomine Compound Tablets 1317
Hycotuss Expectorant Syrup 1318
Lortab 3319
Lortab Elixir 3317
Maxidone Tablets CIII 3399
Norco 5/325 Tablets CIII 3424
Norco 7.5/325 Tablets CIII 3425
Norco 10/325 Tablets CIII 3427
Norco 10/325 Tablets CIII 3425
Vicodin Tablets 516
Vicodin ES Tablets 517
Vicodin HP Tablets 518
Vicodin Tuss Expectorant 519
Vicoprofen Tablets 520
Zydone Tablets 1330

Hydrocodone Polistirex (Phenothiazines may intensify or prolong the action of other central nervous system depressants). Products include:
Tussionex Pennkinetic Extended-Release Suspension 1174

Hydroflumethiazide (Accentuates the orthostatic hypotension that may occur with phenothiazines). Products include:
Diucardin Tablets 3494

Hydromorphone Hydrochloride (Phenothiazines may intensify or prolong the action of other central nervous system depressants). Products include:
Dilaudid 441
Dilaudid Oral Liquid 445
Dilaudid Powder 441
Dilaudid Rectal Suppositories 441
Dilaudid Tablets 441
Dilaudid Tablets - 8 mg 445
Dilaudid-HP 443

Hydroxyurea (Vomiting as a sign of toxicity of antineoplastic agents may be obscured by the antiemetic effect of Compazine). Products include:
Mylocel Tablets 2227

Hydroxyzine Hydrochloride (Phenothiazines may intensify or prolong the action of other central nervous system depressants). Products include:
Atarax Tablets & Syrup 2667
Vistaril Intramuscular Solution 2738

Idarubicin Hydrochloride (Vomiting as a sign of toxicity of antineoplastic agents may be obscured by the antiemetic effect of Compazine). Products include:
Idamycin PFS Injection 2825

Ifosfamide (Vomiting as a sign of toxicity of antineoplastic agents may be obscured by the antiemetic effect of Compazine). Products include:
Ifex for Injection 1123

Interferon alfa-2A, Recombinant (Vomiting as a sign of toxicity of antineoplastic agents may be obscured by the antiemetic effect of Compazine). Products include:
Roferon-A Injection 2996

Interferon alfa-2B, Recombinant (Vomiting as a sign of toxicity of antineoplastic agents may be obscured by the antiemetic effect of Compazine). Products include:
Intron A for Injection 3120

Rebetron Combination Therapy 3153

Irinotecan Hydrochloride (Vomiting as a sign of toxicity of antineoplastic agents may be obscured by the antiemetic effect of Compazine).
No products indexed under this heading.

Isoflurane (Phenothiazines may intensify or prolong the action of other central nervous system depressants).
No products indexed under this heading.

Ketamine Hydrochloride (Phenothiazines may intensify or prolong the action of other central nervous system depressants).
No products indexed under this heading.

Lamotrigine (Phenothiazines may lower convulsive threshold; dosage adjustments of anticonvulsant may be necessary). Products include:
Lamictal 1567

Levamisole Hydrochloride (Vomiting as a sign of toxicity of antineoplastic agents may be obscured by the antiemetic effect of Compazine). Products include:
Ergamisol Tablets 1789

Levetiracetam (Phenothiazines may lower convulsive threshold; dosage adjustments of anticonvulsant may be necessary). Products include:
Keppra Tablets 3314

Levomethadyl Acetate Hydrochloride (Phenothiazines may intensify or prolong the action of other central nervous system depressants).
No products indexed under this heading.

Levorphanol Tartrate (Phenothiazines may intensify or prolong the action of other central nervous system depressants). Products include:
Levo-Dromoran 1734
Levorphanol Tartrate Tablets 3059

Lomustine (CCNU) (Vomiting as a sign of toxicity of antineoplastic agents may be obscured by the antiemetic effect of Compazine).
No products indexed under this heading.

Loratadine (Phenothiazines may intensify or prolong the action of other central nervous system depressants). Products include:
Claritin 3100
Claritin-D 12 Hour Extended Release Tablets 3102
Claritin-D 24 Hour Extended Release Tablets 3104

Lorazepam (Phenothiazines may intensify or prolong the action of other central nervous system depressants). Products include:
Ativan Injection 3478
Ativan Tablets 3482

Loxapine Hydrochloride (Phenothiazines may intensify or prolong the action of other central nervous system depressants).
No products indexed under this heading.

Loxapine Succinate (Phenothiazines may intensify or prolong the action of other central nervous system depressants). Products include:
Loxitane Capsules 3398

Mechlorethamine Hydrochloride (Vomiting as a sign of toxicity of antineoplastic agents may be obscured by the antiemetic effect of Compazine). Products include:
Mustargen for Injection 2142

Megestrol Acetate (Vomiting as a sign of toxicity of antineoplastic agents may be obscured by the antiemetic effect of Compazine). Products include:
Megace Oral Suspension 1124

Melphalan (Vomiting as a sign of toxicity of antineoplastic agents may be obscured by the antiemetic effect of Compazine). Products include:
Alkeran Tablets 1466

Meperidine Hydrochloride (Phenothiazines may intensify or prolong the action of other central nervous system depressants). Products include:
Demerol 3079
Mepergan Injection 3539

Mephenytoin (Phenothiazines may lower convulsive threshold; dosage adjustments of anticonvulsant may be necessary).
No products indexed under this heading.

Mephobarbital (Phenothiazines may intensify or prolong the action of other central nervous system depressants).
No products indexed under this heading.

Meprobamate (Phenothiazines may intensify or prolong the action of other central nervous system depressants). Products include:
Miltown Tablets 3349

Mercaptopurine (Vomiting as a sign of toxicity of antineoplastic agents may be obscured by the antiemetic effect of Compazine). Products include:
Purinethol Tablets 1615

Mesoridazine Besylate (Phenothiazines may intensify or prolong the action of other central nervous system depressants). Products include:
Serentil 1057

Methadone Hydrochloride (Phenothiazines may intensify or prolong the action of other central nervous system depressants). Products include:
Dolophine Hydrochloride Tablets 3056

Methdilazine Hydrochloride (Phenothiazines may intensify or prolong the action of other central nervous system depressants).
No products indexed under this heading.

Methohexital Sodium (Phenothiazines may intensify or prolong the action of other central nervous system depressants). Products include:
Brevital Sodium for Injection, USP .. 1815

Methotrexate Sodium (Vomiting as a sign of toxicity of antineoplastic agents may be obscured by the antiemetic effect of Compazine).
No products indexed under this heading.

Methotrimeprazine (Phenothiazines may intensify or prolong the action of other central nervous system depressants).
No products indexed under this heading.

Methoxyflurane (Phenothiazines may intensify or prolong the action of other central nervous system depressants).
No products indexed under this heading.

Methsuximide (Phenothiazines may lower convulsive threshold; dosage adjustments of anticonvulsant may be necessary). Products include:
Celontin Capsules 2618

Methyclothiazide (Accentuates the orthostatic hypotension that may occur with phenothiazines).
No products indexed under this heading.

Metrizamide (Concurrent use is not recommended; Compazine should be discontinued at least 48 hours before myelography and should not be resumed for at least 24 hours).
No products indexed under this heading.

Midazolam Hydrochloride (Phenothiazines may intensify or prolong the action of other central nervous system depressants). Products include:
Versed Injection 3027
Versed Syrup 3033

Mitomycin (Mitomycin-C) (Vomiting as a sign of toxicity of antineoplastic agents may be obscured by the antiemetic effect of Compazine).
No products indexed under this heading.

Mitotane (Vomiting as a sign of toxicity of antineoplastic agents may be obscured by the antiemetic effect of Compazine).
No products indexed under this heading.

Mitoxantrone Hydrochloride (Vomiting as a sign of toxicity of antineoplastic agents may be obscured by the antiemetic effect of Compazine). Products include:
Novantrone for Injection 1760

Molindone Hydrochloride (Phenothiazines may intensify or prolong the action of other central nervous system depressants). Products include:
Moban 1320

Morphine Sulfate (Phenothiazines may intensify or prolong the action of other central nervous system depressants). Products include:
Astramorph/PF Injection, USP (Preservative-Free) 594
Duramorph Injection 1312
Infumorph 200 and Infumorph 500 Sterile Solutions 1314
Kadian Capsules 1335
MS Contin Tablets 2896
MSIR 2898
Oramorph SR Tablets 3062
Roxanol 3066

Olanzapine (Phenothiazines may intensify or prolong the action of other central nervous system depressants). Products include:
Zyprexa Tablets 1973
Zyprexa ZYDIS Orally Disintegrating Tablets 1973

Oxazepam (Phenothiazines may intensify or prolong the action of other central nervous system depressants).
No products indexed under this heading.

Oxcarbazepine (Phenothiazines may lower convulsive threshold; dosage adjustments of anticonvulsant may be necessary). Products include:
Trileptal Oral Suspension 2407
Trileptal Tablets 2407

Oxycodone Hydrochloride (Phenothiazines may intensify or prolong the action of other central nervous system depressants). Products include:
OxyContin Tablets 2912
OxyFast Oral Concentrate Solution . 2916
OxyIR Capsules 2916
Percocet Tablets 1326
Percodan Tablets 1327
Percolone Tablets 1327
Roxicodone 3067
Tylox Capsules 2597

Paclitaxel (Vomiting as a sign of toxicity of antineoplastic agents may be obscured by the antiemetic effect of Compazine). Products include:
Taxol Injection 1129

Paramethadione (Phenothiazines may lower convulsive threshold; dosage adjustments of anticonvulsant may be necessary).
No products indexed under this heading.

Pentobarbital Sodium (Phenothiazines may intensify or prolong the action of other central nervous system depressants). Products include:
Nembutal Sodium Solution 485

Perphenazine (Phenothiazines may intensify or prolong the action of other central nervous system depressants). Products include:
Etrafon 3115
Trilafon 3160

Phenacemide (Phenothiazines may lower convulsive threshold; dosage adjustments of anticonvulsant may be necessary).
No products indexed under this heading.

Phenobarbital (Phenothiazines may lower convulsive threshold; dosage adjustments of anticonvulsant may be necessary; phenothiazines may intensify or prolong the action of other central nervous system depressants). Products include:
Arco-Lase Plus Tablets 592
Donnatal 2929
Donnatal Extentabs 2930

Phensuximide (Phenothiazines may lower convulsive threshold; dosage adjustments of anticonvulsant may be necessary).
No products indexed under this heading.

Phenytoin (Phenothiazines may lower convulsive threshold; dosage adjustments of anticonvulsant may be necessary; interference with the metabolism of phenytoin precipitating in the phenytoin toxicity). Products include:
Dilantin Infatabs 2624
Dilantin-125 Oral Suspension 2625

Phenytoin Sodium (Phenothiazines may lower convulsive threshold; dosage adjustments of anticonvulsant may be necessary; interference with the metabolism of phenytoin precipitating in the phenytoin toxicity). Products include:
Dilantin Kapseals 2622

Polythiazide (Accentuates the orthostatic hypotension that may occur with phenothiazines). Products include:
Minizide Capsules 2700
Renese Tablets 2712

Prazepam (Phenothiazines may intensify or prolong the action of other central nervous system depressants).
No products indexed under this heading.

Primidone (Phenothiazines may lower convulsive threshold; dosage adjustments of anticonvulsant may be necessary).
No products indexed under this heading.

Procarbazine Hydrochloride (Vomiting as a sign of toxicity of antineoplastic agents may be obscured by the antiemetic effect of Compazine). Products include:
Matulane Capsules 3246

Promethazine Hydrochloride (Phenothiazines may intensify or prolong the action of other central nervous system depressants). Products include:
Mepergan Injection 3539
Phenergan Injection 3553
Phenergan 3556
Phenergan Syrup 3554
Phenergan with Codeine Syrup 3557
Phenergan with Dextromethorphan Syrup 3559
Phenergan VC Syrup 3560
Phenergan VC with Codeine Syrup .. 3561

Propofol (Phenothiazines may intensify or prolong the action of other central nervous system depressants). Products include:
Diprivan Injectable Emulsion 667

Propoxyphene Hydrochloride (Phenothiazines may intensify or prolong the action of other central nervous system depressants). Products include:
Darvon Pulvules 1909
Darvon Compound-65 Pulvules 1910

Propoxyphene Napsylate (Phenothiazines may intensify or prolong the action of other central nervous system depressants). Products include:
- Darvon-N/Darvocet-N 1907
- Darvon-N Tablets 1912

Propranolol Hydrochloride (Co-administration results in increased plasma levels of both drugs). Products include:
- Inderal 3513
- Inderal LA Long-Acting Capsules 3516
- Inderide Tablets 3517
- Inderide LA Long-Acting Capsules .. 3519

Pyrilamine Maleate (Phenothiazines may intensify or prolong the action of other central nervous system depressants). Products include:
- Maximum Strength Midol Menstrual Caplets and Gelcaps.......................... ■D612
- Maximum Strength Midol PMS Caplets and Gelcaps................. ■D613

Pyrilamine Tannate (Phenothiazines may intensify or prolong the action of other central nervous system depressants). Products include:
- Ryna-12 S Suspension 3351

Quazepam (Phenothiazines may intensify or prolong the action of other central nervous system depressants).
No products indexed under this heading.

Quetiapine Fumarate (Phenothiazines may intensify or prolong the action of other central nervous system depressants). Products include:
- Seroquel Tablets 684

Remifentanil Hydrochloride (Phenothiazines may intensify or prolong the action of other central nervous system depressants).
No products indexed under this heading.

Risperidone (Phenothiazines may intensify or prolong the action of other central nervous system depressants). Products include:
- Risperdal 1796

Secobarbital Sodium (Phenothiazines may intensify or prolong the action of other central nervous system depressants).
No products indexed under this heading.

Sevoflurane (Phenothiazines may intensify or prolong the action of other central nervous system depressants).
No products indexed under this heading.

Streptozocin (Vomiting as a sign of toxicity of antineoplastic agents may be obscured by the antiemetic effect of Compazine).
No products indexed under this heading.

Sufentanil Citrate (Phenothiazines may intensify or prolong the action of other central nervous system depressants).
No products indexed under this heading.

Tamoxifen Citrate (Vomiting as a sign of toxicity of antineoplastic agents may be obscured by the antiemetic effect of Compazine). Products include:
- Nolvadex Tablets 678

Temazepam (Phenothiazines may intensify or prolong the action of other central nervous system depressants).
No products indexed under this heading.

Teniposide (Vomiting as a sign of toxicity of antineoplastic agents may be obscured by the antiemetic effect of Compazine).
No products indexed under this heading.

Terfenadine (Phenothiazines may intensify or prolong the action of other central nervous system depressants).
No products indexed under this heading.

Thiamylal Sodium (Phenothiazines may intensify or prolong the action of other central nervous system depressants).
No products indexed under this heading.

Thioguanine (Vomiting as a sign of toxicity of antineoplastic agents may be obscured by the antiemetic effect of Compazine). Products include:
- Tabloid Tablets 1642

Thioridazine Hydrochloride (Phenothiazines may intensify or prolong the action of other central nervous system depressants). Products include:
- Thioridazine Hydrochloride Tablets................................. 2289

Thiotepa (Vomiting as a sign of toxicity of antineoplastic agents may be obscured by the antiemetic effect of Compazine). Products include:
- Thioplex for Injection 1765

Thiothixene (Phenothiazines may intensify or prolong the action of other central nervous system depressants). Products include:
- Navane Capsules 2701
- Thiothixene Capsules 2290

Tiagabine Hydrochloride (Phenothiazines may lower convulsive threshold; dosage adjustments of anticonvulsant may be necessary). Products include:
- Gabitril Tablets 1189

Topiramate (Phenothiazines may lower convulsive threshold; dosage adjustments of anticonvulsant may be necessary). Products include:
- Topamax Sprinkle Capsules 2590
- Topamax Tablets 2590

Topotecan Hydrochloride (Vomiting as a sign of toxicity of antineoplastic agents may be obscured by the antiemetic effect of Compazine). Products include:
- Hycamtin for Injection 1546

Toremifene Citrate (Vomiting as a sign of toxicity of antineoplastic agents may be obscured by the antiemetic effect of Compazine). Products include:
- Fareston Tablets 3237

Triazolam (Phenothiazines may intensify or prolong the action of other central nervous system depressants). Products include:
- Halcion Tablets 2823

Trifluoperazine Hydrochloride (Phenothiazines may intensify or prolong the action of other central nervous system depressants). Products include:
- Stelazine 1640

Trimeprazine Tartrate (Phenothiazines may intensify or prolong the action of other central nervous system depressants).
No products indexed under this heading.

Trimethadione (Phenothiazines may lower convulsive threshold; dosage adjustments of anticonvulsant may be necessary).
No products indexed under this heading.

Tripelennamine Hydrochloride (Phenothiazines may intensify or prolong the action of other central nervous system depressants).
No products indexed under this heading.

Triprolidine Hydrochloride (Phenothiazines may intensify or prolong the action of other central nervous system depressants). Products include:
- Actifed Cold & Allergy Tablets .... ■D688

Valproate Sodium (Phenothiazines may lower convulsive threshold; dosage adjustments of anticonvulsant may be necessary). Products include:
- Depacon Injection 416

Valproic Acid (Phenothiazines may lower convulsive threshold; dosage adjustments of anticonvulsant may be necessary). Products include:
- Depakene 421

Valrubicin (Vomiting as a sign of toxicity of antineoplastic agents may be obscured by the antiemetic effect of Compazine). Products include:
- Valstar Sterile Solution for Intravesical Instillation 1175

Vincristine Sulfate (Vomiting as a sign of toxicity of antineoplastic agents may be obscured by the antiemetic effect of Compazine).
No products indexed under this heading.

Vinorelbine Tartrate (Vomiting as a sign of toxicity of antineoplastic agents may be obscured by the antiemetic effect of Compazine). Products include:
- Navelbine Injection 1604

Warfarin Sodium (Diminished effect of oral anticoagulants). Products include:
- Coumadin for Injection 1243
- Coumadin Tablets 1243
- Warfarin Sodium Tablets, USP 3302

Zaleplon (Phenothiazines may intensify or prolong the action of other central nervous system depressants). Products include:
- Sonata Capsules 3591

Ziprasidone Hydrochloride (Phenothiazines may intensify or prolong the action of other central nervous system depressants). Products include:
- Geodon Capsules 2688

Zolpidem Tartrate (Phenothiazines may intensify or prolong the action of other central nervous system depressants). Products include:
- Ambien Tablets 3191

Zonisamide (Phenothiazines may lower convulsive threshold; dosage adjustments of anticonvulsant may be necessary). Products include:
- Zonegran Capsules 1307

Food Interactions

Alcohol (Phenothiazines may intensify or prolong the action of other central nervous system depressants).

COMPOUND W ONE STEP PADS FOR KIDS

(Salicylic Acid) .... ■D664
None cited in PDR database.

COMPOUND W ONE STEP PLANTAR PADS

(Salicylic Acid) .... ■D664
None cited in PDR database.

COMPOUND W ONE STEP WART REMOVER PADS

(Salicylic Acid) .... ■D664
None cited in PDR database.

COMPOUND W WART REMOVER GEL

(Salicylic Acid) .... ■D665
None cited in PDR database.

COMPOUND W WART REMOVER LIQUID

(Salicylic Acid) .... ■D665
None cited in PDR database.

COMPUTER EYE DROPS

(Glycerin) Q252
None cited in PDR database.

COMTAN TABLETS

(Entacapone) 2328
May interact with central nervous system depressants, drugs metabolized by Catechol-*O*-methyltransferase, erythromycin, nonselective MAO inhibitors, and certain other agents. Compounds in these categories include:

Alfentanil Hydrochloride (Possible additive sedative effects).
No products indexed under this heading.

Alprazolam (Possible additive sedative effects). Products include:
- Xanax Tablets 2865

Ampicillin Sodium (As most entacapone excretion is via bile, co-administration with drugs known to interfere with biliary excretion, glucuronidation, and intestinal beta-glucuronidation, such as ampicillin, requires caution). Products include:
- Unasyn for Injection 2728

Apomorphine (Co-administration of drugs that are metabolized by catechol-O-methyltransferase (COMT) may result in increased heart rates, possibly arrhythmias, and excessive changes in blood pressure).
No products indexed under this heading.

Aprobarbital (Possible additive sedative effects).
No products indexed under this heading.

Bitolterol Mesylate (Co-administration of drugs that are metabolized by catechol-O-methyltransferase (COMT) may result in increased heart rates, possibly arrhythmias, and excessive changes in blood pressure).
No products indexed under this heading.

Buprenorphine Hydrochloride (Possible additive sedative effects). Products include:
- Buprenex Injectable 2918

Buspirone Hydrochloride (Possible additive sedative effects).
No products indexed under this heading.

Butabarbital (Possible additive sedative effects).
No products indexed under this heading.

Butalbital (Possible additive sedative effects). Products include:
- Phrenilin 578
- Sedapap Tablets 50 mg/650 mg 2225

Chloramphenicol Sodium Succinate (As most entacapone excretion is via bile, co-administration with drugs known to interfere with biliary excretion, glucuronidation, and intestinal beta-glucuronidation, such as chloramphenicol, requires caution).
No products indexed under this heading.

Chlordiazepoxide (Possible additive sedative effects). Products include:
- Limbitrol 1738

Chlordiazepoxide Hydrochloride (Possible additive sedative effects). Products include:
- Librium Capsules 1736
- Librium for Injection 1737

Chlorpromazine (Possible additive sedative effects). Products include:
- Thorazine Suppositories 1656

Chlorpromazine Hydrochloride (Possible additive sedative effects). Products include:
- Thorazine 1656

Chlorprothixene (Possible additive sedative effects).
No products indexed under this heading.

Chlorprothixene Hydrochloride (Possible additive sedative effects).
No products indexed under this heading.

Chlorprothixene Lactate (Possible additive sedative effects).
No products indexed under this heading.

Cholestyramine (As most entacapone excretion is via bile, co-administration with drugs known to interfere with biliary excretion, glucuronidation, and intestinal beta-glucuronidation, such as cholestyramine, requires caution).
No products indexed under this heading.

Clorazepate Dipotassium (Possible additive sedative effects). Products include:
Tranxene 511

Clozapine (Possible additive sedative effects). Products include:
Clozaril Tablets 2319

Codeine Phosphate (Possible additive sedative effects). Products include:
Phenergan with Codeine Syrup 3557
Phenergan VC with Codeine Syrup 3561
Robitussin A-C Syrup 2942
Robitussin-DAC Syrup 2942
Ryna-C Liquid .... ▣768
Soma Compound w/Codeine Tablets 3355
Tussi-Organidin NR Liquid 3350
Tussi-Organidin-S NR Liquid 3350
Tylenol with Codeine 2595

Desflurane (Possible additive sedative effects). Products include:
Suprane Liquid for Inhalation 874

Dezocine (Possible additive sedative effects).
No products indexed under this heading.

Diazepam (Possible additive sedative effects). Products include:
Valium Injectable 3026
Valium Tablets 3047

Dobutamine Hydrochloride (Co-administration of drugs that are metabolized by catechol-O-methyltransferase (COMT) may result in increased heart rates, possibly arrhythmias, and excessive changes in blood pressure). Products include:
Dobutrex Solution Vials 1914

Dopamine Hydrochloride (Co-administration of drugs that are metabolized by catechol-O-methyltransferase (COMT) may result in increased heart rates, possibly arrhythmias, and excessive changes in blood pressure).
No products indexed under this heading.

Droperidol (Possible additive sedative effects).
No products indexed under this heading.

Enflurane (Possible additive sedative effects).
No products indexed under this heading.

Epinephrine (Co-administration of drugs that are metabolized by catechol-O-methyltransferase (COMT) may result in increased heart rates, possibly arrhythmias, and excessive changes in blood pressure; concurrent use of epinephrine infusion has resulted in a case report of ventricular tachycardia). Products include:
Epifrin Sterile Ophthalmic Solution .... ⊙235
EpiPen 1236
Primatene Mist .... ▣779
Xylocaine with Epinephrine Injection 653

Epinephrine Bitartrate (Co-administration of drugs that are metabolized by catechol-O-methyltransferase (COMT) may result in increased heart rates, possibly arrhythmias, and excessive changes in blood pressure; concurrent use of epinephrine infusion has resulted in a case report of ventricular tachycardia). Products include:
Sensorcaine 643

Epinephrine Hydrochloride (Co-administration of drugs that are metabolized by catechol-O-methyltransferase (COMT) may result in increased heart rates, possibly arrhythmias, and excessive changes in blood pressure; concurrent use of epinephrine infusion has resulted in a case report of ventricular tachycardia).
No products indexed under this heading.

Erythromycin (As most entacapone excretion is via bile, co-administration with drugs known to interfere with biliary excretion, glucuronidation, and intestinal beta-glucuronidation, such as erythromycin, requires caution). Products include:
Emgel 2% Topical Gel 1285
Ery-Tab Tablets 448
Erythromycin Base Filmtab Tablets 454
Erythromycin Delayed-Release Capsules, USP 455
PCE Dispertab Tablets 498

Erythromycin Estolate (As most entacapone excretion is via bile, co-administration with drugs known to interfere with biliary excretion, glucuronidation, and intestinal beta-glucuronidation, such as erythromycin, requires caution).
No products indexed under this heading.

Erythromycin Ethylsuccinate (As most entacapone excretion is via bile, co-administration with drugs known to interfere with biliary excretion, glucuronidation, and intestinal beta-glucuronidation, such as erythromycin, requires caution). Products include:
E.E.S. 450
EryPed 446
Pediazole Suspension 3050

Erythromycin Gluceptate (As most entacapone excretion is via bile, co-administration with drugs known to interfere with biliary excretion, glucuronidation, and intestinal beta-glucuronidation, such as erythromycin, requires caution).
No products indexed under this heading.

Erythromycin Stearate (As most entacapone excretion is via bile, co-administration with drugs known to interfere with biliary excretion, glucuronidation, and intestinal beta-glucuronidation, such as erythromycin, requires caution). Products include:
Erythrocin Stearate Filmtab Tablets 452

Estazolam (Possible additive sedative effects). Products include:
ProSom Tablets 500

Ethchlorvynol (Possible additive sedative effects).
No products indexed under this heading.

Ethinamate (Possible additive sedative effects).
No products indexed under this heading.

Fentanyl (Possible additive sedative effects). Products include:
Duragesic Transdermal System 1786

Fentanyl Citrate (Possible additive sedative effects). Products include:
Actiq 1184

Fluphenazine Decanoate (Possible additive sedative effects).
No products indexed under this heading.

Fluphenazine Enanthate (Possible additive sedative effects).
No products indexed under this heading.

Fluphenazine Hydrochloride (Possible additive sedative effects).
No products indexed under this heading.

Flurazepam Hydrochloride (Possible additive sedative effects).
No products indexed under this heading.

Glutethimide (Possible additive sedative effects).
No products indexed under this heading.

Haloperidol (Possible additive sedative effects). Products include:
Haldol Injection, Tablets and Concentrate 2533

Haloperidol Decanoate (Possible additive sedative effects). Products include:
Haldol Decanoate 2535

Hydrocodone Bitartrate (Possible additive sedative effects). Products include:
Hycodan 1316
Hycomine Compound Tablets 1317
Hycotuss Expectorant Syrup 1318
Lortab 3319
Lortab Elixir 3317
Maxidone Tablets CIII 3399
Norco 5/325 Tablets CIII 3424
Norco 7.5/325 Tablets CIII 3425
Norco 10/325 Tablets CIII 3427
Norco 10/325 Tablets CIII 3425
Vicodin Tablets 516
Vicodin ES Tablets 517
Vicodin HP Tablets 518
Vicodin Tuss Expectorant 519
Vicoprofen Tablets 520
Zydone Tablets 1330

Hydrocodone Polistirex (Possible additive sedative effects). Products include:
Tussionex Pennkinetic Extended-Release Suspension 1174

Hydromorphone Hydrochloride (Possible additive sedative effects). Products include:
Dilaudid 441
Dilaudid Oral Liquid 445
Dilaudid Powder 441
Dilaudid Rectal Suppositories 441
Dilaudid Tablets 441
Dilaudid Tablets - 8 mg 445
Dilaudid-HP 443

Hydroxyzine Hydrochloride (Possible additive sedative effects). Products include:
Atarax Tablets & Syrup 2667
Vistaril Intramuscular Solution 2738

Isocarboxazid (Co-administration of non-selective MAO inhibitors with entacapone would result in inhibition of the majority of the pathways responsible for normal catecholamine metabolism; concurrent use should be avoided).
No products indexed under this heading.

Isoetharine (Co-administration of drugs that are metabolized by catechol-O-methyltransferase (COMT) may result in increased heart rates, possibly arrhythmias, and excessive changes in blood pressure).
No products indexed under this heading.

Isoflurane (Possible additive sedative effects).
No products indexed under this heading.

Isoproterenol Hydrochloride (Co-administration of drugs that are metabolized by catechol-O-methyltransferase (COMT) may result in increased heart rates, possibly arrhythmias, and excessive changes in blood pressure).
No products indexed under this heading.

Isoproterenol Sulfate (Co-administration of drugs that are metabolized by catechol-O-methyltransferase (COMT) may result in increased heart rates, possibly arrhythmias, and excessive changes in blood pressure).
No products indexed under this heading.

Ketamine Hydrochloride (Possible additive sedative effects).
No products indexed under this heading.

Levodopa (Entacapone enhances levodopa bioavailability and, therefore, might be expected to increase the occurence of orthostatic hypotension). Products include:
Sinemet Tablets 1253
Sinemet CR Tablets 1255

Levomethadyl Acetate Hydrochloride (Possible additive sedative effects).
No products indexed under this heading.

Levorphanol Tartrate (Possible additive sedative effects). Products include:
Levo-Dromoran 1734
Levorphanol Tartrate Tablets 3059

Lorazepam (Possible additive sedative effects). Products include:
Ativan Injection 3478
Ativan Tablets 3482

Loxapine Hydrochloride (Possible additive sedative effects).
No products indexed under this heading.

Loxapine Succinate (Possible additive sedative effects). Products include:
Loxitane Capsules 3398

Meperidine Hydrochloride (Possible additive sedative effects). Products include:
Demerol 3079
Mepergan Injection 3539

Mephobarbital (Possible additive sedative effects).
No products indexed under this heading.

Meprobamate (Possible additive sedative effects). Products include:
Miltown Tablets 3349

Mesoridazine Besylate (Possible additive sedative effects). Products include:
Serentil 1057

Methadone Hydrochloride (Possible additive sedative effects). Products include:
Dolophine Hydrochloride Tablets 3056

Methohexital Sodium (Possible additive sedative effects). Products include:
Brevital Sodium for Injection, USP 1815

Methotrimeprazine (Possible additive sedative effects).
No products indexed under this heading.

Methoxyflurane (Possible additive sedative effects).
No products indexed under this heading.

Methyldopa (Co-administration of drugs that are metabolized by catechol-O-methyltransferase (COMT) may result in increased heart rates, possibly arrhythmias, and excessive changes in blood pressure). Products include:
Aldoclor Tablets 2035
Aldomet Tablets 2037
Aldoril Tablets 2039

Midazolam Hydrochloride (Possible additive sedative effects). Products include:
Versed Injection 3027
Versed Syrup 3033

Molindone Hydrochloride (Possible additive sedative effects). Products include:
Moban 1320

Morphine Sulfate (Possible additive sedative effects). Products include:
Astramorph/PF Injection, USP (Preservative-Free) 594
Duramorph Injection 1312

Infumorph 200 and Infumorph 500 Sterile Solutions 1314
Kadian Capsules 1335
MS Contin Tablets 2896
MSIR 2898
Oramorph SR Tablets 3062
Roxanol 3066

Norepinephrine Bitartrate (Co-administration of drugs that are metabolized by catechol-O-methyltransferase (COMT) may result in increased heart rates, possibly arrhythmias, and excessive changes in blood pressure).
No products indexed under this heading.

Olanzapine (Possible additive sedative effects). Products include:
Zyprexa Tablets 1973
Zyprexa ZYDIS Orally Disintegrating Tablets 1973

Oxazepam (Possible additive sedative effects).
No products indexed under this heading.

Oxycodone Hydrochloride (Possible additive sedative effects). Products include:
OxyContin Tablets 2912
OxyFast Oral Concentrate Solution . 2916
OxyIR Capsules 2916
Percocet Tablets 1326
Percodan Tablets 1327
Percolone Tablets 1327
Roxicodone 3067
Tylox Capsules 2597

Pargyline Hydrochloride (Co-administration of non-selective MAO inhibitors with entacapone would result in inhibition of the majority of the pathways responsible for normal catecholamine metabolism; concurrent use should be avoided).
No products indexed under this heading.

Pentobarbital Sodium (Possible additive sedative effects). Products include:
Nembutal Sodium Solution 485

Perphenazine (Possible additive sedative effects). Products include:
Etrafon 3115
Trilafon 3160

Phenelzine Sulfate (Co-administration of non-selective MAO inhibitors with entacapone would result in inhibition of the majority of the pathways responsible for normal catecholamine metabolism; concurrent use should be avoided). Products include:
Nardil Tablets 2653

Phenobarbital (Possible additive sedative effects). Products include:
Arco-Lase Plus Tablets 592
Donnatal 2929
Donnatal Extentabs 2930

Prazepam (Possible additive sedative effects).
No products indexed under this heading.

Probenecid (As most entacapone excretion is via bile, co-administration with drugs known to interfere with biliary excretion, glucuronidation, and intestinal beta-glucuronidation, such as probenecid, requires caution).
No products indexed under this heading.

Procarbazine Hydrochloride (Co-administration of non-selective MAO inhibitors with entacapone would result in inhibition of the majority of the pathways responsible for normal catecholamine metabolism; concurrent use should be avoided). Products include:
Matulane Capsules 3246

Prochlorperazine (Possible additive sedative effects). Products include:
Compazine 1505

Promethazine Hydrochloride (Possible additive sedative effects). Products include:
Mepergan Injection 3539
Phenergan Injection 3553
Phenergan 3556
Phenergan Syrup 3554
Phenergan with Codeine Syrup 3557
Phenergan with Dextromethorphan Syrup 3559
Phenergan VC Syrup 3560
Phenergan VC with Codeine Syrup .. 3561

Propofol (Possible additive sedative effects). Products include:
Diprivan Injectable Emulsion 667

Propoxyphene Hydrochloride (Possible additive sedative effects). Products include:
Darvon Pulvules 1909
Darvon Compound-65 Pulvules 1910

Propoxyphene Napsylate (Possible additive sedative effects). Products include:
Darvon-N/Darvocet-N 1907
Darvon-N Tablets 1912

Quazepam (Possible additive sedative effects).
No products indexed under this heading.

Quetiapine Fumarate (Possible additive sedative effects). Products include:
Seroquel Tablets 684

Remifentanil Hydrochloride (Possible additive sedative effects).
No products indexed under this heading.

Rifampin (As most entacapone excretion is via bile, co-administration with drugs known to interfere with biliary excretion, glucuronidation, and intestinal beta-glucuronidation, such as rifampin, requires caution). Products include:
Rifadin 765
Rifamate Capsules 767
Rifater Tablets 769

Risperidone (Possible additive sedative effects). Products include:
Risperdal 1796

Secobarbital Sodium (Possible additive sedative effects).
No products indexed under this heading.

Sevoflurane (Possible additive sedative effects).
No products indexed under this heading.

Sufentanil Citrate (Possible additive sedative effects).
No products indexed under this heading.

Temazepam (Possible additive sedative effects).
No products indexed under this heading.

Thiamylal Sodium (Possible additive sedative effects).
No products indexed under this heading.

Thioridazine Hydrochloride (Possible additive sedative effects). Products include:
Thioridazine Hydrochloride Tablets 2289

Thiothixene (Possible additive sedative effects). Products include:
Navane Capsules 2701
Thiothixene Capsules 2290

Tranylcypromine Sulfate (Co-administration of non-selective MAO inhibitors with entacapone would result in inhibition of the majority of the pathways responsible for normal catecholamine metabolism; concurrent use should be avoided). Products include:
Parnate Tablets 1607

Triazolam (Possible additive sedative effects). Products include:
Halcion Tablets 2823

Trifluoperazine Hydrochloride (Possible additive sedative effects). Products include:
Stelazine 1640

Zaleplon (Possible additive sedative effects). Products include:
Sonata Capsules 3591

Ziprasidone Hydrochloride (Possible additive sedative effects). Products include:
Geodon Capsules 2688

Zolpidem Tartrate (Possible additive sedative effects). Products include:
Ambien Tablets 3191

Food Interactions

Alcohol (Possible additive sedative effects).

COMTREX ACUTE HEAD COLD & SINUS PRESSURE RELIEF TABLETS

(Acetaminophen, Brompheniramine Maleate, Pseudoephedrine Hydrochloride) 627
See Comtrex Maximum Strength Multi-Symptom Cold & Cough Relief Tablets and Caplets

COMTREX DEEP CHEST COLD & CONGESTION RELIEF SOFTGELS

(Acetaminophen, Dextromethorphan Hydrobromide, Guaifenesin, Pseudoephedrine Hydrochloride) 627
May interact with monoamine oxidase inhibitors and certain other agents. Compounds in these categories include:

Isocarboxazid (Concurrent and/or sequential use with MAO inhibitors is not recommended).
No products indexed under this heading.

Moclobemide (Concurrent and/or sequential use with MAO inhibitors is not recommended).
No products indexed under this heading.

Pargyline Hydrochloride (Concurrent and/or sequential use with MAO inhibitors is not recommended).
No products indexed under this heading.

Phenelzine Sulfate (Concurrent and/or sequential use with MAO inhibitors is not recommended). Products include:
Nardil Tablets 2653

Procarbazine Hydrochloride (Concurrent and/or sequential use with MAO inhibitors is not recommended). Products include:
Matulane Capsules 3246

Selegiline Hydrochloride (Concurrent and/or sequential use with MAO inhibitors is not recommended). Products include:
Eldepryl Capsules 3266

Tranylcypromine Sulfate (Concurrent and/or sequential use with MAO inhibitors is not recommended). Products include:
Parnate Tablets 1607

Food Interactions

Alcohol (Chronic heavy alcohol users, 3 or more drinks per day, should consult their physicians for advice on when and how they should take pain relievers/fever reducers including acetaminophen).

COMTREX FLU THERAPY & FEVER RELIEF DAYTIME CAPLETS

(Acetaminophen, Pseudoephedrine Hydrochloride) 628
See Comtrex Deep Chest Cold & Congestion Relief Softgels

COMTREX FLU THERAPY & FEVER RELIEF NIGHTTIME TABLETS

(Acetaminophen, Chlorpheniramine Maleate, Pseudoephedrine Hydrochloride) 628
See Comtrex Maximum Strength Multi-Symptom Cold & Cough Relief Tablets and Caplets

COMTREX MAXIMUM STRENGTH MULTI-SYMPTOM COLD & COUGH RELIEF TABLETS AND CAPLETS

(Acetaminophen, Chlorpheniramine Maleate, Dextromethorphan Hydrobromide, Pseudoephedrine Hydrochloride) 626
May interact with hypnotics and sedatives, monoamine oxidase inhibitors, tranquilizers, and certain other agents. Compounds in these categories include:

Alprazolam (May increase drowsiness effect). Products include:
Xanax Tablets 2865

Buspirone Hydrochloride (May increase drowsiness effect).
No products indexed under this heading.

Chlordiazepoxide (May increase drowsiness effect). Products include:
Limbitrol 1738

Chlordiazepoxide Hydrochloride (May increase drowsiness effect). Products include:
Librium Capsules 1736
Librium for Injection 1737

Chlorpromazine (May increase drowsiness effect). Products include:
Thorazine Suppositories 1656

Chlorpromazine Hydrochloride (May increase drowsiness effect). Products include:
Thorazine 1656

Chlorprothixene (May increase drowsiness effect).
No products indexed under this heading.

Chlorprothixene Hydrochloride (May increase drowsiness effect).
No products indexed under this heading.

Clorazepate Dipotassium (May increase drowsiness effect). Products include:
Tranxene 511

Diazepam (May increase drowsiness effect). Products include:
Valium Injectable 3026
Valium Tablets 3047

Droperidol (May increase drowsiness effect).
No products indexed under this heading.

Estazolam (May increase drowsiness effect). Products include:
ProSom Tablets 500

Ethchlorvynol (May increase drowsiness effect).
No products indexed under this heading.

Ethinamate (May increase drowsiness effect).
No products indexed under this heading.

Fluphenazine Decanoate (May increase drowsiness effect).
No products indexed under this heading.

Fluphenazine Enanthate (May increase drowsiness effect).
No products indexed under this heading.

Fluphenazine Hydrochloride (May increase drowsiness effect).
No products indexed under this heading.

Flurazepam Hydrochloride (May increase drowsiness effect).
No products indexed under this heading.

Glutethimide (May increase drowsiness effect).
No products indexed under this heading.

Haloperidol (May increase drowsiness effect). Products include:
Haldol Injection, Tablets and Concentrate 2533

IMPORTANT NOTE: Always consult each drug listing in the patient's regimen for possible interactions.

Haloperidol Decanoate (May increase drowsiness effect). Products include:
Haldol Decanoate 2535

Hydroxyzine Hydrochloride (May increase drowsiness effect). Products include:
Atarax Tablets & Syrup 2667
Vistaril Intramuscular Solution 2738

Isocarboxazid (Concurrent and/or sequential use with MAO inhibitors is not recommended).
No products indexed under this heading.

Lorazepam (May increase drowsiness effect). Products include:
Ativan Injection 3478
Ativan Tablets 3482

Loxapine Hydrochloride (May increase drowsiness effect).
No products indexed under this heading.

Loxapine Succinate (May increase drowsiness effect). Products include:
Loxitane Capsules 3398

Meprobamate (May increase drowsiness effect). Products include:
Miltown Tablets 3349

Mesoridazine Besylate (May increase drowsiness effect). Products include:
Serentil 1057

Midazolam Hydrochloride (May increase drowsiness effect). Products include:
Versed Injection 3027
Versed Syrup 3033

Moclobemide (Concurrent and/or sequential use with MAO inhibitors is not recommended).
No products indexed under this heading.

Molindone Hydrochloride (May increase drowsiness effect). Products include:
Moban 1320

Oxazepam (May increase drowsiness effect).
No products indexed under this heading.

Pargyline Hydrochloride (Concurrent and/or sequential use with MAO inhibitors is not recommended).
No products indexed under this heading.

Perphenazine (May increase drowsiness effect). Products include:
Etrafon 3115
Trilafon 3160

Phenelzine Sulfate (Concurrent and/or sequential use with MAO inhibitors is not recommended). Products include:
Nardil Tablets 2653

Prazepam (May increase drowsiness effect).
No products indexed under this heading.

Procarbazine Hydrochloride (Concurrent and/or sequential use with MAO inhibitors is not recommended). Products include:
Matulane Capsules 3246

Prochlorperazine (May increase drowsiness effect). Products include:
Compazine 1505

Promethazine Hydrochloride (May increase drowsiness effect). Products include:
Mepergan Injection 3539
Phenergan Injection 3553
Phenergan 3556
Phenergan Syrup 3554
Phenergan with Codeine Syrup 3557
Phenergan with Dextromethorphan Syrup 3559
Phenergan VC Syrup 3560
Phenergan VC with Codeine Syrup 3561

Propofol (May increase drowsiness effect). Products include:
Diprivan Injectable Emulsion 667

Quazepam (May increase drowsiness effect).
No products indexed under this heading.

Secobarbital Sodium (May increase drowsiness effect).
No products indexed under this heading.

Selegiline Hydrochloride (Concurrent and/or sequential use with MAO inhibitors is not recommended). Products include:
Eldepryl Capsules 3266

Temazepam (May increase drowsiness effect).
No products indexed under this heading.

Thioridazine Hydrochloride (May increase drowsiness effect). Products include:
Thioridazine Hydrochloride Tablets 2289

Thiothixene (May increase drowsiness effect). Products include:
Navane Capsules 2701
Thiothixene Capsules 2290

Tranylcypromine Sulfate (Concurrent and/or sequential use with MAO inhibitors is not recommended). Products include:
Parnate Tablets 1607

Triazolam (May increase drowsiness effect). Products include:
Halcion Tablets 2823

Trifluoperazine Hydrochloride (May increase drowsiness effect). Products include:
Stelazine 1640

Zaleplon (May increase drowsiness effect). Products include:
Sonata Capsules 3591

Zolpidem Tartrate (May increase drowsiness effect). Products include:
Ambien Tablets 3191

Food Interactions

Alcohol (Chronic heavy alcohol users, 3 or more drinks per day, should consult their physicians for advice on when and how they should take pain relievers/fever reducers; may increase drowsiness).

COMVAX

(Haemophilus B Conjugate Vaccine, Hepatitis B Vaccine, Recombinant) 2056

May interact with immunosuppressive agents. Compounds in these categories include:

Azathioprine (Deferral of immunization may be considered in individuals receiving immunosuppresive therapy).
No products indexed under this heading.

Basiliximab (Deferral of immunization may be considered in individuals receiving immunosuppresive therapy). Products include:
Simulect for Injection 2399

Cyclosporine (Deferral of immunization may be considered in individuals receiving immunosuppresive therapy). Products include:
Gengraf Capsules 457
Neoral Soft Gelatin Capsules 2380
Neoral Oral Solution 2380
Sandimmune 2388

Muromonab-CD3 (Deferral of immunization may be considered in individuals receiving immunosuppresive therapy). Products include:
Orthoclone OKT3 Sterile Solution ... 2498

Mycophenolate Mofetil (Deferral of immunization may be considered in individuals receiving immunosuppresive therapy). Products include:
CellCept Capsules 2951
CellCept Oral Suspension 2951
CellCept Tablets 2951

Sirolimus (Deferral of immunization may be considered in individuals receiving immunosuppresive therapy). Products include:
Rapamune Oral Solution and Tablets 3584

Tacrolimus (Deferral of immunization may be considered in individuals receiving immunosuppresive therapy). Products include:
Prograf 1393
Protopic Ointment 1397

CONCERTA EXTENDED-RELEASE TABLETS

(Methylphenidate Hydrochloride) 1998

May interact with oral anticoagulants, monoamine oxidase inhibitors, phenytoin, selective serotonin reuptake inhibitors, tricyclic antidepressants, vasopressors, and certain other agents. Compounds in these categories include:

Amitriptyline Hydrochloride (Methylphenidate may inhibit the metabolism of certain tricyclic antidepressants; downward dosage adjustment of tricyclic antidepressants may be required). Products include:
Etrafon 3115
Limbitrol 1738

Amoxapine (Methylphenidate may inhibit the metabolism of certain tricyclic antidepressants; downward dosage adjustment of tricyclic antidepressants may be required).
No products indexed under this heading.

Citalopram Hydrobromide (Methylphenidate may inhibit the metabolism of certain selective serotonin reuptake inhibitors; downward dosage adjustment of these drugs may be required). Products include:
Celexa 1365

Clomipramine Hydrochloride (Methylphenidate may inhibit the metabolism of certain tricyclic antidepressants; downward dosage adjustment of tricyclic antidepressants may be required).
No products indexed under this heading.

Desipramine Hydrochloride (Methylphenidate may inhibit the metabolism of certain tricyclic antidepressants; downward dosage adjustment of tricyclic antidepressants may be required). Products include:
Norpramin Tablets 755

Dicumarol (Methylphenidate may inhibit the metabolism of coumarin anticoagulants; downward dosage adjustment of anticoagulants may be required).
No products indexed under this heading.

Dopamine Hydrochloride (Methylphenidate causes rise in blood pressure; co-administration with other pressor agents should be undertaken with caution).
No products indexed under this heading.

Doxepin Hydrochloride (Methylphenidate may inhibit the metabolism of certain tricyclic antidepressants; downward dosage adjustment of tricyclic antidepressants may be required). Products include:
Sinequan 2713

Epinephrine Bitartrate (Methylphenidate causes rise in blood pressure; co-administration with other pressor agents should be undertaken with caution). Products include:
Sensorcaine 643

Epinephrine Hydrochloride (Methylphenidate causes rise in blood pressure; co-administration with other pressor agents should be undertaken with caution).
No products indexed under this heading.

Fluoxetine Hydrochloride (Methylphenidate may inhibit the metabolism of certain selective serotonin reuptake inhibitors; downward dosage adjustment of these drugs may be required). Products include:
Prozac Pulvules, Liquid, and Weekly Capsules 1238
Sarafem Pulvules 1962

Fluvoxamine Maleate (Methylphenidate may inhibit the metabolism of certain selective serotonin reuptake inhibitors; downward dosage adjustment of these drugs may be required). Products include:
Luvox Tablets (25, 50, 100 mg) 3256

Fosphenytoin Sodium (Methylphenidate may inhibit the metabolism of phenytoin; downward dosage adjustment of phenytoin may be required). Products include:
Cerebyx Injection 2619

Imipramine Hydrochloride (Methylphenidate may inhibit the metabolism of certain tricyclic antidepressants; downward dosage adjustment of tricyclic antidepressants may be required).
No products indexed under this heading.

Imipramine Pamoate (Methylphenidate may inhibit the metabolism of certain tricyclic antidepressants; downward dosage adjustment of tricyclic antidepressants may be required).
No products indexed under this heading.

Isocarboxazid (Co-administration with MAO inhibitors may result in hypertensive crises; concurrent and/or sequential use is contraindicated).
No products indexed under this heading.

Maprotiline Hydrochloride (Methylphenidate may inhibit the metabolism of certain tricyclic antidepressants; downward dosage adjustment of tricyclic antidepressants may be required).
No products indexed under this heading.

Metaraminol Bitartrate (Methylphenidate causes rise in blood pressure; co-administration with other pressor agents should be undertaken with caution). Products include:
Aramine Injection 2043

Methoxamine Hydrochloride (Methylphenidate causes rise in blood pressure; co-administration with other pressor agents should be undertaken with caution).
No products indexed under this heading.

Moclobemide (Co-administration with MAO inhibitors may result in hypertensive crises; concurrent and/or sequential use is contraindicated).
No products indexed under this heading.

Norepinephrine Bitartrate (Methylphenidate causes rise in blood pressure; co-administration with other pressor agents should be undertaken with caution).
No products indexed under this heading.

Nortriptyline Hydrochloride (Methylphenidate may inhibit the metabolism of certain tricyclic antidepressants; downward dosage adjustment of tricyclic antidepressants may be required).
No products indexed under this heading.

Pargyline Hydrochloride (Co-administration with MAO inhibitors may result in hypertensive crises; concurrent and/or sequential use is

contraindicated).
No products indexed under this heading.

Paroxetine Hydrochloride (Methylphenidate may inhibit the metabolism of certain selective serotonin reuptake inhibitors; downward dosage adjustment of these drugs may be required). Products include:
Paxil 1609

Phenelzine Sulfate (Co-administration with MAO inhibitors may result in hypertensive crises; concurrent and/or sequential use is contraindicated). Products include:
Nardil Tablets 2653

Phenobarbital (Methylphenidate may inhibit the metabolism of phenobarbital; downward dosage adjustment of phenobarbital may be required). Products include:
Arco-Lase Plus Tablets 592
Donnatal 2929
Donnatal Extentabs 2930

Phenylephrine Hydrochloride (Methylphenidate causes rise in blood pressure; co-administration with other pressor agents should be undertaken with caution). Products include:
Afrin Nasal Decongestant Children's Pump Mist 734
Extendryl 1361
Hycomine Compound Tablets 1317
Neo-Synephrine 614
Phenergan VC Syrup 3560
Phenergan VC with Codeine Syrup . 3561
Preparation H Cream 778
Preparation H Cooling Gel 778
Preparation H 778
Vicks Sinex Nasal Spray and Ultra Fine Mist 729

Phenytoin (Methylphenidate may inhibit the metabolism of phenytoin; downward dosage adjustment of phenytoin may be required). Products include:
Dilantin Infatabs 2624
Dilantin-125 Oral Suspension 2625

Phenytoin Sodium (Methylphenidate may inhibit the metabolism of phenytoin; downward dosage adjustment of phenytoin may be required). Products include:
Dilantin Kapseals 2622

Primidone (Methylphenidate may inhibit the metabolism of primidone; downward dosage adjustment of primidone may be required).
No products indexed under this heading.

Procarbazine Hydrochloride (Co-administration with MAO inhibitors may result in hypertensive crises; concurrent and/or sequential use is contraindicated). Products include:
Matulane Capsules 3246

Protriptyline Hydrochloride (Methylphenidate may inhibit the metabolism of certain tricyclic antidepressants; downward dosage adjustment of tricyclic antidepressants may be required). Products include:
Vivactil Tablets 2446
Vivactil Tablets 2217

Selegiline Hydrochloride (Co-administration with MAO inhibitors may result in hypertensive crises; concurrent and/or sequential use is contraindicated). Products include:
Eldepryl Capsules 3266

Sertraline Hydrochloride (Methylphenidate may inhibit the metabolism of certain selective serotonin reuptake inhibitors; downward dosage adjustment of these drugs may be required). Products include:
Zoloft 2751

Tranylcypromine Sulfate (Co-administration with MAO inhibitors may result in hypertensive crises; concurrent and/or sequential use is contraindicated). Products include:
Parnate Tablets 1607

Trimipramine Maleate (Methylphenidate may inhibit the metabolism of certain tricyclic antidepressants; downward dosage adjustment of tricyclic antidepressants may be required). Products include:
Surmontil Capsules 3595

Warfarin Sodium (Methylphenidate may inhibit the metabolism of coumarin anticoagulants; downward dosage adjustment of anticoagulants may be required). Products include:
Coumadin for Injection 1243
Coumadin Tablets 1243
Warfarin Sodium Tablets, USP 3302

CONCERTA TABLETS

(Methylphenidate Hydrochloride) 561
May interact with oral anticoagulants, monoamine oxidase inhibitors, phenytoin, selective serotonin reuptake inhibitors, tricyclic antidepressants, vasopressors, and certain other agents. Compounds in these categories include:

Amitriptyline Hydrochloride (Methylphenidate may inhibit the metabolism of certain tricyclic antidepressants; downward dosage adjustment of tricyclic antidepressants may be required). Products include:
Etrafon 3115
Limbitrol 1738

Amoxapine (Methylphenidate may inhibit the metabolism of certain tricyclic antidepressants; downward dosage adjustment of tricyclic antidepressants may be required).
No products indexed under this heading.

Citalopram Hydrobromide (Methylphenidate may inhibit the metabolism of certain selective serotonin reuptake inhibitors; downward dosage adjustment of these drugs may be required). Products include:
Celexa 1365

Clomipramine Hydrochloride (Methylphenidate may inhibit the metabolism of certain tricyclic antidepressants; downward dosage adjustment of tricyclic antidepressants may be required).
No products indexed under this heading.

Desipramine Hydrochloride (Methylphenidate may inhibit the metabolism of certain tricyclic antidepressants; downward dosage adjustment of tricyclic antidepressants may be required). Products include:
Norpramin Tablets 755

Dicumarol (Methylphenidate may inhibit the metabolism of coumarin anticoagulants; downward dosage adjustment of anticoagulants may be required).
No products indexed under this heading.

Dopamine Hydrochloride (Methylphenidate causes rise in blood pressure; co-administration with other pressor agents should be undertaken with caution).
No products indexed under this heading.

Doxepin Hydrochloride (Methylphenidate may inhibit the metabolism of certain tricyclic antidepressants; downward dosage adjustment of tricyclic antidepressants may be required). Products include:
Sinequan 2713

Epinephrine Bitartrate (Methylphenidate causes rise in blood pressure; co-administration with other pressor agents should be undertaken with caution). Products include:
Sensorcaine 643

Epinephrine Hydrochloride (Methylphenidate causes rise in blood pressure; co-administration with other pressor agents should be undertaken with caution).
No products indexed under this heading.

Fluoxetine Hydrochloride (Methylphenidate may inhibit the metabolism of certain selective serotonin reuptake inhibitors; downward dosage adjustment of these drugs may be required). Products include:
Prozac Pulvules, Liquid, and Weekly Capsules 1238
Sarafem Pulvules 1962

Fluvoxamine Maleate (Methylphenidate may inhibit the metabolism of certain selective serotonin reuptake inhibitors; downward dosage adjustment of these drugs may be required). Products include:
Luvox Tablets (25, 50, 100 mg) 3256

Fosphenytoin Sodium (Methylphenidate may inhibit the metabolism of phenytoin; downward dosage adjustment of phenytoin may be required). Products include:
Cerebyx Injection 2619

Imipramine Hydrochloride (Methylphenidate may inhibit the metabolism of certain tricyclic antidepressants; downward dosage adjustment of tricyclic antidepressants may be required).
No products indexed under this heading.

Imipramine Pamoate (Methylphenidate may inhibit the metabolism of certain tricyclic antidepressants; downward dosage adjustment of tricyclic antidepressants may be required).
No products indexed under this heading.

Isocarboxazid (Co-administration with MAO inhibitors may result in hypertensive crises; concurrent and/or sequential use is contraindicated).
No products indexed under this heading.

Maprotiline Hydrochloride (Methylphenidate may inhibit the metabolism of certain tricyclic antidepressants; downward dosage adjustment of tricyclic antidepressants may be required).
No products indexed under this heading.

Metaraminol Bitartrate (Methylphenidate causes rise in blood pressure; co-administration with other pressor agents should be undertaken with caution). Products include:
Aramine Injection 2043

Methoxamine Hydrochloride (Methylphenidate causes rise in blood pressure; co-administration with other pressor agents should be undertaken with caution).
No products indexed under this heading.

Moclobemide (Co-administration with MAO inhibitors may result in hypertensive crises; concurrent and/or sequential use is contraindicated).
No products indexed under this heading.

Norepinephrine Bitartrate (Methylphenidate causes rise in blood pressure; co-administration with other pressor agents should be undertaken with caution).
No products indexed under this heading.

Nortriptyline Hydrochloride (Methylphenidate may inhibit the metabolism of certain tricyclic antidepressants; downward dosage adjustment of tricyclic antidepressants may be required).
No products indexed under this heading.

Pargyline Hydrochloride (Co-administration with MAO inhibitors may result in hypertensive crises; concurrent and/or sequential use is

contraindicated).
No products indexed under this heading.

Paroxetine Hydrochloride (Methylphenidate may inhibit the metabolism of certain selective serotonin reuptake inhibitors; downward dosage adjustment of these drugs may be required). Products include:
Paxil 1609

Phenelzine Sulfate (Co-administration with MAO inhibitors may result in hypertensive crises; concurrent and/or sequential use is contraindicated). Products include:
Nardil Tablets 2653

Phenobarbital (Methylphenidate may inhibit the metabolism of phenobarbital; downward dosage adjustment of phenobarbital may be required). Products include:
Arco-Lase Plus Tablets 592
Donnatal 2929
Donnatal Extentabs 2930

Phenylephrine Hydrochloride (Methylphenidate causes rise in blood pressure; co-administration with other pressor agents should be undertaken with caution). Products include:
Afrin Nasal Decongestant Children's Pump Mist 734
Extendryl 1361
Hycomine Compound Tablets 1317
Neo-Synephrine 614
Phenergan VC Syrup 3560
Phenergan VC with Codeine Syrup . 3561
Preparation H Cream 778
Preparation H Cooling Gel 778
Preparation H 778
Vicks Sinex Nasal Spray and Ultra Fine Mist 729

Phenytoin (Methylphenidate may inhibit the metabolism of phenytoin; downward dosage adjustment of phenytoin may be required). Products include:
Dilantin Infatabs 2624
Dilantin-125 Oral Suspension 2625

Phenytoin Sodium (Methylphenidate may inhibit the metabolism of phenytoin; downward dosage adjustment of phenytoin may be required). Products include:
Dilantin Kapseals 2622

Primidone (Methylphenidate may inhibit the metabolism of primidone; downward dosage adjustment of primidone may be required).
No products indexed under this heading.

Procarbazine Hydrochloride (Co-administration with MAO inhibitors may result in hypertensive crises; concurrent and/or sequential use is contraindicated). Products include:
Matulane Capsules 3246

Protriptyline Hydrochloride (Methylphenidate may inhibit the metabolism of certain tricyclic antidepressants; downward dosage adjustment of tricyclic antidepressants may be required). Products include:
Vivactil Tablets 2446
Vivactil Tablets 2217

Selegiline Hydrochloride (Co-administration with MAO inhibitors may result in hypertensive crises; concurrent and/or sequential use is contraindicated). Products include:
Eldepryl Capsules 3266

Sertraline Hydrochloride (Methylphenidate may inhibit the metabolism of certain selective serotonin reuptake inhibitors; downward dosage adjustment of these drugs may be required). Products include:
Zoloft 2751

Tranylcypromine Sulfate (Co-administration with MAO inhibitors may result in hypertensive crises; concurrent and/or sequential use is contraindicated). Products include:
Parnate Tablets 1607

Trimipramine Maleate (Methylphenidate may inhibit the metabolism of certain tricyclic antidepressants; downward dosage adjustment of tricyclic antidepressants may be required). Products include:
Surmontil Capsules 3595

Warfarin Sodium (Methylphenidate may inhibit the metabolism of coumarin anticoagulants; downward dosage adjustment of anticoagulants may be required). Products include:
Coumadin for Injection 1243
Coumadin Tablets 1243
Warfarin Sodium Tablets, USP 3302

CONDYLOX GEL
(Podofilox) 2436
None cited in PDR database.

CONDYLOX TOPICAL SOLUTION
(Podofilox) 2437
None cited in PDR database.

CONTAC NON-DROWSY 12 HOUR COLD CAPLETS
(Pseudoephedrine Hydrochloride) ....■ 745
May interact with monoamine oxidase inhibitors. Compounds in these categories include:

Isocarboxazid (Concurrent and/or sequential use with MAO inhibitors is not recommended).
No products indexed under this heading.

Moclobemide (Concurrent and/or sequential use with MAO inhibitors is not recommended).
No products indexed under this heading.

Pargyline Hydrochloride (Concurrent and/or sequential use with MAO inhibitors is not recommended).
No products indexed under this heading.

Phenelzine Sulfate (Concurrent and/or sequential use with MAO inhibitors is not recommended). Products include:
Nardil Tablets 2653

Procarbazine Hydrochloride (Concurrent and/or sequential use with MAO inhibitors is not recommended). Products include:
Matulane Capsules 3246

Selegiline Hydrochloride (Concurrent and/or sequential use with MAO inhibitors is not recommended). Products include:
Eldepryl Capsules 3266

Tranylcypromine Sulfate (Concurrent and/or sequential use with MAO inhibitors is not recommended). Products include:
Parnate Tablets 1607

CONTAC NON-DROWSY TIMED RELEASE 12 HOUR COLD CAPLETS
(Pseudoephedrine Hydrochloride) ....■ 746
See Contac Non-Drowsy 12 Hour Cold Caplets

CONTAC SEVERE COLD AND FLU CAPLETS MAXIMUM STRENGTH
(Acetaminophen, Chlorpheniramine Maleate, Dextromethorphan Hydrobromide, Pseudoephedrine Hydrochloride) .....■ 746
May interact with hypnotics and sedatives, monoamine oxidase inhibitors, tranquilizers, and certain other agents. Compounds in these categories include:

Alprazolam (May increase drowsiness effect; concurrent use should be avoided). Products include:
Xanax Tablets 2865

Buspirone Hydrochloride (May increase drowsiness effect; concurrent use should be avoided).
No products indexed under this heading.

Chlordiazepoxide (May increase drowsiness effect; concurrent use should be avoided). Products include:
Limbitrol 1738

Chlordiazepoxide Hydrochloride (May increase drowsiness effect; concurrent use should be avoided). Products include:
Librium Capsules 1736
Librium for Injection 1737

Chlorpromazine (May increase drowsiness effect; concurrent use should be avoided). Products include:
Thorazine Suppositories 1656

Chlorpromazine Hydrochloride (May increase drowsiness effect; concurrent use should be avoided). Products include:
Thorazine 1656

Chlorprothixene (May increase drowsiness effect; concurrent use should be avoided).
No products indexed under this heading.

Chlorprothixene Hydrochloride (May increase drowsiness effect; concurrent use should be avoided).
No products indexed under this heading.

Clorazepate Dipotassium (May increase drowsiness effect; concurrent use should be avoided). Products include:
Tranxene 511

Diazepam (May increase drowsiness effect; concurrent use should be avoided). Products include:
Valium Injectable 3026
Valium Tablets 3047

Droperidol (May increase drowsiness effect; concurrent use should be avoided).
No products indexed under this heading.

Estazolam (May increase drowsiness effect; concurrent use should be avoided). Products include:
ProSom Tablets 500

Ethchlorvynol (May increase drowsiness effect; concurrent use should be avoided).
No products indexed under this heading.

Ethinamate (May increase drowsiness effect; concurrent use should be avoided).
No products indexed under this heading.

Fluphenazine Decanoate (May increase drowsiness effect; concurrent use should be avoided).
No products indexed under this heading.

Fluphenazine Enanthate (May increase drowsiness effect; concurrent use should be avoided).
No products indexed under this heading.

Fluphenazine Hydrochloride (May increase drowsiness effect; concurrent use should be avoided).
No products indexed under this heading.

Flurazepam Hydrochloride (May increase drowsiness effect; concurrent use should be avoided).
No products indexed under this heading.

Glutethimide (May increase drowsiness effect; concurrent use should be avoided).
No products indexed under this heading.

Haloperidol (May increase drowsiness effect; concurrent use should be avoided). Products include:
Haldol Injection, Tablets and Concentrate 2533

Haloperidol Decanoate (May increase drowsiness effect; concurrent use should be avoided). Products include:
Haldol Decanoate 2535

Hydroxyzine Hydrochloride (May increase drowsiness effect; concurrent use should be avoided). Products include:
Atarax Tablets & Syrup 2667
Vistaril Intramuscular Solution 2738

Isocarboxazid (Concurrent and/or sequential use is not recommended unless directed by a doctor).
No products indexed under this heading.

Lorazepam (May increase drowsiness effect; concurrent use should be avoided). Products include:
Ativan Injection 3478
Ativan Tablets 3482

Loxapine Hydrochloride (May increase drowsiness effect; concurrent use should be avoided).
No products indexed under this heading.

Loxapine Succinate (May increase drowsiness effect; concurrent use should be avoided). Products include:
Loxitane Capsules 3398

Meprobamate (May increase drowsiness effect; concurrent use should be avoided). Products include:
Miltown Tablets 3349

Mesoridazine Besylate (May increase drowsiness effect; concurrent use should be avoided). Products include:
Serentil 1057

Midazolam Hydrochloride (May increase drowsiness effect; concurrent use should be avoided). Products include:
Versed Injection 3027
Versed Syrup 3033

Moclobemide (Concurrent and/or sequential use is not recommended unless directed by a doctor).
No products indexed under this heading.

Molindone Hydrochloride (May increase drowsiness effect; concurrent use should be avoided). Products include:
Moban 1320

Oxazepam (May increase drowsiness effect; concurrent use should be avoided).
No products indexed under this heading.

Pargyline Hydrochloride (Concurrent and/or sequential use is not recommended unless directed by a doctor).
No products indexed under this heading.

Perphenazine (May increase drowsiness effect; concurrent use should be avoided). Products include:
Etrafon 3115
Trilafon 3160

Phenelzine Sulfate (Concurrent and/or sequential use is not recommended unless directed by a doctor). Products include:
Nardil Tablets 2653

Prazepam (May increase drowsiness effect; concurrent use should be avoided).
No products indexed under this heading.

Procarbazine Hydrochloride (Concurrent and/or sequential use is not recommended unless directed by a doctor). Products include:
Matulane Capsules 3246

Prochlorperazine (May increase drowsiness effect; concurrent use should be avoided). Products include:
Compazine 1505

Promethazine Hydrochloride (May increase drowsiness effect; concurrent use should be avoided). Products include:
Mepergan Injection 3539
Phenergan Injection 3553
Phenergan 3556
Phenergan Syrup 3554
Phenergan with Codeine Syrup 3557
Phenergan with Dextromethorphan Syrup 3559
Phenergan VC Syrup 3560
Phenergan VC with Codeine Syrup .. 3561

Propofol (May increase drowsiness effect; concurrent use should be avoided). Products include:
Diprivan Injectable Emulsion 667

Quazepam (May increase drowsiness effect; concurrent use should be avoided).
No products indexed under this heading.

Secobarbital Sodium (May increase drowsiness effect; concurrent use should be avoided).
No products indexed under this heading.

Selegiline Hydrochloride (Concurrent and/or sequential use is not recommended unless directed by a doctor). Products include:
Eldepryl Capsules 3266

Temazepam (May increase drowsiness effect; concurrent use should be avoided).
No products indexed under this heading.

Thioridazine Hydrochloride (May increase drowsiness effect; concurrent use should be avoided). Products include:
Thioridazine Hydrochloride Tablets 2289

Thiothixene (May increase drowsiness effect; concurrent use should be avoided). Products include:
Navane Capsules 2701
Thiothixene Capsules 2290

Tranylcypromine Sulfate (Concurrent and/or sequential use is not recommended unless directed by a doctor). Products include:
Parnate Tablets 1607

Triazolam (May increase drowsiness effect; concurrent use should be avoided). Products include:
Halcion Tablets 2823

Trifluoperazine Hydrochloride (May increase drowsiness effect; concurrent use should be avoided). Products include:
Stelazine 1640

Zaleplon (May increase drowsiness effect; concurrent use should be avoided). Products include:
Sonata Capsules 3591

Zolpidem Tartrate (May increase drowsiness effect; concurrent use should be avoided). Products include:
Ambien Tablets 3191

Food Interactions

Alcohol (May increase drowsiness effect; concurrent use should be avoided).

CONTAC SEVERE COLD AND FLU CAPLETS NON-DROWSY
(Acetaminophen, Dextromethorphan Hydrobromide, Pseudoephedrine Hydrochloride) .....■ 746
See Contac Severe Cold and Flu Caplets Maximum Strength

COPAXONE FOR INJECTION
(Glatiramer Acetate) 3306
None cited in PDR database.

COQUINONE CAPSULES
(Coenzyme Q-10, Lipoic Acid) 3335
None cited in PDR database.

CORDARONE INTRAVENOUS
(Amiodarone Hydrochloride) 3491
May interact with beta blockers, calcium channel blockers, halogenated hydrocarbon anesthetics, phenytoin, quinidine, and certain other agents. Compounds in these categories include:

Acebutolol Hydrochloride (Amiodarone has weak beta blocking activity, use with beta blocking agents could increase risk of hypotension and bradycardia). Products include:
- Sectral Capsules 3589

Amlodipine Besylate (Amiodarone inhibits atrioventricular conduction and decreases myocardial contractility, increasing the risk of AV block with calcium channel blockers). Products include:
- Lotrel Capsules 2370
- Norvasc Tablets 2704

Atenolol (Amiodarone has weak beta blocking activity, use with beta blocking agents could increase risk of hypotension and bradycardia). Products include:
- Tenoretic Tablets 690
- Tenormin I.V. Injection 692

Bepridil Hydrochloride (Amiodarone inhibits atrioventricular conduction and decreases myocardial contractility, increasing the risk of AV block with calcium channel blockers). Products include:
- Vascor Tablets 2602

Betaxolol Hydrochloride (Amiodarone has weak beta blocking activity, use with beta blocking agents could increase risk of hypotension and bradycardia). Products include:
- Betoptic S Ophthalmic Suspension 537

Bisoprolol Fumarate (Amiodarone has weak beta blocking activity, use with beta blocking agents could increase risk of hypotension and bradycardia). Products include:
- Zebeta Tablets 1885
- Ziac Tablets 1887

Carteolol Hydrochloride (Amiodarone has weak beta blocking activity, use with beta blocking agents could increase risk of hypotension and bradycardia). Products include:
- Carteolol Hydrochloride Ophthalmic Solution USP, 1% .... ⊙258
- Ocupress Ophthalmic Solution, 1% Sterile .... ⊙303

Cholestyramine (Increases enterohepatic elimination of amiodarone and may reduce serum levels and t1/2).
- No products indexed under this heading.

Cimetidine (Co-administration with cimetidine results in increased serum amiodarone levels). Products include:
- Tagamet HB 200 Suspension .... ▣762
- Tagamet HB 200 Tablets .... ▣761
- Tagamet Tablets 1644

Cimetidine Hydrochloride (Co-administration with cimetidine results in increased serum amiodarone levels). Products include:
- Tagamet 1644

Cyclosporine (Amiodarone can inhibit metabolism mediated by cytochrome P-450 enzymes, probably accounting for the significant effects of oral amiodarone on the pharmacokinetics of various agents including cyclosporine; co-administration produces persistently elevated plasma concentrations of cyclosporine resulting in elevated creatinine, despite reduction in dose of cyclosporine). Products include:
- Gengraf Capsules 457
- Neoral Soft Gelatin Capsules 2380
- Neoral Oral Solution 2380
- Sandimmune 2388

Dextromethorphan Hydrobromide (Amiodarone can inhibit metabolism mediated by cytochrome P-450 enzymes, probably accounting for the significant effects of oral amiodarone on the pharmacokinetics of various agents including dextromethorphan; oral amiodarone administration impairs metabolism of dextromethorphan). Products include:
- Alka-Seltzer Plus Liqui-Gels .... ▣604
- Alka-Seltzer Plus Cold & Flu Medicine Liqui-Gels .... ▣604
- Benylin Adult Formula Cough Suppressant Liquid .... ▣696
- Benylin Cough Suppressant/Expectorant Liquid .... ▣697
- Benylin Multi-Symptom Liquid .... ▣697
- Benylin Pediatric Cough Suppressant Liquid .... ▣698
- Comtrex Deep Chest Cold & Congestion Relief Softgels .... ▣627
- Comtrex Maximum Strength Multi-Symptom Cold & Cough Relief Tablets and Caplets .... ▣626
- Contac Severe Cold and Flu Caplets Maximum Strength .... ▣746
- Contac Severe Cold and Flu Caplets Non-Drowsy .... ▣746
- Coricidin HBP Cough & Cold Tablets .... ▣738
- Coricidin HBP Maximum Strength Flu Tablets .... ▣738
- Dimetapp DM Cold & Cough Elixir .... ▣775
- Dimetapp Nighttime Flu Liquid .... ▣776
- Dimetapp Non-Drowsy Flu Syrup .... ▣777
- Dimetapp Infant Drops Decongestant Plus Cough .... ▣776
- PediaCare Cough-Cold Liquid .... ▣719
- PediaCare Infants' Drops Decongestant Plus Cough .... ▣719
- PediaCare NightRest Cough-Cold Liquid .... ▣719
- Phenergan with Dextromethorphan Syrup 3559
- Robitussin Cold Caplets Cold & Congestion .... ▣780
- Robitussin Cold Softgels Cold & Congestion .... ▣780
- Robitussin Cold Caplets Multi-Symptom Cold & Flu .... ▣781
- Robitussin Cold Softgels Multi-Symptom Cold & Flu .... ▣781
- Robitussin Cough & Cold Infant Drops .... ▣782
- Robitussin Maximum Strength Cough & Cold Liquid .... ▣785
- Robitussin Pediatric Cough & Cold Formula Liquid .... ▣785
- Robitussin Maximum Strength Cough Suppressant Liquid .... ▣784
- Robitussin Pediatric Cough Suppressant Liquid .... ▣784
- Robitussin Multi Symptom Honey Flu Liquid .... ▣785
- Robitussin Nighttime Honey Flu Liquid .... ▣786
- Robitussin-CF Liquid .... ▣783
- Robitussin DM Infant Drops .... ▣783
- Robitussin-DM Liquid .... ▣783
- Children's Sudafed Cold & Cough Liquid .... ▣709
- Sudafed Cold & Cough Liquid Caps .... ▣709
- Sudafed Severe Cold .... ▣711
- TheraFlu Regular Strength Cold & Cough Night Time Hot Liquid .... ▣676
- TheraFlu Maximum Strength Flu & Congestion Non-Drowsy Hot Liquid .... ▣677
- TheraFlu Maximum Strength Flu & Cough Night Time Hot Liquid .... ▣678
- TheraFlu Maximum Strength Severe Cold & Congestion Night Time Caplets .... ▣678
- TheraFlu Maximum Strength Severe Cold & Congestion Night Time Hot Liquid .... ▣678
- TheraFlu Maximum Strength Severe Cold & Congestion Non-Drowsy .... ▣679
- Triaminic Cold & Cough Liquid .... ▣681
- Triaminic Cold & Cough Softchews .... ▣683
- Triaminic Cold & Night Time Cough Liquid .... ▣681
- Triaminic Cold, Cough & Fever Liquid .... ▣681
- Triaminic Cough Liquid .... ▣682
- Triaminic Cough Softchews .... ▣684
- Triaminic Cough & Congestion Liquid .... ▣682
- Triaminic Cough & Sore Throat Liquid .... ▣682
- Triaminic Cough & Sore Throat Softchews .... ▣684
- Tussi-Organidin DM NR Liquid 3350
- Tussi-Organidin DM-S NR Liquid 3350
- Children's Tylenol Cold Plus Cough Suspension Liquid and Chewable Tablets 2015
- Children's Tylenol Flu Suspension Liquid 2015
- Infants' Tylenol Cold Decongestant and Fever Reducer Concentrated Drops Plus Cough .. 2015
- Multi-Symptom Tylenol Cold Complete Formula Caplets 2010
- Multi-Symptom Tylenol Cold Non-Drowsy Caplets and Gelcaps 2010
- Multi-Symptom Tylenol Cold Severe Congestion Non-Drowsy Caplets 2011
- Maximum Strength Tylenol Flu NightTime Liquid 2011
- Maximum Strength Tylenol Flu Non-Drowsy Gelcaps 2011
- Vicks 44 Cough Relief Liquid .... ▣724
- Vicks 44D Cough & Head Congestion Relief Liquid .... ▣724
- Vicks 44E Cough & Chest Congestion Relief Liquid .... ▣725
- Pediatric Vicks 44e Cough & Chest Congestion Relief Liquid .... ▣728
- Vicks 44M Cough, Cold & Flu Relief Liquid .... ▣725
- Pediatric Vicks 44m Cough & Cold Relief .... ▣728
- Vicks DayQuil LiquiCaps/Liquid Multi-Symptom Cold/Flu Relief .... ▣727
- Children's Vicks NyQuil Cold/Cough Relief .... ▣726
- Vicks NyQuil LiquiCaps/Liquid Multi-Symptom Cold/Flu Relief, Original and Cherry Flavors .... ▣727

Digoxin (Amiodarone can inhibit metabolism mediated by cytochrome P-450 enzymes, probably accounting for the significant effects of oral amiodarone on the pharmacokinetics of various agents including digoxin; co-administration increases digoxin serum concentration). Products include:
- Digitek Tablets 1003
- Lanoxicaps Capsules 1574
- Lanoxin Injection 1581
- Lanoxin Tablets 1587
- Lanoxin Elixir Pediatric 1578
- Lanoxin Injection Pediatric 1584

Diltiazem Hydrochloride (Amiodarone inhibits atrioventricular conduction and decreases myocardial contractility, increasing the risk of AV block with calcium channel blockers). Products include:
- Cardizem Injectable 1018
- Cardizem Lyo-Ject Syringe 1018
- Cardizem Monovial 1018
- Cardizem CD Capsules 1016
- Tiazac Capsules 1378

Disopyramide Phosphate (Co-administration increases QT prolongation, which could cause arrhythmia).
- No products indexed under this heading.

Enflurane (Patients undergoing general anesthesia who are on amiodarone therapy are potentially more sensitive to the myocardial depressant and conduction effects of halogenated inhalation anesthetic).
- No products indexed under this heading.

Esmolol Hydrochloride (Amiodarone has weak beta blocking activity, use with beta blocking agents could increase risk of hypotension and bradycardia). Products include:
- Brevibloc Injection 858

Felodipine (Amiodarone inhibits atrioventricular conduction and decreases myocardial contractility, increasing the risk of AV block with calcium channel blockers). Products include:
- Lexxel Tablets 608
- Plendil Extended-Release Tablets 623

Fentanyl (Co-administration may cause hypotension, bradycardia, and decreased cardiac output). Products include:
- Duragesic Transdermal System 1786

Fentanyl Citrate (Co-administration may cause hypotension, bradycardia, and decreased cardiac output). Products include:
- Actiq 1184

Flecainide Acetate (Reduces the dose of flecainide needed to maintain therapeutic plasma concentrations). Products include:
- Tambocor Tablets 1990

Fosphenytoin Sodium (Co-administration with phenytoin results in decreased serum amiodarone levels; oral amiodarone administration impairs metabolism of phenytoin). Products include:
- Cerebyx Injection 2619

Halothane (Patients undergoing general anesthesia who are on amiodarone therapy are potentially more sensitive to the myocardial depressant and conduction effects of halogenated inhalation anesthetic). Products include:
- Fluothane Inhalation 3508

Isoflurane (Patients undergoing general anesthesia who are on amiodarone therapy are potentially more sensitive to the myocardial depressant and conduction effects of halogenated inhalation anesthetic).
- No products indexed under this heading.

Isradipine (Amiodarone inhibits atrioventricular conduction and decreases myocardial contractility, increasing the risk of AV block with calcium channel blockers). Products include:
- DynaCirc Capsules 2921
- DynaCirc CR Tablets 2923

Labetalol Hydrochloride (Amiodarone has weak beta blocking activity, use with beta blocking agents could increase risk of hypotension and bradycardia). Products include:
- Normodyne Injection 3135
- Normodyne Tablets 3137

Levobunolol Hydrochloride (Amiodarone has weak beta blocking activity, use with beta blocking agents could increase risk of hypotension and bradycardia). Products include:
- Betagan .... ⊙228

Lidocaine Hydrochloride (Co-administration of oral amiodarone and lidocaine for anesthesia has resulted in sinus bradycardia; seizure associated with increased lidocaine concentrations has resulted when lidocaine is used concurrently with intravenous amiodarone). Products include:
- Bactine First Aid Liquid .... ▣611
- Xylocaine Injections 653

Methotrexate Sodium (Oral amiodarone administration impairs metabolism of methotrexate).
- No products indexed under this heading.

Methoxyflurane (Patients undergoing general anesthesia who are on amiodarone therapy are potentially more sensitive to the myocardial depressant and conduction effects of halogenated inhalation anesthetic).
- No products indexed under this heading.

Metipranolol Hydrochloride (Amiodarone has weak beta blocking activity, use with beta blocking agents could increase risk of hypotension and bradycardia).
- No products indexed under this heading.

Metoprolol Succinate (Amiodarone has weak beta blocking activ-

IMPORTANT NOTE: Always consult each drug listing in the patient's regimen for possible interactions.

ity, use with beta blocking agents could increase risk of hypotension and bradycardia). Products include:

Toprol-XL Tablets 651

Metoprolol Tartrate (Amiodarone has weak beta blocking activity, use with beta blocking agents could increase risk of hypotension and bradycardia).

No products indexed under this heading.

Mibefradil Dihydrochloride (Amiodarone inhibits atrioventricular conduction and decreases myocardial contractility, increasing the risk of AV block with calcium channel blockers).

No products indexed under this heading.

Nadolol (Amiodarone has weak beta blocking activity, use with beta blocking agents could increase risk of hypotension and bradycardia). Products include:

Corgard Tablets 2245
Corzide 40/5 Tablets 2247
Corzide 80/5 Tablets 2247
Nadolol Tablets 2288

Nicardipine Hydrochloride (Amiodarone inhibits atrioventricular conduction and decreases myocardial contractility, increasing the risk of AV block with calcium channel blockers). Products include:

Cardene I.V. 3485

Nifedipine (Amiodarone inhibits atrioventricular conduction and decreases myocardial contractility, increasing the risk of AV block with calcium channel blockers). Products include:

Adalat CC Tablets 877
Procardia Capsules 2708
Procardia XL Extended Release Tablets 2710

Nimodipine (Amiodarone inhibits atrioventricular conduction and decreases myocardial contractility, increasing the risk of AV block with calcium channel blockers). Products include:

Nimotop Capsules 904

Nisoldipine (Amiodarone inhibits atrioventricular conduction and decreases myocardial contractility, increasing the risk of AV block with calcium channel blockers). Products include:

Sular Tablets 688

Penbutolol Sulfate (Amiodarone has weak beta blocking activity, use with beta blocking agents could increase risk of hypotension and bradycardia).

No products indexed under this heading.

Phenytoin (Co-administration with phenytoin results in decreased serum amiodarone levels; oral amiodarone administration impairs metabolism of phenytoin). Products include:

Dilantin Infatabs 2624
Dilantin-125 Oral Suspension 2625

Phenytoin Sodium (Co-administration with phenytoin results in decreased serum amiodarone levels; oral amiodarone administration impairs metabolism of phenytoin). Products include:

Dilantin Kapseals 2622

Pindolol (Amiodarone has weak beta blocking activity, use with beta blocking agents could increase risk of hypotension and bradycardia).

No products indexed under this heading.

Procainamide Hydrochloride (Amiodarone can inhibit metabolism mediated by cytochrome P-450 enzymes, probably accounting for the significant effects of oral amiodarone on the pharmacokinetics of various agents including procainamide; co-administration increases procainamide serum concentration and NAPA concentration). Products include:

Procanbid Extended-Release Tablets 2262

Propranolol Hydrochloride (Amiodarone has weak beta blocking activity, use with beta blocking agents could increase risk of hypotension and bradycardia). Products include:

Inderal 3513
Inderal LA Long-Acting Capsules 3516
Inderide Tablets 3517
Inderide LA Long-Acting Capsules 3519

Quinidine Gluconate (Amiodarone can inhibit metabolism mediated by cytochrome P-450 enzymes, probably accounting for the significant effects of oral amiodarone on the pharmacokinetics of various agents including quinidine; co-administration increases quinidine serum concentration). Products include:

Quinaglute Dura-Tabs Tablets 978

Quinidine Polygalacturonate (Amiodarone can inhibit metabolism mediated by cytochrome P-450 enzymes, probably accounting for the significant effects of oral amiodarone on the pharmacokinetics of various agents including quinidine; co-administration increases quinidine serum concentration).

No products indexed under this heading.

Quinidine Sulfate (Amiodarone can inhibit metabolism mediated by cytochrome P-450 enzymes, probably accounting for the significant effects of oral amiodarone on the pharmacokinetics of various agents including quinidine; co-administration increases quinidine serum concentration). Products include:

Quinidex Extentabs 2933

Sotalol Hydrochloride (Amiodarone has weak beta blocking activity, use with beta blocking agents could increase risk of hypotension and bradycardia). Products include:

Betapace Tablets 950
Betapace AF Tablets 954

Timolol Hemihydrate (Amiodarone has weak beta blocking activity, use with beta blocking agents could increase risk of hypotension and bradycardia). Products include:

Betimol Ophthalmic Solution .... ⊙ 324

Timolol Maleate (Amiodarone has weak beta blocking activity, use with beta blocking agents could increase risk of hypotension and bradycardia). Products include:

Blocadren Tablets 2046
Cosopt Sterile Ophthalmic Solution 2065
Timolide Tablets 2187
Timolol GFS .... ⊙ 266
Timoptic in Ocudose 2192
Timoptic Sterile Ophthalmic Solution 2190
Timoptic-XE Sterile Ophthalmic Gel Forming Solution 2194

Verapamil Hydrochloride (Amiodarone inhibits atrioventricular conduction and decreases myocardial contractility, increasing the risk of AV block with calcium channel blockers). Products include:

Covera-HS Tablets 3199
Isoptin SR Tablets 467
Tarka Tablets 508
Verelan Capsules 3184
Verelan PM Capsules 3186

Warfarin Sodium (Amiodarone can inhibit metabolism mediated by cytochrome P-450 enzymes, probably accounting for the significant effects of oral amiodarone on the pharmacokinetics of various agents including warfarin; co-administration increases prothrombin time). Products include:

Coumadin for Injection 1243
Coumadin Tablets 1243
Warfarin Sodium Tablets, USP 3302

CORDARONE TABLETS

(Amiodarone Hydrochloride) 3487

May interact with antiarrhythmics, beta blockers, calcium channel blockers, oral anticoagulants, cardiac glycosides, halogenated hydrocarbon anesthetics, phenytoin, quinidine, and certain other agents. Compounds in these categories include:

Acebutolol Hydrochloride (Possible potentiation of bradycardia, sinus arrest and AV block). Products include:

Sectral Capsules 3589

Adenosine (Possible increase in serious toxicity when amiodarone is used with other antiarrhythmics). Products include:

Adenocard Injection 1380
Adenoscan 1381

Amlodipine Besylate (Possible potentiation of bradycardia, sinus arrest and AV block). Products include:

Lotrel Capsules 2370
Norvasc Tablets 2704

Atenolol (Possible potentiation of bradycardia, sinus arrest and AV block). Products include:

Tenoretic Tablets 690
Tenormin I.V. Injection 692

Bepridil Hydrochloride (Possible potentiation of bradycardia, sinus arrest and AV block). Products include:

Vascor Tablets 2602

Betaxolol Hydrochloride (Possible potentiation of bradycardia, sinus arrest and AV block). Products include:

Betoptic S Ophthalmic Suspension 537

Bisoprolol Fumarate (Possible potentiation of bradycardia, sinus arrest and AV block). Products include:

Zebeta Tablets 1885
Ziac Tablets 1887

Bretylium Tosylate (Possible increase in serious toxicity when amiodarone is used with other antiarrhythmics).

No products indexed under this heading.

Carteolol Hydrochloride (Possible potentiation of bradycardia, sinus arrest and AV block). Products include:

Carteolol Hydrochloride Ophthalmic Solution USP, 1% .... ⊙ 258
Ocupress Ophthalmic Solution, 1% Sterile .... ⊙ 303

Cyclosporine (Concomitant use has been reported to produce persistently elevated plasma concentrations of cyclosporine resulting in elevated creatinine, despite reduction in dose of cyclosporine). Products include:

Gengraf Capsules 457
Neoral Soft Gelatin Capsules 2380
Neoral Oral Solution 2380
Sandimmune 2388

Deslanoside (Co-administration results in an increase in serum cardiac glycosides concentration that may reach toxic levels with resultant clinical toxicity; discontinue or reduce dose of digitalis by approximately 50%).

No products indexed under this heading.

Dicumarol (Potentiation of warfarin-type anticoagulant resulting in serious or fatal bleeding; the dose of anticoagulant should be reduced by 1/3 to 1/2; monitor prothrombin time closely).

No products indexed under this heading.

Digitoxin (Co-administration results in an increase in serum cardiac glycosides concentration that may reach toxic levels with resultant clinical toxicity; discontinue or reduce dose of digitalis by approximately 50%).

No products indexed under this heading.

Digoxin (Co-administration results in an increase in serum digoxin concentration by 70% with resultant clinical toxicity; discontinue or reduce dose of digoxin by approximately 50%). Products include:

Digitek Tablets 1003
Lanoxicaps Capsules 1574
Lanoxin Injection 1581
Lanoxin Tablets 1587
Lanoxin Elixir Pediatric 1578
Lanoxin Injection Pediatric 1584

Diltiazem Hydrochloride (Possible potentiation of bradycardia, sinus arrest and AV block). Products include:

Cardizem Injectable 1018
Cardizem Lyo-Ject Syringe 1018
Cardizem Monovial 1018
Cardizem CD Capsules 1016
Tiazac Capsules 1378

Disopyramide Phosphate (Possible increase in serious toxicity when amiodarone is used with other antiarrhythmics).

No products indexed under this heading.

Dofetilide (Possible increase in serious toxicity when amiodarone is used with other antiarrhythmics). Products include:

Tikosyn Capsules 2717

Enflurane (Patients may be more sensitive to the myocardial depressant and conduction effects of halogenated inhalational anesthetics with co-administration).

No products indexed under this heading.

Esmolol Hydrochloride (Possible potentiation of bradycardia, sinus arrest and AV block). Products include:

Brevibloc Injection 858

Felodipine (Possible potentiation of bradycardia, sinus arrest and AV block). Products include:

Lexxel Tablets 608
Plendil Extended-Release Tablets 623

Flecainide Acetate (Possible increase in serious toxicity when amiodarone is used with other antiarrhythmics). Products include:

Tambocor Tablets 1990

Fosphenytoin Sodium (Concomitant therapy has resulted in steady-state levels of phenytoin). Products include:

Cerebyx Injection 2619

Halothane (Patients may be more sensitive to the myocardial depressant and conduction effects of halogenated inhalational anesthetics with co-administration). Products include:

Fluothane Inhalation 3508

Isoflurane (Patients may be more sensitive to the myocardial depressant and conduction effects of halogenated inhalational anesthetics with co-administration).

No products indexed under this heading.

Isradipine (Possible potentiation of bradycardia, sinus arrest and AV block). Products include:

DynaCirc Capsules 2921
DynaCirc CR Tablets 2923

Labetalol Hydrochloride (Possible potentiation of bradycardia, sinus arrest and AV block). Products include:

Normodyne Injection 3135
Normodyne Tablets 3137

Levobunolol Hydrochloride (Possible potentiation of bradycardia, sinus arrest and AV block). Products include:

Betagan .... ⊙ 228

Lidocaine Hydrochloride (Possible increase in serious toxicity when amiodarone is used with other antiarrhythmics). Products include:
- Bactine First Aid Liquid .... ◘611
- Xylocaine Injections 653

Methoxyflurane (Patients may be more sensitive to the myocardial depressant and conduction effects of halogenated inhalational anesthetics with co-administration).
No products indexed under this heading.

Metipranolol Hydrochloride (Possible potentiation of bradycardia, sinus arrest and AV block).
No products indexed under this heading.

Metoprolol Succinate (Possible potentiation of bradycardia, sinus arrest and AV block). Products include:
- Toprol-XL Tablets 651

Metoprolol Tartrate (Possible potentiation of bradycardia, sinus arrest and AV block).
No products indexed under this heading.

Mexiletine Hydrochloride (Possible increase in serious toxicity when amiodarone is used with other antiarrhythmics). Products include:
- Mexitil Capsules 1047

Mibefradil Dihydrochloride (Possible potentiation of bradycardia, sinus arrest and AV block).
No products indexed under this heading.

Moricizine Hydrochloride (Possible increase in serious toxicity when amiodarone is used with other antiarrhythmics).
No products indexed under this heading.

Nadolol (Possible potentiation of bradycardia, sinus arrest and AV block). Products include:
- Corgard Tablets 2245
- Corzide 40/5 Tablets 2247
- Corzide 80/5 Tablets 2247
- Nadolol Tablets 2288

Nicardipine Hydrochloride (Possible potentiation of bradycardia, sinus arrest and AV block). Products include:
- Cardene I.V. 3485

Nifedipine (Possible potentiation of bradycardia, sinus arrest and AV block). Products include:
- Adalat CC Tablets 877
- Procardia Capsules 2708
- Procardia XL Extended Release Tablets 2710

Nimodipine (Possible potentiation of bradycardia, sinus arrest and AV block). Products include:
- Nimotop Capsules 904

Nisoldipine (Possible potentiation of bradycardia, sinus arrest and AV block). Products include:
- Sular Tablets 688

Penbutolol Sulfate (Possible potentiation of bradycardia, sinus arrest and AV block).
No products indexed under this heading.

Phenytoin (Concomitant therapy has resulted in steady-state levels of phenytoin). Products include:
- Dilantin Infatabs 2624
- Dilantin-125 Oral Suspension 2625

Phenytoin Sodium (Concomitant therapy has resulted in steady-state levels of phenytoin). Products include:
- Dilantin Kapseals 2622

Pindolol (Possible potentiation of bradycardia, sinus arrest and AV block).
No products indexed under this heading.

Procainamide Hydrochloride (Concomitant therapy has resulted in increased steady-state levels of procainamide; any antiarrhythmic drug therapy, such as procainamide, should be initiated at a lower than usual dose). Products include:
- Procanbid Extended-Release Tablets 2262

Propafenone Hydrochloride (Possible increase in serious toxicity when amiodarone is used with other antiarrhythmics). Products include:
- Rythmol Tablets – 150 mg, 225 mg, 300 mg 502

Propranolol Hydrochloride (Possible potentiation of bradycardia, sinus arrest and AV block). Products include:
- Inderal 3513
- Inderal LA Long-Acting Capsules 3516
- Inderide Tablets 3517
- Inderide LA Long-Acting Capsules 3519

Quinidine Gluconate (Concomitant therapy has resulted in increased steady-state levels of quinidine; any added antiarrhythmic drug therapy, such as quinidine, should be initiated at a lower than usual dose). Products include:
- Quinaglute Dura-Tabs Tablets 978

Quinidine Polygalacturonate (Concomitant therapy has resulted in increased steady-state levels of quinidine; any added antiarrhythmic drug therapy, such as quinidine, should be initiated at a lower than usual dose).
No products indexed under this heading.

Quinidine Sulfate (Concomitant therapy has resulted in increased steady-state levels of quinidine; any added antiarrhythmic drug therapy, such as quinidine, should be initiated at a lower than usual dose). Products include:
- Quinidex Extentabs 2933

Sotalol Hydrochloride (Possible potentiation of bradycardia, sinus arrest and AV block). Products include:
- Betapace Tablets 950
- Betapace AF Tablets 954

Timolol Hemihydrate (Possible potentiation of bradycardia, sinus arrest and AV block). Products include:
- Betimol Ophthalmic Solution .... ⊙324

Timolol Maleate (Possible potentiation of bradycardia, sinus arrest and AV block). Products include:
- Blocadren Tablets 2046
- Cosopt Sterile Ophthalmic Solution 2065
- Timolide Tablets 2187
- Timolol GFS .... ⊙266
- Timoptic in Ocudose 2192
- Timoptic Sterile Ophthalmic Solution 2190
- Timoptic-XE Sterile Ophthalmic Gel Forming Solution 2194

Tocainide Hydrochloride (Possible increase in serious toxicity when amiodarone is used with other antiarrhythmics). Products include:
- Tonocard Tablets 649

Verapamil Hydrochloride (Possible potentiation of bradycardia, sinus arrest and AV block). Products include:
- Covera-HS Tablets 3199
- Isoptin SR Tablets 467
- Tarka Tablets 508
- Verelan Capsules 3184
- Verelan PM Capsules 3186

Warfarin Sodium (Increased prothrombin time by 100%; potentiation of warfarin-type anticoagulant resulting in serious or fatal bleeding; the dose of anticoagulant should be reduced by 1/3 to 1/2; monitor prothrombin time closely). Products include:
- Coumadin for Injection 1243
- Coumadin Tablets 1243
- Warfarin Sodium Tablets, USP 3302

Food Interactions

Food, unspecified (Increases the rate and extent of absorption of amiodarone; because of the food effect on absorption, Cordarone should be administered consistently with regard to meals).

CORDRAN LOTION
(Flurandrenolide) 2438
None cited in PDR database.

CORDRAN TAPE
(Flurandrenolide) 2439
None cited in PDR database.

COREG TABLETS
(Carvedilol) 1508
May interact with oral hypoglycemic agents, insulin, monoamine oxidase inhibitors, quinidine, and certain other agents. Compounds in these categories include:

Acarbose (B-blockers may mask some of the manifestations of hypoglycemia; may enhance the blood-sugar-reducing effect of oral hypoglycemics). Products include:
- Precose Tablets 906

Chlorpropamide (B-blockers may mask some of the manifestations of hypoglycemia; may enhance the blood-sugar-reducing effect of oral hypoglycemics). Products include:
- Diabinese Tablets 2680

Cimetidine (Carvedilol undergoes substantial oxidative metabolism; co-administration has resulted in increased steady-state AUC of carvedilol by about 30% with no change in Cmax). Products include:
- Tagamet HB 200 Suspension .... ◘762
- Tagamet HB 200 Tablets .... ◘761
- Tagamet Tablets 1644

Cimetidine Hydrochloride (Carvedilol undergoes substantial oxidative metabolism; co-administration has resulted in increased steady-state AUC of carvedilol by about 30% with no change in Cmax). Products include:
- Tagamet 1644

Clonidine (Co-administration of clonidine with agents with B-blocking properties may potentiate blood-pressure- and heart-rate-lowering effects). Products include:
- Catapres-TTS 1038

Clonidine Hydrochloride (Co-administration of clonidine with agents with B-blocking properties may potentiate blood-pressure- and heart-rate-lowering effects). Products include:
- Catapres Tablets 1037
- Clorpres Tablets 1002
- Combipres Tablets 1040
- Duraclon Injection 3057

Cyclosporine (Co-administration in renal transplant patients has resulted in modest increase in mean trough cyclosporine concentrations; dose of cyclosporine may need to be reduced in some patients). Products include:
- Gengraf Capsules 457
- Neoral Soft Gelatin Capsules 2380
- Neoral Oral Solution 2380
- Sandimmune 2388

Digoxin (Co-administration has resulted in increased steady-state AUC and trough concentrations of digoxin by 14% and 16% respectively). Products include:
- Digitek Tablets 1003
- Lanoxicaps Capsules 1574
- Lanoxin Injection 1581
- Lanoxin Tablets 1587
- Lanoxin Elixir Pediatric 1578
- Lanoxin Injection Pediatric 1584

Diltiazem Hydrochloride (Co-administration has resulted in isolated cases of conduction disturbances, rarely with hemodynamic compromise). Products include:
- Cardizem Injectable 1018
- Cardizem Lyo-Ject Syringe 1018
- Cardizem Monovial 1018
- Cardizem CD Capsules 1016
- Tiazac Capsules 1378

Epinephrine Hydrochloride (Potential for unresponsiveness to the usual dose of epinephrine used to treat allergic reactions).
No products indexed under this heading.

Fluoxetine Hydrochloride (Co-administration of carvedilol with strong inhibitors of CYP2D6, such as fluoxetine, have not been studied, but fluoxetine would be expected to increase blood levels). Products include:
- Prozac Pulvules, Liquid, and Weekly Capsules 1238
- Sarafem Pulvules 1962

Glimepiride (B-blockers may mask some of the manifestations of hypoglycemia; may enhance the blood-sugar-reducing effect of oral hypoglycemics). Products include:
- Amaryl Tablets 717

Glipizide (B-blockers may mask some of the manifestations of hypoglycemia; may enhance the blood-sugar-reducing effect of oral hypoglycemics). Products include:
- Glucotrol Tablets 2692
- Glucotrol XL Extended Release Tablets 2693

Glyburide (B-blockers may mask some of the manifestations of hypoglycemia; may enhance the blood-sugar-reducing effect of oral hypoglycemics). Products include:
- DiaBeta Tablets 741
- Glucovance Tablets 1086

Insulin, Human, Zinc Suspension (Nonselective β-blockers, such as carvedilol, may potentiate insulin-induced hypoglycemia and delay recovery of serum glucose). Products include:
- Humulin L, 100 Units 1937
- Humulin U, 100 Units 1943
- Novolin L Human Insulin 10 ml Vials 2422

Insulin, Human NPH (Nonselective β-blockers, such as carvedilol, may potentiate insulin-induced hypoglycemia and delay recovery of serum glucose). Products include:
- Humulin N, 100 Units 1939
- Humulin N NPH Pen 1940
- Novolin N Human Insulin 10 ml Vials 2422
- Novolin N PenFill 2423
- Novolin N Prefilled Syringe Disposable Insulin Delivery System 2425

Insulin, Human Regular (Nonselective β-blockers, such as carvedilol, may potentiate insulin-induced hypoglycemia and delay recovery of serum glucose). Products include:
- Humulin R Regular (U-500) 1943
- Humulin R, 100 Units 1941
- Novolin R Human Insulin 10 ml Vials 2423
- Novolin R PenFill 2423
- Novolin R Prefilled Syringe Disposable Insulin Delivery System 2425
- Velosulin BR Human Insulin 10 ml Vials 2435

Insulin, Human Regular and Human NPH Mixture (Nonselective β-blockers, such as carvedilol, may potentiate insulin-induced hypoglycemia and delay recovery of serum glucose). Products include:
- Humulin 50/50, 100 Units 1934
- Humulin 70/30, 100 Units 1935
- Humulin 70/30 Pen 1936
- Novolin 70/30 Human Insulin 10 ml Vials 2421
- Novolin 70/30 PenFill 2423
- Novolin 70/30 Prefilled Disposable Insulin Delivery System 2425

Insulin, NPH (Nonselective β-blockers, such as carvedilol, may

potentiate insulin-induced hypoglycemia and delay recovery of serum glucose). Products include:

Iletin II, NPH (Pork), 100 Units 1946

Insulin, Regular (Nonselective β-blockers, such as carvedilol, may potentiate insulin-induced hypoglycemia and delay recovery of serum glucose). Products include:

Iletin II, Regular (Pork), 100 Units ... 1947

Insulin, Zinc Crystals (Nonselective β-blockers, such as carvedilol, may potentiate insulin-induced hypoglycemia and delay recovery of serum glucose).

No products indexed under this heading.

Insulin, Zinc Suspension (Nonselective β-blockers, such as carvedilol, may potentiate insulin-induced hypoglycemia and delay recovery of serum glucose). Products include:

Iletin II, Lente (Pork), 100 Units 1945

Insulin Aspart, Human Regular (Nonselective β-blockers, such as carvedilol, may potentiate insulin-induced hypoglycemia and delay recovery of serum glucose).

No products indexed under this heading.

Insulin glargine (Nonselective β-blockers, such as carvedilol, may potentiate insulin-induced hypoglycemia and delay recovery of serum glucose). Products include:

Lantus Injection 742

Insulin Lispro, Human (Nonselective β-blockers, such as carvedilol, may potentiate insulin-induced hypoglycemia and delay recovery of serum glucose). Products include:

Humalog 1926
Humalog Mix 75/25 Pen 1928

Insulin Lispro Protamine, Human (Nonselective β-blockers, such as carvedilol, may potentiate insulin-induced hypoglycemia and delay recovery of serum glucose). Products include:

Humalog Mix 75/25 Pen 1928

Isocarboxazid (Co-administration of agents with β-blocking properties and a drug that can deplete catecholamines, such as MAO inhibitors, may result in hypotension and/or severe bradycardia).

No products indexed under this heading.

Metformin Hydrochloride (B-blockers may mask some of the manifestations of hypoglycemia; may enhance the blood-sugar-reducing effect of oral hypoglycemics). Products include:

Glucophage Tablets 1080
Glucophage XR Tablets 1080
Glucovance Tablets 1086

Miglitol (B-blockers may mask some of the manifestations of hypoglycemia; may enhance the blood-sugar-reducing effect of oral hypoglycemics). Products include:

Glyset Tablets 2821

Moclobemide (Co-administration of agents with β-blocking properties and a drug that can deplete catecholamines, such as MAO inhibitors, may result in hypotension and/or severe bradycardia).

No products indexed under this heading.

Pargyline Hydrochloride (Co-administration of agents with β-blocking properties and a drug that can deplete catecholamines, such as MAO inhibitors, may result in hypotension and/or severe bradycardia).

No products indexed under this heading.

Paroxetine Hydrochloride (Co-administration of carvedilol with strong inhibitors of CYP2D6, such as paroxetine, have not been studied, but paroxetine would be expected to increase blood levels). Products include:

Paxil 1609

Phenelzine Sulfate (Co-administration of agents with β-blocking properties and a drug that can deplete catecholamines, such as MAO inhibitors, may result in hypotension and/or severe bradycardia). Products include:

Nardil Tablets 2653

Pioglitazone Hydrochloride (β-blockers may mask some of the manifestations of hypoglycemia; may enhance the blood-sugar-reducing effect of oral hypoglycemics). Products include:

Actos Tablets 3275

Procarbazine Hydrochloride (Co-administration of agents with β-blocking properties and a drug that can deplete catecholamines, such as MAO inhibitors, may result in hypotension and/or severe bradycardia). Products include:

Matulane Capsules 3246

Propafenone Hydrochloride (Co-administration of carvedilol with strong inhibitors of CYP2D6, such as propafenone, have not been studied, but propafenone would be expected to increase blood levels). Products include:

Rythmol Tablets – 150 mg, 225 mg, 300 mg 502

Quinidine Gluconate (Co-administration of carvedilol with strong inhibitors of CYP2D6, such as quinidine, have not been studied, but quinidine would be expected to increase blood levels). Products include:

Quinaglute Dura-Tabs Tablets 978

Quinidine Polygalacturonate (Co-administration of carvedilol with strong inhibitors of CYP2D6, such as quinidine, have not been studied, but quinidine would be expected to increase blood levels).

No products indexed under this heading.

Quinidine Sulfate (Co-administration of carvedilol with strong inhibitors of CYP2D6, such as quinidine, have not been studied, but quinidine would be expected to increase blood levels). Products include:

Quinidex Extentabs 2933

Repaglinide (β-blockers may mask some of the manifestations of hypoglycemia; may enhance the blood-sugar-reducing effect of oral hypoglycemics). Products include:

Prandin Tablets (0.5, 1, and 2 mg) 2432

Reserpine (Co-administration of agents with B-blocking properties and a drug that can deplete catecholamines, such as reserpine, may result in hypotension and/or severe bradycardia).

No products indexed under this heading.

Rifampin (Carvedilol undergoes substantial oxidative metabolism, co-administration has resulted in decreased AUC and Cmax of carvedilol by about 70%). Products include:

Rifadin 765
Rifamate Capsules 767
Rifater Tablets 769

Rosiglitazone Maleate (β-blockers may mask some of the manifestations of hypoglycemia; may enhance the blood-sugar-reducing effect of oral hypoglycemics). Products include:

Avandia Tablets 1490

Selegiline Hydrochloride (Co-administration of agents with β-blocking properties and a drug that can deplete catecholamines, such as MAO inhibitors, may result in hypotension and/or severe bradycardia). Products include:

Eldepryl Capsules 3266

Tolazamide (B-blockers may mask some of the manifestations of hypoglycemia; may enhance the blood-sugar-reducing effect of oral hypoglycemics).

No products indexed under this heading.

Tolbutamide (B-blockers may mask some of the manifestations of hypoglycemia; may enhance the blood-sugar-reducing effect of oral hypoglycemics).

No products indexed under this heading.

Tranylcypromine Sulfate (Co-administration of agents with β-blocking properties and a drug that can deplete catecholamines, such as MAO inhibitors, may result in hypotension and/or severe bradycardia). Products include:

Parnate Tablets 1607

Troglitazone (B-blockers may mask some of the manifestations of hypoglycemia; may enhance the blood-sugar-reducing effect of oral hypoglycemics).

No products indexed under this heading.

Verapamil Hydrochloride (Co-administration has resulted in isolated cases of conduction disturbances, rarely with hemodynamic compromise). Products include:

Covera-HS Tablets 3199
Isoptin SR Tablets 467
Tarka Tablets 508
Verelan Capsules 3184
Verelan PM Capsules 3186

Food Interactions

Food, unspecified (When carvedilol is administered with food, the rate of absorption is slowed, as evidenced by a delay in the time to reach peak plasma levels, with no significant difference in extent of bioavailability; patients should be instructed to take Coreg with food in order to minimize the risk of hypotension).

COREPLEX CAPSULES

(Allium sativum, Ginkgo biloba, Herbals with Vitamins & Minerals) .... ◘796
None cited in PDR database.

CORGARD TABLETS

(Nadolol) 2245
May interact with general anesthetics, oral hypoglycemic agents, insulin, and certain other agents. Compounds in these categories include:

Acarbose (Beta-adrenergic blockade may prevent the appearance of premonitory signs and symptoms of acute hypoglycemia; hypo- or hyperglycemia may occur with concurrent use). Products include:

Precose Tablets 906

Chlorpropamide (Beta-adrenergic blockade may prevent the appearance of premonitory signs and symptoms of acute hypoglycemia; hypo- or hyperglycemia may occur with concurrent use). Products include:

Diabinese Tablets 2680

Enflurane (Co-administration with general anesthetics may exaggerate hypotension).

No products indexed under this heading.

Epinephrine (While taking beta-blocker, patients with a history of anaphylactic reaction may be unresponsive to the usual dose of epinephrine). Products include:

Epifrin Sterile Ophthalmic Solution .... ⊙235
EpiPen 1236
Primatene Mist .... ◘779
Xylocaine with Epinephrine Injection 653

Epinephrine Hydrochloride (While taking beta-blocker, patients with a history of anaphylactic reaction may be unresponsive to the usual dose of epinephrine).

No products indexed under this heading.

Glimepiride (Beta-adrenergic blockade may prevent the appearance of premonitory signs and symptoms of acute hypoglycemia; hypo- or hyperglycemia may occur with concurrent use). Products include:

Amaryl Tablets 717

Glipizide (Beta-adrenergic blockade may prevent the appearance of premonitory signs and symptoms of acute hypoglycemia; hypo- or hyperglycemia may occur with concurrent use). Products include:

Glucotrol Tablets 2692
Glucotrol XL Extended Release Tablets 2693

Glyburide (Beta-adrenergic blockade may prevent the appearance of premonitory signs and symptoms of acute hypoglycemia; hypo- or hyperglycemia may occur with concurrent use). Products include:

DiaBeta Tablets 741
Glucovance Tablets 1086

Insulin, Human, Zinc Suspension (Beta-adrenergic blockade may prevent the appearance of premonitory signs and symptoms of acute hypoglycemia; hypo- or hyperglycemia may occur with concurrent use). Products include:

Humulin L, 100 Units 1937
Humulin U, 100 Units 1943
Novolin L Human Insulin 10 ml Vials 2422

Insulin, Human NPH (Beta-adrenergic blockade may prevent the appearance of premonitory signs and symptoms of acute hypoglycemia; hypo- or hyperglycemia may occur with concurrent use). Products include:

Humulin N, 100 Units 1939
Humulin N NPH Pen 1940
Novolin N Human Insulin 10 ml Vials 2422
Novolin N PenFill 2423
Novolin N Prefilled Syringe Disposable Insulin Delivery System 2425

Insulin, Human Regular (Beta-adrenergic blockade may prevent the appearance of premonitory signs and symptoms of acute hypoglycemia; hypo- or hyperglycemia may occur with concurrent use). Products include:

Humulin R Regular (U-500) 1943
Humulin R, 100 Units 1941
Novolin R Human Insulin 10 ml Vials 2423
Novolin R PenFill 2423
Novolin R Prefilled Syringe Disposable Insulin Delivery System 2425
Velosulin BR Human Insulin 10 ml Vials 2435

Insulin, Human Regular and Human NPH Mixture (Beta-adrenergic blockade may prevent the appearance of premonitory signs and symptoms of acute hypoglycemia; hypo- or hyperglycemia may occur with concurrent use). Products include:

Humulin 50/50, 100 Units 1934
Humulin 70/30, 100 Units 1935
Humulin 70/30 Pen 1936
Novolin 70/30 Human Insulin 10 ml Vials 2421
Novolin 70/30 PenFill 2423
Novolin 70/30 Prefilled Disposable Insulin Delivery System 2425

Insulin, NPH (Beta-adrenergic blockade may prevent the appearance of premonitory signs and symp-

toms of acute hypoglycemia; hypo- or hyperglycemia may occur with concurrent use). Products include:
Iletin II, NPH (Pork), 100 Units 1946

Insulin, Regular (Beta-adrenergic blockade may prevent the appearance of premonitory signs and symptoms of acute hypoglycemia; hypo- or hyperglycemia may occur with concurrent use). Products include:
Iletin II, Regular (Pork), 100 Units ... 1947

Insulin, Zinc Crystals (Beta-adrenergic blockade may prevent the appearance of premonitory signs and symptoms of acute hypoglycemia; hypo- or hyperglycemia may occur with concurrent use).
No products indexed under this heading.

Insulin, Zinc Suspension (Beta-adrenergic blockade may prevent the appearance of premonitory signs and symptoms of acute hypoglycemia; hypo- or hyperglycemia may occur with concurrent use). Products include:
Iletin II, Lente (Pork), 100 Units 1945

Insulin Aspart, Human Regular (Beta-adrenergic blockade may prevent the appearance of premonitory signs and symptoms of acute hypoglycemia; hypo- or hyperglycemia may occur with concurrent use).
No products indexed under this heading.

Insulin glargine (Beta-adrenergic blockade may prevent the appearance of premonitory signs and symptoms of acute hypoglycemia; hypo- or hyperglycemia may occur with concurrent use). Products include:
Lantus Injection 742

Insulin Lispro, Human (Beta-adrenergic blockade may prevent the appearance of premonitory signs and symptoms of acute hypoglycemia; hypo- or hyperglycemia may occur with concurrent use). Products include:
Humalog 1926
Humalog Mix 75/25 Pen 1928

Insulin Lispro Protamine, Human (Beta-adrenergic blockade may prevent the appearance of premonitory signs and symptoms of acute hypoglycemia; hypo- or hyperglycemia may occur with concurrent use). Products include:
Humalog Mix 75/25 Pen 1928

Isoflurane (Co-administration with general anesthetics may exaggerate hypotension).
No products indexed under this heading.

Ketamine Hydrochloride (Co-administration with general anesthetics may exaggerate hypotension).
No products indexed under this heading.

Metformin Hydrochloride (Beta-adrenergic blockade may prevent the appearance of premonitory signs and symptoms of acute hypoglycemia; hypo- or hyperglycemia may occur with concurrent use). Products include:
Glucophage Tablets 1080
Glucophage XR Tablets 1080
Glucovance Tablets 1086

Methohexital Sodium (Co-administration with general anesthetics may exaggerate hypotension). Products include:
Brevital Sodium for Injection, USP .. 1815

Methoxyflurane (Co-administration with general anesthetics may exaggerate hypotension).
No products indexed under this heading.

Miglitol (Beta-adrenergic blockade may prevent the appearance of premonitory signs and symptoms of acute hypoglycemia; hypo- or hyperglycemia may occur with concurrent use). Products include:
Glyset Tablets 2821

Pioglitazone Hydrochloride (Beta-adrenergic blockade may prevent the appearance of premonitory signs and symptoms of acute hypoglycemia; hypo- or hyperglycemia may occur with concurrent use). Products include:
Actos Tablets 3275

Propofol (Co-administration with general anesthetics may exaggerate hypotension). Products include:
Diprivan Injectable Emulsion 667

Repaglinide (Beta-adrenergic blockade may prevent the appearance of premonitory signs and symptoms of acute hypoglycemia; hypo- or hyperglycemia may occur with concurrent use). Products include:
Prandin Tablets (0.5, 1, and 2 mg) 2432

Reserpine (Co-administration may result in additive effect, such as hypotension, and/or excessive bradycardia, vertigo, syncope, and postural hypotension).
No products indexed under this heading.

Rosiglitazone Maleate (Beta-adrenergic blockade may prevent the appearance of premonitory signs and symptoms of acute hypoglycemia; hypo- or hyperglycemia may occur with concurrent use). Products include:
Avandia Tablets 1490

Sevoflurane (Co-administration with general anesthetics may exaggerate hypotension).
No products indexed under this heading.

Tolazamide (Beta-adrenergic blockade may prevent the appearance of premonitory signs and symptoms of acute hypoglycemia; hypo- or hyperglycemia may occur with concurrent use).
No products indexed under this heading.

Tolbutamide (Beta-adrenergic blockade may prevent the appearance of premonitory signs and symptoms of acute hypoglycemia; hypo- or hyperglycemia may occur with concurrent use).
No products indexed under this heading.

Troglitazone (Beta-adrenergic blockade may prevent the appearance of premonitory signs and symptoms of acute hypoglycemia; hypo- or hyperglycemia may occur with concurrent use).
No products indexed under this heading.

CORICIDIN 'D' COLD, FLU & SINUS TABLETS

(Acetaminophen, Chlorpheniramine Maleate, Pseudoephedrine Sulfate)............... 737
May interact with hypnotics and sedatives, monoamine oxidase inhibitors, tranquilizers, and certain other agents. Compounds in these categories include:

Alprazolam (May increase drowsiness effect). Products include:
Xanax Tablets 2865

Buspirone Hydrochloride (May increase drowsiness effect).
No products indexed under this heading.

Chlordiazepoxide (May increase drowsiness effect). Products include:
Limbitrol 1738

Chlordiazepoxide Hydrochloride (May increase drowsiness effect). Products include:
Librium Capsules 1736
Librium for Injection 1737

Chlorpromazine (May increase drowsiness effect). Products include:
Thorazine Suppositories 1656

Chlorpromazine Hydrochloride (May increase drowsiness effect). Products include:
Thorazine 1656

Chlorprothixene (May increase drowsiness effect).
No products indexed under this heading.

Chlorprothixene Hydrochloride (May increase drowsiness effect).
No products indexed under this heading.

Clorazepate Dipotassium (May increase drowsiness effect). Products include:
Tranxene 511

Diazepam (May increase drowsiness effect). Products include:
Valium Injectable 3026
Valium Tablets 3047

Droperidol (May increase drowsiness effect).
No products indexed under this heading.

Estazolam (May increase drowsiness effect). Products include:
ProSom Tablets 500

Ethchlorvynol (May increase drowsiness effect).
No products indexed under this heading.

Ethinamate (May increase drowsiness effect).
No products indexed under this heading.

Fluphenazine Decanoate (May increase drowsiness effect).
No products indexed under this heading.

Fluphenazine Enanthate (May increase drowsiness effect).
No products indexed under this heading.

Fluphenazine Hydrochloride (May increase drowsiness effect).
No products indexed under this heading.

Flurazepam Hydrochloride (May increase drowsiness effect).
No products indexed under this heading.

Glutethimide (May increase drowsiness effect).
No products indexed under this heading.

Haloperidol (May increase drowsiness effect). Products include:
Haldol Injection, Tablets and Concentrate 2533

Haloperidol Decanoate (May increase drowsiness effect). Products include:
Haldol Decanoate 2535

Hydroxyzine Hydrochloride (May increase drowsiness effect). Products include:
Atarax Tablets & Syrup 2667
Vistaril Intramuscular Solution 2738

Isocarboxazid (Concurrent and/or sequential use with MAO inhibitors is not recommended).
No products indexed under this heading.

Lorazepam (May increase drowsiness effect). Products include:
Ativan Injection 3478
Ativan Tablets 3482

Loxapine Hydrochloride (May increase drowsiness effect).
No products indexed under this heading.

Loxapine Succinate (May increase drowsiness effect). Products include:
Loxitane Capsules 3398

Meprobamate (May increase drowsiness effect). Products include:
Miltown Tablets 3349

Mesoridazine Besylate (May increase drowsiness effect). Products include:
Serentil 1057

Midazolam Hydrochloride (May increase drowsiness effect). Products include:
Versed Injection 3027
Versed Syrup 3033

Moclobemide (Concurrent and/or sequential use with MAO inhibitors is not recommended).
No products indexed under this heading.

Molindone Hydrochloride (May increase drowsiness effect). Products include:
Moban 1320

Oxazepam (May increase drowsiness effect).
No products indexed under this heading.

Pargyline Hydrochloride (Concurrent and/or sequential use with MAO inhibitors is not recommended).
No products indexed under this heading.

Perphenazine (May increase drowsiness effect). Products include:
Etrafon 3115
Trilafon 3160

Phenelzine Sulfate (Concurrent and/or sequential use with MAO inhibitors is not recommended). Products include:
Nardil Tablets 2653

Phenylpropanolamine Containing Anorectics (Concurrent use with appetite-controlling medication containing phenylpropanolamine is not recommended).
No products indexed under this heading.

Prazepam (May increase drowsiness effect).
No products indexed under this heading.

Procarbazine Hydrochloride (Concurrent and/or sequential use with MAO inhibitors is not recommended). Products include:
Matulane Capsules 3246

Prochlorperazine (May increase drowsiness effect). Products include:
Compazine 1505

Promethazine Hydrochloride (May increase drowsiness effect). Products include:
Mepergan Injection 3539
Phenergan Injection 3553
Phenergan 3556
Phenergan Syrup 3554
Phenergan with Codeine Syrup 3557
Phenergan with Dextromethorphan Syrup 3559
Phenergan VC Syrup 3560
Phenergan VC with Codeine Syrup .. 3561

Propofol (May increase drowsiness effect). Products include:
Diprivan Injectable Emulsion 667

Quazepam (May increase drowsiness effect).
No products indexed under this heading.

Secobarbital Sodium (May increase drowsiness effect).
No products indexed under this heading.

Selegiline Hydrochloride (Concurrent and/or sequential use with MAO inhibitors is not recommended). Products include:
Eldepryl Capsules 3266

Temazepam (May increase drowsiness effect).
No products indexed under this heading.

Thioridazine Hydrochloride (May increase drowsiness effect). Products include:
Thioridazine Hydrochloride Tablets 2289

Thiothixene (May increase drowsiness effect). Products include:
Navane Capsules 2701
Thiothixene Capsules 2290

Tranylcypromine Sulfate (Concurrent and/or sequential use with MAO inhibitors is not recommended). Products include:
- Parnate Tablets ... 1607

Triazolam (May increase drowsiness effect). Products include:
- Halcion Tablets ... 2823

Trifluoperazine Hydrochloride (May increase drowsiness effect). Products include:
- Stelazine ... 1640

Zaleplon (May increase drowsiness effect). Products include:
- Sonata Capsules ... 3591

Zolpidem Tartrate (May increase drowsiness effect). Products include:
- Ambien Tablets ... 3191

Food Interactions

Alcohol (May increase drowsiness effect; patients consuming 3 or more alcoholic drinks per day should consult their physician on when and how they should take this medication).

CORICIDIN HBP COLD & FLU TABLETS

(Acetaminophen, Chlorpheniramine Maleate) ... ▣738

See Coricidin HBP Maximum Strength Flu Tablets

CORICIDIN HBP COUGH & COLD TABLETS

(Chlorpheniramine Maleate, Dextromethorphan Hydrobromide) ... ▣738

See Coricidin HBP Maximum Strength Flu Tablets

CORICIDIN HBP MAXIMUM STRENGTH FLU TABLETS

(Acetaminophen, Chlorpheniramine Maleate, Dextromethorphan Hydrobromide) ... ▣738

May interact with hypnotics and sedatives, monoamine oxidase inhibitors, tranquilizers, and certain other agents. Compounds in these categories include:

Alprazolam (May increase drowsiness effect). Products include:
- Xanax Tablets ... 2865

Buspirone Hydrochloride (May increase drowsiness effect).
- No products indexed under this heading.

Chlordiazepoxide (May increase drowsiness effect). Products include:
- Limbitrol ... 1738

Chlordiazepoxide Hydrochloride (May increase drowsiness effect). Products include:
- Librium Capsules ... 1736
- Librium for Injection ... 1737

Chlorpromazine (May increase drowsiness effect). Products include:
- Thorazine Suppositories ... 1656

Chlorpromazine Hydrochloride (May increase drowsiness effect). Products include:
- Thorazine ... 1656

Chlorprothixene (May increase drowsiness effect).
- No products indexed under this heading.

Chlorprothixene Hydrochloride (May increase drowsiness effect).
- No products indexed under this heading.

Clorazepate Dipotassium (May increase drowsiness effect). Products include:
- Tranxene ... 511

Diazepam (May increase drowsiness effect). Products include:
- Valium Injectable ... 3026
- Valium Tablets ... 3047

Droperidol (May increase drowsiness effect).
- No products indexed under this heading.

Estazolam (May increase drowsiness effect). Products include:
- ProSom Tablets ... 500

Ethchlorvynol (May increase drowsiness effect).
- No products indexed under this heading.

Ethinamate (May increase drowsiness effect).
- No products indexed under this heading.

Fluphenazine Decanoate (May increase drowsiness effect).
- No products indexed under this heading.

Fluphenazine Enanthate (May increase drowsiness effect).
- No products indexed under this heading.

Fluphenazine Hydrochloride (May increase drowsiness effect).
- No products indexed under this heading.

Flurazepam Hydrochloride (May increase drowsiness effect).
- No products indexed under this heading.

Glutethimide (May increase drowsiness effect).
- No products indexed under this heading.

Haloperidol (May increase drowsiness effect). Products include:
- Haldol Injection, Tablets and Concentrate ... 2533

Haloperidol Decanoate (May increase drowsiness effect). Products include:
- Haldol Decanoate ... 2535

Hydroxyzine Hydrochloride (May increase drowsiness effect). Products include:
- Atarax Tablets & Syrup ... 2667
- Vistaril Intramuscular Solution ... 2738

Isocarboxazid (Concurrent and/or sequential use with MAO inhibitors is not recommended).
- No products indexed under this heading.

Lorazepam (May increase drowsiness effect). Products include:
- Ativan Injection ... 3478
- Ativan Tablets ... 3482

Loxapine Hydrochloride (May increase drowsiness effect).
- No products indexed under this heading.

Loxapine Succinate (May increase drowsiness effect). Products include:
- Loxitane Capsules ... 3398

Meprobamate (May increase drowsiness effect). Products include:
- Miltown Tablets ... 3349

Mesoridazine Besylate (May increase drowsiness effect). Products include:
- Serentil ... 1057

Midazolam Hydrochloride (May increase drowsiness effect). Products include:
- Versed Injection ... 3027
- Versed Syrup ... 3033

Moclobemide (Concurrent and/or sequential use with MAO inhibitors is not recommended).
- No products indexed under this heading.

Molindone Hydrochloride (May increase drowsiness effect). Products include:
- Moban ... 1320

Oxazepam (May increase drowsiness effect).
- No products indexed under this heading.

Pargyline Hydrochloride (Concurrent and/or sequential use with MAO inhibitors is not recommended).
- No products indexed under this heading.

Perphenazine (May increase drowsiness effect). Products include:
- Etrafon ... 3115
- Trilafon ... 3160

Phenelzine Sulfate (Concurrent and/or sequential use with MAO inhibitors is not recommended). Products include:
- Nardil Tablets ... 2653

Prazepam (May increase drowsiness effect).
- No products indexed under this heading.

Procarbazine Hydrochloride (Concurrent and/or sequential use with MAO inhibitors is not recommended). Products include:
- Matulane Capsules ... 3246

Prochlorperazine (May increase drowsiness effect). Products include:
- Compazine ... 1505

Promethazine Hydrochloride (May increase drowsiness effect). Products include:
- Mepergan Injection ... 3539
- Phenergan Injection ... 3553
- Phenergan ... 3556
- Phenergan Syrup ... 3554
- Phenergan with Codeine Syrup ... 3557
- Phenergan with Dextromethorphan Syrup ... 3559
- Phenergan VC Syrup ... 3560
- Phenergan VC with Codeine Syrup ... 3561

Propofol (May increase drowsiness effect). Products include:
- Diprivan Injectable Emulsion ... 667

Quazepam (May increase drowsiness effect).
- No products indexed under this heading.

Secobarbital Sodium (May increase drowsiness effect).
- No products indexed under this heading.

Selegiline Hydrochloride (Concurrent and/or sequential use with MAO inhibitors is not recommended). Products include:
- Eldepryl Capsules ... 3266

Temazepam (May increase drowsiness effect).
- No products indexed under this heading.

Thioridazine Hydrochloride (May increase drowsiness effect). Products include:
- Thioridazine Hydrochloride Tablets ... 2289

Thiothixene (May increase drowsiness effect). Products include:
- Navane Capsules ... 2701
- Thiothixene Capsules ... 2290

Tranylcypromine Sulfate (Concurrent and/or sequential use with MAO inhibitors is not recommended). Products include:
- Parnate Tablets ... 1607

Triazolam (May increase drowsiness effect). Products include:
- Halcion Tablets ... 2823

Trifluoperazine Hydrochloride (May increase drowsiness effect). Products include:
- Stelazine ... 1640

Zaleplon (May increase drowsiness effect). Products include:
- Sonata Capsules ... 3591

Zolpidem Tartrate (May increase drowsiness effect). Products include:
- Ambien Tablets ... 3191

Food Interactions

Alcohol (Chronic heavy alcohol users, 3 or more drinks per day, should consult their physician for advice on when and how they should take pain relievers/fever reducers including acetaminophen; increases drowsiness effect).

CORICIDIN HBP NIGHT-TIME COLD & FLU TABLETS

(Acetaminophen, Diphenhydramine Hydrochloride) ... ▣738

See Coricidin HBP Maximum Strength Flu Tablets

CORLOPAM INJECTION

(Fenoldopam Mesylate) ... 412

None cited in PDR database.

CORMAX CREAM

(Clobetasol Propionate) ... 2440

None cited in PDR database.

CORMAX OINTMENT

(Clobetasol Propionate) ... 2440

None cited in PDR database.

CORMAX SCALP APPLICATION

(Clobetasol Propionate) ... 2441

None cited in PDR database.

CORRECTOL LAXATIVE TABLETS AND CAPLETS

(Bisacodyl) ... ▣739

May interact with antacids and certain other agents. Compounds in these categories include:

Aluminum Carbonate (Concurrent use within one hour after taking antacid is not recommended).
- No products indexed under this heading.

Aluminum Hydroxide (Concurrent use within one hour after taking antacid is not recommended). Products include:
- Amphojel Suspension (Mint Flavor) ... ▣789
- Gaviscon Extra Strength Liquid ... ▣751
- Gaviscon Extra Strength Tablets ... ▣751
- Gaviscon Regular Strength Liquid ... ▣751
- Gaviscon Regular Strength Tablets ... ▣750
- Maalox Antacid/Anti-Gas Oral Suspension ... ▣673
- Maalox Max Maximum Strength Antacid/Anti-Gas Liquid ... 2300
- Maalox Regular Strength Antacid/Antigas Liquid ... 2300
- Mylanta ... 1813
- Vanquish Caplets ... ▣617

Magaldrate (Concurrent use within one hour after taking antacid is not recommended).
- No products indexed under this heading.

Magnesium Hydroxide (Concurrent use within one hour after taking antacid is not recommended). Products include:
- Ex•Lax Milk of Magnesia Liquid ... ▣670
- Maalox Antacid/Anti-Gas Oral Suspension ... ▣673
- Maalox Max Maximum Strength Antacid/Anti-Gas Liquid ... 2300
- Maalox Regular Strength Antacid/Antigas Liquid ... 2300
- Mylanta Fast-Acting ... 1813
- Mylanta ... 1813
- Pepcid Complete Chewable Tablets ... 1815
- Phillips' Chewable Tablets ... ▣615
- Phillips' Milk of Magnesia Liquid (Original, Cherry, & Mint) ... ▣616
- Rolaids Tablets ... ▣706
- Extra Strength Rolaids Tablets ... ▣706
- Vanquish Caplets ... ▣617

Magnesium Oxide (Concurrent use within one hour after taking antacid is not recommended). Products include:
- Beelith Tablets ... 946
- Mag-Ox 400 Tablets ... 1024
- Uro-Mag Capsules ... 1024

Sodium Bicarbonate (Concurrent use within one hour after taking antacid is not recommended). Products include:
- Alka-Seltzer ... ▣603
- Alka-Seltzer Lemon Lime Antacid and Pain Reliever Effervescent Tablets ... ▣603
- Alka-Seltzer Extra Strength Antacid and Pain Reliever Effervescent Tablets ... ▣603
- Alka-Seltzer Heartburn Relief Tablets ... ▣604
- Ceo-Two Evacuant Suppository ... ▣618
- Colyte with Flavor Packs for Oral Solution ... 3170
- GoLYTELY and Pineapple Flavor GoLYTELY for Oral Solution ... 1068

NuLYTELY, Cherry Flavor, Lemon-Lime Flavor, and Orange Flavor NuLYTELY for Oral Solution ... 1068

Food Interactions

Dairy products (Concurrent use within one hour after taking milk is not recommended).

CORTAID INTENSIVE THERAPY CREAM
(Hydrocortisone) ... ■717
None cited in PDR database.

CORTAID MAXIMUM STRENGTH CREAM
(Hydrocortisone) ... ■717
None cited in PDR database.

CORTAID MAXIMUM STRENGTH OINTMENT
(Hydrocortisone Acetate) ... ■717
None cited in PDR database.

CORTAID SENSITIVE SKIN CREAM
(Hydrocortisone Acetate) ... ■717
None cited in PDR database.

CORTIFOAM RECTAL FOAM
(Hydrocortisone Acetate) ... 3170
None cited in PDR database.

CORTISPORIN OPHTHALMIC SUSPENSION STERILE
(Hydrocortisone, Neomycin Sulfate, Polymyxin B Sulfate) ... ⊙297
None cited in PDR database.

CORTISPORIN-TC OTIC SUSPENSION
(Colistin Sulfate, Hydrocortisone Acetate, Neomycin Sulfate, Thonzonium Bromide) ... 2246
None cited in PDR database.

CORTIZONE•5 CREME
(Hydrocortisone) ... ■699
None cited in PDR database.

CORTIZONE•5 OINTMENT
(Hydrocortisone) ... ■699
None cited in PDR database.

CORTIZONE•10 CREME
(Hydrocortisone) ... ■699
None cited in PDR database.

CORTIZONE•10 OINTMENT
(Hydrocortisone) ... ■699
None cited in PDR database.

CORTIZONE•10 PLUS CREME
(Hydrocortisone) ... ■700
None cited in PDR database.

CORTIZONE•10 QUICK SHOT SPRAY
(Hydrocortisone) ... ■699
None cited in PDR database.

CORTIZONE FOR KIDS CREME
(Hydrocortisone) ... ■699
None cited in PDR database.

CORTONE ACETATE INJECTABLE SUSPENSION
(Cortisone Acetate) ... 2059
May interact with oral anticoagulants, oral hypoglycemic agents, insulin, phenytoin, potassium-depleting diuretics, and certain other agents. Compounds in these categories include:

Acarbose (Potential for increased requirements of oral hypoglycemic agents). Products include:
Precose Tablets ... 906

Aspirin (Aspirin should be used cautiously in conjunction with corticosteroids in hypoprothrombinemia). Products include:
Aggrenox Capsules ... 1026
Alka-Seltzer ... ■603
Alka-Seltzer Lemon Lime Antacid and Pain Reliever Effervescent Tablets ... ■603
Alka-Seltzer Extra Strength Antacid and Pain Reliever Effervescent Tablets ... ■603
Alka-Seltzer PM Effervescent Tablets ... ■605
Genuine Bayer Tablets, Caplets and Gelcaps ... ■606
Extra Strength Bayer Caplets and Gelcaps ... ■610
Aspirin Regimen Bayer Children's Chewable Tablets (Orange or Cherry Flavored) ... ■607
Bayer, Aspirin Regimen ... ■606
Aspirin Regimen Bayer 81 mg Caplets with Calcium ... ■607
Genuine Bayer Professional Labeling (Aspirin Regimen Bayer) ... ■608
Extra Strength Bayer Arthritis Caplets ... ■610
Extra Strength Bayer Plus Caplets ... ■610
Extra Strength Bayer PM Caplets ... ■611
BC Powder ... ■619
BC Allergy Sinus Cold Powder ... ■619
Arthritis Strength BC Powder ... ■619
BC Sinus Cold Powder ... ■619
Darvon Compound-65 Pulvules ... 1910
Ecotrin Enteric Coated Aspirin Low, Regular and Maximum Strength Tablets ... 1715
Excedrin Extra-Strength Tablets, Caplets, and Geltabs ... ■629
Excedrin Migraine ... 1070
Goody's Body Pain Formula Powder ... ■620
Goody's Extra Strength Headache Powder ... ■620
Goody's Extra Strength Pain Relief Tablets ... ■620
Percodan Tablets ... 1327
Robaxisal Tablets ... 2939
Soma Compound Tablets ... 3354
Soma Compound w/Codeine Tablets ... 3355
Vanquish Caplets ... ■617

Bendroflumethiazide (Co-administration may result in hypokalemia). Products include:
Corzide 40/5 Tablets ... 2247
Corzide 80/5 Tablets ... 2247

Bumetanide (Co-administration may result in hypokalemia).
No products indexed under this heading.

Chlorothiazide (Co-administration may result in hypokalemia). Products include:
Aldoclor Tablets ... 2035
Diuril Oral ... 2087

Chlorothiazide Sodium (Co-administration may result in hypokalemia). Products include:
Diuril Sodium Intravenous ... 2086

Chlorpropamide (Potential for increased requirements of oral hypoglycemic agents). Products include:
Diabinese Tablets ... 2680

Dicumarol (Potential for altered response to coumarin anticoagulants).
No products indexed under this heading.

Ephedrine Hydrochloride (Co-administration may enhance the metabolic clearance of corticosteroids, resulting in decreased blood levels and lessened physiologic activity; corticosteroid dosage may need to be adjusted). Products include:
Primatene Tablets ... ■780

Ephedrine Sulfate (Co-administration may enhance the metabolic clearance of corticosteroids, resulting in decreased blood levels and lessened physiologic activity; corticosteroid dosage may need to be adjusted).
No products indexed under this heading.

Ephedrine Tannate (Co-administration may enhance the metabolic clearance of corticosteroids, resulting in decreased blood levels and lessened physiologic activity; corticosteroid dosage may need to be adjusted). Products include:
Rynatuss Pediatric Suspension ... 3353
Rynatuss Tablets ... 3353

Ethacrynic Acid (Co-administration may result in hypokalemia). Products include:
Edecrin Tablets ... 2091

Fosphenytoin Sodium (Co-administration may enhance the metabolic clearance of corticosteroids, resulting in decreased blood levels and lessened physiologic activity; corticosteroid dosage may need to be adjusted). Products include:
Cerebyx Injection ... 2619

Furosemide (Co-administration may result in hypokalemia). Products include:
Furosemide Tablets ... 2284

Glimepiride (Potential for increased requirements of oral hypoglycemic agents). Products include:
Amaryl Tablets ... 717

Glipizide (Potential for increased requirements of oral hypoglycemic agents). Products include:
Glucotrol Tablets ... 2692
Glucotrol XL Extended Release Tablets ... 2693

Glyburide (Potential for increased requirements of oral hypoglycemic agents). Products include:
DiaBeta Tablets ... 741
Glucovance Tablets ... 1086

Hydrochlorothiazide (Co-administration may result in hypokalemia). Products include:
Accuretic Tablets ... 2614
Aldoril Tablets ... 2039
Atacand HCT Tablets ... 597
Avalide Tablets ... 1070
Diovan HCT Tablets ... 2338
Dyazide Capsules ... 1515
HydroDIURIL Tablets ... 2108
Hyzaar ... 2109
Inderide Tablets ... 3517
Inderide LA Long-Acting Capsules ... 3519
Lotensin HCT Tablets ... 2367
Maxzide ... 1008
Micardis HCT Tablets ... 1051
Microzide Capsules ... 3414
Moduretic Tablets ... 2138
Monopril HCT ... 1094
Prinzide Tablets ... 2168
Timolide Tablets ... 2187
Uniretic Tablets ... 3178
Vaseretic Tablets ... 2204
Zestoretic Tablets ... 695
Ziac Tablets ... 1887

Hydroflumethiazide (Co-administration may result in hypokalemia). Products include:
Diucardin Tablets ... 3494

Insulin, Human, Zinc Suspension (Potential for increased requirements of insulin). Products include:
Humulin L, 100 Units ... 1937
Humulin U, 100 Units ... 1943
Novolin L Human Insulin 10 ml Vials ... 2422

Insulin, Human NPH (Potential for increased requirements of insulin). Products include:
Humulin N, 100 Units ... 1939
Humulin N NPH Pen ... 1940
Novolin N Human Insulin 10 ml Vials ... 2422
Novolin N PenFill ... 2423
Novolin N Prefilled Syringe Disposable Insulin Delivery System ... 2425

Insulin, Human Regular (Potential for increased requirements of insulin). Products include:
Humulin R Regular (U-500) ... 1943
Humulin R, 100 Units ... 1941
Novolin R Human Insulin 10 ml Vials ... 2423
Novolin R PenFill ... 2423
Novolin R Prefilled Syringe Disposable Insulin Delivery System ... 2425
Velosulin BR Human Insulin 10 ml Vials ... 2435

Insulin, Human Regular and Human NPH Mixture (Potential for increased requirements of insulin). Products include:
Humulin 50/50, 100 Units ... 1934
Humulin 70/30, 100 Units ... 1935
Humulin 70/30 Pen ... 1936
Novolin 70/30 Human Insulin 10 ml Vials ... 2421
Novolin 70/30 PenFill ... 2423
Novolin 70/30 Prefilled Disposable Insulin Delivery System ... 2425

Insulin, NPH (Potential for increased requirements of insulin). Products include:
Iletin II, NPH (Pork), 100 Units ... 1946

Insulin, Regular (Potential for increased requirements of insulin). Products include:
Iletin II, Regular (Pork), 100 Units ... 1947

Insulin, Zinc Crystals (Potential for increased requirements of insulin).
No products indexed under this heading.

Insulin, Zinc Suspension (Potential for increased requirements of insulin). Products include:
Iletin II, Lente (Pork), 100 Units ... 1945

Insulin Aspart, Human Regular (Potential for increased requirements of insulin).
No products indexed under this heading.

Insulin glargine (Potential for increased requirements of insulin). Products include:
Lantus Injection ... 742

Insulin Lispro, Human (Potential for increased requirements of insulin). Products include:
Humalog ... 1926
Humalog Mix 75/25 Pen ... 1928

Insulin Lispro Protamine, Human (Potential for increased requirements of insulin). Products include:
Humalog Mix 75/25 Pen ... 1928

Live Virus Vaccines (Co-administration is contraindicated in patients receiving immunosuppresive doses of corticosteroids).

Metformin Hydrochloride (Potential for increased requirements of oral hypoglycemic agents). Products include:
Glucophage Tablets ... 1080
Glucophage XR Tablets ... 1080
Glucovance Tablets ... 1086

Methyclothiazide (Co-administration may result in hypokalemia).
No products indexed under this heading.

Miglitol (Potential for increased requirements of oral hypoglycemic agents). Products include:
Glyset Tablets ... 2821

Phenobarbital (Co-administration may enhance the metabolic clearance of corticosteroids, resulting in decreased blood levels and lessened physiologic activity; corticosteroid dosage may need to be adjusted). Products include:
Arco-Lase Plus Tablets ... 592
Donnatal ... 2929
Donnatal Extentabs ... 2930

Phenytoin (Co-administration may enhance the metabolic clearance of corticosteroids, resulting in decreased blood levels and lessened physiologic activity; corticosteroid dosage may need to be adjusted). Products include:
Dilantin Infatabs ... 2624
Dilantin-125 Oral Suspension ... 2625

Phenytoin Sodium (Co-administration may enhance the metabolic clearance of corticosteroids, resulting in decreased blood levels and lessened physiologic activity; corticosteroid dosage may need to be adjusted). Products include:

Dilantin Kapseals 2622

Pioglitazone Hydrochloride (Potential for increased requirements of oral hypoglycemic agents). Products include:
Actos Tablets 3275

Polythiazide (Co-administration may result in hypokalemia). Products include:
Minizide Capsules 2700
Renese Tablets 2712

Repaglinide (Potential for increased requirements of oral hypoglycemic agents). Products include:
Prandin Tablets (0.5, 1, and 2 mg) 2432

Rifampin (Co-adminstration may enhance the metabolic clearance of corticosteroids, resulting in decreased blood levels and lessened physiologic activity; corticosteroid dosage may need to be adjusted). Products include:
Rifadin 765
Rifamate Capsules 767
Rifater Tablets 769

Rosiglitazone Maleate (Potential for increased requirements of oral hypoglycemic agents). Products include:
Avandia Tablets 1490

Tolazamide (Potential for increased requirements of oral hypoglycemic agents).
No products indexed under this heading.

Tolbutamide (Potential for increased requirements of oral hypoglycemic agents).
No products indexed under this heading.

Torsemide (Co-administration may result in hypokalemia). Products include:
Demadex Tablets and Injection 2965

Troglitazone (Potential for increased requirements of oral hypoglycemic agents).
No products indexed under this heading.

Warfarin Sodium (Potential for altered response to coumarin anticoagulants). Products include:
Coumadin for Injection 1243
Coumadin Tablets 1243
Warfarin Sodium Tablets, USP 3302

CORTONE ACETATE TABLETS

(Cortisone Acetate) 2061

May interact with oral anticoagulants, oral hypoglycemic agents, insulin, phenytoin, potassium-depleting diuretics, and certain other agents. Compounds in these categories include:

Acarbose (Potential for increased requirements of oral hypoglycemic agents). Products include:
Precose Tablets 906

Aspirin (Aspirin should be used cautiously in conjunction with corticosteroids in hypoprothrombinemia). Products include:
Aggrenox Capsules 1026
Alka-Seltzer .... ■603
Alka-Seltzer Lemon Lime Antacid and Pain Reliever Effervescent Tablets .... ■603
Alka-Seltzer Extra Strength Antacid and Pain Reliever Effervescent Tablets .... ■603
Alka-Seltzer PM Effervescent Tablets .... ■605
Genuine Bayer Tablets, Caplets and Gelcaps .... ■606
Extra Strength Bayer Caplets and Gelcaps .... ■610
Aspirin Regimen Bayer Children's Chewable Tablets (Orange or Cherry Flavored) .... ■607
Bayer, Aspirin Regimen .... ■606
Aspirin Regimen Bayer 81 mg Caplets with Calcium .... ■607
Genuine Bayer Professional Labeling (Aspirin Regimen Bayer) .... ■608
Extra Strength Bayer Arthritis Caplets .... ■610
Extra Strength Bayer Plus Caplets .... ■610
Extra Strength Bayer PM Caplets .. ■611
BC Powder .... ■619
BC Allergy Sinus Cold Powder ...... ■619
Arthritis Strength BC Powder .... ■619
BC Sinus Cold Powder .... ■619
Darvon Compound-65 Pulvules 1910
Ecotrin Enteric Coated Aspirin Low, Regular and Maximum Strength Tablets 1715
Excedrin Extra-Strength Tablets, Caplets, and Geltabs .... ■629
Excedrin Migraine 1070
Goody's Body Pain Formula Powder .... ■620
Goody's Extra Strength Headache Powder .... ■620
Goody's Extra Strength Pain Relief Tablets .... ■620
Percodan Tablets 1327
Robaxisal Tablets 2939
Soma Compound Tablets 3354
Soma Compound w/Codeine Tablets 3355
Vanquish Caplets .... ■617

Bendroflumethiazide (Co-administration may result in hypokalemia). Products include:
Corzide 40/5 Tablets 2247
Corzide 80/5 Tablets 2247

Bumetanide (Co-administration may result in hypokalemia).
No products indexed under this heading.

Chlorothiazide (Co-administration may result in hypokalemia). Products include:
Aldoclor Tablets 2035
Diuril Oral 2087

Chlorothiazide Sodium (Co-administration may result in hypokalemia). Products include:
Diuril Sodium Intravenous 2086

Chlorpropamide (Potential for increased requirements of oral hypoglycemic agents). Products include:
Diabinese Tablets 2680

Dicumarol (Potential for altered response to coumarin anticoagulants).
No products indexed under this heading.

Ephedrine Hydrochloride (Co-administration may enhance the metabolic clearance of corticosteroids, resulting in decreased blood levels and lessened physiologic activity; corticosteroid dosage may need to be adjusted). Products include:
Primatene Tablets .... ■780

Ephedrine Sulfate (Co-administration may enhance the metabolic clearance of corticosteroids, resulting in decreased blood levels and lessened physiologic activity; corticosteroid dosage may need to be adjusted).
No products indexed under this heading.

Ephedrine Tannate (Co-administration may enhance the metabolic clearance of corticosteroids, resulting in decreased blood levels and lessened physiologic activity; corticosteroid dosage may need to be adjusted). Products include:
Rynatuss Pediatric Suspension 3353
Rynatuss Tablets 3353

Ethacrynic Acid (Co-administration may result in hypokalemia). Products include:
Edecrin Tablets 2091

Fosphenytoin Sodium (Co-administration may enhance the metabolic clearance of corticosteroids, resulting in decreased blood levels and lessened physiologic activity; corticosteroid dosage may need to be adjusted). Products include:
Cerebyx Injection 2619

Furosemide (Co-administration may result in hypokalemia). Products include:
Furosemide Tablets 2284

Glimepiride (Potential for increased requirements of oral hypoglycemic agents). Products include:
Amaryl Tablets 717

Glipizide (Potential for increased requirements of oral hypoglycemic agents). Products include:
Glucotrol Tablets 2692
Glucotrol XL Extended Release Tablets 2693

Glyburide (Potential for increased requirements of oral hypoglycemic agents). Products include:
DiaBeta Tablets 741
Glucovance Tablets 1086

Hydrochlorothiazide (Co-administration may result in hypokalemia). Products include:
Accuretic Tablets 2614
Aldoril Tablets 2039
Atacand HCT Tablets 597
Avalide Tablets 1070
Diovan HCT Tablets 2338
Dyazide Capsules 1515
HydroDIURIL Tablets 2108
Hyzaar 2109
Inderide Tablets 3517
Inderide LA Long-Acting Capsules .. 3519
Lotensin HCT Tablets 2367
Maxzide 1008
Micardis HCT Tablets 1051
Microzide Capsules 3414
Moduretic Tablets 2138
Monopril HCT 1094
Prinzide Tablets 2168
Timolide Tablets 2187
Uniretic Tablets 3178
Vaseretic Tablets 2204
Zestoretic Tablets 695
Ziac Tablets 1887

Hydroflumethiazide (Co-administration may result in hypokalemia). Products include:
Diucardin Tablets 3494

Insulin, Human, Zinc Suspension (Potential for increased requirements of insulin). Products include:
Humulin L, 100 Units 1937
Humulin U, 100 Units 1943
Novolin L Human Insulin 10 ml Vials 2422

Insulin, Human NPH (Potential for increased requirements of insulin). Products include:
Humulin N, 100 Units 1939
Humulin N NPH Pen 1940
Novolin N Human Insulin 10 ml Vials 2422
Novolin N PenFill 2423
Novolin N Prefilled Syringe Disposable Insulin Delivery System 2425

Insulin, Human Regular (Potential for increased requirements of insulin). Products include:
Humulin R Regular (U-500) 1943
Humulin R, 100 Units 1941
Novolin R Human Insulin 10 ml Vials 2423
Novolin R PenFill 2423
Novolin R Prefilled Syringe Disposable Insulin Delivery System 2425
Velosulin BR Human Insulin 10 ml Vials 2435

Insulin, Human Regular and Human NPH Mixture (Potential for increased requirements of insulin). Products include:
Humulin 50/50, 100 Units 1934
Humulin 70/30, 100 Units 1935
Humulin 70/30 Pen 1936
Novolin 70/30 Human Insulin 10 ml Vials 2421
Novolin 70/30 PenFill 2423
Novolin 70/30 Prefilled Disposable Insulin Delivery System 2425

Insulin, NPH (Potential for increased requirements of insulin). Products include:
Iletin II, NPH (Pork), 100 Units 1946

Insulin, Regular (Potential for increased requirements of insulin). Products include:
Iletin II, Regular (Pork), 100 Units ... 1947

Insulin, Zinc Crystals (Potential for increased requirements of insulin).
No products indexed under this heading.

Insulin, Zinc Suspension (Potential for increased requirements of insulin). Products include:
Iletin II, Lente (Pork), 100 Units 1945

Insulin Aspart, Human Regular (Potential for increased requirements of insulin).
No products indexed under this heading.

Insulin glargine (Potential for increased requirements of insulin). Products include:
Lantus Injection 742

Insulin Lispro, Human (Potential for increased requirements of insulin). Products include:
Humalog 1926
Humalog Mix 75/25 Pen 1928

Insulin Lispro Protamine, Human (Potential for increased requirements of insulin). Products include:
Humalog Mix 75/25 Pen 1928

Metformin Hydrochloride (Potential for increased requirements of oral hypoglycemic agents). Products include:
Glucophage Tablets 1080
Glucophage XR Tablets 1080
Glucovance Tablets 1086

Methyclothiazide (Co-administration may result in hypokalemia).
No products indexed under this heading.

Miglitol (Potential for increased requirements of oral hypoglycemic agents). Products include:
Glyset Tablets 2821

Phenobarbital (Co-administration may enhance the metabolic clearance of corticosteroids, resulting in decreased blood levels and lessened physiologic activity; corticosteroid dosage may need to be adjusted). Products include:
Arco-Lase Plus Tablets 592
Donnatal 2929
Donnatal Extentabs 2930

Phenytoin (Co-administration may enhance the metabolic clearance of corticosteroids, resulting in decreased blood levels and lessened physiologic activity; corticosteroid dosage may need to be adjusted). Products include:
Dilantin Infatabs 2624
Dilantin-125 Oral Suspension 2625

Phenytoin Sodium (Co-administration may enhance the metabolic clearance of corticosteroids, resulting in decreased blood levels and lessened physiologic activity; corticosteroid dosage may need to be adjusted). Products include:
Dilantin Kapseals 2622

Pioglitazone Hydrochloride (Potential for increased requirements of oral hypoglycemic agents). Products include:
Actos Tablets 3275

Polythiazide (Co-administration may result in hypokalemia). Products include:
Minizide Capsules 2700
Renese Tablets 2712

Repaglinide (Potential for increased requirements of oral hypoglycemic agents). Products include:
Prandin Tablets (0.5, 1, and 2 mg) 2432

Rifampin (Co-administration may enhance the metabolic clearance of corticosteroids, resulting in decreased blood levels and lessened physiologic activity; corticosteroid dosage may need to be adjusted). Products include:
Rifadin 765
Rifamate Capsules 767
Rifater Tablets 769

Rosiglitazone Maleate (Potential for increased requirements of oral hypoglycemic agents). Products include:
Avandia Tablets 1490

Tolazamide (Potential for increased requirements of oral hypoglycemic agents).
No products indexed under this heading.

Tolbutamide (Potential for increased requirements of oral hypoglycemic agents).
No products indexed under this heading.

Torsemide (Co-administration may result in hypokalemia). Products include:
Demadex Tablets and Injection 2965

Troglitazone (Potential for increased requirements of oral hypoglycemic agents).
No products indexed under this heading.

Warfarin Sodium (Potential for altered response to coumarin anticoagulants). Products include:
Coumadin for Injection 1243
Coumadin Tablets 1243
Warfarin Sodium Tablets, USP 3302

CORTROSYN FOR INJECTION

(Cosyntropin) 2449
May interact with diuretics. Compounds in these categories include:

Amiloride Hydrochloride (Corticotropin may accentuate the electrolyte loss associated with diuretic therapy). Products include:
Midamor Tablets 2136
Moduretic Tablets 2138

Bendroflumethiazide (Corticotropin may accentuate the electrolyte loss associated with diuretic therapy). Products include:
Corzide 40/5 Tablets 2247
Corzide 80/5 Tablets 2247

Bumetanide (Corticotropin may accentuate the electrolyte loss associated with diuretic therapy).
No products indexed under this heading.

Chlorothiazide (Corticotropin may accentuate the electrolyte loss associated with diuretic therapy).
Products include:
Aldoclor Tablets 2035
Diuril Oral 2087

Chlorothiazide Sodium (Corticotropin may accentuate the electrolyte loss associated with diuretic therapy). Products include:
Diuril Sodium Intravenous 2086

Chlorthalidone (Corticotropin may accentuate the electrolyte loss associated with diuretic therapy).
Products include:
Clorpres Tablets 1002
Combipres Tablets 1040
Tenoretic Tablets 690

Ethacrynic Acid (Corticotropin may accentuate the electrolyte loss associated with diuretic therapy).
Products include:
Edecrin Tablets 2091

Furosemide (Corticotropin may accentuate the electrolyte loss associated with diuretic therapy).
Products include:
Furosemide Tablets 2284

Hydrochlorothiazide (Corticotropin may accentuate the electrolyte loss associated with diuretic therapy). Products include:
Accuretic Tablets 2614
Aldoril Tablets 2039
Atacand HCT Tablets 597
Avalide Tablets 1070
Diovan HCT Tablets 2338
Dyazide Capsules 1515
HydroDIURIL Tablets 2108
Hyzaar 2109
Inderide Tablets 3517
Inderide LA Long-Acting Capsules .. 3519
Lotensin HCT Tablets 2367
Maxzide 1008
Micardis HCT Tablets 1051
Microzide Capsules 3414
Moduretic Tablets 2138
Monopril HCT 1094
Prinzide Tablets 2168
Timolide Tablets 2187
Uniretic Tablets 3178
Vaseretic Tablets 2204
Zestoretic Tablets 695
Ziac Tablets 1887

Hydroflumethiazide (Corticotropin may accentuate the electrolyte loss associated with diuretic therapy).
Products include:
Diucardin Tablets 3494

Indapamide (Corticotropin may accentuate the electrolyte loss associated with diuretic therapy).
Products include:
Indapamide Tablets 2286

Methyclothiazide (Corticotropin may accentuate the electrolyte loss associated with diuretic therapy).
No products indexed under this heading.

Metolazone (Corticotropin may accentuate the electrolyte loss associated with diuretic therapy).
Products include:
Mykrox Tablets 1168
Zaroxolyn Tablets 1177

Polythiazide (Corticotropin may accentuate the electrolyte loss associated with diuretic therapy).
Products include:
Minizide Capsules 2700
Renese Tablets 2712

Spironolactone (Corticotropin may accentuate the electrolyte loss associated with diuretic therapy).
No products indexed under this heading.

Torsemide (Corticotropin may accentuate the electrolyte loss associated with diuretic therapy).
Products include:
Demadex Tablets and Injection 2965

Triamterene (Corticotropin may accentuate the electrolyte loss associated with diuretic therapy).
Products include:
Dyazide Capsules 1515
Dyrenium Capsules 3458
Maxzide 1008

CORVERT INJECTION

(Ibutilide Fumarate) 2793
May interact with drugs that prolong the QT interval, quinidine, and certain other agents. Compounds in these categories include:

Amiodarone Hydrochloride (Potential for prolonged refractoriness; amiodarone should not be given concomitantly or within 4 hours postinfusion). Products include:
Cordarone Intravenous 3491
Cordarone Tablets 3487
Pacerone Tablets 3331

Amitriptyline Hydrochloride (The potential for proarrhythmia may increase with co-administration of ibutilide to patients who are being treated with drugs that prolong the QT interval). Products include:
Etrafon 3115
Limbitrol 1738

Amoxapine (The potential for proarrhythmia may increase with co-administration of ibutilide to patients who are being treated with drugs that prolong the QT interval).
No products indexed under this heading.

Astemizole (The potential for proarrhythmia may increase with co-administration of ibutilide to patients who are being treated with drugs that prolong the QT interval).
No products indexed under this heading.

Bretylium Tosylate (The potential for proarrhythmia may increase with co-administration of ibutilide to patients who are being treated with drugs that prolong the QT interval).
No products indexed under this heading.

Chlorpromazine (The potential for proarrhythmia may increase with co-administration of ibutilide to patients who are being treated with drugs that prolong the QT interval).
Products include:
Thorazine Suppositories 1656

Chlorpromazine Hydrochloride (The potential for proarrhythmia may increase with co-administration of ibutilide to patients who are being treated with drugs that prolong the QT interval). Products include:
Thorazine 1656

Clomipramine Hydrochloride (The potential for proarrhythmia may increase with co-administration of ibutilide to patients who are being treated with drugs that prolong the QT interval).
No products indexed under this heading.

Desipramine Hydrochloride (The potential for proarrhythmia may increase with co-administration of ibutilide to patients who are being treated with drugs that prolong the QT interval). Products include:
Norpramin Tablets 755

Digoxin (Supraventricular arrhythmias may mask the cardiotoxicity associated with excessive digoxin levels; caution is advised in patients whose plasma digoxin levels are above or suspected to be above the therapeutic range; co-administration did not have effects on the safety or efficacy of ibutilide). Products include:
Digitek Tablets 1003
Lanoxicaps Capsules 1574
Lanoxin Injection 1581
Lanoxin Tablets 1587
Lanoxin Elixir Pediatric 1578
Lanoxin Injection Pediatric 1584

Disopyramide Phosphate (Potential for prolonged refractoriness; disopyramide should not be given concomitantly or within 4 hours postinfusion).
No products indexed under this heading.

Dofetilide (The potential for proarrhythmia may increase with co-administration of ibutilide to patients who are being treated with drugs that prolong the QT interval).
Products include:
Tikosyn Capsules 2717

Doxepin Hydrochloride (The potential for proarrhythmia may increase with co-administration of ibutilide to patients who are being treated with drugs that prolong the QT interval). Products include:
Sinequan 2713

Flecainide Acetate (The potential for proarrhythmia may increase with co-administration of ibutilide to patients who are being treated with drugs that prolong the QT interval).
Products include:
Tambocor Tablets 1990

Fluphenazine Decanoate (The potential for proarrhythmia may increase with co-administration of ibutilide to patients who are being treated with drugs that prolong the QT interval).
No products indexed under this heading.

Fluphenazine Enanthate (The potential for proarrhythmia may increase with co-administration of ibutilide to patients who are being treated with drugs that prolong the QT interval).
No products indexed under this heading.

Fluphenazine Hydrochloride (The potential for proarrhythmia may increase with co-administration of ibutilide to patients who are being treated with drugs that prolong the QT interval).
No products indexed under this heading.

Imipramine Hydrochloride (The potential for proarrhythmia may increase with co-administration of ibutilide to patients who are being treated with drugs that prolong the QT interval).
No products indexed under this heading.

Imipramine Pamoate (The potential for proarrhythmia may increase with co-administration of ibutilide to patients who are being treated with drugs that prolong the QT interval).
No products indexed under this heading.

Lidocaine Hydrochloride (The potential for proarrhythmia may increase with co-administration of ibutilide to patients who are being treated with drugs that prolong the QT interval). Products include:
Bactine First Aid Liquid 611
Xylocaine Injections 653

Maprotiline Hydrochloride (The potential for proarrhythmia may increase with co-administration of ibutilide to patients who are being treated with drugs that prolong the QT interval).
No products indexed under this heading.

Mesoridazine Besylate (The potential for proarrhythmia may increase with co-administration of ibutilide to patients who are being treated with drugs that prolong the QT interval). Products include:
Serentil 1057

Mexiletine Hydrochloride (The potential for proarrhythmia may increase with co-administration of ibutilide to patients who are being treated with drugs that prolong the QT interval). Products include:
Mexitil Capsules 1047

Nortriptyline Hydrochloride (The potential for proarrhythmia may increase with co-administration of ibutilide to patients who are being treated with drugs that prolong the QT interval).
No products indexed under this heading.

Perphenazine (The potential for proarrhythmia may increase with co-administration of ibutilide to patients who are being treated with drugs that prolong the QT interval).
Products include:
Etrafon 3115
Trilafon 3160

Procainamide Hydrochloride (Potential for prolonged refractoriness; procainamide should not be given concomitantly or within 4 hours postinfusion). Products include:
Procanbid Extended-Release Tablets 2262

Prochlorperazine (The potential for proarrhythmia may increase with co-administration of ibutilide to patients who are being treated with drugs that prolong the QT interval).
Products include:
Compazine 1505

Promethazine Hydrochloride (The potential for proarrhythmia may increase with co-administration of ibutilide to patients who are being treated with drugs that prolong the QT interval). Products include:
Mepergan Injection 3539
Phenergan Injection 3553

Phenergan 3556
Phenergan Syrup 3554
Phenergan with Codeine Syrup 3557
Phenergan with Dextromethorphan Syrup 3559
Phenergan VC Syrup 3560
Phenergan VC with Codeine Syrup .. 3561

Propafenone Hydrochloride (The potential for proarrhythmia may increase with co-administration of ibutilide to patients who are being treated with drugs that prolong the QT interval). Products include:
Rythmol Tablets – 150 mg, 225 mg, 300 mg 502

Protriptyline Hydrochloride (The potential for proarrhythmia may increase with co-administration of ibutilide to patients who are being treated with drugs that prolong the QT interval). Products include:
Vivactil Tablets 2446
Vivactil Tablets 2217

Quinidine Gluconate (Potential for prolonged refractoriness; quinidine should not be given concomitantly or within 4 hours postinfusion). Products include:
Quinaglute Dura-Tabs Tablets 978

Quinidine Polygalacturonate (Potential for prolonged refractoriness; quinidine should not be given concomitantly or within 4 hours postinfusion).
No products indexed under this heading.

Quinidine Sulfate (Potential for prolonged refractoriness; quinidine should not be given concomitantly or within 4 hours postinfusion). Products include:
Quinidex Extentabs 2933

Sotalol Hydrochloride (Potential for prolonged refractoriness; sotalol should not be given concomitantly or within 4 hours postinfusion). Products include:
Betapace Tablets 950
Betapace AF Tablets 954

Terfenadine (The potential for proarrhythmia may increase with co-administration of ibutilide to patients who are being treated with drugs that prolong the QT interval).
No products indexed under this heading.

Thioridazine Hydrochloride (The potential for proarrhythmia may increase with co-administration of ibutilide to patients who are being treated with drugs that prolong the QT interval). Products include:
Thioridazine Hydrochloride Tablets 2289

Tocainide Hydrochloride (The potential for proarrhythmia may increase with co-administration of ibutilide to patients who are being treated with drugs that prolong the QT interval). Products include:
Tonocard Tablets 649

Trifluoperazine Hydrochloride (The potential for proarrhythmia may increase with co-administration of ibutilide to patients who are being treated with drugs that prolong the QT interval). Products include:
Stelazine 1640

Trimipramine Maleate (The potential for proarrhythmia may increase with co-administration of ibutilide to patients who are being treated with drugs that prolong the QT interval). Products include:
Surmontil Capsules 3595

Ziprasidone Hydrochloride (The potential for proarrhythmia may increase with co-administration of ibutilide to patients who are being treated with drugs that prolong the QT interval). Products include:
Geodon Capsules 2688

CORZIDE 40/5 TABLETS
(Bendroflumethiazide, Nadolol) 2247
See Corzide 80/5 Tablets

CORZIDE 80/5 TABLETS
(Bendroflumethiazide, Nadolol) 2247
May interact with antihypertensives, barbiturates, calcium preparations, corticosteroids, oral anticoagulants, general anesthetics, cardiac glycosides, oral hypoglycemic agents, insulin, lithium preparations, monoamine oxidase inhibitors, narcotic analgesics, nondepolarizing neuromuscular blocking agents, non-steroidal anti-inflammatory agents, and certain other agents. Compounds in these categories include:

Acarbose (Beta-adrenergic blockade may prevent the appearance of signs and symptoms of acute hypoglycemia; beta-blockade also reduces the release of insulin in response to hyperglycemia, therefore, it may be necessary to adjust the dose of oral antidiabetic drugs). Products include:
Precose Tablets 906

Acebutolol Hydrochloride (Bendroflumethiazide may potentiate the effects of other antihypertensives). Products include:
Sectral Capsules 3589

ACTH (Co-administration with ACTH intensifies electrolyte imbalance, particularly hypokalemia).
No products indexed under this heading.

Alfentanil Hydrochloride (Co-administration may result in potentiation of orthostatic hypotension).
No products indexed under this heading.

Amlodipine Besylate (Bendroflumethiazide may potentiate the effects of other antihypertensives). Products include:
Lotrel Capsules 2370
Norvasc Tablets 2704

Amphotericin B (Co-administration with amphotericin B intensifies electrolyte imbalance, particularly hypokalemia). Products include:
Abelcet Injection 1273
AmBisome for Injection 1383
Amphotec 1774

Aprobarbital (Co-administration may result in potentiation of orthostatic hypotension).
No products indexed under this heading.

Atenolol (Bendroflumethiazide may potentiate the effects of other antihypertensives). Products include:
Tenoretic Tablets 690
Tenormin I.V. Injection 692

Atracurium Besylate (Effects of nondepolarizing muscle relaxants may be potentiated).
No products indexed under this heading.

Benazepril Hydrochloride (Bendroflumethiazide may potentiate the effects of other antihypertensives). Products include:
Lotensin Tablets 2365
Lotensin HCT Tablets 2367
Lotrel Capsules 2370

Betamethasone Acetate (Co-adminsitration with corticosteroids intensifies electrolyte imbalance, particulary hypokalemia). Products include:
Celestone Soluspan Injectable Suspension 3097

Betamethasone Sodium Phosphate (Co-adminsitration with corticosteroids intensifies electrolyte imbalance, particulary hypokalemia). Products include:
Celestone Soluspan Injectable Suspension 3097

Betaxolol Hydrochloride (Bendroflumethiazide may potentiate the effects of other antihypertensives). Products include:
Betoptic S Ophthalmic Suspension 537

Bisoprolol Fumarate (Bendroflumethiazide may potentiate the effects of other antihypertensives). Products include:
Zebeta Tablets 1885
Ziac Tablets 1887

Buprenorphine Hydrochloride (Co-administration may result in potentiation of orthostatic hypotension). Products include:
Buprenex Injectable 2918

Butabarbital (Co-administration may result in potentiation of orthostatic hypotension).
No products indexed under this heading.

Butalbital (Co-administration may result in potentiation of orthostatic hypotension). Products include:
Phrenilin 578
Sedapap Tablets 50 mg/650 mg ... 2225

Calcium Carbonate (Increased calcium levels due to decreased excretion may occur). Products include:
Aspirin Regimen Bayer 81 mg Caplets with Calcium .... ▣607
Extra Strength Bayer Plus Caplets .... ▣610
Caltrate 600 Tablets .... ▣814
Caltrate 600 PLUS .... ▣815
Caltrate 600 + D Tablets .... ▣814
Caltrate 600 + Soy Tablets .... ▣814
D-Cal Chewable Caplets .... ▣794
Florical Capsules and Tablets 2223
Quick Dissolve Maalox Max Maximum Strength Antacid/Antigas Tablets 2301
Quick Dissolve Maalox Regular Strength Antacid Tablets 2301
Marblen Suspension .... ▣633
Monocal Tablets 2223
Mylanta Fast-Acting 1813
Mylanta Calci Tabs .... ▣636
One-A-Day Bedtime & Rest Tablets .... ▣805
One-A-Day Calcium Plus Chewable Tablets .... ▣805
Os-Cal Chewable Tablets .... ▣838
Pepcid Complete Chewable Tablets 1815
ReSource Wellness CalciWise Soft Chews .... ▣824
Rolaids Tablets .... ▣706
Extra Strength Rolaids Tablets .... ▣706
Slow-Mag Tablets .... ▣835
Titralac .... ▣640
3M Titralac Plus Antacid Tablets ... ▣640
Tums .... ▣763

Calcium Chloride (Increased calcium levels due to decreased excretion may occur).
No products indexed under this heading.

Calcium Citrate (Increased calcium levels due to decreased excretion may occur). Products include:
Active Calcium Tablets 3335
Citracal Liquitab Tablets .... ▣823
Citracal Tablets 2231
Citracal Caplets + D .... ▣823

Calcium Glubionate (Increased calcium levels due to decreased excretion may occur).
No products indexed under this heading.

Candesartan Cilexetil (Bendroflumethiazide may potentiate the effects of other antihypertensives). Products include:
Atacand Tablets 595
Atacand HCT Tablets 597

Captopril (Bendroflumethiazide may potentiate the effects of other antihypertensives). Products include:
Captopril Tablets 2281

Carteolol Hydrochloride (Bendroflumethiazide may potentiate the effects of other antihypertensives). Products include:
Carteolol Hydrochloride Ophthalmic Solution USP, 1% ..... ⊙258
Ocupress Ophthalmic Solution, 1% Sterile .... ⊙303

Celecoxib (Co-administration with non-steroidal anti-inflammatory agents can reduce the diuretic, natriuretic, and antihypertensive effect of thiazide diuretics). Products include:
Celebrex Capsules 2676
Celebrex Capsules 2780

Chlorothiazide (Bendroflumethiazide may potentiate the effects of other antihypertensives). Products include:
Aldoclor Tablets 2035
Diuril Oral 2087

Chlorothiazide Sodium (Bendroflumethiazide may potentiate the effects of other antihypertensives). Products include:
Diuril Sodium Intravenous 2086

Chlorpropamide (Beta-adrenergic blockade may prevent the appearance of signs and symptoms of acute hypoglycemia; beta-blockade also reduces the release of insulin in response to hyperglycemia, therefore, it may be necessary to adjust the dose of oral antidiabetic drugs). Products include:
Diabinese Tablets 2680

Chlorthalidone (Bendroflumethiazide may potentiate the effects of other antihypertensives). Products include:
Clorpres Tablets 1002
Combipres Tablets 1040
Tenoretic Tablets 690

Cholestyramine (May delay or decrease absorption of bendroflumethiazide; thiazide diuretics should be taken at least one hour before or four to six hours after cholestyramine).
No products indexed under this heading.

Cisatracurium Besylate (Effects of nondepolarizing muscle relaxants may be potentiated).
No products indexed under this heading.

Clonidine (Bendroflumethiazide may potentiate the effects of other antihypertensives). Products include:
Catapres-TTS 1038

Clonidine Hydrochloride (Bendroflumethiazide may potentiate the effects of other antihypertensives). Products include:
Catapres Tablets 1037
Clorpres Tablets 1002
Combipres Tablets 1040
Duraclon Injection 3057

Codeine Phosphate (Co-administration may result in potentiation of orthostatic hypotension). Products include:
Phenergan with Codeine Syrup 3557
Phenergan VC with Codeine Syrup 3561
Robitussin A-C Syrup 2942
Robitussin-DAC Syrup 2942
Ryna-C Liquid .... ▣768
Soma Compound w/Codeine Tablets 3355
Tussi-Organidin NR Liquid 3350
Tussi-Organidin-S NR Liquid 3350
Tylenol with Codeine 2595

Colestipol Hydrochloride (May delay or decrease absorption of bendroflumethiazide; thiazide diuretics should be taken at least one hour before or four to six hours after colestipol). Products include:
Colestid Tablets 2791

Cortisone Acetate (Co-adminsitration with corticosteroids intensifies electrolyte imbalance, particulary hypokalemia). Products include:
Cortone Acetate Injectable Suspension 2059
Cortone Acetate Tablets 2061

Deserpidine (Bendroflumethiazide may potentiate the effects of other antihypertensives).
No products indexed under this heading.

Deslanoside (Enhanced possibility of digitalis toxicity associated with hypokalemia).
No products indexed under this heading.

Dexamethasone (Co-administration with corticosteroids intensifies electrolyte imbalance, particulary hypokalemia). Products include:
- Decadron Elixir ... 2078
- Decadron Tablets ... 2079
- TobraDex Ophthalmic Ointment ... 542
- TobraDex Ophthalmic Suspension ... 541

Dexamethasone Acetate (Co-administration with corticosteroids intensifies electrolyte imbalance, particulary hypokalemia).
- No products indexed under this heading.

Dexamethasone Sodium Phosphate (Co-administration with corticosteroids intensifies electrolyte imbalance, particulary hypokalemia). Products include:
- Decadron Phosphate Injection ... 2081
- Decadron Phosphate Sterile Ophthalmic Ointment ... 2083
- Decadron Phosphate Sterile Ophthalmic Solution ... 2084
- NeoDecadron Sterile Ophthalmic Solution ... 2144

Dezocine (Co-administration may result in potentiation of orthostatic hypotension).
- No products indexed under this heading.

Diazoxide (Enhanced hyperglycemic, hyperuricemic, and antihypertensive effects).
- No products indexed under this heading.

Diclofenac Potassium (Co-administration with non-steroidal anti-inflammatory agents can reduce the diuretic, natriuretic, and antihypertensive effect of thiazide diuretics). Products include:
- Cataflam Tablets ... 2315

Diclofenac Sodium (Co-administration with non-steroidal anti-inflammatory agents can reduce the diuretic, natriuretic, and antihypertensive effect of thiazide diuretics). Products include:
- Arthrotec Tablets ... 3195
- Voltaren Ophthalmic Sterile Ophthalmic Solution ... ⊙312
- Voltaren Tablets ... 2315
- Voltaren-XR Tablets ... 2315

Dicumarol (Bendroflumethiazide may decrease the effects of oral anticoagulants; dosage adjustment of anticoagulants may be necessary).
- No products indexed under this heading.

Digitoxin (Enhanced possibility of digitalis toxicity associated with hypokalemia).
- No products indexed under this heading.

Digoxin (Enhanced possibility of digitalis toxicity associated with hypokalemia). Products include:
- Digitek Tablets ... 1003
- Lanoxicaps Capsules ... 1574
- Lanoxin Injection ... 1581
- Lanoxin Tablets ... 1587
- Lanoxin Elixir Pediatric ... 1578
- Lanoxin Injection Pediatric ... 1584

Diltiazem Hydrochloride (Bendroflumethiazide may potentiate the effects of other antihypertensives). Products include:
- Cardizem Injectable ... 1018
- Cardizem Lyo-Ject Syringe ... 1018
- Cardizem Monovial ... 1018
- Cardizem CD Capsules ... 1016
- Tiazac Capsules ... 1378

Doxazosin Mesylate (Bendroflumethiazide may potentiate the effects of other antihypertensives). Products include:
- Cardura Tablets ... 2668

Enalapril Maleate (Bendroflumethiazide may potentiate the effects of other antihypertensives). Products include:
- Lexxel Tablets ... 608
- Vaseretic Tablets ... 2204
- Vasotec Tablets ... 2210

Enalaprilat (Bendroflumethiazide may potentiate the effects of other antihypertensives). Products include:
- Enalaprilat Injection ... 863
- Vasotec I.V. Injection ... 2207

Enflurane (Co-administration may result in exaggeration of the hypotension induced by general anesthetics).
- No products indexed under this heading.

Epinephrine (Patients with severe anaphylactic reaction to variety of allergens may be unresponsive to the usual doses of epinephrine used to treat allergic reaction). Products include:
- Epifrin Sterile Ophthalmic Solution ... ⊙235
- EpiPen ... 1236
- Primatene Mist ... ▣779
- Xylocaine with Epinephrine Injection ... 653

Epinephrine Hydrochloride (Patients with severe anaphylactic reaction to variety of allergens may be unresponsive to the usual doses of epinephrine used to treat allergic reaction).
- No products indexed under this heading.

Eprosartan Mesylate (Bendroflumethiazide may potentiate the effects of other antihypertensives). Products include:
- Teveten Tablets ... 3327

Esmolol Hydrochloride (Bendroflumethiazide may potentiate the effects of other antihypertensives). Products include:
- Brevibloc Injection ... 858

Etodolac (Co-administration with non-steroidal anti-inflammatory agents can reduce the diuretic, natriuretic, and antihypertensive effect of thiazide diuretics). Products include:
- Lodine ... 3528
- Lodine XL Extended-Release Tablets ... 3530

Felodipine (Bendroflumethiazide may potentiate the effects of other antihypertensives). Products include:
- Lexxel Tablets ... 608
- Plendil Extended-Release Tablets ... 623

Fenoprofen Calcium (Co-administration with non-steroidal anti-inflammatory agents can reduce the diuretic, natriuretic, and antihypertensive effect of thiazide diuretics).
- No products indexed under this heading.

Fentanyl (Co-administration may result in potentiation of orthostatic hypotension). Products include:
- Duragesic Transdermal System ... 1786

Fentanyl Citrate (Co-administration may result in potentiation of orthostatic hypotension). Products include:
- Actiq ... 1184

Fludrocortisone Acetate (Co-adminsitration with corticosteroids intensifies electrolyte imbalance, particulary hypokalemia). Products include:
- Florinef Acetate Tablets ... 2250

Flurbiprofen (Co-administration with non-steroidal anti-inflammatory agents can reduce the diuretic, natriuretic, and antihypertensive effect of thiazide diuretics).
- No products indexed under this heading.

Fosinopril Sodium (Bendroflumethiazide may potentiate the effects of other antihypertensives). Products include:
- Monopril Tablets ... 1091
- Monopril HCT ... 1094

Furosemide (Bendroflumethiazide may potentiate the effects of other antihypertensives). Products include:
- Furosemide Tablets ... 2284

Gallamine Triethiodide (Effects of muscle relaxants may be potentiated).

Glimepiride (Beta-adrenergic blockade may prevent the appearance of signs and symptoms of acute hypoglycemia; beta-blockade also reduces the release of insulin in response to hyperglycemia, therefore, it may be necessary to adjust the dose of oral antidiabetic drugs). Products include:
- Amaryl Tablets ... 717

Glipizide (Beta-adrenergic blockade may prevent the appearance of signs and symptoms of acute hypoglycemia; beta-blockade also reduces the release of insulin in response to hyperglycemia, therefore, it may be necessary to adjust the dose of oral antidiabetic drugs). Products include:
- Glucotrol Tablets ... 2692
- Glucotrol XL Extended Release Tablets ... 2693

Glyburide (Beta-adrenergic blockade may prevent the appearance of signs and symptoms of acute hypoglycemia; beta-blockade also reduces the release of insulin in response to hyperglycemia, therefore, it may be necessary to adjust the dose of oral antidiabetic drugs). Products include:
- DiaBeta Tablets ... 741
- Glucovance Tablets ... 1086

Guanabenz Acetate (Bendroflumethiazide may potentiate the effects of other antihypertensives).
- No products indexed under this heading.

Guanethidine Monosulfate (Bendroflumethiazide may potentiate the effects of other antihypertensives).
- No products indexed under this heading.

Hydralazine Hydrochloride (Bendroflumethiazide may potentiate the effects of other antihypertensives).
- No products indexed under this heading.

Hydrochlorothiazide (Bendroflumethiazide may potentiate the effects of other antihypertensives). Products include:
- Accuretic Tablets ... 2614
- Aldoril Tablets ... 2039
- Atacand HCT Tablets ... 597
- Avalide Tablets ... 1070
- Diovan HCT Tablets ... 2338
- Dyazide Capsules ... 1515
- HydroDIURIL Tablets ... 2108
- Hyzaar ... 2109
- Inderide Tablets ... 3517
- Inderide LA Long-Acting Capsules ... 3519
- Lotensin HCT Tablets ... 2367
- Maxzide ... 1008
- Micardis HCT Tablets ... 1051
- Microzide Capsules ... 3414
- Moduretic Tablets ... 2138
- Monopril HCT ... 1094
- Prinzide Tablets ... 2168
- Timolide Tablets ... 2187
- Uniretic Tablets ... 3178
- Vaseretic Tablets ... 2204
- Zestoretic Tablets ... 695
- Ziac Tablets ... 1887

Hydrocodone Bitartrate (Co-administration may result in potentiation of orthostatic hypotension). Products include:
- Hycodan ... 1316
- Hycomine Compound Tablets ... 1317
- Hycotuss Expectorant Syrup ... 1318
- Lortab ... 3319
- Lortab Elixir ... 3317
- Maxidone Tablets CIII ... 3399
- Norco 5/325 Tablets CIII ... 3424
- Norco 7.5/325 Tablets CIII ... 3425
- Norco 10/325 Tablets CIII ... 3427
- Norco 10/325 Tablets CIII ... 3425
- Vicodin Tablets ... 516
- Vicodin ES Tablets ... 517
- Vicodin HP Tablets ... 518
- Vicodin Tuss Expectorant ... 519
- Vicoprofen Tablets ... 520
- Zydone Tablets ... 1330

Hydrocodone Polistirex (Co-administration may result in potentiation of orthostatic hypotension). Products include:
- Tussionex Pennkinetic Extended-Release Suspension ... 1174

Hydrocortisone (Co-adminsitration with corticosteroids intensifies electrolyte imbalance, particulary hypokalemia). Products include:
- Anusol-HC Cream 2.5% ... 2237
- Cipro HC Otic Suspension ... 540
- Cortaid Intensive Therapy Cream ... ▣717
- Cortaid Maximum Strength Cream ... ▣717
- Cortisporin Ophthalmic Suspension Sterile ... ⊙297
- Cortizone•5 ... ▣699
- Cortizone•10 ... ▣699
- Cortizone•10 Plus Creme ... ▣700
- Cortizone for Kids Creme ... ▣699
- Hydrocortone Tablets ... 2106
- Massengill Medicated Soft Cloth Towelette ... ▣753
- VōSoL HC Otic Solution ... 3356

Hydrocortisone Acetate (Co-adminsitration with corticosteroids intensifies electrolyte imbalance, particulary hypokalemia). Products include:
- Analpram-HC ... 1338
- Anusol HC-1 Hydrocortisone Anti-Itch Cream ... ▣689
- Anusol-HC Suppositories ... 2238
- Cortaid ... ▣717
- Cortifoam Rectal Foam ... 3170
- Cortisporin-TC Otic Suspension ... 2246
- Hydrocortone Acetate Injectable Suspension ... 2103
- Pramosone ... 1343
- Proctocort Suppositories ... 2264
- ProctoFoam-HC ... 3177
- Terra-Cortril Ophthalmic Suspension ... 2716

Hydrocortisone Sodium Phosphate (Co-adminsitration with corticosteroids intensifies electrolyte imbalance, particulary hypokalemia). Products include:
- Hydrocortone Phosphate Injection, Sterile ... 2105

Hydrocortisone Sodium Succinate (Co-adminsitration with corticosteroids intensifies electrolyte imbalance, particulary hypokalemia).
- No products indexed under this heading.

Hydroflumethiazide (Bendroflumethiazide may potentiate the effects of other antihypertensives). Products include:
- Diucardin Tablets ... 3494

Hydromorphone Hydrochloride (Co-administration may result in potentiation of orthostatic hypotension). Products include:
- Dilaudid ... 441
- Dilaudid Oral Liquid ... 445
- Dilaudid Powder ... 441
- Dilaudid Rectal Suppositories ... 441
- Dilaudid Tablets ... 441
- Dilaudid Tablets - 8 mg ... 445
- Dilaudid-HP ... 443

Ibuprofen (Co-administration with non-steroidal anti-inflammatory agents can reduce the diuretic, natriuretic, and antihypertensive effect of thiazide diuretics). Products include:
- Advil ... ▣771
- Children's Advil Oral Suspension ... ▣773
- Children's Advil Chewable Tablets ... ▣773
- Advil Cold and Sinus Caplets ... ▣771
- Advil Cold and Sinus Tablets ... ▣771
- Advil Flu & Body Ache Caplets ... ▣772
- Infants' Advil Drops ... ▣773
- Junior Strength Advil Tablets ... ▣773
- Junior Strength Advil Chewable Tablets ... ▣773
- Advil Migraine Liquigels ... ▣772
- Children's Motrin Oral Suspension and Chewable Tablets ... 2006
- Children's Motrin Cold Oral Suspension ... 2007
- Children's Motrin Oral Suspension ... ▣643
- Motrin Suspension, Oral Drops, Chewable Tablets, and Caplets ... 2002
- Infants' Motrin Concentrated Drops ... 2006

Junior Strength Motrin Caplets and Chewable Tablets ... 2006
Motrin IB Tablets, Caplets, and Gelcaps ... 2002
Motrin Migraine Pain Caplets ... 2005
Motrin Sinus Headache Caplets ... 2005
Vicoprofen Tablets ... 520

Indapamide (Bendroflumethiazide may potentiate the effects of other antihypertensives). Products include:
Indapamide Tablets ... 2286

Indomethacin (Co-administration with non-steroidal anti-inflammatory agents can reduce the diuretic, natriuretic, and antihypertensive effect of thiazide diuretics). Products include:
Indocin ... 2112

Indomethacin Sodium Trihydrate (Co-administration with non-steroidal anti-inflammatory agents can reduce the diuretic, natriuretic, and antihypertensive effect of thiazide diuretics). Products include:
Indocin I.V. ... 2115

Insulin, Human, Zinc Suspension (Beta-adrenergic blockade may prevent the appearance of signs and symptoms of acute hypoglycemia; beta-blockade also reduces the release of insulin in response to hyperglycemia, therefore, it may be necessary to adjust the dose of insulin). Products include:
Humulin L, 100 Units ... 1937
Humulin U, 100 Units ... 1943
Novolin L Human Insulin 10 ml Vials ... 2422

Insulin, Human NPH (Beta-adrenergic blockade may prevent the appearance of signs and symptoms of acute hypoglycemia; beta-blockade also reduces the release of insulin in response to hyperglycemia, therefore, it may be necessary to adjust the dose of insulin). Products include:
Humulin N, 100 Units ... 1939
Humulin N NPH Pen ... 1940
Novolin N Human Insulin 10 ml Vials ... 2422
Novolin N PenFill ... 2423
Novolin N Prefilled Syringe Disposable Insulin Delivery System ... 2425

Insulin, Human Regular (Beta-adrenergic blockade may prevent the appearance of signs and symptoms of acute hypoglycemia; beta-blockade also reduces the release of insulin in response to hyperglycemia, therefore, it may be necessary to adjust the dose of insulin). Products include:
Humulin R Regular (U-500) ... 1943
Humulin R, 100 Units ... 1941
Novolin R Human Insulin 10 ml Vials ... 2423
Novolin R PenFill ... 2423
Novolin R Prefilled Syringe Disposable Insulin Delivery System ... 2425
Velosulin BR Human Insulin 10 ml Vials ... 2435

Insulin, Human Regular and Human NPH Mixture (Beta-adrenergic blockade may prevent the appearance of signs and symptoms of acute hypoglycemia; beta-blockade also reduces the release of insulin in response to hyperglycemia, therefore, it may be necessary to adjust the dose of insulin). Products include:
Humulin 50/50, 100 Units ... 1934
Humulin 70/30, 100 Units ... 1935
Humulin 70/30 Pen ... 1936
Novolin 70/30 Human Insulin 10 ml Vials ... 2421
Novolin 70/30 PenFill ... 2423
Novolin 70/30 Prefilled Disposable Insulin Delivery System ... 2425

Insulin, NPH (Beta-adrenergic blockade may prevent the appearance of signs and symptoms of acute hypoglycemia; beta-blockade also reduces the release of insulin in response to hyperglycemia, therefore, it may be necessary to adjust the dose of insulin). Products include:
Iletin II, NPH (Pork), 100 Units ... 1946

Insulin, Regular (Beta-adrenergic blockade may prevent the appearance of signs and symptoms of acute hypoglycemia; beta-blockade also reduces the release of insulin in response to hyperglycemia, therefore, it may be necessary to adjust the dose of insulin). Products include:
Iletin II, Regular (Pork), 100 Units ... 1947

Insulin, Zinc Crystals (Beta-adrenergic blockade may prevent the appearance of signs and symptoms of acute hypoglycemia; beta-blockade also reduces the release of insulin in response to hyperglycemia, therefore, it may be necessary to adjust the dose of insulin).
No products indexed under this heading.

Insulin, Zinc Suspension (Beta-adrenergic blockade may prevent the appearance of signs and symptoms of acute hypoglycemia; beta-blockade also reduces the release of insulin in response to hyperglycemia, therefore, it may be necessary to adjust the dose of insulin). Products include:
Iletin II, Lente (Pork), 100 Units ... 1945

Insulin Aspart, Human Regular (Beta-adrenergic blockade may prevent the appearance of signs and symptoms of acute hypoglycemia; beta-blockade also reduces the release of insulin in response to hyperglycemia, therefore, it may be necessary to adjust the dose of insulin).
No products indexed under this heading.

Insulin glargine (Beta-adrenergic blockade may prevent the appearance of signs and symptoms of acute hypoglycemia; beta-blockade also reduces the release of insulin in response to hyperglycemia, therefore, it may be necessary to adjust the dose of insulin). Products include:
Lantus Injection ... 742

Insulin Lispro, Human (Beta-adrenergic blockade may prevent the appearance of signs and symptoms of acute hypoglycemia; beta-blockade also reduces the release of insulin in response to hyperglycemia, therefore, it may be necessary to adjust the dose of insulin). Products include:
Humalog ... 1926
Humalog Mix 75/25 Pen ... 1928

Insulin Lispro Protamine, Human (Beta-adrenergic blockade may prevent the appearance of signs and symptoms of acute hypoglycemia; beta-blockade also reduces the release of insulin in response to hyperglycemia, therefore, it may be necessary to adjust the dose of insulin). Products include:
Humalog Mix 75/25 Pen ... 1928

Irbesartan (Bendroflumethiazide may potentiate the effects of other antihypertensives). Products include:
Avalide Tablets ... 1070
Avapro Tablets ... 1074
Avapro Tablets ... 3076

Isocarboxazid (Enhanced hypotensive effects; dosage adjustments of one or both agents may be necessary).
No products indexed under this heading.

Isoflurane (Co-administration may result in exaggeration of the hypotension induced by general anesthetics).
No products indexed under this heading.

Isradipine (Bendroflumethiazide may potentiate the effects of other antihypertensives). Products include:
DynaCirc Capsules ... 2921
DynaCirc CR Tablets ... 2923

Ketamine Hydrochloride (Co-administration may result in exaggeration of the hypotension induced by general anesthetics).
No products indexed under this heading.

Ketoprofen (Co-administration with non-steroidal anti-inflammatory agents can reduce the diuretic, natriuretic, and antihypertensive effect of thiazide diuretics). Products include:
Orudis Capsules ... 3548
Orudis KT Tablets ... ▣778
Oruvail Capsules ... 3548

Ketorolac Tromethamine (Co-administration with non-steroidal anti-inflammatory agents can reduce the diuretic, natriuretic, and antihypertensive effect of thiazide diuretics). Products include:
Acular Ophthalmic Solution ... 544
Acular PF Ophthalmic Solution ... 544
Toradol ... 3018

Labetalol Hydrochloride (Bendroflumethiazide may potentiate the effects of other antihypertensives). Products include:
Normodyne Injection ... 3135
Normodyne Tablets ... 3137

Levorphanol Tartrate (Co-administration may result in potentiation of orthostatic hypotension). Products include:
Levo-Dromoran ... 1734
Levorphanol Tartrate Tablets ... 3059

Lisinopril (Bendroflumethiazide may potentiate the effects of other antihypertensives). Products include:
Prinivil Tablets ... 2164
Prinzide Tablets ... 2168
Zestoretic Tablets ... 695
Zestril Tablets ... 698

Lithium Carbonate (Diuretics reduce the renal clearance of lithium and add a high risk of lithium toxicity). Products include:
Eskalith ... 1527
Lithium Carbonate ... 3061
Lithobid Slow-Release Tablets ... 3255

Lithium Citrate (Diuretics reduce the renal clearance of lithium and add a high risk of lithium toxicity). Products include:
Lithium Citrate Syrup ... 3061

Losartan Potassium (Bendroflumethiazide may potentiate the effects of other antihypertensives). Products include:
Cozaar Tablets ... 2067
Hyzaar ... 2109

Mecamylamine Hydrochloride (Bendroflumethiazide may potentiate the effects of other antihypertensives). Products include:
Inversine Tablets ... 1850

Meclofenamate Sodium (Co-administration with non-steroidal anti-inflammatory agents can reduce the diuretic, natriuretic, and antihypertensive effect of thiazide diuretics).
No products indexed under this heading.

Mefenamic Acid (Co-administration with non-steroidal anti-inflammatory agents can reduce the diuretic, natriuretic, and antihypertensive effect of thiazide diuretics). Products include:
Ponstel Capsules ... 1356

Meloxicam (Co-administration with non-steroidal anti-inflammatory agents can reduce the diuretic, natriuretic, and antihypertensive effect of thiazide diuretics). Products include:
Mobic Tablets ... 1054

Meperidine Hydrochloride (Co-administration may result in potentiation of orthostatic hypotension). Products include:
Demerol ... 3079
Mepergan Injection ... 3539

Mephobarbital (Co-administration may result in potentiation of orthostatic hypotension).
No products indexed under this heading.

Metformin Hydrochloride (Beta-adrenergic blockade may prevent the appearance of signs and symptoms of acute hypoglycemia; beta-blockade also reduces the release of insulin in response to hyperglycemia, therefore, it may be necessary to adjust the dose of oral antidiabetic drugs). Products include:
Glucophage Tablets ... 1080
Glucophage XR Tablets ... 1080
Glucovance Tablets ... 1086

Methadone Hydrochloride (Co-administration may result in potentiation of orthostatic hypotension). Products include:
Dolophine Hydrochloride Tablets ... 3056

Methenamine (Possible decreased effectiveness of methenamine due to alkalinization of the urine). Products include:
Prosed/DS Tablets ... 3268
Urimax Tablets ... 1769
Urised Tablets ... 2876

Methenamine Hippurate (Possible decreased effectiveness of methenamine due to alkalinization of the urine).
No products indexed under this heading.

Methenamine Mandelate (Possible decreased effectiveness of methenamine due to alkalinization of the urine). Products include:
Uroqid-Acid No. 2 Tablets ... 947

Methohexital Sodium (Co-administration may result in exaggeration of the hypotension induced by general anesthetics). Products include:
Brevital Sodium for Injection, USP ... 1815

Methoxyflurane (Co-administration may result in exaggeration of the hypotension induced by general anesthetics).
No products indexed under this heading.

Methyclothiazide (Bendroflumethiazide may potentiate the effects of other antihypertensives).
No products indexed under this heading.

Methyldopa (Bendroflumethiazide may potentiate the effects of other antihypertensives). Products include:
Aldoclor Tablets ... 2035
Aldomet Tablets ... 2037
Aldoril Tablets ... 2039

Methyldopate Hydrochloride (Bendroflumethiazide may potentiate the effects of other antihypertensives).
No products indexed under this heading.

Methylprednisolone Acetate (Co-adminsitration with corticosteroids intensifies electrolyte imbalance, particulary hypokalemia). Products include:
Depo-Medrol Injectable Suspension ... 2795

Methylprednisolone Sodium Succinate (Co-adminsitration with corticosteroids intensifies electrolyte imbalance, particulary hypokalemia). Products include:
Solu-Medrol Sterile Powder ... 2855

Metocurine Iodide (Effects of non-depolarizing muscle relaxants may be potentiated).
No products indexed under this heading.

Metolazone (Bendroflumethiazide may potentiate the effects of other antihypertensives). Products include:
Mykrox Tablets ... 1168
Zaroxolyn Tablets ... 1177

Metoprolol Succinate (Bendroflumethiazide may potentiate the effects of other antihypertensives).
Products include:
Toprol-XL Tablets 651

Metoprolol Tartrate (Bendroflumethiazide may potentiate the effects of other antihypertensives).
No products indexed under this heading.

Metyrosine (Bendroflumethiazide may potentiate the effects of other antihypertensives). Products include:
Demser Capsules 2085

Mibefradil Dihydrochloride (Bendroflumethiazide may potentiate the effects of other antihypertensives).
No products indexed under this heading.

Miglitol (Beta-adrenergic blockade may prevent the appearance of signs and symptoms of acute hypoglycemia; beta-blockade also reduces the release of insulin in response to hyperglycemia, therefore, it may be necessary to adjust the dose of oral antidiabetic drugs).
Products include:
Glyset Tablets 2821

Minoxidil (Bendroflumethiazide may potentiate the effects of other antihypertensives). Products include:
Rogaine Extra Strength for Men Topical Solution .... ⊞721
Rogaine for Women Topical Solution .... ⊞721

Mivacurium Chloride (Effects of nondepolarizing muscle relaxants may be potentiated).
No products indexed under this heading.

Moclobemide (Enhanced hypotensive effects; dosage adjustments of one or both agents may be necessary).
No products indexed under this heading.

Moexipril Hydrochloride (Bendroflumethiazide may potentiate the effects of other antihypertensives).
Products include:
Uniretic Tablets 3178
Univasc Tablets 3181

Morphine Sulfate (Co-administration may result in potentiation of orthostatic hypotension).
Products include:
Astramorph/PF Injection, USP (Preservative-Free) 594
Duramorph Injection 1312
Infumorph 200 and Infumorph 500 Sterile Solutions 1314
Kadian Capsules 1335
MS Contin Tablets 2896
MSIR 2898
Oramorph SR Tablets 3062
Roxanol 3066

Nabumetone (Co-administration with non-steroidal anti-inflammatory agents can reduce the diuretic, natriuretic, and antihypertensive effect of thiazide diuretics). Products include:
Relafen Tablets 1617

Naproxen (Co-administration with non-steroidal anti-inflammatory agents can reduce the diuretic, natriuretic, and antihypertensive effect of thiazide diuretics). Products include:
EC-Naprosyn Delayed-Release Tablets 2967
Naprosyn Suspension 2967
Naprosyn Tablets 2967

Naproxen Sodium (Co-administration with non-steroidal anti-inflammatory agents can reduce the diuretic, natriuretic, and antihypertensive effect of thiazide diuretics). Products include:
Aleve Tablets, Caplets and Gelcaps .... ⊞602
Aleve Cold & Sinus Caplets .... ⊞603
Anaprox Tablets 2967
Anaprox DS Tablets 2967
Naprelan Tablets 1293

Nicardipine Hydrochloride (Bendroflumethiazide may potentiate the effects of other antihypertensives).
Products include:
Cardene I.V. 3485

Nifedipine (Bendroflumethiazide may potentiate the effects of other antihypertensives). Products include:
Adalat CC Tablets 877
Procardia Capsules 2708
Procardia XL Extended Release Tablets 2710

Nisoldipine (Bendroflumethiazide may potentiate the effects of other antihypertensives). Products include:
Sular Tablets 688

Nitroglycerin (Bendroflumethiazide may potentiate the effects of other antihypertensives). Products include:
Nitro-Dur Transdermal Infusion System 3134
Nitro-Dur Transdermal Infusion System 1834
Nitrolingual Pumpspray 1355
Nitrostat Tablets 2658

Norepinephrine Bitartrate (Thiazide may decrease the arterial responsiveness to norepinephrine).
No products indexed under this heading.

Oxaprozin (Co-administration with non-steroidal anti-inflammatory agents can reduce the diuretic, natriuretic, and antihypertensive effect of thiazide diuretics).
No products indexed under this heading.

Oxycodone Hydrochloride (Co-administration may result in potentiation of orthostatic hypotension).
Products include:
OxyContin Tablets 2912
OxyFast Oral Concentrate Solution 2916
OxyIR Capsules 2916
Percocet Tablets 1326
Percodan Tablets 1327
Percolone Tablets 1327
Roxicodone 3067
Tylox Capsules 2597

Pancuronium Bromide (Effects of nondepolarizing muscle relaxants may be potentiated).
No products indexed under this heading.

Pargyline Hydrochloride (Enhanced hypotensive effects; dosage adjustments of one or both agents may be necessary).
No products indexed under this heading.

Penbutolol Sulfate (Bendroflumethiazide may potentiate the effects of other antihypertensives).
No products indexed under this heading.

Pentobarbital Sodium (Co-administration may result in potentiation of orthostatic hypotension).
Products include:
Nembutal Sodium Solution 485

Perindopril Erbumine (Bendroflumethiazide may potentiate the effects of other antihypertensives).
Products include:
Aceon Tablets (2 mg, 4 mg, 8 mg) 3249

Phenelzine Sulfate (Enhanced hypotensive effects; dosage adjustments of one or both agents may be necessary). Products include:
Nardil Tablets 2653

Phenobarbital (Co-administration may result in potentiation of orthostatic hypotension). Products include:
Arco-Lase Plus Tablets 592
Donnatal 2929
Donnatal Extentabs 2930

Phenoxybenzamine Hydrochloride (Bendroflumethiazide may potentiate the effects of other antihypertensives). Products include:
Dibenzyline Capsules 3457

Phentolamine Mesylate (Bendroflumethiazide may potentiate the effects of other antihypertensives).
No products indexed under this heading.

Phenylbutazone (Co-administration with non-steroidal anti-inflammatory agents can reduce the diuretic, natriuretic, and antihypertensive effect of thiazide diuretics).
No products indexed under this heading.

Pindolol (Bendroflumethiazide may potentiate the effects of other antihypertensives).
No products indexed under this heading.

Pioglitazone Hydrochloride (Beta-adrenergic blockade may prevent the appearance of signs and symptoms of acute hypoglycemia; beta-blockade also reduces the release of insulin in response to hyperglycemia, therefore, it may be necessary to adjust the dose of oral antidiabetic drugs). Products include:
Actos Tablets 3275

Piroxicam (Co-administration with non-steroidal anti-inflammatory agents can reduce the diuretic, natriuretic, and antihypertensive effect of thiazide diuretics). Products include:
Feldene Capsules 2685

Polythiazide (Bendroflumethiazide may potentiate the effects of other antihypertensives). Products include:
Minizide Capsules 2700
Renese Tablets 2712

Prazosin Hydrochloride (Bendroflumethiazide may potentiate the effects of other antihypertensives).
Products include:
Minipress Capsules 2699
Minizide Capsules 2700

Prednisolone Acetate (Co-adminsitration with corticosteroids intensifies electrolyte imbalance, particulary hypokalemia). Products include:
Blephamide Ophthalmic Ointment 547
Blephamide Ophthalmic Suspension 548
Poly-Pred Liquifilm Ophthalmic Suspension .... ⊙245
Pred Forte Ophthalmic Suspension .... ⊙246
Pred Mild Sterile Ophthalmic Suspension .... ⊙249
Pred-G Ophthalmic Suspension .... ⊙247
Pred-G Sterile Ophthalmic Ointment .... ⊙248

Prednisolone Sodium Phosphate (Co-adminsitration with corticosteroids intensifies electrolyte imbalance, particulary hypokalemia).
Products include:
Pediapred Oral Solution 1170

Prednisolone Tebutate (Co-adminsitration with corticosteroids intensifies electrolyte imbalance, particulary hypokalemia).
No products indexed under this heading.

Prednisone (Co-adminsitration with corticosteroids intensifies electrolyte imbalance, particulary hypokalemia).
Products include:
Prednisone 3064

Probenecid (Bendroflumethiazide may raise the level of blood uric acid; dosage adjustment of antigout agents may be necessary).
No products indexed under this heading.

Procarbazine Hydrochloride (Enhanced hypotensive effects; dosage adjustments of one or both agents may be necessary). Products include:
Matulane Capsules 3246

Propofol (Co-administration may result in exaggeration of the hypotension induced by general anesthetics). Products include:
Diprivan Injectable Emulsion 667

Propoxyphene Hydrochloride (Co-administration may result in potentiation of orthostatic hypotension). Products include:
Darvon Pulvules 1909
Darvon Compound-65 Pulvules 1910

Propoxyphene Napsylate (Co-administration may result in potentiation of orthostatic hypotension).
Products include:
Darvon-N/Darvocet-N 1907
Darvon-N Tablets 1912

Propranolol Hydrochloride (Bendroflumethiazide may potentiate the effects of other antihypertensives).
Products include:
Inderal 3513
Inderal LA Long-Acting Capsules 3516
Inderide Tablets 3517
Inderide LA Long-Acting Capsules 3519

Quinapril Hydrochloride (Bendroflumethiazide may potentiate the effects of other antihypertensives).
Products include:
Accupril Tablets 2611
Accuretic Tablets 2614

Ramipril (Bendroflumethiazide may potentiate the effects of other antihypertensives). Products include:
Altace Capsules 2233

Rapacuronium Bromide (Effects of nondepolarizing muscle relaxants may be potentiated).
No products indexed under this heading.

Rauwolfia serpentina (Bendroflumethiazide may potentiate the effects of other antihypertensives).
No products indexed under this heading.

Remifentanil Hydrochloride (Co-administration may result in potentiation of orthostatic hypotension).
No products indexed under this heading.

Repaglinide (Beta-adrenergic blockade may prevent the appearance of signs and symptoms of acute hypoglycemia; beta-blockade also reduces the release of insulin in response to hyperglycemia, therefore, it may be necessary to adjust the dose of oral antidiabetic drugs).
Products include:
Prandin Tablets (0.5, 1, and 2 mg) 2432

Rescinnamine (Bendroflumethiazide may potentiate the effects of other antihypertensives).
No products indexed under this heading.

Reserpine (Co-administration with catecholamine-depleting drugs, such as reserpine, may result in additive effects, such as vertigo, syncope, excessive bradycardia, hypotension and postural hypotension).
No products indexed under this heading.

Rocuronium Bromide (Effects of nondepolarizing muscle relaxants may be potentiated). Products include:
Zemuron Injection 2491

Rofecoxib (Co-administration with non-steroidal anti-inflammatory agents can reduce the diuretic, natriuretic, and antihypertensive effect of thiazide diuretics). Products include:
Vioxx 2213

Rosiglitazone Maleate (Beta-adrenergic blockade may prevent the appearance of signs and symptoms of acute hypoglycemia; beta-blockade also reduces the release of insulin in response to hyperglycemia, therefore, it may be necessary to adjust the dose of oral antidiabetic drugs). Products include:
Avandia Tablets 1490

Secobarbital Sodium (Co-administration may result in potentiation of orthostatic hypotension).
No products indexed under this heading.

Selegiline Hydrochloride (Enhanced hypotensive effects; dosage adjustments of one or both agents may be necessary). Products include:
Eldepryl Capsules 3266

Sevoflurane (Co-administration may result in exaggeration of the hypotension induced by general anesthetics).
No products indexed under this heading.

Sodium Nitroprusside (Bendroflumethiazide may potentiate the effects of other antihypertensives).
No products indexed under this heading.

Sotalol Hydrochloride (Bendroflumethiazide may potentiate the effects of other antihypertensives). Products include:
Betapace Tablets 950
Betapace AF Tablets 954

Spirapril Hydrochloride (Bendroflumethiazide may potentiate the effects of other antihypertensives).
No products indexed under this heading.

Sufentanil Citrate (Co-administration may result in potentiation of orthostatic hypotension).
No products indexed under this heading.

Sulfinpyrazone (Bendroflumethiazide may raise the level of blood uric acid; dosage adjustment of antigout agents may be necessary).
No products indexed under this heading.

Sulindac (Co-administration with non-steroidal anti-inflammatory agents can reduce the diuretic, natriuretic, and antihypertensive effect of thiazide diuretics). Products include:
Clinoril Tablets 2053

Telmisartan (Bendroflumethiazide may potentiate the effects of other antihypertensives). Products include:
Micardis Tablets 1049
Micardis HCT Tablets 1051

Terazosin Hydrochloride (Bendroflumethiazide may potentiate the effects of other antihypertensives). Products include:
Hytrin Capsules 464

Thiamylal Sodium (Co-administration may result in potentiation of orthostatic hypotension).
No products indexed under this heading.

Timolol Maleate (Bendroflumethiazide may potentiate the effects of other antihypertensives). Products include:
Blocadren Tablets 2046
Cosopt Sterile Ophthalmic Solution 2065
Timolide Tablets 2187
Timolol GFS .... ⊙ 266
Timoptic in Ocudose 2192
Timoptic Sterile Ophthalmic Solution 2190
Timoptic-XE Sterile Ophthalmic Gel Forming Solution 2194

Tolazamide (Beta-adrenergic blockade may prevent the appearance of signs and symptoms of acute hypoglycemia; beta-blockade also reduces the release of insulin in response to hyperglycemia, therefore, it may be necessary to adjust the dose of oral antidiabetic drugs).
No products indexed under this heading.

Tolbutamide (Beta-adrenergic blockade may prevent the appearance of signs and symptoms of acute hypoglycemia; beta-blockade also reduces the release of insulin in response to hyperglycemia, therefore, it may be necessary to adjust the dose of oral antidiabetic drugs).
No products indexed under this heading.

Tolmetin Sodium (Co-administration with non-steroidal anti-inflammatory agents can reduce the diuretic, natriuretic, and antihypertensive effect of thiazide diuretics). Products include:
Tolectin 2589

Torsemide (Bendroflumethiazide may potentiate the effects of other antihypertensives). Products include:
Demadex Tablets and Injection 2965

Trandolapril (Bendroflumethiazide may potentiate the effects of other antihypertensives). Products include:
Mavik Tablets 478
Tarka Tablets 508

Tranylcypromine Sulfate (Enhanced hypotensive effects; dosage adjustments of one or both agents may be necessary). Products include:
Parnate Tablets 1607

Triamcinolone (Co-adminsitration with corticosteroids intensifies electrolyte imbalance, particulary hypokalemia).
No products indexed under this heading.

Triamcinolone Acetonide (Co-adminsitration with corticosteroids intensifies electrolyte imbalance, particulary hypokalemia). Products include:
Azmacort Inhalation Aerosol 728
Nasacort Nasal Inhaler 750
Nasacort AQ Nasal Spray 752
Tri-Nasal Spray 2274

Triamcinolone Diacetate (Co-adminsitration with corticosteroids intensifies electrolyte imbalance, particulary hypokalemia).
No products indexed under this heading.

Triamcinolone Hexacetonide (Co-adminsitration with corticosteroids intensifies electrolyte imbalance, particulary hypokalemia).
No products indexed under this heading.

Trimethaphan Camsylate (Bendroflumethiazide may potentiate the effects of other antihypertensives).
No products indexed under this heading.

Troglitazone (Beta-adrenergic blockade may prevent the appearance of signs and symptoms of acute hypoglycemia; beta-blockade also reduces the release of insulin in response to hyperglycemia, therefore, it may be necessary to adjust the dose of oral antidiabetic drugs).
No products indexed under this heading.

Tubocurarine Chloride (Effects of muscle relaxants may be potentiated).
No products indexed under this heading.

Valsartan (Bendroflumethiazide may potentiate the effects of other antihypertensives). Products include:
Diovan Capsules 2337
Diovan HCT Tablets 2338

Vecuronium Bromide (Effects of nondepolarizing muscle relaxants may be potentiated). Products include:
Norcuron for Injection 2478

Verapamil Hydrochloride (Bendroflumethiazide may potentiate the effects of other antihypertensives). Products include:
Covera-HS Tablets 3199
Isoptin SR Tablets 467
Tarka Tablets 508
Verelan Capsules 3184
Verelan PM Capsules 3186

Warfarin Sodium (Bendroflumethiazide may decrease the effects of oral anticoagulants; dosage adjustment of anticoagluants may be necessary). Products include:
Coumadin for Injection 1243
Coumadin Tablets 1243
Warfarin Sodium Tablets, USP 3302

Food Interactions

Alcohol (Co-administration may result in potentiation of orthostatic hypotension).

COSMEGEN FOR INJECTION
(Dactinomycin) 2062
None cited in PDR database.

COSOPT STERILE OPHTHALMIC SOLUTION
(Dorzolamide Hydrochloride, Timolol Maleate) 2065
May interact with beta blockers, carbonic anhydrase inhibitors, calcium channel blockers, cardiac glycosides, quinidine, salicylates, and certain other agents. Compounds in these categories include:

Acebutolol Hydrochloride (Co-administration of oral beta-adrenergic blockers and Cosopt may result in potential additive effects of beta-blockade, both systemic and on intraocular pressure). Products include:
Sectral Capsules 3589

Acetazolamide (Co-administration with oral carbonic anhydrase inhibitor may result in additive carbonic anhydrase inhibition). Products include:
Diamox Sequels Sustained Release Capsules .... ⊙ 270
Diamox Tablets .... ⊙ 269

Amlodipine Besylate (Co-administration of beta-adrenergic blockers and calcium channel blockers may result in possible atrioventricular conduction disturbances, left ventricular failure, and hypotension). Products include:
Lotrel Capsules 2370
Norvasc Tablets 2704

Aspirin (Potential for acid-base and electrolyte disturbances with high-dose salicylate therapy). Products include:
Aggrenox Capsules 1026
Alka-Seltzer .... ▣ 603
Alka-Seltzer Lemon Lime Antacid and Pain Reliever Effervescent Tablets .... ▣ 603
Alka-Seltzer Extra Strength Antacid and Pain Reliever Effervescent Tablets .... ▣ 603
Alka-Seltzer PM Effervescent Tablets .... ▣ 605
Genuine Bayer Tablets, Caplets and Gelcaps .... ▣ 606
Extra Strength Bayer Caplets and Gelcaps .... ▣ 610
Aspirin Regimen Bayer Children's Chewable Tablets (Orange or Cherry Flavored) .... ▣ 607
Bayer, Aspirin Regimen .... ▣ 606
Aspirin Regimen Bayer 81 mg Caplets with Calcium .... ▣ 607
Genuine Bayer Professional Labeling (Aspirin Regimen Bayer) .... ▣ 608
Extra Strength Bayer Arthritis Caplets .... ▣ 610
Extra Strength Bayer Plus Caplets .... ▣ 610
Extra Strength Bayer PM Caplets .... ▣ 611
BC Powder .... ▣ 619
BC Allergy Sinus Cold Powder .... ▣ 619
Arthritis Strength BC Powder .... ▣ 619
BC Sinus Cold Powder .... ▣ 619
Darvon Compound-65 Pulvules 1910
Ecotrin Enteric Coated Aspirin Low, Regular and Maximum Strength Tablets 1715
Excedrin Extra-Strength Tablets, Caplets, and Geltabs .... ▣ 629
Excedrin Migraine 1070
Goody's Body Pain Formula Powder .... ▣ 620
Goody's Extra Strength Headache Powder .... ▣ 620
Goody's Extra Strength Pain Relief Tablets .... ▣ 620
Percodan Tablets 1327
Robaxisal Tablets 2939
Soma Compound Tablets 3354
Soma Compound w/Codeine Tablets 3355
Vanquish Caplets .... ▣ 617

Atenolol (Co-administration of oral beta-adrenergic blockers and Cosopt may result in potential additive effects of beta-blockade, both systemic and on intraocular pressure). Products include:
Tenoretic Tablets 690
Tenormin I.V. Injection 692

Bepridil Hydrochloride (Co-administration of beta-adrenergic blockers and calcium channel blockers may result in possible atrioventricular conduction disturbances, left ventricular failure, and hypotension). Products include:
Vascor Tablets 2602

Betaxolol Hydrochloride (Co-administration of oral beta-adrenergic blockers and Cosopt may result in potential additive effects of beta-blockade, both systemic and on intraocular pressure; the concomitant use of two topical beta-adrenergic agents is not recommended). Products include:
Betoptic S Ophthalmic Suspension 537

Carteolol Hydrochloride (Co-administration of oral beta-adrenergic blockers and Cosopt may result in potential additive effects of beta-blockade, both systemic and on intraocular pressure; the concomitant use of two topical beta-adrenergic agents is not recommended). Products include:
Carteolol Hydrochloride Ophthalmic Solution USP, 1% .... ⊙ 258
Ocupress Ophthalmic Solution, 1% Sterile .... ⊙ 303

Choline Magnesium Trisalicylate (Potential for acid-base and electrolyte disturbances with high-dose salicylate therapy). Products include:
Trilisate 2901

Clonidine (Oral beta-adrenergic blocking agents may exacerbate the rebound hypertension which can follow withdrawal of clonidine; there have been no reports of exacerbation of rebound hypertension with ophthalmic timolol). Products include:
Catapres-TTS 1038

Clonidine Hydrochloride (Oral beta-adrenergic blocking agents may exacerbate the rebound hypertension which can follow withdrawal of clonidine; there have been no reports of exacerbation of rebound hypertension with ophthalmic timolol). Products include:
Catapres Tablets 1037
Clorpres Tablets 1002
Combipres Tablets 1040
Duraclon Injection 3057

Deslanoside (The concomitant use of beta-adrenergic blocking agents with digitalis and calcium antagonists may have additive effects in prolonging atrioventricular conduction time).
No products indexed under this heading.

Dichlorphenamide (Co-administration with oral carbonic anhydrase inhibitor may result in additive carbonic anhydrase inhibition). Products include:
Daranide Tablets 2077

Diflunisal (Potential for acid-base and electrolyte disturbances with high-dose salicylate therapy). Products include:
Dolobid Tablets 2088

Digitoxin (The concomitant use of beta-adrenergic blocking agents with digitalis and calcium antagonists may have additive effects in prolonging atrioventricular conduction time).
No products indexed under this heading.

Digoxin (The concomitant use of beta-adrenergic blocking agents with

digitalis and calcium antagonists may have additive effects in prolonging atrioventricular conduction time). Products include:
Digitek Tablets 1003
Lanoxicaps Capsules 1574
Lanoxin Injection 1581
Lanoxin Tablets 1587
Lanoxin Elixir Pediatric 1578
Lanoxin Injection Pediatric 1584

Diltiazem Hydrochloride (Co-administration of beta-adrenergic blockers and calcium channel blockers may result in possible atrioventricular conduction disturbances, left ventricular failure, and hypotension). Products include:
Cardizem Injectable 1018
Cardizem Lyo-Ject Syringe 1018
Cardizem Monovial 1018
Cardizem CD Capsules 1016
Tiazac Capsules 1378

Epinephrine (Patients with a history of atopy or anaphylactic reactions to a variety of allergens may be unresponsive to the usual dose of injectable epinephrine used to treat allergic reactions). Products include:
Epifrin Sterile Ophthalmic Solution .... ⊙235
EpiPen 1236
Primatene Mist .... ▣779
Xylocaine with Epinephrine Injection 653

Epinephrine Hydrochloride (Patients with a history of atopy or anaphylactic reactions to a variety of allergens may be unresponsive to the usual dose of injectable epinephrine used to treat allergic reactions).
No products indexed under this heading.

Felodipine (Co-administration of beta-adrenergic blockers and calcium channel blockers may result in possible atrioventricular conduction disturbances, left ventricular failure, and hypotension). Products include:
Lexxel Tablets 608
Plendil Extended-Release Tablets 623

Isradipine (Co-administration of beta-adrenergic blockers and calcium channel blockers may result in possible atrioventricular conduction disturbances, left ventricular failure, and hypotension). Products include:
DynaCirc Capsules 2921
DynaCirc CR Tablets 2923

Levobunolol Hydrochloride (Co-administration of oral beta-adrenergic blockers and Cosopt may result in potential additive effects of beta-blockade, both systemic and on intraocular pressure; the concomitant use of two topical beta-adrenergic agents is not recommended). Products include:
Betagan .... ⊙228

Magnesium Salicylate (Potential for acid-base and electrolyte disturbances with high-dose salicylate therapy). Products include:
Momentum Backache Relief Extra Strength Caplets .... ▣666

Methazolamide (Co-administration with oral carbonic anhydrase inhibitor may result in additive carbonic anhydrase inhibition). Products include:
Neptazane Tablets .... ⊙271

Metipranolol Hydrochloride (Co-administration of oral beta-adrenergic blockers and Cosopt may result in potential additive effects of beta-blockade, both systemic and on intraocular pressure; the concomitant use of two topical beta-adrenergic agents is not recommended).
No products indexed under this heading.

Mibefradil Dihydrochloride (Co-administration of beta-adrenergic blockers and calcium channel blockers may result in possible atrioventricular conduction disturbances, left ventricular failure, and hypotension).
No products indexed under this heading.

Nicardipine Hydrochloride (Co-administration of beta-adrenergic blockers and calcium channel blockers may result in possible atrioventricular conduction disturbances, left ventricular failure, and hypotension). Products include:
Cardene I.V. 3485

Nifedipine (Co-administration of beta-adrenergic blockers and calcium channel blockers may result in possible atrioventricular conduction disturbances, left ventricular failure, and hypotension). Products include:
Adalat CC Tablets 877
Procardia Capsules 2708
Procardia XL Extended Release Tablets 2710

Nimodipine (Co-administration of beta-adrenergic blockers and calcium channel blockers may result in possible atrioventricular conduction disturbances, left ventricular failure, and hypotension). Products include:
Nimotop Capsules 904

Nisoldipine (Co-administration of beta-adrenergic blockers and calcium channel blockers may result in possible atrioventricular conduction disturbances, left ventricular failure, and hypotension). Products include:
Sular Tablets 688

Quinidine Gluconate (Potentiated systemic beta-blockade has been reported during combined treatment with quinidine and timolol). Products include:
Quinaglute Dura-Tabs Tablets 978

Quinidine Polygalacturonate (Potentiated systemic beta-blockade has been reported during combined treatment with quinidine and timolol).
No products indexed under this heading.

Quinidine Sulfate (Potentiated systemic beta-blockade has been reported during combined treatment with quinidine and timolol). Products include:
Quinidex Extentabs 2933

Reserpine (Co-administration of catecholamine-depleting drugs and beta-adrenergic blocker may result in possible additive effects and the production of hypotension and/or marked bradycardia).
No products indexed under this heading.

Salsalate (Potential for acid-base and electrolyte disturbances with high-dose salicylate therapy).
No products indexed under this heading.

Timolol Hemihydrate (Co-administration of oral beta-adrenergic blockers and Cosopt may result in potential additive effects of beta-blockade, both systemic and on intraocular pressure; the concomitant use of two topical beta-adrenergic agents is not recommended). Products include:
Betimol Ophthalmic Solution .... ⊙324

Verapamil Hydrochloride (Co-administration of beta-adrenergic blockers and calcium channel blockers may result in possible atrioventricular conduction disturbances, left ventricular failure, and hypotension). Products include:
Covera-HS Tablets 3199
Isoptin SR Tablets 467
Tarka Tablets 508
Verelan Capsules 3184
Verelan PM Capsules 3186

COUMADIN FOR INJECTION

(Warfarin Sodium) 1243
See Coumadin Tablets

COUMADIN TABLETS

(Warfarin Sodium) 1243
May interact with 5-lipoxygenase inhibitors, oral aminoglycosides, androgens, antacids, antihistamines, antiandrogens, barbiturates, corticosteroids, diuretics, erythromycin, fluoroquinolone antibiotics, inhalant anesthetics, leukotriene receptor antagonists, monoamine oxidase inhibitors, narcotic analgesics, nonsteroidal anti-inflammatory agents, oral contraceptives, pyrazolon derivatives, salicylates, selective serotonin reuptake inhibitors, sulfonamides, thyroid preparations, and certain other agents. Compounds in these categories include:

Acetaminophen (May be responsible for increased prothrombin time response). Products include:
Actifed Cold & Sinus Caplets and Tablets .... ▣688
Alka-Seltzer Plus Liqui-Gels .... ▣604
Alka-Seltzer Plus Cold & Flu Medicine Liqui-Gels .... ▣604
Alka-Seltzer Plus Cold & Sinus Medicine Liqui-Gels .... ▣604
Benadryl Allergy/Cold Tablets .... ▣691
Benadryl Allergy Sinus Headache Caplets & Gelcaps .... ▣693
Benadryl Severe Allergy & Sinus Headache Caplets .... ▣694
Children's Cēpacol Sore Throat .... ▣788
Comtrex Acute Head Cold & Sinus Pressure Relief Tablets .... ▣627
Comtrex Deep Chest Cold & Congestion Relief Softgels .... ▣627
Comtrex Flu Therapy & Fever Relief Daytime Caplets .... ▣628
Comtrex Flu Therapy & Fever Relief Nighttime Tablets .... ▣628
Comtrex Maximum Strength Multi-Symptom Cold & Cough Relief Tablets and Caplets .... ▣626
Contac Severe Cold and Flu Caplets Maximum Strength .... ▣746
Contac Severe Cold and Flu Caplets Non-Drowsy .... ▣746
Coricidin 'D' Cold, Flu & Sinus Tablets .... ▣737
Coricidin HBP Cold & Flu Tablets .... ▣738
Coricidin HBP Maximum Strength Flu Tablets .... ▣738
Coricidin HBP Night-Time Cold & Flu Tablets .... ▣738
Darvon-N/Darvocet-N 1907
Dimetapp Cold and Fever Suspension .... ▣775
Dimetapp Nighttime Flu Liquid .... ▣776
Dimetapp Non-Drowsy Flu Syrup .... ▣777
Drixoral Allergy/Sinus Extended-Release Tablets .... ▣741
Drixoral Cold & Flu Extended-Release Tablets .... ▣740
Aspirin Free Excedrin Caplets and Geltabs .... ▣628
Excedrin Extra-Strength Tablets, Caplets, and Geltabs .... ▣629
Excedrin Migraine 1070
Excedrin PM Tablets, Caplets, and Geltabs .... ▣631
Goody's Body Pain Formula Powder .... ▣620
Goody's Extra Strength Headache Powder .... ▣620
Goody's Extra Strength Pain Relief Tablets .... ▣620
Goody's PM Powder .... ▣621
Hycomine Compound Tablets 1317
Lortab 3319
Lortab Elixir 3317
Maxidone Tablets CIII 3399
Maximum Strength Midol Menstrual Caplets and Gelcaps .... ▣612
Maximum Strength Midol PMS Caplets and Gelcaps .... ▣613
Maximum Strength Midol Teen Caplets .... ▣612
Midrin Capsules 3464
Norco 5/325 Tablets CIII 3424
Norco 7.5/325 Tablets CIII 3425
Norco 10/325 Tablets CIII 3427
Norco 10/325 Tablets CIII 3425
Percocet Tablets 1326
Percogesic Aspirin-Free Coated Tablets .... ▣667
Extra Strength Percogesic Aspirin-Free Coated Caplets .... ▣665
Phrenilin 578
Robitussin Cold Caplets Multi-Symptom Cold & Flu .... ▣781
Robitussin Cold Softgels Multi-Symptom Cold & Flu .... ▣781
Robitussin Multi Symptom Honey Flu Liquid .... ▣785
Robitussin Nighttime Honey Flu Liquid .... ▣786
Sedapap Tablets 50 mg/650 mg 2225
Singlet Caplets .... ▣761
Sinutab Sinus Allergy Medication, Maximum Strength Formula, Tablets & Caplets .... ▣707
Sinutab Sinus Medication, Maximum Strength Without Drowsiness Formula, Tablets & Caplets .... ▣707
Sudafed Cold & Cough Liquid Caps .... ▣709
Sudafed Cold & Sinus Liquid Caps .... ▣710
Sudafed Severe Cold .... ▣711
Sudafed Sinus Headache Caplets .... ▣712
Sudafed Sinus Headache Tablets .... ▣712
Tavist Sinus Non-Drowsy Coated Caplets .... ▣676
TheraFlu Regular Strength Cold & Cough Night Time Hot Liquid .... ▣676
TheraFlu Regular Strength Cold & Sore Throat Night Time Hot Liquid .... ▣676
TheraFlu Maximum Strength Flu & Congestion Non-Drowsy Hot Liquid .... ▣677
TheraFlu Maximum Strength Flu & Cough Night Time Hot Liquid .... ▣678
TheraFlu Maximum Strength Flu & Sore Throat Night Time Hot Liquid .... ▣677
TheraFlu Maximum Strength Severe Cold & Congestion Night Time Caplets .... ▣678
TheraFlu Maximum Strength Severe Cold & Congestion Night Time Hot Liquid .... ▣678
TheraFlu Maximum Strength Severe Cold & Congestion Non-Drowsy .... ▣679
Triaminic Cold, Cough & Fever Liquid .... ▣681
Triaminic Cough & Sore Throat Liquid .... ▣682
Triaminic Cough & Sore Throat Softchews .... ▣684
Tylenol, Children's 2014
Children's Tylenol Allergy-D Liquid 2014
Children's Tylenol Cold Suspension Liquid and Chewable Tablets 2015
Children's Tylenol Cold Plus Cough Suspension Liquid and Chewable Tablets 2015
Children's Tylenol Flu Suspension Liquid 2015
Children's Tylenol Sinus Suspension Liquid 2017
Infants' Tylenol Cold Decongestant and Fever Reducer Concentrated Drops 2015
Infants' Tylenol Cold Decongestant and Fever Reducer Concentrated Drops Plus Cough 2015
Junior Strength Tylenol Soft Chews Chewable Tablets 2014
Tylenol 2009
Tylenol Allergy Sinus 2010
Tylenol Severe Allergy Caplets 2010
Multi-Symptom Tylenol Cold Complete Formula Caplets 2010
Multi-Symptom Tylenol Cold Non-Drowsy Caplets and Gelcaps 2010
Multi-Symptom Tylenol Cold Severe Congestion Non-Drowsy Caplets 2011
Maximum Strength Tylenol Flu NightTime Gelcaps 2011
Maximum Strength Tylenol Flu NightTime Liquid 2011
Maximum Strength Tylenol Flu Non-Drowsy Gelcaps 2011
Extra Strength Tylenol PM Caplets, Geltabs, and Gelcaps 2012
Maximum Strength Tylenol Sinus NightTime Caplets 2012
Maximum Strength Tylenol Sinus Non-Drowsy Geltabs, Gelcaps, Caplets, and Tablets 2012
Maximum Strength Tylenol Sore Throat Adult Liquid 2013
Tylenol with Codeine 2595
Women's Tylenol Menstrual Relief Caplets 2013
Tylox Capsules 2597
Ultracet Tablets 2597
Vanquish Caplets .... ▣617
Vicks 44M Cough, Cold & Flu Relief Liquid .... ▣725
Vicks DayQuil LiquiCaps/Liquid Multi-Symptom Cold/Flu Relief .... ▣727

Vicks NyQuil LiquiCaps/Liquid Multi-Symptom Cold/Flu Relief, Original and Cherry Flavors ▣727
Vicodin Tablets 516
Vicodin ES Tablets 517
Vicodin HP Tablets 518
Zydone Tablets 1330

Achillea millefolium (Co-administration with botanicals with coagulant properties, such as yarrow, may affect the anticoagulant effects of warfarin).
No products indexed under this heading.

Acrivastine (Decreased prothrombin time response). Products include:
Semprex-D Capsules 1172

ACTH (Decreased prothrombin time response).
No products indexed under this heading.

Agrimonia eupatoria (Co-administration with botanicals that contain salicylate and/or have antiplatelet properties, such as agrimony, may result in increased anticoagulant effects; agrimony contains salicylate and has coagulant properties).
No products indexed under this heading.

Alatrofloxacin Mesylate (Increased prothrombin time response). Products include:
Trovan I.V. 2722

Alfentanil Hydrochloride (Increased prothrombin time response with prolonged use).
No products indexed under this heading.

Allium cepa (Co-administration with botanicals that contain salicylate and/or have antiplatelet or fibrinolytic properties, such as onion, may result in increased anticoagulant effects).
No products indexed under this heading.

Allium sativum (Co-administration is associated most often with increases in the effects of warfarin; garlic may cause bleeding events when taken alone and may have anticoagulant, antiplatelet, and/or fibrinolytic properties). Products include:
Beta-C Tablets ▣811
Centrum Focused Formulas Heart Tablets ▣816
CorePlex Capsules ▣796
One-A-Day Cholesterol Health Tablets ▣805
System 3-4-3 Capsules ▣800

Allopurinol (Increased prothrombin time response).
No products indexed under this heading.

Aloe Gel (Co-administration with botanicals that contain salicylate and/or have antiplatelet properties, such as aloe gel, may result in increased anticoagulant effects).
No products indexed under this heading.

Alteplase, Recombinant (Increased prothrombin time response). Products include:
Activase I.V. 1410
Cathflo Activase 3611

Aluminum Carbonate (Decreased prothrombin time response).
No products indexed under this heading.

Aluminum Hydroxide (Decreased prothrombin time response). Products include:
Amphojel Suspension (Mint Flavor) ▣789
Gaviscon Extra Strength Liquid ▣751
Gaviscon Extra Strength Tablets ▣751
Gaviscon Regular Strength Liquid ▣751
Gaviscon Regular Strength Tablets ▣750
Maalox Antacid/Anti-Gas Oral Suspension ▣673
Maalox Max Maximum Strength Antacid/Anti-Gas Liquid 2300
Maalox Regular Strength Antacid/Antigas Liquid 2300
Mylanta 1813
Vanquish Caplets ▣617

Amiloride Hydrochloride (Decreased or increased prothrombin time response). Products include:
Midamor Tablets 2136
Moduretic Tablets 2138

Aminoglutethimide (Decreased prothrombin time response).
No products indexed under this heading.

p-Aminosalicylic Acid (Increased prothrombin time response).
No products indexed under this heading.

Amiodarone Hydrochloride (Increased prothrombin time response). Products include:
Cordarone Intravenous 3491
Cordarone Tablets 3487
Pacerone Tablets 3331

Amobarbital (Decreased prothrombin time response).
No products indexed under this heading.

Aniseed (Co-administration with botanicals that contain coumarins, such as aniseed, may result in increased anticoagulant effects).
No products indexed under this heading.

Anistreplase (Increased prothrombin time response).
No products indexed under this heading.

Antibiotics, unspecified (Decreased or increased prothrombin time response).
No products indexed under this heading.

Antipyrine (Increased prothrombin time response). Products include:
Auralgan Otic Solution 3485

Apium graveolens (Co-administration with botanicals that contain coumarins, such as celery, may result in increased anticoagulant effects).
No products indexed under this heading.

Aprobarbital (Decreased prothrombin time response).
No products indexed under this heading.

Ardeparin Sodium (Co-administration has resulted in cases of venous limb ischemia, necrosis, and gangrene in patients with heparin-induced thrombocytopenia and deep venous thrombosis when heparin treatment was discontinued and warfarin therapy was started or continued; sequelae have included amputation of the involved area and/or death).
No products indexed under this heading.

Armoracia rusticana (Co-administration with botanicals that contain coumarins, such as horseradish, may result in increased anticoagulant effects).
No products indexed under this heading.

Arnica montana (Co-administration with botanicals that contain coumarins, such as arnica, may result in increased anticoagulant effects).
No products indexed under this heading.

Aspen (Co-administration with botanicals that contain salicylate and/or have antiplatelet properties, such as aspen, may result in increased anticoagulant effects).
No products indexed under this heading.

Aspirin (Increased prothrombin time response; caution should be observed when used concurrently). Products include:
Aggrenox Capsules 1026
Alka-Seltzer ▣603
Alka-Seltzer Lemon Lime Antacid and Pain Reliever Effervescent Tablets ▣603
Alka-Seltzer Extra Strength Antacid and Pain Reliever Effervescent Tablets ▣603
Alka-Seltzer PM Effervescent Tablets ▣605
Genuine Bayer Tablets, Caplets and Gelcaps ▣606
Extra Strength Bayer Caplets and Gelcaps ▣610
Aspirin Regimen Bayer Children's Chewable Tablets (Orange or Cherry Flavored) ▣607
Bayer, Aspirin Regimen ▣606
Aspirin Regimen Bayer 81 mg Caplets with Calcium ▣607
Genuine Bayer Professional Labeling (Aspirin Regimen Bayer) ▣608
Extra Strength Bayer Arthritis Caplets ▣610
Extra Strength Bayer Plus Caplets ▣610
Extra Strength Bayer PM Caplets ▣611
BC Powder ▣619
BC Allergy Sinus Cold Powder ▣619
Arthritis Strength BC Powder ▣619
BC Sinus Cold Powder ▣619
Darvon Compound-65 Pulvules 1910
Ecotrin Enteric Coated Aspirin Low, Regular and Maximum Strength Tablets 1715
Excedrin Extra-Strength Tablets, Caplets, and Geltabs ▣629
Excedrin Migraine 1070
Goody's Body Pain Formula Powder ▣620
Goody's Extra Strength Headache Powder ▣620
Goody's Extra Strength Pain Relief Tablets ▣620
Percodan Tablets 1327
Robaxisal Tablets 2939
Soma Compound Tablets 3354
Soma Compound w/Codeine Tablets 3355
Vanquish Caplets ▣617

Astemizole (Decreased prothrombin time response).
No products indexed under this heading.

Atorvastatin Calcium (Decreased prothrombin time response). Products include:
Lipitor Tablets 2639
Lipitor Tablets 2696

Azatadine Maleate (Decreased prothrombin time response). Products include:
Rynatan Tablets 3351

Azathioprine (Decreased prothrombin time response).
No products indexed under this heading.

Azithromycin Dihydrate (Increased prothrombin time response). Products include:
Zithromax 2743
Zithromax for IV Infusion 2748
Zithromax for Oral Suspension, 300 mg, 600 mg, 900 mg, 1200 mg 2739
Zithromax Tablets, 250 mg 2739

Bendroflumethiazide (Decreased or increased prothrombin time response). Products include:
Corzide 40/5 Tablets 2247
Corzide 80/5 Tablets 2247

Betamethasone Acetate (Decreased or increased prothrombin time response). Products include:
Celestone Soluspan Injectable Suspension 3097

Betamethasone Sodium Phosphate (Decreased or increased prothrombin time response). Products include:
Celestone Soluspan Injectable Suspension 3097

Bicalutamide (May be responsible, alone or in combination, for increased prothrombin time/international normalized ratio (PT/INR) response). Products include:
Casodex Tablets 662

Black Cohosh (Co-administration with botanicals that contain salicylate and/or have antiplatelet properties, such as black cohosh, may result in increased anticoagulant effects). Products include:
One-A-Day Menopause Health Tablets ▣808
Remifemin Menopause Tablets ▣839

Bromelains (Co-administration is associated most often with increases in the effects of warfarin).
No products indexed under this heading.

Bromodiphenhydramine Hydrochloride (Decreased prothrombin time response).
No products indexed under this heading.

Brompheniramine Maleate (Decreased prothrombin time response). Products include:
Bromfed Capsules (Extended-Release) 2269
Bromfed-PD Capsules (Extended-Release) 2269
Comtrex Acute Head Cold & Sinus Pressure Relief Tablets ▣627
Dimetapp Elixir ▣777
Dimetapp Cold and Fever Suspension ▣775
Dimetapp DM Cold & Cough Elixir ▣775
Dimetapp Nighttime Flu Liquid ▣776

Buchu (Co-administration with botanicals that contain coumarins, such as buchu, may result in increased anticoagulant effects).
No products indexed under this heading.

Bumetanide (Decreased or increased prothrombin time response).
No products indexed under this heading.

Buprenorphine Hydrochloride (Increased prothrombin time response with prolonged use). Products include:
Buprenex Injectable 2918

Butabarbital (Decreased prothrombin time response).
No products indexed under this heading.

Butalbital (Decreased prothrombin time response). Products include:
Phrenilin 578
Sedapap Tablets 50 mg/650 mg 2225

Capecitabine (Increased prothrombin time response). Products include:
Xeloda Tablets 3039

Capsicum annuum (Co-administration with botanicals that contain coumarins, such as capsicum, may result in increased anticoagulant effects; capsicum also has fibrinolytic properties).
No products indexed under this heading.

Carbamazepine (Decreased prothrombin time response). Products include:
Carbatrol Capsules 3234
Tegretol/Tegretol-XR 2404

Cassia angustifolia (Co-administration with botanicals that contain coumarins, such as cassia, may result in increased anticoagulant effects).
No products indexed under this heading.

Cassia fistula (Co-administration with botanicals that contain coumarins, such as cassia, may result in increased anticoagulant effects).
No products indexed under this heading.

Cassia senna (Co-administration with botanicals that contain coumarins, such as cassia, may result in

increased anticoagulant effects).
No products indexed under this heading.

Cefamandole Nafate (Increased prothrombin time response). Products include:
Mandol Vials 1953

Cefazolin Sodium (Increased prothrombin time response). Products include:
Ancef for Injection 1474
Ancef Injection 1474
Kefzol Vials, ADD-Vantage 1951

Cefoperazone Sodium (Increased prothrombin time response). Products include:
Cefobid Pharmacy Bulk Package - Not for Direct Infusion 2673

Cefotetan (Increased prothrombin time response). Products include:
Cefotan 664

Cefoxitin Sodium (Increased prothrombin time response). Products include:
Mefoxin for Injection 2124
Mefoxin Premixed Intravenous Solution 2127

Ceftriaxone Sodium (Increased prothrombin time response). Products include:
Rocephin Injectable Vials, ADD-Vantage, Galaxy, Bulk 2993

Celecoxib (Increased prothrombin time response; caution should be observed when used concurrently). Products include:
Celebrex Capsules 2676
Celebrex Capsules 2780

Cerivastatin Sodium (May be responsible, alone or in combination, for increased prothrombin time/international normalized ratio (PT/INR) response). Products include:
Baycol Tablets 883

Cetirizine Hydrochloride (Decreased prothrombin time response). Products include:
Zyrtec 2756
Zyrtec-D 12 Hour Extended Relief Tablets 2758

Chenodiol (Increased prothrombin time response).
No products indexed under this heading.

Chloral Hydrate (Decreased or increased prothrombin time response).
No products indexed under this heading.

Chloramphenicol (Increased prothrombin time response). Products include:
Chloromycetin Ophthalmic Ointment, 1% ⊙296
Chloromycetin Ophthalmic Solution ⊙297
Chloroptic Sterile Ophthalmic Ointment ⊙234
Chloroptic Sterile Ophthalmic Solution ⊙235

Chloramphenicol Palmitate (Increased prothrombin time response).
No products indexed under this heading.

Chloramphenicol Sodium Succinate (Increased prothrombin time response).
No products indexed under this heading.

Chlordiazepoxide (Decreased prothrombin time response). Products include:
Limbitrol 1738

Chlordiazepoxide Hydrochloride (Decreased prothrombin time response). Products include:
Librium Capsules 1736
Librium for Injection 1737

Chlorothiazide (Decreased or increased prothrombin time response). Products include:
Aldoclor Tablets 2035
Diuril Oral 2087

Chlorothiazide Sodium (Decreased or increased prothrombin time response). Products include:
Diuril Sodium Intravenous 2086

Chlorpheniramine Maleate (Decreased prothrombin time response). Products include:
Actifed Cold & Sinus Caplets and Tablets ▣688
Alka-Seltzer Plus Liqui-Gels ▣604
BC Allergy Sinus Cold Powder ▣619
Chlor-Trimeton Allergy Tablets ▣735
Chlor-Trimeton Allergy/Decongestant Tablets ▣736
Comtrex Flu Therapy & Fever Relief Nighttime Tablets ▣628
Comtrex Maximum Strength Multi-Symptom Cold & Cough Relief Tablets and Caplets ▣626
Contac Severe Cold and Flu Caplets Maximum Strength ▣746
Coricidin 'D' Cold, Flu & Sinus Tablets ▣737
Coricidin/Coricidin D ▣738
Coricidin HBP Maximum Strength Flu Tablets ▣738
Extendryl 1361
Hycomine Compound Tablets 1317
Kronofed-A 1341
PediaCare Cough-Cold Liquid ▣719
PediaCare NightRest Cough-Cold Liquid ▣719
Robitussin Nighttime Honey Flu Liquid ▣786
Ryna ▣768
Singlet Caplets ▣761
Sinutab Sinus Allergy Medication, Maximum Strength Formula, Tablets & Caplets ▣707
Sudafed Cold & Allergy Tablets ▣708
TheraFlu Regular Strength Cold & Cough Night Time Hot Liquid ▣676
TheraFlu Regular Strength Cold & Sore Throat Night Time Hot Liquid ▣676
TheraFlu Maximum Strength Flu & Cough Night Time Hot Liquid ▣678
TheraFlu Maximum Strength Flu & Sore Throat Night Time Hot Liquid ▣677
TheraFlu Maximum Strength Severe Cold & Congestion Night Time Caplets ▣678
TheraFlu Maximum Strength Severe Cold & Congestion Night Time Hot Liquid ▣678
Triaminic Cold & Allergy Liquid ▣681
Triaminic Cold & Allergy Softchews ▣683
Triaminic Cold & Cough Liquid ▣681
Triaminic Cold & Cough Softchews ▣683
Triaminic Cold & Night Time Cough Liquid ▣681
Triaminic Cold, Cough & Fever Liquid ▣681
Children's Tylenol Cold Suspension Liquid and Chewable Tablets 2015
Children's Tylenol Cold Plus Cough Suspension Liquid and Chewable Tablets 2015
Children's Tylenol Flu Suspension Liquid 2015
Maximum Strength Tylenol Allergy Sinus Caplets, Gelcaps, and Geltabs 2010
Multi-Symptom Tylenol Cold Complete Formula Caplets 2010
Vicks 44M Cough, Cold & Flu Relief Liquid ▣725
Pediatric Vicks 44m Cough & Cold Relief ▣728
Children's Vicks NyQuil Cold/Cough Relief ▣726

Chlorpheniramine Polistirex (Decreased prothrombin time response). Products include:
Tussionex Pennkinetic Extended-Release Suspension 1174

Chlorpheniramine Tannate (Decreased prothrombin time response). Products include:
Reformulated Rynatan Pediatric Suspension 3352
Rynatuss Pediatric Suspension 3353
Rynatuss Tablets 3353
Tussi-12 S Suspension 3356
Tussi-12 Tablets 3356

Chlorpropamide (Increased prothrombin time response; accumulation of chlorpropamide). Products include:
Diabinese Tablets 2680

Chlorthalidone (Decreased or increased prothrombin time response). Products include:
Clorpres Tablets 1002
Combipres Tablets 1040
Tenoretic Tablets 690

Cholestyramine (Decreased or increased prothrombin time response).
No products indexed under this heading.

Choline Magnesium Trisalicylate (Increased prothrombin time response; caution should be observed when used concurrently). Products include:
Trilisate 2901

Cimetidine (Increased prothrombin time response). Products include:
Tagamet HB 200 Suspension ▣762
Tagamet HB 200 Tablets ▣761
Tagamet Tablets 1644

Cimetidine Hydrochloride (Increased prothrombin time response). Products include:
Tagamet 1644

Ciprofloxacin (Increased prothrombin time response). Products include:
Cipro I.V. 893
Cipro I.V. Pharmacy Bulk Package 897
Cipro Oral Suspension 887

Ciprofloxacin Hydrochloride (Increased prothrombin time response). Products include:
Ciloxan 538
Cipro HC Otic Suspension 540
Cipro Tablets 887

Cisapride (Increased prothrombin time response).
No products indexed under this heading.

Citalopram Hydrobromide (Increased prothrombin time response). Products include:
Celexa 1365

Clarithromycin (Increased prothrombin time response). Products include:
Biaxin/Biaxin XL 403
PREVPAC 3298

Clemastine Fumarate (Decreased prothrombin time response). Products include:
Tavist 12 Hour Allergy Tablets ▣676

Clofibrate (Increased prothrombin time response). Products include:
Atromid-S Capsules 3483

Clozapine (May be responsible, alone or in combination, for decreased prothrombin time/international normalized ratio (PT/INR) response). Products include:
Clozaril Tablets 2319

Codeine Phosphate (Increased prothrombin time response with prolonged use). Products include:
Phenergan with Codeine Syrup 3557
Phenergan VC with Codeine Syrup 3561
Robitussin A-C Syrup 2942
Robitussin-DAC Syrup 2942
Ryna-C Liquid ▣768
Soma Compound w/Codeine Tablets 3355
Tussi-Organidin NR Liquid 3350
Tussi-Organidin-S NR Liquid 3350
Tylenol with Codeine 2595

Coenzyme Q-10 (Co-administration is associated most often with decreases in the effects of warfarin). Products include:
Cardio Essentials Capsules 3321
Centrum Focused Formulas Heart Tablets ▣816
CoQuinone Capsules 3335

Cortisone Acetate (Decreased or increased prothrombin time response). Products include:
Cortone Acetate Injectable Suspension 2059
Cortone Acetate Tablets 2061

Cyclophosphamide (Increased or decreased prothrombin time response).
No products indexed under this heading.

Cyproheptadine Hydrochloride (Decreased prothrombin time response). Products include:
Periactin Tablets 2155

Dalteparin Sodium (Co-administration has resulted in cases of venous limb ischemia, necrosis, and gangrene in patients with heparin-induced thrombocytopenia and deep venous thrombosis when heparin treatment was discontinued and warfarin therapy was started or continued; sequelae have included amputation of the involved area and/or death). Products include:
Fragmin Injection 2814

Danazol (Increased prothrombin time response).
No products indexed under this heading.

Danshen (Increased prothrombin time response).
No products indexed under this heading.

Daucus carota (Co-administration with botanicals that contain coumarins, such as wild carrots, may result in increased anticoagulant effects).
No products indexed under this heading.

Desflurane (Increased prothrombin time response). Products include:
Suprane Liquid for Inhalation 874

Desogestrel (Decreased prothrombin time response). Products include:
Cyclessa Tablets 2450
Desogen Tablets 2458
Mircette Tablets 2470
Ortho-Cept 21 Tablets 2546
Ortho-Cept 28 Tablets 2546

Dexamethasone (Decreased or increased prothrombin time response). Products include:
Decadron Elixir 2078
Decadron Tablets 2079
TobraDex Ophthalmic Ointment 542
TobraDex Ophthalmic Suspension 541

Dexamethasone Acetate (Decreased or increased prothrombin time response).
No products indexed under this heading.

Dexamethasone Sodium Phosphate (Decreased or increased prothrombin time response). Products include:
Decadron Phosphate Injection 2081
Decadron Phosphate Sterile Ophthalmic Ointment 2083
Decadron Phosphate Sterile Ophthalmic Solution 2084
NeoDecadron Sterile Ophthalmic Solution 2144

Dexchlorpheniramine Maleate (Decreased prothrombin time response).
No products indexed under this heading.

Dextrans (Low Molecular Weight) (Increased prothrombin time response).
No products indexed under this heading.

Dextrothyroxine Sodium (Increased prothrombin time response).
No products indexed under this heading.

Dezocine (Increased prothrombin time response with prolonged use).
No products indexed under this heading.

Diazoxide (Increased prothrombin time response).
No products indexed under this heading.

Diclofenac Potassium (Increased prothrombin time response; caution should be observed when used concurrently). Products include:

Cataflam Tablets 2315

Diclofenac Sodium (Increased prothrombin time response; caution should be observed when used concurrently). Products include:
- Arthrotec Tablets 3195
- Voltaren Ophthalmic Sterile Ophthalmic Solution .... ⊙312
- Voltaren Tablets 2315
- Voltaren-XR Tablets 2315

Dicloxacillin Sodium (Decreased prothrombin time response).
No products indexed under this heading.

Dicumarol (Increased prothrombin time response).
No products indexed under this heading.

Diflunisal (Increased prothrombin time response; caution should be observed when used concurrently). Products include:
- Dolobid Tablets 2088

Diphenhydramine Citrate (Decreased prothrombin time response). Products include:
- Alka-Seltzer PM Effervescent Tablets .... ▣605
- Benadryl Allergy & Sinus Fastmelt Tablets .... ▣693
- Benadryl Children's Allergy/Cold Fastmelt Tablets .... ▣692
- Excedrin PM Tablets, Caplets, and Geltabs .... ▣631
- Goody's PM Powder .... ▣621

Diphenhydramine Hydrochloride (Decreased prothrombin time response). Products include:
- Extra Strength Bayer PM Caplets .... ▣611
- Benadryl Allergy Chewables .... ▣689
- Benadryl Allergy .... ▣691
- Benadryl Allergy Liquid .... ▣690
- Benadryl Allergy/Cold Tablets .... ▣691
- Benadryl Allergy/Congestion Tablets .... ▣692
- Benadryl Allergy & Sinus Liquid .... ▣693
- Benadryl Allergy Sinus Headache Caplets & Gelcaps .... ▣693
- Benadryl Severe Allergy & Sinus Headache Caplets .... ▣694
- Benadryl Dye-Free Allergy Liquid .... ▣690
- Benadryl Dye-Free Allergy Liqui-Gels Softgels .... ▣690
- Benadryl Itch Relief Stick Extra Strength .... ▣695
- Benadryl Cream .... ▣695
- Benadryl Gel .... ▣695
- Benadryl Spray .... ▣696
- Benadryl Parenteral 2617
- Coricidin HBP Night-Time Cold & Flu Tablets .... ▣738
- Nytol QuickCaps Caplets .... ▣622
- Maximum Strength Nytol QuickGels Softgels .... ▣621
- Extra Strength Percogesic Aspirin-Free Coated Caplets .... ▣665
- Simply Sleep Caplets 2008
- Sominex Original Formula Tablets .... ▣761
- Children's Tylenol Allergy-D Liquid 2014
- Maximum Strength Tylenol Allergy Sinus NightTime Caplets 2010
- Tylenol Severe Allergy Caplets 2010
- Maximum Strength Tylenol Flu NightTime Gelcaps 2011
- Extra Strength Tylenol PM Caplets, Geltabs, and Gelcaps 2012
- Unisom Maximum Strength SleepGels .... ▣713

Diphenylpyraline Hydrochloride (Decreased prothrombin time response).
No products indexed under this heading.

Dipteryx odorata (Co-administration with botanicals that contain coumarins, such as tonka beans, may result in increased anticoagulant effects).
No products indexed under this heading.

Disulfiram (Increased prothrombin time response). Products include:
- Antabuse Tablets 2444
- Antabuse Tablets 3474

Divalproex Sodium (Increased prothrombin time response). Products include:
- Depakote Sprinkle Capsules 426
- Depakote Tablets 430
- Depakote ER Tablets 436

Dong Quai (Co-administration with botanicals that contain coumarins, such as dong quai (angelica), may result in increased anticoagulant effects).
No products indexed under this heading.

Doxycycline Calcium (Increased prothrombin time response). Products include:
- Vibramycin Calcium Oral Suspension Syrup 2735

Doxycycline Hyclate (Increased prothrombin time response). Products include:
- Doryx Coated Pellet Filled Capsules 3357
- Periostat Tablets 1208
- Vibramycin Hyclate Capsules 2735
- Vibramycin Hyclate Intravenous 2737
- Vibra-Tabs Film Coated Tablets 2735

Doxycycline Monohydrate (Increased prothrombin time response). Products include:
- Monodox Capsules 2442
- Vibramycin Monohydrate for Oral Suspension 2735

Enflurane (Increased prothrombin time response).
No products indexed under this heading.

Enoxacin (Increased prothrombin time response).
No products indexed under this heading.

Enoxaparin (Co-administration has resulted in cases of venous limb ischemia, necrosis, and gangrene in patients with heparin-induced thrombocytopenia and deep venous thrombosis when heparin treatment was discontinued and warfarin therapy was started or continued; sequelae have included amputation of the involved area and/or death). Products include:
- Lovenox Injection 746

Erythromycin (Increased prothrombin time response). Products include:
- Emgel 2% Topical Gel 1285
- Ery-Tab Tablets 448
- Erythromycin Base Filmtab Tablets 454
- Erythromycin Delayed-Release Capsules, USP 455
- PCE Dispertab Tablets 498

Erythromycin Estolate (Increased prothrombin time response).
No products indexed under this heading.

Erythromycin Ethylsuccinate (Increased prothrombin time response). Products include:
- E.E.S. 450
- EryPed 446
- Pediazole Suspension 3050

Erythromycin Gluceptate (Increased prothrombin time response).
No products indexed under this heading.

Erythromycin Stearate (Increased prothrombin time response). Products include:
- Erythrocin Stearate Filmtab Tablets 452

Ethacrynic Acid (Decreased or increased prothrombin time response). Products include:
- Edecrin Tablets 2091

Ethchlorvynol (Decreased prothrombin time response).
No products indexed under this heading.

Ethinyl Estradiol (Decreased prothrombin time response). Products include:
- Alesse-21 Tablets 3468
- Alesse-28 Tablets 3473
- Brevicon 28-Day Tablets 3380
- Cyclessa Tablets 2450
- Desogen Tablets 2458
- Estinyl Tablets 3112
- Estrostep 2627
- femhrt Tablets 2635
- Levlen 962
- Levlite 21 Tablets 962
- Levlite 28 Tablets 962
- Levora Tablets 3389
- Loestrin 21 Tablets 2642
- Loestrin Fe Tablets 2642
- Lo/Ovral Tablets 3532
- Lo/Ovral-28 Tablets 3538
- Low-Ogestrel-28 Tablets 3392
- Microgestin Fe 1.5/30 Tablets 3407
- Microgestin Fe 1/20 Tablets 3400
- Mircette Tablets 2470
- Modicon 2563
- Necon 3415
- Nordette-28 Tablets 2257
- Norinyl 1 +35 28-Day Tablets 3380
- Ogestrel 0.5/50-28 Tablets 3428
- Ortho-Cept 21 Tablets 2546
- Ortho-Cept 28 Tablets 2546
- Ortho-Cyclen/Ortho Tri-Cyclen 2573
- Ortho-Novum 2563
- Ovcon 3364
- Ovral Tablets 3551
- Ovral-28 Tablets 3552
- Tri-Levlen 962
- Tri-Norinyl-28 Tablets 3433
- Triphasil-21 Tablets 3600
- Triphasil-28 Tablets 3605
- Trivora Tablets 3439
- Yasmin 28 Tablets 980
- Zovia 3449

Ethynodiol Diacetate (Decreased prothrombin time response). Products include:
- Zovia 3449

Etodolac (Increased prothrombin time response; caution should be observed when used concurrently). Products include:
- Lodine 3528
- Lodine XL Extended-Release Tablets 3530

Fenofibrate (Increased prothrombin time response). Products include:
- Tricor Capsules, Micronized 513

Fenoprofen Calcium (Increased prothrombin time response; caution should be observed when used concurrently).
No products indexed under this heading.

Fentanyl (Increased prothrombin time response with prolonged use). Products include:
- Duragesic Transdermal System 1786

Fentanyl Citrate (Increased prothrombin time response with prolonged use). Products include:
- Actiq 1184

Ferula foetida (Co-administration with botanicals that contain coumarins, such as asafoetida, may result in increased anticoagulant effects).
No products indexed under this heading.

Fexofenadine Hydrochloride (Decreased prothrombin time response). Products include:
- Allegra 712
- Allegra-D Extended-Release Tablets 714

Filipendula ulmaria (Co-administration with botanicals that contain coumarins and salicylate, such as meadowsweet, may result in increased anticoagulant effects).
No products indexed under this heading.

Fluconazole (Increased prothrombin time response). Products include:
- Diflucan Tablets, Injection, and Oral Suspension 2681

Fludrocortisone Acetate (Decreased or increased prothrombin time response). Products include:
- Florinef Acetate Tablets 2250

Fluorouracil (Increased prothrombin time response). Products include:
- Carac Cream 1222
- Efudex 1733
- Fluoroplex 552

Fluoxetine Hydrochloride (Increased prothrombin time response). Products include:
- Prozac Pulvules, Liquid, and Weekly Capsules 1238
- Sarafem Pulvules 1962

Fluoxymesterone (Increased prothrombin time response).
No products indexed under this heading.

Flurbiprofen (Increased prothrombin time response; caution should be observed when used concurrently).
No products indexed under this heading.

Flutamide (May be responsible, alone or in combination, for increased prothrombin time/international normalized ratio (PT/INR) response). Products include:
- Eulexin Capsules 3118

Fluvastatin Sodium (Increased prothrombin time response). Products include:
- Lescol Capsules 2361
- Lescol 2925
- Lescol XL Tablets 2361

Fluvoxamine Maleate (Increased prothrombin time response). Products include:
- Luvox Tablets (25, 50, 100 mg) 3256

Fosphenytoin Sodium (Accumulation of phenytoin; decreased or increased prothrombin time response). Products include:
- Cerebyx Injection 2619

Fucus vesiculosus (Concurrent use may result in increased anticoagulant effects).
No products indexed under this heading.

Furosemide (Decreased or increased prothrombin time response). Products include:
- Furosemide Tablets 2284

Galium odoratum (Co-administration with botanicals that contain coumarins, such as sweet woodruff, may result in increased anticoagulant effects).
No products indexed under this heading.

Garlic Extract (Co-administration is associated most often with increases in the effects of warfarin; garlic may cause bleeding events when taken alone and may have anticoagulant, antiplatelet, and/or fibrinolytic properties).
No products indexed under this heading.

Garlic Oil (Co-administration is associated most often with increases in the effects of warfarin; garlic may cause bleeding events when taken alone and may have anticoagulant, antiplatelet, and/or fibrinolytic properties). Products include:
- One-A-Day Garlic Softgels .... ▣806

Gaultheria procumbens (Co-administration with botanicals that contain salicylate and/or have antiplatelet properties, such as wintergreen, may result in increased anticoagulant effects).
No products indexed under this heading.

Gemfibrozil (May be responsible, alone or in combination, for increased prothrombin time/international normalized ratio (PT/INR) response). Products include:
- Lopid Tablets 2650

Ginger (Co-administration with botanicals that contain salicylate and/or have antiplatelet properties, such as ginger, may result in increased anticoagulant effects).
No products indexed under this heading.

Ginkgo biloba (Co-administration is associated most often with increases in the effects of warfarin; Gingko biloba may cause bleeding

events when taken alone and may have anticoagulant, antiplatelet, and/or fibrinolytic properties). Products include:
- BioLean Free Tablets ▣843
- Centrum Focused Formulas Mental Clarity Tablets ▣816
- Centrum Ginkgo Biloba Softgels ▣852
- CorePlex Capsules ▣796
- DHEA Plus Capsules ▣844
- Ginkoba Tablets ▣828
- Ginkoba M/E Suppli-Cap Capsules ▣829
- IntelleQ Capsules ▣797
- One-A-Day Memory & Concentration Tablets ▣807
- Phyto-Vite Tablets ▣849
- ReSource Wellness EnVigor Caplets ▣824
- ReSource Wellness MemorAble Softgels ▣825
- Satiete Tablets ▣846
- StePHan Clarity Capsules ▣844
- StePHan Elixir Capsules ▣848

Ginseng (Co-administration with botanicals that contain salicylate and/or have antiplatelet properties, such as ginseng (Panax) may result in increased anticoagulant effects). Products include:
- BioLean Free Tablets ▣843
- Centrum Focused Formulas Energy Tablets ▣816
- Centrum Ginseng Softgels ▣853
- Ginkoba M/E Suppli-Cap Capsules ▣829
- Ginsana ▣830
- Metabolic Nutrition System ▣798
- One-A-Day Energy Formula Tablets ▣806
- Performance Gold Caplets ▣798
- Performance Optimizer System ▣798
- ReSource Wellness EnVigor Caplets ▣824
- ReSource Wellness ResistEx Capsules ▣826
- ReSource Wellness 2ndWind Capsules ▣826
- Vitasana Gelcaps ▣834

Glipizide (Increased prothrombin time response). Products include:
- Glucotrol Tablets 2692
- Glucotrol XL Extended Release Tablets 2693

Glucagon (Increased prothrombin time response). Products include:
- GlucaGen for Injection Diagnostic Kit 949
- Glucagon for Injection Vials and Emergency Kit 1924

Glutethimide (Decreased prothrombin time response).
- No products indexed under this heading.

Glyburide (Increased prothrombin time response). Products include:
- DiaBeta Tablets 741
- Glucovance Tablets 1086

Grepafloxacin Hydrochloride (Increased prothrombin time response).
- No products indexed under this heading.

Griseofulvin (Decreased prothrombin time response). Products include:
- Grifulvin V Tablets Microsize and Oral Suspension Microsize 2518
- Gris-PEG Tablets 2661

Haloperidol (Decreased prothrombin time response). Products include:
- Haldol Injection, Tablets and Concentrate 2533

Haloperidol Decanoate (Decreased prothrombin time response). Products include:
- Haldol Decanoate 2535

Halothane (Increased prothrombin time response). Products include:
- Fluothane Inhalation 3508

Heparin Sodium (Co-administration has resulted in cases of venous limb ischemia, necrosis, and gangrene in patients with heparin-induced thrombocytopenia and deep venous thrombosis when heparin treatment was discontinued and warfarin therapy was started or continued; sequelae have included amputation of the involved area and/or death). Products include:
- Heparin Lock Flush Solution 3509
- Heparin Sodium Injection 3511

Hepatotoxic Drugs, unspecified (Increased prothrombin time response).
- No products indexed under this heading.

Horse Chestnut Seed Extract (Co-administration with botanicals that contain coumarins, such as horse chestnut, may result in increased anticoagulant effects). Products include:
- Venastat Suppli-Cap Capsules ▣833

Hydrastis canadensis (Co-administration with botanicals with coagulant properties, such as goldenseal, may affect the anticoagulant effects of warfarin).
- No products indexed under this heading.

Hydrochlorothiazide (Decreased or increased prothrombin time response). Products include:
- Accuretic Tablets 2614
- Aldoril Tablets 2039
- Atacand HCT Tablets 597
- Avalide Tablets 1070
- Diovan HCT Tablets 2338
- Dyazide Capsules 1515
- HydroDIURIL Tablets 2108
- Hyzaar 2109
- Inderide Tablets 3517
- Inderide LA Long-Acting Capsules 3519
- Lotensin HCT Tablets 2367
- Maxzide 1008
- Micardis HCT Tablets 1051
- Microzide Capsules 3414
- Moduretic Tablets 2138
- Monopril HCT 1094
- Prinzide Tablets 2168
- Timolide Tablets 2187
- Uniretic Tablets 3178
- Vaseretic Tablets 2204
- Zestoretic Tablets 695
- Ziac Tablets 1887

Hydrocodone Bitartrate (Increased prothrombin time response with prolonged use). Products include:
- Hycodan 1316
- Hycomine Compound Tablets 1317
- Hycotuss Expectorant Syrup 1318
- Lortab 3319
- Lortab Elixir 3317
- Maxidone Tablets CIII 3399
- Norco 5/325 Tablets CIII 3424
- Norco 7.5/325 Tablets CIII 3425
- Norco 10/325 Tablets CIII 3427
- Norco 10/325 Tablets CIII 3425
- Vicodin Tablets 516
- Vicodin ES Tablets 517
- Vicodin HP Tablets 518
- Vicodin Tuss Expectorant 519
- Vicoprofen Tablets 520
- Zydone Tablets 1330

Hydrocodone Polistirex (Increased prothrombin time response with prolonged use). Products include:
- Tussionex Pennkinetic Extended-Release Suspension 1174

Hydrocortisone (Decreased or increased prothrombin time response). Products include:
- Anusol-HC Cream 2.5% 2237
- Cipro HC Otic Suspension 540
- Cortaid Intensive Therapy Cream ▣717
- Cortaid Maximum Strength Cream ▣717
- Cortisporin Ophthalmic Suspension Sterile ⊙297
- Cortizone•5 ▣699
- Cortizone•10 ▣699
- Cortizone•10 Plus Creme ▣700
- Cortizone for Kids Creme ▣699
- Hydrocortone Tablets 2106
- Massengill Medicated Soft Cloth Towelette ▣753
- VōSoL HC Otic Solution 3356

Hydrocortisone Acetate (Decreased or increased prothrombin time response). Products include:
- Analpram-HC 1338
- Anusol HC-1 Hydrocortisone Anti-Itch Cream ▣689
- Anusol-HC Suppositories 2238
- Cortaid ▣717
- Cortifoam Rectal Foam 3170
- Cortisporin-TC Otic Suspension 2246
- Hydrocortone Acetate Injectable Suspension 2103
- Pramosone 1343
- Proctocort Suppositories 2264
- ProctoFoam-HC 3177
- Terra-Cortril Ophthalmic Suspension 2716

Hydrocortisone Sodium Phosphate (Decreased or increased prothrombin time response). Products include:
- Hydrocortone Phosphate Injection, Sterile 2105

Hydrocortisone Sodium Succinate (Decreased or increased prothrombin time response).
- No products indexed under this heading.

Hydroflumethiazide (Decreased or increased prothrombin time response). Products include:
- Diucardin Tablets 3494

Hydromorphone Hydrochloride (Increased prothrombin time response with prolonged use). Products include:
- Dilaudid 441
- Dilaudid Oral Liquid 445
- Dilaudid Powder 441
- Dilaudid Rectal Suppositories 441
- Dilaudid Tablets 441
- Dilaudid Tablets - 8 mg 445
- Dilaudid-HP 443

Hypericum (Co-administration is associated most often with decreases in the effects of warfarin). Products include:
- Brite-Life Caplets ▣795
- Centrum St. John's Wort Softgels ▣853
- Metabolic Nutrition System ▣798
- Movana Tablets ▣832
- One-A-Day Tension & Mood Softgels ▣808
- ReSource Wellness StayCalm Caplets ▣826
- Satiete Tablets ▣846

Ibuprofen (Increased prothrombin time response; caution should be observed when used concurrently). Products include:
- Advil ▣771
- Children's Advil Oral Suspension ▣773
- Children's Advil Chewable Tablets ▣773
- Advil Cold and Sinus Caplets ▣771
- Advil Cold and Sinus Tablets ▣771
- Advil Flu & Body Ache Caplets ▣772
- Infants' Advil Drops ▣773
- Junior Strength Advil Tablets ▣773
- Junior Strength Advil Chewable Tablets ▣773
- Advil Migraine Liquigels ▣772
- Children's Motrin Oral Suspension and Chewable Tablets 2006
- Children's Motrin Cold Oral Suspension 2007
- Children's Motrin Oral Suspension ▣643
- Motrin Suspension, Oral Drops, Chewable Tablets, and Caplets 2002
- Infants' Motrin Concentrated Drops 2006
- Junior Strength Motrin Caplets and Chewable Tablets 2006
- Motrin IB Tablets, Caplets, and Gelcaps 2002
- Motrin Migraine Pain Caplets 2005
- Motrin Sinus Headache Caplets 2005
- Vicoprofen Tablets 520

Ifosfamide (Increased prothrombin time response). Products include:
- Ifex for Injection 1123

Indapamide (Decreased or increased prothrombin time response). Products include:
- Indapamide Tablets 2286

Indomethacin (Increased prothrombin time response; caution should be observed when used concurrently). Products include:
- Indocin 2112

Indomethacin Sodium Trihydrate (Increased prothrombin time response; caution should be observed when used concurrently). Products include:
- Indocin I.V. 2115

Influenza Virus Vaccine (Increased prothrombin time response). Products include:
- FluShield Influenza Vaccine 3521
- Fluzone Vaccine 802

Inositol Nicotinate (Co-administration with botanicals that contain salicylate and/or have antiplatelet properties, such as inositol nicotinate, may result in increased anticoagulant effects).
- No products indexed under this heading.

Isocarboxazid (Increased prothrombin time response).
- No products indexed under this heading.

Isoflurane (Increased prothrombin time response).
- No products indexed under this heading.

Itraconazole (Increased prothrombin time response). Products include:
- Sporanox Capsules 1800
- Sporanox Injection 1804
- Sporanox Injection 2509
- Sporanox Oral Solution 1808
- Sporanox Oral Solution 2512

Kanamycin Sulfate (Increased prothrombin time response with oral aminoglycosides).
- No products indexed under this heading.

Ketoprofen (Increased prothrombin time response; caution should be observed when used concurrently). Products include:
- Orudis Capsules 3548
- Orudis KT Tablets ▣778
- Oruvail Capsules 3548

Ketorolac Tromethamine (Increased prothrombin time response; caution should be observed when used concurrently). Products include:
- Acular Ophthalmic Solution 544
- Acular PF Ophthalmic Solution 544
- Toradol 3018

Levamisole Hydrochloride (Increased prothrombin time response). Products include:
- Ergamisol Tablets 1789

Levonorgestrel (Decreased prothrombin time response). Products include:
- Alesse-21 Tablets 3468
- Alesse-28 Tablets 3473
- Levlen 962
- Levlite 21 Tablets 962
- Levlite 28 Tablets 962
- Levora Tablets 3389
- Mirena Intrauterine System 974
- Nordette-28 Tablets 2257
- Norplant System 3543
- Tri-Levlen 962
- Triphasil-21 Tablets 3600
- Triphasil-28 Tablets 3605
- Trivora Tablets 3439

Levorphanol Tartrate (Increased prothrombin time response with prolonged use). Products include:
- Levo-Dromoran 1734
- Levorphanol Tartrate Tablets 3059

Levothyroxine Sodium (Decreased or increased prothrombin time response). Products include:
- Levothroid Tablets 1373
- Levoxyl Tablets 1819
- Synthroid 505
- Unithroid Tablets 3445

Licorice (Co-administration with botanicals that contain coumarins, such as licorice, may result in increased anticoagulant effects; licorice also has antiplatelet properties).

Liothyronine Sodium (Decreased or increased prothrombin time response). Products include:
- Cytomel Tablets 1817
- Triostat Injection 1825

IMPORTANT NOTE: Always consult each drug listing in the patient's regimen for possible interactions.

Liotrix (Decreased or increased prothrombin time response).
No products indexed under this heading.

Lomefloxacin Hydrochloride (Increased prothrombin time response).
No products indexed under this heading.

Loratadine (Decreased prothrombin time response). Products include:
Claritin ... 3100
Claritin-D 12 Hour Extended Release Tablets ... 3102
Claritin-D 24 Hour Extended Release Tablets ... 3104

Lovastatin (Increased prothrombin time response). Products include:
Mevacor Tablets ... 2132

Magaldrate (Decreased prothrombin time response).
No products indexed under this heading.

Magnesium Hydroxide (Decreased prothrombin time response). Products include:
Ex•Lax Milk of Magnesia Liquid ... ■670
Maalox Antacid/Anti-Gas Oral Suspension ... ■673
Maalox Max Maximum Strength Antacid/Anti-Gas Liquid ... 2300
Maalox Regular Strength Antacid/Antigas Liquid ... 2300
Mylanta Fast-Acting ... 1813
Mylanta ... 1813
Pepcid Complete Chewable Tablets ... 1815
Phillips' Chewable Tablets ... ■615
Phillips' Milk of Magnesia Liquid (Original, Cherry, & Mint) ... ■616
Rolaids Tablets ... ■706
Extra Strength Rolaids Tablets ... ■706
Vanquish Caplets ... ■617

Magnesium Oxide (Decreased prothrombin time response). Products include:
Beelith Tablets ... 946
Mag-Ox 400 Tablets ... 1024
Uro-Mag Capsules ... 1024

Magnesium Salicylate (Increased prothrombin time response; caution should be observed when used concurrently). Products include:
Momentum Backache Relief Extra Strength Caplets ... ■666

Matricaria recutita (Co-administration with botanicals that contain coumarins, such as chamomile, may result in increased anticoagulant effects).
No products indexed under this heading.

Meclofenamate Sodium (Increased prothrombin time response; caution should be observed when used concurrently).
No products indexed under this heading.

Medicago sativa (Co-administration with botanicals that contain coumarins, such as alfalfa, may result in increased anticoagulant effects).
No products indexed under this heading.

Mefenamic Acid (Increased prothrombin time response; caution should be observed when used concurrently). Products include:
Ponstel Capsules ... 1356

Melilotus officinalis (Co-administration with botanicals that contain coumarins, such as sweet clover, may result in increased anticoagulant effects).
No products indexed under this heading.

Meloxicam (Increased prothrombin time response; caution should be observed when used concurrently). Products include:
Mobic Tablets ... 1054

Menyanthes trifoliata (Co-administration with botanicals that contain coumarins, such as bogbean, may result in increased anticoagulant effects).
No products indexed under this heading.

Meperidine Hydrochloride (Increased prothrombin time response with prolonged use). Products include:
Demerol ... 3079
Mepergan Injection ... 3539

Mephobarbital (Decreased prothrombin time response).
No products indexed under this heading.

Meprobamate (Decreased prothrombin time response). Products include:
Miltown Tablets ... 3349

Mercaptopurine (Decreased prothrombin time response). Products include:
Purinethol Tablets ... 1615

Mestranol (Decreased prothrombin time response). Products include:
Necon 1/50 Tablets ... 3415
Norinyl 1 + 50 28-Day Tablets ... 3380
Ortho-Novum 1/50□28 Tablets ... 2556

Methadone Hydrochloride (Increased prothrombin time response with prolonged use). Products include:
Dolophine Hydrochloride Tablets ... 3056

Methdilazine Hydrochloride (Decreased prothrombin time response).
No products indexed under this heading.

Methimazole (Increased or decreased prothrombin time response).
No products indexed under this heading.

Methoxyflurane (Increased or decreased prothrombin time response).
No products indexed under this heading.

Methyclothiazide (Decreased or increased prothrombin time response).
No products indexed under this heading.

Methyl Salicylate (Increased prothrombin time response with topical methyl salicylate ointment). Products include:
BenGay External Analgesic Products ... ■696
Listerine Mouthrinse ... ■702
Cool Mint Listerine Mouthrinse ... ■702
FreshBurst Listerine Mouthrinse ... ■702
Tartar Control Listerine Mouthrinse ... ■702
Thera-Gesic Creme ... 2233

Methyldopa (Increased prothrombin time response). Products include:
Aldoclor Tablets ... 2035
Aldomet Tablets ... 2037
Aldoril Tablets ... 2039

Methyldopate Hydrochloride (Increased prothrombin time response).
No products indexed under this heading.

Methylphenidate Hydrochloride (Increased prothrombin time response). Products include:
Concerta Extended-Release Tablets ... 1998
Concerta Tablets ... 561
Metadate CD Capsules ... 1164
Metadate ER Tablets ... 1167
Methylin Tablets ... 1995
Methylin ER Tablets ... 1995
Ritalin ... 2387

Methylprednisolone Acetate (Decreased or increased prothrombin time response). Products include:
Depo-Medrol Injectable Suspension ... 2795

Methylprednisolone Sodium Succinate (Decreased or increased prothrombin time response). Products include:
Solu-Medrol Sterile Powder ... 2855

Methyltestosterone (Increased prothrombin time response). Products include:
Android Capsules, 10 mg ... 1731
Estratest ... 3252
Testred Capsules, 10 mg ... 1746

Metolazone (Decreased or increased prothrombin time response). Products include:
Mykrox Tablets ... 1168
Zaroxolyn Tablets ... 1177

Metronidazole (Increased prothrombin time response). Products include:
MetroCream ... 1404
MetroGel ... 1405
MetroGel-Vaginal Gel ... 1986
MetroLotion ... 1405
Noritate Cream ... 1224

Metronidazole Hydrochloride (Increased prothrombin time response).
No products indexed under this heading.

Miconazole (Increased prothrombin time response).
No products indexed under this heading.

Mistletoe (Co-administration with botanicals with coagulant properties, such as mistletoe, may affect the anticoagulant effects of warfarin).
No products indexed under this heading.

Moclobemide (Increased prothrombin time response).
No products indexed under this heading.

Montelukast Sodium (May be responsible, alone or in combination, for increased prothrombin time/international normalized ratio (PT/INR) response). Products include:
Singulair ... 2181

Moricizine Hydrochloride (Decreased or increased prothrombin time response).
No products indexed under this heading.

Morphine Sulfate (Increased prothrombin time response with prolonged use). Products include:
Astramorph/PF Injection, USP (Preservative-Free) ... 594
Duramorph Injection ... 1312
Infumorph 200 and Infumorph 500 Sterile Solutions ... 1314
Kadian Capsules ... 1335
MS Contin Tablets ... 2896
MSIR ... 2898
Oramorph SR Tablets ... 3062
Roxanol ... 3066

Moxifloxacin Hydrochloride (Increased prothrombin time response). Products include:
Avelox Tablets ... 879

Nabumetone (Increased prothrombin time response; caution should be observed when used concurrently). Products include:
Relafen Tablets ... 1617

Nafcillin Sodium (Decreased prothrombin time response).
No products indexed under this heading.

Nalidixic Acid (Increased prothrombin time response).
No products indexed under this heading.

Naproxen (Increased prothrombin time response; caution should be observed when used concurrently). Products include:
EC-Naprosyn Delayed-Release Tablets ... 2967
Naprosyn Suspension ... 2967
Naprosyn Tablets ... 2967

Naproxen Sodium (Increased prothrombin time response; caution should be observed when used concurrently). Products include:
Aleve Tablets, Caplets and Gelcaps ... ■602
Aleve Cold & Sinus Caplets ... ■603
Anaprox Tablets ... 2967
Anaprox DS Tablets ... 2967
Naprelan Tablets ... 1293

Neomycin, oral (Increased prothrombin time response with oral aminoglycosides).

Nettle (Co-administration with botanicals that contain coumarins, such as nettle, may result in increased anticoagulant effects).
No products indexed under this heading.

Nilutamide (May be responsible, alone or in combination, for increased prothrombin time/international normalized ratio (PT/INR) response). Products include:
Nilandron Tablets ... 753

Norethindrone (Decreased prothrombin time response). Products include:
Brevicon 28-Day Tablets ... 3380
Micronor Tablets ... 2543
Modicon ... 2563
Necon ... 3415
Norinyl 1 +35 28-Day Tablets ... 3380
Norinyl 1 + 50 28-Day Tablets ... 3380
Nor-QD Tablets ... 3423
Ortho-Novum ... 2563
Ortho-Novum 1/50□28 Tablets ... 2556
Ovcon ... 3364
Tri-Norinyl-28 Tablets ... 3433

Norethynodrel (Decreased prothrombin time response).
No products indexed under this heading.

Norfloxacin (Increased prothrombin time response). Products include:
Chibroxin Sterile Ophthalmic Solution ... 2051
Noroxin Tablets ... 2145

Norgestimate (Decreased prothrombin time response). Products include:
Ortho-Cyclen/Ortho Tri-Cyclen ... 2573
Ortho-Prefest Tablets ... 2570

Norgestrel (Decreased prothrombin time response). Products include:
Lo/Ovral Tablets ... 3532
Lo/Ovral-28 Tablets ... 3538
Low-Ogestrel-28 Tablets ... 3392
Ogestrel 0.5/50-28 Tablets ... 3428
Ovral Tablets ... 3551
Ovral-28 Tablets ... 3552
Ovrette Tablets ... 3552

Ofloxacin (Increased prothrombin time response). Products include:
Floxin I.V. ... 2526
Floxin Otic Solution ... 1219
Floxin Tablets ... 2529
Ocuflox Ophthalmic Solution ... 554

Olsalazine Sodium (Increased prothrombin time response). Products include:
Dipentum Capsules ... 2803

Omeprazole (Increased prothrombin time response). Products include:
Prilosec Delayed-Release Capsules ... 628

Oxandrolone (Increased prothrombin time response). Products include:
Oxandrin Tablets ... 1153

Oxaprozin (Increased prothrombin time response; caution should be observed when used concurrently).
No products indexed under this heading.

Oxycodone Hydrochloride (Increased prothrombin time response with prolonged use). Products include:
OxyContin Tablets ... 2912
OxyFast Oral Concentrate Solution ... 2916
OxyIR Capsules ... 2916
Percocet Tablets ... 1326
Percodan Tablets ... 1327

Percolone Tablets 1327
Roxicodone 3067
Tylox Capsules 2597

Oxymetholone (Increased prothrombin time response). Products include:
Anadrol-50 Tablets 3321

Oxyphenbutazone (Increased prothrombin time response).
No products indexed under this heading.

Paraldehyde (Decreased prothrombin time response).

Pargyline Hydrochloride (Increased prothrombin time response).
No products indexed under this heading.

Paromomycin Sulfate (Increased prothrombin time response with oral aminoglycosides).
No products indexed under this heading.

Paroxetine Hydrochloride (Increased prothrombin time response). Products include:
Paxil 1609

Passiflora incarnata (Co-administration with botanicals that contain coumarins, such as passion flower, may result in increased anticoagulant effects).
No products indexed under this heading.

Pau d'arco (Concurrent use may result in increased anticoagulant effects).
No products indexed under this heading.

Penicillin G Potassium (Increased prothrombin time response with intravenous penicillin G). Products include:
Pfizerpen for Injection 2707

Penicillin G Sodium (Increased prothrombin time response with intravenous penicillin G).
No products indexed under this heading.

Pentobarbital Sodium (Decreased prothrombin time response). Products include:
Nembutal Sodium Solution 485

Pentoxifylline (Increased prothrombin time response). Products include:
Trental Tablets 784

Petroselinum crispum (Co-administration with botanicals that contain coumarins, such as parsley, may result in increased anticoagulant effects).
No products indexed under this heading.

Peumus boldus (Co-administration with botanicals that contain coumarins, such as boldo, may result in increased anticoagulant effects).
No products indexed under this heading.

Phenelzine Sulfate (Increased prothrombin time response). Products include:
Nardil Tablets 2653

Phenobarbital (Decreased prothrombin time response; accumulation of phenobarbital). Products include:
Arco-Lase Plus Tablets 592
Donnatal 2929
Donnatal Extentabs 2930

Phenylbutazone (Increased prothrombin time response; caution should be observed when used concurrently).
No products indexed under this heading.

Phenytoin (Accumulation of phenytoin; decreased or increased prothrombin time response). Products include:
Dilantin Infatabs 2624
Dilantin-125 Oral Suspension 2625

Phenytoin Sodium (Accumulation of phenytoin; decreased or increased prothrombin time response). Products include:
Dilantin Kapseals 2622

Phytonadione (Decreased prothrombin time response).
No products indexed under this heading.

Piperacillin Sodium (Increased prothrombin time response). Products include:
Pipracil 1866
Zosyn 1890
Zosyn in Galaxy Containers 1894

Piroxicam (Increased prothrombin time response; caution should be observed when used concurrently). Products include:
Feldene Capsules 2685

Policosanol (Co-administration with botanicals that contain salicylate and/or have antiplatelet properties, such as policosanol, may result in increased anticoagulant effects).
No products indexed under this heading.

Polythiazide (Decreased or increased prothrombin time response). Products include:
Minizide Capsules 2700
Renese Tablets 2712

Populus species (Co-administration with botanicals that contain salicylate and/or have antiplatelet properties, such as poplar, may result in increased anticoagulant effects).
No products indexed under this heading.

Prednisolone Acetate (Decreased or increased prothrombin time response). Products include:
Blephamide Ophthalmic Ointment 547
Blephamide Ophthalmic Suspension 548
Poly-Pred Liquifilm Ophthalmic Suspension .... ⊙245
Pred Forte Ophthalmic Suspension .... ⊙246
Pred Mild Sterile Ophthalmic Suspension .... ⊙249
Pred-G Ophthalmic Suspension .... ⊙247
Pred-G Sterile Ophthalmic Ointment .... ⊙248

Prednisolone Sodium Phosphate (Decreased or increased prothrombin time response). Products include:
Pediapred Oral Solution 1170

Prednisolone Tebutate (Decreased or increased prothrombin time response).
No products indexed under this heading.

Prednisone (Decreased or increased prothrombin time response). Products include:
Prednisone 3064

Prickly Ash (Co-administration with botanicals that contain coumarins, such as prickly ash, may result in increased anticoagulant effects).
No products indexed under this heading.

Primidone (Decreased prothrombin time response).
No products indexed under this heading.

Procarbazine Hydrochloride (Increased prothrombin time response). Products include:
Matulane Capsules 3246

Promethazine Hydrochloride (Decreased prothrombin time response). Products include:
Mepergan Injection 3539
Phenergan Injection 3553
Phenergan 3556
Phenergan Syrup 3554
Phenergan with Codeine Syrup 3557
Phenergan with Dextromethorphan Syrup 3559
Phenergan VC Syrup 3560
Phenergan VC with Codeine Syrup 3561

Propafenone Hydrochloride (Increased prothrombin time response). Products include:
Rythmol Tablets – 150 mg, 225 mg, 300 mg 502

Propoxyphene Hydrochloride (Increased prothrombin time response with prolonged use). Products include:
Darvon Pulvules 1909
Darvon Compound-65 Pulvules 1910

Propoxyphene Napsylate (Increased prothrombin time response with prolonged use). Products include:
Darvon-N/Darvocet-N 1907
Darvon-N Tablets 1912

Propranolol Hydrochloride (Increased prothrombin time response). Products include:
Inderal 3513
Inderal LA Long-Acting Capsules 3516
Inderide Tablets 3517
Inderide LA Long-Acting Capsules 3519

Propylthiouracil (Increased or decreased prothrombin time response).
No products indexed under this heading.

Pyrazolones (Increased prothrombin time response).

Pyrilamine Maleate (Decreased prothrombin time response). Products include:
Maximum Strength Midol Menstrual Caplets and Gelcaps .... ■612
Maximum Strength Midol PMS Caplets and Gelcaps .... ■613

Pyrilamine Tannate (Decreased prothrombin time response). Products include:
Ryna-12 S Suspension 3351

Quassia amara (Co-administration with botanicals that contain coumarins, such as quassia, may result in increased anticoagulant effects).
No products indexed under this heading.

Quinidine Gluconate (Increased prothrombin time response). Products include:
Quinaglute Dura-Tabs Tablets 978

Quinidine Polygalacturonate (Increased prothrombin time response).
No products indexed under this heading.

Quinidine Sulfate (Increased prothrombin time response). Products include:
Quinidex Extentabs 2933

Quinine Sulfate (Increased prothrombin time response).
No products indexed under this heading.

Raloxifene Hydrochloride (May be responsible, alone or in combination, for decreased prothrombin time/international normalized ratio (PT/INR) response). Products include:
Evista Tablets 1915

Ranitidine Hydrochloride (Decreased or increased prothrombin time response). Products include:
Zantac 1690
Zantac Injection 1688
Zantac 75 Tablets .... ■717

Remifentanil Hydrochloride (Increased prothrombin time response with prolonged use).
No products indexed under this heading.

Rifampin (Decreased prothrombin time response). Products include:
Rifadin 765
Rifamate Capsules 767
Rifater Tablets 769

Rofecoxib (Increased prothrombin time response; caution should be observed when used concurrently). Products include:
Vioxx 2213

Salsalate (Increased prothrombin time response; caution should be observed when used concurrently).
No products indexed under this heading.

Sarsaparilla, German (Co-administration with botanicals that contain salicylate and/or have antiplatelet properties, such as German sarsaparilla, may result in increased anticoagulant effects).
No products indexed under this heading.

Secobarbital Sodium (Decreased prothrombin time response).
No products indexed under this heading.

Selegiline Hydrochloride (Increased prothrombin time response). Products include:
Eldepryl Capsules 3266

Senega (Co-administration with botanicals that contain salicylate and/or have antiplatelet properties, such as senega, may result in increased anticoagulant effects).
No products indexed under this heading.

Sertraline Hydrochloride (Increased prothrombin time response). Products include:
Zoloft 2751

Simvastatin (Increased prothrombin time response). Products include:
Zocor Tablets 2219

Sodium Bicarbonate (Decreased prothrombin time response). Products include:
Alka-Seltzer .... ■603
Alka-Seltzer Lemon Lime Antacid and Pain Reliever Effervescent Tablets .... ■603
Alka-Seltzer Extra Strength Antacid and Pain Reliever Effervescent Tablets .... ■603
Alka-Seltzer Heartburn Relief Tablets .... ■604
Ceo-Two Evacuant Suppository .... ■618
Colyte with Flavor Packs for Oral Solution 3170
GoLYTELY and Pineapple Flavor GoLYTELY for Oral Solution 1068
NuLYTELY, Cherry Flavor, Lemon-Lime Flavor, and Orange Flavor NuLYTELY for Oral Solution 1068

Spironolactone (Decreased or increased prothrombin time response).
No products indexed under this heading.

Stanozolol (Increased prothrombin time response).
No products indexed under this heading.

Streptokinase (Concurrent use is not recommended and may be hazardous; increased prothrombin time response). Products include:
Streptase for Infusion 647

Sucralfate (Decreased prothrombin time response). Products include:
Carafate Suspension 731
Carafate Tablets 730

Sufentanil Citrate (Increased prothrombin time response with prolonged use).
No products indexed under this heading.

Sulfacytine (Increased prothrombin time response).

Sulfamethizole (Increased prothrombin time response). Products include:
Urobiotic-250 Capsules 2731

Sulfamethoxazole (Increased prothrombin time response). Products include:
Bactrim 2949
Septra Suspension 2265
Septra Tablets 2265
Septra DS Tablets 2265

Sulfasalazine (Increased prothrombin time response). Products include:

Azulfidine EN-tabs Tablets 2775

Sulfinpyrazone (Increased prothrombin time response).
No products indexed under this heading.

Sulfisoxazole (Increased prothrombin time response).
No products indexed under this heading.

Sulfisoxazole Acetyl (Increased prothrombin time response). Products include:
Pediazole Suspension 3050

Sulfisoxazole Diolamine (Increased prothrombin time response).
No products indexed under this heading.

Sulindac (Increased prothrombin time response; caution should be observed when used concurrently). Products include:
Clinoril Tablets 2053

Syzygium aromaticum (Co-administration with botanicals that contain salicylate and/or have antiplatelet properties, such as clove, may result in increased anticoagulant effects).
No products indexed under this heading.

Tamarindus indica (Co-administration with botanicals that contain salicylate and/or have antiplatelet properties, such as tamarind, may result in increased anticoagulant effects).
No products indexed under this heading.

Tamoxifen Citrate (Increased prothrombin time response). Products include:
Nolvadex Tablets 678

Tanacetum parthenium (Co-administration with botanicals that contain salicylate and/or have antiplatelet properties, such as feverfew, may result in increased anticoagulant effects).
No products indexed under this heading.

Taraxacum officinale (Co-administration with botanicals that contain coumarins, such as dandelion, may result in increased anticoagulant effects; dandelion also has antiplatelet properties).
No products indexed under this heading.

Terfenadine (Decreased prothrombin time response).
No products indexed under this heading.

Tetracycline Hydrochloride (Increased prothrombin time response).
No products indexed under this heading.

Thiamylal Sodium (Decreased prothrombin time response).
No products indexed under this heading.

Thyroglobulin (Decreased or increased prothrombin time response).
No products indexed under this heading.

Thyroid (Decreased or increased prothrombin time response).
No products indexed under this heading.

Thyroxine (Decreased or increased prothrombin time response).
No products indexed under this heading.

Thyroxine Sodium (Decreased or increased prothrombin time response).
No products indexed under this heading.

Ticarcillin Disodium (Increased prothrombin time response). Products include:
Timentin Injection- ADD-Vantage Vial...................................... 1661
Timentin Injection-Galaxy Container 1664
Timentin Injection-Pharmacy Bulk Package.. 1666
Timentin for Intravenous Administration............................. 1658

Ticlopidine Hydrochloride (Concomitant administration may be associated with cholestatic hepatitis; increased prothrombin time response). Products include:
Ticlid Tablets 3015

Tolazamide (Increased prothrombin time response).
No products indexed under this heading.

Tolbutamide (Increased prothrombin time response; accumulation of tolbutamide).
No products indexed under this heading.

Tolmetin Sodium (Increased prothrombin time response; caution should be observed when used concurrently). Products include:
Tolectin 2589

Torsemide (Decreased or increased prothrombin time response). Products include:
Demadex Tablets and Injection 2965

Tramadol Hydrochloride (Increased prothrombin time response). Products include:
Ultracet Tablets 2597
Ultram Tablets 2600

Tranylcypromine Sulfate (Increased prothrombin time response). Products include:
Parnate Tablets 1607

Trazodone Hydrochloride (Decreased prothrombin time response).
No products indexed under this heading.

Triamcinolone (Decreased or increased prothrombin time response).
No products indexed under this heading.

Triamcinolone Acetonide (Decreased or increased prothrombin time response). Products include:
Azmacort Inhalation Aerosol 728
Nasacort Nasal Inhaler 750
Nasacort AQ Nasal Spray 752
Tri-Nasal Spray 2274

Triamcinolone Diacetate (Decreased or increased prothrombin time response).
No products indexed under this heading.

Triamcinolone Hexacetonide (Decreased or increased prothrombin time response).
No products indexed under this heading.

Triamterene (Decreased or increased prothrombin time response). Products include:
Dyazide Capsules 1515
Dyrenium Capsules 3458
Maxzide 1008

Trifolium pratense (Co-administration with botanicals that contain coumarins, such as red clover, may result in increased anticoagulant effects).
No products indexed under this heading.

Trigonella foenum-graecum (Co-administration with botanicals that contain coumarins, such as fenugreek, may result in increased anticoagulant effects).
No products indexed under this heading.

Trimeprazine Tartrate (Decreased prothrombin time response).
No products indexed under this heading.

Trimethoprim (Increased prothrombin time response). Products include:
Bactrim 2949
Septra Suspension 2265
Septra Tablets 2265
Septra DS Tablets 2265

Tripelennamine Hydrochloride (Decreased prothrombin time response).
No products indexed under this heading.

Triprolidine Hydrochloride (Decreased prothrombin time response). Products include:
Actifed Cold & Allergy Tablets .... ■688

Trovafloxacin Mesylate (Increased prothrombin time response). Products include:
Trovan Tablets 2722

Urokinase (Concurrent use is not recommended and may be hazardous).
No products indexed under this heading.

Valproic Acid (Increased prothrombin time response). Products include:
Depakene 421

Viburnum prunifolium (Co-administration with botanicals that contain salicylate and/or have antiplatelet properties, such as black haw, may result in increased anticoagulant effects).
No products indexed under this heading.

Vitamin C (Decreased prothrombin time response (with high dose)). Products include:
Beta-C Tablets .... ■811
C-Grams Caplets .... ■795
Halls Defense Drops .... ■687
Peridin-C Tablets .... ■618

Vitamin E (Increased prothrombin time response). Products include:
Nutr-E-Sol Liquid 526
One-A-Day Cholesterol Health Tablets .... ■805
One-A-Day Menopause Health Tablets .... ■808
StePHan Bio-Nutritional Daytime Hydrating Creme .... ■770
StePHan Feminine Capsules .... ■848
Unique E Vitamin E Capsules 1723

Wild Lettuce (Co-administration with botanicals that contain coumarins, such as wild lettuce, may result in increased anticoagulant effects).
No products indexed under this heading.

Willow (Co-administration with botanicals that contain salicylate and/or have antiplatelet properties, such as willow, may result in increased anticoagulant effects).
No products indexed under this heading.

Zafirlukast (May be responsible, alone or in combination, for increased prothrombin time/international normalized ratio (PT/INR) response). Products include:
Accolate Tablets 657

Zileuton (May be responsible, alone or in combination, for increased prothrombin time/international normalized ratio (PT/INR) response). Products include:
Zyflo Filmtab Tablets 524

Food Interactions

Alcohol (Decreased or increased prothrombin time response).

Diet high in vitamin K (Decreased prothrombin time).

Vegetables, green leafy (Large amounts of green leafy vegetables may affect Coumadin therapy).

COVERA-HS TABLETS

(Verapamil Hydrochloride) 3199

May interact with ACE inhibitors, antihypertensives, beta blockers, diuretics, cardiac glycosides, inhalant anesthetics, lithium preparations, nondepolarizing neuromuscular blocking agents, vasodilators, and theophylline. Compounds in these categories include:

Acebutolol Hydrochloride (Concomitant therapy may result in additive negative effects on heart rate, atrioventricular conduction and/or cardiac contractility; excessive bradycardia and AV block, including complete heart block). Products include:
Sectral Capsules 3589

Amiloride Hydrochloride (Possible additive effect on lowering of blood pressure). Products include:
Midamor Tablets 2136
Moduretic Tablets 2138

Aminophylline (Verapamil may inhibit the clearance and increase plasma levels of theophylline).
No products indexed under this heading.

Amlodipine Besylate (Possible additive effect on lowering of blood pressure). Products include:
Lotrel Capsules 2370
Norvasc Tablets 2704

Atenolol (Concomitant therapy may result in additive negative effects on heart rate, atrioventricular conduction and/or cardiac contractility; excessive bradycardia and AV block, including complete heart block; a variable effect on atenolol clearance has been observed with concomitant use). Products include:
Tenoretic Tablets 690
Tenormin I.V. Injection 692

Atracurium Besylate (Verapamil may potentiate the activity of neuromuscular blocking agents).
No products indexed under this heading.

Benazepril Hydrochloride (Possible additive effect on lowering of blood pressure). Products include:
Lotensin Tablets 2365
Lotensin HCT Tablets 2367
Lotrel Capsules 2370

Bendroflumethiazide (Possible additive effect on lowering of blood pressure). Products include:
Corzide 40/5 Tablets 2247
Corzide 80/5 Tablets 2247

Betaxolol Hydrochloride (Concomitant therapy may result in additive negative effects on heart rate, atrioventricular conduction and/or cardiac contractility; excessive bradycardia and AV block, including complete heart block). Products include:
Betoptic S Ophthalmic Suspension 537

Bisoprolol Fumarate (Concomitant therapy may result in additive negative effects on heart rate, atrioventricular conduction and/or cardiac contractility; excessive bradycardia and AV block, including complete heart block). Products include:
Zebeta Tablets 1885
Ziac Tablets 1887

Bumetanide (Possible additive effect on lowering of blood pressure).
No products indexed under this heading.

Candesartan Cilexetil (Possible additive effect on lowering of blood pressure). Products include:
Atacand Tablets 595
Atacand HCT Tablets 597

Captopril (Possible additive effect on lowering of blood pressure). Products include:
Captopril Tablets 2281

Carbamazepine (Co-administration may increase carbamazepine concentrations and this may produce side effects such as diplopia, headache, ataxia, or dizziness). Products include:
Carbatrol Capsules 3234
Tegretol/Tegretol-XR 2404

Carteolol Hydrochloride (Concomitant therapy may result in additive negative effects on heart rate, atrioventricular conduction and/or cardiac contractility; excessive

bradycardia and AV block, including complete heart block). Products include:
- Carteolol Hydrochloride Ophthalmic Solution USP, 1% ..... ⊙258
- Ocupress Ophthalmic Solution, 1% Sterile ..... ⊙303

Chlorothiazide (Possible additive effect on lowering of blood pressure). Products include:
- Aldoclor Tablets 2035
- Diuril Oral 2087

Chlorothiazide Sodium (Possible additive effect on lowering of blood pressure). Products include:
- Diuril Sodium Intravenous 2086

Chlorthalidone (Possible additive effect on lowering of blood pressure). Products include:
- Clorpres Tablets 1002
- Combipres Tablets 1040
- Tenoretic Tablets 690

Cimetidine (Variable results on verapamil clearance). Products include:
- Tagamet HB 200 Suspension 762
- Tagamet HB 200 Tablets 761
- Tagamet Tablets 1644

Cimetidine Hydrochloride (Variable results on verapamil clearance). Products include:
- Tagamet 1644

Cisatracurium Besylate (Verapamil may potentiate the activity of neuromuscular blocking agents).
No products indexed under this heading.

Clonidine (Possible additive effect on lowering of blood pressure). Products include:
- Catapres-TTS 1038

Clonidine Hydrochloride (Possible additive effect on lowering of blood pressure). Products include:
- Catapres Tablets 1037
- Clorpres Tablets 1002
- Combipres Tablets 1040
- Duraclon Injection 3057

Cyclosporine (Increased serum levels of cyclosporine). Products include:
- Gengraf Capsules 457
- Neoral Soft Gelatin Capsules 2380
- Neoral Oral Solution 2380
- Sandimmune 2388

Deserpidine (Possible additive effect on lowering of blood pressure).
No products indexed under this heading.

Desflurane (Potential for excessive cardiovascular depression). Products include:
- Suprane Liquid for Inhalation 874

Deslanoside (Chronic verapamil treatment can increase serum digoxin levels by 50% to 75% and this can result in digitalis toxicity).
No products indexed under this heading.

Diazoxide (Possible additive effect on lowering of blood pressure).
No products indexed under this heading.

Digitoxin (Chronic verapamil treatment can increase serum digoxin levels by 50% to 75% and this can result in digitalis toxicity).
No products indexed under this heading.

Digoxin (Chronic verapamil treatment can increase serum digoxin levels by 50% to 75% and this can result in digitalis toxicity). Products include:
- Digitek Tablets 1003
- Lanoxicaps Capsules 1574
- Lanoxin Injection 1581
- Lanoxin Tablets 1587
- Lanoxin Elixir Pediatric 1578
- Lanoxin Injection Pediatric 1584

Diltiazem Hydrochloride (Possible additive effect on lowering of blood pressure). Products include:
- Cardizem Injectable 1018
- Cardizem Lyo-Ject Syringe 1018
- Cardizem Monovial 1018
- Cardizem CD Capsules 1016
- Tiazac Capsules 1378

Disopyramide Phosphate (Concurrent use within 48 hours before or 24 hours after verapamil administration is not recommended).
No products indexed under this heading.

Doxazosin Mesylate (Possible additive effect on lowering of blood pressure). Products include:
- Cardura Tablets 2668

Dyphylline (Verapamil may inhibit the clearance and increase plasma levels of theophylline). Products include:
- Lufyllin Tablets 3347
- Lufyllin-400 Tablets 3347
- Lufyllin-GG Elixir 3348
- Lufyllin-GG Tablets 3348

Enalapril Maleate (Possible additive effect on lowering of blood pressure). Products include:
- Lexxel Tablets 608
- Vaseretic Tablets 2204
- Vasotec Tablets 2210

Enalaprilat (Possible additive effect on lowering of blood pressure). Products include:
- Enalaprilat Injection 863
- Vasotec I.V. Injection 2207

Enflurane (Potential for excessive cardiovascular depression).
No products indexed under this heading.

Epoprostenol Sodium (Possible additive effect on lowering of blood pressure). Products include:
- Flolan for Injection 1528

Eprosartan Mesylate (Possible additive effect on lowering of blood pressure). Products include:
- Teveten Tablets 3327

Esmolol Hydrochloride (Concomitant therapy may result in additive negative effects on heart rate, atrioventricular conduction and/or cardiac contractility; excessive bradycardia and AV block, including complete heart block). Products include:
- Brevibloc Injection 858

Ethacrynic Acid (Possible additive effect on lowering of blood pressure). Products include:
- Edecrin Tablets 2091

Felodipine (Possible additive effect on lowering of blood pressure). Products include:
- Lexxel Tablets 608
- Plendil Extended-Release Tablets 623

Flecainide Acetate (Potential for additive effects on myocardial contractility, AV conduction, and repolarization). Products include:
- Tambocor Tablets 1990

Fosinopril Sodium (Possible additive effect on lowering of blood pressure). Products include:
- Monopril Tablets 1091
- Monopril HCT 1094

Furosemide (Possible additive effect on lowering of blood pressure). Products include:
- Furosemide Tablets 2284

Guanabenz Acetate (Possible additive effect on lowering of blood pressure).
No products indexed under this heading.

Guanethidine Monosulfate (Possible additive effect on lowering of blood pressure).
No products indexed under this heading.

Halothane (Potential for excessive cardiovascular depression). Products include:
- Fluothane Inhalation 3508

Hydralazine Hydrochloride (Possible additive effect on lowering of blood pressure).
No products indexed under this heading.

Hydrochlorothiazide (Possible additive effect on lowering of blood pressure). Products include:
- Accuretic Tablets 2614
- Aldoril Tablets 2039
- Atacand HCT Tablets 597
- Avalide Tablets 1070
- Diovan HCT Tablets 2338
- Dyazide Capsules 1515
- HydroDIURIL Tablets 2108
- Hyzaar 2109
- Inderide Tablets 3517
- Inderide LA Long-Acting Capsules .. 3519
- Lotensin HCT Tablets 2367
- Maxzide 1008
- Micardis HCT Tablets 1051
- Microzide Capsules 3414
- Moduretic Tablets 2138
- Monopril HCT 1094
- Prinzide Tablets 2168
- Timolide Tablets 2187
- Uniretic Tablets 3178
- Vaseretic Tablets 2204
- Zestoretic Tablets 695
- Ziac Tablets 1887

Hydroflumethiazide (Possible additive effect on lowering of blood pressure). Products include:
- Diucardin Tablets 3494

Indapamide (Possible additive effect on lowering of blood pressure). Products include:
- Indapamide Tablets 2286

Irbesartan (Possible additive effect on lowering of blood pressure). Products include:
- Avalide Tablets 1070
- Avapro Tablets 1074
- Avapro Tablets 3076

Isoflurane (Potential for excessive cardiovascular depression).
No products indexed under this heading.

Isradipine (Possible additive effect on lowering of blood pressure). Products include:
- DynaCirc Capsules 2921
- DynaCirc CR Tablets 2923

Labetalol Hydrochloride (Concomitant therapy may result in additive negative effects on heart rate, atrioventricular conduction and/or cardiac contractility; excessive bradycardia and AV block, including complete heart block). Products include:
- Normodyne Injection 3135
- Normodyne Tablets 3137

Levobunolol Hydrochloride (Concomitant therapy may result in additive negative effects on heart rate, atrioventricular conduction and/or cardiac contractility; excessive bradycardia and AV block, including complete heart block). Products include:
- Betagan ..... ⊙228

Lisinopril (Possible additive effect on lowering of blood pressure). Products include:
- Prinivil Tablets 2164
- Prinzide Tablets 2168
- Zestoretic Tablets 695
- Zestril Tablets 698

Lithium Carbonate (Co-administration has resulted in increased sensitivity to the effects of lithium, neurotoxicity; lithium levels have been observed sometimes to increase, decrease, or remain unchanged). Products include:
- Eskalith 1527
- Lithium Carbonate 3061
- Lithobid Slow-Release Tablets 3255

Lithium Citrate (Co-administration has resulted in increased sensitivity to the effects of lithium, neurotoxicity; lithium levels have been observed sometimes to increase, decrease, or remain unchanged). Products include:
- Lithium Citrate Syrup 3061

Losartan Potassium (Possible additive effect on lowering of blood pressure). Products include:
- Cozaar Tablets 2067
- Hyzaar 2109

Mecamylamine Hydrochloride (Possible additive effect on lowering of blood pressure). Products include:
- Inversine Tablets 1850

Methoxyflurane (Potential for excessive cardiovascular depression).
No products indexed under this heading.

Methyclothiazide (Possible additive effect on lowering of blood pressure).
No products indexed under this heading.

Methyldopa (Possible additive effect on lowering of blood pressure). Products include:
- Aldoclor Tablets 2035
- Aldomet Tablets 2037
- Aldoril Tablets 2039

Methyldopate Hydrochloride (Possible additive effect on lowering of blood pressure).
No products indexed under this heading.

Metipranolol Hydrochloride (Concomitant therapy may result in additive negative effects on heart rate, atrioventricular conduction and/or cardiac contractility; excessive bradycardia and AV block, including complete heart block).
No products indexed under this heading.

Metocurine Iodide (Verapamil may potentiate the activity of neuromuscular blocking agents).
No products indexed under this heading.

Metolazone (Possible additive effect on lowering of blood pressure). Products include:
- Mykrox Tablets 1168
- Zaroxolyn Tablets 1177

Metoprolol Succinate (Concomitant therapy may result in additive negative effects on heart rate, atrioventricular conduction and/or cardiac contractility; excessive bradycardia and AV block, including complete heart block; a decrease in metoprolol clearance has been observed with concomitant use). Products include:
- Toprol-XL Tablets 651

Metoprolol Tartrate (Concomitant therapy may result in additive negative effects on heart rate, atrioventricular conduction and/or cardiac contractility; excessive bradycardia and AV block, including complete heart block; a decrease in metoprolol clearance has been observed with concomitant use).
No products indexed under this heading.

Metyrosine (Possible additive effect on lowering of blood pressure). Products include:
- Demser Capsules 2085

Mibefradil Dihydrochloride (Possible additive effect on lowering of blood pressure).
No products indexed under this heading.

Minoxidil (Possible additive effect on lowering of blood pressure). Products include:
- Rogaine Extra Strength for Men Topical Solution 721
- Rogaine for Women Topical Solution 721

Mivacurium Chloride (Verapamil may potentiate the activity of neuromuscular blocking agents).
No products indexed under this heading.

Moexipril Hydrochloride (Possible additive effect on lowering of blood pressure). Products include:

Uniretic Tablets 3178
Univasc Tablets 3181

Nadolol (Concomitant therapy may result in additive negative effects on heart rate, atrioventricular conduction and/or cardiac contractility; excessive bradycardia and AV block, including complete heart block). Products include:
Corgard Tablets 2245
Corzide 40/5 Tablets 2247
Corzide 80/5 Tablets 2247
Nadolol Tablets 2288

Nicardipine Hydrochloride (Possible additive effect on lowering of blood pressure). Products include:
Cardene I.V. 3485

Nifedipine (Possible additive effect on lowering of blood pressure). Products include:
Adalat CC Tablets 877
Procardia Capsules 2708
Procardia XL Extended Release Tablets 2710

Nisoldipine (Possible additive effect on lowering of blood pressure). Products include:
Sular Tablets 688

Nitroglycerin (Possible additive effect on lowering of blood pressure). Products include:
Nitro-Dur Transdermal Infusion System 3134
Nitro-Dur Transdermal Infusion System 1834
Nitrolingual Pumpspray 1355
Nitrostat Tablets 2658

Pancuronium Bromide (Verapamil may potentiate the activity of neuromuscular blocking agents).
No products indexed under this heading.

Penbutolol Sulfate (Concomitant therapy may result in additive negative effects on heart rate, atrioventricular conduction and/or cardiac contractility; excessive bradycardia and AV block, including complete heart block).
No products indexed under this heading.

Perindopril Erbumine (Possible additive effect on lowering of blood pressure). Products include:
Aceon Tablets (2 mg, 4 mg, 8 mg) 3249

Phenobarbital (May increase verapamil clearance). Products include:
Arco-Lase Plus Tablets 592
Donnatal 2929
Donnatal Extentabs 2930

Phenoxybenzamine Hydrochloride (Possible additive effect on lowering of blood pressure). Products include:
Dibenzyline Capsules 3457

Phentolamine Mesylate (Possible additive effect on lowering of blood pressure).
No products indexed under this heading.

Pindolol (Concomitant therapy may result in additive negative effects on heart rate, atrioventricular conduction and/or cardiac contractility; excessive bradycardia and AV block, including complete heart block).
No products indexed under this heading.

Polythiazide (Possible additive effect on lowering of blood pressure). Products include:
Minizide Capsules 2700
Renese Tablets 2712

Prazosin Hydrochloride (Possible additive effect on lowering of blood pressure). Products include:
Minipress Capsules 2699
Minizide Capsules 2700

Propranolol Hydrochloride (Concomitant therapy may result in additive negative effects on heart rate, atrioventricular conduction and/or cardiac contractility; excessive bradycardia and AV block, including complete heart block; a decrease in propranolol clearance has been observed with concomitant use). Products include:
Inderal 3513
Inderal LA Long-Acting Capsules 3516
Inderide Tablets 3517
Inderide LA Long-Acting Capsules 3519

Quinapril Hydrochloride (Possible additive effect on lowering of blood pressure). Products include:
Accupril Tablets 2611
Accuretic Tablets 2614

Quinidine Gluconate (Concomitant use may result in significant hypertension; verapamil significantly counteracts the effects of quinidine on AV conduction; potential for increased quinidine levels with co-administration). Products include:
Quinaglute Dura-Tabs Tablets 978

Quinidine Polygalacturonate (Concomitant use may result in significant hypertension; verapamil significantly counteracts the effects of quinidine on AV conduction; potential for increased quinidine levels with co-administration).
No products indexed under this heading.

Quinidine Sulfate (Concomitant use may result in significant hypertension; verapamil significantly counteracts the effects of quinidine on AV conduction; potential for increased quinidine levels with co-administration). Products include:
Quinidex Extentabs 2933

Ramipril (Possible additive effect on lowering of blood pressure). Products include:
Altace Capsules 2233

Rapacuronium Bromide (Verapamil may potentiate the activity of neuromuscular blocking agents).
No products indexed under this heading.

Rauwolfia serpentina (Possible additive effect on lowering of blood pressure).
No products indexed under this heading.

Rescinnamine (Possible additive effect on lowering of blood pressure).
No products indexed under this heading.

Reserpine (Possible additive effect on lowering of blood pressure).
No products indexed under this heading.

Rifampin (Therapy with rifampin may markedly reduce oral verapamil bioavailability). Products include:
Rifadin 765
Rifamate Capsules 767
Rifater Tablets 769

Rocuronium Bromide (Verapamil may potentiate the activity of neuromuscular blocking agents). Products include:
Zemuron Injection 2491

Sodium Nitroprusside (Possible additive effect on lowering of blood pressure).
No products indexed under this heading.

Sotalol Hydrochloride (Concomitant therapy may result in additive negative effects on heart rate, atrioventricular conduction and/or cardiac contractility; excessive bradycardia and AV block, including complete heart block). Products include:
Betapace Tablets 950
Betapace AF Tablets 954

Spirapril Hydrochloride (Possible additive effect on lowering of blood pressure).
No products indexed under this heading.

Spironolactone (Possible additive effect on lowering of blood pressure).
No products indexed under this heading.

Telmisartan (Possible additive effect on lowering of blood pressure). Products include:
Micardis Tablets 1049
Micardis HCT Tablets 1051

Terazosin Hydrochloride (Possible additive effect on lowering of blood pressure). Products include:
Hytrin Capsules 464

Theophylline (Verapamil may inhibit the clearance and increase plasma levels of theophylline). Products include:
Aerolate 1361
Theo-Dur Extended-Release Tablets 1835
Uni-Dur Extended-Release Tablets 1841
Uniphyl 400 mg and 600 mg Tablets 2903

Theophylline Calcium Salicylate (Verapamil may inhibit the clearance and increase plasma levels of theophylline).
No products indexed under this heading.

Theophylline Sodium Glycinate (Verapamil may inhibit the clearance and increase plasma levels of theophylline).
No products indexed under this heading.

Timolol Hemihydrate (Concomitant therapy may result in additive negative effects on heart rate, atrioventricular conduction and/or cardiac contractility; excessive bradycardia and AV block, including complete heart block; one case of asymptomatic bradycardia with a wandering atrial pacemaker has been observed with timolol eye drops and oral verapamil). Products include:
Betimol Ophthalmic Solution .... ⊙ 324

Timolol Maleate (Concomitant therapy may result in additive negative effects on heart rate, atrioventricular conduction and/or cardiac contractility; excessive bradycardia and AV block, including complete heart block; one case of asymptomatic bradycardia with a wandering atrial pacemaker has been observed with timolol eye drops and oral verapamil). Products include:
Blocadren Tablets 2046
Cosopt Sterile Ophthalmic Solution 2065
Timolide Tablets 2187
Timolol GFS .... ⊙ 266
Timoptic in Ocudose 2192
Timoptic Sterile Ophthalmic Solution 2190
Timoptic-XE Sterile Ophthalmic Gel Forming Solution 2194

Torsemide (Possible additive effect on lowering of blood pressure). Products include:
Demadex Tablets and Injection 2965

Trandolapril (Possible additive effect on lowering of blood pressure). Products include:
Mavik Tablets 478
Tarka Tablets 508

Triamterene (Possible additive effect on lowering of blood pressure). Products include:
Dyazide Capsules 1515
Dyrenium Capsules 3458
Maxzide 1008

Trimethaphan Camsylate (Possible additive effect on lowering of blood pressure).
No products indexed under this heading.

Valsartan (Possible additive effect on lowering of blood pressure). Products include:
Diovan Capsules 2337
Diovan HCT Tablets 2338

Vecuronium Bromide (Verapamil may potentiate the activity of neuromuscular blocking agents). Products include:
Norcuron for Injection 2478

Food Interactions

Alcohol (Verapamil may increase blood alcohol concentrations and prolong its effect).

COZAAR TABLETS

(Losartan Potassium) 2067
May interact with potassium preparations, potassium sparing diuretics, and certain other agents. Compounds in these categories include:

Amiloride Hydrochloride (Concomitant use with potassium-sparing diuretics may lead to hyperkalemia). Products include:
Midamor Tablets 2136
Moduretic Tablets 2138

Cimetidine (Co-administration leads to an increase of about 18% in AUC of losartan with no effect on pharmacokinetics of its active metabolites). Products include:
Tagamet HB 200 Suspension .... ■ 762
Tagamet HB 200 Tablets .... ■ 761
Tagamet Tablets 1644

Cimetidine Hydrochloride (Co-administration leads to an increase of about 18% in AUC of losartan with no effect on pharmacokinetics of its active metabolites). Products include:
Tagamet 1644

Gestodene (*In Vitro* studies show significant inhibition of the formation of the active metabolite by inhibitors of P450 3A4 such as gestodene; pharmacodynamic consequences of concomitant use is undefined).
No products indexed under this heading.

Ketoconazole (*In Vitro* studies show significant inhibition of the formation of the active metabolite by inhibitors of P450 3A4 such as ketoconazole or complete inhibition by the combination of ketoconazole and sulfaphenazole; pharmacodynamic consequences of concomitant use is undefined). Products include:
Nizoral 2% Cream 3620
Nizoral A-D Shampoo 2008
Nizoral 2% Shampoo 2007
Nizoral Tablets 1791

Phenobarbital (Co-administration leads to a reduction of about 20% in AUC of losartan and that of its active metabolites). Products include:
Arco-Lase Plus Tablets 592
Donnatal 2929
Donnatal Extentabs 2930

Potassium Acid Phosphate (Concomitant use with potassium supplements or salt substitute containing potassium may lead to hyperkalemia; patients should be advised to avoid these potassium-containing preparations). Products include:
K-Phos Original (Sodium Free) Tablets 947

Potassium Bicarbonate (Concomitant use with potassium supplements or salt substitute containing potassium may lead to hyperkalemia; patients should be advised to avoid these potassium-containing preparations).
No products indexed under this heading.

Potassium Chloride (Concomitant use with potassium supplements or salt substitute containing potassium may lead to hyperkalemia; patients should be advised to avoid these potassium-containing preparations). Products include:
Chlor-3 1361
Colyte with Flavor Packs for Oral Solution 3170
GoLYTELY and Pineapple Flavor GoLYTELY for Oral Solution 1068
K-Dur Microburst Release System ER Tablets 1832
Klor-Con M20/Klor-Con M10 Tablets 3329

K-Lor Powder Packets 469
K-Tab Filmtab Tablets 470
Micro-K 3311
NuLYTELY, Cherry Flavor, Lemon-Lime Flavor, and Orange Flavor NuLYTELY for Oral Solution 1068
Rum-K 1363

Potassium Citrate (Concomitant use with potassium supplements or salt substitute containing potassium may lead to hyperkalemia; patients should be advised to avoid these potassium-containing preparations). Products include:
Urocit-K Tablets 2232

Potassium Gluconate (Concomitant use with potassium supplements or salt substitute containing potassium may lead to hyperkalemia; patients should be advised to avoid these potassium-containing preparations).
No products indexed under this heading.

Potassium Phosphate (Concomitant use with potassium supplements or salt substitute containing potassium may lead to hyperkalemia; patients should be advised to avoid these potassium-containing preparations). Products include:
K-Phos Neutral Tablets 946

Salt Substitutes (Concomitant use with salt substitutes may lead to hyperkalemia).
No products indexed under this heading.

Spironolactone (Concomitant use with potassium-sparing diuretics may lead to hyperkalemia).
No products indexed under this heading.

Sulfaphenazole (*In Vitro* studies show significant inhibition of the formation of the active metabolite by inhibitors of P450 3A4 such as sulfaphenazole; pharmacodynamic consequences of concomitant use is undefined).
No products indexed under this heading.

Triamterene (Concomitant use with potassium-sparing diuretics may lead to hyperkalemia). Products include:
Dyazide Capsules 1515
Dyrenium Capsules 3458
Maxzide 1008

Troleandomycin (*In Vitro* studies show significant inhibition of the formation of the active metabolite by inhibitors of P450 3A4 such as troleandomycin; pharmacodynamic consequences of concomitant use is undefined). Products include:
Tao Capsules 2716

Food Interactions

Meal, unspecified (Meal slows absorption and decreases Cmax, but has minor effects on losartan AUC or on the AUC of the metabolite).

CREON 5 CAPSULES
(Pancrelipase) 3251

Food Interactions

Food having a pH greater than 5.5 (Can dissolve the protective coating resulting in early release of enzymes, irritation of oral mucosa, and/or loss of enzyme activity).

CREON 10 CAPSULES
(Pancrelipase) 3251
See Creon 5 Capsules

CREON 20 CAPSULES
(Pancrelipase) 3251
See Creon 5 Capsules

CRINONE 4% GEL
(Progesterone) 3213
None cited in PDR database.

CRINONE 8% GEL
(Progesterone) 3213
None cited in PDR database.

CRIXIVAN CAPSULES
(Indinavir Sulfate) 2070
May interact with dexamethasone, ergot-containing drugs, phenytoin, and certain other agents. Compounds in these categories include:

Astemizole (Inhibition of CYP3A4 by indinavir could result in elevated plasma concentrations of astemizole, potentially causing serious or life-threatening reactions; co-administration is contraindicated).
No products indexed under this heading.

Atorvastatin Calcium (The risk of myopathy including rhabdomyolysis may be increased when protease inhibitors, including indinavir, are used in combination with HMG-CoA inhibitors that are metabolized by the CYP3A4 pathway). Products include:
Lipitor Tablets 2639
Lipitor Tablets 2696

Carbamazepine (Could diminish plasma concentrations of indinavir because carbamazepine is an inducer of P450 3A4; caution is advised if co-administered). Products include:
Carbatrol Capsules 3234
Tegretol/Tegretol-XR 2404

Cerivastatin Sodium (The risk of myopathy including rhabdomyolysis may be increased when protease inhibitors, including indinavir, are used in combination with HMG-CoA inhibitors that are metabolized by the CYP3A4 pathway). Products include:
Baycol Tablets 883

Clarithromycin (Co-administration has resulted in a 29% ±42% increase in indinavir AUC and a 53% ±36% increase in clarithromycin AUC). Products include:
Biaxin/Biaxin XL 403
PREVPAC 3298

Delavirdine Mesylate (Co-administration results in inhibition of indinavir metabolism producing an increase in indinavir concentrations; a reduction of indinavir dosage should be considered when used concurrently). Products include:
Rescriptor Tablets 526

Dexamethasone (Could diminish plasma concentrations of indinavir because dexamethasone is an inducer of P450 3A4; caution is advised if co-administered). Products include:
Decadron Elixir 2078
Decadron Tablets 2079
TobraDex Ophthalmic Ointment 542
TobraDex Ophthalmic Suspension .. 541

Dexamethasone Acetate (Could diminish plasma concentrations of indinavir because dexamethasone is an inducer of P450 3A4; caution is advised if co-administered).
No products indexed under this heading.

Dexamethasone Sodium Phosphate (Could diminish plasma concentrations of indinavir because dexamethasone is an inducer of P450 3A4; caution is advised if co-administered). Products include:
Decadron Phosphate Injection 2081
Decadron Phosphate Sterile Ophthalmic Ointment 2083
Decadron Phosphate Sterile Ophthalmic Solution 2084
NeoDecadron Sterile Ophthalmic Solution 2144

Didanosine (Gastric acid rapidly degrades didanosine and a normal (acidic) gastric pH may be necessary for the optimum absorption of indinavir; if administered concomitantly, they should be administered at least one hour apart on an empty stomach). Products include:
Videx 1138
Videx EC Capsules 1143

Dihydroergotamine Mesylate (Inhibition of CYP3A4 by indinavir could result in elevated plasma concentrations of ergot derivatives, potentially causing serious or life-threatening reactions; co-administration is contraindicated). Products include:
D.H.E. 45 Injection 2334
Migranal Nasal Spray 2376

Efavirenz (Co-administration results in a decrease in the plasma concentrations of indinavir; a dosage increase of indinavir is recommended when used concurrently). Products include:
Sustiva Capsules 1258

Ergonovine Maleate (Inhibition of CYP3A4 by indinavir could result in elevated plasma concentrations of ergot derivatives, potentially causing serious or life-threatening reactions; co-administration is contraindicated).
No products indexed under this heading.

Ergotamine Tartrate (Inhibition of CYP3A4 by indinavir could result in elevated plasma concentrations of ergot derivatives, potentially causing serious or life-threatening reactions; co-administration is contraindicated).
No products indexed under this heading.

Ethinyl Estradiol (Co-administration with Ortho-Novum 1/35 has resulted in an increase in ethinyl estradiol AUC). Products include:
Alesse-21 Tablets 3468
Alesse-28 Tablets 3473
Brevicon 28-Day Tablets 3380
Cyclessa Tablets 2450
Desogen Tablets 2458
Estinyl Tablets 3112
Estrostep 2627
femhrt Tablets 2635
Levlen 962
Levlite 21 Tablets 962
Levlite 28 Tablets 962
Levora Tablets 3389
Loestrin 21 Tablets 2642
Loestrin Fe Tablets 2642
Lo/Ovral Tablets 3532
Lo/Ovral-28 Tablets 3538
Low-Ogestrel-28 Tablets 3392
Microgestin Fe 1.5/30 Tablets 3407
Microgestin Fe 1/20 Tablets 3400
Mircette Tablets 2470
Modicon 2563
Necon 3415
Nordette-28 Tablets 2257
Norinyl 1 +35 28-Day Tablets 3380
Ogestrel 0.5/50-28 Tablets 3428
Ortho-Cept 21 Tablets 2546
Ortho-Cept 28 Tablets 2546
Ortho-Cyclen/Ortho Tri-Cyclen 2573
Ortho-Novum 2563
Ovcon 3364
Ovral Tablets 3551
Ovral-28 Tablets 3552
Tri-Levlen 962
Tri-Norinyl-28 Tablets 3433
Triphasil-21 Tablets 3600
Triphasil-28 Tablets 3605
Trivora Tablets 3439
Yasmin 28 Tablets 980
Zovia 3449

Fluconazole (Co-administration has resulted in a 19% ±33% decrease in indinavir AUC). Products include:
Diflucan Tablets, Injection, and Oral Suspension 2681

Fosphenytoin Sodium (Could diminish plasma concentrations of indinavir because phenytoin is an inducer of P450 3A4; caution is advised if co-administered). Products include:
Cerebyx Injection 2619

Hypericum (Co-administration of indinavir and St. John's Wort (hypericum perforatum) or products containing St. John's Wort has been shown to substantially decrease indinavir concentrations and may lead to loss of virologic response and possible resistance to indinavir or to the class of protease inhibitors; co-administration is not recommended). Products include:
Brite-Life Caplets .... ■795
Centrum St. John's Wort Softgels .... ■853
Metabolic Nutrition System .... ■798
Movana Tablets .... ■832
One-A-Day Tension & Mood Softgels .... ■808
ReSource Wellness StayCalm Caplets .... ■826
Satiete Tablets .... ■846

Isoniazid (Co-administration has resulted in a 13% ±15% increase in isoniazid AUC). Products include:
Rifamate Capsules 767
Rifater Tablets 769

Itraconazole (Co-administration results in increased plasma concentrations of indinavir because itraconazole is an inhibitor of P4503A4; a dosage reduction of indinavir is recommended when used concurrently). Products include:
Sporanox Capsules 1800
Sporanox Injection 1804
Sporanox Injection 2509
Sporanox Oral Solution 1808
Sporanox Oral Solution 2512

Ketoconazole (Co-administration results in an increase in the plasma concentrations of indinavir; a dosage reduction of indinavir may be necessary). Products include:
Nizoral 2% Cream 3620
Nizoral A-D Shampoo 2008
Nizoral 2% Shampoo 2007
Nizoral Tablets 1791

Lovastatin (The risk of myopathy including rhabdomyolysis may be increased when protease inhibitors, including indinavir, are used in combination with HMG-CoA inhibitors that are metabolized by the CYP3A4 pathway; concomitant use is not recommended). Products include:
Mevacor Tablets 2132

Methylergonovine Maleate (Inhibition of CYP3A4 by indinavir could result in elevated plasma concentrations of ergot derivatives, potentially causing serious or life-threatening reactions; co-administration is contraindicated).
No products indexed under this heading.

Methysergide Maleate (Inhibition of CYP3A4 by indinavir could result in elevated plasma concentrations of ergot derivatives, potentially causing serious or life-threatening reactions; co-administration is contraindicated).
No products indexed under this heading.

Midazolam Hydrochloride (Inhibition of CYP3A4 by indinavir could result in elevated plasma concentrations of midazolam, potentially causing serious or life-threatening reactions; co-administration is contraindicated). Products include:
Versed Injection 3027
Versed Syrup 3033

Norethindrone (Co-administration with Ortho-Novum 1/35 has resulted in an increase in norethindrone AUC). Products include:
Brevicon 28-Day Tablets 3380
Micronor Tablets 2543
Modicon 2563
Necon 3415
Norinyl 1 +35 28-Day Tablets 3380
Norinyl 1 + 50 28-Day Tablets 3380
Nor-QD Tablets 3423
Ortho-Novum 2563
Ortho-Novum 1/50□28 Tablets 2556
Ovcon 3364
Tri-Norinyl-28 Tablets 3433

Phenobarbital (Could diminish plasma concentrations of indinavir because phenobarbital is an inducer of P450 3A4; caution is advised if co-administered). Products include:
Arco-Lase Plus Tablets 592
Donnatal 2929
Donnatal Extentabs 2930

Phenytoin (Could diminish plasma concentrations of indinavir because phenytoin is an inducer of P450 3A4; caution is advised if co-administered). Products include:
- Dilantin Infatabs 2624
- Dilantin-125 Oral Suspension 2625

Phenytoin Sodium (Could diminish plasma concentrations of indinavir because phenytoin is an inducer of P450 3A4; caution is advised if co-administered). Products include:
- Dilantin Kapseals 2622

Pimozide (Inhibition of CYP3A4 by indinavir could result in elevated plasma concentrations of pimozide, potentially causing serious or life-threatening reactions; co-administration is contraindicated). Products include:
- Orap Tablets 1407

Quinidine Sulfate (Potential for an increase in indinavir AUC). Products include:
- Quinidex Extentabs 2933

Rifabutin (Co-administration results in an increase in the plasma concentrations of rifabutin and a decrease in the plasma concentrations of indinavir; a dosage decrease of rifabutin and a dosage increase of Crixivan are recommended when used concurrently). Products include:
- Mycobutin Capsules 2838

Rifampin (Markedly diminishes plasma concentrations of indinavir because rifampin is a potent inducer of P450 3A4; co-administration is not recommended). Products include:
- Rifadin 765
- Rifamate Capsules 767
- Rifater Tablets 769

Simvastatin (The risk of myopathy including rhabdomyolysis may be increased when protease inhibitors, including indinavir, are used in combination with HMG-CoA inhibitors that are metabolized by the CYP3A4 pathway; concomitant use is not recommended). Products include:
- Zocor Tablets 2219

Stavudine (Co-administration has resulted in a 25% ±26% increase in stavudine AUC and no change in indinavir AUC; co-administration does not require dose modification). Products include:
- Zerit 1147

Terfenadine (Inhibition of CYP3A4 by indinavir could result in elevated plasma concentrations of terfenadine, potentially causing serious or life-threatening reactions; co-administration is contraindicated).
No products indexed under this heading.

Triazolam (Inhibition of CYP3A4 by indinavir could result in elevated plasma concentrations of triazolam, potentially causing serious or life-threatening reactions; co-administration is contraindicated). Products include:
- Halcion Tablets 2823

Trimethoprim (Co-administration with trimethoprim/sulfamethoxazole tablet has resulted in a 19% ±31% increase in trimethoprim AUC). Products include:
- Bactrim 2949
- Septra Suspension 2265
- Septra Tablets 2265
- Septra DS Tablets 2265

Zidovudine (Co-administration has resulted in a 13% ±48% increase in indinavir AUC and a 17% ±23% increase in zidovudine AUC; co-administration does not require dose modification). Products include:
- Combivir Tablets 1502
- Retrovir 1625
- Retrovir IV Infusion 1629
- Trizivir Tablets 1669

Food Interactions

Food, unspecified (Co-administration with a meal high in calories, fat, and protein has resulted in a 77% ±8% reduction in AUC and an 84% ±7% reduction in Cmax; administer without food 1 hour before or 2 hours after a meal).

Grapefruit Juice (Potential for decrease in indinavir AUC).

CROLOM STERILE OPHTHALMIC SOLUTION USP 4%

(Cromolyn Sodium) .... ⊙259
None cited in PDR database.

CUPRIMINE CAPSULES

(Penicillamine) 2075
May interact with antimalarials, cytotoxic drugs, and certain other agents. Compounds in these categories include:

Auranofin (Concurrent use not recommended).
No products indexed under this heading.

Aurothioglucose (Concurrent use not recommended).
No products indexed under this heading.

Bleomycin Sulfate (Concurrent use not recommended).
No products indexed under this heading.

Chloroquine Hydrochloride (Concurrent use not recommended).
No products indexed under this heading.

Chloroquine Phosphate (Concurrent use not recommended). Products include:
- Aralen Tablets 3075

Cyclophosphamide (Concurrent use not recommended).
No products indexed under this heading.

Daunorubicin Hydrochloride (Concurrent use not recommended). Products include:
- Cerubidine for Injection 947

Doxorubicin Hydrochloride (Concurrent use not recommended). Products include:
- Adriamycin PFS/RDF Injection 2767
- Doxil Injection 566

Epirubicin Hydrochloride (Concurrent use not recommended). Products include:
- Ellence Injection 2806

Fluorouracil (Concurrent use not recommended). Products include:
- Carac Cream 1222
- Efudex 1733
- Fluoroplex 552

Hydroxychloroquine Sulfate (Concurrent use not recommended). Products include:
- Plaquenil Tablets 3082

Hydroxyurea (Concurrent use not recommended). Products include:
- Mylocel Tablets 2227

Mefloquine Hydrochloride (Concurrent use not recommended). Products include:
- Lariam Tablets 2989

Methotrexate Sodium (Concurrent use not recommended).
No products indexed under this heading.

Mineral Supplements (Block response).
No products indexed under this heading.

Mitotane (Concurrent use not recommended).
No products indexed under this heading.

Mitoxantrone Hydrochloride (Concurrent use not recommended). Products include:
- Novantrone for Injection 1760

Oxyphenbutazone (Concurrent use not recommended).
No products indexed under this heading.

Phenylbutazone (Concurrent use not recommended).
No products indexed under this heading.

Procarbazine Hydrochloride (Concurrent use not recommended). Products include:
- Matulane Capsules 3246

Pyridoxine (Penicillamine increases pyridoxine requirement).
No products indexed under this heading.

Pyrimethamine (Concurrent use not recommended). Products include:
- Daraprim Tablets 1511

Tamoxifen Citrate (Concurrent use not recommended). Products include:
- Nolvadex Tablets 678

Vincristine Sulfate (Concurrent use not recommended).
No products indexed under this heading.

CUROSURF INTRATRACHEAL SUSPENSION

(Poractant alfa) 1232
None cited in PDR database.

CUTIVATE CREAM

(Fluticasone Propionate) 1282
None cited in PDR database.

CUTIVATE OINTMENT

(Fluticasone Propionate) 1284
None cited in PDR database.

CYCLESSA TABLETS

(Desogestrel, Ethinyl Estradiol) 2450
May interact with barbiturates, phenytoin, prednisolone, protease inhibitors, tetracyclines, theophylline, and certain other agents. Compounds in these categories include:

Acetaminophen (May increase plasma levels of ethinyl estradiol possibly by inhibition of conjugation; co-administration may decrease plasma concentrations of acetaminophen). Products include:
- Actifed Cold & Sinus Caplets and Tablets .... ■688
- Alka-Seltzer Plus Liqui-Gels .... ■604
- Alka-Seltzer Plus Cold & Flu Medicine Liqui-Gels .... ■604
- Alka-Seltzer Plus Cold & Sinus Medicine Liqui-Gels .... ■604
- Benadryl Allergy/Cold Tablets .... ■691
- Benadryl Allergy Sinus Headache Caplets & Gelcaps .... ■693
- Benadryl Severe Allergy & Sinus Headache Caplets .... ■694
- Children's Cēpacol Sore Throat .... ■788
- Comtrex Acute Head Cold & Sinus Pressure Relief Tablets .... ■627
- Comtrex Deep Chest Cold & Congestion Relief Softgels .... ■627
- Comtrex Flu Therapy & Fever Relief Daytime Caplets .... ■628
- Comtrex Flu Therapy & Fever Relief Nighttime Tablets .... ■628
- Comtrex Maximum Strength Multi-Symptom Cold & Cough Relief Tablets and Caplets .... ■626
- Contac Severe Cold and Flu Caplets Maximum Strength .... ■746
- Contac Severe Cold and Flu Caplets Non-Drowsy .... ■746
- Coricidin 'D' Cold, Flu & Sinus Tablets .... ■737
- Coricidin HBP Cold & Flu Tablets .... ■738
- Coricidin HBP Maximum Strength Flu Tablets .... ■738
- Coricidin HBP Night-Time Cold & Flu Tablets .... ■738
- Darvon-N/Darvocet-N 1907
- Dimetapp Cold and Fever Suspension .... ■775
- Dimetapp Nighttime Flu Liquid .... ■776
- Dimetapp Non-Drowsy Flu Syrup .... ■777
- Drixoral Allergy/Sinus Extended-Release Tablets .... ■741
- Drixoral Cold & Flu Extended-Release Tablets .... ■740
- Aspirin Free Excedrin Caplets and Geltabs .... ■628
- Excedrin Extra-Strength Tablets, Caplets, and Geltabs .... ■629
- Excedrin Migraine 1070
- Excedrin PM Tablets, Caplets, and Geltabs .... ■631
- Goody's Body Pain Formula Powder .... ■620
- Goody's Extra Strength Headache Powder .... ■620
- Goody's Extra Strength Pain Relief Tablets .... ■620
- Goody's PM Powder .... ■621
- Hycomine Compound Tablets 1317
- Lortab 3319
- Lortab Elixir 3317
- Maxidone Tablets CIII 3399
- Maximum Strength Midol Menstrual Caplets and Gelcaps .... ■612
- Maximum Strength Midol PMS Caplets and Gelcaps .... ■613
- Maximum Strength Midol Teen Caplets .... ■612
- Midrin Capsules 3464
- Norco 5/325 Tablets CIII 3424
- Norco 7.5/325 Tablets CIII 3425
- Norco 10/325 Tablets CIII 3427
- Norco 10/325 Tablets CIII 3425
- Percocet Tablets 1326
- Percogesic Aspirin-Free Coated Tablets .... ■667
- Extra Strength Percogesic Aspirin-Free Coated Caplets .... ■665
- Phrenilin 578
- Robitussin Cold Caplets Multi-Symptom Cold & Flu .... ■781
- Robitussin Cold Softgels Multi-Symptom Cold & Flu .... ■781
- Robitussin Multi Symptom Honey Flu Liquid .... ■785
- Robitussin Nighttime Honey Flu Liquid .... ■786
- Sedapap Tablets 50 mg/650 mg 2225
- Singlet Caplets .... ■761
- Sinutab Sinus Allergy Medication, Maximum Strength Formula, Tablets & Caplets .... ■707
- Sinutab Sinus Medication, Maximum Strength Without Drowsiness Formula, Tablets & Caplets .... ■707
- Sudafed Cold & Cough Liquid Caps .... ■709
- Sudafed Cold & Sinus Liquid Caps .... ■710
- Sudafed Severe Cold .... ■711
- Sudafed Sinus Headache Caplets .... ■712
- Sudafed Sinus Headache Tablets .... ■712
- Tavist Sinus Non-Drowsy Coated Caplets .... ■676
- TheraFlu Regular Strength Cold & Cough Night Time Hot Liquid .... ■676
- TheraFlu Regular Strength Cold & Sore Throat Night Time Hot Liquid .... ■676
- TheraFlu Maximum Strength Flu & Congestion Non-Drowsy Hot Liquid .... ■677
- TheraFlu Maximum Strength Flu & Cough Night Time Hot Liquid .... ■678
- TheraFlu Maximum Strength Flu & Sore Throat Night Time Hot Liquid .... ■677
- TheraFlu Maximum Strength Severe Cold & Congestion Night Time Caplets .... ■678
- TheraFlu Maximum Strength Severe Cold & Congestion Night Time Hot Liquid .... ■678
- TheraFlu Maximum Strength Severe Cold & Congestion Non-Drowsy .... ■679
- Triaminic Cold, Cough & Fever Liquid .... ■681
- Triaminic Cough & Sore Throat Liquid .... ■682
- Triaminic Cough & Sore Throat Softchews .... ■684
- Tylenol, Children's 2014
- Children's Tylenol Allergy-D Liquid 2014
- Children's Tylenol Cold Suspension Liquid and Chewable Tablets 2015
- Children's Tylenol Cold Plus Cough Suspension Liquid and Chewable Tablets 2015
- Children's Tylenol Flu Suspension Liquid 2015
- Children's Tylenol Sinus Suspension Liquid 2017
- Infants' Tylenol Cold Decongestant and Fever Reducer Concentrated Drops 2015
- Infants' Tylenol Cold Decongestant and Fever Reducer Concentrated Drops Plus Cough 2015

Junior Strength Tylenol Soft Chews Chewable Tablets 2014
Tylenol 2009
Tylenol Allergy Sinus 2010
Tylenol Severe Allergy Caplets 2010
Multi-Symptom Tylenol Cold Complete Formula Caplets 2010
Multi-Symptom Tylenol Cold Non-Drowsy Caplets and Gelcaps 2010
Multi-Symptom Tylenol Cold Severe Congestion Non-Drowsy Caplets 2011
Maximum Strength Tylenol Flu NightTime Gelcaps 2011
Maximum Strength Tylenol Flu NightTime Liquid 2011
Maximum Strength Tylenol Flu Non-Drowsy Gelcaps 2011
Extra Strength Tylenol PM Caplets, Geltabs, and Gelcaps 2012
Maximum Strength Tylenol Sinus NightTime Caplets 2012
Maximum Strength Tylenol Sinus Non-Drowsy Geltabs, Gelcaps, Caplets, and Tablets 2012
Maximum Strength Tylenol Sore Throat Adult Liquid 2013
Tylenol with Codeine 2595
Women's Tylenol Menstrual Relief Caplets 2013
Tylox Capsules 2597
Ultracet Tablets 2597
Vanquish Caplets 617
Vicks 44M Cough, Cold & Flu Relief Liquid 725
Vicks DayQuil LiquiCaps/Liquid Multi-Symptom Cold/Flu Relief 727
Vicks NyQuil LiquiCaps/Liquid Multi-Symptom Cold/Flu Relief, Original and Cherry Flavors 727
Vicodin Tablets 516
Vicodin ES Tablets 517
Vicodin HP Tablets 518
Zydone Tablets 1330

Aminophylline (Co-administration of products containing ethinyl estradiol may inhibit the metabolism of other compounds, such as theophylline, resulting in increased plasma concentrations of theophylline).
No products indexed under this heading.

Ampicillin (Co-administration may result in increased metabolism of contraceptive steroids precipitating a reduction in contraceptive effectiveness and increased incidence of breakthrough bleeding and unintended pregnancy).
No products indexed under this heading.

Ampicillin Sodium (Co-administration may result in increased metabolism of contraceptive steroids precipitating a reduction in contraceptive effectiveness and increased incidence of breakthrough bleeding and unintended pregnancy). Products include:
Unasyn for Injection 2728

Amprenavir (Co-administration of protease inhibitors with some oral contraceptives has resulted in significant changes in the mean AUC of estrogen and progestins; the efficacy of these oral contraceptive products may be affected). Products include:
Agenerase Capsules 1454
Agenerase Oral Solution 1459

Aprobarbital (Co-administration results in increased metabolism of contraceptive steroids precipitating a reduction in contraceptive effectiveness and increased incidence of breakthrough bleeding and unintended pregnancy).
No products indexed under this heading.

Atorvastatin Calcium (Co-administration of atorvastatin and an oral contraceptive increased AUC values for ethinyl estradiol by approximately 20%). Products include:
Lipitor Tablets 2639
Lipitor Tablets 2696

Butabarbital (Co-administration results in increased metabolism of contraceptive steroids precipitating a reduction in contraceptive effectiveness and increased incidence of breakthrough bleeding and unintended pregnancy).
No products indexed under this heading.

Butalbital (Co-administration results in increased metabolism of contraceptive steroids precipitating a reduction in contraceptive effectiveness and increased incidence of breakthrough bleeding and unintended pregnancy). Products include:
Phrenilin 578
Sedapap Tablets 50 mg/650 mg 2225

Carbamazepine (Co-administration results in increased metabolism of contraceptive steroids precipitating a reduction in contraceptive effectiveness and increased incidence of breakthrough bleeding and unintended pregnancy). Products include:
Carbatrol Capsules 3234
Tegretol/Tegretol-XR 2404

Celecoxib (Desogestrel is metabolized by CYP 2C9 to form etonogestrel, the active progestins; there is a possibility of interactions with CYP 2C9 substrates or inhibitors; the clinical significance of this interaction is unknown). Products include:
Celebrex Capsules 2676
Celebrex Capsules 2780

Clofibrate (Co-administration of products containing ethinyl estradiol may increase clearance of clofibric acid). Products include:
Atromid-S Capsules 3483

Cyclosporine (Co-administration of products containing ethinyl estradiol may inhibit the metabolism of other compounds, such as cyclosporine, resulting in increased plasma concentrations of cyclosporine). Products include:
Gengraf Capsules 457
Neoral Soft Gelatin Capsules 2380
Neoral Oral Solution 2380
Sandimmune 2388

Demeclocycline Hydrochloride (Co-administration may result in increased metabolism of contraceptive steroids precipitating a reduction in contraceptive effectiveness and increased incidence of breakthrough bleeding and unintended pregnancy). Products include:
Declomycin Tablets 1855

Diclofenac Potassium (Desogestrel is metabolized by CYP 2C9 to form etonogestrel, the active progestins; there is a possibility of interactions with CYP 2C9 substrates or inhibitors; the clinical significance of this interaction is unknown). Products include:
Cataflam Tablets 2315

Diclofenac Sodium (Desogestrel is metabolized by CYP 2C9 to form etonogestrel, the active progestins; there is a possibility of interactions with CYP 2C9 substrates or inhibitors; the clinical significance of this interaction is unknown). Products include:
Arthrotec Tablets 3195
Voltaren Ophthalmic Sterile Ophthalmic Solution .... ⊙312
Voltaren Tablets 2315
Voltaren-XR Tablets 2315

Doxycycline Calcium (Co-administration may result in increased metabolism of contraceptive steroids precipitating a reduction in contraceptive effectiveness and increased incidence of breakthrough bleeding and unintended pregnancy). Products include:
Vibramycin Calcium Oral Suspension Syrup 2735

Doxycycline Hyclate (Co-administration may result in increased metabolism of contraceptive steroids precipitating a reduction in contraceptive effectiveness and increased incidence of breakthrough bleeding and unintended pregnancy). Products include:
Doryx Coated Pellet Filled Capsules 3357
Periostat Tablets 1208
Vibramycin Hyclate Capsules 2735
Vibramycin Hyclate Intravenous 2737
Vibra-Tabs Film Coated Tablets 2735

Doxycycline Monohydrate (Co-administration may result in increased metabolism of contraceptive steroids precipitating a reduction in contraceptive effectiveness and increased incidence of breakthrough bleeding and unintended pregnancy). Products include:
Monodox Capsules 2442
Vibramycin Monohydrate for Oral Suspension 2735

Dyphylline (Co-administration of products containing ethinyl estradiol may inhibit the metabolism of other compounds, such as theophylline, resulting in increased plasma concentrations of theophylline). Products include:
Lufyllin Tablets 3347
Lufyllin-400 Tablets 3347
Lufyllin-GG Elixir 3348
Lufyllin-GG Tablets 3348

Felbamate (Co-administration results in increased metabolism of contraceptive steroids precipitating a reduction in contraceptive effectiveness and increased incidence of breakthrough bleeding and unintended pregnancy). Products include:
Felbatol 3343

Fluconazole (Desogestrel is metabolized by CYP 2C9 to form etonogestrel, the active progestins; there is a possibility of interactions with CYP 2C9 substrates or inhibitors; the clinical significance of this interaction is unknown). Products include:
Diflucan Tablets, Injection, and Oral Suspension 2681

Fosphenytoin Sodium (Co-administration results in increased metabolism of contraceptive steroids precipitating a reduction in contraceptive effectiveness and increased incidence of breakthrough bleeding and unintended pregnancy). Products include:
Cerebyx Injection 2619

Glipizide (Desogestrel is metabolized by CYP 2C9 to form etonogestrel, the active progestins; there is a possibility of interactions with CYP 2C9 substrates or inhibitors; the clinical significance of this interaction is unknown). Products include:
Glucotrol Tablets 2692
Glucotrol XL Extended Release Tablets 2693

Griseofulvin (Co-administration may result in increased metabolism of contraceptive steroids precipitating a reduction in contraceptive effectiveness and increased incidence of breakthrough bleeding and unintended pregnancy). Products include:
Grifulvin V Tablets Microsize and Oral Suspension Microsize 2518
Gris-PEG Tablets 2661

Hypericum (Herbal products containing St. John's Wort may induce hepatic enzyme and p-glycoprotein transport and may reduce the effectiveness of contraceptive steroids). Products include:
Brite-Life Caplets 795
Centrum St. John's Wort Softgels 853
Metabolic Nutrition System 798
Movana Tablets 832
One-A-Day Tension & Mood Softgels 808
ReSource Wellness StayCalm Caplets 826
Satiete Tablets 846

Ibuprofen (Desogestrel is metabolized by CYP 2C9 to form etonogestrel, the active progestins; there is a possibility of interactions with CYP 2C9 substrates or inhibitors; the clinical significance of this interaction is unknown). Products include:
Advil 771
Children's Advil Oral Suspension 773
Children's Advil Chewable Tablets 773
Advil Cold and Sinus Caplets 771
Advil Cold and Sinus Tablets 771
Advil Flu & Body Ache Caplets 772
Infants' Advil Drops 773
Junior Strength Advil Tablets 773
Junior Strength Advil Chewable Tablets 773
Advil Migraine Liquigels 772
Children's Motrin Oral Suspension and Chewable Tablets 2006
Children's Motrin Cold Oral Suspension 2007
Children's Motrin Oral Suspension 643
Motrin Suspension, Oral Drops, Chewable Tablets, and Caplets 2002
Infants' Motrin Concentrated Drops 2006
Junior Strength Motrin Caplets and Chewable Tablets 2006
Motrin IB Tablets, Caplets, and Gelcaps 2002
Motrin Migraine Pain Caplets 2005
Motrin Sinus Headache Caplets 2005
Vicoprofen Tablets 520

Indinavir Sulfate (Co-administration of protease inhibitors with some oral contraceptives has resulted in significant changes in the mean AUC of estrogen and progestins; the efficacy of these oral contraceptive products may be affected). Products include:
Crixivan Capsules 2070

Irbesartan (Desogestrel is metabolized by CYP 2C9 to form etonogestrel, the active progestins; there is a possibility of interactions with CYP 2C9 substrates or inhibitors; the clinical significance of this interaction is unknown). Products include:
Avalide Tablets 1070
Avapro Tablets 1074
Avapro Tablets 3076

Isoniazid (Desogestrel is metabolized by CYP 2C9 to form etonogestrel, the active progestins; there is a possibility of interactions with CYP 2C9 substrates or inhibitors; the clinical significance of this interaction is unknown). Products include:
Rifamate Capsules 767
Rifater Tablets 769

Itraconazole (May increase plasma hormone levels). Products include:
Sporanox Capsules 1800
Sporanox Injection 1804
Sporanox Injection 2509
Sporanox Oral Solution 1808
Sporanox Oral Solution 2512

Ketoconazole (May increase plasma hormone levels). Products include:
Nizoral 2% Cream 3620
Nizoral A-D Shampoo 2008
Nizoral 2% Shampoo 2007
Nizoral Tablets 1791

Lopinavir (Co-administration of protease inhibitors with some oral contraceptives has resulted in significant changes in the mean AUC of estrogen and progestins; the efficacy of these oral contraceptive products may be affected). Products include:
Kaletra Capsules 471
Kaletra Oral Solution 471

Losartan Potassium (Desogestrel is metabolized by CYP 2C9 to form etonogestrel, the active progestins; there is a possibility of interactions with CYP 2C9 substrates or inhibi-

tors; the clinical significance of this interaction is unknown). Products include:

Cozaar Tablets 2067
Hyzaar 2109

Mephobarbital (Co-administration results in increased metabolism of contraceptive steroids precipitating a reduction in contraceptive effectiveness and increased incidence of breakthrough bleeding and unintended pregnancy).

No products indexed under this heading.

Methacycline Hydrochloride (Co-administration may result in increased metabolism of contraceptive steroids precipitating a reduction in contraceptive effectiveness and increased incidence of breakthrough bleeding and unintended pregnancy).

No products indexed under this heading.

Minocycline Hydrochloride (Co-administration may result in increased metabolism of contraceptive steroids precipitating a reduction in contraceptive effectiveness and increased incidence of breakthrough bleeding and unintended pregnancy). Products include:

Dynacin Capsules 2019
Minocin Intravenous 1862
Minocin Oral Suspension 1865
Minocin Pellet-Filled Capsules 1863

Morphine Sulfate (Co-administration of products containing ethinyl estradiol may increase clearance of morphine). Products include:

Astramorph/PF Injection, USP (Preservative-Free) 594
Duramorph Injection 1312
Infumorph 200 and Infumorph 500 Sterile Solutions 1314
Kadian Capsules 1335
MS Contin Tablets 2896
MSIR 2898
Oramorph SR Tablets 3062
Roxanol 3066

Naproxen (Desogestrel is metabolized by CYP 2C9 to form etonogestrel, the active progestins; there is a possibility of interactions with CYP 2C9 substrates or inhibitors; the clinical significance of this interaction is unknown). Products include:

EC-Naprosyn Delayed-Release Tablets 2967
Naprosyn Suspension 2967
Naprosyn Tablets 2967

Naproxen Sodium (Desogestrel is metabolized by CYP 2C9 to form etonogestrel, the active progestins; there is a possibility of interactions with CYP 2C9 substrates or inhibitors; the clinical significance of this interaction is unknown). Products include:

Aleve Tablets, Caplets and Gelcaps .... ▣602
Aleve Cold & Sinus Caplets .... ▣603
Anaprox Tablets 2967
Anaprox DS Tablets 2967
Naprelan Tablets 1293

Nelfinavir Mesylate (Co-administration of protease inhibitors with some oral contraceptives has resulted in significant changes in the mean AUC of estrogen and progestins; the efficacy of these oral contraceptive products may be affected). Products include:

Viracept 532

Oxcarbazepine (Co-administration results in increased metabolism of contraceptive steroids precipitating a reduction in contraceptive effectiveness and increased incidence of breakthrough bleeding and unintended pregnancy). Products include:

Trileptal Oral Suspension 2407
Trileptal Tablets 2407

Oxytetracycline Hydrochloride (Co-administration may result in increased metabolism of contraceptive steroids precipitating a reduction in contraceptive effectiveness and increased incidence of breakthrough bleeding and unintended pregnancy). Products include:

Terra-Cortril Ophthalmic Suspension 2716
Urobiotic-250 Capsules 2731

Pentobarbital Sodium (Co-administration results in increased metabolism of contraceptive steroids precipitating a reduction in contraceptive effectiveness and increased incidence of breakthrough bleeding and unintended pregnancy). Products include:

Nembutal Sodium Solution 485

Phenobarbital (Co-administration results in increased metabolism of contraceptive steroids precipitating a reduction in contraceptive effectiveness and increased incidence of breakthrough bleeding and unintended pregnancy). Products include:

Arco-Lase Plus Tablets 592
Donnatal 2929
Donnatal Extentabs 2930

Phenylbutazone (Co-administration results in increased metabolism of contraceptive steroids precipitating a reduction in contraceptive effectiveness and increased incidence of breakthrough bleeding and unintended pregnancy).

No products indexed under this heading.

Phenytoin (Co-administration results in increased metabolism of contraceptive steroids precipitating a reduction in contraceptive effectiveness and increased incidence of breakthrough bleeding and unintended pregnancy). Products include:

Dilantin Infatabs 2624
Dilantin-125 Oral Suspension 2625

Phenytoin Sodium (Co-administration results in increased metabolism of contraceptive steroids precipitating a reduction in contraceptive effectiveness and increased incidence of breakthrough bleeding and unintended pregnancy). Products include:

Dilantin Kapseals 2622

Piroxicam (Desogestrel is metabolized by CYP 2C9 to form etonogestrel, the active progestins; there is a possibility of interactions with CYP 2C9 substrates or inhibitors; the clinical significance of this interaction is unknown). Products include:

Feldene Capsules 2685

Prednisolone (Co-administration of products containing ethinyl estradiol may inhibit the metabolism of other compounds, such as prednisolone, resulting in increased plasma concentrations of prednisolone). Products include:

Prelone Syrup 2273

Prednisolone Acetate (Co-administration of products containing ethinyl estradiol may inhibit the metabolism of other compounds, such as prednisolone, resulting in increased plasma concentrations of prednisolone). Products include:

Blephamide Ophthalmic Ointment .. 547
Blephamide Ophthalmic Suspension 548
Poly-Pred Liquifilm Ophthalmic Suspension .... ⊙245
Pred Forte Ophthalmic Suspension .... ⊙246
Pred Mild Sterile Ophthalmic Suspension .... ⊙249
Pred-G Ophthalmic Suspension .... ⊙247
Pred-G Sterile Ophthalmic Ointment .... ⊙248

Prednisolone Sodium Phosphate (Co-administration of products containing ethinyl estradiol may inhibit the metabolism of other compounds, such as prednisolone, resulting in increased plasma concentrations of prednisolone). Products include:

Pediapred Oral Solution 1170

Prednisolone Tebutate (Co-administration of products containing ethinyl estradiol may inhibit the metabolism of other compounds, such as prednisolone, resulting in increased plasma concentrations of prednisolone).

No products indexed under this heading.

Rifampin (Co-administration results in increased metabolism of contraceptive steroids precipitating a reduction in contraceptive effectiveness and increased incidence of breakthrough bleeding and unintended pregnancy). Products include:

Rifadin 765
Rifamate Capsules 767
Rifater Tablets 769

Ritonavir (Co-administration of protease inhibitors with some oral contraceptives has resulted in significant changes in the mean AUC of estrogen and progestins; the efficacy of these oral contraceptive products may be affected). Products include:

Kaletra Capsules 471
Kaletra Oral Solution 471
Norvir Capsules 487
Norvir Oral Solution 487

Salicylic Acid (Co-administration of products containing ethinyl estradiol may increase clearance of salicylic acid). Products include:

Clear Away Gel with Aloe Wart Remover System .... ▣736
Clear Away Liquid Wart Remover System .... ▣736
Clear Away One Step Wart Remover .... ▣737
Clear Away One Step Wart Remover for Kids .... ▣737
Clear Away One Step Plantar Wart Remover .... ▣737
Compound W One Step Pads for Kids .... ▣664
Compound W One Step Plantar Pads .... ▣664
Compound W One Step Wart Remover Pads .... ▣664
Compound W Wart Remover Gel .. ▣665
Compound W Wart Remover Liquid .... ▣665
Wart-Off Liquid .... ▣716

Saquinavir (Co-administration of protease inhibitors with some oral contraceptives has resulted in significant changes in the mean AUC of estrogen and progestins; the efficacy of these oral contraceptive products may be affected). Products include:

Fortovase Capsules 2970

Saquinavir Mesylate (Co-administration of protease inhibitors with some oral contraceptives has resulted in significant changes in the mean AUC of estrogen and progestins; the efficacy of these oral contraceptive products may be affected). Products include:

Invirase Capsules 2979

Secobarbital Sodium (Co-administration results in increased metabolism of contraceptive steroids precipitating a reduction in contraceptive effectiveness and increased incidence of breakthrough bleeding and unintended pregnancy).

No products indexed under this heading.

Sulfamethoxazole (Desogestrel is metabolized by CYP 2C9 to form etonogestrel, the active progestins; there is a possibility of interactions with CYP 2C9 substrates or inhibitors; the clinical significance of this interaction is unknown). Products include:

Bactrim 2949
Septra Suspension 2265
Septra Tablets 2265
Septra DS Tablets 2265

Temazepam (Co-administration of products containing ethinyl estradiol may increase clearance of temazepam).

No products indexed under this heading.

Tetracycline Hydrochloride (Co-administration may result in increased metabolism of contraceptive steroids precipitating a reduction in contraceptive effectiveness and increased incidence of breakthrough bleeding and unintended pregnancy).

No products indexed under this heading.

Theophylline (Co-administration of products containing ethinyl estradiol may inhibit the metabolism of other compounds, such as theophylline, resulting in increased plasma concentrations of theophylline). Products include:

Aerolate 1361
Theo-Dur Extended-Release Tablets 1835
Uni-Dur Extended-Release Tablets .. 1841
Uniphyl 400 mg and 600 mg Tablets 2903

Theophylline Calcium Salicylate (Co-administration of products containing ethinyl estradiol may inhibit the metabolism of other compounds, such as theophylline, resulting in increased plasma concentrations of theophylline).

No products indexed under this heading.

Theophylline Sodium Glycinate (Co-administration of products containing ethinyl estradiol may inhibit the metabolism of other compounds, such as theophylline, resulting in increased plasma concentrations of theophylline).

No products indexed under this heading.

Thiamylal Sodium (Co-administration results in increased metabolism of contraceptive steroids precipitating a reduction in contraceptive effectiveness and increased incidence of breakthrough bleeding and unintended pregnancy).

No products indexed under this heading.

Tolbutamide (Desogestrel is metabolized by CYP 2C9 to form etonogestrel, the active progestins; there is a possibility of interactions with CYP 2C9 substrates or inhibitors; the clinical significance of this interaction is unknown).

No products indexed under this heading.

Topiramate (Co-administration results in increased metabolism of contraceptive steroids precipitating a reduction in contraceptive effectiveness and increased incidence of breakthrough bleeding and unintended pregnancy). Products include:

Topamax Sprinkle Capsules 2590
Topamax Tablets 2590

Torsemide (Desogestrel is metabolized by CYP 2C9 to form etonogestrel, the active progestins; there is a possibility of interactions with CYP 2C9 substrates or inhibitors; the clinical significance of this interaction is unknown). Products include:

Demadex Tablets and Injection 2965

Valsartan (Desogestrel is metabolized by CYP 2C9 to form etonogestrel, the active progestins; there is a possibility of interactions with CYP 2C9 substrates or inhibitors; the clinical significance of this interaction is unknown). Products include:

Diovan Capsules 2337
Diovan HCT Tablets 2338

Vitamin C (May increase plasma levels of ethinyl estradiol possibly by inhibition of conjugation). Products include:
Beta-C Tablets ⊞811
C-Grams Caplets ⊞795
Halls Defense Drops ⊞687
Peridin-C Tablets ⊞618

CYLERT TABLETS
(Pemoline) 415
May interact with anticonvulsants and certain other agents. Compounds in these categories include:

Carbamazepine (Co-administration with antiepileptic medications results in decreased seizure threshold). Products include:
Carbatrol Capsules 3234
Tegretol/Tegretol-XR 2404

Clonazepam (Co-administration with antiepileptic medications results in decreased seizure threshold). Products include:
Klonopin Tablets 2983

CNS-Active Drugs, unspecified (Patients receiving Cylert concurrently with other drugs with CNS activity should be monitored carefully).

Divalproex Sodium (Co-administration with antiepileptic medications results in decreased seizure threshold). Products include:
Depakote Sprinkle Capsules 426
Depakote Tablets 430
Depakote ER Tablets 436

Ethosuximide (Co-administration with antiepileptic medications results in decreased seizure threshold). Products include:
Zarontin Capsules 2659
Zarontin Syrup 2660

Ethotoin (Co-administration with antiepileptic medications results in decreased seizure threshold).
No products indexed under this heading.

Felbamate (Co-administration with antiepileptic medications results in decreased seizure threshold). Products include:
Felbatol 3343

Fosphenytoin Sodium (Co-administration with antiepileptic medications results in decreased seizure threshold). Products include:
Cerebyx Injection 2619

Lamotrigine (Co-administration with antiepileptic medications results in decreased seizure threshold). Products include:
Lamictal 1567

Levetiracetam (Co-administration with antiepileptic medications results in decreased seizure threshold). Products include:
Keppra Tablets 3314

Mephenytoin (Co-administration with antiepileptic medications results in decreased seizure threshold).
No products indexed under this heading.

Methsuximide (Co-administration with antiepileptic medications results in decreased seizure threshold). Products include:
Celontin Capsules 2618

Oxcarbazepine (Co-administration with antiepileptic medications results in decreased seizure threshold). Products include:
Trileptal Oral Suspension 2407
Trileptal Tablets 2407

Paramethadione (Co-administration with antiepileptic medications results in decreased seizure threshold).
No products indexed under this heading.

Phenacemide (Co-administration with antiepileptic medications results in decreased seizure threshold).
No products indexed under this heading.

Phenobarbital (Co-administration with antiepileptic medications results in decreased seizure threshold). Products include:
Arco-Lase Plus Tablets 592
Donnatal 2929
Donnatal Extentabs 2930

Phensuximide (Co-administration with antiepileptic medications results in decreased seizure threshold).
No products indexed under this heading.

Phenytoin (Co-administration with antiepileptic medications results in decreased seizure threshold). Products include:
Dilantin Infatabs 2624
Dilantin-125 Oral Suspension 2625

Phenytoin Sodium (Co-administration with antiepileptic medications results in decreased seizure threshold). Products include:
Dilantin Kapseals 2622

Primidone (Co-administration with antiepileptic medications results in decreased seizure threshold).
No products indexed under this heading.

Tiagabine Hydrochloride (Co-administration with antiepileptic medications results in decreased seizure threshold). Products include:
Gabitril Tablets 1189

Topiramate (Co-administration with antiepileptic medications results in decreased seizure threshold). Products include:
Topamax Sprinkle Capsules 2590
Topamax Tablets 2590

Trimethadione (Co-administration with antiepileptic medications results in decreased seizure threshold).
No products indexed under this heading.

Valproate Sodium (Co-administration with antiepileptic medications results in decreased seizure threshold). Products include:
Depacon Injection 416

Valproic Acid (Co-administration with antiepileptic medications results in decreased seizure threshold). Products include:
Depakene 421

Zonisamide (Co-administration with antiepileptic medications results in decreased seizure threshold). Products include:
Zonegran Capsules 1307

CYLERT CHEWABLE TABLETS
(Pemoline) 415
See Cylert Tablets

CYTOGAM INTRAVENOUS
(Cytomegalovirus Immune Globulin) 2026
May interact with:

Measles, Mumps & Rubella Virus Vaccine, Live (May interfere with the immune response to live virus vaccine). Products include:
M-M-R II 2118

CYTOMEL TABLETS
(Liothyronine Sodium) 1817
May interact with oral anticoagulants, estrogens, cardiac glycosides, oral hypoglycemic agents, insulin, tricyclic antidepressants, and certain other agents. Compounds in these categories include:

Acarbose (Initiating thyroid replacement therapy may cause increases in oral hypoglycemic requirements). Products include:
Precose Tablets 906

Amitriptyline Hydrochloride (Use of thyroid hormones may increase receptor sensitivity and enhance antidepressant activity; transient cardiac arrhythmias; thyroid hormone activity may also be enhanced). Products include:
Etrafon 3115
Limbitrol 1738

Amoxapine (Use of thyroid hormones may increase receptor sensitivity and enhance antidepressant activity; transient cardiac arrhythmias; thyroid hormone activity may also be enhanced).
No products indexed under this heading.

Chlorotrianisene (Estrogens tend to increase serum thyroxine-binding globulin in a patient with a nonfunctioning thyroid gland who is receiving thyroid replacement therapy; patients without functioning thyroid gland who are on thyroid replacement therapy may need to increase their thyroid dose if estrogens or estrogen-containing oral contraceptives are given).
No products indexed under this heading.

Chlorpropamide (Initiating thyroid replacement therapy may cause increases in oral hypoglycemic requirements). Products include:
Diabinese Tablets 2680

Cholestyramine (Binds both T_4 and T_3 in the intestine thus impairing absorption of thyroid hormones; 4 to 5 hours should elapse between administration of thyroid hormone and cholestyramine).
No products indexed under this heading.

Clomipramine Hydrochloride (Use of thyroid hormones may increase receptor sensitivity and enhance antidepressant activity; transient cardiac arrhythmias; thyroid hormone activity may also be enhanced).
No products indexed under this heading.

Desipramine Hydrochloride (Use of thyroid hormones may increase receptor sensitivity and enhance antidepressant activity; transient cardiac arrhythmias; thyroid hormone activity may also be enhanced). Products include:
Norpramin Tablets 755

Deslanoside (Thyroid preparations may potentiate the toxic effects of digitalis; thyroid hormone increase metabolic rate which requires an increase in digitalis dosage).
No products indexed under this heading.

Dicumarol (Thyroid hormones appear to increase catabolism of vitamin K-dependent clotting factor; if oral anticoagulants are also given compensatory increases in clotting factor synthesis are impaired).
No products indexed under this heading.

Dienestrol (Estrogens tend to increase serum thyroxine-binding globulin in a patient with a nonfunctioning thyroid gland who is receiving thyroid replacement therapy; patients without functioning thyroid gland who are on thyroid replacement therapy may need to increase their thyroid dose if estrogens or estrogen-containing oral contraceptives are given). Products include:
Ortho Dienestrol Cream 2554

Diethylstilbestrol (Estrogens tend to increase serum thyroxine-binding globulin in a patient with a nonfunctioning thyroid gland who is receiving thyroid replacement therapy; patients without functioning thyroid gland who are on thyroid replacement therapy may need to increase their thyroid dose if estrogens or estrogen-containing oral contraceptives are given).
No products indexed under this heading.

Digitoxin (Thyroid preparations may potentiate the toxic effects of digitalis; thyroid hormone increase metabolic rate which requires an increase in digitalis dosage).
No products indexed under this heading.

Digoxin (Thyroid preparations may potentiate the toxic effects of digitalis; thyroid hormone increase metabolic rate which requires an increase in digitalis dosage). Products include:
Digitek Tablets 1003
Lanoxicaps Capsules 1574
Lanoxin Injection 1581
Lanoxin Tablets 1587
Lanoxin Elixir Pediatric 1578
Lanoxin Injection Pediatric 1584

Doxepin Hydrochloride (Use of thyroid hormones may increase receptor sensitivity and enhance antidepressant activity; transient cardiac arrhythmias; thyroid hormone activity may also be enhanced). Products include:
Sinequan 2713

Epinephrine (Thyroxine increases the adrenergic effect of catecholamines, such as epinephrine). Products include:
Epifrin Sterile Ophthalmic Solution ⊙235
EpiPen 1236
Primatene Mist ⊞779
Xylocaine with Epinephrine Injection 653

Epinephrine Bitartrate (Thyroxine increases the adrenergic effect of catecholamines, such as epinephrine). Products include:
Sensorcaine 643

Epinephrine Hydrochloride (Thyroxine increases the adrenergic effect of catecholamines, such as epinephrine).
No products indexed under this heading.

Estradiol (Estrogens tend to increase serum thyroxine-binding globulin in a patient with a nonfunctioning thyroid gland who is receiving thyroid replacement therapy; patients without functioning thyroid gland who are on thyroid replacement therapy may need to increase their thyroid dose if estrogens or estrogen-containing oral contraceptives are given). Products include:
Activella Tablets 2764
Alora Transdermal System 3372
Climara Transdermal System 958
CombiPatch Transdermal System 2323
Esclim Transdermal System 3460
Estrace Vaginal Cream 3358
Estrace Tablets 3361
Estring Vaginal Ring 2811
Ortho-Prefest Tablets 2570
Vagifem Tablets 2857
Vivelle Transdermal System 2412
Vivelle-Dot Transdermal System 2416

Estrogens, Conjugated (Estrogens tend to increase serum thyroxine-binding globulin in a patient with a nonfunctioning thyroid gland who is receiving thyroid replacement therapy; patients without functioning thyroid gland who are on thyroid replacement therapy may need to increase their thyroid dose if estrogens or estrogen-containing oral contraceptives are given). Products include:
Premarin Intravenous 3563
Premarin Tablets 3566
Premarin Vaginal Cream 3570
Premphase Tablets 3572
Prempro Tablets 3572

Estrogens, Esterified (Estrogens tend to increase serum thyroxine-binding globulin in a patient with a nonfunctioning thyroid gland who is receiving thyroid replacement therapy; patients without functioning thy-

roid gland who are on thyroid replacement therapy may need to increase their thyroid dose if estrogens or estrogen-containing oral contraceptives are given). Products include:

Estratest ... 3252
Menest Tablets ... 2254

Estropipate (Estrogens tend to increase serum thyroxine-binding globulin in a patient with a nonfunctioning thyroid gland who is receiving thyroid replacement therapy; patients without functioning thyroid gland who are on thyroid replacement therapy may need to increase their thyroid dose if estrogens or estrogen-containing oral contraceptives are given). Products include:

Ogen Tablets ... 2846
Ortho-Est Tablets ... 3464

Ethinyl Estradiol (Estrogens tend to increase serum thyroxine-binding globulin in a patient with a nonfunctioning thyroid gland who is receiving thyroid replacement therapy; patients without functioning thyroid gland who are on thyroid replacement therapy may need to increase their thyroid dose if estrogens or estrogen-containing oral contraceptives are given). Products include:

Alesse-21 Tablets ... 3468
Alesse-28 Tablets ... 3473
Brevicon 28-Day Tablets ... 3380
Cyclessa Tablets ... 2450
Desogen Tablets ... 2458
Estinyl Tablets ... 3112
Estrostep ... 2627
femhrt Tablets ... 2635
Levlen ... 962
Levlite 21 Tablets ... 962
Levlite 28 Tablets ... 962
Levora Tablets ... 3389
Loestrin 21 Tablets ... 2642
Loestrin Fe Tablets ... 2642
Lo/Ovral Tablets ... 3532
Lo/Ovral-28 Tablets ... 3538
Low-Ogestrel-28 Tablets ... 3392
Microgestin Fe 1.5/30 Tablets ... 3407
Microgestin Fe 1/20 Tablets ... 3400
Mircette Tablets ... 2470
Modicon ... 2563
Necon ... 3415
Nordette-28 Tablets ... 2257
Norinyl 1 +35 28-Day Tablets ... 3380
Ogestrel 0.5/50-28 Tablets ... 3428
Ortho-Cept 21 Tablets ... 2546
Ortho-Cept 28 Tablets ... 2546
Ortho-Cyclen/Ortho Tri-Cyclen ... 2573
Ortho-Novum ... 2563
Ovcon ... 3364
Ovral Tablets ... 3551
Ovral-28 Tablets ... 3552
Tri-Levlen ... 962
Tri-Norinyl-28 Tablets ... 3433
Triphasil-21 Tablets ... 3600
Triphasil-28 Tablets ... 3605
Trivora Tablets ... 3439
Yasmin 28 Tablets ... 980
Zovia ... 3449

Glimepiride (Initiating thyroid replacement therapy may cause increases in oral hypoglycemic requirements). Products include:

Amaryl Tablets ... 717

Glipizide (Initiating thyroid replacement therapy may cause increases in oral hypoglycemic requirements). Products include:

Glucotrol Tablets ... 2692
Glucotrol XL Extended Release Tablets ... 2693

Glyburide (Initiating thyroid replacement therapy may cause increases in oral hypoglycemic requirements). Products include:

DiaBeta Tablets ... 741
Glucovance Tablets ... 1086

Imipramine Hydrochloride (Use of thyroid hormones may increase receptor sensitivity and enhance antidepressant activity; transient cardiac arrhythmias; thyroid hormone activity may also be enhanced).

No products indexed under this heading.

Imipramine Pamoate (Use of thyroid hormones may increase receptor sensitivity and enhance antidepressant activity; transient cardiac arrhythmias; thyroid hormone activity may also be enhanced).

No products indexed under this heading.

Insulin, Human, Zinc Suspension (Initiating thyroid replacement therapy may cause increases in insulin requirements). Products include:

Humulin L, 100 Units ... 1937
Humulin U, 100 Units ... 1943
Novolin L Human Insulin 10 ml Vials ... 2422

Insulin, Human NPH (Initiating thyroid replacement therapy may cause increases in insulin requirements). Products include:

Humulin N, 100 Units ... 1939
Humulin N NPH Pen ... 1940
Novolin N Human Insulin 10 ml Vials ... 2422
Novolin N PenFill ... 2423
Novolin N Prefilled Syringe Disposable Insulin Delivery System ... 2425

Insulin, Human Regular (Initiating thyroid replacement therapy may cause increases in insulin requirements). Products include:

Humulin R Regular (U-500) ... 1943
Humulin R, 100 Units ... 1941
Novolin R Human Insulin 10 ml Vials ... 2423
Novolin R PenFill ... 2423
Novolin R Prefilled Syringe Disposable Insulin Delivery System ... 2425
Velosulin BR Human Insulin 10 ml Vials ... 2435

Insulin, Human Regular and Human NPH Mixture (Initiating thyroid replacement therapy may cause increases in insulin requirements). Products include:

Humulin 50/50, 100 Units ... 1934
Humulin 70/30, 100 Units ... 1935
Humulin 70/30 Pen ... 1936
Novolin 70/30 Human Insulin 10 ml Vials ... 2421
Novolin 70/30 PenFill ... 2423
Novolin 70/30 Prefilled Disposable Insulin Delivery System ... 2425

Insulin, NPH (Initiating thyroid replacement therapy may cause increases in insulin requirements). Products include:

Iletin II, NPH (Pork), 100 Units ... 1946

Insulin, Regular (Initiating thyroid replacement therapy may cause increases in insulin requirements). Products include:

Iletin II, Regular (Pork), 100 Units ... 1947

Insulin, Zinc Crystals (Initiating thyroid replacement therapy may cause increases in insulin requirements).

No products indexed under this heading.

Insulin, Zinc Suspension (Initiating thyroid replacement therapy may cause increases in insulin requirements). Products include:

Iletin II, Lente (Pork), 100 Units ... 1945

Insulin Aspart, Human Regular (Initiating thyroid replacement therapy may cause increases in insulin requirements).

No products indexed under this heading.

Insulin glargine (Initiating thyroid replacement therapy may cause increases in insulin requirements). Products include:

Lantus Injection ... 742

Insulin Lispro, Human (Initiating thyroid replacement therapy may cause increases in insulin requirements). Products include:

Humalog ... 1926
Humalog Mix 75/25 Pen ... 1928

Insulin Lispro Protamine, Human (Initiating thyroid replacement therapy may cause increases in insulin requirements). Products include:

Humalog Mix 75/25 Pen ... 1928

Ketamine Hydrochloride (Co-administration may cause hypertension and tachycardia).

No products indexed under this heading.

Maprotiline Hydrochloride (Use of thyroid hormones may increase receptor sensitivity and enhance antidepressant activity; transient cardiac arrhythmias; thyroid hormone activity may also be enhanced).

No products indexed under this heading.

Metformin Hydrochloride (Initiating thyroid replacement therapy may cause increases in oral hypoglycemic requirements). Products include:

Glucophage Tablets ... 1080
Glucophage XR Tablets ... 1080
Glucovance Tablets ... 1086

Miglitol (Initiating thyroid replacement therapy may cause increases in oral hypoglycemic requirements). Products include:

Glyset Tablets ... 2821

Norepinephrine Hydrochloride (Thyroxine increases the adrenergic effect of catecholamines, such as norepinephrine).

No products indexed under this heading.

Nortriptyline Hydrochloride (Use of thyroid hormones may increase receptor sensitivity and enhance antidepressant activity; transient cardiac arrhythmias; thyroid hormone activity may also be enhanced).

No products indexed under this heading.

Pioglitazone Hydrochloride (Initiating thyroid replacement therapy may cause increases in oral hypoglycemic requirements). Products include:

Actos Tablets ... 3275

Polyestradiol Phosphate (Estrogens tend to increase serum thyroxine-binding globulin in a patient with a nonfunctioning thyroid gland who is receiving thyroid replacement therapy; patients without functioning thyroid gland who are on thyroid replacement therapy may need to increase their thyroid dose if estrogens or estrogen-containing oral contraceptives are given).

No products indexed under this heading.

Protriptyline Hydrochloride (Use of thyroid hormones may increase receptor sensitivity and enhance antidepressant activity; transient cardiac arrhythmias; thyroid hormone activity may also be enhanced). Products include:

Vivactil Tablets ... 2446
Vivactil Tablets ... 2217

Quinestrol (Estrogens tend to increase serum thyroxine-binding globulin in a patient with a nonfunctioning thyroid gland who is receiving thyroid replacement therapy; patients without functioning thyroid gland who are on thyroid replacement therapy may need to increase their thyroid dose if estrogens or estrogen-containing oral contraceptives are given).

No products indexed under this heading.

Repaglinide (Initiating thyroid replacement therapy may cause increases in oral hypoglycemic requirements). Products include:

Prandin Tablets (0.5, 1, and 2 mg) ... 2432

Rosiglitazone Maleate (Initiating thyroid replacement therapy may cause increases in oral hypoglycemic requirements). Products include:

Avandia Tablets ... 1490

Tolazamide (Initiating thyroid replacement therapy may cause increases in oral hypoglycemic requirements).

No products indexed under this heading.

Tolbutamide (Initiating thyroid replacement therapy may cause increases in oral hypoglycemic requirements).

No products indexed under this heading.

Trimipramine Maleate (Use of thyroid hormones may increase receptor sensitivity and enhance antidepressant activity; transient cardiac arrhythmias; thyroid hormone activity may also be enhanced). Products include:

Surmontil Capsules ... 3595

Troglitazone (Initiating thyroid replacement therapy may cause increases in oral hypoglycemic requirements).

No products indexed under this heading.

Warfarin Sodium (Thyroid hormones appear to increase catabolism of vitamin K-dependent clotting factor; if oral anticoagulants are also given compensatory increases in clotting factor synthesis are impaired). Products include:

Coumadin for Injection ... 1243
Coumadin Tablets ... 1243
Warfarin Sodium Tablets, USP ... 3302

CYTOTEC TABLETS

(Misoprostol) ... 3202

May interact with antacids containing aluminum, calcium and magnesium and certain other agents. Compounds in these categories include:

Aluminum Carbonate (Total availability of misoprostol is reduced by use of concomitant antacid).

No products indexed under this heading.

Aluminum Hydroxide (Total availability of misoprostol is reduced by use of concomitant antacid). Products include:

Amphojel Suspension (Mint Flavor) ... ▣789
Gaviscon Extra Strength Liquid ... ▣751
Gaviscon Extra Strength Tablets ... ▣751
Gaviscon Regular Strength Liquid ... ▣751
Gaviscon Regular Strength Tablets ... ▣750
Maalox Antacid/Anti-Gas Oral Suspension ... ▣673
Maalox Max Maximum Strength Antacid/Anti-Gas Liquid ... 2300
Maalox Regular Strength Antacid/Antigas Liquid ... 2300
Mylanta ... 1813
Vanquish Caplets ... ▣617

Magaldrate (Avoid co-administration with magnesium-containing antacids; total availability of misoprostol is reduced by use of concomitant antacid).

No products indexed under this heading.

Magnesium Carbonate (Avoid co-administration with magnesium-containing antacids). Products include:

Gaviscon Extra Strength Liquid ... ▣751
Gaviscon Extra Strength Tablets ... ▣751
Gaviscon Regular Strength Liquid ... ▣751
Marblen Suspension ... ▣633
One-A-Day Calcium Plus Chewable Tablets ... ▣805

Magnesium Hydroxide (Avoid co-administration with magnesium-containing antacids; total availability of misoprostol is reduced by use of concomitant antacid). Products include:

Ex•Lax Milk of Magnesia Liquid ... ▣670
Maalox Antacid/Anti-Gas Oral Suspension ... ▣673

Maalox Max Maximum Strength Antacid/Anti-Gas Liquid ... 2300
Maalox Regular Strength Antacid/Antigas Liquid ... 2300
Mylanta Fast-Acting ... 1813
Mylanta ... 1813
Pepcid Complete Chewable Tablets ... 1815
Phillips' Chewable Tablets ... 615
Phillips' Milk of Magnesia Liquid (Original, Cherry, & Mint) ... 616
Rolaids Tablets ... 706
Extra Strength Rolaids Tablets ... 706
Vanquish Caplets ... 617

Magnesium Oxide (Total availability of misoprostol is reduced by use of concomitant antacid). Products include:
Beelith Tablets ... 946
Mag-Ox 400 Tablets ... 1024
Uro-Mag Capsules ... 1024

Food Interactions

Food, unspecified (Diminishes maximum plasma concentrations).

CYTOVENE CAPSULES

(Ganciclovir) ... 2959

May interact with nucleoside analogues, drugs inhibiting replication of cell populations of bone marrow, spermatogonia, and germinal layers, and certain other agents. Compounds in these categories include:

Acyclovir (Potential for additive toxicity). Products include:
Zovirax ... 1706
Zovirax Ointment ... 1707

Acyclovir Sodium (Potential for additive toxicity). Products include:
Zovirax for Injection ... 1708

Amphotericin B (Potential for additive toxicity; increases in serum creatinine and may result in increased nephrotoxicity). Products include:
Abelcet Injection ... 1273
AmBisome for Injection ... 1383
Amphotec ... 1774

Cilastatin Sodium (Co-administration results in generalized seizures). Products include:
Primaxin I.M. ... 2158
Primaxin I.V. ... 2160

Cyclosporine (Increases in serum creatinine and may result in increased nephrotoxicity). Products include:
Gengraf Capsules ... 457
Neoral Soft Gelatin Capsules ... 2380
Neoral Oral Solution ... 2380
Sandimmune ... 2388

Dapsone (Potential for additive toxicity). Products include:
Dapsone Tablets USP ... 1780

Didanosine (When administered concurrently or 2 hours prior to oral Cytovene, the steady-state didanosine AUC 0-12 increased 111 ±114%; a decrease in ganciclovir steady-state AUC of 21 ±17%). Products include:
Videx ... 1138
Videx EC Capsules ... 1143

Doxorubicin Hydrochloride (Potential for additive toxicity). Products include:
Adriamycin PFS/RDF Injection ... 2767
Doxil Injection ... 566

Flucytosine (Potential for additive toxicity). Products include:
Ancobon Capsules ... 1730

Imipenem (Co-administration results in generalized seizures). Products include:
Primaxin I.M. ... 2158
Primaxin I.V. ... 2160

Pentamidine Isethionate (Potential for additive toxicity).
No products indexed under this heading.

Probenecid (Increases AUC 0-8 53 ±91%, decreases renal clearance 22 ±20%).
No products indexed under this heading.

Sulfamethoxazole (Potential for additive toxicity). Products include:
Bactrim ... 2949
Septra Suspension ... 2265
Septra Tablets ... 2265
Septra DS Tablets ... 2265

Trimethoprim (Potential for additive toxicity). Products include:
Bactrim ... 2949
Septra Suspension ... 2265
Septra Tablets ... 2265
Septra DS Tablets ... 2265

Vinblastine Sulfate (Potential for additive toxicity).
No products indexed under this heading.

Vincristine Sulfate (Potential for additive toxicity).
No products indexed under this heading.

Zidovudine (Man steady-state ganciclovir AUC 0-8 decreases 17 ±25% in presence of zidovudine; steady-state zidovudine AUC 0-4 increases 19 ±27%; both have potential to cause anemia and neutropenia). Products include:
Combivir Tablets ... 1502
Retrovir ... 1625
Retrovir IV Infusion ... 1629
Trizivir Tablets ... 1669

Food Interactions

Meal, unspecified (Meal containing 46.5% fat increases the steady-state AUC of oral Cytovene by 22% ±22% and significant prolongation of time Tmax and a higher Cmax; patients should take Cytovene Capsules with food to maximize bioavailability).

CYTOVENE-IV

(Ganciclovir Sodium) ... 2959
See Cytovene Capsules

DANTRIUM CAPSULES

(Dantrolene Sodium) ... 2885

May interact with calcium channel blockers, central nervous system depressants, estrogens, hypnotics and sedatives, tranquilizers, and certain other agents. Compounds in these categories include:

Alfentanil Hydrochloride (Co-administration may result in increased drowsiness; caution should be exercised).
No products indexed under this heading.

Alprazolam (Co-administration may result in increased drowsiness; caution should be exercised). Products include:
Xanax Tablets ... 2865

Amlodipine Besylate (Due to interaction between verapamil and dantrolene, combination of dantrolene and calcium channel blockers is not recommended during the management of malignant hyperthermia). Products include:
Lotrel Capsules ... 2370
Norvasc Tablets ... 2704

Aprobarbital (Co-administration may result in increased drowsiness; caution should be exercised).
No products indexed under this heading.

Bepridil Hydrochloride (Due to interaction between verapamil and dantrolene, combination of dantrolene and calcium channel blockers is not recommended during the management of malignant hyperthermia). Products include:
Vascor Tablets ... 2602

Buprenorphine Hydrochloride (Co-administration may result in increased drowsiness; caution should be exercised). Products include:
Buprenex Injectable ... 2918

Buspirone Hydrochloride (Co-administration may result in increased drowsiness; caution should be exercised).
No products indexed under this heading.

Butabarbital (Co-administration may result in increased drowsiness; caution should be exercised).
No products indexed under this heading.

Butalbital (Co-administration may result in increased drowsiness; caution should be exercised). Products include:
Phrenilin ... 578
Sedapap Tablets 50 mg/650 mg ... 2225

Chlordiazepoxide (Co-administration may result in increased drowsiness; caution should be exercised). Products include:
Limbitrol ... 1738

Chlordiazepoxide Hydrochloride (Co-administration may result in increased drowsiness; caution should be exercised). Products include:
Librium Capsules ... 1736
Librium for Injection ... 1737

Chlorotrianisene (Hepatotoxicity has occurred more often in women over 35 years of age receiving concomitant estrogen therapy).
No products indexed under this heading.

Chlorpromazine (Co-administration may result in increased drowsiness; caution should be exercised). Products include:
Thorazine Suppositories ... 1656

Chlorpromazine Hydrochloride (Co-administration may result in increased drowsiness; caution should be exercised). Products include:
Thorazine ... 1656

Chlorprothixene (Co-administration may result in increased drowsiness; caution should be exercised).
No products indexed under this heading.

Chlorprothixene Hydrochloride (Co-administration may result in increased drowsiness; caution should be exercised).
No products indexed under this heading.

Chlorprothixene Lactate (Co-administration may result in increased drowsiness; caution should be exercised).
No products indexed under this heading.

Clorazepate Dipotassium (Co-administration may result in increased drowsiness; caution should be exercised). Products include:
Tranxene ... 511

Clozapine (Co-administration may result in increased drowsiness; caution should be exercised). Products include:
Clozaril Tablets ... 2319

Codeine Phosphate (Co-administration may result in increased drowsiness; caution should be exercised). Products include:
Phenergan with Codeine Syrup ... 3557
Phenergan VC with Codeine Syrup ... 3561
Robitussin A-C Syrup ... 2942
Robitussin-DAC Syrup ... 2942
Ryna-C Liquid ... 768
Soma Compound w/Codeine Tablets ... 3355
Tussi-Organidin NR Liquid ... 3350
Tussi-Organidin-S NR Liquid ... 3350
Tylenol with Codeine ... 2595

Desflurane (Co-administration may result in increased drowsiness; caution should be exercised). Products include:
Suprane Liquid for Inhalation ... 874

Dezocine (Co-administration may result in increased drowsiness; caution should be exercised).
No products indexed under this heading.

Diazepam (Co-administration may result in increased drowsiness; caution should be exercised). Products include:
Valium Injectable ... 3026
Valium Tablets ... 3047

Dienestrol (Hepatotoxicity has occurred more often in women over 35 years of age receiving concomitant estrogen therapy). Products include:
Ortho Dienestrol Cream ... 2554

Diethylstilbestrol (Hepatotoxicity has occurred more often in women over 35 years of age receiving concomitant estrogen therapy).
No products indexed under this heading.

Diltiazem Hydrochloride (Due to interaction between verapamil and dantrolene, combination of dantrolene and calcium channel blockers is not recommended during the management of malignant hyperthermia). Products include:
Cardizem Injectable ... 1018
Cardizem Lyo-Ject Syringe ... 1018
Cardizem Monovial ... 1018
Cardizem CD Capsules ... 1016
Tiazac Capsules ... 1378

Droperidol (Co-administration may result in increased drowsiness; caution should be exercised).
No products indexed under this heading.

Enflurane (Co-administration may result in increased drowsiness; caution should be exercised).
No products indexed under this heading.

Estazolam (Co-administration may result in increased drowsiness; caution should be exercised). Products include:
ProSom Tablets ... 500

Estradiol (Hepatotoxicity has occurred more often in women over 35 years of age receiving concomitant estrogen therapy). Products include:
Activella Tablets ... 2764
Alora Transdermal System ... 3372
Climara Transdermal System ... 958
CombiPatch Transdermal System ... 2323
Esclim Transdermal System ... 3460
Estrace Vaginal Cream ... 3358
Estrace Tablets ... 3361
Estring Vaginal Ring ... 2811
Ortho-Prefest Tablets ... 2570
Vagifem Tablets ... 2857
Vivelle Transdermal System ... 2412
Vivelle-Dot Transdermal System ... 2416

Estrogens, Conjugated (Hepatotoxicity has occurred more often in women over 35 years of age receiving concomitant estrogen therapy). Products include:
Premarin Intravenous ... 3563
Premarin Tablets ... 3566
Premarin Vaginal Cream ... 3570
Premphase Tablets ... 3572
Prempro Tablets ... 3572

Estrogens, Esterified (Hepatotoxicity has occurred more often in women over 35 years of age receiving concomitant estrogen therapy). Products include:
Estratest ... 3252
Menest Tablets ... 2254

Estropipate (Hepatotoxicity has occurred more often in women over 35 years of age receiving concomitant estrogen therapy). Products include:
Ogen Tablets ... 2846
Ortho-Est Tablets ... 3464

Ethchlorvynol (Co-administration may result in increased drowsiness; caution should be exercised).
No products indexed under this heading.

Ethinamate (Co-administration may result in increased drowsiness; cau-

tion should be exercised).
No products indexed under this heading.

Ethinyl Estradiol (Hepatotoxicity has occurred more often in women over 35 years of age receiving concomitant estrogen therapy). Products include:
Alesse-21 Tablets 3468
Alesse-28 Tablets 3473
Brevicon 28-Day Tablets 3380
Cyclessa Tablets 2450
Desogen Tablets 2458
Estinyl Tablets 3112
Estrostep 2627
femhrt Tablets 2635
Levlen 962
Levlite 21 Tablets 962
Levlite 28 Tablets 962
Levora Tablets 3389
Loestrin 21 Tablets 2642
Loestrin Fe Tablets 2642
Lo/Ovral Tablets 3532
Lo/Ovral-28 Tablets 3538
Low-Ogestrel-28 Tablets 3392
Microgestin Fe 1.5/30 Tablets 3407
Microgestin Fe 1/20 Tablets 3400
Mircette Tablets 2470
Modicon 2563
Necon 3415
Nordette-28 Tablets 2257
Norinyl 1 +35 28-Day Tablets 3380
Ogestrel 0.5/50-28 Tablets 3428
Ortho-Cept 21 Tablets 2546
Ortho-Cept 28 Tablets 2546
Ortho-Cyclen/Ortho Tri-Cyclen 2573
Ortho-Novum 2563
Ovcon 3364
Ovral Tablets 3551
Ovral-28 Tablets 3552
Tri-Levlen 962
Tri-Norinyl-28 Tablets 3433
Triphasil-21 Tablets 3600
Triphasil-28 Tablets 3605
Trivora Tablets 3439
Yasmin 28 Tablets 980
Zovia 3449

Felodipine (Due to interaction between verapamil and dantrolene, combination of dantrolene and calcium channel blockers is not recommended during the management of malignant hyperthermia). Products include:
Lexxel Tablets 608
Plendil Extended-Release Tablets 623

Fentanyl (Co-administration may result in increased drowsiness; caution should be exercised). Products include:
Duragesic Transdermal System 1786

Fentanyl Citrate (Co-administration may result in increased drowsiness; caution should be exercised). Products include:
Actiq 1184

Fluphenazine Decanoate (Co-administration may result in increased drowsiness; caution should be exercised).
No products indexed under this heading.

Fluphenazine Enanthate (Co-administration may result in increased drowsiness; caution should be exercised).
No products indexed under this heading.

Fluphenazine Hydrochloride (Co-administration may result in increased drowsiness; caution should be exercised).
No products indexed under this heading.

Flurazepam Hydrochloride (Co-administration may result in increased drowsiness; caution should be exercised).
No products indexed under this heading.

Glutethimide (Co-administration may result in increased drowsiness; caution should be exercised).
No products indexed under this heading.

Haloperidol (Co-administration may result in increased drowsiness; caution should be exercised). Products include:
Haldol Injection, Tablets and Concentrate 2533

Haloperidol Decanoate (Co-administration may result in increased drowsiness; caution should be exercised). Products include:
Haldol Decanoate 2535

Hydrocodone Bitartrate (Co-administration may result in increased drowsiness; caution should be exercised). Products include:
Hycodan 1316
Hycomine Compound Tablets 1317
Hycotuss Expectorant Syrup 1318
Lortab 3319
Lortab Elixir 3317
Maxidone Tablets CIII 3399
Norco 5/325 Tablets CIII 3424
Norco 7.5/325 Tablets CIII 3425
Norco 10/325 Tablets CIII 3427
Norco 10/325 Tablets CIII 3425
Vicodin Tablets 516
Vicodin ES Tablets 517
Vicodin HP Tablets 518
Vicodin Tuss Expectorant 519
Vicoprofen Tablets 520
Zydone Tablets 1330

Hydrocodone Polistirex (Co-administration may result in increased drowsiness; caution should be exercised). Products include:
Tussionex Pennkinetic Extended-Release Suspension 1174

Hydromorphone Hydrochloride (Co-administration may result in increased drowsiness; caution should be exercised). Products include:
Dilaudid 441
Dilaudid Oral Liquid 445
Dilaudid Powder 441
Dilaudid Rectal Suppositories 441
Dilaudid Tablets 441
Dilaudid Tablets - 8 mg 445
Dilaudid-HP 443

Hydroxyzine Hydrochloride (Co-administration may result in increased drowsiness; caution should be exercised). Products include:
Atarax Tablets & Syrup 2667
Vistaril Intramuscular Solution 2738

Isoflurane (Co-administration may result in increased drowsiness; caution should be exercised).
No products indexed under this heading.

Isradipine (Due to interaction between verapamil and dantrolene, combination of dantrolene and calcium channel blockers is not recommended during the management of malignant hyperthermia). Products include:
DynaCirc Capsules 2921
DynaCirc CR Tablets 2923

Ketamine Hydrochloride (Co-administration may result in increased drowsiness; caution should be exercised).
No products indexed under this heading.

Levomethadyl Acetate Hydrochloride (Co-administration may result in increased drowsiness; caution should be exercised).
No products indexed under this heading.

Levorphanol Tartrate (Co-administration may result in increased drowsiness; caution should be exercised). Products include:
Levo-Dromoran 1734
Levorphanol Tartrate Tablets 3059

Lorazepam (Co-administration may result in increased drowsiness; caution should be exercised). Products include:
Ativan Injection 3478
Ativan Tablets 3482

Loxapine Hydrochloride (Co-administration may result in increased drowsiness; caution should be exercised).
No products indexed under this heading.

Loxapine Succinate (Co-administration may result in increased drowsiness; caution should be exercised). Products include:
Loxitane Capsules 3398

Meperidine Hydrochloride (Co-administration may result in increased drowsiness; caution should be exercised). Products include:
Demerol 3079
Mepergan Injection 3539

Mephobarbital (Co-administration may result in increased drowsiness; caution should be exercised).
No products indexed under this heading.

Meprobamate (Co-administration may result in increased drowsiness; caution should be exercised). Products include:
Miltown Tablets 3349

Mesoridazine Besylate (Co-administration may result in increased drowsiness; caution should be exercised). Products include:
Serentil 1057

Methadone Hydrochloride (Co-administration may result in increased drowsiness; caution should be exercised). Products include:
Dolophine Hydrochloride Tablets 3056

Methohexital Sodium (Co-administration may result in increased drowsiness; caution should be exercised). Products include:
Brevital Sodium for Injection, USP 1815

Methotrimeprazine (Co-administration may result in increased drowsiness; caution should be exercised).
No products indexed under this heading.

Methoxyflurane (Co-administration may result in increased drowsiness; caution should be exercised).
No products indexed under this heading.

Mibefradil Dihydrochloride (Due to interaction between verapamil and dantrolene, combination of dantrolene and calcium channel blockers is not recommended during the management of malignant hyperthermia).
No products indexed under this heading.

Midazolam Hydrochloride (Co-administration may result in increased drowsiness; caution should be exercised). Products include:
Versed Injection 3027
Versed Syrup 3033

Molindone Hydrochloride (Co-administration may result in increased drowsiness; caution should be exercised). Products include:
Moban 1320

Morphine Sulfate (Co-administration may result in increased drowsiness; caution should be exercised). Products include:
Astramorph/PF Injection, USP (Preservative-Free) 594
Duramorph Injection 1312
Infumorph 200 and Infumorph 500 Sterile Solutions 1314
Kadian Capsules 1335
MS Contin Tablets 2896
MSIR 2898
Oramorph SR Tablets 3062
Roxanol 3066

Nicardipine Hydrochloride (Due to interaction between verapamil and dantrolene, combination of dantrolene and calcium channel blockers is not recommended during the management of malignant hyperthermia). Products include:
Cardene I.V. 3485

Nifedipine (Due to interaction between verapamil and dantrolene, combination of dantrolene and calcium channel blockers is not recommended during the management of malignant hyperthermia). Products include:
Adalat CC Tablets 877
Procardia Capsules 2708
Procardia XL Extended Release Tablets 2710

Nimodipine (Due to interaction between verapamil and dantrolene, combination of dantrolene and calcium channel blockers is not recommended during the management of malignant hyperthermia). Products include:
Nimotop Capsules 904

Nisoldipine (Due to interaction between verapamil and dantrolene, combination of dantrolene and calcium channel blockers is not recommended during the management of malignant hyperthermia). Products include:
Sular Tablets 688

Olanzapine (Co-administration may result in increased drowsiness; caution should be exercised). Products include:
Zyprexa Tablets 1973
Zyprexa ZYDIS Orally Disintegrating Tablets 1973

Oxazepam (Co-administration may result in increased drowsiness; caution should be exercised).
No products indexed under this heading.

Oxycodone Hydrochloride (Co-administration may result in increased drowsiness; caution should be exercised). Products include:
OxyContin Tablets 2912
OxyFast Oral Concentrate Solution 2916
OxyIR Capsules 2916
Percocet Tablets 1326
Percodan Tablets 1327
Percolone Tablets 1327
Roxicodone 3067
Tylox Capsules 2597

Pentobarbital Sodium (Co-administration may result in increased drowsiness; caution should be exercised). Products include:
Nembutal Sodium Solution 485

Perphenazine (Co-administration may result in increased drowsiness; caution should be exercised). Products include:
Etrafon 3115
Trilafon 3160

Phenobarbital (Co-administration may result in increased drowsiness; caution should be exercised). Products include:
Arco-Lase Plus Tablets 592
Donnatal 2929
Donnatal Extentabs 2930

Polyestradiol Phosphate (Hepatotoxicity has occurred more often in women over 35 years of age receiving concomitant estrogen therapy).
No products indexed under this heading.

Prazepam (Co-administration may result in increased drowsiness; caution should be exercised).
No products indexed under this heading.

Prochlorperazine (Co-administration may result in increased drowsiness; caution should be exercised). Products include:
Compazine 1505

Promethazine Hydrochloride (Co-administration may result in increased drowsiness; caution should be exercised). Products include:

- Mepergan Injection 3539
- Phenergan Injection 3553
- Phenergan 3556
- Phenergan Syrup 3554
- Phenergan with Codeine Syrup 3557
- Phenergan with Dextromethorphan Syrup 3559
- Phenergan VC Syrup 3560
- Phenergan VC with Codeine Syrup .. 3561

Propofol (Co-administration may result in increased drowsiness; caution should be exercised). Products include:

- Diprivan Injectable Emulsion 667

Propoxyphene Hydrochloride (Co-administration may result in increased drowsiness; caution should be exercised). Products include:

- Darvon Pulvules 1909
- Darvon Compound-65 Pulvules 1910

Propoxyphene Napsylate (Co-administration may result in increased drowsiness; caution should be exercised). Products include:

- Darvon-N/Darvocet-N 1907
- Darvon-N Tablets 1912

Quazepam (Co-administration may result in increased drowsiness; caution should be exercised).

No products indexed under this heading.

Quetiapine Fumarate (Co-administration may result in increased drowsiness; caution should be exercised). Products include:

- Seroquel Tablets 684

Quinestrol (Hepatotoxicity has occurred more often in women over 35 years of age receiving concomitant estrogen therapy).

No products indexed under this heading.

Remifentanil Hydrochloride (Co-administration may result in increased drowsiness; caution should be exercised).

No products indexed under this heading.

Risperidone (Co-administration may result in increased drowsiness; caution should be exercised). Products include:

- Risperdal 1796

Secobarbital Sodium (Co-administration may result in increased drowsiness; caution should be exercised).

No products indexed under this heading.

Sevoflurane (Co-administration may result in increased drowsiness; caution should be exercised).

No products indexed under this heading.

Sufentanil Citrate (Co-administration may result in increased drowsiness; caution should be exercised).

No products indexed under this heading.

Temazepam (Co-administration may result in increased drowsiness; caution should be exercised).

No products indexed under this heading.

Thiamylal Sodium (Co-administration may result in increased drowsiness; caution should be exercised).

No products indexed under this heading.

Thioridazine Hydrochloride (Co-administration may result in increased drowsiness; caution should be exercised). Products include:

- Thioridazine Hydrochloride Tablets 2289

Thiothixene (Co-administration may result in increased drowsiness; caution should be exercised). Products include:

- Navane Capsules 2701
- Thiothixene Capsules 2290

Triazolam (Co-administration may result in increased drowsiness; caution should be exercised). Products include:

- Halcion Tablets 2823

Trifluoperazine Hydrochloride (Co-administration may result in increased drowsiness; caution should be exercised). Products include:

- Stelazine 1640

Vecuronium Bromide (Co-administration may result in potentiation of vecuronium-induced neuromuscular block). Products include:

- Norcuron for Injection 2478

Verapamil Hydrochloride (Simultaneous use has resulted in rare cases of cardiovascular collapse). Products include:

- Covera-HS Tablets 3199
- Isoptin SR Tablets 467
- Tarka Tablets 508
- Verelan Capsules 3184
- Verelan PM Capsules 3186

Zaleplon (Co-administration may result in increased drowsiness; caution should be exercised). Products include:

- Sonata Capsules 3591

Ziprasidone Hydrochloride (Co-administration may result in increased drowsiness; caution should be exercised). Products include:

- Geodon Capsules 2688

Zolpidem Tartrate (Co-administration may result in increased drowsiness; caution should be exercised). Products include:

- Ambien Tablets 3191

Food Interactions

Alcohol (Co-administration may result in increased drowsiness; caution should be exercised).

DANTRIUM INTRAVENOUS

(Dantrolene Sodium) 2886
May interact with:

Clofibrate (Reduces binding of dantrolene to plasma proteins). Products include:

- Atromid-S Capsules 3483

Tolbutamide (Increases binding of dantrolene to plasma proteins).

No products indexed under this heading.

Vecuronium Bromide (Administration of dantrolene may potentiate vecuronium-induced neuromuscular block). Products include:

- Norcuron for Injection 2478

Verapamil Hydrochloride (The combination of therapeutic doses of intravenous dantrolene sodium and verapamil in halothane/alpha-chloralose anesthetized swine has resulted in ventricular fibrillation and cardiovascular collapse in association with hyperkalemia; it is recommended that this combination should not be used during the management of malignant hyperthermia crisis until the human data is available). Products include:

- Covera-HS Tablets 3199
- Isoptin SR Tablets 467
- Tarka Tablets 508
- Verelan Capsules 3184
- Verelan PM Capsules 3186

Warfarin Sodium (Reduces binding of dantrolene to plasma proteins). Products include:

- Coumadin for Injection 1243
- Coumadin Tablets 1243
- Warfarin Sodium Tablets, USP 3302

DAPSONE TABLETS USP

(Dapsone) 1780
May interact with:

Pyrimethamine (Agranulocytosis; increased likelihood of hematological reactions). Products include:

- Daraprim Tablets 1511

Rifampin (Lowered Dapsone levels). Products include:

- Rifadin 765
- Rifamate Capsules 767
- Rifater Tablets 769

Trimethoprim (Mutual interaction between Dapsone and trimethoprim in which each raises the level of the other about 1.5 times). Products include:

- Bactrim 2949
- Septra Suspension 2265
- Septra Tablets 2265
- Septra DS Tablets 2265

DARANIDE TABLETS

(Dichlorphenamide) 2077
May interact with corticosteroids and certain other agents. Compounds in these categories include:

ACTH (Hypokalemia may develop).

No products indexed under this heading.

Aspirin (Concomitant high-dose aspirin may produce anorexia, tachypnea, lethargy and coma). Products include:

- Aggrenox Capsules 1026
- Alka-Seltzer .... ⊞603
- Alka-Seltzer Lemon Lime Antacid and Pain Reliever Effervescent Tablets .... ⊞603
- Alka-Seltzer Extra Strength Antacid and Pain Reliever Effervescent Tablets .... ⊞603
- Alka-Seltzer PM Effervescent Tablets .... ⊞605
- Genuine Bayer Tablets, Caplets and Gelcaps .... ⊞606
- Extra Strength Bayer Caplets and Gelcaps .... ⊞610
- Aspirin Regimen Bayer Children's Chewable Tablets (Orange or Cherry Flavored) .... ⊞607
- Bayer, Aspirin Regimen .... ⊞606
- Aspirin Regimen Bayer 81 mg Caplets with Calcium .... ⊞607
- Genuine Bayer Professional Labeling (Aspirin Regimen Bayer) .... ⊞608
- Extra Strength Bayer Arthritis Caplets .... ⊞610
- Extra Strength Bayer Plus Caplets .... ⊞610
- Extra Strength Bayer PM Caplets .. ⊞611
- BC Powder .... ⊞619
- BC Allergy Sinus Cold Powder .... ⊞619
- Arthritis Strength BC Powder .... ⊞619
- BC Sinus Cold Powder .... ⊞619
- Darvon Compound-65 Pulvules 1910
- Ecotrin Enteric Coated Aspirin Low, Regular and Maximum Strength Tablets 1715
- Excedrin Extra-Strength Tablets, Caplets, and Geltabs .... ⊞629
- Excedrin Migraine 1070
- Goody's Body Pain Formula Powder .... ⊞620
- Goody's Extra Strength Headache Powder .... ⊞620
- Goody's Extra Strength Pain Relief Tablets .... ⊞620
- Percodan Tablets 1327
- Robaxisal Tablets 2939
- Soma Compound Tablets 3354
- Soma Compound w/Codeine Tablets 3355
- Vanquish Caplets .... ⊞617

Aspirin, Enteric Coated (Concomitant high-dose aspirin may produce anorexia, tachypnea, lethargy and coma).

No products indexed under this heading.

Betamethasone Acetate (Hypokalemia may develop). Products include:

- Celestone Soluspan Injectable Suspension 3097

Betamethasone Sodium Phosphate (Hypokalemia may develop). Products include:

- Celestone Soluspan Injectable Suspension 3097

Cortisone Acetate (Hypokalemia may develop). Products include:

- Cortone Acetate Injectable Suspension 2059
- Cortone Acetate Tablets 2061

Dexamethasone (Hypokalemia may develop). Products include:

- Decadron Elixir 2078
- Decadron Tablets 2079
- TobraDex Ophthalmic Ointment 542
- TobraDex Ophthalmic Suspension .. 541

Dexamethasone Acetate (Hypokalemia may develop).

No products indexed under this heading.

Dexamethasone Sodium Phosphate (Hypokalemia may develop). Products include:

- Decadron Phosphate Injection 2081
- Decadron Phosphate Sterile Ophthalmic Ointment 2083
- Decadron Phosphate Sterile Ophthalmic Solution 2084
- NeoDecadron Sterile Ophthalmic Solution 2144

Fludrocortisone Acetate (Hypokalemia may develop). Products include:

- Florinef Acetate Tablets 2250

Hydrocortisone (Hypokalemia may develop). Products include:

- Anusol-HC Cream 2.5% 2237
- Cipro HC Otic Suspension 540
- Cortaid Intensive Therapy Cream .. ⊞717
- Cortaid Maximum Strength Cream .... ⊞717
- Cortisporin Ophthalmic Suspension Sterile .... ⊙297
- Cortizone•5 .... ⊞699
- Cortizone•10 .... ⊞699
- Cortizone•10 Plus Creme .... ⊞700
- Cortizone for Kids Creme .... ⊞699
- Hydrocortone Tablets 2106
- Massengill Medicated Soft Cloth Towelette .... ⊞753
- VōSoL HC Otic Solution 3356

Hydrocortisone Acetate (Hypokalemia may develop). Products include:

- Analpram-HC 1338
- Anusol HC-1 Hydrocortisone Anti-Itch Cream .... ⊞689
- Anusol-HC Suppositories 2238
- Cortaid .... ⊞717
- Cortifoam Rectal Foam 3170
- Cortisporin-TC Otic Suspension 2246
- Hydrocortone Acetate Injectable Suspension 2103
- Pramosone 1343
- Proctocort Suppositories 2264
- ProctoFoam-HC 3177
- Terra-Cortril Ophthalmic Suspension 2716

Hydrocortisone Sodium Phosphate (Hypokalemia may develop). Products include:

- Hydrocortone Phosphate Injection, Sterile 2105

Hydrocortisone Sodium Succinate (Hypokalemia may develop).

No products indexed under this heading.

Methylprednisolone Acetate (Hypokalemia may develop). Products include:

- Depo-Medrol Injectable Suspension 2795

Methylprednisolone Sodium Succinate (Hypokalemia may develop). Products include:

- Solu-Medrol Sterile Powder 2855

Prednisolone Acetate (Hypokalemia may develop). Products include:

- Blephamide Ophthalmic Ointment 547
- Blephamide Ophthalmic Suspension 548
- Poly-Pred Liquifilm Ophthalmic Suspension .... ⊙245
- Pred Forte Ophthalmic Suspension .... ⊙246
- Pred Mild Sterile Ophthalmic Suspension .... ⊙249
- Pred-G Ophthalmic Suspension .... ⊙247
- Pred-G Sterile Ophthalmic Ointment .... ⊙248

Prednisolone Sodium Phosphate (Hypokalemia may develop). Products include:
Pediapred Oral Solution 1170

Prednisolone Tebutate (Hypokalemia may develop).
No products indexed under this heading.

Prednisone (Hypokalemia may develop). Products include:
Prednisone 3064

Triamcinolone (Hypokalemia may develop).
No products indexed under this heading.

Triamcinolone Acetonide (Hypokalemia may develop). Products include:
Azmacort Inhalation Aerosol 728
Nasacort Nasal Inhaler 750
Nasacort AQ Nasal Spray 752
Tri-Nasal Spray 2274

Triamcinolone Diacetate (Hypokalemia may develop).
No products indexed under this heading.

Triamcinolone Hexacetonide (Hypokalemia may develop).
No products indexed under this heading.

DARAPRIM TABLETS

(Pyrimethamine) 1511

May interact with phenytoin and certain other agents. Compounds in these categories include:

Fosphenytoin Sodium (Co-administration with agents that affect folate levels, such as phenytoin, should be undertaken with caution). Products include:
Cerebyx Injection 2619

Lorazepam (Concomitant therapy may result in mild hepatotoxicity). Products include:
Ativan Injection 3478
Ativan Tablets 3482

Phenytoin (Co-administration with agents that affect folate levels, such as phenytoin, should be undertaken with caution). Products include:
Dilantin Infatabs 2624
Dilantin-125 Oral Suspension 2625

Phenytoin Sodium (Co-administration with agents that affect folate levels, such as phenytoin, should be undertaken with caution). Products include:
Dilantin Kapseals 2622

Sulfadoxine (Co-administration of other antifolinic drugs, such as sulfonamides, may increase the risk of bone marrow suppression; potential for hypersensitivity reactions such as Stevens-Johnson syndrome, toxic epidermal necrolysis, erythema multiforme, and anaphylaxis).
No products indexed under this heading.

Sulfamethoxazole (Co-administration of other antifolinic drugs, such as sulfonamides or trimethoprim-sulfamethoxazole combinations, may increase the risk of bone marrow suppression; potential for hypersensitivity reactions such as Stevens-Johnson syndrome, toxic epidermalnecrolysis, erythema multiforme, and anaphylaxis). Products include:
Bactrim 2949
Septra Suspension 2265
Septra Tablets 2265
Septra DS Tablets 2265

Sulfisoxazole Acetyl (Co-administration of other antifolinic drugs, such as sulfonamides, may increase the risk of bone marrow suppression; potential for hypersensitivity reactions such as Stevens-Johnson syndrome, toxic epidermal necrolysis, erythema multiforme, and anaphylaxis). Products include:
Pediazole Suspension 3050

DARVOCET-N 50 TABLETS

(Acetaminophen, Propoxyphene Napsylate).. 1907

May interact with central nervous system depressants, oral anticoagulants, anticonvulsants, tricyclic antidepressants, and certain other agents. Compounds in these categories include:

Alfentanil Hydrochloride (Additive CNS depression).
No products indexed under this heading.

Alprazolam (Additive CNS depression). Products include:
Xanax Tablets 2865

Amitriptyline Hydrochloride (Propoxyphene may slow metabolism). Products include:
Etrafon 3115
Limbitrol 1738

Amoxapine (Propoxyphene may slow metabolism).
No products indexed under this heading.

Aprobarbital (Additive CNS depression).
No products indexed under this heading.

Buprenorphine Hydrochloride (Additive CNS depression). Products include:
Buprenex Injectable 2918

Buspirone Hydrochloride (Additive CNS depression).
No products indexed under this heading.

Butabarbital (Additive CNS depression).
No products indexed under this heading.

Butalbital (Additive CNS depression). Products include:
Phrenilin 578
Sedapap Tablets 50 mg/650 mg ... 2225

Carbamazepine (Concurrent use may result in severe neurological signs, including coma). Products include:
Carbatrol Capsules 3234
Tegretol/Tegretol-XR 2404

Chlordiazepoxide (Additive CNS depression). Products include:
Limbitrol 1738

Chlordiazepoxide Hydrochloride (Additive CNS depression). Products include:
Librium Capsules 1736
Librium for Injection 1737

Chlorpromazine (Additive CNS depression). Products include:
Thorazine Suppositories 1656

Chlorpromazine Hydrochloride (Additive CNS depression). Products include:
Thorazine 1656

Chlorprothixene (Additive CNS depression).
No products indexed under this heading.

Chlorprothixene Hydrochloride (Additive CNS depression).
No products indexed under this heading.

Chlorprothixene Lactate (Additive CNS depression).
No products indexed under this heading.

Clomipramine Hydrochloride (Propoxyphene may slow metabolism).
No products indexed under this heading.

Clorazepate Dipotassium (Additive CNS depression). Products include:
Tranxene 511

Clozapine (Additive CNS depression). Products include:
Clozaril Tablets 2319

Codeine Phosphate (Additive CNS depression). Products include:
Phenergan with Codeine Syrup 3557
Phenergan VC with Codeine Syrup .. 3561
Robitussin A-C Syrup 2942
Robitussin-DAC Syrup 2942
Ryna-C Liquid 768
Soma Compound w/Codeine Tablets 3355
Tussi-Organidin NR Liquid 3350
Tussi-Organidin-S NR Liquid 3350
Tylenol with Codeine 2595

Desflurane (Additive CNS depression). Products include:
Suprane Liquid for Inhalation 874

Desipramine Hydrochloride (Propoxyphene may slow metabolism). Products include:
Norpramin Tablets 755

Dezocine (Additive CNS depression).
No products indexed under this heading.

Diazepam (Additive CNS depression). Products include:
Valium Injectable 3026
Valium Tablets 3047

Dicumarol (Propoxyphene may slow metabolism).
No products indexed under this heading.

Divalproex Sodium (Propoxyphene may slow metabolism). Products include:
Depakote Sprinkle Capsules 426
Depakote Tablets 430
Depakote ER Tablets 436

Doxepin Hydrochloride (Propoxyphene may slow metabolism). Products include:
Sinequan 2713

Droperidol (Additive CNS depression).
No products indexed under this heading.

Enflurane (Additive CNS depression).
No products indexed under this heading.

Estazolam (Additive CNS depression). Products include:
ProSom Tablets 500

Ethchlorvynol (Additive CNS depression).
No products indexed under this heading.

Ethinamate (Additive CNS depression).
No products indexed under this heading.

Ethosuximide (Propoxyphene may slow metabolism). Products include:
Zarontin Capsules 2659
Zarontin Syrup 2660

Ethotoin (Propoxyphene may slow metabolism).
No products indexed under this heading.

Felbamate (Concurrent use may result in severe neurological signs, including coma). Products include:
Felbatol 3343

Fentanyl (Additive CNS depression). Products include:
Duragesic Transdermal System 1786

Fentanyl Citrate (Additive CNS depression). Products include:
Actiq 1184

Fluphenazine Decanoate (Additive CNS depression).
No products indexed under this heading.

Fluphenazine Enanthate (Additive CNS depression).
No products indexed under this heading.

Fluphenazine Hydrochloride (Additive CNS depression).
No products indexed under this heading.

Flurazepam Hydrochloride (Additive CNS depression).
No products indexed under this heading.

Fosphenytoin Sodium (Propoxyphene may slow metabolism). Products include:
Cerebyx Injection 2619

Glutethimide (Additive CNS depression).
No products indexed under this heading.

Haloperidol (Additive CNS depression). Products include:
Haldol Injection, Tablets and Concentrate 2533

Haloperidol Decanoate (Additive CNS depression). Products include:
Haldol Decanoate 2535

Hydrocodone Bitartrate (Additive CNS depression). Products include:
Hycodan 1316
Hycomine Compound Tablets 1317
Hycotuss Expectorant Syrup 1318
Lortab 3319
Lortab Elixir 3317
Maxidone Tablets CIII 3399
Norco 5/325 Tablets CIII 3424
Norco 7.5/325 Tablets CIII 3425
Norco 10/325 Tablets CIII 3427
Norco 10/325 Tablets CIII 3425
Vicodin Tablets 516
Vicodin ES Tablets 517
Vicodin HP Tablets 518
Vicodin Tuss Expectorant 519
Vicoprofen Tablets 520
Zydone Tablets 1330

Hydrocodone Polistirex (Additive CNS depression). Products include:
Tussionex Pennkinetic Extended-Release Suspension 1174

Hydromorphone Hydrochloride (Additive CNS depression). Products include:
Dilaudid 441
Dilaudid Oral Liquid 445
Dilaudid Powder 441
Dilaudid Rectal Suppositories 441
Dilaudid Tablets 441
Dilaudid Tablets - 8 mg 445
Dilaudid-HP 443

Hydroxyzine Hydrochloride (Additive CNS depression). Products include:
Atarax Tablets & Syrup 2667
Vistaril Intramuscular Solution 2738

Imipramine Hydrochloride (Propoxyphene may slow metabolism).
No products indexed under this heading.

Imipramine Pamoate (Propoxyphene may slow metabolism).
No products indexed under this heading.

Isoflurane (Additive CNS depression).
No products indexed under this heading.

Ketamine Hydrochloride (Additive CNS depression).
No products indexed under this heading.

Lamotrigine (Propoxyphene may slow the metabolism of anticonvulsants). Products include:
Lamictal 1567

Levetiracetam (Propoxyphene may slow metabolism). Products include:
Keppra Tablets 3314

Levomethadyl Acetate Hydrochloride (Additive CNS depression).
No products indexed under this heading.

Levorphanol Tartrate (Additive CNS depression). Products include:
Levo-Dromoran 1734
Levorphanol Tartrate Tablets 3059

Lorazepam (Additive CNS depression). Products include:
Ativan Injection 3478
Ativan Tablets 3482

Loxapine Hydrochloride (Additive CNS depression).
No products indexed under this heading.

Loxapine Succinate (Additive CNS depression). Products include:
Loxitane Capsules 3398

Maprotiline Hydrochloride (Propoxyphene may slow metabolism).
No products indexed under this heading.

Meperidine Hydrochloride (Additive CNS depression). Products include:
Demerol 3079
Mepergan Injection 3539

Mephenytoin (Propoxyphene may slow metabolism).
No products indexed under this heading.

Mephobarbital (Additive CNS depression).
No products indexed under this heading.

Meprobamate (Additive CNS depression). Products include:
Miltown Tablets 3349

Mesoridazine Besylate (Additive CNS depression). Products include:
Serentil 1057

Methadone Hydrochloride (Additive CNS depression). Products include:
Dolophine Hydrochloride Tablets 3056

Methohexital Sodium (Additive CNS depression). Products include:
Brevital Sodium for Injection, USP .. 1815

Methotrimeprazine (Additive CNS depression).
No products indexed under this heading.

Methoxyflurane (Additive CNS depression).
No products indexed under this heading.

Methsuximide (Propoxyphene may slow metabolism). Products include:
Celontin Capsules 2618

Midazolam Hydrochloride (Additive CNS depression). Products include:
Versed Injection 3027
Versed Syrup 3033

Molindone Hydrochloride (Additive CNS depression). Products include:
Moban 1320

Morphine Sulfate (Additive CNS depression). Products include:
Astramorph/PF Injection, USP (Preservative-Free) 594
Duramorph Injection 1312
Infumorph 200 and Infumorph 500 Sterile Solutions 1314
Kadian Capsules 1335
MS Contin Tablets 2896
MSIR 2898
Oramorph SR Tablets 3062
Roxanol 3066

Nortriptyline Hydrochloride (Propoxyphene may slow metabolism).
No products indexed under this heading.

Olanzapine (Additive CNS depression). Products include:
Zyprexa Tablets 1973
Zyprexa ZYDIS Orally Disintegrating Tablets 1973

Oxazepam (Additive CNS depression).
No products indexed under this heading.

Oxcarbazepine (Propoxyphene may slow metabolism). Products include:
Trileptal Oral Suspension 2407
Trileptal Tablets 2407

Oxycodone Hydrochloride (Additive CNS depression). Products include:
OxyContin Tablets 2912
OxyFast Oral Concentrate Solution 2916
OxyIR Capsules 2916
Percocet Tablets 1326
Percodan Tablets 1327
Percolone Tablets 1327
Roxicodone 3067
Tylox Capsules 2597

Paramethadione (Propoxyphene may slow metabolism).
No products indexed under this heading.

Pentobarbital Sodium (Additive CNS depression). Products include:
Nembutal Sodium Solution 485

Perphenazine (Additive CNS depression). Products include:
Etrafon 3115
Trilafon 3160

Phenacemide (Propoxyphene may slow metabolism).
No products indexed under this heading.

Phenobarbital (Additive CNS depression; propoxyphene may slow metabolism). Products include:
Arco-Lase Plus Tablets 592
Donnatal 2929
Donnatal Extentabs 2930

Phensuximide (Propoxyphene may slow metabolism).
No products indexed under this heading.

Phenytoin (Propoxyphene may slow metabolism). Products include:
Dilantin Infatabs 2624
Dilantin-125 Oral Suspension 2625

Phenytoin Sodium (Propoxyphene may slow metabolism). Products include:
Dilantin Kapseals 2622

Prazepam (Additive CNS depression).
No products indexed under this heading.

Primidone (Propoxyphene may slow metabolism).
No products indexed under this heading.

Prochlorperazine (Additive CNS depression). Products include:
Compazine 1505

Promethazine Hydrochloride (Additive CNS depression). Products include:
Mepergan Injection 3539
Phenergan Injection 3553
Phenergan 3556
Phenergan Syrup 3554
Phenergan with Codeine Syrup 3557
Phenergan with Dextromethorphan Syrup 3559
Phenergan VC Syrup 3560
Phenergan VC with Codeine Syrup 3561

Propofol (Additive CNS depression). Products include:
Diprivan Injectable Emulsion 667

Propoxyphene Hydrochloride (Additive CNS depression). Products include:
Darvon Pulvules 1909
Darvon Compound-65 Pulvules 1910

Protriptyline Hydrochloride (Propoxyphene may slow metabolism). Products include:
Vivactil Tablets 2446
Vivactil Tablets 2217

Quazepam (Additive CNS depression).
No products indexed under this heading.

Quetiapine Fumarate (Additive CNS depression). Products include:
Seroquel Tablets 684

Remifentanil Hydrochloride (Additive CNS depression).
No products indexed under this heading.

Risperidone (Additive CNS depression). Products include:
Risperdal 1796

Secobarbital Sodium (Additive CNS depression).
No products indexed under this heading.

Sevoflurane (Additive CNS depression).
No products indexed under this heading.

Sufentanil Citrate (Additive CNS depression).
No products indexed under this heading.

Temazepam (Additive CNS depression).
No products indexed under this heading.

Thiamylal Sodium (Additive CNS depression).
No products indexed under this heading.

Thioridazine Hydrochloride (Additive CNS depression). Products include:
Thioridazine Hydrochloride Tablets 2289

Thiothixene (Additive CNS depression). Products include:
Navane Capsules 2701
Thiothixene Capsules 2290

Tiagabine Hydrochloride (Propoxyphene may slow metabolism). Products include:
Gabitril Tablets 1189

Topiramate (Propoxyphene may slow metabolism). Products include:
Topamax Sprinkle Capsules 2590
Topamax Tablets 2590

Triazolam (Additive CNS depression). Products include:
Halcion Tablets 2823

Trifluoperazine Hydrochloride (Additive CNS depression). Products include:
Stelazine 1640

Trimethadione (Propoxyphene may slow metabolism).
No products indexed under this heading.

Trimipramine Maleate (Propoxyphene may slow metabolism). Products include:
Surmontil Capsules 3595

Valproate Sodium (Propoxyphene may slow metabolism). Products include:
Depacon Injection 416

Valproic Acid (Propoxyphene may slow metabolism). Products include:
Depakene 421

Warfarin Sodium (Propoxyphene may slow metabolism). Products include:
Coumadin for Injection 1243
Coumadin Tablets 1243
Warfarin Sodium Tablets, USP 3302

Zaleplon (Additive CNS depression). Products include:
Sonata Capsules 3591

Ziprasidone Hydrochloride (Additive CNS depression). Products include:
Geodon Capsules 2688

Zolpidem Tartrate (Additive CNS depression). Products include:
Ambien Tablets 3191

Zonisamide (Propoxyphene may slow metabolism). Products include:
Zonegran Capsules 1307

Food Interactions

Alcohol (Additive CNS depression).

DARVOCET-N 100 TABLETS

(Acetaminophen, Propoxyphene Napsylate) 1907
See Darvocet-N 50 Tablets

DARVON PULVULES

(Propoxyphene Hydrochloride) 1909
May interact with central nervous system depressants, oral anticoagulants, antidepressant drugs, anticonvulsants, and certain other agents. Compounds in these categories include:

Alfentanil Hydrochloride (The CNS-depressant effect of propoxyphene is additive with that of other CNS depressants).
No products indexed under this heading.

Alprazolam (The CNS-depressant effect of propoxyphene is additive with that of other CNS depressants). Products include:
Xanax Tablets 2865

Amitriptyline Hydrochloride (Propoxyphene may slow the metabolism of antidepressants). Products include:
Etrafon 3115
Limbitrol 1738

Amoxapine (Propoxyphene may slow the metabolism of antidepressants).
No products indexed under this heading.

Aprobarbital (The CNS-depressant effect of propoxyphene is additive with that of other CNS depressants).
No products indexed under this heading.

Buprenorphine Hydrochloride (The CNS-depressant effect of propoxyphene is additive with that of other CNS depressants). Products include:
Buprenex Injectable 2918

Bupropion Hydrochloride (Propoxyphene may slow the metabolism of antidepressants). Products include:
Wellbutrin Tablets 1680
Wellbutrin SR Sustained-Release Tablets 1684
Zyban Sustained-Release Tablets 1710

Buspirone Hydrochloride (The CNS-depressant effect of propoxyphene is additive with that of other CNS depressants).
No products indexed under this heading.

Butabarbital (The CNS-depressant effect of propoxyphene is additive with that of other CNS depressants).
No products indexed under this heading.

Butalbital (The CNS-depressant effect of propoxyphene is additive with that of other CNS depressants). Products include:
Phrenilin 578
Sedapap Tablets 50 mg/650 mg 2225

Carbamazepine (Co-administration has resulted in severe neurological signs, including coma). Products include:
Carbatrol Capsules 3234
Tegretol/Tegretol-XR 2404

Chlordiazepoxide (The CNS-depressant effect of propoxyphene is additive with that of other CNS depressants). Products include:
Limbitrol 1738

Chlordiazepoxide Hydrochloride (The CNS-depressant effect of propoxyphene is additive with that of other CNS depressants). Products include:
Librium Capsules 1736
Librium for Injection 1737

Chlorpromazine (The CNS-depressant effect of propoxyphene is additive with that of other CNS depressants). Products include:
Thorazine Suppositories 1656

Chlorpromazine Hydrochloride (The CNS-depressant effect of propoxyphene is additive with that of other CNS depressants). Products include:
Thorazine 1656

Chlorprothixene (The CNS-depressant effect of propoxyphene is additive with that of other CNS depressants).
No products indexed under this heading.

Chlorprothixene Hydrochloride (The CNS-depressant effect of propoxyphene is additive with that of other CNS depressants).
No products indexed under this heading.

Chlorprothixene Lactate (The CNS-depressant effect of propoxyphene is additive with that of other CNS depressants).
No products indexed under this heading.

Citalopram Hydrobromide (Propoxyphene may slow the metabolism of antidepressants). Products include:
Celexa 1365

Clorazepate Dipotassium (The CNS-depressant effect of propoxyphene is additive with that of other CNS depressants). Products include:
Tranxene 511

Clozapine (The CNS-depressant effect of propoxyphene is additive with that of other CNS depressants). Products include:
Clozaril Tablets 2319

Codeine Phosphate (The CNS-depressant effect of propoxyphene is additive with that of other CNS depressants). Products include:
Phenergan with Codeine Syrup 3557
Phenergan VC with Codeine Syrup 3561
Robitussin A-C Syrup 2942
Robitussin-DAC Syrup 2942
Ryna-C Liquid .... ▣768
Soma Compound w/Codeine Tablets 3355
Tussi-Organidin NR Liquid 3350
Tussi-Organidin-S NR Liquid 3350
Tylenol with Codeine 2595

Desflurane (The CNS-depressant effect of propoxyphene is additive with that of other CNS depressants). Products include:
Suprane Liquid for Inhalation 874

Desipramine Hydrochloride (Propoxyphene may slow the metabolism of antidepressants). Products include:
Norpramin Tablets 755

Dezocine (The CNS-depressant effect of propoxyphene is additive with that of other CNS depressants).
No products indexed under this heading.

Diazepam (The CNS-depressant effect of propoxyphene is additive with that of other CNS depressants). Products include:
Valium Injectable 3026
Valium Tablets 3047

Dicumarol (Propoxyphene may slow the metabolism of warfarin-like drugs).
No products indexed under this heading.

Divalproex Sodium (Propoxyphene may slow the metabolism of anticonvulsants). Products include:
Depakote Sprinkle Capsules 426
Depakote Tablets 430
Depakote ER Tablets 436

Doxepin Hydrochloride (Propoxyphene may slow the metabolism of antidepressants). Products include:
Sinequan 2713

Droperidol (The CNS-depressant effect of propoxyphene is additive with that of other CNS depressants).
No products indexed under this heading.

Enflurane (The CNS-depressant effect of propoxyphene is additive with that of other CNS depressants).
No products indexed under this heading.

Estazolam (The CNS-depressant effect of propoxyphene is additive with that of other CNS depressants). Products include:
ProSom Tablets 500

Ethchlorvynol (The CNS-depressant effect of propoxyphene is additive with that of other CNS depressants).
No products indexed under this heading.

Ethinamate (The CNS-depressant effect of propoxyphene is additive with that of other CNS depressants).
No products indexed under this heading.

Ethosuximide (Propoxyphene may slow the metabolism of anticonvulsants). Products include:
Zarontin Capsules 2659
Zarontin Syrup 2660

Ethotoin (Propoxyphene may slow the metabolism of anticonvulsants).
No products indexed under this heading.

Felbamate (Propoxyphene may slow the metabolism of anticonvulsants). Products include:
Felbatol 3343

Fentanyl (The CNS-depressant effect of propoxyphene is additive with that of other CNS depressants). Products include:
Duragesic Transdermal System 1786

Fentanyl Citrate (The CNS-depressant effect of propoxyphene is additive with that of other CNS depressants). Products include:
Actiq 1184

Fluoxetine Hydrochloride (Propoxyphene may slow the metabolism of antidepressants). Products include:
Prozac Pulvules, Liquid, and Weekly Capsules 1238
Sarafem Pulvules 1962

Fluphenazine Decanoate (The CNS-depressant effect of propoxyphene is additive with that of other CNS depressants).
No products indexed under this heading.

Fluphenazine Enanthate (The CNS-depressant effect of propoxyphene is additive with that of other CNS depressants).
No products indexed under this heading.

Fluphenazine Hydrochloride (The CNS-depressant effect of propoxyphene is additive with that of other CNS depressants).
No products indexed under this heading.

Flurazepam Hydrochloride (The CNS-depressant effect of propoxyphene is additive with that of other CNS depressants).
No products indexed under this heading.

Fosphenytoin Sodium (Propoxyphene may slow the metabolism of anticonvulsants). Products include:
Cerebyx Injection 2619

Glutethimide (The CNS-depressant effect of propoxyphene is additive with that of other CNS depressants).
No products indexed under this heading.

Haloperidol (The CNS-depressant effect of propoxyphene is additive with that of other CNS depressants). Products include:
Haldol Injection, Tablets and Concentrate 2533

Haloperidol Decanoate (The CNS-depressant effect of propoxyphene is additive with that of other CNS depressants). Products include:
Haldol Decanoate 2535

Hydrocodone Bitartrate (The CNS-depressant effect of propoxyphene is additive with that of other CNS depressants). Products include:
Hycodan 1316
Hycomine Compound Tablets 1317
Hycotuss Expectorant Syrup 1318
Lortab 3319
Lortab Elixir 3317
Maxidone Tablets CIII 3399
Norco 5/325 Tablets CIII 3424
Norco 7.5/325 Tablets CIII 3425
Norco 10/325 Tablets CIII 3427
Norco 10/325 Tablets CIII 3425
Vicodin Tablets 516
Vicodin ES Tablets 517
Vicodin HP Tablets 518
Vicodin Tuss Expectorant 519
Vicoprofen Tablets 520
Zydone Tablets 1330

Hydrocodone Polistirex (The CNS-depressant effect of propoxyphene is additive with that of other CNS depressants). Products include:
Tussionex Pennkinetic Extended-Release Suspension 1174

Hydromorphone Hydrochloride (The CNS-depressant effect of propoxyphene is additive with that of other CNS depressants). Products include:
Dilaudid 441
Dilaudid Oral Liquid 445
Dilaudid Powder 441
Dilaudid Rectal Suppositories 441
Dilaudid Tablets 441
Dilaudid Tablets - 8 mg 445
Dilaudid-HP 443

Hydroxyzine Hydrochloride (The CNS-depressant effect of propoxyphene is additive with that of other CNS depressants). Products include:
Atarax Tablets & Syrup 2667
Vistaril Intramuscular Solution 2738

Imipramine Hydrochloride (Propoxyphene may slow the metabolism of antidepressants).
No products indexed under this heading.

Imipramine Pamoate (Propoxyphene may slow the metabolism of antidepressants).
No products indexed under this heading.

Isocarboxazid (Propoxyphene may slow the metabolism of antidepressants).
No products indexed under this heading.

Isoflurane (The CNS-depressant effect of propoxyphene is additive with that of other CNS depressants).
No products indexed under this heading.

Ketamine Hydrochloride (The CNS-depressant effect of propoxyphene is additive with that of other CNS depressants).
No products indexed under this heading.

Lamotrigine (Propoxyphene may slow the metabolism of anticonvulsants). Products include:
Lamictal 1567

Levetiracetam (Propoxyphene may slow the metabolism of anticonvulsants). Products include:
Keppra Tablets 3314

Levomethadyl Acetate Hydrochloride (The CNS-depressant effect of propoxyphene is additive with that of other CNS depressants).
No products indexed under this heading.

Levorphanol Tartrate (The CNS-depressant effect of propoxyphene is additive with that of other CNS depressants). Products include:
Levo-Dromoran 1734
Levorphanol Tartrate Tablets 3059

Lorazepam (The CNS-depressant effect of propoxyphene is additive with that of other CNS depressants). Products include:
Ativan Injection 3478
Ativan Tablets 3482

Loxapine Hydrochloride (The CNS-depressant effect of propoxyphene is additive with that of other CNS depressants).
No products indexed under this heading.

Loxapine Succinate (The CNS-depressant effect of propoxyphene is additive with that of other CNS depressants). Products include:
Loxitane Capsules 3398

Maprotiline Hydrochloride (Propoxyphene may slow the metabolism of antidepressants).
No products indexed under this heading.

Meperidine Hydrochloride (The CNS-depressant effect of propoxyphene is additive with that of other CNS depressants). Products include:
Demerol 3079
Mepergan Injection 3539

Mephenytoin (Propoxyphene may slow the metabolism of anticonvulsants).
No products indexed under this heading.

Mephobarbital (The CNS-depressant effect of propoxyphene is additive with that of other CNS depressants).
No products indexed under this heading.

Meprobamate (The CNS-depressant effect of propoxyphene is additive with that of other CNS depressants). Products include:
Miltown Tablets 3349

Mesoridazine Besylate (The CNS-depressant effect of propoxyphene is additive with that of other CNS depressants). Products include:
Serentil 1057

Methadone Hydrochloride (The CNS-depressant effect of propoxyphene is additive with that of other CNS depressants). Products include:
Dolophine Hydrochloride Tablets 3056

Methohexital Sodium (The CNS-depressant effect of propoxyphene is additive with that of other CNS depressants). Products include:
Brevital Sodium for Injection, USP 1815

Methotrimeprazine (The CNS-depressant effect of propoxyphene is additive with that of other CNS depressants).
No products indexed under this heading.

Methoxyflurane (The CNS-depressant effect of propoxyphene is additive with that of other CNS depressants).
No products indexed under this heading.

Methsuximide (Propoxyphene may slow the metabolism of anticonvulsants). Products include:
Celontin Capsules 2618

Midazolam Hydrochloride (The CNS-depressant effect of propoxyphene is additive with that of other CNS depressants). Products include:
Versed Injection 3027
Versed Syrup 3033

Mirtazapine (Propoxyphene may slow the metabolism of antidepressants). Products include:
Remeron Tablets 2483
Remeron SolTab Tablets 2486

Molindone Hydrochloride (The CNS-depressant effect of propoxyphene is additive with that of other CNS depressants). Products include:
Moban 1320

Morphine Sulfate (The CNS-depressant effect of propoxyphene is additive with that of other CNS depressants). Products include:
Astramorph/PF Injection, USP (Preservative-Free) 594
Duramorph Injection 1312
Infumorph 200 and Infumorph 500 Sterile Solutions 1314
Kadian Capsules 1335
MS Contin Tablets 2896
MSIR 2898
Oramorph SR Tablets 3062
Roxanol 3066

Nefazodone Hydrochloride (Propoxyphene may slow the metabolism of antidepressants). Products include:
Serzone Tablets 1104

Nortriptyline Hydrochloride (Propoxyphene may slow the metabolism of antidepressants).
No products indexed under this heading.

Olanzapine (The CNS-depressant effect of propoxyphene is additive with that of other CNS depressants). Products include:
- Zyprexa Tablets 1973
- Zyprexa ZYDIS Orally Disintegrating Tablets 1973

Oxazepam (The CNS-depressant effect of propoxyphene is additive with that of other CNS depressants).
- No products indexed under this heading.

Oxcarbazepine (Propoxyphene may slow the metabolism of anticonvulsants). Products include:
- Trileptal Oral Suspension 2407
- Trileptal Tablets 2407

Oxycodone Hydrochloride (The CNS-depressant effect of propoxyphene is additive with that of other CNS depressants). Products include:
- OxyContin Tablets 2912
- OxyFast Oral Concentrate Solution . 2916
- OxyIR Capsules 2916
- Percocet Tablets 1326
- Percodan Tablets 1327
- Percolone Tablets 1327
- Roxicodone 3067
- Tylox Capsules 2597

Paramethadione (Propoxyphene may slow the metabolism of anticonvulsants).
- No products indexed under this heading.

Paroxetine Hydrochloride (Propoxyphene may slow the metabolism of antidepressants). Products include:
- Paxil 1609

Pentobarbital Sodium (The CNS-depressant effect of propoxyphene is additive with that of other CNS depressants). Products include:
- Nembutal Sodium Solution 485

Perphenazine (The CNS-depressant effect of propoxyphene is additive with that of other CNS depressants). Products include:
- Etrafon 3115
- Trilafon 3160

Phenacemide (Propoxyphene may slow the metabolism of anticonvulsants).
- No products indexed under this heading.

Phenelzine Sulfate (Propoxyphene may slow the metabolism of antidepressants). Products include:
- Nardil Tablets 2653

Phenobarbital (The CNS-depressant effect of propoxyphene is additive with that of other CNS depressants; propoxyphene may slow the metabolism of anticonvulsants). Products include:
- Arco-Lase Plus Tablets 592
- Donnatal 2929
- Donnatal Extentabs 2930

Phensuximide (Propoxyphene may slow the metabolism of anticonvulsants).
- No products indexed under this heading.

Phenytoin (Propoxyphene may slow the metabolism of anticonvulsants). Products include:
- Dilantin Infatabs 2624
- Dilantin-125 Oral Suspension 2625

Phenytoin Sodium (Propoxyphene may slow the metabolism of anticonvulsants). Products include:
- Dilantin Kapseals 2622

Prazepam (The CNS-depressant effect of propoxyphene is additive with that of other CNS depressants).
- No products indexed under this heading.

Primidone (Propoxyphene may slow the metabolism of anticonvulsants).
- No products indexed under this heading.

Prochlorperazine (The CNS-depressant effect of propoxyphene is additive with that of other CNS depressants). Products include:
- Compazine 1505

Promethazine Hydrochloride (The CNS-depressant effect of propoxyphene is additive with that of other CNS depressants). Products include:
- Mepergan Injection 3539
- Phenergan Injection 3553
- Phenergan 3556
- Phenergan Syrup 3554
- Phenergan with Codeine Syrup 3557
- Phenergan with Dextromethorphan Syrup 3559
- Phenergan VC Syrup 3560
- Phenergan VC with Codeine Syrup .. 3561

Propofol (The CNS-depressant effect of propoxyphene is additive with that of other CNS depressants). Products include:
- Diprivan Injectable Emulsion 667

Propoxyphene Napsylate (The CNS-depressant effect of propoxyphene is additive with that of other CNS depressants). Products include:
- Darvon-N/Darvocet-N 1907
- Darvon-N Tablets 1912

Protriptyline Hydrochloride (Propoxyphene may slow the metabolism of antidepressants). Products include:
- Vivactil Tablets 2446
- Vivactil Tablets 2217

Quazepam (The CNS-depressant effect of propoxyphene is additive with that of other CNS depressants).
- No products indexed under this heading.

Quetiapine Fumarate (The CNS-depressant effect of propoxyphene is additive with that of other CNS depressants). Products include:
- Seroquel Tablets 684

Remifentanil Hydrochloride (The CNS-depressant effect of propoxyphene is additive with that of other CNS depressants).
- No products indexed under this heading.

Risperidone (The CNS-depressant effect of propoxyphene is additive with that of other CNS depressants). Products include:
- Risperdal 1796

Secobarbital Sodium (The CNS-depressant effect of propoxyphene is additive with that of other CNS depressants).
- No products indexed under this heading.

Sertraline Hydrochloride (Propoxyphene may slow the metabolism of antidepressants). Products include:
- Zoloft 2751

Sevoflurane (The CNS-depressant effect of propoxyphene is additive with that of other CNS depressants).
- No products indexed under this heading.

Sufentanil Citrate (The CNS-depressant effect of propoxyphene is additive with that of other CNS depressants).
- No products indexed under this heading.

Temazepam (The CNS-depressant effect of propoxyphene is additive with that of other CNS depressants).
- No products indexed under this heading.

Thiamylal Sodium (The CNS-depressant effect of propoxyphene is additive with that of other CNS depressants).
- No products indexed under this heading.

Thioridazine Hydrochloride (The CNS-depressant effect of propoxyphene is additive with that of other CNS depressants). Products include:
- Thioridazine Hydrochloride Tablets 2289

Thiothixene (The CNS-depressant effect of propoxyphene is additive with that of other CNS depressants). Products include:
- Navane Capsules 2701
- Thiothixene Capsules 2290

Tiagabine Hydrochloride (Propoxyphene may slow the metabolism of anticonvulsants). Products include:
- Gabitril Tablets 1189

Topiramate (Propoxyphene may slow the metabolism of anticonvulsants). Products include:
- Topamax Sprinkle Capsules 2590
- Topamax Tablets 2590

Tranylcypromine Sulfate (Propoxyphene may slow the metabolism of antidepressants). Products include:
- Parnate Tablets 1607

Trazodone Hydrochloride (Propoxyphene may slow the metabolism of antidepressants).
- No products indexed under this heading.

Triazolam (The CNS-depressant effect of propoxyphene is additive with that of other CNS depressants). Products include:
- Halcion Tablets 2823

Trifluoperazine Hydrochloride (The CNS-depressant effect of propoxyphene is additive with that of other CNS depressants). Products include:
- Stelazine 1640

Trimethadione (Propoxyphene may slow the metabolism of anticonvulsants).
- No products indexed under this heading.

Trimipramine Maleate (Propoxyphene may slow the metabolism of antidepressants). Products include:
- Surmontil Capsules 3595

Valproate Sodium (Propoxyphene may slow the metabolism of anticonvulsants). Products include:
- Depacon Injection 416

Valproic Acid (Propoxyphene may slow the metabolism of anticonvulsants). Products include:
- Depakene 421

Venlafaxine Hydrochloride (Propoxyphene may slow the metabolism of antidepressants). Products include:
- Effexor Tablets 3495
- Effexor XR Capsules 3499

Warfarin Sodium (Propoxyphene may slow the metabolism of warfarin-like drugs). Products include:
- Coumadin for Injection 1243
- Coumadin Tablets 1243
- Warfarin Sodium Tablets, USP 3302

Zaleplon (The CNS-depressant effect of propoxyphene is additive with that of other CNS depressants). Products include:
- Sonata Capsules 3591

Ziprasidone Hydrochloride (The CNS-depressant effect of propoxyphene is additive with that of other CNS depressants). Products include:
- Geodon Capsules 2688

Zolpidem Tartrate (The CNS-depressant effect of propoxyphene is additive with that of other CNS depressants). Products include:
- Ambien Tablets 3191

Zonisamide (Propoxyphene may slow the metabolism of anticonvulsants). Products include:
- Zonegran Capsules 1307

Food Interactions

Alcohol (The CNS-depressant effect of propoxyphene is additive with that of alcohol).

DARVON COMPOUND-65 PULVULES

(Aspirin, Caffeine, Propoxyphene Hydrochloride) 1910

May interact with central nervous system depressants, oral anticoagulants, antidepressant drugs, anticonvulsants, hypnotics and sedatives, tranquilizers, and certain other agents. Compounds in these categories include:

Alfentanil Hydrochloride (Co-administration can result in possible additive CNS depressant effects).
- No products indexed under this heading.

Alprazolam (Co-administration can result in possible additive CNS depressant effects). Products include:
- Xanax Tablets 2865

Amitriptyline Hydrochloride (Propoxyphene may slow the metabolism of antidepressants; co-administration may result in higher serum concentrations of antidepressants resulting in increased pharmacologic or adverse effects concurrent use with antidepressants can result in possible additive CNS depressant effects). Products include:
- Etrafon 3115
- Limbitrol 1738

Amoxapine (Propoxyphene may slow the metabolism of antidepressants; co-administration may result in higher serum concentrations of antidepressants resulting in increased pharmacologic or adverse effects concurrent use with antidepressants can result in possible additive CNS depressant effects).
- No products indexed under this heading.

Aprobarbital (Co-administration can result in possible additive CNS depressant effects).
- No products indexed under this heading.

Buprenorphine Hydrochloride (Co-administration can result in possible additive CNS depressant effects). Products include:
- Buprenex Injectable 2918

Bupropion Hydrochloride (Propoxyphene may slow the metabolism of antidepressants; co-administration may result in higher serum concentrations of antidepressants resulting in increased pharmacologic or adverse effects concurrent use with antidepressants can result in possible additive CNS depressant effects). Products include:
- Wellbutrin Tablets 1680
- Wellbutrin SR Sustained-Release Tablets 1684
- Zyban Sustained-Release Tablets ... 1710

Buspirone Hydrochloride (Co-administration can result in possible additive CNS depressant effects).
- No products indexed under this heading.

Butabarbital (Co-administration can result in possible additive CNS depressant effects).
- No products indexed under this heading.

Butalbital (Co-administration can result in possible additive CNS depressant effects). Products include:
- Phrenilin 578
- Sedapap Tablets 50 mg/650 mg ... 2225

Carbamazepine (Propoxyphene may slow the metabolism of anticonvulsants; co-administration may result in higher serum concentrations of anticonvulsants resulting in increased pharmacologic or adverse effects; severe neurologic signs, including coma, have occurred with concurrent carbamazepine). Products include:
- Carbatrol Capsules 3234
- Tegretol/Tegretol-XR 2404

Chlordiazepoxide (Co-administration can result in possible additive CNS depressant effects). Products include:
- Limbitrol 1738

Chlordiazepoxide Hydrochloride (Co-administration can result in possible additive CNS depressant effects). Products include:
- Librium Capsules 1736
- Librium for Injection 1737

Chlorpromazine (Co-administration can result in possible additive CNS depressant effects). Products include:
- Thorazine Suppositories 1656

Chlorpromazine Hydrochloride (Co-administration can result in possible additive CNS depressant effects). Products include:
- Thorazine 1656

Chlorprothixene (Co-administration can result in possible additive CNS depressant effects).
No products indexed under this heading.

Chlorprothixene Hydrochloride (Co-administration can result in possible additive CNS depressant effects).
No products indexed under this heading.

Chlorprothixene Lactate (Co-administration can result in possible additive CNS depressant effects).
No products indexed under this heading.

Citalopram Hydrobromide (Propoxyphene may slow the metabolism of antidepressants; co-administration may result in higher serum concentrations of antidepressants resulting in increased pharmacologic or adverse effects concurrent use with antidepressants can result in possible additive CNS depressant effects). Products include:
- Celexa 1365

Clorazepate Dipotassium (Co-administration can result in possible additive CNS depressant effects). Products include:
- Tranxene 511

Clozapine (Co-administration can result in possible additive CNS depressant effects). Products include:
- Clozaril Tablets 2319

Codeine Phosphate (Co-administration can result in possible additive CNS depressant effects). Products include:
- Phenergan with Codeine Syrup 3557
- Phenergan VC with Codeine Syrup .. 3561
- Robitussin A-C Syrup 2942
- Robitussin-DAC Syrup 2942
- Ryna-C Liquid .... ▣768
- Soma Compound w/Codeine Tablets 3355
- Tussi-Organidin NR Liquid 3350
- Tussi-Organidin-S NR Liquid 3350
- Tylenol with Codeine 2595

Desflurane (Co-administration can result in possible additive CNS depressant effects). Products include:
- Suprane Liquid for Inhalation 874

Desipramine Hydrochloride (Propoxyphene may slow the metabolism of antidepressants; co administration may result in higher serum concentrations of antidepressants resulting in increased pharmacologic or adverse effects concurrent use with antidepressants can result in possible additive CNS depressant effects). Products include:
- Norpramin Tablets 755

Dezocine (Co-administration can result in possible additive CNS depressant effects).
No products indexed under this heading.

Diazepam (Co-administration can result in possible additive CNS depressant effects). Products include:
- Valium Injectable 3026
- Valium Tablets 3047

Dicumarol (Propoxyphene may slow the metabolism of warfarin-like drugs and salicylates may enhance the effects of anticoagulants; co-administration may result in higher serum concentrations of anticoagulants resulting in increased pharmacologic or adverse effects).
No products indexed under this heading.

Doxepin Hydrochloride (Propoxyphene may slow the metabolism of antidepressants; co-administration may result in higher serum concentrations of antidepressants resulting in increased pharmacologic or adverse effects concurrent use with antidepressants can result in possible additive CNS depressant effects). Products include:
- Sinequan 2713

Droperidol (Co-administration can result in possible additive CNS depressant effects).
No products indexed under this heading.

Enflurane (Co-administration can result in possible additive CNS depressant effects).
No products indexed under this heading.

Estazolam (Co-administration can result in possible additive CNS depressant effects). Products include:
- ProSom Tablets 500

Ethchlorvynol (Co-administration can result in possible additive CNS depressant effects).
No products indexed under this heading.

Ethinamate (Co-administration can result in possible additive CNS depressant effects).
No products indexed under this heading.

Fentanyl (Co-administration can result in possible additive CNS depressant effects). Products include:
- Duragesic Transdermal System 1786

Fentanyl Citrate (Co-administration can result in possible additive CNS depressant effects). Products include:
- Actiq 1184

Fluoxetine Hydrochloride (Propoxyphene may slow the metabolism of antidepressants; co-administration may result in higher serum concentrations of antidepressants resulting in increased pharmacologic or adverse effects concurrent use with antidepressants can result in possible additive CNS depressant effects). Products include:
- Prozac Pulvules, Liquid, and Weekly Capsules 1238
- Sarafem Pulvules 1962

Fluphenazine Decanoate (Co-administration can result in possible additive CNS depressant effects).
No products indexed under this heading.

Fluphenazine Enanthate (Co-administration can result in possible additive CNS depressant effects).
No products indexed under this heading.

Fluphenazine Hydrochloride (Co-administration can result in possible additive CNS depressant effects).
No products indexed under this heading.

Flurazepam Hydrochloride (Co-administration can result in possible additive CNS depressant effects).
No products indexed under this heading.

Glutethimide (Co-administration can result in possible additive CNS depressant effects).
No products indexed under this heading.

Haloperidol (Co-administration can result in possible additive CNS depressant effects). Products include:
- Haldol Injection, Tablets and Concentrate 2533

Haloperidol Decanoate (Co-administration can result in possible additive CNS depressant effects). Products include:
- Haldol Decanoate 2535

Hydrocodone Bitartrate (Co-administration can result in possible additive CNS depressant effects). Products include:
- Hycodan 1316
- Hycomine Compound Tablets 1317
- Hycotuss Expectorant Syrup 1318
- Lortab 3319
- Lortab Elixir 3317
- Maxidone Tablets CIII 3399
- Norco 5/325 Tablets CIII 3424
- Norco 7.5/325 Tablets CIII 3425
- Norco 10/325 Tablets CIII 3427
- Norco 10/325 Tablets CIII 3425
- Vicodin Tablets 516
- Vicodin ES Tablets 517
- Vicodin HP Tablets 518
- Vicodin Tuss Expectorant 519
- Vicoprofen Tablets 520
- Zydone Tablets 1330

Hydrocodone Polistirex (Co-administration can result in possible additive CNS depressant effects). Products include:
- Tussionex Pennkinetic Extended-Release Suspension 1174

Hydromorphone Hydrochloride (Co-administration can result in possible additive CNS depressant effects). Products include:
- Dilaudid 441
- Dilaudid Oral Liquid 445
- Dilaudid Powder 441
- Dilaudid Rectal Suppositories 441
- Dilaudid Tablets 441
- Dilaudid Tablets - 8 mg 445
- Dilaudid-HP 443

Hydroxyzine Hydrochloride (Co-administration can result in possible additive CNS depressant effects). Products include:
- Atarax Tablets & Syrup 2667
- Vistaril Intramuscular Solution 2738

Imipramine Hydrochloride (Propoxyphene may slow the metabolism of antidepressants; co-administration may result in higher serum concentrations of antidepressants resulting in increased pharmacologic or adverse effects concurrent use with antidepressants can result in possible additive CNS depressant effects).
No products indexed under this heading.

Imipramine Pamoate (Propoxyphene may slow the metabolism of antidepressants; co-administration may result in higher serum concentrations of antidepressants resulting in increased pharmacologic or adverse effects concurrent use with antidepressants can result in possible additive CNS depressant effects).
No products indexed under this heading.

Isocarboxazid (Propoxyphene may slow the metabolism of antidepressants; co-administration may result in higher serum concentrations of antidepressants resulting in increased pharmacologic or adverse effects concurrent use with antidepressants can result in possible additive CNS depressant effects).
No products indexed under this heading.

Isoflurane (Co-administration can result in possible additive CNS depressant effects).
No products indexed under this heading.

Ketamine Hydrochloride (Co-administration can result in possible additive CNS depressant effects).
No products indexed under this heading.

Levetiracetam (Propoxyphene may slow the metabolism of anticonvulsants; co-administration may result in higher serum concentrations of anticonvulsants resulting in increased pharmacologic or adverse effects). Products include:
- Keppra Tablets 3314

Levomethadyl Acetate Hydrochloride (Co-administration can result in possible additive CNS depressant effects).
No products indexed under this heading.

Levorphanol Tartrate (Co-administration can result in possible additive CNS depressant effects). Products include:
- Levo-Dromoran 1734
- Levorphanol Tartrate Tablets 3059

Lorazepam (Co-administration can result in possible additive CNS depressant effects). Products include:
- Ativan Injection 3478
- Ativan Tablets 3482

Loxapine Hydrochloride (Co-administration can result in possible additive CNS depressant effects).
No products indexed under this heading.

Loxapine Succinate (Co-administration can result in possible additive CNS depressant effects). Products include:
- Loxitane Capsules 3398

Maprotiline Hydrochloride (Propoxyphene may slow the metabolism of antidepressants; co-administration may result in higher serum concentrations of antidepressants resulting in increased pharmacologic or adverse effects concurrent use with antidepressants can result in possible additive CNS depressant effects).
No products indexed under this heading.

Meperidine Hydrochloride (Co-administration can result in possible additive CNS depressant effects). Products include:
- Demerol 3079
- Mepergan Injection 3539

Mephobarbital (Co-administration can result in possible additive CNS depressant effects).
No products indexed under this heading.

Meprobamate (Co-administration can result in possible additive CNS depressant effects). Products include:
- Miltown Tablets 3349

Mesoridazine Besylate (Co-administration can result in possible additive CNS depressant effects). Products include:
- Serentil 1057

Methadone Hydrochloride (Co-administration can result in possible additive CNS depressant effects). Products include:
- Dolophine Hydrochloride Tablets 3056

Methohexital Sodium (Co-administration can result in possible additive CNS depressant effects). Products include:
- Brevital Sodium for Injection, USP .. 1815

Methotrimeprazine (Co-administration can result in possible additive CNS depressant effects).
No products indexed under this heading.

Methoxyflurane (Co-administration can result in possible additive CNS depressant effects).
No products indexed under this heading.

Midazolam Hydrochloride (Co-administration can result in possible additive CNS depressant effects). Products include:
- Versed Injection 3027
- Versed Syrup 3033

Mirtazapine (Propoxyphene may slow the metabolism of antidepres-

sants; co-administration may result in higher serum concentrations of antidepressants resulting in increased pharmacologic or adverse effects concurrent use with antidepressants can result in possible additive CNS depressant effects). Products include:

Remeron Tablets 2483
Remeron SolTab Tablets 2486

Molindone Hydrochloride (Co-administration can result in possible additive CNS depressant effects). Products include:

Moban 1320

Morphine Sulfate (Co-administration can result in possible additive CNS depressant effects). Products include:

Astramorph/PF Injection, USP (Preservative-Free) 594
Duramorph Injection 1312
Infumorph 200 and Infumorph 500 Sterile Solutions 1314
Kadian Capsules 1335
MS Contin Tablets 2896
MSIR 2898
Oramorph SR Tablets 3062
Roxanol 3066

Nefazodone Hydrochloride (Propoxyphene may slow the metabolism of antidepressants; co-administration may result in higher serum concentrations of antidepressants resulting in increased pharmacologic or adverse effects concurrent use with antidepressants can result in possible additive CNS depressant effects). Products include:

Serzone Tablets 1104

Nortriptyline Hydrochloride (Propoxyphene may slow the metabolism of antidepressants; co-administration may result in higher serum concentrations of antidepressants resulting in increased pharmacologic or adverse effects concurrent use with antidepressants can result in possible additive CNS depressant effects).

No products indexed under this heading.

Oxazepam (Co-administration can result in possible additive CNS depressant effects).

No products indexed under this heading.

Oxcarbazepine (Propoxyphene may slow the metabolism of anticonvulsants; co-administration may result in higher serum concentrations of anticonvulsants resulting in increased pharmacologic or adverse effects). Products include:

Trileptal Oral Suspension 2407
Trileptal Tablets 2407

Oxycodone Hydrochloride (Co-administration can result in possible additive CNS depressant effects). Products include:

OxyContin Tablets 2912
OxyFast Oral Concentrate Solution . 2916
OxyIR Capsules 2916
Percocet Tablets 1326
Percodan Tablets 1327
Percolone Tablets 1327
Roxicodone 3067
Tylox Capsules 2597

Paroxetine Hydrochloride (Propoxyphene may slow the metabolism of antidepressants; co-administration may result in higher serum concentrations of antidepressants resulting in increased pharmacologic or adverse effects concurrent use with antidepressants can result in possible additive CNS depressant effects). Products include:

Paxil 1609

Pentobarbital Sodium (Co-administration can result in possible additive CNS depressant effects). Products include:

Nembutal Sodium Solution 485

Perphenazine (Co-administration can result in possible additive CNS depressant effects). Products include:

Etrafon 3115
Trilafon 3160

Phenelzine Sulfate (Propoxyphene may slow the metabolism of antidepressants; co-administration may result in higher serum concentrations of antidepressants resulting in increased pharmacologic or adverse effects concurrent use with antidepressants can result in possible additive CNS depressant effects). Products include:

Nardil Tablets 2653

Phenobarbital (Co-administration can result in possible additive CNS depressant effects; propoxyphene may slow the metabolism of anticonvulsants; co-administration may result in higher serum concentrations of anticonvulsants resulting in increased pharmacologic or adverse effects). Products include:

Arco-Lase Plus Tablets 592
Donnatal 2929
Donnatal Extentabs 2930

Probenecid (Salicylates may inhibit the uricosuric effects of uricosuric agents, such as probencid).

No products indexed under this heading.

Protriptyline Hydrochloride (Propoxyphene may slow the metabolism of antidepressants; co-administration may result in higher serum concentrations of antidepressants resulting in increased pharmacologic or adverse effects concurrent use with antidepressants can result in possible additive CNS depressant effects). Products include:

Vivactil Tablets 2446
Vivactil Tablets 2217

Sertraline Hydrochloride (Propoxyphene may slow the metabolism of antidepressants; co-administration may result in higher serum concentrations of antidepressants resulting in increased pharmacologic or adverse effects concurrent use with antidepressants can result in possible additive CNS depressant effects). Products include:

Zoloft 2751

Sulfinpyrazone (Salicylates may inhibit the uricosuric effects of uricosuric agents, such as sulfinpyrazone).

No products indexed under this heading.

Tiagabine Hydrochloride (Propoxyphene may slow the metabolism of anticonvulsants; co-administration may result in higher serum concentrations of anticonvulsants resulting in increased pharmacologic or adverse effects). Products include:

Gabitril Tablets 1189

Tranylcypromine Sulfate (Propoxyphene may slow the metabolism of antidepressants; co-administration may result in higher serum concentrations of antidepressants resulting in increased pharmacologic or adverse effects concurrent use with antidepressants can result in possible additive CNS depressant effects). Products include:

Parnate Tablets 1607

Trazodone Hydrochloride (Propoxyphene may slow the metabolism of antidepressants; co-administration may result in higher serum concentrations of antidepressants resulting in increased pharmacologic or adverse effects concurrent use with antidepressants can result in possible additive CNS depressant effects).

No products indexed under this heading.

Trimipramine Maleate (Propoxyphene may slow the metabolism of antidepressants; co-administration may result in higher serum concentrations of antidepressants resulting in increased pharmacologic or adverse effects concurrent use with antidepressants can result in possible additive CNS depressant effects). Products include:

Surmontil Capsules 3595

Venlafaxine Hydrochloride (Propoxyphene may slow the metabolism of antidepressants; co-administration may result in higher serum concentrations of antidepressants resulting in increased pharmacologic or adverse effects concurrent use with antidepressants can result in possible additive CNS depressant effects). Products include:

Effexor Tablets 3495
Effexor XR Capsules 3499

Warfarin Sodium (Propoxyphene may slow the metabolism of warfarin-like drugs and salicylates may enhance the effects of anticoagulants; co-administration may result in higher serum concentrations of anticoagulants resulting in increased pharmacologic or adverse effects). Products include:

Coumadin for Injection 1243
Coumadin Tablets 1243
Warfarin Sodium Tablets, USP 3302

Zaleplon (Co-administration can result in possible additive CNS depressant effects). Products include:

Sonata Capsules 3591

Ziprasidone Hydrochloride (Co-administration can result in possible additive CNS depressant effects). Products include:

Geodon Capsules 2688

Zonisamide (Propoxyphene may slow the metabolism of anticonvulsants; co-administration may result in higher serum concentrations of anticonvulsants resulting in increased pharmacologic or adverse effects). Products include:

Zonegran Capsules 1307

Food Interactions

Alcohol (Concurrent use can lead to potentially serious CNS depressant effects).

DARVON-N TABLETS

(Propoxyphene Napsylate) 1912

May interact with central nervous system depressants, oral anticoagulants, antidepressant drugs, anticonvulsants, hypnotics and sedatives, tranquilizers, and certain other agents. Compounds in these categories include:

Alfentanil Hydrochloride (Co-administration can result in possible additive CNS depressant effects).

No products indexed under this heading.

Alprazolam (Co-administration can result in possible additive CNS depressant effects). Products include:

Xanax Tablets 2865

Amitriptyline Hydrochloride (Propoxyphene may slow the metabolism of antidepressants; co-administration may result in higher serum concentrations of antidepressants resulting in increased pharmacologic or adverse effects concurrent use with antidepressants can result in possible additive CNS depressant effects). Products include:

Etrafon 3115
Limbitrol 1738

Amoxapine (Propoxyphene may slow the metabolism of antidepressants; co-administration may result in higher serum concentrations of antidepressants resulting in increased pharmacologic or adverse effects concurrent use with antidepressants can result in possible additive CNS depressant effects).

No products indexed under this heading.

Aprobarbital (Co-administration can result in possible additive CNS depressant effects).

No products indexed under this heading.

Buprenorphine Hydrochloride (Co-administration can result in possible additive CNS depressant effects). Products include:

Buprenex Injectable 2918

Bupropion Hydrochloride (Propoxyphene may slow the metabolism of antidepressants; co-administration may result in higher serum concentrations of antidepressants resulting in increased pharmacologic or adverse effects concurrent use with antidepressants can result in possible additive CNS depressant effects). Products include:

Wellbutrin Tablets 1680
Wellbutrin SR Sustained-Release Tablets 1684
Zyban Sustained-Release Tablets ... 1710

Buspirone Hydrochloride (Co-administration can result in possible additive CNS depressant effects).

No products indexed under this heading.

Butabarbital (Co-administration can result in possible additive CNS depressant effects).

No products indexed under this heading.

Butalbital (Co-administration can result in possible additive CNS depressant effects). Products include:

Phrenilin 578
Sedapap Tablets 50 mg/650 mg ... 2225

Carbamazepine (Propoxyphene may slow the metabolism of anticonvulsants; co-administration may result in higher serum concentrations of anticonvulsants resulting in increased pharmacologic or adverse effects; severe neurologic signs, including coma, have occured with concurrent carbamazepine). Products include:

Carbatrol Capsules 3234
Tegretol/Tegretol-XR 2404

Carisoprodol (Co-administration with muscle relaxants, such as carisoprodol, can result in possible additive CNS depressant effects). Products include:

Soma Tablets 3353
Soma Compound Tablets 3354
Soma Compound w/Codeine Tablets 3355

Chlordiazepoxide (Co-administration can result in possible additive CNS depressant effects). Products include:

Limbitrol 1738

Chlordiazepoxide Hydrochloride (Co-administration can result in possible additive CNS depressant effects). Products include:

Librium Capsules 1736
Librium for Injection 1737

Chlorpromazine (Co-administration can result in possible additive CNS depressant effects). Products include:

Thorazine Suppositories 1656

Chlorpromazine Hydrochloride (Co-administration can result in possible additive CNS depressant effects). Products include:

Thorazine 1656

Chlorprothixene (Co-administration can result in possible additive CNS depressant effects).

No products indexed under this heading.

Chlorprothixene Hydrochloride (Co-administration can result in pos-

sible additive CNS depressant effects).
No products indexed under this heading.

Chlorprothixene Lactate (Co-administration can result in possible additive CNS depressant effects).
No products indexed under this heading.

Chlorzoxazone (Co-administration with muscle relaxants, such as chlorzoxazone, can result in possible additive CNS depressant effects). Products include:
Parafon Forte DSC Caplets 2582

Citalopram Hydrobromide (Propoxyphene may slow the metabolism of antidepressants; co-administration may result in higher serum concentrations of antidepressants resulting in increased pharmacologic or adverse effects concurrent use with antidepressants can result in possible additive CNS depressant effects). Products include:
Celexa 1365

Clorazepate Dipotassium (Co-administration can result in possible additive CNS depressant effects). Products include:
Tranxene 511

Clozapine (Co-administration can result in possible additive CNS depressant effects). Products include:
Clozaril Tablets 2319

Codeine Phosphate (Co-administration can result in possible additive CNS depressant effects). Products include:
Phenergan with Codeine Syrup 3557
Phenergan VC with Codeine Syrup .. 3561
Robitussin A-C Syrup 2942
Robitussin-DAC Syrup 2942
Ryna-C Liquid .... ▣768
Soma Compound w/Codeine Tablets 3355
Tussi-Organidin NR Liquid 3350
Tussi-Organidin-S NR Liquid 3350
Tylenol with Codeine 2595

Cyclobenzaprine Hydrochloride (Co-administration with muscle relaxants, such as cyclobenzaprine, can result in possible additive CNS depressant effects). Products include:
Flexeril Tablets 572
Flexeril Tablets 2094

Desflurane (Co-administration can result in possible additive CNS depressant effects). Products include:
Suprane Liquid for Inhalation 874

Desipramine Hydrochloride (Propoxyphene may slow the metabolism of antidepressants; co-administration may result in higher serum concentrations of antidepressants resulting in increased pharmacologic or adverse effects concurrent use with antidepressants can result in possible additive CNS depressant effects). Products include:
Norpramin Tablets 755

Dezocine (Co-administration can result in possible additive CNS depressant effects).
No products indexed under this heading.

Diazepam (Co-administration can result in possible additive CNS depressant effects). Products include:
Valium Injectable 3026
Valium Tablets 3047

Dicumarol (Propoxyphene may slow the metabolism of warfarin-like drugs; co-administration may result in higher serum concentrations of anticoagulants resulting in increased pharmacologic or adverse effects).
No products indexed under this heading.

Doxepin Hydrochloride (Propoxyphene may slow the metabolism of antidepressants; co-administration may result in higher serum concentrations of antidepressants resulting in increased pharmacologic or adverse effects concurrent use with antidepressants can result in possible additive CNS depressant effects). Products include:
Sinequan 2713

Droperidol (Co-administration can result in possible additive CNS depressant effects).
No products indexed under this heading.

Enflurane (Co-administration can result in possible additive CNS depressant effects).
No products indexed under this heading.

Estazolam (Co-administration can result in possible additive CNS depressant effects). Products include:
ProSom Tablets 500

Ethchlorvynol (Co-administration can result in possible additive CNS depressant effects).
No products indexed under this heading.

Ethinamate (Co-administration can result in possible additive CNS depressant effects).
No products indexed under this heading.

Fentanyl (Co-administration can result in possible additive CNS depressant effects). Products include:
Duragesic Transdermal System 1786

Fentanyl Citrate (Co-administration can result in possible additive CNS depressant effects). Products include:
Actiq 1184

Fluoxetine Hydrochloride (Propoxyphene may slow the metabolism of antidepressants; co-administration may result in higher serum concentrations of antidepressants resulting in increased pharmacologic or adverse effects concurrent use with antidepressants can result in possible additive CNS depressant effects). Products include:
Prozac Pulvules, Liquid, and Weekly Capsules 1238
Sarafem Pulvules 1962

Fluphenazine Decanoate (Co-administration can result in possible additive CNS depressant effects).
No products indexed under this heading.

Fluphenazine Enanthate (Co-administration can result in possible additive CNS depressant effects).
No products indexed under this heading.

Fluphenazine Hydrochloride (Co-administration can result in possible additive CNS depressant effects).
No products indexed under this heading.

Flurazepam Hydrochloride (Co-administration can result in possible additive CNS depressant effects).
No products indexed under this heading.

Glutethimide (Co-administration can result in possible additive CNS depressant effects).
No products indexed under this heading.

Haloperidol (Co-administration can result in possible additive CNS depressant effects). Products include:
Haldol Injection, Tablets and Concentrate 2533

Haloperidol Decanoate (Co-administration can result in possible additive CNS depressant effects). Products include:
Haldol Decanoate 2535

Hydrocodone Bitartrate (Co-administration can result in possible additive CNS depressant effects). Products include:
Hycodan 1316
Hycomine Compound Tablets 1317
Hycotuss Expectorant Syrup 1318
Lortab 3319
Lortab Elixir 3317
Maxidone Tablets CIII 3399
Norco 5/325 Tablets CIII 3424
Norco 7.5/325 Tablets CIII 3425
Norco 10/325 Tablets CIII 3427
Norco 10/325 Tablets CIII 3425
Vicodin Tablets 516
Vicodin ES Tablets 517
Vicodin HP Tablets 518
Vicodin Tuss Expectorant 519
Vicoprofen Tablets 520
Zydone Tablets 1330

Hydrocodone Polistirex (Co-administration can result in possible additive CNS depressant effects). Products include:
Tussionex Pennkinetic Extended-Release Suspension 1174

Hydromorphone Hydrochloride (Co-administration can result in possible additive CNS depressant effects). Products include:
Dilaudid 441
Dilaudid Oral Liquid 445
Dilaudid Powder 441
Dilaudid Rectal Suppositories 441
Dilaudid Tablets 441
Dilaudid Tablets - 8 mg 445
Dilaudid-HP 443

Hydroxyzine Hydrochloride (Co-administration can result in possible additive CNS depressant effects). Products include:
Atarax Tablets & Syrup 2667
Vistaril Intramuscular Solution 2738

Imipramine Hydrochloride (Propoxyphene may slow the metabolism of antidepressants; co-administration may result in higher serum concentrations of antidepressants resulting in increased pharmacologic or adverse effects concurrent use with antidepressants can result in possible additive CNS depressant effects).
No products indexed under this heading.

Imipramine Pamoate (Propoxyphene may slow the metabolism of antidepressants; co-administration may result in higher serum concentrations of antidepressants resulting in increased pharmacologic or adverse effects concurrent use with antidepressants can result in possible additive CNS depressant effects).
No products indexed under this heading.

Isocarboxazid (Propoxyphene may slow the metabolism of antidepressants; co-administration may result in higher serum concentrations of antidepressants resulting in increased pharmacologic or adverse effects concurrent use with antidepressants can result in possible additive CNS depressant effects).
No products indexed under this heading.

Isoflurane (Co-administration can result in possible additive CNS depressant effects).
No products indexed under this heading.

Ketamine Hydrochloride (Co-administration can result in possible additive CNS depressant effects).
No products indexed under this heading.

Levetiracetam (Propoxyphene may slow the metabolism of anticonvulsants; co-administration may result in higher serum concentrations of anticonvulsants resulting in increased pharmacologic or adverse effects). Products include:
Keppra Tablets 3314

Levomethadyl Acetate Hydrochloride (Co-administration can result in possible additive CNS depressant effects).
No products indexed under this heading.

Levorphanol Tartrate (Co-administration can result in possible additive CNS depressant effects). Products include:
Levo-Dromoran 1734
Levorphanol Tartrate Tablets 3059

Lorazepam (Co-administration can result in possible additive CNS depressant effects). Products include:
Ativan Injection 3478
Ativan Tablets 3482

Loxapine Hydrochloride (Co-administration can result in possible additive CNS depressant effects).
No products indexed under this heading.

Loxapine Succinate (Co-administration can result in possible additive CNS depressant effects). Products include:
Loxitane Capsules 3398

Maprotiline Hydrochloride (Propoxyphene may slow the metabolism of antidepressants; co-administration may result in higher serum concentrations of antidepressants resulting in increased pharmacologic or adverse effects concurrent use with antidepressants can result in possible additive CNS depressant effects).
No products indexed under this heading.

Meperidine Hydrochloride (Co-administration can result in possible additive CNS depressant effects). Products include:
Demerol 3079
Mepergan Injection 3539

Mephobarbital (Co-administration can result in possible additive CNS depressant effects).
No products indexed under this heading.

Meprobamate (Co-administration can result in possible additive CNS depressant effects). Products include:
Miltown Tablets 3349

Mesoridazine Besylate (Co-administration can result in possible additive CNS depressant effects). Products include:
Serentil 1057

Methadone Hydrochloride (Co-administration can result in possible additive CNS depressant effects). Products include:
Dolophine Hydrochloride Tablets 3056

Methocarbamol (Co-administration with muscle relaxants, such as methocarbamol, can result in possible additive CNS depressant effects). Products include:
Robaxin Injectable 2938
Robaxin Tablets 2939
Robaxisal Tablets 2939

Methohexital Sodium (Co-administration can result in possible additive CNS depressant effects). Products include:
Brevital Sodium for Injection, USP .. 1815

Methotrimeprazine (Co-administration can result in possible additive CNS depressant effects).
No products indexed under this heading.

Methoxyflurane (Co-administration can result in possible additive CNS depressant effects).
No products indexed under this heading.

Midazolam Hydrochloride (Co-administration can result in possible additive CNS depressant effects). Products include:
Versed Injection 3027

Versed Syrup 3033

Mirtazapine (Propoxyphene may slow the metabolism of antidepressants; co-administration may result in higher serum concentrations of antidepressants resulting in increased pharmacologic or adverse effects concurrent use with antidepressants can result in possible additive CNS depressant effects). Products include:

Remeron Tablets 2483
Remeron SolTab Tablets 2486

Molindone Hydrochloride (Co-administration can result in possible additive CNS depressant effects). Products include:

Moban 1320

Morphine Sulfate (Co-administration can result in possible additive CNS depressant effects). Products include:

Astramorph/PF Injection, USP (Preservative-Free) 594
Duramorph Injection 1312
Infumorph 200 and Infumorph 500 Sterile Solutions 1314
Kadian Capsules 1335
MS Contin Tablets 2896
MSIR 2898
Oramorph SR Tablets 3062
Roxanol 3066

Nefazodone Hydrochloride (Propoxyphene may slow the metabolism of antidepressants; co-administration may result in higher serum concentrations of antidepressants resulting in increased pharmacologic or adverse effects concurrent use with antidepressants can result in possible additive CNS depressant effects). Products include:

Serzone Tablets 1104

Nortriptyline Hydrochloride (Propoxyphene may slow the metabolism of antidepressants; co-administration may result in higher serum concentrations of antidepressants resulting in increased pharmacologic or adverse effects concurrent use with antidepressants can result in possible additive CNS depressant effects).

No products indexed under this heading.

Olanzapine (Co-administration can result in possible additive CNS depressant effects). Products include:

Zyprexa Tablets 1973
Zyprexa ZYDIS Orally Disintegrating Tablets 1973

Oxazepam (Co-administration can result in possible additive CNS depressant effects).

No products indexed under this heading.

Oxcarbazepine (Propoxyphene may slow the metabolism of anticonvulsants; co-administration may result in higher serum concentrations of anticonvulsants resulting in increased pharmacologic or adverse effects). Products include:

Trileptal Oral Suspension 2407
Trileptal Tablets 2407

Oxycodone Hydrochloride (Co-administration can result in possible additive CNS depressant effects). Products include:

OxyContin Tablets 2912
OxyFast Oral Concentrate Solution . 2916
OxyIR Capsules 2916
Percocet Tablets 1326
Percodan Tablets 1327
Percolone Tablets 1327
Roxicodone 3067
Tylox Capsules 2597

Paroxetine Hydrochloride (Propoxyphene may slow the metabolism of antidepressants; co-administration may result in higher serum concentrations of antidepressants resulting in increased pharmacologic or adverse effects concurrent use with antidepressants can result in possible additive CNS depressant effects). Products include:

Paxil 1609

Pentobarbital Sodium (Co-administration can result in possible additive CNS depressant effects). Products include:

Nembutal Sodium Solution 485

Perphenazine (Co-administration can result in possible additive CNS depressant effects). Products include:

Etrafon 3115
Trilafon 3160

Phenelzine Sulfate (Propoxyphene may slow the metabolism of antidepressants; co-administration may result in higher serum concentrations of antidepressants resulting in increased pharmacologic or adverse effects concurrent use with antidepressants can result in possible additive CNS depressant effects). Products include:

Nardil Tablets 2653

Phenobarbital (Co-administration can result in possible additive CNS depressant effects; propoxyphene may slow the metabolism of anticonvulsants; co-administration may result in higher serum concentrations of anticonvulsants resulting in increased pharmacologic or adverse effects). Products include:

Arco-Lase Plus Tablets 592
Donnatal 2929
Donnatal Extentabs 2930

Prazepam (Co-administration can result in possible additive CNS depressant effects).

No products indexed under this heading.

Prochlorperazine (Co-administration can result in possible additive CNS depressant effects). Products include:

Compazine 1505

Promethazine Hydrochloride (Co-administration can result in possible additive CNS depressant effects). Products include:

Mepergan Injection 3539
Phenergan Injection 3553
Phenergan 3556
Phenergan Syrup 3554
Phenergan with Codeine Syrup 3557
Phenergan with Dextromethorphan Syrup 3559
Phenergan VC Syrup 3560
Phenergan VC with Codeine Syrup ... 3561

Propofol (Co-administration can result in possible additive CNS depressant effects). Products include:

Diprivan Injectable Emulsion 667

Propoxyphene Hydrochloride (Co-administration can result in possible additive CNS depressant effects). Products include:

Darvon Pulvules 1909
Darvon Compound-65 Pulvules 1910

Protriptyline Hydrochloride (Propoxyphene may slow the metabolism of antidepressants; co-administration may result in higher serum concentrations of antidepressants resulting in increased pharmacologic or adverse effects concurrent use with antidepressants can result in possible additive CNS depressant effects). Products include:

Vivactil Tablets 2446
Vivactil Tablets 2217

Quazepam (Co-administration can result in possible additive CNS depressant effects).

No products indexed under this heading.

Quetiapine Fumarate (Co-administration can result in possible additive CNS depressant effects). Products include:

Seroquel Tablets 684

Remifentanil Hydrochloride (Co-administration can result in possible additive CNS depressant effects).

No products indexed under this heading.

Risperidone (Co-administration can result in possible additive CNS depressant effects). Products include:

Risperdal 1796

Secobarbital Sodium (Co-administration can result in possible additive CNS depressant effects).

No products indexed under this heading.

Sertraline Hydrochloride (Propoxyphene may slow the metabolism of antidepressants; co-administration may result in higher serum concentrations of antidepressants resulting in increased pharmacologic or adverse effects concurrent use with antidepressants can result in possible additive CNS depressant effects). Products include:

Zoloft 2751

Sevoflurane (Co-administration can result in possible additive CNS depressant effects).

No products indexed under this heading.

Sufentanil Citrate (Co-administration can result in possible additive CNS depressant effects).

No products indexed under this heading.

Temazepam (Co-administration can result in possible additive CNS depressant effects).

No products indexed under this heading.

Thiamylal Sodium (Co-administration can result in possible additive CNS depressant effects).

No products indexed under this heading.

Thioridazine Hydrochloride (Co-administration can result in possible additive CNS depressant effects). Products include:

Thioridazine Hydrochloride Tablets 2289

Thiothixene (Co-administration can result in possible additive CNS depressant effects). Products include:

Navane Capsules 2701
Thiothixene Capsules 2290

Tiagabine Hydrochloride (Propoxyphene may slow the metabolism of anticonvulsants; co-administration may result in higher serum concentrations of anticonvulsants resulting in increased pharmacologic or adverse effects). Products include:

Gabitril Tablets 1189

Tranylcypromine Sulfate (Propoxyphene may slow the metabolism of antidepressants; co-administration may result in higher serum concentrations of antidepressants resulting in increased pharmacologic or adverse effects concurrent use with antidepressants can result in possible additive CNS depressant effects). Products include:

Parnate Tablets 1607

Trazodone Hydrochloride (Propoxyphene may slow the metabolism of antidepressants; co-administration may result in higher serum concentrations of antidepressants resulting in increased pharmacologic or adverse effects concurrent use with antidepressants can result in possible additive CNS depressant effects).

No products indexed under this heading.

Triazolam (Co-administration can result in possible additive CNS depressant effects). Products include:

Halcion Tablets 2823

Trifluoperazine Hydrochloride (Co-administration can result in possible additive CNS depressant effects). Products include:

Stelazine 1640

Trimipramine Maleate (Propoxyphene may slow the metabolism of antidepressants; co-administration may result in higher serum concentrations of antidepressants resulting in increased pharmacologic or adverse effects concurrent use with antidepressants can result in possible additive CNS depressant effects). Products include:

Surmontil Capsules 3595

Venlafaxine Hydrochloride (Propoxyphene may slow the metabolism of antidepressants; co-administration may result in higher serum concentrations of antidepressants resulting in increased pharmacologic or adverse effects concurrent use with antidepressants can result in possible additive CNS depressant effects). Products include:

Effexor Tablets 3495
Effexor XR Capsules 3499

Warfarin Sodium (Propoxyphene may slow the metabolism of warfarin-like drugs; co-administration may result in higher serum concentrations of anticoagulants resulting in increased pharmacologic or adverse effects). Products include:

Coumadin for Injection 1243
Coumadin Tablets 1243
Warfarin Sodium Tablets, USP 3302

Zaleplon (Co-administration can result in possible additive CNS depressant effects). Products include:

Sonata Capsules 3591

Ziprasidone Hydrochloride (Co-administration can result in possible additive CNS depressant effects). Products include:

Geodon Capsules 2688

Zolpidem Tartrate (Co-administration can result in possible additive CNS depressant effects). Products include:

Ambien Tablets 3191

Zonisamide (Propoxyphene may slow the metabolism of anticonvulsants; co-administration may result in higher serum concentrations of anticonvulsants resulting in increased pharmacologic or adverse effects). Products include:

Zonegran Capsules 1307

Food Interactions

Alcohol (Concurrent use can lead to potentially serious CNS depressant effects).

DAUNOXOME INJECTION

(Daunorubicin Citrate) 1442

May interact with anthracycline antibiotics and their derivatives. Compounds in these categories include:

Daunorubicin Hydrochloride (Special attention must be given to the potential cardiac toxicity of DaunoXome, particularly in patients who have received prior anthracyclines). Products include:

Cerubidine for Injection 947

Doxorubicin Hydrochloride (Special attention must be given to the potential cardiac toxicity of DaunoXome, particularly in patients who have received prior anthracyclines). Products include:

Adriamycin PFS/RDF Injection 2767
Doxil Injection 566

Epirubicin Hydrochloride (Special attention must be given to the potential cardiac toxicity of DaunoXome, particularly in patients who have received prior anthracyclines). Products include:

Ellence Injection 2806

Idarubicin Hydrochloride (Special attention must be given to the potential cardiac toxicity of DaunoXome, particularly in patients who have received prior anthracyclines). Products include:

Idamycin PFS Injection 2825

D-CAL CHEWABLE CAPLETS
(Calcium Carbonate, Vitamin D) ...... ▣794
None cited in PDR database.

DDAVP INJECTION 4 MCG/ML
(Desmopressin Acetate) 737
May interact with vasopressors. Compounds in these categories include:

Dopamine Hydrochloride (Co-administration with other pressor agents may result in possible additive pressor activity).
No products indexed under this heading.

Epinephrine Bitartrate (Co-administration with other pressor agents may result in possible additive pressor activity). Products include:
Sensorcaine 643

Epinephrine Hydrochloride (Co-administration with other pressor agents may result in possible additive pressor activity).
No products indexed under this heading.

Metaraminol Bitartrate (Co-administration with other pressor agents may result in possible additive pressor activity). Products include:
Aramine Injection 2043

Methoxamine Hydrochloride (Co-administration with other pressor agents may result in possible additive pressor activity).
No products indexed under this heading.

Norepinephrine Bitartrate (Co-administration with other pressor agents may result in possible additive pressor activity).
No products indexed under this heading.

Phenylephrine Hydrochloride (Co-administration with other pressor agents may result in possible additive pressor activity). Products include:
Afrin Nasal Decongestant Children's Pump Mist .... ▣734
Extendryl 1361
Hycomine Compound Tablets 1317
Neo-Synephrine .... ▣614
Phenergan VC Syrup 3560
Phenergan VC with Codeine Syrup . 3561
Preparation H Cream .... ▣778
Preparation H Cooling Gel .... ▣778
Preparation H .... ▣778
Vicks Sinex Nasal Spray and Ultra Fine Mist .... ▣729

DDAVP NASAL SPRAY
(Desmopressin Acetate) 738
See DDAVP Injection 4 mcg/mL

DDAVP RHINAL TUBE
(Desmopressin Acetate) 738
See DDAVP Injection 4 mcg/mL

DDAVP TABLETS
(Desmopressin Acetate) 739
May interact with vasopressors. Compounds in these categories include:

Dopamine Hydrochloride (Although the pressor activity of DDAVP is very low, large doses of DDAVP tablets should be used with other vasopressor agents only with careful patient monitoring).
No products indexed under this heading.

Epinephrine Bitartrate (Although the pressor activity of DDAVP is very low, large doses of DDAVP tablets should be used with other vasopressor agents only with careful patient monitoring). Products include:
Sensorcaine 643

Epinephrine Hydrochloride (Although the pressor activity of DDAVP is very low, large doses of DDAVP tablets should be used with other vasopressor agents only with careful patient monitoring).
No products indexed under this heading.

Metaraminol Bitartrate (Although the pressor activity of DDAVP is very low, large doses of DDAVP tablets should be used with other vasopressor agents only with careful patient monitoring). Products include:
Aramine Injection 2043

Methoxamine Hydrochloride (Although the pressor activity of DDAVP is very low, large doses of DDAVP tablets should be used with other vasopressor agents only with careful patient monitoring).
No products indexed under this heading.

Norepinephrine Bitartrate (Although the pressor activity of DDAVP is very low, large doses of DDAVP tablets should be used with other vasopressor agents only with careful patient monitoring).
No products indexed under this heading.

Phenylephrine Hydrochloride (Although the pressor activity of DDAVP is very low, large doses of DDAVP tablets should be used with other vasopressor agents only with careful patient monitoring). Products include:
Afrin Nasal Decongestant Children's Pump Mist .... ▣734
Extendryl 1361
Hycomine Compound Tablets 1317
Neo-Synephrine .... ▣614
Phenergan VC Syrup 3560
Phenergan VC with Codeine Syrup . 3561
Preparation H Cream .... ▣778
Preparation H Cooling Gel .... ▣778
Preparation H .... ▣778
Vicks Sinex Nasal Spray and Ultra Fine Mist .... ▣729

DDS-ACIDOPHILUS CAPSULES, TABLETS, AND POWDER
(Lactobacillus Acidophilus) .... ▣767
None cited in PDR database.

DEBROX DROPS
(Carbamide Peroxide) .... ▣747
None cited in PDR database.

DECADRON ELIXIR
(Dexamethasone) 2078
May interact with oral anticoagulants, oral hypoglycemic agents, insulin, potassium-depleting diuretics, and certain other agents. Compounds in these categories include:

Acarbose (Potential for increased requirements of oral hypoglycemic agents). Products include:
Precose Tablets 906

Aspirin (Aspirin should be used cautiously in conjunction with corticosteroids in hypoprothrombinemia). Products include:
Aggrenox Capsules 1026
Alka-Seltzer .... ▣603
Alka-Seltzer Lemon Lime Antacid and Pain Reliever Effervescent Tablets .... ▣603
Alka-Seltzer Extra Strength Antacid and Pain Reliever Effervescent Tablets .... ▣603
Alka-Seltzer PM Effervescent Tablets .... ▣605
Genuine Bayer Tablets, Caplets and Gelcaps .... ▣606
Extra Strength Bayer Caplets and Gelcaps .... ▣610
Aspirin Regimen Bayer Children's Chewable Tablets (Orange or Cherry Flavored) .... ▣607
Bayer, Aspirin Regimen .... ▣606
Aspirin Regimen Bayer 81 mg Caplets with Calcium .... ▣607
Genuine Bayer Professional Labeling (Aspirin Regimen Bayer) .... ▣608
Extra Strength Bayer Arthritis Caplets .... ▣610
Extra Strength Bayer Plus Caplets .... ▣610
Extra Strength Bayer PM Caplets .. ▣611
BC Powder .... ▣619
BC Allergy Sinus Cold Powder ...... ▣619
Arthritis Strength BC Powder .... ▣619
BC Sinus Cold Powder .... ▣619
Darvon Compound-65 Pulvules 1910
Ecotrin Enteric Coated Aspirin Low, Regular and Maximum Strength Tablets 1715
Excedrin Extra-Strength Tablets, Caplets, and Geltabs .... ▣629
Excedrin Migraine 1070
Goody's Body Pain Formula Powder .... ▣620
Goody's Extra Strength Headache Powder .... ▣620
Goody's Extra Strength Pain Relief Tablets .... ▣620
Percodan Tablets 1327
Robaxisal Tablets 2939
Soma Compound Tablets 3354
Soma Compound w/Codeine Tablets 3355
Vanquish Caplets .... ▣617

Bendroflumethiazide (Co-administration may result in hypokalemia). Products include:
Corzide 40/5 Tablets 2247
Corzide 80/5 Tablets 2247

Bumetanide (Co-administration may result in hypokalemia).
No products indexed under this heading.

Chlorothiazide (Co-administration may result in hypokalemia). Products include:
Aldoclor Tablets 2035
Diuril Oral 2087

Chlorothiazide Sodium (Co-administration may result in hypokalemia). Products include:
Diuril Sodium Intravenous 2086

Chlorpropamide (Potential for increased requirements of oral hypoglycemic agents). Products include:
Diabinese Tablets 2680

Dicumarol (Potential for altered response to coumarin anticoagulants).
No products indexed under this heading.

Ephedrine Hydrochloride (Enhanced metabolic clearance of corticosteroids). Products include:
Primatene Tablets .... ▣780

Ephedrine Sulfate (Enhanced metabolic clearance of corticosteroids).
No products indexed under this heading.

Ephedrine Tannate (Enhanced metabolic clearance of corticosteroids). Products include:
Rynatuss Pediatric Suspension 3353
Rynatuss Tablets 3353

Ethacrynic Acid (Co-administration may result in hypokalemia). Products include:
Edecrin Tablets 2091

Fosphenytoin Sodium (Enhanced metabolic clearance of corticosteroids). Products include:
Cerebyx Injection 2619

Furosemide (Co-administration may result in hypokalemia). Products include:
Furosemide Tablets 2284

Glimepiride (Potential for increased requirements of oral hypoglycemic agents). Products include:
Amaryl Tablets 717

Glipizide (Potential for increased requirements of oral hypoglycemic agents). Products include:
Glucotrol Tablets 2692
Glucotrol XL Extended Release Tablets 2693

Glyburide (Potential for increased requirements of oral hypoglycemic agents). Products include:
DiaBeta Tablets 741
Glucovance Tablets 1086

Hydrochlorothiazide (Co-administration may result in hypokalemia). Products include:
Accuretic Tablets 2614
Aldoril Tablets 2039
Atacand HCT Tablets 597
Avalide Tablets 1070
Diovan HCT Tablets 2338
Dyazide Capsules 1515
HydroDIURIL Tablets 2108
Hyzaar 2109
Inderide Tablets 3517
Inderide LA Long-Acting Capsules .. 3519
Lotensin HCT Tablets 2367
Maxzide 1008
Micardis HCT Tablets 1051
Microzide Capsules 3414
Moduretic Tablets 2138
Monopril HCT 1094
Prinzide Tablets 2168
Timolide Tablets 2187
Uniretic Tablets 3178
Vaseretic Tablets 2204
Zestoretic Tablets 695
Ziac Tablets 1887

Hydroflumethiazide (Co-administration may result in hypokalemia). Products include:
Diucardin Tablets 3494

Insulin, Human, Zinc Suspension (Potential for increased requirements of insulin). Products include:
Humulin L, 100 Units 1937
Humulin U, 100 Units 1943
Novolin L Human Insulin 10 ml Vials 2422

Insulin, Human NPH (Potential for increased requirements of insulin). Products include:
Humulin N, 100 Units 1939
Humulin N NPH Pen 1940
Novolin N Human Insulin 10 ml Vials 2422
Novolin N PenFill 2423
Novolin N Prefilled Syringe Disposable Insulin Delivery System 2425

Insulin, Human Regular (Potential for increased requirements of insulin). Products include:
Humulin R Regular (U-500) 1943
Humulin R, 100 Units 1941
Novolin R Human Insulin 10 ml Vials 2423
Novolin R PenFill 2423
Novolin R Prefilled Syringe Disposable Insulin Delivery System 2425
Velosulin BR Human Insulin 10 ml Vials 2435

Insulin, Human Regular and Human NPH Mixture (Potential for increased requirements of insulin). Products include:
Humulin 50/50, 100 Units 1934
Humulin 70/30, 100 Units 1935
Humulin 70/30 Pen 1936
Novolin 70/30 Human Insulin 10 ml Vials 2421
Novolin 70/30 PenFill 2423
Novolin 70/30 Prefilled Disposable Insulin Delivery System 2425

Insulin, NPH (Potential for increased requirements of insulin). Products include:
Iletin II, NPH (Pork), 100 Units 1946

Insulin, Regular (Potential for increased requirements of insulin). Products include:
Iletin II, Regular (Pork), 100 Units ... 1947

Insulin, Zinc Crystals (Potential for increased requirements of insulin).
No products indexed under this heading.

Insulin, Zinc Suspension (Potential for increased requirements of insulin). Products include:
Iletin II, Lente (Pork), 100 Units 1945

Insulin Aspart, Human Regular (Potential for increased requirements of insulin).
No products indexed under this heading.

Insulin glargine (Potential for increased requirements of insulin). Products include:

Lantus Injection 742

Insulin Lispro, Human (Potential for increased requirements of insulin). Products include:

Humalog 1926
Humalog Mix 75/25 Pen 1928

Insulin Lispro Protamine, Human (Potential for increased requirements of insulin). Products include:

Humalog Mix 75/25 Pen 1928

Live Virus Vaccines (Co-administration is contraindicated in patients receiving immunosuppressive doses of corticosteroids).

Metformin Hydrochloride (Potential for increased requirements of oral hypoglycemic agents). Products include:

Glucophage Tablets 1080
Glucophage XR Tablets 1080
Glucovance Tablets 1086

Methyclothiazide (Co-administration may result in hypokalemia).

No products indexed under this heading.

Miglitol (Potential for increased requirements of oral hypoglycemic agents). Products include:

Glyset Tablets 2821

Phenobarbital (Enhanced metabolic clearance of corticosteroids). Products include:

Arco-Lase Plus Tablets 592
Donnatal 2929
Donnatal Extentabs 2930

Phenytoin (Enhanced metabolic clearance of corticosteroids). Products include:

Dilantin Infatabs 2624
Dilantin-125 Oral Suspension 2625

Phenytoin Sodium (Enhanced metabolic clearance of corticosteroids). Products include:

Dilantin Kapseals 2622

Pioglitazone Hydrochloride (Potential for increased requirements of oral hypoglycemic agents). Products include:

Actos Tablets 3275

Polythiazide (Co-administration may result in hypokalemia). Products include:

Minizide Capsules 2700
Renese Tablets 2712

Repaglinide (Potential for increased requirements of oral hypoglycemic agents). Products include:

Prandin Tablets (0.5, 1, and 2 mg) 2432

Rifampin (Enhanced metabolic clearance of corticosteroids). Products include:

Rifadin 765
Rifamate Capsules 767
Rifater Tablets 769

Rosiglitazone Maleate (Potential for increased requirements of oral hypoglycemic agents). Products include:

Avandia Tablets 1490

Tolazamide (Potential for increased requirements of oral hypoglycemic agents).

No products indexed under this heading.

Tolbutamide (Potential for increased requirements of oral hypoglycemic agents).

No products indexed under this heading.

Torsemide (Co-administration may result in hypokalemia). Products include:

Demadex Tablets and Injection 2965

Troglitazone (Potential for increased requirements of oral hypoglycemic agents).

No products indexed under this heading.

Warfarin Sodium (Potential for altered response to coumarin anticoagulants). Products include:

Coumadin for Injection 1243
Coumadin Tablets 1243
Warfarin Sodium Tablets, USP 3302

DECADRON TABLETS

(Dexamethasone) 2079

May interact with oral anticoagulants, oral hypoglycemic agents, insulin, potassium-depleting diuretics, and certain other agents. Compounds in these categories include:

Acarbose (Increased requirements for oral hypoglycemic agents in diabetes). Products include:

Precose Tablets 906

Aspirin (Aspirin should be used cautiously in conjunction with corticosteroids in hypoprothrombinemia). Products include:

Aggrenox Capsules 1026
Alka-Seltzer .... ▣603
Alka-Seltzer Lemon Lime Antacid and Pain Reliever Effervescent Tablets .... ▣603
Alka-Seltzer Extra Strength Antacid and Pain Reliever Effervescent Tablets .... ▣603
Alka-Seltzer PM Effervescent Tablets .... ▣605
Genuine Bayer Tablets, Caplets and Gelcaps .... ▣606
Extra Strength Bayer Caplets and Gelcaps .... ▣610
Aspirin Regimen Bayer Children's Chewable Tablets (Orange or Cherry Flavored) .... ▣607
Bayer, Aspirin Regimen .... ▣606
Aspirin Regimen Bayer 81 mg Caplets with Calcium .... ▣607
Genuine Bayer Professional Labeling (Aspirin Regimen Bayer) .... ▣608
Extra Strength Bayer Arthritis Caplets .... ▣610
Extra Strength Bayer Plus Caplets .... ▣610
Extra Strength Bayer PM Caplets .... ▣611
BC Powder .... ▣619
BC Allergy Sinus Cold Powder .... ▣619
Arthritis Strength BC Powder .... ▣619
BC Sinus Cold Powder .... ▣619
Darvon Compound-65 Pulvules 1910
Ecotrin Enteric Coated Aspirin Low, Regular and Maximum Strength Tablets 1715
Excedrin Extra-Strength Tablets, Caplets, and Geltabs .... ▣629
Excedrin Migraine 1070
Goody's Body Pain Formula Powder .... ▣620
Goody's Extra Strength Headache Powder .... ▣620
Goody's Extra Strength Pain Relief Tablets .... ▣620
Percodan Tablets 1327
Robaxisal Tablets 2939
Soma Compound Tablets 3354
Soma Compound w/Codeine Tablets 3355
Vanquish Caplets .... ▣617

Bendroflumethiazide (Co-administration may result in hypokalemia). Products include:

Corzide 40/5 Tablets 2247
Corzide 80/5 Tablets 2247

Bumetanide (Co-administration may result in hypokalemia).

No products indexed under this heading.

Chlorothiazide (Co-administration may result in hypokalemia). Products include:

Aldoclor Tablets 2035
Diuril Oral 2087

Chlorothiazide Sodium (Co-administration may result in hypokalemia). Products include:

Diuril Sodium Intravenous 2086

Chlorpropamide (Increased requirements for oral hypoglycemic agents in diabetes). Products include:

Diabinese Tablets 2680

Dicumarol (Potential for altered response to coumarin anticoagulants).

No products indexed under this heading.

Ephedrine Hydrochloride (Enhanced metabolic clearance of corticosteroids). Products include:

Primatene Tablets .... ▣780

Ephedrine Sulfate (Enhanced metabolic clearance of corticosteroids).

No products indexed under this heading.

Ephedrine Tannate (Enhanced metabolic clearance of corticosteroids). Products include:

Rynatuss Pediatric Suspension 3353
Rynatuss Tablets 3353

Ethacrynic Acid (Co-administration may result in hypokalemia). Products include:

Edecrin Tablets 2091

Fosphenytoin Sodium (Enhanced metabolic clearance of corticosteroids). Products include:

Cerebyx Injection 2619

Furosemide (Co-administration may result in hypokalemia). Products include:

Furosemide Tablets 2284

Glimepiride (Increased requirements for oral hypoglycemic agents in diabetes). Products include:

Amaryl Tablets 717

Glipizide (Increased requirements for oral hypoglycemic agents in diabetes). Products include:

Glucotrol Tablets 2692
Glucotrol XL Extended Release Tablets 2693

Glyburide (Increased requirements for oral hypoglycemic agents in diabetes). Products include:

DiaBeta Tablets 741
Glucovance Tablets 1086

Hydrochlorothiazide (Co-administration may result in hypokalemia). Products include:

Accuretic Tablets 2614
Aldoril Tablets 2039
Atacand HCT Tablets 597
Avalide Tablets 1070
Diovan HCT Tablets 2338
Dyazide Capsules 1515
HydroDIURIL Tablets 2108
Hyzaar 2109
Inderide Tablets 3517
Inderide LA Long-Acting Capsules 3519
Lotensin HCT Tablets 2367
Maxzide 1008
Micardis HCT Tablets 1051
Microzide Capsules 3414
Moduretic Tablets 2138
Monopril HCT 1094
Prinzide Tablets 2168
Timolide Tablets 2187
Uniretic Tablets 3178
Vaseretic Tablets 2204
Zestoretic Tablets 695
Ziac Tablets 1887

Hydroflumethiazide (Co-administration may result in hypokalemia). Products include:

Diucardin Tablets 3494

Insulin, Human, Zinc Suspension (Increased requirements for insulin in diabetes). Products include:

Humulin L, 100 Units 1937
Humulin U, 100 Units 1943
Novolin L Human Insulin 10 ml Vials 2422

Insulin, Human NPH (Increased requirements for insulin in diabetes). Products include:

Humulin N, 100 Units 1939
Humulin N NPH Pen 1940
Novolin N Human Insulin 10 ml Vials 2422
Novolin N PenFill 2423
Novolin N Prefilled Syringe Disposable Insulin Delivery System 2425

Insulin, Human Regular (Increased requirements for insulin in diabetes). Products include:

Humulin R Regular (U-500) 1943
Humulin R, 100 Units 1941
Novolin R Human Insulin 10 ml Vials 2423
Novolin R PenFill 2423
Novolin R Prefilled Syringe Disposable Insulin Delivery System 2425
Velosulin BR Human Insulin 10 ml Vials 2435

Insulin, Human Regular and Human NPH Mixture (Increased requirements for insulin in diabetes). Products include:

Humulin 50/50, 100 Units 1934
Humulin 70/30, 100 Units 1935
Humulin 70/30 Pen 1936
Novolin 70/30 Human Insulin 10 ml Vials 2421
Novolin 70/30 PenFill 2423
Novolin 70/30 Prefilled Disposable Insulin Delivery System 2425

Insulin, NPH (Increased requirements for insulin in diabetes). Products include:

Iletin II, NPH (Pork), 100 Units 1946

Insulin, Regular (Increased requirements for insulin in diabetes). Products include:

Iletin II, Regular (Pork), 100 Units 1947

Insulin, Zinc Crystals (Increased requirements for insulin in diabetes).

No products indexed under this heading.

Insulin, Zinc Suspension (Increased requirements for insulin in diabetes). Products include:

Iletin II, Lente (Pork), 100 Units 1945

Insulin Aspart, Human Regular (Increased requirements for insulin in diabetes).

No products indexed under this heading.

Insulin glargine (Increased requirements for insulin in diabetes). Products include:

Lantus Injection 742

Insulin Lispro, Human (Increased requirements for insulin in diabetes). Products include:

Humalog 1926
Humalog Mix 75/25 Pen 1928

Insulin Lispro Protamine, Human (Increased requirements for insulin in diabetes). Products include:

Humalog Mix 75/25 Pen 1928

Live Virus Vaccines (Co-administration is contraindicated in patients receiving immunosuppressive doses of corticosteroids).

Metformin Hydrochloride (Increased requirements for oral hypoglycemic agents in diabetes). Products include:

Glucophage Tablets 1080
Glucophage XR Tablets 1080
Glucovance Tablets 1086

Methyclothiazide (Co-administration may result in hypokalemia).

No products indexed under this heading.

Miglitol (Increased requirements for oral hypoglycemic agents in diabetes). Products include:

Glyset Tablets 2821

Phenobarbital (Enhanced metabolic clearance of corticosteroids). Products include:

Arco-Lase Plus Tablets 592
Donnatal 2929
Donnatal Extentabs 2930

Phenytoin (Enhanced metabolic clearance of corticosteroids). Products include:

Dilantin Infatabs 2624
Dilantin-125 Oral Suspension 2625

Phenytoin Sodium (Enhanced metabolic clearance of corticosteroids). Products include:

Dilantin Kapseals 2622

Pioglitazone Hydrochloride (Increased requirements for oral hypoglycemic agents in diabetes). Products include:

Actos Tablets 3275

Polythiazide (Co-administration may result in hypokalemia). Products include:

Minizide Capsules 2700
Renese Tablets 2712

Repaglinide (Increased requirements for oral hypoglycemic agents in diabetes). Products include:

Prandin Tablets (0.5, 1, and 2 mg) ... 2432

Rifampin (Enhanced metabolic clearance of corticosteroids). Products include:
- Rifadin ... 765
- Rifamate Capsules ... 767
- Rifater Tablets ... 769

Rosiglitazone Maleate (Increased requirements for oral hypoglycemic agents in diabetes). Products include:
- Avandia Tablets ... 1490

Tolazamide (Increased requirements for oral hypoglycemic agents in diabetes).
- No products indexed under this heading.

Tolbutamide (Increased requirements for oral hypoglycemic agents in diabetes).
- No products indexed under this heading.

Torsemide (Co-administration may result in hypokalemia). Products include:
- Demadex Tablets and Injection ... 2965

Troglitazone (Increased requirements for oral hypoglycemic agents in diabetes).
- No products indexed under this heading.

Warfarin Sodium (Potential for altered response to coumarin anticoagulants). Products include:
- Coumadin for Injection ... 1243
- Coumadin Tablets ... 1243
- Warfarin Sodium Tablets, USP ... 3302

DECADRON PHOSPHATE INJECTION

(Dexamethasone Sodium Phosphate) ... 2081

May interact with oral anticoagulants, oral hypoglycemic agents, insulin, potassium-depleting diuretics, and certain other agents. Compounds in these categories include:

Acarbose (Potential for increased requirements of oral hypoglycemic agents). Products include:
- Precose Tablets ... 906

Aspirin (Aspirin should be used cautiously in conjunction with corticosteroids in hypoprothrombinemia). Products include:
- Aggrenox Capsules ... 1026
- Alka-Seltzer ... ■603
- Alka-Seltzer Lemon Lime Antacid and Pain Reliever Effervescent Tablets ... ■603
- Alka-Seltzer Extra Strength Antacid and Pain Reliever Effervescent Tablets ... ■603
- Alka-Seltzer PM Effervescent Tablets ... ■605
- Genuine Bayer Tablets, Caplets and Gelcaps ... ■606
- Extra Strength Bayer Caplets and Gelcaps ... ■610
- Aspirin Regimen Bayer Children's Chewable Tablets (Orange or Cherry Flavored) ... ■607
- Bayer, Aspirin Regimen ... ■606
- Aspirin Regimen Bayer 81 mg Caplets with Calcium ... ■607
- Genuine Bayer Professional Labeling (Aspirin Regimen Bayer) ... ■608
- Extra Strength Bayer Arthritis Caplets ... ■610
- Extra Strength Bayer Plus Caplets ... ■610
- Extra Strength Bayer PM Caplets ... ■611
- BC Powder ... ■619
- BC Allergy Sinus Cold Powder ... ■619
- Arthritis Strength BC Powder ... ■619
- BC Sinus Cold Powder ... ■619
- Darvon Compound-65 Pulvules ... 1910
- Ecotrin Enteric Coated Aspirin Low, Regular and Maximum Strength Tablets ... 1715
- Excedrin Extra-Strength Tablets, Caplets, and Geltabs ... ■629
- Excedrin Migraine ... 1070
- Goody's Body Pain Formula Powder ... ■620
- Goody's Extra Strength Headache Powder ... ■620
- Goody's Extra Strength Pain Relief Tablets ... ■620
- Percodan Tablets ... 1327
- Robaxisal Tablets ... 2939
- Soma Compound Tablets ... 3354
- Soma Compound w/Codeine Tablets ... 3355
- Vanquish Caplets ... ■617

Bendroflumethiazide (Co-administration may result in hypokalemia). Products include:
- Corzide 40/5 Tablets ... 2247
- Corzide 80/5 Tablets ... 2247

Bumetanide (Co-administration may result in hypokalemia).
- No products indexed under this heading.

Chlorothiazide (Co-administration may result in hypokalemia). Products include:
- Aldoclor Tablets ... 2035
- Diuril Oral ... 2087

Chlorothiazide Sodium (Co-administration may result in hypokalemia). Products include:
- Diuril Sodium Intravenous ... 2086

Chlorpropamide (Potential for increased requirements of oral hypoglycemic agents). Products include:
- Diabinese Tablets ... 2680

Dicumarol (Potential for altered response to coumarin anticoagulants).
- No products indexed under this heading.

Ephedrine Hydrochloride (Enhanced metabolic clearance of corticosteroids). Products include:
- Primatene Tablets ... ■780

Ephedrine Sulfate (Enhanced metabolic clearance of corticosteroids).
- No products indexed under this heading.

Ephedrine Tannate (Enhanced metabolic clearance of corticosteroids). Products include:
- Rynatuss Pediatric Suspension ... 3353
- Rynatuss Tablets ... 3353

Ethacrynic Acid (Co-administration may result in hypokalemia). Products include:
- Edecrin Tablets ... 2091

Fosphenytoin Sodium (Enhanced metabolic clearance of corticosteroids). Products include:
- Cerebyx Injection ... 2619

Furosemide (Co-administration may result in hypokalemia). Products include:
- Furosemide Tablets ... 2284

Glimepiride (Potential for increased requirements of oral hypoglycemic agents). Products include:
- Amaryl Tablets ... 717

Glipizide (Potential for increased requirements of oral hypoglycemic agents). Products include:
- Glucotrol Tablets ... 2692
- Glucotrol XL Extended Release Tablets ... 2693

Glyburide (Potential for increased requirements of oral hypoglycemic agents). Products include:
- DiaBeta Tablets ... 741
- Glucovance Tablets ... 1086

Hydrochlorothiazide (Co-administration may result in hypokalemia). Products include:
- Accuretic Tablets ... 2614
- Aldoril Tablets ... 2039
- Atacand HCT Tablets ... 597
- Avalide Tablets ... 1070
- Diovan HCT Tablets ... 2338
- Dyazide Capsules ... 1515
- HydroDIURIL Tablets ... 2108
- Hyzaar ... 2109
- Inderide Tablets ... 3517
- Inderide LA Long-Acting Capsules ... 3519
- Lotensin HCT Tablets ... 2367
- Maxzide ... 1008
- Micardis HCT Tablets ... 1051
- Microzide Capsules ... 3414
- Moduretic Tablets ... 2138
- Monopril HCT ... 1094
- Prinzide Tablets ... 2168
- Timolide Tablets ... 2187
- Uniretic Tablets ... 3178
- Vaseretic Tablets ... 2204
- Zestoretic Tablets ... 695
- Ziac Tablets ... 1887

Hydroflumethiazide (Co-administration may result in hypokalemia). Products include:
- Diucardin Tablets ... 3494

Insulin, Human, Zinc Suspension (Potential for increased requirements of insulin). Products include:
- Humulin L, 100 Units ... 1937
- Humulin U, 100 Units ... 1943
- Novolin L Human Insulin 10 ml Vials ... 2422

Insulin, Human NPH (Potential for increased requirements of insulin). Products include:
- Humulin N, 100 Units ... 1939
- Humulin N NPH Pen ... 1940
- Novolin N Human Insulin 10 ml Vials ... 2422
- Novolin N PenFill ... 2423
- Novolin N Prefilled Syringe Disposable Insulin Delivery System ... 2425

Insulin, Human Regular (Potential for increased requirements of insulin). Products include:
- Humulin R Regular (U-500) ... 1943
- Humulin R, 100 Units ... 1941
- Novolin R Human Insulin 10 ml Vials ... 2423
- Novolin R PenFill ... 2423
- Novolin R Prefilled Syringe Disposable Insulin Delivery System ... 2425
- Velosulin BR Human Insulin 10 ml Vials ... 2435

Insulin, Human Regular and Human NPH Mixture (Potential for increased requirements of insulin). Products include:
- Humulin 50/50, 100 Units ... 1934
- Humulin 70/30, 100 Units ... 1935
- Humulin 70/30 Pen ... 1936
- Novolin 70/30 Human Insulin 10 ml Vials ... 2421
- Novolin 70/30 PenFill ... 2423
- Novolin 70/30 Prefilled Disposable Insulin Delivery System ... 2425

Insulin, NPH (Potential for increased requirements of insulin). Products include:
- Iletin II, NPH (Pork), 100 Units ... 1946

Insulin, Regular (Potential for increased requirements of insulin). Products include:
- Iletin II, Regular (Pork), 100 Units ... 1947

Insulin, Zinc Crystals (Potential for increased requirements of insulin).
- No products indexed under this heading.

Insulin, Zinc Suspension (Potential for increased requirements of insulin). Products include:
- Iletin II, Lente (Pork), 100 Units ... 1945

Insulin Aspart, Human Regular (Potential for increased requirements of insulin).
- No products indexed under this heading.

Insulin glargine (Potential for increased requirements of insulin). Products include:
- Lantus Injection ... 742

Insulin Lispro, Human (Potential for increased requirements of insulin). Products include:
- Humalog ... 1926
- Humalog Mix 75/25 Pen ... 1928

Insulin Lispro Protamine, Human (Potential for increased requirements of insulin). Products include:
- Humalog Mix 75/25 Pen ... 1928

Live Virus Vaccines (Co-administration is contraindicated in patients receiving immunosuppressive doses of corticosteroids).

Metformin Hydrochloride (Potential for increased requirements of oral hypoglycemic agents). Products include:
- Glucophage Tablets ... 1080
- Glucophage XR Tablets ... 1080
- Glucovance Tablets ... 1086

Methyclothiazide (Co-administration may result in hypokalemia).
- No products indexed under this heading.

Miglitol (Potential for increased requirements of oral hypoglycemic agents). Products include:
- Glyset Tablets ... 2821

Phenobarbital (Enhanced metabolic clearance of corticosteroids). Products include:
- Arco-Lase Plus Tablets ... 592
- Donnatal ... 2929
- Donnatal Extentabs ... 2930

Phenytoin (Enhanced metabolic clearance of corticosteroids). Products include:
- Dilantin Infatabs ... 2624
- Dilantin-125 Oral Suspension ... 2625

Phenytoin Sodium (Enhanced metabolic clearance of corticosteroids). Products include:
- Dilantin Kapseals ... 2622

Pioglitazone Hydrochloride (Potential for increased requirements of oral hypoglycemic agents). Products include:
- Actos Tablets ... 3275

Polythiazide (Co-administration may result in hypokalemia). Products include:
- Minizide Capsules ... 2700
- Renese Tablets ... 2712

Repaglinide (Potential for increased requirements of oral hypoglycemic agents). Products include:
- Prandin Tablets (0.5, 1, and 2 mg) ... 2432

Rifampin (Enhanced metabolic clearance of corticosteroids). Products include:
- Rifadin ... 765
- Rifamate Capsules ... 767
- Rifater Tablets ... 769

Rosiglitazone Maleate (Potential for increased requirements of oral hypoglycemic agents). Products include:
- Avandia Tablets ... 1490

Tolazamide (Potential for increased requirements of oral hypoglycemic agents).
- No products indexed under this heading.

Tolbutamide (Potential for increased requirements of oral hypoglycemic agents).
- No products indexed under this heading.

Torsemide (Co-administration may result in hypokalemia). Products include:
- Demadex Tablets and Injection ... 2965

Troglitazone (Potential for increased requirements of oral hypoglycemic agents).
- No products indexed under this heading.

Warfarin Sodium (Potential for altered response to coumarin anticoagulants). Products include:
- Coumadin for Injection ... 1243
- Coumadin Tablets ... 1243
- Warfarin Sodium Tablets, USP ... 3302

DECADRON PHOSPHATE STERILE OPHTHALMIC OINTMENT

(Dexamethasone Sodium Phosphate) ... 2083

None cited in PDR database.

DECADRON PHOSPHATE STERILE OPHTHALMIC SOLUTION

(Dexamethasone Sodium Phosphate) ... 2084

None cited in PDR database.

DECLOMYCIN TABLETS
(Demeclocycline Hydrochloride) 1855
May interact with antacids containing aluminum, calcium and magnesium, oral anticoagulants, iron containing oral preparations, oral contraceptives, penicillins, and certain other agents. Compounds in these categories include:

Aluminum Carbonate (Absorption of tetracyclines is impaired by antacids containing aluminum, calcium, and magnesium).
No products indexed under this heading.

Aluminum Hydroxide (Absorption of tetracyclines is impaired by antacids containing aluminum, calcium, and magnesium). Products include:
Amphojel Suspension (Mint Flavor) ■ 789
Gaviscon Extra Strength Liquid ■ 751
Gaviscon Extra Strength Tablets ■ 751
Gaviscon Regular Strength Liquid ■ 751
Gaviscon Regular Strength Tablets ■ 750
Maalox Antacid/Anti-Gas Oral Suspension ■ 673
Maalox Max Maximum Strength Antacid/Anti-Gas Liquid 2300
Maalox Regular Strength Antacid/Antigas Liquid 2300
Mylanta 1813
Vanquish Caplets ■ 617

Amoxicillin Trihydrate (Bacteriostatic drugs may interfere with the bactericidal action of penicillin; avoid giving tetracycline-class drugs in conjunction with penicillin).

Ampicillin (Interference with bactericidal action of penicillin).
No products indexed under this heading.

Ampicillin Sodium (Bacteriostatic drugs may interfere with the bactericidal action of penicillin; avoid giving tetracycline-class drugs in conjunction with penicillin). Products include:
Unasyn for Injection 2728

Ampicillin Trihydrate (Bacteriostatic drugs may interfere with the bactericidal action of penicillin; avoid giving tetracycline-class drugs in conjunction with penicillin).
No products indexed under this heading.

Azlocillin Sodium (Bacteriostatic drugs may interfere with the bactericidal action of penicillin; avoid giving tetracycline-class drugs in conjunction with penicillin).
No products indexed under this heading.

Bacampicillin Hydrochloride (Bacteriostatic drugs may interfere with the bactericidal action of penicillin; avoid giving tetracycline-class drugs in conjunction with penicillin).
No products indexed under this heading.

Calcium Carbonate (Absorption of tetracyclines is impaired by antacids containing aluminum, calcium, and magnesium). Products include:
Aspirin Regimen Bayer 81 mg Caplets with Calcium ■ 607
Extra Strength Bayer Plus Caplets ■ 610
Caltrate 600 Tablets ■ 814
Caltrate 600 PLUS ■ 815
Caltrate 600 + D Tablets ■ 814
Caltrate 600 + Soy Tablets ■ 814
D-Cal Chewable Caplets ■ 794
Florical Capsules and Tablets 2223
Quick Dissolve Maalox Max Maximum Strength Antacid/Antigas Tablets 2301
Quick Dissolve Maalox Regular Strength Antacid Tablets 2301
Marblen Suspension ■ 633
Monocal Tablets 2223
Mylanta Fast-Acting 1813
Mylanta Calci Tabs ■ 636
One-A-Day Bedtime & Rest Tablets ■ 805
One-A-Day Calcium Plus Chewable Tablets ■ 805
Os-Cal Chewable Tablets ■ 838
Pepcid Complete Chewable Tablets 1815
ReSource Wellness CalciWise Soft Chews ■ 824
Rolaids Tablets ■ 706
Extra Strength Rolaids Tablets ■ 706
Slow-Mag Tablets ■ 835
Titralac ■ 640
3M Titralac Plus Antacid Tablets ■ 640
Tums ■ 763

Carbenicillin Disodium (Bacteriostatic drugs may interfere with the bactericidal action of penicillin; avoid giving tetracycline-class drugs in conjunction with penicillin).
No products indexed under this heading.

Carbenicillin Indanyl Sodium (Bacteriostatic drugs may interfere with the bactericidal action of penicillin; avoid giving tetracycline-class drugs in conjunction with penicillin). Products include:
Geocillin Tablets 2687

Desogestrel (Concurrent use of tetracycline with oral contraceptives may render oral contraceptives less effective). Products include:
Cyclessa Tablets 2450
Desogen Tablets 2458
Mircette Tablets 2470
Ortho-Cept 21 Tablets 2546
Ortho-Cept 28 Tablets 2546

Dicloxacillin Sodium (Bacteriostatic drugs may interfere with the bactericidal action of penicillin; avoid giving tetracycline-class drugs in conjunction with penicillin).
No products indexed under this heading.

Dicumarol (Tetracyclines depress the plasma prothrombin activity; downward adjustment of the anticoagulant dosage may be required).
No products indexed under this heading.

Ethinyl Estradiol (Concurrent use of tetracycline with oral contraceptives may render oral contraceptives less effective). Products include:
Alesse-21 Tablets 3468
Alesse-28 Tablets 3473
Brevicon 28-Day Tablets 3380
Cyclessa Tablets 2450
Desogen Tablets 2458
Estinyl Tablets 3112
Estrostep 2627
femhrt Tablets 2635
Levlen 962
Levlite 21 Tablets 962
Levlite 28 Tablets 962
Levora Tablets 3389
Loestrin 21 Tablets 2642
Loestrin Fe Tablets 2642
Lo/Ovral Tablets 3532
Lo/Ovral-28 Tablets 3538
Low-Ogestrel-28 Tablets 3392
Microgestin Fe 1.5/30 Tablets 3407
Microgestin Fe 1/20 Tablets 3400
Mircette Tablets 2470
Modicon 2563
Necon 3415
Nordette-28 Tablets 2257
Norinyl 1 +35 28-Day Tablets 3380
Ogestrel 0.5/50-28 Tablets 3428
Ortho-Cept 21 Tablets 2546
Ortho-Cept 28 Tablets 2546
Ortho-Cyclen/Ortho Tri-Cyclen 2573
Ortho-Novum 2563
Ovcon 3364
Ovral Tablets 3551
Ovral-28 Tablets 3552
Tri-Levlen 962
Tri-Norinyl-28 Tablets 3433
Triphasil-21 Tablets 3600
Triphasil-28 Tablets 3605
Trivora Tablets 3439
Yasmin 28 Tablets 980
Zovia 3449

Ethynodiol Diacetate (Concurrent use of tetracycline with oral contraceptives may render oral contraceptives less effective). Products include:
Zovia 3449

Ferrous Fumarate (Absorption of tetracyclines is impaired by iron-containing preparations). Products include:
New Formulation Chromagen OB Capsules 3094
Loestrin Fe Tablets 2642
NataChew Tablets 3364

Ferrous Gluconate (Absorption of tetracyclines is impaired by iron-containing preparations). Products include:
Fergon Iron Tablets ■ 802

Ferrous Sulfate (Absorption of tetracyclines is impaired by iron-containing preparations). Products include:
Feosol Tablets 1717
Slow Fe Tablets ■ 827
Slow Fe with Folic Acid Tablets ■ 828

Iron (Absorption of tetracyclines is impaired by iron-containing preparations).
No products indexed under this heading.

Levonorgestrel (Concurrent use of tetracycline with oral contraceptives may render oral contraceptives less effective). Products include:
Alesse-21 Tablets 3468
Alesse-28 Tablets 3473
Levlen 962
Levlite 21 Tablets 962
Levlite 28 Tablets 962
Levora Tablets 3389
Mirena Intrauterine System 974
Nordette-28 Tablets 2257
Norplant System 3543
Tri-Levlen 962
Triphasil-21 Tablets 3600
Triphasil-28 Tablets 3605
Trivora Tablets 3439

Magaldrate (Absorption of tetracyclines is impaired by antacids containing aluminum, calcium, and magnesium).
No products indexed under this heading.

Magnesium Hydroxide (Absorption of tetracyclines is impaired by antacids containing aluminum, calcium, and magnesium). Products include:
Ex•Lax Milk of Magnesia Liquid ■ 670
Maalox Antacid/Anti-Gas Oral Suspension ■ 673
Maalox Max Maximum Strength Antacid/Anti-Gas Liquid 2300
Maalox Regular Strength Antacid/Antigas Liquid 2300
Mylanta Fast-Acting 1813
Mylanta 1813
Pepcid Complete Chewable Tablets 1815
Phillips' Chewable Tablets ■ 615
Phillips' Milk of Magnesia Liquid (Original, Cherry, & Mint) ■ 616
Rolaids Tablets ■ 706
Extra Strength Rolaids Tablets ■ 706
Vanquish Caplets ■ 617

Magnesium Oxide (Absorption of tetracyclines is impaired by antacids containing aluminum, calcium, and magnesium). Products include:
Beelith Tablets 946
Mag-Ox 400 Tablets 1024
Uro-Mag Capsules 1024

Mestranol (Concurrent use of tetracycline with oral contraceptives may render oral contraceptives less effective). Products include:
Necon 1/50 Tablets 3415
Norinyl 1 + 50 28-Day Tablets 3380
Ortho-Novum 1/50□28 Tablets 2556

Methoxyflurane (Co-administration results in fatal renal toxicity).
No products indexed under this heading.

Mezlocillin Sodium (Bacteriostatic drugs may interfere with the bactericidal action of penicillin; avoid giving tetracycline-class drugs in conjunction with penicillin).
No products indexed under this heading.

Nafcillin Sodium (Bacteriostatic drugs may interfere with the bactericidal action of penicillin; avoid giving tetracycline-class drugs in conjunction with penicillin).
No products indexed under this heading.

Norethindrone (Concurrent use of tetracycline with oral contraceptives may render oral contraceptives less effective). Products include:
Brevicon 28-Day Tablets 3380
Micronor Tablets 2543
Modicon 2563
Necon 3415
Norinyl 1 +35 28-Day Tablets 3380
Norinyl 1 + 50 28-Day Tablets 3380
Nor-QD Tablets 3423
Ortho-Novum 2563
Ortho-Novum 1/50□28 Tablets 2556
Ovcon 3364
Tri-Norinyl-28 Tablets 3433

Norethynodrel (Concurrent use of tetracycline with oral contraceptives may render oral contraceptives less effective).
No products indexed under this heading.

Norgestimate (Concurrent use of tetracycline with oral contraceptives may render oral contraceptives less effective). Products include:
Ortho-Cyclen/Ortho Tri-Cyclen 2573
Ortho-Prefest Tablets 2570

Norgestrel (Concurrent use of tetracycline with oral contraceptives may render oral contraceptives less effective). Products include:
Lo/Ovral Tablets 3532
Lo/Ovral-28 Tablets 3538
Low-Ogestrel-28 Tablets 3392
Ogestrel 0.5/50-28 Tablets 3428
Ovral Tablets 3551
Ovral-28 Tablets 3552
Ovrette Tablets 3552

Penicillin G Benzathine (Bacteriostatic drugs may interfere with the bactericidal action of penicillin; avoid giving tetracycline-class drugs in conjunction with penicillin). Products include:
Bicillin C-R 900/300 Injection 2240
Bicillin C-R Injection 2238
Bicillin L-A Injection 2242
Permapen Isoject 2706

Penicillin G Potassium (Bacteriostatic drugs may interfere with the bactericidal action of penicillin; avoid giving tetracycline-class drugs in conjunction with penicillin). Products include:
Pfizerpen for Injection 2707

Penicillin G Procaine (Bacteriostatic drugs may interfere with the bactericidal action of penicillin; avoid giving tetracycline-class drugs in conjunction with penicillin). Products include:
Bicillin C-R 900/300 Injection 2240
Bicillin C-R Injection 2238

Penicillin G Sodium (Interference with bactericidal action of penicillin).
No products indexed under this heading.

Penicillin V Potassium (Bacteriostatic drugs may interfere with the bactericidal action of penicillin; avoid giving tetracycline-class drugs in conjunction with penicillin).
No products indexed under this heading.

Polysaccharide-Iron Complex (Absorption of tetracyclines is impaired by iron-containing preparations). Products include:
Niferex 3176
Niferex-150 Capsules 3176
Nu-Iron 150 Capsules 2224

Ticarcillin Disodium (Bacteriostatic drugs may interfere with the bactericidal action of penicillin; avoid giving tetracycline-class drugs in conjunction with penicillin). Products include:
Timentin Injection- ADD-Vantage Vial 1661
Timentin Injection-Galaxy Container 1664
Timentin Injection-Pharmacy Bulk Package 1666
Timentin for Intravenous Administration 1658

Warfarin Sodium (Tetracyclines depress the plasma prothrombin

activity; downward adjustment of the anticoagulant dosage may be required). Products include:
Coumadin for Injection 1243
Coumadin Tablets 1243
Warfarin Sodium Tablets, USP 3302

Food Interactions

Dairy products (Interferes with absorption).

Food, unspecified (Interferes with absorption).

DELATESTRYL INJECTION

(Testosterone Enanthate) 1151

May interact with corticosteroids, oral anticoagulants, oral hypoglycemic agents, insulin, and certain other agents. Compounds in these categories include:

Acarbose (In diabetic patients, the metabolic effects of androgens may decrease blood glucose and, therefore, antidiabetic drug requirements). Products include:
Precose Tablets 906

ACTH (Co-administration of testosterone with ACTH may enhance edema formation).
No products indexed under this heading.

Betamethasone Acetate (Co-administration of testosterone with corticosteroids may enhance edema formation). Products include:
Celestone Soluspan Injectable Suspension 3097

Betamethasone Sodium Phosphate (Co-administration of testosterone with corticosteroids may enhance edema formation). Products include:
Celestone Soluspan Injectable Suspension 3097

Chlorpropamide (In diabetic patients, the metabolic effects of androgens may decrease blood glucose and, therefore, antidiabetic drug requirements). Products include:
Diabinese Tablets 2680

Cortisone Acetate (Co-administration of testosterone with corticosteroids may enhance edema formation). Products include:
Cortone Acetate Injectable Suspension 2059
Cortone Acetate Tablets 2061

Dexamethasone (Co-administration of testosterone with corticosteroids may enhance edema formation). Products include:
Decadron Elixir 2078
Decadron Tablets 2079
TobraDex Ophthalmic Ointment 542
TobraDex Ophthalmic Suspension .. 541

Dexamethasone Acetate (Co-administration of testosterone with corticosteroids may enhance edema formation).
No products indexed under this heading.

Dexamethasone Sodium Phosphate (Co-administration of testosterone with corticosteroids may enhance edema formation). Products include:
Decadron Phosphate Injection 2081
Decadron Phosphate Sterile Ophthalmic Ointment 2083
Decadron Phosphate Sterile Ophthalmic Solution 2084
NeoDecadron Sterile Ophthalmic Solution 2144

Dicumarol (Co-administration of C-17 substituted derivatives of testosterone have been reported to decrease the anticoagulant requirements; concomitant therapy has resulted in bleeding).
No products indexed under this heading.

Fludrocortisone Acetate (Co-administration of testosterone with corticosteroids may enhance edema formation). Products include:
Florinef Acetate Tablets 2250

Glimepiride (In diabetic patients, the metabolic effects of androgens may decrease blood glucose and, therefore, antidiabetic drug requirements). Products include:
Amaryl Tablets 717

Glipizide (In diabetic patients, the metabolic effects of androgens may decrease blood glucose and, therefore, antidiabetic drug requirements). Products include:
Glucotrol Tablets 2692
Glucotrol XL Extended Release Tablets 2693

Glyburide (In diabetic patients, the metabolic effects of androgens may decrease blood glucose and, therefore, antidiabetic drug requirements). Products include:
DiaBeta Tablets 741
Glucovance Tablets 1086

Hydrocortisone (Co-administration of testosterone with corticosteroids may enhance edema formation). Products include:
Anusol-HC Cream 2.5% 2237
Cipro HC Otic Suspension 540
Cortaid Intensive Therapy Cream .. ■ 717
Cortaid Maximum Strength Cream .... ■ 717
Cortisporin Ophthalmic Suspension Sterile .... ⊙ 297
Cortizone•5 .... ■ 699
Cortizone•10 .... ■ 699
Cortizone•10 Plus Creme .... ■ 700
Cortizone for Kids Creme .... ■ 699
Hydrocortone Tablets 2106
Massengill Medicated Soft Cloth Towelette .... ■ 753
VōSoL HC Otic Solution 3356

Hydrocortisone Acetate (Co-administration of testosterone with corticosteroids may enhance edema formation). Products include:
Analpram-HC 1338
Anusol HC-1 Hydrocortisone Anti-Itch Cream .... ■ 689
Anusol-HC Suppositories 2238
Cortaid .... ■ 717
Cortifoam Rectal Foam 3170
Cortisporin-TC Otic Suspension 2246
Hydrocortone Acetate Injectable Suspension 2103
Pramosone 1343
Proctocort Suppositories 2264
ProctoFoam-HC 3177
Terra-Cortril Ophthalmic Suspension 2716

Hydrocortisone Sodium Phosphate (Co-administration of testosterone with corticosteroids may enhance edema formation). Products include:
Hydrocortone Phosphate Injection, Sterile 2105

Hydrocortisone Sodium Succinate (Co-administration of testosterone with corticosteroids may enhance edema formation).
No products indexed under this heading.

Insulin, Human, Zinc Suspension (In diabetic patients, the metabolic effects of androgens may decrease blood glucose and, therefore, insulin requirements). Products include:
Humulin L, 100 Units 1937
Humulin U, 100 Units 1943
Novolin L Human Insulin 10 ml Vials 2422

Insulin, Human NPH (In diabetic patients, the metabolic effects of androgens may decrease blood glucose and, therefore, insulin requirements). Products include:
Humulin N, 100 Units 1939
Humulin N NPH Pen 1940
Novolin N Human Insulin 10 ml Vials 2422
Novolin N PenFill 2423
Novolin N Prefilled Syringe Disposable Insulin Delivery System 2425

Insulin, Human Regular (In diabetic patients, the metabolic effects of androgens may decrease blood glucose and, therefore, insulin requirements). Products include:
Humulin R Regular (U-500) 1943
Humulin R, 100 Units 1941
Novolin R Human Insulin 10 ml Vials 2423
Novolin R PenFill 2423
Novolin R Prefilled Syringe Disposable Insulin Delivery System 2425
Velosulin BR Human Insulin 10 ml Vials 2435

Insulin, Human Regular and Human NPH Mixture (In diabetic patients, the metabolic effects of androgens may decrease blood glucose and, therefore, insulin requirements). Products include:
Humulin 50/50, 100 Units 1934
Humulin 70/30, 100 Units 1935
Humulin 70/30 Pen 1936
Novolin 70/30 Human Insulin 10 ml Vials 2421
Novolin 70/30 PenFill 2423
Novolin 70/30 Prefilled Disposable Insulin Delivery System 2425

Insulin, NPH (In diabetic patients, the metabolic effects of androgens may decrease blood glucose and, therefore, insulin requirements). Products include:
Iletin II, NPH (Pork), 100 Units 1946

Insulin, Regular (In diabetic patients, the metabolic effects of androgens may decrease blood glucose and, therefore, insulin requirements). Products include:
Iletin II, Regular (Pork), 100 Units ... 1947

Insulin, Zinc Crystals (In diabetic patients, the metabolic effects of androgens may decrease blood glucose and, therefore, insulin requirements).
No products indexed under this heading.

Insulin, Zinc Suspension (In diabetic patients, the metabolic effects of androgens may decrease blood glucose and, therefore, insulin requirements). Products include:
Iletin II, Lente (Pork), 100 Units 1945

Insulin Aspart, Human Regular (In diabetic patients, the metabolic effects of androgens may decrease blood glucose and, therefore, insulin requirements).
No products indexed under this heading.

Insulin glargine (In diabetic patients, the metabolic effects of androgens may decrease blood glucose and, therefore, insulin requirements). Products include:
Lantus Injection 742

Insulin Lispro, Human (In diabetic patients, the metabolic effects of androgens may decrease blood glucose and, therefore, insulin requirements). Products include:
Humalog 1926
Humalog Mix 75/25 Pen 1928

Insulin Lispro Protamine, Human (In diabetic patients, the metabolic effects of androgens may decrease blood glucose and, therefore, insulin requirements). Products include:
Humalog Mix 75/25 Pen 1928

Metformin Hydrochloride (In diabetic patients, the metabolic effects of androgens may decrease blood glucose and, therefore, antidiabetic drug requirements). Products include:
Glucophage Tablets 1080
Glucophage XR Tablets 1080
Glucovance Tablets 1086

Methylprednisolone Acetate (Co-administration of testosterone with corticosteroids may enhance edema formation). Products include:
Depo-Medrol Injectable Suspension 2795

Methylprednisolone Sodium Succinate (Co-administration of testosterone with corticosteroids may enhance edema formation). Products include:
Solu-Medrol Sterile Powder 2855

Miglitol (In diabetic patients, the metabolic effects of androgens may decrease blood glucose and, therefore, antidiabetic drug requirements). Products include:
Glyset Tablets 2821

Oxyphenbutazone (Co-administration of androgens and oxyphenbutazone may result in elevated serum levels of oxyphenbutazone).
No products indexed under this heading.

Pioglitazone Hydrochloride (In diabetic patients, the metabolic effects of androgens may decrease blood glucose and, therefore, antidiabetic drug requirements). Products include:
Actos Tablets 3275

Prednisolone Acetate (Co-administration of testosterone with corticosteroids may enhance edema formation). Products include:
Blephamide Ophthalmic Ointment .. 547
Blephamide Ophthalmic Suspension 548
Poly-Pred Liquifilm Ophthalmic Suspension .... ⊙ 245
Pred Forte Ophthalmic Suspension .... ⊙ 246
Pred Mild Sterile Ophthalmic Suspension .... ⊙ 249
Pred-G Ophthalmic Suspension ..... ⊙ 247
Pred-G Sterile Ophthalmic Ointment .... ⊙ 248

Prednisolone Sodium Phosphate (Co-administration of testosterone with corticosteroids may enhance edema formation). Products include:
Pediapred Oral Solution 1170

Prednisolone Tebutate (Co-administration of testosterone with corticosteroids may enhance edema formation).
No products indexed under this heading.

Prednisone (Co-administration of testosterone with corticosteroids may enhance edema formation). Products include:
Prednisone 3064

Repaglinide (In diabetic patients, the metabolic effects of androgens may decrease blood glucose and, therefore, antidiabetic drug requirements). Products include:
Prandin Tablets (0.5, 1, and 2 mg) 2432

Rosiglitazone Maleate (In diabetic patients, the metabolic effects of androgens may decrease blood glucose and, therefore, antidiabetic drug requirements). Products include:
Avandia Tablets 1490

Tolazamide (In diabetic patients, the metabolic effects of androgens may decrease blood glucose and, therefore, antidiabetic drug requirements).
No products indexed under this heading.

Tolbutamide (In diabetic patients, the metabolic effects of androgens may decrease blood glucose and, therefore, antidiabetic drug requirements).
No products indexed under this heading.

Triamcinolone (Co-administration of testosterone with corticosteroids may enhance edema formation).
No products indexed under this heading.

Triamcinolone Acetonide (Co-administration of testosterone with corticosteroids may enhance edema formation). Products include:

Azmacort Inhalation Aerosol 728
Nasacort Nasal Inhaler 750
Nasacort AQ Nasal Spray 752
Tri-Nasal Spray 2274

Triamcinolone Diacetate (Co-administration of testosterone with corticosteroids may enhance edema formation).
No products indexed under this heading.

Triamcinolone Hexacetonide (Co-administration of testosterone with corticosteroids may enhance edema formation).
No products indexed under this heading.

Troglitazone (In diabetic patients, the metabolic effects of androgens may decrease blood glucose and, therefore, antidiabetic drug requirements).
No products indexed under this heading.

Warfarin Sodium (Co-administration of C-17 substituted derivatives of testosterone have been reported to decrease the anti-coagulant requirements; concomitant therapy has resulted in bleeding). Products include:
Coumadin for Injection 1243
Coumadin Tablets 1243
Warfarin Sodium Tablets, USP 3302

DELSYM EXTENDED-RELEASE SUSPENSION

(Dextromethorphan Polistirex) 664
May interact with monoamine oxidase inhibitors. Compounds in these categories include:

Isocarboxazid (Concurrent and/or sequential use is not recommended).
No products indexed under this heading.

Moclobemide (Concurrent and/or sequential use is not recommended).
No products indexed under this heading.

Pargyline Hydrochloride (Concurrent and/or sequential use is not recommended).
No products indexed under this heading.

Phenelzine Sulfate (Concurrent and/or sequential use is not recommended). Products include:
Nardil Tablets 2653

Procarbazine Hydrochloride (Concurrent and/or sequential use is not recommended). Products include:
Matulane Capsules 3246

Selegiline Hydrochloride (Concurrent and/or sequential use is not recommended). Products include:
Eldepryl Capsules 3266

Tranylcypromine Sulfate (Concurrent and/or sequential use is not recommended). Products include:
Parnate Tablets 1607

DEMADEX TABLETS AND INJECTION

(Torsemide) 2965
May interact with aminoglycosides, lithium preparations, non-steroidal anti-inflammatory agents, salicylates, and certain other agents. Compounds in these categories include:

Amikacin Sulfate (Co-administration of other diuretics has been reported to increase the ototoxic potential of aminoglycoside antibiotics, especially in the presence of impaired renal function; concurrent use of aminoglycoside and tosemide has not been studied, however, such combined therapy should be undertaken with great caution).
No products indexed under this heading.

Aspirin (Co-administration in patients receiving high dose of salicylates may be associated with salicylate toxicity due to competition for secretion by renal tubule). Products include:
Aggrenox Capsules 1026
Alka-Seltzer 603
Alka-Seltzer Lemon Lime Antacid and Pain Reliever Effervescent Tablets 603
Alka-Seltzer Extra Strength Antacid and Pain Reliever Effervescent Tablets 603
Alka-Seltzer PM Effervescent Tablets 605
Genuine Bayer Tablets, Caplets and Gelcaps 606
Extra Strength Bayer Caplets and Gelcaps 610
Aspirin Regimen Bayer Children's Chewable Tablets (Orange or Cherry Flavored) 607
Bayer, Aspirin Regimen 606
Aspirin Regimen Bayer 81 mg Caplets with Calcium 607
Genuine Bayer Professional Labeling (Aspirin Regimen Bayer) 608
Extra Strength Bayer Arthritis Caplets 610
Extra Strength Bayer Plus Caplets 610
Extra Strength Bayer PM Caplets 611
BC Powder 619
BC Allergy Sinus Cold Powder 619
Arthritis Strength BC Powder 619
BC Sinus Cold Powder 619
Darvon Compound-65 Pulvules 1910
Ecotrin Enteric Coated Aspirin Low, Regular and Maximum Strength Tablets 1715
Excedrin Extra-Strength Tablets, Caplets, and Geltabs 629
Excedrin Migraine 1070
Goody's Body Pain Formula Powder 620
Goody's Extra Strength Headache Powder 620
Goody's Extra Strength Pain Relief Tablets 620
Percodan Tablets 1327
Robaxisal Tablets 2939
Soma Compound Tablets 3354
Soma Compound w/Codeine Tablets 3355
Vanquish Caplets 617

Celecoxib (Co-administration of another loop diuretic and nonsteroidal anti-inflammatory agents has been associated with renal dysfunction; concurrent use of torsemide and these agents has not been studied, however, such combined therapy should be undertaken with great caution). Products include:
Celebrex Capsules 2676
Celebrex Capsules 2780

Cholestyramine (Possibility of decreased oral absorption of torsemide; simultaneous administration is not recommended).
No products indexed under this heading.

Choline Magnesium Trisalicylate (Co-administration in patients receiving high dose of salicylates may be associated with salicylate toxicity due to competition for secretion by renal tubule). Products include:
Trilisate 2901

Diclofenac Potassium (Co-administration of another loop diuretic and nonsteroidal anti-inflammatory agents has been associated with renal dysfunction; concurrent use of torsemide and these agents has not been studied, however, such combined therapy should be undertaken with great caution). Products include:
Cataflam Tablets 2315

Diclofenac Sodium (Co-administration of another loop diuretic and nonsteroidal anti-inflammatory agents has been associated with renal dysfunction; concurrent use of torsemide and these agents has not been studied, however, such combined therapy should be undertaken with great caution). Products include:
Arthrotec Tablets 3195
Voltaren Ophthalmic Sterile Ophthalmic Solution .... ⊙ 312
Voltaren Tablets 2315
Voltaren-XR Tablets 2315

Diflunisal (Co-administration in patients receiving high dose of salicylates may be associated with salicylate toxicity due to competition for secretion by renal tubule). Products include:
Dolobid Tablets 2088

Digoxin (Co-administration of digoxin is reported to increase the AUC for torsemide by 50%). Products include:
Digitek Tablets 1003
Lanoxicaps Capsules 1574
Lanoxin Injection 1581
Lanoxin Tablets 1587
Lanoxin Elixir Pediatric 1578
Lanoxin Injection Pediatric 1584

Etodolac (Co-administration of another loop diuretic and nonsteroidal anti-inflammatory agents has been associated with renal dysfunction; concurrent use of torsemide and these agents has not been studied, however, such combined therapy should be undertaken with great caution). Products include:
Lodine 3528
Lodine XL Extended-Release Tablets 3530

Fenoprofen Calcium (Co-administration of another loop diuretic and nonsteroidal anti-inflammatory agents has been associated with renal dysfunction; concurrent use of torsemide and these agents has not been studied, however, such combined therapy should be undertaken with great caution).
No products indexed under this heading.

Flurbiprofen (Co-administration of another loop diuretic and nonsteroidal anti-inflammatory agents has been associated with renal dysfunction; concurrent use of torsemide and these agents has not been studied, however, such combined therapy should be undertaken with great caution).
No products indexed under this heading.

Gentamicin Sulfate (Co-administration of other diuretics has been reported to increase the ototoxic potential of aminoglycoside antibiotics, especially in the presence of impaired renal function; concurrent use of aminoglycoside and tosemide has not been studied, however, such combined therapy should be undertaken with great caution). Products include:
Genoptic Ophthalmic Ointment .... ⊙ 239
Genoptic Sterile Ophthalmic Solution .... ⊙ 239
Pred-G Ophthalmic Suspension .... ⊙ 247
Pred-G Sterile Ophthalmic Ointment .... ⊙ 248

Ibuprofen (Co-administration of another loop diuretic and nonsteroidal anti-inflammatory agents has been associated with renal dysfunction; concurrent use of torsemide and these agents has not been studied, however, such combined therapy should be undertaken with great caution). Products include:
Advil 771
Children's Advil Oral Suspension 773
Children's Advil Chewable Tablets 773
Advil Cold and Sinus Caplets 771
Advil Cold and Sinus Tablets 771
Advil Flu & Body Ache Caplets 772
Infants' Advil Drops 773
Junior Strength Advil Tablets 773
Junior Strength Advil Chewable Tablets 773
Advil Migraine Liquigels 772
Children's Motrin Oral Suspension and Chewable Tablets 2006
Children's Motrin Cold Oral Suspension 2007
Children's Motrin Oral Suspension 643
Motrin Suspension, Oral Drops, Chewable Tablets, and Caplets 2002
Infants' Motrin Concentrated Drops 2006
Junior Strength Motrin Caplets and Chewable Tablets 2006
Motrin IB Tablets, Caplets, and Gelcaps 2002
Motrin Migraine Pain Caplets 2005
Motrin Sinus Headache Caplets 2005
Vicoprofen Tablets 520

Indomethacin (The natriuretic effect of torsemide is partially inhibited by the co-administration). Products include:
Indocin 2112

Indomethacin Sodium Trihydrate (The natriuretic effect of torsemide is partially inhibited by the co-administration). Products include:
Indocin I.V. 2115

Kanamycin Sulfate (Co-administration of other diuretics has been reported to increase the ototoxic potential of aminoglycoside antibiotics, especially in the presence of impaired renal function; concurrent use of aminoglycoside and tosemide has not been studied, however, such combined therapy should be undertaken with great caution).
No products indexed under this heading.

Ketoprofen (Co-administration of another loop diuretic and nonsteroidal anti-inflammatory agents has been associated with renal dysfunction; concurrent use of torsemide and these agents has not been studied, however, such combined therapy should be undertaken with great caution). Products include:
Orudis Capsules 3548
Orudis KT Tablets 778
Oruvail Capsules 3548

Ketorolac Tromethamine (Co-administration of another loop diuretic and nonsteroidal anti-inflammatory agents has been associated with renal dysfunction; concurrent use of torsemide and these agents has not been studied, however, such combined therapy should be undertaken with great caution). Products include:
Acular Ophthalmic Solution 544
Acular PF Ophthalmic Solution 544
Toradol 3018

Lithium Carbonate (Co-administration of other diuretics are known to reduce the renal clearance of lithium, inducing a high risk of lithium toxicity; concurrent use of lithium and torsemide has not been studied, however, such combined therapy should be undertaken with great caution). Products include:
Eskalith 1527
Lithium Carbonate 3061
Lithobid Slow-Release Tablets 3255

Lithium Citrate (Co-administration of other diuretics are known to reduce the renal clearance of lithium, inducing a high risk of lithium toxicity; concurrent use of lithium and torsemide has not been studied, however, such combined therapy should be undertaken with great caution). Products include:
Lithium Citrate Syrup 3061

Magnesium Salicylate (Co-administration in patients receiving high dose of salicylates may be associated with salicylate toxicity due to competition for secretion by renal tubule). Products include:
Momentum Backache Relief Extra Strength Caplets 666

Meclofenamate Sodium (Co-administration of another loop diuretic and nonsteroidal anti-inflammatory agents has been associated with renal dysfunction; concurrent use of

torsemide and these agents has not been studied, however, such combined therapy should be undertaken with great caution).
No products indexed under this heading.

Mefenamic Acid (Co-administration of another loop diuretic and nonsteroidal anti-inflammatory agents has been associated with renal dysfunction; concurrent use of torsemide and these agents has not been studied, however, such combined therapy should be undertaken with great caution). Products include:
Ponstel Capsules 1356

Meloxicam (Co-administration of another loop diuretic and nonsteroidal anti-inflammatory agents has been associated with renal dysfunction; concurrent use of torsemide and these agents has not been studied, however, such combined therapy should be undertaken with great caution). Products include:
Mobic Tablets 1054

Nabumetone (Co-administration of another loop diuretic and nonsteroidal anti-inflammatory agents has been associated with renal dysfunction; concurrent use of torsemide and these agents has not been studied, however, such combined therapy should be undertaken with great caution). Products include:
Relafen Tablets 1617

Naproxen (Co-administration of another loop diuretic and nonsteroidal anti-inflammatory agents has been associated with renal dysfunction; concurrent use of torsemide and these agents has not been studied, however, such combined therapy should be undertaken with great caution). Products include:
EC-Naprosyn Delayed-Release Tablets 2967
Naprosyn Suspension 2967
Naprosyn Tablets 2967

Naproxen Sodium (Co-administration of another loop diuretic and nonsteroidal anti-inflammatory agents has been associated with renal dysfunction; concurrent use of torsemide and these agents has not been studied, however, such combined therapy should be undertaken with great caution). Products include:
Aleve Tablets, Caplets and Gelcaps .... ▣602
Aleve Cold & Sinus Caplets .... ▣603
Anaprox Tablets 2967
Anaprox DS Tablets 2967
Naprelan Tablets 1293

Oxaprozin (Co-administration of another loop diuretic and nonsteroidal anti-inflammatory agents has been associated with renal dysfunction; concurrent use of torsemide and these agents has not been studied, however, such combined therapy should be undertaken with great caution).
No products indexed under this heading.

Phenylbutazone (Co-administration of another loop diuretic and nonsteroidal anti-inflammatory agents has been associated with renal dysfunction; concurrent use of torsemide and these agents has not been studied, however, such combined therapy should be undertaken with great caution).
No products indexed under this heading.

Piroxicam (Co-administration of another loop diuretic and nonsteroidal anti-inflammatory agents has been associated with renal dysfunction; concurrent use of torsemide and these agents has not been studied, however, such combined therapy should be undertaken with great caution). Products include:
Feldene Capsules 2685

Probenecid (Reduces secretion of torsemide into the proximal tubule and thereby decreases diuretic effect).
No products indexed under this heading.

Rofecoxib (Co-administration of another loop diuretic and nonsteroidal anti-inflammatory agents has been associated with renal dysfunction; concurrent use of torsemide and these agents has not been studied, however, such combined therapy should be undertaken with great caution). Products include:
Vioxx 2213

Salsalate (Co-administration in patients receiving high dose of salicylates may be associated with salicylate toxicity due to competition for secretion by renal tubule).
No products indexed under this heading.

Spironolactone (Co-administration may be associated with significant reduction in the renal clearance of spironolactone, with corresponding increase in the AUC).
No products indexed under this heading.

Streptomycin Sulfate (Co-administration of other diuretics has been reported to increase the ototoxic potential of aminoglycoside antibiotics, especially in the presence of impaired renal function; concurrent use of aminoglycoside and tosemide has not been studied, however, such combined therapy should be undertaken with great caution). Products include:
Streptomycin Sulfate Injection 2714

Sulindac (Co-administration of another loop diuretic and nonsteroidal anti-inflammatory agents has been associated with renal dysfunction; concurrent use of torsemide and these agents has not been studied, however, such combined therapy should be undertaken with great caution). Products include:
Clinoril Tablets 2053

Tobramycin (Co-administration of other diuretics has been reported to increase the ototoxic potential of aminoglycoside antibiotics, especially in the presence of impaired renal function; concurrent use of aminoglycoside and tosemide has not been studied, however, such combined therapy should be undertaken with great caution). Products include:
TOBI Solution for Inhalation 1206
TobraDex Ophthalmic Ointment 542
TobraDex Ophthalmic Suspension 541
Tobrex Ophthalmic Ointment .... ⊙220
Tobrex Ophthalmic Solution .... ⊙221

Tobramycin Sulfate (Co-administration of other diuretics has been reported to increase the ototoxic potential of aminoglycoside antibiotics, especially in the presence of impaired renal function; concurrent use of aminoglycoside and tosemide has not been studied, however, such combined therapy should be undertaken with great caution). Products include:
Nebcin Vials, Hyporets & ADD-Vantage 1955

Tolmetin Sodium (Co-administration of another loop diuretic and nonsteroidal anti-inflammatory agents has been associated with renal dysfunction; concurrent use of torsemide and these agents has not been studied, however, such combined therapy should be undertaken with great caution). Products include:
Tolectin 2589

Food Interactions

Food, unspecified (Simultaneous food intake delays the time to Cmax by about 30 minutes, but overall bioavailability (AUC) and diuretic activity are unchanged).

DEMEROL SYRUP

(Meperidine Hydrochloride) 3079
See Demerol Tablets

DEMEROL TABLETS

(Meperidine Hydrochloride) 3079
May interact with antihistamines, barbiturates, central nervous system depressants, general anesthetics, hypnotics and sedatives, monoamine oxidase inhibitors, narcotic analgesics, phenothiazines, tranquilizers, tricyclic antidepressants, and certain other agents. Compounds in these categories include:

Acrivastine (Co-administration may result in respiratory depression, hypotension, and profound sedation or coma; reduced dosage of meperidine may be required if given concurrently). Products include:
Semprex-D Capsules 1172

Alfentanil Hydrochloride (Co-administration may result in respiratory depression, hypotension, and profound sedation or coma; reduced dosage of meperidine may be required if given concurrently).
No products indexed under this heading.

Alprazolam (Co-administration may result in respiratory depression, hypotension, and profound sedation or coma; reduced dosage of meperidine may be required if given concurrently). Products include:
Xanax Tablets 2865

Amitriptyline Hydrochloride (Co-administration may result in respiratory depression, hypotension, and profound sedation or coma; reduced dosage of meperidine may be required if given concurrently). Products include:
Etrafon 3115
Limbitrol 1738

Amoxapine (Co-administration may result in respiratory depression, hypotension, and profound sedation or coma; reduced dosage of meperidine may be required if given concurrently).
No products indexed under this heading.

Aprobarbital (Co-administration may result in respiratory depression, hypotension, and profound sedation or coma; reduced dosage of meperidine may be required if given concurrently).
No products indexed under this heading.

Astemizole (Co-administration may result in respiratory depression, hypotension, and profound sedation or coma; reduced dosage of meperidine may be required if given concurrently).
No products indexed under this heading.

Azatadine Maleate (Co-administration may result in respiratory depression, hypotension, and profound sedation or coma; reduced dosage of meperidine may be required if given concurrently). Products include:
Rynatan Tablets 3351

Bromodiphenhydramine Hydrochloride (Co-administration may result in respiratory depression, hypotension, and profound sedation or coma; reduced dosage of meperidine may be required if given concurrently).
No products indexed under this heading.

Brompheniramine Maleate (Co-administration may result in respiratory depression, hypotension, and profound sedation or coma; reduced dosage of meperidine may be required if given concurrently). Products include:
Bromfed Capsules (Extended-Release) 2269
Bromfed-PD Capsules (Extended-Release) 2269
Comtrex Acute Head Cold & Sinus Pressure Relief Tablets .... ▣627
Dimetapp Elixir .... ▣777
Dimetapp Cold and Fever Suspension .... ▣775
Dimetapp DM Cold & Cough Elixir .... ▣775
Dimetapp Nighttime Flu Liquid .... ▣776

Buprenorphine Hydrochloride (Co-administration may result in respiratory depression, hypotension, and profound sedation or coma; reduced dosage of meperidine may be required if given concurrently). Products include:
Buprenex Injectable 2918

Buspirone Hydrochloride (Co-administration may result in respiratory depression, hypotension, and profound sedation or coma; reduced dosage of meperidine may be required if given concurrently).
No products indexed under this heading.

Butabarbital (Co-administration may result in respiratory depression, hypotension, and profound sedation or coma; reduced dosage of meperidine may be required if given concurrently).
No products indexed under this heading.

Butalbital (Co-administration may result in respiratory depression, hypotension, and profound sedation or coma; reduced dosage of meperidine may be required if given concurrently). Products include:
Phrenilin 578
Sedapap Tablets 50 mg/650 mg 2225

Cetirizine Hydrochloride (Co-administration may result in respiratory depression, hypotension, and profound sedation or coma; reduced dosage of meperidine may be required if given concurrently). Products include:
Zyrtec 2756
Zyrtec-D 12 Hour Extended Relief Tablets 2758

Chlordiazepoxide (Co-administration may result in respiratory depression, hypotension, and profound sedation or coma; reduced dosage of meperidine may be required if given concurrently). Products include:
Limbitrol 1738

Chlordiazepoxide Hydrochloride (Co-administration may result in respiratory depression, hypotension, and profound sedation or coma; reduced dosage of meperidine may be required if given concurrently). Products include:
Librium Capsules 1736
Librium for Injection 1737

Chlorpheniramine Maleate (Co-administration may result in respiratory depression, hypotension, and profound sedation or coma; reduced dosage of meperidine may be required if given concurrently). Products include:
Actifed Cold & Sinus Caplets and Tablets .... ▣688
Alka-Seltzer Plus Liqui-Gels .... ▣604
BC Allergy Sinus Cold Powder .... ▣619
Chlor-Trimeton Allergy Tablets .... ▣735
Chlor-Trimeton Allergy/Decongestant Tablets .... ▣736
Comtrex Flu Therapy & Fever Relief Nighttime Tablets .... ▣628
Comtrex Maximum Strength Multi-Symptom Cold & Cough Relief Tablets and Caplets .... ▣626
Contac Severe Cold and Flu Caplets Maximum Strength .... ▣746

Coricidin 'D' Cold, Flu & Sinus Tablets ■ 737
Coricidin/Coricidin D ■ 738
Coricidin HBP Maximum Strength Flu Tablets ■ 738
Extendryl 1361
Hycomine Compound Tablets 1317
Kronofed-A 1341
PediaCare Cough-Cold Liquid ■ 719
PediaCare NightRest Cough-Cold Liquid ■ 719
Robitussin Nighttime Honey Flu Liquid ■ 786
Ryna ■ 768
Singlet Caplets ■ 761
Sinutab Sinus Allergy Medication, Maximum Strength Formula, Tablets & Caplets ■ 707
Sudafed Cold & Allergy Tablets ■ 708
TheraFlu Regular Strength Cold & Cough Night Time Hot Liquid ■ 676
TheraFlu Regular Strength Cold & Sore Throat Night Time Hot Liquid ■ 676
TheraFlu Maximum Strength Flu & Cough Night Time Hot Liquid ■ 678
TheraFlu Maximum Strength Flu & Sore Throat Night Time Hot Liquid ■ 677
TheraFlu Maximum Strength Severe Cold & Congestion Night Time Caplets ■ 678
TheraFlu Maximum Strength Severe Cold & Congestion Night Time Hot Liquid ■ 678
Triaminic Cold & Allergy Liquid ■ 681
Triaminic Cold & Allergy Softchews ■ 683
Triaminic Cold & Cough Liquid ■ 681
Triaminic Cold & Cough Softchews ■ 683
Triaminic Cold & Night Time Cough Liquid ■ 681
Triaminic Cold, Cough & Fever Liquid ■ 681
Children's Tylenol Cold Suspension Liquid and Chewable Tablets 2015
Children's Tylenol Cold Plus Cough Suspension Liquid and Chewable Tablets 2015
Children's Tylenol Flu Suspension Liquid 2015
Maximum Strength Tylenol Allergy Sinus Caplets, Gelcaps, and Geltabs 2010
Multi-Symptom Tylenol Cold Complete Formula Caplets 2010
Vicks 44M Cough, Cold & Flu Relief Liquid ■ 725
Pediatric Vicks 44m Cough & Cold Relief ■ 728
Children's Vicks NyQuil Cold/Cough Relief ■ 726

Chlorpheniramine Polistirex (Co-administration may result in respiratory depression, hypotension, and profound sedation or coma; reduced dosage of meperidine may be required if given concurrently). Products include:
Tussionex Pennkinetic Extended-Release Suspension 1174

Chlorpheniramine Tannate (Co-administration may result in respiratory depression, hypotension, and profound sedation or coma; reduced dosage of meperidine may be required if given concurrently). Products include:
Reformulated Rynatan Pediatric Suspension 3352
Rynatuss Pediatric Suspension 3353
Rynatuss Tablets 3353
Tussi-12 S Suspension 3356
Tussi-12 Tablets 3356

Chlorpromazine (Co-administration may result in respiratory depression, hypotension, and profound sedation or coma; reduced dosage of meperidine may be required if given concurrently). Products include:
Thorazine Suppositories 1656

Chlorpromazine Hydrochloride (Co-administration may result in respiratory depression, hypotension, and profound sedation or coma; reduced dosage of meperidine may be required if given concurrently). Products include:
Thorazine 1656

Chlorprothixene (Co-administration may result in respiratory depression, hypotension, and profound sedation or coma; reduced dosage of meperidine may be required if given concurrently).
No products indexed under this heading.

Chlorprothixene Hydrochloride (Co-administration may result in respiratory depression, hypotension, and profound sedation or coma; reduced dosage of meperidine may be required if given concurrently).
No products indexed under this heading.

Chlorprothixene Lactate (Co-administration may result in respiratory depression, hypotension, and profound sedation or coma; reduced dosage of meperidine may be required if given concurrently).
No products indexed under this heading.

Clemastine Fumarate (Co-administration may result in respiratory depression, hypotension, and profound sedation or coma; reduced dosage of meperidine may be required if given concurrently). Products include:
Tavist 12 Hour Allergy Tablets ■ 676

Clomipramine Hydrochloride (Co-administration may result in respiratory depression, hypotension, and profound sedation or coma; reduced dosage of meperidine may be required if given concurrently).
No products indexed under this heading.

Clorazepate Dipotassium (Co-administration may result in respiratory depression, hypotension, and profound sedation or coma; reduced dosage of meperidine may be required if given concurrently). Products include:
Tranxene 511

Clozapine (Co-administration may result in respiratory depression, hypotension, and profound sedation or coma; reduced dosage of meperidine may be required if given concurrently). Products include:
Clozaril Tablets 2319

Codeine Phosphate (Co-administration may result in respiratory depression, hypotension, and profound sedation or coma; reduced dosage of meperidine may be required if given concurrently). Products include:
Phenergan with Codeine Syrup 3557
Phenergan VC with Codeine Syrup 3561
Robitussin A-C Syrup 2942
Robitussin-DAC Syrup 2942
Ryna-C Liquid ■ 768
Soma Compound w/Codeine Tablets 3355
Tussi-Organidin NR Liquid 3350
Tussi-Organidin-S NR Liquid 3350
Tylenol with Codeine 2595

Cyproheptadine Hydrochloride (Co-administration may result in respiratory depression, hypotension, and profound sedation or coma; reduced dosage of meperidine may be required if given concurrently). Products include:
Periactin Tablets 2155

Desflurane (Co-administration may result in respiratory depression, hypotension, and profound sedation or coma; reduced dosage of meperidine may be required if given concurrently). Products include:
Suprane Liquid for Inhalation 874

Desipramine Hydrochloride (Co-administration may result in respiratory depression, hypotension, and profound sedation or coma; reduced dosage of meperidine may be required if given concurrently). Products include:
Norpramin Tablets 755

Dexchlorpheniramine Maleate (Co-administration may result in respiratory depression, hypotension, and profound sedation or coma; reduced dosage of meperidine may be required if given concurrently).
No products indexed under this heading.

Dezocine (Co-administration may result in respiratory depression, hypotension, and profound sedation or coma; reduced dosage of meperidine may be required if given concurrently).
No products indexed under this heading.

Diazepam (Co-administration may result in respiratory depression, hypotension, and profound sedation or coma; reduced dosage of meperidine may be required if given concurrently). Products include:
Valium Injectable 3026
Valium Tablets 3047

Diphenhydramine Citrate (Co-administration may result in respiratory depression, hypotension, and profound sedation or coma; reduced dosage of meperidine may be required if given concurrently). Products include:
Alka-Seltzer PM Effervescent Tablets ■ 605
Benadryl Allergy & Sinus Fastmelt Tablets ■ 693
Benadryl Children's Allergy/Cold Fastmelt Tablets ■ 692
Excedrin PM Tablets, Caplets, and Geltabs ■ 631
Goody's PM Powder ■ 621

Diphenhydramine Hydrochloride (Co-administration may result in respiratory depression, hypotension, and profound sedation or coma; reduced dosage of meperidine may be required if given concurrently). Products include:
Extra Strength Bayer PM Caplets ■ 611
Benadryl Allergy Chewables ■ 689
Benadryl Allergy ■ 691
Benadryl Allergy Liquid ■ 690
Benadryl Allergy/Cold Tablets ■ 691
Benadryl Allergy/Congestion Tablets ■ 692
Benadryl Allergy & Sinus Liquid ■ 693
Benadryl Allergy Sinus Headache Caplets & Gelcaps ■ 693
Benadryl Severe Allergy & Sinus Headache Caplets ■ 694
Benadryl Dye-Free Allergy Liquid ■ 690
Benadryl Dye-Free Allergy Liqui-Gels Softgels ■ 690
Benadryl Itch Relief Stick Extra Strength ■ 695
Benadryl Cream ■ 695
Benadryl Gel ■ 695
Benadryl Spray ■ 696
Benadryl Parenteral 2617
Coricidin HBP Night-Time Cold & Flu Tablets ■ 738
Nytol QuickCaps Caplets ■ 622
Maximum Strength Nytol QuickGels Softgels ■ 621
Extra Strength Percogesic Aspirin-Free Coated Caplets ■ 665
Simply Sleep Caplets 2008
Sominex Original Formula Tablets ■ 761
Children's Tylenol Allergy-D Liquid 2014
Maximum Strength Tylenol Allergy Sinus NightTime Caplets 2010
Tylenol Severe Allergy Caplets 2010
Maximum Strength Tylenol Flu NightTime Gelcaps 2011
Extra Strength Tylenol PM Caplets, Geltabs, and Gelcaps 2012
Unisom Maximum Strength SleepGels ■ 713

Diphenylpyraline Hydrochloride (Co-administration may result in respiratory depression, hypotension, and profound sedation or coma; reduced dosage of meperidine may be required if given concurrently).
No products indexed under this heading.

Doxepin Hydrochloride (Co-administration may result in respiratory depression, hypotension, and profound sedation or coma; reduced dosage of meperidine may be required if given concurrently). Products include:
Sinequan 2713

Droperidol (Co-administration may result in respiratory depression, hypotension, and profound sedation or coma; reduced dosage of meperidine may be required if given concurrently).
No products indexed under this heading.

Enflurane (Co-administration may result in respiratory depression, hypotension, and profound sedation or coma; reduced dosage of meperidine may be required if given concurrently).
No products indexed under this heading.

Estazolam (Co-administration may result in respiratory depression, hypotension, and profound sedation or coma; reduced dosage of meperidine may be required if given concurrently). Products include:
ProSom Tablets 500

Ethchlorvynol (Co-administration may result in respiratory depression, hypotension, and profound sedation or coma; reduced dosage of meperidine may be required if given concurrently).
No products indexed under this heading.

Ethinamate (Co-administration may result in respiratory depression, hypotension, and profound sedation or coma; reduced dosage of meperidine may be required if given concurrently).
No products indexed under this heading.

Fentanyl (Co-administration may result in respiratory depression, hypotension, and profound sedation or coma; reduced dosage of meperidine may be required if given concurrently). Products include:
Duragesic Transdermal System 1786

Fentanyl Citrate (Co-administration may result in respiratory depression, hypotension, and profound sedation or coma; reduced dosage of meperidine may be required if given concurrently). Products include:
Actiq 1184

Fexofenadine Hydrochloride (Co-administration may result in respiratory depression, hypotension, and profound sedation or coma; reduced dosage of meperidine may be required if given concurrently). Products include:
Allegra 712
Allegra-D Extended-Release Tablets 714

Fluphenazine Decanoate (Co-administration may result in respiratory depression, hypotension, and profound sedation or coma; reduced dosage of meperidine may be required if given concurrently).
No products indexed under this heading.

Fluphenazine Enanthate (Co-administration may result in respiratory depression, hypotension, and profound sedation or coma; reduced dosage of meperidine may be required if given concurrently).
No products indexed under this heading.

Fluphenazine Hydrochloride (Co-administration may result in respiratory depression, hypotension, and profound sedation or coma; reduced dosage of meperidine may be required if given concurrently).
No products indexed under this heading.

Flurazepam Hydrochloride (Co-administration may result in respiratory depression, hypotension, and

profound sedation or coma; reduced dosage of meperidine may be required if given concurrently).

No products indexed under this heading.

Glutethimide (Co-administration may result in respiratory depression, hypotension, and profound sedation or coma; reduced dosage of meperidine may be required if given concurrently).

No products indexed under this heading.

Haloperidol (Co-administration may result in respiratory depression, hypotension, and profound sedation or coma; reduced dosage of meperidine may be required if given concurrently). Products include:

Haldol Injection, Tablets and Concentrate 2533

Haloperidol Decanoate (Co-administration may result in respiratory depression, hypotension, and profound sedation or coma; reduced dosage of meperidine may be required if given concurrently).
Products include:

Haldol Decanoate 2535

Hydrocodone Bitartrate (Co-administration may result in respiratory depression, hypotension, and profound sedation or coma; reduced dosage of meperidine may be required if given concurrently).
Products include:

Hycodan 1316
Hycomine Compound Tablets 1317
Hycotuss Expectorant Syrup 1318
Lortab 3319
Lortab Elixir 3317
Maxidone Tablets CIII 3399
Norco 5/325 Tablets CIII 3424
Norco 7.5/325 Tablets CIII 3425
Norco 10/325 Tablets CIII 3427
Norco 10/325 Tablets CIII 3425
Vicodin Tablets 516
Vicodin ES Tablets 517
Vicodin HP Tablets 518
Vicodin Tuss Expectorant 519
Vicoprofen Tablets 520
Zydone Tablets 1330

Hydrocodone Polistirex (Co-administration may result in respiratory depression, hypotension, and profound sedation or coma; reduced dosage of meperidine may be required if given concurrently).
Products include:

Tussionex Pennkinetic Extended-Release Suspension 1174

Hydromorphone Hydrochloride (Co-administration may result in respiratory depression, hypotension, and profound sedation or coma; reduced dosage of meperidine may be required if given concurrently).
Products include:

Dilaudid 441
Dilaudid Oral Liquid 445
Dilaudid Powder 441
Dilaudid Rectal Suppositories 441
Dilaudid Tablets 441
Dilaudid Tablets - 8 mg 445
Dilaudid-HP 443

Hydroxyzine Hydrochloride (Co-administration may result in respiratory depression, hypotension, and profound sedation or coma; reduced dosage of meperidine may be required if given concurrently).
Products include:

Atarax Tablets & Syrup 2667
Vistaril Intramuscular Solution 2738

Imipramine Hydrochloride (Co-administration may result in respiratory depression, hypotension, and profound sedation or coma; reduced dosage of meperidine may be required if given concurrently).

No products indexed under this heading.

Imipramine Pamoate (Co-administration may result in respiratory depression, hypotension, and profound sedation or coma; reduced dosage of meperidine may be required if given concurrently).

No products indexed under this heading.

Isocarboxazid (Co-administration with the therapeutic doses of meperidine and MAO inhibitors have occasionally precipitated unpredictable, severe, and sometimes fatal reactions; concurrent and/or sequential use is contraindicated).

No products indexed under this heading.

Isoflurane (Co-administration may result in respiratory depression, hypotension, and profound sedation or coma; reduced dosage of meperidine may be required if given concurrently).

No products indexed under this heading.

Ketamine Hydrochloride (Co-administration may result in respiratory depression, hypotension, and profound sedation or coma; reduced dosage of meperidine may be required if given concurrently).

No products indexed under this heading.

Levomethadyl Acetate Hydrochloride (Co-administration may result in respiratory depression, hypotension, and profound sedation or coma; reduced dosage of meperidine may be required if given concurrently).

No products indexed under this heading.

Levorphanol Tartrate (Co-administration may result in respiratory depression, hypotension, and profound sedation or coma ; reduced dosage of meperidine may be required if given concurrently).
Products include:

Levo-Dromoran 1734
Levorphanol Tartrate Tablets 3059

Loratadine (Co-administration may result in respiratory depression, hypotension, and profound sedation or coma; reduced dosage of meperidine may be required if given concurrently). Products include:

Claritin 3100
Claritin-D 12 Hour Extended Release Tablets 3102
Claritin-D 24 Hour Extended Release Tablets 3104

Lorazepam (Co-administration may result in respiratory depression, hypotension, and profound sedation or coma; reduced dosage of meperidine may be required if given concurrently). Products include:

Ativan Injection 3478
Ativan Tablets 3482

Loxapine Hydrochloride (Co-administration may result in respiratory depression, hypotension, and profound sedation or coma; reduced dosage of meperidine may be required if given concurrently).

No products indexed under this heading.

Loxapine Succinate (Co-administration may result in respiratory depression, hypotension, and profound sedation or coma; reduced dosage of meperidine may be required if given concurrently).
Products include:

Loxitane Capsules 3398

Maprotiline Hydrochloride (Co-administration may result in respiratory depression, hypotension, and profound sedation or coma; reduced dosage of meperidine may be required if given concurrently).

No products indexed under this heading.

Mephobarbital (Co-administration may result in respiratory depression, hypotension, and profound sedation or coma; reduced dosage of meperidine may be required if given concurrently).

No products indexed under this heading.

Meprobamate (Co-administration may result in respiratory depression, hypotension, and profound sedation or coma; reduced dosage of meperidine may be required if given concurrently). Products include:

Miltown Tablets 3349

Mesoridazine Besylate (Co-administration may result in respiratory depression, hypotension, and profound sedation or coma; reduced dosage of meperidine may be required if given concurrently).
Products include:

Serentil 1057

Methadone Hydrochloride (Co-administration may result in respiratory depression, hypotension, and profound sedation or coma; reduced dosage of meperidine may be required if given concurrently).
Products include:

Dolophine Hydrochloride Tablets 3056

Methdilazine Hydrochloride (Co-administration may result in respiratory depression, hypotension, and profound sedation or coma; reduced dosage of meperidine may be required if given concurrently).

No products indexed under this heading.

Methohexital Sodium (Co-administration may result in respiratory depression, hypotension, and profound sedation or coma; reduced dosage of meperidine may be required if given concurrently).
Products include:

Brevital Sodium for Injection, USP .. 1815

Methotrimeprazine (Co-administration may result in respiratory depression, hypotension, and profound sedation or coma; reduced dosage of meperidine may be required if given concurrently).

No products indexed under this heading.

Methoxyflurane (Co-administration may result in respiratory depression, hypotension, and profound sedation or coma; reduced dosage of meperidine may be required if given concurrently).

No products indexed under this heading.

Midazolam Hydrochloride (Co-administration may result in respiratory depression, hypotension, and profound sedation or coma; reduced dosage of meperidine may be required if given concurrently).
Products include:

Versed Injection 3027
Versed Syrup 3033

Mirtazapine (Co-administration may result in respiratory depression, hypotension, and profound sedation or coma; reduced dosage of meperidine may be required if given concurrently). Products include:

Remeron Tablets 2483
Remeron SolTab Tablets 2486

Moclobemide (Co-administration with the therapeutic doses of meperidine and MAO inhibitors have occasionally precipitated unpredictable, severe, and sometimes fatal reactions; concurrent and/or sequential use is contraindicated).

No products indexed under this heading.

Molindone Hydrochloride (Co-administration may result in respiratory depression, hypotension, and profound sedation or coma; reduced dosage of meperidine may be required if given concurrently).
Products include:

Moban 1320

Morphine Sulfate (Co-administration may result in respiratory depression, hypotension, and profound sedation or coma; reduced dosage of meperidine may be required if given concurrently).
Products include:

Astramorph/PF Injection, USP (Preservative-Free) 594
Duramorph Injection 1312
Infumorph 200 and Infumorph 500 Sterile Solutions 1314
Kadian Capsules 1335
MS Contin Tablets 2896
MSIR 2898
Oramorph SR Tablets 3062
Roxanol 3066

Nortriptyline Hydrochloride (Co-administration may result in respiratory depression, hypotension, and profound sedation or coma; reduced dosage of meperidine may be required if given concurrently).

No products indexed under this heading.

Olanzapine (Co-administration may result in respiratory depression, hypotension, and profound sedation or coma; reduced dosage of meperidine may be required if given concurrently). Products include:

Zyprexa Tablets 1973
Zyprexa ZYDIS Orally Disintegrating Tablets 1973

Oxazepam (Co-administration may result in respiratory depression, hypotension, and profound sedation or coma; reduced dosage of meperidine may be required if given concurrently).

No products indexed under this heading.

Oxycodone Hydrochloride (Co-administration may result in respiratory depression, hypotension, and profound sedation or coma; reduced dosage of meperidine may be required if given concurrently).
Products include:

OxyContin Tablets 2912
OxyFast Oral Concentrate Solution 2916
OxyIR Capsules 2916
Percocet Tablets 1326
Percodan Tablets 1327
Percolone Tablets 1327
Roxicodone 3067
Tylox Capsules 2597

Pargyline Hydrochloride (Co-administration with the therapeutic doses of meperidine and MAO inhibitors have occasionally precipitated unpredictable, severe, and sometimes fatal reactions; concurrent and/or sequential use is contraindicated).

No products indexed under this heading.

Pentobarbital Sodium (Co-administration may result in respiratory depression, hypotension, and profound sedation or coma; reduced dosage of meperidine may be required if given concurrently).
Products Include:

Nembutal Sodium Solution 485

Perphenazine (Co-administration may result in respiratory depression, hypotension, and profound sedation or coma; reduced dosage of meperidine may be required if given concurrently). Products include:

Etrafon 3115
Trilafon 3160

Phenelzine Sulfate (Co-administration with the therapeutic doses of meperidine and MAO inhibitors have occasionally precipitated unpredictable, severe, and sometimes fatal reactions; concurrent and/or sequential use is contraindicated). Products include:

Nardil Tablets 2653

Phenobarbital (Co-administration may result in respiratory depression, hypotension, and profound sedation or coma; reduced dosage of meperidine may be required if given concurrently). Products include:

Arco-Lase Plus Tablets 592
Donnatal 2929

Donnatal Extentabs 2930

Prazepam (Co-administration may result in respiratory depression, hypotension, and profound sedation or coma; reduced dosage of meperidine may be required if given concurrently).
No products indexed under this heading.

Procarbazine Hydrochloride (Co-administration with the therapeutic doses of meperidine and MAO inhibitors have occasionally precipitated unpredictable, severe, and sometimes fatal reactions; concurrent and/or sequential use is contraindicated). Products include:
Matulane Capsules 3246

Prochlorperazine (Co-administration may result in respiratory depression, hypotension, and profound sedation or coma; reduced dosage of meperidine may be required if given concurrently). Products include:
Compazine 1505

Promethazine Hydrochloride (Co-administration may result in respiratory depression, hypotension, and profound sedation or coma; reduced dosage of meperidine may be required if given concurrently). Products include:
Mepergan Injection 3539
Phenergan Injection 3553
Phenergan 3556
Phenergan Syrup 3554
Phenergan with Codeine Syrup 3557
Phenergan with Dextromethorphan Syrup 3559
Phenergan VC Syrup 3560
Phenergan VC with Codeine Syrup .. 3561

Propofol (Co-administration may result in respiratory depression, hypotension, and profound sedation or coma; reduced dosage of meperidine may be required if given concurrently). Products include:
Diprivan Injectable Emulsion 667

Propoxyphene Hydrochloride (Co-administration may result in respiratory depression, hypotension, and profound sedation or coma; reduced dosage of meperidine may be required if given concurrently). Products include:
Darvon Pulvules 1909
Darvon Compound-65 Pulvules 1910

Propoxyphene Napsylate (Co-administration may result in respiratory depression, hypotension, and profound sedation or coma; reduced dosage of meperidine may be required if given concurrently). Products include:
Darvon-N/Darvocet-N 1907
Darvon-N Tablets 1912

Protriptyline Hydrochloride (Co-administration may result in respiratory depression, hypotension, and profound sedation or coma; reduced dosage of meperidine may be required if given concurrently). Products include:
Vivactil Tablets 2446
Vivactil Tablets 2217

Pyrilamine Maleate (Co-administration may result in respiratory depression, hypotension, and profound sedation or coma; reduced dosage of meperidine may be required if given concurrently). Products include:
Maximum Strength Midol Menstrual Caplets and Gelcaps 612
Maximum Strength Midol PMS Caplets and Gelcaps 613

Pyrilamine Tannate (Co-administration may result in respiratory depression, hypotension, and profound sedation or coma; reduced dosage of meperidine may be required if given concurrently). Products include:
Ryna-12 S Suspension 3351

Quazepam (Co-administration may result in respiratory depression, hypotension, and profound sedation or coma; reduced dosage of meperidine may be required if given concurrently).
No products indexed under this heading.

Quetiapine Fumarate (Co-administration may result in respiratory depression, hypotension, and profound sedation or coma; reduced dosage of meperidine may be required if given concurrently). Products include:
Seroquel Tablets 684

Remifentanil Hydrochloride (Co-administration may result in respiratory depression, hypotension, and profound sedation or coma; reduced dosage of meperidine may be required if given concurrently).
No products indexed under this heading.

Risperidone (Co-administration may result in respiratory depression, hypotension, and profound sedation or coma; reduced dosage of meperidine may be required if given concurrently). Products include:
Risperdal 1796

Secobarbital Sodium (Co-administration may result in respiratory depression, hypotension, and profound sedation or coma; reduced dosage of meperidine may be required if given concurrently).
No products indexed under this heading.

Selegiline Hydrochloride (Co-administration with the therapeutic doses of meperidine and MAO inhibitors have occasionally precipitated unpredictable, severe, and sometimes fatal reactions; concurrent and/or sequential use is contraindicated). Products include:
Eldepryl Capsules 3266

Sevoflurane (Co-administration may result in respiratory depression, hypotension, and profound sedation or coma; reduced dosage of meperidine may be required if given concurrently).
No products indexed under this heading.

Sufentanil Citrate (Co-administration may result in respiratory depression, hypotension, and profound sedation or coma; reduced dosage of meperidine may be required if given concurrently).
No products indexed under this heading.

Temazepam (Co-administration may result in respiratory depression, hypotension, and profound sedation or coma; reduced dosage of meperidine may be required if given concurrently).
No products indexed under this heading.

Terfenadine (Co-administration may result in respiratory depression, hypotension, and profound sedation or coma; reduced dosage of meperidine may be required if given concurrently).
No products indexed under this heading.

Thiamylal Sodium (Co-administration may result in respiratory depression, hypotension, and profound sedation or coma; reduced dosage of meperidine may be required if given concurrently).
No products indexed under this heading.

Thioridazine Hydrochloride (Co-administration may result in respiratory depression, hypotension, and profound sedation or coma; reduced dosage of meperidine may be required if given concurrently). Products include:
Thioridazine Hydrochloride Tablets 2289

Thiothixene (Co-administration may result in respiratory depression, hypotension, and profound sedation or coma; reduced dosage of meperidine may be required if given concurrently). Products include:
Navane Capsules 2701
Thiothixene Capsules 2290

Tranylcypromine Sulfate (Co-administration with the therapeutic doses of meperidine and MAO inhibitors have occasionally precipitated unpredictable, severe, and sometimes fatal reactions; concurrent and/or sequential use is contraindicated). Products include:
Parnate Tablets 1607

Triazolam (Co-administration may result in respiratory depression, hypotension, and profound sedation or coma; reduced dosage of meperidine may be required if given concurrently). Products include:
Halcion Tablets 2823

Trifluoperazine Hydrochloride (Co-administration may result in respiratory depression, hypotension, and profound sedation or coma; reduced dosage of meperidine may be required if given concurrently). Products include:
Stelazine 1640

Trimeprazine Tartrate (Co-administration may result in respiratory depression, hypotension, and profound sedation or coma; reduced dosage of meperidine may be required if given concurrently).
No products indexed under this heading.

Trimipramine Maleate (Co-administration may result in respiratory depression, hypotension, and profound sedation or coma; reduced dosage of meperidine may be required if given concurrently). Products include:
Surmontil Capsules 3595

Tripelennamine Hydrochloride (Co-administration may result in respiratory depression, hypotension, and profound sedation or coma; reduced dosage of meperidine may be required if given concurrently).
No products indexed under this heading.

Triprolidine Hydrochloride (Co-administration may result in respiratory depression, hypotension, and profound sedation or coma; reduced dosage of meperidine may be required if given concurrently). Products include:
Actifed Cold & Allergy Tablets 688

Zaleplon (Co-administration may result in respiratory depression, hypotension, and profound sedation or coma; reduced dosage of meperidine may be required if given concurrently). Products include:
Sonata Capsules 3591

Ziprasidone Hydrochloride (Co-administration may result in respiratory depression, hypotension, and profound sedation or coma; reduced dosage of meperidine may be required if given concurrently). Products include:
Geodon Capsules 2688

Zolpidem Tartrate (Co-administration may result in respiratory depression, hypotension, and profound sedation or coma; reduced dosage of meperidine may be required if given concurrently). Products include:
Ambien Tablets 3191

Food Interactions

Alcohol (Concurrent use may result in respiratory depression, hypotension, and profound sedation or coma).

DEMSER CAPSULES
(Metyrosine) 2085
May interact with central nervous system depressants, phenothiazines, and certain other agents. Compounds in these categories include:

Alfentanil Hydrochloride (Additive sedative effects).
No products indexed under this heading.

Alprazolam (Additive sedative effects). Products include:
Xanax Tablets 2865

Aprobarbital (Additive sedative effects).
No products indexed under this heading.

Buprenorphine Hydrochloride (Additive sedative effects). Products include:
Buprenex Injectable 2918

Buspirone Hydrochloride (Additive sedative effects).
No products indexed under this heading.

Butabarbital (Additive sedative effects).
No products indexed under this heading.

Butalbital (Additive sedative effects). Products include:
Phrenilin 578
Sedapap Tablets 50 mg/650 mg ... 2225

Chlordiazepoxide (Additive sedative effects). Products include:
Limbitrol 1738

Chlordiazepoxide Hydrochloride (Additive sedative effects). Products include:
Librium Capsules 1736
Librium for Injection 1737

Chlorpromazine (Possible potentiation of extrapyramidal effects; additive sedative effects). Products include:
Thorazine Suppositories 1656

Chlorpromazine Hydrochloride (Possible potentiation of extrapyramidal effects; additive sedative effects). Products include:
Thorazine 1656

Chlorprothixene (Additive sedative effects).
No products indexed under this heading.

Chlorprothixene Hydrochloride (Additive sedative effects).
No products indexed under this heading.

Chlorprothixene Lactate (Additive sedative effects).
No products indexed under this heading.

Clorazepate Dipotassium (Additive sedative effects). Products include:
Tranxene 511

Clozapine (Additive sedative effects). Products include:
Clozaril Tablets 2319

Codeine Phosphate (Additive sedative effects). Products include:
Phenergan with Codeine Syrup 3557
Phenergan VC with Codeine Syrup .. 3561
Robitussin A-C Syrup 2942
Robitussin-DAC Syrup 2942
Ryna-C Liquid 768
Soma Compound w/Codeine Tablets 3355
Tussi-Organidin NR Liquid 3350
Tussi-Organidin-S NR Liquid 3350
Tylenol with Codeine 2595

Desflurane (Additive sedative effects). Products include:
Suprane Liquid for Inhalation 874

IMPORTANT NOTE: Always consult each drug listing in the patient's regimen for possible interactions.

Dezocine (Additive sedative effects).
No products indexed under this heading.

Diazepam (Additive sedative effects). Products include:
Valium Injectable 3026
Valium Tablets 3047

Droperidol (Additive sedative effects).
No products indexed under this heading.

Enflurane (Additive sedative effects).
No products indexed under this heading.

Estazolam (Additive sedative effects). Products include:
ProSom Tablets 500

Ethchlorvynol (Additive sedative effects).
No products indexed under this heading.

Ethinamate (Additive sedative effects).
No products indexed under this heading.

Fentanyl (Additive sedative effects). Products include:
Duragesic Transdermal System 1786

Fentanyl Citrate (Additive sedative effects). Products include:
Actiq 1184

Fluphenazine Decanoate (Possible potentiation of extrapyramidal effects; additive sedative effects).
No products indexed under this heading.

Fluphenazine Enanthate (Possible potentiation of extrapyramidal effects; additive sedative effects).
No products indexed under this heading.

Fluphenazine Hydrochloride (Possible potentiation of extrapyramidal effects; additive sedative effects).
No products indexed under this heading.

Flurazepam Hydrochloride (Additive sedative effects).
No products indexed under this heading.

Glutethimide (Additive sedative effects).
No products indexed under this heading.

Haloperidol (Possible potentiation of extrapyramidal effects; additive sedative effects). Products include:
Haldol Injection, Tablets and Concentrate 2533

Haloperidol Decanoate (Possible potentiation of extrapyramidal effects; additive sedative effects). Products include:
Haldol Decanoate 2535

Hydrocodone Bitartrate (Additive sedative effects). Products include:
Hycodan 1316
Hycomine Compound Tablets 1317
Hycotuss Expectorant Syrup 1318
Lortab 3319
Lortab Elixir 3317
Maxidone Tablets CIII 3399
Norco 5/325 Tablets CIII 3424
Norco 7.5/325 Tablets CIII 3425
Norco 10/325 Tablets CIII 3427
Norco 10/325 Tablets CII 3425
Vicodin Tablets 516
Vicodin ES Tablets 517
Vicodin HP Tablets 518
Vicodin Tuss Expectorant 519
Vicoprofen Tablets 520
Zydone Tablets 1330

Hydrocodone Polistirex (Additive sedative effects). Products include:
Tussionex Pennkinetic Extended-Release Suspension 1174

Hydromorphone Hydrochloride (Additive sedative effects). Products include:
Dilaudid 441
Dilaudid Oral Liquid 445
Dilaudid Powder 441
Dilaudid Rectal Suppositories 441
Dilaudid Tablets 441
Dilaudid Tablets - 8 mg 445
Dilaudid-HP 443

Hydroxyzine Hydrochloride (Additive sedative effects). Products include:
Atarax Tablets & Syrup 2667
Vistaril Intramuscular Solution 2738

Isoflurane (Additive sedative effects).
No products indexed under this heading.

Ketamine Hydrochloride (Additive sedative effects).
No products indexed under this heading.

Levomethadyl Acetate Hydrochloride (Additive sedative effects).
No products indexed under this heading.

Levorphanol Tartrate (Additive sedative effects). Products include:
Levo-Dromoran 1734
Levorphanol Tartrate Tablets 3059

Lorazepam (Additive sedative effects). Products include:
Ativan Injection 3478
Ativan Tablets 3482

Loxapine Hydrochloride (Additive sedative effects).
No products indexed under this heading.

Loxapine Succinate (Additive sedative effects). Products include:
Loxitane Capsules 3398

Meperidine Hydrochloride (Additive sedative effects). Products include:
Demerol 3079
Mepergan Injection 3539

Mephobarbital (Additive sedative effects).
No products indexed under this heading.

Meprobamate (Additive sedative effects). Products include:
Miltown Tablets 3349

Mesoridazine Besylate (Possible potentiation of extrapyramidal effects; additive sedative effects). Products include:
Serentil 1057

Methadone Hydrochloride (Additive sedative effects). Products include:
Dolophine Hydrochloride Tablets 3056

Methohexital Sodium (Additive sedative effects). Products include:
Brevital Sodium for Injection, USP 1815

Methotrimeprazine (Possible potentiation of extrapyramidal effects; additive sedative effects).
No products indexed under this heading.

Methoxyflurane (Additive sedative effects).
No products indexed under this heading.

Midazolam Hydrochloride (Additive sedative effects). Products include:
Versed Injection 3027
Versed Syrup 3033

Molindone Hydrochloride (Additive sedative effects). Products include:
Moban 1320

Morphine Sulfate (Additive sedative effects). Products include:
Astramorph/PF Injection, USP (Preservative-Free) 594
Duramorph Injection 1312
Infumorph 200 and Infumorph 500 Sterile Solutions 1314
Kadian Capsules 1335
MS Contin Tablets 2896
MSIR 2898
Oramorph SR Tablets 3062
Roxanol 3066

Olanzapine (Additive sedative effects). Products include:
Zyprexa Tablets 1973
Zyprexa ZYDIS Orally Disintegrating Tablets 1973

Oxazepam (Additive sedative effects).
No products indexed under this heading.

Oxycodone Hydrochloride (Additive sedative effects). Products include:
OxyContin Tablets 2912
OxyFast Oral Concentrate Solution 2916
OxyIR Capsules 2916
Percocet Tablets 1326
Percodan Tablets 1327
Percolone Tablets 1327
Roxicodone 3067
Tylox Capsules 2597

Pentobarbital Sodium (Additive sedative effects). Products include:
Nembutal Sodium Solution 485

Perphenazine (Possible potentiation of extrapyramidal effects of perphenazine; additive sedative effects). Products include:
Etrafon 3115
Trilafon 3160

Phenobarbital (Additive sedative effects). Products include:
Arco-Lase Plus Tablets 592
Donnatal 2929
Donnatal Extentabs 2930

Prazepam (Additive sedative effects).
No products indexed under this heading.

Prochlorperazine (Possible potentiation of extrapyramidal effects; additive sedative effects). Products include:
Compazine 1505

Promethazine Hydrochloride (Possible potentiation of extrapyramidal effects; additive sedative effects). Products include:
Mepergan Injection 3539
Phenergan Injection 3553
Phenergan 3556
Phenergan Syrup 3554
Phenergan with Codeine Syrup 3557
Phenergan with Dextromethorphan Syrup 3559
Phenergan VC Syrup 3560
Phenergan VC with Codeine Syrup 3561

Propofol (Additive sedative effects). Products include:
Diprivan Injectable Emulsion 667

Propoxyphene Hydrochloride (Additive sedative effects). Products include:
Darvon Pulvules 1909
Darvon Compound-65 Pulvules 1910

Propoxyphene Napsylate (Additive sedative effects). Products include:
Darvon-N/Darvocet-N 1907
Darvon-N Tablets 1912

Quazepam (Additive sedative effects).
No products indexed under this heading.

Quetiapine Fumarate (Additive sedative effects). Products include:
Seroquel Tablets 684

Remifentanil Hydrochloride (Additive sedative effects).
No products indexed under this heading.

Risperidone (Additive sedative effects). Products include:
Risperdal 1796

Secobarbital Sodium (Additive sedative effects).
No products indexed under this heading.

Sevoflurane (Additive sedative effects).
No products indexed under this heading.

Sufentanil Citrate (Additive sedative effects).
No products indexed under this heading.

Temazepam (Additive sedative effects).
No products indexed under this heading.

Thiamylal Sodium (Additive sedative effects).
No products indexed under this heading.

Thioridazine Hydrochloride (Possible potentiation of extrapyramidal effects; additive sedative effects). Products include:
Thioridazine Hydrochloride Tablets 2289

Thiothixene (Additive sedative effects). Products include:
Navane Capsules 2701
Thiothixene Capsules 2290

Triazolam (Additive sedative effects). Products include:
Halcion Tablets 2823

Trifluoperazine Hydrochloride (Possible potentiation of extrapyramidal effects; additive sedative effects). Products include:
Stelazine 1640

Zaleplon (Additive sedative effects). Products include:
Sonata Capsules 3591

Ziprasidone Hydrochloride (Additive sedative effects). Products include:
Geodon Capsules 2688

Zolpidem Tartrate (Additive sedative effects). Products include:
Ambien Tablets 3191

Food Interactions

Alcohol (Additive sedative effects).

DENAVIR CREAM
(Penciclovir) 2332
None cited in PDR database.

DEPACON INJECTION
(Valproate Sodium) 416
May interact with central nervous system depressants, phenytoin, and certain other agents. Compounds in these categories include:

Alfentanil Hydrochloride (Co-administration may result in additive CNS depression).
No products indexed under this heading.

Alprazolam (Co-administration may result in additive CNS depression). Products include:
Xanax Tablets 2865

Amitriptyline Hydrochloride (Co-administration has resulted in a 21% decrease in plasma clearance of amitriptyline; this interaction is likely to be clinically unimportant). Products include:
Etrafon 3115
Limbitrol 1738

Aprobarbital (Co-administration may result in additive CNS depression).
No products indexed under this heading.

Aspirin (Co-administration has resulted in decreased protein binding and an inhibition of metabolism of valproate). Products include:
Aggrenox Capsules 1026
Alka-Seltzer .... ▣603
Alka-Seltzer Lemon Lime Antacid and Pain Reliever Effervescent Tablets .... ▣603
Alka-Seltzer Extra Strength Antacid and Pain Reliever Effervescent Tablets .... ▣603
Alka-Seltzer PM Effervescent Tablets .... ▣605
Genuine Bayer Tablets, Caplets and Gelcaps .... ▣606
Extra Strength Bayer Caplets and Gelcaps .... ▣610
Aspirin Regimen Bayer Children's Chewable Tablets (Orange or Cherry Flavored) .... ▣607
Bayer, Aspirin Regimen .... ▣606
Aspirin Regimen Bayer 81 mg Caplets with Calcium .... ▣607

Genuine Bayer Professional Labeling (Aspirin Regimen Bayer) 608
Extra Strength Bayer Arthritis Caplets 610
Extra Strength Bayer Plus Caplets 610
Extra Strength Bayer PM Caplets 611
BC Powder 619
BC Allergy Sinus Cold Powder 619
Arthritis Strength BC Powder 619
BC Sinus Cold Powder 619
Darvon Compound-65 Pulvules 1910
Ecotrin Enteric Coated Aspirin Low, Regular and Maximum Strength Tablets 1715
Excedrin Extra-Strength Tablets, Caplets, and Geltabs 629
Excedrin Migraine 1070
Goody's Body Pain Formula Powder 620
Goody's Extra Strength Headache Powder 620
Goody's Extra Strength Pain Relief Tablets 620
Percodan Tablets 1327
Robaxisal Tablets 2939
Soma Compound Tablets 3354
Soma Compound w/Codeine Tablets 3355
Vanquish Caplets 617

Buprenorphine Hydrochloride (Co-administration may result in additive CNS depression). Products include:
Buprenex Injectable 2918

Buspirone Hydrochloride (Co-administration may result in additive CNS depression).
No products indexed under this heading.

Butabarbital (Co-administration may result in additive CNS depression).
No products indexed under this heading.

Butalbital (Co-administration may result in additive CNS depression). Products include:
Phrenilin 578
Sedapap Tablets 50 mg/650 mg 2225

Carbamazepine (Can double the clearance of valproate; co-administration has resulted in decreased carbamazepine and increased carbamazepine 10,11-epoxide serum levels). Products include:
Carbatrol Capsules 3234
Tegretol/Tegretol-XR 2404

Chlordiazepoxide (Co-administration may result in additive CNS depression). Products include:
Limbitrol 1738

Chlordiazepoxide Hydrochloride (Co-administration may result in additive CNS depression). Products include:
Librium Capsules 1736
Librium for Injection 1737

Chlorpromazine (Co-administration has resulted in a 15% increase in trough plasma levels of valproate; concurrent use may result in additive CNS depression). Products include:
Thorazine Suppositories 1656

Chlorpromazine Hydrochloride (Co-administration has resulted in a 15% increase in trough plasma levels of valproate; concurrent use may result in additive CNS depression). Products include:
Thorazine 1656

Chlorprothixene (Co-administration may result in additive CNS depression).
No products indexed under this heading.

Chlorprothixene Hydrochloride (Co-administration may result in additive CNS depression).
No products indexed under this heading.

Chlorprothixene Lactate (Co-administration may result in additive CNS depression).
No products indexed under this heading.

Clonazepam (Co-administration may induce absence status in patients with a history of absence-type seizures). Products include:
Klonopin Tablets 2983

Clorazepate Dipotassium (Co-administration may result in additive CNS depression). Products include:
Tranxene 511

Clozapine (Co-administration may result in additive CNS depression). Products include:
Clozaril Tablets 2319

Codeine Phosphate (Co-administration may result in additive CNS depression). Products include:
Phenergan with Codeine Syrup 3557
Phenergan VC with Codeine Syrup 3561
Robitussin A-C Syrup 2942
Robitussin-DAC Syrup 2942
Ryna-C Liquid 768
Soma Compound w/Codeine Tablets 3355
Tussi-Organidin NR Liquid 3350
Tussi-Organidin-S NR Liquid 3350
Tylenol with Codeine 2595

Desflurane (Co-administration may result in additive CNS depression). Products include:
Suprane Liquid for Inhalation 874

Dezocine (Co-administration may result in additive CNS depression).
No products indexed under this heading.

Diazepam (Valproate displaces diazepam from its plasma albumin binding sites and inhibits its metabolism; plasma clearance and volume of distribution for free diazepam may be reduced; concurrent use may result in additive CNS depression). Products include:
Valium Injectable 3026
Valium Tablets 3047

Droperidol (Co-administration may result in additive CNS depression).
No products indexed under this heading.

Enflurane (Co-administration may result in additive CNS depression).
No products indexed under this heading.

Estazolam (Co-administration may result in additive CNS depression). Products include:
ProSom Tablets 500

Ethchlorvynol (Co-administration may result in additive CNS depression).
No products indexed under this heading.

Ethinamate (Co-administration may result in additive CNS depression).
No products indexed under this heading.

Ethosuximide (Valproate inhibits the metabolism of ethosuximide). Products include:
Zarontin Capsules 2659
Zarontin Syrup 2660

Felbamate (Co-administration has resulted in an increase in mean valproate peak concentration; a reduction in valproate dosage may be necessary). Products include:
Felbatol 3343

Fentanyl (Co-administration may result in additive CNS depression). Products include:
Duragesic Transdermal System 1786

Fentanyl Citrate (Co-administration may result in additive CNS depression). Products include:
Actiq 1184

Fluphenazine Decanoate (Co-administration may result in additive CNS depression).
No products indexed under this heading.

Fluphenazine Enanthate (Co-administration may result in additive CNS depression).
No products indexed under this heading.

Fluphenazine Hydrochloride (Co-administration may result in additive CNS depression).
No products indexed under this heading.

Flurazepam Hydrochloride (Co-administration may result in additive CNS depression).
No products indexed under this heading.

Fosphenytoin Sodium (Can double the clearance of valproate; valproate displaces phenytoin from its plasma albumin binding sites and inhibits its hepatic metabolism; co-administration has resulted in break-through seizures). Products include:
Cerebyx Injection 2619

Glutethimide (Co-administration may result in additive CNS depression).
No products indexed under this heading.

Haloperidol (Co-administration may result in additive CNS depression). Products include:
Haldol Injection, Tablets and Concentrate 2533

Haloperidol Decanoate (Co-administration may result in additive CNS depression). Products include:
Haldol Decanoate 2535

Hydrocodone Bitartrate (Co-administration may result in additive CNS depression). Products include:
Hycodan 1316
Hycomine Compound Tablets 1317
Hycotuss Expectorant Syrup 1318
Lortab 3319
Lortab Elixir 3317
Maxidone Tablets CIII 3399
Norco 5/325 Tablets CIII 3424
Norco 7.5/325 Tablets CIII 3425
Norco 10/325 Tablets CIII 3427
Norco 10/325 Tablets CIII 3425
Vicodin Tablets 516
Vicodin ES Tablets 517
Vicodin HP Tablets 518
Vicodin Tuss Expectorant 519
Vicoprofen Tablets 520
Zydone Tablets 1330

Hydrocodone Polistirex (Co-administration may result in additive CNS depression). Products include:
Tussionex Pennkinetic Extended-Release Suspension 1174

Hydromorphone Hydrochloride (Co-administration may result in additive CNS depression). Products include:
Dilaudid 441
Dilaudid Oral Liquid 445
Dilaudid Powder 441
Dilaudid Rectal Suppositories 441
Dilaudid Tablets 441
Dilaudid Tablets - 8 mg 445
Dilaudid-HP 443

Hydroxyzine Hydrochloride (Co-administration may result in additive CNS depression). Products include:
Atarax Tablets & Syrup 2667
Vistaril Intramuscular Solution 2738

Isoflurane (Co-administration may result in additive CNS depression).
No products indexed under this heading.

Ketamine Hydrochloride (Co-administration may result in additive CNS depression).
No products indexed under this heading.

Lamotrigine (Co-administration has resulted in increased elimination half-life of lamotrigine; the dose of lamotrigine should be reduced if used concurrently). Products include:
Lamictal 1567

Levomethadyl Acetate Hydrochloride (Co-administration may result in additive CNS depression).
No products indexed under this heading.

Levorphanol Tartrate (Co-administration may result in additive CNS depression). Products include:
Levo-Dromoran 1734
Levorphanol Tartrate Tablets 3059

Lorazepam (Co-administration was accompanied by a 17% decrease in the plasma clearance of lorazepam; this pharmacokinetic interaction is likely to be clinically unimportant; concurrent use may result in additive CNS depression). Products include:
Ativan Injection 3478
Ativan Tablets 3482

Loxapine Hydrochloride (Co-administration may result in additive CNS depression).
No products indexed under this heading.

Loxapine Succinate (Co-administration may result in additive CNS depression). Products include:
Loxitane Capsules 3398

Meperidine Hydrochloride (Co-administration may result in additive CNS depression). Products include:
Demerol 3079
Mepergan Injection 3539

Mephobarbital (Co-administration may result in additive CNS depression).
No products indexed under this heading.

Meprobamate (Co-administration may result in additive CNS depression). Products include:
Miltown Tablets 3349

Mesoridazine Besylate (Co-administration may result in additive CNS depression). Products include:
Serentil 1057

Methadone Hydrochloride (Co-administration may result in additive CNS depression). Products include:
Dolophine Hydrochloride Tablets 3056

Methohexital Sodium (Co-administration may result in additive CNS depression). Products include:
Brevital Sodium for Injection, USP 1815

Methotrimeprazine (Co-administration may result in additive CNS depression).
No products indexed under this heading.

Methoxyflurane (Co-administration may result in additive CNS depression).
No products indexed under this heading.

Midazolam Hydrochloride (Co-administration may result in additive CNS depression). Products include:
Versed Injection 3027
Versed Syrup 3033

Molindone Hydrochloride (Co-administration may result in additive CNS depression). Products include:
Moban 1320

Morphine Sulfate (Co-administration may result in additive CNS depression). Products include:
Astramorph/PF Injection, USP (Preservative-Free) 594
Duramorph Injection 1312
Infumorph 200 and Infumorph 500 Sterile Solutions 1314
Kadian Capsules 1335
MS Contin Tablets 2896
MSIR 2898
Oramorph SR Tablets 3062
Roxanol 3066

Nortriptyline Hydrochloride (Co-administration has resulted in a 34% decrease in the net clearance of nortriptyline; this interaction is likely to be clinically unimportant).
No products indexed under this heading.

Olanzapine (Co-administration may result in additive CNS depression). Products include:
Zyprexa Tablets 1973
Zyprexa ZYDIS Orally Disintegrating Tablets 1973

Oxazepam (Co-administration may result in additive CNS depression).
No products indexed under this heading.

Oxycodone Hydrochloride (Co-administration may result in additive CNS depression). Products include:
OxyContin Tablets ... 2912
OxyFast Oral Concentrate Solution ... 2916
OxyIR Capsules ... 2916
Percocet Tablets ... 1326
Percodan Tablets ... 1327
Percolone Tablets ... 1327
Roxicodone ... 3067
Tylox Capsules ... 2597

Pentobarbital Sodium (Co-administration may result in additive CNS depression). Products include:
Nembutal Sodium Solution ... 485

Perphenazine (Co-administration may result in additive CNS depression). Products include:
Etrafon ... 3115
Trilafon ... 3160

Phenobarbital (Can double the clearance of valproate; co-administration has resulted in inhibition of the metabolism of phenobarbital resulting in increased half-life and decreased plasma clearance; concurrent use may result in additive CNS depression). Products include:
Arco-Lase Plus Tablets ... 592
Donnatal ... 2929
Donnatal Extentabs ... 2930

Phenytoin (Can double the clearance of valproate; valproate displaces phenytoin from its plasma albumin binding sites and inhibits its hepatic metabolism; co-administration has resulted in break-through seizures). Products include:
Dilantin Infatabs ... 2624
Dilantin-125 Oral Suspension ... 2625

Phenytoin Sodium (Can double the clearance of valproate; valproate displaces phenytoin from its plasma albumin binding sites and inhibits its hepatic metabolism; co-administration has resulted in break-through seizures). Products include:
Dilantin Kapseals ... 2622

Prazepam (Co-administration may result in additive CNS depression).
No products indexed under this heading.

Primidone (Can double the clearance of valproate; primidone is metabolized to a barbiturate, therefore, co-administration may result in inhibition of the metabolism of primidone resulting in increased half-life and decreased plasma clearance).
No products indexed under this heading.

Prochlorperazine (Co-administration may result in additive CNS depression). Products include:
Compazine ... 1505

Promethazine Hydrochloride (Co-administration may result in additive CNS depression). Products include:
Mepergan Injection ... 3539
Phenergan Injection ... 3553
Phenergan ... 3556
Phenergan Syrup ... 3554
Phenergan with Codeine Syrup ... 3557
Phenergan with Dextromethorphan Syrup ... 3559
Phenergan VC Syrup ... 3560
Phenergan VC with Codeine Syrup ... 3561

Propofol (Co-administration may result in additive CNS depression). Products include:
Diprivan Injectable Emulsion ... 667

Propoxyphene Hydrochloride (Co-administration may result in additive CNS depression). Products include:
Darvon Pulvules ... 1909
Darvon Compound-65 Pulvules ... 1910

Propoxyphene Napsylate (Co-administration may result in additive CNS depression). Products include:
Darvon-N/Darvocet-N ... 1907
Darvon-N Tablets ... 1912

Quazepam (Co-administration may result in additive CNS depression).
No products indexed under this heading.

Quetiapine Fumarate (Co-administration may result in additive CNS depression). Products include:
Seroquel Tablets ... 684

Remifentanil Hydrochloride (Co-administration may result in additive CNS depression).
No products indexed under this heading.

Rifampin (Co-administration has resulted in a 40% increase in oral clearance of valproate). Products include:
Rifadin ... 765
Rifamate Capsules ... 767
Rifater Tablets ... 769

Risperidone (Co-administration may result in additive CNS depression). Products include:
Risperdal ... 1796

Secobarbital Sodium (Co-administration may result in additive CNS depression).
No products indexed under this heading.

Sevoflurane (Co-administration may result in additive CNS depression).
No products indexed under this heading.

Sufentanil Citrate (Co-administration may result in additive CNS depression).
No products indexed under this heading.

Temazepam (Co-administration may result in additive CNS depression).
No products indexed under this heading.

Thiamylal Sodium (Co-administration may result in additive CNS depression).
No products indexed under this heading.

Thioridazine Hydrochloride (Co-administration may result in additive CNS depression). Products include:
Thioridazine Hydrochloride Tablets ... 2289

Thiothixene (Co-administration may result in additive CNS depression). Products include:
Navane Capsules ... 2701
Thiothixene Capsules ... 2290

Tolbutamide (*In vitro* studies with co-administration has resulted in an increase in unbound fraction of tolbutamide; the clinical relevance of this displacement is unknown).
No products indexed under this heading.

Triazolam (Co-administration may result in additive CNS depression). Products include:
Halcion Tablets ... 2823

Trifluoperazine Hydrochloride (Co-administration may result in additive CNS depression). Products include:
Stelazine ... 1640

Warfarin Sodium (In an *in vitro* study, valproate increased the unbound fraction of warfarin by up to 32.6%; therapeutic relevance of this is unknown). Products include:
Coumadin for Injection ... 1243
Coumadin Tablets ... 1243
Warfarin Sodium Tablets, USP ... 3302

Zaleplon (Co-administration may result in additive CNS depression). Products include:
Sonata Capsules ... 3591

Ziprasidone Hydrochloride (Co-administration may result in additive CNS depression). Products include:
Geodon Capsules ... 2688

Zolpidem Tartrate (Co-administration may result in additive CNS depression). Products include:
Ambien Tablets ... 3191

Food Interactions

Alcohol (Co-administration may result in additive CNS depression).

DEPAKENE CAPSULES

(Valproic Acid) ... 421

May interact with central nervous system depressants, phenytoin, and certain other agents. Compounds in these categories include:

Alfentanil Hydrochloride (Valproate produces CNS depression, especially when combined with another CNS depressant).
No products indexed under this heading.

Alprazolam (Valproate produces CNS depression, especially when combined with another CNS depressant). Products include:
Xanax Tablets ... 2865

Amitriptyline Hydrochloride (Co-administration has resulted in a decrease in plasma clearance of amitriptyline; rare postmarketing reports of increased amitriptyline levels). Products include:
Etrafon ... 3115
Limbitrol ... 1738

Aprobarbital (Valproate produces CNS depression, especially when combined with another CNS depressant).
No products indexed under this heading.

Aspirin (Co-administration has resulted in a decrease in protein binding and an inhibition of metabolism of valproate; valproate free fraction was increased 4-fold in the presence of aspirin compared to valproate alone). Products include:
Aggrenox Capsules ... 1026
Alka-Seltzer ... ▣603
Alka-Seltzer Lemon Lime Antacid and Pain Reliever Effervescent Tablets ... ▣603
Alka-Seltzer Extra Strength Antacid and Pain Reliever Effervescent Tablets ... ▣603
Alka-Seltzer PM Effervescent Tablets ... ▣605
Genuine Bayer Tablets, Caplets and Gelcaps ... ▣606
Extra Strength Bayer Caplets and Gelcaps ... ▣610
Aspirin Regimen Bayer Children's Chewable Tablets (Orange or Cherry Flavored) ... ▣607
Bayer, Aspirin Regimen ... ▣606
Aspirin Regimen Bayer 81 mg Caplets with Calcium ... ▣607
Genuine Bayer Professional Labeling (Aspirin Regimen Bayer) ... ▣608
Extra Strength Bayer Arthritis Caplets ... ▣610
Extra Strength Bayer Plus Caplets ... ▣610
Extra Strength Bayer PM Caplets ... ▣611
BC Powder ... ▣619
BC Allergy Sinus Cold Powder ... ▣619
Arthritis Strength BC Powder ... ▣619
BC Sinus Cold Powder ... ▣619
Darvon Compound-65 Pulvules ... 1910
Ecotrin Enteric Coated Aspirin Low, Regular and Maximum Strength Tablets ... 1715
Excedrin Extra-Strength Tablets, Caplets, and Geltabs ... ▣629
Excedrin Migraine ... 1070
Goody's Body Pain Formula Powder ... ▣620
Goody's Extra Strength Headache Powder ... ▣620
Goody's Extra Strength Pain Relief Tablets ... ▣620
Percodan Tablets ... 1327
Robaxisal Tablets ... 2939
Soma Compound Tablets ... 3354
Soma Compound w/Codeine Tablets ... 3355
Vanquish Caplets ... ▣617

Buprenorphine Hydrochloride (Valproate produces CNS depression, especially when combined with another CNS depressant). Products include:
Buprenex Injectable ... 2918

Buspirone Hydrochloride (Valproate produces CNS depression, especially when combined with another CNS depressant).
No products indexed under this heading.

Butabarbital (Valproate produces CNS depression, especially when combined with another CNS depressant).
No products indexed under this heading.

Butalbital (Valproate produces CNS depression, especially when combined with another CNS depressant). Products include:
Phrenilin ... 578
Sedapap Tablets 50 mg/650 mg ... 2225

Carbamazepine (Co-administration has resulted in decreased serum levels of carbamazepine and increased serum levels of carbamazepine 10, 11-epoxide; drugs that affect the levels of expression of hepatic enzymes, particularly those that elevate levels of glucuronosyltransferases, such as carbamazepine, may increase the clearance of valproate). Products include:
Carbatrol Capsules ... 3234
Tegretol/Tegretol-XR ... 2404

Chlordiazepoxide (Valproate produces CNS depression, especially when combined with another CNS depressant). Products include:
Limbitrol ... 1738

Chlordiazepoxide Hydrochloride (Valproate produces CNS depression, especially when combined with another CNS depressant). Products include:
Librium Capsules ... 1736
Librium for Injection ... 1737

Chlorpromazine (Co-administration has resulted in an increase in trough plasma levels of valproate). Products include:
Thorazine Suppositories ... 1656

Chlorpromazine Hydrochloride (Co-administration has resulted in an increase in trough plasma levels of valproate). Products include:
Thorazine ... 1656

Chlorprothixene (Valproate produces CNS depression, especially when combined with another CNS depressant).
No products indexed under this heading.

Chlorprothixene Hydrochloride (Valproate produces CNS depression, especially when combined with another CNS depressant).
No products indexed under this heading.

Chlorprothixene Lactate (Valproate produces CNS depression, especially when combined with another CNS depressant).
No products indexed under this heading.

Clonazepam (Co-administration may induce absence status in patients with a history of absence type seizures). Products include:
Klonopin Tablets ... 2983

Clorazepate Dipotassium (Valproate produces CNS depression, especially when combined with another CNS depressant). Products include:
Tranxene ... 511

Clozapine (Valproate produces CNS depression, especially when combined with another CNS depressant). Products include:
Clozaril Tablets ... 2319

Codeine Phosphate (Valproate produces CNS depression, especially when combined with another CNS depressant). Products include:

Phenergan with Codeine Syrup 3557
Phenergan VC with Codeine Syrup .. 3561
Robitussin A-C Syrup 2942
Robitussin-DAC Syrup 2942
Ryna-C Liquid 768
Soma Compound w/Codeine Tablets 3355
Tussi-Organidin NR Liquid 3350
Tussi-Organidin-S NR Liquid 3350
Tylenol with Codeine 2595

Desflurane (Valproate produces CNS depression, especially when combined with another CNS depressant). Products include:
Suprane Liquid for Inhalation 874

Dezocine (Valproate produces CNS depression, especially when combined with another CNS depressant).
No products indexed under this heading.

Diazepam (Co-administration increases the free fraction of diazepam by 90% in healthy volunteers; plasma clearance and volume of distribution for diazepam were reduced by 25% and 20%, respectively, in the presence of valproate). Products include:
Valium Injectable 3026
Valium Tablets 3047

Droperidol (Valproate produces CNS depression, especially when combined with another CNS depressant).
No products indexed under this heading.

Enflurane (Valproate produces CNS depression, especially when combined with another CNS depressant).
No products indexed under this heading.

Estazolam (Valproate produces CNS depression, especially when combined with another CNS depressant). Products include:
ProSom Tablets 500

Ethchlorvynol (Valproate produces CNS depression, especially when combined with another CNS depressant).
No products indexed under this heading.

Ethinamate (Valproate produces CNS depression, especially when combined with another CNS depressant).
No products indexed under this heading.

Ethosuximide (Valproate inhibits the metabolism of ethosuximide; co-administration was accompanied by a 25% increase in elimination half-life of ethosuximide and a 15% decrease in its total clearance as compared to ethosuximide alone). Products include:
Zarontin Capsules 2659
Zarontin Syrup 2660

Felbamate (Co-administration has resulted in an increase in mean valproate peak concentration). Products include:
Felbatol 3343

Fentanyl (Valproate produces CNS depression, especially when combined with another CNS depressant). Products include:
Duragesic Transdermal System 1786

Fentanyl Citrate (Valproate produces CNS depression, especially when combined with another CNS depressant). Products include:
Actiq 1184

Fluphenazine Decanoate (Valproate produces CNS depression, especially when combined with another CNS depressant).
No products indexed under this heading.

Fluphenazine Enanthate (Valproate produces CNS depression, especially when combined with another CNS depressant).
No products indexed under this heading.

Fluphenazine Hydrochloride (Valproate produces CNS depression, especially when combined with another CNS depressant).
No products indexed under this heading.

Flurazepam Hydrochloride (Valproate produces CNS depression, especially when combined with another CNS depressant).
No products indexed under this heading.

Fosphenytoin Sodium (Co-administration with drugs that affect the levels of expression of hepatic enzymes, particularly those that elevate levels of glucuronosyltransferases, such as phenytoin, may increase the clearance of valproate; valproate displaces phenytoin from its plasma binding sites and inhibits its hepatic metabolism; concurrent use has resulted in breakthrough seizures). Products include:
Cerebyx Injection 2619

Glutethimide (Valproate produces CNS depression, especially when combined with another CNS depressant).
No products indexed under this heading.

Haloperidol (Valproate produces CNS depression, especially when combined with another CNS depressant). Products include:
Haldol Injection, Tablets and Concentrate 2533

Haloperidol Decanoate (Valproate produces CNS depression, especially when combined with another CNS depressant). Products include:
Haldol Decanoate 2535

Hydrocodone Bitartrate (Valproate produces CNS depression, especially when combined with another CNS depressant). Products include:
Hycodan 1316
Hycomine Compound Tablets 1317
Hycotuss Expectorant Syrup 1318
Lortab 3319
Lortab Elixir 3317
Maxidone Tablets CIII 3399
Norco 5/325 Tablets CIII 3424
Norco 7.5/325 Tablets CIII 3425
Norco 10/325 Tablets CIII 3427
Norco 10/325 Tablets CIII 3425
Vicodin Tablets 516
Vicodin ES Tablets 517
Vicodin HP Tablets 518
Vicodin Tuss Expectorant 519
Vicoprofen Tablets 520
Zydone Tablets 1330

Hydrocodone Polistirex (Valproate produces CNS depression, especially when combined with another CNS depressant). Products include:
Tussionex Pennkinetic Extended-Release Suspension..... 1174

Hydromorphone Hydrochloride (Valproate produces CNS depression, especially when combined with another CNS depressant). Products include:
Dilaudid 441
Dilaudid Oral Liquid 445
Dilaudid Powder 441
Dilaudid Rectal Suppositories 441
Dilaudid Tablets 441
Dilaudid Tablets - 8 mg 445
Dilaudid-HP 443

Hydroxyzine Hydrochloride (Valproate produces CNS depression, especially when combined with another CNS depressant). Products include:
Atarax Tablets & Syrup 2667
Vistaril Intramuscular Solution 2738

Isoflurane (Valproate produces CNS depression, especially when combined with another CNS depressant).
No products indexed under this heading.

Ketamine Hydrochloride (Valproate produces CNS depression, especially when combined with another CNS depressant).
No products indexed under this heading.

Lamotrigine (Co-administration has resulted in increased elimination half-life of lamotrigine from 26 to 72 hours). Products include:
Lamictal 1567

Levomethadyl Acetate Hydrochloride (Valproate produces CNS depression, especially when combined with another CNS depressant).
No products indexed under this heading.

Levorphanol Tartrate (Valproate produces CNS depression, especially when combined with another CNS depressant). Products include:
Levo-Dromoran 1734
Levorphanol Tartrate Tablets 3059

Lorazepam (Co-administration was accompanied by a 17% decrease in the plasma clearance of lorazepam). Products include:
Ativan Injection 3478
Ativan Tablets 3482

Loxapine Hydrochloride (Valproate produces CNS depression, especially when combined with another CNS depressant).
No products indexed under this heading.

Loxapine Succinate (Valproate produces CNS depression, especially when combined with another CNS depressant). Products include:
Loxitane Capsules 3398

Meperidine Hydrochloride (Valproate produces CNS depression, especially when combined with another CNS depressant). Products include:
Demerol 3079
Mepergan Injection 3539

Mephobarbital (Valproate produces CNS depression, especially when combined with another CNS depressant).
No products indexed under this heading.

Meprobamate (Valproate produces CNS depression, especially when combined with another CNS depressant). Products include:
Miltown Tablets 3349

Mesoridazine Besylate (Valproate produces CNS depression, especially when combined with another CNS depressant). Products include:
Serentil 1057

Methadone Hydrochloride (Valproate produces CNS depression, especially when combined with another CNS depressant). Products include:
Dolophine Hydrochloride Tablets 3056

Methohexital Sodium (Valproate produces CNS depression, especially when combined with another CNS depressant). Products include:
Brevital Sodium for Injection, USP .. 1815

Methotrimeprazine (Valproate produces CNS depression, especially when combined with another CNS depressant).
No products indexed under this heading.

Methoxyflurane (Valproate produces CNS depression, especially when combined with another CNS depressant).
No products indexed under this heading.

Midazolam Hydrochloride (Valproate produces CNS depression, especially when combined with another CNS depressant). Products include:
Versed Injection 3027
Versed Syrup 3033

Molindone Hydrochloride (Valproate produces CNS depression, especially when combined with another CNS depressant). Products include:
Moban 1320

Morphine Sulfate (Valproate produces CNS depression, especially when combined with another CNS depressant). Products include:
Astramorph/PF Injection, USP (Preservative-Free)........................ 594
Duramorph Injection 1312
Infumorph 200 and Infumorph 500 Sterile Solutions 1314
Kadian Capsules 1335
MS Contin Tablets 2896
MSIR 2898
Oramorph SR Tablets 3062
Roxanol 3066

Nortriptyline Hydrochloride (Co-administration has resulted in a decrease in the net clearance of nortriptyline).
No products indexed under this heading.

Olanzapine (Valproate produces CNS depression, especially when combined with another CNS depressant). Products include:
Zyprexa Tablets 1973
Zyprexa ZYDIS Orally Disintegrating Tablets.................. 1973

Oxazepam (Valproate produces CNS depression, especially when combined with another CNS depressant).
No products indexed under this heading.

Oxycodone Hydrochloride (Valproate produces CNS depression, especially when combined with another CNS depressant). Products include:
OxyContin Tablets 2912
OxyFast Oral Concentrate Solution . 2916
OxyIR Capsules 2916
Percocet Tablets 1326
Percodan Tablets 1327
Percolone Tablets 1327
Roxicodone 3067
Tylox Capsules 2597

Pentobarbital Sodium (Valproate produces CNS depression, especially when combined with another CNS depressant). Products include:
Nembutal Sodium Solution 485

Perphenazine (Valproate produces CNS depression, especially when combined with another CNS depressant). Products include:
Etrafon 3115
Trilafon 3160

Phenobarbital (Co-administration with drugs that affect the levels of expression of hepatic enzymes, particularly those that elevate levels of glucuronosyltransferases, such as phenobarbital, may increase the clearance of valproate; valproate inhibits the metabolism ofphenobarbital; co-administration has resulted in an increase in half-life and decrease in plasma clearance of phenobarbital; all patients should be monitored for neurological toxicity because of severe CNS depression). Products include:
Arco-Lase Plus Tablets 592
Donnatal 2929
Donnatal Extentabs 2930

Phenytoin (Co-administration with drugs that affect the levels of expression of hepatic enzymes, particularly those that elevate levels of glucuronosyltransferases, such as phenytoin, may increase the clearance of valproate; valproate displaces phenytoin from its plasma binding sites and inhibits its hepatic metabolism; concurrent use has resulted in breakthrough seizures). Products include:
Dilantin Infatabs 2624
Dilantin-125 Oral Suspension 2625

Phenytoin Sodium (Co-administration with drugs that affect the levels of expression of hepatic enzymes, particularly those that ele-

IMPORTANT NOTE: Always consult each drug listing in the patient's regimen for possible interactions.

vate levels of glucuronosyltransferases, such as phenytoin, may increase the clearance of valproate; valproate displaces phenytoin from its plasma binding sites and inhibits its hepatic metabolism; concurrent use has resulted in breakthrough seizures). Products include:
Dilantin Kapseals 2622

Prazepam (Valproate produces CNS depression, especially when combined with another CNS depressant).
No products indexed under this heading.

Primidone (Co-administraion may result in severe CNS depression because primidone is metabolized to a barbiturate; potential for same interaction as phenobarbital and valproate).
No products indexed under this heading.

Prochlorperazine (Valproate produces CNS depression, especially when combined with another CNS depressant). Products include:
Compazine 1505

Promethazine Hydrochloride (Valproate produces CNS depression, especially when combined with another CNS depressant). Products include:
Mepergan Injection 3539
Phenergan Injection 3553
Phenergan 3556
Phenergan Syrup 3554
Phenergan with Codeine Syrup 3557
Phenergan with Dextromethorphan Syrup 3559
Phenergan VC Syrup 3560
Phenergan VC with Codeine Syrup 3561

Propofol (Valproate produces CNS depression, especially when combined with another CNS depressant). Products include:
Diprivan Injectable Emulsion 667

Propoxyphene Hydrochloride (Valproate produces CNS depression, especially when combined with another CNS depressant). Products include:
Darvon Pulvules 1909
Darvon Compound-65 Pulvules 1910

Propoxyphene Napsylate (Valproate produces CNS depression, especially when combined with another CNS depressant). Products include:
Darvon-N/Darvocet-N 1907
Darvon-N Tablets 1912

Quazepam (Valproate produces CNS depression, especially when combined with another CNS depressant).
No products indexed under this heading.

Quetiapine Fumarate (Valproate produces CNS depression, especially when combined with another CNS depressant). Products include:
Seroquel Tablets 684

Remifentanil Hydrochloride (Valproate produces CNS depression, especially when combined with another CNS depressant).
No products indexed under this heading.

Rifampin (Co-administration has resulted in an increase in the oral clearance of valproate). Products include:
Rifadin 765
Rifamate Capsules 767
Rifater Tablets 769

Risperidone (Valproate produces CNS depression, especially when combined with another CNS depressant). Products include:
Risperdal 1796

Secobarbital Sodium (Valproate produces CNS depression, especially when combined with another CNS depressant).
No products indexed under this heading.

Sevoflurane (Valproate produces CNS depression, especially when combined with another CNS depressant).
No products indexed under this heading.

Sufentanil Citrate (Valproate produces CNS depression, especially when combined with another CNS depressant).
No products indexed under this heading.

Temazepam (Valproate produces CNS depression, especially when combined with another CNS depressant).
No products indexed under this heading.

Thiamylal Sodium (Valproate produces CNS depression, especially when combined with another CNS depressant).
No products indexed under this heading.

Thioridazine Hydrochloride (Valproate produces CNS depression, especially when combined with another CNS depressant). Products include:
Thioridazine Hydrochloride Tablets 2289

Thiothixene (Valproate produces CNS depression, especially when combined with another CNS depressant). Products include:
Navane Capsules 2701
Thiothixene Capsules 2290

Tolbutamide (Co-administration in vitro experiments has resulted in increased unbound fraction of tolbutamide).
No products indexed under this heading.

Triazolam (Valproate produces CNS depression, especially when combined with another CNS depressant). Products include:
Halcion Tablets 2823

Trifluoperazine Hydrochloride (Valproate produces CNS depression, especially when combined with another CNS depressant). Products include:
Stelazine 1640

Warfarin Sodium (Co-administration in vitro experiments has resulted in increased unbound fraction of warfarin). Products include:
Coumadin for Injection 1243
Coumadin Tablets 1243
Warfarin Sodium Tablets, USP 3302

Zaleplon (Valproate produces CNS depression, especially when combined with another CNS depressant). Products include:
Sonata Capsules 3591

Ziprasidone Hydrochloride (Valproate produces CNS depression, especially when combined with another CNS depressant). Products include:
Geodon Capsules 2688

Zidovudine (Co-administration has resulted in decreased clearance of zidovudine; the half-life of zidovudine was unaffected). Products include:
Combivir Tablets 1502
Retrovir 1625
Retrovir IV Infusion 1629
Trizivir Tablets 1669

Zolpidem Tartrate (Valproate produces CNS depression, especially when combined with another CNS depressant). Products include:
Ambien Tablets 3191

Food Interactions

Alcohol (Valproate produces CNS depression, especially when combined with another CNS depressant, such as alcohol).

DEPAKENE SYRUP
(Valproic Acid) 421
See Depakene Capsules

DEPAKOTE SPRINKLE CAPSULES
(Divalproex Sodium) 426
See Depakote Tablets

DEPAKOTE TABLETS
(Divalproex Sodium) 430
May interact with central nervous system depressants, phenytoin, and certain other agents. Compounds in these categories include:

Alfentanil Hydrochloride (Valproate produces CNS depression, especially when combined with another CNS depressant).
No products indexed under this heading.

Alprazolam (Valproate produces CNS depression, especially when combined with another CNS depressant). Products include:
Xanax Tablets 2865

Amitriptyline Hydrochloride (Co-administration has resulted in a decrease in plasma clearance of amitriptyline; rare postmarketing reports of increased amitriptyline levels). Products include:
Etrafon 3115
Limbitrol 1738

Aprobarbital (Valproate produces CNS depression, especially when combined with another CNS depressant).
No products indexed under this heading.

Aspirin (Co-administration has resulted in a decrease in protein binding and an inhibition of metabolism of valproate; valproate free fraction was increased 4-fold in the presence of aspirin compared to valproate alone). Products include:
Aggrenox Capsules 1026
Alka-Seltzer .... ▣603
Alka-Seltzer Lemon Lime Antacid and Pain Reliever Effervescent Tablets .... ▣603
Alka-Seltzer Extra Strength Antacid and Pain Reliever Effervescent Tablets .... ▣603
Alka-Seltzer PM Effervescent Tablets .... ▣605
Genuine Bayer Tablets, Caplets and Gelcaps .... ▣606
Extra Strength Bayer Caplets and Gelcaps .... ▣610
Aspirin Regimen Bayer Children's Chewable Tablets (Orange or Cherry Flavored) .... ▣607
Bayer, Aspirin Regimen .... ▣606
Aspirin Regimen Bayer 81 mg Caplets with Calcium .... ▣607
Genuine Bayer Professional Labeling (Aspirin Regimen Bayer) .... ▣608
Extra Strength Bayer Arthritis Caplets .... ▣610
Extra Strength Bayer Plus Caplets .... ▣610
Extra Strength Bayer PM Caplets .... ▣611
BC Powder .... ▣619
BC Allergy Sinus Cold Powder .... ▣619
Arthritis Strength BC Powder .... ▣619
BC Sinus Cold Powder .... ▣619
Darvon Compound-65 Pulvules 1910
Ecotrin Enteric Coated Aspirin Low, Regular and Maximum Strength Tablets 1715
Excedrin Extra-Strength Tablets, Caplets, and Geltabs .... ▣629
Excedrin Migraine 1070
Goody's Body Pain Formula Powder .... ▣620
Goody's Extra Strength Headache Powder .... ▣620
Goody's Extra Strength Pain Relief Tablets .... ▣620
Percodan Tablets 1327
Robaxisal Tablets 2939
Soma Compound Tablets 3354
Soma Compound w/Codeine Tablets 3355
Vanquish Caplets .... ▣617

Buprenorphine Hydrochloride (Valproate produces CNS depression, especially when combined with another CNS depressant). Products include:
Buprenex Injectable 2918

Buspirone Hydrochloride (Valproate produces CNS depression, especially when combined with another CNS depressant).
No products indexed under this heading.

Butabarbital (Valproate produces CNS depression, especially when combined with another CNS depressant).
No products indexed under this heading.

Butalbital (Valproate produces CNS depression, especially when combined with another CNS depressant). Products include:
Phrenilin 578
Sedapap Tablets 50 mg/650 mg 2225

Carbamazepine (Co-administration has resulted in decreased serum levels of carbamazepine and increased serum levels of carbamazepine 10,11-epoxide; drugs that affect the levels of expression of hepatic enzymes, particularly those that elevate levels of glucuronosyltransferases, such as carbamazepine, may increase the clearance of valproate). Products include:
Carbatrol Capsules 3234
Tegretol/Tegretol-XR 2404

Chlordiazepoxide (Valproate produces CNS depression, especially when combined with another CNS depressant). Products include:
Limbitrol 1738

Chlordiazepoxide Hydrochloride (Valproate produces CNS depression, especially when combined with another CNS depressant). Products include:
Librium Capsules 1736
Librium for Injection 1737

Chlorpromazine (Co-administration has resulted in an increase in trough plasma levels of valproate). Products include:
Thorazine Suppositories 1656

Chlorpromazine Hydrochloride (Co-administration has resulted in an increase in trough plasma levels of valproate). Products include:
Thorazine 1656

Chlorprothixene (Valproate produces CNS depression, especially when combined with another CNS depressant).
No products indexed under this heading.

Chlorprothixene Hydrochloride (Valproate produces CNS depression, especially when combined with another CNS depressant).
No products indexed under this heading.

Chlorprothixene Lactate (Valproate produces CNS depression, especially when combined with another CNS depressant).
No products indexed under this heading.

Clonazepam (Co-administration may induce absence status in patients with a history of absence type seizures). Products include:
Klonopin Tablets 2983

Clorazepate Dipotassium (Valproate produces CNS depression, especially when combined with another CNS depressant). Products include:
Tranxene 511

Clozapine (Valproate produces CNS depression, especially when combined with another CNS depressant). Products include:
Clozaril Tablets 2319

Codeine Phosphate (Valproate produces CNS depression, especially when combined with another CNS depressant). Products include:
- Phenergan with Codeine Syrup 3557
- Phenergan VC with Codeine Syrup 3561
- Robitussin A-C Syrup 2942
- Robitussin-DAC Syrup 2942
- Ryna-C Liquid 768
- Soma Compound w/Codeine Tablets 3355
- Tussi-Organidin NR Liquid 3350
- Tussi-Organidin-S NR Liquid 3350
- Tylenol with Codeine 2595

Desflurane (Valproate produces CNS depression, especially when combined with another CNS depressant). Products include:
- Suprane Liquid for Inhalation 874

Dezocine (Valproate produces CNS depression, especially when combined with another CNS depressant).
No products indexed under this heading.

Diazepam (Co-administration increases the free fraction of diazepam by 90% in healthy volunteers; plasma clearance and volume of distribution for diazepam were reduced by 25% and 20%, respectively, in the presence of valproate). Products include:
- Valium Injectable 3026
- Valium Tablets 3047

Droperidol (Valproate produces CNS depression, especially when combined with another CNS depressant).
No products indexed under this heading.

Enflurane (Valproate produces CNS depression, especially when combined with another CNS depressant).
No products indexed under this heading.

Estazolam (Valproate produces CNS depression, especially when combined with another CNS depressant). Products include:
- ProSom Tablets 500

Ethchlorvynol (Valproate produces CNS depression, especially when combined with another CNS depressant).
No products indexed under this heading.

Ethinamate (Valproate produces CNS depression, especially when combined with another CNS depressant).
No products indexed under this heading.

Ethosuximide (Valproate inhibits the metabolism of ethosuximide; co-administration was accompanied by a 25% increase in elimination half-life of ethosuximide and a 15% decrease in its total clearance as compared to ethosuximide alone). Products include:
- Zarontin Capsules 2659
- Zarontin Syrup 2660

Felbamate (Co-administration has resulted in an increase in mean valproate peak concentration). Products include:
- Felbatol 3343

Fentanyl (Valproate produces CNS depression, especially when combined with another CNS depressant). Products include:
- Duragesic Transdermal System 1786

Fentanyl Citrate (Valproate produces CNS depression, especially when combined with another CNS depressant). Products include:
- Actiq 1184

Fluphenazine Decanoate (Valproate produces CNS depression, especially when combined with another CNS depressant).
No products indexed under this heading.

Fluphenazine Enanthate (Valproate produces CNS depression, especially when combined with another CNS depressant).
No products indexed under this heading.

Fluphenazine Hydrochloride (Valproate produces CNS depression, especially when combined with another CNS depressant).
No products indexed under this heading.

Flurazepam Hydrochloride (Valproate produces CNS depression, especially when combined with another CNS depressant).
No products indexed under this heading.

Fosphenytoin Sodium (Co-administration with drugs that affect the levels of expression of hepatic enzymes, particularly those that elevate levels of glucuronosyltransferases, such as phenytoin, may increase the clearance of valproate; valproate displaces phenytoin from its plasma binding sites and inhibits its hepatic metabolism; concurrent use has resulted in breakthrough seizures). Products include:
- Cerebyx Injection 2619

Glutethimide (Valproate produces CNS depression, especially when combined with another CNS depressant).
No products indexed under this heading.

Haloperidol (Valproate produces CNS depression, especially when combined with another CNS depressant). Products include:
- Haldol Injection, Tablets and Concentrate 2533

Haloperidol Decanoate (Valproate produces CNS depression, especially when combined with another CNS depressant). Products include:
- Haldol Decanoate 2535

Hydrocodone Bitartrate (Valproate produces CNS depression, especially when combined with another CNS depressant). Products include:
- Hycodan 1316
- Hycomine Compound Tablets 1317
- Hycotuss Expectorant Syrup 1318
- Lortab 3319
- Lortab Elixir 3317
- Maxidone Tablets CIII 3399
- Norco 5/325 Tablets CIII 3424
- Norco 7.5/325 Tablets CIII 3425
- Norco 10/325 Tablets CIII 3427
- Norco 10/325 Tablets CIII 3425
- Vicodin Tablets 516
- Vicodin ES Tablets 517
- Vicodin HP Tablets 518
- Vicodin Tuss Expectorant 519
- Vicoprofen Tablets 520
- Zydone Tablets 1330

Hydrocodone Polistirex (Valproate produces CNS depression, especially when combined with another CNS depressant). Products include:
- Tussionex Pennkinetic Extended-Release Suspension 1174

Hydromorphone Hydrochloride (Valproate produces CNS depression, especially when combined with another CNS depressant). Products include:
- Dilaudid 441
- Dilaudid Oral Liquid 445
- Dilaudid Powder 441
- Dilaudid Rectal Suppositories 441
- Dilaudid Tablets 441
- Dilaudid Tablets - 8 mg 445
- Dilaudid-HP 443

Hydroxyzine Hydrochloride (Valproate produces CNS depression, especially when combined with another CNS depressant). Products include:
- Atarax Tablets & Syrup 2667
- Vistaril Intramuscular Solution 2738

Isoflurane (Valproate produces CNS depression, especially when combined with another CNS depressant).
No products indexed under this heading.

Ketamine Hydrochloride (Valproate produces CNS depression, especially when combined with another CNS depressant).
No products indexed under this heading.

Lamotrigine (Co-administration has resulted in increased elimination half-life of lamotrigine from 26 to 72 hours). Products include:
- Lamictal 1567

Levomethadyl Acetate Hydrochloride (Valproate produces CNS depression, especially when combined with another CNS depressant).
No products indexed under this heading.

Levorphanol Tartrate (Valproate produces CNS depression, especially when combined with another CNS depressant). Products include:
- Levo-Dromoran 1734
- Levorphanol Tartrate Tablets 3059

Lorazepam (Co-administration was accompanied by a 17% decrease in the plasma clearance of lorazepam). Products include:
- Ativan Injection 3478
- Ativan Tablets 3482

Loxapine Hydrochloride (Valproate produces CNS depression, especially when combined with another CNS depressant).
No products indexed under this heading.

Loxapine Succinate (Valproate produces CNS depression, especially when combined with another CNS depressant). Products include:
- Loxitane Capsules 3398

Meperidine Hydrochloride (Valproate produces CNS depression, especially when combined with another CNS depressant). Products include:
- Demerol 3079
- Mepergan Injection 3539

Mephobarbital (Valproate produces CNS depression, especially when combined with another CNS depressant).
No products indexed under this heading.

Meprobamate (Valproate produces CNS depression, especially when combined with another CNS depressant). Products include:
- Miltown Tablets 3349

Mesoridazine Besylate (Valproate produces CNS depression, especially when combined with another CNS depressant). Products include:
- Serentil 1057

Methadone Hydrochloride (Valproate produces CNS depression, especially when combined with another CNS depressant). Products include:
- Dolophine Hydrochloride Tablets 3056

Methohexital Sodium (Valproate produces CNS depression, especially when combined with another CNS depressant). Products include:
- Brevital Sodium for Injection, USP 1815

Methotrimeprazine (Valproate produces CNS depression, especially when combined with another CNS depressant).
No products indexed under this heading.

Methoxyflurane (Valproate produces CNS depression, especially when combined with another CNS depressant).
No products indexed under this heading.

Midazolam Hydrochloride (Valproate produces CNS depression, especially when combined with another CNS depressant). Products include:
- Versed Injection 3027
- Versed Syrup 3033

Molindone Hydrochloride (Valproate produces CNS depression, especially when combined with another CNS depressant). Products include:
- Moban 1320

Morphine Sulfate (Valproate produces CNS depression, especially when combined with another CNS depressant). Products include:
- Astramorph/PF Injection, USP (Preservative-Free) 594
- Duramorph Injection 1312
- Infumorph 200 and Infumorph 500 Sterile Solutions 1314
- Kadian Capsules 1335
- MS Contin Tablets 2896
- MSIR 2898
- Oramorph SR Tablets 3062
- Roxanol 3066

Nortriptyline Hydrochloride (Co-administration has resulted in a decrease in the net clearance of nortriptyline).
No products indexed under this heading.

Olanzapine (Valproate produces CNS depression, especially when combined with another CNS depressant). Products include:
- Zyprexa Tablets 1973
- Zyprexa ZYDIS Orally Disintegrating Tablets 1973

Oxazepam (Valproate produces CNS depression, especially when combined with another CNS depressant).
No products indexed under this heading.

Oxycodone Hydrochloride (Valproate produces CNS depression, especially when combined with another CNS depressant). Products include:
- OxyContin Tablets 2912
- OxyFast Oral Concentrate Solution 2916
- OxyIR Capsules 2916
- Percocet Tablets 1326
- Percodan Tablets 1327
- Percolone Tablets 1327
- Roxicodone 3067
- Tylox Capsules 2597

Pentobarbital Sodium (Valproate produces CNS depression, especially when combined with another CNS depressant). Products include:
- Nembutal Sodium Solution 485

Perphenazine (Valproate produces CNS depression, especially when combined with another CNS depressant). Products include:
- Etrafon 3115
- Trilafon 3160

Phenobarbital (Co-administration with drugs that affect the levels of expression of hepatic enzymes, particularly those that elevate levels of glucuronosyltransferases, such as phenobarbital, may increase the clearance of valproate; valproate inhibits the metabolism ofphenobarbital; co-administration has resulted in an increase in half-life and a decrease in plasma clearance of phenobarbital; all patients should be monitored for neurological toxicity because of severe CNS depression). Products include:
- Arco-Lase Plus Tablets 592
- Donnatal 2929
- Donnatal Extentabs 2930

Phenytoin (Co-administration with drugs that affect the levels of expression of hepatic enzymes, particularly those that elevate levels of glucuronosyltransferases, such as phenytoin, may increase the clearance of valproate; valproate displaces phenytoin from its plasma binding sites and inhibits its hepatic metabolism; concurrent use has resulted in breakthrough seizures). Products include:
- Dilantin Infatabs 2624
- Dilantin-125 Oral Suspension 2625

IMPORTANT NOTE: Always consult each drug listing in the patient's regimen for possible interactions.

Phenytoin Sodium (Co-administration with drugs that affect the levels of expression of hepatic enzymes, particularly those that elevate levels of glucuronosyltransferases, such as phenytoin, may increase the clearance of valproate; valproate displaces phenytoin from its plasma binding sites and inhibits its hepatic metabolism; concurrent use has resulted in breakthrough seizures). Products include:
- Dilantin Kapseals 2622

Prazepam (Valproate produces CNS depression, especially when combined with another CNS depressant).
- No products indexed under this heading.

Primidone (Co-administration may result in severe CNS depression because primidone is metabolized to a barbiturate; potential for same interaction as phenobarbital and valproate).
- No products indexed under this heading.

Prochlorperazine (Valproate produces CNS depression, especially when combined with another CNS depressant). Products include:
- Compazine 1505

Promethazine Hydrochloride (Valproate produces CNS depression, especially when combined with another CNS depressant). Products include:
- Mepergan Injection 3539
- Phenergan Injection 3553
- Phenergan 3556
- Phenergan Syrup 3554
- Phenergan with Codeine Syrup 3557
- Phenergan with Dextromethorphan Syrup 3559
- Phenergan VC Syrup 3560
- Phenergan VC with Codeine Syrup .. 3561

Propofol (Valproate produces CNS depression, especially when combined with another CNS depressant). Products include:
- Diprivan Injectable Emulsion 667

Propoxyphene Hydrochloride (Valproate produces CNS depression, especially when combined with another CNS depressant). Products include:
- Darvon Pulvules 1909
- Darvon Compound-65 Pulvules 1910

Propoxyphene Napsylate (Valproate produces CNS depression, especially when combined with another CNS depressant). Products include:
- Darvon-N/Darvocet-N 1907
- Darvon-N Tablets 1912

Quazepam (Valproate produces CNS depression, especially when combined with another CNS depressant).
- No products indexed under this heading.

Quetiapine Fumarate (Valproate produces CNS depression, especially when combined with another CNS depressant). Products include:
- Seroquel Tablets 684

Remifentanil Hydrochloride (Valproate produces CNS depression, especially when combined with another CNS depressant).
- No products indexed under this heading.

Rifampin (Co-administration has resulted in a increase in the oral clearance of valproate). Products include:
- Rifadin 765
- Rifamate Capsules 767
- Rifater Tablets 769

Risperidone (Valproate produces CNS depression, especially when combined with another CNS depressant). Products include:
- Risperdal 1796

Secobarbital Sodium (Valproate produces CNS depression, especially when combined with another CNS depressant).
- No products indexed under this heading.

Sevoflurane (Valproate produces CNS depression, especially when combined with another CNS depressant).
- No products indexed under this heading.

Sufentanil Citrate (Valproate produces CNS depression, especially when combined with another CNS depressant).
- No products indexed under this heading.

Temazepam (Valproate produces CNS depression, especially when combined with another CNS depressant).
- No products indexed under this heading.

Thiamylal Sodium (Valproate produces CNS depression, especially when combined with another CNS depressant).
- No products indexed under this heading.

Thioridazine Hydrochloride (Valproate produces CNS depression, especially when combined with another CNS depressant). Products include:
- Thioridazine Hydrochloride Tablets 2289

Thiothixene (Valproate produces CNS depression, especially when combined with another CNS depressant). Products include:
- Navane Capsules 2701
- Thiothixene Capsules 2290

Tolbutamide (Co-administration in in vitro experiments has resulted in increased unbound fraction of tolbutamide).
- No products indexed under this heading.

Triazolam (Valproate produces CNS depression, especially when combined with another CNS depressant). Products include:
- Halcion Tablets 2823

Trifluoperazine Hydrochloride (Valproate produces CNS depression, especially when combined with another CNS depressant). Products include:
- Stelazine 1640

Warfarin Sodium (Co-administration in in vitro experiments has resulted in increased unbound fraction of warfarin). Products include:
- Coumadin for Injection 1243
- Coumadin Tablets 1243
- Warfarin Sodium Tablets, USP 3302

Zaleplon (Valproate produces CNS depression, especially when combined with another CNS depressant). Products include:
- Sonata Capsules 3591

Ziprasidone Hydrochloride (Valproate produces CNS depression, especially when combined with another CNS depressant). Products include:
- Geodon Capsules 2688

Zidovudine (Co-administration has resulted in decreased clearance of zidovudin; the half-life of zidovudine was unaffected). Products include:
- Combivir Tablets 1502
- Retrovir 1625
- Retrovir IV Infusion 1629
- Trizivir Tablets 1669

Zolpidem Tartrate (Valproate produces CNS depression, especially when combined with another CNS depressant). Products include:
- Ambien Tablets 3191

Food Interactions

Alcohol (Valproate produces CNS depression, especially when combined with another CNS depressant, such as alcohol).

DEPAKOTE ER TABLETS

(Divalproex Sodium) 436

See Depakote Tablets

DEPEN TITRATABLE TABLETS

(Penicillamine) 3341

May interact with antimalarials, cytotoxic drugs, iron containing oral preparations, and certain other agents. Compounds in these categories include:

Auranofin (Co-administration should be avoided because gold therapy is also associated with serious hematologic and renal adverse events).
- No products indexed under this heading.

Bleomycin Sulfate (Co-administration should be avoided because cytotoxic drugs are also associated with serious hematologic and renal adverse events).
- No products indexed under this heading.

Chloroquine Hydrochloride (Co-administration should be avoided because antimalarial drugs are also associated with serious hematologic and renal adverse events).
- No products indexed under this heading.

Chloroquine Phosphate (Co-administration should be avoided because antimalarial drugs are also associated with serious hematologic and renal adverse events). Products include:
- Aralen Tablets 3075

Cyclophosphamide (Co-administration should be avoided because cytotoxic drugs are also associated with serious hematologic and renal adverse events).
- No products indexed under this heading.

Daunorubicin Hydrochloride (Co-administration should be avoided because cytotoxic drugs are also associated with serious hematologic and renal adverse events). Products include:
- Cerubidine for Injection 947

Doxorubicin Hydrochloride (Co-administration should be avoided because cytotoxic drugs are also associated with serious hematologic and renal adverse events). Products include:
- Adriamycin PFS/RDF Injection 2767
- Doxil Injection 566

Epirubicin Hydrochloride (Co-administration should be avoided because cytotoxic drugs are also associated with serious hematologic and renal adverse events). Products include:
- Ellence Injection 2806

Ferrous Fumarate (Orally administered iron reduces the effects of penicillamine). Products include:
- New Formulation Chromagen OB Capsules 3094
- Loestrin Fe Tablets 2642
- NataChew Tablets 3364

Ferrous Gluconate (Orally administered iron reduces the effects of penicillamine). Products include:
- Fergon Iron Tablets .... ▭802

Ferrous Sulfate (Orally administered iron reduces the effects of penicillamine). Products include:
- Feosol Tablets 1717
- Slow Fe Tablets .... ▭827
- Slow Fe with Folic Acid Tablets .... ▭828

Fluorouracil (Co-administration should be avoided because cytotoxic drugs are also associated with serious hematologic and renal adverse events). Products include:
- Carac Cream 1222
- Efudex 1733
- Fluoroplex 552

Gold Sodium Thiomalate (Co-administration should be avoided because gold therapy is also associated with serious hematologic and renal adverse events).
- No products indexed under this heading.

Hydroxyurea (Co-administration should be avoided because cytotoxic drugs are also associated with serious hematologic and renal adverse events). Products include:
- Mylocel Tablets 2227

Iron (Orally administered iron reduces the effects of penicillamine).
- No products indexed under this heading.

Mefloquine Hydrochloride (Co-administration should be avoided because antimalarial drugs are also associated with serious hematologic and renal adverse events). Products include:
- Lariam Tablets 2989

Methotrexate Sodium (Co-administration should be avoided because cytotoxic drugs are also associated with serious hematologic and renal adverse events).
- No products indexed under this heading.

Mitotane (Co-administration should be avoided because cytotoxic drugs are also associated with serious hematologic and renal adverse events).
- No products indexed under this heading.

Mitoxantrone Hydrochloride (Co-administration should be avoided because cytotoxic drugs are also associated with serious hematologic and renal adverse events). Products include:
- Novantrone for Injection 1760

Oxyphenbutazone (Co-administration should be avoided because oxyphenbutazone is also associated with serious hematologic and renal adverse events).
- No products indexed under this heading.

Phenylbutazone (Co-administration should be avoided because phenylbutazone is also associated with serious hematologic and renal adverse events).
- No products indexed under this heading.

Polysaccharide-Iron Complex (Orally administered iron reduces the effects of penicillamine). Products include:
- Niferex 3176
- Niferex-150 Capsules 3176
- Nu-Iron 150 Capsules 2224

Procarbazine Hydrochloride (Co-administration should be avoided because cytotoxic drugs are also associated with serious hematologic and renal adverse events). Products include:
- Matulane Capsules 3246

Pyrimethamine (Co-administration should be avoided because antimalarial drugs are also associated with serious hematologic and renal adverse events). Products include:
- Daraprim Tablets 1511

Tamoxifen Citrate (Co-administration should be avoided because cytotoxic drugs are also associated with serious hematologic and renal adverse events). Products include:
- Nolvadex Tablets 678

Vincristine Sulfate (Co-administration should be avoided because cytotoxic drugs are also associated with serious hematologic and renal adverse events).
- No products indexed under this heading.

Food Interactions

Dairy products (Penicillamine should be given on an empty stomach or at least one hour apart from food or milk because this permits maximum absorp-

tion and reduces the likelihood of inactivation by metal binding in the GI tract).

Food, unspecified (Penicillamine should be given on an empty stomach or at least one hour apart from food or milk because this permits maximum absorption and reduces the likelihood of inactivation by metal binding in the GI tract).

DEPOCYT INJECTION

(Cytarabine Liposome) ... 1197
May interact with cytotoxic drugs. Compounds in these categories include:

Bleomycin Sulfate (Co-administration of intrathecal cytarbine and other cytotoxic agents administered intrathecally may enhance neurotoxicity).
No products indexed under this heading.

Cyclophosphamide (Co-administration of intrathecal cytarbine and other cytotoxic agents administered intrathecally may enhance neurotoxicity).
No products indexed under this heading.

Daunorubicin Hydrochloride (Co-administration of intrathecal cytarbine and other cytotoxic agents administered intrathecally may enhance neurotoxicity). Products include:
Cerubidine for Injection ... 947

Doxorubicin Hydrochloride (Co-administration of intrathecal cytarbine and other cytotoxic agents administered intrathecally may enhance neurotoxicity). Products include:
Adriamycin PFS/RDF Injection ... 2767
Doxil Injection ... 566

Epirubicin Hydrochloride (Co-administration of intrathecal cytarbine and other cytotoxic agents administered intrathecally may enhance neurotoxicity). Products include:
Ellence Injection ... 2806

Fluorouracil (Co-administration of intrathecal cytarbine and other cytotoxic agents administered intrathecally may enhance neurotoxicity). Products include:
Carac Cream ... 1222
Efudex ... 1733
Fluoroplex ... 552

Hydroxyurea (Co-administration of intrathecal cytarbine and other cytotoxic agents administered intrathecally may enhance neurotoxicity). Products include:
Mylocel Tablets ... 2227

Methotrexate Sodium (Co-administration of intrathecal cytarbine and other cytotoxic agents administered intrathecally may enhance neurotoxicity).
No products indexed under this heading.

Mitotane (Co-administration of intrathecal cytarbine and other cytotoxic agents administered intrathecally may enhance neurotoxicity).
No products indexed under this heading.

Mitoxantrone Hydrochloride (Co-administration of intrathecal cytarbine and other cytotoxic agents administered intrathecally may enhance neurotoxicity). Products include:
Novantrone for Injection ... 1760

Procarbazine Hydrochloride (Co-administration of intrathecal cytarbine and other cytotoxic agents administered intrathecally may enhance neurotoxicity). Products include:
Matulane Capsules ... 3246

Tamoxifen Citrate (Co-administration of intrathecal cytarbine and other cytotoxic agents administered intrathecally may enhance neurotoxicity). Products include:
Nolvadex Tablets ... 678

Vincristine Sulfate (Co-administration of intrathecal cytarbine and other cytotoxic agents administered intrathecally may enhance neurotoxicity).
No products indexed under this heading.

DEPO-MEDROL INJECTABLE SUSPENSION

(Methylprednisolone Acetate) ... 2795
May interact with oral anticoagulants, phenytoin, and certain other agents. Compounds in these categories include:

Aspirin (Methylprednisolone may increase the clearance of chronic high dose aspirin resulting in decreased salicylate serum levels or increased risk of salicylate toxicity when methylprednisolone is withdrawn; aspirin should be used cautiously in conjunction withcorticosteroids in patients suffering from hypoprothrombinemia). Products include:
Aggrenox Capsules ... 1026
Alka-Seltzer ... 603
Alka-Seltzer Lemon Lime Antacid and Pain Reliever Effervescent Tablets ... 603
Alka-Seltzer Extra Strength Antacid and Pain Reliever Effervescent Tablets ... 603
Alka-Seltzer PM Effervescent Tablets ... 605
Genuine Bayer Tablets, Caplets and Gelcaps ... 606
Extra Strength Bayer Caplets and Gelcaps ... 610
Aspirin Regimen Bayer Children's Chewable Tablets (Orange or Cherry Flavored) ... 607
Bayer, Aspirin Regimen ... 606
Aspirin Regimen Bayer 81 mg Caplets with Calcium ... 607
Genuine Bayer Professional Labeling (Aspirin Regimen Bayer) ... 608
Extra Strength Bayer Arthritis Caplets ... 610
Extra Strength Bayer Plus Caplets ... 610
Extra Strength Bayer PM Caplets ... 611
BC Powder ... 619
BC Allergy Sinus Cold Powder ... 619
Arthritis Strength BC Powder ... 619
BC Sinus Cold Powder ... 619
Darvon Compound-65 Pulvules ... 1910
Ecotrin Enteric Coated Aspirin Low, Regular and Maximum Strength Tablets ... 1715
Excedrin Extra-Strength Tablets, Caplets, and Geltabs ... 629
Excedrin Migraine ... 1070
Goody's Body Pain Formula Powder ... 620
Goody's Extra Strength Headache Powder ... 620
Goody's Extra Strength Pain Relief Tablets ... 620
Percodan Tablets ... 1327
Robaxisal Tablets ... 2939
Soma Compound Tablets ... 3354
Soma Compound w/Codeine Tablets ... 3355
Vanquish Caplets ... 617

Cyclosporine (Co-administration results in mutual inhibition of metabolism, therefore, it is possible that adverse events associated with the individual use of either drug may be more apt to occur; convulsions have been reported with concurrent use). Products include:
Gengraf Capsules ... 457
Neoral Soft Gelatin Capsules ... 2380
Neoral Oral Solution ... 2380
Sandimmune ... 2388

Dicumarol (The effect of methylprednisolone on oral anticoagulants is variable; there are reports of enhanced as well as diminished effects of anticoagulants when given concurrently with corticosteroids).
No products indexed under this heading.

Fosphenytoin Sodium (Co-administration with drugs that induce hepatic metabolism, such as phenytoin, may increase the clearance of methylprednisolone and may require increases in methylprednisolone dose to achieve the desired response). Products include:
Cerebyx Injection ... 2619

Ketoconazole (Co-administration with drugs that inhibit the metabolism of methylprednisolone, such as ketoconazole, may decrease the clearance of methylprednisolone and may require dose titration to avoid steroid toxicity). Products include:
Nizoral 2% Cream ... 3620
Nizoral A-D Shampoo ... 2008
Nizoral 2% Shampoo ... 2007
Nizoral Tablets ... 1791

Phenobarbital (Co-administration with drugs that induce hepatic metabolism, such as phenobarbital, may increase the clearance of methylprednisolone and may require increases in methylprednisolone dose to achieve the desired response). Products include:
Arco-Lase Plus Tablets ... 592
Donnatal ... 2929
Donnatal Extentabs ... 2930

Phenytoin (Co-administration with drugs that induce hepatic metabolism, such as phenytoin, may increase the clearance of methylprednisolone and may require increases in methylprednisolone dose to achieve the desired response). Products include:
Dilantin Infatabs ... 2624
Dilantin-125 Oral Suspension ... 2625

Phenytoin Sodium (Co-administration with drugs that induce hepatic metabolism, such as phenytoin, may increase the clearance of methylprednisolone and may require increases in methylprednisolone dose to achieve the desired response). Products include:
Dilantin Kapseals ... 2622

Rifampin (Co-administration with drugs that induce hepatic metabolism, such as rifampin, may increase the clearance of methylprednisolone and may require increases in methylprednisolone dose to achieve the desired response). Products include:
Rifadin ... 765
Rifamate Capsules ... 767
Rifater Tablets ... 769

Troleandomycin (Co-administration with drugs that inhibit the metabolism of methylprednisolone, such as troleandomycin, may decrease the clearance of methylprednisolone and may require dose titration to avoid steroid toxicity). Products include:
Tao Capsules ... 2716

Warfarin Sodium (The effect of methylprednisolone on oral anticoagulants is variable; there are reports of enhanced as well as diminished effects of anticoagulants when given concurrently with corticosteroids). Products include:
Coumadin for Injection ... 1243
Coumadin Tablets ... 1243
Warfarin Sodium Tablets, USP ... 3302

DEPO-PROVERA CONTRACEPTIVE INJECTION

(Medroxyprogesterone Acetate) ... 2798
May interact with:

Aminoglutethimide (Co-administration may significantly depress the serum concentrations of medroxyprogesterone acetate with the possibility of decreased efficacy).
No products indexed under this heading.

DERMATOP EMOLLIENT CREAM

(Prednicarbate) ... 2517
None cited in PDR database.

DERMOPLAST HOSPITAL STRENGTH SPRAY

(Benzocaine, Menthol) ... 666
None cited in PDR database.

DESENEX LIQUID SPRAY

(Miconazole Nitrate) ... 668
None cited in PDR database.

DESENEX SHAKE POWDER

(Miconazole Nitrate) ... 668
None cited in PDR database.

DESENEX SPRAY POWDER

(Miconazole Nitrate) ... 668
None cited in PDR database.

DESENEX JOCK ITCH SPRAY POWDER

(Miconazole Nitrate) ... 668
None cited in PDR database.

DESFERAL VIALS

(Deferoxamine Mesylate) ... 2333
May interact with:

Aluminum Hydroxide (Treatment with Desferal in the presence of aluminum overload may result in decreased serum calcium and aggravation of hyperparathyroidism). Products include:
Amphojel Suspension (Mint Flavor) ... 789
Gaviscon Extra Strength Liquid ... 751
Gaviscon Extra Strength Tablets ... 751
Gaviscon Regular Strength Liquid ... 751
Gaviscon Regular Strength Tablets ... 750
Maalox Antacid/Anti-Gas Oral Suspension ... 673
Maalox Max Maximum Strength Antacid/Anti-Gas Liquid ... 2300
Maalox Regular Strength Antacid/Antigas Liquid ... 2300
Mylanta ... 1813
Vanquish Caplets ... 617

Gallium-67 (Imaging results may be distorted because of the rapid urinary excretion of Desferal-bound gallium-67).
No products indexed under this heading.

Prochlorperazine (Co-administration may lead to temporary impairment of consciousness). Products include:
Compazine ... 1505

Vitamin C (Co-administration with high doses of vitamin C (more than 500 mg daily in adults) in patients with severe chronic iron overload has resulted in impairment of cardiac function; vitamin C supplements should not be given to patients with cardiac failure; as an adjuvant to iron chelation therapy, vitamin C in doses up to 200 mg/day for adults may be given in divided doses). Products include:
Beta-C Tablets ... 811
C-Grams Caplets ... 795
Halls Defense Drops ... 687
Peridin-C Tablets ... 618

DESITIN BABY POWDER

(Corn Starch, Zinc Oxide) ... 700
None cited in PDR database.

DESITIN CREAMY OINTMENT

(Zinc Oxide) ... 700
None cited in PDR database.

DESITIN OINTMENT

(Cod Liver Oil, Zinc Oxide) ... 700
None cited in PDR database.

DESMOPRESSIN ACETATE INJECTION
(Desmopressin Acetate) 1344
See Desmopressin Acetate Rhinal Tube

DESMOPRESSIN ACETATE RHINAL TUBE
(Desmopressin Acetate) 1345
May interact with vasopressors. Compounds in these categories include:

Dopamine Hydrochloride (The pressor activity of desmopressin is very low, use of large doses of desmopressin with pressor agents should only be done with careful monitoring).
No products indexed under this heading.

Epinephrine Bitartrate (The pressor activity of desmopressin is very low, use of large doses of desmopressin with pressor agents should only be done with careful monitoring). Products include:
Sensorcaine 643

Epinephrine Hydrochloride (The pressor activity of desmopressin is very low, use of large doses of desmopressin with pressor agents should only be done with careful monitoring).
No products indexed under this heading.

Metaraminol Bitartrate (The pressor activity of desmopressin is very low, use of large doses of desmopressin with pressor agents should only be done with careful monitoring). Products include:
Aramine Injection 2043

Methoxamine Hydrochloride (The pressor activity of desmopressin is very low, use of large doses of desmopressin with pressor agents should only be done with careful monitoring).
No products indexed under this heading.

Norepinephrine Bitartrate (The pressor activity of desmopressin is very low, use of large doses of desmopressin with pressor agents should only be done with careful monitoring).
No products indexed under this heading.

Phenylephrine Hydrochloride (The pressor activity of desmopressin is very low, use of large doses of desmopressin with pressor agents should only be done with careful monitoring). Products include:
Afrin Nasal Decongestant Children's Pump Mist ....■ 734
Extendryl 1361
Hycomine Compound Tablets 1317
Neo-Synephrine ....■ 614
Phenergan VC Syrup 3560
Phenergan VC with Codeine Syrup . 3561
Preparation H Cream ....■ 778
Preparation H Cooling Gel ....■ 778
Preparation H ....■ 778
Vicks Sinex Nasal Spray and Ultra Fine Mist ....■ 729

DESOGEN TABLETS
(Desogestrel, Ethinyl Estradiol) 2458
May interact with barbiturates, phenytoin, tetracyclines, and certain other agents. Compounds in these categories include:

Ampicillin (Potential for reduced efficacy and increased incidence of breakthrough bleeding and menstrual irregularities with concomitant use).
No products indexed under this heading.

Ampicillin Sodium (Potential for reduced efficacy and increased incidence of breakthrough bleeding and menstrual irregularities with concomitant use). Products include:
Unasyn for Injection 2728

Aprobarbital (Potential for reduced efficacy and increased incidence of breakthrough bleeding and menstrual irregularities with concomitant use).
No products indexed under this heading.

Butabarbital (Potential for reduced efficacy and increased incidence of breakthrough bleeding and menstrual irregularities with concomitant use).
No products indexed under this heading.

Butalbital (Potential for reduced efficacy and increased incidence of breakthrough bleeding and menstrual irregularities with concomitant use). Products include:
Phrenilin 578
Sedapap Tablets 50 mg/650 mg ... 2225

Demeclocycline Hydrochloride (Potential for reduced efficacy and increased incidence of breakthrough bleeding and menstrual irregularities with concomitant use). Products include:
Declomycin Tablets 1855

Doxycycline Calcium (Potential for reduced efficacy and increased incidence of breakthrough bleeding and menstrual irregularities with concomitant use). Products include:
Vibramycin Calcium Oral Suspension Syrup 2735

Doxycycline Hyclate (Potential for reduced efficacy and increased incidence of breakthrough bleeding and menstrual irregularities with concomitant use). Products include:
Doryx Coated Pellet Filled Capsules 3357
Periostat Tablets 1208
Vibramycin Hyclate Capsules 2735
Vibramycin Hyclate Intravenous 2737
Vibra-Tabs Film Coated Tablets 2735

Doxycycline Monohydrate (Potential for reduced efficacy and increased incidence of breakthrough bleeding and menstrual irregularities with concomitant use). Products include:
Monodox Capsules 2442
Vibramycin Monohydrate for Oral Suspension 2735

Fosphenytoin Sodium (Potential for reduced efficacy and increased incidence of breakthrough bleeding and menstrual irregularities with concomitant use). Products include:
Cerebyx Injection 2619

Griseofulvin (Potential for reduced efficacy and increased incidence of breakthrough bleeding and menstrual irregularities with concomitant use). Products include:
Grifulvin V Tablets Microsize and Oral Suspension Microsize 2518
Gris-PEG Tablets 2661

Mephobarbital (Potential for reduced efficacy and increased incidence of breakthrough bleeding and menstrual irregularities with concomitant use).
No products indexed under this heading.

Methacycline Hydrochloride (Potential for reduced efficacy and increased incidence of breakthrough bleeding and menstrual irregularities with concomitant use).
No products indexed under this heading.

Minocycline Hydrochloride (Potential for reduced efficacy and increased incidence of breakthrough bleeding and menstrual irregularities with concomitant use). Products include:
Dynacin Capsules 2019
Minocin Intravenous 1862
Minocin Oral Suspension 1865
Minocin Pellet-Filled Capsules 1863

Oxytetracycline Hydrochloride (Potential for reduced efficacy and increased incidence of breakthrough bleeding and menstrual irregularities with concomitant use). Products include:
Terra-Cortril Ophthalmic Suspension 2716
Urobiotic-250 Capsules 2731

Pentobarbital Sodium (Potential for reduced efficacy and increased incidence of breakthrough bleeding and menstrual irregularities with concomitant use). Products include:
Nembutal Sodium Solution 485

Phenobarbital (Potential for reduced efficacy and increased incidence of breakthrough bleeding and menstrual irregularities with concomitant use). Products include:
Arco-Lase Plus Tablets 592
Donnatal 2929
Donnatal Extentabs 2930

Phenylbutazone (Potential for reduced efficacy and increased incidence of breakthrough bleeding and menstrual irregularities with concomitant use).
No products indexed under this heading.

Phenytoin (Potential for reduced efficacy and increased incidence of breakthrough bleeding and menstrual irregularities with concomitant use). Products include:
Dilantin Infatabs 2624
Dilantin-125 Oral Suspension 2625

Phenytoin Sodium (Potential for reduced efficacy and increased incidence of breakthrough bleeding and menstrual irregularities with concomitant use). Products include:
Dilantin Kapseals 2622

Rifampin (Co-administration has been associated with reduced efficacy and increased incidence of breakthrough bleeding and menstrual irregularities). Products include:
Rifadin 765
Rifamate Capsules 767
Rifater Tablets 769

Secobarbital Sodium (Potential for reduced efficacy and increased incidence of breakthrough bleeding and menstrual irregularities with concomitant use).
No products indexed under this heading.

Tetracycline Hydrochloride (Potential for reduced efficacy and increased incidence of breakthrough bleeding and menstrual irregularities with concomitant use).
No products indexed under this heading.

Thiamylal Sodium (Potential for reduced efficacy and increased incidence of breakthrough bleeding and menstrual irregularities with concomitant use).
No products indexed under this heading.

DESOWEN CREAM
(Desonide) 1401
None cited in PDR database.

DESOWEN LOTION
(Desonide) 1401
See DesOwen Cream

DESOWEN OINTMENT
(Desonide) 1401
See DesOwen Cream

DESOXYN TABLETS
(Methamphetamine Hydrochloride) 440
May interact with insulin, monoamine oxidase inhibitors, phenothiazines, tricyclic antidepressants, and certain other agents. Compounds in these categories include:

Amitriptyline Hydrochloride (Co-administration of tricyclic antidepressants and indirect-acting sympathomimetic amines such as amphetamines should be closely supervised and dosage carefully adjusted). Products include:
Etrafon 3115
Limbitrol 1738

Amoxapine (Co-administration of tricyclic antidepressants and indirect-acting sympathomimetic amines such as amphetamines should be closely supervised and dosage carefully adjusted).
No products indexed under this heading.

Chlorpromazine (May antagonize the CNS stimulant action of the amphetamine). Products include:
Thorazine Suppositories 1656

Chlorpromazine Hydrochloride (May antagonize the CNS stimulant action of the amphetamine). Products include:
Thorazine 1656

Clomipramine Hydrochloride (Co-administration of tricyclic antidepressants and indirect-acting sympathomimetic amines such as amphetamines should be closely supervised and dosage carefully adjusted).
No products indexed under this heading.

Desipramine Hydrochloride (Co-administration of tricyclic antidepressants and indirect-acting sympathomimetic amines such as amphetamines should be closely supervised and dosage carefully adjusted). Products include:
Norpramin Tablets 755

Doxepin Hydrochloride (Co-administration of tricyclic antidepressants and indirect-acting sympathomimetic amines such as amphetamines should be closely supervised and dosage carefully adjusted). Products include:
Sinequan 2713

Fluphenazine Decanoate (May antagonize the CNS stimulant action of the amphetamine).
No products indexed under this heading.

Fluphenazine Enanthate (May antagonize the CNS stimulant action of the amphetamine).
No products indexed under this heading.

Fluphenazine Hydrochloride (May antagonize the CNS stimulant action of the amphetamine).
No products indexed under this heading.

Guanethidine Monosulfate (Decreased hypotensive effect).
No products indexed under this heading.

Imipramine Hydrochloride (Co-administration of tricyclic antidepressants and indirect-acting sympathomimetic amines such as amphetamines should be closely supervised and dosage carefully adjusted).
No products indexed under this heading.

Imipramine Pamoate (Co-administration of tricyclic antidepressants and indirect-acting sympathomimetic amines such as amphetamines should be closely supervised and dosage carefully adjusted).
No products indexed under this heading.

Insulin, Human, Zinc Suspension (Insulin requirement in diabetics may be altered). Products include:
Humulin L, 100 Units 1937
Humulin U, 100 Units 1943
Novolin L Human Insulin 10 ml Vials 2422

Insulin, Human NPH (Insulin requirement in diabetics may be altered). Products include:

Humulin N, 100 Units 1939
Humulin N NPH Pen 1940
Novolin N Human Insulin 10 ml Vials 2422
Novolin N PenFill 2423
Novolin N Prefilled Syringe Disposable Insulin Delivery System 2425

Insulin, Human Regular (Insulin requirement in diabetics may be altered). Products include:
Humulin R Regular (U-500) 1943
Humulin R, 100 Units 1941
Novolin R Human Insulin 10 ml Vials 2423
Novolin R PenFill 2423
Novolin R Prefilled Syringe Disposable Insulin Delivery System 2425
Velosulin BR Human Insulin 10 ml Vials 2435

Insulin, Human Regular and Human NPH Mixture (Insulin requirement in diabetics may be altered). Products include:
Humulin 50/50, 100 Units 1934
Humulin 70/30, 100 Units 1935
Humulin 70/30 Pen 1936
Novolin 70/30 Human Insulin 10 ml Vials 2421
Novolin 70/30 PenFill 2423
Novolin 70/30 Prefilled Disposable Insulin Delivery System 2425

Insulin, NPH (Insulin requirement in diabetics may be altered). Products include:
Iletin II, NPH (Pork), 100 Units 1946

Insulin, Regular (Insulin requirement in diabetics may be altered). Products include:
Iletin II, Regular (Pork), 100 Units 1947

Insulin, Zinc Crystals (Insulin requirement in diabetics may be altered).
No products indexed under this heading.

Insulin, Zinc Suspension (Insulin requirement in diabetics may be altered). Products include:
Iletin II, Lente (Pork), 100 Units 1945

Insulin Aspart, Human Regular (Insulin requirement in diabetics may be altered).
No products indexed under this heading.

Insulin glargine (Insulin requirement in diabetics may be altered). Products include:
Lantus Injection 742

Insulin Lispro, Human (Insulin requirement in diabetics may be altered). Products include:
Humalog 1926
Humalog Mix 75/25 Pen 1928

Insulin Lispro Protamine, Human (Insulin requirement in diabetics may be altered). Products include:
Humalog Mix 75/25 Pen 1928

Isocarboxazid (Co-administration may result in hypertensive crises; concurrent and/or sequential use is contraindicated).
No products indexed under this heading.

Maprotiline Hydrochloride (Co-administration of tricyclic antidepressants and indirect-acting sympathomimetic amines such as amphetamines should be closely supervised and dosage carefully adjusted).
No products indexed under this heading.

Mesoridazine Besylate (May antagonize the CNS stimulant action of the amphetamine). Products include:
Serentil 1057

Methotrimeprazine (May antagonize the CNS stimulant action of the amphetamine).
No products indexed under this heading.

Moclobemide (Co-administration may result in hypertensive crises; concurrent and/or sequential use is contraindicated).
No products indexed under this heading.

Nortriptyline Hydrochloride (Co-administration of tricyclic antidepressants and indirect-acting sympathomimetic amines such as amphetamines should be closely supervised and dosage carefully adjusted).
No products indexed under this heading.

Pargyline Hydrochloride (Co-administration may result in hypertensive crises; concurrent and/or sequential use is contraindicated).
No products indexed under this heading.

Perphenazine (May antagonize the CNS stimulant action of the amphetamine). Products include:
Etrafon 3115
Trilafon 3160

Phenelzine Sulfate (Co-administration may result in hypertensive crises; concurrent and/or sequential use is contraindicated). Products include:
Nardil Tablets 2653

Procarbazine Hydrochloride (Co-administration may result in hypertensive crises; concurrent and/or sequential use is contraindicated). Products include:
Matulane Capsules 3246

Prochlorperazine (May antagonize the CNS stimulant action of the amphetamine). Products include:
Compazine 1505

Promethazine Hydrochloride (May antagonize the CNS stimulant action of the amphetamine). Products include:
Mepergan Injection 3539
Phenergan Injection 3553
Phenergan 3556
Phenergan Syrup 3554
Phenergan with Codeine Syrup 3557
Phenergan with Dextromethorphan Syrup 3559
Phenergan VC Syrup 3560
Phenergan VC with Codeine Syrup 3561

Protriptyline Hydrochloride (Co-administration of tricyclic antidepressants and indirect-acting sympathomimetic amines such as amphetamines should be closely supervised and dosage carefully adjusted). Products include:
Vivactil Tablets 2446
Vivactil Tablets 2217

Selegiline Hydrochloride (Co-administration may result in hypertensive crises; concurrent and/or sequential use is contraindicated). Products include:
Eldepryl Capsules 3266

Thioridazine Hydrochloride (May antagonize the CNS stimulant action of the amphetamine). Products include:
Thioridazine Hydrochloride Tablets 2289

Tranylcypromine Sulfate (Co-administration may result in hypertensive crises; concurrent and/or sequential use is contraindicated). Products include:
Parnate Tablets 1607

Trifluoperazine Hydrochloride (May antagonize the CNS stimulant action of the amphetamine). Products include:
Stelazine 1640

Trimipramine Maleate (Co-administration of tricyclic antidepressants and indirect-acting sympathomimetic amines such as amphetamines should be closely supervised and dosage carefully adjusted). Products include:
Surmontil Capsules 3595

DETROL TABLETS

(Tolterodine Tartrate) 3623
See Detrol LA Capsules

DETROL LA CAPSULES

(Tolterodine Tartrate) 2801
May interact with erythromycin and certain other agents. Compounds in these categories include:

Clarithromycin (Co-administration with other potent inhibitors of CYP3A4, such as clarithromycin, may lead to increase of tolterodine plasma concentrations; for patients receiving concomitant erythromycin the recommended dose of Detrol LA is 2 mg). Products include:
Biaxin/Biaxin XL 403
PREVPAC 3298

Cyclosporine (Co-administration with other potent inhibitors of CYP3A4, such as cyclosporine, may lead to increase of tolterodine plasma concentrations; for patients receiving concomitant cyclosporine the recommended dose of Detrol LA is 2 mg). Products include:
Gengraf Capsules 457
Neoral Soft Gelatin Capsules 2380
Neoral Oral Solution 2380
Sandimmune 2388

Erythromycin (Co-administration with other potent inhibitors of CYP3A4, such as erythromycin, may lead to increase of tolterodine plasma concentrations; for patients receiving concomitant erythromycin the recommended dose of Detrol LA is 2 mg). Products include:
Emgel 2% Topical Gel 1285
Ery-Tab Tablets 448
Erythromycin Base Filmtab Tablets 454
Erythromycin Delayed-Release Capsules, USP 455
PCE Dispertab Tablets 498

Erythromycin Estolate (Co-administration with other potent inhibitors of CYP3A4, such as erythromycin, may lead to increase of tolterodine plasma concentrations; for patients receiving concomitant erythromycin the recommended dose of Detrol LA is 2 mg).
No products indexed under this heading.

Erythromycin Ethylsuccinate (Co-administration with other potent inhibitors of CYP3A4, such as erythromycin, may lead to increase of tolterodine plasma concentrations; for patients receiving concomitant erythromycin the recommended dose of Detrol LA is 2 mg). Products include:
E.E.S. 450
EryPed 446
Pediazole Suspension 3050

Erythromycin Gluceptate (Co-administration with other potent inhibitors of CYP3A4, such as erythromycin, may lead to increase of tolterodine plasma concentrations; for patients receiving concomitant erythromycin the recommended dose of Detrol LA is 2 mg).
No products indexed under this heading.

Erythromycin Stearate (Co-administration with other potent inhibitors of CYP3A4, such as erythromycin, may lead to increase of tolterodine plasma concentrations; for patients receiving concomitant erythromycin the recommended dose of Detrol LA is 2 mg). Products include:
Erythrocin Stearate Filmtab Tablets 452

Fluoxetine Hydrochloride (Co-administration with a potent inhibitor of CYP2D6, such as fluoxetine, significantly inhibits the metabolism of tolterodine immediate release formulation in extensive metabolizers, resulting in a 4.8-fold increase in tolterodine AUC; the sums of unbound serum concentrations of tolterodine and the 5-hydroxymethyl metabolite are only 25% higher during the interaction; no dose adjustment is required). Products include:
Prozac Pulvules, Liquid, and Weekly Capsules 1238
Sarafem Pulvules 1962

Itraconazole (Co-administration with other potent inhibitors of CYP3A4, such as itraconazole, may lead to increase of tolterodine plasma concentrations; for patients receiving concomitant itraconazole the recommended dose of Detrol LA is 2 mg). Products include:
Sporanox Capsules 1800
Sporanox Injection 1804
Sporanox Injection 2509
Sporanox Oral Solution 1808
Sporanox Oral Solution 2512

Ketoconazole (Co-administration of ketoconazole, an inhibitor of CYP3A4, significantly increased plasma concentrations of tolterodine in subjects who were poor metabolizers; for patients receiving concomitant ketoconazole the recommended dose of Detrol LA is 2 mg). Products include:
Nizoral 2% Cream 3620
Nizoral A-D Shampoo 2008
Nizoral 2% Shampoo 2007
Nizoral Tablets 1791

Miconazole (Co-administration with other potent inhibitors of CYP3A4, such as miconazole, may lead to increase of tolterodine plasma concentrations; for patients receiving concomitant miconazole the recommended dose of Detrol LA is 2 mg).
No products indexed under this heading.

Vinblastine Sulfate (Co-administration with other potent inhibitors of CYP3A4, such as vinblastine, may lead to increase of tolterodine plasma concentrations; for patients receiving concomitant vinblastine the recommended dose of Detrol LA is 2 mg).
No products indexed under this heading.

DEVROM CHEWABLE TABLETS

(Bismuth Subgallate) .... ■685
None cited in PDR database.

DEXEDRINE SPANSULE CAPSULES

(Dextroamphetamine Sulfate) 1512
May interact with antihistamines, antihypertensives, beta blockers, monoamine oxidase inhibitors, phenytoin, thiazides, tricyclic antidepressants, urinary alkalinizing agents, veratrum alkaloids, and certain other agents. Compounds in these categories include:

Acebutolol Hydrochloride (Amphetamine may antagonize the hypotensive effects of antihypertensives; adrenergic blockers are inhibited by amphetamines). Products include:
Sectral Capsules 3589

Acetazolamide (Increases the concentration of the non-ionized species of the amphetamine molecule, thereby decreasing urinary excretion; increases amphetamines blood levels and thereby potentiates the actions of amphetamines). Products include:
Diamox Sequels Sustained Release Capsules .... ⊙270
Diamox Tablets .... ⊙269

Acetazolamide Sodium (Increases the concentration of the non-ionized species of the amphetamine molecule, thereby decreasing urinary excretion; increases amphetamines blood levels and thereby potentiates the actions of amphetamines). Products include:

Diamox Intravenous ⊙269

Acrivastine (Amphetamines may counteract the sedative effect of antihistamine). Products include:
Semprex-D Capsules 1172

Amitriptyline Hydrochloride (Enhanced activity of tricyclic or sympathomimetics; possible increases in the brain concentration of d-amphetamine in the brain; cardiovascular effect may be potentiated). Products include:
Etrafon 3115
Limbitrol 1738

Amlodipine Besylate (Amphetamine may antagonize the hypotensive effects of antihypertensives). Products include:
Lotrel Capsules 2370
Norvasc Tablets 2704

Ammonium Chloride (Increases the concentration of the ionized species of the amphetamine molecule, thereby increasing urinary excretion; lowers amphetamines blood levels and efficacy).
No products indexed under this heading.

Amoxapine (Enhanced activity of tricyclic or sympathomimetics; possible increases in the brain concentration of d-amphetamine in the brain; cardiovascular effect may be potentiated).
No products indexed under this heading.

Astemizole (Amphetamines may counteract the sedative effect of antihistamine).
No products indexed under this heading.

Atenolol (Amphetamine may antagonize the hypotensive effects of antihypertensives; adrenergic blockers are inhibited by amphetamines). Products include:
Tenoretic Tablets 690
Tenormin I.V. Injection 692

Azatadine Maleate (Amphetamines may counteract the sedative effect of antihistamine). Products include:
Rynatan Tablets 3351

Benazepril Hydrochloride (Amphetamine may antagonize the hypotensive effects of antihypertensives). Products include:
Lotensin Tablets 2365
Lotensin HCT Tablets 2367
Lotrel Capsules 2370

Bendroflumethiazide (Increases the concentration of the non-ionized species of the amphetamine molecule, thereby decreasing urinary excretion; increases amphetamines blood levels and thereby potentiates the actions of amphetamines). Products include:
Corzide 40/5 Tablets 2247
Corzide 80/5 Tablets 2247

Betaxolol Hydrochloride (Amphetamine may antagonize the hypotensive effects of antihypertensives; adrenergic blockers are inhibited by amphetamines). Products include:
Betoptic S Ophthalmic Suspension 537

Bisoprolol Fumarate (Amphetamine may antagonize the hypotensive effects of antihypertensives; adrenergic blockers are inhibited by amphetamines). Products include:
Zebeta Tablets 1885
Ziac Tablets 1887

Bromodiphenhydramine Hydrochloride (Amphetamines may counteract the sedative effect of antihistamine).
No products indexed under this heading.

Brompheniramine Maleate (Amphetamines may counteract the sedative effect of antihistamine). Products include:
Bromfed Capsules (Extended-Release) 2269
Bromfed-PD Capsules (Extended-Release) 2269
Comtrex Acute Head Cold & Sinus Pressure Relief Tablets ▣627
Dimetapp Elixir ▣777
Dimetapp Cold and Fever Suspension ▣775
Dimetapp DM Cold & Cough Elixir ▣775
Dimetapp Nighttime Flu Liquid ▣776

Candesartan Cilexetil (Amphetamine may antagonize the hypotensive effects of antihypertensives). Products include:
Atacand Tablets 595
Atacand HCT Tablets 597

Captopril (Amphetamine may antagonize the hypotensive effects of antihypertensives). Products include:
Captopril Tablets 2281

Carteolol Hydrochloride (Amphetamine may antagonize the hypotensive effects of antihypertensives; adrenergic blockers are inhibited by amphetamines). Products include:
Carteolol Hydrochloride Ophthalmic Solution USP, 1% ⊙258
Ocupress Ophthalmic Solution, 1% Sterile ⊙303

Cetirizine Hydrochloride (Amphetamines may counteract the sedative effect of antihistamine). Products include:
Zyrtec 2756
Zyrtec-D 12 Hour Extended Relief Tablets 2758

Chlorothiazide (Increases the concentration of the non-ionized species of the amphetamine molecule, thereby decreasing urinary excretion; increases amphetamines blood levels and thereby potentiates the actions of amphetamines). Products include:
Aldoclor Tablets 2035
Diuril Oral 2087

Chlorothiazide Sodium (Increases the concentration of the non-ionized species of the amphetamine molecule, thereby decreasing urinary excretion; increases amphetamines blood levels and thereby potentiates the actions of amphetamines). Products include:
Diuril Sodium Intravenous 2086

Chlorpheniramine Maleate (Amphetamines may counteract the sedative effect of antihistamine). Products include:
Actifed Cold & Sinus Caplets and Tablets ▣688
Alka-Seltzer Plus Liqui-Gels ▣604
BC Allergy Sinus Cold Powder ▣619
Chlor-Trimeton Allergy Tablets ▣735
Chlor-Trimeton Allergy/Decongestant Tablets ▣736
Comtrex Flu Therapy & Fever Relief Nighttime Tablets ▣628
Comtrex Maximum Strength Multi-Symptom Cold & Cough Relief Tablets and Caplets ▣626
Contac Severe Cold and Flu Caplets Maximum Strength ▣746
Coricidin 'D' Cold, Flu & Sinus Tablets ▣737
Coricidin/Coricidin D ▣738
Coricidin HBP Maximum Strength Flu Tablets ▣738
Extendryl 1361
Hycomine Compound Tablets 1317
Kronofed-A 1341
PediaCare Cough-Cold Liquid ▣719
PediaCare NightRest Cough-Cold Liquid ▣719
Robitussin Nighttime Honey Flu Liquid ▣786
Ryna ▣768
Singlet Caplets ▣761
Sinutab Sinus Allergy Medication, Maximum Strength Formula, Tablets & Caplets ▣707
Sudafed Cold & Allergy Tablets ▣708
TheraFlu Regular Strength Cold & Cough Night Time Hot Liquid ▣676
TheraFlu Regular Strength Cold & Sore Throat Night Time Hot Liquid ▣676
TheraFlu Maximum Strength Flu & Cough Night Time Hot Liquid ▣678
TheraFlu Maximum Strength Flu & Sore Throat Night Time Hot Liquid ▣677
TheraFlu Maximum Strength Severe Cold & Congestion Night Time Caplets ▣678
TheraFlu Maximum Strength Severe Cold & Congestion Night Time Hot Liquid ▣678
Triaminic Cold & Allergy Liquid ▣681
Triaminic Cold & Allergy Softchews ▣683
Triaminic Cold & Cough Liquid ▣681
Triaminic Cold & Cough Softchews ▣683
Triaminic Cold & Night Time Cough Liquid ▣681
Triaminic Cold, Cough & Fever Liquid ▣681
Children's Tylenol Cold Suspension Liquid and Chewable Tablets 2015
Children's Tylenol Cold Plus Cough Suspension Liquid and Chewable Tablets 2015
Children's Tylenol Flu Suspension Liquid 2015
Maximum Strength Tylenol Allergy Sinus Caplets, Gelcaps, and Geltabs 2010
Multi-Symptom Tylenol Cold Complete Formula Caplets 2010
Vicks 44M Cough, Cold & Flu Relief Liquid ▣725
Pediatric Vicks 44m Cough & Cold Relief ▣728
Children's Vicks NyQuil Cold/Cough Relief ▣726

Chlorpheniramine Polistirex (Amphetamines may counteract the sedative effect of antihistamine). Products include:
Tussionex Pennkinetic Extended-Release Suspension 1174

Chlorpheniramine Tannate (Amphetamines may counteract the sedative effect of antihistamine). Products include:
Reformulated Rynatan Pediatric Suspension 3352
Rynatuss Pediatric Suspension 3353
Rynatuss Tablets 3353
Tussi-12 S Suspension 3356
Tussi-12 Tablets 3356

Chlorpromazine (Blocks dopamine and norepinephrine reuptake resulting in inhibition of central stimulating effects). Products include:
Thorazine Suppositories 1656

Chlorpromazine Hydrochloride (Blocks dopamine and norepinephrine reuptake resulting in inhibition of central stimulating effects). Products include:
Thorazine 1656

Chlorthalidone (Amphetamine may antagonize the hypotensive effects of antihypertensives). Products include:
Clorpres Tablets 1002
Combipres Tablets 1040
Tenoretic Tablets 690

Clemastine Fumarate (Amphetamines may counteract the sedative effect of antihistamine). Products include:
Tavist 12 Hour Allergy Tablets ▣676

Clomipramine Hydrochloride (Enhanced activity of tricyclic or sympathomimetics; possible increases in the brain concentration of d-amphetamine in the brain; cardiovascular effect may be potentiated).
No products indexed under this heading.

Clonidine (Amphetamine may antagonize the hypotensive effects of antihypertensives). Products include:
Catapres-TTS 1038

Clonidine Hydrochloride (Amphetamine may antagonize the hypotensive effects of antihypertensives). Products include:
Catapres Tablets 1037
Clorpres Tablets 1002
Combipres Tablets 1040
Duraclon Injection 3057

Cryptenamine Preparations (Amphetamines inhibit the hypotensive effect of veratrum alkaloids).
No products indexed under this heading.

Cyproheptadine Hydrochloride (Amphetamines may counteract the sedative effect of antihistamine). Products include:
Periactin Tablets 2155

Deserpidine (Amphetamine may antagonize the hypotensive effects of antihypertensives).
No products indexed under this heading.

Desipramine Hydrochloride (Enhanced activity of tricyclic or sympathomimetics; possible increases in the brain concentration of d-amphetamine in the brain; cardiovascular effect may be potentiated). Products include:
Norpramin Tablets 755

Dexchlorpheniramine Maleate (Amphetamines may counteract the sedative effect of antihistamine).
No products indexed under this heading.

Diazoxide (Amphetamine may antagonize the hypotensive effects of antihypertensives).
No products indexed under this heading.

Diltiazem Hydrochloride (Amphetamine may antagonize the hypotensive effects of antihypertensives). Products include:
Cardizem Injectable 1018
Cardizem Lyo-Ject Syringe 1018
Cardizem Monovial 1018
Cardizem CD Capsules 1016
Tiazac Capsules 1378

Diphenhydramine Citrate (Amphetamines may counteract the sedative effect of antihistamine). Products include:
Alka-Seltzer PM Effervescent Tablets ▣605
Benadryl Allergy & Sinus Fastmelt Tablets ▣693
Benadryl Children's Allergy/Cold Fastmelt Tablets ▣692
Excedrin PM Tablets, Caplets, and Geltabs ▣631
Goody's PM Powder ▣621

Diphenhydramine Hydrochloride (Amphetamines may counteract the sedative effect of antihistamine). Products include:
Extra Strength Bayer PM Caplets ▣611
Benadryl Allergy Chewables ▣689
Benadryl Allergy ▣691
Benadryl Allergy Liquid ▣690
Benadryl Allergy/Cold Tablets ▣691
Benadryl Allergy/Congestion Tablets ▣692
Benadryl Allergy & Sinus Liquid ▣693
Benadryl Allergy Sinus Headache Caplets & Gelcaps ▣693
Benadryl Severe Allergy & Sinus Headache Caplets ▣694
Benadryl Dye-Free Allergy Liquid ▣690
Benadryl Dye-Free Allergy Liqui-Gels Softgels ▣690
Benadryl Itch Relief Stick Extra Strength ▣695
Benadryl Cream ▣695
Benadryl Gel ▣695
Benadryl Spray ▣696
Benadryl Parenteral 2617
Coricidin HBP Night-Time Cold & Flu Tablets ▣738
Nytol QuickCaps Caplets ▣622
Maximum Strength Nytol QuickGels Softgels ▣621
Extra Strength Percogesic Aspirin-Free Coated Caplets ▣665
Simply Sleep Caplets 2008
Sominex Original Formula Tablets ▣761
Children's Tylenol Allergy-D Liquid 2014
Maximum Strength Tylenol Allergy Sinus NightTime Caplets 2010
Tylenol Severe Allergy Caplets 2010
Maximum Strength Tylenol Flu NightTime Gelcaps 2011
Extra Strength Tylenol PM Caplets, Geltabs, and Gelcaps 2012
Unisom Maximum Strength SleepGels ▣713

Diphenylpyraline Hydrochloride (Amphetamines may counteract the

sedative effect of antihistamine).
No products indexed under this heading.

Doxazosin Mesylate (Amphetamine may antagonize the hypotensive effects of antihypertensives). Products include:
Cardura Tablets ... 2668

Doxepin Hydrochloride (Enhanced activity of tricyclic or sympathomimetics; possible increases in the brain concentration of d-amphetamine in the brain; cardiovascular effect may be potentiated). Products include:
Sinequan ... 2713

Enalapril Maleate (Amphetamine may antagonize the hypotensive effects of antihypertensives). Products include:
Lexxel Tablets ... 608
Vaseretic Tablets ... 2204
Vasotec Tablets ... 2210

Enalaprilat (Amphetamine may antagonize the hypotensive effects of antihypertensives). Products include:
Enalaprilat Injection ... 863
Vasotec I.V. Injection ... 2207

Eprosartan Mesylate (Amphetamine may antagonize the hypotensive effects of antihypertensives). Products include:
Teveten Tablets ... 3327

Esmolol Hydrochloride (Amphetamine may antagonize the hypotensive effects of antihypertensives; adrenergic blockers are inhibited by amphetamines). Products include:
Brevibloc Injection ... 858

Ethosuximide (Amphetamine may delay intestinal absorption of ethosuximide). Products include:
Zarontin Capsules ... 2659
Zarontin Syrup ... 2660

Felodipine (Amphetamine may antagonize the hypotensive effects of antihypertensives). Products include:
Lexxel Tablets ... 608
Plendil Extended-Release Tablets ... 623

Fexofenadine Hydrochloride (Amphetamines may counteract the sedative effect of antihistamine). Products include:
Allegra ... 712
Allegra-D Extended-Release Tablets ... 714

Fosinopril Sodium (Amphetamine may antagonize the hypotensive effects of antihypertensives). Products include:
Monopril Tablets ... 1091
Monopril HCT ... 1094

Fosphenytoin Sodium (Amphetamine delays intestinal absorption of phenytoin; co-administration may produce synergestic anticonvulsant action). Products include:
Cerebyx Injection ... 2619

Furosemide (Amphetamine may antagonize the hypotensive effects of antihypertensives). Products include:
Furosemide Tablets ... 2284

Glutamic Acid Hydrochloride (Lowers absorption of amphetamines).
No products indexed under this heading.

Guanabenz Acetate (Amphetamine may antagonize the hypotensive effects of antihypertensives).
No products indexed under this heading.

Guanethidine Monosulfate (Lowers absorption of amphetamines).
No products indexed under this heading.

Haloperidol (Blocks dopamine and norepinephrine reuptake resulting in inhibition of central stimulating effects). Products include:
Haldol Injection, Tablets and Concentrate ... 2533

Haloperidol Decanoate (Blocks dopamine and norepinephrine reuptake resulting in inhibition of central stimulating effects). Products include:
Haldol Decanoate ... 2535

Hydralazine Hydrochloride (Amphetamine may antagonize the hypotensive effects of antihypertensives).
No products indexed under this heading.

Hydrochlorothiazide (Increases the concentration of the non-ionized species of the amphetamine molecule, thereby decreasing urinary excretion; increases amphetamines blood levels and thereby potentiates the actions of amphetamines). Products include:
Accuretic Tablets ... 2614
Aldoril Tablets ... 2039
Atacand HCT Tablets ... 597
Avalide Tablets ... 1070
Diovan HCT Tablets ... 2338
Dyazide Capsules ... 1515
HydroDIURIL Tablets ... 2108
Hyzaar ... 2109
Inderide Tablets ... 3517
Inderide LA Long-Acting Capsules ... 3519
Lotensin HCT Tablets ... 2367
Maxzide ... 1008
Micardis HCT Tablets ... 1051
Microzide Capsules ... 3414
Moduretic Tablets ... 2138
Monopril HCT ... 1094
Prinzide Tablets ... 2168
Timolide Tablets ... 2187
Uniretic Tablets ... 3178
Vaseretic Tablets ... 2204
Zestoretic Tablets ... 695
Ziac Tablets ... 1887

Hydroflumethiazide (Increases the concentration of the non-ionized species of the amphetamine molecule, thereby decreasing urinary excretion; increases amphetamines blood levels and thereby potentiates the actions of amphetamines). Products include:
Diucardin Tablets ... 3494

Imipramine Hydrochloride (Enhanced activity of tricyclic or sympathomimetics; possible increases in the brain concentration of d-amphetamine in the brain; cardiovascular effect may be potentiated).
No products indexed under this heading.

Imipramine Pamoate (Enhanced activity of tricyclic or sympathomimetics; possible increases in the brain concentration of d-amphetamine in the brain; cardiovascular effect may be potentiated).
No products indexed under this heading.

Indapamide (Amphetamine may antagonize the hypotensive effects of antihypertensives). Products include:
Indapamide Tablets ... 2286

Irbesartan (Amphetamine may antagonize the hypotensive effects of antihypertensives). Products include:
Avalide Tablets ... 1070
Avapro Tablets ... 1074
Avapro Tablets ... 3076

Isocarboxazid (Concurrent and/or sequential use with MAO inhibitors is contraindicated; hypertensive crisis may occur).
No products indexed under this heading.

Isradipine (Amphetamine may antagonize the hypotensive effects of antihypertensives). Products include:
DynaCirc Capsules ... 2921
DynaCirc CR Tablets ... 2923

Labetalol Hydrochloride (Amphetamine may antagonize the hypotensive effects of antihypertensives; adrenergic blockers are inhibited by amphetamines). Products include:
Normodyne Injection ... 3135
Normodyne Tablets ... 3137

Levobunolol Hydrochloride (Amphetamine may antagonize the hypotensive effects of antihypertensives; adrenergic blockers are inhibited by amphetamines). Products include:
Betagan ... ⊙ 228

Lisinopril (Amphetamine may antagonize the hypotensive effects of antihypertensives). Products include:
Prinivil Tablets ... 2164
Prinzide Tablets ... 2168
Zestoretic Tablets ... 695
Zestril Tablets ... 698

Lithium Carbonate (Inhibits stimulatory effects of amphetamines). Products include:
Eskalith ... 1527
Lithium Carbonate ... 3061
Lithobid Slow-Release Tablets ... 3255

Loratadine (Amphetamines may counteract the sedative effect of antihistamine). Products include:
Claritin ... 3100
Claritin-D 12 Hour Extended Release Tablets ... 3102
Claritin-D 24 Hour Extended Release Tablets ... 3104

Losartan Potassium (Amphetamine may antagonize the hypotensive effects of antihypertensives). Products include:
Cozaar Tablets ... 2067
Hyzaar ... 2109

Maprotiline Hydrochloride (Enhanced activity of tricyclic or sympathomimetics; possible increases in the brain concentration of d-amphetamine in the brain; cardiovascular effect may be potentiated).
No products indexed under this heading.

Mecamylamine Hydrochloride (Amphetamine may antagonize the hypotensive effects of antihypertensives). Products include:
Inversine Tablets ... 1850

Meperidine Hydrochloride (Amphetamine potentiates the analgesic effect of meperidine). Products include:
Demerol ... 3079
Mepergan Injection ... 3539

Methdilazine Hydrochloride (Amphetamines may counteract the sedative effect of antihistamine).
No products indexed under this heading.

Methenamine (Acidifying agents used in methenamine therapy increases the urinary excretion and reduces the efficacy of amphetamine). Products include:
Prosed/DS Tablets ... 3268
Urimax Tablets ... 1769
Urised Tablets ... 2876

Methenamine Hippurate (Acidifying agents used in methenamine therapy increases the urinary excretion and reduces the efficacy of amphetamine).
No products indexed under this heading.

Methenamine Mandelate (Acidifying agents used in methenamine therapy increases the urinary excretion and reduces the efficacy of amphetamine). Products include:
Uroqid-Acid No. 2 Tablets ... 947

Methyclothiazide (Increases the concentration of the non-ionized species of the amphetamine molecule, thereby decreasing urinary excretion; increases amphetamines blood levels and thereby potentiates the actions of amphetamines).
No products indexed under this heading.

Methyldopa (Amphetamine may antagonize the hypotensive effects of antihypertensives). Products include:
Aldoclor Tablets ... 2035
Aldomet Tablets ... 2037
Aldoril Tablets ... 2039

Methyldopate Hydrochloride (Amphetamine may antagonize the hypotensive effects of antihypertensives).
No products indexed under this heading.

Metipranolol Hydrochloride (Amphetamine may antagonize the hypotensive effects of antihypertensives; adrenergic blockers are inhibited by amphetamines).
No products indexed under this heading.

Metolazone (Amphetamine may antagonize the hypotensive effects of antihypertensives). Products include:
Mykrox Tablets ... 1168
Zaroxolyn Tablets ... 1177

Metoprolol Succinate (Amphetamine may antagonize the hypotensive effects of antihypertensives; adrenergic blockers are inhibited by amphetamines). Products include:
Toprol-XL Tablets ... 651

Metoprolol Tartrate (Amphetamine may antagonize the hypotensive effects of antihypertensives; adrenergic blockers are inhibited by amphetamines).
No products indexed under this heading.

Metyrosine (Amphetamine may antagonize the hypotensive effects of antihypertensives). Products include:
Demser Capsules ... 2085

Mibefradil Dihydrochloride (Amphetamine may antagonize the hypotensive effects of antihypertensives).
No products indexed under this heading.

Minoxidil (Amphetamine may antagonize the hypotensive effects of antihypertensives). Products include:
Rogaine Extra Strength for Men Topical Solution ... ▣ 721
Rogaine for Women Topical Solution ... ▣ 721

Moclobemide (Concurrent and/or sequential use with MAO inhibitors is contraindicated; hypertensive crisis may occur).
No products indexed under this heading.

Moexipril Hydrochloride (Amphetamine may antagonize the hypotensive effects of antihypertensives). Products include:
Uniretic Tablets ... 3178
Univasc Tablets ... 3181

Nadolol (Amphetamine may antagonize the hypotensive effects of antihypertensives; adrenergic blockers are inhibited by amphetamines). Products include:
Corgard Tablets ... 2245
Corzide 40/5 Tablets ... 2247
Corzide 80/5 Tablets ... 2247
Nadolol Tablets ... 2288

Nicardipine Hydrochloride (Amphetamine may antagonize the hypotensive effects of antihypertensives). Products include:
Cardene I.V. ... 3485

Nifedipine (Amphetamine may antagonize the hypotensive effects of antihypertensives). Products include:
Adalat CC Tablets ... 877
Procardia Capsules ... 2708
Procardia XL Extended Release Tablets ... 2710

Nisoldipine (Amphetamine may antagonize the hypotensive effects of antihypertensives). Products include:

Sular Tablets 688

Nitroglycerin (Amphetamine may antagonize the hypotensive effects of antihypertensives). Products include:
- Nitro-Dur Transdermal Infusion System 3134
- Nitro-Dur Transdermal Infusion System 1834
- Nitrolingual Pumpspray 1355
- Nitrostat Tablets 2658

Norepinephrine Hydrochloride (Enhances adenergic effect of norepinephrine).
No products indexed under this heading.

Nortriptyline Hydrochloride (Enhanced activity of tricyclic or sympathomimetics; possible increases in the brain concentration of d-amphetamine in the brain; cardiovascular effect may be potentiated).
No products indexed under this heading.

Pargyline Hydrochloride (Concurrent and/or sequential use with MAO inhibitors is contraindicated; hypertensive crisis may occur).
No products indexed under this heading.

Penbutolol Sulfate (Amphetamine may antagonize the hypotensive effects of antihypertensives; adrenergic blockers are inhibited by amphetamines).
No products indexed under this heading.

Perindopril Erbumine (Amphetamine may antagonize the hypotensive effects of antihypertensives). Products include:
- Aceon Tablets (2 mg, 4 mg, 8 mg) 3249

Phenelzine Sulfate (Concurrent and/or sequential use with MAO inhibitors is contraindicated; hypertensive crisis may occur). Products include:
- Nardil Tablets 2653

Phenobarbital (Amphetamine delays intestinal absorption of phenobarbital; co-administration may produce synergistic anticonvulsant action). Products include:
- Arco-Lase Plus Tablets 592
- Donnatal 2929
- Donnatal Extentabs 2930

Phenoxybenzamine Hydrochloride (Amphetamine may antagonize the hypotensive effects of antihypertensives). Products include:
- Dibenzyline Capsules 3457

Phentolamine Mesylate (Amphetamine may antagonize the hypotensive effects of antihypertensives).
No products indexed under this heading.

Phenytoin (Amphetamine delays intestinal absorption of phenytoin; co-administration may produce synergistic anticonvulsant action). Products include:
- Dilantin Infatabs 2624
- Dilantin-125 Oral Suspension 2625

Phenytoin Sodium (Amphetamine delays intestinal absorption of phenytoin; co-administration may produce synergistic anticonvulsant action). Products include:
- Dilantin Kapseals 2622

Pindolol (Amphetamine may antagonize the hypotensive effects of antihypertensives; adrenergic blockers are inhibited by amphetamines).
No products indexed under this heading.

Polythiazide (Increases the concentration of the non-ionized species of the amphetamine molecule, thereby decreasing urinary excretion; increases amphetamines blood levels and thereby potentiates the actions of amphetamines). Products include:
- Minizide Capsules 2700
- Renese Tablets 2712

Potassium Citrate (Increases the concentration of the non-ionized species of the amphetamine molecule, thereby decreasing urinary excretion; increases amphetamines blood levels and thereby potentiates the actions of amphetamines). Products include:
- Urocit-K Tablets 2232

Prazosin Hydrochloride (Amphetamine may antagonize the hypotensive effects of antihypertensives). Products include:
- Minipress Capsules 2699
- Minizide Capsules 2700

Procarbazine Hydrochloride (Concurrent and/or sequential use with MAO inhibitors is contraindicated; hypertensive crisis may occur). Products include:
- Matulane Capsules 3246

Promethazine Hydrochloride (Amphetamines may counteract the sedative effect of antihistamine). Products include:
- Mepergan Injection 3539
- Phenergan Injection 3553
- Phenergan 3556
- Phenergan Syrup 3554
- Phenergan with Codeine Syrup 3557
- Phenergan with Dextromethorphan Syrup 3559
- Phenergan VC Syrup 3560
- Phenergan VC with Codeine Syrup 3561

Propoxyphene Hydrochloride (In cases of propoxyphene overdosage, amphetamine CNS stimulation is potentiated and fatal convulsions can occur). Products include:
- Darvon Pulvules 1909
- Darvon Compound-65 Pulvules 1910

Propoxyphene Napsylate (In cases of propoxyphene overdosage, amphetamine CNS stimulation is potentiated and fatal convulsions can occur). Products include:
- Darvon-N/Darvocet-N 1907
- Darvon-N Tablets 1912

Propranolol Hydrochloride (Amphetamine may antagonize the hypotensive effects of antihypertensives; adrenergic blockers are inhibited by amphetamines). Products include:
- Inderal 3513
- Inderal LA Long-Acting Capsules 3516
- Inderide Tablets 3517
- Inderide LA Long-Acting Capsules 3519

Protriptyline Hydrochloride (Enhanced activity of tricyclic or sympathomimetics; possible increases in the brain concentration of d-amphetamine in the brain; cardiovascular effect may be potentiated). Products include:
- Vivactil Tablets 2446
- Vivactil Tablets 2217

Pyrilamine Maleate (Amphetamines may counteract the sedative effect of antihistamine). Products include:
- Maximum Strength Midol Menstrual Caplets and Gelcaps .... ◘612
- Maximum Strength Midol PMS Caplets and Gelcaps .... ◘613

Pyrilamine Tannate (Amphetamines may counteract the sedative effect of antihistamine). Products include:
- Ryna-12 S Suspension 3351

Quinapril Hydrochloride (Amphetamine may antagonize the hypotensive effects of antihypertensives). Products include:
- Accupril Tablets 2611
- Accuretic Tablets 2614

Ramipril (Amphetamine may antagonize the hypotensive effects of antihypertensives). Products include:
- Altace Capsules 2233

Rauwolfia serpentina (Amphetamine may antagonize the hypotensive effects of antihypertensives).
No products indexed under this heading.

Rescinnamine (Amphetamine may antagonize the hypotensive effects of antihypertensives).
No products indexed under this heading.

Reserpine (Lowers absorption of amphetamines).
No products indexed under this heading.

Selegiline Hydrochloride (Concurrent and/or sequential use with MAO inhibitors is contraindicated; hypertensive crisis may occur). Products include:
- Eldepryl Capsules 3266

Sodium Acid Phosphate (Increases the concentration of the ionized species of the amphetamine molecule, thereby increasing urinary excretion; lowers amphetamines blood levels and efficacy). Products include:
- Uroqid-Acid No. 2 Tablets 947

Sodium Bicarbonate (Increases absorption of amphetamines). Products include:
- Alka-Seltzer .... ◘603
- Alka-Seltzer Lemon Lime Antacid and Pain Reliever Effervescent Tablets .... ◘603
- Alka-Seltzer Extra Strength Antacid and Pain Reliever Effervescent Tablets .... ◘603
- Alka-Seltzer Heartburn Relief Tablets .... ◘604
- Ceo-Two Evacuant Suppository .... ◘618
- Colyte with Flavor Packs for Oral Solution 3170
- GoLYTELY and Pineapple Flavor GoLYTELY for Oral Solution 1068
- NuLYTELY, Cherry Flavor, Lemon-Lime Flavor, and Orange Flavor NuLYTELY for Oral Solution 1068

Sodium Citrate (Increases the concentration of the non-ionized species of the amphetamine molecule, thereby decreasing urinary excretion; increases amphetamines blood levels and thereby potentiates the actions of amphetamines).
No products indexed under this heading.

Sodium Nitroprusside (Amphetamine may antagonize the hypotensive effects of antihypertensives).
No products indexed under this heading.

Sotalol Hydrochloride (Amphetamine may antagonize the hypotensive effects of antihypertensives; adrenergic blockers are inhibited by amphetamines). Products include:
- Betapace Tablets 950
- Betapace AF Tablets 954

Spirapril Hydrochloride (Amphetamine may antagonize the hypotensive effects of antihypertensives).
No products indexed under this heading.

Telmisartan (Amphetamine may antagonize the hypotensive effects of antihypertensives). Products include:
- Micardis Tablets 1049
- Micardis HCT Tablets 1051

Terazosin Hydrochloride (Amphetamine may antagonize the hypotensive effects of antihypertensives). Products include:
- Hytrin Capsules 464

Terfenadine (Amphetamines may counteract the sedative effect of antihistamine).
No products indexed under this heading.

Timolol Hemihydrate (Amphetamine may antagonize the hypotensive effects of antihypertensives; adrenergic blockers are inhibited by amphetamines). Products include:
- Betimol Ophthalmic Solution .... ⊙324

Timolol Maleate (Amphetamine may antagonize the hypotensive effects of antihypertensives; adrenergic blockers are inhibited by amphetamines). Products include:
- Blocadren Tablets 2046
- Cosopt Sterile Ophthalmic Solution 2065
- Timolide Tablets 2187
- Timolol GFS .... ⊙266
- Timoptic in Ocudose 2192
- Timoptic Sterile Ophthalmic Solution 2190
- Timoptic-XE Sterile Ophthalmic Gel Forming Solution 2194

Torsemide (Amphetamine may antagonize the hypotensive effects of antihypertensives). Products include:
- Demadex Tablets and Injection 2965

Trandolapril (Amphetamine may antagonize the hypotensive effects of antihypertensives). Products include:
- Mavik Tablets 478
- Tarka Tablets 508

Tranylcypromine Sulfate (Concurrent and/or sequential use with MAO inhibitors is contraindicated; hypertensive crisis may occur). Products include:
- Parnate Tablets 1607

Trimeprazine Tartrate (Amphetamines may counteract the sedative effect of antihistamine).
No products indexed under this heading.

Trimethaphan Camsylate (Amphetamine may antagonize the hypotensive effects of antihypertensives).
No products indexed under this heading.

Trimipramine Maleate (Enhanced activity of tricyclic or sympathomimetics; possible increases in the brain concentration of d-amphetamine in the brain; cardiovascular effect may be potentiated). Products include:
- Surmontil Capsules 3595

Tripelennamine Hydrochloride (Amphetamines may counteract the sedative effect of antihistamine).
No products indexed under this heading.

Triprolidine Hydrochloride (Amphetamines may counteract the sedative effect of antihistamine). Products include:
- Actifed Cold & Allergy Tablets .... ◘688

Valsartan (Amphetamine may antagonize the hypotensive effects of antihypertensives). Products include:
- Diovan Capsules 2337
- Diovan HCT Tablets 2338

Verapamil Hydrochloride (Amphetamine may antagonize the hypotensive effects of antihypertensives). Products include:
- Covera-HS Tablets 3199
- Isoptin SR Tablets 467
- Tarka Tablets 508
- Verelan Capsules 3184
- Verelan PM Capsules 3186

Vitamin C (Lowers absorption of amphetamines). Products include:
- Beta-C Tablets .... ◘811
- C-Grams Caplets .... ◘795
- Halls Defense Drops .... ◘687
- Peridin-C Tablets .... ◘618

Food Interactions

Fruit juices, unspecified (Lowers absorption of amphetamines).

DEXEDRINE TABLETS

(Dextroamphetamine Sulfate) 1512

See Dexedrine Spansule Capsules

DEXTROSTAT TABLETS
(Dextroamphetamine Sulfate) 3236
May interact with alpha adrenergic blockers, antihistamines, antihypertensives, beta blockers, monoamine oxidase inhibitors, sympathomimetics, thiazides, tricyclic antidepressants, urinary alkalinizing agents, veratrum alkaloids, and certain other agents. Compounds in these categories include:

Acebutolol Hydrochloride (Adrenergic blockers are inhibited by amphetamines; amphetamines may antagonize the hypotensive effects of antihypertensives). Products include:
- Sectral Capsules 3589

Acetazolamide (Increases the concentration of the non-ionized species of the amphetamine molecule thereby decreasing urinary excretion; increases blood levels and potentiates the action of amphetamines). Products include:
- Diamox Sequels Sustained Release Capsules .... ⊙270
- Diamox Tablets .... ⊙269

Acetazolamide Sodium (Increases the concentration of the non-ionized species of the amphetamine molecule thereby decreasing urinary excretion; increases blood levels and potentiates the action of amphetamines). Products include:
- Diamox Intravenous .... ⊙269

Acrivastine (Amphetamines may counteract the sedative effect of antihistamines). Products include:
- Semprex-D Capsules 1172

Albuterol (Enhanced activity of sympathomimetics). Products include:
- Proventil Inhalation Aerosol 3142
- Ventolin Inhalation Aerosol and Refill 1679

Albuterol Sulfate (Enhanced activity of sympathomimetics). Products include:
- AccuNeb Inhalation Solution 1230
- Combivent Inhalation Aerosol 1041
- DuoNeb Inhalation Solution 1233
- Proventil Inhalation Solution 0.083% 3146
- Proventil Repetabs Tablets 3148
- Proventil Solution for Inhalation 0.5% 3144
- Proventil HFA Inhalation Aerosol 3150
- Ventolin HFA Inhalation Aerosol 3618
- Volmax Extended-Release Tablets .. 2276

Amitriptyline Hydrochloride (Enhanced activity of tricyclic antidepressants; cardiovascular effects can be potentiated). Products include:
- Etrafon 3115
- Limbitrol 1738

Amlodipine Besylate (Amphetamines may antagonize the hypotensive effects of antihypertensives). Products include:
- Lotrel Capsules 2370
- Norvasc Tablets 2704

Ammonium Chloride (Increases the concentration of ionized species of the amphetamine molecule thereby increasing urinary excretion; lowers blood levels and efficacy of amphetamines).
- No products indexed under this heading.

Amoxapine (Enhanced activity of tricyclic antidepressants; cardiovascular effects can be potentiated).
- No products indexed under this heading.

Astemizole (Amphetamines may counteract the sedative effect of antihistamines).
- No products indexed under this heading.

Atenolol (Adrenergic blockers are inhibited by amphetamines; amphetamines may antagonize the hypotensive effects of antihypertensives). Products include:
- Tenoretic Tablets 690
- Tenormin I.V. Injection 692

Azatadine Maleate (Amphetamines may counteract the sedative effect of antihistamines). Products include:
- Rynatan Tablets 3351

Benazepril Hydrochloride (Amphetamines may antagonize the hypotensive effects of antihypertensives). Products include:
- Lotensin Tablets 2365
- Lotensin HCT Tablets 2367
- Lotrel Capsules 2370

Bendroflumethiazide (Some thiazide diuretics increase concentration of the non-ionized species of the amphetamine molecule thereby decreasing urinary excretion; increases blood levels and potentiates the action of amphetamines; amphetamines may antagonize the hypotensive effects of antihypertensives). Products include:
- Corzide 40/5 Tablets 2247
- Corzide 80/5 Tablets 2247

Betaxolol Hydrochloride (Adrenergic blockers are inhibited by amphetamines; amphetamines may antagonize the hypotensive effects of antihypertensives). Products include:
- Betoptic S Ophthalmic Suspension 537

Bisoprolol Fumarate (Adrenergic blockers are inhibited by amphetamines; amphetamines may antagonize the hypotensive effects of antihypertensives). Products include:
- Zebeta Tablets 1885
- Ziac Tablets 1887

Bromodiphenhydramine Hydrochloride (Amphetamines may counteract the sedative effect of antihistamines).
- No products indexed under this heading.

Brompheniramine Maleate (Amphetamines may counteract the sedative effect of antihistamines). Products include:
- Bromfed Capsules (Extended-Release) 2269
- Bromfed-PD Capsules (Extended-Release) 2269
- Comtrex Acute Head Cold & Sinus Pressure Relief Tablets ..... ▣627
- Dimetapp Elixir .... ▣777
- Dimetapp Cold and Fever Suspension .... ▣775
- Dimetapp DM Cold & Cough Elixir .. ▣775
- Dimetapp Nighttime Flu Liquid .... ▣776

Candesartan Cilexetil (Amphetamines may antagonize the hypotensive effects of antihypertensives). Products include:
- Atacand Tablets 595
- Atacand HCT Tablets 597

Captopril (Amphetamines may antagonize the hypotensive effects of antihypertensives). Products include:
- Captopril Tablets 2281

Carteolol Hydrochloride (Adrenergic blockers are inhibited by amphetamines; amphetamines may antagonize the hypotensive effects of antihypertensives). Products include:
- Carteolol Hydrochloride Ophthalmic Solution USP, 1% ..... ⊙258
- Ocupress Ophthalmic Solution, 1% Sterile .... ⊙303

Cetirizine Hydrochloride (Amphetamines may counteract the sedative effect of antihistamines). Products include:
- Zyrtec 2756
- Zyrtec-D 12 Hour Extended Relief Tablets 2758

Chlorothiazide (Some thiazide diuretics increase concentration of the non-ionized species of the amphetamine molecule thereby decreasing urinary excretion; increases blood levels and potentiates the action of amphetamines; amphetamines may antagonize the hypotensive effects of antihypertensives). Products include:
- Aldoclor Tablets 2035
- Diuril Oral 2087

Chlorothiazide Sodium (Some thiazide diuretics increase concentration of the non-ionized species of the amphetamine molecule thereby decreasing urinary excretion; increases blood levels and potentiates the action of amphetamines; amphetamines may antagonize the hypotensive effects of antihypertensives). Products include:
- Diuril Sodium Intravenous 2086

Chlorpheniramine Maleate (Amphetamines may counteract the sedative effect of antihistamines). Products include:
- Actifed Cold & Sinus Caplets and Tablets .... ▣688
- Alka-Seltzer Plus Liqui-Gels .... ▣604
- BC Allergy Sinus Cold Powder .... ▣619
- Chlor-Trimeton Allergy Tablets ...... ▣735
- Chlor-Trimeton Allergy/Decongestant Tablets .... ▣736
- Comtrex Flu Therapy & Fever Relief Nighttime Tablets .... ▣628
- Comtrex Maximum Strength Multi-Symptom Cold & Cough Relief Tablets and Caplets .... ▣626
- Contac Severe Cold and Flu Caplets Maximum Strength .... ▣746
- Coricidin 'D' Cold, Flu & Sinus Tablets .... ▣737
- Coricidin/Coricidin D .... ▣738
- Coricidin HBP Maximum Strength Flu Tablets .... ▣738
- Extendryl 1361
- Hycomine Compound Tablets 1317
- Kronofed-A 1341
- PediaCare Cough-Cold Liquid .... ▣719
- PediaCare NightRest Cough-Cold Liquid .... ▣719
- Robitussin Nighttime Honey Flu Liquid .... ▣786
- Ryna .... ▣768
- Singlet Caplets .... ▣761
- Sinutab Sinus Allergy Medication, Maximum Strength Formula, Tablets & Caplets .... ▣707
- Sudafed Cold & Allergy Tablets ...... ▣708
- TheraFlu Regular Strength Cold & Cough Night Time Hot Liquid ..... ▣676
- TheraFlu Regular Strength Cold & Sore Throat Night Time Hot Liquid .... ▣676
- TheraFlu Maximum Strength Flu & Cough Night Time Hot Liquid .. ▣678
- TheraFlu Maximum Strength Flu & Sore Throat Night Time Hot Liquid .... ▣677
- TheraFlu Maximum Strength Severe Cold & Congestion Night Time Caplets .... ▣678
- TheraFlu Maximum Strength Severe Cold & Congestion Night Time Hot Liquid .... ▣678
- Triaminic Cold & Allergy Liquid ...... ▣681
- Triaminic Cold & Allergy Softchews .... ▣683
- Triaminic Cold & Cough Liquid .... ▣681
- Triaminic Cold & Cough Softchews .... ▣683
- Triaminic Cold & Night Time Cough Liquid .... ▣681
- Triaminic Cold, Cough & Fever Liquid .... ▣681
- Children's Tylenol Cold Suspension Liquid and Chewable Tablets 2015
- Children's Tylenol Cold Plus Cough Suspension Liquid and Chewable Tablets 2015
- Children's Tylenol Flu Suspension Liquid 2015
- Maximum Strength Tylenol Allergy Sinus Caplets, Gelcaps, and Geltabs 2010
- Multi-Symptom Tylenol Cold Complete Formula Caplets 2010
- Vicks 44M Cough, Cold & Flu Relief Liquid .... ▣725
- Pediatric Vicks 44m Cough & Cold Relief .... ▣728
- Children's Vicks NyQuil Cold/Cough Relief .... ▣726

Chlorpheniramine Polistirex (Amphetamines may counteract the sedative effect of antihistamines). Products include:
- Tussionex Pennkinetic Extended-Release Suspension 1174

Chlorpheniramine Tannate (Amphetamines may counteract the sedative effect of antihistamines). Products include:
- Reformulated Rynatan Pediatric Suspension 3352
- Rynatuss Pediatric Suspension 3353
- Rynatuss Tablets 3353
- Tussi-12 S Suspension 3356
- Tussi-12 Tablets 3356

Chlorpromazine (Inhibits central stimulant effects of amphetamines). Products include:
- Thorazine Suppositories 1656

Chlorpromazine Hydrochloride (Inhibits central stimulant effects of amphetamines). Products include:
- Thorazine 1656

Chlorthalidone (Amphetamines may antagonize the hypotensive effects of antihypertensives). Products include:
- Clorpres Tablets 1002
- Combipres Tablets 1040
- Tenoretic Tablets 690

Clemastine Fumarate (Amphetamines may counteract the sedative effect of antihistamines). Products include:
- Tavist 12 Hour Allergy Tablets .... ▣676

Clomipramine Hydrochloride (Enhanced activity of tricyclic antidepressants; cardiovascular effects can be potentiated).
- No products indexed under this heading.

Clonidine (Amphetamines may antagonize the hypotensive effects of antihypertensives). Products include:
- Catapres-TTS 1038

Clonidine Hydrochloride (Amphetamines may antagonize the hypotensive effects of antihypertensives). Products include:
- Catapres Tablets 1037
- Clorpres Tablets 1002
- Combipres Tablets 1040
- Duraclon Injection 3057

Cryptenamine Preparations (Amphetamines may inhibit the hypotensive effects of veratrum alkaloids).
- No products indexed under this heading.

Cyproheptadine Hydrochloride (Amphetamines may counteract the sedative effect of antihistamines). Products include:
- Periactin Tablets 2155

Deserpidine (Amphetamines may antagonize the hypotensive effects of antihypertensives).
- No products indexed under this heading.

Desipramine Hydrochloride (Enhanced activity of tricyclic antidepressants; cardiovascular effects can be potentiated). Products include:
- Norpramin Tablets 755

Dexchlorpheniramine Maleate (Amphetamines may counteract the sedative effect of antihistamines).
- No products indexed under this heading.

Diazoxide (Amphetamines may antagonize the hypotensive effects of antihypertensives).
- No products indexed under this heading.

Diltiazem Hydrochloride (Amphetamines may antagonize the hypotensive effects of antihypertensives). Products include:
- Cardizem Injectable 1018
- Cardizem Lyo-Ject Syringe 1018
- Cardizem Monovial 1018
- Cardizem CD Capsules 1016
- Tiazac Capsules 1378

Diphenhydramine Citrate (Amphetamines may counteract the sedative effect of antihistamines). Products include:
- Alka-Seltzer PM Effervescent Tablets .... ▣605

Benadryl Allergy & Sinus Fastmelt Tablets ▣693
Benadryl Children's Allergy/Cold Fastmelt Tablets ▣692
Excedrin PM Tablets, Caplets, and Geltabs ▣631
Goody's PM Powder ▣621

Diphenhydramine Hydrochloride (Amphetamines may counteract the sedative effect of antihistamines). Products include:
Extra Strength Bayer PM Caplets ▣611
Benadryl Allergy Chewables ▣689
Benadryl Allergy ▣691
Benadryl Allergy Liquid ▣690
Benadryl Allergy/Cold Tablets ▣691
Benadryl Allergy/Congestion Tablets ▣692
Benadryl Allergy & Sinus Liquid ▣693
Benadryl Allergy Sinus Headache Caplets & Gelcaps ▣693
Benadryl Severe Allergy & Sinus Headache Caplets ▣694
Benadryl Dye-Free Allergy Liquid ▣690
Benadryl Dye-Free Allergy Liqui-Gels Softgels ▣690
Benadryl Itch Relief Stick Extra Strength ▣695
Benadryl Cream ▣695
Benadryl Gel ▣695
Benadryl Spray ▣696
Benadryl Parenteral 2617
Coricidin HBP Night-Time Cold & Flu Tablets ▣738
Nytol QuickCaps Caplets ▣622
Maximum Strength Nytol QuickGels Softgels ▣621
Extra Strength Percogesic Aspirin-Free Coated Caplets ▣665
Simply Sleep Caplets 2008
Sominex Original Formula Tablets ▣761
Children's Tylenol Allergy-D Liquid 2014
Maximum Strength Tylenol Allergy Sinus NightTime Caplets 2010
Tylenol Severe Allergy Caplets 2010
Maximum Strength Tylenol Flu NightTime Gelcaps 2011
Extra Strength Tylenol PM Caplets, Geltabs, and Gelcaps 2012
Unisom Maximum Strength SleepGels ▣713

Diphenylpyraline Hydrochloride (Amphetamines may counteract the sedative effect of antihistamines).
No products indexed under this heading.

Dobutamine Hydrochloride (Enhanced activity of sympathomimetics). Products include:
Dobutrex Solution Vials 1914

Dopamine Hydrochloride (Enhanced activity of sympathomimetics).
No products indexed under this heading.

Doxazosin Mesylate (Adrenergic blockers are inhibited by amphetamines; amphetamines may antagonize the hypotensive effects of antihypertensives). Products include:
Cardura Tablets 2668

Doxepin Hydrochloride (Enhanced activity of tricyclic antidepressants; cardiovascular effects can be potentiated). Products include:
Sinequan 2713

Enalapril Maleate (Amphetamines may antagonize the hypotensive effects of antihypertensives). Products include:
Lexxel Tablets 608
Vaseretic Tablets 2204
Vasotec Tablets 2210

Enalaprilat (Amphetamines may antagonize the hypotensive effects of antihypertensives). Products include:
Enalaprilat Injection 863
Vasotec I.V. Injection 2207

Ephedrine Hydrochloride (Enhanced activity of sympathomimetics). Products include:
Primatene Tablets ▣780

Ephedrine Sulfate (Enhanced activity of sympathomimetics).
No products indexed under this heading.

Ephedrine Tannate (Enhanced activity of sympathomimetics). Products include:
Rynatuss Pediatric Suspension 3353
Rynatuss Tablets 3353

Epinephrine (Enhanced activity of sympathomimetics). Products include:
Epifrin Sterile Ophthalmic Solution ⊙235
EpiPen 1236
Primatene Mist ▣779
Xylocaine with Epinephrine Injection 653

Epinephrine Bitartrate (Enhanced activity of sympathomimetics). Products include:
Sensorcaine 643

Epinephrine Hydrochloride (Enhanced activity of sympathomimetics).
No products indexed under this heading.

Eprosartan Mesylate (Amphetamines may antagonize the hypotensive effects of antihypertensives). Products include:
Teveten Tablets 3327

Esmolol Hydrochloride (Adrenergic blockers are inhibited by amphetamines; amphetamines may antagonize the hypotensive effects of antihypertensives). Products include:
Brevibloc Injection 858

Ethosuximide (Delayed intestinal absorption of ethosuximide). Products include:
Zarontin Capsules 2659
Zarontin Syrup 2660

Felodipine (Amphetamines may antagonize the hypotensive effects of antihypertensives). Products include:
Lexxel Tablets 608
Plendil Extended-Release Tablets 623

Fexofenadine Hydrochloride (Amphetamines may counteract the sedative effect of antihistamines). Products include:
Allegra 712
Allegra-D Extended-Release Tablets 714

Fosinopril Sodium (Amphetamines may antagonize the hypotensive effects of antihypertensives). Products include:
Monopril Tablets 1091
Monopril HCT 1094

Fosphenytoin Sodium (Co-administration may produce synergistic anticonvulsant action). Products include:
Cerebyx Injection 2619

Furosemide (Amphetamines may antagonize the hypotensive effects of antihypertensives). Products include:
Furosemide Tablets 2284

Glutamic Acid Hydrochloride (Lowers absorption of amphetamines by acting as gastrointestinal acidifying agent).
No products indexed under this heading.

Guanabenz Acetate (Amphetamines may antagonize the hypotensive effects of antihypertensives).
No products indexed under this heading.

Guanethidine Monosulfate (Lowers absorption of amphetamines by acting as gastrointestinal acidifying agent; amphetamines may antagonize the hypotensive effects of antihypertensives).
No products indexed under this heading.

Haloperidol (Inhibits central stimulant effects of amphetamines). Products include:
Haldol Injection, Tablets and Concentrate 2533

Haloperidol Decanoate (Inhibits central stimulant effects of amphetamines). Products include:
Haldol Decanoate 2535

Hydralazine Hydrochloride (Amphetamines may antagonize the hypotensive effects of antihypertensives).
No products indexed under this heading.

Hydrochlorothiazide (Some thiazide diuretics increase concentration of the non-ionized species of the amphetamine molecule thereby decreasing urinary excretion; increases blood levels and potentiates the action of amphetamines; amphetamines may antagonize the hypotensive effects of antihypertensives). Products include:
Accuretic Tablets 2614
Aldoril Tablets 2039
Atacand HCT Tablets 597
Avalide Tablets 1070
Diovan HCT Tablets 2338
Dyazide Capsules 1515
HydroDIURIL Tablets 2108
Hyzaar 2109
Inderide Tablets 3517
Inderide LA Long-Acting Capsules 3519
Lotensin HCT Tablets 2367
Maxzide 1008
Micardis HCT Tablets 1051
Microzide Capsules 3414
Moduretic Tablets 2138
Monopril HCT 1094
Prinzide Tablets 2168
Timolide Tablets 2187
Uniretic Tablets 3178
Vaseretic Tablets 2204
Zestoretic Tablets 695
Ziac Tablets 1887

Hydroflumethiazide (Some thiazide diuretics increase concentration of the non-ionized species of the amphetamine molecule thereby decreasing urinary excretion; increases blood levels and potentiates the action of amphetamines; amphetamines may antagonize the hypotensive effects of antihypertensives). Products include:
Diucardin Tablets 3494

Imipramine Hydrochloride (Enhanced activity of tricyclic antidepressants; cardiovascular effects can be potentiated).
No products indexed under this heading.

Imipramine Pamoate (Enhanced activity of tricyclic antidepressants; cardiovascular effects can be potentiated).
No products indexed under this heading.

Indapamide (Amphetamines may antagonize the hypotensive effects of antihypertensives). Products include:
Indapamide Tablets 2286

Irbesartan (Amphetamines may antagonize the hypotensive effects of antihypertensives). Products include:
Avalide Tablets 1070
Avapro Tablets 1074
Avapro Tablets 3076

Isocarboxazid (Potential for hypertensive crisis; slows amphetamine metabolism; concurrent and/or sequential use is contraindicated).
No products indexed under this heading.

Isoproterenol Hydrochloride (Enhanced activity of sympathomimetics).
No products indexed under this heading.

Isoproterenol Sulfate (Enhanced activity of sympathomimetics).
No products indexed under this heading.

Isradipine (Amphetamines may antagonize the hypotensive effects of antihypertensives). Products include:
DynaCirc Capsules 2921
DynaCirc CR Tablets 2923

Labetalol Hydrochloride (Adrenergic blockers are inhibited by amphetamines; amphetamines may antagonize the hypotensive effects of antihypertensives). Products include:
Normodyne Injection 3135
Normodyne Tablets 3137

Levalbuterol Hydrochloride (Enhanced activity of sympathomimetics). Products include:
Xopenex Inhalation Solution 3207

Levobunolol Hydrochloride (Adrenergic blockers are inhibited by amphetamines; amphetamines may antagonize the hypotensive effects of antihypertensives). Products include:
Betagan ⊙228

Lisinopril (Amphetamines may antagonize the hypotensive effects of antihypertensives). Products include:
Prinivil Tablets 2164
Prinzide Tablets 2168
Zestoretic Tablets 695
Zestril Tablets 698

Lithium Carbonate (Inhibits stimulatory effects of amphetamines). Products include:
Eskalith 1527
Lithium Carbonate 3061
Lithobid Slow-Release Tablets 3255

Loratadine (Amphetamines may counteract the sedative effect of antihistamines). Products include:
Claritin 3100
Claritin-D 12 Hour Extended Release Tablets 3102
Claritin-D 24 Hour Extended Release Tablets 3104

Losartan Potassium (Amphetamines may antagonize the hypotensive effects of antihypertensives). Products include:
Cozaar Tablets 2067
Hyzaar 2109

Maprotiline Hydrochloride (Enhanced activity of tricyclic antidepressants; cardiovascular effects can be potentiated).
No products indexed under this heading.

Mecamylamine Hydrochloride (Amphetamines may antagonize the hypotensive effects of antihypertensives). Products include:
Inversine Tablets 1850

Meperidine Hydrochloride (Analgesic effect of meperidine potentiated). Products include:
Demerol 3079
Mepergan Injection 3539

Metaproterenol Sulfate (Enhanced activity of sympathomimetics). Products include:
Alupent 1029

Metaraminol Bitartrate (Enhanced activity of sympathomimetics). Products include:
Aramine Injection 2043

Methdilazine Hydrochloride (Amphetamines may counteract the sedative effect of antihistamines).
No products indexed under this heading.

Methenamine (Increases urinary excretion and efficacy is reduced by acidifying agents used in methenamine therapy). Products include:
Prosed/DS Tablets 3268
Urimax Tablets 1769
Urised Tablets 2876

Methenamine Hippurate (Increases urinary excretion and efficacy is reduced by acidifying agents used in methenamine therapy).
No products indexed under this heading.

Methenamine Mandelate (Increases urinary excretion and efficacy is reduced by acidifying agents used in methenamine therapy). Products include:
Uroqid-Acid No. 2 Tablets 947

Methoxamine Hydrochloride (Enhanced activity of sympathomimetics).
No products indexed under this heading.

Methyclothiazide (Some thiazide diuretics increase concentration of the non-ionized species of the amphetamine molecule thereby decreasing urinary excretion; increases blood levels and potentiates the action of amphetamines; amphetamines may antagonize the hypotensive effects of antihypertensives).
No products indexed under this heading.

Methyldopa (Amphetamines may antagonize the hypotensive effects of antihypertensives). Products include:
Aldoclor Tablets ... 2035
Aldomet Tablets ... 2037
Aldoril Tablets ... 2039

Methyldopate Hydrochloride (Amphetamines may antagonize the hypotensive effects of antihypertensives).
No products indexed under this heading.

Metipranolol Hydrochloride (Adrenergic blockers are inhibited by amphetamines; amphetamines may antagonize the hypotensive effects of antihypertensives).
No products indexed under this heading.

Metolazone (Amphetamines may antagonize the hypotensive effects of antihypertensives). Products include:
Mykrox Tablets ... 1168
Zaroxolyn Tablets ... 1177

Metoprolol Succinate (Adrenergic blockers are inhibited by amphetamines; amphetamines may antagonize the hypotensive effects of antihypertensives). Products include:
Toprol-XL Tablets ... 651

Metoprolol Tartrate (Adrenergic blockers are inhibited by amphetamines; amphetamines may antagonize the hypotensive effects of antihypertensives).
No products indexed under this heading.

Metyrosine (Amphetamines may antagonize the hypotensive effects of antihypertensives). Products include:
Demser Capsules ... 2085

Mibefradil Dihydrochloride (Amphetamines may antagonize the hypotensive effects of antihypertensives).
No products indexed under this heading.

Minoxidil (Amphetamines may antagonize the hypotensive effects of antihypertensives). Products include:
Rogaine Extra Strength for Men Topical Solution ... ■ 721
Rogaine for Women Topical Solution ... ■ 721

Moclobemide (Potential for hypertensive crisis; slows amphetamine metabolism; concurrent and/or sequential use is contraindicated).
No products indexed under this heading.

Moexipril Hydrochloride (Amphetamines may antagonize the hypotensive effects of antihypertensives). Products include:
Uniretic Tablets ... 3178
Univasc Tablets ... 3181

Nadolol (Adrenergic blockers are inhibited by amphetamines; amphetamines may antagonize the hypotensive effects of antihypertensives). Products include:
Corgard Tablets ... 2245
Corzide 40/5 Tablets ... 2247
Corzide 80/5 Tablets ... 2247
Nadolol Tablets ... 2288

Nicardipine Hydrochloride (Amphetamines may antagonize the hypotensive effects of antihypertensives). Products include:
Cardene I.V. ... 3485

Nifedipine (Amphetamines may antagonize the hypotensive effects of antihypertensives). Products include:
Adalat CC Tablets ... 877
Procardia Capsules ... 2708
Procardia XL Extended Release Tablets ... 2710

Nisoldipine (Amphetamines may antagonize the hypotensive effects of antihypertensives). Products include:
Sular Tablets ... 688

Nitroglycerin (Amphetamines may antagonize the hypotensive effects of antihypertensives). Products include:
Nitro-Dur Transdermal Infusion System ... 3134
Nitro-Dur Transdermal Infusion System ... 1834
Nitrolingual Pumpspray ... 1355
Nitrostat Tablets ... 2658

Norepinephrine Bitartrate (Enhanced activity of sympathomimetics).
No products indexed under this heading.

Norepinephrine Hydrochloride (Enhanced adrenergic effect of norepinephrine).
No products indexed under this heading.

Nortriptyline Hydrochloride (Enhanced activity of tricyclic antidepressants; cardiovascular effects can be potentiated).
No products indexed under this heading.

Pargyline Hydrochloride (Potential for hypertensive crisis; slows amphetamine metabolism; concurrent and/or sequential use is contraindicated).
No products indexed under this heading.

Penbutolol Sulfate (Adrenergic blockers are inhibited by amphetamines; amphetamines may antagonize the hypotensive effects of antihypertensives).
No products indexed under this heading.

Perindopril Erbumine (Amphetamines may antagonize the hypotensive effects of antihypertensives). Products include:
Aceon Tablets (2 mg, 4 mg, 8 mg) ... 3249

Phenelzine Sulfate (Potential for hypertensive crisis; slows amphetamine metabolism; concurrent and/or sequential use is contraindicated). Products include:
Nardil Tablets ... 2653

Phenobarbital (Delayed intestinal absorption of phenobarbital; synergistic anticonvulsant action may be produced). Products include:
Arco-Lase Plus Tablets ... 592
Donnatal ... 2929
Donnatal Extentabs ... 2930

Phenoxybenzamine Hydrochloride (Amphetamines may antagonize the hypotensive effects of antihypertensives). Products include:
Dibenzyline Capsules ... 3457

Phentolamine Mesylate (Amphetamines may antagonize the hypotensive effects of antihypertensives).
No products indexed under this heading.

Phenylephrine Bitartrate (Enhanced activity of sympathomimetics).
No products indexed under this heading.

Phenylephrine Hydrochloride (Enhanced activity of sympathomimetics). Products include:
Afrin Nasal Decongestant Children's Pump Mist ... ■ 734
Extendryl ... 1361
Hycomine Compound Tablets ... 1317
Neo-Synephrine ... ■ 614
Phenergan VC Syrup ... 3560
Phenergan VC with Codeine Syrup ... 3561
Preparation H Cream ... ■ 778
Preparation H Cooling Gel ... ■ 778
Preparation H ... ■ 778
Vicks Sinex Nasal Spray and Ultra Fine Mist ... ■ 729

Phenylephrine Tannate (Enhanced activity of sympathomimetics). Products include:
Ryna-12 S Suspension ... 3351
Reformulated Rynatan Pediatric Suspension ... 3352
Rynatuss Pediatric Suspension ... 3353
Rynatuss Tablets ... 3353

Phenylpropanolamine Hydrochloride (Enhanced activity of sympathomimetics).
No products indexed under this heading.

Phenytoin (Delayed intestinal absorption of phenobarbital; synergistic anticonvulsant action may be produced). Products include:
Dilantin Infatabs ... 2624
Dilantin-125 Oral Suspension ... 2625

Phenytoin Sodium (Delayed intestinal absorption of phenobarbital; synergistic anticonvulsant action may be produced). Products include:
Dilantin Kapseals ... 2622

Pindolol (Adrenergic blockers are inhibited by amphetamines; amphetamines may antagonize the hypotensive effects of antihypertensives).
No products indexed under this heading.

Pirbuterol Acetate (Enhanced activity of sympathomimetics). Products include:
Maxair Autohaler ... 1981
Maxair Inhaler ... 1984

Polythiazide (Some thiazide diuretics increase concentration of the non-ionized species of the amphetamine molecule thereby decreasing urinary excretion; increases blood levels and potentiates the action of amphetamines; amphetamines may antagonize the hypotensive effects of antihypertensives). Products include:
Minizide Capsules ... 2700
Renese Tablets ... 2712

Potassium Citrate (Increases the concentration of the non-ionized species of the amphetamine molecule thereby decreasing urinary excretion; increases blood levels and potentiates the action of amphetamines). Products include:
Urocit-K Tablets ... 2232

Prazosin Hydrochloride (Adrenergic blockers are inhibited by amphetamines; amphetamines may antagonize the hypotensive effects of antihypertensives). Products include:
Minipress Capsules ... 2699
Minizide Capsules ... 2700

Procarbazine Hydrochloride (Potential for hypertensive crisis; slows amphetamine metabolism; concurrent and/or sequential use is contraindicated). Products include:
Matulane Capsules ... 3246

Promethazine Hydrochloride (Amphetamines may counteract the sedative effect of antihistamines). Products include:
Mepergan Injection ... 3539
Phenergan Injection ... 3553
Phenergan ... 3556
Phenergan Syrup ... 3554
Phenergan with Codeine Syrup ... 3557
Phenergan with Dextromethorphan Syrup ... 3559
Phenergan VC Syrup ... 3560
Phenergan VC with Codeine Syrup ... 3561

Propoxyphene Hydrochloride (In cases of propoxyphene overdosage, amphetamine CNS stimulation is potentiated and fatal convulsions can occur). Products include:
Darvon Pulvules ... 1909
Darvon Compound-65 Pulvules ... 1910

Propoxyphene Napsylate (In cases of propoxyphene overdosage, amphetamine CNS stimulation is potentiated and fatal convulsions can occur). Products include:
Darvon-N/Darvocet-N ... 1907
Darvon-N Tablets ... 1912

Propranolol Hydrochloride (Adrenergic blockers are inhibited by amphetamines; amphetamines may antagonize the hypotensive effects of antihypertensives). Products include:
Inderal ... 3513
Inderal LA Long-Acting Capsules ... 3516
Inderide Tablets ... 3517
Inderide LA Long-Acting Capsules ... 3519

Protriptyline Hydrochloride (Enhanced activity of tricyclic antidepressants; cardiovascular effects can be potentiated). Products include:
Vivactil Tablets ... 2446
Vivactil Tablets ... 2217

Pseudoephedrine Hydrochloride (Enhanced activity of sympathomimetics). Products include:
Actifed Cold & Allergy Tablets ... ■ 688
Actifed Cold & Sinus Caplets and Tablets ... ■ 688
Advil Cold and Sinus Caplets ... ■ 771
Advil Cold and Sinus Tablets ... ■ 771
Advil Flu & Body Ache Caplets ... ■ 772
Aleve Cold & Sinus Caplets ... ■ 603
Alka-Seltzer Plus Liqui-Gels ... ■ 604
Alka-Seltzer Plus Cold & Flu Medicine Liqui-Gels ... ■ 604
Alka-Seltzer Plus Cold & Sinus Medicine Liqui-Gels ... ■ 604
Allegra-D Extended-Release Tablets ... 714
BC Cold Powder ... ■ 619
Benadryl Allergy/Cold Tablets ... ■ 691
Benadryl Allergy/Congestion Tablets ... ■ 692
Benadryl Allergy & Sinus Liquid ... ■ 693
Benadryl Allergy & Sinus Fastmelt Tablets ... ■ 693
Benadryl Allergy Sinus Headache Caplets & Gelcaps ... ■ 693
Benadryl Severe Allergy & Sinus Headache Caplets ... ■ 694
Benadryl Children's Allergy/Cold Fastmelt Tablets ... ■ 692
Benylin Multi-Symptom Liquid ... ■ 697
Bromfed Capsules (Extended-Release) ... 2269
Bromfed-PD Capsules (Extended-Release) ... 2269
Children's Cēpacol Sore Throat ... ■ 788
Comtrex Acute Head Cold & Sinus Pressure Relief Tablets ... ■ 627
Comtrex Deep Chest Cold & Congestion Relief Softgels ... ■ 627
Comtrex Flu Therapy & Fever Relief Daytime Caplets ... ■ 628
Comtrex Flu Therapy & Fever Relief Nighttime Tablets ... ■ 628
Comtrex Maximum Strength Multi-Symptom Cold & Cough Relief Tablets and Caplets ... ■ 626
Contac Non-Drowsy 12 Hour Cold Caplets ... ■ 745
Contac Non-Drowsy Timed Release 12 Hour Cold Caplets ... ■ 746
Contac Severe Cold and Flu Caplets Maximum Strength ... ■ 746
Contac Severe Cold and Flu Caplets Non-Drowsy ... ■ 746
Dimetapp Elixir ... ■ 777
Dimetapp Cold and Fever Suspension ... ■ 775
Dimetapp DM Cold & Cough Elixir ... ■ 775
Dimetapp Nighttime Flu Liquid ... ■ 776
Dimetapp Non-Drowsy Flu Syrup ... ■ 777
Dimetapp Infant Drops Decongestant ... ■ 775
Dimetapp Infant Drops Decongestant Plus Cough ... ■ 776
Guaifed ... 2272
Kronofed-A ... 1341
Children's Motrin Cold Oral Suspension ... 2007
Motrin Sinus Headache Caplets ... 2005
PediaCare Cough-Cold Liquid ... ■ 719

IMPORTANT NOTE: Always consult each drug listing in the patient's regimen for possible interactions.

PediaCare Infants' Drops Decongestant ▣719
PediaCare Infants' Drops Decongestant Plus Cough ▣719
PediaCare NightRest Cough-Cold Liquid ▣719
Robitussin Cold Caplets Cold & Congestion ▣780
Robitussin Cold Softgels Cold & Congestion ▣780
Robitussin Cold Caplets Multi-Symptom Cold & Flu ▣781
Robitussin Cold Softgels Multi-Symptom Cold & Flu ▣781
Robitussin Cold Softgels Severe Congestion ▣782
Robitussin Cough & Cold Infant Drops ▣782
Robitussin Maximum Strength Cough & Cold Liquid ▣785
Robitussin Pediatric Cough & Cold Formula Liquid ▣785
Robitussin Multi Symptom Honey Flu Liquid ▣785
Robitussin Nighttime Honey Flu Liquid ▣786
Robitussin-CF Liquid ▣783
Robitussin-DAC Syrup 2942
Robitussin-PE Liquid ▣782
Ryna ▣768
Semprex-D Capsules 1172
Singlet Caplets ▣761
Sinutab Non-Drying Liquid Caps ▣706
Sinutab Sinus Allergy Medication, Maximum Strength Formula, Tablets & Caplets ▣707
Sinutab Sinus Medication, Maximum Strength Without Drowsiness Formula, Tablets & Caplets ▣707
Sudafed 12 Hour Tablets ▣708
Sudafed 24 Hour Tablets ▣708
Children's Sudafed Cold & Cough Liquid ▣709
Children's Sudafed Nasal Decongestant Chewables ▣711
Children's Sudafed Nasal Decongestant Liquid Medication ▣711
Sudafed Cold & Allergy Tablets ▣708
Sudafed Cold & Cough Liquid Caps ▣709
Sudafed Cold & Sinus Liquid Caps ▣710
Sudafed Nasal Decongestant Tablets ▣710
Sudafed Non-Drying Sinus Liquid Caps ▣712
Sudafed Severe Cold ▣711
Sudafed Sinus Headache Caplets ▣712
Sudafed Sinus Headache Tablets ▣712
Tavist Sinus Non-Drowsy Coated Caplets ▣676
TheraFlu Regular Strength Cold & Cough Night Time Hot Liquid ▣676
TheraFlu Regular Strength Cold & Sore Throat Night Time Hot Liquid ▣676
TheraFlu Maximum Strength Flu & Congestion Non-Drowsy Hot Liquid ▣677
TheraFlu Maximum Strength Flu & Cough Night Time Hot Liquid ▣678
TheraFlu Maximum Strength Flu & Sore Throat Night Time Hot Liquid ▣677
TheraFlu Maximum Strength Severe Cold & Congestion Night Time Caplets ▣678
TheraFlu Maximum Strength Severe Cold & Congestion Night Time Hot Liquid ▣678
TheraFlu Maximum Strength Severe Cold & Congestion Non-Drowsy ▣679
Triaminic Allergy Congestion Liquid ▣680
Triaminic Chest Congestion Liquid ▣680
Triaminic Cold & Allergy Liquid ▣681
Triaminic Cold & Allergy Softchews ▣683
Triaminic Cold & Cough Liquid ▣681
Triaminic Cold & Cough Softchews ▣683
Triaminic Cold & Night Time Cough Liquid ▣681
Triaminic Cold, Cough & Fever Liquid ▣681
Triaminic Cough Liquid ▣682
Triaminic Cough & Congestion Liquid ▣682
Triaminic Cough & Sore Throat Liquid ▣682
Triaminic Cough & Sore Throat Softchews ▣684
Children's Tylenol Allergy-D Liquid 2014
Children's Tylenol Cold Suspension Liquid and Chewable Tablets 2015
Children's Tylenol Cold Plus Cough Suspension Liquid and Chewable Tablets 2015
Children's Tylenol Flu Suspension Liquid 2015
Children's Tylenol Sinus Suspension Liquid 2017
Infants' Tylenol Cold Decongestant and Fever Reducer Concentrated Drops 2015
Infants' Tylenol Cold Decongestant and Fever Reducer Concentrated Drops Plus Cough 2015
Tylenol Allergy Sinus 2010
Multi-Symptom Tylenol Cold Complete Formula Caplets 2010
Multi-Symptom Tylenol Cold Non-Drowsy Caplets and Gelcaps 2010
Multi-Symptom Tylenol Cold Severe Congestion Non-Drowsy Caplets 2011
Maximum Strength Tylenol Flu NightTime Gelcaps 2011
Maximum Strength Tylenol Flu NightTime Liquid 2011
Maximum Strength Tylenol Flu Non-Drowsy Gelcaps 2011
Maximum Strength Tylenol Sinus NightTime Caplets 2012
Maximum Strength Tylenol Sinus Non-Drowsy Geltabs, Gelcaps, Caplets, and Tablets 2012
Vicks 44D Cough & Head Congestion Relief Liquid ▣724
Vicks 44M Cough, Cold & Flu Relief Liquid ▣725
Pediatric Vicks 44m Cough & Cold Relief ▣728
Vicks DayQuil LiquiCaps/Liquid Multi-Symptom Cold/Flu Relief ▣727
Children's Vicks NyQuil Cold/Cough Relief ▣726
Vicks NyQuil LiquiCaps/Liquid Multi-Symptom Cold/Flu Relief, Original and Cherry Flavors ▣727
Zephrex Tablets 3091
Zephrex LA Tablets 3092
Zyrtec-D 12 Hour Extended Relief Tablets 2758

Pseudoephedrine Sulfate (Enhanced activity of sympathomimetics). Products include:
Chlor-Trimeton Allergy/Decongestant Tablets ▣736
Claritin-D 12 Hour Extended Release Tablets 3102
Claritin-D 24 Hour Extended Release Tablets 3104
Coricidin 'D' Cold, Flu & Sinus Tablets ▣737
Drixoral Allergy/Sinus Extended-Release Tablets ▣741
Drixoral Cold & Allergy Sustained-Action Tablets ▣740
Drixoral Cold & Flu Extended-Release Tablets ▣740
Drixoral Nasal Decongestant Long-Acting Non-Drowsy Tablets ▣740
Rynatan Tablets 3351

Pyrilamine Maleate (Amphetamines may counteract the sedative effect of antihistamines). Products include:
Maximum Strength Midol Menstrual Caplets and Gelcaps ▣612
Maximum Strength Midol PMS Caplets and Gelcaps ▣613

Pyrilamine Tannate (Amphetamines may counteract the sedative effect of antihistamines). Products include:
Ryna-12 S Suspension 3351

Quinapril Hydrochloride (Amphetamines may antagonize the hypotensive effects of antihypertensives). Products include:
Accupril Tablets 2611
Accuretic Tablets 2614

Ramipril (Amphetamines may antagonize the hypotensive effects of antihypertensives). Products include:
Altace Capsules 2233

Rauwolfia serpentina (Amphetamines may antagonize the hypotensive effects of antihypertensives).
No products indexed under this heading.

Rescinnamine (Amphetamines may antagonize the hypotensive effects of antihypertensives).
No products indexed under this heading.

Reserpine (Lowers absorption of amphetamines by acting as gastrointestinal acidifying agent; amphetamines may antagonize the hypotensive effects of antihypertensives).
No products indexed under this heading.

Salmeterol Xinafoate (Enhanced activity of sympathomimetics). Products include:
Advair Diskus 100/50 1448
Advair Diskus 250/50 1448
Advair Diskus 500/50 1448
Serevent Diskus 1637
Serevent Inhalation Aerosol 1633

Selegiline Hydrochloride (Potential for hypertensive crisis; slows amphetamine metabolism; concurrent and/or sequential use is contraindicated). Products include:
Eldepryl Capsules 3266

Sodium Acid Phosphate (Increases the concentration of ionized species of the amphetamine molecule thereby increasing urinary excretion; lowers blood levels and efficacy of amphetamines). Products include:
Uroqid-Acid No. 2 Tablets 947

Sodium Bicarbonate (Increases absorption of amphetamines; increases blood levels and potentiates the action of amphetamines). Products include:
Alka-Seltzer ▣603
Alka-Seltzer Lemon Lime Antacid and Pain Reliever Effervescent Tablets ▣603
Alka-Seltzer Extra Strength Antacid and Pain Reliever Effervescent Tablets ▣603
Alka-Seltzer Heartburn Relief Tablets ▣604
Ceo-Two Evacuant Suppository ▣618
Colyte with Flavor Packs for Oral Solution 3170
GoLYTELY and Pineapple Flavor GoLYTELY for Oral Solution 1068
NuLYTELY, Cherry Flavor, Lemon-Lime Flavor, and Orange Flavor NuLYTELY for Oral Solution 1068

Sodium Citrate (Increases the concentration of the non-ionized species of the amphetamine molecule thereby decreasing urinary excretion; increases blood levels and potentiates the action of amphetamines).
No products indexed under this heading.

Sodium Nitroprusside (Amphetamines may antagonize the hypotensive effects of antihypertensives).
No products indexed under this heading.

Sotalol Hydrochloride (Adrenergic blockers are inhibited by amphetamines; amphetamines may antagonize the hypotensive effects of antihypertensives). Products include:
Betapace Tablets 950
Betapace AF Tablets 954

Spirapril Hydrochloride (Amphetamines may antagonize the hypotensive effects of antihypertensives).
No products indexed under this heading.

Telmisartan (Amphetamines may antagonize the hypotensive effects of antihypertensives). Products include:
Micardis Tablets 1049
Micardis HCT Tablets 1051

Terazosin Hydrochloride (Adrenergic blockers are inhibited by amphetamines; amphetamines may antagonize the hypotensive effects of antihypertensives). Products include:
Hytrin Capsules 464

Terbutaline Sulfate (Enhanced activity of sympathomimetics). Products include:
Brethine Ampuls 2314
Brethine Tablets 2313

Terfenadine (Amphetamines may counteract the sedative effect of antihistamines).
No products indexed under this heading.

Timolol Hemihydrate (Adrenergic blockers are inhibited by amphetamines; amphetamines may antagonize the hypotensive effects of antihypertensives). Products include:
Betimol Ophthalmic Solution ⊙324

Timolol Maleate (Adrenergic blockers are inhibited by amphetamines; amphetamines may antagonize the hypotensive effects of antihypertensives). Products include:
Blocadren Tablets 2046
Cosopt Sterile Ophthalmic Solution 2065
Timolide Tablets 2187
Timolol GFS ⊙266
Timoptic in Ocudose 2192
Timoptic Sterile Ophthalmic Solution 2190
Timoptic-XE Sterile Ophthalmic Gel Forming Solution 2194

Torsemide (Amphetamines may antagonize the hypotensive effects of antihypertensives). Products include:
Demadex Tablets and Injection 2965

Trandolapril (Amphetamines may antagonize the hypotensive effects of antihypertensives). Products include:
Mavik Tablets 478
Tarka Tablets 508

Tranylcypromine Sulfate (Potential for hypertensive crisis; slows amphetamine metabolism; concurrent and/or sequential use is contraindicated). Products include:
Parnate Tablets 1607

Trimeprazine Tartrate (Amphetamines may counteract the sedative effect of antihistamines).
No products indexed under this heading.

Trimethaphan Camsylate (Amphetamines may antagonize the hypotensive effects of antihypertensives).
No products indexed under this heading.

Trimipramine Maleate (Enhanced activity of tricyclic antidepressants; cardiovascular effects can be potentiated). Products include:
Surmontil Capsules 3595

Tripelennamine Hydrochloride (Amphetamines may counteract the sedative effect of antihistamines).
No products indexed under this heading.

Triprolidine Hydrochloride (Amphetamines may counteract the sedative effect of antihistamines). Products include:
Actifed Cold & Allergy Tablets ▣688

Valsartan (Amphetamines may antagonize the hypotensive effects of antihypertensives). Products include:
Diovan Capsules 2337
Diovan HCT Tablets 2338

Verapamil Hydrochloride (Amphetamines may antagonize the hypotensive effects of antihypertensives). Products include:
Covera-HS Tablets 3199
Isoptin SR Tablets 467
Tarka Tablets 508
Verelan Capsules 3184
Verelan PM Capsules 3186

Vitamin C (Lowers absorption of amphetamines by acting as gastrointestinal acidifying agent). Products include:
Beta-C Tablets ▣811

C-Grams Caplets 795
Halls Defense Drops 687
Peridin-C Tablets 618

Food Interactions

Fruit juices, unspecified (Lowers absorption of amphetamines by acting as gastrointestinal acidifying agent).

D.H.E. 45 INJECTION

(Dihydroergotamine Mesylate) 2334
May interact with 5HT1-receptor agonists, macrolide antibiotics, vasopressors, and certain other agents. Compounds in these categories include:

Azithromycin Dihydrate (Co-administration of ergot alkaloids with macrolide antibiotics has resulted in increased plasma levels of unchanged alkaloids and peripheral vasoconstriction; vasospastic reactions have been reported with concurrent use at therapeutic doses). Products include:
- Zithromax 2743
- Zithromax for IV Infusion 2748
- Zithromax for Oral Suspension, 300 mg, 600 mg, 900 mg, 1200 mg 2739
- Zithromax Tablets, 250 mg 2739

Clarithromycin (Co-administration of ergot alkaloids with macrolide antibiotics has resulted in increased plasma levels of unchanged alkaloids and peripheral vasoconstriction; vasospastic reactions have been reported with concurrent use at therapeutic doses). Products include:
- Biaxin/Biaxin XL 403
- PREVPAC 3298

Dirithromycin (Co-administration of ergot alkaloids with macrolide antibiotics has resulted in increased plasma levels of unchanged alkaloids and peripheral vasoconstriction; vasospastic reactions have been reported with concurrent use at therapeutic doses). Products include:
- Dynabac Tablets 2269

Dopamine Hydrochloride (Concurrent use with peripheral and central vasoconstrictors is not recommended because the combination may result in additive or synergistic elevation of blood pressure).
No products indexed under this heading.

Epinephrine Bitartrate (Concurrent use with peripheral and central vasoconstrictors is not recommended because the combination may result in additive or synergistic elevation of blood pressure). Products include:
- Sensorcaine 643

Epinephrine Hydrochloride (Concurrent use with peripheral and central vasoconstrictors is not recommended because the combination may result in additive or synergistic elevation of blood pressure).
No products indexed under this heading.

Erythromycin (Co-administration of ergot alkaloids with macrolide antibiotics has resulted in increased plasma levels of unchanged alkaloids and peripheral vasoconstriction; vasospastic reactions have been reported with concurrent use at therapeutic doses). Products include:
- Emgel 2% Topical Gel 1285
- Ery-Tab Tablets 448
- Erythromycin Base Filmtab Tablets 454
- Erythromycin Delayed-Release Capsules, USP 455
- PCE Dispertab Tablets 498

Erythromycin Estolate (Co-administration of ergot alkaloids with macrolide antibiotics has resulted in increased plasma levels of unchanged alkaloids and peripheral vasoconstriction; vasospastic reactions have been reported with concurrent use at therapeutic doses).
No products indexed under this heading.

Erythromycin Ethylsuccinate (Co-administration of ergot alkaloids with macrolide antibiotics has resulted in increased plasma levels of unchanged alkaloids and peripheral vasoconstriction; vasospastic reactions have been reported with concurrent use at therapeutic doses). Products include:
- E.E.S. 450
- EryPed 446
- Pediazole Suspension 3050

Erythromycin Gluceptate (Co-administration of ergot alkaloids with macrolide antibiotics has resulted in increased plasma levels of unchanged alkaloids and peripheral vasoconstriction; vasospastic reactions have been reported with concurrent use at therapeutic doses).
No products indexed under this heading.

Erythromycin Stearate (Co-administration of ergot alkaloids with macrolide antibiotics has resulted in increased plasma levels of unchanged alkaloids and peripheral vasoconstriction; vasospastic reactions have been reported with concurrent use at therapeutic doses). Products include:
- Erythrocin Stearate Filmtab Tablets 452

Metaraminol Bitartrate (Concurrent use with peripheral and central vasoconstrictors is not recommended because the combination may result in additive or synergistic elevation of blood pressure). Products include:
- Aramine Injection 2043

Methoxamine Hydrochloride (Concurrent use with peripheral and central vasoconstrictors is not recommended because the combination may result in additive or synergistic elevation of blood pressure).
No products indexed under this heading.

Naratriptan Hydrochloride (Concurrent use of 5-HT1 agonists and ergot-containing or ergot-type medications should not be undertaken within 24 hours of each other). Products include:
- Amerge Tablets 1467

Nicotine (May provoke vasoconstriction in some patients, predisposing to a greater ischemic response to ergot). Products include:
- Nicoderm CQ Patch 1717
- Nicotrol Inhaler 2840
- Nicotrol Nasal Spray 2843
- Nicotrol Patch 2840

Nicotine Polacrilex (May provoke vasoconstriction in some patients, predisposing to a greater ischemic response to ergot). Products include:
- Nicorette Gum 1720

Norepinephrine Bitartrate (Concurrent use with peripheral and central vasoconstrictors is not recommended because the combination may result in additive or synergistic elevation of blood pressure).
No products indexed under this heading.

Phenylephrine Hydrochloride (Concurrent use with peripheral and central vasoconstrictors is not recommended because the combination may result in additive or synergistic elevation of blood pressure). Products include:
- Afrin Nasal Decongestant Children's Pump Mist 734
- Extendryl 1361
- Hycomine Compound Tablets 1317
- Neo-Synephrine 614
- Phenergan VC Syrup 3560
- Phenergan VC with Codeine Syrup 3561
- Preparation H Cream 778
- Preparation H Cooling Gel 778
- Preparation H 778
- Vicks Sinex Nasal Spray and Ultra Fine Mist 729

Propranolol Hydrochloride (May potentiate the vasoconstrictive action of ergotamine by blocking the vasodilating property of epinephrine). Products include:
- Inderal 3513
- Inderal LA Long-Acting Capsules 3516
- Inderide Tablets 3517
- Inderide LA Long-Acting Capsules 3519

Rizatriptan Benzoate (Concurrent use of 5-HT1 agonists and ergot-containing or ergot-type medications should not be undertaken within 24 hours of each other). Products include:
- Maxalt Tablets 2120
- Maxalt-MLT Orally Disintegrating Tablets 2120

Sumatriptan (Co-administration could lead to additive coronary artery vasospasm effect; concurrent use should not be undertaken within 24 hours of each other). Products include:
- Imitrex Nasal Spray 1554

Sumatriptan Succinate (Co-administration could lead to additive coronary artery vasospasm effect; concurrent use should not be undertaken within 24 hours of each other). Products include:
- Imitrex Injection 1549
- Imitrex Tablets 1558

Troleandomycin (Co-administration of ergot alkaloids with macrolide antibiotics has resulted in increased plasma levels of unchanged alkaloids and peripheral vasoconstriction; vasospastic reactions have been reported with concurrent use at therapeutic doses). Products include:
- Tao Capsules 2716

Zolmitriptan (Concurrent use of 5-HT1 agonists and ergot-containing or ergot-type medications should not be undertaken within 24 hours of each other). Products include:
- Zomig Tablets 708
- Zomig-ZMT Tablets 708

DHEA PLUS CAPSULES

(Dehydroepiandrosterone (DHEA), Ginkgo biloba) 844
None cited in PDR database.

DIABETA TABLETS

(Glyburide) 741
May interact with beta blockers, calcium channel blockers, corticosteroids, oral anticoagulants, diuretics, estrogens, monoamine oxidase inhibitors, non-steroidal anti-inflammatory agents, oral contraceptives, phenothiazines, highly protein bound drugs (selected), salicylates, sulfonamides, sympathomimetics, thiazides, thyroid preparations, and certain other agents. Compounds in these categories include:

Acebutolol Hydrochloride (Co-administration with beta blockers may result in hypoglycemia). Products include:
- Sectral Capsules 3589

Albuterol (Sympathomimetics tend to produce hyperglycemia and concurrent use may lead to loss of control). Products include:
- Proventil Inhalation Aerosol 3142
- Ventolin Inhalation Aerosol and Refill 1679

Albuterol Sulfate (Sympathomimetics tend to produce hyperglycemia and concurrent use may lead to loss of control). Products include:
- AccuNeb Inhalation Solution 1230
- Combivent Inhalation Aerosol 1041
- DuoNeb Inhalation Solution 1233
- Proventil Inhalation Solution 0.083% 3146
- Proventil Repetabs Tablets 3148
- Proventil Solution for Inhalation 0.5% 3144
- Proventil HFA Inhalation Aerosol 3150
- Ventolin HFA Inhalation Aerosol 3618
- Volmax Extended-Release Tablets 2276

Amiloride Hydrochloride (Diuretics tend to produce hyperglycemia and concurrent use may lead to loss of control). Products include:
- Midamor Tablets 2136
- Moduretic Tablets 2138

Amiodarone Hydrochloride (Co-administration with drugs that are highly protein bound may result in hypoglycemia). Products include:
- Cordarone Intravenous 3491
- Cordarone Tablets 3487
- Pacerone Tablets 3331

Amitriptyline Hydrochloride (Co-administration with drugs that are highly protein bound may result in hypoglycemia). Products include:
- Etrafon 3115
- Limbitrol 1738

Amlodipine Besylate (Calcium channel blockers tend to produce hyperglycemia and concurrent use may lead to loss of control). Products include:
- Lotrel Capsules 2370
- Norvasc Tablets 2704

Aspirin (Co-administration with salicylates may result in hypoglycemia). Products include:
- Aggrenox Capsules 1026
- Alka-Seltzer 603
- Alka-Seltzer Lemon Lime Antacid and Pain Reliever Effervescent Tablets 603
- Alka-Seltzer Extra Strength Antacid and Pain Reliever Effervescent Tablets 603
- Alka-Seltzer PM Effervescent Tablets 605
- Genuine Bayer Tablets, Caplets and Gelcaps 606
- Extra Strength Bayer Caplets and Gelcaps 610
- Aspirin Regimen Bayer Children's Chewable Tablets (Orange or Cherry Flavored) 607
- Bayer, Aspirin Regimen 606
- Aspirin Regimen Bayer 81 mg Caplets with Calcium 607
- Genuine Bayer Professional Labeling (Aspirin Regimen Bayer) 608
- Extra Strength Bayer Arthritis Caplets 610
- Extra Strength Bayer Plus Caplets 610
- Extra Strength Bayer PM Caplets 611
- BC Powder 619
- BC Allergy Sinus Cold Powder 619
- Arthritis Strength BC Powder 619
- BC Sinus Cold Powder 619
- Darvon Compound-65 Pulvules 1910
- Ecotrin Enteric Coated Aspirin Low, Regular and Maximum Strength Tablets 1715
- Excedrin Extra-Strength Tablets, Caplets, and Geltabs 629
- Excedrin Migraine 1070
- Goody's Body Pain Formula Powder 620
- Goody's Extra Strength Headache Powder 620
- Goody's Extra Strength Pain Relief Tablets 620
- Percodan Tablets 1327
- Robaxisal Tablets 2939
- Soma Compound Tablets 3354
- Soma Compound w/Codeine Tablets 3355
- Vanquish Caplets 617

Atenolol (Co-administration with beta blockers may result in hypoglycemia). Products include:
- Tenoretic Tablets 690
- Tenormin I.V. Injection 692

Atovaquone (Co-administration with drugs that are highly protein bound may result in hypoglycemia). Products include:
- Malarone 1596
- Mepron Suspension 1598

Bendroflumethiazide (Thiazides tend to produce hyperglycemia and concurrent use may lead to loss of control). Products include:
- Corzide 40/5 Tablets 2247

Corzide 80/5 Tablets 2247

Bepridil Hydrochloride (Calcium channel blockers tend to produce hyperglycemia and concurrent use may lead to loss of control).
Products include:
Vascor Tablets 2602

Betamethasone Acetate (Corticosteroids tend to produce hyperglycemia and concurrent use may lead to loss of control). Products include:
Celestone Soluspan Injectable Suspension 3097

Betamethasone Sodium Phosphate (Corticosteroids tend to produce hyperglycemia and concurrent use may lead to loss of control).
Products include:
Celestone Soluspan Injectable Suspension 3097

Betaxolol Hydrochloride (Co-administration with beta blockers may result in hypoglycemia).
Products include:
Betoptic S Ophthalmic Suspension 537

Bisoprolol Fumarate (Co-administration with beta blockers may result in hypoglycemia).
Products include:
Zebeta Tablets 1885
Ziac Tablets 1887

Bumetanide (Diuretics tend to produce hyperglycemia and concurrent use may lead to loss of control).
No products indexed under this heading.

Carteolol Hydrochloride (Co-administration with beta blockers may result in hypoglycemia).
Products include:
Carteolol Hydrochloride Ophthalmic Solution USP, 1% .... ⊙258
Ocupress Ophthalmic Solution, 1% Sterile .... ⊙303

Cefonicid Sodium (Co-administration with drugs that are highly protein bound may result in hypoglycemia).
No products indexed under this heading.

Celecoxib (Co-administration with non-steroidal anti-inflammatory agents may result in hypoglycemia).
Products include:
Celebrex Capsules 2676
Celebrex Capsules 2780

Chloramphenicol Palmitate (Co-administration with chloramphenicol may result in hypoglycemia).
No products indexed under this heading.

Chloramphenicol Sodium Succinate (Co-administration with chloramphenicol may result in hypoglycemia).
No products indexed under this heading.

Chlordiazepoxide (Co-administration with drugs that are highly protein bound may result in hypoglycemia). Products include:
Limbitrol 1738

Chlordiazepoxide Hydrochloride (Co-administration with drugs that are highly protein bound may result in hypoglycemia). Products include:
Librium Capsules 1736
Librium for Injection 1737

Chlorothiazide (Thiazides tend to produce hyperglycemia and concurrent use may lead to loss of control).
Products include:
Aldoclor Tablets 2035
Diuril Oral 2087

Chlorothiazide Sodium (Thiazides tend to produce hyperglycemia and concurrent use may lead to loss of control). Products include:
Diuril Sodium Intravenous 2086

Chlorotrianisene (Estrogens tend to produce hyperglycemia and concurrent use may lead to loss of control).
No products indexed under this heading.

Chlorpromazine (Phenothiazines tend to produce hyperglycemia and concurrent use may lead to loss of control). Products include:
Thorazine Suppositories 1656

Chlorpromazine Hydrochloride (Phenothiazines tend to produce hyperglycemia and concurrent use may lead to loss of control).
Products include:
Thorazine 1656

Chlorpropamide (Co-administration with sulfonamides may result in hypoglycemia).
Products include:
Diabinese Tablets 2680

Chlorthalidone (Diuretics tend to produce hyperglycemia and concurrent use may lead to loss of control).
Products include:
Clorpres Tablets 1002
Combipres Tablets 1040
Tenoretic Tablets 690

Choline Magnesium Trisalicylate (Co-administration with salicylates may result in hypoglycemia).
Products include:
Trilisate 2901

Ciprofloxacin (Co-administration has resulted in a potentiation of the hypoglycemic action of glyburide).
Products include:
Cipro I.V. 893
Cipro I.V. Pharmacy Bulk Package .. 897
Cipro Oral Suspension 887

Ciprofloxacin Hydrochloride (Co-administration has resulted in a potentiation of the hypoglycemic action of glyburide). Products include:
Ciloxan 538
Cipro HC Otic Suspension 540
Cipro Tablets 887

Clomipramine Hydrochloride (Co-administration with drugs that are highly protein bound may result in hypoglycemia).
No products indexed under this heading.

Clozapine (Co-administration with drugs that are highly protein bound may result in hypoglycemia).
Products include:
Clozaril Tablets 2319

Cortisone Acetate (Corticosteroids tend to produce hyperglycemia and concurrent use may lead to loss of control). Products include:
Cortone Acetate Injectable Suspension 2059
Cortone Acetate Tablets 2061

Cyclosporine (Co-administration with drugs that are highly protein bound may result in hypoglycemia).
Products include:
Gengraf Capsules 457
Neoral Soft Gelatin Capsules 2380
Neoral Oral Solution 2380
Sandimmune 2388

Desogestrel (Oral contraceptives tend to produce hyperglycemia and concurrent use may lead to loss of control). Products include:
Cyclessa Tablets 2450
Desogen Tablets 2458
Mircette Tablets 2470
Ortho-Cept 21 Tablets 2546
Ortho-Cept 28 Tablets 2546

Dexamethasone (Corticosteroids tend to produce hyperglycemia and concurrent use may lead to loss of control). Products include:
Decadron Elixir 2078
Decadron Tablets 2079
TobraDex Ophthalmic Ointment 542
TobraDex Ophthalmic Suspension .. 541

Dexamethasone Acetate (Corticosteroids tend to produce hyperglycemia and concurrent use may lead to loss of control).
No products indexed under this heading.

Dexamethasone Sodium Phosphate (Corticosteroids tend to produce hyperglycemia and concurrent use may lead to loss of control).
Products include:
Decadron Phosphate Injection 2081
Decadron Phosphate Sterile Ophthalmic Ointment 2083
Decadron Phosphate Sterile Ophthalmic Solution 2084
NeoDecadron Sterile Ophthalmic Solution 2144

Diazepam (Co-administration with drugs that are highly protein bound may result in hypoglycemia).
Products include:
Valium Injectable 3026
Valium Tablets 3047

Diclofenac Potassium (Co-administration with non-steroidal anti-inflammatory agents may result in hypoglycemia). Products include:
Cataflam Tablets 2315

Diclofenac Sodium (Co-administration with non-steroidal anti-inflammatory agents may result in hypoglycemia). Products include:
Arthrotec Tablets 3195
Voltaren Ophthalmic Sterile Ophthalmic Solution .... ⊙312
Voltaren Tablets 2315
Voltaren-XR Tablets 2315

Dicumarol (Co-administration with coumarins may result in hypoglycemia).
No products indexed under this heading.

Dienestrol (Estrogens tend to produce hyperglycemia and concurrent use may lead to loss of control).
Products include:
Ortho Dienestrol Cream 2554

Diethylstilbestrol (Estrogens tend to produce hyperglycemia and concurrent use may lead to loss of control).
No products indexed under this heading.

Diflunisal (Co-administration with salicylates may result in hypoglycemia). Products include:
Dolobid Tablets 2088

Diltiazem Hydrochloride (Calcium channel blockers tend to produce hyperglycemia and concurrent use may lead to loss of control).
Products include:
Cardizem Injectable 1018
Cardizem Lyo-Ject Syringe 1018
Cardizem Monovial 1018
Cardizem CD Capsules 1016
Tiazac Capsules 1378

Dipyridamole (Co-administration with drugs that are highly protein bound may result in hypoglycemia).
Products include:
Aggrenox Capsules 1026
Persantine Tablets 1057

Dobutamine Hydrochloride (Sympathomimetics tend to produce hyperglycemia and concurrent use may lead to loss of control).
Products include:
Dobutrex Solution Vials 1914

Dopamine Hydrochloride (Sympathomimetics tend to produce hyperglycemia and concurrent use may lead to loss of control).
No products indexed under this heading.

Ephedrine Hydrochloride (Sympathomimetics tend to produce hyperglycemia and concurrent use may lead to loss of control).
Products include:
Primatene Tablets .... ▣780

Ephedrine Sulfate (Sympathomimetics tend to produce hyperglycemia and concurrent use may lead to loss of control).
No products indexed under this heading.

Ephedrine Tannate (Sympathomimetics tend to produce hyperglycemia and concurrent use may lead to loss of control). Products include:
Rynatuss Pediatric Suspension 3353
Rynatuss Tablets 3353

Epinephrine (Sympathomimetics tend to produce hyperglycemia and concurrent use may lead to loss of control). Products include:
Epifrin Sterile Ophthalmic Solution .... ⊙235
EpiPen 1236
Primatene Mist .... ▣779
Xylocaine with Epinephrine Injection 653

Epinephrine Bitartrate (Sympathomimetics tend to produce hyperglycemia and concurrent use may lead to loss of control).
Products include:
Sensorcaine 643

Epinephrine Hydrochloride (Sympathomimetics tend to produce hyperglycemia and concurrent use may lead to loss of control).
No products indexed under this heading.

Esmolol Hydrochloride (Co-administration with beta blockers may result in hypoglycemia).
Products include:
Brevibloc Injection 858

Estradiol (Estrogens tend to produce hyperglycemia and concurrent use may lead to loss of control).
Products include:
Activella Tablets 2764
Alora Transdermal System 3372
Climara Transdermal System 958
CombiPatch Transdermal System .. 2323
Esclim Transdermal System 3460
Estrace Vaginal Cream 3358
Estrace Tablets 3361
Estring Vaginal Ring 2811
Ortho-Prefest Tablets 2570
Vagifem Tablets 2857
Vivelle Transdermal System 2412
Vivelle-Dot Transdermal System 2416

Estrogens, Conjugated (Estrogens tend to produce hyperglycemia and concurrent use may lead to loss of control). Products include:
Premarin Intravenous 3563
Premarin Tablets 3566
Premarin Vaginal Cream 3570
Premphase Tablets 3572
Prempro Tablets 3572

Estrogens, Esterified (Estrogens tend to produce hyperglycemia and concurrent use may lead to loss of control). Products include:
Estratest 3252
Menest Tablets 2254

Estropipate (Estrogens tend to produce hyperglycemia and concurrent use may lead to loss of control).
Products include:
Ogen Tablets 2846
Ortho-Est Tablets 3464

Ethacrynic Acid (Diuretics tend to produce hyperglycemia and concurrent use may lead to loss of control).
Products include:
Edecrin Tablets 2091

Ethinyl Estradiol (Estrogens tend to produce hyperglycemia and concurrent use may lead to loss of control). Products include:
Alesse-21 Tablets 3468
Alesse-28 Tablets 3473
Brevicon 28-Day Tablets 3380
Cyclessa Tablets 2450
Desogen Tablets 2458
Estinyl Tablets 3112
Estrostep 2627
femhrt Tablets 2635
Levlen 962
Levlite 21 Tablets 962
Levlite 28 Tablets 962
Levora Tablets 3389
Loestrin 21 Tablets 2642
Loestrin Fe Tablets 2642
Lo/Ovral Tablets 3532
Lo/Ovral-28 Tablets 3538
Low-Ogestrel-28 Tablets 3392
Microgestin Fe 1.5/30 Tablets 3407
Microgestin Fe 1/20 Tablets 3400
Mircette Tablets 2470
Modicon 2563
Necon 3415
Nordette-28 Tablets 2257

Norinyl 1 +35 28-Day Tablets 3380
Ogestrel 0.5/50-28 Tablets 3428
Ortho-Cept 21 Tablets 2546
Ortho-Cept 28 Tablets 2546
Ortho-Cyclen/Ortho Tri-Cyclen 2573
Ortho-Novum 2563
Ovcon 3364
Ovral Tablets 3551
Ovral-28 Tablets 3552
Tri-Levlen 962
Tri-Norinyl-28 Tablets 3433
Triphasil-21 Tablets 3600
Triphasil-28 Tablets 3605
Trivora Tablets 3439
Yasmin 28 Tablets 980
Zovia 3449

Ethynodiol Diacetate (Oral contraceptives tend to produce hyperglycemia and concurrent use may lead to loss of control). Products include:
Zovia 3449

Etodolac (Co-administration with non-steroidal anti-inflammatory agents may result in hypoglycemia). Products include:
Lodine 3528
Lodine XL Extended-Release Tablets 3530

Felodipine (Calcium channel blockers tend to produce hyperglycemia and concurrent use may lead to loss of control). Products include:
Lexxel Tablets 608
Plendil Extended-Release Tablets ... 623

Fenoprofen Calcium (Co-administration with non-steroidal anti-inflammatory agents may result in hypoglycemia).
No products indexed under this heading.

Fludrocortisone Acetate (Corticosteroids tend to produce hyperglycemia and concurrent use may lead to loss of control). Products include:
Florinef Acetate Tablets 2250

Fluphenazine Decanoate (Phenothiazines tend to produce hyperglycemia and concurrent use may lead to loss of control).
No products indexed under this heading.

Fluphenazine Enanthate (Phenothiazines tend to produce hyperglycemia and concurrent use may lead to loss of control).
No products indexed under this heading.

Fluphenazine Hydrochloride (Phenothiazines tend to produce hyperglycemia and concurrent use may lead to loss of control).
No products indexed under this heading.

Flurazepam Hydrochloride (Co-administration with drugs that are highly protein bound may result in hypoglycemia).
No products indexed under this heading.

Flurbiprofen (Co-administration with non-steroidal anti-inflammatory agents may result in hypoglycemia).
No products indexed under this heading.

Fosphenytoin Sodium (Phenytoin tends to produce hyperglycemia and concurrent use may lead to loss of control). Products include:
Cerebyx Injection 2619

Furosemide (Diuretics tend to produce hyperglycemia and concurrent use may lead to loss of control). Products include:
Furosemide Tablets 2284

Glipizide (Co-administration with sulfonamides may result in hypoglycemia). Products include:
Glucotrol Tablets 2692
Glucotrol XL Extended Release Tablets 2693

Hydrochlorothiazide (Thiazides tend to produce hyperglycemia and concurrent use may lead to loss of control). Products include:
Accuretic Tablets 2614
Aldoril Tablets 2039
Atacand HCT Tablets 597
Avalide Tablets 1070
Diovan HCT Tablets 2338
Dyazide Capsules 1515
HydroDIURIL Tablets 2108
Hyzaar 2109
Inderide Tablets 3517
Inderide LA Long-Acting Capsules .. 3519
Lotensin HCT Tablets 2367
Maxzide 1008
Micardis HCT Tablets 1051
Microzide Capsules 3414
Moduretic Tablets 2138
Monopril HCT 1094
Prinzide Tablets 2168
Timolide Tablets 2187
Uniretic Tablets 3178
Vaseretic Tablets 2204
Zestoretic Tablets 695
Ziac Tablets 1887

Hydrocortisone (Corticosteroids tend to produce hyperglycemia and concurrent use may lead to loss of control). Products include:
Anusol-HC Cream 2.5% 2237
Cipro HC Otic Suspension 540
Cortaid Intensive Therapy Cream . ▣717
Cortaid Maximum Strength Cream .... ▣717
Cortisporin Ophthalmic Suspension Sterile .... ⊙297
Cortizone•5 .... ▣699
Cortizone•10 .... ▣699
Cortizone•10 Plus Creme .... ▣700
Cortizone for Kids Creme .... ▣699
Hydrocortone Tablets 2106
Massengill Medicated Soft Cloth Towelette .... ▣753
VōSoL HC Otic Solution 3356

Hydrocortisone Acetate (Corticosteroids tend to produce hyperglycemia and concurrent use may lead to loss of control). Products include:
Analpram-HC 1338
Anusol HC-1 Hydrocortisone Anti-Itch Cream .... ▣689
Anusol-HC Suppositories 2238
Cortaid .... ▣717
Cortifoam Rectal Foam 3170
Cortisporin-TC Otic Suspension 2246
Hydrocortone Acetate Injectable Suspension 2103
Pramosone 1343
Proctocort Suppositories 2264
ProctoFoam-HC 3177
Terra-Cortril Ophthalmic Suspension 2716

Hydrocortisone Sodium Phosphate (Corticosteroids tend to produce hyperglycemia and concurrent use may lead to loss of control). Products include:
Hydrocortone Phosphate Injection, Sterile 2105

Hydrocortisone Sodium Succinate (Corticosteroids tend to produce hyperglycemia and concurrent use may lead to loss of control).
No products indexed under this heading.

Hydroflumethiazide (Thiazides tend to produce hyperglycemia and concurrent use may lead to loss of control). Products include:
Diucardin Tablets 3494

Ibuprofen (Co-administration with non-steroidal anti-inflammatory agents may result in hypoglycemia). Products include:
Advil .... ▣771
Children's Advil Oral Suspension ... ▣773
Children's Advil Chewable Tablets .. ▣773
Advil Cold and Sinus Caplets .... ▣771
Advil Cold and Sinus Tablets .... ▣771
Advil Flu & Body Ache Caplets ...... ▣772
Infants' Advil Drops .... ▣773
Junior Strength Advil Tablets .... ▣773
Junior Strength Advil Chewable Tablets .... ▣773
Advil Migraine Liquigels .... ▣772
Children's Motrin Oral Suspension and Chewable Tablets 2006
Children's Motrin Cold Oral Suspension 2007
Children's Motrin Oral Suspension .... ▣643
Motrin Suspension, Oral Drops, Chewable Tablets, and Caplets 2002
Infants' Motrin Concentrated Drops 2006
Junior Strength Motrin Caplets and Chewable Tablets 2006
Motrin IB Tablets, Caplets, and Gelcaps 2002
Motrin Migraine Pain Caplets 2005
Motrin Sinus Headache Caplets 2005
Vicoprofen Tablets 520

Imipramine Hydrochloride (Co-administration with drugs that are highly protein bound may result in hypoglycemia).
No products indexed under this heading.

Imipramine Pamoate (Co-administration with drugs that are highly protein bound may result in hypoglycemia).
No products indexed under this heading.

Indapamide (Diuretics tend to produce hyperglycemia and concurrent use may lead to loss of control). Products include:
Indapamide Tablets 2286

Indomethacin (Co-administration with non-steroidal anti-inflammatory agents may result in hypoglycemia). Products include:
Indocin 2112

Indomethacin Sodium Trihydrate (Co-administration with non-steroidal anti-inflammatory agents may result in hypoglycemia). Products include:
Indocin I.V. 2115

Isocarboxazid (Co-administration with monoamine oxidase inhibitors may result in hypoglycemia).
No products indexed under this heading.

Isoniazid (Isoniazid tends to produce hyperglycemia and concurrent use may lead to loss of control). Products include:
Rifamate Capsules 767
Rifater Tablets 769

Isoproterenol Hydrochloride (Sympathomimetics tend to produce hyperglycemia and concurrent use may lead to loss of control).
No products indexed under this heading.

Isoproterenol Sulfate (Sympathomimetics tend to produce hyperglycemia and concurrent use may lead to loss of control).
No products indexed under this heading.

Isradipine (Calcium channel blockers tend to produce hyperglycemia and concurrent use may lead to loss of control). Products include:
DynaCirc Capsules 2921
DynaCirc CR Tablets 2923

Ketoprofen (Co-administration with non-steroidal anti-inflammatory agents may result in hypoglycemia). Products include:
Orudis Capsules 3548
Orudis KT Tablets .... ▣778
Oruvail Capsules 3548

Ketorolac Tromethamine (Co-administration with non-steroidal anti-inflammatory agents may result in hypoglycemia). Products include:
Acular Ophthalmic Solution 544
Acular PF Ophthalmic Solution 544
Toradol 3018

Labetalol Hydrochloride (Co-administration with beta blockers may result in hypoglycemia). Products include:
Normodyne Injection 3135
Normodyne Tablets 3137

Levalbuterol Hydrochloride (Sympathomimetics tend to produce hyperglycemia and concurrent use may lead to loss of control). Products include:
Xopenex Inhalation Solution 3207

Levobunolol Hydrochloride (Co-administration with beta blockers may result in hypoglycemia). Products include:
Betagan .... ⊙228

Levonorgestrel (Oral contraceptives tend to produce hyperglycemia and concurrent use may lead to loss of control). Products include:
Alesse-21 Tablets 3468
Alesse-28 Tablets 3473
Levlen 962
Levlite 21 Tablets 962
Levlite 28 Tablets 962
Levora Tablets 3389
Mirena Intrauterine System 974
Nordette-28 Tablets 2257
Norplant System 3543
Tri-Levlen 962
Triphasil-21 Tablets 3600
Triphasil-28 Tablets 3605
Trivora Tablets 3439

Levothyroxine Sodium (Thyroid products tend to produce hyperglycemia and concurrent use may lead to loss of control). Products include:
Levothroid Tablets 1373
Levoxyl Tablets 1819
Synthroid 505
Unithroid Tablets 3445

Liothyronine Sodium (Thyroid products tend to produce hyperglycemia and concurrent use may lead to loss of control). Products include:
Cytomel Tablets 1817
Triostat Injection 1825

Liotrix (Thyroid products tend to produce hyperglycemia and concurrent use may lead to loss of control).
No products indexed under this heading.

Magnesium Salicylate (Co-administration with salicylates may result in hypoglycemia). Products include:
Momentum Backache Relief Extra Strength Caplets .... ▣666

Meclofenamate Sodium (Co-administration with non-steroidal anti-inflammatory agents may result in hypoglycemia).
No products indexed under this heading.

Mefenamic Acid (Co-administration with non-steroidal anti-inflammatory agents may result in hypoglycemia). Products include:
Ponstel Capsules 1356

Meloxicam (Co-administration with non-steroidal anti-inflammatory agents may result in hypoglycemia). Products include:
Mobic Tablets 1054

Mesoridazine Besylate (Phenothiazines tend to produce hyperglycemia and concurrent use may lead to loss of control). Products include:
Serentil 1057

Mestranol (Oral contraceptives tend to produce hyperglycemia and concurrent use may lead to loss of control). Products include:
Necon 1/50 Tablets 3415
Norinyl 1 + 50 28-Day Tablets 3380
Ortho-Novum 1/50▫28 Tablets 2556

Metaproterenol Sulfate (Sympathomimetics tend to produce hyperglycemia and concurrent use may lead to loss of control). Products include:
Alupent 1029

Metaraminol Bitartrate (Sympathomimetics tend to produce hyperglycemia and concurrent use may lead to loss of control). Products include:
Aramine Injection 2043

Methotrimeprazine (Phenothiazines tend to produce hyperglycemia and concurrent use may lead to loss of control).
No products indexed under this heading.

Methoxamine Hydrochloride (Sympathomimetics tend to produce hyperglycemia and concurrent use may lead to loss of control).
No products indexed under this heading.

IMPORTANT NOTE: Always consult each drug listing in the patient's regimen for possible interactions.

Methyclothiazide (Thiazides tend to produce hyperglycemia and concurrent use may lead to loss of control).
No products indexed under this heading.

Methylprednisolone Acetate (Corticosteroids tend to produce hyperglycemia and concurrent use may lead to loss of control).
Products include:
Depo-Medrol Injectable Suspension ... 2795

Methylprednisolone Sodium Succinate (Corticosteroids tend to produce hyperglycemia and concurrent use may lead to loss of control).
Products include:
Solu-Medrol Sterile Powder ... 2855

Metipranolol Hydrochloride (Co-administration with beta blockers may result in hypoglycemia).
No products indexed under this heading.

Metolazone (Diuretics tend to produce hyperglycemia and concurrent use may lead to loss of control).
Products include:
Mykrox Tablets ... 1168
Zaroxolyn Tablets ... 1177

Metoprolol Succinate (Co-administration with beta blockers may result in hypoglycemia).
Products include:
Toprol-XL Tablets ... 651

Metoprolol Tartrate (Co-administration with beta blockers may result in hypoglycemia).
No products indexed under this heading.

Mibefradil Dihydrochloride (Calcium channel blockers tend to produce hyperglycemia and concurrent use may lead to loss of control).
No products indexed under this heading.

Miconazole (Co-administration with oral miconazole and oral hypoglycemic agents has resulted in severe hypoglycemia).
No products indexed under this heading.

Midazolam Hydrochloride (Co-administration with drugs that are highly protein bound may result in hypoglycemia). Products include:
Versed Injection ... 3027
Versed Syrup ... 3033

Moclobemide (Co-administration with monoamine oxidase inhibitors may result in hypoglycemia).
No products indexed under this heading.

Nabumetone (Co-administration with non-steroidal anti-inflammatory agents may result in hypoglycemia).
Products include:
Relafen Tablets ... 1617

Nadolol (Co-administration with beta blockers may result in hypoglycemia). Products include:
Corgard Tablets ... 2245
Corzide 40/5 Tablets ... 2247
Corzide 80/5 Tablets ... 2247
Nadolol Tablets ... 2288

Naproxen (Co-administration with non-steroidal anti-inflammatory agents may result in hypoglycemia).
Products include:
EC-Naprosyn Delayed-Release Tablets ... 2967
Naprosyn Suspension ... 2967
Naprosyn Tablets ... 2967

Naproxen Sodium (Co-administration with non-steroidal anti-inflammatory agents may result in hypoglycemia). Products include:
Aleve Tablets, Caplets and Gelcaps ... ▣602
Aleve Cold & Sinus Caplets ... ▣603
Anaprox Tablets ... 2967
Anaprox DS Tablets ... 2967
Naprelan Tablets ... 1293

Nicardipine Hydrochloride (Calcium channel blockers tend to produce hyperglycemia and concurrent use may lead to loss of control).
Products include:
Cardene I.V. ... 3485

Nicotinic Acid (Nicotinic acid tends to produce hyperglycemia and concurrent use may lead to loss of control).
No products indexed under this heading.

Nifedipine (Calcium channel blockers tend to produce hyperglycemia and concurrent use may lead to loss of control). Products include:
Adalat CC Tablets ... 877
Procardia Capsules ... 2708
Procardia XL Extended Release Tablets ... 2710

Nimodipine (Calcium channel blockers tend to produce hyperglycemia and concurrent use may lead to loss of control). Products include:
Nimotop Capsules ... 904

Nisoldipine (Calcium channel blockers tend to produce hyperglycemia and concurrent use may lead to loss of control). Products include:
Sular Tablets ... 688

Norepinephrine Bitartrate (Sympathomimetics tend to produce hyperglycemia and concurrent use may lead to loss of control).
No products indexed under this heading.

Norethindrone (Oral contraceptives tend to produce hyperglycemia and concurrent use may lead to loss of control). Products include:
Brevicon 28-Day Tablets ... 3380
Micronor Tablets ... 2543
Modicon ... 2563
Necon ... 3415
Norinyl 1 +35 28-Day Tablets ... 3380
Norinyl 1 + 50 28-Day Tablets ... 3380
Nor-QD Tablets ... 3423
Ortho-Novum ... 2563
Ortho-Novum 1/50▫28 Tablets ... 2556
Ovcon ... 3364
Tri-Norinyl-28 Tablets ... 3433

Norethynodrel (Oral contraceptives tend to produce hyperglycemia and concurrent use may lead to loss of control).
No products indexed under this heading.

Norgestimate (Oral contraceptives tend to produce hyperglycemia and concurrent use may lead to loss of control). Products include:
Ortho-Cyclen/Ortho Tri-Cyclen ... 2573
Ortho-Prefest Tablets ... 2570

Norgestrel (Oral contraceptives tend to produce hyperglycemia and concurrent use may lead to loss of control). Products include:
Lo/Ovral Tablets ... 3532
Lo/Ovral-28 Tablets ... 3538
Low-Ogestrel-28 Tablets ... 3392
Ogestrel 0.5/50-28 Tablets ... 3428
Ovral Tablets ... 3551
Ovral-28 Tablets ... 3552
Ovrette Tablets ... 3552

Nortriptyline Hydrochloride (Co-administration with drugs that are highly protein bound may result in hypoglycemia).
No products indexed under this heading.

Oxaprozin (Co-administration with non-steroidal anti-inflammatory agents may result in hypoglycemia).
No products indexed under this heading.

Oxazepam (Co-administration with drugs that are highly protein bound may result in hypoglycemia).
No products indexed under this heading.

Pargyline Hydrochloride (Co-administration with monoamine oxidase inhibitors may result in hypoglycemia).
No products indexed under this heading.

Penbutolol Sulfate (Co-administration with beta blockers may result in hypoglycemia).
No products indexed under this heading.

Perphenazine (Phenothiazines tend to produce hyperglycemia and concurrent use may lead to loss of control). Products include:
Etrafon ... 3115
Trilafon ... 3160

Phenelzine Sulfate (Co-administration with monoamine oxidase inhibitors may result in hypoglycemia). Products include:
Nardil Tablets ... 2653

Phenylbutazone (Co-administration with non-steroidal anti-inflammatory agents may result in hypoglycemia).
No products indexed under this heading.

Phenylephrine Bitartrate (Sympathomimetics tend to produce hyperglycemia and concurrent use may lead to loss of control).
No products indexed under this heading.

Phenylephrine Hydrochloride (Sympathomimetics tend to produce hyperglycemia and concurrent use may lead to loss of control).
Products include:
Afrin Nasal Decongestant Children's Pump Mist ... ▣734
Extendryl ... 1361
Hycomine Compound Tablets ... 1317
Neo-Synephrine ... ▣614
Phenergan VC Syrup ... 3560
Phenergan VC with Codeine Syrup ... 3561
Preparation H Cream ... ▣778
Preparation H Cooling Gel ... ▣778
Preparation H ... ▣778
Vicks Sinex Nasal Spray and Ultra Fine Mist ... ▣729

Phenylephrine Tannate (Sympathomimetics tend to produce hyperglycemia and concurrent use may lead to loss of control).
Products include:
Ryna-12 S Suspension ... 3351
Reformulated Rynatan Pediatric Suspension ... 3352
Rynatuss Pediatric Suspension ... 3353
Rynatuss Tablets ... 3353

Phenylpropanolamine Hydrochloride (Sympathomimetics tend to produce hyperglycemia and concurrent use may lead to loss of control).
No products indexed under this heading.

Phenytoin (Phenytoin tends to produce hyperglycemia and concurrent use may lead to loss of control).
Products include:
Dilantin Infatabs ... 2624
Dilantin-125 Oral Suspension ... 2625

Phenytoin Sodium (Phenytoin tends to produce hyperglycemia and concurrent use may lead to loss of control). Products include:
Dilantin Kapseals ... 2622

Pindolol (Co-administration with beta blockers may result in hypoglycemia).
No products indexed under this heading.

Pirbuterol Acetate (Sympathomimetics tend to produce hyperglycemia and concurrent use may lead to loss of control). Products include:
Maxair Autohaler ... 1981
Maxair Inhaler ... 1984

Piroxicam (Co-administration with non-steroidal anti-inflammatory agents may result in hypoglycemia).
Products include:
Feldene Capsules ... 2685

Polyestradiol Phosphate (Estrogens tend to produce hyperglycemia and concurrent use may lead to loss of control).
No products indexed under this heading.

Polythiazide (Thiazides tend to produce hyperglycemia and concurrent use may lead to loss of control).
Products include:
Minizide Capsules ... 2700
Renese Tablets ... 2712

Prednisolone Acetate (Corticosteroids tend to produce hyperglycemia and concurrent use may lead to loss of control). Products include:
Blephamide Ophthalmic Ointment ... 547
Blephamide Ophthalmic Suspension ... 548
Poly-Pred Liquifilm Ophthalmic Suspension ... ⊙245
Pred Forte Ophthalmic Suspension ... ⊙246
Pred Mild Sterile Ophthalmic Suspension ... ⊙249
Pred-G Ophthalmic Suspension ... ⊙247
Pred-G Sterile Ophthalmic Ointment ... ⊙248

Prednisolone Sodium Phosphate (Corticosteroids tend to produce hyperglycemia and concurrent use may lead to loss of control).
Products include:
Pediapred Oral Solution ... 1170

Prednisolone Tebutate (Corticosteroids tend to produce hyperglycemia and concurrent use may lead to loss of control).
No products indexed under this heading.

Prednisone (Corticosteroids tend to produce hyperglycemia and concurrent use may lead to loss of control). Products include:
Prednisone ... 3064

Probenecid (Co-administration with probenecid may result in hypoglycemia).
No products indexed under this heading.

Procarbazine Hydrochloride (Co-administration with monoamine oxidase inhibitors may result in hypoglycemia). Products include:
Matulane Capsules ... 3246

Prochlorperazine (Phenothiazines tend to produce hyperglycemia and concurrent use may lead to loss of control). Products include:
Compazine ... 1505

Promethazine Hydrochloride (Phenothiazines tend to produce hyperglycemia and concurrent use may lead to loss of control).
Products include:
Mepergan Injection ... 3539
Phenergan Injection ... 3553
Phenergan ... 3556
Phenergan Syrup ... 3554
Phenergan with Codeine Syrup ... 3557
Phenergan with Dextromethorphan Syrup ... 3559
Phenergan VC Syrup ... 3560
Phenergan VC with Codeine Syrup ... 3561

Propranolol Hydrochloride (Co-administration with beta blockers may result in hypoglycemia).
Products include:
Inderal ... 3513
Inderal LA Long-Acting Capsules ... 3516
Inderide Tablets ... 3517
Inderide LA Long-Acting Capsules ... 3519

Pseudoephedrine Hydrochloride (Sympathomimetics tend to produce hyperglycemia and concurrent use may lead to loss of control).
Products include:
Actifed Cold & Allergy Tablets ... ▣688
Actifed Cold & Sinus Caplets and Tablets ... ▣688
Advil Cold and Sinus Caplets ... ▣771
Advil Cold and Sinus Tablets ... ▣771
Advil Flu & Body Ache Caplets ... ▣772
Aleve Cold & Sinus Caplets ... ▣603
Alka-Seltzer Plus Liqui-Gels ... ▣604
Alka-Seltzer Plus Cold & Flu Medicine Liqui-Gels ... ▣604
Alka-Seltzer Plus Cold & Sinus Medicine Liqui-Gels ... ▣604
Allegra-D Extended-Release Tablets ... 714
BC Cold Powder ... ▣619
Benadryl Allergy/Cold Tablets ... ▣691

Benadryl Allergy/Congestion Tablets 692
Benadryl Allergy & Sinus Liquid 693
Benadryl Allergy & Sinus Fastmelt Tablets 693
Benadryl Allergy Sinus Headache Caplets & Gelcaps 693
Benadryl Severe Allergy & Sinus Headache Caplets 694
Benadryl Children's Allergy/Cold Fastmelt Tablets 692
Benylin Multi-Symptom Liquid 697
Bromfed Capsules (Extended-Release) 2269
Bromfed-PD Capsules (Extended-Release) 2269
Children's Cēpacol Sore Throat 788
Comtrex Acute Head Cold & Sinus Pressure Relief Tablets 627
Comtrex Deep Chest Cold & Congestion Relief Softgels 627
Comtrex Flu Therapy & Fever Relief Daytime Caplets 628
Comtrex Flu Therapy & Fever Relief Nighttime Tablets 628
Comtrex Maximum Strength Multi-Symptom Cold & Cough Relief Tablets and Caplets 626
Contac Non-Drowsy 12 Hour Cold Caplets 745
Contac Non-Drowsy Timed Release 12 Hour Cold Caplets 746
Contac Severe Cold and Flu Caplets Maximum Strength 746
Contac Severe Cold and Flu Caplets Non-Drowsy 746
Dimetapp Elixir 777
Dimetapp Cold and Fever Suspension 775
Dimetapp DM Cold & Cough Elixir 775
Dimetapp Nighttime Flu Liquid 776
Dimetapp Non-Drowsy Flu Syrup 777
Dimetapp Infant Drops Decongestant 775
Dimetapp Infant Drops Decongestant Plus Cough 776
Guaifed 2272
Kronofed-A 1341
Children's Motrin Cold Oral Suspension 2007
Motrin Sinus Headache Caplets 2005
PediaCare Cough-Cold Liquid 719
PediaCare Infants' Drops Decongestant 719
PediaCare Infants' Drops Decongestant Plus Cough 719
PediaCare NightRest Cough-Cold Liquid 719
Robitussin Cold Caplets Cold & Congestion 780
Robitussin Cold Softgels Cold & Congestion 780
Robitussin Cold Caplets Multi-Symptom Cold & Flu 781
Robitussin Cold Softgels Multi-Symptom Cold & Flu 781
Robitussin Cold Softgels Severe Congestion 782
Robitussin Cough & Cold Infant Drops 782
Robitussin Maximum Strength Cough & Cold Liquid 785
Robitussin Pediatric Cough & Cold Formula Liquid 785
Robitussin Multi Symptom Honey Flu Liquid 785
Robitussin Nighttime Honey Flu Liquid 786
Robitussin-CF Liquid 783
Robitussin-DAC Syrup 2942
Robitussin-PE Liquid 782
Ryna 768
Semprex-D Capsules 1172
Singlet Caplets 761
Sinutab Non-Drying Liquid Caps 706
Sinutab Sinus Allergy Medication, Maximum Strength Formula, Tablets & Caplets 707
Sinutab Sinus Medication, Maximum Strength Without Drowsiness Formula, Tablets & Caplets 707
Sudafed 12 Hour Tablets 708
Sudafed 24 Hour Tablets 708
Children's Sudafed Cold & Cough Liquid 709
Children's Sudafed Nasal Decongestant Chewables 711
Children's Sudafed Nasal Decongestant Liquid Medication 711
Sudafed Cold & Allergy Tablets 708
Sudafed Cold & Cough Liquid Caps 709
Sudafed Cold & Sinus Liquid Caps 710
Sudafed Nasal Decongestant Tablets 710
Sudafed Non-Drying Sinus Liquid Caps 712
Sudafed Severe Cold 711
Sudafed Sinus Headache Caplets 712
Sudafed Sinus Headache Tablets 712
Tavist Sinus Non-Drowsy Coated Caplets 676
TheraFlu Regular Strength Cold & Cough Night Time Hot Liquid 676
TheraFlu Regular Strength Cold & Sore Throat Night Time Hot Liquid 676
TheraFlu Maximum Strength Flu & Congestion Non-Drowsy Hot Liquid 677
TheraFlu Maximum Strength Flu & Cough Night Time Hot Liquid 678
TheraFlu Maximum Strength Flu & Sore Throat Night Time Hot Liquid 677
TheraFlu Maximum Strength Severe Cold & Congestion Night Time Caplets 678
TheraFlu Maximum Strength Severe Cold & Congestion Night Time Hot Liquid 678
TheraFlu Maximum Strength Severe Cold & Congestion Non-Drowsy 679
Triaminic Allergy Congestion Liquid 680
Triaminic Chest Congestion Liquid 680
Triaminic Cold & Allergy Liquid 681
Triaminic Cold & Allergy Softchews 683
Triaminic Cold & Cough Liquid 681
Triaminic Cold & Cough Softchews 683
Triaminic Cold & Night Time Cough Liquid 681
Triaminic Cold, Cough & Fever Liquid 681
Triaminic Cough Liquid 682
Triaminic Cough & Congestion Liquid 682
Triaminic Cough & Sore Throat Liquid 682
Triaminic Cough & Sore Throat Softchews 684
Children's Tylenol Allergy-D Liquid 2014
Children's Tylenol Cold Suspension Liquid and Chewable Tablets 2015
Children's Tylenol Cold Plus Cough Suspension Liquid and Chewable Tablets 2015
Children's Tylenol Flu Suspension Liquid 2015
Children's Tylenol Sinus Suspension Liquid 2017
Infants' Tylenol Cold Decongestant and Fever Reducer Concentrated Drops 2015
Infants' Tylenol Cold Decongestant and Fever Reducer Concentrated Drops Plus Cough 2015
Tylenol Allergy Sinus 2010
Multi-Symptom Tylenol Cold Complete Formula Caplets 2010
Multi-Symptom Tylenol Cold Non-Drowsy Caplets and Gelcaps 2010
Multi-Symptom Tylenol Cold Severe Congestion Non-Drowsy Caplets 2011
Maximum Strength Tylenol Flu NightTime Gelcaps 2011
Maximum Strength Tylenol Flu NightTime Liquid 2011
Maximum Strength Tylenol Flu Non-Drowsy Gelcaps 2011
Maximum Strength Tylenol Sinus NightTime Caplets 2012
Maximum Strength Tylenol Sinus Non-Drowsy Geltabs, Gelcaps, Caplets, and Tablets 2012
Vicks 44D Cough & Head Congestion Relief Liquid 724
Vicks 44M Cough, Cold & Flu Relief Liquid 725
Pediatric Vicks 44m Cough & Cold Relief 728
Vicks DayQuil LiquiCaps/Liquid Multi-Symptom Cold/Flu Relief 727
Children's Vicks NyQuil Cold/Cough Relief 726
Vicks NyQuil LiquiCaps/Liquid Multi-Symptom Cold/Flu Relief, Original and Cherry Flavors 727
Zephrex Tablets 3091
Zephrex LA Tablets 3092
Zyrtec-D 12 Hour Extended Relief Tablets 2758

Pseudoephedrine Sulfate (Sympathomimetics tend to produce hyperglycemia and concurrent use may lead to loss of control). Products include:
Chlor-Trimeton Allergy/Decongestant Tablets 736
Claritin-D 12 Hour Extended Release Tablets 3102
Claritin-D 24 Hour Extended Release Tablets 3104
Coricidin 'D' Cold, Flu & Sinus Tablets 737
Drixoral Allergy/Sinus Extended-Release Tablets 741
Drixoral Cold & Allergy Sustained-Action Tablets 740
Drixoral Cold & Flu Extended-Release Tablets 740
Drixoral Nasal Decongestant Long-Acting Non-Drowsy Tablets 740
Rynatan Tablets 3351

Quinestrol (Estrogens tend to produce hyperglycemia and concurrent use may lead to loss of control).
No products indexed under this heading.

Rofecoxib (Co-administration with non-steroidal anti-inflammatory agents may result in hypoglycemia). Products include:
Vioxx 2213

Salmeterol Xinafoate (Sympathomimetics tend to produce hyperglycemia and concurrent use may lead to loss of control). Products include:
Advair Diskus 100/50 1448
Advair Diskus 250/50 1448
Advair Diskus 500/50 1448
Serevent Diskus 1637
Serevent Inhalation Aerosol 1633

Salsalate (Co-administration with salicylates may result in hypoglycemia).
No products indexed under this heading.

Selegiline Hydrochloride (Co-administration with monoamine oxidase inhibitors may result in hypoglycemia). Products include:
Eldepryl Capsules 3266

Sotalol Hydrochloride (Co-administration with beta blockers may result in hypoglycemia). Products include:
Betapace Tablets 950
Betapace AF Tablets 954

Spironolactone (Diuretics tend to produce hyperglycemia and concurrent use may lead to loss of control).
No products indexed under this heading.

Sulfacytine (Co-administration with sulfonamides may result in hypoglycemia).
No products indexed under this heading.

Sulfamethizole (Co-administration with sulfonamides may result in hypoglycemia). Products include:
Urobiotic-250 Capsules 2731

Sulfamethoxazole (Co-administration with sulfonamides may result in hypoglycemia). Products include:
Bactrim 2949
Septra Suspension 2265
Septra Tablets 2265
Septra DS Tablets 2265

Sulfasalazine (Co-administration with sulfonamides may result in hypoglycemia). Products include:
Azulfidine EN-tabs Tablets 2775

Sulfinpyrazone (Co-administration with sulfonamides may result in hypoglycemia).
No products indexed under this heading.

Sulfisoxazole (Co-administration with sulfonamides may result in hypoglycemia).
No products indexed under this heading.

Sulfisoxazole Acetyl (Co-administration with sulfonamides may result in hypoglycemia). Products include:
Pediazole Suspension 3050

Sulfisoxazole Diolamine (Co-administration with sulfonamides may result in hypoglycemia).
No products indexed under this heading.

Sulindac (Co-administration with non-steroidal anti-inflammatory agents may result in hypoglycemia). Products include:
Clinoril Tablets 2053

Temazepam (Co-administration with drugs that are highly protein bound may result in hypoglycemia).
No products indexed under this heading.

Terbutaline Sulfate (Sympathomimetics tend to produce hyperglycemia and concurrent use may lead to loss of control). Products include:
Brethine Ampuls 2314
Brethine Tablets 2313

Thioridazine Hydrochloride (Phenothiazines tend to produce hyperglycemia and concurrent use may lead to loss of control). Products include:
Thioridazine Hydrochloride Tablets 2289

Thyroglobulin (Thyroid products tend to produce hyperglycemia and concurrent use may lead to loss of control).
No products indexed under this heading.

Thyroid (Thyroid products tend to produce hyperglycemia and concurrent use may lead to loss of control).
No products indexed under this heading.

Thyroxine (Thyroid products tend to produce hyperglycemia and concurrent use may lead to loss of control).
No products indexed under this heading.

Thyroxine Sodium (Thyroid products tend to produce hyperglycemia and concurrent use may lead to loss of control).
No products indexed under this heading.

Timolol Hemihydrate (Co-administration with beta blockers may result in hypoglycemia). Products include:
Betimol Ophthalmic Solution .... ⊙ 324

Timolol Maleate (Co-administration with beta blockers may result in hypoglycemia). Products include:
Blocadren Tablets 2046
Cosopt Sterile Ophthalmic Solution 2065
Timolide Tablets 2187
Timolol GFS .... ⊙ 266
Timoptic in Ocudose 2192
Timoptic Sterile Ophthalmic Solution 2190
Timoptic-XE Sterile Ophthalmic Gel Forming Solution 2194

Tolazamide (Co-administration with sulfonamides may result in hypoglycemia).
No products indexed under this heading.

Tolbutamide (Co-administration with sulfonamides may result in hypoglycemia).
No products indexed under this heading.

Tolmetin Sodium (Co-administration with non-steroidal anti-inflammatory agents may result in hypoglycemia). Products include:
Tolectin 2589

Torsemide (Diuretics tend to produce hyperglycemia and concurrent use may lead to loss of control). Products include:
Demadex Tablets and Injection 2965

Tranylcypromine Sulfate (Co-administration with monoamine oxidase inhibitors may result in hypoglycemia). Products include:
Parnate Tablets 1607

IMPORTANT NOTE: Always consult each drug listing in the patient's regimen for possible interactions.

Triamcinolone (Corticosteroids tend to produce hyperglycemia and concurrent use may lead to loss of control).
No products indexed under this heading.

Triamcinolone Acetonide (Corticosteroids tend to produce hyperglycemia and concurrent use may lead to loss of control). Products include:
Azmacort Inhalation Aerosol 728
Nasacort Nasal Inhaler 750
Nasacort AQ Nasal Spray 752
Tri-Nasal Spray 2274

Triamcinolone Diacetate (Corticosteroids tend to produce hyperglycemia and concurrent use may lead to loss of control).
No products indexed under this heading.

Triamcinolone Hexacetonide (Corticosteroids tend to produce hyperglycemia and concurrent use may lead to loss of control).
No products indexed under this heading.

Triamterene (Diuretics tend to produce hyperglycemia and concurrent use may lead to loss of control). Products include:
Dyazide Capsules 1515
Dyrenium Capsules 3458
Maxzide 1008

Trifluoperazine Hydrochloride (Phenothiazines tend to produce hyperglycemia and concurrent use may lead to loss of control). Products include:
Stelazine 1640

Trimipramine Maleate (Co-administration with drugs that are highly protein bound may result in hypoglycemia). Products include:
Surmontil Capsules 3595

Verapamil Hydrochloride (Calcium channel blockers tend to produce hyperglycemia and concurrent use may lead to loss of control). Products include:
Covera-HS Tablets 3199
Isoptin SR Tablets 467
Tarka Tablets 508
Verelan Capsules 3184
Verelan PM Capsules 3186

Warfarin Sodium (Co-administration with coumarins may result in hypoglycemia). Products include:
Coumadin for Injection 1243
Coumadin Tablets 1243
Warfarin Sodium Tablets, USP 3302

Food Interactions

Alcohol (Potential for hypoglycemia).

DIABINESE TABLETS

(Chlorpropamide) 2680
May interact with barbiturates, beta blockers, calcium channel blockers, corticosteroids, oral anticoagulants, diuretics, estrogens, monoamine oxidase inhibitors, non-steroidal anti-inflammatory agents, oral contraceptives, phenothiazines, highly protein bound drugs (selected), salicylates, sulfonamides, sympathomimetics, thiazides, thyroid preparations, and certain other agents. Compounds in these categories include:

Acebutolol Hydrochloride (The hypoglycemic action of sulfonylureas may be potentiated by beta adrenergic blockers). Products include:
Sectral Capsules 3589

Albuterol (Sympathomimetics tend to produce hyperglycemia and concurrent use may lead to loss of control). Products include:
Proventil Inhalation Aerosol 3142
Ventolin Inhalation Aerosol and Refill 1679

Albuterol Sulfate (Sympathomimetics tend to produce hyperglycemia and concurrent use may lead to loss of control). Products include:
AccuNeb Inhalation Solution 1230
Combivent Inhalation Aerosol 1041
DuoNeb Inhalation Solution 1233
Proventil Inhalation Solution 0.083% 3146
Proventil Repetabs Tablets 3148
Proventil Solution for Inhalation 0.5% 3144
Proventil HFA Inhalation Aerosol 3150
Ventolin HFA Inhalation Aerosol 3618
Volmax Extended-Release Tablets .. 2276

Amiloride Hydrochloride (Diuretics tend to produce hyperglycemia and concurrent use may lead to loss of control). Products include:
Midamor Tablets 2136
Moduretic Tablets 2138

Amiodarone Hydrochloride (The hypoglycemic action of sulfonylureas may be potentiated by drugs that are highly protein bound). Products include:
Cordarone Intravenous 3491
Cordarone Tablets 3487
Pacerone Tablets 3331

Amitriptyline Hydrochloride (The hypoglycemic action of sulfonylureas may be potentiated by drugs that are highly protein bound). Products include:
Etrafon 3115
Limbitrol 1738

Amlodipine Besylate (Calcium channel blockers tend to produce hyperglycemia and concurrent use may lead to loss of control). Products include:
Lotrel Capsules 2370
Norvasc Tablets 2704

Aprobarbital (The action of barbiturates may be prolonged by therapy with chlorpropamide; barbiturates should be employed with caution).
No products indexed under this heading.

Aspirin (The hypoglycemic action of sulfonylureas may be potentiated by salicylates). Products include:
Aggrenox Capsules 1026
Alka-Seltzer .... ▣ 603
Alka-Seltzer Lemon Lime Antacid and Pain Reliever Effervescent Tablets .... ▣ 603
Alka-Seltzer Extra Strength Antacid and Pain Reliever Effervescent Tablets .... ▣ 603
Alka-Seltzer PM Effervescent Tablets .... ▣ 605
Genuine Bayer Tablets, Caplets and Gelcaps .... ▣ 606
Extra Strength Bayer Caplets and Gelcaps .... ▣ 610
Aspirin Regimen Bayer Children's Chewable Tablets (Orange or Cherry Flavored) .... ▣ 607
Bayer, Aspirin Regimen .... ▣ 606
Aspirin Regimen Bayer 81 mg Caplets with Calcium .... ▣ 607
Genuine Bayer Professional Labeling (Aspirin Regimen Bayer) .... ▣ 608
Extra Strength Bayer Arthritis Caplets .... ▣ 610
Extra Strength Bayer Plus Caplets .... ▣ 610
Extra Strength Bayer PM Caplets .... ▣ 611
BC Powder .... ▣ 619
BC Allergy Sinus Cold Powder .... ▣ 619
Arthritis Strength BC Powder .... ▣ 619
BC Sinus Cold Powder .... ▣ 619
Darvon Compound-65 Pulvules 1910
Ecotrin Enteric Coated Aspirin Low, Regular and Maximum Strength Tablets 1715
Excedrin Extra-Strength Tablets, Caplets, and Geltabs .... ▣ 629
Excedrin Migraine 1070
Goody's Body Pain Formula Powder .... ▣ 620
Goody's Extra Strength Headache Powder .... ▣ 620
Goody's Extra Strength Pain Relief Tablets .... ▣ 620
Percodan Tablets 1327
Robaxisal Tablets 2939
Soma Compound Tablets 3354
Soma Compound w/Codeine Tablets 3355
Vanquish Caplets .... ▣ 617

Atenolol (The hypoglycemic action of sulfonylureas may be potentiated by beta adrenergic blockers). Products include:
Tenoretic Tablets 690
Tenormin I.V. Injection 692

Atovaquone (The hypoglycemic action of sulfonylureas may be potentiated by drugs that are highly protein bound). Products include:
Malarone 1596
Mepron Suspension 1598

Bendroflumethiazide (Thiazides tend to produce hyperglycemia and concurrent use may lead to loss of control). Products include:
Corzide 40/5 Tablets 2247
Corzide 80/5 Tablets 2247

Bepridil Hydrochloride (Calcium channel blockers tend to produce hyperglycemia and concurrent use may lead to loss of control). Products include:
Vascor Tablets 2602

Betamethasone Acetate (Corticosteroids tend to produce hyperglycemia and concurrent use may lead to loss of control). Products include:
Celestone Soluspan Injectable Suspension 3097

Betamethasone Sodium Phosphate (Corticosteroids tend to produce hyperglycemia and concurrent use may lead to loss of control). Products include:
Celestone Soluspan Injectable Suspension 3097

Betaxolol Hydrochloride (The hypoglycemic action of sulfonylureas may be potentiated by beta adrenergic blockers). Products include:
Betoptic S Ophthalmic Suspension 537

Bisoprolol Fumarate (The hypoglycemic action of sulfonylureas may be potentiated by beta adrenergic blockers). Products include:
Zebeta Tablets 1885
Ziac Tablets 1887

Bumetanide (Diuretics tend to produce hyperglycemia and concurrent use may lead to loss of control).
No products indexed under this heading.

Butabarbital (The action of barbiturates may be prolonged by therapy with chlorpropamide; barbiturates should be employed with caution).
No products indexed under this heading.

Butalbital (The action of barbiturates may be prolonged by therapy with chlorpropamide; barbiturates should be employed with caution). Products include:
Phrenilin 578
Sedapap Tablets 50 mg/650 mg 2225

Carteolol Hydrochloride (The hypoglycemic action of sulfonylureas may be potentiated by beta adrenergic blockers). Products include:
Carteolol Hydrochloride Ophthalmic Solution USP, 1% ...... ⊙ 258
Ocupress Ophthalmic Solution, 1% Sterile .... ⊙ 303

Cefonicid Sodium (The hypoglycemic action of sulfonylureas may be potentiated by drugs that are highly protein bound).
No products indexed under this heading.

Celecoxib (The hypoglycemic action of sulfonylureas may be potentiated by nonsteroidal anti-inflammatory agents). Products include:
Celebrex Capsules 2676
Celebrex Capsules 2780

Chloramphenicol (The hypoglycemic action of sulfonylureas may be potentiated by chloramphenicol). Products include:
Chloromycetin Ophthalmic Ointment, 1% .... ⊙ 296
Chloromycetin Ophthalmic Solution .... ⊙ 297
Chloroptic Sterile Ophthalmic Ointment .... ⊙ 234
Chloroptic Sterile Ophthalmic Solution .... ⊙ 235

Chloramphenicol Palmitate (The hypoglycemic action of sulfonylureas may be potentiated by chloramphenicol).
No products indexed under this heading.

Chloramphenicol Sodium Succinate (The hypoglycemic action of sulfonylureas may be potentiated by chloramphenicol).
No products indexed under this heading.

Chlordiazepoxide (The hypoglycemic action of sulfonylureas may be potentiated by drugs that are highly protein bound). Products include:
Limbitrol 1738

Chlordiazepoxide Hydrochloride (The hypoglycemic action of sulfonylureas may be potentiated by drugs that are highly protein bound). Products include:
Librium Capsules 1736
Librium for Injection 1737

Chlorothiazide (Thiazides tend to produce hyperglycemia and concurrent use may lead to loss of control). Products include:
Aldoclor Tablets 2035
Diuril Oral 2087

Chlorothiazide Sodium (Thiazides tend to produce hyperglycemia and concurrent use may lead to loss of control). Products include:
Diuril Sodium Intravenous 2086

Chlorotrianisene (Estrogens tend to produce hyperglycemia and concurrent use may lead to loss of control).
No products indexed under this heading.

Chlorpromazine (Phenothiazines tend to produce hyperglycemia and concurrent use may lead to loss of control). Products include:
Thorazine Suppositories 1656

Chlorpromazine Hydrochloride (Phenothiazines tend to produce hyperglycemia and concurrent use may lead to loss of control). Products include:
Thorazine 1656

Chlorthalidone (Diuretics tend to produce hyperglycemia and concurrent use may lead to loss of control). Products include:
Clorpres Tablets 1002
Combipres Tablets 1040
Tenoretic Tablets 690

Choline Magnesium Trisalicylate (The hypoglycemic action of sulfonylureas may be potentiated by salicylates). Products include:
Trilisate 2901

Clomipramine Hydrochloride (The hypoglycemic action of sulfonylureas may be potentiated by drugs that are highly protein bound).
No products indexed under this heading.

Clozapine (The hypoglycemic action of sulfonylureas may be potentiated by drugs that are highly protein bound). Products include:
Clozaril Tablets 2319

Cortisone Acetate (Corticosteroids tend to produce hyperglycemia and concurrent use may lead to loss of control). Products include:
Cortone Acetate Injectable Suspension 2059
Cortone Acetate Tablets 2061

Cyclosporine (The hypoglycemic action of sulfonylureas may be potentiated by drugs that are highly protein bound). Products include:
Gengraf Capsules 457
Neoral Soft Gelatin Capsules 2380
Neoral Oral Solution 2380
Sandimmune 2388

Desogestrel (Oral contraceptives tend to produce hyperglycemia and concurrent use may lead to loss of control). Products include:
- Cyclessa Tablets ... 2450
- Desogen Tablets ... 2458
- Mircette Tablets ... 2470
- Ortho-Cept 21 Tablets ... 2546
- Ortho-Cept 28 Tablets ... 2546

Dexamethasone (Corticosteroids tend to produce hyperglycemia and concurrent use may lead to loss of control). Products include:
- Decadron Elixir ... 2078
- Decadron Tablets ... 2079
- TobraDex Ophthalmic Ointment ... 542
- TobraDex Ophthalmic Suspension .. 541

Dexamethasone Acetate (Corticosteroids tend to produce hyperglycemia and concurrent use may lead to loss of control).
- No products indexed under this heading.

Dexamethasone Sodium Phosphate (Corticosteroids tend to produce hyperglycemia and concurrent use may lead to loss of control). Products include:
- Decadron Phosphate Injection ... 2081
- Decadron Phosphate Sterile Ophthalmic Ointment ... 2083
- Decadron Phosphate Sterile Ophthalmic Solution ... 2084
- NeoDecadron Sterile Ophthalmic Solution ... 2144

Diazepam (The hypoglycemic action of sulfonylureas may be potentiated by drugs that are highly protein bound). Products include:
- Valium Injectable ... 3026
- Valium Tablets ... 3047

Diclofenac Potassium (The hypoglycemic action of sulfonylureas may be potentiated by nonsteroidal anti-inflammatory agents). Products include:
- Cataflam Tablets ... 2315

Diclofenac Sodium (The hypoglycemic action of sulfonylureas may be potentiated by nonsteroidal anti-inflammatory agents). Products include:
- Arthrotec Tablets ... 3195
- Voltaren Ophthalmic Sterile Ophthalmic Solution ... ⊙312
- Voltaren Tablets ... 2315
- Voltaren-XR Tablets ... 2315

Dicumarol (The hypoglycemic action of sulfonylureas may be potentiated by coumarins).
- No products indexed under this heading.

Dienestrol (Estrogens tend to produce hyperglycemia and concurrent use may lead to loss of control). Products include:
- Ortho Dienestrol Cream ... 2554

Diethylstilbestrol (Estrogens tend to produce hyperglycemia and concurrent use may lead to loss of control).
- No products indexed under this heading.

Diflunisal (The hypoglycemic action of sulfonylureas may be potentiated by salicylates). Products include:
- Dolobid Tablets ... 2088

Diltiazem Hydrochloride (Calcium channel blockers tend to produce hyperglycemia and concurrent use may lead to loss of control). Products include:
- Cardizem Injectable ... 1018
- Cardizem Lyo-Ject Syringe ... 1018
- Cardizem Monovial ... 1018
- Cardizem CD Capsules ... 1016
- Tiazac Capsules ... 1378

Dipyridamole (The hypoglycemic action of sulfonylureas may be potentiated by drugs that are highly protein bound). Products include:
- Aggrenox Capsules ... 1026
- Persantine Tablets ... 1057

Dobutamine Hydrochloride (Sympathomimetics tend to produce hyperglycemia and concurrent use may lead to loss of control). Products include:
- Dobutrex Solution Vials ... 1914

Dopamine Hydrochloride (Sympathomimetics tend to produce hyperglycemia and concurrent use may lead to loss of control).
- No products indexed under this heading.

Ephedrine Hydrochloride (Sympathomimetics tend to produce hyperglycemia and concurrent use may lead to loss of control). Products include:
- Primatene Tablets ... ▣780

Ephedrine Sulfate (Sympathomimetics tend to produce hyperglycemia and concurrent use may lead to loss of control).
- No products indexed under this heading.

Ephedrine Tannate (Sympathomimetics tend to produce hyperglycemia and concurrent use may lead to loss of control). Products include:
- Rynatuss Pediatric Suspension ... 3353
- Rynatuss Tablets ... 3353

Epinephrine (Sympathomimetics tend to produce hyperglycemia and concurrent use may lead to loss of control). Products include:
- Epifrin Sterile Ophthalmic Solution ... ⊙235
- EpiPen ... 1236
- Primatene Mist ... ▣779
- Xylocaine with Epinephrine Injection ... 653

Epinephrine Bitartrate (Sympathomimetics tend to produce hyperglycemia and concurrent use may lead to loss of control). Products include:
- Sensorcaine ... 643

Epinephrine Hydrochloride (Sympathomimetics tend to produce hyperglycemia and concurrent use may lead to loss of control).
- No products indexed under this heading.

Esmolol Hydrochloride (The hypoglycemic action of sulfonylureas may be potentiated by beta adrenergic blockers). Products include:
- Brevibloc Injection ... 858

Estradiol (Estrogens tend to produce hyperglycemia and concurrent use may lead to loss of control). Products include:
- Activella Tablets ... 2764
- Alora Transdermal System ... 3372
- Climara Transdermal System ... 958
- CombiPatch Transdermal System .. 2323
- Esclim Transdermal System ... 3460
- Estrace Vaginal Cream ... 3358
- Estrace Tablets ... 3361
- Estring Vaginal Ring ... 2811
- Ortho-Prefest Tablets ... 2570
- Vagifem Tablets ... 2857
- Vivelle Transdermal System ... 2412
- Vivelle-Dot Transdermal System ... 2416

Estrogens, Conjugated (Estrogens tend to produce hyperglycemia and concurrent use may lead to loss of control). Products include:
- Premarin Intravenous ... 3563
- Premarin Tablets ... 3566
- Premarin Vaginal Cream ... 3570
- Premphase Tablets ... 3572
- Prempro Tablets ... 3572

Estrogens, Esterified (Estrogens tend to produce hyperglycemia and concurrent use may lead to loss of control). Products include:
- Estratest ... 3252
- Menest Tablets ... 2254

Estropipate (Estrogens tend to produce hyperglycemia and concurrent use may lead to loss of control). Products include:
- Ogen Tablets ... 2846
- Ortho-Est Tablets ... 3464

Ethacrynic Acid (Diuretics tend to produce hyperglycemia and concurrent use may lead to loss of control). Products include:
- Edecrin Tablets ... 2091

Ethinyl Estradiol (Estrogens tend to produce hyperglycemia and concurrent use may lead to loss of control). Products include:
- Alesse-21 Tablets ... 3468
- Alesse-28 Tablets ... 3473
- Brevicon 28-Day Tablets ... 3380
- Cyclessa Tablets ... 2450
- Desogen Tablets ... 2458
- Estinyl Tablets ... 3112
- Estrostep ... 2627
- femhrt Tablets ... 2635
- Levlen ... 962
- Levlite 21 Tablets ... 962
- Levlite 28 Tablets ... 962
- Levora Tablets ... 3389
- Loestrin 21 Tablets ... 2642
- Loestrin Fe Tablets ... 2642
- Lo/Ovral Tablets ... 3532
- Lo/Ovral-28 Tablets ... 3538
- Low-Ogestrel-28 Tablets ... 3392
- Microgestin Fe 1.5/30 Tablets ... 3407
- Microgestin Fe 1/20 Tablets ... 3400
- Mircette Tablets ... 2470
- Modicon ... 2563
- Necon ... 3415
- Nordette-28 Tablets ... 2257
- Norinyl 1 +35 28-Day Tablets ... 3380
- Ogestrel 0.5/50-28 Tablets ... 3428
- Ortho-Cept 21 Tablets ... 2546
- Ortho-Cept 28 Tablets ... 2546
- Ortho-Cyclen/Ortho Tri-Cyclen ... 2573
- Ortho-Novum ... 2563
- Ovcon ... 3364
- Ovral Tablets ... 3551
- Ovral-28 Tablets ... 3552
- Tri-Levlen ... 962
- Tri-Norinyl-28 Tablets ... 3433
- Triphasil-21 Tablets ... 3600
- Triphasil-28 Tablets ... 3605
- Trivora Tablets ... 3439
- Yasmin 28 Tablets ... 980
- Zovia ... 3449

Ethynodiol Diacetate (Oral contraceptives tend to produce hyperglycemia and concurrent use may lead to loss of control). Products include:
- Zovia ... 3449

Etodolac (The hypoglycemic action of sulfonylureas may be potentiated by nonsteroidal anti-inflammatory agents). Products include:
- Lodine ... 3528
- Lodine XL Extended-Release Tablets ... 3530

Felodipine (Calcium channel blockers tend to produce hyperglycemia and concurrent use may lead to loss of control). Products include:
- Lexxel Tablets ... 608
- Plendil Extended-Release Tablets ... 623

Fenoprofen Calcium (The hypoglycemic action of sulfonylureas may be potentiated by nonsteroidal anti-inflammatory agents).
- No products indexed under this heading.

Fludrocortisone Acetate (Corticosteroids tend to produce hyperglycemia and concurrent use may lead to loss of control). Products include:
- Florinef Acetate Tablets ... 2250

Fluphenazine Decanoate (Phenothiazines tend to produce hyperglycemia and concurrent use may lead to loss of control).
- No products indexed under this heading.

Fluphenazine Enanthate (Phenothiazines tend to produce hyperglycemia and concurrent use may lead to loss of control).
- No products indexed under this heading.

Fluphenazine Hydrochloride (Phenothiazines tend to produce hyperglycemia and concurrent use may lead to loss of control).
- No products indexed under this heading.

Flurazepam Hydrochloride (The hypoglycemic action of sulfonylureas may be potentiated by drugs that are highly protein bound).
- No products indexed under this heading.

Flurbiprofen (The hypoglycemic action of sulfonylureas may be potentiated by nonsteroidal anti-inflammatory agents).
- No products indexed under this heading.

Furosemide (Diuretics tend to produce hyperglycemia and concurrent use may lead to loss of control). Products include:
- Furosemide Tablets ... 2284

Glipizide (The hypoglycemic action of sulfonylureas may be potentiated by sulfonamides). Products include:
- Glucotrol Tablets ... 2692
- Glucotrol XL Extended Release Tablets ... 2693

Glyburide (The hypoglycemic action of sulfonylureas may be potentiated by sulfonamides). Products include:
- DiaBeta Tablets ... 741
- Glucovance Tablets ... 1086

Hydrochlorothiazide (Thiazides tend to produce hyperglycemia and concurrent use may lead to loss of control). Products include:
- Accuretic Tablets ... 2614
- Aldoril Tablets ... 2039
- Atacand HCT Tablets ... 597
- Avalide Tablets ... 1070
- Diovan HCT Tablets ... 2338
- Dyazide Capsules ... 1515
- HydroDIURIL Tablets ... 2108
- Hyzaar ... 2109
- Inderide Tablets ... 3517
- Inderide LA Long-Acting Capsules .. 3519
- Lotensin HCT Tablets ... 2367
- Maxzide ... 1008
- Micardis HCT Tablets ... 1051
- Microzide Capsules ... 3414
- Moduretic Tablets ... 2138
- Monopril HCT ... 1094
- Prinzide Tablets ... 2168
- Timolide Tablets ... 2187
- Uniretic Tablets ... 3178
- Vaseretic Tablets ... 2204
- Zestoretic Tablets ... 695
- Ziac Tablets ... 1887

Hydrocortisone (Corticosteroids tend to produce hyperglycemia and concurrent use may lead to loss of control). Products include:
- Anusol-HC Cream 2.5% ... 2237
- Cipro HC Otic Suspension ... 540
- Cortaid Intensive Therapy Cream . ▣717
- Cortaid Maximum Strength Cream ... ▣717
- Cortisporin Ophthalmic Suspension Sterile ... ⊙297
- Cortizone•5 ... ▣699
- Cortizone•10 ... ▣699
- Cortizone•10 Plus Creme ... ▣700
- Cortizone for Kids Creme ... ▣699
- Hydrocortone Tablets ... 2106
- Massengill Medicated Soft Cloth Towelette ... ▣753
- VōSoL HC Otic Solution ... 3356

Hydrocortisone Acetate (Corticosteroids tend to produce hyperglycemia and concurrent use may lead to loss of control). Products include:
- Analpram-HC ... 1338
- Anusol HC-1 Hydrocortisone Anti-Itch Cream ... ▣689
- Anusol-HC Suppositories ... 2238
- Cortaid ... ▣717
- Cortifoam Rectal Foam ... 3170
- Cortisporin-TC Otic Suspension ... 2246
- Hydrocortone Acetate Injectable Suspension ... 2103
- Pramosone ... 1343
- Proctocort Suppositories ... 2264
- ProctoFoam-HC ... 3177
- Terra-Cortril Ophthalmic Suspension ... 2716

Hydrocortisone Sodium Phosphate (Corticosteroids tend to produce hyperglycemia and concurrent use may lead to loss of control). Products include:
- Hydrocortone Phosphate Injection, Sterile ... 2105

Hydrocortisone Sodium Succinate (Corticosteroids tend to produce hyperglycemia and concurrent use may lead to loss of control).
- No products indexed under this heading.

Hydroflumethiazide (Thiazides tend to produce hyperglycemia and concurrent use may lead to loss of control). Products include:
Diucardin Tablets 3494

Ibuprofen (The hypoglycemic action of sulfonylureas may be potentiated by nonsteroidal anti-inflammatory agents). Products include:
Advil ..... ▣771
Children's Advil Oral Suspension ..... ▣773
Children's Advil Chewable Tablets ..... ▣773
Advil Cold and Sinus Caplets ..... ▣771
Advil Cold and Sinus Tablets ..... ▣771
Advil Flu & Body Ache Caplets ..... ▣772
Infants' Advil Drops ..... ▣773
Junior Strength Advil Tablets ..... ▣773
Junior Strength Advil Chewable Tablets ..... ▣773
Advil Migraine Liquigels ..... ▣772
Children's Motrin Oral Suspension and Chewable Tablets 2006
Children's Motrin Cold Oral Suspension 2007
Children's Motrin Oral Suspension ..... ▣643
Motrin Suspension, Oral Drops, Chewable Tablets, and Caplets 2002
Infants' Motrin Concentrated Drops 2006
Junior Strength Motrin Caplets and Chewable Tablets 2006
Motrin IB Tablets, Caplets, and Gelcaps 2002
Motrin Migraine Pain Caplets 2005
Motrin Sinus Headache Caplets 2005
Vicoprofen Tablets 520

Imipramine Hydrochloride (The hypoglycemic action of sulfonylureas may be potentiated by drugs that are highly protein bound).
No products indexed under this heading.

Imipramine Pamoate (The hypoglycemic action of sulfonylureas may be potentiated by drugs that are highly protein bound).
No products indexed under this heading.

Indapamide (Diuretics tend to produce hyperglycemia and concurrent use may lead to loss of control). Products include:
Indapamide Tablets 2286

Indomethacin (The hypoglycemic action of sulfonylureas may be potentiated by nonsteroidal anti-inflammatory agents). Products include:
Indocin 2112

Indomethacin Sodium Trihydrate (The hypoglycemic action of sulfonylureas may be potentiated by nonsteroidal anti-inflammatory agents). Products include:
Indocin I.V. 2115

Isocarboxazid (The hypoglycemic action of sulfonylureas may be potentiated by monoamine oxidase inhibitors).
No products indexed under this heading.

Isoniazid (Isoniazid tends to produce hyperglycemia and concurrent use may lead to loss of control). Products include:
Rifamate Capsules 767
Rifater Tablets 769

Isoproterenol Hydrochloride (Sympathomimetics tend to produce hyperglycemia and concurrent use may lead to loss of control).
No products indexed under this heading.

Isoproterenol Sulfate (Sympathomimetics tend to produce hyperglycemia and concurrent use may lead to loss of control).
No products indexed under this heading.

Isradipine (Calcium channel blockers tend to produce hyperglycemia and concurrent use may lead to loss of control). Products include:
DynaCirc Capsules 2921
DynaCirc CR Tablets 2923

Ketoprofen (The hypoglycemic action of sulfonylureas may be potentiated by nonsteroidal anti-inflammatory agents). Products include:
Orudis Capsules 3548
Orudis KT Tablets ..... ▣778
Oruvail Capsules 3548

Ketorolac Tromethamine (The hypoglycemic action of sulfonylureas may be potentiated by nonsteroidal anti-inflammatory agents). Products include:
Acular Ophthalmic Solution 544
Acular PF Ophthalmic Solution 544
Toradol 3018

Labetalol Hydrochloride (The hypoglycemic action of sulfonylureas may be potentiated by beta adrenergic blockers). Products include:
Normodyne Injection 3135
Normodyne Tablets 3137

Levalbuterol Hydrochloride (Sympathomimetics tend to produce hyperglycemia and concurrent use may lead to loss of control). Products include:
Xopenex Inhalation Solution 3207

Levobunolol Hydrochloride (The hypoglycemic action of sulfonylureas may be potentiated by beta adrenergic blockers). Products include:
Betagan ..... ⊙228

Levonorgestrel (Oral contraceptives tend to produce hyperglycemia and concurrent use may lead to loss of control). Products include:
Alesse-21 Tablets 3468
Alesse-28 Tablets 3473
Levlen 962
Levlite 21 Tablets 962
Levlite 28 Tablets 962
Levora Tablets 3389
Mirena Intrauterine System 974
Nordette-28 Tablets 2257
Norplant System 3543
Tri-Levlen 962
Triphasil-21 Tablets 3600
Triphasil-28 Tablets 3605
Trivora Tablets 3439

Levothyroxine Sodium (Thyroid products tend to produce hyperglycemia and concurrent use may lead to loss of control). Products include:
Levothroid Tablets 1373
Levoxyl Tablets 1819
Synthroid 505
Unithroid Tablets 3445

Liothyronine Sodium (Thyroid products tend to produce hyperglycemia and concurrent use may lead to loss of control). Products include:
Cytomel Tablets 1817
Triostat Injection 1825

Liotrix (Thyroid products tend to produce hyperglycemia and concurrent use may lead to loss of control).
No products indexed under this heading.

Magnesium Salicylate (The hypoglycemic action of sulfonylureas may be potentiated by salicylates). Products include:
Momentum Backache Relief Extra Strength Caplets ..... ▣666

Meclofenamate Sodium (The hypoglycemic action of sulfonylureas may be potentiated by nonsteroidal anti-inflammatory agents).
No products indexed under this heading.

Mefenamic Acid (The hypoglycemic action of sulfonylureas may be potentiated by nonsteroidal anti-inflammatory agents). Products include:
Ponstel Capsules 1356

Meloxicam (The hypoglycemic action of sulfonylureas may be potentiated by nonsteroidal anti-inflammatory agents). Products include:
Mobic Tablets 1054

Mephobarbital (The action of barbiturates may be prolonged by therapy with chlorpropamide; barbiturates should be employed with caution).
No products indexed under this heading.

Mesoridazine Besylate (Phenothiazines tend to produce hyperglycemia and concurrent use may lead to loss of control). Products include:
Serentil 1057

Mestranol (Oral contraceptives tend to produce hyperglycemia and concurrent use may lead to loss of control). Products include:
Necon 1/50 Tablets 3415
Norinyl 1 + 50 28-Day Tablets 3380
Ortho-Novum 1/50▫28 Tablets 2556

Metaproterenol Sulfate (Sympathomimetics tend to produce hyperglycemia and concurrent use may lead to loss of control). Products include:
Alupent 1029

Metaraminol Bitartrate (Sympathomimetics tend to produce hyperglycemia and concurrent use may lead to loss of control). Products include:
Aramine Injection 2043

Methotrimeprazine (Phenothiazines tend to produce hyperglycemia and concurrent use may lead to loss of control).
No products indexed under this heading.

Methoxamine Hydrochloride (Sympathomimetics tend to produce hyperglycemia and concurrent use may lead to loss of control).
No products indexed under this heading.

Methyclothiazide (Thiazides tend to produce hyperglycemia and concurrent use may lead to loss of control).
No products indexed under this heading.

Methylprednisolone Acetate (Corticosteroids tend to produce hyperglycemia and concurrent use may lead to loss of control). Products include:
Depo-Medrol Injectable Suspension 2795

Methylprednisolone Sodium Succinate (Corticosteroids tend to produce hyperglycemia and concurrent use may lead to loss of control). Products include:
Solu-Medrol Sterile Powder 2855

Metipranolol Hydrochloride (The hypoglycemic action of sulfonylureas may be potentiated by beta adrenergic blockers).
No products indexed under this heading.

Metolazone (Diuretics tend to produce hyperglycemia and concurrent use may lead to loss of control). Products include:
Mykrox Tablets 1168
Zaroxolyn Tablets 1177

Metoprolol Succinate (The hypoglycemic action of sulfonylureas may be potentiated by beta adrenergic blockers). Products include:
Toprol-XL Tablets 651

Metoprolol Tartrate (The hypoglycemic action of sulfonylureas may be potentiated by beta adrenergic blockers).
No products indexed under this heading.

Mibefradil Dihydrochloride (Calcium channel blockers tend to produce hyperglycemia and concurrent use may lead to loss of control).
No products indexed under this heading.

Miconazole (Co-administration with oral miconazole and oral hypoglycemic agents has resulted in severe hypoglycemia).
No products indexed under this heading.

Midazolam Hydrochloride (The hypoglycemic action of sulfonylureas may be potentiated by drugs that are highly protein bound). Products include:
Versed Injection 3027
Versed Syrup 3033

Moclobemide (The hypoglycemic action of sulfonylureas may be potentiated by monoamine oxidase inhibitors).
No products indexed under this heading.

Nabumetone (The hypoglycemic action of sulfonylureas may be potentiated by nonsteroidal anti-inflammatory agents). Products include:
Relafen Tablets 1617

Nadolol (The hypoglycemic action of sulfonylureas may be potentiated by beta adrenergic blockers). Products include:
Corgard Tablets 2245
Corzide 40/5 Tablets 2247
Corzide 80/5 Tablets 2247
Nadolol Tablets 2288

Naproxen (The hypoglycemic action of sulfonylureas may be potentiated by nonsteroidal anti-inflammatory agents). Products include:
EC-Naprosyn Delayed-Release Tablets 2967
Naprosyn Suspension 2967
Naprosyn Tablets 2967

Naproxen Sodium (The hypoglycemic action of sulfonylureas may be potentiated by nonsteroidal anti-inflammatory agents). Products include:
Aleve Tablets, Caplets and Gelcaps ..... ▣602
Aleve Cold & Sinus Caplets ..... ▣603
Anaprox Tablets 2967
Anaprox DS Tablets 2967
Naprelan Tablets 1293

Niacin (Nicotinic acid tends to produce hyperglycemia and concurrent use may lead to loss of control). Products include:
Niaspan Extended-Release Tablets 1846
Nicotinex Elixir ..... ▣633

Nicardipine Hydrochloride (Calcium channel blockers tend to produce hyperglycemia and concurrent use may lead to loss of control). Products include:
Cardene I.V. 3485

Nifedipine (Calcium channel blockers tend to produce hyperglycemia and concurrent use may lead to loss of control). Products include:
Adalat CC Tablets 877
Procardia Capsules 2708
Procardia XL Extended Release Tablets 2710

Nimodipine (Calcium channel blockers tend to produce hyperglycemia and concurrent use may lead to loss of control). Products include:
Nimotop Capsules 904

Nisoldipine (Calcium channel blockers tend to produce hyperglycemia and concurrent use may lead to loss of control). Products include:
Sular Tablets 688

Norepinephrine Bitartrate (Sympathomimetics tend to produce hyperglycemia and concurrent use may lead to loss of control).
No products indexed under this heading.

Norethindrone (Oral contraceptives tend to produce hyperglycemia and concurrent use may lead to loss of control). Products include:
Brevicon 28-Day Tablets 3380
Micronor Tablets 2543
Modicon 2563
Necon 3415
Norinyl 1 + 35 28-Day Tablets 3380
Norinyl 1 + 50 28-Day Tablets 3380
Nor-QD Tablets 3423
Ortho-Novum 2563
Ortho-Novum 1/50▫28 Tablets 2556

Ovcon 3364
Tri-Norinyl-28 Tablets 3433

Norethynodrel (Oral contraceptives tend to produce hyperglycemia and concurrent use may lead to loss of control).
No products indexed under this heading.

Norgestimate (Oral contraceptives tend to produce hyperglycemia and concurrent use may lead to loss of control). Products include:
Ortho-Cyclen/Ortho Tri-Cyclen 2573
Ortho-Prefest Tablets 2570

Norgestrel (Oral contraceptives tend to produce hyperglycemia and concurrent use may lead to loss of control). Products include:
Lo/Ovral Tablets 3532
Lo/Ovral-28 Tablets 3538
Low-Ogestrel-28 Tablets 3392
Ogestrel 0.5/50-28 Tablets 3428
Ovral Tablets 3551
Ovral-28 Tablets 3552
Ovrette Tablets 3552

Nortriptyline Hydrochloride (The hypoglycemic action of sulfonylureas may be potentiated by drugs that are highly protein bound).
No products indexed under this heading.

Oxaprozin (The hypoglycemic action of sulfonylureas may be potentiated by nonsteroidal anti-inflammatory agents).
No products indexed under this heading.

Oxazepam (The hypoglycemic action of sulfonylureas may be potentiated by drugs that are highly protein bound).
No products indexed under this heading.

Pargyline Hydrochloride (The hypoglycemic action of sulfonylureas may be potentiated by monoamine oxidase inhibitors).
No products indexed under this heading.

Penbutolol Sulfate (The hypoglycemic action of sulfonylureas may be potentiated by beta adrenergic blockers).
No products indexed under this heading.

Pentobarbital Sodium (The action of barbiturates may be prolonged by therapy with chlorpropamide; barbiturates should be employed with caution). Products include:
Nembutal Sodium Solution 485

Perphenazine (Phenothiazines tend to produce hyperglycemia and concurrent use may lead to loss of control). Products include:
Etrafon 3115
Trilafon 3160

Phenelzine Sulfate (The hypoglycemic action of sulfonylureas may be potentiated by monoamine oxidase inhibitors). Products include:
Nardil Tablets 2653

Phenobarbital (The action of barbiturates may be prolonged by therapy with chlorpropamide; barbiturates should be employed with caution). Products include:
Arco-Lase Plus Tablets 592
Donnatal 2929
Donnatal Extentabs 2930

Phenylbutazone (The hypoglycemic action of sulfonylureas may be potentiated by nonsteroidal anti-inflammatory agents).
No products indexed under this heading.

Phenylephrine Bitartrate (Sympathomimetics tend to produce hyperglycemia and concurrent use may lead to loss of control).
No products indexed under this heading.

Phenylephrine Hydrochloride (Sympathomimetics tend to produce hyperglycemia and concurrent use may lead to loss of control). Products include:
Afrin Nasal Decongestant Children's Pump Mist .... ▣734
Extendryl 1361
Hycomine Compound Tablets 1317
Neo-Synephrine .... ▣614
Phenergan VC Syrup 3560
Phenergan VC with Codeine Syrup 3561
Preparation H Cream .... ▣778
Preparation H Cooling Gel .... ▣778
Preparation H .... ▣778
Vicks Sinex Nasal Spray and Ultra Fine Mist .... ▣729

Phenylephrine Tannate (Sympathomimetics tend to produce hyperglycemia and concurrent use may lead to loss of control). Products include:
Ryna-12 S Suspension 3351
Reformulated Rynatan Pediatric Suspension 3352
Rynatuss Pediatric Suspension 3353
Rynatuss Tablets 3353

Phenylpropanolamine Hydrochloride (Sympathomimetics tend to produce hyperglycemia and concurrent use may lead to loss of control).
No products indexed under this heading.

Phenytoin (Phenytoin tends to produce hyperglycemia and concurrent use may lead to loss of control). Products include:
Dilantin Infatabs 2624
Dilantin-125 Oral Suspension 2625

Phenytoin Sodium (Phenytoin tends to produce hyperglycemia and concurrent use may lead to loss of control). Products include:
Dilantin Kapseals 2622

Pindolol (The hypoglycemic action of sulfonylureas may be potentiated by beta adrenergic blockers).
No products indexed under this heading.

Pirbuterol Acetate (Sympathomimetics tend to produce hyperglycemia and concurrent use may lead to loss of control). Products include:
Maxair Autohaler 1981
Maxair Inhaler 1984

Piroxicam (The hypoglycemic action of sulfonylureas may be potentiated by nonsteroidal anti-inflammatory agents). Products include:
Feldene Capsules 2685

Polyestradiol Phosphate (Estrogens tend to produce hyperglycemia and concurrent use may lead to loss of control).
No products indexed under this heading.

Polythiazide (Thiazides tend to produce hyperglycemia and concurrent use may lead to loss of control). Products include:
Minizide Capsules 2700
Renese Tablets 2712

Prednisolone Acetate (Corticosteroids tend to produce hyperglycemia and concurrent use may lead to loss of control). Products include:
Blephamide Ophthalmic Ointment 547
Blephamide Ophthalmic Suspension 548
Poly-Pred Liquifilm Ophthalmic Suspension .... ⊙245
Pred Forte Ophthalmic Suspension .... ⊙246
Pred Mild Sterile Ophthalmic Suspension .... ⊙249
Pred-G Ophthalmic Suspension .... ⊙247
Pred-G Sterile Ophthalmic Ointment .... ⊙248

Prednisolone Sodium Phosphate (Corticosteroids tend to produce hyperglycemia and concurrent use may lead to loss of control). Products include:
Pediapred Oral Solution 1170

Prednisolone Tebutate (Corticosteroids tend to produce hyperglycemia and concurrent use may lead to loss of control).
No products indexed under this heading.

Prednisone (Corticosteroids tend to produce hyperglycemia and concurrent use may lead to loss of control). Products include:
Prednisone 3064

Probenecid (The hypoglycemic action of sulfonylureas may be potentiated by probenecid).
No products indexed under this heading.

Procarbazine Hydrochloride (The hypoglycemic action of sulfonylureas may be potentiated by monoamine oxidase inhibitors). Products include:
Matulane Capsules 3246

Prochlorperazine (Phenothiazines tend to produce hyperglycemia and concurrent use may lead to loss of control). Products include:
Compazine 1505

Promethazine Hydrochloride (Phenothiazines tend to produce hyperglycemia and concurrent use may lead to loss of control). Products include:
Mepergan Injection 3539
Phenergan Injection 3553
Phenergan 3556
Phenergan Syrup 3554
Phenergan with Codeine Syrup 3557
Phenergan with Dextromethorphan Syrup 3559
Phenergan VC Syrup 3560
Phenergan VC with Codeine Syrup 3561

Propranolol Hydrochloride (The hypoglycemic action of sulfonylureas may be potentiated by beta adrenergic blockers). Products include:
Inderal 3513
Inderal LA Long-Acting Capsules 3516
Inderide Tablets 3517
Inderide LA Long-Acting Capsules 3519

Pseudoephedrine Hydrochloride (Sympathomimetics tend to produce hyperglycemia and concurrent use may lead to loss of control). Products include:
Actifed Cold & Allergy Tablets .... ▣688
Actifed Cold & Sinus Caplets and Tablets .... ▣688
Advil Cold and Sinus Caplets .... ▣771
Advil Cold and Sinus Tablets .... ▣771
Advil Flu & Body Ache Caplets .... ▣772
Aleve Cold & Sinus Caplets .... ▣603
Alka-Seltzer Plus Liqui-Gels .... ▣604
Alka-Seltzer Plus Cold & Flu Medicine Liqui-Gels .... ▣604
Alka-Seltzer Plus Cold & Sinus Medicine Liqui-Gels .... ▣604
Allegra-D Extended-Release Tablets 714
BC Cold Powder .... ▣619
Benadryl Allergy/Cold Tablets .... ▣691
Benadryl Allergy/Congestion Tablets .... ▣692
Benadryl Allergy & Sinus Liquid .... ▣693
Benadryl Allergy & Sinus Fastmelt Tablets .... ▣693
Benadryl Allergy Sinus Headache Caplets & Gelcaps .... ▣693
Benadryl Severe Allergy & Sinus Headache Caplets .... ▣694
Benadryl Children's Allergy/Cold Fastmelt Tablets .... ▣692
Benylin Multi-Symptom Liquid .... ▣697
Bromfed Capsules (Extended-Release) 2269
Bromfed-PD Capsules (Extended-Release) 2269
Children's Cēpacol Sore Throat .... ▣788
Comtrex Acute Head Cold & Sinus Pressure Relief Tablets .... ▣627
Comtrex Deep Chest Cold & Congestion Relief Softgels .... ▣627
Comtrex Flu Therapy & Fever Relief Daytime Caplets .... ▣628
Comtrex Flu Therapy & Fever Relief Nighttime Tablets .... ▣628
Comtrex Maximum Strength Multi-Symptom Cold & Cough Relief Tablets and Caplets .... ▣626
Contac Non-Drowsy 12 Hour Cold Caplets .... ▣745
Contac Non-Drowsy Timed Release 12 Hour Cold Caplets .... ▣746
Contac Severe Cold and Flu Caplets Maximum Strength .... ▣746
Contac Severe Cold and Flu Caplets Non-Drowsy .... ▣746
Dimetapp Elixir .... ▣777
Dimetapp Cold and Fever Suspension .... ▣775
Dimetapp DM Cold & Cough Elixir .... ▣775
Dimetapp Nighttime Flu Liquid .... ▣776
Dimetapp Non-Drowsy Flu Syrup .... ▣777
Dimetapp Infant Drops Decongestant .... ▣775
Dimetapp Infant Drops Decongestant Plus Cough .... ▣776
Guaifed 2272
Kronofed-A 1341
Children's Motrin Cold Oral Suspension 2007
Motrin Sinus Headache Caplets 2005
PediaCare Cough-Cold Liquid .... ▣719
PediaCare Infants' Drops Decongestant .... ▣719
PediaCare Infants' Drops Decongestant Plus Cough .... ▣719
PediaCare NightRest Cough-Cold Liquid .... ▣719
Robitussin Cold Caplets Cold & Congestion .... ▣780
Robitussin Cold Softgels Cold & Congestion .... ▣780
Robitussin Cold Caplets Multi-Symptom Cold & Flu .... ▣781
Robitussin Cold Softgels Multi-Symptom Cold & Flu .... ▣781
Robitussin Cold Softgels Severe Congestion .... ▣782
Robitussin Cough & Cold Infant Drops .... ▣782
Robitussin Maximum Strength Cough & Cold Liquid .... ▣785
Robitussin Pediatric Cough & Cold Formula Liquid .... ▣785
Robitussin Multi Symptom Honey Flu Liquid .... ▣785
Robitussin Nighttime Honey Flu Liquid .... ▣786
Robitussin-CF Liquid .... ▣783
Robitussin-DAC Syrup 2942
Robitussin-PE Liquid .... ▣782
Ryna .... ▣768
Semprex-D Capsules 1172
Singlet Caplets .... ▣761
Sinutab Non-Drying Liquid Caps .... ▣706
Sinutab Sinus Allergy Medication, Maximum Strength Formula, Tablets & Caplets .... ▣707
Sinutab Sinus Medication, Maximum Strength Without Drowsiness Formula, Tablets & Caplets .... ▣707
Sudafed 12 Hour Tablets .... ▣708
Sudafed 24 Hour Tablets .... ▣708
Children's Sudafed Cold & Cough Liquid .... ▣709
Children's Sudafed Nasal Decongestant Chewables .... ▣711
Children's Sudafed Nasal Decongestant Liquid Medication .... ▣711
Sudafed Cold & Allergy Tablets .... ▣708
Sudafed Cold & Cough Liquid Caps .... ▣709
Sudafed Cold & Sinus Liquid Caps .... ▣710
Sudafed Nasal Decongestant Tablets .... ▣710
Sudafed Non-Drying Sinus Liquid Caps .... ▣712
Sudafed Severe Cold .... ▣711
Sudafed Sinus Headache Caplets .... ▣712
Sudafed Sinus Headache Tablets .... ▣712
Tavist Sinus Non-Drowsy Coated Caplets .... ▣676
TheraFlu Regular Strength Cold & Cough Night Time Hot Liquid .... ▣676
TheraFlu Regular Strength Cold & Sore Throat Night Time Hot Liquid .... ▣676
TheraFlu Maximum Strength Flu & Congestion Non-Drowsy Hot Liquid .... ▣677
TheraFlu Maximum Strength Flu & Cough Night Time Hot Liquid .... ▣678
TheraFlu Maximum Strength Flu & Sore Throat Night Time Hot Liquid .... ▣677
TheraFlu Maximum Strength Severe Cold & Congestion Night Time Caplets .... ▣678
TheraFlu Maximum Strength Severe Cold & Congestion Night Time Hot Liquid .... ▣678
TheraFlu Maximum Strength Severe Cold & Congestion Non-Drowsy .... ▣679
Triaminic Allergy Congestion Liquid .... ▣680
Triaminic Chest Congestion Liquid .... ▣680

Triaminic Cold & Allergy Liquid ...... ▣681
Triaminic Cold & Allergy Softchews ...... ▣683
Triaminic Cold & Cough Liquid ...... ▣681
Triaminic Cold & Cough Softchews ...... ▣683
Triaminic Cold & Night Time Cough Liquid ...... ▣681
Triaminic Cold, Cough & Fever Liquid ...... ▣681
Triaminic Cough Liquid ...... ▣682
Triaminic Cough & Congestion Liquid ...... ▣682
Triaminic Cough & Sore Throat Liquid ...... ▣682
Triaminic Cough & Sore Throat Softchews ...... ▣684
Children's Tylenol Allergy-D Liquid ... 2014
Children's Tylenol Cold Suspension Liquid and Chewable Tablets 2015
Children's Tylenol Cold Plus Cough Suspension Liquid and Chewable Tablets 2015
Children's Tylenol Flu Suspension Liquid 2015
Children's Tylenol Sinus Suspension Liquid 2017
Infants' Tylenol Cold Decongestant and Fever Reducer Concentrated Drops 2015
Infants' Tylenol Cold Decongestant and Fever Reducer Concentrated Drops Plus Cough .. 2015
Tylenol Allergy Sinus 2010
Multi-Symptom Tylenol Cold Complete Formula Caplets 2010
Multi-Symptom Tylenol Cold Non-Drowsy Caplets and Gelcaps 2010
Multi-Symptom Tylenol Cold Severe Congestion Non-Drowsy Caplets 2011
Maximum Strength Tylenol Flu NightTime Gelcaps 2011
Maximum Strength Tylenol Flu NightTime Liquid 2011
Maximum Strength Tylenol Flu Non-Drowsy Gelcaps 2011
Maximum Strength Tylenol Sinus NightTime Caplets 2012
Maximum Strength Tylenol Sinus Non-Drowsy Geltabs, Gelcaps, Caplets, and Tablets 2012
Vicks 44D Cough & Head Congestion Relief Liquid ...... ▣724
Vicks 44M Cough, Cold & Flu Relief Liquid ...... ▣725
Pediatric Vicks 44m Cough & Cold Relief ...... ▣728
Vicks DayQuil LiquiCaps/Liquid Multi-Symptom Cold/Flu Relief ...... ▣727
Children's Vicks NyQuil Cold/Cough Relief ...... ▣726
Vicks NyQuil LiquiCaps/Liquid Multi-Symptom Cold/Flu Relief, Original and Cherry Flavors ...... ▣727
Zephrex Tablets 3091
Zephrex LA Tablets 3092
Zyrtec-D 12 Hour Extended Relief Tablets 2758

Pseudoephedrine Sulfate (Sympathomimetics tend to produce hyperglycemia and concurrent use may lead to loss of control). Products include:
Chlor-Trimeton Allergy/Decongestant Tablets ...... ▣736
Claritin-D 12 Hour Extended Release Tablets 3102
Claritin-D 24 Hour Extended Release Tablets 3104
Coricidin 'D' Cold, Flu & Sinus Tablets ...... ▣737
Drixoral Allergy/Sinus Extended-Release Tablets ...... ▣741
Drixoral Cold & Allergy Sustained-Action Tablets ...... ▣740
Drixoral Cold & Flu Extended-Release Tablets ...... ▣740
Drixoral Nasal Decongestant Long-Acting Non-Drowsy Tablets ...... ▣740
Rynatan Tablets 3351

Quinestrol (Estrogens tend to produce hyperglycemia and concurrent use may lead to loss of control).
No products indexed under this heading.

Rofecoxib (The hypoglycemic action of sulfonylureas may be potentiated by nonsteroidal anti-inflammatory agents). Products include:
Vioxx 2213

Salmeterol Xinafoate (Sympathomimetics tend to produce hyperglycemia and concurrent use may lead to loss of control). Products include:
Advair Diskus 100/50 1448
Advair Diskus 250/50 1448
Advair Diskus 500/50 1448
Serevent Diskus 1637
Serevent Inhalation Aerosol 1633

Salsalate (The hypoglycemic action of sulfonylureas may be potentiated by salicylates).
No products indexed under this heading.

Secobarbital Sodium (The action of barbiturates may be prolonged by therapy with chlorpropamide; barbiturates should be employed with caution).
No products indexed under this heading.

Selegiline Hydrochloride (The hypoglycemic action of sulfonylureas may be potentiated by monoamine oxidase inhibitors). Products include:
Eldepryl Capsules 3266

Sotalol Hydrochloride (The hypoglycemic action of sulfonylureas may be potentiated by beta adrenergic blockers). Products include:
Betapace Tablets 950
Betapace AF Tablets 954

Spironolactone (Diuretics tend to produce hyperglycemia and concurrent use may lead to loss of control).
No products indexed under this heading.

Sulfacytine (The hypoglycemic action of sulfonylureas may be potentiated by sulfonamides).
No products indexed under this heading.

Sulfamethizole (The hypoglycemic action of sulfonylureas may be potentiated by sulfonamides). Products include:
Urobiotic-250 Capsules 2731

Sulfamethoxazole (The hypoglycemic action of sulfonylureas may be potentiated by sulfonamides). Products include:
Bactrim 2949
Septra Suspension 2265
Septra Tablets 2265
Septra DS Tablets 2265

Sulfasalazine (The hypoglycemic action of sulfonylureas may be potentiated by sulfonamides). Products include:
Azulfidine EN-tabs Tablets 2775

Sulfinpyrazone (The hypoglycemic action of sulfonylureas may be potentiated by sulfonamides).
No products indexed under this heading.

Sulfisoxazole (The hypoglycemic action of sulfonylureas may be potentiated by sulfonamides).
No products indexed under this heading.

Sulfisoxazole Acetyl (The hypoglycemic action of sulfonylureas may be potentiated by sulfonamides). Products include:
Pediazole Suspension 3050

Sulfisoxazole Diolamine (The hypoglycemic action of sulfonylureas may be potentiated by sulfonamides).
No products indexed under this heading.

Sulindac (The hypoglycemic action of sulfonylureas may be potentiated by nonsteroidal anti-inflammatory agents). Products include:
Clinoril Tablets 2053

Temazepam (The hypoglycemic action of sulfonylureas may be potentiated by drugs that are highly protein bound).
No products indexed under this heading.

Terbutaline Sulfate (Sympathomimetics tend to produce hyperglycemia and concurrent use may lead to loss of control). Products include:
Brethine Ampuls 2314
Brethine Tablets 2313

Thiamylal Sodium (The action of barbiturates may be prolonged by therapy with chlorpropamide; barbiturates should be employed with caution).
No products indexed under this heading.

Thioridazine Hydrochloride (Phenothiazines tend to produce hyperglycemia and concurrent use may lead to loss of control). Products include:
Thioridazine Hydrochloride Tablets 2289

Thyroglobulin (Thyroid products tend to produce hyperglycemia and concurrent use may lead to loss of control).
No products indexed under this heading.

Thyroid (Thyroid products tend to produce hyperglycemia and concurrent use may lead to loss of control).
No products indexed under this heading.

Thyroxine (Thyroid products tend to produce hyperglycemia and concurrent use may lead to loss of control).
No products indexed under this heading.

Thyroxine Sodium (Thyroid products tend to produce hyperglycemia and concurrent use may lead to loss of control).
No products indexed under this heading.

Timolol Hemihydrate (The hypoglycemic action of sulfonylureas may be potentiated by beta adrenergic blockers). Products include:
Betimol Ophthalmic Solution ...... ⊙324

Timolol Maleate (The hypoglycemic action of sulfonylureas may be potentiated by beta adrenergic blockers). Products include:
Blocadren Tablets 2046
Cosopt Sterile Ophthalmic Solution 2065
Timolide Tablets 2187
Timolol GFS ...... ⊙266
Timoptic in Ocudose 2192
Timoptic Sterile Ophthalmic Solution 2190
Timoptic-XE Sterile Ophthalmic Gel Forming Solution 2194

Tolazamide (The hypoglycemic action of sulfonylureas may be potentiated by sulfonamides).
No products indexed under this heading.

Tolbutamide (The hypoglycemic action of sulfonylureas may be potentiated by sulfonamides).
No products indexed under this heading.

Tolmetin Sodium (The hypoglycemic action of sulfonylureas may be potentiated by nonsteroidal anti-inflammatory agents). Products include:
Tolectin 2589

Torsemide (Diuretics tend to produce hyperglycemia and concurrent use may lead to loss of control). Products include:
Demadex Tablets and Injection 2965

Tranylcypromine Sulfate (The hypoglycemic action of sulfonylureas may be potentiated by monoamine oxidase inhibitors). Products include:
Parnate Tablets 1607

Triamcinolone (Corticosteroids tend to produce hyperglycemia and concurrent use may lead to loss of control).
No products indexed under this heading.

Triamcinolone Acetonide (Corticosteroids tend to produce hyperglycemia and concurrent use may lead to loss of control). Products include:
Azmacort Inhalation Aerosol 728
Nasacort Nasal Inhaler 750
Nasacort AQ Nasal Spray 752
Tri-Nasal Spray 2274

Triamcinolone Diacetate (Corticosteroids tend to produce hyperglycemia and concurrent use may lead to loss of control).
No products indexed under this heading.

Triamcinolone Hexacetonide (Corticosteroids tend to produce hyperglycemia and concurrent use may lead to loss of control).
No products indexed under this heading.

Triamterene (Diuretics tend to produce hyperglycemia and concurrent use may lead to loss of control). Products include:
Dyazide Capsules 1515
Dyrenium Capsules 3458
Maxzide 1008

Trifluoperazine Hydrochloride (Phenothiazines tend to produce hyperglycemia and concurrent use may lead to loss of control). Products include:
Stelazine 1640

Trimipramine Maleate (The hypoglycemic action of sulfonylureas may be potentiated by drugs that are highly protein bound). Products include:
Surmontil Capsules 3595

Verapamil Hydrochloride (Calcium channel blockers tend to produce hyperglycemia and concurrent use may lead to loss of control). Products include:
Covera-HS Tablets 3199
Isoptin SR Tablets 467
Tarka Tablets 508
Verelan Capsules 3184
Verelan PM Capsules 3186

Warfarin Sodium (The hypoglycemic action of sulfonylureas may be potentiated by coumarins). Products include:
Coumadin for Injection 1243
Coumadin Tablets 1243
Warfarin Sodium Tablets, USP 3302

Food Interactions

Alcohol (In some patients disulfiram-like reaction may be produced by the ingestion of alcohol).

DIAMOX INTRAVENOUS

(Acetazolamide Sodium) ...... ⊙269
See Diamox Tablets

DIAMOX SEQUELS SUSTAINED RELEASE CAPSULES

(Acetazolamide) ...... ⊙270
May interact with:

Aspirin (Concomitant administration with high-dose aspirin may result in anorexia, tachypnea, lethargy, coma and death). Products include:
Aggrenox Capsules 1026
Alka-Seltzer ...... ▣603
Alka-Seltzer Lemon Lime Antacid and Pain Reliever Effervescent Tablets ...... ▣603
Alka-Seltzer Extra Strength Antacid and Pain Reliever Effervescent Tablets ...... ▣603
Alka-Seltzer PM Effervescent Tablets ...... ▣605
Genuine Bayer Tablets, Caplets and Gelcaps ...... ▣606
Extra Strength Bayer Caplets and Gelcaps ...... ▣610
Aspirin Regimen Bayer Children's Chewable Tablets (Orange or Cherry Flavored) ...... ▣607
Bayer, Aspirin Regimen ...... ▣606
Aspirin Regimen Bayer 81 mg Caplets with Calcium ...... ▣607
Genuine Bayer Professional Labeling (Aspirin Regimen Bayer) ...... ▣608
Extra Strength Bayer Arthritis Caplets ...... ▣610
Extra Strength Bayer Plus Caplets ...... ▣610

Extra Strength Bayer PM Caplets .. 611
BC Powder 619
BC Allergy Sinus Cold Powder 619
Arthritis Strength BC Powder 619
BC Sinus Cold Powder 619
Darvon Compound-65 Pulvules 1910
Ecotrin Enteric Coated Aspirin Low, Regular and Maximum Strength Tablets 1715
Excedrin Extra-Strength Tablets, Caplets, and Geltabs 629
Excedrin Migraine 1070
Goody's Body Pain Formula Powder 620
Goody's Extra Strength Headache Powder 620
Goody's Extra Strength Pain Relief Tablets 620
Percodan Tablets 1327
Robaxisal Tablets 2939
Soma Compound Tablets 3354
Soma Compound w/Codeine Tablets 3355
Vanquish Caplets 617

DIAMOX TABLETS

(Acetazolamide) .... ⊙269

May interact with:

Aspirin (Concomitant administration with high-dose aspirin may result in anorexia, tachypnea, lethargy, coma and death). Products include:

Aggrenox Capsules 1026
Alka-Seltzer 603
Alka-Seltzer Lemon Lime Antacid and Pain Reliever Effervescent Tablets 603
Alka-Seltzer Extra Strength Antacid and Pain Reliever Effervescent Tablets 603
Alka-Seltzer PM Effervescent Tablets 605
Genuine Bayer Tablets, Caplets and Gelcaps 606
Extra Strength Bayer Caplets and Gelcaps 610
Aspirin Regimen Bayer Children's Chewable Tablets (Orange or Cherry Flavored) 607
Bayer, Aspirin Regimen 606
Aspirin Regimen Bayer 81 mg Caplets with Calcium 607
Genuine Bayer Professional Labeling (Aspirin Regimen Bayer) 608
Extra Strength Bayer Arthritis Caplets 610
Extra Strength Bayer Plus Caplets 610
Extra Strength Bayer PM Caplets .. 611
BC Powder 619
BC Allergy Sinus Cold Powder 619
Arthritis Strength BC Powder 619
BC Sinus Cold Powder 619
Darvon Compound-65 Pulvules 1910
Ecotrin Enteric Coated Aspirin Low, Regular and Maximum Strength Tablets 1715
Excedrin Extra-Strength Tablets, Caplets, and Geltabs 629
Excedrin Migraine 1070
Goody's Body Pain Formula Powder 620
Goody's Extra Strength Headache Powder 620
Goody's Extra Strength Pain Relief Tablets 620
Percodan Tablets 1327
Robaxisal Tablets 2939
Soma Compound Tablets 3354
Soma Compound w/Codeine Tablets 3355
Vanquish Caplets 617

DIBENZYLINE CAPSULES

(Phenoxybenzamine Hydrochloride) 3457

May interact with:

Alpha and Beta Adrenergic Stimulators (Exaggerated hypotensive response; tachycardia).

No products indexed under this heading.

Epinephrine (Exaggerated hypotensive response; tachycardia). Products include:

Epifrin Sterile Ophthalmic Solution .... ⊙235
EpiPen 1236
Primatene Mist 779
Xylocaine with Epinephrine Injection 653

Epinephrine Bitartrate (Exaggerated hypotensive response; tachycardia). Products include:

Sensorcaine 643

Norepinephrine Bitartrate (Hyperthermia production of levarterenol blocked by dibenzyline).

No products indexed under this heading.

Reserpine (Hypothermia production of reserpine blocked by dibenzyline).

No products indexed under this heading.

DIDRONEL TABLETS

(Etidronate Disodium) 2888

May interact with:

Warfarin Sodium (Co-administration has resulted in isolated reports of increase in prothrombin time without clinically significant sequelae). Products include:

Coumadin for Injection 1243
Coumadin Tablets 1243
Warfarin Sodium Tablets, USP 3302

DIFFERIN CREAM

(Adapalene) 1402

See Differin Gel

DIFFERIN GEL

(Adapalene) 1403

May interact with:

Resorcinol (Increased potential for local irritation).

No products indexed under this heading.

Salicylic Acid (Increased potential for local irritation). Products include:

Clear Away Gel with Aloe Wart Remover System 736
Clear Away Liquid Wart Remover System 736
Clear Away One Step Wart Remover 737
Clear Away One Step Wart Remover for Kids 737
Clear Away One Step Plantar Wart Remover 737
Compound W One Step Pads for Kids 664
Compound W One Step Plantar Pads 664
Compound W One Step Wart Remover Pads 664
Compound W Wart Remover Gel 665
Compound W Wart Remover Liquid 665
Wart-Off Liquid 716

Sulfur (Increased potential for local irritation). Products include:

Plexion 2024

DIFFERIN SOLUTION/PLEDGETS

(Adapalene) 1404

See Differin Gel

DIFLUCAN TABLETS, INJECTION, AND ORAL SUSPENSION

(Fluconazole) 2681

May interact with oral anticoagulants, phenytoin, sulfonylureas, theophylline, and certain other agents. Compounds in these categories include:

Aminophylline (Increased serum concentrations of theophylline).

No products indexed under this heading.

Astemizole (Co-administration of fluconazole in patients taking drugs metabolized by the CYP450 system, such as astemizole, may be associated with elevation in serum astemizole levels).

No products indexed under this heading.

Chlorpropamide (Co-administration with sulfonylurea oral hypoglycemic agent may precipitate clinically significant hypoglycemia). Products include:

Diabinese Tablets 2680

Cimetidine (Potential for significant decrease in fluconazole AUC and Cmax; however, cimetidine given intravenously over a four hour period does not affect pharmacokinetics of fluconazole). Products include:

Tagamet HB 200 Suspension 762
Tagamet HB 200 Tablets 761
Tagamet Tablets 1644

Cimetidine Hydrochloride (Potential for significant decreae in fluconazole AUC and Cmax; however, cimetidine given intravenously over a four hour period does not affect pharmacokinetics of fluconazole). Products include:

Tagamet 1644

Cisapride (Co-administration has resuled in reports of cardiac events including torsade de pointes).

No products indexed under this heading.

Cyclosporine (Fluconazole may significantly increase cyclosporine levels in renal transplant patients with or without renal impairment). Products include:

Gengraf Capsules 457
Neoral Soft Gelatin Capsules 2380
Neoral Oral Solution 2380
Sandimmune 2388

Dicumarol (Increased prothrombin time; monitoring of prothrombin time is recommended).

No products indexed under this heading.

Dyphylline (Increased serum concentrations of theophylline). Products include:

Lufyllin Tablets 3347
Lufyllin-400 Tablets 3347
Lufyllin-GG Elixir 3348
Lufyllin-GG Tablets 3348

Ethinyl Estradiol (Co-administration with ethinyl estradiol and levonorgestrel-containing oral contraceptive produces an overall mean increase in ethinyl estradiol and levonorgestrel levels; however, in some patients there may be a decrease in these levels; clinical significance unknown). Products include:

Alesse-21 Tablets 3468
Alesse-28 Tablets 3473
Brevicon 28-Day Tablets 3380
Cyclessa Tablets 2450
Desogen Tablets 2458
Estinyl Tablets 3112
Estrostep 2627
femhrt Tablets 2635
Levlen 962
Levlite 21 Tablets 962
Levlite 28 Tablets 962
Levora Tablets 3389
Loestrin 21 Tablets 2642
Loestrin Fe Tablets 2642
Lo/Ovral Tablets 3532
Lo/Ovral-28 Tablets 3538
Low-Ogestrel-28 Tablets 3392
Microgestin Fe 1.5/30 Tablets 3407
Microgestin Fe 1/20 Tablets 3400
Mircette Tablets 2470
Modicon 2563
Necon 3415
Nordette-28 Tablets 2257
Norinyl 1 +35 28-Day Tablets 3380
Ogestrel 0.5/50-28 Tablets 3428
Ortho-Cept 21 Tablets 2546
Ortho-Cept 28 Tablets 2546
Ortho-Cyclen/Ortho Tri-Cyclen 2573
Ortho-Novum 2563
Ovcon 3364
Ovral Tablets 3551
Ovral-28 Tablets 3552
Tri-Levlen 962
Tri-Norinyl-28 Tablets 3433
Triphasil-21 Tablets 3600
Triphasil-28 Tablets 3605
Trivora Tablets 3439
Yasmin 28 Tablets 980
Zovia 3449

Fosphenytoin Sodium (Increased plasma concentrations of phenytoin; monitor phenytoin concentration). Products include:

Cerebyx Injection 2619

Glimepiride (Co-administration with sulfonylurea oral hypoglycemic agent may precipitate clinically significant hypoglycemia). Products include:

Amaryl Tablets 717

Glipizide (Co-administration with sulfonylurea oral hypoglycemic agent may precipitate clinically significant hypoglycemia; reduced metabolism of glipizide). Products include:

Glucotrol Tablets 2692
Glucotrol XL Extended Release Tablets 2693

Glyburide (Co-administration with sulfonylurea oral hypoglycemic agent may precipitate clinically significant hypoglycemia; one fatality has been reported with combined use due to hypoglycemia; reduced metabolism of glyburide). Products include:

DiaBeta Tablets 741
Glucovance Tablets 1086

Hydrochlorothiazide (Potential for a significant increase in fluconazole AUC (45% ±31%) and Cmax (43% ±31%) attributable to reduction in renal clearance of 30% ±12%). Products include:

Accuretic Tablets 2614
Aldoril Tablets 2039
Atacand HCT Tablets 597
Avalide Tablets 1070
Diovan HCT Tablets 2338
Dyazide Capsules 1515
HydroDIURIL Tablets 2108
Hyzaar 2109
Inderide Tablets 3517
Inderide LA Long-Acting Capsules .. 3519
Lotensin HCT Tablets 2367
Maxzide 1008
Micardis HCT Tablets 1051
Microzide Capsules 3414
Moduretic Tablets 2138
Monopril HCT 1094
Prinzide Tablets 2168
Timolide Tablets 2187
Uniretic Tablets 3178
Vaseretic Tablets 2204
Zestoretic Tablets 695
Ziac Tablets 1887

Isoniazid (The incidence of abnormally elevated serum transaminase was greater in patients taking Diflucan concomitantly with isoniazid). Products include:

Rifamate Capsules 767
Rifater Tablets 769

Levonorgestrel (Co-administration with ethinyl estradiol and levonorgestrel-containing oral contraceptive produces an overall mean increase in ethinyl estradiol and levonorgestrel levels; however, in some patients there may be a decrease in these levels; clinical significance unknown). Products include:

Alesse-21 Tablets 3468
Alesse-28 Tablets 3473
Levlen 962
Levlite 21 Tablets 962
Levlite 28 Tablets 962
Levora Tablets 3389
Mirena Intrauterine System 974
Nordette-28 Tablets 2257
Norplant System 3543
Tri-Levlen 962
Triphasil-21 Tablets 3600
Triphasil-28 Tablets 3605
Trivora Tablets 3439

Phenytoin (Increased plasma concentrations of phenytoin; monitor phenytoin concentration). Products include:

Dilantin Infatabs 2624
Dilantin-125 Oral Suspension 2625

Phenytoin Sodium (Increased plasma concentrations of phenytoin; monitor phenytoin concentration). Products include:

Dilantin Kapseals 2622

Rifabutin (Co-administration has resulted in uveitis). Products include:

Mycobutin Capsules 2838

IMPORTANT NOTE: Always consult each drug listing in the patient's regimen for possible interactions.

Rifampin (Enhances the metabolism of concurrently administered fluconazole and decreases fluconazole AUC significantly). Products include:
- Rifadin 765
- Rifamate Capsules 767
- Rifater Tablets 769

Tacrolimus (Co-administration has resulted in nephrotoxicity). Products include:
- Prograf 1393
- Protopic Ointment 1397

Terfenadine (Co-administration of fluconazole at a dose of 400 mg per day or greater has resulted in significant increases in plasma levels of terfenadine resulting in prolonged QTc interval; combined use of fluconazole at doses lower than 400 mg/day should be carefully monitored; co-administration of multiple doses of fluconazole at doses of 400 mg or higher is contraindicated).
- No products indexed under this heading.

Theophylline (Increased serum concentrations of theophylline). Products include:
- Aerolate 1361
- Theo-Dur Extended-Release Tablets 1835
- Uni-Dur Extended-Release Tablets .. 1841
- Uniphyl 400 mg and 600 mg Tablets 2903

Theophylline Calcium Salicylate (Increased serum concentrations of theophylline).
- No products indexed under this heading.

Theophylline Sodium Glycinate (Increased serum concentrations of theophylline).
- No products indexed under this heading.

Tolazamide (Co-administration with sulfonylurea oral hypoglycemic agent may precipitate clinically significant hypoglycemia).
- No products indexed under this heading.

Tolbutamide (Co-administration with sulfonylurea oral hypoglycemic agent may precipitate clinically significant hypoglycemia; reduced metabolism of tolbutamide).
- No products indexed under this heading.

Valproic Acid (The incidence of abnormally elevated serum transaminase was greater in patients taking Diflucan concomitantly with isoniazid). Products include:
- Depakene 421

Warfarin Sodium (Co-administration has resulted in a significant increase in prothrombin time response (area under the prothrombin time-time curve); monitoring of prothrombin time is recommended). Products include:
- Coumadin for Injection 1243
- Coumadin Tablets 1243
- Warfarin Sodium Tablets, USP 3302

Zidovudine (Potential for a significant increase in zidovudine AUC (20% ±32%) following the administration of fluconazole). Products include:
- Combivir Tablets 1502
- Retrovir 1625
- Retrovir IV Infusion 1629
- Trizivir Tablets 1669

DIGIBIND POWDER

(Digoxin Immune Fab (Ovine)) 1514
None cited in PDR database.

DIGITEK TABLETS

(Digoxin) 1003

May interact with antacids, beta blockers, calcium channel blockers, corticosteroids, macrolide antibiotics, potassium-depleting diuretics, quinidine, sympathomimetics, tetracyclines, thyroid preparations, and certain other agents. Compounds in these categories include:

Acebutolol Hydrochloride (Co-administration of digoxin and beta blockers may result in the additive effects on AV node conduction). Products include:
- Sectral Capsules 3589

Albuterol (Co-administration of digoxin and sympathomimetics increases the risk of cardiac arrhythmias). Products include:
- Proventil Inhalation Aerosol 3142
- Ventolin Inhalation Aerosol and Refill 1679

Albuterol Sulfate (Co-administration of digoxin and sympathomimetics increases the risk of cardiac arrhythmias). Products include:
- AccuNeb Inhalation Solution 1230
- Combivent Inhalation Aerosol 1041
- DuoNeb Inhalation Solution 1233
- Proventil Inhalation Solution 0.083% 3146
- Proventil Repetabs Tablets 3148
- Proventil Solution for Inhalation 0.5% 3144
- Proventil HFA Inhalation Aerosol 3150
- Ventolin HFA Inhalation Aerosol 3618
- Volmax Extended-Release Tablets .. 2276

Alprazolam (Co-administration of digoxin with alprazolam raises the serum digoxin concentration due to reduction in clearance and/or in volume of distribution of the drug with implication that digitalis toxicity may result). Products include:
- Xanax Tablets 2865

Aluminum Carbonate (Antacids may interfere with intestinal digoxin absorption resulting in unexpectedly low serum concentrations).
- No products indexed under this heading.

Aluminum Hydroxide (Antacids may interfere with intestinal digoxin absorption resulting in unexpectedly low serum concentrations). Products include:
- Amphojel Suspension (Mint Flavor) .... ▣789
- Gaviscon Extra Strength Liquid .... ▣751
- Gaviscon Extra Strength Tablets .... ▣751
- Gaviscon Regular Strength Liquid .... ▣751
- Gaviscon Regular Strength Tablets .... ▣750
- Maalox Antacid/Anti-Gas Oral Suspension .... ▣673
- Maalox Max Maximum Strength Antacid/Anti-Gas Liquid 2300
- Maalox Regular Strength Antacid/Antigas Liquid 2300
- Mylanta 1813
- Vanquish Caplets .... ▣617

Amiodarone Hydrochloride (Co-administration of digoxin with verapamil raises the serum digoxin concentration due to reduction in clearance and/or in volume of distribution of the drug with implication that digitalis toxicity may result). Products include:
- Cordarone Intravenous 3491
- Cordarone Tablets 3487
- Pacerone Tablets 3331

Amlodipine Besylate (Co-administration of digoxin and calcium channel blockers may result in the additive effects on AV node conduction). Products include:
- Lotrel Capsules 2370
- Norvasc Tablets 2704

Amphotericin B (Can cause hypokalemia or hypomagnesemia and potassium or magnesium depletion can sensitize the myocardium to digoxin resulting in digitalis toxicity). Products include:
- Abelcet Injection 1273
- AmBisome for Injection 1383
- Amphotec 1774

Anticancer Drugs, unspecified (Certain anticancer drugs may interfere with intestinal digoxin absorption resulting in unexpectedly low serum concentrations).

Atenolol (Co-administration of digoxin and beta blockers may result in the additive effects on AV node conduction). Products include:
- Tenoretic Tablets 690
- Tenormin I.V. Injection 692

Azithromycin Dihydrate (Co-administration with erythromycin and other macrolide antibiotics may increase digoxin absorption in patients with inactivate digoxin by bacterial metabolism in the lower intestine, so that digitalis intoxication may result). Products include:
- Zithromax 2743
- Zithromax for IV Infusion 2748
- Zithromax for Oral Suspension, 300 mg, 600 mg, 900 mg, 1200 mg 2739
- Zithromax Tablets, 250 mg 2739

Bendroflumethiazide (Potassium-depleting diuretics can cause hypokalemia and co-administration can result in digitalis toxicity). Products include:
- Corzide 40/5 Tablets 2247
- Corzide 80/5 Tablets 2247

Bepridil Hydrochloride (Co-administration of digoxin and calcium channel blockers may result in the additive effects on AV node conduction). Products include:
- Vascor Tablets 2602

Betamethasone Acetate (Corticosteroids can cause hypokalemia or hypomagnesemia and potassium or magnesium depletion can sensitize the myocardium to digoxin resulting in digitalis toxicity). Products include:
- Celestone Soluspan Injectable Suspension 3097

Betamethasone Sodium Phosphate (Corticosteroids can cause hypokalemia or hypomagnesemia and potassium or magnesium depletion can sensitize the myocardium to digoxin resulting in digitalis toxicity). Products include:
- Celestone Soluspan Injectable Suspension 3097

Betaxolol Hydrochloride (Co-administration of digoxin and beta blockers may result in the additive effects on AV node conduction). Products include:
- Betoptic S Ophthalmic Suspension 537

Bisoprolol Fumarate (Co-administration of digoxin and beta blockers may result in the additive effects on AV node conduction). Products include:
- Zebeta Tablets 1885
- Ziac Tablets 1887

Bumetanide (Potassium-depleting diuretics can cause hypokalemia and co-administration can result in digitalis toxicity).
- No products indexed under this heading.

Calcium, intravenous (Co-administration with calcium, particularly if administered rapidly by the intravenous route may produce serious arrhythmias in digitalized patients).
- No products indexed under this heading.

Carteolol Hydrochloride (Co-administration of digoxin and beta blockers may result in the additive effects on AV node conduction). Products include:
- Carteolol Hydrochloride Ophthalmic Solution USP, 1% .... ⊙258
- Ocupress Ophthalmic Solution, 1% Sterile .... ⊙303

Chlorothiazide (Potassium-depleting diuretics can cause hypokalemia and co-administration can result in digitalis toxicity). Products include:
- Aldoclor Tablets 2035
- Diuril Oral 2087

Chlorothiazide Sodium (Potassium-depleting diuretics can cause hypokalemia and co-administration can result in digitalis toxicity). Products include:
- Diuril Sodium Intravenous 2086

Cholestyramine (May interfere with intestinal digoxin absorption resulting in unexpectedly low serum concentrations).
- No products indexed under this heading.

Clarithromycin (Co-administration with erythromycin and other macrolide antibiotics may increase digoxin absorption in patients with inactivate digoxin by bacterial metabolism in the lower intestine, so that digitalis intoxication may result). Products include:
- Biaxin/Biaxin XL 403
- PREVPAC 3298

Cortisone Acetate (Corticosteroids can cause hypokalemia or hypomagnesemia and potassium or magnesium depletion can sensitize the myocardium to digoxin resulting in digitalis toxicity). Products include:
- Cortone Acetate Injectable Suspension 2059
- Cortone Acetate Tablets 2061

Demeclocycline Hydrochloride (Co-administration with tetracyclines may increase digoxin absorption in patients with inactivate digoxin by bacterial metabolism in the lower intestine, so that digitalis intoxication may result). Products include:
- Declomycin Tablets 1855

Dexamethasone (Corticosteroids can cause hypokalemia or hypomagnesemia and potassium or magnesium depletion can sensitize the myocardium to digoxin resulting in digitalis toxicity). Products include:
- Decadron Elixir 2078
- Decadron Tablets 2079
- TobraDex Ophthalmic Ointment 542
- TobraDex Ophthalmic Suspension .. 541

Dexamethasone Acetate (Corticosteroids can cause hypokalemia or hypomagnesemia and potassium or magnesium depletion can sensitize the myocardium to digoxin resulting in digitalis toxicity).
- No products indexed under this heading.

Dexamethasone Sodium Phosphate (Corticosteroids can cause hypokalemia or hypomagnesemia and potassium or magnesium depletion can sensitize the myocardium to digoxin resulting in digitalis toxicity). Products include:
- Decadron Phosphate Injection 2081
- Decadron Phosphate Sterile Ophthalmic Ointment 2083
- Decadron Phosphate Sterile Ophthalmic Solution 2084
- NeoDecadron Sterile Ophthalmic Solution 2144

Diltiazem Hydrochloride (Co-administration of digoxin and calcium channel blockers may result in the additive effects on AV node conduction). Products include:
- Cardizem Injectable 1018
- Cardizem Lyo-Ject Syringe 1018
- Cardizem Monovial 1018
- Cardizem CD Capsules 1016
- Tiazac Capsules 1378

Diphenoxylate Hydrochloride (Decreases gut motility and may increase digoxin absorption).
- No products indexed under this heading.

Dirithromycin (Co-administration with erythromycin and other macrolide antibiotics may increase digoxin absorption in patients with inactivate digoxin by bacterial metabolism in the lower intestine, so that digitalis intoxication may result). Products include:
- Dynabac Tablets 2269

Dobutamine Hydrochloride (Co-administration of digoxin and sympathomimetics increases the risk of cardiac arrhythmias). Products include:
- Dobutrex Solution Vials 1914

Dopamine Hydrochloride (Co-administration of digoxin and sympathomimetics increases the risk of cardiac arrhythmias).
No products indexed under this heading.

Doxycycline Calcium (Co-administration with tetracyclines may increase digoxin absorption in patients with inactivate digoxin by bacterial metabolism in the lower intestine, so that digitalis intoxication may result). Products include:
Vibramycin Calcium Oral Suspension Syrup 2735

Doxycycline Hyclate (Co-administration with tetracyclines may increase digoxin absorption in patients with inactivate digoxin by bacterial metabolism in the lower intestine, so that digitalis intoxication may result). Products include:
Doryx Coated Pellet Filled Capsules 3357
Periostat Tablets 1208
Vibramycin Hyclate Capsules 2735
Vibramycin Hyclate Intravenous 2737
Vibra-Tabs Film Coated Tablets 2735

Doxycycline Monohydrate (Co-administration with tetracyclines may increase digoxin absorption in patients with inactivate digoxin by bacterial metabolism in the lower intestine, so that digitalis intoxication may result). Products include:
Monodox Capsules 2442
Vibramycin Monohydrate for Oral Suspension 2735

Ephedrine Hydrochloride (Co-administration of digoxin and sympathomimetics increases the risk of cardiac arrhythmias). Products include:
Primatene Tablets .... ▣780

Ephedrine Sulfate (Co-administration of digoxin and sympathomimetics increases the risk of cardiac arrhythmias).
No products indexed under this heading.

Ephedrine Tannate (Co-administration of digoxin and sympathomimetics increases the risk of cardiac arrhythmias). Products include:
Rynatuss Pediatric Suspension 3353
Rynatuss Tablets 3353

Epinephrine (Co-administration of digoxin and sympathomimetics increases the risk of cardiac arrhythmias). Products include:
Epifrin Sterile Ophthalmic Solution .... ⊙235
EpiPen 1236
Primatene Mist .... ▣779
Xylocaine with Epinephrine Injection 653

Epinephrine Bitartrate (Co-administration of digoxin and sympathomimetics increases the risk of cardiac arrhythmias). Products include:
Sensorcaine 643

Epinephrine Hydrochloride (Co-administration of digoxin and sympathomimetics increases the risk of cardiac arrhythmias).
No products indexed under this heading.

Erythromycin (Co-administration with erythromycin and other macrolide antibiotics may increase digoxin absorption in patients with inactivate digoxin by bacterial metabolism in the lower intestine, so that digitalis intoxication may result). Products include:
Emgel 2% Topical Gel 1285
Ery-Tab Tablets 448
Erythromycin Base Filmtab Tablets 454
Erythromycin Delayed-Release Capsules, USP 455
PCE Dispertab Tablets 498

Erythromycin Estolate (Co-administration with erythromycin and other macrolide antibiotics may increase digoxin absorption in patients with inactivate digoxin by bacterial metabolism in the lower intestine, so that digitalis intoxication may result).
No products indexed under this heading.

Erythromycin Ethylsuccinate (Co-administration with erythromycin and other macrolide antibiotics may increase digoxin absorption in patients with inactivate digoxin by bacterial metabolism in the lower intestine, so that digitalis intoxication may result). Products include:
E.E.S. 450
EryPed 446
Pediazole Suspension 3050

Erythromycin Gluceptate (Co-administration with erythromycin and other macrolide antibiotics may increase digoxin absorption in patients with inactivate digoxin by bacterial metabolism in the lower intestine, so that digitalis intoxication may result).
No products indexed under this heading.

Erythromycin Stearate (Co-administration with erythromycin and other macrolide antibiotics may increase digoxin absorption in patients with inactivate digoxin by bacterial metabolism in the lower intestine, so that digitalis intoxication may result). Products include:
Erythrocin Stearate Filmtab Tablets 452

Esmolol Hydrochloride (Co-administration of digoxin and beta blockers may result in the additive effects on AV node conduction). Products include:
Brevibloc Injection 858

Ethacrynic Acid (Potassium-depleting diuretics can cause hypokalemia and co-administration can result in digitalis toxicity). Products include:
Edecrin Tablets 2091

Felodipine (Co-administration of digoxin and calcium channel blockers may result in the additive effects on AV node conduction). Products include:
Lexxel Tablets 608
Plendil Extended-Release Tablets 623

Fludrocortisone Acetate (Corticosteroids can cause hypokalemia or hypomagnesemia and potassium or magnesium depletion can sensitize the myocardium to digoxin resulting in digitalis toxicity). Products include:
Florinef Acetate Tablets 2250

Furosemide (Potassium-depleting diuretics can cause hypokalemia and co-administration can result in digitalis toxicity). Products include:
Furosemide Tablets 2284

Hydrochlorothiazide (Potassium-depleting diuretics can cause hypokalemia and co-administration can result in digitalis toxicity). Products include:
Accuretic Tablets 2614
Aldoril Tablets 2039
Atacand HCT Tablets 597
Avalide Tablets 1070
Diovan HCT Tablets 2338
Dyazide Capsules 1515
HydroDIURIL Tablets 2108
Hyzaar 2109
Inderide Tablets 3517
Inderide LA Long-Acting Capsules 3519
Lotensin HCT Tablets 2367
Maxzide 1008
Micardis HCT Tablets 1051
Microzide Capsules 3414
Moduretic Tablets 2138
Monopril HCT 1094
Prinzide Tablets 2168
Timolide Tablets 2187
Uniretic Tablets 3178
Vaseretic Tablets 2204
Zestoretic Tablets 695
Ziac Tablets 1887

Hydrocortisone (Corticosteroids can cause hypokalemia or hypomagnesemia and potassium or magnesium depletion can sensitize the myocardium to digoxin resulting in digitalis toxicity). Products include:
Anusol-HC Cream 2.5% 2237
Cipro HC Otic Suspension 540
Cortaid Intensive Therapy Cream .... ▣717
Cortaid Maximum Strength Cream .... ▣717
Cortisporin Ophthalmic Suspension Sterile .... ⊙297
Cortizone•5 .... ▣699
Cortizone•10 .... ▣699
Cortizone•10 Plus Creme .... ▣700
Cortizone for Kids Creme .... ▣699
Hydrocortone Tablets 2106
Massengill Medicated Soft Cloth Towelette .... ▣753
VōSoL HC Otic Solution 3356

Hydrocortisone Acetate (Corticosteroids can cause hypokalemia or hypomagnesemia and potassium or magnesium depletion can sensitize the myocardium to digoxin resulting in digitalis toxicity). Products include:
Analpram-HC 1338
Anusol HC-1 Hydrocortisone Anti-Itch Cream .... ▣689
Anusol-HC Suppositories 2238
Cortaid .... ▣717
Cortifoam Rectal Foam 3170
Cortisporin-TC Otic Suspension 2246
Hydrocortone Acetate Injectable Suspension 2103
Pramosone 1343
Proctocort Suppositories 2264
ProctoFoam-HC 3177
Terra-Cortril Ophthalmic Suspension 2716

Hydrocortisone Sodium Phosphate (Corticosteroids can cause hypokalemia or hypomagnesemia and potassium or magnesium depletion can sensitize the myocardium to digoxin resulting in digitalis toxicity). Products include:
Hydrocortone Phosphate Injection, Sterile 2105

Hydrocortisone Sodium Succinate (Corticosteroids can cause hypokalemia or hypomagnesemia and potassium or magnesium depletion can sensitize the myocardium to digoxin resulting in digitalis toxicity).
No products indexed under this heading.

Hydroflumethiazide (Potassium-depleting diuretics can cause hypokalemia and co-administration can result in digitalis toxicity). Products include:
Diucardin Tablets 3494

Indomethacin (Co-administration of digoxin with indomethacin raises the serum digoxin concentration due to reduction in clearance and/or in volume of distribution of the drug with implication that digitalis toxicity may result). Products include:
Indocin 2112

Indomethacin Sodium Trihydrate (Co-administration of digoxin with indomethacin raises the serum digoxin concentration due to reduction in clearance and/or in volume of distribution of the drug with implication that digitalis toxicity may result). Products include:
Indocin I.V. 2115

Isoproterenol Hydrochloride (Co-administration of digoxin and sympathomimetics increases the risk of cardiac arrhythmias).
No products indexed under this heading.

Isoproterenol Sulfate (Co-administration of digoxin and sympathomimetics increases the risk of cardiac arrhythmias).
No products indexed under this heading.

Isradipine (Co-administration of digoxin and calcium channel blockers may result in the additive effects on AV node conduction). Products include:
DynaCirc Capsules 2921
DynaCirc CR Tablets 2923

Itraconazole (Co-administration of digoxin with itraconazole raises the serum digoxin concentration due to reduction in clearance and/or in volume of distribution of the drug with implication that digitalis toxicity may result). Products include:
Sporanox Capsules 1800
Sporanox Injection 1804
Sporanox Injection 2509
Sporanox Oral Solution 1808
Sporanox Oral Solution 2512

Kaolin (May interfere with intestinal digoxin absorption resulting in unexpectedly low serum concentrations).
No products indexed under this heading.

Labetalol Hydrochloride (Co-administration of digoxin and beta blockers may result in the additive effects on AV node conduction). Products include:
Normodyne Injection 3135
Normodyne Tablets 3137

Levalbuterol Hydrochloride (Co-administration of digoxin and sympathomimetics increases the risk of cardiac arrhythmias). Products include:
Xopenex Inhalation Solution 3207

Levobunolol Hydrochloride (Co-administration of digoxin and beta blockers may result in the additive effects on AV node conduction). Products include:
Betagan .... ⊙228

Levothyroxine Sodium (Thyroid administration to a digitalized, hypothyroid patient may increase the dose requirement of digoxin). Products include:
Levothroid Tablets 1373
Levoxyl Tablets 1819
Synthroid 505
Unithroid Tablets 3445

Liothyronine Sodium (Thyroid administration to a digitalized, hypothyroid patient may increase the dose requirement of digoxin). Products include:
Cytomel Tablets 1817
Triostat Injection 1825

Liotrix (Thyroid administration to a digitalized, hypothyroid patient may increase the dose requirement of digoxin).
No products indexed under this heading.

Magaldrate (Antacids may interfere with intestinal digoxin absorption resulting in unexpectedly low serum concentrations).
No products indexed under this heading.

Magnesium Hydroxide (Antacids may interfere with intestinal digoxin absorption resulting in unexpectedly low serum concentrations). Products include:
Ex•Lax Milk of Magnesia Liquid .... ▣670
Maalox Antacid/Anti-Gas Oral Suspension .... ▣673
Maalox Max Maximum Strength Antacid/Anti-Gas Liquid 2300
Maalox Regular Strength Antacid/Antigas Liquid 2300
Mylanta Fast-Acting 1813
Mylanta 1813
Pepcid Complete Chewable Tablets 1815
Phillips' Chewable Tablets .... ▣615
Phillips' Milk of Magnesia Liquid (Original, Cherry, & Mint) .... ▣616
Rolaids Tablets .... ▣706
Extra Strength Rolaids Tablets .... ▣706
Vanquish Caplets .... ▣617

Magnesium Oxide (Antacids may interfere with intestinal digoxin absorption resulting in unexpectedly low serum concentrations). Products include:
Beelith Tablets 946

Mag-Ox 400 Tablets 1024
Uro-Mag Capsules 1024

Metaproterenol Sulfate (Co-administration of digoxin and sympathomimetics increases the risk of cardiac arrhythmias). Products include:
Alupent 1029

Metaraminol Bitartrate (Co-administration of digoxin and sympathomimetics increases the risk of cardiac arrhythmias). Products include:
Aramine Injection 2043

Methacycline Hydrochloride (Co-administration with tetracyclines may increase digoxin absorption in patients with inactivate digoxin by bacterial metabolism in the lower intestine, so that digitalis intoxication may result).
No products indexed under this heading.

Methoxamine Hydrochloride (Co-administration of digoxin and sympathomimetics increases the risk of cardiac arrhythmias).
No products indexed under this heading.

Methyclothiazide (Potassium-depleting diuretics can cause hypokalemia and co-administration can result in digitalis toxicity).
No products indexed under this heading.

Methylprednisolone Acetate (Corticosteroids can cause hypokalemia or hypomagnesemia and potassium or magnesium depletion can sensitize the myocardium to digoxin resulting in digitalis toxicity). Products include:
Depo-Medrol Injectable Suspension 2795

Methylprednisolone Sodium Succinate (Corticosteroids can cause hypokalemia or hypomagnesemia and potassium or magnesium depletion can sensitize the myocardium to digoxin resulting in digitalis toxicity). Products include:
Solu-Medrol Sterile Powder 2855

Metipranolol Hydrochloride (Co-administration of digoxin and beta blockers may result in the additive effects on AV node conduction).
No products indexed under this heading.

Metoclopramide Hydrochloride (May interfere with intestinal digoxin absorption resulting in unexpectedly low serum concentrations). Products include:
Reglan 2935

Metoprolol Succinate (Co-administration of digoxin and beta blockers may result in the additive effects on AV node conduction). Products include:
Toprol-XL Tablets 651

Metoprolol Tartrate (Co-administration of digoxin and beta blockers may result in the additive effects on AV node conduction).
No products indexed under this heading.

Mibefradil Dihydrochloride (Co-administration of digoxin and calcium channel blockers may result in the additive effects on AV node conduction).
No products indexed under this heading.

Minocycline Hydrochloride (Co-administration with tetracyclines may increase digoxin absorption in patients with inactivate digoxin by bacterial metabolism in the lower intestine, so that digitalis intoxication may result). Products include:
Dynacin Capsules 2019
Minocin Intravenous 1862
Minocin Oral Suspension 1865
Minocin Pellet-Filled Capsules 1863

Nadolol (Co-administration of digoxin and beta blockers may result in the additive effects on AV node conduction). Products include:
Corgard Tablets 2245
Corzide 40/5 Tablets 2247
Corzide 80/5 Tablets 2247
Nadolol Tablets 2288

Neomycin, oral (May interfere with intestinal digoxin absorption resulting in unexpectedly low serum concentrations).

Nicardipine Hydrochloride (Co-administration of digoxin and calcium channel blockers may result in the additive effects on AV node conduction). Products include:
Cardene I.V. 3485

Nifedipine (Co-administration of digoxin and calcium channel blockers may result in the additive effects on AV node conduction). Products include:
Adalat CC Tablets 877
Procardia Capsules 2708
Procardia XL Extended Release Tablets 2710

Nimodipine (Co-administration of digoxin and calcium channel blockers may result in the additive effects on AV node conduction). Products include:
Nimotop Capsules 904

Nisoldipine (Co-administration of digoxin and calcium channel blockers may result in the additive effects on AV node conduction). Products include:
Sular Tablets 688

Norepinephrine Bitartrate (Co-administration of digoxin and sympathomimetics increases the risk of cardiac arrhythmias).
No products indexed under this heading.

Oxytetracycline Hydrochloride (Co-administration with tetracyclines may increase digoxin absorption in patients with inactivate digoxin by bacterial metabolism in the lower intestine, so that digitalis intoxication may result). Products include:
Terra-Cortril Ophthalmic Suspension 2716
Urobiotic-250 Capsules 2731

Pectin (May interfere with intestinal digoxin absorption resulting in unexpectedly low serum concentrations). Products include:
Celestial Seasonings Soothers Throat Drops .... ■ 685
Halls Plus Cough Drops .... ■ 686

Penbutolol Sulfate (Co-administration of digoxin and beta blockers may result in the additive effects on AV node conduction).
No products indexed under this heading.

Penicillamine (Co-administration has resulted in inconsistent reports regarding the effects of penicillamine on serum digoxin concentration). Products include:
Cuprimine Capsules 2075
Depen Titratable Tablets 3341

Phenylephrine Bitartrate (Co-administration of digoxin and sympathomimetics increases the risk of cardiac arrhythmias).
No products indexed under this heading.

Phenylephrine Hydrochloride (Co-administration of digoxin and sympathomimetics increases the risk of cardiac arrhythmias). Products include:
Afrin Nasal Decongestant Children's Pump Mist .... ■ 734
Extendryl 1361
Hycomine Compound Tablets 1317
Neo-Synephrine .... ■ 614
Phenergan VC Syrup 3560
Phenergan VC with Codeine Syrup 3561
Preparation H Cream .... ■ 778
Preparation H Cooling Gel .... ■ 778
Preparation H .... ■ 778
Vicks Sinex Nasal Spray and Ultra Fine Mist .... ■ 729

Phenylephrine Tannate (Co-administration of digoxin and sympathomimetics increases the risk of cardiac arrhythmias). Products include:
Ryna-12 S Suspension 3351
Reformulated Rynatan Pediatric Suspension 3352
Rynatuss Pediatric Suspension 3353
Rynatuss Tablets 3353

Phenylpropanolamine Hydrochloride (Co-administration of digoxin and sympathomimetics increases the risk of cardiac arrhythmias).
No products indexed under this heading.

Pindolol (Co-administration of digoxin and beta blockers may result in the additive effects on AV node conduction).
No products indexed under this heading.

Pirbuterol Acetate (Co-administration of digoxin and sympathomimetics increases the risk of cardiac arrhythmias). Products include:
Maxair Autohaler 1981
Maxair Inhaler 1984

Polythiazide (Potassium-depleting diuretics can cause hypokalemia and co-administration can result in digitalis toxicity). Products include:
Minizide Capsules 2700
Renese Tablets 2712

Prednisolone Acetate (Corticosteroids can cause hypokalemia or hypomagnesemia and potassium or magnesium depletion can sensitize the myocardium to digoxin resulting in digitalis toxicity). Products include:
Blephamide Ophthalmic Ointment 547
Blephamide Ophthalmic Suspension 548
Poly-Pred Liquifilm Ophthalmic Suspension .... ⊙ 245
Pred Forte Ophthalmic Suspension .... ⊙ 246
Pred Mild Sterile Ophthalmic Suspension .... ⊙ 249
Pred-G Ophthalmic Suspension .... ⊙ 247
Pred-G Sterile Ophthalmic Ointment .... ⊙ 248

Prednisolone Sodium Phosphate (Corticosteroids can cause hypokalemia or hypomagnesemia and potassium or magnesium depletion can sensitize the myocardium to digoxin resulting in digitalis toxicity). Products include:
Pediapred Oral Solution 1170

Prednisolone Tebutate (Corticosteroids can cause hypokalemia or hypomagnesemia and potassium or magnesium depletion can sensitize the myocardium to digoxin resulting in digitalis toxicity).
No products indexed under this heading.

Prednisone (Corticosteroids can cause hypokalemia or hypomagnesemia and potassium or magnesium depletion can sensitize the myocardium to digoxin resulting in digitalis toxicity). Products include:
Prednisone 3064

Propafenone Hydrochloride (Co-administration of digoxin with propafenone raises the serum digoxin concentration due to reduction in clearance and/or in volume of distribution of the drug with implication that digitalis toxicity may result). Products include:
Rythmol Tablets – 150 mg, 225 mg, 300 mg 502

Propantheline Bromide (Decreases gut motility and may increase digoxin absorption).
No products indexed under this heading.

Propranolol Hydrochloride (Co-administration of digoxin and beta blockers may result in the additive effects on AV node conduction). Products include:
Inderal 3513
Inderal LA Long-Acting Capsules 3516
Inderide Tablets 3517
Inderide LA Long-Acting Capsules 3519

Pseudoephedrine Hydrochloride (Co-administration of digoxin and sympathomimetics increases the risk of cardiac arrhythmias). Products include:
Actifed Cold & Allergy Tablets .... ■ 688
Actifed Cold & Sinus Caplets and Tablets .... ■ 688
Advil Cold and Sinus Caplets .... ■ 771
Advil Cold and Sinus Tablets .... ■ 771
Advil Flu & Body Ache Caplets .... ■ 772
Aleve Cold & Sinus Caplets .... ■ 603
Alka-Seltzer Plus Liqui-Gels .... ■ 604
Alka-Seltzer Plus Cold & Flu Medicine Liqui-Gels .... ■ 604
Alka-Seltzer Plus Cold & Sinus Medicine Liqui-Gels .... ■ 604
Allegra-D Extended-Release Tablets 714
BC Cold Powder .... ■ 619
Benadryl Allergy/Cold Tablets .... ■ 691
Benadryl Allergy/Congestion Tablets .... ■ 692
Benadryl Allergy & Sinus Liquid .... ■ 693
Benadryl Allergy & Sinus Fastmelt Tablets .... ■ 693
Benadryl Allergy Sinus Headache Caplets & Gelcaps .... ■ 693
Benadryl Severe Allergy & Sinus Headache Caplets .... ■ 694
Benadryl Children's Allergy/Cold Fastmelt Tablets .... ■ 692
Benylin Multi-Symptom Liquid .... ■ 697
Bromfed Capsules (Extended-Release) 2269
Bromfed-PD Capsules (Extended-Release) 2269
Children's Cēpacol Sore Throat .... ■ 788
Comtrex Acute Head Cold & Sinus Pressure Relief Tablets .... ■ 627
Comtrex Deep Chest Cold & Congestion Relief Softgels .... ■ 627
Comtrex Flu Therapy & Fever Relief Daytime Caplets .... ■ 628
Comtrex Flu Therapy & Fever Relief Nighttime Tablets .... ■ 628
Comtrex Maximum Strength Multi-Symptom Cold & Cough Relief Tablets and Caplets .... ■ 626
Contac Non-Drowsy 12 Hour Cold Caplets .... ■ 745
Contac Non-Drowsy Timed Release 12 Hour Cold Caplets .... ■ 746
Contac Severe Cold and Flu Caplets Maximum Strength .... ■ 746
Contac Severe Cold and Flu Caplets Non-Drowsy .... ■ 746
Dimetapp Elixir .... ■ 777
Dimetapp Cold and Fever Suspension .... ■ 775
Dimetapp DM Cold & Cough Elixir .... ■ 775
Dimetapp Nighttime Flu Liquid .... ■ 776
Dimetapp Non-Drowsy Flu Syrup .... ■ 777
Dimetapp Infant Drops Decongestant .... ■ 775
Dimetapp Infant Drops Decongestant Plus Cough .... ■ 776
Guaifed 2272
Kronofed-A 1341
Children's Motrin Cold Oral Suspension 2007
Motrin Sinus Headache Caplets 2005
PediaCare Cough-Cold Liquid .... ■ 719
PediaCare Infants' Drops Decongestant .... ■ 719
PediaCare Infants' Drops Decongestant Plus Cough .... ■ 719
PediaCare NightRest Cough-Cold Liquid .... ■ 719
Robitussin Cold Caplets Cold & Congestion .... ■ 780
Robitussin Cold Softgels Cold & Congestion .... ■ 780
Robitussin Cold Caplets Multi-Symptom Cold & Flu .... ■ 781
Robitussin Cold Softgels Multi-Symptom Cold & Flu .... ■ 781
Robitussin Cold Softgels Severe Congestion .... ■ 782
Robitussin Cough & Cold Infant Drops .... ■ 782
Robitussin Maximum Strength Cough & Cold Liquid .... ■ 785
Robitussin Pediatric Cough & Cold Formula Liquid .... ■ 785
Robitussin Multi Symptom Honey Flu Liquid .... ■ 785

Robitussin Nighttime Honey Flu Liquid .... ▣786
Robitussin-CF Liquid .... ▣783
Robitussin-DAC Syrup 2942
Robitussin-PE Liquid .... ▣782
Ryna .... ▣768
Semprex-D Capsules 1172
Singlet Caplets .... ▣761
Sinutab Non-Drying Liquid Caps .... ▣706
Sinutab Sinus Allergy Medication, Maximum Strength Formula, Tablets & Caplets .... ▣707
Sinutab Sinus Medication, Maximum Strength Without Drowsiness Formula, Tablets & Caplets .... ▣707
Sudafed 12 Hour Tablets .... ▣708
Sudafed 24 Hour Tablets .... ▣708
Children's Sudafed Cold & Cough Liquid .... ▣709
Children's Sudafed Nasal Decongestant Chewables .... ▣711
Children's Sudafed Nasal Decongestant Liquid Medication .... ▣711
Sudafed Cold & Allergy Tablets .... ▣708
Sudafed Cold & Cough Liquid Caps .... ▣709
Sudafed Cold & Sinus Liquid Caps .... ▣710
Sudafed Nasal Decongestant Tablets .... ▣710
Sudafed Non-Drying Sinus Liquid Caps .... ▣712
Sudafed Severe Cold .... ▣711
Sudafed Sinus Headache Caplets .... ▣712
Sudafed Sinus Headache Tablets .... ▣712
Tavist Sinus Non-Drowsy Coated Caplets .... ▣676
TheraFlu Regular Strength Cold & Cough Night Time Hot Liquid .... ▣676
TheraFlu Regular Strength Cold & Sore Throat Night Time Hot Liquid .... ▣676
TheraFlu Maximum Strength Flu & Congestion Non-Drowsy Hot Liquid .... ▣677
TheraFlu Maximum Strength Flu & Cough Night Time Hot Liquid .... ▣678
TheraFlu Maximum Strength Flu & Sore Throat Night Time Hot Liquid .... ▣677
TheraFlu Maximum Strength Severe Cold & Congestion Night Time Caplets .... ▣678
TheraFlu Maximum Strength Severe Cold & Congestion Night Time Hot Liquid .... ▣678
TheraFlu Maximum Strength Severe Cold & Congestion Non-Drowsy .... ▣679
Triaminic Allergy Congestion Liquid .... ▣680
Triaminic Chest Congestion Liquid .... ▣680
Triaminic Cold & Allergy Liquid .... ▣681
Triaminic Cold & Allergy Softchews .... ▣683
Triaminic Cold & Cough Liquid .... ▣681
Triaminic Cold & Cough Softchews .... ▣683
Triaminic Cold & Night Time Cough Liquid .... ▣681
Triaminic Cold, Cough & Fever Liquid .... ▣681
Triaminic Cough Liquid .... ▣682
Triaminic Cough & Congestion Liquid .... ▣682
Triaminic Cough & Sore Throat Liquid .... ▣682
Triaminic Cough & Sore Throat Softchews .... ▣684
Children's Tylenol Allergy-D Liquid 2014
Children's Tylenol Cold Suspension Liquid and Chewable Tablets 2015
Children's Tylenol Cold Plus Cough Suspension Liquid and Chewable Tablets 2015
Children's Tylenol Flu Suspension Liquid 2015
Children's Tylenol Sinus Suspension Liquid 2017
Infants' Tylenol Cold Decongestant and Fever Reducer Concentrated Drops 2015
Infants' Tylenol Cold Decongestant and Fever Reducer Concentrated Drops Plus Cough 2015
Tylenol Allergy Sinus 2010
Multi-Symptom Tylenol Cold Complete Formula Caplets 2010
Multi-Symptom Tylenol Cold Non-Drowsy Caplets and Gelcaps 2010
Multi-Symptom Tylenol Cold Severe Congestion Non-Drowsy Caplets 2011
Maximum Strength Tylenol Flu NightTime Gelcaps 2011
Maximum Strength Tylenol Flu NightTime Liquid 2011
Maximum Strength Tylenol Flu Non-Drowsy Gelcaps 2011
Maximum Strength Tylenol Sinus NightTime Caplets 2012
Maximum Strength Tylenol Sinus Non-Drowsy Geltabs, Gelcaps, Caplets, and Tablets 2012
Vicks 44D Cough & Head Congestion Relief Liquid .... ▣724
Vicks 44M Cough, Cold & Flu Relief Liquid .... ▣725
Pediatric Vicks 44m Cough & Cold Relief .... ▣728
Vicks DayQuil LiquiCaps/Liquid Multi-Symptom Cold/Flu Relief .... ▣727
Children's Vicks NyQuil Cold/Cough Relief .... ▣726
Vicks NyQuil LiquiCaps/Liquid Multi-Symptom Cold/Flu Relief, Original and Cherry Flavors .... ▣727
Zephrex Tablets 3091
Zephrex LA Tablets 3092
Zyrtec-D 12 Hour Extended Relief Tablets 2758

Pseudoephedrine Sulfate (Co-administration of digoxin and sympathomimetics increases the risk of cardiac arrhythmias). Products include:

Chlor-Trimeton Allergy/Decongestant Tablets .... ▣736
Claritin-D 12 Hour Extended Release Tablets 3102
Claritin-D 24 Hour Extended Release Tablets 3104
Coricidin 'D' Cold, Flu & Sinus Tablets .... ▣737
Drixoral Allergy/Sinus Extended-Release Tablets .... ▣741
Drixoral Cold & Allergy Sustained-Action Tablets .... ▣740
Drixoral Cold & Flu Extended-Release Tablets .... ▣740
Drixoral Nasal Decongestant Long-Acting Non-Drowsy Tablets .... ▣740
Rynatan Tablets 3351

Quinidine Gluconate (Co-administration of digoxin with quinidine raises the serum digoxin concentration due to reduction in clearance and/or in volume of distribution of the drug with implication that digitalis toxicity may result). Products include:

Quinaglute Dura-Tabs Tablets 978

Quinidine Polygalacturonate (Co-administration of digoxin with quinidine raises the serum digoxin concentration due to reduction in clearance and/or in volume of distribution of the drug with implication that digitalis toxicity may result).

No products indexed under this heading.

Quinidine Sulfate (Co-administration of digoxin with quinidine raises the serum digoxin concentration due to reduction in clearance and/or in volume of distribution of the drug with implication that digitalis toxicity may result). Products include:

Quinidex Extentabs 2933

Quinine (Co-administration has resulted in inconsistent reports regarding the effects of quinine on serum digoxin concentration).

No products indexed under this heading.

Rifampin (May decrease serum digoxin concentration, especially in patients with renal dysfunction, by increasing the non-renal clearance of digoxin). Products include:

Rifadin 765
Rifamate Capsules 767
Rifater Tablets 769

Salmeterol Xinafoate (Co-administration of digoxin and sympathomimetics increases the risk of cardiac arrhythmias). Products include:

Advair Diskus 100/50 1448
Advair Diskus 250/50 1448
Advair Diskus 500/50 1448
Serevent Diskus 1637
Serevent Inhalation Aerosol 1633

Sodium Bicarbonate (Antacids may interfere with intestinal digoxin absorption resulting in unexpectedly low serum concentrations). Products include:

Alka-Seltzer .... ▣603
Alka-Seltzer Lemon Lime Antacid and Pain Reliever Effervescent Tablets .... ▣603
Alka-Seltzer Extra Strength Antacid and Pain Reliever Effervescent Tablets .... ▣603
Alka-Seltzer Heartburn Relief Tablets .... ▣604
Ceo-Two Evacuant Suppository .... ▣618
Colyte with Flavor Packs for Oral Solution 3170
GoLYTELY and Pineapple Flavor GoLYTELY for Oral Solution 1068
NuLYTELY, Cherry Flavor, Lemon-Lime Flavor, and Orange Flavor NuLYTELY for Oral Solution 1068

Sotalol Hydrochloride (Co-administration of digoxin and beta blockers may result in the additive effects on AV node conduction). Products include:

Betapace Tablets 950
Betapace AF Tablets 954

Spironolactone (Co-administration of digoxin with spironolactone raises the serum digoxin concentration due to reduction in clearance and/or in volume of distribution of the drug with implication that digitalis toxicity may result).

No products indexed under this heading.

Succinylcholine Chloride (May cause sudden extrusion of potassium from muscle cells, and may thereby cause arrhythmias in digitalized patients). Products include:

Anectine Injection 1476

Sulfasalazine (May interfere with intestinal digoxin absorption resulting in unexpectedly low serum concentrations). Products include:

Azulfidine EN-tabs Tablets 2775

Terbutaline Sulfate (Co-administration of digoxin and sympathomimetics increases the risk of cardiac arrhythmias). Products include:

Brethine Ampuls 2314
Brethine Tablets 2313

Tetracycline Hydrochloride (Co-administration with tetracyclines may increase digoxin absorption in patients with inactivate digoxin by bacterial metabolism in the lower intestine, so that digitalis intoxication may result).

No products indexed under this heading.

Thyroglobulin (Thyroid administration to a digitalized, hypothyroid patient may increase the dose requirement of digoxin).

No products indexed under this heading.

Thyroid (Thyroid administration to a digitalized, hypothyroid patient may increase the dose requirement of digoxin).

No products indexed under this heading.

Thyroxine (Thyroid administration to a digitalized, hypothyroid patient may increase the dose requirement of digoxin).

No products indexed under this heading.

Thyroxine Sodium (Thyroid administration to a digitalized, hypothyroid patient may increase the dose requirement of digoxin).

No products indexed under this heading.

Timolol Hemihydrate (Co-administration of digoxin and beta blockers may result in the additive effects on AV node conduction). Products include:

Betimol Ophthalmic Solution .... ⊙324

Timolol Maleate (Co-administration of digoxin and beta blockers may result in the additive effects on AV node conduction). Products include:

Blocadren Tablets 2046
Cosopt Sterile Ophthalmic Solution 2065
Timolide Tablets 2187
Timolol GFS .... ⊙266
Timoptic in Ocudose 2192
Timoptic Sterile Ophthalmic Solution 2190
Timoptic-XE Sterile Ophthalmic Gel Forming Solution 2194

Torsemide (Potassium-depleting diuretics can cause hypokalemia and co-administration can result in digitalis toxicity). Products include:

Demadex Tablets and Injection 2965

Triamcinolone (Corticosteroids can cause hypokalemia or hypomagnesemia and potassium or magnesium depletion can sensitize the myocardium to digoxin resulting in digitalis toxicity).

No products indexed under this heading.

Triamcinolone Acetonide (Corticosteroids can cause hypokalemia or hypomagnesemia and potassium or magnesium depletion can sensitize the myocardium to digoxin resulting in digitalis toxicity). Products include:

Azmacort Inhalation Aerosol 728
Nasacort Nasal Inhaler 750
Nasacort AQ Nasal Spray 752
Tri-Nasal Spray 2274

Triamcinolone Diacetate (Corticosteroids can cause hypokalemia or hypomagnesemia and potassium or magnesium depletion can sensitize the myocardium to digoxin resulting in digitalis toxicity).

No products indexed under this heading.

Triamcinolone Hexacetonide (Corticosteroids can cause hypokalemia or hypomagnesemia and potassium or magnesium depletion can sensitize the myocardium to digoxin resulting in digitalis toxicity).

No products indexed under this heading.

Troleandomycin (Co-administration with erythromycin and other macrolide antibiotics may increase digoxin absorption in patients with inactivate digoxin by bacterial metabolism in the lower intestine, so that digitalis intoxication may result). Products include:

Tao Capsules 2716

Verapamil Hydrochloride (Co-administration of digoxin with verapamil raises the serum digoxin concentration due to reduction in clearance and/or in volume of distribution of the drug with implication that digitalis toxicity may result). Products include:

Covera-HS Tablets 3199
Isoptin SR Tablets 467
Tarka Tablets 508
Verelan Capsules 3184
Verelan PM Capsules 3186

Food Interactions

Meal, high in bran fiber (The amount of digoxin from an oral dose may be reduced when taken with meal high in bran fiber).

Meal, unspecified (Slows the rate of absorption).

DILANTIN INFATABS

(Phenytoin) 2624

May interact with corticosteroids, oral anticoagulants, estrogens, histamine H_2-receptor antagonists, oral contraceptives, phenothiazines, salicylates, succinimides, sulfonamides, tricyclic antidepressants, theophylline, and certain other agents. Compounds in these categories include:

Aminophylline (Phenytoin impairs efficacy of theophylline).

No products indexed under this heading.

Amiodarone Hydrochloride (May increase serum phenytoin levels). Products include:
- Cordarone Intravenous 3491
- Cordarone Tablets 3487
- Pacerone Tablets 3331

Amitriptyline Hydrochloride (Tricyclic antidepressants may precipitate seizures in susceptible patients and phenytoin dosage may need to be adjusted). Products include:
- Etrafon 3115
- Limbitrol 1738

Amoxapine (Tricyclic antidepressants may precipitate seizures in susceptible patients and phenytoin dosage may need to be adjusted).
- No products indexed under this heading.

Aspirin (May increase serum phenytoin levels). Products include:
- Aggrenox Capsules 1026
- Alka-Seltzer ▣603
- Alka-Seltzer Lemon Lime Antacid and Pain Reliever Effervescent Tablets ▣603
- Alka-Seltzer Extra Strength Antacid and Pain Reliever Effervescent Tablets ▣603
- Alka-Seltzer PM Effervescent Tablets ▣605
- Genuine Bayer Tablets, Caplets and Gelcaps ▣606
- Extra Strength Bayer Caplets and Gelcaps ▣610
- Aspirin Regimen Bayer Children's Chewable Tablets (Orange or Cherry Flavored) ▣607
- Bayer, Aspirin Regimen ▣606
- Aspirin Regimen Bayer 81 mg Caplets with Calcium ▣607
- Genuine Bayer Professional Labeling (Aspirin Regimen Bayer) ▣608
- Extra Strength Bayer Arthritis Caplets ▣610
- Extra Strength Bayer Plus Caplets ▣610
- Extra Strength Bayer PM Caplets ▣611
- BC Powder ▣619
- BC Allergy Sinus Cold Powder ▣619
- Arthritis Strength BC Powder ▣619
- BC Sinus Cold Powder ▣619
- Darvon Compound-65 Pulvules 1910
- Ecotrin Enteric Coated Aspirin Low, Regular and Maximum Strength Tablets 1715
- Excedrin Extra-Strength Tablets, Caplets, and Geltabs ▣629
- Excedrin Migraine 1070
- Goody's Body Pain Formula Powder ▣620
- Goody's Extra Strength Headache Powder ▣620
- Goody's Extra Strength Pain Relief Tablets ▣620
- Percodan Tablets 1327
- Robaxisal Tablets 2939
- Soma Compound Tablets 3354
- Soma Compound w/Codeine Tablets 3355
- Vanquish Caplets ▣617

Bendroflumethiazide (May increase serum phenytoin levels). Products include:
- Corzide 40/5 Tablets 2247
- Corzide 80/5 Tablets 2247

Betamethasone Acetate (Phenytoin impairs efficacy of corticosteroids). Products include:
- Celestone Soluspan Injectable Suspension 3097

Betamethasone Sodium Phosphate (Phenytoin impairs efficacy of corticosteroids). Products include:
- Celestone Soluspan Injectable Suspension 3097

Calcium Carbonate (Calcium ions interfere with the absorption of phenytoin; ingestion times of phenytoin and antacids containing calcium should be staggered in patients with low phenytoin levels). Products include:
- Aspirin Regimen Bayer 81 mg Caplets with Calcium ▣607
- Extra Strength Bayer Plus Caplets ▣610
- Caltrate 600 Tablets ▣814
- Caltrate 600 PLUS ▣815
- Caltrate 600 + D Tablets ▣814
- Caltrate 600 + Soy Tablets ▣814
- D-Cal Chewable Caplets ▣794
- Florical Capsules and Tablets 2223
- Quick Dissolve Maalox Max Maximum Strength Antacid/Antigas Tablets 2301
- Quick Dissolve Maalox Regular Strength Antacid Tablets 2301
- Marblen Suspension ▣633
- Monocal Tablets 2223
- Mylanta Fast-Acting 1813
- Mylanta Calci Tabs ▣636
- One-A-Day Bedtime & Rest Tablets ▣805
- One-A-Day Calcium Plus Chewable Tablets ▣805
- Os-Cal Chewable Tablets ▣838
- Pepcid Complete Chewable Tablets 1815
- ReSource Wellness CalciWise Soft Chews ▣824
- Rolaids Tablets ▣706
- Extra Strength Rolaids Tablets ▣706
- Slow-Mag Tablets ▣835
- Titralac ▣640
- 3M Titralac Plus Antacid Tablets ▣640
- Tums ▣763

Carbamazepine (May decrease serum phenytoin levels). Products include:
- Carbatrol Capsules 3234
- Tegretol/Tegretol-XR 2404

Chloramphenicol (May increase serum phenytoin levels). Products include:
- Chloromycetin Ophthalmic Ointment, 1% ⊙296
- Chloromycetin Ophthalmic Solution ⊙297
- Chloroptic Sterile Ophthalmic Ointment ⊙234
- Chloroptic Sterile Ophthalmic Solution ⊙235

Chloramphenicol Palmitate (May increase serum phenytoin levels).
- No products indexed under this heading.

Chloramphenicol Sodium Succinate (May increase serum phenytoin levels).
- No products indexed under this heading.

Chlordiazepoxide (May increase serum phenytoin levels). Products include:
- Limbitrol 1738

Chlordiazepoxide Hydrochloride (May increase serum phenytoin levels). Products include:
- Librium Capsules 1736
- Librium for Injection 1737

Chlorothiazide (May increase serum phenytoin levels). Products include:
- Aldoclor Tablets 2035
- Diuril Oral 2087

Chlorothiazide Sodium (May increase serum phenytoin levels). Products include:
- Diuril Sodium Intravenous 2086

Chlorotrianisene (May increase serum phenytoin levels; phenytoin impairs efficacy of estrogens).
- No products indexed under this heading.

Chlorpromazine (May increase serum phenytoin levels). Products include:
- Thorazine Suppositories 1656

Chlorpromazine Hydrochloride (May increase serum phenytoin levels). Products include:
- Thorazine 1656

Chlorpropamide (May increase serum phenytoin levels). Products include:
- Diabinese Tablets 2680

Choline Magnesium Trisalicylate (May increase serum phenytoin levels). Products include:
- Trilisate 2901

Cimetidine (May increase serum phenytoin levels). Products include:
- Tagamet HB 200 Suspension ▣762
- Tagamet HB 200 Tablets ▣761
- Tagamet Tablets 1644

Cimetidine Hydrochloride (May increase serum phenytoin levels). Products include:
- Tagamet 1644

Clomipramine Hydrochloride (Tricyclic antidepressants may precipitate seizures in susceptible patients and phenytoin dosage may need to be adjusted).
- No products indexed under this heading.

Cortisone Acetate (Phenytoin impairs efficacy of corticosteroids). Products include:
- Cortone Acetate Injectable Suspension 2059
- Cortone Acetate Tablets 2061

Desipramine Hydrochloride (Tricyclic antidepressants may precipitate seizures in susceptible patients and phenytoin dosage may need to be adjusted). Products include:
- Norpramin Tablets 755

Desogestrel (Phenytoin impairs efficacy of oral contraceptives). Products include:
- Cyclessa Tablets 2450
- Desogen Tablets 2458
- Mircette Tablets 2470
- Ortho-Cept 21 Tablets 2546
- Ortho-Cept 28 Tablets 2546

Dexamethasone (Phenytoin impairs efficacy of corticosteroids). Products include:
- Decadron Elixir 2078
- Decadron Tablets 2079
- TobraDex Ophthalmic Ointment 542
- TobraDex Ophthalmic Suspension 541

Dexamethasone Acetate (Phenytoin impairs efficacy of corticosteroids).
- No products indexed under this heading.

Dexamethasone Sodium Phosphate (Phenytoin impairs efficacy of corticosteroids). Products include:
- Decadron Phosphate Injection 2081
- Decadron Phosphate Sterile Ophthalmic Ointment 2083
- Decadron Phosphate Sterile Ophthalmic Solution 2084
- NeoDecadron Sterile Ophthalmic Solution 2144

Diazepam (May increase serum phenytoin levels). Products include:
- Valium Injectable 3026
- Valium Tablets 3047

Dicumarol (May increase serum phenytoin levels; phenytoin impairs efficacy of coumarin anticoagulants).
- No products indexed under this heading.

Dienestrol (May increase serum phenytoin levels; phenytoin impairs efficacy of estrogens). Products include:
- Ortho Dienestrol Cream 2554

Diethylstilbestrol (May increase serum phenytoin levels; phenytoin impairs efficacy of estrogens).
- No products indexed under this heading.

Diflunisal (May increase serum phenytoin levels). Products include:
- Dolobid Tablets 2088

Digitoxin (Phenytoin impairs efficacy of digitoxin).
- No products indexed under this heading.

Disulfiram (May increase serum phenytoin levels). Products include:
- Antabuse Tablets 2444
- Antabuse Tablets 3474

Divalproex Sodium (May increase or decrease phenytoin serum levels; unpredictable effect on valproate serum levels). Products include:
- Depakote Sprinkle Capsules 426
- Depakote Tablets 430
- Depakote ER Tablets 436

Doxepin Hydrochloride (Tricyclic antidepressants may precipitate seizures in susceptible patients and phenytoin dosage may need to be adjusted). Products include:
- Sinequan 2713

Doxycycline Calcium (Phenytoin impairs efficacy of doxycycline). Products include:
- Vibramycin Calcium Oral Suspension Syrup 2735

Doxycycline Hyclate (Phenytoin impairs efficacy of doxycycline). Products include:
- Doryx Coated Pellet Filled Capsules 3357
- Periostat Tablets 1208
- Vibramycin Hyclate Capsules 2735
- Vibramycin Hyclate Intravenous 2737
- Vibra-Tabs Film Coated Tablets 2735

Doxycycline Monohydrate (Phenytoin impairs efficacy of doxycycline). Products include:
- Monodox Capsules 2442
- Vibramycin Monohydrate for Oral Suspension 2735

Dyphylline (Phenytoin impairs efficacy of theophylline). Products include:
- Lufyllin Tablets 3347
- Lufyllin-400 Tablets 3347
- Lufyllin-GG Elixir 3348
- Lufyllin-GG Tablets 3348

Estradiol (May increase serum phenytoin levels; phenytoin impairs efficacy of estrogens). Products include:
- Activella Tablets 2764
- Alora Transdermal System 3372
- Climara Transdermal System 958
- CombiPatch Transdermal System 2323
- Esclim Transdermal System 3460
- Estrace Vaginal Cream 3358
- Estrace Tablets 3361
- Estring Vaginal Ring 2811
- Ortho-Prefest Tablets 2570
- Vagifem Tablets 2857
- Vivelle Transdermal System 2412
- Vivelle-Dot Transdermal System 2416

Estrogens, Conjugated (May increase serum phenytoin levels; phenytoin impairs efficacy of estrogens). Products include:
- Premarin Intravenous 3563
- Premarin Tablets 3566
- Premarin Vaginal Cream 3570
- Premphase Tablets 3572
- Prempro Tablets 3572

Estrogens, Esterified (May increase serum phenytoin levels; phenytoin impairs efficacy of estrogens). Products include:
- Estratest 3252
- Menest Tablets 2254

Estropipate (May increase serum phenytoin levels; phenytoin impairs efficacy of estrogens). Products include:
- Ogen Tablets 2846
- Ortho-Est Tablets 3464

Ethinyl Estradiol (May increase serum phenytoin levels; phenytoin impairs efficacy of estrogens). Products include:
- Alesse-21 Tablets 3468
- Alesse-28 Tablets 3473
- Brevicon 28-Day Tablets 3380
- Cyclessa Tablets 2450
- Desogen Tablets 2458
- Estinyl Tablets 3112
- Estrostep 2627
- femhrt Tablets 2635
- Levlen 962
- Levlite 21 Tablets 962
- Levlite 28 Tablets 962
- Levora Tablets 3389
- Loestrin 21 Tablets 2642
- Loestrin Fe Tablets 2642
- Lo/Ovral Tablets 3532
- Lo/Ovral-28 Tablets 3538
- Low-Ogestrel-28 Tablets 3392
- Microgestin Fe 1.5/30 Tablets 3407
- Microgestin Fe 1/20 Tablets 3400
- Mircette Tablets 2470
- Modicon 2563
- Necon 3415
- Nordette-28 Tablets 2257
- Norinyl 1 +35 28-Day Tablets 3380
- Ogestrel 0.5/50-28 Tablets 3428
- Ortho-Cept 21 Tablets 2546
- Ortho-Cept 28 Tablets 2546
- Ortho-Cyclen/Ortho Tri-Cyclen 2573
- Ortho-Novum 2563
- Ovcon 3364

Ovral Tablets ... 3551
Ovral-28 Tablets ... 3552
Tri-Levlen ... 962
Tri-Norinyl-28 Tablets ... 3433
Triphasil-21 Tablets ... 3600
Triphasil-28 Tablets ... 3605
Trivora Tablets ... 3439
Yasmin 28 Tablets ... 980
Zovia ... 3449

Ethosuximide (May increase serum phenytoin levels). Products include:
Zarontin Capsules ... 2659
Zarontin Syrup ... 2660

Ethynodiol Diacetate (Phenytoin impairs efficacy of oral contraceptives). Products include:
Zovia ... 3449

Famotidine (May increase serum phenytoin levels). Products include:
Famotidine Injection ... 866
Pepcid AC ... 1814
Pepcid Complete Chewable Tablets ... 1815
Pepcid Injection ... 2153
Pepcid for Oral Suspension ... 2150
Pepcid RPD Orally Disintegrating Tablets ... 2150
Pepcid Tablets ... 2150

Fludrocortisone Acetate (Phenytoin impairs efficacy of corticosteroids). Products include:
Florinef Acetate Tablets ... 2250

Fluphenazine Decanoate (May increase serum phenytoin levels).
No products indexed under this heading.

Fluphenazine Enanthate (May increase serum phenytoin levels).
No products indexed under this heading.

Fluphenazine Hydrochloride (May increase serum phenytoin levels).
No products indexed under this heading.

Furosemide (Phenytoin impairs efficacy of furosemide). Products include:
Furosemide Tablets ... 2284

Glipizide (May increase serum phenytoin levels). Products include:
Glucotrol Tablets ... 2692
Glucotrol XL Extended Release Tablets ... 2693

Glyburide (May increase serum phenytoin levels). Products include:
DiaBeta Tablets ... 741
Glucovance Tablets ... 1086

Halothane (May increase serum phenytoin levels). Products include:
Fluothane Inhalation ... 3508

Hydrochlorothiazide (May increase serum phenytoin levels). Products include:
Accuretic Tablets ... 2614
Aldoril Tablets ... 2039
Atacand HCT Tablets ... 597
Avalide Tablets ... 1070
Diovan HCT Tablets ... 2338
Dyazide Capsules ... 1515
HydroDIURIL Tablets ... 2108
Hyzaar ... 2109
Inderide Tablets ... 3517
Inderide LA Long-Acting Capsules ... 3519
Lotensin HCT Tablets ... 2367
Maxzide ... 1008
Micardis HCT Tablets ... 1051
Microzide Capsules ... 3414
Moduretic Tablets ... 2138
Monopril HCT ... 1094
Prinzide Tablets ... 2168
Timolide Tablets ... 2187
Uniretic Tablets ... 3178
Vaseretic Tablets ... 2204
Zestoretic Tablets ... 695
Ziac Tablets ... 1887

Hydrocortisone (Phenytoin impairs efficacy of corticosteroids). Products include:
Anusol-HC Cream 2.5% ... 2237
Cipro HC Otic Suspension ... 540
Cortaid Intensive Therapy Cream ... ▣717
Cortaid Maximum Strength Cream ... ▣717
Cortisporin Ophthalmic Suspension Sterile ... ⊙297
Cortizone•5 ... ▣699
Cortizone•10 ... ▣699
Cortizone•10 Plus Creme ... ▣700
Cortizone for Kids Creme ... ▣699
Hydrocortone Tablets ... 2106
Massengill Medicated Soft Cloth Towelette ... ▣753
VōSoL HC Otic Solution ... 3356

Hydrocortisone Acetate (Phenytoin impairs efficacy of corticosteroids). Products include:
Analpram-HC ... 1338
Anusol HC-1 Hydrocortisone Anti-Itch Cream ... ▣689
Anusol-HC Suppositories ... 2238
Cortaid ... ▣717
Cortifoam Rectal Foam ... 3170
Cortisporin-TC Otic Suspension ... 2246
Hydrocortone Acetate Injectable Suspension ... 2103
Pramosone ... 1343
Proctocort Suppositories ... 2264
ProctoFoam-HC ... 3177
Terra-Cortril Ophthalmic Suspension ... 2716

Hydrocortisone Sodium Phosphate (Phenytoin impairs efficacy of corticosteroids). Products include:
Hydrocortone Phosphate Injection, Sterile ... 2105

Hydrocortisone Sodium Succinate (Phenytoin impairs efficacy of corticosteroids).
No products indexed under this heading.

Hydroflumethiazide (May increase serum phenytoin levels). Products include:
Diucardin Tablets ... 3494

Imipramine Hydrochloride (Tricyclic antidepressants may precipitate seizures in susceptible patients and phenytoin dosage may need to be adjusted).
No products indexed under this heading.

Imipramine Pamoate (Tricyclic antidepressants may precipitate seizures in susceptible patients and phenytoin dosage may need to be adjusted).
No products indexed under this heading.

Isoniazid (May increase serum phenytoin levels). Products include:
Rifamate Capsules ... 767
Rifater Tablets ... 769

Levonorgestrel (Phenytoin impairs efficacy of oral contraceptives). Products include:
Alesse-21 Tablets ... 3468
Alesse-28 Tablets ... 3473
Levlen ... 962
Levlite 21 Tablets ... 962
Levlite 28 Tablets ... 962
Levora Tablets ... 3389
Mirena Intrauterine System ... 974
Nordette-28 Tablets ... 2257
Norplant System ... 3543
Tri-Levlen ... 962
Triphasil-21 Tablets ... 3600
Triphasil-28 Tablets ... 3605
Trivora Tablets ... 3439

Magnesium Salicylate (May increase serum phenytoin levels). Products include:
Momentum Backache Relief Extra Strength Caplets ... ▣666

Maprotiline Hydrochloride (Tricyclic antidepressants may precipitate seizures in susceptible patients and phenytoin dosage may need to be adjusted).
No products indexed under this heading.

Mesoridazine Besylate (May increase serum phenytoin levels). Products include:
Serentil ... 1057

Mestranol (Phenytoin impairs efficacy of oral contraceptives). Products include:
Necon 1/50 Tablets ... 3415
Norinyl 1 + 50 28-Day Tablets ... 3380
Ortho-Novum 1/50□28 Tablets ... 2556

Methotrimeprazine (May increase serum phenytoin levels).
No products indexed under this heading.

Methsuximide (May increase serum phenytoin levels). Products include:
Celontin Capsules ... 2618

Methyclothiazide (May increase serum phenytoin levels).
No products indexed under this heading.

Methylphenidate Hydrochloride (May increase serum phenytoin levels). Products include:
Concerta Extended-Release Tablets ... 1998
Concerta Tablets ... 561
Metadate CD Capsules ... 1164
Metadate ER Tablets ... 1167
Methylin Tablets ... 1995
Methylin ER Tablets ... 1995
Ritalin ... 2387

Methylprednisolone Acetate (Phenytoin impairs efficacy of corticosteroids). Products include:
Depo-Medrol Injectable Suspension ... 2795

Methylprednisolone Sodium Succinate (Phenytoin impairs efficacy of corticosteroids). Products include:
Solu-Medrol Sterile Powder ... 2855

Molindone Hydrochloride (Moban brand of molindone contains calcium ions which interfere with the absorption of phenytoin). Products include:
Moban ... 1320

Nizatidine (May increase serum phenytoin levels). Products include:
Axid Pulvules ... 1903
Axid Pulvules ... 2919

Norethindrone (Phenytoin impairs efficacy of oral contraceptives). Products include:
Brevicon 28-Day Tablets ... 3380
Micronor Tablets ... 2543
Modicon ... 2563
Necon ... 3415
Norinyl 1 +35 28-Day Tablets ... 3380
Norinyl 1 + 50 28-Day Tablets ... 3380
Nor-QD Tablets ... 3423
Ortho-Novum ... 2563
Ortho-Novum 1/50□28 Tablets ... 2556
Ovcon ... 3364
Tri-Norinyl-28 Tablets ... 3433

Norethynodrel (Phenytoin impairs efficacy of oral contraceptives).
No products indexed under this heading.

Norgestimate (Phenytoin impairs efficacy of oral contraceptives). Products include:
Ortho-Cyclen/Ortho Tri-Cyclen ... 2573
Ortho-Prefest Tablets ... 2570

Norgestrel (Phenytoin impairs efficacy of oral contraceptives). Products include:
Lo/Ovral Tablets ... 3532
Lo/Ovral-28 Tablets ... 3538
Low-Ogestrel-28 Tablets ... 3392
Ogestrel 0.5/50-28 Tablets ... 3428
Ovral Tablets ... 3551
Ovral-28 Tablets ... 3552
Ovrette Tablets ... 3552

Nortriptyline Hydrochloride (Tricyclic antidepressants may precipitate seizures in susceptible patients and phenytoin dosage may need to be adjusted).
No products indexed under this heading.

Perphenazine (May increase serum phenytoin levels). Products include:
Etrafon ... 3115
Trilafon ... 3160

Phenobarbital (May increase or decrease phenytoin serum levels; unpredictable effect on phenobarbital serum levels). Products include:
Arco-Lase Plus Tablets ... 592
Donnatal ... 2929
Donnatal Extentabs ... 2930

Phensuximide (May increase serum phenytoin levels).
No products indexed under this heading.

Phenylbutazone (May increase serum phenytoin levels).
No products indexed under this heading.

Polyestradiol Phosphate (May increase serum phenytoin levels; phenytoin impairs efficacy of estrogens).
No products indexed under this heading.

Polythiazide (May increase serum phenytoin levels). Products include:
Minizide Capsules ... 2700
Renese Tablets ... 2712

Prednisolone Acetate (Phenytoin impairs efficacy of corticosteroids). Products include:
Blephamide Ophthalmic Ointment ... 547
Blephamide Ophthalmic Suspension ... 548
Poly-Pred Liquifilm Ophthalmic Suspension ... ⊙245
Pred Forte Ophthalmic Suspension ... ⊙246
Pred Mild Sterile Ophthalmic Suspension ... ⊙249
Pred-G Ophthalmic Suspension ... ⊙247
Pred-G Sterile Ophthalmic Ointment ... ⊙248

Prednisolone Sodium Phosphate (Phenytoin impairs efficacy of corticosteroids). Products include:
Pediapred Oral Solution ... 1170

Prednisolone Tebutate (Phenytoin impairs efficacy of corticosteroids).
No products indexed under this heading.

Prednisone (Phenytoin impairs efficacy of corticosteroids). Products include:
Prednisone ... 3064

Prochlorperazine (May increase serum phenytoin levels). Products include:
Compazine ... 1505

Promethazine Hydrochloride (May increase serum phenytoin levels). Products include:
Mepergan Injection ... 3539
Phenergan Injection ... 3553
Phenergan ... 3556
Phenergan Syrup ... 3554
Phenergan with Codeine Syrup ... 3557
Phenergan with Dextromethorphan Syrup ... 3559
Phenergan VC Syrup ... 3560
Phenergan VC with Codeine Syrup ... 3561

Protriptyline Hydrochloride (Tricyclic antidepressants may precipitate seizures in susceptible patients and phenytoin dosage may need to be adjusted). Products include:
Vivactil Tablets ... 2446
Vivactil Tablets ... 2217

Quinestrol (May increase serum phenytoin levels; phenytoin impairs efficacy of estrogens).
No products indexed under this heading.

Quinidine Gluconate (Phenytoin impairs efficacy of quinidine). Products include:
Quinaglute Dura-Tabs Tablets ... 978

Quinidine Polygalacturonate (Phenytoin impairs efficacy of quinidine).
No products indexed under this heading.

Quinidine Sulfate (Phenytoin impairs efficacy of quinidine). Products include:
Quinidex Extentabs ... 2933

Ranitidine Bismuth Citrate (May increase serum phenytoin levels).
No products indexed under this heading.

Ranitidine Hydrochloride (May increase serum phenytoin levels). Products include:
Zantac ... 1690
Zantac Injection ... 1688
Zantac 75 Tablets ... ▣717

Reserpine (May decrease serum phenytoin levels).
No products indexed under this heading.

IMPORTANT NOTE: Always consult each drug listing in the patient's regimen for possible interactions.

Rifampin (Phenytoin impairs efficacy of rifampin). Products include:
Rifadin ... 765
Rifamate Capsules ... 767
Rifater Tablets ... 769

Salsalate (May increase serum phenytoin levels).
No products indexed under this heading.

Sucralfate (May decrease serum phenytoin levels). Products include:
Carafate Suspension ... 731
Carafate Tablets ... 730

Sulfacytine (May increase serum phenytoin levels).

Sulfamethizole (May increase serum phenytoin levels). Products include:
Urobiotic-250 Capsules ... 2731

Sulfamethoxazole (May increase serum phenytoin levels). Products include:
Bactrim ... 2949
Septra Suspension ... 2265
Septra Tablets ... 2265
Septra DS Tablets ... 2265

Sulfasalazine (May increase serum phenytoin levels). Products include:
Azulfidine EN-tabs Tablets ... 2775

Sulfinpyrazone (May increase serum phenytoin levels).
No products indexed under this heading.

Sulfisoxazole (May increase serum phenytoin levels).
No products indexed under this heading.

Sulfisoxazole Acetyl (May increase serum phenytoin levels). Products include:
Pediazole Suspension ... 3050

Sulfisoxazole Diolamine (May increase serum phenytoin levels).
No products indexed under this heading.

Theophylline (Phenytoin impairs efficacy of theophylline). Products include:
Aerolate ... 1361
Theo-Dur Extended-Release Tablets ... 1835
Uni-Dur Extended-Release Tablets .. 1841
Uniphyl 400 mg and 600 mg Tablets ... 2903

Theophylline Calcium Salicylate (Phenytoin impairs efficacy of theophylline).
No products indexed under this heading.

Theophylline Sodium Glycinate (Phenytoin impairs efficacy of theophylline).
No products indexed under this heading.

Thioridazine Hydrochloride (May increase serum phenytoin levels). Products include:
Thioridazine Hydrochloride Tablets ... 2289

Tolazamide (May increase serum phenytoin levels).
No products indexed under this heading.

Tolbutamide (May increase serum phenytoin levels).
No products indexed under this heading.

Trazodone Hydrochloride (May increase serum phenytoin levels).
No products indexed under this heading.

Triamcinolone (Phenytoin impairs efficacy of corticosteroids).
No products indexed under this heading.

Triamcinolone Acetonide (Phenytoin impairs efficacy of corticosteroids). Products include:
Azmacort Inhalation Aerosol ... 728
Nasacort Nasal Inhaler ... 750
Nasacort AQ Nasal Spray ... 752
Tri-Nasal Spray ... 2274

Triamcinolone Diacetate (Phenytoin impairs efficacy of corticosteroids).
No products indexed under this heading.

Triamcinolone Hexacetonide (Phenytoin impairs efficacy of corticosteroids).
No products indexed under this heading.

Trifluoperazine Hydrochloride (May increase serum phenytoin levels). Products include:
Stelazine ... 1640

Trimipramine Maleate (Tricyclic antidepressants may precipitate seizures in susceptible patients and phenytoin dosage may need to be adjusted). Products include:
Surmontil Capsules ... 3595

Valproic Acid (May increase or decrease phenytoin serum levels; unpredictable effect on valproic serum levels). Products include:
Depakene ... 421

Vitamin D (Phenytoin impairs efficacy of vitamin D). Products include:
Active Calcium Tablets ... 3335
Caltrate 600 PLUS ... ■815
Caltrate 600 + D Tablets ... ■814
Centrum Focused Formulas Bone Health Tablets ... ■815
Citracal Caplets + D ... ■823
D-Cal Chewable Caplets ... ■794
One-A-Day Calcium Plus Chewable Tablets ... ■805
Os-Cal 250 + D Tablets ... ■838
Os-Cal 500 + D Tablets ... ■839

Warfarin Sodium (Phenytoin impairs efficacy of coumarin anticoagulants). Products include:
Coumadin for Injection ... 1243
Coumadin Tablets ... 1243
Warfarin Sodium Tablets, USP ... 3302

Food Interactions

Alcohol (Acute alcohol intake increases serum phenytoin levels; chronic alcohol intake decreases serum phenytoin levels).

DILANTIN KAPSEALS

(Phenytoin Sodium) ... 2622

May interact with corticosteroids, oral anticoagulants, estrogens, histamine H_2-receptor antagonists, oral contraceptives, phenothiazines, salicylates, succinimides, sulfonamides, tricyclic antidepressants, theophylline, and certain other agents. Compounds in these categories include:

Aminophylline (Phenytoin impairs efficacy of theophylline).
No products indexed under this heading.

Amiodarone Hydrochloride (May increase serum phenytoin levels). Products include:
Cordarone Intravenous ... 3491
Cordarone Tablets ... 3487
Pacerone Tablets ... 3331

Amitriptyline Hydrochloride (Tricyclic antidepressants may precipitate seizures in susceptible patients and phenytoin dosage may need to be adjusted). Products include:
Etrafon ... 3115
Limbitrol ... 1738

Amoxapine (Tricyclic antidepressants may precipitate seizures in susceptible patients and phenytoin dosage may need to be adjusted).
No products indexed under this heading.

Aspirin (May increase serum phenytoin levels). Products include:
Aggrenox Capsules ... 1026
Alka-Seltzer ... ■603
Alka-Seltzer Lemon Lime Antacid and Pain Reliever Effervescent Tablets ... ■603
Alka-Seltzer Extra Strength Antacid and Pain Reliever Effervescent Tablets ... ■603
Alka-Seltzer PM Effervescent Tablets ... ■605
Genuine Bayer Tablets, Caplets and Gelcaps ... ■606
Extra Strength Bayer Caplets and Gelcaps ... ■610
Aspirin Regimen Bayer Children's Chewable Tablets (Orange or Cherry Flavored) ... ■607
Bayer, Aspirin Regimen ... ■606
Aspirin Regimen Bayer 81 mg Caplets with Calcium ... ■607
Genuine Bayer Professional Labeling (Aspirin Regimen Bayer) ... ■608
Extra Strength Bayer Arthritis Caplets ... ■610
Extra Strength Bayer Plus Caplets ... ■610
Extra Strength Bayer PM Caplets .. ■611
BC Powder ... ■619
BC Allergy Sinus Cold Powder ... ■619
Arthritis Strength BC Powder ... ■619
BC Sinus Cold Powder ... ■619
Darvon Compound-65 Pulvules ... 1910
Ecotrin Enteric Coated Aspirin Low, Regular and Maximum Strength Tablets ... 1715
Excedrin Extra-Strength Tablets, Caplets, and Geltabs ... ■629
Excedrin Migraine ... 1070
Goody's Body Pain Formula Powder ... ■620
Goody's Extra Strength Headache Powder ... ■620
Goody's Extra Strength Pain Relief Tablets ... ■620
Percodan Tablets ... 1327
Robaxisal Tablets ... 2939
Soma Compound Tablets ... 3354
Soma Compound w/Codeine Tablets ... 3355
Vanquish Caplets ... ■617

Bendroflumethiazide (May increase serum phenytoin levels). Products include:
Corzide 40/5 Tablets ... 2247
Corzide 80/5 Tablets ... 2247

Betamethasone Acetate (Phenytoin impairs efficacy of corticosteroids). Products include:
Celestone Soluspan Injectable Suspension ... 3097

Betamethasone Sodium Phosphate (Phenytoin impairs efficacy of corticosteroids). Products include:
Celestone Soluspan Injectable Suspension ... 3097

Calcium Carbonate (Calcium ions interfere with the absorption of phenytoin; ingestion times of phenytoin and antacids containing calcium should be staggered in patients with low phenytoin levels). Products include:
Aspirin Regimen Bayer 81 mg Caplets with Calcium ... ■607
Extra Strength Bayer Plus Caplets ... ■610
Caltrate 600 Tablets ... ■814
Caltrate 600 PLUS ... ■815
Caltrate 600 + D Tablets ... ■814
Caltrate 600 + Soy Tablets ... ■814
D-Cal Chewable Caplets ... ■794
Florical Capsules and Tablets ... 2223
Quick Dissolve Maalox Max Maximum Strength Antacid/Antigas Tablets ... 2301
Quick Dissolve Maalox Regular Strength Antacid Tablets ... 2301
Marblen Suspension ... ■633
Monocal Tablets ... 2223
Mylanta Fast-Acting ... 1813
Mylanta Calci Tabs ... ■636
One-A-Day Bedtime & Rest Tablets ... ■805
One-A-Day Calcium Plus Chewable Tablets ... ■805
Os-Cal Chewable Tablets ... ■838
Pepcid Complete Chewable Tablets ... 1815
ReSource Wellness CalciWise Soft Chews ... ■824
Rolaids Tablets ... ■706
Extra Strength Rolaids Tablets ... ■706
Slow-Mag Tablets ... ■835
Titralac ... ■640
3M Titralac Plus Antacid Tablets ... ■640
Tums ... ■763

Carbamazepine (May decrease serum phenytoin levels). Products include:
Carbatrol Capsules ... 3234
Tegretol/Tegretol-XR ... 2404

Chloramphenicol (May increase serum phenytoin levels). Products include:
Chloromycetin Ophthalmic Ointment, 1% ... ⊙296
Chloromycetin Ophthalmic Solution ... ⊙297
Chloroptic Sterile Ophthalmic Ointment ... ⊙234
Chloroptic Sterile Ophthalmic Solution ... ⊙235

Chloramphenicol Palmitate (May increase serum phenytoin levels).
No products indexed under this heading.

Chloramphenicol Sodium Succinate (May increase serum phenytoin levels).
No products indexed under this heading.

Chlordiazepoxide (May increase serum phenytoin levels). Products include:
Limbitrol ... 1738

Chlordiazepoxide Hydrochloride (May increase serum phenytoin levels). Products include:
Librium Capsules ... 1736
Librium for Injection ... 1737

Chlorothiazide (May increase serum phenytoin levels). Products include:
Aldoclor Tablets ... 2035
Diuril Oral ... 2087

Chlorothiazide Sodium (May increase serum phenytoin levels). Products include:
Diuril Sodium Intravenous ... 2086

Chlorotrianisene (May increase serum phenytoin levels; phenytoin impairs efficacy of estrogens).
No products indexed under this heading.

Chlorpromazine (May increase serum phenytoin levels). Products include:
Thorazine Suppositories ... 1656

Chlorpromazine Hydrochloride (May increase serum phenytoin levels). Products include:
Thorazine ... 1656

Chlorpropamide (May increase serum phenytoin levels). Products include:
Diabinese Tablets ... 2680

Choline Magnesium Trisalicylate (May increase serum phenytoin levels). Products include:
Trilisate ... 2901

Cimetidine (May increase serum phenytoin levels). Products include:
Tagamet HB 200 Suspension ... ■762
Tagamet HB 200 Tablets ... ■761
Tagamet Tablets ... 1644

Cimetidine Hydrochloride (May increase serum phenytoin levels). Products include:
Tagamet ... 1644

Clomipramine Hydrochloride (Tricyclic antidepressants may precipitate seizures in susceptible patients and phenytoin dosage may need to be adjusted).
No products indexed under this heading.

Cortisone Acetate (Phenytoin impairs efficacy of corticosteroids). Products include:
Cortone Acetate Injectable Suspension ... 2059
Cortone Acetate Tablets ... 2061

Desipramine Hydrochloride (Tricyclic antidepressants may precipitate seizures in susceptible patients and phenytoin dosage may need to be adjusted). Products include:
Norpramin Tablets ... 755

Desogestrel (Phenytoin impairs efficacy of oral contraceptives). Products include:
Cyclessa Tablets ... 2450
Desogen Tablets ... 2458
Mircette Tablets ... 2470
Ortho-Cept 21 Tablets ... 2546
Ortho-Cept 28 Tablets ... 2546

Dexamethasone (Phenytoin impairs efficacy of corticosteroids). Products include:
- Decadron Elixir 2078
- Decadron Tablets 2079
- TobraDex Ophthalmic Ointment 542
- TobraDex Ophthalmic Suspension 541

Dexamethasone Acetate (Phenytoin impairs efficacy of corticosteroids).
- No products indexed under this heading.

Dexamethasone Sodium Phosphate (Phenytoin impairs efficacy of corticosteroids). Products include:
- Decadron Phosphate Injection 2081
- Decadron Phosphate Sterile Ophthalmic Ointment 2083
- Decadron Phosphate Sterile Ophthalmic Solution 2084
- NeoDecadron Sterile Ophthalmic Solution 2144

Diazepam (May increase serum phenytoin levels). Products include:
- Valium Injectable 3026
- Valium Tablets 3047

Dicumarol (May increase serum phenytoin levels; phenytoin impairs efficacy of coumarin anticoagulants).
- No products indexed under this heading.

Dienestrol (May increase serum phenytoin levels; phenytoin impairs efficacy of estrogens). Products include:
- Ortho Dienestrol Cream 2554

Diethylstilbestrol (May increase serum phenytoin levels; phenytoin impairs efficacy of estrogens).
- No products indexed under this heading.

Diflunisal (May increase serum phenytoin levels). Products include:
- Dolobid Tablets 2088

Digitoxin (Phenytoin impairs efficacy of digitoxin).
- No products indexed under this heading.

Disulfiram (May increase serum phenytoin levels). Products include:
- Antabuse Tablets 2444
- Antabuse Tablets 3474

Divalproex Sodium (May increase or decrease phenytoin serum levels; unpredictable effect on valproate serum levels). Products include:
- Depakote Sprinkle Capsules 426
- Depakote Tablets 430
- Depakote ER Tablets 436

Doxepin Hydrochloride (Tricyclic antidepressants may precipitate seizures in susceptible patients and phenytoin dosage may need to be adjusted). Products include:
- Sinequan 2713

Doxycycline Calcium (Phenytoin impairs efficacy of doxycycline). Products include:
- Vibramycin Calcium Oral Suspension Syrup 2735

Doxycycline Hyclate (Phenytoin impairs efficacy of doxycycline). Products include:
- Doryx Coated Pellet Filled Capsules 3357
- Periostat Tablets 1208
- Vibramycin Hyclate Capsules 2735
- Vibramycin Hyclate Intravenous 2737
- Vibra-Tabs Film Coated Tablets 2735

Doxycycline Monohydrate (Phenytoin impairs efficacy of doxycycline). Products include:
- Monodox Capsules 2442
- Vibramycin Monohydrate for Oral Suspension 2735

Dyphylline (Phenytoin impairs efficacy of theophylline). Products include:
- Lufyllin Tablets 3347
- Lufyllin-400 Tablets 3347
- Lufyllin-GG Elixir 3348
- Lufyllin-GG Tablets 3348

Estradiol (May increase serum phenytoin levels; phenytoin impairs efficacy of estrogens). Products include:
- Activella Tablets 2764
- Alora Transdermal System 3372
- Climara Transdermal System 958
- CombiPatch Transdermal System 2323
- Esclim Transdermal System 3460
- Estrace Vaginal Cream 3358
- Estrace Tablets 3361
- Estring Vaginal Ring 2811
- Ortho-Prefest Tablets 2570
- Vagifem Tablets 2857
- Vivelle Transdermal System 2412
- Vivelle-Dot Transdermal System 2416

Estrogens, Conjugated (May increase serum phenytoin levels; phenytoin impairs efficacy of estrogens). Products include:
- Premarin Intravenous 3563
- Premarin Tablets 3566
- Premarin Vaginal Cream 3570
- Premphase Tablets 3572
- Prempro Tablets 3572

Estrogens, Esterified (May increase serum phenytoin levels; phenytoin impairs efficacy of estrogens). Products include:
- Estratest 3252
- Menest Tablets 2254

Estropipate (May increase serum phenytoin levels; phenytoin impairs efficacy of estrogens). Products include:
- Ogen Tablets 2846
- Ortho-Est Tablets 3464

Ethinyl Estradiol (May increase serum phenytoin levels; phenytoin impairs efficacy of estrogens). Products include:
- Alesse-21 Tablets 3468
- Alesse-28 Tablets 3473
- Brevicon 28-Day Tablets 3380
- Cyclessa Tablets 2450
- Desogen Tablets 2458
- Estinyl Tablets 3112
- Estrostep 2627
- femhrt Tablets 2635
- Levlen 962
- Levlite 21 Tablets 962
- Levlite 28 Tablets 962
- Levora Tablets 3389
- Loestrin 21 Tablets 2642
- Loestrin Fe Tablets 2642
- Lo/Ovral Tablets 3532
- Lo/Ovral-28 Tablets 3538
- Low-Ogestrel-28 Tablets 3392
- Microgestin Fe 1.5/30 Tablets 3407
- Microgestin Fe 1/20 Tablets 3400
- Mircette Tablets 2470
- Modicon 2563
- Necon 3415
- Nordette-28 Tablets 2257
- Norinyl 1 +35 28-Day Tablets 3380
- Ogestrel 0.5/50-28 Tablets 3428
- Ortho-Cept 21 Tablets 2546
- Ortho-Cept 28 Tablets 2546
- Ortho-Cyclen/Ortho Tri-Cyclen 2573
- Ortho-Novum 2563
- Ovcon 3364
- Ovral Tablets 3551
- Ovral-28 Tablets 3552
- Tri-Levlen 962
- Tri-Norinyl-28 Tablets 3433
- Triphasil-21 Tablets 3600
- Triphasil-28 Tablets 3605
- Trivora Tablets 3439
- Yasmin 28 Tablets 980
- Zovia 3449

Ethosuximide (May increase serum phenytoin levels). Products include:
- Zarontin Capsules 2659
- Zarontin Syrup 2660

Ethynodiol Diacetate (Phenytoin impairs efficacy of oral contraceptives). Products include:
- Zovia 3449

Famotidine (May increase serum phenytoin levels). Products include:
- Famotidine Injection 866
- Pepcid AC 1814
- Pepcid Complete Chewable Tablets 1815
- Pepcid Injection 2153
- Pepcid for Oral Suspension 2150
- Pepcid RPD Orally Disintegrating Tablets 2150
- Pepcid Tablets 2150

Fludrocortisone Acetate (Phenytoin impairs efficacy of corticosteroids). Products include:
- Florinef Acetate Tablets 2250

Fluphenazine Decanoate (May increase serum phenytoin levels).
- No products indexed under this heading.

Fluphenazine Enanthate (May increase serum phenytoin levels).
- No products indexed under this heading.

Fluphenazine Hydrochloride (May increase serum phenytoin levels).
- No products indexed under this heading.

Furosemide (Phenytoin impairs efficacy of furosemide). Products include:
- Furosemide Tablets 2284

Glipizide (May increase serum phenytoin levels). Products include:
- Glucotrol Tablets 2692
- Glucotrol XL Extended Release Tablets 2693

Glyburide (May increase serum phenytoin levels). Products include:
- DiaBeta Tablets 741
- Glucovance Tablets 1086

Halothane (May increase serum phenytoin levels). Products include:
- Fluothane Inhalation 3508

Hydrochlorothiazide (May increase serum phenytoin levels). Products include:
- Accuretic Tablets 2614
- Aldoril Tablets 2039
- Atacand HCT Tablets 597
- Avalide Tablets 1070
- Diovan HCT Tablets 2338
- Dyazide Capsules 1515
- HydroDIURIL Tablets 2108
- Hyzaar 2109
- Inderide Tablets 3517
- Inderide LA Long-Acting Capsules 3519
- Lotensin HCT Tablets 2367
- Maxzide 1008
- Micardis HCT Tablets 1051
- Microzide Capsules 3414
- Moduretic Tablets 2138
- Monopril HCT 1094
- Prinzide Tablets 2168
- Timolide Tablets 2187
- Uniretic Tablets 3178
- Vaseretic Tablets 2204
- Zestoretic Tablets 695
- Ziac Tablets 1887

Hydrocortisone (Phenytoin impairs efficacy of corticosteroids). Products include:
- Anusol-HC Cream 2.5% 2237
- Cipro HC Otic Suspension 540
- Cortaid Intensive Therapy Cream ▣717
- Cortaid Maximum Strength Cream ▣717
- Cortisporin Ophthalmic Suspension Sterile ⊙297
- Cortizone•5 ▣699
- Cortizone•10 ▣699
- Cortizone•10 Plus Creme ▣700
- Cortizone for Kids Creme ▣699
- Hydrocortone Tablets 2106
- Massengill Medicated Soft Cloth Towelette ▣753
- VōSoL HC Otic Solution 3356

Hydrocortisone Acetate (Phenytoin impairs efficacy of corticosteroids). Products include:
- Analpram-HC 1338
- Anusol HC-1 Hydrocortisone Anti-Itch Cream ▣689
- Anusol-HC Suppositories 2238
- Cortaid ▣717
- Cortifoam Rectal Foam 3170
- Cortisporin-TC Otic Suspension 2246
- Hydrocortone Acetate Injectable Suspension 2103
- Pramosone 1343
- Proctocort Suppositories 2264
- ProctoFoam-HC 3177
- Terra-Cortril Ophthalmic Suspension 2716

Hydrocortisone Sodium Phosphate (Phenytoin impairs efficacy of corticosteroids). Products include:
- Hydrocortone Phosphate Injection, Sterile 2105

Hydrocortisone Sodium Succinate (Phenytoin impairs efficacy of corticosteroids).
- No products indexed under this heading.

Hydroflumethiazide (May increase serum phenytoin levels). Products include:
- Diucardin Tablets 3494

Imipramine Hydrochloride (Tricyclic antidepressants may precipitate seizures in susceptible patients and phenytoin dosage may need to be adjusted).
- No products indexed under this heading.

Imipramine Pamoate (Tricyclic antidepressants may precipitate seizures in susceptible patients and phenytoin dosage may need to be adjusted).
- No products indexed under this heading.

Isoniazid (May increase serum phenytoin levels). Products include:
- Rifamate Capsules 767
- Rifater Tablets 769

Levonorgestrel (Phenytoin impairs efficacy of oral contraceptives). Products include:
- Alesse-21 Tablets 3468
- Alesse-28 Tablets 3473
- Levlen 962
- Levlite 21 Tablets 962
- Levlite 28 Tablets 962
- Levora Tablets 3389
- Mirena Intrauterine System 974
- Nordette-28 Tablets 2257
- Norplant System 3543
- Tri-Levlen 962
- Triphasil-21 Tablets 3600
- Triphasil-28 Tablets 3605
- Trivora Tablets 3439

Magnesium Salicylate (May increase serum phenytoin levels). Products include:
- Momentum Backache Relief Extra Strength Caplets ▣666

Maprotiline Hydrochloride (Tricyclic antidepressants may precipitate seizures in susceptible patients and phenytoin dosage may need to be adjusted).
- No products indexed under this heading.

Mesoridazine Besylate (May increase serum phenytoin levels). Products include:
- Serentil 1057

Mestranol (Phenytoin impairs efficacy of oral contraceptives). Products include:
- Necon 1/50 Tablets 3415
- Norinyl 1 + 50 28-Day Tablets 3380
- Ortho-Novum 1/50□28 Tablets 2556

Methotrimeprazine (May increase serum phenytoin levels).
- No products indexed under this heading.

Methsuximide (May increase serum phenytoin levels). Products include:
- Celontin Capsules 2618

Methyclothiazide (May increase serum phenytoin levels).
- No products indexed under this heading.

Methylphenidate Hydrochloride (May increase serum phenytoin levels). Products include:
- Concerta Extended-Release Tablets 1998
- Concerta Tablets 561
- Metadate CD Capsules 1164
- Metadate ER Tablets 1167
- Methylin Tablets 1995
- Methylin ER Tablets 1995
- Ritalin 2387

Methylprednisolone Acetate (Phenytoin impairs efficacy of corticosteroids). Products include:
- Depo-Medrol Injectable Suspension 2795

Methylprednisolone Sodium Succinate (Phenytoin impairs efficacy of corticosteroids). Products include:
- Solu-Medrol Sterile Powder 2855

Molindone Hydrochloride (Moban brand of molindone contains calcium

ions which interfere with the absorption of phenytoin). Products include:
Moban 1320

Nizatidine (May increase serum phenytoin levels). Products include:
Axid Pulvules 1903
Axid Pulvules 2919

Norethindrone (Phenytoin impairs efficacy of oral contraceptives). Products include:
Brevicon 28-Day Tablets 3380
Micronor Tablets 2543
Modicon 2563
Necon 3415
Norinyl 1 +35 28-Day Tablets 3380
Norinyl 1 + 50 28-Day Tablets 3380
Nor-QD Tablets 3423
Ortho-Novum 2563
Ortho-Novum 1/50□28 Tablets 2556
Ovcon 3364
Tri-Norinyl-28 Tablets 3433

Norethynodrel (Phenytoin impairs efficacy of oral contraceptives).
No products indexed under this heading.

Norgestimate (Phenytoin impairs efficacy of oral contraceptives). Products include:
Ortho-Cyclen/Ortho Tri-Cyclen 2573
Ortho-Prefest Tablets 2570

Norgestrel (Phenytoin impairs efficacy of oral contraceptives). Products include:
Lo/Ovral Tablets 3532
Lo/Ovral-28 Tablets 3538
Low-Ogestrel-28 Tablets 3392
Ogestrel 0.5/50-28 Tablets 3428
Ovral Tablets 3551
Ovral-28 Tablets 3552
Ovrette Tablets 3552

Nortriptyline Hydrochloride (Tricyclic antidepressants may precipitate seizures in susceptible patients and phenytoin dosage may need to be adjusted).
No products indexed under this heading.

Perphenazine (May increase serum phenytoin levels). Products include:
Etrafon 3115
Trilafon 3160

Phenobarbital (May increase or decrease phenytoin serum levels; unpredictable effect on phenobarbital serum levels). Products include:
Arco-Lase Plus Tablets 592
Donnatal 2929
Donnatal Extentabs 2930

Phensuximide (May increase serum phenytoin levels).
No products indexed under this heading.

Phenylbutazone (May increase serum phenytoin levels).
No products indexed under this heading.

Polyestradiol Phosphate (May increase serum phenytoin levels; phenytoin impairs efficacy of estrogens).
No products indexed under this heading.

Polythiazide (May increase serum phenytoin levels). Products include:
Minizide Capsules 2700
Renese Tablets 2712

Prednisolone Acetate (Phenytoin impairs efficacy of corticosteroids). Products include:
Blephamide Ophthalmic Ointment 547
Blephamide Ophthalmic Suspension 548
Poly-Pred Liquifilm Ophthalmic Suspension .... ⊙245
Pred Forte Ophthalmic Suspension .... ⊙246
Pred Mild Sterile Ophthalmic Suspension .... ⊙249
Pred-G Ophthalmic Suspension .... ⊙247
Pred-G Sterile Ophthalmic Ointment .... ⊙248

Prednisolone Sodium Phosphate (Phenytoin impairs efficacy of corticosteroids). Products include:
Pediapred Oral Solution 1170

Prednisolone Tebutate (Phenytoin impairs efficacy of corticosteroids).
No products indexed under this heading.

Prednisone (Phenytoin impairs efficacy of corticosteroids). Products include:
Prednisone 3064

Prochlorperazine (May increase serum phenytoin levels). Products include:
Compazine 1505

Promethazine Hydrochloride (May increase serum phenytoin levels). Products include:
Mepergan Injection 3539
Phenergan Injection 3553
Phenergan 3556
Phenergan Syrup 3554
Phenergan with Codeine Syrup 3557
Phenergan with Dextromethorphan Syrup 3559
Phenergan VC Syrup 3560
Phenergan VC with Codeine Syrup 3561

Protriptyline Hydrochloride (Tricyclic antidepressants may precipitate seizures in susceptible patients and phenytoin dosage may need to be adjusted). Products include:
Vivactil Tablets 2446
Vivactil Tablets 2217

Quinestrol (May increase serum phenytoin levels; phenytoin impairs efficacy of estrogens).
No products indexed under this heading.

Quinidine Gluconate (Phenytoin impairs efficacy of quinidine). Products include:
Quinaglute Dura-Tabs Tablets 978

Quinidine Polygalacturonate (Phenytoin impairs efficacy of quinidine).
No products indexed under this heading.

Quinidine Sulfate (Phenytoin impairs efficacy of quinidine). Products include:
Quinidex Extentabs 2933

Ranitidine Bismuth Citrate (May increase serum phenytoin levels).
No products indexed under this heading.

Ranitidine Hydrochloride (May increase serum phenytoin levels). Products include:
Zantac 1690
Zantac Injection 1688
Zantac 75 Tablets .... ▣717

Reserpine (May decrease serum phenytoin levels).
No products indexed under this heading.

Rifampin (Phenytoin impairs efficacy of rifampin). Products include:
Rifadin 765
Rifamate Capsules 767
Rifater Tablets 769

Salsalate (May increase serum phenytoin levels).
No products indexed under this heading.

Sucralfate (May decrease serum phenytoin levels). Products include:
Carafate Suspension 731
Carafate Tablets 730

Sulfacytine (May increase serum phenytoin levels).

Sulfamethizole (May increase serum phenytoin levels). Products include:
Urobiotic-250 Capsules 2731

Sulfamethoxazole (May increase serum phenytoin levels). Products include:
Bactrim 2949
Septra Suspension 2265
Septra Tablets 2265
Septra DS Tablets 2265

Sulfasalazine (May increase serum phenytoin levels). Products include:
Azulfidine EN-tabs Tablets 2775

Sulfinpyrazone (May increase serum phenytoin levels).
No products indexed under this heading.

Sulfisoxazole (May increase serum phenytoin levels).
No products indexed under this heading.

Sulfisoxazole Acetyl (May increase serum phenytoin levels). Products include:
Pediazole Suspension 3050

Sulfisoxazole Diolamine (May increase serum phenytoin levels).
No products indexed under this heading.

Theophylline (Phenytoin impairs efficacy of theophylline). Products include:
Aerolate 1361
Theo-Dur Extended-Release Tablets 1835
Uni-Dur Extended-Release Tablets 1841
Uniphyl 400 mg and 600 mg Tablets 2903

Theophylline Calcium Salicylate (Phenytoin impairs efficacy of theophylline).
No products indexed under this heading.

Theophylline Sodium Glycinate (Phenytoin impairs efficacy of theophylline).
No products indexed under this heading.

Thioridazine Hydrochloride (May increase serum phenytoin levels). Products include:
Thioridazine Hydrochloride Tablets 2289

Tolazamide (May increase serum phenytoin levels).
No products indexed under this heading.

Tolbutamide (May increase serum phenytoin levels).
No products indexed under this heading.

Trazodone Hydrochloride (May increase serum phenytoin levels).
No products indexed under this heading.

Triamcinolone (Phenytoin impairs efficacy of corticosteroids).
No products indexed under this heading.

Triamcinolone Acetonide (Phenytoin impairs efficacy of corticosteroids). Products include:
Azmacort Inhalation Aerosol 728
Nasacort Nasal Inhaler 750
Nasacort AQ Nasal Spray 752
Tri-Nasal Spray 2274

Triamcinolone Diacetate (Phenytoin impairs efficacy of corticosteroids).
No products indexed under this heading.

Triamcinolone Hexacetonide (Phenytoin impairs efficacy of corticosteroids).
No products indexed under this heading.

Trifluoperazine Hydrochloride (May increase serum phenytoin levels). Products include:
Stelazine 1640

Trimipramine Maleate (Tricyclic antidepressants may precipitate seizures in susceptible patients and phenytoin dosage may need to be adjusted). Products include:
Surmontil Capsules 3595

Valproic Acid (May increase or decrease phenytoin serum levels; unpredictable effect on valproic serum levels). Products include:
Depakene 421

Vitamin D (Phenytoin impairs efficacy of vitamin D). Products include:
Active Calcium Tablets 3335
Caltrate 600 PLUS .... ▣815
Caltrate 600 + D Tablets .... ▣814
Centrum Focused Formulas Bone Health Tablets .... ▣815
Citracal Caplets + D .... ▣823
D-Cal Chewable Caplets .... ▣794
One-A-Day Calcium Plus Chewable Tablets .... ▣805
Os-Cal 250 + D Tablets .... ▣838
Os-Cal 500 + D Tablets .... ▣839

Warfarin Sodium (Phenytoin impairs efficacy of coumarin anticoagulants). Products include:
Coumadin for Injection 1243
Coumadin Tablets 1243
Warfarin Sodium Tablets, USP 3302

Food Interactions

Alcohol (Acute alcohol intake increases serum phenytoin levels; chronic alcohol intake decreases serum phenytoin levels).

DILANTIN-125 ORAL SUSPENSION

(Phenytoin) 2625

May interact with corticosteroids, oral anticoagulants, estrogens, histamine H_2-receptor antagonists, oral contraceptives, phenothiazines, salicylates, succinimides, sulfonamides, tricyclic antidepressants, theophylline, and certain other agents. Compounds in these categories include:

Aminophylline (Phenytoin impairs efficacy of theophylline).
No products indexed under this heading.

Amiodarone Hydrochloride (May increase serum phenytoin levels). Products include:
Cordarone Intravenous 3491
Cordarone Tablets 3487
Pacerone Tablets 3331

Amitriptyline Hydrochloride (Tricyclic antidepressants may precipitate seizures in susceptible patients and phenytoin dosage may need to be adjusted). Products include:
Etrafon 3115
Limbitrol 1738

Amoxapine (Tricyclic antidepressants may precipitate seizures in susceptible patients and phenytoin dosage may need to be adjusted).
No products indexed under this heading.

Aspirin (May increase serum phenytoin levels). Products include:
Aggrenox Capsules 1026
Alka-Seltzer .... ▣603
Alka-Seltzer Lemon Lime Antacid and Pain Reliever Effervescent Tablets .... ▣603
Alka-Seltzer Extra Strength Antacid and Pain Reliever Effervescent Tablets .... ▣603
Alka-Seltzer PM Effervescent Tablets .... ▣605
Genuine Bayer Tablets, Caplets and Gelcaps .... ▣606
Extra Strength Bayer Caplets and Gelcaps .... ▣610
Aspirin Regimen Bayer Children's Chewable Tablets (Orange or Cherry Flavored) .... ▣607
Bayer, Aspirin Regimen .... ▣606
Aspirin Regimen Bayer 81 mg Caplets with Calcium .... ▣607
Genuine Bayer Professional Labeling (Aspirin Regimen Bayer) .... ▣608
Extra Strength Bayer Arthritis Caplets .... ▣610
Extra Strength Bayer Plus Caplets .... ▣610
Extra Strength Bayer PM Caplets .... ▣611
BC Powder .... ▣619
BC Allergy Sinus Cold Powder .... ▣619
Arthritis Strength BC Powder .... ▣619
BC Sinus Cold Powder .... ▣619
Darvon Compound-65 Pulvules 1910
Ecotrin Enteric Coated Aspirin Low, Regular and Maximum Strength Tablets 1715
Excedrin Extra-Strength Tablets, Caplets, and Geltabs .... ▣629
Excedrin Migraine 1070
Goody's Body Pain Formula Powder .... ▣620
Goody's Extra Strength Headache Powder .... ▣620

Goody's Extra Strength Pain Relief Tablets ... ■620
Percodan Tablets ... 1327
Robaxisal Tablets ... 2939
Soma Compound Tablets ... 3354
Soma Compound w/Codeine Tablets ... 3355
Vanquish Caplets ... ■617

Bendroflumethiazide (May increase serum phenytoin levels). Products include:
Corzide 40/5 Tablets ... 2247
Corzide 80/5 Tablets ... 2247

Betamethasone Acetate (Phenytoin impairs efficacy of corticosteroids). Products include:
Celestone Soluspan Injectable Suspension ... 3097

Betamethasone Sodium Phosphate (Phenytoin impairs efficacy of corticosteroids). Products include:
Celestone Soluspan Injectable Suspension ... 3097

Calcium Carbonate (Calcium ions interfere with the absorption of phenytoin; ingestion times of phenytoin and antacids containing calcium should be staggered in patients with low phenytoin levels). Products include:
Aspirin Regimen Bayer 81 mg Caplets with Calcium ... ■607
Extra Strength Bayer Plus Caplets ... ■610
Caltrate 600 Tablets ... ■814
Caltrate 600 PLUS ... ■815
Caltrate 600 + D Tablets ... ■814
Caltrate 600 + Soy Tablets ... ■814
D-Cal Chewable Caplets ... ■794
Florical Capsules and Tablets ... 2223
Quick Dissolve Maalox Max Maximum Strength Antacid/Antigas Tablets ... 2301
Quick Dissolve Maalox Regular Strength Antacid Tablets ... 2301
Marblen Suspension ... ■633
Monocal Tablets ... 2223
Mylanta Fast-Acting ... 1813
Mylanta Calci Tabs ... ■636
One-A-Day Bedtime & Rest Tablets ... ■805
One-A-Day Calcium Plus Chewable Tablets ... ■805
Os-Cal Chewable Tablets ... ■838
Pepcid Complete Chewable Tablets ... 1815
ReSource Wellness CalciWise Soft Chews ... ■824
Rolaids Tablets ... ■706
Extra Strength Rolaids Tablets ... ■706
Slow-Mag Tablets ... ■835
Titralac ... ■640
3M Titralac Plus Antacid Tablets ... ■640
Tums ... ■763

Carbamazepine (May decrease serum phenytoin levels). Products include:
Carbatrol Capsules ... 3234
Tegretol/Tegretol-XR ... 2404

Chloramphenicol (May increase serum phenytoin levels). Products include:
Chloromycetin Ophthalmic Ointment, 1% ... ⊙296
Chloromycetin Ophthalmic Solution ... ⊙297
Chloroptic Sterile Ophthalmic Ointment ... ⊙234
Chloroptic Sterile Ophthalmic Solution ... ⊙235

Chloramphenicol Palmitate (May increase serum phenytoin levels).
No products indexed under this heading.

Chloramphenicol Sodium Succinate (May increase serum phenytoin levels).
No products indexed under this heading.

Chlordiazepoxide (May increase serum phenytoin levels). Products include:
Limbitrol ... 1738

Chlordiazepoxide Hydrochloride (May increase serum phenytoin levels). Products include:
Librium Capsules ... 1736
Librium for Injection ... 1737

Chlorothiazide (May increase serum phenytoin levels). Products include:
Aldoclor Tablets ... 2035
Diuril Oral ... 2087

Chlorothiazide Sodium (May increase serum phenytoin levels). Products include:
Diuril Sodium Intravenous ... 2086

Chlorotrianisene (May increase serum phenytoin levels; phenytoin impairs efficacy of estrogens).
No products indexed under this heading.

Chlorpromazine (May increase serum phenytoin levels). Products include:
Thorazine Suppositories ... 1656

Chlorpromazine Hydrochloride (May increase serum phenytoin levels). Products include:
Thorazine ... 1656

Chlorpropamide (May increase serum phenytoin levels). Products include:
Diabinese Tablets ... 2680

Choline Magnesium Trisalicylate (May increase serum phenytoin levels). Products include:
Trilisate ... 2901

Cimetidine (May increase serum phenytoin levels). Products include:
Tagamet HB 200 Suspension ... ■762
Tagamet HB 200 Tablets ... ■761
Tagamet Tablets ... 1644

Cimetidine Hydrochloride (May increase serum phenytoin levels). Products include:
Tagamet ... 1644

Clomipramine Hydrochloride (Tricyclic antidepressants may precipitate seizures in susceptible patients and phenytoin dosage may need to be adjusted).
No products indexed under this heading.

Cortisone Acetate (Phenytoin impairs efficacy of corticosteroids). Products include:
Cortone Acetate Injectable Suspension ... 2059
Cortone Acetate Tablets ... 2061

Desipramine Hydrochloride (Tricyclic antidepressants may precipitate seizures in susceptible patients and phenytoin dosage may need to be adjusted). Products include:
Norpramin Tablets ... 755

Desogestrel (Phenytoin impairs efficacy of oral contraceptives). Products include:
Cyclessa Tablets ... 2450
Desogen Tablets ... 2458
Mircette Tablets ... 2470
Ortho-Cept 21 Tablets ... 2546
Ortho-Cept 28 Tablets ... 2546

Dexamethasone (Phenytoin impairs efficacy of corticosteroids). Products include:
Decadron Elixir ... 2078
Decadron Tablets ... 2079
TobraDex Ophthalmic Ointment ... 542
TobraDex Ophthalmic Suspension ... 541

Dexamethasone Acetate (Phenytoin impairs efficacy of corticosteroids).
No products indexed under this heading.

Dexamethasone Sodium Phosphate (Phenytoin impairs efficacy of corticosteroids). Products include:
Decadron Phosphate Injection ... 2081
Decadron Phosphate Sterile Ophthalmic Ointment ... 2083
Decadron Phosphate Sterile Ophthalmic Solution ... 2084
NeoDecadron Sterile Ophthalmic Solution ... 2144

Diazepam (May increase serum phenytoin levels). Products include:
Valium Injectable ... 3026
Valium Tablets ... 3047

Dicumarol (May increase serum phenytoin levels; phenytoin impairs efficacy of coumarin anticoagulants).
No products indexed under this heading.

Dienestrol (May increase serum phenytoin levels; phenytoin impairs efficacy of estrogens). Products include:
Ortho Dienestrol Cream ... 2554

Diethylstilbestrol (May increase serum phenytoin levels; phenytoin impairs efficacy of estrogens).
No products indexed under this heading.

Diflunisal (May increase serum phenytoin levels). Products include:
Dolobid Tablets ... 2088

Digitoxin (Phenytoin impairs efficacy of digitoxin).
No products indexed under this heading.

Disulfiram (May increase serum phenytoin levels). Products include:
Antabuse Tablets ... 2444
Antabuse Tablets ... 3474

Divalproex Sodium (May increase or decrease phenytoin serum levels; unpredictable effect on valproate serum levels). Products include:
Depakote Sprinkle Capsules ... 426
Depakote Tablets ... 430
Depakote ER Tablets ... 436

Doxepin Hydrochloride (Tricyclic antidepressants may precipitate seizures in susceptible patients and phenytoin dosage may need to be adjusted). Products include:
Sinequan ... 2713

Doxycycline Calcium (Phenytoin impairs efficacy of doxycycline). Products include:
Vibramycin Calcium Oral Suspension Syrup ... 2735

Doxycycline Hyclate (Phenytoin impairs efficacy of doxycycline). Products include:
Doryx Coated Pellet Filled Capsules ... 3357
Periostat Tablets ... 1208
Vibramycin Hyclate Capsules ... 2735
Vibramycin Hyclate Intravenous ... 2737
Vibra-Tabs Film Coated Tablets ... 2735

Doxycycline Monohydrate (Phenytoin impairs efficacy of doxycycline). Products include:
Monodox Capsules ... 2442
Vibramycin Monohydrate for Oral Suspension ... 2735

Dyphylline (Phenytoin impairs efficacy of theophylline). Products include:
Lufyllin Tablets ... 3347
Lufyllin-400 Tablets ... 3347
Lufyllin-GG Elixir ... 3348
Lufyllin-GG Tablets ... 3348

Estradiol (May increase serum phenytoin levels; phenytoin impairs efficacy of estrogens). Products include:
Activella Tablets ... 2764
Alora Transdermal System ... 3372
Climara Transdermal System ... 958
CombiPatch Transdermal System ... 2323
Esclim Transdermal System ... 3460
Estrace Vaginal Cream ... 3358
Estrace Tablets ... 3361
Estring Vaginal Ring ... 2811
Ortho-Prefest Tablets ... 2570
Vagifem Tablets ... 2857
Vivelle Transdermal System ... 2412
Vivelle-Dot Transdermal System ... 2416

Estrogens, Conjugated (May increase serum phenytoin levels; phenytoin impairs efficacy of estrogens). Products include:
Premarin Intravenous ... 3563
Premarin Tablets ... 3566
Premarin Vaginal Cream ... 3570
Premphase Tablets ... 3572
Prempro Tablets ... 3572

Estrogens, Esterified (May increase serum phenytoin levels; phenytoin impairs efficacy of estrogens). Products include:
Estratest ... 3252
Menest Tablets ... 2254

Estropipate (May increase serum phenytoin levels; phenytoin impairs efficacy of estrogens). Products include:
Ogen Tablets ... 2846
Ortho-Est Tablets ... 3464

Ethinyl Estradiol (May increase serum phenytoin levels; phenytoin impairs efficacy of estrogens). Products include:
Alesse-21 Tablets ... 3468
Alesse-28 Tablets ... 3473
Brevicon 28-Day Tablets ... 3380
Cyclessa Tablets ... 2450
Desogen Tablets ... 2458
Estinyl Tablets ... 3112
Estrostep ... 2627
femhrt Tablets ... 2635
Levlen ... 962
Levlite 21 Tablets ... 962
Levlite 28 Tablets ... 962
Levora Tablets ... 3389
Loestrin 21 Tablets ... 2642
Loestrin Fe Tablets ... 2642
Lo/Ovral Tablets ... 3532
Lo/Ovral-28 Tablets ... 3538
Low-Ogestrel-28 Tablets ... 3392
Microgestin Fe 1.5/30 Tablets ... 3407
Microgestin Fe 1/20 Tablets ... 3400
Mircette Tablets ... 2470
Modicon ... 2563
Necon ... 3415
Nordette-28 Tablets ... 2257
Norinyl 1 +35 28-Day Tablets ... 3380
Ogestrel 0.5/50-28 Tablets ... 3428
Ortho-Cept 21 Tablets ... 2546
Ortho-Cept 28 Tablets ... 2546
Ortho-Cyclen/Ortho Tri-Cyclen ... 2573
Ortho-Novum ... 2563
Ovcon ... 3364
Ovral Tablets ... 3551
Ovral-28 Tablets ... 3552
Tri-Levlen ... 962
Tri-Norinyl-28 Tablets ... 3433
Triphasil-21 Tablets ... 3600
Triphasil-28 Tablets ... 3605
Trivora Tablets ... 3439
Yasmin 28 Tablets ... 980
Zovia ... 3449

Ethosuximide (May increase serum phenytoin levels). Products include:
Zarontin Capsules ... 2659
Zarontin Syrup ... 2660

Ethynodiol Diacetate (Phenytoin impairs efficacy of oral contraceptives). Products include:
Zovia ... 3449

Famotidine (May increase serum phenytoin levels). Products include:
Famotidine Injection ... 866
Pepcid AC ... 1814
Pepcid Complete Chewable Tablets ... 1815
Pepcid Injection ... 2153
Pepcid for Oral Suspension ... 2150
Pepcid RPD Orally Disintegrating Tablets ... 2150
Pepcid Tablets ... 2150

Fludrocortisone Acetate (Phenytoin impairs efficacy of corticosteroids). Products include:
Florinef Acetate Tablets ... 2250

Fluphenazine Decanoate (May increase serum phenytoin levels).
No products indexed under this heading.

Fluphenazine Enanthate (May increase serum phenytoin levels).
No products indexed under this heading.

Fluphenazine Hydrochloride (May increase serum phenytoin levels).
No products indexed under this heading.

Furosemide (Phenytoin impairs efficacy of furosemide). Products include:
Furosemide Tablets ... 2284

Glipizide (May increase serum phenytoin levels). Products include:
Glucotrol Tablets ... 2692
Glucotrol XL Extended Release Tablets ... 2693

Glyburide (May increase serum phenytoin levels). Products include:
DiaBeta Tablets ... 741
Glucovance Tablets ... 1086

Halothane (May increase serum phenytoin levels). Products include:
Fluothane Inhalation ... 3508

Hydrochlorothiazide (May increase serum phenytoin levels). Products include:
Accuretic Tablets ... 2614
Aldoril Tablets ... 2039
Atacand HCT Tablets ... 597
Avalide Tablets ... 1070
Diovan HCT Tablets ... 2338
Dyazide Capsules ... 1515
HydroDIURIL Tablets ... 2108
Hyzaar ... 2109
Inderide Tablets ... 3517
Inderide LA Long-Acting Capsules ... 3519
Lotensin HCT Tablets ... 2367
Maxzide ... 1008
Micardis HCT Tablets ... 1051
Microzide Capsules ... 3414
Moduretic Tablets ... 2138
Monopril HCT ... 1094
Prinzide Tablets ... 2168
Timolide Tablets ... 2187
Uniretic Tablets ... 3178
Vaseretic Tablets ... 2204
Zestoretic Tablets ... 695
Ziac Tablets ... 1887

Hydrocortisone (Phenytoin impairs efficacy of corticosteroids). Products include:
Anusol-HC Cream 2.5% ... 2237
Cipro HC Otic Suspension ... 540
Cortaid Intensive Therapy Cream ... ▣717
Cortaid Maximum Strength Cream ... ▣717
Cortisporin Ophthalmic Suspension Sterile ... ⊙297
Cortizone•5 ... ▣699
Cortizone•10 ... ▣699
Cortizone•10 Plus Creme ... ▣700
Cortizone for Kids Creme ... ▣699
Hydrocortone Tablets ... 2106
Massengill Medicated Soft Cloth Towelette ... ▣753
VōSoL HC Otic Solution ... 3356

Hydrocortisone Acetate (Phenytoin impairs efficacy of corticosteroids). Products include:
Analpram-HC ... 1338
Anusol HC-1 Hydrocortisone Anti-Itch Cream ... ▣689
Anusol-HC Suppositories ... 2238
Cortaid ... ▣717
Cortifoam Rectal Foam ... 3170
Cortisporin-TC Otic Suspension ... 2246
Hydrocortone Acetate Injectable Suspension ... 2103
Pramosone ... 1343
Proctocort Suppositories ... 2264
ProctoFoam-HC ... 3177
Terra-Cortril Ophthalmic Suspension ... 2716

Hydrocortisone Sodium Phosphate (Phenytoin impairs efficacy of corticosteroids). Products include:
Hydrocortone Phosphate Injection, Sterile ... 2105

Hydrocortisone Sodium Succinate (Phenytoin impairs efficacy of corticosteroids).
No products indexed under this heading.

Hydroflumethiazide (May increase serum phenytoin levels). Products include:
Diucardin Tablets ... 3494

Imipramine Hydrochloride (Tricyclic antidepressants may precipitate seizures in susceptible patients and phenytoin dosage may need to be adjusted).
No products indexed under this heading.

Imipramine Pamoate (Tricyclic antidepressants may precipitate seizures in susceptible patients and phenytoin dosage may need to be adjusted).
No products indexed under this heading.

Isoniazid (May increase serum phenytoin levels). Products include:
Rifamate Capsules ... 767
Rifater Tablets ... 769

Levonorgestrel (Phenytoin impairs efficacy of oral contraceptives). Products include:
Alesse-21 Tablets ... 3468
Alesse-28 Tablets ... 3473
Levlen ... 962
Levlite 21 Tablets ... 962
Levlite 28 Tablets ... 962
Levora Tablets ... 3389
Mirena Intrauterine System ... 974
Nordette-28 Tablets ... 2257
Norplant System ... 3543
Tri-Levlen ... 962
Triphasil-21 Tablets ... 3600
Triphasil-28 Tablets ... 3605
Trivora Tablets ... 3439

Magnesium Salicylate (May increase serum phenytoin levels). Products include:
Momentum Backache Relief Extra Strength Caplets ... ▣666

Maprotiline Hydrochloride (Tricyclic antidepressants may precipitate seizures in susceptible patients and phenytoin dosage may need to be adjusted).
No products indexed under this heading.

Mesoridazine Besylate (May increase serum phenytoin levels). Products include:
Serentil ... 1057

Mestranol (Phenytoin impairs efficacy of oral contraceptives). Products include:
Necon 1/50 Tablets ... 3415
Norinyl 1 + 50 28-Day Tablets ... 3380
Ortho-Novum 1/50□28 Tablets ... 2556

Methotrimeprazine (May increase serum phenytoin levels).
No products indexed under this heading.

Methsuximide (May increase serum phenytoin levels). Products include:
Celontin Capsules ... 2618

Methyclothiazide (May increase serum phenytoin levels).
No products indexed under this heading.

Methylphenidate Hydrochloride (May increase serum phenytoin levels). Products include:
Concerta Extended-Release Tablets ... 1998
Concerta Tablets ... 561
Metadate CD Capsules ... 1164
Metadate ER Tablets ... 1167
Methylin Tablets ... 1995
Methylin ER Tablets ... 1995
Ritalin ... 2387

Methylprednisolone Acetate (Phenytoin impairs efficacy of corticosteroids). Products include:
Depo-Medrol Injectable Suspension ... 2795

Methylprednisolone Sodium Succinate (Phenytoin impairs efficacy of corticosteroids). Products include:
Solu-Medrol Sterile Powder ... 2855

Molindone Hydrochloride (Moban brand of molindone contains calcium ions which interfere with the absorption of phenytoin). Products include:
Moban ... 1320

Nizatidine (May increase serum phenytoin levels). Products include:
Axid Pulvules ... 1903
Axid Pulvules ... 2919

Norethindrone (Phenytoin impairs efficacy of oral contraceptives). Products include:
Brevicon 28-Day Tablets ... 3380
Micronor Tablets ... 2543
Modicon ... 2563
Necon ... 3415
Norinyl 1 +35 28-Day Tablets ... 3380
Norinyl 1 + 50 28-Day Tablets ... 3380
Nor-QD Tablets ... 3423
Ortho-Novum ... 2563
Ortho-Novum 1/50□28 Tablets ... 2556
Ovcon ... 3364
Tri-Norinyl-28 Tablets ... 3433

Norethynodrel (Phenytoin impairs efficacy of oral contraceptives).
No products indexed under this heading.

Norgestimate (Phenytoin impairs efficacy of oral contraceptives). Products include:
Ortho-Cyclen/Ortho Tri-Cyclen ... 2573
Ortho-Prefest Tablets ... 2570

Norgestrel (Phenytoin impairs efficacy of oral contraceptives). Products include:
Lo/Ovral Tablets ... 3532
Lo/Ovral-28 Tablets ... 3538
Low-Ogestrel-28 Tablets ... 3392
Ogestrel 0.5/50-28 Tablets ... 3428
Ovral Tablets ... 3551
Ovral-28 Tablets ... 3552
Ovrette Tablets ... 3552

Nortriptyline Hydrochloride (Tricyclic antidepressants may precipitate seizures in susceptible patients and phenytoin dosage may need to be adjusted).
No products indexed under this heading.

Perphenazine (May increase serum phenytoin levels). Products include:
Etrafon ... 3115
Trilafon ... 3160

Phenobarbital (May increase or decrease phenytoin serum levels; unpredictable effect on phenobarbital serum levels). Products include:
Arco-Lase Plus Tablets ... 592
Donnatal ... 2929
Donnatal Extentabs ... 2930

Phensuximide (May increase serum phenytoin levels).
No products indexed under this heading.

Phenylbutazone (May increase serum phenytoin levels).
No products indexed under this heading.

Polyestradiol Phosphate (May increase serum phenytoin levels; phenytoin impairs efficacy of estrogens).
No products indexed under this heading.

Polythiazide (May increase serum phenytoin levels). Products include:
Minizide Capsules ... 2700
Renese Tablets ... 2712

Prednisolone Acetate (Phenytoin impairs efficacy of corticosteroids). Products include:
Blephamide Ophthalmic Ointment ... 547
Blephamide Ophthalmic Suspension ... 548
Poly-Pred Liquifilm Ophthalmic Suspension ... ⊙245
Pred Forte Ophthalmic Suspension ... ⊙246
Pred Mild Sterile Ophthalmic Suspension ... ⊙249
Pred-G Ophthalmic Suspension ... ⊙247
Pred-G Sterile Ophthalmic Ointment ... ⊙248

Prednisolone Sodium Phosphate (Phenytoin impairs efficacy of corticosteroids). Products include:
Pediapred Oral Solution ... 1170

Prednisolone Tebutate (Phenytoin impairs efficacy of corticosteroids).
No products indexed under this heading.

Prednisone (Phenytoin impairs efficacy of corticosteroids). Products include:
Prednisone ... 3064

Prochlorperazine (May increase serum phenytoin levels). Products include:
Compazine ... 1505

Promethazine Hydrochloride (May increase serum phenytoin levels). Products include:
Mepergan Injection ... 3539
Phenergan Injection ... 3553
Phenergan ... 3556
Phenergan Syrup ... 3554
Phenergan with Codeine Syrup ... 3557
Phenergan with Dextromethorphan Syrup ... 3559
Phenergan VC Syrup ... 3560
Phenergan VC with Codeine Syrup ... 3561

Protriptyline Hydrochloride (Tricyclic antidepressants may precipitate seizures in susceptible patients and phenytoin dosage may need to be adjusted). Products include:
Vivactil Tablets ... 2446
Vivactil Tablets ... 2217

Quinestrol (May increase serum phenytoin levels; phenytoin impairs efficacy of estrogens).
No products indexed under this heading.

Quinidine Gluconate (Phenytoin impairs efficacy of quinidine). Products include:
Quinaglute Dura-Tabs Tablets ... 978

Quinidine Polygalacturonate (Phenytoin impairs efficacy of quinidine).
No products indexed under this heading.

Quinidine Sulfate (Phenytoin impairs efficacy of quinidine). Products include:
Quinidex Extentabs ... 2933

Ranitidine Bismuth Citrate (May increase serum phenytoin levels).
No products indexed under this heading.

Ranitidine Hydrochloride (May increase serum phenytoin levels). Products include:
Zantac ... 1690
Zantac Injection ... 1688
Zantac 75 Tablets ... ▣717

Reserpine (May decrease serum phenytoin levels).
No products indexed under this heading.

Rifampin (Phenytoin impairs efficacy of rifampin). Products include:
Rifadin ... 765
Rifamate Capsules ... 767
Rifater Tablets ... 769

Salsalate (May increase serum phenytoin levels).
No products indexed under this heading.

Sucralfate (May decrease serum phenytoin levels). Products include:
Carafate Suspension ... 731
Carafate Tablets ... 730

Sulfacytine (May increase serum phenytoin levels).

Sulfamethizole (May increase serum phenytoin levels). Products include:
Urobiotic-250 Capsules ... 2731

Sulfamethoxazole (May increase serum phenytoin levels). Products include:
Bactrim ... 2949
Septra Suspension ... 2265
Septra Tablets ... 2265
Septra DS Tablets ... 2265

Sulfasalazine (May increase serum phenytoin levels). Products include:
Azulfidine EN-tabs Tablets ... 2775

Sulfinpyrazone (May increase serum phenytoin levels).
No products indexed under this heading.

Sulfisoxazole (May increase serum phenytoin levels).
No products indexed under this heading.

Sulfisoxazole Acetyl (May increase serum phenytoin levels). Products include:
Pediazole Suspension ... 3050

Sulfisoxazole Diolamine (May increase serum phenytoin levels).
No products indexed under this heading.

Theophylline (Phenytoin impairs efficacy of theophylline). Products include:
Aerolate ... 1361
Theo-Dur Extended-Release Tablets ... 1835
Uni-Dur Extended-Release Tablets ... 1841
Uniphyl 400 mg and 600 mg Tablets ... 2903

Theophylline Calcium Salicylate (Phenytoin impairs efficacy of theo-

phylline).
No products indexed under this heading.

Theophylline Sodium Glycinate (Phenytoin impairs efficacy of theophylline).
No products indexed under this heading.

Thioridazine Hydrochloride (May increase serum phenytoin levels). Products include:
Thioridazine Hydrochloride Tablets 2289

Tolazamide (May increase serum phenytoin levels).
No products indexed under this heading.

Tolbutamide (May increase serum phenytoin levels).
No products indexed under this heading.

Trazodone Hydrochloride (May increase serum phenytoin levels).
No products indexed under this heading.

Triamcinolone (Phenytoin impairs efficacy of corticosteroids).
No products indexed under this heading.

Triamcinolone Acetonide (Phenytoin impairs efficacy of corticosteroids). Products include:
Azmacort Inhalation Aerosol 728
Nasacort Nasal Inhaler 750
Nasacort AQ Nasal Spray 752
Tri-Nasal Spray 2274

Triamcinolone Diacetate (Phenytoin impairs efficacy of corticosteroids).
No products indexed under this heading.

Triamcinolone Hexacetonide (Phenytoin impairs efficacy of corticosteroids).
No products indexed under this heading.

Trifluoperazine Hydrochloride (May increase serum phenytoin levels). Products include:
Stelazine 1640

Trimipramine Maleate (Tricyclic antidepressants may precipitate seizures in susceptible patients and phenytoin dosage may need to be adjusted). Products include:
Surmontil Capsules 3595

Valproic Acid (May increase or decrease phenytoin serum levels; unpredictable effect on valproic serum levels). Products include:
Depakene 421

Vitamin D (Phenytoin impairs efficacy of vitamin D). Products include:
Active Calcium Tablets 3335
Caltrate 600 PLUS 815
Caltrate 600 + D Tablets 814
Centrum Focused Formulas Bone Health Tablets 815
Citracal Caplets + D 823
D-Cal Chewable Caplets 794
One-A-Day Calcium Plus Chewable Tablets 805
Os-Cal 250 + D Tablets 838
Os-Cal 500 + D Tablets 839

Warfarin Sodium (Phenytoin impairs efficacy of coumarin anticoagulants). Products include:
Coumadin for Injection 1243
Coumadin Tablets 1243
Warfarin Sodium Tablets, USP 3302

Food Interactions

Alcohol (Acute alcohol intake increases serum phenytoin levels; chronic alcohol intake decreases serum phenytoin levels).

DILAUDID AMPULES

(Hydromorphone Hydrochloride) 441
May interact with central nervous system depressants, tricyclic antidepressants, and certain other agents. Compounds in these categories include:

Alfentanil Hydrochloride (Additive CNS depression).
No products indexed under this heading.

Alprazolam (Additive CNS depression). Products include:
Xanax Tablets 2865

Amitriptyline Hydrochloride (Additive CNS depression). Products include:
Etrafon 3115
Limbitrol 1738

Amoxapine (Additive CNS depression).
No products indexed under this heading.

Aprobarbital (Additive CNS depression).
No products indexed under this heading.

Buprenorphine Hydrochloride (Additive CNS depression). Products include:
Buprenex Injectable 2918

Buspirone Hydrochloride (Additive CNS depression).
No products indexed under this heading.

Butabarbital (Additive CNS depression).
No products indexed under this heading.

Butalbital (Additive CNS depression). Products include:
Phrenilin 578
Sedapap Tablets 50 mg/650 mg 2225

Chlordiazepoxide (Additive CNS depression). Products include:
Limbitrol 1738

Chlordiazepoxide Hydrochloride (Additive CNS depression). Products include:
Librium Capsules 1736
Librium for Injection 1737

Chlorpromazine (Additive CNS depression). Products include:
Thorazine Suppositories 1656

Chlorpromazine Hydrochloride (Additive CNS depression). Products include:
Thorazine 1656

Chlorprothixene (Additive CNS depression).
No products indexed under this heading.

Chlorprothixene Hydrochloride (Additive CNS depression).
No products indexed under this heading.

Chlorprothixene Lactate (Additive CNS depression).
No products indexed under this heading.

Clomipramine Hydrochloride (Additive CNS depression).
No products indexed under this heading.

Clorazepate Dipotassium (Additive CNS depression). Products include:
Tranxene 511

Clozapine (Additive CNS depression). Products include:
Clozaril Tablets 2319

Codeine Phosphate (Additive CNS depression). Products include:
Phenergan with Codeine Syrup 3557
Phenergan VC with Codeine Syrup 3561
Robitussin A-C Syrup 2942
Robitussin-DAC Syrup 2942
Ryna-C Liquid 768
Soma Compound w/Codeine Tablets 3355
Tussi-Organidin NR Liquid 3350
Tussi-Organidin-S NR Liquid 3350
Tylenol with Codeine 2595

Desflurane (Additive CNS depression). Products include:
Suprane Liquid for Inhalation 874

Desipramine Hydrochloride (Additive CNS depression). Products include:
Norpramin Tablets 755

Dezocine (Additive CNS depression).
No products indexed under this heading.

Diazepam (Additive CNS depression). Products include:
Valium Injectable 3026
Valium Tablets 3047

Doxepin Hydrochloride (Additive CNS depression). Products include:
Sinequan 2713

Droperidol (Additive CNS depression).
No products indexed under this heading.

Enflurane (Additive CNS depression).
No products indexed under this heading.

Estazolam (Additive CNS depression). Products include:
ProSom Tablets 500

Ethchlorvynol (Additive CNS depression).
No products indexed under this heading.

Ethinamate (Additive CNS depression).
No products indexed under this heading.

Fentanyl (Additive CNS depression). Products include:
Duragesic Transdermal System 1786

Fentanyl Citrate (Additive CNS depression). Products include:
Actiq 1184

Fluphenazine Decanoate (Additive CNS depression).
No products indexed under this heading.

Fluphenazine Enanthate (Additive CNS depression).
No products indexed under this heading.

Fluphenazine Hydrochloride (Additive CNS depression).
No products indexed under this heading.

Flurazepam Hydrochloride (Additive CNS depression).
No products indexed under this heading.

Glutethimide (Additive CNS depression).
No products indexed under this heading.

Haloperidol (Additive CNS depression). Products include:
Haldol Injection, Tablets and Concentrate 2533

Haloperidol Decanoate (Additive CNS depression). Products include:
Haldol Decanoate 2535

Hydrocodone Bitartrate (Additive CNS depression). Products include:
Hycodan 1316
Hycomine Compound Tablets 1317
Hycotuss Expectorant Syrup 1318
Lortab 3319
Lortab Elixir 3317
Maxidone Tablets CIII 3399
Norco 5/325 Tablets CIII 3424
Norco 7.5/325 Tablets CIII 3425
Norco 10/325 Tablets CIII 3427
Norco 10/325 Tablets CIII 3425
Vicodin Tablets 516
Vicodin ES Tablets 517
Vicodin HP Tablets 518
Vicodin Tuss Expectorant 519
Vicoprofen Tablets 520
Zydone Tablets 1330

Hydrocodone Polistirex (Additive CNS depression). Products include:
Tussionex Pennkinetic Extended-Release Suspension 1174

Hydroxyzine Hydrochloride (Additive CNS depression). Products include:
Atarax Tablets & Syrup 2667
Vistaril Intramuscular Solution 2738

Imipramine Hydrochloride (Additive CNS depression).
No products indexed under this heading.

Imipramine Pamoate (Additive CNS depression).
No products indexed under this heading.

Isoflurane (Additive CNS depression).
No products indexed under this heading.

Ketamine Hydrochloride (Additive CNS depression).
No products indexed under this heading.

Levomethadyl Acetate Hydrochloride (Additive CNS depression).
No products indexed under this heading.

Levorphanol Tartrate (Additive CNS depression). Products include:
Levo-Dromoran 1734
Levorphanol Tartrate Tablets 3059

Lorazepam (Additive CNS depression). Products include:
Ativan Injection 3478
Ativan Tablets 3482

Loxapine Hydrochloride (Additive CNS depression).
No products indexed under this heading.

Loxapine Succinate (Additive CNS depression). Products include:
Loxitane Capsules 3398

Maprotiline Hydrochloride (Additive CNS depression).
No products indexed under this heading.

Meperidine Hydrochloride (Additive CNS depression). Products include:
Demerol 3079
Mepergan Injection 3539

Mephobarbital (Additive CNS depression).
No products indexed under this heading.

Meprobamate (Additive CNS depression). Products include:
Miltown Tablets 3349

Mesoridazine Besylate (Additive CNS depression). Products include:
Serentil 1057

Methadone Hydrochloride (Additive CNS depression). Products include:
Dolophine Hydrochloride Tablets 3056

Methohexital Sodium (Additive CNS depression). Products include:
Brevital Sodium for Injection, USP 1815

Methotrimeprazine (Additive CNS depression).
No products indexed under this heading.

Methoxyflurane (Additive CNS depression).
No products indexed under this heading.

Midazolam Hydrochloride (Additive CNS depression). Products include:
Versed Injection 3027
Versed Syrup 3033

Molindone Hydrochloride (Additive CNS depression). Products include:
Moban 1320

Morphine Sulfate (Additive CNS depression). Products include:
Astramorph/PF Injection, USP (Preservative-Free) 594
Duramorph Injection 1312
Infumorph 200 and Infumorph 500 Sterile Solutions 1314
Kadian Capsules 1335
MS Contin Tablets 2896
MSIR 2898
Oramorph SR Tablets 3062
Roxanol 3066

Nortriptyline Hydrochloride (Additive CNS depression).
No products indexed under this heading.

Olanzapine (Additive CNS depression). Products include:
Zyprexa Tablets 1973
Zyprexa ZYDIS Orally Disintegrating Tablets 1973

IMPORTANT NOTE: Always consult each drug listing in the patient's regimen for possible interactions.

Oxazepam (Additive CNS depression).
No products indexed under this heading.

Oxycodone Hydrochloride (Additive CNS depression). Products include:
- OxyContin Tablets 2912
- OxyFast Oral Concentrate Solution . 2916
- OxyIR Capsules 2916
- Percocet Tablets 1326
- Percodan Tablets 1327
- Percolone Tablets 1327
- Roxicodone 3067
- Tylox Capsules 2597

Pentobarbital Sodium (Additive CNS depression). Products include:
- Nembutal Sodium Solution 485

Perphenazine (Additive CNS depression). Products include:
- Etrafon 3115
- Trilafon 3160

Phenobarbital (Additive CNS depression). Products include:
- Arco-Lase Plus Tablets 592
- Donnatal 2929
- Donnatal Extentabs 2930

Prazepam (Additive CNS depression).
No products indexed under this heading.

Prochlorperazine (Additive CNS depression). Products include:
- Compazine 1505

Promethazine Hydrochloride (Additive CNS depression). Products include:
- Mepergan Injection 3539
- Phenergan Injection 3553
- Phenergan 3556
- Phenergan Syrup 3554
- Phenergan with Codeine Syrup 3557
- Phenergan with Dextromethorphan Syrup 3559
- Phenergan VC Syrup 3560
- Phenergan VC with Codeine Syrup .. 3561

Propofol (Additive CNS depression). Products include:
- Diprivan Injectable Emulsion 667

Propoxyphene Hydrochloride (Additive CNS depression). Products include:
- Darvon Pulvules 1909
- Darvon Compound-65 Pulvules 1910

Propoxyphene Napsylate (Additive CNS depression). Products include:
- Darvon-N/Darvocet-N 1907
- Darvon-N Tablets 1912

Protriptyline Hydrochloride (Additive CNS depression). Products include:
- Vivactil Tablets 2446
- Vivactil Tablets 2217

Quazepam (Additive CNS depression).
No products indexed under this heading.

Quetiapine Fumarate (Additive CNS depression). Products include:
- Seroquel Tablets 684

Remifentanil Hydrochloride (Additive CNS depression).
No products indexed under this heading.

Risperidone (Additive CNS depression). Products include:
- Risperdal 1796

Secobarbital Sodium (Additive CNS depression).
No products indexed under this heading.

Sevoflurane (Additive CNS depression).
No products indexed under this heading.

Sufentanil Citrate (Additive CNS depression).
No products indexed under this heading.

Temazepam (Additive CNS depression).
No products indexed under this heading.

Thiamylal Sodium (Additive CNS depression).
No products indexed under this heading.

Thioridazine Hydrochloride (Additive CNS depression). Products include:
- Thioridazine Hydrochloride Tablets 2289

Thiothixene (Additive CNS depression). Products include:
- Navane Capsules 2701
- Thiothixene Capsules 2290

Triazolam (Additive CNS depression). Products include:
- Halcion Tablets 2823

Trifluoperazine Hydrochloride (Additive CNS depression). Products include:
- Stelazine 1640

Trimipramine Maleate (Additive CNS depression). Products include:
- Surmontil Capsules 3595

Zaleplon (Additive CNS depression). Products include:
- Sonata Capsules 3591

Ziprasidone Hydrochloride (Additive CNS depression). Products include:
- Geodon Capsules 2688

Zolpidem Tartrate (Additive CNS depression). Products include:
- Ambien Tablets 3191

Food Interactions

Alcohol (Additive CNS depression).

DILAUDID INJECTION

(Hydromorphone Hydrochloride) 441
See Dilaudid Ampules

DILAUDID MULTIPLE DOSE VIALS (STERILE SOLUTION)

(Hydromorphone Hydrochloride) 441
See Dilaudid Ampules

DILAUDID ORAL LIQUID

(Hydromorphone Hydrochloride) 445
May interact with central nervous system depressants, general anesthetics, hypnotics and sedatives, neuromuscular blocking agents, phenothiazines, tranquilizers, and certain other agents. Compounds in these categories include:

Alfentanil Hydrochloride (May produce additive depressant effects; respiratory depression, hypotension and profound sedation or coma may occur; the dose of one or both agents should be reduced).
No products indexed under this heading.

Alprazolam (May produce additive depressant effects; respiratory depression, hypotension and profound sedation or coma may occur; the dose of one or both agents should be reduced). Products include:
- Xanax Tablets 2865

Aprobarbital (May produce additive depressant effects; respiratory depression, hypotension and profound sedation or coma may occur; the dose of one or both agents should be reduced).
No products indexed under this heading.

Atracurium Besylate (Enhanced action of neuromuscular blocking agents and produce an excessive degree of respiratory depression).
No products indexed under this heading.

Buprenorphine Hydrochloride (May produce additive depressant effects; respiratory depression, hypotension and profound sedation or coma may occur; the dose of one or both agents should be reduced). Products include:
- Buprenex Injectable 2918

Buspirone Hydrochloride (May produce additive depressant effects; respiratory depression, hypotension and profound sedation or coma may occur; the dose of one or both agents should be reduced).
No products indexed under this heading.

Butabarbital (May produce additive depressant effects; respiratory depression, hypotension and profound sedation or coma may occur; the dose of one or both agents should be reduced).
No products indexed under this heading.

Butalbital (May produce additive depressant effects; respiratory depression, hypotension and profound sedation or coma may occur; the dose of one or both agents should be reduced). Products include:
- Phrenilin 578
- Sedapap Tablets 50 mg/650 mg ... 2225

Chlordiazepoxide (May produce additive depressant effects; respiratory depression, hypotension and profound sedation or coma may occur; the dose of one or both agents should be reduced). Products include:
- Limbitrol 1738

Chlordiazepoxide Hydrochloride (May produce additive depressant effects; respiratory depression, hypotension and profound sedation or coma may occur; the dose of one or both agents should be reduced). Products include:
- Librium Capsules 1736
- Librium for Injection 1737

Chlorpromazine (May produce additive depressant effects; respiratory depression, hypotension and profound sedation or coma may occur; the dose of one or both agents should be reduced). Products include:
- Thorazine Suppositories 1656

Chlorpromazine Hydrochloride (May produce additive depressant effects; respiratory depression, hypotension and profound sedation or coma may occur; the dose of one or both agents should be reduced). Products include:
- Thorazine 1656

Chlorprothixene (May produce additive depressant effects; respiratory depression, hypotension and profound sedation or coma may occur; the dose of one or both agents should be reduced).
No products indexed under this heading.

Chlorprothixene Hydrochloride (May produce additive depressant effects; respiratory depression, hypotension and profound sedation or coma may occur; the dose of one or both agents should be reduced).
No products indexed under this heading.

Chlorprothixene Lactate (May produce additive depressant effects; respiratory depression, hypotension and profound sedation or coma may occur; the dose of one or both agents should be reduced).
No products indexed under this heading.

Cisatracurium Besylate (Enhanced action of neuromuscular blocking agents and produce an excessive degree of respiratory depression).
No products indexed under this heading.

Clorazepate Dipotassium (May produce additive depressant effects; respiratory depression, hypotension and profound sedation or coma may occur; the dose of one or both agents should be reduced). Products include:
- Tranxene 511

Clozapine (May produce additive depressant effects; respiratory depression, hypotension and profound sedation or coma may occur; the dose of one or both agents should be reduced). Products include:
- Clozaril Tablets 2319

Codeine Phosphate (May produce additive depressant effects; respiratory depression, hypotension and profound sedation or coma may occur; the dose of one or both agents should be reduced). Products include:
- Phenergan with Codeine Syrup 3557
- Phenergan VC with Codeine Syrup .. 3561
- Robitussin A-C Syrup 2942
- Robitussin-DAC Syrup 2942
- Ryna-C Liquid .... ■768
- Soma Compound w/Codeine Tablets 3355
- Tussi-Organidin NR Liquid 3350
- Tussi-Organidin-S NR Liquid 3350
- Tylenol with Codeine 2595

Desflurane (May produce additive depressant effects; respiratory depression, hypotension and profound sedation or coma may occur; the dose of one or both agents should be reduced). Products include:
- Suprane Liquid for Inhalation 874

Dezocine (May produce additive depressant effects; respiratory depression, hypotension and profound sedation or coma may occur; the dose of one or both agents should be reduced).
No products indexed under this heading.

Diazepam (May produce additive depressant effects; respiratory depression, hypotension and profound sedation or coma may occur; the dose of one or both agents should be reduced). Products include:
- Valium Injectable 3026
- Valium Tablets 3047

Doxacurium Chloride (Enhanced action of neuromuscular blocking agents and produce an excessive degree of respiratory depression).
No products indexed under this heading.

Droperidol (May produce additive depressant effects; respiratory depression, hypotension and profound sedation or coma may occur; the dose of one or both agents should be reduced).
No products indexed under this heading.

Enflurane (May produce additive depressant effects; respiratory depression, hypotension and profound sedation or coma may occur; the dose of one or both agents should be reduced).
No products indexed under this heading.

Estazolam (May produce additive depressant effects; respiratory depression, hypotension and profound sedation or coma may occur; the dose of one or both agents should be reduced). Products include:
- ProSom Tablets 500

Ethchlorvynol (May produce additive depressant effects; respiratory depression, hypotension and profound sedation or coma may occur; the dose of one or both agents should be reduced).
No products indexed under this heading.

Ethinamate (May produce additive depressant effects; respiratory depression, hypotension and pro-

found sedation or coma may occur; the dose of one or both agents should be reduced).
No products indexed under this heading.

Fentanyl (May produce additive depressant effects; respiratory depression, hypotension and profound sedation or coma may occur; the dose of one or both agents should be reduced). Products include:
Duragesic Transdermal System 1786

Fentanyl Citrate (May produce additive depressant effects; respiratory depression, hypotension and profound sedation or coma may occur; the dose of one or both agents should be reduced). Products include:
Actiq 1184

Fluphenazine Decanoate (May produce additive depressant effects; respiratory depression, hypotension and profound sedation or coma may occur; the dose of one or both agents should be reduced).
No products indexed under this heading.

Fluphenazine Enanthate (May produce additive depressant effects; respiratory depression, hypotension and profound sedation or coma may occur; the dose of one or both agents should be reduced).
No products indexed under this heading.

Fluphenazine Hydrochloride (May produce additive depressant effects; respiratory depression, hypotension and profound sedation or coma may occur; the dose of one or both agents should be reduced).
No products indexed under this heading.

Flurazepam Hydrochloride (May produce additive depressant effects; respiratory depression, hypotension and profound sedation or coma may occur; the dose of one or both agents should be reduced).
No products indexed under this heading.

Glutethimide (May produce additive depressant effects; respiratory depression, hypotension and profound sedation or coma may occur; the dose of one or both agents should be reduced).
No products indexed under this heading.

Haloperidol (May produce additive depressant effects; respiratory depression, hypotension and profound sedation or coma may occur; the dose of one or both agents should be reduced). Products include:
Haldol Injection, Tablets and Concentrate 2533

Haloperidol Decanoate (May produce additive depressant effects; respiratory depression, hypotension and profound sedation or coma may occur; the dose of one or both agents should be reduced). Products include:
Haldol Decanoate 2535

Hydrocodone Bitartrate (May produce additive depressant effects; respiratory depression, hypotension and profound sedation or coma may occur; the dose of one or both agents should be reduced). Products include:
Hycodan 1316
Hycomine Compound Tablets 1317
Hycotuss Expectorant Syrup 1318
Lortab 3319
Lortab Elixir 3317
Maxidone Tablets CIII 3399
Norco 5/325 Tablets CIII 3424
Norco 7.5/325 Tablets CIII 3425
Norco 10/325 Tablets CIII 3427
Norco 10/325 Tablets CIII 3425
Vicodin Tablets 516
Vicodin ES Tablets 517
Vicodin HP Tablets 518
Vicodin Tuss Expectorant 519
Vicoprofen Tablets 520
Zydone Tablets 1330

Hydrocodone Polistirex (May produce additive depressant effects; respiratory depression, hypotension and profound sedation or coma may occur; the dose of one or both agents should be reduced). Products include:
Tussionex Pennkinetic Extended-Release Suspension 1174

Hydromorphone Hydrochloride (May produce additive depressant effects; respiratory depression, hypotension and profound sedation or coma may occur; the dose of one or both agents should be reduced). Products include:
Dilaudid 441
Dilaudid Oral Liquid 445
Dilaudid Powder 441
Dilaudid Rectal Suppositories 441
Dilaudid Tablets 441
Dilaudid Tablets - 8 mg 445
Dilaudid-HP 443

Hydroxyzine Hydrochloride (May produce additive depressant effects; respiratory depression, hypotension and profound sedation or coma may occur; the dose of one or both agents should be reduced). Products include:
Atarax Tablets & Syrup 2667
Vistaril Intramuscular Solution 2738

Isoflurane (May produce additive depressant effects; respiratory depression, hypotension and profound sedation or coma may occur; the dose of one or both agents should be reduced).
No products indexed under this heading.

Ketamine Hydrochloride (May produce additive depressant effects; respiratory depression, hypotension and profound sedation or coma may occur; the dose of one or both agents should be reduced).
No products indexed under this heading.

Levomethadyl Acetate Hydrochloride (May produce additive depressant effects; respiratory depression, hypotension and profound sedation or coma may occur; the dose of one or both agents should be reduced).
No products indexed under this heading.

Levorphanol Tartrate (May produce additive depressant effects; respiratory depression, hypotension and profound sedation or coma may occur; the dose of one or both agents should be reduced). Products include:
Levo-Dromoran 1734
Levorphanol Tartrate Tablets 3059

Lorazepam (May produce additive depressant effects; respiratory depression, hypotension and profound sedation or coma may occur; the dose of one or both agents should be reduced). Products include:
Ativan Injection 3478
Ativan Tablets 3482

Loxapine Hydrochloride (May produce additive depressant effects; respiratory depression, hypotension and profound sedation or coma may occur; the dose of one or both agents should be reduced).
No products indexed under this heading.

Loxapine Succinate (May produce additive depressant effects; respiratory depression, hypotension and profound sedation or coma may occur; the dose of one or both agents should be reduced). Products include:
Loxitane Capsules 3398

Meperidine Hydrochloride (May produce additive depressant effects; respiratory depression, hypotension and profound sedation or coma may occur; the dose of one or both agents should be reduced). Products include:
Demerol 3079
Mepergan Injection 3539

Mephobarbital (May produce additive depressant effects; respiratory depression, hypotension and profound sedation or coma may occur; the dose of one or both agents should be reduced).
No products indexed under this heading.

Meprobamate (May produce additive depressant effects; respiratory depression, hypotension and profound sedation or coma may occur; the dose of one or both agents should be reduced). Products include:
Miltown Tablets 3349

Mesoridazine Besylate (May produce additive depressant effects; respiratory depression, hypotension and profound sedation or coma may occur; the dose of one or both agents should be reduced). Products include:
Serentil 1057

Methadone Hydrochloride (May produce additive depressant effects; respiratory depression, hypotension and profound sedation or coma may occur; the dose of one or both agents should be reduced). Products include:
Dolophine Hydrochloride Tablets 3056

Methohexital Sodium (May produce additive depressant effects; respiratory depression, hypotension and profound sedation or coma may occur; the dose of one or both agents should be reduced). Products include:
Brevital Sodium for Injection, USP .. 1815

Methotrimeprazine (May produce additive depressant effects; respiratory depression, hypotension and profound sedation or coma may occur; the dose of one or both agents should be reduced).
No products indexed under this heading.

Methoxyflurane (May produce additive depressant effects; respiratory depression, hypotension and profound sedation or coma may occur; the dose of one or both agents should be reduced).
No products indexed under this heading.

Metocurine Iodide (Enhanced action of neuromuscular blocking agents and produce an excessive degree of respiratory depression).
No products indexed under this heading.

Midazolam Hydrochloride (May produce additive depressant effects; respiratory depression, hypotension and profound sedation or coma may occur; the dose of one or both agents should be reduced). Products include:
Versed Injection 3027
Versed Syrup 3033

Mivacurium Chloride (Enhanced action of neuromuscular blocking agents and produce an excessive degree of respiratory depression).
No products indexed under this heading.

Molindone Hydrochloride (May produce additive depressant effects; respiratory depression, hypotension and profound sedation or coma may occur; the dose of one or both agents should be reduced). Products include:
Moban 1320

Morphine Sulfate (May produce additive depressant effects; respiratory depression, hypotension and profound sedation or coma may occur; the dose of one or both agents should be reduced). Products include:
Astramorph/PF Injection, USP (Preservative-Free) 594
Duramorph Injection 1312
Infumorph 200 and Infumorph 500 Sterile Solutions 1314
Kadian Capsules 1335
MS Contin Tablets 2896
MSIR 2898
Oramorph SR Tablets 3062
Roxanol 3066

Olanzapine (May produce additive depressant effects; respiratory depression, hypotension and profound sedation or coma may occur; the dose of one or both agents should be reduced). Products include:
Zyprexa Tablets 1973
Zyprexa ZYDIS Orally Disintegrating Tablets 1973

Oxazepam (May produce additive depressant effects; respiratory depression, hypotension and profound sedation or coma may occur; the dose of one or both agents should be reduced).
No products indexed under this heading.

Oxycodone Hydrochloride (May produce additive depressant effects; respiratory depression, hypotension and profound sedation or coma may occur; the dose of one or both agents should be reduced). Products include:
OxyContin Tablets 2912
OxyFast Oral Concentrate Solution . 2916
OxyIR Capsules 2916
Percocet Tablets 1326
Percodan Tablets 1327
Percolone Tablets 1327
Roxicodone 3067
Tylox Capsules 2597

Pancuronium Bromide (Enhanced action of neuromuscular blocking agents and produce an excessive degree of respiratory depression).
No products indexed under this heading.

Pentobarbital Sodium (May produce additive depressant effects; respiratory depression, hypotension and profound sedation or coma may occur; the dose of one or both agents should be reduced). Products include:
Nembutal Sodium Solution 485

Perphenazine (May produce additive depressant effects; respiratory depression, hypotension and profound sedation or coma may occur; the dose of one or both agents should be reduced). Products include:
Etrafon 3115
Trilafon 3160

Phenobarbital (May produce additive depressant effects; respiratory depression, hypotension and profound sedation or coma may occur; the dose of one or both agents should be reduced). Products include:
Arco-Lase Plus Tablets 592
Donnatal 2929
Donnatal Extentabs 2930

Prazepam (May produce additive depressant effects; respiratory depression, hypotension and profound sedation or coma may occur; the dose of one or both agents should be reduced).
No products indexed under this heading.

Prochlorperazine (May produce additive depressant effects; respiratory depression, hypotension and profound sedation or coma may

occur; the dose of one or both agents should be reduced). Products include:
- Compazine 1505

Promethazine Hydrochloride (May produce additive depressant effects; respiratory depression, hypotension and profound sedation or coma may occur; the dose of one or both agents should be reduced). Products include:
- Mepergan Injection 3539
- Phenergan Injection 3553
- Phenergan 3556
- Phenergan Syrup 3554
- Phenergan with Codeine Syrup 3557
- Phenergan with Dextromethorphan Syrup 3559
- Phenergan VC Syrup 3560
- Phenergan VC with Codeine Syrup .. 3561

Propofol (May produce additive depressant effects; respiratory depression, hypotension and profound sedation or coma may occur; the dose of one or both agents should be reduced). Products include:
- Diprivan Injectable Emulsion 667

Propoxyphene Hydrochloride (May produce additive depressant effects; respiratory depression, hypotension and profound sedation or coma may occur; the dose of one or both agents should be reduced). Products include:
- Darvon Pulvules 1909
- Darvon Compound-65 Pulvules 1910

Propoxyphene Napsylate (May produce additive depressant effects; respiratory depression, hypotension and profound sedation or coma may occur; the dose of one or both agents should be reduced). Products include:
- Darvon-N/Darvocet-N 1907
- Darvon-N Tablets 1912

Quazepam (May produce additive depressant effects; respiratory depression, hypotension and profound sedation or coma may occur; the dose of one or both agents should be reduced).
No products indexed under this heading.

Quetiapine Fumarate (May produce additive depressant effects; respiratory depression, hypotension and profound sedation or coma may occur; the dose of one or both agents should be reduced). Products include:
- Seroquel Tablets 684

Rapacuronium Bromide (Enhanced action of neuromuscular blocking agents and produce an excessive degree of respiratory depression).
No products indexed under this heading.

Remifentanil Hydrochloride (May produce additive depressant effects; respiratory depression, hypotension and profound sedation or coma may occur; the dose of one or both agents should be reduced).
No products indexed under this heading.

Risperidone (May produce additive depressant effects; respiratory depression, hypotension and profound sedation or coma may occur; the dose of one or both agents should be reduced). Products include:
- Risperdal 1796

Rocuronium Bromide (Enhanced action of neuromuscular blocking agents and produce an excessive degree of respiratory depression). Products include:
- Zemuron Injection 2491

Secobarbital Sodium (May produce additive depressant effects; respiratory depression, hypotension and profound sedation or coma may occur; the dose of one or both agents should be reduced).
No products indexed under this heading.

Sevoflurane (May produce additive depressant effects; respiratory depression, hypotension and profound sedation or coma may occur; the dose of one or both agents should be reduced).
No products indexed under this heading.

Succinylcholine Chloride (Enhanced action of neuromuscular blocking agents and produce an excessive degree of respiratory depression). Products include:
- Anectine Injection 1476

Sufentanil Citrate (May produce additive depressant effects; respiratory depression, hypotension and profound sedation or coma may occur; the dose of one or both agents should be reduced).
No products indexed under this heading.

Temazepam (May produce additive depressant effects; respiratory depression, hypotension and profound sedation or coma may occur; the dose of one or both agents should be reduced).
No products indexed under this heading.

Thiamylal Sodium (May produce additive depressant effects; respiratory depression, hypotension and profound sedation or coma may occur; the dose of one or both agents should be reduced).
No products indexed under this heading.

Thioridazine Hydrochloride (May produce additive depressant effects; respiratory depression, hypotension and profound sedation or coma may occur; the dose of one or both agents should be reduced). Products include:
- Thioridazine Hydrochloride Tablets 2289

Thiothixene (May produce additive depressant effects; respiratory depression, hypotension and profound sedation or coma may occur; the dose of one or both agents should be reduced). Products include:
- Navane Capsules 2701
- Thiothixene Capsules 2290

Triazolam (May produce additive depressant effects; respiratory depression, hypotension and profound sedation or coma may occur; the dose of one or both agents should be reduced). Products include:
- Halcion Tablets 2823

Trifluoperazine Hydrochloride (May produce additive depressant effects; respiratory depression, hypotension and profound sedation or coma may occur; the dose of one or both agents should be reduced). Products include:
- Stelazine 1640

Vecuronium Bromide (Enhanced action of neuromuscular blocking agents and produce an excessive degree of respiratory depression). Products include:
- Norcuron for Injection 2478

Zaleplon (May produce additive depressant effects; respiratory depression, hypotension and profound sedation or coma may occur; the dose of one or both agents should be reduced). Products include:
- Sonata Capsules 3591

Ziprasidone Hydrochloride (May produce additive depressant effects; respiratory depression, hypotension and profound sedation or coma may occur; the dose of one or both agents should be reduced). Products include:
- Geodon Capsules 2688

Zolpidem Tartrate (May produce additive depressant effects; respiratory depression, hypotension and profound sedation or coma may occur; the dose of one or both agents should be reduced). Products include:
- Ambien Tablets 3191

Food Interactions

Alcohol (May exhibit an additive CNS depression).

DILAUDID POWDER
(Hydromorphone Hydrochloride) 441
See Dilaudid Ampules

DILAUDID RECTAL SUPPOSITORIES
(Hydromorphone Hydrochloride) 441
See Dilaudid Ampules

DILAUDID TABLETS
(Hydromorphone Hydrochloride) 441
See Dilaudid Ampules

DILAUDID TABLETS - 8 MG
(Hydromorphone Hydrochloride) 445
See Dilaudid Oral Liquid

DILAUDID-HP INJECTION
(Hydromorphone Hydrochloride) 443
See Dilaudid Oral Liquid

DILAUDID-HP LYOPHILIZED POWDER 250 MG
(Hydromorphone Hydrochloride) 443
See Dilaudid Oral Liquid

DIMETAPP ELIXIR
(Brompheniramine Maleate, Pseudoephedrine Hydrochloride) .... ▭ 777

May interact with hypnotics and sedatives, monoamine oxidase inhibitors, tranquilizers, and certain other agents. Compounds in these categories include:

Alprazolam (May increase drowsiness effect). Products include:
- Xanax Tablets 2865

Buspirone Hydrochloride (May increase drowsiness effect).
No products indexed under this heading.

Chlordiazepoxide (May increase drowsiness effect). Products include:
- Limbitrol 1738

Chlordiazepoxide Hydrochloride (May increase drowsiness effect). Products include:
- Librium Capsules 1736
- Librium for Injection 1737

Chlorpromazine (May increase drowsiness effect). Products include:
- Thorazine Suppositories 1656

Chlorpromazine Hydrochloride (May increase drowsiness effect). Products include:
- Thorazine 1656

Chlorprothixene (May increase drowsiness effect).
No products indexed under this heading.

Chlorprothixene Hydrochloride (May increase drowsiness effect).
No products indexed under this heading.

Clorazepate Dipotassium (May increase drowsiness effect). Products include:
- Tranxene 511

Diazepam (May increase drowsiness effect). Products include:
- Valium Injectable 3026
- Valium Tablets 3047

Droperidol (May increase drowsiness effect).
No products indexed under this heading.

Estazolam (May increase drowsiness effect). Products include:
- ProSom Tablets 500

Ethchlorvynol (May increase drowsiness effect).
No products indexed under this heading.

Ethinamate (May increase drowsiness effect).
No products indexed under this heading.

Fluphenazine Decanoate (May increase drowsiness effect).
No products indexed under this heading.

Fluphenazine Enanthate (May increase drowsiness effect).
No products indexed under this heading.

Fluphenazine Hydrochloride (May increase drowsiness effect).
No products indexed under this heading.

Flurazepam Hydrochloride (May increase drowsiness effect).
No products indexed under this heading.

Glutethimide (May increase drowsiness effect).
No products indexed under this heading.

Haloperidol (May increase drowsiness effect). Products include:
- Haldol Injection, Tablets and Concentrate 2533

Haloperidol Decanoate (May increase drowsiness effect). Products include:
- Haldol Decanoate 2535

Hydroxyzine Hydrochloride (May increase drowsiness effect). Products include:
- Atarax Tablets & Syrup 2667
- Vistaril Intramuscular Solution 2738

Isocarboxazid (Concurrent and/or sequential use with MAO inhibitors is not recommended).
No products indexed under this heading.

Lorazepam (May increase drowsiness effect). Products include:
- Ativan Injection 3478
- Ativan Tablets 3482

Loxapine Hydrochloride (May increase drowsiness effect).
No products indexed under this heading.

Loxapine Succinate (May increase drowsiness effect). Products include:
- Loxitane Capsules 3398

Meprobamate (May increase drowsiness effect). Products include:
- Miltown Tablets 3349

Mesoridazine Besylate (May increase drowsiness effect). Products include:
- Serentil 1057

Midazolam Hydrochloride (May increase drowsiness effect). Products include:
- Versed Injection 3027
- Versed Syrup 3033

Moclobemide (Concurrent and/or sequential use with MAO inhibitors is not recommended).
No products indexed under this heading.

Molindone Hydrochloride (May increase drowsiness effect). Products include:
- Moban 1320

Oxazepam (May increase drowsiness effect).
No products indexed under this heading.

Pargyline Hydrochloride (Concurrent and/or sequential use with MAO inhibitors is not recommended).
No products indexed under this heading.

Perphenazine (May increase drowsiness effect). Products include:

Etrafon 3115
Trilafon 3160

Phenelzine Sulfate (Concurrent and/or sequential use with MAO inhibitors is not recommended). Products include:
Nardil Tablets 2653

Prazepam (May increase drowsiness effect).
No products indexed under this heading.

Procarbazine Hydrochloride (Concurrent and/or sequential use with MAO inhibitors is not recommended). Products include:
Matulane Capsules 3246

Prochlorperazine (May increase drowsiness effect). Products include:
Compazine 1505

Promethazine Hydrochloride (May increase drowsiness effect). Products include:
Mepergan Injection 3539
Phenergan Injection 3553
Phenergan 3556
Phenergan Syrup 3554
Phenergan with Codeine Syrup 3557
Phenergan with Dextromethorphan Syrup 3559
Phenergan VC Syrup 3560
Phenergan VC with Codeine Syrup 3561

Propofol (May increase drowsiness effect). Products include:
Diprivan Injectable Emulsion 667

Quazepam (May increase drowsiness effect).
No products indexed under this heading.

Secobarbital Sodium (May increase drowsiness effect).
No products indexed under this heading.

Selegiline Hydrochloride (Concurrent and/or sequential use with MAO inhibitors is not recommended). Products include:
Eldepryl Capsules 3266

Temazepam (May increase drowsiness effect).
No products indexed under this heading.

Thioridazine Hydrochloride (May increase drowsiness effect). Products include:
Thioridazine Hydrochloride Tablets 2289

Thiothixene (May increase drowsiness effect). Products include:
Navane Capsules 2701
Thiothixene Capsules 2290

Tranylcypromine Sulfate (Concurrent and/or sequential use with MAO inhibitors is not recommended). Products include:
Parnate Tablets 1607

Triazolam (May increase drowsiness effect). Products include:
Halcion Tablets 2823

Trifluoperazine Hydrochloride (May increase drowsiness effect). Products include:
Stelazine 1640

Zaleplon (May increase drowsiness effect). Products include:
Sonata Capsules 3591

Zolpidem Tartrate (May increase drowsiness effect). Products include:
Ambien Tablets 3191

Food Interactions

Alcohol (May increase drowsiness effect).

DIMETAPP COLD AND FEVER SUSPENSION

(Acetaminophen, Brompheniramine Maleate, Pseudoephedrine Hydrochloride) 775
May interact with hypnotics and sedatives, monoamine oxidase inhibitors, tranquilizers, and certain other agents. Compounds in these categories include:

Alprazolam (May increase drowsiness effect). Products include:
Xanax Tablets 2865

Buspirone Hydrochloride (May increase drowsiness effect).
No products indexed under this heading.

Chlordiazepoxide (May increase drowsiness effect). Products include:
Limbitrol 1738

Chlordiazepoxide Hydrochloride (May increase drowsiness effect). Products include:
Librium Capsules 1736
Librium for Injection 1737

Chlorpromazine (May increase drowsiness effect). Products include:
Thorazine Suppositories 1656

Chlorpromazine Hydrochloride (May increase drowsiness effect). Products include:
Thorazine 1656

Chlorprothixene (May increase drowsiness effect).
No products indexed under this heading.

Chlorprothixene Hydrochloride (May increase drowsiness effect).
No products indexed under this heading.

Clorazepate Dipotassium (May increase drowsiness effect). Products include:
Tranxene 511

Diazepam (May increase drowsiness effect). Products include:
Valium Injectable 3026
Valium Tablets 3047

Droperidol (May increase drowsiness effect).
No products indexed under this heading.

Estazolam (May increase drowsiness effect). Products include:
ProSom Tablets 500

Ethchlorvynol (May increase drowsiness effect).
No products indexed under this heading.

Ethinamate (May increase drowsiness effect).
No products indexed under this heading.

Fluphenazine Decanoate (May increase drowsiness effect).
No products indexed under this heading.

Fluphenazine Enanthate (May increase drowsiness effect).
No products indexed under this heading.

Fluphenazine Hydrochloride (May increase drowsiness effect).
No products indexed under this heading.

Flurazepam Hydrochloride (May increase drowsiness effect).
No products indexed under this heading.

Glutethimide (May increase drowsiness effect).
No products indexed under this heading.

Haloperidol (May increase drowsiness effect). Products include:
Haldol Injection, Tablets and Concentrate 2533

Haloperidol Decanoate (May increase drowsiness effect). Products include:
Haldol Decanoate 2535

Hydroxyzine Hydrochloride (May increase drowsiness effect). Products include:
Atarax Tablets & Syrup 2667
Vistaril Intramuscular Solution 2738

Isocarboxazid (Concurrent and/or sequential use with MAO inhibitors is not recommended).
No products indexed under this heading.

Lorazepam (May increase drowsiness effect). Products include:
Ativan Injection 3478
Ativan Tablets 3482

Loxapine Hydrochloride (May increase drowsiness effect).
No products indexed under this heading.

Loxapine Succinate (May increase drowsiness effect). Products include:
Loxitane Capsules 3398

Meprobamate (May increase drowsiness effect). Products include:
Miltown Tablets 3349

Mesoridazine Besylate (May increase drowsiness effect). Products include:
Serentil 1057

Midazolam Hydrochloride (May increase drowsiness effect). Products include:
Versed Injection 3027
Versed Syrup 3033

Moclobemide (Concurrent and/or sequential use with MAO inhibitors is not recommended).
No products indexed under this heading.

Molindone Hydrochloride (May increase drowsiness effect). Products include:
Moban 1320

Oxazepam (May increase drowsiness effect).
No products indexed under this heading.

Pargyline Hydrochloride (Concurrent and/or sequential use with MAO inhibitors is not recommended).
No products indexed under this heading.

Perphenazine (May increase drowsiness effect). Products include:
Etrafon 3115
Trilafon 3160

Phenelzine Sulfate (Concurrent and/or sequential use with MAO inhibitors is not recommended). Products include:
Nardil Tablets 2653

Prazepam (May increase drowsiness effect).
No products indexed under this heading.

Procarbazine Hydrochloride (Concurrent and/or sequential use with MAO inhibitors is not recommended). Products include:
Matulane Capsules 3246

Prochlorperazine (May increase drowsiness effect). Products include:
Compazine 1505

Promethazine Hydrochloride (May increase drowsiness effect). Products include:
Mepergan Injection 3539
Phenergan Injection 3553
Phenergan 3556
Phenergan Syrup 3554
Phenergan with Codeine Syrup 3557
Phenergan with Dextromethorphan Syrup 3559
Phenergan VC Syrup 3560
Phenergan VC with Codeine Syrup 3561

Propofol (May increase drowsiness effect). Products include:
Diprivan Injectable Emulsion 667

Quazepam (May increase drowsiness effect).
No products indexed under this heading.

Secobarbital Sodium (May increase drowsiness effect).
No products indexed under this heading.

Selegiline Hydrochloride (Concurrent and/or sequential use with MAO inhibitors is not recommended). Products include:
Eldepryl Capsules 3266

Temazepam (May increase drowsiness effect).
No products indexed under this heading.

Thioridazine Hydrochloride (May increase drowsiness effect). Products include:
Thioridazine Hydrochloride Tablets 2289

Thiothixene (May increase drowsiness effect). Products include:
Navane Capsules 2701
Thiothixene Capsules 2290

Tranylcypromine Sulfate (Concurrent and/or sequential use with MAO inhibitors is not recommended). Products include:
Parnate Tablets 1607

Triazolam (May increase drowsiness effect). Products include:
Halcion Tablets 2823

Trifluoperazine Hydrochloride (May increase drowsiness effect). Products include:
Stelazine 1640

Zaleplon (May increase drowsiness effect). Products include:
Sonata Capsules 3591

Zolpidem Tartrate (May increase drowsiness effect). Products include:
Ambien Tablets 3191

Food Interactions

Alcohol (May increase drowsiness effect).

DIMETAPP DM COLD & COUGH ELIXIR

(Brompheniramine Maleate, Dextromethorphan Hydrobromide, Pseudoephedrine Hydrochloride) 775
May interact with hypnotics and sedatives, monoamine oxidase inhibitors, tranquilizers, and certain other agents. Compounds in these categories include:

Alprazolam (Increases drowsiness effect). Products include:
Xanax Tablets 2865

Buspirone Hydrochloride (Increases drowsiness effect).
No products indexed under this heading.

Chlordiazepoxide (Increases drowsiness effect). Products include:
Limbitrol 1738

Chlordiazepoxide Hydrochloride (Increases drowsiness effect). Products include:
Librium Capsules 1736
Librium for Injection 1737

Chlorpromazine (Increases drowsiness effect). Products include:
Thorazine Suppositories 1656

Chlorpromazine Hydrochloride (Increases drowsiness effect). Products include:
Thorazine 1656

Chlorprothixene (Increases drowsiness effect).
No products indexed under this heading.

Chlorprothixene Hydrochloride (Increases drowsiness effect).
No products indexed under this heading.

Clorazepate Dipotassium (Increases drowsiness effect). Products include:
Tranxene 511

Diazepam (Increases drowsiness effect). Products include:
Valium Injectable 3026
Valium Tablets 3047

Droperidol (Increases drowsiness effect).
No products indexed under this heading.

Estazolam (Increases drowsiness effect). Products include:
ProSom Tablets 500

Ethchlorvynol (Increases drowsiness effect).
No products indexed under this heading.

Ethinamate (Increases drowsiness effect).
No products indexed under this heading.

Fluphenazine Decanoate (Increases drowsiness effect).
No products indexed under this heading.

Fluphenazine Enanthate (Increases drowsiness effect).
No products indexed under this heading.

Fluphenazine Hydrochloride (Increases drowsiness effect).
No products indexed under this heading.

Flurazepam Hydrochloride (Increases drowsiness effect).
No products indexed under this heading.

Glutethimide (Increases drowsiness effect).
No products indexed under this heading.

Haloperidol (Increases drowsiness effect). Products include:
Haldol Injection, Tablets and Concentrate 2533

Haloperidol Decanoate (Increases drowsiness effect). Products include:
Haldol Decanoate 2535

Hydroxyzine Hydrochloride (Increases drowsiness effect). Products include:
Atarax Tablets & Syrup 2667
Vistaril Intramuscular Solution 2738

Isocarboxazid (Concurrent and/or sequential use with MAO inhibitors is contraindicated).
No products indexed under this heading.

Lorazepam (Increases drowsiness effect). Products include:
Ativan Injection 3478
Ativan Tablets 3482

Loxapine Hydrochloride (Increases drowsiness effect).
No products indexed under this heading.

Loxapine Succinate (Increases drowsiness effect). Products include:
Loxitane Capsules 3398

Meprobamate (Increases drowsiness effect). Products include:
Miltown Tablets 3349

Mesoridazine Besylate (Increases drowsiness effect). Products include:
Serentil 1057

Midazolam Hydrochloride (Increases drowsiness effect). Products include:
Versed Injection 3027
Versed Syrup 3033

Moclobemide (Concurrent and/or sequential use with MAO inhibitors is contraindicated).
No products indexed under this heading.

Molindone Hydrochloride (Increases drowsiness effect). Products include:
Moban 1320

Oxazepam (Increases drowsiness effect).
No products indexed under this heading.

Pargyline Hydrochloride (Concurrent and/or sequential use with MAO inhibitors is contraindicated).
No products indexed under this heading.

Perphenazine (Increases drowsiness effect). Products include:
Etrafon 3115
Trilafon 3160

Phenelzine Sulfate (Concurrent and/or sequential use with MAO inhibitors is contraindicated). Products include:
Nardil Tablets 2653

Prazepam (Increases drowsiness effect).
No products indexed under this heading.

Procarbazine Hydrochloride (Concurrent and/or sequential use with MAO inhibitors is contraindicated). Products include:
Matulane Capsules 3246

Prochlorperazine (Increases drowsiness effect). Products include:
Compazine 1505

Promethazine Hydrochloride (Increases drowsiness effect). Products include:
Mepergan Injection 3539
Phenergan Injection 3553
Phenergan 3556
Phenergan Syrup 3554
Phenergan with Codeine Syrup 3557
Phenergan with Dextromethorphan Syrup 3559
Phenergan VC Syrup 3560
Phenergan VC with Codeine Syrup 3561

Propofol (Increases drowsiness effect). Products include:
Diprivan Injectable Emulsion 667

Quazepam (Increases drowsiness effect).
No products indexed under this heading.

Secobarbital Sodium (Increases drowsiness effect).
No products indexed under this heading.

Selegiline Hydrochloride (Concurrent and/or sequential use with MAO inhibitors is contraindicated). Products include:
Eldepryl Capsules 3266

Temazepam (Increases drowsiness effect).
No products indexed under this heading.

Thioridazine Hydrochloride (Increases drowsiness effect). Products include:
Thioridazine Hydrochloride Tablets 2289

Thiothixene (Increases drowsiness effect). Products include:
Navane Capsules 2701
Thiothixene Capsules 2290

Tranylcypromine Sulfate (Concurrent and/or sequential use with MAO inhibitors is contraindicated). Products include:
Parnate Tablets 1607

Triazolam (Increases drowsiness effect). Products include:
Halcion Tablets 2823

Trifluoperazine Hydrochloride (Increases drowsiness effect). Products include:
Stelazine 1640

Zaleplon (Increases drowsiness effect). Products include:
Sonata Capsules 3591

Zolpidem Tartrate (Increases drowsiness effect). Products include:
Ambien Tablets 3191

Food Interactions

Alcohol (Increases drowsiness effect; avoid concurrent use).

DIMETAPP NIGHTTIME FLU LIQUID

(Acetaminophen, Brompheniramine Maleate, Dextromethorphan Hydrobromide, Pseudoephedrine Hydrochloride) .... ■ 776
May interact with hypnotics and sedatives, monoamine oxidase inhibitors, tranquilizers, and certain other agents. Compounds in these categories include:

Alprazolam (May increase drowsiness). Products include:
Xanax Tablets 2865

Buspirone Hydrochloride (May increase drowsiness).
No products indexed under this heading.

Chlordiazepoxide (May increase drowsiness). Products include:
Limbitrol 1738

Chlordiazepoxide Hydrochloride (May increase drowsiness). Products include:
Librium Capsules 1736
Librium for Injection 1737

Chlorpromazine (May increase drowsiness). Products include:
Thorazine Suppositories 1656

Chlorpromazine Hydrochloride (May increase drowsiness). Products include:
Thorazine 1656

Chlorprothixene (May increase drowsiness).
No products indexed under this heading.

Chlorprothixene Hydrochloride (May increase drowsiness).
No products indexed under this heading.

Clorazepate Dipotassium (May increase drowsiness). Products include:
Tranxene 511

Diazepam (May increase drowsiness). Products include:
Valium Injectable 3026
Valium Tablets 3047

Droperidol (May increase drowsiness).
No products indexed under this heading.

Estazolam (May increase drowsiness). Products include:
ProSom Tablets 500

Ethchlorvynol (May increase drowsiness).
No products indexed under this heading.

Ethinamate (May increase drowsiness).
No products indexed under this heading.

Fluphenazine Decanoate (May increase drowsiness).
No products indexed under this heading.

Fluphenazine Enanthate (May increase drowsiness).
No products indexed under this heading.

Fluphenazine Hydrochloride (May increase drowsiness).
No products indexed under this heading.

Flurazepam Hydrochloride (May increase drowsiness).
No products indexed under this heading.

Glutethimide (May increase drowsiness).
No products indexed under this heading.

Haloperidol (May increase drowsiness). Products include:
Haldol Injection, Tablets and Concentrate 2533

Haloperidol Decanoate (May increase drowsiness). Products include:
Haldol Decanoate 2535

Hydroxyzine Hydrochloride (May increase drowsiness). Products include:
Atarax Tablets & Syrup 2667
Vistaril Intramuscular Solution 2738

Isocarboxazid (Concurrent and/or sequential use with MAO inhibitors is not recommended).
No products indexed under this heading.

Lorazepam (May increase drowsiness). Products include:
Ativan Injection 3478
Ativan Tablets 3482

Loxapine Hydrochloride (May increase drowsiness).
No products indexed under this heading.

Loxapine Succinate (May increase drowsiness). Products include:
Loxitane Capsules 3398

Meprobamate (May increase drowsiness). Products include:
Miltown Tablets 3349

Mesoridazine Besylate (May increase drowsiness). Products include:
Serentil 1057

Midazolam Hydrochloride (May increase drowsiness). Products include:
Versed Injection 3027
Versed Syrup 3033

Moclobemide (Concurrent and/or sequential use with MAO inhibitors is not recommended).
No products indexed under this heading.

Molindone Hydrochloride (May increase drowsiness). Products include:
Moban 1320

Oxazepam (May increase drowsiness).
No products indexed under this heading.

Pargyline Hydrochloride (Concurrent and/or sequential use with MAO inhibitors is not recommended).
No products indexed under this heading.

Perphenazine (May increase drowsiness). Products include:
Etrafon 3115
Trilafon 3160

Phenelzine Sulfate (Concurrent and/or sequential use with MAO inhibitors is not recommended). Products include:
Nardil Tablets 2653

Prazepam (May increase drowsiness).
No products indexed under this heading.

Procarbazine Hydrochloride (Concurrent and/or sequential use with MAO inhibitors is not recommended). Products include:
Matulane Capsules 3246

Prochlorperazine (May increase drowsiness). Products include:
Compazine 1505

Promethazine Hydrochloride (May increase drowsiness). Products include:
Mepergan Injection 3539
Phenergan Injection 3553
Phenergan 3556
Phenergan Syrup 3554
Phenergan with Codeine Syrup 3557
Phenergan with Dextromethorphan Syrup 3559
Phenergan VC Syrup 3560
Phenergan VC with Codeine Syrup 3561

Propofol (May increase drowsiness). Products include:
Diprivan Injectable Emulsion 667

Quazepam (May increase drowsiness).
No products indexed under this heading.

Secobarbital Sodium (May increase drowsiness).
No products indexed under this heading.

Selegiline Hydrochloride (Concurrent and/or sequential use with MAO inhibitors is not recommended). Products include:
Eldepryl Capsules 3266

Temazepam (May increase drowsiness).
No products indexed under this heading.

Thioridazine Hydrochloride (May increase drowsiness). Products include:
Thioridazine Hydrochloride Tablets 2289

Thiothixene (May increase drowsiness). Products include:
Navane Capsules 2701

Thiothixene Capsules 2290

Tranylcypromine Sulfate (Concurrent and/or sequential use with MAO inhibitors is not recommended). Products include:
Parnate Tablets 1607

Triazolam (May increase drowsiness). Products include:
Halcion Tablets 2823

Trifluoperazine Hydrochloride (May increase drowsiness). Products include:
Stelazine 1640

Zaleplon (May increase drowsiness). Products include:
Sonata Capsules 3591

Zolpidem Tartrate (May increase drowsiness). Products include:
Ambien Tablets 3191

Food Interactions

Alcohol (Chronic heavy alcohol users, 3 or more drinks per day, should consult their physician for advice on when and how they should take pain relievers/fever reducers including acetaminophen; increases drowsiness effect).

DIMETAPP NON-DROWSY FLU SYRUP
(Acetaminophen, Dextromethorphan Hydrobromide, Pseudoephedrine Hydrochloride) ..... ▣777
May interact with monoamine oxidase inhibitors and certain other agents. Compounds in these categories include:

Isocarboxazid (Concurrent and/or sequential use with MAO inhibitor is not recommended).
No products indexed under this heading.

Moclobemide (Concurrent and/or sequential use with MAO inhibitor is not recommended).
No products indexed under this heading.

Pargyline Hydrochloride (Concurrent and/or sequential use with MAO inhibitor is not recommended).
No products indexed under this heading.

Phenelzine Sulfate (Concurrent and/or sequential use with MAO inhibitor is not recommended). Products include:
Nardil Tablets 2653

Procarbazine Hydrochloride (Concurrent and/or sequential use with MAO inhibitor is not recommended). Products include:
Matulane Capsules 3246

Selegiline Hydrochloride (Concurrent and/or sequential use with MAO inhibitor is not recommended). Products include:
Eldepryl Capsules 3266

Tranylcypromine Sulfate (Concurrent and/or sequential use with MAO inhibitor is not recommended). Products include:
Parnate Tablets 1607

Food Interactions

Alcohol (Patients consuming three or more alcohol-containing drinks every day should consult their doctor for advice on when and how they should take acetaminophen-containing products).

DIMETAPP INFANT DROPS DECONGESTANT
(Pseudoephedrine Hydrochloride) .... ▣775
May interact with monoamine oxidase inhibitors. Compounds in these categories include:

Isocarboxazid (Concurrent and/or sequential use with MAO inhibitors is not recommended).
No products indexed under this heading.

Moclobemide (Concurrent and/or sequential use with MAO inhibitors is not recommended).
No products indexed under this heading.

Pargyline Hydrochloride (Concurrent and/or sequential use with MAO inhibitors is not recommended).
No products indexed under this heading.

Phenelzine Sulfate (Concurrent and/or sequential use with MAO inhibitors is not recommended). Products include:
Nardil Tablets 2653

Procarbazine Hydrochloride (Concurrent and/or sequential use with MAO inhibitors is not recommended). Products include:
Matulane Capsules 3246

Selegiline Hydrochloride (Concurrent and/or sequential use with MAO inhibitors is not recommended). Products include:
Eldepryl Capsules 3266

Tranylcypromine Sulfate (Concurrent and/or sequential use with MAO inhibitors is not recommended). Products include:
Parnate Tablets 1607

DIMETAPP INFANT DROPS DECONGESTANT PLUS COUGH
(Dextromethorphan Hydrobromide, Pseudoephedrine Hydrochloride) ..... ▣776
May interact with monoamine oxidase inhibitors. Compounds in these categories include:

Isocarboxazid (Concurrent and/or sequential use with MAO inhibitors is not recommended).
No products indexed under this heading.

Moclobemide (Concurrent and/or sequential use with MAO inhibitors is not recommended).
No products indexed under this heading.

Pargyline Hydrochloride (Concurrent and/or sequential use with MAO inhibitors is not recommended).
No products indexed under this heading.

Phenelzine Sulfate (Concurrent and/or sequential use with MAO inhibitors is not recommended). Products include:
Nardil Tablets 2653

Procarbazine Hydrochloride (Concurrent and/or sequential use with MAO inhibitors is not recommended). Products include:
Matulane Capsules 3246

Selegiline Hydrochloride (Concurrent and/or sequential use with MAO inhibitors is not recommended). Products include:
Eldepryl Capsules 3266

Tranylcypromine Sulfate (Concurrent and/or sequential use with MAO inhibitors is not recommended). Products include:
Parnate Tablets 1607

DIOVAN CAPSULES
(Valsartan) 2337
May interact with:

Atenolol (Combination therapy is more antihypertensive than either component, but does not lower the heart rate more than atenolol alone). Products include:
Tenoretic Tablets 690
Tenormin I.V. Injection 692

Food Interactions

Food, unspecified (Decreases the exposure (as measured by AUC) to valsartan about 40% and peak plasma concentration by about 50%).

DIOVAN HCT TABLETS
(Hydrochlorothiazide, Valsartan) 2338
May interact with antihypertensives, barbiturates, corticosteroids, cardiac glycosides, oral hypoglycemic agents, insulin, lithium preparations, narcotic analgesics, nondepolarizing neuromuscular blocking agents, nonsteroidal anti-inflammatory agents, potassium preparations, and certain other agents. Compounds in these categories include:

Acarbose (Dosage adjustment of the antidiabetic drug may be required). Products include:
Precose Tablets 906

Acebutolol Hydrochloride (Co-administration with other antihypertensives may result in additive effect or potentiation). Products include:
Sectral Capsules 3589

ACTH (Co-administration of thiazide diuretics and ACTH may intensify electrolyte depletion, particularly hypokalemia).
No products indexed under this heading.

Alfentanil Hydrochloride (Co-administration of thiazide diuretics and narcotics may result in potentiation of orthostatic hypotension).
No products indexed under this heading.

Amlodipine Besylate (Co-administration with other antihypertensives may result in additive effect or potentiation). Products include:
Lotrel Capsules 2370
Norvasc Tablets 2704

Aprobarbital (Co-administration of thiazide diuretics and barbiturates may result in potentiation of orthostatic hypotension).
No products indexed under this heading.

Atenolol (Co-administration with other antihypertensives may result in additive effect or potentiation). Products include:
Tenoretic Tablets 690
Tenormin I.V. Injection 692

Atracurium Besylate (Co-administration of thiazide diuretics and nondepolarizing skeletal muscle relaxants increases responsiveness to the muscle relaxants).
No products indexed under this heading.

Benazepril Hydrochloride (Co-administration with other antihypertensives may result in additive effect or potentiation). Products include:
Lotensin Tablets 2365
Lotensin HCT Tablets 2367
Lotrel Capsules 2370

Bendroflumethiazide (Co-administration with other antihypertensives may result in additive effect or potentiation). Products include:
Corzide 40/5 Tablets 2247
Corzide 80/5 Tablets 2247

Betamethasone Acetate (Co-administration of thiazide diuretics and corticosteroids may intensify electrolyte depletion, particularly hypokalemia). Products include:
Celestone Soluspan Injectable Suspension 3097

Betamethasone Sodium Phosphate (Co-administration of thiazide diuretics and corticosteroids may intensify electrolyte depletion, particularly hypokalemia). Products include:
Celestone Soluspan Injectable Suspension 3097

Betaxolol Hydrochloride (Co-administration with other antihypertensives may result in additive effect or potentiation). Products include:
Betoptic S Ophthalmic Suspension 537

Bisoprolol Fumarate (Co-administration with other antihypertensives may result in additive effect or potentiation). Products include:
Zebeta Tablets 1885
Ziac Tablets 1887

Buprenorphine Hydrochloride (Co-administration of thiazide diuretics and narcotics may result in potentiation of orthostatic hypotension). Products include:
Buprenex Injectable 2918

Butabarbital (Co-administration of thiazide diuretics and barbiturates may result in potentiation of orthostatic hypotension).
No products indexed under this heading.

Butalbital (Co-administration of thiazide diuretics and barbiturates may result in potentiation of orthostatic hypotension). Products include:
Phrenilin 578
Sedapap Tablets 50 mg/650 mg 2225

Candesartan Cilexetil (Co-administration with other antihypertensives may result in additive effect or potentiation). Products include:
Atacand Tablets 595
Atacand HCT Tablets 597

Captopril (Co-administration with other antihypertensives may result in additive effect or potentiation). Products include:
Captopril Tablets 2281

Carteolol Hydrochloride (Co-administration with other antihypertensives may result in additive effect or potentiation). Products include:
Carteolol Hydrochloride Ophthalmic Solution USP, 1% ..... ⊙258
Ocupress Ophthalmic Solution, 1% Sterile .... ⊙303

Celecoxib (Co-administration of thiazide diuretics and non-steroidal anti-inflammatory agents can reduce the diuretic, natiuretic, and antihypertensive effects). Products include:
Celebrex Capsules 2676
Celebrex Capsules 2780

Chlorothiazide (Co-administration with other antihypertensives may result in additive effect or potentiation). Products include:
Aldoclor Tablets 2035
Diuril Oral 2087

Chlorothiazide Sodium (Co-administration with other antihypertensives may result in additive effect or potentiation). Products include:
Diuril Sodium Intravenous 2086

Chlorpropamide (Dosage adjustment of the antidiabetic drug may be required). Products include:
Diabinese Tablets 2680

Chlorthalidone (Co-administration with other antihypertensives may result in additive effect or potentiation). Products include:
Clorpres Tablets 1002
Combipres Tablets 1040
Tenoretic Tablets 690

Cholestyramine (Absorption of hydrochlorothiazide is impaired in the presence of anionic exchange resins, such as cholestyramine resulting in binding of the hydrochlorothiazide resulting in reduced absorption from GI tract by 85%).
No products indexed under this heading.

Cisatracurium Besylate (Co-administration of thiazide diuretics and nondepolarizing skeletal muscle relaxants increases responsiveness to the muscle relaxants).
No products indexed under this heading.

Clonidine (Co-administration with other antihypertensives may result in additive effect or potentiation). Products include:
Catapres-TTS 1038

Clonidine Hydrochloride (Co-administration with other antihypertensives may result in additive effect or potentiation). Products include:
Catapres Tablets 1037
Clorpres Tablets 1002

Combipres Tablets 1040
Duraclon Injection 3057

Codeine Phosphate (Co-administration of thiazide diuretics and narcotics may result in potentiation of orthostatic hypotension). Products include:
Phenergan with Codeine Syrup 3557
Phenergan VC with Codeine Syrup .. 3561
Robitussin A-C Syrup 2942
Robitussin-DAC Syrup 2942
Ryna-C Liquid .... ■768
Soma Compound w/Codeine Tablets 3355
Tussi-Organidin NR Liquid 3350
Tussi-Organidin-S NR Liquid 3350
Tylenol with Codeine 2595

Colestipol Hydrochloride (Absorption of hydrochlorothiazide is impaired in the presence of anionic exchange resins, such as colestipol resulting in binding of the hydrochlorothiazide resulting in reduced absorption from GI tract by 43%). Products include:
Colestid Tablets 2791

Cortisone Acetate (Co-administration of thiazide diuretics and corticosteroids may intensify electrolyte depletion, particularly hypokalemia). Products include:
Cortone Acetate Injectable Suspension 2059
Cortone Acetate Tablets 2061

Deserpidine (Co-administration with other antihypertensives may result in additive effect or potentiation).
No products indexed under this heading.

Deslanoside (Hypokalemia induced by thiazides may cause cardiac arrhythmia and may sensitize or exaggerate the response of the heart to the toxic effects of digitalis, such as increased ventricular irritability).
No products indexed under this heading.

Dexamethasone (Co-administration of thiazide diuretics and corticosteroids may intensify electrolyte depletion, particularly hypokalemia). Products include:
Decadron Elixir 2078
Decadron Tablets 2079
TobraDex Ophthalmic Ointment 542
TobraDex Ophthalmic Suspension .. 541

Dexamethasone Acetate (Co-administration of thiazide diuretics and corticosteroids may intensify electrolyte depletion, particularly hypokalemia).
No products indexed under this heading.

Dexamethasone Sodium Phosphate (Co-administration of thiazide diuretics and corticosteroids may intensify electrolyte depletion, particularly hypokalemia). Products include:
Decadron Phosphate Injection 2081
Decadron Phosphate Sterile Ophthalmic Ointment 2083
Decadron Phosphate Sterile Ophthalmic Solution 2084
NeoDecadron Sterile Ophthalmic Solution 2144

Dezocine (Co-administration of thiazide diuretics and narcotics may result in potentiation of orthostatic hypotension).
No products indexed under this heading.

Diazoxide (Co-administration with other antihypertensives may result in additive effect or potentiation).
No products indexed under this heading.

Diclofenac Potassium (Co-administration of thiazide diuretics and non-steroidal anti-inflammatory agents can reduce the diuretic, natiuretic, and antihypertensive effects). Products include:
Cataflam Tablets 2315

Diclofenac Sodium (Co-administration of thiazide diuretics and non-steroidal anti-inflammatory agents can reduce the diuretic, natiuretic, and antihypertensive effects). Products include:
Arthrotec Tablets 3195
Voltaren Ophthalmic Sterile Ophthalmic Solution .... ⊙312
Voltaren Tablets 2315
Voltaren-XR Tablets 2315

Digitoxin (Hypokalemia induced by thiazides may cause cardiac arrhythmia and may sensitize or exaggerate the response of the heart to the toxic effects of digitalis, such as increased ventricular irritability).
No products indexed under this heading.

Digoxin (Hypokalemia induced by thiazides may cause cardiac arrhythmia and may sensitize or exaggerate the response of the heart to the toxic effects of digitalis, such as increased ventricular irritability). Products include:
Digitek Tablets 1003
Lanoxicaps Capsules 1574
Lanoxin Injection 1581
Lanoxin Tablets 1587
Lanoxin Elixir Pediatric 1578
Lanoxin Injection Pediatric 1584

Diltiazem Hydrochloride (Co-administration with other antihypertensives may result in additive effect or potentiation). Products include:
Cardizem Injectable 1018
Cardizem Lyo-Ject Syringe 1018
Cardizem Monovial 1018
Cardizem CD Capsules 1016
Tiazac Capsules 1378

Doxazosin Mesylate (Co-administration with other antihypertensives may result in additive effect or potentiation). Products include:
Cardura Tablets 2668

Enalapril Maleate (Co-administration with other antihypertensives may result in additive effect or potentiation). Products include:
Lexxel Tablets 608
Vaseretic Tablets 2204
Vasotec Tablets 2210

Enalaprilat (Co-administration with other antihypertensives may result in additive effect or potentiation). Products include:
Enalaprilat Injection 863
Vasotec I.V. Injection 2207

Eprosartan Mesylate (Co-administration with other antihypertensives may result in additive effect or potentiation). Products include:
Teveten Tablets 3327

Esmolol Hydrochloride (Co-administration with other antihypertensives may result in additive effect or potentiation). Products include:
Brevibloc Injection 858

Etodolac (Co-administration of thiazide diuretics and non-steroidal anti-inflammatory agents can reduce the diuretic, natiuretic, and antihypertensive effects). Products include:
Lodine 3528
Lodine XL Extended-Release Tablets 3530

Felodipine (Co-administration with other antihypertensives may result in additive effect or potentiation). Products include:
Lexxel Tablets 608
Plendil Extended-Release Tablets ... 623

Fenoprofen Calcium (Co-administration of thiazide diuretics and non-steroidal anti-inflammatory agents can reduce the diuretic, natiuretic, and antihypertensive effects).
No products indexed under this heading.

Fentanyl (Co-administration of thiazide diuretics and narcotics may result in potentiation of orthostatic hypotension). Products include:
Duragesic Transdermal System 1786

Fentanyl Citrate (Co-administration of thiazide diuretics and narcotics may result in potentiation of orthostatic hypotension). Products include:
Actiq 1184

Fludrocortisone Acetate (Co-administration of thiazide diuretics and corticosteroids may intensify electrolyte depletion, particularly hypokalemia). Products include:
Florinef Acetate Tablets 2250

Flurbiprofen (Co-administration of thiazide diuretics and non-steroidal anti-inflammatory agents can reduce the diuretic, natiuretic, and antihypertensive effects).
No products indexed under this heading.

Fosinopril Sodium (Co-administration with other antihypertensives may result in additive effect or potentiation). Products include:
Monopril Tablets 1091
Monopril HCT 1094

Furosemide (Co-administration with other antihypertensives may result in additive effect or potentiation). Products include:
Furosemide Tablets 2284

Glimepiride (Dosage adjustment of the antidiabetic drug may be required). Products include:
Amaryl Tablets 717

Glipizide (Dosage adjustment of the antidiabetic drug may be required). Products include:
Glucotrol Tablets 2692
Glucotrol XL Extended Release Tablets 2693

Glyburide (Dosage adjustment of the antidiabetic drug may be required). Products include:
DiaBeta Tablets 741
Glucovance Tablets 1086

Guanabenz Acetate (Co-administration with other antihypertensives may result in additive effect or potentiation).
No products indexed under this heading.

Guanethidine Monosulfate (Co-administration with other antihypertensives may result in additive effect or potentiation).
No products indexed under this heading.

Hydralazine Hydrochloride (Co-administration with other antihypertensives may result in additive effect or potentiation).
No products indexed under this heading.

Hydrocodone Bitartrate (Co-administration of thiazide diuretics and narcotics may result in potentiation of orthostatic hypotension). Products include:
Hycodan 1316
Hycomine Compound Tablets 1317
Hycotuss Expectorant Syrup 1318
Lortab 3319
Lortab Elixir 3317
Maxidone Tablets CIII 3399
Norco 5/325 Tablets CIII 3424
Norco 7.5/325 Tablets CIII 3425
Norco 10/325 Tablets CIII 3427
Norco 10/325 Tablets CIII 3425
Vicodin Tablets 516
Vicodin ES Tablets 517
Vicodin HP Tablets 518
Vicodin Tuss Expectorant 519
Vicoprofen Tablets 520
Zydone Tablets 1330

Hydrocodone Polistirex (Co-administration of thiazide diuretics and narcotics may result in potentiation of orthostatic hypotension). Products include:
Tussionex Pennkinetic Extended-Release Suspension 1174

Hydrocortisone (Co-administration of thiazide diuretics and corticosteroids may intensify electrolyte depletion, particularly hypokalemia). Products include:
Anusol-HC Cream 2.5% 2237
Cipro HC Otic Suspension 540
Cortaid Intensive Therapy Cream .. ■717
Cortaid Maximum Strength Cream .... ■717
Cortisporin Ophthalmic Suspension Sterile .... ⊙297
Cortizone•5 .... ■699
Cortizone•10 .... ■699
Cortizone•10 Plus Creme .... ■700
Cortizone for Kids Creme .... ■699
Hydrocortone Tablets 2106
Massengill Medicated Soft Cloth Towelette .... ■753
VōSoL HC Otic Solution 3356

Hydrocortisone Acetate (Co-administration of thiazide diuretics and corticosteroids may intensify electrolyte depletion, particularly hypokalemia). Products include:
Analpram-HC 1338
Anusol HC-1 Hydrocortisone Anti-Itch Cream .... ■689
Anusol-HC Suppositories 2238
Cortaid .... ■717
Cortifoam Rectal Foam 3170
Cortisporin-TC Otic Suspension 2246
Hydrocortone Acetate Injectable Suspension 2103
Pramosone 1343
Proctocort Suppositories 2264
ProctoFoam-HC 3177
Terra-Cortril Ophthalmic Suspension 2716

Hydrocortisone Sodium Phosphate (Co-administration of thiazide diuretics and corticosteroids may intensify electrolyte depletion, particularly hypokalemia). Products include:
Hydrocortone Phosphate Injection, Sterile 2105

Hydrocortisone Sodium Succinate (Co-administration of thiazide diuretics and corticosteroids may intensify electrolyte depletion, particularly hypokalemia).
No products indexed under this heading.

Hydroflumethiazide (Co-administration with other antihypertensives may result in additive effect or potentiation). Products include:
Diucardin Tablets 3494

Hydromorphone Hydrochloride (Co-administration of thiazide diuretics and narcotics may result in potentiation of orthostatic hypotension). Products include:
Dilaudid 441
Dilaudid Oral Liquid 445
Dilaudid Powder 441
Dilaudid Rectal Suppositories 441
Dilaudid Tablets 441
Dilaudid Tablets - 8 mg 445
Dilaudid-HP 443

Ibuprofen (Co-administration of thiazide diuretics and non-steroidal anti-inflammatory agents can reduce the diuretic, natiuretic, and antihypertensive effects). Products include:
Advil .... ■771
Children's Advil Oral Suspension .. ■773
Children's Advil Chewable Tablets .. ■773
Advil Cold and Sinus Caplets .... ■771
Advil Cold and Sinus Tablets .... ■771
Advil Flu & Body Ache Caplets ...... ■772
Infants' Advil Drops .... ■773
Junior Strength Advil Tablets .... ■773
Junior Strength Advil Chewable Tablets .... ■773
Advil Migraine Liquigels .... ■772
Children's Motrin Oral Suspension and Chewable Tablets 2006
Children's Motrin Cold Oral Suspension 2007
Children's Motrin Oral Suspension .... ■643
Motrin Suspension, Oral Drops, Chewable Tablets, and Caplets 2002
Infants' Motrin Concentrated Drops 2006
Junior Strength Motrin Caplets and Chewable Tablets 2006
Motrin IB Tablets, Caplets, and Gelcaps 2002
Motrin Migraine Pain Caplets 2005
Motrin Sinus Headache Caplets 2005
Vicoprofen Tablets 520

Indapamide (Co-administration with other antihypertensives may result in additive effect or potentiation). Products include:
- Indapamide Tablets 2286

Indomethacin (Co-administration of thiazide diuretics and non-steroidal anti-inflammatory agents can reduce the diuretic, natiuretic, and antihypertensive effects). Products include:
- Indocin 2112

Indomethacin Sodium Trihydrate (Co-administration of thiazide diuretics and non-steroidal anti-inflammatory agents can reduce the diuretic, natiuretic, and antihypertensive effects). Products include:
- Indocin I.V. 2115

Insulin, Human, Zinc Suspension (Dosage adjustment of the antidiabetic drug may be required). Products include:
- Humulin L, 100 Units 1937
- Humulin U, 100 Units 1943
- Novolin L Human Insulin 10 ml Vials 2422

Insulin, Human NPH (Dosage adjustment of the antidiabetic drug may be required). Products include:
- Humulin N, 100 Units 1939
- Humulin N NPH Pen 1940
- Novolin N Human Insulin 10 ml Vials 2422
- Novolin N PenFill 2423
- Novolin N Prefilled Syringe Disposable Insulin Delivery System 2425

Insulin, Human Regular (Dosage adjustment of the antidiabetic drug may be required). Products include:
- Humulin R Regular (U-500) 1943
- Humulin R, 100 Units 1941
- Novolin R Human Insulin 10 ml Vials 2423
- Novolin R PenFill 2423
- Novolin R Prefilled Syringe Disposable Insulin Delivery System 2425
- Velosulin BR Human Insulin 10 ml Vials 2435

Insulin, Human Regular and Human NPH Mixture (Dosage adjustment of the antidiabetic drug may be required). Products include:
- Humulin 50/50, 100 Units 1934
- Humulin 70/30, 100 Units 1935
- Humulin 70/30 Pen 1936
- Novolin 70/30 Human Insulin 10 ml Vials 2421
- Novolin 70/30 PenFill 2423
- Novolin 70/30 Prefilled Disposable Insulin Delivery System 2425

Insulin, NPH (Dosage adjustment of the antidiabetic drug may be required). Products include:
- Iletin II, NPH (Pork), 100 Units 1946

Insulin, Regular (Dosage adjustment of the antidiabetic drug may be required). Products include:
- Iletin II, Regular (Pork), 100 Units ... 1947

Insulin, Zinc Crystals (Dosage adjustment of the antidiabetic drug may be required).
No products indexed under this heading.

Insulin, Zinc Suspension (Dosage adjustment of the antidiabetic drug may be required). Products include:
- Iletin II, Lente (Pork), 100 Units 1945

Insulin Aspart, Human Regular (Dosage adjustment of the antidiabetic drug may be required).
No products indexed under this heading.

Insulin glargine (Dosage adjustment of the antidiabetic drug may be required). Products include:
- Lantus Injection 742

Insulin Lispro, Human (Dosage adjustment of the antidiabetic drug may be required). Products include:
- Humalog 1926
- Humalog Mix 75/25 Pen 1928

Insulin Lispro Protamine, Human (Dosage adjustment of the antidiabetic drug may be required). Products include:
- Humalog Mix 75/25 Pen 1928

Irbesartan (Co-administration with other antihypertensives may result in additive effect or potentiation). Products include:
- Avalide Tablets 1070
- Avapro Tablets 1074
- Avapro Tablets 3076

Isradipine (Co-administration with other antihypertensives may result in additive effect or potentiation). Products include:
- DynaCirc Capsules 2921
- DynaCirc CR Tablets 2923

Ketoprofen (Co-administration of thiazide diuretics and non-steroidal anti-inflammatory agents can reduce the diuretic, natiuretic, and antihypertensive effects). Products include:
- Orudis Capsules 3548
- Orudis KT Tablets .... ▣778
- Oruvail Capsules 3548

Ketorolac Tromethamine (Co-administration of thiazide diuretics and non-steroidal anti-inflammatory agents can reduce the diuretic, natiuretic, and antihypertensive effects). Products include:
- Acular Ophthalmic Solution 544
- Acular PF Ophthalmic Solution 544
- Toradol 3018

Labetalol Hydrochloride (Co-administration with other antihypertensives may result in additive effect or potentiation). Products include:
- Normodyne Injection 3135
- Normodyne Tablets 3137

Levorphanol Tartrate (Co-administration of thiazide diuretics and narcotics may result in potentiation of orthostatic hypotension). Products include:
- Levo-Dromoran 1734
- Levorphanol Tartrate Tablets 3059

Lisinopril (Co-administration with other antihypertensives may result in additive effect or potentiation). Products include:
- Prinivil Tablets 2164
- Prinzide Tablets 2168
- Zestoretic Tablets 695
- Zestril Tablets 698

Lithium Carbonate (Diuretics reduce the renal clearance of lithium and add a high risk of lithium toxicity; concurrent use should be avoided). Products include:
- Eskalith 1527
- Lithium Carbonate 3061
- Lithobid Slow-Release Tablets 3255

Lithium Citrate (Diuretics reduce the renal clearance of lithium and add a high risk of lithium toxicity; concurrent use should be avoided). Products include:
- Lithium Citrate Syrup 3061

Losartan Potassium (Co-administration with other antihypertensives may result in additive effect or potentiation). Products include:
- Cozaar Tablets 2067
- Hyzaar 2109

Mecamylamine Hydrochloride (Co-administration with other antihypertensives may result in additive effect or potentiation). Products include:
- Inversine Tablets 1850

Meclofenamate Sodium (Co-administration of thiazide diuretics and non-steroidal anti-inflammatory agents can reduce the diuretic, natiuretic, and antihypertensive effects).
No products indexed under this heading.

Mefenamic Acid (Co-administration of thiazide diuretics and non-steroidal anti-inflammatory agents can reduce the diuretic, natiuretic, and antihypertensive effects). Products include:
- Ponstel Capsules 1356

Meloxicam (Co-administration of thiazide diuretics and non-steroidal anti-inflammatory agents can reduce the diuretic, natiuretic, and antihypertensive effects). Products include:
- Mobic Tablets 1054

Meperidine Hydrochloride (Co-administration of thiazide diuretics and narcotics may result in potentiation of orthostatic hypotension). Products include:
- Demerol 3079
- Mepergan Injection 3539

Mephobarbital (Co-administration of thiazide diuretics and barbiturates may result in potentiation of orthostatic hypotension).
No products indexed under this heading.

Metformin Hydrochloride (Dosage adjustment of the antidiabetic drug may be required). Products include:
- Glucophage Tablets 1080
- Glucophage XR Tablets 1080
- Glucovance Tablets 1086

Methadone Hydrochloride (Co-administration of thiazide diuretics and narcotics may result in potentiation of orthostatic hypotension). Products include:
- Dolophine Hydrochloride Tablets 3056

Methyclothiazide (Co-administration with other antihypertensives may result in additive effect or potentiation).
No products indexed under this heading.

Methyldopa (Co-administration with other antihypertensives may result in additive effect or potentiation). Products include:
- Aldoclor Tablets 2035
- Aldomet Tablets 2037
- Aldoril Tablets 2039

Methyldopate Hydrochloride (Co-administration with other antihypertensives may result in additive effect or potentiation).
No products indexed under this heading.

Methylprednisolone Acetate (Co-administration of thiazide diuretics and corticosteroids may intensify electrolyte depletion, particularly hypokalemia). Products include:
- Depo-Medrol Injectable Suspension 2795

Methylprednisolone Sodium Succinate (Co-administration of thiazide diuretics and corticosteroids may intensify electrolyte depletion, particularly hypokalemia). Products include:
- Solu-Medrol Sterile Powder 2855

Metocurine Iodide (Co-administration of thiazide diuretics and nondepolarizing skeletal muscle relaxants increases responsiveness to the muscle relaxants).
No products indexed under this heading.

Metolazone (Co-administration with other antihypertensives may result in additive effect or potentiation). Products include:
- Mykrox Tablets 1168
- Zaroxolyn Tablets 1177

Metoprolol Succinate (Co-administration with other antihypertensives may result in additive effect or potentiation). Products include:
- Toprol-XL Tablets 651

Metoprolol Tartrate (Co-administration with other antihypertensives may result in additive effect or potentiation).
No products indexed under this heading.

Metyrosine (Co-administration with other antihypertensives may result in additive effect or potentiation). Products include:
- Demser Capsules 2085

Mibefradil Dihydrochloride (Co-administration with other antihypertensives may result in additive effect or potentiation).
No products indexed under this heading.

Miglitol (Dosage adjustment of the antidiabetic drug may be required). Products include:
- Glyset Tablets 2821

Minoxidil (Co-administration with other antihypertensives may result in additive effect or potentiation). Products include:
- Rogaine Extra Strength for Men Topical Solution .... ▣721
- Rogaine for Women Topical Solution .... ▣721

Mivacurium Chloride (Co-administration of thiazide diuretics and nondepolarizing skeletal muscle relaxants increases responsiveness to the muscle relaxants).
No products indexed under this heading.

Moexipril Hydrochloride (Co-administration with other antihypertensives may result in additive effect or potentiation). Products include:
- Uniretic Tablets 3178
- Univasc Tablets 3181

Morphine Sulfate (Co-administration of thiazide diuretics and narcotics may result in potentiation of orthostatic hypotension). Products include:
- Astramorph/PF Injection, USP (Preservative-Free) 594
- Duramorph Injection 1312
- Infumorph 200 and Infumorph 500 Sterile Solutions 1314
- Kadian Capsules 1335
- MS Contin Tablets 2896
- MSIR 2898
- Oramorph SR Tablets 3062
- Roxanol 3066

Nabumetone (Co-administration of thiazide diuretics and non-steroidal anti-inflammatory agents can reduce the diuretic, natiuretic, and antihypertensive effects). Products include:
- Relafen Tablets 1617

Nadolol (Co-administration with other antihypertensives may result in additive effect or potentiation). Products include:
- Corgard Tablets 2245
- Corzide 40/5 Tablets 2247
- Corzide 80/5 Tablets 2247
- Nadolol Tablets 2288

Naproxen (Co-administration of thiazide diuretics and non-steroidal anti-inflammatory agents can reduce the diuretic, natiuretic, and antihypertensive effects). Products include:
- EC-Naprosyn Delayed-Release Tablets 2967
- Naprosyn Suspension 2967
- Naprosyn Tablets 2967

Naproxen Sodium (Co-administration of thiazide diuretics and non-steroidal anti-inflammatory agents can reduce the diuretic, natiuretic, and antihypertensive effects). Products include:
- Aleve Tablets, Caplets and Gelcaps .... ▣602
- Aleve Cold & Sinus Caplets .... ▣603
- Anaprox Tablets 2967
- Anaprox DS Tablets 2967
- Naprelan Tablets 1293

Nicardipine Hydrochloride (Co-administration with other antihypertensives may result in additive effect or potentiation). Products include:
- Cardene I.V. 3485

Nifedipine (Co-administration with other antihypertensives may result in additive effect or potentiation). Products include:
- Adalat CC Tablets 877
- Procardia Capsules 2708
- Procardia XL Extended Release Tablets 2710

IMPORTANT NOTE: Always consult each drug listing in the patient's regimen for possible interactions.

Nisoldipine (Co-administration with other antihypertensives may result in additive effect or potentiation). Products include:
Sular Tablets 688

Nitroglycerin (Co-administration with other antihypertensives may result in additive effect or potentiation). Products include:
Nitro-Dur Transdermal Infusion System 3134
Nitro-Dur Transdermal Infusion System 1834
Nitrolingual Pumpspray 1355
Nitrostat Tablets 2658

Norepinephrine Bitartrate (Possible decreased response to pressor amines but not sufficient to preclude their use).
No products indexed under this heading.

Oxaprozin (Co-administration of thiazide diuretics and non-steroidal anti-inflammatory agents can reduce the diuretic, natiuretic, and antihypertensive effects).
No products indexed under this heading.

Oxycodone Hydrochloride (Co-administration of thiazide diuretics and narcotics may result in potentiation of orthostatic hypotension). Products include:
OxyContin Tablets 2912
OxyFast Oral Concentrate Solution 2916
OxyIR Capsules 2916
Percocet Tablets 1326
Percodan Tablets 1327
Percolone Tablets 1327
Roxicodone 3067
Tylox Capsules 2597

Pancuronium Bromide (Co-administration of thiazide diuretics and nondepolarizing skeletal muscle relaxants increases responsiveness to the muscle relaxants).
No products indexed under this heading.

Penbutolol Sulfate (Co-administration with other antihypertensives may result in additive effect or potentiation).
No products indexed under this heading.

Pentobarbital Sodium (Co-administration of thiazide diuretics and barbiturates may result in potentiation of orthostatic hypotension). Products include:
Nembutal Sodium Solution 485

Perindopril Erbumine (Co-administration with other antihypertensives may result in additive effect or potentiation). Products include:
Aceon Tablets (2 mg, 4 mg, 8 mg) 3249

Phenobarbital (Co-administration of thiazide diuretics and barbiturates may result in potentiation of orthostatic hypotension). Products include:
Arco-Lase Plus Tablets 592
Donnatal 2929
Donnatal Extentabs 2930

Phenoxybenzamine Hydrochloride (Co-administration with other antihypertensives may result in additive effect or potentiation). Products include:
Dibenzyline Capsules 3457

Phentolamine Mesylate (Co-administration with other antihypertensives may result in additive effect or potentiation).
No products indexed under this heading.

Phenylbutazone (Co-administration of thiazide diuretics and non-steroidal anti-inflammatory agents can reduce the diuretic, natiuretic, and antihypertensive effects).
No products indexed under this heading.

Pindolol (Co-administration with other antihypertensives may result in additive effect or potentiation).
No products indexed under this heading.

Pioglitazone Hydrochloride (Dosage adjustment of the antidiabetic drug may be required). Products include:
Actos Tablets 3275

Piroxicam (Co-administration of thiazide diuretics and non-steroidal anti-inflammatory agents can reduce the diuretic, natiuretic, and antihypertensive effects). Products include:
Feldene Capsules 2685

Polythiazide (Co-administration with other antihypertensives may result in additive effect or potentiation). Products include:
Minizide Capsules 2700
Renese Tablets 2712

Potassium Acid Phosphate (Concurrent use with potassium salt substitutes or potassium supplements should be avoided unless directed by a prescriber). Products include:
K-Phos Original (Sodium Free) Tablets 947

Potassium Bicarbonate (Concurrent use with potassium salt substitutes or potassium supplements should be avoided unless directed by a prescriber).
No products indexed under this heading.

Potassium Chloride (Concurrent use with potassium salt substitutes or potassium supplements should be avoided unless directed by a prescriber). Products include:
Chlor-3 1361
Colyte with Flavor Packs for Oral Solution 3170
GoLYTELY and Pineapple Flavor GoLYTELY for Oral Solution 1068
K-Dur Microburst Release System ER Tablets 1832
Klor-Con M20/Klor-Con M10 Tablets 3329
K-Lor Powder Packets 469
K-Tab Filmtab Tablets 470
Micro-K 3311
NuLYTELY, Cherry Flavor, Lemon-Lime Flavor, and Orange Flavor NuLYTELY for Oral Solution 1068
Rum-K 1363

Potassium Citrate (Concurrent use with potassium salt substitutes or potassium supplements should be avoided unless directed by a prescriber). Products include:
Urocit-K Tablets 2232

Potassium Gluconate (Concurrent use with potassium salt substitutes or potassium supplements should be avoided unless directed by a prescriber).
No products indexed under this heading.

Potassium Phosphate (Concurrent use with potassium salt substitutes or potassium supplements should be avoided unless directed by a prescriber). Products include:
K-Phos Neutral Tablets 946

Prazosin Hydrochloride (Co-administration with other antihypertensives may result in additive effect or potentiation). Products include:
Minipress Capsules 2699
Minizide Capsules 2700

Prednisolone Acetate (Co-administration of thiazide diuretics and corticosteroids may intensify electrolyte depletion, particularly hypokalemia). Products include:
Blephamide Ophthalmic Ointment 547
Blephamide Ophthalmic Suspension 548
Poly-Pred Liquifilm Ophthalmic Suspension .... ⊙245
Pred Forte Ophthalmic Suspension .... ⊙246
Pred Mild Sterile Ophthalmic Suspension .... ⊙249
Pred-G Ophthalmic Suspension .... ⊙247
Pred-G Sterile Ophthalmic Ointment .... ⊙248

Prednisolone Sodium Phosphate (Co-administration of thiazide diuretics and corticosteroids may intensify electrolyte depletion, particularly hypokalemia). Products include:
Pediapred Oral Solution 1170

Prednisolone Tebutate (Co-administration of thiazide diuretics and corticosteroids may intensify electrolyte depletion, particularly hypokalemia).
No products indexed under this heading.

Prednisone (Co-administration of thiazide diuretics and corticosteroids may intensify electrolyte depletion, particularly hypokalemia). Products include:
Prednisone 3064

Propoxyphene Hydrochloride (Co-administration of thiazide diuretics and narcotics may result in potentiation of orthostatic hypotension). Products include:
Darvon Pulvules 1909
Darvon Compound-65 Pulvules 1910

Propoxyphene Napsylate (Co-administration of thiazide diuretics and narcotics may result in potentiation of orthostatic hypotension). Products include:
Darvon-N/Darvocet-N 1907
Darvon-N Tablets 1912

Propranolol Hydrochloride (Co-administration with other antihypertensives may result in additive effect or potentiation). Products include:
Inderal 3513
Inderal LA Long-Acting Capsules 3516
Inderide Tablets 3517
Inderide LA Long-Acting Capsules 3519

Quinapril Hydrochloride (Co-administration with other antihypertensives may result in additive effect or potentiation). Products include:
Accupril Tablets 2611
Accuretic Tablets 2614

Ramipril (Co-administration with other antihypertensives may result in additive effect or potentiation). Products include:
Altace Capsules 2233

Rapacuronium Bromide (Co-administration of thiazide diuretics and nondepolarizing skeletal muscle relaxants increases responsiveness to the muscle relaxants).
No products indexed under this heading.

Rauwolfia serpentina (Co-administration with other antihypertensives may result in additive effect or potentiation).
No products indexed under this heading.

Remifentanil Hydrochloride (Co-administration of thiazide diuretics and narcotics may result in potentiation of orthostatic hypotension).
No products indexed under this heading.

Repaglinide (Dosage adjustment of the antidiabetic drug may be required). Products include:
Prandin Tablets (0.5, 1, and 2 mg) 2432

Rescinnamine (Co-administration with other antihypertensives may result in additive effect or potentiation).
No products indexed under this heading.

Reserpine (Co-administration with other antihypertensives may result in additive effect or potentiation).
No products indexed under this heading.

Rocuronium Bromide (Co-administration of thiazide diuretics and nondepolarizing skeletal muscle relaxants increases responsiveness to the muscle relaxants). Products include:
Zemuron Injection 2491

Rofecoxib (Co-administration of thiazide diuretics and non-steroidal anti-inflammatory agents can reduce the diuretic, natiuretic, and antihypertensive effects). Products include:
Vioxx 2213

Rosiglitazone Maleate (Dosage adjustment of the antidiabetic drug may be required). Products include:
Avandia Tablets 1490

Secobarbital Sodium (Co-administration of thiazide diuretics and barbiturates may result in potentiation of orthostatic hypotension).
No products indexed under this heading.

Sodium Nitroprusside (Co-administration with other antihypertensives may result in additive effect or potentiation).
No products indexed under this heading.

Sotalol Hydrochloride (Co-administration with other antihypertensives may result in additive effect or potentiation). Products include:
Betapace Tablets 950
Betapace AF Tablets 954

Spirapril Hydrochloride (Co-administration with other antihypertensives may result in additive effect or potentiation).
No products indexed under this heading.

Sufentanil Citrate (Co-administration of thiazide diuretics and narcotics may result in potentiation of orthostatic hypotension).
No products indexed under this heading.

Sulindac (Co-administration of thiazide diuretics and non-steroidal anti-inflammatory agents can reduce the diuretic, natiuretic, and antihypertensive effects). Products include:
Clinoril Tablets 2053

Telmisartan (Co-administration with other antihypertensives may result in additive effect or potentiation). Products include:
Micardis Tablets 1049
Micardis HCT Tablets 1051

Terazosin Hydrochloride (Co-administration with other antihypertensives may result in additive effect or potentiation). Products include:
Hytrin Capsules 464

Thiamylal Sodium (Co-administration of thiazide diuretics and barbiturates may result in potentiation of orthostatic hypotension).
No products indexed under this heading.

Timolol Maleate (Co-administration with other antihypertensives may result in additive effect or potentiation). Products include:
Blocadren Tablets 2046
Cosopt Sterile Ophthalmic Solution 2065
Timolide Tablets 2187
Timolol GFS .... ⊙266
Timoptic in Ocudose 2192
Timoptic Sterile Ophthalmic Solution 2190
Timoptic-XE Sterile Ophthalmic Gel Forming Solution 2194

Tolazamide (Dosage adjustment of the antidiabetic drug may be required).
No products indexed under this heading.

Tolbutamide (Dosage adjustment of the antidiabetic drug may be required).
No products indexed under this heading.

Tolmetin Sodium (Co-administration of thiazide diuretics and non-steroidal anti-inflammatory agents can reduce the diuretic, natiuretic, and antihypertensive effects). Products include:
Tolectin 2589

Torsemide (Co-administration with other antihypertensives may result in additive effect or potentiation). Products include:
- Demadex Tablets and Injection 2965

Trandolapril (Co-administration with other antihypertensives may result in additive effect or potentiation). Products include:
- Mavik Tablets 478
- Tarka Tablets 508

Triamcinolone (Co-administration of thiazide diuretics and corticosteroids may intensify electrolyte depletion, particularly hypokalemia).
- No products indexed under this heading.

Triamcinolone Acetonide (Co-administration of thiazide diuretics and corticosteroids may intensify electrolyte depletion, particularly hypokalemia). Products include:
- Azmacort Inhalation Aerosol 728
- Nasacort Nasal Inhaler 750
- Nasacort AQ Nasal Spray 752
- Tri-Nasal Spray 2274

Triamcinolone Diacetate (Co-administration of thiazide diuretics and corticosteroids may intensify electrolyte depletion, particularly hypokalemia).
- No products indexed under this heading.

Triamcinolone Hexacetonide (Co-administration of thiazide diuretics and corticosteroids may intensify electrolyte depletion, particularly hypokalemia).
- No products indexed under this heading.

Trimethaphan Camsylate (Co-administration with other antihypertensives may result in additive effect or potentiation).
- No products indexed under this heading.

Troglitazone (Dosage adjustment of the antidiabetic drug may be required).
- No products indexed under this heading.

Tubocurarine Chloride (Co-administration of thiazide diuretics and nondepolarizing skeletal muscle relaxants increases responsiveness to the muscle relaxants).
- No products indexed under this heading.

Vecuronium Bromide (Co-administration of thiazide diuretics and nondepolarizing skeletal muscle relaxants increases responsiveness to the muscle relaxants). Products include:
- Norcuron for Injection 2478

Verapamil Hydrochloride (Co-administration with other antihypertensives may result in additive effect or potentiation). Products include:
- Covera-HS Tablets 3199
- Isoptin SR Tablets 467
- Tarka Tablets 508
- Verelan Capsules 3184
- Verelan PM Capsules 3186

Food Interactions

Alcohol (Co-administration of thiazide diuretics and alcohol may result in potentiation of orthostatic hypotension).

DIPENTUM CAPSULES

(Olsalazine Sodium) 2803

May interact with oral anticoagulants. Compounds in these categories include:

Dicumarol (Potential for increased prothrombin time).
- No products indexed under this heading.

Warfarin Sodium (Potential for increased prothrombin time). Products include:
- Coumadin for Injection 1243
- Coumadin Tablets 1243
- Warfarin Sodium Tablets, USP 3302

DIPHTHERIA & TETANUS TOXOIDS ADSORBED PUROGENATED FOR PEDIATRIC USE

(Diphtheria & Tetanus Toxoids Adsorbed, (For Pediatric Use)) 1857

See Tetanus & Diphtheria Toxoids Adsorbed for Adult Use

DIPRIVAN INJECTABLE EMULSION

(Propofol) 667

May interact with barbiturates, benzodiazepines, hypnotics and sedatives, inhalant anesthetics, narcotic analgesics, and certain other agents. Compounds in these categories include:

Alfentanil Hydrochloride (Increases anesthetic or sedative effects; may also result in pronounced decreases in systolic, diastolic, and mean arterial pressure and cardiac output).
- No products indexed under this heading.

Alprazolam (Increases anesthetic or sedative effects; may also result in pronounced decreases in systolic, diastolic, and mean arterial pressure and cardiac output). Products include:
- Xanax Tablets 2865

Aprobarbital (Increases anesthetic or sedative effects; may also result in pronounced decreases in systolic, diastolic, and mean arterial pressure and cardiac output).
- No products indexed under this heading.

Buprenorphine Hydrochloride (Increases anesthetic or sedative effects; may also result in pronounced decreases in systolic, diastolic, and mean arterial pressure and cardiac output). Products include:
- Buprenex Injectable 2918

Butabarbital (Increases anesthetic or sedative effects; may also result in pronounced decreases in systolic, diastolic, and mean arterial pressure and cardiac output).
- No products indexed under this heading.

Butalbital (Increases anesthetic or sedative effects; may also result in pronounced decreases in systolic, diastolic, and mean arterial pressure and cardiac output). Products include:
- Phrenilin 578
- Sedapap Tablets 50 mg/650 mg 2225

Chloral Hydrate (Increases anesthetic or sedative effects; may also result in pronounced decreases in systolic, diastolic, and mean arterial pressure and cardiac output).
- No products indexed under this heading.

Chlordiazepoxide (Increases anesthetic or sedative effects; may also result in pronounced decreases in systolic, diastolic, and mean arterial pressure and cardiac output). Products include:
- Limbitrol 1738

Chlordiazepoxide Hydrochloride (Increases anesthetic or sedative effects; may also result in pronounced decreases in systolic, diastolic, and mean arterial pressure and cardiac output). Products include:
- Librium Capsules 1736
- Librium for Injection 1737

Clonazepam (Increases anesthetic or sedative effects; may also result in pronounced decreases in systolic, diastolic, and mean arterial pressure and cardiac output). Products include:
- Klonopin Tablets 2983

Clorazepate Dipotassium (Increases anesthetic or sedative effects; may also result in pronounced decreases in systolic, diastolic, and mean arterial pressure and cardiac output). Products include:
- Tranxene 511

Codeine Phosphate (Increases anesthetic or sedative effects; may also result in pronounced decreases in systolic, diastolic, and mean arterial pressure and cardiac output). Products include:
- Phenergan with Codeine Syrup 3557
- Phenergan VC with Codeine Syrup 3561
- Robitussin A-C Syrup 2942
- Robitussin-DAC Syrup 2942
- Ryna-C Liquid 768
- Soma Compound w/Codeine Tablets 3355
- Tussi-Organidin NR Liquid 3350
- Tussi-Organidin-S NR Liquid 3350
- Tylenol with Codeine 2595

Desflurane (Increases anesthetic or sedative and cardiorespiratory effects). Products include:
- Suprane Liquid for Inhalation 874

Dezocine (Increases anesthetic or sedative effects; may also result in pronounced decreases in systolic, diastolic, and mean arterial pressure and cardiac output).
- No products indexed under this heading.

Diazepam (Increases anesthetic or sedative effects; may also result in pronounced decreases in systolic, diastolic, and mean arterial pressure and cardiac output). Products include:
- Valium Injectable 3026
- Valium Tablets 3047

Droperidol (Increases anesthetic or sedative effects; may also result in pronounced decreases in systolic, diastolic, and mean arterial pressure and cardiac output).
- No products indexed under this heading.

Enflurane (Increases anesthetic or sedative and cardiorespiratory effects).
- No products indexed under this heading.

Estazolam (Increases anesthetic or sedative effects; may also result in pronounced decreases in systolic, diastolic, and mean arterial pressure and cardiac output). Products include:
- ProSom Tablets 500

Ethchlorvynol (Increases anesthetic or sedative effects; may also result in pronounced decreases in systolic, diastolic, and mean arterial pressure and cardiac output).
- No products indexed under this heading.

Ethinamate (Increases anesthetic or sedative effects; may also result in pronounced decreases in systolic, diastolic, and mean arterial pressure and cardiac output).
- No products indexed under this heading.

Fentanyl (Co-administration in pediatric patients may result in serious bradycardia; increases anesthetic or sedative effects; may also result in pronounced decreases in systolic, diastolic, and mean arterial pressure and cardiac output). Products include:
- Duragesic Transdermal System 1786

Fentanyl Citrate (Co-administration in pediatric patients may result in serious bradycardia; increases anesthetic or sedative effects; may also result in pronounced decreases in systolic, diastolic, and mean arterial pressure and cardiac output). Products include:
- Actiq 1184

Flurazepam Hydrochloride (Increases anesthetic or sedative effects; may also result in pronounced decreases in systolic, diastolic, and mean arterial pressure and cardiac output).
- No products indexed under this heading.

Glutethimide (Increases anesthetic or sedative effects; may also result in pronounced decreases in systolic, diastolic, and mean arterial pressure and cardiac output).
- No products indexed under this heading.

Halazepam (Increases anesthetic or sedative effects; may also result in pronounced decreases in systolic, diastolic, and mean arterial pressure and cardiac output).
- No products indexed under this heading.

Halothane (Increases anesthetic or sedative and cardiorespiratory effects). Products include:
- Fluothane Inhalation 3508

Hydrocodone Bitartrate (Increases anesthetic or sedative effects; may also result in pronounced decreases in systolic, diastolic, and mean arterial pressure and cardiac output). Products include:
- Hycodan 1316
- Hycomine Compound Tablets 1317
- Hycotuss Expectorant Syrup 1318
- Lortab 3319
- Lortab Elixir 3317
- Maxidone Tablets CIII 3399
- Norco 5/325 Tablets CIII 3424
- Norco 7.5/325 Tablets CIII 3425
- Norco 10/325 Tablets CIII 3427
- Norco 10/325 Tablets CIII 3425
- Vicodin Tablets 516
- Vicodin ES Tablets 517
- Vicodin HP Tablets 518
- Vicodin Tuss Expectorant 519
- Vicoprofen Tablets 520
- Zydone Tablets 1330

Hydrocodone Polistirex (Increases anesthetic or sedative effects; may also result in pronounced decreases in systolic, diastolic, and mean arterial pressure and cardiac output). Products include:
- Tussionex Pennkinetic Extended-Release Suspension 1174

Hydromorphone Hydrochloride (Increases anesthetic or sedative effects; may also result in pronounced decreases in systolic, diastolic, and mean arterial pressure and cardiac output). Products include:
- Dilaudid 441
- Dilaudid Oral Liquid 445
- Dilaudid Powder 441
- Dilaudid Rectal Suppositories 441
- Dilaudid Tablets 441
- Dilaudid Tablets - 8 mg 445
- Dilaudid-HP 443

Isoflurane (Increases anesthetic or sedative and cardiorespiratory effects).
- No products indexed under this heading.

Levorphanol Tartrate (Increases anesthetic or sedative effects; may also result in pronounced decreases in systolic, diastolic, and mean arterial pressure and cardiac output). Products include:
- Levo-Dromoran 1734
- Levorphanol Tartrate Tablets 3059

Lorazepam (Increases anesthetic or sedative effects; may also result in pronounced decreases in systolic, diastolic, and mean arterial pressure and cardiac output). Products include:
- Ativan Injection 3478
- Ativan Tablets 3482

Meperidine Hydrochloride (Increases anesthetic or sedative effects; may also result in pro-

nounced decreases in systolic, diastolic, and mean arterial pressure and cardiac output). Products include:

Demerol 3079
Mepergan Injection 3539

Mephobarbital (Increases anesthetic or sedative effects; may also result in pronounced decreases in systolic, diastolic, and mean arterial pressure and cardiac output).

No products indexed under this heading.

Methadone Hydrochloride (Increases anesthetic or sedative effects; may also result in pronounced decreases in systolic, diastolic, and mean arterial pressure and cardiac output). Products include:

Dolophine Hydrochloride Tablets 3056

Methoxyflurane (Increases anesthetic or sedative and cardiorespiratory effects).

No products indexed under this heading.

Midazolam Hydrochloride (Increases anesthetic or sedative effects; may also result in pronounced decreases in systolic, diastolic, and mean arterial pressure and cardiac output). Products include:

Versed Injection 3027
Versed Syrup 3033

Morphine Sulfate (Increases anesthetic or sedative effects; may also result in pronounced decreases in systolic, diastolic, and mean arterial pressure and cardiac output). Products include:

Astramorph/PF Injection, USP (Preservative-Free) 594
Duramorph Injection 1312
Infumorph 200 and Infumorph 500 Sterile Solutions 1314
Kadian Capsules 1335
MS Contin Tablets 2896
MSIR 2898
Oramorph SR Tablets 3062
Roxanol 3066

Nitrous Oxide (Rate of administration requires adjustment).

No products indexed under this heading.

Oxazepam (Increases anesthetic or sedative effects; may also result in pronounced decreases in systolic, diastolic, and mean arterial pressure and cardiac output).

No products indexed under this heading.

Oxycodone Hydrochloride (Increases anesthetic or sedative effects; may also result in pronounced decreases in systolic, diastolic, and mean arterial pressure and cardiac output). Products include:

OxyContin Tablets 2912
OxyFast Oral Concentrate Solution . 2916
OxyIR Capsules 2916
Percocet Tablets 1326
Percodan Tablets 1327
Percolone Tablets 1327
Roxicodone 3067
Tylox Capsules 2597

Pentobarbital Sodium (Increases anesthetic or sedative effects; may also result in pronounced decreases in systolic, diastolic, and mean arterial pressure and cardiac output). Products include:

Nembutal Sodium Solution 485

Phenobarbital (Increases anesthetic or sedative effects; may also result in pronounced decreases in systolic, diastolic, and mean arterial pressure and cardiac output). Products include:

Arco-Lase Plus Tablets 592
Donnatal 2929
Donnatal Extentabs 2930

Prazepam (Increases anesthetic or sedative effects; may also result in pronounced decreases in systolic, diastolic, and mean arterial pressure and cardiac output).

No products indexed under this heading.

Propoxyphene Hydrochloride (Increases anesthetic or sedative effects; may also result in pronounced decreases in systolic, diastolic, and mean arterial pressure and cardiac output). Products include:

Darvon Pulvules 1909
Darvon Compound-65 Pulvules 1910

Propoxyphene Napsylate (Increases anesthetic or sedative effects; may also result in pronounced decreases in systolic, diastolic, and mean arterial pressure and cardiac output). Products include:

Darvon-N/Darvocet-N 1907
Darvon-N Tablets 1912

Quazepam (Increases anesthetic or sedative effects; may also result in pronounced decreases in systolic, diastolic, and mean arterial pressure and cardiac output).

No products indexed under this heading.

Remifentanil Hydrochloride (Increases anesthetic or sedative effects; may also result in pronounced decreases in systolic, diastolic, and mean arterial pressure and cardiac output).

No products indexed under this heading.

Secobarbital Sodium (Increases anesthetic or sedative effects; may also result in pronounced decreases in systolic, diastolic, and mean arterial pressure and cardiac output).

No products indexed under this heading.

Sufentanil Citrate (Increases anesthetic or sedative effects; may also result in pronounced decreases in systolic, diastolic, and mean arterial pressure and cardiac output).

No products indexed under this heading.

Temazepam (Increases anesthetic or sedative effects; may also result in pronounced decreases in systolic, diastolic, and mean arterial pressure and cardiac output).

No products indexed under this heading.

Thiamylal Sodium (Increases anesthetic or sedative effects; may also result in pronounced decreases in systolic, diastolic, and mean arterial pressure and cardiac output).

No products indexed under this heading.

Triazolam (Increases anesthetic or sedative effects; may also result in pronounced decreases in systolic, diastolic, and mean arterial pressure and cardiac output). Products include:

Halcion Tablets 2823

Zaleplon (Increases anesthetic or sedative effects; may also result in pronounced decreases in systolic, diastolic, and mean arterial pressure and cardiac output). Products include:

Sonata Capsules 3591

Zolpidem Tartrate (Increases anesthetic or sedative effects; may also result in pronounced decreases in systolic, diastolic, and mean arterial pressure and cardiac output). Products include:

Ambien Tablets 3191

DIPROLENE GEL 0.05%

(Betamethasone Dipropionate) 3107
None cited in PDR database.

DIPROLENE LOTION 0.05%

(Betamethasone Dipropionate) 3107
None cited in PDR database.

DIPROLENE OINTMENT 0.05%

(Betamethasone Dipropionate) 3108
None cited in PDR database.

DIPROLENE AF CREAM 0.05%

(Betamethasone Dipropionate) 3106
None cited in PDR database.

DIPROSONE CREAM

(Betamethasone Dipropionate) 3109
None cited in PDR database.

DIPROSONE LOTION

(Betamethasone Dipropionate) 3109
None cited in PDR database.

DIPROSONE OINTMENT

(Betamethasone Dipropionate) 3109
None cited in PDR database.

DITROPAN XL EXTENDED RELEASE TABLETS

(Oxybutynin Chloride) 564
May interact with anticholinergics, bisphosphonates, hypnotics and sedatives, potassium preparations, and certain other agents. Compounds in these categories include:

Alendronate Sodium (Concurrent use with drugs that can cause or exacerbate esophagitis, such as biphosphonates, should be undertaken with caution). Products include:

Fosamax Tablets 2095

Atropine Sulfate (Co-administration of oxybutynin with other anticholinergic drugs may increase the frequency and/or severity of anticholinergic side effects such as dry mouth, constipation, drowsiness and others). Products include:

Donnatal 2929
Donnatal Extentabs 2930
Motofen Tablets 577
Prosed/DS Tablets 3268
Urised Tablets 2876

Belladonna Alkaloids (Co-administration of oxybutynin with other anticholinergic drugs may increase the frequency and/or severity of anticholinergic side effects such as dry mouth, constipation, drowsiness and others). Products include:

Hyland's Teething Tablets .... ▣ 766
Urimax Tablets 1769

Benztropine Mesylate (Co-administration of oxybutynin with other anticholinergic drugs may increase the frequency and/or severity of anticholinergic side effects such as dry mouth, constipation, drowsiness and others). Products include:

Cogentin 2055

Biperiden Hydrochloride (Co-administration of oxybutynin with other anticholinergic drugs may increase the frequency and/or severity of anticholinergic side effects such as dry mouth, constipation, drowsiness and others). Products include:

Akineton 402

Cisapride (Co-administration of cisapride with anticholinergic agents would be expected to compromise the beneficial effects of cisapride).

No products indexed under this heading.

Clidinium Bromide (Co-administration of oxybutynin with other anticholinergic drugs may increase the frequency and/or severity of anticholinergic side effects such as dry mouth, constipation, drowsiness and others).

No products indexed under this heading.

Dicyclomine Hydrochloride (Co-administration of oxybutynin with other anticholinergic drugs may increase the frequency and/or severity of anticholinergic side effects such as dry mouth, constipation, drowsiness and others).

No products indexed under this heading.

Estazolam (Sedatives enhance the drowsiness effect caused by anticholinergic agents such as oxybutynin). Products include:

ProSom Tablets 500

Ethchlorvynol (Sedatives enhance the drowsiness effect caused by anticholinergic agents such as oxybutynin).

No products indexed under this heading.

Ethinamate (Sedatives enhance the drowsiness effect caused by anticholinergic agents such as oxybutynin).

No products indexed under this heading.

Etidronate Disodium (Concurrent use with drugs that can cause or exacerbate esophagitis, such as biphosphonates, should be undertaken with caution). Products include:

Didronel Tablets 2888

Flurazepam Hydrochloride (Sedatives enhance the drowsiness effect caused by anticholinergic agents such as oxybutynin).

No products indexed under this heading.

Glutethimide (Sedatives enhance the drowsiness effect caused by anticholinergic agents such as oxybutynin).

No products indexed under this heading.

Glycopyrrolate (Co-administration of oxybutynin with other anticholinergic drugs may increase the frequency and/or severity of anticholinergic side effects such as dry mouth, constipation, drowsiness and others). Products include:

Robinul Forte Tablets 1358
Robinul Injectable 2940
Robinul Tablets 1358

Hyoscyamine (Co-administration of oxybutynin with other anticholinergic drugs may increase the frequency and/or severity of anticholinergic side effects such as dry mouth, constipation, drowsiness and others). Products include:

Urised Tablets 2876

Hyoscyamine Sulfate (Co-administration of oxybutynin with other anticholinergic drugs may increase the frequency and/or severity of anticholinergic side effects such as dry mouth, constipation, drowsiness and others). Products include:

Arco-Lase Plus Tablets 592
Donnatal 2929
Donnatal Extentabs 2930
Levsin/Levsinex/Levbid 3172
NuLev Orally Disintegrating Tablets 3176
Prosed/DS Tablets 3268
Urimax Tablets 1769

Ipratropium Bromide (Co-administration of oxybutynin with other anticholinergic drugs may increase the frequency and/or severity of anticholinergic side effects such as dry mouth, constipation, drowsiness and others). Products include:

Atrovent Inhalation Aerosol 1030
Atrovent Inhalation Solution 1031
Atrovent Nasal Spray 0.03% 1032
Atrovent Nasal Spray 0.06% 1033
Combivent Inhalation Aerosol 1041
DuoNeb Inhalation Solution 1233

Lorazepam (Sedatives enhance the drowsiness effect caused by anticholinergic agents such as oxybutynin). Products include:

Ativan Injection 3478
Ativan Tablets 3482

Mepenzolate Bromide (Co-administration of oxybutynin with

other anticholinergic drugs may increase the frequency and/or severity of anticholinergic side effects such as dry mouth, constipation, drowsiness and others).
No products indexed under this heading.

Midazolam Hydrochloride (Sedatives enhance the drowsiness effect caused by anticholinergic agents such as oxybutynin). Products include:
Versed Injection 3027
Versed Syrup 3033

Oxybutynin Chloride (Co-administration of oxybutynin with other anticholinergic drugs may increase the frequency and/or severity of anticholinergic side effects such as dry mouth, constipation, drowsiness and others). Products include:
Ditropan XL Extended Release Tablets 564

Potassium Acid Phosphate (Anticholinergic agents may potentially alter the absorption of some concomitantly administered drugs, such as potassium supplements, due to anticholinergic effects on GI motility, especially arrest or delay in these formulations passage through the GI tract). Products include:
K-Phos Original (Sodium Free) Tablets 947

Potassium Bicarbonate (Anticholinergic agents may potentially alter the absorption of some concomitantly administered drugs, such as potassium supplements, due to anticholinergic effects on GI motility, especially arrest or delay in these formulations passage through the GI tract).
No products indexed under this heading.

Potassium Chloride (Anticholinergic agents may potentially alter the absorption of some concomitantly administered drugs, such as potassium supplements, due to anticholinergic effects on GI motility, especially arrest or delay in these formulations passage through the GI tract). Products include:
Chlor-3 1361
Colyte with Flavor Packs for Oral Solution 3170
GoLYTELY and Pineapple Flavor GoLYTELY for Oral Solution 1068
K-Dur Microburst Release System ER Tablets 1832
Klor-Con M20/Klor-Con M10 Tablets 3329
K-Lor Powder Packets 469
K-Tab Filmtab Tablets 470
Micro-K 3311
NuLYTELY, Cherry Flavor, Lemon-Lime Flavor, and Orange Flavor NuLYTELY for Oral Solution 1068
Rum-K 1363

Potassium Citrate (Anticholinergic agents may potentially alter the absorption of some concomitantly administered drugs, such as potassium supplements, due to anticholinergic effects on GI motility, especially arrest or delay in these formulations passage through the GI tract). Products include:
Urocit-K Tablets 2232

Potassium Gluconate (Anticholinergic agents may potentially alter the absorption of some concomitantly administered drugs, such as potassium supplements, due to anticholinergic effects on GI motility, especially arrest or delay in these formulations passage through the GI tract).
No products indexed under this heading.

Potassium Phosphate (Anticholinergic agents may potentially alter the absorption of some concomitantly administered drugs, such as potassium supplements, due to anticholinergic effects on GI motility, especially arrest or delay in these formulations passage through the GI tract). Products include:
K-Phos Neutral Tablets 946

Procyclidine Hydrochloride (Co-administration of oxybutynin with other anticholinergic drugs may increase the frequency and/or severity of anticholinergic side effects such as dry mouth, constipation, drowsiness and others).
No products indexed under this heading.

Propantheline Bromide (Co-administration of oxybutynin with other anticholinergic drugs may increase the frequency and/or severity of anticholinergic side effects such as dry mouth, constipation, drowsiness and others).
No products indexed under this heading.

Propofol (Sedatives enhance the drowsiness effect caused by anticholinergic agents such as oxybutynin). Products include:
Diprivan Injectable Emulsion 667

Quazepam (Sedatives enhance the drowsiness effect caused by anticholinergic agents such as oxybutynin).
No products indexed under this heading.

Risedronate Sodium (Concurrent use with drugs that can cause or exacerbate esophagitis, such as biphosphonates, should be undertaken with caution). Products include:
Actonel Tablets 2879

Scopolamine (Co-administration of oxybutynin with other anticholinergic drugs may increase the frequency and/or severity of anticholinergic side effects such as dry mouth, constipation, drowsiness and others). Products include:
Transderm Scōp Transdermal Therapeutic System 2302

Scopolamine Hydrobromide (Co-administration of oxybutynin with other anticholinergic drugs may increase the frequency and/or severity of anticholinergic side effects such as dry mouth, constipation, drowsiness and others). Products include:
Donnatal 2929
Donnatal Extentabs 2930

Secobarbital Sodium (Sedatives enhance the drowsiness effect caused by anticholinergic agents such as oxybutynin).
No products indexed under this heading.

Temazepam (Sedatives enhance the drowsiness effect caused by anticholinergic agents such as oxybutynin).
No products indexed under this heading.

Tiludronate Disodium (Concurrent use with drugs that can cause or exacerbate esophagitis, such as biphosphonates, should be undertaken with caution). Products include:
Skelid Tablets 3088

Tolterodine Tartrate (Co-administration of oxybutynin with other anticholinergic drugs may increase the frequency and/or severity of anticholinergic side effects such as dry mouth, constipation, drowsiness and others). Products include:
Detrol Tablets 3623
Detrol LA Capsules 2801

Triazolam (Sedatives enhance the drowsiness effect caused by anticholinergic agents such as oxybutynin). Products include:
Halcion Tablets 2823

Tridihexethyl Chloride (Co-administration of oxybutynin with other anticholinergic drugs may increase the frequency and/or severity of anticholinergic side effects such as dry mouth, constipation, drowsiness and others).
No products indexed under this heading.

Trihexyphenidyl Hydrochloride (Co-administration of oxybutynin with other anticholinergic drugs may increase the frequency and/or severity of anticholinergic side effects such as dry mouth, constipation, drowsiness and others). Products include:
Artane 1855

Zaleplon (Sedatives enhance the drowsiness effect caused by anticholinergic agents such as oxybutynin). Products include:
Sonata Capsules 3591

Zolpidem Tartrate (Sedatives enhance the drowsiness effect caused by anticholinergic agents such as oxybutynin). Products include:
Ambien Tablets 3191

Food Interactions

Alcohol (Enhances the drowsiness effect caused by anticholinergic agents such as oxybutynin).

DIUCARDIN TABLETS

(Hydroflumethiazide) 3494
May interact with antihypertensives, barbiturates, corticosteroids, oral anticoagulants, general anesthetics, cardiac glycosides, antigout agents, oral hypoglycemic agents, insulin, lithium preparations, narcotic analgesics, non-steroidal anti-inflammatory agents, and certain other agents. Compounds in these categories include:

Acarbose (Hyperglycemia may occur with thiazide diuretics; dosage adjustment of the oral antidiabetic drug may be required). Products include:
Precose Tablets 906

Acebutolol Hydrochloride (Antihypertensive effects may be potentiated when used concurrently with thiazide diuretics; dosage adjustment may be necessary). Products include:
Sectral Capsules 3589

ACTH (Intensified electrolyte depletion, particularly hypokalemia).
No products indexed under this heading.

Alfentanil Hydrochloride (Thiazide-induced orthostatic hypotension may be potentiated).
No products indexed under this heading.

Allopurinol (Thiazide diuretics may raise the levels of blood uric acid; dosage adjustment of antigout medication may be necessary to control gout and hyperuricemia).
No products indexed under this heading.

Amlodipine Besylate (Antihypertensive effects may be potentiated when used concurrently with thiazide diuretics; dosage adjustment may be necessary). Products include:
Lotrel Capsules 2370
Norvasc Tablets 2704

Amphotericin B (Intensified electrolyte depletion, particularly hypokalemia). Products include:
Abelcet Injection 1273
AmBisome for Injection 1383
Amphotec 1774

Aprobarbital (Thiazide-induced orthostatic hypotension may be potentiated).
No products indexed under this heading.

Atenolol (Antihypertensive effects may be potentiated when used concurrently with thiazide diuretics; dosage adjustment may be necessary). Products include:
Tenoretic Tablets 690
Tenormin I.V. Injection 692

Benazepril Hydrochloride (Antihypertensive effects may be potentiated when used concurrently with thiazide diuretics; dosage adjustment may be necessary). Products include:
Lotensin Tablets 2365
Lotensin HCT Tablets 2367
Lotrel Capsules 2370

Bendroflumethiazide (Antihypertensive effects may be potentiated when used concurrently with thiazide diuretics; dosage adjustment may be necessary). Products include:
Corzide 40/5 Tablets 2247
Corzide 80/5 Tablets 2247

Betamethasone Acetate (Intensified electrolyte depletion, particularly hypokalemia). Products include:
Celestone Soluspan Injectable Suspension 3097

Betamethasone Sodium Phosphate (Intensified electrolyte depletion, particularly hypokalemia). Products include:
Celestone Soluspan Injectable Suspension 3097

Betaxolol Hydrochloride (Antihypertensive effects may be potentiated when used concurrently with thiazide diuretics; dosage adjustment may be necessary). Products include:
Betoptic S Ophthalmic Suspension 537

Bisoprolol Fumarate (Antihypertensive effects may be potentiated when used concurrently with thiazide diuretics; dosage adjustment may be necessary). Products include:
Zebeta Tablets 1885
Ziac Tablets 1887

Buprenorphine Hydrochloride (Thiazide-induced orthostatic hypotension may be potentiated). Products include:
Buprenex Injectable 2918

Butabarbital (Thiazide-induced orthostatic hypotension may be potentiated).
No products indexed under this heading.

Butalbital (Thiazide-induced orthostatic hypotension may be potentiated). Products include:
Phrenilin 578
Sedapap Tablets 50 mg/650 mg 2225

Candesartan Cilexetil (Antihypertensive effects may be potentiated when used concurrently with thiazide diuretics; dosage adjustment may be necessary). Products include:
Atacand Tablets 595
Atacand HCT Tablets 597

Captopril (Antihypertensive effects may be potentiated when used concurrently with thiazide diuretics; dosage adjustment may be necessary). Products include:
Captopril Tablets 2281

Carteolol Hydrochloride (Antihypertensive effects may be potentiated when used concurrently with thiazide diuretics; dosage adjustment may be necessary). Products include:
Carteolol Hydrochloride Ophthalmic Solution USP, 1% .... ⊙258
Ocupress Ophthalmic Solution, 1% Sterile .... ⊙303

Celecoxib (Concurrent use of non-steroidal anti-inflammatory agents in some patients may reduce the diuretic, natriuretic and antihypertensive effects of thiazide diuretics). Products include:
Celebrex Capsules 2676
Celebrex Capsules 2780

Chlorothiazide (Antihypertensive effects may be potentiated when

used concurrently with thiazide diuretics; dosage adjustment may be necessary). Products include:
- Aldoclor Tablets 2035
- Diuril Oral 2087

Chlorothiazide Sodium (Antihypertensive effects may be potentiated when used concurrently with thiazide diuretics; dosage adjustment may be necessary). Products include:
- Diuril Sodium Intravenous 2086

Chlorpropamide (Hyperglycemia may occur with thiazide diuretics; dosage adjustment of the oral antidiabetic drug may be required). Products include:
- Diabinese Tablets 2680

Chlorthalidone (Antihypertensive effects may be potentiated when used concurrently with thiazide diuretics; dosage adjustment may be necessary). Products include:
- Clorpres Tablets 1002
- Combipres Tablets 1040
- Tenoretic Tablets 690

Clonidine (Antihypertensive effects may be potentiated when used concurrently with thiazide diuretics; dosage adjustment may be necessary). Products include:
- Catapres-TTS 1038

Clonidine Hydrochloride (Antihypertensive effects may be potentiated when used concurrently with thiazide diuretics; dosage adjustment may be necessary). Products include:
- Catapres Tablets 1037
- Clorpres Tablets 1002
- Combipres Tablets 1040
- Duraclon Injection 3057

Codeine Phosphate (Thiazide-induced orthostatic hypotension may be potentiated). Products include:
- Phenergan with Codeine Syrup 3557
- Phenergan VC with Codeine Syrup 3561
- Robitussin A-C Syrup 2942
- Robitussin-DAC Syrup 2942
- Ryna-C Liquid .... ■768
- Soma Compound w/Codeine Tablets 3355
- Tussi-Organidin NR Liquid 3350
- Tussi-Organidin-S NR Liquid 3350
- Tylenol with Codeine 2595

Colestipol Hydrochloride (May inhibit gastrointestinal absorption of the thiazide diuretics; administration 1 hour before or 4 hours after colestipol is recommended). Products include:
- Colestid Tablets 2791

Cortisone Acetate (Intensified electrolyte depletion, particularly hypokalemia). Products include:
- Cortone Acetate Injectable Suspension 2059
- Cortone Acetate Tablets 2061

Deserpidine (Antihypertensive effects may be potentiated when used concurrently with thiazide diuretics; dosage adjustment may be necessary).
No products indexed under this heading.

Deslanoside (Thiazide-induced hypokalemia may exaggerate or sensitize the response of heart to the toxic effect of digitalis).
No products indexed under this heading.

Dexamethasone (Intensified electrolyte depletion, particularly hypokalemia). Products include:
- Decadron Elixir 2078
- Decadron Tablets 2079
- TobraDex Ophthalmic Ointment 542
- TobraDex Ophthalmic Suspension 541

Dexamethasone Acetate (Intensified electrolyte depletion, particularly hypokalemia).
No products indexed under this heading.

Dexamethasone Sodium Phosphate (Intensified electrolyte depletion, particularly hypokalemia). Products include:
- Decadron Phosphate Injection 2081
- Decadron Phosphate Sterile Ophthalmic Ointment 2083
- Decadron Phosphate Sterile Ophthalmic Solution 2084
- NeoDecadron Sterile Ophthalmic Solution 2144

Dezocine (Thiazide-induced orthostatic hypotension may be potentiated).
No products indexed under this heading.

Diazoxide (Antihypertensive effects may be potentiated when used concurrently with thiazide diuretics; dosage adjustment may be necessary).
No products indexed under this heading.

Diclofenac Potassium (Concurrent use of nonsteroidal anti-inflammatory agents in some patients may reduce the diuretic, natriuretic and antihypertensive effects of thiazide diuretics). Products include:
- Cataflam Tablets 2315

Diclofenac Sodium (Concurrent use of nonsteroidal anti-inflammatory agents in some patients may reduce the diuretic, natriuretic and antihypertensive effects of thiazide diuretics). Products include:
- Arthrotec Tablets 3195
- Voltaren Ophthalmic Sterile Ophthalmic Solution .... ⊙312
- Voltaren Tablets 2315
- Voltaren-XR Tablets 2315

Dicumarol (Thiazide diuretics may decrease the effects of oral anticoagulants).
No products indexed under this heading.

Digitoxin (Thiazide-induced hypokalemia may exaggerate or sensitize the response of heart to the toxic effect of digitalis).
No products indexed under this heading.

Digoxin (Thiazide-induced hypokalemia may exaggerate or sensitize the response of heart to the toxic effect of digitalis). Products include:
- Digitek Tablets 1003
- Lanoxicaps Capsules 1574
- Lanoxin Injection 1581
- Lanoxin Tablets 1587
- Lanoxin Elixir Pediatric 1578
- Lanoxin Injection Pediatric 1584

Diltiazem Hydrochloride (Antihypertensive effects may be potentiated when used concurrently with thiazide diuretics; dosage adjustment may be necessary). Products include:
- Cardizem Injectable 1018
- Cardizem Lyo-Ject Syringe 1018
- Cardizem Monovial 1018
- Cardizem CD Capsules 1016
- Tiazac Capsules 1378

Doxazosin Mesylate (Antihypertensive effects may be potentiated when used concurrently with thiazide diuretics; dosage adjustment may be necessary). Products include:
- Cardura Tablets 2668

Enalapril Maleate (Antihypertensive effects may be potentiated when used concurrently with thiazide diuretics; dosage adjustment may be necessary). Products include:
- Lexxel Tablets 608
- Vaseretic Tablets 2204
- Vasotec Tablets 2210

Enalaprilat (Antihypertensive effects may be potentiated when used concurrently with thiazide diuretics; dosage adjustment may be necessary). Products include:
- Enalaprilat Injection 863
- Vasotec I.V. Injection 2207

Enflurane (Effects may be potentiated when used concurrently with thiazide diuretics; dosage adjustment may be necessary).
No products indexed under this heading.

Eprosartan Mesylate (Antihypertensive effects may be potentiated when used concurrently with thiazide diuretics; dosage adjustment may be necessary). Products include:
- Teveten Tablets 3327

Esmolol Hydrochloride (Antihypertensive effects may be potentiated when used concurrently with thiazide diuretics; dosage adjustment may be necessary). Products include:
- Brevibloc Injection 858

Etodolac (Concurrent use of nonsteroidal anti-inflammatory agents in some patients may reduce the diuretic, natriuretic and antihypertensive effects of thiazide diuretics). Products include:
- Lodine 3528
- Lodine XL Extended-Release Tablets 3530

Felodipine (Antihypertensive effects may be potentiated when used concurrently with thiazide diuretics; dosage adjustment may be necessary). Products include:
- Lexxel Tablets 608
- Plendil Extended-Release Tablets 623

Fenoprofen Calcium (Concurrent use of nonsteroidal anti-inflammatory agents in some patients may reduce the diuretic, natriuretic and antihypertensive effects of thiazide diuretics).
No products indexed under this heading.

Fentanyl (Thiazide-induced orthostatic hypotension may be potentiated). Products include:
- Duragesic Transdermal System 1786

Fentanyl Citrate (Thiazide-induced orthostatic hypotension may be potentiated). Products include:
- Actiq 1184

Fludrocortisone Acetate (Intensified electrolyte depletion, particularly hypokalemia). Products include:
- Florinef Acetate Tablets 2250

Flurbiprofen (Concurrent use of nonsteroidal anti-inflammatory agents in some patients may reduce the diuretic, natriuretic and antihypertensive effects of thiazide diuretics).
No products indexed under this heading.

Fosinopril Sodium (Antihypertensive effects may be potentiated when used concurrently with thiazide diuretics; dosage adjustment may be necessary). Products include:
- Monopril Tablets 1091
- Monopril HCT 1094

Furosemide (Antihypertensive effects may be potentiated when used concurrently with thiazide diuretics; dosage adjustment may be necessary). Products include:
- Furosemide Tablets 2284

Glimepiride (Hyperglycemia may occur with thiazide diuretics; dosage adjustment of the oral antidiabetic drug may be required). Products include:
- Amaryl Tablets 717

Glipizide (Hyperglycemia may occur with thiazide diuretics; dosage adjustment of the oral antidiabetic drug may be required). Products include:
- Glucotrol Tablets 2692
- Glucotrol XL Extended Release Tablets 2693

Glyburide (Hyperglycemia may occur with thiazide diuretics; dosage adjustment of the oral antidiabetic drug may be required). Products include:
- DiaBeta Tablets 741
- Glucovance Tablets 1086

Guanabenz Acetate (Antihypertensive effects may be potentiated when used concurrently with thiazide diuretics; dosage adjustment may be necessary).
No products indexed under this heading.

Guanethidine Monosulfate (Antihypertensive effects may be potentiated when used concurrently with thiazide diuretics; dosage adjustment may be necessary).
No products indexed under this heading.

Hydralazine Hydrochloride (Antihypertensive effects may be potentiated when used concurrently with thiazide diuretics; dosage adjustment may be necessary).
No products indexed under this heading.

Hydrochlorothiazide (Antihypertensive effects may be potentiated when used concurrently with thiazide diuretics; dosage adjustment may be necessary). Products include:
- Accuretic Tablets 2614
- Aldoril Tablets 2039
- Atacand HCT Tablets 597
- Avalide Tablets 1070
- Diovan HCT Tablets 2338
- Dyazide Capsules 1515
- HydroDIURIL Tablets 2108
- Hyzaar 2109
- Inderide Tablets 3517
- Inderide LA Long-Acting Capsules 3519
- Lotensin HCT Tablets 2367
- Maxzide 1008
- Micardis HCT Tablets 1051
- Microzide Capsules 3414
- Moduretic Tablets 2138
- Monopril HCT 1094
- Prinzide Tablets 2168
- Timolide Tablets 2187
- Uniretic Tablets 3178
- Vaseretic Tablets 2204
- Zestoretic Tablets 695
- Ziac Tablets 1887

Hydrocodone Bitartrate (Thiazide-induced orthostatic hypotension may be potentiated). Products include:
- Hycodan 1316
- Hycomine Compound Tablets 1317
- Hycotuss Expectorant Syrup 1318
- Lortab 3319
- Lortab Elixir 3317
- Maxidone Tablets CIII 3399
- Norco 5/325 Tablets CIII 3424
- Norco 7.5/325 Tablets CIII 3425
- Norco 10/325 Tablets CIII 3427
- Norco 10/325 Tablets CIII 3425
- Vicodin Tablets 516
- Vicodin ES Tablets 517
- Vicodin HP Tablets 518
- Vicodin Tuss Expectorant 519
- Vicoprofen Tablets 520
- Zydone Tablets 1330

Hydrocodone Polistirex (Thiazide-induced orthostatic hypotension may be potentiated). Products include:
- Tussionex Pennkinetic Extended-Release Suspension 1174

Hydrocortisone (Intensified electrolyte depletion, particularly hypokalemia). Products include:
- AnusoI-H IC Cream 2.5% 2237
- Cipro HC Otic Suspension 540
- Cortaid Intensive Therapy Cream .... ■717
- Cortaid Maximum Strength Cream .... ■717
- Cortisporin Ophthalmic Suspension Sterile .... ⊙297
- Cortizone•5 .... ■699
- Cortizone•10 .... ■699
- Cortizone•10 Plus Creme .... ■700
- Cortizone for Kids Creme .... ■699
- Hydrocortone Tablets 2106
- Massengill Medicated Soft Cloth Towelette .... ■753
- VōSoL HC Otic Solution 3356

Hydrocortisone Acetate (Intensified electrolyte depletion, particularly hypokalemia). Products include:
- Analpram-HC 1338
- Anusol HC-1 Hydrocortisone Anti-Itch Cream .... ■689
- Anusol-HC Suppositories 2238
- Cortaid .... ■717
- Cortifoam Rectal Foam 3170
- Cortisporin-TC Otic Suspension 2246
- Hydrocortone Acetate Injectable Suspension 2103
- Pramosone 1343
- Proctocort Suppositories 2264

ProctoFoam-HC 3177
Terra-Cortril Ophthalmic Suspension 2716

Hydrocortisone Sodium Phosphate (Intensified electrolyte depletion, particularly hypokalemia). Products include:
Hydrocortone Phosphate Injection, Sterile 2105

Hydrocortisone Sodium Succinate (Intensified electrolyte depletion, particularly hypokalemia).
No products indexed under this heading.

Hydromorphone Hydrochloride (Thiazide-induced orthostatic hypotension may be potentiated). Products include:
Dilaudid 441
Dilaudid Oral Liquid 445
Dilaudid Powder 441
Dilaudid Rectal Suppositories 441
Dilaudid Tablets 441
Dilaudid Tablets - 8 mg 445
Dilaudid-HP 443

Ibuprofen (Concurrent use of nonsteroidal anti-inflammatory agents in some patients may reduce the diuretic, natriuretic and antihypertensive effects of thiazide diuretics). Products include:
Advil 771
Children's Advil Oral Suspension 773
Children's Advil Chewable Tablets 773
Advil Cold and Sinus Caplets 771
Advil Cold and Sinus Tablets 771
Advil Flu & Body Ache Caplets 772
Infants' Advil Drops 773
Junior Strength Advil Tablets 773
Junior Strength Advil Chewable Tablets 773
Advil Migraine Liquigels 772
Children's Motrin Oral Suspension and Chewable Tablets 2006
Children's Motrin Cold Oral Suspension 2007
Children's Motrin Oral Suspension 643
Motrin Suspension, Oral Drops, Chewable Tablets, and Caplets 2002
Infants' Motrin Concentrated Drops 2006
Junior Strength Motrin Caplets and Chewable Tablets 2006
Motrin IB Tablets, Caplets, and Gelcaps 2002
Motrin Migraine Pain Caplets 2005
Motrin Sinus Headache Caplets 2005
Vicoprofen Tablets 520

Indapamide (Antihypertensive effects may be potentiated when used concurrently with thiazide diuretics; dosage adjustment may be necessary). Products include:
Indapamide Tablets 2286

Indomethacin (Concurrent use of nonsteroidal anti-inflammatory agents in some patients may reduce the diuretic, natriuretic and antihypertensive effects of thiazide diuretics). Products include:
Indocin 2112

Indomethacin Sodium Trihydrate (Concurrent use of nonsteroidal anti-inflammatory agents in some patients may reduce the diuretic, natriuretic and antihypertensive effects of thiazide diuretics). Products include:
Indocin I.V. 2115

Insulin, Human, Zinc Suspension (Hyperglycemia may occur with thiazide diuretics; dosage adjustment of insulin may be required). Products include:
Humulin L, 100 Units 1937
Humulin U, 100 Units 1943
Novolin L Human Insulin 10 ml Vials 2422

Insulin, Human NPH (Hyperglycemia may occur with thiazide diuretics; dosage adjustment of insulin may be required). Products include:
Humulin N, 100 Units 1939
Humulin N NPH Pen 1940
Novolin N Human Insulin 10 ml Vials 2422
Novolin N PenFill 2423
Novolin N Prefilled Syringe Disposable Insulin Delivery System 2425

Insulin, Human Regular (Hyperglycemia may occur with thiazide diuretics; dosage adjustment of insulin may be required). Products include:
Humulin R Regular (U-500) 1943
Humulin R, 100 Units 1941
Novolin R Human Insulin 10 ml Vials 2423
Novolin R PenFill 2423
Novolin R Prefilled Syringe Disposable Insulin Delivery System 2425
Velosulin BR Human Insulin 10 ml Vials 2435

Insulin, Human Regular and Human NPH Mixture (Hyperglycemia may occur with thiazide diuretics; dosage adjustment of insulin may be required). Products include:
Humulin 50/50, 100 Units 1934
Humulin 70/30, 100 Units 1935
Humulin 70/30 Pen 1936
Novolin 70/30 Human Insulin 10 ml Vials 2421
Novolin 70/30 PenFill 2423
Novolin 70/30 Prefilled Disposable Insulin Delivery System 2425

Insulin, NPH (Hyperglycemia may occur with thiazide diuretics; dosage adjustment of insulin may be required). Products include:
Iletin II, NPH (Pork), 100 Units 1946

Insulin, Regular (Hyperglycemia may occur with thiazide diuretics; dosage adjustment of insulin may be required). Products include:
Iletin II, Regular (Pork), 100 Units 1947

Insulin, Zinc Crystals (Hyperglycemia may occur with thiazide diuretics; dosage adjustment of insulin may be required).
No products indexed under this heading.

Insulin, Zinc Suspension (Hyperglycemia may occur with thiazide diuretics; dosage adjustment of insulin may be required). Products include:
Iletin II, Lente (Pork), 100 Units 1945

Insulin Aspart, Human Regular (Hyperglycemia may occur with thiazide diuretics; dosage adjustment of insulin may be required).
No products indexed under this heading.

Insulin glargine (Hyperglycemia may occur with thiazide diuretics; dosage adjustment of insulin may be required). Products include:
Lantus Injection 742

Insulin Lispro, Human (Hyperglycemia may occur with thiazide diuretics; dosage adjustment of insulin may be required). Products include:
Humalog 1926
Humalog Mix 75/25 Pen 1928

Insulin Lispro Protamine, Human (Hyperglycemia may occur with thiazide diuretics; dosage adjustment of insulin may be required). Products include:
Humalog Mix 75/25 Pen 1928

Irbesartan (Antihypertensive effects may be potentiated when used concurrently with thiazide diuretics; dosage adjustment may be necessary). Products include:
Avalide Tablets 1070
Avapro Tablets 1074
Avapro Tablets 3076

Isoflurane (Effects may be potentiated when used concurrently with thiazide diuretics; dosage adjustment may be necessary).
No products indexed under this heading.

Isradipine (Antihypertensive effects may be potentiated when used concurrently with thiazide diuretics; dosage adjustment may be necessary). Products include:
DynaCirc Capsules 2921
DynaCirc CR Tablets 2923

Ketamine Hydrochloride (Effects may be potentiated when used concurrently with thiazide diuretics; dosage adjustment may be necessary).
No products indexed under this heading.

Ketoprofen (Concurrent use of nonsteroidal anti-inflammatory agents in some patients may reduce the diuretic, natriuretic and antihypertensive effects of thiazide diuretics). Products include:
Orudis Capsules 3548
Orudis KT Tablets 778
Oruvail Capsules 3548

Ketorolac Tromethamine (Concurrent use of nonsteroidal anti-inflammatory agents in some patients may reduce the diuretic, natriuretic and antihypertensive effects of thiazide diuretics). Products include:
Acular Ophthalmic Solution 544
Acular PF Ophthalmic Solution 544
Toradol 3018

Labetalol Hydrochloride (Antihypertensive effects may be potentiated when used concurrently with thiazide diuretics; dosage adjustment may be necessary). Products include:
Normodyne Injection 3135
Normodyne Tablets 3137

Levorphanol Tartrate (Thiazide-induced orthostatic hypotension may be potentiated). Products include:
Levo-Dromoran 1734
Levorphanol Tartrate Tablets 3059

Lisinopril (Antihypertensive effects may be potentiated when used concurrently with thiazide diuretics; dosage adjustment may be necessary). Products include:
Prinivil Tablets 2164
Prinzide Tablets 2168
Zestoretic Tablets 695
Zestril Tablets 698

Lithium Carbonate (Diuretics reduce the renal clearance of lithium and add a high risk of lithium toxicity). Products include:
Eskalith 1527
Lithium Carbonate 3061
Lithobid Slow-Release Tablets 3255

Lithium Citrate (Diuretics reduce the renal clearance of lithium and add a high risk of lithium toxicity). Products include:
Lithium Citrate Syrup 3061

Losartan Potassium (Antihypertensive effects may be potentiated when used concurrently with thiazide diuretics; dosage adjustment may be necessary). Products include:
Cozaar Tablets 2067
Hyzaar 2109

Mecamylamine Hydrochloride (Antihypertensive effects may be potentiated when used concurrently with thiazide diuretics; dosage adjustment may be necessary). Products include:
Inversine Tablets 1850

Meclofenamate Sodium (Concurrent use of nonsteroidal anti-inflammatory agents in some patients may reduce the diuretic, natriuretic and antihypertensive effects of thiazide diuretics).
No products indexed under this heading.

Mefenamic Acid (Concurrent use of nonsteroidal anti-inflammatory agents in some patients may reduce the diuretic, natriuretic and antihypertensive effects of thiazide diuretics). Products include:
Ponstel Capsules 1356

Meloxicam (Concurrent use of nonsteroidal anti-inflammatory agents in some patients may reduce the diuretic, natriuretic and antihypertensive effects of thiazide diuretics). Products include:
Mobic Tablets 1054

Meperidine Hydrochloride (Thiazide-induced orthostatic hypotension may be potentiated). Products include:
Demerol 3079
Mepergan Injection 3539

Mephobarbital (Thiazide-induced orthostatic hypotension may be potentiated).
No products indexed under this heading.

Metformin Hydrochloride (Hyperglycemia may occur with thiazide diuretics; dosage adjustment of the oral antidiabetic drug may be required). Products include:
Glucophage Tablets 1080
Glucophage XR Tablets 1080
Glucovance Tablets 1086

Methadone Hydrochloride (Thiazide-induced orthostatic hypotension may be potentiated). Products include:
Dolophine Hydrochloride Tablets 3056

Methenamine (Effectiveness of methenamine may be decreased when used concurrently with thiazide diuretics because of alkalinization of the urine). Products include:
Prosed/DS Tablets 3268
Urimax Tablets 1769
Urised Tablets 2876

Methenamine Hippurate (Effectiveness of methenamine may be decreased when used concurrently with thiazide diuretics because of alkalinization of the urine).
No products indexed under this heading.

Methenamine Mandelate (Effectiveness of methenamine may be decreased when used concurrently with thiazide diuretics because of alkalinization of the urine). Products include:
Uroqid-Acid No. 2 Tablets 947

Methohexital Sodium (Effects may be potentiated when used concurrently with thiazide diuretics; dosage adjustment may be necessary). Products include:
Brevital Sodium for Injection, USP 1815

Methoxyflurane (Effects may be potentiated when used concurrently with thiazide diuretics; dosage adjustment may be necessary).
No products indexed under this heading.

Methyclothiazide (Antihypertensive effects may be potentiated when used concurrently with thiazide diuretics; dosage adjustment may be necessary).
No products indexed under this heading.

Methyldopa (Antihypertensive effects may be potentiated when used concurrently with thiazide diuretics; dosage adjustment may be necessary). Products include:
Aldoclor Tablets 2035
Aldomet Tablets 2037
Aldoril Tablets 2039

Methyldopate Hydrochloride (Antihypertensive effects may be potentiated when used concurrently with thiazide diuretics; dosage adjustment may be necessary).
No products indexed under this heading.

Methylprednisolone Acetate (Intensified electrolyte depletion, particularly hypokalemia). Products include:
Depo-Medrol Injectable Suspension 2795

Methylprednisolone Sodium Succinate (Intensified electrolyte depletion, particularly hypokalemia). Products include:
Solu-Medrol Sterile Powder 2855

Metolazone (Antihypertensive effects may be potentiated when

used concurrently with thiazide diuretics; dosage adjustment may be necessary). Products include:
Mykrox Tablets 1168
Zaroxolyn Tablets 1177

Metoprolol Succinate (Antihypertensive effects may be potentiated when used concurrently with thiazide diuretics; dosage adjustment may be necessary). Products include:
Toprol-XL Tablets 651

Metoprolol Tartrate (Antihypertensive effects may be potentiated when used concurrently with thiazide diuretics; dosage adjustment may be necessary).
No products indexed under this heading.

Metyrosine (Antihypertensive effects may be potentiated when used concurrently with thiazide diuretics; dosage adjustment may be necessary). Products include:
Demser Capsules 2085

Mibefradil Dihydrochloride (Antihypertensive effects may be potentiated when used concurrently with thiazide diuretics; dosage adjustment may be necessary).
No products indexed under this heading.

Miglitol (Hyperglycemia may occur with thiazide diuretics; dosage adjustment of the oral antidiabetic drug may be required). Products include:
Glyset Tablets 2821

Minoxidil (Antihypertensive effects may be potentiated when used concurrently with thiazide diuretics; dosage adjustment may be necessary). Products include:
Rogaine Extra Strength for Men Topical Solution .... ▣721
Rogaine for Women Topical Solution .... ▣721

Moexipril Hydrochloride (Antihypertensive effects may be potentiated when used concurrently with thiazide diuretics; dosage adjustment may be necessary). Products include:
Uniretic Tablets 3178
Univasc Tablets 3181

Morphine Sulfate (Thiazide-induced orthostatic hypotension may be potentiated). Products include:
Astramorph/PF Injection, USP (Preservative-Free) 594
Duramorph Injection 1312
Infumorph 200 and Infumorph 500 Sterile Solutions 1314
Kadian Capsules 1335
MS Contin Tablets 2896
MSIR 2898
Oramorph SR Tablets 3062
Roxanol 3066

Nabumetone (Concurrent use of nonsteroidal anti-inflammatory agents in some patients may reduce the diuretic, natriuretic and antihypertensive effects of thiazide diuretics). Products include:
Relafen Tablets 1617

Nadolol (Antihypertensive effects may be potentiated when used concurrently with thiazide diuretics; dosage adjustment may be necessary). Products include:
Corgard Tablets 2245
Corzide 40/5 Tablets 2247
Corzide 80/5 Tablets 2247
Nadolol Tablets 2288

Naproxen (Concurrent use of nonsteroidal anti-inflammatory agents in some patients may reduce the diuretic, natriuretic and antihypertensive effects of thiazide diuretics). Products include:
EC-Naprosyn Delayed-Release Tablets 2967
Naprosyn Suspension 2967
Naprosyn Tablets 2967

Naproxen Sodium (Concurrent use of nonsteroidal anti-inflammatory agents in some patients may reduce the diuretic, natriuretic and antihypertensive effects of thiazide diuretics). Products include:
Aleve Tablets, Caplets and Gelcaps .... ▣602
Aleve Cold & Sinus Caplets .... ▣603
Anaprox Tablets 2967
Anaprox DS Tablets 2967
Naprelan Tablets 1293

Nicardipine Hydrochloride (Antihypertensive effects may be potentiated when used concurrently with thiazide diuretics; dosage adjustment may be necessary). Products include:
Cardene I.V. 3485

Nifedipine (Antihypertensive effects may be potentiated when used concurrently with thiazide diuretics; dosage adjustment may be necessary). Products include:
Adalat CC Tablets 877
Procardia Capsules 2708
Procardia XL Extended Release Tablets 2710

Nisoldipine (Antihypertensive effects may be potentiated when used concurrently with thiazide diuretics; dosage adjustment may be necessary). Products include:
Sular Tablets 688

Nitroglycerin (Antihypertensive effects may be potentiated when used concurrently with thiazide diuretics; dosage adjustment may be necessary). Products include:
Nitro-Dur Transdermal Infusion System 3134
Nitro-Dur Transdermal Infusion System 1834
Nitrolingual Pumpspray 1355
Nitrostat Tablets 2658

Norepinephrine Bitartrate (Thiazides may decrease the arterial responsiveness to norepinephrine).
No products indexed under this heading.

Oxaprozin (Concurrent use of nonsteroidal anti-inflammatory agents in some patients may reduce the diuretic, natriuretic and antihypertensive effects of thiazide diuretics).
No products indexed under this heading.

Oxycodone Hydrochloride (Thiazide-induced orthostatic hypotension may be potentiated). Products include:
OxyContin Tablets 2912
OxyFast Oral Concentrate Solution .. 2916
OxyIR Capsules 2916
Percocet Tablets 1326
Percodan Tablets 1327
Percolone Tablets 1327
Roxicodone 3067
Tylox Capsules 2597

Penbutolol Sulfate (Antihypertensive effects may be potentiated when used concurrently with thiazide diuretics; dosage adjustment may be necessary).
No products indexed under this heading.

Pentobarbital Sodium (Thiazide-induced orthostatic hypotension may be potentiated). Products include:
Nembutal Sodium Solution 485

Perindopril Erbumine (Antihypertensive effects may be potentiated when used concurrently with thiazide diuretics; dosage adjustment may be necessary). Products include:
Aceon Tablets (2 mg, 4 mg, 8 mg) 3249

Phenobarbital (Thiazide-induced orthostatic hypotension may be potentiated). Products include:
Arco-Lase Plus Tablets 592
Donnatal 2929
Donnatal Extentabs 2930

Phenoxybenzamine Hydrochloride (Antihypertensive effects may be potentiated when used concurrently with thiazide diuretics; dosage adjustment may be necessary). Products include:
Dibenzyline Capsules 3457

Phentolamine Mesylate (Antihypertensive effects may be potentiated when used concurrently with thiazide diuretics; dosage adjustment may be necessary).
No products indexed under this heading.

Phenylbutazone (Concurrent use of nonsteroidal anti-inflammatory agents in some patients may reduce the diuretic, natriuretic and antihypertensive effects of thiazide diuretics).
No products indexed under this heading.

Pindolol (Antihypertensive effects may be potentiated when used concurrently with thiazide diuretics; dosage adjustment may be necessary).
No products indexed under this heading.

Pioglitazone Hydrochloride (Hyperglycemia may occur with thiazide diuretics; dosage adjustment of the oral antidiabetic drug may be required). Products include:
Actos Tablets 3275

Piroxicam (Concurrent use of nonsteroidal anti-inflammatory agents in some patients may reduce the diuretic, natriuretic and antihypertensive effects of thiazide diuretics). Products include:
Feldene Capsules 2685

Polythiazide (Antihypertensive effects may be potentiated when used concurrently with thiazide diuretics; dosage adjustment may be necessary). Products include:
Minizide Capsules 2700
Renese Tablets 2712

Prazosin Hydrochloride (Antihypertensive effects may be potentiated when used concurrently with thiazide diuretics; dosage adjustment may be necessary). Products include:
Minipress Capsules 2699
Minizide Capsules 2700

Prednisolone Acetate (Intensified electrolyte depletion, particularly hypokalemia). Products include:
Blephamide Ophthalmic Ointment .. 547
Blephamide Ophthalmic Suspension 548
Poly-Pred Liquifilm Ophthalmic Suspension .... ⊙245
Pred Forte Ophthalmic Suspension .... ⊙246
Pred Mild Sterile Ophthalmic Suspension .... ⊙249
Pred-G Ophthalmic Suspension ..... ⊙247
Pred-G Sterile Ophthalmic Ointment .... ⊙248

Prednisolone Sodium Phosphate (Intensified electrolyte depletion, particularly hypokalemia). Products include:
Pediapred Oral Solution 1170

Prednisolone Tebutate (Intensified electrolyte depletion, particularly hypokalemia).
No products indexed under this heading.

Prednisone (Intensified electrolyte depletion, particularly hypokalemia). Products include:
Prednisone 3064

Probenecid (Thiazide diuretics may raise the levels of blood uric acid; dosage adjustment of antigout medication may be necessary to control gout and hyperuricemia).
No products indexed under this heading.

Propofol (Effects may be potentiated when used concurrently with thiazide diuretics; dosage adjustment may be necessary). Products include:
Diprivan Injectable Emulsion 667

Propoxyphene Hydrochloride (Thiazide-induced orthostatic hypotension may be potentiated). Products include:
Darvon Pulvules 1909
Darvon Compound-65 Pulvules 1910

Propoxyphene Napsylate (Thiazide-induced orthostatic hypotension may be potentiated). Products include:
Darvon-N/Darvocet-N 1907
Darvon-N Tablets 1912

Propranolol Hydrochloride (Antihypertensive effects may be potentiated when used concurrently with thiazide diuretics; dosage adjustment may be necessary). Products include:
Inderal 3513
Inderal LA Long-Acting Capsules 3516
Inderide Tablets 3517
Inderide LA Long-Acting Capsules .. 3519

Quinapril Hydrochloride (Antihypertensive effects may be potentiated when used concurrently with thiazide diuretics; dosage adjustment may be necessary). Products include:
Accupril Tablets 2611
Accuretic Tablets 2614

Ramipril (Antihypertensive effects may be potentiated when used concurrently with thiazide diuretics; dosage adjustment may be necessary). Products include:
Altace Capsules 2233

Rauwolfia serpentina (Antihypertensive effects may be potentiated when used concurrently with thiazide diuretics; dosage adjustment may be necessary).
No products indexed under this heading.

Remifentanil Hydrochloride (Thiazide-induced orthostatic hypotension may be potentiated).
No products indexed under this heading.

Repaglinide (Hyperglycemia may occur with thiazide diuretics; dosage adjustment of the oral antidiabetic drug may be required). Products include:
Prandin Tablets (0.5, 1, and 2 mg) 2432

Rescinnamine (Antihypertensive effects may be potentiated when used concurrently with thiazide diuretics; dosage adjustment may be necessary).
No products indexed under this heading.

Reserpine (Antihypertensive effects may be potentiated when used concurrently with thiazide diuretics; dosage adjustment may be necessary).
No products indexed under this heading.

Rofecoxib (Concurrent use of nonsteroidal anti-inflammatory agents in some patients may reduce the diuretic, natriuretic and antihypertensive effects of thiazide diuretics). Products include:
Vioxx 2213

Rosiglitazone Maleate (Hyperglycemia may occur with thiazide diuretics; dosage adjustment of the oral antidiabetic drug may be required). Products include:
Avandia Tablets 1490

Secobarbital Sodium (Thiazide-induced orthostatic hypotension may be potentiated).
No products indexed under this heading.

Sevoflurane (Effects may be potentiated when used concurrently with thiazide diuretics; dosage adjustment may be necessary).
No products indexed under this heading.

Sodium Nitroprusside (Antihypertensive effects may be potentiated when used concurrently with thiazide diuretics; dosage adjustment may be necessary).
No products indexed under this heading.

Sotalol Hydrochloride (Antihypertensive effects may be potentiated when used concurrently with thiazide diuretics; dosage adjustment may be necessary). Products include:
Betapace Tablets ... 950
Betapace AF Tablets ... 954

Spirapril Hydrochloride (Antihypertensive effects may be potentiated when used concurrently with thiazide diuretics; dosage adjustment may be necessary).
No products indexed under this heading.

Sufentanil Citrate (Thiazide-induced orthostatic hypotension may be potentiated).
No products indexed under this heading.

Sulfinpyrazone (Thiazide diuretics may raise the levels of blood uric acid; dosage adjustment of antigout medication may be necessary to control gout and hyperuricemia).
No products indexed under this heading.

Sulindac (Concurrent use of nonsteroidal anti-inflammatory agents in some patients may reduce the diuretic, natriuretic and antihypertensive effects of thiazide diuretics). Products include:
Clinoril Tablets ... 2053

Telmisartan (Antihypertensive effects may be potentiated when used concurrently with thiazide diuretics; dosage adjustment may be necessary). Products include:
Micardis Tablets ... 1049
Micardis HCT Tablets ... 1051

Terazosin Hydrochloride (Antihypertensive effects may be potentiated when used concurrently with thiazide diuretics; dosage adjustment may be necessary). Products include:
Hytrin Capsules ... 464

Thiamylal Sodium (Thiazide-induced orthostatic hypotension may be potentiated).
No products indexed under this heading.

Timolol Maleate (Antihypertensive effects may be potentiated when used concurrently with thiazide diuretics; dosage adjustment may be necessary). Products include:
Blocadren Tablets ... 2046
Cosopt Sterile Ophthalmic Solution ... 2065
Timolide Tablets ... 2187
Timolol GFS ... ⊙266
Timoptic in Ocudose ... 2192
Timoptic Sterile Ophthalmic Solution ... 2190
Timoptic-XE Sterile Ophthalmic Gel Forming Solution ... 2194

Tolazamide (Hyperglycemia may occur with thiazide diuretics; dosage adjustment of the oral antidiabetic drug may be required).
No products indexed under this heading.

Tolbutamide (Hyperglycemia may occur with thiazide diuretics; dosage adjustment of the oral antidiabetic drug may be required).
No products indexed under this heading.

Tolmetin Sodium (Concurrent use of nonsteroidal anti-inflammatory agents in some patients may reduce the diuretic, natriuretic and antihypertensive effects of thiazide diuretics). Products include:
Tolectin ... 2589

Torsemide (Antihypertensive effects may be potentiated when used concurrently with thiazide diuretics; dosage adjustment may be necessary). Products include:
Demadex Tablets and Injection ... 2965

Trandolapril (Antihypertensive effects may be potentiated when used concurrently with thiazide diuretics; dosage adjustment may be necessary). Products include:
Mavik Tablets ... 478
Tarka Tablets ... 508

Triamcinolone (Intensified electrolyte depletion, particularly hypokalemia).
No products indexed under this heading.

Triamcinolone Acetonide (Intensified electrolyte depletion, particularly hypokalemia). Products include:
Azmacort Inhalation Aerosol ... 728
Nasacort Nasal Inhaler ... 750
Nasacort AQ Nasal Spray ... 752
Tri-Nasal Spray ... 2274

Triamcinolone Diacetate (Intensified electrolyte depletion, particularly hypokalemia).
No products indexed under this heading.

Triamcinolone Hexacetonide (Intensified electrolyte depletion, particularly hypokalemia).
No products indexed under this heading.

Trimethaphan Camsylate (Antihypertensive effects may be potentiated when used concurrently with thiazide diuretics; dosage adjustment may be necessary).
No products indexed under this heading.

Troglitazone (Hyperglycemia may occur with thiazide diuretics; dosage adjustment of the oral antidiabetic drug may be required).
No products indexed under this heading.

Tubocurarine Chloride (Thiazides may increase the responsiveness to tubocurarine).
No products indexed under this heading.

Valsartan (Antihypertensive effects may be potentiated when used concurrently with thiazide diuretics; dosage adjustment may be necessary). Products include:
Diovan Capsules ... 2337
Diovan HCT Tablets ... 2338

Verapamil Hydrochloride (Antihypertensive effects may be potentiated when used concurrently with thiazide diuretics; dosage adjustment may be necessary). Products include:
Covera-HS Tablets ... 3199
Isoptin SR Tablets ... 467
Tarka Tablets ... 508
Verelan Capsules ... 3184
Verelan PM Capsules ... 3186

Warfarin Sodium (Thiazide diuretics may decrease the effects of oral anticoagulants). Products include:
Coumadin for Injection ... 1243
Coumadin Tablets ... 1243
Warfarin Sodium Tablets, USP ... 3302

Food Interactions

Alcohol (Thiazide-induced orthostatic hypotension may be potentiated).

DIURIL ORAL SUSPENSION

(Chlorothiazide) ... 2087

May interact with antihypertensives, barbiturates, bile acid sequestering agents, corticosteroids, cardiac glycosides, oral hypoglycemic agents, insulin, lithium preparations, narcotic analgesics, nondepolarizing neuromuscular blocking agents, non-steroidal anti-inflammatory agents, and certain other agents. Compounds in these categories include:

Acarbose (Thiazide-induced hyperglycemia may require dosage adjustment of hypoglycemic agents). Products include:
Precose Tablets ... 906

Acebutolol Hydrochloride (Concurrent use with other antihypertensive agents may result in additive effect or potentiation). Products include:
Sectral Capsules ... 3589

ACTH (Intensified electrolyte depletion particularly hypokalemia).
No products indexed under this heading.

Alfentanil Hydrochloride (Potentiation of orthostatic hypotension may occur).
No products indexed under this heading.

Amlodipine Besylate (Concurrent use with other antihypertensive agents may result in additive effect or potentiation). Products include:
Lotrel Capsules ... 2370
Norvasc Tablets ... 2704

Aprobarbital (Potentiation of orthostatic hypotension may occur).
No products indexed under this heading.

Atenolol (Concurrent use with other antihypertensive agents may result in additive effect or potentiation). Products include:
Tenoretic Tablets ... 690
Tenormin I.V. Injection ... 692

Atracurium Besylate (Possible increased responsiveness to the muscle relaxants).
No products indexed under this heading.

Benazepril Hydrochloride (Concurrent use with other antihypertensive agents may result in additive effect or potentiation). Products include:
Lotensin Tablets ... 2365
Lotensin HCT Tablets ... 2367
Lotrel Capsules ... 2370

Bendroflumethiazide (Concurrent use with other antihypertensive agents may result in additive effect or potentiation). Products include:
Corzide 40/5 Tablets ... 2247
Corzide 80/5 Tablets ... 2247

Betamethasone Acetate (Intensified electrolyte depletion particularly hypokalemia). Products include:
Celestone Soluspan Injectable Suspension ... 3097

Betamethasone Sodium Phosphate (Intensified electrolyte depletion particularly hypokalemia). Products include:
Celestone Soluspan Injectable Suspension ... 3097

Betaxolol Hydrochloride (Concurrent use with other antihypertensive agents may result in additive effect or potentiation). Products include:
Betoptic S Ophthalmic Suspension ... 537

Bisoprolol Fumarate (Concurrent use with other antihypertensive agents may result in additive effect or potentiation). Products include:
Zebeta Tablets ... 1885
Ziac Tablets ... 1887

Buprenorphine Hydrochloride (Potentiation of orthostatic hypotension may occur). Products include:
Buprenex Injectable ... 2918

Butabarbital (Potentiation of orthostatic hypotension may occur).
No products indexed under this heading.

Butalbital (Potentiation of orthostatic hypotension may occur). Products include:
Phrenilin ... 578
Sedapap Tablets 50 mg/650 mg ... 2225

Candesartan Cilexetil (Concurrent use with other antihypertensive agents may result in additive effect or potentiation). Products include:
Atacand Tablets ... 595
Atacand HCT Tablets ... 597

Captopril (Concurrent use with other antihypertensive agents may result in additive effect or potentiation). Products include:
Captopril Tablets ... 2281

Carteolol Hydrochloride (Concurrent use with other antihypertensive agents may result in additive effect or potentiation). Products include:
Carteolol Hydrochloride Ophthalmic Solution USP, 1% ... ⊙258
Ocupress Ophthalmic Solution, 1% Sterile ... ⊙303

Celecoxib (Reduces diuretic, natriuretic, and antihypertensive effects). Products include:
Celebrex Capsules ... 2676
Celebrex Capsules ... 2780

Chlorothiazide Sodium (Concurrent use with other antihypertensive agents may result in additive effect or potentiation). Products include:
Diuril Sodium Intravenous ... 2086

Chlorpropamide (Thiazide-induced hyperglycemia may require dosage adjustment of hypoglycemic agents). Products include:
Diabinese Tablets ... 2680

Chlorthalidone (Concurrent use with other antihypertensive agents may result in additive effect or potentiation). Products include:
Clorpres Tablets ... 1002
Combipres Tablets ... 1040
Tenoretic Tablets ... 690

Cholestyramine (Resins have potential to bind thiazide diuretics and reduce their absorption from the gastrointestinal tract).
No products indexed under this heading.

Cisatracurium Besylate (Possible increased responsiveness to the muscle relaxants).
No products indexed under this heading.

Clonidine (Concurrent use with other antihypertensive agents may result in additive effect or potentiation). Products include:
Catapres-TTS ... 1038

Clonidine Hydrochloride (Concurrent use with other antihypertensive agents may result in additive effect or potentiation). Products include:
Catapres Tablets ... 1037
Clorpres Tablets ... 1002
Combipres Tablets ... 1040
Duraclon Injection ... 3057

Codeine Phosphate (Potentiation of orthostatic hypotension may occur). Products include:
Phenergan with Codeine Syrup ... 3557
Phenergan VC with Codeine Syrup ... 3561
Robitussin A-C Syrup ... 2942
Robitussin-DAC Syrup ... 2942
Ryna-C Liquid ... ⊡768
Soma Compound w/Codeine Tablets ... 3355
Tussi-Organidin NR Liquid ... 3350
Tussi-Organidin-S NR Liquid ... 3350
Tylenol with Codeine ... 2595

Colestipol Hydrochloride (Resins have potential to bind thiazide diuretics and reduce their absorption from the gastrointestinal tract). Products include:
Colestid Tablets ... 2791

Cortisone Acetate (Intensified electrolyte depletion particularly hypokalemia). Products include:
Cortone Acetate Injectable Suspension ... 2059
Cortone Acetate Tablets ... 2061

Deserpidine (Concurrent use with other antihypertensive agents may result in additive effect or potentiation).
No products indexed under this heading.

Deslanoside (Thiazide-induced hypokalemia may sensitize or exaggerate the response of the heart to the toxic effects of digitalis).
No products indexed under this heading.

Dexamethasone (Intensified electrolyte depletion particularly hypokalemia). Products include:
Decadron Elixir ... 2078

Decadron Tablets 2079
TobraDex Ophthalmic Ointment 542
TobraDex Ophthalmic Suspension .. 541

Dexamethasone Acetate (Intensified electrolyte depletion particularly hypokalemia).
No products indexed under this heading.

Dexamethasone Sodium Phosphate (Intensified electrolyte depletion particularly hypokalemia). Products include:
Decadron Phosphate Injection 2081
Decadron Phosphate Sterile Ophthalmic Ointment 2083
Decadron Phosphate Sterile Ophthalmic Solution 2084
NeoDecadron Sterile Ophthalmic Solution 2144

Dezocine (Potentiation of orthostatic hypotension may occur).
No products indexed under this heading.

Diazoxide (Concurrent use with other antihypertensive agents may result in additive effect or potentiation).
No products indexed under this heading.

Diclofenac Potassium (Reduces diuretic, natriuretic, and antihypertensive effects). Products include:
Cataflam Tablets 2315

Diclofenac Sodium (Reduces diuretic, natriuretic, and antihypertensive effects). Products include:
Arthrotec Tablets 3195
Voltaren Ophthalmic Sterile Ophthalmic Solution .... ⊙ 312
Voltaren Tablets 2315
Voltaren-XR Tablets 2315

Digitoxin (Thiazide-induced hypokalemia may sensitize or exaggerate the response of the heart to the toxic effects of digitalis).
No products indexed under this heading.

Digoxin (Thiazide-induced hypokalemia may sensitize or exaggerate the response of the heart to the toxic effects of digitalis). Products include:
Digitek Tablets 1003
Lanoxicaps Capsules 1574
Lanoxin Injection 1581
Lanoxin Tablets 1587
Lanoxin Elixir Pediatric 1578
Lanoxin Injection Pediatric 1584

Diltiazem Hydrochloride (Concurrent use with other antihypertensive agents may result in additive effect or potentiation). Products include:
Cardizem Injectable 1018
Cardizem Lyo-Ject Syringe 1018
Cardizem Monovial 1018
Cardizem CD Capsules 1016
Tiazac Capsules 1378

Doxazosin Mesylate (Concurrent use with other antihypertensive agents may result in additive effect or potentiation). Products include:
Cardura Tablets 2668

Enalapril Maleate (Concurrent use with other antihypertensive agents may result in additive effect or potentiation). Products include:
Lexxel Tablets 608
Vaseretic Tablets 2204
Vasotec Tablets 2210

Enalaprilat (Concurrent use with other antihypertensive agents may result in additive effect or potentiation). Products include:
Enalaprilat Injection 863
Vasotec I.V. Injection 2207

Eprosartan Mesylate (Concurrent use with other antihypertensive agents may result in additive effect or potentiation). Products include:
Teveten Tablets 3327

Esmolol Hydrochloride (Concurrent use with other antihypertensive agents may result in additive effect or potentiation). Products include:
Brevibloc Injection 858

Etodolac (Reduces diuretic, natriuretic, and antihypertensive effects). Products include:
Lodine 3528
Lodine XL Extended-Release Tablets 3530

Felodipine (Concurrent use with other antihypertensive agents may result in additive effect or potentiation). Products include:
Lexxel Tablets 608
Plendil Extended-Release Tablets ... 623

Fenoprofen Calcium (Reduces diuretic, natriuretic, and antihypertensive effects).
No products indexed under this heading.

Fentanyl (Potentiation of orthostatic hypotension may occur). Products include:
Duragesic Transdermal System 1786

Fentanyl Citrate (Potentiation of orthostatic hypotension may occur). Products include:
Actiq 1184

Fludrocortisone Acetate (Intensified electrolyte depletion particularly hypokalemia). Products include:
Florinef Acetate Tablets 2250

Flurbiprofen (Reduces diuretic, natriuretic, and antihypertensive effects).
No products indexed under this heading.

Fosinopril Sodium (Concurrent use with other antihypertensive agents may result in additive effect or potentiation). Products include:
Monopril Tablets 1091
Monopril HCT 1094

Furosemide (Concurrent use with other antihypertensive agents may result in additive effect or potentiation). Products include:
Furosemide Tablets 2284

Glimepiride (Thiazide-induced hyperglycemia may require dosage adjustment of hypoglycemic agents). Products include:
Amaryl Tablets 717

Glipizide (Thiazide-induced hyperglycemia may require dosage adjustment of hypoglycemic agents). Products include:
Glucotrol Tablets 2692
Glucotrol XL Extended Release Tablets 2693

Glyburide (Thiazide-induced hyperglycemia may require dosage adjustment of hypoglycemic agents). Products include:
DiaBeta Tablets 741
Glucovance Tablets 1086

Guanabenz Acetate (Concurrent use with other antihypertensive agents may result in additive effect or potentiation).
No products indexed under this heading.

Guanethidine Monosulfate (Concurrent use with other antihypertensive agents may result in additive effect or potentiation).
No products indexed under this heading.

Hydralazine Hydrochloride (Concurrent use with other antihypertensive agents may result in additive effect or potentiation).
No products indexed under this heading.

Hydrochlorothiazide (Concurrent use with other antihypertensive agents may result in additive effect or potentiation). Products include:
Accuretic Tablets 2614
Aldoril Tablets 2039
Atacand HCT Tablets 597
Avalide Tablets 1070
Diovan HCT Tablets 2338
Dyazide Capsules 1515
HydroDIURIL Tablets 2108
Hyzaar 2109
Inderide Tablets 3517
Inderide LA Long-Acting Capsules .. 3519
Lotensin HCT Tablets 2367
Maxzide 1008
Micardis HCT Tablets 1051
Microzide Capsules 3414
Moduretic Tablets 2138
Monopril HCT 1094
Prinzide Tablets 2168
Timolide Tablets 2187
Uniretic Tablets 3178
Vaseretic Tablets 2204
Zestoretic Tablets 695
Ziac Tablets 1887

Hydrocodone Bitartrate (Potentiation of orthostatic hypotension may occur). Products include:
Hycodan 1316
Hycomine Compound Tablets 1317
Hycotuss Expectorant Syrup 1318
Lortab 3319
Lortab Elixir 3317
Maxidone Tablets CIII 3399
Norco 5/325 Tablets CIII 3424
Norco 7.5/325 Tablets CIII 3425
Norco 10/325 Tablets CIII 3427
Norco 10/325 Tablets CIII 3425
Vicodin Tablets 516
Vicodin ES Tablets 517
Vicodin HP Tablets 518
Vicodin Tuss Expectorant 519
Vicoprofen Tablets 520
Zydone Tablets 1330

Hydrocodone Polistirex (Potentiation of orthostatic hypotension may occur). Products include:
Tussionex Pennkinetic Extended-Release Suspension 1174

Hydrocortisone (Intensified electrolyte depletion particularly hypokalemia). Products include:
Anusol-HC Cream 2.5% 2237
Cipro HC Otic Suspension 540
Cortaid Intensive Therapy Cream . ▣ 717
Cortaid Maximum Strength Cream .... ▣ 717
Cortisporin Ophthalmic Suspension Sterile .... ⊙ 297
Cortizone•5 .... ▣ 699
Cortizone•10 .... ▣ 699
Cortizone•10 Plus Creme .... ▣ 700
Cortizone for Kids Creme .... ▣ 699
Hydrocortone Tablets 2106
Massengill Medicated Soft Cloth Towelette .... ▣ 753
VōSoL HC Otic Solution 3356

Hydrocortisone Acetate (Intensified electrolyte depletion particularly hypokalemia). Products include:
Analpram-HC 1338
Anusol HC-1 Hydrocortisone Anti-Itch Cream .... ▣ 689
Anusol-HC Suppositories 2238
Cortaid .... ▣ 717
Cortifoam Rectal Foam 3170
Cortisporin-TC Otic Suspension 2246
Hydrocortone Acetate Injectable Suspension 2103
Pramosone 1343
Proctocort Suppositories 2264
ProctoFoam-HC 3177
Terra-Cortril Ophthalmic Suspension 2716

Hydrocortisone Sodium Phosphate (Intensified electrolyte depletion particularly hypokalemia). Products include:
Hydrocortone Phosphate Injection, Sterile 2105

Hydrocortisone Sodium Succinate (Intensified electrolyte depletion particularly hypokalemia).
No products indexed under this heading.

Hydroflumethiazide (Concurrent use with other antihypertensive agents may result in additive effect or potentiation). Products include:
Diucardin Tablets 3494

Hydromorphone Hydrochloride (Potentiation of orthostatic hypotension may occur). Products include:
Dilaudid 441
Dilaudid Oral Liquid 445
Dilaudid Powder 441
Dilaudid Rectal Suppositories 441
Dilaudid Tablets 441
Dilaudid Tablets - 8 mg 445
Dilaudid-HP 443

Ibuprofen (Reduces diuretic, natriuretic, and antihypertensive effects). Products include:
Advil .... ▣ 771
Children's Advil Oral Suspension ... ▣ 773
Children's Advil Chewable Tablets . ▣ 773
Advil Cold and Sinus Caplets .... ▣ 771
Advil Cold and Sinus Tablets .... ▣ 771
Advil Flu & Body Ache Caplets .... ▣ 772
Infants' Advil Drops .... ▣ 773
Junior Strength Advil Tablets .... ▣ 773
Junior Strength Advil Chewable Tablets .... ▣ 773
Advil Migraine Liquigels .... ▣ 772
Children's Motrin Oral Suspension and Chewable Tablets 2006
Children's Motrin Cold Oral Suspension 2007
Children's Motrin Oral Suspension .... ▣ 643
Motrin Suspension, Oral Drops, Chewable Tablets, and Caplets 2002
Infants' Motrin Concentrated Drops 2006
Junior Strength Motrin Caplets and Chewable Tablets 2006
Motrin IB Tablets, Caplets, and Gelcaps 2002
Motrin Migraine Pain Caplets 2005
Motrin Sinus Headache Caplets 2005
Vicoprofen Tablets 520

Indapamide (Concurrent use with other antihypertensive agents may result in additive effect or potentiation). Products include:
Indapamide Tablets 2286

Indomethacin (Reduces diuretic, natriuretic, and antihypertensive effects). Products include:
Indocin 2112

Indomethacin Sodium Trihydrate (Reduces diuretic, natriuretic, and antihypertensive effects). Products include:
Indocin I.V. 2115

Insulin, Human, Zinc Suspension (Thiazide-induce hyperglycemia may require dosage adjustment of hypoglycemic agents). Products include:
Humulin L, 100 Units 1937
Humulin U, 100 Units 1943
Novolin L Human Insulin 10 ml Vials 2422

Insulin, Human NPH (Thiazide-induce hyperglycemia may require dosage adjustment of hypoglycemic agents). Products include:
Humulin N, 100 Units 1939
Humulin N NPH Pen 1940
Novolin N Human Insulin 10 ml Vials 2422
Novolin N PenFill 2423
Novolin N Prefilled Syringe Disposable Insulin Delivery System 2425

Insulin, Human Regular (Thiazide-induce hyperglycemia may require dosage adjustment of hypoglycemic agents). Products include:
Humulin R Regular (U-500) 1943
Humulin R, 100 Units 1941
Novolin R Human Insulin 10 ml Vials 2423
Novolin R PenFill 2423
Novolin R Prefilled Syringe Disposable Insulin Delivery System 2425
Velosulin BR Human Insulin 10 ml Vials 2435

Insulin, Human Regular and Human NPH Mixture (Thiazide-induce hyperglycemia may require dosage adjustment of hypoglycemic agents). Products include:
Humulin 50/50, 100 Units 1934
Humulin 70/30, 100 Units 1935
Humulin 70/30 Pen 1936
Novolin 70/30 Human Insulin 10 ml Vials 2421
Novolin 70/30 PenFill 2423
Novolin 70/30 Prefilled Disposable Insulin Delivery System 2425

Insulin, NPH (Thiazide-induce hyperglycemia may require dosage adjustment of hypoglycemic agents). Products include:
Iletin II, NPH (Pork), 100 Units 1946

Insulin, Regular (Thiazide-induce hyperglycemia may require dosage adjustment of hypoglycemic agents). Products include:
Iletin II, Regular (Pork), 100 Units ... 1947

Insulin, Zinc Crystals (Thiazide-induce hyperglycemia may require dosage adjustment of hypoglycemic agents).
No products indexed under this heading.

Insulin, Zinc Suspension (Thiazide-induce hyperglycemia may require dosage adjustment of hypoglycemic agents). Products include:
Iletin II, Lente (Pork), 100 Units 1945

Insulin Aspart, Human Regular (Thiazide-induce hyperglycemia may require dosage adjustment of hypoglycemic agents).
No products indexed under this heading.

Insulin glargine (Thiazide-induce hyperglycemia may require dosage adjustment of hypoglycemic agents). Products include:
Lantus Injection 742

Insulin Lispro, Human (Thiazide-induce hyperglycemia may require dosage adjustment of hypoglycemic agents). Products include:
Humalog 1926
Humalog Mix 75/25 Pen 1928

Insulin Lispro Protamine, Human (Thiazide-induce hyperglycemia may require dosage adjustment of hypoglycemic agents). Products include:
Humalog Mix 75/25 Pen 1928

Irbesartan (Concurrent use with other antihypertensive agents may result in additive effect or potentiation). Products include:
Avalide Tablets 1070
Avapro Tablets 1074
Avapro Tablets 3076

Isradipine (Concurrent use with other antihypertensive agents may result in additive effect or potentiation). Products include:
DynaCirc Capsules 2921
DynaCirc CR Tablets 2923

Ketoprofen (Reduces diuretic, natriuretic, and antihypertensive effects). Products include:
Orudis Capsules 3548
Orudis KT Tablets .... ■ 778
Oruvail Capsules 3548

Ketorolac Tromethamine (Reduces diuretic, natriuretic, and antihypertensive effects). Products include:
Acular Ophthalmic Solution 544
Acular PF Ophthalmic Solution 544
Toradol 3018

Labetalol Hydrochloride (Concurrent use with other antihypertensive agents may result in additive effect or potentiation). Products include:
Normodyne Injection 3135
Normodyne Tablets 3137

Levorphanol Tartrate (Potentiation of orthostatic hypotension may occur). Products include:
Levo-Dromoran 1734
Levorphanol Tartrate Tablets 3059

Lisinopril (Concurrent use with other antihypertensive agents may result in additive effect or potentiation). Products include:
Prinivil Tablets 2164
Prinzide Tablets 2168
Zestoretic Tablets 695
Zestril Tablets 698

Lithium Carbonate (Diuretics reduce the renal clearance of lithium and this may lead to lithium toxicity). Products include:
Eskalith 1527
Lithium Carbonate 3061
Lithobid Slow-Release Tablets 3255

Lithium Citrate (Diuretics reduce the renal clearance of lithium and this may lead to lithium toxicity). Products include:
Lithium Citrate Syrup 3061

Losartan Potassium (Concurrent use with other antihypertensive agents may result in additive effect or potentiation). Products include:
Cozaar Tablets 2067
Hyzaar 2109

Mecamylamine Hydrochloride (Concurrent use with other antihypertensive agents may result in additive effect or potentiation). Products include:
Inversine Tablets 1850

Meclofenamate Sodium (Reduces diuretic, natriuretic, and antihypertensive effects).
No products indexed under this heading.

Mefenamic Acid (Reduces diuretic, natriuretic, and antihypertensive effects). Products include:
Ponstel Capsules 1356

Meloxicam (Reduces diuretic, natriuretic, and antihypertensive effects). Products include:
Mobic Tablets 1054

Meperidine Hydrochloride (Potentiation of orthostatic hypotension may occur). Products include:
Demerol 3079
Mepergan Injection 3539

Mephobarbital (Potentiation of orthostatic hypotension may occur).
No products indexed under this heading.

Metformin Hydrochloride (Thiazide-induced hyperglycemia may require dosage adjustment of hypoglycemic agents). Products include:
Glucophage Tablets 1080
Glucophage XR Tablets 1080
Glucovance Tablets 1086

Methadone Hydrochloride (Potentiation of orthostatic hypotension may occur). Products include:
Dolophine Hydrochloride Tablets 3056

Methyclothiazide (Concurrent use with other antihypertensive agents may result in additive effect or potentiation).
No products indexed under this heading.

Methyldopa (Concurrent use with other antihypertensive agents may result in additive effect or potentiation). Products include:
Aldoclor Tablets 2035
Aldomet Tablets 2037
Aldoril Tablets 2039

Methyldopate Hydrochloride (Concurrent use with other antihypertensive agents may result in additive effect or potentiation).
No products indexed under this heading.

Methylprednisolone Acetate (Intensified electrolyte depletion particularly hypokalemia). Products include:
Depo-Medrol Injectable Suspension 2795

Methylprednisolone Sodium Succinate (Intensified electrolyte depletion particularly hypokalemia). Products include:
Solu-Medrol Sterile Powder 2855

Metipranolol Hydrochloride (Concurrent use with other antihypertensive agents may result in additive effect or potentiation).
No products indexed under this heading.

Metocurine Iodide (Possible increased responsiveness to the muscle relaxants).
No products indexed under this heading.

Metolazone (Concurrent use with other antihypertensive agents may result in additive effect or potentiation). Products include:
Mykrox Tablets 1168
Zaroxolyn Tablets 1177

Metoprolol Succinate (Concurrent use with other antihypertensive agents may result in additive effect or potentiation). Products include:
Toprol-XL Tablets 651

Metoprolol Tartrate (Concurrent use with other antihypertensive agents may result in additive effect or potentiation).
No products indexed under this heading.

Metyrosine (Concurrent use with other antihypertensive agents may result in additive effect or potentiation). Products include:
Demser Capsules 2085

Mibefradil Dihydrochloride (Concurrent use with other antihypertensive agents may result in additive effect or potentiation).
No products indexed under this heading.

Miglitol (Thiazide-induced hyperglycemia may require dosage adjustment of hypoglycemic agents). Products include:
Glyset Tablets 2821

Minoxidil (Concurrent use with other antihypertensive agents may result in additive effect or potentiation). Products include:
Rogaine Extra Strength for Men Topical Solution .... ■ 721
Rogaine for Women Topical Solution .... ■ 721

Mivacurium Chloride (Possible increased responsiveness to the muscle relaxants).
No products indexed under this heading.

Moexipril Hydrochloride (Concurrent use with other antihypertensive agents may result in additive effect or potentiation). Products include:
Uniretic Tablets 3178
Univasc Tablets 3181

Morphine Sulfate (Potentiation of orthostatic hypotension may occur). Products include:
Astramorph/PF Injection, USP (Preservative-Free) 594
Duramorph Injection 1312
Infumorph 200 and Infumorph 500 Sterile Solutions 1314
Kadian Capsules 1335
MS Contin Tablets 2896
MSIR 2898
Oramorph SR Tablets 3062
Roxanol 3066

Nabumetone (Reduces diuretic, natriuretic, and antihypertensive effects). Products include:
Relafen Tablets 1617

Nadolol (Concurrent use with other antihypertensive agents may result in additive effect or potentiation). Products include:
Corgard Tablets 2245
Corzide 40/5 Tablets 2247
Corzide 80/5 Tablets 2247
Nadolol Tablets 2288

Naproxen (Reduces diuretic, natriuretic, and antihypertensive effects). Products include:
EC-Naprosyn Delayed-Release Tablets 2967
Naprosyn Suspension 2967
Naprosyn Tablets 2967

Naproxen Sodium (Reduces diuretic, natriuretic, and antihypertensive effects). Products include:
Aleve Tablets, Caplets and Gelcaps .... ■ 602
Aleve Cold & Sinus Caplets .... ■ 603
Anaprox Tablets 2967
Anaprox DS Tablets 2967
Naprelan Tablets 1293

Nicardipine Hydrochloride (Concurrent use with other antihypertensive agents may result in additive effect or potentiation). Products include:
Cardene I.V. 3485

Nifedipine (Concurrent use with other antihypertensive agents may result in additive effect or potentiation). Products include:
Adalat CC Tablets 877
Procardia Capsules 2708
Procardia XL Extended Release Tablets 2710

Nisoldipine (Concurrent use with other antihypertensive agents may result in additive effect or potentiation). Products include:
Sular Tablets 688

Nitroglycerin (Concurrent use with other antihypertensive agents may result in additive effect or potentiation). Products include:
Nitro-Dur Transdermal Infusion System 3134
Nitro-Dur Transdermal Infusion System 1834
Nitrolingual Pumpspray 1355
Nitrostat Tablets 2658

Norepinephrine Hydrochloride (Decreased arterial responsiveness to pressor amine).
No products indexed under this heading.

Oxaprozin (Reduces diuretic, natriuretic, and antihypertensive effects).
No products indexed under this heading.

Oxycodone Hydrochloride (Potentiation of orthostatic hypotension may occur). Products include:
OxyContin Tablets 2912
OxyFast Oral Concentrate Solution . 2916
OxyIR Capsules 2916
Percocet Tablets 1326
Percodan Tablets 1327
Percolone Tablets 1327
Roxicodone 3067
Tylox Capsules 2597

Pancuronium Bromide (Possible increased responsiveness to the muscle relaxants).
No products indexed under this heading.

Penbutolol Sulfate (Concurrent use with other antihypertensive agents may result in additive effect or potentiation).
No products indexed under this heading.

Pentobarbital Sodium (Potentiation of orthostatic hypotension may occur). Products include:
Nembutal Sodium Solution 485

Perindopril Erbumine (Concurrent use with other antihypertensive agents may result in additive effect or potentiation). Products include:
Aceon Tablets (2 mg, 4 mg, 8 mg) 3249

Phenobarbital (Potentiation of orthostatic hypotension may occur). Products include:
Arco-Lase Plus Tablets 592
Donnatal 2929
Donnatal Extentabs 2930

Phenoxybenzamine Hydrochloride (Concurrent use with other antihypertensive agents may result in additive effect or potentiation). Products include:
Dibenzyline Capsules 3457

Phentolamine Mesylate (Concurrent use with other antihypertensive agents may result in additive effect or potentiation).
No products indexed under this heading.

Phenylbutazone (Reduces diuretic, natriuretic, and antihypertensive effects).
No products indexed under this heading.

Pindolol (Concurrent use with other antihypertensive agents may result in additive effect or potentiation).
No products indexed under this heading.

Pioglitazone Hydrochloride (Thiazide-induced hyperglycemia may require dosage adjustment of hypoglycemic agents). Products include:
Actos Tablets 3275

Piroxicam (Reduces diuretic, natriuretic, and antihypertensive effects). Products include:
Feldene Capsules 2685

Polythiazide (Concurrent use with other antihypertensive agents may result in additive effect or potentiation). Products include:
Minizide Capsules 2700
Renese Tablets 2712

Prazosin Hydrochloride (Concurrent use with other antihypertensive agents may result in additive effect or potentiation). Products include:
Minipress Capsules 2699
Minizide Capsules 2700

Prednisolone Acetate (Intensified electrolyte depletion particularly hypokalemia). Products include:
Blephamide Ophthalmic Ointment 547
Blephamide Ophthalmic Suspension 548
Poly-Pred Liquifilm Ophthalmic Suspension .... ⊙245
Pred Forte Ophthalmic Suspension .... ⊙246
Pred Mild Sterile Ophthalmic Suspension .... ⊙249
Pred-G Ophthalmic Suspension .... ⊙247
Pred-G Sterile Ophthalmic Ointment .... ⊙248

Prednisolone Sodium Phosphate (Intensified electrolyte depletion particularly hypokalemia). Products include:
Pediapred Oral Solution 1170

Prednisolone Tebutate (Intensified electrolyte depletion particularly hypokalemia).
No products indexed under this heading.

Prednisone (Intensified electrolyte depletion particularly hypokalemia). Products include:
Prednisone 3064

Propoxyphene Hydrochloride (Potentiation of orthostatic hypotension may occur). Products include:
Darvon Pulvules 1909
Darvon Compound-65 Pulvules 1910

Propoxyphene Napsylate (Potentiation of orthostatic hypotension may occur). Products include:
Darvon-N/Darvocet-N 1907
Darvon-N Tablets 1912

Propranolol Hydrochloride (Concurrent use with other antihypertensive agents may result in additive effect or potentiation). Products include:
Inderal 3513
Inderal LA Long-Acting Capsules 3516
Inderide Tablets 3517
Inderide LA Long-Acting Capsules 3519

Quinapril Hydrochloride (Concurrent use with other antihypertensive agents may result in additive effect or potentiation). Products include:
Accupril Tablets 2611
Accuretic Tablets 2614

Ramipril (Concurrent use with other antihypertensive agents may result in additive effect or potentiation). Products include:
Altace Capsules 2233

Rapacuronium Bromide (Possible increased responsiveness to the muscle relaxants).
No products indexed under this heading.

Rauwolfia serpentina (Concurrent use with other antihypertensive agents may result in additive effect or potentiation).
No products indexed under this heading.

Remifentanil Hydrochloride (Potentiation of orthostatic hypotension may occur).
No products indexed under this heading.

Repaglinide (Thiazide-induced hyperglycemia may require dosage adjustment of hypoglycemic agents). Products include:
Prandin Tablets (0.5, 1, and 2 mg) 2432

Rescinnamine (Concurrent use with other antihypertensive agents may result in additive effect or potentiation).
No products indexed under this heading.

Reserpine (Concurrent use with other antihypertensive agents may result in additive effect or potentiation).
No products indexed under this heading.

Rocuronium Bromide (Possible increased responsiveness to the muscle relaxants). Products include:
Zemuron Injection 2491

Rofecoxib (Reduces diuretic, natriuretic, and antihypertensive effects). Products include:
Vioxx 2213

Rosiglitazone Maleate (Thiazide-induced hyperglycemia may require dosage adjustment of hypoglycemic agents). Products include:
Avandia Tablets 1490

Secobarbital Sodium (Potentiation of orthostatic hypotension may occur).
No products indexed under this heading.

Sodium Nitroprusside (Concurrent use with other antihypertensive agents may result in additive effect or potentiation).
No products indexed under this heading.

Sotalol Hydrochloride (Concurrent use with other antihypertensive agents may result in additive effect or potentiation). Products include:
Betapace Tablets 950
Betapace AF Tablets 954

Spirapril Hydrochloride (Concurrent use with other antihypertensive agents may result in additive effect or potentiation).
No products indexed under this heading.

Sufentanil Citrate (Potentiation of orthostatic hypotension may occur).
No products indexed under this heading.

Sulindac (Reduces diuretic, natriuretic, and antihypertensive effects). Products include:
Clinoril Tablets 2053

Telmisartan (Concurrent use with other antihypertensive agents may result in additive effect or potentiation). Products include:
Micardis Tablets 1049
Micardis HCT Tablets 1051

Terazosin Hydrochloride (Concurrent use with other antihypertensive agents may result in additive effect or potentiation). Products include:
Hytrin Capsules 464

Thiamylal Sodium (Potentiation of orthostatic hypotension may occur).
No products indexed under this heading.

Timolol Maleate (Concurrent use with other antihypertensive agents may result in additive effect or potentiation). Products include:
Blocadren Tablets 2046
Cosopt Sterile Ophthalmic Solution 2065
Timolide Tablets 2187
Timolol GFS .... ⊙266
Timoptic in Ocudose 2192
Timoptic Sterile Ophthalmic Solution 2190
Timoptic-XE Sterile Ophthalmic Gel Forming Solution 2194

Tolazamide (Thiazide-induced hyperglycemia may require dosage adjustment of hypoglycemic agents).
No products indexed under this heading.

Tolbutamide (Thiazide-induced hyperglycemia may require dosage adjustment of hypoglycemic agents).
No products indexed under this heading.

Tolmetin Sodium (Reduces diuretic, natriuretic, and antihypertensive effects). Products include:
Tolectin 2589

Torsemide (Concurrent use with other antihypertensive agents may result in additive effect or potentiation). Products include:
Demadex Tablets and Injection 2965

Trandolapril (Concurrent use with other antihypertensive agents may result in additive effect or potentiation). Products include:
Mavik Tablets 478
Tarka Tablets 508

Triamcinolone (Intensified electrolyte depletion particularly hypokalemia).
No products indexed under this heading.

Triamcinolone Acetonide (Intensified electrolyte depletion particularly hypokalemia). Products include:
Azmacort Inhalation Aerosol 728
Nasacort Nasal Inhaler 750
Nasacort AQ Nasal Spray 752
Tri-Nasal Spray 2274

Triamcinolone Diacetate (Intensified electrolyte depletion particularly hypokalemia).
No products indexed under this heading.

Triamcinolone Hexacetonide (Intensified electrolyte depletion particularly hypokalemia).
No products indexed under this heading.

Trimethaphan Camsylate (Concurrent use with other antihypertensive agents may result in additive effect or potentiation).
No products indexed under this heading.

Troglitazone (Thiazide-induced hyperglycemia may require dosage adjustment of hypoglycemic agents).
No products indexed under this heading.

Tubocurarine Chloride (Possible increased responsiveness to the muscle relaxants).
No products indexed under this heading.

Valsartan (Concurrent use with other antihypertensive agents may result in additive effect or potentiation). Products include:
Diovan Capsules 2337
Diovan HCT Tablets 2338

Vecuronium Bromide (Possible increased responsiveness to the muscle relaxants). Products include:
Norcuron for Injection 2478

Verapamil Hydrochloride (Concurrent use with other antihypertensive agents may result in additive effect or potentiation). Products include:
Covera-HS Tablets 3199
Isoptin SR Tablets 467
Tarka Tablets 508
Verelan Capsules 3184
Verelan PM Capsules 3186

Food Interactions

Alcohol (Potentiation of orthostatic hypotension may occur).

DIURIL TABLETS
(Chlorothiazide) 2087
See Diuril Oral Suspension

DIURIL SODIUM INTRAVENOUS
(Chlorothiazide Sodium) 2086
May interact with antihypertensives, barbiturates, corticosteroids, cardiac glycosides, oral hypoglycemic agents, insulin, lithium preparations, narcotic analgesics, nondepolarizing neuromuscular blocking agents, nonsteroidal anti-inflammatory agents, and certain other agents. Compounds in these categories include:

Acarbose (Thiazide-induced hyperglycemia may require dosage adjustment of hypoglycemic agents). Products include:
Precose Tablets 906

Acebutolol Hydrochloride (Concurrent use with other antihypertensive agents may result in additive effect or potentiation). Products include:
Sectral Capsules 3589

ACTH (Intensified electrolyte depletion particularly hypokalemia).
No products indexed under this heading.

Alfentanil Hydrochloride (Potentiation of orthostatic hypotension may occur).
No products indexed under this heading.

Amlodipine Besylate (Concurrent use with other antihypertensive agents may result in additive effect or potentiation). Products include:
Lotrel Capsules 2370
Norvasc Tablets 2704

Aprobarbital (Potentiation of orthostatic hypotension may occur).
No products indexed under this heading.

Atenolol (Concurrent use with other antihypertensive agents may result in additive effect or potentiation). Products include:
Tenoretic Tablets 690
Tenormin I.V. Injection 692

Atracurium Besylate (Possible increased responsiveness to the muscle relaxants).
No products indexed under this heading.

Benazepril Hydrochloride (Concurrent use with other antihypertensive agents may result in additive effect or potentiation). Products include:
Lotensin Tablets 2365
Lotensin HCT Tablets 2367
Lotrel Capsules 2370

Bendroflumethiazide (Concurrent use with other antihypertensive agents may result in additive effect or potentiation). Products include:
Corzide 40/5 Tablets 2247
Corzide 80/5 Tablets 2247

Betamethasone Acetate (Intensified electrolyte depletion particularly hypokalemia). Products include:
Celestone Soluspan Injectable Suspension 3097

Betamethasone Sodium Phosphate (Intensified electrolyte depletion particularly hypokalemia). Products include:
Celestone Soluspan Injectable Suspension 3097

Betaxolol Hydrochloride (Concurrent use with other antihypertensive agents may result in additive effect or potentiation). Products include:
Betoptic S Ophthalmic Suspension 537

Bisoprolol Fumarate (Concurrent use with other antihypertensive agents may result in additive effect or potentiation). Products include:
Zebeta Tablets 1885
Ziac Tablets 1887

Buprenorphine Hydrochloride (Potentiation of orthostatic hypotension may occur). Products include:
Buprenex Injectable 2918

Butabarbital (Potentiation of orthostatic hypotension may occur).
No products indexed under this heading.

Butalbital (Potentiation of orthostatic hypotension may occur). Products include:
Phrenilin 578
Sedapap Tablets 50 mg/650 mg 2225

Candesartan Cilexetil (Concurrent use with other antihypertensive agents may result in additive effect or potentiation). Products include:
Atacand Tablets 595
Atacand HCT Tablets 597

Captopril (Concurrent use with other antihypertensive agents may result in additive effect or potentiation). Products include:
Captopril Tablets 2281

Carteolol Hydrochloride (Concurrent use with other antihypertensive agents may result in additive effect or potentiation). Products include:
Carteolol Hydrochloride Ophthalmic Solution USP, 1% .... ⊙258
Ocupress Ophthalmic Solution, 1% Sterile .... ⊙303

Celecoxib (Reduces diuretic, natriuretic, and antihypertensive effects). Products include:
Celebrex Capsules 2676
Celebrex Capsules 2780

Chlorothiazide (Concurrent use with other antihypertensive agents may result in additive effect or potentiation). Products include:
Aldoclor Tablets 2035
Diuril Oral 2087

Chlorpropamide (Thiazide-induced hyperglycemia may require dosage adjustment of hypoglycemic agents). Products include:
Diabinese Tablets 2680

Chlorthalidone (Concurrent use with other antihypertensive agents may result in additive effect or potentiation). Products include:
Clorpres Tablets 1002
Combipres Tablets 1040
Tenoretic Tablets 690

Cisatracurium Besylate (Possible increased responsiveness to the muscle relaxants).
No products indexed under this heading.

Clonidine (Concurrent use with other antihypertensive agents may result in additive effect or potentiation). Products include:
Catapres-TTS 1038

Clonidine Hydrochloride (Concurrent use with other antihypertensive agents may result in additive effect or potentiation). Products include:
Catapres Tablets 1037
Clorpres Tablets 1002
Combipres Tablets 1040
Duraclon Injection 3057

Codeine Phosphate (Potentiation of orthostatic hypotension may occur). Products include:
Phenergan with Codeine Syrup 3557
Phenergan VC with Codeine Syrup 3561
Robitussin A-C Syrup 2942
Robitussin-DAC Syrup 2942
Ryna-C Liquid .... ▣768
Soma Compound w/Codeine Tablets 3355
Tussi-Organidin NR Liquid 3350
Tussi-Organidin-S NR Liquid 3350
Tylenol with Codeine 2595

Cortisone Acetate (Intensified electrolyte depletion particularly hypokalemia). Products include:
Cortone Acetate Injectable Suspension 2059
Cortone Acetate Tablets 2061

Deserpidine (Concurrent use with other antihypertensive agents may result in additive effect or potentiation).
No products indexed under this heading.

Deslanoside (Thiazide-induced hypokalemia may sensitize or exaggerate the response of the heart to the toxic effects of digitalis).
No products indexed under this heading.

Dexamethasone (Intensified electrolyte depletion particularly hypokalemia). Products include:
Decadron Elixir 2078
Decadron Tablets 2079
TobraDex Ophthalmic Ointment 542
TobraDex Ophthalmic Suspension 541

Dexamethasone Acetate (Intensified electrolyte depletion particularly hypokalemia).
No products indexed under this heading.

Dexamethasone Sodium Phosphate (Intensified electrolyte depletion particularly hypokalemia). Products include:
Decadron Phosphate Injection 2081
Decadron Phosphate Sterile Ophthalmic Ointment 2083
Decadron Phosphate Sterile Ophthalmic Solution 2084
NeoDecadron Sterile Ophthalmic Solution 2144

Dezocine (Potentiation of orthostatic hypotension may occur).
No products indexed under this heading.

Diazoxide (Concurrent use with other antihypertensive agents may result in additive effect or potentiation).
No products indexed under this heading.

Diclofenac Potassium (Reduces diuretic, natriuretic, and antihypertensive effects). Products include:
Cataflam Tablets 2315

Diclofenac Sodium (Reduces diuretic, natriuretic, and antihypertensive effects). Products include:
Arthrotec Tablets 3195
Voltaren Ophthalmic Sterile Ophthalmic Solution .... ⊙312
Voltaren Tablets 2315
Voltaren-XR Tablets 2315

Digitoxin (Thiazide-induced hypokalemia may sensitize or exaggerate the response of the heart to the toxic effects of digitalis).
No products indexed under this heading.

Digoxin (Thiazide-induced hypokalemia may sensitize or exaggerate the response of the heart to the toxic effects of digitalis). Products include:
Digitek Tablets 1003
Lanoxicaps Capsules 1574
Lanoxin Injection 1581
Lanoxin Tablets 1587
Lanoxin Elixir Pediatric 1578
Lanoxin Injection Pediatric 1584

Diltiazem Hydrochloride (Concurrent use with other antihypertensive agents may result in additive effect or potentiation). Products include:
Cardizem Injectable 1018
Cardizem Lyo-Ject Syringe 1018
Cardizem Monovial 1018
Cardizem CD Capsules 1016
Tiazac Capsules 1378

Doxazosin Mesylate (Concurrent use with other antihypertensive agents may result in additive effect or potentiation). Products include:
Cardura Tablets 2668

Enalapril Maleate (Concurrent use with other antihypertensive agents may result in additive effect or potentiation). Products include:
Lexxel Tablets 608
Vaseretic Tablets 2204
Vasotec Tablets 2210

Enalaprilat (Concurrent use with other antihypertensive agents may result in additive effect or potentiation). Products include:
Enalaprilat Injection 863
Vasotec I.V. Injection 2207

Eprosartan Mesylate (Concurrent use with other antihypertensive agents may result in additive effect or potentiation). Products include:
Teveten Tablets 3327

Esmolol Hydrochloride (Concurrent use with other antihypertensive agents may result in additive effect or potentiation). Products include:
Brevibloc Injection 858

Etodolac (Reduces diuretic, natriuretic, and antihypertensive effects). Products include:
Lodine 3528
Lodine XL Extended-Release Tablets 3530

Felodipine (Concurrent use with other antihypertensive agents may result in additive effect or potentiation). Products include:
Lexxel Tablets 608
Plendil Extended-Release Tablets 623

Fenoprofen Calcium (Reduces diuretic, natriuretic, and antihypertensive effects).
No products indexed under this heading.

Fentanyl (Potentiation of orthostatic hypotension may occur). Products include:
Duragesic Transdermal System 1786

Fentanyl Citrate (Potentiation of orthostatic hypotension may occur). Products include:
Actiq 1184

Fludrocortisone Acetate (Intensified electrolyte depletion particularly hypokalemia). Products include:
Florinef Acetate Tablets 2250

Flurbiprofen (Reduces diuretic, natriuretic, and antihypertensive effects).
No products indexed under this heading.

Fosinopril Sodium (Concurrent use with other antihypertensive agents may result in additive effect or potentiation). Products include:
Monopril Tablets 1091
Monopril HCT 1094

Furosemide (Concurrent use with other antihypertensive agents may result in additive effect or potentiation). Products include:
Furosemide Tablets 2284

Glimepiride (Thiazide-induced hyperglycemia may require dosage adjustment of hypoglycemic agents). Products include:
Amaryl Tablets 717

Glipizide (Thiazide-induced hyperglycemia may require dosage adjustment of hypoglycemic agents). Products include:
Glucotrol Tablets 2692
Glucotrol XL Extended Release Tablets 2693

Glyburide (Thiazide-induced hyperglycemia may require dosage adjustment of hypoglycemic agents). Products include:
DiaBeta Tablets 741
Glucovance Tablets 1086

Guanabenz Acetate (Concurrent use with other antihypertensive agents may result in additive effect or potentiation).
No products indexed under this heading.

Guanethidine Monosulfate (Concurrent use with other antihypertensive agents may result in additive effect or potentiation).
No products indexed under this heading.

Hydralazine Hydrochloride (Concurrent use with other antihypertensive agents may result in additive effect or potentiation).
No products indexed under this heading.

Hydrochlorothiazide (Concurrent use with other antihypertensive agents may result in additive effect or potentiation). Products include:
Accuretic Tablets 2614
Aldoril Tablets 2039
Atacand HCT Tablets 597
Avalide Tablets 1070
Diovan HCT Tablets 2338
Dyazide Capsules 1515
HydroDIURIL Tablets 2108
Hyzaar 2109
Inderide Tablets 3517
Inderide LA Long-Acting Capsules 3519
Lotensin HCT Tablets 2367
Maxzide 1008
Micardis HCT Tablets 1051
Microzide Capsules 3414
Moduretic Tablets 2138
Monopril HCT 1094
Prinzide Tablets 2168
Timolide Tablets 2187
Uniretic Tablets 3178
Vaseretic Tablets 2204
Zestoretic Tablets 695
Ziac Tablets 1887

Hydrocodone Bitartrate (Potentiation of orthostatic hypotension may occur). Products include:
Hycodan 1316
Hycomine Compound Tablets 1317
Hycotuss Expectorant Syrup 1318
Lortab 3319
Lortab Elixir 3317
Maxidone Tablets CIII 3399
Norco 5/325 Tablets CIII 3424
Norco 7.5/325 Tablets CIII 3425
Norco 10/325 Tablets CIII 3427
Norco 10/325 Tablets CIII 3425
Vicodin Tablets 516
Vicodin ES Tablets 517
Vicodin HP Tablets 518
Vicodin Tuss Expectorant 519
Vicoprofen Tablets 520
Zydone Tablets 1330

Hydrocodone Polistirex (Potentiation of orthostatic hypotension may occur). Products include:
Tussionex Pennkinetic Extended-Release Suspension 1174

Hydrocortisone (Intensified electrolyte depletion particularly hypokalemia). Products include:
Anusol-HC Cream 2.5% 2237
Cipro HC Otic Suspension 540
Cortaid Intensive Therapy Cream .... ▣717
Cortaid Maximum Strength Cream .... ▣717
Cortisporin Ophthalmic Suspension Sterile .... ⊙297
Cortizone•5 .... ▣699
Cortizone•10 .... ▣699
Cortizone•10 Plus Creme .... ▣700
Cortizone for Kids Creme .... ▣699
Hydrocortone Tablets 2106
Massengill Medicated Soft Cloth Towelette .... ▣753
VōSoL HC Otic Solution 3356

Hydrocortisone Acetate (Intensified electrolyte depletion particularly hypokalemia). Products include:
Analpram-HC 1338
Anusol HC-1 Hydrocortisone Anti-Itch Cream .... ▣689
Anusol-HC Suppositories 2238
Cortaid .... ▣717
Cortifoam Rectal Foam 3170
Cortisporin-TC Otic Suspension 2246
Hydrocortone Acetate Injectable Suspension 2103
Pramosone 1343
Proctocort Suppositories 2264
ProctoFoam-HC 3177
Terra-Cortril Ophthalmic Suspension 2716

Hydrocortisone Sodium Phosphate (Intensified electrolyte depletion particularly hypokalemia). Products include:
Hydrocortone Phosphate Injection, Sterile 2105

Hydrocortisone Sodium Succinate (Intensified electrolyte depletion particularly hypokalemia).
No products indexed under this heading.

Hydroflumethiazide (Concurrent use with other antihypertensive agents may result in additive effect or potentiation). Products include:
Diucardin Tablets 3494

Hydromorphone Hydrochloride (Potentiation of orthostatic hypotension may occur). Products include:
Dilaudid 441
Dilaudid Oral Liquid 445
Dilaudid Powder 441
Dilaudid Rectal Suppositories 441
Dilaudid Tablets 441
Dilaudid Tablets - 8 mg 445
Dilaudid-HP 443

Ibuprofen (Reduces diuretic, natriuretic, and antihypertensive effects). Products include:
Advil .... ▣771
Children's Advil Oral Suspension .... ▣773
Children's Advil Chewable Tablets .... ▣773
Advil Cold and Sinus Caplets .... ▣771
Advil Cold and Sinus Tablets .... ▣771
Advil Flu & Body Ache Caplets .... ▣772
Infants' Advil Drops .... ▣773

Junior Strength Advil Tablets .... ■ 773
Junior Strength Advil Chewable Tablets .... ■ 773
Advil Migraine Liquigels .... ■ 772
Children's Motrin Oral Suspension and Chewable Tablets 2006
Children's Motrin Cold Oral Suspension 2007
Children's Motrin Oral Suspension .... ■ 643
Motrin Suspension, Oral Drops, Chewable Tablets, and Caplets 2002
Infants' Motrin Concentrated Drops 2006
Junior Strength Motrin Caplets and Chewable Tablets 2006
Motrin IB Tablets, Caplets, and Gelcaps 2002
Motrin Migraine Pain Caplets 2005
Motrin Sinus Headache Caplets 2005
Vicoprofen Tablets 520

Indapamide (Concurrent use with other antihypertensive agents may result in additive effect or potentiation). Products include:
Indapamide Tablets 2286

Indomethacin (Reduces diuretic, natriuretic, and antihypertensive effects). Products include:
Indocin 2112

Indomethacin Sodium Trihydrate (Reduces diuretic, natriuretic, and antihypertensive effects). Products include:
Indocin I.V. 2115

Insulin, Human, Zinc Suspension (Thiazide-induced hyperglycemia may require dosage adjustment of hypoglycemic agents). Products include:
Humulin L, 100 Units 1937
Humulin U, 100 Units 1943
Novolin L Human Insulin 10 ml Vials 2422

Insulin, Human NPH (Thiazide-induced hyperglycemia may require dosage adjustment of hypoglycemic agents). Products include:
Humulin N, 100 Units 1939
Humulin N NPH Pen 1940
Novolin N Human Insulin 10 ml Vials 2422
Novolin N PenFill 2423
Novolin N Prefilled Syringe Disposable Insulin Delivery System 2425

Insulin, Human Regular (Thiazide-induced hyperglycemia may require dosage adjustment of hypoglycemic agents). Products include:
Humulin R Regular (U-500) 1943
Humulin R, 100 Units 1941
Novolin R Human Insulin 10 ml Vials 2423
Novolin R PenFill 2423
Novolin R Prefilled Syringe Disposable Insulin Delivery System 2425
Velosulin BR Human Insulin 10 ml Vials 2435

Insulin, Human Regular and Human NPH Mixture (Thiazide-induced hyperglycemia may require dosage adjustment of hypoglycemic agents). Products include:
Humulin 50/50, 100 Units 1934
Humulin 70/30, 100 Units 1935
Humulin 70/30 Pen 1936
Novolin 70/30 Human Insulin 10 ml Vials 2421
Novolin 70/30 PenFill 2423
Novolin 70/30 Prefilled Disposable Insulin Delivery System 2425

Insulin, NPH (Thiazide-induced hyperglycemia may require dosage adjustment of hypoglycemic agents). Products include:
Iletin II, NPH (Pork), 100 Units 1946

Insulin, Regular (Thiazide-induced hyperglycemia may require dosage adjustment of hypoglycemic agents). Products include:
Iletin II, Regular (Pork), 100 Units 1947

Insulin, Zinc Crystals (Thiazide-induced hyperglycemia may require dosage adjustment of hypoglycemic agents).
No products indexed under this heading.

Insulin, Zinc Suspension (Thiazide-induced hyperglycemia may require dosage adjustment of hypoglycemic agents). Products include:
Iletin II, Lente (Pork), 100 Units 1945

Insulin Aspart, Human Regular (Thiazide-induced hyperglycemia may require dosage adjustment of hypoglycemic agents).
No products indexed under this heading.

Insulin glargine (Thiazide-induced hyperglycemia may require dosage adjustment of hypoglycemic agents). Products include:
Lantus Injection 742

Insulin Lispro, Human (Thiazide-induced hyperglycemia may require dosage adjustment of hypoglycemic agents). Products include:
Humalog 1926
Humalog Mix 75/25 Pen 1928

Insulin Lispro Protamine, Human (Thiazide-induced hyperglycemia may require dosage adjustment of hypoglycemic agents). Products include:
Humalog Mix 75/25 Pen 1928

Irbesartan (Concurrent use with other antihypertensive agents may result in additive effect or potentiation). Products include:
Avalide Tablets 1070
Avapro Tablets 1074
Avapro Tablets 3076

Isradipine (Concurrent use with other antihypertensive agents may result in additive effect or potentiation). Products include:
DynaCirc Capsules 2921
DynaCirc CR Tablets 2923

Ketoprofen (Reduces diuretic, natriuretic, and antihypertensive effects). Products include:
Orudis Capsules 3548
Orudis KT Tablets .... ■ 778
Oruvail Capsules 3548

Ketorolac Tromethamine (Reduces diuretic, natriuretic, and antihypertensive effects). Products include:
Acular Ophthalmic Solution 544
Acular PF Ophthalmic Solution 544
Toradol 3018

Labetalol Hydrochloride (Concurrent use with other antihypertensive agents may result in additive effect or potentiation). Products include:
Normodyne Injection 3135
Normodyne Tablets 3137

Levobunolol Hydrochloride (Concurrent use with other antihypertensive agents may result in additive effect or potentiation). Products include:
Betagan .... ⊙ 228

Levorphanol Tartrate (Potentiation of orthostatic hypotension may occur). Products include:
Levo-Dromoran 1734
Levorphanol Tartrate Tablets 3059

Lisinopril (Concurrent use with other antihypertensive agents may result in additive effect or potentiation). Products include:
Prinivil Tablets 2164
Prinzide Tablets 2168
Zestoretic Tablets 695
Zestril Tablets 698

Lithium Carbonate (Diuretics reduce the renal clearance of lithium and this may lead to lithium toxicity). Products include:
Eskalith 1527
Lithium Carbonate 3061
Lithobid Slow-Release Tablets 3255

Lithium Citrate (Diuretics reduce the renal clearance of lithium and this may lead to lithium toxicity). Products include:
Lithium Citrate Syrup 3061

Losartan Potassium (Concurrent use with other antihypertensive agents may result in additive effect or potentiation). Products include:
Cozaar Tablets 2067
Hyzaar 2109

Mecamylamine Hydrochloride (Concurrent use with other antihypertensive agents may result in additive effect or potentiation). Products include:
Inversine Tablets 1850

Meclofenamate Sodium (Reduces diuretic, natriuretic, and antihypertensive effects).
No products indexed under this heading.

Mefenamic Acid (Reduces diuretic, natriuretic, and antihypertensive effects). Products include:
Ponstel Capsules 1356

Meloxicam (Reduces diuretic, natriuretic, and antihypertensive effects). Products include:
Mobic Tablets 1054

Meperidine Hydrochloride (Potentiation of orthostatic hypotension may occur). Products include:
Demerol 3079
Mepergan Injection 3539

Mephobarbital (Potentiation of orthostatic hypotension may occur).
No products indexed under this heading.

Metformin Hydrochloride (Thiazide-induced hyperglycemia may require dosage adjustment of hypoglycemic agents). Products include:
Glucophage Tablets 1080
Glucophage XR Tablets 1080
Glucovance Tablets 1086

Methadone Hydrochloride (Potentiation of orthostatic hypotension may occur). Products include:
Dolophine Hydrochloride Tablets 3056

Methyclothiazide (Concurrent use with other antihypertensive agents may result in additive effect or potentiation).
No products indexed under this heading.

Methyldopa (Concurrent use with other antihypertensive agents may result in additive effect or potentiation). Products include:
Aldoclor Tablets 2035
Aldomet Tablets 2037
Aldoril Tablets 2039

Methyldopate Hydrochloride (Concurrent use with other antihypertensive agents may result in additive effect or potentiation).
No products indexed under this heading.

Methylprednisolone Acetate (Intensified electrolyte depletion particularly hypokalemia). Products include:
Depo-Medrol Injectable Suspension 2795

Methylprednisolone Sodium Succinate (Intensified electrolyte depletion particularly hypokalemia). Products include:
Solu-Medrol Sterile Powder 2855

Metipranolol Hydrochloride (Concurrent use with other antihypertensive agents may result in additive effect or potentiation).
No products indexed under this heading.

Metocurine Iodide (Possible increased responsiveness to the muscle relaxants).
No products indexed under this heading.

Metolazone (Concurrent use with other antihypertensive agents may result in additive effect or potentiation). Products include:
Mykrox Tablets 1168
Zaroxolyn Tablets 1177

Metoprolol Succinate (Concurrent use with other antihypertensive agents may result in additive effect or potentiation). Products include:
Toprol-XL Tablets 651

Metoprolol Tartrate (Concurrent use with other antihypertensive agents may result in additive effect or potentiation).
No products indexed under this heading.

Metyrosine (Concurrent use with other antihypertensive agents may result in additive effect or potentiation). Products include:
Demser Capsules 2085

Mibefradil Dihydrochloride (Concurrent use with other antihypertensive agents may result in additive effect or potentiation).
No products indexed under this heading.

Miglitol (Thiazide-induced hyperglycemia may require dosage adjustment of hypoglycemic agents). Products include:
Glyset Tablets 2821

Minoxidil (Concurrent use with other antihypertensive agents may result in additive effect or potentiation). Products include:
Rogaine Extra Strength for Men Topical Solution .... ■ 721
Rogaine for Women Topical Solution .... ■ 721

Mivacurium Chloride (Possible increased responsiveness to the muscle relaxants).
No products indexed under this heading.

Moexipril Hydrochloride (Concurrent use with other antihypertensive agents may result in additive effect or potentiation). Products include:
Uniretic Tablets 3178
Univasc Tablets 3181

Morphine Sulfate (Potentiation of orthostatic hypotension may occur). Products include:
Astramorph/PF Injection, USP (Preservative-Free) 594
Duramorph Injection 1312
Infumorph 200 and Infumorph 500 Sterile Solutions 1314
Kadian Capsules 1335
MS Contin Tablets 2896
MSIR 2898
Oramorph SR Tablets 3062
Roxanol 3066

Nabumetone (Reduces diuretic, natriuretic, and antihypertensive effects). Products include:
Relafen Tablets 1617

Nadolol (Concurrent use with other antihypertensive agents may result in additive effect or potentiation). Products include:
Corgard Tablets 2245
Corzide 40/5 Tablets 2247
Corzide 80/5 Tablets 2247
Nadolol Tablets 2288

Naproxen (Reduces diuretic, natriuretic, and antihypertensive effects). Products include:
EC-Naprosyn Delayed-Release Tablets 2967
Naprosyn Suspension 2967
Naprosyn Tablets 2967

Naproxen Sodium (Reduces diuretic, natriuretic, and antihypertensive effects). Products include:
Aleve Tablets, Caplets and Gelcaps .... ■ 602
Aleve Cold & Sinus Caplets .... ■ 603
Anaprox Tablets 2967
Anaprox DS Tablets 2967
Naprelan Tablets 1293

Nicardipine Hydrochloride (Concurrent use with other antihypertensive agents may result in additive effect or potentiation). Products include:
Cardene I.V. 3485

Nifedipine (Concurrent use with other antihypertensive agents may result in additive effect or potentiation). Products include:
Adalat CC Tablets 877
Procardia Capsules 2708
Procardia XL Extended Release Tablets 2710

Nisoldipine (Concurrent use with other antihypertensive agents may result in additive effect or potentiation). Products include:
Sular Tablets 688

Nitroglycerin (Concurrent use with other antihypertensive agents may result in additive effect or potentiation). Products include:
Nitro-Dur Transdermal Infusion System 3134
Nitro-Dur Transdermal Infusion System 1834
Nitrolingual Pumpspray 1355
Nitrostat Tablets 2658

Norepinephrine Hydrochloride (Decreased arterial responsiveness to pressor amine).
No products indexed under this heading.

Oxaprozin (Reduces diuretic, natriuretic, and antihypertensive effects).
No products indexed under this heading.

Oxycodone Hydrochloride (Potentiation of orthostatic hypotension may occur). Products include:
OxyContin Tablets 2912
OxyFast Oral Concentrate Solution .. 2916
OxyIR Capsules 2916
Percocet Tablets 1326
Percodan Tablets 1327
Percolone Tablets 1327
Roxicodone 3067
Tylox Capsules 2597

Pancuronium Bromide (Possible increased responsiveness to the muscle relaxants).
No products indexed under this heading.

Penbutolol Sulfate (Concurrent use with other antihypertensive agents may result in additive effect or potentiation).
No products indexed under this heading.

Pentobarbital Sodium (Potentiation of orthostatic hypotension may occur). Products include:
Nembutal Sodium Solution 485

Perindopril Erbumine (Concurrent use with other antihypertensive agents may result in additive effect or potentiation). Products include:
Aceon Tablets (2 mg, 4 mg, 8 mg) 3249

Phenobarbital (Potentiation of orthostatic hypotension may occur). Products include:
Arco-Lase Plus Tablets 592
Donnatal 2929
Donnatal Extentabs 2930

Phenoxybenzamine Hydrochloride (Concurrent use with other antihypertensive agents may result in additive effect or potentiation). Products include:
Dibenzyline Capsules 3457

Phentolamine Mesylate (Concurrent use with other antihypertensive agents may result in additive effect or potentiation).
No products indexed under this heading.

Phenylbutazone (Reduces diuretic, natriuretic, and antihypertensive effects).
No products indexed under this heading.

Pindolol (Concurrent use with other antihypertensive agents may result in additive effect or potentiation).
No products indexed under this heading.

Pioglitazone Hydrochloride (Thiazide-induced hyperglycemia may require dosage adjustment of hypoglycemic agents). Products include:
Actos Tablets 3275

Piroxicam (Reduces diuretic, natriuretic, and antihypertensive effects). Products include:
Feldene Capsules 2685

Polythiazide (Concurrent use with other antihypertensive agents may result in additive effect or potentiation). Products include:
Minizide Capsules 2700
Renese Tablets 2712

Prazosin Hydrochloride (Concurrent use with other antihypertensive agents may result in additive effect or potentiation). Products include:
Minipress Capsules 2699
Minizide Capsules 2700

Prednisolone Acetate (Intensified electrolyte depletion particularly hypokalemia). Products include:
Blephamide Ophthalmic Ointment .. 547
Blephamide Ophthalmic Suspension 548
Poly-Pred Liquifilm Ophthalmic Suspension .... ⊙ 245
Pred Forte Ophthalmic Suspension .... ⊙ 246
Pred Mild Sterile Ophthalmic Suspension .... ⊙ 249
Pred-G Ophthalmic Suspension .... ⊙ 247
Pred-G Sterile Ophthalmic Ointment .... ⊙ 248

Prednisolone Sodium Phosphate (Intensified electrolyte depletion particularly hypokalemia). Products include:
Pediapred Oral Solution 1170

Prednisolone Tebutate (Intensified electrolyte depletion particularly hypokalemia).
No products indexed under this heading.

Prednisone (Intensified electrolyte depletion particularly hypokalemia). Products include:
Prednisone 3064

Propoxyphene Hydrochloride (Potentiation of orthostatic hypotension may occur). Products include:
Darvon Pulvules 1909
Darvon Compound-65 Pulvules 1910

Propoxyphene Napsylate (Potentiation of orthostatic hypotension may occur). Products include:
Darvon-N/Darvocet-N 1907
Darvon-N Tablets 1912

Propranolol Hydrochloride (Concurrent use with other antihypertensive agents may result in additive effect or potentiation). Products include:
Inderal 3513
Inderal LA Long-Acting Capsules 3516
Inderide Tablets 3517
Inderide LA Long-Acting Capsules .. 3519

Quinapril Hydrochloride (Concurrent use with other antihypertensive agents may result in additive effect or potentiation). Products include:
Accupril Tablets 2611
Accuretic Tablets 2614

Ramipril (Concurrent use with other antihypertensive agents may result in additive effect or potentiation). Products include:
Altace Capsules 2233

Rapacuronium Bromide (Possible increased responsiveness to the muscle relaxants).
No products indexed under this heading.

Rauwolfia serpentina (Concurrent use with other antihypertensive agents may result in additive effect or potentiation).
No products indexed under this heading.

Remifentanil Hydrochloride (Potentiation of orthostatic hypotension may occur).
No products indexed under this heading.

Repaglinide (Thiazide-induced hyperglycemia may require dosage adjustment of hypoglycemic agents). Products include:
Prandin Tablets (0.5, 1, and 2 mg) 2432

Rescinnamine (Concurrent use with other antihypertensive agents may result in additive effect or potentiation).
No products indexed under this heading.

Reserpine (Concurrent use with other antihypertensive agents may result in additive effect or potentiation).
No products indexed under this heading.

Rocuronium Bromide (Possible increased responsiveness to the muscle relaxants). Products include:
Zemuron Injection 2491

Rofecoxib (Reduces diuretic, natriuretic, and antihypertensive effects). Products include:
Vioxx 2213

Rosiglitazone Maleate (Thiazide-induced hyperglycemia may require dosage adjustment of hypoglycemic agents). Products include:
Avandia Tablets 1490

Secobarbital Sodium (Potentiation of orthostatic hypotension may occur).
No products indexed under this heading.

Sodium Nitroprusside (Concurrent use with other antihypertensive agents may result in additive effect or potentiation).
No products indexed under this heading.

Sotalol Hydrochloride (Concurrent use with other antihypertensive agents may result in additive effect or potentiation). Products include:
Betapace Tablets 950
Betapace AF Tablets 954

Spirapril Hydrochloride (Concurrent use with other antihypertensive agents may result in additive effect or potentiation).
No products indexed under this heading.

Sufentanil Citrate (Potentiation of orthostatic hypotension may occur).
No products indexed under this heading.

Sulindac (Reduces diuretic, natriuretic, and antihypertensive effects). Products include:
Clinoril Tablets 2053

Telmisartan (Concurrent use with other antihypertensive agents may result in additive effect or potentiation). Products include:
Micardis Tablets 1049
Micardis HCT Tablets 1051

Terazosin Hydrochloride (Concurrent use with other antihypertensive agents may result in additive effect or potentiation). Products include:
Hytrin Capsules 464

Thiamylal Sodium (Potentiation of orthostatic hypotension may occur).
No products indexed under this heading.

Timolol Maleate (Concurrent use with other antihypertensive agents may result in additive effect or potentiation). Products include:
Blocadren Tablets 2046
Cosopt Sterile Ophthalmic Solution 2065
Timolide Tablets 2187
Timolol GFS .... ⊙ 266
Timoptic in Ocudose 2192
Timoptic Sterile Ophthalmic Solution 2190
Timoptic-XE Sterile Ophthalmic Gel Forming Solution 2194

Tolazamide (Thiazide-induced hyperglycemia may require dosage adjustment of hypoglycemic agents).
No products indexed under this heading.

Tolbutamide (Thiazide-induced hyperglycemia may require dosage adjustment of hypoglycemic agents).
No products indexed under this heading.

Tolmetin Sodium (Reduces diuretic, natriuretic, and antihypertensive effects). Products include:
Tolectin 2589

Torsemide (Concurrent use with other antihypertensive agents may result in additive effect or potentiation). Products include:
Demadex Tablets and Injection 2965

Trandolapril (Concurrent use with other antihypertensive agents may result in additive effect or potentiation). Products include:
Mavik Tablets 478
Tarka Tablets 508

Triamcinolone (Intensified electrolyte depletion particularly hypokalemia).
No products indexed under this heading.

Triamcinolone Acetonide (Intensified electrolyte depletion particularly hypokalemia). Products include:
Azmacort Inhalation Aerosol 728
Nasacort Nasal Inhaler 750
Nasacort AQ Nasal Spray 752
Tri-Nasal Spray 2274

Triamcinolone Diacetate (Intensified electrolyte depletion particularly hypokalemia).
No products indexed under this heading.

Triamcinolone Hexacetonide (Intensified electrolyte depletion particularly hypokalemia).
No products indexed under this heading.

Trimethaphan Camsylate (Concurrent use with other antihypertensive agents may result in additive effect or potentiation).
No products indexed under this heading.

Troglitazone (Thiazide-induced hyperglycemia may require dosage adjustment of hypoglycemic agents).
No products indexed under this heading.

Tubocurarine Chloride (Possible increased responsiveness to the muscle relaxants).
No products indexed under this heading.

Valsartan (Concurrent use with other antihypertensive agents may result in additive effect or potentiation). Products include:
Diovan Capsules 2337
Diovan HCT Tablets 2338

Vecuronium Bromide (Possible increased responsiveness to the muscle relaxants). Products include:
Norcuron for Injection 2478

Verapamil Hydrochloride (Concurrent use with other antihypertensive agents may result in additive effect or potentiation). Products include:
Covera-HS Tablets 3199
Isoptin SR Tablets 467
Tarka Tablets 508
Verelan Capsules 3184
Verelan PM Capsules 3186

Food Interactions

Alcohol (Potentiation of orthostatic hypotension may occur).

DOBUTREX SOLUTION VIALS
(Dobutamine Hydrochloride) 1914
May interact with beta blockers and certain other agents. Compounds in these categories include:

Acebutolol Hydrochloride (Based on animal studies, dobutamine may

be ineffective in patients recently on beta blocker; potential for increased peripheral vascular resistance). Products include:

Sectral Capsules ... 3589

Atenolol (Based on animal studies, dobutamine may be ineffective in patients recently on beta blocker; potential for increased peripheral vascular resistance). Products include:

Tenoretic Tablets ... 690
Tenormin I.V. Injection ... 692

Betaxolol Hydrochloride (Based on animal studies, dobutamine may be ineffective in patients recently on beta blocker; potential for increased peripheral vascular resistance). Products include:

Betoptic S Ophthalmic Suspension ... 537

Bisoprolol Fumarate (Based on animal studies, dobutamine may be ineffective in patients recently on beta blocker; potential for increased peripheral vascular resistance). Products include:

Zebeta Tablets ... 1885
Ziac Tablets ... 1887

Carteolol Hydrochloride (Based on animal studies, dobutamine may be ineffective in patients recently on beta blocker; potential for increased peripheral vascular resistance). Products include:

Carteolol Hydrochloride Ophthalmic Solution USP, 1% ... ⊙ 258
Ocupress Ophthalmic Solution, 1% Sterile ... ⊙ 303

Esmolol Hydrochloride (Based on animal studies, dobutamine may be ineffective in patients recently on beta blocker; potential for increased peripheral vascular resistance). Products include:

Brevibloc Injection ... 858

Labetalol Hydrochloride (Based on animal studies, dobutamine may be ineffective in patients recently on beta blocker; potential for increased peripheral vascular resistance). Products include:

Normodyne Injection ... 3135
Normodyne Tablets ... 3137

Levobunolol Hydrochloride (Based on animal studies, dobutamine may be ineffective in patients recently on beta blocker; potential for increased peripheral vascular resistance). Products include:

Betagan ... ⊙ 228

Metipranolol Hydrochloride (Based on animal studies, dobutamine may be ineffective in patients recently on beta blocker; potential for increased peripheral vascular resistance).

No products indexed under this heading.

Metoprolol Succinate (Based on animal studies, dobutamine may be ineffective in patients recently on beta blocker; potential for increased peripheral vascular resistance). Products include:

Toprol-XL Tablets ... 651

Metoprolol Tartrate (Based on animal studies, dobutamine may be ineffective in patients recently on beta blocker; potential for increased peripheral vascular resistance).

No products indexed under this heading.

Nadolol (Based on animal studies, dobutamine may be ineffective in patients recently on beta blocker; potential for increased peripheral vascular resistance). Products include:

Corgard Tablets ... 2245
Corzide 40/5 Tablets ... 2247
Corzide 80/5 Tablets ... 2247
Nadolol Tablets ... 2288

Penbutolol Sulfate (Based on animal studies, dobutamine may be ineffective in patients recently on beta blocker; potential for increased peripheral vascular resistance).

No products indexed under this heading.

Pindolol (Based on animal studies, dobutamine may be ineffective in patients recently on beta blocker; potential for increased peripheral vascular resistance).

No products indexed under this heading.

Propranolol Hydrochloride (Based on animal studies, dobutamine may be ineffective in patients recently on beta blocker; potential for increased peripheral vascular resistance). Products include:

Inderal ... 3513
Inderal LA Long-Acting Capsules ... 3516
Inderide Tablets ... 3517
Inderide LA Long-Acting Capsules ... 3519

Sodium Nitroprusside (Concomitant use results in a higher cardiac output and, usually, a lower pulmonary wedge pressure).

No products indexed under this heading.

Sotalol Hydrochloride (Based on animal studies, dobutamine may be ineffective in patients recently on beta blocker; potential for increased peripheral vascular resistance). Products include:

Betapace Tablets ... 950
Betapace AF Tablets ... 954

Timolol Hemihydrate (Based on animal studies, dobutamine may be ineffective in patients recently on beta blocker; potential for increased peripheral vascular resistance). Products include:

Betimol Ophthalmic Solution ... ⊙ 324

Timolol Maleate (Based on animal studies, dobutamine may be ineffective in patients recently on beta blocker; potential for increased peripheral vascular resistance). Products include:

Blocadren Tablets ... 2046
Cosopt Sterile Ophthalmic Solution ... 2065
Timolide Tablets ... 2187
Timolol GFS ... ⊙ 266
Timoptic in Ocudose ... 2192
Timoptic Sterile Ophthalmic Solution ... 2190
Timoptic-XE Sterile Ophthalmic Gel Forming Solution ... 2194

DOLOBID TABLETS

(Diflunisal) ... 2088

May interact with antacids, oral anticoagulants, non-steroidal anti-inflammatory agents, and certain other agents. Compounds in these categories include:

Acetaminophen (Increased plasma levels of acetaminophen). Products include:

Actifed Cold & Sinus Caplets and Tablets ... ▣ 688
Alka-Seltzer Plus Liqui-Gels ... ▣ 604
Alka-Seltzer Plus Cold & Flu Medicine Liqui-Gels ... ▣ 604
Alka-Seltzer Plus Cold & Sinus Medicine Liqui-Gels ... ▣ 604
Benadryl Allergy/Cold Tablets ... ▣ 691
Benadryl Allergy Sinus Headache Caplets & Gelcaps ... ▣ 693
Benadryl Severe Allergy & Sinus Headache Caplets ... ▣ 694
Children's Cēpacol Sore Throat ... ▣ 788
Comtrex Acute Head Cold & Sinus Pressure Relief Tablets ... ▣ 627
Comtrex Deep Chest Cold & Congestion Relief Softgels ... ▣ 627
Comtrex Flu Therapy & Fever Relief Daytime Caplets ... ▣ 628
Comtrex Flu Therapy & Fever Relief Nighttime Tablets ... ▣ 628
Comtrex Maximum Strength Multi-Symptom Cold & Cough Relief Tablets and Caplets ... ▣ 626
Contac Severe Cold and Flu Caplets Maximum Strength ... ▣ 746
Contac Severe Cold and Flu Caplets Non-Drowsy ... ▣ 746
Coricidin 'D' Cold, Flu & Sinus Tablets ... ▣ 737
Coricidin HBP Cold & Flu Tablets ... ▣ 738
Coricidin HBP Maximum Strength Flu Tablets ... ▣ 738
Coricidin HBP Night-Time Cold & Flu Tablets ... ▣ 738
Darvon-N/Darvocet-N ... 1907
Dimetapp Cold and Fever Suspension ... ▣ 775
Dimetapp Nighttime Flu Liquid ... ▣ 776
Dimetapp Non-Drowsy Flu Syrup ... ▣ 777
Drixoral Allergy/Sinus Extended-Release Tablets ... ▣ 741
Drixoral Cold & Flu Extended-Release Tablets ... ▣ 740
Aspirin Free Excedrin Caplets and Geltabs ... ▣ 628
Excedrin Extra-Strength Tablets, Caplets, and Geltabs ... ▣ 629
Excedrin Migraine ... 1070
Excedrin PM Tablets, Caplets, and Geltabs ... ▣ 631
Goody's Body Pain Formula Powder ... ▣ 620
Goody's Extra Strength Headache Powder ... ▣ 620
Goody's Extra Strength Pain Relief Tablets ... ▣ 620
Goody's PM Powder ... ▣ 621
Hycomine Compound Tablets ... 1317
Lortab ... 3319
Lortab Elixir ... 3317
Maxidone Tablets CIII ... 3399
Maximum Strength Midol Menstrual Caplets and Gelcaps ... ▣ 612
Maximum Strength Midol PMS Caplets and Gelcaps ... ▣ 613
Maximum Strength Midol Teen Caplets ... ▣ 612
Midrin Capsules ... 3464
Norco 5/325 Tablets CIII ... 3424
Norco 7.5/325 Tablets CIII ... 3425
Norco 10/325 Tablets CIII ... 3427
Norco 10/325 Tablets CIII ... 3425
Percocet Tablets ... 1326
Percogesic Aspirin-Free Coated Tablets ... ▣ 667
Extra Strength Percogesic Aspirin-Free Coated Caplets ... ▣ 665
Phrenilin ... 578
Robitussin Cold Caplets Multi-Symptom Cold & Flu ... ▣ 781
Robitussin Cold Softgels Multi-Symptom Cold & Flu ... ▣ 781
Robitussin Multi Symptom Honey Flu Liquid ... ▣ 785
Robitussin Nighttime Honey Flu Liquid ... ▣ 786
Sedapap Tablets 50 mg/650 mg ... 2225
Singlet Caplets ... ▣ 761
Sinutab Sinus Allergy Medication, Maximum Strength Formula, Tablets & Caplets ... ▣ 707
Sinutab Sinus Medication, Maximum Strength Without Drowsiness Formula, Tablets & Caplets ... ▣ 707
Sudafed Cold & Cough Liquid Caps ... ▣ 709
Sudafed Cold & Sinus Liquid Caps ... ▣ 710
Sudafed Severe Cold ... ▣ 711
Sudafed Sinus Headache Caplets ... ▣ 712
Sudafed Sinus Headache Tablets ... ▣ 712
Tavist Sinus Non-Drowsy Coated Caplets ... ▣ 676
TheraFlu Regular Strength Cold & Cough Night Time Hot Liquid ... ▣ 676
TheraFlu Regular Strength Cold & Sore Throat Night Time Hot Liquid ... ▣ 676
TheraFlu Maximum Strength Flu & Congestion Non-Drowsy Hot Liquid ... ▣ 677
TheraFlu Maximum Strength Flu & Cough Night Time Hot Liquid ... ▣ 678
TheraFlu Maximum Strength Flu & Sore Throat Night Time Hot Liquid ... ▣ 677
TheraFlu Maximum Strength Severe Cold & Congestion Night Time Caplets ... ▣ 678
TheraFlu Maximum Strength Severe Cold & Congestion Night Time Hot Liquid ... ▣ 678
TheraFlu Maximum Strength Severe Cold & Congestion Non-Drowsy ... ▣ 679
Triaminic Cold, Cough & Fever Liquid ... ▣ 681
Triaminic Cough & Sore Throat Liquid ... ▣ 682
Triaminic Cough & Sore Throat Softchews ... ▣ 684
Tylenol, Children's ... 2014
Children's Tylenol Allergy-D Liquid ... 2014
Children's Tylenol Cold Suspension Liquid and Chewable Tablets ... 2015
Children's Tylenol Cold Plus Cough Suspension Liquid and Chewable Tablets ... 2015
Children's Tylenol Flu Suspension Liquid ... 2015
Children's Tylenol Sinus Suspension Liquid ... 2017
Infants' Tylenol Cold Decongestant and Fever Reducer Concentrated Drops ... 2015
Infants' Tylenol Cold Decongestant and Fever Reducer Concentrated Drops Plus Cough ... 2015
Junior Strength Tylenol Soft Chews Chewable Tablets ... 2014
Tylenol ... 2009
Tylenol Allergy Sinus ... 2010
Tylenol Severe Allergy Caplets ... 2010
Multi-Symptom Tylenol Cold Complete Formula Caplets ... 2010
Multi-Symptom Tylenol Cold Non-Drowsy Caplets and Gelcaps ... 2010
Multi-Symptom Tylenol Cold Severe Congestion Non-Drowsy Caplets ... 2011
Maximum Strength Tylenol Flu NightTime Gelcaps ... 2011
Maximum Strength Tylenol Flu NightTime Liquid ... 2011
Maximum Strength Tylenol Flu Non-Drowsy Gelcaps ... 2011
Extra Strength Tylenol PM Caplets, Geltabs, and Gelcaps ... 2012
Maximum Strength Tylenol Sinus NightTime Caplets ... 2012
Maximum Strength Tylenol Sinus Non-Drowsy Geltabs, Gelcaps, Caplets, and Tablets ... 2012
Maximum Strength Tylenol Sore Throat Adult Liquid ... 2013
Tylenol with Codeine ... 2595
Women's Tylenol Menstrual Relief Caplets ... 2013
Tylox Capsules ... 2597
Ultracet Tablets ... 2597
Vanquish Caplets ... ▣ 617
Vicks 44M Cough, Cold & Flu Relief Liquid ... ▣ 725
Vicks DayQuil LiquiCaps/Liquid Multi-Symptom Cold/Flu Relief ... ▣ 727
Vicks NyQuil LiquiCaps/Liquid Multi-Symptom Cold/Flu Relief, Original and Cherry Flavors ... ▣ 727
Vicodin Tablets ... 516
Vicodin ES Tablets ... 517
Vicodin HP Tablets ... 518
Zydone Tablets ... 1330

Aluminum Carbonate (Reduced plasma levels of Dolobid).

No products indexed under this heading.

Aluminum Hydroxide (Reduced plasma levels of Dolobid). Products include:

Amphojel Suspension (Mint Flavor) ... ▣ 789
Gaviscon Extra Strength Liquid ... ▣ 751
Gaviscon Extra Strength Tablets ... ▣ 751
Gaviscon Regular Strength Liquid ... ▣ 751
Gaviscon Regular Strength Tablets ... ▣ 750
Maalox Antacid/Anti-Gas Oral Suspension ... ▣ 673
Maalox Max Maximum Strength Antacid/Anti-Gas Liquid ... 2300
Maalox Regular Strength Antacid/Antigas Liquid ... 2300
Mylanta ... 1813
Vanquish Caplets ... ▣ 617

Aspirin (Small decrease in diflunisal levels). Products include:

Aggrenox Capsules ... 1026
Alka-Seltzer ... ▣ 603
Alka-Seltzer Lemon Lime Antacid and Pain Reliever Effervescent Tablets ... ▣ 603
Alka-Seltzer Extra Strength Antacid and Pain Reliever Effervescent Tablets ... ▣ 603
Alka-Seltzer PM Effervescent Tablets ... ▣ 605
Genuine Bayer Tablets, Caplets and Gelcaps ... ▣ 606
Extra Strength Bayer Caplets and Gelcaps ... ▣ 610
Aspirin Regimen Bayer Children's Chewable Tablets (Orange or Cherry Flavored) ... ▣ 607
Bayer, Aspirin Regimen ... ▣ 606
Aspirin Regimen Bayer 81 mg Caplets with Calcium ... ▣ 607

Genuine Bayer Professional Labeling (Aspirin Regimen Bayer) 608
Extra Strength Bayer Arthritis Caplets 610
Extra Strength Bayer Plus Caplets 610
Extra Strength Bayer PM Caplets 611
BC Powder 619
BC Allergy Sinus Cold Powder 619
Arthritis Strength BC Powder 619
BC Sinus Cold Powder 619
Darvon Compound-65 Pulvules 1910
Ecotrin Enteric Coated Aspirin Low, Regular and Maximum Strength Tablets 1715
Excedrin Extra-Strength Tablets, Caplets, and Geltabs 629
Excedrin Migraine 1070
Goody's Body Pain Formula Powder 620
Goody's Extra Strength Headache Powder 620
Goody's Extra Strength Pain Relief Tablets 620
Percodan Tablets 1327
Robaxisal Tablets 2939
Soma Compound Tablets 3354
Soma Compound w/Codeine Tablets 3355
Vanquish Caplets 617

Celecoxib (Concomitant use with other NSAIDs is not recommended due to the increased possibility of gastrointestinal toxicity, with little or no increase in efficacy). Products include:
Celebrex Capsules 2676
Celebrex Capsules 2780

Cyclosporine (Increased cyclosporine-induced toxicity). Products include:
Gengraf Capsules 457
Neoral Soft Gelatin Capsules 2380
Neoral Oral Solution 2380
Sandimmune 2388

Diclofenac Potassium (Concomitant use with other NSAIDs is not recommended due to the increased possibility of gastrointestinal toxicity, with little or no increase in efficacy). Products include:
Cataflam Tablets 2315

Diclofenac Sodium (Concomitant use with other NSAIDs is not recommended due to the increased possibility of gastrointestinal toxicity, with little or no increase in efficacy). Products include:
Arthrotec Tablets 3195
Voltaren Ophthalmic Sterile Ophthalmic Solution 312
Voltaren Tablets 2315
Voltaren-XR Tablets 2315

Dicumarol (Prolonged prothrombin time; adjustment of dosage of oral anticoagulants may be required).
No products indexed under this heading.

Etodolac (Concomitant use with other NSAIDs is not recommended due to the increased possibility of gastrointestinal toxicity, with little or no increase in efficacy). Products include:
Lodine 3528
Lodine XL Extended-Release Tablets 3530

Fenoprofen Calcium (Concomitant use with other NSAIDs is not recommended due to the increased possibility of gastrointestinal toxicity, with little or no increase in efficacy).
No products indexed under this heading.

Flurbiprofen (Concomitant use with other NSAIDs is not recommended due to the increased possibility of gastrointestinal toxicity, with little or no increase in efficacy).
No products indexed under this heading.

Furosemide (Decreased hyperuricemic effect). Products include:
Furosemide Tablets 2284

Hydrochlorothiazide (Decreased hyperuricemic effect; increased plasma levels). Products include:
Accuretic Tablets 2614
Aldoril Tablets 2039
Atacand HCT Tablets 597
Avalide Tablets 1070
Diovan HCT Tablets 2338
Dyazide Capsules 1515
HydroDIURIL Tablets 2108
Hyzaar 2109
Inderide Tablets 3517
Inderide LA Long-Acting Capsules 3519
Lotensin HCT Tablets 2367
Maxzide 1008
Micardis HCT Tablets 1051
Microzide Capsules 3414
Moduretic Tablets 2138
Monopril HCT 1094
Prinzide Tablets 2168
Timolide Tablets 2187
Uniretic Tablets 3178
Vaseretic Tablets 2204
Zestoretic Tablets 695
Ziac Tablets 1887

Ibuprofen (Concomitant use with other NSAIDs is not recommended due to the increased possibility of gastrointestinal toxicity, with little or no increase in efficacy). Products include:
Advil 771
Children's Advil Oral Suspension 773
Children's Advil Chewable Tablets 773
Advil Cold and Sinus Caplets 771
Advil Cold and Sinus Tablets 771
Advil Flu & Body Ache Caplets 772
Infants' Advil Drops 773
Junior Strength Advil Tablets 773
Junior Strength Advil Chewable Tablets 773
Advil Migraine Liquigels 772
Children's Motrin Oral Suspension and Chewable Tablets 2006
Children's Motrin Cold Oral Suspension 2007
Children's Motrin Oral Suspension 643
Motrin Suspension, Oral Drops, Chewable Tablets, and Caplets 2002
Infants' Motrin Concentrated Drops 2006
Junior Strength Motrin Caplets and Chewable Tablets 2006
Motrin IB Tablets, Caplets, and Gelcaps 2002
Motrin Migraine Pain Caplets 2005
Motrin Sinus Headache Caplets 2005
Vicoprofen Tablets 520

Indomethacin (Decreased renal clearance and significantly increased plasma levels of indomethacin; potential for fatal gastrointestinal hemorrhage; concomitant use with indomethacin is not recommended). Products include:
Indocin 2112

Indomethacin Sodium Trihydrate (Decreased renal clearance and significantly increased plasma levels of indomethacin; potential for fatal gastrointestinal hemorrhage; concomitant use with indomethacin is not recommended). Products include:
Indocin I.V. 2115

Ketoprofen (Concomitant use with other NSAIDs is not recommended due to the increased possibility of gastrointestinal toxicity, with little or no increase in efficacy). Products include:
Orudis Capsules 3548
Orudis KT Tablets 778
Oruvail Capsules 3548

Ketorolac Tromethamine (Concomitant use with other NSAIDs is not recommended due to the increased possibility of gastrointestinal toxicity, with little or no increase in efficacy). Products include:
Acular Ophthalmic Solution 544
Acular PF Ophthalmic Solution 544
Toradol 3018

Magaldrate (Reduced plasma levels of Dolobid).
No products indexed under this heading.

Magnesium Hydroxide (Reduced plasma levels of Dolobid). Products include:
Ex•Lax Milk of Magnesia Liquid 670
Maalox Antacid/Anti-Gas Oral Suspension 673
Maalox Max Maximum Strength Antacid/Anti-Gas Liquid 2300
Maalox Regular Strength Antacid/Antigas Liquid 2300
Mylanta Fast-Acting 1813
Mylanta 1813
Pepcid Complete Chewable Tablets 1815
Phillips' Chewable Tablets 615
Phillips' Milk of Magnesia Liquid (Original, Cherry, & Mint) 616
Rolaids Tablets 706
Extra Strength Rolaids Tablets 706
Vanquish Caplets 617

Magnesium Oxide (Reduced plasma levels of Dolobid). Products include:
Beelith Tablets 946
Mag-Ox 400 Tablets 1024
Uro-Mag Capsules 1024

Meclofenamate Sodium (Concomitant use with other NSAIDs is not recommended due to the increased possibility of gastrointestinal toxicity, with little or no increase in efficacy).
No products indexed under this heading.

Mefenamic Acid (Concomitant use with other NSAIDs is not recommended due to the increased possibility of gastrointestinal toxicity, with little or no increase in efficacy). Products include:
Ponstel Capsules 1356

Meloxicam (Concomitant use with other NSAIDs is not recommended due to the increased possibility of gastrointestinal toxicity, with little or no increase in efficacy). Products include:
Mobic Tablets 1054

Methotrexate Sodium (Decreased tubular secretion of methotrexate and potentiation of its toxicity).
No products indexed under this heading.

Nabumetone (Concomitant use with other NSAIDs is not recommended due to the increased possibility of gastrointestinal toxicity, with little or no increase in efficacy). Products include:
Relafen Tablets 1617

Naproxen (Significant decrease in urinary excretion of naproxen and its glucuronide metabolite; concomitant use with other NSAIDs is not recommended due to the increased possibility of gastrointestinal toxicity, with little or no increase in efficacy). Products include:
EC-Naprosyn Delayed-Release Tablets 2967
Naprosyn Suspension 2967
Naprosyn Tablets 2967

Naproxen Sodium (Significant decrease in urinary excretion of naproxen and its glucuronide metabolite; concomitant use with other NSAIDs is not recommended due to the increased possibility of gastrointestinal toxicity, with little or no increase in efficacy). Products include:
Aleve Tablets, Caplets and Gelcaps 602
Aleve Cold & Sinus Caplets 603
Anaprox Tablets 2967
Anaprox DS Tablets 2967
Naprelan Tablets 1293

Nephrotoxic Drugs (Overt renal decompensation).

Oxaprozin (Concomitant use with other NSAIDs is not recommended due to the increased possibility of gastrointestinal toxicity, with little or no increase in efficacy).
No products indexed under this heading.

Phenprocoumon (Prolonged prothrombin time).
No products indexed under this heading.

Phenylbutazone (Concomitant use with other NSAIDs is not recommended due to the increased possibility of gastrointestinal toxicity, with little or no increase in efficacy).
No products indexed under this heading.

Piroxicam (Concomitant use with other NSAIDs is not recommended due to the increased possibility of gastrointestinal toxicity, with little or no increase in efficacy). Products include:
Feldene Capsules 2685

Rofecoxib (Concomitant use with other NSAIDs is not recommended due to the increased possibility of gastrointestinal toxicity, with little or no increase in efficacy). Products include:
Vioxx 2213

Sodium Bicarbonate (Reduced plasma levels of Dolobid). Products include:
Alka-Seltzer 603
Alka-Seltzer Lemon Lime Antacid and Pain Reliever Effervescent Tablets 603
Alka-Seltzer Extra Strength Antacid and Pain Reliever Effervescent Tablets 603
Alka-Seltzer Heartburn Relief Tablets 604
Ceo-Two Evacuant Suppository 618
Colyte with Flavor Packs for Oral Solution 3170
GoLYTELY and Pineapple Flavor GoLYTELY for Oral Solution 1068
NuLYTELY, Cherry Flavor, Lemon-Lime Flavor, and Orange Flavor NuLYTELY for Oral Solution 1068

Sulindac (Lowering of the plasma levels of active sulindac sulfide metabolite by approximately one-third; concomitant use with other NSAIDs is not recommended due to the increased possibility of gastrointestinal toxicity, with little or no increase in efficacy). Products include:
Clinoril Tablets 2053

Tolmetin Sodium (Concomitant use with other NSAIDs is not recommended due to the increased possibility of gastrointestinal toxicity, with little or no increase in efficacy). Products include:
Tolectin 2589

Warfarin Sodium (Prolonged prothrombin time; adjustment of dosage of oral anticoagulants may be required). Products include:
Coumadin for Injection 1243
Coumadin Tablets 1243
Warfarin Sodium Tablets, USP 3302

DOLOPHINE HYDROCHLORIDE TABLETS

(Methadone Hydrochloride) 3056
May interact with central nervous system depressants, monoamine oxidase inhibitors, tricyclic antidepressants, and certain other agents. Compounds in these categories include:

Alfentanil Hydrochloride (Co-administration with other CNS depressants may result in respiratory depression, hypotension, and profound sedation or coma).
No products indexed under this heading.

Alprazolam (Co-administration with other CNS depressants may result in respiratory depression, hypotension, and profound sedation or coma). Products include:
Xanax Tablets 2865

Amitriptyline Hydrochloride (Co-administration with other CNS depressants, including tricyclic antidepressants may result in respiratory depression, hypotension, and profound sedation or coma). Products include:

Etrafon 3115
Limbitrol 1738

Amoxapine (Co-administration with other CNS depressants, including tricyclic antidepressants may result in respiratory depression, hypotension, and profound sedation or coma).
No products indexed under this heading.

Aprobarbital (Co-administration with other CNS depressants may result in respiratory depression, hypotension, and profound sedation or coma).
No products indexed under this heading.

Buprenorphine Hydrochloride (Co-administration with other CNS depressants may result in respiratory depression, hypotension, and profound sedation or coma).
Products include:
Buprenex Injectable 2918

Buspirone Hydrochloride (Co-administration with other CNS depressants may result in respiratory depression, hypotension, and profound sedation or coma).
No products indexed under this heading.

Butabarbital (Co-administration with other CNS depressants may result in respiratory depression, hypotension, and profound sedation or coma).
No products indexed under this heading.

Butalbital (Co-administration with other CNS depressants may result in respiratory depression, hypotension, and profound sedation or coma).
Products include:
Phrenilin 578
Sedapap Tablets 50 mg/650 mg ... 2225

Chlordiazepoxide (Co-administration with other CNS depressants may result in respiratory depression, hypotension, and profound sedation or coma).
Products include:
Limbitrol 1738

Chlordiazepoxide Hydrochloride (Co-administration with other CNS depressants may result in respiratory depression, hypotension, and profound sedation or coma).
Products include:
Librium Capsules 1736
Librium for Injection 1737

Chlorpromazine (Co-administration with other CNS depressants may result in respiratory depression, hypotension, and profound sedation or coma). Products include:
Thorazine Suppositories 1656

Chlorpromazine Hydrochloride (Co-administration with other CNS depressants may result in respiratory depression, hypotension, and profound sedation or coma).
Products include:
Thorazine 1656

Chlorprothixene (Co-administration with other CNS depressants may result in respiratory depression, hypotension, and profound sedation or coma).
No products indexed under this heading.

Chlorprothixene Hydrochloride (Co-administration with other CNS depressants may result in respiratory depression, hypotension, and profound sedation or coma).
No products indexed under this heading.

Chlorprothixene Lactate (Co-administration with other CNS depressants may result in respiratory depression, hypotension, and profound sedation or coma).
No products indexed under this heading.

Clomipramine Hydrochloride (Co-administration with other CNS depressants, including tricyclic antidepressants may result in respiratory depression, hypotension, and profound sedation or coma).
No products indexed under this heading.

Clorazepate Dipotassium (Co-administration with other CNS depressants may result in respiratory depression, hypotension, and profound sedation or coma).
Products include:
Tranxene 511

Clozapine (Co-administration with other CNS depressants may result in respiratory depression, hypotension, and profound sedation or coma).
Products include:
Clozaril Tablets 2319

Codeine Phosphate (Co-administration with other CNS depressants may result in respiratory depression, hypotension, and profound sedation or coma).
Products include:
Phenergan with Codeine Syrup 3557
Phenergan VC with Codeine Syrup .. 3561
Robitussin A-C Syrup 2942
Robitussin-DAC Syrup 2942
Ryna-C Liquid .... ■■ 768
Soma Compound w/Codeine Tablets 3355
Tussi-Organidin NR Liquid 3350
Tussi-Organidin-S NR Liquid 3350
Tylenol with Codeine 2595

Desflurane (Co-administration with other CNS depressants may result in respiratory depression, hypotension, and profound sedation or coma).
Products include:
Suprane Liquid for Inhalation 874

Desipramine Hydrochloride (Co-administration has produced increased blood levels of desipramine). Products include:
Norpramin Tablets 755

Dezocine (Co-administration with other CNS depressants may result in respiratory depression, hypotension, and profound sedation or coma).
No products indexed under this heading.

Diazepam (Co-administration with other CNS depressants may result in respiratory depression, hypotension, and profound sedation or coma).
Products include:
Valium Injectable 3026
Valium Tablets 3047

Doxepin Hydrochloride (Co-administration with other CNS depressants, including tricyclic antidepressants may result in respiratory depression, hypotension, and profound sedation or coma).
Products include:
Sinequan 2713

Droperidol (Co-administration with other CNS depressants may result in respiratory depression, hypotension, and profound sedation or coma).
No products indexed under this heading.

Enflurane (Co-administration with other CNS depressants may result in respiratory depression, hypotension, and profound sedation or coma).
No products indexed under this heading.

Estazolam (Co-administration with other CNS depressants may result in respiratory depression, hypotension, and profound sedation or coma).
Products include:
ProSom Tablets 500

Ethchlorvynol (Co-administration with other CNS depressants may result in respiratory depression, hypotension, and profound sedation or coma).
No products indexed under this heading.

Ethinamate (Co-administration with other CNS depressants may result in respiratory depression, hypotension, and profound sedation or coma).
No products indexed under this heading.

Fentanyl (Co-administration with other CNS depressants may result in respiratory depression, hypotension, and profound sedation or coma).
Products include:
Duragesic Transdermal System 1786

Fentanyl Citrate (Co-administration with other CNS depressants may result in respiratory depression, hypotension, and profound sedation or coma). Products include:
Actiq 1184

Fluphenazine Decanoate (Co-administration with other CNS depressants may result in respiratory depression, hypotension, and profound sedation or coma).
No products indexed under this heading.

Fluphenazine Enanthate (Co-administration with other CNS depressants may result in respiratory depression, hypotension, and profound sedation or coma).
No products indexed under this heading.

Fluphenazine Hydrochloride (Co-administration with other CNS depressants may result in respiratory depression, hypotension, and profound sedation or coma).
No products indexed under this heading.

Flurazepam Hydrochloride (Co-administration with other CNS depressants may result in respiratory depression, hypotension, and profound sedation or coma).
No products indexed under this heading.

Glutethimide (Co-administration with other CNS depressants may result in respiratory depression, hypotension, and profound sedation or coma).
No products indexed under this heading.

Haloperidol (Co-administration with other CNS depressants may result in respiratory depression, hypotension, and profound sedation or coma).
Products include:
Haldol Injection, Tablets and Concentrate 2533

Haloperidol Decanoate (Co-administration with other CNS depressants may result in respiratory depression, hypotension, and profound sedation or coma).
Products include:
Haldol Decanoate 2535

Hydrocodone Bitartrate (Co-administration with other CNS depressants may result in respiratory depression, hypotension, and profound sedation or coma).
Products include:
Hycodan 1316
Hycomine Compound Tablets 1317
Hycotuss Expectorant Syrup 1318
Lortab 3319
Lortab Elixir 3317
Maxidone Tablets CIII 3399
Norco 5/325 Tablets CIII 3424
Norco 7.5/325 Tablets CIII 3425
Norco 10/325 Tablets CIII 3427
Norco 10/325 Tablets CIII 3425
Vicodin Tablets 516
Vicodin ES Tablets 517
Vicodin HP Tablets 518
Vicodin Tuss Expectorant 519
Vicoprofen Tablets 520
Zydone Tablets 1330

Hydrocodone Polistirex (Co-administration with other CNS depressants may result in respiratory depression, hypotension, and profound sedation or coma).
Products include:
Tussionex Pennkinetic Extended-Release Suspension 1174

Hydromorphone Hydrochloride (Co-administration with other CNS depressants may result in respiratory depression, hypotension, and profound sedation or coma).
Products include:
Dilaudid 441
Dilaudid Oral Liquid 445
Dilaudid Powder 441
Dilaudid Rectal Suppositories 441
Dilaudid Tablets 441
Dilaudid Tablets - 8 mg 445
Dilaudid-HP 443

Hydroxyzine Hydrochloride (Co-administration with other CNS depressants may result in respiratory depression, hypotension, and profound sedation or coma).
Products include:
Atarax Tablets & Syrup 2667
Vistaril Intramuscular Solution 2738

Imipramine Hydrochloride (Co-administration with other CNS depressants, including tricyclic antidepressants may result in respiratory depression, hypotension, and profound sedation or coma).
No products indexed under this heading.

Imipramine Pamoate (Co-administration with other CNS depressants, including tricyclic antidepressants may result in respiratory depression, hypotension, and profound sedation or coma).
No products indexed under this heading.

Isocarboxazid (Co-administration with other narcotic analgesics, such as meperidine, has precipitated severe reactions; similar reactions have not been reported with methadone, however, the possibility does exist).
No products indexed under this heading.

Isoflurane (Co-administration with other CNS depressants may result in respiratory depression, hypotension, and profound sedation or coma).
No products indexed under this heading.

Ketamine Hydrochloride (Co-administration with other CNS depressants may result in respiratory depression, hypotension, and profound sedation or coma).
No products indexed under this heading.

Levomethadyl Acetate Hydrochloride (Co-administration with other CNS depressants may result in respiratory depression, hypotension, and profound sedation or coma).
No products indexed under this heading.

Levorphanol Tartrate (Co-administration with other CNS depressants may result in respiratory depression, hypotension, and profound sedation or coma).
Products include:
Levo-Dromoran 1734
Levorphanol Tartrate Tablets 3059

Lorazepam (Co-administration with other CNS depressants may result in respiratory depression, hypotension, and profound sedation or coma).
Products include:
Ativan Injection 3478
Ativan Tablets 3482

Loxapine Hydrochloride (Co-administration with other CNS depressants may result in respiratory depression, hypotension, and profound sedation or coma).
No products indexed under this heading.

Loxapine Succinate (Co-administration with other CNS depressants may result in respira-

tory depression, hypotension, and profound sedation or coma). Products include:
Loxitane Capsules ... 3398

Maprotiline Hydrochloride (Co-administration with other CNS depressants, including tricyclic anti-depressants may result in respiratory depression, hypotension, and profound sedation or coma).
No products indexed under this heading.

Meperidine Hydrochloride (Co-administration with other CNS depressants may result in respiratory depression, hypotension, and profound sedation or coma). Products include:
Demerol ... 3079
Mepergan Injection ... 3539

Mephobarbital (Co-administration with other CNS depressants may result in respiratory depression, hypotension, and profound sedation or coma).
No products indexed under this heading.

Meprobamate (Co-administration with other CNS depressants may result in respiratory depression, hypotension, and profound sedation or coma). Products include:
Miltown Tablets ... 3349

Mesoridazine Besylate (Co-administration with other CNS depressants may result in respiratory depression, hypotension, and profound sedation or coma). Products include:
Serentil ... 1057

Methohexital Sodium (Co-administration with other CNS depressants may result in respiratory depression, hypotension, and profound sedation or coma). Products include:
Brevital Sodium for Injection, USP .. 1815

Methotrimeprazine (Co-administration with other CNS depressants may result in respiratory depression, hypotension, and profound sedation or coma).
No products indexed under this heading.

Methoxyflurane (Co-administration with other CNS depressants may result in respiratory depression, hypotension, and profound sedation or coma).
No products indexed under this heading.

Midazolam Hydrochloride (Co-administration with other CNS depressants may result in respiratory depression, hypotension, and profound sedation or coma). Products include:
Versed Injection ... 3027
Versed Syrup ... 3033

Moclobemide (Co-administration with other narcotic analgesics, such as meperidine, has precipitated severe reactions; similar reactions have not been reported with methadone, however, the possibility does exist).
No products indexed under this heading.

Molindone Hydrochloride (Co-administration with other CNS depressants may result in respiratory depression, hypotension, and profound sedation or coma). Products include:
Moban ... 1320

Morphine Sulfate (Co-administration with other CNS depressants may result in respiratory depression, hypotension, and profound sedation or coma). Products include:
Astramorph/PF Injection, USP (Preservative-Free) ... 594
Duramorph Injection ... 1312
Infumorph 200 and Infumorph 500 Sterile Solutions ... 1314
Kadian Capsules ... 1335
MS Contin Tablets ... 2896
MSIR ... 2898
Oramorph SR Tablets ... 3062
Roxanol ... 3066

Nortriptyline Hydrochloride (Co-administration with other CNS depressants, including tricyclic anti-depressants may result in respiratory depression, hypotension, and profound sedation or coma).
No products indexed under this heading.

Olanzapine (Co-administration with other CNS depressants may result in respiratory depression, hypotension, and profound sedation or coma). Products include:
Zyprexa Tablets ... 1973
Zyprexa ZYDIS Orally Disintegrating Tablets ... 1973

Oxazepam (Co-administration with other CNS depressants may result in respiratory depression, hypotension, and profound sedation or coma).
No products indexed under this heading.

Oxycodone Hydrochloride (Co-administration with other CNS depressants may result in respiratory depression, hypotension, and profound sedation or coma). Products include:
OxyContin Tablets ... 2912
OxyFast Oral Concentrate Solution . 2916
OxyIR Capsules ... 2916
Percocet Tablets ... 1326
Percodan Tablets ... 1327
Percolone Tablets ... 1327
Roxicodone ... 3067
Tylox Capsules ... 2597

Pargyline Hydrochloride (Co-administration with other narcotic analgesics, such as meperidine, has precipitated severe reactions; similar reactions have not been reported with methadone, however, the possibility does exist).
No products indexed under this heading.

Pentobarbital Sodium (Co-administration with other CNS depressants may result in respiratory depression, hypotension, and profound sedation or coma). Products include:
Nembutal Sodium Solution ... 485

Perphenazine (Co-administration with other CNS depressants may result in respiratory depression, hypotension, and profound sedation or coma). Products include:
Etrafon ... 3115
Trilafon ... 3160

Phenelzine Sulfate (Co-administration with other narcotic analgesics, such as meperidine, has precipitated severe reactions; similar reactions have not been reported with methadone, however, the possibility does exist). Products include:
Nardil Tablets ... 2653

Phenobarbital (Co-administration with other CNS depressants may result in respiratory depression, hypotension, and profound sedation or coma). Products include:
Arco-Lase Plus Tablets ... 592
Donnatal ... 2929
Donnatal Extentabs ... 2930

Prazepam (Co-administration with other CNS depressants may result in respiratory depression, hypotension, and profound sedation or coma).
No products indexed under this heading.

Procarbazine Hydrochloride (Co-administration with other narcotic analgesics, such as meperidine, has precipitated severe reactions; similar reactions have not been reported with methadone, however, the possibility does exist). Products include:
Matulane Capsules ... 3246

Prochlorperazine (Co-administration with other CNS depressants may result in respiratory depression, hypotension, and profound sedation or coma). Products include:
Compazine ... 1505

Promethazine Hydrochloride (Co-administration with other CNS depressants may result in respiratory depression, hypotension, and profound sedation or coma). Products include:
Mepergan Injection ... 3539
Phenergan Injection ... 3553
Phenergan ... 3556
Phenergan Syrup ... 3554
Phenergan with Codeine Syrup ... 3557
Phenergan with Dextromethorphan Syrup ... 3559
Phenergan VC Syrup ... 3560
Phenergan VC with Codeine Syrup .. 3561

Propofol (Co-administration with other CNS depressants may result in respiratory depression, hypotension, and profound sedation or coma). Products include:
Diprivan Injectable Emulsion ... 667

Propoxyphene Hydrochloride (Co-administration with other CNS depressants may result in respiratory depression, hypotension, and profound sedation or coma). Products include:
Darvon Pulvules ... 1909
Darvon Compound-65 Pulvules ... 1910

Propoxyphene Napsylate (Co-administration with other CNS depressants may result in respiratory depression, hypotension, and profound sedation or coma). Products include:
Darvon-N/Darvocet-N ... 1907
Darvon-N Tablets ... 1912

Protriptyline Hydrochloride (Co-administration with other CNS depressants, including tricyclic anti-depressants may result in respiratory depression, hypotension, and profound sedation or coma). Products include:
Vivactil Tablets ... 2446
Vivactil Tablets ... 2217

Quazepam (Co-administration with other CNS depressants may result in respiratory depression, hypotension, and profound sedation or coma).
No products indexed under this heading.

Quetiapine Fumarate (Co-administration with other CNS depressants may result in respiratory depression, hypotension, and profound sedation or coma). Products include:
Seroquel Tablets ... 684

Remifentanil Hydrochloride (Co-administration with other CNS depressants may result in respiratory depression, hypotension, and profound sedation or coma).
No products indexed under this heading.

Rifampin (Co-administration may possibly reduce the blood concentration of methadone to a degree sufficient to produce withdrawal symptoms). Products include:
Rifadin ... 765
Rifamate Capsules ... 767
Rifater Tablets ... 769

Risperidone (Co-administration with other CNS depressants may result in respiratory depression, hypotension, and profound sedation or coma). Products include:
Risperdal ... 1796

Secobarbital Sodium (Co-administration with other CNS depressants may result in respiratory depression, hypotension, and profound sedation or coma).
No products indexed under this heading.

Selegiline Hydrochloride (Co-administration with other narcotic analgesics, such as meperidine, has precipitated severe reactions; similar reactions have not been reported with methadone, however, the possibility does exist). Products include:
Eldepryl Capsules ... 3266

Sevoflurane (Co-administration with other CNS depressants may result in respiratory depression, hypotension, and profound sedation or coma).
No products indexed under this heading.

Sufentanil Citrate (Co-administration with other CNS depressants may result in respiratory depression, hypotension, and profound sedation or coma).
No products indexed under this heading.

Temazepam (Co-administration with other CNS depressants may result in respiratory depression, hypotension, and profound sedation or coma).
No products indexed under this heading.

Thiamylal Sodium (Co-administration with other CNS depressants may result in respiratory depression, hypotension, and profound sedation or coma).
No products indexed under this heading.

Thioridazine Hydrochloride (Co-administration with other CNS depressants may result in respiratory depression, hypotension, and profound sedation or coma). Products include:
Thioridazine Hydrochloride Tablets ... 2289

Thiothixene (Co-administration with other CNS depressants may result in respiratory depression, hypotension, and profound sedation or coma). Products include:
Navane Capsules ... 2701
Thiothixene Capsules ... 2290

Tranylcypromine Sulfate (Co-administration with other narcotic analgesics, such as meperidine, has precipitated severe reactions; similar reactions have not been reported with methadone, however, the possibility does exist). Products include:
Parnate Tablets ... 1607

Triazolam (Co-administration with other CNS depressants may result in respiratory depression, hypotension, and profound sedation or coma). Products include:
Halcion Tablets ... 2823

Trifluoperazine Hydrochloride (Co-administration with other CNS depressants may result in respiratory depression, hypotension, and profound sedation or coma). Products include:
Stelazine ... 1640

Trimipramine Maleate (Co-administration with other CNS depressants, including tricyclic anti-depressants may result in respiratory depression, hypotension, and profound sedation or coma). Products include:
Surmontil Capsules ... 3595

Zaleplon (Co-administration with other CNS depressants may result in respiratory depression, hypotension, and profound sedation or coma). Products include:
Sonata Capsules ... 3591

Ziprasidone Hydrochloride (Co-administration with other CNS depressants may result in respiratory depression, hypotension, and profound sedation or coma). Products include:
Geodon Capsules ... 2688

Zolpidem Tartrate (Co-administration with other CNS depressants may result in respiratory depression, hypotension, and profound sedation or coma). Products include:

Ambien Tablets 3191

Food Interactions

Alcohol (Concurrent use with other CNS depressants may result in respiratory depression, hypotension, and profound sedation or coma).

DOMEBORO POWDER PACKETS

(Aluminum Sulfate) ..... ▣611
None cited in PDR database.

DOMEBORO EFFERVESCENT TABLETS

(Aluminum Sulfate) ..... ▣611
None cited in PDR database.

DONNAGEL LIQUID

(Attapulgite) ..... ▣789
None cited in PDR database.

DONNATAL CAPSULES

(Atropine Sulfate, Hyoscyamine Sulfate, Phenobarbital, Scopolamine Hydrobromide) 2929
May interact with oral anticoagulants. Compounds in these categories include:

Dicumarol (Decreased phenobarbital effect).
No products indexed under this heading.

Warfarin Sodium (Decreased phenobarbital effect). Products include:
Coumadin for Injection 1243
Coumadin Tablets 1243
Warfarin Sodium Tablets, USP 3302

DONNATAL ELIXIR

(Atropine Sulfate, Hyoscyamine Sulfate, Phenobarbital, Scopolamine Hydrobromide) 2929
See Donnatal Capsules

DONNATAL EXTENTABS

(Atropine Sulfate, Hyoscyamine Sulfate, Phenobarbital, Scopolamine Hydrobromide) 2930
May interact with oral anticoagulants. Compounds in these categories include:

Dicumarol (Decreased phenobarbital effect).
No products indexed under this heading.

Warfarin Sodium (Decreased phenobarbital effect). Products include:
Coumadin for Injection 1243
Coumadin Tablets 1243
Warfarin Sodium Tablets, USP 3302

DONNATAL TABLETS

(Atropine Sulfate, Hyoscyamine Sulfate, Phenobarbital, Scopolamine Hydrobromide) 2929
See Donnatal Capsules

DONNAZYME TABLETS

(Pancreatin) 2931
None cited in PDR database.

DOPRAM INJECTABLE

(Doxapram Hydrochloride) 2931
May interact with inhalant anesthetics, monoamine oxidase inhibitors, muscle relaxants, sympathomimetics, and certain other agents. Compounds in these categories include:

Albuterol (Additive pressor effect). Products include:
Proventil Inhalation Aerosol 3142
Ventolin Inhalation Aerosol and Refill 1679

Albuterol Sulfate (Additive pressor effect). Products include:
AccuNeb Inhalation Solution 1230
Combivent Inhalation Aerosol 1041
DuoNeb Inhalation Solution 1233
Proventil Inhalation Solution 0.083% 3146
Proventil Repetabs Tablets 3148
Proventil Solution for Inhalation 0.5% 3144
Proventil HFA Inhalation Aerosol 3150
Ventolin HFA Inhalation Aerosol 3618
Volmax Extended-Release Tablets 2276

Atracurium Besylate (Residual effects masked by Dopram).
No products indexed under this heading.

Baclofen (Residual effects masked by Dopram).
No products indexed under this heading.

Carisoprodol (Residual effects masked by Dopram). Products include:
Soma Tablets 3353
Soma Compound Tablets 3354
Soma Compound w/Codeine Tablets 3355

Chlorzoxazone (Residual effects masked by Dopram). Products include:
Parafon Forte DSC Caplets 2582

Cisatracurium Besylate (Residual effects masked by Dopram).
No products indexed under this heading.

Cyclobenzaprine Hydrochloride (Residual effects masked by Dopram). Products include:
Flexeril Tablets 572
Flexeril Tablets 2094

Dantrolene Sodium (Residual effects masked by Dopram). Products include:
Dantrium Capsules 2885
Dantrium Intravenous 2886

Desflurane (Increased epinephrine release). Products include:
Suprane Liquid for Inhalation 874

Dobutamine Hydrochloride (Additive pressor effect). Products include:
Dobutrex Solution Vials 1914

Dopamine Hydrochloride (Additive pressor effect).
No products indexed under this heading.

Doxacurium Chloride (Residual effects masked by Dopram).
No products indexed under this heading.

Enflurane (Increased epinephrine release).
No products indexed under this heading.

Ephedrine Hydrochloride (Additive pressor effect). Products include:
Primatene Tablets ..... ▣780

Ephedrine Sulfate (Additive pressor effect).
No products indexed under this heading.

Ephedrine Tannate (Additive pressor effect). Products include:
Rynatuss Pediatric Suspension 3353
Rynatuss Tablets 3353

Epinephrine (Additive pressor effect). Products include:
Epifrin Sterile Ophthalmic Solution ..... ⊙235
EpiPen 1236
Primatene Mist ..... ▣779
Xylocaine with Epinephrine Injection 653

Epinephrine Bitartrate (Additive pressor effect). Products include:
Sensorcaine 643

Epinephrine Hydrochloride (Additive pressor effect).
No products indexed under this heading.

Halothane (Increased epinephrine release). Products include:
Fluothane Inhalation 3508

Isocarboxazid (Additive pressor effect).
No products indexed under this heading.

Isoflurane (Increased epinephrine release).
No products indexed under this heading.

Isoproterenol Hydrochloride (Additive pressor effect).
No products indexed under this heading.

Isoproterenol Sulfate (Additive pressor effect).
No products indexed under this heading.

Levalbuterol Hydrochloride (Additive pressor effect). Products include:
Xopenex Inhalation Solution 3207

Metaproterenol Sulfate (Additive pressor effect). Products include:
Alupent 1029

Metaraminol Bitartrate (Additive pressor effect). Products include:
Aramine Injection 2043

Metaxalone (Residual effects masked by Dopram). Products include:
Skelaxin Tablets 1301

Methocarbamol (Residual effects masked by Dopram). Products include:
Robaxin Injectable 2938
Robaxin Tablets 2939
Robaxisal Tablets 2939

Methoxamine Hydrochloride (Additive pressor effect).
No products indexed under this heading.

Methoxyflurane (Increased epinephrine release).
No products indexed under this heading.

Metocurine Iodide (Residual effects masked by Dopram).
No products indexed under this heading.

Mivacurium Chloride (Residual effects masked by Dopram).
No products indexed under this heading.

Moclobemide (Additive pressor effect).
No products indexed under this heading.

Norepinephrine Bitartrate (Additive pressor effect).
No products indexed under this heading.

Orphenadrine Citrate (Residual effects masked by Dopram). Products include:
Norflex 1987

Pancuronium Bromide (Residual effects masked by Dopram).
No products indexed under this heading.

Pargyline Hydrochloride (Additive pressor effect).
No products indexed under this heading.

Phenelzine Sulfate (Additive pressor effect). Products include:
Nardil Tablets 2653

Phenylephrine Bitartrate (Additive pressor effect).
No products indexed under this heading.

Phenylephrine Hydrochloride (Additive pressor effect). Products include:
Afrin Nasal Decongestant Children's Pump Mist ..... ▣734
Extendryl 1361
Hycomine Compound Tablets 1317
Neo-Synephrine ..... ▣614
Phenergan VC Syrup 3560
Phenergan VC with Codeine Syrup 3561
Preparation H Cream ..... ▣778
Preparation H Cooling Gel ..... ▣778
Preparation H ..... ▣778
Vicks Sinex Nasal Spray and Ultra Fine Mist ..... ▣729

Phenylephrine Tannate (Additive pressor effect). Products include:
Ryna-12 S Suspension 3351
Reformulated Rynatan Pediatric Suspension 3352
Rynatuss Pediatric Suspension 3353
Rynatuss Tablets 3353

Phenylpropanolamine Hydrochloride (Additive pressor effect).
No products indexed under this heading.

Pirbuterol Acetate (Additive pressor effect). Products include:
Maxair Autohaler 1981
Maxair Inhaler 1984

Procarbazine Hydrochloride (Additive pressor effect). Products include:
Matulane Capsules 3246

Pseudoephedrine Hydrochloride (Additive pressor effect). Products include:
Actifed Cold & Allergy Tablets ..... ▣688
Actifed Cold & Sinus Caplets and Tablets ..... ▣688
Advil Cold and Sinus Caplets ..... ▣771
Advil Cold and Sinus Tablets ..... ▣771
Advil Flu & Body Ache Caplets ..... ▣772
Aleve Cold & Sinus Caplets ..... ▣603
Alka-Seltzer Plus Liqui-Gels ..... ▣604
Alka-Seltzer Plus Cold & Flu Medicine Liqui-Gels ..... ▣604
Alka-Seltzer Plus Cold & Sinus Medicine Liqui-Gels ..... ▣604
Allegra-D Extended-Release Tablets 714
BC Cold Powder ..... ▣619
Benadryl Allergy/Cold Tablets ..... ▣691
Benadryl Allergy/Congestion Tablets ..... ▣692
Benadryl Allergy & Sinus Liquid ..... ▣693
Benadryl Allergy & Sinus Fastmelt Tablets ..... ▣693
Benadryl Allergy Sinus Headache Caplets & Gelcaps ..... ▣693
Benadryl Severe Allergy & Sinus Headache Caplets ..... ▣694
Benadryl Children's Allergy/Cold Fastmelt Tablets ..... ▣692
Benylin Multi-Symptom Liquid ..... ▣697
Bromfed Capsules (Extended-Release) 2269
Bromfed-PD Capsules (Extended-Release) 2269
Children's Cēpacol Sore Throat ..... ▣788
Comtrex Acute Head Cold & Sinus Pressure Relief Tablets ..... ▣627
Comtrex Deep Chest Cold & Congestion Relief Softgels ..... ▣627
Comtrex Flu Therapy & Fever Relief Daytime Caplets ..... ▣628
Comtrex Flu Therapy & Fever Relief Nighttime Tablets ..... ▣628
Comtrex Maximum Strength Multi-Symptom Cold & Cough Relief Tablets and Caplets ..... ▣626
Contac Non-Drowsy 12 Hour Cold Caplets ..... ▣745
Contac Non-Drowsy Timed Release 12 Hour Cold Caplets ..... ▣746
Contac Severe Cold and Flu Caplets Maximum Strength ..... ▣746
Contac Severe Cold and Flu Caplets Non-Drowsy ..... ▣746
Dimetapp Elixir ..... ▣777
Dimetapp Cold and Fever Suspension ..... ▣775
Dimetapp DM Cold & Cough Elixir ..... ▣775
Dimetapp Nighttime Flu Liquid ..... ▣776
Dimetapp Non-Drowsy Flu Syrup ..... ▣777
Dimetapp Infant Drops Decongestant ..... ▣775
Dimetapp Infant Drops Decongestant Plus Cough ..... ▣776
Guaifed 2272
Kronofed-A 1341
Children's Motrin Cold Oral Suspension 2007
Motrin Sinus Headache Caplets 2005
PediaCare Cough-Cold Liquid ..... ▣719
PediaCare Infants' Drops Decongestant ..... ▣719
PediaCare Infants' Drops Decongestant Plus Cough ..... ▣719
PediaCare NightRest Cough-Cold Liquid ..... ▣719
Robitussin Cold Caplets Cold & Congestion ..... ▣780
Robitussin Cold Softgels Cold & Congestion ..... ▣780
Robitussin Cold Caplets Multi-Symptom Cold & Flu ..... ▣781
Robitussin Cold Softgels Multi-Symptom Cold & Flu ..... ▣781
Robitussin Cold Softgels Severe Congestion ..... ▣782

Robitussin Cough & Cold Infant Drops ▣782
Robitussin Maximum Strength Cough & Cold Liquid ▣785
Robitussin Pediatric Cough & Cold Formula Liquid ▣785
Robitussin Multi Symptom Honey Flu Liquid ▣785
Robitussin Nighttime Honey Flu Liquid ▣786
Robitussin-CF Liquid ▣783
Robitussin-DAC Syrup 2942
Robitussin-PE Liquid ▣782
Ryna ▣768
Semprex-D Capsules 1172
Singlet Caplets ▣761
Sinutab Non-Drying Liquid Caps ▣706
Sinutab Sinus Allergy Medication, Maximum Strength Formula, Tablets & Caplets ▣707
Sinutab Sinus Medication, Maximum Strength Without Drowsiness Formula, Tablets & Caplets ▣707
Sudafed 12 Hour Tablets ▣708
Sudafed 24 Hour Tablets ▣708
Children's Sudafed Cold & Cough Liquid ▣709
Children's Sudafed Nasal Decongestant Chewables ▣711
Children's Sudafed Nasal Decongestant Liquid Medication ▣711
Sudafed Cold & Allergy Tablets ▣708
Sudafed Cold & Cough Liquid Caps ▣709
Sudafed Cold & Sinus Liquid Caps ▣710
Sudafed Nasal Decongestant Tablets ▣710
Sudafed Non-Drying Sinus Liquid Caps ▣712
Sudafed Severe Cold ▣711
Sudafed Sinus Headache Caplets ▣712
Sudafed Sinus Headache Tablets ▣712
Tavist Sinus Non-Drowsy Coated Caplets ▣676
TheraFlu Regular Strength Cold & Cough Night Time Hot Liquid ▣676
TheraFlu Regular Strength Cold & Sore Throat Night Time Hot Liquid ▣676
TheraFlu Maximum Strength Flu & Congestion Non-Drowsy Hot Liquid ▣677
TheraFlu Maximum Strength Flu & Cough Night Time Hot Liquid ▣678
TheraFlu Maximum Strength Flu & Sore Throat Night Time Hot Liquid ▣677
TheraFlu Maximum Strength Severe Cold & Congestion Night Time Caplets ▣678
TheraFlu Maximum Strength Severe Cold & Congestion Night Time Hot Liquid ▣678
TheraFlu Maximum Strength Severe Cold & Congestion Non-Drowsy ▣679
Triaminic Allergy Congestion Liquid ▣680
Triaminic Chest Congestion Liquid ▣680
Triaminic Cold & Allergy Liquid ▣681
Triaminic Cold & Allergy Softchews ▣683
Triaminic Cold & Cough Liquid ▣681
Triaminic Cold & Cough Softchews ▣683
Triaminic Cold & Night Time Cough Liquid ▣681
Triaminic Cold, Cough & Fever Liquid ▣681
Triaminic Cough Liquid ▣682
Triaminic Cough & Congestion Liquid ▣682
Triaminic Cough & Sore Throat Liquid ▣682
Triaminic Cough & Sore Throat Softchews ▣684
Children's Tylenol Allergy-D Liquid 2014
Children's Tylenol Cold Suspension Liquid and Chewable Tablets 2015
Children's Tylenol Cold Plus Cough Suspension Liquid and Chewable Tablets 2015
Children's Tylenol Flu Suspension Liquid 2015
Children's Tylenol Sinus Suspension Liquid 2017
Infants' Tylenol Cold Decongestant and Fever Reducer Concentrated Drops 2015
Infants' Tylenol Cold Decongestant and Fever Reducer Concentrated Drops Plus Cough 2015
Tylenol Allergy Sinus 2010
Multi-Symptom Tylenol Cold Complete Formula Caplets 2010
Multi-Symptom Tylenol Cold Non-Drowsy Caplets and Gelcaps 2010
Multi-Symptom Tylenol Cold Severe Congestion Non-Drowsy Caplets 2011
Maximum Strength Tylenol Flu NightTime Gelcaps 2011
Maximum Strength Tylenol Flu NightTime Liquid 2011
Maximum Strength Tylenol Flu Non-Drowsy Gelcaps 2011
Maximum Strength Tylenol Sinus NightTime Caplets 2012
Maximum Strength Tylenol Sinus Non-Drowsy Geltabs, Gelcaps, Caplets, and Tablets 2012
Vicks 44D Cough & Head Congestion Relief Liquid ▣724
Vicks 44M Cough, Cold & Flu Relief Liquid ▣725
Pediatric Vicks 44m Cough & Cold Relief ▣728
Vicks DayQuil LiquiCaps/Liquid Multi-Symptom Cold/Flu Relief ▣727
Children's Vicks NyQuil Cold/Cough Relief ▣726
Vicks NyQuil LiquiCaps/Liquid Multi-Symptom Cold/Flu Relief, Original and Cherry Flavors ▣727
Zephrex Tablets 3091
Zephrex LA Tablets 3092
Zyrtec-D 12 Hour Extended Relief Tablets 2758

Pseudoephedrine Sulfate (Additive pressor effect). Products include:
Chlor-Trimeton Allergy/Decongestant Tablets ▣736
Claritin-D 12 Hour Extended Release Tablets 3102
Claritin-D 24 Hour Extended Release Tablets 3104
Coricidin 'D' Cold, Flu & Sinus Tablets ▣737
Drixoral Allergy/Sinus Extended-Release Tablets ▣741
Drixoral Cold & Allergy Sustained-Action Tablets ▣740
Drixoral Cold & Flu Extended-Release Tablets ▣740
Drixoral Nasal Decongestant Long-Acting Non-Drowsy Tablets ▣740
Rynatan Tablets 3351

Rapacuronium Bromide (Residual effects masked by Dopram).
No products indexed under this heading.

Rocuronium Bromide (Residual effects masked by Dopram). Products include:
Zemuron Injection 2491

Salmeterol Xinafoate (Additive pressor effect). Products include:
Advair Diskus 100/50 1448
Advair Diskus 250/50 1448
Advair Diskus 500/50 1448
Serevent Diskus 1637
Serevent Inhalation Aerosol 1633

Selegiline Hydrochloride (Additive pressor effect). Products include:
Eldepryl Capsules 3266

Succinylcholine Chloride (Residual effects masked by Dopram). Products include:
Anectine Injection 1476

Terbutaline Sulfate (Additive pressor effect). Products include:
Brethine Ampuls 2314
Brethine Tablets 2313

Tranylcypromine Sulfate (Additive pressor effect). Products include:
Parnate Tablets 1607

Vecuronium Bromide (Residual effects masked by Dopram). Products include:
Norcuron for Injection 2478

DORYX COATED PELLET FILLED CAPSULES

(Doxycycline Hyclate) 3357

May interact with antacids, oral anticoagulants, iron containing oral preparations, and penicillins. Compounds in these categories include:

Aluminum Carbonate (Co-administration with antacids may interfere with the oral absorption of tetracyclines; concurrent use should be avoided).
No products indexed under this heading.

Aluminum Hydroxide (Co-administration with antacids may interfere with the oral absorption of tetracyclines; concurrent use should be avoided). Products include:
Amphojel Suspension (Mint Flavor) ▣789
Gaviscon Extra Strength Liquid ▣751
Gaviscon Extra Strength Tablets ▣751
Gaviscon Regular Strength Liquid ▣751
Gaviscon Regular Strength Tablets ▣750
Maalox Antacid/Anti-Gas Oral Suspension ▣673
Maalox Max Maximum Strength Antacid/Anti-Gas Liquid 2300
Maalox Regular Strength Antacid/Antigas Liquid 2300
Mylanta 1813
Vanquish Caplets ▣617

Amoxicillin Trihydrate (Bacteriostatic drugs may interfere with the bactericidal action of penicillin; co-administration of tetracyclines with penicillin should be avoided).

Ampicillin (Bacteriostatic drugs may interfere with the bactericidal action of penicillin; co-administration of tetracyclines with penicillin should be avoided).
No products indexed under this heading.

Ampicillin Sodium (Bacteriostatic drugs may interfere with the bactericidal action of penicillin; co-administration of tetracyclines with penicillin should be avoided). Products include:
Unasyn for Injection 2728

Ampicillin Trihydrate (Bacteriostatic drugs may interfere with the bactericidal action of penicillin; co-administration of tetracyclines with penicillin should be avoided).
No products indexed under this heading.

Azlocillin Sodium (Bacteriostatic drugs may interfere with the bactericidal action of penicillin; co-administration of tetracyclines with penicillin should be avoided).
No products indexed under this heading.

Bacampicillin Hydrochloride (Bacteriostatic drugs may interfere with the bactericidal action of penicillin; co-administration of tetracyclines with penicillin should be avoided).
No products indexed under this heading.

Carbenicillin Disodium (Bacteriostatic drugs may interfere with the bactericidal action of penicillin; co-administration of tetracyclines with penicillin should be avoided).
No products indexed under this heading.

Carbenicillin Indanyl Sodium (Bacteriostatic drugs may interfere with the bactericidal action of penicillin; co-administration of tetracyclines with penicillin should be avoided). Products include:
Geocillin Tablets 2687

Dicloxacillin Sodium (Bacteriostatic drugs may interfere with the bactericidal action of penicillin; co-administration of tetracyclines with penicillin should be avoided).
No products indexed under this heading.

Dicumarol (Tetracyclines have been shown to depress plasma prothrombin activity, patients on anticoagulant therapy may require downward adjustment of their anticoagulant dosage).
No products indexed under this heading.

Ferrous Fumarate (Co-administration with iron-containing preparations may interfere with the oral absorption of tetracyclines; concurrent use should be avoided). Products include:
New Formulation Chromagen OB Capsules 3094
Loestrin Fe Tablets 2642
NataChew Tablets 3364

Ferrous Gluconate (Co-administration with iron-containing preparations may interfere with the oral absorption of tetracyclines; concurrent use should be avoided). Products include:
Fergon Iron Tablets ▣802

Ferrous Sulfate (Co-administration with iron-containing preparations may interfere with the oral absorption of tetracyclines; concurrent use should be avoided). Products include:
Feosol Tablets 1717
Slow Fe Tablets ▣827
Slow Fe with Folic Acid Tablets ▣828

Iron (Co-administration with iron-containing preparations may interfere with the oral absorption of tetracyclines; concurrent use should be avoided).
No products indexed under this heading.

Magaldrate (Co-administration with antacids may interfere with the oral absorption of tetracyclines; concurrent use should be avoided).
No products indexed under this heading.

Magnesium Hydroxide (Co-administration with antacids may interfere with the oral absorption of tetracyclines; concurrent use should be avoided). Products include:
Ex•Lax Milk of Magnesia Liquid ▣670
Maalox Antacid/Anti-Gas Oral Suspension ▣673
Maalox Max Maximum Strength Antacid/Anti-Gas Liquid 2300
Maalox Regular Strength Antacid/Antigas Liquid 2300
Mylanta Fast-Acting 1813
Mylanta 1813
Pepcid Complete Chewable Tablets 1815
Phillips' Chewable Tablets ▣615
Phillips' Milk of Magnesia Liquid (Original, Cherry, & Mint) ▣616
Rolaids Tablets ▣706
Extra Strength Rolaids Tablets ▣706
Vanquish Caplets ▣617

Magnesium Oxide (Co-administration with antacids may interfere with the oral absorption of tetracyclines; concurrent use should be avoided). Products include:
Beelith Tablets 946
Mag-Ox 400 Tablets 1024
Uro-Mag Capsules 1024

Mezlocillin Sodium (Bacteriostatic drugs may interfere with the bactericidal action of penicillin; co-administration of tetracyclines with penicillin should be avoided).
No products indexed under this heading.

Nafcillin Sodium (Bacteriostatic drugs may interfere with the bactericidal action of penicillin; co-administration of tetracyclines with penicillin should be avoided).
No products indexed under this heading.

Penicillin G Benzathine (Bacteriostatic drugs may interfere with the bactericidal action of penicillin; co-administration of tetracyclines with penicillin should be avoided). Products include:
Bicillin C-R 900/300 Injection 2240
Bicillin C-R Injection 2238
Bicillin L-A Injection 2242
Permapen Isoject 2706

Penicillin G Potassium (Bacteriostatic drugs may interfere with the bactericidal action of penicillin; co-

administration of tetracyclines with penicillin should be avoided). Products include:
- Pfizerpen for Injection 2707

Penicillin G Procaine (Bacteriostatic drugs may interfere with the bactericidal action of penicillin; co-administration of tetracyclines with penicillin should be avoided). Products include:
- Bicillin C-R 900/300 Injection 2240
- Bicillin C-R Injection 2238

Penicillin G Sodium (Bacteriostatic drugs may interfere with the bactericidal action of penicillin; co-administration of tetracyclines with penicillin should be avoided).
No products indexed under this heading.

Penicillin V Potassium (Bacteriostatic drugs may interfere with the bactericidal action of penicillin; co-administration of tetracyclines with penicillin should be avoided).
No products indexed under this heading.

Polysaccharide-Iron Complex (Co-administration with iron-containing preparations may interfere with the oral absorption of tetracyclines; concurrent use should be avoided). Products include:
- Niferex 3176
- Niferex-150 Capsules 3176
- Nu-Iron 150 Capsules 2224

Sodium Bicarbonate (Co-administration with antacids may interfere with the oral absorption of tetracyclines; concurrent use should be avoided). Products include:
- Alka-Seltzer ....▣603
- Alka-Seltzer Lemon Lime Antacid and Pain Reliever Effervescent Tablets ....▣603
- Alka-Seltzer Extra Strength Antacid and Pain Reliever Effervescent Tablets ....▣603
- Alka-Seltzer Heartburn Relief Tablets ....▣604
- Ceo-Two Evacuant Suppository ....▣618
- Colyte with Flavor Packs for Oral Solution 3170
- GoLYTELY and Pineapple Flavor GoLYTELY for Oral Solution 1068
- NuLYTELY, Cherry Flavor, Lemon-Lime Flavor, and Orange Flavor NuLYTELY for Oral Solution 1068

Ticarcillin Disodium (Bacteriostatic drugs may interfere with the bactericidal action of penicillin; co-administration of tetracyclines with penicillin should be avoided). Products include:
- Timentin Injection- ADD-Vantage Vial 1661
- Timentin Injection-Galaxy Container 1664
- Timentin Injection-Pharmacy Bulk Package 1666
- Timentin for Intravenous Administration 1658

Warfarin Sodium (Tetracyclines have been shown to depress plasma prothrombin activity, patients on anticoagulant therapy may require downward adjustment of their anticoagulant dosage). Products include:
- Coumadin for Injection 1243
- Coumadin Tablets 1243
- Warfarin Sodium Tablets, USP 3302

DOSTINEX TABLETS

(Cabergoline) 2804
May interact with dopamine D2 antagonists. Compounds in these categories include:

Chlorpromazine (Cabergoline is a dopamine receptor antagonist with a high affinity for D2 receptors; concurrent use with dopamine D2-antagonists is not recommended). Products include:
- Thorazine Suppositories 1656

Chlorpromazine Hydrochloride (Cabergoline is a dopamine receptor antagonist with a high affinity for D2 receptors; concurrent use with dopamine D2-antagonists is not recommended). Products include:
- Thorazine 1656

Chlorprothixene (Cabergoline is a dopamine receptor antagonist with a high affinity for D2 receptors; concurrent use with dopamine D2-antagonists is not recommended).
No products indexed under this heading.

Chlorprothixene Hydrochloride (Cabergoline is a dopamine receptor antagonist with a high affinity for D2 receptors; concurrent use with dopamine D2-antagonists is not recommended).
No products indexed under this heading.

Fluphenazine Decanoate (Cabergoline is a dopamine receptor antagonist with a high affinity for D2 receptors; concurrent use with dopamine D2-antagonists is not recommended).
No products indexed under this heading.

Fluphenazine Enanthate (Cabergoline is a dopamine receptor antagonist with a high affinity for D2 receptors; concurrent use with dopamine D2-antagonists is not recommended).
No products indexed under this heading.

Fluphenazine Hydrochloride (Cabergoline is a dopamine receptor antagonist with a high affinity for D2 receptors; concurrent use with dopamine D2-antagonists is not recommended).
No products indexed under this heading.

Haloperidol (Cabergoline is a dopamine receptor antagonist with a high affinity for D2 receptors; concurrent use with dopamine D2-antagonists is not recommended). Products include:
- Haldol Injection, Tablets and Concentrate 2533

Haloperidol Decanoate (Cabergoline is a dopamine receptor antagonist with a high affinity for D2 receptors; concurrent use with dopamine D2-antagonists is not recommended). Products include:
- Haldol Decanoate 2535

Loxapine Hydrochloride (Cabergoline is a dopamine receptor antagonist with a high affinity for D2 receptors; concurrent use with dopamine D2-antagonists is not recommended).
No products indexed under this heading.

Loxapine Succinate (Cabergoline is a dopamine receptor antagonist with a high affinity for D2 receptors; concurrent use with dopamine D2-antagonists is not recommended). Products include:
- Loxitane Capsules 3398

Mesoridazine Besylate (Cabergoline is a dopamine receptor antagonist with a high affinity for D2 receptors; concurrent use with dopamine D2-antagonists is not recommended). Products include:
- Serentil 1057

Methotrimeprazine (Cabergoline is a dopamine receptor antagonist with a high affinity for D2 receptors; concurrent use with dopamine D2-antagonists is not recommended).
No products indexed under this heading.

Metoclopramide Hydrochloride (Cabergoline is a dopamine receptor antagonist with a high affinity for D2 receptors; concurrent use with dopamine D2-antagonists is not recommended). Products include:
- Reglan 2935

Molindone Hydrochloride (Cabergoline is a dopamine receptor antagonist with a high affinity for D2 receptors; concurrent use with dopamine D2-antagonists is not recommended). Products include:
- Moban 1320

Perphenazine (Cabergoline is a dopamine receptor antagonist with a high affinity for D2 receptors; concurrent use with dopamine D2-antagonists is not recommended). Products include:
- Etrafon 3115
- Trilafon 3160

Prochlorperazine (Cabergoline is a dopamine receptor antagonist with a high affinity for D2 receptors; concurrent use with dopamine D2-antagonists is not recommended). Products include:
- Compazine 1505

Promethazine Hydrochloride (Cabergoline is a dopamine receptor antagonist with a high affinity for D2 receptors; concurrent use with dopamine D2-antagonists is not recommended). Products include:
- Mepergan Injection 3539
- Phenergan Injection 3553
- Phenergan 3556
- Phenergan Syrup 3554
- Phenergan with Codeine Syrup 3557
- Phenergan with Dextromethorphan Syrup 3559
- Phenergan VC Syrup 3560
- Phenergan VC with Codeine Syrup . 3561

Quetiapine Fumarate (Cabergoline is a dopamine receptor antagonist with a high affinity for D2 receptors; concurrent use with dopamine D2-antagonists is not recommended). Products include:
- Seroquel Tablets 684

Risperidone (Cabergoline is a dopamine receptor antagonist with a high affinity for D2 receptors; concurrent use with dopamine D2-antagonists is not recommended). Products include:
- Risperdal 1796

Thioridazine Hydrochloride (Cabergoline is a dopamine receptor antagonist with a high affinity for D2 receptors; concurrent use with dopamine D2-antagonists is not recommended). Products include:
- Thioridazine Hydrochloride Tablets 2289

Thiothixene (Cabergoline is a dopamine receptor antagonist with a high affinity for D2 receptors; concurrent use with dopamine D2-antagonists is not recommended). Products include:
- Navane Capsules 2701
- Thiothixene Capsules 2290

Trifluoperazine Hydrochloride (Cabergoline is a dopamine receptor antagonist with a high affinity for D2 receptors; concurrent use with dopamine D2-antagonists is not recommended). Products include:
- Stelazine 1640

DOVONEX CREAM

(Calcipotriene) 1116
None cited in PDR database.

DOVONEX OINTMENT

(Calcipotriene) 1117
None cited in PDR database.

DOVONEX SCALP SOLUTION

(Calcipotriene) 1118
None cited in PDR database.

DOXIL INJECTION

(Doxorubicin Hydrochloride) 566
May interact with antineoplastics and certain other agents. Compounds in these categories include:

Altretamine (Co-administration with the conventional formulation of doxorubicin results in potentiation of the toxicity of other anticancer therapies; this interaction may occur with Doxil). Products include:
- Hexalen Capsules 2226

Anastrozole (Co-administration with the conventional formulation of doxorubicin results in potentiation of the toxicity of other anticancer therapies; this interaction may occur with Doxil). Products include:
- Arimidex Tablets 659

Asparaginase (Co-administration with the conventional formulation of doxorubicin results in potentiation of the toxicity of other anticancer therapies; this interaction may occur with Doxil). Products include:
- Elspar for Injection 2092

Bicalutamide (Co-administration with the conventional formulation of doxorubicin results in potentiation of the toxicity of other anticancer therapies; this interaction may occur with Doxil). Products include:
- Casodex Tablets 662

Bleomycin Sulfate (Co-administration with the conventional formulation of doxorubicin results in potentiation of the toxicity of other anticancer therapies; this interaction may occur with Doxil).
No products indexed under this heading.

Busulfan (Co-administration with the conventional formulation of doxorubicin results in potentiation of the toxicity of other anticancer therapies; this interaction may occur with Doxil). Products include:
- Myleran Tablets 1603

Carboplatin (Co-administration with the conventional formulation of doxorubicin results in potentiation of the toxicity of other anticancer therapies; this interaction may occur with Doxil). Products include:
- Paraplatin for Injection 1126

Carmustine (BCNU) (Co-administration with the conventional formulation of doxorubicin results in potentiation of the toxicity of other anticancer therapies; this interaction may occur with Doxil). Products include:
- Gliadel Wafer 1723

Chlorambucil (Co-administration with the conventional formulation of doxorubicin results in potentiation of the toxicity of other anticancer therapies; this interaction may occur with Doxil). Products include:
- Leukeran Tablets 1591

Cisplatin (Co-administration with the conventional formulation of doxorubicin results in potentiation of the toxicity of other anticancer therapies; this interaction may occur with Doxil).
No products indexed under this heading.

Cyclophosphamide (Co-administration of conventional formulation of doxorubicin with cyclophosphamide has resulted in exacerbation of cyclophosphamide-induced hemorrhagic cystitis; cardiac toxicity may occur at lower cumulative doses in patients who are receiving cyclophosphamide).
No products indexed under this heading.

Cyclosporine (Co-administration of conventional formulation of doxorubicin may result in increases in AUC for both doxorubicin and doxorubicinol possibly due to a decrease in

clearance of parent drug and a decrease in metabolism of doxorubicin; potential for more profound and prolonged hematologic toxicity is associated with combined use; coma and seizures have also been reported). Products include:

- Gengraf Capsules 457
- Neoral Soft Gelatin Capsules 2380
- Neoral Oral Solution 2380
- Sandimmune 2388

Dacarbazine (Co-administration with the conventional formulation of doxorubicin results in potentiation of the toxicity of other anticancer therapies; this interaction may occur with Doxil). Products include:

- DTIC-Dome 902

Daunorubicin Citrate (Co-administration with the conventional formulation of doxorubicin results in potentiation of the toxicity of other anticancer therapies; this interaction may occur with Doxil). Products include:

- DaunoXome Injection 1442

Daunorubicin Hydrochloride (Co-administration with the conventional formulation of doxorubicin results in potentiation of the toxicity of other anticancer therapies; this interaction may occur with Doxil). Products include:

- Cerubidine for Injection 947

Denileukin Diftitox (Co-administration with the conventional formulation of doxorubicin results in potentiation of the toxicity of other anticancer therapies; this interaction may occur with Doxil).

No products indexed under this heading.

Docetaxel (Co-administration with the conventional formulation of doxorubicin results in potentiation of the toxicity of other anticancer therapies; this interaction may occur with Doxil). Products include:

- Taxotere for Injection Concentrate 778

Epirubicin Hydrochloride (Co-administration with the conventional formulation of doxorubicin results in potentiation of the toxicity of other anticancer therapies; this interaction may occur with Doxil). Products include:

- Ellence Injection 2806

Estramustine Phosphate Sodium (Co-administration with the conventional formulation of doxorubicin results in potentiation of the toxicity of other anticancer therapies; this interaction may occur with Doxil). Products include:

- Emcyt Capsules 2810

Etoposide (Co-administration with the conventional formulation of doxorubicin results in potentiation of the toxicity of other anticancer therapies; this interaction may occur with Doxil).

No products indexed under this heading.

Exemestane (Co-administration with the conventional formulation of doxorubicin results in potentiation of the toxicity of other anticancer therapies; this interaction may occur with Doxil). Products include:

- Aromasin Tablets 2769

Floxuridine (Co-administration with the conventional formulation of doxorubicin results in potentiation of the toxicity of other anticancer therapies; this interaction may occur with Doxil). Products include:

- Sterile FUDR 2974

Fluorouracil (Co-administration with the conventional formulation of doxorubicin results in potentiation of the toxicity of other anticancer therapies; this interaction may occur with Doxil). Products include:

- Carac Cream 1222
- Efudex 1733
- Fluoroplex 552

Flutamide (Co-administration with the conventional formulation of doxorubicin results in potentiation of the toxicity of other anticancer therapies; this interaction may occur with Doxil). Products include:

- Eulexin Capsules 3118

Gemcitabine Hydrochloride (Co-administration with the conventional formulation of doxorubicin results in potentiation of the toxicity of other anticancer therapies; this interaction may occur with Doxil). Products include:

- Gemzar for Injection 1919

Hydroxyurea (Co-administration with the conventional formulation of doxorubicin results in potentiation of the toxicity of other anticancer therapies; this interaction may occur with Doxil). Products include:

- Mylocel Tablets 2227

Idarubicin Hydrochloride (Co-administration with the conventional formulation of doxorubicin results in potentiation of the toxicity of other anticancer therapies; this interaction may occur with Doxil). Products include:

- Idamycin PFS Injection 2825

Ifosfamide (Co-administration with the conventional formulation of doxorubicin results in potentiation of the toxicity of other anticancer therapies; this interaction may occur with Doxil). Products include:

- Ifex for Injection 1123

Interferon alfa-2A, Recombinant (Co-administration with the conventional formulation of doxorubicin results in potentiation of the toxicity of other anticancer therapies; this interaction may occur with Doxil). Products include:

- Roferon-A Injection 2996

Interferon alfa-2B, Recombinant (Co-administration with the conventional formulation of doxorubicin results in potentiation of the toxicity of other anticancer therapies; this interaction may occur with Doxil). Products include:

- Intron A for Injection 3120
- Rebetron Combination Therapy 3153

Irinotecan Hydrochloride (Co-administration with the conventional formulation of doxorubicin results in potentiation of the toxicity of other anticancer therapies; this interaction may occur with Doxil).

No products indexed under this heading.

Levamisole Hydrochloride (Co-administration with the conventional formulation of doxorubicin results in potentiation of the toxicity of other anticancer therapies; this interaction may occur with Doxil). Products include:

- Ergamisol Tablets 1789

Lomustine (CCNU) (Co-administration with the conventional formulation of doxorubicin results in potentiation of the toxicity of other anticancer therapies; this interaction may occur with Doxil).

No products indexed under this heading.

Mechlorethamine Hydrochloride (Co-administration with the conventional formulation of doxorubicin results in potentiation of the toxicity of other anticancer therapies; this interaction may occur with Doxil). Products include:

- Mustargen for Injection 2142

Medroxyprogesterone Acetate (Co-administration of intravenous progesterone to patients with advanced malignancies at high doses with conventional formulation of fixed doxorubicin dose via bolus enhances doxorubicin-induced neutropenia and thrombocytopenia; this interaction may occur with Doxil). Products include:

- Depo-Provera Contraceptive Injection ... 2798
- Lunelle Monthly Injection 2827
- Premphase Tablets 3572
- Prempro Tablets 3572
- Provera Tablets 2853

Megestrol Acetate (Co-administration with the conventional formulation of doxorubicin results in potentiation of the toxicity of other anticancer therapies; this interaction may occur with Doxil). Products include:

- Megace Oral Suspension 1124

Melphalan (Co-administration with the conventional formulation of doxorubicin results in potentiation of the toxicity of other anticancer therapies; this interaction may occur with Doxil). Products include:

- Alkeran Tablets 1466

Mercaptopurine (Co-administration of conventional formulation of doxorubicin with 6-mercaptopurine has resulted in enhancement of hepatotoxicity of 6-mercaptopurine). Products include:

- Purinethol Tablets 1615

Methotrexate Sodium (Co-administration with the conventional formulation of doxorubicin results in potentiation of the toxicity of other anticancer therapies; this interaction may occur with Doxil).

No products indexed under this heading.

Mitomycin (Mitomycin-C) (Co-administration with the conventional formulation of doxorubicin results in potentiation of the toxicity of other anticancer therapies; this interaction may occur with Doxil).

No products indexed under this heading.

Mitotane (Co-administration with the conventional formulation of doxorubicin results in potentiation of the toxicity of other anticancer therapies; this interaction may occur with Doxil).

No products indexed under this heading.

Mitoxantrone Hydrochloride (Co-administration with the conventional formulation of doxorubicin results in potentiation of the toxicity of other anticancer therapies; this interaction may occur with Doxil). Products include:

- Novantrone for Injection 1760

Paclitaxel (Administration of paclitaxel infused over 24 hours followed by conventional formulation of doxorubicin administered over 48 hours resulted in a significant decrease in doxorubicin clearance with more profound neutropenic and stomatitis episodes than the reverse sequence of administration; this interaction may occur with Doxil). Products include:

- Taxol Injection 1129

Phenobarbital (Co-administration with the conventional formulation of doxorubicin results in increased elimination of doxorubicin; this interaction may occur with Doxil). Products include:

- Arco-Lase Plus Tablets 592
- Donnatal 2929
- Donnatal Extentabs 2930

Phenytoin (Co-administration with the conventional formulation of doxorubicin results in decreased phenytoin levels; this interaction may occur with Doxil). Products include:

- Dilantin Infatabs 2624
- Dilantin-125 Oral Suspension 2625

Phenytoin Sodium (Co-administration with the conventional formulation of doxorubicin results in decreased phenytoin levels; this interaction may occur with Doxil). Products include:

- Dilantin Kapseals 2622

Procarbazine Hydrochloride (Co-administration with the conventional formulation of doxorubicin results in potentiation of the toxicity of other anticancer therapies; this interaction may occur with Doxil). Products include:

- Matulane Capsules 3246

Progesterone (Co-administration of intravenous progesterone to patients with advanced malignancies at high doses with conventional formulation of fixed doxorubicin dose via bolus enhances doxorubicin-induced neutropenia and thrombocytopenia; this interaction may occur with Doxil). Products include:

- Crinone 3213
- Prometrium Capsules (100 mg, 200 mg) ... 3261

Streptozocin (Co-administration with the conventional formulation of doxorubicin results in inhibition of hepatic metabolism; this interaction may occur with Doxil).

No products indexed under this heading.

Tamoxifen Citrate (Co-administration with the conventional formulation of doxorubicin results in potentiation of the toxicity of other anticancer therapies; this interaction may occur with Doxil). Products include:

- Nolvadex Tablets 678

Teniposide (Co-administration with the conventional formulation of doxorubicin results in potentiation of the toxicity of other anticancer therapies; this interaction may occur with Doxil).

No products indexed under this heading.

Thioguanine (Co-administration with the conventional formulation of doxorubicin results in potentiation of the toxicity of other anticancer therapies; this interaction may occur with Doxil). Products include:

- Tabloid Tablets 1642

Thiotepa (Co-administration with the conventional formulation of doxorubicin results in potentiation of the toxicity of other anticancer therapies; this interaction may occur with Doxil). Products include:

- Thioplex for Injection 1765

Topotecan Hydrochloride (Co-administration with the conventional formulation of doxorubicin results in potentiation of the toxicity of other anticancer therapies; this interaction may occur with Doxil). Products include:

- Hycamtin for Injection 1546

Toremifene Citrate (Co-administration with the conventional formulation of doxorubicin results in potentiation of the toxicity of other anticancer therapies; this interaction may occur with Doxil). Products include:

- Fareston Tablets 3237

Valrubicin (Co-administration with the conventional formulation of doxorubicin results in potentiation of the toxicity of other anticancer therapies; this interaction may occur with Doxil). Products include:

- Valstar Sterile Solution for Intravesical Instillation ... 1175

Verapamil Hydrochloride (Co-administration of conventional formulation of doxorubicin in animal studies has resulted in higher initial peak concentrations of doxorubicin in the heart with a higher incidence and severity of degenerative changes in cardiac tissue resulting in a shorter survival; this interaction may occur with Doxil). Products include:

Covera-HS Tablets ... 3199
Isoptin SR Tablets ... 467
Tarka Tablets ... 508
Verelan Capsules ... 3184
Verelan PM Capsules ... 3186

Vincristine Sulfate (Co-administration with the conventional formulation of doxorubicin results in potentiation of the toxicity of other anticancer therapies; this interaction may occur with Doxil).
No products indexed under this heading.

Vinorelbine Tartrate (Co-administration with the conventional formulation of doxorubicin results in potentiation of the toxicity of other anticancer therapies; this interaction may occur with Doxil). Products include:
Navelbine Injection ... 1604

DRAMAMINE ORIGINAL FORMULA TABLETS

(Dimenhydrinate) ... ▣718
May interact with hypnotics and sedatives, tranquilizers, and certain other agents. Compounds in these categories include:

Alprazolam (May increase drowsiness effect). Products include:
Xanax Tablets ... 2865

Buspirone Hydrochloride (May increase drowsiness effect).
No products indexed under this heading.

Chlordiazepoxide (May increase drowsiness effect). Products include:
Limbitrol ... 1738

Chlordiazepoxide Hydrochloride (May increase drowsiness effect). Products include:
Librium Capsules ... 1736
Librium for Injection ... 1737

Chlorpromazine (May increase drowsiness effect). Products include:
Thorazine Suppositories ... 1656

Chlorpromazine Hydrochloride (May increase drowsiness effect). Products include:
Thorazine ... 1656

Chlorprothixene (May increase drowsiness effect).
No products indexed under this heading.

Chlorprothixene Hydrochloride (May increase drowsiness effect).
No products indexed under this heading.

Clorazepate Dipotassium (May increase drowsiness effect). Products include:
Tranxene ... 511

Diazepam (May increase drowsiness effect). Products include:
Valium Injectable ... 3026
Valium Tablets ... 3047

Droperidol (May increase drowsiness effect).
No products indexed under this heading.

Estazolam (May increase drowsiness effect). Products include:
ProSom Tablets ... 500

Ethchlorvynol (May increase drowsiness effect).
No products indexed under this heading.

Ethinamate (May increase drowsiness effect).
No products indexed under this heading.

Fluphenazine Decanoate (May increase drowsiness effect).
No products indexed under this heading.

Fluphenazine Enanthate (May increase drowsiness effect).
No products indexed under this heading.

Fluphenazine Hydrochloride (May increase drowsiness effect).
No products indexed under this heading.

Flurazepam Hydrochloride (May increase drowsiness effect).
No products indexed under this heading.

Glutethimide (May increase drowsiness effect).
No products indexed under this heading.

Haloperidol (May increase drowsiness effect). Products include:
Haldol Injection, Tablets and Concentrate ... 2533

Haloperidol Decanoate (May increase drowsiness effect). Products include:
Haldol Decanoate ... 2535

Hydroxyzine Hydrochloride (May increase drowsiness effect). Products include:
Atarax Tablets & Syrup ... 2667
Vistaril Intramuscular Solution ... 2738

Lorazepam (May increase drowsiness effect). Products include:
Ativan Injection ... 3478
Ativan Tablets ... 3482

Loxapine Hydrochloride (May increase drowsiness effect).
No products indexed under this heading.

Loxapine Succinate (May increase drowsiness effect). Products include:
Loxitane Capsules ... 3398

Meprobamate (May increase drowsiness effect). Products include:
Miltown Tablets ... 3349

Mesoridazine Besylate (May increase drowsiness effect). Products include:
Serentil ... 1057

Midazolam Hydrochloride (May increase drowsiness effect). Products include:
Versed Injection ... 3027
Versed Syrup ... 3033

Molindone Hydrochloride (May increase drowsiness effect). Products include:
Moban ... 1320

Oxazepam (May increase drowsiness effect).
No products indexed under this heading.

Perphenazine (May increase drowsiness effect). Products include:
Etrafon ... 3115
Trilafon ... 3160

Prazepam (May increase drowsiness effect).
No products indexed under this heading.

Prochlorperazine (May increase drowsiness effect). Products include:
Compazine ... 1505

Promethazine Hydrochloride (May increase drowsiness effect). Products include:
Mepergan Injection ... 3539
Phenergan Injection ... 3553
Phenergan ... 3556
Phenergan Syrup ... 3554
Phenergan with Codeine Syrup ... 3557
Phenergan with Dextromethorphan Syrup ... 3559
Phenergan VC Syrup ... 3560
Phenergan VC with Codeine Syrup ... 3561

Propofol (May increase drowsiness effect). Products include:
Diprivan Injectable Emulsion ... 667

Quazepam (May increase drowsiness effect).
No products indexed under this heading.

Secobarbital Sodium (May increase drowsiness effect).
No products indexed under this heading.

Temazepam (May increase drowsiness effect).
No products indexed under this heading.

Thioridazine Hydrochloride (May increase drowsiness effect). Products include:
Thioridazine Hydrochloride Tablets ... 2289

Thiothixene (May increase drowsiness effect). Products include:
Navane Capsules ... 2701
Thiothixene Capsules ... 2290

Triazolam (May increase drowsiness effect). Products include:
Halcion Tablets ... 2823

Trifluoperazine Hydrochloride (May increase drowsiness effect). Products include:
Stelazine ... 1640

Zaleplon (May increase drowsiness effect). Products include:
Sonata Capsules ... 3591

Zolpidem Tartrate (May increase drowsiness effect). Products include:
Ambien Tablets ... 3191

Food Interactions

Alcohol (May increase drowsiness effect).

DRAMAMINE CHEWABLE FORMULA TABLETS

(Dimenhydrinate) ... ▣718
See Dramamine Original Formula Tablets

DRAMAMINE LESS DROWSY TABLETS

(Meclizine Hydrochloride) ... ▣718
May interact with hypnotics and sedatives, tranquilizers, and certain other agents. Compounds in these categories include:

Alprazolam (May increase drowsiness effect). Products include:
Xanax Tablets ... 2865

Buspirone Hydrochloride (May increase drowsiness effect).
No products indexed under this heading.

Chlordiazepoxide (May increase drowsiness effect). Products include:
Limbitrol ... 1738

Chlordiazepoxide Hydrochloride (May increase drowsiness effect). Products include:
Librium Capsules ... 1736
Librium for Injection ... 1737

Chlorpromazine (May increase drowsiness effect). Products include:
Thorazine Suppositories ... 1656

Chlorpromazine Hydrochloride (May increase drowsiness effect). Products include:
Thorazine ... 1656

Chlorprothixene (May increase drowsiness effect).
No products indexed under this heading.

Chlorprothixene Hydrochloride (May increase drowsiness effect).
No products indexed under this heading.

Clorazepate Dipotassium (May increase drowsiness effect). Products include:
Tranxene ... 511

Diazepam (May increase drowsiness effect). Products include:
Valium Injectable ... 3026
Valium Tablets ... 3047

Droperidol (May increase drowsiness effect).
No products indexed under this heading.

Estazolam (May increase drowsiness effect). Products include:
ProSom Tablets ... 500

Ethchlorvynol (May increase drowsiness effect).
No products indexed under this heading.

Ethinamate (May increase drowsiness effect).
No products indexed under this heading.

Fluphenazine Decanoate (May increase drowsiness effect).
No products indexed under this heading.

Fluphenazine Enanthate (May increase drowsiness effect).
No products indexed under this heading.

Fluphenazine Hydrochloride (May increase drowsiness effect).
No products indexed under this heading.

Flurazepam Hydrochloride (May increase drowsiness effect).
No products indexed under this heading.

Glutethimide (May increase drowsiness effect).
No products indexed under this heading.

Haloperidol (May increase drowsiness effect). Products include:
Haldol Injection, Tablets and Concentrate ... 2533

Haloperidol Decanoate (May increase drowsiness effect). Products include:
Haldol Decanoate ... 2535

Hydroxyzine Hydrochloride (May increase drowsiness effect). Products include:
Atarax Tablets & Syrup ... 2667
Vistaril Intramuscular Solution ... 2738

Lorazepam (May increase drowsiness effect). Products include:
Ativan Injection ... 3478
Ativan Tablets ... 3482

Loxapine Hydrochloride (May increase drowsiness effect).
No products indexed under this heading.

Loxapine Succinate (May increase drowsiness effect). Products include:
Loxitane Capsules ... 3398

Meprobamate (May increase drowsiness effect). Products include:
Miltown Tablets ... 3349

Mesoridazine Besylate (May increase drowsiness effect). Products include:
Serentil ... 1057

Midazolam Hydrochloride (May increase drowsiness effect). Products include:
Versed Injection ... 3027
Versed Syrup ... 3033

Molindone Hydrochloride (May increase drowsiness effect). Products include:
Moban ... 1320

Oxazepam (May increase drowsiness effect).
No products indexed under this heading.

Perphenazine (May increase drowsiness effect). Products include:
Etrafon ... 3115
Trilafon ... 3160

Prazepam (May increase drowsiness effect).
No products indexed under this heading.

Prochlorperazine (May increase drowsiness effect). Products include:
Compazine ... 1505

Promethazine Hydrochloride (May increase drowsiness effect). Products include:
Mepergan Injection ... 3539
Phenergan Injection ... 3553
Phenergan ... 3556
Phenergan Syrup ... 3554
Phenergan with Codeine Syrup ... 3557
Phenergan with Dextromethorphan Syrup ... 3559
Phenergan VC Syrup ... 3560
Phenergan VC with Codeine Syrup ... 3561

Propofol (May increase drowsiness effect). Products include:
Diprivan Injectable Emulsion ... 667

Quazepam (May increase drowsiness effect).
No products indexed under this heading.

Secobarbital Sodium (May increase drowsiness effect).
No products indexed under this heading.

Temazepam (May increase drowsiness effect).
No products indexed under this heading.

Thioridazine Hydrochloride (May increase drowsiness effect). Products include:
Thioridazine Hydrochloride Tablets 2289

Thiothixene (May increase drowsiness effect). Products include:
Navane Capsules 2701
Thiothixene Capsules 2290

Triazolam (May increase drowsiness effect). Products include:
Halcion Tablets 2823

Trifluoperazine Hydrochloride (May increase drowsiness effect). Products include:
Stelazine 1640

Zaleplon (May increase drowsiness effect). Products include:
Sonata Capsules 3591

Zolpidem Tartrate (May increase drowsiness effect). Products include:
Ambien Tablets 3191

Food Interactions

Alcohol (May increase drowsiness effect).

DRIXORAL ALLERGY/ SINUS EXTENDED-RELEASE TABLETS

(Acetaminophen, Dexbrompheniramine Maleate, Pseudoephedrine Sulfate) 741
May interact with hypnotics and sedatives, monoamine oxidase inhibitors, tranquilizers, and certain other agents. Compounds in these categories include:

Alprazolam (May increase the drowsiness effect). Products include:
Xanax Tablets 2865

Buspirone Hydrochloride (May increase the drowsiness effect).
No products indexed under this heading.

Chlordiazepoxide (May increase the drowsiness effect). Products include:
Limbitrol 1738

Chlordiazepoxide Hydrochloride (May increase the drowsiness effect). Products include:
Librium Capsules 1736
Librium for Injection 1737

Chlorpromazine (May increase the drowsiness effect). Products include:
Thorazine Suppositories 1656

Chlorpromazine Hydrochloride (May increase the drowsiness effect). Products include:
Thorazine 1656

Chlorprothixene (May increase the drowsiness effect).
No products indexed under this heading.

Chlorprothixene Hydrochloride (May increase the drowsiness effect).
No products indexed under this heading.

Clorazepate Dipotassium (May increase the drowsiness effect). Products include:
Tranxene 511

Diazepam (May increase the drowsiness effect). Products include:
Valium Injectable 3026
Valium Tablets 3047

Droperidol (May increase the drowsiness effect).
No products indexed under this heading.

Estazolam (May increase the drowsiness effect). Products include:
ProSom Tablets 500

Ethchlorvynol (May increase the drowsiness effect).
No products indexed under this heading.

Ethinamate (May increase the drowsiness effect).
No products indexed under this heading.

Fluphenazine Decanoate (May increase the drowsiness effect).
No products indexed under this heading.

Fluphenazine Enanthate (May increase the drowsiness effect).
No products indexed under this heading.

Fluphenazine Hydrochloride (May increase the drowsiness effect).
No products indexed under this heading.

Flurazepam Hydrochloride (May increase the drowsiness effect).
No products indexed under this heading.

Glutethimide (May increase the drowsiness effect).
No products indexed under this heading.

Haloperidol (May increase the drowsiness effect). Products include:
Haldol Injection, Tablets and Concentrate 2533

Haloperidol Decanoate (May increase the drowsiness effect). Products include:
Haldol Decanoate 2535

Hydroxyzine Hydrochloride (May increase the drowsiness effect). Products include:
Atarax Tablets & Syrup 2667
Vistaril Intramuscular Solution 2738

Isocarboxazid (Concurrent and/or sequential use is not recommended).
No products indexed under this heading.

Lorazepam (May increase the drowsiness effect). Products include:
Ativan Injection 3478
Ativan Tablets 3482

Loxapine Hydrochloride (May increase the drowsiness effect).
No products indexed under this heading.

Loxapine Succinate (May increase the drowsiness effect). Products include:
Loxitane Capsules 3398

Meprobamate (May increase the drowsiness effect). Products include:
Miltown Tablets 3349

Mesoridazine Besylate (May increase the drowsiness effect). Products include:
Serentil 1057

Midazolam Hydrochloride (May increase the drowsiness effect). Products include:
Versed Injection 3027
Versed Syrup 3033

Moclobemide (Concurrent and/or sequential use is not recommended).
No products indexed under this heading.

Molindone Hydrochloride (May increase the drowsiness effect). Products include:
Moban 1320

Oxazepam (May increase the drowsiness effect).
No products indexed under this heading.

Pargyline Hydrochloride (Concurrent and/or sequential use is not recommended).
No products indexed under this heading.

Perphenazine (May increase the drowsiness effect). Products include:
Etrafon 3115
Trilafon 3160

Phenelzine Sulfate (Concurrent and/or sequential use is not recommended). Products include:
Nardil Tablets 2653

Prazepam (May increase the drowsiness effect).
No products indexed under this heading.

Procarbazine Hydrochloride (Concurrent and/or sequential use is not recommended). Products include:
Matulane Capsules 3246

Prochlorperazine (May increase the drowsiness effect). Products include:
Compazine 1505

Promethazine Hydrochloride (May increase the drowsiness effect). Products include:
Mepergan Injection 3539
Phenergan Injection 3553
Phenergan 3556
Phenergan Syrup 3554
Phenergan with Codeine Syrup 3557
Phenergan with Dextromethorphan Syrup 3559
Phenergan VC Syrup 3560
Phenergan VC with Codeine Syrup 3561

Propofol (May increase the drowsiness effect). Products include:
Diprivan Injectable Emulsion 667

Quazepam (May increase the drowsiness effect).
No products indexed under this heading.

Secobarbital Sodium (May increase the drowsiness effect).
No products indexed under this heading.

Selegiline Hydrochloride (Concurrent and/or sequential use is not recommended). Products include:
Eldepryl Capsules 3266

Temazepam (May increase the drowsiness effect).
No products indexed under this heading.

Thioridazine Hydrochloride (May increase the drowsiness effect). Products include:
Thioridazine Hydrochloride Tablets 2289

Thiothixene (May increase the drowsiness effect). Products include:
Navane Capsules 2701
Thiothixene Capsules 2290

Tranylcypromine Sulfate (Concurrent and/or sequential use is not recommended). Products include:
Parnate Tablets 1607

Triazolam (May increase the drowsiness effect). Products include:
Halcion Tablets 2823

Trifluoperazine Hydrochloride (May increase the drowsiness effect). Products include:
Stelazine 1640

Zaleplon (May increase the drowsiness effect). Products include:
Sonata Capsules 3591

Zolpidem Tartrate (May increase the drowsiness effect). Products include:
Ambien Tablets 3191

Food Interactions

Alcohol (May increase drowsiness effect; individuals who consume 3 or more alcohol containing drinks per day should consult their doctor on when and how they should take this product).

DRIXORAL COLD & ALLERGY SUSTAINED-ACTION TABLETS

(Dexbrompheniramine Maleate, Pseudoephedrine Sulfate) 740
May interact with hypnotics and sedatives, monoamine oxidase inhibitors, tranquilizers, and certain other agents. Compounds in these categories include:

Alprazolam (May increase drowsiness effect). Products include:
Xanax Tablets 2865

Buspirone Hydrochloride (May increase drowsiness effect).
No products indexed under this heading.

Chlordiazepoxide (May increase drowsiness effect). Products include:
Limbitrol 1738

Chlordiazepoxide Hydrochloride (May increase drowsiness effect). Products include:
Librium Capsules 1736
Librium for Injection 1737

Chlorpromazine (May increase drowsiness effect). Products include:
Thorazine Suppositories 1656

Chlorpromazine Hydrochloride (May increase drowsiness effect). Products include:
Thorazine 1656

Chlorprothixene (May increase drowsiness effect).
No products indexed under this heading.

Chlorprothixene Hydrochloride (May increase drowsiness effect).
No products indexed under this heading.

Clorazepate Dipotassium (May increase drowsiness effect). Products include:
Tranxene 511

Diazepam (May increase drowsiness effect). Products include:
Valium Injectable 3026
Valium Tablets 3047

Droperidol (May increase drowsiness effect).
No products indexed under this heading.

Estazolam (May increase drowsiness effect). Products include:
ProSom Tablets 500

Ethchlorvynol (May increase drowsiness effect).
No products indexed under this heading.

Ethinamate (May increase drowsiness effect).
No products indexed under this heading.

Fluphenazine Decanoate (May increase drowsiness effect).
No products indexed under this heading.

Fluphenazine Enanthate (May increase drowsiness effect).
No products indexed under this heading.

Fluphenazine Hydrochloride (May increase drowsiness effect).
No products indexed under this heading.

Flurazepam Hydrochloride (May increase drowsiness effect).
No products indexed under this heading.

Glutethimide (May increase drowsiness effect).
No products indexed under this heading.

Haloperidol (May increase drowsiness effect). Products include:
Haldol Injection, Tablets and Concentrate 2533

Haloperidol Decanoate (May increase drowsiness effect). Products include:
Haldol Decanoate 2535

Hydroxyzine Hydrochloride (May increase drowsiness effect). Products include:
Atarax Tablets & Syrup 2667
Vistaril Intramuscular Solution 2738

Isocarboxazid (Concurrent and/or sequential use is not recommended).
No products indexed under this heading.

Lorazepam (May increase drowsiness effect). Products include:
Ativan Injection 3478
Ativan Tablets 3482

Loxapine Hydrochloride (May increase drowsiness effect).
No products indexed under this heading.

Loxapine Succinate (May increase drowsiness effect). Products include:
Loxitane Capsules 3398

Meprobamate (May increase drowsiness effect). Products include:
Miltown Tablets 3349

Mesoridazine Besylate (May increase drowsiness effect). Products include:
Serentil 1057

Midazolam Hydrochloride (May increase drowsiness effect). Products include:
Versed Injection 3027
Versed Syrup 3033

Moclobemide (Concurrent and/or sequential use is not recommended).
No products indexed under this heading.

Molindone Hydrochloride (May increase drowsiness effect). Products include:
Moban 1320

Oxazepam (May increase drowsiness effect).
No products indexed under this heading.

Pargyline Hydrochloride (Concurrent and/or sequential use is not recommended).
No products indexed under this heading.

Perphenazine (May increase drowsiness effect). Products include:
Etrafon 3115
Trilafon 3160

Phenelzine Sulfate (Concurrent and/or sequential use is not recommended). Products include:
Nardil Tablets 2653

Prazepam (May increase drowsiness effect).
No products indexed under this heading.

Procarbazine Hydrochloride (Concurrent and/or sequential use is not recommended). Products include:
Matulane Capsules 3246

Prochlorperazine (May increase drowsiness effect). Products include:
Compazine 1505

Promethazine Hydrochloride (May increase drowsiness effect). Products include:
Mepergan Injection 3539
Phenergan Injection 3553
Phenergan 3556
Phenergan Syrup 3554
Phenergan with Codeine Syrup 3557
Phenergan with Dextromethorphan Syrup 3559
Phenergan VC Syrup 3560
Phenergan VC with Codeine Syrup . 3561

Propofol (May increase drowsiness effect). Products include:
Diprivan Injectable Emulsion 667

Quazepam (May increase drowsiness effect).
No products indexed under this heading.

Secobarbital Sodium (May increase drowsiness effect).
No products indexed under this heading.

Selegiline Hydrochloride (Concurrent and/or sequential use is not recommended). Products include:
Eldepryl Capsules 3266

Temazepam (May increase drowsiness effect).
No products indexed under this heading.

Thioridazine Hydrochloride (May increase drowsiness effect). Products include:
Thioridazine Hydrochloride Tablets 2289

Thiothixene (May increase drowsiness effect). Products include:
Navane Capsules 2701
Thiothixene Capsules 2290

Tranylcypromine Sulfate (Concurrent and/or sequential use is not recommended). Products include:
Parnate Tablets 1607

Triazolam (May increase drowsiness effect). Products include:
Halcion Tablets 2823

Trifluoperazine Hydrochloride (May increase drowsiness effect). Products include:
Stelazine 1640

Zaleplon (May increase drowsiness effect). Products include:
Sonata Capsules 3591

Zolpidem Tartrate (May increase drowsiness effect). Products include:
Ambien Tablets 3191

Food Interactions

Alcohol (May increase drowsiness effect).

DRIXORAL COLD & FLU EXTENDED-RELEASE TABLETS

(Acetaminophen, Dexbrompheniramine Maleate, Pseudoephedrine Sulfate) .... ▣740

May interact with hypnotics and sedatives, monoamine oxidase inhibitors, tranquilizers, and certain other agents. Compounds in these categories include:

Alprazolam (May increase drowsiness effect). Products include:
Xanax Tablets 2865

Buspirone Hydrochloride (May increase drowsiness effect).
No products indexed under this heading.

Chlordiazepoxide (May increase drowsiness effect). Products include:
Limbitrol 1738

Chlordiazepoxide Hydrochloride (May increase drowsiness effect). Products include:
Librium Capsules 1736
Librium for Injection 1737

Chlorpromazine (May increase drowsiness effect). Products include:
Thorazine Suppositories 1656

Chlorpromazine Hydrochloride (May increase drowsiness effect). Products include:
Thorazine 1656

Chlorprothixene (May increase drowsiness effect).
No products indexed under this heading.

Chlorprothixene Hydrochloride (May increase drowsiness effect).
No products indexed under this heading.

Clorazepate Dipotassium (May increase drowsiness effect) Products include:
Tranxene 511

Diazepam (May increase drowsiness effect). Products include:
Valium Injectable 3026
Valium Tablets 3047

Droperidol (May increase drowsiness effect).
No products indexed under this heading.

Estazolam (May increase drowsiness effect). Products include:
ProSom Tablets 500

Ethchlorvynol (May increase drowsiness effect).
No products indexed under this heading.

Ethinamate (May increase drowsiness effect).
No products indexed under this heading.

Fluphenazine Decanoate (May increase drowsiness effect).
No products indexed under this heading.

Fluphenazine Enanthate (May increase drowsiness effect).
No products indexed under this heading.

Fluphenazine Hydrochloride (May increase drowsiness effect).
No products indexed under this heading.

Flurazepam Hydrochloride (May increase drowsiness effect).
No products indexed under this heading.

Glutethimide (May increase drowsiness effect).
No products indexed under this heading.

Haloperidol (May increase drowsiness effect). Products include:
Haldol Injection, Tablets and Concentrate 2533

Haloperidol Decanoate (May increase drowsiness effect). Products include:
Haldol Decanoate 2535

Hydroxyzine Hydrochloride (May increase drowsiness effect). Products include:
Atarax Tablets & Syrup 2667
Vistaril Intramuscular Solution 2738

Isocarboxazid (Concurrent and/or sequential use is not recommended).
No products indexed under this heading.

Lorazepam (May increase drowsiness effect). Products include:
Ativan Injection 3478
Ativan Tablets 3482

Loxapine Hydrochloride (May increase drowsiness effect).
No products indexed under this heading.

Loxapine Succinate (May increase drowsiness effect). Products include:
Loxitane Capsules 3398

Meprobamate (May increase drowsiness effect). Products include:
Miltown Tablets 3349

Mesoridazine Besylate (May increase drowsiness effect). Products include:
Serentil 1057

Midazolam Hydrochloride (May increase drowsiness effect). Products include:
Versed Injection 3027
Versed Syrup 3033

Moclobemide (Concurrent and/or sequential use is not recommended).
No products indexed under this heading.

Molindone Hydrochloride (May increase drowsiness effect). Products include:
Moban 1320

Oxazepam (May increase drowsiness effect).
No products indexed under this heading.

Pargyline Hydrochloride (Concurrent and/or sequential use is not recommended).
No products indexed under this heading.

Perphenazine (May increase drowsiness effect). Products include:
Etrafon 3115
Trilafon 3160

Phenelzine Sulfate (Concurrent and/or sequential use is not recommended). Products include:
Nardil Tablets 2653

Prazepam (May increase drowsiness effect).
No products indexed under this heading.

Procarbazine Hydrochloride (Concurrent and/or sequential use is not recommended). Products include:
Matulane Capsules 3246

Prochlorperazine (May increase drowsiness effect). Products include:
Compazine 1505

Promethazine Hydrochloride (May increase drowsiness effect). Products include:
Mepergan Injection 3539
Phenergan Injection 3553
Phenergan 3556
Phenergan Syrup 3554
Phenergan with Codeine Syrup 3557
Phenergan with Dextromethorphan Syrup 3559
Phenergan VC Syrup 3560
Phenergan VC with Codeine Syrup .. 3561

Propofol (May increase drowsiness effect). Products include:
Diprivan Injectable Emulsion 667

Quazepam (May increase drowsiness effect).
No products indexed under this heading.

Secobarbital Sodium (May increase drowsiness effect).
No products indexed under this heading.

Selegiline Hydrochloride (Concurrent and/or sequential use is not recommended). Products include:
Eldepryl Capsules 3266

Temazepam (May increase drowsiness effect).
No products indexed under this heading.

Thioridazine Hydrochloride (May increase drowsiness effect). Products include:
Thioridazine Hydrochloride Tablets 2289

Thiothixene (May increase drowsiness effect). Products include:
Navane Capsules 2701
Thiothixene Capsules 2290

Tranylcypromine Sulfate (Concurrent and/or sequential use is not recommended). Products include:
Parnate Tablets 1607

Triazolam (May increase drowsiness effect). Products include:
Halcion Tablets 2823

Trifluoperazine Hydrochloride (May increase drowsiness effect). Products include:
Stelazine 1640

Zaleplon (May increase drowsiness effect). Products include:
Sonata Capsules 3591

Zolpidem Tartrate (May increase drowsiness effect). Products include:
Ambien Tablets 3191

Food Interactions

Alcohol (May increase drowsiness effect; individuals who consume 3 or more alcohol containing drinks per day should consult their doctor on when and how they should take this product).

DRIXORAL NASAL DECONGESTANT LONG-ACTING NON-DROWSY TABLETS

(Pseudoephedrine Sulfate) .... ▣740

May interact with monoamine oxidase inhibitors. Compounds in these categories include:

Isocarboxazid (Concurrent and/or sequential use is not recommended).
No products indexed under this heading.

Moclobemide (Concurrent and/or sequential use is not recommended).
No products indexed under this heading.

Pargyline Hydrochloride (Concurrent and/or sequential use is not recommended).
No products indexed under this heading.

Phenelzine Sulfate (Concurrent and/or sequential use is not recommended). Products include:
Nardil Tablets 2653

Procarbazine Hydrochloride (Concurrent and/or sequential use is not recommended). Products include:

Matulane Capsules 3246

Selegiline Hydrochloride (Concurrent and/or sequential use is not recommended). Products include:
Eldepryl Capsules 3266

Tranylcypromine Sulfate (Concurrent and/or sequential use is not recommended). Products include:
Parnate Tablets 1607

DRYSOL SOLUTION
(Aluminum Chloride) 2663
None cited in PDR database.

DTIC-DOME
(Dacarbazine) 902
May interact with antineoplastics. Compounds in these categories include:

Altretamine (Hepatic toxicity). Products include:
Hexalen Capsules 2226

Anastrozole (Hepatic toxicity). Products include:
Arimidex Tablets 659

Asparaginase (Hepatic toxicity). Products include:
Elspar for Injection 2092

Bicalutamide (Hepatic toxicity). Products include:
Casodex Tablets 662

Bleomycin Sulfate (Hepatic toxicity).
No products indexed under this heading.

Busulfan (Hepatic toxicity). Products include:
Myleran Tablets 1603

Carboplatin (Hepatic toxicity). Products include:
Paraplatin for Injection 1126

Carmustine (BCNU) (Hepatic toxicity). Products include:
Gliadel Wafer 1723

Chlorambucil (Hepatic toxicity). Products include:
Leukeran Tablets 1591

Cisplatin (Hepatic toxicity).
No products indexed under this heading.

Cyclophosphamide (Hepatic toxicity).
No products indexed under this heading.

Daunorubicin Citrate (Hepatic toxicity). Products include:
DaunoXome Injection 1442

Daunorubicin Hydrochloride (Hepatic toxicity). Products include:
Cerubidine for Injection 947

Denileukin Diftitox (Hepatic toxicity).
No products indexed under this heading.

Docetaxel (Hepatic toxicity). Products include:
Taxotere for Injection Concentrate 778

Doxorubicin Hydrochloride (Hepatic toxicity). Products include:
Adriamycin PFS/RDF Injection 2767
Doxil Injection 566

Epirubicin Hydrochloride (Hepatic toxicity). Products include:
Ellence Injection 2806

Estramustine Phosphate Sodium (Hepatic toxicity). Products include:
Emcyt Capsules 2810

Etoposide (Hepatic toxicity).
No products indexed under this heading.

Exemestane (Hepatic toxicity). Products include:
Aromasin Tablets 2769

Floxuridine (Hepatic toxicity). Products include:
Sterile FUDR 2974

Fluorouracil (Hepatic toxicity). Products include:
Carac Cream 1222
Efudex 1733
Fluoroplex 552

Flutamide (Hepatic toxicity). Products include:
Eulexin Capsules 3118

Gemcitabine Hydrochloride (Hepatic toxicity). Products include:
Gemzar for Injection 1919

Hydroxyurea (Hepatic toxicity). Products include:
Mylocel Tablets 2227

Idarubicin Hydrochloride (Hepatic toxicity). Products include:
Idamycin PFS Injection 2825

Ifosfamide (Hepatic toxicity). Products include:
Ifex for Injection 1123

Interferon alfa-2A, Recombinant (Hepatic toxicity). Products include:
Roferon-A Injection 2996

Interferon alfa-2B, Recombinant (Hepatic toxicity). Products include:
Intron A for Injection 3120
Rebetron Combination Therapy 3153

Irinotecan Hydrochloride (Hepatic toxicity).
No products indexed under this heading.

Levamisole Hydrochloride (Hepatic toxicity). Products include:
Ergamisol Tablets 1789

Lomustine (CCNU) (Hepatic toxicity).
No products indexed under this heading.

Mechlorethamine Hydrochloride (Hepatic toxicity). Products include:
Mustargen for Injection 2142

Megestrol Acetate (Hepatic toxicity). Products include:
Megace Oral Suspension 1124

Melphalan (Hepatic toxicity). Products include:
Alkeran Tablets 1466

Mercaptopurine (Hepatic toxicity). Products include:
Purinethol Tablets 1615

Methotrexate Sodium (Hepatic toxicity).
No products indexed under this heading.

Mitomycin (Mitomycin-C) (Hepatic toxicity).
No products indexed under this heading.

Mitotane (Hepatic toxicity).
No products indexed under this heading.

Mitoxantrone Hydrochloride (Hepatic toxicity). Products include:
Novantrone for Injection 1760

Paclitaxel (Hepatic toxicity). Products include:
Taxol Injection 1129

Procarbazine Hydrochloride (Hepatic toxicity). Products include:
Matulane Capsules 3246

Streptozocin (Hepatic toxicity).
No products indexed under this heading.

Tamoxifen Citrate (Hepatic toxicity). Products include:
Nolvadex Tablets 678

Teniposide (Hepatic toxicity).
No products indexed under this heading.

Thioguanine (Hepatic toxicity). Products include:
Tabloid Tablets 1642

Thiotepa (Hepatic toxicity). Products include:
Thioplex for Injection 1765

Topotecan Hydrochloride (Hepatic toxicity). Products include:
Hycamtin for Injection 1546

Toremifene Citrate (Hepatic toxicity). Products include:
Fareston Tablets 3237

Valrubicin (Hepatic toxicity). Products include:
Valstar Sterile Solution for Intravesical Instillation 1175

Vincristine Sulfate (Hepatic toxicity).
No products indexed under this heading.

Vinorelbine Tartrate (Hepatic toxicity). Products include:
Navelbine Injection 1604

DULCOLAX SUPPOSITORIES
(Bisacodyl) .... ▣668
None cited in PDR database.

DULCOLAX TABLETS
(Bisacodyl) .... ▣668
None cited in PDR database.

DUONEB INHALATION SOLUTION
(Albuterol Sulfate, Ipratropium Bromide) 1233
May interact with anticholinergics, beta blockers, monoamine oxidase inhibitors, potassium-depleting diuretics, sympathomimetics, and tricyclic antidepressants. Compounds in these categories include:

Acebutolol Hydrochloride (Co-administration with beta blockers inhibits the effects of each other). Products include:
Sectral Capsules 3589

Albuterol (Co-administration with other sympathomimetic agents increases the risk of adverse cardiovascular effects). Products include:
Proventil Inhalation Aerosol 3142
Ventolin Inhalation Aerosol and Refill 1679

Amitriptyline Hydrochloride (Co-administration with tricyclic antidepressants can potentiate the action of albuterol on the cardiovascular system). Products include:
Etrafon 3115
Limbitrol 1738

Amoxapine (Co-administration with tricyclic antidepressants can potentiate the action of albuterol on the cardiovascular system).
No products indexed under this heading.

Atenolol (Co-administration with beta blockers inhibits the effects of each other). Products include:
Tenoretic Tablets 690
Tenormin I.V. Injection 692

Atropine Sulfate (Co-administration has some potential for additive anticholinergic effects; caution is advised). Products include:
Donnatal 2929
Donnatal Extentabs 2930
Motofen Tablets 577
Prosed/DS Tablets 3268
Urised Tablets 2876

Belladonna Alkaloids (Co-administration has some potential for additive anticholinergic effects; caution is advised). Products include:
Hyland's Teething Tablets .... ▣766
Urimax Tablets 1769

Bendroflumethiazide (Co-administration with non-potassium sparing diuretics can result in acute worsening of ECG changes and/or hypokalemia, especially when recommended dose of the beta agonist is exceeded; clinical significance of this interaction is unknown). Products include:
Corzide 40/5 Tablets 2247
Corzide 80/5 Tablets 2247

Benztropine Mesylate (Co-administration has some potential for additive anticholinergic effects; caution is advised). Products include:
Cogentin 2055

Betaxolol Hydrochloride (Co-administration with beta blockers inhibits the effects of each other). Products include:
Betoptic S Ophthalmic Suspension 537

Biperiden Hydrochloride (Co-administration has some potential for additive anticholinergic effects; caution is advised). Products include:
Akineton 402

Bisoprolol Fumarate (Co-administration with beta blockers inhibits the effects of each other). Products include:
Zebeta Tablets 1885
Ziac Tablets 1887

Bumetanide (Co-administration with non-potassium sparing diuretics can result in acute worsening of ECG changes and/or hypokalemia, especially when recommended dose of the beta agonist is exceeded; clinical significance of this interaction is unknown).
No products indexed under this heading.

Carteolol Hydrochloride (Co-administration with beta blockers inhibits the effects of each other). Products include:
Carteolol Hydrochloride Ophthalmic Solution USP, 1% .... ⊙258
Ocupress Ophthalmic Solution, 1% Sterile .... ⊙303

Chlorothiazide (Co-administration with non-potassium sparing diuretics can result in acute worsening of ECG changes and/or hypokalemia, especially when recommended dose of the beta agonist is exceeded; clinical significance of this interaction is unknown). Products include:
Aldoclor Tablets 2035
Diuril Oral 2087

Chlorothiazide Sodium (Co-administration with non-potassium sparing diuretics can result in acute worsening of ECG changes and/or hypokalemia, especially when recommended dose of the beta agonist is exceeded; clinical significance of this interaction is unknown). Products include:
Diuril Sodium Intravenous 2086

Clidinium Bromide (Co-administration has some potential for additive anticholinergic effects; caution is advised).
No products indexed under this heading.

Clomipramine Hydrochloride (Co-administration with tricyclic antidepressants can potentiate the action of albuterol on the cardiovascular system).
No products indexed under this heading.

Desipramine Hydrochloride (Co-administration with tricyclic antidepressants can potentiate the action of albuterol on the cardiovascular system). Products include:
Norpramin Tablets 755

Dicyclomine Hydrochloride (Co-administration has some potential for additive anticholinergic effects; caution is advised).
No products indexed under this heading.

Dobutamine Hydrochloride (Co-administration with other sympathomimetic agents increases the risk of adverse cardiovascular effects). Products include:
Dobutrex Solution Vials 1914

Dopamine Hydrochloride (Co-administration with other sympathomimetic agents increases the risk of adverse cardiovascular effects).
No products indexed under this heading.

Doxepin Hydrochloride (Co-administration with tricyclic antidepressants can potentiate the action of albuterol on the cardiovascular system). Products include:
Sinequan 2713

Ephedrine Hydrochloride (Co-administration with other sympathomimetic agents increases the risk of adverse cardiovascular effects). Products include:
- Primatene Tablets ▣ 780

Ephedrine Sulfate (Co-administration with other sympathomimetic agents increases the risk of adverse cardiovascular effects).
- No products indexed under this heading.

Ephedrine Tannate (Co-administration with other sympathomimetic agents increases the risk of adverse cardiovascular effects). Products include:
- Rynatuss Pediatric Suspension 3353
- Rynatuss Tablets 3353

Epinephrine (Co-administration with other sympathomimetic agents increases the risk of adverse cardiovascular effects). Products include:
- Epifrin Sterile Ophthalmic Solution ...... ⊙ 235
- EpiPen 1236
- Primatene Mist ...... ▣ 779
- Xylocaine with Epinephrine Injection 653

Epinephrine Bitartrate (Co-administration with other sympathomimetic agents increases the risk of adverse cardiovascular effects). Products include:
- Sensorcaine 643

Epinephrine Hydrochloride (Co-administration with other sympathomimetic agents increases the risk of adverse cardiovascular effects).
- No products indexed under this heading.

Esmolol Hydrochloride (Co-administration with beta blockers inhibits the effects of each other). Products include:
- Brevibloc Injection 858

Ethacrynic Acid (Co-administration with non-potassium sparing diuretics can result in acute worsening of ECG changes and/or hypokalemia, especially when recommended dose of the beta agonist is exceeded; clinical significance of this interaction is unknown). Products include:
- Edecrin Tablets 2091

Furosemide (Co-administration with non-potassium sparing diuretics can result in acute worsening of ECG changes and/or hypokalemia, especially when recommended dose of the beta agonist is exceeded; clinical significance of this interaction is unknown). Products include:
- Furosemide Tablets 2284

Glycopyrrolate (Co-administration has some potential for additive anticholinergic effects; caution is advised). Products include:
- Robinul Forte Tablets 1358
- Robinul Injectable 2940
- Robinul Tablets 1358

Hydrochlorothiazide (Co-administration with non-potassium sparing diuretics can result in acute worsening of ECG changes and/or hypokalemia, especially when recommended dose of the beta agonist is exceeded; clinical significance of this interaction is unknown). Products include:
- Accuretic Tablets 2614
- Aldoril Tablets 2039
- Atacand HCT Tablets 597
- Avalide Tablets 1070
- Diovan HCT Tablets 2338
- Dyazide Capsules 1515
- HydroDIURIL Tablets 2108
- Hyzaar 2109
- Inderide Tablets 3517
- Inderide LA Long-Acting Capsules .. 3519
- Lotensin HCT Tablets 2367
- Maxzide 1008
- Micardis HCT Tablets 1051
- Microzide Capsules 3414
- Moduretic Tablets 2138
- Monopril HCT 1094
- Prinzide Tablets 2168
- Timolide Tablets 2187
- Uniretic Tablets 3178
- Vaseretic Tablets 2204
- Zestoretic Tablets 695
- Ziac Tablets 1887

Hydroflumethiazide (Co-administration with non-potassium sparing diuretics can result in acute worsening of ECG changes and/or hypokalemia, especially when recommended dose of the beta agonist is exceeded; clinical significance of this interaction is unknown). Products include:
- Diucardin Tablets 3494

Hyoscyamine (Co-administration has some potential for additive anticholinergic effects; caution is advised). Products include:
- Urised Tablets 2876

Hyoscyamine Sulfate (Co-administration has some potential for additive anticholinergic effects; caution is advised). Products include:
- Arco-Lase Plus Tablets 592
- Donnatal 2929
- Donnatal Extentabs 2930
- Levsin/Levsinex/Levbid 3172
- NuLev Orally Disintegrating Tablets 3176
- Prosed/DS Tablets 3268
- Urimax Tablets 1769

Imipramine Hydrochloride (Co-administration with tricyclic antidepressants can potentiate the action of albuterol on the cardiovascular system).
- No products indexed under this heading.

Imipramine Pamoate (Co-administration with tricyclic antidepressants can potentiate the action of albuterol on the cardiovascular system).
- No products indexed under this heading.

Isocarboxazid (Co-administration with MAO inhibitors can potentiate the action of albuterol on the cardiovascular system).
- No products indexed under this heading.

Isoproterenol Hydrochloride (Co-administration with other sympathomimetic agents increases the risk of adverse cardiovascular effects).
- No products indexed under this heading.

Isoproterenol Sulfate (Co-administration with other sympathomimetic agents increases the risk of adverse cardiovascular effects).
- No products indexed under this heading.

Labetalol Hydrochloride (Co-administration with beta blockers inhibits the effects of each other). Products include:
- Normodyne Injection 3135
- Normodyne Tablets 3137

Levalbuterol Hydrochloride (Co-administration with other sympathomimetic agents increases the risk of adverse cardiovascular effects). Products include:
- Xopenex Inhalation Solution 3207

Levobunolol Hydrochloride (Co-administration with beta blockers inhibits the effects of each other). Products include:
- Betagan ...... ⊙ 228

Maprotiline Hydrochloride (Co-administration with tricyclic antidepressants can potentiate the action of albuterol on the cardiovascular system).
- No products indexed under this heading.

Mepenzolate Bromide (Co-administration has some potential for additive anticholinergic effects; caution is advised).
- No products indexed under this heading.

Metaproterenol Sulfate (Co-administration with other sympathomimetic agents increases the risk of adverse cardiovascular effects). Products include:
- Alupent 1029

Metaraminol Bitartrate (Co-administration with other sympathomimetic agents increases the risk of adverse cardiovascular effects). Products include:
- Aramine Injection 2043

Methoxamine Hydrochloride (Co-administration with other sympathomimetic agents increases the risk of adverse cardiovascular effects).
- No products indexed under this heading.

Methyclothiazide (Co-administration with non-potassium sparing diuretics can result in acute worsening of ECG changes and/or hypokalemia, especially when recommended dose of the beta agonist is exceeded; clinical significance of this interaction is unknown).
- No products indexed under this heading.

Metipranolol Hydrochloride (Co-administration with beta blockers inhibits the effects of each other).
- No products indexed under this heading.

Metoprolol Succinate (Co-administration with beta blockers inhibits the effects of each other). Products include:
- Toprol-XL Tablets 651

Metoprolol Tartrate (Co-administration with beta blockers inhibits the effects of each other).
- No products indexed under this heading.

Moclobemide (Co-administration with MAO inhibitors can potentiate the action of albuterol on the cardiovascular system).
- No products indexed under this heading.

Nadolol (Co-administration with beta blockers inhibits the effects of each other). Products include:
- Corgard Tablets 2245
- Corzide 40/5 Tablets 2247
- Corzide 80/5 Tablets 2247
- Nadolol Tablets 2288

Norepinephrine Bitartrate (Co-administration with other sympathomimetic agents increases the risk of adverse cardiovascular effects).
- No products indexed under this heading.

Nortriptyline Hydrochloride (Co-administration with tricyclic antidepressants can potentiate the action of albuterol on the cardiovascular system).
- No products indexed under this heading.

Oxybutynin Chloride (Co-administration has some potential for additive anticholinergic effects; caution is advised). Products include:
- Ditropan XL Extended Release Tablets 564

Pargyline Hydrochloride (Co-administration with MAO inhibitors can potentiate the action of albuterol on the cardiovascular system).
- No products indexed under this heading.

Penbutolol Sulfate (Co-administration with beta blockers inhibits the effects of each other).
- No products indexed under this heading.

Phenelzine Sulfate (Co-administration with MAO inhibitors can potentiate the action of albuterol on the cardiovascular system). Products include:
- Nardil Tablets 2653

Phenylephrine Bitartrate (Co-administration with other sympathomimetic agents increases the risk of adverse cardiovascular effects).
- No products indexed under this heading.

Phenylephrine Hydrochloride (Co-administration with other sympathomimetic agents increases the risk of adverse cardiovascular effects). Products include:
- Afrin Nasal Decongestant Children's Pump Mist ...... ▣ 734
- Extendryl 1361
- Hycomine Compound Tablets 1317
- Neo-Synephrine ...... ▣ 614
- Phenergan VC Syrup 3560
- Phenergan VC with Codeine Syrup .. 3561
- Preparation H Cream ...... ▣ 778
- Preparation H Cooling Gel ...... ▣ 778
- Preparation H ...... ▣ 778
- Vicks Sinex Nasal Spray and Ultra Fine Mist ...... ▣ 729

Phenylephrine Tannate (Co-administration with other sympathomimetic agents increases the risk of adverse cardiovascular effects). Products include:
- Ryna-12 S Suspension 3351
- Reformulated Rynatan Pediatric Suspension 3352
- Rynatuss Pediatric Suspension 3353
- Rynatuss Tablets 3353

Phenylpropanolamine Hydrochloride (Co-administration with other sympathomimetic agents increases the risk of adverse cardiovascular effects).
- No products indexed under this heading.

Pindolol (Co-administration with beta blockers inhibits the effects of each other).
- No products indexed under this heading.

Pirbuterol Acetate (Co-administration with other sympathomimetic agents increases the risk of adverse cardiovascular effects). Products include:
- Maxair Autohaler 1981
- Maxair Inhaler 1984

Polythiazide (Co-administration with non-potassium sparing diuretics can result in acute worsening of ECG changes and/or hypokalemia, especially when recommended dose of the beta agonist is exceeded; clinical significance of this interaction is unknown). Products include:
- Minizide Capsules 2700
- Renese Tablets 2712

Procarbazine Hydrochloride (Co-administration with MAO inhibitors can potentiate the action of albuterol on the cardiovascular system). Products include:
- Matulane Capsules 3246

Procyclidine Hydrochloride (Co-administration has some potential for additive anticholinergic effects; caution is advised).
- No products indexed under this heading.

Propantheline Bromide (Co-administration has some potential for additive anticholinergic effects; caution is advised).
- No products indexed under this heading.

Propranolol Hydrochloride (Co-administration with beta blockers inhibits the effects of each other). Products include:
- Inderal 3513
- Inderal LA Long-Acting Capsules 3516
- Inderide Tablets 3517
- Inderide LA Long-Acting Capsules 3519

Protriptyline Hydrochloride (Co-administration with tricyclic antidepressants can potentiate the action of albuterol on the cardiovascular system). Products include:
- Vivactil Tablets 2446
- Vivactil Tablets 2217

Pseudoephedrine Hydrochloride (Co-administration with other sympathomimetic agents increases the risk of adverse cardiovascular effects). Products include:

- Actifed Cold & Allergy Tablets 688
- Actifed Cold & Sinus Caplets and Tablets 688
- Advil Cold and Sinus Caplets 771
- Advil Cold and Sinus Tablets 771
- Advil Flu & Body Ache Caplets 772
- Aleve Cold & Sinus Caplets 603
- Alka-Seltzer Plus Liqui-Gels 604
- Alka-Seltzer Plus Cold & Flu Medicine Liqui-Gels 604
- Alka-Seltzer Plus Cold & Sinus Medicine Liqui-Gels 604
- Allegra-D Extended-Release Tablets 714
- BC Cold Powder 619
- Benadryl Allergy/Cold Tablets 691
- Benadryl Allergy/Congestion Tablets 692
- Benadryl Allergy & Sinus Liquid 693
- Benadryl Allergy & Sinus Fastmelt Tablets 693
- Benadryl Allergy Sinus Headache Caplets & Gelcaps 693
- Benadryl Severe Allergy & Sinus Headache Caplets 694
- Benadryl Children's Allergy/Cold Fastmelt Tablets 692
- Benylin Multi-Symptom Liquid 697
- Bromfed Capsules (Extended-Release) 2269
- Bromfed-PD Capsules (Extended-Release) 2269
- Children's Cēpacol Sore Throat 788
- Comtrex Acute Head Cold & Sinus Pressure Relief Tablets 627
- Comtrex Deep Chest Cold & Congestion Relief Softgels 627
- Comtrex Flu Therapy & Fever Relief Daytime Caplets 628
- Comtrex Flu Therapy & Fever Relief Nighttime Tablets 628
- Comtrex Maximum Strength Multi-Symptom Cold & Cough Relief Tablets and Caplets 626
- Contac Non-Drowsy 12 Hour Cold Caplets 745
- Contac Non-Drowsy Timed Release 12 Hour Cold Caplets 746
- Contac Severe Cold and Flu Caplets Maximum Strength 746
- Contac Severe Cold and Flu Caplets Non-Drowsy 746
- Dimetapp Elixir 777
- Dimetapp Cold and Fever Suspension 775
- Dimetapp DM Cold & Cough Elixir 775
- Dimetapp Nighttime Flu Liquid 776
- Dimetapp Non-Drowsy Flu Syrup 777
- Dimetapp Infant Drops Decongestant 775
- Dimetapp Infant Drops Decongestant Plus Cough 776
- Guaifed 2272
- Kronofed-A 1341
- Children's Motrin Cold Oral Suspension 2007
- Motrin Sinus Headache Caplets 2005
- PediaCare Cough-Cold Liquid 719
- PediaCare Infants' Drops Decongestant 719
- PediaCare Infants' Drops Decongestant Plus Cough 719
- PediaCare NightRest Cough-Cold Liquid 719
- Robitussin Cold Caplets Cold & Congestion 780
- Robitussin Cold Softgels Cold & Congestion 780
- Robitussin Cold Caplets Multi-Symptom Cold & Flu 781
- Robitussin Cold Softgels Multi-Symptom Cold & Flu 781
- Robitussin Cold Softgels Severe Congestion 782
- Robitussin Cough & Cold Infant Drops 782
- Robitussin Maximum Strength Cough & Cold Liquid 785
- Robitussin Pediatric Cough & Cold Formula Liquid 785
- Robitussin Multi Symptom Honey Flu Liquid 785
- Robitussin Nighttime Honey Flu Liquid 786
- Robitussin-CF Liquid 783
- Robitussin-DAC Syrup 2942
- Robitussin-PE Liquid 782
- Ryna 768
- Semprex-D Capsules 1172
- Singlet Caplets 761
- Sinutab Non-Drying Liquid Caps 706
- Sinutab Sinus Allergy Medication, Maximum Strength Formula, Tablets & Caplets 707
- Sinutab Sinus Medication, Maximum Strength Without Drowsiness Formula, Tablets & Caplets 707
- Sudafed 12 Hour Tablets 708
- Sudafed 24 Hour Tablets 708
- Children's Sudafed Cold & Cough Liquid 709
- Children's Sudafed Nasal Decongestant Chewables 711
- Children's Sudafed Nasal Decongestant Liquid Medication 711
- Sudafed Cold & Allergy Tablets 708
- Sudafed Cold & Cough Liquid Caps 709
- Sudafed Cold & Sinus Liquid Caps 710
- Sudafed Nasal Decongestant Tablets 710
- Sudafed Non-Drying Sinus Liquid Caps 712
- Sudafed Severe Cold 711
- Sudafed Sinus Headache Caplets 712
- Sudafed Sinus Headache Tablets 712
- Tavist Sinus Non-Drowsy Coated Caplets 676
- TheraFlu Regular Strength Cold & Cough Night Time Hot Liquid 676
- TheraFlu Regular Strength Cold & Sore Throat Night Time Hot Liquid 676
- TheraFlu Maximum Strength Flu & Congestion Non-Drowsy Hot Liquid 677
- TheraFlu Maximum Strength Flu & Cough Night Time Hot Liquid 678
- TheraFlu Maximum Strength Flu & Sore Throat Night Time Hot Liquid 677
- TheraFlu Maximum Strength Severe Cold & Congestion Night Time Caplets 678
- TheraFlu Maximum Strength Severe Cold & Congestion Night Time Hot Liquid 678
- TheraFlu Maximum Strength Severe Cold & Congestion Non-Drowsy 679
- Triaminic Allergy Congestion Liquid 680
- Triaminic Chest Congestion Liquid 680
- Triaminic Cold & Allergy Liquid 681
- Triaminic Cold & Allergy Softchews 683
- Triaminic Cold & Cough Liquid 681
- Triaminic Cold & Cough Softchews 683
- Triaminic Cold & Night Time Cough Liquid 681
- Triaminic Cold, Cough & Fever Liquid 681
- Triaminic Cough Liquid 682
- Triaminic Cough & Congestion Liquid 682
- Triaminic Cough & Sore Throat Liquid 682
- Triaminic Cough & Sore Throat Softchews 684
- Children's Tylenol Allergy-D Liquid 2014
- Children's Tylenol Cold Suspension Liquid and Chewable Tablets 2015
- Children's Tylenol Cold Plus Cough Suspension Liquid and Chewable Tablets 2015
- Children's Tylenol Flu Suspension Liquid 2015
- Children's Tylenol Sinus Suspension Liquid 2017
- Infants' Tylenol Cold Decongestant and Fever Reducer Concentrated Drops 2015
- Infants' Tylenol Cold Decongestant and Fever Reducer Concentrated Drops Plus Cough 2015
- Tylenol Allergy Sinus 2010
- Multi-Symptom Tylenol Cold Complete Formula Caplets 2010
- Multi-Symptom Tylenol Cold Non-Drowsy Caplets and Gelcaps 2010
- Multi-Symptom Tylenol Cold Severe Congestion Non-Drowsy Caplets 2011
- Maximum Strength Tylenol Flu NightTime Gelcaps 2011
- Maximum Strength Tylenol Flu NightTime Liquid 2011
- Maximum Strength Tylenol Flu Non-Drowsy Gelcaps 2011
- Maximum Strength Tylenol Sinus NightTime Caplets 2012
- Maximum Strength Tylenol Sinus Non-Drowsy Geltabs, Gelcaps, Caplets, and Tablets 2012
- Vicks 44D Cough & Head Congestion Relief Liquid 724
- Vicks 44M Cough, Cold & Flu Relief Liquid 725
- Pediatric Vicks 44m Cough & Cold Relief 728
- Vicks DayQuil LiquiCaps/Liquid Multi-Symptom Cold/Flu Relief 727
- Children's Vicks NyQuil Cold/Cough Relief 726
- Vicks NyQuil LiquiCaps/Liquid Multi-Symptom Cold/Flu Relief, Original and Cherry Flavors 727
- Zephrex Tablets 3091
- Zephrex LA Tablets 3092
- Zyrtec-D 12 Hour Extended Relief Tablets 2758

Pseudoephedrine Sulfate (Co-administration with other sympathomimetic agents increases the risk of adverse cardiovascular effects). Products include:

- Chlor-Trimeton Allergy/Decongestant Tablets 736
- Claritin-D 12 Hour Extended Release Tablets 3102
- Claritin-D 24 Hour Extended Release Tablets 3104
- Coricidin 'D' Cold, Flu & Sinus Tablets 737
- Drixoral Allergy/Sinus Extended-Release Tablets 741
- Drixoral Cold & Allergy Sustained-Action Tablets 740
- Drixoral Cold & Flu Extended-Release Tablets 740
- Drixoral Nasal Decongestant Long-Acting Non-Drowsy Tablets 740
- Rynatan Tablets 3351

Salmeterol Xinafoate (Co-administration with other sympathomimetic agents increases the risk of adverse cardiovascular effects). Products include:

- Advair Diskus 100/50 1448
- Advair Diskus 250/50 1448
- Advair Diskus 500/50 1448
- Serevent Diskus 1637
- Serevent Inhalation Aerosol 1633

Scopolamine (Co-administration has some potential for additive anticholinergic effects; caution is advised). Products include:

- Transderm Scōp Transdermal Therapeutic System 2302

Scopolamine Hydrobromide (Co-administration has some potential for additive anticholinergic effects; caution is advised). Products include:

- Donnatal 2929
- Donnatal Extentabs 2930

Selegiline Hydrochloride (Co-administration with MAO inhibitors can potentiate the action of albuterol on the cardiovascular system). Products include:

- Eldepryl Capsules 3266

Sotalol Hydrochloride (Co-administration with beta blockers inhibits the effects of each other). Products include:

- Betapace Tablets 950
- Betapace AF Tablets 954

Terbutaline Sulfate (Co-administration with other sympathomimetic agents increases the risk of adverse cardiovascular effects). Products include:

- Brethine Ampuls 2314
- Brethine Tablets 2313

Timolol Hemihydrate (Co-administration with beta blockers inhibits the effects of each other). Products include:

- Betimol Ophthalmic Solution .... ⊙ 324

Timolol Maleate (Co-administration with beta blockers inhibits the effects of each other). Products include:

- Blocadren Tablets 2046
- Cosopt Sterile Ophthalmic Solution 2065
- Timolide Tablets 2187
- Timolol GFS .... ⊙ 266
- Timoptic in Ocudose 2192
- Timoptic Sterile Ophthalmic Solution 2190
- Timoptic-XE Sterile Ophthalmic Gel Forming Solution 2194

Tolterodine Tartrate (Co-administration has some potential for additive anticholinergic effects; caution is advised). Products include:

- Detrol Tablets 3623
- Detrol LA Capsules 2801

Torsemide (Co-administration with non-potassium sparing diuretics can result in acute worsening of ECG changes and/or hypokalemia, especially when recommended dose of the beta agonist is exceeded; clinical significance of this interaction is unknown). Products include:

- Demadex Tablets and Injection 2965

Tranylcypromine Sulfate (Co-administration with MAO inhibitors can potentiate the action of albuterol on the cardiovascular system). Products include:

- Parnate Tablets 1607

Tridihexethyl Chloride (Co-administration has some potential for additive anticholinergic effects; caution is advised).

No products indexed under this heading.

Trihexyphenidyl Hydrochloride (Co-administration has some potential for additive anticholinergic effects; caution is advised). Products include:

- Artane 1855

Trimipramine Maleate (Co-administration with tricyclic antidepressants can potentiate the action of albuterol on the cardiovascular system). Products include:

- Surmontil Capsules 3595

DURACLON INJECTION

(Clonidine Hydrochloride) 3057

May interact with barbiturates, beta blockers, calcium channel blockers, cardiac glycosides, hypnotics and sedatives, narcotic analgesics, tricyclic antidepressants, and certain other agents. Compounds in these categories include:

Acebutolol Hydrochloride (Beta blockers may exacerbate the hypertensive response seen with clonidine withdrawal; potential additive effects such as bradycardia and AV block). Products include:

- Sectral Capsules 3589

Alfentanil Hydrochloride (Narcotic analgesics may potentiate the hypotensive effects of clonidine).

No products indexed under this heading.

Amitriptyline Hydrochloride (Tricyclic antidepressants may antagonize the hypotensive effects of clonidine). Products include:

- Etrafon 3115
- Limbitrol 1738

Amlodipine Besylate (Co-administration with agents known to affect sinus node function or AV nodal conduction, such as calcium channel blockers, may result in a potential for additive effects such as bradycardia and AV block). Products include:

- Lotrel Capsules 2370
- Norvasc Tablets 2704

Amoxapine (Tricyclic antidepressants may antagonize the hypotensive effects of clonidine).

No products indexed under this heading.

Aprobarbital (Clonidine may potentiate the CNS-depressive effects).

No products indexed under this heading.

Atenolol (Beta blockers may exacerbate the hypertensive response seen with clonidine withdrawal;

IMPORTANT NOTE: Always consult each drug listing in the patient's regimen for possible interactions.

potential additive effects such as bradycardia and AV block). Products include:

Tenoretic Tablets 690
Tenormin I.V. Injection 692

Bepridil Hydrochloride (Co-administration with agents known to affect sinus node function or AV nodal conduction, such as calcium channel blockers, may result in a potential for additive effects such as bradycardia and AV block). Products include:

Vascor Tablets 2602

Betaxolol Hydrochloride (Beta blockers may exacerbate the hypertensive response seen with clonidine withdrawal; potential additive effects such as bradycardia and AV block). Products include:

Betoptic S Ophthalmic Suspension 537

Bisoprolol Fumarate (Beta blockers may exacerbate the hypertensive response seen with clonidine withdrawal; potential additive effects such as bradycardia and AV block). Products include:

Zebeta Tablets 1885
Ziac Tablets 1887

Buprenorphine Hydrochloride (Narcotic analgesics may potentiate the hypotensive effects of clonidine). Products include:

Buprenex Injectable 2918

Butabarbital (Clonidine may potentiate the CNS-depressive effects).

No products indexed under this heading.

Butalbital (Clonidine may potentiate the CNS-depressive effects). Products include:

Phrenilin 578
Sedapap Tablets 50 mg/650 mg 2225

Carteolol Hydrochloride (Beta blockers may exacerbate the hypertensive response seen with clonidine withdrawal; potential additive effects such as bradycardia and AV block). Products include:

Carteolol Hydrochloride Ophthalmic Solution USP, 1% .... ⊙258
Ocupress Ophthalmic Solution, 1% Sterile .... ⊙303

Clomipramine Hydrochloride (Tricyclic antidepressants may antagonize the hypotensive effects of clonidine).

No products indexed under this heading.

Codeine Phosphate (Narcotic analgesics may potentiate the hypotensive effects of clonidine). Products include:

Phenergan with Codeine Syrup 3557
Phenergan VC with Codeine Syrup 3561
Robitussin A-C Syrup 2942
Robitussin-DAC Syrup 2942
Ryna-C Liquid .... ▣768
Soma Compound w/Codeine Tablets 3355
Tussi-Organidin NR Liquid 3350
Tussi-Organidin-S NR Liquid 3350
Tylenol with Codeine 2595

Desipramine Hydrochloride (Tricyclic antidepressants may antagonize the hypotensive effects of clonidine). Products include:

Norpramin Tablets 755

Deslanoside (Co-administration with agents known to affect sinus node function or AV nodal conduction, such as digitalis, may result in a potential for additive effects such as bradycardia and AV block).

No products indexed under this heading.

Dezocine (Narcotic analgesics may potentiate the hypotensive effects of clonidine).

No products indexed under this heading.

Digitoxin (Co-administration with agents known to affect sinus node function or AV nodal conduction, such as digitalis, may result in a potential for additive effects such as bradycardia and AV block).

No products indexed under this heading.

Digoxin (Co-administration with agents known to affect sinus node function or AV nodal conduction, such as digitalis, may result in a potential for additive effects such as bradycardia and AV block). Products include:

Digitek Tablets 1003
Lanoxicaps Capsules 1574
Lanoxin Injection 1581
Lanoxin Tablets 1587
Lanoxin Elixir Pediatric 1578
Lanoxin Injection Pediatric 1584

Diltiazem Hydrochloride (Co-administration with agents known to affect sinus node function or AV nodal conduction, such as calcium channel blockers, may result in a potential for additive effects such as bradycardia and AV block). Products include:

Cardizem Injectable 1018
Cardizem Lyo-Ject Syringe 1018
Cardizem Monovial 1018
Cardizem CD Capsules 1016
Tiazac Capsules 1378

Doxepin Hydrochloride (Tricyclic antidepressants may antagonize the hypotensive effects of clonidine). Products include:

Sinequan 2713

Esmolol Hydrochloride (Beta blockers may exacerbate the hypertensive response seen with clonidine withdrawal; potential additive effects such as bradycardia and AV block). Products include:

Brevibloc Injection 858

Estazolam (Clonidine may potentiate the CNS-depressive effects). Products include:

ProSom Tablets 500

Ethchlorvynol (Clonidine may potentiate the CNS-depressive effects).

No products indexed under this heading.

Ethinamate (Clonidine may potentiate the CNS-depressive effects).

No products indexed under this heading.

Felodipine (Co-administration with agents known to affect sinus node function or AV nodal conduction, such as calcium channel blockers, may result in a potential for additive effects such as bradycardia and AV block). Products include:

Lexxel Tablets 608
Plendil Extended-Release Tablets 623

Fentanyl (Narcotic analgesics may potentiate the hypotensive effects of clonidine). Products include:

Duragesic Transdermal System 1786

Fentanyl Citrate (Narcotic analgesics may potentiate the hypotensive effects of clonidine). Products include:

Actiq 1184

Fluphenazine Decanoate (Co-administration of oral clonidine and fluphenazine has resulted in a case of acute delirium).

No products indexed under this heading.

Fluphenazine Enanthate (Co-administration of oral clonidine and fluphenazine has resulted in a case of acute delirium).

No products indexed under this heading.

Flurazepam Hydrochloride (Clonidine may potentiate the CNS-depressive effects).

No products indexed under this heading.

Glutethimide (Clonidine may potentiate the CNS-depressive effects).

No products indexed under this heading.

Hydrocodone Bitartrate (Narcotic analgesics may potentiate the hypotensive effects of clonidine). Products include:

Hycodan 1316
Hycomine Compound Tablets 1317
Hycotuss Expectorant Syrup 1318
Lortab 3319
Lortab Elixir 3317
Maxidone Tablets CIII 3399
Norco 5/325 Tablets CIII 3424
Norco 7.5/325 Tablets CIII 3425
Norco 10/325 Tablets CIII 3427
Norco 10/325 Tablets CIII 3425
Vicodin Tablets 516
Vicodin ES Tablets 517
Vicodin HP Tablets 518
Vicodin Tuss Expectorant 519
Vicoprofen Tablets 520
Zydone Tablets 1330

Hydrocodone Polistirex (Narcotic analgesics may potentiate the hypotensive effects of clonidine). Products include:

Tussionex Pennkinetic Extended-Release Suspension 1174

Hydromorphone Hydrochloride (Narcotic analgesics may potentiate the hypotensive effects of clonidine). Products include:

Dilaudid 441
Dilaudid Oral Liquid 445
Dilaudid Powder 441
Dilaudid Rectal Suppositories 441
Dilaudid Tablets 441
Dilaudid Tablets - 8 mg 445
Dilaudid-HP 443

Imipramine Hydrochloride (Tricyclic antidepressants may antagonize the hypotensive effects of clonidine).

No products indexed under this heading.

Imipramine Pamoate (Tricyclic antidepressants may antagonize the hypotensive effects of clonidine).

No products indexed under this heading.

Isradipine (Co-administration with agents known to affect sinus node function or AV nodal conduction, such as calcium channel blockers, may result in a potential for additive effects such as bradycardia and AV block). Products include:

DynaCirc Capsules 2921
DynaCirc CR Tablets 2923

Labetalol Hydrochloride (Beta blockers may exacerbate the hypertensive response seen with clonidine withdrawal; potential additive effects such as bradycardia and AV block). Products include:

Normodyne Injection 3135
Normodyne Tablets 3137

Levobunolol Hydrochloride (Beta blockers may exacerbate the hypertensive response seen with clonidine withdrawal; potential additive effects such as bradycardia and AV block). Products include:

Betagan .... ⊙228

Levorphanol Tartrate (Narcotic analgesics may potentiate the hypotensive effects of clonidine). Products include:

Levo-Dromoran 1734
Levorphanol Tartrate Tablets 3059

Lorazepam (Clonidine may potentiate the CNS-depressive effects). Products include:

Ativan Injection 3478
Ativan Tablets 3482

Maprotiline Hydrochloride (Tricyclic antidepressants may antagonize the hypotensive effects of clonidine).

No products indexed under this heading.

Meperidine Hydrochloride (Narcotic analgesics may potentiate the hypotensive effects of clonidine). Products include:

Demerol 3079
Mepergan Injection 3539

Mephobarbital (Clonidine may potentiate the CNS-depressive effects).

No products indexed under this heading.

Methadone Hydrochloride (Narcotic analgesics may potentiate the hypotensive effects of clonidine). Products include:

Dolophine Hydrochloride Tablets 3056

Metipranolol Hydrochloride (Beta blockers may exacerbate the hypertensive response seen with clonidine withdrawal; potential additive effects such as bradycardia and AV block).

No products indexed under this heading.

Metoprolol Succinate (Beta blockers may exacerbate the hypertensive response seen with clonidine withdrawal; potential additive effects such as bradycardia and AV block). Products include:

Toprol-XL Tablets 651

Metoprolol Tartrate (Beta blockers may exacerbate the hypertensive response seen with clonidine withdrawal; potential additive effects such as bradycardia and AV block).

No products indexed under this heading.

Mibefradil Dihydrochloride (Co-administration with agents known to affect sinus node function or AV nodal conduction, such as calcium channel blockers, may result in a potential for additive effects such as bradycardia and AV block).

No products indexed under this heading.

Midazolam Hydrochloride (Clonidine may potentiate the CNS-depressive effects). Products include:

Versed Injection 3027
Versed Syrup 3033

Morphine Sulfate (Narcotic analgesics may potentiate the hypotensive effects of clonidine). Products include:

Astramorph/PF Injection, USP (Preservative-Free) 594
Duramorph Injection 1312
Infumorph 200 and Infumorph 500 Sterile Solutions 1314
Kadian Capsules 1335
MS Contin Tablets 2896
MSIR 2898
Oramorph SR Tablets 3062
Roxanol 3066

Nadolol (Beta blockers may exacerbate the hypertensive response seen with clonidine withdrawal; potential additive effects such as bradycardia and AV block). Products include:

Corgard Tablets 2245
Corzide 40/5 Tablets 2247
Corzide 80/5 Tablets 2247
Nadolol Tablets 2288

Nicardipine Hydrochloride (Co-administration with agents known to affect sinus node function or AV nodal conduction, such as calcium channel blockers, may result in a potential for additive effects such as bradycardia and AV block). Products include:

Cardene I.V. 3485

Nifedipine (Co-administration with agents known to affect sinus node function or AV nodal conduction, such as calcium channel blockers, may result in a potential for additive effects such as bradycardia and AV block). Products include:

Adalat CC Tablets 877
Procardia Capsules 2708
Procardia XL Extended Release Tablets 2710

Nimodipine (Co-administration with agents known to affect sinus node function or AV nodal conduction, such as calcium channel blockers, may result in a potential for additive effects such as bradycardia and AV block). Products include:

Nimotop Capsules 904

Nisoldipine (Co-administration with agents known to affect sinus node function or AV nodal conduction, such as calcium channel blockers, may result in a potential for additive effects such as bradycardia and AV block). Products include:
- Sular Tablets ... 688

Nortriptyline Hydrochloride (Tricyclic antidepressants may antagonize the hypotensive effects of clonidine).
- No products indexed under this heading.

Oxycodone Hydrochloride (Narcotic analgesics may potentiate the hypotensive effects of clonidine). Products include:
- OxyContin Tablets ... 2912
- OxyFast Oral Concentrate Solution ... 2916
- OxyIR Capsules ... 2916
- Percocet Tablets ... 1326
- Percodan Tablets ... 1327
- Percolone Tablets ... 1327
- Roxicodone ... 3067
- Tylox Capsules ... 2597

Penbutolol Sulfate (Beta blockers may exacerbate the hypertensive response seen with clonidine withdrawal; potential additive effects such as bradycardia and AV block).
- No products indexed under this heading.

Pentobarbital Sodium (Clonidine may potentiate the CNS-depressive effects). Products include:
- Nembutal Sodium Solution ... 485

Phenobarbital (Clonidine may potentiate the CNS-depressive effects). Products include:
- Arco-Lase Plus Tablets ... 592
- Donnatal ... 2929
- Donnatal Extentabs ... 2930

Pindolol (Beta blockers may exacerbate the hypertensive response seen with clonidine withdrawal; potential additive effects such as bradycardia and AV block).
- No products indexed under this heading.

Propofol (Clonidine may potentiate the CNS-depressive effects). Products include:
- Diprivan Injectable Emulsion ... 667

Propoxyphene Hydrochloride (Narcotic analgesics may potentiate the hypotensive effects of clonidine). Products include:
- Darvon Pulvules ... 1909
- Darvon Compound-65 Pulvules ... 1910

Propoxyphene Napsylate (Narcotic analgesics may potentiate the hypotensive effects of clonidine). Products include:
- Darvon-N/Darvocet-N ... 1907
- Darvon-N Tablets ... 1912

Propranolol Hydrochloride (Beta blockers may exacerbate the hypertensive response seen with clonidine withdrawal; potential additive effects such as bradycardia and AV block). Products include:
- Inderal ... 3513
- Inderal LA Long-Acting Capsules ... 3516
- Inderide Tablets ... 3517
- Inderide LA Long-Acting Capsules ... 3519

Protriptyline Hydrochloride (Tricyclic antidepressants may antagonize the hypotensive effects of clonidine). Products include:
- Vivactil Tablets ... 2446
- Vivactil Tablets ... 2217

Quazepam (Clonidine may potentiate the CNS-depressive effects).
- No products indexed under this heading.

Remifentanil Hydrochloride (Narcotic analgesics may potentiate the hypotensive effects of clonidine).
- No products indexed under this heading.

Secobarbital Sodium (Clonidine may potentiate the CNS-depressive effects).
- No products indexed under this heading.

Sotalol Hydrochloride (Beta blockers may exacerbate the hypertensive response seen with clonidine withdrawal; potential additive effects such as bradycardia and AV block). Products include:
- Betapace Tablets ... 950
- Betapace AF Tablets ... 954

Sufentanil Citrate (Narcotic analgesics may potentiate the hypotensive effects of clonidine).
- No products indexed under this heading.

Temazepam (Clonidine may potentiate the CNS-depressive effects).
- No products indexed under this heading.

Thiamylal Sodium (Clonidine may potentiate the CNS-depressive effects).
- No products indexed under this heading.

Timolol Hemihydrate (Beta blockers may exacerbate the hypertensive response seen with clonidine withdrawal; potential additive effects such as bradycardia and AV block). Products include:
- Betimol Ophthalmic Solution ... ⊙ 324

Timolol Maleate (Beta blockers may exacerbate the hypertensive response seen with clonidine withdrawal; potential additive effects such as bradycardia and AV block). Products include:
- Blocadren Tablets ... 2046
- Cosopt Sterile Ophthalmic Solution ... 2065
- Timolide Tablets ... 2187
- Timolol GFS ... ⊙ 266
- Timoptic in Ocudose ... 2192
- Timoptic Sterile Ophthalmic Solution ... 2190
- Timoptic-XE Sterile Ophthalmic Gel Forming Solution ... 2194

Triazolam (Clonidine may potentiate the CNS-depressive effects). Products include:
- Halcion Tablets ... 2823

Trimipramine Maleate (Tricyclic antidepressants may antagonize the hypotensive effects of clonidine). Products include:
- Surmontil Capsules ... 3595

Verapamil Hydrochloride (Co-administration with agents known to affect sinus node function or AV nodal conduction, such as calcium channel blockers, may result in a potential for additive effects such as bradycardia and AV block). Products include:
- Covera-HS Tablets ... 3199
- Isoptin SR Tablets ... 467
- Tarka Tablets ... 508
- Verelan Capsules ... 3184
- Verelan PM Capsules ... 3186

Zaleplon (Clonidine may potentiate the CNS-depressive effects). Products include:
- Sonata Capsules ... 3591

Zolpidem Tartrate (Clonidine may potentiate the CNS-depressive effects). Products include:
- Ambien Tablets ... 3191

Food Interactions

Alcohol (Clonidine may potentiate the CNS-depressive effects of alcohol).

DURAGESIC TRANSDERMAL SYSTEM

(Fentanyl) ... 1786

May interact with antihistamines, central nervous system depressants, CYP450 3A4 isoenzyme inhibitors (selected), CYP450 3A4 isoenzyme inducers (selected), hypnotics and sedatives, narcotic analgesics, phenothiazines, tranquilizers, and certain other agents. Compounds in these categories include:

Acrivastine (May produce additive depressant effects, hypoventilation, hypotension and profound sedation or coma may occur). Products include:
- Semprex-D Capsules ... 1172

Alfentanil Hydrochloride (May produce additive depressant effects, hypoventilation, hypotension and profound sedation or coma may occur).
- No products indexed under this heading.

Alprazolam (May produce additive depressant effects, hypoventilation, hypotension and profound sedation or coma may occur). Products include:
- Xanax Tablets ... 2865

Amiodarone Hydrochloride (Fentanyl is metabolized by CYP450 3A4 isoenzyme system; co-administration with drugs that inhibit this enzyme system may result in increased plasma concentrations of fentanyl and increased risk of adverse events). Products include:
- Cordarone Intravenous ... 3491
- Cordarone Tablets ... 3487
- Pacerone Tablets ... 3331

Amprenavir (Fentanyl is metabolized by CYP450 3A4 isoenzyme system; co-administration with drugs that inhibit this enzyme system may result in increased plasma concentrations of fentanyl and increased risk of adverse events). Products include:
- Agenerase Capsules ... 1454
- Agenerase Oral Solution ... 1459

Aprobarbital (May produce additive depressant effects, hypoventilation, hypotension and profound sedation or coma may occur).
- No products indexed under this heading.

Astemizole (May produce additive depressant effects, hypoventilation, hypotension and profound sedation or coma may occur).
- No products indexed under this heading.

Azatadine Maleate (May produce additive depressant effects, hypoventilation, hypotension and profound sedation or coma may occur). Products include:
- Rynatan Tablets ... 3351

Bromodiphenhydramine Hydrochloride (May produce additive depressant effects, hypoventilation, hypotension and profound sedation or coma may occur).
- No products indexed under this heading.

Brompheniramine Maleate (May produce additive depressant effects, hypoventilation, hypotension and profound sedation or coma may occur). Products include:
- Bromfed Capsules (Extended-Release) ... 2269
- Bromfed-PD Capsules (Extended-Release) ... 2269
- Comtrex Acute Head Cold & Sinus Pressure Relief Tablets ... 627
- Dimetapp Elixir ... 777
- Dimetapp Cold and Fever Suspension ... 775
- Dimetapp DM Cold & Cough Elixir ... 775
- Dimetapp Nighttime Flu Liquid ... 776

Buprenorphine Hydrochloride (May produce additive depressant effects, hypoventilation, hypotension and profound sedation or coma may occur). Products include:
- Buprenex Injectable ... 2918

Buspirone Hydrochloride (May produce additive depressant effects, hypoventilation, hypotension and profound sedation or coma may occur).
- No products indexed under this heading.

Butabarbital (May produce additive depressant effects, hypoventilation, hypotension and profound sedation or coma may occur).
- No products indexed under this heading.

Butalbital (May produce additive depressant effects, hypoventilation, hypotension and profound sedation or coma may occur). Products include:
- Phrenilin ... 578
- Sedapap Tablets 50 mg/650 mg ... 2225

Carbamazepine (Fentanyl is metabolized by CYP450 3A4 isoenzyme system; co-administration with drugs that induce this enzyme system may result in decreased plasma concentrations of fentanyl and decrease in therapeutic effect). Products include:
- Carbatrol Capsules ... 3234
- Tegretol/Tegretol-XR ... 2404

Cetirizine Hydrochloride (May produce additive depressant effects, hypoventilation, hypotension and profound sedation or coma may occur). Products include:
- Zyrtec ... 2756
- Zyrtec-D 12 Hour Extended Relief Tablets ... 2758

Chlordiazepoxide (May produce additive depressant effects, hypoventilation, hypotension and profound sedation or coma may occur). Products include:
- Limbitrol ... 1738

Chlordiazepoxide Hydrochloride (May produce additive depressant effects, hypoventilation, hypotension and profound sedation or coma may occur). Products include:
- Librium Capsules ... 1736
- Librium for Injection ... 1737

Chlorpheniramine Maleate (May produce additive depressant effects, hypoventilation, hypotension and profound sedation or coma may occur). Products include:
- Actifed Cold & Sinus Caplets and Tablets ... 688
- Alka-Seltzer Plus Liqui-Gels ... 604
- BC Allergy Sinus Cold Powder ... 619
- Chlor-Trimeton Allergy Tablets ... 735
- Chlor-Trimeton Allergy/Decongestant Tablets ... 736
- Comtrex Flu Therapy & Fever Relief Nighttime Tablets ... 628
- Comtrex Maximum Strength Multi-Symptom Cold & Cough Relief Tablets and Caplets ... 626
- Contac Severe Cold and Flu Caplets Maximum Strength ... 746
- Coricidin 'D' Cold, Flu & Sinus Tablets ... 737
- Coricidin/Coricidin D ... 738
- Coricidin HBP Maximum Strength Flu Tablets ... 738
- Extendryl ... 1361
- Hycomine Compound Tablets ... 1317
- Kronofed-A ... 1341
- PediaCare Cough-Cold Liquid ... 719
- PediaCare NightRest Cough-Cold Liquid ... 719
- Robitussin Nighttime Honey Flu Liquid ... 786
- Ryna ... 768
- Singlet Caplets ... 761
- Sinutab Sinus Allergy Medication, Maximum Strength Formula, Tablets & Caplets ... 707
- Sudafed Cold & Allergy Tablets ... 708
- TheraFlu Regular Strength Cold & Cough Night Time Hot Liquid ... 676
- TheraFlu Regular Strength Cold & Sore Throat Night Time Hot Liquid ... 676
- TheraFlu Maximum Strength Flu & Cough Night Time Hot Liquid ... 678
- TheraFlu Maximum Strength Flu & Sore Throat Night Time Hot Liquid ... 677
- TheraFlu Maximum Strength Severe Cold & Congestion Night Time Caplets ... 678
- TheraFlu Maximum Strength Severe Cold & Congestion Night Time Hot Liquid ... 678
- Triaminic Cold & Allergy Liquid ... 681
- Triaminic Cold & Allergy Softchews ... 683
- Triaminic Cold & Cough Liquid ... 681
- Triaminic Cold & Cough Softchews ... 683

Triaminic Cold & Night Time Cough Liquid ■ 681
Triaminic Cold, Cough & Fever Liquid ■ 681
Children's Tylenol Cold Suspension Liquid and Chewable Tablets 2015
Children's Tylenol Cold Plus Cough Suspension Liquid and Chewable Tablets 2015
Children's Tylenol Flu Suspension Liquid 2015
Maximum Strength Tylenol Allergy Sinus Caplets, Gelcaps, and Geltabs 2010
Multi-Symptom Tylenol Cold Complete Formula Caplets 2010
Vicks 44M Cough, Cold & Flu Relief Liquid ■ 725
Pediatric Vicks 44m Cough & Cold Relief ■ 728
Children's Vicks NyQuil Cold/Cough Relief ■ 726

Chlorpheniramine Polistirex (May produce additive depressant effects, hypoventilation, hypotension and profound sedation or coma may occur). Products include:
Tussionex Pennkinetic Extended-Release Suspension 1174

Chlorpheniramine Tannate (May produce additive depressant effects, hypoventilation, hypotension and profound sedation or coma may occur). Products include:
Reformulated Rynatan Pediatric Suspension 3352
Rynatuss Pediatric Suspension 3353
Rynatuss Tablets 3353
Tussi-12 S Suspension 3356
Tussi-12 Tablets 3356

Chlorpromazine (May produce additive depressant effects, hypoventilation, hypotension and profound sedation or coma may occur). Products include:
Thorazine Suppositories 1656

Chlorpromazine Hydrochloride (May produce additive depressant effects, hypoventilation, hypotension and profound sedation or coma may occur). Products include:
Thorazine 1656

Chlorprothixene (May produce additive depressant effects, hypoventilation, hypotension and profound sedation or coma may occur).
No products indexed under this heading.

Chlorprothixene Hydrochloride (May produce additive depressant effects, hypoventilation, hypotension and profound sedation or coma may occur).
No products indexed under this heading.

Chlorprothixene Lactate (May produce additive depressant effects, hypoventilation, hypotension and profound sedation or coma may occur).
No products indexed under this heading.

Cimetidine (Fentanyl is metabolized by CYP450 3A4 isoenzyme system; co-administration with drugs that inhibit this enzyme system may result in increased plasma concentrations of fentanyl and increased risk of adverse events). Products include:
Tagamet HB 200 Suspension ■ 762
Tagamet HB 200 Tablets ■ 761
Tagamet Tablets 1644

Cimetidine Hydrochloride (Fentanyl is metabolized by CYP450 3A4 isoenzyme system; co-administration with drugs that inhibit this enzyme system may result in increased plasma concentrations of fentanyl and increased risk of adverse events). Products include:
Tagamet 1644

Clarithromycin (Fentanyl is metabolized by CYP450 3A4 isoenzyme system; co-administration with drugs that inhibit this enzyme system may result in increased plasma concentrations of fentanyl and increased risk of adverse events). Products include:
Biaxin/Biaxin XL 403
PREVPAC 3298

Clemastine Fumarate (May produce additive depressant effects, hypoventilation, hypotension and profound sedation or coma may occur). Products include:
Tavist 12 Hour Allergy Tablets ■ 676

Clorazepate Dipotassium (May produce additive depressant effects, hypoventilation, hypotension and profound sedation or coma may occur). Products include:
Tranxene 511

Clozapine (May produce additive depressant effects, hypoventilation, hypotension and profound sedation or coma may occur). Products include:
Clozaril Tablets 2319

Codeine Phosphate (May produce additive depressant effects, hypoventilation, hypotension and profound sedation or coma may occur). Products include:
Phenergan with Codeine Syrup 3557
Phenergan VC with Codeine Syrup 3561
Robitussin A-C Syrup 2942
Robitussin-DAC Syrup 2942
Ryna-C Liquid ■ 768
Soma Compound w/Codeine Tablets 3355
Tussi-Organidin NR Liquid 3350
Tussi-Organidin-S NR Liquid 3350
Tylenol with Codeine 2595

Cyproheptadine Hydrochloride (May produce additive depressant effects, hypoventilation, hypotension and profound sedation or coma may occur). Products include:
Periactin Tablets 2155

Desflurane (May produce additive depressant effects, hypoventilation, hypotension and profound sedation or coma may occur). Products include:
Suprane Liquid for Inhalation 874

Dexchlorpheniramine Maleate (May produce additive depressant effects, hypoventilation, hypotension and profound sedation or coma may occur).
No products indexed under this heading.

Dezocine (May produce additive depressant effects, hypoventilation, hypotension and profound sedation or coma may occur).
No products indexed under this heading.

Diazepam (May produce additive depressant effects, hypoventilation, hypotension and profound sedation or coma may occur). Products include:
Valium Injectable 3026
Valium Tablets 3047

Diphenhydramine Citrate (May produce additive depressant effects, hypoventilation, hypotension and profound sedation or coma may occur). Products include:
Alka-Seltzer PM Effervescent Tablets ■ 605
Benadryl Allergy & Sinus Fastmelt Tablets ■ 693
Benadryl Children's Allergy/Cold Fastmelt Tablets ■ 692
Excedrin PM Tablets, Caplets, and Geltabs ■ 631
Goody's PM Powder ■ 621

Diphenhydramine Hydrochloride (May produce additive depressant effects, hypoventilation, hypotension and profound sedation or coma may occur). Products include:
Extra Strength Bayer PM Caplets ■ 611
Benadryl Allergy Chewables ■ 689
Benadryl Allergy ■ 691
Benadryl Allergy Liquid ■ 690
Benadryl Allergy/Cold Tablets ■ 691
Benadryl Allergy/Congestion Tablets ■ 692
Benadryl Allergy & Sinus Liquid ■ 693
Benadryl Allergy Sinus Headache Caplets & Gelcaps ■ 693
Benadryl Severe Allergy & Sinus Headache Caplets ■ 694
Benadryl Dye-Free Allergy Liquid ■ 690
Benadryl Dye-Free Allergy Liqui-Gels Softgels ■ 690
Benadryl Itch Relief Stick Extra Strength ■ 695
Benadryl Cream ■ 695
Benadryl Gel ■ 695
Benadryl Spray ■ 696
Benadryl Parenteral 2617
Coricidin HBP Night-Time Cold & Flu Tablets ■ 738
Nytol QuickCaps Caplets ■ 622
Maximum Strength Nytol QuickGels Softgels ■ 621
Extra Strength Percogesic Aspirin-Free Coated Caplets ■ 665
Simply Sleep Caplets 2008
Sominex Original Formula Tablets ■ 761
Children's Tylenol Allergy-D Liquid 2014
Maximum Strength Tylenol Allergy Sinus NightTime Caplets 2010
Tylenol Severe Allergy Caplets 2010
Maximum Strength Tylenol Flu NightTime Gelcaps 2011
Extra Strength Tylenol PM Caplets, Geltabs, and Gelcaps 2012
Unisom Maximum Strength SleepGels ■ 713

Diphenylpyraline Hydrochloride (May produce additive depressant effects, hypoventilation, hypotension and profound sedation or coma may occur).
No products indexed under this heading.

Droperidol (May produce additive depressant effects, hypoventilation, hypotension and profound sedation or coma may occur).
No products indexed under this heading.

Enflurane (May produce additive depressant effects, hypoventilation, hypotension and profound sedation or coma may occur).
No products indexed under this heading.

Erythromycin (Fentanyl is metabolized by CYP450 3A4 isoenzyme system; co-administration with drugs that inhibit this enzyme system may result in increased plasma concentrations of fentanyl and increased risk of adverse events). Products include:
Emgel 2% Topical Gel 1285
Ery-Tab Tablets 448
Erythromycin Base Filmtab Tablets 454
Erythromycin Delayed-Release Capsules, USP 455
PCE Dispertab Tablets 498

Erythromycin Estolate (Fentanyl is metabolized by CYP450 3A4 isoenzyme system; co-administration with drugs that inhibit this enzyme system may result in increased plasma concentrations of fentanyl and increased risk of adverse events).
No products indexed under this heading.

Erythromycin Ethylsuccinate (Fentanyl is metabolized by CYP450 3A4 isoenzyme system; co-administration with drugs that inhibit this enzyme system may result in increased plasma concentrations of fentanyl and increased risk of adverse events). Products include:
E.E.S. 450
EryPed 446
Pediazole Suspension 3050

Erythromycin Gluceptate (Fentanyl is metabolized by CYP450 3A4 isoenzyme system; co-administration with drugs that inhibit this enzyme system may result in increased plasma concentrations of fentanyl and increased risk of adverse events).
No products indexed under this heading.

Erythromycin Stearate (Fentanyl is metabolized by CYP450 3A4 isoenzyme system; co-administration with drugs that inhibit this enzyme system may result in increased plasma concentrations of fentanyl and increased risk of adverse events). Products include:
Erythrocin Stearate Filmtab Tablets 452

Estazolam (May produce additive depressant effects, hypoventilation, hypotension and profound sedation or coma may occur). Products include:
ProSom Tablets 500

Ethchlorvynol (May produce additive depressant effects, hypoventilation, hypotension and profound sedation or coma may occur).
No products indexed under this heading.

Ethinamate (May produce additive depressant effects, hypoventilation, hypotension and profound sedation or coma may occur).
No products indexed under this heading.

Fentanyl Citrate (May produce additive depressant effects, hypoventilation, hypotension and profound sedation or coma may occur). Products include:
Actiq 1184

Fexofenadine Hydrochloride (May produce additive depressant effects, hypoventilation, hypotension and profound sedation or coma may occur). Products include:
Allegra 712
Allegra-D Extended-Release Tablets 714

Fluconazole (Fentanyl is metabolized by CYP450 3A4 isoenzyme system; co-administration with drugs that inhibit this enzyme system may result in increased plasma concentrations of fentanyl and increased risk of adverse events). Products include:
Diflucan Tablets, Injection, and Oral Suspension 2681

Fluphenazine Decanoate (May produce additive depressant effects, hypoventilation, hypotension and profound sedation or coma may occur).
No products indexed under this heading.

Fluphenazine Enanthate (May produce additive depressant effects, hypoventilation, hypotension and profound sedation or coma may occur).
No products indexed under this heading.

Fluphenazine Hydrochloride (May produce additive depressant effects, hypoventilation, hypotension and profound sedation or coma may occur).
No products indexed under this heading.

Flurazepam Hydrochloride (May produce additive depressant effects, hypoventilation, hypotension and profound sedation or coma may occur).
No products indexed under this heading.

Fluvoxamine Maleate (Fentanyl is metabolized by CYP450 3A4 isoenzyme system; co-administration with drugs that inhibit this enzyme system may result in increased plasma concentrations of fentanyl and increased risk of adverse events). Products include:
Luvox Tablets (25, 50, 100 mg) 3256

Fosphenytoin Sodium (Fentanyl is metabolized by CYP450 3A4 isoenzyme system; co-administration with drugs that induce this enzyme system may result in decreased plasma concentrations of fentanyl and decrease in therapeutic effect). Products include:
Cerebyx Injection 2619

Glutethimide (May produce additive depressant effects, hypoventilation, hypotension and profound sedation or coma may occur).
No products indexed under this heading.

Haloperidol (May produce additive depressant effects, hypoventilation, hypotension and profound sedation or coma may occur). Products include:
Haldol Injection, Tablets and Concentrate 2533

Haloperidol Decanoate (May produce additive depressant effects, hypoventilation, hypotension and profound sedation or coma may occur). Products include:
Haldol Decanoate 2535

Hydrocodone Bitartrate (May produce additive depressant effects, hypoventilation, hypotension and profound sedation or coma may occur). Products include:
Hycodan 1316
Hycomine Compound Tablets 1317
Hycotuss Expectorant Syrup 1318
Lortab 3319
Lortab Elixir 3317
Maxidone Tablets CIII 3399
Norco 5/325 Tablets CIII 3424
Norco 7.5/325 Tablets CIII 3425
Norco 10/325 Tablets CIII 3427
Norco 10/325 Tablets CIII 3425
Vicodin Tablets 516
Vicodin ES Tablets 517
Vicodin HP Tablets 518
Vicodin Tuss Expectorant 519
Vicoprofen Tablets 520
Zydone Tablets 1330

Hydrocodone Polistirex (May produce additive depressant effects, hypoventilation, hypotension and profound sedation or coma may occur). Products include:
Tussionex Pennkinetic Extended-Release Suspension 1174

Hydromorphone Hydrochloride (May produce additive depressant effects, hypoventilation, hypotension and profound sedation or coma may occur). Products include:
Dilaudid 441
Dilaudid Oral Liquid 445
Dilaudid Powder 441
Dilaudid Rectal Suppositories 441
Dilaudid Tablets 441
Dilaudid Tablets - 8 mg 445
Dilaudid-HP 443

Hydroxyzine Hydrochloride (May produce additive depressant effects, hypoventilation, hypotension and profound sedation or coma may occur). Products include:
Atarax Tablets & Syrup 2667
Vistaril Intramuscular Solution 2738

Indinavir Sulfate (Fentanyl is metabolized by CYP450 3A4 isoenzyme system; co-administration with drugs that inhibit this enzyme system may result in increased plasma concentrations of fentanyl and increased risk of adverse events). Products include:
Crixivan Capsules 2070

Isoflurane (May produce additive depressant effects, hypoventilation, hypotension and profound sedation or coma may occur).
No products indexed under this heading.

Itraconazole (Fentanyl is metabolized by CYP450 3A4 isoenzyme system; co-administration with drugs that inhibit this enzyme system may result in increased plasma concentrations of fentanyl and increased risk of adverse events). Products include:
Sporanox Capsules 1800
Sporanox Injection 1804
Sporanox Injection 2509
Sporanox Oral Solution 1808
Sporanox Oral Solution 2512

Ketamine Hydrochloride (May produce additive depressant effects, hypoventilation, hypotension and profound sedation or coma may occur).
No products indexed under this heading.

Ketoconazole (Fentanyl is metabolized by CYP450 3A4 isoenzyme system; co-administration with drugs that inhibit this enzyme system may result in increased plasma concentrations of fentanyl and increased risk of adverse events). Products include:
Nizoral 2% Cream 3620
Nizoral A-D Shampoo 2008
Nizoral 2% Shampoo 2007
Nizoral Tablets 1791

Levomethadyl Acetate Hydrochloride (May produce additive depressant effects, hypoventilation, hypotension and profound sedation or coma may occur).
No products indexed under this heading.

Levorphanol Tartrate (May produce additive depressant effects, hypoventilation, hypotension and profound sedation or coma may occur). Products include:
Levo-Dromoran 1734
Levorphanol Tartrate Tablets 3059

Loratadine (May produce additive depressant effects, hypoventilation, hypotension and profound sedation or coma may occur). Products include:
Claritin 3100
Claritin-D 12 Hour Extended Release Tablets 3102
Claritin-D 24 Hour Extended Release Tablets 3104

Lorazepam (May produce additive depressant effects, hypoventilation, hypotension and profound sedation or coma may occur). Products include:
Ativan Injection 3478
Ativan Tablets 3482

Loxapine Hydrochloride (May produce additive depressant effects, hypoventilation, hypotension and profound sedation or coma may occur).
No products indexed under this heading.

Loxapine Succinate (May produce additive depressant effects, hypoventilation, hypotension and profound sedation or coma may occur). Products include:
Loxitane Capsules 3398

Meperidine Hydrochloride (May produce additive depressant effects, hypoventilation, hypotension and profound sedation or coma may occur). Products include:
Demerol 3079
Mepergan Injection 3539

Mephobarbital (May produce additive depressant effects, hypoventilation, hypotension and profound sedation or coma may occur).
No products indexed under this heading.

Meprobamate (May produce additive depressant effects, hypoventilation, hypotension and profound sedation or coma may occur). Products include:
Miltown Tablets 3349

Mesoridazine Besylate (May produce additive depressant effects, hypoventilation, hypotension and profound sedation or coma may occur). Products include:
Serentil 1057

Methadone Hydrochloride (May produce additive depressant effects, hypoventilation, hypotension and profound sedation or coma may occur). Products include:
Dolophine Hydrochloride Tablets 3056

Methdilazine Hydrochloride (May produce additive depressant effects, hypoventilation, hypotension and profound sedation or coma may occur).
No products indexed under this heading.

Methohexital Sodium (May produce additive depressant effects, hypoventilation, hypotension and profound sedation or coma may occur). Products include:
Brevital Sodium for Injection, USP 1815

Methotrimeprazine (May produce additive depressant effects, hypoventilation, hypotension and profound sedation or coma may occur).
No products indexed under this heading.

Methoxyflurane (May produce additive depressant effects, hypoventilation, hypotension and profound sedation or coma may occur).
No products indexed under this heading.

Midazolam Hydrochloride (May produce additive depressant effects, hypoventilation, hypotension and profound sedation or coma may occur). Products include:
Versed Injection 3027
Versed Syrup 3033

Molindone Hydrochloride (May produce additive depressant effects, hypoventilation, hypotension and profound sedation or coma may occur). Products include:
Moban 1320

Morphine Sulfate (May produce additive depressant effects, hypoventilation, hypotension and profound sedation or coma may occur). Products include:
Astramorph/PF Injection, USP (Preservative-Free) 594
Duramorph Injection 1312
Infumorph 200 and Infumorph 500 Sterile Solutions 1314
Kadian Capsules 1335
MS Contin Tablets 2896
MSIR 2898
Oramorph SR Tablets 3062
Roxanol 3066

Nefazodone Hydrochloride (Fentanyl is metabolized by CYP450 3A4 isoenzyme system; co-administration with drugs that inhibit this enzyme system may result in increased plasma concentrations of fentanyl and increased risk of adverse events). Products include:
Serzone Tablets 1104

Nelfinavir Mesylate (Fentanyl is metabolized by CYP450 3A4 isoenzyme system; co-administration with drugs that inhibit this enzyme system may result in increased plasma concentrations of fentanyl and increased risk of adverse events). Products include:
Viracept 532

Olanzapine (May produce additive depressant effects, hypoventilation, hypotension and profound sedation or coma may occur). Products include:
Zyprexa Tablets 1973
Zyprexa ZYDIS Orally Disintegrating Tablets 1973

Oxazepam (May produce additive depressant effects, hypoventilation, hypotension and profound sedation or coma may occur).
No products indexed under this heading.

Oxycodone Hydrochloride (May produce additive depressant effects, hypoventilation, hypotension and profound sedation or coma may occur). Products include:
OxyContin Tablets 2912
OxyFast Oral Concentrate Solution 2916
OxyIR Capsules 2916
Percocet Tablets 1326
Percodan Tablets 1327
Percolone Tablets 1327
Roxicodone 3067
Tylox Capsules 2597

Pentobarbital Sodium (May produce additive depressant effects, hypoventilation, hypotension and profound sedation or coma may occur). Products include:
Nembutal Sodium Solution 485

Perphenazine (May produce additive depressant effects, hypoventilation, hypotension and profound sedation or coma may occur). Products include:
Etrafon 3115
Trilafon 3160

Phenobarbital (May produce additive depressant effects, hypoventilation, hypotension and profound sedation or coma may occur). Products include:
Arco-Lase Plus Tablets 592
Donnatal 2929
Donnatal Extentabs 2930

Phenytoin (Fentanyl is metabolized by CYP450 3A4 isoenzyme system; co-administration with drugs that induce this enzyme system may result in decreased plasma concentrations of fentanyl and decrease in therapeutic effect). Products include:
Dilantin Infatabs 2624
Dilantin-125 Oral Suspension 2625

Phenytoin Sodium (Fentanyl is metabolized by CYP450 3A4 isoenzyme system; co-administration with drugs that induce this enzyme system may result in decreased plasma concentrations of fentanyl and decrease in therapeutic effect). Products include:
Dilantin Kapseals 2622

Prazepam (May produce additive depressant effects, hypoventilation, hypotension and profound sedation or coma may occur).
No products indexed under this heading.

Prochlorperazine (May produce additive depressant effects, hypoventilation, hypotension and profound sedation or coma may occur). Products include:
Compazine 1505

Promethazine Hydrochloride (May produce additive depressant effects, hypoventilation, hypotension and profound sedation or coma may occur). Products include:
Mepergan Injection 3539
Phenergan Injection 3553
Phenergan 3556
Phenergan Syrup 3554
Phenergan with Codeine Syrup 3557
Phenergan with Dextromethorphan Syrup 3559
Phenergan VC Syrup 3560
Phenergan VC with Codeine Syrup 3561

Propofol (May produce additive depressant effects, hypoventilation, hypotension and profound sedation or coma may occur). Products include:
Diprivan Injectable Emulsion 667

Propoxyphene Hydrochloride (May produce additive depressant effects, hypoventilation, hypotension and profound sedation or coma may occur). Products include:
Darvon Pulvules 1909
Darvon Compound-65 Pulvules 1910

Propoxyphene Napsylate (May produce additive depressant effects, hypoventilation, hypotension and profound sedation or coma may occur). Products include:
Darvon-N/Darvocet-N 1907
Darvon-N Tablets 1912

Pyrilamine Maleate (May produce additive depressant effects, hypoventilation, hypotension and profound sedation or coma may occur). Products include:
Maximum Strength Midol Menstrual Caplets and Gelcaps 612
Maximum Strength Midol PMS Caplets and Gelcaps 613

Pyrilamine Tannate (May produce additive depressant effects, hypo-

IMPORTANT NOTE: Always consult each drug listing in the patient's regimen for possible interactions.

ventilation, hypotension and profound sedation or coma may occur). Products include:

Ryna-12 S Suspension 3351

Quazepam (May produce additive depressant effects, hypoventilation, hypotension and profound sedation or coma may occur).

No products indexed under this heading.

Quetiapine Fumarate (May produce additive depressant effects, hypoventilation, hypotension and profound sedation or coma may occur). Products include:

Seroquel Tablets 684

Remifentanil Hydrochloride (May produce additive depressant effects, hypoventilation, hypotension and profound sedation or coma may occur).

No products indexed under this heading.

Rifabutin (Fentanyl is metabolized by CYP450 3A4 isoenzyme system; co-administration with drugs that induce this enzyme system may result in decreased plasma concentrations of fentanyl and decrease in therapeutic effect). Products include:

Mycobutin Capsules 2838

Rifampin (Fentanyl is metabolized by CYP450 3A4 isoenzyme system; co-administration with drugs that induce this enzyme system may result in decreased plasma concentrations of fentanyl and decrease in therapeutic effect). Products include:

Rifadin 765
Rifamate Capsules 767
Rifater Tablets 769

Risperidone (May produce additive depressant effects, hypoventilation, hypotension and profound sedation or coma may occur). Products include:

Risperdal 1796

Ritonavir (Fentanyl is metabolized by CYP450 3A4 isoenzyme system; co-administration with drugs that inhibit this enzyme system may result in increased plasma concentrations of fentanyl and increased risk of adverse events). Products include:

Kaletra Capsules 471
Kaletra Oral Solution 471
Norvir Capsules 487
Norvir Oral Solution 487

Saquinavir (Fentanyl is metabolized by CYP450 3A4 isoenzyme system; co-administration with drugs that inhibit this enzyme system may result in increased plasma concentrations of fentanyl and increased risk of adverse events). Products include:

Fortovase Capsules 2970

Saquinavir Mesylate (Fentanyl is metabolized by CYP450 3A4 isoenzyme system; co-administration with drugs that inhibit this enzyme system may result in increased plasma concentrations of fentanyl and increased risk of adverse events). Products include:

Invirase Capsules 2979

Secobarbital Sodium (May produce additive depressant effects, hypoventilation, hypotension and profound sedation or coma may occur).

No products indexed under this heading.

Sevoflurane (May produce additive depressant effects, hypoventilation, hypotension and profound sedation or coma may occur).

No products indexed under this heading.

Sufentanil Citrate (May produce additive depressant effects, hypoventilation, hypotension and profound sedation or coma may occur).

No products indexed under this heading.

Temazepam (May produce additive depressant effects, hypoventilation, hypotension and profound sedation or coma may occur).

No products indexed under this heading.

Terfenadine (May produce additive depressant effects, hypoventilation, hypotension and profound sedation or coma may occur).

No products indexed under this heading.

Thiamylal Sodium (May produce additive depressant effects, hypoventilation, hypotension and profound sedation or coma may occur).

No products indexed under this heading.

Thioridazine Hydrochloride (May produce additive depressant effects, hypoventilation, hypotension and profound sedation or coma may occur). Products include:

Thioridazine Hydrochloride Tablets 2289

Thiothixene (May produce additive depressant effects, hypoventilation, hypotension and profound sedation or coma may occur). Products include:

Navane Capsules 2701
Thiothixene Capsules 2290

Triazolam (May produce additive depressant effects, hypoventilation, hypotension and profound sedation or coma may occur). Products include:

Halcion Tablets 2823

Trifluoperazine Hydrochloride (May produce additive depressant effects, hypoventilation, hypotension and profound sedation or coma may occur). Products include:

Stelazine 1640

Trimeprazine Tartrate (May produce additive depressant effects, hypoventilation, hypotension and profound sedation or coma may occur).

No products indexed under this heading.

Tripelennamine Hydrochloride (May produce additive depressant effects, hypoventilation, hypotension and profound sedation or coma may occur).

No products indexed under this heading.

Triprolidine Hydrochloride (May produce additive depressant effects, hypoventilation, hypotension and profound sedation or coma may occur). Products include:

Actifed Cold & Allergy Tablets .... ▣688

Troglitazone (Fentanyl is metabolized by CYP450 3A4 isoenzyme system; co-administration with drugs that induce this enzyme system may result in decreased plasma concentrations of fentanyl and decrease in therapeutic effect).

No products indexed under this heading.

Troleandomycin (Fentanyl is metabolized by CYP450 3A4 isoenzyme system; co-administration with drugs that inhibit this enzyme system may result in increased plasma concentrations of fentanyl and increased risk of adverse events). Products include:

Tao Capsules 2716

Zaleplon (May produce additive depressant effects, hypoventilation, hypotension and profound sedation or coma may occur). Products include:

Sonata Capsules 3591

Ziprasidone Hydrochloride (May produce additive depressant effects, hypoventilation, hypotension and profound sedation or coma may occur). Products include:

Geodon Capsules 2688

Zolpidem Tartrate (May produce additive depressant effects, hypoventilation, hypotension and profound sedation or coma may occur). Products include:

Ambien Tablets 3191

Food Interactions

Alcohol (May produce additive depressant effects).

DURAMORPH INJECTION

(Morphine Sulfate) 1312

May interact with antihistamines, butyrophenones, anticoagulants, hypnotics and sedatives, monoamine oxidase inhibitors, antipsychotic agents, phenothiazines, psychotropics, tricyclic antidepressants, and certain other agents. Compounds in these categories include:

Acrivastine (Potentiation of depressant effect). Products include:

Semprex-D Capsules 1172

Alfentanil Hydrochloride (Potentiation of depressant effect).

No products indexed under this heading.

Alprazolam (Potentiation of depressant effect). Products include:

Xanax Tablets 2865

Amitriptyline Hydrochloride (Potentiation of depressant effect). Products include:

Etrafon 3115
Limbitrol 1738

Amoxapine (Potentiation of depressant effect).

No products indexed under this heading.

Aprobarbital (Potentiation of depressant effect).

No products indexed under this heading.

Ardeparin Sodium (Concurrent use by epidural or intrathecal route is contraindicated with anticoagulant therapy).

No products indexed under this heading.

Astemizole (Potentiation of depressant effect).

No products indexed under this heading.

Azatadine Maleate (Potentiation of depressant effect). Products include:

Rynatan Tablets 3351

Bromodiphenhydramine Hydrochloride (Potentiation of depressant effect).

No products indexed under this heading.

Brompheniramine Maleate (Potentiation of depressant effect). Products include:

Bromfed Capsules (Extended-Release) 2269
Bromfed-PD Capsules (Extended-Release) 2269
Comtrex Acute Head Cold & Sinus Pressure Relief Tablets .... ▣627
Dimetapp Elixir .... ▣777
Dimetapp Cold and Fever Suspension .... ▣775
Dimetapp DM Cold & Cough Elixir .... ▣775
Dimetapp Nighttime Flu Liquid .... ▣776

Buprenorphine Hydrochloride (Potentiation of depressant effect). Products include:

Buprenex Injectable 2918

Buspirone Hydrochloride (Potentiation of depressant effect).

No products indexed under this heading.

Butabarbital (Potentiation of depressant effect).

No products indexed under this heading.

Butalbital (Potentiation of depressant effect). Products include:

Phrenilin 578
Sedapap Tablets 50 mg/650 mg 2225

Cetirizine Hydrochloride (Potentiation of depressant effect). Products include:

Zyrtec 2756
Zyrtec-D 12 Hour Extended Relief Tablets 2758

Chlordiazepoxide (Potentiation of depressant effect). Products include:

Limbitrol 1738

Chlordiazepoxide Hydrochloride (Potentiation of depressant effect). Products include:

Librium Capsules 1736
Librium for Injection 1737

Chlorpheniramine Maleate (Potentiation of depressant effect). Products include:

Actifed Cold & Sinus Caplets and Tablets .... ▣688
Alka-Seltzer Plus Liqui-Gels .... ▣604
BC Allergy Sinus Cold Powder .... ▣619
Chlor-Trimeton Allergy Tablets .... ▣735
Chlor-Trimeton Allergy/Decongestant Tablets .... ▣736
Comtrex Flu Therapy & Fever Relief Nighttime Tablets .... ▣628
Comtrex Maximum Strength Multi-Symptom Cold & Cough Relief Tablets and Caplets .... ▣626
Contac Severe Cold and Flu Caplets Maximum Strength .... ▣746
Coricidin 'D' Cold, Flu & Sinus Tablets .... ▣737
Coricidin/Coricidin D .... ▣738
Coricidin HBP Maximum Strength Flu Tablets .... ▣738
Extendryl 1361
Hycomine Compound Tablets 1317
Kronofed-A 1341
PediaCare Cough-Cold Liquid .... ▣719
PediaCare NightRest Cough-Cold Liquid .... ▣719
Robitussin Nighttime Honey Flu Liquid .... ▣786
Ryna .... ▣768
Singlet Caplets .... ▣761
Sinutab Sinus Allergy Medication, Maximum Strength Formula, Tablets & Caplets .... ▣707
Sudafed Cold & Allergy Tablets .... ▣708
TheraFlu Regular Strength Cold & Cough Night Time Hot Liquid .... ▣676
TheraFlu Regular Strength Cold & Sore Throat Night Time Hot Liquid .... ▣676
TheraFlu Maximum Strength Flu & Cough Night Time Hot Liquid .... ▣678
TheraFlu Maximum Strength Flu & Sore Throat Night Time Hot Liquid .... ▣677
TheraFlu Maximum Strength Severe Cold & Congestion Night Time Caplets .... ▣678
TheraFlu Maximum Strength Severe Cold & Congestion Night Time Hot Liquid .... ▣678
Triaminic Cold & Allergy Liquid .... ▣681
Triaminic Cold & Allergy Softchews .... ▣683
Triaminic Cold & Cough Liquid .... ▣681
Triaminic Cold & Cough Softchews .... ▣683
Triaminic Cold & Night Time Cough Liquid .... ▣681
Triaminic Cold, Cough & Fever Liquid .... ▣681
Children's Tylenol Cold Suspension Liquid and Chewable Tablets 2015
Children's Tylenol Cold Plus Cough Suspension Liquid and Chewable Tablets 2015
Children's Tylenol Flu Suspension Liquid 2015
Maximum Strength Tylenol Allergy Sinus Caplets, Gelcaps, and Geltabs 2010
Multi-Symptom Tylenol Cold Complete Formula Caplets 2010
Vicks 44M Cough, Cold & Flu Relief Liquid .... ▣725
Pediatric Vicks 44m Cough & Cold Relief .... ▣728
Children's Vicks NyQuil Cold/Cough Relief .... ▣726

Chlorpheniramine Polistirex (Potentiation of depressant effect). Products include:

Tussionex Pennkinetic Extended-Release Suspension 1174

Chlorpheniramine Tannate (Potentiation of depressant effect). Products include:

Reformulated Rynatan Pediatric Suspension 3352
Rynatuss Pediatric Suspension 3353
Rynatuss Tablets 3353
Tussi-12 S Suspension 3356
Tussi-12 Tablets 3356

Chlorpromazine (Potentiation of depressant effect; increased risk of respiratory depression). Products include:
Thorazine Suppositories 1656

Chlorpromazine Hydrochloride (Potentiation of depressant effect; increased risk of respiratory depression). Products include:
Thorazine 1656

Chlorprothixene (Potentiation of depressant effect; increased risk of respiratory depression).
No products indexed under this heading.

Chlorprothixene Hydrochloride (Potentiation of depressant effect; increased risk of respiratory depression).
No products indexed under this heading.

Clemastine Fumarate (Potentiation of depressant effect). Products include:
Tavist 12 Hour Allergy Tablets 676

Clomipramine Hydrochloride (Potentiation of depressant effect).
No products indexed under this heading.

Clorazepate Dipotassium (Potentiation of depressant effect). Products include:
Tranxene 511

Clozapine (Potentiation of depressant effect; increased risk of respiratory depression). Products include:
Clozaril Tablets 2319

Codeine Phosphate (Potentiation of depressant effect). Products include:
Phenergan with Codeine Syrup 3557
Phenergan VC with Codeine Syrup 3561
Robitussin A-C Syrup 2942
Robitussin-DAC Syrup 2942
Ryna-C Liquid 768
Soma Compound w/Codeine Tablets 3355
Tussi-Organidin NR Liquid 3350
Tussi-Organidin-S NR Liquid 3350
Tylenol with Codeine 2595

Cyproheptadine Hydrochloride (Potentiation of depressant effect). Products include:
Periactin Tablets 2155

Dalteparin Sodium (Concurrent use by epidural or intrathecal route is contraindicated with anticoagulant therapy). Products include:
Fragmin Injection 2814

Danaparoid Sodium (Concurrent use by epidural or intrathecal route is contraindicated with anticoagulant therapy). Products include:
Orgaran Injection 2480

Desipramine Hydrochloride (Potentiation of depressant effect). Products include:
Norpramin Tablets 755

Dexchlorpheniramine Maleate (Potentiation of depressant effect).
No products indexed under this heading.

Diazepam (Potentiation of depressant effect). Products include:
Valium Injectable 3026
Valium Tablets 3047

Dicumarol (Concurrent use by epidural or intrathecal route is contraindicated with anticoagulant therapy).
No products indexed under this heading.

Diphenhydramine Citrate (Potentiation of depressant effect). Products include:
Alka-Seltzer PM Effervescent Tablets 605
Benadryl Allergy & Sinus Fastmelt Tablets 693
Benadryl Children's Allergy/Cold Fastmelt Tablets 692
Excedrin PM Tablets, Caplets, and Geltabs 631
Goody's PM Powder 621

Diphenhydramine Hydrochloride (Potentiation of depressant effect). Products include:
Extra Strength Bayer PM Caplets 611
Benadryl Allergy Chewables 689
Benadryl Allergy 691
Benadryl Allergy Liquid 690
Benadryl Allergy/Cold Tablets 691
Benadryl Allergy/Congestion Tablets 692
Benadryl Allergy & Sinus Liquid 693
Benadryl Allergy Sinus Headache Caplets & Gelcaps 693
Benadryl Severe Allergy & Sinus Headache Caplets 694
Benadryl Dye-Free Allergy Liquid 690
Benadryl Dye-Free Allergy Liqui-Gels Softgels 690
Benadryl Itch Relief Stick Extra Strength 695
Benadryl Cream 695
Benadryl Gel 695
Benadryl Spray 696
Benadryl Parenteral 2617
Coricidin HBP Night-Time Cold & Flu Tablets 738
Nytol QuickCaps Caplets 622
Maximum Strength Nytol QuickGels Softgels 621
Extra Strength Percogesic Aspirin-Free Coated Caplets 665
Simply Sleep Caplets 2008
Sominex Original Formula Tablets 761
Children's Tylenol Allergy-D Liquid 2014
Maximum Strength Tylenol Allergy Sinus NightTime Caplets 2010
Tylenol Severe Allergy Caplets 2010
Maximum Strength Tylenol Flu NightTime Gelcaps 2011
Extra Strength Tylenol PM Caplets, Geltabs, and Gelcaps 2012
Unisom Maximum Strength SleepGels 713

Diphenylpyraline Hydrochloride (Potentiation of depressant effect).
No products indexed under this heading.

Doxepin Hydrochloride (Potentiation of depressant effect). Products include:
Sinequan 2713

Droperidol (Potentiation of depressant effect).
No products indexed under this heading.

Enflurane (Potentiation of depressant effect).
No products indexed under this heading.

Enoxaparin (Concurrent use by epidural or intrathecal route is contraindicated with anticoagulant therapy). Products include:
Lovenox Injection 746

Estazolam (Potentiation of depressant effect). Products include:
ProSom Tablets 500

Ethchlorvynol (Potentiation of depressant effect).
No products indexed under this heading.

Ethinamate (Potentiation of depressant effect).
No products indexed under this heading.

Fentanyl Citrate (Potentiation of depressant effect). Products include:
Actiq 1184

Fexofenadine Hydrochloride (Potentiation of depressant effect). Products include:
Allegra 712
Allegra-D Extended-Release Tablets 714

Fluphenazine Decanoate (Potentiation of depressant effect; increased risk of respiratory depression).
No products indexed under this heading.

Fluphenazine Enanthate (Potentiation of depressant effect; increased risk of respiratory depression).
No products indexed under this heading.

Fluphenazine Hydrochloride (Potentiation of depressant effect; increased risk of respiratory depression).
No products indexed under this heading.

Flurazepam Hydrochloride (Potentiation of depressant effect).
No products indexed under this heading.

Glutethimide (Potentiation of depressant effect).
No products indexed under this heading.

Haloperidol (Potentiation of depressant effect; increased risk of respiratory depression). Products include:
Haldol Injection, Tablets and Concentrate 2533

Haloperidol Decanoate (Potentiation of depressant effect; increased risk of respiratory depression). Products include:
Haldol Decanoate 2535

Heparin Sodium (Concurrent use by epidural or intrathecal route is contraindicated with anticoagulant therapy). Products include:
Heparin Lock Flush Solution 3509
Heparin Sodium Injection 3511

Hydrocodone Bitartrate (Potentiation of depressant effect). Products include:
Hycodan 1316
Hycomine Compound Tablets 1317
Hycotuss Expectorant Syrup 1318
Lortab 3319
Lortab Elixir 3317
Maxidone Tablets CIII 3399
Norco 5/325 Tablets CIII 3424
Norco 7.5/325 Tablets CIII 3425
Norco 10/325 Tablets CIII 3427
Norco 10/325 Tablets CIII 3425
Vicodin Tablets 516
Vicodin ES Tablets 517
Vicodin HP Tablets 518
Vicodin Tuss Expectorant 519
Vicoprofen Tablets 520
Zydone Tablets 1330

Hydrocodone Polistirex (Potentiation of depressant effect). Products include:
Tussionex Pennkinetic Extended-Release Suspension 1174

Hydroxyzine Hydrochloride (Potentiation of depressant effect). Products include:
Atarax Tablets & Syrup 2667
Vistaril Intramuscular Solution 2738

Imipramine Hydrochloride (Potentiation of depressant effect).
No products indexed under this heading.

Imipramine Pamoate (Potentiation of depressant effect).
No products indexed under this heading.

Isocarboxazid (Potentiation of depressant effect).
No products indexed under this heading.

Isoflurane (Potentiation of depressant effect).
No products indexed under this heading.

Ketamine Hydrochloride (Potentiation of depressant effect).
No products indexed under this heading.

Levorphanol Tartrate (Potentiation of depressant effect). Products include:
Levo-Dromoran 1734
Levorphanol Tartrate Tablets 3059

Lithium Carbonate (Potentiation of depressant effect; increased risk of respiratory depression). Products include:
Eskalith 1527
Lithium Carbonate 3061
Lithobid Slow-Release Tablets 3255

Lithium Citrate (Potentiation of depressant effect; increased risk of respiratory depression). Products include:
Lithium Citrate Syrup 3061

Loratadine (Potentiation of depressant effect). Products include:
Claritin 3100
Claritin-D 12 Hour Extended Release Tablets 3102
Claritin-D 24 Hour Extended Release Tablets 3104

Lorazepam (Potentiation of depressant effect). Products include:
Ativan Injection 3478
Ativan Tablets 3482

Loxapine Hydrochloride (Potentiation of depressant effect; increased risk of respiratory depression).
No products indexed under this heading.

Loxapine Succinate (Potentiation of depressant effect; increased risk of respiratory depression). Products include:
Loxitane Capsules 3398

Maprotiline Hydrochloride (Potentiation of depressant effect).
No products indexed under this heading.

Meperidine Hydrochloride (Potentiation of depressant effect). Products include:
Demerol 3079
Mepergan Injection 3539

Mephobarbital (Potentiation of depressant effect).
No products indexed under this heading.

Meprobamate (Potentiation of depressant effect). Products include:
Miltown Tablets 3349

Mesoridazine Besylate (Potentiation of depressant effect; increased risk of respiratory depression). Products include:
Serentil 1057

Methadone Hydrochloride (Potentiation of depressant effect). Products include:
Dolophine Hydrochloride Tablets 3056

Methdilazine Hydrochloride (Potentiation of depressant effect).
No products indexed under this heading.

Methohexital Sodium (Potentiation of depressant effect). Products include:
Brevital Sodium for Injection, USP 1815

Methotrimeprazine (Potentiation of depressant effect; increased risk of respiratory depression).
No products indexed under this heading.

Methoxyflurane (Potentiation of depressant effect).
No products indexed under this heading.

Midazolam Hydrochloride (Potentiation of depressant effect). Products include:
Versed Injection 3027
Versed Syrup 3033

Moclobemide (Potentiation of depressant effect).
No products indexed under this heading.

Molindone Hydrochloride (Potentiation of depressant effect; increased risk of respiratory depression). Products include:
Moban 1320

Nortriptyline Hydrochloride (Potentiation of depressant effect).
No products indexed under this heading.

Olanzapine (Potentiation of depressant effect). Products include:
Zyprexa Tablets 1973
Zyprexa ZYDIS Orally Disintegrating Tablets 1973

Oxazepam (Potentiation of depressant effect).
No products indexed under this heading.

Oxycodone Hydrochloride (Potentiation of depressant effect). Products include:
OxyContin Tablets 2912
OxyFast Oral Concentrate Solution . 2916
OxyIR Capsules 2916
Percocet Tablets 1326
Percodan Tablets 1327
Percolone Tablets 1327
Roxicodone 3067
Tylox Capsules 2597

Pargyline Hydrochloride (Potentiation of depressant effect).
No products indexed under this heading.

Pentobarbital Sodium (Potentiation of depressant effect). Products include:
Nembutal Sodium Solution 485

Perphenazine (Potentiation of depressant effect; increased risk of respiratory depression). Products include:
Etrafon 3115
Trilafon 3160

Phenelzine Sulfate (Potentiation of depressant effect). Products include:
Nardil Tablets 2653

Phenobarbital (Potentiation of depressant effect). Products include:
Arco-Lase Plus Tablets 592
Donnatal 2929
Donnatal Extentabs 2930

Pimozide (Potentiation of depressant effect; increased risk of respiratory depression). Products include:
Orap Tablets 1407

Prazepam (Potentiation of depressant effect).
No products indexed under this heading.

Procarbazine Hydrochloride (Potentiation of depressant effect). Products include:
Matulane Capsules 3246

Prochlorperazine (Potentiation of depressant effect; increased risk of respiratory depression). Products include:
Compazine 1505

Promethazine Hydrochloride (Potentiation of depressant effect; increased risk of respiratory depression). Products include:
Mepergan Injection 3539
Phenergan Injection 3553
Phenergan 3556
Phenergan Syrup 3554
Phenergan with Codeine Syrup 3557
Phenergan with Dextromethorphan Syrup 3559
Phenergan VC Syrup 3560
Phenergan VC with Codeine Syrup .. 3561

Propofol (Potentiation of depressant effect). Products include:
Diprivan Injectable Emulsion 667

Propoxyphene Hydrochloride (Potentiation of depressant effect). Products include:
Darvon Pulvules 1909
Darvon Compound-65 Pulvules 1910

Propoxyphene Napsylate (Potentiation of depressant effect). Products include:
Darvon-N/Darvocet-N 1907
Darvon-N Tablets 1912

Protriptyline Hydrochloride (Potentiation of depressant effect). Products include:
Vivactil Tablets 2446
Vivactil Tablets 2217

Pyrilamine Maleate (Potentiation of depressant effect). Products include:
Maximum Strength Midol Menstrual Caplets and Gelcaps........ ▣612
Maximum Strength Midol PMS Caplets and Gelcaps........ ▣613

Pyrilamine Tannate (Potentiation of depressant effect). Products include:
Ryna-12 S Suspension 3351

Quazepam (Potentiation of depressant effect).
No products indexed under this heading.

Quetiapine Fumarate (Potentiation of depressant effect; increased risk of respiratory depression). Products include:
Seroquel Tablets 684

Risperidone (Potentiation of depressant effect; increased risk of respiratory depression). Products include:
Risperdal 1796

Secobarbital Sodium (Potentiation of depressant effect).
No products indexed under this heading.

Selegiline Hydrochloride (Potentiation of depressant effect). Products include:
Eldepryl Capsules 3266

Sufentanil Citrate (Potentiation of depressant effect).
No products indexed under this heading.

Temazepam (Potentiation of depressant effect).
No products indexed under this heading.

Terfenadine (Potentiation of depressant effect).
No products indexed under this heading.

Thiamylal Sodium (Potentiation of depressant effect).
No products indexed under this heading.

Thioridazine Hydrochloride (Potentiation of depressant effect; increased risk of respiratory depression). Products include:
Thioridazine Hydrochloride Tablets 2289

Thiothixene (Potentiation of depressant effect; increased risk of respiratory depression). Products include:
Navane Capsules 2701
Thiothixene Capsules 2290

Tinzaparin sodium (Concurrent use by epidural or intrathecal route is contraindicated with anticoagulant therapy). Products include:
Innohep Injection 1248

Tranylcypromine Sulfate (Potentiation of depressant effect). Products include:
Parnate Tablets 1607

Triazolam (Potentiation of depressant effect). Products include:
Halcion Tablets 2823

Trifluoperazine Hydrochloride (Potentiation of depressant effect; increased risk of respiratory depression). Products include:
Stelazine 1640

Trimeprazine Tartrate (Potentiation of depressant effect).
No products indexed under this heading.

Trimipramine Maleate (Potentiation of depressant effect). Products include:
Surmontil Capsules 3595

Tripelennamine Hydrochloride (Potentiation of depressant effect).
No products indexed under this heading.

Triprolidine Hydrochloride (Potentiation of depressant effect). Products include:
Actifed Cold & Allergy Tablets .... ▣688

Warfarin Sodium (Concurrent use by epidural or intrathecal route is contraindicated with anticoagulant therapy). Products include:
Coumadin for Injection 1243
Coumadin Tablets 1243
Warfarin Sodium Tablets, USP 3302

Zaleplon (Potentiation of depressant effect). Products include:
Sonata Capsules 3591

Ziprasidone Hydrochloride (Potentiation of depressant effect; increased risk of respiratory depression). Products include:
Geodon Capsules 2688

Zolpidem Tartrate (Potentiation of depressant effect). Products include:
Ambien Tablets 3191

Food Interactions

Alcohol (Potentiation of depressant effect).

DURANEST INJECTIONS

(Etidocaine Hydrochloride) 600
May interact with ergot-type oxytocic drugs, monoamine oxidase inhibitors, phenothiazines, and tricyclic antidepressants. Compounds in these categories include:

Amitriptyline Hydrochloride (Concurrent use of Duranest Injection containing epinephrine with tricyclic antidepressant may produce severe, prolonged hypotension or hypertension; concurrent use should be avoided). Products include:
Etrafon 3115
Limbitrol 1738

Amoxapine (Concurrent use of Duranest Injection containing epinephrine with tricyclic antidepressant may produce severe, prolonged hypotension or hypertension; concurrent use should be avoided).
No products indexed under this heading.

Chlorpromazine (Concurrent use of Duranest Injection containing epinephrine with phenothiazine may produce severe, prolonged hypotension or hypertension; concurrent use should be avoided). Products include:
Thorazine Suppositories 1656

Chlorpromazine Hydrochloride (Concurrent use of Duranest Injection containing epinephrine with phenothiazine may produce severe, prolonged hypotension or hypertension; concurrent use should be avoided). Products include:
Thorazine 1656

Clomipramine Hydrochloride (Concurrent use of Duranest Injection containing epinephrine with tricyclic antidepressant may produce severe, prolonged hypotension or hypertension; concurrent use should be avoided).
No products indexed under this heading.

Desipramine Hydrochloride (Concurrent use of Duranest Injection containing epinephrine with tricyclic antidepressant may produce severe, prolonged hypotension or hypertension; concurrent use should be avoided). Products include:
Norpramin Tablets 755

Doxepin Hydrochloride (Concurrent use of Duranest Injection containing epinephrine with tricyclic antidepressant may produce severe, prolonged hypotension or hypertension; concurrent use should be avoided). Products include:
Sinequan 2713

Fluphenazine Decanoate (Concurrent use of Duranest Injection containing epinephrine with phenothiazine may produce severe, prolonged hypotension or hypertension; concurrent use should be avoided).
No products indexed under this heading.

Fluphenazine Enanthate (Concurrent use of Duranest Injection containing epinephrine with phenothiazine may produce severe, prolonged hypotension or hypertension; concurrent use should be avoided).
No products indexed under this heading.

Fluphenazine Hydrochloride (Concurrent use of Duranest Injection containing epinephrine with phenothiazine may produce severe, prolonged hypotension or hypertension; concurrent use should be avoided).
No products indexed under this heading.

Imipramine Hydrochloride (Concurrent use of Duranest Injection containing epinephrine with tricyclic antidepressant may produce severe, prolonged hypotension or hypertension; concurrent use should be avoided).
No products indexed under this heading.

Imipramine Pamoate (Concurrent use of Duranest Injection containing epinephrine with tricyclic antidepressant may produce severe, prolonged hypotension or hypertension; concurrent use should be avoided).
No products indexed under this heading.

Isocarboxazid (Concurrent use of Duranest Injection containing epinephrine with MAOI may produce severe, prolonged hypotension or hypertension; concurrent use should be avoided).
No products indexed under this heading.

Maprotiline Hydrochloride (Concurrent use of Duranest Injection containing epinephrine with tricyclic antidepressant may produce severe, prolonged hypotension or hypertension; concurrent use should be avoided).
No products indexed under this heading.

Mesoridazine Besylate (Concurrent use of Duranest Injection containing epinephrine with phenothiazine may produce severe, prolonged hypotension or hypertension; concurrent use should be avoided). Products include:
Serentil 1057

Methotrimeprazine (Concurrent use of Duranest Injection containing epinephrine with phenothiazine may produce severe, prolonged hypotension or hypertension; concurrent use should be avoided).
No products indexed under this heading.

Methylergonovine Maleate (Concurrent use of vasopressor drugs, for the treatment of hypotension related to epidural blocks, and ergot-type oxytocic drugs may cause severe, persistent hypertension or cerebrovascular accidents).
No products indexed under this heading.

Moclobemide (Concurrent use of Duranest Injection containing epinephrine with MAOI may produce severe, prolonged hypotension or hypertension; concurrent use should be avoided).
No products indexed under this heading.

Nortriptyline Hydrochloride (Concurrent use of Duranest Injection containing epinephrine with tricyclic antidepressant may produce severe, prolonged hypotension or hypertension; concurrent use should be avoided).
No products indexed under this heading.

Pargyline Hydrochloride (Concurrent use of Duranest Injection containing epinephrine with MAOI may produce severe, prolonged hypotension or hypertension; concurrent use should be avoided).
No products indexed under this heading.

Perphenazine (Concurrent use of Duranest Injection containing epi-

nephrine with phenothiazine may produce severe, prolonged hypotension or hypertension; concurrent use should be avoided). Products include:
- Etrafon 3115
- Trilafon 3160

Phenelzine Sulfate (Concurrent use of Duranest Injection containing epinephrine with MAOI may produce severe, prolonged hypotension or hypertension; concurrent use should be avoided). Products include:
- Nardil Tablets 2653

Procarbazine Hydrochloride (Concurrent use of Duranest Injection containing epinephrine with MAOI may produce severe, prolonged hypotension or hypertension; concurrent use should be avoided). Products include:
- Matulane Capsules 3246

Prochlorperazine (Concurrent use of Duranest Injection containing epinephrine with phenothiazine may produce severe, prolonged hypotension or hypertension; concurrent use should be avoided). Products include:
- Compazine 1505

Promethazine Hydrochloride (Concurrent use of Duranest Injection containing epinephrine with phenothiazine may produce severe, prolonged hypotension or hypertension; concurrent use should be avoided). Products include:
- Mepergan Injection 3539
- Phenergan Injection 3553
- Phenergan 3556
- Phenergan Syrup 3554
- Phenergan with Codeine Syrup 3557
- Phenergan with Dextromethorphan Syrup 3559
- Phenergan VC Syrup 3560
- Phenergan VC with Codeine Syrup . 3561

Protriptyline Hydrochloride (Concurrent use of Duranest Injection containing epinephrine with tricyclic antidepressant may produce severe, prolonged hypotension or hypertension; concurrent use should be avoided). Products include:
- Vivactil Tablets 2446
- Vivactil Tablets 2217

Selegiline Hydrochloride (Concurrent use of Duranest Injection containing epinephrine with MAOI may produce severe, prolonged hypotension or hypertension; concurrent use should be avoided). Products include:
- Eldepryl Capsules 3266

Thioridazine Hydrochloride (Concurrent use of Duranest Injection containing epinephrine with phenothiazine may produce severe, prolonged hypotension or hypertension; concurrent use should be avoided). Products include:
- Thioridazine Hydrochloride Tablets 2289

Tranylcypromine Sulfate (Concurrent use of Duranest Injection containing epinephrine with MAOI may produce severe, prolonged hypotension or hypertension; concurrent use should be avoided). Products include:
- Parnate Tablets 1607

Trifluoperazine Hydrochloride (Concurrent use of Duranest Injection containing epinephrine with phenothiazine may produce severe, prolonged hypotension or hypertension; concurrent use should be avoided). Products include:
- Stelazine 1640

Trimipramine Maleate (Concurrent use of Duranest Injection containing epinephrine with tricyclic antidepressant may produce severe, prolonged hypotension or hypertension; concurrent use should be avoided). Products include:
- Surmontil Capsules 3595

DURICEF CAPSULES
(Cefadroxil) 1079
None cited in PDR database.

DURICEF ORAL SUSPENSION
(Cefadroxil) 1079
None cited in PDR database.

DURICEF TABLETS
(Cefadroxil) 1079
None cited in PDR database.

DYAZIDE CAPSULES
(Hydrochlorothiazide, Triamterene) 1515
May interact with ACE inhibitors, antihypertensives, corticosteroids, oral anticoagulants, antigout agents, oral hypoglycemic agents, insulin, lithium preparations, nondepolarizing neuromuscular blocking agents, nonsteroidal anti-inflammatory agents, potassium preparations, potassium sparing diuretics, and certain other agents. Compounds in these categories include:

Acarbose (Increased risk of severe hyponatremia). Products include:
- Precose Tablets 906

Acebutolol Hydrochloride (May add to potentiate the action of other hypertensives). Products include:
- Sectral Capsules 3589

ACTH (May intensify electrolyte imbalance, particularly hypokalemia).
No products indexed under this heading.

Allopurinol (Dyazide may raise the level of blood uric acid; may require dosage adjustment of antigout agent).
No products indexed under this heading.

Amiloride Hydrochloride (Concurrent use is contraindicated). Products include:
- Midamor Tablets 2136
- Moduretic Tablets 2138

Amlodipine Besylate (May add to potentiate the action of other hypertensives). Products include:
- Lotrel Capsules 2370
- Norvasc Tablets 2704

Amphotericin B (May intensify electrolyte imbalance, particularly hypokalemia). Products include:
- Abelcet Injection 1273
- AmBisome for Injection 1383
- Amphotec 1774

Atenolol (May add to potentiate the action of other hypertensives). Products include:
- Tenoretic Tablets 690
- Tenormin I.V. Injection 692

Atracurium Besylate (Increased paralyzing effect).
No products indexed under this heading.

Benazepril Hydrochloride (May add to potentiate the action of other hypertensives; increased risk of hyperkalemia). Products include:
- Lotensin Tablets 2365
- Lotensin HCT Tablets 2367
- Lotrel Capsules 2370

Bendroflumethiazide (May add to potentiate the action of other hypertensives). Products include:
- Corzide 40/5 Tablets 2247
- Corzide 80/5 Tablets 2247

Betamethasone Acetate (May intensify electrolyte imbalance, particularly hypokalemia). Products include:
- Celestone Soluspan Injectable Suspension 3097

Betamethasone Sodium Phosphate (May intensify electrolyte imbalance, particularly hypokalemia). Products include:
- Celestone Soluspan Injectable Suspension 3097

Betaxolol Hydrochloride (May add to potentiate the action of other hypertensives). Products include:
- Betoptic S Ophthalmic Suspension 537

Bisoprolol Fumarate (May add to potentiate the action of other hypertensives). Products include:
- Zebeta Tablets 1885
- Ziac Tablets 1887

Blood, whole (Concurrent use of whole blood from blood bank with triamterene may result in hyperkalemia, especially in patients with renal insufficiency).
No products indexed under this heading.

Candesartan Cilexetil (May add to potentiate the action of other hypertensives). Products include:
- Atacand Tablets 595
- Atacand HCT Tablets 597

Captopril (May add to potentiate the action of other hypertensives; increased risk of hyperkalemia). Products include:
- Captopril Tablets 2281

Carteolol Hydrochloride (May add to potentiate the action of other hypertensives). Products include:
- Carteolol Hydrochloride Ophthalmic Solution USP, 1% ..... ⊙ 258
- Ocupress Ophthalmic Solution, 1% Sterile .... ⊙ 303

Celecoxib (Potential for acute renal failure). Products include:
- Celebrex Capsules 2676
- Celebrex Capsules 2780

Chlorothiazide (May add to potentiate the action of other hypertensives). Products include:
- Aldoclor Tablets 2035
- Diuril Oral 2087

Chlorothiazide Sodium (May add to potentiate the action of other hypertensives). Products include:
- Diuril Sodium Intravenous 2086

Chlorpropamide (Increased risk of severe hyponatremia). Products include:
- Diabinese Tablets 2680

Chlorthalidone (May add to potentiate the action of other hypertensives). Products include:
- Clorpres Tablets 1002
- Combipres Tablets 1040
- Tenoretic Tablets 690

Cisatracurium Besylate (Increased paralyzing effect).
No products indexed under this heading.

Clonidine (May add to potentiate the action of other hypertensives). Products include:
- Catapres-TTS 1038

Clonidine Hydrochloride (May add to potentiate the action of other hypertensives). Products include:
- Catapres Tablets 1037
- Clorpres Tablets 1002
- Combipres Tablets 1040
- Duraclon Injection 3057

Cortisone Acetate (May intensify electrolyte imbalance, particularly hypokalemia). Products include:
- Cortone Acetate Injectable Suspension 2059
- Cortone Acetate Tablets 2061

Deserpidine (May add to potentiate the action of other hypertensives).
No products indexed under this heading.

Dexamethasone (May intensify electrolyte imbalance, particularly hypokalemia). Products include:
- Decadron Elixir 2078
- Decadron Tablets 2079
- TobraDex Ophthalmic Ointment 542
- TobraDex Ophthalmic Suspension .. 541

Dexamethasone Acetate (May intensify electrolyte imbalance, particularly hypokalemia).
No products indexed under this heading.

Dexamethasone Sodium Phosphate (May intensify electrolyte imbalance, particularly hypokalemia). Products include:
- Decadron Phosphate Injection 2081
- Decadron Phosphate Sterile Ophthalmic Ointment 2083
- Decadron Phosphate Sterile Ophthalmic Solution 2084
- NeoDecadron Sterile Ophthalmic Solution 2144

Diazoxide (May add to potentiate the action of other hypertensives).
No products indexed under this heading.

Diclofenac Potassium (Potential for acute renal failure). Products include:
- Cataflam Tablets 2315

Diclofenac Sodium (Potential for acute renal failure). Products include:
- Arthrotec Tablets 3195
- Voltaren Ophthalmic Sterile Ophthalmic Solution .... ⊙ 312
- Voltaren Tablets 2315
- Voltaren-XR Tablets 2315

Dicumarol (Effects of oral anticoagulants may be decreased).
No products indexed under this heading.

Diltiazem Hydrochloride (May add to potentiate the action of other hypertensives). Products include:
- Cardizem Injectable 1018
- Cardizem Lyo-Ject Syringe 1018
- Cardizem Monovial 1018
- Cardizem CD Capsules 1016
- Tiazac Capsules 1378

Doxazosin Mesylate (May add to potentiate the action of other hypertensives). Products include:
- Cardura Tablets 2668

Enalapril Maleate (May add to potentiate the action of other hypertensives; increased risk of hyperkalemia). Products include:
- Lexxel Tablets 608
- Vaseretic Tablets 2204
- Vasotec Tablets 2210

Enalaprilat (May add to potentiate the action of other hypertensives; increased risk of hyperkalemia). Products include:
- Enalaprilat Injection 863
- Vasotec I.V. Injection 2207

Eprosartan Mesylate (May add to potentiate the action of other hypertensives). Products include:
- Teveten Tablets 3327

Esmolol Hydrochloride (May add to potentiate the action of other hypertensives). Products include:
- Brevibloc Injection 858

Etodolac (Potential for acute renal failure). Products include:
- Lodine 3528
- Lodine XL Extended-Release Tablets 3530

Felodipine (May add to potentiate the action of other hypertensives). Products include:
- Lexxel Tablets 608
- Plendil Extended-Release Tablets ... 623

Fenoprofen Calcium (Potential for acute renal failure).
No products indexed under this heading.

Fludrocortisone Acetate (May intensify electrolyte imbalance, particularly hypokalemia). Products include:
- Florinef Acetate Tablets 2250

Flurbiprofen (Potential for acute renal failure).
No products indexed under this heading.

Fosinopril Sodium (May add to potentiate the action of other hypertensives; increased risk of hyperkalemia). Products include:
- Monopril Tablets 1091
- Monopril HCT 1094

Furosemide (May add to potentiate the action of other hypertensives). Products include:

Furosemide Tablets 2284

Glimepiride (Thiazides may cause hyperglycemia and glycosuria; dosage alteration of oral antidiabetic agents may be required). Products include:
- Amaryl Tablets 717

Glipizide (Thiazides may cause hyperglycemia and glycosuria; dosage alteration of oral antidiabetic agents may be required). Products include:
- Glucotrol Tablets 2692
- Glucotrol XL Extended Release Tablets 2693

Glyburide (Thiazides may cause hyperglycemia and glycosuria; dosage alteration of oral antidiabetic agents may be required). Products include:
- DiaBeta Tablets 741
- Glucovance Tablets 1086

Guanabenz Acetate (May add to potentiate the action of other hypertensives).
- No products indexed under this heading.

Guanethidine Monosulfate (May add to potentiate the action of other hypertensives).
- No products indexed under this heading.

Hydralazine Hydrochloride (May add to potentiate the action of other hypertensives).
- No products indexed under this heading.

Hydrocortisone (May intensify electrolyte imbalance, particularly hypokalemia). Products include:
- Anusol-HC Cream 2.5% 2237
- Cipro HC Otic Suspension 540
- Cortaid Intensive Therapy Cream .... ▣717
- Cortaid Maximum Strength Cream .... ▣717
- Cortisporin Ophthalmic Suspension Sterile .... ⊙297
- Cortizone•5 .... ▣699
- Cortizone•10 .... ▣699
- Cortizone•10 Plus Creme .... ▣700
- Cortizone for Kids Creme .... ▣699
- Hydrocortone Tablets 2106
- Massengill Medicated Soft Cloth Towelette .... ▣753
- VōSoL HC Otic Solution 3356

Hydrocortisone Acetate (May intensify electrolyte imbalance, particularly hypokalemia). Products include:
- Analpram-HC 1338
- Anusol HC-1 Hydrocortisone Anti-Itch Cream .... ▣689
- Anusol-HC Suppositories 2238
- Cortaid .... ▣717
- Cortifoam Rectal Foam 3170
- Cortisporin-TC Otic Suspension 2246
- Hydrocortone Acetate Injectable Suspension 2103
- Pramosone 1343
- Proctocort Suppositories 2264
- ProctoFoam-HC 3177
- Terra-Cortril Ophthalmic Suspension 2716

Hydrocortisone Sodium Phosphate (May intensify electrolyte imbalance, particularly hypokalemia). Products include:
- Hydrocortone Phosphate Injection, Sterile 2105

Hydrocortisone Sodium Succinate (May intensify electrolyte imbalance, particularly hypokalemia).
- No products indexed under this heading.

Hydroflumethiazide (May add to potentiate the action of other hypertensives). Products include:
- Diucardin Tablets 3494

Ibuprofen (Potential for acute renal failure). Products include:
- Advil .... ▣771
- Children's Advil Oral Suspension .... ▣773
- Children's Advil Chewable Tablets .... ▣773
- Advil Cold and Sinus Caplets .... ▣771
- Advil Cold and Sinus Tablets .... ▣771
- Advil Flu & Body Ache Caplets .... ▣772
- Infants' Advil Drops .... ▣773
- Junior Strength Advil Tablets .... ▣773
- Junior Strength Advil Chewable Tablets .... ▣773
- Advil Migraine Liquigels .... ▣772
- Children's Motrin Oral Suspension and Chewable Tablets 2006
- Children's Motrin Cold Oral Suspension 2007
- Children's Motrin Oral Suspension .... ▣643
- Motrin Suspension, Oral Drops, Chewable Tablets, and Caplets 2002
- Infants' Motrin Concentrated Drops 2006
- Junior Strength Motrin Caplets and Chewable Tablets 2006
- Motrin IB Tablets, Caplets, and Gelcaps 2002
- Motrin Migraine Pain Caplets 2005
- Motrin Sinus Headache Caplets 2005
- Vicoprofen Tablets 520

Indapamide (May add to potentiate the action of other hypertensives). Products include:
- Indapamide Tablets 2286

Indomethacin (Potential for acute renal failure). Products include:
- Indocin 2112

Indomethacin Sodium Trihydrate (Potential for acute renal failure). Products include:
- Indocin I.V. 2115

Insulin, Human, Zinc Suspension (Thiazides may cause hyperglycemia, glycosuria and alter insulin requirements in diabetes; diabetes mellitus may become manifest during thiazide administration). Products include:
- Humulin L, 100 Units 1937
- Humulin U, 100 Units 1943
- Novolin L Human Insulin 10 ml Vials 2422

Insulin, Human NPH (Thiazides may cause hyperglycemia, glycosuria and alter insulin requirements in diabetes; diabetes mellitus may become manifest during thiazide administration). Products include:
- Humulin N, 100 Units 1939
- Humulin N NPH Pen 1940
- Novolin N Human Insulin 10 ml Vials 2422
- Novolin N PenFill 2423
- Novolin N Prefilled Syringe Disposable Insulin Delivery System 2425

Insulin, Human Regular (Thiazides may cause hyperglycemia, glycosuria and alter insulin requirements in diabetes; diabetes mellitus may become manifest during thiazide administration). Products include:
- Humulin R Regular (U-500) 1943
- Humulin R, 100 Units 1941
- Novolin R Human Insulin 10 ml Vials 2423
- Novolin R PenFill 2423
- Novolin R Prefilled Syringe Disposable Insulin Delivery System 2425
- Velosulin BR Human Insulin 10 ml Vials 2435

Insulin, Human Regular and Human NPH Mixture (Thiazides may cause hyperglycemia, glycosuria and alter insulin requirements in diabetes; diabetes mellitus may become manifest during thiazide administration). Products include:
- Humulin 50/50, 100 Units 1934
- Humulin 70/30, 100 Units 1935
- Humulin 70/30 Pen 1936
- Novolin 70/30 Human Insulin 10 ml Vials 2421
- Novolin 70/30 PenFill 2423
- Novolin 70/30 Prefilled Disposable Insulin Delivery System 2425

Insulin, NPH (Thiazides may cause hyperglycemia, glycosuria and alter insulin requirements in diabetes; diabetes mellitus may become manifest during thiazide administration). Products include:
- Iletin II, NPH (Pork), 100 Units 1946

Insulin, Regular (Thiazides may cause hyperglycemia, glycosuria and alter insulin requirements in diabetes; diabetes mellitus may become manifest during thiazide administration). Products include:
- Iletin II, Regular (Pork), 100 Units 1947

Insulin, Zinc Crystals (Thiazides may cause hyperglycemia, glycosuria and alter insulin requirements in diabetes; diabetes mellitus may become manifest during thiazide administration).
- No products indexed under this heading.

Insulin, Zinc Suspension (Thiazides may cause hyperglycemia, glycosuria and alter insulin requirements in diabetes; diabetes mellitus may become manifest during thiazide administration). Products include:
- Iletin II, Lente (Pork), 100 Units 1945

Insulin Aspart, Human Regular (Thiazides may cause hyperglycemia, glycosuria and alter insulin requirements in diabetes; diabetes mellitus may become manifest during thiazide administration).
- No products indexed under this heading.

Insulin glargine (Thiazides may cause hyperglycemia, glycosuria and alter insulin requirements in diabetes; diabetes mellitus may become manifest during thiazide administration). Products include:
- Lantus Injection 742

Insulin Lispro, Human (Thiazides may cause hyperglycemia, glycosuria and alter insulin requirements in diabetes; diabetes mellitus may become manifest during thiazide administration). Products include:
- Humalog 1926
- Humalog Mix 75/25 Pen 1928

Insulin Lispro Protamine, Human (Thiazides may cause hyperglycemia, glycosuria and alter insulin requirements in diabetes; diabetes mellitus may become manifest during thiazide administration). Products include:
- Humalog Mix 75/25 Pen 1928

Irbesartan (May add to potentiate the action of other hypertensives). Products include:
- Avalide Tablets 1070
- Avapro Tablets 1074
- Avapro Tablets 3076

Isradipine (May add to potentiate the action of other hypertensives). Products include:
- DynaCirc Capsules 2921
- DynaCirc CR Tablets 2923

Ketoprofen (Potential for acute renal failure). Products include:
- Orudis Capsules 3548
- Orudis KT Tablets .... ▣778
- Oruvail Capsules 3548

Ketorolac Tromethamine (Potential for acute renal failure). Products include:
- Acular Ophthalmic Solution 544
- Acular PF Ophthalmic Solution 544
- Toradol 3018

Labetalol Hydrochloride (May add to potentiate the action of other hypertensives). Products include:
- Normodyne Injection 3135
- Normodyne Tablets 3137

Laxatives, unspecified (Interferes with the potassium-retaining effects of triamterene; chronic or overuse of laxatives may reduce serum potassium).
- No products indexed under this heading.

Lisinopril (May add to potentiate the action of other hypertensives; increased risk of hyperkalemia). Products include:
- Prinivil Tablets 2164
- Prinzide Tablets 2168
- Zestoretic Tablets 695
- Zestril Tablets 698

Lithium Carbonate (Reduced renal clearance and increased risk of lithium toxicity). Products include:
- Eskalith 1527
- Lithium Carbonate 3061
- Lithobid Slow-Release Tablets 3255

Lithium Citrate (Reduced renal clearance and increased risk of lithium toxicity). Products include:
- Lithium Citrate Syrup 3061

Losartan Potassium (May add to potentiate the action of other hypertensives). Products include:
- Cozaar Tablets 2067
- Hyzaar 2109

Mecamylamine Hydrochloride (May add to potentiate the action of other hypertensives). Products include:
- Inversine Tablets 1850

Meclofenamate Sodium (Potential for acute renal failure).
- No products indexed under this heading.

Mefenamic Acid (Potential for acute renal failure). Products include:
- Ponstel Capsules 1356

Meloxicam (Potential for acute renal failure). Products include:
- Mobic Tablets 1054

Metformin Hydrochloride (Increased risk of severe hyponatremia). Products include:
- Glucophage Tablets 1080
- Glucophage XR Tablets 1080
- Glucovance Tablets 1086

Methenamine (Decreased effectiveness of methenamine due to alkalinization of urine). Products include:
- Prosed/DS Tablets 3268
- Urimax Tablets 1769
- Urised Tablets 2876

Methenamine Hippurate (Decreased effectiveness of methenamine due to alkalinization of urine).
- No products indexed under this heading.

Methenamine Mandelate (Decreased effectiveness of methenamine due to alkalinization of urine). Products include:
- Uroqid-Acid No. 2 Tablets 947

Methyclothiazide (May add to potentiate the action of other hypertensives).
- No products indexed under this heading.

Methyldopa (May add to potentiate the action of other hypertensives). Products include:
- Aldoclor Tablets 2035
- Aldomet Tablets 2037
- Aldoril Tablets 2039

Methyldopate Hydrochloride (May add to potentiate the action of other hypertensives).
- No products indexed under this heading.

Methylprednisolone Acetate (May intensify electrolyte imbalance, particularly hypokalemia). Products include:
- Depo-Medrol Injectable Suspension 2795

Methylprednisolone Sodium Succinate (May intensify electrolyte imbalance, particularly hypokalemia). Products include:
- Solu-Medrol Sterile Powder 2855

Metocurine Iodide (Increased paralyzing effect).
- No products indexed under this heading.

Metolazone (May add to potentiate the action of other hypertensives). Products include:
- Mykrox Tablets 1168
- Zaroxolyn Tablets 1177

Metoprolol Succinate (May add to potentiate the action of other hypertensives). Products include:
- Toprol-XL Tablets 651

Metoprolol Tartrate (May add to potentiate the action of other hypertensives).
No products indexed under this heading.

Metyrosine (May add to potentiate the action of other hypertensives). Products include:
Demser Capsules 2085

Mibefradil Dihydrochloride (May add to potentiate the action of other hypertensives).
No products indexed under this heading.

Miglitol (Thiazides may cause hyperglycemia and glycosuria; dosage alteration of oral antidiabetic agents may be required). Products include:
Glyset Tablets 2821

Minoxidil (May add to potentiate the action of other hypertensives). Products include:
Rogaine Extra Strength for Men Topical Solution ....▣ 721
Rogaine for Women Topical Solution ....▣ 721

Mivacurium Chloride (Increased paralyzing effect).
No products indexed under this heading.

Moexipril Hydrochloride (May add to potentiate the action of other hypertensives; increased risk of hyperkalemia). Products include:
Uniretic Tablets 3178
Univasc Tablets 3181

Nabumetone (Potential for acute renal failure). Products include:
Relafen Tablets 1617

Nadolol (May add to potentiate the action of other hypertensives). Products include:
Corgard Tablets 2245
Corzide 40/5 Tablets 2247
Corzide 80/5 Tablets 2247
Nadolol Tablets 2288

Naproxen (Potential for acute renal failure). Products include:
EC-Naprosyn Delayed-Release Tablets 2967
Naprosyn Suspension 2967
Naprosyn Tablets 2967

Naproxen Sodium (Potential for acute renal failure). Products include:
Aleve Tablets, Caplets and Gelcaps ....▣ 602
Aleve Cold & Sinus Caplets ....▣ 603
Anaprox Tablets 2967
Anaprox DS Tablets 2967
Naprelan Tablets 1293

Nicardipine Hydrochloride (May add to potentiate the action of other hypertensives). Products include:
Cardene I.V. 3485

Nifedipine (May add to potentiate the action of other hypertensives). Products include:
Adalat CC Tablets 877
Procardia Capsules 2708
Procardia XL Extended Release Tablets 2710

Nisoldipine (May add to potentiate the action of other hypertensives). Products include:
Sular Tablets 688

Nitroglycerin (May add to potentiate the action of other hypertensives). Products include:
Nitro-Dur Transdermal Infusion System 3134
Nitro-Dur Transdermal Infusion System 1834
Nitrolingual Pumpspray 1355
Nitrostat Tablets 2658

Norepinephrine Bitartrate (Decreased arterial responsiveness to norepinephrine).
No products indexed under this heading.

Oxaprozin (Potential for acute renal failure).
No products indexed under this heading.

Pancuronium Bromide (Increased paralyzing effect).
No products indexed under this heading.

Penbutolol Sulfate (May add to potentiate the action of other hypertensives).
No products indexed under this heading.

Penicillin G Potassium (Concurrent use of parenteral penicillin G potassium with triamterene may result in hyperkalemia, especially in patients with renal insufficiency). Products include:
Pfizerpen for Injection 2707

Perindopril Erbumine (May add to potentiate the action of other hypertensives; increased risk of hyperkalemia). Products include:
Aceon Tablets (2 mg, 4 mg, 8 mg) 3249

Phenoxybenzamine Hydrochloride (May add to potentiate the action of other hypertensives). Products include:
Dibenzyline Capsules 3457

Phentolamine Mesylate (May add to potentiate the action of other hypertensives).
No products indexed under this heading.

Phenylbutazone (Potential for acute renal failure).
No products indexed under this heading.

Pindolol (May add to potentiate the action of other hypertensives).
No products indexed under this heading.

Pioglitazone Hydrochloride (Thiazides may cause hyperglycemia and glycosuria; dosage alteration of oral antidiabetic agents may be required). Products include:
Actos Tablets 3275

Piroxicam (Potential for acute renal failure). Products include:
Feldene Capsules 2685

Polythiazide (May add to potentiate the action of other hypertensives). Products include:
Minizide Capsules 2700
Renese Tablets 2712

Potassium Acid Phosphate (Potential for hyperkalemia; concomitant use should be avoided). Products include:
K-Phos Original (Sodium Free) Tablets 947

Potassium Bicarbonate (Potential for hyperkalemia; concomitant use should be avoided).
No products indexed under this heading.

Potassium Chloride (Potential for hyperkalemia; concomitant use should be avoided). Products include:
Chlor-3 1361
Colyte with Flavor Packs for Oral Solution 3170
GoLYTELY and Pineapple Flavor GoLYTELY for Oral Solution 1068
K-Dur Microburst Release System ER Tablets 1832
Klor-Con M20/Klor-Con M10 Tablets 3329
K-Lor Powder Packets 469
K-Tab Filmtab Tablets 470
Micro-K 3311
NuLYTELY, Cherry Flavor, Lemon-Lime Flavor, and Orange Flavor NuLYTELY for Oral Solution 1068
Rum-K 1363

Potassium Citrate (Potential for hyperkalemia; concomitant use should be avoided). Products include:
Urocit-K Tablets 2232

Potassium Gluconate (Potential for hyperkalemia; concomitant use should be avoided).
No products indexed under this heading.

Potassium Phosphate (Potential for hyperkalemia; concomitant use should be avoided). Products include:
K-Phos Neutral Tablets 946

Prazosin Hydrochloride (May add to potentiate the action of other hypertensives). Products include:
Minipress Capsules 2699
Minizide Capsules 2700

Prednisolone Acetate (May intensify electrolyte imbalance, particularly hypokalemia). Products include:
Blephamide Ophthalmic Ointment ... 547
Blephamide Ophthalmic Suspension 548
Poly-Pred Liquifilm Ophthalmic Suspension ....⊙ 245
Pred Forte Ophthalmic Suspension ....⊙ 246
Pred Mild Sterile Ophthalmic Suspension ....⊙ 249
Pred-G Ophthalmic Suspension .....⊙ 247
Pred-G Sterile Ophthalmic Ointment ....⊙ 248

Prednisolone Sodium Phosphate (May intensify electrolyte imbalance, particularly hypokalemia). Products include:
Pediapred Oral Solution 1170

Prednisolone Tebutate (May intensify electrolyte imbalance, particularly hypokalemia).
No products indexed under this heading.

Prednisone (May intensify electrolyte imbalance, particularly hypokalemia). Products include:
Prednisone 3064

Probenecid (Dyazide may raise the level of blood uric acid; may require dosage adjustment of antigout agent).
No products indexed under this heading.

Propranolol Hydrochloride (May add to potentiate the action of other hypertensives). Products include:
Inderal 3513
Inderal LA Long-Acting Capsules 3516
Inderide Tablets 3517
Inderide LA Long-Acting Capsules .. 3519

Quinapril Hydrochloride (May add to potentiate the action of other hypertensives; increased risk of hyperkalemia). Products include:
Accupril Tablets 2611
Accuretic Tablets 2614

Ramipril (May add to potentiate the action of other hypertensives; increased risk of hyperkalemia). Products include:
Altace Capsules 2233

Rapacuronium Bromide (Increased paralyzing effect).
No products indexed under this heading.

Rauwolfia serpentina (May add to potentiate the action of other hypertensives).
No products indexed under this heading.

Repaglinide (Thiazides may cause hyperglycemia and glycosuria; dosage alteration of oral antidiabetic agents may be required). Products include:
Prandin Tablets (0.5, 1, and 2 mg) 2432

Rescinnamine (May add to potentiate the action of other hypertensives).
No products indexed under this heading.

Reserpine (May add to potentiate the action of other hypertensives).
No products indexed under this heading.

Rocuronium Bromide (Increased paralyzing effect). Products include:
Zemuron Injection 2491

Rofecoxib (Potential for acute renal failure). Products include:
Vioxx 2213

Rosiglitazone Maleate (Thiazides may cause hyperglycemia and glycosuria; dosage alteration of oral antidiabetic agents may be required). Products include:
Avandia Tablets 1490

Salt Substitutes (Concurrent use of salt substitues with triamterene may result in hyperkalemia, especially in patients with renal insufficiency).
No products indexed under this heading.

Sodium Nitroprusside (May add to potentiate the action of other hypertensives).
No products indexed under this heading.

Sodium Polystyrene Sulfonate (May result in fluid retention).
No products indexed under this heading.

Sotalol Hydrochloride (May add to potentiate the action of other hypertensives). Products include:
Betapace Tablets 950
Betapace AF Tablets 954

Spirapril Hydrochloride (May add to potentiate the action of other hypertensives; increased risk of hyperkalemia).
No products indexed under this heading.

Spironolactone (Concurrent use is contraindicated).
No products indexed under this heading.

Sulfinpyrazone (Dyazide may raise the level of blood uric acid; may require dosage adjustment of antigout agent).
No products indexed under this heading.

Sulindac (Potential for acute renal failure). Products include:
Clinoril Tablets 2053

Telmisartan (May add to potentiate the action of other hypertensives). Products include:
Micardis Tablets 1049
Micardis HCT Tablets 1051

Terazosin Hydrochloride (May add to potentiate the action of other hypertensives). Products include:
Hytrin Capsules 464

Timolol Maleate (May add to potentiate the action of other hypertensives). Products include:
Blocadren Tablets 2046
Cosopt Sterile Ophthalmic Solution 2065
Timolide Tablets 2187
Timolol GFS ....⊙ 266
Timoptic in Ocudose 2192
Timoptic Sterile Ophthalmic Solution 2190
Timoptic-XE Sterile Ophthalmic Gel Forming Solution 2194

Tolazamide (Thiazides may cause hyperglycemia and glycosuria; dosage alteration of oral antidiabetic agents may be required).
No products indexed under this heading.

Tolbutamide (Thiazides may cause hyperglycemia and glycosuria; dosage alteration of oral antidiabetic agents may be required).
No products indexed under this heading.

Tolmetin Sodium (Potential for acute renal failure). Products include:
Tolectin 2589

Torsemide (May add to potentiate the action of other hypertensives). Products include:
Demadex Tablets and Injection 2965

Trandolapril (May add to potentiate the action of other hypertensives; increased risk of hyperkalemia). Products include:
Mavik Tablets 478
Tarka Tablets 508

Triamcinolone (May intensify electrolyte imbalance, particularly hypo-

kalemia).
No products indexed under this heading.

Triamcinolone Acetonide (May intensify electrolyte imbalance, particularly hypokalemia). Products include:
Azmacort Inhalation Aerosol 728
Nasacort Nasal Inhaler 750
Nasacort AQ Nasal Spray 752
Tri-Nasal Spray 2274

Triamcinolone Diacetate (May intensify electrolyte imbalance, particularly hypokalemia).
No products indexed under this heading.

Triamcinolone Hexacetonide (May intensify electrolyte imbalance, particularly hypokalemia).
No products indexed under this heading.

Trimethaphan Camsylate (May add to potentiate the action of other hypertensives).
No products indexed under this heading.

Troglitazone (Thiazides may cause hyperglycemia and glycosuria; dosage alteration of oral antidiabetic agents may be required).
No products indexed under this heading.

Tubocurarine Chloride (Increased paralyzing effect).
No products indexed under this heading.

Valsartan (May add to potentiate the action of other hypertensives). Products include:
Diovan Capsules 2337
Diovan HCT Tablets 2338

Vecuronium Bromide (Increased paralyzing effect). Products include:
Norcuron for Injection 2478

Verapamil Hydrochloride (May add to potentiate the action of other hypertensives). Products include:
Covera-HS Tablets 3199
Isoptin SR Tablets 467
Tarka Tablets 508
Verelan Capsules 3184
Verelan PM Capsules 3186

Warfarin Sodium (Effects of oral anticoagulants may be decreased). Products include:
Coumadin for Injection 1243
Coumadin Tablets 1243
Warfarin Sodium Tablets, USP 3302

Food Interactions

Milk, low fat (Concurrent use of low-salt milk with triamterene may result in hyperkalemia, especially in patients with renal insufficiency).

DYNABAC TABLETS

(Dirithromycin) 2269

May interact with antacids containing aluminum, calcium and magnesium, oral anticoagulants, histamine H_2-receptor antagonists, phenytoin, valproate, theophylline, and certain other agents. Compounds in these categories include:

Alfentanil Hydrochloride (Caution is advised since erythromycin, a macrolide antibiotic, and alfentanil co-administration is associated with elevation in alfentanil serum levels).
No products indexed under this heading.

Aluminum Carbonate (When dirithromycin is administered immediately following antacids, the absorption of dirithromycin is slightly enhanced).
No products indexed under this heading.

Aluminum Hydroxide (When dirithromycin is administered immediately following antacids, the absorption of dirithromycin is slightly enhanced). Products include:
Amphojel Suspension (Mint Flavor) .... ▣789
Gaviscon Extra Strength Liquid ..... ▣751
Gaviscon Extra Strength Tablets ... ▣751
Gaviscon Regular Strength Liquid . ▣751
Gaviscon Regular Strength Tablets .... ▣750
Maalox Antacid/Anti-Gas Oral Suspension .... ▣673
Maalox Max Maximum Strength Antacid/Anti-Gas Liquid 2300
Maalox Regular Strength Antacid/Antigas Liquid 2300
Mylanta 1813
Vanquish Caplets .... ▣617

Aminophylline (Steady-state plasma concentration is not significantly affected, however, patients with theophylline concentrations at the higher end of the therapeutic range should be monitored for dosage adjustment).
No products indexed under this heading.

Astemizole (Caution is advised since erythromycin, a macrolide antibiotic, and astemizole co-administration is associated with elevation of astemizole serum levels).
No products indexed under this heading.

Bromocriptine Mesylate (Caution is advised since erythromycin, a macrolide antibiotic, and bromocriptine co-administration is associated with elevation in bromocriptine serum levels).
No products indexed under this heading.

Carbamazepine (Caution is advised since erythromycin, a macrolide antibiotic, and carbamazepine co-administration is associated with elevation in carbamazepine serum levels). Products include:
Carbatrol Capsules 3234
Tegretol/Tegretol-XR 2404

Cimetidine (When dirithromycin is administered immediately following H_2-receptor antagonists, the absorption of dirithromycin is slightly enhanced). Products include:
Tagamet HB 200 Suspension .... ▣762
Tagamet HB 200 Tablets .... ▣761
Tagamet Tablets 1644

Cimetidine Hydrochloride (When dirithromycin is administered immediately following H_2-receptor antagonists, the absorption of dirithromycin is slightly enhanced). Products include:
Tagamet 1644

Cyclosporine (Caution is advised since erythromycin, a macrolide antibiotic, and cyclosporine co-administration is associated with elevation in cyclosporine serum levels). Products include:
Gengraf Capsules 457
Neoral Soft Gelatin Capsules 2380
Neoral Oral Solution 2380
Sandimmune 2388

Dicumarol (Caution is advised since erythromycin, a macrolide antibiotic, increases anticoagulant effect).
No products indexed under this heading.

Digoxin (Caution is advised since erythromycin, a macrolide antibiotic, elevates digoxin serum levels). Products include:
Digitek Tablets 1003
Lanoxicaps Capsules 1574
Lanoxin Injection 1581
Lanoxin Tablets 1587
Lanoxin Elixir Pediatric 1578
Lanoxin Injection Pediatric 1584

Dihydroergotamine Mesylate (Caution is advised since erythromycin, a macrolide antibiotic, and ergotamine co-administration is associated with acute ergot toxicity). Products include:
D.H.E. 45 Injection 2334
Migranal Nasal Spray 2376

Disopyramide Phosphate (Caution is advised since erythromycin, a macrolide antibiotic, and disopyramide co-administration is associated with elevation in disopyramide serum levels).
No products indexed under this heading.

Divalproex Sodium (Caution is advised since erythromycin, a macrolide antibiotic, and valproate co-administration is associated with elevation of valproate serum levels). Products include:
Depakote Sprinkle Capsules 426
Depakote Tablets 430
Depakote ER Tablets 436

Dyphylline (Steady-state plasma concentration is not significantly affected, however, patients with theophylline concentrations at the higher end of the therapeutic range should be monitored for dosage adjustment). Products include:
Lufyllin Tablets 3347
Lufyllin-400 Tablets 3347
Lufyllin-GG Elixir 3348
Lufyllin-GG Tablets 3348

Ergotamine Tartrate (Caution is advised since erythromycin, a macrolide antibiotic, and ergotamine co-administration is associated with acute ergot toxicity).
No products indexed under this heading.

Famotidine (When dirithromycin is administered immediately following H_2-receptor antagonists, the absorption of dirithromycin is slightly enhanced). Products include:
Famotidine Injection 866
Pepcid AC 1814
Pepcid Complete Chewable Tablets 1815
Pepcid Injection 2153
Pepcid for Oral Suspension 2150
Pepcid RPD Orally Disintegrating Tablets 2150
Pepcid Tablets 2150

Fosphenytoin Sodium (Caution is advised since erythromycin, a macrolide antibiotic, and phenytoin co-administration is associated with elevation in phenytoin serum levels). Products include:
Cerebyx Injection 2619

Hexobarbital (Caution is advised since erythromycin, a macrolide antibiotic, and hexobarbital co-administration is associated with elevation in hexobarbital serum levels).
No products indexed under this heading.

Lovastatin (Caution is advised since erythromycin, a macrolide antibiotic, and lovastatin co-administration is associated with elevation in lovastatin serum levels). Products include:
Mevacor Tablets 2132

Magaldrate (When dirithromycin is administered immediately following antacids, the absorption of dirithromycin is slightly enhanced).
No products indexed under this heading.

Magnesium Hydroxide (When dirithromycin is administered immediately following antacids, the absorption of dirithromycin is slightly enhanced). Products include:
Ex•Lax Milk of Magnesia Liquid .... ▣670
Maalox Antacid/Anti-Gas Oral Suspension .... ▣673
Maalox Max Maximum Strength Antacid/Anti-Gas Liquid 2300
Maalox Regular Strength Antacid/Antigas Liquid 2300
Mylanta Fast-Acting 1813
Mylanta 1813
Pepcid Complete Chewable Tablets 1815
Phillips' Chewable Tablets .... ▣615
Phillips' Milk of Magnesia Liquid (Original, Cherry, & Mint) .... ▣616
Rolaids Tablets .... ▣706
Extra Strength Rolaids Tablets ...... ▣706
Vanquish Caplets .... ▣617

Magnesium Oxide (When dirithromycin is administered immediately following antacids, the absorption of dirithromycin is slightly enhanced). Products include:
Beelith Tablets 946
Mag-Ox 400 Tablets 1024
Uro-Mag Capsules 1024

Nizatidine (When dirithromycin is administered immediately following H_2-receptor antagonists, the absorption of dirithromycin is slightly enhanced). Products include:
Axid Pulvules 1903
Axid Pulvules 2919

Phenytoin (Caution is advised since erythromycin, a macrolide antibiotic, and phenytoin co-administration is associated with elevation in phenytoin serum levels). Products include:
Dilantin Infatabs 2624
Dilantin-125 Oral Suspension 2625

Phenytoin Sodium (Caution is advised since erythromycin, a macrolide antibiotic, and phenytoin co-administration is associated with elevation in phenytoin serum levels). Products include:
Dilantin Kapseals 2622

Ranitidine Bismuth Citrate (When dirithromycin is administered immediately following H_2-receptor antagonists, the absorption of dirithromycin is slightly enhanced).
No products indexed under this heading.

Ranitidine Hydrochloride (When dirithromycin is administered immediately following H_2-receptor antagonists, the absorption of dirithromycin is slightly enhanced). Products include:
Zantac 1690
Zantac Injection 1688
Zantac 75 Tablets .... ▣717

Terfenadine (Serious cardiac dysrhythmias have occurred in patients receiving terfenadine with other macrolide antibiotics; in a prospective study dirithromycin did not affect the metabolism of terfenadine; it is prudent to monitor the terfenadine levels when dirithromycin and terfenadine are co-administered).
No products indexed under this heading.

Theophylline (Steady-state plasma concentration is not significantly affected, however, patients with theophylline concentrations at the higher end of the therapeutic range should be monitored for dosage adjustment). Products include:
Aerolate 1361
Theo-Dur Extended-Release Tablets 1835
Uni-Dur Extended-Release Tablets .. 1841
Uniphyl 400 mg and 600 mg Tablets 2903

Theophylline Calcium Salicylate (Steady-state plasma concentration is not significantly affected, however, patients with theophylline concentrations at the higher end of the therapeutic range should be monitored for dosage adjustment).
No products indexed under this heading.

Theophylline Sodium Glycinate (Steady-state plasma concentration is not significantly affected, however, patients with theophylline concentrations at the higher end of the therapeutic range should be monitored for dosage adjustment).
No products indexed under this heading.

Triazolam (Caution is advised since erythromycin, a macrolide antibiotic, decreases the clearance of triazolam and thereby increasing the pharmacologic effect of triazolam). Products include:
Halcion Tablets 2823

Valproate Sodium (Caution is advised since erythromycin, a macrolide antibiotic, and valproate co-

administration is associated with elevation of valproate serum levels). Products include:

Depacon Injection 416

Valproic Acid (Caution is advised since erythromycin, a macrolide antibiotic, and valproate co-administration is associated with elevation of valproate serum levels). Products include:

Depakene 421

Warfarin Sodium (Caution is advised since erythromycin, a macrolide antibiotic, increases anticoagulant effect). Products include:

Coumadin for Injection 1243
Coumadin Tablets 1243
Warfarin Sodium Tablets, USP 3302

Food Interactions

Food, unspecified (Slight increase in the absorption of erythromycyclamine when dirithromycin tablets were administered after food; significant decrease in Cmax (33%) and AUC (31%) occurs when administered one hour before food; administer with food or within an hour of having eaten).

DYNACIN CAPSULES

(Minocycline Hydrochloride) 2019
May interact with antacids containing aluminum, calcium and magnesium, oral anticoagulants, iron containing oral preparations, oral contraceptives, penicillins, and certain other agents. Compounds in these categories include:

Aluminum Carbonate (Absorption of tetracyclines is impaired by antacids).

No products indexed under this heading.

Aluminum Hydroxide (Absorption of tetracyclines is impaired by antacids). Products include:

Amphojel Suspension (Mint Flavor) .... ▣789
Gaviscon Extra Strength Liquid .... ▣751
Gaviscon Extra Strength Tablets .... ▣751
Gaviscon Regular Strength Liquid .... ▣751
Gaviscon Regular Strength Tablets .... ▣750
Maalox Antacid/Anti-Gas Oral Suspension .... ▣673
Maalox Max Maximum Strength Antacid/Anti-Gas Liquid 2300
Maalox Regular Strength Antacid/Antigas Liquid 2300
Mylanta 1813
Vanquish Caplets .... ▣617

Amoxicillin Trihydrate (Interference with bactericidal action of penicillin; avoid giving tetracycline-class drugs in conjunction with penicillin).

No products indexed under this heading.

Ampicillin (Interference with bactericidal action of penicillin; avoid giving tetracycline-class drugs in conjunction with penicillin).

No products indexed under this heading.

Ampicillin Sodium (Interference with bactericidal action of penicillin; avoid giving tetracycline-class drugs in conjunction with penicillin). Products include:

Unasyn for Injection 2728

Ampicillin Trihydrate (Interference with bactericidal action of penicillin; avoid giving tetracycline-class drugs in conjunction with penicillin).

No products indexed under this heading.

Azlocillin Sodium (Interference with bactericidal action of penicillin; avoid giving tetracycline-class drugs in conjunction with penicillin).

No products indexed under this heading.

Bacampicillin Hydrochloride (Interference with bactericidal action of penicillin; avoid giving tetracycline-class drugs in conjunction with penicillin).

No products indexed under this heading.

Carbenicillin Disodium (Interference with bactericidal action of penicillin; avoid giving tetracycline-class drugs in conjunction with penicillin).

No products indexed under this heading.

Carbenicillin Indanyl Sodium (Interference with bactericidal action of penicillin; avoid giving tetracycline-class drugs in conjunction with penicillin). Products include:

Geocillin Tablets 2687

Desogestrel (Concurrent use of tetracyclines may render oral contraceptives less effective). Products include:

Cyclessa Tablets 2450
Desogen Tablets 2458
Mircette Tablets 2470
Ortho-Cept 21 Tablets 2546
Ortho-Cept 28 Tablets 2546

Dicloxacillin Sodium (Interference with bactericidal action of penicillin; avoid giving tetracycline-class drugs in conjunction with penicillin).

No products indexed under this heading.

Dicumarol (Tetracyclines have shown to depress plasma prothrombin activity; patients on anticoagulant may require downward adjustments of their anticoagulant dosage).

No products indexed under this heading.

Ethinyl Estradiol (Concurrent use of tetracyclines may render oral contraceptives less effective). Products include:

Alesse-21 Tablets 3468
Alesse-28 Tablets 3473
Brevicon 28-Day Tablets 3380
Cyclessa Tablets 2450
Desogen Tablets 2458
Estinyl Tablets 3112
Estrostep 2627
femhrt Tablets 2635
Levlen 962
Levlite 21 Tablets 962
Levlite 28 Tablets 962
Levora Tablets 3389
Loestrin 21 Tablets 2642
Loestrin Fe Tablets 2642
Lo/Ovral Tablets 3532
Lo/Ovral-28 Tablets 3538
Low-Ogestrel-28 Tablets 3392
Microgestin Fe 1.5/30 Tablets 3407
Microgestin Fe 1/20 Tablets 3400
Mircette Tablets 2470
Modicon 2563
Necon 3415
Nordette-28 Tablets 2257
Norinyl 1 +35 28-Day Tablets 3380
Ogestrel 0.5/50-28 Tablets 3428
Ortho-Cept 21 Tablets 2546
Ortho-Cept 28 Tablets 2546
Ortho-Cyclen/Ortho Tri-Cyclen 2573
Ortho-Novum 2563
Ovcon 3364
Ovral Tablets 3551
Ovral-28 Tablets 3552
Tri-Levlen 962
Tri-Norinyl-28 Tablets 3433
Triphasil-21 Tablets 3600
Triphasil-28 Tablets 3605
Trivora Tablets 3439
Yasmin 28 Tablets 980
Zovia 3449

Ethynodiol Diacetate (Concurrent use of tetracyclines may render oral contraceptives less effective). Products include:

Zovia 3449

Ferrous Fumarate (Absorption of tetracyclines is impaired by iron-containing preparations). Products include:

New Formulation Chromagen OB Capsules 3094
Loestrin Fe Tablets 2642
NataChew Tablets 3364

Ferrous Gluconate (Absorption of tetracyclines is impaired by iron-containing preparations). Products include:

Fergon Iron Tablets .... ▣802

Ferrous Sulfate (Absorption of tetracyclines is impaired by iron-containing preparations). Products include:

Feosol Tablets 1717
Slow Fe Tablets .... ▣827
Slow Fe with Folic Acid Tablets .... ▣828

Iron (Absorption of tetracyclines is impaired by iron-containing preparations).

No products indexed under this heading.

Levonorgestrel (Concurrent use of tetracyclines may render oral contraceptives less effective). Products include:

Alesse-21 Tablets 3468
Alesse-28 Tablets 3473
Levlen 962
Levlite 21 Tablets 962
Levlite 28 Tablets 962
Levora Tablets 3389
Mirena Intrauterine System 974
Nordette-28 Tablets 2257
Norplant System 3543
Tri-Levlen 962
Triphasil-21 Tablets 3600
Triphasil-28 Tablets 3605
Trivora Tablets 3439

Magaldrate (Absorption of tetracyclines is impaired by antacids).

No products indexed under this heading.

Magnesium Hydroxide (Absorption of tetracyclines is impaired by antacids). Products include:

Ex•Lax Milk of Magnesia Liquid .... ▣670
Maalox Antacid/Anti-Gas Oral Suspension .... ▣673
Maalox Max Maximum Strength Antacid/Anti-Gas Liquid 2300
Maalox Regular Strength Antacid/Antigas Liquid 2300
Mylanta Fast-Acting 1813
Mylanta 1813
Pepcid Complete Chewable Tablets 1815
Phillips' Chewable Tablets .... ▣615
Phillips' Milk of Magnesia Liquid (Original, Cherry, & Mint) .... ▣616
Rolaids Tablets .... ▣706
Extra Strength Rolaids Tablets .... ▣706
Vanquish Caplets .... ▣617

Magnesium Oxide (Absorption of tetracyclines is impaired by antacids). Products include:

Beelith Tablets 946
Mag-Ox 400 Tablets 1024
Uro-Mag Capsules 1024

Mestranol (Concurrent use of tetracyclines may render oral contraceptives less effective). Products include:

Necon 1/50 Tablets 3415
Norinyl 1 + 50 28-Day Tablets 3380
Ortho-Novum 1/50□28 Tablets 2556

Methoxyflurane (Potential for fatal renal toxicity).

No products indexed under this heading.

Mezlocillin Sodium (Interference with bactericidal action of penicillin; avoid giving tetracycline-class drugs in conjunction with penicillin).

No products indexed under this heading.

Nafcillin Sodium (Interference with bactericidal action of penicillin; avoid giving tetracycline-class drugs in conjunction with penicillin).

No products indexed under this heading.

Norethindrone (Concurrent use of tetracyclines may render oral contraceptives less effective). Products include:

Brevicon 28-Day Tablets 3380
Micronor Tablets 2543
Modicon 2563
Necon 3415
Norinyl 1 +35 28-Day Tablets 3380
Norinyl 1 + 50 28-Day Tablets 3380
Nor-QD Tablets 3423
Ortho-Novum 2563
Ortho-Novum 1/50□28 Tablets 2556
Ovcon 3364
Tri-Norinyl-28 Tablets 3433

Norethynodrel (Concurrent use of tetracyclines may render oral contraceptives less effective).

No products indexed under this heading.

Norgestimate (Concurrent use of tetracyclines may render oral contraceptives less effective). Products include:

Ortho-Cyclen/Ortho Tri-Cyclen 2573
Ortho-Prefest Tablets 2570

Norgestrel (Concurrent use of tetracyclines may render oral contraceptives less effective). Products include:

Lo/Ovral Tablets 3532
Lo/Ovral-28 Tablets 3538
Low-Ogestrel-28 Tablets 3392
Ogestrel 0.5/50-28 Tablets 3428
Ovral Tablets 3551
Ovral-28 Tablets 3552
Ovrette Tablets 3552

Penicillin G Benzathine (Interference with bactericidal action of penicillin; avoid giving tetracycline-class drugs in conjunction with penicillin). Products include:

Bicillin C-R 900/300 Injection 2240
Bicillin C-R Injection 2238
Bicillin L-A Injection 2242
Permapen Isoject 2706

Penicillin G Potassium (Interference with bactericidal action of penicillin; avoid giving tetracycline-class drugs in conjunction with penicillin). Products include:

Pfizerpen for Injection 2707

Penicillin G Procaine (Interference with bactericidal action of penicillin; avoid giving tetracycline-class drugs in conjunction with penicillin). Products include:

Bicillin C-R 900/300 Injection 2240
Bicillin C-R Injection 2238

Penicillin G Sodium (Interference with bactericidal action of penicillin; avoid giving tetracycline-class drugs in conjunction with penicillin).

No products indexed under this heading.

Penicillin V Potassium (Interference with bactericidal action of penicillin; avoid giving tetracycline-class drugs in conjunction with penicillin).

No products indexed under this heading.

Polysaccharide-Iron Complex (Absorption of tetracyclines is impaired by iron-containing preparations). Products include:

Niferex 3176
Niferex-150 Capsules 3176
Nu-Iron 150 Capsules 2224

Ticarcillin Disodium (Interference with bactericidal action of penicillin; avoid giving tetracycline-class drugs in conjunction with penicillin). Products include:

Timentin Injection- ADD-Vantage Vial 1661
Timentin Injection-Galaxy Container 1664
Timentin Injection-Pharmacy Bulk Package 1666
Timentin for Intravenous Administration 1658

Warfarin Sodium (Tetracyclines have shown to depress plasma prothrombin activity; patients on anticoagulant may require downward adjustments of their anticoagulant dosage). Products include:

Coumadin for Injection 1243
Coumadin Tablets 1243
Warfarin Sodium Tablets, USP 3302

Food Interactions

Food, unspecified (The peak plasma concentrations were slightly decreased and delayed by one hour when administered with a meal which included dairy products; extent of absorption was not noticeably influenced).

DYNACIRC CAPSULES

(Isradipine) 2921
May interact with:

Cimetidine (Co-administration has resulted in increase in isradipine mean peak plasma concentrations and significant increase in the AUC). Products include:
Tagamet HB 200 Suspension .... ▣762
Tagamet HB 200 Tablets .... ▣761
Tagamet Tablets 1644

Cimetidine Hydrochloride (Co-administration has resulted in increase in isradipine mean peak plasma concentrations and significant increase in the AUC). Products include:
Tagamet 1644

Fentanyl (Severe hypotension has been reported during fentanyl anesthesia with concomitant use of beta-blocker and a calcium channel blocker). Products include:
Duragesic Transdermal System 1786

Fentanyl Citrate (Severe hypotension has been reported during fentanyl anesthesia with concomitant use of beta-blocker and a calcium channel blocker). Products include:
Actiq 1184

Hydrochlorothiazide (Additive antihypertensive effect). Products include:
Accuretic Tablets 2614
Aldoril Tablets 2039
Atacand HCT Tablets 597
Avalide Tablets 1070
Diovan HCT Tablets 2338
Dyazide Capsules 1515
HydroDIURIL Tablets 2108
Hyzaar 2109
Inderide Tablets 3517
Inderide LA Long-Acting Capsules .. 3519
Lotensin HCT Tablets 2367
Maxzide 1008
Micardis HCT Tablets 1051
Microzide Capsules 3414
Moduretic Tablets 2138
Monopril HCT 1094
Prinzide Tablets 2168
Timolide Tablets 2187
Uniretic Tablets 3178
Vaseretic Tablets 2204
Zestoretic Tablets 695
Ziac Tablets 1887

Propranolol Hydrochloride (Co-administration has resulted in a small effect on the rate but no effect on the extent of isradipine bioavailability; significant increases in AUC and Cmax and decreases in tmax of propranolol were noted). Products include:
Inderal 3513
Inderal LA Long-Acting Capsules 3516
Inderide Tablets 3517
Inderide LA Long-Acting Capsules .. 3519

Rifampin (Co-administration has resulted in increased metabolism and higher clearance of isradipine; a reduction in isradipine levels to below the detectable limits has been noted). Products include:
Rifadin 765
Rifamate Capsules 767
Rifater Tablets 769

DYNACIRC CR TABLETS

(Isradipine) 2923
See DynaCirc Capsules

DYRENIUM CAPSULES

(Triamterene) 3458
May interact with ACE inhibitors, anesthetics, antihypertensives, diuretics, oral hypoglycemic agents, lithium preparations, nondepolarizing neuromuscular blocking agents, potassium preparations, preanesthetic medications, potassium sparing diuretics, and certain other agents. Compounds in these categories include:

Acarbose (Triamterene may raise blood glucose levels; for adult onset diabetes, dosage adjustments of hypoglycemic agents may be necessary during and after therapy). Products include:
Precose Tablets 906

Acebutolol Hydrochloride (The effects of antihypertensive agents may be potentiated when given concurrently). Products include:
Sectral Capsules 3589

Alfentanil Hydrochloride (The effects of anesthetics may be potentiated when given concurrently).
No products indexed under this heading.

Amiloride Hydrochloride (Co-administration with other potassium-sparing agents has resulted in fatalities; these agents should not be given concomitantly). Products include:
Midamor Tablets 2136
Moduretic Tablets 2138

Amlodipine Besylate (The effects of antihypertensive agents may be potentiated when given concurrently). Products include:
Lotrel Capsules 2370
Norvasc Tablets 2704

Atenolol (The effects of antihypertensive agents may be potentiated when given concurrently). Products include:
Tenoretic Tablets 690
Tenormin I.V. Injection 692

Atracurium Besylate (The effects of nondepolarizing skeletal muscle relaxants may be potentiated when given concurrently).
No products indexed under this heading.

Benazepril Hydrochloride (Co-administration with potassium-sparing agents and angiotensin-coverting enzyme inhibitors increases the risk of hyperkalemia). Products include:
Lotensin Tablets 2365
Lotensin HCT Tablets 2367
Lotrel Capsules 2370

Bendroflumethiazide (The effects of other diuretics may be potentiated when given concurrently). Products include:
Corzide 40/5 Tablets 2247
Corzide 80/5 Tablets 2247

Betaxolol Hydrochloride (The effects of antihypertensive agents may be potentiated when given concurrently). Products include:
Betoptic S Ophthalmic Suspension 537

Bisoprolol Fumarate (The effects of antihypertensive agents may be potentiated when given concurrently). Products include:
Zebeta Tablets 1885
Ziac Tablets 1887

Blood, whole (Co-administration with blood from blood banks may promote serum potassium accumulation and possibly result in hyperkalemia).
No products indexed under this heading.

Bumetanide (The effects of other diuretics may be potentiated when given concurrently).
No products indexed under this heading.

Candesartan Cilexetil (The effects of antihypertensive agents may be potentiated when given concurrently). Products include:
Atacand Tablets 595
Atacand HCT Tablets 597

Captopril (Co-administration with potassium-sparing agents and angiotensin-coverting enzyme inhibitors increases the risk of hyperkalemia). Products include:
Captopril Tablets 2281

Carteolol Hydrochloride (The effects of antihypertensive agents may be potentiated when given concurrently). Products include:
Carteolol Hydrochloride Ophthalmic Solution USP, 1% ..... ⊙258
Ocupress Ophthalmic Solution, 1% Sterile .... ⊙303

Chlorothiazide (The effects of other diuretics may be potentiated when given concurrently). Products include:
Aldoclor Tablets 2035
Diuril Oral 2087

Chlorothiazide Sodium (The effects of other diuretics may be potentiated when given concurrently). Products include:
Diuril Sodium Intravenous 2086

Chlorpropamide (Triamterene may raise blood glucose levels; for adult onset diabetes, dosage adjustments of hypoglycemic agents may be necessary during and after therapy; increased risk of severe hyponatremia with concurrent use). Products include:
Diabinese Tablets 2680

Chlorthalidone (The effects of other diuretics may be potentiated when given concurrently). Products include:
Clorpres Tablets 1002
Combipres Tablets 1040
Tenoretic Tablets 690

Cisatracurium Besylate (The effects of nondepolarizing skeletal muscle relaxants may be potentiated when given concurrently).
No products indexed under this heading.

Clonidine (The effects of antihypertensive agents may be potentiated when given concurrently). Products include:
Catapres-TTS 1038

Clonidine Hydrochloride (The effects of antihypertensive agents may be potentiated when given concurrently). Products include:
Catapres Tablets 1037
Clorpres Tablets 1002
Combipres Tablets 1040
Duraclon Injection 3057

Deserpidine (The effects of antihypertensive agents may be potentiated when given concurrently).
No products indexed under this heading.

Diazepam (The effects of preanesthetic agents may be potentiated when given concurrently). Products include:
Valium Injectable 3026
Valium Tablets 3047

Diazoxide (The effects of antihypertensive agents may be potentiated when given concurrently).
No products indexed under this heading.

Diltiazem Hydrochloride (The effects of antihypertensive agents may be potentiated when given concurrently). Products include:
Cardizem Injectable 1018
Cardizem Lyo-Ject Syringe 1018
Cardizem Monovial 1018
Cardizem CD Capsules 1016
Tiazac Capsules 1378

Doxazosin Mesylate (The effects of antihypertensive agents may be potentiated when given concurrently). Products include:
Cardura Tablets 2668

Droperidol (The effects of preanesthetic agents may be potentiated when given concurrently).
No products indexed under this heading.

Enalapril Maleate (Co-administration with potassium-sparing agents and angiotensin-coverting enzyme inhibitors increases the risk of hyperkalemia). Products include:
Lexxel Tablets 608
Vaseretic Tablets 2204
Vasotec Tablets 2210

Enalaprilat (Co-administration with potassium-sparing agents and angiotensin-coverting enzyme inhibitors increases the risk of hyperkalemia). Products include:
Enalaprilat Injection 863
Vasotec I.V. Injection 2207

Enflurane (The effects of anesthetics may be potentiated when given concurrently).
No products indexed under this heading.

Eprosartan Mesylate (The effects of antihypertensive agents may be potentiated when given concurrently). Products include:
Teveten Tablets 3327

Esmolol Hydrochloride (The effects of antihypertensive agents may be potentiated when given concurrently). Products include:
Brevibloc Injection 858

Ethacrynic Acid (The effects of other diuretics may be potentiated when given concurrently). Products include:
Edecrin Tablets 2091

Felodipine (The effects of antihypertensive agents may be potentiated when given concurrently). Products include:
Lexxel Tablets 608
Plendil Extended-Release Tablets ... 623

Fentanyl Citrate (The effects of anesthetics may be potentiated when given concurrently). Products include:
Actiq 1184

Fosinopril Sodium (Co-administration with potassium-sparing agents and angiotensin-coverting enzyme inhibitors increases the risk of hyperkalemia). Products include:
Monopril Tablets 1091
Monopril HCT 1094

Furosemide (The effects of other diuretics may be potentiated when given concurrently). Products include:
Furosemide Tablets 2284

Glimepiride (Triamterene may raise blood glucose levels; for adult onset diabetes, dosage adjustments of hypoglycemic agents may be necessary during and after therapy). Products include:
Amaryl Tablets 717

Glipizide (Triamterene may raise blood glucose levels; for adult onset diabetes, dosage adjustments of hypoglycemic agents may be necessary during and after therapy). Products include:
Glucotrol Tablets 2692
Glucotrol XL Extended Release Tablets 2693

Glyburide (Triamterene may raise blood glucose levels; for adult onset diabetes, dosage adjustments of hypoglycemic agents may be necessary during and after therapy). Products include:
DiaBeta Tablets 741
Glucovance Tablets 1086

Guanabenz Acetate (The effects of antihypertensive agents may be potentiated when given concurrently).
No products indexed under this heading.

Guanethidine Monosulfate (The effects of antihypertensive agents may be potentiated when given concurrently).
No products indexed under this heading.

Halothane (The effects of anesthetics may be potentiated when given concurrently). Products include:
Fluothane Inhalation 3508

Hydralazine Hydrochloride (The effects of antihypertensive agents may be potentiated when given con-

currently).
No products indexed under this heading.

Hydrochlorothiazide (The effects of other diuretics may be potentiated when given concurrently). Products include:
Accuretic Tablets 2614
Aldoril Tablets 2039
Atacand HCT Tablets 597
Avalide Tablets 1070
Diovan HCT Tablets 2338
Dyazide Capsules 1515
HydroDIURIL Tablets 2108
Hyzaar 2109
Inderide Tablets 3517
Inderide LA Long-Acting Capsules .. 3519
Lotensin HCT Tablets 2367
Maxzide 1008
Micardis HCT Tablets 1051
Microzide Capsules 3414
Moduretic Tablets 2138
Monopril HCT 1094
Prinzide Tablets 2168
Timolide Tablets 2187
Uniretic Tablets 3178
Vaseretic Tablets 2204
Zestoretic Tablets 695
Ziac Tablets 1887

Hydroflumethiazide (The effects of other diuretics may be potentiated when given concurrently). Products include:
Diucardin Tablets 3494

Hydroxyzine Hydrochloride (The effects of pre-anesthetic agents may be potentiated when given concurrently). Products include:
Atarax Tablets & Syrup 2667
Vistaril Intramuscular Solution 2738

Indapamide (The effects of other diuretics may be potentiated when given concurrently). Products include:
Indapamide Tablets 2286

Indomethacin (Co-administration has resulted in acute renal failure). Products include:
Indocin 2112

Irbesartan (The effects of antihypertensive agents may be potentiated when given concurrently). Products include:
Avalide Tablets 1070
Avapro Tablets 1074
Avapro Tablets 3076

Isoflurane (The effects of anesthetics may be potentiated when given concurrently).
No products indexed under this heading.

Isradipine (The effects of antihypertensive agents may be potentiated when given concurrently). Products include:
DynaCirc Capsules 2921
DynaCirc CR Tablets 2923

Ketamine Hydrochloride (The effects of anesthetics may be potentiated when given concurrently).
No products indexed under this heading.

Labetalol Hydrochloride (The effects of antihypertensive agents may be potentiated when given concurrently). Products include:
Normodyne Injection 3135
Normodyne Tablets 3137

Lisinopril (Co-administration with potassium-sparing agents and angiotensin-coverting enzyme inhibitors increases the risk of hyperkalemia). Products include:
Prinivil Tablets 2164
Prinzide Tablets 2168
Zestoretic Tablets 695
Zestril Tablets 698

Lithium Carbonate (Co-administration of lithium and diuretics results in diuretic-induced sodium loss that may reduce renal clearance of lithium and increase serum lithium levels with risk of lithium toxicity). Products include:
Eskalith 1527
Lithium Carbonate 3061
Lithobid Slow-Release Tablets 3255

Lithium Citrate (Co-administration of lithium and diuretics results in diuretic-induced sodium loss that may reduce renal clearance of lithium and increase serum lithium levels with risk of lithium toxicity). Products include:
Lithium Citrate Syrup 3061

Lorazepam (The effects of pre-anesthetic agents may be potentiated when given concurrently). Products include:
Ativan Injection 3478
Ativan Tablets 3482

Losartan Potassium (The effects of antihypertensive agents may be potentiated when given concurrently). Products include:
Cozaar Tablets 2067
Hyzaar 2109

Mecamylamine Hydrochloride (The effects of antihypertensive agents may be potentiated when given concurrently). Products include:
Inversine Tablets 1850

Meperidine Hydrochloride (The effects of pre-anesthetic agents may be potentiated when given concurrently). Products include:
Demerol 3079
Mepergan Injection 3539

Metformin Hydrochloride (Triamterene may raise blood glucose levels; for adult onset diabetes, dosage adjustments of hypoglycemic agents may be necessary during and after therapy). Products include:
Glucophage Tablets 1080
Glucophage XR Tablets 1080
Glucovance Tablets 1086

Methohexital Sodium (The effects of anesthetics may be potentiated when given concurrently). Products include:
Brevital Sodium for Injection, USP .. 1815

Methyclothiazide (The effects of other diuretics may be potentiated when given concurrently).
No products indexed under this heading.

Methyldopa (The effects of antihypertensive agents may be potentiated when given concurrently). Products include:
Aldoclor Tablets 2035
Aldomet Tablets 2037
Aldoril Tablets 2039

Methyldopate Hydrochloride (The effects of antihypertensive agents may be potentiated when given concurrently).
No products indexed under this heading.

Metocurine Iodide (The effects of nondepolarizing skeletal muscle relaxants may be potentiated when given concurrently).
No products indexed under this heading.

Metolazone (The effects of other diuretics may be potentiated when given concurrently). Products include:
Mykrox Tablets 1168
Zaroxolyn Tablets 1177

Metoprolol Succinate (The effects of antihypertensive agents may be potentiated when given concurrently). Products include:
Toprol-XL Tablets 651

Metoprolol Tartrate (The effects of antihypertensive agents may be potentiated when given concurrently).
No products indexed under this heading.

Metyrosine (The effects of antihypertensive agents may be potentiated when given concurrently). Products include:
Demser Capsules 2085

Mibefradil Dihydrochloride (The effects of antihypertensive agents may be potentiated when given concurrently).
No products indexed under this heading.

Midazolam Hydrochloride (The effects of anesthetics may be potentiated when given concurrently). Products include:
Versed Injection 3027
Versed Syrup 3033

Miglitol (Triamterene may raise blood glucose levels; for adult onset diabetes, dosage adjustments of hypoglycemic agents may be necessary during and after therapy). Products include:
Glyset Tablets 2821

Minoxidil (The effects of antihypertensive agents may be potentiated when given concurrently). Products include:
Rogaine Extra Strength for Men Topical Solution .... ▣721
Rogaine for Women Topical Solution .... ▣721

Mivacurium Chloride (The effects of nondepolarizing skeletal muscle relaxants may be potentiated when given concurrently).
No products indexed under this heading.

Moexipril Hydrochloride (Co-administration with potassium-sparing agents and angiotensin-coverting enzyme inhibitors increases the risk of hyperkalemia). Products include:
Uniretic Tablets 3178
Univasc Tablets 3181

Morphine Sulfate (The effects of pre-anesthetic agents may be potentiated when given concurrently). Products include:
Astramorph/PF Injection, USP (Preservative-Free) 594
Duramorph Injection 1312
Infumorph 200 and Infumorph 500 Sterile Solutions 1314
Kadian Capsules 1335
MS Contin Tablets 2896
MSIR 2898
Oramorph SR Tablets 3062
Roxanol 3066

Nadolol (The effects of antihypertensive agents may be potentiated when given concurrently). Products include:
Corgard Tablets 2245
Corzide 40/5 Tablets 2247
Corzide 80/5 Tablets 2247
Nadolol Tablets 2288

Nicardipine Hydrochloride (The effects of antihypertensive agents may be potentiated when given concurrently). Products include:
Cardene I.V. 3485

Nifedipine (The effects of antihypertensive agents may be potentiated when given concurrently). Products include:
Adalat CC Tablets 877
Procardia Capsules 2708
Procardia XL Extended Release Tablets 2710

Nisoldipine (The effects of antihypertensive agents may be potentiated when given concurrently). Products include:
Sular Tablets 688

Nitroglycerin (The effects of antihypertensive agents may be potentiated when given concurrently). Products include:
Nitro-Dur Transdermal Infusion System 3134
Nitro-Dur Transdermal Infusion System 1834
Nitrolingual Pumpspray 1355
Nitrostat Tablets 2658

Pancuronium Bromide (The effects of nondepolarizing skeletal muscle relaxants may be potentiated when given concurrently).
No products indexed under this heading.

Penbutolol Sulfate (The effects of antihypertensive agents may be potentiated when given concurrently).
No products indexed under this heading.

Penicillin G Potassium (Co-administration may promote serum potassium accumulation and possibly result in hyperkalemia). Products include:
Pfizerpen for Injection 2707

Pentobarbital Sodium (The effects of pre-anesthetic agents may be potentiated when given concurrently). Products include:
Nembutal Sodium Solution 485

Perindopril Erbumine (Co-administration with potassium-sparing agents and angiotensin-coverting enzyme inhibitors increases the risk of hyperkalemia). Products include:
Aceon Tablets (2 mg, 4 mg, 8 mg) 3249

Phenoxybenzamine Hydrochloride (The effects of antihypertensive agents may be potentiated when given concurrently). Products include:
Dibenzyline Capsules 3457

Phentolamine Mesylate (The effects of antihypertensive agents may be potentiated when given concurrently).
No products indexed under this heading.

Pindolol (The effects of antihypertensive agents may be potentiated when given concurrently).
No products indexed under this heading.

Pioglitazone Hydrochloride (Triamterene may raise blood glucose levels; for adult onset diabetes, dosage adjustments of hypoglycemic agents may be necessary during and after therapy). Products include:
Actos Tablets 3275

Polythiazide (The effects of other diuretics may be potentiated when given concurrently). Products include:
Minizide Capsules 2700
Renese Tablets 2712

Potassium Acid Phosphate (Co-administration with dietary potassium supplements increases the risk of hyperkalemia; concurrent use is contraindicated). Products include:
K-Phos Original (Sodium Free) Tablets 947

Potassium Bicarbonate (Co-administration with dietary potassium supplements increases the risk of hyperkalemia; concurrent use is contraindicated).
No products indexed under this heading.

Potassium Chloride (Co-administration with dietary potassium supplements increases the risk of hyperkalemia; concurrent use is contraindicated). Products include:
Chlor-3 1361
Colyte with Flavor Packs for Oral Solution 3170
GoLYTELY and Pineapple Flavor GoLYTELY for Oral Solution 1068
K-Dur Microburst Release System ER Tablets 1832
Klor-Con M20/Klor-Con M10 Tablets 3329
K-Lor Powder Packets 469
K-Tab Filmtab Tablets 470
Micro-K 3311
NuLYTELY, Cherry Flavor, Lemon-Lime Flavor, and Orange Flavor NuLYTELY for Oral Solution 1068
Rum-K 1363

Potassium Citrate (Co-administration with dietary potassium supplements increases the risk of hyperkalemia; concurrent use is contraindicated). Products include:
Urocit-K Tablets 2232

Potassium Gluconate (Co-administration with dietary potassium supplements increases the risk of hyperkalemia; concurrent use is contraindicated).
No products indexed under this heading.

Potassium Phosphate (Co-administration with dietary potassium supplements increases the risk of hyperkalemia; concurrent use is contraindicated). Products include:
K-Phos Neutral Tablets 946

Prazosin Hydrochloride (The effects of antihypertensive agents may be potentiated when given concurrently). Products include:
Minipress Capsules 2699
Minizide Capsules 2700

Promethazine Hydrochloride (The effects of pre-anesthetic agents may be potentiated when given concurrently). Products include:
Mepergan Injection 3539
Phenergan Injection 3553
Phenergan 3556
Phenergan Syrup 3554
Phenergan with Codeine Syrup 3557
Phenergan with Dextromethorphan Syrup 3559
Phenergan VC Syrup 3560
Phenergan VC with Codeine Syrup . 3561

Propofol (The effects of anesthetics may be potentiated when given concurrently). Products include:
Diprivan Injectable Emulsion 667

Propranolol Hydrochloride (The effects of antihypertensive agents may be potentiated when given concurrently). Products include:
Inderal 3513
Inderal LA Long-Acting Capsules 3516
Inderide Tablets 3517
Inderide LA Long-Acting Capsules .. 3519

Quinapril Hydrochloride (Co-administration with potassium-sparing agents and angiotensin-coverting enzyme inhibitors increases the risk of hyperkalemia). Products include:
Accupril Tablets 2611
Accuretic Tablets 2614

Ramipril (Co-administration with potassium-sparing agents and angiotensin-coverting enzyme inhibitors increases the risk of hyperkalemia). Products include:
Altace Capsules 2233

Rapacuronium Bromide (The effects of nondepolarizing skeletal muscle relaxants may be potentiated when given concurrently).
No products indexed under this heading.

Rauwolfia serpentina (The effects of antihypertensive agents may be potentiated when given concurrently).
No products indexed under this heading.

Remifentanil Hydrochloride (The effects of anesthetics may be potentiated when given concurrently).
No products indexed under this heading.

Repaglinide (Triamterene may raise blood glucose levels; for adult onset diabetes, dosage adjustments of hypoglycemic agents may be necessary during and after therapy). Products include:
Prandin Tablets (0.5, 1, and 2 mg) 2432

Rescinnamine (The effects of antihypertensive agents may be potentiated when given concurrently).
No products indexed under this heading.

Reserpine (The effects of antihypertensive agents may be potentiated when given concurrently).
No products indexed under this heading.

Rocuronium Bromide (The effects of nondepolarizing skeletal muscle relaxants may be potentiated when given concurrently). Products include:
Zemuron Injection 2491

Rosiglitazone Maleate (Triamterene may raise blood glucose levels; for adult onset diabetes, dosage adjustments of hypoglycemic agents may be necessary during and after therapy). Products include:
Avandia Tablets 1490

Secobarbital Sodium (The effects of pre-anesthetic agents may be potentiated when given concurrently).
No products indexed under this heading.

Sodium Nitroprusside (The effects of antihypertensive agents may be potentiated when given concurrently).
No products indexed under this heading.

Sotalol Hydrochloride (The effects of antihypertensive agents may be potentiated when given concurrently). Products include:
Betapace Tablets 950
Betapace AF Tablets 954

Spirapril Hydrochloride (Co-administration with potassium-sparing agents and angiotensin-coverting enzyme inhibitors increases the risk of hyperkalemia).
No products indexed under this heading.

Spironolactone (Co-administration with other potassium-sparing agents has resulted in fatalities; these agents should not be given concomitantly).
No products indexed under this heading.

Sufentanil Citrate (The effects of anesthetics may be potentiated when given concurrently).
No products indexed under this heading.

Telmisartan (The effects of antihypertensive agents may be potentiated when given concurrently). Products include:
Micardis Tablets 1049
Micardis HCT Tablets 1051

Terazosin Hydrochloride (The effects of antihypertensive agents may be potentiated when given concurrently). Products include:
Hytrin Capsules 464

Thiamylal Sodium (The effects of anesthetics may be potentiated when given concurrently).
No products indexed under this heading.

Timolol Maleate (The effects of antihypertensive agents may be potentiated when given concurrently). Products include:
Blocadren Tablets 2046
Cosopt Sterile Ophthalmic Solution 2065
Timolide Tablets 2187
Timolol GFS .... ⊙266
Timoptic in Ocudose 2192
Timoptic Sterile Ophthalmic Solution 2190
Timoptic-XE Sterile Ophthalmic Gel Forming Solution 2194

Tolazamide (Triamterene may raise blood glucose levels; for adult onset diabetes, dosage adjustments of hypoglycemic agents may be necessary during and after therapy).
No products indexed under this heading.

Tolbutamide (Triamterene may raise blood glucose levels; for adult onset diabetes, dosage adjustments of hypoglycemic agents may be necessary during and after therapy).
No products indexed under this heading.

Torsemide (The effects of other diuretics may be potentiated when given concurrently). Products include:
Demadex Tablets and Injection 2965

Trandolapril (Co-administration with potassium-sparing agents and angiotensin-coverting enzyme inhibitors increases the risk of hyperkalemia). Products include:
Mavik Tablets 478
Tarka Tablets 508

Trimethaphan Camsylate (The effects of antihypertensive agents may be potentiated when given concurrently).
No products indexed under this heading.

Troglitazone (Triamterene may raise blood glucose levels; for adult onset diabetes, dosage adjustments of hypoglycemic agents may be necessary during and after therapy).
No products indexed under this heading.

Valsartan (The effects of antihypertensive agents may be potentiated when given concurrently). Products include:
Diovan Capsules 2337
Diovan HCT Tablets 2338

Vecuronium Bromide (The effects of nondepolarizing skeletal muscle relaxants may be potentiated when given concurrently). Products include:
Norcuron for Injection 2478

Verapamil Hydrochloride (The effects of antihypertensive agents may be potentiated when given concurrently). Products include:
Covera-HS Tablets 3199
Isoptin SR Tablets 467
Tarka Tablets 508
Verelan Capsules 3184
Verelan PM Capsules 3186

Food Interactions

Milk, low salt (Co-administration may promote serum potassium accumulation and possibly result in hyperkalemia).

EC-NAPROSYN DELAYED-RELEASE TABLETS

(Naproxen) 2967
May interact with ACE inhibitors, antacids containing aluminum, calcium and magnesium, beta blockers, oral anticoagulants, histamine H_2-receptor antagonists, hydantoin anticonvulsants, lithium preparations, sulfonylureas, and certain other agents. Compounds in these categories include:

Acebutolol Hydrochloride (Reduced antihypertensive effect of beta blockers). Products include:
Sectral Capsules 3589

Aluminum Carbonate (Due to the gastric pH elevating effects of intensive antacids therapy, concomitant administration of EC-Naprosyn is not recommended).
No products indexed under this heading.

Aluminum Hydroxide (Due to the gastric pH elevating effects of intensive antacids therapy, concomitant administration of EC-Naprosyn is not recommended). Products include:
Amphojel Suspension (Mint Flavor) .... ▣789
Gaviscon Extra Strength Liquid ..... ▣751
Gaviscon Extra Strength Tablets .... ▣751
Gaviscon Regular Strength Liquid . ▣751
Gaviscon Regular Strength Tablets .... ▣750
Maalox Antacid/Anti-Gas Oral Suspension .... ▣673
Maalox Max Maximum Strength Antacid/Anti-Gas Liquid 2300
Maalox Regular Strength Antacid/Antigas Liquid 2300
Mylanta 1813
Vanquish Caplets .... ▣617

Aspirin (Naproxen is displaced from its binding sites during the concomitant administration of aspirin resulting in lower plasma concentrations and peak plasma levels; concurrent use is not recommended). Products include:
Aggrenox Capsules 1026
Alka-Seltzer .... ▣603
Alka-Seltzer Lemon Lime Antacid and Pain Reliever Effervescent Tablets .... ▣603
Alka-Seltzer Extra Strength Antacid and Pain Reliever Effervescent Tablets .... ▣603
Alka-Seltzer PM Effervescent Tablets .... ▣605
Genuine Bayer Tablets, Caplets and Gelcaps .... ▣606
Extra Strength Bayer Caplets and Gelcaps .... ▣610
Aspirin Regimen Bayer Children's Chewable Tablets (Orange or Cherry Flavored) .... ▣607
Bayer, Aspirin Regimen .... ▣606
Aspirin Regimen Bayer 81 mg Caplets with Calcium .... ▣607
Genuine Bayer Professional Labeling (Aspirin Regimen Bayer) .... ▣608
Extra Strength Bayer Arthritis Caplets .... ▣610
Extra Strength Bayer Plus Caplets .... ▣610
Extra Strength Bayer PM Caplets . ▣611
BC Powder .... ▣619
BC Allergy Sinus Cold Powder ...... ▣619
Arthritis Strength BC Powder .... ▣619
BC Sinus Cold Powder .... ▣619
Darvon Compound-65 Pulvules 1910
Ecotrin Enteric Coated Aspirin Low, Regular and Maximum Strength Tablets 1715
Excedrin Extra-Strength Tablets, Caplets, and Geltabs .... ▣629
Excedrin Migraine 1070
Goody's Body Pain Formula Powder .... ▣620
Goody's Extra Strength Headache Powder .... ▣620
Goody's Extra Strength Pain Relief Tablets .... ▣620
Percodan Tablets 1327
Robaxisal Tablets 2939
Soma Compound Tablets 3354
Soma Compound w/Codeine Tablets 3355
Vanquish Caplets .... ▣617

Atenolol (Reduced antihypertensive effect of beta blockers). Products include:
Tenoretic Tablets 690
Tenormin I.V. Injection 692

Benazepril Hydrochloride (Co-administration of NSAIDs and ACE inhibitors may potentiate renal disease states). Products include:
Lotensin Tablets 2365
Lotensin HCT Tablets 2367
Lotrel Capsules 2370

Betaxolol Hydrochloride (Reduced antihypertensive effect of beta blockers). Products include:
Betoptic S Ophthalmic Suspension 537

Bisoprolol Fumarate (Reduced antihypertensive effect of beta blockers). Products include:
Zebeta Tablets 1885
Ziac Tablets 1887

Captopril (Co-administration of NSAIDs and ACE inhibitors may potentiate renal disease states). Products include:
Captopril Tablets 2281

Carteolol Hydrochloride (Reduced antihypertensive effect of beta blockers). Products include:
Carteolol Hydrochloride Ophthalmic Solution USP, 1% ..... ⊙258
Ocupress Ophthalmic Solution, 1% Sterile .... ⊙303

Chlorpropamide (Potential for sulfonylurea toxicity). Products include:
Diabinese Tablets 2680

Cimetidine (Due to the gastric pH elevating effects of H_2-blockers concomitant administration of EC-Naprosyn is not recommended). Products include:
Tagamet HB 200 Suspension .... ▣762
Tagamet HB 200 Tablets .... ▣761
Tagamet Tablets 1644

Cimetidine Hydrochloride (Due to the gastric pH elevating effects of

H_2-blockers concomitant administration of EC-Naprosyn is not recommended). Products include:
- Tagamet 1644

Dicumarol (Short-term studies have failed to show any significant effect of concurrent use on prothrombin time; caution is advised since interactions have been seen with other NSAIDs).
- No products indexed under this heading.

Enalapril Maleate (Co-administration of NSAIDs and ACE inhibitors may potentiate renal disease states). Products include:
- Lexxel Tablets 608
- Vaseretic Tablets 2204
- Vasotec Tablets 2210

Enalaprilat (Co-administration of NSAIDs and ACE inhibitors may potentiate renal disease states). Products include:
- Enalaprilat Injection 863
- Vasotec I.V. Injection 2207

Esmolol Hydrochloride (Reduced antihypertensive effect of beta blockers). Products include:
- Brevibloc Injection 858

Ethotoin (Potential for hydantoin toxicity).
- No products indexed under this heading.

Famotidine (Due to the gastric pH elevating effects of H_2-blockers concomitant administration of EC-Naprosyn is not recommended). Products include:
- Famotidine Injection 866
- Pepcid AC 1814
- Pepcid Complete Chewable Tablets 1815
- Pepcid Injection 2153
- Pepcid for Oral Suspension 2150
- Pepcid RPD Orally Disintegrating Tablets 2150
- Pepcid Tablets 2150

Fosinopril Sodium (Co-administration of NSAIDs and ACE inhibitors may potentiate renal disease states). Products include:
- Monopril Tablets 1091
- Monopril HCT 1094

Fosphenytoin Sodium (Potential for hydantoin toxicity). Products include:
- Cerebyx Injection 2619

Furosemide (Inhibition of natriuretic effect of furosemide). Products include:
- Furosemide Tablets 2284

Glimepiride (Potential for sulfonylurea toxicity). Products include:
- Amaryl Tablets 717

Glipizide (Potential for sulfonylurea toxicity). Products include:
- Glucotrol Tablets 2692
- Glucotrol XL Extended Release Tablets 2693

Glyburide (Potential for sulfonylurea toxicity). Products include:
- DiaBeta Tablets 741
- Glucovance Tablets 1086

Labetalol Hydrochloride (Reduced antihypertensive effect of beta blockers). Products include:
- Normodyne Injection 3135
- Normodyne Tablets 3137

Levobunolol Hydrochloride (Reduced antihypertensive effect of beta blockers). Products include:
- Betagan .... ⊙ 228

Lisinopril (Co-administration of NSAIDs and ACE inhibitors may potentiate renal disease states). Products include:
- Prinivil Tablets 2164
- Prinzide Tablets 2168
- Zestoretic Tablets 695
- Zestril Tablets 698

Lithium Carbonate (Inhibition of lithium renal clearance leading to increase in plasma lithium concentrations). Products include:
- Eskalith 1527
- Lithium Carbonate 3061
- Lithobid Slow-Release Tablets 3255

Lithium Citrate (Inhibition of lithium renal clearance leading to increase in plasma lithium concentrations). Products include:
- Lithium Citrate Syrup 3061

Magaldrate (Due to the gastric pH elevating effects of intensive antacids therapy, concomitant administration of EC-Naprosyn is not recommended).
- No products indexed under this heading.

Magnesium Hydroxide (Due to the gastric pH elevating effects of intensive antacids therapy, concomitant administration of EC-Naprosyn is not recommended). Products include:
- Ex•Lax Milk of Magnesia Liquid .... ▣ 670
- Maalox Antacid/Anti-Gas Oral Suspension .... ▣ 673
- Maalox Max Maximum Strength Antacid/Anti-Gas Liquid 2300
- Maalox Regular Strength Antacid/Antigas Liquid 2300
- Mylanta Fast-Acting 1813
- Mylanta 1813
- Pepcid Complete Chewable Tablets 1815
- Phillips' Chewable Tablets .... ▣ 615
- Phillips' Milk of Magnesia Liquid (Original, Cherry, & Mint) .... ▣ 616
- Rolaids Tablets .... ▣ 706
- Extra Strength Rolaids Tablets .... ▣ 706
- Vanquish Caplets .... ▣ 617

Magnesium Oxide (Due to the gastric pH elevating effects of intensive antacids therapy, concomitant administration of EC-Naprosyn is not recommended). Products include:
- Beelith Tablets 946
- Mag-Ox 400 Tablets 1024
- Uro-Mag Capsules 1024

Mephenytoin (Potential for hydantoin toxicity).
- No products indexed under this heading.

Methotrexate Sodium (Potential for reduced tubular secretion of methotrexate and possible increased methotrexate toxicity as shown in animal model; caution is recommended).
- No products indexed under this heading.

Metipranolol Hydrochloride (Reduced antihypertensive effect of beta blockers).
- No products indexed under this heading.

Metoprolol Succinate (Reduced antihypertensive effect of beta blockers). Products include:
- Toprol-XL Tablets 651

Metoprolol Tartrate (Reduced antihypertensive effect of beta blockers).
- No products indexed under this heading.

Moexipril Hydrochloride (Co-administration of NSAIDs and ACE inhibitors may potentiate renal disease states). Products include:
- Uniretic Tablets 3178
- Univasc Tablets 3181

Nadolol (Reduced antihypertensive effect of beta blockers). Products include:
- Corgard Tablets 2245
- Corzide 40/5 Tablets 2247
- Corzide 80/5 Tablets 2247
- Nadolol Tablets 2288

Naproxen Sodium (Concurrent use of naproxen or naproxen sodium in any dosage form is not recommended since they all circulate in the plasma as the naproxen anion). Products include:
- Aleve Tablets, Caplets and Gelcaps .... ▣ 602
- Aleve Cold & Sinus Caplets .... ▣ 603
- Anaprox Tablets 2967
- Anaprox DS Tablets 2967
- Naprelan Tablets 1293

Nizatidine (Due to the gastric pH elevating effects of H_2-blockers concomitant administration of EC-Naprosyn is not recommended). Products include:
- Axid Pulvules 1903
- Axid Pulvules 2919

Penbutolol Sulfate (Reduced antihypertensive effect of beta blockers).
- No products indexed under this heading.

Perindopril Erbumine (Co-administration of NSAIDs and ACE inhibitors may potentiate renal disease states). Products include:
- Aceon Tablets (2 mg, 4 mg, 8 mg) 3249

Phenytoin (Potential for hydantoin toxicity). Products include:
- Dilantin Infatabs 2624
- Dilantin-125 Oral Suspension 2625

Phenytoin Sodium (Potential for hydantoin toxicity). Products include:
- Dilantin Kapseals 2622

Pindolol (Reduced antihypertensive effect of beta blockers).
- No products indexed under this heading.

Probenecid (Probenecid given concurrently increases naproxen anion plasma levels and extends its plasma half-life significantly).
- No products indexed under this heading.

Propranolol Hydrochloride (Reduced antihypertensive effect of beta blockers). Products include:
- Inderal 3513
- Inderal LA Long-Acting Capsules 3516
- Inderide Tablets 3517
- Inderide LA Long-Acting Capsules 3519

Quinapril Hydrochloride (Co-administration of NSAIDs and ACE inhibitors may potentiate renal disease states). Products include:
- Accupril Tablets 2611
- Accuretic Tablets 2614

Ramipril (Co-administration of NSAIDs and ACE inhibitors may potentiate renal disease states). Products include:
- Altace Capsules 2233

Ranitidine Bismuth Citrate (Due to the gastric pH elevating effects of H_2-blockers concomitant administration of EC-Naprosyn is not recommended).
- No products indexed under this heading.

Ranitidine Hydrochloride (Due to the gastric pH elevating effects of H_2-blockers concomitant administration of EC-Naprosyn is not recommended). Products include:
- Zantac 1690
- Zantac Injection 1688
- Zantac 75 Tablets .... ▣ 717

Sotalol Hydrochloride (Reduced antihypertensive effect of beta blockers). Products include:
- Betapace Tablets 950
- Betapace AF Tablets 954

Spirapril Hydrochloride (Co-administration of NSAIDs and ACE inhibitors may potentiate renal disease states).
- No products indexed under this heading.

Sucralfate (Due to the gastric pH elevating effects of sucralfate, concomitant administration of EC-Naprosyn is not recommended). Products include:
- Carafate Suspension 731
- Carafate Tablets 730

Sulfamethoxazole (Potential for sulfonamide toxicity). Products include:
- Bactrim 2949
- Septra Suspension 2265
- Septra Tablets 2265
- Septra DS Tablets 2265

Sulfisoxazole Acetyl (Potential for sulfonamide toxicity). Products include:
- Pediazole Suspension 3050

Timolol Hemihydrate (Reduced antihypertensive effect of beta blockers). Products include:
- Betimol Ophthalmic Solution .... ⊙ 324

Timolol Maleate (Reduced antihypertensive effect of beta blockers). Products include:
- Blocadren Tablets 2046
- Cosopt Sterile Ophthalmic Solution 2065
- Timolide Tablets 2187
- Timolol GFS .... ⊙ 266
- Timoptic in Ocudose 2192
- Timoptic Sterile Ophthalmic Solution 2190
- Timoptic-XE Sterile Ophthalmic Gel Forming Solution 2194

Tolazamide (Potential for sulfonylurea toxicity).
- No products indexed under this heading.

Tolbutamide (Potential for sulfonylurea toxicity).
- No products indexed under this heading.

Trandolapril (Co-administration of NSAIDs and ACE inhibitors may potentiate renal disease states). Products include:
- Mavik Tablets 478
- Tarka Tablets 508

Warfarin Sodium (Short-term studies have failed to show any significant effect of concurrent use on prothrombin time; caution is advised since interactions have been seen with other NSAIDs). Products include:
- Coumadin for Injection 1243
- Coumadin Tablets 1243
- Warfarin Sodium Tablets, USP 3302

Food Interactions

Food, unspecified (The presence of food prolonged the time the EC-Naprosyn remained in the stomach, time to first detectable serum naproxen levels, and time to maximal naproxen levels (Tmax), but did not affect peak naproxen levels (Cmax)).

ECOTRIN ENTERIC COATED ASPIRIN LOW, REGULAR AND MAXIMUM STRENGTH TABLETS

(Aspirin) 1715

May interact with ACE inhibitors, beta blockers, anticoagulants, diuretics, oral hypoglycemic agents, non-steroidal anti-inflammatory agents, phenytoin, valproate, and certain other agents. Compounds in these categories include:

Acarbose (Moderate doses of aspirin may increase the effectiveness of oral hypoglycemic drugs, leading to hypoglycemia). Products include:
- Precose Tablets 906

Acebutolol Hydrochloride (Co-administration of beta blockers with aspirin may diminish the hypotensive effects of beta blockers due to inhibition of renal prostaglandins, leading to decreased renal blood flow, and salt and fluid retention). Products include:
- Sectral Capsules 3589

Acetazolamide (Co-administration can lead to high serum concentrations of acetazolamide (and toxicity) due to competition at the renal tubule for secretion). Products include:
- Diamox Sequels Sustained Release Capsules .... ⊙ 270
- Diamox Tablets .... ⊙ 269

Acetazolamide Sodium (Co-administration can lead to high serum concentrations of acetazolamide (and toxicity) due to competition at the renal tubule for secretion). Products include:

Diamox Intravenous .... ⊙ 269

Amiloride Hydrochloride (Co-administration of diuretics with aspirin may diminish the effectiveness of diuretics due to inhibition of renal prostaglandins, leading to decreased renal blood flow, and salt and fluid retention). Products include:
- Midamor Tablets 2136
- Moduretic Tablets 2138

Ardeparin Sodium (Patients on anticoagulant therapy are at increased risk for bleeding).
- No products indexed under this heading.

Atenolol (Co-administration of beta blockers with aspirin may diminish the hypotensive effects of beta blockers due to inhibition of renal prostaglandins, leading to decreased renal blood flow, and salt and fluid retention). Products include:
- Tenoretic Tablets 690
- Tenormin I.V. Injection 692

Benazepril Hydrochloride (Co-administration of aspirin with ACE inhibitors may result in hyponatremic and hypotensive effects of ACE inhibitors due to aspirin's direct effect on the renin-angiotensin conversion pathway). Products include:
- Lotensin Tablets 2365
- Lotensin HCT Tablets 2367
- Lotrel Capsules 2370

Bendroflumethiazide (Co-administration of diuretics with aspirin may diminish the effectiveness of diuretics due to inhibition of renal prostaglandins, leading to decreased renal blood flow, and salt and fluid retention). Products include:
- Corzide 40/5 Tablets 2247
- Corzide 80/5 Tablets 2247

Betaxolol Hydrochloride (Co-administration of beta blockers with aspirin may diminish the hypotensive effects of beta blockers due to inhibition of renal prostaglandins, leading to decreased renal blood flow, and salt and fluid retention). Products include:
- Betoptic S Ophthalmic Suspension 537

Bisoprolol Fumarate (Co-administration of beta blockers with aspirin may diminish the hypotensive effects of beta blockers due to inhibition of renal prostaglandins, leading to decreased renal blood flow, and salt and fluid retention). Products include:
- Zebeta Tablets 1885
- Ziac Tablets 1887

Bumetanide (Co-administration of diuretics with aspirin may diminish the effectiveness of diuretics due to inhibition of renal prostaglandins, leading to decreased renal blood flow, and salt and fluid retention).
- No products indexed under this heading.

Captopril (Co-administration of aspirin with ACE inhibitors may result in hyponatremic and hypotensive effects of ACE inhibitors due to aspirin's direct effect on the renin-angiotensin conversion pathway). Products include:
- Captopril Tablets 2281

Carteolol Hydrochloride (Co-administration of beta blockers with aspirin may diminish the hypotensive effects of beta blockers due to inhibition of renal prostaglandins, leading to decreased renal blood flow, and salt and fluid retention). Products include:
- Carteolol Hydrochloride Ophthalmic Solution USP, 1% .... ⊙ 258
- Ocupress Ophthalmic Solution, 1% Sterile .... ⊙ 303

Celecoxib (Co-administration may increase bleeding or lead to decreased renal function). Products include:
- Celebrex Capsules 2676
- Celebrex Capsules 2780

Chlorothiazide (Co-administration of diuretics with aspirin may diminish the effectiveness of diuretics due to inhibition of renal prostaglandins, leading to decreased renal blood flow, and salt and fluid retention). Products include:
- Aldoclor Tablets 2035
- Diuril Oral 2087

Chlorothiazide Sodium (Co-administration of diuretics with aspirin may diminish the effectiveness of diuretics due to inhibition of renal prostaglandins, leading to decreased renal blood flow, and salt and fluid retention). Products include:
- Diuril Sodium Intravenous 2086

Chlorpropamide (Moderate doses of aspirin may increase the effectiveness of oral hypoglycemic drugs, leading to hypoglycemia). Products include:
- Diabinese Tablets 2680

Chlorthalidone (Co-administration of diuretics with aspirin may diminish the effectiveness of diuretics due to inhibition of renal prostaglandins, leading to decreased renal blood flow, and salt and fluid retention). Products include:
- Clorpres Tablets 1002
- Combipres Tablets 1040
- Tenoretic Tablets 690

Dalteparin Sodium (Patients on anticoagulant therapy are at increased risk for bleeding). Products include:
- Fragmin Injection 2814

Danaparoid Sodium (Patients on anticoagulant therapy are at increased risk for bleeding). Products include:
- Orgaran Injection 2480

Diclofenac Potassium (Co-administration may increase bleeding or lead to decreased renal function). Products include:
- Cataflam Tablets 2315

Diclofenac Sodium (Co-administration may increase bleeding or lead to decreased renal function). Products include:
- Arthrotec Tablets 3195
- Voltaren Ophthalmic Sterile Ophthalmic Solution .... ⊙ 312
- Voltaren Tablets 2315
- Voltaren-XR Tablets 2315

Dicumarol (Patients on anticoagulant therapy are at increased risk for bleeding).
- No products indexed under this heading.

Divalproex Sodium (Salicylate can displace protein-bound valproic acid leading to an increase in serum valproic acid levels). Products include:
- Depakote Sprinkle Capsules 426
- Depakote Tablets 430
- Depakote ER Tablets 436

Enalapril Maleate (Co-administration of aspirin with ACE inhibitors may result in hyponatremic and hypotensive effects of ACE inhibitors due to aspirin's direct effect on the renin-angiotensin conversion pathway). Products include:
- Lexxel Tablets 608
- Vaseretic Tablets 2204
- Vasotec Tablets 2210

Enalaprilat (Co-administration of aspirin with ACE inhibitors may result in hyponatremic and hypotensive effects of ACE inhibitors due to aspirin's direct effect on the renin-angiotensin conversion pathway). Products include:
- Enalaprilat Injection 863
- Vasotec I.V. Injection 2207

Enoxaparin (Patients on anticoagulant therapy are at increased risk for bleeding). Products include:
- Lovenox Injection 746

Esmolol Hydrochloride (Co-administration of beta blockers with aspirin may diminish the hypotensive effects of beta blockers due to inhibition of renal prostaglandins, leading to decreased renal blood flow, and salt and fluid retention). Products include:
- Brevibloc Injection 858

Ethacrynic Acid (Co-administration of diuretics with aspirin may diminish the effectiveness of diuretics due to inhibition of renal prostaglandins, leading to decreased renal blood flow, and salt and fluid retention). Products include:
- Edecrin Tablets 2091

Etodolac (Co-administration may increase bleeding or lead to decreased renal function). Products include:
- Lodine 3528
- Lodine XL Extended-Release Tablets 3530

Fenoprofen Calcium (Co-administration may increase bleeding or lead to decreased renal function).
- No products indexed under this heading.

Flurbiprofen (Co-administration may increase bleeding or lead to decreased renal function).
- No products indexed under this heading.

Fosinopril Sodium (Co-administration of aspirin with ACE inhibitors may result in hyponatremic and hypotensive effects of ACE inhibitors due to aspirin's direct effect on the renin-angiotensin conversion pathway). Products include:
- Monopril Tablets 1091
- Monopril HCT 1094

Fosphenytoin Sodium (Salicylate can displace protein-bound phenytoin leading to a decrease in the total concentration of phenytoin). Products include:
- Cerebyx Injection 2619

Furosemide (Co-administration of diuretics with aspirin may diminish the effectiveness of diuretics due to inhibition of renal prostaglandins, leading to decreased renal blood flow, and salt and fluid retention). Products include:
- Furosemide Tablets 2284

Glimepiride (Moderate doses of aspirin may increase the effectiveness of oral hypoglycemic drugs, leading to hypoglycemia). Products include:
- Amaryl Tablets 717

Glipizide (Moderate doses of aspirin may increase the effectiveness of oral hypoglycemic drugs, leading to hypoglycemia). Products include:
- Glucotrol Tablets 2692
- Glucotrol XL Extended Release Tablets 2693

Glyburide (Moderate doses of aspirin may increase the effectiveness of oral hypoglycemic drugs, leading to hypoglycemia). Products include:
- DiaBeta Tablets 741
- Glucovance Tablets 1086

Heparin Sodium (Patients on anticoagulant therapy are at increased risk for bleeding). Products include:
- Heparin Lock Flush Solution 3509
- Heparin Sodium Injection 3511

Hydrochlorothiazide (Co-administration of diuretics with aspirin may diminish the effectiveness of diuretics due to inhibition of renal prostaglandins, leading to decreased renal blood flow, and salt and fluid retention). Products include:
- Accuretic Tablets 2614
- Aldoril Tablets 2039
- Atacand HCT Tablets 597
- Avalide Tablets 1070
- Diovan HCT Tablets 2338
- Dyazide Capsules 1515
- HydroDIURIL Tablets 2108
- Hyzaar 2109
- Inderide Tablets 3517
- Inderide LA Long-Acting Capsules 3519
- Lotensin HCT Tablets 2367
- Maxzide 1008
- Micardis HCT Tablets 1051
- Microzide Capsules 3414
- Moduretic Tablets 2138
- Monopril HCT 1094
- Prinzide Tablets 2168
- Timolide Tablets 2187
- Uniretic Tablets 3178
- Vaseretic Tablets 2204
- Zestoretic Tablets 695
- Ziac Tablets 1887

Hydroflumethiazide (Co-administration of diuretics with aspirin may diminish the effectiveness of diuretics due to inhibition of renal prostaglandins, leading to decreased renal blood flow, and salt and fluid retention). Products include:
- Diucardin Tablets 3494

Ibuprofen (Co-administration may increase bleeding or lead to decreased renal function). Products include:
- Advil .... ▣ 771
- Children's Advil Oral Suspension .... ▣ 773
- Children's Advil Chewable Tablets .... ▣ 773
- Advil Cold and Sinus Caplets .... ▣ 771
- Advil Cold and Sinus Tablets .... ▣ 771
- Advil Flu & Body Ache Caplets .... ▣ 772
- Infants' Advil Drops .... ▣ 773
- Junior Strength Advil Tablets .... ▣ 773
- Junior Strength Advil Chewable Tablets .... ▣ 773
- Advil Migraine Liquigels .... ▣ 772
- Children's Motrin Oral Suspension and Chewable Tablets 2006
- Children's Motrin Cold Oral Suspension 2007
- Children's Motrin Oral Suspension .... ▣ 643
- Motrin Suspension, Oral Drops, Chewable Tablets, and Caplets 2002
- Infants' Motrin Concentrated Drops 2006
- Junior Strength Motrin Caplets and Chewable Tablets 2006
- Motrin IB Tablets, Caplets, and Gelcaps 2002
- Motrin Migraine Pain Caplets 2005
- Motrin Sinus Headache Caplets 2005
- Vicoprofen Tablets 520

Indapamide (Co-administration of diuretics with aspirin may diminish the effectiveness of diuretics due to inhibition of renal prostaglandins, leading to decreased renal blood flow, and salt and fluid retention). Products include:
- Indapamide Tablets 2286

Indomethacin (Co-administration may increase bleeding or lead to decreased renal function). Products include:
- Indocin 2112

Indomethacin Sodium Trihydrate (Co-administration may increase bleeding or lead to decreased renal function). Products include:
- Indocin I.V. 2115

Ketoprofen (Co-administration may increase bleeding or lead to decreased renal function). Products include:
- Orudis Capsules 3548
- Orudis KT Tablets .... ▣ 778
- Oruvail Capsules 3548

Ketorolac Tromethamine (Co-administration may increase bleeding or lead to decreased renal function). Products include:
- Acular Ophthalmic Solution 544
- Acular PF Ophthalmic Solution 544
- Toradol 3018

Labetalol Hydrochloride (Co-administration of beta blockers with aspirin may diminish the hypotensive effects of beta blockers due to inhi-

bition of renal prostaglandins, leading to decreased renal blood flow, and salt and fluid retention). Products include:
- Normodyne Injection 3135
- Normodyne Tablets 3137

Levobunolol Hydrochloride (Co-administration of beta blockers with aspirin may diminish the hypotensive effects of beta blockers due to inhibition of renal prostaglandins, leading to decreased renal blood flow, and salt and fluid retention). Products include:
- Betagan .... ⊙228

Lisinopril (Co-administration of aspirin with ACE inhibitors may result in hyponatremic and hypotensive effects of ACE inhibitors due to aspirin's direct effect on the renin-angiotensin conversion pathway). Products include:
- Prinivil Tablets 2164
- Prinzide Tablets 2168
- Zestoretic Tablets 695
- Zestril Tablets 698

Meclofenamate Sodium (Co-administration may increase bleeding or lead to decreased renal function).
No products indexed under this heading.

Mefenamic Acid (Co-administration may increase bleeding or lead to decreased renal function). Products include:
- Ponstel Capsules 1356

Meloxicam (Co-administration may increase bleeding or lead to decreased renal function). Products include:
- Mobic Tablets 1054

Metformin Hydrochloride (Moderate doses of aspirin may increase the effectiveness of oral hypoglycemic drugs, leading to hypoglycemia). Products include:
- Glucophage Tablets 1080
- Glucophage XR Tablets 1080
- Glucovance Tablets 1086

Methotrexate Sodium (Salicylate can inhibit renal clearance of methotrexate, leading to bone marrow toxicity, especially in the elderly or renal impaired).
No products indexed under this heading.

Methyclothiazide (Co-administration of diuretics with aspirin may diminish the effectiveness of diuretics due to inhibition of renal prostaglandins, leading to decreased renal blood flow, and salt and fluid retention).
No products indexed under this heading.

Metipranolol Hydrochloride (Co-administration of beta blockers with aspirin may diminish the hypotensive effects of beta blockers due to inhibition of renal prostaglandins, leading to decreased renal blood flow, and salt and fluid retention).
No products indexed under this heading.

Metolazone (Co-administration of diuretics with aspirin may diminish the effectiveness of diuretics due to inhibition of renal prostaglandins, leading to decreased renal blood flow, and salt and fluid retention). Products include:
- Mykrox Tablets 1168
- Zaroxolyn Tablets 1177

Metoprolol Succinate (Co-administration of beta blockers with aspirin may diminish the hypotensive effects of beta blockers due to inhibition of renal prostaglandins, leading to decreased renal blood flow, and salt and fluid retention). Products include:
- Toprol-XL Tablets 651

Metoprolol Tartrate (Co-administration of beta blockers with aspirin may diminish the hypotensive effects of beta blockers due to inhibition of renal prostaglandins, leading to decreased renal blood flow, and salt and fluid retention).
No products indexed under this heading.

Miglitol (Moderate doses of aspirin may increase the effectiveness of oral hypoglycemic drugs, leading to hypoglycemia). Products include:
- Glyset Tablets 2821

Moexipril Hydrochloride (Co-administration of aspirin with ACE inhibitors may result in hyponatremic and hypotensive effects of ACE inhibitors due to aspirin's direct effect on the renin-angiotensin conversion pathway). Products include:
- Uniretic Tablets 3178
- Univasc Tablets 3181

Nabumetone (Co-administration may increase bleeding or lead to decreased renal function). Products include:
- Relafen Tablets 1617

Nadolol (Co-administration of beta blockers with aspirin may diminish the hypotensive effects of beta blockers due to inhibition of renal prostaglandins, leading to decreased renal blood flow, and salt and fluid retention). Products include:
- Corgard Tablets 2245
- Corzide 40/5 Tablets 2247
- Corzide 80/5 Tablets 2247
- Nadolol Tablets 2288

Naproxen (Co-administration may increase bleeding or lead to decreased renal function). Products include:
- EC-Naprosyn Delayed-Release Tablets 2967
- Naprosyn Suspension 2967
- Naprosyn Tablets 2967

Naproxen Sodium (Co-administration may increase bleeding or lead to decreased renal function). Products include:
- Aleve Tablets, Caplets and Gelcaps .... ▣602
- Aleve Cold & Sinus Caplets .... ▣603
- Anaprox Tablets 2967
- Anaprox DS Tablets 2967
- Naprelan Tablets 1293

Oxaprozin (Co-administration may increase bleeding or lead to decreased renal function).
No products indexed under this heading.

Penbutolol Sulfate (Co-administration of beta blockers with aspirin may diminish the hypotensive effects of beta blockers due to inhibition of renal prostaglandins, leading to decreased renal blood flow, and salt and fluid retention).
No products indexed under this heading.

Perindopril Erbumine (Co-administration of aspirin with ACE inhibitors may result in hyponatremic and hypotensive effects of ACE inhibitors due to aspirin's direct effect on the renin-angiotensin conversion pathway). Products include:
- Aceon Tablets (2 mg, 4 mg, 8 mg) 3249

Phenylbutazone (Co-administration may increase bleeding or lead to decreased renal function).
No products indexed under this heading.

Phenytoin (Salicylate can displace protein-bound phenytoin leading to a decrease in the total concentration of phenytoin). Products include:
- Dilantin Infatabs 2624
- Dilantin-125 Oral Suspension 2625

Phenytoin Sodium (Salicylate can displace protein-bound phenytoin leading to a decrease in the total concentration of phenytoin). Products include:
- Dilantin Kapseals 2622

Pindolol (Co-administration of beta blockers with aspirin may diminish the hypotensive effects of beta blockers due to inhibition of renal prostaglandins, leading to decreased renal blood flow, and salt and fluid retention).
No products indexed under this heading.

Pioglitazone Hydrochloride (Moderate doses of aspirin may increase the effectiveness of oral hypoglycemic drugs, leading to hypoglycemia). Products include:
- Actos Tablets 3275

Piroxicam (Co-administration may increase bleeding or lead to decreased renal function). Products include:
- Feldene Capsules 2685

Polythiazide (Co-administration of diuretics with aspirin may diminish the effectiveness of diuretics due to inhibition of renal prostaglandins, leading to decreased renal blood flow, and salt and fluid retention). Products include:
- Minizide Capsules 2700
- Renese Tablets 2712

Probenecid (Salicylate can antagonize the uricosuric action of uricosuric agents).
No products indexed under this heading.

Propranolol Hydrochloride (Co-administration of beta blockers with aspirin may diminish the hypotensive effects of beta blockers due to inhibition of renal prostaglandins, leading to decreased renal blood flow, and salt and fluid retention). Products include:
- Inderal 3513
- Inderal LA Long-Acting Capsules 3516
- Inderide Tablets 3517
- Inderide LA Long-Acting Capsules 3519

Quinapril Hydrochloride (Co-administration of aspirin with ACE inhibitors may result in hyponatremic and hypotensive effects of ACE inhibitors due to aspirin's direct effect on the renin-angiotensin conversion pathway). Products include:
- Accupril Tablets 2611
- Accuretic Tablets 2614

Ramipril (Co-administration of aspirin with ACE inhibitors may result in hyponatremic and hypotensive effects of ACE inhibitors due to aspirin's direct effect on the renin-angiotensin conversion pathway). Products include:
- Altace Capsules 2233

Repaglinide (Moderate doses of aspirin may increase the effectiveness of oral hypoglycemic drugs, leading to hypoglycemia). Products include:
- Prandin Tablets (0.5, 1, and 2 mg) 2432

Rofecoxib (Co-administration may increase bleeding or lead to decreased renal function). Products include:
- Vioxx 2213

Rosiglitazone Maleate (Moderate doses of aspirin may increase the effectiveness of oral hypoglycemic drugs, leading to hypoglycemia). Products include:
- Avandia Tablets 1490

Sotalol Hydrochloride (Co-administration of beta blockers with aspirin may diminish the hypotensive effects of beta blockers due to inhibition of renal prostaglandins, leading to decreased renal blood flow, and salt and fluid retention). Products include:
- Betapace Tablets 950
- Betapace AF Tablets 954

Spirapril Hydrochloride (Co-administration of aspirin with ACE inhibitors may result in hyponatremic and hypotensive effects of ACE inhibitors due to aspirin's direct effect on the renin-angiotensin conversion pathway).
No products indexed under this heading.

Spironolactone (Co-administration of diuretics with aspirin may diminish the effectiveness of diuretics due to inhibition of renal prostaglandins, leading to decreased renal blood flow, and salt and fluid retention).
No products indexed under this heading.

Sulfinpyrazone (Salicylate can antagonize the uricosuric action of uricosuric agents).
No products indexed under this heading.

Sulindac (Co-administration may increase bleeding or lead to decreased renal function). Products include:
- Clinoril Tablets 2053

Timolol Hemihydrate (Co-administration of beta blockers with aspirin may diminish the hypotensive effects of beta blockers due to inhibition of renal prostaglandins, leading to decreased renal blood flow, and salt and fluid retention). Products include:
- Betimol Ophthalmic Solution .... ⊙324

Timolol Maleate (Co-administration of beta blockers with aspirin may diminish the hypotensive effects of beta blockers due to inhibition of renal prostaglandins, leading to decreased renal blood flow, and salt and fluid retention). Products include:
- Blocadren Tablets 2046
- Cosopt Sterile Ophthalmic Solution 2065
- Timolide Tablets 2187
- Timolol GFS .... ⊙266
- Timoptic in Ocudose 2192
- Timoptic Sterile Ophthalmic Solution 2190
- Timoptic-XE Sterile Ophthalmic Gel Forming Solution 2194

Tinzaparin sodium (Patients on anticoagulant therapy are at increased risk for bleeding). Products include:
- Innohep Injection 1248

Tolazamide (Moderate doses of aspirin may increase the effectiveness of oral hypoglycemic drugs, leading to hypoglycemia).
No products indexed under this heading.

Tolbutamide (Moderate doses of aspirin may increase the effectiveness of oral hypoglycemic drugs, leading to hypoglycemia).
No products indexed under this heading.

Tolmetin Sodium (Co-administration may increase bleeding or lead to decreased renal function). Products include:
- Tolectin 2589

Torsemide (Co-administration of diuretics with aspirin may diminish the effectiveness of diuretics due to inhibition of renal prostaglandins, leading to decreased renal blood flow, and salt and fluid retention). Products include:
- Demadex Tablets and Injection 2965

Trandolapril (Co-administration of aspirin with ACE inhibitors may result in hyponatremic and hypotensive effects of ACE inhibitors due to aspirin's direct effect on the renin-angiotensin conversion pathway). Products include:
- Mavik Tablets 478
- Tarka Tablets 508

Triamterene (Co-administration of diuretics with aspirin may diminish the effectiveness of diuretics due to inhibition of renal prostaglandins, leading to decreased renal blood flow, and salt and fluid retention). Products include:

Dyazide Capsules 1515
Dyrenium Capsules 3458
Maxzide 1008

Troglitazone (Moderate doses of aspirin may increase the effectiveness of oral hypoglycemic drugs, leading to hypoglycemia).
No products indexed under this heading.

Valproate Sodium (Salicylate can displace protein-bound valproic acid leading to an increase in serum valproic acid levels). Products include:
Depacon Injection 416

Valproic Acid (Salicylate can displace protein-bound valproic acid leading to an increase in serum valproic acid levels). Products include:
Depakene 421

Warfarin Sodium (Aspirin can displace warfarin from protein binding sites, leading to prolongation of both the prothrombin time and the bleeding time). Products include:
Coumadin for Injection 1243
Coumadin Tablets 1243
Warfarin Sodium Tablets, USP 3302

Food Interactions

Alcohol (Chronic heavy alcohol users, 3 or more drinks per day, in combination with analgesic/antipyretic drug products containing aspirin increases the risk of adverse GI events, including stomach bleeding).

EDECRIN TABLETS

(Ethacrynic Acid) 2091
See Edecrin Sodium Intravenous

EDECRIN SODIUM INTRAVENOUS

(Ethacrynate Sodium) 2091
May interact with aminoglycosides, cephalosporins, cardiac glycosides, non-steroidal anti-inflammatory agents, and certain other agents. Compounds in these categories include:

Amikacin Sulfate (Increased ototoxic potential of aminoglycosides).
No products indexed under this heading.

Cefaclor (Increased ototoxic potential of cephalosporins). Products include:
Ceclor CD Tablets 1279
Ceclor 1905

Cefadroxil (Increased ototoxic potential of cephalosporins). Products include:
Duricef 1079

Cefamandole Nafate (Increased ototoxic potential of cephalosporins). Products include:
Mandol Vials 1953

Cefazolin Sodium (Increased ototoxic potential of cephalosporins). Products include:
Ancef for Injection 1474
Ancef Injection 1474
Kefzol Vials, ADD-Vantage 1951

Cefdinir (Increased ototoxic potential of cephalosporins). Products include:
Omnicef 493

Cefepime Hydrochloride (Increased ototoxic potential of cephalosporins). Products include:
Maxipime for Injection 1285

Cefixime (Increased ototoxic potential of cephalosporins). Products include:
Suprax 1877

Cefmetazole Sodium (Increased ototoxic potential of cephalosporins).
No products indexed under this heading.

Cefonicid Sodium (Increased ototoxic potential of cephalosporins).
No products indexed under this heading.

Cefoperazone Sodium (Increased ototoxic potential of cephalosporins). Products include:
Cefobid Pharmacy Bulk Package - Not for Direct Infusion 2673

Ceforanide (Increased ototoxic potential of cephalosporins).
No products indexed under this heading.

Cefotaxime Sodium (Increased ototoxic potential of cephalosporins). Products include:
Claforan Injection 732

Cefotetan (Increased ototoxic potential of cephalosporins). Products include:
Cefotan 664

Cefoxitin Sodium (Increased ototoxic potential of cephalosporins). Products include:
Mefoxin for Injection 2124
Mefoxin Premixed Intravenous Solution 2127

Cefpodoxime Proxetil (Increased ototoxic potential of cephalosporins). Products include:
Vantin Tablets and Oral Suspension 2860

Cefprozil (Increased ototoxic potential of cephalosporins). Products include:
Cefzil 1076

Ceftazidime (Increased ototoxic potential of cephalosporins). Products include:
Ceptaz for Injection 1499
Fortaz for Injection 1541
Tazicef for Injection 1647
Tazicef Pharmacy Bulk Package 1653
Tazidime Vials, Faspak & ADD-Vantage 1966

Ceftizoxime Sodium (Increased ototoxic potential of cephalosporins). Products include:
Cefizox for Intramuscular or Intravenous Use 1390

Ceftriaxone Sodium (Increased ototoxic potential of cephalosporins). Products include:
Rocephin Injectable Vials, ADD-Vantage, Galaxy, Bulk 2993

Cefuroxime Axetil (Increased ototoxic potential of cephalosporins). Products include:
Ceftin 1898

Cefuroxime Sodium (Increased ototoxic potential of cephalosporins). Products include:
Kefurox Vials, ADD-Vantage 1948

Celecoxib (Reduces diuretic, natriuretic, and antihypertensive effects). Products include:
Celebrex Capsules 2676
Celebrex Capsules 2780

Cephalexin (Increased ototoxic potential of cephalosporins). Products include:
Keflex 1237

Cephalothin Sodium (Increased ototoxic potential of cephalosporins).

Cephapirin Sodium (Increased ototoxic potential of cephalosporins).
No products indexed under this heading.

Cephradine (Increased ototoxic potential of cephalosporins).
No products indexed under this heading.

Deslanoside (Excessive potassium loss may precipitate digitalis toxicity).
No products indexed under this heading.

Diclofenac Potassium (Reduces diuretic, natriuretic, and antihypertensive effects). Products include:
Cataflam Tablets 2315

Diclofenac Sodium (Reduces diuretic, natriuretic, and antihypertensive effects). Products include:
Arthrotec Tablets 3195
Voltaren Ophthalmic Sterile Ophthalmic Solution .... ⊙ 312
Voltaren Tablets 2315
Voltaren-XR Tablets 2315

Digitoxin (Excessive potassium loss may precipitate digitalis toxicity).
No products indexed under this heading.

Digoxin (Excessive potassium loss may precipitate digitalis toxicity). Products include:
Digitek Tablets 1003
Lanoxicaps Capsules 1574
Lanoxin Injection 1581
Lanoxin Tablets 1587
Lanoxin Elixir Pediatric 1578
Lanoxin Injection Pediatric 1584

Etodolac (Reduces diuretic, natriuretic, and antihypertensive effects). Products include:
Lodine 3528
Lodine XL Extended-Release Tablets 3530

Fenoprofen Calcium (Reduces diuretic, natriuretic, and antihypertensive effects).
No products indexed under this heading.

Flurbiprofen (Reduces diuretic, natriuretic, and antihypertensive effects).
No products indexed under this heading.

Gentamicin Sulfate (Increased ototoxic potential of aminoglycosides). Products include:
Genoptic Ophthalmic Ointment ..... ⊙ 239
Genoptic Sterile Ophthalmic Solution .... ⊙ 239
Pred-G Ophthalmic Suspension ..... ⊙ 247
Pred-G Sterile Ophthalmic Ointment .... ⊙ 248

Ibuprofen (Reduces diuretic, natriuretic, and antihypertensive effects). Products include:
Advil .... ▣ 771
Children's Advil Oral Suspension ... ▣ 773
Children's Advil Chewable Tablets . ▣ 773
Advil Cold and Sinus Caplets .... ▣ 771
Advil Cold and Sinus Tablets .... ▣ 771
Advil Flu & Body Ache Caplets ...... ▣ 772
Infants' Advil Drops .... ▣ 773
Junior Strength Advil Tablets .... ▣ 773
Junior Strength Advil Chewable Tablets .... ▣ 773
Advil Migraine Liquigels .... ▣ 772
Children's Motrin Oral Suspension and Chewable Tablets 2006
Children's Motrin Cold Oral Suspension 2007
Children's Motrin Oral Suspension .... ▣ 643
Motrin Suspension, Oral Drops, Chewable Tablets, and Caplets 2002
Infants' Motrin Concentrated Drops 2006
Junior Strength Motrin Caplets and Chewable Tablets 2006
Motrin IB Tablets, Caplets, and Gelcaps 2002
Motrin Migraine Pain Caplets 2005
Motrin Sinus Headache Caplets 2005
Vicoprofen Tablets 520

Indomethacin (Reduces diuretic, natriuretic, and antihypertensive effects). Products include:
Indocin 2112

Indomethacin Sodium Trihydrate (Reduces diuretic, natriuretic, and antihypertensive effects). Products include:
Indocin I.V. 2115

Isoproterenol Hydrochloride (Careful adjustment of dosages required).
No products indexed under this heading.

Kanamycin Sulfate (Increased ototoxic potential of aminoglycosides).
No products indexed under this heading.

Ketoprofen (Reduces diuretic, natriuretic, and antihypertensive effects). Products include:
Orudis Capsules 3548
Orudis KT Tablets .... ▣ 778
Oruvail Capsules 3548

Ketorolac Tromethamine (Reduces diuretic, natriuretic, and antihypertensive effects). Products include:
Acular Ophthalmic Solution 544
Acular PF Ophthalmic Solution 544
Toradol 3018

Lithium Carbonate (High risk of lithium toxicity). Products include:
Eskalith 1527
Lithium Carbonate 3061
Lithobid Slow-Release Tablets 3255

Lithium Citrate (High risk of lithium toxicity). Products include:
Lithium Citrate Syrup 3061

Loracarbef (Increased ototoxic potential of cephalosporins). Products include:
Lorabid Suspension and Pulvules ... 2251

Meclofenamate Sodium (Reduces diuretic, natriuretic, and antihypertensive effects).
No products indexed under this heading.

Mefenamic Acid (Reduces diuretic, natriuretic, and antihypertensive effects). Products include:
Ponstel Capsules 1356

Meloxicam (Reduces diuretic, natriuretic, and antihypertensive effects). Products include:
Mobic Tablets 1054

Nabumetone (Reduces diuretic, natriuretic, and antihypertensive effects). Products include:
Relafen Tablets 1617

Naproxen (Reduces diuretic, natriuretic, and antihypertensive effects). Products include:
EC-Naprosyn Delayed-Release Tablets 2967
Naprosyn Suspension 2967
Naprosyn Tablets 2967

Naproxen Sodium (Reduces diuretic, natriuretic, and antihypertensive effects). Products include:
Aleve Tablets, Caplets and Gelcaps .... ▣ 602
Aleve Cold & Sinus Caplets .... ▣ 603
Anaprox Tablets 2967
Anaprox DS Tablets 2967
Naprelan Tablets 1293

Oxaprozin (Reduces diuretic, natriuretic, and antihypertensive effects).
No products indexed under this heading.

Phenylbutazone (Reduces diuretic, natriuretic, and antihypertensive effects).
No products indexed under this heading.

Piroxicam (Reduces diuretic, natriuretic, and antihypertensive effects). Products include:
Feldene Capsules 2685

Rofecoxib (Reduces diuretic, natriuretic, and antihypertensive effects). Products include:
Vioxx 2213

Streptomycin Sulfate (Increased ototoxic potential of aminoglycosides). Products include:
Streptomycin Sulfate Injection 2714

Sulindac (Reduces diuretic, natriuretic, and antihypertensive effects). Products include:
Clinoril Tablets 2053

Tobramycin (Increased ototoxic potential of aminoglycosides). Products include:
TOBI Solution for Inhalation 1206
TobraDex Ophthalmic Ointment 542
TobraDex Ophthalmic Suspension .. 541
Tobrex Ophthalmic Ointment .... ⊙ 220
Tobrex Ophthalmic Solution .... ⊙ 221

Tobramycin Sulfate (Increased ototoxic potential of aminoglycosides). Products include:
Nebcin Vials, Hyporets & ADD-Vantage 1955

Tolmetin Sodium (Reduces diuretic, natriuretic, and antihypertensive effects). Products include:
Tolectin 2589

Warfarin Sodium (Warfarin displaced from plasma protein; reduction in warfarin dosage may be required). Products include:
- Coumadin for Injection 1243
- Coumadin Tablets 1243
- Warfarin Sodium Tablets, USP 3302

E.E.S. 200 LIQUID
(Erythromycin Ethylsuccinate) 450
See E.E.S. 400 Filmtab Tablets

E.E.S. 400 LIQUID
(Erythromycin Ethylsuccinate) 450
See E.E.S. 400 Filmtab Tablets

E.E.S. 400 FILMTAB TABLETS
(Erythromycin Ethylsuccinate) 450
May interact with oral anticoagulants, phenytoin, valproate, theophylline, and certain other agents. Compounds in these categories include:

Alfentanil Hydrochloride (Concurrent use of erythromycin in patients receiving drugs metabolized by the cytochrome P450 system may be associated with elevation in serum levels of alfentanil).
No products indexed under this heading.

Aminophylline (Co-administration in patients who are receiving high doses of theophylline may be associated with an increase in serum theophylline levels and potential theophylline toxicity).
No products indexed under this heading.

Astemizole (Concurrent use of erythromycin in patients receiving astemizole has been reported to significantly alter the metabolism of astemizole; rare cases of cardiovascular adverse events, including prolonged QT interval, cardiac arrest, torsade de pointes, and other ventricular arrhythmias have been reported; co-administration is contraindicated).
No products indexed under this heading.

Bromocriptine Mesylate (Concurrent use of erythromycin in patients receiving drugs metabolized by the cytochrome P450 system may be associated with elevation in serum levels of bromocriptine).
No products indexed under this heading.

Carbamazepine (Concurrent use of erythromycin in patients receiving drugs metabolized by the cytochrome P450 system may be associated with elevation in serum levels of carbamazepine). Products include:
- Carbatrol Capsules 3234
- Tegretol/Tegretol-XR 2404

Cisapride (Concurrent use of erythromycin in patients receiving cisapride has been reported to inhibit the metabolism of cisapride; cases of cardiovascular adverse events, including prolonged QT interval, torsade de pointes, ventricular tachycardia, and ventricular fibrillation have been reported; co-administration is contraindicated).
No products indexed under this heading.

Cyclosporine (Concurrent use of erythromycin in patients receiving drugs metabolized by the cytochrome P450 system may be associated with elevation in serum levels of cyclosporine). Products include:
- Gengraf Capsules 457
- Neoral Soft Gelatin Capsules 2380
- Neoral Oral Solution 2380
- Sandimmune 2388

Dicumarol (Co-administration has resulted in increased anticoagulant effects).
No products indexed under this heading.

Digoxin (Co-administration has been reported to result in elevated digoxin serum levels). Products include:
- Digitek Tablets 1003
- Lanoxicaps Capsules 1574
- Lanoxin Injection 1581
- Lanoxin Tablets 1587
- Lanoxin Elixir Pediatric 1578
- Lanoxin Injection Pediatric 1584

Dihydroergotamine Mesylate (Co-administration has been associated in some patients with acute ergot toxicity characterized by severe peripheral vasospasm and dysesthesia). Products include:
- D.H.E. 45 Injection 2334
- Migranal Nasal Spray 2376

Disopyramide Phosphate (Concurrent use of erythromycin in patients receiving drugs metabolized by the cytochrome P450 system may be associated with elevation in serum levels of disopyramide).
No products indexed under this heading.

Divalproex Sodium (Concurrent use of erythromycin in patients receiving drugs metabolized by the cytochrome P450 system may be associated with elevation in serum levels of valproate). Products include:
- Depakote Sprinkle Capsules 426
- Depakote Tablets 430
- Depakote ER Tablets 436

Dyphylline (Co-administration in patients who are receiving high doses of theophylline may be associated with an increase in serum theophylline levels and potential theophylline toxicity). Products include:
- Lufyllin Tablets 3347
- Lufyllin-400 Tablets 3347
- Lufyllin-GG Elixir 3348
- Lufyllin-GG Tablets 3348

Ergotamine Tartrate (Co-administration has been associated in some patients with acute ergot toxicity characterized by severe peripheral vasospasm and dysesthesia).
No products indexed under this heading.

Fosphenytoin Sodium (Concurrent use of erythromycin in patients receiving drugs metabolized by the cytochrome P450 system may be associated with elevation in serum levels of phenytoin). Products include:
- Cerebyx Injection 2619

Hexobarbital (Concurrent use of erythromycin in patients receiving drugs metabolized by the cytochrome P450 system may be associated with elevation in serum levels of hexobarbital).

Lovastatin (Co-administration in seriously ill patients has resulted in rhabdomyolysis with or without renal impairment). Products include:
- Mevacor Tablets 2132

Midazolam Hydrochloride (Erythromycin has been reported to decrease the clearance of triazolam and, thus, may increase the pharmacologic effect of the benzodiazepine). Products include:
- Versed Injection 3027
- Versed Syrup 3033

Phenytoin (Concurrent use of erythromycin in patients receiving drugs metabolized by the cytochrome P450 system may be associated with elevation in serum levels of phenytoin). Products include:
- Dilantin Infatabs 2624
- Dilantin-125 Oral Suspension 2625

Phenytoin Sodium (Concurrent use of erythromycin in patients receiving drugs metabolized by the cytochrome P450 system may be associated with elevation in serum levels of phenytoin). Products include:
- Dilantin Kapseals 2622

Tacrolimus (Concurrent use of erythromycin in patients receiving drugs metabolized by the cytochrome P450 system may be associated with elevation in serum levels of tacrolimus). Products include:
- Prograf 1393
- Protopic Ointment 1397

Terfenadine (Concurrent use of erythromycin in patients receiving terfenadine has been reported to significantly alter the metabolism of terfenadine; rare cases of cardiovascular adverse events, including prolonged QT interval, cardiac arrest, torsade de pointes, other ventricular arrhythmias, and death have been reported; co-administration is contraindicated).
No products indexed under this heading.

Theophylline (Co-administration in patients who are receiving high doses of theophylline may be associated with an increase in serum theophylline levels and potential theophylline toxicity). Products include:
- Aerolate 1361
- Theo-Dur Extended-Release Tablets 1835
- Uni-Dur Extended-Release Tablets .. 1841
- Uniphyl 400 mg and 600 mg Tablets 2903

Theophylline Calcium Salicylate (Co-administration in patients who are receiving high doses of theophylline may be associated with an increase in serum theophylline levels and potential theophylline toxicity).
No products indexed under this heading.

Theophylline Sodium Glycinate (Co-administration in patients who are receiving high doses of theophylline may be associated with an increase in serum theophylline levels and potential theophylline toxicity).
No products indexed under this heading.

Triazolam (Erythromycin has been reported to decrease the clearance of triazolam and, thus, may increase the pharmacologic effect of the benzodiazepine). Products include:
- Halcion Tablets 2823

Valproate Sodium (Concurrent use of erythromycin in patients receiving drugs metabolized by the cytochrome P450 system may be associated with elevation in serum levels of valproate). Products include:
- Depacon Injection 416

Valproic Acid (Concurrent use of erythromycin in patients receiving drugs metabolized by the cytochrome P450 system may be associated with elevation in serum levels of valproate). Products include:
- Depakene 421

Warfarin Sodium (Co-administration has resulted in increased anticoagulant effects). Products include:
- Coumadin for Injection 1243
- Coumadin Tablets 1243
- Warfarin Sodium Tablets, USP 3302

E.E.S. GRANULES
(Erythromycin Ethylsuccinate) 450
See E.E.S. 400 Filmtab Tablets

EFFEXOR TABLETS
(Venlafaxine Hydrochloride) 3495
See Effexor XR Capsules

EFFEXOR XR CAPSULES
(Venlafaxine Hydrochloride) 3499
May interact with monoamine oxidase inhibitors, quinidine, and certain other agents. Compounds in these categories include:

Cimetidine (Co-administration in a steady-state study for both drugs has resulted in inhibition of first-pass metabolism of venlafaxine; the oral clearance of venlafaxine was reduced by 43% and AUC and Cmax were increased by about 60%). Products include:
- Tagamet HB 200 Suspension 762
- Tagamet HB 200 Tablets 761
- Tagamet Tablets 1644

Cimetidine Hydrochloride (Co-administration in a steady-state study for both drugs has resulted in inhibition of first-pass metabolism of venlafaxine; the oral clearance of venlafaxine was reduced by 43% and AUC and Cmax were increased by about 60%). Products include:
- Tagamet 1644

Clozapine (There have been reports of elevated clozapine levels that were temporarily associated with adverse events including seizures, following the addition of venlafaxine). Products include:
- Clozaril Tablets 2319

Desipramine Hydrochloride (Co-administration has resulted in increased desipramine AUC, Cmax, and Cmin by 35%; the 2-OH-desipramine AUC's increased by at least 2.5 to 4.5 fold; the clinical significance of this elevation is unknown). Products include:
- Norpramin Tablets 755

Haloperidol (Venlafaxine administered under steady-state conditions in healthy subjects decreased total oral-dose clearance of a single dose of haloperidol by 42%, which resulted in a 70% increase in haloperidol AUC and Cmax increased by 88%). Products include:
- Haldol Injection, Tablets and Concentrate 2533

Haloperidol Decanoate (Venlafaxine administered under steady-state conditions in healthy subjects decreased total oral-dose clearance of a single dose of haloperidol by 42%, which resulted in a 70% increase in haloperidol AUC and Cmax increased by 88%). Products include:
- Haldol Decanoate 2535

Indinavir Sulfate (Co-administration has resulted in a 28% decrease in the AUC and 36% decrease in the indinavir Cmax; the clinical significance of this finding is unknown). Products include:
- Crixivan Capsules 2070

Isocarboxazid (Adverse reactions, some of which were serious, have been reported in patients who have recently been discontinued from an MAO inhibitor and started on venlafaxine, or who have recently had venlafaxine therapy discontinued prior to initiation of an MAO inhibitor; concurrent and/or sequential use is contraindicated).
No products indexed under this heading.

Moclobemide (Adverse reactions, some of which were serious, have been reported in patients who have recently been discontinued from an MAO inhibitor and started on venlafaxine, or who have recently had venlafaxine therapy discontinued prior to initiation of an MAO inhibitor; concurrent and/or sequential use is contraindicated).
No products indexed under this heading.

Pargyline Hydrochloride (Adverse reactions, some of which were serious, have been reported in patients who have recently been discontinued from an MAO inhibitor and started on venlafaxine, or who have recently had venlafaxine therapy discontinued prior to initiation of an MAO inhibitor; concurrent and/or sequential use is

contraindicated).
No products indexed under this heading.

Phenelzine Sulfate (Adverse reactions, some of which were serious, have been reported in patients who have recently been discontinued from an MAO inhibitor and started on venlafaxine, or who have recently had venlafaxine therapy discontinued prior to initiation of an MAO inhibitor; concurrent and/or sequential use is contraindicated). Products include:
Nardil Tablets 2653

Procarbazine Hydrochloride (Adverse reactions, some of which were serious, have been reported in patients who have recently been discontinued from an MAO inhibitor and started on venlafaxine, or who have recently had venlafaxine therapy discontinued prior to initiation of an MAO inhibitor; concurrent and/or sequential use is contraindicated). Products include:
Matulane Capsules 3246

Quinidine Gluconate (Venlafaxine is metabolized to its active metabolite, ODV, by CYP2D6, therefore, the potential exists for a drug interaction between the inhibitors of CYP2D6, such as quinidine, and venlafaxine resulting in increased plasma concentrations of venlafaxine and decreased concentrations of the active metabolite). Products include:
Quinaglute Dura-Tabs Tablets 978

Quinidine Polygalacturonate (Venlafaxine is metabolized to its active metabolite, ODV, by CYP2D6, therefore, the potential exists for a drug interaction between the inhibitors of CYP2D6, such as quinidine, and venlafaxine resulting in increased plasma concentrations of venlafaxine and decreased concentrations of the active metabolite).
No products indexed under this heading.

Quinidine Sulfate (Venlafaxine is metabolized to its active metabolite, ODV, by CYP2D6, therefore, the potential exists for a drug interaction between the inhibitors of CYP2D6, such as quinidine, and venlafaxine resulting in increased plasma concentrations of venlafaxine and decreased concentrations of the active metabolite). Products include:
Quinidex Extentabs 2933

Risperidone (Venlafaxine slightly inhibits the CYP2D6-mediated metabolism of risperidone resulting in an approximate 32% increase in risperidone AUC). Products include:
Risperdal 1796

Selegiline Hydrochloride (Adverse reactions, some of which were serious, have been reported in patients who have recently been discontinued from an MAO inhibitor and started on venlafaxine, or who have recently had venlafaxine therapy discontinued prior to initiation of an MAO inhibitor; concurrent and/or sequential use is contraindicated). Products include:
Eldepryl Capsules 3266

Tranylcypromine Sulfate (Adverse reactions, some of which were serious, have been reported in patients who have recently been discontinued from an MAO inhibitor and started on venlafaxine, or who have recently had venlafaxine therapy discontinued prior to initiation of an MAO inhibitor; concurrent and/or sequential use is contraindicated). Products include:
Parnate Tablets 1607

Warfarin Sodium (There have been reports of increases in prothrombin time, partial thromboplastin time, or INR when venlafaxine was given to patients receiving warfarin therapy). Products include:
Coumadin for Injection 1243
Coumadin Tablets 1243
Warfarin Sodium Tablets, USP 3302

Food Interactions

Alcohol (Co-administration of venlafaxine as a stable regimen did not exaggerate the psychomotor and psychometric effects of alcohol; however, patients should be advised to avoid alcohol while taking venlafaxine).

EFUDEX CREAM
(Fluorouracil) 1733
None cited in PDR database.

EFUDEX TOPICAL SOLUTIONS
(Fluorouracil) 1733
None cited in PDR database.

ELA-MAX CREAM
(Lidocaine) 1340
See ELA-Max 5 Cream

ELA-MAX 5 CREAM
(Lidocaine) 1340
May interact with:

Mexiletine Hydrochloride (ELA-Max should be used with caution in patients receiving Class 1 antiarrhythmic drugs, such as mexilitine, since the toxic effects are additive and generally synergistic). Products include:
Mexitil Capsules 1047

Tocainide Hydrochloride (ELA-Max should be used with caution in patients receiving Class 1 antiarrhythmic drugs, such as tocainide, since the toxic effects are additive and generally synergistic). Products include:
Tonocard Tablets 649

ELDEPRYL CAPSULES
(Selegiline Hydrochloride) 3266
May interact with narcotic analgesics, selective serotonin reuptake inhibitors, tricyclic antidepressants, and certain other agents. Compounds in these categories include:

Alfentanil Hydrochloride (Contraindication warning for meperidine is extended to other opioids).
No products indexed under this heading.

Amitriptyline Hydrochloride (Co-administraton has resulted in severe CNS toxicity associated with hyperpyrexia and fatality; concurrent use in some patients may result in hypertension, syncope, asystole, diaphoresis seizures, changes in behavioral and mental status, and muscular rigidity; concurrent and/or sequential use is not recommended). Products include:
Etrafon 3115
Limbitrol 1738

Amoxapine (Co-administration may result in hypertension, syncope, asystole, diaphoresis seizures, changes in behavioral and mental status, and muscular rigidity; concurrent and/or sequential use is not recommended).
No products indexed under this heading.

Buprenorphine Hydrochloride (Contraindication warning for meperidine is extended to other opioids). Products include:
Buprenex Injectable 2918

Citalopram Hydrobromide (Potential for serious, sometimes fatal, reactions including hyperthermia, rigidity, myoclonus, autonomic instability, extreme agitation progressing to delirium and coma; concurrent and/or sequential use is not recommended). Products include:
Celexa 1365

Clomipramine Hydrochloride (Co-administration may result in hypertension, syncope, asystole, diaphoresis seizures, changes in behavioral and mental status, and muscular rigidity; concurrent and/or sequential use is not recommended).
No products indexed under this heading.

Codeine Phosphate (Contraindication warning for meperidine is extended to other opioids). Products include:
Phenergan with Codeine Syrup 3557
Phenergan VC with Codeine Syrup 3561
Robitussin A-C Syrup 2942
Robitussin-DAC Syrup 2942
Ryna-C Liquid .... ▣768
Soma Compound w/Codeine Tablets 3355
Tussi-Organidin NR Liquid 3350
Tussi-Organidin-S NR Liquid 3350
Tylenol with Codeine 2595

Desipramine Hydrochloride (Co-administration may result in hypertension, syncope, asystole, diaphoresis seizures, changes in behavioral and mental status, and muscular rigidity; concurrent and/or sequential use is not recommended). Products include:
Norpramin Tablets 755

Dezocine (Contraindication warning for meperidine is extended to other opioids).
No products indexed under this heading.

Doxepin Hydrochloride (Co-administration may result in hypertension, syncope, asystole, diaphoresis seizures, changes in behavioral and mental status, and muscular rigidity; concurrent and/or sequential use is not recommended). Products include:
Sinequan 2713

Ephedrine Hydrochloride (Co-administration has resulted in one case of hypertensive crisis). Products include:
Primatene Tablets .... ▣780

Ephedrine Sulfate (Co-administration has resulted in one case of hypertensive crisis).
No products indexed under this heading.

Ephedrine Tannate (Co-administration has resulted in one case of hypertensive crisis). Products include:
Rynatuss Pediatric Suspension 3353
Rynatuss Tablets 3353

Fentanyl (Contraindication warning for meperidine is extended to other opioids). Products include:
Duragesic Transdermal System 1786

Fentanyl Citrate (Contraindication warning for meperidine is extended to other opioids). Products include:
Actiq 1184

Fluoxetine Hydrochloride (Co-administration has resulted in serious, sometimes fatal, reactions including hyperthermia, rigidity, myoclonus, autonomic instability, extreme agitation progressing to delirium and coma; concurrent and/or sequential use is not recommended; because of long half-life of fluoxetine, at least 5 weeks or longer should elapse between discontinuation of fluoxetine and initiation of Eldepryl). Products include:
Prozac Pulvules, Liquid, and Weekly Capsules 1238
Sarafem Pulvules 1962

Fluvoxamine Maleate (Potential for serious, sometimes fatal, reactions including hyperthermia, rigidity, myoclonus, autonomic instability, extreme agitation progressing to delirium and coma; concurrent and/or sequential use is not recommended). Products include:
Luvox Tablets (25, 50, 100 mg) 3256

Hydrocodone Bitartrate (Contraindication warning for meperidine is extended to other opioids). Products include:
Hycodan 1316
Hycomine Compound Tablets 1317
Hycotuss Expectorant Syrup 1318
Lortab 3319
Lortab Elixir 3317
Maxidone Tablets CIII 3399
Norco 5/325 Tablets CIII 3424
Norco 7.5/325 Tablets CIII 3425
Norco 10/325 Tablets CIII 3427
Norco 10/325 Tablets CIII 3425
Vicodin Tablets 516
Vicodin ES Tablets 517
Vicodin HP Tablets 518
Vicodin Tuss Expectorant 519
Vicoprofen Tablets 520
Zydone Tablets 1330

Hydrocodone Polistirex (Contraindication warning for meperidine is extended to other opioids). Products include:
Tussionex Pennkinetic Extended-Release Suspension 1174

Hydromorphone Hydrochloride (Contraindication warning for meperidine is extended to other opioids). Products include:
Dilaudid 441
Dilaudid Oral Liquid 445
Dilaudid Powder 441
Dilaudid Rectal Suppositories 441
Dilaudid Tablets 441
Dilaudid Tablets - 8 mg 445
Dilaudid-HP 443

Imipramine Hydrochloride (Co-administration may result in hypertension, syncope, asystole, diaphoresis seizures, changes in behavioral and mental status, and muscular rigidity; concurrent and/or sequential use is not recommended).
No products indexed under this heading.

Imipramine Pamoate (Co-administration may result in hypertension, syncope, asystole, diaphoresis seizures, changes in behavioral and mental status, and muscular rigidity; concurrent and/or sequential use is not recommended).
No products indexed under this heading.

Levodopa (Co-administration in some patients may exacerbate levodopa-associated side effects). Products include:
Sinemet Tablets 1253
Sinemet CR Tablets 1255

Levorphanol Tartrate (Contraindication warning for meperidine is extended to other opioids). Products include:
Levo-Dromoran 1734
Levorphanol Tartrate Tablets 3059

Maprotiline Hydrochloride (Co-administration may result in hypertension, syncope, asystole, diaphoresis seizures, changes in behavioral and mental status, and muscular rigidity; concurrent and/or sequential use is not recommended).
No products indexed under this heading.

Meperidine Hydrochloride (Co-administration has resulted in stupor, muscular rigidity, severe agitation, hallucination, and hyperpyrexia; concurrent use is contraindicated). Products include:
Demerol 3079
Mepergan Injection 3539

Methadone Hydrochloride (Contraindication warning for meperidine is extended to other opioids). Products include:
Dolophine Hydrochloride Tablets 3056

Morphine Sulfate (Contraindication warning for meperidine is extended to other opioids). Products include:
Astramorph/PF Injection, USP (Preservative-Free) 594
Duramorph Injection 1312
Infumorph 200 and Infumorph 500 Sterile Solutions 1314

Kadian Capsules 1335
MS Contin Tablets 2896
MSIR 2898
Oramorph SR Tablets 3062
Roxanol 3066

Nortriptyline Hydrochloride (Co-administration may result in hypertension, syncope, asystole, diaphoresis seizures, changes in behavioral and mental status, and muscular rigidity; concurrent and/or sequential use is not recommended).
No products indexed under this heading.

Oxycodone Hydrochloride (Contraindication warning for meperidine is extended to other opioids). Products include:
OxyContin Tablets 2912
OxyFast Oral Concentrate Solution . 2916
OxyIR Capsules 2916
Percocet Tablets 1326
Percodan Tablets 1327
Percolone Tablets 1327
Roxicodone 3067
Tylox Capsules 2597

Paroxetine Hydrochloride (Potential for serious, sometimes fatal, reactions including hyperthermia, rigidity, myoclonus, autonomic instability, extreme agitation progressing to delirium and coma; concurrent and/or sequential use is not recommended). Products include:
Paxil 1609

Propoxyphene Hydrochloride (Contraindication warning for meperidine is extended to other opioids). Products include:
Darvon Pulvules 1909
Darvon Compound-65 Pulvules 1910

Propoxyphene Napsylate (Contraindication warning for meperidine is extended to other opioids). Products include:
Darvon-N/Darvocet-N 1907
Darvon-N Tablets 1912

Protriptyline Hydrochloride (Co-administration has resulted in tremors, agitation, and restlessness followed by unresponsiveness and fatality; concurrent use in some patients may result in hypertension, syncope, asystole, diaphoresis seizures, changes in behavioral and mental status, and muscular rigidity; concurrent and/or sequential use is not recommended). Products include:
Vivactil Tablets 2446
Vivactil Tablets 2217

Sertraline Hydrochloride (Potential for serious, sometimes fatal, reactions including hyperthermia, rigidity, myoclonus, autonomic instability, extreme agitation progressing to delirium and coma; concurrent and/or sequential use is not recommended). Products include:
Zoloft 2751

Sufentanil Citrate (Contraindication warning for meperidine is extended to other opioids).
No products indexed under this heading.

Trimipramine Maleate (Co-administration may result in hypertension, syncope, asystole, diaphoresis seizures, changes in behavioral and mental status, and muscular rigidity; concurrent and/or sequential use is not recommended).
Products include:
Surmontil Capsules 3595

Venlafaxine Hydrochloride (Potential for serious, sometimes fatal, reactions including hyperthermia, rigidity, myoclonus, autonomic instability, extreme agitation progressing to delirium and coma; concurrent and/or sequential use is not recommended). Products include:
Effexor Tablets 3495
Effexor XR Capsules 3499

Food Interactions

Food, unspecified (The bioavailability of selegiline is increased 3 to 4 fold when it is taken with food).

ELDERTONIC
(Vitamins with Minerals) 2223
None cited in PDR database.

ELDOPAQUE FORTE 4% CREAM
(Hydroquinone) 1734
None cited in PDR database.

ELDOQUIN FORTE 4% CREAM
(Hydroquinone) 1734
None cited in PDR database.

ELECARE POWDER
(Amino Acid Preparations, Vitamins with Minerals)........ 3049
None cited in PDR database.

ELIMITE CREAM
(Permethrin) 552
None cited in PDR database.

ELLENCE INJECTION
(Epirubicin Hydrochloride) 2806
May interact with calcium channel blockers, cytotoxic drugs, and certain other agents. Compounds in these categories include:

Amlodipine Besylate (Co-administration with other cardioactive agents that cause heart failure, such as calcium channel blockers, requires close monitoring of cardiac function throughout treatment).
Products include:
Lotrel Capsules 2370
Norvasc Tablets 2704

Bepridil Hydrochloride (Co-administration with other cardioactive agents that cause heart failure, such as calcium channel blockers, requires close monitoring of cardiac function throughout treatment).
Products include:
Vascor Tablets 2602

Bleomycin Sulfate (Combination therapy with other cytotoxic drugs may show on-treatment additive toxicity, especially hematologic and gastrointestinal effects).
No products indexed under this heading.

Cimetidine (Co-administration increases the AUC of epirubicin by 50%; cimetidine treatment should be stopped during treatment with Ellence). Products include:
Tagamet HB 200 Suspension 762
Tagamet HB 200 Tablets 761
Tagamet Tablets 1644

Cimetidine Hydrochloride (Co-administration increases the AUC of epirubicin by 50%; cimetidine treatment should be stopped during treatment with Ellence). Products include:
Tagamet 1644

Cyclophosphamide (Combination therapy with other cytotoxic drugs may show on-treatment additive toxicity, especially hematologic and gastrointestinal effects).
No products indexed under this heading.

Daunorubicin Hydrochloride (Combination therapy with other cytotoxic drugs may show on-treatment additive toxicity, especially hematologic and gastrointestinal effects). Products include:
Cerubidine for Injection 947

Diltiazem Hydrochloride (Co-administration with other cardioactive agents that cause heart failure, such as calcium channel blockers, requires close monitoring of cardiac function throughout treatment).
Products include:
Cardizem Injectable 1018
Cardizem Lyo-Ject Syringe 1018
Cardizem Monovial 1018
Cardizem CD Capsules 1016
Tiazac Capsules 1378

Doxorubicin Hydrochloride (Combination therapy with other cytotoxic drugs may show on-treatment additive toxicity, especially hematologic and gastrointestinal effects).
Products include:
Adriamycin PFS/RDF Injection 2767
Doxil Injection 566

Felodipine (Co-administration with other cardioactive agents that cause heart failure, such as calcium channel blockers, requires close monitoring of cardiac function throughout treatment). Products include:
Lexxel Tablets 608
Plendil Extended-Release Tablets ... 623

Fluorouracil (Combination therapy with other cytotoxic drugs may show on-treatment additive toxicity, especially hematologic and gastrointestinal effects). Products include:
Carac Cream 1222
Efudex 1733
Fluoroplex 552

Hydroxyurea (Combination therapy with other cytotoxic drugs may show on-treatment additive toxicity, especially hematologic and gastrointestinal effects). Products include:
Mylocel Tablets 2227

Isradipine (Co-administration with other cardioactive agents that cause heart failure, such as calcium channel blockers, requires close monitoring of cardiac function throughout treatment). Products include:
DynaCirc Capsules 2921
DynaCirc CR Tablets 2923

Methotrexate Sodium (Combination therapy with other cytotoxic drugs may show on-treatment additive toxicity, especially hematologic and gastrointestinal effects).
No products indexed under this heading.

Mibefradil Dihydrochloride (Co-administration with other cardioactive agents that cause heart failure, such as calcium channel blockers, requires close monitoring of cardiac function throughout treatment).
No products indexed under this heading.

Mitotane (Combination therapy with other cytotoxic drugs may show on-treatment additive toxicity, especially hematologic and gastrointestinal effects).
No products indexed under this heading.

Mitoxantrone Hydrochloride (Combination therapy with other cytotoxic drugs may show on-treatment additive toxicity, especially hematologic and gastrointestinal effects). Products include:
Novantrone for Injection 1760

Nicardipine Hydrochloride (Co-administration with other cardioactive agents that cause heart failure, such as calcium channel blockers, requires close monitoring of cardiac function throughout treatment).
Products include:
Cardene I.V. 3485

Nifedipine (Co-administration with other cardioactive agents that cause heart failure, such as calcium channel blockers, requires close monitoring of cardiac function throughout treatment). Products include:
Adalat CC Tablets 877
Procardia Capsules 2708
Procardia XL Extended Release Tablets 2710

Nimodipine (Co-administration with other cardioactive agents that cause heart failure, such as calcium channel blockers, requires close monitoring of cardiac function throughout treatment). Products include:
Nimotop Capsules 904

Nisoldipine (Co-administration with other cardioactive agents that cause heart failure, such as calcium channel blockers, requires close monitoring of cardiac function throughout treatment). Products include:
Sular Tablets 688

Procarbazine Hydrochloride (Combination therapy with other cytotoxic drugs may show on-treatment additive toxicity, especially hematologic and gastrointestinal effects). Products include:
Matulane Capsules 3246

Tamoxifen Citrate (Combination therapy with other cytotoxic drugs may show on-treatment additive toxicity, especially hematologic and gastrointestinal effects). Products include:
Nolvadex Tablets 678

Verapamil Hydrochloride (Co-administration with other cardioactive agents that cause heart failure, such as calcium channel blockers, requires close monitoring of cardiac function throughout treatment).
Products include:
Covera-HS Tablets 3199
Isoptin SR Tablets 467
Tarka Tablets 508
Verelan Capsules 3184
Verelan PM Capsules 3186

Vincristine Sulfate (Combination therapy with other cytotoxic drugs may show on-treatment additive toxicity, especially hematologic and gastrointestinal effects).
No products indexed under this heading.

ELMIRON CAPSULES
(Pentosan Polysulfate Sodium) 570
May interact with anticoagulants, thrombolytics, and certain other agents. Compounds in these categories include:

Alteplase, Recombinant (Pentosan polysulfate sodium is a weak anticoagulant and bleeding complications of ecchymosis, epistaxis and gum hemorrhage have been reported with its use; caution should be exercised in patients with increased risk of bleeding due to other concomitant therapies, such as thrombolytics). Products include:
Activase I.V. 1410
Cathflo Activase 3611

Anistreplase (Pentosan polysulfate sodium is a weak anticoagulant and bleeding complications of ecchymosis, epistaxis and gum hemorrhage have been reported with its use; caution should be exercised in patients with increased risk of bleeding due to other concomitant therapies, such as thrombolytics).
No products indexed under this heading.

Ardeparin Sodium (Pentosan polysulfate sodium is a weak anticoagulant and bleeding complications of ecchymosis, epistaxis and gum hemorrhage have been reported with its use; caution should be exercised in patients with increased risk of bleeding due to other concomitant therapies, such as anticoagulants).
No products indexed under this heading.

Aspirin (Pentosan polysulfate sodium is a weak anticoagulant and bleeding complications of ecchymosis, epistaxis and gum hemorrhage have been reported with its use; caution should be exercised in patients with increased risk of bleeding due to other concomitant therapies, such as high dose aspirin). Products include:
Aggrenox Capsules 1026
Alka-Seltzer 603

Alka-Seltzer Lemon Lime Antacid and Pain Reliever Effervescent Tablets .... ▣603
Alka-Seltzer Extra Strength Antacid and Pain Reliever Effervescent Tablets .... ▣603
Alka-Seltzer PM Effervescent Tablets .... ▣605
Genuine Bayer Tablets, Caplets and Gelcaps .... ▣606
Extra Strength Bayer Caplets and Gelcaps .... ▣610
Aspirin Regimen Bayer Children's Chewable Tablets (Orange or Cherry Flavored) .... ▣607
Bayer, Aspirin Regimen .... ▣606
Aspirin Regimen Bayer 81 mg Caplets with Calcium .... ▣607
Genuine Bayer Professional Labeling (Aspirin Regimen Bayer) .... ▣608
Extra Strength Bayer Arthritis Caplets .... ▣610
Extra Strength Bayer Plus Caplets .... ▣610
Extra Strength Bayer PM Caplets .... ▣611
BC Powder .... ▣619
BC Allergy Sinus Cold Powder .... ▣619
Arthritis Strength BC Powder .... ▣619
BC Sinus Cold Powder .... ▣619
Darvon Compound-65 Pulvules 1910
Ecotrin Enteric Coated Aspirin Low, Regular and Maximum Strength Tablets 1715
Excedrin Extra-Strength Tablets, Caplets, and Geltabs .... ▣629
Excedrin Migraine 1070
Goody's Body Pain Formula Powder .... ▣620
Goody's Extra Strength Headache Powder .... ▣620
Goody's Extra Strength Pain Relief Tablets .... ▣620
Percodan Tablets 1327
Robaxisal Tablets 2939
Soma Compound Tablets 3354
Soma Compound w/Codeine Tablets 3355
Vanquish Caplets .... ▣617

Dalteparin Sodium (Pentosan polysulfate sodium is a weak anticoagulant and bleeding complications of ecchymosis, epistaxis and gum hemorrhage have been reported with its use; caution should be exercised in patients with increased risk of bleeding due to other concomitant therapies, such as anticoagulants). Products include:
Fragmin Injection 2814

Danaparoid Sodium (Pentosan polysulfate sodium is a weak anticoagulant and bleeding complications of ecchymosis, epistaxis and gum hemorrhage have been reported with its use; caution should be exercised in patients with increased risk of bleeding due to other concomitant therapies, such as anticoagulants). Products include:
Orgaran Injection 2480

Dicumarol (Pentosan polysulfate sodium is a weak anticoagulant and bleeding complications of ecchymosis, epistaxis and gum hemorrhage have been reported with its use; caution should be exercised in patients with increased risk of bleeding due to other concomitant therapies, such as anticoagulants).
No products indexed under this heading.

Enoxaparin (Pentosan polysulfate sodium is a weak anticoagulant and bleeding complications of ecchymosis, epistaxis and gum hemorrhage have been reported with its use; caution should be exercised in patients with increased risk of bleeding due to other concomitant therapies, such as anticoagulants). Products include:
Lovenox Injection 746

Heparin Sodium (Pentosan polysulfate sodium is a weak anticoagulant and bleeding complications of ecchymosis, epistaxis and gum hemorrhage have been reported with its use; caution should be exercised in patients with increased risk of bleeding due to other concomitant therapies, such as anticoagulants). Products include:
Heparin Lock Flush Solution 3509
Heparin Sodium Injection 3511

Reteplase (Pentosan polysulfate sodium is a weak anticoagulant and bleeding complications of ecchymosis, epistaxis and gum hemorrhage have been reported with its use; caution should be exercised in patients with increased risk of bleeding due to other concomitant therapies, such as thrombolytics). Products include:
Retavase Vials 1182

Streptokinase (Pentosan polysulfate sodium is a weak anticoagulant and bleeding complications of ecchymosis, epistaxis and gum hemorrhage have been reported with its use; caution should be exercised in patients with increased risk of bleeding due to other concomitant therapies, such as thrombolytics). Products include:
Streptase for Infusion 647

Tinzaparin sodium (Pentosan polysulfate sodium is a weak anticoagulant and bleeding complications of ecchymosis, epistaxis and gum hemorrhage have been reported with its use; caution should be exercised in patients with increased risk of bleeding due to other concomitant therapies, such as anticoagulants). Products include:
Innohep Injection 1248

Urokinase (Pentosan polysulfate sodium is a weak anticoagulant and bleeding complications of ecchymosis, epistaxis and gum hemorrhage have been reported with its use; caution should be exercised in patients with increased risk of bleeding due to other concomitant therapies, such as thrombolytics).
No products indexed under this heading.

Warfarin Sodium (Pentosan polysulfate sodium is a weak anticoagulant and bleeding complications of ecchymosis, epistaxis and gum hemorrhage have been reported with its use; caution should be exercised in patients with increased risk of bleeding due to other concomitant therapies, such as anticoagulants). Products include:
Coumadin for Injection 1243
Coumadin Tablets 1243
Warfarin Sodium Tablets, USP 3302

ELOCON CREAM 0.1%
(Mometasone Furoate) 3110
None cited in PDR database.

ELOCON LOTION 0.1%
(Mometasone Furoate) 3111
None cited in PDR database.

ELOCON OINTMENT 0.1%
(Mometasone Furoate) 3112
None cited in PDR database.

ELSPAR FOR INJECTION
(Asparaginase) 2092
May interact with:

Methotrexate Sodium (Tissue culture and animal studies indicate that asparaginase can diminish or abolish the effect of methotrexate on malignant cells).
No products indexed under this heading.

Prednisone (The administration of asparaginase intravenously and concurrently with or immediately before a course of prednisone may be associated with increased toxicity). Products include:
Prednisone 3064

Vincristine Sulfate (The administration of asparaginase intravenously and concurrently with or immediately before a course of prednisone may be associated with increased toxicity).
No products indexed under this heading.

EMADINE OPHTHALMIC SOLUTION
(Emedastine Difumarate) .... ⊙211
None cited in PDR database.

EMCYT CAPSULES
(Estramustine Phosphate Sodium) 2810
May interact with calcium preparations and certain other agents. Compounds in these categories include:

Calcium Carbonate (Calcium-rich drugs may impair the absorption of estramustine). Products include:
Aspirin Regimen Bayer 81 mg Caplets with Calcium .... ▣607
Extra Strength Bayer Plus Caplets .... ▣610
Caltrate 600 Tablets .... ▣814
Caltrate 600 PLUS .... ▣815
Caltrate 600 + D Tablets .... ▣814
Caltrate 600 + Soy Tablets .... ▣814
D-Cal Chewable Caplets .... ▣794
Florical Capsules and Tablets 2223
Quick Dissolve Maalox Max Maximum Strength Antacid/Antigas Tablets 2301
Quick Dissolve Maalox Regular Strength Antacid Tablets 2301
Marblen Suspension .... ▣633
Monocal Tablets 2223
Mylanta Fast-Acting 1813
Mylanta Calci Tabs .... ▣636
One-A-Day Bedtime & Rest Tablets .... ▣805
One-A-Day Calcium Plus Chewable Tablets .... ▣805
Os-Cal Chewable Tablets .... ▣838
Pepcid Complete Chewable Tablets 1815
ReSource Wellness CalciWise Soft Chews .... ▣824
Rolaids Tablets .... ▣706
Extra Strength Rolaids Tablets .... ▣706
Slow-Mag Tablets .... ▣835
Titralac .... ▣640
3M Titralac Plus Antacid Tablets .... ▣640
Tums .... ▣763

Calcium Chloride (Calcium-rich drugs may impair the absorption of estramustine).
No products indexed under this heading.

Calcium Citrate (Calcium-rich drugs may impair the absorption of estramustine). Products include:
Active Calcium Tablets 3335
Citracal Liquitab Tablets .... ▣823
Citracal Tablets 2231
Citracal Caplets + D .... ▣823

Calcium Glubionate (Calcium-rich drugs may impair the absorption of estramustine).
No products indexed under this heading

Food Interactions

Dairy products (Calcium-rich foods may impair the absorption of estramustine).

Food, calcium-rich (Calcium-rich foods may impair the absorption of estramustine).

EMETROL ORAL SOLUTION (LEMON-MINT & CHERRY FLAVORS)
(Dextrose, Levulose, Phosphoric Acid) .... ▣718
None cited in PDR database.

EMGEL 2% TOPICAL GEL
(Erythromycin) 1285
May interact with:

Concomitant Topical Acne Therapy (Possible cumulative irritancy effect).
No products indexed under this heading.

EMLA CREAM
(Lidocaine, Prilocaine) 602
May interact with methemoglobinemia-inducing drugs and certain other agents. Compounds in these categories include:

Acetaminophen (Potential for greater risk of developing methemoglobinemia). Products include:
Actifed Cold & Sinus Caplets and Tablets .... ▣688
Alka-Seltzer Plus Liqui-Gels .... ▣604
Alka-Seltzer Plus Cold & Flu Medicine Liqui-Gels .... ▣604
Alka-Seltzer Plus Cold & Sinus Medicine Liqui-Gels .... ▣604
Benadryl Allergy/Cold Tablets .... ▣691
Benadryl Allergy Sinus Headache Caplets & Gelcaps .... ▣693
Benadryl Severe Allergy & Sinus Headache Caplets .... ▣694
Children's Cēpacol Sore Throat .... ▣788
Comtrex Acute Head Cold & Sinus Pressure Relief Tablets .... ▣627
Comtrex Deep Chest Cold & Congestion Relief Softgels .... ▣627
Comtrex Flu Therapy & Fever Relief Daytime Caplets .... ▣628
Comtrex Flu Therapy & Fever Relief Nighttime Tablets .... ▣628
Comtrex Maximum Strength Multi-Symptom Cold & Cough Relief Tablets and Caplets .... ▣626
Contac Severe Cold and Flu Caplets Maximum Strength .... ▣746
Contac Severe Cold and Flu Caplets Non-Drowsy .... ▣746
Coricidin 'D' Cold, Flu & Sinus Tablets .... ▣737
Coricidin HBP Cold & Flu Tablets .... ▣738
Coricidin HBP Maximum Strength Flu Tablets .... ▣738
Coricidin HBP Night-Time Cold & Flu Tablets .... ▣738
Darvon-N/Darvocet-N 1907
Dimetapp Cold and Fever Suspension .... ▣775
Dimetapp Nighttime Flu Liquid .... ▣776
Dimetapp Non-Drowsy Flu Syrup .... ▣777
Drixoral Allergy/Sinus Extended-Release Tablets .... ▣741
Drixoral Cold & Flu Extended-Release Tablets .... ▣740
Aspirin Free Excedrin Caplets and Geltabs .... ▣628
Excedrin Extra-Strength Tablets, Caplets, and Geltabs .... ▣629
Excedrin Migraine 1070
Excedrin PM Tablets, Caplets, and Geltabs .... ▣631
Goody's Body Pain Formula Powder .... ▣620
Goody's Extra Strength Headache Powder .... ▣620
Goody's Extra Strength Pain Relief Tablets .... ▣620
Goody's PM Powder .... ▣621
Hycomine Compound Tablets 1317
Lortab 3319
Lortab Elixir 3317
Maxidone Tablets CIII 3399
Maximum Strength Midol Menstrual Caplets and Gelcaps .... ▣612
Maximum Strength Midol PMS Caplets and Gelcaps .... ▣613
Maximum Strength Midol Teen Caplets .... ▣612
Midrin Capsules 3464
Norco 5/325 Tablets CIII 3424
Norco 7.5/325 Tablets CIII 3425
Norco 10/325 Tablets CIII 3427
Norco 10/325 Tablets CIII 3425
Percocet Tablets 1326
Percogesic Aspirin-Free Coated Tablets .... ▣667
Extra Strength Percogesic Aspirin-Free Coated Caplets .... ▣665
Phrenilin 578
Robitussin Cold Caplets Multi-Symptom Cold & Flu .... ▣781
Robitussin Cold Softgels Multi-Symptom Cold & Flu .... ▣781
Robitussin Multi Symptom Honey Flu Liquid .... ▣785
Robitussin Nighttime Honey Flu Liquid .... ▣786
Sedapap Tablets 50 mg/650 mg 2225
Singlet Caplets .... ▣761
Sinutab Sinus Allergy Medication, Maximum Strength Formula, Tablets & Caplets .... ▣707
Sinutab Sinus Medication, Maximum Strength Without Drowsiness Formula, Tablets & Caplets .... ▣707

Sudafed Cold & Cough Liquid Caps ■709
Sudafed Cold & Sinus Liquid Caps ■710
Sudafed Severe Cold ■711
Sudafed Sinus Headache Caplets ■712
Sudafed Sinus Headache Tablets ■712
Tavist Sinus Non-Drowsy Coated Caplets ■676
TheraFlu Regular Strength Cold & Cough Night Time Hot Liquid ■676
TheraFlu Regular Strength Cold & Sore Throat Night Time Hot Liquid ■676
TheraFlu Maximum Strength Flu & Congestion Non-Drowsy Hot Liquid ■677
TheraFlu Maximum Strength Flu & Cough Night Time Hot Liquid ■678
TheraFlu Maximum Strength Flu & Sore Throat Night Time Hot Liquid ■677
TheraFlu Maximum Strength Severe Cold & Congestion Night Time Caplets ■678
TheraFlu Maximum Strength Severe Cold & Congestion Night Time Hot Liquid ■678
TheraFlu Maximum Strength Severe Cold & Congestion Non-Drowsy ■679
Triaminic Cold, Cough & Fever Liquid ■681
Triaminic Cough & Sore Throat Liquid ■682
Triaminic Cough & Sore Throat Softchews ■684
Tylenol, Children's 2014
Children's Tylenol Allergy-D Liquid 2014
Children's Tylenol Cold Suspension Liquid and Chewable Tablets 2015
Children's Tylenol Cold Plus Cough Suspension Liquid and Chewable Tablets 2015
Children's Tylenol Flu Suspension Liquid 2015
Children's Tylenol Sinus Suspension Liquid 2017
Infants' Tylenol Cold Decongestant and Fever Reducer Concentrated Drops 2015
Infants' Tylenol Cold Decongestant and Fever Reducer Concentrated Drops Plus Cough 2015
Junior Strength Tylenol Soft Chews Chewable Tablets 2014
Tylenol 2009
Tylenol Allergy Sinus 2010
Tylenol Severe Allergy Caplets 2010
Multi-Symptom Tylenol Cold Complete Formula Caplets 2010
Multi-Symptom Tylenol Cold Non-Drowsy Caplets and Gelcaps 2010
Multi-Symptom Tylenol Cold Severe Congestion Non-Drowsy Caplets 2011
Maximum Strength Tylenol Flu NightTime Gelcaps 2011
Maximum Strength Tylenol Flu NightTime Liquid 2011
Maximum Strength Tylenol Flu Non-Drowsy Gelcaps 2011
Extra Strength Tylenol PM Caplets, Geltabs, and Gelcaps 2012
Maximum Strength Tylenol Sinus NightTime Caplets 2012
Maximum Strength Tylenol Sinus Non-Drowsy Geltabs, Gelcaps, Caplets, and Tablets 2012
Maximum Strength Tylenol Sore Throat Adult Liquid 2013
Tylenol with Codeine 2595
Women's Tylenol Menstrual Relief Caplets 2013
Tylox Capsules 2597
Ultracet Tablets 2597
Vanquish Caplets ■617
Vicks 44M Cough, Cold & Flu Relief Liquid ■725
Vicks DayQuil LiquiCaps/Liquid Multi-Symptom Cold/Flu Relief ■727
Vicks NyQuil LiquiCaps/Liquid Multi-Symptom Cold/Flu Relief, Original and Cherry Flavors ■727
Vicodin Tablets 516
Vicodin ES Tablets 517
Vicodin HP Tablets 518
Zydone Tablets 1330

Amyl Nitrite (Potential for greater risk of developing methemoglobinemia).
No products indexed under this heading.

Bendroflumethiazide (Potential for greater risk of developing methemoglobinemia). Products include:
Corzide 40/5 Tablets 2247
Corzide 80/5 Tablets 2247

Benzocaine (Potential for greater risk of developing methemoglobinemia). Products include:
Americaine Anesthetic Lubricant 1162
Americaine Otic Topical Anesthetic Ear Drops 1162
Baby Anbesol Gel ■774
Junior Anbesol Gel ■774
Anbesol ■774
Auralgan Otic Solution 3485
Cēpacol Maximum Strength Sugar Free Sore Throat Lozenges, Cherry Flavor ■787
Cēpacol Maximum Strength Sugar Free Sore Throat Lozenges, Cool Mint Flavor ■787
Cēpacol Maximum Strength Sore Throat Lozenges, Cherry Flavor ■787
Cēpacol Maximum Strength Sore Throat Lozenges, Mint Flavor ■787
Cetacaine Topical Anesthetic 1196
Dermoplast Hospital Strength Spray ■666
Hurricaine Topical Anesthetic Gel, 1 oz. Fresh Mint, Wild Cherry, Pina Colada, Watermelon, 1/6 oz. Wild Cherry, Watermelon ■618
Hurricaine Topical Anesthetic Liquid, 1 oz. Wild Cherry, Pina Colada, .25 ml Dry Handle Swab Wild Cherry, 1/6 oz. Wild Cherry ■618
Hurricaine Topical Anesthetic Spray Extension Tubes (200) ■618
Hurricaine Topical Anesthetic Spray Kit, 2 oz. Wild Cherry ■618
Hurricaine Topical Anesthetic Spray, 2 oz. Wild Cherry ■618
Zilactin Baby Gel ■791
Zilactin-B Gel ■790

Chloroquine (Potential for greater risk of developing methemoglobinemia).

Chloroquine Hydrochloride (Potential for greater risk of developing methemoglobinemia).
No products indexed under this heading.

Chloroquine Phosphate (Potential for greater risk of developing methemoglobinemia). Products include:
Aralen Tablets 3075

Chlorothiazide (Potential for greater risk of developing methemoglobinemia). Products include:
Aldoclor Tablets 2035
Diuril Oral 2087

Chlorothiazide Sodium (Potential for greater risk of developing methemoglobinemia). Products include:
Diuril Sodium Intravenous 2086

Chlorpropamide (Potential for greater risk of developing methemoglobinemia). Products include:
Diabinese Tablets 2680

Dapsone (Potential for greater risk of developing methemoglobinemia). Products include:
Dapsone Tablets USP 1780

Erythrityl Tetranitrate (Potential for greater risk of developing methemoglobinemia).
No products indexed under this heading.

Fosphenytoin Sodium (Potential for greater risk of developing methemoglobinemia). Products include:
Cerebyx Injection 2619

Glipizide (Potential for greater risk of developing methemoglobinemia). Products include:
Glucotrol Tablets 2692
Glucotrol XL Extended Release Tablets 2693

Glyburide (Potential for greater risk of developing methemoglobinemia). Products include:
DiaBeta Tablets 741
Glucovance Tablets 1086

Hydrochlorothiazide (Potential for greater risk of developing methemoglobinemia). Products include:
Accuretic Tablets 2614
Aldoril Tablets 2039
Atacand HCT Tablets 597
Avalide Tablets 1070
Diovan HCT Tablets 2338
Dyazide Capsules 1515
HydroDIURIL Tablets 2108
Hyzaar 2109
Inderide Tablets 3517
Inderide LA Long-Acting Capsules 3519
Lotensin HCT Tablets 2367
Maxzide 1008
Micardis HCT Tablets 1051
Microzide Capsules 3414
Moduretic Tablets 2138
Monopril HCT 1094
Prinzide Tablets 2168
Timolide Tablets 2187
Uniretic Tablets 3178
Vaseretic Tablets 2204
Zestoretic Tablets 695
Ziac Tablets 1887

Hydroflumethiazide (Potential for greater risk of developing methemoglobinemia). Products include:
Diucardin Tablets 3494

Isosorbide Dinitrate (Potential for greater risk of developing methemoglobinemia). Products include:
Isordil Sublingual Tablets 3525
Isordil Titradose Tablets 3526

Isosorbide Mononitrate (Potential for greater risk of developing methemoglobinemia). Products include:
Imdur Tablets 1826
Ismo Tablets 3524

Methyclothiazide (Potential for greater risk of developing methemoglobinemia).
No products indexed under this heading.

Mexiletine Hydrochloride (Potential for additive or synergistic toxic effects). Products include:
Mexitil Capsules 1047

Nitrofurantoin (Potential for greater risk of developing methemoglobinemia). Products include:
Macrodantin Capsules 2891

Nitrofurantoin Monohydrate (Potential for greater risk of developing methemoglobinemia). Products include:
Macrobid Capsules 2889

Nitroglycerin (Potential for greater risk of developing methemoglobinemia). Products include:
Nitro-Dur Transdermal Infusion System 3134
Nitro-Dur Transdermal Infusion System 1834
Nitrolingual Pumpspray 1355
Nitrostat Tablets 2658

Para-Aminosalicylic Acid (Potential for greater risk of developing methemoglobinemia).
No products indexed under this heading.

Pentaerythritol Tetranitrate (Potential for greater risk of developing methemoglobinemia).
No products indexed under this heading.

Phenacetin (Potential for greater risk of developing methemoglobinemia).
No products indexed under this heading.

Phenobarbital (Potential for greater risk of developing methemoglobinemia). Products include:
Arco-Lase Plus Tablets 592
Donnatal 2929
Donnatal Extentabs 2930

Phenytoin (Potential for greater risk of developing methemoglobinemia). Products include:
Dilantin Infatabs 2624
Dilantin-125 Oral Suspension 2625

Phenytoin Sodium (Potential for greater risk of developing methemoglobinemia). Products include:
Dilantin Kapseals 2622

Polythiazide (Potential for greater risk of developing methemoglobinemia). Products include:
Minizide Capsules 2700
Renese Tablets 2712

Primaquine Phosphate (Potential for greater risk of developing methemoglobinemia).
No products indexed under this heading.

Quinine Sulfate (Potential for greater risk of developing methemoglobinemia).
No products indexed under this heading.

Sodium Nitroprusside (Potential for greater risk of developing methemoglobinemia).
No products indexed under this heading.

Sulfacytine (Potential for greater risk of developing methemoglobinemia).
No products indexed under this heading.

Sulfamethizole (Potential for greater risk of developing methemoglobinemia). Products include:
Urobiotic-250 Capsules 2731

Sulfamethoxazole (Potential for greater risk of developing methemoglobinemia). Products include:
Bactrim 2949
Septra Suspension 2265
Septra Tablets 2265
Septra DS Tablets 2265

Sulfasalazine (Potential for greater risk of developing methemoglobinemia). Products include:
Azulfidine EN-tabs Tablets 2775

Sulfinpyrazone (Potential for greater risk of developing methemoglobinemia).
No products indexed under this heading.

Sulfisoxazole (Potential for greater risk of developing methemoglobinemia).
No products indexed under this heading.

Sulfisoxazole Diolamine (Potential for greater risk of developing methemoglobinemia).
No products indexed under this heading.

Tocainide Hydrochloride (Potential for additive or synergistic toxic effects). Products include:
Tonocard Tablets 649

Tolazamide (Potential for greater risk of developing methemoglobinemia).
No products indexed under this heading.

Tolbutamide (Potential for greater risk of developing methemoglobinemia).
No products indexed under this heading.

EMLA ANESTHETIC DISC

(Lidocaine, Prilocaine) 602
See EMLA Cream

ENALAPRILAT INJECTION

(Enalaprilat) 863
May interact with diuretics, lithium preparations, non-steroidal anti-inflammatory agents, potassium preparations, and potassium sparing diuretics. Compounds in these categories include:

Amiloride Hydrochloride (Enalaprilat attenuates diuretic-induced potassium loss; concomitant use can lead to hyperkalemia; frequent monitoring of serum potassium is recommended if used concurrently; co-administration can result in excessive hypotension). Products include:
Midamor Tablets 2136
Moduretic Tablets 2138

Bendroflumethiazide (Co-administration of enalaprilat in patients on diuretics, especially those in whom diuretic therapy was recently instituted, may occasionally experience excessive hypotension; antihypertensive effects of enalaprilat are augmented by antihypertensive agents that cause rennin release). Products include:
Corzide 40/5 Tablets 2247

Corzide 80/5 Tablets 2247

Bumetanide (Co-administration of enalaprilat in patients on diuretics, especially those in whom diuretic therapy was recently instituted, may occasionally experience excessive hypotension; antihypertensive effects of enalaprilat are augmented by antihypertensive agents that cause rennin release).

No products indexed under this heading.

Celecoxib (Co-administration in some patients with compromised renal function who are being treated with NSAIDs may result in a further deterioration of renal function). Products include:

Celebrex Capsules 2676
Celebrex Capsules 2780

Chlorothiazide (Co-administration of enalaprilat in patients on diuretics, especially those in whom diuretic therapy was recently instituted, may occasionally experience excessive hypotension; antihypertensive effects of enalaprilat are augmented by antihypertensive agents that cause rennin release). Products include:

Aldoclor Tablets 2035
Diuril Oral 2087

Chlorothiazide Sodium (Co-administration of enalaprilat in patients on diuretics, especially those in whom diuretic therapy was recently instituted, may occasionally experience excessive hypotension; antihypertensive effects of enalaprilat are augmented by antihypertensive agents that cause rennin release). Products include:

Diuril Sodium Intravenous 2086

Chlorthalidone (Co-administration of enalaprilat in patients on diuretics, especially those in whom diuretic therapy was recently instituted, may occasionally experience excessive hypotension; antihypertensive effects of enalaprilat are augmented by antihypertensive agents that cause rennin release). Products include:

Clorpres Tablets 1002
Combipres Tablets 1040
Tenoretic Tablets 690

Diclofenac Potassium (Co-administration in some patients with compromised renal function who are being treated with NSAIDs may result in a further deterioration of renal function). Products include:

Cataflam Tablets 2315

Diclofenac Sodium (Co-administration in some patients with compromised renal function who are being treated with NSAIDs may result in a further deterioration of renal function). Products include:

Arthrotec Tablets 3195
Voltaren Ophthalmic Sterile Ophthalmic Solution .... ⊙312
Voltaren Tablets 2315
Voltaren-XR Tablets 2315

Ethacrynic Acid (Co-administration of enalaprilat in patients on diuretics, especially those in whom diuretic therapy was recently instituted, may occasionally experience excessive hypotension; antihypertensive effects of enalaprilat are augmented by antihypertensive agents that cause rennin release). Products include:

Edecrin Tablets 2091

Etodolac (Co-administration in some patients with compromised renal function who are being treated with NSAIDs may result in a further deterioration of renal function). Products include:

Lodine 3528
Lodine XL Extended-Release Tablets 3530

Fenoprofen Calcium (Co-administration in some patients with compromised renal function who are being treated with NSAIDs may result in a further deterioration of renal function).

No products indexed under this heading.

Flurbiprofen (Co-administration in some patients with compromised renal function who are being treated with NSAIDs may result in a further deterioration of renal function).

No products indexed under this heading.

Furosemide (Co-administration of enalaprilat in patients on diuretics, especially those in whom diuretic therapy was recently instituted, may occasionally experience excessive hypotension; antihypertensive effects of enalaprilat are augmented by antihypertensive agents that cause rennin release). Products include:

Furosemide Tablets 2284

Hydrochlorothiazide (Co-administration of enalaprilat in patients on diuretics, especially those in whom diuretic therapy was recently instituted, may occasionally experience excessive hypotension; antihypertensive effects of enalaprilat are augmented by antihypertensive agents that cause rennin release). Products include:

Accuretic Tablets 2614
Aldoril Tablets 2039
Atacand HCT Tablets 597
Avalide Tablets 1070
Diovan HCT Tablets 2338
Dyazide Capsules 1515
HydroDIURIL Tablets 2108
Hyzaar 2109
Inderide Tablets 3517
Inderide LA Long-Acting Capsules .. 3519
Lotensin HCT Tablets 2367
Maxzide 1008
Micardis HCT Tablets 1051
Microzide Capsules 3414
Moduretic Tablets 2138
Monopril HCT 1094
Prinzide Tablets 2168
Timolide Tablets 2187
Uniretic Tablets 3178
Vaseretic Tablets 2204
Zestoretic Tablets 695
Ziac Tablets 1887

Hydroflumethiazide (Co-administration of enalaprilat in patients on diuretics, especially those in whom diuretic therapy was recently instituted, may occasionally experience excessive hypotension; antihypertensive effects of enalaprilat are augmented by antihypertensive agents that cause rennin release). Products include:

Diucardin Tablets 3494

Ibuprofen (Co-administration in some patients with compromised renal function who are being treated with NSAIDs may result in a further deterioration of renal function). Products include:

Advil .... ▣771
Children's Advil Oral Suspension ... ▣773
Children's Advil Chewable Tablets . ▣773
Advil Cold and Sinus Caplets .... ▣771
Advil Cold and Sinus Tablets .... ▣771
Advil Flu & Body Ache Caplets ...... ▣772
Infants' Advil Drops .... ▣773
Junior Strength Advil Tablets .... ▣773
Junior Strength Advil Chewable Tablets .... ▣773
Advil Migraine Liquigels .... ▣772
Children's Motrin Oral Suspension and Chewable Tablets 2006
Children's Motrin Cold Oral Suspension 2007
Children's Motrin Oral Suspension .... ▣643
Motrin Suspension, Oral Drops, Chewable Tablets, and Caplets 2002
Infants' Motrin Concentrated Drops 2006
Junior Strength Motrin Caplets and Chewable Tablets 2006
Motrin IB Tablets, Caplets, and Gelcaps 2002
Motrin Migraine Pain Caplets 2005
Motrin Sinus Headache Caplets 2005
Vicoprofen Tablets 520

Indapamide (Co-administration of enalaprilat in patients on diuretics, especially those in whom diuretic therapy was recently instituted, may occasionally experience excessive hypotension; antihypertensive effects of enalaprilat are augmented by antihypertensive agents that cause rennin release). Products include:

Indapamide Tablets 2286

Indomethacin (Co-administration in some patients with compromised renal function who are being treated with NSAIDs may result in a further deterioration of renal function). Products include:

Indocin 2112

Indomethacin Sodium Trihydrate (Co-administration in some patients with compromised renal function who are being treated with NSAIDs may result in a further deterioration of renal function). Products include:

Indocin I.V. 2115

Ketoprofen (Co-administration in some patients with compromised renal function who are being treated with NSAIDs may result in a further deterioration of renal function). Products include:

Orudis Capsules 3548
Orudis KT Tablets .... ▣778
Oruvail Capsules 3548

Ketorolac Tromethamine (Co-administration in some patients with compromised renal function who are being treated with NSAIDs may result in a further deterioration of renal function). Products include:

Acular Ophthalmic Solution 544
Acular PF Ophthalmic Solution 544
Toradol 3018

Lithium Carbonate (Co-administration of lithium with drugs that cause elimination of sodium, including ACE inhibitors, can lead to lithium toxicity). Products include:

Eskalith 1527
Lithium Carbonate 3061
Lithobid Slow-Release Tablets 3255

Lithium Citrate (Co-administration of lithium with drugs that cause elimination of sodium, including ACE inhibitors, can lead to lithium toxicity). Products include:

Lithium Citrate Syrup 3061

Meclofenamate Sodium (Co-administration in some patients with compromised renal function who are being treated with NSAIDs may result in a further deterioration of renal function).

No products indexed under this heading.

Mefenamic Acid (Co-administration in some patients with compromised renal function who are being treated with NSAIDs may result in a further deterioration of renal function). Products include:

Ponstel Capsules 1356

Meloxicam (Co-administration in some patients with compromised renal function who are being treated with NSAIDs may result in a further deterioration of renal function). Products include:

Mobic Tablets 1054

Methyclothiazide (Co-administration of enalaprilat in patients on diuretics, especially those in whom diuretic therapy was recently instituted, may occasionally experience excessive hypotension; antihypertensive effects of enalaprilat are augmented by antihypertensive agents that cause rennin release).

No products indexed under this heading.

Metolazone (Co-administration of enalaprilat in patients on diuretics, especially those in whom diuretic therapy was recently instituted, may occasionally experience excessive hypotension; antihypertensive effects of enalaprilat are augmented by antihypertensive agents that cause rennin release). Products include:

Mykrox Tablets 1168
Zaroxolyn Tablets 1177

Nabumetone (Co-administration in some patients with compromised renal function who are being treated with NSAIDs may result in a further deterioration of renal function). Products include:

Relafen Tablets 1617

Naproxen (Co-administration in some patients with compromised renal function who are being treated with NSAIDs may result in a further deterioration of renal function). Products include:

EC-Naprosyn Delayed-Release Tablets 2967
Naprosyn Suspension 2967
Naprosyn Tablets 2967

Naproxen Sodium (Co-administration in some patients with compromised renal function who are being treated with NSAIDs may result in a further deterioration of renal function). Products include:

Aleve Tablets, Caplets and Gelcaps .... ▣602
Aleve Cold & Sinus Caplets .... ▣603
Anaprox Tablets 2967
Anaprox DS Tablets 2967
Naprelan Tablets 1293

Oxaprozin (Co-administration in some patients with compromised renal function who are being treated with NSAIDs may result in a further deterioration of renal function).

No products indexed under this heading.

Phenylbutazone (Co-administration in some patients with compromised renal function who are being treated with NSAIDs may result in a further deterioration of renal function).

No products indexed under this heading.

Piroxicam (Co-administration in some patients with compromised renal function who are being treated with NSAIDs may result in a further deterioration of renal function). Products include:

Feldene Capsules 2685

Polythiazide (Co-administration of enalaprilat in patients on diuretics, especially those in whom diuretic therapy was recently instituted, may occasionally experience excessive hypotension; antihypertensive effects of enalaprilat are augmented by antihypertensive agents that cause rennin release). Products include:

Minizide Capsules 2700
Renese Tablets 2712

Potassium Acid Phosphate (Concomitant use of potassium-containing salt substitute or potassium supplements can lead to hyperkalemia; frequent monitoring of serum potassium is recommended if used concurrently). Products include:

K-Phos Original (Sodium Free) Tablets 947

Potassium Bicarbonate (Concomitant use of potassium-containing salt substitute or potassium supplements can lead to hyperkalemia; frequent monitoring of serum potassium is recommended if used concurrently).

No products indexed under this heading.

Potassium Chloride (Concomitant use of potassium-containing salt substitute or potassium supplements

can lead to hyperkalemia; frequent monitoring of serum potassium is recommended if used concurrently). Products include:

Chlor-3 1361
Colyte with Flavor Packs for Oral Solution 3170
GoLYTELY and Pineapple Flavor GoLYTELY for Oral Solution 1068
K-Dur Microburst Release System ER Tablets 1832
Klor-Con M20/Klor-Con M10 Tablets 3329
K-Lor Powder Packets 469
K-Tab Filmtab Tablets 470
Micro-K 3311
NuLYTELY, Cherry Flavor, Lemon-Lime Flavor, and Orange Flavor NuLYTELY for Oral Solution 1068
Rum-K 1363

Potassium Citrate (Concomitant use of potassium-containing salt substitute or potassium supplements can lead to hyperkalemia; frequent monitoring of serum potassium is recommended if used concurrently). Products include:

Urocit-K Tablets 2232

Potassium Gluconate (Concomitant use of potassium-containing salt substitute or potassium supplements can lead to hyperkalemia; frequent monitoring of serum potassium is recommended if used concurrently).

No products indexed under this heading.

Potassium Phosphate (Concomitant use of potassium-containing salt substitute or potassium supplements can lead to hyperkalemia; frequent monitoring of serum potassium is recommended if used concurrently). Products include:

K-Phos Neutral Tablets 946

Rofecoxib (Co-administration in some patients with compromised renal function who are being treated with NSAIDs may result in a further deterioration of renal function). Products include:

Vioxx 2213

Spironolactone (Enalaprilat attenuates diuretic-induced potassium loss; concomitant use can lead to hyperkalemia; frequent monitoring of serum potassium is recommended if used concurrently; co-administration can result in excessive hypotension).

No products indexed under this heading.

Sulindac (Co-administration in some patients with compromised renal function who are being treated with NSAIDs may result in a further deterioration of renal function). Products include:

Clinoril Tablets 2053

Tolmetin Sodium (Co-administration in some patients with compromised renal function who are being treated with NSAIDs may result in a further deterioration of renal function). Products include:

Tolectin 2589

Torsemide (Co-administration of enalaprilat in patients on diuretics, especially those in whom diuretic therapy was recently instituted, may occasionally experience excessive hypotension; antihypertensive effects of enalaprilat are augmented by antihypertensive agents that cause rennin release). Products include:

Demadex Tablets and Injection 2965

Triamterene (Enalaprilat attenuates diuretic-induced potassium loss; concomitant use can lead to hyperkalemia; frequent monitoring of serum potassium is recommended if used concurrently; co-administration can result in excessive hypotension). Products include:

Dyazide Capsules 1515
Dyrenium Capsules 3458
Maxzide 1008

ENBREL FOR INJECTION

(Etanercept) 3504
None cited in PDR database.

ENBREL FOR INJECTION

(Etanercept) 1752
None cited in PDR database.

ENGERIX-B VACCINE

(Hepatitis B Vaccine, Recombinant) 1517
None cited in PDR database.

EPIFRIN STERILE OPHTHALMIC SOLUTION

(Epinephrine) .... ⊙235
None cited in PDR database.

EPIPEN AUTO-INJECTOR

(Epinephrine) 1236
May interact with cardiac glycosides, monoamine oxidase inhibitors, quinidine, tricyclic antidepressants, and certain other agents. Compounds in these categories include:

Amitriptyline Hydrochloride (Co-administration with tricyclic antidepressants may potentiate the effects of epinephrine). Products include:

Etrafon 3115
Limbitrol 1738

Amoxapine (Co-administration with tricyclic antidepressants may potentiate the effects of epinephrine).

No products indexed under this heading.

Clomipramine Hydrochloride (Co-administration with tricyclic antidepressants may potentiate the effects of epinephrine).

No products indexed under this heading.

Desipramine Hydrochloride (Co-administration with tricyclic antidepressants may potentiate the effects of epinephrine). Products include:

Norpramin Tablets 755

Deslanoside (Co-administration with drugs that may sensitize the heart to arrhythmias, such as digitalis, is not recommended).

No products indexed under this heading.

Digitoxin (Co-administration with drugs that may sensitize the heart to arrhythmias, such as digitalis, is not recommended).

No products indexed under this heading.

Digoxin (Co-administration with drugs that may sensitize the heart to arrhythmias, such as digitalis, is not recommended). Products include:

Digitek Tablets 1003
Lanoxicaps Capsules 1574
Lanoxin Injection 1581
Lanoxin Tablets 1587
Lanoxin Elixir Pediatric 1578
Lanoxin Injection Pediatric 1584

Doxepin Hydrochloride (Co-administration with tricyclic antidepressants may potentiate the effects of epinephrine). Products include:

Sinequan 2713

Imipramine Hydrochloride (Co-administration with tricyclic antidepressants may potentiate the effects of epinephrine).

No products indexed under this heading.

Imipramine Pamoate (Co-administration with tricyclic antidepressants may potentiate the effects of epinephrine).

No products indexed under this heading.

Isocarboxazid (Co-administration with MAO inhibitors may potentiate the effects of epinephrine).

No products indexed under this heading.

Maprotiline Hydrochloride (Co-administration with tricyclic antidepressants may potentiate the effects of epinephrine).

No products indexed under this heading.

Mercurial Diuretics (Co-administration with drugs that may sensitize the heart to arrhythmias, such as mercurial diuretics, is not recommended).

Moclobemide (Co-administration with MAO inhibitors may potentiate the effects of epinephrine).

No products indexed under this heading.

Nortriptyline Hydrochloride (Co-administration with tricyclic antidepressants may potentiate the effects of epinephrine).

No products indexed under this heading.

Pargyline Hydrochloride (Co-administration with MAO inhibitors may potentiate the effects of epinephrine).

No products indexed under this heading.

Phenelzine Sulfate (Co-administration with MAO inhibitors may potentiate the effects of epinephrine). Products include:

Nardil Tablets 2653

Procarbazine Hydrochloride (Co-administration with MAO inhibitors may potentiate the effects of epinephrine). Products include:

Matulane Capsules 3246

Protriptyline Hydrochloride (Co-administration with tricyclic antidepressants may potentiate the effects of epinephrine). Products include:

Vivactil Tablets 2446
Vivactil Tablets 2217

Quinidine Gluconate (Co-administration with drugs that may sensitize the heart to arrhythmias, such as quinidine, is not recommended). Products include:

Quinaglute Dura-Tabs Tablets 978

Quinidine Polygalacturonate (Co-administration with drugs that may sensitize the heart to arrhythmias, such as quinidine, is not recommended).

No products indexed under this heading.

Quinidine Sulfate (Co-administration with drugs that may sensitize the heart to arrhythmias, such as quinidine, is not recommended). Products include:

Quinidex Extentabs 2933

Selegiline Hydrochloride (Co-administration with MAO inhibitors may potentiate the effects of epinephrine). Products include:

Eldepryl Capsules 3266

Tranylcypromine Sulfate (Co-administration with MAO inhibitors may potentiate the effects of epinephrine). Products include:

Parnate Tablets 1607

Trimipramine Maleate (Co-administration with tricyclic antidepressants may potentiate the effects of epinephrine). Products include:

Surmontil Capsules 3595

EPIPEN JR. AUTO-INJECTOR

(Epinephrine) 1236
See EpiPen Auto-Injector

EPIVIR ORAL SOLUTION

(Lamivudine) 1520
See Epivir Tablets

EPIVIR TABLETS

(Lamivudine) 1520
May interact with:

Sulfamethoxazole (Co-administration of lamivudine with 160 mg of trimethoprim and 800 mg of sulfamethoxazole once daily has been shown to increase lamivudine exposure (AUC); the effect of higher doses of TMP/SMX on lamivudine pharmacokinetics has not been investigated; no change in dose of either drug is recommended). Products include:

Bactrim 2949
Septra Suspension 2265
Septra Tablets 2265
Septra DS Tablets 2265

Trimethoprim (Co-administration of lamivudine with 160 mg of trimethoprim and 800 mg of sulfamethoxazole once daily has been shown to increase lamivudine exposure (AUC); the effect of higher doses of TMP/SMX on lamivudine pharmacokinetics has not been investigated; no change in dose of either drug is recommended). Products include:

Bactrim 2949
Septra Suspension 2265
Septra Tablets 2265
Septra DS Tablets 2265

Zalcitabine (Lamivudine and zalcitabine may inhibit the intracellular phosphorylation of one another; concurrent use is not recommended). Products include:

Hivid Tablets 2975

Food Interactions

Food, unspecified (Absorption of lamivudine was slower in the fed state compared with fasted state; there was no significant difference in systemic exposure in the fed state and fasted states; Epivir may be given with or without food).

EPIVIR-HBV ORAL SOLUTION

(Lamivudine) 1524
See Epivir-HBV Tablets

EPIVIR-HBV TABLETS

(Lamivudine) 1524
May interact with:

Sulfamethoxazole (Co-administration with TMP 160 mg/SMX 800 mg once daily has been shown to increase lamivudine exposure). Products include:

Bactrim 2949
Septra Suspension 2265
Septra Tablets 2265
Septra DS Tablets 2265

Trimethoprim (Co-administration with TMP 160 mg/SMX 800 mg once daily has been shown to increase lamivudine exposure). Products include:

Bactrim 2949
Septra Suspension 2265
Septra Tablets 2265
Septra DS Tablets 2265

EPOGEN FOR INJECTION

(Epoetin Alfa) 582
None cited in PDR database.

E.P.T. PREGNANCY TEST

(HCG Monoclonal Antibody) .... ▣701
None cited in PDR database.

ERGAMISOL TABLETS

(Levamisole Hydrochloride) 1789
May interact with oral anticoagulants, phenytoin, and certain other agents. Compounds in these categories include:

Dicumarol (Prolongation of the prothrombin time beyond the therapeutic range when co-administered; monitor PT and the dose of warfarin or other coumarin-like drugs should be adjusted accordingly).

No products indexed under this heading.

Fluorouracil (Combination therapy has been associated with frequent neutropenia, anemia, and thrombocytopenia). Products include:

Carac Cream 1222
Efudex 1733
Fluoroplex 552

Fosphenytoin Sodium (Co-administration of phenytoin and levamisole plus fluorouracil has led to increased plasma levels of phenytoin; monitor plasma phenytoin levels and decrease the dose if necessary). Products include:
Cerebyx Injection 2619

Phenytoin (Co-administration of phenytoin and levamisole plus fluorouracil has led to increased plasma levels of phenytoin; monitor plasma phenytoin levels and decrease the dose if necessary). Products include:
Dilantin Infatabs 2624
Dilantin-125 Oral Suspension 2625

Phenytoin Sodium (Co-administration of phenytoin and levamisole plus fluorouracil has led to increased plasma levels of phenytoin; monitor plasma phenytoin levels and decrease the dose if necessary). Products include:
Dilantin Kapseals 2622

Warfarin Sodium (Prolongation of the prothrombin time beyond the therapeutic range when co-administered; monitor PT and the dose of warfarin or other coumarin-like drugs should be adjusted accordingly). Products include:
Coumadin for Injection 1243
Coumadin Tablets 1243
Warfarin Sodium Tablets, USP 3302

Food Interactions

Alcohol (May result in Antabuse-like side effects).

ERYPED 200 & ERYPED 400

(Erythromycin Ethylsuccinate) 446
See EryPed Drops

ERYPED DROPS

(Erythromycin Ethylsuccinate) 446
May interact with oral anticoagulants, phenytoin, valproate, theophylline, and certain other agents. Compounds in these categories include:

Alfentanil Hydrochloride (Concurrent use of erythromycin in patients receiving drugs metabolized by the cytochrome P450 system may be associated with elevation in serum levels of alfentanil).
No products indexed under this heading.

Aminophylline (Co-administration in patients who are receiving high doses of theophylline may be associated with an increase in serum theophylline levels and potential theophylline toxicity).
No products indexed under this heading.

Astemizole (Concurrent use of erythromycin in patients receiving drugs metabolized by the cytochrome P450 system may be associated with elevation in serum levels of astemizole; co-administration is contraindicated).
No products indexed under this heading.

Bromocriptine Mesylate (Concurrent use of erythromycin in patients receiving drugs metabolized by the cytochrome P450 system may be associated with elevation in serum levels of bromocriptine).
No products indexed under this heading.

Carbamazepine (Concurrent use of erythromycin in patients receiving drugs metabolized by the cytochrome P450 system may be associated with elevation in serum levels of carbamazepine). Products include:
Carbatrol Capsules 3234
Tegretol/Tegretol-XR 2404

Cisapride (Concurrent use of erythromycin in patients receiving drugs metabolized by the cytochrome P450 system may be associated with elevation in serum levels of cisapride; co-administration is contraindicated).
No products indexed under this heading.

Cyclosporine (Concurrent use of erythromycin in patients receiving drugs metabolized by the cytochrome P450 system may be associated with elevation in serum levels of cyclosporine). Products include:
Gengraf Capsules 457
Neoral Soft Gelatin Capsules 2380
Neoral Oral Solution 2380
Sandimmune 2388

Dicumarol (Co-administration has resulted in increased anticoagulant effects).
No products indexed under this heading.

Digoxin (Co-administration has been reported to result in elevated digoxin serum levels). Products include:
Digitek Tablets 1003
Lanoxicaps Capsules 1574
Lanoxin Injection 1581
Lanoxin Tablets 1587
Lanoxin Elixir Pediatric 1578
Lanoxin Injection Pediatric 1584

Dihydroergotamine Mesylate (Co-administration has been associated in some patients with acute ergot toxicity characterized by severe peripheral vasospasm and dysesthesia). Products include:
D.H.E. 45 Injection 2334
Migranal Nasal Spray 2376

Disopyramide Phosphate (Concurrent use of erythromycin in patients receiving drugs metabolized by the cytochrome P450 system may be associated with elevation in serum levels of disopyramide).
No products indexed under this heading.

Divalproex Sodium (Concurrent use of erythromycin in patients receiving drugs metabolized by the cytochrome P450 system may be associated with elevation in serum levels of valproate). Products include:
Depakote Sprinkle Capsules 426
Depakote Tablets 430
Depakote ER Tablets 436

Dyphylline (Co-administration in patients who are receiving high doses of theophylline may be associated with an increase in serum theophylline levels and potential theophylline toxicity). Products include:
Lufyllin Tablets 3347
Lufyllin-400 Tablets 3347
Lufyllin-GG Elixir 3348
Lufyllin-GG Tablets 3348

Ergotamine Tartrate (Co-administration has been associated in some patients with acute ergot toxicity characterized by severe peripheral vasospasm and dysesthesia).
No products indexed under this heading.

Fosphenytoin Sodium (Concurrent use of erythromycin in patients receiving drugs metabolized by the cytochrome P450 system may be associated with elevation in serum levels of phenytoin). Products include:
Cerebyx Injection 2619

Hexobarbital (Concurrent use of erythromycin in patients receiving drugs metabolized by the cytochrome P450 system may be associated with elevation in serum levels of hexobarbital).
No products indexed under this heading.

Lovastatin (Co-administration in seriously ill patients has resulted in rhabdomyolysis with or without renal impairment). Products include:
Mevacor Tablets 2132

Midazolam Hydrochloride (Erythromycin has been reported to decrease the clearance of triazolam and, thus, may increase the pharmacologic effect of the benzodiazepine). Products include:
Versed Injection 3027
Versed Syrup 3033

Phenytoin (Concurrent use of erythromycin in patients receiving drugs metabolized by the cytochrome P450 system may be associated with elevation in serum levels of phenytoin). Products include:
Dilantin Infatabs 2624
Dilantin-125 Oral Suspension 2625

Phenytoin Sodium (Concurrent use of erythromycin in patients receiving drugs metabolized by the cytochrome P450 system may be associated with elevation in serum levels of phenytoin). Products include:
Dilantin Kapseals 2622

Tacrolimus (Concurrent use of erythromycin in patients receiving drugs metabolized by the cytochrome P450 system may be associated with elevation in serum levels of tacrolimus). Products include:
Prograf 1393
Protopic Ointment 1397

Terfenadine (Concurrent use of erythromycin in patients receiving drugs metabolized by the cytochrome P450 system may be associated with elevation in serum levels of terfenadine; co-administration is contraindicated).
No products indexed under this heading.

Theophylline (Co-administration in patients who are receiving high doses of theophylline may be associated with an increase in serum theophylline levels and potential theophylline toxicity). Products include:
Aerolate 1361
Theo-Dur Extended-Release Tablets 1835
Uni-Dur Extended-Release Tablets .. 1841
Uniphyl 400 mg and 600 mg Tablets 2903

Theophylline Calcium Salicylate (Co-administration in patients who are receiving high doses of theophylline may be associated with an increase in serum theophylline levels and potential theophylline toxicity).
No products indexed under this heading.

Theophylline Sodium Glycinate (Co-administration in patients who are receiving high doses of theophylline may be associated with an increase in serum theophylline levels and potential theophylline toxicity).
No products indexed under this heading.

Triazolam (Erythromycin has been reported to decrease the clearance of triazolam and, thus, may increase the pharmacologic effect of the benzodiazepine). Products include:
Halcion Tablets 2823

Valproate Sodium (Concurrent use of erythromycin in patients receiving drugs metabolized by the cytochrome P450 system may be associated with elevation in serum levels of valproate). Products include:
Depacon Injection 416

Valproic Acid (Concurrent use of erythromycin in patients receiving drugs metabolized by the cytochrome P450 system may be associated with elevation in serum levels of valproate). Products include:
Depakene 421

Warfarin Sodium (Co-administration has resulted in increased anticoagulant effects). Products include:
Coumadin for Injection 1243
Coumadin Tablets 1243
Warfarin Sodium Tablets, USP 3302

ERYPED CHEWABLE TABLETS

(Erythromycin Ethylsuccinate) 446
See EryPed Drops

ERY-TAB TABLETS

(Erythromycin) 448
May interact with oral anticoagulants, phenytoin, valproate, theophylline, and certain other agents. Compounds in these categories include:

Alfentanil Hydrochloride (Concurrent use of erythromycin in patients receiving drugs metabolized by the cytochrome P450 system may be associated with elevation in serum levels of alfentanil).
No products indexed under this heading.

Aminophylline (Co-administration in patients who are receiving high doses of theophylline may be associated with an increase in serum theophylline levels and potential theophylline toxicity).
No products indexed under this heading.

Astemizole (Concurrent use of erythromycin in patients receiving astemizole has been reported to significantly alter the metabolism of astemizole; rare cases of cardiovascular adverse events, including prolonged QT interval, cardiac arrest, torsade de pointes, and other ventricular arrhythmias have been reported; co-administration is contraindicated).
No products indexed under this heading.

Bromocriptine Mesylate (Concurrent use of erythromycin in patients receiving drugs metabolized by the cytochrome P450 system may be associated with elevation in serum levels of bromocriptine).
No products indexed under this heading.

Carbamazepine (Concurrent use of erythromycin in patients receiving drugs metabolized by the cytochrome P450 system may be associated with elevation in serum levels of carbamazepine). Products include:
Carbatrol Capsules 3234
Tegretol/Tegretol-XR 2404

Cisapride (Concurrent use of erythromycin in patients receiving cisapride has been reported to inhibit the metabolism of cisapride; cases of cardiovascular adverse events, including prolonged QT interval, cardiac arrest, torsade de pointes, ventricular tachycardia,ventricular fibrillation and fatalities have been reported; co-administration is contraindicated).
No products indexed under this heading.

Cyclosporine (Concurrent use of erythromycin in patients receiving drugs metabolized by the cytochrome P450 system may be associated with elevation in serum levels of cyclosporine). Products include:
Gengraf Capsules 457
Neoral Soft Gelatin Capsules 2380
Neoral Oral Solution 2380
Sandimmune 2388

Dicumarol (Co-administration has resulted in increased anticoagulant effects; these effects may be pronounced in the elderly).
No products indexed under this heading.

Digoxin (Co-administration has been reported to result in elevated digoxin serum levels). Products include:
Digitek Tablets 1003
Lanoxicaps Capsules 1574
Lanoxin Injection 1581
Lanoxin Tablets 1587
Lanoxin Elixir Pediatric 1578
Lanoxin Injection Pediatric 1584

Dihydroergotamine Mesylate (Co-administration has been associated in some patients with acute ergot toxicity characterized by severe peripheral vasospasm and dysethesia). Products include:
- D.H.E. 45 Injection 2334
- Migranal Nasal Spray 2376

Disopyramide Phosphate (Concurrent use of erythromycin in patients receiving drugs metabolized by the cytochrome P450 system may be associated with elevation in serum levels of disopyramide).
- No products indexed under this heading.

Divalproex Sodium (Concurrent use of erythromycin in patients receiving drugs metabolized by the cytochrome P450 system may be associated with elevation in serum levels of valproate). Products include:
- Depakote Sprinkle Capsules 426
- Depakote Tablets 430
- Depakote ER Tablets 436

Dyphylline (Co-administration in patients who are receiving high doses of theophylline may be associated with an increase in serum theophylline levels and potential theophylline toxicity). Products include:
- Lufyllin Tablets 3347
- Lufyllin-400 Tablets 3347
- Lufyllin-GG Elixir 3348
- Lufyllin-GG Tablets 3348

Ergotamine Tartrate (Co-administration has been associated in some patients with acute ergot toxicity characterized by severe peripheral vasospasm and dysethesia).
- No products indexed under this heading.

Fosphenytoin Sodium (Concurrent use of erythromycin in patients receiving drugs metabolized by the cytochrome P450 system may be associated with elevation in serum levels of phenytoin). Products include:
- Cerebyx Injection 2619

Hexobarbital (Concurrent use of erythromycin in patients receiving drugs metabolized by the cytochrome P450 system may be associated with elevation in serum levels of hexobarbital).

Lovastatin (Concurrent use of erythromycin in patients receiving drugs metabolized by the cytochrome P450 system may be associated with elevation in serum levels of lovastatin). Products include:
- Mevacor Tablets 2132

Midazolam Hydrochloride (Erythromycin has been reported to decrease clearance of midazolam and, thus, may increase the pharmacologic effect of the benzodiazepines). Products include:
- Versed Injection 3027
- Versed Syrup 3033

Phenytoin (Concurrent use of erythromycin in patients receiving drugs metabolized by the cytochrome P450 system may be associated with elevation in serum levels of phenytoin). Products include:
- Dilantin Infatabs 2624
- Dilantin-125 Oral Suspension 2625

Phenytoin Sodium (Concurrent use of erythromycin in patients receiving drugs metabolized by the cytochrome P450 system may be associated with elevation in serum levels of phenytoin). Products include:
- Dilantin Kapseals 2622

Tacrolimus (Concurrent use of erythromycin in patients receiving drugs metabolized by the cytochrome P450 system may be associated with elevation in serum levels of tacrolimus). Products include:
- Prograf 1393
- Protopic Ointment 1397

Terfenadine (Concurrent use of erythromycin in patients receiving terfenadine has been reported to significantly alter the metabolism of terfenadine; rare cases of cardiovascular adverse events, including prolonged QT interval, cardiac arrest, torsade de pointes, other ventricular arrhythmias, and death have been reported; co-administration is contraindicated).
- No products indexed under this heading.

Theophylline (Co-administration in patients who are receiving high doses of theophylline may be associated with an increase in serum theophylline levels and potential theophylline toxicity). Products include:
- Aerolate 1361
- Theo-Dur Extended-Release Tablets 1835
- Uni-Dur Extended-Release Tablets 1841
- Uniphyl 400 mg and 600 mg Tablets 2903

Theophylline Calcium Salicylate (Co-administration in patients who are receiving high doses of theophylline may be associated with an increase in serum theophylline levels and potential theophylline toxicity).
- No products indexed under this heading.

Theophylline Sodium Glycinate (Co-administration in patients who are receiving high doses of theophylline may be associated with an increase in serum theophylline levels and potential theophylline toxicity).
- No products indexed under this heading.

Triazolam (Erythromycin has been reported to decrease clearance of triazolam and, thus, may increase the pharmacologic effect of the benzodiazepines). Products include:
- Halcion Tablets 2823

Valproate Sodium (Concurrent use of erythromycin in patients receiving drugs metabolized by the cytochrome P450 system may be associated with elevation in serum levels of valproate). Products include:
- Depacon Injection 416

Valproic Acid (Concurrent use of erythromycin in patients receiving drugs metabolized by the cytochrome P450 system may be associated with elevation in serum levels of valproate). Products include:
- Depakene 421

Warfarin Sodium (Co-administration has resulted in increased anticoagulant effects; these effects may be pronounced in the elderly). Products include:
- Coumadin for Injection 1243
- Coumadin Tablets 1243
- Warfarin Sodium Tablets, USP 3302

ERYTHROCIN STEARATE FILMTAB TABLETS

(Erythromycin Stearate) 452

May interact with oral anticoagulants, phenytoin, valproate, theophylline, and certain other agents. Compounds in these categories include:

Alfentanil Hydrochloride (Potential for elevated serum alfentanil levels).
- No products indexed under this heading.

Aminophylline (Co-administration in patients who are receiving high doses of theophylline may be associated with an increase in serum theophylline levels and potential theophylline toxicity).
- No products indexed under this heading.

Astemizole (Co-administration has produced a significant alteration in astemizole metabolism resulting in rare cases of serious cardiovascular adverse events, including QT prolongation, cardiac arrest, torsade de pointes and death; concurrent use is contraindicated).
- No products indexed under this heading.

Bromocriptine Mesylate (Potential for elevated serum bromocriptine levels).
- No products indexed under this heading.

Carbamazepine (Potential for elevated serum carbamazepine levels). Products include:
- Carbatrol Capsules 3234
- Tegretol/Tegretol-XR 2404

Cisapride (Co-administration has produced an inhibition of hepatic metabolism of cisapride metabolism resulting in QT prolongation, cardiac arrhythmias, ventricular tachycardia, ventricular fibrillation, and torsade de pointes; concurrent use is contraindicated).
- No products indexed under this heading.

Cyclosporine (Potential for elevated serum cyclosporine levels). Products include:
- Gengraf Capsules 457
- Neoral Soft Gelatin Capsules 2380
- Neoral Oral Solution 2380
- Sandimmune 2388

Dicumarol (Co-administration has been reported to result in increased anticoagulant effects).
- No products indexed under this heading.

Digoxin (Co-administration has been reported to result in elevated digoxin serum levels). Products include:
- Digitek Tablets 1003
- Lanoxicaps Capsules 1574
- Lanoxin Injection 1581
- Lanoxin Tablets 1587
- Lanoxin Elixir Pediatric 1578
- Lanoxin Injection Pediatric 1584

Dihydroergotamine Mesylate (Co-administration has been reported to result in acute ergot toxicity characterized by severe peripheral vasospasm and dysesthesia). Products include:
- D.H.E. 45 Injection 2334
- Migranal Nasal Spray 2376

Disopyramide Phosphate (Potential for elevated serum disopyramide levels).
- No products indexed under this heading.

Divalproex Sodium (Potential for elevated serum valproate levels). Products include:
- Depakote Sprinkle Capsules 426
- Depakote Tablets 430
- Depakote ER Tablets 436

Dyphylline (Co-administration in patients who are receiving high doses of theophylline may be associated with an increase in serum theophylline levels and potential theophylline toxicity). Products include:
- Lufyllin Tablets 3347
- Lufyllin-400 Tablets 3347
- Lufyllin-GG Elixir 3348
- Lufyllin-GG Tablets 3348

Ergotamine Tartrate (Co-administration has been reported to result in acute ergot toxicity characterized by severe peripheral vasospasm and dysesthesia).
- No products indexed under this heading.

Fosphenytoin Sodium (Potential for elevated serum phenytoin levels). Products include:
- Cerebyx Injection 2619

Hexobarbital (Potential for elevated serum hexobarbital levels).
- No products indexed under this heading.

Lovastatin (Potential for elevated serum lovastatin levels). Products include:
- Mevacor Tablets 2132

Midazolam Hydrochloride (Erythromycin has been reported to decrease the clearance of midazolam and may increase the pharmacologic effect of the benzodiazepine). Products include:
- Versed Injection 3027
- Versed Syrup 3033

Phenytoin (Potential for elevated serum phenytoin levels). Products include:
- Dilantin Infatabs 2624
- Dilantin-125 Oral Suspension 2625

Phenytoin Sodium (Potential for elevated serum phenytoin levels). Products include:
- Dilantin Kapseals 2622

Tacrolimus (Potential for elevated serum tacrolimus levels). Products include:
- Prograf 1393
- Protopic Ointment 1397

Terfenadine (Co-administration has produced a significant alteration in terfenadine metabolism resulting in rare cases of serious cardiovascular adverse events, including QT prolongation, cardiac arrest, torsade de pointes and death; concurrent use is contraindicated).
- No products indexed under this heading.

Theophylline (Co-administration in patients who are receiving high doses of theophylline may be associated with an increase in serum theophylline levels and potential theophylline toxicity). Products include:
- Aerolate 1361
- Theo-Dur Extended-Release Tablets 1835
- Uni-Dur Extended-Release Tablets 1841
- Uniphyl 400 mg and 600 mg Tablets 2903

Theophylline Calcium Salicylate (Co-administration in patients who are receiving high doses of theophylline may be associated with an increase in serum theophylline levels and potential theophylline toxicity).
- No products indexed under this heading.

Theophylline Sodium Glycinate (Co-administration in patients who are receiving high doses of theophylline may be associated with an increase in serum theophylline levels and potential theophylline toxicity).
- No products indexed under this heading.

Triazolam (Erythromycin has been reported to decrease the clearance of triazolam and may increase the pharmacologic effect of the benzodiazepine). Products include:
- Halcion Tablets 2823

Valproate Sodium (Potential for elevated serum valproate levels). Products include:
- Depacon Injection 416

Valproic Acid (Potential for elevated serum valproate levels). Products include:
- Depakene 421

Warfarin Sodium (Co-administration has been reported to result in increased anticoagulant effects). Products include:
- Coumadin for Injection 1243
- Coumadin Tablets 1243
- Warfarin Sodium Tablets, USP 3302

ERYTHROMYCIN BASE FILMTAB TABLETS

(Erythromycin) 454

May interact with oral anticoagulants, phenytoin, valproate, theophylline, and certain other agents. Compounds in these categories include:

Alfentanil Hydrochloride (Potential for elevated serum alfentanil levels).
- No products indexed under this heading.

Aminophylline (Co-administration in patients who are receiving high doses of theophylline may be associated with an increase in serum theophylline levels and potential theophylline toxicity).
No products indexed under this heading.

Astemizole (Co-administration has produced a significant alteration in astemizole metabolism resulting in rare cases of serious cardiovascular adverse events, including QT prolongation, cardiac arrest, torsade de pointes and death; concurrent use is contraindicated).
No products indexed under this heading.

Bromocriptine Mesylate (Potential for elevated serum bromocriptine levels).
No products indexed under this heading.

Carbamazepine (Potential for elevated serum carbamazepine levels). Products include:
Carbatrol Capsules ... 3234
Tegretol/Tegretol-XR ... 2404

Cisapride (Co-administration has produced an inhibition of hepatic metabolism of cisapride metabolism resulting in QT prolongation, cardiac arrhythmias, ventricular fibrillation, and torsade de pointes; concurrent use is contraindicated).
No products indexed under this heading.

Cyclosporine (Potential for elevated serum cyclosporine levels). Products include:
Gengraf Capsules ... 457
Neoral Soft Gelatin Capsules ... 2380
Neoral Oral Solution ... 2380
Sandimmune ... 2388

Dicumarol (Co-administration has been reported to result in increased anticoagulant effects).
No products indexed under this heading.

Digoxin (Co-administration has been reported to result in elevated digoxin serum levels). Products include:
Digitek Tablets ... 1003
Lanoxicaps Capsules ... 1574
Lanoxin Injection ... 1581
Lanoxin Tablets ... 1587
Lanoxin Elixir Pediatric ... 1578
Lanoxin Injection Pediatric ... 1584

Dihydroergotamine Mesylate (Co-administration has been reported to result in acute ergot toxicity characterized by severe peripheral vasospasm and dysesthesia). Products include:
D.H.E. 45 Injection ... 2334
Migranal Nasal Spray ... 2376

Disopyramide Phosphate (Potential for elevated serum disopyramide levels).
No products indexed under this heading.

Divalproex Sodium (Potential for elevated serum valproate levels). Products include:
Depakote Sprinkle Capsules ... 426
Depakote Tablets ... 430
Depakote ER Tablets ... 436

Dyphylline (Co-administration in patients who are receiving high doses of theophylline may be associated with an increase in serum theophylline levels and potential theophylline toxicity). Products include:
Lufyllin Tablets ... 3347
Lufyllin-400 Tablets ... 3347
Lufyllin-GG Elixir ... 3348
Lufyllin-GG Tablets ... 3348

Ergotamine Tartrate (Co-administration has been reported to result in acute ergot toxicity characterized by severe peripheral vasospasm and dysesthesia).
No products indexed under this heading.

Fosphenytoin Sodium (Potential for elevated serum phenytoin levels). Products include:
Cerebyx Injection ... 2619

Hexobarbital (Potential for elevated serum hexobarbital levels).
No products indexed under this heading.

Lovastatin (Potential for elevated serum lovastatin levels). Products include:
Mevacor Tablets ... 2132

Midazolam Hydrochloride (Erythromycin has been reported to decrease the clearance of midazolam and may increase the pharmacologic effect of benzodiazepine). Products include:
Versed Injection ... 3027
Versed Syrup ... 3033

Phenytoin (Potential for elevated serum phenytoin levels). Products include:
Dilantin Infatabs ... 2624
Dilantin-125 Oral Suspension ... 2625

Phenytoin Sodium (Potential for elevated serum phenytoin levels). Products include:
Dilantin Kapseals ... 2622

Tacrolimus (Potential for elevated serum tacrolimus levels). Products include:
Prograf ... 1393
Protopic Ointment ... 1397

Terfenadine (Co-administration has produced a significant alteration in terfenadine metabolism resulting in rare cases of serious cardiovascular events, including QT prolongation, cardiac arrest, torsade de pointes and death; concurrent use is contraindicated).
No products indexed under this heading.

Theophylline (Co-administration in patients who are receiving high doses of theophylline may be associated with an increase in serum theophylline levels and potential theophylline toxicity). Products include:
Aerolate ... 1361
Theo-Dur Extended-Release Tablets ... 1835
Uni-Dur Extended-Release Tablets .. 1841
Uniphyl 400 mg and 600 mg Tablets ... 2903

Theophylline Calcium Salicylate (Co-administration in patients who are receiving high doses of theophylline may be associated with an increase in serum theophylline levels and potential theophylline toxicity).
No products indexed under this heading.

Theophylline Sodium Glycinate (Co-administration in patients who are receiving high doses of theophylline may be associated with an increase in serum theophylline levels and potential theophylline toxicity).
No products indexed under this heading.

Triazolam (Erythromycin has been reported to decrease the clearance of triazolam and may increase the pharmacologic effect of the benzodiazepine). Products include:
Halcion Tablets ... 2823

Valproate Sodium (Potential for elevated serum valproate levels). Products include:
Depacon Injection ... 416

Valproic Acid (Potential for elevated serum valproate levels). Products include:
Depakene ... 421

Warfarin Sodium (Co-administration has been reported to result in increased anticoagulant effects). Products include:
Coumadin for Injection ... 1243
Coumadin Tablets ... 1243
Warfarin Sodium Tablets, USP ... 3302

ERYTHROMYCIN DELAYED-RELEASE CAPSULES, USP

(Erythromycin) ... 455
May interact with oral anticoagulants, theophylline, and certain other agents. Compounds in these categories include:

Aminophylline (Concomitant administration with high doses of theophylline may be associated with increased theophylline levels and potential toxicity).
No products indexed under this heading.

Carbamazepine (Elevations in serum erythromycin and carbamazepine concentration). Products include:
Carbatrol Capsules ... 3234
Tegretol/Tegretol-XR ... 2404

Cyclosporine (Elevations in serum erythromycin and cyclosporine concentration). Products include:
Gengraf Capsules ... 457
Neoral Soft Gelatin Capsules ... 2380
Neoral Oral Solution ... 2380
Sandimmune ... 2388

Dicumarol (Increased anticoagulant effects).
No products indexed under this heading.

Digoxin (Elevated digoxin serum levels). Products include:
Digitek Tablets ... 1003
Lanoxicaps Capsules ... 1574
Lanoxin Injection ... 1581
Lanoxin Tablets ... 1587
Lanoxin Elixir Pediatric ... 1578
Lanoxin Injection Pediatric ... 1584

Dihydroergotamine Mesylate (Potential for acute ergot toxicity characterized by severe peripheral vasospasm and dysesthesia). Products include:
D.H.E. 45 Injection ... 2334
Migranal Nasal Spray ... 2376

Drugs that Undergo Biotransformation by Cytochrome P-450 Mixed Function Oxidase (Potential for elevation in serum levels).
No products indexed under this heading.

Dyphylline (Concomitant administration with high doses of theophylline may be associated with increased theophylline levels and potential toxicity). Products include:
Lufyllin Tablets ... 3347
Lufyllin-400 Tablets ... 3347
Lufyllin-GG Elixir ... 3348
Lufyllin-GG Tablets ... 3348

Ergotamine Tartrate (Potential for acute ergot toxicity characterized by severe peripheral vasospasm and dysesthesia).
No products indexed under this heading.

Hexobarbital (Elevations in serum erythromycin and hexobarbital concentration).
No products indexed under this heading.

Lovastatin (Potential for rhabdomyolysis in seriously ill patients). Products include:
Mevacor Tablets ... 2132

Phenytoin (Elevations in serum erythromycin and phenytoin concentration). Products include:
Dilantin Infatabs ... 2624
Dilantin-125 Oral Suspension ... 2625

Phenytoin Sodium (Elevations in serum erythromycin and phenytoin concentration). Products include:
Dilantin Kapseals ... 2622

Terfenadine (Potential for altered terfenadine metabolism).
No products indexed under this heading.

Theophylline (Concomitant administration with high doses of theophylline may be associated with increased theophylline levels and potential toxicity). Products include:
Aerolate ... 1361
Theo-Dur Extended-Release Tablets ... 1835
Uni-Dur Extended-Release Tablets .. 1841
Uniphyl 400 mg and 600 mg Tablets ... 2903

Theophylline Calcium Salicylate (Concomitant administration with high doses of theophylline may be associated with increased theophylline levels and potential toxicity).
No products indexed under this heading.

Theophylline Sodium Glycinate (Concomitant administration with high doses of theophylline may be associated with increased theophylline levels and potential toxicity).
No products indexed under this heading.

Triazolam (Decreased clearance of triazolam and increased the pharmacologic effect of triazolam). Products include:
Halcion Tablets ... 2823

Warfarin Sodium (Increased anticoagulant effects). Products include:
Coumadin for Injection ... 1243
Coumadin Tablets ... 1243
Warfarin Sodium Tablets, USP ... 3302

Food Interactions

Food, unspecified (Lowers the blood levels of systemically available erythromycin).

ESCLIM TRANSDERMAL SYSTEM

(Estradiol) ... 3460
None cited in PDR database.

ESKALITH CAPSULES

(Lithium Carbonate) ... 1527
May interact with ACE inhibitors, calcium channel blockers, diuretics, antipsychotic agents, neuromuscular blocking agents, non-steroidal anti-inflammatory agents, selective serotonin reuptake inhibitors, urinary alkalinizing agents, theophylline, and certain other agents. Compounds in these categories include:

Acetazolamide (Increases urinary lithium excretion). Products include:
Diamox Sequels Sustained Release Capsules ... ⊙270
Diamox Tablets ... ⊙269

Amiloride Hydrochloride (Diuretic-induced sodium loss may reduce the renal clearance of lithium and increase serum lithium levels with risk of lithium toxicity). Products include:
Midamor Tablets ... 2136
Moduretic Tablets ... 2138

Aminophylline (Lowers serum lithium concentrations).
No products indexed under this heading.

Amlodipine Besylate (Increases the risk of neurotoxicity). Products include:
Lotrel Capsules ... 2370
Norvasc Tablets ... 2704

Atracurium Besylate (Lithium may prolong the effect of neuromuscular blocking agents).
No products indexed under this heading.

Benazepril Hydrochloride (May substantially increase steady-state plasma lithium levels resulting in lithium toxicity). Products include:
Lotensin Tablets ... 2365
Lotensin HCT Tablets ... 2367
Lotrel Capsules ... 2370

Bendroflumethiazide (Diuretic-induced sodium loss may reduce the renal clearance of lithium and increase serum lithium levels with risk of lithium toxicity). Products include:
Corzide 40/5 Tablets ... 2247
Corzide 80/5 Tablets ... 2247

Bepridil Hydrochloride (Increases the risk of neurotoxicity). Products include:
Vascor Tablets ... 2602

Bumetanide (Diuretic-induced sodium loss may reduce the renal clearance of lithium and increase serum lithium levels with risk of lithium toxicity).
No products indexed under this heading.

Captopril (May substantially increase steady-state plasma lithium levels resulting in lithium toxicity). Products include:
Captopril Tablets ... 2281

Carbamazepine (Effect of co-administration not specified in the current prescribing information). Products include:
Carbatrol Capsules ... 3234
Tegretol/Tegretol-XR ... 2404

Celecoxib (Lithium-indomethacin-type interaction may occur with other nonsteroidal anti-inflammatory agents; potential for increase in steady-state plasma lithium levels). Products include:
Celebrex Capsules ... 2676
Celebrex Capsules ... 2780

Chlorothiazide (Diuretic-induced sodium loss may reduce the renal clearance of lithium and increase serum lithium levels with risk of lithium toxicity). Products include:
Aldoclor Tablets ... 2035
Diuril Oral ... 2087

Chlorothiazide Sodium (Diuretic-induced sodium loss may reduce the renal clearance of lithium and increase serum lithium levels with risk of lithium toxicity). Products include:
Diuril Sodium Intravenous ... 2086

Chlorpromazine (Potential for an encephalopathic syndrome with possible irreversible brain damage with co-administration of lithium with a neuroleptic). Products include:
Thorazine Suppositories ... 1656

Chlorpromazine Hydrochloride (Potential for an encephalopathic syndrome with possible irreversible brain damage with co-administration of lithium with a neuroleptic). Products include:
Thorazine ... 1656

Chlorprothixene (Potential for an encephalopathic syndrome with possible irreversible brain damage with co-administration of lithium with a neuroleptic).
No products indexed under this heading.

Chlorprothixene Hydrochloride (Potential for an encephalopathic syndrome with possible irreversible brain damage with co-administration of lithium with a neuroleptic).
No products indexed under this heading.

Chlorthalidone (Diuretic-induced sodium loss may reduce the renal clearance of lithium and increase serum lithium levels with risk of lithium toxicity). Products include:
Clorpres Tablets ... 1002
Combipres Tablets ... 1040
Tenoretic Tablets ... 690

Cisatracurium Besylate (Lithium may prolong the effect of neuromuscular blocking agents).
No products indexed under this heading.

Citalopram Hydrobromide (Co-administration with selective serotonin reuptake inhibitors has been reported to result in diarrhea, confusion, tremor, dizziness and agitation). Products include:
Celexa ... 1365

Clozapine (Potential for an encephalopathic syndrome with possible irreversible brain damage with co-administration of lithium with a neuroleptic). Products include:
Clozaril Tablets ... 2319

Diclofenac Potassium (Lithium-indomethacin-type interaction may occur with other nonsteroidal anti-inflammatory agents; potential for increase in steady-state plasma lithium levels). Products include:
Cataflam Tablets ... 2315

Diclofenac Sodium (Lithium-indomethacin-type interaction may occur with other nonsteroidal anti-inflammatory agents; potential for increase in steady-state plasma lithium levels). Products include:
Arthrotec Tablets ... 3195
Voltaren Ophthalmic Sterile Ophthalmic Solution ... ⊙312
Voltaren Tablets ... 2315
Voltaren-XR Tablets ... 2315

Diltiazem Hydrochloride (Increases the risk of neurotoxicity). Products include:
Cardizem Injectable ... 1018
Cardizem Lyo-Ject Syringe ... 1018
Cardizem Monovial ... 1018
Cardizem CD Capsules ... 1016
Tiazac Capsules ... 1378

Doxacurium Chloride (Lithium may prolong the effect of neuromuscular blocking agents).
No products indexed under this heading.

Dyphylline (Lowers serum lithium concentrations). Products include:
Lufyllin Tablets ... 3347
Lufyllin-400 Tablets ... 3347
Lufyllin-GG Elixir ... 3348
Lufyllin-GG Tablets ... 3348

Enalapril Maleate (May substantially increase steady-state plasma lithium levels resulting in lithium toxicity). Products include:
Lexxel Tablets ... 608
Vaseretic Tablets ... 2204
Vasotec Tablets ... 2210

Enalaprilat (May substantially increase steady-state plasma lithium levels resulting in lithium toxicity). Products include:
Enalaprilat Injection ... 863
Vasotec I.V. Injection ... 2207

Ethacrynic Acid (Diuretic-induced sodium loss may reduce the renal clearance of lithium and increase serum lithium levels with risk of lithium toxicity). Products include:
Edecrin Tablets ... 2091

Etodolac (Lithium-indomethacin-type interaction may occur with other nonsteroidal anti-inflammatory agents; potential for increase in steady-state plasma lithium levels). Products include:
Lodine ... 3528
Lodine XL Extended-Release Tablets ... 3530

Felodipine (Increases the risk of neurotoxicity). Products include:
Lexxel Tablets ... 608
Plendil Extended-Release Tablets ... 623

Fenoprofen Calcium (Lithium-indomethacin-type interaction may occur with other nonsteroidal anti-inflammatory agents; potential for increase in steady-state plasma lithium levels).
No products indexed under this heading.

Fluoxetine Hydrochloride (Co-administration with selective serotonin reuptake inhibitors has been reported to result in diarrhea, confusion, tremor, dizziness and agitation). Products include:
Prozac Pulvules, Liquid, and Weekly Capsules ... 1238
Sarafem Pulvules ... 1962

Fluphenazine Decanoate (Potential for an encephalopathic syndrome with possible irreversible brain damage with co-administration of lithium with a neuroleptic).
No products indexed under this heading.

Fluphenazine Enanthate (Potential for an encephalopathic syndrome with possible irreversible brain damage with co-administration of lithium with a neuroleptic).
No products indexed under this heading.

Fluphenazine Hydrochloride (Potential for an encephalopathic syndrome with possible irreversible brain damage with co-administration of lithium with a neuroleptic).
No products indexed under this heading.

Flurbiprofen (Lithium-indomethacin-type interaction may occur with other nonsteroidal anti-inflammatory agents; potential for increase in steady-state plasma lithium levels).
No products indexed under this heading.

Fluvoxamine Maleate (Co-administration with selective serotonin reuptake inhibitors has been reported to result in diarrhea, confusion, tremor, dizziness and agitation). Products include:
Luvox Tablets (25, 50, 100 mg) ... 3256

Fosinopril Sodium (May substantially increase steady-state plasma lithium levels resulting in lithium toxicity). Products include:
Monopril Tablets ... 1091
Monopril HCT ... 1094

Fosphenytoin Sodium (Effect of co-administration not specified in the current prescribing information). Products include:
Cerebyx Injection ... 2619

Furosemide (Diuretic-induced sodium loss may reduce the renal clearance of lithium and increase serum lithium levels with risk of lithium toxicity). Products include:
Furosemide Tablets ... 2284

Haloperidol (Potential for an encephalopathic syndrome with possible irreversible brain damage with co-administration of lithium with a neuroleptic). Products include:
Haldol Injection, Tablets and Concentrate ... 2533

Haloperidol Decanoate (Potential for an encephalopathic syndrome with possible irreversible brain damage with co-administration of lithium with a neuroleptic). Products include:
Haldol Decanoate ... 2535

Hydrochlorothiazide (Diuretic-induced sodium loss may reduce the renal clearance of lithium and increase serum lithium levels with risk of lithium toxicity). Products include:
Accuretic Tablets ... 2614
Aldoril Tablets ... 2039
Atacand HCT Tablets ... 597
Avalide Tablets ... 1070
Diovan HCT Tablets ... 2338
Dyazide Capsules ... 1515
HydroDIURIL Tablets ... 2108
Hyzaar ... 2109
Inderide Tablets ... 3517
Inderide LA Long-Acting Capsules ... 3519
Lotensin HCT Tablets ... 2367
Maxzide ... 1008
Micardis HCT Tablets ... 1051
Microzide Capsules ... 3414
Moduretic Tablets ... 2138
Monopril HCT ... 1094
Prinzide Tablets ... 2168
Timolide Tablets ... 2187
Uniretic Tablets ... 3178
Vaseretic Tablets ... 2204
Zestoretic Tablets ... 695
Ziac Tablets ... 1887

Hydroflumethiazide (Diuretic-induced sodium loss may reduce the renal clearance of lithium and increase serum lithium levels with risk of lithium toxicity). Products include:
Diucardin Tablets ... 3494

Ibuprofen (Lithium-indomethacin-type interaction may occur with other nonsteroidal anti-inflammatory agents; potential for increase in steady-state plasma lithium levels). Products include:
Advil ... 771
Children's Advil Oral Suspension ... 773
Children's Advil Chewable Tablets ... 773
Advil Cold and Sinus Caplets ... 771
Advil Cold and Sinus Tablets ... 771
Advil Flu & Body Ache Caplets ... 772
Infants' Advil Drops ... 773
Junior Strength Advil Tablets ... 773
Junior Strength Advil Chewable Tablets ... 773
Advil Migraine Liquigels ... 772
Children's Motrin Oral Suspension and Chewable Tablets ... 2006
Children's Motrin Cold Oral Suspension ... 2007
Children's Motrin Oral Suspension ... 643
Motrin Suspension, Oral Drops, Chewable Tablets, and Caplets ... 2002
Infants' Motrin Concentrated Drops ... 2006
Junior Strength Motrin Caplets and Chewable Tablets ... 2006
Motrin IB Tablets, Caplets, and Gelcaps ... 2002
Motrin Migraine Pain Caplets ... 2005
Motrin Sinus Headache Caplets ... 2005
Vicoprofen Tablets ... 520

Indapamide (Diuretic-induced sodium loss may reduce the renal clearance of lithium and increase serum lithium levels with risk of lithium toxicity). Products include:
Indapamide Tablets ... 2286

Indomethacin (Co-administration has resulted in significant increase in steady-state plasma lithium levels with risk of lithium toxicity). Products include:
Indocin ... 2112

Indomethacin Sodium Trihydrate (Co-administration has resulted in significant increase in steady-state plasma lithium levels with risk of lithium toxicity). Products include:
Indocin I.V. ... 2115

Isradipine (Increases the risk of neurotoxicity). Products include:
DynaCirc Capsules ... 2921
DynaCirc CR Tablets ... 2923

Ketoprofen (Lithium-indomethacin-type interaction may occur with other nonsteroidal anti-inflammatory agents; potential for increase in steady-state plasma lithium levels). Products include:
Orudis Capsules ... 3548
Orudis KT Tablets ... 778
Oruvail Capsules ... 3548

Ketorolac Tromethamine (Lithium-indomethacin-type interaction may occur with other nonsteroidal anti-inflammatory agents; potential for increase in steady-state plasma lithium levels). Products include:
Acular Ophthalmic Solution ... 544
Acular PF Ophthalmic Solution ... 544
Toradol ... 3018

Lisinopril (May substantially increase steady-state plasma lithium levels resulting in lithium toxicity). Products include:
Prinivil Tablets ... 2164
Prinzide Tablets ... 2168
Zestoretic Tablets ... 695
Zestril Tablets ... 698

Loxapine Hydrochloride (Potential for an encephalopathic syndrome with possible irreversible brain damage with co-administration of lithium with a neuroleptic).
No products indexed under this heading.

Loxapine Succinate (Potential for an encephalopathic syndrome with possible irreversible brain damage with co-administration of lithium with a neuroleptic). Products include:
Loxitane Capsules ... 3398

Meclofenamate Sodium (Lithium-indomethacin-type interaction may occur with other nonsteroidal anti-inflammatory agents; potential for increase in steady-state plasma lithium levels).
No products indexed under this heading.

Mefenamic Acid (Lithium-indomethacin-type interaction may occur with other nonsteroidal anti-inflammatory agents; potential for increase in steady-state plasma lithium levels). Products include:
Ponstel Capsules 1356

Meloxicam (Lithium-indomethacin-type interaction may occur with other nonsteroidal anti-inflammatory agents; potential for increase in steady-state plasma lithium levels). Products include:
Mobic Tablets 1054

Mesoridazine Besylate (Potential for an encephalopathic syndrome with possible irreversible brain damage with co-administration of lithium with a neuroleptic). Products include:
Serentil 1057

Methotrimeprazine (Potential for an encephalopathic syndrome with possible irreversible brain damage with co-administration of lithium with a neuroleptic).
No products indexed under this heading.

Methyclothiazide (Diuretic-induced sodium loss may reduce the renal clearance of lithium and increase serum lithium levels with risk of lithium toxicity).
No products indexed under this heading.

Methyldopa (Effect of co-administration not specified in the current prescribing information). Products include:
Aldoclor Tablets 2035
Aldomet Tablets 2037
Aldoril Tablets 2039

Metocurine Iodide (Lithium may prolong the effect of neuromuscular blocking agents).
No products indexed under this heading.

Metolazone (Diuretic-induced sodium loss may reduce the renal clearance of lithium and increase serum lithium levels with risk of lithium toxicity). Products include:
Mykrox Tablets 1168
Zaroxolyn Tablets 1177

Metronidazole (May provoke lithium toxicity due to reduced renal clearance). Products include:
MetroCream 1404
MetroGel 1405
MetroGel-Vaginal Gel 1986
MetroLotion 1405
Noritate Cream 1224

Metronidazole Hydrochloride (May provoke lithium toxicity due to reduced renal clearance).
No products indexed under this heading.

Mibefradil Dihydrochloride (Increases the risk of neurotoxicity).
No products indexed under this heading.

Mivacurium Chloride (Lithium may prolong the effect of neuromuscular blocking agents).
No products indexed under this heading.

Moexipril Hydrochloride (May substantially increase steady-state plasma lithium levels resulting in lithium toxicity). Products include:
Uniretic Tablets 3178
Univasc Tablets 3181

Molindone Hydrochloride (Potential for an encephalopathic syndrome with possible irreversible brain damage with co-administration of lithium with a neuroleptic). Products include:
Moban 1320

Nabumetone (Lithium-indomethacin-type interaction may occur with other nonsteroidal anti-inflammatory agents; potential for increase in steady-state plasma lithium levels). Products include:
Relafen Tablets 1617

Naproxen (Lithium-indomethacin-type interaction may occur with other nonsteroidal anti-inflammatory agents; potential for increase in steady-state plasma lithium levels). Products include:
EC-Naprosyn Delayed-Release Tablets 2967
Naprosyn Suspension 2967
Naprosyn Tablets 2967

Naproxen Sodium (Lithium-indomethacin-type interaction may occur with other nonsteroidal anti-inflammatory agents; potential for increase in steady-state plasma lithium levels). Products include:
Aleve Tablets, Caplets and Gelcaps .... ▣602
Aleve Cold & Sinus Caplets .... ▣603
Anaprox Tablets 2967
Anaprox DS Tablets 2967
Naprelan Tablets 1293

Nicardipine Hydrochloride (Increases the risk of neurotoxicity). Products include:
Cardene I.V. 3485

Nifedipine (Increases the risk of neurotoxicity). Products include:
Adalat CC Tablets 877
Procardia Capsules 2708
Procardia XL Extended Release Tablets 2710

Nimodipine (Increases the risk of neurotoxicity). Products include:
Nimotop Capsules 904

Nisoldipine (Increases the risk of neurotoxicity). Products include:
Sular Tablets 688

Olanzapine (Potential for an encephalopathic syndrome with possible irreversible brain damage with co-administration of lithium with a neuroleptic). Products include:
Zyprexa Tablets 1973
Zyprexa ZYDIS Orally Disintegrating Tablets 1973

Oxaprozin (Lithium-indomethacin-type interaction may occur with other nonsteroidal anti-inflammatory agents; potential for increase in steady-state plasma lithium levels).
No products indexed under this heading.

Pancuronium Bromide (Lithium may prolong the effect of neuromuscular blocking agents).
No products indexed under this heading.

Paroxetine Hydrochloride (Co-administration with selective serotonin reuptake inhibitors has been reported to result in diarrhea, confusion, tremor, dizziness and agitation). Products include:
Paxil 1609

Perindopril Erbumine (May substantially increase steady-state plasma lithium levels resulting in lithium toxicity). Products include:
Aceon Tablets (2 mg, 4 mg, 8 mg) 3249

Perphenazine (Potential for an encephalopathic syndrome with possible irreversible brain damage with co-administration of lithium with a neuroleptic). Products include:
Etrafon 3115
Trilafon 3160

Phenylbutazone (Lithium-indomethacin-type interaction may occur with other nonsteroidal anti-inflammatory agents; potential for increase in steady-state plasma lithium levels).
No products indexed under this heading.

Phenytoin (Effect of co-administration not specified in the current prescribing information). Products include:
Dilantin Infatabs 2624
Dilantin-125 Oral Suspension 2625

Phenytoin Sodium (Effect of co-administration not specified in the current prescribing information). Products include:
Dilantin Kapseals 2622

Pimozide (Potential for an encephalopathic syndrome with possible irreversible brain damage with co-administration of lithium with a neuroleptic). Products include:
Orap Tablets 1407

Piroxicam (Co-administration has resulted in significant increase in steady-state plasma lithium levels with risk of lithium toxicity). Products include:
Feldene Capsules 2685

Polythiazide (Diuretic-induced sodium loss may reduce the renal clearance of lithium and increase serum lithium levels with risk of lithium toxicity). Products include:
Minizide Capsules 2700
Renese Tablets 2712

Potassium Citrate (Increases urinary lithium excretion). Products include:
Urocit-K Tablets 2232

Prochlorperazine (Potential for an encephalopathic syndrome with possible irreversible brain damage with co-administration of lithium with a neuroleptic). Products include:
Compazine 1505

Promethazine Hydrochloride (Potential for an encephalopathic syndrome with possible irreversible brain damage with co-administration of lithium with a neuroleptic). Products include:
Mepergan Injection 3539
Phenergan Injection 3553
Phenergan 3556
Phenergan Syrup 3554
Phenergan with Codeine Syrup 3557
Phenergan with Dextromethorphan Syrup 3559
Phenergan VC Syrup 3560
Phenergan VC with Codeine Syrup 3561

Quetiapine Fumarate (Potential for an encephalopathic syndrome with possible irreversible brain damage with co-administration of lithium with a neuroleptic). Products include:
Seroquel Tablets 684

Quinapril Hydrochloride (May substantially increase steady-state plasma lithium levels resulting in lithium toxicity). Products include:
Accupril Tablets 2611
Accuretic Tablets 2614

Ramipril (May substantially increase steady-state plasma lithium levels resulting in lithium toxicity). Products include:
Altace Capsules 2233

Rapacuronium Bromide (Lithium may prolong the effect of neuromuscular blocking agents).
No products indexed under this heading.

Risperidone (Potential for an encephalopathic syndrome with possible irreversible brain damage with co-administration of lithium with a neuroleptic). Products include:
Risperdal 1796

Rocuronium Bromide (Lithium may prolong the effect of neuromuscular blocking agents). Products include:
Zemuron Injection 2491

Rofecoxib (Lithium-indomethacin-type interaction may occur with other nonsteroidal anti-inflammatory agents; potential for increase in steady-state plasma lithium levels). Products include:
Vioxx 2213

Sertraline Hydrochloride (Co-administration with selective serotonin reuptake inhibitors has been reported to result in diarrhea, confusion, tremor, dizziness and agitation). Products include:
Zoloft 2751

Sodium Bicarbonate (Increases urinary lithium excretion). Products include:
Alka-Seltzer .... ▣603
Alka-Seltzer Lemon Lime Antacid and Pain Reliever Effervescent Tablets .... ▣603
Alka-Seltzer Extra Strength Antacid and Pain Reliever Effervescent Tablets .... ▣603
Alka-Seltzer Heartburn Relief Tablets .... ▣604
Ceo-Two Evacuant Suppository .... ▣618
Colyte with Flavor Packs for Oral Solution 3170
GoLYTELY and Pineapple Flavor GoLYTELY for Oral Solution 1068
NuLYTELY, Cherry Flavor, Lemon-Lime Flavor, and Orange Flavor NuLYTELY for Oral Solution 1068

Sodium Citrate (Increases urinary lithium excretion).
No products indexed under this heading.

Spirapril Hydrochloride (May substantially increase steady-state plasma lithium levels resulting in lithium toxicity).
No products indexed under this heading.

Spironolactone (Diuretic-induced sodium loss may reduce the renal clearance of lithium and increase serum lithium levels with risk of lithium toxicity).
No products indexed under this heading.

Succinylcholine Chloride (Lithium may prolong the effect of neuromuscular blocking agents). Products include:
Anectine Injection 1476

Sulindac (Lithium-indomethacin-type interaction may occur with other nonsteroidal anti-inflammatory agents; potential for increase in steady-state plasma lithium levels). Products include:
Clinoril Tablets 2053

Theophylline (Lowers serum lithium concentrations). Products include:
Aerolate 1361
Theo-Dur Extended-Release Tablets 1835
Uni-Dur Extended-Release Tablets 1841
Uniphyl 400 mg and 600 mg Tablets 2903

Theophylline Calcium Salicylate (Lowers serum lithium concentrations).
No products indexed under this heading.

Theophylline Sodium Glycinate (Lowers serum lithium concentrations).
No products indexed under this heading.

Thioridazine Hydrochloride (Potential for an encephalopathic syndrome with possible irreversible brain damage with co-administration of lithium with a neuroleptic). Products include:
Thioridazine Hydrochloride Tablets 2289

Thiothixene (Potential for an encephalopathic syndrome with possible irreversible brain damage with co-administration of lithium with a neuroleptic). Products include:
Navane Capsules 2701
Thiothixene Capsules 2290

Tolmetin Sodium (Lithium-indomethacin-type interaction may occur with other nonsteroidal anti-inflammatory agents; potential for increase in steady-state plasma lithium levels). Products include:
Tolectin 2589

Torsemide (Diuretic-induced sodium loss may reduce the renal clearance of lithium and increase serum lithium levels with risk of lithium toxicity). Products include:
Demadex Tablets and Injection 2965

Trandolapril (May substantially increase steady-state plasma lithium levels resulting in lithium toxicity). Products include:
- Mavik Tablets 478
- Tarka Tablets 508

Triamterene (Diuretic-induced sodium loss may reduce the renal clearance of lithium and increase serum lithium levels with risk of lithium toxicity). Products include:
- Dyazide Capsules 1515
- Dyrenium Capsules 3458
- Maxzide 1008

Trifluoperazine Hydrochloride (Potential for an encephalopathic syndrome with possible irreversible brain damage with co-administration of lithium with a neuroleptic). Products include:
- Stelazine 1640

Urea (Systemic administration of urea with lithium therapy can lower serum lithium concentration by increasing urinary lithium excretion). Products include:
- Accuzyme Debriding Ointment 1725
- Amino-Cerv Creme 2231
- Panafil Ointment 1726

Vecuronium Bromide (Lithium may prolong the effect of neuromuscular blocking agents). Products include:
- Norcuron for Injection 2478

Verapamil Hydrochloride (Increases the risk of neurotoxicity). Products include:
- Covera-HS Tablets 3199
- Isoptin SR Tablets 467
- Tarka Tablets 508
- Verelan Capsules 3184
- Verelan PM Capsules 3186

Ziprasidone Hydrochloride (Potential for an encephalopathic syndrome with possible irreversible brain damage with co-administration of lithium with a neuroleptic). Products include:
- Geodon Capsules 2688

ESKALITH CR CONTROLLED RELEASE TABLETS

(Lithium Carbonate) 1527

See Eskalith Capsules

ESTINYL TABLETS

(Ethinyl Estradiol) 3112

None cited in PDR database.

ESTRACE VAGINAL CREAM

(Estradiol) 3358

None cited in PDR database.

ESTRACE TABLETS

(Estradiol) 3361

None cited in PDR database.

ESTRATEST TABLETS

(Estrogens, Esterified, Methyltestosterone) 3252

See Estratest H.S. Tablets

ESTRATEST H.S. TABLETS

(Estrogens, Esterified, Methyltestosterone) 3252

May interact with oral anticoagulants, insulin, and certain other agents. Compounds in these categories include:

Dicumarol (Decreased anticoagulant requirements).
- No products indexed under this heading.

Insulin, Human, Zinc Suspension (Decreased blood glucose and insulin requirements). Products include:
- Humulin L, 100 Units 1937
- Humulin U, 100 Units 1943
- Novolin L Human Insulin 10 ml Vials 2422

Insulin, Human NPH (Decreased blood glucose and insulin requirements). Products include:
- Humulin N, 100 Units 1939
- Humulin N NPH Pen 1940
- Novolin N Human Insulin 10 ml Vials 2422
- Novolin N PenFill 2423
- Novolin N Prefilled Syringe Disposable Insulin Delivery System 2425

Insulin, Human Regular (Decreased blood glucose and insulin requirements). Products include:
- Humulin R Regular (U-500) 1943
- Humulin R, 100 Units 1941
- Novolin R Human Insulin 10 ml Vials 2423
- Novolin R PenFill 2423
- Novolin R Prefilled Syringe Disposable Insulin Delivery System 2425
- Velosulin BR Human Insulin 10 ml Vials 2435

Insulin, Human Regular and Human NPH Mixture (Decreased blood glucose and insulin requirements). Products include:
- Humulin 50/50, 100 Units 1934
- Humulin 70/30, 100 Units 1935
- Humulin 70/30 Pen 1936
- Novolin 70/30 Human Insulin 10 ml Vials 2421
- Novolin 70/30 PenFill 2423
- Novolin 70/30 Prefilled Disposable Insulin Delivery System 2425

Insulin, NPH (Decreased blood glucose and insulin requirements). Products include:
- Iletin II, NPH (Pork), 100 Units 1946

Insulin, Regular (Decreased blood glucose and insulin requirements). Products include:
- Iletin II, Regular (Pork), 100 Units ... 1947

Insulin, Zinc Crystals (Decreased blood glucose and insulin requirements).
- No products indexed under this heading.

Insulin, Zinc Suspension (Decreased blood glucose and insulin requirements). Products include:
- Iletin II, Lente (Pork), 100 Units 1945

Insulin Aspart, Human Regular (Decreased blood glucose and insulin requirements).
- No products indexed under this heading.

Insulin glargine (Decreased blood glucose and insulin requirements). Products include:
- Lantus Injection 742

Insulin Lispro, Human (Decreased blood glucose and insulin requirements). Products include:
- Humalog 1926
- Humalog Mix 75/25 Pen 1928

Insulin Lispro Protamine, Human (Decreased blood glucose and insulin requirements). Products include:
- Humalog Mix 75/25 Pen 1928

Oxyphenbutazone (Concurrent use may result in elevated serum levels of oxyphenbutazone).
- No products indexed under this heading.

Warfarin Sodium (Decreased anticoagulant requirements). Products include:
- Coumadin for Injection 1243
- Coumadin Tablets 1243
- Warfarin Sodium Tablets, USP 3302

ESTRING VAGINAL RING

(Estradiol) 2811

May interact with:

Vaginally administered preparations, unspecified (It is recommended that Estring be removed during treatment with other vaginally administered preparations).
- No products indexed under this heading.

ESTROSTEP 21 TABLETS

(Ethinyl Estradiol, Norethindrone Acetate) 2627

May interact with methylprednisolone, phenytoin, prednisolone, tetracyclines, theophylline, and certain other agents. Compounds in these categories include:

Acetaminophen (May increase plasma ethinyl estradiol concentrations, possibly by inhibition of conjugation; oral contraceptives may induce the conjugation of other compounds, such as acetaminophen, resulting in decreased plasma concentrations of acetaminophen). Products include:
- Actifed Cold & Sinus Caplets and Tablets 688
- Alka-Seltzer Plus Liqui-Gels 604
- Alka-Seltzer Plus Cold & Flu Medicine Liqui-Gels 604
- Alka-Seltzer Plus Cold & Sinus Medicine Liqui-Gels 604
- Benadryl Allergy/Cold Tablets 691
- Benadryl Allergy Sinus Headache Caplets & Gelcaps 693
- Benadryl Severe Allergy & Sinus Headache Caplets 694
- Children's Cēpacol Sore Throat 788
- Comtrex Acute Head Cold & Sinus Pressure Relief Tablets 627
- Comtrex Deep Chest Cold & Congestion Relief Softgels 627
- Comtrex Flu Therapy & Fever Relief Daytime Caplets 628
- Comtrex Flu Therapy & Fever Relief Nighttime Tablets 628
- Comtrex Maximum Strength Multi-Symptom Cold & Cough Relief Tablets and Caplets 626
- Contac Severe Cold and Flu Caplets Maximum Strength 746
- Contac Severe Cold and Flu Caplets Non-Drowsy 746
- Coricidin 'D' Cold, Flu & Sinus Tablets 737
- Coricidin HBP Cold & Flu Tablets 738
- Coricidin HBP Maximum Strength Flu Tablets 738
- Coricidin HBP Night-Time Cold & Flu Tablets 738
- Darvon-N/Darvocet-N 1907
- Dimetapp Cold and Fever Suspension 775
- Dimetapp Nighttime Flu Liquid 776
- Dimetapp Non-Drowsy Flu Syrup 777
- Drixoral Allergy/Sinus Extended-Release Tablets 741
- Drixoral Cold & Flu Extended-Release Tablets 740
- Aspirin Free Excedrin Caplets and Geltabs 628
- Excedrin Extra-Strength Tablets, Caplets, and Geltabs 629
- Excedrin Migraine 1070
- Excedrin PM Tablets, Caplets, and Geltabs 631
- Goody's Body Pain Formula Powder 620
- Goody's Extra Strength Headache Powder 620
- Goody's Extra Strength Pain Relief Tablets 620
- Goody's PM Powder 621
- Hycomine Compound Tablets 1317
- Lortab 3319
- Lortab Elixir 3317
- Maxidone Tablets CIII 3399
- Maximum Strength Midol Menstrual Caplets and Gelcaps 612
- Maximum Strength Midol PMS Caplets and Gelcaps 613
- Maximum Strength Midol Teen Caplets 612
- Midrin Capsules 3464
- Norco 5/325 Tablets CIII 3424
- Norco 7.5/325 Tablets CIII 3425
- Norco 10/325 Tablets CIII 3427
- Norco 10/325 Tablets CIII 3425
- Percocet Tablets 1326
- Percogesic Aspirin-Free Coated Tablets 667
- Extra Strength Percogesic Aspirin-Free Coated Caplets 665
- Phrenilin 578
- Robitussin Cold Caplets Multi-Symptom Cold & Flu 781
- Robitussin Cold Softgels Multi-Symptom Cold & Flu 781
- Robitussin Multi Symptom Honey Flu Liquid 785
- Robitussin Nighttime Honey Flu Liquid 786
- Sedapap Tablets 50 mg/650 mg ... 2225
- Singlet Caplets 761
- Sinutab Sinus Allergy Medication, Maximum Strength Formula, Tablets & Caplets 707
- Sinutab Sinus Medication, Maximum Strength Without Drowsiness Formula, Tablets & Caplets 707
- Sudafed Cold & Cough Liquid Caps 709
- Sudafed Cold & Sinus Liquid Caps 710
- Sudafed Severe Cold 711
- Sudafed Sinus Headache Caplets 712
- Sudafed Sinus Headache Tablets 712
- Tavist Sinus Non-Drowsy Coated Caplets 676
- TheraFlu Regular Strength Cold & Cough Night Time Hot Liquid 676
- TheraFlu Regular Strength Cold & Sore Throat Night Time Hot Liquid 676
- TheraFlu Maximum Strength Flu & Congestion Non-Drowsy Hot Liquid 677
- TheraFlu Maximum Strength Flu & Cough Night Time Hot Liquid 678
- TheraFlu Maximum Strength Flu & Sore Throat Night Time Hot Liquid 677
- TheraFlu Maximum Strength Severe Cold & Congestion Night Time Caplets 678
- TheraFlu Maximum Strength Severe Cold & Congestion Night Time Hot Liquid 678
- TheraFlu Maximum Strength Severe Cold & Congestion Non-Drowsy 679
- Triaminic Cold, Cough & Fever Liquid 681
- Triaminic Cough & Sore Throat Liquid 682
- Triaminic Cough & Sore Throat Softchews 684
- Tylenol, Children's 2014
- Children's Tylenol Allergy-D Liquid ... 2014
- Children's Tylenol Cold Suspension Liquid and Chewable Tablets 2015
- Children's Tylenol Cold Plus Cough Suspension Liquid and Chewable Tablets 2015
- Children's Tylenol Flu Suspension Liquid 2015
- Children's Tylenol Sinus Suspension Liquid 2017
- Infants' Tylenol Cold Decongestant and Fever Reducer Concentrated Drops 2015
- Infants' Tylenol Cold Decongestant and Fever Reducer Concentrated Drops Plus Cough ... 2015
- Junior Strength Tylenol Soft Chews Chewable Tablets 2014
- Tylenol 2009
- Tylenol Allergy Sinus 2010
- Tylenol Severe Allergy Caplets 2010
- Multi-Symptom Tylenol Cold Complete Formula Caplets 2010
- Multi-Symptom Tylenol Cold Non-Drowsy Caplets and Gelcaps 2010
- Multi-Symptom Tylenol Cold Severe Congestion Non-Drowsy Caplets 2011
- Maximum Strength Tylenol Flu NightTime Gelcaps 2011
- Maximum Strength Tylenol Flu NightTime Liquid 2011
- Maximum Strength Tylenol Flu Non-Drowsy Gelcaps 2011
- Extra Strength Tylenol PM Caplets, Geltabs, and Gelcaps 2012
- Maximum Strength Tylenol Sinus NightTime Caplets 2012
- Maximum Strength Tylenol Sinus Non-Drowsy Geltabs, Gelcaps, Caplets, and Tablets 2012
- Maximum Strength Tylenol Sore Throat Adult Liquid 2013
- Tylenol with Codeine 2595
- Women's Tylenol Menstrual Relief Caplets 2013
- Tylox Capsules 2597
- Ultracet Tablets 2597
- Vanquish Caplets 617
- Vicks 44M Cough, Cold & Flu Relief Liquid 725
- Vicks DayQuil LiquiCaps/Liquid Multi-Symptom Cold/Flu Relief ... 727
- Vicks NyQuil LiquiCaps/Liquid Multi-Symptom Cold/Flu Relief, Original and Cherry Flavors 727
- Vicodin Tablets 516
- Vicodin ES Tablets 517
- Vicodin HP Tablets 518
- Zydone Tablets 1330

Aminophylline (Co-administration of oral contraceptives containing ethinyl estradiol may inhibit metabolism of theophylline resulting in increased plasma concentrations of theophylline).
- No products indexed under this heading.

Ampicillin (Pregnancy while taking oral contraceptives has been reported when oral contraceptives were administered with ampicillin; clinical pharmacokinetic studies have not demonstrated any consistent effect of antibiotics on plasma concentrations of synthetic steroids).
No products indexed under this heading.

Ampicillin Sodium (Pregnancy while taking oral contraceptives has been reported when oral contraceptives were administered with ampicillin; clinical pharmacokinetic studies have not demonstrated any consistent effect of antibiotics on plasma concentrations of synthetic steroids). Products include:
Unasyn for Injection 2728

Atorvastatin Calcium (Co-administration has resulted in increased AUC values for norethindrone and ethinyl estradiol by approximately 30% and 20% respectively). Products include:
Lipitor Tablets 2639
Lipitor Tablets 2696

Carbamazepine (Anticonvulsants such as carbamazepine have been shown to increase the metabolism of ethinyl estradiol and/or norethindrone which could result in a reduction of contraceptive effectiveness). Products include:
Carbatrol Capsules 3234
Tegretol/Tegretol-XR 2404

Clofibrate (Co-administration of oral contraceptives has resulted in increased clearance of clofibric acid). Products include:
Atromid-S Capsules 3483

Cyclosporine (Co-administration of oral contraceptives containing ethinyl estradiol may inhibit metabolism of cyclosporine resulting in increased plasma concentrations of cyclosporine). Products include:
Gengraf Capsules 457
Neoral Soft Gelatin Capsules 2380
Neoral Oral Solution 2380
Sandimmune 2388

Demeclocycline Hydrochloride (Pregnancy while taking oral contraceptives has been reported when oral contraceptives were administered with tetracyclines; clinical pharmacokinetic studies have not demonstrated any consistent effect of antibiotics on plasma concentrations of synthetic steroids). Products include:
Declomycin Tablets 1855

Doxycycline Calcium (Pregnancy while taking oral contraceptives has been reported when oral contraceptives were administered with tetracyclines; clinical pharmacokinetic studies have not demonstrated any consistent effect of antibiotics on plasma concentrations of synthetic steroids). Products include:
Vibramycin Calcium Oral Suspension Syrup 2735

Doxycycline Hyclate (Pregnancy while taking oral contraceptives has been reported when oral contraceptives were administered with tetracyclines; clinical pharmacokinetic studies have not demonstrated any consistent effect of antibiotics on plasma concentrations of synthetic steroids). Products include:
Doryx Coated Pellet Filled Capsules 3357
Periostat Tablets 1208
Vibramycin Hyclate Capsules 2735
Vibramycin Hyclate Intravenous 2737
Vibra-Tabs Film Coated Tablets 2735

Doxycycline Monohydrate (Pregnancy while taking oral contraceptives has been reported when oral contraceptives were administered with tetracyclines; clinical pharmacokinetic studies have not demonstrated any consistent effect of antibiotics on plasma concentrations of synthetic steroids). Products include:
Monodox Capsules 2442
Vibramycin Monohydrate for Oral Suspension 2735

Dyphylline (Co-administration of oral contraceptives containing ethinyl estradiol may inhibit metabolism of theophylline resulting in increased plasma concentrations of theophylline). Products include:
Lufyllin Tablets 3347
Lufyllin-400 Tablets 3347
Lufyllin-GG Elixir 3348
Lufyllin-GG Tablets 3348

Fosphenytoin Sodium (Anticonvulsants such as phenytoin have been shown to increase the metabolism of ethinyl estradiol and/or norethindrone which could result in a reduction of contraceptive effectiveness). Products include:
Cerebyx Injection 2619

Griseofulvin (Pregnancy while taking oral contraceptives has been reported when oral contraceptives were administered with griseofulvin; clinical pharmacokinetic studies have not demonstrated any consistent effect of antibiotics on plasma concentrations of synthetic steroids). Products include:
Grifulvin V Tablets Microsize and Oral Suspension Microsize 2518
Gris-PEG Tablets 2661

Hypericum (Herbal products containing St. John's Wort may induce CYP450 and p-glycoprotein transporter and may reduce the effectiveness of oral contraceptives; may result in breakthrough bleeding). Products include:
Brite-Life Caplets .... ▣795
Centrum St. John's Wort Softgels .... ▣853
Metabolic Nutrition System .... ▣798
Movana Tablets .... ▣832
One-A-Day Tension & Mood Softgels .... ▣808
ReSource Wellness StayCalm Caplets .... ▣826
Satiete Tablets .... ▣846

Methacycline Hydrochloride (Pregnancy while taking oral contraceptives has been reported when oral contraceptives were administered with tetracyclines; clinical pharmacokinetic studies have not demonstrated any consistent effect of antibiotics on plasma concentrations of synthetic steroids).
No products indexed under this heading.

Methylprednisolone (Co-administration of oral contraceptives containing ethinyl estradiol may inhibit metabolism of prednisolone resulting in increased plasma concentrations of prednisolone).
No products indexed under this heading.

Methylprednisolone Acetate (Co-administration of oral contraceptives containing ethinyl estradiol may inhibit metabolism of prednisolone resulting in increased plasma concentrations of prednisolone). Products include:
Depo-Medrol Injectable Suspension 2795

Methylprednisolone Sodium Succinate (Co-administration of oral contraceptives containing ethinyl estradiol may inhibit metabolism of prednisolone resulting in increased plasma concentrations of prednisolone). Products include:
Solu-Medrol Sterile Powder 2855

Minocycline Hydrochloride (Pregnancy while taking oral contraceptives has been reported when oral contraceptives were administered with tetracyclines; clinical pharmacokinetic studies have not demonstrated any consistent effect of antibiotics on plasma concentrations of synthetic steroids). Products include:
Dynacin Capsules 2019
Minocin Intravenous 1862
Minocin Oral Suspension 1865
Minocin Pellet-Filled Capsules 1863

Morphine Sulfate (Co-administration of oral contraceptives has resulted in increased clearance of morphine). Products include:
Astramorph/PF Injection, USP (Preservative-Free) 594
Duramorph Injection 1312
Infumorph 200 and Infumorph 500 Sterile Solutions 1314
Kadian Capsules 1335
MS Contin Tablets 2896
MSIR 2898
Oramorph SR Tablets 3062
Roxanol 3066

Oxytetracycline Hydrochloride (Pregnancy while taking oral contraceptives has been reported when oral contraceptives were administered with tetracyclines; clinical pharmacokinetic studies have not demonstrated any consistent effect of antibiotics on plasma concentrations of synthetic steroids). Products include:
Terra-Cortril Ophthalmic Suspension 2716
Urobiotic-250 Capsules 2731

Phenobarbital (Anticonvulsants such as phenobarbital have been shown to increase the metabolism of ethinyl estradiol and/or norethindrone which could result in a reduction of contraceptive effectiveness). Products include:
Arco-Lase Plus Tablets 592
Donnatal 2929
Donnatal Extentabs 2930

Phenylbutazone (Co-administration has resulted in a reduction in contraceptive effectiveness and increased incidence of breakthrough bleeding).
No products indexed under this heading.

Phenytoin (Anticonvulsants such as phenytoin have been shown to increase the metabolism of ethinyl estradiol and/or norethindrone which could result in a reduction of contraceptive effectiveness). Products include:
Dilantin Infatabs 2624
Dilantin-125 Oral Suspension 2625

Phenytoin Sodium (Anticonvulsants such as phenytoin have been shown to increase the metabolism of ethinyl estradiol and/or norethindrone which could result in a reduction of contraceptive effectiveness). Products include:
Dilantin Kapseals 2622

Prednisolone (Co-administration of oral contraceptives containing ethinyl estradiol may inhibit metabolism of prednisolone resulting in increased plasma concentrations of prednisolone). Products include:
Prelone Syrup 2273

Prednisolone Acetate (Co-administration of oral contraceptives containing ethinyl estradiol may inhibit metabolism of prednisolone resulting in increased plasma concentrations of prednisolone). Products include:
Blephamide Ophthalmic Ointment 547
Blephamide Ophthalmic Suspension 548
Poly-Pred Liquifilm Ophthalmic Suspension .... ⊙245
Pred Forte Ophthalmic Suspension .... ⊙246
Pred Mild Sterile Ophthalmic Suspension .... ⊙249
Pred-G Ophthalmic Suspension .... ⊙247
Pred-G Sterile Ophthalmic Ointment .... ⊙248

Prednisolone Sodium Phosphate (Co-administration of oral contraceptives containing ethinyl estradiol may inhibit metabolism of prednisolone resulting in increased plasma concentrations of prednisolone). Products include:
Pediapred Oral Solution 1170

Prednisolone Tebutate (Co-administration of oral contraceptives containing ethinyl estradiol may inhibit metabolism of prednisolone resulting in increased plasma concentrations of prednisolone).
No products indexed under this heading.

Rifampin (Metabolism of both norethindrone and ethinyl estradiol is increased by rifampin; co-administration has resulted in a reduction of contraceptive effectiveness and increased incidence of breakthrough bleeding and menstrual irregularities). Products include:
Rifadin 765
Rifamate Capsules 767
Rifater Tablets 769

Salicylic Acid (Co-administration of oral contraceptives has resulted in increased clearance of salicylic acid). Products include:
Clear Away Gel with Aloe Wart Remover System .... ▣736
Clear Away Liquid Wart Remover System .... ▣736
Clear Away One Step Wart Remover .... ▣737
Clear Away One Step Wart Remover for Kids .... ▣737
Clear Away One Step Plantar Wart Remover .... ▣737
Compound W One Step Pads for Kids .... ▣664
Compound W One Step Plantar Pads .... ▣664
Compound W One Step Wart Remover Pads .... ▣664
Compound W Wart Remover Gel .... ▣665
Compound W Wart Remover Liquid .... ▣665
Wart-Off Liquid .... ▣716

Temazepam (Co-administration of oral contraceptives has resulted in increased clearance of temazepam).
No products indexed under this heading.

Tetracycline Hydrochloride (Pregnancy while taking oral contraceptives has been reported when oral contraceptives were administered with tetracyclines; clinical pharmacokinetic studies have not demonstrated any consistent effect of antibiotics on plasma concentrations of synthetic steroids).
No products indexed under this heading.

Theophylline (Co-administration of oral contraceptives containing ethinyl estradiol may inhibit metabolism of theophylline resulting in increased plasma concentrations of theophylline). Products include:
Aerolate 1361
Theo-Dur Extended-Release Tablets 1835
Uni-Dur Extended-Release Tablets 1841
Uniphyl 400 mg and 600 mg Tablets 2903

Theophylline Calcium Salicylate (Co-administration of oral contraceptives containing ethinyl estradiol may inhibit metabolism of theophylline resulting in increased plasma concentrations of theophylline).
No products indexed under this heading.

Theophylline Sodium Glycinate (Co-administration of oral contraceptives containing ethinyl estradiol may inhibit metabolism of theophylline resulting in increased plasma concentrations of theophylline).
No products indexed under this heading.

Troglitazone (Co-administration has reduced the plasma concentrations of both norethindrone and ethinyl estradiol by approximately 30%, which could result in a reduction of contraceptive effectiveness).
No products indexed under this heading.

Vitamin C (May increase plasma ethinyl estradiol concentrations, possibly by inhibition of conjugation). Products include:

Beta-C Tablets ... 811
C-Grams Caplets ... 795
Halls Defense Drops ... 687
Peridin-C Tablets ... 618

ESTROSTEP FE TABLETS
(Ethinyl Estradiol, Norethindrone Acetate) ... 2627
See Estrostep 21 Tablets

ETHIODOL INJECTION
(Ethiodized Oil) ... 3095
None cited in PDR database.

ETHYOL FOR INJECTION
(Amifostine) ... 2029
May interact with antihypertensives. Compounds in these categories include:

Acebutolol Hydrochloride (Amifostine produces transient hypotension; caution is advised if it is used with other antihypertensive agents). Products include:

Sectral Capsules ... 3589

Amlodipine Besylate (Amifostine produces transient hypotension; caution is advised if it is used with other antihypertensive agents). Products include:

Lotrel Capsules ... 2370
Norvasc Tablets ... 2704

Atenolol (Amifostine produces transient hypotension; caution is advised if it is used with other antihypertensive agents). Products include:

Tenoretic Tablets ... 690
Tenormin I.V. Injection ... 692

Benazepril Hydrochloride (Amifostine produces transient hypotension; caution is advised if it is used with other antihypertensive agents). Products include:

Lotensin Tablets ... 2365
Lotensin HCT Tablets ... 2367
Lotrel Capsules ... 2370

Bendroflumethiazide (Amifostine produces transient hypotension; caution is advised if it is used with other antihypertensive agents). Products include:

Corzide 40/5 Tablets ... 2247
Corzide 80/5 Tablets ... 2247

Betaxolol Hydrochloride (Amifostine produces transient hypotension; caution is advised if it is used with other antihypertensive agents). Products include:

Betoptic S Ophthalmic Suspension ... 537

Bisoprolol Fumarate (Amifostine produces transient hypotension; caution is advised if it is used with other antihypertensive agents). Products include:

Zebeta Tablets ... 1885
Ziac Tablets ... 1887

Candesartan Cilexetil (Amifostine produces transient hypotension; caution is advised if it is used with other antihypertensive agents). Products include:

Atacand Tablets ... 595
Atacand HCT Tablets ... 597

Captopril (Amifostine produces transient hypotension; caution is advised if it is used with other antihypertensive agents). Products include:

Captopril Tablets ... 2281

Carteolol Hydrochloride (Amifostine produces transient hypotension; caution is advised if it is used with other antihypertensive agents). Products include:

Carteolol Hydrochloride Ophthalmic Solution USP, 1% ... ⊙258
Ocupress Ophthalmic Solution, 1% Sterile ... ⊙303

Chlorothiazide (Amifostine produces transient hypotension; caution is advised if it is used with other antihypertensive agents). Products include:

Aldoclor Tablets ... 2035
Diuril Oral ... 2087

Chlorothiazide Sodium (Amifostine produces transient hypotension; caution is advised if it is used with other antihypertensive agents). Products include:

Diuril Sodium Intravenous ... 2086

Chlorthalidone (Amifostine produces transient hypotension; caution is advised if it is used with other antihypertensive agents). Products include:

Clorpres Tablets ... 1002
Combipres Tablets ... 1040
Tenoretic Tablets ... 690

Clonidine (Amifostine produces transient hypotension; caution is advised if it is used with other antihypertensive agents). Products include:

Catapres-TTS ... 1038

Clonidine Hydrochloride (Amifostine produces transient hypotension; caution is advised if it is used with other antihypertensive agents). Products include:

Catapres Tablets ... 1037
Clorpres Tablets ... 1002
Combipres Tablets ... 1040
Duraclon Injection ... 3057

Deserpidine (Amifostine produces transient hypotension; caution is advised if it is used with other antihypertensive agents).

No products indexed under this heading.

Diazoxide (Amifostine produces transient hypotension; caution is advised if it is used with other antihypertensive agents).

No products indexed under this heading.

Diltiazem Hydrochloride (Amifostine produces transient hypotension; caution is advised if it is used with other antihypertensive agents). Products include:

Cardizem Injectable ... 1018
Cardizem Lyo-Ject Syringe ... 1018
Cardizem Monovial ... 1018
Cardizem CD Capsules ... 1016
Tiazac Capsules ... 1378

Doxazosin Mesylate (Amifostine produces transient hypotension; caution is advised if it is used with other antihypertensive agents). Products include:

Cardura Tablets ... 2668

Enalapril Maleate (Amifostine produces transient hypotension; caution is advised if it is used with other antihypertensive agents). Products include:

Lexxel Tablets ... 608
Vaseretic Tablets ... 2204
Vasotec Tablets ... 2210

Enalaprilat (Amifostine produces transient hypotension; caution is advised if it is used with other antihypertensive agents). Products include:

Enalaprilat Injection ... 863
Vasotec I.V. Injection ... 2207

Eprosartan Mesylate (Amifostine produces transient hypotension; caution is advised if it is used with other antihypertensive agents). Products include:

Teveten Tablets ... 3327

Esmolol Hydrochloride (Amifostine produces transient hypotension; caution is advised if it is used with other antihypertensive agents). Products include:

Brevibloc Injection ... 858

Felodipine (Amifostine produces transient hypotension; caution is advised if it is used with other antihypertensive agents). Products include:

Lexxel Tablets ... 608
Plendil Extended-Release Tablets ... 623

Fosinopril Sodium (Amifostine produces transient hypotension; caution is advised if it is used with other antihypertensive agents). Products include:

Monopril Tablets ... 1091
Monopril HCT ... 1094

Furosemide (Amifostine produces transient hypotension; caution is advised if it is used with other antihypertensive agents). Products include:

Furosemide Tablets ... 2284

Guanabenz Acetate (Amifostine produces transient hypotension; caution is advised if it is used with other antihypertensive agents).

No products indexed under this heading.

Guanethidine Monosulfate (Amifostine produces transient hypotension; caution is advised if it is used with other antihypertensive agents).

No products indexed under this heading.

Hydralazine Hydrochloride (Amifostine produces transient hypotension; caution is advised if it is used with other antihypertensive agents).

No products indexed under this heading.

Hydrochlorothiazide (Amifostine produces transient hypotension; caution is advised if it is used with other antihypertensive agents). Products include:

Accuretic Tablets ... 2614
Aldoril Tablets ... 2039
Atacand HCT Tablets ... 597
Avalide Tablets ... 1070
Diovan HCT Tablets ... 2338
Dyazide Capsules ... 1515
HydroDIURIL Tablets ... 2108
Hyzaar ... 2109
Inderide Tablets ... 3517
Inderide LA Long-Acting Capsules ... 3519
Lotensin HCT Tablets ... 2367
Maxzide ... 1008
Micardis HCT Tablets ... 1051
Microzide Capsules ... 3414
Moduretic Tablets ... 2138
Monopril HCT ... 1094
Prinzide Tablets ... 2168
Timolide Tablets ... 2187
Uniretic Tablets ... 3178
Vaseretic Tablets ... 2204
Zestoretic Tablets ... 695
Ziac Tablets ... 1887

Hydroflumethiazide (Amifostine produces transient hypotension; caution is advised if it is used with other antihypertensive agents). Products include:

Diucardin Tablets ... 3494

Indapamide (Amifostine produces transient hypotension; caution is advised if it is used with other antihypertensive agents). Products include:

Indapamide Tablets ... 2286

Irbesartan (Amifostine produces transient hypotension; caution is advised if it is used with other antihypertensive agents). Products include:

Avalide Tablets ... 1070
Avapro Tablets ... 1074
Avapro Tablets ... 3076

Isradipine (Amifostine produces transient hypotension; caution is advised if it is used with other antihypertensive agents). Products include:

DynaCirc Capsules ... 2921
DynaCirc CR Tablets ... 2923

Labetalol Hydrochloride (Amifostine produces transient hypotension; caution is advised if it is used with other antihypertensive agents). Products include:

Normodyne Injection ... 3135
Normodyne Tablets ... 3137

Lisinopril (Amifostine produces transient hypotension; caution is advised if it is used with other antihypertensive agents). Products include:

Prinivil Tablets ... 2164
Prinzide Tablets ... 2168
Zestoretic Tablets ... 695
Zestril Tablets ... 698

Losartan Potassium (Amifostine produces transient hypotension; caution is advised if it is used with other antihypertensive agents). Products include:

Cozaar Tablets ... 2067
Hyzaar ... 2109

Mecamylamine Hydrochloride (Amifostine produces transient hypotension; caution is advised if it is used with other antihypertensive agents). Products include:

Inversine Tablets ... 1850

Methyclothiazide (Amifostine produces transient hypotension; caution is advised if it is used with other antihypertensive agents).

No products indexed under this heading.

Methyldopa (Amifostine produces transient hypotension; caution is advised if it is used with other antihypertensive agents). Products include:

Aldoclor Tablets ... 2035
Aldomet Tablets ... 2037
Aldoril Tablets ... 2039

Methyldopate Hydrochloride (Amifostine produces transient hypotension; caution is advised if it is used with other antihypertensive agents).

No products indexed under this heading.

Metolazone (Amifostine produces transient hypotension; caution is advised if it is used with other antihypertensive agents). Products include:

Mykrox Tablets ... 1168
Zaroxolyn Tablets ... 1177

Metoprolol Succinate (Amifostine produces transient hypotension; caution is advised if it is used with other antihypertensive agents). Products include:

Toprol-XL Tablets ... 651

Metoprolol Tartrate (Amifostine produces transient hypotension; caution is advised if it is used with other antihypertensive agents).

No products indexed under this heading.

Metyrosine (Amifostine produces transient hypotension; caution is advised if it is used with other antihypertensive agents). Products include:

Demser Capsules ... 2085

Mibefradil Dihydrochloride (Amifostine produces transient hypotension; caution is advised if it is used with other antihypertensive agents).

No products indexed under this heading.

Minoxidil (Amifostine produces transient hypotension; caution is advised if it is used with other antihypertensive agents). Products include:

Rogaine Extra Strength for Men Topical Solution ... 721
Rogaine for Women Topical Solution ... 721

Moexipril Hydrochloride (Amifostine produces transient hypotension; caution is advised if it is used with other antihypertensive agents). Products include:

Uniretic Tablets ... 3178
Univasc Tablets ... 3181

Nadolol (Amifostine produces transient hypotension; caution is advised if it is used with other antihypertensive agents). Products include:

Corgard Tablets ... 2245
Corzide 40/5 Tablets ... 2247
Corzide 80/5 Tablets ... 2247

Nadolol Tablets 2288

Nicardipine Hydrochloride (Amifostine produces transient hypotension; caution is advised if it is used with other antihypertensive agents). Products include:
Cardene I.V. 3485

Nifedipine (Amifostine produces transient hypotension; caution is advised if it is used with other antihypertensive agents). Products include:
Adalat CC Tablets 877
Procardia Capsules 2708
Procardia XL Extended Release Tablets 2710

Nisoldipine (Amifostine produces transient hypotension; caution is advised if it is used with other antihypertensive agents). Products include:
Sular Tablets 688

Nitroglycerin (Amifostine produces transient hypotension; caution is advised if it is used with other antihypertensive agents). Products include:
Nitro-Dur Transdermal Infusion System 3134
Nitro-Dur Transdermal Infusion System 1834
Nitrolingual Pumpspray 1355
Nitrostat Tablets 2658

Penbutolol Sulfate (Amifostine produces transient hypotension; caution is advised if it is used with other antihypertensive agents).
No products indexed under this heading.

Perindopril Erbumine (Amifostine produces transient hypotension; caution is advised if it is used with other antihypertensive agents). Products include:
Aceon Tablets (2 mg, 4 mg, 8 mg) 3249

Phenoxybenzamine Hydrochloride (Amifostine produces transient hypotension; caution is advised if it is used with other antihypertensive agents). Products include:
Dibenzyline Capsules 3457

Phentolamine Mesylate (Amifostine produces transient hypotension; caution is advised if it is used with other antihypertensive agents).
No products indexed under this heading.

Pindolol (Amifostine produces transient hypotension; caution is advised if it is used with other antihypertensive agents).
No products indexed under this heading.

Polythiazide (Amifostine produces transient hypotension; caution is advised if it is used with other antihypertensive agents). Products include:
Minizide Capsules 2700
Renese Tablets 2712

Prazosin Hydrochloride (Amifostine produces transient hypotension; caution is advised if it is used with other antihypertensive agents). Products include:
Minipress Capsules 2699
Minizide Capsules 2700

Propranolol Hydrochloride (Amifostine produces transient hypotension; caution is advised if it is used with other antihypertensive agents). Products include:
Inderal 3513
Inderal LA Long-Acting Capsules 3516
Inderide Tablets 3517
Inderide LA Long-Acting Capsules .. 3519

Quinapril Hydrochloride (Amifostine produces transient hypotension; caution is advised if it is used with other antihypertensive agents). Products include:
Accupril Tablets 2611
Accuretic Tablets 2614

Ramipril (Amifostine produces transient hypotension; caution is advised if it is used with other antihypertensive agents). Products include:
Altace Capsules 2233

Rauwolfia serpentina (Amifostine produces transient hypotension; caution is advised if it is used with other antihypertensive agents).
No products indexed under this heading.

Rescinnamine (Amifostine produces transient hypotension; caution is advised if it is used with other antihypertensive agents).
No products indexed under this heading.

Reserpine (Amifostine produces transient hypotension; caution is advised if it is used with other antihypertensive agents).
No products indexed under this heading.

Sodium Nitroprusside (Amifostine produces transient hypotension; caution is advised if it is used with other antihypertensive agents).
No products indexed under this heading.

Sotalol Hydrochloride (Amifostine produces transient hypotension; caution is advised if it is used with other antihypertensive agents). Products include:
Betapace Tablets 950
Betapace AF Tablets 954

Spirapril Hydrochloride (Amifostine produces transient hypotension; caution is advised if it is used with other antihypertensive agents).
No products indexed under this heading.

Telmisartan (Amifostine produces transient hypotension; caution is advised if it is used with other antihypertensive agents). Products include:
Micardis Tablets 1049
Micardis HCT Tablets 1051

Terazosin Hydrochloride (Amifostine produces transient hypotension; caution is advised if it is used with other antihypertensive agents). Products include:
Hytrin Capsules 464

Timolol Maleate (Amifostine produces transient hypotension; caution is advised if it is used with other antihypertensive agents). Products include:
Blocadren Tablets 2046
Cosopt Sterile Ophthalmic Solution 2065
Timolide Tablets 2187
Timolol GFS .... ⊙266
Timoptic in Ocudose 2192
Timoptic Sterile Ophthalmic Solution 2190
Timoptic-XE Sterile Ophthalmic Gel Forming Solution 2194

Torsemide (Amifostine produces transient hypotension; caution is advised if it is used with other antihypertensive agents). Products include:
Demadex Tablets and Injection 2965

Trandolapril (Amifostine produces transient hypotension; caution is advised if it is used with other antihypertensive agents). Products include:
Mavik Tablets 478
Tarka Tablets 508

Trimethaphan Camsylate (Amifostine produces transient hypotension; caution is advised if it is used with other antihypertensive agents).
No products indexed under this heading.

Valsartan (Amifostine produces transient hypotension; caution is advised if it is used with other antihypertensive agents). Products include:
Diovan Capsules 2337
Diovan HCT Tablets 2338

Verapamil Hydrochloride (Amifostine produces transient hypotension; caution is advised if it is used with other antihypertensive agents). Products include:
Covera-HS Tablets 3199
Isoptin SR Tablets 467
Tarka Tablets 508
Verelan Capsules 3184
Verelan PM Capsules 3186

ETRAFON 2-10 TABLETS (2-10)

(Amitriptyline Hydrochloride, Perphenazine)................................ 3115
See Etrafon Tablets (2-25)

ETRAFON TABLETS (2-25)

(Amitriptyline Hydrochloride, Perphenazine)................................ 3115
May interact with anticholinergics, antihistamines, barbiturates, central nervous system depressants, antidepressant drugs, monoamine oxidase inhibitors, narcotic analgesics, quinidine, selective serotonin reuptake inhibitors, sympathomimetics, thyroid preparations, and certain other agents. Compounds in these categories include:

Acrivastine (Co-administration can result in enhanced CNS depression). Products include:
Semprex-D Capsules 1172

Albuterol (Effects of concurrent use not specified; close supervision and careful adjustment of dosages are required). Products include:
Proventil Inhalation Aerosol 3142
Ventolin Inhalation Aerosol and Refill 1679

Albuterol Sulfate (Effects of concurrent use not specified; close supervision and careful adjustment of dosages are required). Products include:
AccuNeb Inhalation Solution 1230
Combivent Inhalation Aerosol 1041
DuoNeb Inhalation Solution 1233
Proventil Inhalation Solution 0.083%.. 3146
Proventil Repetabs Tablets 3148
Proventil Solution for Inhalation 0.5%.. 3144
Proventil HFA Inhalation Aerosol 3150
Ventolin HFA Inhalation Aerosol 3618
Volmax Extended-Release Tablets .. 2276

Alfentanil Hydrochloride (Co-administration can result in enhanced CNS depression).
No products indexed under this heading.

Alprazolam (Co-administration can result in enhanced CNS depression). Products include:
Xanax Tablets 2865

Amoxapine (Co-administration with drugs that are substrate for P450IID6 isoenzyme, such as many other antidepressants, may increase plasma AUC of the tricyclic antidepressant).
No products indexed under this heading.

Aprobarbital (Co-administration can result in enhanced CNS depression).
No products indexed under this heading.

Astemizole (Co-administration can result in enhanced CNS depression).
No products indexed under this heading.

Atropine Sulfate (Co-administration with anticholinergic agents may result in additive anticholinergic effects, including paralytic ileus). Products include:
Donnatal 2929
Donnatal Extentabs 2930
Motofen Tablets 577
Prosed/DS Tablets 3268
Urised Tablets 2876

Azatadine Maleate (Co-administration can result in enhanced CNS depression). Products include:
Rynatan Tablets 3351

Belladonna Alkaloids (Co-administration with anticholinergic agents may result in additive anticholinergic effects, including paralytic ileus). Products include:
Hyland's Teething Tablets .... ◘766
Urimax Tablets 1769

Benztropine Mesylate (Co-administration with anticholinergic agents may result in additive anticholinergic effects, including paralytic ileus). Products include:
Cogentin 2055

Biperiden Hydrochloride (Co-administration with anticholinergic agents may result in additive anticholinergic effects, including paralytic ileus). Products include:
Akineton 402

Bromodiphenhydramine Hydrochloride (Co-administration can result in enhanced CNS depression).
No products indexed under this heading.

Brompheniramine Maleate (Co-administration can result in enhanced CNS depression). Products include:
Bromfed Capsules (Extended-Release).......................... 2269
Bromfed-PD Capsules (Extended-Release).......................... 2269
Comtrex Acute Head Cold & Sinus Pressure Relief Tablets..... ◘627
Dimetapp Elixir .... ◘777
Dimetapp Cold and Fever Suspension.................................. ◘775
Dimetapp DM Cold & Cough Elixir . ◘775
Dimetapp Nighttime Flu Liquid ...... ◘776

Buprenorphine Hydrochloride (Co-administration can result in enhanced CNS depression). Products include:
Buprenex Injectable 2918

Bupropion Hydrochloride (Co-administration with drugs that are substrate for P450IID6 isoenzyme, such as many other antidepressants, may increase plasma AUC of the tricyclic antidepressant). Products include:
Wellbutrin Tablets 1680
Wellbutrin SR Sustained-Release Tablets 1684
Zyban Sustained-Release Tablets ... 1710

Buspirone Hydrochloride (Co-administration can result in enhanced CNS depression).
No products indexed under this heading.

Butabarbital (Co-administration can result in enhanced CNS depression).
No products indexed under this heading.

Butalbital (Co-administration can result in enhanced CNS depression). Products include:
Phrenilin 578
Sedapap Tablets 50 mg/650 mg ... 2225

Cetirizine Hydrochloride (Co-administration can result in enhanced CNS depression). Products include:
Zyrtec 2756
Zyrtec-D 12 Hour Extended Relief Tablets 2758

Chlordiazepoxide (Co-administration can result in enhanced CNS depression). Products include:
Limbitrol 1738

Chlordiazepoxide Hydrochloride (Co-administration can result in enhanced CNS depression). Products include:
Librium Capsules 1736
Librium for Injection 1737

Chlorpheniramine Maleate (Co-administration can result in enhanced CNS depression). Products include:

Actifed Cold & Sinus Caplets and Tablets .... ▣688
Alka-Seltzer Plus Liqui-Gels .... ▣604
BC Allergy Sinus Cold Powder .... ▣619
Chlor-Trimeton Allergy Tablets .... ▣735
Chlor-Trimeton Allergy/Decongestant Tablets .... ▣736
Comtrex Flu Therapy & Fever Relief Nighttime Tablets .... ▣628
Comtrex Maximum Strength Multi-Symptom Cold & Cough Relief Caplets and Tablets .... ▣626
Contac Severe Cold and Flu Caplets Maximum Strength .... ▣746
Coricidin 'D' Cold, Flu & Sinus Tablets .... ▣737
Coricidin/Coricidin D .... ▣738
Coricidin HBP Maximum Strength Flu Tablets .... ▣738
Extendryl 1361
Hycomine Compound Tablets 1317
Kronofed-A 1341
PediaCare Cough-Cold Liquid .... ▣719
PediaCare NightRest Cough-Cold Liquid .... ▣719
Robitussin Nighttime Honey Flu Liquid .... ▣786
Ryna .... ▣768
Singlet Caplets .... ▣761
Sinutab Sinus Allergy Medication, Maximum Strength Formula, Tablets & Caplets .... ▣707
Sudafed Cold & Allergy Tablets .... ▣708
TheraFlu Regular Strength Cold & Cough Night Time Hot Liquid .... ▣676
TheraFlu Regular Strength Cold & Sore Throat Night Time Hot Liquid .... ▣676
TheraFlu Maximum Strength Flu & Cough Night Time Hot Liquid .... ▣678
TheraFlu Maximum Strength Flu & Sore Throat Night Time Hot Liquid .... ▣677
TheraFlu Maximum Strength Severe Cold & Congestion Night Time Caplets .... ▣678
TheraFlu Maximum Strength Severe Cold & Congestion Night Time Hot Liquid .... ▣678
Triaminic Cold & Allergy Liquid .... ▣681
Triaminic Cold & Allergy Softchews .... ▣683
Triaminic Cold & Cough Liquid .... ▣681
Triaminic Cold & Cough Softchews .... ▣683
Triaminic Cold & Night Time Cough Liquid .... ▣681
Triaminic Cold, Cough & Fever Liquid .... ▣681
Children's Tylenol Cold Suspension Liquid and Chewable Tablets 2015
Children's Tylenol Cold Plus Cough Suspension Liquid and Chewable Tablets 2015
Children's Tylenol Flu Suspension Liquid 2015
Maximum Strength Tylenol Allergy Sinus Caplets, Gelcaps, and Geltabs 2010
Multi-Symptom Tylenol Cold Complete Formula Caplets 2010
Vicks 44M Cough, Cold & Flu Relief Liquid .... ▣725
Pediatric Vicks 44m Cough & Cold Relief .... ▣728
Children's Vicks NyQuil Cold/Cough Relief .... ▣726

Chlorpheniramine Polistirex (Co-administration can result in enhanced CNS depression). Products include:
Tussionex Pennkinetic Extended-Release Suspension 1174

Chlorpheniramine Tannate (Co-administration can result in enhanced CNS depression). Products include:
Reformulated Rynatan Pediatric Suspension 3352
Rynatuss Pediatric Suspension 3353
Rynatuss Tablets 3353
Tussi-12 S Suspension 3356
Tussi-12 Tablets 3356

Chlorpromazine (Co-administration can result in enhanced CNS depression). Products include:
Thorazine Suppositories 1656

Chlorpromazine Hydrochloride (Co-administration can result in enhanced CNS depression). Products include:
Thorazine 1656

Chlorprothixene (Co-administration can result in enhanced CNS depression).
No products indexed under this heading.

Chlorprothixene Hydrochloride (Co-administration can result in enhanced CNS depression).
No products indexed under this heading.

Chlorprothixene Lactate (Co-administration can result in enhanced CNS depression).
No products indexed under this heading.

Cimetidine (Co-administration of tricyclic antidepressants and cimetidine can produce clinically significant increases in the plasma concentrations of tricyclic antidepressant resulting in anticholinergic symptoms, such as severe dry mouth, urinary retention, and blurred vision). Products include:
Tagamet HB 200 Suspension .... ▣762
Tagamet HB 200 Tablets .... ▣761
Tagamet Tablets 1644

Cimetidine Hydrochloride (Co-administration of tricyclic antidepressants and cimetidine can produce clinically significant increases in the plasma concentrations of tricyclic antidepressant resulting in anticholinergic symptoms, such as severe dry mouth, urinary retention, and blurred vision; initiation and discontinuation of cimetidine therapy should be closely monitored). Products include:
Tagamet 1644

Citalopram Hydrobromide (Co-administration with drugs that are substrate for P450IID6 isoenzyme, such as selective serotonin reuptake inhibitors, may increase plasma AUC of the tricyclic antidepressant; due to variation in the extent of inhibition, caution is indicated if co-administered and sufficient time must elapse for sequential therapy). Products include:
Celexa 1365

Clemastine Fumarate (Co-administration can result in enhanced CNS depression). Products include:
Tavist 12 Hour Allergy Tablets .... ▣676

Clidinium Bromide (Co-administration with anticholinergic agents may result in additive anticholinergic effects, including paralytic ileus).
No products indexed under this heading.

Clorazepate Dipotassium (Co-administration can result in enhanced CNS depression). Products include:
Tranxene 511

Clozapine (Co-administration can result in enhanced CNS depression). Products include:
Clozaril Tablets 2319

Codeine Phosphate (Co-administration can result in enhanced CNS depression). Products include:
Phenergan with Codeine Syrup 3557
Phenergan VC with Codeine Syrup 3561
Robitussin A-C Syrup 2942
Robitussin-DAC Syrup 2942
Ryna-C Liquid .... ▣768
Soma Compound w/Codeine Tablets 3355
Tussi-Organidin NR Liquid 3350
Tussi-Organidin-S NR Liquid 3350
Tylenol with Codeine 2595

Cyproheptadine Hydrochloride (Co-administration can result in enhanced CNS depression). Products include:
Periactin Tablets 2155

Desflurane (Co-administration can result in enhanced CNS depression). Products include:
Suprane Liquid for Inhalation 874

Desipramine Hydrochloride (Co-administration with drugs that are substrate for P450IID6 isoenzyme, such as many other antidepressants, may increase plasma AUC of the tricyclic antidepressant). Products include:
Norpramin Tablets 755

Dexchlorpheniramine Maleate (Co-administration can result in enhanced CNS depression).
No products indexed under this heading.

Dezocine (Co-administration can result in enhanced CNS depression).
No products indexed under this heading.

Diazepam (Co-administration can result in enhanced CNS depression). Products include:
Valium Injectable 3026
Valium Tablets 3047

Dicyclomine Hydrochloride (Co-administration with anticholinergic agents may result in additive anticholinergic effects, including paralytic ileus).
No products indexed under this heading.

Diphenhydramine Citrate (Co-administration can result in enhanced CNS depression). Products include:
Alka-Seltzer PM Effervescent Tablets .... ▣605
Benadryl Allergy & Sinus Fastmelt Tablets .... ▣693
Benadryl Children's Allergy/Cold Fastmelt Tablets .... ▣692
Excedrin PM Tablets, Caplets, and Geltabs .... ▣631
Goody's PM Powder .... ▣621

Diphenhydramine Hydrochloride (Co-administration can result in enhanced CNS depression). Products include:
Extra Strength Bayer PM Caplets .... ▣611
Benadryl Allergy Chewables .... ▣689
Benadryl Allergy .... ▣691
Benadryl Allergy Liquid .... ▣690
Benadryl Allergy/Cold Tablets .... ▣691
Benadryl Allergy/Congestion Tablets .... ▣692
Benadryl Allergy & Sinus Liquid .... ▣693
Benadryl Allergy Sinus Headache Caplets & Gelcaps .... ▣693
Benadryl Severe Allergy & Sinus Headache Caplets .... ▣694
Benadryl Dye-Free Allergy Liquid .... ▣690
Benadryl Dye-Free Allergy Liqui-Gels Softgels .... ▣690
Benadryl Itch Relief Stick Extra Strength .... ▣695
Benadryl Cream .... ▣695
Benadryl Gel .... ▣695
Benadryl Spray .... ▣696
Benadryl Parenteral 2617
Coricidin HBP Night-Time Cold & Flu Tablets .... ▣738
Nytol QuickCaps Caplets .... ▣622
Maximum Strength Nytol QuickGels Softgels .... ▣621
Extra Strength Percogesic Aspirin-Free Coated Caplets .... ▣665
Simply Sleep Caplets 2008
Sominex Original Formula Tablets .... ▣761
Children's Tylenol Allergy-D Liquid 2014
Maximum Strength Tylenol Allergy Sinus NightTime Caplets 2010
Tylenol Severe Allergy Caplets 2010
Maximum Strength Tylenol Flu NightTime Gelcaps 2011
Extra Strength Tylenol PM Caplets, Geltabs, and Gelcaps 2012
Unisom Maximum Strength SleepGels .... ▣713

Diphenylpyraline Hydrochloride (Co-administration can result in enhanced CNS depression).
No products indexed under this heading.

Dobutamine Hydrochloride (Effects of concurrent use not specified; close supervision and careful adjustment of dosages are required). Products include:
Dobutrex Solution Vials 1914

Dopamine Hydrochloride (Effects of concurrent use not specified; close supervision and careful adjustment of dosages are required).
No products indexed under this heading.

Doxepin Hydrochloride (Co-administration with drugs that are substrate for P450IID6 isoenzyme, such as many other antidepressants, may increase plasma AUC of the tricyclic antidepressant). Products include:
Sinequan 2713

Droperidol (Co-administration can result in enhanced CNS depression).
No products indexed under this heading.

Enflurane (Co-administration can result in enhanced CNS depression).
No products indexed under this heading.

Ephedrine Hydrochloride (Effects of concurrent use not specified; close supervision and careful adjustment of dosages are required). Products include:
Primatene Tablets .... ▣780

Ephedrine Sulfate (Effects of concurrent use not specified; close supervision and careful adjustment of dosages are required).
No products indexed under this heading.

Ephedrine Tannate (Effects of concurrent use not specified; close supervision and careful adjustment of dosages are required). Products include:
Rynatuss Pediatric Suspension 3353
Rynatuss Tablets 3353

Epinephrine (Effects of concurrent use not specified; close supervision and careful adjustment of dosages are required). Products include:
Epifrin Sterile Ophthalmic Solution .... ⊙235
EpiPen 1236
Primatene Mist .... ▣779
Xylocaine with Epinephrine Injection 653

Epinephrine Bitartrate (Effects of concurrent use not specified; close supervision and careful adjustment of dosages are required). Products include:
Sensorcaine 643

Epinephrine Hydrochloride (Effects of concurrent use not specified; close supervision and careful adjustment of dosages are required).
No products indexed under this heading.

Estazolam (Co-administration can result in enhanced CNS depression). Products include:
ProSom Tablets 500

Ethchlorvynol (Concurrent use of ethchlorvynol and amitriptyline has resulted in transient delirium).
No products indexed under this heading.

Ethinamate (Co-administration can result in enhanced CNS depression).
No products indexed under this heading.

Fentanyl (Co-administration can result in enhanced CNS depression). Products include:
Duragesic Transdermal System 1786

Fentanyl Citrate (Co-administration can result in enhanced CNS depression). Products include:
Actiq 1184

Fexofenadine Hydrochloride (Co-administration can result in enhanced CNS depression). Products include:
Allegra 712
Allegra-D Extended-Release Tablets 714

Flecainide Acetate (Co-administration with drugs that are substrate for P450IID6 isoenzyme,

such as flecainide, may increase plasma AUC of the tricyclic antidepressant). Products include:
- Tambocor Tablets 1990

Fluoxetine Hydrochloride (Co-administration with drugs that are substrate for P450IID6 isoenzyme, such as selective serotonin reuptake inhibitors, may increase plasma AUC of the tricyclic antidepressant; due to variation in the extent of inhibition, caution is indicated if co-administered and sufficient time must elapse for sequential therapy). Products include:
- Prozac Pulvules, Liquid, and Weekly Capsules 1238
- Sarafem Pulvules 1962

Fluphenazine Decanoate (Co-administration can result in enhanced CNS depression).
No products indexed under this heading.

Fluphenazine Enanthate (Co-administration can result in enhanced CNS depression).
No products indexed under this heading.

Fluphenazine Hydrochloride (Co-administration can result in enhanced CNS depression).
No products indexed under this heading.

Flurazepam Hydrochloride (Co-administration can result in enhanced CNS depression).
No products indexed under this heading.

Fluvoxamine Maleate (Co-administration with drugs that are substrate for P450IID6 isoenzyme, such as selective serotonin reuptake inhibitors, may increase plasma AUC of the tricyclic antidepressant; due to variation in the extent of inhibition, caution is indicated if co-administered and sufficient time must elapse for sequential therapy). Products include:
- Luvox Tablets (25, 50, 100 mg) 3256

Glutethimide (Co-administration can result in enhanced CNS depression).
No products indexed under this heading.

Glycopyrrolate (Co-administration with anticholinergic agents may result in additive anticholinergic effects, including paralytic ileus). Products include:
- Robinul Forte Tablets 1358
- Robinul Injectable 2940
- Robinul Tablets 1358

Guanadrel Sulfate (Amitriptyline may block the antihypertensive effect).
No products indexed under this heading.

Guanethidine Monosulfate (Amitriptyline may block the antihypertensive effect of guanethidine or similarly acting compounds).
No products indexed under this heading.

Haloperidol (Co-administration can result in enhanced CNS depression). Products include:
- Haldol Injection, Tablets and Concentrate 2533

Haloperidol Decanoate (Co-administration can result in enhanced CNS depression). Products include:
- Haldol Decanoate 2535

Hydrocodone Bitartrate (Co-administration can result in enhanced CNS depression). Products include:
- Hycodan 1316
- Hycomine Compound Tablets 1317
- Hycotuss Expectorant Syrup 1318
- Lortab 3319
- Lortab Elixir 3317
- Maxidone Tablets CIII 3399
- Norco 5/325 Tablets CIII 3424
- Norco 7.5/325 Tablets CIII 3425
- Norco 10/325 Tablets CIII 3427
- Norco 10/325 Tablets CIII 3425
- Vicodin Tablets 516
- Vicodin ES Tablets 517
- Vicodin HP Tablets 518
- Vicodin Tuss Expectorant 519
- Vicoprofen Tablets 520
- Zydone Tablets 1330

Hydrocodone Polistirex (Co-administration can result in enhanced CNS depression). Products include:
- Tussionex Pennkinetic Extended-Release Suspension 1174

Hydromorphone Hydrochloride (Co-administration can result in enhanced CNS depression). Products include:
- Dilaudid 441
- Dilaudid Oral Liquid 445
- Dilaudid Powder 441
- Dilaudid Rectal Suppositories 441
- Dilaudid Tablets 441
- Dilaudid Tablets - 8 mg 445
- Dilaudid-HP 443

Hydroxyzine Hydrochloride (Co-administration can result in enhanced CNS depression). Products include:
- Atarax Tablets & Syrup 2667
- Vistaril Intramuscular Solution 2738

Hyoscyamine (Co-administration with anticholinergic agents may result in additive anticholinergic effects, including paralytic ileus). Products include:
- Urised Tablets 2876

Hyoscyamine Sulfate (Co-administration with anticholinergic agents may result in additive anticholinergic effects, including paralytic ileus). Products include:
- Arco-Lase Plus Tablets 592
- Donnatal 2929
- Donnatal Extentabs 2930
- Levsin/Levsinex/Levbid 3172
- NuLev Orally Disintegrating Tablets 3176
- Prosed/DS Tablets 3268
- Urimax Tablets 1769

Imipramine Hydrochloride (Co-administration with drugs that are substrate for P450IID6 isoenzyme, such as many other antidepressants, may increase plasma AUC of the tricyclic antidepressant).
No products indexed under this heading.

Imipramine Pamoate (Co-administration with drugs that are substrate for P450IID6 isoenzyme, such as many other antidepressants, may increase plasma AUC of the tricyclic antidepressant).
No products indexed under this heading.

Ipratropium Bromide (Co-administration with anticholinergic agents may result in additive anticholinergic effects, including paralytic ileus). Products include:
- Atrovent Inhalation Aerosol 1030
- Atrovent Inhalation Solution 1031
- Atrovent Nasal Spray 0.03% 1032
- Atrovent Nasal Spray 0.06% 1033
- Combivent Inhalation Aerosol 1041
- DuoNeb Inhalation Solution 1233

Isocarboxazid (Co-administration of tricyclic antidepressants and MAO inhibitors has resulted in hyperpyretic crises, severe convulsions, and death; concurrent and/or sequential use is contraindicated).
No products indexed under this heading.

Isoflurane (Co-administration can result in enhanced CNS depression).
No products indexed under this heading.

Isoproterenol Hydrochloride (Effects of concurrent use not specified; close supervision and careful adjustment of dosages are required).
No products indexed under this heading.

Isoproterenol Sulfate (Effects of concurrent use not specified; close supervision and careful adjustment of dosages are required).
No products indexed under this heading.

Ketamine Hydrochloride (Co-administration can result in enhanced CNS depression).
No products indexed under this heading.

Levalbuterol Hydrochloride (Effects of concurrent use not specified; close supervision and careful adjustment of dosages are required). Products include:
- Xopenex Inhalation Solution 3207

Levomethadyl Acetate Hydrochloride (Co-administration can result in enhanced CNS depression).
No products indexed under this heading.

Levorphanol Tartrate (Co-administration can result in enhanced CNS depression). Products include:
- Levo-Dromoran 1734
- Levorphanol Tartrate Tablets 3059

Levothyroxine Sodium (On rare occasions, co-administration may produce arrhythmias). Products include:
- Levothroid Tablets 1373
- Levoxyl Tablets 1819
- Synthroid 505
- Unithroid Tablets 3445

Liothyronine Sodium (On rare occasions, co-administration may produce arrhythmias). Products include:
- Cytomel Tablets 1817
- Triostat Injection 1825

Liotrix (On rare occasions, co-administration may produce arrhythmias).
No products indexed under this heading.

Loratadine (Co-administration can result in enhanced CNS depression). Products include:
- Claritin 3100
- Claritin-D 12 Hour Extended Release Tablets 3102
- Claritin-D 24 Hour Extended Release Tablets 3104

Lorazepam (Co-administration can result in enhanced CNS depression). Products include:
- Ativan Injection 3478
- Ativan Tablets 3482

Loxapine Hydrochloride (Co-administration can result in enhanced CNS depression).
No products indexed under this heading.

Loxapine Succinate (Co-administration can result in enhanced CNS depression). Products include:
- Loxitane Capsules 3398

Maprotiline Hydrochloride (Co-administration with drugs that are substrate for P450IID6 isoenzyme, such as many other antidepressants, may increase plasma AUC of the tricyclic antidepressant).
No products indexed under this heading.

Mepenzolate Bromide (Co-administration with anticholinergic agents may result in additive anticholinergic effects, including paralytic ileus).
No products indexed under this heading.

Meperidine Hydrochloride (Co-administration can result in enhanced CNS depression). Products include:
- Demerol 3079
- Mepergan Injection 3539

Mephobarbital (Co-administration can result in enhanced CNS depression).
No products indexed under this heading.

Meprobamate (Co-administration can result in enhanced CNS depression). Products include:
- Miltown Tablets 3349

Mesoridazine Besylate (Co-administration can result in enhanced CNS depression). Products include:
- Serentil 1057

Metaproterenol Sulfate (Effects of concurrent use not specified; close supervision and careful adjustment of dosages are required). Products include:
- Alupent 1029

Metaraminol Bitartrate (Effects of concurrent use not specified; close supervision and careful adjustment of dosages are required). Products include:
- Aramine Injection 2043

Methadone Hydrochloride (Co-administration can result in enhanced CNS depression). Products include:
- Dolophine Hydrochloride Tablets 3056

Methdilazine Hydrochloride (Co-administration can result in enhanced CNS depression).
No products indexed under this heading.

Methohexital Sodium (Co-administration can result in enhanced CNS depression). Products include:
- Brevital Sodium for Injection, USP 1815

Methotrimeprazine (Co-administration can result in enhanced CNS depression).
No products indexed under this heading.

Methoxamine Hydrochloride (Effects of concurrent use not specified; close supervision and careful adjustment of dosages are required).
No products indexed under this heading.

Methoxyflurane (Co-administration can result in enhanced CNS depression).
No products indexed under this heading.

Midazolam Hydrochloride (Co-administration can result in enhanced CNS depression). Products include:
- Versed Injection 3027
- Versed Syrup 3033

Mirtazapine (Co-administration with drugs that are substrate for P450IID6 isoenzyme, such as many other antidepressants, may increase plasma AUC of the tricyclic antidepressant). Products include:
- Remeron Tablets 2483
- Remeron SolTab Tablets 2486

Moclobemide (Co-administration of tricyclic antidepressants and MAO inhibitors has resulted in hyperpyretic crises, severe convulsions, and death; concurrent and/or sequential use is contraindicated).
No products indexed under this heading.

Molindone Hydrochloride (Co-administration can result in enhanced CNS depression). Products include:
- Moban 1320

Morphine Sulfate (Co-administration can result in enhanced CNS depression). Products include:
- Astramorph/PF Injection, USP (Preservative-Free) 594
- Duramorph Injection 1312
- Infumorph 200 and Infumorph 500 Sterile Solutions 1314
- Kadian Capsules 1335
- MS Contin Tablets 2896
- MSIR 2898
- Oramorph SR Tablets 3062

Roxanol 3066

Nefazodone Hydrochloride (Co-administration with drugs that are substrate for P450IID6 isoenzyme, such as many other antidepressants, may increase plasma AUC of the tricyclic antidepressant). Products include:
- Serzone Tablets 1104

Norepinephrine Bitartrate (Effects of concurrent use not specified; close supervision and careful adjustment of dosages are required).
- No products indexed under this heading.

Nortriptyline Hydrochloride (Co-administration with drugs that are substrate for P450IID6 isoenzyme, such as many other antidepressants, may increase plasma AUC of the tricyclic antidepressant).
- No products indexed under this heading.

Olanzapine (Co-administration can result in enhanced CNS depression). Products include:
- Zyprexa Tablets 1973
- Zyprexa ZYDIS Orally Disintegrating Tablets................ 1973

Oxazepam (Co-administration can result in enhanced CNS depression).
- No products indexed under this heading.

Oxybutynin Chloride (Co-administration with anticholinergic agents may result in additive anticholinergic effects, including paralytic ileus). Products include:
- Ditropan XL Extended Release Tablets.................................... 564

Oxycodone Hydrochloride (Co-administration can result in enhanced CNS depression). Products include:
- OxyContin Tablets 2912
- OxyFast Oral Concentrate Solution . 2916
- OxyIR Capsules 2916
- Percocet Tablets 1326
- Percodan Tablets 1327
- Percolone Tablets 1327
- Roxicodone 3067
- Tylox Capsules 2597

Pargyline Hydrochloride (Co-administration of tricyclic antidepressants and MAO inhibitors has resulted in hyperpyretic crises, severe convulsions, and death; concurrent and/or sequential use is contraindicated).
- No products indexed under this heading.

Paroxetine Hydrochloride (Co-administration with drugs that are substrate for P450IID6 isoenzyme, such as selective serotonin reuptake inhibitors, may increase plasma AUC of the tricyclic antidepressant; due to variation in the extent of inhibition, caution is indicated if co-administered and sufficient time must elapse for sequential therapy). Products include:
- Paxil 1609

Pentobarbital Sodium (Co-administration can result in enhanced CNS depression). Products include:
- Nembutal Sodium Solution 485

Phenelzine Sulfate (Co-administration of tricyclic antidepressants and MAO inhibitors has resulted in hyperpyretic crises, severe convulsions, and death; concurrent and/or sequential use is contraindicated). Products include:
- Nardil Tablets 2653

Phenobarbital (Co-administration can result in enhanced CNS depression). Products include:
- Arco-Lase Plus Tablets 592
- Donnatal 2929
- Donnatal Extentabs 2930

Phenylephrine Bitartrate (Effects of concurrent use not specified; close supervision and careful adjustment of dosages are required).
- No products indexed under this heading.

Phenylephrine Hydrochloride (Effects of concurrent use not specified; close supervision and careful adjustment of dosages are required). Products include:
- Afrin Nasal Decongestant Children's Pump Mist................ 734
- Extendryl 1361
- Hycomine Compound Tablets 1317
- Neo-Synephrine 614
- Phenergan VC Syrup 3560
- Phenergan VC with Codeine Syrup .. 3561
- Preparation H Cream 778
- Preparation H Cooling Gel 778
- Preparation H 778
- Vicks Sinex Nasal Spray and Ultra Fine Mist............................ 729

Phenylephrine Tannate (Effects of concurrent use not specified; close supervision and careful adjustment of dosages are required). Products include:
- Ryna-12 S Suspension 3351
- Reformulated Rynatan Pediatric Suspension.................................. 3352
- Rynatuss Pediatric Suspension 3353
- Rynatuss Tablets 3353

Phenylpropanolamine Hydrochloride (Effects of concurrent use not specified; close supervision and careful adjustment of dosages are required).
- No products indexed under this heading.

Pirbuterol Acetate (Effects of concurrent use not specified; close supervision and careful adjustment of dosages are required). Products include:
- Maxair Autohaler 1981
- Maxair Inhaler 1984

Prazepam (Co-administration can result in enhanced CNS depression).
- No products indexed under this heading.

Procarbazine Hydrochloride (Co-administration of tricyclic antidepressants and MAO inhibitors has resulted in hyperpyretic crises, severe convulsions, and death; concurrent and/or sequential use is contraindicated). Products include:
- Matulane Capsules 3246

Prochlorperazine (Co-administration can result in enhanced CNS depression). Products include:
- Compazine 1505

Procyclidine Hydrochloride (Co-administration with anticholinergic agents may result in additive anticholinergic effects, including paralytic ileus).
- No products indexed under this heading.

Promethazine Hydrochloride (Co-administration can result in enhanced CNS depression). Products include:
- Mepergan Injection 3539
- Phenergan Injection 3553
- Phenergan 3556
- Phenergan Syrup 3554
- Phenergan with Codeine Syrup 3557
- Phenergan with Dextromethorphan Syrup 3559
- Phenergan VC Syrup 3560
- Phenergan VC with Codeine Syrup .. 3561

Propafenone Hydrochloride (Co-administration with drugs that are substrate for P450IID6 isoenzyme, such as propafenone, may increase plasma AUC of the tricyclic antidepressant). Products include:
- Rythmol Tablets – 150 mg, 225 mg, 300 mg 502

Propantheline Bromide (Co-administration with anticholinergic agents may result in additive anticholinergic effects, including paralytic ileus).
- No products indexed under this heading.

Propofol (Co-administration can result in enhanced CNS depression). Products include:
- Diprivan Injectable Emulsion 667

Propoxyphene Hydrochloride (Co-administration can result in enhanced CNS depression). Products include:
- Darvon Pulvules 1909
- Darvon Compound-65 Pulvules 1910

Propoxyphene Napsylate (Co-administration can result in enhanced CNS depression). Products include:
- Darvon-N/Darvocet-N 1907
- Darvon-N Tablets 1912

Protriptyline Hydrochloride (Co-administration with drugs that are substrate for P450IID6 isoenzyme, such as many other antidepressants, may increase plasma AUC of the tricyclic antidepressant). Products include:
- Vivactil Tablets 2446
- Vivactil Tablets 2217

Pseudoephedrine Hydrochloride (Effects of concurrent use not specified; close supervision and careful adjustment of dosages are required). Products include:
- Actifed Cold & Allergy Tablets 688
- Actifed Cold & Sinus Caplets and Tablets 688
- Advil Cold and Sinus Caplets 771
- Advil Cold and Sinus Tablets 771
- Advil Flu & Body Ache Caplets 772
- Aleve Cold & Sinus Caplets 603
- Alka-Seltzer Plus Liqui-Gels 604
- Alka-Seltzer Plus Cold & Flu Medicine Liqui-Gels.................... 604
- Alka-Seltzer Plus Cold & Sinus Medicine Liqui-Gels.................... 604
- Allegra-D Extended-Release Tablets 714
- BC Cold Powder 619
- Benadryl Allergy/Cold Tablets 691
- Benadryl Allergy/Congestion Tablets 692
- Benadryl Allergy & Sinus Liquid 693
- Benadryl Allergy & Sinus Fastmelt Tablets 693
- Benadryl Allergy Sinus Headache Caplets & Gelcaps....................... 693
- Benadryl Severe Allergy & Sinus Headache Caplets 694
- Benadryl Children's Allergy/Cold Fastmelt Tablets 692
- Benylin Multi-Symptom Liquid 697
- Bromfed Capsules (Extended-Release)........................ 2269
- Bromfed-PD Capsules (Extended-Release)........................ 2269
- Children's Cēpacol Sore Throat 788
- Comtrex Acute Head Cold & Sinus Pressure Relief Tablets....... 627
- Comtrex Deep Chest Cold & Congestion Relief Softgels........... 627
- Comtrex Flu Therapy & Fever Relief Daytime Caplets............... 628
- Comtrex Flu Therapy & Fever Relief Nighttime Tablets............... 628
- Comtrex Maximum Strength Multi-Symptom Cold & Cough Relief Tablets and Caplets............ 626
- Contac Non-Drowsy 12 Hour Cold Caplets................................. 745
- Contac Non-Drowsy Timed Release 12 Hour Cold Caplets..... 746
- Contac Severe Cold and Flu Caplets Maximum Strength........ 746
- Contac Severe Cold and Flu Caplets Non-Drowsy 746
- Dimetapp Elixir 777
- Dimetapp Cold and Fever Suspension.................................. 775
- Dimetapp DM Cold & Cough Elixir . 775
- Dimetapp Nighttime Flu Liquid 776
- Dimetapp Non-Drowsy Flu Syrup ... 777
- Dimetapp Infant Drops Decongestant............................... 775
- Dimetapp Infant Drops Decongestant Plus Cough.............. 776
- Guaifed 2272
- Kronofed-A 1341
- Children's Motrin Cold Oral Suspension.................................. 2007
- Motrin Sinus Headache Caplets 2005
- PediaCare Cough-Cold Liquid 719
- PediaCare Infants' Drops Decongestant............................... 719
- PediaCare Infants' Drops Decongestant Plus Cough............. 719
- PediaCare NightRest Cough-Cold Liquid 719
- Robitussin Cold Caplets Cold & Congestion................................. 780
- Robitussin Cold Softgels Cold & Congestion................................. 780
- Robitussin Cold Caplets Multi-Symptom Cold & Flu............ 781
- Robitussin Cold Softgels Multi-Symptom Cold & Flu............ 781
- Robitussin Cold Softgels Severe Congestion................................. 782
- Robitussin Cough & Cold Infant Drops 782
- Robitussin Maximum Strength Cough & Cold Liquid.................. 785
- Robitussin Pediatric Cough & Cold Formula Liquid................... 785
- Robitussin Multi Symptom Honey Flu Liquid 785
- Robitussin Nighttime Honey Flu Liquid 786
- Robitussin-CF Liquid 783
- Robitussin-DAC Syrup 2942
- Robitussin-PE Liquid 782
- Ryna 768
- Semprex-D Capsules 1172
- Singlet Caplets 761
- Sinutab Non-Drying Liquid Caps 706
- Sinutab Sinus Allergy Medication, Maximum Strength Formula, Tablets & Caplets......................... 707
- Sinutab Sinus Medication, Maximum Strength Without Drowsiness Formula, Tablets & Caplets.................................... 707
- Sudafed 12 Hour Tablets 708
- Sudafed 24 Hour Tablets 708
- Children's Sudafed Cold & Cough Liquid 709
- Children's Sudafed Nasal Decongestant Chewables........... 711
- Children's Sudafed Nasal Decongestant Liquid Medication.................................. 711
- Sudafed Cold & Allergy Tablets 708
- Sudafed Cold & Cough Liquid Caps 709
- Sudafed Cold & Sinus Liquid Caps 710
- Sudafed Nasal Decongestant Tablets 710
- Sudafed Non-Drying Sinus Liquid Caps 712
- Sudafed Severe Cold 711
- Sudafed Sinus Headache Caplets .. 712
- Sudafed Sinus Headache Tablets .. 712
- Tavist Sinus Non-Drowsy Coated Caplets...................................... 676
- TheraFlu Regular Strength Cold & Cough Night Time Hot Liquid...... 676
- TheraFlu Regular Strength Cold & Sore Throat Night Time Hot Liquid 676
- TheraFlu Maximum Strength Flu & Congestion Non-Drowsy Hot Liquid 677
- TheraFlu Maximum Strength Flu & Cough Night Time Hot Liquid.. 678
- TheraFlu Maximum Strength Flu & Sore Throat Night Time Hot Liquid 677
- TheraFlu Maximum Strength Severe Cold & Congestion Night Time Caplets................... 678
- TheraFlu Maximum Strength Severe Cold & Congestion Night Time Hot Liquid 678
- TheraFlu Maximum Strength Severe Cold & Congestion Non-Drowsy................................ 679
- Triaminic Allergy Congestion Liquid 680
- Triaminic Chest Congestion Liquid 680
- Triaminic Cold & Allergy Liquid 681
- Triaminic Cold & Allergy Softchews 683
- Triaminic Cold & Cough Liquid 681
- Triaminic Cold & Cough Softchews 683
- Triaminic Cold & Night Time Cough Liquid 681
- Triaminic Cold, Cough & Fever Liquid 681
- Triaminic Cough Liquid 682
- Triaminic Cough & Congestion Liquid 682
- Triaminic Cough & Sore Throat Liquid 682
- Triaminic Cough & Sore Throat Softchews 684
- Children's Tylenol Allergy-D Liquid .. 2014
- Children's Tylenol Cold Suspension Liquid and Chewable Tablets.......................... 2015

IMPORTANT NOTE: Always consult each drug listing in the patient's regimen for possible interactions.

Children's Tylenol Cold Plus Cough Suspension Liquid and Chewable Tablets 2015
Children's Tylenol Flu Suspension Liquid 2015
Children's Tylenol Sinus Suspension Liquid 2017
Infants' Tylenol Cold Decongestant and Fever Reducer Concentrated Drops 2015
Infants' Tylenol Cold Decongestant and Fever Reducer Concentrated Drops Plus Cough.. 2015
Tylenol Allergy Sinus 2010
Multi-Symptom Tylenol Cold Complete Formula Caplets 2010
Multi-Symptom Tylenol Cold Non-Drowsy Caplets and Gelcaps 2010
Multi-Symptom Tylenol Cold Severe Congestion Non-Drowsy Caplets 2011
Maximum Strength Tylenol Flu NightTime Gelcaps 2011
Maximum Strength Tylenol Flu NightTime Liquid 2011
Maximum Strength Tylenol Flu Non-Drowsy Gelcaps 2011
Maximum Strength Tylenol Sinus NightTime Caplets 2012
Maximum Strength Tylenol Sinus Non-Drowsy Geltabs, Gelcaps, Caplets, and Tablets 2012
Vicks 44D Cough & Head Congestion Relief Liquid .... ■724
Vicks 44M Cough, Cold & Flu Relief Liquid .... ■725
Pediatric Vicks 44m Cough & Cold Relief .... ■728
Vicks DayQuil LiquiCaps/Liquid Multi-Symptom Cold/Flu Relief ... ■727
Children's Vicks NyQuil Cold/Cough Relief .... ■726
Vicks NyQuil LiquiCaps/Liquid Multi-Symptom Cold/Flu Relief, Original and Cherry Flavors .... ■727
Zephrex Tablets 3091
Zephrex LA Tablets 3092
Zyrtec-D 12 Hour Extended Relief Tablets 2758

Pseudoephedrine Sulfate (Effects of concurrent use not specified; close supervision and careful adjustment of dosages are required). Products include:
Chlor-Trimeton Allergy/Decongestant Tablets .... ■736
Claritin-D 12 Hour Extended Release Tablets 3102
Claritin-D 24 Hour Extended Release Tablets 3104
Coricidin 'D' Cold, Flu & Sinus Tablets .... ■737
Drixoral Allergy/Sinus Extended-Release Tablets .... ■741
Drixoral Cold & Allergy Sustained-Action Tablets .... ■740
Drixoral Cold & Flu Extended-Release Tablets .... ■740
Drixoral Nasal Decongestant Long-Acting Non-Drowsy Tablets .... ■740
Rynatan Tablets 3351

Pyrilamine Maleate (Co-administration can result in enhanced CNS depression). Products include:
Maximum Strength Midol Menstrual Caplets and Gelcaps .... ■612
Maximum Strength Midol PMS Caplets and Gelcaps .... ■613

Pyrilamine Tannate (Co-administration can result in enhanced CNS depression). Products include:
Ryna-12 S Suspension 3351

Quazepam (Co-administration can result in enhanced CNS depression).
No products indexed under this heading.

Quetiapine Fumarate (Co-administration can result in enhanced CNS depression). Products include:
Seroquel Tablets 684

Quinidine Gluconate (Co-administration with drugs that inhibit P450IID6 isoenzyme, such as quinidine, may increase plasma AUC of the tricyclic antidepressant). Products include:
Quinaglute Dura-Tabs Tablets 978

Quinidine Polygalacturonate (Co-administration with drugs that inhibit P450IID6 isoenzyme, such as quinidine, may increase plasma AUC of the tricyclic antidepressant).
No products indexed under this heading.

Quinidine Sulfate (Co-administration with drugs that inhibit P450IID6 isoenzyme, such as quinidine, may increase plasma AUC of the tricyclic antidepressant). Products include:
Quinidex Extentabs 2933

Remifentanil Hydrochloride (Co-administration can result in enhanced CNS depression).
No products indexed under this heading.

Risperidone (Co-administration can result in enhanced CNS depression). Products include:
Risperdal 1796

Salmeterol Xinafoate (Effects of concurrent use not specified; close supervision and careful adjustment of dosages are required). Products include:
Advair Diskus 100/50 1448
Advair Diskus 250/50 1448
Advair Diskus 500/50 1448
Serevent Diskus 1637
Serevent Inhalation Aerosol 1633

Scopolamine (Co-administration with anticholinergic agents may result in additive anticholinergic effects, including paralytic ileus). Products include:
Transderm Scōp Transdermal Therapeutic System 2302

Scopolamine Hydrobromide (Co-administration with anticholinergic agents may result in additive anticholinergic effects, including paralytic ileus). Products include:
Donnatal 2929
Donnatal Extentabs 2930

Secobarbital Sodium (Co-administration can result in enhanced CNS depression).
No products indexed under this heading.

Selegiline Hydrochloride (Co-administration of tricyclic antidepressants and MAO inhibitors has resulted in hyperpyretic crises, severe convulsions, and death; concurrent and/or sequential use is contraindicated). Products include:
Eldepryl Capsules 3266

Sertraline Hydrochloride (Co-administration with drugs that are substrate for P450IID6 isoenzyme, such as selective serotonin reuptake inhibitors, may increase plasma AUC of the tricyclic antidepressant; due to variation in the extent of inhibition, caution is indicated if co-administered and sufficient time must elapse for sequential therapy). Products include:
Zoloft 2751

Sevoflurane (Co-administration can result in enhanced CNS depression).
No products indexed under this heading.

Sufentanil Citrate (Co-administration can result in enhanced CNS depression).
No products indexed under this heading.

Temazepam (Co-administration can result in enhanced CNS depression).
No products indexed under this heading.

Terbutaline Sulfate (Effects of concurrent use not specified; close supervision and careful adjustment of dosages are required). Products include:
Brethine Ampuls 2314
Brethine Tablets 2313

Terfenadine (Co-administration can result in enhanced CNS depression).
No products indexed under this heading.

Thiamylal Sodium (Co-administration can result in enhanced CNS depression).
No products indexed under this heading.

Thioridazine Hydrochloride (Co-administration can result in enhanced CNS depression). Products include:
Thioridazine Hydrochloride Tablets 2289

Thiothixene (Co-administration can result in enhanced CNS depression). Products include:
Navane Capsules 2701
Thiothixene Capsules 2290

Thyroglobulin (On rare occasions, co-administration may produce arrhythmias).
No products indexed under this heading.

Thyroid (On rare occasions, co-administration may produce arrhythmias).
No products indexed under this heading.

Thyroxine (On rare occasions, co-administration may produce arrhythmias).
No products indexed under this heading.

Thyroxine Sodium (On rare occasions, co-administration may produce arrhythmias).
No products indexed under this heading.

Tolterodine Tartrate (Co-administration with anticholinergic agents may result in additive anticholinergic effects, including paralytic ileus). Products include:
Detrol Tablets 3623
Detrol LA Capsules 2801

Tranylcypromine Sulfate (Co-administration of tricyclic antidepressants and MAO inhibitors has resulted in hyperpyretic crises, severe convulsions, and death; concurrent and/or sequential use is contraindicated). Products include:
Parnate Tablets 1607

Trazodone Hydrochloride (Co-administration with drugs that are substrate for P450IID6 isoenzyme, such as many other antidepressants, may increase plasma AUC of the tricyclic antidepressant).
No products indexed under this heading.

Triazolam (Co-administration can result in enhanced CNS depression). Products include:
Halcion Tablets 2823

Tridihexethyl Chloride (Co-administration with anticholinergic agents may result in additive anticholinergic effects, including paralytic ileus).
No products indexed under this heading.

Trifluoperazine Hydrochloride (Co-administration can result in enhanced CNS depression). Products include:
Stelazine 1640

Trihexyphenidyl Hydrochloride (Co-administration with anticholinergic agents may result in additive anticholinergic effects, including paralytic ileus). Products include:
Artane 1855

Trimeprazine Tartrate (Co-administration can result in enhanced CNS depression).
No products indexed under this heading.

Trimipramine Maleate (Co-administration with drugs that are substrate for P450IID6 isoenzyme, such as many other antidepressants, may increase plasma AUC of the tricyclic antidepressant). Products include:
Surmontil Capsules 3595

Tripelennamine Hydrochloride (Co-administration can result in enhanced CNS depression).
No products indexed under this heading.

Triprolidine Hydrochloride (Co-administration can result in enhanced CNS depression). Products include:
Actifed Cold & Allergy Tablets .... ■688

Venlafaxine Hydrochloride (Co-administration with drugs that are substrate for P450IID6 isoenzyme, such as many other antidepressants, may increase plasma AUC of the tricyclic antidepressant). Products include:
Effexor Tablets 3495
Effexor XR Capsules 3499

Zaleplon (Co-administration can result in enhanced CNS depression). Products include:
Sonata Capsules 3591

Ziprasidone Hydrochloride (Co-administration can result in enhanced CNS depression). Products include:
Geodon Capsules 2688

Zolpidem Tartrate (Co-administration can result in enhanced CNS depression). Products include:
Ambien Tablets 3191

Food Interactions

Alcohol (Amitriptyline may enhance the response to alcohol; potential for additive effects and hypotension; concurrent use should be avoided).

ETRAFON-FORTE TABLETS (4-25)

(Amitriptyline Hydrochloride, Perphenazine) 3115
See Etrafon Tablets (2-25)

EULEXIN CAPSULES

(Flutamide) 3118
May interact with:

Warfarin Sodium (Increases in prothrombin time have been noted in patients receiving long-term warfarin therapy after flutamide was initiated). Products include:
Coumadin for Injection 1243
Coumadin Tablets 1243
Warfarin Sodium Tablets, USP 3302

EVISTA TABLETS

(Raloxifene Hydrochloride) 1915
May interact with:

Cholestyramine (Co-administration causes a 60% reduction in the absorption and enterohepatic cycling of raloxifene; concurrent use should be avoided).
No products indexed under this heading.

Warfarin Sodium (Co-administration has resulted in a 10% decrease in prothrombin time in single-dose studies; if used concurrently, prothrombin time should be monitored). Products include:
Coumadin for Injection 1243
Coumadin Tablets 1243
Warfarin Sodium Tablets, USP 3302

Food Interactions

Food, unspecified (Administration of raloxifene with a standardized, high fat meal increases the absorption of raloxifene, but does not lead to clinically meaningful changes in systemic exposure; Evista can be administered without regard to meals).

EVOXAC CAPSULES

(Cevimeline Hydrochloride) 1217
May interact with antimuscarinic drugs, beta blockers, erythromycin, parasympathomimetics, quinidine, and certain other agents. Compounds in these categories include:

Acebutolol Hydrochloride (Possibility of conduction disturbances);

co-administration with beta adrenergic antagonists requires caution). Products include:

Sectral Capsules ... 3589

Amiodarone Hydrochloride (Co-administration with drugs which inhibit CYP2D6, such as amiodarone, may inhibit the metabolism of cevimeline resulting in a higher risk of adverse events). Products include:

Cordarone Intravenous ... 3491
Cordarone Tablets ... 3487
Pacerone Tablets ... 3331

Atenolol (Possibility of conduction disturbances; co-administration with beta adrenergic antagonists requires caution). Products include:

Tenoretic Tablets ... 690
Tenormin I.V. Injection ... 692

Atropine Sulfate (Cevimeline might interfere with the desirable antimuscarinic effects of drugs used concomitantly). Products include:

Donnatal ... 2929
Donnatal Extentabs ... 2930
Motofen Tablets ... 577
Prosed/DS Tablets ... 3268
Urised Tablets ... 2876

Belladonna Alkaloids (Cevimeline might interfere with the desirable antimuscarinic effects of drugs used concomitantly). Products include:

Hyland's Teething Tablets ... ▣766
Urimax Tablets ... 1769

Betaxolol Hydrochloride (Possibility of conduction disturbances; co-administration with beta adrenergic antagonists requires caution). Products include:

Betoptic S Ophthalmic Suspension ... 537

Bisoprolol Fumarate (Possibility of conduction disturbances; co-administration with beta adrenergic antagonists requires caution). Products include:

Zebeta Tablets ... 1885
Ziac Tablets ... 1887

Carteolol Hydrochloride (Possibility of conduction disturbances; co-administration with beta adrenergic antagonists requires caution). Products include:

Carteolol Hydrochloride Ophthalmic Solution USP, 1% ... ⊙258
Ocupress Ophthalmic Solution, 1% Sterile ... ⊙303

Cimetidine (Co-administration with drugs which inhibit CYP2D6, such as cimetidine, may inhibit the metabolism of cevimeline resulting in a higher risk of adverse events). Products include:

Tagamet HB 200 Suspension ... ▣762
Tagamet HB 200 Tablets ... ▣761
Tagamet Tablets ... 1644

Cimetidine Hydrochloride (Co-administration with drugs which inhibit CYP2D6, such as cimetidine, may inhibit the metabolism of cevimeline resulting in a higher risk of adverse events). Products include:

Tagamet ... 1644

Clarithromycin (Co-administration with drugs which inhibit CYP3A3/4, such as clarithromycin, may inhibit the metabolism of cevimeline resulting in a higher risk of adverse events). Products include:

Biaxin/Biaxin XL ... 403
PREVPAC ... 3298

Clidinium Bromide (Cevimeline might interfere with the desirable antimuscarinic effects of drugs used concomitantly).

No products indexed under this heading.

Dicyclomine Hydrochloride (Cevimeline might interfere with the desirable antimuscarinic effects of drugs used concomitantly).

No products indexed under this heading.

Diltiazem Hydrochloride (Co-administration with drugs which inhibit CYP3A3/4, such as diltiazem, may inhibit the metabolism of cevimeline resulting in a higher risk of adverse events). Products include:

Cardizem Injectable ... 1018
Cardizem Lyo-Ject Syringe ... 1018
Cardizem Monovial ... 1018
Cardizem CD Capsules ... 1016
Tiazac Capsules ... 1378

Edrophonium Chloride (Co-administration with parasympathomimetic drugs can be expected to have additive effects). Products include:

Tensilon Injectable ... 1745

Erythromycin (Co-administration with drugs which inhibit CYP3A3/4, such as erythromycin, may inhibit the metabolism of cevimeline resulting in a higher risk of adverse events). Products include:

Emgel 2% Topical Gel ... 1285
Ery-Tab Tablets ... 448
Erythromycin Base Filmtab Tablets . 454
Erythromycin Delayed-Release Capsules, USP ... 455
PCE Dispertab Tablets ... 498

Erythromycin Estolate (Co-administration with drugs which inhibit CYP3A3/4, such as erythromycin, may inhibit the metabolism of cevimeline resulting in a higher risk of adverse events).

No products indexed under this heading.

Erythromycin Ethylsuccinate (Co-administration with drugs which inhibit CYP3A3/4, such as erythromycin, may inhibit the metabolism of cevimeline resulting in a higher risk of adverse events). Products include:

E.E.S. ... 450
EryPed ... 446
Pediazole Suspension ... 3050

Erythromycin Gluceptate (Co-administration with drugs which inhibit CYP3A3/4, such as erythromycin, may inhibit the metabolism of cevimeline resulting in a higher risk of adverse events).

No products indexed under this heading.

Erythromycin Stearate (Co-administration with drugs which inhibit CYP3A3/4, such as erythromycin, may inhibit the metabolism of cevimeline resulting in a higher risk of adverse events). Products include:

Erythrocin Stearate Filmtab Tablets ... 452

Esmolol Hydrochloride (Possibility of conduction disturbances; co-administration with beta adrenergic antagonists requires caution). Products include:

Brevibloc Injection ... 858

Fluoxetine Hydrochloride (Co-administration with drugs which inhibit CYP2D6, such as fluoxetine, may inhibit the metabolism of cevimeline resulting in a higher risk of adverse events). Products include:

Prozac Pulvules, Liquid, and Weekly Capsules ... 1238
Sarafem Pulvules ... 1962

Glycopyrrolate (Cevimeline might interfere with the desirable antimuscarinic effects of drugs used concomitantly). Products include:

Robinul Forte Tablets ... 1358
Robinul Injectable ... 2940
Robinul Tablets ... 1358

Hyoscyamine (Cevimeline might interfere with the desirable antimuscarinic effects of drugs used concomitantly). Products include:

Urised Tablets ... 2876

Hyoscyamine Sulfate (Cevimeline might interfere with the desirable antimuscarinic effects of drugs used concomitantly). Products include:

Arco-Lase Plus Tablets ... 592
Donnatal ... 2929
Donnatal Extentabs ... 2930
Levsin/Levsinex/Levbid ... 3172
NuLev Orally Disintegrating Tablets ... 3176
Prosed/DS Tablets ... 3268
Urimax Tablets ... 1769

Indinavir Sulfate (Co-administration with drugs which inhibit CYP3A3/4, such as indinavir, may inhibit the metabolism of cevimeline resulting in a higher risk of adverse events). Products include:

Crixivan Capsules ... 2070

Ipratropium Bromide (Cevimeline might interfere with the desirable antimuscarinic effects of drugs used concomitantly). Products include:

Atrovent Inhalation Aerosol ... 1030
Atrovent Inhalation Solution ... 1031
Atrovent Nasal Spray 0.03% ... 1032
Atrovent Nasal Spray 0.06% ... 1033
Combivent Inhalation Aerosol ... 1041
DuoNeb Inhalation Solution ... 1233

Itraconazole (Co-administration with drugs which inhibit CYP3A3/4, such as itraconazole, may inhibit the metabolism of cevimeline resulting in a higher risk of adverse events). Products include:

Sporanox Capsules ... 1800
Sporanox Injection ... 1804
Sporanox Injection ... 2509
Sporanox Oral Solution ... 1808
Sporanox Oral Solution ... 2512

Ketoconazole (Co-administration with drugs which inhibit CYP3A3/4, such as ketoconazole, may inhibit the metabolism of cevimeline resulting in a higher risk of adverse events). Products include:

Nizoral 2% Cream ... 3620
Nizoral A-D Shampoo ... 2008
Nizoral 2% Shampoo ... 2007
Nizoral Tablets ... 1791

Labetalol Hydrochloride (Possibility of conduction disturbances; co-administration with beta adrenergic antagonists requires caution). Products include:

Normodyne Injection ... 3135
Normodyne Tablets ... 3137

Levobunolol Hydrochloride (Possibility of conduction disturbances; co-administration with beta adrenergic antagonists requires caution). Products include:

Betagan ... ⊙228

Mepenzolate Bromide (Cevimeline might interfere with the desirable antimuscarinic effects of drugs used concomitantly).

No products indexed under this heading.

Metipranolol Hydrochloride (Possibility of conduction disturbances; co-administration with beta adrenergic antagonists requires caution).

No products indexed under this heading.

Metoprolol Succinate (Possibility of conduction disturbances; co-administration with beta adrenergic antagonists requires caution). Products include:

Toprol-XL Tablets ... 651

Metoprolol Tartrate (Possibility of conduction disturbances; co-administration with beta adrenergic antagonists requires caution).

No products indexed under this heading.

Nadolol (Possibility of conduction disturbances; co-administration with beta adrenergic antagonists requires caution). Products include:

Corgard Tablets ... 2245
Corzide 40/5 Tablets ... 2247
Corzide 80/5 Tablets ... 2247
Nadolol Tablets ... 2288

Nefazodone Hydrochloride (Co-administration with drugs which inhibit CYP3A3/4, such as nefazodone, may inhibit the metabolism of cevimeline resulting in a higher risk of adverse events). Products include:

Serzone Tablets ... 1104

Nelfinavir Mesylate (Co-administration with drugs which inhibit CYP3A3/4, such as nelfinavir, may inhibit the metabolism of cevimeline resulting in a higher risk of adverse events). Products include:

Viracept ... 532

Neostigmine Bromide (Co-administration with parasympathomimetic drugs can be expected to have additive effects). Products include:

Prostigmin Tablets ... 1744

Neostigmine Methylsulfate (Co-administration with parasympathomimetic drugs can be expected to have additive effects). Products include:

Prostigmin Injectable ... 1744

Oxyphenonium Bromide (Cevimeline might interfere with the desirable antimuscarinic effects of drugs used concomitantly).

No products indexed under this heading.

Paroxetine Hydrochloride (Co-administration with drugs which inhibit CYP2D6, such as paroxetine, may inhibit the metabolism of cevimeline resulting in a higher risk of adverse events). Products include:

Paxil ... 1609

Penbutolol Sulfate (Possibility of conduction disturbances; co-administration with beta adrenergic antagonists requires caution).

No products indexed under this heading.

Pindolol (Possibility of conduction disturbances; co-administration with beta adrenergic antagonists requires caution).

No products indexed under this heading.

Propantheline Bromide (Cevimeline might interfere with the desirable antimuscarinic effects of drugs used concomitantly).

No products indexed under this heading.

Propranolol Hydrochloride (Possibility of conduction disturbances; co-administration with beta adrenergic antagonists requires caution). Products include:

Inderal ... 3513
Inderal LA Long-Acting Capsules ... 3516
Inderide Tablets ... 3517
Inderide LA Long-Acting Capsules ... 3519

Pyridostigmine Bromide (Co-administration with parasympathomimetic drugs can be expected to have additive effects). Products include:

Mestinon ... 1740

Quinidine Gluconate (Co-administration with drugs which inhibit CYP2D6, such as quinidine, may inhibit the metabolism of cevimeline resulting in a higher risk of adverse events). Products include:

Quinaglute Dura-Tabs Tablets ... 978

Quinidine Polygalacturonate (Co-administration with drugs which inhibit CYP2D6, such as quinidine, may inhibit the metabolism of cevimeline resulting in a higher risk of adverse events).

No products indexed under this heading.

Quinidine Sulfate (Co-administration with drugs which inhibit CYP2D6, such as quinidine, may inhibit the metabolism of

cevimeline resulting in a higher risk of adverse events). Products include:

Quinidex Extentabs 2933

Ritonavir (Co-administration with drugs which inhibit CYP2D6 and/or CYP3A3/4, such as ritonavir, may inhibit the metabolism of cevimeline resulting in a higher risk of adverse events). Products include:

Kaletra Capsules 471
Kaletra Oral Solution 471
Norvir Capsules 487
Norvir Oral Solution 487

Scopolamine (Cevimeline might interfere with the desirable antimuscarinic effects of drugs used concomitantly). Products include:

Transderm Scōp Transdermal Therapeutic System 2302

Scopolamine Hydrobromide (Cevimeline might interfere with the desirable antimuscarinic effects of drugs used concomitantly). Products include:

Donnatal 2929
Donnatal Extentabs 2930

Sertraline Hydrochloride (Co-administration with drugs which inhibit CYP2D6, such as sertraline, may inhibit the metabolism of cevimeline resulting in a higher risk of adverse events). Products include:

Zoloft 2751

Sotalol Hydrochloride (Possibility of conduction disturbances; co-administration with beta adrenergic antagonists requires caution). Products include:

Betapace Tablets 950
Betapace AF Tablets 954

Timolol Hemihydrate (Possibility of conduction disturbances; co-administration with beta adrenergic antagonists requires caution). Products include:

Betimol Ophthalmic Solution .... ⊙324

Timolol Maleate (Possibility of conduction disturbances; co-administration with beta adrenergic antagonists requires caution). Products include:

Blocadren Tablets 2046
Cosopt Sterile Ophthalmic Solution 2065
Timolide Tablets 2187
Timolol GFS .... ⊙266
Timoptic in Ocudose 2192
Timoptic Sterile Ophthalmic Solution 2190
Timoptic-XE Sterile Ophthalmic Gel Forming Solution 2194

Tolterodine Tartrate (Cevimeline might interfere with the desirable antimuscarinic effects of drugs used concomitantly). Products include:

Detrol Tablets 3623
Detrol LA Capsules 2801

Tridihexethyl Chloride (Cevimeline might interfere with the desirable antimuscarinic effects of drugs used concomitantly).

No products indexed under this heading.

Verapamil Hydrochloride (Co-administration with drugs which inhibit CYP3A3/4, such as verapamil, may inhibit the metabolism of cevimeline resulting in a higher risk of adverse events). Products include:

Covera-HS Tablets 3199
Isoptin SR Tablets 467
Tarka Tablets 508
Verelan Capsules 3184
Verelan PM Capsules 3186

Food Interactions

Food, unspecified (Co-administration with food decreases the rate of absorption, with a fasting Tmax of 1.53 hours and a Tmax of 2.86 hours after a meal; the peak concentration is reduced by 17.3%).

Grapefruit Juice (Co-administration with drugs which inhibit CYP3A3/4, such as grapefruit juice, may inhibit the metabolism of cevimeline resulting in a higher risk of adverse events).

ASPIRIN FREE EXCEDRIN CAPLETS AND GELTABS

(Acetaminophen, Caffeine) .... ▣628

Food Interactions

Alcohol (Chronic heavy alcohol users, 3 or more drinks per day, should consult their physicians for advice on when and how they should take pain relievers/fever reducers including acetaminophen).

EXCEDRIN EXTRA-STRENGTH TABLETS, CAPLETS, AND GELTABS

(Acetaminophen, Aspirin, Caffeine) .... ▣629

May interact with oral anticoagulants, antigout agents, and oral hypoglycemic agents. Compounds in these categories include:

Acarbose (Co-administration is not recommended unless directed by a doctor). Products include:

Precose Tablets 906

Allopurinol (Co-administration is not recommended unless directed by a doctor).

No products indexed under this heading.

Chlorpropamide (Co-administration is not recommended unless directed by a doctor). Products include:

Diabinese Tablets 2680

Dicumarol (Co-administration is not recommended unless directed by a doctor).

No products indexed under this heading.

Glimepiride (Co-administration is not recommended unless directed by a doctor). Products include:

Amaryl Tablets 717

Glipizide (Co-administration is not recommended unless directed by a doctor). Products include:

Glucotrol Tablets 2692
Glucotrol XL Extended Release Tablets 2693

Glyburide (Co-administration is not recommended unless directed by a doctor). Products include:

DiaBeta Tablets 741
Glucovance Tablets 1086

Metformin Hydrochloride (Co-administration is not recommended unless directed by a doctor). Products include:

Glucophage Tablets 1080
Glucophage XR Tablets 1080
Glucovance Tablets 1086

Miglitol (Co-administration is not recommended unless directed by a doctor). Products include:

Glyset Tablets 2821

Pioglitazone Hydrochloride (Co-administration is not recommended unless directed by a doctor). Products include:

Actos Tablets 3275

Probenecid (Co-administration is not recommended unless directed by a doctor).

No products indexed under this heading.

Repaglinide (Co-administration is not recommended unless directed by a doctor). Products include:

Prandin Tablets (0.5, 1, and 2 mg) 2432

Rosiglitazone Maleate (Co-administration is not recommended unless directed by a doctor). Products include:

Avandia Tablets 1490

Sulfinpyrazone (Co-administration is not recommended unless directed by a doctor).

No products indexed under this heading.

Tolazamide (Co-administration is not recommended unless directed by a doctor).

No products indexed under this heading.

Tolbutamide (Co-administration is not recommended unless directed by a doctor).

No products indexed under this heading.

Troglitazone (Co-administration is not recommended unless directed by a doctor).

No products indexed under this heading.

Warfarin Sodium (Co-administration is not recommended unless directed by a doctor). Products include:

Coumadin for Injection 1243
Coumadin Tablets 1243
Warfarin Sodium Tablets, USP 3302

Food Interactions

Alcohol (Chronic heavy alcohol users, 3 or more drinks per day, should consult their physicians for advice on when and how they should take pain relievers/fever reducers including acetaminophen).

EXCEDRIN MIGRAINE CAPLETS

(Acetaminophen, Aspirin, Caffeine) 1070

May interact with oral anticoagulants, oral hypoglycemic agents, and certain other agents. Compounds in these categories include:

Acarbose (Concurrent use with diabetes drugs should be avoided unless directed by a doctor). Products include:

Precose Tablets 906

Antiarthritic Drugs, unspecified (Concurrent use with arthritis medications should be avoided unless directed by a doctor).

Caffeine-containing medications (Concomitant use may cause nervousness, irritability, sleeplessness, and occasionally, rapid heart beat).

No products indexed under this heading.

Chlorpropamide (Concurrent use with diabetes drugs should be avoided unless directed by a doctor). Products include:

Diabinese Tablets 2680

Dicumarol (Concurrent use with anticoagulants should be avoided unless directed by a doctor).

No products indexed under this heading.

Glimepiride (Concurrent use with diabetes drugs should be avoided unless directed by a doctor). Products include:

Amaryl Tablets 717

Glipizide (Concurrent use with diabetes drugs should be avoided unless directed by a doctor). Products include:

Glucotrol Tablets 2692
Glucotrol XL Extended Release Tablets 2693

Glyburide (Concurrent use with diabetes drugs should be avoided unless directed by a doctor). Products include:

DiaBeta Tablets 741
Glucovance Tablets 1086

Metformin Hydrochloride (Concurrent use with diabetes drugs should be avoided unless directed by a doctor). Products include:

Glucophage Tablets 1080
Glucophage XR Tablets 1080
Glucovance Tablets 1086

Miglitol (Concurrent use with diabetes drugs should be avoided unless directed by a doctor). Products include:

Glyset Tablets 2821

Pioglitazone Hydrochloride (Concurrent use with diabetes drugs should be avoided unless directed by a doctor). Products include:

Actos Tablets 3275

Probenecid (Concurrent use with gout medications should be avoided unless directed by a doctor).

No products indexed under this heading.

Repaglinide (Concurrent use with diabetes drugs should be avoided unless directed by a doctor). Products include:

Prandin Tablets (0.5, 1, and 2 mg) 2432

Rosiglitazone Maleate (Concurrent use with diabetes drugs should be avoided unless directed by a doctor). Products include:

Avandia Tablets 1490

Sulfinpyrazone (Concurrent use with gout medications should be avoided unless directed by a doctor).

No products indexed under this heading.

Tolazamide (Concurrent use with diabetes drugs should be avoided unless directed by a doctor).

No products indexed under this heading.

Tolbutamide (Concurrent use with diabetes drugs should be avoided unless directed by a doctor).

No products indexed under this heading.

Troglitazone (Concurrent use with diabetes drugs should be avoided unless directed by a doctor).

No products indexed under this heading.

Warfarin Sodium (Concurrent use with anticoagulants should be avoided unless directed by a doctor). Products include:

Coumadin for Injection 1243
Coumadin Tablets 1243
Warfarin Sodium Tablets, USP 3302

Food Interactions

Alcohol (Chronic heavy alcohol users, 3 or more drinks per day, should consult their physicians for advice on when and how they should take pain relievers/fever reducers including acetaminophen and aspirin).

Beverages, caffeine-containing (Concomitant use may cause nervousness, irritability, sleeplessness, and occasionally, rapid heart beat).

Food, caffeine-containing (Concomitant use may cause nervousness, irritability, sleeplessness, and occasionally, rapid heart beat).

EXCEDRIN MIGRAINE GELTABS

(Acetaminophen, Aspirin, Caffeine) 1070

See Excedrin Migraine Caplets

EXCEDRIN MIGRAINE TABLETS

(Acetaminophen, Aspirin, Caffeine) 1070

See Excedrin Migraine Caplets

EXCEDRIN PM TABLETS, CAPLETS, AND GELTABS

(Acetaminophen, Diphenhydramine Citrate) .... ▣631

May interact with hypnotics and sedatives, tranquilizers, and certain other agents. Compounds in these categories include:

Alprazolam (Excedrine P.M. contains diphenhydramine that causes

drowsiness, therefore, concomitant use should be avoided). Products include:

Xanax Tablets 2865

Buspirone Hydrochloride (Excedrine P.M. contains diphenhydramine that causes drowsiness, therefore, concomitant use should be avoided).

No products indexed under this heading.

Chlordiazepoxide (Excedrine P.M. contains diphenhydramine that causes drowsiness, therefore, concomitant use should be avoided). Products include:

Limbitrol 1738

Chlordiazepoxide Hydrochloride (Excedrine P.M. contains diphenhydramine that causes drowsiness, therefore, concomitant use should be avoided). Products include:

Librium Capsules 1736
Librium for Injection 1737

Chlorpromazine (Excedrine P.M. contains diphenhydramine that causes drowsiness, therefore, concomitant use should be avoided). Products include:

Thorazine Suppositories 1656

Chlorpromazine Hydrochloride (Excedrine P.M. contains diphenhydramine that causes drowsiness, therefore, concomitant use should be avoided). Products include:

Thorazine 1656

Chlorprothixene (Excedrine P.M. contains diphenhydramine that causes drowsiness, therefore, concomitant use should be avoided).

No products indexed under this heading.

Chlorprothixene Hydrochloride (Excedrine P.M. contains diphenhydramine that causes drowsiness, therefore, concomitant use should be avoided).

No products indexed under this heading.

Clorazepate Dipotassium (Excedrine P.M. contains diphenhydramine that causes drowsiness, therefore, concomitant use should be avoided). Products include:

Tranxene 511

Diazepam (Excedrine P.M. contains diphenhydramine that causes drowsiness, therefore, concomitant use should be avoided). Products include:

Valium Injectable 3026
Valium Tablets 3047

Droperidol (Excedrine P.M. contains diphenhydramine that causes drowsiness, therefore, concomitant use should be avoided).

No products indexed under this heading.

Estazolam (Excedrine P.M. contains diphenhydramine that causes drowsiness, therefore, concomitant use should be avoided). Products include:

ProSom Tablets 500

Ethchlorvynol (Excedrine P.M. contains diphenhydramine that causes drowsiness, therefore, concomitant use should be avoided).

No products indexed under this heading.

Ethinamate (Excedrine P.M. contains diphenhydramine that causes drowsiness, therefore, concomitant use should be avoided).

No products indexed under this heading.

Fluphenazine Decanoate (Excedrine P.M. contains diphenhydramine that causes drowsiness, therefore, concomitant use should be avoided).

No products indexed under this heading.

Fluphenazine Enanthate (Excedrine P.M. contains diphenhydramine that causes drowsiness, therefore, concomitant use should be avoided).

No products indexed under this heading.

Fluphenazine Hydrochloride (Excedrine P.M. contains diphenhydramine that causes drowsiness, therefore, concomitant use should be avoided).

No products indexed under this heading.

Flurazepam Hydrochloride (Excedrine P.M. contains diphenhydramine that causes drowsiness, therefore, concomitant use should be avoided).

No products indexed under this heading.

Glutethimide (Excedrine P.M. contains diphenhydramine that causes drowsiness, therefore, concomitant use should be avoided).

No products indexed under this heading.

Haloperidol (Excedrine P.M. contains diphenhydramine that causes drowsiness, therefore, concomitant use should be avoided). Products include:

Haldol Injection, Tablets and Concentrate 2533

Haloperidol Decanoate (Excedrine P.M. contains diphenhydramine that causes drowsiness, therefore, concomitant use should be avoided). Products include:

Haldol Decanoate 2535

Hydroxyzine Hydrochloride (Excedrine P.M. contains diphenhydramine that causes drowsiness, therefore, concomitant use should be avoided). Products include:

Atarax Tablets & Syrup 2667
Vistaril Intramuscular Solution 2738

Lorazepam (Excedrine P.M. contains diphenhydramine that causes drowsiness, therefore, concomitant use should be avoided). Products include:

Ativan Injection 3478
Ativan Tablets 3482

Loxapine Hydrochloride (Excedrine P.M. contains diphenhydramine that causes drowsiness, therefore, concomitant use should be avoided).

No products indexed under this heading.

Loxapine Succinate (Excedrine P.M. contains diphenhydramine that causes drowsiness, therefore, concomitant use should be avoided). Products include:

Loxitane Capsules 3398

Meprobamate (Excedrine P.M. contains diphenhydramine that causes drowsiness, therefore, concomitant use should be avoided). Products include:

Miltown Tablets 3349

Mesoridazine Besylate (Excedrine P.M. contains diphenhydramine that causes drowsiness, therefore, concomitant use should be avoided). Products include:

Serentil 1057

Midazolam Hydrochloride (Excedrine P.M. contains diphenhydramine that causes drowsiness, therefore, concomitant use should be avoided). Products include:

Versed Injection 3027
Versed Syrup 3033

Molindone Hydrochloride (Excedrine P.M. contains diphenhydramine that causes drowsiness, therefore, concomitant use should be avoided). Products include:

Moban 1320

Oxazepam (Excedrine P.M. contains diphenhydramine that causes drowsiness, therefore, concomitant use should be avoided).

No products indexed under this heading.

Perphenazine (Excedrine P.M. contains diphenhydramine that causes drowsiness, therefore, concomitant use should be avoided). Products include:

Etrafon 3115
Trilafon 3160

Prazepam (Excedrine P.M. contains diphenhydramine that causes drowsiness, therefore, concomitant use should be avoided).

No products indexed under this heading.

Prochlorperazine (Excedrine P.M. contains diphenhydramine that causes drowsiness, therefore, concomitant use should be avoided). Products include:

Compazine 1505

Promethazine Hydrochloride (Excedrine P.M. contains diphenhydramine that causes drowsiness, therefore, concomitant use should be avoided). Products include:

Mepergan Injection 3539
Phenergan Injection 3553
Phenergan 3556
Phenergan Syrup 3554
Phenergan with Codeine Syrup 3557
Phenergan with Dextromethorphan Syrup 3559
Phenergan VC Syrup 3560
Phenergan VC with Codeine Syrup . 3561

Propofol (Excedrine P.M. contains diphenhydramine that causes drowsiness, therefore, concomitant use should be avoided). Products include:

Diprivan Injectable Emulsion 667

Quazepam (Excedrine P.M. contains diphenhydramine that causes drowsiness, therefore, concomitant use should be avoided).

No products indexed under this heading.

Secobarbital Sodium (Excedrine P.M. contains diphenhydramine that causes drowsiness, therefore, concomitant use should be avoided).

No products indexed under this heading.

Temazepam (Excedrine P.M. contains diphenhydramine that causes drowsiness, therefore, concomitant use should be avoided).

No products indexed under this heading.

Thioridazine Hydrochloride (Excedrine P.M. contains diphenhydramine that causes drowsiness, therefore, concomitant use should be avoided). Products include:

Thioridazine Hydrochloride Tablets 2289

Thiothixene (Excedrine P.M. contains diphenhydramine that causes drowsiness, therefore, concomitant use should be avoided). Products include:

Navane Capsules 2701
Thiothixene Capsules 2290

Triazolam (Excedrine P.M. contains diphenhydramine that causes drowsiness, therefore, concomitant use should be avoided). Products include:

Halcion Tablets 2823

Trifluoperazine Hydrochloride (Excedrine P.M. contains diphenhydramine that causes drowsiness, therefore, concomitant use should be avoided). Products include:

Stelazine 1640

Zaleplon (Excedrine P.M. contains diphenhydramine that causes drowsiness, therefore, concomitant use should be avoided). Products include:

Sonata Capsules 3591

Zolpidem Tartrate (Excedrine P.M. contains diphenhydramine that causes drowsiness, therefore, concomitant use should be avoided). Products include:

Ambien Tablets 3191

Food Interactions

Alcohol (Chronic heavy alcohol users, 3 or more drinks per day, should consult their physicians for advice on when and how they should take pain relievers/fever reducers including acetaminophen; Excedrine P.M. contains diphenhydramine that causes drowsiness, therefore, concomitant use should be avoided).

EXELON CAPSULES

(Rivastigmine Tartrate) 2342
See Exelon Oral Solution

EXELON ORAL SOLUTION

(Rivastigmine Tartrate) 2345
May interact with anticholinergics and certain other agents. Compounds in these categories include:

Atropine Sulfate (Rivastigmine, a cholinesterase inhibitor, has the potential to interfere with the activity of anticholinergic medications). Products include:

Donnatal 2929
Donnatal Extentabs 2930
Motofen Tablets 577
Prosed/DS Tablets 3268
Urised Tablets 2876

Belladonna Alkaloids (Rivastigmine, a cholinesterase inhibitor, has the potential to interfere with the activity of anticholinergic medications). Products include:

Hyland's Teething Tablets 766
Urimax Tablets 1769

Benztropine Mesylate (Rivastigmine, a cholinesterase inhibitor, has the potential to interfere with the activity of anticholinergic medications). Products include:

Cogentin 2055

Bethanechol Chloride (Coadministration with cholinergic agonist, such as bethanechol, can be expected to result in a synergistic effect). Products include:

Urecholine 2198
Urecholine Tablets 2445

Biperiden Hydrochloride (Rivastigmine, a cholinesterase inhibitor, has the potential to interfere with the activity of anticholinergic medications). Products include:

Akineton 402

Clidinium Bromide (Rivastigmine, a cholinesterase inhibitor, has the potential to interfere with the activity of anticholinergic medications).

No products indexed under this heading.

Dicyclomine Hydrochloride (Rivastigmine, a cholinesterase inhibitor, has the potential to interfere with the activity of anticholinergic medications).

No products indexed under this heading.

Glycopyrrolate (Rivastigmine, a cholinesterase inhibitor, has the potential to interfere with the activity of anticholinergic medications). Products include:

Robinul Forte Tablets 1358
Robinul Injectable 2940
Robinul Tablets 1358

Hyoscyamine (Rivastigmine, a cholinesterase inhibitor, has the potential to interfere with the activity of anticholinergic medications). Products include:

Urised Tablets 2876

Hyoscyamine Sulfate (Rivastigmine, a cholinesterase inhibitor, has the potential to interfere with the activity of anticholinergic medications). Products include:

Arco-Lase Plus Tablets 592
Donnatal 2929
Donnatal Extentabs 2930

Levsin/Levsinex/Levbid 3172
NuLev Orally Disintegrating Tablets 3176
Prosed/DS Tablets 3268
Urimax Tablets 1769

Ipratropium Bromide (Rivastigmine, a cholinesterase inhibitor, has the potential to interfere with the activity of anticholinergic medications). Products include:
Atrovent Inhalation Aerosol 1030
Atrovent Inhalation Solution 1031
Atrovent Nasal Spray 0.03% 1032
Atrovent Nasal Spray 0.06% 1033
Combivent Inhalation Aerosol 1041
DuoNeb Inhalation Solution 1233

Mepenzolate Bromide (Rivastigmine, a cholinesterase inhibitor, has the potential to interfere with the activity of anticholinergic medications).
No products indexed under this heading.

Oxybutynin Chloride (Rivastigmine, a cholinesterase inhibitor, has the potential to interfere with the activity of anticholinergic medications). Products include:
Ditropan XL Extended Release Tablets 564

Procyclidine Hydrochloride (Rivastigmine, a cholinesterase inhibitor, has the potential to interfere with the activity of anticholinergic medications).
No products indexed under this heading.

Propantheline Bromide (Rivastigmine, a cholinesterase inhibitor, has the potential to interfere with the activity of anticholinergic medications).
No products indexed under this heading.

Scopolamine (Rivastigmine, a cholinesterase inhibitor, has the potential to interfere with the activity of anticholinergic medications). Products include:
Transderm Scōp Transdermal Therapeutic System 2302

Scopolamine Hydrobromide (Rivastigmine, a cholinesterase inhibitor, has the potential to interfere with the activity of anticholinergic medications). Products include:
Donnatal 2929
Donnatal Extentabs 2930

Succinylcholine Chloride (Co-administration with succinylcholine can be expected to result in a synergistic effect). Products include:
Anectine Injection 1476

Tolterodine Tartrate (Rivastigmine, a cholinesterase inhibitor, has the potential to interfere with the activity of anticholinergic medications). Products include:
Detrol Tablets 3623
Detrol LA Capsules 2801

Tridihexethyl Chloride (Rivastigmine, a cholinesterase inhibitor, has the potential to interfere with the activity of anticholinergic medications).
No products indexed under this heading.

Trihexyphenidyl Hydrochloride (Rivastigmine, a cholinesterase inhibitor, has the potential to interfere with the activity of anticholinergic medications). Products include:
Artane 1855

Food Interactions

Food, unspecified (Co-administration with food delays absorption (tmax) by 90 minutes, lowers Cmax by approximately 30% and increases AUC by approximately 30%).

EX•LAX GENTLE STRENGTH CAPLETS

(Docusate Sodium, Sennosides) ..... ▣670
None cited in PDR database.

EX•LAX REGULAR STRENGTH PILLS

(Sennosides) .... ▣670
None cited in PDR database.

EX•LAX REGULAR STRENGTH CHOCOLATED PIECES

(Sennosides) .... ▣669
None cited in PDR database.

EX•LAX MAXIMUM STRENGTH PILLS

(Sennosides) .... ▣670
None cited in PDR database.

EX•LAX MILK OF MAGNESIA LIQUID

(Magnesium Hydroxide) .... ▣670
May interact with:

Prescription Drugs, unspecified (Antacids may interact with certain unspecified prescription drugs).

EX•LAX STOOL SOFTENER CAPLETS

(Docusate Sodium) .... ▣671
May interact with:

Mineral Oil (Concurrent use with oral mineral oil-containing products is not recommended). Products include:
Anusol Ointment .... ▣688
Fleet Mineral Oil Enema 1360
Lubriderm Advanced Therapy Creamy Lotion .... ▣703
Lubriderm Seriously Sensitive Lotion .... ▣703
Lubriderm Skin Therapy Moisturizing Lotion .... ▣703
Moisture Eyes PM Preservative Free Eye Ointment .... ⊙253
Preparation H Ointment .... ▣778
Refresh P.M. Lubricant Eye Ointment .... ⊙251

EXTENDRYL CHEWABLE TABLETS

(Chlorpheniramine Maleate, Methscopolamine Nitrate, Phenylephrine Hydrochloride)........... 1361
See Extendryl Syrup

EXTENDRYL SR & JR CAPSULES

(Chlorpheniramine Maleate, Methscopolamine Nitrate, Phenylephrine Hydrochloride)........... 1361
See Extendryl Syrup

EXTENDRYL SYRUP

(Chlorpheniramine Maleate, Methscopolamine Nitrate, Phenylephrine Hydrochloride)........... 1361
May interact with beta blockers, central nervous system depressants, monoamine oxidase inhibitors, veratrum alkaloids, and certain other agents. Compounds in these categories include:

Acebutolol Hydrochloride (Concurrent use with beta adrenergic blocker increases the effects of sympathomimetics). Products include:
Sectral Capsules 3589

Alfentanil Hydrochloride (Concomitant use of antihistamines with CNS depressants may have an additive effect).
No products indexed under this heading.

Alprazolam (Concomitant use of antihistamines with CNS depressants may have an additive effect). Products include:
Xanax Tablets 2865

Aprobarbital (Concomitant use of antihistamines with CNS depressants may have an additive effect).
No products indexed under this heading.

Atenolol (Concurrent use with beta adrenergic blocker increases the effects of sympathomimetics). Products include:
Tenoretic Tablets 690
Tenormin I.V. Injection 692

Betaxolol Hydrochloride (Concurrent use with beta adrenergic blocker increases the effects of sympathomimetics). Products include:
Betoptic S Ophthalmic Suspension 537

Bisoprolol Fumarate (Concurrent use with beta adrenergic blocker increases the effects of sympathomimetics). Products include:
Zebeta Tablets 1885
Ziac Tablets 1887

Buprenorphine Hydrochloride (Concomitant use of antihistamines with CNS depressants may have an additive effect). Products include:
Buprenex Injectable 2918

Buspirone Hydrochloride (Concomitant use of antihistamines with CNS depressants may have an additive effect).
No products indexed under this heading.

Butabarbital (Concomitant use of antihistamines with CNS depressants may have an additive effect).
No products indexed under this heading.

Butalbital (Concomitant use of antihistamines with CNS depressants may have an additive effect). Products include:
Phrenilin 578
Sedapap Tablets 50 mg/650 mg ... 2225

Carteolol Hydrochloride (Concurrent use with beta adrenergic blocker increases the effects of sympathomimetics). Products include:
Carteolol Hydrochloride Ophthalmic Solution USP, 1% ..... ⊙258
Ocupress Ophthalmic Solution, 1% Sterile .... ⊙303

Chlordiazepoxide (Concomitant use of antihistamines with CNS depressants may have an additive effect). Products include:
Limbitrol 1738

Chlordiazepoxide Hydrochloride (Concomitant use of antihistamines with CNS depressants may have an additive effect). Products include:
Librium Capsules 1736
Librium for Injection 1737

Chlorpromazine (Concomitant use of antihistamines with CNS depressants may have an additive effect). Products include:
Thorazine Suppositories 1656

Chlorpromazine Hydrochloride (Concomitant use of antihistamines with CNS depressants may have an additive effect). Products include:
Thorazine 1656

Chlorprothixene (Concomitant use of antihistamines with CNS depressants may have an additive effect).
No products indexed under this heading.

Chlorprothixene Hydrochloride (Concomitant use of antihistamines with CNS depressants may have an additive effect).
No products indexed under this heading.

Chlorprothixene Lactate (Concomitant use of antihistamines with CNS depressants may have an additive effect).
No products indexed under this heading.

Clorazepate Dipotassium (Concomitant use of antihistamines with CNS depressants may have an additive effect). Products include:
Tranxene 511

Clozapine (Concomitant use of antihistamines with CNS depressants may have an additive effect). Products include:
Clozaril Tablets 2319

Codeine Phosphate (Concomitant use of antihistamines with CNS depressants may have an additive effect). Products include:
Phenergan with Codeine Syrup 3557
Phenergan VC with Codeine Syrup .. 3561
Robitussin A-C Syrup 2942
Robitussin-DAC Syrup 2942
Ryna-C Liquid .... ▣768
Soma Compound w/Codeine Tablets 3355
Tussi-Organidin NR Liquid 3350
Tussi-Organidin-S NR Liquid 3350
Tylenol with Codeine 2595

Cryptenamine Preparations (Sympathomimetics may reduce the antihypertensive effects of veratrum alkaloids).

Desflurane (Concomitant use of antihistamines with CNS depressants may have an additive effect). Products include:
Suprane Liquid for Inhalation 874

Dezocine (Concomitant use of antihistamines with CNS depressants may have an additive effect).
No products indexed under this heading.

Diazepam (Concomitant use of antihistamines with CNS depressants may have an additive effect). Products include:
Valium Injectable 3026
Valium Tablets 3047

Droperidol (Concomitant use of antihistamines with CNS depressants may have an additive effect).
No products indexed under this heading.

Enflurane (Concomitant use of antihistamines with CNS depressants may have an additive effect).
No products indexed under this heading.

Esmolol Hydrochloride (Concurrent use with beta adrenergic blocker increases the effects of sympathomimetics). Products include:
Brevibloc Injection 858

Estazolam (Concomitant use of antihistamines with CNS depressants may have an additive effect). Products include:
ProSom Tablets 500

Ethchlorvynol (Concomitant use of antihistamines with CNS depressants may have an additive effect).
No products indexed under this heading.

Ethinamate (Concomitant use of antihistamines with CNS depressants may have an additive effect).
No products indexed under this heading.

Fentanyl (Concomitant use of antihistamines with CNS depressants may have an additive effect). Products include:
Duragesic Transdermal System 1786

Fentanyl Citrate (Concomitant use of antihistamines with CNS depressants may have an additive effect). Products include:
Actiq 1184

Fluphenazine Decanoate (Concomitant use of antihistamines with CNS depressants may have an additive effect).
No products indexed under this heading.

Fluphenazine Enanthate (Concomitant use of antihistamines with CNS depressants may have an additive effect).
No products indexed under this heading.

Fluphenazine Hydrochloride (Concomitant use of antihistamines with CNS depressants may have an additive effect).
No products indexed under this heading.

Flurazepam Hydrochloride (Concomitant use of antihistamines with CNS depressants may have an additive effect).
No products indexed under this heading.

Glutethimide (Concomitant use of antihistamines with CNS depressants may have an additive effect).
No products indexed under this heading.

Guanethidine Monosulfate (Sympathomimetics may reduce the antihypertensive effects of guanethidine).
No products indexed under this heading.

Haloperidol (Concomitant use of antihistamines with CNS depressants may have an additive effect).
Products include:
Haldol Injection, Tablets and Concentrate 2533

Haloperidol Decanoate (Concomitant use of antihistamines with CNS depressants may have an additive effect). Products include:
Haldol Decanoate 2535

Hydrocodone Bitartrate (Concomitant use of antihistamines with CNS depressants may have an additive effect). Products include:
Hycodan 1316
Hycomine Compound Tablets 1317
Hycotuss Expectorant Syrup 1318
Lortab 3319
Lortab Elixir 3317
Maxidone Tablets CIII 3399
Norco 5/325 Tablets CIII 3424
Norco 7.5/325 Tablets CIII 3425
Norco 10/325 Tablets CIII 3427
Norco 10/325 Tablets CIII 3425
Vicodin Tablets 516
Vicodin ES Tablets 517
Vicodin HP Tablets 518
Vicodin Tuss Expectorant 519
Vicoprofen Tablets 520
Zydone Tablets 1330

Hydrocodone Polistirex (Concomitant use of antihistamines with CNS depressants may have an additive effect). Products include:
Tussionex Pennkinetic Extended-Release Suspension 1174

Hydromorphone Hydrochloride (Concomitant use of antihistamines with CNS depressants may have an additive effect). Products include:
Dilaudid 441
Dilaudid Oral Liquid 445
Dilaudid Powder 441
Dilaudid Rectal Suppositories 441
Dilaudid Tablets 441
Dilaudid Tablets - 8 mg 445
Dilaudid-HP 443

Hydroxyzine Hydrochloride (Concomitant use of antihistamines with CNS depressants may have an additive effect). Products include:
Atarax Tablets & Syrup 2667
Vistaril Intramuscular Solution 2738

Isocarboxazid (Concurrent use with MAO inhibitor increases the effects of sympathomimetics; co-administration is contraindicated).
No products indexed under this heading.

Isoflurane (Concomitant use of antihistamines with CNS depressants may have an additive effect).
No products indexed under this heading.

Ketamine Hydrochloride (Concomitant use of antihistamines with CNS depressants may have an additive effect).
No products indexed under this heading.

Labetalol Hydrochloride (Concurrent use with beta adrenergic blocker increases the effects of sympathomimetics). Products include:
Normodyne Injection 3135
Normodyne Tablets 3137

Levobunolol Hydrochloride (Concurrent use with beta adrenergic blocker increases the effects of sympathomimetics). Products include:
Betagan .... ⊙228

Levomethadyl Acetate Hydrochloride (Concomitant use of antihistamines with CNS depressants may have an additive effect).
No products indexed under this heading.

Levorphanol Tartrate (Concomitant use of antihistamines with CNS depressants may have an additive effect). Products include:
Levo-Dromoran 1734
Levorphanol Tartrate Tablets 3059

Lorazepam (Concomitant use of antihistamines with CNS depressants may have an additive effect). Products include:
Ativan Injection 3478
Ativan Tablets 3482

Loxapine Hydrochloride (Concomitant use of antihistamines with CNS depressants may have an additive effect).
No products indexed under this heading.

Loxapine Succinate (Concomitant use of antihistamines with CNS depressants may have an additive effect). Products include:
Loxitane Capsules 3398

Meperidine Hydrochloride (Concomitant use of antihistamines with CNS depressants may have an additive effect). Products include:
Demerol 3079
Mepergan Injection 3539

Mephobarbital (Concomitant use of antihistamines with CNS depressants may have an additive effect).
No products indexed under this heading.

Meprobamate (Concomitant use of antihistamines with CNS depressants may have an additive effect).
Products include:
Miltown Tablets 3349

Mesoridazine Besylate (Concomitant use of antihistamines with CNS depressants may have an additive effect). Products include:
Serentil 1057

Methadone Hydrochloride (Concomitant use of antihistamines with CNS depressants may have an additive effect). Products include:
Dolophine Hydrochloride Tablets 3056

Methohexital Sodium (Concomitant use of antihistamines with CNS depressants may have an additive effect). Products include:
Brevital Sodium for Injection, USP 1815

Methotrimeprazine (Concomitant use of antihistamines with CNS depressants may have an additive effect).
No products indexed under this heading.

Methoxyflurane (Concomitant use of antihistamines with CNS depressants may have an additive effect).
No products indexed under this heading.

Methyldopa (Sympathomimetics may reduce the antihypertensive effects of methyldopa). Products include:
Aldoclor Tablets 2035
Aldomet Tablets 2037
Aldoril Tablets 2039

Metipranolol Hydrochloride (Concurrent use with beta adrenergic blocker increases the effects of sympathomimetics).
No products indexed under this heading.

Metoprolol Succinate (Concurrent use with beta adrenergic blocker increases the effects of sympathomimetics). Products include:
Toprol-XL Tablets 651

Metoprolol Tartrate (Concurrent use with beta adrenergic blocker increases the effects of sympathomimetics).
No products indexed under this heading.

Midazolam Hydrochloride (Concomitant use of antihistamines with CNS depressants may have an additive effect). Products include:
Versed Injection 3027
Versed Syrup 3033

Moclobemide (Concurrent use with MAO inhibitor increases the effects of sympathomimetics; co-administration is contraindicated).
No products indexed under this heading.

Molindone Hydrochloride (Concomitant use of antihistamines with CNS depressants may have an additive effect). Products include:
Moban 1320

Morphine Sulfate (Concomitant use of antihistamines with CNS depressants may have an additive effect). Products include:
Astramorph/PF Injection, USP (Preservative-Free) 594
Duramorph Injection 1312
Infumorph 200 and Infumorph 500 Sterile Solutions 1314
Kadian Capsules 1335
MS Contin Tablets 2896
MSIR 2898
Oramorph SR Tablets 3062
Roxanol 3066

Nadolol (Concurrent use with beta adrenergic blocker increases the effects of sympathomimetics).
Products include:
Corgard Tablets 2245
Corzide 40/5 Tablets 2247
Corzide 80/5 Tablets 2247
Nadolol Tablets 2288

Olanzapine (Concomitant use of antihistamines with CNS depressants may have an additive effect).
Products include:
Zyprexa Tablets 1973
Zyprexa ZYDIS Orally Disintegrating Tablets 1973

Oxazepam (Concomitant use of antihistamines with CNS depressants may have an additive effect).
No products indexed under this heading.

Oxycodone Hydrochloride (Concomitant use of antihistamines with CNS depressants may have an additive effect). Products include:
OxyContin Tablets 2912
OxyFast Oral Concentrate Solution 2916
OxyIR Capsules 2916
Percocet Tablets 1326
Percodan Tablets 1327
Percolone Tablets 1327
Roxicodone 3067
Tylox Capsules 2597

Pargyline Hydrochloride (Concurrent use with MAO inhibitor increases the effects of sympathomimetics; co-administration is contraindicated).
No products indexed under this heading.

Penbutolol Sulfate (Concurrent use with beta adrenergic blocker increases the effects of sympathomimetics).
No products indexed under this heading.

Pentobarbital Sodium (Concomitant use of antihistamines with CNS depressants may have an additive effect). Products include:
Nembutal Sodium Solution 485

Perphenazine (Concomitant use of antihistamines with CNS depressants may have an additive effect).
Products include:
Etrafon 3115
Trilafon 3160

Phenelzine Sulfate (Concurrent use with MAO inhibitor increases the effects of sympathomimetics; co-administration is contraindicated).
Products include:
Nardil Tablets 2653

Phenobarbital (Concomitant use of antihistamines with CNS depressants may have an additive effect).
Products include:
Arco-Lase Plus Tablets 592
Donnatal 2929
Donnatal Extentabs 2930

Pindolol (Concurrent use with beta adrenergic blocker increases the effects of sympathomimetics).
No products indexed under this heading.

Prazepam (Concomitant use of antihistamines with CNS depressants may have an additive effect).
No products indexed under this heading.

Procarbazine Hydrochloride (Concurrent use with MAO inhibitor increases the effects of sympathomimetics; co-administration is contraindicated). Products include:
Matulane Capsules 3246

Prochlorperazine (Concomitant use of antihistamines with CNS depressants may have an additive effect). Products include:
Compazine 1505

Promethazine Hydrochloride (Concomitant use of antihistamines with CNS depressants may have an additive effect). Products include:
Mepergan Injection 3539
Phenergan Injection 3553
Phenergan 3556
Phenergan Syrup 3554
Phenergan with Codeine Syrup 3557
Phenergan with Dextromethorphan Syrup 3559
Phenergan VC Syrup 3560
Phenergan VC with Codeine Syrup 3561

Propofol (Concomitant use of antihistamines with CNS depressants may have an additive effect).
Products include:
Diprivan Injectable Emulsion 667

Propoxyphene Hydrochloride (Concomitant use of antihistamines with CNS depressants may have an additive effect). Products include:
Darvon Pulvules 1909
Darvon Compound-65 Pulvules 1910

Propoxyphene Napsylate (Concomitant use of antihistamines with CNS depressants may have an additive effect). Products include:
Darvon-N/Darvocet-N 1907
Darvon-N Tablets 1912

Propranolol Hydrochloride (Concurrent use with beta adrenergic blocker increases the effects of sympathomimetics). Products include:
Inderal 3513
Inderal LA Long-Acting Capsules 3516
Inderide Tablets 3517
Inderide LA Long-Acting Capsules 3519

Quazepam (Concomitant use of antihistamines with CNS depressants may have an additive effect).
No products indexed under this heading.

Quetiapine Fumarate (Concomitant use of antihistamines with CNS depressants may have an additive effect). Products include:
Seroquel Tablets 684

Remifentanil Hydrochloride (Concomitant use of antihistamines with CNS depressants may have an additive effect).
No products indexed under this heading.

Reserpine (Sympathomimetics may reduce the antihypertensive effects of reserpine).
No products indexed under this heading.

Risperidone (Concomitant use of antihistamines with CNS depressants may have an additive effect).
Products include:

Risperdal 1796

Secobarbital Sodium (Concomitant use of antihistamines with CNS depressants may have an additive effect).
No products indexed under this heading.

Selegiline Hydrochloride (Concurrent use with MAO inhibitor increases the effects of sympathomimetics; co-administration is contraindicated). Products include:
Eldepryl Capsules 3266

Sevoflurane (Concomitant use of antihistamines with CNS depressants may have an additive effect).
No products indexed under this heading.

Sotalol Hydrochloride (Concurrent use with beta adrenergic blocker increases the effects of sympathomimetics). Products include:
Betapace Tablets 950
Betapace AF Tablets 954

Sufentanil Citrate (Concomitant use of antihistamines with CNS depressants may have an additive effect).
No products indexed under this heading.

Temazepam (Concomitant use of antihistamines with CNS depressants may have an additive effect).
No products indexed under this heading.

Thiamylal Sodium (Concomitant use of antihistamines with CNS depressants may have an additive effect).
No products indexed under this heading.

Thioridazine Hydrochloride (Concomitant use of antihistamines with CNS depressants may have an additive effect). Products include:
Thioridazine Hydrochloride Tablets 2289

Thiothixene (Concomitant use of antihistamines with CNS depressants may have an additive effect). Products include:
Navane Capsules 2701
Thiothixene Capsules 2290

Timolol Hemihydrate (Concurrent use with beta adrenergic blocker increases the effects of sympathomimetics). Products include:
Betimol Ophthalmic Solution .... ⊙324

Timolol Maleate (Concurrent use with beta adrenergic blocker increases the effects of sympathomimetics). Products include:
Blocadren Tablets 2046
Cosopt Sterile Ophthalmic Solution 2065
Timolide Tablets 2187
Timolol GFS .... ⊙266
Timoptic in Ocudose 2192
Timoptic Sterile Ophthalmic Solution 2190
Timoptic-XE Sterile Ophthalmic Gel Forming Solution 2194

Tranylcypromine Sulfate (Concurrent use with MAO inhibitor increases the effects of sympathomimetics; co-administration is contraindicated). Products include:
Parnate Tablets 1607

Triazolam (Concomitant use of antihistamines with CNS depressants may have an additive effect). Products include:
Halcion Tablets 2823

Trifluoperazine Hydrochloride (Concomitant use of antihistamines with CNS depressants may have an additive effect). Products include:
Stelazine 1640

Zaleplon (Concomitant use of antihistamines with CNS depressants may have an additive effect). Products include:
Sonata Capsules 3591

Ziprasidone Hydrochloride (Concomitant use of antihistamines with CNS depressants may have an additive effect). Products include:
Geodon Capsules 2688

Zolpidem Tartrate (Concomitant use of antihistamines with CNS depressants may have an additive effect). Products include:
Ambien Tablets 3191

Food Interactions

Alcohol (Concomitant use of antihistamines with alcohol may have an additive effect).

EYE WASH SOLUTION
(Boric Acid, Sodium Borate, Sodium Chloride) .... ⊙252
None cited in PDR database.

EYE•SCRUB PADS
(PEG-200 Glyceryl Tallowate) .... ⊙304
None cited in PDR database.

FACTREL
(Gonadorelin Hydrochloride) 3633
May interact with androgens, dopamine antagonists, corticosteroids, estrogens, oral contraceptives, phenothiazines, progestins, and certain other agents. Compounds in these categories include:

Betamethasone Acetate (Pituitary secretion of gonadotropins affected). Products include:
Celestone Soluspan Injectable Suspension 3097

Betamethasone Sodium Phosphate (Pituitary secretion of gonadotropins affected). Products include:
Celestone Soluspan Injectable Suspension 3097

Chlorotrianisene (Pituitary secretion of gonadotropins affected).
No products indexed under this heading.

Chlorpromazine (Rise in prolactin; response to Factrel may be blunted). Products include:
Thorazine Suppositories 1656

Chlorpromazine Hydrochloride (Rise in prolactin; response to Factrel may be blunted). Products include:
Thorazine 1656

Clozapine (Rise in prolactin; response to Factrel may be blunted). Products include:
Clozaril Tablets 2319

Cortisone Acetate (Pituitary secretion of gonadotropins affected). Products include:
Cortone Acetate Injectable Suspension 2059
Cortone Acetate Tablets 2061

Desogestrel (Pituitary secretion of gonadotropins affected; gonadotropin levels suppressed). Products include:
Cyclessa Tablets 2450
Desogen Tablets 2458
Mircette Tablets 2470
Ortho-Cept 21 Tablets 2546
Ortho-Cept 28 Tablets 2546

Dexamethasone (Pituitary secretion of gonadotropins affected). Products include:
Decadron Elixir 2078
Decadron Tablets 2079
TobraDex Ophthalmic Ointment 542
TobraDex Ophthalmic Suspension 541

Dexamethasone Acetate (Pituitary secretion of gonadotropins affected).
No products indexed under this heading.

Dexamethasone Sodium Phosphate (Pituitary secretion of gonadotropins affected). Products include:
Decadron Phosphate Injection 2081
Decadron Phosphate Sterile Ophthalmic Ointment 2083
Decadron Phosphate Sterile Ophthalmic Solution 2084
NeoDecadron Sterile Ophthalmic Solution 2144

Dienestrol (Pituitary secretion of gonadotropins affected). Products include:
Ortho Dienestrol Cream 2554

Diethylstilbestrol (Pituitary secretion of gonadotropins affected).
No products indexed under this heading.

Digitoxin (Gonadotropin levels suppressed).
No products indexed under this heading.

Digoxin (Gonadotropin levels suppressed). Products include:
Digitek Tablets 1003
Lanoxicaps Capsules 1574
Lanoxin Injection 1581
Lanoxin Tablets 1587
Lanoxin Elixir Pediatric 1578
Lanoxin Injection Pediatric 1584

Estradiol (Pituitary secretion of gonadotropins affected). Products include:
Activella Tablets 2764
Alora Transdermal System 3372
Climara Transdermal System 958
CombiPatch Transdermal System 2323
Esclim Transdermal System 3460
Estrace Vaginal Cream 3358
Estrace Tablets 3361
Estring Vaginal Ring 2811
Ortho-Prefest Tablets 2570
Vagifem Tablets 2857
Vivelle Transdermal System 2412
Vivelle-Dot Transdermal System 2416

Estrogens, Conjugated (Pituitary secretion of gonadotropins affected). Products include:
Premarin Intravenous 3563
Premarin Tablets 3566
Premarin Vaginal Cream 3570
Premphase Tablets 3572
Prempro Tablets 3572

Estrogens, Esterified (Pituitary secretion of gonadotropins affected). Products include:
Estratest 3252
Menest Tablets 2254

Estropipate (Pituitary secretion of gonadotropins affected). Products include:
Ogen Tablets 2846
Ortho-Est Tablets 3464

Ethinyl Estradiol (Pituitary secretion of gonadotropins affected; gonadotropin levels suppressed). Products include:
Alesse-21 Tablets 3468
Alesse-28 Tablets 3473
Brevicon 28-Day Tablets 3380
Cyclessa Tablets 2450
Desogen Tablets 2458
Estinyl Tablets 3112
Estrostep 2627
femhrt Tablets 2635
Levlen 962
Levlite 21 Tablets 962
Levlite 28 Tablets 962
Levora Tablets 3389
Loestrin 21 Tablets 2642
Loestrin Fe Tablets 2642
Lo/Ovral Tablets 3532
Lo/Ovral-28 Tablets 3538
Low-Ogestrel-28 Tablets 3392
Microgestin Fe 1.5/30 Tablets 3407
Microgestin Fe 1/20 Tablets 3400
Mircette Tablets 2470
Modicon 2563
Necon 3415
Nordette-28 Tablets 2257
Norinyl 1 +35 28-Day Tablets 3380
Ogestrel 0.5/50-28 Tablets 3428
Ortho-Cept 21 Tablets 2546
Ortho-Cept 28 Tablets 2546
Ortho-Cyclen/Ortho Tri-Cyclen 2573
Ortho-Novum 2563
Ovcon 3364
Ovral Tablets 3551
Ovral-28 Tablets 3552
Tri-Levlen 962
Tri-Norinyl-28 Tablets 3433
Triphasil-21 Tablets 3600
Triphasil-28 Tablets 3605
Trivora Tablets 3439
Yasmin 28 Tablets 980
Zovia 3449

Ethynodiol Diacetate (Gonadotropin levels suppressed). Products include:
Zovia 3449

Fludrocortisone Acetate (Pituitary secretion of gonadotropins affected). Products include:
Florinef Acetate Tablets 2250

Fluoxymesterone (Pituitary secretion of gonadotropins affected).
No products indexed under this heading.

Fluphenazine Decanoate (Rise in prolactin; response to Factrel may be blunted).
No products indexed under this heading.

Fluphenazine Enanthate (Rise in prolactin; response to Factrel may be blunted).
No products indexed under this heading.

Fluphenazine Hydrochloride (Rise in prolactin; response to Factrel may be blunted).
No products indexed under this heading.

Haloperidol (Rise in prolactin; response to Factrel may be blunted). Products include:
Haldol Injection, Tablets and Concentrate 2533

Haloperidol Decanoate (Rise in prolactin; response to Factrel may be blunted). Products include:
Haldol Decanoate 2535

Hydrocortisone (Pituitary secretion of gonadotropins affected). Products include:
Anusol-HC Cream 2.5% 2237
Cipro HC Otic Suspension 540
Cortaid Intensive Therapy Cream .... ▣717
Cortaid Maximum Strength Cream .... ▣717
Cortisporin Ophthalmic Suspension Sterile .... ⊙297
Cortizone•5 .... ▣699
Cortizone•10 .... ▣699
Cortizone•10 Plus Creme .... ▣700
Cortizone for Kids Creme .... ▣699
Hydrocortone Tablets 2106
Massengill Medicated Soft Cloth Towelette .... ▣753
VōSoL HC Otic Solution 3356

Hydrocortisone Acetate (Pituitary secretion of gonadotropins affected). Products include:
Analpram-HC 1338
Anusol HC-1 Hydrocortisone Anti-Itch Cream .... ▣689
Anusol-HC Suppositories 2238
Cortaid .... ▣717
Cortifoam Rectal Foam 3170
Cortisporin-TC Otic Suspension 2246
Hydrocortone Acetate Injectable Suspension 2103
Pramosone 1343
Proctocort Suppositories 2264
ProctoFoam-HC 3177
Terra-Cortril Ophthalmic Suspension 2716

Hydrocortisone Sodium Phosphate (Pituitary secretion of gonadotropins affected). Products include:
Hydrocortone Phosphate Injection, Sterile 2105

Hydrocortisone Sodium Succinate (Pituitary secretion of gonadotropins affected).
No products indexed under this heading.

Levodopa (Minimal elevation of gonadotropin levels). Products include:
Sinemet Tablets 1253
Sinemet CR Tablets 1255

Levonorgestrel (Gonadotropin levels suppressed). Products include:
Alesse-21 Tablets 3468
Alesse-28 Tablets 3473
Levlen 962
Levlite 21 Tablets 962
Levlite 28 Tablets 962
Levora Tablets 3389
Mirena Intrauterine System 974
Nordette-28 Tablets 2257
Norplant System 3543
Tri-Levlen 962
Triphasil-21 Tablets 3600

Triphasil-28 Tablets 3605
Trivora Tablets 3439

Medroxyprogesterone Acetate (Pituitary secretion of gonadotropins affected). Products include:
Depo-Provera Contraceptive Injection 2798
Lunelle Monthly Injection 2827
Premphase Tablets 3572
Prempro Tablets 3572
Provera Tablets 2853

Megestrol Acetate (Pituitary secretion of gonadotropins affected). Products include:
Megace Oral Suspension 1124

Mesoridazine Besylate (Rise in prolactin; response to Factrel may be blunted). Products include:
Serentil 1057

Mestranol (Gonadotropin levels suppressed). Products include:
Necon 1/50 Tablets 3415
Norinyl 1 + 50 28-Day Tablets 3380
Ortho-Novum 1/50□28 Tablets 2556

Methotrimeprazine (Rise in prolactin; response to Factrel may be blunted).
No products indexed under this heading.

Methylprednisolone Acetate (Pituitary secretion of gonadotropins affected). Products include:
Depo-Medrol Injectable Suspension 2795

Methylprednisolone Sodium Succinate (Pituitary secretion of gonadotropins affected). Products include:
Solu-Medrol Sterile Powder 2855

Methyltestosterone (Pituitary secretion of gonadotropins affected). Products include:
Android Capsules, 10 mg 1731
Estratest 3252
Testred Capsules, 10 mg 1746

Metoclopramide Hydrochloride (Rise in prolactin; response to Factrel may be blunted). Products include:
Reglan 2935

Norethindrone (Gonadotropin levels suppressed). Products include:
Brevicon 28-Day Tablets 3380
Micronor Tablets 2543
Modicon 2563
Necon 3415
Norinyl 1 +35 28-Day Tablets 3380
Norinyl 1 + 50 28-Day Tablets 3380
Nor-QD Tablets 3423
Ortho-Novum 2563
Ortho-Novum 1/50□28 Tablets 2556
Ovcon 3364
Tri-Norinyl-28 Tablets 3433

Norethynodrel (Gonadotropin levels suppressed).
No products indexed under this heading.

Norgestimate (Pituitary secretion of gonadotropins affected; gonadotropin levels suppressed). Products include:
Ortho-Cyclen/Ortho Tri-Cyclen 2573
Ortho-Prefest Tablets 2570

Norgestrel (Gonadotropin levels suppressed). Products include:
Lo/Ovral Tablets 3532
Lo/Ovral-28 Tablets 3538
Low-Ogestrel-28 Tablets 3392
Ogestrel 0.5/50-28 Tablets 3428
Ovral Tablets 3551
Ovral-28 Tablets 3552
Ovrette Tablets 3552

Olanzapine (Rise in prolactin; response to Factrel may be blunted). Products include:
Zyprexa Tablets 1973
Zyprexa ZYDIS Orally Disintegrating Tablets 1973

Oxandrolone (Pituitary secretion of gonadotropins affected). Products include:
Oxandrin Tablets 1153

Oxymetholone (Pituitary secretion of gonadotropins affected). Products include:
Anadrol-50 Tablets 3321

Perphenazine (Rise in prolactin; response to Factrel may be blunted). Products include:
Etrafon 3115
Trilafon 3160

Pimozide (Rise in prolactin; response to Factrel may be blunted). Products include:
Orap Tablets 1407

Polyestradiol Phosphate (Pituitary secretion of gonadotropins affected).
No products indexed under this heading.

Prednisolone Acetate (Pituitary secretion of gonadotropins affected). Products include:
Blephamide Ophthalmic Ointment 547
Blephamide Ophthalmic Suspension 548
Poly-Pred Liquifilm Ophthalmic Suspension .... ⊙ 245
Pred Forte Ophthalmic Suspension .... ⊙ 246
Pred Mild Sterile Ophthalmic Suspension .... ⊙ 249
Pred-G Ophthalmic Suspension .... ⊙ 247
Pred-G Sterile Ophthalmic Ointment .... ⊙ 248

Prednisolone Sodium Phosphate (Pituitary secretion of gonadotropins affected). Products include:
Pediapred Oral Solution 1170

Prednisolone Tebutate (Pituitary secretion of gonadotropins affected).
No products indexed under this heading.

Prednisone (Pituitary secretion of gonadotropins affected). Products include:
Prednisone 3064

Prochlorperazine (Rise in prolactin; response to Factrel may be blunted). Products include:
Compazine 1505

Promethazine Hydrochloride (Rise in prolactin; response to Factrel may be blunted). Products include:
Mepergan Injection 3539
Phenergan Injection 3553
Phenergan 3556
Phenergan Syrup 3554
Phenergan with Codeine Syrup 3557
Phenergan with Dextromethorphan Syrup 3559
Phenergan VC Syrup 3560
Phenergan VC with Codeine Syrup 3561

Quetiapine Fumarate (Rise in prolactin; response to Factrel may be blunted). Products include:
Seroquel Tablets 684

Quinestrol (Pituitary secretion of gonadotropins affected).
No products indexed under this heading.

Spironolactone (Gonadotropin levels transiently elevated).
No products indexed under this heading.

Stanozolol (Pituitary secretion of gonadotropins affected).
No products indexed under this heading.

Thioridazine Hydrochloride (Rise in prolactin; response to Factrel may be blunted). Products include:
Thioridazine Hydrochloride Tablets 2289

Triamcinolone (Pituitary secretion of gonadotropins affected).
No products indexed under this heading.

Triamcinolone Acetonide (Pituitary secretion of gonadotropins affected). Products include:
Azmacort Inhalation Aerosol 728
Nasacort Nasal Inhaler 750
Nasacort AQ Nasal Spray 752
Tri-Nasal Spray 2274

Triamcinolone Diacetate (Pituitary secretion of gonadotropins affected).
No products indexed under this heading.

Triamcinolone Hexacetonide (Pituitary secretion of gonadotropins affected).
No products indexed under this heading.

Trifluoperazine Hydrochloride (Rise in prolactin; response to Factrel may be blunted). Products include:
Stelazine 1640

FAMOTIDINE INJECTION
(Famotidine) 866
None cited in PDR database.

FAMVIR TABLETS
(Famciclovir) 2348
May interact with:

Probenecid (Concurrent use may result in increased plasma concentration of penciclovir).
No products indexed under this heading.

Food Interactions

Meal, unspecified (Penciclovir Cmax decreased approximately 50% and Tmax was delayed by 1.5 hours when a capsule formulation of famciclovir was administered with food; there is no effect on the extent of availability (AUC) of penciclovir).

FARESTON TABLETS
(Toremifene Citrate) 3237
May interact with erythromycin, phenytoin, thiazides, and certain other agents. Compounds in these categories include:

Bendroflumethiazide (Drugs that decrease renal calcium excretion, such as thiazide diuretics, may increase the risk of hypercalcemia with concurrent use). Products include:
Corzide 40/5 Tablets 2247
Corzide 80/5 Tablets 2247

Carbamazepine (Cytochrome P450 3A4 enzyme inducers, such as carbamazepine, increase the rate of toremifene metabolism, lowering the steady-state concentration in serum). Products include:
Carbatrol Capsules 3234
Tegretol/Tegretol-XR 2404

Chlorothiazide (Drugs that decrease renal calcium excretion, such as thiazide diuretics, may increase the risk of hypercalcemia with concurrent use). Products include:
Aldoclor Tablets 2035
Diuril Oral 2087

Chlorothiazide Sodium (Drugs that decrease renal calcium excretion, such as thiazide diuretics, may increase the risk of hypercalcemia with concurrent use). Products include:
Diuril Sodium Intravenous 2086

Erythromycin (Metabolism of toremifene may be inhibited by drugs known to inhibit CYP3A4-6 enzymes, such as erythromycin; clinical relevance of this interaction is uncertain). Products include:
Emgel 2% Topical Gel 1285
Ery-Tab Tablets 448
Erythromycin Base Filmtab Tablets 454
Erythromycin Delayed-Release Capsules, USP 455
PCE Dispertab Tablets 498

Erythromycin Estolate (Metabolism of toremifene may be inhibited by drugs known to inhibit CYP3A4-6 enzymes, such as erythromycin; clinical relevance of this interaction is uncertain).
No products indexed under this heading.

Erythromycin Ethylsuccinate (Metabolism of toremifene may be inhibited by drugs known to inhibit CYP3A4-6 enzymes, such as erythromycin; clinical relevance of this interaction is uncertain). Products include:
E.E.S. 450
EryPed 446
Pediazole Suspension 3050

Erythromycin Gluceptate (Metabolism of toremifene may be inhibited by drugs known to inhibit CYP3A4-6 enzymes, such as erythromycin; clinical relevance of this interaction is uncertain).
No products indexed under this heading.

Erythromycin Stearate (Metabolism of toremifene may be inhibited by drugs known to inhibit CYP3A4-6 enzymes, such as erythromycin; clinical relevance of this interaction is uncertain). Products include:
Erythrocin Stearate Filmtab Tablets 452

Fosphenytoin Sodium (Cytochrome P450 3A4 enzyme inducers, such as phenytoin, increase the rate of toremifene metabolism, lowering the steady-state concentration in serum). Products include:
Cerebyx Injection 2619

Hydrochlorothiazide (Drugs that decrease renal calcium excretion, such as thiazide diuretics, may increase the risk of hypercalcemia with concurrent use). Products include:
Accuretic Tablets 2614
Aldoril Tablets 2039
Atacand HCT Tablets 597
Avalide Tablets 1070
Diovan HCT Tablets 2338
Dyazide Capsules 1515
HydroDIURIL Tablets 2108
Hyzaar 2109
Inderide Tablets 3517
Inderide LA Long-Acting Capsules 3519
Lotensin HCT Tablets 2367
Maxzide 1008
Micardis HCT Tablets 1051
Microzide Capsules 3414
Moduretic Tablets 2138
Monopril HCT 1094
Prinzide Tablets 2168
Timolide Tablets 2187
Uniretic Tablets 3178
Vaseretic Tablets 2204
Zestoretic Tablets 695
Ziac Tablets 1887

Hydroflumethiazide (Drugs that decrease renal calcium excretion, such as thiazide diuretics, may increase the risk of hypercalcemia with concurrent use). Products include:
Diucardin Tablets 3494

Ketoconazole (Metabolism of toremifene may be inhibited by drugs known to inhibit CYP3A4-6 enzymes, such as ketoconazole; clinical relevance of this interaction is uncertain). Products include:
Nizoral 2% Cream 3620
Nizoral A-D Shampoo 2008
Nizoral 2% Shampoo 2007
Nizoral Tablets 1791

Methyclothiazide (Drugs that decrease renal calcium excretion, such as thiazide diuretics, may increase the risk of hypercalcemia with concurrent use).
No products indexed under this heading.

Phenobarbital (Cytochrome P450 3A4 enzyme inducers, such as phenobarbital, increase the rate of toremifene metabolism, lowering the steady-state concentration in serum). Products include:
Arco-Lase Plus Tablets 592
Donnatal 2929
Donnatal Extentabs 2930

Phenytoin (Cytochrome P450 3A4 enzyme inducers, such as phenytoin, increase the rate of toremifene metabolism, lowering the steady-state concentration in serum). Products include:
Dilantin Infatabs 2624

Dilantin-125 Oral Suspension 2625

Phenytoin Sodium (Cytochrome P450 3A4 enzyme inducers, such as phenytoin, increase the rate of toremifene metabolism, lowering the steady-state concentration in serum). Products include:

Dilantin Kapseals 2622

Polythiazide (Drugs that decrease renal calcium excretion, such as thiazide diuretics, may increase the risk of hypercalcemia with concurrent use). Products include:

Minizide Capsules 2700
Renese Tablets 2712

Warfarin Sodium (Co-administration of antiestrogenic compounds and coumarin-type anticoagulant has resulted in an increased prothrombin time). Products include:

Coumadin for Injection 1243
Coumadin Tablets 1243
Warfarin Sodium Tablets, USP 3302

FAT METABOLIZER + CAPSULES

(Herbals with Minerals) .... ▣ 854
None cited in PDR database.

FEIBA VH

(Anti-Inhibitor Coagulant Complex) 843
None cited in PDR database.

FELBATOL ORAL SUSPENSION

(Felbamate) 3343
See Felbatol Tablets

FELBATOL TABLETS

(Felbamate) 3343
May interact with phenytoin, valproate, and certain other agents. Compounds in these categories include:

Carbamazepine (Causes an approximate 50% increase in the clearance of felbamate; decrease in steady-state carbamazepine plasma concentration and an increase in the steady-state carbamazepine epoxide plasma concentration caused by felbamate). Products include:

Carbatrol Capsules 3234
Tegretol/Tegretol-XR 2404

Divalproex Sodium (Felbamate causes an increase in steady-state valproate concentrations; no significant effect of valproate on the clearance of felbamate). Products include:

Depakote Sprinkle Capsules 426
Depakote Tablets 430
Depakote ER Tablets 436

Fosphenytoin Sodium (Co-administration causes an increase in steady-state phenytoin plasma concentrations; phenytoin causes an approximate doubling of the clearance of felbamate at steady-state and, therefore, the addition of phenytoin causes an approximate 45% decrease in the steady-state trough concentration of felbamate). Products include:

Cerebyx Injection 2619

Gestodene (Co-administration with low-dose combination oral contraceptive containing gestodene and ethinyl estradiol has resulted in a 42% decrease in the gestodene AUC 0-24, but no clinically relevant effect was observed on the pharmacokinetic parameters of ethinyl estradiol; one case of intermenstrual bleeding has been reported).

No products indexed under this heading.

Phenobarbital (May reduce plasma felbamate concentrations; felbamate causes an increase in phenobarbital plasma concentrations). Products include:

Arco-Lase Plus Tablets 592
Donnatal 2929
Donnatal Extentabs 2930

Phenytoin (Co-administration causes an increase in steady-state phenytoin plasma concentrations; phenytoin causes an approximate doubling of the clearance of felbamate at steady-state and, therefore, the addition of phenytoin causes an approximate 45% decrease in the steady-state trough concentration of felbamate). Products include:

Dilantin Infatabs 2624
Dilantin-125 Oral Suspension 2625

Phenytoin Sodium (Co-administration causes an increase in steady-state phenytoin plasma concentrations; phenytoin causes an approximate doubling of the clearance of felbamate at steady-state and, therefore, the addition of phenytoin causes an approximate 45% decrease in the steady-state trough concentration of felbamate). Products include:

Dilantin Kapseals 2622

Valproate Sodium (Felbamate causes an increase in steady-state valproate concentrations; no significant effect of valproate on the clearance of felbamate). Products include:

Depacon Injection 416

Valproic Acid (Felbamate causes an increase in steady-state valproate concentrations; no significant effect of valproate on the clearance of felbamate). Products include:

Depakene 421

FELDENE CAPSULES

(Piroxicam) 2685
May interact with ACE inhibitors, lithium preparations, highly protein bound drugs (selected), thiazides, and certain other agents. Compounds in these categories include:

Amiodarone Hydrochloride (Piroxicam is highly protein bound and, therefore, might be expected to displace other protein bound drugs). Products include:

Cordarone Intravenous 3491
Cordarone Tablets 3487
Pacerone Tablets 3331

Amitriptyline Hydrochloride (Piroxicam is highly protein bound and, therefore, might be expected to displace other protein bound drugs). Products include:

Etrafon 3115
Limbitrol 1738

Aspirin (Co-administration of piroxicam (20 mg/day) with 3900 mg/day of aspirin depresses plasma levels of piroxicam by 80%; concurrent use is not recommended). Products include:

Aggrenox Capsules 1026
Alka-Seltzer .... ▣ 603
Alka-Seltzer Lemon Lime Antacid and Pain Reliever Effervescent Tablets .... ▣ 603
Alka-Seltzer Extra Strength Antacid and Pain Reliever Effervescent Tablets .... ▣ 603
Alka-Seltzer PM Effervescent Tablets .... ▣ 605
Genuine Bayer Tablets, Caplets and Gelcaps .... ▣ 606
Extra Strength Bayer Caplets and Gelcaps .... ▣ 610
Aspirin Regimen Bayer Children's Chewable Tablets (Orange or Cherry Flavored) .... ▣ 607
Bayer, Aspirin Regimen .... ▣ 606
Aspirin Regimen Bayer 81 mg Caplets with Calcium .... ▣ 607
Genuine Bayer Professional Labeling (Aspirin Regimen Bayer) .... ▣ 608
Extra Strength Bayer Arthritis Caplets .... ▣ 610
Extra Strength Bayer Plus Caplets .... ▣ 610
Extra Strength Bayer PM Caplets . ▣ 611
BC Powder .... ▣ 619
BC Allergy Sinus Cold Powder ...... ▣ 619
Arthritis Strength BC Powder ...... ▣ 619
BC Sinus Cold Powder .... ▣ 619
Darvon Compound-65 Pulvules 1910
Ecotrin Enteric Coated Aspirin Low, Regular and Maximum Strength Tablets 1715
Excedrin Extra-Strength Tablets, Caplets, and Geltabs .... ▣ 629
Excedrin Migraine 1070
Goody's Body Pain Formula Powder .... ▣ 620
Goody's Extra Strength Headache Powder .... ▣ 620
Goody's Extra Strength Pain Relief Tablets .... ▣ 620
Percodan Tablets 1327
Robaxisal Tablets 2939
Soma Compound Tablets 3354
Soma Compound w/Codeine Tablets 3355
Vanquish Caplets .... ▣ 617

Atovaquone (Piroxicam is highly protein bound and, therefore, might be expected to displace other protein bound drugs). Products include:

Malarone 1596
Mepron Suspension 1598

Benazepril Hydrochloride (NSAIDs may diminish the antihypertensive effect of ACE inhibitors). Products include:

Lotensin Tablets 2365
Lotensin HCT Tablets 2367
Lotrel Capsules 2370

Bendroflumethiazide (Piroxicam can reduce natriuretic effect of thiazides possibly due to inhibition of prostaglandin synthesis; if used concurrently, patients should be observed closely for signs of renal failure). Products include:

Corzide 40/5 Tablets 2247
Corzide 80/5 Tablets 2247

Captopril (NSAIDs may diminish the antihypertensive effect of ACE inhibitors). Products include:

Captopril Tablets 2281

Cefonicid Sodium (Piroxicam is highly protein bound and, therefore, might be expected to displace other protein bound drugs).

No products indexed under this heading.

Celecoxib (Piroxicam is highly protein bound and, therefore, might be expected to displace other protein bound drugs). Products include:

Celebrex Capsules 2676
Celebrex Capsules 2780

Chlordiazepoxide (Piroxicam is highly protein bound and, therefore, might be expected to displace other protein bound drugs). Products include:

Limbitrol 1738

Chlordiazepoxide Hydrochloride (Piroxicam is highly protein bound and, therefore, might be expected to displace other protein bound drugs). Products include:

Librium Capsules 1736
Librium for Injection 1737

Chlorothiazide (Piroxicam can reduce natriuretic effect of thiazides possibly due to inhibition of prostaglandin synthesis; if used concurrently, patients should be observed closely for signs of renal failure). Products include:

Aldoclor Tablets 2035
Diuril Oral 2087

Chlorothiazide Sodium (Piroxicam can reduce natriuretic effect of thiazides possibly due to inhibition of prostaglandin synthesis; if used concurrently, patients should be observed closely for signs of renal failure). Products include:

Diuril Sodium Intravenous 2086

Chlorpromazine (Piroxicam is highly protein bound and, therefore, might be expected to displace other protein bound drugs). Products include:

Thorazine Suppositories 1656

Chlorpromazine Hydrochloride (Piroxicam is highly protein bound and, therefore, might be expected to displace other protein bound drugs). Products include:

Thorazine 1656

Clomipramine Hydrochloride (Piroxicam is highly protein bound and, therefore, might be expected to displace other protein bound drugs).

No products indexed under this heading.

Clozapine (Piroxicam is highly protein bound and, therefore, might be expected to displace other protein bound drugs). Products include:

Clozaril Tablets 2319

Cyclosporine (Piroxicam is highly protein bound and, therefore, might be expected to displace other protein bound drugs). Products include:

Gengraf Capsules 457
Neoral Soft Gelatin Capsules 2380
Neoral Oral Solution 2380
Sandimmune 2388

Diazepam (Piroxicam is highly protein bound and, therefore, might be expected to displace other protein bound drugs). Products include:

Valium Injectable 3026
Valium Tablets 3047

Diclofenac Potassium (Piroxicam is highly protein bound and, therefore, might be expected to displace other protein bound drugs). Products include:

Cataflam Tablets 2315

Diclofenac Sodium (Piroxicam is highly protein bound and, therefore, might be expected to displace other protein bound drugs). Products include:

Arthrotec Tablets 3195
Voltaren Ophthalmic Sterile Ophthalmic Solution .... ⊙ 312
Voltaren Tablets 2315
Voltaren-XR Tablets 2315

Dipyridamole (Piroxicam is highly protein bound and, therefore, might be expected to displace other protein bound drugs). Products include:

Aggrenox Capsules 1026
Persantine Tablets 1057

Enalapril Maleate (NSAIDs may diminish the antihypertensive effect of ACE inhibitors). Products include:

Lexxel Tablets 608
Vaseretic Tablets 2204
Vasotec Tablets 2210

Enalaprilat (NSAIDs may diminish the antihypertensive effect of ACE inhibitors). Products include:

Enalaprilat Injection 863
Vasotec I.V. Injection 2207

Fenoprofen Calcium (Piroxicam is highly protein bound and, therefore, might be expected to displace other protein bound drugs).

No products indexed under this heading.

Flurazepam Hydrochloride (Piroxicam is highly protein bound and, therefore, might be expected to displace other protein bound drugs).

No products indexed under this heading.

Flurbiprofen (Piroxicam is highly protein bound and, therefore, might be expected to displace other protein bound drugs).

No products indexed under this heading.

Fosinopril Sodium (NSAIDs may diminish the antihypertensive effect of ACE inhibitors). Products include:

Monopril Tablets 1091
Monopril HCT 1094

Furosemide (Piroxicam can reduce natriuretic effect of furosemide possibly due to inhibition of prostaglandin synthesis; if used concurrently, patients should be observed closely for signs of renal failure). Products include:

Furosemide Tablets 2284

Glipizide (Piroxicam is highly protein bound and, therefore, might be expected to displace other protein bound drugs). Products include:
- Glucotrol Tablets 2692
- Glucotrol XL Extended Release Tablets 2693

Hydrochlorothiazide (Piroxicam can reduce natriuretic effect of thiazides possibly due to inhibition of prostaglandin synthesis; if used concurrently, patients should be observed closely for signs of renal failure). Products include:
- Accuretic Tablets 2614
- Aldoril Tablets 2039
- Atacand HCT Tablets 597
- Avalide Tablets 1070
- Diovan HCT Tablets 2338
- Dyazide Capsules 1515
- HydroDIURIL Tablets 2108
- Hyzaar 2109
- Inderide Tablets 3517
- Inderide LA Long-Acting Capsules .. 3519
- Lotensin HCT Tablets 2367
- Maxzide 1008
- Micardis HCT Tablets 1051
- Microzide Capsules 3414
- Moduretic Tablets 2138
- Monopril HCT 1094
- Prinzide Tablets 2168
- Timolide Tablets 2187
- Uniretic Tablets 3178
- Vaseretic Tablets 2204
- Zestoretic Tablets 695
- Ziac Tablets 1887

Hydroflumethiazide (Piroxicam can reduce natriuretic effect of thiazides possibly due to inhibition of prostaglandin synthesis; if used concurrently, patients should be observed closely for signs of renal failure). Products include:
- Diucardin Tablets 3494

Ibuprofen (Piroxicam is highly protein bound and, therefore, might be expected to displace other protein bound drugs). Products include:
- Advil .... ■771
- Children's Advil Oral Suspension ... ■773
- Children's Advil Chewable Tablets . ■773
- Advil Cold and Sinus Caplets .... ■771
- Advil Cold and Sinus Tablets .... ■771
- Advil Flu & Body Ache Caplets .... ■772
- Infants' Advil Drops .... ■773
- Junior Strength Advil Tablets .... ■773
- Junior Strength Advil Chewable Tablets .... ■773
- Advil Migraine Liquigels .... ■772
- Children's Motrin Oral Suspension and Chewable Tablets 2006
- Children's Motrin Cold Oral Suspension 2007
- Children's Motrin Oral Suspension .... ■643
- Motrin Suspension, Oral Drops, Chewable Tablets, and Caplets 2002
- Infants' Motrin Concentrated Drops 2006
- Junior Strength Motrin Caplets and Chewable Tablets 2006
- Motrin IB Tablets, Caplets, and Gelcaps 2002
- Motrin Migraine Pain Caplets 2005
- Motrin Sinus Headache Caplets 2005
- Vicoprofen Tablets 520

Imipramine Hydrochloride (Piroxicam is highly protein bound and, therefore, might be expected to displace other protein bound drugs).
No products indexed under this heading.

Imipramine Pamoate (Piroxicam is highly protein bound and, therefore, might be expected to displace other protein bound drugs).
No products indexed under this heading.

Indomethacin (Piroxicam is highly protein bound and, therefore, might be expected to displace other protein bound drugs). Products include:
- Indocin 2112

Indomethacin Sodium Trihydrate (Piroxicam is highly protein bound and, therefore, might be expected to displace other protein bound drugs). Products include:
- Indocin I.V. 2115

Ketoprofen (Piroxicam is highly protein bound and, therefore, might be expected to displace other protein bound drugs). Products include:
- Orudis Capsules 3548
- Orudis KT Tablets .... ■778
- Oruvail Capsules 3548

Ketorolac Tromethamine (Piroxicam is highly protein bound and, therefore, might be expected to displace other protein bound drugs). Products include:
- Acular Ophthalmic Solution 544
- Acular PF Ophthalmic Solution 544
- Toradol 3018

Lisinopril (NSAIDs may diminish the antihypertensive effect of ACE inhibitors). Products include:
- Prinivil Tablets 2164
- Prinzide Tablets 2168
- Zestoretic Tablets 695
- Zestril Tablets 698

Lithium Carbonate (NSAIDs have produced an elevation of plasma lithium levels and a reduction in renal lithium clearance possibly due to inhibition of prostaglandin synthesis by NSAID; if used concurrently, patients should be observed closely for signs of lithium toxicity). Products include:
- Eskalith 1527
- Lithium Carbonate 3061
- Lithobid Slow-Release Tablets 3255

Lithium Citrate (NSAIDs have produced an elevation of plasma lithium levels and a reduction in renal lithium clearance possibly due to inhibition of prostaglandin synthesis by NSAID; if used concurrently, patients should be observed closely for signs of lithium toxicity). Products include:
- Lithium Citrate Syrup 3061

Meclofenamate Sodium (Piroxicam is highly protein bound and, therefore, might be expected to displace other protein bound drugs).
No products indexed under this heading.

Mefenamic Acid (Piroxicam is highly protein bound and, therefore, might be expected to displace other protein bound drugs). Products include:
- Ponstel Capsules 1356

Methotrexate Sodium (Co-administration of NSAIDs with methotrexate has been reported to competitively inhibit methotrexate accumulation in animal model).
No products indexed under this heading.

Methyclothiazide (Piroxicam can reduce natriuretic effect of thiazides possibly due to inhibition of prostaglandin synthesis; if used concurrently, patients should be observed closely for signs of renal failure).
No products indexed under this heading.

Midazolam Hydrochloride (Piroxicam is highly protein bound and, therefore, might be expected to displace other protein bound drugs). Products include:
- Versed Injection 3027
- Versed Syrup 3033

Moexipril Hydrochloride (NSAIDs may diminish the antihypertensive effect of ACE inhibitors). Products include:
- Uniretic Tablets 3178
- Univasc Tablets 3181

Naproxen (Piroxicam is highly protein bound and, therefore, might be expected to displace other protein bound drugs). Products include:
- EC-Naprosyn Delayed-Release Tablets 2967
- Naprosyn Suspension 2967
- Naprosyn Tablets 2967

Naproxen Sodium (Piroxicam is highly protein bound and, therefore, might be expected to displace other protein bound drugs). Products include:
- Aleve Tablets, Caplets and Gelcaps .... ■602
- Aleve Cold & Sinus Caplets .... ■603
- Anaprox Tablets 2967
- Anaprox DS Tablets 2967
- Naprelan Tablets 1293

Nortriptyline Hydrochloride (Piroxicam is highly protein bound and, therefore, might be expected to displace other protein bound drugs).
No products indexed under this heading.

Oxaprozin (Piroxicam is highly protein bound and, therefore, might be expected to displace other protein bound drugs).
No products indexed under this heading.

Oxazepam (Piroxicam is highly protein bound and, therefore, might be expected to displace other protein bound drugs).
No products indexed under this heading.

Perindopril Erbumine (NSAIDs may diminish the antihypertensive effect of ACE inhibitors). Products include:
- Aceon Tablets (2 mg, 4 mg, 8 mg) 3249

Phenylbutazone (Piroxicam is highly protein bound and, therefore, might be expected to displace other protein bound drugs).
No products indexed under this heading.

Polythiazide (Piroxicam can reduce natriuretic effect of thiazides possibly due to inhibition of prostaglandin synthesis; if used concurrently, patients should be observed closely for signs of renal failure). Products include:
- Minizide Capsules 2700
- Renese Tablets 2712

Propranolol Hydrochloride (Piroxicam is highly protein bound and, therefore, might be expected to displace other protein bound drugs). Products include:
- Inderal 3513
- Inderal LA Long-Acting Capsules 3516
- Inderide Tablets 3517
- Inderide LA Long-Acting Capsules .. 3519

Quinapril Hydrochloride (NSAIDs may diminish the antihypertensive effect of ACE inhibitors). Products include:
- Accupril Tablets 2611
- Accuretic Tablets 2614

Ramipril (NSAIDs may diminish the antihypertensive effect of ACE inhibitors). Products include:
- Altace Capsules 2233

Spirapril Hydrochloride (NSAIDs may diminish the antihypertensive effect of ACE inhibitors).
No products indexed under this heading.

Sulindac (Piroxicam is highly protein bound and, therefore, might be expected to displace other protein bound drugs). Products include:
- Clinoril Tablets 2053

Temazepam (Piroxicam is highly protein bound and, therefore, might be expected to displace other protein bound drugs).
No products indexed under this heading.

Tolbutamide (Piroxicam is highly protein bound and, therefore, might be expected to displace other protein bound drugs).
No products indexed under this heading.

Tolmetin Sodium (Piroxicam is highly protein bound and, therefore, might be expected to displace other protein bound drugs). Products include:
- Tolectin 2589

Trandolapril (NSAIDs may diminish the antihypertensive effect of ACE inhibitors). Products include:
- Mavik Tablets 478
- Tarka Tablets 508

Trimipramine Maleate (Piroxicam is highly protein bound and, therefore, might be expected to displace other protein bound drugs). Products include:
- Surmontil Capsules 3595

Warfarin Sodium (The effects of warfarin and NSAIDs on GI bleeding are synergistic). Products include:
- Coumadin for Injection 1243
- Coumadin Tablets 1243
- Warfarin Sodium Tablets, USP 3302

Food Interactions

Food, unspecified (With food there is a slight delay in the rate but not the extent of absorption).

FEMARA TABLETS

(Letrozole) 2351
None cited in PDR database.

FEMHRT TABLETS

(Ethinyl Estradiol, Norethindrone Acetate) 2635
May interact with phenytoin, prednisolone, theophylline, and certain other agents. Compounds in these categories include:

Acetaminophen (May increase AUC and/or plasma concentrations of ethinyl estradiol; co-administration may decrease plasma concentrations of acetaminophen). Products include:
- Actifed Cold & Sinus Caplets and Tablets .... ■688
- Alka-Seltzer Plus Liqui-Gels .... ■604
- Alka-Seltzer Plus Cold & Flu Medicine Liqui-Gels .... ■604
- Alka-Seltzer Plus Cold & Sinus Medicine Liqui-Gels .... ■604
- Benadryl Allergy/Cold Tablets .... ■691
- Benadryl Allergy Sinus Headache Caplets & Gelcaps .... ■693
- Benadryl Severe Allergy & Sinus Headache Caplets .... ■694
- Children's Cēpacol Sore Throat .... ■788
- Comtrex Acute Head Cold & Sinus Pressure Relief Tablets .... ■627
- Comtrex Deep Chest Cold & Congestion Relief Softgels .... ■627
- Comtrex Flu Therapy & Fever Relief Daytime Caplets .... ■628
- Comtrex Flu Therapy & Fever Relief Nighttime Tablets .... ■628
- Comtrex Maximum Strength Multi-Symptom Cold & Cough Relief Tablets and Caplets .... ■626
- Contac Severe Cold and Flu Caplets Maximum Strength .... ■746
- Contac Severe Cold and Flu Caplets Non-Drowsy .... ■746
- Coricidin 'D' Cold, Flu & Sinus Tablets .... ■737
- Coricidin HBP Cold & Flu Tablets .. ■738
- Coricidin HBP Maximum Strength Flu Tablets .... ■738
- Coricidin HBP Night-Time Cold & Flu Tablets .... ■738
- Darvon-N/Darvocet-N 1907
- Dimetapp Cold and Fever Suspension .... ■775
- Dimetapp Nighttime Flu Liquid .... ■776
- Dimetapp Non-Drowsy Flu Syrup .. ■777
- Drixoral Allergy/Sinus Extended-Release Tablets .... ■741
- Drixoral Cold & Flu Extended-Release Tablets .... ■740
- Aspirin Free Excedrin Caplets and Geltabs .... ■628
- Excedrin Extra-Strength Tablets, Caplets, and Geltabs .... ■629
- Excedrin Migraine 1070
- Excedrin PM Tablets, Caplets, and Geltabs .... ■631
- Goody's Body Pain Formula Powder .... ■620
- Goody's Extra Strength Headache Powder .... ■620
- Goody's Extra Strength Pain Relief Tablets .... ■620
- Goody's PM Powder .... ■621
- Hycomine Compound Tablets 1317
- Lortab 3319
- Lortab Elixir 3317
- Maxidone Tablets CIII 3399
- Maximum Strength Midol Menstrual Caplets and Gelcaps .. ■612

Maximum Strength Midol PMS Caplets and Gelcaps ◘613
Maximum Strength Midol Teen Caplets ◘612
Midrin Capsules 3464
Norco 5/325 Tablets CIII 3424
Norco 7.5/325 Tablets CIII 3425
Norco 10/325 Tablets CIII 3427
Norco 10/325 Tablets CIII 3425
Percocet Tablets 1326
Percogesic Aspirin-Free Coated Tablets ◘667
Extra Strength Percogesic Aspirin-Free Coated Caplets ◘665
Phrenilin 578
Robitussin Cold Caplets Multi-Symptom Cold & Flu ◘781
Robitussin Cold Softgels Multi-Symptom Cold & Flu ◘781
Robitussin Multi Symptom Honey Flu Liquid ◘785
Robitussin Nighttime Honey Flu Liquid ◘786
Sedapap Tablets 50 mg/650 mg 2225
Singlet Caplets ◘761
Sinutab Sinus Allergy Medication, Maximum Strength Formula, Tablets & Caplets ◘707
Sinutab Sinus Medication, Maximum Strength Without Drowsiness Formula, Tablets & Caplets ◘707
Sudafed Cold & Cough Liquid Caps ◘709
Sudafed Cold & Sinus Liquid Caps ◘710
Sudafed Severe Cold ◘711
Sudafed Sinus Headache Caplets ◘712
Sudafed Sinus Headache Tablets ◘712
Tavist Sinus Non-Drowsy Coated Caplets ◘676
TheraFlu Regular Strength Cold & Cough Night Time Hot Liquid ◘676
TheraFlu Regular Strength Cold & Sore Throat Night Time Hot Liquid ◘676
TheraFlu Maximum Strength Flu & Congestion Non-Drowsy Hot Liquid ◘677
TheraFlu Maximum Strength Flu & Cough Night Time Hot Liquid ◘678
TheraFlu Maximum Strength Flu & Sore Throat Night Time Hot Liquid ◘677
TheraFlu Maximum Strength Severe Cold & Congestion Night Time Caplets ◘678
TheraFlu Maximum Strength Severe Cold & Congestion Night Time Hot Liquid ◘678
TheraFlu Maximum Strength Severe Cold & Congestion Non-Drowsy ◘679
Triaminic Cold, Cough & Fever Liquid ◘681
Triaminic Cough & Sore Throat Liquid ◘682
Triaminic Cough & Sore Throat Softchews ◘684
Tylenol, Children's 2014
Children's Tylenol Allergy-D Liquid 2014
Children's Tylenol Cold Suspension Liquid and Chewable Tablets 2015
Children's Tylenol Cold Plus Cough Suspension Liquid and Chewable Tablets 2015
Children's Tylenol Flu Suspension Liquid 2015
Children's Tylenol Sinus Suspension Liquid 2017
Infants' Tylenol Cold Decongestant and Fever Reducer Concentrated Drops 2015
Infants' Tylenol Cold Decongestant and Fever Reducer Concentrated Drops Plus Cough 2015
Junior Strength Tylenol Soft Chews Chewable Tablets 2014
Tylenol 2009
Tylenol Allergy Sinus 2010
Tylenol Severe Allergy Caplets 2010
Multi-Symptom Tylenol Cold Complete Formula Caplets 2010
Multi-Symptom Tylenol Cold Non-Drowsy Caplets and Gelcaps 2010
Multi-Symptom Tylenol Cold Severe Congestion Non-Drowsy Caplets 2011
Maximum Strength Tylenol Flu NightTime Gelcaps 2011
Maximum Strength Tylenol Flu NightTime Liquid 2011
Maximum Strength Tylenol Flu Non-Drowsy Gelcaps 2011
Extra Strength Tylenol PM Caplets, Geltabs, and Gelcaps 2012
Maximum Strength Tylenol Sinus NightTime Caplets 2012
Maximum Strength Tylenol Sinus Non-Drowsy Geltabs, Gelcaps, Caplets, and Tablets 2012
Maximum Strength Tylenol Sore Throat Adult Liquid 2013
Tylenol with Codeine 2595
Women's Tylenol Menstrual Relief Caplets 2013
Tylox Capsules 2597
Ultracet Tablets 2597
Vanquish Caplets ◘617
Vicks 44M Cough, Cold & Flu Relief Liquid ◘725
Vicks DayQuil LiquiCaps/Liquid Multi-Symptom Cold/Flu Relief ◘727
Vicks NyQuil LiquiCaps/Liquid Multi-Symptom Cold/Flu Relief, Original and Cherry Flavors ◘727
Vicodin Tablets 516
Vicodin ES Tablets 517
Vicodin HP Tablets 518
Zydone Tablets 1330

Aminophylline (Co-administration of products containing ethinyl estradiol may inhibit the metabolism of other compounds, such as theophylline, resulting in increased plasma concentrations of theophylline).
No products indexed under this heading.

Atorvastatin Calcium (Co-administration of atorvastatin and certain ethinyl estradiol containing products increases the AUC values for ethinyl estradiol by 20%). Products include:
Lipitor Tablets 2639
Lipitor Tablets 2696

Carbamazepine (Co-administration of ethinyl estradiol with carbamazepine results in increased metabolism of ethinyl estradiol). Products include:
Carbatrol Capsules 3234
Tegretol/Tegretol-XR 2404

Clofibrate (Co-administration of products containing ethinyl estradiol may increase clearance of clofibric acid). Products include:
Atromid-S Capsules 3483

Cyclosporine (Co-administration of products containing ethinyl estradiol may inhibit the metabolism of other compounds, such as cyclosporine, resulting in increased plasma concentrations of cyclosporine). Products include:
Gengraf Capsules 457
Neoral Soft Gelatin Capsules 2380
Neoral Oral Solution 2380
Sandimmune 2388

Dyphylline (Co-administration of products containing ethinyl estradiol may inhibit the metabolism of other compounds, such as theophylline, resulting in increased plasma concentrations of theophylline). Products include:
Lufyllin Tablets 3347
Lufyllin-400 Tablets 3347
Lufyllin-GG Elixir 3348
Lufyllin-GG Tablets 3348

Fosphenytoin Sodium (Co-administration of ethinyl estradiol with phenytoin results in increased metabolism of ethinyl estradiol). Products include:
Cerebyx Injection 2619

Morphine Sulfate (Co-administration of products containing ethinyl estradiol may increase clearance of morphine). Products include:
Astramorph/PF Injection, USP (Preservative-Free) 594
Duramorph Injection 1312
Infumorph 200 and Infumorph 500 Sterile Solutions 1314
Kadian Capsules 1335
MS Contin Tablets 2896
MSIR 2898
Oramorph SR Tablets 3062
Roxanol 3066

Phenobarbital (Co-administration of ethinyl estradiol with phenobarbital results in increased metabolism of ethinyl estradiol). Products include:
Arco-Lase Plus Tablets 592
Donnatal 2929
Donnatal Extentabs 2930

Phenytoin (Co-administration of ethinyl estradiol with phenytoin results in increased metabolism of ethinyl estradiol). Products include:
Dilantin Infatabs 2624
Dilantin-125 Oral Suspension 2625

Phenytoin Sodium (Co-administration of ethinyl estradiol with phenytoin results in increased metabolism of ethinyl estradiol). Products include:
Dilantin Kapseals 2622

Prednisolone (Co-administration of products containing ethinyl estradiol may inhibit the metabolism of other compounds, such as prednisolone, resulting in increased plasma concentrations of prednisolone). Products include:
Prelone Syrup 2273

Prednisolone Acetate (Co-administration of products containing ethinyl estradiol may inhibit the metabolism of other compounds, such as prednisolone, resulting in increased plasma concentrations of prednisolone). Products include:
Blephamide Ophthalmic Ointment 547
Blephamide Ophthalmic Suspension 548
Poly-Pred Liquifilm Ophthalmic Suspension ⊙245
Pred Forte Ophthalmic Suspension ⊙246
Pred Mild Sterile Ophthalmic Suspension ⊙249
Pred-G Ophthalmic Suspension ⊙247
Pred-G Sterile Ophthalmic Ointment ⊙248

Prednisolone Sodium Phosphate (Co-administration of products containing ethinyl estradiol may inhibit the metabolism of other compounds, such as prednisolone, resulting in increased plasma concentrations of prednisolone). Products include:
Pediapred Oral Solution 1170

Prednisolone Tebutate (Co-administration of products containing ethinyl estradiol may inhibit the metabolism of other compounds, such as prednisolone, resulting in increased plasma concentrations of prednisolone).
No products indexed under this heading.

Prednisone (Co-administration of products containing ethinyl estradiol may inhibit the metabolism of other compounds, such as prednisone, resulting in increased plasma concentrations of prednisone). Products include:
Prednisone 3064

Rifampin (Co-administration of ethinyl estradiol with rifampin results in increased metabolism of ethinyl estradiol). Products include:
Rifadin 765
Rifamate Capsules 767
Rifater Tablets 769

Salicylic Acid (Co-administration of products containing ethinyl estradiol may increase clearance of salicylic acid). Products include:
Clear Away Gel with Aloe Wart Remover System ◘736
Clear Away Liquid Wart Remover System ◘736
Clear Away One Step Wart Remover ◘737
Clear Away One Step Wart Remover for Kids ◘737
Clear Away One Step Plantar Wart Remover ◘737
Compound W One Step Pads for Kids ◘664
Compound W One Step Plantar Pads ◘664
Compound W One Step Wart Remover Pads ◘664
Compound W Wart Remover Gel ◘665
Compound W Wart Remover Liquid ◘665
Wart-Off Liquid ◘716

Temazepam (Co-administration of products containing ethinyl estradiol may increase clearance of temazepam).
No products indexed under this heading.

Theophylline (Co-administration of products containing ethinyl estradiol may inhibit the metabolism of other compounds, such as theophylline, resulting in increased plasma concentrations of theophylline). Products include:
Aerolate 1361
Theo-Dur Extended-Release Tablets 1835
Uni-Dur Extended-Release Tablets 1841
Uniphyl 400 mg and 600 mg Tablets 2903

Theophylline Calcium Salicylate (Co-administration of products containing ethinyl estradiol may inhibit the metabolism of other compounds, such as theophylline, resulting in increased plasma concentrations of theophylline).
No products indexed under this heading.

Theophylline Sodium Glycinate (Co-administration of products containing ethinyl estradiol may inhibit the metabolism of other compounds, such as theophylline, resulting in increased plasma concentrations of theophylline).
No products indexed under this heading.

Troglitazone (Co-administration of troglitazone and certain ethinyl estradiol containing products reduces the plasma concentrations of ethinyl estradiol by 30%).
No products indexed under this heading.

Vitamin C (May increase AUC and/or plasma concentrations of ethinyl estradiol). Products include:
Beta-C Tablets ◘811
C-Grams Caplets ◘795
Halls Defense Drops ◘687
Peridin-C Tablets ◘618

FEOSOL CAPLETS

(Iron Carbonyl) 1717
May interact with tetracyclines. Compounds in these categories include:

Demeclocycline Hydrochloride (Oral iron products interfere with absorption of oral tetracyclines; these products should not be taken within two hours of each other). Products include:
Declomycin Tablets 1855

Doxycycline Calcium (Oral iron products interfere with absorption of oral tetracyclines; these products should not be taken within two hours of each other). Products include:
Vibramycin Calcium Oral Suspension Syrup 2735

Doxycycline Hyclate (Oral iron products interfere with absorption of oral tetracyclines; these products should not be taken within two hours of each other). Products include:
Doryx Coated Pellet Filled Capsules 3357
Periostat Tablets 1208
Vibramycin Hyclate Capsules 2735
Vibramycin Hyclate Intravenous 2737
Vibra-Tabs Film Coated Tablets 2735

Doxycycline Monohydrate (Oral iron products interfere with absorption of oral tetracyclines; these products should not be taken within two hours of each other). Products include:
Monodox Capsules 2442
Vibramycin Monohydrate for Oral Suspension 2735

Methacycline Hydrochloride (Oral iron products interfere with

absorption of oral tetracyclines; these products should not be taken within two hours of each other).
No products indexed under this heading.

Minocycline Hydrochloride (Oral iron products interfere with absorption of oral tetracyclines; these products should not be taken within two hours of each other). Products include:
Dynacin Capsules ... 2019
Minocin Intravenous ... 1862
Minocin Oral Suspension ... 1865
Minocin Pellet-Filled Capsules ... 1863

Oxytetracycline Hydrochloride (Oral iron products interfere with absorption of oral tetracyclines; these products should not be taken within two hours of each other). Products include:
Terra-Cortril Ophthalmic Suspension ... 2716
Urobiotic-250 Capsules ... 2731

Tetracycline Hydrochloride (Oral iron products interfere with absorption of oral tetracyclines; these products should not be taken within two hours of each other).
No products indexed under this heading.

FEOSOL TABLETS
(Ferrous Sulfate) ... 1717
See Feosol Caplets

FERGON IRON TABLETS
(Ferrous Gluconate) ... ▣802
None cited in PDR database.

FERRLECIT INJECTION
(Sodium Ferric Gluconate) ... 3386
May interact with ACE inhibitors. Compounds in these categories include:

Benazepril Hydrochloride (Co-administration with ACE inhibitor has resulted in increased incidence of both drug intolerance or suspected allergic events). Products include:
Lotensin Tablets ... 2365
Lotensin HCT Tablets ... 2367
Lotrel Capsules ... 2370

Captopril (Co-administration with ACE inhibitor has resulted in increased incidence of both drug intolerance or suspected allergic events). Products include:
Captopril Tablets ... 2281

Enalapril Maleate (Co-administration with ACE inhibitor has resulted in increased incidence of both drug intolerance or suspected allergic events). Products include:
Lexxel Tablets ... 608
Vaseretic Tablets ... 2204
Vasotec Tablets ... 2210

Enalaprilat (Co-administration with ACE inhibitor has resulted in increased incidence of both drug intolerance or suspected allergic events). Products include:
Enalaprilat Injection ... 863
Vasotec I.V. Injection ... 2207

Fosinopril Sodium (Co-administration with ACE inhibitor has resulted in increased incidence of both drug intolerance or suspected allergic events). Products include:
Monopril Tablets ... 1091
Monopril HCT ... 1094

Lisinopril (Co-administration with ACE inhibitor has resulted in increased incidence of both drug intolerance or suspected allergic events). Products include:
Prinivil Tablets ... 2164
Prinzide Tablets ... 2168
Zestoretic Tablets ... 695
Zestril Tablets ... 698

Moexipril Hydrochloride (Co-administration with ACE inhibitor has resulted in increased incidence of both drug intolerance or suspected allergic events). Products include:
Uniretic Tablets ... 3178
Univasc Tablets ... 3181

Perindopril Erbumine (Co-administration with ACE inhibitor has resulted in increased incidence of both drug intolerance or suspected allergic events). Products include:
Aceon Tablets (2 mg, 4 mg, 8 mg) ... 3249

Quinapril Hydrochloride (Co-administration with ACE inhibitor has resulted in increased incidence of both drug intolerance or suspected allergic events). Products include:
Accupril Tablets ... 2611
Accuretic Tablets ... 2614

Ramipril (Co-administration with ACE inhibitor has resulted in increased incidence of both drug intolerance or suspected allergic events). Products include:
Altace Capsules ... 2233

Spirapril Hydrochloride (Co-administration with ACE inhibitor has resulted in increased incidence of both drug intolerance or suspected allergic events).
No products indexed under this heading.

Trandolapril (Co-administration with ACE inhibitor has resulted in increased incidence of both drug intolerance or suspected allergic events). Products include:
Mavik Tablets ... 478
Tarka Tablets ... 508

FIBER 10 PACKETS
(Carboxymethylcellulose Sodium, Herbals, Multiple, Lactobacillus Acidophilus, Psyllium Preparations) ... ▣797
None cited in PDR database.

FIBERCON CAPLETS
(Calcium Polycarbophil) ... ▣639
May interact with tetracyclines. Compounds in these categories include:

Demeclocycline Hydrochloride (Fibercon should be taken at least one hour before or two hours after you have taken any form of tetracycline). Products include:
Declomycin Tablets ... 1855

Doxycycline Calcium (Fibercon should be taken at least one hour before or two hours after you have taken any form of tetracycline). Products include:
Vibramycin Calcium Oral Suspension Syrup ... 2735

Doxycycline Hyclate (Fibercon should be taken at least one hour before or two hours after you have taken any form of tetracycline). Products include:
Doryx Coated Pellet Filled Capsules ... 3357
Periostat Tablets ... 1208
Vibramycin Hyclate Capsules ... 2735
Vibramycin Hyclate Intravenous ... 2737
Vibra-Tabs Film Coated Tablets ... 2735

Doxycycline Monohydrate (Fibercon should be taken at least one hour before or two hours after you have taken any form of tetracycline). Products include:
Monodox Capsules ... 2442
Vibramycin Monohydrate for Oral Suspension ... 2735

Methacycline Hydrochloride (Fibercon should be taken at least one hour before or two hours after you have taken any form of tetracycline).
No products indexed under this heading.

Minocycline Hydrochloride (Fibercon should be taken at least one hour before or two hours after you have taken any form of tetracycline). Products include:
Dynacin Capsules ... 2019
Minocin Intravenous ... 1862
Minocin Oral Suspension ... 1865
Minocin Pellet-Filled Capsules ... 1863

Oxytetracycline Hydrochloride (Fibercon should be taken at least one hour before or two hours after you have taken any form of tetracycline). Products include:
Terra-Cortril Ophthalmic Suspension ... 2716
Urobiotic-250 Capsules ... 2731

Tetracycline Hydrochloride (Fibercon should be taken at least one hour before or two hours after you have taken any form of tetracycline).
No products indexed under this heading.

FINEVIN CREAM
(Azelaic Acid) ... 962
None cited in PDR database.

FLEET BISACODYL LAXATIVES
(Bisacodyl) ... 1359
None cited in PDR database.

FLEET ENEMA
(Sodium Phosphate) ... 1359
May interact with:

Diuretics, Unspecified (Effect not specified).

FLEET ENEMA FOR CHILDREN
(Sodium Phosphate) ... 1359
See Fleet Enema

FLEET GLYCERIN LAXATIVES
(Glycerin) ... 1359
None cited in PDR database.

FLEET MINERAL OIL ENEMA
(Mineral Oil) ... 1360
None cited in PDR database.

FLEET PHOSPHO-SODA
(Sodium Phosphate) ... 1360
None cited in PDR database.

FLEET PREP KITS
(Sodium Phosphate) ... 1361
May interact with antacids and certain other agents. Compounds in these categories include:

Aluminum Carbonate (Concurrent use within one-hour should be avoided).
No products indexed under this heading.

Aluminum Hydroxide (Concurrent use within one-hour should be avoided). Products include:
Amphojel Suspension (Mint Flavor) ... ▣789
Gaviscon Extra Strength Liquid ... ▣751
Gaviscon Extra Strength Tablets ... ▣751
Gaviscon Regular Strength Liquid ... ▣751
Gaviscon Regular Strength Tablets ... ▣750
Maalox Antacid/Anti-Gas Oral Suspension ... ▣673
Maalox Max Maximum Strength Antacid/Anti-Gas Liquid ... 2300
Maalox Regular Strength Antacid/Antigas Liquid ... 2300
Mylanta ... 1813
Vanquish Caplets ... ▣617

Magaldrate (Concurrent use within one-hour should be avoided).
No products indexed under this heading.

Magnesium Hydroxide (Concurrent use within one-hour should be avoided). Products include:
Ex•Lax Milk of Magnesia Liquid ... ▣670
Maalox Antacid/Anti-Gas Oral Suspension ... ▣673
Maalox Max Maximum Strength Antacid/Anti-Gas Liquid ... 2300
Maalox Regular Strength Antacid/Antigas Liquid ... 2300
Mylanta Fast-Acting ... 1813
Mylanta ... 1813
Pepcid Complete Chewable Tablets ... 1815
Phillips' Chewable Tablets ... ▣615
Phillips' Milk of Magnesia Liquid (Original, Cherry, & Mint) ... ▣616
Rolaids Tablets ... ▣706
Extra Strength Rolaids Tablets ... ▣706
Vanquish Caplets ... ▣617

Magnesium Oxide (Concurrent use within one-hour should be avoided). Products include:
Beelith Tablets ... 946
Mag-Ox 400 Tablets ... 1024
Uro-Mag Capsules ... 1024

Sodium Bicarbonate (Concurrent use within one-hour should be avoided). Products include:
Alka-Seltzer ... ▣603
Alka-Seltzer Lemon Lime Antacid and Pain Reliever Effervescent Tablets ... ▣603
Alka-Seltzer Extra Strength Antacid and Pain Reliever Effervescent Tablets ... ▣603
Alka-Seltzer Heartburn Relief Tablets ... ▣604
Ceo-Two Evacuant Suppository ... ▣618
Colyte with Flavor Packs for Oral Solution ... 3170
GoLYTELY and Pineapple Flavor GoLYTELY for Oral Solution ... 1068
NuLYTELY, Cherry Flavor, Lemon-Lime Flavor, and Orange Flavor NuLYTELY for Oral Solution ... 1068

Food Interactions

Dairy products (Concurrent use within one-hour should be avoided).

FLEXERIL TABLETS
(Cyclobenzaprine Hydrochloride) ... 572
May interact with anticholinergics, barbiturates, central nervous system depressants, monoamine oxidase inhibitors, and certain other agents. Compounds in these categories include:

Alfentanil Hydrochloride (Co-administration results in enhanced effects).
No products indexed under this heading.

Alprazolam (Co-administration results in enhanced effects). Products include:
Xanax Tablets ... 2865

Aprobarbital (Co-administration results in enhanced effects).
No products indexed under this heading.

Atropine Sulfate (Caution is advised when co-administered due to cyclobenzaprine-induced atropine-like actions). Products include:
Donnatal ... 2929
Donnatal Extentabs ... 2930
Motofen Tablets ... 577
Prosed/DS Tablets ... 3268
Urised Tablets ... 2876

Belladonna Alkaloids (Caution is advised when co-administered due to cyclobenzaprine-induced atropine-like actions). Products include:
Hyland's Teething Tablets ... ▣766
Urimax Tablets ... 1769

Benztropine Mesylate (Caution is advised when co-administered due to cyclobenzaprine-induced atropine-like actions). Products include:
Cogentin ... 2055

Biperiden Hydrochloride (Caution is advised when co-administered due to cyclobenzaprine-induced atropine-like actions). Products include:
Akineton ... 402

Buprenorphine Hydrochloride (Co-administration results in enhanced effects). Products include:
Buprenex Injectable ... 2918

Buspirone Hydrochloride (Co-administration results in enhanced effects).
No products indexed under this heading.

IMPORTANT NOTE: Always consult each drug listing in the patient's regimen for possible interactions.

Butabarbital (Co-administration results in enhanced effects).
No products indexed under this heading.

Butalbital (Co-administration results in enhanced effects). Products include:
Phrenilin ... 578
Sedapap Tablets 50 mg/650 mg ... 2225

Chlordiazepoxide (Co-administration results in enhanced effects). Products include:
Limbitrol ... 1738

Chlordiazepoxide Hydrochloride (Co-administration results in enhanced effects). Products include:
Librium Capsules ... 1736
Librium for Injection ... 1737

Chlorpromazine (Co-administration results in enhanced effects). Products include:
Thorazine Suppositories ... 1656

Chlorpromazine Hydrochloride (Co-administration results in enhanced effects). Products include:
Thorazine ... 1656

Chlorprothixene (Co-administration results in enhanced effects).
No products indexed under this heading.

Chlorprothixene Hydrochloride (Co-administration results in enhanced effects).
No products indexed under this heading.

Chlorprothixene Lactate (Co-administration results in enhanced effects).
No products indexed under this heading.

Clidinium Bromide (Caution is advised when co-administered due to cyclobenzaprine-induced atropine-like actions).
No products indexed under this heading.

Clorazepate Dipotassium (Co-administration results in enhanced effects). Products include:
Tranxene ... 511

Clozapine (Co-administration results in enhanced effects). Products include:
Clozaril Tablets ... 2319

Codeine Phosphate (Co-administration results in enhanced effects). Products include:
Phenergan with Codeine Syrup ... 3557
Phenergan VC with Codeine Syrup .. 3561
Robitussin A-C Syrup ... 2942
Robitussin-DAC Syrup ... 2942
Ryna-C Liquid ... ▣768
Soma Compound w/Codeine Tablets ... 3355
Tussi-Organidin NR Liquid ... 3350
Tussi-Organidin-S NR Liquid ... 3350
Tylenol with Codeine ... 2595

Desflurane (Co-administration results in enhanced effects). Products include:
Suprane Liquid for Inhalation ... 874

Dezocine (Co-administration results in enhanced effects).
No products indexed under this heading.

Diazepam (Co-administration results in enhanced effects). Products include:
Valium Injectable ... 3026
Valium Tablets ... 3047

Dicyclomine Hydrochloride (Caution is advised when co-administered due to cyclobenzaprine-induced atropine-like actions).
No products indexed under this heading.

Droperidol (Co-administration results in enhanced effects).
No products indexed under this heading.

Enflurane (Co-administration results in enhanced effects).
No products indexed under this heading.

Estazolam (Co-administration results in enhanced effects). Products include:
ProSom Tablets ... 500

Ethchlorvynol (Co-administration results in enhanced effects).
No products indexed under this heading.

Ethinamate (Co-administration results in enhanced effects).
No products indexed under this heading.

Fentanyl (Co-administration results in enhanced effects). Products include:
Duragesic Transdermal System ... 1786

Fentanyl Citrate (Co-administration results in enhanced effects). Products include:
Actiq ... 1184

Fluphenazine Decanoate (Co-administration results in enhanced effects).
No products indexed under this heading.

Fluphenazine Enanthate (Co-administration results in enhanced effects).
No products indexed under this heading.

Fluphenazine Hydrochloride (Co-administration results in enhanced effects).
No products indexed under this heading.

Flurazepam Hydrochloride (Co-administration results in enhanced effects).
No products indexed under this heading.

Glutethimide (Co-administration results in enhanced effects).
No products indexed under this heading.

Glycopyrrolate (Caution is advised when co-administered due to cyclobenzaprine-induced atropine-like actions). Products include:
Robinul Forte Tablets ... 1358
Robinul Injectable ... 2940
Robinul Tablets ... 1358

Guanethidine Monosulfate (Cyclobenzaprine is closely related to tricyclic antidepressants and potential exists for cyclobenzaprine to block antihypertensive effects).
No products indexed under this heading.

Haloperidol (Co-administration results in enhanced effects). Products include:
Haldol Injection, Tablets and Concentrate ... 2533

Haloperidol Decanoate (Co-administration results in enhanced effects). Products include:
Haldol Decanoate ... 2535

Hydrocodone Bitartrate (Co-administration results in enhanced effects). Products include:
Hycodan ... 1316
Hycomine Compound Tablets ... 1317
Hycotuss Expectorant Syrup ... 1318
Lortab ... 3319
Lortab Elixir ... 3317
Maxidone Tablets CIII ... 3399
Norco 5/325 Tablets CIII ... 3424
Norco 7.5/325 Tablets CIII ... 3425
Norco 10/325 Tablets CIII ... 3427
Norco 10/325 Tablets CIII ... 3425
Vicodin Tablets ... 516
Vicodin ES Tablets ... 517
Vicodin HP Tablets ... 518
Vicodin Tuss Expectorant ... 519
Vicoprofen Tablets ... 520
Zydone Tablets ... 1330

Hydrocodone Polistirex (Co-administration results in enhanced effects). Products include:
Tussionex Pennkinetic Extended-Release Suspension ... 1174

Hydromorphone Hydrochloride (Co-administration results in enhanced effects). Products include:
Dilaudid ... 441
Dilaudid Oral Liquid ... 445
Dilaudid Powder ... 441
Dilaudid Rectal Suppositories ... 441
Dilaudid Tablets ... 441
Dilaudid Tablets - 8 mg ... 445
Dilaudid-HP ... 443

Hydroxyzine Hydrochloride (Co-administration results in enhanced effects). Products include:
Atarax Tablets & Syrup ... 2667
Vistaril Intramuscular Solution ... 2738

Hyoscyamine (Caution is advised when co-administered due to cyclobenzaprine-induced atropine-like actions). Products include:
Urised Tablets ... 2876

Hyoscyamine Sulfate (Caution is advised when co-administered due to cyclobenzaprine-induced atropine-like actions). Products include:
Arco-Lase Plus Tablets ... 592
Donnatal ... 2929
Donnatal Extentabs ... 2930
Levsin/Levsinex/Levbid ... 3172
NuLev Orally Disintegrating Tablets ... 3176
Prosed/DS Tablets ... 3268
Urimax Tablets ... 1769

Ipratropium Bromide (Caution is advised when co-administered due to cyclobenzaprine-induced atropine-like actions). Products include:
Atrovent Inhalation Aerosol ... 1030
Atrovent Inhalation Solution ... 1031
Atrovent Nasal Spray 0.03% ... 1032
Atrovent Nasal Spray 0.06% ... 1033
Combivent Inhalation Aerosol ... 1041
DuoNeb Inhalation Solution ... 1233

Isocarboxazid (Cyclobenzaprine is closely related to tricyclic antidepressants and hyperpyretic crises, severe convulsions and death have occurred in patients taking these agents concurrently; cyclobenzaprine may interact in the same fashion with MAO inhibitors hence concurrent and/or sequential use is contraindicated).
No products indexed under this heading.

Isoflurane (Co-administration results in enhanced effects).
No products indexed under this heading.

Ketamine Hydrochloride (Co-administration results in enhanced effects).
No products indexed under this heading.

Levomethadyl Acetate Hydrochloride (Co-administration results in enhanced effects).
No products indexed under this heading.

Levorphanol Tartrate (Co-administration results in enhanced effects). Products include:
Levo-Dromoran ... 1734
Levorphanol Tartrate Tablets ... 3059

Lorazepam (Co-administration results in enhanced effects). Products include:
Ativan Injection ... 3478
Ativan Tablets ... 3482

Loxapine Hydrochloride (Co-administration results in enhanced effects).
No products indexed under this heading.

Loxapine Succinate (Co-administration results in enhanced effects). Products include:
Loxitane Capsules ... 3398

Mepenzolate Bromide (Caution is advised when co-administered due to cyclobenzaprine-induced atropine-like actions).
No products indexed under this heading.

Meperidine Hydrochloride (Co-administration results in enhanced effects). Products include:
Demerol ... 3079
Mepergan Injection ... 3539

Mephobarbital (Co-administration results in enhanced effects).
No products indexed under this heading.

Meprobamate (Co-administration results in enhanced effects). Products include:
Miltown Tablets ... 3349

Mesoridazine Besylate (Co-administration results in enhanced effects). Products include:
Serentil ... 1057

Methadone Hydrochloride (Co-administration results in enhanced effects). Products include:
Dolophine Hydrochloride Tablets ... 3056

Methohexital Sodium (Co-administration results in enhanced effects). Products include:
Brevital Sodium for Injection, USP .. 1815

Methotrimeprazine (Co-administration results in enhanced effects).
No products indexed under this heading.

Methoxyflurane (Co-administration results in enhanced effects).
No products indexed under this heading.

Midazolam Hydrochloride (Co-administration results in enhanced effects). Products include:
Versed Injection ... 3027
Versed Syrup ... 3033

Moclobemide (Cyclobenzaprine is closely related to tricyclic antidepressants and hyperpyretic crises, severe convulsions and death have occurred in patients taking these agents concurrently; cyclobenzaprine may interact in the same fashion with MAO inhibitors hence concurrent and/or sequential use is contraindicated).
No products indexed under this heading.

Molindone Hydrochloride (Co-administration results in enhanced effects). Products include:
Moban ... 1320

Morphine Sulfate (Co-administration results in enhanced effects). Products include:
Astramorph/PF Injection, USP (Preservative-Free) ... 594
Duramorph Injection ... 1312
Infumorph 200 and Infumorph 500 Sterile Solutions ... 1314
Kadian Capsules ... 1335
MS Contin Tablets ... 2896
MSIR ... 2898
Oramorph SR Tablets ... 3062
Roxanol ... 3066

Olanzapine (Co-administration results in enhanced effects). Products include:
Zyprexa Tablets ... 1973
Zyprexa ZYDIS Orally Disintegrating Tablets ... 1973

Oxazepam (Co-administration results in enhanced effects).
No products indexed under this heading.

Oxybutynin Chloride (Caution is advised when co-administered due to cyclobenzaprine-induced atropine-like actions). Products include:
Ditropan XL Extended Release Tablets ... 564

Oxycodone Hydrochloride (Co-administration results in enhanced effects). Products include:
OxyContin Tablets ... 2912
OxyFast Oral Concentrate Solution . 2916
OxyIR Capsules ... 2916
Percocet Tablets ... 1326
Percodan Tablets ... 1327
Percolone Tablets ... 1327
Roxicodone ... 3067
Tylox Capsules ... 2597

Pargyline Hydrochloride (Cyclobenzaprine is closely related to tricyclic antidepressants and hyperpyretic crises, severe convulsions and death have occurred in

patients taking these agents concurrently; cyclobenzaprine may interact in the same fashion with MAO inhibitors hence concurrent and/or sequential use is contraindicated).
No products indexed under this heading.

Pentobarbital Sodium (Co-administration results in enhanced effects). Products include:
Nembutal Sodium Solution 485

Perphenazine (Co-administration results in enhanced effects). Products include:
Etrafon 3115
Trilafon 3160

Phenelzine Sulfate (Cyclobenzaprine is closely related to tricyclic antidepressants and hyperpyretic crises, severe convulsions and death have occurred in patients taking these agents concurrently; cyclobenzaprine may interact in the same fashion with MAO inhibitors hence concurrent and/or sequential use is contraindicated). Products include:
Nardil Tablets 2653

Phenobarbital (Co-administration results in enhanced effects). Products include:
Arco-Lase Plus Tablets 592
Donnatal 2929
Donnatal Extentabs 2930

Prazepam (Co-administration results in enhanced effects).
No products indexed under this heading.

Procarbazine Hydrochloride (Cyclobenzaprine is closely related to tricyclic antidepressants and hyperpyretic crises, severe convulsions and death have occurred in patients taking these agents concurrently; cyclobenzaprine may interact in the same fashion with MAO inhibitors hence concurrent and/or sequential use is contraindicated). Products include:
Matulane Capsules 3246

Prochlorperazine (Co-administration results in enhanced effects). Products include:
Compazine 1505

Procyclidine Hydrochloride (Caution is advised when co-administered due to cyclobenzaprine-induced atropine-like actions).
No products indexed under this heading.

Promethazine Hydrochloride (Co-administration results in enhanced effects). Products include:
Mepergan Injection 3539
Phenergan Injection 3553
Phenergan 3556
Phenergan Syrup 3554
Phenergan with Codeine Syrup 3557
Phenergan with Dextromethorphan Syrup 3559
Phenergan VC Syrup 3560
Phenergan VC with Codeine Syrup 3561

Propantheline Bromide (Caution is advised when co-administered due to cyclobenzaprine-induced atropine-like actions).
No products indexed under this heading.

Propofol (Co-administration results in enhanced effects). Products include:
Diprivan Injectable Emulsion 667

Propoxyphene Hydrochloride (Co-administration results in enhanced effects). Products include:
Darvon Pulvules 1909
Darvon Compound-65 Pulvules 1910

Propoxyphene Napsylate (Co-administration results in enhanced effects). Products include:
Darvon-N/Darvocet-N 1907
Darvon-N Tablets 1912

Quazepam (Co-administration results in enhanced effects).
No products indexed under this heading.

Quetiapine Fumarate (Co-administration results in enhanced effects). Products include:
Seroquel Tablets 684

Remifentanil Hydrochloride (Co-administration results in enhanced effects).
No products indexed under this heading.

Risperidone (Co-administration results in enhanced effects). Products include:
Risperdal 1796

Scopolamine (Caution is advised when co-administered due to cyclobenzaprine-induced atropine-like actions). Products include:
Transderm Scōp Transdermal Therapeutic System 2302

Scopolamine Hydrobromide (Caution is advised when co-administered due to cyclobenzaprine-induced atropine-like actions). Products include:
Donnatal 2929
Donnatal Extentabs 2930

Secobarbital Sodium (Co-administration results in enhanced effects).
No products indexed under this heading.

Selegiline Hydrochloride (Cyclobenzaprine is closely related to tricyclic antidepressants and hyperpyretic crises, severe convulsions and death have occurred in patients taking these agents concurrently; cyclobenzaprine may interact in the same fashion with MAO inhibitors hence concurrent and/or sequential use is contraindicated). Products include:
Eldepryl Capsules 3266

Sevoflurane (Co-administration results in enhanced effects).
No products indexed under this heading.

Sufentanil Citrate (Co-administration results in enhanced effects).
No products indexed under this heading.

Temazepam (Co-administration results in enhanced effects).
No products indexed under this heading.

Thiamylal Sodium (Co-administration results in enhanced effects).
No products indexed under this heading.

Thioridazine Hydrochloride (Co-administration results in enhanced effects). Products include:
Thioridazine Hydrochloride Tablets 2289

Thiothixene (Co-administration results in enhanced effects). Products include:
Navane Capsules 2701
Thiothixene Capsules 2290

Tolterodine Tartrate (Caution is advised when co-administered due to cyclobenzaprine-induced atropine-like actions). Products include:
Detrol Tablets 3623
Detrol LA Capsules 2801

Tramadol Hydrochloride (Cyclobenzaprine is closely related to tricyclic antidepressants, hence, may enhance the seizure risk in patients taking tramadol). Products include:
Ultracet Tablets 2597
Ultram Tablets 2600

Tranylcypromine Sulfate (Cyclobenzaprine is closely related to tricyclic antidepressants and hyperpyretic crises, severe convulsions and death have occurred in patients taking these agents concurrently; cyclobenzaprine may interact in the same fashion with MAO inhibitors hence concurrent and/or sequential use is contraindicated). Products include:
Parnate Tablets 1607

Triazolam (Co-administration results in enhanced effects). Products include:
Halcion Tablets 2823

Tridihexethyl Chloride (Caution is advised when co-administered due to cyclobenzaprine-induced atropine-like actions).
No products indexed under this heading.

Trifluoperazine Hydrochloride (Co-administration results in enhanced effects). Products include:
Stelazine 1640

Trihexyphenidyl Hydrochloride (Caution is advised when co-administered due to cyclobenzaprine-induced atropine-like actions). Products include:
Artane 1855

Zaleplon (Co-administration results in enhanced effects). Products include:
Sonata Capsules 3591

Ziprasidone Hydrochloride (Co-administration results in enhanced effects). Products include:
Geodon Capsules 2688

Zolpidem Tartrate (Co-administration results in enhanced effects). Products include:
Ambien Tablets 3191

Food Interactions

Alcohol (Concurrent use results in enhanced effects).

FLEXERIL TABLETS

(Cyclobenzaprine Hydrochloride) 2094
May interact with anticholinergics, barbiturates, central nervous system depressants, monoamine oxidase inhibitors, and certain other agents. Compounds in these categories include:

Alfentanil Hydrochloride (Co-administration results in enhanced effects).
No products indexed under this heading.

Alprazolam (Co-administration results in enhanced effects). Products include:
Xanax Tablets 2865

Aprobarbital (Co-administration results in enhanced effects).
No products indexed under this heading.

Atropine Sulfate (Caution is advised when co-administered due to cyclobenzaprine-induced atropine-like actions). Products include:
Donnatal 2929
Donnatal Extentabs 2930
Motofen Tablets 577
Prosed/DS Tablets 3268
Urised Tablets 2876

Belladonna Alkaloids (Caution is advised when co-administered due to cyclobenzaprine-induced atropine-like actions). Products include:
Hyland's Teething Tablets 766
Urimax Tablets 1769

Benztropine Mesylate (Caution is advised when co-administered due to cyclobenzaprine-induced atropine-like actions). Products include:
Cogentin 2055

Biperiden Hydrochloride (Caution is advised when co-administered due to cyclobenzaprine-induced atropine-like actions). Products include:
Akineton 402

Buprenorphine Hydrochloride (Co-administration results in enhanced effects). Products include:
Buprenex Injectable 2918

Buspirone Hydrochloride (Co-administration results in enhanced effects).
No products indexed under this heading.

Butabarbital (Co-administration results in enhanced effects).
No products indexed under this heading.

Butalbital (Co-administration results in enhanced effects). Products include:
Phrenilin 578
Sedapap Tablets 50 mg/650 mg 2225

Chlordiazepoxide (Co-administration results in enhanced effects). Products include:
Limbitrol 1738

Chlordiazepoxide Hydrochloride (Co-administration results in enhanced effects). Products include:
Librium Capsules 1736
Librium for Injection 1737

Chlorpromazine (Co-administration results in enhanced effects). Products include:
Thorazine Suppositories 1656

Chlorpromazine Hydrochloride (Co-administration results in enhanced effects). Products include:
Thorazine 1656

Chlorprothixene (Co-administration results in enhanced effects).
No products indexed under this heading.

Chlorprothixene Hydrochloride (Co-administration results in enhanced effects).
No products indexed under this heading.

Chlorprothixene Lactate (Co-administration results in enhanced effects).
No products indexed under this heading.

Clidinium Bromide (Caution is advised when co-administered due to cyclobenzaprine-induced atropine-like actions).
No products indexed under this heading.

Clorazepate Dipotassium (Co-administration results in enhanced effects). Products include:
Tranxene 511

Clozapine (Co-administration results in enhanced effects). Products include:
Clozaril Tablets 2319

Codeine Phosphate (Co-administration results in enhanced effects). Products include:
Phenergan with Codeine Syrup 3557
Phenergan VC with Codeine Syrup 3561
Robitussin A-C Syrup 2942
Robitussin-DAC Syrup 2942
Ryna-C Liquid 768
Soma Compound w/Codeine Tablets 3355
Tussi-Organidin NR Liquid 3350
Tussi-Organidin-S NR Liquid 3350
Tylenol with Codeine 2595

Desflurane (Co-administration results in enhanced effects). Products include:
Suprane Liquid for Inhalation 874

Dezocine (Co-administration results in enhanced effects).
No products indexed under this heading.

Diazepam (Co-administration results in enhanced effects). Products include:
Valium Injectable 3026
Valium Tablets 3047

Dicyclomine Hydrochloride (Caution is advised when co-administered due to cyclobenzaprine-induced atropine-like actions).
No products indexed under this heading.

Droperidol (Co-administration results in enhanced effects).
No products indexed under this heading.

IMPORTANT NOTE: Always consult each drug listing in the patient's regimen for possible interactions.

Enflurane (Co-administration results in enhanced effects).
No products indexed under this heading.

Estazolam (Co-administration results in enhanced effects). Products include:
ProSom Tablets 500

Ethchlorvynol (Co-administration results in enhanced effects).
No products indexed under this heading.

Ethinamate (Co-administration results in enhanced effects).
No products indexed under this heading.

Fentanyl (Co-administration results in enhanced effects). Products include:
Duragesic Transdermal System 1786

Fentanyl Citrate (Co-administration results in enhanced effects). Products include:
Actiq 1184

Fluphenazine Decanoate (Co-administration results in enhanced effects).
No products indexed under this heading.

Fluphenazine Enanthate (Co-administration results in enhanced effects).
No products indexed under this heading.

Fluphenazine Hydrochloride (Co-administration results in enhanced effects).
No products indexed under this heading.

Flurazepam Hydrochloride (Co-administration results in enhanced effects).
No products indexed under this heading.

Glutethimide (Co-administration results in enhanced effects).
No products indexed under this heading.

Glycopyrrolate (Caution is advised when co-administered due to cyclobenzaprine-induced atropine-like actions). Products include:
Robinul Forte Tablets 1358
Robinul Injectable 2940
Robinul Tablets 1358

Guanethidine Monosulfate (Cyclobenzaprine is closely related to tricyclic antidepressants and potential exists for cyclobenzaprine to block antihypertensive effects).
No products indexed under this heading.

Haloperidol (Co-administration results in enhanced effects). Products include:
Haldol Injection, Tablets and Concentrate 2533

Haloperidol Decanoate (Co-administration results in enhanced effects). Products include:
Haldol Decanoate 2535

Hydrocodone Bitartrate (Co-administration results in enhanced effects). Products include:
Hycodan 1316
Hycomine Compound Tablets 1317
Hycotuss Expectorant Syrup 1318
Lortab 3319
Lortab Elixir 3317
Maxidone Tablets CIII 3399
Norco 5/325 Tablets CIII 3424
Norco 7.5/325 Tablets CIII 3425
Norco 10/325 Tablets CIII 3427
Norco 10/325 Tablets CIII 3425
Vicodin Tablets 516
Vicodin ES Tablets 517
Vicodin HP Tablets 518
Vicodin Tuss Expectorant 519
Vicoprofen Tablets 520
Zydone Tablets 1330

Hydrocodone Polistirex (Co-administration results in enhanced effects). Products include:
Tussionex Pennkinetic Extended-Release Suspension 1174

Hydromorphone Hydrochloride (Co-administration results in enhanced effects). Products include:
Dilaudid 441
Dilaudid Oral Liquid 445
Dilaudid Powder 441
Dilaudid Rectal Suppositories 441
Dilaudid Tablets 441
Dilaudid Tablets - 8 mg 445
Dilaudid-HP 443

Hydroxyzine Hydrochloride (Co-administration results in enhanced effects). Products include:
Atarax Tablets & Syrup 2667
Vistaril Intramuscular Solution 2738

Hyoscyamine (Caution is advised when co-administered due to cyclobenzaprine-induced atropine-like actions). Products include:
Urised Tablets 2876

Hyoscyamine Sulfate (Caution is advised when co-administered due to cyclobenzaprine-induced atropine-like actions). Products include:
Arco-Lase Plus Tablets 592
Donnatal 2929
Donnatal Extentabs 2930
Levsin/Levsinex/Levbid 3172
NuLev Orally Disintegrating Tablets 3176
Prosed/DS Tablets 3268
Urimax Tablets 1769

Ipratropium Bromide (Caution is advised when co-administered due to cyclobenzaprine-induced atropine-like actions). Products include:
Atrovent Inhalation Aerosol 1030
Atrovent Inhalation Solution 1031
Atrovent Nasal Spray 0.03% 1032
Atrovent Nasal Spray 0.06% 1033
Combivent Inhalation Aerosol 1041
DuoNeb Inhalation Solution 1233

Isocarboxazid (Cyclobenzaprine is closely related to tricyclic antidepressants and hyperpyretic crises, severe convulsions and death have occurred in patients taking these agents concurrently; cyclobenzaprine may interact in the same fashion with MAO inhibitors hence concurrent and/or sequential use is contraindicated).
No products indexed under this heading.

Isoflurane (Co-administration results in enhanced effects).
No products indexed under this heading.

Ketamine Hydrochloride (Co-administration results in enhanced effects).
No products indexed under this heading.

Levomethadyl Acetate Hydrochloride (Co-administration results in enhanced effects).
No products indexed under this heading.

Levorphanol Tartrate (Co-administration results in enhanced effects). Products include:
Levo-Dromoran 1734
Levorphanol Tartrate Tablets 3059

Lorazepam (Co-administration results in enhanced effects). Products include:
Ativan Injection 3478
Ativan Tablets 3482

Loxapine Hydrochloride (Co-administration results in enhanced effects).
No products indexed under this heading.

Loxapine Succinate (Co-administration results in enhanced effects). Products include:
Loxitane Capsules 3398

Mepenzolate Bromide (Caution is advised when co-administered due to cyclobenzaprine-induced atropine-like actions).
No products indexed under this heading.

Meperidine Hydrochloride (Co-administration results in enhanced effects). Products include:
Demerol 3079
Mepergan Injection 3539

Mephobarbital (Co-administration results in enhanced effects).
No products indexed under this heading.

Meprobamate (Co-administration results in enhanced effects). Products include:
Miltown Tablets 3349

Mesoridazine Besylate (Co-administration results in enhanced effects). Products include:
Serentil 1057

Methadone Hydrochloride (Co-administration results in enhanced effects). Products include:
Dolophine Hydrochloride Tablets 3056

Methohexital Sodium (Co-administration results in enhanced effects). Products include:
Brevital Sodium for Injection, USP 1815

Methotrimeprazine (Co-administration results in enhanced effects).
No products indexed under this heading.

Methoxyflurane (Co-administration results in enhanced effects).
No products indexed under this heading.

Midazolam Hydrochloride (Co-administration results in enhanced effects). Products include:
Versed Injection 3027
Versed Syrup 3033

Moclobemide (Cyclobenzaprine is closely related to tricyclic antidepressants and hyperpyretic crises, severe convulsions and death have occurred in patients taking these agents concurrently; cyclobenzaprine may interact in the same fashion with MAO inhibitors hence concurrent and/or sequential use is contraindicated).
No products indexed under this heading.

Molindone Hydrochloride (Co-administration results in enhanced effects). Products include:
Moban 1320

Morphine Sulfate (Co-administration results in enhanced effects). Products include:
Astramorph/PF Injection, USP (Preservative-Free) 594
Duramorph Injection 1312
Infumorph 200 and Infumorph 500 Sterile Solutions 1314
Kadian Capsules 1335
MS Contin Tablets 2896
MSIR 2898
Oramorph SR Tablets 3062
Roxanol 3066

Olanzapine (Co-administration results in enhanced effects). Products include:
Zyprexa Tablets 1973
Zyprexa ZYDIS Orally Disintegrating Tablets 1973

Oxazepam (Co-administration results in enhanced effects).
No products indexed under this heading.

Oxybutynin Chloride (Caution is advised when co-administered due to cyclobenzaprine-induced atropine-like actions). Products include:
Ditropan XL Extended Release Tablets 564

Oxycodone Hydrochloride (Co-administration results in enhanced effects). Products include:
OxyContin Tablets 2912
OxyFast Oral Concentrate Solution 2916
OxyIR Capsules 2916
Percocet Tablets 1326
Percodan Tablets 1327
Percolone Tablets 1327
Roxicodone 3067
Tylox Capsules 2597

Pargyline Hydrochloride (Cyclobenzaprine is closely related to tricyclic antidepressants and hyperpyretic crises, severe convulsions and death have occurred in patients taking these agents concurrently; cyclobenzaprine may interact in the same fashion with MAO inhibitors hence concurrent and/or sequential use is contraindicated).
No products indexed under this heading.

Pentobarbital Sodium (Co-administration results in enhanced effects). Products include:
Nembutal Sodium Solution 485

Perphenazine (Co-administration results in enhanced effects). Products include:
Etrafon 3115
Trilafon 3160

Phenelzine Sulfate (Cyclobenzaprine is closely related to tricyclic antidepressants and hyperpyretic crises, severe convulsions and death have occurred in patients taking these agents concurrently; cyclobenzaprine may interact in the same fashion with MAO inhibitors hence concurrent and/or sequential use is contraindicated). Products include:
Nardil Tablets 2653

Phenobarbital (Co-administration results in enhanced effects). Products include:
Arco-Lase Plus Tablets 592
Donnatal 2929
Donnatal Extentabs 2930

Prazepam (Co-administration results in enhanced effects).
No products indexed under this heading.

Procarbazine Hydrochloride (Cyclobenzaprine is closely related to tricyclic antidepressants and hyperpyretic crises, severe convulsions and death have occurred in patients taking these agents concurrently; cyclobenzaprine may interact in the same fashion with MAO inhibitors hence concurrent and/or sequential use is contraindicated). Products include:
Matulane Capsules 3246

Prochlorperazine (Co-administration results in enhanced effects). Products include:
Compazine 1505

Procyclidine Hydrochloride (Caution is advised when co-administered due to cyclobenzaprine-induced atropine-like actions).
No products indexed under this heading.

Promethazine Hydrochloride (Co-administration results in enhanced effects). Products include:
Mepergan Injection 3539
Phenergan Injection 3553
Phenergan 3556
Phenergan Syrup 3554
Phenergan with Codeine Syrup 3557
Phenergan with Dextromethorphan Syrup 3559
Phenergan VC Syrup 3560
Phenergan VC with Codeine Syrup 3561

Propantheline Bromide (Caution is advised when co-administered due to cyclobenzaprine-induced atropine-like actions).
No products indexed under this heading.

Propofol (Co-administration results in enhanced effects). Products include:
Diprivan Injectable Emulsion 667

Propoxyphene Hydrochloride (Co-administration results in enhanced effects). Products include:
Darvon Pulvules 1909
Darvon Compound-65 Pulvules 1910

Propoxyphene Napsylate (Co-administration results in enhanced effects). Products include:
Darvon-N/Darvocet-N 1907
Darvon-N Tablets 1912

Quazepam (Co-administration results in enhanced effects).
No products indexed under this heading.

Quetiapine Fumarate (Co-administration results in enhanced effects). Products include:
Seroquel Tablets 684

Remifentanil Hydrochloride (Co-administration results in enhanced effects).
No products indexed under this heading.

Risperidone (Co-administration results in enhanced effects). Products include:
Risperdal 1796

Scopolamine (Caution is advised when co-administered due to cyclobenzaprine-induced atropine-like actions). Products include:
Transderm Scōp Transdermal Therapeutic System 2302

Scopolamine Hydrobromide (Caution is advised when co-administered due to cyclobenzaprine-induced atropine-like actions). Products include:
Donnatal 2929
Donnatal Extentabs 2930

Secobarbital Sodium (Co-administration results in enhanced effects).
No products indexed under this heading.

Selegiline Hydrochloride (Cyclobenzaprine is closely related to tricyclic antidepressants and hyperpyretic crises, severe convulsions and death have occurred in patients taking these agents concurrently; cyclobenzaprine may interact in the same fashion with MAO inhibitors hence concurrent and/or sequential use is contraindicated). Products include:
Eldepryl Capsules 3266

Sevoflurane (Co-administration results in enhanced effects).
No products indexed under this heading.

Sufentanil Citrate (Co-administration results in enhanced effects).
No products indexed under this heading.

Temazepam (Co-administration results in enhanced effects).
No products indexed under this heading.

Thiamylal Sodium (Co-administration results in enhanced effects).
No products indexed under this heading.

Thioridazine Hydrochloride (Co-administration results in enhanced effects). Products include:
Thioridazine Hydrochloride Tablets 2289

Thiothixene (Co-administration results in enhanced effects). Products include:
Navane Capsules 2701
Thiothixene Capsules 2290

Tolterodine Tartrate (Caution is advised when co-administered due to cyclobenzaprine-induced atropine-like actions). Products include:
Detrol Tablets 3623
Detrol LA Capsules 2801

Tramadol Hydrochloride (Cyclobenzaprine is closely related to tricyclic antidepressants, hence, may enhance the seizure risk in patients taking tramadol). Products include:
Ultracet Tablets 2597
Ultram Tablets 2600

Tranylcypromine Sulfate (Cyclobenzaprine is closely related to tricyclic antidepressants and hyperpyretic crises, severe convulsions and death have occurred in patients taking these agents concurrently; cyclobenzaprine may interact in the same fashion with MAO inhibitors hence concurrent and/or sequential use is contraindicated). Products include:
Parnate Tablets 1607

Triazolam (Co-administration results in enhanced effects). Products include:
Halcion Tablets 2823

Tridihexethyl Chloride (Caution is advised when co-administered due to cyclobenzaprine-induced atropine-like actions).
No products indexed under this heading.

Trifluoperazine Hydrochloride (Co-administration results in enhanced effects). Products include:
Stelazine 1640

Trihexyphenidyl Hydrochloride (Caution is advised when co-administered due to cyclobenzaprine-induced atropine-like actions). Products include:
Artane 1855

Zaleplon (Co-administration results in enhanced effects). Products include:
Sonata Capsules 3591

Ziprasidone Hydrochloride (Co-administration results in enhanced effects). Products include:
Geodon Capsules 2688

Zolpidem Tartrate (Co-administration results in enhanced effects). Products include:
Ambien Tablets 3191

Food Interactions

Alcohol (Concurrent use results in enhanced effects).

FLINTSTONES ORIGINAL CHILDREN'S MULTIVITAMIN CHEWABLE TABLETS

(Vitamins, Multiple) .... ▣802
None cited in PDR database.

FLINTSTONES CHILDREN'S MULTIVITAMIN PLUS CALCIUM CHEWABLE TABLETS

(Vitamins with Minerals) .... ▣804
None cited in PDR database.

FLINTSTONES CHILDREN'S MULTIVITAMIN PLUS EXTRA C CHEWABLE TABLETS

(Vitamins, Multiple) .... ▣804
None cited in PDR database.

FLINTSTONES CHILDREN'S MULTIVITAMIN PLUS IRON CHEWABLE TABLETS

(Vitamins with Iron) .... ▣802
None cited in PDR database.

FLINTSTONES COMPLETE CHILDREN'S MUTIVITAMIN/ MULTIMINERAL CHEWABLE TABLETS

(Vitamins with Minerals) .... ▣803
None cited in PDR database.

FLOLAN FOR INJECTION

(Epoprostenol Sodium) 1528
May interact with antihypertensives, oral anticoagulants, diuretics, platelet inhibitors, vasodilators, and certain other agents. Compounds in these categories include:

Acebutolol Hydrochloride (Additional reductions in blood pressure may occur). Products include:
Sectral Capsules 3589

Amiloride Hydrochloride (Additional reductions in blood pressure may occur). Products include:
Midamor Tablets 2136
Moduretic Tablets 2138

Amlodipine Besylate (Additional reductions in blood pressure may occur). Products include:
Lotrel Capsules 2370
Norvasc Tablets 2704

Aspirin (Potential for increased risk of bleeding). Products include:
Aggrenox Capsules 1026
Alka-Seltzer .... ▣603
Alka-Seltzer Lemon Lime Antacid and Pain Reliever Effervescent Tablets .... ▣603
Alka-Seltzer Extra Strength Antacid and Pain Reliever Effervescent Tablets .... ▣603
Alka-Seltzer PM Effervescent Tablets .... ▣605
Genuine Bayer Tablets, Caplets and Gelcaps .... ▣606
Extra Strength Bayer Caplets and Gelcaps .... ▣610
Aspirin Regimen Bayer Children's Chewable Tablets (Orange or Cherry Flavored) .... ▣607
Bayer, Aspirin Regimen .... ▣606
Aspirin Regimen Bayer 81 mg Caplets with Calcium .... ▣607
Genuine Bayer Professional Labeling (Aspirin Regimen Bayer) .... ▣608
Extra Strength Bayer Arthritis Caplets .... ▣610
Extra Strength Bayer Plus Caplets .... ▣610
Extra Strength Bayer PM Caplets .... ▣611
BC Powder .... ▣619
BC Allergy Sinus Cold Powder .... ▣619
Arthritis Strength BC Powder .... ▣619
BC Sinus Cold Powder .... ▣619
Darvon Compound-65 Pulvules 1910
Ecotrin Enteric Coated Aspirin Low, Regular and Maximum Strength Tablets 1715
Excedrin Extra-Strength Tablets, Caplets, and Geltabs .... ▣629
Excedrin Migraine 1070
Goody's Body Pain Formula Powder .... ▣620
Goody's Extra Strength Headache Powder .... ▣620
Goody's Extra Strength Pain Relief Tablets .... ▣620
Percodan Tablets 1327
Robaxisal Tablets 2939
Soma Compound Tablets 3354
Soma Compound w/Codeine Tablets 3355
Vanquish Caplets .... ▣617

Atenolol (Additional reductions in blood pressure may occur). Products include:
Tenoretic Tablets 690
Tenormin I.V. Injection 692

Azlocillin Sodium (Potential for increased risk of bleeding).
No products indexed under this heading.

Benazepril Hydrochloride (Additional reductions in blood pressure may occur). Products include:
Lotensin Tablets 2365
Lotensin HCT Tablets 2367
Lotrel Capsules 2370

Bendroflumethiazide (Additional reductions in blood pressure may occur). Products include:
Corzide 40/5 Tablets 2247
Corzide 80/5 Tablets 2247

Betaxolol Hydrochloride (Additional reductions in blood pressure may occur). Products include:
Betoptic S Ophthalmic Suspension 537

Bisoprolol Fumarate (Additional reductions in blood pressure may occur). Products include:
Zebeta Tablets 1885
Ziac Tablets 1887

Bumetanide (Additional reductions in blood pressure may occur).
No products indexed under this heading.

Candesartan Cilexetil (Additional reductions in blood pressure may occur). Products include:
Atacand Tablets 595
Atacand HCT Tablets 597

Captopril (Additional reductions in blood pressure may occur). Products include:
Captopril Tablets 2281

Carbenicillin Indanyl Sodium (Potential for increased risk of bleeding). Products include:
Geocillin Tablets 2687

Carteolol Hydrochloride (Additional reductions in blood pressure may occur). Products include:
Carteolol Hydrochloride Ophthalmic Solution USP, 1% .... ⊙258
Ocupress Ophthalmic Solution, 1% Sterile .... ⊙303

Chlorothiazide (Additional reductions in blood pressure may occur). Products include:
Aldoclor Tablets 2035
Diuril Oral 2087

Chlorothiazide Sodium (Additional reductions in blood pressure may occur). Products include:
Diuril Sodium Intravenous 2086

Chlorthalidone (Additional reductions in blood pressure may occur). Products include:
Clorpres Tablets 1002
Combipres Tablets 1040
Tenoretic Tablets 690

Choline Magnesium Trisalicylate (Potential for increased risk of bleeding). Products include:
Trilisate 2901

Clonidine (Additional reductions in blood pressure may occur). Products include:
Catapres-TTS 1038

Clonidine Hydrochloride (Additional reductions in blood pressure may occur). Products include:
Catapres Tablets 1037
Clorpres Tablets 1002
Combipres Tablets 1040
Duraclon Injection 3057

Clopidogrel Bisulfate (Potential for increased risk of bleeding). Products include:
Plavix Tablets 1097
Plavix Tablets 3084

Deserpidine (Additional reductions in blood pressure may occur).
No products indexed under this heading.

Diazoxide (Additional reductions in blood pressure may occur).
No products indexed under this heading.

Diclofenac Potassium (Potential for increased risk of bleeding). Products include:
Cataflam Tablets 2315

Diclofenac Sodium (Potential for increased risk of bleeding). Products include:
Arthrotec Tablets 3195
Voltaren Ophthalmic Sterile Ophthalmic Solution .... ⊙312
Voltaren Tablets 2315
Voltaren-XR Tablets 2315

Dicumarol (Potential for increased risk of bleeding).
No products indexed under this heading.

Diflunisal (Potential for increased risk of bleeding). Products include:
Dolobid Tablets 2088

Digoxin (Co-administration of epoprostenol with digoxin in patients with congestive heart failure has resulted in decreased apparent oral clearance values of digoxin by 15%; patients on digoxin may show elevations of digoxin concentrations after initiation of epoprostenol therapy, which may be clinically significant in patients prone to digoxin toxicity.). Products include:
Digitek Tablets 1003
Lanoxicaps Capsules 1574

Lanoxin Injection 1581
Lanoxin Tablets 1587
Lanoxin Elixir Pediatric 1578
Lanoxin Injection Pediatric 1584

Diltiazem Hydrochloride (Additional reductions in blood pressure may occur). Products include:
Cardizem Injectable 1018
Cardizem Lyo-Ject Syringe 1018
Cardizem Monovial 1018
Cardizem CD Capsules 1016
Tiazac Capsules 1378

Dipyridamole (Potential for increased risk of bleeding). Products include:
Aggrenox Capsules 1026
Persantine Tablets 1057

Doxazosin Mesylate (Additional reductions in blood pressure may occur). Products include:
Cardura Tablets 2668

Enalapril Maleate (Additional reductions in blood pressure may occur). Products include:
Lexxel Tablets 608
Vaseretic Tablets 2204
Vasotec Tablets 2210

Enalaprilat (Additional reductions in blood pressure may occur). Products include:
Enalaprilat Injection 863
Vasotec I.V. Injection 2207

Eprosartan Mesylate (Additional reductions in blood pressure may occur). Products include:
Teveten Tablets 3327

Esmolol Hydrochloride (Additional reductions in blood pressure may occur). Products include:
Brevibloc Injection 858

Ethacrynic Acid (Additional reductions in blood pressure may occur). Products include:
Edecrin Tablets 2091

Felodipine (Additional reductions in blood pressure may occur). Products include:
Lexxel Tablets 608
Plendil Extended-Release Tablets 623

Fenoprofen Calcium (Potential for increased risk of bleeding).
No products indexed under this heading.

Flurbiprofen (Potential for increased risk of bleeding).
No products indexed under this heading.

Fosinopril Sodium (Additional reductions in blood pressure may occur). Products include:
Monopril Tablets 1091
Monopril HCT 1094

Furosemide (Co-administration in patients with congestive heart failure receiving furosemide apparent oral clearance values for furosemide were decreased by 13% on the second day of therapy and had returned to baseline values by day 87). Products include:
Furosemide Tablets 2284

Guanabenz Acetate (Additional reductions in blood pressure may occur).
No products indexed under this heading.

Guanethidine Monosulfate (Additional reductions in blood pressure may occur).
No products indexed under this heading.

Hydralazine Hydrochloride (Additional reductions in blood pressure may occur).
No products indexed under this heading.

Hydrochlorothiazide (Additional reductions in blood pressure may occur). Products include:
Accuretic Tablets 2614
Aldoril Tablets 2039
Atacand HCT Tablets 597
Avalide Tablets 1070
Diovan HCT Tablets 2338
Dyazide Capsules 1515
HydroDIURIL Tablets 2108
Hyzaar 2109
Inderide Tablets 3517
Inderide LA Long-Acting Capsules 3519
Lotensin HCT Tablets 2367
Maxzide 1008
Micardis HCT Tablets 1051
Microzide Capsules 3414
Moduretic Tablets 2138
Monopril HCT 1094
Prinzide Tablets 2168
Timolide Tablets 2187
Uniretic Tablets 3178
Vaseretic Tablets 2204
Zestoretic Tablets 695
Ziac Tablets 1887

Hydroflumethiazide (Additional reductions in blood pressure may occur). Products include:
Diucardin Tablets 3494

Ibuprofen (Potential for increased risk of bleeding). Products include:
Advil .... ◘771
Children's Advil Oral Suspension .... ◘773
Children's Advil Chewable Tablets .... ◘773
Advil Cold and Sinus Caplets .... ◘771
Advil Cold and Sinus Tablets .... ◘771
Advil Flu & Body Ache Caplets .... ◘772
Infants' Advil Drops .... ◘773
Junior Strength Advil Tablets .... ◘773
Junior Strength Advil Chewable Tablets .... ◘773
Advil Migraine Liquigels .... ◘772
Children's Motrin Oral Suspension and Chewable Tablets 2006
Children's Motrin Cold Oral Suspension 2007
Children's Motrin Oral Suspension .... ◘643
Motrin Suspension, Oral Drops, Chewable Tablets, and Caplets 2002
Infants' Motrin Concentrated Drops 2006
Junior Strength Motrin Caplets and Chewable Tablets 2006
Motrin IB Tablets, Caplets, and Gelcaps 2002
Motrin Migraine Pain Caplets 2005
Motrin Sinus Headache Caplets 2005
Vicoprofen Tablets 520

Indapamide (Additional reductions in blood pressure may occur). Products include:
Indapamide Tablets 2286

Indomethacin (Potential for increased risk of bleeding). Products include:
Indocin 2112

Indomethacin Sodium Trihydrate (Potential for increased risk of bleeding). Products include:
Indocin I.V. 2115

Irbesartan (Additional reductions in blood pressure may occur). Products include:
Avalide Tablets 1070
Avapro Tablets 1074
Avapro Tablets 3076

Isradipine (Additional reductions in blood pressure may occur). Products include:
DynaCirc Capsules 2921
DynaCirc CR Tablets 2923

Ketoprofen (Potential for increased risk of bleeding). Products include:
Orudis Capsules 3548
Orudis KT Tablets .... ◘778
Oruvail Capsules 3548

Labetalol Hydrochloride (Additional reductions in blood pressure may occur). Products include:
Normodyne Injection 3135
Normodyne Tablets 3137

Lisinopril (Additional reductions in blood pressure may occur). Products include:
Prinivil Tablets 2164
Prinzide Tablets 2168
Zestoretic Tablets 695
Zestril Tablets 698

Losartan Potassium (Additional reductions in blood pressure may occur). Products include:
Cozaar Tablets 2067
Hyzaar 2109

Magnesium Salicylate (Potential for increased risk of bleeding). Products include:
Momentum Backache Relief Extra Strength Caplets .... ◘666

Mecamylamine Hydrochloride (Additional reductions in blood pressure may occur). Products include:
Inversine Tablets 1850

Meclofenamate Sodium (Potential for increased risk of bleeding).
No products indexed under this heading.

Mefenamic Acid (Potential for increased risk of bleeding). Products include:
Ponstel Capsules 1356

Methyclothiazide (Additional reductions in blood pressure may occur).
No products indexed under this heading.

Methyldopa (Additional reductions in blood pressure may occur). Products include:
Aldoclor Tablets 2035
Aldomet Tablets 2037
Aldoril Tablets 2039

Methyldopate Hydrochloride (Additional reductions in blood pressure may occur).
No products indexed under this heading.

Metolazone (Additional reductions in blood pressure may occur). Products include:
Mykrox Tablets 1168
Zaroxolyn Tablets 1177

Metoprolol Succinate (Additional reductions in blood pressure may occur). Products include:
Toprol-XL Tablets 651

Metoprolol Tartrate (Additional reductions in blood pressure may occur).
No products indexed under this heading.

Metyrosine (Additional reductions in blood pressure may occur). Products include:
Demser Capsules 2085

Mezlocillin Sodium (Potential for increased risk of bleeding).
No products indexed under this heading.

Mibefradil Dihydrochloride (Additional reductions in blood pressure may occur).
No products indexed under this heading.

Minoxidil (Additional reductions in blood pressure may occur). Products include:
Rogaine Extra Strength for Men Topical Solution .... ◘721
Rogaine for Women Topical Solution .... ◘721

Moexipril Hydrochloride (Additional reductions in blood pressure may occur). Products include:
Uniretic Tablets 3178
Univasc Tablets 3181

Nadolol (Additional reductions in blood pressure may occur). Products include:
Corgard Tablets 2245
Corzide 40/5 Tablets 2247
Corzide 80/5 Tablets 2247
Nadolol Tablets 2288

Nafcillin Sodium (Potential for increased risk of bleeding).
No products indexed under this heading.

Naproxen (Potential for increased risk of bleeding). Products include:
EC-Naprosyn Delayed-Release Tablets 2967
Naprosyn Suspension 2967
Naprosyn Tablets 2967

Naproxen Sodium (Potential for increased risk of bleeding). Products include:
Aleve Tablets, Caplets and Gelcaps .... ◘602
Aleve Cold & Sinus Caplets .... ◘603
Anaprox Tablets 2967
Anaprox DS Tablets 2967
Naprelan Tablets 1293

Nicardipine Hydrochloride (Additional reductions in blood pressure may occur). Products include:
Cardene I.V. 3485

Nifedipine (Additional reductions in blood pressure may occur). Products include:
Adalat CC Tablets 877
Procardia Capsules 2708
Procardia XL Extended Release Tablets 2710

Nisoldipine (Additional reductions in blood pressure may occur). Products include:
Sular Tablets 688

Nitroglycerin (Additional reductions in blood pressure may occur). Products include:
Nitro-Dur Transdermal Infusion System 3134
Nitro-Dur Transdermal Infusion System 1834
Nitrolingual Pumpspray 1355
Nitrostat Tablets 2658

Penbutolol Sulfate (Additional reductions in blood pressure may occur).
No products indexed under this heading.

Penicillin G Benzathine (Potential for increased risk of bleeding). Products include:
Bicillin C-R 900/300 Injection 2240
Bicillin C-R Injection 2238
Bicillin L-A Injection 2242
Permapen Isoject 2706

Penicillin G Procaine (Potential for increased risk of bleeding). Products include:
Bicillin C-R 900/300 Injection 2240
Bicillin C-R Injection 2238

Perindopril Erbumine (Additional reductions in blood pressure may occur). Products include:
Aceon Tablets (2 mg, 4 mg, 8 mg) 3249

Phenoxybenzamine Hydrochloride (Additional reductions in blood pressure may occur). Products include:
Dibenzyline Capsules 3457

Phentolamine Mesylate (Additional reductions in blood pressure may occur).
No products indexed under this heading.

Phenylbutazone (Potential for increased risk of bleeding).
No products indexed under this heading.

Pindolol (Additional reductions in blood pressure may occur).
No products indexed under this heading.

Piroxicam (Potential for increased risk of bleeding). Products include:
Feldene Capsules 2685

Polythiazide (Additional reductions in blood pressure may occur). Products include:
Minizide Capsules 2700
Renese Tablets 2712

Prazosin Hydrochloride (Additional reductions in blood pressure may occur). Products include:
Minipress Capsules 2699
Minizide Capsules 2700

Propranolol Hydrochloride (Additional reductions in blood pressure may occur). Products include:
Inderal 3513
Inderal LA Long-Acting Capsules 3516
Inderide Tablets 3517
Inderide LA Long-Acting Capsules 3519

Quinapril Hydrochloride (Additional reductions in blood pressure may occur). Products include:
Accupril Tablets 2611
Accuretic Tablets 2614

Ramipril (Additional reductions in blood pressure may occur). Products include:
Altace Capsules 2233

Rauwolfia serpentina (Additional reductions in blood pressure may

occur).
No products indexed under this heading.

Rescinnamine (Additional reductions in blood pressure may occur).
No products indexed under this heading.

Reserpine (Additional reductions in blood pressure may occur).
No products indexed under this heading.

Salsalate (Potential for increased risk of bleeding).
No products indexed under this heading.

Sodium Nitroprusside (Additional reductions in blood pressure may occur).
No products indexed under this heading.

Sotalol Hydrochloride (Additional reductions in blood pressure may occur). Products include:
Betapace Tablets 950
Betapace AF Tablets 954

Spirapril Hydrochloride (Additional reductions in blood pressure may occur).
No products indexed under this heading.

Spironolactone (Additional reductions in blood pressure may occur).
No products indexed under this heading.

Sulindac (Potential for increased risk of bleeding). Products include:
Clinoril Tablets 2053

Telmisartan (Additional reductions in blood pressure may occur). Products include:
Micardis Tablets 1049
Micardis HCT Tablets 1051

Terazosin Hydrochloride (Additional reductions in blood pressure may occur). Products include:
Hytrin Capsules 464

Ticarcillin Disodium (Potential for increased risk of bleeding). Products include:
Timentin Injection- ADD-Vantage Vial 1661
Timentin Injection-Galaxy Container 1664
Timentin Injection-Pharmacy Bulk Package 1666
Timentin for Intravenous Administration 1658

Ticlopidine Hydrochloride (Potential for increased risk of bleeding). Products include:
Ticlid Tablets 3015

Timolol Maleate (Additional reductions in blood pressure may occur). Products include:
Blocadren Tablets 2046
Cosopt Sterile Ophthalmic Solution 2065
Timolide Tablets 2187
Timolol GFS .... ⊙266
Timoptic in Ocudose 2192
Timoptic Sterile Ophthalmic Solution 2190
Timoptic-XE Sterile Ophthalmic Gel Forming Solution 2194

Tolmetin Sodium (Potential for increased risk of bleeding). Products include:
Tolectin 2589

Torsemide (Additional reductions in blood pressure may occur). Products include:
Demadex Tablets and Injection 2965

Trandolapril (Additional reductions in blood pressure may occur). Products include:
Mavik Tablets 478
Tarka Tablets 508

Triamterene (Additional reductions in blood pressure may occur). Products include:
Dyazide Capsules 1515
Dyrenium Capsules 3458
Maxzide 1008

Trimethaphan Camsylate (Additional reductions in blood pressure may occur).
No products indexed under this heading.

Valsartan (Additional reductions in blood pressure may occur). Products include:
Diovan Capsules 2337
Diovan HCT Tablets 2338

Verapamil Hydrochloride (Additional reductions in blood pressure may occur). Products include:
Covera-HS Tablets 3199
Isoptin SR Tablets 467
Tarka Tablets 508
Verelan Capsules 3184
Verelan PM Capsules 3186

Warfarin Sodium (Potential for increased risk of bleeding). Products include:
Coumadin for Injection 1243
Coumadin Tablets 1243
Warfarin Sodium Tablets, USP 3302

FLOMAX CAPSULES

(Tamsulosin Hydrochloride) 1044
May interact with alpha adrenergic blockers and certain other agents. Compounds in these categories include:

Cimetidine (Co-administration with highest recommended dose of cimetidine has resulted in a significant decrease (26%) in the clearance of tamsulosin which resulted in a moderate increase in tamsulosin AUC (44%)). Products include:
Tagamet HB 200 Suspension .... ▣762
Tagamet HB 200 Tablets .... ▣761
Tagamet Tablets 1644

Cimetidine Hydrochloride (Co-administration with highest recommended dose of cimetidine has resulted in a significant decrease (26%) in the clearance of tamsulosin which resulted in a moderate increase in tamsulosin AUC (44%)). Products include:
Tagamet 1644

Doxazosin Mesylate (The pharmacokinetic and pharmacodynamic interactions between tamsulosin and other alpha-adrenergic blockers have not been determined, however, interactions may be expected and co-administration should be avoided). Products include:
Cardura Tablets 2668

Furosemide (Co-administration produces an 11% to 12% reduction in tamsulosin Cmax and AUC; these changes are expected to be clinically insignificant). Products include:
Furosemide Tablets 2284

Prazosin Hydrochloride (The pharmacokinetic and pharmacodynamic interactions between tamsulosin and other alpha-adrenergic blockers have not been determined, however, interactions may be expected and co-administration should be avoided). Products include:
Minipress Capsules 2699
Minizide Capsules 2700

Terazosin Hydrochloride (The pharmacokinetic and pharmacodynamic interactions between tamsulosin and other alpha-adrenergic blockers have not been determined, however, interactions may be expected and co-administration should be avoided). Products include:
Hytrin Capsules 464

Warfarin Sodium (Results from *in vitro* and *in vivo* interaction studies are inconclusive, therefore, caution should be exercised with concomitant use). Products include:
Coumadin for Injection 1243
Coumadin Tablets 1243
Warfarin Sodium Tablets, USP 3302

Food Interactions

Food, unspecified (Tmax is reached by 4 to 5 hours under fasting conditions and by 6 to 7 hours when tamsulosin is administered with food; taking tamsulosin under fasted conditions results in a 30% increase in AUC and 40% to 70% increase in Cmax compared to fed conditions; Flomax should be taken approximately 30 minutes following the meal).

FLONASE NASAL SPRAY

(Fluticasone Propionate) 1533
May interact with:

Ketoconazole (Co-administration of a single dose of orally inhaled fluticasone (1000 mcg) with multiple doses of ketoconazole (200 mg) to steady state has resulted in increased mean fluticasone concentrations and reduction in plasma cortisol AUC). Products include:
Nizoral 2% Cream 3620
Nizoral A-D Shampoo 2008
Nizoral 2% Shampoo 2007
Nizoral Tablets 1791

Ritonavir (Fluticasone is a substrate of CYP4503A4; co-administration with ritonavir could result in increased plasma concentrations of fluticasone). Products include:
Kaletra Capsules 471
Kaletra Oral Solution 471
Norvir Capsules 487
Norvir Oral Solution 487

FLORICAL CAPSULES AND TABLETS

(Calcium Carbonate, Sodium Fluoride) 2223
None cited in PDR database.

FLORINEF ACETATE TABLETS

(Fludrocortisone Acetate) 2250
May interact with barbiturates, oral anticoagulants, estrogens, cardiac glycosides, oral hypoglycemic agents, insulin, loop diuretics, phenytoin, thiazides, and certain other agents. Compounds in these categories include:

Acarbose (Diminished antidiabetic effect). Products include:
Precose Tablets 906

Amphotericin B (Co-administration results in enhanced hypokalemia). Products include:
Abelcet Injection 1273
AmBisome for Injection 1383
Amphotec 1774

Aprobarbital (Increased metabolic clearance of fludrocortisone because of the induction of hepatic enzymes).
No products indexed under this heading.

Aspirin (Increased ulcerogenic effect; decreased pharmacologic effect of aspirin; rarely salicylate toxicity may occur in patients who discontinue steroids after concurrent high-dose aspirin therapy). Products include:
Aggrenox Capsules 1026
Alka-Seltzer .... ▣603
Alka-Seltzer Lemon Lime Antacid and Pain Reliever Effervescent Tablets .... ▣603
Alka-Seltzer Extra Strength Antacid and Pain Reliever Effervescent Tablets .... ▣603
Alka-Seltzer PM Effervescent Tablets .... ▣605
Genuine Bayer Tablets, Caplets and Gelcaps .... ▣606
Extra Strength Bayer Caplets and Gelcaps .... ▣610
Aspirin Regimen Bayer Children's Chewable Tablets (Orange or Cherry Flavored) .... ▣607
Bayer, Aspirin Regimen .... ▣606
Aspirin Regimen Bayer 81 mg Caplets with Calcium .... ▣607
Genuine Bayer Professional Labeling (Aspirin Regimen Bayer) .... ▣608
Extra Strength Bayer Arthritis Caplets .... ▣610
Extra Strength Bayer Plus Caplets .... ▣610
Extra Strength Bayer PM Caplets .... ▣611
BC Powder .... ▣619
BC Allergy Sinus Cold Powder .... ▣619
Arthritis Strength BC Powder .... ▣619
BC Sinus Cold Powder .... ▣619
Darvon Compound-65 Pulvules 1910
Ecotrin Enteric Coated Aspirin Low, Regular and Maximum Strength Tablets 1715
Excedrin Extra-Strength Tablets, Caplets, and Geltabs .... ▣629
Excedrin Migraine 1070
Goody's Body Pain Formula Powder .... ▣620
Goody's Extra Strength Headache Powder .... ▣620
Goody's Extra Strength Pain Relief Tablets .... ▣620
Percodan Tablets 1327
Robaxisal Tablets 2939
Soma Compound Tablets 3354
Soma Compound w/Codeine Tablets 3355
Vanquish Caplets .... ▣617

Bendroflumethiazide (Co-administration results in enhanced hypokalemia). Products include:
Corzide 40/5 Tablets 2247
Corzide 80/5 Tablets 2247

Bumetanide (Co-administration results in enhanced hypokalemia).
No products indexed under this heading.

Butabarbital (Increased metabolic clearance of fludrocortisone because of the induction of hepatic enzymes).
No products indexed under this heading.

Butalbital (Increased metabolic clearance of fludrocortisone because of the induction of hepatic enzymes). Products include:
Phrenilin 578
Sedapap Tablets 50 mg/650 mg 2225

Chlorothiazide (Co-administration results in enhanced hypokalemia). Products include:
Aldoclor Tablets 2035
Diuril Oral 2087

Chlorothiazide Sodium (Co-administration results in enhanced hypokalemia). Products include:
Diuril Sodium Intravenous 2086

Chlorotrianisene (Increased levels of corticosteroid-binding globulin, thereby increasing the bound (inactive) fraction).
No products indexed under this heading.

Chlorpropamide (Diminished antidiabetic effect). Products include:
Diabinese Tablets 2680

Deslanoside (Enhanced possibility of arrhythmias or digitalis toxicity associated with hypokalemia).
No products indexed under this heading.

Dicumarol (Decreased prothrombin time response).
No products indexed under this heading.

Dienestrol (Increased levels of corticosteroid-binding globulin, thereby increasing the bound (inactive) fraction). Products include:
Ortho Dienestrol Cream 2554

Diethylstilbestrol (Increased levels of corticosteroid-binding globulin, thereby increasing the bound (inactive) fraction).
No products indexed under this heading.

Digitoxin (Enhanced possibility of arrhythmias or digitalis toxicity associated with hypokalemia).
No products indexed under this heading.

Digoxin (Enhanced possibility of arrhythmias or digitalis toxicity associated with hypokalemia). Products include:

Digitek Tablets ... 1003
Lanoxicaps Capsules ... 1574
Lanoxin Injection ... 1581
Lanoxin Tablets ... 1587
Lanoxin Elixir Pediatric ... 1578
Lanoxin Injection Pediatric ... 1584

Estradiol (Increased levels of corticosteroid-binding globulin, thereby increasing the bound (inactive) fraction). Products include:
Activella Tablets ... 2764
Alora Transdermal System ... 3372
Climara Transdermal System ... 958
CombiPatch Transdermal System ... 2323
Esclim Transdermal System ... 3460
Estrace Vaginal Cream ... 3358
Estrace Tablets ... 3361
Estring Vaginal Ring ... 2811
Ortho-Prefest Tablets ... 2570
Vagifem Tablets ... 2857
Vivelle Transdermal System ... 2412
Vivelle-Dot Transdermal System ... 2416

Estrogens, Conjugated (Increased levels of corticosteroid-binding globulin, thereby increasing the bound (inactive) fraction). Products include:
Premarin Intravenous ... 3563
Premarin Tablets ... 3566
Premarin Vaginal Cream ... 3570
Premphase Tablets ... 3572
Prempro Tablets ... 3572

Estrogens, Esterified (Increased levels of corticosteroid-binding globulin, thereby increasing the bound (inactive) fraction). Products include:
Estratest ... 3252
Menest Tablets ... 2254

Estropipate (Increased levels of corticosteroid-binding globulin, thereby increasing the bound (inactive) fraction). Products include:
Ogen Tablets ... 2846
Ortho-Est Tablets ... 3464

Ethacrynic Acid (Co-administration results in enhanced hypokalemia). Products include:
Edecrin Tablets ... 2091

Ethinyl Estradiol (Increased levels of corticosteroid-binding globulin, thereby increasing the bound (inactive) fraction). Products include:
Alesse-21 Tablets ... 3468
Alesse-28 Tablets ... 3473
Brevicon 28-Day Tablets ... 3380
Cyclessa Tablets ... 2450
Desogen Tablets ... 2458
Estinyl Tablets ... 3112
Estrostep ... 2627
femhrt Tablets ... 2635
Levlen ... 962
Levlite 21 Tablets ... 962
Levlite 28 Tablets ... 962
Levora Tablets ... 3389
Loestrin 21 Tablets ... 2642
Loestrin Fe Tablets ... 2642
Lo/Ovral Tablets ... 3532
Lo/Ovral-28 Tablets ... 3538
Low-Ogestrel-28 Tablets ... 3392
Microgestin Fe 1.5/30 Tablets ... 3407
Microgestin Fe 1/20 Tablets ... 3400
Mircette Tablets ... 2470
Modicon ... 2563
Necon ... 3415
Nordette-28 Tablets ... 2257
Norinyl 1 +35 28-Day Tablets ... 3380
Ogestrel 0.5/50-28 Tablets ... 3428
Ortho-Cept 21 Tablets ... 2546
Ortho-Cept 28 Tablets ... 2546
Ortho-Cyclen/Ortho Tri-Cyclen ... 2573
Ortho-Novum ... 2563
Ovcon ... 3364
Ovral Tablets ... 3551
Ovral-28 Tablets ... 3552
Tri-Levlen ... 962
Tri-Norinyl-28 Tablets ... 3433
Triphasil-21 Tablets ... 3600
Triphasil-28 Tablets ... 3605
Trivora Tablets ... 3439
Yasmin 28 Tablets ... 980
Zovia ... 3449

Fosphenytoin Sodium (Increased metabolic clearance of fludrocortisone because of the induction of hepatic enzymes). Products include:
Cerebyx Injection ... 2619

Furosemide (Co-administration results in enhanced hypokalemia). Products include:
Furosemide Tablets ... 2284

Glimepiride (Diminished antidiabetic effect). Products include:
Amaryl Tablets ... 717

Glipizide (Diminished antidiabetic effect). Products include:
Glucotrol Tablets ... 2692
Glucotrol XL Extended Release Tablets ... 2693

Glyburide (Diminished antidiabetic effect). Products include:
DiaBeta Tablets ... 741
Glucovance Tablets ... 1086

Hydrochlorothiazide (Co-administration results in enhanced hypokalemia). Products include:
Accuretic Tablets ... 2614
Aldoril Tablets ... 2039
Atacand HCT Tablets ... 597
Avalide Tablets ... 1070
Diovan HCT Tablets ... 2338
Dyazide Capsules ... 1515
HydroDIURIL Tablets ... 2108
Hyzaar ... 2109
Inderide Tablets ... 3517
Inderide LA Long-Acting Capsules ... 3519
Lotensin HCT Tablets ... 2367
Maxzide ... 1008
Micardis HCT Tablets ... 1051
Microzide Capsules ... 3414
Moduretic Tablets ... 2138
Monopril HCT ... 1094
Prinzide Tablets ... 2168
Timolide Tablets ... 2187
Uniretic Tablets ... 3178
Vaseretic Tablets ... 2204
Zestoretic Tablets ... 695
Ziac Tablets ... 1887

Hydroflumethiazide (Co-administration results in enhanced hypokalemia). Products include:
Diucardin Tablets ... 3494

Insulin, Human, Zinc Suspension (Diminished antidiabetic effect). Products include:
Humulin L, 100 Units ... 1937
Humulin U, 100 Units ... 1943
Novolin L Human Insulin 10 ml Vials ... 2422

Insulin, Human NPH (Diminished antidiabetic effect). Products include:
Humulin N, 100 Units ... 1939
Humulin N NPH Pen ... 1940
Novolin N Human Insulin 10 ml Vials ... 2422
Novolin N PenFill ... 2423
Novolin N Prefilled Syringe Disposable Insulin Delivery System ... 2425

Insulin, Human Regular (Diminished antidiabetic effect). Products include:
Humulin R Regular (U-500) ... 1943
Humulin R, 100 Units ... 1941
Novolin R Human Insulin 10 ml Vials ... 2423
Novolin R PenFill ... 2423
Novolin R Prefilled Syringe Disposable Insulin Delivery System ... 2425
Velosulin BR Human Insulin 10 ml Vials ... 2435

Insulin, Human Regular and Human NPH Mixture (Diminished antidiabetic effect). Products include:
Humulin 50/50, 100 Units ... 1934
Humulin 70/30, 100 Units ... 1935
Humulin 70/30 Pen ... 1936
Novolin 70/30 Human Insulin 10 ml Vials ... 2421
Novolin 70/30 PenFill ... 2423
Novolin 70/30 Prefilled Disposable Insulin Delivery System ... 2425

Insulin, NPH (Diminished antidiabetic effect). Products include:
Iletin II, NPH (Pork), 100 Units ... 1946

Insulin, Regular (Diminished antidiabetic effect). Products include:
Iletin II, Regular (Pork), 100 Units ... 1947

Insulin, Zinc Crystals (Diminished antidiabetic effect).
No products indexed under this heading.

Insulin, Zinc Suspension (Diminished antidiabetic effect). Products include:
Iletin II, Lente (Pork), 100 Units ... 1945

Insulin Aspart, Human Regular (Diminished antidiabetic effect).
No products indexed under this heading.

Insulin glargine (Diminished antidiabetic effect). Products include:
Lantus Injection ... 742

Insulin Lispro, Human (Diminished antidiabetic effect). Products include:
Humalog ... 1926
Humalog Mix 75/25 Pen ... 1928

Insulin Lispro Protamine, Human (Diminished antidiabetic effect). Products include:
Humalog Mix 75/25 Pen ... 1928

Mephobarbital (Increased metabolic clearance of fludrocortisone because of the induction of hepatic enzymes).
No products indexed under this heading.

Metformin Hydrochloride (Diminished antidiabetic effect). Products include:
Glucophage Tablets ... 1080
Glucophage XR Tablets ... 1080
Glucovance Tablets ... 1086

Methandrostinolone (Enhanced tendency towards edema).
No products indexed under this heading.

Methyclothiazide (Co-administration results in enhanced hypokalemia).
No products indexed under this heading.

Miglitol (Diminished antidiabetic effect). Products include:
Glyset Tablets ... 2821

Norethandrolone (Enhanced tendency towards edema).
No products indexed under this heading.

Oxymetholone (Enhanced tendency towards edema). Products include:
Anadrol-50 Tablets ... 3321

Pentobarbital Sodium (Increased metabolic clearance of fludrocortisone because of the induction of hepatic enzymes). Products include:
Nembutal Sodium Solution ... 485

Phenobarbital (Increased metabolic clearance of fludrocortisone because of the induction of hepatic enzymes). Products include:
Arco-Lase Plus Tablets ... 592
Donnatal ... 2929
Donnatal Extentabs ... 2930

Phenytoin (Increased metabolic clearance of fludrocortisone because of the induction of hepatic enzymes). Products include:
Dilantin Infatabs ... 2624
Dilantin-125 Oral Suspension ... 2625

Phenytoin Sodium (Increased metabolic clearance of fludrocortisone because of the induction of hepatic enzymes). Products include:
Dilantin Kapseals ... 2622

Pioglitazone Hydrochloride (Diminished antidiabetic effect). Products include:
Actos Tablets ... 3275

Polyestradiol Phosphate (Increased levels of corticosteroid-binding globulin, thereby increasing the bound (inactive) fraction).
No products indexed under this heading.

Polythiazide (Co-administration results in enhanced hypokalemia). Products include:
Minizide Capsules ... 2700
Renese Tablets ... 2712

Quinestrol (Increased levels of corticosteroid-binding globulin, thereby increasing the bound (inactive) fraction).
No products indexed under this heading.

Repaglinide (Diminished antidiabetic effect). Products include:
Prandin Tablets (0.5, 1, and 2 mg) ... 2432

Rifampin (Increased metabolic clearance of fludrocortisone because of the induction of hepatic enzymes). Products include:
Rifadin ... 765
Rifamate Capsules ... 767
Rifater Tablets ... 769

Rosiglitazone Maleate (Diminished antidiabetic effect). Products include:
Avandia Tablets ... 1490

Secobarbital Sodium (Increased metabolic clearance of fludrocortisone because of the induction of hepatic enzymes).
No products indexed under this heading.

Thiamylal Sodium (Increased metabolic clearance of fludrocortisone because of the induction of hepatic enzymes).
No products indexed under this heading.

Tolazamide (Diminished antidiabetic effect).
No products indexed under this heading.

Tolbutamide (Diminished antidiabetic effect).
No products indexed under this heading.

Torsemide (Co-administration results in enhanced hypokalemia). Products include:
Demadex Tablets and Injection ... 2965

Troglitazone (Diminished antidiabetic effect).
No products indexed under this heading.

Warfarin Sodium (Decreased prothrombin time response). Products include:
Coumadin for Injection ... 1243
Coumadin Tablets ... 1243
Warfarin Sodium Tablets, USP ... 3302

FLOVENT DISKUS 50 MCG
(Fluticasone Propionate) ... 3614
See Flovent Rotadisk 250 mcg

FLOVENT DISKUS 100 MCG
(Fluticasone Propionate) ... 3614
See Flovent Rotadisk 250 mcg

FLOVENT DISKUS 250 MCG
(Fluticasone Propionate) ... 3614
See Flovent Rotadisk 250 mcg

FLOVENT 44 MCG INHALATION AEROSOL
(Fluticasone Propionate) ... 1535
None cited in PDR database.

FLOVENT 110 MCG INHALATION AEROSOL
(Fluticasone Propionate) ... 1535
None cited in PDR database.

FLOVENT 220 MCG INHALATION AEROSOL
(Fluticasone Propionate) ... 1535
None cited in PDR database.

FLOVENT ROTADISK 50 MCG
(Fluticasone Propionate) ... 1537
See Flovent Rotadisk 250 mcg

FLOVENT ROTADISK 100 MCG
(Fluticasone Propionate) ... 1537
See Flovent Rotadisk 250 mcg

FLOVENT ROTADISK 250 MCG
(Fluticasone Propionate) ... 1537
May interact with:

Ketoconazole (Co-administration of a single dose of fluticasone (1000

mcg) with multiple doses of ketoconazole (200 mg) to steady state has resulted in increased mean fluticasone concentrations and reduction in plasma cortisol AUC). Products include:
Nizoral 2% Cream ... 3620
Nizoral A-D Shampoo ... 2008
Nizoral 2% Shampoo ... 2007
Nizoral Tablets ... 1791

FLOXIN I.V.
(Ofloxacin) ... 2526
See Floxin Tablets

FLOXIN OTIC SOLUTION
(Ofloxacin) ... 1219
None cited in PDR database.

FLOXIN TABLETS
(Ofloxacin) ... 2529
May interact with antacids containing aluminum, calcium and magnesium, oral anticoagulants, oral hypoglycemic agents, insulin, iron containing oral preparations, nonsteroidal anti-inflammatory agents, theophylline, and certain other agents. Compounds in these categories include:

Acarbose (Potentiation of hypoglycemic action). Products include:
Precose Tablets ... 906

Aluminum Carbonate (Co-administration with antacids containing calcium, aluminum, or magnesium may substantially interfere with the oral absorption of quinolones; these preparations should not be taken within the two-hour period before or within the two-hour period after taking ofloxacin).
No products indexed under this heading.

Aluminum Hydroxide (Co-administration with antacids containing calcium, aluminum, or magnesium may substantially interfere with the oral absorption of quinolones; these preparations should not be taken within the two-hour period before or within the two-hour period after taking ofloxacin). Products include:
Amphojel Suspension (Mint Flavor) ... ■789
Gaviscon Extra Strength Liquid ... ■751
Gaviscon Extra Strength Tablets ... ■751
Gaviscon Regular Strength Liquid ... ■751
Gaviscon Regular Strength Tablets ... ■750
Maalox Antacid/Anti-Gas Oral Suspension ... ■673
Maalox Max Maximum Strength Antacid/Anti-Gas Liquid ... 2300
Maalox Regular Strength Antacid/Antigas Liquid ... 2300
Mylanta ... 1813
Vanquish Caplets ... ■617

Aminophylline (Increased steady-state theophylline levels; concurrent therapy may prolong the half-life of theophylline, elevate serum theophylline levels, and increase the risk of theophylline-related adverse reactions).
No products indexed under this heading.

Calcium Carbonate (Co-administration with antacids containing calcium, aluminum, or magnesium may substantially interfere with the oral absorption of quinolones; these preparations should not be taken within the two-hour period before or within the two-hour period after taking ofloxacin). Products include:
Aspirin Regimen Bayer 81 mg Caplets with Calcium ... ■607
Extra Strength Bayer Plus Caplets ... ■610
Caltrate 600 Tablets ... ■814
Caltrate 600 PLUS ... ■815
Caltrate 600 + D Tablets ... ■814
Caltrate 600 + Soy Tablets ... ■814
D-Cal Chewable Caplets ... ■794
Florical Capsules and Tablets ... 2223
Quick Dissolve Maalox Max Maximum Strength Antacid/Antigas Tablets ... 2301
Quick Dissolve Maalox Regular Strength Antacid Tablets ... 2301
Marblen Suspension ... ■633
Monocal Tablets ... 2223
Mylanta Fast-Acting ... 1813
Mylanta Calci Tabs ... ■636
One-A-Day Bedtime & Rest Tablets ... ■805
One-A-Day Calcium Plus Chewable Tablets ... ■805
Os-Cal Chewable Tablets ... ■838
Pepcid Complete Chewable Tablets ... 1815
ReSource Wellness CalciWise Soft Chews ... ■824
Rolaids Tablets ... ■706
Extra Strength Rolaids Tablets ... ■706
Slow-Mag Tablets ... ■835
Titralac ... ■640
3M Titralac Plus Antacid Tablets ... ■640
Tums ... ■763

Celecoxib (Co-administration with a non-steroidal anti-inflammatory agent may increase the risk of CNS stimulation and convulsive seizures). Products include:
Celebrex Capsules ... 2676
Celebrex Capsules ... 2780

Chlorpropamide (Potentiation of hypoglycemic action). Products include:
Diabinese Tablets ... 2680

Cimetidine (May interfere with the elimination of quinolones resulting in significant increase in half-life and AUC of some quinolones; this interaction has not been studied with ofloxacin). Products include:
Tagamet HB 200 Suspension ... ■762
Tagamet HB 200 Tablets ... ■761
Tagamet Tablets ... 1644

Cimetidine Hydrochloride (May interfere with the elimination of quinolones resulting in significant increase in half-life and AUC of some quinolones; this interaction has not been studied with ofloxacin). Products include:
Tagamet ... 1644

Cyclosporine (Potential for prolonged half-life and elevated serum levels of cyclosporine). Products include:
Gengraf Capsules ... 457
Neoral Soft Gelatin Capsules ... 2380
Neoral Oral Solution ... 2380
Sandimmune ... 2388

Diclofenac Potassium (Co-administration with a non-steroidal anti-inflammatory agent may increase the risk of CNS stimulation and convulsive seizures). Products include:
Cataflam Tablets ... 2315

Diclofenac Sodium (Co-administration with a non-steroidal anti-inflammatory agent may increase the risk of CNS stimulation and convulsive seizures). Products include:
Arthrotec Tablets ... 3195
Voltaren Ophthalmic Sterile Ophthalmic Solution ... ⊙312
Voltaren Tablets ... 2315
Voltaren-XR Tablets ... 2315

Dicumarol (Potential for enhanced effects of the oral anticoagulant).
No products indexed under this heading.

Didanosine (Didanosine (Videx) chewable tablets or pediatric powder for oral solution contains aluminum- magnesium-based antacid; co-administration may interfere with Floxin oral absorption; these preparations should not be taken within the two-hour period before or within the two-hour period after taking ofloxacin). Products include:
Videx ... 1138
Videx EC Capsules ... 1143

Dyphylline (Increased steady-state theophylline levels; concurrent therapy may prolong the half-life of theophylline, elevate serum theophylline levels, and increase the risk of theophylline-related adverse reactions). Products include:
Lufyllin Tablets ... 3347
Lufyllin-400 Tablets ... 3347
Lufyllin-GG Elixir ... 3348
Lufyllin-GG Tablets ... 3348

Etodolac (Co-administration with a non-steroidal anti-inflammatory agent may increase the risk of CNS stimulation and convulsive seizures). Products include:
Lodine ... 3528
Lodine XL Extended-Release Tablets ... 3530

Fenoprofen Calcium (Co-administration with a non-steroidal anti-inflammatory agent may increase the risk of CNS stimulation and convulsive seizures).
No products indexed under this heading.

Ferrous Fumarate (Co-administration with iron-containing products may substantially interfere with the oral absorption of quinolones; these preparations should not be taken within the two-hour period before or within the two-hour period after taking ofloxacin). Products include:
New Formulation Chromagen OB Capsules ... 3094
Loestrin Fe Tablets ... 2642
NataChew Tablets ... 3364

Ferrous Gluconate (Co-administration with iron-containing products may substantially interfere with the oral absorption of quinolones; these preparations should not be taken within the two-hour period before or within the two-hour period after taking ofloxacin). Products include:
Fergon Iron Tablets ... ■802

Ferrous Sulfate (Co-administration with iron-containing products may substantially interfere with the oral absorption of quinolones; these preparations should not be taken within the two-hour period before or within the two-hour period after taking ofloxacin). Products include:
Feosol Tablets ... 1717
Slow Fe Tablets ... ■827
Slow Fe with Folic Acid Tablets ... ■828

Flurbiprofen (Co-administration with a non-steroidal anti-inflammatory agent may increase the risk of CNS stimulation and convulsive seizures).
No products indexed under this heading.

Glimepiride (Potentiation of hypoglycemic action). Products include:
Amaryl Tablets ... 717

Glipizide (Potentiation of hypoglycemic action). Products include:
Glucotrol Tablets ... 2692
Glucotrol XL Extended Release Tablets ... 2693

Glyburide (Potentiation of hypoglycemic action). Products include:
DiaBeta Tablets ... 741
Glucovance Tablets ... 1086

Ibuprofen (Co-administration with a non-steroidal anti-inflammatory agent may increase the risk of CNS stimulation and convulsive seizures). Products include:
Advil ... ■771
Children's Advil Oral Suspension ... ■773
Children's Advil Chewable Tablets ... ■773
Advil Cold and Sinus Caplets ... ■771
Advil Cold and Sinus Tablets ... ■771
Advil Flu & Body Ache Caplets ... ■772
Infants' Advil Drops ... ■773
Junior Strength Advil Tablets ... ■773
Junior Strength Advil Chewable Tablets ... ■773
Advil Migraine Liquigels ... ■772
Children's Motrin Oral Suspension and Chewable Tablets ... 2006
Children's Motrin Cold Oral Suspension ... 2007
Children's Motrin Oral Suspension ... ■643
Motrin Suspension, Oral Drops, Chewable Tablets, and Caplets ... 2002
Infants' Motrin Concentrated Drops ... 2006
Junior Strength Motrin Caplets and Chewable Tablets ... 2006
Motrin IB Tablets, Caplets, and Gelcaps ... 2002
Motrin Migraine Pain Caplets ... 2005
Motrin Sinus Headache Caplets ... 2005
Vicoprofen Tablets ... 520

Indomethacin (Co-administration with a non-steroidal anti-inflammatory agent may increase the risk of CNS stimulation and convulsive seizures). Products include:
Indocin ... 2112

Indomethacin Sodium Trihydrate (Co-administration with a non-steroidal anti-inflammatory agent may increase the risk of CNS stimulation and convulsive seizures). Products include:
Indocin I.V. ... 2115

Insulin, Human, Zinc Suspension (Potentiation of hypoglycemic action). Products include:
Humulin L, 100 Units ... 1937
Humulin U, 100 Units ... 1943
Novolin L Human Insulin 10 ml Vials ... 2422

Insulin, Human NPH (Potentiation of hypoglycemic action). Products include:
Humulin N, 100 Units ... 1939
Humulin N NPH Pen ... 1940
Novolin N Human Insulin 10 ml Vials ... 2422
Novolin N PenFill ... 2423
Novolin N Prefilled Syringe Disposable Insulin Delivery System ... 2425

Insulin, Human Regular (Potentiation of hypoglycemic action). Products include:
Humulin R Regular (U-500) ... 1943
Humulin R, 100 Units ... 1941
Novolin R Human Insulin 10 ml Vials ... 2423
Novolin R PenFill ... 2423
Novolin R Prefilled Syringe Disposable Insulin Delivery System ... 2425
Velosulin BR Human Insulin 10 ml Vials ... 2435

Insulin, Human Regular and Human NPH Mixture (Potentiation of hypoglycemic action). Products include:
Humulin 50/50, 100 Units ... 1934
Humulin 70/30, 100 Units ... 1935
Humulin 70/30 Pen ... 1936
Novolin 70/30 Human Insulin 10 ml Vials ... 2421
Novolin 70/30 PenFill ... 2423
Novolin 70/30 Prefilled Disposable Insulin Delivery System ... 2425

Insulin, NPH (Potentiation of hypoglycemic action). Products include:
Iletin II, NPH (Pork), 100 Units ... 1946

Insulin, Regular (Potentiation of hypoglycemic action). Products include:
Iletin II, Regular (Pork), 100 Units ... 1947

Insulin, Zinc Crystals (Potentiation of hypoglycemic action).
No products indexed under this heading.

Insulin, Zinc Suspension (Potentiation of hypoglycemic action). Products include:
Iletin II, Lente (Pork), 100 Units ... 1945

Insulin Aspart, Human Regular (Potentiation of hypoglycemic action).
No products indexed under this heading.

Insulin glargine (Potentiation of hypoglycemic action). Products include:
Lantus Injection ... 742

Insulin Lispro, Human (Potentiation of hypoglycemic action). Products include:
Humalog ... 1926
Humalog Mix 75/25 Pen ... 1928

Insulin Lispro Protamine, Human (Potentiation of hypoglycemic action). Products include:

Humalog Mix 75/25 Pen 1928

Iron (Co-administration with iron-containing products may substantially interfere with the oral absorption of quinolones; these preparations should not be taken within the two-hour period before or within the two-hour period after taking ofloxacin).
No products indexed under this heading.

Ketoprofen (Co-administration with a non-steroidal anti-inflammatory agent may increase the risk of CNS stimulation and convulsive seizures). Products include:
Orudis Capsules 3548
Orudis KT Tablets .... ■778
Oruvail Capsules 3548

Ketorolac Tromethamine (Co-administration with a non-steroidal anti-inflammatory agent may increase the risk of CNS stimulation and convulsive seizures). Products include:
Acular Ophthalmic Solution 544
Acular PF Ophthalmic Solution 544
Toradol 3018

Magaldrate (Co-administration with antacids containing calcium, aluminum, or magnesium may substantially interfere with the oral absorption of quinolones; these preparations should not be taken within the two-hour period before or within the two-hour period after taking ofloxacin).
No products indexed under this heading.

Magnesium Hydroxide (Co-administration with antacids containing calcium, aluminum, or magnesium may substantially interfere with the oral absorption of quinolones; these preparations should not be taken within the two-hour period before or within the two-hour period after taking ofloxacin). Products include:
Ex•Lax Milk of Magnesia Liquid .... ■670
Maalox Antacid/Anti-Gas Oral Suspension .... ■673
Maalox Max Maximum Strength Antacid/Anti-Gas Liquid 2300
Maalox Regular Strength Antacid/Antigas Liquid 2300
Mylanta Fast-Acting 1813
Mylanta 1813
Pepcid Complete Chewable Tablets 1815
Phillips' Chewable Tablets .... ■615
Phillips' Milk of Magnesia Liquid (Original, Cherry, & Mint) .... ■616
Rolaids Tablets .... ■706
Extra Strength Rolaids Tablets ...... ■706
Vanquish Caplets .... ■617

Magnesium Oxide (Co-administration with antacids containing calcium, aluminum, or magnesium may substantially interfere with the oral absorption of quinolones; these preparations should not be taken within the two-hour period before or within the two-hour period after taking ofloxacin). Products include:
Beelith Tablets 946
Mag-Ox 400 Tablets 1024
Uro-Mag Capsules 1024

Meclofenamate Sodium (Co-administration with a non-steroidal anti-inflammatory agent may increase the risk of CNS stimulation and convulsive seizures).
No products indexed under this heading.

Mefenamic Acid (Co-administration with a non-steroidal anti-inflammatory agent may increase the risk of CNS stimulation and convulsive seizures). Products include:
Ponstel Capsules 1356

Meloxicam (Co-administration with a non-steroidal anti-inflammatory agent may increase the risk of CNS stimulation and convulsive seizures). Products include:
Mobic Tablets 1054

Metformin Hydrochloride (Potentiation of hypoglycemic action). Products include:
Glucophage Tablets 1080
Glucophage XR Tablets 1080
Glucovance Tablets 1086

Miglitol (Potentiation of hypoglycemic action). Products include:
Glyset Tablets 2821

Nabumetone (Co-administration with a non-steroidal anti-inflammatory agent may increase the risk of CNS stimulation and convulsive seizures). Products include:
Relafen Tablets 1617

Naproxen (Co-administration with a non-steroidal anti-inflammatory agent may increase the risk of CNS stimulation and convulsive seizures). Products include:
EC-Naprosyn Delayed-Release Tablets 2967
Naprosyn Suspension 2967
Naprosyn Tablets 2967

Naproxen Sodium (Co-administration with a non-steroidal anti-inflammatory agent may increase the risk of CNS stimulation and convulsive seizures). Products include:
Aleve Tablets, Caplets and Gelcaps .... ■602
Aleve Cold & Sinus Caplets .... ■603
Anaprox Tablets 2967
Anaprox DS Tablets 2967
Naprelan Tablets 1293

Oxaprozin (Co-administration with a non-steroidal anti-inflammatory agent may increase the risk of CNS stimulation and convulsive seizures).
No products indexed under this heading.

Phenylbutazone (Co-administration with a non-steroidal anti-inflammatory agent may increase the risk of CNS stimulation and convulsive seizures).
No products indexed under this heading.

Pioglitazone Hydrochloride (Potentiation of hypoglycemic action). Products include:
Actos Tablets 3275

Piroxicam (Co-administration with a non-steroidal anti-inflammatory agent may increase the risk of CNS stimulation and convulsive seizures). Products include:
Feldene Capsules 2685

Polysaccharide-Iron Complex (Co-administration with iron-containing products may substantially interfere with the oral absorption of quinolones; these preparations should not be taken within the two-hour period before or within the two-hour period after taking ofloxacin). Products include:
Niferex 3176
Niferex-150 Capsules 3176
Nu-Iron 150 Capsules 2224

Probenecid (Potential to affect renal tubular secretion; this interaction has not been studied with ofloxacin).
No products indexed under this heading.

Repaglinide (Potentiation of hypoglycemic action). Products include:
Prandin Tablets (0.5, 1, and 2 mg) 2432

Rofecoxib (Co-administration with a non-steroidal anti-inflammatory agent may increase the risk of CNS stimulation and convulsive seizures). Products include:
Vioxx 2213

Rosiglitazone Maleate (Potentiation of hypoglycemic action). Products include:
Avandia Tablets 1490

Sucralfate (Co-administration with sucralfate may substantially interfere with the oral absorption of quinolones; these preparations should not be taken within the two-hour period before or within the two-hour period after taking ofloxacin). Products include:
Carafate Suspension 731
Carafate Tablets 730

Sulindac (Co-administration with a non-steroidal anti-inflammatory agent may increase the risk of CNS stimulation and convulsive seizures). Products include:
Clinoril Tablets 2053

Theophylline (Increased steady-state theophylline levels; concurrent therapy may prolong the half-life of theophylline, elevate serum theophylline levels, and increase the risk of theophylline-related adverse reactions). Products include:
Aerolate 1361
Theo-Dur Extended-Release Tablets 1835
Uni-Dur Extended-Release Tablets .. 1841
Uniphyl 400 mg and 600 mg Tablets 2903

Theophylline Calcium Salicylate (Increased steady-state theophylline levels; concurrent therapy may prolong the half-life of theophylline, elevate serum theophylline levels, and increase the risk of theophylline-related adverse reactions).
No products indexed under this heading.

Theophylline Sodium Glycinate (Increased steady-state theophylline levels; concurrent therapy may prolong the half-life of theophylline, elevate serum theophylline levels, and increase the risk of theophylline-related adverse reactions).
No products indexed under this heading.

Tolazamide (Potentiation of hypoglycemic action).
No products indexed under this heading.

Tolbutamide (Potentiation of hypoglycemic action).
No products indexed under this heading.

Tolmetin Sodium (Co-administration with a non-steroidal anti-inflammatory agent may increase the risk of CNS stimulation and convulsive seizures). Products include:
Tolectin 2589

Troglitazone (Potentiation of hypoglycemic action).
No products indexed under this heading.

Warfarin Sodium (Potential for enhanced effects of the oral anticoagulant). Products include:
Coumadin for Injection 1243
Coumadin Tablets 1243
Warfarin Sodium Tablets, USP 3302

Zinc Sulfate (Co-administration with multivitamins containing zinc may substantially interfere with the oral absorption of quinolones; these preparations should not be taken within the two-hour period before or within the two-hour period after taking ofloxacin). Products include:
Clear Eyes ACR Astringent/Lubricant Eye Redness Reliever .... ⊙322
Visine A.C. Seasonal Relief From Pollen & Dust Eye Drops .... ⊙314

Food Interactions

Food, unspecified (Food does not affect the Cmax and AUC∞ of the drug, but Tmax is prolonged).

FLUDARA FOR INJECTION
(Fludarabine Phosphate) 995
May interact with:

Pentostatin (Co-administration may produce severe pulmonary toxicity; the use of Fludara in combination with pentostatin is not recommended). Products include:
Nipent for Injection 3272

FLUMADINE SYRUP
(Rimantadine Hydrochloride) 1370
See Flumadine Tablets

FLUMADINE TABLETS
(Rimantadine Hydrochloride) 1370
May interact with:

Acetaminophen (Coadministration reduces the peak concentration and AUC values for rimantadine). Products include:
Actifed Cold & Sinus Caplets and Tablets .... ■688
Alka-Seltzer Plus Liqui-Gels .... ■604
Alka-Seltzer Plus Cold & Flu Medicine Liqui-Gels .... ■604
Alka-Seltzer Plus Cold & Sinus Medicine Liqui-Gels .... ■604
Benadryl Allergy/Cold Tablets .... ■691
Benadryl Allergy Sinus Headache Caplets & Gelcaps .... ■693
Benadryl Severe Allergy & Sinus Headache Caplets .... ■694
Children's Cēpacol Sore Throat .... ■788
Comtrex Acute Head Cold & Sinus Pressure Relief Tablets ..... ■627
Comtrex Deep Chest Cold & Congestion Relief Softgels .... ■627
Comtrex Flu Therapy & Fever Relief Daytime Caplets .... ■628
Comtrex Flu Therapy & Fever Relief Nighttime Tablets .... ■628
Comtrex Maximum Strength Multi-Symptom Cold & Cough Relief Tablets and Caplets .... ■626
Contac Severe Cold and Flu Caplets Maximum Strength .... ■746
Contac Severe Cold and Flu Caplets Non-Drowsy .... ■746
Coricidin 'D' Cold, Flu & Sinus Tablets .... ■737
Coricidin HBP Cold & Flu Tablets .. ■738
Coricidin HBP Maximum Strength Flu Tablets .... ■738
Coricidin HBP Night-Time Cold & Flu Tablets .... ■738
Darvon-N/Darvocet-N 1907
Dimetapp Cold and Fever Suspension .... ■775
Dimetapp Nighttime Flu Liquid ...... ■776
Dimetapp Non-Drowsy Flu Syrup .. ■777
Drixoral Allergy/Sinus Extended-Release Tablets .... ■741
Drixoral Cold & Flu Extended-Release Tablets .... ■740
Aspirin Free Excedrin Caplets and Geltabs .... ■628
Excedrin Extra-Strength Tablets, Caplets, and Geltabs .... ■629
Excedrin Migraine 1070
Excedrin PM Tablets, Caplets, and Geltabs .... ■631
Goody's Body Pain Formula Powder .... ■620
Goody's Extra Strength Headache Powder .... ■620
Goody's Extra Strength Pain Relief Tablets .... ■620
Goody's PM Powder .... ■621
Hycomine Compound Tablets 1317
Lortab 3319
Lortab Elixir 3317
Maxidone Tablets CIII 3399
Maximum Strength Midol Menstrual Caplets and Gelcaps .. ■612
Maximum Strength Midol PMS Caplets and Gelcaps .... ■613
Maximum Strength Midol Teen Caplets .... ■612
Midrin Capsules 3464
Norco 5/325 Tablets CIII 3424
Norco 7.5/325 Tablets CIII 3425
Norco 10/325 Tablets CIII 3427
Norco 10/325 Tablets CIII 3425
Percocet Tablets 1326
Percogesic Aspirin-Free Coated Tablets .... ■667
Extra Strength Percogesic Aspirin-Free Coated Caplets .... ■665
Phrenilin 578
Robitussin Cold Caplets Multi-Symptom Cold & Flu .... ■781
Robitussin Cold Softgels Multi-Symptom Cold & Flu .... ■781
Robitussin Multi Symptom Honey Flu Liquid .... ■785
Robitussin Nighttime Honey Flu Liquid .... ■786
Sedapap Tablets 50 mg/650 mg ... 2225
Singlet Caplets .... ■761
Sinutab Sinus Allergy Medication, Maximum Strength Formula, Tablets & Caplets .... ■707

Sinutab Sinus Medication, Maximum Strength Without Drowsiness Formula, Tablets & Caplets 707
Sudafed Cold & Cough Liquid Caps 709
Sudafed Cold & Sinus Liquid Caps 710
Sudafed Severe Cold 711
Sudafed Sinus Headache Caplets .. 712
Sudafed Sinus Headache Tablets .. 712
Tavist Sinus Non-Drowsy Coated Caplets 676
TheraFlu Regular Strength Cold & Cough Night Time Hot Liquid 676
TheraFlu Regular Strength Cold & Sore Throat Night Time Hot Liquid 676
TheraFlu Maximum Strength Flu & Congestion Non-Drowsy Hot Liquid 677
TheraFlu Maximum Strength Flu & Cough Night Time Hot Liquid .. 678
TheraFlu Maximum Strength Flu & Sore Throat Night Time Hot Liquid 677
TheraFlu Maximum Strength Severe Cold & Congestion Night Time Caplets 678
TheraFlu Maximum Strength Severe Cold & Congestion Night Time Hot Liquid 678
TheraFlu Maximum Strength Severe Cold & Congestion Non-Drowsy 679
Triaminic Cold, Cough & Fever Liquid 681
Triaminic Cough & Sore Throat Liquid 682
Triaminic Cough & Sore Throat Softchews 684
Tylenol, Children's 2014
Children's Tylenol Allergy-D Liquid 2014
Children's Tylenol Cold Suspension Liquid and Chewable Tablets 2015
Children's Tylenol Cold Plus Cough Suspension Liquid and Chewable Tablets 2015
Children's Tylenol Flu Suspension Liquid 2015
Children's Tylenol Sinus Suspension Liquid 2017
Infants' Tylenol Cold Decongestant and Fever Reducer Concentrated Drops 2015
Infants' Tylenol Cold Decongestant and Fever Reducer Concentrated Drops Plus Cough .. 2015
Junior Strength Tylenol Soft Chews Chewable Tablets 2014
Tylenol 2009
Tylenol Allergy Sinus 2010
Tylenol Severe Allergy Caplets 2010
Multi-Symptom Tylenol Cold Complete Formula Caplets 2010
Multi-Symptom Tylenol Cold Non-Drowsy Caplets and Gelcaps 2010
Multi-Symptom Tylenol Cold Severe Congestion Non-Drowsy Caplets 2011
Maximum Strength Tylenol Flu NightTime Gelcaps 2011
Maximum Strength Tylenol Flu NightTime Liquid 2011
Maximum Strength Tylenol Flu Non-Drowsy Gelcaps 2011
Extra Strength Tylenol PM Caplets, Geltabs, and Gelcaps 2012
Maximum Strength Tylenol Sinus NightTime Caplets 2012
Maximum Strength Tylenol Sinus Non-Drowsy Geltabs, Gelcaps, Caplets, and Tablets 2012
Maximum Strength Tylenol Sore Throat Adult Liquid 2013
Tylenol with Codeine 2595
Women's Tylenol Menstrual Relief Caplets 2013
Tylox Capsules 2597
Ultracet Tablets 2597
Vanquish Caplets 617
Vicks 44M Cough, Cold & Flu Relief Liquid 725
Vicks DayQuil LiquiCaps/Liquid Multi-Symptom Cold/Flu Relief ... 727
Vicks NyQuil LiquiCaps/Liquid Multi-Symptom Cold/Flu Relief, Original and Cherry Flavors 727
Vicodin Tablets 516
Vicodin ES Tablets 517
Vicodin HP Tablets 518
Zydone Tablets 1330

Aspirin (Coadministration reduces the peak concentration and AUC values for rimantadine). Products include:
Aggrenox Capsules 1026
Alka-Seltzer 603
Alka-Seltzer Lemon Lime Antacid and Pain Reliever Effervescent Tablets 603
Alka-Seltzer Extra Strength Antacid and Pain Reliever Effervescent Tablets 603
Alka-Seltzer PM Effervescent Tablets 605
Genuine Bayer Tablets, Caplets and Gelcaps 606
Extra Strength Bayer Caplets and Gelcaps 610
Aspirin Regimen Bayer Children's Chewable Tablets (Orange or Cherry Flavored) 607
Bayer, Aspirin Regimen 606
Aspirin Regimen Bayer 81 mg Caplets with Calcium 607
Genuine Bayer Professional Labeling (Aspirin Regimen Bayer) 608
Extra Strength Bayer Arthritis Caplets 610
Extra Strength Bayer Plus Caplets 610
Extra Strength Bayer PM Caplets .. 611
BC Powder 619
BC Allergy Sinus Cold Powder 619
Arthritis Strength BC Powder 619
BC Sinus Cold Powder 619
Darvon Compound-65 Pulvules 1910
Ecotrin Enteric Coated Aspirin Low, Regular and Maximum Strength Tablets 1715
Excedrin Extra-Strength Tablets, Caplets, and Geltabs 629
Excedrin Migraine 1070
Goody's Body Pain Formula Powder 620
Goody's Extra Strength Headache Powder 620
Goody's Extra Strength Pain Relief Tablets 620
Percodan Tablets 1327
Robaxisal Tablets 2939
Soma Compound Tablets 3354
Soma Compound w/Codeine Tablets 3355
Vanquish Caplets 617

Cimetidine (Potential for reduced clearance of total rimantadine). Products include:
Tagamet HB 200 Suspension 762
Tagamet HB 200 Tablets 761
Tagamet Tablets 1644

Cimetidine Hydrochloride (Potential for reduced clearance of total rimantadine). Products include:
Tagamet 1644

FLUORESCITE INJECTION

(Fluorescein Sodium) .... ⊙ 211
None cited in PDR database.

FLUOR-I-STRIP A.T. OPHTHALMIC STRIPS 1 MG

(Fluorescein Sodium) .... ⊙ 260
None cited in PDR database.

FLUOR-I-STRIP OPHTHALMIC STRIPS 9 MG

(Fluorescein Sodium) .... ⊙ 260
None cited in PDR database.

FLUOROPLEX TOPICAL CREAM

(Fluorouracil) 552
None cited in PDR database.

FLUOROPLEX TOPICAL SOLUTION

(Fluorouracil) 552

See Fluoroplex Topical Cream

FLUOTHANE INHALATION

(Halothane) 3508

May interact with ganglionic blocking agents, nondepolarizing neuromuscular blocking agents, phenytoin, drugs that prolong the QT interval, sympathomimetics, theophylline, and certain other agents. Compounds in these categories include:

Albuterol (Co-administration with sympathomimetics may induce ventricular tachycardia or fibrillation). Products include:
Proventil Inhalation Aerosol 3142
Ventolin Inhalation Aerosol and Refill 1679

Albuterol Sulfate (Co-administration with sympathomimetics may induce ventricular tachycardia or fibrillation). Products include:
AccuNeb Inhalation Solution 1230
Combivent Inhalation Aerosol 1041
DuoNeb Inhalation Solution 1233
Proventil Inhalation Solution 0.083% 3146
Proventil Repetabs Tablets 3148
Proventil Solution for Inhalation 0.5% 3144
Proventil HFA Inhalation Aerosol 3150
Ventolin HFA Inhalation Aerosol 3618
Volmax Extended-Release Tablets .. 2276

Aminophylline (Co-administration may increase the risk of ventricular arrhythmias and cardiac arrest).
No products indexed under this heading.

Amiodarone Hydrochloride (Halothane has been reported to prolong the Q-T interval; co-administration with other drugs known to prolong the Q-T interval should be undertaken with caution). Products include:
Cordarone Intravenous 3491
Cordarone Tablets 3487
Pacerone Tablets 3331

Amitriptyline Hydrochloride (Halothane has been reported to prolong the Q-T interval; co-administration with other drugs known to prolong the Q-T interval should be undertaken with caution). Products include:
Etrafon 3115
Limbitrol 1738

Amoxapine (Halothane has been reported to prolong the Q-T interval; co-administration with other drugs known to prolong the Q-T interval should be undertaken with caution).
No products indexed under this heading.

Astemizole (Halothane has been reported to prolong the Q-T interval; co-administration with other drugs known to prolong the Q-T interval should be undertaken with caution).
No products indexed under this heading.

Atracurium Besylate (Actions augmented by halothane).
No products indexed under this heading.

Bretylium Tosylate (Halothane has been reported to prolong the Q-T interval; co-administration with other drugs known to prolong the Q-T interval should be undertaken with caution).
No products indexed under this heading.

Chlorpromazine (Halothane has been reported to prolong the Q-T interval; co-administration with other drugs known to prolong the Q-T interval should be undertaken with caution). Products include:
Thorazine Suppositories 1656

Chlorpromazine Hydrochloride (Halothane has been reported to prolong the Q-T interval; co-administration with other drugs known to prolong the Q-T interval should be undertaken with caution). Products include:
Thorazine 1656

Cisatracurium Besylate (Actions augmented by halothane).
No products indexed under this heading.

Clomipramine Hydrochloride (Halothane has been reported to prolong the Q-T interval; co-administration with other drugs known to prolong the Q-T interval should be undertaken with caution).
No products indexed under this heading.

Desipramine Hydrochloride (Halothane has been reported to prolong the Q-T interval; co-administration with other drugs known to prolong the Q-T interval should be undertaken with caution). Products include:
Norpramin Tablets 755

Disopyramide Phosphate (Halothane has been reported to prolong the Q-T interval; co-administration with other drugs known to prolong the Q-T interval should be undertaken with caution).
No products indexed under this heading.

Dobutamine Hydrochloride (Co-administration with sympathomimetics may induce ventricular tachycardia or fibrillation). Products include:
Dobutrex Solution Vials 1914

Dofetilide (Halothane has been reported to prolong the Q-T interval; co-administration with other drugs known to prolong the Q-T interval should be undertaken with caution). Products include:
Tikosyn Capsules 2717

Dopamine Hydrochloride (Co-administration with sympathomimetics may induce ventricular tachycardia or fibrillation).
No products indexed under this heading.

Doxepin Hydrochloride (Halothane has been reported to prolong the Q-T interval; co-administration with other drugs known to prolong the Q-T interval should be undertaken with caution). Products include:
Sinequan 2713

Dyphylline (Co-administration may increase the risk of ventricular arrhythmias and cardiac arrest). Products include:
Lufyllin Tablets 3347
Lufyllin-400 Tablets 3347
Lufyllin-GG Elixir 3348
Lufyllin-GG Tablets 3348

Ephedrine Hydrochloride (Co-administration with sympathomimetics may induce ventricular tachycardia or fibrillation). Products include:
Primatene Tablets 780

Ephedrine Sulfate (Co-administration with sympathomimetics may induce ventricular tachycardia or fibrillation).
No products indexed under this heading.

Ephedrine Tannate (Co-administration with sympathomimetics may induce ventricular tachycardia or fibrillation). Products include:
Rynatuss Pediatric Suspension 3353
Rynatuss Tablets 3353

Epinephrine (Co-administration with sympathomimetics may induce ventricular tachycardia or fibrillation). Products include:
Epifrin Sterile Ophthalmic Solution .... ⊙ 235
EpiPen 1236
Primatene Mist 779
Xylocaine with Epinephrine Injection 653

Epinephrine Bitartrate (Co-administration with sympathomimetics may induce ventricular tachycardia or fibrillation). Products include:
Sensorcaine 643

Epinephrine Hydrochloride (Co-administration with sympathomimetics may induce ventricular tachycardia or fibrillation).
No products indexed under this heading.

Fentanyl (Chronic exposure to trace concentrations of halothane have been reported to increase hepatic microsomal enzyme activity and can inhibit the metabolism of drugs eliminated by the liver microsomal enzyme system such as fentanyl). Products include:
Duragesic Transdermal System 1786

Fentanyl Citrate (Chronic exposure to trace concentrations of halothane

have been reported to increase hepatic microsomal enzyme activity and can inhibit the metabolism of drugs eliminated by the liver microsomal enzyme system such as fentanyl). Products include:
Actiq 1184

Flecainide Acetate (Halothane has been reported to prolong the Q-T interval; co-administration with other drugs known to prolong the Q-T interval should be undertaken with caution). Products include:
Tambocor Tablets 1990

Fluphenazine Decanoate (Halothane has been reported to prolong the Q-T interval; co-administration with other drugs known to prolong the Q-T interval should be undertaken with caution).
No products indexed under this heading.

Fluphenazine Enanthate (Halothane has been reported to prolong the Q-T interval; co-administration with other drugs known to prolong the Q-T interval should be undertaken with caution).
No products indexed under this heading.

Fluphenazine Hydrochloride (Halothane has been reported to prolong the Q-T interval; co-administration with other drugs known to prolong the Q-T interval should be undertaken with caution).
No products indexed under this heading.

Fosphenytoin Sodium (Co-administration may increase the risk of hepatotoxicity; halothane-induced hepatic function impairment may increase the risk of phenytoin toxicity). Products include:
Cerebyx Injection 2619

Imipramine Hydrochloride (Halothane has been reported to prolong the Q-T interval; co-administration with other drugs known to prolong the Q-T interval should be undertaken with caution).
No products indexed under this heading.

Imipramine Pamoate (Halothane has been reported to prolong the Q-T interval; co-administration with other drugs known to prolong the Q-T interval should be undertaken with caution).
No products indexed under this heading.

Isoniazid (Co-administration with drugs known to elevate hepatic levels of CYP450 enzyme, such as isoniazid, enhances the metabolism of volatile anesthetics). Products include:
Rifamate Capsules 767
Rifater Tablets 769

Isoproterenol Hydrochloride (Co-administration with sympathomimetics may induce ventricular tachycardia or fibrillation).
No products indexed under this heading.

Isoproterenol Sulfate (Co-administration with sympathomimetics may induce ventricular tachycardia or fibrillation).
No products indexed under this heading.

Ketamine Hydrochloride (Chronic exposure to trace concentrations of halothane have been reported to increase hepatic microsomal enzyme activity and can inhibit the metabolism of drugs eliminated by the liver microsomal enzyme system such as ketamine).
No products indexed under this heading.

Levalbuterol Hydrochloride (Co-administration with sympathomimetics may induce ventricular tachycardia or fibrillation). Products include:
Xopenex Inhalation Solution 3207

Lidocaine Hydrochloride (Chronic exposure to trace concentrations of halothane have been reported to increase hepatic microsomal enzyme activity and can inhibit the metabolism of drugs eliminated by the liver microsomal enzyme system such as lidocaine). Products include:
Bactine First Aid Liquid .... ▣611
Xylocaine Injections 653

Maprotiline Hydrochloride (Halothane has been reported to prolong the Q-T interval; co-administration with other drugs known to prolong the Q-T interval should be undertaken with caution).
No products indexed under this heading.

Mecamylamine Hydrochloride (Actions augmented by halothane). Products include:
Inversine Tablets 1850

Meperidine Hydrochloride (Chronic exposure to trace concentrations of halothane have been reported to increase hepatic microsomal enzyme activity and can inhibit the metabolism of drugs eliminated by the liver microsomal enzyme system such as meperidine). Products include:
Demerol 3079
Mepergan Injection 3539

Mesoridazine Besylate (Halothane has been reported to prolong the Q-T interval; co-administration with other drugs known to prolong the Q-T interval should be undertaken with caution). Products include:
Serentil 1057

Metaproterenol Sulfate (Co-administration with sympathomimetics may induce ventricular tachycardia or fibrillation). Products include:
Alupent 1029

Metaraminol Bitartrate (Co-administration with sympathomimetics may induce ventricular tachycardia or fibrillation). Products include:
Aramine Injection 2043

Methoxamine Hydrochloride (Co-administration with sympathomimetics may induce ventricular tachycardia or fibrillation).
No products indexed under this heading.

Metocurine Iodide (Actions augmented by halothane).
No products indexed under this heading.

Mexiletine Hydrochloride (Halothane has been reported to prolong the Q-T interval; co-administration with other drugs known to prolong the Q-T interval should be undertaken with caution). Products include:
Mexitil Capsules 1047

Mivacurium Chloride (Actions augmented by halothane).
No products indexed under this heading.

Norepinephrine Bitartrate (Co-administration with sympathomimetics may induce ventricular tachycardia or fibrillation).
No products indexed under this heading.

Nortriptyline Hydrochloride (Halothane has been reported to prolong the Q-T interval; co-administration with other drugs known to prolong the Q-T interval should be undertaken with caution).
No products indexed under this heading.

Pancuronium Bromide (Co-administration in patients on chronic tricyclic antidepressants therapy who are anesthetized with halothane may result in ventricular arrhythmias).
No products indexed under this heading.

Perphenazine (Halothane has been reported to prolong the Q-T interval; co-administration with other drugs known to prolong the Q-T interval should be undertaken with caution). Products include:
Etrafon 3115
Trilafon 3160

Phenylephrine Bitartrate (Co-administration with sympathomimetics may induce ventricular tachycardia or fibrillation).
No products indexed under this heading.

Phenylephrine Hydrochloride (Co-administration with sympathomimetics may induce ventricular tachycardia or fibrillation). Products include:
Afrin Nasal Decongestant Children's Pump Mist .... ▣734
Extendryl 1361
Hycomine Compound Tablets 1317
Neo-Synephrine .... ▣614
Phenergan VC Syrup 3560
Phenergan VC with Codeine Syrup .. 3561
Preparation H Cream .... ▣778
Preparation H Cooling Gel .... ▣778
Preparation H .... ▣778
Vicks Sinex Nasal Spray and Ultra Fine Mist .... ▣729

Phenylephrine Tannate (Co-administration with sympathomimetics may induce ventricular tachycardia or fibrillation). Products include:
Ryna-12 S Suspension 3351
Reformulated Rynatan Pediatric Suspension 3352
Rynatuss Pediatric Suspension 3353
Rynatuss Tablets 3353

Phenylpropanolamine Hydrochloride (Co-administration with sympathomimetics may induce ventricular tachycardia or fibrillation).
No products indexed under this heading.

Phenytoin (Co-administration may increase the risk of hepatotoxicity; halothane-induced hepatic function impairment may increase the risk of phenytoin toxicity). Products include:
Dilantin Infatabs 2624
Dilantin-125 Oral Suspension 2625

Phenytoin Sodium (Co-administration may increase the risk of hepatotoxicity; halothane-induced hepatic function impairment may increase the risk of phenytoin toxicity). Products include:
Dilantin Kapseals 2622

Pirbuterol Acetate (Co-administration with sympathomimetics may induce ventricular tachycardia or fibrillation). Products include:
Maxair Autohaler 1981
Maxair Inhaler 1984

Procainamide Hydrochloride (Halothane has been reported to prolong the Q-T interval; co-administration with other drugs known to prolong the Q-T interval should be undertaken with caution). Products include:
Procanbid Extended-Release Tablets 2262

Prochlorperazine (Halothane has been reported to prolong the Q-T interval; co-administration with other drugs known to prolong the Q-T interval should be undertaken with caution). Products include:
Compazine 1505

Promethazine Hydrochloride (Halothane has been reported to prolong the Q-T interval; co-administration with other drugs known to prolong the Q-T interval should be undertaken with caution). Products include:
Mepergan Injection 3539
Phenergan Injection 3553
Phenergan 3556
Phenergan Syrup 3554
Phenergan with Codeine Syrup 3557
Phenergan with Dextromethorphan Syrup 3559
Phenergan VC Syrup 3560
Phenergan VC with Codeine Syrup .. 3561

Propafenone Hydrochloride (Halothane has been reported to prolong the Q-T interval; co-administration with other drugs known to prolong the Q-T interval should be undertaken with caution). Products include:
Rythmol Tablets – 150 mg, 225 mg, 300 mg 502

Propranolol Hydrochloride (Chronic exposure to trace concentrations of halothane have been reported to increase hepatic microsomal enzyme activity and can inhibit the metabolism of drugs eliminated by the liver microsomal enzyme system such as propranolol). Products include:
Inderal 3513
Inderal LA Long-Acting Capsules 3516
Inderide Tablets 3517
Inderide LA Long-Acting Capsules .. 3519

Protriptyline Hydrochloride (Halothane has been reported to prolong the Q-T interval; co-administration with other drugs known to prolong the Q-T interval should be undertaken with caution). Products include:
Vivactil Tablets 2446
Vivactil Tablets 2217

Pseudoephedrine Hydrochloride (Co-administration with sympathomimetics may induce ventricular tachycardia or fibrillation). Products include:
Actifed Cold & Allergy Tablets .... ▣688
Actifed Cold & Sinus Caplets and Tablets .... ▣688
Advil Cold and Sinus Caplets .... ▣771
Advil Cold and Sinus Tablets .... ▣771
Advil Flu & Body Ache Caplets .... ▣772
Aleve Cold & Sinus Caplets .... ▣603
Alka-Seltzer Plus Liqui-Gels .... ▣604
Alka-Seltzer Plus Cold & Flu Medicine Liqui-Gels .... ▣604
Alka-Seltzer Plus Cold & Sinus Medicine Liqui-Gels .... ▣604
Allegra-D Extended-Release Tablets 714
BC Cold Powder .... ▣619
Benadryl Allergy/Cold Tablets .... ▣691
Benadryl Allergy/Congestion Tablets .... ▣692
Benadryl Allergy & Sinus Liquid .... ▣693
Benadryl Allergy & Sinus Fastmelt Tablets .... ▣693
Benadryl Allergy Sinus Headache Caplets & Gelcaps .... ▣693
Benadryl Severe Allergy & Sinus Headache Caplets .... ▣694
Benadryl Children's Allergy/Cold Fastmelt Tablets .... ▣692
Benylin Multi-Symptom Liquid .... ▣697
Bromfed Capsules (Extended-Release) 2269
Bromfed-PD Capsules (Extended-Release) 2269
Children's Cēpacol Sore Throat .... ▣788
Comtrex Acute Head Cold & Sinus Pressure Relief Tablets .... ▣627
Comtrex Deep Chest Cold & Congestion Relief Softgels .... ▣627
Comtrex Flu Therapy & Fever Relief Daytime Caplets .... ▣628
Comtrex Flu Therapy & Fever Relief Nighttime Tablets .... ▣628
Comtrex Maximum Strength Multi-Symptom Cold & Cough Relief Tablets and Caplets .... ▣626
Contac Non-Drowsy 12 Hour Cold Caplets .... ▣745
Contac Non-Drowsy Timed Release 12 Hour Cold Caplets .... ▣746
Contac Severe Cold and Flu Caplets Maximum Strength .... ▣746
Contac Severe Cold and Flu Caplets Non-Drowsy .... ▣746
Dimetapp Elixir .... ▣777
Dimetapp Cold and Fever Suspension .... ▣775
Dimetapp DM Cold & Cough Elixir . ▣775
Dimetapp Nighttime Flu Liquid .... ▣776
Dimetapp Non-Drowsy Flu Syrup .... ▣777
Dimetapp Infant Drops Decongestant .... ▣775
Dimetapp Infant Drops Decongestant Plus Cough .... ▣776
Guaifed 2272
Kronofed-A 1341

Children's Motrin Cold Oral Suspension ... 2007
Motrin Sinus Headache Caplets ... 2005
PediaCare Cough-Cold Liquid ... 719
PediaCare Infants' Drops Decongestant ... 719
PediaCare Infants' Drops Decongestant Plus Cough ... 719
PediaCare NightRest Cough-Cold Liquid ... 719
Robitussin Cold Caplets Cold & Congestion ... 780
Robitussin Cold Softgels Cold & Congestion ... 780
Robitussin Cold Caplets Multi-Symptom Cold & Flu ... 781
Robitussin Cold Softgels Multi-Symptom Cold & Flu ... 781
Robitussin Cold Softgels Severe Congestion ... 782
Robitussin Cough & Cold Infant Drops ... 782
Robitussin Maximum Strength Cough & Cold Liquid ... 785
Robitussin Pediatric Cough & Cold Formula Liquid ... 785
Robitussin Multi Symptom Honey Flu Liquid ... 785
Robitussin Nighttime Honey Flu Liquid ... 786
Robitussin-CF Liquid ... 783
Robitussin-DAC Syrup ... 2942
Robitussin-PE Liquid ... 782
Ryna ... 768
Semprex-D Capsules ... 1172
Singlet Caplets ... 761
Sinutab Non-Drying Liquid Caps ... 706
Sinutab Sinus Allergy Medication, Maximum Strength Formula, Tablets & Caplets ... 707
Sinutab Sinus Medication, Maximum Strength Without Drowsiness Formula, Tablets & Caplets ... 707
Sudafed 12 Hour Tablets ... 708
Sudafed 24 Hour Tablets ... 708
Children's Sudafed Cold & Cough Liquid ... 709
Children's Sudafed Nasal Decongestant Chewables ... 711
Children's Sudafed Nasal Decongestant Liquid Medication ... 711
Sudafed Cold & Allergy Tablets ... 708
Sudafed Cold & Cough Liquid Caps ... 709
Sudafed Cold & Sinus Liquid Caps ... 710
Sudafed Nasal Decongestant Tablets ... 710
Sudafed Non-Drying Sinus Liquid Caps ... 712
Sudafed Severe Cold ... 711
Sudafed Sinus Headache Caplets ... 712
Sudafed Sinus Headache Tablets ... 712
Tavist Sinus Non-Drowsy Coated Caplets ... 676
TheraFlu Regular Strength Cold & Cough Night Time Hot Liquid ... 676
TheraFlu Regular Strength Cold & Sore Throat Night Time Hot Liquid ... 676
TheraFlu Maximum Strength Flu & Congestion Non-Drowsy Hot Liquid ... 677
TheraFlu Maximum Strength Flu & Cough Night Time Hot Liquid ... 678
TheraFlu Maximum Strength Flu & Sore Throat Night Time Hot Liquid ... 677
TheraFlu Maximum Strength Severe Cold & Congestion Night Time Caplets ... 678
TheraFlu Maximum Strength Severe Cold & Congestion Night Time Hot Liquid ... 678
TheraFlu Maximum Strength Severe Cold & Congestion Non-Drowsy ... 679
Triaminic Allergy Congestion Liquid ... 680
Triaminic Chest Congestion Liquid ... 680
Triaminic Cold & Allergy Liquid ... 681
Triaminic Cold & Allergy Softchews ... 683
Triaminic Cold & Cough Liquid ... 681
Triaminic Cold & Cough Softchews ... 683
Triaminic Cold & Night Time Cough Liquid ... 681
Triaminic Cold, Cough & Fever Liquid ... 681
Triaminic Cough Liquid ... 682
Triaminic Cough & Congestion Liquid ... 682
Triaminic Cough & Sore Throat Liquid ... 682
Triaminic Cough & Sore Throat Softchews ... 684
Children's Tylenol Allergy-D Liquid ... 2014
Children's Tylenol Cold Suspension Liquid and Chewable Tablets ... 2015
Children's Tylenol Cold Plus Cough Suspension Liquid and Chewable Tablets ... 2015
Children's Tylenol Flu Suspension Liquid ... 2015
Children's Tylenol Sinus Suspension Liquid ... 2017
Infants' Tylenol Cold Decongestant and Fever Reducer Concentrated Drops ... 2015
Infants' Tylenol Cold Decongestant and Fever Reducer Concentrated Drops Plus Cough ... 2015
Tylenol Allergy Sinus ... 2010
Multi-Symptom Tylenol Cold Complete Formula Caplets ... 2010
Multi-Symptom Tylenol Cold Non-Drowsy Caplets and Gelcaps ... 2010
Multi-Symptom Tylenol Cold Severe Congestion Non-Drowsy Caplets ... 2011
Maximum Strength Tylenol Flu NightTime Gelcaps ... 2011
Maximum Strength Tylenol Flu NightTime Liquid ... 2011
Maximum Strength Tylenol Flu Non-Drowsy Gelcaps ... 2011
Maximum Strength Tylenol Sinus NightTime Caplets ... 2012
Maximum Strength Tylenol Sinus Non-Drowsy Geltabs, Gelcaps, Caplets, and Tablets ... 2012
Vicks 44D Cough & Head Congestion Relief Liquid ... 724
Vicks 44M Cough, Cold & Flu Relief Liquid ... 725
Pediatric Vicks 44m Cough & Cold Relief ... 728
Vicks DayQuil LiquiCaps/Liquid Multi-Symptom Cold/Flu Relief ... 727
Children's Vicks NyQuil Cold/Cough Relief ... 726
Vicks NyQuil LiquiCaps/Liquid Multi-Symptom Cold/Flu Relief, Original and Cherry Flavors ... 727
Zephrex Tablets ... 3091
Zephrex LA Tablets ... 3092
Zyrtec-D 12 Hour Extended Relief Tablets ... 2758

Pseudoephedrine Sulfate (Co-administration with sympathomimetics may induce ventricular tachycardia or fibrillation). Products include:
Chlor-Trimeton Allergy/Decongestant Tablets ... 736
Claritin-D 12 Hour Extended Release Tablets ... 3102
Claritin-D 24 Hour Extended Release Tablets ... 3104
Coricidin 'D' Cold, Flu & Sinus Tablets ... 737
Drixoral Allergy/Sinus Extended-Release Tablets ... 741
Drixoral Cold & Allergy Sustained-Action Tablets ... 740
Drixoral Cold & Flu Extended-Release Tablets ... 740
Drixoral Nasal Decongestant Long-Acting Non-Drowsy Tablets ... 740
Rynatan Tablets ... 3351

Quinidine Gluconate (Halothane has been reported to prolong the Q-T interval; co-administration with other drugs known to prolong the Q-T interval should be undertaken with caution). Products include:
Quinaglute Dura-Tabs Tablets ... 978

Quinidine Polygalacturonate (Halothane has been reported to prolong the Q-T interval; co-administration with other drugs known to prolong the Q-T interval should be undertaken with caution).
No products indexed under this heading.

Quinidine Sulfate (Halothane has been reported to prolong the Q-T interval; co-administration with other drugs known to prolong the Q-T interval should be undertaken with caution). Products include:
Quinidex Extentabs ... 2933

Rapacuronium Bromide (Actions augmented by halothane).
No products indexed under this heading.

Rocuronium Bromide (Actions augmented by halothane). Products include:
Zemuron Injection ... 2491

Salmeterol Xinafoate (Co-administration with sympathomimetics may induce ventricular tachycardia or fibrillation). Products include:
Advair Diskus 100/50 ... 1448
Advair Diskus 250/50 ... 1448
Advair Diskus 500/50 ... 1448
Serevent Diskus ... 1637
Serevent Inhalation Aerosol ... 1633

Terbutaline Sulfate (Co-administration with sympathomimetics may induce ventricular tachycardia or fibrillation). Products include:
Brethine Ampuls ... 2314
Brethine Tablets ... 2313

Terfenadine (Halothane has been reported to prolong the Q-T interval; co-administration with other drugs known to prolong the Q-T interval should be undertaken with caution).
No products indexed under this heading.

Theophylline (Co-administration may increase the risk of ventricular arrhythmias and cardiac arrest). Products include:
Aerolate ... 1361
Theo-Dur Extended-Release Tablets ... 1835
Uni-Dur Extended-Release Tablets ... 1841
Uniphyl 400 mg and 600 mg Tablets ... 2903

Theophylline Calcium Salicylate (Co-administration may increase the risk of ventricular arrhythmias and cardiac arrest).
No products indexed under this heading.

Theophylline Sodium Glycinate (Co-administration may increase the risk of ventricular arrhythmias and cardiac arrest).
No products indexed under this heading.

Thioridazine Hydrochloride (Halothane has been reported to prolong the Q-T interval; co-administration with other drugs known to prolong the Q-T interval should be undertaken with caution). Products include:
Thioridazine Hydrochloride Tablets ... 2289

Tocainide Hydrochloride (Halothane has been reported to prolong the Q-T interval; co-administration with other drugs known to prolong the Q-T interval should be undertaken with caution). Products include:
Tonocard Tablets ... 649

Trifluoperazine Hydrochloride (Halothane has been reported to prolong the Q-T interval; co-administration with other drugs known to prolong the Q-T interval should be undertaken with caution). Products include:
Stelazine ... 1640

Trimethaphan Camsylate (Actions augmented by halothane).
No products indexed under this heading.

Trimipramine Maleate (Halothane has been reported to prolong the Q-T interval; co-administration with other drugs known to prolong the Q-T interval should be undertaken with caution). Products include:
Surmontil Capsules ... 3595

Vecuronium Bromide (Actions augmented by halothane). Products include:
Norcuron for Injection ... 2478

Verapamil Hydrochloride (Chronic exposure to trace concentrations of halothane have been reported to increase hepatic microsomal enzyme activity and can inhibit the metabolism of drugs eliminated by the liver microsomal enzyme system such as verapamil). Products include:
Covera-HS Tablets ... 3199
Isoptin SR Tablets ... 467
Tarka Tablets ... 508
Verelan Capsules ... 3184
Verelan PM Capsules ... 3186

Ziprasidone Hydrochloride (Halothane has been reported to prolong the Q-T interval; co-administration with other drugs known to prolong the Q-T interval should be undertaken with caution). Products include:
Geodon Capsules ... 2688

Food Interactions

Alcohol (Co-administration with agents known to elevate hepatic levels of CYP450 enzyme, such as alcohol, enhances the metabolism of volatile anesthetics).

FLUSHIELD INFLUENZA VACCINE

(Influenza Virus Vaccine) ... 3521
May interact with alkylating agents, corticosteroids, cytotoxic drugs, theophylline, and certain other agents. Compounds in these categories include:

Aminophylline (Potential for elevated theophylline serum concentrations resulting in possible enhanced effects or toxicity).
No products indexed under this heading.

Betamethasone Acetate (Individual receiving large amount of corticosteroids as immunosuppressive agents may not respond optimally to active immunization procedures). Products include:
Celestone Soluspan Injectable Suspension ... 3097

Betamethasone Sodium Phosphate (Individual receiving large amount of corticosteroids as immunosuppressive agents may not respond optimally to active immunization procedures). Products include:
Celestone Soluspan Injectable Suspension ... 3097

Bleomycin Sulfate (Individual receiving large amount of cytotoxic agents may not respond optimally to active immunization procedures).
No products indexed under this heading.

Busulfan (Individual receiving large amount of alkylating agents may not respond optimally to active immunization procedures). Products include:
Myleran Tablets ... 1603

Carmustine (BCNU) (Individual receiving large amount of alkylating agents may not respond optimally to active immunization procedures). Products include:
Gliadel Wafer ... 1723

Chlorambucil (Individual receiving large amount of alkylating agents may not respond optimally to active immunization procedures). Products include:
Leukeran Tablets ... 1591

Cortisone Acetate (Individual receiving large amount of corticosteroids as immunosuppressive agents may not respond optimally to active immunization procedures). Products include:
Cortone Acetate Injectable Suspension ... 2059
Cortone Acetate Tablets ... 2061

Cyclophosphamide (Individual receiving large amount of cytotoxic agents may not respond optimally to active immunization procedures).
No products indexed under this heading.

Dacarbazine (Individual receiving large amount of alkylating agents

IMPORTANT NOTE: Always consult each drug listing in the patient's regimen for possible interactions.

may not respond optimally to active immunization procedures). Products include:

- DTIC-Dome 902

Daunorubicin Hydrochloride (Individual receiving large amount of cytotoxic agents may not respond optimally to active immunization procedures). Products include:

- Cerubidine for Injection 947

Dexamethasone (Individual receiving large amount of corticosteroids as immunosuppressive agents may not respond optimally to active immunization procedures). Products include:

- Decadron Elixir 2078
- Decadron Tablets 2079
- TobraDex Ophthalmic Ointment 542
- TobraDex Ophthalmic Suspension .. 541

Dexamethasone Acetate (Individual receiving large amount of corticosteroids as immunosuppressive agents may not respond optimally to active immunization procedures).

No products indexed under this heading.

Dexamethasone Sodium Phosphate (Individual receiving large amount of corticosteroids as immunosuppressive agents may not respond optimally to active immunization procedures). Products include:

- Decadron Phosphate Injection 2081
- Decadron Phosphate Sterile Ophthalmic Ointment 2083
- Decadron Phosphate Sterile Ophthalmic Solution 2084
- NeoDecadron Sterile Ophthalmic Solution 2144

Doxorubicin Hydrochloride (Individual receiving large amount of cytotoxic agents may not respond optimally to active immunization procedures). Products include:

- Adriamycin PFS/RDF Injection 2767
- Doxil Injection 566

Dyphylline (Potential for elevated theophylline serum concentrations resulting in possible enhanced effects or toxicity). Products include:

- Lufyllin Tablets 3347
- Lufyllin-400 Tablets 3347
- Lufyllin-GG Elixir 3348
- Lufyllin-GG Tablets 3348

Epirubicin Hydrochloride (Individual receiving large amount of cytotoxic agents may not respond optimally to active immunization procedures). Products include:

- Ellence Injection 2806

Fludrocortisone Acetate (Individual receiving large amount of corticosteroids as immunosuppressive agents may not respond optimally to active immunization procedures). Products include:

- Florinef Acetate Tablets 2250

Fluorouracil (Individual receiving large amount of cytotoxic agents may not respond optimally to active immunization procedures). Products include:

- Carac Cream 1222
- Efudex 1733
- Fluoroplex 552

Hydrocortisone (Individual receiving large amount of corticosteroids as immunosuppressive agents may not respond optimally to active immunization procedures). Products include:

- Anusol-HC Cream 2.5% 2237
- Cipro HC Otic Suspension 540
- Cortaid Intensive Therapy Cream .. ▣717
- Cortaid Maximum Strength Cream .... ▣717
- Cortisporin Ophthalmic Suspension Sterile .... ⊙297
- Cortizone•5 .... ▣699
- Cortizone•10 .... ▣699
- Cortizone•10 Plus Creme .... ▣700
- Cortizone for Kids Creme .... ▣699
- Hydrocortone Tablets 2106
- Massengill Medicated Soft Cloth Towelette .... ▣753
- VōSoL HC Otic Solution 3356

Hydrocortisone Acetate (Individual receiving large amount of corticosteroids as immunosuppressive agents may not respond optimally to active immunization procedures). Products include:

- Analpram-HC 1338
- Anusol HC-1 Hydrocortisone Anti-Itch Cream .... ▣689
- Anusol-HC Suppositories 2238
- Cortaid .... ▣717
- Cortifoam Rectal Foam 3170
- Cortisporin-TC Otic Suspension 2246
- Hydrocortone Acetate Injectable Suspension 2103
- Pramosone 1343
- Proctocort Suppositories 2264
- ProctoFoam-HC 3177
- Terra-Cortril Ophthalmic Suspension 2716

Hydrocortisone Sodium Phosphate (Individual receiving large amount of corticosteroids as immunosuppressive agents may not respond optimally to active immunization procedures). Products include:

- Hydrocortone Phosphate Injection, Sterile 2105

Hydrocortisone Sodium Succinate (Individual receiving large amount of corticosteroids as immunosuppressive agents may not respond optimally to active immunization procedures).

No products indexed under this heading.

Hydroxyurea (Individual receiving large amount of cytotoxic agents may not respond optimally to active immunization procedures). Products include:

- Mylocel Tablets 2227

Lomustine (CCNU) (Individual receiving large amount of alkylating agents may not respond optimally to active immunization procedures).

No products indexed under this heading.

Mechlorethamine Hydrochloride (Individual receiving large amount of alkylating agents may not respond optimally to active immunization procedures). Products include:

- Mustargen for Injection 2142

Melphalan (Individual receiving large amount of alkylating agents may not respond optimally to active immunization procedures). Products include:

- Alkeran Tablets 1466

Methotrexate Sodium (Individual receiving large amount of cytotoxic agents may not respond optimally to active immunization procedures).

No products indexed under this heading.

Methylprednisolone Acetate (Individual receiving large amount of corticosteroids as immunosuppressive agents may not respond optimally to active immunization procedures). Products include:

- Depo-Medrol Injectable Suspension 2795

Methylprednisolone Sodium Succinate (Individual receiving large amount of corticosteroids as immunosuppressive agents may not respond optimally to active immunization procedures). Products include:

- Solu-Medrol Sterile Powder 2855

Mitotane (Individual receiving large amount of cytotoxic agents may not respond optimally to active immunization procedures).

No products indexed under this heading.

Mitoxantrone Hydrochloride (Individual receiving large amount of cytotoxic agents may not respond optimally to active immunization procedures). Products include:

- Novantrone for Injection 1760

Prednisolone Acetate (Individual receiving large amount of corticosteroids as immunosuppressive agents may not respond optimally to active immunization procedures). Products include:

- Blephamide Ophthalmic Ointment 547
- Blephamide Ophthalmic Suspension 548
- Poly-Pred Liquifilm Ophthalmic Suspension .... ⊙245
- Pred Forte Ophthalmic Suspension .... ⊙246
- Pred Mild Sterile Ophthalmic Suspension .... ⊙249
- Pred-G Ophthalmic Suspension .... ⊙247
- Pred-G Sterile Ophthalmic Ointment .... ⊙248

Prednisolone Sodium Phosphate (Individual receiving large amount of corticosteroids as immunosuppressive agents may not respond optimally to active immunization procedures). Products include:

- Pediapred Oral Solution 1170

Prednisolone Tebutate (Individual receiving large amount of corticosteroids as immunosuppressive agents may not respond optimally to active immunization procedures).

No products indexed under this heading.

Prednisone (Individual receiving large amount of corticosteroids as immunosuppressive agents may not respond optimally to active immunization procedures). Products include:

- Prednisone 3064

Procarbazine Hydrochloride (Individual receiving large amount of cytotoxic agents may not respond optimally to active immunization procedures). Products include:

- Matulane Capsules 3246

Tamoxifen Citrate (Individual receiving large amount of cytotoxic agents may not respond optimally to active immunization procedures). Products include:

- Nolvadex Tablets 678

Theophylline (Potential for elevated theophylline serum concentrations resulting in possible enhanced effects or toxicity). Products include:

- Aerolate 1361
- Theo-Dur Extended-Release Tablets 1835
- Uni-Dur Extended-Release Tablets .. 1841
- Uniphyl 400 mg and 600 mg Tablets 2903

Theophylline Calcium Salicylate (Potential for elevated theophylline serum concentrations resulting in possible enhanced effects or toxicity).

No products indexed under this heading.

Theophylline Sodium Glycinate (Potential for elevated theophylline serum concentrations resulting in possible enhanced effects or toxicity).

No products indexed under this heading.

Thiotepa (Individual receiving large amount of alkylating agents may not respond optimally to active immunization procedures). Products include:

- Thioplex for Injection 1765

Triamcinolone (Individual receiving large amount of corticosteroids as immunosuppressive agents may not respond optimally to active immunization procedures).

No products indexed under this heading.

Triamcinolone Acetonide (Individual receiving large amount of corticosteroids as immunosuppressive agents may not respond optimally to active immunization procedures). Products include:

- Azmacort Inhalation Aerosol 728
- Nasacort Nasal Inhaler 750
- Nasacort AQ Nasal Spray 752
- Tri-Nasal Spray 2274

Triamcinolone Diacetate (Individual receiving large amount of corticosteroids as immunosuppressive agents may not respond optimally to active immunization procedures).

No products indexed under this heading.

Triamcinolone Hexacetonide (Individual receiving large amount of corticosteroids as immunosuppressive agents may not respond optimally to active immunization procedures).

No products indexed under this heading.

Vincristine Sulfate (Individual receiving large amount of cytotoxic agents may not respond optimally to active immunization procedures).

No products indexed under this heading.

Warfarin Sodium (Potential for hypoprothrombinemia resulting in possible enhanced effects or toxicity). Products include:

- Coumadin for Injection 1243
- Coumadin Tablets 1243
- Warfarin Sodium Tablets, USP 3302

FLUZONE VACCINE

(Influenza Virus Vaccine) 802

May interact with antineoplastics, corticosteroids, immunosuppressive agents, phenytoin, theophylline, and certain other agents. Compounds in these categories include:

Altretamine (The expected antibody response may not be obtained in patients with compromised immune system resulting from chemotherapy). Products include:

- Hexalen Capsules 2226

Aminophylline (Influenza vaccination can inhibit the clearance of theophylline, however, studies have failed to show any adverse clinical effects attributable to co-administration).

No products indexed under this heading.

Anastrozole (The expected antibody response may not be obtained in patients with compromised immune system resulting from chemotherapy). Products include:

- Arimidex Tablets 659

Asparaginase (The expected antibody response may not be obtained in patients with compromised immune system resulting from chemotherapy). Products include:

- Elspar for Injection 2092

Azathioprine (The expected antibody response may not be obtained in patients on immunosuppressive therapy).

No products indexed under this heading.

Basiliximab (The expected antibody response may not be obtained in patients on immunosuppressive therapy). Products include:

- Simulect for Injection 2399

Betamethasone Acetate (The expected antibody response may not be obtained in patients with compromised immune system resulting from corticosteroid therapy). Products include:

- Celestone Soluspan Injectable Suspension 3097

Betamethasone Sodium Phosphate (The expected antibody response may not be obtained in patients with compromised immune system resulting from corticosteroid therapy). Products include:

- Celestone Soluspan Injectable Suspension 3097

Bicalutamide (The expected antibody response may not be obtained in patients with compromised immune system resulting from chemotherapy). Products include:

Casodex Tablets 662

Bleomycin Sulfate (The expected antibody response may not be obtained in patients with compromised immune system resulting from chemotherapy).
No products indexed under this heading.

Busulfan (The expected antibody response may not be obtained in patients with compromised immune system resulting from chemotherapy). Products include:
Myleran Tablets 1603

Carboplatin (The expected antibody response may not be obtained in patients with compromised immune system resulting from chemotherapy). Products include:
Paraplatin for Injection 1126

Carmustine (BCNU) (The expected antibody response may not be obtained in patients with compromised immune system resulting from chemotherapy). Products include:
Gliadel Wafer 1723

Chlorambucil (The expected antibody response may not be obtained in patients with compromised immune system resulting from chemotherapy). Products include:
Leukeran Tablets 1591

Cisplatin (The expected antibody response may not be obtained in patients with compromised immune system resulting from chemotherapy).
No products indexed under this heading.

Cortisone Acetate (The expected antibody response may not be obtained in patients with compromised immune system resulting from corticosteroid therapy). Products include:
Cortone Acetate Injectable Suspension 2059
Cortone Acetate Tablets 2061

Cyclophosphamide (The expected antibody response may not be obtained in patients with compromised immune system resulting from chemotherapy).
No products indexed under this heading.

Cyclosporine (The expected antibody response may not be obtained in patients on immunosuppressive therapy). Products include:
Gengraf Capsules 457
Neoral Soft Gelatin Capsules 2380
Neoral Oral Solution 2380
Sandimmune 2388

Dacarbazine (The expected antibody response may not be obtained in patients with compromised immune system resulting from chemotherapy). Products include:
DTIC-Dome 902

Daunorubicin Citrate (The expected antibody response may not be obtained in patients with compromised immune system resulting from chemotherapy). Products include:
DaunoXome Injection 1442

Daunorubicin Hydrochloride (The expected antibody response may not be obtained in patients with compromised immune system resulting from chemotherapy). Products include:
Cerubidine for Injection 947

Denileukin Diftitox (The expected antibody response may not be obtained in patients with compromised immune system resulting from chemotherapy).
No products indexed under this heading.

Dexamethasone (The expected antibody response may not be obtained in patients with compromised immune system resulting from corticosteroid therapy). Products include:
Decadron Elixir 2078
Decadron Tablets 2079
TobraDex Ophthalmic Ointment 542
TobraDex Ophthalmic Suspension .. 541

Dexamethasone Acetate (The expected antibody response may not be obtained in patients with compromised immune system resulting from corticosteroid therapy).
No products indexed under this heading.

Dexamethasone Sodium Phosphate (The expected antibody response may not be obtained in patients with compromised immune system resulting from corticosteroid therapy). Products include:
Decadron Phosphate Injection 2081
Decadron Phosphate Sterile Ophthalmic Ointment 2083
Decadron Phosphate Sterile Ophthalmic Solution 2084
NeoDecadron Sterile Ophthalmic Solution 2144

Docetaxel (The expected antibody response may not be obtained in patients with compromised immune system resulting from chemotherapy). Products include:
Taxotere for Injection Concentrate 778

Doxorubicin Hydrochloride (The expected antibody response may not be obtained in patients with compromised immune system resulting from chemotherapy). Products include:
Adriamycin PFS/RDF Injection 2767
Doxil Injection 566

Dyphylline (Influenza vaccination can inhibit the clearance of theophylline, however, studies have failed to show any adverse clinical effects attributable to co-administration). Products include:
Lufyllin Tablets 3347
Lufyllin-400 Tablets 3347
Lufyllin-GG Elixir 3348
Lufyllin-GG Tablets 3348

Epirubicin Hydrochloride (The expected antibody response may not be obtained in patients with compromised immune system resulting from chemotherapy). Products include:
Ellence Injection 2806

Estramustine Phosphate Sodium (The expected antibody response may not be obtained in patients with compromised immune system resulting from chemotherapy). Products include:
Emcyt Capsules 2810

Etoposide (The expected antibody response may not be obtained in patients with compromised immune system resulting from chemotherapy).
No products indexed under this heading.

Exemestane (The expected antibody response may not be obtained in patients with compromised immune system resulting from chemotherapy). Products include:
Aromasin Tablets 2769

Floxuridine (The expected antibody response may not be obtained in patients with compromised immune system resulting from chemotherapy). Products include:
Sterile FUDR 2974

Fludrocortisone Acetate (The expected antibody response may not be obtained in patients with compromised immune system resulting from corticosteroid therapy). Products include:
Florinef Acetate Tablets 2250

Fluorouracil (The expected antibody response may not be obtained in patients with compromised immune system resulting from chemotherapy). Products include:
Carac Cream 1222
Efudex 1733
Fluoroplex 552

Flutamide (The expected antibody response may not be obtained in patients with compromised immune system resulting from chemotherapy). Products include:
Eulexin Capsules 3118

Fosphenytoin Sodium (Influenza vaccination can inhibit the clearance of phenytoin, however, studies have failed to show any adverse clinical effects attributable to co-administration). Products include:
Cerebyx Injection 2619

Gemcitabine Hydrochloride (The expected antibody response may not be obtained in patients with compromised immune system resulting from chemotherapy). Products include:
Gemzar for Injection 1919

Hydrocortisone (The expected antibody response may not be obtained in patients with compromised immune system resulting from corticosteroid therapy). Products include:
Anusol-HC Cream 2.5% 2237
Cipro HC Otic Suspension 540
Cortaid Intensive Therapy Cream .◘ 717
Cortaid Maximum Strength Cream .... ◘ 717
Cortisporin Ophthalmic Suspension Sterile .... ⊙ 297
Cortizone•5 .... ◘ 699
Cortizone•10 .... ◘ 699
Cortizone•10 Plus Creme .... ◘ 700
Cortizone for Kids Creme .... ◘ 699
Hydrocortone Tablets 2106
Massengill Medicated Soft Cloth Towelette .... ◘ 753
VōSoL HC Otic Solution 3356

Hydrocortisone Acetate (The expected antibody response may not be obtained in patients with compromised immune system resulting from corticosteroid therapy). Products include:
Analpram-HC 1338
Anusol HC-1 Hydrocortisone Anti-Itch Cream .... ◘ 689
Anusol-HC Suppositories 2238
Cortaid .... ◘ 717
Cortifoam Rectal Foam 3170
Cortisporin-TC Otic Suspension 2246
Hydrocortone Acetate Injectable Suspension 2103
Pramosone 1343
Proctocort Suppositories 2264
ProctoFoam-HC 3177
Terra-Cortril Ophthalmic Suspension 2716

Hydrocortisone Sodium Phosphate (The expected antibody response may not be obtained in patients with compromised immune system resulting from corticosteroid therapy). Products include:
Hydrocortone Phosphate Injection, Sterile 2105

Hydrocortisone Sodium Succinate (The expected antibody response may not be obtained in patients with compromised immune system resulting from corticosteroid therapy).
No products indexed under this heading.

Hydroxyurea (The expected antibody response may not be obtained in patients with compromised immune system resulting from chemotherapy). Products include:
Mylocel Tablets 2227

Idarubicin Hydrochloride (The expected antibody response may not be obtained in patients with compromised immune system resulting from chemotherapy). Products include:
Idamycin PFS Injection 2825

Ifosfamide (The expected antibody response may not be obtained in patients with compromised immune system resulting from chemotherapy). Products include:
Ifex for Injection 1123

Interferon alfa-2A, Recombinant (The expected antibody response may not be obtained in patients with compromised immune system resulting from chemotherapy). Products include:
Roferon-A Injection 2996

Interferon alfa-2B, Recombinant (The expected antibody response may not be obtained in patients with compromised immune system resulting from chemotherapy). Products include:
Intron A for Injection 3120
Rebetron Combination Therapy 3153

Irinotecan Hydrochloride (The expected antibody response may not be obtained in patients with compromised immune system resulting from chemotherapy).
No products indexed under this heading.

Levamisole Hydrochloride (The expected antibody response may not be obtained in patients with compromised immune system resulting from chemotherapy). Products include:
Ergamisol Tablets 1789

Lomustine (CCNU) (The expected antibody response may not be obtained in patients with compromised immune system resulting from chemotherapy).
No products indexed under this heading.

Mechlorethamine Hydrochloride (The expected antibody response may not be obtained in patients with compromised immune system resulting from chemotherapy). Products include:
Mustargen for Injection 2142

Megestrol Acetate (The expected antibody response may not be obtained in patients with compromised immune system resulting from chemotherapy). Products include:
Megace Oral Suspension 1124

Melphalan (The expected antibody response may not be obtained in patients with compromised immune system resulting from chemotherapy). Products include:
Alkeran Tablets 1466

Mercaptopurine (The expected antibody response may not be obtained in patients with compromised immune system resulting from chemotherapy). Products include:
Purinethol Tablets 1615

Methotrexate Sodium (The expected antibody response may not be obtained in patients with compromised immune system resulting from chemotherapy).
No products indexed under this heading.

Methylprednisolone Acetate (The expected antibody response may not be obtained in patients with compromised immune system resulting from corticosteroid therapy). Products include:
Depo-Medrol Injectable Suspension 2795

Methylprednisolone Sodium Succinate (The expected antibody response may not be obtained in patients with compromised immune system resulting from corticosteroid therapy). Products include:
Solu-Medrol Sterile Powder 2855

Mitomycin (Mitomycin-C) (The expected antibody response may not be obtained in patients with compromised immune system resulting from chemotherapy).
No products indexed under this heading.

Mitotane (The expected antibody response may not be obtained in patients with compromised immune system resulting from chemotherapy).
No products indexed under this heading.

Mitoxantrone Hydrochloride (The expected antibody response may not

be obtained in patients with compromised immune system resulting from chemotherapy). Products include:

Novantrone for Injection 1760

Muromonab-CD3 (The expected antibody response may not be obtained in patients on immunosuppressive therapy). Products include:

Orthoclone OKT3 Sterile Solution ... 2498

Mycophenolate Mofetil (The expected antibody response may not be obtained in patients on immunosuppressive therapy). Products include:

CellCept Capsules 2951
CellCept Oral Suspension 2951
CellCept Tablets 2951

Paclitaxel (The expected antibody response may not be obtained in patients with compromised immune system resulting from chemotherapy). Products include:

Taxol Injection 1129

Phenytoin (Influenza vaccination can inhibit the clearance of phenytoin, however, studies have failed to show any adverse clinical effects attributable to co-administration). Products include:

Dilantin Infatabs 2624
Dilantin-125 Oral Suspension 2625

Phenytoin Sodium (Influenza vaccination can inhibit the clearance of phenytoin, however, studies have failed to show any adverse clinical effects attributable to co-administration). Products include:

Dilantin Kapseals 2622

Prednisolone Acetate (The expected antibody response may not be obtained in patients with compromised immune system resulting from corticosteroid therapy). Products include:

Blephamide Ophthalmic Ointment ... 547
Blephamide Ophthalmic Suspension 548
Poly-Pred Liquifilm Ophthalmic Suspension .... ⊙245
Pred Forte Ophthalmic Suspension .... ⊙246
Pred Mild Sterile Ophthalmic Suspension .... ⊙249
Pred-G Ophthalmic Suspension ..... ⊙247
Pred-G Sterile Ophthalmic Ointment .... ⊙248

Prednisolone Sodium Phosphate (The expected antibody response may not be obtained in patients with compromised immune system resulting from corticosteroid therapy). Products include:

Pediapred Oral Solution 1170

Prednisolone Tebutate (The expected antibody response may not be obtained in patients with compromised immune system resulting from corticosteroid therapy).

No products indexed under this heading.

Prednisone (The expected antibody response may not be obtained in patients with compromised immune system resulting from corticosteroid therapy). Products include:

Prednisone 3064

Procarbazine Hydrochloride (The expected antibody response may not be obtained in patients with compromised immune system resulting from chemotherapy). Products include:

Matulane Capsules 3246

Sirolimus (The expected antibody response may not be obtained in patients on immunosuppressive therapy). Products include:

Rapamune Oral Solution and Tablets 3584

Streptozocin (The expected antibody response may not be obtained in patients with compromised immune system resulting from chemotherapy).

No products indexed under this heading.

Tacrolimus (The expected antibody response may not be obtained in patients on immunosuppressive therapy). Products include:

Prograf 1393
Protopic Ointment 1397

Tamoxifen Citrate (The expected antibody response may not be obtained in patients with compromised immune system resulting from chemotherapy). Products include:

Nolvadex Tablets 678

Teniposide (The expected antibody response may not be obtained in patients with compromised immune system resulting from chemotherapy).

No products indexed under this heading.

Theophylline (Influenza vaccination can inhibit the clearance of theophylline, however, studies have failed to show any adverse clinical effects attributable to co-administration). Products include:

Aerolate 1361
Theo-Dur Extended-Release Tablets 1835
Uni-Dur Extended-Release Tablets .. 1841
Uniphyl 400 mg and 600 mg Tablets 2903

Theophylline Calcium Salicylate (Influenza vaccination can inhibit the clearance of theophylline, however, studies have failed to show any adverse clinical effects attributable to co-administration).

No products indexed under this heading.

Theophylline Sodium Glycinate (Influenza vaccination can inhibit the clearance of theophylline, however, studies have failed to show any adverse clinical effects attributable to co-administration).

No products indexed under this heading.

Thioguanine (The expected antibody response may not be obtained in patients with compromised immune system resulting from chemotherapy). Products include:

Tabloid Tablets 1642

Thiotepa (The expected antibody response may not be obtained in patients with compromised immune system resulting from chemotherapy). Products include:

Thioplex for Injection 1765

Topotecan Hydrochloride (The expected antibody response may not be obtained in patients with compromised immune system resulting from chemotherapy). Products include:

Hycamtin for Injection 1546

Toremifene Citrate (The expected antibody response may not be obtained in patients with compromised immune system resulting from chemotherapy). Products include:

Fareston Tablets 3237

Triamcinolone (The expected antibody response may not be obtained in patients with compromised immune system resulting from corticosteroid therapy).

No products indexed under this heading.

Triamcinolone Acetonide (The expected antibody response may not be obtained in patients with compromised immune system resulting from corticosteroid therapy). Products include:

Azmacort Inhalation Aerosol 728
Nasacort Nasal Inhaler 750
Nasacort AQ Nasal Spray 752
Tri-Nasal Spray 2274

Triamcinolone Diacetate (The expected antibody response may not be obtained in patients with compromised immune system resulting from corticosteroid therapy).

No products indexed under this heading.

Triamcinolone Hexacetonide (The expected antibody response may not be obtained in patients with compromised immune system resulting from corticosteroid therapy).

No products indexed under this heading.

Valrubicin (The expected antibody response may not be obtained in patients with compromised immune system resulting from chemotherapy). Products include:

Valstar Sterile Solution for Intravesical Instillation 1175

Vincristine Sulfate (The expected antibody response may not be obtained in patients with compromised immune system resulting from chemotherapy).

No products indexed under this heading.

Vinorelbine Tartrate (The expected antibody response may not be obtained in patients with compromised immune system resulting from chemotherapy). Products include:

Navelbine Injection 1604

Warfarin Sodium (Influenza vaccination can inhibit the clearance of warfarin, however, studies have failed to show any adverse clinical effects attributable to co-administration). Products include:

Coumadin for Injection 1243
Coumadin Tablets 1243
Warfarin Sodium Tablets, USP 3302

FML OPHTHALMIC OINTMENT

(Fluorometholone) .... ⊙237
None cited in PDR database.

FML OPHTHALMIC SUSPENSION

(Fluorometholone) .... ⊙236
None cited in PDR database.

FML FORTE OPHTHALMIC SUSPENSION

(Fluorometholone) .... ⊙235
None cited in PDR database.

FML-S LIQUIFILM STERILE OPHTHALMIC SUSPENSION

(Fluorometholone, Sulfacetamide Sodium) .... ⊙238
May interact with silver preparations. Compounds in these categories include:

Silver Nitrate (Sulfacetamide preparations are incompatible with silver preparations).

No products indexed under this heading.

FOLLISTIM FOR INJECTION

(Follitropin Beta) 2465
None cited in PDR database.

FOOD FOR THOUGHT DRINK MIX

(Amino Acid Preparations, Vitamins with Minerals) .... ▣844
May interact with:

Aluminum Carbonate (Concomitant use with aluminum-containing antacids should be avoided).

No products indexed under this heading.

Aluminum Hydroxide (Concomitant use with aluminum-containing antacids should be avoided). Products include:

Amphojel Suspension (Mint Flavor) .... ▣789
Gaviscon Extra Strength Liquid ...... ▣751
Gaviscon Extra Strength Tablets .... ▣751
Gaviscon Regular Strength Liquid . ▣751
Gaviscon Regular Strength Tablets .... ▣750
Maalox Antacid/Anti-Gas Oral Suspension .... ▣673
Maalox Max Maximum Strength Antacid/Anti-Gas Liquid 2300
Maalox Regular Strength Antacid/Antigas Liquid 2300
Mylanta 1813
Vanquish Caplets .... ▣617

FORADIL AEROLIZER

(Formoterol Fumarate) 2354
May interact with beta blockers, glucocorticoids, monoamine oxidase inhibitors, potassium-depleting diuretics, drugs that prolong the QT interval, sympathomimetics, tricyclic antidepressants, and theophylline. Compounds in these categories include:

Acebutolol Hydrochloride (Co-administration with beta-blockers may inhibit the effect of each other, beta-blockers not only block the therapeutic effect of beta-agonists, such as formoterol, but may produce severe bronchospasm in patients with asthma). Products include:

Sectral Capsules 3589

Albuterol (Co-administration with additional adrenergic drugs may potentiate the sympathetic effects of formoterol). Products include:

Proventil Inhalation Aerosol 3142
Ventolin Inhalation Aerosol and Refill 1679

Albuterol Sulfate (Co-administration with additional adrenergic drugs may potentiate the sympathetic effects of formoterol). Products include:

AccuNeb Inhalation Solution 1230
Combivent Inhalation Aerosol 1041
DuoNeb Inhalation Solution 1233
Proventil Inhalation Solution 0.083% 3146
Proventil Repetabs Tablets 3148
Proventil Solution for Inhalation 0.5% 3144
Proventil HFA Inhalation Aerosol 3150
Ventolin HFA Inhalation Aerosol 3618
Volmax Extended-Release Tablets .. 2276

Aminophylline (Co-administration with xanthine derivatives may potentiate hypokalemic effect of adrenergic agonists).

No products indexed under this heading.

Amiodarone Hydrochloride (Co-administration with drugs known to prolong the QTc interval have an increased risk of ventricular arrhythmias). Products include:

Cordarone Intravenous 3491
Cordarone Tablets 3487
Pacerone Tablets 3331

Amitriptyline Hydrochloride (Concurrent and/or sequential administration with tricyclic antidepressants may potentiate the action of salmeterol on vascular system). Products include:

Etrafon 3115
Limbitrol 1738

Amoxapine (Concurrent and/or sequential administration with tricyclic antidepressants may potentiate the action of salmeterol on vascular system).

No products indexed under this heading.

Astemizole (Co-administration with drugs known to prolong the QTc interval have an increased risk of ventricular arrhythmias).

No products indexed under this heading.

Atenolol (Co-administration with beta-blockers may inhibit the effect of each other, beta-blockers not only block the therapeutic effect of beta-agonists, such as formoterol, but may produce severe bronchospasm in patients with asthma). Products include:

Tenoretic Tablets 690
Tenormin I.V. Injection 692

Bendroflumethiazide (The ECG changes and/or hypokalemia that may result from the administration of non-potassium sparing diuretics can be acutely worsened by beta-agonists, especially when the recommended dose of beta-agonist is exceeded). Products include:
- Corzide 40/5 Tablets 2247
- Corzide 80/5 Tablets 2247

Betamethasone Acetate (Co-administration with glucocorticosteroids may potentiate hypokalemic effect of adrenergic agonists). Products include:
- Celestone Soluspan Injectable Suspension 3097

Betamethasone Sodium Phosphate (Co-administration with glucocorticosteroids may potentiate hypokalemic effect of adrenergic agonists). Products include:
- Celestone Soluspan Injectable Suspension 3097

Betaxolol Hydrochloride (Co-administration with beta-blockers may inhibit the effect of each other, beta-blockers not only block the therapeutic effect of beta-agonists, such as formoterol, but may produce severe bronchospasm in patients with asthma). Products include:
- Betoptic S Ophthalmic Suspension 537

Bisoprolol Fumarate (Co-administration with beta-blockers may inhibit the effect of each other, beta-blockers not only block the therapeutic effect of beta-agonists, such as formoterol, but may produce severe bronchospasm in patients with asthma). Products include:
- Zebeta Tablets 1885
- Ziac Tablets 1887

Bretylium Tosylate (Co-administration with drugs known to prolong the QTc interval have an increased risk of ventricular arrhythmias).
- No products indexed under this heading.

Bumetanide (The ECG changes and/or hypokalemia that may result from the administration of non-potassium sparing diuretics can be acutely worsened by beta-agonists, especially when the recommended dose of beta-agonist is exceeded).
- No products indexed under this heading.

Carteolol Hydrochloride (Co-administration with beta-blockers may inhibit the effect of each other, beta-blockers not only block the therapeutic effect of beta-agonists, such as formoterol, but may produce severe bronchospasm in patients with asthma). Products include:
- Carteolol Hydrochloride Ophthalmic Solution USP, 1% .... ⊙258
- Ocupress Ophthalmic Solution, 1% Sterile .... ⊙303

Chlorothiazide (The ECG changes and/or hypokalemia that may result from the administration of non-potassium sparing diuretics can be acutely worsened by beta-agonists, especially when the recommended dose of beta-agonist is exceeded). Products include:
- Aldoclor Tablets 2035
- Diuril Oral 2087

Chlorothiazide Sodium (The ECG changes and/or hypokalemia that may result from the administration of non-potassium sparing diuretics can be acutely worsened by beta-agonists, especially when the recommended dose of beta-agonist is exceeded). Products include:
- Diuril Sodium Intravenous 2086

Chlorpromazine (Co-administration with drugs known to prolong the QTc interval have an increased risk of ventricular arrhythmias). Products include:
- Thorazine Suppositories 1656

Chlorpromazine Hydrochloride (Co-administration with drugs known to prolong the QTc interval have an increased risk of ventricular arrhythmias). Products include:
- Thorazine 1656

Clomipramine Hydrochloride (Concurrent and/or sequential administration with tricyclic antidepressants may potentiate the action of salmeterol on vascular system).
- No products indexed under this heading.

Cortisone Acetate (Co-administration with glucocorticosteroids may potentiate hypokalemic effect of adrenergic agonists). Products include:
- Cortone Acetate Injectable Suspension 2059
- Cortone Acetate Tablets 2061

Desipramine Hydrochloride (Concurrent and/or sequential administration with tricyclic antidepressants may potentiate the action of salmeterol on vascular system). Products include:
- Norpramin Tablets 755

Dexamethasone (Co-administration with glucocorticosteroids may potentiate hypokalemic effect of adrenergic agonists). Products include:
- Decadron Elixir 2078
- Decadron Tablets 2079
- TobraDex Ophthalmic Ointment 542
- TobraDex Ophthalmic Suspension 541

Dexamethasone Acetate (Co-administration with glucocorticosteroids may potentiate hypokalemic effect of adrenergic agonists).
- No products indexed under this heading.

Dexamethasone Sodium Phosphate (Co-administration with glucocorticosteroids may potentiate hypokalemic effect of adrenergic agonists). Products include:
- Decadron Phosphate Injection 2081
- Decadron Phosphate Sterile Ophthalmic Ointment 2083
- Decadron Phosphate Sterile Ophthalmic Solution 2084
- NeoDecadron Sterile Ophthalmic Solution 2144

Disopyramide Phosphate (Co-administration with drugs known to prolong the QTc interval have an increased risk of ventricular arrhythmias).
- No products indexed under this heading.

Dobutamine Hydrochloride (Co-administration with additional adrenergic drugs may potentiate the sympathetic effects of formoterol). Products include:
- Dobutrex Solution Vials 1914

Dofetilide (Co-administration with drugs known to prolong the QTc interval have an increased risk of ventricular arrhythmias). Products include:
- Tikosyn Capsules 2717

Dopamine Hydrochloride (Co-administration with additional adrenergic drugs may potentiate the sympathetic effects of formoterol).
- No products indexed under this heading.

Doxepin Hydrochloride (Concurrent and/or sequential administration with tricyclic antidepressants may potentiate the action of salmeterol on vascular system). Products include:
- Sinequan 2713

Dyphylline (Co-administration with xanthine derivatives may potentiate hypokalemic effect of adrenergic agonists). Products include:
- Lufyllin Tablets 3347
- Lufyllin-400 Tablets 3347
- Lufyllin-GG Elixir 3348
- Lufyllin-GG Tablets 3348

Ephedrine Hydrochloride (Co-administration with additional adrenergic drugs may potentiate the sympathetic effects of formoterol). Products include:
- Primatene Tablets .... ▣780

Ephedrine Sulfate (Co-administration with additional adrenergic drugs may potentiate the sympathetic effects of formoterol).
- No products indexed under this heading.

Ephedrine Tannate (Co-administration with additional adrenergic drugs may potentiate the sympathetic effects of formoterol). Products include:
- Rynatuss Pediatric Suspension 3353
- Rynatuss Tablets 3353

Epinephrine (Co-administration with additional adrenergic drugs may potentiate the sympathetic effects of formoterol). Products include:
- Epifrin Sterile Ophthalmic Solution .... ⊙235
- EpiPen 1236
- Primatene Mist .... ▣779
- Xylocaine with Epinephrine Injection 653

Epinephrine Bitartrate (Co-administration with additional adrenergic drugs may potentiate the sympathetic effects of formoterol). Products include:
- Sensorcaine 643

Epinephrine Hydrochloride (Co-administration with additional adrenergic drugs may potentiate the sympathetic effects of formoterol).
- No products indexed under this heading.

Esmolol Hydrochloride (Co-administration with beta-blockers may inhibit the effect of each other, beta-blockers not only block the therapeutic effect of beta-agonists, such as formoterol, but may produce severe bronchospasm in patients with asthma). Products include:
- Brevibloc Injection 858

Ethacrynic Acid (The ECG changes and/or hypokalemia that may result from the administration of non-potassium sparing diuretics can be acutely worsened by beta-agonists, especially when the recommended dose of beta-agonist is exceeded). Products include:
- Edecrin Tablets 2091

Flecainide Acetate (Co-administration with drugs known to prolong the QTc interval have an increased risk of ventricular arrhythmias). Products include:
- Tambocor Tablets 1990

Fludrocortisone Acetate (Co-administration with glucocorticosteroids may potentiate hypokalemic effect of adrenergic agonists). Products include:
- Florinef Acetate Tablets 2250

Fluphenazine Decanoate (Co-administration with drugs known to prolong the QTc interval have an increased risk of ventricular arrhythmias).
- No products indexed under this heading.

Fluphenazine Enanthate (Co-administration with drugs known to prolong the QTc interval have an increased risk of ventricular arrhythmias).
- No products indexed under this heading.

Fluphenazine Hydrochloride (Co-administration with drugs known to prolong the QTc interval have an increased risk of ventricular arrhythmias).
- No products indexed under this heading.

Furosemide (The ECG changes and/or hypokalemia that may result from the administration of non-potassium sparing diuretics can be acutely worsened by beta-agonists, especially when the recommended dose of beta-agonist is exceeded). Products include:
- Furosemide Tablets 2284

Hydrochlorothiazide (The ECG changes and/or hypokalemia that may result from the administration of non-potassium sparing diuretics can be acutely worsened by beta-agonists, especially when the recommended dose of beta-agonist is exceeded). Products include:
- Accuretic Tablets 2614
- Aldoril Tablets 2039
- Atacand HCT Tablets 597
- Avalide Tablets 1070
- Diovan HCT Tablets 2338
- Dyazide Capsules 1515
- HydroDIURIL Tablets 2108
- Hyzaar 2109
- Inderide Tablets 3517
- Inderide LA Long-Acting Capsules 3519
- Lotensin HCT Tablets 2367
- Maxzide 1008
- Micardis HCT Tablets 1051
- Microzide Capsules 3414
- Moduretic Tablets 2138
- Monopril HCT 1094
- Prinzide Tablets 2168
- Timolide Tablets 2187
- Uniretic Tablets 3178
- Vaseretic Tablets 2204
- Zestoretic Tablets 695
- Ziac Tablets 1887

Hydrocortisone (Co-administration with glucocorticosteroids may potentiate hypokalemic effect of adrenergic agonists). Products include:
- Anusol-HC Cream 2.5% 2237
- Cipro HC Otic Suspension 540
- Cortaid Intensive Therapy Cream .... ▣717
- Cortaid Maximum Strength Cream .... ▣717
- Cortisporin Ophthalmic Suspension Sterile .... ⊙297
- Cortizone•5 .... ▣699
- Cortizone•10 .... ▣699
- Cortizone•10 Plus Creme .... ▣700
- Cortizone for Kids Creme .... ▣699
- Hydrocortone Tablets 2106
- Massengill Medicated Soft Cloth Towelette .... ▣753
- VōSoL HC Otic Solution 3356

Hydrocortisone Acetate (Co-administration with glucocorticosteroids may potentiate hypokalemic effect of adrenergic agonists). Products include:
- Analpram-HC 1338
- Anusol HC-1 Hydrocortisone Anti-Itch Cream .... ▣689
- Anusol-HC Suppositories 2238
- Cortaid .... ▣717
- Cortifoam Rectal Foam 3170
- Cortisporin-TC Otic Suspension 2246
- Hydrocortone Acetate Injectable Suspension 2103
- Pramosone 1343
- Proctocort Suppositories 2264
- ProctoFoam-HC 3177
- Terra-Cortril Ophthalmic Suspension 2716

Hydrocortisone Sodium Phosphate (Co-administration with glucocorticosteroids may potentiate hypokalemic effect of adrenergic agonists). Products include:
- Hydrocortone Phosphate Injection, Sterile 2105

Hydrocortisone Sodium Succinate (Co-administration with glucocorticosteroids may potentiate hypokalemic effect of adrenergic agonists).
- No products indexed under this heading.

Hydroflumethiazide (The ECG changes and/or hypokalemia that may result from the administration of non-potassium sparing diuretics can be acutely worsened by beta-agonists, especially when the recommended dose of beta-agonist is exceeded). Products include:
- Diucardin Tablets 3494

Imipramine Hydrochloride (Concurrent and/or sequential administration with tricyclic antidepressants

may potentiate the action of salmeterol on vascular system).
No products indexed under this heading.

Imipramine Pamoate (Concurrent and/or sequential administration with tricyclic antidepressants may potentiate the action of salmeterol on vascular system).
No products indexed under this heading.

Isocarboxazid (Concurrent and/or sequential administration with MAO inhibitors may potentiate the action of salmeterol on vascular system).
No products indexed under this heading.

Isoproterenol Hydrochloride (Co-administration with additional adrenergic drugs may potentiate the sympathetic effects of formoterol).
No products indexed under this heading.

Isoproterenol Sulfate (Co-administration with additional adrenergic drugs may potentiate the sympathetic effects of formoterol).
No products indexed under this heading.

Labetalol Hydrochloride (Co-administration with beta-blockers may inhibit the effect of each other, beta-blockers not only block the therapeutic effect of beta-agonists, such as formoterol, but may produce severe bronchospasm in patients with asthma). Products include:
Normodyne Injection **3135**
Normodyne Tablets **3137**

Levalbuterol Hydrochloride (Co-administration with additional adrenergic drugs may potentiate the sympathetic effects of formoterol). Products include:
Xopenex Inhalation Solution **3207**

Levobunolol Hydrochloride (Co-administration with beta-blockers may inhibit the effect of each other, beta-blockers not only block the therapeutic effect of beta-agonists, such as formoterol, but may produce severe bronchospasm in patients with asthma). Products include:
Betagan .... ⊙**228**

Lidocaine Hydrochloride (Co-administration with drugs known to prolong the QTc interval have an increased risk of ventricular arrhythmias). Products include:
Bactine First Aid Liquid .... ▣**611**
Xylocaine Injections **653**

Maprotiline Hydrochloride (Concurrent and/or sequential administration with tricyclic antidepressants may potentiate the action of salmeterol on vascular system).
No products indexed under this heading.

Mesoridazine Besylate (Co-administration with drugs known to prolong the QTc interval have an increased risk of ventricular arrhythmias). Products include:
Serentil **1057**

Metaproterenol Sulfate (Co-administration with additional adrenergic drugs may potentiate the sympathetic effects of formoterol). Products include:
Alupent **1029**

Metaraminol Bitartrate (Co-administration with additional adrenergic drugs may potentiate the sympathetic effects of formoterol). Products include:
Aramine Injection **2043**

Methoxamine Hydrochloride (Co-administration with additional adrenergic drugs may potentiate the sympathetic effects of formoterol).
No products indexed under this heading.

Methyclothiazide (The ECG changes and/or hypokalemia that may result from the administration of non-potassium sparing diuretics can be acutely worsened by beta-agonists, especially when the recommended dose of beta-agonist is exceeded).
No products indexed under this heading.

Methylprednisolone Acetate (Co-administration with glucocorticosteroids may potentiate hypokalemic effect of adrenergic agonists). Products include:
Depo-Medrol Injectable Suspension **2795**

Methylprednisolone Sodium Succinate (Co-administration with glucocorticosteroids may potentiate hypokalemic effect of adrenergic agonists). Products include:
Solu-Medrol Sterile Powder **2855**

Metipranolol Hydrochloride (Co-administration with beta-blockers may inhibit the effect of each other, beta-blockers not only block the therapeutic effect of beta-agonists, such as formoterol, but may produce severe bronchospasm in patients with asthma).
No products indexed under this heading.

Metoprolol Succinate (Co-administration with beta-blockers may inhibit the effect of each other, beta-blockers not only block the therapeutic effect of beta-agonists, such as formoterol, but may produce severe bronchospasm in patients with asthma). Products include:
Toprol-XL Tablets **651**

Metoprolol Tartrate (Co-administration with beta-blockers may inhibit the effect of each other, beta-blockers not only block the therapeutic effect of beta-agonists, such as formoterol, but may produce severe bronchospasm in patients with asthma).
No products indexed under this heading.

Mexiletine Hydrochloride (Co-administration with drugs known to prolong the QTc interval have an increased risk of ventricular arrhythmias). Products include:
Mexitil Capsules **1047**

Moclobemide (Concurrent and/or sequential administration with MAO inhibitors may potentiate the action of salmeterol on vascular system).
No products indexed under this heading.

Nadolol (Co-administration with beta-blockers may inhibit the effect of each other, beta-blockers not only block the therapeutic effect of beta-agonists, such as formoterol, but may produce severe bronchospasm in patients with asthma). Products include:
Corgard Tablets **2245**
Corzide 40/5 Tablets **2247**
Corzide 80/5 Tablets **2247**
Nadolol Tablets **2288**

Norepinephrine Bitartrate (Co-administration with additional adrenergic drugs may potentiate the sympathetic effects of formoterol).
No products indexed under this heading.

Nortriptyline Hydrochloride (Concurrent and/or sequential administration with tricyclic antidepressants may potentiate the action of salmeterol on vascular system).
No products indexed under this heading.

Pargyline Hydrochloride (Concurrent and/or sequential administration with MAO inhibitors may potentiate the action of salmeterol on vascular system).
No products indexed under this heading.

Penbutolol Sulfate (Co-administration with beta-blockers may inhibit the effect of each other, beta-blockers not only block the therapeutic effect of beta-agonists, such as formoterol, but may produce severe bronchospasm in patients with asthma).
No products indexed under this heading.

Perphenazine (Co-administration with drugs known to prolong the QTc interval have an increased risk of ventricular arrhythmias). Products include:
Etrafon **3115**
Trilafon **3160**

Phenelzine Sulfate (Concurrent and/or sequential administration with MAO inhibitors may potentiate the action of salmeterol on vascular system). Products include:
Nardil Tablets **2653**

Phenylephrine Bitartrate (Co-administration with additional adrenergic drugs may potentiate the sympathetic effects of formoterol).
No products indexed under this heading.

Phenylephrine Hydrochloride (Co-administration with additional adrenergic drugs may potentiate the sympathetic effects of formoterol). Products include:
Afrin Nasal Decongestant Children's Pump Mist .... ▣**734**
Extendryl **1361**
Hycomine Compound Tablets **1317**
Neo-Synephrine .... ▣**614**
Phenergan VC Syrup **3560**
Phenergan VC with Codeine Syrup .. **3561**
Preparation H Cream .... ▣**778**
Preparation H Cooling Gel .... ▣**778**
Preparation H .... ▣**778**
Vicks Sinex Nasal Spray and Ultra Fine Mist .... ▣**729**

Phenylephrine Tannate (Co-administration with additional adrenergic drugs may potentiate the sympathetic effects of formoterol). Products include:
Ryna-12 S Suspension **3351**
Reformulated Rynatan Pediatric Suspension **3352**
Rynatuss Pediatric Suspension **3353**
Rynatuss Tablets **3353**

Phenylpropanolamine Hydrochloride (Co-administration with additional adrenergic drugs may potentiate the sympathetic effects of formoterol).
No products indexed under this heading.

Pindolol (Co-administration with beta-blockers may inhibit the effect of each other, beta-blockers not only block the therapeutic effect of beta-agonists, such as formoterol, but may produce severe bronchospasm in patients with asthma).
No products indexed under this heading.

Pirbuterol Acetate (Co-administration with additional adrenergic drugs may potentiate the sympathetic effects of formoterol). Products include:
Maxair Autohaler **1981**
Maxair Inhaler **1984**

Polythiazide (The ECG changes and/or hypokalemia that may result from the administration of non-potassium sparing diuretics can be acutely worsened by beta-agonists, especially when the recommended dose of beta-agonist is exceeded). Products include:
Minizide Capsules **2700**
Renese Tablets **2712**

Prednisolone Acetate (Co-administration with glucocorticosteroids may potentiate hypokalemic effect of adrenergic agonists). Products include:
Blephamide Ophthalmic Ointment .. **547**
Blephamide Ophthalmic Suspension **548**
Poly-Pred Liquifilm Ophthalmic Suspension .... ⊙**245**
Pred Forte Ophthalmic Suspension .... ⊙**246**
Pred Mild Sterile Ophthalmic Suspension .... ⊙**249**
Pred-G Ophthalmic Suspension .... ⊙**247**
Pred-G Sterile Ophthalmic Ointment .... ⊙**248**

Prednisolone Sodium Phosphate (Co-administration with glucocorticosteroids may potentiate hypokalemic effect of adrenergic agonists). Products include:
Pediapred Oral Solution **1170**

Prednisolone Tebutate (Co-administration with glucocorticosteroids may potentiate hypokalemic effect of adrenergic agonists).
No products indexed under this heading.

Prednisone (Co-administration with glucocorticosteroids may potentiate hypokalemic effect of adrenergic agonists). Products include:
Prednisone **3064**

Procainamide Hydrochloride (Co-administration with drugs known to prolong the QTc interval have an increased risk of ventricular arrhythmias). Products include:
Procanbid Extended-Release Tablets **2262**

Procarbazine Hydrochloride (Concurrent and/or sequential administration with MAO inhibitors may potentiate the action of salmeterol on vascular system). Products include:
Matulane Capsules **3246**

Prochlorperazine (Co-administration with drugs known to prolong the QTc interval have an increased risk of ventricular arrhythmias). Products include:
Compazine **1505**

Promethazine Hydrochloride (Co-administration with drugs known to prolong the QTc interval have an increased risk of ventricular arrhythmias). Products include:
Mepergan Injection **3539**
Phenergan Injection **3553**
Phenergan **3556**
Phenergan Syrup **3554**
Phenergan with Codeine Syrup **3557**
Phenergan with Dextromethorphan Syrup **3559**
Phenergan VC Syrup **3560**
Phenergan VC with Codeine Syrup .. **3561**

Propafenone Hydrochloride (Co-administration with drugs known to prolong the QTc interval have an increased risk of ventricular arrhythmias). Products include:
Rythmol Tablets – 150 mg, 225 mg, 300 mg **502**

Propranolol Hydrochloride (Co-administration with beta-blockers may inhibit the effect of each other, beta-blockers not only block the therapeutic effect of beta-agonists, such as formoterol, but may produce severe bronchospasm in patients with asthma). Products include:
Inderal **3513**
Inderal LA Long-Acting Capsules **3516**
Inderide Tablets **3517**
Inderide LA Long-Acting Capsules .. **3519**

Protriptyline Hydrochloride (Concurrent and/or sequential administration with tricyclic antidepressants may potentiate the action of salmeterol on vascular system). Products include:
Vivactil Tablets **2446**
Vivactil Tablets **2217**

Pseudoephedrine Hydrochloride (Co-administration with additional adrenergic drugs may potentiate the sympathetic effects of formoterol). Products include:
Actifed Cold & Allergy Tablets .... ▣**688**
Actifed Cold & Sinus Caplets and Tablets .... ▣**688**
Advil Cold and Sinus Caplets .... ▣**771**
Advil Cold and Sinus Tablets .... ▣**771**
Advil Flu & Body Ache Caplets .... ▣**772**
Aleve Cold & Sinus Caplets .... ▣**603**

Alka-Seltzer Plus Liqui-Gels 604
Alka-Seltzer Plus Cold & Flu Medicine Liqui-Gels 604
Alka-Seltzer Plus Cold & Sinus Medicine Liqui-Gels 604
Allegra-D Extended-Release Tablets 714
BC Cold Powder 619
Benadryl Allergy/Cold Tablets 691
Benadryl Allergy/Congestion Tablets 692
Benadryl Allergy & Sinus Liquid 693
Benadryl Allergy & Sinus Fastmelt Tablets 693
Benadryl Allergy Sinus Headache Caplets & Gelcaps 693
Benadryl Severe Allergy & Sinus Headache Caplets 694
Benadryl Children's Allergy/Cold Fastmelt Tablets 692
Benylin Multi-Symptom Liquid 697
Bromfed Capsules (Extended-Release) 2269
Bromfed-PD Capsules (Extended-Release) 2269
Children's Cēpacol Sore Throat 788
Comtrex Acute Head Cold & Sinus Pressure Relief Tablets 627
Comtrex Deep Chest Cold & Congestion Relief Softgels 627
Comtrex Flu Therapy & Fever Relief Daytime Caplets 628
Comtrex Flu Therapy & Fever Relief Nighttime Tablets 628
Comtrex Maximum Strength Multi-Symptom Cold & Cough Relief Tablets and Caplets 626
Contac Non-Drowsy 12 Hour Cold Caplets 745
Contac Non-Drowsy Timed Release 12 Hour Cold Caplets 746
Contac Severe Cold and Flu Caplets Maximum Strength 746
Contac Severe Cold and Flu Caplets Non-Drowsy 746
Dimetapp Elixir 777
Dimetapp Cold and Fever Suspension 775
Dimetapp DM Cold & Cough Elixir 775
Dimetapp Nighttime Flu Liquid 776
Dimetapp Non-Drowsy Flu Syrup 777
Dimetapp Infant Drops Decongestant 775
Dimetapp Infant Drops Decongestant Plus Cough 776
Guaifed 2272
Kronofed-A 1341
Children's Motrin Cold Oral Suspension 2007
Motrin Sinus Headache Caplets 2005
PediaCare Cough-Cold Liquid 719
PediaCare Infants' Drops Decongestant 719
PediaCare Infants' Drops Decongestant Plus Cough 719
PediaCare NightRest Cough-Cold Liquid 719
Robitussin Cold Caplets Cold & Congestion 780
Robitussin Cold Softgels Cold & Congestion 780
Robitussin Cold Caplets Multi-Symptom Cold & Flu 781
Robitussin Cold Softgels Multi-Symptom Cold & Flu 781
Robitussin Cold Softgels Severe Congestion 782
Robitussin Cough & Cold Infant Drops 782
Robitussin Maximum Strength Cough & Cold Liquid 785
Robitussin Pediatric Cough & Cold Formula Liquid 785
Robitussin Multi Symptom Honey Flu Liquid 785
Robitussin Nighttime Honey Flu Liquid 786
Robitussin-CF Liquid 783
Robitussin-DAC Syrup 2942
Robitussin-PE Liquid 782
Ryna 768
Semprex-D Capsules 1172
Singlet Caplets 761
Sinutab Non-Drying Liquid Caps 706
Sinutab Sinus Allergy Medication, Maximum Strength Formula, Tablets & Caplets 707
Sinutab Sinus Medication, Maximum Strength Without Drowsiness Formula, Tablets & Caplets 707
Sudafed 12 Hour Tablets 708
Sudafed 24 Hour Tablets 708
Children's Sudafed Cold & Cough Liquid 709
Children's Sudafed Nasal Decongestant Chewables 711
Children's Sudafed Nasal Decongestant Liquid Medication 711
Sudafed Cold & Allergy Tablets 708
Sudafed Cold & Cough Liquid Caps 709
Sudafed Cold & Sinus Liquid Caps 710
Sudafed Nasal Decongestant Tablets 710
Sudafed Non-Drying Sinus Liquid Caps 712
Sudafed Severe Cold 711
Sudafed Sinus Headache Caplets 712
Sudafed Sinus Headache Tablets 712
Tavist Sinus Non-Drowsy Coated Caplets 676
TheraFlu Regular Strength Cold & Cough Night Time Hot Liquid 676
TheraFlu Regular Strength Cold & Sore Throat Night Time Hot Liquid 676
TheraFlu Maximum Strength Flu & Congestion Non-Drowsy Hot Liquid 677
TheraFlu Maximum Strength Flu & Cough Night Time Hot Liquid 678
TheraFlu Maximum Strength Flu & Sore Throat Night Time Hot Liquid 677
TheraFlu Maximum Strength Severe Cold & Congestion Night Time Caplets 678
TheraFlu Maximum Strength Severe Cold & Congestion Night Time Hot Liquid 678
TheraFlu Maximum Strength Severe Cold & Congestion Non-Drowsy 679
Triaminic Allergy Congestion Liquid 680
Triaminic Chest Congestion Liquid 680
Triaminic Cold & Allergy Liquid 681
Triaminic Cold & Allergy Softchews 683
Triaminic Cold & Cough Liquid 681
Triaminic Cold & Cough Softchews 683
Triaminic Cold & Night Time Cough Liquid 681
Triaminic Cold, Cough & Fever Liquid 681
Triaminic Cough Liquid 682
Triaminic Cough & Congestion Liquid 682
Triaminic Cough & Sore Throat Liquid 682
Triaminic Cough & Sore Throat Softchews 684
Children's Tylenol Allergy-D Liquid 2014
Children's Tylenol Cold Suspension Liquid and Chewable Tablets 2015
Children's Tylenol Cold Plus Cough Suspension Liquid and Chewable Tablets 2015
Children's Tylenol Flu Suspension Liquid 2015
Children's Tylenol Sinus Suspension Liquid 2017
Infants' Tylenol Cold Decongestant and Fever Reducer Concentrated Drops 2015
Infants' Tylenol Cold Decongestant and Fever Reducer Concentrated Drops Plus Cough 2015
Tylenol Allergy Sinus 2010
Multi-Symptom Tylenol Cold Complete Formula Caplets 2010
Multi-Symptom Tylenol Cold Non-Drowsy Caplets and Gelcaps 2010
Multi-Symptom Tylenol Cold Severe Congestion Non-Drowsy Caplets 2011
Maximum Strength Tylenol Flu NightTime Gelcaps 2011
Maximum Strength Tylenol Flu NightTime Liquid 2011
Maximum Strength Tylenol Flu Non-Drowsy Gelcaps 2011
Maximum Strength Tylenol Sinus NightTime Caplets 2012
Maximum Strength Tylenol Sinus Non-Drowsy Geltabs, Gelcaps, Caplets, and Tablets 2012
Vicks 44D Cough & Head Congestion Relief Liquid 724
Vicks 44M Cough, Cold & Flu Relief Liquid 725
Pediatric Vicks 44m Cough & Cold Relief 728
Vicks DayQuil LiquiCaps/Liquid Multi-Symptom Cold/Flu Relief 727
Children's Vicks NyQuil Cold/Cough Relief 726
Vicks NyQuil LiquiCaps/Liquid Multi-Symptom Cold/Flu Relief, Original and Cherry Flavors 727
Zephrex Tablets 3091
Zephrex LA Tablets 3092
Zyrtec-D 12 Hour Extended Relief Tablets 2758

Pseudoephedrine Sulfate (Co-administration with additional adrenergic drugs may potentiate the sympathetic effects of formoterol). Products include:
Chlor-Trimeton Allergy/Decongestant Tablets 736
Claritin-D 12 Hour Extended Release Tablets 3102
Claritin-D 24 Hour Extended Release Tablets 3104
Coricidin 'D' Cold, Flu & Sinus Tablets 737
Drixoral Allergy/Sinus Extended-Release Tablets 741
Drixoral Cold & Allergy Sustained-Action Tablets 740
Drixoral Cold & Flu Extended-Release Tablets 740
Drixoral Nasal Decongestant Long-Acting Non-Drowsy Tablets 740
Rynatan Tablets 3351

Quinidine Gluconate (Co-administration with drugs known to prolong the QTc interval have an increased risk of ventricular arrhythmias). Products include:
Quinaglute Dura-Tabs Tablets 978

Quinidine Polygalacturonate (Co-administration with drugs known to prolong the QTc interval have an increased risk of ventricular arrhythmias).
No products indexed under this heading.

Quinidine Sulfate (Co-administration with drugs known to prolong the QTc interval have an increased risk of ventricular arrhythmias). Products include:
Quinidex Extentabs 2933

Salmeterol Xinafoate (Co-administration with additional adrenergic drugs may potentiate the sympathetic effects of formoterol). Products include:
Advair Diskus 100/50 1448
Advair Diskus 250/50 1448
Advair Diskus 500/50 1448
Serevent Diskus 1637
Serevent Inhalation Aerosol 1633

Selegiline Hydrochloride (Concurrent and/or sequential administration with MAO inhibitors may potentiate the action of salmeterol on vascular system). Products include:
Eldepryl Capsules 3266

Sotalol Hydrochloride (Co-administration with beta-blockers may inhibit the effect of each other, beta-blockers not only block the therapeutic effect of beta-agonists, such as formoterol, but may produce severe bronchospasm in patients with asthma). Products include:
Betapace Tablets 950
Betapace AF Tablets 954

Terbutaline Sulfate (Co-administration with additional adrenergic drugs may potentiate the sympathetic effects of formoterol). Products include:
Brethine Ampuls 2314
Brethine Tablets 2313

Terfenadine (Co-administration with drugs known to prolong the QTc interval have an increased risk of ventricular arrhythmias).
No products indexed under this heading.

Theophylline (Co-administration with xanthine derivatives may potentiate hypokalemic effect of adrenergic agonists). Products include:
Aerolate 1361
Theo-Dur Extended-Release Tablets 1835
Uni-Dur Extended-Release Tablets 1841
Uniphyl 400 mg and 600 mg Tablets 2903

Theophylline Calcium Salicylate (Co-administration with xanthine derivatives may potentiate hypokalemic effect of adrenergic agonists).
No products indexed under this heading.

Theophylline Sodium Glycinate (Co-administration with xanthine derivatives may potentiate hypokalemic effect of adrenergic agonists).
No products indexed under this heading.

Thioridazine Hydrochloride (Co-administration with drugs known to prolong the QTc interval have an increased risk of ventricular arrhythmias). Products include:
Thioridazine Hydrochloride Tablets 2289

Timolol Hemihydrate (Co-administration with beta-blockers may inhibit the effect of each other, beta-blockers not only block the therapeutic effect of beta-agonists, such as formoterol, but may produce severe bronchospasm in patients with asthma). Products include:
Betimol Ophthalmic Solution .... ⊙ 324

Timolol Maleate (Co-administration with beta-blockers may inhibit the effect of each other, beta-blockers not only block the therapeutic effect of beta-agonists, such as formoterol, but may produce severe bronchospasm in patients with asthma). Products include:
Blocadren Tablets 2046
Cosopt Sterile Ophthalmic Solution 2065
Timolide Tablets 2187
Timolol GFS .... ⊙ 266
Timoptic in Ocudose 2192
Timoptic Sterile Ophthalmic Solution 2190
Timoptic-XE Sterile Ophthalmic Gel Forming Solution 2194

Tocainide Hydrochloride (Co-administration with drugs known to prolong the QTc interval have an increased risk of ventricular arrhythmias). Products include:
Tonocard Tablets 649

Torsemide (The ECG changes and/or hypokalemia that may result from the administration of non-potassium sparing diuretics can be acutely worsened by beta-agonists, especially when the recommended dose of beta-agonist is exceeded). Products include:
Demadex Tablets and Injection 2965

Tranylcypromine Sulfate (Concurrent and/or sequential administration with MAO inhibitors may potentiate the action of salmeterol on vascular system). Products include:
Parnate Tablets 1607

Triamcinolone (Co-administration with glucocorticosteroids may potentiate hypokalemic effect of adrenergic agonists).
No products indexed under this heading.

Triamcinolone Acetonide (Co-administration with glucocorticosteroids may potentiate hypokalemic effect of adrenergic agonists). Products include:
Azmacort Inhalation Aerosol 728
Nasacort Nasal Inhaler 750
Nasacort AQ Nasal Spray 752
Tri-Nasal Spray 2274

Triamcinolone Diacetate (Co-administration with glucocorticosteroids may potentiate hypokalemic effect of adrenergic agonists).
No products indexed under this heading.

Triamcinolone Hexacetonide (Co-administration with glucocorticosteroids may potentiate hypokalemic effect of adrenergic agonists).
No products indexed under this heading.

Trifluoperazine Hydrochloride (Co-administration with drugs known to prolong the QTc interval have an increased risk of ventricular arrhythmias). Products include:
Stelazine 1640
Trimipramine Maleate (Concurrent and/or sequential administration with tricyclic antidepressants may potentiate the action of salmeterol on vascular system). Products include:
Surmontil Capsules 3595
Ziprasidone Hydrochloride (Co-administration with drugs known to prolong the QTc interval have an increased risk of ventricular arrhythmias). Products include:
Geodon Capsules 2688

FORTAZ INJECTION
(Ceftazidime Sodium) 1541
See Fortaz for Injection

FORTAZ FOR INJECTION
(Ceftazidime) 1541
May interact with aminoglycosides and certain other agents. Compounds in these categories include:

Amikacin Sulfate (Potential for nephrotoxicity following concomitant administration).
No products indexed under this heading.
Chloramphenicol (Possibility of antagonism *in vivo*, particularly when bactericidal activity is desired; avoid this combination). Products include:
Chloromycetin Ophthalmic Ointment, 1% .... ⊙296
Chloromycetin Ophthalmic Solution .... ⊙297
Chloroptic Sterile Ophthalmic Ointment .... ⊙234
Chloroptic Sterile Ophthalmic Solution .... ⊙235
Chloramphenicol Palmitate (Possibility of antagonism *in vivo*, particularly when bactericidal activity is desired; avoid this combination).
No products indexed under this heading.
Chloramphenicol Sodium Succinate (Possibility of antagonism *in vivo*, particularly when bactericidal activity is desired; avoid this combination).
No products indexed under this heading.
Furosemide (Potential for nephrotoxicity following concomitant administration). Products include:
Furosemide Tablets 2284
Gentamicin Sulfate (Potential for nephrotoxicity following concomitant administration). Products include:
Genoptic Ophthalmic Ointment .... ⊙239
Genoptic Sterile Ophthalmic Solution .... ⊙239
Pred-G Ophthalmic Suspension ..... ⊙247
Pred-G Sterile Ophthalmic Ointment .... ⊙248
Kanamycin Sulfate (Potential for nephrotoxicity following concomitant administration).
No products indexed under this heading.
Streptomycin Sulfate (Potential for nephrotoxicity following concomitant administration). Products include:
Streptomycin Sulfate Injection 2714
Tobramycin (Potential for nephrotoxicity following concomitant administration). Products include:
TOBI Solution for Inhalation 1206
TobraDex Ophthalmic Ointment 542
TobraDex Ophthalmic Suspension .. 541
Tobrex Ophthalmic Ointment .... ⊙220
Tobrex Ophthalmic Solution .... ⊙221
Tobramycin Sulfate (Potential for nephrotoxicity following concomitant administration). Products include:
Nebcin Vials, Hyporets & ADD-Vantage 1955

FORTOVASE CAPSULES
(Saquinavir) 2970
May interact with dexamethasone, ergot-containing drugs, phenytoin, and certain other agents. Compounds in these categories include:

Astemizole (Competition for CYP3A by saquinavir could result in inhibition of the metabolism of astemizole and create the potential for serious and/or life-threatening reactions such as cardiac arrhythmias; concurrent use is contraindicated).
No products indexed under this heading.
Atorvastatin Calcium (Co-administration of Fortovase and other HMG-CoA reductase inhibitors that are metabolized by the CYP3A4 pathway, such as atorvastatin may result in increased concentrations of statins; potential for, in rare cases, severe adverse events such as myopathyincluding rhabdomyolysis). Products include:
Lipitor Tablets 2639
Lipitor Tablets 2696
Carbamazepine (May decrease saquinavir plasma concentrations). Products include:
Carbatrol Capsules 3234
Tegretol/Tegretol-XR 2404
Cerivastatin Sodium (Co-administration of Fortovase and other HMG-CoA reductase inhibitors that are metabolized by the CYP3A4 pathway, such as cerivastatin, may result in increased concentrations of statins; potential for, in rare cases, severe adverse events such as myopathy including rhabdomyolysis). Products include:
Baycol Tablets 883
Cisapride (Competition for CYP3A by saquinavir could result in inhibition of the metabolism of cisapride and create the potential for serious and/or life-threatening reactions such as cardiac arrhythmias; concurrent use is contraindicated).
No products indexed under this heading.
Clarithromycin (Co-administration has resulted in a 117% increase in saquinavir plasma AUC, a 48% decrease in clarithromycin AUC and a 24% decrease in clarithromycin 14-OH metabolite AUC). Products include:
Biaxin/Biaxin XL 403
PREVPAC 3298
Delavirdine Mesylate (Co-administration has resulted in a 5-fold increase in saquinavir plasma AUC; currently, there are no safety and efficacy data available from use of this combination; hepatocellular enzyme elevations have occured in some patients). Products include:
Rescriptor Tablets 526
Dexamethasone (May decrease saquinavir plasma concentrations). Products include:
Decadron Elixir 2078
Decadron Tablets 2079
TobraDex Ophthalmic Ointment 542
TobraDex Ophthalmic Suspension .. 541
Dexamethasone Acetate (May decrease saquinavir plasma concentrations).
No products indexed under this heading.
Dexamethasone Sodium Phosphate (May decrease saquinavir plasma concentrations). Products include:
Decadron Phosphate Injection 2081
Decadron Phosphate Sterile Ophthalmic Ointment 2083
Decadron Phosphate Sterile Ophthalmic Solution 2084
NeoDecadron Sterile Ophthalmic Solution 2144
Dihydroergotamine Mesylate (Competition for CYP3A by saquinavir could result in inhibition of the metabolism of ergot derivatives and create the potential for serious and/or life-threatening reactions such as cardiac arrhythmias; concurrent use is contraindicated). Products include:
D.H.E. 45 Injection 2334
Migranal Nasal Spray 2376
Ergonovine Maleate (Competition for CYP3A by saquinavir could result in inhibition of the metabolism of ergot derivatives and create the potential for serious and/or life-threatening reactions such as cardiac arrhythmias; concurrent use is contraindicated).
No products indexed under this heading.
Ergotamine Tartrate (Competition for CYP3A by saquinavir could result in inhibition of the metabolism of ergot derivatives and create the potential for serious and/or life-threatening reactions such as cardiac arrhythmias; concurrent use is contraindicated).
No products indexed under this heading.
Fosphenytoin Sodium (May decrease saquinavir plasma concentrations). Products include:
Cerebyx Injection 2619
Indinavir Sulfate (Co-administration has resulted in a 364% increase in saquinavir plasma AUC; currently, there are no safety and efficacy data available from use of this combination). Products include:
Crixivan Capsules 2070
Ketoconazole (Co-administration has resulted in a 130% increase in saquinavir plasma AUC). Products include:
Nizoral 2% Cream 3620
Nizoral A-D Shampoo 2008
Nizoral 2% Shampoo 2007
Nizoral Tablets 1791
Lovastatin (Co-administration of Fortovase and lovastatin may result in increased concentrations of statins; potential for, in rare cases, severe adverse events such as myopathy including rhabdomyolysis; concomitant use is not recommended). Products include:
Mevacor Tablets 2132
Methylergonovine Maleate (Competition for CYP3A by saquinavir could result in inhibition of the metabolism of ergot derivatives and create the potential for serious and/or life-threatening reactions such as cardiac arrhythmias; concurrent use is contraindicated).
No products indexed under this heading.
Methysergide Maleate (Competition for CYP3A by saquinavir could result in inhibition of the metabolism of ergot derivatives and create the potential for serious and/or life-threatening reactions such as cardiac arrhythmias; concurrent use is contraindicated).
No products indexed under this heading.
Midazolam Hydrochloride (Competition for CYP3A by saquinavir could result in inhibition of the metabolism of midazolam and create the potential for serious and/or life-threatening reactions such as prolonged sedation; concurrent use is contraindicated). Products include:
Versed Injection 3027
Versed Syrup 3033
Nevirapine (Co-administration has resulted in a 24% decrease in saquinavir plasma AUC; currently, there are no safety and efficacy data available from use of this combination). Products include:
Viramune Oral Suspension 1060
Viramune Tablets 1060
Phenobarbital (Anticonvulsants, such as phenobarbital, may decrease saquinavir plasma concentrations). Products include:
Arco-Lase Plus Tablets 592
Donnatal 2929
Donnatal Extentabs 2930
Phenytoin (May decrease saquinavir plasma concentrations). Products include:
Dilantin Infatabs 2624
Dilantin-125 Oral Suspension 2625
Phenytoin Sodium (May decrease saquinavir plasma concentrations). Products include:
Dilantin Kapseals 2622
Rifabutin (Co-administration has resulted in a 43% decrease in saquinavir plasma AUC; prescriber should consider using an alternative to rifabutin). Products include:
Mycobutin Capsules 2838
Rifampin (Co-administration has resulted in a 84% decrease in saquinavir plasma AUC; prescriber should consider using an alternative to rifampin). Products include:
Rifadin 765
Rifamate Capsules 767
Rifater Tablets 769
Ritonavir (Combination therapy in HIV-infected patients has resulted in AUC values which were at least 17-fold greater than historical AUC values from patients who received saquinavir without ritonavir). Products include:
Kaletra Capsules 471
Kaletra Oral Solution 471
Norvir Capsules 487
Norvir Oral Solution 487
Sildenafil Citrate (Co-administration has resulted in a 140% increase in sildenafil Cmax and a 210% increase in sildenafil AUC; when sildenafil is administered concomitantly with saquinavir a starting dose of 25 mg of sildenafil should be considered). Products include:
Viagra Tablets 2732
Simvastatin (Co-administration of Fortovase and simvastatin may result in increased concentrations of statins; potential for, in rare cases, severe adverse events such as myopathy including rhabdomyolysis; concomitant use is not recommended). Products include:
Zocor Tablets 2219
Terfenadine (Co-administration has resulted in increased terfenadine plasma levels; competition for CYP3A by saquinavir could result in inhibition of the metabolism of terfenadine and create the potential for serious and/or life-threatening reactions such as cardiac arrhythmias; concurrent use is contraindicated).
No products indexed under this heading.
Triazolam (Competition for CYP3A by saquinavir could result in inhibition of the metabolism of triazolam and create the potential for serious and/or life-threatening reactions such as prolonged sedation; concurrent use is contraindicated). Products include:
Halcion Tablets 2823

Food Interactions

Food, unspecified (The mean 12-hour AUC is increased in fed condition; Fortovase should be taken with a meal or up to 2 hours after a meal).

FOSAMAX TABLETS
(Alendronate Sodium) 2095
May interact with antacids containing aluminum, calcium and magnesium, calcium preparations, non-steroidal anti-inflammatory agents, and certain other agents. Compounds in these categories include:

Aluminum Carbonate (May interfere with the absorption of alendronate; patient must wait at least one-half hour after taking alendronate before taking any drug).
No products indexed under this heading.

Aluminum Hydroxide (May interfere with the absorption of alendronate; patient must wait at least one-half hour after taking alendronate before taking any drug). Products include:
- Amphojel Suspension (Mint Flavor) 789
- Gaviscon Extra Strength Liquid 751
- Gaviscon Extra Strength Tablets 751
- Gaviscon Regular Strength Liquid 751
- Gaviscon Regular Strength Tablets 750
- Maalox Antacid/Anti-Gas Oral Suspension 673
- Maalox Max Maximum Strength Antacid/Anti-Gas Liquid 2300
- Maalox Regular Strength Antacid/Antigas Liquid 2300
- Mylanta 1813
- Vanquish Caplets 617

Aspirin (Co-administration with doses of alendronate greater than 10 mg/day and aspirin-containing compounds can increase the incidence of gastrointestinal adverse events; one case of anastomotic ulcer with mild hemorrhage has been reported in a patient with history of peptic ulcer disease and gastrectomy on alendronate 10 mg/day plus aspirin). Products include:
- Aggrenox Capsules 1026
- Alka-Seltzer 603
- Alka-Seltzer Lemon Lime Antacid and Pain Reliever Effervescent Tablets 603
- Alka-Seltzer Extra Strength Antacid and Pain Reliever Effervescent Tablets 603
- Alka-Seltzer PM Effervescent Tablets 605
- Genuine Bayer Tablets, Caplets and Gelcaps 606
- Extra Strength Bayer Caplets and Gelcaps 610
- Aspirin Regimen Bayer Children's Chewable Tablets (Orange or Cherry Flavored) 607
- Bayer, Aspirin Regimen 606
- Aspirin Regimen Bayer 81 mg Caplets with Calcium 607
- Genuine Bayer Professional Labeling (Aspirin Regimen Bayer) 608
- Extra Strength Bayer Arthritis Caplets 610
- Extra Strength Bayer Plus Caplets 610
- Extra Strength Bayer PM Caplets 611
- BC Powder 619
- BC Allergy Sinus Cold Powder 619
- Arthritis Strength BC Powder 619
- BC Sinus Cold Powder 619
- Darvon Compound-65 Pulvules 1910
- Ecotrin Enteric Coated Aspirin Low, Regular and Maximum Strength Tablets 1715
- Excedrin Extra-Strength Tablets, Caplets, and Geltabs 629
- Excedrin Migraine 1070
- Goody's Body Pain Formula Powder 620
- Goody's Extra Strength Headache Powder 620
- Goody's Extra Strength Pain Relief Tablets 620
- Percodan Tablets 1327
- Robaxisal Tablets 2939
- Soma Compound Tablets 3354
- Soma Compound w/Codeine Tablets 3355
- Vanquish Caplets 617

Calcium Carbonate (May interfere with the absorption of alendronate; patient must wait at least one-half hour after taking alendronate before taking any drug). Products include:
- Aspirin Regimen Bayer 81 mg Caplets with Calcium 607
- Extra Strength Bayer Plus Caplets 610
- Caltrate 600 Tablets 814
- Caltrate 600 PLUS 815
- Caltrate 600 + D Tablets 814
- Caltrate 600 + Soy Tablets 814
- D-Cal Chewable Caplets 794
- Florical Capsules and Tablets 2223
- Quick Dissolve Maalox Max Maximum Strength Antacid/Antigas Tablets 2301
- Quick Dissolve Maalox Regular Strength Antacid Tablets 2301
- Marblen Suspension 633
- Monocal Tablets 2223
- Mylanta Fast-Acting 1813
- Mylanta Calci Tabs 636
- One-A-Day Bedtime & Rest Tablets 805
- One-A-Day Calcium Plus Chewable Tablets 805
- Os-Cal Chewable Tablets 838
- Pepcid Complete Chewable Tablets 1815
- ReSource Wellness CalciWise Soft Chews 824
- Rolaids Tablets 706
- Extra Strength Rolaids Tablets 706
- Slow-Mag Tablets 835
- Titralac 640
- 3M Titralac Plus Antacid Tablets 640
- Tums 763

Calcium Chloride (May interfere with the absorption of alendronate; patient must wait at least one-half hour after taking alendronate before taking any drug).
No products indexed under this heading.

Calcium Citrate (May interfere with the absorption of alendronate; patient must wait at least one-half hour after taking alendronate before taking any drug). Products include:
- Active Calcium Tablets 3335
- Citracal Liquitab Tablets 823
- Citracal Tablets 2231
- Citracal Caplets + D 823

Calcium Glubionate (May interfere with the absorption of alendronate; patient must wait at least one-half hour after taking alendronate before taking any drug).
No products indexed under this heading.

Celecoxib (Since NSAID use is associated with gastrointestinal irritation, caution should be used during concomitant use; no increase in the incidence of gastrointestinal irritation was reported in clinical trials). Products include:
- Celebrex Capsules 2676
- Celebrex Capsules 2780

Diclofenac Potassium (Since NSAID use is associated with gastrointestinal irritation, caution should be used during concomitant use; no increase in the incidence of gastrointestinal irritation was reported in clinical trials). Products include:
- Cataflam Tablets 2315

Diclofenac Sodium (Since NSAID use is associated with gastrointestinal irritation, caution should be used during concomitant use; no increase in the incidence of gastrointestinal irritation was reported in clinical trials). Products include:
- Arthrotec Tablets 3195
- Voltaren Ophthalmic Sterile Ophthalmic Solution .... ⊙312
- Voltaren Tablets 2315
- Voltaren-XR Tablets 2315

Etodolac (Since NSAID use is associated with gastrointestinal irritation, caution should be used during concomitant use; no increase in the incidence of gastrointestinal irritation was reported in clinical trials). Products include:
- Lodine 3528
- Lodine XL Extended-Release Tablets 3530

Fenoprofen Calcium (Since NSAID use is associated with gastrointestinal irritation, caution should be used during concomitant use; no increase in the incidence of gastrointestinal irritation was reported in clinical trials).
No products indexed under this heading.

Flurbiprofen (Since NSAID use is associated with gastrointestinal irritation, caution should be used during concomitant use; no increase in the incidence of gastrointestinal irritation was reported in clinical trials).
No products indexed under this heading.

Ibuprofen (Since NSAID use is associated with gastrointestinal irritation, caution should be used during concomitant use; no increase in the incidence of gastrointestinal irritation was reported in clinical trials). Products include:
- Advil 771
- Children's Advil Oral Suspension 773
- Children's Advil Chewable Tablets 773
- Advil Cold and Sinus Caplets 771
- Advil Cold and Sinus Tablets 771
- Advil Flu & Body Ache Caplets 772
- Infants' Advil Drops 773
- Junior Strength Advil Tablets 773
- Junior Strength Advil Chewable Tablets 773
- Advil Migraine Liquigels 772
- Children's Motrin Oral Suspension and Chewable Tablets 2006
- Children's Motrin Cold Oral Suspension 2007
- Children's Motrin Oral Suspension 643
- Motrin Suspension, Oral Drops, Chewable Tablets, and Caplets 2002
- Infants' Motrin Concentrated Drops 2006
- Junior Strength Motrin Caplets and Chewable Tablets 2006
- Motrin IB Tablets, Caplets, and Gelcaps 2002
- Motrin Migraine Pain Caplets 2005
- Motrin Sinus Headache Caplets 2005
- Vicoprofen Tablets 520

Indomethacin (Since NSAID use is associated with gastrointestinal irritation, caution should be used during concomitant use; no increase in the incidence of gastrointestinal irritation was reported in clinical trials). Products include:
- Indocin 2112

Indomethacin Sodium Trihydrate (Since NSAID use is associated with gastrointestinal irritation, caution should be used during concomitant use; no increase in the incidence of gastrointestinal irritation was reported in clinical trials). Products include:
- Indocin I.V. 2115

Ketoprofen (Since NSAID use is associated with gastrointestinal irritation, caution should be used during concomitant use; no increase in the incidence of gastrointestinal irritation was reported in clinical trials). Products include:
- Orudis Capsules 3548
- Orudis KT Tablets 778
- Oruvail Capsules 3548

Ketorolac Tromethamine (Since NSAID use is associated with gastrointestinal irritation, caution should be used during concomitant use; no increase in the incidence of gastrointestinal irritation was reported in clinical trials). Products include:
- Acular Ophthalmic Solution 544
- Acular PF Ophthalmic Solution 544
- Toradol 3018

Magaldrate (May interfere with the absorption of alendronate; patient must wait at least one-half hour after taking alendronate before taking any drug).
No products indexed under this heading.

Magnesium Hydroxide (May interfere with the absorption of alendronate; patient must wait at least one-half hour after taking alendronate before taking any drug). Products include:
- Ex•Lax Milk of Magnesia Liquid 670
- Maalox Antacid/Anti-Gas Oral Suspension 673
- Maalox Max Maximum Strength Antacid/Anti-Gas Liquid 2300
- Maalox Regular Strength Antacid/Antigas Liquid 2300
- Mylanta Fast-Acting 1813
- Mylanta 1813
- Pepcid Complete Chewable Tablets 1815
- Phillips' Chewable Tablets 615
- Phillips' Milk of Magnesia Liquid (Original, Cherry, & Mint) 616
- Rolaids Tablets 706
- Extra Strength Rolaids Tablets 706
- Vanquish Caplets 617

Magnesium Oxide (May interfere with the absorption of alendronate; patient must wait at least one-half hour after taking alendronate before taking any drug). Products include:
- Beelith Tablets 946
- Mag-Ox 400 Tablets 1024
- Uro-Mag Capsules 1024

Meclofenamate Sodium (Since NSAID use is associated with gastrointestinal irritation, caution should be used during concomitant use; no increase in the incidence of gastrointestinal irritation was reported in clinical trials).
No products indexed under this heading.

Mefenamic Acid (Since NSAID use is associated with gastrointestinal irritation, caution should be used during concomitant use; no increase in the incidence of gastrointestinal irritation was reported in clinical trials). Products include:
- Ponstel Capsules 1356

Meloxicam (Since NSAID use is associated with gastrointestinal irritation, caution should be used during concomitant use; no increase in the incidence of gastrointestinal irritation was reported in clinical trials). Products include:
- Mobic Tablets 1054

Nabumetone (Since NSAID use is associated with gastrointestinal irritation, caution should be used during concomitant use; no increase in the incidence of gastrointestinal irritation was reported in clinical trials). Products include:
- Relafen Tablets 1617

Naproxen (Since NSAID use is associated with gastrointestinal irritation, caution should be used during concomitant use; no increase in the incidence of gastrointestinal irritation was reported in clinical trials). Products include:
- EC-Naprosyn Delayed-Release Tablets 2967
- Naprosyn Suspension 2967
- Naprosyn Tablets 2967

Naproxen Sodium (Since NSAID use is associated with gastrointestinal irritation, caution should be used during concomitant use; no increase in the incidence of gastrointestinal irritation was reported in clinical trials). Products include:
- Aleve Tablets, Caplets and Gelcaps 602
- Aleve Cold & Sinus Caplets 603
- Anaprox Tablets 2967
- Anaprox DS Tablets 2967
- Naprelan Tablets 1293

Oxaprozin (Since NSAID use is associated with gastrointestinal irritation, caution should be used during concomitant use; no increase in the incidence of gastrointestinal irritation was reported in clinical trials).
No products indexed under this heading.

Phenylbutazone (Since NSAID use is associated with gastrointestinal irritation, caution should be used

during concomitant use; no increase in the incidence of gastrointestinal irritation was reported in clinical trials).
No products indexed under this heading.

Piroxicam (Since NSAID use is associated with gastrointestinal irritation, caution should be used during concomitant use; no increase in the incidence of gastrointestinal irritation was reported in clinical trials). Products include:
Feldene Capsules ... 2685

Ranitidine Hydrochloride (Intravenous ranitidine has shown to double the bioavailability of oral alendronate; clinical significance of this increased bioavailability and whether similar increases will occur with oral ranitidine is unknown). Products include:
Zantac ... 1690
Zantac Injection ... 1688
Zantac 75 Tablets ... ▣717

Rofecoxib (Since NSAID use is associated with gastrointestinal irritation, caution should be used during concomitant use; no increase in the incidence of gastrointestinal irritation was reported in clinical trials). Products include:
Vioxx ... 2213

Sulindac (Since NSAID use is associated with gastrointestinal irritation, caution should be used during concomitant use; no increase in the incidence of gastrointestinal irritation was reported in clinical trials). Products include:
Clinoril Tablets ... 2053

Tolmetin Sodium (Since NSAID use is associated with gastrointestinal irritation, caution should be used during concomitant use; no increase in the incidence of gastrointestinal irritation was reported in clinical trials). Products include:
Tolectin ... 2589

Food Interactions

Beverages, caffeine-containing (Concomitant administration of alendronate with coffee reduces bioavailability by approximately 60%).

Meal, unspecified (Standardized breakfast decreases bioavailability by approximately 40% when alendronate is administered either 0.5 or 1 hour before breakfast).

Orange Juice (Concomitant administration of alendronate with orange juice reduces bioavailability by approximately 60%).

FOSCAVIR INJECTION
(Foscarnet Sodium) ... 605
May interact with aminoglycosides, drugs known to influence serum calcium levels (selected), inhibitors of renal tubular secretion or resorption, and certain other agents. Compounds in these categories include:

Aldesleukin (Foscarnet decreases serum concentrations of ionized calcium; concurrent treatment with other drugs known to influence serum calcium concentrations, such as aldesleukin, should be used with particular caution). Products include:
Proleukin for Injection ... 1199

Alendronate Sodium (Foscarnet decreases serum concentrations of ionized calcium; concurrent treatment with other drugs known to influence serum calcium concentrations, such as alendronate, should be used with particular caution). Products include:
Fosamax Tablets ... 2095

Amikacin Sulfate (Concurrent administration should be avoided because of foscarnet's tendency to cause renal impairment).
No products indexed under this heading.

Amphotericin B (Concurrent administration should be avoided because of foscarnet's tendency to cause renal impairment). Products include:
Abelcet Injection ... 1273
AmBisome for Injection ... 1383
Amphotec ... 1774

Carboplatin (Foscarnet decreases serum concentrations of ionized calcium; concurrent treatment with other drugs known to influence serum calcium concentrations, such as carboplatin, should be used with particular caution). Products include:
Paraplatin for Injection ... 1126

Cisplatin (Potential for increased hypocalcemia).
No products indexed under this heading.

Furosemide (Foscarnet decreases serum concentrations of ionized calcium; concurrent treatment with other drugs known to influence serum calcium concentrations, such as furosemide, should be used with particular caution). Products include:
Furosemide Tablets ... 2284

Gallium Nitrate (Potential for increased hypocalcemia).
No products indexed under this heading.

Gentamicin Sulfate (Concurrent administration should be avoided because of foscarnet's tendency to cause renal impairment). Products include:
Genoptic Ophthalmic Ointment ... ⊙239
Genoptic Sterile Ophthalmic Solution ... ⊙239
Pred-G Ophthalmic Suspension ... ⊙247
Pred-G Sterile Ophthalmic Ointment ... ⊙248

Interferon alfa-2A, Recombinant (Foscarnet decreases serum concentrations of ionized calcium; concurrent treatment with other drugs known to influence serum calcium concentrations, such as interferon alfa-2A, should be used with particular caution). Products include:
Roferon-A Injection ... 2996

Kanamycin Sulfate (Concurrent administration should be avoided because of foscarnet's tendency to cause renal impairment).
No products indexed under this heading.

Pamidronate Disodium (Foscarnet decreases serum concentrations of ionized calcium; concurrent treatment with other drugs known to influence serum calcium concentrations, such as pamidronate, should be used with particular caution). Products include:
Aredia for Injection ... 2309

Pentamidine Isethionate (Co-administration with intravenous pentamidine may cause hypocalcemia; one patient died with severe hypocalcemia; toxicity associated with concomitant use of aerosolized pentamidine has not been reported).
No products indexed under this heading.

Probenecid (Elimination of foscarnet may be impaired).
No products indexed under this heading.

Ritonavir (Co-administration of foscarnet with ritonavir or saquinavir and ritonavir has resulted in abnormal renal function). Products include:
Kaletra Capsules ... 471
Kaletra Oral Solution ... 471
Norvir Capsules ... 487
Norvir Oral Solution ... 487

Saquinavir (Co-administration of foscarnet with ritonavir or saquinavir and ritonavir has resulted in abnormal renal function). Products include:
Fortovase Capsules ... 2970

Saquinavir Mesylate (Co-administration of foscarnet with ritonavir or saquinavir and ritonavir has resulted in abnormal renal function). Products include:
Invirase Capsules ... 2979

Sodium Polystyrene Sulfonate (Foscarnet decreases serum concentrations of ionized calcium; concurrent treatment with other drugs known to influence serum calcium concentrations, such as sodium polystyrene sulfonate, should be used with particular caution).
No products indexed under this heading.

Streptomycin Sulfate (Concurrent administration should be avoided because of foscarnet's tendency to cause renal impairment). Products include:
Streptomycin Sulfate Injection ... 2714

Sulfinpyrazone (Elimination of foscarnet may be impaired).
No products indexed under this heading.

Tobramycin (Concurrent administration should be avoided because of foscarnet's tendency to cause renal impairment). Products include:
TOBI Solution for Inhalation ... 1206
TobraDex Ophthalmic Ointment ... 542
TobraDex Ophthalmic Suspension ... 541
Tobrex Ophthalmic Ointment ... ⊙220
Tobrex Ophthalmic Solution ... ⊙221

Tobramycin Sulfate (Concurrent administration should be avoided because of foscarnet's tendency to cause renal impairment). Products include:
Nebcin Vials, Hyporets & ADD-Vantage ... 1955

Zidovudine (Potential for additive effects on anemia). Products include:
Combivir Tablets ... 1502
Retrovir ... 1625
Retrovir IV Infusion ... 1629
Trizivir Tablets ... 1669

FRAGMIN INJECTION
(Dalteparin Sodium) ... 2814
May interact with oral anticoagulants, non-steroidal anti-inflammatory agents, salicylates, and certain other agents. Compounds in these categories include:

Abciximab (Drugs that alter platelet function, such as abciximab, may increase the risk of bleeding). Products include:
ReoPro Vials ... 1958

Aspirin (Concomitant use with platelet inhibitors, such as salicylates, may increase the risk of bleeding). Products include:
Aggrenox Capsules ... 1026
Alka-Seltzer ... ▣603
Alka-Seltzer Lemon Lime Antacid and Pain Reliever Effervescent Tablets ... ▣603
Alka-Seltzer Extra Strength Antacid and Pain Reliever Effervescent Tablets ... ▣603
Alka-Seltzer PM Effervescent Tablets ... ▣605
Genuine Bayer Tablets, Caplets and Gelcaps ... ▣606
Extra Strength Bayer Caplets and Gelcaps ... ▣610
Aspirin Regimen Bayer Children's Chewable Tablets (Orange or Cherry Flavored) ... ▣607
Bayer, Aspirin Regimen ... ▣606
Aspirin Regimen Bayer 81 mg Caplets with Calcium ... ▣607
Genuine Bayer Professional Labeling (Aspirin Regimen Bayer) ... ▣608
Extra Strength Bayer Arthritis Caplets ... ▣610
Extra Strength Bayer Plus Caplets ... ▣610
Extra Strength Bayer PM Caplets ... ▣611
BC Powder ... ▣619
BC Allergy Sinus Cold Powder ... ▣619
Arthritis Strength BC Powder ... ▣619
BC Sinus Cold Powder ... ▣619
Darvon Compound-65 Pulvules ... 1910
Ecotrin Enteric Coated Aspirin Low, Regular and Maximum Strength Tablets ... 1715
Excedrin Extra-Strength Tablets, Caplets, and Geltabs ... ▣629
Excedrin Migraine ... 1070
Goody's Body Pain Formula Powder ... ▣620
Goody's Extra Strength Headache Powder ... ▣620
Goody's Extra Strength Pain Relief Tablets ... ▣620
Percodan Tablets ... 1327
Robaxisal Tablets ... 2939
Soma Compound Tablets ... 3354
Soma Compound w/Codeine Tablets ... 3355
Vanquish Caplets ... ▣617

Celecoxib (Concomitant use with platelet inhibitors, such as NSAIDs, may increase the risk of bleeding). Products include:
Celebrex Capsules ... 2676
Celebrex Capsules ... 2780

Choline Magnesium Trisalicylate (Concomitant use with platelet inhibitors, such as salicylates, may increase the risk of bleeding). Products include:
Trilisate ... 2901

Clopidogrel Bisulfate (Drugs that alter platelet function, such as clopidogrel, may increase the risk of bleeding). Products include:
Plavix Tablets ... 1097
Plavix Tablets ... 3084

Diclofenac Potassium (Concomitant use with platelet inhibitors, such as NSAIDs, may increase the risk of bleeding). Products include:
Cataflam Tablets ... 2315

Diclofenac Sodium (Concomitant use with platelet inhibitors, such as NSAIDs, may increase the risk of bleeding). Products include:
Arthrotec Tablets ... 3195
Voltaren Ophthalmic Sterile Ophthalmic Solution ... ⊙312
Voltaren Tablets ... 2315
Voltaren-XR Tablets ... 2315

Dicumarol (Concomitant use with oral anticoagulants may increase the risk of bleeding).
No products indexed under this heading.

Diflunisal (Concomitant use with platelet inhibitors, such as salicylates, may increase the risk of bleeding). Products include:
Dolobid Tablets ... 2088

Dipyridamole (Concomitant use with platelet inhibitors, such as dipyridamole, may increase the risk of bleeding). Products include:
Aggrenox Capsules ... 1026
Persantine Tablets ... 1057

Eptifibatide (Drugs that alter platelet function, such as eptifibatide, may increase the risk of bleeding). Products include:
Integrilin Injection ... 1213
Integrilin Injection ... 1828

Etodolac (Concomitant use with platelet inhibitors, such as NSAIDs, may increase the risk of bleeding). Products include:
Lodine ... 3528
Lodine XL Extended-Release Tablets ... 3530

Fenoprofen Calcium (Concomitant use with platelet inhibitors, such as NSAIDs, may increase the risk of bleeding).
No products indexed under this heading.

Flurbiprofen (Concomitant use with platelet inhibitors, such as NSAIDs, may increase the risk of bleeding).
No products indexed under this heading.

Ibuprofen (Concomitant use with platelet inhibitors, such as NSAIDs, may increase the risk of bleeding). Products include:
Advil ... ▣771

Children's Advil Oral Suspension ... 773
Children's Advil Chewable Tablets ... 773
Advil Cold and Sinus Caplets ... 771
Advil Cold and Sinus Tablets ... 771
Advil Flu & Body Ache Caplets ... 772
Infants' Advil Drops ... 773
Junior Strength Advil Tablets ... 773
Junior Strength Advil Chewable Tablets ... 773
Advil Migraine Liquigels ... 772
Children's Motrin Oral Suspension and Chewable Tablets ... 2006
Children's Motrin Cold Oral Suspension ... 2007
Children's Motrin Oral Suspension ... 643
Motrin Suspension, Oral Drops, Chewable Tablets, and Caplets ... 2002
Infants' Motrin Concentrated Drops ... 2006
Junior Strength Motrin Caplets and Chewable Tablets ... 2006
Motrin IB Tablets, Caplets, and Gelcaps ... 2002
Motrin Migraine Pain Caplets ... 2005
Motrin Sinus Headache Caplets ... 2005
Vicoprofen Tablets ... 520

Indomethacin (Concomitant use with platelet inhibitors, such as NSAIDs, may increase the risk of bleeding). Products include:
Indocin ... 2112

Indomethacin Sodium Trihydrate (Concomitant use with platelet inhibitors, such as NSAIDs, may increase the risk of bleeding). Products include:
Indocin I.V. ... 2115

Ketoprofen (Concomitant use with platelet inhibitors, such as NSAIDs, may increase the risk of bleeding). Products include:
Orudis Capsules ... 3548
Orudis KT Tablets ... 778
Oruvail Capsules ... 3548

Ketorolac Tromethamine (Concomitant use with platelet inhibitors, such as NSAIDs, may increase the risk of bleeding). Products include:
Acular Ophthalmic Solution ... 544
Acular PF Ophthalmic Solution ... 544
Toradol ... 3018

Magnesium Salicylate (Concomitant use with platelet inhibitors, such as salicylates, may increase the risk of bleeding). Products include:
Momentum Backache Relief Extra Strength Caplets ... 666

Meclofenamate Sodium (Concomitant use with platelet inhibitors, such as NSAIDs, may increase the risk of bleeding).
No products indexed under this heading.

Mefenamic Acid (Concomitant use with platelet inhibitors, such as NSAIDs, may increase the risk of bleeding). Products include:
Ponstel Capsules ... 1356

Meloxicam (Concomitant use with platelet inhibitors, such as NSAIDs, may increase the risk of bleeding). Products include:
Mobic Tablets ... 1054

Nabumetone (Concomitant use with platelet inhibitors, such as NSAIDs, may increase the risk of bleeding). Products include:
Relafen Tablets ... 1617

Naproxen (Concomitant use with platelet inhibitors, such as NSAIDs, may increase the risk of bleeding). Products include:
EC-Naprosyn Delayed-Release Tablets ... 2967
Naprosyn Suspension ... 2967
Naprosyn Tablets ... 2967

Naproxen Sodium (Concomitant use with platelet inhibitors, such as NSAIDs, may increase the risk of bleeding). Products include:
Aleve Tablets, Caplets and Gelcaps ... 602
Aleve Cold & Sinus Caplets ... 603
Anaprox Tablets ... 2967
Anaprox DS Tablets ... 2967
Naprelan Tablets ... 1293

Oxaprozin (Concomitant use with platelet inhibitors, such as NSAIDs, may increase the risk of bleeding).
No products indexed under this heading.

Phenylbutazone (Concomitant use with platelet inhibitors, such as NSAIDs, may increase the risk of bleeding).
No products indexed under this heading.

Piroxicam (Concomitant use with platelet inhibitors, such as NSAIDs, may increase the risk of bleeding). Products include:
Feldene Capsules ... 2685

Rofecoxib (Concomitant use with platelet inhibitors, such as NSAIDs, may increase the risk of bleeding). Products include:
Vioxx ... 2213

Salsalate (Concomitant use with platelet inhibitors, such as salicylates, may increase the risk of bleeding).
No products indexed under this heading.

Sulindac (Concomitant use with platelet inhibitors, such as NSAIDs, may increase the risk of bleeding). Products include:
Clinoril Tablets ... 2053

Ticlopidine Hydrochloride (Drugs that alter platelet function, such as ticlopidine, may increase the risk of bleeding). Products include:
Ticlid Tablets ... 3015

Tirofiban Hydrochloride (Drugs that alter platelet function, such as tirofiban, may increase the risk of bleeding). Products include:
Aggrastat ... 2031

Tolmetin Sodium (Concomitant use with platelet inhibitors, such as NSAIDs, may increase the risk of bleeding). Products include:
Tolectin ... 2589

Warfarin Sodium (Concomitant use with oral anticoagulants may increase the risk of bleeding). Products include:
Coumadin for Injection ... 1243
Coumadin Tablets ... 1243
Warfarin Sodium Tablets, USP ... 3302

STERILE FUDR
(Floxuridine) ... 2974
May interact with alkylating agents. Compounds in these categories include:

Bone Marrow Depressants, unspecified (Increased toxicity of FUDR).

Busulfan (FUDR should be used with extreme caution in patients with previous use of alkylating agents). Products include:
Myleran Tablets ... 1603

Carmustine (BCNU) (FUDR should be used with extreme caution in patients with previous use of alkylating agents). Products include:
Gliadel Wafer ... 1723

Chlorambucil (FUDR should be used with extreme caution in patients with previous use of alkylating agents). Products include:
Leukeran Tablets ... 1591

Cyclophosphamide (FUDR should be used with extreme caution in patients with previous use of alkylating agents).
No products indexed under this heading.

Dacarbazine (FUDR should be used with extreme caution in patients with previous use of alkylating agents). Products include:
DTIC-Dome ... 902

Lomustine (CCNU) (FUDR should be used with extreme caution in patients with previous use of alkylating agents).
No products indexed under this heading.

Mechlorethamine Hydrochloride (FUDR should be used with extreme caution in patients with previous use of alkylating agents). Products include:
Mustargen for Injection ... 2142

Melphalan (FUDR should be used with extreme caution in patients with previous use of alkylating agents). Products include:
Alkeran Tablets ... 1466

Thiotepa (FUDR should be used with extreme caution in patients with previous use of alkylating agents). Products include:
Thioplex for Injection ... 1765

FUROSEMIDE TABLETS
(Furosemide) ... 2284
May interact with aminoglycosides, antihypertensives, barbiturates, corticosteroids, cardiac glycosides, lithium preparations, narcotic analgesics, non-steroidal anti-inflammatory agents, salicylates, and certain other agents. Compounds in these categories include:

Acebutolol Hydrochloride (Furosemide may add to or potentiate the therapeutic effect of other antihypertensive drugs). Products include:
Sectral Capsules ... 3589

ACTH (Co-administration with ACTH may increase the risk of hypokalemia).
No products indexed under this heading.

Alfentanil Hydrochloride (Aggravates orthostatic hypotension).
No products indexed under this heading.

Amikacin Sulfate (Potential for increased risk of ototoxicity with concomitant therapy, especially in the presence of impaired renal function; avoid concurrent use except in presence of life threatening situations).
No products indexed under this heading.

Amlodipine Besylate (Furosemide may add to or potentiate the therapeutic effect of other antihypertensive drugs). Products include:
Lotrel Capsules ... 2370
Norvasc Tablets ... 2704

Aprobarbital (Aggravates orthostatic hypotension).
No products indexed under this heading.

Aspirin (Combination of furosemide and aspirin temporarily reduced creatinine clearance in patients with chronic renal insufficiency; co-administration in patients receiving high doses of salicylates may experience salicylate toxicity). Products include:
Aggrenox Capsules ... 1026
Alka-Seltzer ... 603
Alka-Seltzer Lemon Lime Antacid and Pain Reliever Effervescent Tablets ... 603
Alka-Seltzer Extra Strength Antacid and Pain Reliever Effervescent Tablets ... 603
Alka-Seltzer PM Effervescent Tablets ... 605
Genuine Bayer Tablets, Caplets and Gelcaps ... 606
Extra Strength Bayer Caplets and Gelcaps ... 610
Aspirin Regimen Bayer Children's Chewable Tablets (Orange or Cherry Flavored) ... 607
Bayer, Aspirin Regimen ... 606
Aspirin Regimen Bayer 81 mg Caplets with Calcium ... 607
Genuine Bayer Professional Labeling (Aspirin Regimen Bayer) ... 608
Extra Strength Bayer Arthritis Caplets ... 610
Extra Strength Bayer Plus Caplets ... 610
Extra Strength Bayer PM Caplets ... 611
BC Powder ... 619
BC Allergy Sinus Cold Powder ... 619
Arthritis Strength BC Powder ... 619
BC Sinus Cold Powder ... 619
Darvon Compound-65 Pulvules ... 1910
Ecotrin Enteric Coated Aspirin Low, Regular and Maximum Strength Tablets ... 1715
Excedrin Extra-Strength Tablets, Caplets, and Geltabs ... 629
Excedrin Migraine ... 1070
Goody's Body Pain Formula Powder ... 620
Goody's Extra Strength Headache Powder ... 620
Goody's Extra Strength Pain Relief Tablets ... 620
Percodan Tablets ... 1327
Robaxisal Tablets ... 2939
Soma Compound Tablets ... 3354
Soma Compound w/Codeine Tablets ... 3355
Vanquish Caplets ... 617

Atenolol (Furosemide may add to or potentiate the therapeutic effect of other antihypertensive drugs). Products include:
Tenoretic Tablets ... 690
Tenormin I.V. Injection ... 692

Benazepril Hydrochloride (Furosemide may add to or potentiate the therapeutic effect of other antihypertensive drugs). Products include:
Lotensin Tablets ... 2365
Lotensin HCT Tablets ... 2367
Lotrel Capsules ... 2370

Bendroflumethiazide (Furosemide may add to or potentiate the therapeutic effect of other antihypertensive drugs). Products include:
Corzide 40/5 Tablets ... 2247
Corzide 80/5 Tablets ... 2247

Betamethasone Acetate (Co-administration with corticosteroids may increase the risk of hypokalemia). Products include:
Celestone Soluspan Injectable Suspension ... 3097

Betamethasone Sodium Phosphate (Co-administration with corticosteroids may increase the risk of hypokalemia). Products include:
Celestone Soluspan Injectable Suspension ... 3097

Betaxolol Hydrochloride (Furosemide may add to or potentiate the therapeutic effect of other antihypertensive drugs). Products include:
Betoptic S Ophthalmic Suspension ... 537

Bisoprolol Fumarate (Furosemide may add to or potentiate the therapeutic effect of other antihypertensive drugs). Products include:
Zebeta Tablets ... 1885
Ziac Tablets ... 1887

Buprenorphine Hydrochloride (Aggravates orthostatic hypotension). Products include:
Buprenex Injectable ... 2918

Butabarbital (Aggravates orthostatic hypotension).
No products indexed under this heading.

Butalbital (Aggravates orthostatic hypotension). Products include:
Phrenilin ... 578
Sedapap Tablets 50 mg/650 mg ... 2225

Candesartan Cilexetil (Furosemide may add to or potentiate the therapeutic effect of other antihypertensive drugs). Products include:
Atacand Tablets ... 595
Atacand HCT Tablets ... 597

Captopril (Furosemide may add to or potentiate the therapeutic effect of other antihypertensive drugs). Products include:
Captopril Tablets ... 2281

Carteolol Hydrochloride (Furosemide may add to or potentiate the therapeutic effect of other antihypertensive drugs). Products include:
Carteolol Hydrochloride Ophthalmic Solution USP, 1% ... ⊙258

IMPORTANT NOTE: Always consult each drug listing in the patient's regimen for possible interactions.

Ocupress Ophthalmic Solution, 1% Sterile ⊙ 303

Celecoxib (Co-administration with NSAIDs has resulted in increased BUN, serum creatinine and serum potassium levels, and weight gain). Products include:
Celebrex Capsules 2676
Celebrex Capsules 2780

Chlorothiazide (Furosemide may add to or potentiate the therapeutic effect of other antihypertensive drugs). Products include:
Aldoclor Tablets 2035
Diuril Oral 2087

Chlorothiazide Sodium (Furosemide may add to or potentiate the therapeutic effect of other antihypertensive drugs). Products include:
Diuril Sodium Intravenous 2086

Chlorthalidone (Furosemide may add to or potentiate the therapeutic effect of other antihypertensive drugs). Products include:
Clorpres Tablets 1002
Combipres Tablets 1040
Tenoretic Tablets 690

Choline Magnesium Trisalicylate (Co-administration in patients receiving high doses of salicylates may experience salicylate toxicity). Products include:
Trilisate 2901

Clonidine (Furosemide may add to or potentiate the therapeutic effect of other antihypertensive drugs). Products include:
Catapres-TTS 1038

Clonidine Hydrochloride (Furosemide may add to or potentiate the therapeutic effect of other antihypertensive drugs). Products include:
Catapres Tablets 1037
Clorpres Tablets 1002
Combipres Tablets 1040
Duraclon Injection 3057

Codeine Phosphate (Aggravates orthostatic hypotension). Products include:
Phenergan with Codeine Syrup 3557
Phenergan VC with Codeine Syrup 3561
Robitussin A-C Syrup 2942
Robitussin-DAC Syrup 2942
Ryna-C Liquid ▣ 768
Soma Compound w/Codeine Tablets 3355
Tussi-Organidin NR Liquid 3350
Tussi-Organidin-S NR Liquid 3350
Tylenol with Codeine 2595

Cortisone Acetate (Co-administration with corticosteroids may increase the risk of hypokalemia). Products include:
Cortone Acetate Injectable Suspension 2059
Cortone Acetate Tablets 2061

Deserpidine (Furosemide may add to or potentiate the therapeutic effect of other antihypertensive drugs).
No products indexed under this heading.

Deslanoside (Concurrent digitalis therapy may exaggerate metabolic effects of hypokalemia, especially myocardial effects).
No products indexed under this heading.

Dexamethasone (Co-administration with corticosteroids may increase the risk of hypokalemia). Products include:
Decadron Elixir 2078
Decadron Tablets 2079
TobraDex Ophthalmic Ointment 542
TobraDex Ophthalmic Suspension 541

Dexamethasone Acetate (Co-administration with corticosteroids may increase the risk of hypokalemia).
No products indexed under this heading.

Dexamethasone Sodium Phosphate (Co-administration with corticosteroids may increase the risk of hypokalemia). Products include:
Decadron Phosphate Injection 2081
Decadron Phosphate Sterile Ophthalmic Ointment 2083
Decadron Phosphate Sterile Ophthalmic Solution 2084
NeoDecadron Sterile Ophthalmic Solution 2144

Dezocine (Aggravates orthostatic hypotension).
No products indexed under this heading.

Diazoxide (Furosemide may add to or potentiate the therapeutic effect of other antihypertensive drugs).
No products indexed under this heading.

Diclofenac Potassium (Co-administration with NSAIDs has resulted in increased BUN, serum creatinine and serum potassium levels, and weight gain). Products include:
Cataflam Tablets 2315

Diclofenac Sodium (Co-administration with NSAIDs has resulted in increased BUN, serum creatinine and serum potassium levels, and weight gain). Products include:
Arthrotec Tablets 3195
Voltaren Ophthalmic Sterile Ophthalmic Solution ⊙ 312
Voltaren Tablets 2315
Voltaren-XR Tablets 2315

Diflunisal (Co-administration in patients receiving high doses of salicylates may experience salicylate toxicity). Products include:
Dolobid Tablets 2088

Digitoxin (Concurrent digitalis therapy may exaggerate metabolic effects of hypokalemia, especially myocardial effects).
No products indexed under this heading.

Digoxin (Concurrent digitalis therapy may exaggerate metabolic effects of hypokalemia, especially myocardial effects). Products include:
Digitek Tablets 1003
Lanoxicaps Capsules 1574
Lanoxin Injection 1581
Lanoxin Tablets 1587
Lanoxin Elixir Pediatric 1578
Lanoxin Injection Pediatric 1584

Diltiazem Hydrochloride (Furosemide may add to or potentiate the therapeutic effect of other antihypertensive drugs). Products include:
Cardizem Injectable 1018
Cardizem Lyo-Ject Syringe 1018
Cardizem Monovial 1018
Cardizem CD Capsules 1016
Tiazac Capsules 1378

Doxazosin Mesylate (Furosemide may add to or potentiate the therapeutic effect of other antihypertensive drugs). Products include:
Cardura Tablets 2668

Enalapril Maleate (Furosemide may add to or potentiate the therapeutic effect of other antihypertensive drugs). Products include:
Lexxel Tablets 608
Vaseretic Tablets 2204
Vasotec Tablets 2210

Enalaprilat (Furosemide may add to or potentiate the therapeutic effect of other antihypertensive drugs). Products include:
Enalaprilat Injection 863
Vasotec I.V. Injection 2207

Eprosartan Mesylate (Furosemide may add to or potentiate the therapeutic effect of other antihypertensive drugs). Products include:
Teveten Tablets 3327

Esmolol Hydrochloride (Furosemide may add to or potentiate the therapeutic effect of other antihypertensive drugs). Products include:
Brevibloc Injection 858

Ethacrynic Acid (Potential for increased risk of ototoxicity with concomitant therapy; concurrent use should be avoided). Products include:
Edecrin Tablets 2091

Etodolac (Co-administration with NSAIDs has resulted in increased BUN, serum creatinine and serum potassium levels, and weight gain). Products include:
Lodine 3528
Lodine XL Extended-Release Tablets 3530

Felodipine (Furosemide may add to or potentiate the therapeutic effect of other antihypertensive drugs). Products include:
Lexxel Tablets 608
Plendil Extended-Release Tablets 623

Fenoprofen Calcium (Co-administration with NSAIDs has resulted in increased BUN, serum creatinine and serum potassium levels, and weight gain).
No products indexed under this heading.

Fentanyl (Aggravates orthostatic hypotension). Products include:
Duragesic Transdermal System 1786

Fentanyl Citrate (Aggravates orthostatic hypotension). Products include:
Actiq 1184

Fludrocortisone Acetate (Co-administration with corticosteroids may increase the risk of hypokalemia). Products include:
Florinef Acetate Tablets 2250

Flurbiprofen (Co-administration with NSAIDs has resulted in increased BUN, serum creatinine and serum potassium levels, and weight gain).
No products indexed under this heading.

Fosinopril Sodium (Furosemide may add to or potentiate the therapeutic effect of other antihypertensive drugs). Products include:
Monopril Tablets 1091
Monopril HCT 1094

Gentamicin Sulfate (Potential for increased risk of ototoxicity with concomitant therapy, especially in the presence of impaired renal function; avoid concurrent use except in presence of life threatening situations). Products include:
Genoptic Ophthalmic Ointment ⊙ 239
Genoptic Sterile Ophthalmic Solution ⊙ 239
Pred-G Ophthalmic Suspension ⊙ 247
Pred-G Sterile Ophthalmic Ointment ⊙ 248

Guanabenz Acetate (Furosemide may add to or potentiate the therapeutic effect of other antihypertensive drugs).
No products indexed under this heading.

Guanethidine Monosulfate (Furosemide may add to or potentiate the therapeutic effect of other antihypertensive drugs).
No products indexed under this heading.

Hydralazine Hydrochloride (Furosemide may add to or potentiate the therapeutic effect of other antihypertensive drugs).
No products indexed under this heading.

Hydrochlorothiazide (Furosemide may add to or potentiate the therapeutic effect of other antihypertensive drugs). Products include:
Accuretic Tablets 2614
Aldoril Tablets 2039
Atacand HCT Tablets 597
Avalide Tablets 1070
Diovan HCT Tablets 2338
Dyazide Capsules 1515
HydroDIURIL Tablets 2108
Hyzaar 2109
Inderide Tablets 3517
Inderide LA Long-Acting Capsules 3519
Lotensin HCT Tablets 2367
Maxzide 1008
Micardis HCT Tablets 1051
Microzide Capsules 3414
Moduretic Tablets 2138
Monopril HCT 1094
Prinzide Tablets 2168
Timolide Tablets 2187
Uniretic Tablets 3178
Vaseretic Tablets 2204
Zestoretic Tablets 695
Ziac Tablets 1887

Hydrocodone Bitartrate (Aggravates orthostatic hypotension). Products include:
Hycodan 1316
Hycomine Compound Tablets 1317
Hycotuss Expectorant Syrup 1318
Lortab 3319
Lortab Elixir 3317
Maxidone Tablets CIII 3399
Norco 5/325 Tablets CIII 3424
Norco 7.5/325 Tablets CIII 3425
Norco 10/325 Tablets CIII 3427
Norco 10/325 Tablets CIII 3425
Vicodin Tablets 516
Vicodin ES Tablets 517
Vicodin HP Tablets 518
Vicodin Tuss Expectorant 519
Vicoprofen Tablets 520
Zydone Tablets 1330

Hydrocodone Polistirex (Aggravates orthostatic hypotension). Products include:
Tussionex Pennkinetic Extended-Release Suspension 1174

Hydrocortisone (Co-administration with corticosteroids may increase the risk of hypokalemia). Products include:
Anusol-HC Cream 2.5% 2237
Cipro HC Otic Suspension 540
Cortaid Intensive Therapy Cream ▣ 717
Cortaid Maximum Strength Cream ▣ 717
Cortisporin Ophthalmic Suspension Sterile ⊙ 297
Cortizone•5 ▣ 699
Cortizone•10 ▣ 699
Cortizone•10 Plus Creme ▣ 700
Cortizone for Kids Creme ▣ 699
Hydrocortone Tablets 2106
Massengill Medicated Soft Cloth Towelette ▣ 753
VōSoL HC Otic Solution 3356

Hydrocortisone Acetate (Co-administration with corticosteroids may increase the risk of hypokalemia). Products include:
Analpram-HC 1338
Anusol HC-1 Hydrocortisone Anti-Itch Cream ▣ 689
Anusol-HC Suppositories 2238
Cortaid ▣ 717
Cortifoam Rectal Foam 3170
Cortisporin-TC Otic Suspension 2246
Hydrocortone Acetate Injectable Suspension 2103
Pramosone 1343
Proctocort Suppositories 2264
ProctoFoam-HC 3177
Terra-Cortril Ophthalmic Suspension 2716

Hydrocortisone Sodium Phosphate (Co-administration with corticosteroids may increase the risk of hypokalemia). Products include:
Hydrocortone Phosphate Injection, Sterile 2105

Hydrocortisone Sodium Succinate (Co-administration with corticosteroids may increase the risk of hypokalemia).
No products indexed under this heading.

Hydroflumethiazide (Furosemide may add to or potentiate the therapeutic effect of other antihypertensive drugs). Products include:
Diucardin Tablets 3494

Hydromorphone Hydrochloride (Aggravates orthostatic hypotension). Products include:
Dilaudid 441
Dilaudid Oral Liquid 445
Dilaudid Powder 441
Dilaudid Rectal Suppositories 441
Dilaudid Tablets 441
Dilaudid Tablets - 8 mg 445
Dilaudid-HP 443

Ibuprofen (Co-administration with NSAIDs has resulted in increased BUN, serum creatinine and serum potassium levels, and weight gain). Products include:
- Advil ... 771
- Children's Advil Oral Suspension ... 773
- Children's Advil Chewable Tablets ... 773
- Advil Cold and Sinus Caplets ... 771
- Advil Cold and Sinus Tablets ... 771
- Advil Flu & Body Ache Caplets ... 772
- Infants' Advil Drops ... 773
- Junior Strength Advil Tablets ... 773
- Junior Strength Advil Chewable Tablets ... 773
- Advil Migraine Liquigels ... 772
- Children's Motrin Oral Suspension and Chewable Tablets ... 2006
- Children's Motrin Cold Oral Suspension ... 2007
- Children's Motrin Oral Suspension ... 643
- Motrin Suspension, Oral Drops, Chewable Tablets, and Caplets ... 2002
- Infants' Motrin Concentrated Drops ... 2006
- Junior Strength Motrin Caplets and Chewable Tablets ... 2006
- Motrin IB Tablets, Caplets, and Gelcaps ... 2002
- Motrin Migraine Pain Caplets ... 2005
- Motrin Sinus Headache Caplets ... 2005
- Vicoprofen Tablets ... 520

Indapamide (Furosemide may add to or potentiate the therapeutic effect of other antihypertensive drugs). Products include:
- Indapamide Tablets ... 2286

Indomethacin (Co-administration may educe the natriuretic and antihypertensive effects of furosemide in some patients by inhibiting prostaglandin synthesis). Products include:
- Indocin ... 2112

Indomethacin Sodium Trihydrate (Co-administration with NSAIDs has resulted in increased BUN, serum creatinine and serum potassium levels, and weight gain). Products include:
- Indocin I.V. ... 2115

Irbesartan (Furosemide may add to or potentiate the therapeutic effect of other antihypertensive drugs). Products include:
- Avalide Tablets ... 1070
- Avapro Tablets ... 1074
- Avapro Tablets ... 3076

Isradipine (Furosemide may add to or potentiate the therapeutic effect of other antihypertensive drugs). Products include:
- DynaCirc Capsules ... 2921
- DynaCirc CR Tablets ... 2923

Kanamycin Sulfate (Potential for increased risk of ototoxicity with concomitant therapy, especially in the presence of impaired renal function; avoid concurrent use except in presence of life threatening situations).
- No products indexed under this heading.

Ketoprofen (Co-administration with NSAIDs has resulted in increased BUN, serum creatinine and serum potassium levels, and weight gain). Products include:
- Orudis Capsules ... 3548
- Orudis KT Tablets ... 778
- Oruvail Capsules ... 3548

Ketorolac Tromethamine (Co-administration with NSAIDs has resulted in increased BUN, serum creatinine and serum potassium levels, and weight gain). Products include:
- Acular Ophthalmic Solution ... 544
- Acular PF Ophthalmic Solution ... 544
- Toradol ... 3018

Labetalol Hydrochloride (Furosemide may add to or potentiate the therapeutic effect of other antihypertensive drugs). Products include:
- Normodyne Injection ... 3135
- Normodyne Tablets ... 3137

Levorphanol Tartrate (Aggravates orthostatic hypotension). Products include:
- Levo-Dromoran ... 1734
- Levorphanol Tartrate Tablets ... 3059

Lisinopril (Furosemide may add to or potentiate the therapeutic effect of other antihypertensive drugs). Products include:
- Prinivil Tablets ... 2164
- Prinzide Tablets ... 2168
- Zestoretic Tablets ... 695
- Zestril Tablets ... 698

Lithium Carbonate (Diuretics reduce lithium's renal clearance and add a high risk of lithium toxicity). Products include:
- Eskalith ... 1527
- Lithium Carbonate ... 3061
- Lithobid Slow-Release Tablets ... 3255

Lithium Citrate (Diuretics reduce lithium's renal clearance and add a high risk of lithium toxicity). Products include:
- Lithium Citrate Syrup ... 3061

Losartan Potassium (Furosemide may add to or potentiate the therapeutic effect of other antihypertensive drugs). Products include:
- Cozaar Tablets ... 2067
- Hyzaar ... 2109

Magnesium Salicylate (Co-administration in patients receiving high doses of salicylates may experience salicylate toxicity). Products include:
- Momentum Backache Relief Extra Strength Caplets ... 666

Mecamylamine Hydrochloride (Furosemide may add to or potentiate the therapeutic effect of other antihypertensive drugs). Products include:
- Inversine Tablets ... 1850

Meclofenamate Sodium (Co-administration with NSAIDs has resulted in increased BUN, serum creatinine and serum potassium levels, and weight gain).
- No products indexed under this heading.

Mefenamic Acid (Co-administration with NSAIDs has resulted in increased BUN, serum creatinine and serum potassium levels, and weight gain). Products include:
- Ponstel Capsules ... 1356

Meloxicam (Co-administration with NSAIDs has resulted in increased BUN, serum creatinine and serum potassium levels, and weight gain). Products include:
- Mobic Tablets ... 1054

Meperidine Hydrochloride (Aggravates orthostatic hypotension). Products include:
- Demerol ... 3079
- Mepergan Injection ... 3539

Mephobarbital (Aggravates orthostatic hypotension).
- No products indexed under this heading.

Methadone Hydrochloride (Aggravates orthostatic hypotension). Products include:
- Dolophine Hydrochloride Tablets ... 3056

Methyclothiazide (Furosemide may add to or potentiate the therapeutic effect of other antihypertensive drugs).
- No products indexed under this heading.

Methyldopa (Furosemide may add to or potentiate the therapeutic effect of other antihypertensive drugs). Products include:
- Aldoclor Tablets ... 2035
- Aldomet Tablets ... 2037
- Aldoril Tablets ... 2039

Methyldopate Hydrochloride (Furosemide may add to or potentiate the therapeutic effect of other antihypertensive drugs).
- No products indexed under this heading.

Methylprednisolone Acetate (Co-administration with corticosteroids may increase the risk of hypokalemia). Products include:
- Depo-Medrol Injectable Suspension ... 2795

Methylprednisolone Sodium Succinate (Co-administration with corticosteroids may increase the risk of hypokalemia). Products include:
- Solu-Medrol Sterile Powder ... 2855

Metolazone (Furosemide may add to or potentiate the therapeutic effect of other antihypertensive drugs). Products include:
- Mykrox Tablets ... 1168
- Zaroxolyn Tablets ... 1177

Metoprolol Succinate (Furosemide may add to or potentiate the therapeutic effect of other antihypertensive drugs). Products include:
- Toprol-XL Tablets ... 651

Metoprolol Tartrate (Furosemide may add to or potentiate the therapeutic effect of other antihypertensive drugs).
- No products indexed under this heading.

Metyrosine (Furosemide may add to or potentiate the therapeutic effect of other antihypertensive drugs). Products include:
- Demser Capsules ... 2085

Mibefradil Dihydrochloride (Furosemide may add to or potentiate the therapeutic effect of other antihypertensive drugs).
- No products indexed under this heading.

Minoxidil (Furosemide may add to or potentiate the therapeutic effect of other antihypertensive drugs). Products include:
- Rogaine Extra Strength for Men Topical Solution ... 721
- Rogaine for Women Topical Solution ... 721

Moexipril Hydrochloride (Furosemide may add to or potentiate the therapeutic effect of other antihypertensive drugs). Products include:
- Uniretic Tablets ... 3178
- Univasc Tablets ... 3181

Morphine Sulfate (Aggravates orthostatic hypotension). Products include:
- Astramorph/PF Injection, USP (Preservative-Free) ... 594
- Duramorph Injection ... 1312
- Infumorph 200 and Infumorph 500 Sterile Solutions ... 1314
- Kadian Capsules ... 1335
- MS Contin Tablets ... 2896
- MSIR ... 2898
- Oramorph SR Tablets ... 3062
- Roxanol ... 3066

Nabumetone (Co-administration with NSAIDs has resulted in increased BUN, serum creatinine and serum potassium levels, and weight gain). Products include:
- Relafen Tablets ... 1617

Nadolol (Furosemide may add to or potentiate the therapeutic effect of other antihypertensive drugs). Products include:
- Corgard Tablets ... 2245
- Corzide 40/5 Tablets ... 2247
- Corzide 80/5 Tablets ... 2247
- Nadolol Tablets ... 2288

Naproxen (Co-administration with NSAIDs has resulted in increased BUN, serum creatinine and serum potassium levels, and weight gain). Products include:
- EC-Naprosyn Delayed-Release Tablets ... 2967
- Naprosyn Suspension ... 2967
- Naprosyn Tablets ... 2967

Naproxen Sodium (Co-administration with NSAIDs has resulted in increased BUN, serum creatinine and serum potassium levels, and weight gain). Products include:
- Aleve Tablets, Caplets and Gelcaps ... 602
- Aleve Cold & Sinus Caplets ... 603
- Anaprox Tablets ... 2967
- Anaprox DS Tablets ... 2967
- Naprelan Tablets ... 1293

Nicardipine Hydrochloride (Furosemide may add to or potentiate the therapeutic effect of other antihypertensive drugs). Products include:
- Cardene I.V. ... 3485

Nifedipine (Furosemide may add to or potentiate the therapeutic effect of other antihypertensive drugs). Products include:
- Adalat CC Tablets ... 877
- Procardia Capsules ... 2708
- Procardia XL Extended Release Tablets ... 2710

Nisoldipine (Furosemide may add to or potentiate the therapeutic effect of other antihypertensive drugs). Products include:
- Sular Tablets ... 688

Nitroglycerin (Furosemide may add to or potentiate the therapeutic effect of other antihypertensive drugs). Products include:
- Nitro-Dur Transdermal Infusion System ... 3134
- Nitro-Dur Transdermal Infusion System ... 1834
- Nitrolingual Pumpspray ... 1355
- Nitrostat Tablets ... 2658

Norepinephrine Bitartrate (Furosemide may decrease arterial responsiveness to norepinephrine).
- No products indexed under this heading.

Oxaprozin (Co-administration with NSAIDs has resulted in increased BUN, serum creatinine and serum potassium levels, and weight gain).
- No products indexed under this heading.

Oxycodone Hydrochloride (Aggravates orthostatic hypotension). Products include:
- OxyContin Tablets ... 2912
- OxyFast Oral Concentrate Solution ... 2916
- OxyIR Capsules ... 2916
- Percocet Tablets ... 1326
- Percodan Tablets ... 1327
- Percolone Tablets ... 1327
- Roxicodone ... 3067
- Tylox Capsules ... 2597

Penbutolol Sulfate (Furosemide may add to or potentiate the therapeutic effect of other antihypertensive drugs).
- No products indexed under this heading.

Pentobarbital Sodium (Aggravates orthostatic hypotension). Products include:
- Nembutal Sodium Solution ... 485

Perindopril Erbumine (Furosemide may add to or potentiate the therapeutic effect of other antihypertensive drugs). Products include:
- Aceon Tablets (2 mg, 4 mg, 8 mg) ... 3249

Phenobarbital (Aggravates orthostatic hypotension). Products include:
- Arco-Lase Plus Tablets ... 592
- Donnatal ... 2929
- Donnatal Extentabs ... 2930

Phenoxybenzamine Hydrochloride (Furosemide may add to or potentiate the therapeutic effect of other antihypertensive drugs). Products include:
- Dibenzyline Capsules ... 3457

Phentolamine Mesylate (Furosemide may add to or potentiate the therapeutic effect of other antihypertensive drugs).
- No products indexed under this heading.

Phenylbutazone (Co-administration with NSAIDs has resulted in increased BUN, serum creatinine

and serum potassium levels, and weight gain).
No products indexed under this heading.

Pindolol (Furosemide may add to or potentiate the therapeutic effect of other antihypertensive drugs).
No products indexed under this heading.

Piroxicam (Co-administration with NSAIDs has resulted in increased BUN, serum creatinine and serum potassium levels, and weight gain). Products include:
Feldene Capsules 2685

Polythiazide (Furosemide may add to or potentiate the therapeutic effect of other antihypertensive drugs). Products include:
Minizide Capsules 2700
Renese Tablets 2712

Prazosin Hydrochloride (Furosemide may add to or potentiate the therapeutic effect of other antihypertensive drugs). Products include:
Minipress Capsules 2699
Minizide Capsules 2700

Prednisolone Acetate (Co-administration with corticosteroids may increase the risk of hypokalemia). Products include:
Blephamide Ophthalmic Ointment ... 547
Blephamide Ophthalmic Suspension 548
Poly-Pred Liquifilm Ophthalmic Suspension .... ⊙245
Pred Forte Ophthalmic Suspension .... ⊙246
Pred Mild Sterile Ophthalmic Suspension .... ⊙249
Pred-G Ophthalmic Suspension ..... ⊙247
Pred-G Sterile Ophthalmic Ointment .... ⊙248

Prednisolone Sodium Phosphate (Co-administration with corticosteroids may increase the risk of hypokalemia). Products include:
Pediapred Oral Solution 1170

Prednisolone Tebutate (Co-administration with corticosteroids may increase the risk of hypokalemia).
No products indexed under this heading.

Prednisone (Co-administration with corticosteroids may increase the risk of hypokalemia). Products include:
Prednisone 3064

Propoxyphene Hydrochloride (Aggravates orthostatic hypotension). Products include:
Darvon Pulvules 1909
Darvon Compound-65 Pulvules 1910

Propoxyphene Napsylate (Aggravates orthostatic hypotension). Products include:
Darvon-N/Darvocet-N 1907
Darvon-N Tablets 1912

Propranolol Hydrochloride (Furosemide may add to or potentiate the therapeutic effect of other antihypertensive drugs). Products include:
Inderal 3513
Inderal LA Long-Acting Capsules 3516
Inderide Tablets 3517
Inderide LA Long-Acting Capsules .. 3519

Quinapril Hydrochloride (Furosemide may add to or potentiate the therapeutic effect of other antihypertensive drugs). Products include:
Accupril Tablets 2611
Accuretic Tablets 2614

Ramipril (Furosemide may add to or potentiate the therapeutic effect of other antihypertensive drugs). Products include:
Altace Capsules 2233

Rauwolfia serpentina (Furosemide may add to or potentiate the therapeutic effect of other antihypertensive drugs).
No products indexed under this heading.

Remifentanil Hydrochloride (Aggravates orthostatic hypotension).
No products indexed under this heading.

Rescinnamine (Furosemide may add to or potentiate the therapeutic effect of other antihypertensive drugs).
No products indexed under this heading.

Reserpine (Furosemide may add to or potentiate the therapeutic effect of other antihypertensive drugs).
No products indexed under this heading.

Rofecoxib (Co-administration with NSAIDs has resulted in increased BUN, serum creatinine and serum potassium levels, and weight gain). Products include:
Vioxx 2213

Salsalate (Co-administration in patients receiving high doses of salicylates may experience salicylate toxicity).
No products indexed under this heading.

Secobarbital Sodium (Aggravates orthostatic hypotension).
No products indexed under this heading.

Sodium Nitroprusside (Furosemide may add to or potentiate the therapeutic effect of other antihypertensive drugs).
No products indexed under this heading.

Sotalol Hydrochloride (Furosemide may add to or potentiate the therapeutic effect of other antihypertensive drugs). Products include:
Betapace Tablets 950
Betapace AF Tablets 954

Spirapril Hydrochloride (Furosemide may add to or potentiate the therapeutic effect of other antihypertensive drugs).
No products indexed under this heading.

Streptomycin Sulfate (Potential for increased risk of ototoxicity with concomitant therapy, especially in the presence of impaired renal function; avoid concurrent use except in presence of life threatening situations). Products include:
Streptomycin Sulfate Injection 2714

Succinylcholine Chloride (Furosemide has a tendency to potentiate the action of succinylcholine). Products include:
Anectine Injection 1476

Sucralfate (Simultaneous administration of sucralfate and furosemide may reduce the natriuretic and antihypertensive effects of furosemide; the intake of these two drugs should be separated by at least two hours). Products include:
Carafate Suspension 731
Carafate Tablets 730

Sufentanil Citrate (Aggravates orthostatic hypotension).
No products indexed under this heading.

Sulindac (Co-administration with NSAIDs has resulted in increased BUN, serum creatinine and serum potassium levels, and weight gain). Products include:
Clinoril Tablets 2053

Telmisartan (Furosemide may add to or potentiate the therapeutic effect of other antihypertensive drugs). Products include:
Micardis Tablets 1049
Micardis HCT Tablets 1051

Terazosin Hydrochloride (Furosemide may add to or potentiate the therapeutic effect of other antihypertensive drugs). Products include:
Hytrin Capsules 464

Thiamylal Sodium (Aggravates orthostatic hypotension).
No products indexed under this heading.

Timolol Maleate (Furosemide may add to or potentiate the therapeutic effect of other antihypertensive drugs). Products include:
Blocadren Tablets 2046
Cosopt Sterile Ophthalmic Solution 2065
Timolide Tablets 2187
Timolol GFS .... ⊙266
Timoptic in Ocudose 2192
Timoptic Sterile Ophthalmic Solution 2190
Timoptic-XE Sterile Ophthalmic Gel Forming Solution 2194

Tobramycin (Potential for increased risk of ototoxicity with concomitant therapy, especially in the presence of impaired renal function; avoid concurrent use except in presence of life threatening situations). Products include:
TOBI Solution for Inhalation 1206
TobraDex Ophthalmic Ointment 542
TobraDex Ophthalmic Suspension .. 541
Tobrex Ophthalmic Ointment .... ⊙220
Tobrex Ophthalmic Solution .... ⊙221

Tobramycin Sulfate (Potential for increased risk of ototoxicity with concomitant therapy, especially in the presence of impaired renal function; avoid concurrent use except in presence of life threatening situations). Products include:
Nebcin Vials, Hyporets & ADD-Vantage 1955

Tolmetin Sodium (Co-administration with NSAIDs has resulted in increased BUN, serum creatinine and serum potassium levels, and weight gain). Products include:
Tolectin 2589

Torsemide (Furosemide may add to or potentiate the therapeutic effect of other antihypertensive drugs). Products include:
Demadex Tablets and Injection 2965

Trandolapril (Furosemide may add to or potentiate the therapeutic effect of other antihypertensive drugs). Products include:
Mavik Tablets 478
Tarka Tablets 508

Triamcinolone (Co-administration with corticosteroids may increase the risk of hypokalemia).
No products indexed under this heading.

Triamcinolone Acetonide (Co-administration with corticosteroids may increase the risk of hypokalemia). Products include:
Azmacort Inhalation Aerosol 728
Nasacort Nasal Inhaler 750
Nasacort AQ Nasal Spray 752
Tri-Nasal Spray 2274

Triamcinolone Diacetate (Co-administration with corticosteroids may increase the risk of hypokalemia).
No products indexed under this heading.

Triamcinolone Hexacetonide (Co-administration with corticosteroids may increase the risk of hypokalemia).
No products indexed under this heading.

Trimethaphan Camsylate (Furosemide may add to or potentiate the therapeutic effect of other antihypertensive drugs).
No products indexed under this heading.

Tubocurarine Chloride (Furosemide has a tendency to antagonize the skeletal muscle relaxing effects of tubocurarine).
No products indexed under this heading.

Valsartan (Furosemide may add to or potentiate the therapeutic effect of other antihypertensive drugs). Products include:
Diovan Capsules 2337
Diovan HCT Tablets 2338

Verapamil Hydrochloride (Furosemide may add to or potentiate the therapeutic effect of other antihypertensive drugs). Products include:
Covera-HS Tablets 3199
Isoptin SR Tablets 467
Tarka Tablets 508
Verelan Capsules 3184
Verelan PM Capsules 3186

Food Interactions

Alcohol (Aggravates orthostatic hypotension).

GABITRIL TABLETS

(Tiagabine Hydrochloride) 1189
May interact with central nervous system depressants. Compounds in these categories include:

Alfentanil Hydrochloride (Possible additive depressive effects).
No products indexed under this heading.

Alprazolam (Possible additive depressive effects). Products include:
Xanax Tablets 2865

Aprobarbital (Possible additive depressive effects).
No products indexed under this heading.

Buprenorphine Hydrochloride (Possible additive depressive effects). Products include:
Buprenex Injectable 2918

Buspirone Hydrochloride (Possible additive depressive effects).
No products indexed under this heading.

Butabarbital (Possible additive depressive effects).
No products indexed under this heading.

Butalbital (Possible additive depressive effects). Products include:
Phrenilin 578
Sedapap Tablets 50 mg/650 mg ... 2225

Carbamazepine (Population pharmacokinetic analyses indicate that tiagabine clearance is 60% greater in patients taking carbamazepine with or without other enzyme-inducing antiepileptic drugs; tiagabine had no effect on the steady-state plasma concentrations of carbamazepine or its epoxide metabolite in patients with epilepsy). Products include:
Carbatrol Capsules 3234
Tegretol/Tegretol-XR 2404

Chlordiazepoxide (Possible additive depressive effects). Products include:
Limbitrol 1738

Chlordiazepoxide Hydrochloride (Possible additive depressive effects). Products include:
Librium Capsules 1736
Librium for Injection 1737

Chlorpromazine (Possible additive depressive effects). Products include:
Thorazine Suppositories 1656

Chlorpromazine Hydrochloride (Possible additive depressive effects). Products include:
Thorazine 1656

Chlorprothixene (Possible additive depressive effects).
No products indexed under this heading.

Chlorprothixene Hydrochloride (Possible additive depressive effects).
No products indexed under this heading.

Chlorprothixene Lactate (Possible additive depressive effects).
No products indexed under this heading.

Clorazepate Dipotassium (Possible additive depressive effects). Products include:
Tranxene ... 511

Clozapine (Possible additive depressive effects). Products include:
Clozaril Tablets ... 2319

Codeine Phosphate (Possible additive depressive effects). Products include:
Phenergan with Codeine Syrup ... 3557
Phenergan VC with Codeine Syrup .. 3561
Robitussin A-C Syrup ... 2942
Robitussin-DAC Syrup ... 2942
Ryna-C Liquid ... 768
Soma Compound w/Codeine Tablets ... 3355
Tussi-Organidin NR Liquid ... 3350
Tussi-Organidin-S NR Liquid ... 3350
Tylenol with Codeine ... 2595

Desflurane (Possible additive depressive effects). Products include:
Suprane Liquid for Inhalation ... 874

Dezocine (Possible additive depressive effects).
No products indexed under this heading.

Diazepam (Possible additive depressive effects). Products include:
Valium Injectable ... 3026
Valium Tablets ... 3047

Divalproex Sodium (Co-administration of tiagabine in patients taking valproate chronically had no effect on tiagabine pharmacokinetics, but valproate significantly decreased tiagabine binding in vitro from 96.3% to 94.8% which resulted in an increase of approximately 40% in the tiagabine concentrations; the clinical relevance of this in vitro finding is unknown). Products include:
Depakote Sprinkle Capsules ... 426
Depakote Tablets ... 430
Depakote ER Tablets ... 436

Droperidol (Possible additive depressive effects).
No products indexed under this heading.

Enflurane (Possible additive depressive effects).
No products indexed under this heading.

Estazolam (Possible additive depressive effects). Products include:
ProSom Tablets ... 500

Ethchlorvynol (Possible additive depressive effects).
No products indexed under this heading.

Ethinamate (Possible additive depressive effects).
No products indexed under this heading.

Fentanyl (Possible additive depressive effects). Products include:
Duragesic Transdermal System ... 1786

Fentanyl Citrate (Possible additive depressive effects). Products include:
Actiq ... 1184

Fluphenazine Decanoate (Possible additive depressive effects).
No products indexed under this heading.

Fluphenazine Enanthate (Possible additive depressive effects).
No products indexed under this heading.

Fluphenazine Hydrochloride (Possible additive depressive effects).
No products indexed under this heading.

Flurazepam Hydrochloride (Possible additive depressive effects).
No products indexed under this heading.

Fosphenytoin Sodium (Population pharmacokinetic analyses indicate that tiagabine clearance is 60% greater in patients taking phenytoin with or without other enzyme-inducing antiepileptic drugs; tiagabine had no effect on the steady-state plasma concentrations of phenytoin in patients with epilepsy). Products include:
Cerebyx Injection ... 2619

Glutethimide (Possible additive depressive effects).
No products indexed under this heading.

Haloperidol (Possible additive depressive effects). Products include:
Haldol Injection, Tablets and Concentrate ... 2533

Haloperidol Decanoate (Possible additive depressive effects). Products include:
Haldol Decanoate ... 2535

Hydrocodone Bitartrate (Possible additive depressive effects). Products include:
Hycodan ... 1316
Hycomine Compound Tablets ... 1317
Hycotuss Expectorant Syrup ... 1318
Lortab ... 3319
Lortab Elixir ... 3317
Maxidone Tablets CIII ... 3399
Norco 5/325 Tablets CIII ... 3424
Norco 7.5/325 Tablets CIII ... 3425
Norco 10/325 Tablets CIII ... 3427
Norco 10/325 Tablets CIII ... 3425
Vicodin Tablets ... 516
Vicodin ES Tablets ... 517
Vicodin HP Tablets ... 518
Vicodin Tuss Expectorant ... 519
Vicoprofen Tablets ... 520
Zydone Tablets ... 1330

Hydrocodone Polistirex (Possible additive depressive effects). Products include:
Tussionex Pennkinetic Extended-Release Suspension ... 1174

Hydromorphone Hydrochloride (Possible additive depressive effects). Products include:
Dilaudid ... 441
Dilaudid Oral Liquid ... 445
Dilaudid Powder ... 441
Dilaudid Rectal Suppositories ... 441
Dilaudid Tablets ... 441
Dilaudid Tablets - 8 mg ... 445
Dilaudid-HP ... 443

Hydroxyzine Hydrochloride (Possible additive depressive effects). Products include:
Atarax Tablets & Syrup ... 2667
Vistaril Intramuscular Solution ... 2738

Isoflurane (Possible additive depressive effects).
No products indexed under this heading.

Ketamine Hydrochloride (Possible additive depressive effects).
No products indexed under this heading.

Levomethadyl Acetate Hydrochloride (Possible additive depressive effects).
No products indexed under this heading.

Levorphanol Tartrate (Possible additive depressive effects). Products include:
Levo-Dromoran ... 1734
Levorphanol Tartrate Tablets ... 3059

Lorazepam (Possible additive depressive effects). Products include:
Ativan Injection ... 3478
Ativan Tablets ... 3482

Loxapine Hydrochloride (Possible additive depressive effects).
No products indexed under this heading.

Loxapine Succinate (Possible additive depressive effects). Products include:
Loxitane Capsules ... 3398

Meperidine Hydrochloride (Possible additive depressive effects). Products include:
Demerol ... 3079
Mepergan Injection ... 3539

Mephobarbital (Possible additive depressive effects).
No products indexed under this heading.

Meprobamate (Possible additive depressive effects). Products include:
Miltown Tablets ... 3349

Mesoridazine Besylate (Possible additive depressive effects). Products include:
Serentil ... 1057

Methadone Hydrochloride (Possible additive depressive effects). Products include:
Dolophine Hydrochloride Tablets ... 3056

Methohexital Sodium (Possible additive depressive effects). Products include:
Brevital Sodium for Injection, USP .. 1815

Methotrimeprazine (Possible additive depressive effects).
No products indexed under this heading.

Methoxyflurane (Possible additive depressive effects).
No products indexed under this heading.

Midazolam Hydrochloride (Possible additive depressive effects). Products include:
Versed Injection ... 3027
Versed Syrup ... 3033

Molindone Hydrochloride (Possible additive depressive effects). Products include:
Moban ... 1320

Morphine Sulfate (Possible additive depressive effects). Products include:
Astramorph/PF Injection, USP (Preservative-Free) ... 594
Duramorph Injection ... 1312
Infumorph 200 and Infumorph 500 Sterile Solutions ... 1314
Kadian Capsules ... 1335
MS Contin Tablets ... 2896
MSIR ... 2898
Oramorph SR Tablets ... 3062
Roxanol ... 3066

Olanzapine (Possible additive depressive effects). Products include:
Zyprexa Tablets ... 1973
Zyprexa ZYDIS Orally Disintegrating Tablets ... 1973

Oxazepam (Possible additive depressive effects).
No products indexed under this heading.

Oxycodone Hydrochloride (Possible additive depressive effects). Products include:
OxyContin Tablets ... 2912
OxyFast Oral Concentrate Solution . 2916
OxyIR Capsules ... 2916
Percocet Tablets ... 1326
Percodan Tablets ... 1327
Percolone Tablets ... 1327
Roxicodone ... 3067
Tylox Capsules ... 2597

Pentobarbital Sodium (Possible additive depressive effects). Products include:
Nembutal Sodium Solution ... 485

Perphenazine (Possible additive depressive effects). Products include:
Etrafon ... 3115
Trilafon ... 3160

Phenobarbital (Population pharmacokinetic analyses indicate that tiagabine clearance is 60% greater in patients taking phenobarbital with or without other enzyme-inducing antiepileptic drugs; possible additive depressive effects). Products include:
Arco-Lase Plus Tablets ... 592
Donnatal ... 2929
Donnatal Extentabs ... 2930

Phenytoin (Population pharmacokinetic analyses indicate that tiagabine clearance is 60% greater in patients taking phenytoin with or without other enzyme-inducing antiepileptic drugs; tiagabine had no effect on the steady-state plasma concentrations of phenytoin in patients with epilepsy). Products include:
Dilantin Infatabs ... 2624
Dilantin-125 Oral Suspension ... 2625

Phenytoin Sodium (Population pharmacokinetic analyses indicate that tiagabine clearance is 60% greater in patients taking phenytoin with or without other enzyme-inducing antiepileptic drugs; tiagabine had no effect on the steady-state plasma concentrations of phenytoin in patients with epilepsy). Products include:
Dilantin Kapseals ... 2622

Prazepam (Possible additive depressive effects).
No products indexed under this heading.

Prochlorperazine (Possible additive depressive effects). Products include:
Compazine ... 1505

Promethazine Hydrochloride (Possible additive depressive effects). Products include:
Mepergan Injection ... 3539
Phenergan Injection ... 3553
Phenergan ... 3556
Phenergan Syrup ... 3554
Phenergan with Codeine Syrup ... 3557
Phenergan with Dextromethorphan Syrup ... 3559
Phenergan VC Syrup ... 3560
Phenergan VC with Codeine Syrup .. 3561

Propofol (Possible additive depressive effects). Products include:
Diprivan Injectable Emulsion ... 667

Propoxyphene Hydrochloride (Possible additive depressive effects). Products include:
Darvon Pulvules ... 1909
Darvon Compound-65 Pulvules ... 1910

Propoxyphene Napsylate (Possible additive depressive effects). Products include:
Darvon-N/Darvocet-N ... 1907
Darvon-N Tablets ... 1912

Quazepam (Possible additive depressive effects).
No products indexed under this heading.

Quetiapine Fumarate (Possible additive depressive effects). Products include:
Seroquel Tablets ... 684

Remifentanil Hydrochloride (Possible additive depressive effects).
No products indexed under this heading.

Risperidone (Possible additive depressive effects). Products include:
Risperdal ... 1796

Secobarbital Sodium (Possible additive depressive effects).
No products indexed under this heading.

Sevoflurane (Possible additive depressive effects).
No products indexed under this heading.

Sufentanil Citrate (Possible additive depressive effects).
No products indexed under this heading.

Temazepam (Possible additive depressive effects).
No products indexed under this heading.

IMPORTANT NOTE: Always consult each drug listing in the patient's regimen for possible interactions.

Thiamylal Sodium (Possible additive depressive effects).
No products indexed under this heading.

Thioridazine Hydrochloride (Possible additive depressive effects). Products include:
Thioridazine Hydrochloride Tablets 2289

Thiothixene (Possible additive depressive effects). Products include:
Navane Capsules 2701
Thiothixene Capsules 2290

Triazolam (Possible additive depressive effects). Products include:
Halcion Tablets 2823

Trifluoperazine Hydrochloride (Possible additive depressive effects). Products include:
Stelazine 1640

Valproate Sodium (Co-administration of tiagabine in patients taking valproate chronically had no effect on tiagabine pharmacokinetics, but valproate significantly decreased tiagabine binding in vitro from 96.3% to 94.8% which resulted in an increase of approximately 40% in the tiagabine concentrations; the clinical relevance of this in vitro finding is unknown). Products include:
Depacon Injection 416

Valproic Acid (Co-administration of tiagabine in patients taking valproate chronically had no effect on tiagabine pharmacokinetics, but valproate significantly decreased tiagabine binding in vitro from 96.3% to 94.8% which resulted in an increase of approximately 40% in the tiagabine concentrations; the clinical relevance of this in vitro finding is unknown). Products include:
Depakene 421

Zaleplon (Possible additive depressive effects). Products include:
Sonata Capsules 3591

Ziprasidone Hydrochloride (Possible additive depressive effects). Products include:
Geodon Capsules 2688

Zolpidem Tartrate (Possible additive depressive effects). Products include:
Ambien Tablets 3191

Food Interactions

Alcohol (Possible additive depressive effects).

Food, unspecified (A high fat meal decreases the rate (mean Tmax was prolonged to 2.5 hours, and Cmax was reduced by about 40%) but not the extent (AUC) of tiagabine).

GAMIMUNE N, 5% SOLVENT/DETERGENT TREATED
(Globulin, Immune (Human)) 925
May interact with:

Measles, Mumps & Rubella Virus Vaccine, Live (Antibodies in Gamimune N, 5% may interfere with the response to live virus vaccine; use of such vaccines should be deferred until approximately 6 months after Gamimune N, 10% administration). Products include:
M-M-R II 2118

GAMIMUNE N, 10% SOLVENT/DETERGENT TREATED
(Globulin, Immune (Human)) 928
See Gamimune N, 5% Solvent/Detergent Treated

GAMMAGARD S/D
(Globulin, Immune (Human)) 845
May interact with:

Measles, Mumps & Rubella Virus Vaccine, Live (Antibodies in immune globulin may interfere with patient response to vaccine). Products include:
M-M-R II 2118

GAMMAR-P I.V.
(Immune Globulin (Human)) 787
May interact with:

Measles, Mumps & Rubella Virus Vaccine, Live (Antibodies in the globulin preparation may interfere with the response to live viral vaccines). Products include:
M-M-R II 2118

MAXIMUM STRENGTH GAS AID SOFTGELS
(Simethicone) 2001
None cited in PDR database.

GASTROCROM ORAL CONCENTRATE
(Cromolyn Sodium) 1162
May interact with:

Isoproterenol Hydrochloride (Concurrent use at extremely high doses of both drugs appears to have increased resorptions and malformations in animal studies).
No products indexed under this heading.

GAS-X CHEWABLE TABLETS
(Simethicone) .... ▣671
None cited in PDR database.

EXTRA STRENGTH GAS-X LIQUID
(Simethicone) .... ▣671
None cited in PDR database.

EXTRA STRENGTH GAS-X SOFTGELS
(Simethicone) .... ▣671
None cited in PDR database.

EXTRA STRENGTH GAS-X CHEWABLE TABLETS
(Simethicone) .... ▣671
None cited in PDR database.

MAXIMUM STRENGTH GAS-X SOFTGELS
(Simethicone) .... ▣671
None cited in PDR database.

GAVISCON EXTRA STRENGTH LIQUID
(Aluminum Hydroxide, Magnesium Carbonate) .... ▣751
May interact with:

Prescription Drugs, unspecified (Concurrent use with certain unspecified drugs is not recommended; consult your physicians).

GAVISCON EXTRA STRENGTH TABLETS
(Aluminum Hydroxide, Magnesium Carbonate) .... ▣751
May interact with:

Prescription Drugs, unspecified (Concurrent use with certain unspecified drugs is not recommended; consult your physicians).

GAVISCON REGULAR STRENGTH LIQUID
(Aluminum Hydroxide, Magnesium Carbonate) .... ▣751
May interact with:

Prescription Drugs, unspecified (Concurrent use with certain unspecified drugs is not recommended; consult your physicians).

GAVISCON REGULAR STRENGTH TABLETS
(Aluminum Hydroxide, Magnesium Trisilicate) .... ▣750
May interact with:

Prescription Drugs, unspecified (Concurrent use with certain unspecified drugs is not recommended; consult your physicians).

GEBAUER'S ETHYL CHLORIDE
(Ethyl Chloride) 1409
None cited in PDR database.

GEMZAR FOR INJECTION
(Gemcitabine Hydrochloride) 1919
None cited in PDR database.

GENGRAF CAPSULES
(Cyclosporine) 457
May interact with erythromycin, immunosuppressive agents, methylprednisolone, non-steroidal anti-inflammatory agents, phenytoin, prednisolone, protease inhibitors, potassium sparing diuretics, and certain other agents. Compounds in these categories include:

Allopurinol (Co-administration with drugs that inhibit CYP4503A, such as allopurinol, could decrease metabolism of cyclosporine and increase its concentrations).
No products indexed under this heading.

Amiloride Hydrochloride (Cyclosporine causes hyperkalemia; concurrent use with potassium-sparing diuretics can result in increased risk of hyperkalemia; co-administration should be avoided). Products include:
Midamor Tablets 2136
Moduretic Tablets 2138

Amphotericin B (May potentiate renal dysfunction). Products include:
Abelcet Injection 1273
AmBisome for Injection 1383
Amphotec 1774

Amprenavir (The HIV inhibitors are known to inhibit CYP4503A and increase the concentration of drugs metabolized by this system; cyclosporine is extensively metabolized by CYP4503A system, therefore, caution should be exercised). Products include:
Agenerase Capsules 1454
Agenerase Oral Solution 1459

Azapropazon (May potentiate renal dysfunction).

Azathioprine (Co-administration with other immunosuppressive agents increases the possibility of excessive immunosuppression).
No products indexed under this heading.

Basiliximab (Co-administration with other immunosuppressive agents increases the possibility of excessive immunosuppression). Products include:
Simulect for Injection 2399

Bromocriptine Mesylate (Co-administration with drugs that inhibit CYP4503A, such as bromocriptine, could decrease metabolism of cyclosporine and increase its concentrations).
No products indexed under this heading.

Carbamazepine (Co-administration with drugs that are inducers of CYP4503A, such as carbamazepine, could increase metabolism of cyclosporine and decrease its concentrations). Products include:
Carbatrol Capsules 3234
Tegretol/Tegretol-XR 2404

Celecoxib (Cyclosporine can cause nephrotoxicity; clinical status and serum creatinine should be closely monitored when cyclosporine is used with NSAIDs in rheumatoid arthritis patients). Products include:
Celebrex Capsules 2676
Celebrex Capsules 2780

Cimetidine (May potentiate renal dysfunction). Products include:
Tagamet HB 200 Suspension .... ▣762
Tagamet HB 200 Tablets .... ▣761
Tagamet Tablets 1644

Cimetidine Hydrochloride (May potentiate renal dysfunction). Products include:
Tagamet 1644

Clarithromycin (Co-administration with drugs that inhibit CYP4503A, such as clarithromycin, could decrease metabolism of cyclosporine and increase its concentrations). Products include:
Biaxin/Biaxin XL 403
PREVPAC 3298

Danazol (Co-administration with drugs that inhibit CYP4503A, such as danazol, could decrease metabolism of cyclosporine and increase its concentrations).
No products indexed under this heading.

Diclofenac Potassium (May potentiate renal dysfunction; potential for doubling of diclofenac blood levels and occasional reports of reversible decreases in renal function has been reported with concurrent use). Products include:
Cataflam Tablets 2315

Diclofenac Sodium (May potentiate renal dysfunction; potential for doubling of diclofenac blood levels and occasional reports of reversible decreases in renal function has been reported with concurrent use). Products include:
Arthrotec Tablets 3195
Voltaren Ophthalmic Sterile Ophthalmic Solution .... ⊙312
Voltaren Tablets 2315
Voltaren-XR Tablets 2315

Digoxin (Co-administration results in reduced clearance of digoxin; decrease in the apparent volume of distribution of digoxin has reported with concurrent use along with digitalis toxicity). Products include:
Digitek Tablets 1003
Lanoxicaps Capsules 1574
Lanoxin Injection 1581
Lanoxin Tablets 1587
Lanoxin Elixir Pediatric 1578
Lanoxin Injection Pediatric 1584

Diltiazem Hydrochloride (Co-administration with drugs that inhibit CYP4503A, such as diltiazem, could decrease metabolism of cyclosporine and increase its concentrations). Products include:
Cardizem Injectable 1018
Cardizem Lyo-Ject Syringe 1018
Cardizem Monovial 1018
Cardizem CD Capsules 1016
Tiazac Capsules 1378

Diltiazem Malate (Co-administration with drugs that inhibit CYP4503A, such as diltiazem, could decrease metabolism of cyclosporine and increase its concentrations).
No products indexed under this heading.

Erythromycin (Co-administration with drugs that inhibit CYP4503A, such as erythromycin, could decrease metabolism of cyclosporine and increase its concentrations). Products include:
Emgel 2% Topical Gel 1285
Ery-Tab Tablets 448
Erythromycin Base Filmtab Tablets 454
Erythromycin Delayed-Release Capsules, USP 455
PCE Dispertab Tablets 498

Erythromycin Estolate (Co-administration with drugs that inhibit CYP4503A, such as erythromycin, could decrease metabolism of cyclosporine and increase its con-

centrations).
No products indexed under this heading.

Erythromycin Ethylsuccinate (Co-administration with drugs that inhibit CYP4503A, such as erythromycin, could decrease metabolism of cyclosporine and increase its concentrations). Products include:
E.E.S. ... 450
EryPed ... 446
Pediazole Suspension ... 3050

Erythromycin Gluceptate (Co-administration with drugs that inhibit CYP4503A, such as erythromycin, could decrease metabolism of cyclosporine and increase its concentrations).
No products indexed under this heading.

Erythromycin Stearate (Co-administration with drugs that inhibit CYP4503A, such as erythromycin, could decrease metabolism of cyclosporine and increase its concentrations). Products include:
Erythrocin Stearate Filmtab Tablets ... 452

Etodolac (Cyclosporine can cause nephrotoxicity; clinical status and serum creatinine should be closely monitored when cyclosporine is used with NSAIDs in rheumatoid arthritis patients). Products include:
Lodine ... 3528
Lodine XL Extended-Release Tablets ... 3530

Fenoprofen Calcium (Cyclosporine can cause nephrotoxicity; clinical status and serum creatinine should be closely monitored when cyclosporine is used with NSAIDs in rheumatoid arthritis patients).
No products indexed under this heading.

Fluconazole (Co-administration with drugs that inhibit CYP4503A, such as fluconazole, could decrease metabolism of cyclosporine and increase its concentrations). Products include:
Diflucan Tablets, Injection, and Oral Suspension ... 2681

Flurbiprofen (Cyclosporine can cause nephrotoxicity; clinical status and serum creatinine should be closely monitored when cyclosporine is used with NSAIDs in rheumatoid arthritis patients).
No products indexed under this heading.

Fosphenytoin Sodium (Co-administration with drugs that are inducers of CYP4503A, such as phenytoin, could increase metabolism of cyclosporine and decrease its concentrations). Products include:
Cerebyx Injection ... 2619

Gentamicin Sulfate (May potentiate renal dysfunction). Products include:
Genoptic Ophthalmic Ointment ... ⊙ 239
Genoptic Sterile Ophthalmic Solution ... ⊙ 239
Pred-G Ophthalmic Suspension ... ⊙ 247
Pred-G Sterile Ophthalmic Ointment ... ⊙ 248

Ibuprofen (Cyclosporine can cause nephrotoxicity; clinical status and serum creatinine should be closely monitored when cyclosporine is used with NSAIDs in rheumatoid arthritis patients). Products include:
Advil ... 771
Children's Advil Oral Suspension ... 773
Children's Advil Chewable Tablets ... 773
Advil Cold and Sinus Caplets ... 771
Advil Cold and Sinus Tablets ... 771
Advil Flu & Body Ache Caplets ... 772
Infants' Advil Drops ... 773
Junior Strength Advil Tablets ... 773
Junior Strength Advil Chewable Tablets ... 773
Advil Migraine Liquigels ... 772
Children's Motrin Oral Suspension and Chewable Tablets ... 2006
Children's Motrin Cold Oral Suspension ... 2007
Children's Motrin Oral Suspension ... 643
Motrin Suspension, Oral Drops, Chewable Tablets, and Caplets ... 2002
Infants' Motrin Concentrated Drops ... 2006
Junior Strength Motrin Caplets and Chewable Tablets ... 2006
Motrin IB Tablets, Caplets, and Gelcaps ... 2002
Motrin Migraine Pain Caplets ... 2005
Motrin Sinus Headache Caplets ... 2005
Vicoprofen Tablets ... 520

Indinavir Sulfate (The HIV inhibitors are known to inhibit CYP4503A and increase the concentration of drugs metabolized by this system; cyclosporine is extensively metabolized by CYP4503A system, therefore, caution should be exercised). Products include:
Crixivan Capsules ... 2070

Indomethacin (Cyclosporine can cause nephrotoxicity; clinical status and serum creatinine should be closely monitored when cyclosporine is used with NSAIDs in rheumatoid arthritis patients). Products include:
Indocin ... 2112

Indomethacin Sodium Trihydrate (Cyclosporine can cause nephrotoxicity; clinical status and serum creatinine should be closely monitored when cyclosporine is used with NSAIDs in rheumatoid arthritis patients). Products include:
Indocin I.V. ... 2115

Itraconazole (Co-administration with drugs that inhibit CYP4503A, such as itraconazole, could decrease metabolism of cyclosporine and increase its concentrations). Products include:
Sporanox Capsules ... 1800
Sporanox Injection ... 1804
Sporanox Injection ... 2509
Sporanox Oral Solution ... 1808
Sporanox Oral Solution ... 2512

Ketoconazole (May potentiate renal dysfunction; co-administration with drugs that inhibit CYP4503A, such as ketoconazole, could decrease metabolism of cyclosporine and increase its concentrations). Products include:
Nizoral 2% Cream ... 3620
Nizoral A-D Shampoo ... 2008
Nizoral 2% Shampoo ... 2007
Nizoral Tablets ... 1791

Ketoprofen (Cyclosporine can cause nephrotoxicity; clinical status and serum creatinine should be closely monitored when cyclosporine is used with NSAIDs in rheumatoid arthritis patients). Products include:
Orudis Capsules ... 3548
Orudis KT Tablets ... 778
Oruvail Capsules ... 3548

Ketorolac Tromethamine (Cyclosporine can cause nephrotoxicity; clinical status and serum creatinine should be closely monitored when cyclosporine is used with NSAIDs in rheumatoid arthritis patients). Products include:
Acular Ophthalmic Solution ... 544
Acular PF Ophthalmic Solution ... 544
Toradol ... 3018

Lopinavir (The HIV inhibitors are known to inhibit CYP4503A and increase the concentration of drugs metabolized by this system; cyclosporine is extensively metabolized by CYP4503A system, therefore, caution should be exercised). Products include:
Kaletra Capsules ... 471
Kaletra Oral Solution ... 471

Lovastatin (Co-administration results in reduced clearance of lovastatin; myositis has been reported with concurrent use). Products include:
Mevacor Tablets ... 2132

Meclofenamate Sodium (Cyclosporine can cause nephrotoxicity; clinical status and serum creatinine should be closely monitored when cyclosporine is used with NSAIDs in rheumatoid arthritis patients).
No products indexed under this heading.

Mefenamic Acid (Cyclosporine can cause nephrotoxicity; clinical status and serum creatinine should be closely monitored when cyclosporine is used with NSAIDs in rheumatoid arthritis patients). Products include:
Ponstel Capsules ... 1356

Meloxicam (Cyclosporine can cause nephrotoxicity; clinical status and serum creatinine should be closely monitored when cyclosporine is used with NSAIDs in rheumatoid arthritis patients). Products include:
Mobic Tablets ... 1054

Melphalan (May potentiate renal dysfunction). Products include:
Alkeran Tablets ... 1466

Methotrexate Sodium (Co-administration in rheumatoid arthritis patients has resulted in increased concentrations (AUC) of methotrexate by approximately 30% and the concentrations of its metabolite, 7-hydroxymethotrexate, were decreased by approximately 80%; the clinical significance of this outcome is not known).
No products indexed under this heading.

Methylprednisolone (Co-administration with drugs that inhibit CYP4503A, such as methylprednisolone, could decrease metabolism of cyclosporine and increase its concentrations; convulsions have been reported with concurrent high dose methylprednisolone).
No products indexed under this heading.

Methylprednisolone Acetate (Co-administration with drugs that inhibit CYP4503A, such as methylprednisolone, could decrease metabolism of cyclosporine and increase its concentrations; convulsions have been reported with concurrent high dose methylprednisolone). Products include:
Depo-Medrol Injectable Suspension ... 2795

Methylprednisolone Sodium Succinate (Co-administration with drugs that inhibit CYP4503A, such as methylprednisolone, could decrease metabolism of cyclosporine and increase its concentrations; convulsions have been reported with concurrent high dose methylprednisolone). Products include:
Solu-Medrol Sterile Powder ... 2855

Metoclopramide Hydrochloride (Co-administration with drugs that inhibit CYP4503A, such as metoclopramide, could decrease metabolism of cyclosporine and increase its concentrations). Products include:
Reglan ... 2935

Muromonab-CD3 (Co-administration with other immunosuppressive agents increases the possibility of excessive immunosuppression). Products include:
Orthoclone OKT3 Sterile Solution ... 2498

Mycophenolate Mofetil (Co-administration with other immunosuppressive agents increases the possibility of excessive immunosuppression). Products include:
CellCept Capsules ... 2951
CellCept Oral Suspension ... 2951
CellCept Tablets ... 2951

Nabumetone (Cyclosporine can cause nephrotoxicity; clinical status and serum creatinine should be closely monitored when cyclosporine is used with NSAIDs in rheumatoid arthritis patients). Products include:
Relafen Tablets ... 1617

Nafcillin Sodium (Co-administration with drugs that are inducers of CYP4503A, such as nafcillin, could increase metabolism of cyclosporine and decrease its concentrations).
No products indexed under this heading.

Naproxen (May potentiate renal dysfunction; co-administration is associated with additive decreases in renal function). Products include:
EC-Naprosyn Delayed-Release Tablets ... 2967
Naprosyn Suspension ... 2967
Naprosyn Tablets ... 2967

Naproxen Sodium (May potentiate renal dysfunction; co-administration is associated with additive decreases in renal function). Products include:
Aleve Tablets, Caplets and Gelcaps ... 602
Aleve Cold & Sinus Caplets ... 603
Anaprox Tablets ... 2967
Anaprox DS Tablets ... 2967
Naprelan Tablets ... 1293

Nelfinavir Mesylate (The HIV inhibitors are known to inhibit CYP4503A and increase the concentration of drugs metabolized by this system; cyclosporine is extensively metabolized by CYP4503A system, therefore, caution should be exercised). Products include:
Viracept ... 532

Nicardipine Hydrochloride (Co-administration with drugs that inhibit CYP4503A, such as nicardipine, could decrease metabolism of cyclosporine and increase its concentrations). Products include:
Cardene I.V. ... 3485

Nifedipine (Co-administration results in frequent episodes of gingival hyperplasia). Products include:
Adalat CC Tablets ... 877
Procardia Capsules ... 2708
Procardia XL Extended Release Tablets ... 2710

Octreotide Acetate (Co-administration with drugs that are inducers of CYP4503A, such as octreotide, could increase metabolism of cyclosporine and decrease its concentrations). Products include:
Sandostatin LAR Depot ... 2395

Oxaprozin (Cyclosporine can cause nephrotoxicity; clinical status and serum creatinine should be closely monitored when cyclosporine is used with NSAIDs in rheumatoid arthritis patients).
No products indexed under this heading.

Phenobarbital (Co-administration with drugs that are inducers of CYP4503A, such as phenobarbital, could increase metabolism of cyclosporine and decrease its concentrations). Products include:
Arco-Lase Plus Tablets ... 592
Donnatal ... 2929
Donnatal Extentabs ... 2930

Phenylbutazone (Cyclosporine can cause nephrotoxicity; clinical status and serum creatinine should be closely monitored when cyclosporine is used with NSAIDs in rheumatoid arthritis patients).
No products indexed under this heading.

Phenytoin (Co-administration with drugs that are inducers of CYP4503A, such as phenytoin, could increase metabolism of cyclosporine and decrease its concentrations). Products include:
Dilantin Infatabs ... 2624
Dilantin-125 Oral Suspension ... 2625

Phenytoin Sodium (Co-administration with drugs that are inducers of CYP4503A, such as

phenytoin, could increase metabolism of cyclosporine and decrease its concentrations). Products include:
- Dilantin Kapseals 2622

Piroxicam (Cyclosporine can cause nephrotoxicity; clinical status and serum creatinine should be closely monitored when cyclosporine is used with NSAIDs in rheumatoid arthritis patients). Products include:
- Feldene Capsules 2685

Prednisolone (Co-administration results in reduced clearance of prednisolone). Products include:
- Prelone Syrup 2273

Prednisolone Acetate (Co-administration results in reduced clearance of prednisolone). Products include:
- Blephamide Ophthalmic Ointment ... 547
- Blephamide Ophthalmic Suspension 548
- Poly-Pred Liquifilm Ophthalmic Suspension .... ⊙245
- Pred Forte Ophthalmic Suspension .... ⊙246
- Pred Mild Sterile Ophthalmic Suspension .... ⊙249
- Pred-G Ophthalmic Suspension .... ⊙247
- Pred-G Sterile Ophthalmic Ointment .... ⊙248

Prednisolone Sodium Phosphate (Co-administration results in reduced clearance of prednisolone). Products include:
- Pediapred Oral Solution 1170

Prednisolone Tebutate (Co-administration results in reduced clearance of prednisolone).
No products indexed under this heading.

Ranitidine Hydrochloride (May potentiate renal dysfunction). Products include:
- Zantac 1690
- Zantac Injection 1688
- Zantac 75 Tablets .... ■717

Rifabutin (Rifabutin is known to increase the metabolism of other drugs metabolized by CYP450 system; cyclosporine is extensively metabolized by CYP4503A system, therefore, caution should be exercised). Products include:
- Mycobutin Capsules 2838

Rifampin (Co-administration with drugs that are inducers of CYP4503A, such as rifampin, could increase metabolism of cyclosporine and decrease its concentrations). Products include:
- Rifadin 765
- Rifamate Capsules 767
- Rifater Tablets 769

Ritonavir (The HIV inhibitors are known to inhibit CYP4503A and increase the concentration of drugs metabolized by this system; cyclosporine is extensively metabolized by CYP4503A system, therefore, caution should be exercised). Products include:
- Kaletra Capsules 471
- Kaletra Oral Solution 471
- Norvir Capsules 487
- Norvir Oral Solution 487

Rofecoxib (Cyclosporine can cause nephrotoxicity; clinical status and serum creatinine should be closely monitored when cyclosporine is used with NSAIDs in rheumatoid arthritis patients). Products include:
- Vioxx 2213

Saquinavir (The HIV inhibitors are known to inhibit CYP4503A and increase the concentration of drugs metabolized by this system; cyclosporine is extensively metabolized by CYP4503A system, therefore, caution should be exercised). Products include:
- Fortovase Capsules 2970

Saquinavir Mesylate (The HIV inhibitors are known to inhibit CYP4503A and increase the concentration of drugs metabolized by this system; cyclosporine is extensively metabolized by CYP4503A system, therefore, caution should be exercised). Products include:
- Invirase Capsules 2979

Sirolimus (Co-administration with other immunosuppressive agents increases the possibility of excessive immunosuppression). Products include:
- Rapamune Oral Solution and Tablets 3584

Spironolactone (Cyclosporine causes hyperkalemia; concurrent use with potassium-sparing diuretics can result in increased risk of hyperkalemia; co-administration should be avoided).
No products indexed under this heading.

Sulfamethoxazole (May potentiate renal dysfunction). Products include:
- Bactrim 2949
- Septra Suspension 2265
- Septra Tablets 2265
- Septra DS Tablets 2265

Sulindac (May potentiate renal dysfunction; co-administration is associated with additive decreases in renal function). Products include:
- Clinoril Tablets 2053

Tacrolimus (May potentiate renal dysfunction; co-administration with other immunosuppressive agents increases the possibility of excessive immunosuppression). Products include:
- Prograf 1393
- Protopic Ointment 1397

Ticlopidine Hydrochloride (Co-administration with drugs that are inducers of CYP4503A, such as ticlopidine, could increase metabolism of cyclosporine and decrease its concentrations). Products include:
- Ticlid Tablets 3015

Tobramycin (May potentiate renal dysfunction). Products include:
- TOBI Solution for Inhalation 1206
- TobraDex Ophthalmic Ointment 542
- TobraDex Ophthalmic Suspension .. 541
- Tobrex Ophthalmic Ointment .... ⊙220
- Tobrex Ophthalmic Solution .... ⊙221

Tobramycin Sulfate (May potentiate renal dysfunction). Products include:
- Nebcin Vials, Hyporets & ADD-Vantage 1955

Tolmetin Sodium (Cyclosporine can cause nephrotoxicity; clinical status and serum creatinine should be closely monitored when cyclosporine is used with NSAIDs in rheumatoid arthritis patients). Products include:
- Tolectin 2589

Triamterene (Cyclosporine causes hyperkalemia; concurrent use with potassium-sparing diuretics can result in increased risk of hyperkalemia; co-administration should be avoided). Products include:
- Dyazide Capsules 1515
- Dyrenium Capsules 3458
- Maxzide 1008

Trimethoprim (May potentiate renal dysfunction). Products include:
- Bactrim 2949
- Septra Suspension 2265
- Septra Tablets 2265
- Septra DS Tablets 2265

Vaccines (Live) (During treatment with cyclosporine, vaccination may be less effective and the use of live attenuated vaccines should be avoided).
No products indexed under this heading.

Vancomycin Hydrochloride (May potentiate renal dysfunction). Products include:
- Vancocin HCl Capsules & Pulvules .. 1972
- Vancocin HCl Oral Solution 1971
- Vancocin HCl, Vials & ADD-Vantage 1970

Verapamil Hydrochloride (Co-administration with drugs that inhibit CYP4503A, such as verapamil, could decrease metabolism of cyclosporine and increase its concentrations). Products include:
- Covera-HS Tablets 3199
- Isoptin SR Tablets 467
- Tarka Tablets 508
- Verelan Capsules 3184
- Verelan PM Capsules 3186

Food Interactions

Diet, high-lipid (A high fat meal within one-half hour before cyclosporine administration decreases the AUC by 13% and Cmax by 33%).

Food, unspecified (The administration of food with Gengraf decreases the cyclosporine AUC and Cmax).

Grapefruit (Affects the metabolism of cyclosporine by increasing blood concentration of cyclosporine; concurrent use should be avoided).

Grapefruit Juice (Affects the metabolism of cyclosporine by increasing blood concentration of cyclosporine; concurrent use should be avoided).

GENOPTIC OPHTHALMIC OINTMENT

(Gentamicin Sulfate) .... ⊙239
None cited in PDR database.

GENOPTIC STERILE OPHTHALMIC SOLUTION

(Gentamicin Sulfate) .... ⊙239
None cited in PDR database.

GENOTROPIN LYOPHILIZED POWDER

(Somatropin) 2818
May interact with glucocorticoids. Compounds in these categories include:

Betamethasone Acetate (Concomitant glucocorticoid therapy may inhibit human growth promoting effect). Products include:
- Celestone Soluspan Injectable Suspension 3097

Betamethasone Sodium Phosphate (Concomitant glucocorticoid therapy may inhibit human growth promoting effect). Products include:
- Celestone Soluspan Injectable Suspension 3097

Cortisone Acetate (Concomitant glucocorticoid therapy may inhibit human growth promoting effect). Products include:
- Cortone Acetate Injectable Suspension 2059
- Cortone Acetate Tablets 2061

Dexamethasone (Concomitant glucocorticoid therapy may inhibit human growth promoting effect). Products include:
- Decadron Elixir 2078
- Decadron Tablets 2079
- TobraDex Ophthalmic Ointment 542
- TobraDex Ophthalmic Suspension .. 541

Dexamethasone Acetate (Concomitant glucocorticoid therapy may inhibit human growth promoting effect).
No products indexed under this heading.

Dexamethasone Sodium Phosphate (Concomitant glucocorticoid therapy may inhibit human growth promoting effect). Products include:
- Decadron Phosphate Injection 2081
- Decadron Phosphate Sterile Ophthalmic Ointment 2083
- Decadron Phosphate Sterile Ophthalmic Solution 2084
- NeoDecadron Sterile Ophthalmic Solution 2144

Fludrocortisone Acetate (Concomitant glucocorticoid therapy may inhibit human growth promoting effect). Products include:
- Florinef Acetate Tablets 2250

Hydrocortisone (Concomitant glucocorticoid therapy may inhibit human growth promoting effect). Products include:
- Anusol-HC Cream 2.5% 2237
- Cipro HC Otic Suspension 540
- Cortaid Intensive Therapy Cream .. ■717
- Cortaid Maximum Strength Cream .... ■717
- Cortisporin Ophthalmic Suspension Sterile .... ⊙297
- Cortizone•5 .... ■699
- Cortizone•10 .... ■699
- Cortizone•10 Plus Creme .... ■700
- Cortizone for Kids Creme .... ■699
- Hydrocortone Tablets 2106
- Massengill Medicated Soft Cloth Towelette .... ■753
- VōSoL HC Otic Solution 3356

Hydrocortisone Acetate (Concomitant glucocorticoid therapy may inhibit human growth promoting effect). Products include:
- Analpram-HC 1338
- Anusol HC-1 Hydrocortisone Anti-Itch Cream .... ■689
- Anusol-HC Suppositories 2238
- Cortaid .... ■717
- Cortifoam Rectal Foam 3170
- Cortisporin-TC Otic Suspension 2246
- Hydrocortone Acetate Injectable Suspension 2103
- Pramosone 1343
- Proctocort Suppositories 2264
- ProctoFoam-HC 3177
- Terra-Cortril Ophthalmic Suspension 2716

Hydrocortisone Sodium Phosphate (Concomitant glucocorticoid therapy may inhibit human growth promoting effect). Products include:
- Hydrocortone Phosphate Injection, Sterile 2105

Hydrocortisone Sodium Succinate (Concomitant glucocorticoid therapy may inhibit human growth promoting effect).
No products indexed under this heading.

Methylprednisolone Acetate (Concomitant glucocorticoid therapy may inhibit human growth promoting effect). Products include:
- Depo-Medrol Injectable Suspension 2795

Methylprednisolone Sodium Succinate (Concomitant glucocorticoid therapy may inhibit human growth promoting effect). Products include:
- Solu-Medrol Sterile Powder 2855

Prednisolone Acetate (Concomitant glucocorticoid therapy may inhibit human growth promoting effect). Products include:
- Blephamide Ophthalmic Ointment .. 547
- Blephamide Ophthalmic Suspension 548
- Poly-Pred Liquifilm Ophthalmic Suspension .... ⊙245
- Pred Forte Ophthalmic Suspension .... ⊙246
- Pred Mild Sterile Ophthalmic Suspension .... ⊙249
- Pred-G Ophthalmic Suspension .... ⊙247
- Pred-G Sterile Ophthalmic Ointment .... ⊙248

Prednisolone Sodium Phosphate (Concomitant glucocorticoid therapy may inhibit human growth promoting effect). Products include:
- Pediapred Oral Solution 1170

Prednisolone Tebutate (Concomitant glucocorticoid therapy may inhibit human growth promoting effect).
No products indexed under this heading.

Prednisone (Concomitant glucocorticoid therapy may inhibit human growth promoting effect). Products include:
- Prednisone 3064

Triamcinolone (Concomitant glucocorticoid therapy may inhibit human growth promoting effect).
No products indexed under this heading.

Triamcinolone Acetonide (Concomitant glucocorticoid therapy may inhibit human growth promoting effect). Products include:
- Azmacort Inhalation Aerosol 728
- Nasacort Nasal Inhaler 750
- Nasacort AQ Nasal Spray 752
- Tri-Nasal Spray 2274

Triamcinolone Diacetate (Concomitant glucocorticoid therapy may inhibit human growth promoting effect).
No products indexed under this heading.

Triamcinolone Hexacetonide (Concomitant glucocorticoid therapy may inhibit human growth promoting effect).
No products indexed under this heading.

GENTEAL EYE DROPS
(Hydroxypropyl Methylcellulose) ......⊙304
None cited in PDR database.

GENTEAL GEL
(Hydroxypropyl Methylcellulose) ......⊙304
None cited in PDR database.

GENTEAL MILD EYE DROPS
(Polyethylene Glycol, Polyvinyl Alcohol) ......⊙304
None cited in PDR database.

GEOCILLIN TABLETS
(Carbenicillin Indanyl Sodium) 2687
May interact with:

Probenecid (Geocillin blood levels may be increased and prolonged).
No products indexed under this heading.

GEODON CAPSULES
(Ziprasidone Hydrochloride) 2688
May interact with antihypertensives, central nervous system depressants, dopamine agonists, erythromycin, quinidine, and certain other agents. Compounds in these categories include:

Acebutolol Hydrochloride (Ziprasidone may induce orthostatic hypotension; co-administration with certain antihypertensive drugs may enhance the hypotensive effects). Products include:
- Sectral Capsules 3589

Alfentanil Hydrochloride (Somnolence was a commonly reported adverse event in patients treated with ziprasidone; concurrent use with other CNS active drugs, such as depressants, should be undertaken with caution).
No products indexed under this heading.

Alprazolam (Somnolence was a commonly reported adverse event in patients treated with ziprasidone; concurrent use with other CNS active drugs, such as depressants, should be undertaken with caution). Products include:
- Xanax Tablets 2865

Amlodipine Besylate (Ziprasidone may induce orthostatic hypotension; co-administration with certain antihypertensive drugs may enhance the hypotensive effects). Products include:
- Lotrel Capsules 2370
- Norvasc Tablets 2704

Aprobarbital (Somnolence was a commonly reported adverse event in patients treated with ziprasidone; concurrent use with other CNS active drugs, such as depressants, should be undertaken with caution).
No products indexed under this heading.

Atenolol (Ziprasidone may induce orthostatic hypotension; co-administration with certain antihypertensive drugs may enhance the hypotensive effects). Products include:
- Tenoretic Tablets 690
- Tenormin I.V. Injection 692

Benazepril Hydrochloride (Ziprasidone may induce orthostatic hypotension; co-administration with certain antihypertensive drugs may enhance the hypotensive effects). Products include:
- Lotensin Tablets 2365
- Lotensin HCT Tablets 2367
- Lotrel Capsules 2370

Bendroflumethiazide (Ziprasidone may induce orthostatic hypotension; co-administration with certain antihypertensive drugs may enhance the hypotensive effects). Products include:
- Corzide 40/5 Tablets 2247
- Corzide 80/5 Tablets 2247

Betaxolol Hydrochloride (Ziprasidone may induce orthostatic hypotension; co-administration with certain antihypertensive drugs may enhance the hypotensive effects). Products include:
- Betoptic S Ophthalmic Suspension 537

Bisoprolol Fumarate (Ziprasidone may induce orthostatic hypotension; co-administration with certain antihypertensive drugs may enhance the hypotensive effects). Products include:
- Zebeta Tablets 1885
- Ziac Tablets 1887

Bromocriptine Mesylate (Ziprasidone may antagonize the effects of dopamine agonists).
No products indexed under this heading.

Buprenorphine Hydrochloride (Somnolence was a commonly reported adverse event in patients treated with ziprasidone; concurrent use with other CNS active drugs, such as depressants, should be undertaken with caution). Products include:
- Buprenex Injectable 2918

Buspirone Hydrochloride (Somnolence was a commonly reported adverse event in patients treated with ziprasidone; concurrent use with other CNS active drugs, such as depressants, should be undertaken with caution).
No products indexed under this heading.

Butabarbital (Somnolence was a commonly reported adverse event in patients treated with ziprasidone; concurrent use with other CNS active drugs, such as depressants, should be undertaken with caution).
No products indexed under this heading.

Butalbital (Somnolence was a commonly reported adverse event in patients treated with ziprasidone; concurrent use with other CNS active drugs, such as depressants, should be undertaken with caution). Products include:
- Phrenilin 578
- Sedapap Tablets 50 mg/650 mg 2225

Candesartan Cilexetil (Ziprasidone may induce orthostatic hypotension; co-administration with certain antihypertensive drugs may enhance the hypotensive effects). Products include:
- Atacand Tablets 595
- Atacand HCT Tablets 597

Captopril (Ziprasidone may induce orthostatic hypotension; co-administration with certain antihypertensive drugs may enhance the hypotensive effects). Products include:
- Captopril Tablets 2281

Carbamazepine (Co-administration with carbamazepine, an inducer of CYP3A4, has resulted in a decrease of approximately 35% in AUC of ziprasidone; this effect may be greater when higher doses of carbamazepine are administered). Products include:
- Carbatrol Capsules 3234
- Tegretol/Tegretol-XR 2404

Carteolol Hydrochloride (Ziprasidone may induce orthostatic hypotension; co-administration with certain antihypertensive drugs may enhance the hypotensive effects). Products include:
- Carteolol Hydrochloride Ophthalmic Solution USP, 1% .... ⊙258
- Ocupress Ophthalmic Solution, 1% Sterile .... ⊙303

Chlordiazepoxide (Somnolence was a commonly reported adverse event in patients treated with ziprasidone; concurrent use with other CNS active drugs, such as depressants, should be undertaken with caution). Products include:
- Limbitrol 1738

Chlordiazepoxide Hydrochloride (Somnolence was a commonly reported adverse event in patients treated with ziprasidone; concurrent use with other CNS active drugs, such as depressants, should be undertaken with caution). Products include:
- Librium Capsules 1736
- Librium for Injection 1737

Chlorothiazide (Ziprasidone may induce orthostatic hypotension; co-administration with certain antihypertensive drugs may enhance the hypotensive effects). Products include:
- Aldoclor Tablets 2035
- Diuril Oral 2087

Chlorothiazide Sodium (Ziprasidone may induce orthostatic hypotension; co-administration with certain antihypertensive drugs may enhance the hypotensive effects). Products include:
- Diuril Sodium Intravenous 2086

Chlorpromazine (Somnolence was a commonly reported adverse event in patients treated with ziprasidone; concurrent use with other CNS active drugs, such as depressants, should be undertaken with caution). Products include:
- Thorazine Suppositories 1656

Chlorpromazine Hydrochloride (Somnolence was a commonly reported adverse event in patients treated with ziprasidone; concurrent use with other CNS active drugs, such as depressants, should be undertaken with caution). Products include:
- Thorazine 1656

Chlorprothixene (Somnolence was a commonly reported adverse event in patients treated with ziprasidone; concurrent use with other CNS active drugs, such as depressants, should be undertaken with caution).
No products indexed under this heading.

Chlorprothixene Hydrochloride (Somnolence was a commonly reported adverse event in patients treated with ziprasidone; concurrent use with other CNS active drugs, such as depressants, should be undertaken with caution).
No products indexed under this heading.

Chlorprothixene Lactate (Somnolence was a commonly reported adverse event in patients treated with ziprasidone; concurrent use with other CNS active drugs, such as depressants, should be undertaken with caution).
No products indexed under this heading.

Chlorthalidone (Ziprasidone may induce orthostatic hypotension; co-administration with certain antihypertensive drugs may enhance the hypotensive effects). Products include:
- Clorpres Tablets 1002
- Combipres Tablets 1040
- Tenoretic Tablets 690

Clonidine (Ziprasidone may induce orthostatic hypotension; co-administration with certain antihypertensive drugs may enhance the hypotensive effects). Products include:
- Catapres-TTS 1038

Clonidine Hydrochloride (Ziprasidone may induce orthostatic hypotension; co-administration with certain antihypertensive drugs may enhance the hypotensive effects). Products include:
- Catapres Tablets 1037
- Clorpres Tablets 1002
- Combipres Tablets 1040
- Duraclon Injection 3057

Clorazepate Dipotassium (Somnolence was a commonly reported adverse event in patients treated with ziprasidone; concurrent use with other CNS active drugs, such as depressants, should be undertaken with caution). Products include:
- Tranxene 511

Clozapine (Somnolence was a commonly reported adverse event in patients treated with ziprasidone; concurrent use with other CNS active drugs, such as depressants, should be undertaken with caution). Products include:
- Clozaril Tablets 2319

Codeine Phosphate (Somnolence was a commonly reported adverse event in patients treated with ziprasidone; concurrent use with other CNS active drugs, such as depressants, should be undertaken with caution). Products include:
- Phenergan with Codeine Syrup 3557
- Phenergan VC with Codeine Syrup 3561
- Robitussin A-C Syrup 2942
- Robitussin-DAC Syrup 2942
- Ryna-C Liquid 768
- Soma Compound w/Codeine Tablets 3355
- Tussi-Organidin NR Liquid 3350
- Tussi-Organidin-S NR Liquid 3350
- Tylenol with Codeine 2595

Deserpidine (Ziprasidone may induce orthostatic hypotension; co-administration with certain antihypertensive drugs may enhance the hypotensive effects).
No products indexed under this heading.

Desflurane (Somnolence was a commonly reported adverse event in patients treated with ziprasidone; concurrent use with other CNS active drugs, such as depressants, should be undertaken with caution). Products include:
- Suprane Liquid for Inhalation 874

Dezocine (Somnolence was a commonly reported adverse event in patients treated with ziprasidone; concurrent use with other CNS active drugs, such as depressants, should be undertaken with caution).
No products indexed under this heading.

Diazepam (Somnolence was a commonly reported adverse event in patients treated with ziprasidone; concurrent use with other CNS active drugs, such as depressants, should be undertaken with caution). Products include:
- Valium Injectable 3026
- Valium Tablets 3047

Diazoxide (Ziprasidone may induce orthostatic hypotension; co-administration with certain antihypertensive drugs may enhance the

hypotensive effects).
No products indexed under this heading.

Diltiazem Hydrochloride (Ziprasidone may induce orthostatic hypotension; co-administration with certain antihypertensive drugs may enhance the hypotensive effects). Products include:
Cardizem Injectable ... 1018
Cardizem Lyo-Ject Syringe ... 1018
Cardizem Monovial ... 1018
Cardizem CD Capsules ... 1016
Tiazac Capsules ... 1378

Dofetilide (Ziprasidone produces dose-related prolongation of the QT interval; co-administration with drugs that prolong the QT interval, such as dofetilide, may increase the risk of torsade de pointes and/or sudden death; concurrent use is not recommended). Products include:
Tikosyn Capsules ... 2717

Dopamine Hydrochloride (Ziprasidone may antagonize the effects of dopamine agonists).
No products indexed under this heading.

Doxazosin Mesylate (Ziprasidone may induce orthostatic hypotension; co-administration with certain antihypertensive drugs may enhance the hypotensive effects). Products include:
Cardura Tablets ... 2668

Droperidol (Somnolence was a commonly reported adverse event in patients treated with ziprasidone; concurrent use with other CNS active drugs, such as depressants, should be undertaken with caution).
No products indexed under this heading.

Enalapril Maleate (Ziprasidone may induce orthostatic hypotension; co-administration with certain antihypertensive drugs may enhance the hypotensive effects). Products include:
Lexxel Tablets ... 608
Vaseretic Tablets ... 2204
Vasotec Tablets ... 2210

Enalaprilat (Ziprasidone may induce orthostatic hypotension; co-administration with certain antihypertensive drugs may enhance the hypotensive effects). Products include:
Enalaprilat Injection ... 863
Vasotec I.V. Injection ... 2207

Enflurane (Somnolence was a commonly reported adverse event in patients treated with ziprasidone; concurrent use with other CNS active drugs, such as depressants, should be undertaken with caution).
No products indexed under this heading.

Eprosartan Mesylate (Ziprasidone may induce orthostatic hypotension; co-administration with certain antihypertensive drugs may enhance the hypotensive effects). Products include:
Teveten Tablets ... 3327

Erythromycin (Co-administration with inhibitors of CYP3A4, such as erythromycin, may result in increased AUC and Cmax of ziprasidone). Products include:
Emgel 2% Topical Gel ... 1285
Ery-Tab Tablets ... 448
Erythromycin Base Filmtab Tablets . 454
Erythromycin Delayed-Release Capsules, USP ... 455
PCE Dispertab Tablets ... 498

Erythromycin Estolate (Co-administration with inhibitors of CYP3A4, such as erythromycin, may result in increased AUC and Cmax of ziprasidone).
No products indexed under this heading.

Erythromycin Ethylsuccinate (Co-administration with inhibitors of CYP3A4, such as erythromycin, may result in increased AUC and Cmax of ziprasidone). Products include:
E.E.S. ... 450
EryPed ... 446
Pediazole Suspension ... 3050

Erythromycin Gluceptate (Co-administration with inhibitors of CYP3A4, such as erythromycin, may result in increased AUC and Cmax of ziprasidone).
No products indexed under this heading.

Erythromycin Stearate (Co-administration with inhibitors of CYP3A4, such as erythromycin, may result in increased AUC and Cmax of ziprasidone). Products include:
Erythrocin Stearate Filmtab Tablets ... 452

Esmolol Hydrochloride (Ziprasidone may induce orthostatic hypotension; co-administration with certain antihypertensive drugs may enhance the hypotensive effects). Products include:
Brevibloc Injection ... 858

Estazolam (Somnolence was a commonly reported adverse event in patients treated with ziprasidone; concurrent use with other CNS active drugs, such as depressants, should be undertaken with caution). Products include:
ProSom Tablets ... 500

Ethchlorvynol (Somnolence was a commonly reported adverse event in patients treated with ziprasidone; concurrent use with other CNS active drugs, such as depressants, should be undertaken with caution).
No products indexed under this heading.

Ethinamate (Somnolence was a commonly reported adverse event in patients treated with ziprasidone; concurrent use with other CNS active drugs, such as depressants, should be undertaken with caution).
No products indexed under this heading.

Felodipine (Ziprasidone may induce orthostatic hypotension; co-administration with certain antihypertensive drugs may enhance the hypotensive effects). Products include:
Lexxel Tablets ... 608
Plendil Extended-Release Tablets ... 623

Fentanyl (Somnolence was a commonly reported adverse event in patients treated with ziprasidone; concurrent use with other CNS active drugs, such as depressants, should be undertaken with caution). Products include:
Duragesic Transdermal System ... 1786

Fentanyl Citrate (Somnolence was a commonly reported adverse event in patients treated with ziprasidone; concurrent use with other CNS active drugs, such as depressants, should be undertaken with caution). Products include:
Actiq ... 1184

Fluphenazine Decanoate (Somnolence was a commonly reported adverse event in patients treated with ziprasidone; concurrent use with other CNS active drugs, such as depressants, should be undertaken with caution).
No products indexed under this heading.

Fluphenazine Enanthate (Somnolence was a commonly reported adverse event in patients treated with ziprasidone; concurrent use with other CNS active drugs, such as depressants, should be undertaken with caution).
No products indexed under this heading.

Fluphenazine Hydrochloride (Somnolence was a commonly reported adverse event in patients treated with ziprasidone; concurrent use with other CNS active drugs, such as depressants, should be undertaken with caution).
No products indexed under this heading.

Flurazepam Hydrochloride (Somnolence was a commonly reported adverse event in patients treated with ziprasidone; concurrent use with other CNS active drugs, such as depressants, should be undertaken with caution).
No products indexed under this heading.

Fosinopril Sodium (Ziprasidone may induce orthostatic hypotension; co-administration with certain antihypertensive drugs may enhance the hypotensive effects). Products include:
Monopril Tablets ... 1091
Monopril HCT ... 1094

Furosemide (Ziprasidone may induce orthostatic hypotension; co-administration with certain antihypertensive drugs may enhance the hypotensive effects). Products include:
Furosemide Tablets ... 2284

Glutethimide (Somnolence was a commonly reported adverse event in patients treated with ziprasidone; concurrent use with other CNS active drugs, such as depressants, should be undertaken with caution).
No products indexed under this heading.

Guanabenz Acetate (Ziprasidone may induce orthostatic hypotension; co-administration with certain antihypertensive drugs may enhance the hypotensive effects).
No products indexed under this heading.

Guanethidine Monosulfate (Ziprasidone may induce orthostatic hypotension; co-administration with certain antihypertensive drugs may enhance the hypotensive effects).
No products indexed under this heading.

Haloperidol (Somnolence was a commonly reported adverse event in patients treated with ziprasidone; concurrent use with other CNS active drugs, such as depressants, should be undertaken with caution). Products include:
Haldol Injection, Tablets and Concentrate ... 2533

Haloperidol Decanoate (Somnolence was a commonly reported adverse event in patients treated with ziprasidone; concurrent use with other CNS active drugs, such as depressants, should be undertaken with caution). Products include:
Haldol Decanoate ... 2535

Hydralazine Hydrochloride (Ziprasidone may induce orthostatic hypotension; co-administration with certain antihypertensive drugs may enhance the hypotensive effects).
No products indexed under this heading.

Hydrochlorothiazide (Ziprasidone may induce orthostatic hypotension; co-administration with certain antihypertensive drugs may enhance the hypotensive effects). Products include:
Accuretic Tablets ... 2614
Aldoril Tablets ... 2039
Atacand HCT Tablets ... 597
Avalide Tablets ... 1070
Diovan HCT Tablets ... 2338
Dyazide Capsules ... 1515
HydroDIURIL Tablets ... 2108
Hyzaar ... 2109
Inderide Tablets ... 3517
Inderide LA Long-Acting Capsules .. 3519
Lotensin HCT Tablets ... 2367
Maxzide ... 1008
Micardis HCT Tablets ... 1051
Microzide Capsules ... 3414
Moduretic Tablets ... 2138
Monopril HCT ... 1094
Prinzide Tablets ... 2168
Timolide Tablets ... 2187
Uniretic Tablets ... 3178
Vaseretic Tablets ... 2204
Zestoretic Tablets ... 695
Ziac Tablets ... 1887

Hydrocodone Bitartrate (Somnolence was a commonly reported adverse event in patients treated with ziprasidone; concurrent use with other CNS active drugs, such as depressants, should be undertaken with caution). Products include:
Hycodan ... 1316
Hycomine Compound Tablets ... 1317
Hycotuss Expectorant Syrup ... 1318
Lortab ... 3319
Lortab Elixir ... 3317
Maxidone Tablets CIII ... 3399
Norco 5/325 Tablets CIII ... 3424
Norco 7.5/325 Tablets CIII ... 3425
Norco 10/325 Tablets CIII ... 3427
Norco 10/325 Tablets CIII ... 3425
Vicodin Tablets ... 516
Vicodin ES Tablets ... 517
Vicodin HP Tablets ... 518
Vicodin Tuss Expectorant ... 519
Vicoprofen Tablets ... 520
Zydone Tablets ... 1330

Hydrocodone Polistirex (Somnolence was a commonly reported adverse event in patients treated with ziprasidone; concurrent use with other CNS active drugs, such as depressants, should be undertaken with caution). Products include:
Tussionex Pennkinetic Extended-Release Suspension ... 1174

Hydroflumethiazide (Ziprasidone may induce orthostatic hypotension; co-administration with certain antihypertensive drugs may enhance the hypotensive effects). Products include:
Diucardin Tablets ... 3494

Hydromorphone Hydrochloride (Somnolence was a commonly reported adverse event in patients treated with ziprasidone; concurrent use with other CNS active drugs, such as depressants, should be undertaken with caution). Products include:
Dilaudid ... 441
Dilaudid Oral Liquid ... 445
Dilaudid Powder ... 441
Dilaudid Rectal Suppositories ... 441
Dilaudid Tablets ... 441
Dilaudid Tablets - 8 mg ... 445
Dilaudid-HP ... 443

Hydroxyzine Hydrochloride (Somnolence was a commonly reported adverse event in patients treated with ziprasidone; concurrent use with other CNS active drugs, such as depressants, should be undertaken with caution). Products include:
Atarax Tablets & Syrup ... 2667
Vistaril Intramuscular Solution ... 2738

Indapamide (Ziprasidone may induce orthostatic hypotension; co-administration with certain antihypertensive drugs may enhance the hypotensive effects). Products include:
Indapamide Tablets ... 2286

Irbesartan (Ziprasidone may induce orthostatic hypotension; co-administration with certain antihypertensive drugs may enhance the hypotensive effects). Products include:
Avalide Tablets ... 1070
Avapro Tablets ... 1074
Avapro Tablets ... 3076

Isoflurane (Somnolence was a commonly reported adverse event in patients treated with ziprasidone; concurrent use with other CNS active drugs, such as depressants, should be undertaken with caution).
No products indexed under this heading.

Isradipine (Ziprasidone may induce orthostatic hypotension; co-administration with certain antihypertensive drugs may enhance the hypotensive effects). Products include:

DynaCirc Capsules 2921
DynaCirc CR Tablets 2923

Itraconazole (Co-administration with inhibitors of CYP3A4, such as itraconazole, may result in increased AUC and Cmax of ziprasidone). Products include:

Sporanox Capsules 1800
Sporanox Injection 1804
Sporanox Injection 2509
Sporanox Oral Solution 1808
Sporanox Oral Solution 2512

Ketamine Hydrochloride (Somnolence was a commonly reported adverse event in patients treated with ziprasidone; concurrent use with other CNS active drugs, such as depressants, should be undertaken with caution).

No products indexed under this heading.

Ketoconazole (Co-administration with ketoconazole, a potent inhibitor of CYP3A4, has resulted in increased AUC and Cmax of ziprasidone by about 35-40%). Products include:

Nizoral 2% Cream 3620
Nizoral A-D Shampoo 2008
Nizoral 2% Shampoo 2007
Nizoral Tablets 1791

Labetalol Hydrochloride (Ziprasidone may induce orthostatic hypotension; co-administration with certain antihypertensive drugs may enhance the hypotensive effects). Products include:

Normodyne Injection 3135
Normodyne Tablets 3137

Levodopa (Ziprasidone may antagonize the effects of levodopa). Products include:

Sinemet Tablets 1253
Sinemet CR Tablets 1255

Levomethadyl Acetate Hydrochloride (Somnolence was a commonly reported adverse event in patients treated with ziprasidone; concurrent use with other CNS active drugs, such as depressants, should be undertaken with caution).

No products indexed under this heading.

Levorphanol Tartrate (Somnolence was a commonly reported adverse event in patients treated with ziprasidone; concurrent use with other CNS active drugs, such as depressants, should be undertaken with caution). Products include:

Levo-Dromoran 1734
Levorphanol Tartrate Tablets 3059

Lisinopril (Ziprasidone may induce orthostatic hypotension; co-administration with certain antihypertensive drugs may enhance the hypotensive effects). Products include:

Prinivil Tablets 2164
Prinzide Tablets 2168
Zestoretic Tablets 695
Zestril Tablets 698

Lorazepam (Somnolence was a commonly reported adverse event in patients treated with ziprasidone; concurrent use with other CNS active drugs, such as depressants, should be undertaken with caution). Products include:

Ativan Injection 3478
Ativan Tablets 3482

Losartan Potassium (Ziprasidone may induce orthostatic hypotension; co-administration with certain antihypertensive drugs may enhance the hypotensive effects). Products include:

Cozaar Tablets 2067
Hyzaar 2109

Loxapine Hydrochloride (Somnolence was a commonly reported adverse event in patients treated with ziprasidone; concurrent use with other CNS active drugs, such as depressants, should be undertaken with caution).

No products indexed under this heading.

Loxapine Succinate (Somnolence was a commonly reported adverse event in patients treated with ziprasidone; concurrent use with other CNS active drugs, such as depressants, should be undertaken with caution). Products include:

Loxitane Capsules 3398

Mecamylamine Hydrochloride (Ziprasidone may induce orthostatic hypotension; co-administration with certain antihypertensive drugs may enhance the hypotensive effects). Products include:

Inversine Tablets 1850

Meperidine Hydrochloride (Somnolence was a commonly reported adverse event in patients treated with ziprasidone; concurrent use with other CNS active drugs, such as depressants, should be undertaken with caution). Products include:

Demerol 3079
Mepergan Injection 3539

Mephobarbital (Somnolence was a commonly reported adverse event in patients treated with ziprasidone; concurrent use with other CNS active drugs, such as depressants, should be undertaken with caution).

No products indexed under this heading.

Meprobamate (Somnolence was a commonly reported adverse event in patients treated with ziprasidone; concurrent use with other CNS active drugs, such as depressants, should be undertaken with caution). Products include:

Miltown Tablets 3349

Mesoridazine Besylate (Somnolence was a commonly reported adverse event in patients treated with ziprasidone; concurrent use with other CNS active drugs, such as depressants, should be undertaken with caution). Products include:

Serentil 1057

Methadone Hydrochloride (Somnolence was a commonly reported adverse event in patients treated with ziprasidone; concurrent use with other CNS active drugs, such as depressants, should be undertaken with caution). Products include:

Dolophine Hydrochloride Tablets 3056

Methohexital Sodium (Somnolence was a commonly reported adverse event in patients treated with ziprasidone; concurrent use with other CNS active drugs, such as depressants, should be undertaken with caution). Products include:

Brevital Sodium for Injection, USP 1815

Methotrimeprazine (Somnolence was a commonly reported adverse event in patients treated with ziprasidone; concurrent use with other CNS active drugs, such as depressants, should be undertaken with caution).

No products indexed under this heading.

Methoxyflurane (Somnolence was a commonly reported adverse event in patients treated with ziprasidone; concurrent use with other CNS active drugs, such as depressants, should be undertaken with caution).

No products indexed under this heading.

Methyclothiazide (Ziprasidone may induce orthostatic hypotension; co-administration with certain antihypertensive drugs may enhance the hypotensive effects).

No products indexed under this heading.

Methyldopa (Ziprasidone may induce orthostatic hypotension; co-administration with certain antihypertensive drugs may enhance the hypotensive effects). Products include:

Aldoclor Tablets 2035
Aldomet Tablets 2037
Aldoril Tablets 2039

Methyldopate Hydrochloride (Ziprasidone may induce orthostatic hypotension; co-administration with certain antihypertensive drugs may enhance the hypotensive effects).

No products indexed under this heading.

Metolazone (Ziprasidone may induce orthostatic hypotension; co-administration with certain antihypertensive drugs may enhance the hypotensive effects). Products include:

Mykrox Tablets 1168
Zaroxolyn Tablets 1177

Metoprolol Succinate (Ziprasidone may induce orthostatic hypotension; co-administration with certain antihypertensive drugs may enhance the hypotensive effects). Products include:

Toprol-XL Tablets 651

Metoprolol Tartrate (Ziprasidone may induce orthostatic hypotension; co-administration with certain antihypertensive drugs may enhance the hypotensive effects).

No products indexed under this heading.

Metyrosine (Ziprasidone may induce orthostatic hypotension; co-administration with certain antihypertensive drugs may enhance the hypotensive effects). Products include:

Demser Capsules 2085

Mibefradil Dihydrochloride (Ziprasidone may induce orthostatic hypotension; co-administration with certain antihypertensive drugs may enhance the hypotensive effects).

No products indexed under this heading.

Midazolam Hydrochloride (Somnolence was a commonly reported adverse event in patients treated with ziprasidone; concurrent use with other CNS active drugs, such as depressants, should be undertaken with caution). Products include:

Versed Injection 3027
Versed Syrup 3033

Minoxidil (Ziprasidone may induce orthostatic hypotension; co-administration with certain antihypertensive drugs may enhance the hypotensive effects). Products include:

Rogaine Extra Strength for Men Topical Solution 721
Rogaine for Women Topical Solution 721

Moexipril Hydrochloride (Ziprasidone may induce orthostatic hypotension; co-administration with certain antihypertensive drugs may enhance the hypotensive effects). Products include:

Uniretic Tablets 3178
Univasc Tablets 3181

Molindone Hydrochloride (Somnolence was a commonly reported adverse event in patients treated with ziprasidone; concurrent use with other CNS active drugs, such as depressants, should be undertaken with caution). Products include:

Moban 1320

Morphine Sulfate (Somnolence was a commonly reported adverse event in patients treated with ziprasidone; concurrent use with other CNS active drugs, such as depressants, should be undertaken with caution). Products include:

Astramorph/PF Injection, USP (Preservative-Free) 594
Duramorph Injection 1312
Infumorph 200 and Infumorph 500 Sterile Solutions 1314
Kadian Capsules 1335
MS Contin Tablets 2896
MSIR 2898
Oramorph SR Tablets 3062
Roxanol 3066

Moxifloxacin Hydrochloride (Ziprasidone produces dose-related prolongation of the QT interval; co-administration with drugs that prolong the QT interval, such as moxifloxacin, may increase the risk of torsade de pointes and/or sudden death; concurrent use is not recommended). Products include:

Avelox Tablets 879

Nadolol (Ziprasidone may induce orthostatic hypotension; co-administration with certain antihypertensive drugs may enhance the hypotensive effects). Products include:

Corgard Tablets 2245
Corzide 40/5 Tablets 2247
Corzide 80/5 Tablets 2247
Nadolol Tablets 2288

Nicardipine Hydrochloride (Ziprasidone may induce orthostatic hypotension; co-administration with certain antihypertensive drugs may enhance the hypotensive effects). Products include:

Cardene I.V. 3485

Nifedipine (Ziprasidone may induce orthostatic hypotension; co-administration with certain antihypertensive drugs may enhance the hypotensive effects). Products include:

Adalat CC Tablets 877
Procardia Capsules 2708
Procardia XL Extended Release Tablets 2710

Nisoldipine (Ziprasidone may induce orthostatic hypotension; co-administration with certain antihypertensive drugs may enhance the hypotensive effects). Products include:

Sular Tablets 688

Nitroglycerin (Ziprasidone may induce orthostatic hypotension; co-administration with certain antihypertensive drugs may enhance the hypotensive effects). Products include:

Nitro-Dur Transdermal Infusion System 3134
Nitro-Dur Transdermal Infusion System 1834
Nitrolingual Pumpspray 1355
Nitrostat Tablets 2658

Olanzapine (Somnolence was a commonly reported adverse event in patients treated with ziprasidone; concurrent use with other CNS active drugs, such as depressants, should be undertaken with caution). Products include:

Zyprexa Tablets 1973
Zyprexa ZYDIS Orally Disintegrating Tablets 1973

Oxazepam (Somnolence was a commonly reported adverse event in patients treated with ziprasidone; concurrent use with other CNS active drugs, such as depressants, should be undertaken with caution).

No products indexed under this heading.

Oxycodone Hydrochloride (Somnolence was a commonly reported adverse event in patients treated with ziprasidone; concurrent use with other CNS active drugs, such as depressants, should be undertaken with caution). Products include:

OxyContin Tablets 2912
OxyFast Oral Concentrate Solution 2916
OxyIR Capsules 2916

Percocet Tablets 1326
Percodan Tablets 1327
Percolone Tablets 1327
Roxicodone 3067
Tylox Capsules 2597

Penbutolol Sulfate (Ziprasidone may induce orthostatic hypotension; co-administration with certain antihypertensive drugs may enhance the hypotensive effects).
No products indexed under this heading.

Pentobarbital Sodium (Somnolence was a commonly reported adverse event in patients treated with ziprasidone; concurrent use with other CNS active drugs, such as depressants, should be undertaken with caution). Products include:
Nembutal Sodium Solution 485

Pergolide Mesylate (Ziprasidone may antagonize the effects of dopamine agonists). Products include:
Permax Tablets 1299

Perindopril Erbumine (Ziprasidone may induce orthostatic hypotension; co-administration with certain antihypertensive drugs may enhance the hypotensive effects). Products include:
Aceon Tablets (2 mg, 4 mg, 8 mg) 3249

Perphenazine (Somnolence was a commonly reported adverse event in patients treated with ziprasidone; concurrent use with other CNS active drugs, such as depressants, should be undertaken with caution). Products include:
Etrafon 3115
Trilafon 3160

Phenobarbital (Somnolence was a commonly reported adverse event in patients treated with ziprasidone; concurrent use with other CNS active drugs, such as depressants, should be undertaken with caution). Products include:
Arco-Lase Plus Tablets 592
Donnatal 2929
Donnatal Extentabs 2930

Phenoxybenzamine Hydrochloride (Ziprasidone may induce orthostatic hypotension; co-administration with certain antihypertensive drugs may enhance the hypotensive effects). Products include:
Dibenzyline Capsules 3457

Phentolamine Mesylate (Ziprasidone may induce orthostatic hypotension; co-administration with certain antihypertensive drugs may enhance the hypotensive effects).
No products indexed under this heading.

Pimozide (Ziprasidone produces dose-related prolongation of the QT interval; co-administration with drugs that prolong the QT interval, such as pimozide, may increase the risk of torsade de pointes and/or sudden death; concurrent use is not recommended). Products include:
Orap Tablets 1407

Pindolol (Ziprasidone may induce orthostatic hypotension; co-administration with certain antihypertensive drugs may enhance the hypotensive effects).
No products indexed under this heading.

Polythiazide (Ziprasidone may induce orthostatic hypotension; co-administration with certain antihypertensive drugs may enhance the hypotensive effects). Products include:
Minizide Capsules 2700
Renese Tablets 2712

Pramipexole Dihydrochloride (Ziprasidone may antagonize the effects of dopamine agonists). Products include:
Mirapex Tablets 2834

Prazepam (Somnolence was a commonly reported adverse event in patients treated with ziprasidone; concurrent use with other CNS active drugs, such as depressants, should be undertaken with caution).
No products indexed under this heading.

Prazosin Hydrochloride (Ziprasidone may induce orthostatic hypotension; co-administration with certain antihypertensive drugs may enhance the hypotensive effects). Products include:
Minipress Capsules 2699
Minizide Capsules 2700

Prochlorperazine (Somnolence was a commonly reported adverse event in patients treated with ziprasidone; concurrent use with other CNS active drugs, such as depressants, should be undertaken with caution). Products include:
Compazine 1505

Promethazine Hydrochloride (Somnolence was a commonly reported adverse event in patients treated with ziprasidone; concurrent use with other CNS active drugs, such as depressants, should be undertaken with caution). Products include:
Mepergan Injection 3539
Phenergan Injection 3553
Phenergan 3556
Phenergan Syrup 3554
Phenergan with Codeine Syrup 3557
Phenergan with Dextromethorphan Syrup 3559
Phenergan VC Syrup 3560
Phenergan VC with Codeine Syrup 3561

Propofol (Somnolence was a commonly reported adverse event in patients treated with ziprasidone; concurrent use with other CNS active drugs, such as depressants, should be undertaken with caution). Products include:
Diprivan Injectable Emulsion 667

Propoxyphene Hydrochloride (Somnolence was a commonly reported adverse event in patients treated with ziprasidone; concurrent use with other CNS active drugs, such as depressants, should be undertaken with caution). Products include:
Darvon Pulvules 1909
Darvon Compound-65 Pulvules 1910

Propoxyphene Napsylate (Somnolence was a commonly reported adverse event in patients treated with ziprasidone; concurrent use with other CNS active drugs, such as depressants, should be undertaken with caution). Products include:
Darvon-N/Darvocet-N 1907
Darvon-N Tablets 1912

Propranolol Hydrochloride (Ziprasidone may induce orthostatic hypotension; co-administration with certain antihypertensive drugs may enhance the hypotensive effects). Products include:
Inderal 3513
Inderal LA Long-Acting Capsules 3516
Inderide Tablets 3517
Inderide LA Long-Acting Capsules 3519

Quazepam (Somnolence was a commonly reported adverse event in patients treated with ziprasidone; concurrent use with other CNS active drugs, such as depressants, should be undertaken with caution).
No products indexed under this heading.

Quetiapine Fumarate (Somnolence was a commonly reported adverse event in patients treated with ziprasidone; concurrent use with other CNS active drugs, such as depressants, should be undertaken with caution). Products include:
Seroquel Tablets 684

Quinapril Hydrochloride (Ziprasidone may induce orthostatic hypotension; co-administration with certain antihypertensive drugs may enhance the hypotensive effects). Products include:
Accupril Tablets 2611
Accuretic Tablets 2614

Quinidine Gluconate (Ziprasidone produces dose-related prolongation of the QT interval; co-administration with drugs that prolong the QT interval, such as quinidine, may increase the risk of torsade de pointes and/or sudden death; concurrent use is not recommended). Products include:
Quinaglute Dura-Tabs Tablets 978

Quinidine Polygalacturonate (Ziprasidone produces dose-related prolongation of the QT interval; co-administration with drugs that prolong the QT interval, such as quinidine, may increase the risk of torsade de pointes and/or sudden death; concurrent use is not recommended).
No products indexed under this heading.

Quinidine Sulfate (Ziprasidone produces dose-related prolongation of the QT interval; co-administration with drugs that prolong the QT interval, such as quinidine, may increase the risk of torsade de pointes and/or sudden death; concurrent use is not recommended). Products include:
Quinidex Extentabs 2933

Ramipril (Ziprasidone may induce orthostatic hypotension; co-administration with certain antihypertensive drugs may enhance the hypotensive effects). Products include:
Altace Capsules 2233

Rauwolfia serpentina (Ziprasidone may induce orthostatic hypotension; co-administration with certain antihypertensive drugs may enhance the hypotensive effects).
No products indexed under this heading.

Remifentanil Hydrochloride (Somnolence was a commonly reported adverse event in patients treated with ziprasidone; concurrent use with other CNS active drugs, such as depressants, should be undertaken with caution).
No products indexed under this heading.

Rescinnamine (Ziprasidone may induce orthostatic hypotension; co-administration with certain antihypertensive drugs may enhance the hypotensive effects).
No products indexed under this heading.

Reserpine (Ziprasidone may induce orthostatic hypotension; co-administration with certain antihypertensive drugs may enhance the hypotensive effects).
No products indexed under this heading.

Risperidone (Somnolence was a commonly reported adverse event in patients treated with ziprasidone; concurrent use with other CNS active drugs, such as depressants, should be undertaken with caution). Products include:
Risperdal 1796

Ropinirole Hydrochloride (Ziprasidone may antagonize the effects of dopamine agonists). Products include:
Requip Tablets 1621

Secobarbital Sodium (Somnolence was a commonly reported adverse event in patients treated with ziprasidone; concurrent use with other CNS active drugs, such as depressants, should be undertaken with caution).
No products indexed under this heading.

Sevoflurane (Somnolence was a commonly reported adverse event in patients treated with ziprasidone; concurrent use with other CNS active drugs, such as depressants, should be undertaken with caution).
No products indexed under this heading.

Sodium Nitroprusside (Ziprasidone may induce orthostatic hypotension; co-administration with certain antihypertensive drugs may enhance the hypotensive effects).
No products indexed under this heading.

Sotalol Hydrochloride (Ziprasidone produces dose-related prolongation of the QT interval; co-administration with drugs that prolong the QT interval, such as sotalol, may increase the risk of torsade de pointes and/or sudden death; concurrent use is not recommended). Products include:
Betapace Tablets 950
Betapace AF Tablets 954

Sparfloxacin (Ziprasidone produces dose-related prolongation of the QT interval; co-administration with drugs that prolong the QT interval, such as sparfloxacin, may increase the risk of torsade de pointes and/or sudden death; concurrent use is not recommended).
No products indexed under this heading.

Spirapril Hydrochloride (Ziprasidone may induce orthostatic hypotension; co-administration with certain antihypertensive drugs may enhance the hypotensive effects).
No products indexed under this heading.

Sufentanil Citrate (Somnolence was a commonly reported adverse event in patients treated with ziprasidone; concurrent use with other CNS active drugs, such as depressants, should be undertaken with caution).
No products indexed under this heading.

Telmisartan (Ziprasidone may induce orthostatic hypotension; co-administration with certain antihypertensive drugs may enhance the hypotensive effects). Products include:
Micardis Tablets 1049
Micardis HCT Tablets 1051

Temazepam (Somnolence was a commonly reported adverse event in patients treated with ziprasidone; concurrent use with other CNS active drugs, such as depressants, should be undertaken with caution).
No products indexed under this heading.

Terazosin Hydrochloride (Ziprasidone may induce orthostatic hypotension; co-administration with certain antihypertensive drugs may enhance the hypotensive effects). Products include:
Hytrin Capsules 464

Thiamylal Sodium (Somnolence was a commonly reported adverse event in patients treated with ziprasidone; concurrent use with other CNS active drugs, such as depressants, should be undertaken with caution).
No products indexed under this heading.

Thioridazine Hydrochloride (Ziprasidone produces dose-related prolongation of the QT interval; co-administration with drugs that prolong the QT interval, such as thioridazine, may increase the risk of torsade de pointes and/or sudden death; concurrent use is not recommended). Products include:
Thioridazine Hydrochloride Tablets 2289

Thiothixene (Somnolence was a commonly reported adverse event in

patients treated with ziprasidone; concurrent use with other CNS active drugs, such as depressants, should be undertaken with caution). Products include:
Navane Capsules 2701
Thiothixene Capsules 2290

Timolol Maleate (Ziprasidone may induce orthostatic hypotension; co-administration with certain antihypertensive drugs may enhance the hypotensive effects). Products include:
Blocadren Tablets 2046
Cosopt Sterile Ophthalmic Solution 2065
Timolide Tablets 2187
Timolol GFS .... ⊙ 266
Timoptic in Ocudose 2192
Timoptic Sterile Ophthalmic Solution 2190
Timoptic-XE Sterile Ophthalmic Gel Forming Solution 2194

Torsemide (Ziprasidone may induce orthostatic hypotension; co-administration with certain antihypertensive drugs may enhance the hypotensive effects). Products include:
Demadex Tablets and Injection 2965

Trandolapril (Ziprasidone may induce orthostatic hypotension; co-administration with certain antihypertensive drugs may enhance the hypotensive effects). Products include:
Mavik Tablets 478
Tarka Tablets 508

Triazolam (Somnolence was a commonly reported adverse event in patients treated with ziprasidone; concurrent use with other CNS active drugs, such as depressants, should be undertaken with caution). Products include:
Halcion Tablets 2823

Trifluoperazine Hydrochloride (Somnolence was a commonly reported adverse event in patients treated with ziprasidone; concurrent use with other CNS active drugs, such as depressants, should be undertaken with caution). Products include:
Stelazine 1640

Trimethaphan Camsylate (Ziprasidone may induce orthostatic hypotension; co-administration with certain antihypertensive drugs may enhance the hypotensive effects).
No products indexed under this heading.

Valsartan (Ziprasidone may induce orthostatic hypotension; co-administration with certain antihypertensive drugs may enhance the hypotensive effects). Products include:
Diovan Capsules 2337
Diovan HCT Tablets 2338

Verapamil Hydrochloride (Ziprasidone may induce orthostatic hypotension; co-administration with certain antihypertensive drugs may enhance the hypotensive effects). Products include:
Covera-HS Tablets 3199
Isoptin SR Tablets 467
Tarka Tablets 508
Verelan Capsules 3184
Verelan PM Capsules 3186

Zaleplon (Somnolence was a commonly reported adverse event in patients treated with ziprasidone; concurrent use with other CNS active drugs, such as depressants, should be undertaken with caution). Products include:
Sonata Capsules 3591

Zolpidem Tartrate (Somnolence was a commonly reported adverse event in patients treated with ziprasidone; concurrent use with other CNS active drugs, such as depressants, should be undertaken with caution). Products include:
Ambien Tablets 3191

Food Interactions

Alcohol (Somnolence was a commonly reported adverse event in patients treated with ziprasidone; concurrent use with alcohol or other CNS active drugs, such as depressants, should be undertaken with caution).

GEREF FOR INJECTION

(Sermorelin Acetate) 3215
May interact with glucocorticoids. Compounds in these categories include:

Betamethasone Acetate (Concomitant glucocorticoid therapy may inhibit the response to Geref). Products include:
Celestone Soluspan Injectable Suspension 3097

Betamethasone Sodium Phosphate (Concomitant glucocorticoid therapy may inhibit the response to Geref). Products include:
Celestone Soluspan Injectable Suspension 3097

Cortisone Acetate (Concomitant glucocorticoid therapy may inhibit the response to Geref). Products include:
Cortone Acetate Injectable Suspension 2059
Cortone Acetate Tablets 2061

Dexamethasone (Concomitant glucocorticoid therapy may inhibit the response to Geref). Products include:
Decadron Elixir 2078
Decadron Tablets 2079
TobraDex Ophthalmic Ointment 542
TobraDex Ophthalmic Suspension 541

Dexamethasone Acetate (Concomitant glucocorticoid therapy may inhibit the response to Geref).
No products indexed under this heading.

Dexamethasone Sodium Phosphate (Concomitant glucocorticoid therapy may inhibit the response to Geref). Products include:
Decadron Phosphate Injection 2081
Decadron Phosphate Sterile Ophthalmic Ointment 2083
Decadron Phosphate Sterile Ophthalmic Solution 2084
NeoDecadron Sterile Ophthalmic Solution 2144

Fludrocortisone Acetate (Concomitant glucocorticoid therapy may inhibit the response to Geref). Products include:
Florinef Acetate Tablets 2250

Hydrocortisone (Concomitant glucocorticoid therapy may inhibit the response to Geref). Products include:
Anusol-HC Cream 2.5% 2237
Cipro HC Otic Suspension 540
Cortaid Intensive Therapy Cream .... ▣ 717
Cortaid Maximum Strength Cream .... ▣ 717
Cortisporin Ophthalmic Suspension Sterile .... ⊙ 297
Cortizone•5 .... ▣ 699
Cortizone•10 .... ▣ 699
Cortizone•10 Plus Creme .... ▣ 700
Cortizone for Kids Creme .... ▣ 699
Hydrocortone Tablets 2106
Massengill Medicated Soft Cloth Towelette .... ▣ 753
VōSoL HC Otic Solution 3356

Hydrocortisone Acetate (Concomitant glucocorticoid therapy may inhibit the response to Geref). Products include:
Analpram-HC 1338
Anusol HC-1 Hydrocortisone Anti-Itch Cream .... ▣ 689
Anusol-HC Suppositories 2238
Cortaid .... ▣ 717
Cortifoam Rectal Foam 3170
Cortisporin-TC Otic Suspension 2246
Hydrocortone Acetate Injectable Suspension 2103
Pramosone 1343
Proctocort Suppositories 2264
ProctoFoam-HC 3177
Terra-Cortril Ophthalmic Suspension 2716

Hydrocortisone Sodium Phosphate (Concomitant glucocorticoid therapy may inhibit the response to Geref). Products include:
Hydrocortone Phosphate Injection, Sterile 2105

Hydrocortisone Sodium Succinate (Concomitant glucocorticoid therapy may inhibit the response to Geref).
No products indexed under this heading.

Methylprednisolone Acetate (Concomitant glucocorticoid therapy may inhibit the response to Geref). Products include:
Depo-Medrol Injectable Suspension 2795

Methylprednisolone Sodium Succinate (Concomitant glucocorticoid therapy may inhibit the response to Geref). Products include:
Solu-Medrol Sterile Powder 2855

Prednisolone Acetate (Concomitant glucocorticoid therapy may inhibit the response to Geref). Products include:
Blephamide Ophthalmic Ointment 547
Blephamide Ophthalmic Suspension 548
Poly-Pred Liquifilm Ophthalmic Suspension .... ⊙ 245
Pred Forte Ophthalmic Suspension .... ⊙ 246
Pred Mild Sterile Ophthalmic Suspension .... ⊙ 249
Pred-G Ophthalmic Suspension .... ⊙ 247
Pred-G Sterile Ophthalmic Ointment .... ⊙ 248

Prednisolone Sodium Phosphate (Concomitant glucocorticoid therapy may inhibit the response to Geref). Products include:
Pediapred Oral Solution 1170

Prednisolone Tebutate (Concomitant glucocorticoid therapy may inhibit the response to Geref).
No products indexed under this heading.

Prednisone (Concomitant glucocorticoid therapy may inhibit the response to Geref). Products include:
Prednisone 3064

Triamcinolone (Concomitant glucocorticoid therapy may inhibit the response to Geref).
No products indexed under this heading.

Triamcinolone Acetonide (Concomitant glucocorticoid therapy may inhibit the response to Geref). Products include:
Azmacort Inhalation Aerosol 728
Nasacort Nasal Inhaler 750
Nasacort AQ Nasal Spray 752
Tri-Nasal Spray 2274

Triamcinolone Diacetate (Concomitant glucocorticoid therapy may inhibit the response to Geref).
No products indexed under this heading.

Triamcinolone Hexacetonide (Concomitant glucocorticoid therapy may inhibit the response to Geref).
No products indexed under this heading.

GINKOBA TABLETS

(Ginkgo biloba) .... ▣ 828
May interact with oral anticoagulants. Compounds in these categories include:

Dicumarol (Cocurrent use with anticoagulant agents is not recommended).
No products indexed under this heading.

Warfarin Sodium (Cocurrent use with anticoagulant agents is not recommended). Products include:
Coumadin for Injection 1243
Coumadin Tablets 1243
Warfarin Sodium Tablets, USP 3302

GINKOBA M/E SUPPLI-CAP CAPSULES

(Ginkgo biloba, Ginseng) .... ▣ 829
May interact with oral anticoagulants. Compounds in these categories include:

Dicumarol (Concurrent use with anticoagulent agents is not recommended).
No products indexed under this heading.

Warfarin Sodium (Concurrent use with anticoagulent agents is not recommended). Products include:
Coumadin for Injection 1243
Coumadin Tablets 1243
Warfarin Sodium Tablets, USP 3302

GINSANA CAPSULES

(Ginseng) .... ▣ 830
None cited in PDR database.

GINSANA CHEWY SQUARES

(Ginseng) .... ▣ 830
None cited in PDR database.

GLEEVEC CAPSULES

(Imatinib mesylate) 2357
May interact with dexamethasone, dihydrofolate reductase inhibitors, erythromycin, phenytoin, triazolobenzodiazepines, and certain other agents. Compounds in these categories include:

Alprazolam (Imatinib will increase the plasma concentrations of triazolobenzodiazepines by inhibiting CYP3A4). Products include:
Xanax Tablets 2865

Atorvastatin Calcium (Imatinib will increase the plasma concentrations of certain HMG-CoA reductase inhibitors by inhibiting CYP3A4). Products include:
Lipitor Tablets 2639
Lipitor Tablets 2696

Carbamazepine (Co-administration with inducers of CYP3A4, such as carbamazepine, may increase the metabolism and decrease imatinib concentrations). Products include:
Carbatrol Capsules 3234
Tegretol/Tegretol-XR 2404

Cerivastatin Sodium (Imatinib will increase the plasma concentrations of certain HMG-CoA reductase inhibitors by inhibiting CYP3A4). Products include:
Baycol Tablets 883

Clarithromycin (Co-administration with CYP3A4 inhibitors, such as clarithromycin, may decrease the metabolism and increase imatinib concentrations). Products include:
Biaxin/Biaxin XL 403
PREVPAC 3298

Cyclosporine (Co-administration of cyclosporine, a CYP3A4 substrate with a narrow therapeutic window, may have its plasma concentration altered by imatinib). Products include:
Gengraf Capsules 457
Neoral Soft Gelatin Capsules 2380
Neoral Oral Solution 2380
Sandimmune 2388

Dexamethasone (Co-administration with inducers of CYP3A4, such as dexamethasone, may increase the metabolism and decrease imatinib concentrations). Products include:
Decadron Elixir 2078
Decadron Tablets 2079
TobraDex Ophthalmic Ointment 542
TobraDex Ophthalmic Suspension 541

Dexamethasone Acetate (Co-administration with inducers of CYP3A4, such as dexamethasone, may increase the metabolism and

decrease imatinib concentrations).
No products indexed under this heading.

Dexamethasone Sodium Phosphate (Co-administration with inducers of CYP3A4, such as dexamethasone, may increase the metabolism and decrease imatinib concentrations). Products include:
- Decadron Phosphate Injection 2081
- Decadron Phosphate Sterile Ophthalmic Ointment 2083
- Decadron Phosphate Sterile Ophthalmic Solution 2084
- NeoDecadron Sterile Ophthalmic Solution 2144

Erythromycin (Co-administration with CYP3A4 inhibitors, such as erythromycin, may decrease the metabolism and increase imatinib concentrations). Products include:
- Emgel 2% Topical Gel 1285
- Ery-Tab Tablets 448
- Erythromycin Base Filmtab Tablets . 454
- Erythromycin Delayed-Release Capsules, USP 455
- PCE Dispertab Tablets 498

Erythromycin Estolate (Co-administration with CYP3A4 inhibitors, such as erythromycin, may decrease the metabolism and increase imatinib concentrations).
No products indexed under this heading.

Erythromycin Ethylsuccinate (Co-administration with CYP3A4 inhibitors, such as erythromycin, may decrease the metabolism and increase imatinib concentrations). Products include:
- E.E.S. 450
- EryPed 446
- Pediazole Suspension 3050

Erythromycin Gluceptate (Co-administration with CYP3A4 inhibitors, such as erythromycin, may decrease the metabolism and increase imatinib concentrations).
No products indexed under this heading.

Erythromycin Stearate (Co-administration with CYP3A4 inhibitors, such as erythromycin, may decrease the metabolism and increase imatinib concentrations). Products include:
- Erythrocin Stearate Filmtab Tablets 452

Fosphenytoin Sodium (Co-administration with inducers of CYP3A4, such as phenytoin, may increase the metabolism and decrease imatinib concentrations). Products include:
- Cerebyx Injection 2619

Hypericum (Co-administration with inducers of CYP3A4, such as St. John's Wort, may increase the metabolism and decrease imatinib concentrations). Products include:
- Brite-Life Caplets .... ◙795
- Centrum St. John's Wort Softgels . ◙853
- Metabolic Nutrition System .... ◙798
- Movana Tablets .... ◙832
- One-A-Day Tension & Mood Softgels .... ◙808
- ReSource Wellness StayCalm Caplets .... ◙826
- Satiete Tablets .... ◙846

Itraconazole (Co-administration with CYP3A4 inhibitors, such as itraconazole, may decrease the metabolism and increase imatinib concentrations). Products include:
- Sporanox Capsules 1800
- Sporanox Injection 1804
- Sporanox Injection 2509
- Sporanox Oral Solution 1808
- Sporanox Oral Solution 2512

Ketoconazole (Co-administration with CYP3A4 inhibitors, such as ketoconazole, may decrease the metabolism and increase imatinib concentrations). Products include:
- Nizoral 2% Cream 3620
- Nizoral A-D Shampoo 2008
- Nizoral 2% Shampoo 2007
- Nizoral Tablets 1791

Lovastatin (Imatinib will increase the plasma concentrations of certain HMG-CoA reductase inhibitors by inhibiting CYP3A4). Products include:
- Mevacor Tablets 2132

Methotrexate Sodium (Imatinib will increase the plasma concentrations of dihydropyridine calcium channel blockers by inhibiting CYP3A4).
No products indexed under this heading.

Midazolam Hydrochloride (Imatinib will increase the plasma concentrations of triazolobenzodiazepines by inhibiting CYP3A4). Products include:
- Versed Injection 3027
- Versed Syrup 3033

Phenobarbital (Co-administration with inducers of CYP3A4, such as phenobarbital, may increase the metabolism and decrease imatinib concentrations). Products include:
- Arco-Lase Plus Tablets 592
- Donnatal 2929
- Donnatal Extentabs 2930

Phenytoin (Co-administration with inducers of CYP3A4, such as phenytoin, may increase the metabolism and decrease imatinib concentrations). Products include:
- Dilantin Infatabs 2624
- Dilantin-125 Oral Suspension 2625

Phenytoin Sodium (Co-administration with inducers of CYP3A4, such as phenytoin, may increase the metabolism and decrease imatinib concentrations). Products include:
- Dilantin Kapseals 2622

Pimozide (Co-administration of pimozide, a CYP3A4 substrate with a narrow therapeutic window, may have its plasma concentration altered by imatinib). Products include:
- Orap Tablets 1407

Rifampin (Co-administration with inducers of CYP3A4, such as rifampin, may increase the metabolism and decrease imatinib concentrations). Products include:
- Rifadin 765
- Rifamate Capsules 767
- Rifater Tablets 769

Simvastatin (Imatinib increases the mean Cmax and AUC of simvastatin 2- and 3.5-fold, respectively by inhibiting CYP3A4). Products include:
- Zocor Tablets 2219

Triazolam (Imatinib will increase the plasma concentrations of triazolobenzodiazepines by inhibiting CYP3A4). Products include:
- Halcion Tablets 2823

Trimethoprim (Imatinib will increase the plasma concentrations of dihydropyridine calcium channel blockers by inhibiting CYP3A4). Products include:
- Bactrim 2949
- Septra Suspension 2265
- Septra Tablets 2265
- Septra DS Tablets 2265

Trimetrexate Glucuronate (Imatinib will increase the plasma concentrations of dihydropyridine calcium channel blockers by inhibiting CYP3A4).
No products indexed under this heading.

Warfarin Sodium (Imatinib is a potent competitive inhibitor of CYP2C9; warfarin is metabolized by CYP2C9, therefore, patients who require anticoagulation should receive low-molecular weight or standard heparin). Products include:
- Coumadin for Injection 1243
- Coumadin Tablets 1243
- Warfarin Sodium Tablets, USP 3302

GLIADEL WAFER

(Carmustine (BCNU)) 1723
None cited in PDR database.

GLUCA-BALANCE CAPSULES

(Amino Acid Preparations) 2269
None cited in PDR database.

GLUCAGEN FOR INJECTION DIAGNOSTIC KIT

(Glucagon) 949
May interact with beta blockers. Compounds in these categories include:

Acebutolol Hydrochloride (Patients taking beta blockers might be expected to have a greater increase in both pulse and blood pressure). Products include:
- Sectral Capsules 3589

Atenolol (Patients taking beta blockers might be expected to have a greater increase in both pulse and blood pressure). Products include:
- Tenoretic Tablets 690
- Tenormin I.V. Injection 692

Betaxolol Hydrochloride (Patients taking beta blockers might be expected to have a greater increase in both pulse and blood pressure). Products include:
- Betoptic S Ophthalmic Suspension 537

Bisoprolol Fumarate (Patients taking beta blockers might be expected to have a greater increase in both pulse and blood pressure). Products include:
- Zebeta Tablets 1885
- Ziac Tablets 1887

Carteolol Hydrochloride (Patients taking beta blockers might be expected to have a greater increase in both pulse and blood pressure). Products include:
- Carteolol Hydrochloride Ophthalmic Solution USP, 1% ..... ⊙258
- Ocupress Ophthalmic Solution, 1% Sterile .... ⊙303

Esmolol Hydrochloride (Patients taking beta blockers might be expected to have a greater increase in both pulse and blood pressure). Products include:
- Brevibloc Injection 858

Labetalol Hydrochloride (Patients taking beta blockers might be expected to have a greater increase in both pulse and blood pressure). Products include:
- Normodyne Injection 3135
- Normodyne Tablets 3137

Levobunolol Hydrochloride (Patients taking beta blockers might be expected to have a greater increase in both pulse and blood pressure). Products include:
- Betagan .... ⊙228

Metipranolol Hydrochloride (Patients taking beta blockers might be expected to have a greater increase in both pulse and blood pressure).
No products indexed under this heading.

Metoprolol Succinate (Patients taking beta blockers might be expected to have a greater increase in both pulse and blood pressure). Products include:
- Toprol-XL Tablets 651

Metoprolol Tartrate (Patients taking beta blockers might be expected to have a greater increase in both pulse and blood pressure).
No products indexed under this heading.

Nadolol (Patients taking beta blockers might be expected to have a greater increase in both pulse and blood pressure). Products include:
- Corgard Tablets 2245
- Corzide 40/5 Tablets 2247
- Corzide 80/5 Tablets 2247
- Nadolol Tablets 2288

Penbutolol Sulfate (Patients taking beta blockers might be expected to have a greater increase in both pulse and blood pressure).
No products indexed under this heading.

Pindolol (Patients taking beta blockers might be expected to have a greater increase in both pulse and blood pressure).
No products indexed under this heading.

Propranolol Hydrochloride (Patients taking beta blockers might be expected to have a greater increase in both pulse and blood pressure). Products include:
- Inderal 3513
- Inderal LA Long-Acting Capsules 3516
- Inderide Tablets 3517
- Inderide LA Long-Acting Capsules .. 3519

Sotalol Hydrochloride (Patients taking beta blockers might be expected to have a greater increase in both pulse and blood pressure). Products include:
- Betapace Tablets 950
- Betapace AF Tablets 954

Timolol Hemihydrate (Patients taking beta blockers might be expected to have a greater increase in both pulse and blood pressure). Products include:
- Betimol Ophthalmic Solution .... ⊙324

Timolol Maleate (Patients taking beta blockers might be expected to have a greater increase in both pulse and blood pressure). Products include:
- Blocadren Tablets 2046
- Cosopt Sterile Ophthalmic Solution 2065
- Timolide Tablets 2187
- Timolol GFS .... ⊙266
- Timoptic in Ocudose 2192
- Timoptic Sterile Ophthalmic Solution 2190
- Timoptic-XE Sterile Ophthalmic Gel Forming Solution 2194

GLUCAGON FOR INJECTION VIALS AND EMERGENCY KIT

(Glucagon) 1924
None cited in PDR database.

GLUCOPHAGE TABLETS

(Metformin Hydrochloride) 1080
May interact with cationic drugs that are eliminated by renal tubular, calcium channel blockers, corticosteroids, diuretics, estrogens, oral contraceptives, phenothiazines, phenytoin, quinidine, radiographic iodinated contrast media, sympathomimetics, thiazides, thyroid preparations, and certain other agents. Compounds in these categories include:

Albuterol (Certain drugs, such as sympathomimetics, tend to produce hyperglycemia and may lead to loss of glycemic control). Products include:
- Proventil Inhalation Aerosol 3142
- Ventolin Inhalation Aerosol and Refill 1679

Albuterol Sulfate (Certain drugs, such as sympathomimetics, tend to produce hyperglycemia and may lead to loss of glycemic control). Products include:
- AccuNeb Inhalation Solution 1230
- Combivent Inhalation Aerosol 1041
- DuoNeb Inhalation Solution 1233
- Proventil Inhalation Solution 0.083% 3146
- Proventil Repetabs Tablets 3148
- Proventil Solution for Inhalation 0.5% 3144
- Proventil HFA Inhalation Aerosol 3150
- Ventolin HFA Inhalation Aerosol 3618
- Volmax Extended-Release Tablets .. 2276

Amiloride Hydrochloride (Potential for loss of glycemic control; the-

oretical potential for interaction with metformin by competing for common renal tubular transport system). Products include:

Midamor Tablets 2136
Moduretic Tablets 2138

Amlodipine Besylate (Certain drugs, such as calcium channel blockers, tend to produce hyperglycemia and may lead to loss of glycemic control). Products include:

Lotrel Capsules 2370
Norvasc Tablets 2704

Bendroflumethiazide (Certain drugs, such as thiazides and other diuretics, tend to produce hyperglycemia and may lead to loss of glycemic control). Products include:

Corzide 40/5 Tablets 2247
Corzide 80/5 Tablets 2247

Bepridil Hydrochloride (Certain drugs, such as calcium channel blockers, tend to produce hyperglycemia and may lead to loss of glycemic control). Products include:

Vascor Tablets 2602

Betamethasone Acetate (Certain drugs, such as corticosteroids, tend to produce hyperglycemia and may lead to loss of glycemic control). Products include:

Celestone Soluspan Injectable Suspension 3097

Betamethasone Sodium Phosphate (Certain drugs, such as corticosteroids, tend to produce hyperglycemia and may lead to loss of glycemic control). Products include:

Celestone Soluspan Injectable Suspension 3097

Bumetanide (Certain drugs, such as diuretics, tend to produce hyperglycemia and may lead to loss of glycemic control).

No products indexed under this heading.

Chlorothiazide (Certain drugs, such as thiazides and other diuretics, tend to produce hyperglycemia and may lead to loss of glycemic control). Products include:

Aldoclor Tablets 2035
Diuril Oral 2087

Chlorothiazide Sodium (Certain drugs, such as thiazides and other diuretics, tend to produce hyperglycemia and may lead to loss of glycemic control). Products include:

Diuril Sodium Intravenous 2086

Chlorotrianisene (Certain drugs, such as estrogens, tend to produce hyperglycemia and may lead to loss of glycemic control).

No products indexed under this heading.

Chlorpromazine (Certain drugs, such as phenothiazines, tend to produce hyperglycemia and may lead to loss of glycemic control). Products include:

Thorazine Suppositories 1656

Chlorpromazine Hydrochloride (Certain drugs, such as phenothiazines, tend to produce hyperglycemia and may lead to loss of glycemic control). Products include:

Thorazine 1656

Chlorthalidone (Certain drugs, such as diuretics, tend to produce hyperglycemia and may lead to loss of glycemic control). Products include:

Clorpres Tablets 1002
Combipres Tablets 1040
Tenoretic Tablets 690

Cimetidine (Co-administered with oral cimetidine may increase peak metformin plasma and whole blood concentrations by 60% and a 40% increase in plasma and whole blood metformin AUC). Products include:

Tagamet HB 200 Suspension 762
Tagamet HB 200 Tablets 761
Tagamet Tablets 1644

Cortisone Acetate (Certain drugs, such as corticosteroids, tend to produce hyperglycemia and may lead to loss of glycemic control). Products include:

Cortone Acetate Injectable Suspension 2059
Cortone Acetate Tablets 2061

Desogestrel (Certain drugs, such as oral contraceptives, tend to produce hyperglycemia and may lead to loss of glycemic control). Products include:

Cyclessa Tablets 2450
Desogen Tablets 2458
Mircette Tablets 2470
Ortho-Cept 21 Tablets 2546
Ortho-Cept 28 Tablets 2546

Dexamethasone (Certain drugs, such as corticosteroids, tend to produce hyperglycemia and may lead to loss of glycemic control). Products include:

Decadron Elixir 2078
Decadron Tablets 2079
TobraDex Ophthalmic Ointment 542
TobraDex Ophthalmic Suspension 541

Dexamethasone Acetate (Certain drugs, such as corticosteroids, tend to produce hyperglycemia and may lead to loss of glycemic control).

No products indexed under this heading.

Dexamethasone Sodium Phosphate (Certain drugs, such as corticosteroids, tend to produce hyperglycemia and may lead to loss of glycemic control). Products include:

Decadron Phosphate Injection 2081
Decadron Phosphate Sterile Ophthalmic Ointment 2083
Decadron Phosphate Sterile Ophthalmic Solution 2084
NeoDecadron Sterile Ophthalmic Solution 2144

Diatrizoate Meglumine (Potential for acute alteration of renal function; metformin should be temporarily withheld in patients undergoing radiologic studies involving parenteral iodinated contrast material).

No products indexed under this heading.

Diatrizoate Sodium (Potential for acute alteration of renal function; metformin should be temporarily withheld in patients undergoing radiologic studies involving parenteral iodinated contrast material).

No products indexed under this heading.

Dienestrol (Certain drugs, such as estrogens, tend to produce hyperglycemia and may lead to loss of glycemic control). Products include:

Ortho Dienestrol Cream 2554

Diethylstilbestrol (Certain drugs, such as estrogens, tend to produce hyperglycemia and may lead to loss of glycemic control).

No products indexed under this heading.

Digoxin (Theoretical potential for interaction with metformin by competing for common renal tubular transport system). Products include:

Digitek Tablets 1003
Lanoxicaps Capsules 1574
Lanoxin Injection 1581
Lanoxin Tablets 1587
Lanoxin Elixir Pediatric 1578
Lanoxin Injection Pediatric 1584

Diltiazem Hydrochloride (Certain drugs, such as calcium channel blockers, tend to produce hyperglycemia and may lead to loss of glycemic control). Products include:

Cardizem Injectable 1018
Cardizem Lyo-Ject Syringe 1018
Cardizem Monovial 1018
Cardizem CD Capsules 1016
Tiazac Capsules 1378

Dobutamine Hydrochloride (Certain drugs, such as sympathomimetics, tend to produce hyperglycemia and may lead to loss of glycemic control). Products include:

Dobutrex Solution Vials 1914

Dopamine Hydrochloride (Certain drugs, such as sympathomimetics, tend to produce hyperglycemia and may lead to loss of glycemic control).

No products indexed under this heading.

Ephedrine Hydrochloride (Certain drugs, such as sympathomimetics, tend to produce hyperglycemia and may lead to loss of glycemic control). Products include:

Primatene Tablets 780

Ephedrine Sulfate (Certain drugs, such as sympathomimetics, tend to produce hyperglycemia and may lead to loss of glycemic control).

No products indexed under this heading.

Ephedrine Tannate (Certain drugs, such as sympathomimetics, tend to produce hyperglycemia and may lead to loss of glycemic control). Products include:

Rynatuss Pediatric Suspension 3353
Rynatuss Tablets 3353

Epinephrine (Certain drugs, such as sympathomimetics, tend to produce hyperglycemia and may lead to loss of glycemic control). Products include:

Epifrin Sterile Ophthalmic Solution .... ⊙235
EpiPen 1236
Primatene Mist 779
Xylocaine with Epinephrine Injection 653

Epinephrine Bitartrate (Certain drugs, such as sympathomimetics, tend to produce hyperglycemia and may lead to loss of glycemic control). Products include:

Sensorcaine 643

Epinephrine Hydrochloride (Certain drugs, such as sympathomimetics, tend to produce hyperglycemia and may lead to loss of glycemic control).

No products indexed under this heading.

Estradiol (Certain drugs, such as estrogens, tend to produce hyperglycemia and may lead to loss of glycemic control). Products include:

Activella Tablets 2764
Alora Transdermal System 3372
Climara Transdermal System 958
CombiPatch Transdermal System 2323
Esclim Transdermal System 3460
Estrace Vaginal Cream 3358
Estrace Tablets 3361
Estring Vaginal Ring 2811
Ortho-Prefest Tablets 2570
Vagifem Tablets 2857
Vivelle Transdermal System 2412
Vivelle-Dot Transdermal System 2416

Estrogens, Conjugated (Certain drugs, such as estrogens, tend to produce hyperglycemia and may lead to loss of glycemic control). Products include:

Premarin Intravenous 3563
Premarin Tablets 3566
Premarin Vaginal Cream 3570
Premphase Tablets 3572
Prempro Tablets 3572

Estrogens, Esterified (Certain drugs, such as estrogens, tend to produce hyperglycemia and may lead to loss of glycemic control). Products include:

Estratest 3252
Menest Tablets 2254

Estropipate (Certain drugs, such as estrogens, tend to produce hyperglycemia and may lead to loss of glycemic control). Products include:

Ogen Tablets 2846
Ortho-Est Tablets 3464

Ethacrynic Acid (Certain drugs, such as diuretics, tend to produce hyperglycemia and may lead to loss of glycemic control). Products include:

Edecrin Tablets 2091

Ethinyl Estradiol (Certain drugs, such as estrogens, tend to produce hyperglycemia and may lead to loss of glycemic control). Products include:

Alesse-21 Tablets 3468
Alesse-28 Tablets 3473
Brevicon 28-Day Tablets 3380
Cyclessa Tablets 2450
Desogen Tablets 2458
Estinyl Tablets 3112
Estrostep 2627
femhrt Tablets 2635
Levlen 962
Levlite 21 Tablets 962
Levlite 28 Tablets 962
Levora Tablets 3389
Loestrin 21 Tablets 2642
Loestrin Fe Tablets 2642
Lo/Ovral Tablets 3532
Lo/Ovral-28 Tablets 3538
Low-Ogestrel-28 Tablets 3392
Microgestin Fe 1.5/30 Tablets 3407
Microgestin Fe 1/20 Tablets 3400
Mircette Tablets 2470
Modicon 2563
Necon 3415
Nordette-28 Tablets 2257
Norinyl 1 +35 28-Day Tablets 3380
Ogestrel 0.5/50-28 Tablets 3428
Ortho-Cept 21 Tablets 2546
Ortho-Cept 28 Tablets 2546
Ortho-Cyclen/Ortho Tri-Cyclen 2573
Ortho-Novum 2563
Ovcon 3364
Ovral Tablets 3551
Ovral-28 Tablets 3552
Tri-Levlen 962
Tri-Norinyl-28 Tablets 3433
Triphasil-21 Tablets 3600
Triphasil-28 Tablets 3605
Trivora Tablets 3439
Yasmin 28 Tablets 980
Zovia 3449

Ethiodized Oil (Potential for acute alteration of renal function; metformin should be temporarily withheld in patients undergoing radiologic studies involving parenteral iodinated contrast material). Products include:

Ethiodol Injection 3095

Ethynodiol Diacetate (Certain drugs, such as oral contraceptives, tend to produce hyperglycemia and may lead to loss of glycemic control). Products include:

Zovia 3449

Felodipine (Certain drugs, such as calcium channel blockers, tend to produce hyperglycemia and may lead to loss of glycemic control). Products include:

Lexxel Tablets 608
Plendil Extended-Release Tablets 623

Fludrocortisone Acetate (Certain drugs, such as corticosteroids, tend to produce hyperglycemia and may lead to loss of glycemic control). Products include:

Florinef Acetate Tablets 2250

Fluphenazine Decanoate (Certain drugs, such as phenothiazines, tend to produce hyperglycemia and may lead to loss of glycemic control).

No products indexed under this heading.

Fluphenazine Enanthate (Certain drugs, such as phenothiazines, tend to produce hyperglycemia and may lead to loss of glycemic control).

No products indexed under this heading.

Fluphenazine Hydrochloride (Certain drugs, such as phenothiazines, tend to produce hyperglycemia and may lead to loss of glycemic control).

No products indexed under this heading.

Fosphenytoin Sodium (Certain drugs, such as phenytoin, tend to produce hyperglycemia and may lead to loss of glycemic control). Products include:

Cerebyx Injection 2619

Furosemide (Increases metformin plasma and blood Cmax by 22% and blood AUC by 15%; the Cmax and AUC of furosemide were 31% and

12% smaller when co-administered; potential for loss of glycemic control). Products include:
Furosemide Tablets 2284

Gadopentetate Dimeglumine (Potential for acute alteration of renal function; metformin should be temporarily withheld in patients undergoing radiologic studies involving parenteral iodinated contrast material).
No products indexed under this heading.

Glyburide (Decrease in glyburide AUC and Cmax have been observed, but were highly variable). Products include:
DiaBeta Tablets 741
Glucovance Tablets 1086

Hydrochlorothiazide (Certain drugs, such as thiazides and other diuretics, tend to produce hyperglycemia and may lead to loss of glycemic control). Products include:
Accuretic Tablets 2614
Aldoril Tablets 2039
Atacand HCT Tablets 597
Avalide Tablets 1070
Diovan HCT Tablets 2338
Dyazide Capsules 1515
HydroDIURIL Tablets 2108
Hyzaar 2109
Inderide Tablets 3517
Inderide LA Long-Acting Capsules .. 3519
Lotensin HCT Tablets 2367
Maxzide 1008
Micardis HCT Tablets 1051
Microzide Capsules 3414
Moduretic Tablets 2138
Monopril HCT 1094
Prinzide Tablets 2168
Timolide Tablets 2187
Uniretic Tablets 3178
Vaseretic Tablets 2204
Zestoretic Tablets 695
Ziac Tablets 1887

Hydrocortisone (Certain drugs, such as corticosteroids, tend to produce hyperglycemia and may lead to loss of glycemic control). Products include:
Anusol-HC Cream 2.5% 2237
Cipro HC Otic Suspension 540
Cortaid Intensive Therapy Cream ... ▣717
Cortaid Maximum Strength Cream .... ▣717
Cortisporin Ophthalmic Suspension Sterile .... ⊙297
Cortizone•5 .... ▣699
Cortizone•10 .... ▣699
Cortizone•10 Plus Creme .... ▣700
Cortizone for Kids Creme .... ▣699
Hydrocortone Tablets 2106
Massengill Medicated Soft Cloth Towelette .... ▣753
VōSoL HC Otic Solution 3356

Hydrocortisone Acetate (Certain drugs, such as corticosteroids, tend to produce hyperglycemia and may lead to loss of glycemic control). Products include:
Analpram-HC 1338
Anusol HC-1 Hydrocortisone Anti-Itch Cream .... ▣689
Anusol-HC Suppositories 2238
Cortaid .... ▣717
Cortifoam Rectal Foam 3170
Cortisporin-TC Otic Suspension 2246
Hydrocortone Acetate Injectable Suspension 2103
Pramosone 1343
Proctocort Suppositories 2264
ProctoFoam-HC 3177
Terra-Cortril Ophthalmic Suspension 2716

Hydrocortisone Sodium Phosphate (Certain drugs, such as corticosteroids, tend to produce hyperglycemia and may lead to loss of glycemic control). Products include:
Hydrocortone Phosphate Injection, Sterile 2105

Hydrocortisone Sodium Succinate (Certain drugs, such as corticosteroids, tend to produce hyperglycemia and may lead to loss of glycemic control).
No products indexed under this heading.

Hydroflumethiazide (Certain drugs, such as thiazides and other diuretics, tend to produce hyperglycemia and may lead to loss of glycemic control). Products include:
Diucardin Tablets 3494

Indapamide (Certain drugs, such as diuretics, tend to produce hyperglycemia and may lead to loss of glycemic control). Products include:
Indapamide Tablets 2286

Iodamide Meglumine (Potential for acute alteration of renal function; metformin should be temporarily withheld in patients undergoing radiologic studies involving parenteral iodinated contrast material).
No products indexed under this heading.

Iohexol (Potential for acute alteration of renal function; metformin should be temporarily withheld in patients undergoing radiologic studies involving parenteral iodinated contrast material).
No products indexed under this heading.

Iopamidol (Potential for acute alteration of renal function; metformin should be temporarily withheld in patients undergoing radiologic studies involving parenteral iodinated contrast material).
No products indexed under this heading.

Iopanoic Acid (Potential for acute alteration of renal function; metformin should be temporarily withheld in patients undergoing radiologic studies involving parenteral iodinated contrast material).
No products indexed under this heading.

Iothalamate Meglumine (Potential for acute alteration of renal function; metformin should be temporarily withheld in patients undergoing radiologic studies involving parenteral iodinated contrast material).
No products indexed under this heading.

Ioxaglate Meglumine (Potential for acute alteration of renal function; metformin should be temporarily withheld in patients undergoing radiologic studies involving parenteral iodinated contrast material).
No products indexed under this heading.

Ioxaglate Sodium (Potential for acute alteration of renal function; metformin should be temporarily withheld in patients undergoing radiologic studies involving parenteral iodinated contrast material).
No products indexed under this heading.

Isoniazid (Certain drugs, such as isoniazid, tend to produce hyperglycemia and may lead to loss of glycemic control). Products include:
Rifamate Capsules 767
Rifater Tablets 769

Isoproterenol Hydrochloride (Certain drugs, such as sympathomimetics, tend to produce hyperglycemia and may lead to loss of glycemic control).
No products indexed under this heading.

Isoproterenol Sulfate (Certain drugs, such as sympathomimetics, tend to produce hyperglycemia and may lead to loss of glycemic control).
No products indexed under this heading.

Isradipine (Certain drugs, such as calcium channel blockers, tend to produce hyperglycemia and may lead to loss of glycemic control). Products include:
DynaCirc Capsules 2921
DynaCirc CR Tablets 2923

Levalbuterol Hydrochloride (Certain drugs, such as sympathomimetics, tend to produce hyperglycemia and may lead to loss of glycemic control). Products include:
Xopenex Inhalation Solution 3207

Levonorgestrel (Certain drugs, such as oral contraceptives, tend to produce hyperglycemia and may lead to loss of glycemic control). Products include:
Alesse-21 Tablets 3468
Alesse-28 Tablets 3473
Levlen 962
Levlite 21 Tablets 962
Levlite 28 Tablets 962
Levora Tablets 3389
Mirena Intrauterine System 974
Nordette-28 Tablets 2257
Norplant System 3543
Tri-Levlen 962
Triphasil-21 Tablets 3600
Triphasil-28 Tablets 3605
Trivora Tablets 3439

Levothyroxine Sodium (Certain drugs, such as thyroid products, tend to produce hyperglycemia and may lead to loss of glycemic control). Products include:
Levothroid Tablets 1373
Levoxyl Tablets 1819
Synthroid 505
Unithroid Tablets 3445

Liothyronine Sodium (Certain drugs, such as thyroid products, tend to produce hyperglycemia and may lead to loss of glycemic control). Products include:
Cytomel Tablets 1817
Triostat Injection 1825

Liotrix (Certain drugs, such as thyroid products, tend to produce hyperglycemia and may lead to loss of glycemic control).
No products indexed under this heading.

Mesoridazine Besylate (Certain drugs, such as phenothiazines, tend to produce hyperglycemia and may lead to loss of glycemic control). Products include:
Serentil 1057

Mestranol (Certain drugs, such as oral contraceptives, tend to produce hyperglycemia and may lead to loss of glycemic control). Products include:
Necon 1/50 Tablets 3415
Norinyl 1 + 50 28-Day Tablets 3380
Ortho-Novum 1/50□28 Tablets 2556

Metaproterenol Sulfate (Certain drugs, such as sympathomimetics, tend to produce hyperglycemia and may lead to loss of glycemic control). Products include:
Alupent 1029

Metaraminol Bitartrate (Certain drugs, such as sympathomimetics, tend to produce hyperglycemia and may lead to loss of glycemic control). Products include:
Aramine Injection 2043

Methotrimeprazine (Certain drugs, such as phenothiazines, tend to produce hyperglycemia and may lead to loss of glycemic control).
No products indexed under this heading.

Methoxamine Hydrochloride (Certain drugs, such as sympathomimetics, tend to produce hyperglycemia and may lead to loss of glycemic control).
No products indexed under this heading.

Methyclothiazide (Certain drugs, such as thiazides and other diuretics, tend to produce hyperglycemia and may lead to loss of glycemic control).
No products indexed under this heading.

Methylprednisolone Acetate (Certain drugs, such as corticosteroids, tend to produce hyperglycemia and may lead to loss of glycemic control). Products include:
Depo-Medrol Injectable Suspension 2795

Methylprednisolone Sodium Succinate (Certain drugs, such as corticosteroids, tend to produce hyperglycemia and may lead to loss of glycemic control). Products include:
Solu-Medrol Sterile Powder 2855

Metolazone (Certain drugs, such as diuretics, tend to produce hyperglycemia and may lead to loss of glycemic control). Products include:
Mykrox Tablets 1168
Zaroxolyn Tablets 1177

Mibefradil Dihydrochloride (Certain drugs, such as calcium channel blockers, tend to produce hyperglycemia and may lead to loss of glycemic control).
No products indexed under this heading.

Morphine Sulfate (Theoretical potential for interaction with metformin by competing for common renal tubular transport system). Products include:
Astramorph/PF Injection, USP (Preservative-Free) 594
Duramorph Injection 1312
Infumorph 200 and Infumorph 500 Sterile Solutions 1314
Kadian Capsules 1335
MS Contin Tablets 2896
MSIR 2898
Oramorph SR Tablets 3062
Roxanol 3066

Niacin (Certain drugs, such as niacin, tend to produce hyperglycemia and may lead to loss of glycemic control). Products include:
Niaspan Extended-Release Tablets 1846
Nicotinex Elixir .... ▣633

Nicardipine Hydrochloride (Certain drugs, such as calcium channel blockers, tend to produce hyperglycemia and may lead to loss of glycemic control). Products include:
Cardene I.V. 3485

Nicotinic Acid (Potential for loss of glycemic control).
No products indexed under this heading.

Nifedipine (Enhances the absorption of metformin by increasing plasma metformin Cmax and AUC; potential for loss of glycemic control). Products include:
Adalat CC Tablets 877
Procardia Capsules 2708
Procardia XL Extended Release Tablets 2710

Nimodipine (Certain drugs, such as calcium channel blockers, tend to produce hyperglycemia and may lead to loss of glycemic control). Products include:
Nimotop Capsules 904

Nisoldipine (Certain drugs, such as calcium channel blockers, tend to produce hyperglycemia and may lead to loss of glycemic control). Products include:
Sular Tablets 688

Norepinephrine Bitartrate (Certain drugs, such as sympathomimetics, tend to produce hyperglycemia and may lead to loss of glycemic control).
No products indexed under this heading.

Norethindrone (Certain drugs, such as oral contraceptives, tend to produce hyperglycemia and may lead to loss of glycemic control). Products include:
Brevicon 28-Day Tablets 3380
Micronor Tablets 2543
Modicon 2563
Necon 3415
Norinyl 1 +35 28-Day Tablets 3380
Norinyl 1 + 50 28-Day Tablets 3380
Nor-QD Tablets 3423
Ortho-Novum 2563
Ortho-Novum 1/50□28 Tablets 2556
Ovcon 3364

Tri-Norinyl-28 Tablets 3433

Norethynodrel (Certain drugs, such as oral contraceptives, tend to produce hyperglycemia and may lead to loss of glycemic control).

No products indexed under this heading.

Norgestimate (Certain drugs, such as oral contraceptives, tend to produce hyperglycemia and may lead to loss of glycemic control). Products include:

Ortho-Cyclen/Ortho Tri-Cyclen 2573
Ortho-Prefest Tablets 2570

Norgestrel (Certain drugs, such as oral contraceptives, tend to produce hyperglycemia and may lead to loss of glycemic control). Products include:

Lo/Ovral Tablets 3532
Lo/Ovral-28 Tablets 3538
Low-Ogestrel-28 Tablets 3392
Ogestrel 0.5/50-28 Tablets 3428
Ovral Tablets 3551
Ovral-28 Tablets 3552
Ovrette Tablets 3552

Perphenazine (Certain drugs, such as phenothiazines, tend to produce hyperglycemia and may lead to loss of glycemic control). Products include:

Etrafon 3115
Trilafon 3160

Phenylephrine Bitartrate (Certain drugs, such as sympathomimetics, tend to produce hyperglycemia and may lead to loss of glycemic control).

No products indexed under this heading.

Phenylephrine Hydrochloride (Certain drugs, such as sympathomimetics, tend to produce hyperglycemia and may lead to loss of glycemic control). Products include:

Afrin Nasal Decongestant Children's Pump Mist .... ■734
Extendryl 1361
Hycomine Compound Tablets 1317
Neo-Synephrine .... ■614
Phenergan VC Syrup 3560
Phenergan VC with Codeine Syrup . 3561
Preparation H Cream .... ■778
Preparation H Cooling Gel .... ■778
Preparation H .... ■778
Vicks Sinex Nasal Spray and Ultra Fine Mist .... ■729

Phenylephrine Tannate (Certain drugs, such as sympathomimetics, tend to produce hyperglycemia and may lead to loss of glycemic control). Products include:

Ryna-12 S Suspension 3351
Reformulated Rynatan Pediatric Suspension 3352
Rynatuss Pediatric Suspension 3353
Rynatuss Tablets 3353

Phenylpropanolamine Hydrochloride (Certain drugs, such as sympathomimetics, tend to produce hyperglycemia and may lead to loss of glycemic control).

No products indexed under this heading.

Phenytoin (Certain drugs, such as phenytoin, tend to produce hyperglycemia and may lead to loss of glycemic control). Products include:

Dilantin Infatabs 2624
Dilantin-125 Oral Suspension 2625

Phenytoin Sodium (Certain drugs, such as phenytoin, tend to produce hyperglycemia and may lead to loss of glycemic control). Products include:

Dilantin Kapseals 2622

Pirbuterol Acetate (Certain drugs, such as sympathomimetics, tend to produce hyperglycemia and may lead to loss of glycemic control). Products include:

Maxair Autohaler 1981
Maxair Inhaler 1984

Polyestradiol Phosphate (Certain drugs, such as estrogens, tend to produce hyperglycemia and may lead to loss of glycemic control).

No products indexed under this heading.

Polythiazide (Certain drugs, such as thiazides and other diuretics, tend to produce hyperglycemia and may lead to loss of glycemic control). Products include:

Minizide Capsules 2700
Renese Tablets 2712

Prednisolone Acetate (Certain drugs, such as corticosteroids, tend to produce hyperglycemia and may lead to loss of glycemic control). Products include:

Blephamide Ophthalmic Ointment ... 547
Blephamide Ophthalmic Suspension 548
Poly-Pred Liquifilm Ophthalmic Suspension .... ⊙245
Pred Forte Ophthalmic Suspension .... ⊙246
Pred Mild Sterile Ophthalmic Suspension .... ⊙249
Pred-G Ophthalmic Suspension ..... ⊙247
Pred-G Sterile Ophthalmic Ointment .... ⊙248

Prednisolone Sodium Phosphate (Certain drugs, such as corticosteroids, tend to produce hyperglycemia and may lead to loss of glycemic control). Products include:

Pediapred Oral Solution 1170

Prednisolone Tebutate (Certain drugs, such as corticosteroids, tend to produce hyperglycemia and may lead to loss of glycemic control).

No products indexed under this heading.

Prednisone (Certain drugs, such as corticosteroids, tend to produce hyperglycemia and may lead to loss of glycemic control). Products include:

Prednisone 3064

Procainamide Hydrochloride (Theoretical potential for interaction with metformin by competing for common renal tubular transport system). Products include:

Procanbid Extended-Release Tablets 2262

Prochlorperazine (Certain drugs, such as phenothiazines, tend to produce hyperglycemia and may lead to loss of glycemic control). Products include:

Compazine 1505

Promethazine Hydrochloride (Certain drugs, such as phenothiazines, tend to produce hyperglycemia and may lead to loss of glycemic control). Products include:

Mepergan Injection 3539
Phenergan Injection 3553
Phenergan 3556
Phenergan Syrup 3554
Phenergan with Codeine Syrup 3557
Phenergan with Dextromethorphan Syrup 3559
Phenergan VC Syrup 3560
Phenergan VC with Codeine Syrup . 3561

Pseudoephedrine Hydrochloride (Certain drugs, such as sympathomimetics, tend to produce hyperglycemia and may lead to loss of glycemic control). Products include:

Actifed Cold & Allergy Tablets .... ■688
Actifed Cold & Sinus Caplets and Tablets .... ■688
Advil Cold and Sinus Caplets .... ■771
Advil Cold and Sinus Tablets .... ■771
Advil Flu & Body Ache Caplets ...... ■772
Aleve Cold & Sinus Caplets .... ■603
Alka-Seltzer Plus Liqui-Gels .... ■604
Alka-Seltzer Plus Cold & Flu Medicine Liqui-Gels .... ■604
Alka-Seltzer Plus Cold & Sinus Medicine Liqui-Gels .... ■604
Allegra-D Extended-Release Tablets 714
BC Cold Powder .... ■619
Benadryl Allergy/Cold Tablets .... ■691
Benadryl Allergy/Congestion Tablets .... ■692
Benadryl Allergy & Sinus Liquid .... ■693
Benadryl Allergy & Sinus Fastmelt Tablets .... ■693
Benadryl Allergy Sinus Headache Caplets & Gelcaps .... ■693
Benadryl Severe Allergy & Sinus Headache Caplets .... ■694
Benadryl Children's Allergy/Cold Fastmelt Tablets .... ■692
Benylin Multi-Symptom Liquid .... ■697
Bromfed Capsules (Extended-Release) 2269
Bromfed-PD Capsules (Extended-Release) 2269
Children's Cēpacol Sore Throat .... ■788
Comtrex Acute Head Cold & Sinus Pressure Relief Tablets ..... ■627
Comtrex Deep Chest Cold & Congestion Relief Softgels .... ■627
Comtrex Flu Therapy & Fever Relief Daytime Caplets .... ■628
Comtrex Flu Therapy & Fever Relief Nighttime Tablets .... ■628
Comtrex Maximum Strength Multi-Symptom Cold & Cough Relief Tablets and Caplets .... ■626
Contac Non-Drowsy 12 Hour Cold Caplets .... ■745
Contac Non-Drowsy Timed Release 12 Hour Cold Caplets .. ■746
Contac Severe Cold and Flu Caplets Maximum Strength .... ■746
Contac Severe Cold and Flu Caplets Non-Drowsy .... ■746
Dimetapp Elixir .... ■777
Dimetapp Cold and Fever Suspension .... ■775
Dimetapp DM Cold & Cough Elixir . ■775
Dimetapp Nighttime Flu Liquid ...... ■776
Dimetapp Non-Drowsy Flu Syrup .. ■777
Dimetapp Infant Drops Decongestant .... ■775
Dimetapp Infant Drops Decongestant Plus Cough .... ■776
Guaifed 2272
Kronofed-A 1341
Children's Motrin Cold Oral Suspension 2007
Motrin Sinus Headache Caplets 2005
PediaCare Cough-Cold Liquid .... ■719
PediaCare Infants' Drops Decongestant .... ■719
PediaCare Infants' Drops Decongestant Plus Cough .... ■719
PediaCare NightRest Cough-Cold Liquid .... ■719
Robitussin Cold Caplets Cold & Congestion .... ■780
Robitussin Cold Softgels Cold & Congestion .... ■780
Robitussin Cold Caplets Multi-Symptom Cold & Flu .... ■781
Robitussin Cold Softgels Multi-Symptom Cold & Flu .... ■781
Robitussin Cold Softgels Severe Congestion .... ■782
Robitussin Cough & Cold Infant Drops .... ■782
Robitussin Maximum Strength Cough & Cold Liquid .... ■785
Robitussin Pediatric Cough & Cold Formula Liquid .... ■785
Robitussin Multi Symptom Honey Flu Liquid .... ■785
Robitussin Nighttime Honey Flu Liquid .... ■786
Robitussin-CF Liquid .... ■783
Robitussin-DAC Syrup 2942
Robitussin-PE Liquid .... ■782
Ryna .... ■768
Semprex-D Capsules 1172
Singlet Caplets .... ■761
Sinutab Non-Drying Liquid Caps .... ■706
Sinutab Sinus Allergy Medication, Maximum Strength Formula, Tablets & Caplets .... ■707
Sinutab Sinus Medication, Maximum Strength Without Drowsiness Formula, Tablets & Caplets .... ■707
Sudafed 12 Hour Tablets .... ■708
Sudafed 24 Hour Tablets .... ■708
Children's Sudafed Cold & Cough Liquid .... ■709
Children's Sudafed Nasal Decongestant Chewables .... ■711
Children's Sudafed Nasal Decongestant Liquid Medication .... ■711
Sudafed Cold & Allergy Tablets ..... ■708
Sudafed Cold & Cough Liquid Caps .... ■709
Sudafed Cold & Sinus Liquid Caps .... ■710
Sudafed Nasal Decongestant Tablets .... ■710
Sudafed Non-Drying Sinus Liquid Caps .... ■712
Sudafed Severe Cold .... ■711
Sudafed Sinus Headache Caplets . ■712
Sudafed Sinus Headache Tablets .. ■712
Tavist Sinus Non-Drowsy Coated Caplets .... ■676
TheraFlu Regular Strength Cold & Cough Night Time Hot Liquid .... ■676
TheraFlu Regular Strength Cold & Sore Throat Night Time Hot Liquid .... ■676
TheraFlu Maximum Strength Flu & Congestion Non-Drowsy Hot Liquid .... ■677
TheraFlu Maximum Strength Flu & Cough Night Time Hot Liquid .. ■678
TheraFlu Maximum Strength Flu & Sore Throat Night Time Hot Liquid .... ■677
TheraFlu Maximum Strength Severe Cold & Congestion Night Time Caplets .... ■678
TheraFlu Maximum Strength Severe Cold & Congestion Night Time Hot Liquid .... ■678
TheraFlu Maximum Strength Severe Cold & Congestion Non-Drowsy .... ■679
Triaminic Allergy Congestion Liquid .... ■680
Triaminic Chest Congestion Liquid .... ■680
Triaminic Cold & Allergy Liquid ...... ■681
Triaminic Cold & Allergy Softchews .... ■683
Triaminic Cold & Cough Liquid ...... ■681
Triaminic Cold & Cough Softchews .... ■683
Triaminic Cold & Night Time Cough Liquid .... ■681
Triaminic Cold, Cough & Fever Liquid .... ■681
Triaminic Cough Liquid .... ■682
Triaminic Cough & Congestion Liquid .... ■682
Triaminic Cough & Sore Throat Liquid .... ■682
Triaminic Cough & Sore Throat Softchews .... ■684
Children's Tylenol Allergy-D Liquid .. 2014
Children's Tylenol Cold Suspension Liquid and Chewable Tablets 2015
Children's Tylenol Cold Plus Cough Suspension Liquid and Chewable Tablets 2015
Children's Tylenol Flu Suspension Liquid 2015
Children's Tylenol Sinus Suspension Liquid 2017
Infants' Tylenol Cold Decongestant and Fever Reducer Concentrated Drops 2015
Infants' Tylenol Cold Decongestant and Fever Reducer Concentrated Drops Plus Cough .. 2015
Tylenol Allergy Sinus 2010
Multi-Symptom Tylenol Cold Complete Formula Caplets 2010
Multi-Symptom Tylenol Cold Non-Drowsy Caplets and Gelcaps 2010
Multi-Symptom Tylenol Cold Severe Congestion Non-Drowsy Caplets 2011
Maximum Strength Tylenol Flu NightTime Gelcaps 2011
Maximum Strength Tylenol Flu NightTime Liquid 2011
Maximum Strength Tylenol Flu Non-Drowsy Gelcaps 2011
Maximum Strength Tylenol Sinus NightTime Caplets 2012
Maximum Strength Tylenol Sinus Non-Drowsy Geltabs, Gelcaps, Caplets, and Tablets 2012
Vicks 44D Cough & Head Congestion Relief Liquid .... ■724
Vicks 44M Cough, Cold & Flu Relief Liquid .... ■725
Pediatric Vicks 44m Cough & Cold Relief .... ■728
Vicks DayQuil LiquiCaps/Liquid Multi-Symptom Cold/Flu Relief ... ■727
Children's Vicks NyQuil Cold/Cough Relief .... ■726
Vicks NyQuil LiquiCaps/Liquid Multi-Symptom Cold/Flu Relief, Original and Cherry Flavors .... ■727
Zephrex Tablets 3091
Zephrex LA Tablets 3092
Zyrtec-D 12 Hour Extended Relief Tablets 2758

Pseudoephedrine Sulfate (Certain drugs, such as sympathomimetics, tend to produce hyperglycemia and may lead to loss of glycemic control). Products include:

Chlor-Trimeton Allergy/Decongestant Tablets .... ■736

IMPORTANT NOTE: Always consult each drug listing in the patient's regimen for possible interactions.

Claritin-D 12 Hour Extended Release Tablets ... 3102
Claritin-D 24 Hour Extended Release Tablets ... 3104
Coricidin 'D' Cold, Flu & Sinus Tablets ... ▣737
Drixoral Allergy/Sinus Extended-Release Tablets ... ▣741
Drixoral Cold & Allergy Sustained-Action Tablets ... ▣740
Drixoral Cold & Flu Extended-Release Tablets ... ▣740
Drixoral Nasal Decongestant Long-Acting Non-Drowsy Tablets ... ▣740
Rynatan Tablets ... 3351

Quinestrol (Certain drugs, such as estrogens, tend to produce hyperglycemia and may lead to loss of glycemic control).
No products indexed under this heading.

Quinidine Gluconate (Theoretical potential for interaction with metformin by competing for common renal tubular transport system). Products include:
Quinaglute Dura-Tabs Tablets ... 978

Quinidine Polygalacturonate (Theoretical potential for interaction with metformin by competing for common renal tubular transport system).
No products indexed under this heading.

Quinidine Sulfate (Theoretical potential for interaction with metformin by competing for common renal tubular transport system). Products include:
Quinidex Extentabs ... 2933

Quinine Sulfate (Theoretical potential for interaction with metformin by competing for common renal tubular transport system).
No products indexed under this heading.

Ranitidine Hydrochloride (Theoretical potential for interaction with metformin by competing for common renal tubular transport system). Products include:
Zantac ... 1690
Zantac Injection ... 1688
Zantac 75 Tablets ... ▣717

Salmeterol Xinafoate (Certain drugs, such as sympathomimetics, tend to produce hyperglycemia and may lead to loss of glycemic control). Products include:
Advair Diskus 100/50 ... 1448
Advair Diskus 250/50 ... 1448
Advair Diskus 500/50 ... 1448
Serevent Diskus ... 1637
Serevent Inhalation Aerosol ... 1633

Spironolactone (Certain drugs, such as diuretics, tend to produce hyperglycemia and may lead to loss of glycemic control).
No products indexed under this heading.

Terbutaline Sulfate (Certain drugs, such as sympathomimetics, tend to produce hyperglycemia and may lead to loss of glycemic control). Products include:
Brethine Ampuls ... 2314
Brethine Tablets ... 2313

Thioridazine Hydrochloride (Certain drugs, such as phenothiazines, tend to produce hyperglycemia and may lead to loss of glycemic control). Products include:
Thioridazine Hydrochloride Tablets ... 2289

Thyroglobulin (Certain drugs, such as thyroid products, tend to produce hyperglycemia and may lead to loss of glycemic control).
No products indexed under this heading.

Thyroid (Certain drugs, such as thyroid products, tend to produce hyperglycemia and may lead to loss of glycemic control).
No products indexed under this heading.

Thyroxine (Certain drugs, such as thyroid products, tend to produce hyperglycemia and may lead to loss of glycemic control).
No products indexed under this heading.

Thyroxine Sodium (Certain drugs, such as thyroid products, tend to produce hyperglycemia and may lead to loss of glycemic control).
No products indexed under this heading.

Torsemide (Certain drugs, such as diuretics, tend to produce hyperglycemia and may lead to loss of glycemic control). Products include:
Demadex Tablets and Injection ... 2965

Triamcinolone (Certain drugs, such as corticosteroids, tend to produce hyperglycemia and may lead to loss of glycemic control).
No products indexed under this heading.

Triamcinolone Acetonide (Certain drugs, such as corticosteroids, tend to produce hyperglycemia and may lead to loss of glycemic control). Products include:
Azmacort Inhalation Aerosol ... 728
Nasacort Nasal Inhaler ... 750
Nasacort AQ Nasal Spray ... 752
Tri-Nasal Spray ... 2274

Triamcinolone Diacetate (Certain drugs, such as corticosteroids, tend to produce hyperglycemia and may lead to loss of glycemic control).
No products indexed under this heading.

Triamcinolone Hexacetonide (Certain drugs, such as corticosteroids, tend to produce hyperglycemia and may lead to loss of glycemic control).
No products indexed under this heading.

Triamterene (Potential for loss of glycemic control; theoretical potential for interaction with metformin by competing for common renal tubular transport system). Products include:
Dyazide Capsules ... 1515
Dyrenium Capsules ... 3458
Maxzide ... 1008

Trifluoperazine Hydrochloride (Certain drugs, such as phenothiazines, tend to produce hyperglycemia and may lead to loss of glycemic control). Products include:
Stelazine ... 1640

Trimethoprim (Theoretical potential for interaction with metformin by competing for common renal tubular transport system). Products include:
Bactrim ... 2949
Septra Suspension ... 2265
Septra Tablets ... 2265
Septra DS Tablets ... 2265

Trimethoprim Sulfate (Theoretical potential for interaction with metformin by competing for common renal tubular transport system). Products include:
Polytrim Ophthalmic Solution ... 556

Tyropanoate Sodium (Potential for acute alteration of renal function; metformin should be temporarily withheld in patients undergoing radiologic studies involving parenteral iodinated contrast material).
No products indexed under this heading.

Vancomycin Hydrochloride (Theoretical potential for interaction with metformin by competing for common renal tubular transport system). Products include:
Vancocin HCl Capsules & Pulvules ... 1972
Vancocin HCl Oral Solution ... 1971
Vancocin HCl, Vials & ADD-Vantage ... 1970

Verapamil Hydrochloride (Certain drugs, such as calcium channel blockers, tend to produce hyperglycemia and may lead to loss of glycemic control). Products include:
Covera-HS Tablets ... 3199
Isoptin SR Tablets ... 467
Tarka Tablets ... 508
Verelan Capsules ... 3184
Verelan PM Capsules ... 3186

Food Interactions

Alcohol (Alcohol potentiates the effect of metformin on lactate metabolism; patients should be warned against excessive alcohol intake, acute or chronic).

Food, unspecified (Food decreases the extent and slightly delays the absorption of metformin).

GLUCOPHAGE XR TABLETS

(Metformin Hydrochloride) ... 1080
See Glucophage Tablets

GLUCOTROL TABLETS

(Glipizide) ... 2692
May interact with beta blockers, calcium channel blockers, corticosteroids, oral anticoagulants, diuretics, and estrogens. Compounds in these categories include:

Acebutolol Hydrochloride (Co-administration with beta blockers may result in hypoglycemia). Products include:
Sectral Capsules ... 3589

Albuterol (Sympathomimetics tend to produce hyperglycemia and concurrent use may lead to loss of control). Products include:
Proventil Inhalation Aerosol ... 3142
Ventolin Inhalation Aerosol and Refill ... 1679

Albuterol Sulfate (Sympathomimetics tend to produce hyperglycemia and concurrent use may lead to loss of control). Products include:
AccuNeb Inhalation Solution ... 1230
Combivent Inhalation Aerosol ... 1041
DuoNeb Inhalation Solution ... 1233
Proventil Inhalation Solution 0.083% ... 3146
Proventil Repetabs Tablets ... 3148
Proventil Solution for Inhalation 0.5% ... 3144
Proventil HFA Inhalation Aerosol ... 3150
Ventolin HFA Inhalation Aerosol ... 3618
Volmax Extended-Release Tablets ... 2276

Amiloride Hydrochloride (Diuretics tend to produce hyperglycemia and concurrent use may lead to loss of control). Products include:
Midamor Tablets ... 2136
Moduretic Tablets ... 2138

Amiodarone Hydrochloride (Co-administration with drugs that are highly protein bound may result in hypoglycemia). Products include:
Cordarone Intravenous ... 3491
Cordarone Tablets ... 3487
Pacerone Tablets ... 3331

Amitriptyline Hydrochloride (Co-administration with drugs that are highly protein bound may result in hypoglycemia). Products include:
Etrafon ... 3115
Limbitrol ... 1738

Amlodipine Besylate (Calcium channel blockers tend to produce hyperglycemia and concurrent use may lead to loss of control). Products include:
Lotrel Capsules ... 2370
Norvasc Tablets ... 2704

Aspirin (Co-administration with salicylates may result in hypoglycemia). Products include:
Aggrenox Capsules ... 1026
Alka-Seltzer ... ▣603
Alka-Seltzer Lemon Lime Antacid and Pain Reliever Effervescent Tablets ... ▣603
Alka-Seltzer Extra Strength Antacid and Pain Reliever Effervescent Tablets ... ▣603
Alka-Seltzer PM Effervescent Tablets ... ▣605
Genuine Bayer Tablets, Caplets and Gelcaps ... ▣606
Extra Strength Bayer Caplets and Gelcaps ... ▣610
Aspirin Regimen Bayer Children's Chewable Tablets (Orange or Cherry Flavored) ... ▣607
Bayer, Aspirin Regimen ... ▣606
Aspirin Regimen Bayer 81 mg Caplets with Calcium ... ▣607
Genuine Bayer Professional Labeling (Aspirin Regimen Bayer) ... ▣608
Extra Strength Bayer Arthritis Caplets ... ▣610
Extra Strength Bayer Plus Caplets ... ▣610
Extra Strength Bayer PM Caplets ... ▣611
BC Powder ... ▣619
BC Allergy Sinus Cold Powder ... ▣619
Arthritis Strength BC Powder ... ▣619
BC Sinus Cold Powder ... ▣619
Darvon Compound-65 Pulvules ... 1910
Ecotrin Enteric Coated Aspirin Low, Regular and Maximum Strength Tablets ... 1715
Excedrin Extra-Strength Tablets, Caplets, and Geltabs ... ▣629
Excedrin Migraine ... 1070
Goody's Body Pain Formula Powder ... ▣620
Goody's Extra Strength Headache Powder ... ▣620
Goody's Extra Strength Pain Relief Tablets ... ▣620
Percodan Tablets ... 1327
Robaxisal Tablets ... 2939
Soma Compound Tablets ... 3354
Soma Compound w/Codeine Tablets ... 3355
Vanquish Caplets ... ▣617

Atenolol (Co-administration with beta blockers may result in hypoglycemia). Products include:
Tenoretic Tablets ... 690
Tenormin I.V. Injection ... 692

Atovaquone (Co-administration with drugs that are highly protein bound may result in hypoglycemia). Products include:
Malarone ... 1596
Mepron Suspension ... 1598

Bendroflumethiazide (Thiazides tend to produce hyperglycemia and concurrent use may lead to loss of control). Products include:
Corzide 40/5 Tablets ... 2247
Corzide 80/5 Tablets ... 2247

Bepridil Hydrochloride (Calcium channel blockers tend to produce hyperglycemia and concurrent use may lead to loss of control). Products include:
Vascor Tablets ... 2602

Betamethasone Acetate (Corticosteroids tend to produce hyperglycemia and concurrent use may lead to loss of control). Products include:
Celestone Soluspan Injectable Suspension ... 3097

Betamethasone Sodium Phosphate (Corticosteroids tend to produce hyperglycemia and concurrent use may lead to loss of control). Products include:
Celestone Soluspan Injectable Suspension ... 3097

Betaxolol Hydrochloride (Co-administration with beta blockers may result in hypoglycemia). Products include:
Betoptic S Ophthalmic Suspension ... 537

Bisoprolol Fumarate (Co-administration with beta blockers may result in hypoglycemia). Products include:
Zebeta Tablets ... 1885
Ziac Tablets ... 1887

Bumetanide (Diuretics tend to produce hyperglycemia and concurrent use may lead to loss of control).
No products indexed under this heading.

Carteolol Hydrochloride (Co-administration with beta blockers may result in hypoglycemia). Products include:
Carteolol Hydrochloride Ophthalmic Solution USP, 1% ... ⊙258
Ocupress Ophthalmic Solution, 1% Sterile ... ⊙303

Cefonicid Sodium (Co-administration with drugs that are highly protein bound may result in hypoglycemia).
No products indexed under this heading.

Celecoxib (Co-administration with nonsteroidal anti-inflammatory agents may result in hypoglycemia). Products include:
Celebrex Capsules 2676
Celebrex Capsules 2780

Chloramphenicol (Co-administration with chloramphenicol may result in hypoglycemia). Products include:
Chloromycetin Ophthalmic Ointment, 1% .... ⊙296
Chloromycetin Ophthalmic Solution .... ⊙297
Chloroptic Sterile Ophthalmic Ointment .... ⊙234
Chloroptic Sterile Ophthalmic Solution .... ⊙235

Chloramphenicol Palmitate (Co-administration with chloramphenicol may result in hypoglycemia).
No products indexed under this heading.

Chloramphenicol Sodium Succinate (Co-administration with chloramphenicol may result in hypoglycemia).
No products indexed under this heading.

Chlordiazepoxide (Co-administration with drugs that are highly protein bound may result in hypoglycemia). Products include:
Limbitrol 1738

Chlordiazepoxide Hydrochloride (Co-administration with drugs that are highly protein bound may result in hypoglycemia). Products include:
Librium Capsules 1736
Librium for Injection 1737

Chlorothiazide (Thiazides tend to produce hyperglycemia and concurrent use may lead to loss of control). Products include:
Aldoclor Tablets 2035
Diuril Oral 2087

Chlorothiazide Sodium (Thiazides tend to produce hyperglycemia and concurrent use may lead to loss of control). Products include:
Diuril Sodium Intravenous 2086

Chlorotrianisene (Estrogens tend to produce hyperglycemia and concurrent use may lead to loss of control).
No products indexed under this heading.

Chlorpromazine (Phenothiazines tend to produce hyperglycemia and concurrent use may lead to loss of control). Products include:
Thorazine Suppositories 1656

Chlorpromazine Hydrochloride (Phenothiazines tend to produce hyperglycemia and concurrent use may lead to loss of control). Products include:
Thorazine 1656

Chlorpropamide (Co-administration with sulfonamides may result in hypoglycemia). Products include:
Diabinese Tablets 2680

Chlorthalidone (Diuretics tend to produce hyperglycemia and concurrent use may lead to loss of control). Products include:
Clorpres Tablets 1002
Combipres Tablets 1040
Tenoretic Tablets 690

Choline Magnesium Trisalicylate (Co-administration with salicylates may result in hypoglycemia). Products include:
Trilisate 2901

Clomipramine Hydrochloride (Co-administration with drugs that are highly protein bound may result in hypoglycemia).
No products indexed under this heading.

Clozapine (Co-administration with drugs that are highly protein bound may result in hypoglycemia). Products include:
Clozaril Tablets 2319

Cortisone Acetate (Corticosteroids tend to produce hyperglycemia and concurrent use may lead to loss of control). Products include:
Cortone Acetate Injectable Suspension 2059
Cortone Acetate Tablets 2061

Cyclosporine (Co-administration with drugs that are highly protein bound may result in hypoglycemia). Products include:
Gengraf Capsules 457
Neoral Soft Gelatin Capsules 2380
Neoral Oral Solution 2380
Sandimmune 2388

Desogestrel (Oral contraceptives tend to produce hyperglycemia and concurrent use may lead to loss of control). Products include:
Cyclessa Tablets 2450
Desogen Tablets 2458
Mircette Tablets 2470
Ortho-Cept 21 Tablets 2546
Ortho-Cept 28 Tablets 2546

Dexamethasone (Corticosteroids tend to produce hyperglycemia and concurrent use may lead to loss of control). Products include:
Decadron Elixir 2078
Decadron Tablets 2079
TobraDex Ophthalmic Ointment 542
TobraDex Ophthalmic Suspension 541

Dexamethasone Acetate (Corticosteroids tend to produce hyperglycemia and concurrent use may lead to loss of control).
No products indexed under this heading.

Dexamethasone Sodium Phosphate (Corticosteroids tend to produce hyperglycemia and concurrent use may lead to loss of control). Products include:
Decadron Phosphate Injection 2081
Decadron Phosphate Sterile Ophthalmic Ointment 2083
Decadron Phosphate Sterile Ophthalmic Solution 2084
NeoDecadron Sterile Ophthalmic Solution 2144

Diazepam (Co-administration with drugs that are highly protein bound may result in hypoglycemia). Products include:
Valium Injectable 3026
Valium Tablets 3047

Diclofenac Potassium (Co-administration with nonsteroidal anti-inflammatory agents may result in hypoglycemia). Products include:
Cataflam Tablets 2315

Diclofenac Sodium (Co-administration with nonsteroidal anti-inflammatory agents may result in hypoglycemia). Products include:
Arthrotec Tablets 3195
Voltaren Ophthalmic Sterile Ophthalmic Solution .... ⊙312
Voltaren Tablets 2315
Voltaren-XR Tablets 2315

Dicumarol (Co-administration with coumarins may result in hypoglycemia).
No products indexed under this heading.

Dienestrol (Estrogens tend to produce hyperglycemia and concurrent use may lead to loss of control). Products include:
Ortho Dienestrol Cream 2554

Diethylstilbestrol (Estrogens tend to produce hyperglycemia and concurrent use may lead to loss of control).
No products indexed under this heading.

Diflunisal (Co-administration with salicylates may result in hypoglycemia). Products include:
Dolobid Tablets 2088

Diltiazem Hydrochloride (Calcium channel blockers tend to produce hyperglycemia and concurrent use may lead to loss of control). Products include:
Cardizem Injectable 1018
Cardizem Lyo-Ject Syringe 1018
Cardizem Monovial 1018
Cardizem CD Capsules 1016
Tiazac Capsules 1378

Dipyridamole (Co-administration with drugs that are highly protein bound may result in hypoglycemia). Products include:
Aggrenox Capsules 1026
Persantine Tablets 1057

Dobutamine Hydrochloride (Sympathomimetics tend to produce hyperglycemia and concurrent use may lead to loss of control). Products include:
Dobutrex Solution Vials 1914

Dopamine Hydrochloride (Sympathomimetics tend to produce hyperglycemia and concurrent use may lead to loss of control).
No products indexed under this heading.

Ephedrine Hydrochloride (Sympathomimetics tend to produce hyperglycemia and concurrent use may lead to loss of control). Products include:
Primatene Tablets .... ▣780

Ephedrine Sulfate (Sympathomimetics tend to produce hyperglycemia and concurrent use may lead to loss of control).
No products indexed under this heading.

Ephedrine Tannate (Sympathomimetics tend to produce hyperglycemia and concurrent use may lead to loss of control). Products include:
Rynatuss Pediatric Suspension 3353
Rynatuss Tablets 3353

Epinephrine (Sympathomimetics tend to produce hyperglycemia and concurrent use may lead to loss of control). Products include:
Epifrin Sterile Ophthalmic Solution .... ⊙235
EpiPen 1236
Primatene Mist .... ▣779
Xylocaine with Epinephrine Injection 653

Epinephrine Bitartrate (Sympathomimetics tend to produce hyperglycemia and concurrent use may lead to loss of control). Products include:
Sensorcaine 643

Epinephrine Hydrochloride (Sympathomimetics tend to produce hyperglycemia and concurrent use may lead to loss of control).
No products indexed under this heading.

Esmolol Hydrochloride (Co-administration with beta blockers may result in hypoglycemia). Products include:
Brevibloc Injection 858

Estradiol (Estrogens tend to produce hyperglycemia and concurrent use may lead to loss of control). Products include:
Activella Tablets 2764
Alora Transdermal System 3372
Climara Transdermal System 958
CombiPatch Transdermal System 2323
Esclim Transdermal System 3460
Estrace Vaginal Cream 3358
Estrace Tablets 3361
Estring Vaginal Ring 2811
Ortho-Prefest Tablets 2570
Vagifem Tablets 2857
Vivelle Transdermal System 2412
Vivelle-Dot Transdermal System 2416

Estrogens, Conjugated (Estrogens tend to produce hyperglycemia and concurrent use may lead to loss of control). Products include:
Premarin Intravenous 3563
Premarin Tablets 3566
Premarin Vaginal Cream 3570
Premphase Tablets 3572
Prempro Tablets 3572

Estrogens, Esterified (Estrogens tend to produce hyperglycemia and concurrent use may lead to loss of control). Products include:
Estratest 3252
Menest Tablets 2254

Estropipate (Estrogens tend to produce hyperglycemia and concurrent use may lead to loss of control). Products include:
Ogen Tablets 2846
Ortho-Est Tablets 3464

Ethacrynic Acid (Diuretics tend to produce hyperglycemia and concurrent use may lead to loss of control). Products include:
Edecrin Tablets 2091

Ethinyl Estradiol (Estrogens tend to produce hyperglycemia and concurrent use may lead to loss of control). Products include:
Alesse-21 Tablets 3468
Alesse-28 Tablets 3473
Brevicon 28-Day Tablets 3380
Cyclessa Tablets 2450
Desogen Tablets 2458
Estinyl Tablets 3112
Estrostep 2627
femhrt Tablets 2635
Levlen 962
Levlite 21 Tablets 962
Levlite 28 Tablets 962
Levora Tablets 3389
Loestrin 21 Tablets 2642
Loestrin Fe Tablets 2642
Lo/Ovral Tablets 3532
Lo/Ovral-28 Tablets 3538
Low-Ogestrel-28 Tablets 3392
Microgestin Fe 1.5/30 Tablets 3407
Microgestin Fe 1/20 Tablets 3400
Mircette Tablets 2470
Modicon 2563
Necon 3415
Nordette-28 Tablets 2257
Norinyl 1 +35 28-Day Tablets 3380
Ogestrel 0.5/50-28 Tablets 3428
Ortho-Cept 21 Tablets 2546
Ortho-Cept 28 Tablets 2546
Ortho-Cyclen/Ortho Tri-Cyclen 2573
Ortho-Novum 2563
Ovcon 3364
Ovral Tablets 3551
Ovral-28 Tablets 3552
Tri-Levlen 962
Tri-Norinyl-28 Tablets 3433
Triphasil-21 Tablets 3600
Triphasil-28 Tablets 3605
Trivora Tablets 3439
Yasmin 28 Tablets 980
Zovia 3449

Ethynodiol Diacetate (Oral contraceptives tend to produce hyperglycemia and concurrent use may lead to loss of control). Products include:
Zovia 3449

Etodolac (Co-administration with nonsteroidal anti-inflammatory agents may result in hypoglycemia). Products include:
Lodine 3528
Lodine XL Extended-Release Tablets 3530

Felodipine (Calcium channel blockers tend to produce hyperglycemia and concurrent use may lead to loss of control). Products include:
Lexxel Tablets 608
Plendil Extended-Release Tablets 623

Fenoprofen Calcium (Co-administration with nonsteroidal anti-inflammatory agents may result in hypoglycemia).
No products indexed under this heading.

Fluconazole (Co-administration with oral fluconazole has resulted in an increase in Glucotrol AUC by 56.9%). Products include:

Diflucan Tablets, Injection, and Oral Suspension ... 2681

Fludrocortisone Acetate (Corticosteroids tend to produce hyperglycemia and concurrent use may lead to loss of control). Products include:
Florinef Acetate Tablets ... 2250

Fluphenazine Decanoate (Phenothiazines tend to produce hyperglycemia and concurrent use may lead to loss of control).
No products indexed under this heading.

Fluphenazine Enanthate (Phenothiazines tend to produce hyperglycemia and concurrent use may lead to loss of control).
No products indexed under this heading.

Fluphenazine Hydrochloride (Phenothiazines tend to produce hyperglycemia and concurrent use may lead to loss of control).
No products indexed under this heading.

Flurazepam Hydrochloride (Co-administration with drugs that are highly protein bound may result in hypoglycemia).
No products indexed under this heading.

Flurbiprofen (Co-administration with nonsteroidal anti-inflammatory agents may result in hypoglycemia).
No products indexed under this heading.

Furosemide (Diuretics tend to produce hyperglycemia and concurrent use may lead to loss of control). Products include:
Furosemide Tablets ... 2284

Glyburide (Co-administration with sulfonamides may result in hypoglycemia). Products include:
DiaBeta Tablets ... 741
Glucovance Tablets ... 1086

Hydrochlorothiazide (Thiazides tend to produce hyperglycemia and concurrent use may lead to loss of control). Products include:
Accuretic Tablets ... 2614
Aldoril Tablets ... 2039
Atacand HCT Tablets ... 597
Avalide Tablets ... 1070
Diovan HCT Tablets ... 2338
Dyazide Capsules ... 1515
HydroDIURIL Tablets ... 2108
Hyzaar ... 2109
Inderide Tablets ... 3517
Inderide LA Long-Acting Capsules ... 3519
Lotensin HCT Tablets ... 2367
Maxzide ... 1008
Micardis HCT Tablets ... 1051
Microzide Capsules ... 3414
Moduretic Tablets ... 2138
Monopril HCT ... 1094
Prinzide Tablets ... 2168
Timolide Tablets ... 2187
Uniretic Tablets ... 3178
Vaseretic Tablets ... 2204
Zestoretic Tablets ... 695
Ziac Tablets ... 1887

Hydrocortisone (Corticosteroids tend to produce hyperglycemia and concurrent use may lead to loss of control). Products include:
Anusol-HC Cream 2.5% ... 2237
Cipro HC Otic Suspension ... 540
Cortaid Intensive Therapy Cream ... ▣717
Cortaid Maximum Strength Cream ... ▣717
Cortisporin Ophthalmic Suspension Sterile ... ⊙297
Cortizone•5 ... ▣699
Cortizone•10 ... ▣699
Cortizone•10 Plus Creme ... ▣700
Cortizone for Kids Creme ... ▣699
Hydrocortone Tablets ... 2106
Massengill Medicated Soft Cloth Towelette ... ▣753
VōSoL HC Otic Solution ... 3356

Hydrocortisone Acetate (Corticosteroids tend to produce hyperglycemia and concurrent use may lead to loss of control). Products include:
Analpram-HC ... 1338
Anusol HC-1 Hydrocortisone Anti-Itch Cream ... ▣689
Anusol-HC Suppositories ... 2238
Cortaid ... ▣717
Cortifoam Rectal Foam ... 3170
Cortisporin-TC Otic Suspension ... 2246
Hydrocortone Acetate Injectable Suspension ... 2103
Pramosone ... 1343
Proctocort Suppositories ... 2264
ProctoFoam-HC ... 3177
Terra-Cortril Ophthalmic Suspension ... 2716

Hydrocortisone Sodium Phosphate (Corticosteroids tend to produce hyperglycemia and concurrent use may lead to loss of control). Products include:
Hydrocortone Phosphate Injection, Sterile ... 2105

Hydrocortisone Sodium Succinate (Corticosteroids tend to produce hyperglycemia and concurrent use may lead to loss of control).
No products indexed under this heading.

Hydroflumethiazide (Thiazides tend to produce hyperglycemia and concurrent use may lead to loss of control). Products include:
Diucardin Tablets ... 3494

Ibuprofen (Co-administration with nonsteroidal anti-inflammatory agents may result in hypoglycemia). Products include:
Advil ... ▣771
Children's Advil Oral Suspension ... ▣773
Children's Advil Chewable Tablets ... ▣773
Advil Cold and Sinus Caplets ... ▣771
Advil Cold and Sinus Tablets ... ▣771
Advil Flu & Body Ache Caplets ... ▣772
Infants' Advil Drops ... ▣773
Junior Strength Advil Tablets ... ▣773
Junior Strength Advil Chewable Tablets ... ▣773
Advil Migraine Liquigels ... ▣772
Children's Motrin Oral Suspension and Chewable Tablets ... 2006
Children's Motrin Cold Oral Suspension ... 2007
Children's Motrin Oral Suspension ... ▣643
Motrin Suspension, Oral Drops, Chewable Tablets, and Caplets ... 2002
Infants' Motrin Concentrated Drops ... 2006
Junior Strength Motrin Caplets and Chewable Tablets ... 2006
Motrin IB Tablets, Caplets, and Gelcaps ... 2002
Motrin Migraine Pain Caplets ... 2005
Motrin Sinus Headache Caplets ... 2005
Vicoprofen Tablets ... 520

Imipramine Hydrochloride (Co-administration with drugs that are highly protein bound may result in hypoglycemia).
No products indexed under this heading.

Imipramine Pamoate (Co-administration with drugs that are highly protein bound may result in hypoglycemia).
No products indexed under this heading.

Indapamide (Diuretics tend to produce hyperglycemia and concurrent use may lead to loss of control). Products include:
Indapamide Tablets ... 2286

Indomethacin (Co-administration with nonsteroidal anti-inflammatory agents may result in hypoglycemia). Products include:
Indocin ... 2112

Indomethacin Sodium Trihydrate (Co-administration with nonsteroidal anti-inflammatory agents may result in hypoglycemia). Products include:
Indocin I.V. ... 2115

Isocarboxazid (Co-administration with monamine oxidase inhibitors may result in hypoglycemia).
No products indexed under this heading.

Isoniazid (Isoniazid tends to produce hyperglycemia and concurrent use may lead to loss of control). Products include:
Rifamate Capsules ... 767
Rifater Tablets ... 769

Isoproterenol Hydrochloride (Sympathomimetics tend to produce hyperglycemia and concurrent use may lead to loss of control).
No products indexed under this heading.

Isoproterenol Sulfate (Sympathomimetics tend to produce hyperglycemia and concurrent use may lead to loss of control).
No products indexed under this heading.

Isradipine (Calcium channel blockers tend to produce hyperglycemia and concurrent use may lead to loss of control). Products include:
DynaCirc Capsules ... 2921
DynaCirc CR Tablets ... 2923

Ketoprofen (Co-administration with nonsteroidal anti-inflammatory agents may result in hypoglycemia). Products include:
Orudis Capsules ... 3548
Orudis KT Tablets ... ▣778
Oruvail Capsules ... 3548

Ketorolac Tromethamine (Co-administration with nonsteroidal anti-inflammatory agents may result in hypoglycemia). Products include:
Acular Ophthalmic Solution ... 544
Acular PF Ophthalmic Solution ... 544
Toradol ... 3018

Labetalol Hydrochloride (Co-administration with beta blockers may result in hypoglycemia). Products include:
Normodyne Injection ... 3135
Normodyne Tablets ... 3137

Levalbuterol Hydrochloride (Sympathomimetics tend to produce hyperglycemia and concurrent use may lead to loss of control). Products include:
Xopenex Inhalation Solution ... 3207

Levobunolol Hydrochloride (Co-administration with beta blockers may result in hypoglycemia). Products include:
Betagan ... ⊙228

Levonorgestrel (Oral contraceptives tend to produce hyperglycemia and concurrent use may lead to loss of control). Products include:
Alesse-21 Tablets ... 3468
Alesse-28 Tablets ... 3473
Levlen ... 962
Levlite 21 Tablets ... 962
Levlite 28 Tablets ... 962
Levora Tablets ... 3389
Mirena Intrauterine System ... 974
Nordette-28 Tablets ... 2257
Norplant System ... 3543
Tri-Levlen ... 962
Triphasil-21 Tablets ... 3600
Triphasil-28 Tablets ... 3605
Trivora Tablets ... 3439

Levothyroxine Sodium (Thyroid products tend to produce hyperglycemia and concurrent use may lead to loss of control). Products include:
Levothroid Tablets ... 1373
Levoxyl Tablets ... 1819
Synthroid ... 505
Unithroid Tablets ... 3445

Liothyronine Sodium (Thyroid products tend to produce hyperglycemia and concurrent use may lead to loss of control). Products include:
Cytomel Tablets ... 1817
Triostat Injection ... 1825

Liotrix (Thyroid products tend to produce hyperglycemia and concurrent use may lead to loss of control).
No products indexed under this heading.

Magnesium Salicylate (Co-administration with salicylates may result in hypoglycemia). Products include:
Momentum Backache Relief Extra Strength Caplets ... ▣666

Meclofenamate Sodium (Co-administration with nonsteroidal anti-inflammatory agents may result in hypoglycemia).
No products indexed under this heading.

Mefenamic Acid (Co-administration with nonsteroidal anti-inflammatory agents may result in hypoglycemia). Products include:
Ponstel Capsules ... 1356

Meloxicam (Co-administration with nonsteroidal anti-inflammatory agents may result in hypoglycemia). Products include:
Mobic Tablets ... 1054

Mesoridazine Besylate (Phenothiazines tend to produce hyperglycemia and concurrent use may lead to loss of control). Products include:
Serentil ... 1057

Mestranol (Oral contraceptives tend to produce hyperglycemia and concurrent use may lead to loss of control). Products include:
Necon 1/50 Tablets ... 3415
Norinyl 1 + 50 28-Day Tablets ... 3380
Ortho-Novum 1/50□28 Tablets ... 2556

Metaproterenol Sulfate (Sympathomimetics tend to produce hyperglycemia and concurrent use may lead to loss of control). Products include:
Alupent ... 1029

Metaraminol Bitartrate (Sympathomimetics tend to produce hyperglycemia and concurrent use may lead to loss of control). Products include:
Aramine Injection ... 2043

Methotrimeprazine (Phenothiazines tend to produce hyperglycemia and concurrent use may lead to loss of control).
No products indexed under this heading.

Methoxamine Hydrochloride (Sympathomimetics tend to produce hyperglycemia and concurrent use may lead to loss of control).
No products indexed under this heading.

Methyclothiazide (Thiazides tend to produce hyperglycemia and concurrent use may lead to loss of control).
No products indexed under this heading.

Methylprednisolone Acetate (Corticosteroids tend to produce hyperglycemia and concurrent use may lead to loss of control). Products include:
Depo-Medrol Injectable Suspension ... 2795

Methylprednisolone Sodium Succinate (Corticosteroids tend to produce hyperglycemia and concurrent use may lead to loss of control). Products include:
Solu-Medrol Sterile Powder ... 2855

Metipranolol Hydrochloride (Co-administration with beta blockers may result in hypoglycemia).
No products indexed under this heading.

Metolazone (Diuretics tend to produce hyperglycemia and concurrent use may lead to loss of control). Products include:
Mykrox Tablets ... 1168
Zaroxolyn Tablets ... 1177

Metoprolol Succinate (Co-administration with beta blockers may result in hypoglycemia). Products include:
Toprol-XL Tablets ... 651

Metoprolol Tartrate (Co-administration with beta blockers may result in hypoglycemia).
No products indexed under this heading.

Mibefradil Dihydrochloride (Calcium channel blockers tend to produce hyperglycemia and concurrent

use may lead to loss of control).
No products indexed under this heading.

Miconazole (Co-administration with oral miconazole and oral hypoglycemic agents has resulted in severe hypoglycemia).
No products indexed under this heading.

Midazolam Hydrochloride (Co-administration with drugs that are highly protein bound may result in hypoglycemia). Products include:
Versed Injection 3027
Versed Syrup 3033

Moclobemide (Co-administration with monamine oxidase inhibitors may result in hypoglycemia).
No products indexed under this heading.

Nabumetone (Co-administration with nonsteroidal anti-inflammatory agents may result in hypoglycemia). Products include:
Relafen Tablets 1617

Nadolol (Co-administration with beta blockers may result in hypoglycemia). Products include:
Corgard Tablets 2245
Corzide 40/5 Tablets 2247
Corzide 80/5 Tablets 2247
Nadolol Tablets 2288

Naproxen (Co-administration with nonsteroidal anti-inflammatory agents may result in hypoglycemia). Products include:
EC-Naprosyn Delayed-Release Tablets 2967
Naprosyn Suspension 2967
Naprosyn Tablets 2967

Naproxen Sodium (Co-administration with nonsteroidal anti-inflammatory agents may result in hypoglycemia). Products include:
Aleve Tablets, Caplets and Gelcaps .... ▣602
Aleve Cold & Sinus Caplets .... ▣603
Anaprox Tablets 2967
Anaprox DS Tablets 2967
Naprelan Tablets 1293

Nicardipine Hydrochloride (Calcium channel blockers tend to produce hyperglycemia and concurrent use may lead to loss of control). Products include:
Cardene I.V. 3485

Nicotinic Acid (Nicotinic acid tends to produce hyperglycemia and concurrent use may lead to loss of control).
No products indexed under this heading.

Nifedipine (Calcium channel blockers tend to produce hyperglycemia and concurrent use may lead to loss of control). Products include:
Adalat CC Tablets 877
Procardia Capsules 2708
Procardia XL Extended Release Tablets 2710

Nimodipine (Calcium channel blockers tend to produce hyperglycemia and concurrent use may lead to loss of control). Products include:
Nimotop Capsules 904

Nisoldipine (Calcium channel blockers tend to produce hyperglycemia and concurrent use may lead to loss of control). Products include:
Sular Tablets 688

Norepinephrine Bitartrate (Sympathomimetics tend to produce hyperglycemia and concurrent use may lead to loss of control).
No products indexed under this heading.

Norethindrone (Oral contraceptives tend to produce hyperglycemia and concurrent use may lead to loss of control). Products include:
Brevicon 28-Day Tablets 3380
Micronor Tablets 2543
Modicon 2563
Necon 3415
Norinyl 1 +35 28-Day Tablets 3380
Norinyl 1 + 50 28-Day Tablets 3380
Nor-QD Tablets 3423
Ortho-Novum 2563
Ortho-Novum 1/50▫28 Tablets 2556
Ovcon 3364
Tri-Norinyl-28 Tablets 3433

Norethynodrel (Oral contraceptives tend to produce hyperglycemia and concurrent use may lead to loss of control).
No products indexed under this heading.

Norgestimate (Oral contraceptives tend to produce hyperglycemia and concurrent use may lead to loss of control). Products include:
Ortho-Cyclen/Ortho Tri-Cyclen 2573
Ortho-Prefest Tablets 2570

Norgestrel (Oral contraceptives tend to produce hyperglycemia and concurrent use may lead to loss of control). Products include:
Lo/Ovral Tablets 3532
Lo/Ovral-28 Tablets 3538
Low-Ogestrel-28 Tablets 3392
Ogestrel 0.5/50-28 Tablets 3428
Ovral Tablets 3551
Ovral-28 Tablets 3552
Ovrette Tablets 3552

Nortriptyline Hydrochloride (Co-administration with drugs that are highly protein bound may result in hypoglycemia).
No products indexed under this heading.

Oxaprozin (Co-administration with nonsteroidal anti-inflammatory agents may result in hypoglycemia).
No products indexed under this heading.

Oxazepam (Co-administration with drugs that are highly protein bound may result in hypoglycemia).
No products indexed under this heading.

Pargyline Hydrochloride (Co-administration with monamine oxidase inhibitors may result in hypoglycemia).
No products indexed under this heading.

Penbutolol Sulfate (Co-administration with beta blockers may result in hypoglycemia).
No products indexed under this heading.

Perphenazine (Phenothiazines tend to produce hyperglycemia and concurrent use may lead to loss of control). Products include:
Etrafon 3115
Trilafon 3160

Phenelzine Sulfate (Co-administration with monamine oxidase inhibitors may result in hypoglycemia). Products include:
Nardil Tablets 2653

Phenylbutazone (Co-administration with nonsteroidal anti-inflammatory agents may result in hypoglycemia).
No products indexed under this heading.

Phenylephrine Bitartrate (Sympathomimetics tend to produce hyperglycemia and concurrent use may lead to loss of control).
No products indexed under this heading.

Phenylephrine Hydrochloride (Sympathomimetics tend to produce hyperglycemia and concurrent use may lead to loss of control). Products include:
Afrin Nasal Decongestant Children's Pump Mist .... ▣734
Extendryl 1361
Hycomine Compound Tablets 1317
Neo-Synephrine .... ▣614
Phenergan VC Syrup 3560
Phenergan VC with Codeine Syrup . 3561
Preparation H Cream .... ▣778
Preparation H Cooling Gel .... ▣778
Preparation H .... ▣778
Vicks Sinex Nasal Spray and Ultra Fine Mist .... ▣729

Phenylephrine Tannate (Sympathomimetics tend to produce hyperglycemia and concurrent use may lead to loss of control). Products include:
Ryna-12 S Suspension 3351
Reformulated Rynatan Pediatric Suspension 3352
Rynatuss Pediatric Suspension 3353
Rynatuss Tablets 3353

Phenylpropanolamine Hydrochloride (Sympathomimetics tend to produce hyperglycemia and concurrent use may lead to loss of control).
No products indexed under this heading.

Phenytoin (Phenytoin tends to produce hyperglycemia and concurrent use may lead to loss of control). Products include:
Dilantin Infatabs 2624
Dilantin-125 Oral Suspension 2625

Phenytoin Sodium (Phenytoin tends to produce hyperglycemia and concurrent use may lead to loss of control). Products include:
Dilantin Kapseals 2622

Pindolol (Co-administration with beta blockers may result in hypoglycemia).
No products indexed under this heading.

Pirbuterol Acetate (Sympathomimetics tend to produce hyperglycemia and concurrent use may lead to loss of control). Products include:
Maxair Autohaler 1981
Maxair Inhaler 1984

Piroxicam (Co-administration with nonsteroidal anti-inflammatory agents may result in hypoglycemia). Products include:
Feldene Capsules 2685

Polyestradiol Phosphate (Estrogens tend to produce hyperglycemia and concurrent use may lead to loss of control).
No products indexed under this heading.

Polythiazide (Thiazides tend to produce hyperglycemia and concurrent use may lead to loss of control). Products include:
Minizide Capsules 2700
Renese Tablets 2712

Prednisolone Acetate (Corticosteroids tend to produce hyperglycemia and concurrent use may lead to loss of control). Products include:
Blephamide Ophthalmic Ointment .. 547
Blephamide Ophthalmic Suspension 548
Poly-Pred Liquifilm Ophthalmic Suspension .... ⊙245
Pred Forte Ophthalmic Suspension .... ⊙246
Pred Mild Sterile Ophthalmic Suspension .... ⊙249
Pred-G Ophthalmic Suspension .... ⊙247
Pred-G Sterile Ophthalmic Ointment .... ⊙248

Prednisolone Sodium Phosphate (Corticosteroids tend to produce hyperglycemia and concurrent use may lead to loss of control). Products include:
Pediapred Oral Solution 1170

Prednisolone Tebutate (Corticosteroids tend to produce hyperglycemia and concurrent use may lead to loss of control).
No products indexed under this heading.

Prednisone (Corticosteroids tend to produce hyperglycemia and concurrent use may lead to loss of control). Products include:
Prednisone 3064

Probenecid (Co-administration with probenecid may result in hypoglycemia).
No products indexed under this heading.

Procarbazine Hydrochloride (Co-administration with monamine oxidase inhibitors may result in hypoglycemia). Products include:
Matulane Capsules 3246

Prochlorperazine (Phenothiazines tend to produce hyperglycemia and concurrent use may lead to loss of control). Products include:
Compazine 1505

Promethazine Hydrochloride (Phenothiazines tend to produce hyperglycemia and concurrent use may lead to loss of control). Products include:
Mepergan Injection 3539
Phenergan Injection 3553
Phenergan 3556
Phenergan Syrup 3554
Phenergan with Codeine Syrup 3557
Phenergan with Dextromethorphan Syrup 3559
Phenergan VC Syrup 3560
Phenergan VC with Codeine Syrup .. 3561

Propranolol Hydrochloride (Co-administration with beta blockers may result in hypoglycemia). Products include:
Inderal 3513
Inderal LA Long-Acting Capsules 3516
Inderide Tablets 3517
Inderide LA Long-Acting Capsules .. 3519

Pseudoephedrine Hydrochloride (Sympathomimetics tend to produce hyperglycemia and concurrent use may lead to loss of control). Products include:
Actifed Cold & Allergy Tablets .... ▣688
Actifed Cold & Sinus Caplets and Tablets .... ▣688
Advil Cold and Sinus Caplets .... ▣771
Advil Cold and Sinus Tablets .... ▣771
Advil Flu & Body Ache Caplets .... ▣772
Aleve Cold & Sinus Caplets .... ▣603
Alka-Seltzer Plus Liqui-Gels .... ▣604
Alka-Seltzer Plus Cold & Flu Medicine Liqui-Gels .... ▣604
Alka-Seltzer Plus Cold & Sinus Medicine Liqui-Gels .... ▣604
Allegra-D Extended-Release Tablets 714
BC Cold Powder .... ▣619
Benadryl Allergy/Cold Tablets .... ▣691
Benadryl Allergy/Congestion Tablets .... ▣692
Benadryl Allergy & Sinus Liquid .... ▣693
Benadryl Allergy & Sinus Fastmelt Tablets .... ▣693
Benadryl Allergy Sinus Headache Caplets & Gelcaps .... ▣693
Benadryl Severe Allergy & Sinus Headache Caplets .... ▣694
Benadryl Children's Allergy/Cold Fastmelt Tablets .... ▣692
Benylin Multi-Symptom Liquid .... ▣697
Bromfed Capsules (Extended-Release) 2269
Bromfed-PD Capsules (Extended-Release) 2269
Children's Cēpacol Sore Throat .... ▣788
Comtrex Acute Head Cold & Sinus Pressure Relief Tablets .... ▣627
Comtrex Deep Chest Cold & Congestion Relief Softgels .... ▣627
Comtrex Flu Therapy & Fever Relief Daytime Caplets .... ▣628
Comtrex Flu Therapy & Fever Relief Nighttime Tablets .... ▣628
Comtrex Maximum Strength Multi-Symptom Cold & Cough Relief Tablets and Caplets .... ▣626
Contac Non-Drowsy 12 Hour Cold Caplets .... ▣745
Contac Non-Drowsy Timed Release 12 Hour Cold Caplets ... ▣746
Contac Severe Cold and Flu Caplets Maximum Strength .... ▣746
Contac Severe Cold and Flu Caplets Non-Drowsy .... ▣746
Dimetapp Elixir .... ▣777
Dimetapp Cold and Fever Suspension .... ▣775
Dimetapp DM Cold & Cough Elixir . ▣775
Dimetapp Nighttime Flu Liquid .... ▣776
Dimetapp Non-Drowsy Flu Syrup ... ▣777
Dimetapp Infant Drops Decongestant .... ▣775
Dimetapp Infant Drops Decongestant Plus Cough .... ▣776
Guaifed 2272
Kronofed-A 1341
Children's Motrin Cold Oral Suspension 2007
Motrin Sinus Headache Caplets 2005
PediaCare Cough-Cold Liquid .... ▣719
PediaCare Infants' Drops Decongestant .... ▣719

PediaCare Infants' Drops
Decongestant Plus Cough.......... ▭719
PediaCare NightRest Cough-Cold
Liquid.................................... ▭719
Robitussin Cold Caplets Cold &
Congestion................................ ▭780
Robitussin Cold Softgels Cold &
Congestion................................ ▭780
Robitussin Cold Caplets
Multi-Symptom Cold & Flu.......... ▭781
Robitussin Cold Softgels
Multi-Symptom Cold & Flu.......... ▭781
Robitussin Cold Softgels Severe
Congestion................................ ▭782
Robitussin Cough & Cold Infant
Drops...................................... ▭782
Robitussin Maximum Strength
Cough & Cold Liquid.................. ▭785
Robitussin Pediatric Cough &
Cold Formula Liquid.................. ▭785
Robitussin Multi Symptom Honey
Flu Liquid .... ▭785
Robitussin Nighttime Honey Flu
Liquid .... ▭786
Robitussin-CF Liquid .... ▭783
Robitussin-DAC Syrup 2942
Robitussin-PE Liquid .... ▭782
Ryna .... ▭768
Semprex-D Capsules 1172
Singlet Caplets .... ▭761
Sinutab Non-Drying Liquid Caps .... ▭706
Sinutab Sinus Allergy Medication,
Maximum Strength Formula,
Tablets & Caplets .... ▭707
Sinutab Sinus Medication,
Maximum Strength Without
Drowsiness Formula, Tablets &
Caplets .... ▭707
Sudafed 12 Hour Tablets .... ▭708
Sudafed 24 Hour Tablets .... ▭708
Children's Sudafed Cold & Cough
Liquid .... ▭709
Children's Sudafed Nasal
Decongestant Chewables .... ▭711
Children's Sudafed Nasal
Decongestant Liquid
Medication .... ▭711
Sudafed Cold & Allergy Tablets ..... ▭708
Sudafed Cold & Cough Liquid
Caps .... ▭709
Sudafed Cold & Sinus Liquid
Caps .... ▭710
Sudafed Nasal Decongestant
Tablets .... ▭710
Sudafed Non-Drying Sinus Liquid
Caps .... ▭712
Sudafed Severe Cold .... ▭711
Sudafed Sinus Headache Caplets . ▭712
Sudafed Sinus Headache Tablets . ▭712
Tavist Sinus Non-Drowsy Coated
Caplets .... ▭676
TheraFlu Regular Strength Cold &
Cough Night Time Hot Liquid ...... ▭676
TheraFlu Regular Strength Cold &
Sore Throat Night Time Hot
Liquid .... ▭676
TheraFlu Maximum Strength Flu
& Congestion Non-Drowsy Hot
Liquid .... ▭677
TheraFlu Maximum Strength Flu
& Cough Night Time Hot Liquid .. ▭678
TheraFlu Maximum Strength Flu
& Sore Throat Night Time Hot
Liquid .... ▭677
TheraFlu Maximum Strength
Severe Cold & Congestion
Night Time Caplets .... ▭678
TheraFlu Maximum Strength
Severe Cold & Congestion
Night Time Hot Liquid .... ▭678
TheraFlu Maximum Strength
Severe Cold & Congestion
Non-Drowsy .... ▭679
Triaminic Allergy Congestion
Liquid .... ▭680
Triaminic Chest Congestion
Liquid .... ▭680
Triaminic Cold & Allergy Liquid ...... ▭681
Triaminic Cold & Allergy
Softchews .... ▭683
Triaminic Cold & Cough Liquid ...... ▭681
Triaminic Cold & Cough
Softchews .... ▭683
Triaminic Cold & Night Time
Cough Liquid .... ▭681
Triaminic Cold, Cough & Fever
Liquid .... ▭681
Triaminic Cough Liquid .... ▭682
Triaminic Cough & Congestion
Liquid .... ▭682
Triaminic Cough & Sore Throat
Liquid .... ▭682
Triaminic Cough & Sore Throat
Softchews .... ▭684
Children's Tylenol Allergy-D Liquid ... 2014
Children's Tylenol Cold
Suspension Liquid and
Chewable Tablets 2015
Children's Tylenol Cold Plus Cough
Suspension Liquid and
Chewable Tablets 2015
Children's Tylenol Flu Suspension
Liquid 2015
Children's Tylenol Sinus
Suspension Liquid 2017
Infants' Tylenol Cold Decongestant
and Fever Reducer
Concentrated Drops 2015
Infants' Tylenol Cold Decongestant
and Fever Reducer
Concentrated Drops Plus Cough.. 2015
Tylenol Allergy Sinus 2010
Multi-Symptom Tylenol Cold
Complete Formula Caplets.......... 2010
Multi-Symptom Tylenol Cold
Non-Drowsy Caplets and
Gelcaps.................................... 2010
Multi-Symptom Tylenol Cold
Severe Congestion Non-Drowsy
Caplets 2011
Maximum Strength Tylenol Flu
NightTime Gelcaps 2011
Maximum Strength Tylenol Flu
NightTime Liquid 2011
Maximum Strength Tylenol Flu
Non-Drowsy Gelcaps 2011
Maximum Strength Tylenol Sinus
NightTime Caplets 2012
Maximum Strength Tylenol Sinus
Non-Drowsy Geltabs, Gelcaps,
Caplets, and Tablets 2012
Vicks 44D Cough & Head
Congestion Relief Liquid .... ▭724
Vicks 44M Cough, Cold & Flu
Relief Liquid .... ▭725
Pediatric Vicks 44m Cough &
Cold Relief .... ▭728
Vicks DayQuil LiquiCaps/Liquid
Multi-Symptom Cold/Flu Relief ... ▭727
Children's Vicks NyQuil
Cold/Cough Relief .... ▭726
Vicks NyQuil LiquiCaps/Liquid
Multi-Symptom Cold/Flu Relief,
Original and Cherry Flavors .... ▭727
Zephrex Tablets 3091
Zephrex LA Tablets 3092
Zyrtec-D 12 Hour Extended Relief
Tablets 2758

Pseudoephedrine Sulfate (Sympathomimetics tend to produce hyperglycemia and concurrent use may lead to loss of control). Products include:
Chlor-Trimeton
Allergy/Decongestant Tablets .... ▭736
Claritin-D 12 Hour Extended
Release Tablets 3102
Claritin-D 24 Hour Extended
Release Tablets 3104
Coricidin 'D' Cold, Flu & Sinus
Tablets .... ▭737
Drixoral Allergy/Sinus
Extended-Release Tablets .... ▭741
Drixoral Cold & Allergy
Sustained-Action Tablets .... ▭740
Drixoral Cold & Flu
Extended-Release Tablets .... ▭740
Drixoral Nasal Decongestant
Long-Acting Non-Drowsy
Tablets .... ▭740
Rynatan Tablets 3351

Quinestrol (Estrogens tend to produce hyperglycemia and concurrent use may lead to loss of control).
No products indexed under this heading.

Rofecoxib (Co-administration with nonsteroidal anti-inflammatory agents may result in hypoglycemia). Products include:
Vioxx 2213

Salmeterol Xinafoate (Sympathomimetics tend to produce hyperglycemia and concurrent use may lead to loss of control). Products include:
Advair Diskus 100/50 1448
Advair Diskus 250/50 1448
Advair Diskus 500/50 1448
Serevent Diskus 1637
Serevent Inhalation Aerosol 1633

Salsalate (Co-administration with salicylates may result in hypoglycemia).
No products indexed under this heading.

Selegiline Hydrochloride (Co-administration with monamine oxidase inhibitors may result in hypoglycemia). Products include:
Eldepryl Capsules 3266

Sotalol Hydrochloride (Co-administration with beta blockers may result in hypoglycemia). Products include:
Betapace Tablets 950
Betapace AF Tablets 954

Spironolactone (Diuretics tend to produce hyperglycemia and concurrent use may lead to loss of control).
No products indexed under this heading.

Sulfacytine (Co-administration with sulfonamides may result in hypoglycemia).

Sulfamethizole (Co-administration with sulfonamides may result in hypoglycemia). Products include:
Urobiotic-250 Capsules 2731

Sulfamethoxazole (Co-administration with sulfonamides may result in hypoglycemia). Products include:
Bactrim 2949
Septra Suspension 2265
Septra Tablets 2265
Septra DS Tablets 2265

Sulfasalazine (Co-administration with sulfonamides may result in hypoglycemia). Products include:
Azulfidine EN-tabs Tablets 2775

Sulfinpyrazone (Co-administration with sulfonamides may result in hypoglycemia).
No products indexed under this heading.

Sulfisoxazole (Co-administration with sulfonamides may result in hypoglycemia).
No products indexed under this heading.

Sulfisoxazole Acetyl (Co-administration with sulfonamides may result in hypoglycemia). Products include:
Pediazole Suspension 3050

Sulfisoxazole Diolamine (Co-administration with sulfonamides may result in hypoglycemia).
No products indexed under this heading.

Sulindac (Co-administration with nonsteroidal anti-inflammatory agents may result in hypoglycemia). Products include:
Clinoril Tablets 2053

Temazepam (Co-administration with drugs that are highly protein bound may result in hypoglycemia).
No products indexed under this heading.

Terbutaline Sulfate (Sympathomimetics tend to produce hyperglycemia and concurrent use may lead to loss of control). Products include:
Brethine Ampuls 2314
Brethine Tablets 2313

Thioridazine Hydrochloride (Phenothiazines tend to produce hyperglycemia and concurrent use may lead to loss of control). Products include:
Thioridazine Hydrochloride
Tablets 2289

Thyroglobulin (Thyroid products tend to produce hyperglycemia and concurrent use may lead to loss of control).
No products indexed under this heading.

Thyroid (Thyroid products tend to produce hyperglycemia and concurrent use may lead to loss of control).
No products indexed under this heading.

Thyroxine (Thyroid products tend to produce hyperglycemia and concurrent use may lead to loss of control).
No products indexed under this heading.

Thyroxine Sodium (Thyroid products tend to produce hyperglycemia and concurrent use may lead to loss of control).
No products indexed under this heading.

Timolol Hemihydrate (Co-administration with beta blockers may result in hypoglycemia). Products include:
Betimol Ophthalmic Solution .... ⊙324

Timolol Maleate (Co-administration with beta blockers may result in hypoglycemia). Products include:
Blocadren Tablets 2046
Cosopt Sterile Ophthalmic
Solution.................................... 2065
Timolide Tablets 2187
Timolol GFS .... ⊙266
Timoptic in Ocudose 2192
Timoptic Sterile Ophthalmic
Solution.................................... 2190
Timoptic-XE Sterile Ophthalmic
Gel Forming Solution 2194

Tolazamide (Co-administration with sulfonamides may result in hypoglycemia).
No products indexed under this heading.

Tolbutamide (Co-administration with drugs that are highly protein bound may result in hypoglycemia).
No products indexed under this heading.

Tolmetin Sodium (Co-administration with nonsteroidal anti-inflammatory agents may result in hypoglycemia). Products include:
Tolectin 2589

Torsemide (Diuretics tend to produce hyperglycemia and concurrent use may lead to loss of control). Products include:
Demadex Tablets and Injection 2965

Tranylcypromine Sulfate (Co-administration with monamine oxidase inhibitors may result in hypoglycemia). Products include:
Parnate Tablets 1607

Triamcinolone (Corticosteroids tend to produce hyperglycemia and concurrent use may lead to loss of control).
No products indexed under this heading.

Triamcinolone Acetonide (Corticosteroids tend to produce hyperglycemia and concurrent use may lead to loss of control). Products include:
Azmacort Inhalation Aerosol 728
Nasacort Nasal Inhaler 750
Nasacort AQ Nasal Spray 752
Tri-Nasal Spray 2274

Triamcinolone Diacetate (Corticosteroids tend to produce hyperglycemia and concurrent use may lead to loss of control).
No products indexed under this heading.

Triamcinolone Hexacetonide (Corticosteroids tend to produce hyperglycemia and concurrent use may lead to loss of control).
No products indexed under this heading.

Triamterene (Diuretics tend to produce hyperglycemia and concurrent use may lead to loss of control). Products include:
Dyazide Capsules 1515
Dyrenium Capsules 3458
Maxzide 1008

Trifluoperazine Hydrochloride (Phenothiazines tend to produce hyperglycemia and concurrent use may lead to loss of control). Products include:
Stelazine 1640

Trimipramine Maleate (Co-administration with drugs that are highly protein bound may result in hypoglycemia). Products include:

Surmontil Capsules ... 3595

Verapamil Hydrochloride (Calcium channel blockers tend to produce hyperglycemia and concurrent use may lead to loss of control). Products include:
- Covera-HS Tablets ... 3199
- Isoptin SR Tablets ... 467
- Tarka Tablets ... 508
- Verelan Capsules ... 3184
- Verelan PM Capsules ... 3186

Warfarin Sodium (Co-administration with coumarins may result in hypoglycemia). Products include:
- Coumadin for Injection ... 1243
- Coumadin Tablets ... 1243
- Warfarin Sodium Tablets, USP ... 3302

Food Interactions

Alcohol (Co-administration with alcohol may result in hypoglycemia).

Food, unspecified (Delays absorption by 40 minutes; administer 30 minutes prior to meals).

GLUCOTROL XL EXTENDED RELEASE TABLETS

(Glipizide) ... 2693

May interact with beta blockers, calcium channel blockers, corticosteroids, oral anticoagulants, diuretics, estrogens, monoamine oxidase inhibitors, non-steroidal anti-inflammatory agents, oral contraceptives, phenothiazines, highly protein bound drugs (selected), salicylates, sulfonamides, sympathomimetics, thiazides, thyroid preparations, and certain other agents. Compounds in these categories include:

Acebutolol Hydrochloride (Co-administration with beta blockers may result in hypoglycemia). Products include:
- Sectral Capsules ... 3589

Albuterol (Sympathomimetics tend to produce hyperglycemia and concurrent use may lead to loss of control). Products include:
- Proventil Inhalation Aerosol ... 3142
- Ventolin Inhalation Aerosol and Refill ... 1679

Albuterol Sulfate (Sympathomimetics tend to produce hyperglycemia and concurrent use may lead to loss of control). Products include:
- AccuNeb Inhalation Solution ... 1230
- Combivent Inhalation Aerosol ... 1041
- DuoNeb Inhalation Solution ... 1233
- Proventil Inhalation Solution 0.083% ... 3146
- Proventil Repetabs Tablets ... 3148
- Proventil Solution for Inhalation 0.5% ... 3144
- Proventil HFA Inhalation Aerosol ... 3150
- Ventolin HFA Inhalation Aerosol ... 3618
- Volmax Extended-Release Tablets ... 2276

Amiloride Hydrochloride (Diuretics tend to produce hyperglycemia and concurrent use may lead to loss of control). Products include:
- Midamor Tablets ... 2136
- Moduretic Tablets ... 2138

Amiodarone Hydrochloride (Co-administration with drugs that are highly protein bound may result in hypoglycemia). Products include:
- Cordarone Intravenous ... 3491
- Cordarone Tablets ... 3487
- Pacerone Tablets ... 3331

Amitriptyline Hydrochloride (Co-administration with drugs that are highly protein bound may result in hypoglycemia). Products include:
- Etrafon ... 3115
- Limbitrol ... 1738

Amlodipine Besylate (Calcium channel blockers tend to produce hyperglycemia and concurrent use may lead to loss of control). Products include:
- Lotrel Capsules ... 2370
- Norvasc Tablets ... 2704

Aspirin (Co-administration with salicylates may result in hypoglycemia). Products include:
- Aggrenox Capsules ... 1026
- Alka-Seltzer ... ■603
- Alka-Seltzer Lemon Lime Antacid and Pain Reliever Effervescent Tablets ... ■603
- Alka-Seltzer Extra Strength Antacid and Pain Reliever Effervescent Tablets ... ■603
- Alka-Seltzer PM Effervescent Tablets ... ■605
- Genuine Bayer Tablets, Caplets and Gelcaps ... ■606
- Extra Strength Bayer Caplets and Gelcaps ... ■610
- Aspirin Regimen Bayer Children's Chewable Tablets (Orange or Cherry Flavored) ... ■607
- Bayer, Aspirin Regimen ... ■606
- Aspirin Regimen Bayer 81 mg Caplets with Calcium ... ■607
- Genuine Bayer Professional Labeling (Aspirin Regimen Bayer) ... ■608
- Extra Strength Bayer Arthritis Caplets ... ■610
- Extra Strength Bayer Plus Caplets ... ■610
- Extra Strength Bayer PM Caplets ... ■611
- BC Powder ... ■619
- BC Allergy Sinus Cold Powder ... ■619
- Arthritis Strength BC Powder ... ■619
- BC Sinus Cold Powder ... ■619
- Darvon Compound-65 Pulvules ... 1910
- Ecotrin Enteric Coated Aspirin Low, Regular and Maximum Strength Tablets ... 1715
- Excedrin Extra-Strength Tablets, Caplets, and Geltabs ... ■629
- Excedrin Migraine ... 1070
- Goody's Body Pain Formula Powder ... ■620
- Goody's Extra Strength Headache Powder ... ■620
- Goody's Extra Strength Pain Relief Tablets ... ■620
- Percodan Tablets ... 1327
- Robaxisal Tablets ... 2939
- Soma Compound Tablets ... 3354
- Soma Compound w/Codeine Tablets ... 3355
- Vanquish Caplets ... ■617

Atenolol (Co-administration with beta blockers may result in hypoglycemia). Products include:
- Tenoretic Tablets ... 690
- Tenormin I.V. Injection ... 692

Atovaquone (Co-administration with drugs that are highly protein bound may result in hypoglycemia). Products include:
- Malarone ... 1596
- Mepron Suspension ... 1598

Bendroflumethiazide (Thiazides tend to produce hyperglycemia and concurrent use may lead to loss of control). Products include:
- Corzide 40/5 Tablets ... 2247
- Corzide 80/5 Tablets ... 2247

Bepridil Hydrochloride (Calcium channel blockers tend to produce hyperglycemia and concurrent use may lead to loss of control). Products include:
- Vascor Tablets ... 2602

Betamethasone Acetate (Corticosteroids tend to produce hyperglycemia and concurrent use may lead to loss of control). Products include:
- Celestone Soluspan Injectable Suspension ... 3097

Betamethasone Sodium Phosphate (Corticosteroids tend to produce hyperglycemia and concurrent use may lead to loss of control). Products include:
- Celestone Soluspan Injectable Suspension ... 3097

Betaxolol Hydrochloride (Co-administration with beta blockers may result in hypoglycemia). Products include:
- Betoptic S Ophthalmic Suspension ... 537

Bisoprolol Fumarate (Co-administration with beta blockers may result in hypoglycemia). Products include:
- Zebeta Tablets ... 1885
- Ziac Tablets ... 1887

Bumetanide (Diuretics tend to produce hyperglycemia and concurrent use may lead to loss of control).
No products indexed under this heading.

Carteolol Hydrochloride (Co-administration with beta blockers may result in hypoglycemia). Products include:
- Carteolol Hydrochloride Ophthalmic Solution USP, 1% ... ⊙258
- Ocupress Ophthalmic Solution, 1% Sterile ... ⊙303

Cefonicid Sodium (Co-administration with drugs that are highly protein bound may result in hypoglycemia).
No products indexed under this heading.

Celecoxib (Co-administration with nonsteroidal anti-inflammatory agents may result in hypoglycemia). Products include:
- Celebrex Capsules ... 2676
- Celebrex Capsules ... 2780

Chloramphenicol (Co-administration with chloramphenicol may result in hypoglycemia). Products include:
- Chloromycetin Ophthalmic Ointment, 1% ... ⊙296
- Chloromycetin Ophthalmic Solution ... ⊙297
- Chloroptic Sterile Ophthalmic Ointment ... ⊙234
- Chloroptic Sterile Ophthalmic Solution ... ⊙235

Chloramphenicol Palmitate (Co-administration with chloramphenicol may result in hypoglycemia).
No products indexed under this heading.

Chloramphenicol Sodium Succinate (Co-administration with chloramphenicol may result in hypoglycemia).
No products indexed under this heading.

Chlordiazepoxide (Co-administration with drugs that are highly protein bound may result in hypoglycemia). Products include:
- Limbitrol ... 1738

Chlordiazepoxide Hydrochloride (Co-administration with drugs that are highly protein bound may result in hypoglycemia). Products include:
- Librium Capsules ... 1736
- Librium for Injection ... 1737

Chlorothiazide (Thiazides tend to produce hyperglycemia and concurrent use may lead to loss of control). Products include:
- Aldoclor Tablets ... 2035
- Diuril Oral ... 2087

Chlorothiazide Sodium (Thiazides tend to produce hyperglycemia and concurrent use may lead to loss of control). Products include:
- Diuril Sodium Intravenous ... 2086

Chlorotrianisene (Estrogens tend to produce hyperglycemia and concurrent use may lead to loss of control).
No products indexed under this heading.

Chlorpromazine (Phenothiazines tend to produce hyperglycemia and concurrent use may lead to loss of control). Products include:
- Thorazine Suppositories ... 1656

Chlorpromazine Hydrochloride (Phenothiazines tend to produce hyperglycemia and concurrent use may lead to loss of control). Products include:
- Thorazine ... 1656

Chlorpropamide (Co-administration with sulfonamides may result in hypoglycemia). Products include:
- Diabinese Tablets ... 2680

Chlorthalidone (Diuretics tend to produce hyperglycemia and concurrent use may lead to loss of control). Products include:
- Clorpres Tablets ... 1002
- Combipres Tablets ... 1040
- Tenoretic Tablets ... 690

Choline Magnesium Trisalicylate (Co-administration with salicylates may result in hypoglycemia). Products include:
- Trilisate ... 2901

Clomipramine Hydrochloride (Co-administration with drugs that are highly protein bound may result in hypoglycemia).
No products indexed under this heading.

Clozapine (Co-administration with drugs that are highly protein bound may result in hypoglycemia). Products include:
- Clozaril Tablets ... 2319

Cortisone Acetate (Corticosteroids tend to produce hyperglycemia and concurrent use may lead to loss of control). Products include:
- Cortone Acetate Injectable Suspension ... 2059
- Cortone Acetate Tablets ... 2061

Cyclosporine (Co-administration with drugs that are highly protein bound may result in hypoglycemia). Products include:
- Gengraf Capsules ... 457
- Neoral Soft Gelatin Capsules ... 2380
- Neoral Oral Solution ... 2380
- Sandimmune ... 2388

Desogestrel (Oral contraceptives tend to produce hyperglycemia and concurrent use may lead to loss of control). Products include:
- Cyclessa Tablets ... 2450
- Desogen Tablets ... 2458
- Mircette Tablets ... 2470
- Ortho-Cept 21 Tablets ... 2546
- Ortho-Cept 28 Tablets ... 2546

Dexamethasone (Corticosteroids tend to produce hyperglycemia and concurrent use may lead to loss of control). Products include:
- Decadron Elixir ... 2078
- Decadron Tablets ... 2079
- TobraDex Ophthalmic Ointment ... 542
- TobraDex Ophthalmic Suspension ... 541

Dexamethasone Acetate (Corticosteroids tend to produce hyperglycemia and concurrent use may lead to loss of control).
No products indexed under this heading.

Dexamethasone Sodium Phosphate (Corticosteroids tend to produce hyperglycemia and concurrent use may lead to loss of control). Products include:
- Decadron Phosphate Injection ... 2081
- Decadron Phosphate Sterile Ophthalmic Ointment ... 2083
- Decadron Phosphate Sterile Ophthalmic Solution ... 2084
- NeoDecadron Sterile Ophthalmic Solution ... 2144

Diazepam (Co-administration with drugs that are highly protein bound may result in hypoglycemia). Products include:
- Valium Injectable ... 3026
- Valium Tablets ... 3047

Diclofenac Potassium (Co-administration with nonsteroidal anti-inflammatory agents may result in hypoglycemia). Products include:
- Cataflam Tablets ... 2315

Diclofenac Sodium (Co-administration with nonsteroidal anti-inflammatory agents may result in hypoglycemia). Products include:
- Arthrotec Tablets ... 3195
- Voltaren Ophthalmic Sterile Ophthalmic Solution ... ⊙312
- Voltaren Tablets ... 2315
- Voltaren-XR Tablets ... 2315

Dicumarol (Co-administration with coumarins may result in hypoglyce-

mia).
No products indexed under this heading.

Dienestrol (Estrogens tend to produce hyperglycemia and concurrent use may lead to loss of control). Products include:
Ortho Dienestrol Cream 2554

Diethylstilbestrol (Estrogens tend to produce hyperglycemia and concurrent use may lead to loss of control).
No products indexed under this heading.

Diflunisal (Co-administration with salicylates may result in hypoglycemia). Products include:
Dolobid Tablets 2088

Diltiazem Hydrochloride (Calcium channel blockers tend to produce hyperglycemia and concurrent use may lead to loss of control). Products include:
Cardizem Injectable 1018
Cardizem Lyo-Ject Syringe 1018
Cardizem Monovial 1018
Cardizem CD Capsules 1016
Tiazac Capsules 1378

Dipyridamole (Co-administration with drugs that are highly protein bound may result in hypoglycemia). Products include:
Aggrenox Capsules 1026
Persantine Tablets 1057

Dobutamine Hydrochloride (Sympathomimetics tend to produce hyperglycemia and concurrent use may lead to loss of control). Products include:
Dobutrex Solution Vials 1914

Dopamine Hydrochloride (Sympathomimetics tend to produce hyperglycemia and concurrent use may lead to loss of control).
No products indexed under this heading.

Ephedrine Hydrochloride (Sympathomimetics tend to produce hyperglycemia and concurrent use may lead to loss of control). Products include:
Primatene Tablets .... ▣780

Ephedrine Sulfate (Sympathomimetics tend to produce hyperglycemia and concurrent use may lead to loss of control).
No products indexed under this heading.

Ephedrine Tannate (Sympathomimetics tend to produce hyperglycemia and concurrent use may lead to loss of control). Products include:
Rynatuss Pediatric Suspension 3353
Rynatuss Tablets 3353

Epinephrine (Sympathomimetics tend to produce hyperglycemia and concurrent use may lead to loss of control). Products include:
Epifrin Sterile Ophthalmic Solution .... ⊙235
EpiPen 1236
Primatene Mist .... ▣779
Xylocaine with Epinephrine Injection 653

Epinephrine Bitartrate (Sympathomimetics tend to produce hyperglycemia and concurrent use may lead to loss of control). Products include:
Sensorcaine 643

Epinephrine Hydrochloride (Sympathomimetics tend to produce hyperglycemia and concurrent use may lead to loss of control).
No products indexed under this heading.

Esmolol Hydrochloride (Co-administration with beta blockers may result in hypoglycemia). Products include:
Brevibloc Injection 858

Estradiol (Estrogens tend to produce hyperglycemia and concurrent use may lead to loss of control). Products include:
Activella Tablets 2764
Alora Transdermal System 3372
Climara Transdermal System 958
CombiPatch Transdermal System 2323
Esclim Transdermal System 3460
Estrace Vaginal Cream 3358
Estrace Tablets 3361
Estring Vaginal Ring 2811
Ortho-Prefest Tablets 2570
Vagifem Tablets 2857
Vivelle Transdermal System 2412
Vivelle-Dot Transdermal System 2416

Estrogens, Conjugated (Estrogens tend to produce hyperglycemia and concurrent use may lead to loss of control). Products include:
Premarin Intravenous 3563
Premarin Tablets 3566
Premarin Vaginal Cream 3570
Premphase Tablets 3572
Prempro Tablets 3572

Estrogens, Esterified (Estrogens tend to produce hyperglycemia and concurrent use may lead to loss of control). Products include:
Estratest 3252
Menest Tablets 2254

Estropipate (Estrogens tend to produce hyperglycemia and concurrent use may lead to loss of control). Products include:
Ogen Tablets 2846
Ortho-Est Tablets 3464

Ethacrynic Acid (Diuretics tend to produce hyperglycemia and concurrent use may lead to loss of control). Products include:
Edecrin Tablets 2091

Ethinyl Estradiol (Estrogens tend to produce hyperglycemia and concurrent use may lead to loss of control). Products include:
Alesse-21 Tablets 3468
Alesse-28 Tablets 3473
Brevicon 28-Day Tablets 3380
Cyclessa Tablets 2450
Desogen Tablets 2458
Estinyl Tablets 3112
Estrostep 2627
femhrt Tablets 2635
Levlen 962
Levlite 21 Tablets 962
Levlite 28 Tablets 962
Levora Tablets 3389
Loestrin 21 Tablets 2642
Loestrin Fe Tablets 2642
Lo/Ovral Tablets 3532
Lo/Ovral-28 Tablets 3538
Low-Ogestrel-28 Tablets 3392
Microgestin Fe 1.5/30 Tablets 3407
Microgestin Fe 1/20 Tablets 3400
Mircette Tablets 2470
Modicon 2563
Necon 3415
Nordette-28 Tablets 2257
Norinyl 1 +35 28-Day Tablets 3380
Ogestrel 0.5/50-28 Tablets 3428
Ortho-Cept 21 Tablets 2546
Ortho-Cept 28 Tablets 2546
Ortho-Cyclen/Ortho Tri-Cyclen 2573
Ortho-Novum 2563
Ovcon 3364
Ovral Tablets 3551
Ovral-28 Tablets 3552
Tri-Levlen 962
Tri-Norinyl-28 Tablets 3433
Triphasil-21 Tablets 3600
Triphasil-28 Tablets 3605
Trivora Tablets 3439
Yasmin 28 Tablets 980
Zovia 3449

Ethynodiol Diacetate (Oral contraceptives tend to produce hyperglycemia and concurrent use may lead to loss of control). Products include:
Zovia 3449

Etodolac (Co-administration with nonsteroidal anti-inflammatory agents may result in hypoglycemia). Products include:
Lodine 3528
Lodine XL Extended-Release Tablets 3530

Felodipine (Calcium channel blockers tend to produce hyperglycemia and concurrent use may lead to loss of control). Products include:
Lexxel Tablets 608
Plendil Extended-Release Tablets 623

Fenoprofen Calcium (Co-administration with nonsteroidal anti-inflammatory agents may result in hypoglycemia).
No products indexed under this heading.

Fluconazole (Co-administration with oral fluconazole has resulted in an increase in Glucotrol AUC by 56.9%). Products include:
Diflucan Tablets, Injection, and Oral Suspension 2681

Fludrocortisone Acetate (Corticosteroids tend to produce hyperglycemia and concurrent use may lead to loss of control). Products include:
Florinef Acetate Tablets 2250

Fluphenazine Decanoate (Phenothiazines tend to produce hyperglycemia and concurrent use may lead to loss of control).
No products indexed under this heading.

Fluphenazine Enanthate (Phenothiazines tend to produce hyperglycemia and concurrent use may lead to loss of control).
No products indexed under this heading.

Fluphenazine Hydrochloride (Phenothiazines tend to produce hyperglycemia and concurrent use may lead to loss of control).
No products indexed under this heading.

Flurazepam Hydrochloride (Co-administration with drugs that are highly protein bound may result in hypoglycemia).
No products indexed under this heading.

Flurbiprofen (Co-administration with nonsteroidal anti-inflammatory agents may result in hypoglycemia).
No products indexed under this heading.

Furosemide (Diuretics tend to produce hyperglycemia and concurrent use may lead to loss of control). Products include:
Furosemide Tablets 2284

Glyburide (Co-administration with sulfonamides may result in hypoglycemia). Products include:
DiaBeta Tablets 741
Glucovance Tablets 1086

Hydrochlorothiazide (Thiazides tend to produce hyperglycemia and concurrent use may lead to loss of control). Products include:
Accuretic Tablets 2614
Aldoril Tablets 2039
Atacand HCT Tablets 597
Avalide Tablets 1070
Diovan HCT Tablets 2338
Dyazide Capsules 1515
HydroDIURIL Tablets 2108
Hyzaar 2109
Inderide Tablets 3517
Inderide LA Long-Acting Capsules 3519
Lotensin HCT Tablets 2367
Maxzide 1008
Micardis HCT Tablets 1051
Microzide Capsules 3414
Moduretic Tablets 2138
Monopril HCT 1094
Prinzide Tablets 2168
Timolide Tablets 2187
Uniretic Tablets 3178
Vaseretic Tablets 2204
Zestoretic Tablets 695
Ziac Tablets 1887

Hydrocortisone (Corticosteroids tend to produce hyperglycemia and concurrent use may lead to loss of control). Products include:
AnusoI-HC Cream 2.5% 2237
Cipro HC Otic Suspension 540
Cortaid Intensive Therapy Cream .... ▣717
Cortaid Maximum Strength Cream .... ▣717
Cortisporin Ophthalmic Suspension Sterile .... ⊙297
Cortizone•5 .... ▣699
Cortizone•10 .... ▣699
Cortizone•10 Plus Creme .... ▣700
Cortizone for Kids Creme .... ▣699
Hydrocortone Tablets 2106
Massengill Medicated Soft Cloth Towelette .... ▣753
VōSoL HC Otic Solution 3356

Hydrocortisone Acetate (Corticosteroids tend to produce hyperglycemia and concurrent use may lead to loss of control). Products include:
Analpram-HC 1338
Anusol HC-1 Hydrocortisone Anti-Itch Cream .... ▣689
Anusol-HC Suppositories 2238
Cortaid .... ▣717
Cortifoam Rectal Foam 3170
Cortisporin-TC Otic Suspension 2246
Hydrocortone Acetate Injectable Suspension 2103
Pramosone 1343
Proctocort Suppositories 2264
ProctoFoam-HC 3177
Terra-Cortril Ophthalmic Suspension 2716

Hydrocortisone Sodium Phosphate (Corticosteroids tend to produce hyperglycemia and concurrent use may lead to loss of control). Products include:
Hydrocortone Phosphate Injection, Sterile 2105

Hydrocortisone Sodium Succinate (Corticosteroids tend to produce hyperglycemia and concurrent use may lead to loss of control).
No products indexed under this heading.

Hydroflumethiazide (Thiazides tend to produce hyperglycemia and concurrent use may lead to loss of control). Products include:
Diucardin Tablets 3494

Ibuprofen (Co-administration with nonsteroidal anti-inflammatory agents may result in hypoglycemia). Products include:
Advil .... ▣771
Children's Advil Oral Suspension .... ▣773
Children's Advil Chewable Tablets .... ▣773
Advil Cold and Sinus Caplets .... ▣771
Advil Cold and Sinus Tablets .... ▣771
Advil Flu & Body Ache Caplets .... ▣772
Infants' Advil Drops .... ▣773
Junior Strength Advil Tablets .... ▣773
Junior Strength Advil Chewable Tablets .... ▣773
Advil Migraine Liquigels .... ▣772
Children's Motrin Oral Suspension and Chewable Tablets 2006
Children's Motrin Cold Oral Suspension 2007
Children's Motrin Oral Suspension .... ▣643
Motrin Suspension, Oral Drops, Chewable Tablets, and Caplets 2002
Infants' Motrin Concentrated Drops 2006
Junior Strength Motrin Caplets and Chewable Tablets 2006
Motrin IB Tablets, Caplets, and Gelcaps 2002
Motrin Migraine Pain Caplets 2005
Motrin Sinus Headache Caplets 2005
Vicoprofen Tablets 520

Imipramine Hydrochloride (Co-administration with drugs that are highly protein bound may result in hypoglycemia).
No products indexed under this heading.

Imipramine Pamoate (Co-administration with drugs that are highly protein bound may result in hypoglycemia).
No products indexed under this heading.

Indapamide (Diuretics tend to produce hyperglycemia and concurrent use may lead to loss of control). Products include:
Indapamide Tablets 2286

Indomethacin (Co-administration with nonsteroidal anti-inflammatory agents may result in hypoglycemia). Products include:
Indocin 2112

Indomethacin Sodium Trihydrate (Co-administration with nonsteroidal anti-inflammatory agents may result in hypoglycemia). Products include:

Indocin I.V. 2115

Isocarboxazid (Co-administration with monamine oxidase inhibitors may result in hypoglycemia).
No products indexed under this heading.

Isoniazid (Isoniazid tends to produce hyperglycemia and concurrent use may lead to loss of control). Products include:
Rifamate Capsules 767
Rifater Tablets 769

Isoproterenol Hydrochloride (Sympathomimetics tend to produce hyperglycemia and concurrent use may lead to loss of control).
No products indexed under this heading.

Isoproterenol Sulfate (Sympathomimetics tend to produce hyperglycemia and concurrent use may lead to loss of control).
No products indexed under this heading.

Isradipine (Calcium channel blockers tend to produce hyperglycemia and concurrent use may lead to loss of control). Products include:
DynaCirc Capsules 2921
DynaCirc CR Tablets 2923

Ketoprofen (Co-administration with nonsteroidal anti-inflammatory agents may result in hypoglycemia). Products include:
Orudis Capsules 3548
Orudis KT Tablets .... ▣778
Oruvail Capsules 3548

Ketorolac Tromethamine (Co-administration with nonsteroidal anti-inflammatory agents may result in hypoglycemia). Products include:
Acular Ophthalmic Solution 544
Acular PF Ophthalmic Solution 544
Toradol 3018

Labetalol Hydrochloride (Co-administration with beta blockers may result in hypoglycemia). Products include:
Normodyne Injection 3135
Normodyne Tablets 3137

Levalbuterol Hydrochloride (Sympathomimetics tend to produce hyperglycemia and concurrent use may lead to loss of control). Products include:
Xopenex Inhalation Solution 3207

Levobunolol Hydrochloride (Co-administration with beta blockers may result in hypoglycemia). Products include:
Betagan .... ⊙228

Levonorgestrel (Oral contraceptives tend to produce hyperglycemia and concurrent use may lead to loss of control). Products include:
Alesse-21 Tablets 3468
Alesse-28 Tablets 3473
Levlen 962
Levlite 21 Tablets 962
Levlite 28 Tablets 962
Levora Tablets 3389
Mirena Intrauterine System 974
Nordette-28 Tablets 2257
Norplant System 3543
Tri-Levlen 962
Triphasil-21 Tablets 3600
Triphasil-28 Tablets 3605
Trivora Tablets 3439

Levothyroxine Sodium (Thyroid products tend to produce hyperglycemia and concurrent use may lead to loss of control). Products include:
Levothroid Tablets 1373
Levoxyl Tablets 1819
Synthroid 505
Unithroid Tablets 3445

Liothyronine Sodium (Thyroid products tend to produce hyperglycemia and concurrent use may lead to loss of control). Products include:
Cytomel Tablets 1817
Triostat Injection 1825

Liotrix (Thyroid products tend to produce hyperglycemia and concurrent use may lead to loss of control).
No products indexed under this heading.

Magnesium Salicylate (Co-administration with salicylates may result in hypoglycemia). Products include:
Momentum Backache Relief Extra Strength Caplets .... ▣666

Meclofenamate Sodium (Co-administration with nonsteroidal anti-inflammatory agents may result in hypoglycemia).
No products indexed under this heading.

Mefenamic Acid (Co-administration with nonsteroidal anti-inflammatory agents may result in hypoglycemia). Products include:
Ponstel Capsules 1356

Meloxicam (Co-administration with nonsteroidal anti-inflammatory agents may result in hypoglycemia). Products include:
Mobic Tablets 1054

Mesoridazine Besylate (Phenothiazines tend to produce hyperglycemia and concurrent use may lead to loss of control). Products include:
Serentil 1057

Mestranol (Oral contraceptives tend to produce hyperglycemia and concurrent use may lead to loss of control). Products include:
Necon 1/50 Tablets 3415
Norinyl 1 + 50 28-Day Tablets 3380
Ortho-Novum 1/50□28 Tablets 2556

Metaproterenol Sulfate (Sympathomimetics tend to produce hyperglycemia and concurrent use may lead to loss of control). Products include:
Alupent 1029

Metaraminol Bitartrate (Sympathomimetics tend to produce hyperglycemia and concurrent use may lead to loss of control). Products include:
Aramine Injection 2043

Methotrimeprazine (Phenothiazines tend to produce hyperglycemia and concurrent use may lead to loss of control).
No products indexed under this heading.

Methoxamine Hydrochloride (Sympathomimetics tend to produce hyperglycemia and concurrent use may lead to loss of control).
No products indexed under this heading.

Methyclothiazide (Thiazides tend to produce hyperglycemia and concurrent use may lead to loss of control).
No products indexed under this heading.

Methylprednisolone Acetate (Corticosteroids tend to produce hyperglycemia and concurrent use may lead to loss of control). Products include:
Depo-Medrol Injectable Suspension 2795

Methylprednisolone Sodium Succinate (Corticosteroids tend to produce hyperglycemia and concurrent use may lead to loss of control). Products include:
Solu-Medrol Sterile Powder 2855

Metipranolol Hydrochloride (Co-administration with beta blockers may result in hypoglycemia).
No products indexed under this heading.

Metolazone (Diuretics tend to produce hyperglycemia and concurrent use may lead to loss of control). Products include:
Mykrox Tablets 1168
Zaroxolyn Tablets 1177

Metoprolol Succinate (Co-administration with beta blockers may result in hypoglycemia). Products include:
Toprol-XL Tablets 651

Metoprolol Tartrate (Co-administration with beta blockers may result in hypoglycemia).
No products indexed under this heading.

Mibefradil Dihydrochloride (Calcium channel blockers tend to produce hyperglycemia and concurrent use may lead to loss of control).
No products indexed under this heading.

Miconazole (Co-administration with oral miconazole and oral hypoglycemic agents has resulted in severe hypoglycemia).
No products indexed under this heading.

Midazolam Hydrochloride (Co-administration with drugs that are highly protein bound may result in hypoglycemia). Products include:
Versed Injection 3027
Versed Syrup 3033

Moclobemide (Co-administration with monamine oxidase inhibitors may result in hypoglycemia).
No products indexed under this heading.

Nabumetone (Co-administration with nonsteroidal anti-inflammatory agents may result in hypoglycemia). Products include:
Relafen Tablets 1617

Nadolol (Co-administration with beta blockers may result in hypoglycemia). Products include:
Corgard Tablets 2245
Corzide 40/5 Tablets 2247
Corzide 80/5 Tablets 2247
Nadolol Tablets 2288

Naproxen (Co-administration with nonsteroidal anti-inflammatory agents may result in hypoglycemia). Products include:
EC-Naprosyn Delayed-Release Tablets 2967
Naprosyn Suspension 2967
Naprosyn Tablets 2967

Naproxen Sodium (Co-administration with nonsteroidal anti-inflammatory agents may result in hypoglycemia). Products include:
Aleve Tablets, Caplets and Gelcaps .... ▣602
Aleve Cold & Sinus Caplets .... ▣603
Anaprox Tablets 2967
Anaprox DS Tablets 2967
Naprelan Tablets 1293

Nicardipine Hydrochloride (Calcium channel blockers tend to produce hyperglycemia and concurrent use may lead to loss of control). Products include:
Cardene I.V. 3485

Nicotinic Acid (Nicotinic acid tends to produce hyperglycemia and concurrent use may lead to loss of control).
No products indexed under this heading.

Nifedipine (Calcium channel blockers tend to produce hyperglycemia and concurrent use may lead to loss of control). Products include:
Adalat CC Tablets 877
Procardia Capsules 2708
Procardia XL Extended Release Tablets 2710

Nimodipine (Calcium channel blockers tend to produce hyperglycemia and concurrent use may lead to loss of control). Products include:
Nimotop Capsules 904

Nisoldipine (Calcium channel blockers tend to produce hyperglycemia and concurrent use may lead to loss of control). Products include:
Sular Tablets 688

Norepinephrine Bitartrate (Sympathomimetics tend to produce hyperglycemia and concurrent use may lead to loss of control).
No products indexed under this heading.

Norethindrone (Oral contraceptives tend to produce hyperglycemia and concurrent use may lead to loss of control). Products include:
Brevicon 28-Day Tablets 3380
Micronor Tablets 2543
Modicon 2563
Necon 3415
Norinyl 1 +35 28-Day Tablets 3380
Norinyl 1 + 50 28-Day Tablets 3380
Nor-QD Tablets 3423
Ortho-Novum 2563
Ortho-Novum 1/50□28 Tablets 2556
Ovcon 3364
Tri-Norinyl-28 Tablets 3433

Norethynodrel (Oral contraceptives tend to produce hyperglycemia and concurrent use may lead to loss of control).
No products indexed under this heading.

Norgestimate (Oral contraceptives tend to produce hyperglycemia and concurrent use may lead to loss of control). Products include:
Ortho-Cyclen/Ortho Tri-Cyclen 2573
Ortho-Prefest Tablets 2570

Norgestrel (Oral contraceptives tend to produce hyperglycemia and concurrent use may lead to loss of control). Products include:
Lo/Ovral Tablets 3532
Lo/Ovral-28 Tablets 3538
Low-Ogestrel-28 Tablets 3392
Ogestrel 0.5/50-28 Tablets 3428
Ovral Tablets 3551
Ovral-28 Tablets 3552
Ovrette Tablets 3552

Nortriptyline Hydrochloride (Co-administration with drugs that are highly protein bound may result in hypoglycemia).
No products indexed under this heading.

Oxaprozin (Co-administration with nonsteroidal anti-inflammatory agents may result in hypoglycemia).
No products indexed under this heading.

Oxazepam (Co-administration with drugs that are highly protein bound may result in hypoglycemia).
No products indexed under this heading.

Pargyline Hydrochloride (Co-administration with monamine oxidase inhibitors may result in hypoglycemia).
No products indexed under this heading.

Penbutolol Sulfate (Co-administration with beta blockers may result in hypoglycemia).
No products indexed under this heading.

Perphenazine (Phenothiazines tend to produce hyperglycemia and concurrent use may lead to loss of control). Products include:
Etrafon 3115
Trilafon 3160

Phenelzine Sulfate (Co-administration with monamine oxidase inhibitors may result in hypoglycemia). Products include:
Nardil Tablets 2653

Phenylbutazone (Co-administration with nonsteroidal anti-inflammatory agents may result in hypoglycemia).
No products indexed under this heading.

Phenylephrine Bitartrate (Sympathomimetics tend to produce hyperglycemia and concurrent use may lead to loss of control).
No products indexed under this heading.

Phenylephrine Hydrochloride (Sympathomimetics tend to produce hyperglycemia and concurrent use may lead to loss of control). Products include:
Afrin Nasal Decongestant Children's Pump Mist .... ▣734
Extendryl 1361
Hycomine Compound Tablets 1317

Neo-Synephrine ▣614
Phenergan VC Syrup 3560
Phenergan VC with Codeine Syrup 3561
Preparation H Cream ▣778
Preparation H Cooling Gel ▣778
Preparation H ▣778
Vicks Sinex Nasal Spray and Ultra Fine Mist ▣729

Phenylephrine Tannate (Sympathomimetics tend to produce hyperglycemia and concurrent use may lead to loss of control). Products include:
Ryna-12 S Suspension 3351
Reformulated Rynatan Pediatric Suspension 3352
Rynatuss Pediatric Suspension 3353
Rynatuss Tablets 3353

Phenylpropanolamine Hydrochloride (Sympathomimetics tend to produce hyperglycemia and concurrent use may lead to loss of control).
No products indexed under this heading.

Phenytoin (Phenytoin tends to produce hyperglycemia and concurrent use may lead to loss of control). Products include:
Dilantin Infatabs 2624
Dilantin-125 Oral Suspension 2625

Phenytoin Sodium (Phenytoin tends to produce hyperglycemia and concurrent use may lead to loss of control). Products include:
Dilantin Kapseals 2622

Pindolol (Co-administration with beta blockers may result in hypoglycemia).
No products indexed under this heading.

Pirbuterol Acetate (Sympathomimetics tend to produce hyperglycemia and concurrent use may lead to loss of control). Products include:
Maxair Autohaler 1981
Maxair Inhaler 1984

Piroxicam (Co-administration with nonsteroidal anti-inflammatory agents may result in hypoglycemia). Products include:
Feldene Capsules 2685

Polyestradiol Phosphate (Estrogens tend to produce hyperglycemia and concurrent use may lead to loss of control).
No products indexed under this heading.

Polythiazide (Thiazides tend to produce hyperglycemia and concurrent use may lead to loss of control). Products include:
Minizide Capsules 2700
Renese Tablets 2712

Prednisolone Acetate (Corticosteroids tend to produce hyperglycemia and concurrent use may lead to loss of control). Products include:
Blephamide Ophthalmic Ointment 547
Blephamide Ophthalmic Suspension 548
Poly-Pred Liquifilm Ophthalmic Suspension ⊙245
Pred Forte Ophthalmic Suspension ⊙246
Pred Mild Sterile Ophthalmic Suspension ⊙249
Pred-G Ophthalmic Suspension ⊙247
Pred-G Sterile Ophthalmic Ointment ⊙248

Prednisolone Sodium Phosphate (Corticosteroids tend to produce hyperglycemia and concurrent use may lead to loss of control). Products include:
Pediapred Oral Solution 1170

Prednisolone Tebutate (Corticosteroids tend to produce hyperglycemia and concurrent use may lead to loss of control).
No products indexed under this heading.

Prednisone (Corticosteroids tend to produce hyperglycemia and concurrent use may lead to loss of control). Products include:
Prednisone 3064

Probenecid (Co-administration with probenecid may result in hypoglycemia).
No products indexed under this heading.

Procarbazine Hydrochloride (Co-administration with monamine oxidase inhibitors may result in hypoglycemia). Products include:
Matulane Capsules 3246

Prochlorperazine (Phenothiazines tend to produce hyperglycemia and concurrent use may lead to loss of control). Products include:
Compazine 1505

Promethazine Hydrochloride (Phenothiazines tend to produce hyperglycemia and concurrent use may lead to loss of control). Products include:
Mepergan Injection 3539
Phenergan Injection 3553
Phenergan 3556
Phenergan Syrup 3554
Phenergan with Codeine Syrup 3557
Phenergan with Dextromethorphan Syrup 3559
Phenergan VC Syrup 3560
Phenergan VC with Codeine Syrup 3561

Propranolol Hydrochloride (Co-administration with beta blockers may result in hypoglycemia). Products include:
Inderal 3513
Inderal LA Long-Acting Capsules 3516
Inderide Tablets 3517
Inderide LA Long-Acting Capsules 3519

Pseudoephedrine Hydrochloride (Sympathomimetics tend to produce hyperglycemia and concurrent use may lead to loss of control). Products include:
Actifed Cold & Allergy Tablets ▣688
Actifed Cold & Sinus Caplets and Tablets ▣688
Advil Cold and Sinus Caplets ▣771
Advil Cold and Sinus Tablets ▣771
Advil Flu & Body Ache Caplets ▣772
Aleve Cold & Sinus Caplets ▣603
Alka-Seltzer Plus Liqui-Gels ▣604
Alka-Seltzer Plus Cold & Flu Medicine Liqui-Gels ▣604
Alka-Seltzer Plus Cold & Sinus Medicine Liqui-Gels ▣604
Allegra-D Extended-Release Tablets 714
BC Cold Powder ▣619
Benadryl Allergy/Cold Tablets ▣691
Benadryl Allergy/Congestion Tablets ▣692
Benadryl Allergy & Sinus Liquid ▣693
Benadryl Allergy & Sinus Fastmelt Tablets ▣693
Benadryl Allergy Sinus Headache Caplets & Gelcaps ▣693
Benadryl Severe Allergy & Sinus Headache Caplets ▣694
Benadryl Children's Allergy/Cold Fastmelt Tablets ▣692
Benylin Multi-Symptom Liquid ▣697
Bromfed Capsules (Extended-Release) 2269
Bromfed-PD Capsules (Extended-Release) 2269
Children's Cēpacol Sore Throat ▣788
Comtrex Acute Head Cold & Sinus Pressure Relief Tablets ▣627
Comtrex Deep Chest Cold & Congestion Relief Softgels ▣627
Comtrex Flu Therapy & Fever Relief Daytime Caplets ▣628
Comtrex Flu Therapy & Fever Relief Nighttime Tablets ▣628
Comtrex Maximum Strength Multi-Symptom Cold & Cough Relief Tablets and Caplets ▣626
Contac Non-Drowsy 12 Hour Cold Caplets ▣745
Contac Non-Drowsy Timed Release 12 Hour Cold Caplets ▣746
Contac Severe Cold and Flu Caplets Maximum Strength ▣746
Contac Severe Cold and Flu Caplets Non-Drowsy ▣746
Dimetapp Elixir ▣777
Dimetapp Cold and Fever Suspension ▣775
Dimetapp DM Cold & Cough Elixir ▣775
Dimetapp Nighttime Flu Liquid ▣776
Dimetapp Non-Drowsy Flu Syrup ▣777
Dimetapp Infant Drops Decongestant ▣775
Dimetapp Infant Drops Decongestant Plus Cough ▣776
Guaifed 2272
Kronofed-A 1341
Children's Motrin Cold Oral Suspension 2007
Motrin Sinus Headache Caplets 2005
PediaCare Cough-Cold Liquid ▣719
PediaCare Infants' Drops Decongestant ▣719
PediaCare Infants' Drops Decongestant Plus Cough ▣719
PediaCare NightRest Cough-Cold Liquid ▣719
Robitussin Cold Caplets Cold & Congestion ▣780
Robitussin Cold Softgels Cold & Congestion ▣780
Robitussin Cold Caplets Multi-Symptom Cold & Flu ▣781
Robitussin Cold Softgels Multi-Symptom Cold & Flu ▣781
Robitussin Cold Softgels Severe Congestion ▣782
Robitussin Cough & Cold Infant Drops ▣782
Robitussin Maximum Strength Cough & Cold Liquid ▣785
Robitussin Pediatric Cough & Cold Formula Liquid ▣785
Robitussin Multi Symptom Honey Flu Liquid ▣785
Robitussin Nighttime Honey Flu Liquid ▣786
Robitussin-CF Liquid ▣783
Robitussin-DAC Syrup 2942
Robitussin-PE Liquid ▣782
Ryna ▣768
Semprex-D Capsules 1172
Singlet Caplets ▣761
Sinutab Non-Drying Liquid Caps ▣706
Sinutab Sinus Allergy Medication, Maximum Strength Formula, Tablets & Caplets ▣707
Sinutab Sinus Medication, Maximum Strength Without Drowsiness Formula, Tablets & Caplets ▣707
Sudafed 12 Hour Tablets ▣708
Sudafed 24 Hour Tablets ▣708
Children's Sudafed Cold & Cough Liquid ▣709
Children's Sudafed Nasal Decongestant Chewables ▣711
Children's Sudafed Nasal Decongestant Liquid Medication ▣711
Sudafed Cold & Allergy Tablets ▣708
Sudafed Cold & Cough Liquid Caps ▣709
Sudafed Cold & Sinus Liquid Caps ▣710
Sudafed Nasal Decongestant Tablets ▣710
Sudafed Non-Drying Sinus Liquid Caps ▣712
Sudafed Severe Cold ▣711
Sudafed Sinus Headache Caplets ▣712
Sudafed Sinus Headache Tablets ▣712
Tavist Sinus Non-Drowsy Coated Caplets ▣676
TheraFlu Regular Strength Cold & Cough Night Time Hot Liquid ▣676
TheraFlu Regular Strength Cold & Sore Throat Night Time Hot Liquid ▣676
TheraFlu Maximum Strength Flu & Congestion Non-Drowsy Hot Liquid ▣677
TheraFlu Maximum Strength Flu & Cough Night Time Hot Liquid ▣678
TheraFlu Maximum Strength Flu & Sore Throat Night Time Hot Liquid ▣677
TheraFlu Maximum Strength Severe Cold & Congestion Night Time Caplets ▣678
TheraFlu Maximum Strength Severe Cold & Congestion Night Time Hot Liquid ▣678
TheraFlu Maximum Strength Severe Cold & Congestion Non-Drowsy ▣679
Triaminic Allergy Congestion Liquid ▣680
Triaminic Chest Congestion Liquid ▣680
Triaminic Cold & Allergy Liquid ▣681
Triaminic Cold & Allergy Softchews ▣683
Triaminic Cold & Cough Liquid ▣681
Triaminic Cold & Cough Softchews ▣683
Triaminic Cold & Night Time Cough Liquid ▣681
Triaminic Cold, Cough & Fever Liquid ▣681
Triaminic Cough Liquid ▣682
Triaminic Cough & Congestion Liquid ▣682
Triaminic Cough & Sore Throat Liquid ▣682
Triaminic Cough & Sore Throat Softchews ▣684
Children's Tylenol Allergy-D Liquid 2014
Children's Tylenol Cold Suspension Liquid and Chewable Tablets 2015
Children's Tylenol Cold Plus Cough Suspension Liquid and Chewable Tablets 2015
Children's Tylenol Flu Suspension Liquid 2015
Children's Tylenol Sinus Suspension Liquid 2017
Infants' Tylenol Cold Decongestant and Fever Reducer Concentrated Drops 2015
Infants' Tylenol Cold Decongestant and Fever Reducer Concentrated Drops Plus Cough 2015
Tylenol Allergy Sinus 2010
Multi-Symptom Tylenol Cold Complete Formula Caplets 2010
Multi-Symptom Tylenol Cold Non-Drowsy Caplets and Gelcaps 2010
Multi-Symptom Tylenol Cold Severe Congestion Non-Drowsy Caplets 2011
Maximum Strength Tylenol Flu NightTime Gelcaps 2011
Maximum Strength Tylenol Flu NightTime Liquid 2011
Maximum Strength Tylenol Flu Non-Drowsy Gelcaps 2011
Maximum Strength Tylenol Sinus NightTime Caplets 2012
Maximum Strength Tylenol Sinus Non-Drowsy Geltabs, Gelcaps, Caplets, and Tablets 2012
Vicks 44D Cough & Head Congestion Relief Liquid ▣724
Vicks 44M Cough, Cold & Flu Relief Liquid ▣725
Pediatric Vicks 44m Cough & Cold Relief ▣728
Vicks DayQuil LiquiCaps/Liquid Multi-Symptom Cold/Flu Relief ▣727
Children's Vicks NyQuil Cold/Cough Relief ▣726
Vicks NyQuil LiquiCaps/Liquid Multi-Symptom Cold/Flu Relief, Original and Cherry Flavors ▣727
Zephrex Tablets 3091
Zephrex LA Tablets 3092
Zyrtec-D 12 Hour Extended Relief Tablets 2758

Pseudoephedrine Sulfate (Sympathomimetics tend to produce hyperglycemia and concurrent use may lead to loss of control). Products include:
Chlor-Trimeton Allergy/Decongestant Tablets ▣736
Claritin-D 12 Hour Extended Release Tablets 3102
Claritin-D 24 Hour Extended Release Tablets 3104
Coricidin 'D' Cold, Flu & Sinus Tablets ▣737
Drixoral Allergy/Sinus Extended-Release Tablets ▣741
Drixoral Cold & Allergy Sustained-Action Tablets ▣740
Drixoral Cold & Flu Extended-Release Tablets ▣740
Drixoral Nasal Decongestant Long-Acting Non-Drowsy Tablets ▣740
Rynatan Tablets 3351

Quinestrol (Estrogens tend to produce hyperglycemia and concurrent use may lead to loss of control).
No products indexed under this heading.

Rofecoxib (Co-administration with nonsteroidal anti-inflammatory agents may result in hypoglycemia). Products include:
Vioxx 2213

Salmeterol Xinafoate (Sympathomimetics tend to produce hyperglycemia and concurrent use may lead to loss of control). Products include:
Advair Diskus 100/50 1448
Advair Diskus 250/50 1448
Advair Diskus 500/50 1448
Serevent Diskus 1637

(▣ Described in PDR For Nonprescription Drugs) (⊙ Described in PDR For Ophthalmic Medicines™)

Serevent Inhalation Aerosol 1633

Salsalate (Co-administration with salicylates may result in hypoglycemia).
No products indexed under this heading.

Selegiline Hydrochloride (Co-administration with monamine oxidase inhibitors may result in hypoglycemia). Products include:
Eldepryl Capsules 3266

Sotalol Hydrochloride (Co-administration with beta blockers may result in hypoglycemia). Products include:
Betapace Tablets 950
Betapace AF Tablets 954

Spironolactone (Diuretics tend to produce hyperglycemia and concurrent use may lead to loss of control).
No products indexed under this heading.

Sulfacytine (Co-administration with sulfonamides may result in hypoglycemia).
No products indexed under this heading.

Sulfamethizole (Co-administration with sulfonamides may result in hypoglycemia). Products include:
Urobiotic-250 Capsules 2731

Sulfamethoxazole (Co-administration with sulfonamides may result in hypoglycemia). Products include:
Bactrim 2949
Septra Suspension 2265
Septra Tablets 2265
Septra DS Tablets 2265

Sulfasalazine (Co-administration with sulfonamides may result in hypoglycemia). Products include:
Azulfidine EN-tabs Tablets 2775

Sulfinpyrazone (Co-administration with sulfonamides may result in hypoglycemia).
No products indexed under this heading.

Sulfisoxazole (Co-administration with sulfonamides may result in hypoglycemia).
No products indexed under this heading.

Sulfisoxazole Acetyl (Co-administration with sulfonamides may result in hypoglycemia). Products include:
Pediazole Suspension 3050

Sulfisoxazole Diolamine (Co-administration with sulfonamides may result in hypoglycemia).
No products indexed under this heading.

Sulindac (Co-administration with nonsteroidal anti-inflammatory agents may result in hypoglycemia). Products include:
Clinoril Tablets 2053

Temazepam (Co-administration with drugs that are highly protein bound may result in hypoglycemia).
No products indexed under this heading.

Terbutaline Sulfate (Sympathomimetics tend to produce hyperglycemia and concurrent use may lead to loss of control). Products include:
Brethine Ampuls 2314
Brethine Tablets 2313

Thioridazine Hydrochloride (Phenothiazines tend to produce hyperglycemia and concurrent use may lead to loss of control). Products include:
Thioridazine Hydrochloride Tablets 2289

Thyroglobulin (Thyroid products tend to produce hyperglycemia and concurrent use may lead to loss of control).
No products indexed under this heading.

Thyroid (Thyroid products tend to produce hyperglycemia and concurrent use may lead to loss of control).
No products indexed under this heading.

Thyroxine (Thyroid products tend to produce hyperglycemia and concurrent use may lead to loss of control).
No products indexed under this heading.

Thyroxine Sodium (Thyroid products tend to produce hyperglycemia and concurrent use may lead to loss of control).
No products indexed under this heading.

Timolol Hemihydrate (Co-administration with beta blockers may result in hypoglycemia). Products include:
Betimol Ophthalmic Solution .... ⊙324

Timolol Maleate (Co-administration with beta blockers may result in hypoglycemia). Products include:
Blocadren Tablets 2046
Cosopt Sterile Ophthalmic Solution 2065
Timolide Tablets 2187
Timolol GFS .... ⊙266
Timoptic in Ocudose 2192
Timoptic Sterile Ophthalmic Solution 2190
Timoptic-XE Sterile Ophthalmic Gel Forming Solution 2194

Tolazamide (Co-administration with sulfonamides may result in hypoglycemia).
No products indexed under this heading.

Tolbutamide (Co-administration with sulfonamides may result in hypoglycemia).
No products indexed under this heading.

Tolmetin Sodium (Co-administration with nonsteroidal anti-inflammatory agents may result in hypoglycemia). Products include:
Tolectin 2589

Torsemide (Diuretics tend to produce hyperglycemia and concurrent use may lead to loss of control). Products include:
Demadex Tablets and Injection 2965

Tranylcypromine Sulfate (Co-administration with monamine oxidase inhibitors may result in hypoglycemia). Products include:
Parnate Tablets 1607

Triamcinolone (Corticosteroids tend to produce hyperglycemia and concurrent use may lead to loss of control).
No products indexed under this heading.

Triamcinolone Acetonide (Corticosteroids tend to produce hyperglycemia and concurrent use may lead to loss of control). Products include:
Azmacort Inhalation Aerosol 728
Nasacort Nasal Inhaler 750
Nasacort AQ Nasal Spray 752
Tri-Nasal Spray 2274

Triamcinolone Diacetate (Corticosteroids tend to produce hyperglycemia and concurrent use may lead to loss of control).
No products indexed under this heading.

Triamcinolone Hexacetonide (Corticosteroids tend to produce hyperglycemia and concurrent use may lead to loss of control).
No products indexed under this heading.

Triamterene (Diuretics tend to produce hyperglycemia and concurrent use may lead to loss of control). Products include:
Dyazide Capsules 1515
Dyrenium Capsules 3458
Maxzide 1008

Trifluoperazine Hydrochloride (Phenothiazines tend to produce hyperglycemia and concurrent use may lead to loss of control). Products include:
Stelazine 1640

Trimipramine Maleate (Co-administration with drugs that are highly protein bound may result in hypoglycemia). Products include:
Surmontil Capsules 3595

Verapamil Hydrochloride (Calcium channel blockers tend to produce hyperglycemia and concurrent use may lead to loss of control). Products include:
Covera-HS Tablets 3199
Isoptin SR Tablets 467
Tarka Tablets 508
Verelan Capsules 3184
Verelan PM Capsules 3186

Warfarin Sodium (Co-administration with coumarins may result in hypoglycemia). Products include:
Coumadin for Injection 1243
Coumadin Tablets 1243
Warfarin Sodium Tablets, USP 3302

Food Interactions

Alcohol (Co-administration with alcohol may result in hypoglycemia).

GLUCOVANCE TABLETS

(Glyburide, Metformin Hydrochloride) 1086

May interact with beta blockers, cationic drugs that are eliminated by renal tubular, calcium channel blockers, corticosteroids, oral anticoagulants, diuretics, estrogens, monoamine oxidase inhibitors, nonsteroidal anti-inflammatory agents, oral contraceptives, phenothiazines, phenytoin, radiographic iodinated contrast media, salicylates, sulfonamides, sympathomimetics, thiazides, thyroid preparations, and certain other agents. Compounds in these categories include:

Acebutolol Hydrochloride (The hypoglycemic action of sulfonylureas may be potentiated by beta adrenergic agents). Products include:
Sectral Capsules 3589

Albuterol (Co-administration with drugs that tend to produce hyperglycemia, such as sympathomimetics, may lead to loss of blood glucose control). Products include:
Proventil Inhalation Aerosol 3142
Ventolin Inhalation Aerosol and Refill 1679

Albuterol Sulfate (Co-administration with drugs that tend to produce hyperglycemia, such as sympathomimetics, may lead to loss of blood glucose control). Products include:
AccuNeb Inhalation Solution 1230
Combivent Inhalation Aerosol 1041
DuoNeb Inhalation Solution 1233
Proventil Inhalation Solution 0.083% 3146
Proventil Repetabs Tablets 3148
Proventil Solution for Inhalation 0.5% 3144
Proventil HFA Inhalation Aerosol 3150
Ventolin HFA Inhalation Aerosol 3618
Volmax Extended-Release Tablets .. 2276

Amiloride Hydrochloride (Co-administration with cationic drugs that are eliminated by renal tubular secretion, such as amiloride, have the theoretical potential for interacting with metformin by competing for common renal tubular transport systems; concurrent use with drugs thattend to produce hyperglycemia, such as diuretics, may lead to loss of blood glucose control). Products include:
Midamor Tablets 2136
Moduretic Tablets 2138

Amlodipine Besylate (Co-administration with drugs that tend to produce hyperglycemia, such as calcium channel blockers, may lead to loss of blood glucose control). Products include:
Lotrel Capsules 2370
Norvasc Tablets 2704

Aspirin (The hypoglycemic action of sulfonylureas may be potentiated by salicylates). Products include:
Aggrenox Capsules 1026
Alka-Seltzer 603
Alka-Seltzer Lemon Lime Antacid and Pain Reliever Effervescent Tablets 603
Alka-Seltzer Extra Strength Antacid and Pain Reliever Effervescent Tablets 603
Alka-Seltzer PM Effervescent Tablets 605
Genuine Bayer Tablets, Caplets and Gelcaps 606
Extra Strength Bayer Caplets and Gelcaps 610
Aspirin Regimen Bayer Children's Chewable Tablets (Orange or Cherry Flavored) 607
Bayer, Aspirin Regimen 606
Aspirin Regimen Bayer 81 mg Caplets with Calcium 607
Genuine Bayer Professional Labeling (Aspirin Regimen Bayer) 608
Extra Strength Bayer Arthritis Caplets 610
Extra Strength Bayer Plus Caplets 610
Extra Strength Bayer PM Caplets ... 611
BC Powder 619
BC Allergy Sinus Cold Powder 619
Arthritis Strength BC Powder 619
BC Sinus Cold Powder 619
Darvon Compound-65 Pulvules 1910
Ecotrin Enteric Coated Aspirin Low, Regular and Maximum Strength Tablets 1715
Excedrin Extra-Strength Tablets, Caplets, and Geltabs 629
Excedrin Migraine 1070
Goody's Body Pain Formula Powder 620
Goody's Extra Strength Headache Powder 620
Goody's Extra Strength Pain Relief Tablets 620
Percodan Tablets 1327
Robaxisal Tablets 2939
Soma Compound Tablets 3354
Soma Compound w/Codeine Tablets 3355
Vanquish Caplets 617

Atenolol (The hypoglycemic action of sulfonylureas may be potentiated by beta adrenergic agents). Products include:
Tenoretic Tablets 690
Tenormin I.V. Injection 692

Bendroflumethiazide (Co-administration with drugs that tend to produce hyperglycemia, such as thiazides, may lead to loss of blood glucose control). Products include:
Corzide 40/5 Tablets 2247
Corzide 80/5 Tablets 2247

Bepridil Hydrochloride (Co-administration with drugs that tend to produce hyperglycemia, such as calcium channel blockers, may lead to loss of blood glucose control). Products include:
Vascor Tablets 2602

Betamethasone Acetate (Co-administration with drugs that tend to produce hyperglycemia, such as corticosteroids, may lead to loss of blood glucose control). Products include:
Celestone Soluspan Injectable Suspension 3097

Betamethasone Sodium Phosphate (Co-administration with drugs that tend to produce hyperglycemia, such as corticosteroids, may lead to loss of blood glucose control). Products include:
Celestone Soluspan Injectable Suspension 3097

Betaxolol Hydrochloride (The hypoglycemic action of sulfonylureas may be potentiated by beta adrenergic agents). Products include:
Betoptic S Ophthalmic Suspension 537

IMPORTANT NOTE: Always consult each drug listing in the patient's regimen for possible interactions.

Bisoprolol Fumarate (The hypoglycemic action of sulfonylureas may be potentiated by beta adrenergic agents). Products include:
Zebeta Tablets 1885
Ziac Tablets 1887

Bumetanide (Co-administration with drugs that tend to produce hyperglycemia, such as diuretics, may lead to loss of blood glucose control).
No products indexed under this heading.

Carteolol Hydrochloride (The hypoglycemic action of sulfonylureas may be potentiated by beta adrenergic agents). Products include:
Carteolol Hydrochloride Ophthalmic Solution USP, 1% .... ⊙258
Ocupress Ophthalmic Solution, 1% Sterile .... ⊙303

Celecoxib (The hypoglycemic action of sulfonylureas may be potentiated by non-steroidal anti-inflammatory agents). Products include:
Celebrex Capsules 2676
Celebrex Capsules 2780

Chloramphenicol (The hypoglycemic action of sulfonylureas may be potentiated by chloramphenicol). Products include:
Chloromycetin Ophthalmic Ointment, 1% .... ⊙296
Chloromycetin Ophthalmic Solution .... ⊙297
Chloroptic Sterile Ophthalmic Ointment .... ⊙234
Chloroptic Sterile Ophthalmic Solution .... ⊙235

Chlorothiazide (Co-administration with drugs that tend to produce hyperglycemia, such as thiazides, may lead to loss of blood glucose control). Products include:
Aldoclor Tablets 2035
Diuril Oral 2087

Chlorothiazide Sodium (Co-administration with drugs that tend to produce hyperglycemia, such as thiazides, may lead to loss of blood glucose control). Products include:
Diuril Sodium Intravenous 2086

Chlorotrianisene (Co-administration with drugs that tend to produce hyperglycemia, such as estrogens, may lead to loss of blood glucose control).
No products indexed under this heading.

Chlorpromazine (Co-administration with drugs that tend to produce hyperglycemia, such as phenothiazines, may lead to loss of blood glucose control). Products include:
Thorazine Suppositories 1656

Chlorpromazine Hydrochloride (Co-administration with drugs that tend to produce hyperglycemia, such as phenothiazines, may lead to loss of blood glucose control). Products include:
Thorazine 1656

Chlorpropamide (The hypoglycemic action of sulfonylureas may be potentiated by sulfonamides). Products include:
Diabinese Tablets 2680

Chlorthalidone (Co-administration with drugs that tend to produce hyperglycemia, such as diuretics, may lead to loss of blood glucose control). Products include:
Clorpres Tablets 1002
Combipres Tablets 1040
Tenoretic Tablets 690

Choline Magnesium Trisalicylate (The hypoglycemic action of sulfonylureas may be potentiated by salicylates). Products include:
Trilisate 2901

Cimetidine (Co-administration of metformin with oral cimetidine has resulted in a 60% increase in peak metformin plasma and whole blood concentrations and a 40% increase in plasma and whole blood metformin AUC). Products include:
Tagamet HB 200 Suspension .... ▣762
Tagamet HB 200 Tablets .... ▣761
Tagamet Tablets 1644

Cimetidine Hydrochloride (Co-administration of metformin with oral cimetidine has resulted in a 60% increase in peak metformin plasma and whole blood concentrations and a 40% increase in plasma and whole blood metformin AUC). Products include:
Tagamet 1644

Ciprofloxacin (Co-administration of glyburide and ciprofloxacin has resulted in potentiation of hypoglycemic action). Products include:
Cipro I.V. 893
Cipro I.V. Pharmacy Bulk Package .. 897
Cipro Oral Suspension 887

Ciprofloxacin Hydrochloride (Co-administration of glyburide and ciprofloxacin has resulted in potentiation of hypoglycemic action). Products include:
Ciloxan 538
Cipro HC Otic Suspension 540
Cipro Tablets 887

Cortisone Acetate (Co-administration with drugs that tend to produce hyperglycemia, such as corticosteroids, may lead to loss of blood glucose control). Products include:
Cortone Acetate Injectable Suspension 2059
Cortone Acetate Tablets 2061

Desogestrel (Co-administration with drugs that tend to produce hyperglycemia, such as oral contraceptives, may lead to loss of blood glucose control). Products include:
Cyclessa Tablets 2450
Desogen Tablets 2458
Mircette Tablets 2470
Ortho-Cept 21 Tablets 2546
Ortho-Cept 28 Tablets 2546

Dexamethasone (Co-administration with drugs that tend to produce hyperglycemia, such as corticosteroids, may lead to loss of blood glucose control). Products include:
Decadron Elixir 2078
Decadron Tablets 2079
TobraDex Ophthalmic Ointment 542
TobraDex Ophthalmic Suspension .. 541

Dexamethasone Acetate (Co-administration with drugs that tend to produce hyperglycemia, such as corticosteroids, may lead to loss of blood glucose control).
No products indexed under this heading.

Dexamethasone Sodium Phosphate (Co-administration with drugs that tend to produce hyperglycemia, such as corticosteroids, may lead to loss of blood glucose control). Products include:
Decadron Phosphate Injection 2081
Decadron Phosphate Sterile Ophthalmic Ointment 2083
Decadron Phosphate Sterile Ophthalmic Solution 2084
NeoDecadron Sterile Ophthalmic Solution 2144

Diatrizoate Meglumine (Potential for acute alteration of renal function; metformin should be temporarily withheld in patients undergoing radiologic studies involving iodinated contrast material).
No products indexed under this heading.

Diatrizoate Sodium (Potential for acute alteration of renal function; metformin should be temporarily withheld in patients undergoing radiologic studies involving iodinated contrast material).
No products indexed under this heading.

Diclofenac Potassium (The hypoglycemic action of sulfonylureas may be potentiated by non-steroidal anti-inflammatory agents). Products include:
Cataflam Tablets 2315

Diclofenac Sodium (The hypoglycemic action of sulfonylureas may be potentiated by non-steroidal anti-inflammatory agents). Products include:
Arthrotec Tablets 3195
Voltaren Ophthalmic Sterile Ophthalmic Solution .... ⊙312
Voltaren Tablets 2315
Voltaren-XR Tablets 2315

Dicumarol (The hypoglycemic action of sulfonylureas may be potentiated by coumarins).
No products indexed under this heading.

Dienestrol (Co-administration with drugs that tend to produce hyperglycemia, such as estrogens, may lead to loss of blood glucose control). Products include:
Ortho Dienestrol Cream 2554

Diethylstilbestrol (Co-administration with drugs that tend to produce hyperglycemia, such as estrogens, may lead to loss of blood glucose control).
No products indexed under this heading.

Diflunisal (The hypoglycemic action of sulfonylureas may be potentiated by salicylates). Products include:
Dolobid Tablets 2088

Digoxin (Co-administration with cationic drugs that are eliminated by renal tubular secretion have the theoretical potential for interacting with metformin by competing for common renal tubular transport systems). Products include:
Digitek Tablets 1003
Lanoxicaps Capsules 1574
Lanoxin Injection 1581
Lanoxin Tablets 1587
Lanoxin Elixir Pediatric 1578
Lanoxin Injection Pediatric 1584

Diltiazem Hydrochloride (Co-administration with drugs that tend to produce hyperglycemia, such as calcium channel blockers, may lead to loss of blood glucose control). Products include:
Cardizem Injectable 1018
Cardizem Lyo-Ject Syringe 1018
Cardizem Monovial 1018
Cardizem CD Capsules 1016
Tiazac Capsules 1378

Dobutamine Hydrochloride (Co-administration with drugs that tend to produce hyperglycemia, such as sympathomimetics, may lead to loss of blood glucose control). Products include:
Dobutrex Solution Vials 1914

Dopamine Hydrochloride (Co-administration with drugs that tend to produce hyperglycemia, such as sympathomimetics, may lead to loss of blood glucose control).
No products indexed under this heading.

Ephedrine Hydrochloride (Co-administration with drugs that tend to produce hyperglycemia, such as sympathomimetics, may lead to loss of blood glucose control). Products include:
Primatene Tablets .... ▣780

Ephedrine Sulfate (Co-administration with drugs that tend to produce hyperglycemia, such as sympathomimetics, may lead to loss of blood glucose control).
No products indexed under this heading.

Ephedrine Tannate (Co-administration with drugs that tend to produce hyperglycemia, such as sympathomimetics, may lead to loss of blood glucose control). Products include:
Rynatuss Pediatric Suspension 3353
Rynatuss Tablets 3353

Epinephrine (Co-administration with drugs that tend to produce hyperglycemia, such as sympathomimetics, may lead to loss of blood glucose control). Products include:
Epifrin Sterile Ophthalmic Solution .... ⊙235
EpiPen 1236
Primatene Mist .... ▣779
Xylocaine with Epinephrine Injection 653

Epinephrine Bitartrate (Co-administration with drugs that tend to produce hyperglycemia, such as sympathomimetics, may lead to loss of blood glucose control). Products include:
Sensorcaine 643

Epinephrine Hydrochloride (Co-administration with drugs that tend to produce hyperglycemia, such as sympathomimetics, may lead to loss of blood glucose control).
No products indexed under this heading.

Esmolol Hydrochloride (The hypoglycemic action of sulfonylureas may be potentiated by beta adrenergic agents). Products include:
Brevibloc Injection 858

Estradiol (Co-administration with drugs that tend to produce hyperglycemia, such as estrogens, may lead to loss of blood glucose control). Products include:
Activella Tablets 2764
Alora Transdermal System 3372
Climara Transdermal System 958
CombiPatch Transdermal System .. 2323
Esclim Transdermal System 3460
Estrace Vaginal Cream 3358
Estrace Tablets 3361
Estring Vaginal Ring 2811
Ortho-Prefest Tablets 2570
Vagifem Tablets 2857
Vivelle Transdermal System 2412
Vivelle-Dot Transdermal System 2416

Estrogens, Conjugated (Co-administration with drugs that tend to produce hyperglycemia, such as estrogens, may lead to loss of blood glucose control). Products include:
Premarin Intravenous 3563
Premarin Tablets 3566
Premarin Vaginal Cream 3570
Premphase Tablets 3572
Prempro Tablets 3572

Estrogens, Esterified (Co-administration with drugs that tend to produce hyperglycemia, such as estrogens, may lead to loss of blood glucose control). Products include:
Estratest 3252
Menest Tablets 2254

Estropipate (Co-administration with drugs that tend to produce hyperglycemia, such as estrogens, may lead to loss of blood glucose control). Products include:
Ogen Tablets 2846
Ortho-Est Tablets 3464

Ethacrynic Acid (Co-administration with drugs that tend to produce hyperglycemia, such as diuretics, may lead to loss of blood glucose control). Products include:
Edecrin Tablets 2091

Ethinyl Estradiol (Co-administration with drugs that tend to produce hyperglycemia, such as oral contraceptives, may lead to loss of blood glucose control). Products include:
Alesse-21 Tablets 3468
Alesse-28 Tablets 3473
Brevicon 28-Day Tablets 3380
Cyclessa Tablets 2450
Desogen Tablets 2458
Estinyl Tablets 3112
Estrostep 2627
femhrt Tablets 2635
Levlen 962
Levlite 21 Tablets 962
Levlite 28 Tablets 962
Levora Tablets 3389
Loestrin 21 Tablets 2642
Loestrin Fe Tablets 2642
Lo/Ovral Tablets 3532
Lo/Ovral-28 Tablets 3538
Low-Ogestrel-28 Tablets 3392

Microgestin Fe 1.5/30 Tablets 3407
Microgestin Fe 1/20 Tablets 3400
Mircette Tablets 2470
Modicon 2563
Necon 3415
Nordette-28 Tablets 2257
Norinyl 1 +35 28-Day Tablets 3380
Ogestrel 0.5/50-28 Tablets 3428
Ortho-Cept 21 Tablets 2546
Ortho-Cept 28 Tablets 2546
Ortho-Cyclen/Ortho Tri-Cyclen 2573
Ortho-Novum 2563
Ovcon 3364
Ovral Tablets 3551
Ovral-28 Tablets 3552
Tri-Levlen 962
Tri-Norinyl-28 Tablets 3433
Triphasil-21 Tablets 3600
Triphasil-28 Tablets 3605
Trivora Tablets 3439
Yasmin 28 Tablets 980
Zovia 3449

Ethiodized Oil (Potential for acute alteration of renal function; metformin should be temporarily withheld in patients undergoing radiologic studies involving iodinated contrast material). Products include:
Ethiodol Injection 3095

Ethynodiol Diacetate (Co-administration with drugs that tend to produce hyperglycemia, such as oral contraceptives, may lead to loss of blood glucose control). Products include:
Zovia 3449

Etodolac (The hypoglycemic action of sulfonylureas may be potentiated by non-steroidal anti-inflammatory agents). Products include:
Lodine 3528
Lodine XL Extended-Release Tablets 3530

Felodipine (Co-administration with drugs that tend to produce hyperglycemia, such as calcium channel blockers, may lead to loss of blood glucose control). Products include:
Lexxel Tablets 608
Plendil Extended-Release Tablets 623

Fenoprofen Calcium (The hypoglycemic action of sulfonylureas may be potentiated by non-steroidal anti-inflammatory agents).
No products indexed under this heading.

Fludrocortisone Acetate (Co-administration with drugs that tend to produce hyperglycemia, such as corticosteroids, may lead to loss of blood glucose control). Products include:
Florinef Acetate Tablets 2250

Fluphenazine Decanoate (Co-administration with drugs that tend to produce hyperglycemia, such as phenothiazines, may lead to loss of blood glucose control).
No products indexed under this heading.

Fluphenazine Enanthate (Co-administration with drugs that tend to produce hyperglycemia, such as phenothiazines, may lead to loss of blood glucose control).
No products indexed under this heading.

Fluphenazine Hydrochloride (Co-administration with drugs that tend to produce hyperglycemia, such as phenothiazines, may lead to loss of blood glucose control).
No products indexed under this heading.

Flurbiprofen (The hypoglycemic action of sulfonylureas may be potentiated by non-steroidal anti-inflammatory agents).
No products indexed under this heading.

Fosphenytoin Sodium (Co-administration with drugs that tend to produce hyperglycemia, such as phenytoin, may lead to loss of blood glucose control). Products include:
Cerebyx Injection 2619

Furosemide (Co-administration of furosemide with metformin has resulted in increased plasma and blood Cmax and AUC of metformin; furosemide's Cmax and AUC were smaller and terminal half-life was decreased). Products include:
Furosemide Tablets 2284

Gadopentetate Dimeglumine (Potential for acute alteration of renal function; metformin should be temporarily withheld in patients undergoing radiologic studies involving iodinated contrast material).
No products indexed under this heading.

Glipizide (The hypoglycemic action of sulfonylureas may be potentiated by sulfonamides). Products include:
Glucotrol Tablets 2692
Glucotrol XL Extended Release Tablets 2693

Hydrochlorothiazide (Co-administration with drugs that tend to produce hyperglycemia, such as thiazides, may lead to loss of blood glucose control). Products include:
Accuretic Tablets 2614
Aldoril Tablets 2039
Atacand HCT Tablets 597
Avalide Tablets 1070
Diovan HCT Tablets 2338
Dyazide Capsules 1515
HydroDIURIL Tablets 2108
Hyzaar 2109
Inderide Tablets 3517
Inderide LA Long-Acting Capsules .. 3519
Lotensin HCT Tablets 2367
Maxzide 1008
Micardis HCT Tablets 1051
Microzide Capsules 3414
Moduretic Tablets 2138
Monopril HCT 1094
Prinzide Tablets 2168
Timolide Tablets 2187
Uniretic Tablets 3178
Vaseretic Tablets 2204
Zestoretic Tablets 695
Ziac Tablets 1887

Hydrocortisone (Co-administration with drugs that tend to produce hyperglycemia, such as corticosteroids, may lead to loss of blood glucose control). Products include:
Anusol-HC Cream 2.5% 2237
Cipro HC Otic Suspension 540
Cortaid Intensive Therapy Cream . ■717
Cortaid Maximum Strength Cream .... ■717
Cortisporin Ophthalmic Suspension Sterile .... ⊙297
Cortizone•5 .... ■699
Cortizone•10 .... ■699
Cortizone•10 Plus Creme .... ■700
Cortizone for Kids Creme .... ■699
Hydrocortone Tablets 2106
Massengill Medicated Soft Cloth Towelette .... ■753
VōSoL HC Otic Solution 3356

Hydrocortisone Acetate (Co-administration with drugs that tend to produce hyperglycemia, such as corticosteroids, may lead to loss of blood glucose control). Products include:
Analpram-HC 1338
Anusol HC-1 Hydrocortisone Anti-Itch Cream .... ■689
Anusol-HC Suppositories 2238
Cortaid .... ■717
Cortifoam Rectal Foam 3170
Cortisporin-TC Otic Suspension 2246
Hydrocortone Acetate Injectable Suspension 2103
Pramosone 1343
Proctocort Suppositories 2264
ProctoFoam-HC 3177
Terra-Cortril Ophthalmic Suspension 2716

Hydrocortisone Sodium Phosphate (Co-administration with drugs that tend to produce hyperglycemia, such as corticosteroids, may lead to loss of blood glucose control). Products include:
Hydrocortone Phosphate Injection, Sterile 2105

Hydrocortisone Sodium Succinate (Co-administration with drugs that tend to produce hyperglycemia, such as corticosteroids, may lead to loss of blood glucose control).
No products indexed under this heading.

Hydroflumethiazide (Co-administration with drugs that tend to produce hyperglycemia, such as thiazides, may lead to loss of blood glucose control). Products include:
Diucardin Tablets 3494

Ibuprofen (The hypoglycemic action of sulfonylureas may be potentiated by non-steroidal anti-inflammatory agents). Products include:
Advil .... ■771
Children's Advil Oral Suspension ... ■773
Children's Advil Chewable Tablets . ■773
Advil Cold and Sinus Caplets .... ■771
Advil Cold and Sinus Tablets .... ■771
Advil Flu & Body Ache Caplets ...... ■772
Infants' Advil Drops .... ■773
Junior Strength Advil Tablets .... ■773
Junior Strength Advil Chewable Tablets .... ■773
Advil Migraine Liquigels .... ■772
Children's Motrin Oral Suspension and Chewable Tablets 2006
Children's Motrin Cold Oral Suspension 2007
Children's Motrin Oral Suspension .... ■643
Motrin Suspension, Oral Drops, Chewable Tablets, and Caplets 2002
Infants' Motrin Concentrated Drops 2006
Junior Strength Motrin Caplets and Chewable Tablets 2006
Motrin IB Tablets, Caplets, and Gelcaps 2002
Motrin Migraine Pain Caplets 2005
Motrin Sinus Headache Caplets 2005
Vicoprofen Tablets 520

Indapamide (Co-administration with drugs that tend to produce hyperglycemia, such as diuretics, may lead to loss of blood glucose control). Products include:
Indapamide Tablets 2286

Indomethacin (The hypoglycemic action of sulfonylureas may be potentiated by non-steroidal anti-inflammatory agents). Products include:
Indocin 2112

Indomethacin Sodium Trihydrate (The hypoglycemic action of sulfonylureas may be potentiated by non-steroidal anti-inflammatory agents). Products include:
Indocin I.V. 2115

Iodamide Meglumine (Potential for acute alteration of renal function; metformin should be temporarily withheld in patients undergoing radiologic studies involving iodinated contrast material).
No products indexed under this heading.

Iohexol (Potential for acute alteration of renal function; metformin should be temporarily withheld in patients undergoing radiologic studies involving iodinated contrast material).
No products indexed under this heading.

Iopamidol (Potential for acute alteration of renal function; metformin should be temporarily withheld in patients undergoing radiologic studies involving iodinated contrast material).
No products indexed under this heading.

Iopanoic Acid (Potential for acute alteration of renal function; metformin should be temporarily withheld in patients undergoing radiologic studies involving iodinated contrast material).
No products indexed under this heading.

Iothalamate Meglumine (Potential for acute alteration of renal function; metformin should be temporarily withheld in patients undergoing radiologic studies involving iodinated contrast material).
No products indexed under this heading.

Ioxaglate Meglumine (Potential for acute alteration of renal function; metformin should be temporarily withheld in patients undergoing radiologic studies involving iodinated contrast material).
No products indexed under this heading.

Ioxaglate Sodium (Potential for acute alteration of renal function; metformin should be temporarily withheld in patients undergoing radiologic studies involving iodinated contrast material).
No products indexed under this heading.

Isocarboxazid (The hypoglycemic action of sulfonylureas may be potentiated by MAO inhibitors).
No products indexed under this heading.

Isoniazid (Co-administration with drugs that tend to produce hyperglycemia, such as isoniazid, may lead to loss of blood glucose control). Products include:
Rifamate Capsules 767
Rifater Tablets 769

Isoproterenol Hydrochloride (Co-administration with drugs that tend to produce hyperglycemia, such as sympathomimetics, may lead to loss of blood glucose control).
No products indexed under this heading.

Isoproterenol Sulfate (Co-administration with drugs that tend to produce hyperglycemia, such as sympathomimetics, may lead to loss of blood glucose control).
No products indexed under this heading.

Isradipine (Co-administration with drugs that tend to produce hyperglycemia, such as calcium channel blockers, may lead to loss of blood glucose control). Products include:
DynaCirc Capsules 2921
DynaCirc CR Tablets 2923

Ketoprofen (The hypoglycemic action of sulfonylureas may be potentiated by non-steroidal anti-inflammatory agents). Products include:
Orudis Capsules 3548
Orudis KT Tablets .... ■778
Oruvail Capsules 3548

Ketorolac Tromethamine (The hypoglycemic action of sulfonylureas may be potentiated by non-steroidal anti-inflammatory agents). Products include:
Acular Ophthalmic Solution 544
Acular PF Ophthalmic Solution 544
Toradol 3018

Labetalol Hydrochloride (The hypoglycemic action of sulfonylureas may be potentiated by beta adrenergic agents). Products include:
Normodyne Injection 3135
Normodyne Tablets 3137

Levalbuterol Hydrochloride (Co-administration with drugs that tend to produce hyperglycemia, such as sympathomimetics, may lead to loss of blood glucose control). Products include:
Xopenex Inhalation Solution 3207

Levobunolol Hydrochloride (The hypoglycemic action of sulfonylureas may be potentiated by beta adrenergic agents). Products include:
Betagan .... ⊙228

Levonorgestrel (Co-administration with drugs that tend to produce hyperglycemia, such as oral contraceptives, may lead to loss of blood glucose control). Products include:
Alesse-21 Tablets 3468
Alesse-28 Tablets 3473
Levlen 962
Levlite 21 Tablets 962

Levlite 28 Tablets 962
Levora Tablets 3389
Mirena Intrauterine System 974
Nordette-28 Tablets 2257
Norplant System 3543
Tri-Levlen 962
Triphasil-21 Tablets 3600
Triphasil-28 Tablets 3605
Trivora Tablets 3439

Levothyroxine Sodium (Co-administration with drugs that tend to produce hyperglycemia, such as thyroid products, may lead to loss of blood glucose control). Products include:
Levothroid Tablets 1373
Levoxyl Tablets 1819
Synthroid 505
Unithroid Tablets 3445

Liothyronine Sodium (Co-administration with drugs that tend to produce hyperglycemia, such as thyroid products, may lead to loss of blood glucose control). Products include:
Cytomel Tablets 1817
Triostat Injection 1825

Liotrix (Co-administration with drugs that tend to produce hyperglycemia, such as thyroid products, may lead to loss of blood glucose control).
No products indexed under this heading.

Magnesium Salicylate (The hypoglycemic action of sulfonylureas may be potentiated by salicylates). Products include:
Momentum Backache Relief Extra Strength Caplets .... ■666

Meclofenamate Sodium (The hypoglycemic action of sulfonylureas may be potentiated by non-steroidal anti-inflammatory agents).
No products indexed under this heading.

Mefenamic Acid (The hypoglycemic action of sulfonylureas may be potentiated by non-steroidal anti-inflammatory agents). Products include:
Ponstel Capsules 1356

Meloxicam (The hypoglycemic action of sulfonylureas may be potentiated by non-steroidal anti-inflammatory agents). Products include:
Mobic Tablets 1054

Mesoridazine Besylate (Co-administration with drugs that tend to produce hyperglycemia, such as phenothiazines, may lead to loss of blood glucose control). Products include:
Serentil 1057

Mestranol (Co-administration with drugs that tend to produce hyperglycemia, such as oral contraceptives, may lead to loss of blood glucose control). Products include:
Necon 1/50 Tablets 3415
Norinyl 1 + 50 28-Day Tablets 3380
Ortho-Novum 1/50□28 Tablets 2556

Metaproterenol Sulfate (Co-administration with drugs that tend to produce hyperglycemia, such as sympathomimetics, may lead to loss of blood glucose control). Products include:
Alupent 1029

Metaraminol Bitartrate (Co-administration with drugs that tend to produce hyperglycemia, such as sympathomimetics, may lead to loss of blood glucose control). Products include:
Aramine Injection 2043

Methotrimeprazine (Co-administration with drugs that tend to produce hyperglycemia, such as phenothiazines, may lead to loss of blood glucose control).
No products indexed under this heading.

Methoxamine Hydrochloride (Co-administration with drugs that tend to produce hyperglycemia, such as sympathomimetics, may lead to loss of blood glucose control).
No products indexed under this heading.

Methyclothiazide (Co-administration with drugs that tend to produce hyperglycemia, such as thiazides, may lead to loss of blood glucose control).
No products indexed under this heading.

Methylprednisolone Acetate (Co-administration with drugs that tend to produce hyperglycemia, such as corticosteroids, may lead to loss of blood glucose control). Products include:
Depo-Medrol Injectable Suspension 2795

Methylprednisolone Sodium Succinate (Co-administration with drugs that tend to produce hyperglycemia, such as corticosteroids, may lead to loss of blood glucose control). Products include:
Solu-Medrol Sterile Powder 2855

Metipranolol Hydrochloride (The hypoglycemic action of sulfonylureas may be potentiated by beta adrenergic agents).
No products indexed under this heading.

Metolazone (Co-administration with drugs that tend to produce hyperglycemia, such as diuretics, may lead to loss of blood glucose control). Products include:
Mykrox Tablets 1168
Zaroxolyn Tablets 1177

Metoprolol Succinate (The hypoglycemic action of sulfonylureas may be potentiated by beta adrenergic agents). Products include:
Toprol-XL Tablets 651

Metoprolol Tartrate (The hypoglycemic action of sulfonylureas may be potentiated by beta adrenergic agents).
No products indexed under this heading.

Mibefradil Dihydrochloride (Co-administration with drugs that tend to produce hyperglycemia, such as calcium channel blockers, may lead to loss of blood glucose control).
No products indexed under this heading.

Miconazole (Co-administration of oral hypoglycemic agents and oral miconazole has resulted in severe hypoglycemia).
No products indexed under this heading.

Moclobemide (The hypoglycemic action of sulfonylureas may be potentiated by MAO inhibitors).
No products indexed under this heading.

Morphine Sulfate (Co-administration with cationic drugs that are eliminated by renal tubular secretion have the theoretical potential for interacting with metformin by competing for common renal tubular transport systems). Products include:
Astramorph/PF Injection, USP (Preservative-Free) 594
Duramorph Injection 1312
Infumorph 200 and Infumorph 500 Sterile Solutions 1314
Kadian Capsules 1335
MS Contin Tablets 2896
MSIR 2898
Oramorph SR Tablets 3062
Roxanol 3066

Nabumetone (The hypoglycemic action of sulfonylureas may be potentiated by non-steroidal anti-inflammatory agents). Products include:
Relafen Tablets 1617

Nadolol (The hypoglycemic action of sulfonylureas may be potentiated by beta adrenergic agents). Products include:
Corgard Tablets 2245
Corzide 40/5 Tablets 2247
Corzide 80/5 Tablets 2247
Nadolol Tablets 2288

Naproxen (The hypoglycemic action of sulfonylureas may be potentiated by non-steroidal anti-inflammatory agents). Products include:
EC-Naprosyn Delayed-Release Tablets 2967
Naprosyn Suspension 2967
Naprosyn Tablets 2967

Naproxen Sodium (The hypoglycemic action of sulfonylureas may be potentiated by non-steroidal anti-inflammatory agents). Products include:
Aleve Tablets, Caplets and Gelcaps .... ■602
Aleve Cold & Sinus Caplets .... ■603
Anaprox Tablets 2967
Anaprox DS Tablets 2967
Naprelan Tablets 1293

Niacin (Co-administration with drugs that tend to produce hyperglycemia, such as niacin, may lead to loss of blood glucose control). Products include:
Niaspan Extended-Release Tablets 1846
Nicotinex Elixir .... ■633

Nicardipine Hydrochloride (Co-administration with drugs that tend to produce hyperglycemia, such as calcium channel blockers, may lead to loss of blood glucose control). Products include:
Cardene I.V. 3485

Nicotinic Acid (Co-administration with drugs that tend to produce hyperglycemia, such as nicotinic acid, may lead to loss of blood glucose control).
No products indexed under this heading.

Nifedipine (Co-administration with nifedipine has resulted in increased plasma metformin Cmax and AUC and increased the amount excreted in the urine). Products include:
Adalat CC Tablets 877
Procardia Capsules 2708
Procardia XL Extended Release Tablets 2710

Nimodipine (Co-administration with drugs that tend to produce hyperglycemia, such as calcium channel blockers, may lead to loss of blood glucose control). Products include:
Nimotop Capsules 904

Nisoldipine (Co-administration with drugs that tend to produce hyperglycemia, such as calcium channel blockers, may lead to loss of blood glucose control). Products include:
Sular Tablets 688

Norepinephrine Bitartrate (Co-administration with drugs that tend to produce hyperglycemia, such as sympathomimetics, may lead to loss of blood glucose control).
No products indexed under this heading.

Norethindrone (Co-administration with drugs that tend to produce hyperglycemia, such as oral contraceptives, may lead to loss of blood glucose control). Products include:
Brevicon 28-Day Tablets 3380
Micronor Tablets 2543
Modicon 2563
Necon 3415
Norinyl 1 +35 28-Day Tablets 3380
Norinyl 1 + 50 28-Day Tablets 3380
Nor-QD Tablets 3423
Ortho-Novum 2563
Ortho-Novum 1/50□28 Tablets 2556
Ovcon 3364
Tri-Norinyl-28 Tablets 3433

Norethynodrel (Co-administration with drugs that tend to produce hyperglycemia, such as oral contraceptives, may lead to loss of blood glucose control).
No products indexed under this heading.

Norgestimate (Co-administration with drugs that tend to produce hyperglycemia, such as oral contraceptives, may lead to loss of blood glucose control). Products include:
Ortho-Cyclen/Ortho Tri-Cyclen 2573
Ortho-Prefest Tablets 2570

Norgestrel (Co-administration with drugs that tend to produce hyperglycemia, such as oral contraceptives, may lead to loss of blood glucose control). Products include:
Lo/Ovral Tablets 3532
Lo/Ovral-28 Tablets 3538
Low-Ogestrel-28 Tablets 3392
Ogestrel 0.5/50-28 Tablets 3428
Ovral Tablets 3551
Ovral-28 Tablets 3552
Ovrette Tablets 3552

Oxaprozin (The hypoglycemic action of sulfonylureas may be potentiated by non-steroidal anti-inflammatory agents).
No products indexed under this heading.

Pargyline Hydrochloride (The hypoglycemic action of sulfonylureas may be potentiated by MAO inhibitors).
No products indexed under this heading.

Penbutolol Sulfate (The hypoglycemic action of sulfonylureas may be potentiated by beta adrenergic agents).
No products indexed under this heading.

Perphenazine (Co-administration with drugs that tend to produce hyperglycemia, such as phenothiazines, may lead to loss of blood glucose control). Products include:
Etrafon 3115
Trilafon 3160

Phenelzine Sulfate (The hypoglycemic action of sulfonylureas may be potentiated by MAO inhibitors). Products include:
Nardil Tablets 2653

Phenylbutazone (The hypoglycemic action of sulfonylureas may be potentiated by non-steroidal anti-inflammatory agents).
No products indexed under this heading.

Phenylephrine Bitartrate (Co-administration with drugs that tend to produce hyperglycemia, such as sympathomimetics, may lead to loss of blood glucose control).
No products indexed under this heading.

Phenylephrine Hydrochloride (Co-administration with drugs that tend to produce hyperglycemia, such as sympathomimetics, may lead to loss of blood glucose control). Products include:
Afrin Nasal Decongestant Children's Pump Mist .... ■734
Extendryl 1361
Hycomine Compound Tablets 1317
Neo-Synephrine .... ■614
Phenergan VC Syrup 3560
Phenergan VC with Codeine Syrup 3561
Preparation H Cream .... ■778
Preparation H Cooling Gel .... ■778
Preparation H .... ■778
Vicks Sinex Nasal Spray and Ultra Fine Mist .... ■729

Phenylephrine Tannate (Co-administration with drugs that tend to produce hyperglycemia, such as sympathomimetics, may lead to loss of blood glucose control). Products include:
Ryna-12 S Suspension 3351
Reformulated Rynatan Pediatric Suspension 3352
Rynatuss Pediatric Suspension 3353
Rynatuss Tablets 3353

Phenylpropanolamine Hydrochloride (Co-administration with drugs that tend to produce hyperglycemia, such as sympathomimetics, may lead to loss of blood glucose control).
No products indexed under this heading.

Phenytoin (Co-administration with drugs that tend to produce hyperglycemia, such as phenytoin, may lead to loss of blood glucose control). Products include:
Dilantin Infatabs ... 2624
Dilantin-125 Oral Suspension ... 2625

Phenytoin Sodium (Co-administration with drugs that tend to produce hyperglycemia, such as phenytoin, may lead to loss of blood glucose control). Products include:
Dilantin Kapseals ... 2622

Pindolol (The hypoglycemic action of sulfonylureas may be potentiated by beta adrenergic agents).
No products indexed under this heading.

Pirbuterol Acetate (Co-administration with drugs that tend to produce hyperglycemia, such as sympathomimetics, may lead to loss of blood glucose control). Products include:
Maxair Autohaler ... 1981
Maxair Inhaler ... 1984

Piroxicam (The hypoglycemic action of sulfonylureas may be potentiated by non-steroidal anti-inflammatory agents). Products include:
Feldene Capsules ... 2685

Polyestradiol Phosphate (Co-administration with drugs that tend to produce hyperglycemia, such as estrogens, may lead to loss of blood glucose control).
No products indexed under this heading.

Polythiazide (Co-administration with drugs that tend to produce hyperglycemia, such as thiazides, may lead to loss of blood glucose control). Products include:
Minizide Capsules ... 2700
Renese Tablets ... 2712

Prednisolone Acetate (Co-administration with drugs that tend to produce hyperglycemia, such as corticosteroids, may lead to loss of blood glucose control). Products include:
Blephamide Ophthalmic Ointment ... 547
Blephamide Ophthalmic Suspension ... 548
Poly-Pred Liquifilm Ophthalmic Suspension ... ⊙245
Pred Forte Ophthalmic Suspension ... ⊙246
Pred Mild Sterile Ophthalmic Suspension ... ⊙249
Pred-G Ophthalmic Suspension ... ⊙247
Pred-G Sterile Ophthalmic Ointment ... ⊙248

Prednisolone Sodium Phosphate (Co-administration with drugs that tend to produce hyperglycemia, such as corticosteroids, may lead to loss of blood glucose control). Products include:
Pediapred Oral Solution ... 1170

Prednisolone Tebutate (Co-administration with drugs that tend to produce hyperglycemia, such as corticosteroids, may lead to loss of blood glucose control).
No products indexed under this heading.

Prednisone (Co-administration with drugs that tend to produce hyperglycemia, such as corticosteroids, may lead to loss of blood glucose control). Products include:
Prednisone ... 3064

Probenecid (The hypoglycemic action of sulfonylureas may be potentiated by probenecid).
No products indexed under this heading.

Procainamide Hydrochloride (Co-administration with cationic drugs that are eliminated by renal tubular secretion have the theoretical potential for interacting with metformin by competing for common renal tubular transport systems). Products include:
Procanbid Extended-Release Tablets ... 2262

Procarbazine Hydrochloride (The hypoglycemic action of sulfonylureas may be potentiated by MAO inhibitors). Products include:
Matulane Capsules ... 3246

Prochlorperazine (Co-administration with drugs that tend to produce hyperglycemia, such as phenothiazines, may lead to loss of blood glucose control). Products include:
Compazine ... 1505

Promethazine Hydrochloride (Co-administration with drugs that tend to produce hyperglycemia, such as phenothiazines, may lead to loss of blood glucose control). Products include:
Mepergan Injection ... 3539
Phenergan Injection ... 3553
Phenergan ... 3556
Phenergan Syrup ... 3554
Phenergan with Codeine Syrup ... 3557
Phenergan with Dextromethorphan Syrup ... 3559
Phenergan VC Syrup ... 3560
Phenergan VC with Codeine Syrup ... 3561

Propranolol Hydrochloride (The hypoglycemic action of sulfonylureas may be potentiated by beta adrenergic agents). Products include:
Inderal ... 3513
Inderal LA Long-Acting Capsules ... 3516
Inderide Tablets ... 3517
Inderide LA Long-Acting Capsules ... 3519

Pseudoephedrine Hydrochloride (Co-administration with drugs that tend to produce hyperglycemia, such as sympathomimetics, may lead to loss of blood glucose control). Products include:
Actifed Cold & Allergy Tablets ... 688
Actifed Cold & Sinus Caplets and Tablets ... 688
Advil Cold and Sinus Caplets ... 771
Advil Cold and Sinus Tablets ... 771
Advil Flu & Body Ache Caplets ... 772
Aleve Cold & Sinus Caplets ... 603
Alka-Seltzer Plus Liqui-Gels ... 604
Alka-Seltzer Plus Cold & Flu Medicine Liqui-Gels ... 604
Alka-Seltzer Plus Cold & Sinus Medicine Liqui-Gels ... 604
Allegra-D Extended-Release Tablets ... 714
BC Cold Powder ... 619
Benadryl Allergy/Cold Tablets ... 691
Benadryl Allergy/Congestion Tablets ... 692
Benadryl Allergy & Sinus Liquid ... 693
Benadryl Allergy & Sinus Fastmelt Tablets ... 693
Benadryl Allergy Sinus Headache Caplets & Gelcaps ... 693
Benadryl Severe Allergy & Sinus Headache Caplets ... 694
Benadryl Children's Allergy/Cold Fastmelt Tablets ... 692
Benylin Multi-Symptom Liquid ... 697
Bromfed Capsules (Extended-Release) ... 2269
Bromfed-PD Capsules (Extended-Release) ... 2269
Children's Cēpacol Sore Throat ... 788
Comtrex Acute Head Cold & Sinus Pressure Relief Tablets ... 627
Comtrex Deep Chest Cold & Congestion Relief Softgels ... 627
Comtrex Flu Therapy & Fever Relief Daytime Caplets ... 628
Comtrex Flu Therapy & Fever Relief Nighttime Tablets ... 628
Comtrex Maximum Strength Multi-Symptom Cold & Cough Relief Tablets and Caplets ... 626
Contac Non-Drowsy 12 Hour Cold Caplets ... 745
Contac Non-Drowsy Timed Release 12 Hour Cold Caplets ... 746
Contac Severe Cold and Flu Caplets Maximum Strength ... 746
Contac Severe Cold and Flu Caplets Non-Drowsy ... 746
Dimetapp Elixir ... 777
Dimetapp Cold and Fever Suspension ... 775
Dimetapp DM Cold & Cough Elixir ... 775
Dimetapp Nighttime Flu Liquid ... 776
Dimetapp Non-Drowsy Flu Syrup ... 777
Dimetapp Infant Drops Decongestant ... 775
Dimetapp Infant Drops Decongestant Plus Cough ... 776
Guaifed ... 2272
Kronofed-A ... 1341
Children's Motrin Cold Oral Suspension ... 2007
Motrin Sinus Headache Caplets ... 2005
PediaCare Cough-Cold Liquid ... 719
PediaCare Infants' Drops Decongestant ... 719
PediaCare Infants' Drops Decongestant Plus Cough ... 719
PediaCare NightRest Cough-Cold Liquid ... 719
Robitussin Cold Caplets Cold & Congestion ... 780
Robitussin Cold Softgels Cold & Congestion ... 780
Robitussin Cold Caplets Multi-Symptom Cold & Flu ... 781
Robitussin Cold Softgels Multi-Symptom Cold & Flu ... 781
Robitussin Cold Softgels Severe Congestion ... 782
Robitussin Cough & Cold Infant Drops ... 782
Robitussin Maximum Strength Cough & Cold Liquid ... 785
Robitussin Pediatric Cough & Cold Formula Liquid ... 785
Robitussin Multi Symptom Honey Flu Liquid ... 785
Robitussin Nighttime Honey Flu Liquid ... 786
Robitussin-CF Liquid ... 783
Robitussin-DAC Syrup ... 2942
Robitussin-PE Liquid ... 782
Ryna ... 768
Semprex-D Capsules ... 1172
Singlet Caplets ... 761
Sinutab Non-Drying Liquid Caps ... 706
Sinutab Sinus Allergy Medication, Maximum Strength Formula, Tablets & Caplets ... 707
Sinutab Sinus Medication, Maximum Strength Without Drowsiness Formula, Tablets & Caplets ... 707
Sudafed 12 Hour Tablets ... 708
Sudafed 24 Hour Tablets ... 708
Children's Sudafed Cold & Cough Liquid ... 709
Children's Sudafed Nasal Decongestant Chewables ... 711
Children's Sudafed Nasal Decongestant Liquid Medication ... 711
Sudafed Cold & Allergy Tablets ... 708
Sudafed Cold & Cough Liquid Caps ... 709
Sudafed Cold & Sinus Liquid Caps ... 710
Sudafed Nasal Decongestant Tablets ... 710
Sudafed Non-Drying Sinus Liquid Caps ... 712
Sudafed Severe Cold ... 711
Sudafed Sinus Headache Caplets ... 712
Sudafed Sinus Headache Tablets ... 712
Tavist Sinus Non-Drowsy Coated Caplets ... 676
TheraFlu Regular Strength Cold & Cough Night Time Hot Liquid ... 676
TheraFlu Regular Strength Cold & Sore Throat Night Time Hot Liquid ... 676
TheraFlu Maximum Strength Flu & Congestion Non-Drowsy Hot Liquid ... 677
TheraFlu Maximum Strength Flu & Cough Night Time Hot Liquid ... 678
TheraFlu Maximum Strength Flu & Sore Throat Night Time Hot Liquid ... 677
TheraFlu Maximum Strength Severe Cold & Congestion Night Time Caplets ... 678
TheraFlu Maximum Strength Severe Cold & Congestion Night Time Hot Liquid ... 678
TheraFlu Maximum Strength Severe Cold & Congestion Non-Drowsy ... 679
Triaminic Allergy Congestion Liquid ... 680
Triaminic Chest Congestion Liquid ... 680
Triaminic Cold & Allergy Liquid ... 681
Triaminic Cold & Allergy Softchews ... 683
Triaminic Cold & Cough Liquid ... 681
Triaminic Cold & Cough Softchews ... 683
Triaminic Cold & Night Time Cough Liquid ... 681
Triaminic Cold, Cough & Fever Liquid ... 681
Triaminic Cough Liquid ... 682
Triaminic Cough & Congestion Liquid ... 682
Triaminic Cough & Sore Throat Liquid ... 682
Triaminic Cough & Sore Throat Softchews ... 684
Children's Tylenol Allergy-D Liquid ... 2014
Children's Tylenol Cold Suspension Liquid and Chewable Tablets ... 2015
Children's Tylenol Cold Plus Cough Suspension Liquid and Chewable Tablets ... 2015
Children's Tylenol Flu Suspension Liquid ... 2015
Children's Tylenol Sinus Suspension Liquid ... 2017
Infants' Tylenol Cold Decongestant and Fever Reducer Concentrated Drops ... 2015
Infants' Tylenol Cold Decongestant and Fever Reducer Concentrated Drops Plus Cough ... 2015
Tylenol Allergy Sinus ... 2010
Multi-Symptom Tylenol Cold Complete Formula Caplets ... 2010
Multi-Symptom Tylenol Cold Non-Drowsy Caplets and Gelcaps ... 2010
Multi-Symptom Tylenol Cold Severe Congestion Non-Drowsy Caplets ... 2011
Maximum Strength Tylenol Flu NightTime Gelcaps ... 2011
Maximum Strength Tylenol Flu NightTime Liquid ... 2011
Maximum Strength Tylenol Flu Non-Drowsy Gelcaps ... 2011
Maximum Strength Tylenol Sinus NightTime Caplets ... 2012
Maximum Strength Tylenol Sinus Non-Drowsy Geltabs, Gelcaps, Caplets, and Tablets ... 2012
Vicks 44D Cough & Head Congestion Relief Liquid ... 724
Vicks 44M Cough, Cold & Flu Relief Liquid ... 725
Pediatric Vicks 44m Cough & Cold Relief ... 728
Vicks DayQuil LiquiCaps/Liquid Multi-Symptom Cold/Flu Relief ... 727
Children's Vicks NyQuil Cold/Cough Relief ... 726
Vicks NyQuil LiquiCaps/Liquid Multi-Symptom Cold/Flu Relief, Original and Cherry Flavors ... 727
Zephrex Tablets ... 3091
Zephrex LA Tablets ... 3092
Zyrtec-D 12 Hour Extended Relief Tablets ... 2758

Pseudoephedrine Sulfate (Co-administration with drugs that tend to produce hyperglycemia, such as sympathomimetics, may lead to loss of blood glucose control). Products include:
Chlor-Trimeton Allergy/Decongestant Tablets ... 736
Claritin-D 12 Hour Extended Release Tablets ... 3102
Claritin-D 24 Hour Extended Release Tablets ... 3104
Coricidin 'D' Cold, Flu & Sinus Tablets ... 737
Drixoral Allergy/Sinus Extended-Release Tablets ... 741
Drixoral Cold & Allergy Sustained-Action Tablets ... 740
Drixoral Cold & Flu Extended-Release Tablets ... 740
Drixoral Nasal Decongestant Long-Acting Non-Drowsy Tablets ... 740
Rynatan Tablets ... 3351

Quinestrol (Co-administration with drugs that tend to produce hyperglycemia, such as estrogens, may lead to loss of blood glucose control).
No products indexed under this heading.

IMPORTANT NOTE: Always consult each drug listing in the patient's regimen for possible interactions.

Quinidine Gluconate (Co-administration with cationic drugs that are eliminated by renal tubular secretion have the theoretical potential for interacting with metformin by competing for common renal tubular transport systems). Products include:
Quinaglute Dura-Tabs Tablets 978

Quinidine Polygalacturonate (Co-administration with cationic drugs that are eliminated by renal tubular secretion have the theoretical potential for interacting with metformin by competing for common renal tubular transport systems).
No products indexed under this heading.

Quinidine Sulfate (Co-administration with cationic drugs that are eliminated by renal tubular secretion have the theoretical potential for interacting with metformin by competing for common renal tubular transport systems). Products include:
Quinidex Extentabs 2933

Quinine Sulfate (Co-administration with cationic drugs that are eliminated by renal tubular secretion have the theoretical potential for interacting with metformin by competing for common renal tubular transport systems).
No products indexed under this heading.

Ranitidine Hydrochloride (Co-administration with cationic drugs that are eliminated by renal tubular secretion have the theoretical potential for interacting with metformin by competing for common renal tubular transport systems). Products include:
Zantac 1690
Zantac Injection 1688
Zantac 75 Tablets .... ▣717

Rofecoxib (The hypoglycemic action of sulfonylureas may be potentiated by non-steroidal anti-inflammatory agents). Products include:
Vioxx 2213

Salmeterol Xinafoate (Co-administration with drugs that tend to produce hyperglycemia, such as sympathomimetics, may lead to loss of blood glucose control). Products include:
Advair Diskus 100/50 1448
Advair Diskus 250/50 1448
Advair Diskus 500/50 1448
Serevent Diskus 1637
Serevent Inhalation Aerosol 1633

Salsalate (The hypoglycemic action of sulfonylureas may be potentiated by salicylates).
No products indexed under this heading.

Selegiline Hydrochloride (The hypoglycemic action of sulfonylureas may be potentiated by MAO inhibitors). Products include:
Eldepryl Capsules 3266

Sotalol Hydrochloride (The hypoglycemic action of sulfonylureas may be potentiated by beta adrenergic agents). Products include:
Betapace Tablets 950
Betapace AF Tablets 954

Spironolactone (Co-administration with drugs that tend to produce hyperglycemia, such as diuretics, may lead to loss of blood glucose control).
No products indexed under this heading.

Sulfacytine (The hypoglycemic action of sulfonylureas may be potentiated by sulfonamides).
No products indexed under this heading.

Sulfamethizole (The hypoglycemic action of sulfonylureas may be potentiated by sulfonamides). Products include:
Urobiotic-250 Capsules 2731

Sulfamethoxazole (The hypoglycemic action of sulfonylureas may be potentiated by sulfonamides). Products include:
Bactrim 2949
Septra Suspension 2265
Septra Tablets 2265
Septra DS Tablets 2265

Sulfasalazine (The hypoglycemic action of sulfonylureas may be potentiated by sulfonamides). Products include:
Azulfidine EN-tabs Tablets 2775

Sulfinpyrazone (The hypoglycemic action of sulfonylureas may be potentiated by sulfonamides).
No products indexed under this heading.

Sulfisoxazole (The hypoglycemic action of sulfonylureas may be potentiated by sulfonamides).
No products indexed under this heading.

Sulfisoxazole Acetyl (The hypoglycemic action of sulfonylureas may be potentiated by sulfonamides). Products include:
Pediazole Suspension 3050

Sulfisoxazole Diolamine (The hypoglycemic action of sulfonylureas may be potentiated by sulfonamides).
No products indexed under this heading.

Sulindac (The hypoglycemic action of sulfonylureas may be potentiated by non-steroidal anti-inflammatory agents). Products include:
Clinoril Tablets 2053

Terbutaline Sulfate (Co-administration with drugs that tend to produce hyperglycemia, such as sympathomimetics, may lead to loss of blood glucose control). Products include:
Brethine Ampuls 2314
Brethine Tablets 2313

Thioridazine Hydrochloride (Co-administration with drugs that tend to produce hyperglycemia, such as phenothiazines, may lead to loss of blood glucose control). Products include:
Thioridazine Hydrochloride Tablets 2289

Thyroglobulin (Co-administration with drugs that tend to produce hyperglycemia, such as thyroid products, may lead to loss of blood glucose control).
No products indexed under this heading.

Thyroid (Co-administration with drugs that tend to produce hyperglycemia, such as thyroid products, may lead to loss of blood glucose control).
No products indexed under this heading.

Thyroxine (Co-administration with drugs that tend to produce hyperglycemia, such as thyroid products, may lead to loss of blood glucose control).
No products indexed under this heading.

Thyroxine Sodium (Co-administration with drugs that tend to produce hyperglycemia, such as thyroid products, may lead to loss of blood glucose control).
No products indexed under this heading.

Timolol Hemihydrate (The hypoglycemic action of sulfonylureas may be potentiated by beta adrenergic agents). Products include:
Betimol Ophthalmic Solution .... ⊙324

Timolol Maleate (The hypoglycemic action of sulfonylureas may be potentiated by beta adrenergic agents). Products include:
Blocadren Tablets 2046
Cosopt Sterile Ophthalmic Solution 2065
Timolide Tablets 2187
Timolol GFS .... ⊙266
Timoptic in Ocudose 2192
Timoptic Sterile Ophthalmic Solution 2190
Timoptic-XE Sterile Ophthalmic Gel Forming Solution 2194

Tolazamide (The hypoglycemic action of sulfonylureas may be potentiated by sulfonamides).
No products indexed under this heading.

Tolbutamide (The hypoglycemic action of sulfonylureas may be potentiated by sulfonamides).
No products indexed under this heading.

Tolmetin Sodium (The hypoglycemic action of sulfonylureas may be potentiated by non-steroidal anti-inflammatory agents). Products include:
Tolectin 2589

Torsemide (Co-administration with drugs that tend to produce hyperglycemia, such as diuretics, may lead to loss of blood glucose control). Products include:
Demadex Tablets and Injection 2965

Tranylcypromine Sulfate (The hypoglycemic action of sulfonylureas may be potentiated by MAO inhibitors). Products include:
Parnate Tablets 1607

Triamcinolone (Co-administration with drugs that tend to produce hyperglycemia, such as corticosteroids, may lead to loss of blood glucose control).
No products indexed under this heading.

Triamcinolone Acetonide (Co-administration with drugs that tend to produce hyperglycemia, such as corticosteroids, may lead to loss of blood glucose control). Products include:
Azmacort Inhalation Aerosol 728
Nasacort Nasal Inhaler 750
Nasacort AQ Nasal Spray 752
Tri-Nasal Spray 2274

Triamcinolone Diacetate (Co-administration with drugs that tend to produce hyperglycemia, such as corticosteroids, may lead to loss of blood glucose control).
No products indexed under this heading.

Triamcinolone Hexacetonide (Co-administration with drugs that tend to produce hyperglycemia, such as corticosteroids, may lead to loss of blood glucose control).
No products indexed under this heading.

Triamterene (Co-administration with drugs that tend to produce hyperglycemia, such as diuretics, may lead to loss of blood glucose control). Products include:
Dyazide Capsules 1515
Dyrenium Capsules 3458
Maxzide 1008

Trifluoperazine Hydrochloride (Co-administration with drugs that tend to produce hyperglycemia, such as phenothiazines, may lead to loss of blood glucose control). Products include:
Stelazine 1640

Trimethoprim (Co-administration with cationic drugs that are eliminated by renal tubular secretion have the theoretical potential for interacting with metformin by competing for common renal tubular transport systems). Products include:
Bactrim 2949
Septra Suspension 2265
Septra Tablets 2265
Septra DS Tablets 2265

Trimethoprim Sulfate (Co-administration with cationic drugs that are eliminated by renal tubular secretion have the theoretical potential for interacting with metformin by competing for common renal tubular transport systems). Products include:
Polytrim Ophthalmic Solution 556

Tyropanoate Sodium (Potential for acute alteration of renal function; metformin should be temporarily withheld in patients undergoing radiologic studies involving iodinated contrast material).
No products indexed under this heading.

Vancomycin Hydrochloride (Co-administration with cationic drugs that are eliminated by renal tubular secretion have the theoretical potential for interacting with metformin by competing for common renal tubular transport systems). Products include:
Vancocin HCl Capsules & Pulvules .. 1972
Vancocin HCl Oral Solution 1971
Vancocin HCl, Vials & ADD-Vantage 1970

Verapamil Hydrochloride (Co-administration with drugs that tend to produce hyperglycemia, such as calcium channel blockers, may lead to loss of blood glucose control). Products include:
Covera-HS Tablets 3199
Isoptin SR Tablets 467
Tarka Tablets 508
Verelan Capsules 3184
Verelan PM Capsules 3186

Warfarin Sodium (The hypoglycemic action of sulfonylureas may be potentiated by coumarins). Products include:
Coumadin for Injection 1243
Coumadin Tablets 1243
Warfarin Sodium Tablets, USP 3302

GLY-OXIDE LIQUID

(Carbamide Peroxide) .... ▣751
None cited in PDR database.

GLYSET TABLETS

(Miglitol) 2821
May interact with:

Amylase (May reduce the effect of miglitol; concomitant use should be avoided). Products include:
Arco-Lase Tablets 592
Arco-Lase Plus Tablets 592

Charcoal, Activated (May reduce the effect of miglitol; concomitant use should be avoided).
No products indexed under this heading.

Digoxin (Co-administration has resulted in reduced plasma concentrations of digoxin). Products include:
Digitek Tablets 1003
Lanoxicaps Capsules 1574
Lanoxin Injection 1581
Lanoxin Tablets 1587
Lanoxin Elixir Pediatric 1578
Lanoxin Injection Pediatric 1584

Glyburide (Potential for lower Cmax and AUC values for glyburide; these differences are statistically insignificant). Products include:
DiaBeta Tablets 741
Glucovance Tablets 1086

Metformin (Potential for lower Cmax and AUC values for metformin; these differences are statistically insignificant).

Pancreatin (May reduce the effect of miglitol; concomitant use should be avoided). Products include:
Donnazyme Tablets 2931

Propranolol Hydrochloride (Co-administration may significantly reduce the bioavailability of propranolol). Products include:
Inderal 3513
Inderal LA Long-Acting Capsules .. 3516
Inderide Tablets 3517
Inderide LA Long-Acting Capsules .. 3519

Ranitidine Hydrochloride (Co-administration may significantly reduce the bioavailability of ranitidine). Products include:
Zantac 1690
Zantac Injection 1688
Zantac 75 Tablets .... ■717

GOLYTELY AND PINEAPPLE FLAVOR GOLYTELY FOR ORAL SOLUTION
(Polyethylene Glycol, Potassium Chloride, Sodium Bicarbonate, Sodium Chloride, Sodium Sulfate).......... 1068
May interact with:

Oral Medications, unspecified (Those administered within one hour of GoLYTELY usage may be flushed from the gastrointestinal tract and not absorbed).

Food Interactions

Food, unspecified (For best results, no solid food should be consumed during 3 to 4 hour period before drinking solution).

GONAL-F FOR INJECTION
(Follitropin Alfa) 3216
None cited in PDR database.

GOODY'S BODY PAIN FORMULA POWDER
(Acetaminophen, Aspirin) .... ■620

Food Interactions

Alcohol (Individuals consuming 3 or more alcohol-containing drinks per day should consult their physicians for advice on when and how they should take this product).

GOODY'S EXTRA STRENGTH HEADACHE POWDER
(Acetaminophen, Aspirin, Caffeine) .... ■620

Food Interactions

Alcohol (Individuals consuming 3 or more alcohol-containing drinks per day should consult their physicians for advice on when and how they should take this product).

GOODY'S EXTRA STRENGTH PAIN RELIEF TABLETS
(Acetaminophen, Aspirin, Caffeine) .... ■620

Food Interactions

Alcohol (Individuals consuming 3 or more alcohol-containing drinks per day should consult their physicians for advice on when and how they should take this product).

GOODY'S PM POWDER
(Acetaminophen, Diphenhydramine Citrate) .... ■621
May interact with hypnotics and sedatives, tranquilizers, and certain other agents. Compounds in these categories include:

Alprazolam (Concurrent use is not recommended). Products include:
Xanax Tablets 2865

Buspirone Hydrochloride (Concurrent use is not recommended).
No products indexed under this heading.

Chlordiazepoxide (Concurrent use is not recommended). Products include:
Limbitrol 1738

Chlordiazepoxide Hydrochloride (Concurrent use is not recommended). Products include:
Librium Capsules 1736
Librium for Injection 1737

Chlorpromazine (Concurrent use is not recommended). Products include:
Thorazine Suppositories 1656

Chlorpromazine Hydrochloride (Concurrent use is not recommended). Products include:
Thorazine 1656

Chlorprothixene (Concurrent use is not recommended).
No products indexed under this heading.

Chlorprothixene Hydrochloride (Concurrent use is not recommended).
No products indexed under this heading.

Clorazepate Dipotassium (Concurrent use is not recommended). Products include:
Tranxene 511

Diazepam (Concurrent use is not recommended). Products include:
Valium Injectable 3026
Valium Tablets 3047

Diphenhydramine Hydrochloride (Concurrent use with any other product containing diphenhydramine, including topical preparations, should be avoided). Products include:
Extra Strength Bayer PM Caplets .... ■611
Benadryl Allergy Chewables .... ■689
Benadryl Allergy .... ■691
Benadryl Allergy Liquid .... ■690
Benadryl Allergy/Cold Tablets .... ■691
Benadryl Allergy/Congestion Tablets .... ■692
Benadryl Allergy & Sinus Liquid .... ■693
Benadryl Allergy Sinus Headache Caplets & Gelcaps .... ■693
Benadryl Severe Allergy & Sinus Headache Caplets .... ■694
Benadryl Dye-Free Allergy Liquid .... ■690
Benadryl Dye-Free Allergy Liqui-Gels Softgels .... ■690
Benadryl Itch Relief Stick Extra Strength .... ■695
Benadryl Cream .... ■695
Benadryl Gel .... ■695
Benadryl Spray .... ■696
Benadryl Parenteral 2617
Coricidin HBP Night-Time Cold & Flu Tablets .... ■738
Nytol QuickCaps Caplets .... ■622
Maximum Strength Nytol QuickGels Softgels .... ■621
Extra Strength Percogesic Aspirin-Free Coated Caplets .... ■665
Simply Sleep Caplets 2008
Sominex Original Formula Tablets .... ■761
Children's Tylenol Allergy-D Liquid 2014
Maximum Strength Tylenol Allergy Sinus NightTime Caplets 2010
Tylenol Severe Allergy Caplets 2010
Maximum Strength Tylenol Flu NightTime Gelcaps 2011
Extra Strength Tylenol PM Caplets, Geltabs, and Gelcaps 2012
Unisom Maximum Strength SleepGels .... ■713

Droperidol (Concurrent use is not recommended).
No products indexed under this heading.

Estazolam (Concurrent use is not recommended). Products include:
ProSom Tablets 500

Ethchlorvynol (Concurrent use is not recommended).
No products indexed under this heading.

Ethinamate (Concurrent use is not recommended).
No products indexed under this heading.

Fluphenazine Decanoate (Concurrent use is not recommended).
No products indexed under this heading.

Fluphenazine Enanthate (Concurrent use is not recommended).
No products indexed under this heading.

Fluphenazine Hydrochloride (Concurrent use is not recommended).
No products indexed under this heading.

Flurazepam Hydrochloride (Concurrent use is not recommended).
No products indexed under this heading.

Glutethimide (Concurrent use is not recommended).
No products indexed under this heading.

Haloperidol (Concurrent use is not recommended). Products include:
Haldol Injection, Tablets and Concentrate 2533

Haloperidol Decanoate (Concurrent use is not recommended). Products include:
Haldol Decanoate 2535

Hydroxyzine Hydrochloride (Concurrent use is not recommended). Products include:
Atarax Tablets & Syrup 2667
Vistaril Intramuscular Solution 2738

Lorazepam (Concurrent use is not recommended). Products include:
Ativan Injection 3478
Ativan Tablets 3482

Loxapine Hydrochloride (Concurrent use is not recommended).
No products indexed under this heading.

Loxapine Succinate (Concurrent use is not recommended). Products include:
Loxitane Capsules 3398

Meprobamate (Concurrent use is not recommended). Products include:
Miltown Tablets 3349

Mesoridazine Besylate (Concurrent use is not recommended). Products include:
Serentil 1057

Midazolam Hydrochloride (Concurrent use is not recommended). Products include:
Versed Injection 3027
Versed Syrup 3033

Molindone Hydrochloride (Concurrent use is not recommended). Products include:
Moban 1320

Oxazepam (Concurrent use is not recommended).
No products indexed under this heading.

Perphenazine (Concurrent use is not recommended). Products include:
Etrafon 3115
Trilafon 3160

Prazepam (Concurrent use is not recommended).
No products indexed under this heading.

Prochlorperazine (Concurrent use is not recommended). Products include:
Compazine 1505

Promethazine Hydrochloride (Concurrent use is not recommended). Products include:
Mepergan Injection 3539
Phenergan Injection 3553
Phenergan 3556
Phenergan Syrup 3554
Phenergan with Codeine Syrup 3557
Phenergan with Dextromethorphan Syrup 3559
Phenergan VC Syrup 3560
Phenergan VC with Codeine Syrup 3561

Propofol (Concurrent use is not recommended). Products include:
Diprivan Injectable Emulsion 667

Quazepam (Concurrent use is not recommended).
No products indexed under this heading.

Secobarbital Sodium (Concurrent use is not recommended).
No products indexed under this heading.

Temazepam (Concurrent use is not recommended).
No products indexed under this heading.

Thioridazine Hydrochloride (Concurrent use is not recommended). Products include:
Thioridazine Hydrochloride Tablets 2289

Thiothixene (Concurrent use is not recommended). Products include:
Navane Capsules 2701
Thiothixene Capsules 2290

Triazolam (Concurrent use is not recommended). Products include:
Halcion Tablets 2823

Trifluoperazine Hydrochloride (Concurrent use is not recommended). Products include:
Stelazine 1640

Zaleplon (Concurrent use is not recommended). Products include:
Sonata Capsules 3591

Zolpidem Tartrate (Concurrent use is not recommended). Products include:
Ambien Tablets 3191

Food Interactions

Alcohol (Individuals consuming 3 or more alcohol-containing drinks per day should consult their physicians for advice on when and how they should take this product; avoid alcoholic beverages since diphenhydramine causes drowsiness).

GORDOCHOM SOLUTION
(Chloroxylenol, Undecylenic Acid) 1722
None cited in PDR database.

GRANULEX AEROSOL
(Balsam Peru, Castor Oil, Trypsin) 1007
None cited in PDR database.

GRIFULVIN V TABLETS MICROSIZE AND ORAL SUSPENSION MICROSIZE
(Griseofulvin) 2518
May interact with barbiturates, oral anticoagulants, and oral contraceptives. Compounds in these categories include:

Aprobarbital (Usually depresses griseofulvin activity; may necessitate dosage increase).
No products indexed under this heading.

Butabarbital (Usually depresses griseofulvin activity; may necessitate dosage increase).
No products indexed under this heading.

Butalbital (Usually depresses griseofulvin activity; may necessitate dosage increase). Products include:
Phrenilin 578
Sedapap Tablets 50 mg/650 mg 2225

Desogestrel (Reduced contraceptive efficacy; increased incidence of breakthrough bleeding). Products include:
Cyclessa Tablets 2450
Desogen Tablets 2458
Mircette Tablets 2470
Ortho-Cept 21 Tablets 2546
Ortho-Cept 28 Tablets 2546

Dicumarol (Dosage adjustment of anticoagulant may be necessary).
No products indexed under this heading.

Ethinyl Estradiol (Reduced contraceptive efficacy; increased incidence of breakthrough bleeding). Products include:
Alesse-21 Tablets 3468
Alesse-28 Tablets 3473
Brevicon 28-Day Tablets 3380
Cyclessa Tablets 2450
Desogen Tablets 2458
Estinyl Tablets 3112
Estrostep 2627
femhrt Tablets 2635
Levlen 962

Levlite 21 Tablets 962
Levlite 28 Tablets 962
Levora Tablets 3389
Loestrin 21 Tablets 2642
Loestrin Fe Tablets 2642
Lo/Ovral Tablets 3532
Lo/Ovral-28 Tablets 3538
Low-Ogestrel-28 Tablets 3392
Microgestin Fe 1.5/30 Tablets 3407
Microgestin Fe 1/20 Tablets 3400
Mircette Tablets 2470
Modicon 2563
Necon 3415
Nordette-28 Tablets 2257
Norinyl 1 +35 28-Day Tablets 3380
Ogestrel 0.5/50-28 Tablets 3428
Ortho-Cept 21 Tablets 2546
Ortho-Cept 28 Tablets 2546
Ortho-Cyclen/Ortho Tri-Cyclen 2573
Ortho-Novum 2563
Ovcon 3364
Ovral Tablets 3551
Ovral-28 Tablets 3552
Tri-Levlen 962
Tri-Norinyl-28 Tablets 3433
Triphasil-21 Tablets 3600
Triphasil-28 Tablets 3605
Trivora Tablets 3439
Yasmin 28 Tablets 980
Zovia 3449

Ethynodiol Diacetate (Reduced contraceptive efficacy; increased incidence of breakthrough bleeding). Products include:
Zovia 3449

Levonorgestrel (Reduced contraceptive efficacy; increased incidence of breakthrough bleeding). Products include:
Alesse-21 Tablets 3468
Alesse-28 Tablets 3473
Levlen 962
Levlite 21 Tablets 962
Levlite 28 Tablets 962
Levora Tablets 3389
Mirena Intrauterine System 974
Nordette-28 Tablets 2257
Norplant System 3543
Tri-Levlen 962
Triphasil-21 Tablets 3600
Triphasil-28 Tablets 3605
Trivora Tablets 3439

Mephobarbital (Usually depresses griseofulvin activity; may necessitate dosage increase).
No products indexed under this heading.

Mestranol (Reduced contraceptive efficacy; increased incidence of breakthrough bleeding). Products include:
Necon 1/50 Tablets 3415
Norinyl 1 + 50 28-Day Tablets 3380
Ortho-Novum 1/50□28 Tablets 2556

Norethindrone (Reduced contraceptive efficacy; increased incidence of breakthrough bleeding). Products include:
Brevicon 28-Day Tablets 3380
Micronor Tablets 2543
Modicon 2563
Necon 3415
Norinyl 1 +35 28-Day Tablets 3380
Norinyl 1 + 50 28-Day Tablets 3380
Nor-QD Tablets 3423
Ortho-Novum 2563
Ortho-Novum 1/50□28 Tablets 2556
Ovcon 3364
Tri-Norinyl-28 Tablets 3433

Norethynodrel (Reduced contraceptive efficacy; increased incidence of breakthrough bleeding).
No products indexed under this heading.

Norgestimate (Reduced contraceptive efficacy; increased incidence of breakthrough bleeding). Products include:
Ortho-Cyclen/Ortho Tri-Cyclen 2573
Ortho-Prefest Tablets 2570

Norgestrel (Reduced contraceptive efficacy; increased incidence of breakthrough bleeding). Products include:
Lo/Ovral Tablets 3532
Lo/Ovral-28 Tablets 3538
Low-Ogestrel-28 Tablets 3392
Ogestrel 0.5/50-28 Tablets 3428
Ovral Tablets 3551
Ovral-28 Tablets 3552
Ovrette Tablets 3552

Pentobarbital Sodium (Usually depresses griseofulvin activity; may necessitate dosage increase). Products include:
Nembutal Sodium Solution 485

Phenobarbital (Usually depresses griseofulvin activity; may necessitate dosage increase). Products include:
Arco-Lase Plus Tablets 592
Donnatal 2929
Donnatal Extentabs 2930

Secobarbital Sodium (Usually depresses griseofulvin activity; may necessitate dosage increase).
No products indexed under this heading.

Thiamylal Sodium (Usually depresses griseofulvin activity; may necessitate dosage increase).
No products indexed under this heading.

Warfarin Sodium (Dosage adjustment of anticoagulant may be necessary). Products include:
Coumadin for Injection 1243
Coumadin Tablets 1243
Warfarin Sodium Tablets, USP 3302

GRIS-PEG TABLETS

(Griseofulvin) 2661
May interact with barbiturates, oral contraceptives, and certain other agents. Compounds in these categories include:

Aprobarbital (Barbiturates usually depress griseofulvin activity and co-administration requires a dosage adjustment of the antifungal agent).
No products indexed under this heading.

Butabarbital (Barbiturates usually depress griseofulvin activity and co-administration requires a dosage adjustment of the antifungal agent).
No products indexed under this heading.

Butalbital (Barbiturates usually depress griseofulvin activity and co-administration requires a dosage adjustment of the antifungal agent). Products include:
Phrenilin 578
Sedapap Tablets 50 mg/650 mg 2225

Desogestrel (There have been reports in the literature of possible interactions between griseofulvin and oral contraceptives). Products include:
Cyclessa Tablets 2450
Desogen Tablets 2458
Mircette Tablets 2470
Ortho-Cept 21 Tablets 2546
Ortho-Cept 28 Tablets 2546

Ethinyl Estradiol (There have been reports in the literature of possible interactions between griseofulvin and oral contraceptives). Products include:
Alesse-21 Tablets 3468
Alesse-28 Tablets 3473
Brevicon 28-Day Tablets 3380
Cyclessa Tablets 2450
Desogen Tablets 2458
Estinyl Tablets 3112
Estrostep 2627
femhrt Tablets 2635
Levlen 962
Levlite 21 Tablets 962
Levlite 28 Tablets 962
Levora Tablets 3389
Loestrin 21 Tablets 2642
Loestrin Fe Tablets 2642
Lo/Ovral Tablets 3532
Lo/Ovral-28 Tablets 3538
Low-Ogestrel-28 Tablets 3392
Microgestin Fe 1.5/30 Tablets 3407
Microgestin Fe 1/20 Tablets 3400
Mircette Tablets 2470
Modicon 2563
Necon 3415
Nordette-28 Tablets 2257
Norinyl 1 +35 28-Day Tablets 3380
Ogestrel 0.5/50-28 Tablets 3428
Ortho-Cept 21 Tablets 2546
Ortho-Cept 28 Tablets 2546
Ortho-Cyclen/Ortho Tri-Cyclen 2573
Ortho-Novum 2563
Ovcon 3364
Ovral Tablets 3551
Ovral-28 Tablets 3552
Tri-Levlen 962
Tri-Norinyl-28 Tablets 3433
Triphasil-21 Tablets 3600
Triphasil-28 Tablets 3605
Trivora Tablets 3439
Yasmin 28 Tablets 980
Zovia 3449

Ethynodiol Diacetate (There have been reports in the literature of possible interactions between griseofulvin and oral contraceptives). Products include:
Zovia 3449

Levonorgestrel (There have been reports in the literature of possible interactions between griseofulvin and oral contraceptives). Products include:
Alesse-21 Tablets 3468
Alesse-28 Tablets 3473
Levlen 962
Levlite 21 Tablets 962
Levlite 28 Tablets 962
Levora Tablets 3389
Mirena Intrauterine System 974
Nordette-28 Tablets 2257
Norplant System 3543
Tri-Levlen 962
Triphasil-21 Tablets 3600
Triphasil-28 Tablets 3605
Trivora Tablets 3439

Mephobarbital (Barbiturates usually depress griseofulvin activity and co-administration requires a dosage adjustment of the antifungal agent).
No products indexed under this heading.

Mestranol (There have been reports in the literature of possible interactions between griseofulvin and oral contraceptives). Products include:
Necon 1/50 Tablets 3415
Norinyl 1 + 50 28-Day Tablets 3380
Ortho-Novum 1/50□28 Tablets 2556

Norethindrone (There have been reports in the literature of possible interactions between griseofulvin and oral contraceptives). Products include:
Brevicon 28-Day Tablets 3380
Micronor Tablets 2543
Modicon 2563
Necon 3415
Norinyl 1 +35 28-Day Tablets 3380
Norinyl 1 + 50 28-Day Tablets 3380
Nor-QD Tablets 3423
Ortho-Novum 2563
Ortho-Novum 1/50□28 Tablets 2556
Ovcon 3364
Tri-Norinyl-28 Tablets 3433

Norethynodrel (There have been reports in the literature of possible interactions between griseofulvin and oral contraceptives).
No products indexed under this heading.

Norgestimate (There have been reports in the literature of possible interactions between griseofulvin and oral contraceptives). Products include:
Ortho-Cyclen/Ortho Tri-Cyclen 2573
Ortho-Prefest Tablets 2570

Norgestrel (There have been reports in the literature of possible interactions between griseofulvin and oral contraceptives). Products include:
Lo/Ovral Tablets 3532
Lo/Ovral-28 Tablets 3538
Low-Ogestrel-28 Tablets 3392
Ogestrel 0.5/50-28 Tablets 3428
Ovral Tablets 3551
Ovral-28 Tablets 3552
Ovrette Tablets 3552

Pentobarbital Sodium (Barbiturates usually depress griseofulvin activity and co-administration requires a dosage adjustment of the antifungal agent). Products include:
Nembutal Sodium Solution 485

Phenobarbital (Barbiturates usually depress griseofulvin activity and co-administration requires a dosage adjustment of the antifungal agent). Products include:
Arco-Lase Plus Tablets 592
Donnatal 2929
Donnatal Extentabs 2930

Secobarbital Sodium (Barbiturates usually depress griseofulvin activity and co-administration requires a dosage adjustment of the antifungal agent).
No products indexed under this heading.

Thiamylal Sodium (Barbiturates usually depress griseofulvin activity and co-administration requires a dosage adjustment of the antifungal agent).
No products indexed under this heading.

Warfarin Sodium (Griseofulvin decreases the activity of warfarin-type anticoagulants). Products include:
Coumadin for Injection 1243
Coumadin Tablets 1243
Warfarin Sodium Tablets, USP 3302

Food Interactions

Alcohol (The effects of alcohol may be potentiated by griseofulvin, producing such effects as tachycardia and flushing).

GUAIFED CAPSULES

(Guaifenesin, Pseudoephedrine Hydrochloride) 2272
May interact with beta blockers, cardiac glycosides, monoamine oxidase inhibitors, veratrum alkaloids, and certain other agents. Compounds in these categories include:

Acebutolol Hydrochloride (Concurrent use with beta adrenergic blocker increases the effects of sympathomimetics). Products include:
Sectral Capsules 3589

Atenolol (Concurrent use with beta adrenergic blocker increases the effects of sympathomimetics). Products include:
Tenoretic Tablets 690
Tenormin I.V. Injection 692

Betaxolol Hydrochloride (Concurrent use with beta adrenergic blocker increases the effects of sympathomimetics). Products include:
Betoptic S Ophthalmic Suspension 537

Bisoprolol Fumarate (Concurrent use with beta adrenergic blocker increases the effects of sympathomimetics). Products include:
Zebeta Tablets 1885
Ziac Tablets 1887

Carteolol Hydrochloride (Concurrent use with beta adrenergic blocker increases the effects of sympathomimetics). Products include:
Carteolol Hydrochloride Ophthalmic Solution USP, 1% .... ⊙258
Ocupress Ophthalmic Solution, 1% Sterile .... ⊙303

Cryptenamine Preparations (Sympathomimetics may reduce the antihypertensive effects of veratrum alkaloids).
No products indexed under this heading.

Deslanoside (Pseudoephedrine may increase the possibility of cardiac arrhythmias in patients taking digitalis glycosides).
No products indexed under this heading.

Digitoxin (Pseudoephedrine may increase the possibility of cardiac arrhythmias in patients taking digitalis glycosides).
No products indexed under this heading.

Digoxin (Pseudoephedrine may increase the possibility of cardiac arrhythmias in patients taking digitalis glycosides). Products include:

Digitek Tablets 1003
Lanoxicaps Capsules 1574
Lanoxin Injection 1581
Lanoxin Tablets 1587
Lanoxin Elixir Pediatric 1578
Lanoxin Injection Pediatric 1584

Esmolol Hydrochloride (Concurrent use with beta adrenergic blocker increases the effects of sympathomimetics). Products include:
Brevibloc Injection 858

Guanethidine Monosulfate (Sympathomimetics may reduce the antihypertensive effects of guanethidine).
No products indexed under this heading.

Isocarboxazid (Concurrent and/or sequential use with MAO inhibitors is contraindicated; MAO inhibitors may increase the effect of sympathomimetics).
No products indexed under this heading.

Labetalol Hydrochloride (Concurrent use with beta adrenergic blocker increases the effects of sympathomimetics). Products include:
Normodyne Injection 3135
Normodyne Tablets 3137

Levobunolol Hydrochloride (Concurrent use with beta adrenergic blocker increases the effects of sympathomimetics). Products include:
Betagan .... ⊙228

Methyldopa (Sympathomimetics may reduce the antihypertensive effects of methyldopa). Products include:
Aldoclor Tablets 2035
Aldomet Tablets 2037
Aldoril Tablets 2039

Methyldopate Hydrochloride (Reduced antihypertensive effects).
No products indexed under this heading.

Metipranolol Hydrochloride (Concurrent use with beta adrenergic blocker increases the effects of sympathomimetics).
No products indexed under this heading.

Metoprolol Succinate (Concurrent use with beta adrenergic blocker increases the effects of sympathomimetics). Products include:
Toprol-XL Tablets 651

Metoprolol Tartrate (Concurrent use with beta adrenergic blocker increases the effects of sympathomimetics).
No products indexed under this heading.

Moclobemide (Concurrent and/or sequential use with MAO inhibitors is contraindicated; MAO inhibitors may increase the effect of sympathomimetics).
No products indexed under this heading.

Nadolol (Concurrent use with beta adrenergic blocker increases the effects of sympathomimetics). Products include:
Corgard Tablets 2245
Corzide 40/5 Tablets 2247
Corzide 80/5 Tablets 2247
Nadolol Tablets 2288

Pargyline Hydrochloride (Concurrent and/or sequential use with MAO inhibitors is contraindicated; MAO inhibitors may increase the effect of sympathomimetics).
No products indexed under this heading.

Penbutolol Sulfate (Concurrent use with beta adrenergic blocker increases the effects of sympathomimetics).
No products indexed under this heading.

Phenelzine Sulfate (Concurrent and/or sequential use with MAO inhibitors is contraindicated; MAO inhibitors may increase the effect of sympathomimetics). Products include:
Nardil Tablets 2653

Pindolol (Concurrent use with beta adrenergic blocker increases the effects of sympathomimetics).
No products indexed under this heading.

Procarbazine Hydrochloride (Concurrent and/or sequential use with MAO inhibitors is contraindicated; MAO inhibitors may increase the effect of sympathomimetics). Products include:
Matulane Capsules 3246

Propranolol Hydrochloride (Concurrent use with beta adrenergic blocker increases the effects of sympathomimetics). Products include:
Inderal 3513
Inderal LA Long-Acting Capsules 3516
Inderide Tablets 3517
Inderide LA Long-Acting Capsules 3519

Reserpine (Sympathomimetics may reduce the antihypertensive effects of reserpine).
No products indexed under this heading.

Selegiline Hydrochloride (Concurrent and/or sequential use with MAO inhibitors is contraindicated; MAO inhibitors may increase the effect of sympathomimetics). Products include:
Eldepryl Capsules 3266

Sotalol Hydrochloride (Concurrent use with beta adrenergic blocker increases the effects of sympathomimetics). Products include:
Betapace Tablets 950
Betapace AF Tablets 954

Timolol Hemihydrate (Concurrent use with beta adrenergic blocker increases the effects of sympathomimetics). Products include:
Betimol Ophthalmic Solution .... ⊙324

Timolol Maleate (Concurrent use with beta adrenergic blocker increases the effects of sympathomimetics). Products include:
Blocadren Tablets 2046
Cosopt Sterile Ophthalmic Solution 2065
Timolide Tablets 2187
Timolol GFS .... ⊙266
Timoptic in Ocudose 2192
Timoptic Sterile Ophthalmic Solution 2190
Timoptic-XE Sterile Ophthalmic Gel Forming Solution 2194

Tranylcypromine Sulfate (Concurrent and/or sequential use with MAO inhibitors is contraindicated; MAO inhibitors may increase the effect of sympathomimetics). Products include:
Parnate Tablets 1607

GUAIFED-PD CAPSULES
(Guaifenesin, Pseudoephedrine Hydrochloride) 2272
See Guaifed Capsules

GYNAZOLE-1 VAGINAL CREAM
(Butoconazole Nitrate) 3310
None cited in PDR database.

GYNE-LOTRIMIN 3, 3-DAY CREAM
(Clotrimazole) .... ▣741
None cited in PDR database.

HALCION TABLETS
(Triazolam) 2823
May interact with antihistamines, azole antifungals, central nervous system depressants, anticonvulsants, erythromycin, macrolide antibiotics, oral contraceptives, and certain other agents. Compounds in these categories include:

Acrivastine (Co-administration results in additive CNS depressant effects). Products include:
Semprex-D Capsules 1172

Alfentanil Hydrochloride (Co-administration results in additive CNS depressant effects).
No products indexed under this heading.

Alprazolam (Co-administration results in additive CNS depressant effects). Products include:
Xanax Tablets 2865

Amiodarone Hydrochloride (Data from in vitro studies of benzodiazepines other than triazolam suggest a possible interaction; caution is recommended during co-administration). Products include:
Cordarone Intravenous 3491
Cordarone Tablets 3487
Pacerone Tablets 3331

Aprobarbital (Co-administration results in additive CNS depressant effects).
No products indexed under this heading.

Astemizole (Co-administration results in additive CNS depressant effects).
No products indexed under this heading.

Azatadine Maleate (Co-administration results in additive CNS depressant effects). Products include:
Rynatan Tablets 3351

Azithromycin Dihydrate (Co-administration with other macrolides, erythromycin, has resulted in increased maximum plasma concentration of triazolam, decreased clearance, and increased half-life; caution and consideration of appropriate triazolam dose reduction are recommended). Products include:
Zithromax 2743
Zithromax for IV Infusion 2748
Zithromax for Oral Suspension, 300 mg, 600 mg, 900 mg, 1200 mg 2739
Zithromax Tablets, 250 mg 2739

Bromodiphenhydramine Hydrochloride (Co-administration results in additive CNS depressant effects).
No products indexed under this heading.

Brompheniramine Maleate (Co-administration results in additive CNS depressant effects). Products include:
Bromfed Capsules (Extended-Release) 2269
Bromfed-PD Capsules (Extended-Release) 2269
Comtrex Acute Head Cold & Sinus Pressure Relief Tablets .... ▣627
Dimetapp Elixir .... ▣777
Dimetapp Cold and Fever Suspension .... ▣775
Dimetapp DM Cold & Cough Elixir .... ▣775
Dimetapp Nighttime Flu Liquid .... ▣776

Buprenorphine Hydrochloride (Co-administration results in additive CNS depressant effects). Products include:
Buprenex Injectable 2918

Buspirone Hydrochloride (Co-administration results in additive CNS depressant effects).
No products indexed under this heading.

Butabarbital (Co-administration results in additive CNS depressant effects).
No products indexed under this heading.

Butalbital (Co-administration results in additive CNS depressant effects). Products include:
Phrenilin 578
Sedapap Tablets 50 mg/650 mg 2225

Carbamazepine (Co-administration results in additive CNS depressant effects). Products include:
Carbatrol Capsules 3234
Tegretol/Tegretol-XR 2404

Cetirizine Hydrochloride (Co-administration results in additive CNS depressant effects). Products include:
Zyrtec 2756
Zyrtec-D 12 Hour Extended Relief Tablets 2758

Chlordiazepoxide (Co-administration results in additive CNS depressant effects). Products include:
Limbitrol 1738

Chlordiazepoxide Hydrochloride (Co-administration results in additive CNS depressant effects). Products include:
Librium Capsules 1736
Librium for Injection 1737

Chlorpheniramine Maleate (Co-administration results in additive CNS depressant effects). Products include:
Actifed Cold & Sinus Caplets and Tablets .... ▣688
Alka-Seltzer Plus Liqui-Gels .... ▣604
BC Allergy Sinus Cold Powder .... ▣619
Chlor-Trimeton Allergy Tablets .... ▣735
Chlor-Trimeton Allergy/Decongestant Tablets .... ▣736
Comtrex Flu Therapy & Fever Relief Nighttime Tablets .... ▣628
Comtrex Maximum Strength Multi-Symptom Cold & Cough Relief Tablets and Caplets .... ▣626
Contac Severe Cold and Flu Caplets Maximum Strength .... ▣746
Coricidin 'D' Cold, Flu & Sinus Tablets .... ▣737
Coricidin/Coricidin D .... ▣738
Coricidin HBP Maximum Strength Flu Tablets .... ▣738
Extendryl 1361
Hycomine Compound Tablets 1317
Kronofed-A 1341
PediaCare Cough-Cold Liquid .... ▣719
PediaCare NightRest Cough-Cold Liquid .... ▣719
Robitussin Nighttime Honey Flu Liquid .... ▣786
Ryna .... ▣768
Singlet Caplets .... ▣761
Sinutab Sinus Allergy Medication, Maximum Strength Formula, Tablets & Caplets .... ▣707
Sudafed Cold & Allergy Tablets .... ▣708
TheraFlu Regular Strength Cold & Cough Night Time Hot Liquid .... ▣676
TheraFlu Regular Strength Cold & Sore Throat Night Time Hot Liquid .... ▣676
TheraFlu Maximum Strength Flu & Cough Night Time Hot Liquid .... ▣678
TheraFlu Maximum Strength Flu & Sore Throat Night Time Hot Liquid .... ▣677
TheraFlu Maximum Strength Severe Cold & Congestion Night Time Caplets .... ▣678
TheraFlu Maximum Strength Severe Cold & Congestion Night Time Hot Liquid .... ▣678
Triaminic Cold & Allergy Liquid .... ▣681
Triaminic Cold & Allergy Softchews .... ▣683
Triaminic Cold & Cough Liquid .... ▣681
Triaminic Cold & Cough Softchews .... ▣683
Triaminic Cold & Night Time Cough Liquid .... ▣681
Triaminic Cold, Cough & Fever Liquid .... ▣681
Children's Tylenol Cold Suspension Liquid and Chewable Tablets 2015
Children's Tylenol Cold Plus Cough Suspension Liquid and Chewable Tablets 2015
Children's Tylenol Flu Suspension Liquid 2015
Maximum Strength Tylenol Allergy Sinus Caplets, Gelcaps, and Geltabs 2010
Multi-Symptom Tylenol Cold Complete Formula Caplets 2010
Vicks 44M Cough, Cold & Flu Relief Liquid .... ▣725
Pediatric Vicks 44m Cough & Cold Relief .... ▣728
Children's Vicks NyQuil Cold/Cough Relief .... ▣726

Chlorpheniramine Polistirex (Co-administration results in additive CNS depressant effects). Products include:

Tussionex Pennkinetic Extended-Release Suspension..... 1174

Chlorpheniramine Tannate (Co-administration results in additive CNS depressant effects). Products include:
Reformulated Rynatan Pediatric Suspension..... 3352
Rynatuss Pediatric Suspension..... 3353
Rynatuss Tablets..... 3353
Tussi-12 S Suspension..... 3356
Tussi-12 Tablets..... 3356

Chlorpromazine (Co-administration results in additive CNS depressant effects). Products include:
Thorazine Suppositories..... 1656

Chlorpromazine Hydrochloride (Co-administration results in additive CNS depressant effects). Products include:
Thorazine..... 1656

Chlorprothixene (Co-administration results in additive CNS depressant effects).
No products indexed under this heading.

Chlorprothixene Hydrochloride (Co-administration results in additive CNS depressant effects).
No products indexed under this heading.

Chlorprothixene Lactate (Co-administration results in additive CNS depressant effects).
No products indexed under this heading.

Cimetidine (Co-administration of cimetidine increased the maximum plasma concentration of triazolam by 51%; decreased the clearance by 55%, increased the half-life by 68%; caution and consideration of appropriate triazolam dose reduction are recommended). Products include:
Tagamet HB 200 Suspension..... ▣762
Tagamet HB 200 Tablets..... ▣761
Tagamet Tablets..... 1644

Cimetidine Hydrochloride (Co-administration of cimetidine increased the maximum plasma concentration of triazolam by 51%; decreased the clearance by 55%, increased the half-life by 68%; caution and consideration of appropriate triazolam dose reduction are recommended). Products include:
Tagamet..... 1644

Clarithromycin (Co-administration with other macrolides, erythromycin, has resulted in increased maximum plasma concentration of triazolam, decreased clearance, and increased half-life; caution and consideration of appropriate triazolam dose reduction are recommended). Products include:
Biaxin/Biaxin XL..... 403
PREVPAC..... 3298

Clemastine Fumarate (Co-administration results in additive CNS depressant effects). Products include:
Tavist 12 Hour Allergy Tablets..... ▣676

Clorazepate Dipotassium (Co-administration results in additive CNS depressant effects). Products include:
Tranxene..... 511

Clotrimazole (Other azole-type antifungals, such as ketoconazole or itraconazole, have demonstrated to be potent CYP 3A inhibitors with a potential for a profound effect on the clearance of triazolam; although data concerning the effect of other azole-type antifungals are not available, concurrent use is not recommended). Products include:
Gyne-Lotrimin 3, 3-Day Cream..... ▣741
Lotrimin AF Cream, Lotion, Solution, and Jock Itch Cream..... ▣742
Lotrimin..... 3128
Lotrisone..... 3129
Mycelex Troche..... 573
Mycelex-7 Combination-Pack Vaginal Inserts & External Vulvar Cream..... ▣614
Mycelex-7 Vaginal Cream..... ▣614
Mycelex-7 Vaginal Cream with 7 Disposable Applicators..... ▣614

Clozapine (Co-administration results in additive CNS depressant effects). Products include:
Clozaril Tablets..... 2319

Codeine Phosphate (Co-administration results in additive CNS depressant effects). Products include:
Phenergan with Codeine Syrup..... 3557
Phenergan VC with Codeine Syrup..... 3561
Robitussin A-C Syrup..... 2942
Robitussin-DAC Syrup..... 2942
Ryna-C Liquid..... ▣768
Soma Compound w/Codeine Tablets..... 3355
Tussi-Organidin NR Liquid..... 3350
Tussi-Organidin-S NR Liquid..... 3350
Tylenol with Codeine..... 2595

Cyclosporine (Data from in vitro studies of benzodiazepines other than triazolam suggest a possible interaction; caution is recommended during co-administration). Products include:
Gengraf Capsules..... 457
Neoral Soft Gelatin Capsules..... 2380
Neoral Oral Solution..... 2380
Sandimmune..... 2388

Cyproheptadine Hydrochloride (Co-administration results in additive CNS depressant effects). Products include:
Periactin Tablets..... 2155

Desflurane (Co-administration results in additive CNS depressant effects). Products include:
Suprane Liquid for Inhalation..... 874

Desogestrel (Co-administration of oral contraceptives increased the maximum plasma concentration of triazolam by 6%; decreased the clearance by 32%, increased the half-life by 16%). Products include:
Cyclessa Tablets..... 2450
Desogen Tablets..... 2458
Mircette Tablets..... 2470
Ortho-Cept 21 Tablets..... 2546
Ortho-Cept 28 Tablets..... 2546

Dexchlorpheniramine Maleate (Co-administration results in additive CNS depressant effects).
No products indexed under this heading.

Dezocine (Co-administration results in additive CNS depressant effects).
No products indexed under this heading.

Diazepam (Co-administration results in additive CNS depressant effects). Products include:
Valium Injectable..... 3026
Valium Tablets..... 3047

Dihydroergotamine Mesylate (Data from in vitro studies of benzodiazepines other than triazolam suggest a possible interaction; caution is recommended during co-administration). Products include:
D.H.E. 45 Injection..... 2334
Migranal Nasal Spray..... 2376

Diltiazem Hydrochloride (Co-administration of drugs demonstrated to be CYP 3A inhibitors on the basis of clinical studies involving benzodiazepine metabolized similarly to triazolam, such as diltiazem, may result in possible drug interaction with triazolam). Products include:
Cardizem Injectable..... 1018
Cardizem Lyo-Ject Syringe..... 1018
Cardizem Monovial..... 1018
Cardizem CD Capsules..... 1016
Tiazac Capsules..... 1378

Diphenhydramine Citrate (Co-administration results in additive CNS depressant effects). Products include:
Alka-Seltzer PM Effervescent Tablets..... ▣605
Benadryl Allergy & Sinus Fastmelt Tablets..... ▣693
Benadryl Children's Allergy/Cold Fastmelt Tablets..... ▣692
Excedrin PM Tablets, Caplets, and Geltabs..... ▣631
Goody's PM Powder..... ▣621

Diphenhydramine Hydrochloride (Co-administration results in additive CNS depressant effects). Products include:
Extra Strength Bayer PM Caplets..... ▣611
Benadryl Allergy Chewables..... ▣689
Benadryl Allergy..... ▣691
Benadryl Allergy Liquid..... ▣690
Benadryl Allergy/Cold Tablets..... ▣691
Benadryl Allergy/Congestion Tablets..... ▣692
Benadryl Allergy & Sinus Liquid..... ▣693
Benadryl Allergy Sinus Headache Caplets & Gelcaps..... ▣693
Benadryl Severe Allergy & Sinus Headache Caplets..... ▣694
Benadryl Dye-Free Allergy Liquid..... ▣690
Benadryl Dye-Free Allergy Liqui-Gels Softgels..... ▣690
Benadryl Itch Relief Stick Extra Strength..... ▣695
Benadryl Cream..... ▣695
Benadryl Gel..... ▣695
Benadryl Spray..... ▣696
Benadryl Parenteral..... 2617
Coricidin HBP Night-Time Cold & Flu Tablets..... ▣738
Nytol QuickCaps Caplets..... ▣622
Maximum Strength Nytol QuickGels Softgels..... ▣621
Extra Strength Percogesic Aspirin-Free Coated Caplets..... ▣665
Simply Sleep Caplets..... 2008
Sominex Original Formula Tablets..... ▣761
Children's Tylenol Allergy-D Liquid..... 2014
Maximum Strength Tylenol Allergy Sinus NightTime Caplets..... 2010
Tylenol Severe Allergy Caplets..... 2010
Maximum Strength Tylenol Flu NightTime Gelcaps..... 2011
Extra Strength Tylenol PM Caplets, Geltabs, and Gelcaps..... 2012
Unisom Maximum Strength SleepGels..... ▣713

Diphenylpyraline Hydrochloride (Co-administration results in additive CNS depressant effects).
No products indexed under this heading.

Dirithromycin (Co-administration with other macrolides, erythromycin, has resulted in increased maximum plasma concentration of triazolam, decreased clearance, and increased half-life; caution and consideration of appropriate triazolam dose reduction are recommended). Products include:
Dynabac Tablets..... 2269

Divalproex Sodium (Co-administration results in additive CNS depressant effects). Products include:
Depakote Sprinkle Capsules..... 426
Depakote Tablets..... 430
Depakote ER Tablets..... 436

Droperidol (Co-administration results in additive CNS depressant effects).
No products indexed under this heading.

Enflurane (Co-administration results in additive CNS depressant effects).
No products indexed under this heading.

Ergotamine Tartrate (Data from in vitro studies of benzodiazepines other than triazolam suggest a possible interaction; caution is recommended during co-administration).
No products indexed under this heading.

Erythromycin (Co-administration of erythromycin increased the maximum plasma concentration of triazolam by 46%; decreased the clearance by 53%, increased the half-life by 35%; caution and consideration of appropriate triazolam dose reduction are recommended). Products include:
Emgel 2% Topical Gel..... 1285
Ery-Tab Tablets..... 448
Erythromycin Base Filmtab Tablets..... 454
Erythromycin Delayed-Release Capsules, USP..... 455
PCE Dispertab Tablets..... 498

Erythromycin Estolate (Co-administration of erythromycin increased the maximum plasma concentration of triazolam by 46%; decreased the clearance by 53%, increased the half-life by 35%; caution and consideration of appropriate triazolam dose reduction are recommended).
No products indexed under this heading.

Erythromycin Ethylsuccinate (Co-administration of erythromycin increased the maximum plasma concentration of triazolam by 46%; decreased the clearance by 53%, increased the half-life by 35%; caution and consideration of appropriate triazolam dose reduction are recommended). Products include:
E.E.S...... 450
EryPed..... 446
Pediazole Suspension..... 3050

Erythromycin Gluceptate (Co-administration of erythromycin increased the maximum plasma concentration of triazolam by 46%; decreased the clearance by 53%, increased the half-life by 35%; caution and consideration of appropriate triazolam dose reduction are recommended).
No products indexed under this heading.

Erythromycin Stearate (Co-administration of erythromycin increased the maximum plasma concentration of triazolam by 46%; decreased the clearance by 53%, increased the half-life by 35%; caution and consideration of appropriate triazolam dose reduction are recommended). Products include:
Erythrocin Stearate Filmtab Tablets..... 452

Estazolam (Co-administration results in additive CNS depressant effects). Products include:
ProSom Tablets..... 500

Ethchlorvynol (Co-administration results in additive CNS depressant effects).
No products indexed under this heading.

Ethinamate (Co-administration results in additive CNS depressant effects).
No products indexed under this heading.

Ethinyl Estradiol (Co-administration of oral contraceptives increased the maximum plasma concentration of triazolam by 6%; decreased the clearance by 32%, increased the half-life by 16%). Products include:
Alesse-21 Tablets..... 3468
Alesse-28 Tablets..... 3473
Brevicon 28-Day Tablets..... 3380
Cyclessa Tablets..... 2450
Desogen Tablets..... 2458
Estinyl Tablets..... 3112
Estrostep..... 2627
femhrt Tablets..... 2635
Levlen..... 962
Levlite 21 Tablets..... 962
Levlite 28 Tablets..... 962
Levora Tablets..... 3389
Loestrin 21 Tablets..... 2642
Loestrin Fe Tablets..... 2642
Lo/Ovral Tablets..... 3532
Lo/Ovral-28 Tablets..... 3538
Low-Ogestrel-28 Tablets..... 3392
Microgestin Fe 1.5/30 Tablets..... 3407
Microgestin Fe 1/20 Tablets..... 3400
Mircette Tablets..... 2470
Modicon..... 2563
Necon..... 3415
Nordette-28 Tablets..... 2257
Norinyl 1 +35 28-Day Tablets..... 3380
Ogestrel 0.5/50-28 Tablets..... 3428
Ortho-Cept 21 Tablets..... 2546

Ortho-Cept 28 Tablets 2546
Ortho-Cyclen/Ortho Tri-Cyclen 2573
Ortho-Novum 2563
Ovcon 3364
Ovral Tablets 3551
Ovral-28 Tablets 3552
Tri-Levlen 962
Tri-Norinyl-28 Tablets 3433
Triphasil-21 Tablets 3600
Triphasil-28 Tablets 3605
Trivora Tablets 3439
Yasmin 28 Tablets 980
Zovia 3449

Ethosuximide (Co-administration results in additive CNS depressant effects). Products include:
Zarontin Capsules 2659
Zarontin Syrup 2660

Ethotoin (Co-administration results in additive CNS depressant effects).
No products indexed under this heading.

Ethynodiol Diacetate (Co-administration of oral contraceptives increased the maximum plasma concentration of triazolam by 6%; decreased the clearance by 32%, increased the half-life by 16%). Products include:
Zovia 3449

Felbamate (Co-administration results in additive CNS depressant effects). Products include:
Felbatol 3343

Fentanyl (Co-administration results in additive CNS depressant effects). Products include:
Duragesic Transdermal System 1786

Fentanyl Citrate (Co-administration results in additive CNS depressant effects). Products include:
Actiq 1184

Fexofenadine Hydrochloride (Co-administration results in additive CNS depressant effects). Products include:
Allegra 712
Allegra-D Extended-Release Tablets 714

Fluconazole (Other azole-type antifungals, such as ketoconazole or itraconazole, have demonstrated to be potent CYP 3A inhibitors with a potential for a profound effect on the clearance of triazolam; although data concerning the effect of other azole-type antifungals are not available, concurrent use is not recommended). Products include:
Diflucan Tablets, Injection, and Oral Suspension 2681

Fluphenazine Decanoate (Co-administration results in additive CNS depressant effects).
No products indexed under this heading.

Fluphenazine Enanthate (Co-administration results in additive CNS depressant effects).
No products indexed under this heading.

Fluphenazine Hydrochloride (Co-administration results in additive CNS depressant effects).
No products indexed under this heading.

Flurazepam Hydrochloride (Co-administration results in additive CNS depressant effects).
No products indexed under this heading.

Fluvoxamine Maleate (Co-administration of drugs demonstrated to be CYP 3A inhibitors on the basis of clinical studies involving benzodiazepine metabolized similarly to triazolam, such as fluvoxamine, may result in possible drug interaction with triazolam). Products include:
Luvox Tablets (25, 50, 100 mg) 3256

Fosphenytoin Sodium (Co-administration results in additive CNS depressant effects). Products include:
Cerebyx Injection 2619

Glutethimide (Co-administration results in additive CNS depressant effects).
No products indexed under this heading.

Haloperidol (Co-administration results in additive CNS depressant effects). Products include:
Haldol Injection, Tablets and Concentrate 2533

Haloperidol Decanoate (Co-administration results in additive CNS depressant effects). Products include:
Haldol Decanoate 2535

Hydrocodone Bitartrate (Co-administration results in additive CNS depressant effects). Products include:
Hycodan 1316
Hycomine Compound Tablets 1317
Hycotuss Expectorant Syrup 1318
Lortab 3319
Lortab Elixir 3317
Maxidone Tablets CIII 3399
Norco 5/325 Tablets CIII 3424
Norco 7.5/325 Tablets CIII 3425
Norco 10/325 Tablets CIII 3427
Norco 10/325 Tablets CIII 3425
Vicodin Tablets 516
Vicodin ES Tablets 517
Vicodin HP Tablets 518
Vicodin Tuss Expectorant 519
Vicoprofen Tablets 520
Zydone Tablets 1330

Hydrocodone Polistirex (Co-administration results in additive CNS depressant effects). Products include:
Tussionex Pennkinetic Extended-Release Suspension..... 1174

Hydromorphone Hydrochloride (Co-administration results in additive CNS depressant effects). Products include:
Dilaudid 441
Dilaudid Oral Liquid 445
Dilaudid Powder 441
Dilaudid Rectal Suppositories 441
Dilaudid Tablets 441
Dilaudid Tablets - 8 mg 445
Dilaudid-HP 443

Hydroxyzine Hydrochloride (Co-administration results in additive CNS depressant effects). Products include:
Atarax Tablets & Syrup 2667
Vistaril Intramuscular Solution 2738

Isoflurane (Co-administration results in additive CNS depressant effects).
No products indexed under this heading.

Isoniazid (Co-administration of isoniazid increased the maximum plasma concentration of triazolam by 20%; decreased the clearance by 42%, increased the half-life by 31%). Products include:
Rifamate Capsules 767
Rifater Tablets 769

Itraconazole (The initial step in triazolam metabolism is hydroxylation catalyzed by cytochrome P450 3A, therefore, inhibitors of this metabolic pathway, such as itraconazole, may have a profound effect on the clearance of triazolam; concurrent use is contraindicated). Products include:
Sporanox Capsules 1800
Sporanox Injection 1804
Sporanox Injection 2509
Sporanox Oral Solution 1808
Sporanox Oral Solution 2512

Ketamine Hydrochloride (Co-administration results in additive CNS depressant effects).
No products indexed under this heading.

Ketoconazole (The initial step in triazolam metabolism is hydroxylation catalyzed by cytochrome P450 3A, therefore, inhibitors of this metabolic pathway, such as ketoconazole, may have a profound effect on the clearance of triazolam; concurrent use is contraindicated). Products include:
Nizoral 2% Cream 3620
Nizoral A-D Shampoo 2008
Nizoral 2% Shampoo 2007
Nizoral Tablets 1791

Lamotrigine (Co-administration results in additive CNS depressant effects). Products include:
Lamictal 1567

Levetiracetam (Co-administration results in additive CNS depressant effects). Products include:
Keppra Tablets 3314

Levomethadyl Acetate Hydrochloride (Co-administration results in additive CNS depressant effects).
No products indexed under this heading.

Levonorgestrel (Co-administration of oral contraceptives increased the maximum plasma concentration of triazolam by 6%; decreased the clearance by 32%, increased the half-life by 16%). Products include:
Alesse-21 Tablets 3468
Alesse-28 Tablets 3473
Levlen 962
Levlite 21 Tablets 962
Levlite 28 Tablets 962
Levora Tablets 3389
Mirena Intrauterine System 974
Nordette-28 Tablets 2257
Norplant System 3543
Tri-Levlen 962
Triphasil-21 Tablets 3600
Triphasil-28 Tablets 3605
Trivora Tablets 3439

Levorphanol Tartrate (Co-administration results in additive CNS depressant effects). Products include:
Levo-Dromoran 1734
Levorphanol Tartrate Tablets 3059

Loratadine (Co-administration results in additive CNS depressant effects). Products include:
Claritin 3100
Claritin-D 12 Hour Extended Release Tablets 3102
Claritin-D 24 Hour Extended Release Tablets 3104

Lorazepam (Co-administration results in additive CNS depressant effects). Products include:
Ativan Injection 3478
Ativan Tablets 3482

Loxapine Hydrochloride (Co-administration results in additive CNS depressant effects).
No products indexed under this heading.

Loxapine Succinate (Co-administration results in additive CNS depressant effects). Products include:
Loxitane Capsules 3398

Meperidine Hydrochloride (Co-administration results in additive CNS depressant effects). Products include:
Demerol 3079
Mepergan Injection 3539

Mephenytoin (Co-administration results in additive CNS depressant effects).
No products indexed under this heading.

Mephobarbital (Co-administration results in additive CNS depressant effects).
No products indexed under this heading.

Meprobamate (Co-administration results in additive CNS depressant effects). Products include:
Miltown Tablets 3349

Mesoridazine Besylate (Co-administration results in additive CNS depressant effects). Products include:
Serentil 1057

Mestranol (Co-administration of oral contraceptives increased the maximum plasma concentration of triazolam by 6%; decreased the clearance by 32%, increased the half-life by 16%). Products include:
Necon 1/50 Tablets 3415
Norinyl 1 + 50 28-Day Tablets 3380
Ortho-Novum 1/50□28 Tablets 2556

Methadone Hydrochloride (Co-administration results in additive CNS depressant effects). Products include:
Dolophine Hydrochloride Tablets 3056

Methdilazine Hydrochloride (Co-administration results in additive CNS depressant effects).
No products indexed under this heading.

Methohexital Sodium (Co-administration results in additive CNS depressant effects). Products include:
Brevital Sodium for Injection, USP .. 1815

Methotrimeprazine (Co-administration results in additive CNS depressant effects).
No products indexed under this heading.

Methoxyflurane (Co-administration results in additive CNS depressant effects).
No products indexed under this heading.

Methsuximide (Co-administration results in additive CNS depressant effects). Products include:
Celontin Capsules 2618

Miconazole (Other azole-type antifungals, such as ketoconazole or itraconazole, have demonstrated to be potent CYP 3A inhibitors with a potential for a profound effect on the clearance of triazolam; although data concerning the effect of other azole-type antifungals are not available, concurrent use is not recommended).
No products indexed under this heading.

Midazolam Hydrochloride (Co-administration results in additive CNS depressant effects). Products include:
Versed Injection 3027
Versed Syrup 3033

Molindone Hydrochloride (Co-administration results in additive CNS depressant effects). Products include:
Moban 1320

Morphine Sulfate (Co-administration results in additive CNS depressant effects). Products include:
Astramorph/PF Injection, USP (Preservative-Free)......................... 594
Duramorph Injection 1312
Infumorph 200 and Infumorph 500 Sterile Solutions 1314
Kadian Capsules 1335
MS Contin Tablets 2896
MSIR 2898
Oramorph SR Tablets 3062
Roxanol 3066

Nefazodone Hydrochloride (The initial step in triazolam metabolism is hydroxylation catalyzed by cytochrome P450 3A, therefore, inhibitors of this metabolic pathway, such as nefazadone, may have a profound effect on the clearance of triazolam; concurrent use is contraindicated). Products include:
Serzone Tablets 1104

Nicardipine Hydrochloride (Data from in vitro studies of benzodiazepines other than triazolam suggest a possible interaction; caution is recommended during co-administration). Products include:
Cardene I.V. 3485

Nifedipine (Data from in vitro studies of benzodiazepines other than triazolam suggest a possible interaction; caution is recommended during co-administration). Products include:

IMPORTANT NOTE: Always consult each drug listing in the patient's regimen for possible interactions.

Adalat CC Tablets 877
Procardia Capsules 2708
Procardia XL Extended Release Tablets 2710

Norethindrone (Co-administration of oral contraceptives increased the maximum plasma concentration of triazolam by 6%; decreased the clearance by 32%, increased the half-life by 16%). Products include:
Brevicon 28-Day Tablets 3380
Micronor Tablets 2543
Modicon 2563
Necon 3415
Norinyl 1 +35 28-Day Tablets 3380
Norinyl 1 + 50 28-Day Tablets 3380
Nor-QD Tablets 3423
Ortho-Novum 2563
Ortho-Novum 1/50▫28 Tablets 2556
Ovcon 3364
Tri-Norinyl-28 Tablets 3433

Norethynodrel (Co-administration of oral contraceptives increased the maximum plasma concentration of triazolam by 6%; decreased the clearance by 32%, increased the half-life by 16%).
No products indexed under this heading.

Norgestimate (Co-administration of oral contraceptives increased the maximum plasma concentration of triazolam by 6%; decreased the clearance by 32%, increased the half-life by 16%). Products include:
Ortho-Cyclen/Ortho Tri-Cyclen 2573
Ortho-Prefest Tablets 2570

Norgestrel (Co-administration of oral contraceptives increased the maximum plasma concentration of triazolam by 6%; decreased the clearance by 32%, increased the half-life by 16%). Products include:
Lo/Ovral Tablets 3532
Lo/Ovral-28 Tablets 3538
Low-Ogestrel-28 Tablets 3392
Ogestrel 0.5/50-28 Tablets 3428
Ovral Tablets 3551
Ovral-28 Tablets 3552
Ovrette Tablets 3552

Olanzapine (Co-administration results in additive CNS depressant effects). Products include:
Zyprexa Tablets 1973
Zyprexa ZYDIS Orally Disintegrating Tablets 1973

Oxazepam (Co-administration results in additive CNS depressant effects).
No products indexed under this heading.

Oxcarbazepine (Co-administration results in additive CNS depressant effects). Products include:
Trileptal Oral Suspension 2407
Trileptal Tablets 2407

Oxiconazole Nitrate (Other azole-type antifungals, such as ketoconazole or itraconazole, have demonstrated to be potent CYP 3A inhibitors with a potential for a profound effect on the clearance of triazolam; although data concerning the effect of other azole-type antifungals are not available, concurrent use is not recommended). Products include:
Oxistat 1298

Oxycodone Hydrochloride (Co-administration results in additive CNS depressant effects). Products include:
OxyContin Tablets 2912
OxyFast Oral Concentrate Solution 2916
OxyIR Capsules 2916
Percocet Tablets 1326
Percodan Tablets 1327
Percolone Tablets 1327
Roxicodone 3067
Tylox Capsules 2597

Paramethadione (Co-administration results in additive CNS depressant effects).
No products indexed under this heading.

Paroxetine Hydrochloride (Data from in vitro studies of triazolam suggest a possible interaction; caution is recommended during co-administration). Products include:
Paxil 1609

Pentobarbital Sodium (Co-administration results in additive CNS depressant effects). Products include:
Nembutal Sodium Solution 485

Perphenazine (Co-administration results in additive CNS depressant effects). Products include:
Etrafon 3115
Trilafon 3160

Phenacemide (Co-administration results in additive CNS depressant effects).
No products indexed under this heading.

Phenobarbital (Co-administration results in additive CNS depressant effects). Products include:
Arco-Lase Plus Tablets 592
Donnatal 2929
Donnatal Extentabs 2930

Phensuximide (Co-administration results in additive CNS depressant effects).
No products indexed under this heading.

Phenytoin (Co-administration results in additive CNS depressant effects). Products include:
Dilantin Infatabs 2624
Dilantin-125 Oral Suspension 2625

Phenytoin Sodium (Co-administration results in additive CNS depressant effects). Products include:
Dilantin Kapseals 2622

Prazepam (Co-administration results in additive CNS depressant effects).
No products indexed under this heading.

Primidone (Co-administration results in additive CNS depressant effects).
No products indexed under this heading.

Prochlorperazine (Co-administration results in additive CNS depressant effects). Products include:
Compazine 1505

Promethazine Hydrochloride (Co-administration results in additive CNS depressant effects). Products include:
Mepergan Injection 3539
Phenergan Injection 3553
Phenergan 3556
Phenergan Syrup 3554
Phenergan with Codeine Syrup 3557
Phenergan with Dextromethorphan Syrup 3559
Phenergan VC Syrup 3560
Phenergan VC with Codeine Syrup 3561

Propofol (Co-administration results in additive CNS depressant effects). Products include:
Diprivan Injectable Emulsion 667

Propoxyphene Hydrochloride (Co-administration results in additive CNS depressant effects). Products include:
Darvon Pulvules 1909
Darvon Compound-65 Pulvules 1910

Propoxyphene Napsylate (Co-administration results in additive CNS depressant effects). Products include:
Darvon-N/Darvocet-N 1907
Darvon-N Tablets 1912

Pyrilamine Maleate (Co-administration results in additive CNS depressant effects). Products include:
Maximum Strength Midol Menstrual Caplets and Gelcaps .... ■612
Maximum Strength Midol PMS Caplets and Gelcaps .... ■613

Pyrilamine Tannate (Co-administration results in additive CNS depressant effects). Products include:
Ryna-12 S Suspension 3351

Quazepam (Co-administration results in additive CNS depressant effects).
No products indexed under this heading.

Quetiapine Fumarate (Co-administration results in additive CNS depressant effects). Products include:
Seroquel Tablets 684

Ranitidine Hydrochloride (Co-administration of ranitidine increased the maximum plasma concentration of triazolam by 30%; increased the AUC by 27%, increased the half-life by 3.3%; caution is recommended during co-administration). Products include:
Zantac 1690
Zantac Injection 1688
Zantac 75 Tablets .... ■717

Remifentanil Hydrochloride (Co-administration results in additive CNS depressant effects).
No products indexed under this heading.

Risperidone (Co-administration results in additive CNS depressant effects). Products include:
Risperdal 1796

Secobarbital Sodium (Co-administration results in additive CNS depressant effects).
No products indexed under this heading.

Sertraline Hydrochloride (Data from in vitro studies of triazolam suggest a possible interaction; caution is recommended during co-administration). Products include:
Zoloft 2751

Sevoflurane (Co-administration results in additive CNS depressant effects).
No products indexed under this heading.

Sufentanil Citrate (Co-administration results in additive CNS depressant effects).
No products indexed under this heading.

Temazepam (Co-administration results in additive CNS depressant effects).
No products indexed under this heading.

Terconazole (Other azole-type antifungals, such as ketoconazole or itraconazole, have demonstrated to be potent CYP 3A inhibitors with a potential for a profound effect on the clearance of triazolam; although data concerning the effect of other azole-type antifungals are not available, concurrent use is not recommended). Products include:
Terazol 3 Vaginal Cream 2587
Terazol 3 Vaginal Suppositories 2587
Terazol 7 Vaginal Cream 2587

Terfenadine (Co-administration results in additive CNS depressant effects).
No products indexed under this heading.

Thiamylal Sodium (Co-administration results in additive CNS depressant effects).
No products indexed under this heading.

Thioridazine Hydrochloride (Co-administration results in additive CNS depressant effects). Products include:
Thioridazine Hydrochloride Tablets 2289

Thiothixene (Co-administration results in additive CNS depressant effects). Products include:
Navane Capsules 2701
Thiothixene Capsules 2290

Tiagabine Hydrochloride (Co-administration results in additive CNS depressant effects). Products include:
Gabitril Tablets 1189

Topiramate (Co-administration results in additive CNS depressant effects). Products include:
Topamax Sprinkle Capsules 2590
Topamax Tablets 2590

Trifluoperazine Hydrochloride (Co-administration results in additive CNS depressant effects). Products include:
Stelazine 1640

Trimeprazine Tartrate (Co-administration results in additive CNS depressant effects).
No products indexed under this heading.

Trimethadione (Co-administration results in additive CNS depressant effects).
No products indexed under this heading.

Tripelennamine Hydrochloride (Co-administration results in additive CNS depressant effects).
No products indexed under this heading.

Triprolidine Hydrochloride (Co-administration results in additive CNS depressant effects). Products include:
Actifed Cold & Allergy Tablets .... ■688

Troleandomycin (Co-administration with other macrolides, erythromycin, has resulted in increased maximum plasma concentration of triazolam, decreased clearance, and increased half-life; caution and consideration of appropriate triazolam dose reduction are recommended). Products include:
Tao Capsules 2716

Valproate Sodium (Co-administration results in additive CNS depressant effects). Products include:
Depacon Injection 416

Valproic Acid (Co-administration results in additive CNS depressant effects). Products include:
Depakene 421

Verapamil Hydrochloride (Co-administration of drugs demonstrated to be CYP 3A inhibitors on the basis of clinical studies involving benzodiazepine metabolized similarly to triazolam, such as verapamil, may result in possible drug interaction with triazolam). Products include:
Covera-HS Tablets 3199
Isoptin SR Tablets 467
Tarka Tablets 508
Verelan Capsules 3184
Verelan PM Capsules 3186

Zaleplon (Co-administration results in additive CNS depressant effects). Products include:
Sonata Capsules 3591

Ziprasidone Hydrochloride (Co-administration results in additive CNS depressant effects). Products include:
Geodon Capsules 2688

Zolpidem Tartrate (Co-administration results in additive CNS depressant effects). Products include:
Ambien Tablets 3191

Zonisamide (Co-administration results in additive CNS depressant effects). Products include:
Zonegran Capsules 1307

Food Interactions

Alcohol (Concurrent use results in additive CNS depressant effects).

Grapefruit Juice (Co-administration of grapefruit juice increased the maximum plasma concentration of triazolam by 25%; increased the AUC by 48%, and increased the half-life by 18%).

HALDOL DECANOATE 50 INJECTION
(Haloperidol Decanoate) 2535
See Haldol Injection, Tablets and Concentrate

HALDOL DECANOATE 100 INJECTION
(Haloperidol Decanoate) 2535
See Haldol Injection, Tablets and Concentrate

HALDOL INJECTION, TABLETS AND CONCENTRATE
(Haloperidol) 2533
May interact with anticholinergics, anticholinergic-type antiparkinsonism drugs, central nervous system depressants, oral anticoagulants, anticonvulsants, lithium preparations, and certain other agents. Compounds in these categories include:

Alfentanil Hydrochloride (Potentiation of CNS depressant effects).
No products indexed under this heading.

Alprazolam (Potentiation of CNS depressant effects). Products include:
Xanax Tablets 2865

Aprobarbital (Potentiation of CNS depressant effects).
No products indexed under this heading.

Atropine Sulfate (Co-administration with anticholinergic drugs, including antiparkinson agents, may result in possible increase in intraocular pressure). Products include:
Donnatal 2929
Donnatal Extentabs 2930
Motofen Tablets 577
Prosed/DS Tablets 3268
Urised Tablets 2876

Belladonna Alkaloids (Co-administration with anticholinergic drugs, including antiparkinson agents, may result in possible increase in intraocular pressure). Products include:
Hyland's Teething Tablets .... ▣766
Urimax Tablets 1769

Benztropine Mesylate (Co-administration with anticholinergic drugs, including antiparkinson agents, may result in possible increase in intraocular pressure). Products include:
Cogentin 2055

Biperiden Hydrochloride (Co-administration with anticholinergic drugs, including antiparkinson agents, may result in possible increase in intraocular pressure). Products include:
Akineton 402

Buprenorphine Hydrochloride (Potentiation of CNS depressant effects). Products include:
Buprenex Injectable 2918

Buspirone Hydrochloride (Potentiation of CNS depressant effects).
No products indexed under this heading.

Butabarbital (Potentiation of CNS depressant effects).
No products indexed under this heading.

Butalbital (Potentiation of CNS depressant effects). Products include:
Phrenilin 578
Sedapap Tablets 50 mg/650 mg ... 2225

Carbamazepine (Haloperidol may lower the convulsive threshold; adequate anticonvulsant therapy is indicated if co-administered). Products include:
Carbatrol Capsules 3234
Tegretol/Tegretol-XR 2404

Chlordiazepoxide (Potentiation of CNS depressant effects). Products include:
Limbitrol 1738

Chlordiazepoxide Hydrochloride (Potentiation of CNS depressant effects). Products include:
Librium Capsules 1736
Librium for Injection 1737

Chlorpromazine (Potentiation of CNS depressant effects). Products include:
Thorazine Suppositories 1656

Chlorpromazine Hydrochloride (Potentiation of CNS depressant effects). Products include:
Thorazine 1656

Chlorprothixene (Potentiation of CNS depressant effects).
No products indexed under this heading.

Chlorprothixene Hydrochloride (Potentiation of CNS depressant effects).
No products indexed under this heading.

Chlorprothixene Lactate (Potentiation of CNS depressant effects).
No products indexed under this heading.

Clidinium Bromide (Co-administration with anticholinergic drugs, including antiparkinson agents, may result in possible increase in intraocular pressure).
No products indexed under this heading.

Clorazepate Dipotassium (Potentiation of CNS depressant effects). Products include:
Tranxene 511

Clozapine (Potentiation of CNS depressant effects). Products include:
Clozaril Tablets 2319

Codeine Phosphate (Potentiation of CNS depressant effects). Products include:
Phenergan with Codeine Syrup 3557
Phenergan VC with Codeine Syrup .. 3561
Robitussin A-C Syrup 2942
Robitussin-DAC Syrup 2942
Ryna-C Liquid .... ▣768
Soma Compound w/Codeine Tablets 3355
Tussi-Organidin NR Liquid 3350
Tussi-Organidin-S NR Liquid 3350
Tylenol with Codeine 2595

Desflurane (Potentiation of CNS depressant effects). Products include:
Suprane Liquid for Inhalation 874

Dezocine (Potentiation of CNS depressant effects).
No products indexed under this heading.

Diazepam (Potentiation of CNS depressant effects). Products include:
Valium Injectable 3026
Valium Tablets 3047

Dicumarol (Co-administration with one anticoagulant, phenindione, has resulted in an isolated instance of interference with anticoagulation effect).
No products indexed under this heading.

Dicyclomine Hydrochloride (Co-administration with anticholinergic drugs, including antiparkinson agents, may result in possible increase in intraocular pressure).
No products indexed under this heading.

Diphenhydramine Hydrochloride (Co-administration with antiparkinson agents may result in possible increase in intraocular pressure). Products include:
Extra Strength Bayer PM Caplets .... ▣611
Benadryl Allergy Chewables .... ▣689
Benadryl Allergy .... ▣691
Benadryl Allergy Liquid .... ▣690
Benadryl Allergy/Cold Tablets .... ▣691
Benadryl Allergy/Congestion Tablets .... ▣692
Benadryl Allergy & Sinus Liquid ..... ▣693
Benadryl Allergy Sinus Headache Caplets & Gelcaps .... ▣693
Benadryl Severe Allergy & Sinus Headache Caplets .... ▣694
Benadryl Dye-Free Allergy Liquid ... ▣690
Benadryl Dye-Free Allergy Liqui-Gels Softgels .... ▣690
Benadryl Itch Relief Stick Extra Strength .... ▣695
Benadryl Cream .... ▣695
Benadryl Gel .... ▣695
Benadryl Spray .... ▣696
Benadryl Parenteral 2617
Coricidin HBP Night-Time Cold & Flu Tablets .... ▣738
Nytol QuickCaps Caplets .... ▣622
Maximum Strength Nytol QuickGels Softgels .... ▣621
Extra Strength Percogesic Aspirin-Free Coated Caplets .... ▣665
Simply Sleep Caplets 2008
Sominex Original Formula Tablets . ▣761
Children's Tylenol Allergy-D Liquid ... 2014
Maximum Strength Tylenol Allergy Sinus NightTime Caplets 2010
Tylenol Severe Allergy Caplets 2010
Maximum Strength Tylenol Flu NightTime Gelcaps 2011
Extra Strength Tylenol PM Caplets, Geltabs, and Gelcaps 2012
Unisom Maximum Strength SleepGels .... ▣713

Divalproex Sodium (Haloperidol may lower the convulsive threshold; adequate anticonvulsant therapy is indicated if co-administered). Products include:
Depakote Sprinkle Capsules 426
Depakote Tablets 430
Depakote ER Tablets 436

Droperidol (Potentiation of CNS depressant effects).
No products indexed under this heading.

Enflurane (Potentiation of CNS depressant effects).
No products indexed under this heading.

Estazolam (Potentiation of CNS depressant effects). Products include:
ProSom Tablets 500

Ethchlorvynol (Potentiation of CNS depressant effects).
No products indexed under this heading.

Ethinamate (Potentiation of CNS depressant effects).
No products indexed under this heading.

Ethosuximide (Haloperidol may lower the convulsive threshold; adequate anticonvulsant therapy is indicated if co-administered). Products include:
Zarontin Capsules 2659
Zarontin Syrup 2660

Ethotoin (Haloperidol may lower the convulsive threshold; adequate anticonvulsant therapy is indicated if co-administered).
No products indexed under this heading.

Felbamate (Haloperidol may lower the convulsive threshold; adequate anticonvulsant therapy is indicated if co-administered). Products include:
Felbatol 3343

Fentanyl (Potentiation of CNS depressant effects). Products include:
Duragesic Transdermal System 1786

Fentanyl Citrate (Potentiation of CNS depressant effects). Products include:
Actiq 1184

Fluphenazine Decanoate (Potentiation of CNS depressant effects).
No products indexed under this heading.

Fluphenazine Enanthate (Potentiation of CNS depressant effects).
No products indexed under this heading.

Fluphenazine Hydrochloride (Potentiation of CNS depressant effects).
No products indexed under this heading.

Flurazepam Hydrochloride (Potentiation of CNS depressant effects).
No products indexed under this heading.

Fosphenytoin Sodium (Haloperidol may lower the convulsive threshold; adequate anticonvulsant therapy is indicated if co-administered). Products include:
Cerebyx Injection 2619

Glutethimide (Potentiation of CNS depressant effects).
No products indexed under this heading.

Glycopyrrolate (Co-administration with anticholinergic drugs, including antiparkinson agents, may result in possible increase in intraocular pressure). Products include:
Robinul Forte Tablets 1358
Robinul Injectable 2940
Robinul Tablets 1358

Haloperidol Decanoate (Potentiation of CNS depressant effects). Products include:
Haldol Decanoate 2535

Hydrocodone Bitartrate (Potentiation of CNS depressant effects). Products include:
Hycodan 1316
Hycomine Compound Tablets 1317
Hycotuss Expectorant Syrup 1318
Lortab 3319
Lortab Elixir 3317
Maxidone Tablets CIII 3399
Norco 5/325 Tablets CIII 3424
Norco 7.5/325 Tablets CIII 3425
Norco 10/325 Tablets CIII 3427
Norco 10/325 Tablets CIII 3425
Vicodin Tablets 516
Vicodin ES Tablets 517
Vicodin HP Tablets 518
Vicodin Tuss Expectorant 519
Vicoprofen Tablets 520
Zydone Tablets 1330

Hydrocodone Polistirex (Potentiation of CNS depressant effects). Products include:
Tussionex Pennkinetic Extended-Release Suspension 1174

Hydromorphone Hydrochloride (Potentiation of CNS depressant effects). Products include:
Dilaudid 441
Dilaudid Oral Liquid 445
Dilaudid Powder 441
Dilaudid Rectal Suppositories 441
Dilaudid Tablets 441
Dilaudid Tablets - 8 mg 445
Dilaudid-HP 443

Hydroxyzine Hydrochloride (Potentiation of CNS depressant effects). Products include:
Atarax Tablets & Syrup 2667
Vistaril Intramuscular Solution 2738

Hyoscyamine (Co-administration with anticholinergic drugs, including antiparkinson agents, may result in possible increase in intraocular pressure). Products include:
Urised Tablets 2876

Hyoscyamine Sulfate (Co-administration with anticholinergic drugs, including antiparkinson agents, may result in possible increase in intraocular pressure). Products include:
Arco-Lase Plus Tablets 592
Donnatal 2929
Donnatal Extentabs 2930
Levsin/Levsinex/Levbid 3172
NuLev Orally Disintegrating Tablets 3176
Prosed/DS Tablets 3268
Urimax Tablets 1769

Ipratropium Bromide (Co-administration with anticholinergic drugs, including antiparkinson agents, may result in possible increase in intraocular pressure). Products include:
Atrovent Inhalation Aerosol 1030
Atrovent Inhalation Solution 1031

IMPORTANT NOTE: Always consult each drug listing in the patient's regimen for possible interactions.

Atrovent Nasal Spray 0.03% 1032
Atrovent Nasal Spray 0.06% 1033
Combivent Inhalation Aerosol 1041
DuoNeb Inhalation Solution 1233

Isoflurane (Potentiation of CNS depressant effects).
No products indexed under this heading.

Ketamine Hydrochloride (Potentiation of CNS depressant effects).
No products indexed under this heading.

Lamotrigine (Haloperidol may lower the convulsive threshold; adequate anticonvulsant therapy is indicated if co-administered). Products include:
Lamictal 1567

Levetiracetam (Haloperidol may lower the convulsive threshold; adequate anticonvulsant therapy is indicated if co-administered). Products include:
Keppra Tablets 3314

Levomethadyl Acetate Hydrochloride (Potentiation of CNS depressant effects).
No products indexed under this heading.

Levorphanol Tartrate (Potentiation of CNS depressant effects). Products include:
Levo-Dromoran 1734
Levorphanol Tartrate Tablets 3059

Lithium Carbonate (Co-administration has resulted in an encephalopathic syndrome characterized by weakness, lethargy, fever, tremulousness and confusion, extrapyramidal symptoms, leukocytosis, elevated BUN and FBS followed by irreversible brain damage in a few patients). Products include:
Eskalith 1527
Lithium Carbonate 3061
Lithobid Slow-Release Tablets 3255

Lithium Citrate (Co-administration has resulted in an encephalopathic syndrome characterized by weakness, lethargy, fever, tremulousness and confusion, extrapyramidal symptoms, leukocytosis, elevated BUN and FBS followed by irreversible brain damage in a few patients). Products include:
Lithium Citrate Syrup 3061

Lorazepam (Potentiation of CNS depressant effects). Products include:
Ativan Injection 3478
Ativan Tablets 3482

Loxapine Hydrochloride (Potentiation of CNS depressant effects).
No products indexed under this heading.

Loxapine Succinate (Potentiation of CNS depressant effects). Products include:
Loxitane Capsules 3398

Mepenzolate Bromide (Co-administration with anticholinergic drugs, including antiparkinson agents, may result in possible increase in intraocular pressure).
No products indexed under this heading.

Meperidine Hydrochloride (Potentiation of CNS depressant effects). Products include:
Demerol 3079
Mepergan Injection 3539

Mephenytoin (Haloperidol may lower the convulsive threshold; adequate anticonvulsant therapy is indicated if co-administered).
No products indexed under this heading.

Mephobarbital (Potentiation of CNS depressant effects).
No products indexed under this heading.

Meprobamate (Potentiation of CNS depressant effects). Products include:
Miltown Tablets 3349

Mesoridazine Besylate (Potentiation of CNS depressant effects). Products include:
Serentil 1057

Methadone Hydrochloride (Potentiation of CNS depressant effects). Products include:
Dolophine Hydrochloride Tablets 3056

Methohexital Sodium (Potentiation of CNS depressant effects). Products include:
Brevital Sodium for Injection, USP .. 1815

Methotrimeprazine (Potentiation of CNS depressant effects).
No products indexed under this heading.

Methoxyflurane (Potentiation of CNS depressant effects).
No products indexed under this heading.

Methsuximide (Haloperidol may lower the convulsive threshold; adequate anticonvulsant therapy is indicated if co-administered). Products include:
Celontin Capsules 2618

Midazolam Hydrochloride (Potentiation of CNS depressant effects). Products include:
Versed Injection 3027
Versed Syrup 3033

Molindone Hydrochloride (Potentiation of CNS depressant effects). Products include:
Moban 1320

Morphine Sulfate (Potentiation of CNS depressant effects). Products include:
Astramorph/PF Injection, USP (Preservative-Free)...................... 594
Duramorph Injection 1312
Infumorph 200 and Infumorph 500 Sterile Solutions........................ 1314
Kadian Capsules 1335
MS Contin Tablets 2896
MSIR 2898
Oramorph SR Tablets 3062
Roxanol 3066

Olanzapine (Potentiation of CNS depressant effects). Products include:
Zyprexa Tablets 1973
Zyprexa ZYDIS Orally Disintegrating Tablets................ 1973

Oxazepam (Potentiation of CNS depressant effects).
No products indexed under this heading.

Oxcarbazepine (Haloperidol may lower the convulsive threshold; adequate anticonvulsant therapy is indicated if co-administered). Products include:
Trileptal Oral Suspension 2407
Trileptal Tablets 2407

Oxybutynin Chloride (Co-administration with anticholinergic drugs, including antiparkinson agents, may result in possible increase in intraocular pressure). Products include:
Ditropan XL Extended Release Tablets 564

Oxycodone Hydrochloride (Potentiation of CNS depressant effects). Products include:
OxyContin Tablets 2912
OxyFast Oral Concentrate Solution . 2916
OxyIR Capsules 2916
Percocet Tablets 1326
Percodan Tablets 1327
Percolone Tablets 1327
Roxicodone 3067
Tylox Capsules 2597

Paramethadione (Haloperidol may lower the convulsive threshold; adequate anticonvulsant therapy is indicated if co-administered).
No products indexed under this heading.

Pentobarbital Sodium (Potentiation of CNS depressant effects). Products include:
Nembutal Sodium Solution 485

Perphenazine (Potentiation of CNS depressant effects). Products include:
Etrafon 3115
Trilafon 3160

Phenacemide (Haloperidol may lower the convulsive threshold; adequate anticonvulsant therapy is indicated if co-administered).
No products indexed under this heading.

Phenobarbital (Haloperidol may lower the convulsive threshold; adequate anticonvulsant therapy is indicated if co-administered; potentiation of CNS depressant effects). Products include:
Arco-Lase Plus Tablets 592
Donnatal 2929
Donnatal Extentabs 2930

Phensuximide (Haloperidol may lower the convulsive threshold; adequate anticonvulsant therapy is indicated if co-administered).
No products indexed under this heading.

Phenytoin (Haloperidol may lower the convulsive threshold; adequate anticonvulsant therapy is indicated if co-administered). Products include:
Dilantin Infatabs 2624
Dilantin-125 Oral Suspension 2625

Phenytoin Sodium (Haloperidol may lower the convulsive threshold; adequate anticonvulsant therapy is indicated if co-administered). Products include:
Dilantin Kapseals 2622

Prazepam (Potentiation of CNS depressant effects).
No products indexed under this heading.

Primidone (Haloperidol may lower the convulsive threshold; adequate anticonvulsant therapy is indicated if co-administered).
No products indexed under this heading.

Prochlorperazine (Potentiation of CNS depressant effects). Products include:
Compazine 1505

Procyclidine Hydrochloride (Co-administration with anticholinergic drugs, including antiparkinson agents, may result in possible increase in intraocular pressure).
No products indexed under this heading.

Promethazine Hydrochloride (Potentiation of CNS depressant effects). Products include:
Mepergan Injection 3539
Phenergan Injection 3553
Phenergan 3556
Phenergan Syrup 3554
Phenergan with Codeine Syrup 3557
Phenergan with Dextromethorphan Syrup 3559
Phenergan VC Syrup 3560
Phenergan VC with Codeine Syrup .. 3561

Propantheline Bromide (Co-administration with anticholinergic drugs, including antiparkinson agents, may result in possible increase in intraocular pressure).
No products indexed under this heading.

Propofol (Potentiation of CNS depressant effects). Products include:
Diprivan Injectable Emulsion 667

Propoxyphene Hydrochloride (Potentiation of CNS depressant effects). Products include:
Darvon Pulvules 1909
Darvon Compound-65 Pulvules 1910

Propoxyphene Napsylate (Potentiation of CNS depressant effects). Products include:
Darvon-N/Darvocet-N 1907
Darvon-N Tablets 1912

Quazepam (Potentiation of CNS depressant effects).
No products indexed under this heading.

Quetiapine Fumarate (Potentiation of CNS depressant effects). Products include:
Seroquel Tablets 684

Remifentanil Hydrochloride (Potentiation of CNS depressant effects).
No products indexed under this heading.

Rifampin (Co-administration has resulted in decreased plasma haloperidol levels by a mean of 70% and increased mean scores on the Brief Psychiatric Rating Scales from baseline; careful monitoring of clinical status is warranted when used concurrently). Products include:
Rifadin 765
Rifamate Capsules 767
Rifater Tablets 769

Risperidone (Potentiation of CNS depressant effects). Products include:
Risperdal 1796

Scopolamine (Co-administration with anticholinergic drugs, including antiparkinson agents, may result in possible increase in intraocular pressure). Products include:
Transderm Scōp Transdermal Therapeutic System...................... 2302

Scopolamine Hydrobromide (Co-administration with anticholinergic drugs, including antiparkinson agents, may result in possible increase in intraocular pressure). Products include:
Donnatal 2929
Donnatal Extentabs 2930

Secobarbital Sodium (Potentiation of CNS depressant effects).
No products indexed under this heading.

Sevoflurane (Potentiation of CNS depressant effects).
No products indexed under this heading.

Sufentanil Citrate (Potentiation of CNS depressant effects).
No products indexed under this heading.

Temazepam (Potentiation of CNS depressant effects).
No products indexed under this heading.

Thiamylal Sodium (Potentiation of CNS depressant effects).
No products indexed under this heading.

Thioridazine Hydrochloride (Potentiation of CNS depressant effects). Products include:
Thioridazine Hydrochloride Tablets.. 2289

Thiothixene (Potentiation of CNS depressant effects). Products include:
Navane Capsules 2701
Thiothixene Capsules 2290

Tiagabine Hydrochloride (Haloperidol may lower the convulsive threshold; adequate anticonvulsant therapy is indicated if co-administered). Products include:
Gabitril Tablets 1189

Tolterodine Tartrate (Co-administration with anticholinergic drugs, including antiparkinson agents, may result in possible increase in intraocular pressure). Products include:
Detrol Tablets 3623
Detrol LA Capsules 2801

Topiramate (Haloperidol may lower the convulsive threshold; adequate anticonvulsant therapy is indicated if co-administered). Products include:
Topamax Sprinkle Capsules 2590
Topamax Tablets 2590

Triazolam (Potentiation of CNS depressant effects). Products include:
- Halcion Tablets 2823

Tridihexethyl Chloride (Co-administration with anticholinergic drugs, including antiparkinson agents, may result in possible increase in intraocular pressure).
- No products indexed under this heading.

Trifluoperazine Hydrochloride (Potentiation of CNS depressant effects). Products include:
- Stelazine 1640

Trihexyphenidyl Hydrochloride (Co-administration with anticholinergic drugs, including antiparkinson agents, may result in possible increase in intraocular pressure). Products include:
- Artane 1855

Trimethadione (Haloperidol may lower the convulsive threshold; adequate anticonvulsant therapy is indicated if co-administered).
- No products indexed under this heading.

Valproate Sodium (Haloperidol may lower the convulsive threshold; adequate anticonvulsant therapy is indicated if co-administered). Products include:
- Depacon Injection 416

Valproic Acid (Haloperidol may lower the convulsive threshold; adequate anticonvulsant therapy is indicated if co-administered). Products include:
- Depakene 421

Warfarin Sodium (Co-administration with one anticoagulant, phenindione, has resulted in an isolated instance of interference with anticoagulation effect). Products include:
- Coumadin for Injection 1243
- Coumadin Tablets 1243
- Warfarin Sodium Tablets, USP 3302

Zaleplon (Potentiation of CNS depressant effects). Products include:
- Sonata Capsules 3591

Ziprasidone Hydrochloride (Potentiation of CNS depressant effects). Products include:
- Geodon Capsules 2688

Zolpidem Tartrate (Potentiation of CNS depressant effects). Products include:
- Ambien Tablets 3191

Zonisamide (Haloperidol may lower the convulsive threshold; adequate anticonvulsant therapy is indicated if co-administered). Products include:
- Zonegran Capsules 1307

Food Interactions

Alcohol (Potentiation of CNS depressant effects).

HALLS DEFENSE DROPS
(Vitamin C) .... ◘ 687
None cited in PDR database.

HALLS MENTHO-LYPTUS DROPS
(Menthol) .... ◘ 686
None cited in PDR database.

HALLS SUGAR FREE MENTHO-LYPTUS DROPS
(Menthol) .... ◘ 686
None cited in PDR database.

HALLS SUGAR FREE SQUARES
(Menthol) .... ◘ 686
None cited in PDR database.

HALLS PLUS COUGH DROPS
(Menthol, Pectin) .... ◘ 686
None cited in PDR database.

HAVRIX VACCINE
(Hepatitis A Vaccine, Inactivated) 1544
May interact with anticoagulants. Compounds in these categories include:

Ardeparin Sodium (Havrix should be given with caution to individuals on anticoagulant therapy).
- No products indexed under this heading.

Dalteparin Sodium (Havrix should be given with caution to individuals on anticoagulant therapy). Products include:
- Fragmin Injection 2814

Danaparoid Sodium (Havrix should be given with caution to individuals on anticoagulant therapy). Products include:
- Orgaran Injection 2480

Dicumarol (Havrix should be given with caution to individuals on anticoagulant therapy).
- No products indexed under this heading.

Enoxaparin (Havrix should be given with caution to individuals on anticoagulant therapy). Products include:
- Lovenox Injection 746

Heparin Sodium (Havrix should be given with caution to individuals on anticoagulant therapy). Products include:
- Heparin Lock Flush Solution 3509
- Heparin Sodium Injection 3511

Tinzaparin sodium (Havrix should be given with caution to individuals on anticoagulant therapy). Products include:
- Innohep Injection 1248

Warfarin Sodium (Havrix should be given with caution to individuals on anticoagulant therapy). Products include:
- Coumadin for Injection 1243
- Coumadin Tablets 1243
- Warfarin Sodium Tablets, USP 3302

HEAD & SHOULDERS DANDRUFF SHAMPOO
(Pyrithione Zinc) 2876
None cited in PDR database.

HEAD & SHOULDERS DANDRUFF SHAMPOO DRY SCALP
(Pyrithione Zinc) 2876
None cited in PDR database.

HEAD & SHOULDERS INTENSIVE TREATMENT DANDRUFF AND SEBORRHEIC DERMATITIS SHAMPOO
(Selenium Sulfide) 2877
None cited in PDR database.

HEALON
(Sodium Hyaluronate) .... ⊙ 316
None cited in PDR database.

HEALON 5
(Sodium Hyaluronate) .... ⊙ 317
None cited in PDR database.

HEALON GV
(Sodium Hyaluronate) .... ⊙ 320
None cited in PDR database.

HEARTBAR
(Amino Acid Preparations, Vitamins, Multiple) 1212
None cited in PDR database.

HEARTBAR ORANGE DRINK
(Amino Acid Preparations, Vitamins, Multiple) 1212
None cited in PDR database.

HECTOROL CAPSULES
(Doxercalciferol) 1064
May interact with phenytoin and certain other agents. Compounds in these categories include:

Cholestyramine (Reduces the intestinal absorption of fat-soluble vitamins; therefore, it may impair absorption of doxercalciferol).
- No products indexed under this heading.

Fosphenytoin Sodium (Co-administration with enzyme inhibitors, such as phenytoin, may affect the 25-hydroxylation of Hectorol and may necessitate dosage adjustment). Products include:
- Cerebyx Injection 2619

Glutethimide (Co-administration with enzyme inducers, such as glutethimide, may affect the 25-hydroxylation of Hectorol and may necessitate dosage adjustment).
- No products indexed under this heading.

Magnesium Hydroxide (Co-administration with magnesium-containing antacids and Hectorol may lead to the development of hypermagnesemia; concurrent use should be avoided). Products include:
- Ex•Lax Milk of Magnesia Liquid .... ◘ 670
- Maalox Antacid/Anti-Gas Oral Suspension .... ◘ 673
- Maalox Max Maximum Strength Antacid/Anti-Gas Liquid 2300
- Maalox Regular Strength Antacid/Antigas Liquid 2300
- Mylanta Fast-Acting 1813
- Mylanta 1813
- Pepcid Complete Chewable Tablets 1815
- Phillips' Chewable Tablets .... ◘ 615
- Phillips' Milk of Magnesia Liquid (Original, Cherry, & Mint) .... ◘ 616
- Rolaids Tablets .... ◘ 706
- Extra Strength Rolaids Tablets .... ◘ 706
- Vanquish Caplets .... ◘ 617

Magnesium Oxide (Co-administration with magnesium-containing antacids and Hectorol may lead to the development of hypermagnesemia; concurrent use should be avoided). Products include:
- Beelith Tablets 946
- Mag-Ox 400 Tablets 1024
- Uro-Mag Capsules 1024

Mineral Oil (The use of mineral oil or other substances that affect absorption of the fat may influence the absorption and availability of Hectorol). Products include:
- Anusol Ointment .... ◘ 688
- Fleet Mineral Oil Enema 1360
- Lubriderm Advanced Therapy Creamy Lotion .... ◘ 703
- Lubriderm Seriously Sensitive Lotion .... ◘ 703
- Lubriderm Skin Therapy Moisturizing Lotion .... ◘ 703
- Moisture Eyes PM Preservative Free Eye Ointment .... ⊙ 253
- Preparation H Ointment .... ◘ 778
- Refresh P.M. Lubricant Eye Ointment .... ⊙ 251

Phenobarbital (Co-administration with enzyme inducers, such as phenobarbital, may affect the 25-hydroxylation of Hectorol and may necessitate dosage adjustment). Products include:
- Arco-Lase Plus Tablets 592
- Donnatal 2929
- Donnatal Extentabs 2930

Phenytoin (Co-administration with enzyme inhibitors, such as phenytoin, may affect the 25-hydroxylation of Hectorol and may necessitate dosage adjustment). Products include:
- Dilantin Infatabs 2624
- Dilantin-125 Oral Suspension 2625

Phenytoin Sodium (Co-administration with enzyme inhibitors, such as phenytoin, may affect the 25-hydroxylation of Hectorol and may necessitate dosage adjustment). Products include:
- Dilantin Kapseals 2622

HELIXATE CONCENTRATE
(Antihemophilic Factor (Recombinant)) 788
None cited in PDR database.

HEMOFIL M
(Antihemophilic Factor (Human)) 847
None cited in PDR database.

HEPARIN LOCK FLUSH SOLUTION
(Heparin Sodium) 3509
May interact with antihistamines, cardiac glycosides, non-steroidal anti-inflammatory agents, platelet inhibitors, tetracyclines, and certain other agents. Compounds in these categories include:

Acrivastine (Anticoagulant action partially counteracted). Products include:
- Semprex-D Capsules 1172

Aspirin (Interferes with platelet-aggregation reactions and may induce bleeding). Products include:
- Aggrenox Capsules 1026
- Alka-Seltzer .... ◘ 603
- Alka-Seltzer Lemon Lime Antacid and Pain Reliever Effervescent Tablets .... ◘ 603
- Alka-Seltzer Extra Strength Antacid and Pain Reliever Effervescent Tablets .... ◘ 603
- Alka-Seltzer PM Effervescent Tablets .... ◘ 605
- Genuine Bayer Tablets, Caplets and Gelcaps .... ◘ 606
- Extra Strength Bayer Caplets and Gelcaps .... ◘ 610
- Aspirin Regimen Bayer Children's Chewable Tablets (Orange or Cherry Flavored) .... ◘ 607
- Bayer, Aspirin Regimen .... ◘ 606
- Aspirin Regimen Bayer 81 mg Caplets with Calcium .... ◘ 607
- Genuine Bayer Professional Labeling (Aspirin Regimen Bayer) .... ◘ 608
- Extra Strength Bayer Arthritis Caplets .... ◘ 610
- Extra Strength Bayer Plus Caplets .... ◘ 610
- Extra Strength Bayer PM Caplets .... ◘ 611
- BC Powder .... ◘ 619
- BC Allergy Sinus Cold Powder .... ◘ 619
- Arthritis Strength BC Powder .... ◘ 619
- BC Sinus Cold Powder .... ◘ 619
- Darvon Compound-65 Pulvules 1910
- Ecotrin Enteric Coated Aspirin Low, Regular and Maximum Strength Tablets 1715
- Excedrin Extra-Strength Tablets, Caplets, and Geltabs .... ◘ 629
- Excedrin Migraine 1070
- Goody's Body Pain Formula Powder .... ◘ 620
- Goody's Extra Strength Headache Powder .... ◘ 620
- Goody's Extra Strength Pain Relief Tablets .... ◘ 620
- Percodan Tablets 1327
- Robaxisal Tablets 2939
- Soma Compound Tablets 3354
- Soma Compound w/Codeine Tablets 3355
- Vanquish Caplets .... ◘ 617

Astemizole (Anticoagulant action partially counteracted).
- No products indexed under this heading.

Azatadine Maleate (Anticoagulant action partially counteracted). Products include:
- Rynatan Tablets 3351

Azlocillin Sodium (Interferes with platelet-aggregation reactions and may induce bleeding).
- No products indexed under this heading.

Bromodiphenhydramine Hydrochloride (Anticoagulant action partially counteracted).
- No products indexed under this heading.

Brompheniramine Maleate (Anticoagulant action partially counteracted). Products include:
- Bromfed Capsules (Extended-Release) 2269

Bromfed-PD Capsules (Extended-Release) 2269
Comtrex Acute Head Cold & Sinus Pressure Relief Tablets .... ▣627
Dimetapp Elixir .... ▣777
Dimetapp Cold and Fever Suspension .... ▣775
Dimetapp DM Cold & Cough Elixir .... ▣775
Dimetapp Nighttime Flu Liquid .... ▣776

Carbenicillin Indanyl Sodium (Interferes with platelet-aggregation reactions and may induce bleeding). Products include:
Geocillin Tablets 2687

Celecoxib (Interferes with platelet-aggregation reactions and may induce bleeding). Products include:
Celebrex Capsules 2676
Celebrex Capsules 2780

Cetirizine Hydrochloride (Anticoagulant action partially counteracted). Products include:
Zyrtec 2756
Zyrtec-D 12 Hour Extended Relief Tablets 2758

Chlorpheniramine Maleate (Anticoagulant action partially counteracted). Products include:
Actifed Cold & Sinus Caplets and Tablets .... ▣688
Alka-Seltzer Plus Liqui-Gels .... ▣604
BC Allergy Sinus Cold Powder .... ▣619
Chlor-Trimeton Allergy Tablets .... ▣735
Chlor-Trimeton Allergy/Decongestant Tablets .... ▣736
Comtrex Flu Therapy & Fever Relief Nighttime Tablets .... ▣628
Comtrex Maximum Strength Multi-Symptom Cold & Cough Relief Tablets and Caplets .... ▣626
Contac Severe Cold and Flu Caplets Maximum Strength .... ▣746
Coricidin 'D' Cold, Flu & Sinus Tablets .... ▣737
Coricidin/Coricidin D .... ▣738
Coricidin HBP Maximum Strength Flu Tablets .... ▣738
Extendryl 1361
Hycomine Compound Tablets 1317
Kronofed-A 1341
PediaCare Cough-Cold Liquid .... ▣719
PediaCare NightRest Cough-Cold Liquid .... ▣719
Robitussin Nighttime Honey Flu Liquid .... ▣786
Ryna .... ▣768
Singlet Caplets .... ▣761
Sinutab Sinus Allergy Medication, Maximum Strength Formula, Tablets & Caplets .... ▣707
Sudafed Cold & Allergy Tablets .... ▣708
TheraFlu Regular Strength Cold & Cough Night Time Hot Liquid .... ▣676
TheraFlu Regular Strength Cold & Sore Throat Night Time Hot Liquid .... ▣676
TheraFlu Maximum Strength Flu & Cough Night Time Hot Liquid .... ▣678
TheraFlu Maximum Strength Flu & Sore Throat Night Time Hot Liquid .... ▣677
TheraFlu Maximum Strength Severe Cold & Congestion Night Time Caplets .... ▣678
TheraFlu Maximum Strength Severe Cold & Congestion Night Time Hot Liquid .... ▣678
Triaminic Cold & Allergy Liquid .... ▣681
Triaminic Cold & Allergy Softchews .... ▣683
Triaminic Cold & Cough Liquid .... ▣681
Triaminic Cold & Cough Softchews .... ▣683
Triaminic Cold & Night Time Cough Liquid .... ▣681
Triaminic Cold, Cough & Fever Liquid .... ▣681
Children's Tylenol Cold Suspension Liquid and Chewable Tablets 2015
Children's Tylenol Cold Plus Cough Suspension Liquid and Chewable Tablets 2015
Children's Tylenol Flu Suspension Liquid 2015
Maximum Strength Tylenol Allergy Sinus Caplets, Gelcaps, and Geltabs 2010
Multi-Symptom Tylenol Cold Complete Formula Caplets 2010
Vicks 44M Cough, Cold & Flu Relief Liquid .... ▣725
Pediatric Vicks 44m Cough & Cold Relief .... ▣728
Children's Vicks NyQuil Cold/Cough Relief .... ▣726

Chlorpheniramine Polistirex (Anticoagulant action partially counteracted). Products include:
Tussionex Pennkinetic Extended-Release Suspension 1174

Chlorpheniramine Tannate (Anticoagulant action partially counteracted). Products include:
Reformulated Rynatan Pediatric Suspension 3352
Rynatuss Pediatric Suspension 3353
Rynatuss Tablets 3353
Tussi-12 S Suspension 3356
Tussi-12 Tablets 3356

Choline Magnesium Trisalicylate (Interferes with platelet-aggregation reactions and may induce bleeding). Products include:
Trilisate 2901

Clemastine Fumarate (Anticoagulant action partially counteracted). Products include:
Tavist 12 Hour Allergy Tablets .... ▣676

Clopidogrel Bisulfate (Interferes with platelet-aggregation reactions and may induce bleeding). Products include:
Plavix Tablets 1097
Plavix Tablets 3084

Cyproheptadine Hydrochloride (Anticoagulant action partially counteracted). Products include:
Periactin Tablets 2155

Demeclocycline Hydrochloride (Anticoagulant action partially counteracted). Products include:
Declomycin Tablets 1855

Deslanoside (Anticoagulant action partially counteracted).
No products indexed under this heading.

Dexchlorpheniramine Maleate (Anticoagulant action partially counteracted).
No products indexed under this heading.

Dextran 40 (Interferes with platelet-aggregation reactions and may induce bleeding).
No products indexed under this heading.

Diclofenac Potassium (Interferes with platelet-aggregation reactions and may induce bleeding). Products include:
Cataflam Tablets 2315

Diclofenac Sodium (Interferes with platelet-aggregation reactions and may induce bleeding). Products include:
Arthrotec Tablets 3195
Voltaren Ophthalmic Sterile Ophthalmic Solution .... ⊙312
Voltaren Tablets 2315
Voltaren-XR Tablets 2315

Diflunisal (Interferes with platelet-aggregation reactions and may induce bleeding). Products include:
Dolobid Tablets 2088

Digitoxin (Anticoagulant action partially counteracted).
No products indexed under this heading.

Digoxin (Anticoagulant action partially counteracted). Products include:
Digitek Tablets 1003
Lanoxicaps Capsules 1574
Lanoxin Injection 1581
Lanoxin Tablets 1587
Lanoxin Elixir Pediatric 1578
Lanoxin Injection Pediatric 1584

Diphenhydramine Citrate (Anticoagulant action partially counteracted). Products include:
Alka-Seltzer PM Effervescent Tablets .... ▣605
Benadryl Allergy & Sinus Fastmelt Tablets .... ▣693
Benadryl Children's Allergy/Cold Fastmelt Tablets .... ▣692
Excedrin PM Tablets, Caplets, and Geltabs .... ▣631
Goody's PM Powder .... ▣621

Diphenhydramine Hydrochloride (Anticoagulant action partially counteracted). Products include:
Extra Strength Bayer PM Caplets .... ▣611
Benadryl Allergy Chewables .... ▣689
Benadryl Allergy .... ▣691
Benadryl Allergy Liquid .... ▣690
Benadryl Allergy/Cold Tablets .... ▣691
Benadryl Allergy/Congestion Tablets .... ▣692
Benadryl Allergy & Sinus Liquid .... ▣693
Benadryl Allergy Sinus Headache Caplets & Gelcaps .... ▣693
Benadryl Severe Allergy & Sinus Headache Caplets .... ▣694
Benadryl Dye-Free Allergy Liquid .... ▣690
Benadryl Dye-Free Allergy Liqui-Gels Softgels .... ▣690
Benadryl Itch Relief Stick Extra Strength .... ▣695
Benadryl Cream .... ▣695
Benadryl Gel .... ▣695
Benadryl Spray .... ▣696
Benadryl Parenteral 2617
Coricidin HBP Night-Time Cold & Flu Tablets .... ▣738
Nytol QuickCaps Caplets .... ▣622
Maximum Strength Nytol QuickGels Softgels .... ▣621
Extra Strength Percogesic Aspirin-Free Coated Caplets .... ▣665
Simply Sleep Caplets 2008
Sominex Original Formula Tablets .... ▣761
Children's Tylenol Allergy-D Liquid 2014
Maximum Strength Tylenol Allergy Sinus NightTime Caplets 2010
Tylenol Severe Allergy Caplets 2010
Maximum Strength Tylenol Flu NightTime Gelcaps 2011
Extra Strength Tylenol PM Caplets, Geltabs, and Gelcaps 2012
Unisom Maximum Strength SleepGels .... ▣713

Diphenylpyraline Hydrochloride (Anticoagulant action partially counteracted).
No products indexed under this heading.

Dipyridamole (Interferes with platelet-aggregation reactions and may induce bleeding). Products include:
Aggrenox Capsules 1026
Persantine Tablets 1057

Doxycycline Calcium (Anticoagulant action partially counteracted). Products include:
Vibramycin Calcium Oral Suspension Syrup 2735

Doxycycline Hyclate (Anticoagulant action partially counteracted). Products include:
Doryx Coated Pellet Filled Capsules 3357
Periostat Tablets 1208
Vibramycin Hyclate Capsules 2735
Vibramycin Hyclate Intravenous 2737
Vibra-Tabs Film Coated Tablets 2735

Doxycycline Monohydrate (Anticoagulant action partially counteracted). Products include:
Monodox Capsules 2442
Vibramycin Monohydrate for Oral Suspension 2735

Etodolac (Interferes with platelet-aggregation reactions and may induce bleeding). Products include:
Lodine 3528
Lodine XL Extended-Release Tablets 3530

Fenoprofen Calcium (Interferes with platelet-aggregation reactions and may induce bleeding).
No products indexed under this heading.

Fexofenadine Hydrochloride (Anticoagulant action partially counteracted). Products include:
Allegra 712
Allegra-D Extended-Release Tablets 714

Flurbiprofen (Interferes with platelet-aggregation reactions and may induce bleeding).
No products indexed under this heading.

Hydroxychloroquine Sulfate (Interferes with platelet-aggregation reactions and may induce bleeding). Products include:
Plaquenil Tablets 3082

Ibuprofen (Interferes with platelet-aggregation reactions and may induce bleeding). Products include:
Advil .... ▣771
Children's Advil Oral Suspension .... ▣773
Children's Advil Chewable Tablets .... ▣773
Advil Cold and Sinus Caplets .... ▣771
Advil Cold and Sinus Tablets .... ▣771
Advil Flu & Body Ache Caplets .... ▣772
Infants' Advil Drops .... ▣773
Junior Strength Advil Tablets .... ▣773
Junior Strength Advil Chewable Tablets .... ▣773
Advil Migraine Liquigels .... ▣772
Children's Motrin Oral Suspension and Chewable Tablets 2006
Children's Motrin Cold Oral Suspension 2007
Children's Motrin Oral Suspension .... ▣643
Motrin Suspension, Oral Drops, Chewable Tablets, and Caplets 2002
Infants' Motrin Concentrated Drops 2006
Junior Strength Motrin Caplets and Chewable Tablets 2006
Motrin IB Tablets, Caplets, and Gelcaps 2002
Motrin Migraine Pain Caplets 2005
Motrin Sinus Headache Caplets 2005
Vicoprofen Tablets 520

Indomethacin (Interferes with platelet-aggregation reactions and may induce bleeding). Products include:
Indocin 2112

Indomethacin Sodium Trihydrate (Interferes with platelet-aggregation reactions and may induce bleeding). Products include:
Indocin I.V. 2115

Ketoprofen (Interferes with platelet-aggregation reactions and may induce bleeding). Products include:
Orudis Capsules 3548
Orudis KT Tablets .... ▣778
Oruvail Capsules 3548

Ketorolac Tromethamine (Interferes with platelet-aggregation reactions and may induce bleeding). Products include:
Acular Ophthalmic Solution 544
Acular PF Ophthalmic Solution 544
Toradol 3018

Loratadine (Anticoagulant action partially counteracted). Products include:
Claritin 3100
Claritin-D 12 Hour Extended Release Tablets 3102
Claritin-D 24 Hour Extended Release Tablets 3104

Magnesium Salicylate (Interferes with platelet-aggregation reactions and may induce bleeding). Products include:
Momentum Backache Relief Extra Strength Caplets .... ▣666

Meclofenamate Sodium (Interferes with platelet-aggregation reactions and may induce bleeding).
No products indexed under this heading.

Mefenamic Acid (Interferes with platelet-aggregation reactions and may induce bleeding). Products include:
Ponstel Capsules 1356

Meloxicam (Interferes with platelet-aggregation reactions and may induce bleeding). Products include:
Mobic Tablets 1054

Methacycline Hydrochloride (Anticoagulant action partially counteracted).
No products indexed under this heading.

Methdilazine Hydrochloride (Anticoagulant action partially counteracted).
No products indexed under this heading.

Mezlocillin Sodium (Interferes with platelet-aggregation reactions and may induce bleeding).
No products indexed under this heading.

Minocycline Hydrochloride (Anticoagulant action partially counteracted). Products include:
Dynacin Capsules 2019
Minocin Intravenous 1862
Minocin Oral Suspension 1865
Minocin Pellet-Filled Capsules 1863

Nabumetone (Interferes with platelet-aggregation reactions and may induce bleeding). Products include:
Relafen Tablets 1617

Nafcillin Sodium (Interferes with platelet-aggregation reactions and may induce bleeding).
No products indexed under this heading.

Naproxen (Interferes with platelet-aggregation reactions and may induce bleeding). Products include:
EC-Naprosyn Delayed-Release Tablets 2967
Naprosyn Suspension 2967
Naprosyn Tablets 2967

Naproxen Sodium (Interferes with platelet-aggregation reactions and may induce bleeding). Products include:
Aleve Tablets, Caplets and Gelcaps .... ■602
Aleve Cold & Sinus Caplets .... ■603
Anaprox Tablets 2967
Anaprox DS Tablets 2967
Naprelan Tablets 1293

Nicotine Polacrilex (Anticoagulant action partially counteracted). Products include:
Nicorette Gum 1720

Oxaprozin (Interferes with platelet-aggregation reactions and may induce bleeding).
No products indexed under this heading.

Oxytetracycline (Anticoagulant action partially counteracted).
No products indexed under this heading.

Oxytetracycline Hydrochloride (Anticoagulant action partially counteracted). Products include:
Terra-Cortril Ophthalmic Suspension 2716
Urobiotic-250 Capsules 2731

Penicillin G Benzathine (Interferes with platelet-aggregation reactions and may induce bleeding). Products include:
Bicillin C-R 900/300 Injection 2240
Bicillin C-R Injection 2238
Bicillin L-A Injection 2242
Permapen Isoject 2706

Penicillin G Procaine (Interferes with platelet-aggregation reactions and may induce bleeding). Products include:
Bicillin C-R 900/300 Injection 2240
Bicillin C-R Injection 2238

Phenylbutazone (Interferes with platelet-aggregation reactions and may induce bleeding).
No products indexed under this heading.

Piroxicam (Interferes with platelet-aggregation reactions and may induce bleeding). Products include:
Feldene Capsules 2685

Promethazine Hydrochloride (Anticoagulant action partially counteracted). Products include:
Mepergan Injection 3539
Phenergan Injection 3553
Phenergan 3556
Phenergan Syrup 3554
Phenergan with Codeine Syrup 3557
Phenergan with Dextromethorphan Syrup 3559
Phenergan VC Syrup 3560
Phenergan VC with Codeine Syrup 3561

Pyrilamine Maleate (Anticoagulant action partially counteracted). Products include:
Maximum Strength Midol Menstrual Caplets and Gelcaps .... ■612
Maximum Strength Midol PMS Caplets and Gelcaps .... ■613

Pyrilamine Tannate (Anticoagulant action partially counteracted). Products include:
Ryna-12 S Suspension 3351

Rofecoxib (Interferes with platelet-aggregation reactions and may induce bleeding). Products include:
Vioxx 2213

Salsalate (Interferes with platelet-aggregation reactions and may induce bleeding).
No products indexed under this heading.

Sulindac (Interferes with platelet-aggregation reactions and may induce bleeding). Products include:
Clinoril Tablets 2053

Terfenadine (Anticoagulant action partially counteracted).
No products indexed under this heading.

Tetracycline Hydrochloride (Anticoagulant action partially counteracted).
No products indexed under this heading.

Ticarcillin Disodium (Interferes with platelet-aggregation reactions and may induce bleeding). Products include:
Timentin Injection- ADD-Vantage Vial 1661
Timentin Injection-Galaxy Container 1664
Timentin Injection-Pharmacy Bulk Package 1666
Timentin for Intravenous Administration 1658

Ticlopidine Hydrochloride (Interferes with platelet-aggregation reactions and may induce bleeding). Products include:
Ticlid Tablets 3015

Tolmetin Sodium (Interferes with platelet-aggregation reactions and may induce bleeding). Products include:
Tolectin 2589

Trimeprazine Tartrate (Anticoagulant action partially counteracted).
No products indexed under this heading.

Tripelennamine Hydrochloride (Anticoagulant action partially counteracted).
No products indexed under this heading.

Triprolidine Hydrochloride (Anticoagulant action partially counteracted). Products include:
Actifed Cold & Allergy Tablets .... ■688

HEPARIN SODIUM INJECTION

(Heparin Sodium) 3511
See Heparin Lock Flush Solution

HEP-FORTE CAPSULES

(Vitamins with Minerals) 1997
None cited in PDR database.

HERCEPTIN I.V.

(Trastuzumab) 1414
May interact with anthracycline antibiotics and their derivatives and certain other agents. Compounds in these categories include:

Cyclophosphamide (The increase and severity of cardiac dysfunction is particularly high in patients who receive trastuzumab in combination with cyclophosphamide).
No products indexed under this heading.

Daunorubicin Hydrochloride (The increase and severity of cardiac dysfunction is particularly high in patients who receive trastuzumab in combination with anthracyclines). Products include:
Cerubidine for Injection 947

Doxorubicin Hydrochloride (The increase and severity of cardiac dysfunction is particularly high in patients who receive trastuzumab in combination with anthracyclines). Products include:
Adriamycin PFS/RDF Injection 2767
Doxil Injection 566

Epirubicin Hydrochloride (The increase and severity of cardiac dysfunction is particularly high in patients who receive trastuzumab in combination with anthracyclines). Products include:
Ellence Injection 2806

Idarubicin Hydrochloride (The increase and severity of cardiac dysfunction is particularly high in patients who receive trastuzumab in combination with anthracyclines). Products include:
Idamycin PFS Injection 2825

Paclitaxel (Co-administration has resulted in a two-fold decrease in trastuzumab clearance in a non-human primate study and in a 1.5-fold increase in trastuzumab serum levels in clinical studies). Products include:
Taxol Injection 1129

HEXALEN CAPSULES

(Altretamine) 2226
May interact with monoamine oxidase inhibitors and certain other agents. Compounds in these categories include:

Cimetidine (Increases altretamine's half-life and toxicity in a rat model). Products include:
Tagamet HB 200 Suspension .... ■762
Tagamet HB 200 Tablets .... ■761
Tagamet Tablets 1644

Cimetidine Hydrochloride (Increases altretamine's half-life and toxicity in a rat model). Products include:
Tagamet 1644

Isocarboxazid (Potential for severe orthostatic hypotension).
No products indexed under this heading.

Moclobemide (Potential for severe orthostatic hypotension).
No products indexed under this heading.

Pargyline Hydrochloride (Potential for severe orthostatic hypotension).
No products indexed under this heading.

Phenelzine Sulfate (Potential for severe orthostatic hypotension). Products include:
Nardil Tablets 2653

Procarbazine Hydrochloride (Potential for severe orthostatic hypotension). Products include:
Matulane Capsules 3246

Pyridoxine Hydrochloride (May adversely affect response duration; should not be administered with Hexalen and/or Cisplatin).
No products indexed under this heading.

Selegiline Hydrochloride (Potential for severe orthostatic hypotension). Products include:
Eldepryl Capsules 3266

Tranylcypromine Sulfate (Potential for severe orthostatic hypotension). Products include:
Parnate Tablets 1607

HGH-TURN BACK THE HANDS OF TIME CAPSULES

(Amino Acid Preparations, Minerals, Multiple) .... ■854
None cited in PDR database.

HIBTITER

(Haemophilus B Conjugate Vaccine) 1859
May interact with alkylating agents, anticoagulants, corticosteroids, cytotoxic drugs, and immunosuppressive agents. Compounds in these categories include:

Ardeparin Sodium (HibTITER should be given with caution to children on anticoagulant therapy).
No products indexed under this heading.

Azathioprine (Reduces antibody response to active immunization procedures).
No products indexed under this heading.

Basiliximab (Reduces antibody response to active immunization procedures). Products include:
Simulect for Injection 2399

Betamethasone Acetate (Reduces antibody response to active immunization procedures). Products include:
Celestone Soluspan Injectable Suspension 3097

Betamethasone Sodium Phosphate (Reduces antibody response to active immunization procedures). Products include:
Celestone Soluspan Injectable Suspension 3097

Bleomycin Sulfate (Reduces antibody response to active immunization procedures).
No products indexed under this heading.

Busulfan (Reduces antibody response to active immunization procedures). Products include:
Myleran Tablets 1603

Carmustine (BCNU) (Reduces antibody response to active immunization procedures). Products include:
Gliadel Wafer 1723

Chlorambucil (Reduces antibody response to active immunization procedures). Products include:
Leukeran Tablets 1591

Cortisone Acetate (Reduces antibody response to active immunization procedures). Products include:
Cortone Acetate Injectable Suspension 2059
Cortone Acetate Tablets 2061

Cyclophosphamide (Reduces antibody response to active immunization procedures).
No products indexed under this heading.

Cyclosporine (Reduces antibody response to active immunization procedures). Products include:
Gengraf Capsules 457
Neoral Soft Gelatin Capsules 2380
Neoral Oral Solution 2380
Sandimmune 2388

Dacarbazine (Reduces antibody response to active immunization procedures). Products include:
DTIC-Dome 902

Dalteparin Sodium (HibTITER should be given with caution to children on anticoagulant therapy). Products include:
Fragmin Injection 2814

Danaparoid Sodium (HibTITER should be given with caution to children on anticoagulant therapy). Products include:
Orgaran Injection 2480

Daunorubicin Hydrochloride (Reduces antibody response to active immunization procedures). Products include:
Cerubidine for Injection 947

Dexamethasone (Reduces antibody response to active immunization procedures). Products include:
Decadron Elixir 2078
Decadron Tablets 2079
TobraDex Ophthalmic Ointment 542

TobraDex Ophthalmic Suspension .. 541

Dexamethasone Acetate (Reduces antibody response to active immunization procedures).
No products indexed under this heading.

Dexamethasone Sodium Phosphate (Reduces antibody response to active immunization procedures). Products include:
Decadron Phosphate Injection 2081
Decadron Phosphate Sterile Ophthalmic Ointment.................. 2083
Decadron Phosphate Sterile Ophthalmic Solution.................. 2084
NeoDecadron Sterile Ophthalmic Solution.............................. 2144

Dicumarol (HibTITER should be given with caution to children on anticoagulant therapy).
No products indexed under this heading.

Doxorubicin Hydrochloride (Reduces antibody response to active immunization procedures). Products include:
Adriamycin PFS/RDF Injection 2767
Doxil Injection 566

Enoxaparin (HibTITER should be given with caution to children on anticoagulant therapy). Products include:
Lovenox Injection 746

Epirubicin Hydrochloride (Reduces antibody response to active immunization procedures). Products include:
Ellence Injection 2806

Fludrocortisone Acetate (Reduces antibody response to active immunization procedures). Products include:
Florinef Acetate Tablets 2250

Fluorouracil (Reduces antibody response to active immunization procedures). Products include:
Carac Cream 1222
Efudex 1733
Fluoroplex 552

Heparin Sodium (HibTITER should be given with caution to children on anticoagulant therapy). Products include:
Heparin Lock Flush Solution 3509
Heparin Sodium Injection 3511

Hydrocortisone (Reduces antibody response to active immunization procedures). Products include:
Anusol-HC Cream 2.5% 2237
Cipro HC Otic Suspension 540
Cortaid Intensive Therapy Cream . ▣717
Cortaid Maximum Strength Cream .... ▣717
Cortisporin Ophthalmic Suspension Sterile .... ⊙297
Cortizone•5 .... ▣699
Cortizone•10 .... ▣699
Cortizone•10 Plus Creme .... ▣700
Cortizone for Kids Creme .... ▣699
Hydrocortone Tablets 2106
Massengill Medicated Soft Cloth Towelette .... ▣753
VōSoL HC Otic Solution 3356

Hydrocortisone Acetate (Reduces antibody response to active immunization procedures). Products include:
Analpram-HC 1338
Anusol HC-1 Hydrocortisone Anti-Itch Cream .... ▣689
Anusol-HC Suppositories 2238
Cortaid .... ▣717
Cortifoam Rectal Foam 3170
Cortisporin-TC Otic Suspension 2246
Hydrocortone Acetate Injectable Suspension 2103
Pramosone 1343
Proctocort Suppositories 2264
ProctoFoam-HC 3177
Terra-Cortril Ophthalmic Suspension 2716

Hydrocortisone Sodium Phosphate (Reduces antibody response to active immunization procedures). Products include:
Hydrocortone Phosphate Injection, Sterile 2105

Hydrocortisone Sodium Succinate (Reduces antibody response to active immunization procedures).
No products indexed under this heading.

Hydroxyurea (Reduces antibody response to active immunization procedures). Products include:
Mylocel Tablets 2227

Immune Globulin Intravenous (Human) (Reduces antibody response to active immunization procedures).
No products indexed under this heading.

Lomustine (CCNU) (Reduces antibody response to active immunization procedures).
No products indexed under this heading.

Mechlorethamine Hydrochloride (Reduces antibody response to active immunization procedures). Products include:
Mustargen for Injection 2142

Melphalan (Reduces antibody response to active immunization procedures). Products include:
Alkeran Tablets 1466

Methotrexate Sodium (Reduces antibody response to active immunization procedures).
No products indexed under this heading.

Methylprednisolone Acetate (Reduces antibody response to active immunization procedures). Products include:
Depo-Medrol Injectable Suspension 2795

Methylprednisolone Sodium Succinate (Reduces antibody response to active immunization procedures). Products include:
Solu-Medrol Sterile Powder 2855

Mitotane (Reduces antibody response to active immunization procedures).
No products indexed under this heading.

Mitoxantrone Hydrochloride (Reduces antibody response to active immunization procedures). Products include:
Novantrone for Injection 1760

Muromonab-CD3 (Reduces antibody response to active immunization procedures). Products include:
Orthoclone OKT3 Sterile Solution ... 2498

Mycophenolate Mofetil (Reduces antibody response to active immunization procedures). Products include:
CellCept Capsules 2951
CellCept Oral Suspension 2951
CellCept Tablets 2951

Prednisolone Acetate (Reduces antibody response to active immunization procedures). Products include:
Blephamide Ophthalmic Ointment .. 547
Blephamide Ophthalmic Suspension 548
Poly-Pred Liquifilm Ophthalmic Suspension .... ⊙245
Pred Forte Ophthalmic Suspension .... ⊙246
Pred Mild Sterile Ophthalmic Suspension .... ⊙249
Pred-G Ophthalmic Suspension ..... ⊙247
Pred-G Sterile Ophthalmic Ointment .... ⊙248

Prednisolone Sodium Phosphate (Reduces antibody response to active immunization procedures). Products include:
Pediapred Oral Solution 1170

Prednisolone Tebutate (Reduces antibody response to active immunization procedures).
No products indexed under this heading.

Prednisone (Reduces antibody response to active immunization procedures). Products include:
Prednisone 3064

Procarbazine Hydrochloride (Reduces antibody response to active immunization procedures). Products include:
Matulane Capsules 3246

Sirolimus (Reduces antibody response to active immunization procedures). Products include:
Rapamune Oral Solution and Tablets 3584

Tacrolimus (Reduces antibody response to active immunization procedures). Products include:
Prograf 1393
Protopic Ointment 1397

Tamoxifen Citrate (Reduces antibody response to active immunization procedures). Products include:
Nolvadex Tablets 678

Thiotepa (Reduces antibody response to active immunization procedures). Products include:
Thioplex for Injection 1765

Tinzaparin sodium (HibTITER should be given with caution to children on anticoagulant therapy). Products include:
Innohep Injection 1248

Triamcinolone (Reduces antibody response to active immunization procedures).
No products indexed under this heading.

Triamcinolone Acetonide (Reduces antibody response to active immunization procedures). Products include:
Azmacort Inhalation Aerosol 728
Nasacort Nasal Inhaler 750
Nasacort AQ Nasal Spray 752
Tri-Nasal Spray 2274

Triamcinolone Diacetate (Reduces antibody response to active immunization procedures).
No products indexed under this heading.

Triamcinolone Hexacetonide (Reduces antibody response to active immunization procedures).
No products indexed under this heading.

Vincristine Sulfate (Reduces antibody response to active immunization procedures).
No products indexed under this heading.

Warfarin Sodium (HibTITER should be given with caution to children on anticoagulant therapy). Products include:
Coumadin for Injection 1243
Coumadin Tablets 1243
Warfarin Sodium Tablets, USP 3302

HIVID TABLETS
(Zalcitabine) 2975
May interact with aminoglycosides, antacids containing aluminum, calcium and magnesium, drugs that are known to cause peripheral neuropathy and pancreatitis (selected), and certain other agents. Compounds in these categories include:

Altretamine (Potential for increased peripheral neuropathy; concomitant use should be avoided). Products include:
Hexalen Capsules 2226

Aluminum Carbonate (Absorption of zalcitabine is moderately reduced (approximately 25%) when coadministered with magnesium/aluminum containing antacids).
No products indexed under this heading.

Aluminum Hydroxide (Absorption of zalcitabine is moderately reduced (approximately 25%) when coadministered with magnesium/aluminum containing antacids). Products include:
Amphojel Suspension (Mint Flavor) .... ▣789
Gaviscon Extra Strength Liquid ..... ▣751
Gaviscon Extra Strength Tablets ... ▣751
Gaviscon Regular Strength Liquid . ▣751
Gaviscon Regular Strength Tablets .... ▣750
Maalox Antacid/Anti-Gas Oral Suspension .... ▣673
Maalox Max Maximum Strength Antacid/Anti-Gas Liquid 2300
Maalox Regular Strength Antacid/Antigas Liquid 2300
Mylanta 1813
Vanquish Caplets .... ▣617

Amikacin Sulfate (Increases the risk of developing peripheral neuropathy or other Hivid-associated toxicities by interfering with the renal clearance of zalcitabine).
No products indexed under this heading.

Amphotericin B (Increases the risk of developing peripheral neuropathy or other Hivid-associated toxicities by interfering with the renal clearance of zalcitabine). Products include:
Abelcet Injection 1273
AmBisome for Injection 1383
Amphotec 1774

Auranofin (Potential for increased peripheral neuropathy; concomitant use should be avoided).
No products indexed under this heading.

Carboplatin (Potential for increased peripheral neuropathy; concomitant use should be avoided). Products include:
Paraplatin for Injection 1126

Chloramphenicol (Potential for increased peripheral neuropathy; concomitant use should be avoided). Products include:
Chloromycetin Ophthalmic Ointment, 1% .... ⊙296
Chloromycetin Ophthalmic Solution .... ⊙297
Chloroptic Sterile Ophthalmic Ointment .... ⊙234
Chloroptic Sterile Ophthalmic Solution .... ⊙235

Chloramphenicol Palmitate (Potential for increased peripheral neuropathy; concomitant use should be avoided).
No products indexed under this heading.

Chloramphenicol Sodium Succinate (Potential for increased peripheral neuropathy; concomitant use should be avoided).
No products indexed under this heading.

Cimetidine (Concomitant administration decreases the elimination of zalcitabine, most likely by inhibition of renal tubular secretion of zalcitabine). Products include:
Tagamet HB 200 Suspension .... ▣762
Tagamet HB 200 Tablets .... ▣761
Tagamet Tablets 1644

Cimetidine Hydrochloride (Concomitant administration decreases the elimination of zalcitabine, most likely by inhibition of renal tubular secretion of zalcitabine). Products include:
Tagamet 1644

Cisplatin (Potential for increased peripheral neuropathy; concomitant use should be avoided).
No products indexed under this heading.

Dapsone (Potential for increased peripheral neuropathy; concomitant use should be avoided). Products include:
Dapsone Tablets USP 1780

Didanosine (Concomitant use is not recommended). Products include:
Videx 1138
Videx EC Capsules 1143

Disulfiram (Potential for increased peripheral neuropathy; concomitant use should be avoided). Products include:
Antabuse Tablets 2444

Antabuse Tablets 3474

Doxorubicin Hydrochloride (Co-administration results in a decrease in zalcitabine phosphorylation in U937/Molt 4 cells; the clinical relevance of these in vitro results is not known). Products include:

Adriamycin PFS/RDF Injection 2767
Doxil Injection 566

Ethionamide (Potential for increased peripheral neuropathy; concomitant use should be avoided). Products include:

Trecator-SC Tablets 3598

Foscarnet Sodium (Increases the risk of developing peripheral neuropathy or other Hivid-associated toxicities by interfering with the renal clearance of zalcitabine). Products include:

Foscavir Injection 605

Gentamicin Sulfate (Increases the risk of developing peripheral neuropathy or other Hivid-associated toxicities by interfering with the renal clearance of zalcitabine). Products include:

Genoptic Ophthalmic Ointment .... ⊙239
Genoptic Sterile Ophthalmic Solution .... ⊙239
Pred-G Ophthalmic Suspension .... ⊙247
Pred-G Sterile Ophthalmic Ointment .... ⊙248

Glutethimide (Potential for increased peripheral neuropathy; concomitant use should be avoided).

No products indexed under this heading.

Gold Sodium Thiomalate (Potential for increased peripheral neuropathy; concomitant use should be avoided).

No products indexed under this heading.

Hydralazine Hydrochloride (Potential for increased peripheral neuropathy; concomitant use should be avoided).

No products indexed under this heading.

Iodoquinol (Potential for increased peripheral neuropathy; concomitant use should be avoided). Products include:

Yodoxin Tablets 1722

Isoniazid (Potential for increased peripheral neuropathy; concomitant use should be avoided). Products include:

Rifamate Capsules 767
Rifater Tablets 769

Kanamycin Sulfate (Increases the risk of developing peripheral neuropathy or other Hivid-associated toxicities by interfering with the renal clearance of zalcitabine).

No products indexed under this heading.

Leuprolide Acetate (Potential for increased peripheral neuropathy; concomitant use should be avoided). Products include:

Lupron Depot 3.75 mg 3281
Lupron Depot 7.5 mg 3284
Lupron Depot–3 Month 11.25 mg 3285
Lupron Depot–3 Month 22.5 mg 3288
Lupron Depot–4 Month 30 mg 3289
Lupron Depot-PED 7.5 mg, 11.25 mg and 15 mg 3291
Lupron Injection 3279
Lupron Injection Pediatric 3280
Viadur Implant 912

Magaldrate (Absorption of zalcitabine is moderately reduced (approximately 25%) when coadministered with magnesium/aluminum containing antacids).

No products indexed under this heading.

Magnesium Hydroxide (Absorption of zalcitabine is moderately reduced (approximately 25%) when coadministered with magnesium/aluminum containing antacids). Products include:

Ex•Lax Milk of Magnesia Liquid .... ▣670
Maalox Antacid/Anti-Gas Oral Suspension .... ▣673
Maalox Max Maximum Strength Antacid/Anti-Gas Liquid 2300
Maalox Regular Strength Antacid/Antigas Liquid 2300
Mylanta Fast-Acting 1813
Mylanta 1813
Pepcid Complete Chewable Tablets 1815
Phillips' Chewable Tablets .... ▣615
Phillips' Milk of Magnesia Liquid (Original, Cherry, & Mint) .... ▣616
Rolaids Tablets .... ▣706
Extra Strength Rolaids Tablets .... ▣706
Vanquish Caplets .... ▣617

Magnesium Oxide (Absorption of zalcitabine is moderately reduced (approximately 25%) when coadministered with magnesium/aluminum containing antacids). Products include:

Beelith Tablets 946
Mag-Ox 400 Tablets 1024
Uro-Mag Capsules 1024

Metoclopramide Hydrochloride (Co-administration may reduce bioavailability (approximately 10%)). Products include:

Reglan 2935

Metronidazole (Potential for increased peripheral neuropathy; concomitant use should be avoided). Products include:

MetroCream 1404
MetroGel 1405
MetroGel-Vaginal Gel 1986
MetroLotion 1405
Noritate Cream 1224

Nitrofurantoin (Potential for increased peripheral neuropathy; concomitant use should be avoided). Products include:

Macrodantin Capsules 2891

Pentamidine Isethionate (Death due to fulminant pancreatitis possibly related to intravenous pentamidine and Hivid has been reported; treatment with Hivid should be interrupted if intravenous pentamidine is required to treat Pneumocystis carinii pneumonia).

No products indexed under this heading.

Phenytoin (Potential for increased peripheral neuropathy; concomitant use should be avoided). Products include:

Dilantin Infatabs 2624
Dilantin-125 Oral Suspension 2625

Phenytoin Sodium (Potential for increased peripheral neuropathy; concomitant use should be avoided). Products include:

Dilantin Kapseals 2622

Probenecid (Concomitant administration decreases the elimination of zalcitabine, most likely by inhibition of renal tubular secretion of zalcitabine).

No products indexed under this heading.

Ribavirin (Potential for increased peripheral neuropathy; concomitant use should be avoided). Products include:

Rebetron Combination Therapy 3153
Virazole for Inhalation Solution 1747

Streptomycin Sulfate (Increases the risk of developing peripheral neuropathy or other Hivid-associated toxicities by interfering with the renal clearance of zalcitabine). Products include:

Streptomycin Sulfate Injection 2714

Sulfamethoxazole (Potential for increased peripheral neuropathy; concomitant use should be avoided). Products include:

Bactrim 2949
Septra Suspension 2265
Septra Tablets 2265
Septra DS Tablets 2265

Tobramycin (Increases the risk of developing peripheral neuropathy or other Hivid-associated toxicities by interfering with the renal clearance of zalcitabine). Products include:

TOBI Solution for Inhalation 1206
TobraDex Ophthalmic Ointment 542
TobraDex Ophthalmic Suspension 541
Tobrex Ophthalmic Ointment .... ⊙220
Tobrex Ophthalmic Solution .... ⊙221

Tobramycin Sulfate (Increases the risk of developing peripheral neuropathy or other Hivid-associated toxicities by interfering with the renal clearance of zalcitabine). Products include:

Nebcin Vials, Hyporets & ADD-Vantage 1955

Vincristine Sulfate (Potential for increased peripheral neuropathy; concomitant use should be avoided).

No products indexed under this heading.

Food Interactions

Food, unspecified (The absorption rate of a 15mg oral dose of zalactabine was reduced when administered with food).

HMS STERILE OPHTHALMIC SUSPENSION

(Medrysone) .... ⊙240
None cited in PDR database.

HUMALOG

(Insulin Lispro, Human) 1926
May interact with ACE inhibitors, beta blockers, corticosteroids, estrogens, oral hypoglycemic agents, oral contraceptives, phenothiazines, salicylates, thyroid preparations, and certain other agents. Compounds in these categories include:

Acarbose (Co-administration with drugs with hypoglycemic activity, such as oral hypoglycemic agents, may result in decreased insulin requirements). Products include:

Precose Tablets 906

Acebutolol Hydrochloride (Co-administration with drugs with hypoglycemic activity, such as beta blockers, may result in decreased insulin requirements; beta blockers may mask the symptoms of hypoglycemia in some patients). Products include:

Sectral Capsules 3589

Aspirin (Co-administration with drugs with hypoglycemic activity, such as salicylates, may result in decreased insulin requirements). Products include:

Aggrenox Capsules 1026
Alka-Seltzer .... ▣603
Alka-Seltzer Lemon Lime Antacid and Pain Reliever Effervescent Tablets .... ▣603
Alka-Seltzer Extra Strength Antacid and Pain Reliever Effervescent Tablets .... ▣603
Alka-Seltzer PM Effervescent Tablets .... ▣605
Genuine Bayer Tablets, Caplets and Gelcaps .... ▣606
Extra Strength Bayer Caplets and Gelcaps .... ▣610
Aspirin Regimen Bayer Children's Chewable Tablets (Orange or Cherry Flavored) .... ▣607
Bayer, Aspirin Regimen .... ▣606
Aspirin Regimen Bayer 81 mg Caplets with Calcium .... ▣607
Genuine Bayer Professional Labeling (Aspirin Regimen Bayer) .... ▣608
Extra Strength Bayer Arthritis Caplets .... ▣610
Extra Strength Bayer Plus Caplets .... ▣610
Extra Strength Bayer PM Caplets .... ▣611
BC Powder .... ▣619
BC Allergy Sinus Cold Powder .... ▣619
Arthritis Strength BC Powder .... ▣619
BC Sinus Cold Powder .... ▣619
Darvon Compound-65 Pulvules 1910
Ecotrin Enteric Coated Aspirin Low, Regular and Maximum Strength Tablets 1715
Excedrin Extra-Strength Tablets, Caplets, and Geltabs .... ▣629
Excedrin Migraine 1070
Goody's Body Pain Formula Powder .... ▣620
Goody's Extra Strength Headache Powder .... ▣620
Goody's Extra Strength Pain Relief Tablets .... ▣620
Percodan Tablets 1327
Robaxisal Tablets 2939
Soma Compound Tablets 3354
Soma Compound w/Codeine Tablets 3355
Vanquish Caplets .... ▣617

Atenolol (Co-administration with drugs with hypoglycemic activity, such as beta blockers, may result in decreased insulin requirements; beta blockers may mask the symptoms of hypoglycemia in some patients). Products include:

Tenoretic Tablets 690
Tenormin I.V. Injection 692

Benazepril Hydrochloride (Co-administration with drugs with hypoglycemic activity, such as certain ACE inhibitors, may result in decreased insulin requirements). Products include:

Lotensin Tablets 2365
Lotensin HCT Tablets 2367
Lotrel Capsules 2370

Betamethasone Acetate (Co-administration may result in increased insulin requirements). Products include:

Celestone Soluspan Injectable Suspension 3097

Betamethasone Sodium Phosphate (Co-administration may result in increased insulin requirements). Products include:

Celestone Soluspan Injectable Suspension 3097

Betaxolol Hydrochloride (Co-administration with drugs with hypoglycemic activity, such as beta blockers, may result in decreased insulin requirements; beta blockers may mask the symptoms of hypoglycemia in some patients). Products include:

Betoptic S Ophthalmic Suspension 537

Bisoprolol Fumarate (Co-administration with drugs with hypoglycemic activity, such as beta blockers, may result in decreased insulin requirements; beta blockers may mask the symptoms of hypoglycemia in some patients). Products include:

Zebeta Tablets 1885
Ziac Tablets 1887

Captopril (Co-administration with drugs with hypoglycemic activity, such as certain ACE inhibitors, may result in decreased insulin requirements). Products include:

Captopril Tablets 2281

Carteolol Hydrochloride (Co-administration with drugs with hypoglycemic activity, such as beta blockers, may result in decreased insulin requirements; beta blockers may mask the symptoms of hypoglycemia in some patients). Products include:

Carteolol Hydrochloride Ophthalmic Solution USP, 1% .... ⊙258
Ocupress Ophthalmic Solution, 1% Sterile .... ⊙303

Chlorotrianisene (Co-administration may result in increased insulin requirements).

No products indexed under this heading.

Chlorpromazine (Co-administration with phenothiazines may result in increased insulin requirements). Products include:

Thorazine Suppositories 1656

Chlorpromazine Hydrochloride (Co-administration with phenothiazines may result in increased insulin requirements). Products include:

Thorazine ... 1656

Chlorpropamide (Co-administration with drugs with hypoglycemic activity, such as oral hypoglycemic agents, may result in decreased insulin requirements). Products include:

Diabinese Tablets ... 2680

Choline Magnesium Trisalicylate (Co-administration with drugs with hypoglycemic activity, such as salicylates, may result in decreased insulin requirements). Products include:

Trilisate ... 2901

Cortisone Acetate (Co-administration may result in increased insulin requirements). Products include:

Cortone Acetate Injectable Suspension ... 2059
Cortone Acetate Tablets ... 2061

Desogestrel (Co-admininstration with oral contraceptives may result in increased insulin requirements). Products include:

Cyclessa Tablets ... 2450
Desogen Tablets ... 2458
Mircette Tablets ... 2470
Ortho-Cept 21 Tablets ... 2546
Ortho-Cept 28 Tablets ... 2546

Dexamethasone (Co-administration may result in increased insulin requirements). Products include:

Decadron Elixir ... 2078
Decadron Tablets ... 2079
TobraDex Ophthalmic Ointment ... 542
TobraDex Ophthalmic Suspension .. 541

Dexamethasone Acetate (Co-administration may result in increased insulin requirements).

No products indexed under this heading.

Dexamethasone Sodium Phosphate (Co-administration may result in increased insulin requirements). Products include:

Decadron Phosphate Injection ... 2081
Decadron Phosphate Sterile Ophthalmic Ointment ... 2083
Decadron Phosphate Sterile Ophthalmic Solution ... 2084
NeoDecadron Sterile Ophthalmic Solution ... 2144

Dienestrol (Co-administration may result in increased insulin requirements). Products include:

Ortho Dienestrol Cream ... 2554

Diethylstilbestrol (Co-administration may result in increased insulin requirements).

No products indexed under this heading.

Diflunisal (Co-administration with drugs with hypoglycemic activity, such as salicylates, may result in decreased insulin requirements). Products include:

Dolobid Tablets ... 2088

Enalapril Maleate (Co-administration with drugs with hypoglycemic activity, such as certain ACE inhibitors, may result in decreased insulin requirements). Products include:

Lexxel Tablets ... 608
Vaseretic Tablets ... 2204
Vasotec Tablets ... 2210

Enalaprilat (Co-administration with drugs with hypoglycemic activity, such as certain ACE inhibitors, may result in decreased insulin requirements). Products include:

Enalaprilat Injection ... 863
Vasotec I.V. Injection ... 2207

Esmolol Hydrochloride (Co-administration with drugs with hypoglycemic activity, such as beta blockers, may result in decreased insulin requirements; beta blockers may mask the symptoms of hypoglycemia in some patients). Products include:

Brevibloc Injection ... 858

Estradiol (Co-administration may result in increased insulin requirements). Products include:

Activella Tablets ... 2764
Alora Transdermal System ... 3372
Climara Transdermal System ... 958
CombiPatch Transdermal System .. 2323
Esclim Transdermal System ... 3460
Estrace Vaginal Cream ... 3358
Estrace Tablets ... 3361
Estring Vaginal Ring ... 2811
Ortho-Prefest Tablets ... 2570
Vagifem Tablets ... 2857
Vivelle Transdermal System ... 2412
Vivelle-Dot Transdermal System ... 2416

Estrogens, Conjugated (Co-administration may result in increased insulin requirements). Products include:

Premarin Intravenous ... 3563
Premarin Tablets ... 3566
Premarin Vaginal Cream ... 3570
Premphase Tablets ... 3572
Prempro Tablets ... 3572

Estrogens, Esterified (Co-administration may result in increased insulin requirements). Products include:

Estratest ... 3252
Menest Tablets ... 2254

Estropipate (Co-administration may result in increased insulin requirements). Products include:

Ogen Tablets ... 2846
Ortho-Est Tablets ... 3464

Ethinyl Estradiol (Co-administration may result in increased insulin requirements). Products include:

Alesse-21 Tablets ... 3468
Alesse-28 Tablets ... 3473
Brevicon 28-Day Tablets ... 3380
Cyclessa Tablets ... 2450
Desogen Tablets ... 2458
Estinyl Tablets ... 3112
Estrostep ... 2627
femhrt Tablets ... 2635
Levlen ... 962
Levlite 21 Tablets ... 962
Levlite 28 Tablets ... 962
Levora Tablets ... 3389
Loestrin 21 Tablets ... 2642
Loestrin Fe Tablets ... 2642
Lo/Ovral Tablets ... 3532
Lo/Ovral-28 Tablets ... 3538
Low-Ogestrel-28 Tablets ... 3392
Microgestin Fe 1.5/30 Tablets ... 3407
Microgestin Fe 1/20 Tablets ... 3400
Mircette Tablets ... 2470
Modicon ... 2563
Necon ... 3415
Nordette-28 Tablets ... 2257
Norinyl 1 +35 28-Day Tablets ... 3380
Ogestrel 0.5/50-28 Tablets ... 3428
Ortho-Cept 21 Tablets ... 2546
Ortho-Cept 28 Tablets ... 2546
Ortho-Cyclen/Ortho Tri-Cyclen ... 2573
Ortho-Novum ... 2563
Ovcon ... 3364
Ovral Tablets ... 3551
Ovral-28 Tablets ... 3552
Tri-Levlen ... 962
Tri-Norinyl-28 Tablets ... 3433
Triphasil-21 Tablets ... 3600
Triphasil-28 Tablets ... 3605
Trivora Tablets ... 3439
Yasmin 28 Tablets ... 980
Zovia ... 3449

Ethynodiol Diacetate (Co-admininstration with oral contraceptives may result in increased insulin requirements). Products include:

Zovia ... 3449

Fludrocortisone Acetate (Co-administration may result in increased insulin requirements). Products include:

Florinef Acetate Tablets ... 2250

Fluphenazine Decanoate (Co-administration with phenothiazines may result in increased insulin requirements).

No products indexed under this heading.

Fluphenazine Enanthate (Co-administration with phenothiazines may result in increased insulin requirements).

No products indexed under this heading.

Fluphenazine Hydrochloride (Co-administration with phenothiazines may result in increased insulin requirements).

No products indexed under this heading.

Fosinopril Sodium (Co-administration with drugs with hypoglycemic activity, such as certain ACE inhibitors, may result in decreased insulin requirements). Products include:

Monopril Tablets ... 1091
Monopril HCT ... 1094

Glimepiride (Co-administration with drugs with hypoglycemic activity, such as oral hypoglycemic agents, may result in decreased insulin requirements). Products include:

Amaryl Tablets ... 717

Glipizide (Co-administration with drugs with hypoglycemic activity, such as oral hypoglycemic agents, may result in decreased insulin requirements). Products include:

Glucotrol Tablets ... 2692
Glucotrol XL Extended Release Tablets ... 2693

Glyburide (Co-administration with drugs with hypoglycemic activity, such as oral hypoglycemic agents, may result in decreased insulin requirements). Products include:

DiaBeta Tablets ... 741
Glucovance Tablets ... 1086

Hydrocortisone (Co-administration may result in increased insulin requirements). Products include:

Anusol-HC Cream 2.5% ... 2237
Cipro HC Otic Suspension ... 540
Cortaid Intensive Therapy Cream . ⊡ 717
Cortaid Maximum Strength Cream ... ⊡ 717
Cortisporin Ophthalmic Suspension Sterile ... ⊙ 297
Cortizone•5 ... ⊡ 699
Cortizone•10 ... ⊡ 699
Cortizone•10 Plus Creme ... ⊡ 700
Cortizone for Kids Creme ... ⊡ 699
Hydrocortone Tablets ... 2106
Massengill Medicated Soft Cloth Towelette ... ⊡ 753
VōSoL HC Otic Solution ... 3356

Hydrocortisone Acetate (Co-administration may result in increased insulin requirements). Products include:

Analpram-HC ... 1338
Anusol HC-1 Hydrocortisone Anti-Itch Cream ... ⊡ 689
Anusol-HC Suppositories ... 2238
Cortaid ... ⊡ 717
Cortifoam Rectal Foam ... 3170
Cortisporin-TC Otic Suspension ... 2246
Hydrocortone Acetate Injectable Suspension ... 2103
Pramosone ... 1343
Proctocort Suppositories ... 2264
ProctoFoam-HC ... 3177
Terra-Cortril Ophthalmic Suspension ... 2716

Hydrocortisone Sodium Phosphate (Co-administration may result in increased insulin requirements). Products include:

Hydrocortone Phosphate Injection, Sterile ... 2105

Hydrocortisone Sodium Succinate (Co-administration may result in increased insulin requirements).

No products indexed under this heading.

Isoniazid (Co-administration may result in increased insulin requirements). Products include:

Rifamate Capsules ... 767
Rifater Tablets ... 769

Labetalol Hydrochloride (Co-administration with drugs with hypoglycemic activity, such as beta blockers, may result in decreased insulin requirements; beta blockers may mask the symptoms of hypoglycemia in some patients). Products include:

Normodyne Injection ... 3135
Normodyne Tablets ... 3137

Levobunolol Hydrochloride (Co-administration with drugs with hypoglycemic activity, such as beta blockers, may result in decreased insulin requirements; beta blockers may mask the symptoms of hypoglycemia in some patients). Products include:

Betagan ... ⊙ 228

Levonorgestrel (Co-admininstration with oral contraceptives may result in increased insulin requirements). Products include:

Alesse-21 Tablets ... 3468
Alesse-28 Tablets ... 3473
Levlen ... 962
Levlite 21 Tablets ... 962
Levlite 28 Tablets ... 962
Levora Tablets ... 3389
Mirena Intrauterine System ... 974
Nordette-28 Tablets ... 2257
Norplant System ... 3543
Tri-Levlen ... 962
Triphasil-21 Tablets ... 3600
Triphasil-28 Tablets ... 3605
Trivora Tablets ... 3439

Levothyroxine Sodium (Co-administration with thyroid replacement therapy may result in increased insulin requirements). Products include:

Levothroid Tablets ... 1373
Levoxyl Tablets ... 1819
Synthroid ... 505
Unithroid Tablets ... 3445

Liothyronine Sodium (Co-administration with thyroid replacement therapy may result in increased insulin requirements). Products include:

Cytomel Tablets ... 1817
Triostat Injection ... 1825

Liotrix (Co-administration with thyroid replacement therapy may result in increased insulin requirements).

No products indexed under this heading.

Lisinopril (Co-administration with drugs with hypoglycemic activity, such as certain ACE inhibitors, may result in decreased insulin requirements). Products include:

Prinivil Tablets ... 2164
Prinzide Tablets ... 2168
Zestoretic Tablets ... 695
Zestril Tablets ... 698

Magnesium Salicylate (Co-administration with drugs with hypoglycemic activity, such as salicylates, may result in decreased insulin requirements). Products include:

Momentum Backache Relief Extra Strength Caplets ... ⊡ 666

Mesoridazine Besylate (Co-administration with phenothiazines may result in increased insulin requirements). Products include:

Serentil ... 1057

Mestranol (Co-admininstration with oral contraceptives may result in increased insulin requirements). Products include:

Necon 1/50 Tablets ... 3415
Norinyl 1 + 50 28-Day Tablets ... 3380
Ortho-Novum 1/50□28 Tablets ... 2556

Metformin Hydrochloride (Co-administration with drugs with hypoglycemic activity, such as oral hypoglycemic agents, may result in decreased insulin requirements). Products include:

Glucophage Tablets ... 1080
Glucophage XR Tablets ... 1080
Glucovance Tablets ... 1086

Methotrimeprazine (Co-administration with phenothiazines may result in increased insulin requirements).

No products indexed under this heading.

Methylprednisolone Acetate (Co-administration may result in increased insulin requirements). Products include:

Depo-Medrol Injectable Suspension 2795

Methylprednisolone Sodium Succinate (Co-administration may result in increased insulin requirements). Products include:
Solu-Medrol Sterile Powder 2855

Metipranolol Hydrochloride (Co-administration with drugs with hypoglycemic activity, such as beta blockers, may result in decreased insulin requirements; beta blockers may mask the symptoms of hypoglycemia in some patients).
No products indexed under this heading.

Metoprolol Succinate (Co-administration with drugs with hypoglycemic activity, such as beta blockers, may result in decreased insulin requirements; beta blockers may mask the symptoms of hypoglycemia in some patients). Products include:
Toprol-XL Tablets 651

Metoprolol Tartrate (Co-administration with drugs with hypoglycemic activity, such as beta blockers, may result in decreased insulin requirements; beta blockers may mask the symptoms of hypoglycemia in some patients).
No products indexed under this heading.

Miglitol (Co-administration with drugs with hypoglycemic activity, such as oral hypoglycemic agents, may result in decreased insulin requirements). Products include:
Glyset Tablets 2821

Moexipril Hydrochloride (Co-administration with drugs with hypoglycemic activity, such as certain ACE inhibitors, may result in decreased insulin requirements). Products include:
Uniretic Tablets 3178
Univasc Tablets 3181

Nadolol (Co-administration with drugs with hypoglycemic activity, such as beta blockers, may result in decreased insulin requirements; beta blockers may mask the symptoms of hypoglycemia in some patients). Products include:
Corgard Tablets 2245
Corzide 40/5 Tablets 2247
Corzide 80/5 Tablets 2247
Nadolol Tablets 2288

Niacin (Co-administration may result in increased insulin requirements). Products include:
Niaspan Extended-Release Tablets 1846
Nicotinex Elixir .... ▣633

Norethindrone (Co-admininstration with oral contraceptives may result in increased insulin requirements). Products include:
Brevicon 28-Day Tablets 3380
Micronor Tablets 2543
Modicon 2563
Necon 3415
Norinyl 1 +35 28-Day Tablets 3380
Norinyl 1 + 50 28-Day Tablets 3380
Nor-QD Tablets 3423
Ortho-Novum 2563
Ortho-Novum 1/50▫28 Tablets 2556
Ovcon 3364
Tri-Norinyl-28 Tablets 3433

Norethynodrel (Co-admininstration with oral contraceptives may result in increased insulin requirements).
No products indexed under this heading.

Norgestimate (Co-admininstration with oral contraceptives may result in increased insulin requirements). Products include:
Ortho-Cyclen/Ortho Tri-Cyclen 2573
Ortho-Prefest Tablets 2570

Norgestrel (Co-admininstration with oral contraceptives may result in increased insulin requirements). Products include:
Lo/Ovral Tablets 3532
Lo/Ovral-28 Tablets 3538
Low-Ogestrel-28 Tablets 3392
Ogestrel 0.5/50-28 Tablets 3428
Ovral Tablets 3551
Ovral-28 Tablets 3552
Ovrette Tablets 3552

Octreotide Acetate (Co-administration with drugs with hypoglycemic activity, such as inhibitors of pancreatic function, may result in decreased insulin requirements). Products include:
Sandostatin LAR Depot 2395

Penbutolol Sulfate (Co-administration with drugs with hypoglycemic activity, such as beta blockers, may result in decreased insulin requirements; beta blockers may mask the symptoms of hypoglycemia in some patients).
No products indexed under this heading.

Perindopril Erbumine (Co-administration with drugs with hypoglycemic activity, such as certain ACE inhibitors, may result in decreased insulin requirements). Products include:
Aceon Tablets (2 mg, 4 mg, 8 mg) 3249

Perphenazine (Co-administration with phenothiazines may result in increased insulin requirements). Products include:
Etrafon 3115
Trilafon 3160

Phenelzine Sulfate (Co-administration with drugs with hypoglycemic activity, such as certain MAO inhibitor antidepressants, may result in decreased insulin requirements). Products include:
Nardil Tablets 2653

Pindolol (Co-administration with drugs with hypoglycemic activity, such as beta blockers, may result in decreased insulin requirements; beta blockers may mask the symptoms of hypoglycemia in some patients).
No products indexed under this heading.

Pioglitazone Hydrochloride (Co-administration with drugs with hypoglycemic activity, such as oral hypoglycemic agents, may result in decreased insulin requirements). Products include:
Actos Tablets 3275

Polyestradiol Phosphate (Co-administration may result in increased insulin requirements).
No products indexed under this heading.

Prednisolone Acetate (Co-administration may result in increased insulin requirements). Products include:
Blephamide Ophthalmic Ointment 547
Blephamide Ophthalmic Suspension 548
Poly-Pred Liquifilm Ophthalmic Suspension .... ⊙245
Pred Forte Ophthalmic Suspension .... ⊙246
Pred Mild Sterile Ophthalmic Suspension .... ⊙249
Pred-G Ophthalmic Suspension .... ⊙247
Pred-G Sterile Ophthalmic Ointment .... ⊙248

Prednisolone Sodium Phosphate (Co-administration may result in increased insulin requirements). Products include:
Pediapred Oral Solution 1170

Prednisolone Tebutate (Co-administration may result in increased insulin requirements).
No products indexed under this heading.

Prednisone (Co-administration may result in increased insulin requirements). Products include:
Prednisone 3064

Prochlorperazine (Co-administration with phenothiazines may result in increased insulin requirements). Products include:
Compazine 1505

Promethazine Hydrochloride (Co-administration with phenothiazines may result in increased insulin requirements). Products include:
Mepergan Injection 3539
Phenergan Injection 3553
Phenergan 3556
Phenergan Syrup 3554
Phenergan with Codeine Syrup 3557
Phenergan with Dextromethorphan Syrup 3559
Phenergan VC Syrup 3560
Phenergan VC with Codeine Syrup 3561

Propranolol Hydrochloride (Co-administration with drugs with hypoglycemic activity, such as beta blockers, may result in decreased insulin requirements; beta blockers may mask the symptoms of hypoglycemia in some patients). Products include:
Inderal 3513
Inderal LA Long-Acting Capsules 3516
Inderide Tablets 3517
Inderide LA Long-Acting Capsules 3519

Quinapril Hydrochloride (Co-administration with drugs with hypoglycemic activity, such as certain ACE inhibitors, may result in decreased insulin requirements). Products include:
Accupril Tablets 2611
Accuretic Tablets 2614

Quinestrol (Co-administration may result in increased insulin requirements).
No products indexed under this heading.

Ramipril (Co-administration with drugs with hypoglycemic activity, such as certain ACE inhibitors, may result in decreased insulin requirements). Products include:
Altace Capsules 2233

Repaglinide (Co-administration with drugs with hypoglycemic activity, such as oral hypoglycemic agents, may result in decreased insulin requirements). Products include:
Prandin Tablets (0.5, 1, and 2 mg) 2432

Rosiglitazone Maleate (Co-administration with drugs with hypoglycemic activity, such as oral hypoglycemic agents, may result in decreased insulin requirements). Products include:
Avandia Tablets 1490

Salsalate (Co-administration with drugs with hypoglycemic activity, such as salicylates, may result in decreased insulin requirements).
No products indexed under this heading.

Sotalol Hydrochloride (Co-administration with drugs with hypoglycemic activity, such as beta blockers, may result in decreased insulin requirements; beta blockers may mask the symptoms of hypoglycemia in some patients). Products include:
Betapace Tablets 950
Betapace AF Tablets 954

Spirapril Hydrochloride (Co-administration with drugs with hypoglycemic activity, such as certain ACE inhibitors, may result in decreased insulin requirements).
No products indexed under this heading.

Sulfacytine (Co-administration with drugs with hypoglycemic activity, such as sulfa antibiotics, may result in decreased insulin requirements).

Sulfamethizole (Co-administration with drugs with hypoglycemic activity, such as sulfa antibiotics, may result in decreased insulin requirements). Products include:
Urobiotic-250 Capsules 2731

Sulfamethoxazole (Co-administration with drugs with hypoglycemic activity, such as sulfa antibiotics, may result in decreased insulin requirements). Products include:
Bactrim 2949
Septra Suspension 2265
Septra Tablets 2265
Septra DS Tablets 2265

Sulfasalazine (Co-administration with drugs with hypoglycemic activity, such as sulfa antibiotics, may result in decreased insulin requirements). Products include:
Azulfidine EN-tabs Tablets 2775

Sulfisoxazole (Co-administration with drugs with hypoglycemic activity, such as sulfa antibiotics, may result in decreased insulin requirements).
No products indexed under this heading.

Thioridazine Hydrochloride (Co-administration with phenothiazines may result in increased insulin requirements). Products include:
Thioridazine Hydrochloride Tablets 2289

Thyroglobulin (Co-administration with thyroid replacement therapy may result in increased insulin requirements).
No products indexed under this heading.

Thyroid (Co-administration with thyroid replacement therapy may result in increased insulin requirements).
No products indexed under this heading.

Thyroxine (Co-administration with thyroid replacement therapy may result in increased insulin requirements).
No products indexed under this heading.

Thyroxine Sodium (Co-administration with thyroid replacement therapy may result in increased insulin requirements).
No products indexed under this heading.

Timolol Hemihydrate (Co-administration with drugs with hypoglycemic activity, such as beta blockers, may result in decreased insulin requirements; beta blockers may mask the symptoms of hypoglycemia in some patients). Products include:
Betimol Ophthalmic Solution .... ⊙324

Timolol Maleate (Co-administration with drugs with hypoglycemic activity, such as beta blockers, may result in decreased insulin requirements; beta blockers may mask the symptoms of hypoglycemia in some patients). Products include:
Blocadren Tablets 2046
Cosopt Sterile Ophthalmic Solution 2065
Timolide Tablets 2187
Timolol GFS .... ⊙266
Timoptic in Ocudose 2192
Timoptic Sterile Ophthalmic Solution 2190
Timoptic-XE Sterile Ophthalmic Gel Forming Solution 2194

Tolazamide (Co-administration with drugs with hypoglycemic activity, such as oral hypoglycemic agents, may result in decreased insulin requirements).
No products indexed under this heading.

Tolbutamide (Co-administration with drugs with hypoglycemic activity, such as oral hypoglycemic agents, may result in decreased insulin requirements).
No products indexed under this heading.

Trandolapril (Co-administration with drugs with hypoglycemic activity,

such as certain ACE inhibitors, may result in decreased insulin requirements). Products include:
Mavik Tablets 478
Tarka Tablets 508

Tranylcypromine Sulfate (Co-administration with drugs with hypoglycemic activity, such as certain MAO inhibitor antidepressants, may result in decreased insulin requirements). Products include:
Parnate Tablets 1607

Triamcinolone (Co-administration may result in increased insulin requirements).
No products indexed under this heading.

Triamcinolone Acetonide (Co-administration may result in increased insulin requirements).
Products include:
Azmacort Inhalation Aerosol 728
Nasacort Nasal Inhaler 750
Nasacort AQ Nasal Spray 752
Tri-Nasal Spray 2274

Triamcinolone Diacetate (Co-administration may result in increased insulin requirements).
No products indexed under this heading.

Triamcinolone Hexacetonide (Co-administration may result in increased insulin requirements).
No products indexed under this heading.

Trifluoperazine Hydrochloride (Co-administration with phenothiazines may result in increased insulin requirements). Products include:
Stelazine 1640

Troglitazone (Co-administration with drugs with hypoglycemic activity, such as oral hypoglycemic agents, may result in decreased insulin requirements).
No products indexed under this heading.

Food Interactions

Alcohol (Co-administration with drugs with hypoglycemic activity may result in decreased insulin requirements).

HUMALOG MIX 75/25 PEN

(Insulin Lispro, Human, Insulin Lispro Protamine, Human) 1928
See Humalog

HUMATE-P CONCENTRATE

(Antihemophilic Factor (Human)) 790
None cited in PDR database.

HUMATRIX MICROCLYSMIC BURN/ WOUND HEALING GEL

(Chondroitin Sulfate, Collagen) .... ▣632
None cited in PDR database.

HUMATROPE VIALS AND CARTRIDGES

(Somatropin) 1930
May interact with glucocorticoids, insulin, sex steroids, and certain other agents. Compounds in these categories include:

ACTH (Excessive glucocorticoid therapy will inhibit the growth promoting effect of somatropin; growth hormone administration may alter the clearance of compounds known to be metabolized by cytochrome P450 liver enzymes; such as corticosteroids).
No products indexed under this heading.

Betamethasone Acetate (Excessive glucocorticoid therapy will inhibit the growth promoting effect of somatropin; growth hormone administration may alter the clearance of compounds known to be metabolized by cytochrome P450 liver enzymes; such as corticosteroids). Products include:
Celestone Soluspan Injectable Suspension 3097

Betamethasone Sodium Phosphate (Excessive glucocorticoid therapy will inhibit the growth promoting effect of somatropin; growth hormone administration may alter the clearance of compounds known to be metabolized by cytochrome P450 liver enzymes; such as corticosteroids). Products include:
Celestone Soluspan Injectable Suspension 3097

Cortisone Acetate (Excessive glucocorticoid therapy will inhibit the growth promoting effect of somatropin; growth hormone administration may alter the clearance of compounds known to be metabolized by cytochrome P450 liver enzymes; such as corticosteroids). Products include:
Cortone Acetate Injectable Suspension 2059
Cortone Acetate Tablets 2061

Cyclosporine (Growth hormone administration may alter the clearance of compounds known to be metabolized by cytochrome P450 liver enzymes, such as cyclosporine). Products include:
Gengraf Capsules 457
Neoral Soft Gelatin Capsules 2380
Neoral Oral Solution 2380
Sandimmune 2388

Desogestrel (Growth hormone administration may alter the clearance of compounds known to be metabolized by cytochrome P450 liver enzymes, such as sex steroids). Products include:
Cyclessa Tablets 2450
Desogen Tablets 2458
Mircette Tablets 2470
Ortho-Cept 21 Tablets 2546
Ortho-Cept 28 Tablets 2546

Dexamethasone (Excessive glucocorticoid therapy will inhibit the growth promoting effect of somatropin; growth hormone administration may alter the clearance of compounds known to be metabolized by cytochrome P450 liver enzymes; such as corticosteroids). Products include:
Decadron Elixir 2078
Decadron Tablets 2079
TobraDex Ophthalmic Ointment 542
TobraDex Ophthalmic Suspension .. 541

Dexamethasone Acetate (Excessive glucocorticoid therapy will inhibit the growth promoting effect of somatropin; growth hormone administration may alter the clearance of compounds known to be metabolized by cytochrome P450 liver enzymes; such as corticosteroids).
No products indexed under this heading.

Dexamethasone Sodium Phosphate (Excessive glucocorticoid therapy will inhibit the growth promoting effect of somatropin; growth hormone administration may alter the clearance of compounds known to be metabolized by cytochrome P450 liver enzymes; such as corticosteroids). Products include:
Decadron Phosphate Injection 2081
Decadron Phosphate Sterile Ophthalmic Ointment 2083
Decadron Phosphate Sterile Ophthalmic Solution 2084
NeoDecadron Sterile Ophthalmic Solution 2144

Estradiol (Growth hormone administration may alter the clearance of compounds known to be metabolized by cytochrome P450 liver enzymes, such as sex steroids). Products include:
Activella Tablets 2764
Alora Transdermal System 3372
Climara Transdermal System 958
CombiPatch Transdermal System .. 2323
Esclim Transdermal System 3460
Estrace Vaginal Cream 3358
Estrace Tablets 3361
Estring Vaginal Ring 2811
Ortho-Prefest Tablets 2570
Vagifem Tablets 2857
Vivelle Transdermal System 2412
Vivelle-Dot Transdermal System 2416

Estrogens, Conjugated (Growth hormone administration may alter the clearance of compounds known to be metabolized by cytochrome P450 liver enzymes, such as sex steroids). Products include:
Premarin Intravenous 3563
Premarin Tablets 3566
Premarin Vaginal Cream 3570
Premphase Tablets 3572
Prempro Tablets 3572

Ethinyl Estradiol (Growth hormone administration may alter the clearance of compounds known to be metabolized by cytochrome P450 liver enzymes, such as sex steroids). Products include:
Alesse-21 Tablets 3468
Alesse-28 Tablets 3473
Brevicon 28-Day Tablets 3380
Cyclessa Tablets 2450
Desogen Tablets 2458
Estinyl Tablets 3112
Estrostep 2627
femhrt Tablets 2635
Levlen 962
Levlite 21 Tablets 962
Levlite 28 Tablets 962
Levora Tablets 3389
Loestrin 21 Tablets 2642
Loestrin Fe Tablets 2642
Lo/Ovral Tablets 3532
Lo/Ovral-28 Tablets 3538
Low-Ogestrel-28 Tablets 3392
Microgestin Fe 1.5/30 Tablets 3407
Microgestin Fe 1/20 Tablets 3400
Mircette Tablets 2470
Modicon 2563
Necon 3415
Nordette-28 Tablets 2257
Norinyl 1 +35 28-Day Tablets 3380
Ogestrel 0.5/50-28 Tablets 3428
Ortho-Cept 21 Tablets 2546
Ortho-Cept 28 Tablets 2546
Ortho-Cyclen/Ortho Tri-Cyclen 2573
Ortho-Novum 2563
Ovcon 3364
Ovral Tablets 3551
Ovral-28 Tablets 3552
Tri-Levlen 962
Tri-Norinyl-28 Tablets 3433
Triphasil-21 Tablets 3600
Triphasil-28 Tablets 3605
Trivora Tablets 3439
Yasmin 28 Tablets 980
Zovia 3449

Ethynodiol Diacetate (Growth hormone administration may alter the clearance of compounds known to be metabolized by cytochrome P450 liver enzymes, such as sex steroids). Products include:
Zovia 3449

Fludrocortisone Acetate (Excessive glucocorticoid therapy will inhibit the growth promoting effect of somatropin; growth hormone administration may alter the clearance of compounds known to be metabolized by cytochrome P450 liver enzymes; such as corticosteroids). Products include:
Florinef Acetate Tablets 2250

Fluoxymesterone (Growth hormone administration may alter the clearance of compounds known to be metabolized by cytochrome P450 liver enzymes, such as sex steroids).
No products indexed under this heading.

Hydrocortisone (Excessive glucocorticoid therapy will inhibit the growth promoting effect of somatropin; growth hormone administration may alter the clearance of compounds known to be metabolized by cytochrome P450 liver enzymes; such as corticosteroids). Products include:
Anusol-HC Cream 2.5% 2237
Cipro HC Otic Suspension 540
Cortaid Intensive Therapy Cream .. ▣717
Cortaid Maximum Strength Cream .... ▣717
Cortisporin Ophthalmic Suspension Sterile .... ⊙297
Cortizone•5 .... ▣699
Cortizone•10 .... ▣699
Cortizone•10 Plus Creme .... ▣700
Cortizone for Kids Creme .... ▣699
Hydrocortone Tablets 2106
Massengill Medicated Soft Cloth Towelette .... ▣753
VōSoL HC Otic Solution 3356

Hydrocortisone Acetate (Excessive glucocorticoid therapy will inhibit the growth promoting effect of somatropin; growth hormone administration may alter the clearance of compounds known to be metabolized by cytochrome P450 liver enzymes; such as corticosteroids). Products include:
Analpram-HC 1338
Anusol HC-1 Hydrocortisone Anti-Itch Cream .... ▣689
Anusol-HC Suppositories 2238
Cortaid .... ▣717
Cortifoam Rectal Foam 3170
Cortisporin-TC Otic Suspension 2246
Hydrocortone Acetate Injectable Suspension 2103
Pramosone 1343
Proctocort Suppositories 2264
ProctoFoam-HC 3177
Terra-Cortril Ophthalmic Suspension 2716

Hydrocortisone Sodium Phosphate (Excessive glucocorticoid therapy will inhibit the growth promoting effect of somatropin; growth hormone administration may alter the clearance of compounds known to be metabolized by cytochrome P450 liver enzymes; such as corticosteroids). Products include:
Hydrocortone Phosphate Injection, Sterile 2105

Hydrocortisone Sodium Succinate (Excessive glucocorticoid therapy will inhibit the growth promoting effect of somatropin; growth hormone administration may alter the clearance of compounds known to be metabolized by cytochrome P450 liver enzymes; such as corticosteroids).
No products indexed under this heading.

Insulin, Human, Zinc Suspension (For diabetics, the insulin dose may require adjustment when somatropin therapy is instituted; growth hormone may induce a state insulin resistance; patients should be observed for evidence of glucose intolerance). Products include:
Humulin L, 100 Units 1937
Humulin U, 100 Units 1943
Novolin L Human Insulin 10 ml Vials 2422

Insulin, Human NPH (For diabetics, the insulin dose may require adjustment when somatropin therapy is instituted; growth hormone may induce a state insulin resistance; patients should be observed for evidence of glucose intolerance). Products include:
Humulin N, 100 Units 1939
Humulin N NPH Pen 1940
Novolin N Human Insulin 10 ml Vials 2422
Novolin N PenFill 2423
Novolin N Prefilled Syringe Disposable Insulin Delivery System 2425

Insulin, Human Regular (For diabetics, the insulin dose may require adjustment when somatropin therapy is instituted; growth hormone may induce a state insulin resistance; patients should be observed for evidence of glucose intolerance). Products include:
Humulin R Regular (U-500) 1943
Humulin R, 100 Units 1941

Novolin R Human Insulin 10 ml Vials 2423
Novolin R PenFill 2423
Novolin R Prefilled Syringe Disposable Insulin Delivery System 2425
Velosulin BR Human Insulin 10 ml Vials 2435

Insulin, Human Regular and Human NPH Mixture (For diabetics, the insulin dose may require adjustment when somatropin therapy is instituted; growth hormone may induce a state insulin resistance; patients should be observed for evidence of glucose intolerance). Products include:
Humulin 50/50, 100 Units 1934
Humulin 70/30, 100 Units 1935
Humulin 70/30 Pen 1936
Novolin 70/30 Human Insulin 10 ml Vials 2421
Novolin 70/30 PenFill 2423
Novolin 70/30 Prefilled Disposable Insulin Delivery System 2425

Insulin, NPH (For diabetics, the insulin dose may require adjustment when somatropin therapy is instituted; growth hormone may induce a state insulin resistance; patients should be observed for evidence of glucose intolerance). Products include:
Iletin II, NPH (Pork), 100 Units 1946

Insulin, Regular (For diabetics, the insulin dose may require adjustment when somatropin therapy is instituted; growth hormone may induce a state insulin resistance; patients should be observed for evidence of glucose intolerance). Products include:
Iletin II, Regular (Pork), 100 Units 1947

Insulin, Zinc Crystals (For diabetics, the insulin dose may require adjustment when somatropin therapy is instituted; growth hormone may induce a state insulin resistance; patients should be observed for evidence of glucose intolerance).
No products indexed under this heading.

Insulin, Zinc Suspension (For diabetics, the insulin dose may require adjustment when somatropin therapy is instituted; growth hormone may induce a state insulin resistance; patients should be observed for evidence of glucose intolerance). Products include:
Iletin II, Lente (Pork), 100 Units 1945

Insulin Aspart, Human Regular (For diabetics, the insulin dose may require adjustment when somatropin therapy is instituted; growth hormone may induce a state insulin resistance; patients should be observed for evidence of glucose intolerance).
No products indexed under this heading.

Insulin glargine (For diabetics, the insulin dose may require adjustment when somatropin therapy is instituted; growth hormone may induce a state insulin resistance; patients should be observed for evidence of glucose intolerance). Products include:
Lantus Injection 742

Insulin Lispro, Human (For diabetics, the insulin dose may require adjustment when somatropin therapy is instituted; growth hormone may induce a state insulin resistance; patients should be observed for evidence of glucose intolerance). Products include:
Humalog 1926
Humalog Mix 75/25 Pen 1928

Insulin Lispro Protamine, Human (For diabetics, the insulin dose may require adjustment when somatropin therapy is instituted; growth hormone may induce a state insulin resistance; patients should be observed for evidence of glucose intolerance). Products include:
Humalog Mix 75/25 Pen 1928

Levonorgestrel (Growth hormone administration may alter the clearance of compounds known to be metabolized by cytochrome P450 liver enzymes, such as sex steroids). Products include:
Alesse-21 Tablets 3468
Alesse-28 Tablets 3473
Levlen 962
Levlite 21 Tablets 962
Levlite 28 Tablets 962
Levora Tablets 3389
Mirena Intrauterine System 974
Nordette-28 Tablets 2257
Norplant System 3543
Tri-Levlen 962
Triphasil-21 Tablets 3600
Triphasil-28 Tablets 3605
Trivora Tablets 3439

Mestranol (Growth hormone administration may alter the clearance of compounds known to be metabolized by cytochrome P450 liver enzymes, such as sex steroids). Products include:
Necon 1/50 Tablets 3415
Norinyl 1 + 50 28-Day Tablets 3380
Ortho-Novum 1/50□28 Tablets 2556

Methylprednisolone Acetate (Excessive glucocorticoid therapy will inhibit the growth promoting effect of somatropin; growth hormone administration may alter the clearance of compounds known to be metabolized by cytochrome P450 liver enzymes; such as corticosteroids). Products include:
Depo-Medrol Injectable Suspension 2795

Methylprednisolone Sodium Succinate (Excessive glucocorticoid therapy will inhibit the growth promoting effect of somatropin; growth hormone administration may alter the clearance of compounds known to be metabolized by cytochrome P450 liver enzymes; such as corticosteroids). Products include:
Solu-Medrol Sterile Powder 2855

Methyltestosterone (Growth hormone administration may alter the clearance of compounds known to be metabolized by cytochrome P450 liver enzymes, such as sex steroids). Products include:
Android Capsules, 10 mg 1731
Estratest 3252
Testred Capsules, 10 mg 1746

Norethindrone (Growth hormone administration may alter the clearance of compounds known to be metabolized by cytochrome P450 liver enzymes, such as sex steroids). Products include:
Brevicon 28-Day Tablets 3380
Micronor Tablets 2543
Modicon 2563
Necon 3415
Norinyl 1 +35 28-Day Tablets 3380
Norinyl 1 + 50 28-Day Tablets 3380
Nor-QD Tablets 3423
Ortho-Novum 2563
Ortho-Novum 1/50□28 Tablets 2556
Ovcon 3364
Tri-Norinyl-28 Tablets 3433

Norethindrone Acetate (Growth hormone administration may alter the clearance of compounds known to be metabolized by cytochrome P450 liver enzymes, such as sex steroids). Products include:
Activella Tablets 2764
Aygestin Tablets 1333
CombiPatch Transdermal System 2323
Estrostep 2627
femhrt Tablets 2635
Loestrin 21 Tablets 2642
Loestrin Fe Tablets 2642
Microgestin Fe 1.5/30 Tablets 3407
Microgestin Fe 1/20 Tablets 3400

Norgestimate (Growth hormone administration may alter the clearance of compounds known to be metabolized by cytochrome P450 liver enzymes, such as sex steroids). Products include:
Ortho-Cyclen/Ortho Tri-Cyclen 2573
Ortho-Prefest Tablets 2570

Prednisolone Acetate (Excessive glucocorticoid therapy will inhibit the growth promoting effect of somatropin; growth hormone administration may alter the clearance of compounds known to be metabolized by cytochrome P450 liver enzymes; such as corticosteroids). Products include:
Blephamide Ophthalmic Ointment 547
Blephamide Ophthalmic Suspension 548
Poly-Pred Liquifilm Ophthalmic Suspension .... ⊙245
Pred Forte Ophthalmic Suspension .... ⊙246
Pred Mild Sterile Ophthalmic Suspension .... ⊙249
Pred-G Ophthalmic Suspension .... ⊙247
Pred-G Sterile Ophthalmic Ointment .... ⊙248

Prednisolone Sodium Phosphate (Excessive glucocorticoid therapy will inhibit the growth promoting effect of somatropin; growth hormone administration may alter the clearance of compounds known to be metabolized by cytochrome P450 liver enzymes; such as corticosteroids). Products include:
Pediapred Oral Solution 1170

Prednisolone Tebutate (Excessive glucocorticoid therapy will inhibit the growth promoting effect of somatropin; growth hormone administration may alter the clearance of compounds known to be metabolized by cytochrome P450 liver enzymes; such as corticosteroids).
No products indexed under this heading.

Prednisone (Excessive glucocorticoid therapy will inhibit the growth promoting effect of somatropin; growth hormone administration may alter the clearance of compounds known to be metabolized by cytochrome P450 liver enzymes; such as corticosteroids). Products include:
Prednisone 3064

Testosterone (Growth hormone administration may alter the clearance of compounds known to be metabolized by cytochrome P450 liver enzymes, such as sex steroids). Products include:
Androderm Transdermal System CIII 3377
AndroGel 3322
Testoderm Transdermal Systems 574
Testopel Pellets 3610

Triamcinolone (Excessive glucocorticoid therapy will inhibit the growth promoting effect of somatropin; growth hormone administration may alter the clearance of compounds known to be metabolized by cytochrome P450 liver enzymes; such as corticosteroids).
No products indexed under this heading.

Triamcinolone Acetonide (Excessive glucocorticoid therapy will inhibit the growth promoting effect of somatropin; growth hormone administration may alter the clearance of compounds known to be metabolized by cytochrome P450 liver enzymes; such as corticosteroids). Products include:
Azmacort Inhalation Aerosol 728
Nasacort Nasal Inhaler 750
Nasacort AQ Nasal Spray 752
Tri-Nasal Spray 2274

Triamcinolone Diacetate (Excessive glucocorticoid therapy will inhibit the growth promoting effect of somatropin; growth hormone administration may alter the clearance of compounds known to be metabolized by cytochrome P450 liver enzymes; such as corticosteroids).
No products indexed under this heading.

Triamcinolone Hexacetonide (Excessive glucocorticoid therapy will inhibit the growth promoting effect of somatropin; growth hormone administration may alter the clearance of compounds known to be metabolized by cytochrome P450 liver enzymes; such as corticosteroids).
No products indexed under this heading.

HUMEGON FOR INJECTION

(Menotropins) 2468
None cited in PDR database.

HUMORSOL STERILE OPHTHALMIC SOLUTION

(Demecarium Bromide) 2102
May interact with cholinergic agents and certain other agents. Compounds in these categories include:

Bethanechol Chloride (Additive adverse effects). Products include:
Urecholine 2198
Urecholine Tablets 2445

Cevimeline Hydrochloride (Additive adverse effects). Products include:
Evoxac Capsules 1217

Donepezil Hydrochloride (Additive adverse effects). Products include:
Aricept Tablets 1270
Aricept Tablets 2665

Edrophonium Chloride (Additive adverse effects). Products include:
Tensilon Injectable 1745

Galantamine Hydrobromide (Additive adverse effects). Products include:
Reminyl Oral Solution 1792
Reminyl Tablets 1792

Neostigmine Bromide (Additive adverse effects). Products include:
Prostigmin Tablets 1744

Neostigmine Methylsulfate (Additive adverse effects). Products include:
Prostigmin Injectable 1744

Pyridostigmine Bromide (Additive adverse effects). Products include:
Mestinon 1740

Rivastigmine Tartrate (Additive adverse effects). Products include:
Exelon Capsules 2342
Exelon Oral Solution 2345

Succinylcholine Chloride (Possible respiratory and cardiovascular collapse). Products include:
Anectine Injection 1476

Tacrine Hydrochloride (Additive adverse effects). Products include:
Cognex Capsules 1351

HUMULIN 50/50, 100 UNITS

(Insulin, Human Regular and Human NPH Mixture) 1934
See Iletin II, Regular (Pork), 100 Units

HUMULIN 70/30, 100 UNITS

(Insulin, Human Regular and Human NPH Mixture) 1935
See Iletin II, Regular (Pork), 100 Units

HUMULIN 70/30 PEN

(Insulin, Human Regular and Human NPH Mixture) 1936
See Iletin II, Regular (Pork), 100 Units

HUMULIN L, 100 UNITS

(Insulin, Human, Zinc Suspension) 1937
See Iletin II, Regular (Pork), 100 Units

HUMULIN N, 100 UNITS

(Insulin, Human NPH) 1939
See Iletin II, Regular (Pork), 100 Units

HUMULIN R REGULAR (U-500)
(Insulin, Human Regular) 1943
May interact with beta blockers and oral hypoglycemic agents. Compounds in these categories include:

Acarbose (Concurrent use of oral hypoglycemic agents with Humulin R (U-500) is not recommended since there are no data to support such use). Products include:
Precose Tablets 906

Acebutolol Hydrochloride (Early warning symptoms of hypoglycemia may be different or less pronounced under certain conditions, such as concurrent beta blocker therapy). Products include:
Sectral Capsules 3589

Atenolol (Early warning symptoms of hypoglycemia may be different or less pronounced under certain conditions, such as concurrent beta blocker therapy). Products include:
Tenoretic Tablets 690
Tenormin I.V. Injection 692

Betaxolol Hydrochloride (Early warning symptoms of hypoglycemia may be different or less pronounced under certain conditions, such as concurrent beta blocker therapy). Products include:
Betoptic S Ophthalmic Suspension 537

Bisoprolol Fumarate (Early warning symptoms of hypoglycemia may be different or less pronounced under certain conditions, such as concurrent beta blocker therapy). Products include:
Zebeta Tablets 1885
Ziac Tablets 1887

Carteolol Hydrochloride (Early warning symptoms of hypoglycemia may be different or less pronounced under certain conditions, such as concurrent beta blocker therapy). Products include:
Carteolol Hydrochloride Ophthalmic Solution USP, 1% ..... ⊙258
Ocupress Ophthalmic Solution, 1% Sterile .... ⊙303

Chlorpropamide (Concurrent use of oral hypoglycemic agents with Humulin R (U-500) is not recommended since there are no data to support such use). Products include:
Diabinese Tablets 2680

Esmolol Hydrochloride (Early warning symptoms of hypoglycemia may be different or less pronounced under certain conditions, such as concurrent beta blocker therapy). Products include:
Brevibloc Injection 858

Glimepiride (Concurrent use of oral hypoglycemic agents with Humulin R (U-500) is not recommended since there are no data to support such use). Products include:
Amaryl Tablets 717

Glipizide (Concurrent use of oral hypoglycemic agents with Humulin R (U-500) is not recommended since there are no data to support such use). Products include:
Glucotrol Tablets 2692
Glucotrol XL Extended Release Tablets 2693

Glyburide (Concurrent use of oral hypoglycemic agents with Humulin R (U-500) is not recommended since there are no data to support such use). Products include:
DiaBeta Tablets 741
Glucovance Tablets 1086

Labetalol Hydrochloride (Early warning symptoms of hypoglycemia may be different or less pronounced under certain conditions, such as concurrent beta blocker therapy). Products include:
Normodyne Injection 3135
Normodyne Tablets 3137

Levobunolol Hydrochloride (Early warning symptoms of hypoglycemia may be different or less pronounced under certain conditions, such as concurrent beta blocker therapy). Products include:
Betagan .... ⊙228

Metformin Hydrochloride (Concurrent use of oral hypoglycemic agents with Humulin R (U-500) is not recommended since there are no data to support such use). Products include:
Glucophage Tablets 1080
Glucophage XR Tablets 1080
Glucovance Tablets 1086

Metipranolol Hydrochloride (Early warning symptoms of hypoglycemia may be different or less pronounced under certain conditions, such as concurrent beta blocker therapy).
No products indexed under this heading.

Metoprolol Succinate (Early warning symptoms of hypoglycemia may be different or less pronounced under certain conditions, such as concurrent beta blocker therapy). Products include:
Toprol-XL Tablets 651

Metoprolol Tartrate (Early warning symptoms of hypoglycemia may be different or less pronounced under certain conditions, such as concurrent beta blocker therapy).
No products indexed under this heading.

Miglitol (Concurrent use of oral hypoglycemic agents with Humulin R (U-500) is not recommended since there are no data to support such use). Products include:
Glyset Tablets 2821

Nadolol (Early warning symptoms of hypoglycemia may be different or less pronounced under certain conditions, such as concurrent beta blocker therapy). Products include:
Corgard Tablets 2245
Corzide 40/5 Tablets 2247
Corzide 80/5 Tablets 2247
Nadolol Tablets 2288

Penbutolol Sulfate (Early warning symptoms of hypoglycemia may be different or less pronounced under certain conditions, such as concurrent beta blocker therapy).
No products indexed under this heading.

Pindolol (Early warning symptoms of hypoglycemia may be different or less pronounced under certain conditions, such as concurrent beta blocker therapy).
No products indexed under this heading.

Pioglitazone Hydrochloride (Concurrent use of oral hypoglycemic agents with Humulin R (U-500) is not recommended since there are no data to support such use). Products include:
Actos Tablets 3275

Propranolol Hydrochloride (Early warning symptoms of hypoglycemia may be different or less pronounced under certain conditions, such as concurrent beta blocker therapy). Products include:
Inderal 3513
Inderal LA Long-Acting Capsules 3516
Inderide Tablets 3517
Inderide LA Long-Acting Capsules .. 3519

Repaglinide (Concurrent use of oral hypoglycemic agents with Humulin R (U-500) is not recommended since there are no data to support such use). Products include:
Prandin Tablets (0.5, 1, and 2 mg) 2432

Rosiglitazone Maleate (Concurrent use of oral hypoglycemic agents with Humulin R (U-500) is not recommended since there are no data to support such use). Products include:
Avandia Tablets 1490

Sotalol Hydrochloride (Early warning symptoms of hypoglycemia may be different or less pronounced under certain conditions, such as concurrent beta blocker therapy). Products include:
Betapace Tablets 950
Betapace AF Tablets 954

Timolol Hemihydrate (Early warning symptoms of hypoglycemia may be different or less pronounced under certain conditions, such as concurrent beta blocker therapy). Products include:
Betimol Ophthalmic Solution .... ⊙324

Timolol Maleate (Early warning symptoms of hypoglycemia may be different or less pronounced under certain conditions, such as concurrent beta blocker therapy). Products include:
Blocadren Tablets 2046
Cosopt Sterile Ophthalmic Solution 2065
Timolide Tablets 2187
Timolol GFS .... ⊙266
Timoptic in Ocudose 2192
Timoptic Sterile Ophthalmic Solution 2190
Timoptic-XE Sterile Ophthalmic Gel Forming Solution 2194

Tolazamide (Concurrent use of oral hypoglycemic agents with Humulin R (U-500) is not recommended since there are no data to support such use).
No products indexed under this heading.

Tolbutamide (Concurrent use of oral hypoglycemic agents with Humulin R (U-500) is not recommended since there are no data to support such use).
No products indexed under this heading.

Troglitazone (Concurrent use of oral hypoglycemic agents with Humulin R (U-500) is not recommended since there are no data to support such use).
No products indexed under this heading.

HUMULIN R, 100 UNITS
(Insulin, Human Regular) 1941
See Iletin II, Regular (Pork), 100 Units

HUMULIN U, 100 UNITS
(Insulin, Human, Zinc Suspension) 1943
See Iletin II, Regular (Pork), 100 Units

HUMULIN N NPH PEN
(Insulin, Human NPH) 1940
See Iletin II, Regular (Pork), 100 Units

HURRICAINE TOPICAL ANESTHETIC GEL, 1 OZ. FRESH MINT, WILD CHERRY, PINA COLADA, WATERMELON, 1/6 OZ. WILD CHERRY, WATERMELON
(Benzocaine) .... ▣618
None cited in PDR database.

HURRICAINE TOPICAL ANESTHETIC LIQUID, 1 OZ. WILD CHERRY, PINA COLADA, .25 ML DRY HANDLE SWAB WILD CHERRY, 1/6 OZ. WILD CHERRY
(Benzocaine) .... ▣618
None cited in PDR database.

HURRICAINE TOPICAL ANESTHETIC SPRAY EXTENSION TUBES (200)
(Benzocaine) .... ▣618
None cited in PDR database.

HURRICAINE TOPICAL ANESTHETIC SPRAY KIT, 2 OZ. WILD CHERRY
(Benzocaine) .... ▣618
None cited in PDR database.

HURRICAINE TOPICAL ANESTHETIC SPRAY, 2 OZ. WILD CHERRY
(Benzocaine) .... ▣618
None cited in PDR database.

HYALGAN SOLUTION
(Sodium Hyaluronate) 3080
None cited in PDR database.

HYCAMTIN FOR INJECTION
(Topotecan Hydrochloride) 1546
May interact with:

Cisplatin (Co-administration has resulted in severe myelosuppression; case of neutropenia and fatal neutropenic sepsis has been reported).
No products indexed under this heading.

Filgrastim (Co-administration of G-CSF can prolong the duration of neutropenia, so if G-CSF is to be used, it should not be initiated until day 6 of the course of therapy). Products include:
Neupogen for Injection 587

HYCODAN SYRUP
(Homatropine Methylbromide, Hydrocodone Bitartrate) 1316
See Hycodan Tablets

HYCODAN TABLETS
(Homatropine Methylbromide, Hydrocodone Bitartrate) 1316
May interact with antihistamines, central nervous system depressants, monoamine oxidase inhibitors, narcotic analgesics, antipsychotic agents, tranquilizers, tricyclic antidepressants, and certain other agents. Compounds in these categories include:

Acrivastine (Exhibits an additive CNS depression). Products include:
Semprex-D Capsules 1172

Alfentanil Hydrochloride (Exhibits an additive CNS depression).
No products indexed under this heading.

Alprazolam (Exhibits an additive CNS depression). Products include:
Xanax Tablets 2865

Amitriptyline Hydrochloride (Increased effect of either the antidepressant or hydrocodone). Products include:
Etrafon 3115
Limbitrol 1738

Amoxapine (Increased effect of either the antidepressant or hydrocodone).
No products indexed under this heading.

Aprobarbital (Exhibits an additive CNS depression).
No products indexed under this heading.

Astemizole (Exhibits an additive CNS depression).
No products indexed under this heading.

Azatadine Maleate (Exhibits an additive CNS depression). Products include:
Rynatan Tablets 3351

Bromodiphenhydramine Hydrochloride (Exhibits an additive CNS depression).
No products indexed under this heading.

Brompheniramine Maleate (Exhibits an additive CNS depression). Products include:

Bromfed Capsules (Extended-Release) 2269
Bromfed-PD Capsules (Extended-Release) 2269
Comtrex Acute Head Cold & Sinus Pressure Relief Tablets 627
Dimetapp Elixir 777
Dimetapp Cold and Fever Suspension 775
Dimetapp DM Cold & Cough Elixir 775
Dimetapp Nighttime Flu Liquid 776

Buprenorphine Hydrochloride (Exhibits an additive CNS depression). Products include:
Buprenex Injectable 2918

Buspirone Hydrochloride (Exhibits an additive CNS depression).
No products indexed under this heading.

Butabarbital (Exhibits an additive CNS depression).
No products indexed under this heading.

Butalbital (Exhibits an additive CNS depression). Products include:
Phrenilin 578
Sedapap Tablets 50 mg/650 mg 2225

Cetirizine Hydrochloride (Exhibits an additive CNS depression). Products include:
Zyrtec 2756
Zyrtec-D 12 Hour Extended Relief Tablets 2758

Chlordiazepoxide (Exhibits an additive CNS depression). Products include:
Limbitrol 1738

Chlordiazepoxide Hydrochloride (Exhibits an additive CNS depression). Products include:
Librium Capsules 1736
Librium for Injection 1737

Chlorpheniramine Maleate (Exhibits an additive CNS depression). Products include:
Actifed Cold & Sinus Caplets and Tablets 688
Alka-Seltzer Plus Liqui-Gels 604
BC Allergy Sinus Cold Powder 619
Chlor-Trimeton Allergy Tablets 735
Chlor-Trimeton Allergy/Decongestant Tablets 736
Comtrex Flu Therapy & Fever Relief Nighttime Tablets 628
Comtrex Maximum Strength Multi-Symptom Cold & Cough Relief Tablets and Caplets 626
Contac Severe Cold and Flu Caplets Maximum Strength 746
Coricidin 'D' Cold, Flu & Sinus Tablets 737
Coricidin/Coricidin D 738
Coricidin HBP Maximum Strength Flu Tablets 738
Extendryl 1361
Hycomine Compound Tablets 1317
Kronofed-A 1341
PediaCare Cough-Cold Liquid 719
PediaCare NightRest Cough-Cold Liquid 719
Robitussin Nighttime Honey Flu Liquid 786
Ryna 768
Singlet Caplets 761
Sinutab Sinus Allergy Medication, Maximum Strength Formula, Tablets & Caplets 707
Sudafed Cold & Allergy Tablets 708
TheraFlu Regular Strength Cold & Cough Night Time Hot Liquid 676
TheraFlu Regular Strength Cold & Sore Throat Night Time Hot Liquid 676
TheraFlu Maximum Strength Flu & Cough Night Time Hot Liquid 678
TheraFlu Maximum Strength Flu & Sore Throat Night Time Hot Liquid 677
TheraFlu Maximum Strength Severe Cold & Congestion Night Time Caplets 678
TheraFlu Maximum Strength Severe Cold & Congestion Night Time Hot Liquid 678
Triaminic Cold & Allergy Liquid 681
Triaminic Cold & Allergy Softchews 683
Triaminic Cold & Cough Liquid 681
Triaminic Cold & Cough Softchews 683
Triaminic Cold & Night Time Cough Liquid 681
Triaminic Cold, Cough & Fever Liquid 681
Children's Tylenol Cold Suspension Liquid and Chewable Tablets 2015
Children's Tylenol Cold Plus Cough Suspension Liquid and Chewable Tablets 2015
Children's Tylenol Flu Suspension Liquid 2015
Maximum Strength Tylenol Allergy Sinus Caplets, Gelcaps, and Geltabs 2010
Multi-Symptom Tylenol Cold Complete Formula Caplets 2010
Vicks 44M Cough, Cold & Flu Relief Liquid 725
Pediatric Vicks 44m Cough & Cold Relief 728
Children's Vicks NyQuil Cold/Cough Relief 726

Chlorpheniramine Polistirex (Exhibits an additive CNS depression). Products include:
Tussionex Pennkinetic Extended-Release Suspension 1174

Chlorpheniramine Tannate (Exhibits an additive CNS depression). Products include:
Reformulated Rynatan Pediatric Suspension 3352
Rynatuss Pediatric Suspension 3353
Rynatuss Tablets 3353
Tussi-12 S Suspension 3356
Tussi-12 Tablets 3356

Chlorpromazine (Exhibits an additive CNS depression). Products include:
Thorazine Suppositories 1656

Chlorpromazine Hydrochloride (Exhibits an additive CNS depression). Products include:
Thorazine 1656

Chlorprothixene (Exhibits an additive CNS depression).
No products indexed under this heading.

Chlorprothixene Hydrochloride (Exhibits an additive CNS depression).
No products indexed under this heading.

Chlorprothixene Lactate (Exhibits an additive CNS depression).
No products indexed under this heading.

Clemastine Fumarate (Exhibits an additive CNS depression). Products include:
Tavist 12 Hour Allergy Tablets 676

Clomipramine Hydrochloride (Increased effect of either the antidepressant or hydrocodone).
No products indexed under this heading.

Clorazepate Dipotassium (Exhibits an additive CNS depression). Products include:
Tranxene 511

Clozapine (Exhibits an additive CNS depression). Products include:
Clozaril Tablets 2319

Codeine Phosphate (Exhibits an additive CNS depression). Products include:
Phenergan with Codeine Syrup 3557
Phenergan VC with Codeine Syrup 3561
Robitussin A-C Syrup 2942
Robitussin-DAC Syrup 2942
Ryna-C Liquid 768
Soma Compound w/Codeine Tablets 3355
Tussi-Organidin NR Liquid 3350
Tussi-Organidin-S NR Liquid 3350
Tylenol with Codeine 2595

Cyproheptadine Hydrochloride (Exhibits an additive CNS depression). Products include:
Periactin Tablets 2155

Desflurane (Exhibits an additive CNS depression). Products include:
Suprane Liquid for Inhalation 874

Desipramine Hydrochloride (Increased effect of either the antidepressant or hydrocodone). Products include:
Norpramin Tablets 755

Dexchlorpheniramine Maleate (Exhibits an additive CNS depression).
No products indexed under this heading.

Dezocine (Exhibits an additive CNS depression).
No products indexed under this heading.

Diazepam (Exhibits an additive CNS depression). Products include:
Valium Injectable 3026
Valium Tablets 3047

Diphenhydramine Citrate (Exhibits an additive CNS depression). Products include:
Alka-Seltzer PM Effervescent Tablets 605
Benadryl Allergy & Sinus Fastmelt Tablets 693
Benadryl Children's Allergy/Cold Fastmelt Tablets 692
Excedrin PM Tablets, Caplets, and Geltabs 631
Goody's PM Powder 621

Diphenhydramine Hydrochloride (Exhibits an additive CNS depression). Products include:
Extra Strength Bayer PM Caplets 611
Benadryl Allergy Chewables 689
Benadryl Allergy 691
Benadryl Allergy Liquid 690
Benadryl Allergy/Cold Tablets 691
Benadryl Allergy/Congestion Tablets 692
Benadryl Allergy & Sinus Liquid 693
Benadryl Allergy Sinus Headache Caplets & Gelcaps 693
Benadryl Severe Allergy & Sinus Headache Caplets 694
Benadryl Dye-Free Allergy Liquid 690
Benadryl Dye-Free Allergy Liqui-Gels Softgels 690
Benadryl Itch Relief Stick Extra Strength 695
Benadryl Cream 695
Benadryl Gel 695
Benadryl Spray 696
Benadryl Parenteral 2617
Coricidin HBP Night-Time Cold & Flu Tablets 738
Nytol QuickCaps Caplets 622
Maximum Strength Nytol QuickGels Softgels 621
Extra Strength Percogesic Aspirin-Free Coated Caplets 665
Simply Sleep Caplets 2008
Sominex Original Formula Tablets 761
Children's Tylenol Allergy-D Liquid 2014
Maximum Strength Tylenol Allergy Sinus NightTime Caplets 2010
Tylenol Severe Allergy Caplets 2010
Maximum Strength Tylenol Flu NightTime Gelcaps 2011
Extra Strength Tylenol PM Caplets, Geltabs, and Gelcaps 2012
Unisom Maximum Strength SleepGels 713

Diphenylpyraline Hydrochloride (Exhibits an additive CNS depression).
No products indexed under this heading.

Doxepin Hydrochloride (Increased effect of either the antidepressant or hydrocodone). Products include:
Sinequan 2713

Droperidol (Exhibits an additive CNS depression).
No products indexed under this heading.

Enflurane (Exhibits an additive CNS depression).
No products indexed under this heading.

Estazolam (Exhibits an additive CNS depression). Products include:
ProSom Tablets 500

Ethchlorvynol (Exhibits an additive CNS depression).
No products indexed under this heading.

Ethinamate (Exhibits an additive CNS depression).
No products indexed under this heading.

Fentanyl (Exhibits an additive CNS depression). Products include:
Duragesic Transdermal System 1786

Fentanyl Citrate (Exhibits an additive CNS depression). Products include:
Actiq 1184

Fexofenadine Hydrochloride (Exhibits an additive CNS depression). Products include:
Allegra 712
Allegra-D Extended-Release Tablets 714

Fluphenazine Decanoate (Exhibits an additive CNS depression).
No products indexed under this heading.

Fluphenazine Enanthate (Exhibits an additive CNS depression).
No products indexed under this heading.

Fluphenazine Hydrochloride (Exhibits an additive CNS depression).
No products indexed under this heading.

Flurazepam Hydrochloride (Exhibits an additive CNS depression).
No products indexed under this heading.

Glutethimide (Exhibits an additive CNS depression).
No products indexed under this heading.

Haloperidol (Exhibits an additive CNS depression). Products include:
Haldol Injection, Tablets and Concentrate 2533

Haloperidol Decanoate (Exhibits an additive CNS depression). Products include:
Haldol Decanoate 2535

Hydrocodone Polistirex (Exhibits an additive CNS depression). Products include:
Tussionex Pennkinetic Extended-Release Suspension 1174

Hydromorphone Hydrochloride (Exhibits an additive CNS depression). Products include:
Dilaudid 441
Dilaudid Oral Liquid 445
Dilaudid Powder 441
Dilaudid Rectal Suppositories 441
Dilaudid Tablets 441
Dilaudid Tablets - 8 mg 445
Dilaudid-HP 443

Hydroxyzine Hydrochloride (Exhibits an additive CNS depression). Products include:
Atarax Tablets & Syrup 2667
Vistaril Intramuscular Solution 2738

Imipramine Hydrochloride (Increased effect of either the antidepressant or hydrocodone).
No products indexed under this heading.

Imipramine Pamoate (Increased effect of either the antidepressant or hydrocodone).
No products indexed under this heading.

Isocarboxazid (May increase the effect of either MAO inhibitor or hydrocodone).
No products indexed under this heading.

Isoflurane (Exhibits an additive CNS depression).
No products indexed under this heading.

Ketamine Hydrochloride (Exhibits an additive CNS depression).
No products indexed under this heading.

Levomethadyl Acetate Hydrochloride (Exhibits an additive CNS depression).
No products indexed under this heading.

Levorphanol Tartrate (Exhibits an additive CNS depression). Products include:

Levo-Dromoran 1734
Levorphanol Tartrate Tablets 3059

Lithium Carbonate (Exhibits an additive CNS depression). Products include:
Eskalith 1527
Lithium Carbonate 3061
Lithobid Slow-Release Tablets 3255

Lithium Citrate (Exhibits an additive CNS depression). Products include:
Lithium Citrate Syrup 3061

Loratadine (Exhibits an additive CNS depression). Products include:
Claritin 3100
Claritin-D 12 Hour Extended Release Tablets 3102
Claritin-D 24 Hour Extended Release Tablets 3104

Lorazepam (Exhibits an additive CNS depression). Products include:
Ativan Injection 3478
Ativan Tablets 3482

Loxapine Hydrochloride (Exhibits an additive CNS depression).
No products indexed under this heading.

Loxapine Succinate (Exhibits an additive CNS depression). Products include:
Loxitane Capsules 3398

Maprotiline Hydrochloride (Increased effect of either the antidepressant or hydrocodone).
No products indexed under this heading.

Meperidine Hydrochloride (Exhibits an additive CNS depression). Products include:
Demerol 3079
Mepergan Injection 3539

Mephobarbital (Exhibits an additive CNS depression).
No products indexed under this heading.

Meprobamate (Exhibits an additive CNS depression). Products include:
Miltown Tablets 3349

Mesoridazine Besylate (Exhibits an additive CNS depression). Products include:
Serentil 1057

Methadone Hydrochloride (Exhibits an additive CNS depression). Products include:
Dolophine Hydrochloride Tablets 3056

Methdilazine Hydrochloride (Exhibits an additive CNS depression).
No products indexed under this heading.

Methohexital Sodium (Exhibits an additive CNS depression). Products include:
Brevital Sodium for Injection, USP 1815

Methotrimeprazine (Exhibits an additive CNS depression).
No products indexed under this heading.

Methoxyflurane (Exhibits an additive CNS depression).
No products indexed under this heading.

Midazolam Hydrochloride (Exhibits an additive CNS depression). Products include:
Versed Injection 3027
Versed Syrup 3033

Moclobemide (May increase the effect of either MAO inhibitor or hydrocodone).
No products indexed under this heading.

Molindone Hydrochloride (Exhibits an additive CNS depression). Products include:
Moban 1320

Morphine Sulfate (Exhibits an additive CNS depression). Products include:
Astramorph/PF Injection, USP (Preservative-Free) 594
Duramorph Injection 1312
Infumorph 200 and Infumorph 500 Sterile Solutions 1314
Kadian Capsules 1335
MS Contin Tablets 2896
MSIR 2898
Oramorph SR Tablets 3062
Roxanol 3066

Nortriptyline Hydrochloride (Increased effect of either the antidepressant or hydrocodone).
No products indexed under this heading.

Olanzapine (Exhibits an additive CNS depression). Products include:
Zyprexa Tablets 1973
Zyprexa ZYDIS Orally Disintegrating Tablets 1973

Oxazepam (Exhibits an additive CNS depression).
No products indexed under this heading.

Oxycodone Hydrochloride (Exhibits an additive CNS depression). Products include:
OxyContin Tablets 2912
OxyFast Oral Concentrate Solution 2916
OxyIR Capsules 2916
Percocet Tablets 1326
Percodan Tablets 1327
Percolone Tablets 1327
Roxicodone 3067
Tylox Capsules 2597

Pargyline Hydrochloride (May increase the effect of either MAO inhibitor or hydrocodone).
No products indexed under this heading.

Pentobarbital Sodium (Exhibits an additive CNS depression). Products include:
Nembutal Sodium Solution 485

Perphenazine (Exhibits an additive CNS depression). Products include:
Etrafon 3115
Trilafon 3160

Phenelzine Sulfate (May increase the effect of either MAO inhibitor or hydrocodone). Products include:
Nardil Tablets 2653

Phenobarbital (Exhibits an additive CNS depression). Products include:
Arco-Lase Plus Tablets 592
Donnatal 2929
Donnatal Extentabs 2930

Pimozide (Exhibits an additive CNS depression). Products include:
Orap Tablets 1407

Prazepam (Exhibits an additive CNS depression).
No products indexed under this heading.

Procarbazine Hydrochloride (May increase the effect of either MAO inhibitor or hydrocodone). Products include:
Matulane Capsules 3246

Prochlorperazine (Exhibits an additive CNS depression). Products include:
Compazine 1505

Promethazine Hydrochloride (Exhibits an additive CNS depression). Products include:
Mepergan Injection 3539
Phenergan Injection 3553
Phenergan 3556
Phenergan Syrup 3554
Phenergan with Codeine Syrup 3557
Phenergan with Dextromethorphan Syrup 3559
Phenergan VC Syrup 3560
Phenergan VC with Codeine Syrup 3561

Propofol (Exhibits an additive CNS depression). Products include:
Diprivan Injectable Emulsion 667

Propoxyphene Hydrochloride (Exhibits an additive CNS depression). Products include:
Darvon Pulvules 1909
Darvon Compound-65 Pulvules 1910

Propoxyphene Napsylate (Exhibits an additive CNS depression). Products include:
Darvon-N/Darvocet-N 1907
Darvon-N Tablets 1912

Protriptyline Hydrochloride (Increased effect of either the antidepressant or hydrocodone). Products include:
Vivactil Tablets 2446
Vivactil Tablets 2217

Pyrilamine Maleate (Exhibits an additive CNS depression). Products include:
Maximum Strength Midol Menstrual Caplets and Gelcaps .... ▣612
Maximum Strength Midol PMS Caplets and Gelcaps .... ▣613

Pyrilamine Tannate (Exhibits an additive CNS depression). Products include:
Ryna-12 S Suspension 3351

Quazepam (Exhibits an additive CNS depression).
No products indexed under this heading.

Quetiapine Fumarate (Exhibits an additive CNS depression). Products include:
Seroquel Tablets 684

Remifentanil Hydrochloride (Exhibits an additive CNS depression).
No products indexed under this heading.

Risperidone (Exhibits an additive CNS depression). Products include:
Risperdal 1796

Secobarbital Sodium (Exhibits an additive CNS depression).
No products indexed under this heading.

Selegiline Hydrochloride (May increase the effect of either MAO inhibitor or hydrocodone). Products include:
Eldepryl Capsules 3266

Sevoflurane (Exhibits an additive CNS depression).
No products indexed under this heading.

Sufentanil Citrate (Exhibits an additive CNS depression).
No products indexed under this heading.

Temazepam (Exhibits an additive CNS depression).
No products indexed under this heading.

Terfenadine (Exhibits an additive CNS depression).
No products indexed under this heading.

Thiamylal Sodium (Exhibits an additive CNS depression).
No products indexed under this heading.

Thioridazine Hydrochloride (Exhibits an additive CNS depression). Products include:
Thioridazine Hydrochloride Tablets 2289

Thiothixene (Exhibits an additive CNS depression). Products include:
Navane Capsules 2701
Thiothixene Capsules 2290

Tranylcypromine Sulfate (May increase the effect of either MAO inhibitor or hydrocodone). Products include:
Parnate Tablets 1607

Triazolam (Exhibits an additive CNS depression). Products include:
Halcion Tablets 2823

Trifluoperazine Hydrochloride (Exhibits an additive CNS depression). Products include:
Stelazine 1640

Trimeprazine Tartrate (Exhibits an additive CNS depression).
No products indexed under this heading.

Trimipramine Maleate (Increased effect of either the antidepressant or hydrocodone). Products include:
Surmontil Capsules 3595

Tripelennamine Hydrochloride (Exhibits an additive CNS depression).
No products indexed under this heading.

Triprolidine Hydrochloride (Exhibits an additive CNS depression). Products include:
Actifed Cold & Allergy Tablets .... ▣688

Zaleplon (Exhibits an additive CNS depression). Products include:
Sonata Capsules 3591

Ziprasidone Hydrochloride (Exhibits an additive CNS depression). Products include:
Geodon Capsules 2688

Zolpidem Tartrate (Exhibits an additive CNS depression). Products include:
Ambien Tablets 3191

Food Interactions

Alcohol (Exhibits an additive CNS depression).

HYCOMINE COMPOUND TABLETS

(Acetaminophen, Caffeine, Chlorpheniramine Maleate, Hydrocodone Bitartrate, Phenylephrine Hydrochloride) 1317
May interact with beta blockers, central nervous system depressants, general anesthetics, hypnotics and sedatives, monoamine oxidase inhibitors, narcotic analgesics, phenothiazines, sympathomimetics, tranquilizers, and certain other agents. Compounds in these categories include:

Acebutolol Hydrochloride (Concurrent use of phenylephrine with beta blockers may result in hypertensive crises). Products include:
Sectral Capsules 3589

Albuterol (Additive elevation of blood pressure). Products include:
Proventil Inhalation Aerosol 3142
Ventolin Inhalation Aerosol and Refill 1679

Albuterol Sulfate (Additive elevation of blood pressure). Products include:
AccuNeb Inhalation Solution 1230
Combivent Inhalation Aerosol 1041
DuoNeb Inhalation Solution 1233
Proventil Inhalation Solution 0.083% 3146
Proventil Repetabs Tablets 3148
Proventil Solution for Inhalation 0.5% 3144
Proventil HFA Inhalation Aerosol 3150
Ventolin HFA Inhalation Aerosol 3618
Volmax Extended-Release Tablets 2276

Alfentanil Hydrochloride (Exhibits an additive CNS depression).
No products indexed under this heading.

Alprazolam (Exhibits an additive CNS depression). Products include:
Xanax Tablets 2865

Aprobarbital (Exhibits an additive CNS depression).
No products indexed under this heading.

Atenolol (Concurrent use of phenylephrine with beta blockers may result in hypertensive crises). Products include:
Tenoretic Tablets 690
Tenormin I.V. Injection 692

Betaxolol Hydrochloride (Concurrent use of phenylephrine with beta blockers may result in hypertensive crises). Products include:
Betoptic S Ophthalmic Suspension 537

Bisoprolol Fumarate (Concurrent use of phenylephrine with beta blockers may result in hypertensive crises). Products include:
Zebeta Tablets 1885
Ziac Tablets 1887

Buprenorphine Hydrochloride (Exhibits an additive CNS depression). Products include:
Buprenex Injectable 2918

Buspirone Hydrochloride (Exhibits an additive CNS depression).
No products indexed under this heading.

Butabarbital (Exhibits an additive CNS depression).
No products indexed under this heading.

Butalbital (Exhibits an additive CNS depression). Products include:
Phrenilin 578
Sedapap Tablets 50 mg/650 mg ... 2225

Carteolol Hydrochloride (Concurrent use of phenylephrine with beta blockers may result in hypertensive crises). Products include:
Carteolol Hydrochloride Ophthalmic Solution USP, 1% ..... ⊙258
Ocupress Ophthalmic Solution, 1% Sterile .... ⊙303

Chlordiazepoxide (Exhibits an additive CNS depression). Products include:
Limbitrol 1738

Chlordiazepoxide Hydrochloride (Exhibits an additive CNS depression). Products include:
Librium Capsules 1736
Librium for Injection 1737

Chlorpromazine (Exhibits an additive CNS depression). Products include:
Thorazine Suppositories 1656

Chlorpromazine Hydrochloride (Exhibits an additive CNS depression). Products include:
Thorazine 1656

Chlorprothixene (Exhibits an additive CNS depression).
No products indexed under this heading.

Chlorprothixene Hydrochloride (Exhibits an additive CNS depression).
No products indexed under this heading.

Chlorprothixene Lactate (Exhibits an additive CNS depression).
No products indexed under this heading.

Clorazepate Dipotassium (Exhibits an additive CNS depression). Products include:
Tranxene 511

Clozapine (Exhibits an additive CNS depression). Products include:
Clozaril Tablets 2319

Codeine Phosphate (Exhibits an additive CNS depression). Products include:
Phenergan with Codeine Syrup 3557
Phenergan VC with Codeine Syrup .. 3561
Robitussin A-C Syrup 2942
Robitussin-DAC Syrup 2942
Ryna-C Liquid .... ◙768
Soma Compound w/Codeine Tablets 3355
Tussi-Organidin NR Liquid 3350
Tussi-Organidin-S NR Liquid 3350
Tylenol with Codeine 2595

Desflurane (Exhibits an additive CNS depression). Products include:
Suprane Liquid for Inhalation 874

Dezocine (Exhibits an additive CNS depression).
No products indexed under this heading.

Diazepam (Exhibits an additive CNS depression). Products include:
Valium Injectable 3026
Valium Tablets 3047

Dobutamine Hydrochloride (Additive elevation of blood pressure). Products include:
Dobutrex Solution Vials 1914

Dopamine Hydrochloride (Additive elevation of blood pressure).
No products indexed under this heading.

Droperidol (Exhibits an additive CNS depression).
No products indexed under this heading.

Enflurane (Exhibits an additive CNS depression).
No products indexed under this heading.

Ephedrine Hydrochloride (Additive elevation of blood pressure). Products include:
Primatene Tablets .... ◙780

Ephedrine Sulfate (Additive elevation of blood pressure).
No products indexed under this heading.

Ephedrine Tannate (Additive elevation of blood pressure). Products include:
Rynatuss Pediatric Suspension 3353
Rynatuss Tablets 3353

Epinephrine (Additive elevation of blood pressure). Products include:
Epifrin Sterile Ophthalmic Solution .... ⊙235
EpiPen 1236
Primatene Mist .... ◙779
Xylocaine with Epinephrine Injection 653

Epinephrine Bitartrate (Additive elevation of blood pressure). Products include:
Sensorcaine 643

Epinephrine Hydrochloride (Additive elevation of blood pressure).
No products indexed under this heading.

Esmolol Hydrochloride (Concurrent use of phenylephrine with beta blockers may result in hypertensive crises). Products include:
Brevibloc Injection 858

Estazolam (Exhibits an additive CNS depression). Products include:
ProSom Tablets 500

Ethchlorvynol (Exhibits an additive CNS depression).
No products indexed under this heading.

Ethinamate (Exhibits an additive CNS depression).
No products indexed under this heading.

Fentanyl (Exhibits an additive CNS depression). Products include:
Duragesic Transdermal System 1786

Fentanyl Citrate (Exhibits an additive CNS depression). Products include:
Actiq 1184

Fluphenazine Decanoate (Exhibits an additive CNS depression).
No products indexed under this heading.

Fluphenazine Enanthate (Exhibits an additive CNS depression).
No products indexed under this heading.

Fluphenazine Hydrochloride (Exhibits an additive CNS depression).
No products indexed under this heading.

Flurazepam Hydrochloride (Exhibits an additive CNS depression).
No products indexed under this heading.

Glutethimide (Exhibits an additive CNS depression).
No products indexed under this heading.

Haloperidol (Exhibits an additive CNS depression). Products include:
Haldol Injection, Tablets and Concentrate 2533

Haloperidol Decanoate (Exhibits an additive CNS depression). Products include:
Haldol Decanoate 2535

Hydrocodone Polistirex (Exhibits an additive CNS depression). Products include:
Tussionex Pennkinetic Extended-Release Suspension 1174

Hydromorphone Hydrochloride (Exhibits an additive CNS depression). Products include:
Dilaudid 441
Dilaudid Oral Liquid 445
Dilaudid Powder 441
Dilaudid Rectal Suppositories 441
Dilaudid Tablets 441
Dilaudid Tablets - 8 mg 445
Dilaudid-HP 443

Hydroxyzine Hydrochloride (Exhibits an additive CNS depression). Products include:
Atarax Tablets & Syrup 2667
Vistaril Intramuscular Solution 2738

Indomethacin (Concurrent use of indomethacin with beta blockers may result in hypertensive crises). Products include:
Indocin 2112

Isocarboxazid (Co-administration of sympathomimetics and MAO inhibitors may produce an additive elevation of blood pressure leading to hypertensive crises; MAO inhibitors may prolong the anticholinergic effects of antihistamines; concurrent use is contraindicated).
No products indexed under this heading.

Isoflurane (Exhibits an additive CNS depression).
No products indexed under this heading.

Isoproterenol Hydrochloride (Additive elevation of blood pressure).
No products indexed under this heading.

Isoproterenol Sulfate (Additive elevation of blood pressure).
No products indexed under this heading.

Ketamine Hydrochloride (Exhibits an additive CNS depression).
No products indexed under this heading.

Labetalol Hydrochloride (Concurrent use of phenylephrine with beta blockers may result in hypertensive crises). Products include:
Normodyne Injection 3135
Normodyne Tablets 3137

Levalbuterol Hydrochloride (Additive elevation of blood pressure). Products include:
Xopenex Inhalation Solution 3207

Levobunolol Hydrochloride (Concurrent use of phenylephrine with beta blockers may result in hypertensive crises). Products include:
Betagan .... ⊙228

Levomethadyl Acetate Hydrochloride (Exhibits an additive CNS depression).
No products indexed under this heading.

Levorphanol Tartrate (Exhibits an additive CNS depression). Products include:
Levo-Dromoran 1734
Levorphanol Tartrate Tablets 3059

Lorazepam (Exhibits an additive CNS depression). Products include:
Ativan Injection 3478
Ativan Tablets 3482

Loxapine Hydrochloride (Exhibits an additive CNS depression).
No products indexed under this heading.

Loxapine Succinate (Exhibits an additive CNS depression). Products include:
Loxitane Capsules 3398

Meperidine Hydrochloride (Exhibits an additive CNS depression). Products include:
Demerol 3079
Mepergan Injection 3539

Mephobarbital (Exhibits an additive CNS depression).
No products indexed under this heading.

Meprobamate (Exhibits an additive CNS depression). Products include:
Miltown Tablets 3349

Mesoridazine Besylate (Exhibits an additive CNS depression). Products include:
Serentil 1057

Metaproterenol Sulfate (Additive elevation of blood pressure). Products include:
Alupent 1029

Metaraminol Bitartrate (Additive elevation of blood pressure). Products include:
Aramine Injection 2043

Methadone Hydrochloride (Exhibits an additive CNS depression). Products include:
Dolophine Hydrochloride Tablets 3056

Methohexital Sodium (Exhibits an additive CNS depression). Products include:
Brevital Sodium for Injection, USP .. 1815

Methotrimeprazine (Exhibits an additive CNS depression).
No products indexed under this heading.

Methoxamine Hydrochloride (Additive elevation of blood pressure).
No products indexed under this heading.

Methoxyflurane (Exhibits an additive CNS depression).
No products indexed under this heading.

Methyldopa (Concurrent use of methyldopa with beta blockers may result in hypertensive crises). Products include:
Aldoclor Tablets 2035
Aldomet Tablets 2037
Aldoril Tablets 2039

Metipranolol Hydrochloride (Concurrent use of phenylephrine with beta blockers may result in hypertensive crises).
No products indexed under this heading.

Metoprolol Succinate (Concurrent use of phenylephrine with beta blockers may result in hypertensive crises). Products include:
Toprol-XL Tablets 651

Metoprolol Tartrate (Concurrent use of phenylephrine with beta blockers may result in hypertensive crises).
No products indexed under this heading.

Midazolam Hydrochloride (Exhibits an additive CNS depression). Products include:
Versed Injection 3027
Versed Syrup 3033

Moclobemide (Co-administration of sympathomimetics and MAO inhibitors may produce an additive elevation of blood pressure leading to hypertensive crises; MAO inhibitors may prolong the anticholinergic effects of antihistamines; concurrent use is contraindicated).
No products indexed under this heading.

Molindone Hydrochloride (Exhibits an additive CNS depression). Products include:
Moban 1320

Morphine Sulfate (Exhibits an additive CNS depression). Products include:
Astramorph/PF Injection, USP (Preservative-Free) 594
Duramorph Injection 1312
Infumorph 200 and Infumorph 500 Sterile Solutions 1314
Kadian Capsules 1335
MS Contin Tablets 2896
MSIR 2898
Oramorph SR Tablets 3062
Roxanol 3066

Nadolol (Concurrent use of phenylephrine with beta blockers may result in hypertensive crises). Products include:
Corgard Tablets 2245
Corzide 40/5 Tablets 2247

IMPORTANT NOTE: Always consult each drug listing in the patient's regimen for possible interactions.

Corzide 80/5 Tablets 2247
Nadolol Tablets 2288

Norepinephrine Bitartrate (Additive elevation of blood pressure).
No products indexed under this heading.

Olanzapine (Exhibits an additive CNS depression). Products include:
Zyprexa Tablets 1973
Zyprexa ZYDIS Orally Disintegrating Tablets................. 1973

Oxazepam (Exhibits an additive CNS depression).
No products indexed under this heading.

Oxycodone Hydrochloride (Exhibits an additive CNS depression). Products include:
OxyContin Tablets 2912
OxyFast Oral Concentrate Solution . 2916
OxyIR Capsules 2916
Percocet Tablets 1326
Percodan Tablets 1327
Percolone Tablets 1327
Roxicodone 3067
Tylox Capsules 2597

Pargyline Hydrochloride (Co-administration of sympathomimetics and MAO inhibitors may produce an additive elevation of blood pressure leading to hypertensive crises; MAO inhibitors may prolong the anticholinergic effects of antihistamines; concurrent use is contraindicated).
No products indexed under this heading.

Penbutolol Sulfate (Concurrent use of phenylephrine with beta blockers may result in hypertensive crises).
No products indexed under this heading.

Pentobarbital Sodium (Exhibits an additive CNS depression). Products include:
Nembutal Sodium Solution 485

Perphenazine (Exhibits an additive CNS depression). Products include:
Etrafon 3115
Trilafon 3160

Phenelzine Sulfate (Co-administration of sympathomimetics and MAO inhibitors may produce an additive elevation of blood pressure leading to hypertensive crises; MAO inhibitors may prolong the anticholinergic effects of antihistamines; concurrent use is contraindicated). Products include:
Nardil Tablets 2653

Phenobarbital (Exhibits an additive CNS depression). Products include:
Arco-Lase Plus Tablets 592
Donnatal 2929
Donnatal Extentabs 2930

Phenylephrine Bitartrate (Additive elevation of blood pressure).
No products indexed under this heading.

Phenylephrine Tannate (Additive elevation of blood pressure). Products include:
Ryna-12 S Suspension 3351
Reformulated Rynatan Pediatric Suspension 3352
Rynatuss Pediatric Suspension 3353
Rynatuss Tablets 3353

Phenylpropanolamine Hydrochloride (Additive elevation of blood pressure).
No products indexed under this heading.

Pindolol (Concurrent use of phenylephrine with beta blockers may result in hypertensive crises).
No products indexed under this heading.

Pirbuterol Acetate (Additive elevation of blood pressure). Products include:
Maxair Autohaler 1981
Maxair Inhaler 1984

Prazepam (Exhibits an additive CNS depression).
No products indexed under this heading.

Procarbazine Hydrochloride (Co-administration of sympathomimetics and MAO inhibitors may produce an additive elevation of blood pressure leading to hypertensive crises; MAO inhibitors may prolong the anticholinergic effects of antihistamines; concurrent use is contraindicated). Products include:
Matulane Capsules 3246

Prochlorperazine (Exhibits an additive CNS depression). Products include:
Compazine 1505

Promethazine Hydrochloride (Exhibits an additive CNS depression). Products include:
Mepergan Injection 3539
Phenergan Injection 3553
Phenergan 3556
Phenergan Syrup 3554
Phenergan with Codeine Syrup 3557
Phenergan with Dextromethorphan Syrup 3559
Phenergan VC Syrup 3560
Phenergan VC with Codeine Syrup .. 3561

Propofol (Exhibits an additive CNS depression). Products include:
Diprivan Injectable Emulsion 667

Propoxyphene Hydrochloride (Exhibits an additive CNS depression). Products include:
Darvon Pulvules 1909
Darvon Compound-65 Pulvules 1910

Propoxyphene Napsylate (Exhibits an additive CNS depression). Products include:
Darvon-N/Darvocet-N 1907
Darvon-N Tablets 1912

Propranolol Hydrochloride (Concurrent use of phenylephrine with beta blockers may result in hypertensive crises). Products include:
Inderal 3513
Inderal LA Long-Acting Capsules 3516
Inderide Tablets 3517
Inderide LA Long-Acting Capsules .. 3519

Pseudoephedrine Hydrochloride (Additive elevation of blood pressure). Products include:
Actifed Cold & Allergy Tablets .... ▣688
Actifed Cold & Sinus Caplets and Tablets .... ▣688
Advil Cold and Sinus Caplets .... ▣771
Advil Cold and Sinus Tablets .... ▣771
Advil Flu & Body Ache Caplets ...... ▣772
Aleve Cold & Sinus Caplets .... ▣603
Alka-Seltzer Plus Liqui-Gels .... ▣604
Alka-Seltzer Plus Cold & Flu Medicine Liqui-Gels .... ▣604
Alka-Seltzer Plus Cold & Sinus Medicine Liqui-Gels .... ▣604
Allegra-D Extended-Release Tablets 714
BC Cold Powder .... ▣619
Benadryl Allergy/Cold Tablets .... ▣691
Benadryl Allergy/Congestion Tablets .... ▣692
Benadryl Allergy & Sinus Liquid ..... ▣693
Benadryl Allergy & Sinus Fastmelt Tablets .... ▣693
Benadryl Allergy Sinus Headache Caplets & Gelcaps .... ▣693
Benadryl Severe Allergy & Sinus Headache Caplets .... ▣694
Benadryl Children's Allergy/Cold Fastmelt Tablets .... ▣692
Benylin Multi-Symptom Liquid .... ▣697
Bromfed Capsules (Extended-Release)........................ 2269
Bromfed-PD Capsules (Extended-Release)........................ 2269
Children's Cēpacol Sore Throat ..... ▣788
Comtrex Acute Head Cold & Sinus Pressure Relief Tablets...... ▣627
Comtrex Deep Chest Cold & Congestion Relief Softgels........ ▣627
Comtrex Flu Therapy & Fever Relief Daytime Caplets............... ▣628
Comtrex Flu Therapy & Fever Relief Nighttime Tablets............. ▣628
Comtrex Maximum Strength Multi-Symptom Cold & Cough Relief Tablets and Caplets.......... ▣626
Contac Non-Drowsy 12 Hour Cold Caplets................................. ▣745
Contac Non-Drowsy Timed Release 12 Hour Cold Caplets ... ▣746
Contac Severe Cold and Flu Caplets Maximum Strength........ ▣746
Contac Severe Cold and Flu Caplets Non-Drowsy .... ▣746
Dimetapp Elixir .... ▣777
Dimetapp Cold and Fever Suspension................................. ▣775
Dimetapp DM Cold & Cough Elixir . ▣775
Dimetapp Nighttime Flu Liquid ...... ▣776
Dimetapp Non-Drowsy Flu Syrup ... ▣777
Dimetapp Infant Drops Decongestant............................. ▣775
Dimetapp Infant Drops Decongestant Plus Cough.......... ▣776
Guaifed 2272
Kronofed-A 1341
Children's Motrin Cold Oral Suspension 2007
Motrin Sinus Headache Caplets 2005
PediaCare Cough-Cold Liquid .... ▣719
PediaCare Infants' Drops Decongestant............................. ▣719
PediaCare Infants' Drops Decongestant Plus Cough.......... ▣719
PediaCare NightRest Cough-Cold Liquid .... ▣719
Robitussin Cold Caplets Cold & Congestion................................. ▣780
Robitussin Cold Softgels Cold & Congestion................................. ▣780
Robitussin Cold Caplets Multi-Symptom Cold & Flu.......... ▣781
Robitussin Cold Softgels Multi-Symptom Cold & Flu.......... ▣781
Robitussin Cold Softgels Severe Congestion................................. ▣782
Robitussin Cough & Cold Infant Drops.. ▣782
Robitussin Maximum Strength Cough & Cold Liquid.................. ▣785
Robitussin Pediatric Cough & Cold Formula Liquid.................. ▣785
Robitussin Multi Symptom Honey Flu Liquid................................. ▣785
Robitussin Nighttime Honey Flu Liquid .... ▣786
Robitussin-CF Liquid .... ▣783
Robitussin-DAC Syrup 2942
Robitussin-PE Liquid .... ▣782
Ryna .... ▣768
Semprex-D Capsules 1172
Singlet Caplets .... ▣761
Sinutab Non-Drying Liquid Caps .... ▣706
Sinutab Sinus Allergy Medication, Maximum Strength Formula, Tablets & Caplets........................ ▣707
Sinutab Sinus Medication, Maximum Strength Without Drowsiness Formula, Tablets & Caplets.. ▣707
Sudafed 12 Hour Tablets .... ▣708
Sudafed 24 Hour Tablets .... ▣708
Children's Sudafed Cold & Cough Liquid .... ▣709
Children's Sudafed Nasal Decongestant Chewables .... ▣711
Children's Sudafed Nasal Decongestant Liquid Medication.................................. ▣711
Sudafed Cold & Allergy Tablets ..... ▣708
Sudafed Cold & Cough Liquid Caps .... ▣709
Sudafed Cold & Sinus Liquid Caps .... ▣710
Sudafed Nasal Decongestant Tablets .... ▣710
Sudafed Non-Drying Sinus Liquid Caps .... ▣712
Sudafed Severe Cold .... ▣711
Sudafed Sinus Headache Caplets . ▣712
Sudafed Sinus Headache Tablets .. ▣712
Tavist Sinus Non-Drowsy Coated Caplets....................................... ▣676
TheraFlu Regular Strength Cold & Cough Night Time Hot Liquid...... ▣676
TheraFlu Regular Strength Cold & Sore Throat Night Time Hot Liquid .... ▣676
TheraFlu Maximum Strength Flu & Congestion Non-Drowsy Hot Liquid .... ▣677
TheraFlu Maximum Strength Flu & Cough Night Time Hot Liquid.. ▣678
TheraFlu Maximum Strength Flu & Sore Throat Night Time Hot Liquid .... ▣677
TheraFlu Maximum Strength Severe Cold & Congestion Night Time Caplets .... ▣678
TheraFlu Maximum Strength Severe Cold & Congestion Night Time Hot Liquid .... ▣678
TheraFlu Maximum Strength Severe Cold & Congestion Non-Drowsy................................. ▣679
Triaminic Allergy Congestion Liquid .... ▣680
Triaminic Chest Congestion Liquid .... ▣680
Triaminic Cold & Allergy Liquid ...... ▣681
Triaminic Cold & Allergy Softchews .... ▣683
Triaminic Cold & Cough Liquid ...... ▣681
Triaminic Cold & Cough Softchews .... ▣683
Triaminic Cold & Night Time Cough Liquid .... ▣681
Triaminic Cold, Cough & Fever Liquid .... ▣681
Triaminic Cough Liquid .... ▣682
Triaminic Cough & Congestion Liquid .... ▣682
Triaminic Cough & Sore Throat Liquid .... ▣682
Triaminic Cough & Sore Throat Softchews .... ▣684
Children's Tylenol Allergy-D Liquid ... 2014
Children's Tylenol Cold Suspension Liquid and Chewable Tablets 2015
Children's Tylenol Cold Plus Cough Suspension Liquid and Chewable Tablets 2015
Children's Tylenol Flu Suspension Liquid 2015
Children's Tylenol Sinus Suspension Liquid 2017
Infants' Tylenol Cold Decongestant and Fever Reducer Concentrated Drops.................. 2015
Infants' Tylenol Cold Decongestant and Fever Reducer Concentrated Drops Plus Cough.. 2015
Tylenol Allergy Sinus 2010
Multi-Symptom Tylenol Cold Complete Formula Caplets 2010
Multi-Symptom Tylenol Cold Non-Drowsy Caplets and Gelcaps.. 2010
Multi-Symptom Tylenol Cold Severe Congestion Non-Drowsy Caplets 2011
Maximum Strength Tylenol Flu NightTime Gelcaps..................... 2011
Maximum Strength Tylenol Flu NightTime Liquid......................... 2011
Maximum Strength Tylenol Flu Non-Drowsy Gelcaps.................... 2011
Maximum Strength Tylenol Sinus NightTime Caplets....................... 2012
Maximum Strength Tylenol Sinus Non-Drowsy Geltabs, Gelcaps, Caplets, and Tablets................... 2012
Vicks 44D Cough & Head Congestion Relief Liquid .... ▣724
Vicks 44M Cough, Cold & Flu Relief Liquid................................ ▣725
Pediatric Vicks 44m Cough & Cold Relief................................... ▣728
Vicks DayQuil LiquiCaps/Liquid Multi-Symptom Cold/Flu Relief ... ▣727
Children's Vicks NyQuil Cold/Cough Relief.......................... ▣726
Vicks NyQuil LiquiCaps/Liquid Multi-Symptom Cold/Flu Relief, Original and Cherry Flavors......... ▣727
Zephrex Tablets 3091
Zephrex LA Tablets 3092
Zyrtec-D 12 Hour Extended Relief Tablets 2758

Pseudoephedrine Sulfate (Additive elevation of blood pressure). Products include:
Chlor-Trimeton Allergy/Decongestant Tablets.... ▣736
Claritin-D 12 Hour Extended Release Tablets........................... 3102
Claritin-D 24 Hour Extended Release Tablets........................... 3104
Coricidin 'D' Cold, Flu & Sinus Tablets .... ▣737
Drixoral Allergy/Sinus Extended-Release Tablets............ ▣741
Drixoral Cold & Allergy Sustained-Action Tablets............ ▣740
Drixoral Cold & Flu Extended-Release Tablets............ ▣740
Drixoral Nasal Decongestant Long-Acting Non-Drowsy Tablets .... ▣740
Rynatan Tablets 3351

Quazepam (Exhibits an additive CNS depression).
No products indexed under this heading.

Quetiapine Fumarate (Exhibits an additive CNS depression). Products include:
Seroquel Tablets 684

Remifentanil Hydrochloride (Exhibits an additive CNS depression).
No products indexed under this heading.

Risperidone (Exhibits an additive CNS depression). Products include:
Risperdal ... 1796

Salmeterol Xinafoate (Additive elevation of blood pressure). Products include:
Advair Diskus 100/50 ... 1448
Advair Diskus 250/50 ... 1448
Advair Diskus 500/50 ... 1448
Serevent Diskus ... 1637
Serevent Inhalation Aerosol ... 1633

Secobarbital Sodium (Exhibits an additive CNS depression).
No products indexed under this heading.

Selegiline Hydrochloride (Co-administration of sympathomimetics and MAO inhibitors may produce an additive elevation of blood pressure leading to hypertensive crises; MAO inhibitors may prolong the anticholinergic effects of antihistamines; concurrent use is contraindicated). Products include:
Eldepryl Capsules ... 3266

Sevoflurane (Exhibits an additive CNS depression).
No products indexed under this heading.

Sotalol Hydrochloride (Concurrent use of phenylephrine with beta blockers may result in hypertensive crises). Products include:
Betapace Tablets ... 950
Betapace AF Tablets ... 954

Sufentanil Citrate (Exhibits an additive CNS depression).
No products indexed under this heading.

Temazepam (Exhibits an additive CNS depression).
No products indexed under this heading.

Terbutaline Sulfate (Additive elevation of blood pressure). Products include:
Brethine Ampuls ... 2314
Brethine Tablets ... 2313

Thiamylal Sodium (Exhibits an additive CNS depression).
No products indexed under this heading.

Thioridazine Hydrochloride (Exhibits an additive CNS depression). Products include:
Thioridazine Hydrochloride Tablets ... 2289

Thiothixene (Exhibits an additive CNS depression). Products include:
Navane Capsules ... 2701
Thiothixene Capsules ... 2290

Timolol Hemihydrate (Concurrent use of phenylephrine with beta blockers may result in hypertensive crises). Products include:
Betimol Ophthalmic Solution ... ⊙324

Timolol Maleate (Concurrent use of phenylephrine with beta blockers may result in hypertensive crises). Products include:
Blocadren Tablets ... 2046
Cosopt Sterile Ophthalmic Solution ... 2065
Timolide Tablets ... 2187
Timolol GFS ... ⊙266
Timoptic in Ocudose ... 2192
Timoptic Sterile Ophthalmic Solution ... 2190
Timoptic-XE Sterile Ophthalmic Gel Forming Solution ... 2194

Tranylcypromine Sulfate (Co-administration of sympathomimetics and MAO inhibitors may produce an additive elevation of blood pressure leading to hypertensive crises; MAO inhibitors may prolong the anticholinergic effects of antihistamines; concurrent use is contraindicated). Products include:
Parnate Tablets ... 1607

Triazolam (Exhibits an additive CNS depression). Products include:
Halcion Tablets ... 2823

Trifluoperazine Hydrochloride (Exhibits an additive CNS depression). Products include:
Stelazine ... 1640

Zaleplon (Exhibits an additive CNS depression). Products include:
Sonata Capsules ... 3591

Ziprasidone Hydrochloride (Exhibits an additive CNS depression). Products include:
Geodon Capsules ... 2688

Zolpidem Tartrate (Exhibits an additive CNS depression). Products include:
Ambien Tablets ... 3191

Food Interactions

Alcohol (Exhibits an additive CNS depression).

HYCOTUSS EXPECTORANT SYRUP

(Guaifenesin, Hydrocodone Bitartrate) ... 1318

May interact with central nervous system depressants, narcotic analgesics, antipsychotic agents, tranquilizers, and certain other agents. Compounds in these categories include:

Alfentanil Hydrochloride (Exhibits an additive CNS depression).
No products indexed under this heading.

Alprazolam (Exhibits an additive CNS depression). Products include:
Xanax Tablets ... 2865

Aprobarbital (Exhibits an additive CNS depression).
No products indexed under this heading.

Buprenorphine Hydrochloride (Exhibits an additive CNS depression). Products include:
Buprenex Injectable ... 2918

Buspirone Hydrochloride (Exhibits an additive CNS depression).
No products indexed under this heading.

Butabarbital (Exhibits an additive CNS depression).
No products indexed under this heading.

Butalbital (Exhibits an additive CNS depression). Products include:
Phrenilin ... 578
Sedapap Tablets 50 mg/650 mg ... 2225

Chlordiazepoxide (Exhibits an additive CNS depression). Products include:
Limbitrol ... 1738

Chlordiazepoxide Hydrochloride (Exhibits an additive CNS depression). Products include:
Librium Capsules ... 1736
Librium for Injection ... 1737

Chlorpromazine (Exhibits an additive CNS depression). Products include:
Thorazine Suppositories ... 1656

Chlorpromazine Hydrochloride (Exhibits an additive CNS depression). Products include:
Thorazine ... 1656

Chlorprothixene (Exhibits an additive CNS depression).
No products indexed under this heading.

Chlorprothixene Hydrochloride (Exhibits an additive CNS depression).
No products indexed under this heading.

Chlorprothixene Lactate (Exhibits an additive CNS depression).
No products indexed under this heading.

Clorazepate Dipotassium (Exhibits an additive CNS depression). Products include:
Tranxene ... 511

Clozapine (Exhibits an additive CNS depression). Products include:
Clozaril Tablets ... 2319

Codeine Phosphate (Exhibits an additive CNS depression). Products include:
Phenergan with Codeine Syrup ... 3557
Phenergan VC with Codeine Syrup ... 3561
Robitussin A-C Syrup ... 2942
Robitussin-DAC Syrup ... 2942
Ryna-C Liquid ... ▣768
Soma Compound w/Codeine Tablets ... 3355
Tussi-Organidin NR Liquid ... 3350
Tussi-Organidin-S NR Liquid ... 3350
Tylenol with Codeine ... 2595

Desflurane (Exhibits an additive CNS depression). Products include:
Suprane Liquid for Inhalation ... 874

Dezocine (Exhibits an additive CNS depression).
No products indexed under this heading.

Diazepam (Exhibits an additive CNS depression). Products include:
Valium Injectable ... 3026
Valium Tablets ... 3047

Droperidol (Exhibits an additive CNS depression).
No products indexed under this heading.

Enflurane (Exhibits an additive CNS depression).
No products indexed under this heading.

Estazolam (Exhibits an additive CNS depression). Products include:
ProSom Tablets ... 500

Ethchlorvynol (Exhibits an additive CNS depression).
No products indexed under this heading.

Ethinamate (Exhibits an additive CNS depression).
No products indexed under this heading.

Fentanyl (Exhibits an additive CNS depression). Products include:
Duragesic Transdermal System ... 1786

Fentanyl Citrate (Exhibits an additive CNS depression). Products include:
Actiq ... 1184

Fluphenazine Decanoate (Exhibits an additive CNS depression).
No products indexed under this heading.

Fluphenazine Enanthate (Exhibits an additive CNS depression).
No products indexed under this heading.

Fluphenazine Hydrochloride (Exhibits an additive CNS depression).
No products indexed under this heading.

Flurazepam Hydrochloride (Exhibits an additive CNS depression).
No products indexed under this heading.

Glutethimide (Exhibits an additive CNS depression).
No products indexed under this heading.

Haloperidol (Exhibits an additive CNS depression). Products include:
Haldol Injection, Tablets and Concentrate ... 2533

Haloperidol Decanoate (Exhibits an additive CNS depression). Products include:
Haldol Decanoate ... 2535

Hydrocodone Polistirex (Exhibits an additive CNS depression). Products include:
Tussionex Pennkinetic Extended-Release Suspension ... 1174

Hydromorphone Hydrochloride (Exhibits an additive CNS depression). Products include:
Dilaudid ... 441
Dilaudid Oral Liquid ... 445
Dilaudid Powder ... 441
Dilaudid Rectal Suppositories ... 441
Dilaudid Tablets ... 441
Dilaudid Tablets - 8 mg ... 445
Dilaudid-HP ... 443

Hydroxyzine Hydrochloride (Exhibits an additive CNS depression). Products include:
Atarax Tablets & Syrup ... 2667
Vistaril Intramuscular Solution ... 2738

Isoflurane (Exhibits an additive CNS depression).
No products indexed under this heading.

Ketamine Hydrochloride (Exhibits an additive CNS depression).
No products indexed under this heading.

Levomethadyl Acetate Hydrochloride (Exhibits an additive CNS depression).
No products indexed under this heading.

Levorphanol Tartrate (Exhibits an additive CNS depression). Products include:
Levo-Dromoran ... 1734
Levorphanol Tartrate Tablets ... 3059

Lithium Carbonate (Exhibits an additive CNS depression). Products include:
Eskalith ... 1527
Lithium Carbonate ... 3061
Lithobid Slow-Release Tablets ... 3255

Lithium Citrate (Exhibits an additive CNS depression). Products include:
Lithium Citrate Syrup ... 3061

Lorazepam (Exhibits an additive CNS depression). Products include:
Ativan Injection ... 3478
Ativan Tablets ... 3482

Loxapine Hydrochloride (Exhibits an additive CNS depression).
No products indexed under this heading.

Loxapine Succinate (Exhibits an additive CNS depression). Products include:
Loxitane Capsules ... 3398

Meperidine Hydrochloride (Exhibits an additive CNS depression). Products include:
Demerol ... 3079
Mepergan Injection ... 3539

Mephobarbital (Exhibits an additive CNS depression).
No products indexed under this heading.

Meprobamate (Exhibits an additive CNS depression). Products include:
Miltown Tablets ... 3349

Mesoridazine Besylate (Exhibits an additive CNS depression). Products include:
Serentil ... 1057

Methadone Hydrochloride (Exhibits an additive CNS depression). Products include:
Dolophine Hydrochloride Tablets ... 3056

Methohexital Sodium (Exhibits an additive CNS depression). Products include:
Brevital Sodium for Injection, USP ... 1815

Methotrimeprazine (Exhibits an additive CNS depression).
No products indexed under this heading.

Methoxyflurane (Exhibits an additive CNS depression).
No products indexed under this heading.

Midazolam Hydrochloride (Exhibits an additive CNS depression). Products include:
Versed Injection ... 3027
Versed Syrup ... 3033

Molindone Hydrochloride (Exhibits an additive CNS depression). Products include:
Moban ... 1320

Morphine Sulfate (Exhibits an additive CNS depression). Products include:

Astramorph/PF Injection, USP (Preservative-Free) 594
Duramorph Injection 1312
Infumorph 200 and Infumorph 500 Sterile Solutions 1314
Kadian Capsules 1335
MS Contin Tablets 2896
MSIR 2898
Oramorph SR Tablets 3062
Roxanol 3066

Olanzapine (Exhibits an additive CNS depression). Products include:
Zyprexa Tablets 1973
Zyprexa ZYDIS Orally Disintegrating Tablets 1973

Oxazepam (Exhibits an additive CNS depression).
No products indexed under this heading.

Oxycodone Hydrochloride (Exhibits an additive CNS depression). Products include:
OxyContin Tablets 2912
OxyFast Oral Concentrate Solution 2916
OxyIR Capsules 2916
Percocet Tablets 1326
Percodan Tablets 1327
Percolone Tablets 1327
Roxicodone 3067
Tylox Capsules 2597

Pentobarbital Sodium (Exhibits an additive CNS depression). Products include:
Nembutal Sodium Solution 485

Perphenazine (Exhibits an additive CNS depression). Products include:
Etrafon 3115
Trilafon 3160

Phenobarbital (Exhibits an additive CNS depression). Products include:
Arco-Lase Plus Tablets 592
Donnatal 2929
Donnatal Extentabs 2930

Pimozide (Exhibits an additive CNS depression). Products include:
Orap Tablets 1407

Prazepam (Exhibits an additive CNS depression).
No products indexed under this heading.

Prochlorperazine (Exhibits an additive CNS depression). Products include:
Compazine 1505

Promethazine Hydrochloride (Exhibits an additive CNS depression). Products include:
Mepergan Injection 3539
Phenergan Injection 3553
Phenergan 3556
Phenergan Syrup 3554
Phenergan with Codeine Syrup 3557
Phenergan with Dextromethorphan Syrup 3559
Phenergan VC Syrup 3560
Phenergan VC with Codeine Syrup 3561

Propofol (Exhibits an additive CNS depression). Products include:
Diprivan Injectable Emulsion 667

Propoxyphene Hydrochloride (Exhibits an additive CNS depression). Products include:
Darvon Pulvules 1909
Darvon Compound-65 Pulvules 1910

Propoxyphene Napsylate (Exhibits an additive CNS depression). Products include:
Darvon-N/Darvocet-N 1907
Darvon-N Tablets 1912

Quazepam (Exhibits an additive CNS depression).
No products indexed under this heading.

Quetiapine Fumarate (Exhibits an additive CNS depression). Products include:
Seroquel Tablets 684

Remifentanil Hydrochloride (Exhibits an additive CNS depression).
No products indexed under this heading.

Risperidone (Exhibits an additive CNS depression). Products include:
Risperdal 1796

Secobarbital Sodium (Exhibits an additive CNS depression).
No products indexed under this heading.

Sevoflurane (Exhibits an additive CNS depression).
No products indexed under this heading.

Sufentanil Citrate (Exhibits an additive CNS depression).
No products indexed under this heading.

Temazepam (Exhibits an additive CNS depression).
No products indexed under this heading.

Thiamylal Sodium (Exhibits an additive CNS depression).
No products indexed under this heading.

Thioridazine Hydrochloride (Exhibits an additive CNS depression). Products include:
Thioridazine Hydrochloride Tablets 2289

Thiothixene (Exhibits an additive CNS depression). Products include:
Navane Capsules 2701
Thiothixene Capsules 2290

Triazolam (Exhibits an additive CNS depression). Products include:
Halcion Tablets 2823

Trifluoperazine Hydrochloride (Exhibits an additive CNS depression). Products include:
Stelazine 1640

Zaleplon (Exhibits an additive CNS depression). Products include:
Sonata Capsules 3591

Ziprasidone Hydrochloride (Exhibits an additive CNS depression). Products include:
Geodon Capsules 2688

Zolpidem Tartrate (Exhibits an additive CNS depression). Products include:
Ambien Tablets 3191

Food Interactions

Alcohol (Exhibits an additive CNS depression).

HYDROCORTONE TABLETS

(Hydrocortisone) 2106

May interact with oral anticoagulants, oral hypoglycemic agents, insulin, potassium-depleting diuretics, and certain other agents. Compounds in these categories include:

Acarbose (Potential for increased requirements of oral hypoglycemic agents). Products include:
Precose Tablets 906

Aspirin (Aspirin should be used cautiously in conjunction with corticosteroids in hypoprothrombinemia). Products include:
Aggrenox Capsules 1026
Alka-Seltzer .... ■603
Alka-Seltzer Lemon Lime Antacid and Pain Reliever Effervescent Tablets .... ■603
Alka-Seltzer Extra Strength Antacid and Pain Reliever Effervescent Tablets .... ■603
Alka-Seltzer PM Effervescent Tablets .... ■605
Genuine Bayer Tablets, Caplets and Gelcaps .... ■606
Extra Strength Bayer Caplets and Gelcaps .... ■610
Aspirin Regimen Bayer Children's Chewable Tablets (Orange or Cherry Flavored) .... ■607
Bayer, Aspirin Regimen .... ■606
Aspirin Regimen Bayer 81 mg Caplets with Calcium .... ■607
Genuine Bayer Professional Labeling (Aspirin Regimen Bayer) .... ■608
Extra Strength Bayer Arthritis Caplets .... ■610
Extra Strength Bayer Plus Caplets .... ■610
Extra Strength Bayer PM Caplets .... ■611
BC Powder .... ■619
BC Allergy Sinus Cold Powder .... ■619
Arthritis Strength BC Powder .... ■619
BC Sinus Cold Powder .... ■619
Darvon Compound-65 Pulvules 1910
Ecotrin Enteric Coated Aspirin Low, Regular and Maximum Strength Tablets 1715
Excedrin Extra-Strength Tablets, Caplets, and Geltabs .... ■629
Excedrin Migraine 1070
Goody's Body Pain Formula Powder .... ■620
Goody's Extra Strength Headache Powder .... ■620
Goody's Extra Strength Pain Relief Tablets .... ■620
Percodan Tablets 1327
Robaxisal Tablets 2939
Soma Compound Tablets 3354
Soma Compound w/Codeine Tablets 3355
Vanquish Caplets .... ■617

Bendroflumethiazide (Co-administration may result in hypokalemia). Products include:
Corzide 40/5 Tablets 2247
Corzide 80/5 Tablets 2247

Bumetanide (Co-administration may result in hypokalemia).
No products indexed under this heading.

Chlorothiazide (Co-administration may result in hypokalemia). Products include:
Aldoclor Tablets 2035
Diuril Oral 2087

Chlorothiazide Sodium (Co-administration may result in hypokalemia). Products include:
Diuril Sodium Intravenous 2086

Chlorpropamide (Potential for increased requirements of oral hypoglycemic agents). Products include:
Diabinese Tablets 2680

Dicumarol (Potential for altered response to coumarin anticoagulants).
No products indexed under this heading.

Ephedrine Hydrochloride (Enhances metabolic clearance of corticosteroids resulting in decreased blood levels and lessened physiologic activity). Products include:
Primatene Tablets .... ■780

Ephedrine Sulfate (Enhances metabolic clearance of corticosteroids resulting in decreased blood levels and lessened physiologic activity).
No products indexed under this heading.

Ephedrine Tannate (Enhances metabolic clearance of corticosteroids resulting in decreased blood levels and lessened physiologic activity). Products include:
Rynatuss Pediatric Suspension 3353
Rynatuss Tablets 3353

Ethacrynic Acid (Co-administration may result in hypokalemia). Products include:
Edecrin Tablets 2091

Fosphenytoin Sodium (Enhances metabolic clearance of corticosteroids resulting in decreased blood levels and lessened physiologic activity). Products include:
Cerebyx Injection 2619

Furosemide (Co-administration may result in hypokalemia). Products include:
Furosemide Tablets 2284

Glimepiride (Potential for increased requirements of oral hypoglycemic agents). Products include:
Amaryl Tablets 717

Glipizide (Potential for increased requirements of oral hypoglycemic agents). Products include:
Glucotrol Tablets 2692
Glucotrol XL Extended Release Tablets 2693

Glyburide (Potential for increased requirements of oral hypoglycemic agents). Products include:
DiaBeta Tablets 741
Glucovance Tablets 1086

Hydrochlorothiazide (Co-administration may result in hypokalemia). Products include:
Accuretic Tablets 2614
Aldoril Tablets 2039
Atacand HCT Tablets 597
Avalide Tablets 1070
Diovan HCT Tablets 2338
Dyazide Capsules 1515
HydroDIURIL Tablets 2108
Hyzaar 2109
Inderide Tablets 3517
Inderide LA Long-Acting Capsules 3519
Lotensin HCT Tablets 2367
Maxzide 1008
Micardis HCT Tablets 1051
Microzide Capsules 3414
Moduretic Tablets 2138
Monopril HCT 1094
Prinzide Tablets 2168
Timolide Tablets 2187
Uniretic Tablets 3178
Vaseretic Tablets 2204
Zestoretic Tablets 695
Ziac Tablets 1887

Hydroflumethiazide (Co-administration may result in hypokalemia). Products include:
Diucardin Tablets 3494

Insulin, Human, Zinc Suspension (Potential for increased requirements of insulin). Products include:
Humulin L, 100 Units 1937
Humulin U, 100 Units 1943
Novolin L Human Insulin 10 ml Vials 2422

Insulin, Human NPH (Potential for increased requirements of insulin). Products include:
Humulin N, 100 Units 1939
Humulin N NPH Pen 1940
Novolin N Human Insulin 10 ml Vials 2422
Novolin N PenFill 2423
Novolin N Prefilled Syringe Disposable Insulin Delivery System 2425

Insulin, Human Regular (Potential for increased requirements of insulin). Products include:
Humulin R Regular (U-500) 1943
Humulin R, 100 Units 1941
Novolin R Human Insulin 10 ml Vials 2423
Novolin R PenFill 2423
Novolin R Prefilled Syringe Disposable Insulin Delivery System 2425
Velosulin BR Human Insulin 10 ml Vials 2435

Insulin, Human Regular and Human NPH Mixture (Potential for increased requirements of insulin). Products include:
Humulin 50/50, 100 Units 1934
Humulin 70/30, 100 Units 1935
Humulin 70/30 Pen 1936
Novolin 70/30 Human Insulin 10 ml Vials 2421
Novolin 70/30 PenFill 2423
Novolin 70/30 Prefilled Disposable Insulin Delivery System 2425

Insulin, NPH (Potential for increased requirements of insulin). Products include:
Iletin II, NPH (Pork), 100 Units 1946

Insulin, Regular (Potential for increased requirements of insulin). Products include:
Iletin II, Regular (Pork), 100 Units 1947

Insulin, Zinc Crystals (Potential for increased requirements of insulin).
No products indexed under this heading.

Insulin, Zinc Suspension (Potential for increased requirements of insulin). Products include:
- Iletin II, Lente (Pork), 100 Units 1945

Insulin Aspart, Human Regular (Potential for increased requirements of insulin).
- No products indexed under this heading.

Insulin glargine (Potential for increased requirements of insulin). Products include:
- Lantus Injection 742

Insulin Lispro, Human (Potential for increased requirements of insulin). Products include:
- Humalog 1926
- Humalog Mix 75/25 Pen 1928

Insulin Lispro Protamine, Human (Potential for increased requirements of insulin). Products include:
- Humalog Mix 75/25 Pen 1928

Live Virus Vaccines (Co-administration is contraindicated in patients receiving immunosuppressive doses of corticosteroids).
- No products indexed under this heading.

Metformin Hydrochloride (Potential for increased requirements of oral hypoglycemic agents). Products include:
- Glucophage Tablets 1080
- Glucophage XR Tablets 1080
- Glucovance Tablets 1086

Methyclothiazide (Co-administration may result in hypokalemia).
- No products indexed under this heading.

Miglitol (Potential for increased requirements of oral hypoglycemic agents). Products include:
- Glyset Tablets 2821

Phenobarbital (Enhances metabolic clearance of corticosteroids resulting in decreased blood levels and lessened physiologic activity). Products include:
- Arco-Lase Plus Tablets 592
- Donnatal 2929
- Donnatal Extentabs 2930

Phenytoin (Enhances metabolic clearance of corticosteroids resulting in decreased blood levels and lessened physiologic activity). Products include:
- Dilantin Infatabs 2624
- Dilantin-125 Oral Suspension 2625

Phenytoin Sodium (Enhances metabolic clearance of corticosteroids resulting in decreased blood levels and lessened physiologic activity). Products include:
- Dilantin Kapseals 2622

Pioglitazone Hydrochloride (Potential for increased requirements of oral hypoglycemic agents). Products include:
- Actos Tablets 3275

Polythiazide (Co-administration may result in hypokalemia). Products include:
- Minizide Capsules 2700
- Renese Tablets 2712

Repaglinide (Potential for increased requirements of oral hypoglycemic agents). Products include:
- Prandin Tablets (0.5, 1, and 2 mg) 2432

Rifampin (Enhances metabolic clearance of corticosteroids resulting in decreased blood levels and lessened physiologic activity). Products include:
- Rifadin 765
- Rifamate Capsules 767
- Rifater Tablets 769

Rosiglitazone Maleate (Potential for increased requirements of oral hypoglycemic agents). Products include:
- Avandia Tablets 1490

Tolazamide (Potential for increased requirements of oral hypoglycemic agents).
- No products indexed under this heading.

Tolbutamide (Potential for increased requirements of oral hypoglycemic agents).
- No products indexed under this heading.

Torsemide (Co-administration may result in hypokalemia). Products include:
- Demadex Tablets and Injection 2965

Troglitazone (Potential for increased requirements of oral hypoglycemic agents).
- No products indexed under this heading.

Warfarin Sodium (Potential for altered response to coumarin anticoagulants). Products include:
- Coumadin for Injection 1243
- Coumadin Tablets 1243
- Warfarin Sodium Tablets, USP 3302

HYDROCORTONE ACETATE INJECTABLE SUSPENSION

(Hydrocortisone Acetate) 2103

May interact with oral anticoagulants, oral hypoglycemic agents, insulin, potassium-depleting diuretics, and certain other agents. Compounds in these categories include:

Acarbose (Potential for increased requirements of oral hypoglycemic agents). Products include:
- Precose Tablets 906

Aspirin (Aspirin should be used cautiously in conjunction with corticosteroids in hypoprothrombinemia). Products include:
- Aggrenox Capsules 1026
- Alka-Seltzer 603
- Alka-Seltzer Lemon Lime Antacid and Pain Reliever Effervescent Tablets 603
- Alka-Seltzer Extra Strength Antacid and Pain Reliever Effervescent Tablets 603
- Alka-Seltzer PM Effervescent Tablets 605
- Genuine Bayer Tablets, Caplets and Gelcaps 606
- Extra Strength Bayer Caplets and Gelcaps 610
- Aspirin Regimen Bayer Children's Chewable Tablets (Orange or Cherry Flavored) 607
- Bayer, Aspirin Regimen 606
- Aspirin Regimen Bayer 81 mg Caplets with Calcium 607
- Genuine Bayer Professional Labeling (Aspirin Regimen Bayer) 608
- Extra Strength Bayer Arthritis Caplets 610
- Extra Strength Bayer Plus Caplets 610
- Extra Strength Bayer PM Caplets 611
- BC Powder 619
- BC Allergy Sinus Cold Powder 619
- Arthritis Strength BC Powder 619
- BC Sinus Cold Powder 619
- Darvon Compound-65 Pulvules 1910
- Ecotrin Enteric Coated Aspirin Low, Regular and Maximum Strength Tablets 1715
- Excedrin Extra-Strength Tablets, Caplets, and Geltabs 629
- Excedrin Migraine 1070
- Goody's Body Pain Formula Powder 620
- Goody's Extra Strength Headache Powder 620
- Goody's Extra Strength Pain Relief Tablets 620
- Percodan Tablets 1327
- Robaxisal Tablets 2939
- Soma Compound Tablets 3354
- Soma Compound w/Codeine Tablets 3355
- Vanquish Caplets 617

Bendroflumethiazide (Co-administration may result in hypokalemia). Products include:
- Corzide 40/5 Tablets 2247
- Corzide 80/5 Tablets 2247

Bumetanide (Co-administration may result in hypokalemia).
- No products indexed under this heading.

Chlorothiazide (Co-administration may result in hypokalemia). Products include:
- Aldoclor Tablets 2035
- Diuril Oral 2087

Chlorothiazide Sodium (Co-administration may result in hypokalemia). Products include:
- Diuril Sodium Intravenous 2086

Chlorpropamide (Potential for increased requirements of oral hypoglycemic agents). Products include:
- Diabinese Tablets 2680

Dicumarol (Potential for altered response to coumarin anticoagulants).
- No products indexed under this heading.

Ephedrine Hydrochloride (Enhances metabolic clearance of corticosteroids resulting in decreased blood levels and lessened physiologic activity). Products include:
- Primatene Tablets 780

Ephedrine Sulfate (Enhances metabolic clearance of corticosteroids resulting in decreased blood levels and lessened physiologic activity).
- No products indexed under this heading.

Ephedrine Tannate (Enhances metabolic clearance of corticosteroids resulting in decreased blood levels and lessened physiologic activity). Products include:
- Rynatuss Pediatric Suspension 3353
- Rynatuss Tablets 3353

Ethacrynic Acid (Co-administration may result in hypokalemia). Products include:
- Edecrin Tablets 2091

Fosphenytoin Sodium (Enhances metabolic clearance of corticosteroids resulting in decreased blood levels and lessened physiologic activity). Products include:
- Cerebyx Injection 2619

Furosemide (Co-administration may result in hypokalemia). Products include:
- Furosemide Tablets 2284

Glimepiride (Potential for increased requirements of oral hypoglycemic agents). Products include:
- Amaryl Tablets 717

Glipizide (Potential for increased requirements of oral hypoglycemic agents). Products include:
- Glucotrol Tablets 2692
- Glucotrol XL Extended Release Tablets 2693

Glyburide (Potential for increased requirements of oral hypoglycemic agents). Products include:
- DiaBeta Tablets 741
- Glucovance Tablets 1086

Hydrochlorothiazide (Co-administration may result in hypokalemia). Products include:
- Accuretic Tablets 2614
- Aldoril Tablets 2039
- Atacand HCT Tablets 597
- Avalide Tablets 1070
- Diovan HCT Tablets 2338
- Dyazide Capsules 1515
- HydroDIURIL Tablets 2108
- Hyzaar 2109
- Inderide Tablets 3517
- Inderide LA Long-Acting Capsules 3519
- Lotensin HCT Tablets 2367
- Maxzide 1008
- Micardis HCT Tablets 1051
- Microzide Capsules 3414
- Moduretic Tablets 2138
- Monopril HCT 1094
- Prinzide Tablets 2168
- Timolide Tablets 2187
- Uniretic Tablets 3178
- Vaseretic Tablets 2204
- Zestoretic Tablets 695
- Ziac Tablets 1887

Hydroflumethiazide (Co-administration may result in hypokalemia). Products include:
- Diucardin Tablets 3494

Insulin, Human, Zinc Suspension (Potential for increased requirements of insulin). Products include:
- Humulin L, 100 Units 1937
- Humulin U, 100 Units 1943
- Novolin L Human Insulin 10 ml Vials 2422

Insulin, Human NPH (Potential for increased requirements of insulin). Products include:
- Humulin N, 100 Units 1939
- Humulin N NPH Pen 1940
- Novolin N Human Insulin 10 ml Vials 2422
- Novolin N PenFill 2423
- Novolin N Prefilled Syringe Disposable Insulin Delivery System 2425

Insulin, Human Regular (Potential for increased requirements of insulin). Products include:
- Humulin R Regular (U-500) 1943
- Humulin R, 100 Units 1941
- Novolin R Human Insulin 10 ml Vials 2423
- Novolin R PenFill 2423
- Novolin R Prefilled Syringe Disposable Insulin Delivery System 2425
- Velosulin BR Human Insulin 10 ml Vials 2435

Insulin, Human Regular and Human NPH Mixture (Potential for increased requirements of insulin). Products include:
- Humulin 50/50, 100 Units 1934
- Humulin 70/30, 100 Units 1935
- Humulin 70/30 Pen 1936
- Novolin 70/30 Human Insulin 10 ml Vials 2421
- Novolin 70/30 PenFill 2423
- Novolin 70/30 Prefilled Disposable Insulin Delivery System 2425

Insulin, NPH (Potential for increased requirements of insulin). Products include:
- Iletin II, NPH (Pork), 100 Units 1946

Insulin, Regular (Potential for increased requirements of insulin). Products include:
- Iletin II, Regular (Pork), 100 Units 1947

Insulin, Zinc Crystals (Potential for increased requirements of insulin).
- No products indexed under this heading.

Insulin, Zinc Suspension (Potential for increased requirements of insulin). Products include:
- Iletin II, Lente (Pork), 100 Units 1945

Insulin Aspart, Human Regular (Potential for increased requirements of insulin).
- No products indexed under this heading.

Insulin glargine (Potential for increased requirements of insulin). Products include:
- Lantus Injection 742

Insulin Lispro, Human (Potential for increased requirements of insulin). Products include:
- Humalog 1926
- Humalog Mix 75/25 Pen 1928

Insulin Lispro Protamine, Human (Potential for increased requirements of insulin). Products include:
- Humalog Mix 75/25 Pen 1928

Live Virus Vaccines (Co-administration is contraindicated in patients receiving immunosuppressive doses of corticosteroids).
- No products indexed under this heading.

Metformin Hydrochloride (Potential for increased requirements of oral hypoglycemic agents). Products include:
- Glucophage Tablets 1080
- Glucophage XR Tablets 1080
- Glucovance Tablets 1086

Methyclothiazide (Co-administration may result in hypoka-

lemia).
No products indexed under this heading.

Miglitol (Potential for increased requirements of oral hypoglycemic agents). Products include:
Glyset Tablets 2821

Phenobarbital (Enhances metabolic clearance of corticosteroids resulting in decreased blood levels and lessened physiologic activity). Products include:
Arco-Lase Plus Tablets 592
Donnatal 2929
Donnatal Extentabs 2930

Phenytoin (Enhances metabolic clearance of corticosteroids resulting in decreased blood levels and lessened physiologic activity). Products include:
Dilantin Infatabs 2624
Dilantin-125 Oral Suspension 2625

Phenytoin Sodium (Enhances metabolic clearance of corticosteroids resulting in decreased blood levels and lessened physiologic activity). Products include:
Dilantin Kapseals 2622

Pioglitazone Hydrochloride (Potential for increased requirements of oral hypoglycemic agents). Products include:
Actos Tablets 3275

Polythiazide (Co-administration may result in hypokalemia). Products include:
Minizide Capsules 2700
Renese Tablets 2712

Repaglinide (Potential for increased requirements of oral hypoglycemic agents). Products include:
Prandin Tablets (0.5, 1, and 2 mg) 2432

Rifampin (Enhances metabolic clearance of corticosteroids resulting in decreased blood levels and lessened physiologic activity). Products include:
Rifadin 765
Rifamate Capsules 767
Rifater Tablets 769

Rosiglitazone Maleate (Potential for increased requirements of oral hypoglycemic agents). Products include:
Avandia Tablets 1490

Tolazamide (Potential for increased requirements of oral hypoglycemic agents).
No products indexed under this heading.

Tolbutamide (Potential for increased requirements of oral hypoglycemic agents).
No products indexed under this heading.

Torsemide (Co-administration may result in hypokalemia). Products include:
Demadex Tablets and Injection 2965

Troglitazone (Potential for increased requirements of oral hypoglycemic agents).
No products indexed under this heading.

Warfarin Sodium (Potential for altered response to coumarin anticoagulants). Products include:
Coumadin for Injection 1243
Coumadin Tablets 1243
Warfarin Sodium Tablets, USP 3302

HYDROCORTONE PHOSPHATE INJECTION, STERILE

(Hydrocortisone Sodium Phosphate) 2105

May interact with oral anticoagulants, oral hypoglycemic agents, insulin, potassium-depleting diuretics, and certain other agents. Compounds in these categories include:

Acarbose (Potential for increased requirements of oral hypoglycemic agents). Products include:
Precose Tablets 906

Aspirin (Aspirin should be used cautiously in conjunction with corticosteroids in hypoprothrombinemia). Products include:
Aggrenox Capsules 1026
Alka-Seltzer ..... ▣603
Alka-Seltzer Lemon Lime Antacid and Pain Reliever Effervescent Tablets ..... ▣603
Alka-Seltzer Extra Strength Antacid and Pain Reliever Effervescent Tablets ..... ▣603
Alka-Seltzer PM Effervescent Tablets ..... ▣605
Genuine Bayer Tablets, Caplets and Gelcaps ..... ▣606
Extra Strength Bayer Caplets and Gelcaps ..... ▣610
Aspirin Regimen Bayer Children's Chewable Tablets (Orange or Cherry Flavored) ..... ▣607
Bayer, Aspirin Regimen ..... ▣606
Aspirin Regimen Bayer 81 mg Caplets with Calcium ..... ▣607
Genuine Bayer Professional Labeling (Aspirin Regimen Bayer) ..... ▣608
Extra Strength Bayer Arthritis Caplets ..... ▣610
Extra Strength Bayer Plus Caplets ..... ▣610
Extra Strength Bayer PM Caplets ..... ▣611
BC Powder ..... ▣619
BC Allergy Sinus Cold Powder ..... ▣619
Arthritis Strength BC Powder ..... ▣619
BC Sinus Cold Powder ..... ▣619
Darvon Compound-65 Pulvules 1910
Ecotrin Enteric Coated Aspirin Low, Regular and Maximum Strength Tablets 1715
Excedrin Extra-Strength Tablets, Caplets, and Geltabs ..... ▣629
Excedrin Migraine 1070
Goody's Body Pain Formula Powder ..... ▣620
Goody's Extra Strength Headache Powder ..... ▣620
Goody's Extra Strength Pain Relief Tablets ..... ▣620
Percodan Tablets 1327
Robaxisal Tablets 2939
Soma Compound Tablets 3354
Soma Compound w/Codeine Tablets 3355
Vanquish Caplets ..... ▣617

Bendroflumethiazide (Co-administration may result in hypokalemia). Products include:
Corzide 40/5 Tablets 2247
Corzide 80/5 Tablets 2247

Bumetanide (Co-administration may result in hypokalemia).
No products indexed under this heading.

Chlorothiazide (Co-administration may result in hypokalemia). Products include:
Aldoclor Tablets 2035
Diuril Oral 2087

Chlorothiazide Sodium (Co-administration may result in hypokalemia). Products include:
Diuril Sodium Intravenous 2086

Chlorpropamide (Potential for increased requirements of oral hypoglycemic agents). Products include:
Diabinese Tablets 2680

Dicumarol (Potential for altered response to coumarin anticoagulants).
No products indexed under this heading.

Ephedrine Hydrochloride (Enhances metabolic clearance of corticosteroids resulting in decreased blood levels and lessened physiologic activity). Products include:
Primatene Tablets ..... ▣780

Ephedrine Sulfate (Enhances metabolic clearance of corticosteroids resulting in decreased blood levels and lessened physiologic activity).
No products indexed under this heading.

Ephedrine Tannate (Enhances metabolic clearance of corticosteroids resulting in decreased blood levels and lessened physiologic activity). Products include:
Rynatuss Pediatric Suspension 3353
Rynatuss Tablets 3353

Ethacrynic Acid (Co-administration may result in hypokalemia). Products include:
Edecrin Tablets 2091

Fosphenytoin Sodium (Enhances metabolic clearance of corticosteroids resulting in decreased blood levels and lessened physiologic activity). Products include:
Cerebyx Injection 2619

Furosemide (Co-administration may result in hypokalemia). Products include:
Furosemide Tablets 2284

Glimepiride (Potential for increased requirements of oral hypoglycemic agents). Products include:
Amaryl Tablets 717

Glipizide (Potential for increased requirements of oral hypoglycemic agents). Products include:
Glucotrol Tablets 2692
Glucotrol XL Extended Release Tablets 2693

Glyburide (Potential for increased requirements of oral hypoglycemic agents). Products include:
DiaBeta Tablets 741
Glucovance Tablets 1086

Hydrochlorothiazide (Co-administration may result in hypokalemia). Products include:
Accuretic Tablets 2614
Aldoril Tablets 2039
Atacand HCT Tablets 597
Avalide Tablets 1070
Diovan HCT Tablets 2338
Dyazide Capsules 1515
HydroDIURIL Tablets 2108
Hyzaar 2109
Inderide Tablets 3517
Inderide LA Long-Acting Capsules 3519
Lotensin HCT Tablets 2367
Maxzide 1008
Micardis HCT Tablets 1051
Microzide Capsules 3414
Moduretic Tablets 2138
Monopril HCT 1094
Prinzide Tablets 2168
Timolide Tablets 2187
Uniretic Tablets 3178
Vaseretic Tablets 2204
Zestoretic Tablets 695
Ziac Tablets 1887

Hydroflumethiazide (Co-administration may result in hypokalemia). Products include:
Diucardin Tablets 3494

Insulin, Human, Zinc Suspension (Potential for increased requirements of insulin). Products include:
Humulin L, 100 Units 1937
Humulin U, 100 Units 1943
Novolin L Human Insulin 10 ml Vials 2422

Insulin, Human NPH (Potential for increased requirements of insulin). Products include:
Humulin N, 100 Units 1939
Humulin N NPH Pen 1940
Novolin N Human Insulin 10 ml Vials 2422
Novolin N PenFill 2423
Novolin N Prefilled Syringe Disposable Insulin Delivery System 2425

Insulin, Human Regular (Potential for increased requirements of insulin). Products include:
Humulin R Regular (U-500) 1943
Humulin R, 100 Units 1941
Novolin R Human Insulin 10 ml Vials 2423
Novolin R PenFill 2423
Novolin R Prefilled Syringe Disposable Insulin Delivery System 2425
Velosulin BR Human Insulin 10 ml Vials 2435

Insulin, Human Regular and Human NPH Mixture (Potential for increased requirements of insulin). Products include:
Humulin 50/50, 100 Units 1934
Humulin 70/30, 100 Units 1935
Humulin 70/30 Pen 1936
Novolin 70/30 Human Insulin 10 ml Vials 2421
Novolin 70/30 PenFill 2423
Novolin 70/30 Prefilled Disposable Insulin Delivery System 2425

Insulin, NPH (Potential for increased requirements of insulin). Products include:
Iletin II, NPH (Pork), 100 Units 1946

Insulin, Regular (Potential for increased requirements of insulin). Products include:
Iletin II, Regular (Pork), 100 Units 1947

Insulin, Zinc Crystals (Potential for increased requirements of insulin).
No products indexed under this heading.

Insulin, Zinc Suspension (Potential for increased requirements of insulin). Products include:
Iletin II, Lente (Pork), 100 Units 1945

Insulin Aspart, Human Regular (Potential for increased requirements of insulin).
No products indexed under this heading.

Insulin glargine (Potential for increased requirements of insulin). Products include:
Lantus Injection 742

Insulin Lispro, Human (Potential for increased requirements of insulin). Products include:
Humalog 1926
Humalog Mix 75/25 Pen 1928

Insulin Lispro Protamine, Human (Potential for increased requirements of insulin). Products include:
Humalog Mix 75/25 Pen 1928

Live Virus Vaccines (Co-administration is contraindicated in patients receiving immunosuppressive doses of corticosteroids).
No products indexed under this heading.

Metformin Hydrochloride (Potential for increased requirements of oral hypoglycemic agents). Products include:
Glucophage Tablets 1080
Glucophage XR Tablets 1080
Glucovance Tablets 1086

Methyclothiazide (Co-administration may result in hypokalemia).
No products indexed under this heading.

Miglitol (Potential for increased requirements of oral hypoglycemic agents). Products include:
Glyset Tablets 2821

Phenobarbital (Enhances metabolic clearance of corticosteroids resulting in decreased blood levels and lessened physiologic activity). Products include:
Arco-Lase Plus Tablets 592
Donnatal 2929
Donnatal Extentabs 2930

Phenytoin (Enhances metabolic clearance of corticosteroids resulting in decreased blood levels and lessened physiologic activity). Products include:
Dilantin Infatabs 2624
Dilantin-125 Oral Suspension 2625

Phenytoin Sodium (Enhances metabolic clearance of corticosteroids resulting in decreased blood levels and lessened physiologic activity). Products include:
Dilantin Kapseals 2622

Pioglitazone Hydrochloride (Potential for increased requirements of oral hypoglycemic agents). Products include:
Actos Tablets 3275

Polythiazide (Co-administration may result in hypokalemia). Products include:
Minizide Capsules 2700
Renese Tablets 2712

Repaglinide (Potential for increased requirements of oral hypoglycemic agents). Products include:
Prandin Tablets (0.5, 1, and 2 mg) ... 2432

Rifampin (Enhances metabolic clearance of corticosteroids resulting in decreased blood levels and lessened physiologic activity). Products include:
Rifadin ... 765
Rifamate Capsules ... 767
Rifater Tablets ... 769

Rosiglitazone Maleate (Potential for increased requirements of oral hypoglycemic agents). Products include:
Avandia Tablets ... 1490

Tolazamide (Potential for increased requirements of oral hypoglycemic agents).
No products indexed under this heading.

Tolbutamide (Potential for increased requirements of oral hypoglycemic agents).
No products indexed under this heading.

Torsemide (Co-administration may result in hypokalemia). Products include:
Demadex Tablets and Injection ... 2965

Troglitazone (Potential for increased requirements of oral hypoglycemic agents).
No products indexed under this heading.

Warfarin Sodium (Potential for altered response to coumarin anticoagulants). Products include:
Coumadin for Injection ... 1243
Coumadin Tablets ... 1243
Warfarin Sodium Tablets, USP ... 3302

HYDRODIURIL TABLETS

(Hydrochlorothiazide) ... 2108
May interact with antihypertensives, barbiturates, bile acid sequestering agents, corticosteroids, cardiac glycosides, oral hypoglycemic agents, insulin, lithium preparations, narcotic analgesics, nondepolarizing neuromuscular blocking agents, non-steroidal anti-inflammatory agents, and certain other agents. Compounds in these categories include:

Acarbose (Hyperglycemia may occur with thiazide diuretics; dosage adjustment of the oral antidiabetic drug may be required). Products include:
Precose Tablets ... 906

Acebutolol Hydrochloride (Potentiation of antihypertensive drugs). Products include:
Sectral Capsules ... 3589

ACTH (Intensified electrolyte depletion, particularly hypokalemia).
No products indexed under this heading.

Alfentanil Hydrochloride (Potentiation of orthostatic hypotension).
No products indexed under this heading.

Amlodipine Besylate (Potentiation of antihypertensive drugs). Products include:
Lotrel Capsules ... 2370
Norvasc Tablets ... 2704

Aprobarbital (Potentiation of orthostatic hypotension).
No products indexed under this heading.

Atenolol (Potentiation of antihypertensive drugs). Products include:
Tenoretic Tablets ... 690
Tenormin I.V. Injection ... 692

Atracurium Besylate (Possible increased responsiveness to the muscle relaxants).
No products indexed under this heading.

Benazepril Hydrochloride (Potentiation of antihypertensive drugs). Products include:
Lotensin Tablets ... 2365
Lotensin HCT Tablets ... 2367
Lotrel Capsules ... 2370

Bendroflumethiazide (Potentiation of antihypertensive drugs). Products include:
Corzide 40/5 Tablets ... 2247
Corzide 80/5 Tablets ... 2247

Betamethasone Acetate (Intensified electrolyte depletion, particularly hypokalemia). Products include:
Celestone Soluspan Injectable Suspension ... 3097

Betamethasone Sodium Phosphate (Intensified electrolyte depletion, particularly hypokalemia). Products include:
Celestone Soluspan Injectable Suspension ... 3097

Betaxolol Hydrochloride (Potentiation of antihypertensive drugs). Products include:
Betoptic S Ophthalmic Suspension ... 537

Bisoprolol Fumarate (Potentiation of antihypertensive drugs). Products include:
Zebeta Tablets ... 1885
Ziac Tablets ... 1887

Buprenorphine Hydrochloride (Potentiation of orthostatic hypotension). Products include:
Buprenex Injectable ... 2918

Butabarbital (Potentiation of orthostatic hypotension).
No products indexed under this heading.

Butalbital (Potentiation of orthostatic hypotension). Products include:
Phrenilin ... 578
Sedapap Tablets 50 mg/650 mg ... 2225

Candesartan Cilexetil (Potentiation of antihypertensive drugs). Products include:
Atacand Tablets ... 595
Atacand HCT Tablets ... 597

Captopril (Potentiation of antihypertensive drugs). Products include:
Captopril Tablets ... 2281

Carteolol Hydrochloride (Potentiation of antihypertensive drugs). Products include:
Carteolol Hydrochloride Ophthalmic Solution USP, 1% ... ⊙ 258
Ocupress Ophthalmic Solution, 1% Sterile ... ⊙ 303

Celecoxib (Reduced diuretic, natriuretic, and antihypertensive effects). Products include:
Celebrex Capsules ... 2676
Celebrex Capsules ... 2780

Chlorothiazide (Potentiation of antihypertensive drugs). Products include:
Aldoclor Tablets ... 2035
Diuril Oral ... 2087

Chlorothiazide Sodium (Potentiation of antihypertensive drugs). Products include:
Diuril Sodium Intravenous ... 2086

Chlorpropamide (Hyperglycemia may occur with thiazide diuretics; dosage adjustment of the oral antidiabetic drug may be required). Products include:
Diabinese Tablets ... 2680

Chlorthalidone (Potentiation of antihypertensive drugs). Products include:
Clorpres Tablets ... 1002
Combipres Tablets ... 1040
Tenoretic Tablets ... 690

Cholestyramine (Cholestyramine resin has potential of binding hydrochlorothiazide and reducing its absorption from the GI tract by up to 85%).
No products indexed under this heading.

Cisatracurium Besylate (Possible increased responsiveness to the muscle relaxants).
No products indexed under this heading.

Clonidine (Potentiation of antihypertensive drugs). Products include:
Catapres-TTS ... 1038

Clonidine Hydrochloride (Potentiation of antihypertensive drugs). Products include:
Catapres Tablets ... 1037
Clorpres Tablets ... 1002
Combipres Tablets ... 1040
Duraclon Injection ... 3057

Codeine Phosphate (Potentiation of orthostatic hypotension). Products include:
Phenergan with Codeine Syrup ... 3557
Phenergan VC with Codeine Syrup ... 3561
Robitussin A-C Syrup ... 2942
Robitussin-DAC Syrup ... 2942
Ryna-C Liquid ... ⊠ 768
Soma Compound w/Codeine Tablets ... 3355
Tussi-Organidin NR Liquid ... 3350
Tussi-Organidin-S NR Liquid ... 3350
Tylenol with Codeine ... 2595

Colestipol Hydrochloride (Colestipol resin has potential of binding hydrochlorothiazide and reducing its absorption from the GI tract by up to 43%). Products include:
Colestid Tablets ... 2791

Cortisone Acetate (Intensified electrolyte depletion, particularly hypokalemia). Products include:
Cortone Acetate Injectable Suspension ... 2059
Cortone Acetate Tablets ... 2061

Deserpidine (Potentiation of antihypertensive drugs).
No products indexed under this heading.

Deslanoside (Resultant hypokalemia may exaggerate cardiac toxicity of digitalis).
No products indexed under this heading.

Dexamethasone (Intensified electrolyte depletion, particularly hypokalemia). Products include:
Decadron Elixir ... 2078
Decadron Tablets ... 2079
TobraDex Ophthalmic Ointment ... 542
TobraDex Ophthalmic Suspension ... 541

Dexamethasone Acetate (Intensified electrolyte depletion, particularly hypokalemia).
No products indexed under this heading.

Dexamethasone Sodium Phosphate (Intensified electrolyte depletion, particularly hypokalemia). Products include:
Decadron Phosphate Injection ... 2081
Decadron Phosphate Sterile Ophthalmic Ointment ... 2083
Decadron Phosphate Sterile Ophthalmic Solution ... 2084
NeoDecadron Sterile Ophthalmic Solution ... 2144

Dezocine (Potentiation of orthostatic hypotension).
No products indexed under this heading.

Diazoxide (Potentiation of antihypertensive drugs).
No products indexed under this heading.

Diclofenac Potassium (Reduced diuretic, natriuretic, and antihypertensive effects). Products include:
Cataflam Tablets ... 2315

Diclofenac Sodium (Reduced diuretic, natriuretic, and antihypertensive effects). Products include:
Arthrotec Tablets ... 3195
Voltaren Ophthalmic Sterile Ophthalmic Solution ... ⊙ 312
Voltaren Tablets ... 2315
Voltaren-XR Tablets ... 2315

Digitoxin (Resultant hypokalemia may exaggerate cardiac toxicity of digitalis).
No products indexed under this heading.

Digoxin (Resultant hypokalemia may exaggerate cardiac toxicity of digitalis). Products include:
Digitek Tablets ... 1003
Lanoxicaps Capsules ... 1574
Lanoxin Injection ... 1581
Lanoxin Tablets ... 1587
Lanoxin Elixir Pediatric ... 1578
Lanoxin Injection Pediatric ... 1584

Diltiazem Hydrochloride (Potentiation of antihypertensive drugs). Products include:
Cardizem Injectable ... 1018
Cardizem Lyo-Ject Syringe ... 1018
Cardizem Monovial ... 1018
Cardizem CD Capsules ... 1016
Tiazac Capsules ... 1378

Doxazosin Mesylate (Potentiation of antihypertensive drugs). Products include:
Cardura Tablets ... 2668

Enalapril Maleate (Potentiation of antihypertensive drugs). Products include:
Lexxel Tablets ... 608
Vaseretic Tablets ... 2204
Vasotec Tablets ... 2210

Enalaprilat (Potentiation of antihypertensive drugs). Products include:
Enalaprilat Injection ... 863
Vasotec I.V. Injection ... 2207

Eprosartan Mesylate (Potentiation of antihypertensive drugs). Products include:
Teveten Tablets ... 3327

Esmolol Hydrochloride (Potentiation of antihypertensive drugs). Products include:
Brevibloc Injection ... 858

Etodolac (Reduced diuretic, natriuretic, and antihypertensive effects). Products include:
Lodine ... 3528
Lodine XL Extended-Release Tablets ... 3530

Felodipine (Potentiation of antihypertensive drugs). Products include:
Lexxel Tablets ... 608
Plendil Extended-Release Tablets ... 623

Fenoprofen Calcium (Reduced diuretic, natriuretic, and antihypertensive effects).
No products indexed under this heading.

Fentanyl (Potentiation of orthostatic hypotension). Products include:
Duragesic Transdermal System ... 1786

Fentanyl Citrate (Potentiation of orthostatic hypotension). Products include:
Actiq ... 1184

Fludrocortisone Acetate (Intensified electrolyte depletion, particularly hypokalemia). Products include:
Florinef Acetate Tablets ... 2250

Flurbiprofen (Reduced diuretic, natriuretic, and antihypertensive effects).
No products indexed under this heading.

Fosinopril Sodium (Potentiation of antihypertensive drugs). Products include:
Monopril Tablets ... 1091
Monopril HCT ... 1094

Furosemide (Potentiation of antihypertensive drugs). Products include:
Furosemide Tablets ... 2284

Glimepiride (Hyperglycemia may occur with thiazide diuretics; dosage adjustment of the oral antidiabetic drug may be required). Products include:
Amaryl Tablets ... 717

Glipizide (Hyperglycemia may occur with thiazide diuretics; dosage adjustment of the oral antidiabetic drug may be required). Products include:
Glucotrol Tablets ... 2692
Glucotrol XL Extended Release Tablets ... 2693

Glyburide (Hyperglycemia may occur with thiazide diuretics; dosage adjustment of the oral antidiabetic drug may be required). Products include:
DiaBeta Tablets ... 741
Glucovance Tablets ... 1086

IMPORTANT NOTE: Always consult each drug listing in the patient's regimen for possible interactions.

Guanabenz Acetate (Potentiation of antihypertensive drugs).
No products indexed under this heading.

Guanethidine Monosulfate (Potentiation of antihypertensive drugs).
No products indexed under this heading.

Hydralazine Hydrochloride (Potentiation of antihypertensive drugs).
No products indexed under this heading.

Hydrocodone Bitartrate (Potentiation of orthostatic hypotension). Products include:
Hycodan ... 1316
Hycomine Compound Tablets ... 1317
Hycotuss Expectorant Syrup ... 1318
Lortab ... 3319
Lortab Elixir ... 3317
Maxidone Tablets CIII ... 3399
Norco 5/325 Tablets CIII ... 3424
Norco 7.5/325 Tablets CIII ... 3425
Norco 10/325 Tablets CIII ... 3427
Norco 10/325 Tablets CIII ... 3425
Vicodin Tablets ... 516
Vicodin ES Tablets ... 517
Vicodin HP Tablets ... 518
Vicodin Tuss Expectorant ... 519
Vicoprofen Tablets ... 520
Zydone Tablets ... 1330

Hydrocodone Polistirex (Potentiation of orthostatic hypotension). Products include:
Tussionex Pennkinetic Extended-Release Suspension ... 1174

Hydrocortisone (Intensified electrolyte depletion, particularly hypokalemia). Products include:
Anusol-HC Cream 2.5% ... 2237
Cipro HC Otic Suspension ... 540
Cortaid Intensive Therapy Cream ... ▣717
Cortaid Maximum Strength Cream ... ▣717
Cortisporin Ophthalmic Suspension Sterile ... ⊙297
Cortizone•5 ... ▣699
Cortizone•10 ... ▣699
Cortizone•10 Plus Creme ... ▣700
Cortizone for Kids Creme ... ▣699
Hydrocortone Tablets ... 2106
Massengill Medicated Soft Cloth Towelette ... ▣753
VōSoL HC Otic Solution ... 3356

Hydrocortisone Acetate (Intensified electrolyte depletion, particularly hypokalemia). Products include:
Analpram-HC ... 1338
Anusol HC-1 Hydrocortisone Anti-Itch Cream ... ▣689
Anusol-HC Suppositories ... 2238
Cortaid ... ▣717
Cortifoam Rectal Foam ... 3170
Cortisporin-TC Otic Suspension ... 2246
Hydrocortone Acetate Injectable Suspension ... 2103
Pramosone ... 1343
Proctocort Suppositories ... 2264
ProctoFoam-HC ... 3177
Terra Cortril Ophthalmic Suspension ... 2716

Hydrocortisone Sodium Phosphate (Intensified electrolyte depletion, particularly hypokalemia). Products include:
Hydrocortone Phosphate Injection, Sterile ... 2105

Hydrocortisone Sodium Succinate (Intensified electrolyte depletion, particularly hypokalemia).
No products indexed under this heading.

Hydroflumethiazide (Potentiation of antihypertensive drugs). Products include:
Diucardin Tablets ... 3494

Hydromorphone Hydrochloride (Potentiation of orthostatic hypotension). Products include:
Dilaudid ... 441
Dilaudid Oral Liquid ... 445
Dilaudid Powder ... 441
Dilaudid Rectal Suppositories ... 441
Dilaudid Tablets ... 441
Dilaudid Tablets - 8 mg ... 445
Dilaudid-HP ... 443

Ibuprofen (Reduced diuretic, natriuretic, and antihypertensive effects). Products include:
Advil ... ▣771
Children's Advil Oral Suspension ... ▣773
Children's Advil Chewable Tablets ... ▣773
Advil Cold and Sinus Caplets ... ▣771
Advil Cold and Sinus Tablets ... ▣771
Advil Flu & Body Ache Caplets ... ▣772
Infants' Advil Drops ... ▣773
Junior Strength Advil Tablets ... ▣773
Junior Strength Advil Chewable Tablets ... ▣773
Advil Migraine Liquigels ... ▣772
Children's Motrin Oral Suspension and Chewable Tablets ... 2006
Children's Motrin Cold Oral Suspension ... 2007
Children's Motrin Oral Suspension ... ▣643
Motrin Suspension, Oral Drops, Chewable Tablets, and Caplets ... 2002
Infants' Motrin Concentrated Drops ... 2006
Junior Strength Motrin Caplets and Chewable Tablets ... 2006
Motrin IB Tablets, Caplets, and Gelcaps ... 2002
Motrin Migraine Pain Caplets ... 2005
Motrin Sinus Headache Caplets ... 2005
Vicoprofen Tablets ... 520

Indapamide (Potentiation of antihypertensive drugs). Products include:
Indapamide Tablets ... 2286

Indomethacin (Reduced diuretic, natriuretic, and antihypertensive effects). Products include:
Indocin ... 2112

Indomethacin Sodium Trihydrate (Reduced diuretic, natriuretic, and antihypertensive effects). Products include:
Indocin I.V. ... 2115

Insulin, Human, Zinc Suspension (Hyperglycemia may occur with thiazide diuretics; dosage adjustment of insulin may be required). Products include:
Humulin L, 100 Units ... 1937
Humulin U, 100 Units ... 1943
Novolin L Human Insulin 10 ml Vials ... 2422

Insulin, Human NPH (Hyperglycemia may occur with thiazide diuretics; dosage adjustment of insulin may be required). Products include:
Humulin N, 100 Units ... 1939
Humulin N NPH Pen ... 1940
Novolin N Human Insulin 10 ml Vials ... 2422
Novolin N PenFill ... 2423
Novolin N Prefilled Syringe Disposable Insulin Delivery System ... 2425

Insulin, Human Regular (Hyperglycemia may occur with thiazide diuretics; dosage adjustment of insulin may be required). Products include:
Humulin R Regular (U-500) ... 1943
Humulin R, 100 Units ... 1941
Novolin R Human Insulin 10 ml Vials ... 2423
Novolin R PenFill ... 2423
Novolin R Prefilled Syringe Disposable Insulin Delivery System ... 2425
Velosulin BR Human Insulin 10 ml Vials ... 2435

Insulin, Human Regular and Human NPH Mixture (Hyperglycemia may occur with thiazide diuretics; dosage adjustment of insulin may be required). Products include:
Humulin 50/50, 100 Units ... 1934
Humulin 70/30, 100 Units ... 1935
Humulin 70/30 Pen ... 1936
Novolin 70/30 Human Insulin 10 ml Vials ... 2421
Novolin 70/30 PenFill ... 2423
Novolin 70/30 Prefilled Disposable Insulin Delivery System ... 2425

Insulin, NPH (Hyperglycemia may occur with thiazide diuretics; dosage adjustment of insulin may be required). Products include:
Iletin II, NPH (Pork), 100 Units ... 1946

Insulin, Regular (Hyperglycemia may occur with thiazide diuretics; dosage adjustment of insulin may be required). Products include:
Iletin II, Regular (Pork), 100 Units ... 1947

Insulin, Zinc Crystals (Hyperglycemia may occur with thiazide diuretics; dosage adjustment of insulin may be required).
No products indexed under this heading.

Insulin, Zinc Suspension (Hyperglycemia may occur with thiazide diuretics; dosage adjustment of insulin may be required). Products include:
Iletin II, Lente (Pork), 100 Units ... 1945

Insulin Aspart, Human Regular (Hyperglycemia may occur with thiazide diuretics; dosage adjustment of insulin may be required).
No products indexed under this heading.

Insulin glargine (Hyperglycemia may occur with thiazide diuretics; dosage adjustment of insulin may be required). Products include:
Lantus Injection ... 742

Insulin Lispro, Human (Hyperglycemia may occur with thiazide diuretics; dosage adjustment of insulin may be required). Products include:
Humalog ... 1926
Humalog Mix 75/25 Pen ... 1928

Insulin Lispro Protamine, Human (Hyperglycemia may occur with thiazide diuretics; dosage adjustment of insulin may be required). Products include:
Humalog Mix 75/25 Pen ... 1928

Irbesartan (Potentiation of antihypertensive drugs). Products include:
Avalide Tablets ... 1070
Avapro Tablets ... 1074
Avapro Tablets ... 3076

Isradipine (Potentiation of antihypertensive drugs). Products include:
DynaCirc Capsules ... 2921
DynaCirc CR Tablets ... 2923

Ketoprofen (Reduced diuretic, natriuretic, and antihypertensive effects). Products include:
Orudis Capsules ... 3548
Orudis KT Tablets ... ▣778
Oruvail Capsules ... 3548

Ketorolac Tromethamine (Reduced diuretic, natriuretic, and antihypertensive effects). Products include:
Acular Ophthalmic Solution ... 544
Acular PF Ophthalmic Solution ... 544
Toradol ... 3018

Labetalol Hydrochloride (Potentiation of antihypertensive drugs). Products include:
Normodyne Injection ... 3135
Normodyne Tablets ... 3137

Levorphanol Tartrate (Potentiation of orthostatic hypotension). Products include:
Levo-Dromoran ... 1734
Levorphanol Tartrate Tablets ... 3059

Lisinopril (Potentiation of antihypertensive drugs). Products include:
Prinivil Tablets ... 2164
Prinzide Tablets ... 2168
Zestoretic Tablets ... 695
Zestril Tablets ... 698

Lithium Carbonate (Diuretics reduce the renal clearance of lithium and add a high risk of lithium toxicity). Products include:
Eskalith ... 1527
Lithium Carbonate ... 3061
Lithobid Slow-Release Tablets ... 3255

Lithium Citrate (Diuretics reduce the renal clearance of lithium and add a high risk of lithium toxicity). Products include:
Lithium Citrate Syrup ... 3061

Losartan Potassium (Potentiation of antihypertensive drugs). Products include:
Cozaar Tablets ... 2067
Hyzaar ... 2109

Mecamylamine Hydrochloride (Potentiation of antihypertensive drugs). Products include:
Inversine Tablets ... 1850

Meclofenamate Sodium (Reduced diuretic, natriuretic, and antihypertensive effects).
No products indexed under this heading.

Mefenamic Acid (Reduced diuretic, natriuretic, and antihypertensive effects). Products include:
Ponstel Capsules ... 1356

Meloxicam (Reduced diuretic, natriuretic, and antihypertensive effects). Products include:
Mobic Tablets ... 1054

Meperidine Hydrochloride (Potentiation of orthostatic hypotension). Products include:
Demerol ... 3079
Mepergan Injection ... 3539

Mephobarbital (Potentiation of orthostatic hypotension).
No products indexed under this heading.

Metformin Hydrochloride (Hyperglycemia may occur with thiazide diuretics; dosage adjustment of the oral antidiabetic drug may be required). Products include:
Glucophage Tablets ... 1080
Glucophage XR Tablets ... 1080
Glucovance Tablets ... 1086

Methadone Hydrochloride (Potentiation of orthostatic hypotension). Products include:
Dolophine Hydrochloride Tablets ... 3056

Methyclothiazide (Potentiation of antihypertensive drugs).
No products indexed under this heading.

Methyldopa (Potentiation of antihypertensive drugs). Products include:
Aldoclor Tablets ... 2035
Aldomet Tablets ... 2037
Aldoril Tablets ... 2039

Methyldopate Hydrochloride (Potentiation of antihypertensive drugs).
No products indexed under this heading.

Methylprednisolone Acetate (Intensified electrolyte depletion, particularly hypokalemia). Products include:
Depo-Medrol Injectable Suspension ... 2795

Methylprednisolone Sodium Succinate (Intensified electrolyte depletion, particularly hypokalemia). Products include:
Solu-Medrol Sterile Powder ... 2855

Metocurine Iodide (Possible increased responsiveness to the muscle relaxants).
No products indexed under this heading.

Metolazone (Potentiation of antihypertensive drugs). Products include:
Mykrox Tablets ... 1168
Zaroxolyn Tablets ... 1177

Metoprolol Succinate (Potentiation of antihypertensive drugs). Products include:
Toprol-XL Tablets ... 651

Metoprolol Tartrate (Potentiation of antihypertensive drugs).
No products indexed under this heading.

Metyrosine (Potentiation of antihypertensive drugs). Products include:
Demser Capsules ... 2085

Mibefradil Dihydrochloride (Potentiation of antihypertensive drugs).
No products indexed under this heading.

Miglitol (Hyperglycemia may occur with thiazide diuretics; dosage adjustment of the oral antidiabetic drug may be required). Products include:
Glyset Tablets ... 2821

Minoxidil (Potentiation of antihypertensive drugs). Products include:
- Rogaine Extra Strength for Men Topical Solution .... ▣721
- Rogaine for Women Topical Solution .... ▣721

Mivacurium Chloride (Possible increased responsiveness to the muscle relaxants).
- No products indexed under this heading.

Moexipril Hydrochloride (Potentiation of antihypertensive drugs). Products include:
- Uniretic Tablets 3178
- Univasc Tablets 3181

Morphine Sulfate (Potentiation of orthostatic hypotension). Products include:
- Astramorph/PF Injection, USP (Preservative-Free) 594
- Duramorph Injection 1312
- Infumorph 200 and Infumorph 500 Sterile Solutions 1314
- Kadian Capsules 1335
- MS Contin Tablets 2896
- MSIR 2898
- Oramorph SR Tablets 3062
- Roxanol 3066

Nabumetone (Reduced diuretic, natriuretic, and antihypertensive effects). Products include:
- Relafen Tablets 1617

Nadolol (Potentiation of antihypertensive drugs). Products include:
- Corgard Tablets 2245
- Corzide 40/5 Tablets 2247
- Corzide 80/5 Tablets 2247
- Nadolol Tablets 2288

Naproxen (Reduced diuretic, natriuretic, and antihypertensive effects). Products include:
- EC-Naprosyn Delayed-Release Tablets 2967
- Naprosyn Suspension 2967
- Naprosyn Tablets 2967

Naproxen Sodium (Reduced diuretic, natriuretic, and antihypertensive effects). Products include:
- Aleve Tablets, Caplets and Gelcaps .... ▣602
- Aleve Cold & Sinus Caplets .... ▣603
- Anaprox Tablets 2967
- Anaprox DS Tablets 2967
- Naprelan Tablets 1293

Nicardipine Hydrochloride (Potentiation of antihypertensive drugs). Products include:
- Cardene I.V. 3485

Nifedipine (Potentiation of antihypertensive drugs). Products include:
- Adalat CC Tablets 877
- Procardia Capsules 2708
- Procardia XL Extended Release Tablets 2710

Nisoldipine (Potentiation of antihypertensive drugs). Products include:
- Sular Tablets 688

Nitroglycerin (Potentiation of antihypertensive drugs). Products include:
- Nitro-Dur Transdermal Infusion System 3134
- Nitro-Dur Transdermal Infusion System 1834
- Nitrolingual Pumpspray 1355
- Nitrostat Tablets 2658

Norepinephrine Bitartrate (Decreased arterial responsiveness to norepinephrine).
- No products indexed under this heading.

Oxaprozin (Reduced diuretic, natriuretic, and antihypertensive effects).
- No products indexed under this heading.

Oxycodone Hydrochloride (Potentiation of orthostatic hypotension). Products include:
- OxyContin Tablets 2912
- OxyFast Oral Concentrate Solution 2916
- OxyIR Capsules 2916
- Percocet Tablets 1326
- Percodan Tablets 1327
- Percolone Tablets 1327
- Roxicodone 3067
- Tylox Capsules 2597

Pancuronium Bromide (Possible increased responsiveness to the muscle relaxants).
- No products indexed under this heading.

Penbutolol Sulfate (Potentiation of antihypertensive drugs).
- No products indexed under this heading.

Pentobarbital Sodium (Potentiation of orthostatic hypotension). Products include:
- Nembutal Sodium Solution 485

Perindopril Erbumine (Potentiation of antihypertensive drugs). Products include:
- Aceon Tablets (2 mg, 4 mg, 8 mg) 3249

Phenobarbital (Potentiation of orthostatic hypotension). Products include:
- Arco-Lase Plus Tablets 592
- Donnatal 2929
- Donnatal Extentabs 2930

Phenoxybenzamine Hydrochloride (Potentiation of antihypertensive drugs). Products include:
- Dibenzyline Capsules 3457

Phentolamine Mesylate (Potentiation of antihypertensive drugs).
- No products indexed under this heading.

Phenylbutazone (Reduced diuretic, natriuretic, and antihypertensive effects).
- No products indexed under this heading.

Pindolol (Potentiation of antihypertensive drugs).
- No products indexed under this heading.

Pioglitazone Hydrochloride (Hyperglycemia may occur with thiazide diuretics; dosage adjustment of the oral antidiabetic drug may be required). Products include:
- Actos Tablets 3275

Piroxicam (Reduced diuretic, natriuretic, and antihypertensive effects). Products include:
- Feldene Capsules 2685

Polythiazide (Potentiation of antihypertensive drugs). Products include:
- Minizide Capsules 2700
- Renese Tablets 2712

Prazosin Hydrochloride (Potentiation of antihypertensive drugs). Products include:
- Minipress Capsules 2699
- Minizide Capsules 2700

Prednisolone Acetate (Intensified electrolyte depletion, particularly hypokalemia). Products include:
- Blephamide Ophthalmic Ointment 547
- Blephamide Ophthalmic Suspension 548
- Poly-Pred Liquifilm Ophthalmic Suspension .... ⊙245
- Pred Forte Ophthalmic Suspension .... ⊙246
- Pred Mild Sterile Ophthalmic Suspension .... ⊙249
- Pred-G Ophthalmic Suspension .... ⊙247
- Pred-G Sterile Ophthalmic Ointment .... ⊙248

Prednisolone Sodium Phosphate (Intensified electrolyte depletion, particularly hypokalemia). Products include:
- Pediapred Oral Solution 1170

Prednisolone Tebutate (Intensified electrolyte depletion, particularly hypokalemia).
- No products indexed under this heading.

Prednisone (Intensified electrolyte depletion, particularly hypokalemia). Products include:
- Prednisone 3064

Propoxyphene Hydrochloride (Potentiation of orthostatic hypotension). Products include:
- Darvon Pulvules 1909
- Darvon Compound-65 Pulvules 1910

Propoxyphene Napsylate (Potentiation of orthostatic hypotension). Products include:
- Darvon-N/Darvocet-N 1907
- Darvon-N Tablets 1912

Propranolol Hydrochloride (Potentiation of antihypertensive drugs). Products include:
- Inderal 3513
- Inderal LA Long-Acting Capsules 3516
- Inderide Tablets 3517
- Inderide LA Long-Acting Capsules 3519

Quinapril Hydrochloride (Potentiation of antihypertensive drugs). Products include:
- Accupril Tablets 2611
- Accuretic Tablets 2614

Ramipril (Potentiation of antihypertensive drugs). Products include:
- Altace Capsules 2233

Rapacuronium Bromide (Possible increased responsiveness to the muscle relaxants).
- No products indexed under this heading.

Rauwolfia serpentina (Potentiation of antihypertensive drugs).
- No products indexed under this heading.

Remifentanil Hydrochloride (Potentiation of orthostatic hypotension).
- No products indexed under this heading.

Repaglinide (Hyperglycemia may occur with thiazide diuretics; dosage adjustment of the oral antidiabetic drug may be required). Products include:
- Prandin Tablets (0.5, 1, and 2 mg) 2432

Rescinnamine (Potentiation of antihypertensive drugs).
- No products indexed under this heading.

Reserpine (Potentiation of antihypertensive drugs).
- No products indexed under this heading.

Rocuronium Bromide (Possible increased responsiveness to the muscle relaxants). Products include:
- Zemuron Injection 2491

Rofecoxib (Reduced diuretic, natriuretic, and antihypertensive effects). Products include:
- Vioxx 2213

Rosiglitazone Maleate (Hyperglycemia may occur with thiazide diuretics; dosage adjustment of the oral antidiabetic drug may be required). Products include:
- Avandia Tablets 1490

Secobarbital Sodium (Potentiation of orthostatic hypotension).
- No products indexed under this heading.

Sodium Nitroprusside (Potentiation of antihypertensive drugs).
- No products indexed under this heading.

Sotalol Hydrochloride (Potentiation of antihypertensive drugs). Products include:
- Betapace Tablets 950
- Betapace AF Tablets 954

Spirapril Hydrochloride (Potentiation of antihypertensive drugs).
- No products indexed under this heading.

Sufentanil Citrate (Potentiation of orthostatic hypotension).
- No products indexed under this heading.

Sulindac (Reduced diuretic, natriuretic, and antihypertensive effects). Products include:
- Clinoril Tablets 2053

Telmisartan (Potentiation of antihypertensive drugs). Products include:
- Micardis Tablets 1049
- Micardis HCT Tablets 1051

Terazosin Hydrochloride (Potentiation of antihypertensive drugs). Products include:
- Hytrin Capsules 464

Thiamylal Sodium (Potentiation of orthostatic hypotension).
- No products indexed under this heading.

Timolol Maleate (Potentiation of antihypertensive drugs). Products include:
- Blocadren Tablets 2046
- Cosopt Sterile Ophthalmic Solution 2065
- Timolide Tablets 2187
- Timolol GFS .... ⊙266
- Timoptic in Ocudose 2192
- Timoptic Sterile Ophthalmic Solution 2190
- Timoptic-XE Sterile Ophthalmic Gel Forming Solution 2194

Tolazamide (Hyperglycemia may occur with thiazide diuretics; dosage adjustment of the oral antidiabetic drug may be required).
- No products indexed under this heading.

Tolbutamide (Hyperglycemia may occur with thiazide diuretics; dosage adjustment of the oral antidiabetic drug may be required).
- No products indexed under this heading.

Tolmetin Sodium (Reduced diuretic, natriuretic, and antihypertensive effects). Products include:
- Tolectin 2589

Torsemide (Potentiation of antihypertensive drugs). Products include:
- Demadex Tablets and Injection 2965

Trandolapril (Potentiation of antihypertensive drugs). Products include:
- Mavik Tablets 478
- Tarka Tablets 508

Triamcinolone (Intensified electrolyte depletion, particularly hypokalemia).
- No products indexed under this heading.

Triamcinolone Acetonide (Intensified electrolyte depletion, particularly hypokalemia). Products include:
- Azmacort Inhalation Aerosol 728
- Nasacort Nasal Inhaler 750
- Nasacort AQ Nasal Spray 752
- Tri-Nasal Spray 2274

Triamcinolone Diacetate (Intensified electrolyte depletion, particularly hypokalemia).
- No products indexed under this heading.

Triamcinolone Hexacetonide (Intensified electrolyte depletion, particularly hypokalemia).
- No products indexed under this heading.

Trimethaphan Camsylate (Potentiation of antihypertensive drugs).
- No products indexed under this heading.

Troglitazone (Hyperglycemia may occur with thiazide diuretics; dosage adjustment of the oral antidiabetic drug may be required).
- No products indexed under this heading.

Tubocurarine Chloride (Increased responsiveness to tubocurarine).
- No products indexed under this heading.

Valsartan (Potentiation of antihypertensive drugs). Products include:
- Diovan Capsules 2337
- Diovan HCT Tablets 2338

Vecuronium Bromide (Possible increased responsiveness to the muscle relaxants). Products include:
- Norcuron for Injection 2478

Verapamil Hydrochloride (Potentiation of antihypertensive drugs). Products include:
- Covera-HS Tablets 3199
- Isoptin SR Tablets 467
- Tarka Tablets 508
- Verelan Capsules 3184

IMPORTANT NOTE: Always consult each drug listing in the patient's regimen for possible interactions.

Verelan PM Capsules 3186

Food Interactions

Alcohol (Potentiation of orthostatic hypotension).

HYLAND'S ARNISPORT TABLETS

(Homeopathic Formulations) .... ▣764
None cited in PDR database.

HYLAND'S CALMS FORTE TABLETS AND CAPLETS

(Homeopathic Formulations) .... ▣764
None cited in PDR database.

HYLAND'S COLD TABLETS WITH ZINC

(Homeopathic Formulations) .... ▣765
None cited in PDR database.

HYLAND'S COLIC TABLETS

(Disocorea, Homeopathic Formulations)................................ ▣765
None cited in PDR database.

HYLAND'S EARACHE TABLETS

(Homeopathic Formulations) .... ▣765
None cited in PDR database.

HYLAND'S LEG CRAMPS WITH QUININE TABLETS

(Homeopathic Formulations) .... ▣765
None cited in PDR database.

HYLAND'S MENOCALM TABLETS

(Homeopathic Formulations) .... ▣765
None cited in PDR database.

HYLAND'S NERVE TONIC TABLETS AND CAPLETS

(Homeopathic Formulations) .... ▣766
None cited in PDR database.

HYLAND'S TEETHING GEL

(Homeopathic Formulations) .... ▣766
None cited in PDR database.

HYLAND'S TEETHING TABLETS

(Belladonna Alkaloids, Homeopathic Formulations) .... ▣766
None cited in PDR database.

HYTRIN CAPSULES

(Terazosin Hydrochloride) 464

May interact with antihypertensives and certain other agents. Compounds in these categories include:

Acebutolol Hydrochloride (Possibility of significant hypotension; dosage adjustment may be necessary). Products include:
Sectral Capsules 3589

Amlodipine Besylate (Possibility of significant hypotension; dosage adjustment may be necessary). Products include:
Lotrel Capsules 2370
Norvasc Tablets 2704

Atenolol (Possibility of significant hypotension; dosage adjustment may be necessary). Products include:
Tenoretic Tablets 690
Tenormin I.V. Injection 692

Benazepril Hydrochloride (Possibility of significant hypotension; dosage adjustment may be necessary). Products include:
Lotensin Tablets 2365
Lotensin HCT Tablets 2367
Lotrel Capsules 2370

Bendroflumethiazide (Possibility of significant hypotension; dosage adjustment may be necessary). Products include:
Corzide 40/5 Tablets 2247
Corzide 80/5 Tablets 2247

Betaxolol Hydrochloride (Possibility of significant hypotension; dosage adjustment may be necessary). Products include:
Betoptic S Ophthalmic Suspension 537

Bisoprolol Fumarate (Possibility of significant hypotension; dosage adjustment may be necessary). Products include:
Zebeta Tablets 1885
Ziac Tablets 1887

Candesartan Cilexetil (Possibility of significant hypotension; dosage adjustment may be necessary). Products include:
Atacand Tablets 595
Atacand HCT Tablets 597

Captopril (Co-administration increases terazosin's maximum plasma concentrations linearly with dose at steady-state after administration of terazosin plus captopril). Products include:
Captopril Tablets 2281

Carteolol Hydrochloride (Possibility of significant hypotension; dosage adjustment may be necessary). Products include:
Carteolol Hydrochloride Ophthalmic Solution USP, 1% ..... ⊙258
Ocupress Ophthalmic Solution, 1% Sterile .... ⊙303

Chlorothiazide (Possibility of significant hypotension; dosage adjustment may be necessary). Products include:
Aldoclor Tablets 2035
Diuril Oral 2087

Chlorothiazide Sodium (Possibility of significant hypotension; dosage adjustment may be necessary). Products include:
Diuril Sodium Intravenous 2086

Chlorthalidone (Possibility of significant hypotension; dosage adjustment may be necessary). Products include:
Clorpres Tablets 1002
Combipres Tablets 1040
Tenoretic Tablets 690

Clonidine (Possibility of significant hypotension; dosage adjustment may be necessary). Products include:
Catapres-TTS 1038

Clonidine Hydrochloride (Possibility of significant hypotension; dosage adjustment may be necessary). Products include:
Catapres Tablets 1037
Clorpres Tablets 1002
Combipres Tablets 1040
Duraclon Injection 3057

Deserpidine (Possibility of significant hypotension; dosage adjustment may be necessary).
No products indexed under this heading.

Diazoxide (Possibility of significant hypotension; dosage adjustment may be necessary).
No products indexed under this heading.

Diltiazem Hydrochloride (Possibility of significant hypotension; dosage adjustment may be necessary). Products include:
Cardizem Injectable 1018
Cardizem Lyo-Ject Syringe 1018
Cardizem Monovial 1018
Cardizem CD Capsules 1016
Tiazac Capsules 1378

Doxazosin Mesylate (Possibility of significant hypotension; dosage adjustment may be necessary). Products include:
Cardura Tablets 2668

Enalapril Maleate (Possibility of significant hypotension; dosage adjustment may be necessary). Products include:
Lexxel Tablets 608
Vaseretic Tablets 2204
Vasotec Tablets 2210

Enalaprilat (Possibility of significant hypotension; dosage adjustment may be necessary). Products include:
Enalaprilat Injection 863
Vasotec I.V. Injection 2207

Eprosartan Mesylate (Possibility of significant hypotension; dosage adjustment may be necessary). Products include:
Teveten Tablets 3327

Esmolol Hydrochloride (Possibility of significant hypotension; dosage adjustment may be necessary). Products include:
Brevibloc Injection 858

Felodipine (Possibility of significant hypotension; dosage adjustment may be necessary). Products include:
Lexxel Tablets 608
Plendil Extended-Release Tablets ... 623

Fosinopril Sodium (Possibility of significant hypotension; dosage adjustment may be necessary). Products include:
Monopril Tablets 1091
Monopril HCT 1094

Furosemide (Possibility of significant hypotension; dosage adjustment may be necessary). Products include:
Furosemide Tablets 2284

Guanabenz Acetate (Possibility of significant hypotension; dosage adjustment may be necessary).
No products indexed under this heading.

Guanethidine Monosulfate (Possibility of significant hypotension; dosage adjustment may be necessary).
No products indexed under this heading.

Hydralazine Hydrochloride (Possibility of significant hypotension; dosage adjustment may be necessary).
No products indexed under this heading.

Hydrochlorothiazide (Possibility of significant hypotension; dosage adjustment may be necessary). Products include:
Accuretic Tablets 2614
Aldoril Tablets 2039
Atacand HCT Tablets 597
Avalide Tablets 1070
Diovan HCT Tablets 2338
Dyazide Capsules 1515
HydroDIURIL Tablets 2108
Hyzaar 2109
Inderide Tablets 3517
Inderide LA Long-Acting Capsules .. 3519
Lotensin HCT Tablets 2367
Maxzide 1008
Micardis HCT Tablets 1051
Microzide Capsules 3414
Moduretic Tablets 2138
Monopril HCT 1094
Prinzide Tablets 2168
Timolide Tablets 2187
Uniretic Tablets 3178
Vaseretic Tablets 2204
Zestoretic Tablets 695
Ziac Tablets 1887

Hydroflumethiazide (Possibility of significant hypotension; dosage adjustment may be necessary). Products include:
Diucardin Tablets 3494

Indapamide (Possibility of significant hypotension; dosage adjustment may be necessary). Products include:
Indapamide Tablets 2286

Irbesartan (Possibility of significant hypotension; dosage adjustment may be necessary). Products include:
Avalide Tablets 1070
Avapro Tablets 1074
Avapro Tablets 3076

Isradipine (Possibility of significant hypotension; dosage adjustment may be necessary). Products include:
DynaCirc Capsules 2921
DynaCirc CR Tablets 2923

Labetalol Hydrochloride (Possibility of significant hypotension; dosage adjustment may be necessary). Products include:
Normodyne Injection 3135
Normodyne Tablets 3137

Lisinopril (Possibility of significant hypotension; dosage adjustment may be necessary). Products include:
Prinivil Tablets 2164
Prinzide Tablets 2168
Zestoretic Tablets 695
Zestril Tablets 698

Losartan Potassium (Possibility of significant hypotension; dosage adjustment may be necessary). Products include:
Cozaar Tablets 2067
Hyzaar 2109

Mecamylamine Hydrochloride (Possibility of significant hypotension; dosage adjustment may be necessary). Products include:
Inversine Tablets 1850

Methyclothiazide (Possibility of significant hypotension; dosage adjustment may be necessary).
No products indexed under this heading.

Methyldopa (Possibility of significant hypotension; dosage adjustment may be necessary). Products include:
Aldoclor Tablets 2035
Aldomet Tablets 2037
Aldoril Tablets 2039

Methyldopate Hydrochloride (Possibility of significant hypotension; dosage adjustment may be necessary).
No products indexed under this heading.

Metipranolol Hydrochloride (Possibility of significant hypotension; dosage adjustment may be necessary).
No products indexed under this heading.

Metolazone (Possibility of significant hypotension; dosage adjustment may be necessary). Products include:
Mykrox Tablets 1168
Zaroxolyn Tablets 1177

Metoprolol Succinate (Possibility of significant hypotension; dosage adjustment may be necessary). Products include:
Toprol-XL Tablets 651

Metoprolol Tartrate (Possibility of significant hypotension; dosage adjustment may be necessary).
No products indexed under this heading.

Metyrosine (Possibility of significant hypotension; dosage adjustment may be necessary). Products include:
Demser Capsules 2085

Mibefradil Dihydrochloride (Possibility of significant hypotension; dosage adjustment may be necessary).
No products indexed under this heading.

Minoxidil (Possibility of significant hypotension; dosage adjustment may be necessary). Products include:
Rogaine Extra Strength for Men Topical Solution .... ▣721
Rogaine for Women Topical Solution .... ▣721

Moexipril Hydrochloride (Possibility of significant hypotension; dosage adjustment may be necessary). Products include:
Uniretic Tablets 3178
Univasc Tablets 3181

Nadolol (Possibility of significant hypotension; dosage adjustment may be necessary). Products include:
- Corgard Tablets 2245
- Corzide 40/5 Tablets 2247
- Corzide 80/5 Tablets 2247
- Nadolol Tablets 2288

Nicardipine Hydrochloride (Possibility of significant hypotension; dosage adjustment may be necessary). Products include:
- Cardene I.V. 3485

Nifedipine (Possibility of significant hypotension; dosage adjustment may be necessary). Products include:
- Adalat CC Tablets 877
- Procardia Capsules 2708
- Procardia XL Extended Release Tablets 2710

Nisoldipine (Possibility of significant hypotension; dosage adjustment may be necessary). Products include:
- Sular Tablets 688

Nitroglycerin (Possibility of significant hypotension; dosage adjustment may be necessary). Products include:
- Nitro-Dur Transdermal Infusion System 3134
- Nitro-Dur Transdermal Infusion System 1834
- Nitrolingual Pumpspray 1355
- Nitrostat Tablets 2658

Penbutolol Sulfate (Possibility of significant hypotension; dosage adjustment may be necessary).
No products indexed under this heading.

Perindopril Erbumine (Possibility of significant hypotension; dosage adjustment may be necessary). Products include:
- Aceon Tablets (2 mg, 4 mg, 8 mg) 3249

Phenoxybenzamine Hydrochloride (Possibility of significant hypotension; dosage adjustment may be necessary). Products include:
- Dibenzyline Capsules 3457

Phentolamine Mesylate (Possibility of significant hypotension; dosage adjustment may be necessary).
No products indexed under this heading.

Pindolol (Possibility of significant hypotension; dosage adjustment may be necessary).
No products indexed under this heading.

Polythiazide (Possibility of significant hypotension; dosage adjustment may be necessary). Products include:
- Minizide Capsules 2700
- Renese Tablets 2712

Prazosin Hydrochloride (Possibility of significant hypotension; dosage adjustment may be necessary). Products include:
- Minipress Capsules 2699
- Minizide Capsules 2700

Propranolol Hydrochloride (Possibility of significant hypotension; dosage adjustment may be necessary). Products include:
- Inderal 3513
- Inderal LA Long-Acting Capsules 3516
- Inderide Tablets 3517
- Inderide LA Long-Acting Capsules .. 3519

Quinapril Hydrochloride (Possibility of significant hypotension; dosage adjustment may be necessary). Products include:
- Accupril Tablets 2611
- Accuretic Tablets 2614

Ramipril (Possibility of significant hypotension; dosage adjustment may be necessary). Products include:
- Altace Capsules 2233

Rauwolfia serpentina (Possibility of significant hypotension; dosage adjustment may be necessary).
No products indexed under this heading.

Rescinnamine (Possibility of significant hypotension; dosage adjustment may be necessary).
No products indexed under this heading.

Reserpine (Possibility of significant hypotension; dosage adjustment may be necessary).
No products indexed under this heading.

Sodium Nitroprusside (Possibility of significant hypotension; dosage adjustment may be necessary).
No products indexed under this heading.

Sotalol Hydrochloride (Possibility of significant hypotension; dosage adjustment may be necessary). Products include:
- Betapace Tablets 950
- Betapace AF Tablets 954

Spirapril Hydrochloride (Possibility of significant hypotension; dosage adjustment may be necessary).
No products indexed under this heading.

Telmisartan (Possibility of significant hypotension; dosage adjustment may be necessary). Products include:
- Micardis Tablets 1049
- Micardis HCT Tablets 1051

Timolol Maleate (Possibility of significant hypotension; dosage adjustment may be necessary). Products include:
- Blocadren Tablets 2046
- Cosopt Sterile Ophthalmic Solution 2065
- Timolide Tablets 2187
- Timolol GFS .... ⊙266
- Timoptic in Ocudose 2192
- Timoptic Sterile Ophthalmic Solution 2190
- Timoptic-XE Sterile Ophthalmic Gel Forming Solution 2194

Torsemide (Possibility of significant hypotension; dosage adjustment may be necessary). Products include:
- Demadex Tablets and Injection 2965

Trandolapril (Possibility of significant hypotension; dosage adjustment may be necessary). Products include:
- Mavik Tablets 478
- Tarka Tablets 508

Trimethaphan Camsylate (Possibility of significant hypotension; dosage adjustment may be necessary).
No products indexed under this heading.

Valsartan (Possibility of significant hypotension; dosage adjustment may be necessary). Products include:
- Diovan Capsules 2337
- Diovan HCT Tablets 2338

Verapamil Hydrochloride (Co-administration increases terazosin's mean AUC0-24 by 11% to 24% with associated increase in Cmax (25%) and Cmin (32%)). Products include:
- Covera-HS Tablets 3199
- Isoptin SR Tablets 467
- Tarka Tablets 508
- Verelan Capsules 3184
- Verelan PM Capsules 3186

Food Interactions

Food, unspecified (Delays the time to peak concentration by about 40 minutes; minimal effect on the extent of absorption).

HYZAAR 50-12.5 TABLETS

(Hydrochlorothiazide, Losartan Potassium) 2109

May interact with antihypertensives, barbiturates, corticosteroids, oral hypoglycemic agents, insulin, lithium preparations, narcotic analgesics, nondepolarizing neuromuscular blocking agents, non-steroidal anti-inflammatory agents, potassium preparations, potassium sparing diuretics, and certain other agents. Compounds in these categories include:

Acarbose (Hyperglycemia may occur with thiazide diuretics; dosage adjustment of the antidiabetic drug may be required). Products include:
- Precose Tablets 906

Acebutolol Hydrochloride (Additive effect or potentiation of other antihypertensives). Products include:
- Sectral Capsules 3589

ACTH (Potential for intensified electrolyte depletion particularly hypokalemia).
No products indexed under this heading.

Alfentanil Hydrochloride (Potentiation of orthostatic hypotension).
No products indexed under this heading.

Amiloride Hydrochloride (Concomitant use with potassium-sparing diuretics may lead to hyperkalemia). Products include:
- Midamor Tablets 2136
- Moduretic Tablets 2138

Amlodipine Besylate (Additive effect or potentiation of other antihypertensives). Products include:
- Lotrel Capsules 2370
- Norvasc Tablets 2704

Aprobarbital (Potentiation of orthostatic hypotension).
No products indexed under this heading.

Atenolol (Additive effect or potentiation of other antihypertensives). Products include:
- Tenoretic Tablets 690
- Tenormin I.V. Injection 692

Atracurium Besylate (Possible increased responsiveness to the muscle relaxant).
No products indexed under this heading.

Benazepril Hydrochloride (Additive effect or potentiation of other antihypertensives). Products include:
- Lotensin Tablets 2365
- Lotensin HCT Tablets 2367
- Lotrel Capsules 2370

Bendroflumethiazide (Additive effect or potentiation of other antihypertensives). Products include:
- Corzide 40/5 Tablets 2247
- Corzide 80/5 Tablets 2247

Betamethasone Acetate (Potential for intensified electrolyte depletion particularly hypokalemia). Products include:
- Celestone Soluspan Injectable Suspension 3097

Betamethasone Sodium Phosphate (Potential for intensified electrolyte depletion particularly hypokalemia). Products include:
- Celestone Soluspan Injectable Suspension 3097

Betaxolol Hydrochloride (Additive effect or potentiation of other antihypertensives). Products include:
- Betoptic S Ophthalmic Suspension 537

Bisoprolol Fumarate (Additive effect or potentiation of other antihypertensives). Products include:
- Zebeta Tablets 1885
- Ziac Tablets 1887

Buprenorphine Hydrochloride (Potentiation of orthostatic hypotension). Products include:
- Buprenex Injectable 2918

Butabarbital (Potentiation of orthostatic hypotension).
No products indexed under this heading.

Butalbital (Potentiation of orthostatic hypotension). Products include:
- Phrenilin 578
- Sedapap Tablets 50 mg/650 mg 2225

Candesartan Cilexetil (Additive effect or potentiation of other antihypertensives). Products include:
- Atacand Tablets 595
- Atacand HCT Tablets 597

Captopril (Additive effect or potentiation of other antihypertensives). Products include:
- Captopril Tablets 2281

Carteolol Hydrochloride (Additive effect or potentiation of other antihypertensives). Products include:
- Carteolol Hydrochloride Ophthalmic Solution USP, 1% .... ⊙258
- Ocupress Ophthalmic Solution, 1% Sterile .... ⊙303

Celecoxib (Potential reduced diuretic, natriuretic, and antihypertensive effects). Products include:
- Celebrex Capsules 2676
- Celebrex Capsules 2780

Chlorothiazide (Additive effect or potentiation of other antihypertensives). Products include:
- Aldoclor Tablets 2035
- Diuril Oral 2087

Chlorothiazide Sodium (Additive effect or potentiation of other antihypertensives). Products include:
- Diuril Sodium Intravenous 2086

Chlorpropamide (Hyperglycemia may occur with thiazide diuretics; dosage adjustment of the antidiabetic drug may be required). Products include:
- Diabinese Tablets 2680

Chlorthalidone (Additive effect or potentiation of other antihypertensives). Products include:
- Clorpres Tablets 1002
- Combipres Tablets 1040
- Tenoretic Tablets 690

Cholestyramine (Absorption of hydrochlorothiazide is impaired in the presence of anionic exchange resins; cholestyramine binds hydrochlorothiazide and reduces its absorption from GI tract by up to 85%).
No products indexed under this heading.

Cimetidine (Co-administration may lead to an increase of about 18% in AUC of losartan but did not affect the pharmacokinetics of its active metabolite). Products include:
- Tagamet HB 200 Suspension .... ▣762
- Tagamet HB 200 Tablets .... ▣761
- Tagamet Tablets 1644

Cimetidine Hydrochloride (Co-administration may lead to an increase of about 18% in AUC of losartan but did not affect the pharmacokinetics of its active metabolite). Products include:
- Tagamet 1644

Cisatracurium Besylate (Possible increased responsiveness to the muscle relaxant).
No products indexed under this heading.

Clonidine (Additive effect or potentiation of other antihypertensives). Products include:
- Catapres-TTS 1038

Clonidine Hydrochloride (Additive effect or potentiation of other antihypertensives). Products include:
- Catapres Tablets 1037
- Clorpres Tablets 1002
- Combipres Tablets 1040
- Duraclon Injection 3057

Codeine Phosphate (Potentiation of orthostatic hypotension). Products include:
- Phenergan with Codeine Syrup 3557
- Phenergan VC with Codeine Syrup .. 3561
- Robitussin A-C Syrup 2942
- Robitussin-DAC Syrup 2942
- Ryna-C Liquid .... ▣768
- Soma Compound w/Codeine Tablets 3355
- Tussi-Organidin NR Liquid 3350
- Tussi-Organidin-S NR Liquid 3350
- Tylenol with Codeine 2595

Colestipol Hydrochloride (Absorption of hydrochlorothiazide is impaired in the presence of anionic exchange resins; cholestyramine

IMPORTANT NOTE: Always consult each drug listing in the patient's regimen for possible interactions.

binds hydrochlorothiazide and reduces its absorption from GI tract by up to 85%). Products include:
Colestid Tablets 2791

Cortisone Acetate (Potential for intensified electrolyte depletion particularly hypokalemia). Products include:
Cortone Acetate Injectable Suspension 2059
Cortone Acetate Tablets 2061

Deserpidine (Additive effect or potentiation of other antihypertensives).
No products indexed under this heading.

Dexamethasone (Potential for intensified electrolyte depletion particularly hypokalemia). Products include:
Decadron Elixir 2078
Decadron Tablets 2079
TobraDex Ophthalmic Ointment 542
TobraDex Ophthalmic Suspension 541

Dexamethasone Acetate (Potential for intensified electrolyte depletion particularly hypokalemia).
No products indexed under this heading.

Dexamethasone Sodium Phosphate (Potential for intensified electrolyte depletion particularly hypokalemia). Products include:
Decadron Phosphate Injection 2081
Decadron Phosphate Sterile Ophthalmic Ointment 2083
Decadron Phosphate Sterile Ophthalmic Solution 2084
NeoDecadron Sterile Ophthalmic Solution 2144

Dezocine (Potentiation of orthostatic hypotension).
No products indexed under this heading.

Diazoxide (Additive effect or potentiation of other antihypertensives).
No products indexed under this heading.

Diclofenac Potassium (Potential reduced diuretic, natriuretic, and antihypertensive effects). Products include:
Cataflam Tablets 2315

Diclofenac Sodium (Potential reduced diuretic, natriuretic, and antihypertensive effects). Products include:
Arthrotec Tablets 3195
Voltaren Ophthalmic Sterile Ophthalmic Solution .... ⊙312
Voltaren Tablets 2315
Voltaren-XR Tablets 2315

Diltiazem Hydrochloride (Additive effect or potentiation of other antihypertensives). Products include:
Cardizem Injectable 1018
Cardizem Lyo-Ject Syringe 1018
Cardizem Monovial 1018
Cardizem CD Capsules 1016
Tiazac Capsules 1378

Doxazosin Mesylate (Additive effect or potentiation of other antihypertensives). Products include:
Cardura Tablets 2668

Enalapril Maleate (Additive effect or potentiation of other antihypertensives). Products include:
Lexxel Tablets 608
Vaseretic Tablets 2204
Vasotec Tablets 2210

Enalaprilat (Additive effect or potentiation of other antihypertensives). Products include:
Enalaprilat Injection 863
Vasotec I.V. Injection 2207

Eprosartan Mesylate (Additive effect or potentiation of other antihypertensives). Products include:
Teveten Tablets 3327

Esmolol Hydrochloride (Additive effect or potentiation of other antihypertensives). Products include:
Brevibloc Injection 858

Etodolac (Potential reduced diuretic, natriuretic, and antihypertensive effects). Products include:
Lodine 3528
Lodine XL Extended-Release Tablets 3530

Felodipine (Additive effect or potentiation of other antihypertensives). Products include:
Lexxel Tablets 608
Plendil Extended-Release Tablets 623

Fenoprofen Calcium (Potential reduced diuretic, natriuretic, and antihypertensive effects).
No products indexed under this heading.

Fentanyl (Potentiation of orthostatic hypotension). Products include:
Duragesic Transdermal System 1786

Fentanyl Citrate (Potentiation of orthostatic hypotension). Products include:
Actiq 1184

Fludrocortisone Acetate (Potential for intensified electrolyte depletion particularly hypokalemia). Products include:
Florinef Acetate Tablets 2250

Flurbiprofen (Potential reduced diuretic, natriuretic, and antihypertensive effects).
No products indexed under this heading.

Fosinopril Sodium (Additive effect or potentiation of other antihypertensives). Products include:
Monopril Tablets 1091
Monopril HCT 1094

Furosemide (Additive effect or potentiation of other antihypertensives). Products include:
Furosemide Tablets 2284

Gestodene (*In Vitro* studies show significant inhibition of the formation of the active metabolite by inhibitors of P4503A4 such as gestodene; pharmacodynamic consequences of concomitant use is undefined).
No products indexed under this heading.

Glimepiride (Hyperglycemia may occur with thiazide diuretics; dosage adjustment of the antidiabetic drug may be required). Products include:
Amaryl Tablets 717

Glipizide (Hyperglycemia may occur with thiazide diuretics; dosage adjustment of the antidiabetic drug may be required). Products include:
Glucotrol Tablets 2692
Glucotrol XL Extended Release Tablets 2693

Glyburide (Hyperglycemia may occur with thiazide diuretics; dosage adjustment of the antidiabetic drug may be required). Products include:
DiaBeta Tablets 741
Glucovance Tablets 1086

Guanabenz Acetate (Additive effect or potentiation of other antihypertensives).
No products indexed under this heading.

Guanethidine Monosulfate (Additive effect or potentiation of other antihypertensives).
No products indexed under this heading.

Hydralazine Hydrochloride (Additive effect or potentiation of other antihypertensives).
No products indexed under this heading.

Hydrocodone Bitartrate (Potentiation of orthostatic hypotension). Products include:
Hycodan 1316
Hycomine Compound Tablets 1317
Hycotuss Expectorant Syrup 1318
Lortab 3319
Lortab Elixir 3317
Maxidone Tablets CIII 3399
Norco 5/325 Tablets CIII 3424
Norco 7.5/325 Tablets CIII 3425
Norco 10/325 Tablets CIII 3427
Norco 10/325 Tablets CIII 3425
Vicodin Tablets 516
Vicodin ES Tablets 517
Vicodin HP Tablets 518
Vicodin Tuss Expectorant 519
Vicoprofen Tablets 520
Zydone Tablets 1330

Hydrocodone Polistirex (Potentiation of orthostatic hypotension). Products include:
Tussionex Pennkinetic Extended-Release Suspension 1174

Hydrocortisone (Potential for intensified electrolyte depletion particularly hypokalemia). Products include:
Anusol-HC Cream 2.5% 2237
Cipro HC Otic Suspension 540
Cortaid Intensive Therapy Cream .... ■717
Cortaid Maximum Strength Cream .... ■717
Cortisporin Ophthalmic Suspension Sterile .... ⊙297
Cortizone•5 .... ■699
Cortizone•10 .... ■699
Cortizone•10 Plus Creme .... ■700
Cortizone for Kids Creme .... ■699
Hydrocortone Tablets 2106
Massengill Medicated Soft Cloth Towelette .... ■753
VōSoL HC Otic Solution 3356

Hydrocortisone Acetate (Potential for intensified electrolyte depletion particularly hypokalemia). Products include:
Analpram-HC 1338
Anusol HC-1 Hydrocortisone Anti-Itch Cream .... ■689
Anusol-HC Suppositories 2238
Cortaid .... ■717
Cortifoam Rectal Foam 3170
Cortisporin-TC Otic Suspension 2246
Hydrocortone Acetate Injectable Suspension 2103
Pramosone 1343
Proctocort Suppositories 2264
ProctoFoam-HC 3177
Terra-Cortril Ophthalmic Suspension 2716

Hydrocortisone Sodium Phosphate (Potential for intensified electrolyte depletion particularly hypokalemia). Products include:
Hydrocortone Phosphate Injection, Sterile 2105

Hydrocortisone Sodium Succinate (Potential for intensified electrolyte depletion particularly hypokalemia).
No products indexed under this heading.

Hydroflumethiazide (Additive effect or potentiation of other antihypertensives). Products include:
Diucardin Tablets 3494

Hydromorphone Hydrochloride (Potentiation of orthostatic hypotension). Products include:
Dilaudid 441
Dilaudid Oral Liquid 445
Dilaudid Powder 441
Dilaudid Rectal Suppositories 441
Dilaudid Tablets 441
Dilaudid Tablets - 8 mg 445
Dilaudid-HP 443

Ibuprofen (Potential reduced diuretic, natriuretic, and antihypertensive effects). Products include:
Advil .... ■771
Children's Advil Oral Suspension .... ■773
Children's Advil Chewable Tablets .... ■773
Advil Cold and Sinus Caplets .... ■771
Advil Cold and Sinus Tablets .... ■771
Advil Flu & Body Ache Caplets .... ■772
Infants' Advil Drops .... ■773
Junior Strength Advil Tablets .... ■773
Junior Strength Advil Chewable Tablets .... ■773
Advil Migraine Liquigels .... ■772
Children's Motrin Oral Suspension and Chewable Tablets 2006
Children's Motrin Cold Oral Suspension 2007
Children's Motrin Oral Suspension .... ■643
Motrin Suspension, Oral Drops, Chewable Tablets, and Caplets 2002
Infants' Motrin Concentrated Drops 2006
Junior Strength Motrin Caplets and Chewable Tablets 2006
Motrin IB Tablets, Caplets, and Gelcaps 2002
Motrin Migraine Pain Caplets 2005
Motrin Sinus Headache Caplets 2005
Vicoprofen Tablets 520

Indapamide (Additive effect or potentiation of other antihypertensives). Products include:
Indapamide Tablets 2286

Indomethacin (Potential reduced diuretic, natriuretic, and antihypertensive effects). Products include:
Indocin 2112

Indomethacin Sodium Trihydrate (Potential reduced diuretic, natriuretic, and antihypertensive effects). Products include:
Indocin I.V. 2115

Insulin, Human, Zinc Suspension (Hyperglycemia may occur with thiazide diuretics; dosage adjustment of the antidiabetic drug may be required). Products include:
Humulin L, 100 Units 1937
Humulin U, 100 Units 1943
Novolin L Human Insulin 10 ml Vials 2422

Insulin, Human NPH (Hyperglycemia may occur with thiazide diuretics; dosage adjustment of the antidiabetic drug may be required). Products include:
Humulin N, 100 Units 1939
Humulin N NPH Pen 1940
Novolin N Human Insulin 10 ml Vials 2422
Novolin N PenFill 2423
Novolin N Prefilled Syringe Disposable Insulin Delivery System 2425

Insulin, Human Regular (Hyperglycemia may occur with thiazide diuretics; dosage adjustment of the antidiabetic drug may be required). Products include:
Humulin R Regular (U-500) 1943
Humulin R, 100 Units 1941
Novolin R Human Insulin 10 ml Vials 2423
Novolin R PenFill 2423
Novolin R Prefilled Syringe Disposable Insulin Delivery System 2425
Velosulin BR Human Insulin 10 ml Vials 2435

Insulin, Human Regular and Human NPH Mixture (Hyperglycemia may occur with thiazide diuretics; dosage adjustment of the antidiabetic drug may be required). Products include:
Humulin 50/50, 100 Units 1934
Humulin 70/30, 100 Units 1935
Humulin 70/30 Pen 1936
Novolin 70/30 Human Insulin 10 ml Vials 2421
Novolin 70/30 PenFill 2423
Novolin 70/30 Prefilled Disposable Insulin Delivery System 2425

Insulin, NPH (Hyperglycemia may occur with thiazide diuretics; dosage adjustment of the antidiabetic drug may be required). Products include:
Iletin II, NPH (Pork), 100 Units 1946

Insulin, Regular (Hyperglycemia may occur with thiazide diuretics; dosage adjustment of the antidiabetic drug may be required). Products include:
Iletin II, Regular (Pork), 100 Units 1947

Insulin, Zinc Crystals (Hyperglycemia may occur with thiazide diuretics; dosage adjustment of the antidiabetic drug may be required).
No products indexed under this heading.

Insulin, Zinc Suspension (Hyperglycemia may occur with thiazide diuretics; dosage adjustment of the antidiabetic drug may be required). Products include:
Iletin II, Lente (Pork), 100 Units 1945

Insulin Aspart, Human Regular (Hyperglycemia may occur with thiazide diuretics; dosage adjustment of the antidiabetic drug may be required).
No products indexed under this heading.

Insulin glargine (Hyperglycemia may occur with thiazide diuretics; dosage adjustment of the antidiabetic drug may be required). Products include:
Lantus Injection 742

Insulin Lispro, Human (Hyperglycemia may occur with thiazide diuretics; dosage adjustment of the antidiabetic drug may be required). Products include:
Humalog 1926
Humalog Mix 75/25 Pen 1928

Insulin Lispro Protamine, Human (Hyperglycemia may occur with thiazide diuretics; dosage adjustment of the antidiabetic drug may be required). Products include:
Humalog Mix 75/25 Pen 1928

Irbesartan (Additive effect or potentiation of other antihypertensives). Products include:
Avalide Tablets 1070
Avapro Tablets 1074
Avapro Tablets 3076

Isradipine (Additive effect or potentiation of other antihypertensives). Products include:
DynaCirc Capsules 2921
DynaCirc CR Tablets 2923

Ketoconazole (*In Vitro* studies show significant inhibition of the formation of the active metabolite by inhibitors of P4503A4 such as ketoconazole or complete inhibition by the combination of ketoconazole and sulfaphenazole; pharmacodynamic consequences of concomitantuse are undefined). Products include:
Nizoral 2% Cream 3620
Nizoral A-D Shampoo 2008
Nizoral 2% Shampoo 2007
Nizoral Tablets 1791

Ketoprofen (Potential reduced diuretic, natriuretic, and antihypertensive effects). Products include:
Orudis Capsules 3548
Orudis KT Tablets 778
Oruvail Capsules 3548

Ketorolac Tromethamine (Potential reduced diuretic, natriuretic, and antihypertensive effects). Products include:
Acular Ophthalmic Solution 544
Acular PF Ophthalmic Solution 544
Toradol 3018

Labetalol Hydrochloride (Additive effect or potentiation of other antihypertensives). Products include:
Normodyne Injection 3135
Normodyne Tablets 3137

Levobunolol Hydrochloride (Additive effect or potentiation of other antihypertensives). Products include:
Betagan .... ⊙ 228

Levorphanol Tartrate (Potentiation of orthostatic hypotension). Products include:
Levo-Dromoran 1734
Levorphanol Tartrate Tablets 3059

Lisinopril (Additive effect or potentiation of other antihypertensives). Products include:
Prinivil Tablets 2164
Prinzide Tablets 2168
Zestoretic Tablets 695
Zestril Tablets 698

Lithium Carbonate (Diuretics reduce the renal clearance of lithium and add a high risk of lithium toxicity; concurrent use should be avoided). Products include:
Eskalith 1527
Lithium Carbonate 3061
Lithobid Slow-Release Tablets 3255

Lithium Citrate (Diuretics reduce the renal clearance of lithium and add a high risk of lithium toxicity; concurrent use should be avoided). Products include:
Lithium Citrate Syrup 3061

Mecamylamine Hydrochloride (Additive effect or potentiation of other antihypertensives). Products include:
Inversine Tablets 1850

Meclofenamate Sodium (Potential reduced diuretic, natriuretic, and antihypertensive effects).
No products indexed under this heading.

Mefenamic Acid (Potential reduced diuretic, natriuretic, and antihypertensive effects). Products include:
Ponstel Capsules 1356

Meloxicam (Potential reduced diuretic, natriuretic, and antihypertensive effects). Products include:
Mobic Tablets 1054

Meperidine Hydrochloride (Potentiation of orthostatic hypotension). Products include:
Demerol 3079
Mepergan Injection 3539

Mephobarbital (Potentiation of orthostatic hypotension).
No products indexed under this heading.

Metformin Hydrochloride (Hyperglycemia may occur with thiazide diuretics; dosage adjustment of the antidiabetic drug may be required). Products include:
Glucophage Tablets 1080
Glucophage XR Tablets 1080
Glucovance Tablets 1086

Methadone Hydrochloride (Potentiation of orthostatic hypotension). Products include:
Dolophine Hydrochloride Tablets 3056

Methyclothiazide (Additive effect or potentiation of other antihypertensives).
No products indexed under this heading.

Methyldopa (Additive effect or potentiation of other antihypertensives). Products include:
Aldoclor Tablets 2035
Aldomet Tablets 2037
Aldoril Tablets 2039

Methyldopate Hydrochloride (Additive effect or potentiation of other antihypertensives).
No products indexed under this heading.

Methylprednisolone Acetate (Potential for intensified electrolyte depletion particularly hypokalemia). Products include:
Depo-Medrol Injectable Suspension 2795

Methylprednisolone Sodium Succinate (Potential for intensified electrolyte depletion particularly hypokalemia). Products include:
Solu-Medrol Sterile Powder 2855

Metipranolol Hydrochloride (Additive effect or potentiation of other antihypertensives).
No products indexed under this heading.

Metocurine Iodide (Possible increased responsiveness to the muscle relaxant).
No products indexed under this heading.

Metolazone (Additive effect or potentiation of other antihypertensives). Products include:
Mykrox Tablets 1168
Zaroxolyn Tablets 1177

Metoprolol Succinate (Additive effect or potentiation of other antihypertensives). Products include:
Toprol-XL Tablets 651

Metoprolol Tartrate (Additive effect or potentiation of other antihypertensives).
No products indexed under this heading.

Metyrosine (Additive effect or potentiation of other antihypertensives). Products include:
Demser Capsules 2085

Mibefradil Dihydrochloride (Additive effect or potentiation of other antihypertensives).
No products indexed under this heading.

Miglitol (Hyperglycemia may occur with thiazide diuretics; dosage adjustment of the antidiabetic drug may be required). Products include:
Glyset Tablets 2821

Minoxidil (Additive effect or potentiation of other antihypertensives). Products include:
Rogaine Extra Strength for Men Topical Solution 721
Rogaine for Women Topical Solution 721

Mivacurium Chloride (Possible increased responsiveness to the muscle relaxant).
No products indexed under this heading.

Moexipril Hydrochloride (Additive effect or potentiation of other antihypertensives). Products include:
Uniretic Tablets 3178
Univasc Tablets 3181

Morphine Sulfate (Potentiation of orthostatic hypotension). Products include:
Astramorph/PF Injection, USP (Preservative-Free) 594
Duramorph Injection 1312
Infumorph 200 and Infumorph 500 Sterile Solutions 1314
Kadian Capsules 1335
MS Contin Tablets 2896
MSIR 2898
Oramorph SR Tablets 3062
Roxanol 3066

Nabumetone (Potential reduced diuretic, natriuretic, and antihypertensive effects). Products include:
Relafen Tablets 1617

Nadolol (Additive effect or potentiation of other antihypertensives). Products include:
Corgard Tablets 2245
Corzide 40/5 Tablets 2247
Corzide 80/5 Tablets 2247
Nadolol Tablets 2288

Naproxen (Potential reduced diuretic, natriuretic, and antihypertensive effects). Products include:
EC-Naprosyn Delayed-Release Tablets 2967
Naprosyn Suspension 2967
Naprosyn Tablets 2967

Naproxen Sodium (Potential reduced diuretic, natriuretic, and antihypertensive effects). Products include:
Aleve Tablets, Caplets and Gelcaps 602
Aleve Cold & Sinus Caplets 603
Anaprox Tablets 2967
Anaprox DS Tablets 2967
Naprelan Tablets 1293

Nicardipine Hydrochloride (Additive effect or potentiation of other antihypertensives). Products include:
Cardene I.V. 3485

Nifedipine (Additive effect or potentiation of other antihypertensives). Products include:
Adalat CC Tablets 877
Procardia Capsules 2708
Procardia XL Extended Release Tablets 2710

Nisoldipine (Additive effect or potentiation of other antihypertensives). Products include:
Sular Tablets 688

Nitroglycerin (Additive effect or potentiation of other antihypertensives). Products include:
Nitro-Dur Transdermal Infusion System 3134
Nitro-Dur Transdermal Infusion System 1834
Nitrolingual Pumpspray 1355
Nitrostat Tablets 2658

Norepinephrine Bitartrate (Possible decreased response to pressor amines).
No products indexed under this heading.

Oxaprozin (Potential reduced diuretic, natriuretic, and antihypertensive effects).
No products indexed under this heading.

Oxycodone Hydrochloride (Potentiation of orthostatic hypotension). Products include:
OxyContin Tablets 2912
OxyFast Oral Concentrate Solution 2916
OxyIR Capsules 2916
Percocet Tablets 1326
Percodan Tablets 1327
Percolone Tablets 1327
Roxicodone 3067
Tylox Capsules 2597

Pancuronium Bromide (Possible increased responsiveness to the muscle relaxant).
No products indexed under this heading.

Penbutolol Sulfate (Additive effect or potentiation of other antihypertensives).
No products indexed under this heading.

Pentobarbital Sodium (Potentiation of orthostatic hypotension). Products include:
Nembutal Sodium Solution 485

Perindopril Erbumine (Additive effect or potentiation of other antihypertensives). Products include:
Aceon Tablets (2 mg, 4 mg, 8 mg) 3249

Phenobarbital (Co-administration may lead to a reduction of about 20% in AUC of losartan and its active metabolite; potentiation of orthostatic hypotension). Products include:
Arco-Lase Plus Tablets 592
Donnatal 2929
Donnatal Extentabs 2930

Phenoxybenzamine Hydrochloride (Additive effect or potentiation of other antihypertensives). Products include:
Dibenzyline Capsules 3457

Phentolamine Mesylate (Additive effect or potentiation of other antihypertensives).
No products indexed under this heading.

Phenylbutazone (Potential reduced diuretic, natriuretic, and antihypertensive effects).
No products indexed under this heading.

Pindolol (Additive effect or potentiation of other antihypertensives).
No products indexed under this heading.

Pioglitazone Hydrochloride (Hyperglycemia may occur with thiazide diuretics; dosage adjustment of the antidiabetic drug may be required). Products include:
Actos Tablets 3275

Piroxicam (Potential reduced diuretic, natriuretic, and antihypertensive effects). Products include:
Feldene Capsules 2685

Polythiazide (Additive effect or potentiation of other antihypertensives). Products include:
Minizide Capsules 2700
Renese Tablets 2712

Potassium Acid Phosphate (Concomitant use with potassium supplements may lead to hyperkalemia). Products include:
K-Phos Original (Sodium Free) Tablets 947

Potassium Bicarbonate (Concomitant use with potassium supplements may lead to hyperkalemia).
No products indexed under this heading.

Potassium Chloride (Concomitant use with potassium supplements may lead to hyperkalemia). Products include:
Chlor-3 1361
Colyte with Flavor Packs for Oral Solution 3170

IMPORTANT NOTE: Always consult each drug listing in the patient's regimen for possible interactions.

GoLYTELY and Pineapple Flavor GoLYTELY for Oral Solution 1068
K-Dur Microburst Release System ER Tablets 1832
Klor-Con M20/Klor-Con M10 Tablets 3329
K-Lor Powder Packets 469
K-Tab Filmtab Tablets 470
Micro-K 3311
NuLYTELY, Cherry Flavor, Lemon-Lime Flavor, and Orange Flavor NuLYTELY for Oral Solution 1068
Rum-K 1363

Potassium Citrate (Concomitant use with potassium supplements may lead to hyperkalemia). Products include:
Urocit-K Tablets 2232

Potassium Gluconate (Concomitant use with potassium supplements may lead to hyperkalemia).
No products indexed under this heading.

Potassium Phosphate (Concomitant use with potassium supplements may lead to hyperkalemia). Products include:
K-Phos Neutral Tablets 946

Prazosin Hydrochloride (Additive effect or potentiation of other antihypertensives). Products include:
Minipress Capsules 2699
Minizide Capsules 2700

Prednisolone Acetate (Potential for intensified electrolyte depletion particularly hypokalemia). Products include:
Blephamide Ophthalmic Ointment 547
Blephamide Ophthalmic Suspension 548
Poly-Pred Liquifilm Ophthalmic Suspension .... ⊙245
Pred Forte Ophthalmic Suspension .... ⊙246
Pred Mild Sterile Ophthalmic Suspension .... ⊙249
Pred-G Ophthalmic Suspension .... ⊙247
Pred-G Sterile Ophthalmic Ointment .... ⊙248

Prednisolone Sodium Phosphate (Potential for intensified electrolyte depletion particularly hypokalemia). Products include:
Pediapred Oral Solution 1170

Prednisolone Tebutate (Potential for intensified electrolyte depletion particularly hypokalemia).
No products indexed under this heading.

Prednisone (Potential for intensified electrolyte depletion particularly hypokalemia). Products include:
Prednisone 3064

Propoxyphene Hydrochloride (Potentiation of orthostatic hypotension). Products include:
Darvon Pulvules 1909
Darvon Compound-65 Pulvules 1910

Propoxyphene Napsylate (Potentiation of orthostatic hypotension). Products include:
Darvon-N/Darvocet-N 1907
Darvon-N Tablets 1912

Propranolol Hydrochloride (Additive effect or potentiation of other antihypertensives). Products include:
Inderal 3513
Inderal LA Long-Acting Capsules 3516
Inderide Tablets 3517
Inderide LA Long-Acting Capsules 3519

Quinapril Hydrochloride (Additive effect or potentiation of other antihypertensives). Products include:
Accupril Tablets 2611
Accuretic Tablets 2614

Ramipril (Additive effect or potentiation of other antihypertensives). Products include:
Altace Capsules 2233

Rapacuronium Bromide (Possible increased responsiveness to the muscle relaxant).
No products indexed under this heading.

Rauwolfia serpentina (Additive effect or potentiation of other antihypertensives).
No products indexed under this heading.

Remifentanil Hydrochloride (Potentiation of orthostatic hypotension).
No products indexed under this heading.

Repaglinide (Hyperglycemia may occur with thiazide diuretics; dosage adjustment of the antidiabetic drug may be required). Products include:
Prandin Tablets (0.5, 1, and 2 mg) 2432

Rescinnamine (Additive effect or potentiation of other antihypertensives).
No products indexed under this heading.

Reserpine (Additive effect or potentiation of other antihypertensives).
No products indexed under this heading.

Rocuronium Bromide (Possible increased responsiveness to the muscle relaxant). Products include:
Zemuron Injection 2491

Rofecoxib (Potential reduced diuretic, natriuretic, and antihypertensive effects). Products include:
Vioxx 2213

Rosiglitazone Maleate (Hyperglycemia may occur with thiazide diuretics; dosage adjustment of the antidiabetic drug may be required). Products include:
Avandia Tablets 1490

Salt Substitutes (Concomitant use with salt substitutes may lead to hyperkalemia).
No products indexed under this heading.

Secobarbital Sodium (Potentiation of orthostatic hypotension).
No products indexed under this heading.

Sodium Nitroprusside (Additive effect or potentiation of other antihypertensives).
No products indexed under this heading.

Sotalol Hydrochloride (Additive effect or potentiation of other antihypertensives). Products include:
Betapace Tablets 950
Betapace AF Tablets 954

Spirapril Hydrochloride (Additive effect or potentiation of other antihypertensives).
No products indexed under this heading.

Spironolactone (Concomitant use with potassium-sparing diuretics may lead to hyperkalemia).
No products indexed under this heading.

Sufentanil Citrate (Potentiation of orthostatic hypotension).
No products indexed under this heading.

Sulfaphenazole (*In Vitro* studies show significant inhibition of the formation of the active metabolite by inhibitors of P4503A4 such as sulfaphenazole; pharmacodynamic consequences of concomitant use are undefined).
No products indexed under this heading.

Sulindac (Potential reduced diuretic, natriuretic, and antihypertensive effects). Products include:
Clinoril Tablets 2053

Telmisartan (Additive effect or potentiation of other antihypertensives). Products include:
Micardis Tablets 1049
Micardis HCT Tablets 1051

Terazosin Hydrochloride (Additive effect or potentiation of other antihypertensives). Products include:
Hytrin Capsules 464

Thiamylal Sodium (Potentiation of orthostatic hypotension).
No products indexed under this heading.

Timolol Maleate (Additive effect or potentiation of other antihypertensives). Products include:
Blocadren Tablets 2046
Cosopt Sterile Ophthalmic Solution 2065
Timolide Tablets 2187
Timolol GFS .... ⊙266
Timoptic in Ocudose 2192
Timoptic Sterile Ophthalmic Solution 2190
Timoptic-XE Sterile Ophthalmic Gel Forming Solution 2194

Tolazamide (Hyperglycemia may occur with thiazide diuretics; dosage adjustment of the antidiabetic drug may be required).
No products indexed under this heading.

Tolbutamide (Hyperglycemia may occur with thiazide diuretics; dosage adjustment of the antidiabetic drug may be required).
No products indexed under this heading.

Tolmetin Sodium (Potential reduced diuretic, natriuretic, and antihypertensive effects). Products include:
Tolectin 2589

Torsemide (Additive effect or potentiation of other antihypertensives). Products include:
Demadex Tablets and Injection 2965

Trandolapril (Additive effect or potentiation of other antihypertensives). Products include:
Mavik Tablets 478
Tarka Tablets 508

Triamcinolone (Potential for intensified electrolyte depletion particularly hypokalemia).
No products indexed under this heading.

Triamcinolone Acetonide (Potential for intensified electrolyte depletion particularly hypokalemia). Products include:
Azmacort Inhalation Aerosol 728
Nasacort Nasal Inhaler 750
Nasacort AQ Nasal Spray 752
Tri-Nasal Spray 2274

Triamcinolone Diacetate (Potential for intensified electrolyte depletion particularly hypokalemia).
No products indexed under this heading.

Triamcinolone Hexacetonide (Potential for intensified electrolyte depletion particularly hypokalemia).
No products indexed under this heading.

Triamterene (Concomitant use with potassium-sparing diuretics may lead to hyperkalemia). Products include:
Dyazide Capsules 1515
Dyrenium Capsules 3458
Maxzide 1008

Trimethaphan Camsylate (Additive effect or potentiation of other antihypertensives).
No products indexed under this heading.

Troglitazone (Hyperglycemia may occur with thiazide diuretics; dosage adjustment of the antidiabetic drug may be required).
No products indexed under this heading.

Troleandomycin (*In Vitro* studies show significant inhibition of the formation of the active metabolite by inhibitors of P4503A4 such as troleandomycin; pharmacodynamic consequences of concomitant use are undefined). Products include:
Tao Capsules 2716

Valsartan (Additive effect or potentiation of other antihypertensives). Products include:
Diovan Capsules 2337
Diovan HCT Tablets 2338

Vecuronium Bromide (Possible increased responsiveness to the muscle relaxant). Products include:
Norcuron for Injection 2478

Verapamil Hydrochloride (Additive effect or potentiation of other antihypertensives). Products include:
Covera-HS Tablets 3199
Isoptin SR Tablets 467
Tarka Tablets 508
Verelan Capsules 3184
Verelan PM Capsules 3186

Food Interactions

Alcohol (Potentiation of orthostatic hypotension).

Meal, unspecified (Meal slows absorption and decreases Cmax but has minor effects on losartan AUC or on the AUC of the metabolite).

HYZAAR 100-25 TABLETS
(Hydrochlorothiazide, Losartan Potassium) 2109
See Hyzaar 50-12.5 Tablets

IDAMYCIN PFS INJECTION
(Idarubicin Hydrochloride) 2825
May interact with anthracyclines. Compounds in these categories include:

Daunorubicin Citrate (Previous therapy with anthracyclines is co-factor for increased cardiac toxicity). Products include:
DaunoXome Injection 1442

Daunorubicin Hydrochloride (Previous therapy with anthracyclines is co-factor for increased cardiac toxicity). Products include:
Cerubidine for Injection 947

Doxorubicin Hydrochloride (Previous therapy with anthracyclines is co-factor for increased cardiac toxicity). Products include:
Adriamycin PFS/RDF Injection 2767
Doxil Injection 566

Epirubicin Hydrochloride (Previous therapy with anthracyclines is co-factor for increased cardiac toxicity). Products include:
Ellence Injection 2806

Valrubicin (Previous therapy with anthracyclines is co-factor for increased cardiac toxicity). Products include:
Valstar Sterile Solution for Intravesical Instillation 1175

IFEX FOR INJECTION
(Ifosfamide) 1123
May interact with:

Bone Marrow Depressants, unspecified (Adjustments in dosing may be necessary).

ILETIN II, LENTE (PORK), 100 UNITS
(Insulin, Zinc Suspension) 1945
See Iletin II, Regular (Pork), 100 Units

ILETIN II, NPH (PORK), 100 UNITS
(Insulin, NPH) 1946
See Iletin II, Regular (Pork), 100 Units

ILETIN II, REGULAR (PORK), 100 UNITS
(Insulin, Regular) 1947
May interact with corticosteroids, oral hypoglycemic agents, oral contraceptives, salicylates, thyroid preparations, and certain other agents. Compounds in these categories include:

Acarbose (Co-administration with drugs with hypoglycemic activity, such as oral hypoglycemic agents, may result in decreased insulin requirements). Products include:
Precose Tablets 906

Aspirin (Co-administration with drugs with hypoglycemic activity,

such as salicylates, may result in decreased insulin requirements). Products include:

Aggrenox Capsules 1026
Alka-Seltzer □603
Alka-Seltzer Lemon Lime Antacid and Pain Reliever Effervescent Tablets □603
Alka-Seltzer Extra Strength Antacid and Pain Reliever Effervescent Tablets □603
Alka-Seltzer PM Effervescent Tablets □605
Genuine Bayer Tablets, Caplets and Gelcaps □606
Extra Strength Bayer Caplets and Gelcaps □610
Aspirin Regimen Bayer Children's Chewable Tablets (Orange or Cherry Flavored) □607
Bayer, Aspirin Regimen □606
Aspirin Regimen Bayer 81 mg Caplets with Calcium □607
Genuine Bayer Professional Labeling (Aspirin Regimen Bayer) □608
Extra Strength Bayer Arthritis Caplets □610
Extra Strength Bayer Plus Caplets □610
Extra Strength Bayer PM Caplets □611
BC Powder □619
BC Allergy Sinus Cold Powder □619
Arthritis Strength BC Powder □619
BC Sinus Cold Powder □619
Darvon Compound-65 Pulvules 1910
Ecotrin Enteric Coated Aspirin Low, Regular and Maximum Strength Tablets 1715
Excedrin Extra-Strength Tablets, Caplets, and Geltabs □629
Excedrin Migraine 1070
Goody's Body Pain Formula Powder □620
Goody's Extra Strength Headache Powder □620
Goody's Extra Strength Pain Relief Tablets □620
Percodan Tablets 1327
Robaxisal Tablets 2939
Soma Compound Tablets 3354
Soma Compound w/Codeine Tablets 3355
Vanquish Caplets □617

Betamethasone Acetate (Co-administration may result in increased insulin requirements). Products include:

Celestone Soluspan Injectable Suspension 3097

Betamethasone Sodium Phosphate (Co-administration may result in increased insulin requirements). Products include:

Celestone Soluspan Injectable Suspension 3097

Chlorpropamide (Co-administration with drugs with hypoglycemic activity, such as oral hypoglycemic agents, may result in decreased insulin requirements). Products include:

Diabinese Tablets 2680

Choline Magnesium Trisalicylate (Co-administration with drugs with hypoglycemic activity, such as salicylates, may result in decreased insulin requirements). Products include:

Trilisate 2901

Cortisone Acetate (Co-administration may result in increased insulin requirements). Products include:

Cortone Acetate Injectable Suspension 2059
Cortone Acetate Tablets 2061

Desogestrel (Co-administration with oral contraceptives may result in increased insulin requirements). Products include:

Cyclessa Tablets 2450
Desogen Tablets 2458
Mircette Tablets 2470
Ortho-Cept 21 Tablets 2546
Ortho-Cept 28 Tablets 2546

Dexamethasone (Co-administration may result in increased insulin requirements). Products include:

Decadron Elixir 2078
Decadron Tablets 2079
TobraDex Ophthalmic Ointment 542
TobraDex Ophthalmic Suspension 541

Dexamethasone Acetate (Co-administration may result in increased insulin requirements).

No products indexed under this heading.

Dexamethasone Sodium Phosphate (Co-administration may result in increased insulin requirements). Products include:

Decadron Phosphate Injection 2081
Decadron Phosphate Sterile Ophthalmic Ointment 2083
Decadron Phosphate Sterile Ophthalmic Solution 2084
NeoDecadron Sterile Ophthalmic Solution 2144

Diflunisal (Co-administration with drugs with hypoglycemic activity, such as salicylates, may result in decreased insulin requirements). Products include:

Dolobid Tablets 2088

Ethinyl Estradiol (Co-administration with oral contraceptives may result in increased insulin requirements). Products include:

Alesse-21 Tablets 3468
Alesse-28 Tablets 3473
Brevicon 28-Day Tablets 3380
Cyclessa Tablets 2450
Desogen Tablets 2458
Estinyl Tablets 3112
Estrostep 2627
femhrt Tablets 2635
Levlen 962
Levlite 21 Tablets 962
Levlite 28 Tablets 962
Levora Tablets 3389
Loestrin 21 Tablets 2642
Loestrin Fe Tablets 2642
Lo/Ovral Tablets 3532
Lo/Ovral-28 Tablets 3538
Low-Ogestrel-28 Tablets 3392
Microgestin Fe 1.5/30 Tablets 3407
Microgestin Fe 1/20 Tablets 3400
Mircette Tablets 2470
Modicon 2563
Necon 3415
Nordette-28 Tablets 2257
Norinyl 1 +35 28-Day Tablets 3380
Ogestrel 0.5/50-28 Tablets 3428
Ortho-Cept 21 Tablets 2546
Ortho-Cept 28 Tablets 2546
Ortho-Cyclen/Ortho Tri-Cyclen 2573
Ortho-Novum 2563
Ovcon 3364
Ovral Tablets 3551
Ovral-28 Tablets 3552
Tri-Levlen 962
Tri-Norinyl-28 Tablets 3433
Triphasil-21 Tablets 3600
Triphasil-28 Tablets 3605
Trivora Tablets 3439
Yasmin 28 Tablets 980
Zovia 3449

Ethynodiol Diacetate (Co-administration with oral contraceptives may result in increased insulin requirements). Products include:

Zovia 3449

Fludrocortisone Acetate (Co-administration may result in increased insulin requirements). Products include:

Florinef Acetate Tablets 2250

Glimepiride (Co-administration with drugs with hypoglycemic activity, such as oral hypoglycemic agents, may result in decreased insulin requirements). Products include:

Amaryl Tablets 717

Glipizide (Co-administration with drugs with hypoglycemic activity, such as oral hypoglycemic agents, may result in decreased insulin requirements). Products include:

Glucotrol Tablets 2692
Glucotrol XL Extended Release Tablets 2693

Glyburide (Co-administration with drugs with hypoglycemic activity, such as oral hypoglycemic agents, may result in decreased insulin requirements). Products include:

DiaBeta Tablets 741
Glucovance Tablets 1086

Hydrocortisone (Co-administration may result in increased insulin requirements). Products include:

Anusol-HC Cream 2.5% 2237
Cipro HC Otic Suspension 540
Cortaid Intensive Therapy Cream □717
Cortaid Maximum Strength Cream □717
Cortisporin Ophthalmic Suspension Sterile ⊙297
Cortizone•5 □699
Cortizone•10 □699
Cortizone•10 Plus Creme □700
Cortizone for Kids Creme □699
Hydrocortone Tablets 2106
Massengill Medicated Soft Cloth Towelette □753
VōSoL HC Otic Solution 3356

Hydrocortisone Acetate (Co-administration may result in increased insulin requirements). Products include:

Analpram-HC 1338
Anusol HC-1 Hydrocortisone Anti-Itch Cream □689
Anusol-HC Suppositories 2238
Cortaid □717
Cortifoam Rectal Foam 3170
Cortisporin-TC Otic Suspension 2246
Hydrocortone Acetate Injectable Suspension 2103
Pramosone 1343
Proctocort Suppositories 2264
ProctoFoam-HC 3177
Terra-Cortril Ophthalmic Suspension 2716

Hydrocortisone Sodium Phosphate (Co-administration may result in increased insulin requirements). Products include:

Hydrocortone Phosphate Injection, Sterile 2105

Hydrocortisone Sodium Succinate (Co-administration may result in increased insulin requirements).

No products indexed under this heading.

Levonorgestrel (Co-administration with oral contraceptives may result in increased insulin requirements). Products include:

Alesse-21 Tablets 3468
Alesse-28 Tablets 3473
Levlen 962
Levlite 21 Tablets 962
Levlite 28 Tablets 962
Levora Tablets 3389
Mirena Intrauterine System 974
Nordette-28 Tablets 2257
Norplant System 3543
Tri-Levlen 962
Triphasil-21 Tablets 3600
Triphasil-28 Tablets 3605
Trivora Tablets 3439

Levothyroxine Sodium (Co-administration with thyroid replacement therapy may result in increased insulin requirements). Products include:

Levothroid Tablets 1373
Levoxyl Tablets 1819
Synthroid 505
Unithroid Tablets 3445

Liothyronine Sodium (Co-administration with thyroid replacement therapy may result in increased insulin requirements). Products include:

Cytomel Tablets 1817
Triostat Injection 1825

Liotrix (Co-administration with thyroid replacement therapy may result in increased insulin requirements).

No products indexed under this heading.

Magnesium Salicylate (Co-administration with drugs with hypoglycemic activity, such as salicylates, may result in decreased insulin requirements). Products include:

Momentum Backache Relief Extra Strength Caplets □666

Mestranol (Co-administration with oral contraceptives may result in increased insulin requirements). Products include:

Necon 1/50 Tablets 3415
Norinyl 1 + 50 28-Day Tablets 3380
Ortho-Novum 1/50□28 Tablets 2556

Metformin Hydrochloride (Co-administration with drugs with hypoglycemic activity, such as oral hypoglycemic agents, may result in decreased insulin requirements). Products include:

Glucophage Tablets 1080
Glucophage XR Tablets 1080
Glucovance Tablets 1086

Methylprednisolone Acetate (Co-administration may result in increased insulin requirements). Products include:

Depo-Medrol Injectable Suspension 2795

Methylprednisolone Sodium Succinate (Co-administration may result in increased insulin requirements). Products include:

Solu-Medrol Sterile Powder 2855

Miglitol (Co-administration with drugs with hypoglycemic activity, such as oral hypoglycemic agents, may result in decreased insulin requirements). Products include:

Glyset Tablets 2821

Norethindrone (Co-administration with oral contraceptives may result in increased insulin requirements). Products include:

Brevicon 28-Day Tablets 3380
Micronor Tablets 2543
Modicon 2563
Necon 3415
Norinyl 1 +35 28-Day Tablets 3380
Norinyl 1 + 50 28-Day Tablets 3380
Nor-QD Tablets 3423
Ortho-Novum 2563
Ortho-Novum 1/50□28 Tablets 2556
Ovcon 3364
Tri-Norinyl-28 Tablets 3433

Norethynodrel (Co-administration with oral contraceptives may result in increased insulin requirements).

No products indexed under this heading.

Norgestimate (Co-administration with oral contraceptives may result in increased insulin requirements). Products include:

Ortho-Cyclen/Ortho Tri-Cyclen 2573
Ortho-Prefest Tablets 2570

Norgestrel (Co-administration with oral contraceptives may result in increased insulin requirements). Products include:

Lo/Ovral Tablets 3532
Lo/Ovral-28 Tablets 3538
Low-Ogestrel-28 Tablets 3392
Ogestrel 0.5/50-28 Tablets 3428
Ovral Tablets 3551
Ovral-28 Tablets 3552
Ovrette Tablets 3552

Phenelzine Sulfate (Co-administration with drugs with hypoglycemic activity, such as certain MAO inhibitor antidepressants, may result in decreased insulin requirements). Products include:

Nardil Tablets 2653

Pioglitazone Hydrochloride (Co-administration with drugs with hypoglycemic activity, such as oral hypoglycemic agents, may result in decreased insulin requirements). Products include:

Actos Tablets 3275

Prednisolone Acetate (Co-administration may result in increased insulin requirements). Products include:

Blephamide Ophthalmic Ointment 547
Blephamide Ophthalmic Suspension 548
Poly-Pred Liquifilm Ophthalmic Suspension ⊙245
Pred Forte Ophthalmic Suspension ⊙246
Pred Mild Sterile Ophthalmic Suspension ⊙249
Pred-G Ophthalmic Suspension ⊙247
Pred-G Sterile Ophthalmic Ointment ⊙248

Prednisolone Sodium Phosphate (Co-administration may result in increased insulin requirements). Products include:

Pediapred Oral Solution 1170

Prednisolone Tebutate (Co-administration may result in increased insulin requirements).
No products indexed under this heading.

Prednisone (Co-administration may result in increased insulin requirements). Products include:
Prednisone 3064

Repaglinide (Co-administration with drugs with hypoglycemic activity, such as oral hypoglycemic agents, may result in decreased insulin requirements). Products include:
Prandin Tablets (0.5, 1, and 2 mg).. 2432

Rosiglitazone Maleate (Co-administration with drugs with hypoglycemic activity, such as oral hypoglycemic agents, may result in decreased insulin requirements). Products include:
Avandia Tablets 1490

Salsalate (Co-administration with drugs with hypoglycemic activity, such as salicylates, may result in decreased insulin requirements).
No products indexed under this heading.

Sulfacytine (Co-administration with drugs with hypoglycemic activity, such as sulfa antibiotics, may result in decreased insulin requirements).

Sulfamethizole (Co-administration with drugs with hypoglycemic activity, such as sulfa antibiotics, may result in decreased insulin requirements). Products include:
Urobiotic-250 Capsules 2731

Sulfamethoxazole (Co-administration with drugs with hypoglycemic activity, such as sulfa antibiotics, may result in decreased insulin requirements). Products include:
Bactrim 2949
Septra Suspension 2265
Septra Tablets 2265
Septra DS Tablets 2265

Sulfasalazine (Co-administration with drugs with hypoglycemic activity, such as sulfa antibiotics, may result in decreased insulin requirements). Products include:
Azulfidine EN-tabs Tablets 2775

Sulfisoxazole (Co-administration with drugs with hypoglycemic activity, such as sulfa antibiotics, may result in decreased insulin requirements).
No products indexed under this heading.

Thyroglobulin (Co-administration with thyroid replacement therapy may result in increased insulin requirements).
No products indexed under this heading.

Thyroid (Co-administration with thyroid replacement therapy may result in increased insulin requirements).
No products indexed under this heading.

Thyroxine (Co-administration with thyroid replacement therapy may result in increased insulin requirements).
No products indexed under this heading.

Thyroxine Sodium (Co-administration with thyroid replacement therapy may result in increased insulin requirements).
No products indexed under this heading.

Tolazamide (Co-administration with drugs with hypoglycemic activity, such as oral hypoglycemic agents, may result in decreased insulin requirements).
No products indexed under this heading.

Tolbutamide (Co-administration with drugs with hypoglycemic activity, such as oral hypoglycemic agents, may result in decreased insulin requirements).
No products indexed under this heading.

Tranylcypromine Sulfate (Co-administration with drugs with hypoglycemic activity, such as certain MAO inhibitor antidepressants, may result in decreased insulin requirements). Products include:
Parnate Tablets 1607

Triamcinolone (Co-administration may result in increased insulin requirements).
No products indexed under this heading.

Triamcinolone Acetonide (Co-administration may result in increased insulin requirements). Products include:
Azmacort Inhalation Aerosol 728
Nasacort Nasal Inhaler 750
Nasacort AQ Nasal Spray 752
Tri-Nasal Spray 2274

Triamcinolone Diacetate (Co-administration may result in increased insulin requirements).
No products indexed under this heading.

Triamcinolone Hexacetonide (Co-administration may result in increased insulin requirements).
No products indexed under this heading.

Troglitazone (Co-administration with drugs with hypoglycemic activity, such as oral hypoglycemic agents, may result in decreased insulin requirements).
No products indexed under this heading.

IMDUR TABLETS

(Isosorbide Mononitrate) 1826
May interact with calcium channel blockers, vasodilators, and certain other agents. Compounds in these categories include:

Amlodipine Besylate (Marked symptomatic orthostatic hypotension has been reported when calcium channel blockers and organic nitrates were used in combination). Products include:
Lotrel Capsules 2370
Norvasc Tablets 2704

Bepridil Hydrochloride (Marked symptomatic orthostatic hypotension has been reported when calcium channel blockers and organic nitrates were used in combination). Products include:
Vascor Tablets 2602

Diazoxide (Additive vasodilating effects).
No products indexed under this heading.

Diltiazem Hydrochloride (Marked symptomatic orthostatic hypotension has been reported when calcium channel blockers and organic nitrates were used in combination). Products include:
Cardizem Injectable 1018
Cardizem Lyo-Ject Syringe 1018
Cardizem Monovial 1018
Cardizem CD Capsules 1016
Tiazac Capsules 1378

Epoprostenol Sodium (Additive vasodilating effects). Products include:
Flolan for Injection 1528

Felodipine (Marked symptomatic orthostatic hypotension has been reported when calcium channel blockers and organic nitrates were used in combination). Products include:
Lexxel Tablets 608
Plendil Extended-Release Tablets ... 623

Hydralazine Hydrochloride (Additive vasodilating effects).
No products indexed under this heading.

Isradipine (Marked symptomatic orthostatic hypotension has been reported when calcium channel blockers and organic nitrates were used in combination). Products include:
DynaCirc Capsules 2921
DynaCirc CR Tablets 2923

Mibefradil Dihydrochloride (Marked symptomatic orthostatic hypotension has been reported when calcium channel blockers and organic nitrates were used in combination).
No products indexed under this heading.

Minoxidil (Additive vasodilating effects). Products include:
Rogaine Extra Strength for Men Topical Solution .... ⊡721
Rogaine for Women Topical Solution .... ⊡721

Nicardipine Hydrochloride (Marked symptomatic orthostatic hypotension has been reported when calcium channel blockers and organic nitrates were used in combination). Products include:
Cardene I.V. 3485

Nifedipine (Marked symptomatic orthostatic hypotension has been reported when calcium channel blockers and organic nitrates were used in combination). Products include:
Adalat CC Tablets 877
Procardia Capsules 2708
Procardia XL Extended Release Tablets.. 2710

Nimodipine (Marked symptomatic orthostatic hypotension has been reported when calcium channel blockers and organic nitrates were used in combination). Products include:
Nimotop Capsules 904

Nisoldipine (Marked symptomatic orthostatic hypotension has been reported when calcium channel blockers and organic nitrates were used in combination). Products include:
Sular Tablets 688

Sildenafil Citrate (Amplification of the vasodilatory effects of Imdur by sildenafil can result in severe hypotension). Products include:
Viagra Tablets 2732

Verapamil Hydrochloride (Marked symptomatic orthostatic hypotension has been reported when calcium channel blockers and organic nitrates were used in combination). Products include:
Covera-HS Tablets 3199
Isoptin SR Tablets 467
Tarka Tablets 508
Verelan Capsules 3184
Verelan PM Capsules 3186

Food Interactions

Alcohol (Additive vasodilating effects).

Food, unspecified (May decrease the rate (increase in Tmax) but not the extent (AUC) of absorption).

IMITREX INJECTION

(Sumatriptan Succinate) 1549
See Imitrex Tablets

IMITREX NASAL SPRAY

(Sumatriptan) 1554
See Imitrex Tablets

IMITREX TABLETS

(Sumatriptan Succinate) 1558
May interact with 5HT1-receptor agonists, ergot-containing drugs, nonselective MAO inhibitors, selective serotonin reuptake inhibitors, and certain other agents. Compounds in these categories include:

Citalopram Hydrobromide (Co-administration of sumatriptan with selective serotonin reuptake inhibitors (SSRIs) has resulted, rarely, in hyperreflexia, weakness, and incoordination). Products include:
Celexa 1365

Dihydroergotamine Mesylate (Ergot-containing drugs have been reported to cause prolonged vasospastic reactions; because there is a theoretical basis that these effects may be additive, use of ergot-type agents and sumatriptan within 24 hours is contraindicated). Products include:
D.H.E. 45 Injection 2334
Migranal Nasal Spray 2376

Ergonovine Maleate (Ergot-containing drugs have been reported to cause prolonged vasospastic reactions; because there is a theoretical basis that these effects may be additive, use of ergot-type agents and sumatriptan within 24 hours is contraindicated).
No products indexed under this heading.

Ergotamine Tartrate (Ergot-containing drugs have been reported to cause prolonged vasospastic reactions; because there is a theoretical basis that these effects may be additive, use of ergot-type agents and sumatriptan within 24 hours is contraindicated).
No products indexed under this heading.

Fluoxetine Hydrochloride (Co-administration of sumatriptan with selective serotonin reuptake inhibitors (SSRIs) has resulted, rarely, in hyperreflexia, weakness, and incoordination). Products include:
Prozac Pulvules, Liquid, and Weekly Capsules 1238
Sarafem Pulvules 1962

Fluvoxamine Maleate (Co-administration of sumatriptan with selective serotonin reuptake inhibitors (SSRIs) has resulted, rarely, in hyperreflexia, weakness, and incoordination). Products include:
Luvox Tablets (25, 50, 100 mg) 3256

Isocarboxazid (MAO-A inhibitors reduce sumatriptan clearance and significantly increasing systemic exposure; concurrent and/or sequential use is contraindicated).
No products indexed under this heading.

Methylergonovine Maleate (Ergot-containing drugs have been reported to cause prolonged vasospastic reactions; because there is a theoretical basis that these effects may be additive, use of ergot-type agents and sumatriptan within 24 hours is contraindicated).
No products indexed under this heading.

Methysergide Maleate (Ergot-containing drugs have been reported to cause prolonged vasospastic reactions; because there is a theoretical basis that these effects may be additive, use of ergot-type agents and sumatriptan within 24 hours is contraindicated).
No products indexed under this heading.

Naratriptan Hydrochloride (Co-administration with other 5-HT_1 agonists within 24 hours of each other is contraindicated because the vasospastic effects may be additive). Products include:
Amerge Tablets 1467

Pargyline Hydrochloride (MAO-A inhibitors reduce sumatriptan clearance and significantly increasing systemic exposure; concurrent and/or sequential use is contraindicated).
No products indexed under this heading.

Paroxetine Hydrochloride (Co-administration of sumatriptan with

selective serotonin reuptake inhibitors (SSRIs) has resulted, rarely, in hyperreflexia, weakness, and incoordination). Products include:

Paxil 1609

Phenelzine Sulfate (MAO-A inhibitors reduce sumatriptan clearance and significantly increasing systemic exposure; concurrent and/or sequential use is contraindicated). Products include:

Nardil Tablets 2653

Procarbazine Hydrochloride (MAO-A inhibitors reduce sumatriptan clearance and significantly increasing systemic exposure; concurrent and/or sequential use is contraindicated). Products include:

Matulane Capsules 3246

Rizatriptan Benzoate (Co-administration with other 5-HT_1 agonists within 24 hours of each other is contraindicated because the vasospastic effects may be additive). Products include:

Maxalt Tablets 2120
Maxalt-MLT Orally Disintegrating Tablets 2120

Sertraline Hydrochloride (Co-administration of sumatriptan with selective serotonin reuptake inhibitors (SSRIs) has resulted, rarely, in hyperreflexia, weakness, and incoordination). Products include:

Zoloft 2751

Sumatriptan (Co-administration with other 5-HT_1 agonists within 24 hours of each other is contraindicated because the vasospastic effects may be additive). Products include:

Imitrex Nasal Spray 1554

Tranylcypromine Sulfate (MAO-A inhibitors reduce sumatriptan clearance and significantly increasing systemic exposure; concurrent and/or sequential use is contraindicated). Products include:

Parnate Tablets 1607

Zolmitriptan (Co-administration with other 5-HT_1 agonists within 24 hours of each other is contraindicated because the vasospastic effects may be additive). Products include:

Zomig Tablets 708
Zomig-ZMT Tablets 708

Food Interactions

Food, unspecified (Delays the Tmax slightly by about 0.5 hour with no significant effect on the bioavailability).

IMMUNOCAL POWDER SACHETS

(Whey Protein Isolate) 1766
None cited in PDR database.

IMODIUM A-D LIQUID AND CAPLETS

(Loperamide Hydrochloride) 2001
None cited in PDR database.

IMODIUM ADVANCED CAPLETS AND CHEWABLE TABLETS

(Loperamide Hydrochloride, Simethicone) 2001
None cited in PDR database.

IMOGAM RABIES - HT

(Rabies Immune Globulin (Human)) ... 805
May interact with:

Measles Virus Vaccine Live (Antibodies may interfere with the immune response to the vaccine). Products include:

Attenuvax 2044

IMOVAX RABIES VACCINE

(Rabies Vaccine) 807
May interact with corticosteroids, immunosuppressive agents, and certain other agents. Compounds in these categories include:

Azathioprine (Can interfere with the development of active immunity and predispose the patient to develop rabies).

No products indexed under this heading.

Basiliximab (Can interfere with the development of active immunity and predispose the patient to develop rabies). Products include:

Simulect for Injection 2399

Betamethasone Acetate (Can interfere with the development of active immunity and predispose the patient to develop rabies). Products include:

Celestone Soluspan Injectable Suspension 3097

Betamethasone Sodium Phosphate (Can interfere with the development of active immunity and predispose the patient to develop rabies). Products include:

Celestone Soluspan Injectable Suspension 3097

Cortisone Acetate (Can interfere with the development of active immunity and predispose the patient to develop rabies). Products include:

Cortone Acetate Injectable Suspension 2059
Cortone Acetate Tablets 2061

Cyclosporine (Can interfere with the development of active immunity and predispose the patient to develop rabies). Products include:

Gengraf Capsules 457
Neoral Soft Gelatin Capsules 2380
Neoral Oral Solution 2380
Sandimmune 2388

Dexamethasone (Can interfere with the development of active immunity and predispose the patient to develop rabies). Products include:

Decadron Elixir 2078
Decadron Tablets 2079
TobraDex Ophthalmic Ointment 542
TobraDex Ophthalmic Suspension .. 541

Dexamethasone Acetate (Can interfere with the development of active immunity and predispose the patient to develop rabies).

No products indexed under this heading.

Dexamethasone Sodium Phosphate (Can interfere with the development of active immunity and predispose the patient to develop rabies). Products include:

Decadron Phosphate Injection 2081
Decadron Phosphate Sterile Ophthalmic Ointment 2083
Decadron Phosphate Sterile Ophthalmic Solution 2084
NeoDecadron Sterile Ophthalmic Solution 2144

Fludrocortisone Acetate (Can interfere with the development of active immunity and predispose the patient to develop rabies). Products include:

Florinef Acetate Tablets 2250

Hydrocortisone (Can interfere with the development of active immunity and predispose the patient to develop rabies). Products include:

Anusol-HC Cream 2.5% 2237
Cipro HC Otic Suspension 540
Cortaid Intensive Therapy Cream .■717
Cortaid Maximum Strength Cream .... ■717
Cortisporin Ophthalmic Suspension Sterile .... ⊙297
Cortizone•5 .... ■699
Cortizone•10 .... ■699
Cortizone•10 Plus Creme .... ■700
Cortizone for Kids Creme .... ■699
Hydrocortone Tablets 2106
Massengill Medicated Soft Cloth Towelette .... ■753
VōSoL HC Otic Solution 3356

Hydrocortisone Acetate (Can interfere with the development of active immunity and predispose the patient to develop rabies). Products include:

Analpram-HC 1338
Anusol HC-1 Hydrocortisone Anti-Itch Cream .... ■689
Anusol-HC Suppositories 2238
Cortaid .... ■717
Cortifoam Rectal Foam 3170
Cortisporin-TC Otic Suspension 2246
Hydrocortone Acetate Injectable Suspension 2103
Pramosone 1343
Proctocort Suppositories 2264
ProctoFoam-HC 3177
Terra-Cortril Ophthalmic Suspension 2716

Hydrocortisone Sodium Phosphate (Can interfere with the development of active immunity and predispose the patient to develop rabies). Products include:

Hydrocortone Phosphate Injection, Sterile 2105

Hydrocortisone Sodium Succinate (Can interfere with the development of active immunity and predispose the patient to develop rabies).

No products indexed under this heading.

Immune Globulin Intravenous (Human) (Can interfere with the development of active immunity and predispose the patient to develop rabies).

No products indexed under this heading.

Methylprednisolone Acetate (Can interfere with the development of active immunity and predispose the patient to develop rabies). Products include:

Depo-Medrol Injectable Suspension 2795

Methylprednisolone Sodium Succinate (Can interfere with the development of active immunity and predispose the patient to develop rabies). Products include:

Solu-Medrol Sterile Powder 2855

Muromonab-CD3 (Can interfere with the development of active immunity and predispose the patient to develop rabies). Products include:

Orthoclone OKT3 Sterile Solution 2498

Mycophenolate Mofetil (Can interfere with the development of active immunity and predispose the patient to develop rabies). Products include:

CellCept Capsules 2951
CellCept Oral Suspension 2951
CellCept Tablets 2951

Prednisolone Acetate (Can interfere with the development of active immunity and predispose the patient to develop rabies). Products include:

Blephamide Ophthalmic Ointment .. 547
Blephamide Ophthalmic Suspension 548
Poly-Pred Liquifilm Ophthalmic Suspension .... ⊙245
Pred Forte Ophthalmic Suspension .... ⊙246
Pred Mild Sterile Ophthalmic Suspension .... ⊙249
Pred-G Ophthalmic Suspension .... ⊙247
Pred-G Sterile Ophthalmic Ointment .... ⊙248

Prednisolone Sodium Phosphate (Can interfere with the development of active immunity and predispose the patient to develop rabies). Products include:

Pediapred Oral Solution 1170

Prednisolone Tebutate (Can interfere with the development of active immunity and predispose the patient to develop rabies).

No products indexed under this heading.

Prednisone (Can interfere with the development of active immunity and predispose the patient to develop rabies). Products include:

Prednisone 3064

Sirolimus (Can interfere with the development of active immunity and predispose the patient to develop rabies). Products include:

Rapamune Oral Solution and Tablets 3584

Tacrolimus (Can interfere with the development of active immunity and predispose the patient to develop rabies). Products include:

Prograf 1393
Protopic Ointment 1397

Triamcinolone (Can interfere with the development of active immunity and predispose the patient to develop rabies).

No products indexed under this heading.

Triamcinolone Acetonide (Can interfere with the development of active immunity and predispose the patient to develop rabies). Products include:

Azmacort Inhalation Aerosol 728
Nasacort Nasal Inhaler 750
Nasacort AQ Nasal Spray 752
Tri-Nasal Spray 2274

Triamcinolone Diacetate (Can interfere with the development of active immunity and predispose the patient to develop rabies).

No products indexed under this heading.

Triamcinolone Hexacetonide (Can interfere with the development of active immunity and predispose the patient to develop rabies).

No products indexed under this heading.

IMUPLUS FORMULA

(Whey Protein Isolate) 3274
None cited in PDR database.

INDAPAMIDE TABLETS

(Indapamide) 2286
May interact with antihypertensives, barbiturates, corticosteroids, cardiac glycosides, insulin, lithium preparations, narcotic analgesics, and certain other agents. Compounds in these categories include:

Acebutolol Hydrochloride (Indapamide may add to or potentiate the therapeutic effect of other antihypertensive drugs). Products include:

Sectral Capsules 3589

ACTH (Co-administration with ACTH may increase the risk of hypokalemia).

No products indexed under this heading.

Alfentanil Hydrochloride (Aggravates orthostatic hypotension).

No products indexed under this heading.

Amlodipine Besylate (Indapamide may add to or potentiate the therapeutic effect of other antihypertensive drugs). Products include:

Lotrel Capsules 2370
Norvasc Tablets 2704

Aprobarbital (Aggravates orthostatic hypotension).

No products indexed under this heading.

Atenolol (Indapamide may add to or potentiate the therapeutic effect of other antihypertensive drugs). Products include:

Tenoretic Tablets 690
Tenormin I.V. Injection 692

Benazepril Hydrochloride (Indapamide may add to or potentiate the therapeutic effect of other antihypertensive drugs). Products include:

Lotensin Tablets 2365
Lotensin HCT Tablets 2367
Lotrel Capsules 2370

Bendroflumethiazide (Indapamide may add to or potentiate the therapeutic effect of other antihypertensive drugs). Products include:

Corzide 40/5 Tablets 2247
Corzide 80/5 Tablets 2247

Betamethasone Acetate (Co-administration with corticosteroids may increase the risk of hypokalemia). Products include:

Celestone Soluspan Injectable Suspension 3097

Betamethasone Sodium Phosphate (Co-administration with corticosteroids may increase the risk of hypokalemia). Products include:

Celestone Soluspan Injectable Suspension 3097

Betaxolol Hydrochloride (Indapamide may add to or potentiate the therapeutic effect of other antihypertensive drugs). Products include:

Betoptic S Ophthalmic Suspension 537

Bisoprolol Fumarate (Indapamide may add to or potentiate the therapeutic effect of other antihypertensive drugs). Products include:

Zebeta Tablets 1885
Ziac Tablets 1887

Buprenorphine Hydrochloride (Aggravates orthostatic hypotension). Products include:

Buprenex Injectable 2918

Butabarbital (Aggravates orthostatic hypotension).

No products indexed under this heading.

Butalbital (Aggravates orthostatic hypotension). Products include:

Phrenilin 578
Sedapap Tablets 50 mg/650 mg 2225

Candesartan Cilexetil (Indapamide may add to or potentiate the therapeutic effect of other antihypertensive drugs). Products include:

Atacand Tablets 595
Atacand HCT Tablets 597

Captopril (Indapamide may add to or potentiate the therapeutic effect of other antihypertensive drugs). Products include:

Captopril Tablets 2281

Carteolol Hydrochloride (Indapamide may add to or potentiate the therapeutic effect of other antihypertensive drugs). Products include:

Carteolol Hydrochloride Ophthalmic Solution USP, 1% ⊙258
Ocupress Ophthalmic Solution, 1% Sterile ⊙303

Chlorothiazide (Indapamide may add to or potentiate the therapeutic effect of other antihypertensive drugs). Products include:

Aldoclor Tablets 2035
Diuril Oral 2087

Chlorothiazide Sodium (Indapamide may add to or potentiate the therapeutic effect of other antihypertensive drugs). Products include:

Diuril Sodium Intravenous 2086

Chlorthalidone (Indapamide may add to or potentiate the therapeutic effect of other antihypertensive drugs). Products include:

Clorpres Tablets 1002
Combipres Tablets 1040
Tenoretic Tablets 690

Clonidine (Indapamide may add to or potentiate the therapeutic effect of other antihypertensive drugs). Products include:

Catapres-TTS 1038

Clonidine Hydrochloride (Indapamide may add to or potentiate the therapeutic effect of other antihypertensive drugs). Products include:

Catapres Tablets 1037
Clorpres Tablets 1002
Combipres Tablets 1040
Duraclon Injection 3057

Codeine Phosphate (Aggravates orthostatic hypotension). Products include:

Phenergan with Codeine Syrup 3557
Phenergan VC with Codeine Syrup 3561
Robitussin A-C Syrup 2942
Robitussin-DAC Syrup 2942
Ryna-C Liquid ▣768
Soma Compound w/Codeine Tablets 3355
Tussi-Organidin NR Liquid 3350
Tussi-Organidin-S NR Liquid 3350
Tylenol with Codeine 2595

Cortisone Acetate (Co-administration with corticosteroids may increase the risk of hypokalemia). Products include:

Cortone Acetate Injectable Suspension 2059
Cortone Acetate Tablets 2061

Deserpidine (Indapamide may add to or potentiate the therapeutic effect of other antihypertensive drugs).

No products indexed under this heading.

Deslanoside (Concurrent digitalis therapy may exaggerate metabolic effects of hypokalemia; especially myocardial effects such as increase ventricular irritability).

No products indexed under this heading.

Dexamethasone (Co-administration with corticosteroids may increase the risk of hypokalemia). Products include:

Decadron Elixir 2078
Decadron Tablets 2079
TobraDex Ophthalmic Ointment 542
TobraDex Ophthalmic Suspension 541

Dexamethasone Acetate (Co-administration with corticosteroids may increase the risk of hypokalemia).

No products indexed under this heading.

Dexamethasone Sodium Phosphate (Co-administration with corticosteroids may increase the risk of hypokalemia). Products include:

Decadron Phosphate Injection 2081
Decadron Phosphate Sterile Ophthalmic Ointment 2083
Decadron Phosphate Sterile Ophthalmic Solution 2084
NeoDecadron Sterile Ophthalmic Solution 2144

Dezocine (Aggravates orthostatic hypotension).

No products indexed under this heading.

Diazoxide (Indapamide may add to or potentiate the therapeutic effect of other antihypertensive drugs).

No products indexed under this heading.

Digitoxin (Concurrent digitalis therapy may exaggerate metabolic effects of hypokalemia; especially myocardial effects such as increase ventricular irritability).

No products indexed under this heading.

Digoxin (Concurrent digitalis therapy may exaggerate metabolic effects of hypokalemia; especially myocardial effects such as increase ventricular irritability). Products include:

Digitek Tablets 1003
Lanoxicaps Capsules 1574
Lanoxin Injection 1581
Lanoxin Tablets 1587
Lanoxin Elixir Pediatric 1578
Lanoxin Injection Pediatric 1584

Diltiazem Hydrochloride (Indapamide may add to or potentiate the therapeutic effect of other antihypertensive drugs). Products include:

Cardizem Injectable 1018
Cardizem Lyo-Ject Syringe 1018
Cardizem Monovial 1018
Cardizem CD Capsules 1016
Tiazac Capsules 1378

Doxazosin Mesylate (Indapamide may add to or potentiate the therapeutic effect of other antihypertensive drugs). Products include:

Cardura Tablets 2668

Enalapril Maleate (Indapamide may add to or potentiate the therapeutic effect of other antihypertensive drugs). Products include:

Lexxel Tablets 608
Vaseretic Tablets 2204
Vasotec Tablets 2210

Enalaprilat (Indapamide may add to or potentiate the therapeutic effect of other antihypertensive drugs). Products include:

Enalaprilat Injection 863
Vasotec I.V. Injection 2207

Eprosartan Mesylate (Indapamide may add to or potentiate the therapeutic effect of other antihypertensive drugs). Products include:

Teveten Tablets 3327

Esmolol Hydrochloride (Indapamide may add to or potentiate the therapeutic effect of other antihypertensive drugs). Products include:

Brevibloc Injection 858

Felodipine (Indapamide may add to or potentiate the therapeutic effect of other antihypertensive drugs). Products include:

Lexxel Tablets 608
Plendil Extended-Release Tablets 623

Fentanyl (Aggravates orthostatic hypotension). Products include:

Duragesic Transdermal System 1786

Fentanyl Citrate (Aggravates orthostatic hypotension). Products include:

Actiq 1184

Fludrocortisone Acetate (Co-administration with corticosteroids may increase the risk of hypokalemia). Products include:

Florinef Acetate Tablets 2250

Fosinopril Sodium (Indapamide may add to or potentiate the therapeutic effect of other antihypertensive drugs). Products include:

Monopril Tablets 1091
Monopril HCT 1094

Furosemide (Indapamide may add to or potentiate the therapeutic effect of other antihypertensive drugs). Products include:

Furosemide Tablets 2284

Guanabenz Acetate (Indapamide may add to or potentiate the therapeutic effect of other antihypertensive drugs).

No products indexed under this heading.

Guanethidine Monosulfate (Indapamide may add to or potentiate the therapeutic effect of other antihypertensive drugs).

No products indexed under this heading.

Hydralazine Hydrochloride (Indapamide may add to or potentiate the therapeutic effect of other antihypertensive drugs).

No products indexed under this heading.

Hydrochlorothiazide (Indapamide may add to or potentiate the therapeutic effect of other antihypertensive drugs). Products include:

Accuretic Tablets 2614
Aldoril Tablets 2039
Atacand HCT Tablets 597
Avalide Tablets 1070
Diovan HCT Tablets 2338
Dyazide Capsules 1515
HydroDIURIL Tablets 2108
Hyzaar 2109
Inderide Tablets 3517
Inderide LA Long-Acting Capsules 3519
Lotensin HCT Tablets 2367
Maxzide 1008
Micardis HCT Tablets 1051
Microzide Capsules 3414
Moduretic Tablets 2138
Monopril HCT 1094
Prinzide Tablets 2168
Timolide Tablets 2187
Uniretic Tablets 3178
Vaseretic Tablets 2204
Zestoretic Tablets 695
Ziac Tablets 1887

Hydrocodone Bitartrate (Aggravates orthostatic hypotension). Products include:

Hycodan 1316
Hycomine Compound Tablets 1317
Hycotuss Expectorant Syrup 1318
Lortab 3319
Lortab Elixir 3317
Maxidone Tablets CIII 3399
Norco 5/325 Tablets CIII 3424
Norco 7.5/325 Tablets CIII 3425
Norco 10/325 Tablets CIII 3427
Norco 10/325 Tablets CIII 3425
Vicodin Tablets 516
Vicodin ES Tablets 517
Vicodin HP Tablets 518
Vicodin Tuss Expectorant 519
Vicoprofen Tablets 520
Zydone Tablets 1330

Hydrocodone Polistirex (Aggravates orthostatic hypotension). Products include:

Tussionex Pennkinetic Extended-Release Suspension 1174

Hydrocortisone (Co-administration with corticosteroids may increase the risk of hypokalemia). Products include:

Anusol-HC Cream 2.5% 2237
Cipro HC Otic Suspension 540
Cortaid Intensive Therapy Cream ▣717
Cortaid Maximum Strength Cream ▣717
Cortisporin Ophthalmic Suspension Sterile ⊙297
Cortizone•5 ▣699
Cortizone•10 ▣699
Cortizone•10 Plus Creme ▣700
Cortizone for Kids Creme ▣699
Hydrocortone Tablets 2106
Massengill Medicated Soft Cloth Towelette ▣753
VōSoL HC Otic Solution 3356

Hydrocortisone Acetate (Co-administration with corticosteroids may increase the risk of hypokalemia). Products include:

Analpram-HC 1338
Anusol HC-1 Hydrocortisone Anti-Itch Cream ▣689
Anusol-HC Suppositories 2238
Cortaid ▣717
Cortifoam Rectal Foam 3170
Cortisporin-TC Otic Suspension 2246
Hydrocortone Acetate Injectable Suspension 2103
Pramosone 1343
Proctocort Suppositories 2264
ProctoFoam-HC 3177
Terra-Cortril Ophthalmic Suspension 2716

Hydrocortisone Sodium Phosphate (Co-administration with corticosteroids may increase the risk of hypokalemia). Products include:

Hydrocortone Phosphate Injection, Sterile 2105

Hydrocortisone Sodium Succinate (Co-administration with corticosteroids may increase the risk of hypokalemia).

No products indexed under this heading.

Hydroflumethiazide (Indapamide may add to or potentiate the therapeutic effect of other antihypertensive drugs). Products include:

Diucardin Tablets 3494

Hydromorphone Hydrochloride (Aggravates orthostatic hypotension). Products include:

Dilaudid 441
Dilaudid Oral Liquid 445
Dilaudid Powder 441
Dilaudid Rectal Suppositories 441
Dilaudid Tablets 441
Dilaudid Tablets - 8 mg 445
Dilaudid-HP 443

Insulin, Human, Zinc Suspension (Hyperglycemia has been reported with the use of indapamide; co-administration may require adjustment in insulin dosage in diabetic patients). Products include:

Humulin L, 100 Units 1937
Humulin U, 100 Units 1943
Novolin L Human Insulin 10 ml Vials 2422

Insulin, Human NPH (Hyperglycemia has been reported with the use of indapamide; co-administration may require adjustment in insulin dosage in diabetic patients). Products include:

Humulin N, 100 Units 1939
Humulin N NPH Pen 1940

- Novolin N Human Insulin 10 ml Vials 2422
- Novolin N PenFill 2423
- Novolin N Prefilled Syringe Disposable Insulin Delivery System 2425

Insulin, Human Regular (Hyperglycemia has been reported with the use of indapamide; co-administration may require adjustment in insulin dosage in diabetic patients). Products include:
- Humulin R Regular (U-500) 1943
- Humulin R, 100 Units 1941
- Novolin R Human Insulin 10 ml Vials 2423
- Novolin R PenFill 2423
- Novolin R Prefilled Syringe Disposable Insulin Delivery System 2425
- Velosulin BR Human Insulin 10 ml Vials 2435

Insulin, Human Regular and Human NPH Mixture (Hyperglycemia has been reported with the use of indapamide; co-administration may require adjustment in insulin dosage in diabetic patients). Products include:
- Humulin 50/50, 100 Units 1934
- Humulin 70/30, 100 Units 1935
- Humulin 70/30 Pen 1936
- Novolin 70/30 Human Insulin 10 ml Vials 2421
- Novolin 70/30 PenFill 2423
- Novolin 70/30 Prefilled Disposable Insulin Delivery System 2425

Insulin, NPH (Hyperglycemia has been reported with the use of indapamide; co-administration may require adjustment in insulin dosage in diabetic patients). Products include:
- Iletin II, NPH (Pork), 100 Units 1946

Insulin, Regular (Hyperglycemia has been reported with the use of indapamide; co-administration may require adjustment in insulin dosage in diabetic patients). Products include:
- Iletin II, Regular (Pork), 100 Units 1947

Insulin, Zinc Crystals (Hyperglycemia has been reported with the use of indapamide; co-administration may require adjustment in insulin dosage in diabetic patients).
- No products indexed under this heading.

Insulin, Zinc Suspension (Hyperglycemia has been reported with the use of indapamide; co-administration may require adjustment in insulin dosage in diabetic patients). Products include:
- Iletin II, Lente (Pork), 100 Units 1945

Insulin Aspart, Human Regular (Hyperglycemia has been reported with the use of indapamide; co-administration may require adjustment in insulin dosage in diabetic patients).
- No products indexed under this heading.

Insulin glargine (Hyperglycemia has been reported with the use of indapamide; co-administration may require adjustment in insulin dosage in diabetic patients). Products include:
- Lantus Injection 742

Insulin Lispro, Human (Hyperglycemia has been reported with the use of indapamide; co-administration may require adjustment in insulin dosage in diabetic patients). Products include:
- Humalog 1926
- Humalog Mix 75/25 Pen 1928

Insulin Lispro Protamine, Human (Hyperglycemia has been reported with the use of indapamide; co-administration may require adjustment in insulin dosage in diabetic patients). Products include:
- Humalog Mix 75/25 Pen 1928

Irbesartan (Indapamide may add to or potentiate the therapeutic effect of other antihypertensive drugs). Products include:
- Avalide Tablets 1070
- Avapro Tablets 1074
- Avapro Tablets 3076

Isradipine (Indapamide may add to or potentiate the therapeutic effect of other antihypertensive drugs). Products include:
- DynaCirc Capsules 2921
- DynaCirc CR Tablets 2923

Labetalol Hydrochloride (Indapamide may add to or potentiate the therapeutic effect of other antihypertensive drugs). Products include:
- Normodyne Injection 3135
- Normodyne Tablets 3137

Levorphanol Tartrate (Aggravates orthostatic hypotension). Products include:
- Levo-Dromoran 1734
- Levorphanol Tartrate Tablets 3059

Lisinopril (Indapamide may add to or potentiate the therapeutic effect of other antihypertensive drugs). Products include:
- Prinivil Tablets 2164
- Prinzide Tablets 2168
- Zestoretic Tablets 695
- Zestril Tablets 698

Lithium Carbonate (Diuretics reduce lithium's renal clearance and add a high risk of lithium toxicity). Products include:
- Eskalith 1527
- Lithium Carbonate 3061
- Lithobid Slow-Release Tablets 3255

Lithium Citrate (Diuretics reduce lithium's renal clearance and add a high risk of lithium toxicity). Products include:
- Lithium Citrate Syrup 3061

Losartan Potassium (Indapamide may add to or potentiate the therapeutic effect of other antihypertensive drugs). Products include:
- Cozaar Tablets 2067
- Hyzaar 2109

Mecamylamine Hydrochloride (Indapamide may add to or potentiate the therapeutic effect of other antihypertensive drugs). Products include:
- Inversine Tablets 1850

Meperidine Hydrochloride (Aggravates orthostatic hypotension). Products include:
- Demerol 3079
- Mepergan Injection 3539

Mephobarbital (Aggravates orthostatic hypotension).
- No products indexed under this heading.

Methadone Hydrochloride (Aggravates orthostatic hypotension). Products include:
- Dolophine Hydrochloride Tablets 3056

Methyclothiazide (Indapamide may add to or potentiate the therapeutic effect of other antihypertensive drugs).
- No products indexed under this heading.

Methyldopa (Indapamide may add to or potentiate the therapeutic effect of other antihypertensive drugs). Products include:
- Aldoclor Tablets 2035
- Aldomet Tablets 2037
- Aldoril Tablets 2039

Methyldopate Hydrochloride (Indapamide may add to or potentiate the therapeutic effect of other antihypertensive drugs).
- No products indexed under this heading.

Methylprednisolone Acetate (Co-administration with corticosteroids may increase the risk of hypokalemia). Products include:
- Depo-Medrol Injectable Suspension 2795

Methylprednisolone Sodium Succinate (Co-administration with corticosteroids may increase the risk of hypokalemia). Products include:
- Solu-Medrol Sterile Powder 2855

Metolazone (Indapamide may add to or potentiate the therapeutic effect of other antihypertensive drugs). Products include:
- Mykrox Tablets 1168
- Zaroxolyn Tablets 1177

Metoprolol Succinate (Indapamide may add to or potentiate the therapeutic effect of other antihypertensive drugs). Products include:
- Toprol-XL Tablets 651

Metoprolol Tartrate (Indapamide may add to or potentiate the therapeutic effect of other antihypertensive drugs).
- No products indexed under this heading.

Metyrosine (Indapamide may add to or potentiate the therapeutic effect of other antihypertensive drugs). Products include:
- Demser Capsules 2085

Mibefradil Dihydrochloride (Indapamide may add to or potentiate the therapeutic effect of other antihypertensive drugs).
- No products indexed under this heading.

Minoxidil (Indapamide may add to or potentiate the therapeutic effect of other antihypertensive drugs). Products include:
- Rogaine Extra Strength for Men Topical Solution .... ⊡721
- Rogaine for Women Topical Solution .... ⊡721

Moexipril Hydrochloride (Indapamide may add to or potentiate the therapeutic effect of other antihypertensive drugs). Products include:
- Uniretic Tablets 3178
- Univasc Tablets 3181

Morphine Sulfate (Aggravates orthostatic hypotension). Products include:
- Astramorph/PF Injection, USP (Preservative-Free) 594
- Duramorph Injection 1312
- Infumorph 200 and Infumorph 500 Sterile Solutions 1314
- Kadian Capsules 1335
- MS Contin Tablets 2896
- MSIR 2898
- Oramorph SR Tablets 3062
- Roxanol 3066

Nadolol (Indapamide may add to or potentiate the therapeutic effect of other antihypertensive drugs). Products include:
- Corgard Tablets 2245
- Corzide 40/5 Tablets 2247
- Corzide 80/5 Tablets 2247
- Nadolol Tablets 2288

Nicardipine Hydrochloride (Indapamide may add to or potentiate the therapeutic effect of other antihypertensive drugs). Products include:
- Cardene I.V. 3485

Nifedipine (Indapamide may add to or potentiate the therapeutic effect of other antihypertensive drugs). Products include:
- Adalat CC Tablets 877
- Procardia Capsules 2708
- Procardia XL Extended Release Tablets 2710

Nisoldipine (Indapamide may add to or potentiate the therapeutic effect of other antihypertensive drugs). Products include:
- Sular Tablets 688

Nitroglycerin (Indapamide may add to or potentiate the therapeutic effect of other antihypertensive drugs). Products include:
- Nitro-Dur Transdermal Infusion System 3134
- Nitro-Dur Transdermal Infusion System 1834
- Nitrolingual Pumpspray 1355
- Nitrostat Tablets 2658

Norepinephrine Bitartrate (Indapamide may decrease arterial responsiveness to norepinephrine).
- No products indexed under this heading.

Oxycodone Hydrochloride (Aggravates orthostatic hypotension). Products include:
- OxyContin Tablets 2912
- OxyFast Oral Concentrate Solution 2916
- OxyIR Capsules 2916
- Percocet Tablets 1326
- Percodan Tablets 1327
- Percolone Tablets 1327
- Roxicodone 3067
- Tylox Capsules 2597

Penbutolol Sulfate (Indapamide may add to or potentiate the therapeutic effect of other antihypertensive drugs).
- No products indexed under this heading.

Pentobarbital Sodium (Aggravates orthostatic hypotension). Products include:
- Nembutal Sodium Solution 485

Perindopril Erbumine (Indapamide may add to or potentiate the therapeutic effect of other antihypertensive drugs). Products include:
- Aceon Tablets (2 mg, 4 mg, 8 mg) 3249

Phenobarbital (Aggravates orthostatic hypotension). Products include:
- Arco-Lase Plus Tablets 592
- Donnatal 2929
- Donnatal Extentabs 2930

Phenoxybenzamine Hydrochloride (Indapamide may add to or potentiate the therapeutic effect of other antihypertensive drugs). Products include:
- Dibenzyline Capsules 3457

Phentolamine Mesylate (Indapamide may add to or potentiate the therapeutic effect of other antihypertensive drugs).
- No products indexed under this heading.

Pindolol (Indapamide may add to or potentiate the therapeutic effect of other antihypertensive drugs).
- No products indexed under this heading.

Polythiazide (Indapamide may add to or potentiate the therapeutic effect of other antihypertensive drugs). Products include:
- Minizide Capsules 2700
- Renese Tablets 2712

Prazosin Hydrochloride (Indapamide may add to or potentiate the therapeutic effect of other antihypertensive drugs). Products include:
- Minipress Capsules 2699
- Minizide Capsules 2700

Prednisolone Acetate (Co-administration with corticosteroids may increase the risk of hypokalemia). Products include:
- Blephamide Ophthalmic Ointment 547
- Blephamide Ophthalmic Suspension 548
- Poly-Pred Liquifilm Ophthalmic Suspension .... ⊙245
- Pred Forte Ophthalmic Suspension .... ⊙246
- Pred Mild Sterile Ophthalmic Suspension .... ⊙249
- Pred-G Ophthalmic Suspension .... ⊙247
- Pred-G Sterile Ophthalmic Ointment .... ⊙248

Prednisolone Sodium Phosphate (Co-administration with corticosteroids may increase the risk of hypokalemia). Products include:
- Pediapred Oral Solution 1170

Prednisolone Tebutate (Co-administration with corticosteroids may increase the risk of hypokalemia).
- No products indexed under this heading.

IMPORTANT NOTE: Always consult each drug listing in the patient's regimen for possible interactions.

Prednisone (Co-administration with corticosteroids may increase the risk of hypokalemia). Products include:
- Prednisone 3064

Propoxyphene Hydrochloride (Aggravates orthostatic hypotension). Products include:
- Darvon Pulvules 1909
- Darvon Compound-65 Pulvules 1910

Propoxyphene Napsylate (Aggravates orthostatic hypotension). Products include:
- Darvon-N/Darvocet-N 1907
- Darvon-N Tablets 1912

Propranolol Hydrochloride (Indapamide may add to or potentiate the therapeutic effect of other antihypertensive drugs). Products include:
- Inderal 3513
- Inderal LA Long-Acting Capsules 3516
- Inderide Tablets 3517
- Inderide LA Long-Acting Capsules .. 3519

Quinapril Hydrochloride (Indapamide may add to or potentiate the therapeutic effect of other antihypertensive drugs). Products include:
- Accupril Tablets 2611
- Accuretic Tablets 2614

Ramipril (Indapamide may add to or potentiate the therapeutic effect of other antihypertensive drugs). Products include:
- Altace Capsules 2233

Rauwolfia serpentina (Indapamide may add to or potentiate the therapeutic effect of other antihypertensive drugs).
- No products indexed under this heading.

Remifentanil Hydrochloride (Aggravates orthostatic hypotension).
- No products indexed under this heading.

Rescinnamine (Indapamide may add to or potentiate the therapeutic effect of other antihypertensive drugs).
- No products indexed under this heading.

Reserpine (Indapamide may add to or potentiate the therapeutic effect of other antihypertensive drugs).
- No products indexed under this heading.

Secobarbital Sodium (Aggravates orthostatic hypotension).
- No products indexed under this heading.

Sodium Nitroprusside (Indapamide may add to or potentiate the therapeutic effect of other antihypertensive drugs).
- No products indexed under this heading.

Sotalol Hydrochloride (Indapamide may add to or potentiate the therapeutic effect of other antihypertensive drugs). Products include:
- Betapace Tablets 950
- Betapace AF Tablets 954

Spirapril Hydrochloride (Indapamide may add to or potentiate the therapeutic effect of other antihypertensive drugs).
- No products indexed under this heading.

Sufentanil Citrate (Aggravates orthostatic hypotension).
- No products indexed under this heading.

Telmisartan (Indapamide may add to or potentiate the therapeutic effect of other antihypertensive drugs). Products include:
- Micardis Tablets 1049
- Micardis HCT Tablets 1051

Terazosin Hydrochloride (Indapamide may add to or potentiate the therapeutic effect of other antihypertensive drugs). Products include:
- Hytrin Capsules 464

Thiamylal Sodium (Aggravates orthostatic hypotension).
- No products indexed under this heading.

Timolol Maleate (Indapamide may add to or potentiate the therapeutic effect of other antihypertensive drugs). Products include:
- Blocadren Tablets 2046
- Cosopt Sterile Ophthalmic Solution 2065
- Timolide Tablets 2187
- Timolol GFS .... ⊙266
- Timoptic in Ocudose 2192
- Timoptic Sterile Ophthalmic Solution 2190
- Timoptic-XE Sterile Ophthalmic Gel Forming Solution 2194

Torsemide (Indapamide may add to or potentiate the therapeutic effect of other antihypertensive drugs). Products include:
- Demadex Tablets and Injection 2965

Trandolapril (Indapamide may add to or potentiate the therapeutic effect of other antihypertensive drugs). Products include:
- Mavik Tablets 478
- Tarka Tablets 508

Triamcinolone (Co-administration with corticosteroids may increase the risk of hypokalemia).
- No products indexed under this heading.

Triamcinolone Acetonide (Co-administration with corticosteroids may increase the risk of hypokalemia). Products include:
- Azmacort Inhalation Aerosol 728
- Nasacort Nasal Inhaler 750
- Nasacort AQ Nasal Spray 752
- Tri-Nasal Spray 2274

Triamcinolone Diacetate (Co-administration with corticosteroids may increase the risk of hypokalemia).
- No products indexed under this heading.

Triamcinolone Hexacetonide (Co-administration with corticosteroids may increase the risk of hypokalemia).
- No products indexed under this heading.

Trimethaphan Camsylate (Indapamide may add to or potentiate the therapeutic effect of other antihypertensive drugs).
- No products indexed under this heading.

Valsartan (Indapamide may add to or potentiate the therapeutic effect of other antihypertensive drugs). Products include:
- Diovan Capsules 2337
- Diovan HCT Tablets 2338

Verapamil Hydrochloride (Indapamide may add to or potentiate the therapeutic effect of other antihypertensive drugs). Products include:
- Covera-HS Tablets 3199
- Isoptin SR Tablets 467
- Tarka Tablets 508
- Verelan Capsules 3184
- Verelan PM Capsules 3186

Food Interactions

Alcohol (Aggravates orthostatic hypotension).

INDERAL INJECTABLE

(Propranolol Hydrochloride) 3513

May interact with beta-adrenergic stimulating agents, calcium channel blockers, oral hypoglycemic agents, insulin, non-steroidal anti-inflammatory agents, phenytoin, theophylline, and certain other agents. Compounds in these categories include:

Acarbose (Beta-adrenergic blockade may prevent the appearance of certain premonitory signs and symptoms of acute hypoglycemia in labile insulin-dependent diabetes). Products include:
- Precose Tablets 906

Albuterol (Propranolol may block bronchodilation produced by exogenous catecholamine stimulation of beta receptors). Products include:
- Proventil Inhalation Aerosol 3142
- Ventolin Inhalation Aerosol and Refill 1679

Albuterol Sulfate (Propranolol may block bronchodilation produced by exogenous catecholamine stimulation of beta receptors). Products include:
- AccuNeb Inhalation Solution 1230
- Combivent Inhalation Aerosol 1041
- DuoNeb Inhalation Solution 1233
- Proventil Inhalation Solution 0.083% 3146
- Proventil Repetabs Tablets 3148
- Proventil Solution for Inhalation 0.5% 3144
- Proventil HFA Inhalation Aerosol 3150
- Ventolin HFA Inhalation Aerosol 3618
- Volmax Extended-Release Tablets .. 2276

Aluminum Hydroxide (Greatly reduces intestinal absorption of propranolol). Products include:
- Amphojel Suspension (Mint Flavor) .... ▣789
- Gaviscon Extra Strength Liquid ...... ▣751
- Gaviscon Extra Strength Tablets .... ▣751
- Gaviscon Regular Strength Liquid .. ▣751
- Gaviscon Regular Strength Tablets .... ▣750
- Maalox Antacid/Anti-Gas Oral Suspension .... ▣673
- Maalox Max Maximum Strength Antacid/Anti-Gas Liquid 2300
- Maalox Regular Strength Antacid/Antigas Liquid 2300
- Mylanta 1813
- Vanquish Caplets .... ▣617

Aminophylline (Co-administration of theophylline with propranolol results in reduced theophylline clearance).
- No products indexed under this heading.

Amlodipine Besylate (Both agents may depress myocardial contractility or AV conduction resulting in increased adverse reactions). Products include:
- Lotrel Capsules 2370
- Norvasc Tablets 2704

Antipyrine (Reduced clearance of antipyrine). Products include:
- Auralgan Otic Solution 3485

Bepridil Hydrochloride (Both agents may depress myocardial contractility or AV conduction resulting in increased adverse reactions). Products include:
- Vascor Tablets 2602

Bitolterol Mesylate (Propranolol may block bronchodilation produced by exogenous catecholamine stimulation of beta receptors).
- No products indexed under this heading.

Celecoxib (Blunts antihypertensive effect of beta blocker). Products include:
- Celebrex Capsules 2676
- Celebrex Capsules 2780

Chlorpromazine (Increased plasma levels of both drugs). Products include:
- Thorazine Suppositories 1656

Chlorpromazine Hydrochloride (Increased plasma levels of both drugs). Products include:
- Thorazine 1656

Chlorpropamide (Beta-adrenergic blockade may prevent the appearance of certain premonitory signs and symptoms of acute hypoglycemia in labile insulin-dependent diabetes). Products include:
- Diabinese Tablets 2680

Cimetidine (Decreases hepatic metabolism of propranolol resulting in increased blood levels). Products include:
- Tagamet HB 200 Suspension .... ▣762
- Tagamet HB 200 Tablets .... ▣761
- Tagamet Tablets 1644

Cimetidine Hydrochloride (Decreases hepatic metabolism of propranolol resulting in increased blood levels). Products include:
- Tagamet 1644

Diclofenac Potassium (Blunts antihypertensive effect of beta blocker). Products include:
- Cataflam Tablets 2315

Diclofenac Sodium (Blunts antihypertensive effect of beta blocker). Products include:
- Arthrotec Tablets 3195
- Voltaren Ophthalmic Sterile Ophthalmic Solution .... ⊙312
- Voltaren Tablets 2315
- Voltaren-XR Tablets 2315

Diltiazem Hydrochloride (Both agents may depress myocardial contractility or AV conduction resulting in increased adverse reactions). Products include:
- Cardizem Injectable 1018
- Cardizem Lyo-Ject Syringe 1018
- Cardizem Monovial 1018
- Cardizem CD Capsules 1016
- Tiazac Capsules 1378

Dobutamine Hydrochloride (Reversed effects of propranolol). Products include:
- Dobutrex Solution Vials 1914

Dyphylline (Co-administration of theophylline with propranolol results in reduced theophylline clearance). Products include:
- Lufyllin Tablets 3347
- Lufyllin-400 Tablets 3347
- Lufyllin-GG Elixir 3348
- Lufyllin-GG Tablets 3348

Ephedrine Hydrochloride (Propranolol may block bronchodilation produced by exogenous catecholamine stimulation of beta receptors). Products include:
- Primatene Tablets .... ▣780

Ephedrine Sulfate (Propranolol may block bronchodilation produced by exogenous catecholamine stimulation of beta receptors).
- No products indexed under this heading.

Ephedrine Tannate (Propranolol may block bronchodilation produced by exogenous catecholamine stimulation of beta receptors). Products include:
- Rynatuss Pediatric Suspension 3353
- Rynatuss Tablets 3353

Epinephrine (Potential for unresponsiveness to the usual dose of epinephrine to treat allergic reaction). Products include:
- Epifrin Sterile Ophthalmic Solution .... ⊙235
- EpiPen 1236
- Primatene Mist .... ▣779
- Xylocaine with Epinephrine Injection 653

Epinephrine Hydrochloride (Potential for unresponsiveness to the usual dose of epinephrine to treat allergic reaction).
- No products indexed under this heading.

Etodolac (Blunts antihypertensive effect of beta blocker). Products include:
- Lodine 3528
- Lodine XL Extended-Release Tablets 3530

Felodipine (Both agents may depress myocardial contractility or AV conduction resulting in increased adverse reactions). Products include:
- Lexxel Tablets 608
- Plendil Extended-Release Tablets ... 623

Fenoprofen Calcium (Blunts antihypertensive effect of beta blocker).
- No products indexed under this heading.

Flurbiprofen (Blunts antihypertensive effect of beta blocker).
- No products indexed under this heading.

Fosphenytoin Sodium (Accelerates propranolol clearance). Products include:
- Cerebyx Injection 2619

Glimepiride (Beta-adrenergic blockade may prevent the appearance of certain premonitory signs and symptoms of acute hypoglycemia in labile insulin-dependent diabetes). Products include:
- Amaryl Tablets 717

Glipizide (Beta-adrenergic blockade may prevent the appearance of certain premonitory signs and symptoms of acute hypoglycemia in labile insulin-dependent diabetes). Products include:
- Glucotrol Tablets 2692
- Glucotrol XL Extended Release Tablets 2693

Glyburide (Beta-adrenergic blockade may prevent the appearance of certain premonitory signs and symptoms of acute hypoglycemia in labile insulin-dependent diabetes). Products include:
- DiaBeta Tablets 741
- Glucovance Tablets 1086

Haloperidol (Hypotension and cardiac arrest have been reported with the concomitant use of propranolol and haloperidol). Products include:
- Haldol Injection, Tablets and Concentrate 2533

Haloperidol Decanoate (Hypotension and cardiac arrest have been reported with the concomitant use of propranolol and haloperidol). Products include:
- Haldol Decanoate 2535

Ibuprofen (Blunts antihypertensive effect of beta blocker). Products include:
- Advil 771
- Children's Advil Oral Suspension 773
- Children's Advil Chewable Tablets 773
- Advil Cold and Sinus Caplets 771
- Advil Cold and Sinus Tablets 771
- Advil Flu & Body Ache Caplets 772
- Infants' Advil Drops 773
- Junior Strength Advil Tablets 773
- Junior Strength Advil Chewable Tablets 773
- Advil Migraine Liquigels 772
- Children's Motrin Oral Suspension and Chewable Tablets 2006
- Children's Motrin Cold Oral Suspension 2007
- Children's Motrin Oral Suspension 643
- Motrin Suspension, Oral Drops, Chewable Tablets, and Caplets 2002
- Infants' Motrin Concentrated Drops 2006
- Junior Strength Motrin Caplets and Chewable Tablets 2006
- Motrin IB Tablets, Caplets, and Gelcaps 2002
- Motrin Migraine Pain Caplets 2005
- Motrin Sinus Headache Caplets 2005
- Vicoprofen Tablets 520

Indomethacin (Blunts antihypertensive effect of beta blocker). Products include:
- Indocin 2112

Indomethacin Sodium Trihydrate (Blunts antihypertensive effect of beta blocker). Products include:
- Indocin I.V. 2115

Insulin, Human, Zinc Suspension (Beta-adrenergic blockade may prevent the appearance of certain premonitory signs and symptoms of acute hypoglycemia in labile insulin-dependent diabetes; acute increases in blood pressure occurred after insulin-induced hypoglycemia in patients of propranolol). Products include:
- Humulin L, 100 Units 1937
- Humulin U, 100 Units 1943
- Novolin L Human Insulin 10 ml Vials 2422

Insulin, Human NPH (Beta-adrenergic blockade may prevent the appearance of certain premonitory signs and symptoms of acute hypoglycemia in labile insulin-dependent diabetes; acute increases in blood pressure occurred after insulin-induced hypoglycemia in patients of propranolol). Products include:
- Humulin N, 100 Units 1939
- Humulin N NPH Pen 1940
- Novolin N Human Insulin 10 ml Vials 2422
- Novolin N PenFill 2423
- Novolin N Prefilled Syringe Disposable Insulin Delivery System 2425

Insulin, Human Regular (Beta-adrenergic blockade may prevent the appearance of certain premonitory signs and symptoms of acute hypoglycemia in labile insulin-dependent diabetes; acute increases in blood pressure occurred after insulin-induced hypoglycemia in patients of propranolol). Products include:
- Humulin R Regular (U-500) 1943
- Humulin R, 100 Units 1941
- Novolin R Human Insulin 10 ml Vials 2423
- Novolin R PenFill 2423
- Novolin R Prefilled Syringe Disposable Insulin Delivery System 2425
- Velosulin BR Human Insulin 10 ml Vials 2435

Insulin, Human Regular and Human NPH Mixture (Beta-adrenergic blockade may prevent the appearance of certain premonitory signs and symptoms of acute hypoglycemia in labile insulin-dependent diabetes; acute increases in blood pressure occurred after insulin-induced hypoglycemia in patients of propranolol). Products include:
- Humulin 50/50, 100 Units 1934
- Humulin 70/30, 100 Units 1935
- Humulin 70/30 Pen 1936
- Novolin 70/30 Human Insulin 10 ml Vials 2421
- Novolin 70/30 PenFill 2423
- Novolin 70/30 Prefilled Disposable Insulin Delivery System 2425

Insulin, NPH (Beta-adrenergic blockade may prevent the appearance of certain premonitory signs and symptoms of acute hypoglycemia in labile insulin-dependent diabetes; acute increases in blood pressure occurred after insulin-induced hypoglycemia in patients of propranolol). Products include:
- Iletin II, NPH (Pork), 100 Units 1946

Insulin, Regular (Beta-adrenergic blockade may prevent the appearance of certain premonitory signs and symptoms of acute hypoglycemia in labile insulin-dependent diabetes; acute increases in blood pressure occurred after insulin-induced hypoglycemia in patients of propranolol). Products include:
- Iletin II, Regular (Pork), 100 Units 1947

Insulin, Zinc Crystals (Beta-adrenergic blockade may prevent the appearance of certain premonitory signs and symptoms of acute hypoglycemia in labile insulin-dependent diabetes; acute increases in blood pressure occurred after insulin-induced hypoglycemia in patients of propranolol).
- No products indexed under this heading.

Insulin, Zinc Suspension (Beta-adrenergic blockade may prevent the appearance of certain premonitory signs and symptoms of acute hypoglycemia in labile insulin-dependent diabetes; acute increases in blood pressure occurred after insulin-induced hypoglycemia in patients of propranolol). Products include:
- Iletin II, Lente (Pork), 100 Units 1945

Insulin Aspart, Human Regular (Beta-adrenergic blockade may prevent the appearance of certain premonitory signs and symptoms of acute hypoglycemia in labile insulin-dependent diabetes; acute increases in blood pressure occurred after insulin-induced hypoglycemia in patients of propranolol).
- No products indexed under this heading.

Insulin glargine (Beta-adrenergic blockade may prevent the appearance of certain premonitory signs and symptoms of acute hypoglycemia in labile insulin-dependent diabetes; acute increases in blood pressure occurred after insulin-induced hypoglycemia in patients of propranolol). Products include:
- Lantus Injection 742

Insulin Lispro, Human (Beta-adrenergic blockade may prevent the appearance of certain premonitory signs and symptoms of acute hypoglycemia in labile insulin-dependent diabetes; acute increases in blood pressure occurred after insulin-induced hypoglycemia in patients of propranolol). Products include:
- Humalog 1926
- Humalog Mix 75/25 Pen 1928

Insulin Lispro Protamine, Human (Beta-adrenergic blockade may prevent the appearance of certain premonitory signs and symptoms of acute hypoglycemia in labile insulin-dependent diabetes; acute increases in blood pressure occurred after insulin-induced hypoglycemia in patients of propranolol). Products include:
- Humalog Mix 75/25 Pen 1928

Isoetharine (Propranolol may block bronchodilation produced by exogenous catecholamine stimulation of beta receptors).
- No products indexed under this heading.

Isoproterenol Hydrochloride (Propranolol may block bronchodilation produced by exogenous catecholamine stimulation of beta receptors).
- No products indexed under this heading.

Isoproterenol Sulfate (Propranolol may block bronchodilation produced by exogenous catecholamine stimulation of beta receptors).
- No products indexed under this heading.

Isradipine (Both agents may depress myocardial contractility or AV conduction resulting in increased adverse reactions). Products include:
- DynaCirc Capsules 2921
- DynaCirc CR Tablets 2923

Ketoprofen (Blunts antihypertensive effect of beta blocker). Products include:
- Orudis Capsules 3548
- Orudis KT Tablets 778
- Oruvail Capsules 3548

Ketorolac Tromethamine (Blunts antihypertensive effect of beta blocker). Products include:
- Acular Ophthalmic Solution 544
- Acular PF Ophthalmic Solution 544
- Toradol 3018

Levalbuterol Hydrochloride (Propranolol may block bronchodilation produced by exogenous catecholamine stimulation of beta receptors). Products include:
- Xopenex Inhalation Solution 3207

Levothyroxine Sodium (Concurrent use may result in lower than expected T_3 concentration). Products include:
- Levothroid Tablets 1373
- Levoxyl Tablets 1819
- Synthroid 505
- Unithroid Tablets 3445

Lidocaine Hydrochloride (Reduced clearance of lidocaine). Products include:
- Bactine First Aid Liquid 611
- Xylocaine Injections 653

Meclofenamate Sodium (Blunts antihypertensive effect of beta blocker).
- No products indexed under this heading.

Mefenamic Acid (Blunts antihypertensive effect of beta blocker). Products include:
- Ponstel Capsules 1356

Meloxicam (Blunts antihypertensive effect of beta blocker). Products include:
- Mobic Tablets 1054

Metaproterenol Sulfate (Propranolol may block bronchodilation produced by exogenous catecholamine stimulation of beta receptors). Products include:
- Alupent 1029

Metformin Hydrochloride (Beta-adrenergic blockade may prevent the appearance of certain premonitory signs and symptoms of acute hypoglycemia in labile insulin-dependent diabetes). Products include:
- Glucophage Tablets 1080
- Glucophage XR Tablets 1080
- Glucovance Tablets 1086

Mibefradil Dihydrochloride (Both agents may depress myocardial contractility or AV conduction resulting in increased adverse reactions).
- No products indexed under this heading.

Miglitol (Beta-adrenergic blockade may prevent the appearance of certain premonitory signs and symptoms of acute hypoglycemia in labile insulin-dependent diabetes). Products include:
- Glyset Tablets 2821

Nabumetone (Blunts antihypertensive effect of beta blocker). Products include:
- Relafen Tablets 1617

Naproxen (Blunts antihypertensive effect of beta blocker). Products include:
- EC-Naprosyn Delayed-Release Tablets 2967
- Naprosyn Suspension 2967
- Naprosyn Tablets 2967

Naproxen Sodium (Blunts antihypertensive effect of beta blocker). Products include:
- Aleve Tablets, Caplets and Gelcaps 602
- Aleve Cold & Sinus Caplets 603
- Anaprox Tablets 2967
- Anaprox DS Tablets 2967
- Naprelan Tablets 1293

Nicardipine Hydrochloride (Both agents may depress myocardial contractility or AV conduction resulting in increased adverse reactions). Products include:
- Cardene I.V. 3485

Nifedipine (Both agents may depress myocardial contractility or AV conduction resulting in increased adverse reactions). Products include:
- Adalat CC Tablets 877
- Procardia Capsules 2708
- Procardia XL Extended Release Tablets 2710

Nimodipine (Both agents may depress myocardial contractility or AV conduction resulting in increased adverse reactions). Products include:
- Nimotop Capsules 904

Nisoldipine (Both agents may depress myocardial contractility or AV conduction resulting in increased adverse reactions). Products include:
- Sular Tablets 688

Oxaprozin (Blunts antihypertensive effect of beta blocker).
- No products indexed under this heading.

Phenobarbital (Accelerates propranolol clearance). Products include:
- Arco-Lase Plus Tablets 592

IMPORTANT NOTE: Always consult each drug listing in the patient's regimen for possible interactions.

Donnatal 2929
Donnatal Extentabs 2930

Phenylbutazone (Blunts antihypertensive effect of beta blocker).
No products indexed under this heading.

Phenytoin (Accelerates propranolol clearance). Products include:
Dilantin Infatabs 2624
Dilantin-125 Oral Suspension 2625

Phenytoin Sodium (Accelerates propranolol clearance). Products include:
Dilantin Kapseals 2622

Pioglitazone Hydrochloride (Beta-adrenergic blockade may prevent the appearance of certain premonitory signs and symptoms of acute hypoglycemia in labile insulin-dependent diabetes). Products include:
Actos Tablets 3275

Pirbuterol Acetate (Propranolol may block bronchodilation produced by exogenous catecholamine stimulation of beta receptors). Products include:
Maxair Autohaler 1981
Maxair Inhaler 1984

Piroxicam (Blunts antihypertensive effect of beta blocker). Products include:
Feldene Capsules 2685

Repaglinide (Beta-adrenergic blockade may prevent the appearance of certain premonitory signs and symptoms of acute hypoglycemia in labile insulin-dependent diabetes). Products include:
Prandin Tablets (0.5, 1, and 2 mg) 2432

Reserpine (Co-administration of catecholamine-depleting drugs, such as reserpine, may produce an excessive reduction of resting sympathetic nervous activity, which may result in hypotension, vertigo, marked bradycardia, syncopal attacks or orthostatic hypotension).
No products indexed under this heading.

Rifampin (Accelerates propranolol clearance). Products include:
Rifadin 765
Rifamate Capsules 767
Rifater Tablets 769

Rofecoxib (Blunts antihypertensive effect of beta blocker). Products include:
Vioxx 2213

Rosiglitazone Maleate (Beta-adrenergic blockade may prevent the appearance of certain premonitory signs and symptoms of acute hypoglycemia in labile insulin-dependent diabetes). Products include:
Avandia Tablets 1490

Salmeterol Xinafoate (Propranolol may block bronchodilation produced by exogenous catecholamine stimulation of beta receptors). Products include:
Advair Diskus 100/50 1448
Advair Diskus 250/50 1448
Advair Diskus 500/50 1448
Serevent Diskus 1637
Serevent Inhalation Aerosol 1633

Sulindac (Blunts antihypertensive effect of beta blocker). Products include:
Clinoril Tablets 2053

Terbutaline Sulfate (Propranolol may block bronchodilation produced by exogenous catecholamine stimulation of beta receptors). Products include:
Brethine Ampuls 2314
Brethine Tablets 2313

Theophylline (Co-administration of theophylline with propranolol results in reduced theophylline clearance). Products include:
Aerolate 1361
Theo-Dur Extended-Release Tablets 1835
Uni-Dur Extended-Release Tablets .. 1841
Uniphyl 400 mg and 600 mg Tablets 2903

Theophylline Calcium Salicylate (Co-administration of theophylline with propranolol results in reduced theophylline clearance).
No products indexed under this heading.

Theophylline Sodium Glycinate (Co-administration of theophylline with propranolol results in reduced theophylline clearance).
No products indexed under this heading.

Tolazamide (Beta-adrenergic blockade may prevent the appearance of certain premonitory signs and symptoms of acute hypoglycemia in labile insulin-dependent diabetes).
No products indexed under this heading.

Tolbutamide (Beta-adrenergic blockade may prevent the appearance of certain premonitory signs and symptoms of acute hypoglycemia in labile insulin-dependent diabetes).
No products indexed under this heading.

Tolmetin Sodium (Blunts antihypertensive effect of beta blocker). Products include:
Tolectin 2589

Troglitazone (Beta-adrenergic blockade may prevent the appearance of certain premonitory signs and symptoms of acute hypoglycemia in labile insulin-dependent diabetes).
No products indexed under this heading.

Verapamil Hydrochloride (Co-administration of intravenous beta-blocker and verapamil, on rare occasion, has resulted in serious adverse reactions, especially in patients with severe cardiomyopathy, congestive heart failure or recent myocardial infarction; calcium channel blockers and beta-blockers may depress myocardial contractility or AV conduction). Products include:
Covera-HS Tablets 3199
Isoptin SR Tablets 467
Tarka Tablets 508
Verelan Capsules 3184
Verelan PM Capsules 3186

Food Interactions

Alcohol (Slows the rate of absorption of propranolol).

INDERAL TABLETS
(Propranolol Hydrochloride) 3513
See Inderal Injectable

INDERAL LA LONG-ACTING CAPSULES
(Propranolol Hydrochloride) 3516
See Inderal Injectable

INDERIDE TABLETS
(Hydrochlorothiazide, Propranolol Hydrochloride) 3517

May interact with antihypertensives, barbiturates, calcium channel blockers, corticosteroids, cardiac glycosides, oral hypoglycemic agents, insulin, narcotic analgesics, non-steroidal anti-inflammatory agents, phenytoin, theophylline, and certain other agents. Compounds in these categories include:

Acarbose (Beta-adrenergic blockade may prevent the appearance of certain premonitory signs and symptoms of acute hypoglycemia in labile insulin-dependent diabetes). Products include:
Precose Tablets 906

Acebutolol Hydrochloride (Potentiated or additive action). Products include:
Sectral Capsules 3589

ACTH (Hypokalemia may develop with concomitant use).
No products indexed under this heading.

Alfentanil Hydrochloride (Aggravates orthostatic hypotension).
No products indexed under this heading.

Aluminum Hydroxide (Greatly reduces intestinal absorption of propranolol). Products include:
Amphojel Suspension (Mint Flavor) .... ■789
Gaviscon Extra Strength Liquid ..... ■751
Gaviscon Extra Strength Tablets .... ■751
Gaviscon Regular Strength Liquid . ■751
Gaviscon Regular Strength Tablets .... ■750
Maalox Antacid/Anti-Gas Oral Suspension .... ■673
Maalox Max Maximum Strength Antacid/Anti-Gas Liquid 2300
Maalox Regular Strength Antacid/Antigas Liquid 2300
Mylanta 1813
Vanquish Caplets .... ■617

Aminophylline (Co-administration of theophylline with propranolol results in reduced theophylline clearance).
No products indexed under this heading.

Amlodipine Besylate (Both agents may depress myocardial contractility or AV conduction resulting in increased adverse reactions). Products include:
Lotrel Capsules 2370
Norvasc Tablets 2704

Antipyrine (Reduced clearance of antipyrine). Products include:
Auralgan Otic Solution 3485

Aprobarbital (Aggravates orthostatic hypotension).
No products indexed under this heading.

Atenolol (Potentiated or additive action). Products include:
Tenoretic Tablets 690
Tenormin I.V. Injection 692

Benazepril Hydrochloride (Potentiated or additive action). Products include:
Lotensin Tablets 2365
Lotensin HCT Tablets 2367
Lotrel Capsules 2370

Bendroflumethiazide (Potentiated or additive action). Products include:
Corzide 40/5 Tablets 2247
Corzide 80/5 Tablets 2247

Bepridil Hydrochloride (Both agents may depress myocardial contractility or AV conduction resulting in increased adverse reactions). Products include:
Vascor Tablets 2602

Betamethasone Acetate (Hypokalemia may develop with concomitant use). Products include:
Celestone Soluspan Injectable Suspension 3097

Betamethasone Sodium Phosphate (Hypokalemia may develop with concomitant use). Products include:
Celestone Soluspan Injectable Suspension 3097

Betaxolol Hydrochloride (Potentiated or additive action). Products include:
Betoptic S Ophthalmic Suspension 537

Bisoprolol Fumarate (Potentiated or additive action). Products include:
Zebeta Tablets 1885
Ziac Tablets 1887

Buprenorphine Hydrochloride (Aggravates orthostatic hypotension). Products include:
Buprenex Injectable 2918

Butabarbital (Aggravates orthostatic hypotension).
No products indexed under this heading.

Butalbital (Aggravates orthostatic hypotension). Products include:
Phrenilin 578
Sedapap Tablets 50 mg/650 mg ... 2225

Candesartan Cilexetil (Potentiated or additive action). Products include:
Atacand Tablets 595
Atacand HCT Tablets 597

Captopril (Potentiated or additive action). Products include:
Captopril Tablets 2281

Carteolol Hydrochloride (Potentiated or additive action). Products include:
Carteolol Hydrochloride Ophthalmic Solution USP, 1% ..... ⊙258
Ocupress Ophthalmic Solution, 1% Sterile .... ⊙303

Celecoxib (Blunting of the antihypertensive effect). Products include:
Celebrex Capsules 2676
Celebrex Capsules 2780

Chlorothiazide (Potentiated or additive action). Products include:
Aldoclor Tablets 2035
Diuril Oral 2087

Chlorothiazide Sodium (Potentiated or additive action). Products include:
Diuril Sodium Intravenous 2086

Chlorpromazine (Increased plasma levels of both drugs). Products include:
Thorazine Suppositories 1656

Chlorpropamide (Beta-adrenergic blockade may prevent the appearance of certain premonitory signs and symptoms of acute hypoglycemia in labile insulin-dependent diabetes). Products include:
Diabinese Tablets 2680

Chlorthalidone (Potentiated or additive action). Products include:
Clorpres Tablets 1002
Combipres Tablets 1040
Tenoretic Tablets 690

Cimetidine (Decreases hepatic metabolism of propranolol resulting in increased blood levels). Products include:
Tagamet HB 200 Suspension .... ■762
Tagamet HB 200 Tablets .... ■761
Tagamet Tablets 1644

Cimetidine Hydrochloride (Decreases hepatic metabolism of propranolol resulting in increased blood levels). Products include:
Tagamet 1644

Clonidine (Potentiated or additive action). Products include:
Catapres-TTS 1038

Clonidine Hydrochloride (Potentiated or additive action). Products include:
Catapres Tablets 1037
Clorpres Tablets 1002
Combipres Tablets 1040
Duraclon Injection 3057

Codeine Phosphate (Aggravates orthostatic hypotension). Products include:
Phenergan with Codeine Syrup 3557
Phenergan VC with Codeine Syrup . 3561
Robitussin A-C Syrup 2942
Robitussin-DAC Syrup 2942
Ryna-C Liquid .... ■768
Soma Compound w/Codeine Tablets 3355
Tussi-Organidin NR Liquid 3350
Tussi-Organidin-S NR Liquid 3350
Tylenol with Codeine 2595

Cortisone Acetate (Hypokalemia may develop with concomitant use). Products include:
Cortone Acetate Injectable Suspension 2059
Cortone Acetate Tablets 2061

Deserpidine (Potentiated or additive action).
No products indexed under this heading.

Deslanoside (Hypokalemia can sensitize or exaggerate the response of

the heart to digitalis toxicity).
No products indexed under this heading.

Dexamethasone (Hypokalemia may develop with concomitant use). Products include:
Decadron Elixir 2078
Decadron Tablets 2079
TobraDex Ophthalmic Ointment 542
TobraDex Ophthalmic Suspension 541

Dexamethasone Acetate (Hypokalemia may develop with concomitant use).
No products indexed under this heading.

Dexamethasone Sodium Phosphate (Hypokalemia may develop with concomitant use). Products include:
Decadron Phosphate Injection 2081
Decadron Phosphate Sterile Ophthalmic Ointment 2083
Decadron Phosphate Sterile Ophthalmic Solution 2084
NeoDecadron Sterile Ophthalmic Solution 2144

Dezocine (Aggravates orthostatic hypotension).
No products indexed under this heading.

Diazoxide (Potentiated or additive action).
No products indexed under this heading.

Diclofenac Potassium (Blunting of the antihypertensive effect). Products include:
Cataflam Tablets 2315

Diclofenac Sodium (Blunting of the antihypertensive effect). Products include:
Arthrotec Tablets 3195
Voltaren Ophthalmic Sterile Ophthalmic Solution .... ⊙ 312
Voltaren Tablets 2315
Voltaren-XR Tablets 2315

Digitoxin (Hypokalemia can sensitize or exaggerate the response of the heart to digitalis toxicity).
No products indexed under this heading.

Digoxin (Hypokalemia can sensitize or exaggerate the response of the heart to digitalis toxicity). Products include:
Digitek Tablets 1003
Lanoxicaps Capsules 1574
Lanoxin Injection 1581
Lanoxin Tablets 1587
Lanoxin Elixir Pediatric 1578
Lanoxin Injection Pediatric 1584

Diltiazem Hydrochloride (Both agents may depress myocardial contractility or AV conduction resulting in increased adverse reactions). Products include:
Cardizem Injectable 1018
Cardizem Lyo-Ject Syringe 1018
Cardizem Monovial 1018
Cardizem CD Capsules 1016
Tiazac Capsules 1378

Doxazosin Mesylate (Potentiated or additive action). Products include:
Cardura Tablets 2668

Dyphylline (Co-administration of theophylline with propranolol results in reduced theophylline clearance). Products include:
Lufyllin Tablets 3347
Lufyllin-400 Tablets 3347
Lufyllin-GG Elixir 3348
Lufyllin-GG Tablets 3348

Enalapril Maleate (Potentiated or additive action). Products include:
Lexxel Tablets 608
Vaseretic Tablets 2204
Vasotec Tablets 2210

Enalaprilat (Potentiated or additive action). Products include:
Enalaprilat Injection 863
Vasotec I.V. Injection 2207

Eprosartan Mesylate (Potentiated or additive action). Products include:
Teveten Tablets 3327

Esmolol Hydrochloride (Potentiated or additive action). Products include:
Brevibloc Injection 858

Etodolac (Blunting of the antihypertensive effect). Products include:
Lodine 3528
Lodine XL Extended-Release Tablets 3530

Felodipine (Both agents may depress myocardial contractility or AV conduction resulting in increased adverse reactions). Products include:
Lexxel Tablets 608
Plendil Extended-Release Tablets 623

Fenoprofen Calcium (Blunting of the antihypertensive effect).
No products indexed under this heading.

Fentanyl (Aggravates orthostatic hypotension). Products include:
Duragesic Transdermal System 1786

Fentanyl Citrate (Aggravates orthostatic hypotension). Products include:
Actiq 1184

Fludrocortisone Acetate (Hypokalemia may develop with concomitant use). Products include:
Florinef Acetate Tablets 2250

Flurbiprofen (Blunting of the antihypertensive effect).
No products indexed under this heading.

Fosinopril Sodium (Potentiated or additive action). Products include:
Monopril Tablets 1091
Monopril HCT 1094

Fosphenytoin Sodium (Accelarate propranolol clearance). Products include:
Cerebyx Injection 2619

Furosemide (Potentiated or additive action). Products include:
Furosemide Tablets 2284

Glimepiride (Beta-adrenergic blockade may prevent the appearance of certain premonitory signs and symptoms of acute hypoglycemia in labile insulin-dependent diabetes). Products include:
Amaryl Tablets 717

Glipizide (Beta-adrenergic blockade may prevent the appearance of certain premonitory signs and symptoms of acute hypoglycemia in labile insulin-dependent diabetes). Products include:
Glucotrol Tablets 2692
Glucotrol XL Extended Release Tablets 2693

Glyburide (Beta-adrenergic blockade may prevent the appearance of certain premonitory signs and symptoms of acute hypoglycemia in labile insulin-dependent diabetes). Products include:
DiaBeta Tablets 741
Glucovance Tablets 1086

Guanabenz Acetate (Potentiated or additive action).
No products indexed under this heading.

Guanethidine Monosulfate (Potentiated or additive action).
No products indexed under this heading.

Haloperidol (Concomitant use may result in hypotension and coronary arrest). Products include:
Haldol Injection, Tablets and Concentrate 2533

Haloperidol Decanoate (Concomitant use may result in hypotension and coronary arrest). Products include:
Haldol Decanoate 2535

Hydralazine Hydrochloride (Potentiated or additive action).
No products indexed under this heading.

Hydrocodone Bitartrate (Aggravates orthostatic hypotension). Products include:
Hycodan 1316
Hycomine Compound Tablets 1317
Hycotuss Expectorant Syrup 1318
Lortab 3319
Lortab Elixir 3317
Maxidone Tablets CIII 3399
Norco 5/325 Tablets CIII 3424
Norco 7.5/325 Tablets CIII 3425
Norco 10/325 Tablets CIII 3427
Norco 10/325 Tablets CIII 3425
Vicodin Tablets 516
Vicodin ES Tablets 517
Vicodin HP Tablets 518
Vicodin Tuss Expectorant 519
Vicoprofen Tablets 520
Zydone Tablets 1330

Hydrocodone Polistirex (Aggravates orthostatic hypotension). Products include:
Tussionex Pennkinetic Extended-Release Suspension 1174

Hydrocortisone (Hypokalemia may develop with concomitant use). Products include:
Anusol-HC Cream 2.5% 2237
Cipro HC Otic Suspension 540
Cortaid Intensive Therapy Cream 717
Cortaid Maximum Strength Cream 717
Cortisporin Ophthalmic Suspension Sterile .... ⊙ 297
Cortizone•5 699
Cortizone•10 699
Cortizone•10 Plus Creme 700
Cortizone for Kids Creme 699
Hydrocortone Tablets 2106
Massengill Medicated Soft Cloth Towelette 753
VōSoL HC Otic Solution 3356

Hydrocortisone Acetate (Hypokalemia may develop with concomitant use). Products include:
Analpram-HC 1338
Anusol HC-1 Hydrocortisone Anti-Itch Cream 689
Anusol-HC Suppositories 2238
Cortaid 717
Cortifoam Rectal Foam 3170
Cortisporin-TC Otic Suspension 2246
Hydrocortone Acetate Injectable Suspension 2103
Pramosone 1343
Proctocort Suppositories 2264
ProctoFoam-HC 3177
Terra-Cortril Ophthalmic Suspension 2716

Hydrocortisone Sodium Phosphate (Hypokalemia may develop with concomitant use). Products include:
Hydrocortone Phosphate Injection, Sterile 2105

Hydrocortisone Sodium Succinate (Hypokalemia may develop with concomitant use).
No products indexed under this heading.

Hydroflumethiazide (Potentiated or additive action). Products include:
Diucardin Tablets 3494

Hydromorphone Hydrochloride (Aggravates orthostatic hypotension). Products include:
Dilaudid 441
Dilaudid Oral Liquid 445
Dilaudid Powder 441
Dilaudid Rectal Suppositories 441
Dilaudid Tablets 441
Dilaudid Tablets - 8 mg 445
Dilaudid-HP 443

Ibuprofen (Blunting of the antihypertensive effect). Products include:
Advil 771
Children's Advil Oral Suspension 773
Children's Advil Chewable Tablets 773
Advil Cold and Sinus Caplets 771
Advil Cold and Sinus Tablets 771
Advil Flu & Body Ache Caplets 772
Infants' Advil Drops 773
Junior Strength Advil Tablets 773
Junior Strength Advil Chewable Tablets 773
Advil Migraine Liquigels 772
Children's Motrin Oral Suspension and Chewable Tablets 2006
Children's Motrin Cold Oral Suspension 2007
Children's Motrin Oral Suspension 643
Motrin Suspension, Oral Drops, Chewable Tablets, and Caplets 2002
Infants' Motrin Concentrated Drops 2006
Junior Strength Motrin Caplets and Chewable Tablets 2006
Motrin IB Tablets, Caplets, and Gelcaps 2002
Motrin Migraine Pain Caplets 2005
Motrin Sinus Headache Caplets 2005
Vicoprofen Tablets 520

Indapamide (Potentiated or additive action). Products include:
Indapamide Tablets 2286

Indomethacin (Blunting of the antihypertensive effect). Products include:
Indocin 2112

Indomethacin Sodium Trihydrate (Blunting of the antihypertensive effect). Products include:
Indocin I.V. 2115

Insulin, Human, Zinc Suspension (Beta-adrenergic blockers may prevent the appearance of certain premonitory signs and symptoms of acute hypoglycemia in labile insulin-dependent diabetes; acute increases in blood pressure have occured after insulin-induced hypoglycemia in patients on propranolol). Products include:
Humulin L, 100 Units 1937
Humulin U, 100 Units 1943
Novolin L Human Insulin 10 ml Vials 2422

Insulin, Human NPH (Beta-adrenergic blockers may prevent the appearance of certain premonitory signs and symptoms of acute hypoglycemia in labile insulin-dependent diabetes; acute increases in blood pressure have occured after insulin-induced hypoglycemia in patients on propranolol). Products include:
Humulin N, 100 Units 1939
Humulin N NPH Pen 1940
Novolin N Human Insulin 10 ml Vials 2422
Novolin N PenFill 2423
Novolin N Prefilled Syringe Disposable Insulin Delivery System 2425

Insulin, Human Regular (Beta-adrenergic blockers may prevent the appearance of certain premonitory signs and symptoms of acute hypoglycemia in labile insulin-dependent diabetes; acute increases in blood pressure have occured after insulin-induced hypoglycemia in patients on propranolol). Products include:
Humulin R Regular (U-500) 1943
Humulin R, 100 Units 1941
Novolin R Human Insulin 10 ml Vials 2423
Novolin R PenFill 2423
Novolin R Prefilled Syringe Disposable Insulin Delivery System 2425
Velosulin BR Human Insulin 10 ml Vials 2435

Insulin, Human Regular and Human NPH Mixture (Beta-adrenergic blockers may prevent the appearance of certain premonitory signs and symptoms of acute hypoglycemia in labile insulin-dependent diabetes; acute increases in blood pressure have occured after insulin-induced hypoglycemia in patients on propranolol). Products include:
Humulin 50/50, 100 Units 1934
Humulin 70/30, 100 Units 1935
Humulin 70/30 Pen 1936
Novolin 70/30 Human Insulin 10 ml Vials 2421
Novolin 70/30 PenFill 2423
Novolin 70/30 Prefilled Disposable Insulin Delivery System 2425

Insulin, NPH (Beta-adrenergic blockers may prevent the appearance of certain premonitory signs and symptoms of acute hypoglycemia in labile insulin-dependent diabetes; acute increases in blood pres-

sure have occured after insulin-induced hypoglycemia in patients on propranolol). Products include:
Iletin II, NPH (Pork), 100 Units 1946

Insulin, Regular (Beta-adrenergic blockers may prevent the appearance of certain premonitory signs and symptoms of acute hypoglycemia in labile insulin-dependent diabetes; acute increases in blood pressure have occured after insulin-induced hypoglycemia in patients on propranolol). Products include:
Iletin II, Regular (Pork), 100 Units ... 1947

Insulin, Zinc Crystals (Beta-adrenergic blockers may prevent the appearance of certain premonitory signs and symptoms of acute hypoglycemia in labile insulin-dependent diabetes; acute increases in blood pressure have occured after insulin-induced hypoglycemia in patients on propranolol).
No products indexed under this heading.

Insulin, Zinc Suspension (Beta-adrenergic blockers may prevent the appearance of certain premonitory signs and symptoms of acute hypoglycemia in labile insulin-dependent diabetes; acute increases in blood pressure have occured after insulin-induced hypoglycemia in patients on propranolol). Products include:
Iletin II, Lente (Pork), 100 Units 1945

Insulin Aspart, Human Regular (Beta-adrenergic blockers may prevent the appearance of certain premonitory signs and symptoms of acute hypoglycemia in labile insulin-dependent diabetes; acute increases in blood pressure have occured after insulin-induced hypoglycemia in patients on propranolol).
No products indexed under this heading.

Insulin glargine (Beta-adrenergic blockers may prevent the appearance of certain premonitory signs and symptoms of acute hypoglycemia in labile insulin-dependent diabetes; acute increases in blood pressure have occured after insulin-induced hypoglycemia in patients on propranolol). Products include:
Lantus Injection 742

Insulin Lispro, Human (Beta-adrenergic blockers may prevent the appearance of certain premonitory signs and symptoms of acute hypoglycemia in labile insulin-dependent diabetes; acute increases in blood pressure have occured after insulin-induced hypoglycemia in patients on propranolol). Products include:
Humalog 1926
Humalog Mix 75/25 Pen 1928

Insulin Lispro Protamine, Human (Beta-adrenergic blockers may prevent the appearance of certain premonitory signs and symptoms of acute hypoglycemia in labile insulin-dependent diabetes; acute increases in blood pressure have occured after insulin-induced hypoglycemia in patients on propranolol). Products include:
Humalog Mix 75/25 Pen 1928

Irbesartan (Potentiated or additive action). Products include:
Avalide Tablets 1070
Avapro Tablets 1074
Avapro Tablets 3076

Isradipine (Both agents may depress myocardial contractility or AV conduction resulting in increased adverse reactions). Products include:
DynaCirc Capsules 2921
DynaCirc CR Tablets 2923

Ketoprofen (Blunting of the antihypertensive effect). Products include:
Orudis Capsules 3548
Orudis KT Tablets .... ▣778
Oruvail Capsules 3548

Ketorolac Tromethamine (Blunting of the antihypertensive effect). Products include:
Acular Ophthalmic Solution 544
Acular PF Ophthalmic Solution 544
Toradol 3018

Labetalol Hydrochloride (Potentiated or additive action). Products include:
Normodyne Injection 3135
Normodyne Tablets 3137

Levorphanol Tartrate (Aggravates orthostatic hypotension). Products include:
Levo-Dromoran 1734
Levorphanol Tartrate Tablets 3059

Levothyroxine Sodium (Coadministration may result in lower than expected T3 concentration). Products include:
Levothroid Tablets 1373
Levoxyl Tablets 1819
Synthroid 505
Unithroid Tablets 3445

Lidocaine Hydrochloride (Reduced clearance of lidocaine). Products include:
Bactine First Aid Liquid .... ▣611
Xylocaine Injections 653

Lisinopril (Potentiated or additive action). Products include:
Prinivil Tablets 2164
Prinzide Tablets 2168
Zestoretic Tablets 695
Zestril Tablets 698

Losartan Potassium (Potentiated or additive action). Products include:
Cozaar Tablets 2067
Hyzaar 2109

Mecamylamine Hydrochloride (Potentiated or additive action). Products include:
Inversine Tablets 1850

Meclofenamate Sodium (Blunting of the antihypertensive effect).
No products indexed under this heading.

Mefenamic Acid (Blunting of the antihypertensive effect). Products include:
Ponstel Capsules 1356

Meloxicam (Blunting of the antihypertensive effect). Products include:
Mobic Tablets 1054

Meperidine Hydrochloride (Aggravates orthostatic hypotension). Products include:
Demerol 3079
Mepergan Injection 3539

Mephobarbital (Aggravates orthostatic hypotension).
No products indexed under this heading.

Metformin Hydrochloride (Beta-adrenergic blockade may prevent the appearance of certain premonitory signs and symptoms of acute hypoglycemia in labile insulin-dependent diabetes). Products include:
Glucophage Tablets 1080
Glucophage XR Tablets 1080
Glucovance Tablets 1086

Methadone Hydrochloride (Aggravates orthostatic hypotension). Products include:
Dolophine Hydrochloride Tablets 3056

Methyclothiazide (Potentiated or additive action).
No products indexed under this heading.

Methyldopa (Potentiated or additive action). Products include:
Aldoclor Tablets 2035
Aldomet Tablets 2037
Aldoril Tablets 2039

Methyldopate Hydrochloride (Potentiated or additive action).
No products indexed under this heading.

Methylprednisolone Acetate (Hypokalemia may develop with concomitant use). Products include:
Depo-Medrol Injectable Suspension 2795

Methylprednisolone Sodium Succinate (Hypokalemia may develop with concomitant use). Products include:
Solu-Medrol Sterile Powder 2855

Metolazone (Potentiated or additive action). Products include:
Mykrox Tablets 1168
Zaroxolyn Tablets 1177

Metoprolol Succinate (Potentiated or additive action). Products include:
Toprol-XL Tablets 651

Metoprolol Tartrate (Potentiated or additive action).
No products indexed under this heading.

Metyrosine (Potentiated or additive action). Products include:
Demser Capsules 2085

Mibefradil Dihydrochloride (Both agents may depress myocardial contractility or AV conduction resulting in increased adverse reactions).
No products indexed under this heading.

Miglitol (Beta-adrenergic blockade may prevent the appearance of certain premonitory signs and symptoms of acute hypoglycemia in labile insulin-dependent diabetes). Products include:
Glyset Tablets 2821

Minoxidil (Potentiated or additive action). Products include:
Rogaine Extra Strength for Men Topical Solution .... ▣721
Rogaine for Women Topical Solution .... ▣721

Moexipril Hydrochloride (Potentiated or additive action). Products include:
Uniretic Tablets 3178
Univasc Tablets 3181

Morphine Sulfate (Aggravates orthostatic hypotension). Products include:
Astramorph/PF Injection, USP (Preservative-Free) 594
Duramorph Injection 1312
Infumorph 200 and Infumorph 500 Sterile Solutions 1314
Kadian Capsules 1335
MS Contin Tablets 2896
MSIR 2898
Oramorph SR Tablets 3062
Roxanol 3066

Nabumetone (Blunting of the antihypertensive effect). Products include:
Relafen Tablets 1617

Nadolol (Potentiated or additive action). Products include:
Corgard Tablets 2245
Corzide 40/5 Tablets 2247
Corzide 80/5 Tablets 2247
Nadolol Tablets 2288

Naproxen (Blunting of the antihypertensive effect). Products include:
EC-Naprosyn Delayed-Release Tablets 2967
Naprosyn Suspension 2967
Naprosyn Tablets 2967

Naproxen Sodium (Blunting of the antihypertensive effect). Products include:
Aleve Tablets, Caplets and Gelcaps .... ▣602
Aleve Cold & Sinus Caplets .... ▣603
Anaprox Tablets 2967
Anaprox DS Tablets 2967
Naprelan Tablets 1293

Nicardipine Hydrochloride (Both agents may depress myocardial contractility or AV conduction resulting in increased adverse reactions). Products include:
Cardene I.V. 3485

Nifedipine (Both agents may depress myocardial contractility or AV conduction resulting in increased adverse reactions). Products include:
Adalat CC Tablets 877
Procardia Capsules 2708
Procardia XL Extended Release Tablets 2710

Nimodipine (Both agents may depress myocardial contractility or AV conduction resulting in increased adverse reactions). Products include:
Nimotop Capsules 904

Nisoldipine (Both agents may depress myocardial contractility or AV conduction resulting in increased adverse reactions). Products include:
Sular Tablets 688

Nitroglycerin (Potentiated or additive action). Products include:
Nitro-Dur Transdermal Infusion System 3134
Nitro-Dur Transdermal Infusion System 1834
Nitrolingual Pumpspray 1355
Nitrostat Tablets 2658

Norepinephrine Bitartrate (Decreased arterial responsiveness to norepinephrine).
No products indexed under this heading.

Oxaprozin (Blunting of the antihypertensive effect).
No products indexed under this heading.

Oxycodone Hydrochloride (Aggravates orthostatic hypotension). Products include:
OxyContin Tablets 2912
OxyFast Oral Concentrate Solution . 2916
OxyIR Capsules 2916
Percocet Tablets 1326
Percodan Tablets 1327
Percolone Tablets 1327
Roxicodone 3067
Tylox Capsules 2597

Penbutolol Sulfate (Potentiated or additive action).
No products indexed under this heading.

Pentobarbital Sodium (Aggravates orthostatic hypotension). Products include:
Nembutal Sodium Solution 485

Perindopril Erbumine (Potentiated or additive action). Products include:
Aceon Tablets (2 mg, 4 mg, 8 mg) 3249

Phenobarbital (Accelerates propranolol clearance). Products include:
Arco-Lase Plus Tablets 592
Donnatal 2929
Donnatal Extentabs 2930

Phenoxybenzamine Hydrochloride (Potentiated or additive action). Products include:
Dibenzyline Capsules 3457

Phentolamine Mesylate (Potentiated or additive action).
No products indexed under this heading.

Phenylbutazone (Blunting of the antihypertensive effect).
No products indexed under this heading.

Phenytoin (Accelarate propranolol clearance). Products include:
Dilantin Infatabs 2624
Dilantin-125 Oral Suspension 2625

Phenytoin Sodium (Accelarate propranolol clearance). Products include:
Dilantin Kapseals 2622

Pindolol (Potentiated or additive action).
No products indexed under this heading.

Pioglitazone Hydrochloride (Beta-adrenergic blockade may prevent the appearance of certain premonitory signs and symptoms of

acute hypoglycemia in labile insulin-dependent diabetes). Products include:
- Actos Tablets ... 3275

Piroxicam (Blunting of the antihypertensive effect). Products include:
- Feldene Capsules ... 2685

Polythiazide (Potentiated or additive action). Products include:
- Minizide Capsules ... 2700
- Renese Tablets ... 2712

Prazosin Hydrochloride (Potentiated or additive action). Products include:
- Minipress Capsules ... 2699
- Minizide Capsules ... 2700

Prednisolone Acetate (Hypokalemia may develop with concomitant use). Products include:
- Blephamide Ophthalmic Ointment ... 547
- Blephamide Ophthalmic Suspension ... 548
- Poly-Pred Liquifilm Ophthalmic Suspension ... ⊙245
- Pred Forte Ophthalmic Suspension ... ⊙246
- Pred Mild Sterile Ophthalmic Suspension ... ⊙249
- Pred-G Ophthalmic Suspension ... ⊙247
- Pred-G Sterile Ophthalmic Ointment ... ⊙248

Prednisolone Sodium Phosphate (Hypokalemia may develop with concomitant use). Products include:
- Pediapred Oral Solution ... 1170

Prednisolone Tebutate (Hypokalemia may develop with concomitant use).
No products indexed under this heading.

Prednisone (Hypokalemia may develop with concomitant use). Products include:
- Prednisone ... 3064

Propoxyphene Hydrochloride (Aggravates orthostatic hypotension). Products include:
- Darvon Pulvules ... 1909
- Darvon Compound-65 Pulvules ... 1910

Propoxyphene Napsylate (Aggravates orthostatic hypotension). Products include:
- Darvon-N/Darvocet-N ... 1907
- Darvon-N Tablets ... 1912

Quinapril Hydrochloride (Potentiated or additive action). Products include:
- Accupril Tablets ... 2611
- Accuretic Tablets ... 2614

Ramipril (Potentiated or additive action). Products include:
- Altace Capsules ... 2233

Rauwolfia serpentina (Potentiated or additive action).
No products indexed under this heading.

Remifentanil Hydrochloride (Aggravates orthostatic hypotension).
No products indexed under this heading.

Repaglinide (Beta-adrenergic blockade may prevent the appearance of certain premonitory signs and symptoms of acute hypoglycemia in labile insulin-dependent diabetes). Products include:
- Prandin Tablets (0.5, 1, and 2 mg) ... 2432

Rescinnamine (Potentiated or additive action).
No products indexed under this heading.

Reserpine (Co-administration of catecholamine-depleting drugs, such as reserpine, may produce an excessive reduction of resting sympathetic nervous activity, which may result in hypotension, vertigo, marked bradycardia, syncopal attacks or orthostatic hypotension).
No products indexed under this heading.

Rifampin (Accelerates propranolol clearance). Products include:
- Rifadin ... 765
- Rifamate Capsules ... 767
- Rifater Tablets ... 769

Rofecoxib (Blunting of the antihypertensive effect). Products include:
- Vioxx ... 2213

Rosiglitazone Maleate (Beta-adrenergic blockade may prevent the appearance of certain premonitory signs and symptoms of acute hypoglycemia in labile insulin-dependent diabetes). Products include:
- Avandia Tablets ... 1490

Secobarbital Sodium (Aggravates orthostatic hypotension).
No products indexed under this heading.

Sodium Nitroprusside (Potentiated or additive action).
No products indexed under this heading.

Sotalol Hydrochloride (Potentiated or additive action). Products include:
- Betapace Tablets ... 950
- Betapace AF Tablets ... 954

Spirapril Hydrochloride (Potentiated or additive action).
No products indexed under this heading.

Sufentanil Citrate (Aggravates orthostatic hypotension).
No products indexed under this heading.

Sulindac (Blunting of the antihypertensive effect). Products include:
- Clinoril Tablets ... 2053

Telmisartan (Potentiated or additive action). Products include:
- Micardis Tablets ... 1049
- Micardis HCT Tablets ... 1051

Terazosin Hydrochloride (Potentiated or additive action). Products include:
- Hytrin Capsules ... 464

Theophylline (Co-administration of theophylline with propranolol results in reduced theophylline clearance). Products include:
- Aerolate ... 1361
- Theo-Dur Extended-Release Tablets ... 1835
- Uni-Dur Extended-Release Tablets ... 1841
- Uniphyl 400 mg and 600 mg Tablets ... 2903

Theophylline Calcium Salicylate (Co-administration of theophylline with propranolol results in reduced theophylline clearance).
No products indexed under this heading.

Theophylline Sodium Glycinate (Co-administration of theophylline with propranolol results in reduced theophylline clearance).
No products indexed under this heading.

Thiamylal Sodium (Aggravates orthostatic hypotension).
No products indexed under this heading.

Timolol Maleate (Potentiated or additive action). Products include:
- Blocadren Tablets ... 2046
- Cosopt Sterile Ophthalmic Solution ... 2065
- Timolide Tablets ... 2187
- Timolol GFS ... ⊙266
- Timoptic in Ocudose ... 2192
- Timoptic Sterile Ophthalmic Solution ... 2190
- Timoptic-XE Sterile Ophthalmic Gel Forming Solution ... 2194

Tolazamide (Beta-adrenergic blockade may prevent the appearance of certain premonitory signs and symptoms of acute hypoglycemia in labile insulin-dependent diabetes).
No products indexed under this heading.

Tolbutamide (Beta-adrenergic blockade may prevent the appearance of certain premonitory signs and symptoms of acute hypoglycemia in labile insulin-dependent diabetes).
No products indexed under this heading.

Tolmetin Sodium (Blunting of the antihypertensive effect). Products include:
- Tolectin ... 2589

Torsemide (Potentiated or additive action). Products include:
- Demadex Tablets and Injection ... 2965

Trandolapril (Potentiated or additive action). Products include:
- Mavik Tablets ... 478
- Tarka Tablets ... 508

Triamcinolone (Hypokalemia may develop with concomitant use).
No products indexed under this heading.

Triamcinolone Acetonide (Hypokalemia may develop with concomitant use). Products include:
- Azmacort Inhalation Aerosol ... 728
- Nasacort Nasal Inhaler ... 750
- Nasacort AQ Nasal Spray ... 752
- Tri-Nasal Spray ... 2274

Triamcinolone Diacetate (Hypokalemia may develop with concomitant use).
No products indexed under this heading.

Triamcinolone Hexacetonide (Hypokalemia may develop with concomitant use).
No products indexed under this heading.

Trimethaphan Camsylate (Potentiated or additive action).
No products indexed under this heading.

Troglitazone (Beta-adrenergic blockade may prevent the appearance of certain premonitory signs and symptoms of acute hypoglycemia in labile insulin-dependent diabetes).
No products indexed under this heading.

Tubocurarine Chloride (Increased responsiveness to tubocurarine).
No products indexed under this heading.

Valsartan (Potentiated or additive action). Products include:
- Diovan Capsules ... 2337
- Diovan HCT Tablets ... 2338

Verapamil Hydrochloride (Co-administration of intravenous beta-blocker and verapamil, on rare occasion, has resulted in serious adverse reactions, especially in patients with severe cardiomyopathy, congestive heart failure or recent myocardial infarction; calcium channel blockers and beta-blockers may depress myocardial contractility or A-V conduction). Products include:
- Covera-HS Tablets ... 3199
- Isoptin SR Tablets ... 467
- Tarka Tablets ... 508
- Verelan Capsules ... 3184
- Verelan PM Capsules ... 3186

Food Interactions

Alcohol (Slows the rate of absorption of propranolol).

INDERIDE LA LONG-ACTING CAPSULES

(Hydrochlorothiazide, Propranolol Hydrochloride) ... 3519
See Inderide Tablets

INDOCIN CAPSULES

(Indomethacin) ... 2112

May interact with beta blockers, oral anticoagulants, lithium preparations, loop diuretics, non-steroidal anti-inflammatory agents, potassium sparing diuretics, thiazides, and certain other agents. Compounds in these categories include:

Acebutolol Hydrochloride (Blunting of antihypertensive effect of beta blockers). Products include:
- Sectral Capsules ... 3589

Amiloride Hydrochloride (Reduced diuretic, natriuretic and antihypertensive effects of increased serum potassium levels). Products include:
- Midamor Tablets ... 2136
- Moduretic Tablets ... 2138

Aspirin (Decreases indomethacin blood levels). Products include:
- Aggrenox Capsules ... 1026
- Alka-Seltzer ... ▣603
- Alka-Seltzer Lemon Lime Antacid and Pain Reliever Effervescent Tablets ... ▣603
- Alka-Seltzer Extra Strength Antacid and Pain Reliever Effervescent Tablets ... ▣603
- Alka-Seltzer PM Effervescent Tablets ... ▣605
- Genuine Bayer Tablets, Caplets and Gelcaps ... ▣606
- Extra Strength Bayer Caplets and Gelcaps ... ▣610
- Aspirin Regimen Bayer Children's Chewable Tablets (Orange or Cherry Flavored) ... ▣607
- Bayer, Aspirin Regimen ... ▣606
- Aspirin Regimen Bayer 81 mg Caplets with Calcium ... ▣607
- Genuine Bayer Professional Labeling (Aspirin Regimen Bayer) ... ▣608
- Extra Strength Bayer Arthritis Caplets ... ▣610
- Extra Strength Bayer Plus Caplets ... ▣610
- Extra Strength Bayer PM Caplets ... ▣611
- BC Powder ... ▣619
- BC Allergy Sinus Cold Powder ... ▣619
- Arthritis Strength BC Powder ... ▣619
- BC Sinus Cold Powder ... ▣619
- Darvon Compound-65 Pulvules ... 1910
- Ecotrin Enteric Coated Aspirin Low, Regular and Maximum Strength Tablets ... 1715
- Excedrin Extra-Strength Tablets, Caplets, and Geltabs ... ▣629
- Excedrin Migraine ... 1070
- Goody's Body Pain Formula Powder ... ▣620
- Goody's Extra Strength Headache Powder ... ▣620
- Goody's Extra Strength Pain Relief Tablets ... ▣620
- Percodan Tablets ... 1327
- Robaxisal Tablets ... 2939
- Soma Compound Tablets ... 3354
- Soma Compound w/Codeine Tablets ... 3355
- Vanquish Caplets ... ▣617

Atenolol (Blunting of antihypertensive effect of beta blockers). Products include:
- Tenoretic Tablets ... 690
- Tenormin I.V. Injection ... 692

Bendroflumethiazide (Reduced diuretic, natriuretic, and antihypertensive effects of thiazide diuretics). Products include:
- Corzide 40/5 Tablets ... 2247
- Corzide 80/5 Tablets ... 2247

Betaxolol Hydrochloride (Blunting of antihypertensive effect of beta blockers). Products include:
- Betoptic S Ophthalmic Suspension ... 537

Bisoprolol Fumarate (Blunting of antihypertensive effect of beta blockers). Products include:
- Zebeta Tablets ... 1885
- Ziac Tablets ... 1887

Bumetanide (Reduced diuretic, natriuretic, and antihypertensive effects of loop diuretics).
No products indexed under this heading.

Captopril (Reduced antihypertensive effect of captopril). Products include:
- Captopril Tablets ... 2281

Carteolol Hydrochloride (Blunting of antihypertensive effect of beta blockers). Products include:
- Carteolol Hydrochloride Ophthalmic Solution USP, 1% ... ⊙258
- Ocupress Ophthalmic Solution, 1% Sterile ... ⊙303

Celecoxib (Concomitant use is not recommended due to the increased

possibility of gastrointestinal toxicity, with little or no increase in efficacy). Products include:
- Celebrex Capsules 2676
- Celebrex Capsules 2780

Chlorothiazide (Reduced diuretic, natriuretic, and antihypertensive effects of thiazide diuretics). Products include:
- Aldoclor Tablets 2035
- Diuril Oral 2087

Chlorothiazide Sodium (Reduced diuretic, natriuretic, and antihypertensive effects of thiazide diuretics). Products include:
- Diuril Sodium Intravenous 2086

Cyclosporine (Increase in cyclosporine-induced toxicity). Products include:
- Gengraf Capsules 457
- Neoral Soft Gelatin Capsules 2380
- Neoral Oral Solution 2380
- Sandimmune 2388

Dexamethasone (False-negative results in dexamethasone suppression test). Products include:
- Decadron Elixir 2078
- Decadron Tablets 2079
- TobraDex Ophthalmic Ointment 542
- TobraDex Ophthalmic Suspension .. 541

Dexamethasone Acetate (False-negative results in dexamethasone suppression test).
- No products indexed under this heading.

Dexamethasone Sodium Phosphate (False-negative results in dexamethasone suppression test). Products include:
- Decadron Phosphate Injection 2081
- Decadron Phosphate Sterile Ophthalmic Ointment 2083
- Decadron Phosphate Sterile Ophthalmic Solution 2084
- NeoDecadron Sterile Ophthalmic Solution 2144

Diclofenac Potassium (Concomitant use is not recommended due to the increased possibility of gastrointestinal toxicity, with little or no increase in efficacy). Products include:
- Cataflam Tablets 2315

Diclofenac Sodium (Concomitant use is not recommended due to the increased possibility of gastrointestinal toxicity, with little or no increase in efficacy). Products include:
- Arthrotec Tablets 3195
- Voltaren Ophthalmic Sterile Ophthalmic Solution .... ⊙312
- Voltaren Tablets 2315
- Voltaren-XR Tablets 2315

Dicumarol (Possible alterations of the prothrombin time; clinical studies have shown that indomethacin does not influence the hypoprothrombinemia).
- No products indexed under this heading.

Diflunisal (Co-administration results in decreased renal clearance and significant increase in the plasma levels of indomethacin; in some patients combined therapy has been associated with fatal gastrointestinal hemorrhage; concurrent use is not recommended). Products include:
- Dolobid Tablets 2088

Digoxin (Increased serum digoxin concentration and prolonged half-life). Products include:
- Digitek Tablets 1003
- Lanoxicaps Capsules 1574
- Lanoxin Injection 1581
- Lanoxin Tablets 1587
- Lanoxin Elixir Pediatric 1578
- Lanoxin Injection Pediatric 1584

Esmolol Hydrochloride (Blunting of antihypertensive effect of beta blockers). Products include:
- Brevibloc Injection 858

Ethacrynic Acid (Reduced diuretic, natriuretic, and antihypertensive effects of loop diuretics). Products include:
- Edecrin Tablets 2091

Etodolac (Concomitant use is not recommended due to the increased possibility of gastrointestinal toxicity, with little or no increase in efficacy). Products include:
- Lodine 3528
- Lodine XL Extended-Release Tablets 3530

Fenoprofen Calcium (Concomitant use is not recommended due to the increased possibility of gastrointestinal toxicity, with little or no increase in efficacy).
- No products indexed under this heading.

Flurbiprofen (Concomitant use is not recommended due to the increased possibility of gastrointestinal toxicity, with little or no increase in efficacy).
- No products indexed under this heading.

Furosemide (Indomethacin reduces basal plasma renin activity (PRA) induced by furosemide; reduced diuretic, natriuretic, and antihypertensive effects of loop diuretics). Products include:
- Furosemide Tablets 2284

Hydrochlorothiazide (Reduced diuretic, natriuretic, and antihypertensive effects of thiazide diuretics). Products include:
- Accuretic Tablets 2614
- Aldoril Tablets 2039
- Atacand HCT Tablets 597
- Avalide Tablets 1070
- Diovan HCT Tablets 2338
- Dyazide Capsules 1515
- HydroDIURIL Tablets 2108
- Hyzaar 2109
- Inderide Tablets 3517
- Inderide LA Long-Acting Capsules .. 3519
- Lotensin HCT Tablets 2367
- Maxzide 1008
- Micardis HCT Tablets 1051
- Microzide Capsules 3414
- Moduretic Tablets 2138
- Monopril HCT 1094
- Prinzide Tablets 2168
- Timolide Tablets 2187
- Uniretic Tablets 3178
- Vaseretic Tablets 2204
- Zestoretic Tablets 695
- Ziac Tablets 1887

Hydroflumethiazide (Reduced diuretic, natriuretic, and antihypertensive effects of thiazide diuretics). Products include:
- Diucardin Tablets 3494

Ibuprofen (Concomitant use is not recommended due to the increased possibility of gastrointestinal toxicity, with little or no increase in efficacy). Products include:
- Advil .... ▣771
- Children's Advil Oral Suspension .... ▣773
- Children's Advil Chewable Tablets .... ▣773
- Advil Cold and Sinus Caplets .... ▣771
- Advil Cold and Sinus Tablets .... ▣771
- Advil Flu & Body Ache Caplets .... ▣772
- Infants' Advil Drops .... ▣773
- Junior Strength Advil Tablets .... ▣773
- Junior Strength Advil Chewable Tablets .... ▣773
- Advil Migraine Liquigels .... ▣772
- Children's Motrin Oral Suspension and Chewable Tablets 2006
- Children's Motrin Cold Oral Suspension 2007
- Children's Motrin Oral Suspension .... ▣643
- Motrin Suspension, Oral Drops, Chewable Tablets, and Caplets 2002
- Infants' Motrin Concentrated Drops 2006
- Junior Strength Motrin Caplets and Chewable Tablets 2006
- Motrin IB Tablets, Caplets, and Gelcaps 2002
- Motrin Migraine Pain Caplets 2005
- Motrin Sinus Headache Caplets 2005
- Vicoprofen Tablets 520

Ketoprofen (Concomitant use is not recommended due to the increased possibility of gastrointestinal toxicity, with little or no increase in efficacy). Products include:
- Orudis Capsules 3548
- Orudis KT Tablets .... ▣778
- Oruvail Capsules 3548

Ketorolac Tromethamine (Concomitant use is not recommended due to the increased possibility of gastrointestinal toxicity, with little or no increase in efficacy). Products include:
- Acular Ophthalmic Solution 544
- Acular PF Ophthalmic Solution 544
- Toradol 3018

Labetalol Hydrochloride (Blunting of antihypertensive effect of beta blockers). Products include:
- Normodyne Injection 3135
- Normodyne Tablets 3137

Levobunolol Hydrochloride (Blunting of antihypertensive effect of beta blockers). Products include:
- Betagan .... ⊙228

Lithium Carbonate (Co-administration produces a clinically relevant elevation of plasma lithium and reduction in renal lithium clearance with a potential for lithium toxicity). Products include:
- Eskalith 1527
- Lithium Carbonate 3061
- Lithobid Slow-Release Tablets 3255

Lithium Citrate (Co-administration produces a clinically relevant elevation of plasma lithium and reduction in renal lithium clearance with a potential for lithium toxicity). Products include:
- Lithium Citrate Syrup 3061

Meclofenamate Sodium (Concomitant use is not recommended due to the increased possibility of gastrointestinal toxicity, with little or no increase in efficacy).
- No products indexed under this heading.

Mefenamic Acid (Concomitant use is not recommended due to the increased possibility of gastrointestinal toxicity, with little or no increase in efficacy). Products include:
- Ponstel Capsules 1356

Meloxicam (Concomitant use is not recommended due to the increased possibility of gastrointestinal toxicity, with little or no increase in efficacy). Products include:
- Mobic Tablets 1054

Methotrexate Sodium (Potentiation of methotrexate toxicity).
- No products indexed under this heading.

Methyclothiazide (Reduced diuretic, natriuretic, and antihypertensive effects of thiazide diuretics).
- No products indexed under this heading.

Metipranolol Hydrochloride (Blunting of antihypertensive effect of beta blockers).
- No products indexed under this heading.

Metoprolol Succinate (Blunting of antihypertensive effect of beta blockers). Products include:
- Toprol-XL Tablets 651

Metoprolol Tartrate (Blunting of antihypertensive effect of beta blockers).
- No products indexed under this heading.

Nabumetone (Concomitant use is not recommended due to the increased possibility of gastrointestinal toxicity, with little or no increase in efficacy). Products include:
- Relafen Tablets 1617

Nadolol (Blunting of antihypertensive effect of beta blockers). Products include:
- Corgard Tablets 2245
- Corzide 40/5 Tablets 2247
- Corzide 80/5 Tablets 2247
- Nadolol Tablets 2288

Naproxen (Concomitant use is not recommended due to the increased possibility of gastrointestinal toxicity, with little or no increase in efficacy). Products include:
- EC-Naprosyn Delayed-Release Tablets 2967
- Naprosyn Suspension 2967
- Naprosyn Tablets 2967

Naproxen Sodium (Concomitant use is not recommended due to the increased possibility of gastrointestinal toxicity, with little or no increase in efficacy). Products include:
- Aleve Tablets, Caplets and Gelcaps .... ▣602
- Aleve Cold & Sinus Caplets .... ▣603
- Anaprox Tablets 2967
- Anaprox DS Tablets 2967
- Naprelan Tablets 1293

Nephrotoxic Drugs (Overt renal decompensation).
- No products indexed under this heading.

Oxaprozin (Concomitant use is not recommended due to the increased possibility of gastrointestinal toxicity, with little or no increase in efficacy).
- No products indexed under this heading.

Penbutolol Sulfate (Blunting of antihypertensive effect of beta blockers).
- No products indexed under this heading.

Phenylbutazone (Concomitant use is not recommended due to the increased possibility of gastrointestinal toxicity, with little or no increase in efficacy).
- No products indexed under this heading.

Pindolol (Blunting of antihypertensive effect of beta blockers).
- No products indexed under this heading.

Piroxicam (Concomitant use is not recommended due to the increased possibility of gastrointestinal toxicity, with little or no increase in efficacy). Products include:
- Feldene Capsules 2685

Polythiazide (Reduced diuretic, natriuretic, and antihypertensive effects of thiazide diuretics). Products include:
- Minizide Capsules 2700
- Renese Tablets 2712

Probenecid (Increased plasma levels of indomethacin).
- No products indexed under this heading.

Propranolol Hydrochloride (Blunting of antihypertensive effect of beta blockers). Products include:
- Inderal 3513
- Inderal LA Long-Acting Capsules 3516
- Inderide Tablets 3517
- Inderide LA Long-Acting Capsules .. 3519

Rofecoxib (Concomitant use is not recommended due to the increased possibility of gastrointestinal toxicity, with little or no increase in efficacy). Products include:
- Vioxx 2213

Sotalol Hydrochloride (Blunting of antihypertensive effect of beta blockers). Products include:
- Betapace Tablets 950
- Betapace AF Tablets 954

Spironolactone (Reduced diuretic, natriuretic and antihypertensive effects of increased serum potassium levels).
- No products indexed under this heading.

Sulindac (Concomitant use is not recommended due to the increased possibility of gastrointestinal toxicity, with little or no increase in efficacy). Products include:
- Clinoril Tablets 2053

Timolol Hemihydrate (Blunting of antihypertensive effect of beta blockers). Products include:
- Betimol Ophthalmic Solution .... ⊙324

Timolol Maleate (Blunting of antihypertensive effect of beta blockers). Products include:

Blocadren Tablets 2046
Cosopt Sterile Ophthalmic Solution 2065
Timolide Tablets 2187
Timolol GFS ⊙266
Timoptic in Ocudose 2192
Timoptic Sterile Ophthalmic Solution 2190
Timoptic-XE Sterile Ophthalmic Gel Forming Solution 2194

Tolmetin Sodium (Concomitant use is not recommended due to the increased possibility of gastrointestinal toxicity, with little or no increase in efficacy). Products include:
Tolectin 2589

Torsemide (Reduced diuretic, natriuretic, and antihypertensive effects of loop diuretics). Products include:
Demadex Tablets and Injection 2965

Triamterene (The addition of triamterene to maintenance schedule of indomethacin has resulted in reversible acute renal failure; potential for increased hyperkalemia; concurrent therapy should be avoided). Products include:
Dyazide Capsules 1515
Dyrenium Capsules 3458
Maxzide 1008

Warfarin Sodium (Possible alterations of the prothrombin time; clinical studies have shown that indomethacin does not influence the hypoprothrombinemia). Products include:
Coumadin for Injection 1243
Coumadin Tablets 1243
Warfarin Sodium Tablets, USP 3302

INDOCIN I.V.

(Indomethacin Sodium Trihydrate) 2115
May interact with cardiac glycosides and certain other agents. Compounds in these categories include:

Amikacin Sulfate (Serum levels of amikacin significantly elevated).
No products indexed under this heading.

Deslanoside (Half-life of digitalis may be prolonged when given concomitantly).
No products indexed under this heading.

Digitoxin (Half-life of digitalis may be prolonged when given concomitantly).
No products indexed under this heading.

Digoxin (Half-life of digitalis may be prolonged when given concomitantly). Products include:
Digitek Tablets 1003
Lanoxicaps Capsules 1574
Lanoxin Injection 1581
Lanoxin Tablets 1587
Lanoxin Elixir Pediatric 1578
Lanoxin Injection Pediatric 1584

Furosemide (Blunted natriuretic effect of furosemide). Products include:
Furosemide Tablets 2284

Gentamicin Sulfate (Serum levels of gentamicin significantly elevated). Products include:
Genoptic Ophthalmic Ointment ⊙239
Genoptic Sterile Ophthalmic Solution ⊙239
Pred-G Ophthalmic Suspension ⊙247
Pred-G Sterile Ophthalmic Ointment ⊙248

INDOCIN ORAL SUSPENSION

(Indomethacin) 2112
See Indocin Capsules

INDOCIN SUPPOSITORIES

(Indomethacin) 2112
See Indocin Capsules

INFANRIX VACCINE

(Diphtheria & Tetanus Toxoids and Acellular Pertussis Vaccine Adsorbed) 1562
May interact with alkylating agents, corticosteroids, cytotoxic drugs, and immunosuppressive agents. Compounds in these categories include:

Azathioprine (Concurrent immunosuppressive therapy may reduce the immune response to vaccine).
No products indexed under this heading.

Basiliximab (Concurrent immunosuppressive therapy may reduce the immune response to vaccine). Products include:
Simulect for Injection 2399

Betamethasone Acetate (Concurrent immunosuppressive therapy with greater than physiologic doses of corticosteroids may reduce the immune response to vaccine). Products include:
Celestone Soluspan Injectable Suspension 3097

Betamethasone Sodium Phosphate (Concurrent immunosuppressive therapy with greater than physiologic doses of corticosteroids may reduce the immune response to vaccine). Products include:
Celestone Soluspan Injectable Suspension 3097

Bleomycin Sulfate (Cytotoxic drugs may reduce the immune response to vaccine).
No products indexed under this heading.

Busulfan (Alkylating drugs may reduce the immune response to vaccine). Products include:
Myleran Tablets 1603

Carmustine (BCNU) (Alkylating drugs may reduce the immune response to vaccine). Products include:
Gliadel Wafer 1723

Chlorambucil (Alkylating drugs may reduce the immune response to vaccine). Products include:
Leukeran Tablets 1591

Cortisone Acetate (Concurrent immunosuppressive therapy with greater than physiologic doses of corticosteroids may reduce the immune response to vaccine). Products include:
Cortone Acetate Injectable Suspension 2059
Cortone Acetate Tablets 2061

Cyclophosphamide (Alkylating drugs may reduce the immune response to vaccine).
No products indexed under this heading.

Cyclosporine (Concurrent immunosuppressive therapy may reduce the immune response to vaccine). Products include:
Gengraf Capsules 457
Neoral Soft Gelatin Capsules 2380
Neoral Oral Solution 2380
Sandimmune 2388

Dacarbazine (Alkylating drugs may reduce the immune response to vaccine). Products include:
DTIC-Dome 902

Daunorubicin Hydrochloride (Cytotoxic drugs may reduce the immune response to vaccine). Products include:
Cerubidine for Injection 947

Dexamethasone (Concurrent immunosuppressive therapy with greater than physiologic doses of corticosteroids may reduce the immune response to vaccine). Products include:
Decadron Elixir 2078
Decadron Tablets 2079
TobraDex Ophthalmic Ointment 542
TobraDex Ophthalmic Suspension 541

Dexamethasone Acetate (Concurrent immunosuppressive therapy with greater than physiologic doses of corticosteroids may reduce the immune response to vaccine).
No products indexed under this heading.

Dexamethasone Sodium Phosphate (Concurrent immunosuppressive therapy with greater than physiologic doses of corticosteroids may reduce the immune response to vaccine). Products include:
Decadron Phosphate Injection 2081
Decadron Phosphate Sterile Ophthalmic Ointment 2083
Decadron Phosphate Sterile Ophthalmic Solution 2084
NeoDecadron Sterile Ophthalmic Solution 2144

Doxorubicin Hydrochloride (Cytotoxic drugs may reduce the immune response to vaccine). Products include:
Adriamycin PFS/RDF Injection 2767
Doxil Injection 566

Epirubicin Hydrochloride (Cytotoxic drugs may reduce the immune response to vaccine). Products include:
Ellence Injection 2806

Fludrocortisone Acetate (Concurrent immunosuppressive therapy with greater than physiologic doses of corticosteroids may reduce the immune response to vaccine). Products include:
Florinef Acetate Tablets 2250

Fluorouracil (Cytotoxic drugs may reduce the immune response to vaccine). Products include:
Carac Cream 1222
Efudex 1733
Fluoroplex 552

Hydrocortisone (Concurrent immunosuppressive therapy with greater than physiologic doses of corticosteroids may reduce the immune response to vaccine). Products include:
Anusol-HC Cream 2.5% 2237
Cipro HC Otic Suspension 540
Cortaid Intensive Therapy Cream ▣717
Cortaid Maximum Strength Cream ▣717
Cortisporin Ophthalmic Suspension Sterile ⊙297
Cortizone•5 ▣699
Cortizone•10 ▣699
Cortizone•10 Plus Creme ▣700
Cortizone for Kids Creme ▣699
Hydrocortone Tablets 2106
Massengill Medicated Soft Cloth Towelette ▣753
VōSoL HC Otic Solution 3356

Hydrocortisone Acetate (Concurrent immunosuppressive therapy with greater than physiologic doses of corticosteroids may reduce the immune response to vaccine). Products include:
Analpram-HC 1338
Anusol HC-1 Hydrocortisone Anti-Itch Cream ▣689
Anusol-HC Suppositories 2238
Cortaid ▣717
Cortifoam Rectal Foam 3170
Cortisporin-TC Otic Suspension 2246
Hydrocortone Acetate Injectable Suspension 2103
Pramosone 1343
Proctocort Suppositories 2264
ProctoFoam-HC 3177
Terra-Cortril Ophthalmic Suspension 2716

Hydrocortisone Sodium Phosphate (Concurrent immunosuppressive therapy with greater than physiologic doses of corticosteroids may reduce the immune response to vaccine). Products include:
Hydrocortone Phosphate Injection, Sterile 2105

Hydrocortisone Sodium Succinate (Concurrent immunosuppressive therapy with greater than physiologic doses of corticosteroids may reduce the immune response to vaccine).
No products indexed under this heading.

Hydroxyurea (Cytotoxic drugs may reduce the immune response to vaccine). Products include:
Mylocel Tablets 2227

Lomustine (CCNU) (Alkylating drugs may reduce the immune response to vaccine).
No products indexed under this heading.

Mechlorethamine Hydrochloride (Alkylating drugs may reduce the immune response to vaccine). Products include:
Mustargen for Injection 2142

Melphalan (Alkylating drugs may reduce the immune response to vaccine). Products include:
Alkeran Tablets 1466

Methotrexate Sodium (Cytotoxic drugs may reduce the immune response to vaccine).
No products indexed under this heading.

Methylprednisolone Acetate (Concurrent immunosuppressive therapy with greater than physiologic doses of corticosteroids may reduce the immune response to vaccine). Products include:
Depo-Medrol Injectable Suspension 2795

Methylprednisolone Sodium Succinate (Concurrent immunosuppressive therapy with greater than physiologic doses of corticosteroids may reduce the immune response to vaccine). Products include:
Solu-Medrol Sterile Powder 2855

Mitotane (Cytotoxic drugs may reduce the immune response to vaccine).
No products indexed under this heading.

Mitoxantrone Hydrochloride (Cytotoxic drugs may reduce the immune response to vaccine). Products include:
Novantrone for Injection 1760

Muromonab-CD3 (Concurrent immunosuppressive therapy may reduce the immune response to vaccine). Products include:
Orthoclone OKT3 Sterile Solution 2498

Mycophenolate Mofetil (Concurrent immunosuppressive therapy may reduce the immune response to vaccine). Products include:
CellCept Capsules 2951
CellCept Oral Suspension 2951
CellCept Tablets 2951

Prednisolone Acetate (Concurrent immunosuppressive therapy with greater than physiologic doses of corticosteroids may reduce the immune response to vaccine). Products include:
Blephamide Ophthalmic Ointment 547
Blephamide Ophthalmic Suspension 548
Poly-Pred Liquifilm Ophthalmic Suspension ⊙245
Pred Forte Ophthalmic Suspension ⊙246
Pred Mild Sterile Ophthalmic Suspension ⊙249
Pred-G Ophthalmic Suspension ⊙247
Pred-G Sterile Ophthalmic Ointment ⊙248

Prednisolone Sodium Phosphate (Concurrent immunosuppressive therapy with greater than physiologic doses of corticosteroids may reduce the immune response to vaccine). Products include:
Pediapred Oral Solution 1170

Prednisolone Tebutate (Concurrent immunosuppressive therapy with greater than physiologic doses of corticosteroids may reduce the immune response to vaccine).
No products indexed under this heading.

IMPORTANT NOTE: Always consult each drug listing in the patient's regimen for possible interactions.

Prednisone (Concurrent immunosuppressive therapy with greater than physiologic doses of corticosteroids may reduce the immune response to vaccine). Products include:
Prednisone ... 3064

Procarbazine Hydrochloride (Cytotoxic drugs may reduce the immune response to vaccine). Products include:
Matulane Capsules ... 3246

Sirolimus (Concurrent immunosuppressive therapy may reduce the immune response to vaccine). Products include:
Rapamune Oral Solution and Tablets ... 3584

Tacrolimus (Concurrent immunosuppressive therapy may reduce the immune response to vaccine). Products include:
Prograf ... 1393
Protopic Ointment ... 1397

Tamoxifen Citrate (Cytotoxic drugs may reduce the immune response to vaccine). Products include:
Nolvadex Tablets ... 678

Thiotepa (Alkylating drugs may reduce the immune response to vaccine). Products include:
Thioplex for Injection ... 1765

Triamcinolone (Concurrent immunosuppressive therapy with greater than physiologic doses of corticosteroids may reduce the immune response to vaccine).
No products indexed under this heading.

Triamcinolone Acetonide (Concurrent immunosuppressive therapy with greater than physiologic doses of corticosteroids may reduce the immune response to vaccine). Products include:
Azmacort Inhalation Aerosol ... 728
Nasacort Nasal Inhaler ... 750
Nasacort AQ Nasal Spray ... 752
Tri-Nasal Spray ... 2274

Triamcinolone Diacetate (Concurrent immunosuppressive therapy with greater than physiologic doses of corticosteroids may reduce the immune response to vaccine).
No products indexed under this heading.

Triamcinolone Hexacetonide (Concurrent immunosuppressive therapy with greater than physiologic doses of corticosteroids may reduce the immune response to vaccine).
No products indexed under this heading.

Vincristine Sulfate (Cytotoxic drugs may reduce the immune response to vaccine).
No products indexed under this heading.

INFASURF INTRATRACHEAL SUSPENSION

(Calfactant) ... 1372
None cited in PDR database.

INFED INJECTION

(Iron Dextran) ... 3388
None cited in PDR database.

INFERGEN

(Interferon Alfacon-1) ... 1777
May interact with drugs which undergo biotransformation by cytochrome p-450 mixed function oxidase and certain other agents. Compounds in these categories include:

Bone Marrow Depressants, unspecified (Concurrent use with agents known to cause myelosuppression requires caution).
No products indexed under this heading.

Drugs that Undergo Biotransformation by Cytochrome P-450 Mixed Function Oxidase (Concurrent use with agents known to be metabolized via cytochrome P450 pathway requires caution).

INFUMORPH 200 AND INFUMORPH 500 STERILE SOLUTIONS

(Morphine Sulfate) ... 1314
May interact with antihistamines, central nervous system depressants, antipsychotic agents, and certain other agents. Compounds in these categories include:

Acrivastine (Potentiates CNS depressant effects). Products include:
Semprex-D Capsules ... 1172

Alfentanil Hydrochloride (Potentiates CNS depressant effects).
No products indexed under this heading.

Alprazolam (Potentiates CNS depressant effects). Products include:
Xanax Tablets ... 2865

Aprobarbital (Potentiates CNS depressant effects).
No products indexed under this heading.

Astemizole (Potentiates CNS depressant effects).
No products indexed under this heading.

Azatadine Maleate (Potentiates CNS depressant effects). Products include:
Rynatan Tablets ... 3351

Bromodiphenhydramine Hydrochloride (Potentiates CNS depressant effects).
No products indexed under this heading.

Brompheniramine Maleate (Potentiates CNS depressant effects). Products include:
Bromfed Capsules (Extended-Release) ... 2269
Bromfed-PD Capsules (Extended-Release) ... 2269
Comtrex Acute Head Cold & Sinus Pressure Relief Tablets ... ■ 627
Dimetapp Elixir ... ■ 777
Dimetapp Cold and Fever Suspension ... ■ 775
Dimetapp DM Cold & Cough Elixir ... ■ 775
Dimetapp Nighttime Flu Liquid ... ■ 776

Buprenorphine Hydrochloride (Potentiates CNS depressant effects). Products include:
Buprenex Injectable ... 2918

Buspirone Hydrochloride (Potentiates CNS depressant effects).
No products indexed under this heading.

Butabarbital (Potentiates CNS depressant effects).
No products indexed under this heading.

Butalbital (Potentiates CNS depressant effects). Products include:
Phrenilin ... 578
Sedapap Tablets 50 mg/650 mg ... 2225

Cetirizine Hydrochloride (Potentiates CNS depressant effects). Products include:
Zyrtec ... 2756
Zyrtec-D 12 Hour Extended Relief Tablets ... 2758

Chlordiazepoxide (Potentiates CNS depressant effects). Products include:
Limbitrol ... 1738

Chlordiazepoxide Hydrochloride (Potentiates CNS depressant effects). Products include:
Librium Capsules ... 1736
Librium for Injection ... 1737

Chlorpheniramine Maleate (Potentiates CNS depressant effects). Products include:
Actifed Cold & Sinus Caplets and Tablets ... ■ 688
Alka-Seltzer Plus Liqui-Gels ... ■ 604
BC Allergy Sinus Cold Powder ... ■ 619
Chlor-Trimeton Allergy Tablets ... ■ 735
Chlor-Trimeton Allergy/Decongestant Tablets ... ■ 736
Comtrex Flu Therapy & Fever Relief Nighttime Tablets ... ■ 628
Comtrex Maximum Strength Multi-Symptom Cold & Cough Relief Tablets and Caplets ... ■ 626
Contac Severe Cold and Flu Caplets Maximum Strength ... ■ 746
Coricidin 'D' Cold, Flu & Sinus Tablets ... ■ 737
Coricidin/Coricidin D ... ■ 738
Coricidin HBP Maximum Strength Flu Tablets ... ■ 738
Extendryl ... 1361
Hycomine Compound Tablets ... 1317
Kronofed-A ... 1341
PediaCare Cough-Cold Liquid ... ■ 719
PediaCare NightRest Cough-Cold Liquid ... ■ 719
Robitussin Nighttime Honey Flu Liquid ... ■ 786
Ryna ... ■ 768
Singlet Caplets ... ■ 761
Sinutab Sinus Allergy Medication, Maximum Strength Formula, Tablets & Caplets ... ■ 707
Sudafed Cold & Allergy Tablets ... ■ 708
TheraFlu Regular Strength Cold & Cough Night Time Hot Liquid ... ■ 676
TheraFlu Regular Strength Cold & Sore Throat Night Time Hot Liquid ... ■ 676
TheraFlu Maximum Strength Flu & Cough Night Time Hot Liquid ... ■ 678
TheraFlu Maximum Strength Flu & Sore Throat Night Time Hot Liquid ... ■ 677
TheraFlu Maximum Strength Severe Cold & Congestion Night Time Caplets ... ■ 678
TheraFlu Maximum Strength Severe Cold & Congestion Night Time Hot Liquid ... ■ 678
Triaminic Cold & Allergy Liquid ... ■ 681
Triaminic Cold & Allergy Softchews ... ■ 683
Triaminic Cold & Cough Liquid ... ■ 681
Triaminic Cold & Cough Softchews ... ■ 683
Triaminic Cold & Night Time Cough Liquid ... ■ 681
Triaminic Cold, Cough & Fever Liquid ... ■ 681
Children's Tylenol Cold Suspension Liquid and Chewable Tablets ... 2015
Children's Tylenol Cold Plus Cough Suspension Liquid and Chewable Tablets ... 2015
Children's Tylenol Flu Suspension Liquid ... 2015
Maximum Strength Tylenol Allergy Sinus Caplets, Gelcaps, and Geltabs ... 2010
Multi-Symptom Tylenol Cold Complete Formula Caplets ... 2010
Vicks 44M Cough, Cold & Flu Relief Liquid ... ■ 725
Pediatric Vicks 44m Cough & Cold Relief ... ■ 728
Children's Vicks NyQuil Cold/Cough Relief ... ■ 726

Chlorpheniramine Polistirex (Potentiates CNS depressant effects). Products include:
Tussionex Pennkinetic Extended-Release Suspension ... 1174

Chlorpheniramine Tannate (Potentiates CNS depressant effects). Products include:
Reformulated Rynatan Pediatric Suspension ... 3352
Rynatuss Pediatric Suspension ... 3353
Rynatuss Tablets ... 3353
Tussi-12 S Suspension ... 3356
Tussi-12 Tablets ... 3356

Chlorpromazine (Potentiates CNS depressant effects; increases the risk of respiratory depression). Products include:
Thorazine Suppositories ... 1656

Chlorpromazine Hydrochloride (Potentiates CNS depressant effects; increases the risk of respiratory depression). Products include:
Thorazine ... 1656

Chlorprothixene (Potentiates CNS depressant effects; increases the risk of respiratory depression).
No products indexed under this heading.

Chlorprothixene Hydrochloride (Potentiates CNS depressant effects; increases the risk of respiratory depression).
No products indexed under this heading.

Chlorprothixene Lactate (Potentiates CNS depressant effects).
No products indexed under this heading.

Clemastine Fumarate (Potentiates CNS depressant effects). Products include:
Tavist 12 Hour Allergy Tablets ... ■ 676

Clorazepate Dipotassium (Potentiates CNS depressant effects). Products include:
Tranxene ... 511

Clozapine (Potentiates CNS depressant effects; increases the risk of respiratory depression). Products include:
Clozaril Tablets ... 2319

Codeine Phosphate (Potentiates CNS depressant effects). Products include:
Phenergan with Codeine Syrup ... 3557
Phenergan VC with Codeine Syrup ... 3561
Robitussin A-C Syrup ... 2942
Robitussin-DAC Syrup ... 2942
Ryna-C Liquid ... ■ 768
Soma Compound w/Codeine Tablets ... 3355
Tussi-Organidin NR Liquid ... 3350
Tussi-Organidin-S NR Liquid ... 3350
Tylenol with Codeine ... 2595

Cyproheptadine Hydrochloride (Potentiates CNS depressant effects). Products include:
Periactin Tablets ... 2155

Desflurane (Potentiates CNS depressant effects). Products include:
Suprane Liquid for Inhalation ... 874

Dexchlorpheniramine Maleate (Potentiates CNS depressant effects).
No products indexed under this heading.

Dezocine (Potentiates CNS depressant effects).
No products indexed under this heading.

Diazepam (Potentiates CNS depressant effects). Products include:
Valium Injectable ... 3026
Valium Tablets ... 3047

Diphenhydramine Citrate (Potentiates CNS depressant effects). Products include:
Alka-Seltzer PM Effervescent Tablets ... ■ 605
Benadryl Allergy & Sinus Fastmelt Tablets ... ■ 693
Benadryl Children's Allergy/Cold Fastmelt Tablets ... ■ 692
Excedrin PM Tablets, Caplets, and Geltabs ... ■ 631
Goody's PM Powder ... ■ 621

Diphenhydramine Hydrochloride (Potentiates CNS depressant effects). Products include:
Extra Strength Bayer PM Caplets ... ■ 611
Benadryl Allergy Chewables ... ■ 689
Benadryl Allergy ... ■ 691
Benadryl Allergy Liquid ... ■ 690
Benadryl Allergy/Cold Tablets ... ■ 691
Benadryl Allergy/Congestion Tablets ... ■ 692
Benadryl Allergy & Sinus Liquid ... ■ 693
Benadryl Allergy Sinus Headache Caplets & Gelcaps ... ■ 693
Benadryl Severe Allergy & Sinus Headache Caplets ... ■ 694
Benadryl Dye-Free Allergy Liquid ... ■ 690
Benadryl Dye-Free Allergy Liqui-Gels Softgels ... ■ 690
Benadryl Itch Relief Stick Extra Strength ... ■ 695
Benadryl Cream ... ■ 695
Benadryl Gel ... ■ 695
Benadryl Spray ... ■ 696
Benadryl Parenteral ... 2617
Coricidin HBP Night-Time Cold & Flu Tablets ... ■ 738
Nytol QuickCaps Caplets ... ■ 622

Maximum Strength Nytol QuickGels Softgels ... 621
Extra Strength Percogesic Aspirin-Free Coated Caplets ... 665
Simply Sleep Caplets ... 2008
Sominex Original Formula Tablets ... 761
Children's Tylenol Allergy-D Liquid ... 2014
Maximum Strength Tylenol Allergy Sinus NightTime Caplets ... 2010
Tylenol Severe Allergy Caplets ... 2010
Maximum Strength Tylenol Flu NightTime Gelcaps ... 2011
Extra Strength Tylenol PM Caplets, Geltabs, and Gelcaps ... 2012
Unisom Maximum Strength SleepGels ... 713

Diphenylpyraline Hydrochloride (Potentiates CNS depressant effects).
No products indexed under this heading.

Droperidol (Potentiates CNS depressant effects).
No products indexed under this heading.

Enflurane (Potentiates CNS depressant effects).
No products indexed under this heading.

Estazolam (Potentiates CNS depressant effects). Products include:
ProSom Tablets ... 500

Ethchlorvynol (Potentiates CNS depressant effects).
No products indexed under this heading.

Ethinamate (Potentiates CNS depressant effects).
No products indexed under this heading.

Fentanyl (Potentiates CNS depressant effects). Products include:
Duragesic Transdermal System ... 1786

Fentanyl Citrate (Potentiates CNS depressant effects). Products include:
Actiq ... 1184

Fexofenadine Hydrochloride (Potentiates CNS depressant effects). Products include:
Allegra ... 712
Allegra-D Extended-Release Tablets ... 714

Fluphenazine Decanoate (Potentiates CNS depressant effects; increases the risk of respiratory depression).
No products indexed under this heading.

Fluphenazine Enanthate (Potentiates CNS depressant effects; increases the risk of respiratory depression).
No products indexed under this heading.

Fluphenazine Hydrochloride (Potentiates CNS depressant effects; increases the risk of respiratory depression).
No products indexed under this heading.

Flurazepam Hydrochloride (Potentiates CNS depressant effects).
No products indexed under this heading.

Glutethimide (Potentiates CNS depressant effects).
No products indexed under this heading.

Haloperidol (Potentiates CNS depressant effects; increases the risk of respiratory depression). Products include:
Haldol Injection, Tablets and Concentrate ... 2533

Haloperidol Decanoate (Potentiates CNS depressant effects; increases the risk of respiratory depression). Products include:
Haldol Decanoate ... 2535

Hydrocodone Bitartrate (Potentiates CNS depressant effects). Products include:
Hycodan ... 1316
Hycomine Compound Tablets ... 1317
Hycotuss Expectorant Syrup ... 1318
Lortab ... 3319
Lortab Elixir ... 3317
Maxidone Tablets CIII ... 3399
Norco 5/325 Tablets CIII ... 3424
Norco 7.5/325 Tablets CIII ... 3425
Norco 10/325 Tablets CIII ... 3427
Norco 10/325 Tablets CIII ... 3425
Vicodin Tablets ... 516
Vicodin ES Tablets ... 517
Vicodin HP Tablets ... 518
Vicodin Tuss Expectorant ... 519
Vicoprofen Tablets ... 520
Zydone Tablets ... 1330

Hydrocodone Polistirex (Potentiates CNS depressant effects). Products include:
Tussionex Pennkinetic Extended-Release Suspension ... 1174

Hydromorphone Hydrochloride (Potentiates CNS depressant effects). Products include:
Dilaudid ... 441
Dilaudid Oral Liquid ... 445
Dilaudid Powder ... 441
Dilaudid Rectal Suppositories ... 441
Dilaudid Tablets ... 441
Dilaudid Tablets - 8 mg ... 445
Dilaudid-HP ... 443

Hydroxyzine Hydrochloride (Potentiates CNS depressant effects). Products include:
Atarax Tablets & Syrup ... 2667
Vistaril Intramuscular Solution ... 2738

Isoflurane (Potentiates CNS depressant effects).
No products indexed under this heading.

Ketamine Hydrochloride (Potentiates CNS depressant effects).
No products indexed under this heading.

Levomethadyl Acetate Hydrochloride (Potentiates CNS depressant effects).
No products indexed under this heading.

Levorphanol Tartrate (Potentiates CNS depressant effects). Products include:
Levo-Dromoran ... 1734
Levorphanol Tartrate Tablets ... 3059

Lithium Carbonate (Potentiates CNS depressant effects; increases the risk of respiratory depression). Products include:
Eskalith ... 1527
Lithium Carbonate ... 3061
Lithobid Slow-Release Tablets ... 3255

Lithium Citrate (Potentiates CNS depressant effects; increases the risk of respiratory depression). Products include:
Lithium Citrate Syrup ... 3061

Loratadine (Potentiates CNS depressant effects). Products include:
Claritin ... 3100
Claritin-D 12 Hour Extended Release Tablets ... 3102
Claritin-D 24 Hour Extended Release Tablets ... 3104

Lorazepam (Potentiates CNS depressant effects). Products include:
Ativan Injection ... 3478
Ativan Tablets ... 3482

Loxapine Hydrochloride (Potentiates CNS depressant effects; increases the risk of respiratory depression).
No products indexed under this heading.

Loxapine Succinate (Potentiates CNS depressant effects; increases the risk of respiratory depression). Products include:
Loxitane Capsules ... 3398

Meperidine Hydrochloride (Potentiates CNS depressant effects). Products include:
Demerol ... 3079
Mepergan Injection ... 3539

Mephobarbital (Potentiates CNS depressant effects).
No products indexed under this heading.

Meprobamate (Potentiates CNS depressant effects). Products include:
Miltown Tablets ... 3349

Mesoridazine Besylate (Potentiates CNS depressant effects; increases the risk of respiratory depression). Products include:
Serentil ... 1057

Methadone Hydrochloride (Potentiates CNS depressant effects). Products include:
Dolophine Hydrochloride Tablets ... 3056

Methdilazine Hydrochloride (Potentiates CNS depressant effects).
No products indexed under this heading.

Methohexital Sodium (Potentiates CNS depressant effects). Products include:
Brevital Sodium for Injection, USP ... 1815

Methotrimeprazine (Potentiates CNS depressant effects; increases the risk of respiratory depression).
No products indexed under this heading.

Methoxyflurane (Potentiates CNS depressant effects).
No products indexed under this heading.

Midazolam Hydrochloride (Potentiates CNS depressant effects). Products include:
Versed Injection ... 3027
Versed Syrup ... 3033

Molindone Hydrochloride (Potentiates CNS depressant effects; increases the risk of respiratory depression). Products include:
Moban ... 1320

Olanzapine (Potentiates CNS depressant effects). Products include:
Zyprexa Tablets ... 1973
Zyprexa ZYDIS Orally Disintegrating Tablets ... 1973

Oxazepam (Potentiates CNS depressant effects).
No products indexed under this heading.

Oxycodone Hydrochloride (Potentiates CNS depressant effects). Products include:
OxyContin Tablets ... 2912
OxyFast Oral Concentrate Solution ... 2916
OxyIR Capsules ... 2916
Percocet Tablets ... 1326
Percodan Tablets ... 1327
Percolone Tablets ... 1327
Roxicodone ... 3067
Tylox Capsules ... 2597

Pentobarbital Sodium (Potentiates CNS depressant effects). Products include:
Nembutal Sodium Solution ... 485

Perphenazine (Potentiates CNS depressant effects; increases the risk of respiratory depression). Products include:
Etrafon ... 3115
Trilafon ... 3160

Phenobarbital (Potentiates CNS depressant effects). Products include:
Arco-Lase Plus Tablets ... 592
Donnatal ... 2929
Donnatal Extentabs ... 2930

Pimozide (Potentiates CNS depressant effects; increases the risk of respiratory depression). Products include:
Orap Tablets ... 1407

Prazepam (Potentiates CNS depressant effects).
No products indexed under this heading.

Prochlorperazine (Potentiates CNS depressant effects; increases the risk of respiratory depression). Products include:
Compazine ... 1505

Promethazine Hydrochloride (Potentiates CNS depressant effects; increases the risk of respiratory depression). Products include:
Mepergan Injection ... 3539
Phenergan Injection ... 3553
Phenergan ... 3556
Phenergan Syrup ... 3554
Phenergan with Codeine Syrup ... 3557
Phenergan with Dextromethorphan Syrup ... 3559
Phenergan VC Syrup ... 3560
Phenergan VC with Codeine Syrup ... 3561

Propofol (Potentiates CNS depressant effects). Products include:
Diprivan Injectable Emulsion ... 667

Propoxyphene Hydrochloride (Potentiates CNS depressant effects). Products include:
Darvon Pulvules ... 1909
Darvon Compound-65 Pulvules ... 1910

Propoxyphene Napsylate (Potentiates CNS depressant effects). Products include:
Darvon-N/Darvocet-N ... 1907
Darvon-N Tablets ... 1912

Pyrilamine Maleate (Potentiates CNS depressant effects). Products include:
Maximum Strength Midol Menstrual Caplets and Gelcaps ... 612
Maximum Strength Midol PMS Caplets and Gelcaps ... 613

Pyrilamine Tannate (Potentiates CNS depressant effects). Products include:
Ryna-12 S Suspension ... 3351

Quazepam (Potentiates CNS depressant effects).
No products indexed under this heading.

Quetiapine Fumarate (Potentiates CNS depressant effects; increases the risk of respiratory depression). Products include:
Seroquel Tablets ... 684

Remifentanil Hydrochloride (Potentiates CNS depressant effects).
No products indexed under this heading.

Risperidone (Potentiates CNS depressant effects; increases the risk of respiratory depression). Products include:
Risperdal ... 1796

Secobarbital Sodium (Potentiates CNS depressant effects).
No products indexed under this heading.

Sevoflurane (Potentiates CNS depressant effects).
No products indexed under this heading.

Sufentanil Citrate (Potentiates CNS depressant effects).
No products indexed under this heading.

Temazepam (Potentiates CNS depressant effects).
No products indexed under this heading.

Terfenadine (Potentiates CNS depressant effects).
No products indexed under this heading.

Thiamylal Sodium (Potentiates CNS depressant effects).
No products indexed under this heading.

Thioridazine Hydrochloride (Potentiates CNS depressant effects; increases the risk of respiratory depression). Products include:
Thioridazine Hydrochloride Tablets ... 2289

Thiothixene (Potentiates CNS depressant effects; increases the risk of respiratory depression). Products include:
Navane Capsules ... 2701
Thiothixene Capsules ... 2290

Triazolam (Potentiates CNS depressant effects). Products include:
Halcion Tablets ... 2823

Trifluoperazine Hydrochloride (Potentiates CNS depressant effects; increases the risk of respiratory depression). Products include:
Stelazine ... 1640

Trimeprazine Tartrate (Potentiates CNS depressant effects).
No products indexed under this heading.

Tripelennamine Hydrochloride (Potentiates CNS depressant effects).
No products indexed under this heading.

Triprolidine Hydrochloride (Potentiates CNS depressant effects). Products include:
Actifed Cold & Allergy Tablets ... ▣688

Zaleplon (Potentiates CNS depressant effects). Products include:
Sonata Capsules ... 3591

Ziprasidone Hydrochloride (Potentiates CNS depressant effects; increases the risk of respiratory depression). Products include:
Geodon Capsules ... 2688

Zolpidem Tartrate (Potentiates CNS depressant effects). Products include:
Ambien Tablets ... 3191

Food Interactions

Alcohol (Potentiates CNS depressant effects).

INNOHEP INJECTION

(Tinzaparin sodium) ... 1248
May interact with oral anticoagulants, non-steroidal anti-inflammatory agents, salicylates, thrombolytics, and certain other agents. Compounds in these categories include:

Alteplase, Recombinant (Co-administration with thrombolytics can result in increased risk of bleeding). Products include:
Activase I.V. ... 1410
Cathflo Activase ... 3611

Anistreplase (Co-administration with thrombolytics can result in increased risk of bleeding).
No products indexed under this heading.

Aspirin (Co-administration with platelet inhibitors, such as salicylates, can result in increased risk of bleeding). Products include:
Aggrenox Capsules ... 1026
Alka-Seltzer ... ▣603
Alka-Seltzer Lemon Lime Antacid and Pain Reliever Effervescent Tablets ... ▣603
Alka-Seltzer Extra Strength Antacid and Pain Reliever Effervescent Tablets ... ▣603
Alka-Seltzer PM Effervescent Tablets ... ▣605
Genuine Bayer Tablets, Caplets and Gelcaps ... ▣606
Extra Strength Bayer Caplets and Gelcaps ... ▣610
Aspirin Regimen Bayer Children's Chewable Tablets (Orange or Cherry Flavored) ... ▣607
Bayer, Aspirin Regimen ... ▣606
Aspirin Regimen Bayer 81 mg Caplets with Calcium ... ▣607
Genuine Bayer Professional Labeling (Aspirin Regimen Bayer) ... ▣608
Extra Strength Bayer Arthritis Caplets ... ▣610
Extra Strength Bayer Plus Caplets ... ▣610
Extra Strength Bayer PM Caplets ... ▣611
BC Powder ... ▣619
BC Allergy Sinus Cold Powder ... ▣619
Arthritis Strength BC Powder ... ▣619
BC Sinus Cold Powder ... ▣619
Darvon Compound-65 Pulvules ... 1910
Ecotrin Enteric Coated Aspirin Low, Regular and Maximum Strength Tablets ... 1715
Excedrin Extra-Strength Tablets, Caplets, and Geltabs ... ▣629
Excedrin Migraine ... 1070
Goody's Body Pain Formula Powder ... ▣620
Goody's Extra Strength Headache Powder ... ▣620
Goody's Extra Strength Pain Relief Tablets ... ▣620
Percodan Tablets ... 1327
Robaxisal Tablets ... 2939
Soma Compound Tablets ... 3354
Soma Compound w/Codeine Tablets ... 3355
Vanquish Caplets ... ▣617

Celecoxib (Co-administration with platelet inhibitors, such as NSAIDs, can result in increased risk of bleeding). Products include:
Celebrex Capsules ... 2676
Celebrex Capsules ... 2780

Choline Magnesium Trisalicylate (Co-administration with platelet inhibitors, such as salicylates, can result in increased risk of bleeding). Products include:
Trilisate ... 2901

Clopidogrel Bisulfate (Co-administration with platelet inhibitors, such as clopidogrel, can result in increased risk of bleeding). Products include:
Plavix Tablets ... 1097
Plavix Tablets ... 3084

Dextran (Co-administration with platelet inhibitors, such as dextran, can result in increased risk of bleeding).
No products indexed under this heading.

Diclofenac Potassium (Co-administration with platelet inhibitors, such as NSAIDs, can result in increased risk of bleeding). Products include:
Cataflam Tablets ... 2315

Diclofenac Sodium (Co-administration with platelet inhibitors, such as NSAIDs, can result in increased risk of bleeding). Products include:
Arthrotec Tablets ... 3195
Voltaren Ophthalmic Sterile Ophthalmic Solution ... ⊙312
Voltaren Tablets ... 2315
Voltaren-XR Tablets ... 2315

Dicumarol (Co-administration can result in increased risk of bleeding).
No products indexed under this heading.

Diflunisal (Co-administration with platelet inhibitors, such as salicylates, can result in increased risk of bleeding). Products include:
Dolobid Tablets ... 2088

Dipyridamole (Co-adminstration with platelet inhibitors, such as dipyridamole, can result in increased risk of bleeding). Products include:
Aggrenox Capsules ... 1026
Persantine Tablets ... 1057

Etodolac (Co-administration with platelet inhibitors, such as NSAIDs, can result in increased risk of bleeding). Products include:
Lodine ... 3528
Lodine XL Extended-Release Tablets ... 3530

Fenoprofen Calcium (Co-administration with platelet inhibitors, such as NSAIDs, can result in increased risk of bleeding).
No products indexed under this heading.

Flurbiprofen (Co-administration with platelet inhibitors, such as NSAIDs, can result in increased risk of bleeding).
No products indexed under this heading.

Ibuprofen (Co-administration with platelet inhibitors, such as NSAIDs, can result in increased risk of bleeding). Products include:
Advil ... ▣771
Children's Advil Oral Suspension ... ▣773
Children's Advil Chewable Tablets ... ▣773
Advil Cold and Sinus Caplets ... ▣771
Advil Cold and Sinus Tablets ... ▣771
Advil Flu & Body Ache Caplets ... ▣772
Infants' Advil Drops ... ▣773
Junior Strength Advil Tablets ... ▣773
Junior Strength Advil Chewable Tablets ... ▣773
Advil Migraine Liquigels ... ▣772
Children's Motrin Oral Suspension and Chewable Tablets ... 2006
Children's Motrin Cold Oral Suspension ... 2007
Children's Motrin Oral Suspension ... ▣643
Motrin Suspension, Oral Drops, Chewable Tablets, and Caplets ... 2002
Infants' Motrin Concentrated Drops ... 2006
Junior Strength Motrin Caplets and Chewable Tablets ... 2006
Motrin IB Tablets, Caplets, and Gelcaps ... 2002
Motrin Migraine Pain Caplets ... 2005
Motrin Sinus Headache Caplets ... 2005
Vicoprofen Tablets ... 520

Indomethacin (Co-administration with platelet inhibitors, such as NSAIDs, can result in increased risk of bleeding). Products include:
Indocin ... 2112

Indomethacin Sodium Trihydrate (Co-administration with platelet inhibitors, such as NSAIDs, can result in increased risk of bleeding). Products include:
Indocin I.V. ... 2115

Ketoprofen (Co-administration with platelet inhibitors, such as NSAIDs, can result in increased risk of bleeding). Products include:
Orudis Capsules ... 3548
Orudis KT Tablets ... ▣778
Oruvail Capsules ... 3548

Ketorolac Tromethamine (Co-administration with platelet inhibitors, such as NSAIDs, can result in increased risk of bleeding). Products include:
Acular Ophthalmic Solution ... 544
Acular PF Ophthalmic Solution ... 544
Toradol ... 3018

Magnesium Salicylate (Co-administration with platelet inhibitors, such as salicylates, can result in increased risk of bleeding). Products include:
Momentum Backache Relief Extra Strength Caplets ... ▣666

Meclofenamate Sodium (Co-administration with platelet inhibitors, such as NSAIDs, can result in increased risk of bleeding).
No products indexed under this heading.

Mefenamic Acid (Co-administration with platelet inhibitors, such as NSAIDs, can result in increased risk of bleeding). Products include:
Ponstel Capsules ... 1356

Meloxicam (Co-administration with platelet inhibitors, such as NSAIDs, can result in increased risk of bleeding). Products include:
Mobic Tablets ... 1054

Nabumetone (Co-administration with platelet inhibitors, such as NSAIDs, can result in increased risk of bleeding). Products include:
Relafen Tablets ... 1617

Naproxen (Co-administration with platelet inhibitors, such as NSAIDs, can result in increased risk of bleeding). Products include:
EC-Naprosyn Delayed-Release Tablets ... 2967
Naprosyn Suspension ... 2967
Naprosyn Tablets ... 2967

Naproxen Sodium (Co-administration with platelet inhibitors, such as NSAIDs, can result in increased risk of bleeding). Products include:
Aleve Tablets, Caplets and Gelcaps ... ▣602
Aleve Cold & Sinus Caplets ... ▣603
Anaprox Tablets ... 2967
Anaprox DS Tablets ... 2967
Naprelan Tablets ... 1293

Oxaprozin (Co-administration with platelet inhibitors, such as NSAIDs, can result in increased risk of bleeding).
No products indexed under this heading.

Phenylbutazone (Co-administration with platelet inhibitors, such as NSAIDs, can result in increased risk of bleeding).
No products indexed under this heading.

Piroxicam (Co-administration with platelet inhibitors, such as NSAIDs, can result in increased risk of bleeding). Products include:
Feldene Capsules ... 2685

Reteplase (Co-administration with thrombolytics can result in increased risk of bleeding). Products include:
Retavase Vials ... 1182

Rofecoxib (Co-administration with platelet inhibitors, such as NSAIDs, can result in increased risk of bleeding). Products include:
Vioxx ... 2213

Salsalate (Co-administration with platelet inhibitors, such as salicylates, can result in increased risk of bleeding).
No products indexed under this heading.

Streptokinase (Co-administration with thrombolytics can result in increased risk of bleeding). Products include:
Streptase for Infusion ... 647

Sulfinpyrazone (Co-administration with platelet inhibitors, such as sulfinpyrazone, can result in increased risk of bleeding).
No products indexed under this heading.

Sulindac (Co-administration with platelet inhibitors, such as NSAIDs, can result in increased risk of bleeding). Products include:
Clinoril Tablets ... 2053

Tolmetin Sodium (Co-administration with platelet inhibitors, such as NSAIDs, can result in increased risk of bleeding). Products include:
Tolectin ... 2589

Urokinase (Co-administration with thrombolytics can result in increased risk of bleeding).
No products indexed under this heading.

Warfarin Sodium (Co-administration can result in increased risk of bleeding). Products include:
Coumadin for Injection ... 1243
Coumadin Tablets ... 1243
Warfarin Sodium Tablets, USP ... 3302

INTEGRILIN INJECTION

(Eptifibatide) ... 1828
May interact with oral anticoagulants, glycoprotein (GP) IIb/IIIa inhibitors, non-steroidal anti-inflammatory agents, and certain other agents. Compounds in these categories include:

Abciximab (Current or planned administration of another parenteral GP IIb/IIIa inhibitor is contraindicated). Products include:
ReoPro Vials ... 1958

Celecoxib (Potential for additive pharmacologic effects because eptifibatide inhibits platelet aggregation; concurrent use requires caution). Products include:
Celebrex Capsules ... 2676
Celebrex Capsules ... 2780

Clopidogrel Bisulfate (Potential for additive pharmacologic effects because eptifibatide inhibits platelet

aggregation; concurrent use requires caution). Products include:
- Plavix Tablets 1097
- Plavix Tablets 3084

Diclofenac Potassium (Potential for additive pharmacologic effects because eptifibatide inhibits platelet aggregation; concurrent use requires caution). Products include:
- Cataflam Tablets 2315

Diclofenac Sodium (Potential for additive pharmacologic effects because eptifibatide inhibits platelet aggregation; concurrent use requires caution). Products include:
- Arthrotec Tablets 3195
- Voltaren Ophthalmic Sterile Ophthalmic Solution .... ⊙312
- Voltaren Tablets 2315
- Voltaren-XR Tablets 2315

Dicumarol (Potential for additive pharmacologic effects because eptifibatide inhibits platelet aggregation; concurrent use requires caution).
No products indexed under this heading.

Dipyridamole (Potential for additive pharmacologic effects because eptifibatide inhibits platelet aggregation; concurrent use requires caution). Products include:
- Aggrenox Capsules 1026
- Persantine Tablets 1057

Etodolac (Potential for additive pharmacologic effects because eptifibatide inhibits platelet aggregation; concurrent use requires caution). Products include:
- Lodine 3528
- Lodine XL Extended-Release Tablets 3530

Fenoprofen Calcium (Potential for additive pharmacologic effects because eptifibatide inhibits platelet aggregation; concurrent use requires caution).
No products indexed under this heading.

Flurbiprofen (Potential for additive pharmacologic effects because eptifibatide inhibits platelet aggregation; concurrent use requires caution).
No products indexed under this heading.

Ibuprofen (Potential for additive pharmacologic effects because eptifibatide inhibits platelet aggregation; concurrent use requires caution). Products include:
- Advil .... ◙771
- Children's Advil Oral Suspension .... ◙773
- Children's Advil Chewable Tablets .... ◙773
- Advil Cold and Sinus Caplets .... ◙771
- Advil Cold and Sinus Tablets .... ◙771
- Advil Flu & Body Ache Caplets .... ◙772
- Infants' Advil Drops .... ◙773
- Junior Strength Advil Tablets .... ◙773
- Junior Strength Advil Chewable Tablets .... ◙773
- Advil Migraine Liquigels .... ◙772
- Children's Motrin Oral Suspension and Chewable Tablets 2006
- Children's Motrin Cold Oral Suspension 2007
- Children's Motrin Oral Suspension .... ◙643
- Motrin Suspension, Oral Drops, Chewable Tablets, and Caplets 2002
- Infants' Motrin Concentrated Drops 2006
- Junior Strength Motrin Caplets and Chewable Tablets 2006
- Motrin IB Tablets, Caplets, and Gelcaps 2002
- Motrin Migraine Pain Caplets 2005
- Motrin Sinus Headache Caplets 2005
- Vicoprofen Tablets 520

Indomethacin (Potential for additive pharmacologic effects because eptifibatide inhibits platelet aggregation; concurrent use requires caution). Products include:
- Indocin 2112

Indomethacin Sodium Trihydrate (Potential for additive pharmacologic effects because eptifibatide inhibits platelet aggregation; concurrent use requires caution). Products include:
- Indocin I.V. 2115

Ketoprofen (Potential for additive pharmacologic effects because eptifibatide inhibits platelet aggregation; concurrent use requires caution). Products include:
- Orudis Capsules 3548
- Orudis KT Tablets .... ◙778
- Oruvail Capsules 3548

Ketorolac Tromethamine (Potential for additive pharmacologic effects because eptifibatide inhibits platelet aggregation; concurrent use requires caution). Products include:
- Acular Ophthalmic Solution 544
- Acular PF Ophthalmic Solution 544
- Toradol 3018

Meclofenamate Sodium (Potential for additive pharmacologic effects because eptifibatide inhibits platelet aggregation; concurrent use requires caution).
No products indexed under this heading.

Mefenamic Acid (Potential for additive pharmacologic effects because eptifibatide inhibits platelet aggregation; concurrent use requires caution). Products include:
- Ponstel Capsules 1356

Meloxicam (Potential for additive pharmacologic effects because eptifibatide inhibits platelet aggregation; concurrent use requires caution). Products include:
- Mobic Tablets 1054

Nabumetone (Potential for additive pharmacologic effects because eptifibatide inhibits platelet aggregation; concurrent use requires caution). Products include:
- Relafen Tablets 1617

Naproxen (Potential for additive pharmacologic effects because eptifibatide inhibits platelet aggregation; concurrent use requires caution). Products include:
- EC-Naprosyn Delayed-Release Tablets 2967
- Naprosyn Suspension 2967
- Naprosyn Tablets 2967

Naproxen Sodium (Potential for additive pharmacologic effects because eptifibatide inhibits platelet aggregation; concurrent use requires caution). Products include:
- Aleve Tablets, Caplets and Gelcaps .... ◙602
- Aleve Cold & Sinus Caplets .... ◙603
- Anaprox Tablets 2967
- Anaprox DS Tablets 2967
- Naprelan Tablets 1293

Oxaprozin (Potential for additive pharmacologic effects because eptifibatide inhibits platelet aggregation; concurrent use requires caution).
No products indexed under this heading.

Phenylbutazone (Potential for additive pharmacologic effects because eptifibatide inhibits platelet aggregation; concurrent use requires caution).
No products indexed under this heading.

Piroxicam (Potential for additive pharmacologic effects because eptifibatide inhibits platelet aggregation; concurrent use requires caution). Products include:
- Feldene Capsules 2685

Rofecoxib (Potential for additive pharmacologic effects because eptifibatide inhibits platelet aggregation; concurrent use requires caution). Products include:
- Vioxx 2213

Sulindac (Potential for additive pharmacologic effects because eptifibatide inhibits platelet aggregation; concurrent use requires caution). Products include:
- Clinoril Tablets 2053

Ticlopidine Hydrochloride (Potential for additive pharmacologic effects because eptifibatide inhibits platelet aggregation; concurrent use requires caution). Products include:
- Ticlid Tablets 3015

Tirofiban Hydrochloride (Current or planned administration of another parenteral GP IIb/IIIa inhibitor is contraindicated). Products include:
- Aggrastat 2031

Tolmetin Sodium (Potential for additive pharmacologic effects because eptifibatide inhibits platelet aggregation; concurrent use requires caution). Products include:
- Tolectin 2589

Warfarin Sodium (Potential for additive pharmacologic effects because eptifibatide inhibits platelet aggregation; concurrent use requires caution). Products include:
- Coumadin for Injection 1243
- Coumadin Tablets 1243
- Warfarin Sodium Tablets, USP 3302

INTEGRILIN INJECTION

(Eptifibatide) 1213

May interact with oral anticoagulants, glycoprotein (GP) IIb/IIIa inhibitors, non-steroidal anti-inflammatory agents, and certain other agents. Compounds in these categories include:

Abciximab (Current or planned administration of another parenteral GP IIb/IIIa inhibitor is contraindicated). Products include:
- ReoPro Vials 1958

Aspirin (Co-administration of eptifibatide with heparin and aspirin has resulted in cerebral, GI and pulmonary hemorrhage). Products include:
- Aggrenox Capsules 1026
- Alka-Seltzer .... ◙603
- Alka-Seltzer Lemon Lime Antacid and Pain Reliever Effervescent Tablets .... ◙603
- Alka-Seltzer Extra Strength Antacid and Pain Reliever Effervescent Tablets .... ◙603
- Alka-Seltzer PM Effervescent Tablets .... ◙605
- Genuine Bayer Tablets, Caplets and Gelcaps .... ◙606
- Extra Strength Bayer Caplets and Gelcaps .... ◙610
- Aspirin Regimen Bayer Children's Chewable Tablets (Orange or Cherry Flavored) .... ◙607
- Bayer, Aspirin Regimen .... ◙606
- Aspirin Regimen Bayer 81 mg Caplets with Calcium .... ◙607
- Genuine Bayer Professional Labeling (Aspirin Regimen Bayer) .... ◙608
- Extra Strength Bayer Arthritis Caplets .... ◙610
- Extra Strength Bayer Plus Caplets .... ◙610
- Extra Strength Bayer PM Caplets .... ◙611
- BC Powder .... ◙619
- BC Allergy Sinus Cold Powder .... ◙619
- Arthritis Strength BC Powder .... ◙619
- BC Sinus Cold Powder .... ◙619
- Darvon Compound-65 Pulvules 1910
- Ecotrin Enteric Coated Aspirin Low, Regular and Maximum Strength Tablets 1715
- Excedrin Extra-Strength Tablets, Caplets, and Geltabs .... ◙629
- Excedrin Migraine 1070
- Goody's Body Pain Formula Powder .... ◙620
- Goody's Extra Strength Headache Powder .... ◙620
- Goody's Extra Strength Pain Relief Tablets .... ◙620
- Percodan Tablets 1327
- Robaxisal Tablets 2939
- Soma Compound Tablets 3354
- Soma Compound w/Codeine Tablets 3355
- Vanquish Caplets .... ◙617

Celecoxib (Potential for additive pharmacologic effects because eptifibatide inhibits platelet aggregation; concurrent use requires caution). Products include:
- Celebrex Capsules 2676
- Celebrex Capsules 2780

Clopidogrel Bisulfate (Potential for additive pharmacologic effects because eptifibatide inhibits platelet aggregation; concurrent use requires caution). Products include:
- Plavix Tablets 1097
- Plavix Tablets 3084

Diclofenac Potassium (Potential for additive pharmacologic effects because eptifibatide inhibits platelet aggregation; concurrent use requires caution). Products include:
- Cataflam Tablets 2315

Diclofenac Sodium (Potential for additive pharmacologic effects because eptifibatide inhibits platelet aggregation; concurrent use requires caution). Products include:
- Arthrotec Tablets 3195
- Voltaren Ophthalmic Sterile Ophthalmic Solution .... ⊙312
- Voltaren Tablets 2315
- Voltaren-XR Tablets 2315

Dicumarol (Potential for additive pharmacologic effects because eptifibatide inhibits platelet aggregation; concurrent use requires caution).
No products indexed under this heading.

Dipyridamole (Potential for additive pharmacologic effects because eptifibatide inhibits platelet aggregation; concurrent use requires caution). Products include:
- Aggrenox Capsules 1026
- Persantine Tablets 1057

Etodolac (Potential for additive pharmacologic effects because eptifibatide inhibits platelet aggregation; concurrent use requires caution). Products include:
- Lodine 3528
- Lodine XL Extended-Release Tablets 3530

Fenoprofen Calcium (Potential for additive pharmacologic effects because eptifibatide inhibits platelet aggregation; concurrent use requires caution).
No products indexed under this heading.

Flurbiprofen (Potential for additive pharmacologic effects because eptifibatide inhibits platelet aggregation; concurrent use requires caution).
No products indexed under this heading.

Heparin Sodium (Co-administration of eptifibatide with heparin and aspirin has resulted in cerebral, GI and pulmonary hemorrhage). Products include:
- Heparin Lock Flush Solution 3509
- Heparin Sodium Injection 3511

Ibuprofen (Potential for additive pharmacologic effects because eptifibatide inhibits platelet aggregation; concurrent use requires caution). Products include:
- Advil .... ◙771
- Children's Advil Oral Suspension .... ◙773
- Children's Advil Chewable Tablets .... ◙773
- Advil Cold and Sinus Caplets .... ◙771
- Advil Cold and Sinus Tablets .... ◙771
- Advil Flu & Body Ache Caplets .... ◙772
- Infants' Advil Drops .... ◙773
- Junior Strength Advil Tablets .... ◙773
- Junior Strength Advil Chewable Tablets .... ◙773
- Advil Migraine Liquigels .... ◙772
- Children's Motrin Oral Suspension and Chewable Tablets 2006
- Children's Motrin Cold Oral Suspension 2007
- Children's Motrin Oral Suspension .... ◙643
- Motrin Suspension, Oral Drops, Chewable Tablets, and Caplets 2002
- Infants' Motrin Concentrated Drops 2006
- Junior Strength Motrin Caplets and Chewable Tablets 2006
- Motrin IB Tablets, Caplets, and Gelcaps 2002
- Motrin Migraine Pain Caplets 2005
- Motrin Sinus Headache Caplets 2005

Vicoprofen Tablets 520

Indomethacin (Potential for additive pharmacologic effects because eptifibatide inhibits platelet aggregation; concurrent use requires caution). Products include:
Indocin 2112

Indomethacin Sodium Trihydrate (Potential for additive pharmacologic effects because eptifibatide inhibits platelet aggregation; concurrent use requires caution). Products include:
Indocin I.V. 2115

Ketoprofen (Potential for additive pharmacologic effects because eptifibatide inhibits platelet aggregation; concurrent use requires caution). Products include:
Orudis Capsules 3548
Orudis KT Tablets .... ▣778
Oruvail Capsules 3548

Ketorolac Tromethamine (Potential for additive pharmacologic effects because eptifibatide inhibits platelet aggregation; concurrent use requires caution). Products include:
Acular Ophthalmic Solution 544
Acular PF Ophthalmic Solution 544
Toradol 3018

Meclofenamate Sodium (Potential for additive pharmacologic effects because eptifibatide inhibits platelet aggregation; concurrent use requires caution).
No products indexed under this heading.

Mefenamic Acid (Potential for additive pharmacologic effects because eptifibatide inhibits platelet aggregation; concurrent use requires caution). Products include:
Ponstel Capsules 1356

Meloxicam (Potential for additive pharmacologic effects because eptifibatide inhibits platelet aggregation; concurrent use requires caution). Products include:
Mobic Tablets 1054

Nabumetone (Potential for additive pharmacologic effects because eptifibatide inhibits platelet aggregation; concurrent use requires caution). Products include:
Relafen Tablets 1617

Naproxen (Potential for additive pharmacologic effects because eptifibatide inhibits platelet aggregation; concurrent use requires caution). Products include:
EC-Naprosyn Delayed-Release Tablets 2967
Naprosyn Suspension 2967
Naprosyn Tablets 2967

Naproxen Sodium (Potential for additive pharmacologic effects because eptifibatide inhibits platelet aggregation; concurrent use requires caution). Products include:
Aleve Tablets, Caplets and Gelcaps .... ▣602
Aleve Cold & Sinus Caplets .... ▣603
Anaprox Tablets 2967
Anaprox DS Tablets 2967
Naprelan Tablets 1293

Oxaprozin (Potential for additive pharmacologic effects because eptifibatide inhibits platelet aggregation; concurrent use requires caution).
No products indexed under this heading.

Phenylbutazone (Potential for additive pharmacologic effects because eptifibatide inhibits platelet aggregation; concurrent use requires caution).
No products indexed under this heading.

Piroxicam (Potential for additive pharmacologic effects because eptifibatide inhibits platelet aggregation; concurrent use requires caution). Products include:
Feldene Capsules 2685

Rofecoxib (Potential for additive pharmacologic effects because eptifibatide inhibits platelet aggregation; concurrent use requires caution). Products include:
Vioxx 2213

Sulindac (Potential for additive pharmacologic effects because eptifibatide inhibits platelet aggregation; concurrent use requires caution). Products include:
Clinoril Tablets 2053

Ticlopidine Hydrochloride (Potential for additive pharmacologic effects because eptifibatide inhibits platelet aggregation; concurrent use requires caution). Products include:
Ticlid Tablets 3015

Tirofiban Hydrochloride (Current or planned administration of another parenteral GP IIb/IIIa inhibitor is contraindicated). Products include:
Aggrastat 2031

Tolmetin Sodium (Potential for additive pharmacologic effects because eptifibatide inhibits platelet aggregation; concurrent use requires caution). Products include:
Tolectin 2589

Warfarin Sodium (Potential for additive pharmacologic effects because eptifibatide inhibits platelet aggregation; concurrent use requires caution). Products include:
Coumadin for Injection 1243
Coumadin Tablets 1243
Warfarin Sodium Tablets, USP 3302

INTELECTOL TABLETS

(Vinpocetine) .... ▣813
None cited in PDR database.

INTELLEQ CAPSULES

(Amino Acid Preparations, Ginkgo biloba, Herbals with Vitamins) .... ▣797
None cited in PDR database.

INTRON A FOR INJECTION

(Interferon alfa-2B, Recombinant) 3120
May interact with theophylline and certain other agents. Compounds in these categories include:

Aminophylline (Co-administration results in decreased theophylline clearance resulting in a 100% increase in serum theophylline levels).
No products indexed under this heading.

Bone Marrow Depressants, unspecified (Careful monitoring of the WBC count is indicated).

Dyphylline (Co-administration results in decreased theophylline clearance resulting in a 100% increase in serum theophylline levels). Products include:
Lufyllin Tablets 3347
Lufyllin-400 Tablets 3347
Lufyllin-GG Elixir 3348
Lufyllin-GG Tablets 3348

Theophylline (Co-administration results in decreased theophylline clearance resulting in a 100% increase in serum theophylline levels). Products include:
Aerolate 1361
Theo-Dur Extended-Release Tablets 1835
Uni-Dur Extended-Release Tablets .. 1841
Uniphyl 400 mg and 600 mg Tablets 2903

Theophylline Calcium Salicylate (Co-administration results in decreased theophylline clearance resulting in a 100% increase in serum theophylline levels).
No products indexed under this heading.

Theophylline Sodium Glycinate (Co-administration results in decreased theophylline clearance resulting in a 100% increase in serum theophylline levels).
No products indexed under this heading.

Zidovudine (Concomitant administration may result in a higher incidence of neutropenia). Products include:
Combivir Tablets 1502
Retrovir 1625
Retrovir IV Infusion 1629
Trizivir Tablets 1669

INVERSINE TABLETS

(Mecamylamine Hydrochloride) 1850
May interact with anesthetics, antihypertensives, and certain other agents. Compounds in these categories include:

Acebutolol Hydrochloride (The action of mecamylamine may be potentiated by other antihypertensives). Products include:
Sectral Capsules 3589

Alfentanil Hydrochloride (The action of mecamylamine may be potentiated by anesthetics).
No products indexed under this heading.

Amlodipine Besylate (The action of mecamylamine may be potentiated by other antihypertensives). Products include:
Lotrel Capsules 2370
Norvasc Tablets 2704

Antibiotics, unspecified (Concurrent use of ganglionic blockers in patients receiving antibiotics should be avoided).

Atenolol (The action of mecamylamine may be potentiated by other antihypertensives). Products include:
Tenoretic Tablets 690
Tenormin I.V. Injection 692

Benazepril Hydrochloride (The action of mecamylamine may be potentiated by other antihypertensives). Products include:
Lotensin Tablets 2365
Lotensin HCT Tablets 2367
Lotrel Capsules 2370

Bendroflumethiazide (The action of mecamylamine may be potentiated by other antihypertensives). Products include:
Corzide 40/5 Tablets 2247
Corzide 80/5 Tablets 2247

Betaxolol Hydrochloride (The action of mecamylamine may be potentiated by other antihypertensives). Products include:
Betoptic S Ophthalmic Suspension 537

Bisoprolol Fumarate (The action of mecamylamine may be potentiated by other antihypertensives). Products include:
Zebeta Tablets 1885
Ziac Tablets 1887

Candesartan Cilexetil (The action of mecamylamine may be potentiated by other antihypertensives). Products include:
Atacand Tablets 595
Atacand HCT Tablets 597

Captopril (The action of mecamylamine may be potentiated by other antihypertensives). Products include:
Captopril Tablets 2281

Carteolol Hydrochloride (The action of mecamylamine may be potentiated by other antihypertensives). Products include:
Carteolol Hydrochloride Ophthalmic Solution USP, 1% ..... ⊙258
Ocupress Ophthalmic Solution, 1% Sterile .... ⊙303

Chlorothiazide (The action of mecamylamine may be potentiated by other antihypertensives). Products include:
Aldoclor Tablets 2035
Diuril Oral 2087

Chlorothiazide Sodium (The action of mecamylamine may be potentiated by other antihypertensives). Products include:
Diuril Sodium Intravenous 2086

Chlorthalidone (The action of mecamylamine may be potentiated by other antihypertensives). Products include:
Clorpres Tablets 1002
Combipres Tablets 1040
Tenoretic Tablets 690

Clonidine (The action of mecamylamine may be potentiated by other antihypertensives). Products include:
Catapres-TTS 1038

Clonidine Hydrochloride (The action of mecamylamine may be potentiated by other antihypertensives). Products include:
Catapres Tablets 1037
Clorpres Tablets 1002
Combipres Tablets 1040
Duraclon Injection 3057

Deserpidine (The action of mecamylamine may be potentiated by other antihypertensives).
No products indexed under this heading.

Diazoxide (The action of mecamylamine may be potentiated by other antihypertensives).
No products indexed under this heading.

Diltiazem Hydrochloride (The action of mecamylamine may be potentiated by other antihypertensives). Products include:
Cardizem Injectable 1018
Cardizem Lyo-Ject Syringe 1018
Cardizem Monovial 1018
Cardizem CD Capsules 1016
Tiazac Capsules 1378

Doxazosin Mesylate (The action of mecamylamine may be potentiated by other antihypertensives). Products include:
Cardura Tablets 2668

Enalapril Maleate (The action of mecamylamine may be potentiated by other antihypertensives). Products include:
Lexxel Tablets 608
Vaseretic Tablets 2204
Vasotec Tablets 2210

Enalaprilat (The action of mecamylamine may be potentiated by other antihypertensives). Products include:
Enalaprilat Injection 863
Vasotec I.V. Injection 2207

Enflurane (The action of mecamylamine may be potentiated by anesthetics).
No products indexed under this heading.

Eprosartan Mesylate (The action of mecamylamine may be potentiated by other antihypertensives). Products include:
Teveten Tablets 3327

Esmolol Hydrochloride (The action of mecamylamine may be potentiated by other antihypertensives). Products include:
Brevibloc Injection 858

Felodipine (The action of mecamylamine may be potentiated by other antihypertensives). Products include:
Lexxel Tablets 608
Plendil Extended-Release Tablets ... 623

Fentanyl Citrate (The action of mecamylamine may be potentiated by anesthetics). Products include:
Actiq 1184

Fosinopril Sodium (The action of mecamylamine may be potentiated by other antihypertensives). Products include:
Monopril Tablets 1091
Monopril HCT 1094

Furosemide (The action of mecamylamine may be potentiated by other antihypertensives). Products include:
Furosemide Tablets 2284

Guanabenz Acetate (The action of mecamylamine may be potentiated by other antihypertensives).
No products indexed under this heading.

Guanethidine Monosulfate (The action of mecamylamine may be potentiated by other antihypertensives).
No products indexed under this heading.

Halothane (The action of mecamylamine may be potentiated by anesthetics). Products include:
Fluothane Inhalation 3508

Hydralazine Hydrochloride (The action of mecamylamine may be potentiated by other antihypertensives).
No products indexed under this heading.

Hydrochlorothiazide (The action of mecamylamine may be potentiated by other antihypertensives).
Products include:
Accuretic Tablets 2614
Aldoril Tablets 2039
Atacand HCT Tablets 597
Avalide Tablets 1070
Diovan HCT Tablets 2338
Dyazide Capsules 1515
HydroDIURIL Tablets 2108
Hyzaar 2109
Inderide Tablets 3517
Inderide LA Long-Acting Capsules .. 3519
Lotensin HCT Tablets 2367
Maxzide 1008
Micardis HCT Tablets 1051
Microzide Capsules 3414
Moduretic Tablets 2138
Monopril HCT 1094
Prinzide Tablets 2168
Timolide Tablets 2187
Uniretic Tablets 3178
Vaseretic Tablets 2204
Zestoretic Tablets 695
Ziac Tablets 1887

Hydroflumethiazide (The action of mecamylamine may be potentiated by other antihypertensives).
Products include:
Diucardin Tablets 3494

Indapamide (The action of mecamylamine may be potentiated by other antihypertensives). Products include:
Indapamide Tablets 2286

Irbesartan (The action of mecamylamine may be potentiated by other antihypertensives). Products include:
Avalide Tablets 1070
Avapro Tablets 1074
Avapro Tablets 3076

Isoflurane (The action of mecamylamine may be potentiated by anesthetics).
No products indexed under this heading.

Isradipine (The action of mecamylamine may be potentiated by other antihypertensives). Products include:
DynaCirc Capsules 2921
DynaCirc CR Tablets 2923

Ketamine Hydrochloride (The action of mecamylamine may be potentiated by anesthetics).
No products indexed under this heading.

Labetalol Hydrochloride (The action of mecamylamine may be potentiated by other antihypertensives). Products include:
Normodyne Injection 3135
Normodyne Tablets 3137

Lisinopril (The action of mecamylamine may be potentiated by other antihypertensives). Products include:
Prinivil Tablets 2164
Prinzide Tablets 2168
Zestoretic Tablets 695
Zestril Tablets 698

Losartan Potassium (The action of mecamylamine may be potentiated by other antihypertensives).
Products include:
Cozaar Tablets 2067
Hyzaar 2109

Methohexital Sodium (The action of mecamylamine may be potentiated by anesthetics). Products include:
Brevital Sodium for Injection, USP .. 1815

Methyclothiazide (The action of mecamylamine may be potentiated by other antihypertensives).
No products indexed under this heading.

Methyldopa (The action of mecamylamine may be potentiated by other antihypertensives). Products include:
Aldoclor Tablets 2035
Aldomet Tablets 2037
Aldoril Tablets 2039

Methyldopate Hydrochloride (The action of mecamylamine may be potentiated by other antihypertensives).
No products indexed under this heading.

Metolazone (The action of mecamylamine may be potentiated by other antihypertensives). Products include:
Mykrox Tablets 1168
Zaroxolyn Tablets 1177

Metoprolol Succinate (The action of mecamylamine may be potentiated by other antihypertensives).
Products include:
Toprol-XL Tablets 651

Metoprolol Tartrate (The action of mecamylamine may be potentiated by other antihypertensives).
No products indexed under this heading.

Metyrosine (The action of mecamylamine may be potentiated by other antihypertensives). Products include:
Demser Capsules 2085

Mibefradil Dihydrochloride (The action of mecamylamine may be potentiated by other antihypertensives).
No products indexed under this heading.

Midazolam Hydrochloride (The action of mecamylamine may be potentiated by anesthetics).
Products include:
Versed Injection 3027
Versed Syrup 3033

Minoxidil (The action of mecamylamine may be potentiated by other antihypertensives). Products include:
Rogaine Extra Strength for Men Topical Solution .... ▣ 721
Rogaine for Women Topical Solution .... ▣ 721

Moexipril Hydrochloride (The action of mecamylamine may be potentiated by other antihypertensives). Products include:
Uniretic Tablets 3178
Univasc Tablets 3181

Nadolol (The action of mecamylamine may be potentiated by other antihypertensives). Products include:
Corgard Tablets 2245
Corzide 40/5 Tablets 2247
Corzide 80/5 Tablets 2247
Nadolol Tablets 2288

Nicardipine Hydrochloride (The action of mecamylamine may be potentiated by other antihypertensives). Products include:
Cardene I.V. 3485

Nifedipine (The action of mecamylamine may be potentiated by other antihypertensives). Products include:
Adalat CC Tablets 877
Procardia Capsules 2708
Procardia XL Extended Release Tablets 2710

Nisoldipine (The action of mecamylamine may be potentiated by other antihypertensives). Products include:
Sular Tablets 688

Nitroglycerin (The action of mecamylamine may be potentiated by other antihypertensives). Products include:
Nitro-Dur Transdermal Infusion System 3134
Nitro-Dur Transdermal Infusion System 1834
Nitrolingual Pumpspray 1355
Nitrostat Tablets 2658

Penbutolol Sulfate (The action of mecamylamine may be potentiated by other antihypertensives).
No products indexed under this heading.

Perindopril Erbumine (The action of mecamylamine may be potentiated by other antihypertensives).
Products include:
Aceon Tablets (2 mg, 4 mg, 8 mg) 3249

Phenoxybenzamine Hydrochloride (The action of mecamylamine may be potentiated by other antihypertensives). Products include:
Dibenzyline Capsules 3457

Phentolamine Mesylate (The action of mecamylamine may be potentiated by other antihypertensives).
No products indexed under this heading.

Pindolol (The action of mecamylamine may be potentiated by other antihypertensives).
No products indexed under this heading.

Polythiazide (The action of mecamylamine may be potentiated by other antihypertensives). Products include:
Minizide Capsules 2700
Renese Tablets 2712

Prazosin Hydrochloride (The action of mecamylamine may be potentiated by other antihypertensives). Products include:
Minipress Capsules 2699
Minizide Capsules 2700

Propofol (The action of mecamylamine may be potentiated by anesthetics). Products include:
Diprivan Injectable Emulsion 667

Propranolol Hydrochloride (The action of mecamylamine may be potentiated by other antihypertensives). Products include:
Inderal 3513
Inderal LA Long-Acting Capsules 3516
Inderide Tablets 3517
Inderide LA Long-Acting Capsules .. 3519

Quinapril Hydrochloride (The action of mecamylamine may be potentiated by other antihypertensives). Products include:
Accupril Tablets 2611
Accuretic Tablets 2614

Ramipril (The action of mecamylamine may be potentiated by other antihypertensives). Products include:
Altace Capsules 2233

Rauwolfia serpentina (The action of mecamylamine may be potentiated by other antihypertensives).
No products indexed under this heading.

Remifentanil Hydrochloride (The action of mecamylamine may be potentiated by anesthetics).
No products indexed under this heading.

Rescinnamine (The action of mecamylamine may be potentiated by other antihypertensives).
No products indexed under this heading.

Reserpine (The action of mecamylamine may be potentiated by other antihypertensives).
No products indexed under this heading.

Sodium Nitroprusside (The action of mecamylamine may be potentiated by other antihypertensives).
No products indexed under this heading.

Sotalol Hydrochloride (The action of mecamylamine may be potentiated by other antihypertensives).
Products include:
Betapace Tablets 950
Betapace AF Tablets 954

Spirapril Hydrochloride (The action of mecamylamine may be potentiated by other antihypertensives).
No products indexed under this heading.

Sufentanil Citrate (The action of mecamylamine may be potentiated by anesthetics).
No products indexed under this heading.

Sulfamethoxazole (Concurrent use of ganglionic blockers in patients receiving sulfonamides should be avoided). Products include:
Bactrim 2949
Septra Suspension 2265
Septra Tablets 2265
Septra DS Tablets 2265

Sulfisoxazole Acetyl (Concurrent use of ganglionic blockers in patients receiving sulfonamides should be avoided). Products include:
Pediazole Suspension 3050

Telmisartan (The action of mecamylamine may be potentiated by other antihypertensives). Products include:
Micardis Tablets 1049
Micardis HCT Tablets 1051

Terazosin Hydrochloride (The action of mecamylamine may be potentiated by other antihypertensives). Products include:
Hytrin Capsules 464

Thiamylal Sodium (The action of mecamylamine may be potentiated by anesthetics).
No products indexed under this heading.

Timolol Maleate (The action of mecamylamine may be potentiated by other antihypertensives).
Products include:
Blocadren Tablets 2046
Cosopt Sterile Ophthalmic Solution 2065
Timolide Tablets 2187
Timolol GFS .... ⊙ 266
Timoptic in Ocudose 2192
Timoptic Sterile Ophthalmic Solution 2190
Timoptic-XE Sterile Ophthalmic Gel Forming Solution 2194

Torsemide (The action of mecamylamine may be potentiated by other antihypertensives). Products include:
Demadex Tablets and Injection 2965

Trandolapril (The action of mecamylamine may be potentiated by other antihypertensives). Products include:
Mavik Tablets 478
Tarka Tablets 508

Trimethaphan Camsylate (The action of mecamylamine may be potentiated by other antihypertensives).
No products indexed under this heading.

Valsartan (The action of mecamylamine may be potentiated by other antihypertensives). Products include:
Diovan Capsules 2337
Diovan HCT Tablets 2338

Verapamil Hydrochloride (The action of mecamylamine may be potentiated by other antihypertensives). Products include:
Covera-HS Tablets 3199
Isoptin SR Tablets 467
Tarka Tablets 508
Verelan Capsules 3184
Verelan PM Capsules 3186

IMPORTANT NOTE: Always consult each drug listing in the patient's regimen for possible interactions.

Food Interactions

Alcohol (The action of mecamylamine may be potentiated by alcohol).

INVIRASE CAPSULES

(Saquinavir Mesylate) 2979

May interact with calcium channel blockers, dexamethasone, ergot-containing drugs, phenytoin, quinidine, and certain other agents. Compounds in these categories include:

Amlodipine Besylate (Potential for elevated plasma concentrations of compounds that are substrate of CYP3A4, such as calcium channel blockers). Products include:
- Lotrel Capsules 2370
- Norvasc Tablets 2704

Astemizole (Inhibition of CYP3A by saquinavir could result in increased astemizole plasma levels and create the potential for serious and/or life-threatening reactions such as rare cases of serious cardiovascular adverse events; concurrent use is contraindicated).
No products indexed under this heading.

Bepridil Hydrochloride (Potential for elevated plasma concentrations of compounds that are substrate of CYP3A4, such as calcium channel blockers). Products include:
- Vascor Tablets 2602

Carbamazepine (May decrease saquinavir plasma concentrations). Products include:
- Carbatrol Capsules 3234
- Tegretol/Tegretol-XR 2404

Cisapride (Inhibition of CYP3A by saquinavir could result in increased cisapride plasma levels and create the potential for serious and/or life-threatening reactions such as rare cases of serious cardiovascular adverse events; concurrent use is contraindicated).
No products indexed under this heading.

Clindamycin Hydrochloride (Potential for elevated plasma concentrations of compounds that are substrate of CYP3A4, such as clindamycin). Products include:
- Cleocin HCl Capsules 2784

Clindamycin Palmitate Hydrochloride (Potential for elevated plasma concentrations of compounds that are substrate of CYP3A4, such as clindamycin).
No products indexed under this heading.

Clindamycin Phosphate (Potential for elevated plasma concentrations of compounds that are substrate of CYP3A4, such as clindamycin). Products include:
- Benzaclin Topical Gel 1220
- Cleocin Phosphate Sterile Solution .. 2785
- Cleocin T Topical 2790
- Cleocin Vaginal Cream 2788
- Cleocin Vaginal Ovules 2789
- Clindagel 1401
- Clindets Pledgets 3270

Dapsone (Potential for elevated plasma concentrations of compounds that are substrate of CYP3A4, such as dapsone). Products include:
- Dapsone Tablets USP 1780

Delavirdine Mesylate (Co-administration has resulted in a 5-fold increase in saquinavir plasma AUC; currently, there are no safety and efficacy data available from use of this combination; hepatocellular enzyme elevations have occurred in some patients). Products include:
- Rescriptor Tablets 526

Dexamethasone (May decrease saquinavir plasma concentrations). Products include:
- Decadron Elixir 2078
- Decadron Tablets 2079
- TobraDex Ophthalmic Ointment 542
- TobraDex Ophthalmic Suspension ... 541

Dexamethasone Acetate (May decrease saquinavir plasma concentrations).
No products indexed under this heading.

Dexamethasone Sodium Phosphate (May decrease saquinavir plasma concentrations). Products include:
- Decadron Phosphate Injection 2081
- Decadron Phosphate Sterile Ophthalmic Ointment 2083
- Decadron Phosphate Sterile Ophthalmic Solution 2084
- NeoDecadron Sterile Ophthalmic Solution 2144

Dihydroergotamine Mesylate (Inhibition of CYP3A by saquinavir could result in increased ergot derivatives plasma levels and create the potential for serious and/or life-threatening reactions; concurrent use is contraindicated). Products include:
- D.H.E. 45 Injection 2334
- Migranal Nasal Spray 2376

Diltiazem Hydrochloride (Potential for elevated plasma concentrations of compounds that are substrate of CYP3A4, such as calcium channel blockers). Products include:
- Cardizem Injectable 1018
- Cardizem Lyo-Ject Syringe 1018
- Cardizem Monovial 1018
- Cardizem CD Capsules 1016
- Tiazac Capsules 1378

Ergonovine Maleate (Inhibition of CYP3A by saquinavir could result in increased ergot derivatives plasma levels and create the potential for serious and/or life-threatening reactions; concurrent use is contraindicated).
No products indexed under this heading.

Ergotamine Tartrate (Inhibition of CYP3A by saquinavir could result in increased ergot derivatives plasma levels and create the potential for serious and/or life-threatening reactions; concurrent use is contraindicated).
No products indexed under this heading.

Felodipine (Potential for elevated plasma concentrations of compounds that are substrate of CYP3A4, such as calcium channel blockers). Products include:
- Lexxel Tablets 608
- Plendil Extended-Release Tablets ... 623

Fosphenytoin Sodium (May decrease saquinavir plasma concentrations). Products include:
- Cerebyx Injection 2619

Isradipine (Potential for elevated plasma concentrations of compounds that are substrate of CYP3A4, such as calcium channel blockers). Products include:
- DynaCirc Capsules 2921
- DynaCirc CR Tablets 2923

Ketoconazole (Co-administration has resulted in a 130% increase in saquinavir plasma AUC). Products include:
- Nizoral 2% Cream 3620
- Nizoral A-D Shampoo 2008
- Nizoral 2% Shampoo 2007
- Nizoral Tablets 1791

Methylergonovine Maleate (Inhibition of CYP3A by saquinavir could result in increased ergot derivatives plasma levels and create the potential for serious and/or life-threatening reactions; concurrent use is contraindicated).
No products indexed under this heading.

Methysergide Maleate (Inhibition of CYP3A by saquinavir could result in increased ergot derivatives plasma levels and create the potential for serious and/or life-threatening reactions; concurrent use is contraindicated).
No products indexed under this heading.

Mibefradil Dihydrochloride (Potential for elevated plasma concentrations of compounds that are substrate of CYP3A4, such as calcium channel blockers).
No products indexed under this heading.

Midazolam Hydrochloride (Inhibition of CYP3A by saquinavir could result in increased midazolam plasma levels and create the potential for serious and/or life-threatening reactions; concurrent use is contraindicated). Products include:
- Versed Injection 3027
- Versed Syrup 3033

Nelfinavir Mesylate (Co-administration has resulted in an 18% increase in nelfinavir plasma AUC and a 392% increase in saquinavir plasma AUC; currently, there are no safety and efficacy data available from use of this combination). Products include:
- Viracept 532

Nevirapine (Co-administration has resulted in a 24% decrease in saquinavir plasma AUC; currently, there are no safety and efficacy data available from use of this combination). Products include:
- Viramune Oral Suspension 1060
- Viramune Tablets 1060

Nicardipine Hydrochloride (Potential for elevated plasma concentrations of compounds that are substrate of CYP3A4, such as calcium channel blockers). Products include:
- Cardene I.V. 3485

Nifedipine (Potential for elevated plasma concentrations of compounds that are substrate of CYP3A4, such as calcium channel blockers). Products include:
- Adalat CC Tablets 877
- Procardia Capsules 2708
- Procardia XL Extended Release Tablets 2710

Nimodipine (Potential for elevated plasma concentrations of compounds that are substrate of CYP3A4, such as calcium channel blockers). Products include:
- Nimotop Capsules 904

Nisoldipine (Potential for elevated plasma concentrations of compounds that are substrate of CYP3A4, such as calcium channel blockers). Products include:
- Sular Tablets 688

Phenobarbital (Anticonvulsants, such as phenobarbital, may decrease saquinavir plasma concentrations). Products include:
- Arco-Lase Plus Tablets 592
- Donnatal 2929
- Donnatal Extentabs 2930

Phenytoin (May decrease saquinavir plasma concentrations). Products include:
- Dilantin Infatabs 2624
- Dilantin-125 Oral Suspension 2625

Phenytoin Sodium (May decrease saquinavir plasma concentrations). Products include:
- Dilantin Kapseals 2622

Quinidine Gluconate (Potential for elevated plasma concentrations of compounds that are substrate of CYP3A4, such as quinidine). Products include:
- Quinaglute Dura-Tabs Tablets 978

Quinidine Polygalacturonate (Potential for elevated plasma concentrations of compounds that are substrate of CYP3A4, such as quinidine).
No products indexed under this heading.

Quinidine Sulfate (Potential for elevated plasma concentrations of compounds that are substrate of CYP3A4, such as quinidine). Products include:
- Quinidex Extentabs 2933

Rifabutin (Co-administration has resulted in a 43% decrease in saquinavir plasma AUC; prescriber should condsider using an alternative to rifabutin). Products include:
- Mycobutin Capsules 2838

Rifampin (Co-administration has resulted in an 84% decrease in saquinavir plasma AUC; prescriber should consider using an alternative to rifampin). Products include:
- Rifadin 765
- Rifamate Capsules 767
- Rifater Tablets 769

Ritonavir (Combination therapy in HIV-infected patients has resulted in AUC values which were at least 17-fold greater than historical AUC values from patients who received saquinavir without ritonavir). Products include:
- Kaletra Capsules 471
- Kaletra Oral Solution 471
- Norvir Capsules 487
- Norvir Oral Solution 487

Terfenadine (Inhibition of CYP3A by saquinavir could result in increased terfenadine plasma levels and create the potential for serious and/or life-threatening reactions such as rare cases of serious cardiovascular adverse events; concurrent use is contraindicated).
No products indexed under this heading.

Triazolam (Inhibition of CYP3A by saquinavir could result in increased triazolam plasma levels and create the potential for serious and/or life-threatening reactions; concurrent use is contraindicated). Products include:
- Halcion Tablets 2823

Verapamil Hydrochloride (Potential for elevated plasma concentrations of compounds that are substrate of CYP3A4, such as calcium channel blockers). Products include:
- Covera-HS Tablets 3199
- Isoptin SR Tablets 467
- Tarka Tablets 508
- Verelan Capsules 3184
- Verelan PM Capsules 3186

Food Interactions

Food, unspecified (Saquinavir 24-hour AUC and Cmax following the administration of a high calorie meal were an average two times higher than after a lower calorie, lower fat meal; the effect of food has been shown to persist for up to 2 hours).

IONAMIN CAPSULES

(Phentermine Resin) 1163

May interact with anorexiants, insulin, monoamine oxidase inhibitors, selective serotonin reuptake inhibitors, and certain other agents. Compounds in these categories include:

Amphetamine Resins (The safety and efficacy of combination therapy with phentermine and other products for weight loss have not been established; co-administration of these products for weight loss is not recommended).
No products indexed under this heading.

Benzphetamine Hydrochloride (The safety and efficacy of combination therapy with phentermine and other products for weight loss have not been established; co-administration of these products for weight loss is not recommended).
No products indexed under this heading.

Citalopram Hydrobromide (The safety and efficacy of combination therapy with phentermine and SSRIs

have not been established; co-administration of these products for weight loss is not recommended). Products include:
Celexa 1365

Dextroamphetamine Sulfate (The safety and efficacy of combination therapy with phentermine and other products for weight loss have not been established; co-administration of these products for weight loss is not recommended). Products include:
Adderall Tablets 3231
Adderall XR Capsules ....
Dexedrine 1512
DextroStat Tablets 3236

Diethylpropion Hydrochloride (The safety and efficacy of combination therapy with phentermine and other products for weight loss have not been established; co-administration of these products for weight loss is not recommended).
No products indexed under this heading.

Fenfluramine Hydrochloride (Combination therapy has been reported to be associated with the occurrence of serious regurgitant cardiac valvular disease).
No products indexed under this heading.

Fluoxetine Hydrochloride (The safety and efficacy of combination therapy with phentermine and SSRIs have not been established; co-administration of these products for weight loss is not recommended). Products include:
Prozac Pulvules, Liquid, and Weekly Capsules 1238
Sarafem Pulvules 1962

Fluvoxamine Maleate (The safety and efficacy of combination therapy with phentermine and SSRIs have not been established; co-administration of these products for weight loss is not recommended). Products include:
Luvox Tablets (25, 50, 100 mg) 3256

Guanethidine Monosulfate (Decreased hypotensive effect of adrenergic neuron blocking drugs, such as guanethidine).
No products indexed under this heading.

Insulin, Human, Zinc Suspension (Insulin requirements in diabetic patients may be altered in association with the use of phentermine and the concomitant dietary regimen). Products include:
Humulin L, 100 Units 1937
Humulin U, 100 Units 1943
Novolin L Human Insulin 10 ml Vials 2422

Insulin, Human NPH (Insulin requirements in diabetic patients may be altered in association with the use of phentermine and the concomitant dietary regimen). Products include:
Humulin N, 100 Units 1939
Humulin N NPH Pen 1940
Novolin N Human Insulin 10 ml Vials 2422
Novolin N PenFill 2423
Novolin N Prefilled Syringe Disposable Insulin Delivery System 2425

Insulin, Human Regular (Insulin requirements in diabetic patients may be altered in association with the use of phentermine and the concomitant dietary regimen). Products include:
Humulin R Regular (U-500) 1943
Humulin R, 100 Units 1941
Novolin R Human Insulin 10 ml Vials 2423
Novolin R PenFill 2423
Novolin R Prefilled Syringe Disposable Insulin Delivery System 2425
Velosulin BR Human Insulin 10 ml Vials 2435

Insulin, Human Regular and Human NPH Mixture (Insulin requirements in diabetic patients may be altered in association with the use of phentermine and the concomitant dietary regimen). Products include:
Humulin 50/50, 100 Units 1934
Humulin 70/30, 100 Units 1935
Humulin 70/30 Pen 1936
Novolin 70/30 Human Insulin 10 ml Vials 2421
Novolin 70/30 PenFill 2423
Novolin 70/30 Prefilled Disposable Insulin Delivery System 2425

Insulin, NPH (Insulin requirements in diabetic patients may be altered in association with the use of phentermine and the concomitant dietary regimen). Products include:
Iletin II, NPH (Pork), 100 Units 1946

Insulin, Regular (Insulin requirements in diabetic patients may be altered in association with the use of phentermine and the concomitant dietary regimen). Products include:
Iletin II, Regular (Pork), 100 Units ... 1947

Insulin, Zinc Crystals (Insulin requirements in diabetic patients may be altered in association with the use of phentermine and the concomitant dietary regimen).
No products indexed under this heading.

Insulin, Zinc Suspension (Insulin requirements in diabetic patients may be altered in association with the use of phentermine and the concomitant dietary regimen). Products include:
Iletin II, Lente (Pork), 100 Units 1945

Insulin Aspart, Human Regular (Insulin requirements in diabetic patients may be altered in association with the use of phentermine and the concomitant dietary regimen).
No products indexed under this heading.

Insulin glargine (Insulin requirements in diabetic patients may be altered in association with the use of phentermine and the concomitant dietary regimen). Products include:
Lantus Injection 742

Insulin Lispro, Human (Insulin requirements in diabetic patients may be altered in association with the use of phentermine and the concomitant dietary regimen). Products include:
Humalog 1926
Humalog Mix 75/25 Pen 1928

Insulin Lispro Protamine, Human (Insulin requirements in diabetic patients may be altered in association with the use of phentermine and the concomitant dietary regimen). Products include:
Humalog Mix 75/25 Pen 1928

Isocarboxazid (Co-administration with MAO inhibitors may result in hypertensive crises; concurrent and/or sequential use is contraindicated).
No products indexed under this heading.

Mazindol (The safety and efficacy of combination therapy with phentermine and other products for weight loss have not been established; co-administration of these products for weight loss is not recommended).
No products indexed under this heading.

Methamphetamine Hydrochloride (The safety and efficacy of combination therapy with phentermine and other products for weight loss have not been established; co-administration of these products for weight loss is not recommended). Products include:
Desoxyn Tablets 440

Moclobemide (Co-administration with MAO inhibitors may result in hypertensive crises; concurrent and/or sequential use is contraindicated).
No products indexed under this heading.

Pargyline Hydrochloride (Co-administration with MAO inhibitors may result in hypertensive crises; concurrent and/or sequential use is contraindicated).
No products indexed under this heading.

Paroxetine Hydrochloride (The safety and efficacy of combination therapy with phentermine and SSRIs have not been established; co-administration of these products for weight loss is not recommended). Products include:
Paxil 1609

Phendimetrazine Tartrate (The safety and efficacy of combination therapy with phentermine and other products for weight loss have not been established; co-administration of these products for weight loss is not recommended). Products include:
Bontril Slow-Release Capsules 576

Phenelzine Sulfate (Co-administration with MAO inhibitors may result in hypertensive crises; concurrent and/or sequential use is contraindicated). Products include:
Nardil Tablets 2653

Phenmetrazine Hydrochloride (The safety and efficacy of combination therapy with phentermine and other products for weight loss have not been established; co-administration of these products for weight loss is not recommended).
No products indexed under this heading.

Phentermine Hydrochloride (The safety and efficacy of combination therapy with phentermine and other products for weight loss have not been established; co-administration of these products for weight loss is not recommended). Products include:
Adipex-P 1406

Procarbazine Hydrochloride (Co-administration with MAO inhibitors may result in hypertensive crises; concurrent and/or sequential use is contraindicated). Products include:
Matulane Capsules 3246

Selegiline Hydrochloride (Co-administration with MAO inhibitors may result in hypertensive crises; concurrent and/or sequential use is contraindicated). Products include:
Eldepryl Capsules 3266

Sertraline Hydrochloride (The safety and efficacy of combination therapy with phentermine and SSRIs have not been established; co-administration of these products for weight loss is not recommended). Products include:
Zoloft 2751

Sibutramine Hydrochloride Monohydrate (The safety and efficacy of combination therapy with phentermine and other products for weight loss have not been established; co-administration of these products for weight loss is not recommended). Products include:
Meridia Capsules 481

Tranylcypromine Sulfate (Co-administration with MAO inhibitors may result in hypertensive crises; concurrent and/or sequential use is contraindicated). Products include:
Parnate Tablets 1607

Food Interactions

Alcohol (Possible adverse interactions with alcohol).

IOPIDINE 0.5% OPHTHALMIC SOLUTION

(Apraclonidine Hydrochloride) .... ⊙213
May interact with antihypertensives, barbiturates, beta blockers, central nervous system depressants, general anesthetics, cardiac glycosides, hypnotics and sedatives, insulin, monoamine oxidase inhibitors, narcotic analgesics, antipsychotic agents, tricyclic antidepressants, and certain other agents. Compounds in these categories include:

Acebutolol Hydrochloride (Apraclonidine reduces pulse and blood pressure, caution is advised when used concurrently). Products include:
Sectral Capsules 3589

Alfentanil Hydrochloride (Possible additive or potentiating effect with CNS depressant).
No products indexed under this heading.

Alprazolam (Possible additive or potentiating effect with CNS depressant). Products include:
Xanax Tablets 2865

Amitriptyline Hydrochloride (Tricyclic antidepressants have been reported to blunt the hypotensive effect of clonidine; it is not known whether the concurrent use with apraclonidine can lead to reduction in IOP lowering effect). Products include:
Etrafon 3115
Limbitrol 1738

Amlodipine Besylate (Apraclonidine reduces pulse and blood pressure, caution is advised when used concurrently). Products include:
Lotrel Capsules 2370
Norvasc Tablets 2704

Amoxapine (Tricyclic antidepressants have been reported to blunt the hypotensive effect of clonidine; it is not known whether the concurrent use with apraclonidine can lead to reduction in IOP lowering effect).
No products indexed under this heading.

Aprobarbital (Possible additive or potentiating effect with CNS depressant).
No products indexed under this heading.

Atenolol (Apraclonidine reduces pulse and blood pressure, caution is advised when used concurrently). Products include:
Tenoretic Tablets 690
Tenormin I.V. Injection 692

Benazepril Hydrochloride (Apraclonidine reduces pulse and blood pressure, caution is advised when used concurrently). Products include:
Lotensin Tablets 2365
Lotensin HCT Tablets 2367
Lotrel Capsules 2370

Bendroflumethiazide (Apraclonidine reduces pulse and blood pressure, caution is advised when used concurrently). Products include:
Corzide 40/5 Tablets 2247
Corzide 80/5 Tablets 2247

Betaxolol Hydrochloride (Apraclonidine reduces pulse and blood pressure, caution is advised when used concurrently). Products include:
Betoptic S Ophthalmic Suspension 537

Bisoprolol Fumarate (Apraclonidine reduces pulse and blood pressure, caution is advised when used concurrently). Products include:
Zebeta Tablets 1885
Ziac Tablets 1887

Buprenorphine Hydrochloride (Possible additive or potentiating effect with CNS depressant). Products include:
Buprenex Injectable 2918

IMPORTANT NOTE: Always consult each drug listing in the patient's regimen for possible interactions.

Buspirone Hydrochloride (Possible additive or potentiating effect with CNS depressant).
No products indexed under this heading.

Butabarbital (Possible additive or potentiating effect with CNS depressant).
No products indexed under this heading.

Butalbital (Possible additive or potentiating effect with CNS depressant). Products include:
Phrenilin 578
Sedapap Tablets 50 mg/650 mg ... 2225

Candesartan Cilexetil (Apraclonidine reduces pulse and blood pressure, caution is advised when used concurrently). Products include:
Atacand Tablets 595
Atacand HCT Tablets 597

Captopril (Apraclonidine reduces pulse and blood pressure, caution is advised when used concurrently). Products include:
Captopril Tablets 2281

Carteolol Hydrochloride (Apraclonidine reduces pulse and blood pressure, caution is advised when used concurrently). Products include:
Carteolol Hydrochloride Ophthalmic Solution USP, 1% ..... ⊙258
Ocupress Ophthalmic Solution, 1% Sterile .... ⊙303

Chlordiazepoxide (Possible additive or potentiating effect with CNS depressant). Products include:
Limbitrol 1738

Chlordiazepoxide Hydrochloride (Possible additive or potentiating effect with CNS depressant). Products include:
Librium Capsules 1736
Librium for Injection 1737

Chlorothiazide (Apraclonidine reduces pulse and blood pressure, caution is advised when used concurrently). Products include:
Aldoclor Tablets 2035
Diuril Oral 2087

Chlorothiazide Sodium (Apraclonidine reduces pulse and blood pressure, caution is advised when used concurrently). Products include:
Diuril Sodium Intravenous 2086

Chlorpromazine (An additive hypotensive effect has been reported with the combination of systemic clonidine and neuroleptic therapy; possible additive or potentiating effect with CNS depressant). Products include:
Thorazine Suppositories 1656

Chlorpromazine Hydrochloride (An additive hypotensive effect has been reported with the combination of systemic clonidine and neuroleptic therapy; possible additive or potentiating effect with CNS depressant). Products include:
Thorazine 1656

Chlorprothixene (An additive hypotensive effect has been reported with the combination of systemic clonidine and neuroleptic therapy; possible additive or potentiating effect with CNS depressant).
No products indexed under this heading.

Chlorprothixene Hydrochloride (An additive hypotensive effect has been reported with the combination of systemic clonidine and neuroleptic therapy; possible additive or potentiating effect with CNS depressant).
No products indexed under this heading.

Chlorprothixene Lactate (Possible additive or potentiating effect with CNS depressant).
No products indexed under this heading.

Chlorthalidone (Apraclonidine reduces pulse and blood pressure, caution is advised when used concurrently). Products include:
Clorpres Tablets 1002
Combipres Tablets 1040
Tenoretic Tablets 690

Clomipramine Hydrochloride (Tricyclic antidepressants have been reported to blunt the hypotensive effect of clonidine; it is not known whether the concurrent use with apraclonidine can lead to reduction in IOP lowering effect).
No products indexed under this heading.

Clonidine (Apraclonidine reduces pulse and blood pressure, caution is advised when used concurrently). Products include:
Catapres-TTS 1038

Clonidine Hydrochloride (Apraclonidine reduces pulse and blood pressure, caution is advised when used concurrently). Products include:
Catapres Tablets 1037
Clorpres Tablets 1002
Combipres Tablets 1040
Duraclon Injection 3057

Clorazepate Dipotassium (Possible additive or potentiating effect with CNS depressant). Products include:
Tranxene 511

Clozapine (An additive hypotensive effect has been reported with the combination of systemic clonidine and neuroleptic therapy; possible additive or potentiating effect with CNS depressant). Products include:
Clozaril Tablets 2319

Codeine Phosphate (Possible additive or potentiating effect with CNS depressant). Products include:
Phenergan with Codeine Syrup 3557
Phenergan VC with Codeine Syrup .. 3561
Robitussin A-C Syrup 2942
Robitussin-DAC Syrup 2942
Ryna-C Liquid .... ■□768
Soma Compound w/Codeine Tablets 3355
Tussi-Organidin NR Liquid 3350
Tussi-Organidin-S NR Liquid 3350
Tylenol with Codeine 2595

Deserpidine (Apraclonidine reduces pulse and blood pressure, caution is advised when used concurrently).
No products indexed under this heading.

Desflurane (Possible additive or potentiating effect with CNS depressant). Products include:
Suprane Liquid for Inhalation 874

Desipramine Hydrochloride (Tricyclic antidepressants have been reported to blunt the hypotensive effect of clonidine; it is not known whether the concurrent use with apraclonidine can lead to reduction in IOP lowering effect). Products include:
Norpramin Tablets 755

Deslanoside (Apraclonidine reduces pulse and blood pressure, caution is advised when used concurrently).
No products indexed under this heading.

Dezocine (Possible additive or potentiating effect with CNS depressant).
No products indexed under this heading.

Diazepam (Possible additive or potentiating effect with CNS depressant). Products include:
Valium Injectable 3026
Valium Tablets 3047

Diazoxide (Apraclonidine reduces pulse and blood pressure, caution is advised when used concurrently).
No products indexed under this heading.

Digitoxin (Apraclonidine reduces pulse and blood pressure, caution is advised when used concurrently).
No products indexed under this heading.

Digoxin (Apraclonidine reduces pulse and blood pressure, caution is advised when used concurrently). Products include:
Digitek Tablets 1003
Lanoxicaps Capsules 1574
Lanoxin Injection 1581
Lanoxin Tablets 1587
Lanoxin Elixir Pediatric 1578
Lanoxin Injection Pediatric 1584

Diltiazem Hydrochloride (Apraclonidine reduces pulse and blood pressure, caution is advised when used concurrently). Products include:
Cardizem Injectable 1018
Cardizem Lyo-Ject Syringe 1018
Cardizem Monovial 1018
Cardizem CD Capsules 1016
Tiazac Capsules 1378

Doxazosin Mesylate (Apraclonidine reduces pulse and blood pressure, caution is advised when used concurrently). Products include:
Cardura Tablets 2668

Doxepin Hydrochloride (Tricyclic antidepressants have been reported to blunt the hypotensive effect of clonidine; it is not known whether the concurrent use with apraclonidine can lead to reduction in IOP lowering effect). Products include:
Sinequan 2713

Droperidol (Possible additive or potentiating effect with CNS depressant).
No products indexed under this heading.

Enalapril Maleate (Apraclonidine reduces pulse and blood pressure, caution is advised when used concurrently). Products include:
Lexxel Tablets 608
Vaseretic Tablets 2204
Vasotec Tablets 2210

Enalaprilat (Apraclonidine reduces pulse and blood pressure, caution is advised when used concurrently). Products include:
Enalaprilat Injection 863
Vasotec I.V. Injection 2207

Enflurane (Possible additive or potentiating effect with CNS depressant).
No products indexed under this heading.

Eprosartan Mesylate (Apraclonidine reduces pulse and blood pressure, caution is advised when used concurrently). Products include:
Teveten Tablets 3327

Esmolol Hydrochloride (Apraclonidine reduces pulse and blood pressure, caution is advised when used concurrently). Products include:
Brevibloc Injection 858

Estazolam (Possible additive or potentiating effect with CNS depressant). Products include:
ProSom Tablets 500

Ethchlorvynol (Possible additive or potentiating effect with CNS depressant).
No products indexed under this heading.

Ethinamate (Possible additive or potentiating effect with CNS depressant).
No products indexed under this heading.

Felodipine (Apraclonidine reduces pulse and blood pressure, caution is advised when used concurrently). Products include:
Lexxel Tablets 608
Plendil Extended-Release Tablets ... 623

Fentanyl (Possible additive or potentiating effect with CNS depressant). Products include:
Duragesic Transdermal System 1786

Fentanyl Citrate (Possible additive or potentiating effect with CNS depressant). Products include:
Actiq 1184

Fluphenazine Decanoate (An additive hypotensive effect has been reported with the combination of systemic clonidine and neuroleptic therapy; possible additive or potentiating effect with CNS depressant).
No products indexed under this heading.

Fluphenazine Enanthate (An additive hypotensive effect has been reported with the combination of systemic clonidine and neuroleptic therapy; possible additive or potentiating effect with CNS depressant).
No products indexed under this heading.

Fluphenazine Hydrochloride (An additive hypotensive effect has been reported with the combination of systemic clonidine and neuroleptic therapy; possible additive or potentiating effect with CNS depressant).
No products indexed under this heading.

Flurazepam Hydrochloride (Possible additive or potentiating effect with CNS depressant).
No products indexed under this heading.

Fosinopril Sodium (Apraclonidine reduces pulse and blood pressure, caution is advised when used concurrently). Products include:
Monopril Tablets 1091
Monopril HCT 1094

Furosemide (Apraclonidine reduces pulse and blood pressure, caution is advised when used concurrently). Products include:
Furosemide Tablets 2284

Glutethimide (Possible additive or potentiating effect with CNS depressant).
No products indexed under this heading.

Guanabenz Acetate (Apraclonidine reduces pulse and blood pressure, caution is advised when used concurrently).
No products indexed under this heading.

Guanethidine Monosulfate (Apraclonidine reduces pulse and blood pressure, caution is advised when used concurrently).
No products indexed under this heading.

Haloperidol (An additive hypotensive effect has been reported with the combination of systemic clonidine and neuroleptic therapy; possible additive or potentiating effect with CNS depressant). Products include:
Haldol Injection, Tablets and Concentrate 2533

Haloperidol Decanoate (An additive hypotensive effect has been reported with the combination of systemic clonidine and neuroleptic therapy; possible additive or potentiating effect with CNS depressant). Products include:
Haldol Decanoate 2535

Hydralazine Hydrochloride (Apraclonidine reduces pulse and blood pressure, caution is advised when used concurrently).
No products indexed under this heading.

Hydrochlorothiazide (Apraclonidine reduces pulse and blood pressure, caution is advised when used concurrently). Products include:
Accuretic Tablets 2614
Aldoril Tablets 2039
Atacand HCT Tablets 597
Avalide Tablets 1070
Diovan HCT Tablets 2338
Dyazide Capsules 1515
HydroDIURIL Tablets 2108

Hyzaar 2109
Inderide Tablets 3517
Inderide LA Long-Acting Capsules .. 3519
Lotensin HCT Tablets 2367
Maxzide 1008
Micardis HCT Tablets 1051
Microzide Capsules 3414
Moduretic Tablets 2138
Monopril HCT 1094
Prinzide Tablets 2168
Timolide Tablets 2187
Uniretic Tablets 3178
Vaseretic Tablets 2204
Zestoretic Tablets 695
Ziac Tablets 1887

Hydrocodone Bitartrate (Possible additive or potentiating effect with CNS depressant). Products include:
Hycodan 1316
Hycomine Compound Tablets 1317
Hycotuss Expectorant Syrup 1318
Lortab 3319
Lortab Elixir 3317
Maxidone Tablets CIII 3399
Norco 5/325 Tablets CIII 3424
Norco 7.5/325 Tablets CIII 3425
Norco 10/325 Tablets CIII 3427
Norco 10/325 Tablets CIII 3425
Vicodin Tablets 516
Vicodin ES Tablets 517
Vicodin HP Tablets 518
Vicodin Tuss Expectorant 519
Vicoprofen Tablets 520
Zydone Tablets 1330

Hydrocodone Polistirex (Possible additive or potentiating effect with CNS depressant). Products include:
Tussionex Pennkinetic Extended-Release Suspension..... 1174

Hydroflumethiazide (Apraclonidine reduces pulse and blood pressure, caution is advised when used concurrently). Products include:
Diucardin Tablets 3494

Hydromorphone Hydrochloride (Possible additive or potentiating effect with CNS depressant). Products include:
Dilaudid 441
Dilaudid Oral Liquid 445
Dilaudid Powder 441
Dilaudid Rectal Suppositories 441
Dilaudid Tablets 441
Dilaudid Tablets - 8 mg 445
Dilaudid-HP 443

Hydroxyzine Hydrochloride (Possible additive or potentiating effect with CNS depressant). Products include:
Atarax Tablets & Syrup 2667
Vistaril Intramuscular Solution 2738

Imipramine Hydrochloride (Tricyclic antidepressants have been reported to blunt the hypotensive effect of clonidine; it is not known whether the concurrent use with apraclonidine can lead to reduction in IOP lowering effect).
No products indexed under this heading.

Imipramine Pamoate (Tricyclic antidepressants have been reported to blunt the hypotensive effect of clonidine; it is not known whether the concurrent use with apraclonidine can lead to reduction in IOP lowering effect).
No products indexed under this heading.

Indapamide (Apraclonidine reduces pulse and blood pressure, caution is advised when used concurrently). Products include:
Indapamide Tablets 2286

Insulin, Human, Zinc Suspension (Systemic clonidine may inhibit the production of catecholamines in response to insulin-induced hypoglycemia and mask the signs and symptoms of hypoglycemia). Products include:
Humulin L, 100 Units 1937
Humulin U, 100 Units 1943
Novolin L Human Insulin 10 ml Vials 2422

Insulin, Human NPH (Systemic clonidine may inhibit the production of catecholamines in response to insulin-induced hypoglycemia and mask the signs and symptoms of hypoglycemia). Products include:
Humulin N, 100 Units 1939
Humulin N NPH Pen 1940
Novolin N Human Insulin 10 ml Vials 2422
Novolin N PenFill 2423
Novolin N Prefilled Syringe Disposable Insulin Delivery System 2425

Insulin, Human Regular (Systemic clonidine may inhibit the production of catecholamines in response to insulin-induced hypoglycemia and mask the signs and symptoms of hypoglycemia). Products include:
Humulin R Regular (U-500) 1943
Humulin R, 100 Units 1941
Novolin R Human Insulin 10 ml Vials 2423
Novolin R PenFill 2423
Novolin R Prefilled Syringe Disposable Insulin Delivery System 2425
Velosulin BR Human Insulin 10 ml Vials 2435

Insulin, Human Regular and Human NPH Mixture (Systemic clonidine may inhibit the production of catecholamines in response to insulin-induced hypoglycemia and mask the signs and symptoms of hypoglycemia). Products include:
Humulin 50/50, 100 Units 1934
Humulin 70/30, 100 Units 1935
Humulin 70/30 Pen 1936
Novolin 70/30 Human Insulin 10 ml Vials 2421
Novolin 70/30 PenFill 2423
Novolin 70/30 Prefilled Disposable Insulin Delivery System 2425

Insulin, NPH (Systemic clonidine may inhibit the production of catecholamines in response to insulin-induced hypoglycemia and mask the signs and symptoms of hypoglycemia). Products include:
Iletin II, NPH (Pork), 100 Units 1946

Insulin, Regular (Systemic clonidine may inhibit the production of catecholamines in response to insulin-induced hypoglycemia and mask the signs and symptoms of hypoglycemia). Products include:
Iletin II, Regular (Pork), 100 Units ... 1947

Insulin, Zinc Crystals (Systemic clonidine may inhibit the production of catecholamines in response to insulin-induced hypoglycemia and mask the signs and symptoms of hypoglycemia).
No products indexed under this heading.

Insulin, Zinc Suspension (Systemic clonidine may inhibit the production of catecholamines in response to insulin-induced hypoglycemia and mask the signs and symptoms of hypoglycemia). Products include:
Iletin II, Lente (Pork), 100 Units 1945

Insulin Aspart, Human Regular (Systemic clonidine may inhibit the production of catecholamines in response to insulin-induced hypoglycemia and mask the signs and symptoms of hypoglycemia).
No products indexed under this heading.

Insulin glargine (Systemic clonidine may inhibit the production of catecholamines in response to insulin-induced hypoglycemia and mask the signs and symptoms of hypoglycemia). Products include:
Lantus Injection 742

Insulin Lispro, Human (Systemic clonidine may inhibit the production of catecholamines in response to insulin-induced hypoglycemia and mask the signs and symptoms of hypoglycemia). Products include:
Humalog 1926
Humalog Mix 75/25 Pen 1928

Insulin Lispro Protamine, Human (Systemic clonidine may inhibit the production of catecholamines in response to insulin-induced hypoglycemia and mask the signs and symptoms of hypoglycemia). Products include:
Humalog Mix 75/25 Pen 1928

Irbesartan (Apraclonidine reduces pulse and blood pressure, caution is advised when used concurrently). Products include:
Avalide Tablets 1070
Avapro Tablets 1074
Avapro Tablets 3076

Isocarboxazid (Concurrent use is contraindicated).
No products indexed under this heading.

Isoflurane (Possible additive or potentiating effect with CNS depressant).
No products indexed under this heading.

Isradipine (Apraclonidine reduces pulse and blood pressure, caution is advised when used concurrently). Products include:
DynaCirc Capsules 2921
DynaCirc CR Tablets 2923

Ketamine Hydrochloride (Possible additive or potentiating effect with CNS depressant).
No products indexed under this heading.

Labetalol Hydrochloride (Apraclonidine reduces pulse and blood pressure, caution is advised when used concurrently). Products include:
Normodyne Injection 3135
Normodyne Tablets 3137

Levobunolol Hydrochloride (Apraclonidine reduces pulse and blood pressure, caution is advised when used concurrently). Products include:
Betagan .... ⊙228

Levomethadyl Acetate Hydrochloride (Possible additive or potentiating effect with CNS depressant).
No products indexed under this heading.

Levorphanol Tartrate (Possible additive or potentiating effect with CNS depressant). Products include:
Levo-Dromoran 1734
Levorphanol Tartrate Tablets 3059

Lisinopril (Apraclonidine reduces pulse and blood pressure, caution is advised when used concurrently). Products include:
Prinivil Tablets 2164
Prinzide Tablets 2168
Zestoretic Tablets 695
Zestril Tablets 698

Lithium Carbonate (An additive hypotensive effect has been reported with the combination of systemic clonidine and neuroleptic therapy). Products include:
Eskalith 1527
Lithium Carbonate 3061
Lithobid Slow-Release Tablets 3255

Lithium Citrate (An additive hypotensive effect has been reported with the combination of systemic clonidine and neuroleptic therapy). Products include:
Lithium Citrate Syrup 3061

Lorazepam (Possible additive or potentiating effect with CNS depressant). Products include:
Ativan Injection 3478
Ativan Tablets 3482

Losartan Potassium (Apraclonidine reduces pulse and blood pressure, caution is advised when used concurrently). Products include:
Cozaar Tablets 2067
Hyzaar 2109

Loxapine Hydrochloride (An additive hypotensive effect has been reported with the combination of systemic clonidine and neuroleptic therapy; possible additive or potentiating effect with CNS depressant).
No products indexed under this heading.

Loxapine Succinate (An additive hypotensive effect has been reported with the combination of systemic clonidine and neuroleptic therapy; possible additive or potentiating effect with CNS depressant). Products include:
Loxitane Capsules 3398

Maprotiline Hydrochloride (Tricyclic antidepressants have been reported to blunt the hypotensive effect of clonidine; it is not known whether the concurrent use with apraclonidine can lead to reduction in IOP lowering effect).
No products indexed under this heading.

Mecamylamine Hydrochloride (Apraclonidine reduces pulse and blood pressure, caution is advised when used concurrently). Products include:
Inversine Tablets 1850

Meperidine Hydrochloride (Possible additive or potentiating effect with CNS depressant). Products include:
Demerol 3079
Mepergan Injection 3539

Mephobarbital (Possible additive or potentiating effect with CNS depressant).
No products indexed under this heading.

Meprobamate (Possible additive or potentiating effect with CNS depressant). Products include:
Miltown Tablets 3349

Mesoridazine Besylate (An additive hypotensive effect has been reported with the combination of systemic clonidine and neuroleptic therapy; possible additive or potentiating effect with CNS depressant). Products include:
Serentil 1057

Methadone Hydrochloride (Possible additive or potentiating effect with CNS depressant). Products include:
Dolophine Hydrochloride Tablets 3056

Methohexital Sodium (Possible additive or potentiating effect with CNS depressant). Products include:
Brevital Sodium for Injection, USP .. 1815

Methotrimeprazine (An additive hypotensive effect has been reported with the combination of systemic clonidine and neuroleptic therapy; possible additive or potentiating effect with CNS depressant).
No products indexed under this heading.

Methoxyflurane (Possible additive or potentiating effect with CNS depressant).
No products indexed under this heading.

Methyclothiazide (Apraclonidine reduces pulse and blood pressure, caution is advised when used concurrently).
No products indexed under this heading.

Methyldopa (Apraclonidine reduces pulse and blood pressure, caution is advised when used concurrently). Products include:
Aldoclor Tablets 2035
Aldomet Tablets 2037
Aldoril Tablets 2039

Methyldopate Hydrochloride (Apraclonidine reduces pulse and blood pressure, caution is advised when used concurrently).
No products indexed under this heading.

Metipranolol Hydrochloride (Apraclonidine reduces pulse and blood pressure, caution is advised

when used concurrently).
No products indexed under this heading.

Metolazone (Apraclonidine reduces pulse and blood pressure, caution is advised when used concurrently). Products include:
Mykrox Tablets 1168
Zaroxolyn Tablets 1177

Metoprolol Succinate (Apraclonidine reduces pulse and blood pressure, caution is advised when used concurrently). Products include:
Toprol-XL Tablets 651

Metoprolol Tartrate (Apraclonidine reduces pulse and blood pressure, caution is advised when used concurrently).
No products indexed under this heading.

Metyrosine (Apraclonidine reduces pulse and blood pressure, caution is advised when used concurrently). Products include:
Demser Capsules 2085

Mibefradil Dihydrochloride (Apraclonidine reduces pulse and blood pressure, caution is advised when used concurrently).
No products indexed under this heading.

Midazolam Hydrochloride (Possible additive or potentiating effect with CNS depressant). Products include:
Versed Injection 3027
Versed Syrup 3033

Minoxidil (Apraclonidine reduces pulse and blood pressure, caution is advised when used concurrently). Products include:
Rogaine Extra Strength for Men Topical Solution ..... ▣721
Rogaine for Women Topical Solution ..... ▣721

Moclobemide (Concurrent use is contraindicated).
No products indexed under this heading.

Moexipril Hydrochloride (Apraclonidine reduces pulse and blood pressure, caution is advised when used concurrently). Products include:
Uniretic Tablets 3178
Univasc Tablets 3181

Molindone Hydrochloride (An additive hypotensive effect has been reported with the combination of systemic clonidine and neuroleptic therapy; possible additive or potentiating effect with CNS depressant). Products include:
Moban 1320

Morphine Sulfate (Possible additive or potentiating effect with CNS depressant). Products include:
Astramorph/PF Injection, USP (Preservative-Free) 594
Duramorph Injection 1312
Infumorph 200 and Infumorph 500 Sterile Solutions 1314
Kadian Capsules 1335
MS Contin Tablets 2896
MSIR 2898
Oramorph SR Tablets 3062
Roxanol 3066

Nadolol (Apraclonidine reduces pulse and blood pressure, caution is advised when used concurrently). Products include:
Corgard Tablets 2245
Corzide 40/5 Tablets 2247
Corzide 80/5 Tablets 2247
Nadolol Tablets 2288

Nicardipine Hydrochloride (Apraclonidine reduces pulse and blood pressure, caution is advised when used concurrently). Products include:
Cardene I.V. 3485

Nifedipine (Apraclonidine reduces pulse and blood pressure, caution is advised when used concurrently). Products include:
Adalat CC Tablets 877
Procardia Capsules 2708
Procardia XL Extended Release Tablets 2710

Nisoldipine (Apraclonidine reduces pulse and blood pressure, caution is advised when used concurrently). Products include:
Sular Tablets 688

Nitroglycerin (Apraclonidine reduces pulse and blood pressure, caution is advised when used concurrently). Products include:
Nitro-Dur Transdermal Infusion System 3134
Nitro-Dur Transdermal Infusion System 1834
Nitrolingual Pumpspray 1355
Nitrostat Tablets 2658

Nortriptyline Hydrochloride (Tricyclic antidepressants have been reported to blunt the hypotensive effect of clonidine; it is not known whether the concurrent use with apraclonidine can lead to reduction in IOP lowering effect).
No products indexed under this heading.

Olanzapine (An additive hypotensive effect has been reported with the combination of systemic clonidine and neuroleptic therapy). Products include:
Zyprexa Tablets 1973
Zyprexa ZYDIS Orally Disintegrating Tablets 1973

Oxazepam (Possible additive or potentiating effect with CNS depressant).
No products indexed under this heading.

Oxycodone Hydrochloride (Possible additive or potentiating effect with CNS depressant). Products include:
OxyContin Tablets 2912
OxyFast Oral Concentrate Solution . 2916
OxyIR Capsules 2916
Percocet Tablets 1326
Percodan Tablets 1327
Percolone Tablets 1327
Roxicodone 3067
Tylox Capsules 2597

Pargyline Hydrochloride (Concurrent use is contraindicated).
No products indexed under this heading.

Penbutolol Sulfate (Apraclonidine reduces pulse and blood pressure, caution is advised when used concurrently).
No products indexed under this heading.

Pentobarbital Sodium (Possible additive or potentiating effect with CNS depressant). Products include:
Nembutal Sodium Solution 485

Perindopril Erbumine (Apraclonidine reduces pulse and blood pressure, caution is advised when used concurrently). Products include:
Aceon Tablets (2 mg, 4 mg, 8 mg) 3249

Perphenazine (An additive hypotensive effect has been reported with the combination of systemic clonidine and neuroleptic therapy; possible additive or potentiating effect with CNS depressant). Products include:
Etrafon 3115
Trilafon 3160

Phenelzine Sulfate (Concurrent use is contraindicated). Products include:
Nardil Tablets 2653

Phenobarbital (Possible additive or potentiating effect with CNS depressant). Products include:
Arco-Lase Plus Tablets 592
Donnatal 2929
Donnatal Extentabs 2930

Phenoxybenzamine Hydrochloride (Apraclonidine reduces pulse and blood pressure, caution is advised when used concurrently). Products include:
Dibenzyline Capsules 3457

Phentolamine Mesylate (Apraclonidine reduces pulse and blood pressure, caution is advised when used concurrently).
No products indexed under this heading.

Pimozide (An additive hypotensive effect has been reported with the combination of systemic clonidine and neuroleptic therapy). Products include:
Orap Tablets 1407

Pindolol (Apraclonidine reduces pulse and blood pressure, caution is advised when used concurrently).
No products indexed under this heading.

Polythiazide (Apraclonidine reduces pulse and blood pressure, caution is advised when used concurrently). Products include:
Minizide Capsules 2700
Renese Tablets 2712

Prazepam (Possible additive or potentiating effect with CNS depressant).
No products indexed under this heading.

Prazosin Hydrochloride (Apraclonidine reduces pulse and blood pressure, caution is advised when used concurrently). Products include:
Minipress Capsules 2699
Minizide Capsules 2700

Procarbazine Hydrochloride (Concurrent use is contraindicated). Products include:
Matulane Capsules 3246

Prochlorperazine (An additive hypotensive effect has been reported with the combination of systemic clonidine and neuroleptic therapy; possible additive or potentiating effect with CNS depressant). Products include:
Compazine 1505

Promethazine Hydrochloride (An additive hypotensive effect has been reported with the combination of systemic clonidine and neuroleptic therapy; possible additive or potentiating effect with CNS depressant). Products include:
Mepergan Injection 3539
Phenergan Injection 3553
Phenergan 3556
Phenergan Syrup 3554
Phenergan with Codeine Syrup 3557
Phenergan with Dextromethorphan Syrup 3559
Phenergan VC Syrup 3560
Phenergan VC with Codeine Syrup .. 3561

Propofol (Possible additive or potentiating effect with CNS depressant). Products include:
Diprivan Injectable Emulsion 667

Propoxyphene Hydrochloride (Possible additive or potentiating effect with CNS depressant). Products include:
Darvon Pulvules 1909
Darvon Compound-65 Pulvules 1910

Propoxyphene Napsylate (Possible additive or potentiating effect with CNS depressant). Products include:
Darvon-N/Darvocet-N 1907
Darvon-N Tablets 1912

Propranolol Hydrochloride (Apraclonidine reduces pulse and blood pressure, caution is advised when used concurrently). Products include:
Inderal 3513
Inderal LA Long-Acting Capsules 3516
Inderide Tablets 3517
Inderide LA Long-Acting Capsules .. 3519

Protriptyline Hydrochloride (Tricyclic antidepressants have been reported to blunt the hypotensive effect of clonidine; it is not known whether the concurrent use with apraclonidine can lead to reduction in IOP lowering effect). Products include:
Vivactil Tablets 2446
Vivactil Tablets 2217

Quazepam (Possible additive or potentiating effect with CNS depressant).
No products indexed under this heading.

Quetiapine Fumarate (An additive hypotensive effect has been reported with the combination of systemic clonidine and neuroleptic therapy). Products include:
Seroquel Tablets 684

Quinapril Hydrochloride (Apraclonidine reduces pulse and blood pressure, caution is advised when used concurrently). Products include:
Accupril Tablets 2611
Accuretic Tablets 2614

Ramipril (Apraclonidine reduces pulse and blood pressure, caution is advised when used concurrently). Products include:
Altace Capsules 2233

Rauwolfia serpentina (Apraclonidine reduces pulse and blood pressure, caution is advised when used concurrently).
No products indexed under this heading.

Remifentanil Hydrochloride (Possible additive or potentiating effect with CNS depressant).
No products indexed under this heading.

Rescinnamine (Apraclonidine reduces pulse and blood pressure, caution is advised when used concurrently).
No products indexed under this heading.

Reserpine (Apraclonidine reduces pulse and blood pressure, caution is advised when used concurrently).
No products indexed under this heading.

Risperidone (An additive hypotensive effect has been reported with the combination of systemic clonidine and neuroleptic therapy; possible additive or potentiating effect with CNS depressant). Products include:
Risperdal 1796

Secobarbital Sodium (Possible additive or potentiating effect with CNS depressant).
No products indexed under this heading.

Selegiline Hydrochloride (Concurrent use is contraindicated). Products include:
Eldepryl Capsules 3266

Sevoflurane (Possible additive or potentiating effect with CNS depressant).
No products indexed under this heading.

Sodium Nitroprusside (Apraclonidine reduces pulse and blood pressure, caution is advised when used concurrently).
No products indexed under this heading.

Sotalol Hydrochloride (Apraclonidine reduces pulse and blood pressure, caution is advised when used concurrently). Products include:
Betapace Tablets 950
Betapace AF Tablets 954

Spirapril Hydrochloride (Apraclonidine reduces pulse and blood pressure, caution is advised when used concurrently).
No products indexed under this heading.

Sufentanil Citrate (Possible additive or potentiating effect with CNS

depressant).
No products indexed under this heading.

Telmisartan (Apraclonidine reduces pulse and blood pressure, caution is advised when used concurrently). Products include:
Micardis Tablets 1049
Micardis HCT Tablets 1051

Temazepam (Possible additive or potentiating effect with CNS depressant).
No products indexed under this heading.

Terazosin Hydrochloride (Apraclonidine reduces pulse and blood pressure, caution is advised when used concurrently). Products include:
Hytrin Capsules 464

Thiamylal Sodium (Possible additive or potentiating effect with CNS depressant).
No products indexed under this heading.

Thioridazine Hydrochloride (An additive hypotensive effect has been reported with the combination of systemic clonidine and neuroleptic therapy; possible additive or potentiating effect with CNS depressant). Products include:
Thioridazine Hydrochloride Tablets 2289

Thiothixene (An additive hypotensive effect has been reported with the combination of systemic clonidine and neuroleptic therapy; possible additive or potentiating effect with CNS depressant). Products include:
Navane Capsules 2701
Thiothixene Capsules 2290

Timolol Hemihydrate (Apraclonidine reduces pulse and blood pressure, caution is advised when used concurrently). Products include:
Betimol Ophthalmic Solution .... ⊙ 324

Timolol Maleate (Apraclonidine reduces pulse and blood pressure, caution is advised when used concurrently). Products include:
Blocadren Tablets 2046
Cosopt Sterile Ophthalmic Solution 2065
Timolide Tablets 2187
Timolol GFS .... ⊙ 266
Timoptic in Ocudose 2192
Timoptic Sterile Ophthalmic Solution 2190
Timoptic-XE Sterile Ophthalmic Gel Forming Solution 2194

Torsemide (Apraclonidine reduces pulse and blood pressure, caution is advised when used concurrently). Products include:
Demadex Tablets and Injection 2965

Trandolapril (Apraclonidine reduces pulse and blood pressure, caution is advised when used concurrently). Products include:
Mavik Tablets 478
Tarka Tablets 508

Tranylcypromine Sulfate (Concurrent use is contraindicated). Products include:
Parnate Tablets 1607

Triazolam (Possible additive or potentiating effect with CNS depressant). Products include:
Halcion Tablets 2823

Trifluoperazine Hydrochloride (An additive hypotensive effect has been reported with the combination of systemic clonidine and neuroleptic therapy; possible additive or potentiating effect with CNS depressant). Products include:
Stelazine 1640

Trimethaphan Camsylate (Apraclonidine reduces pulse and blood pressure, caution is advised when used concurrently).
No products indexed under this heading.

Trimipramine Maleate (Tricyclic antidepressants have been reported to blunt the hypotensive effect of clonidine; it is not known whether the concurrent use with apraclonidine can lead to reduction in IOP lowering effect). Products include:
Surmontil Capsules 3595

Valsartan (Apraclonidine reduces pulse and blood pressure, caution is advised when used concurrently). Products include:
Diovan Capsules 2337
Diovan HCT Tablets 2338

Verapamil Hydrochloride (Apraclonidine reduces pulse and blood pressure, caution is advised when used concurrently). Products include:
Covera-HS Tablets 3199
Isoptin SR Tablets 467
Tarka Tablets 508
Verelan Capsules 3184
Verelan PM Capsules 3186

Zaleplon (Possible additive or potentiating effect with CNS depressant). Products include:
Sonata Capsules 3591

Ziprasidone Hydrochloride (An additive hypotensive effect has been reported with the combination of systemic clonidine and neuroleptic therapy). Products include:
Geodon Capsules 2688

Zolpidem Tartrate (Possible additive or potentiating effect with CNS depressant). Products include:
Ambien Tablets 3191

IOPIDINE STERILE OPHTHALMIC SOLUTION
(Apraclonidine Hydrochloride) .... ⊙ 212
May interact with monoamine oxidase inhibitors. Compounds in these categories include:

Isocarboxazid (Co-administration with MAO inhibitor is contraindicated).
No products indexed under this heading.

Moclobemide (Co-administration with MAO inhibitor is contraindicated).
No products indexed under this heading.

Pargyline Hydrochloride (Co-administration with MAO inhibitor is contraindicated).
No products indexed under this heading.

Phenelzine Sulfate (Co-administration with MAO inhibitor is contraindicated). Products include:
Nardil Tablets 2653

Procarbazine Hydrochloride (Co-administration with MAO inhibitor is contraindicated). Products include:
Matulane Capsules 3246

Selegiline Hydrochloride (Co-administration with MAO inhibitor is contraindicated). Products include:
Eldepryl Capsules 3266

Tranylcypromine Sulfate (Co-administration with MAO inhibitor is contraindicated). Products include:
Parnate Tablets 1607

IPOL VACCINE
(Poliovirus Vaccine Inactivated, Trivalent Types 1,2,3) 809
May interact with immunosuppressive agents. Compounds in these categories include:

Azathioprine (An adequate immunologic response may not be obtained if given concomitantly to persons receiving immunosuppressive therapy).
No products indexed under this heading.

Basiliximab (An adequate immunologic response may not be obtained if given concomitantly to persons receiving immunosuppressive therapy). Products include:
Simulect for Injection 2399

Cyclosporine (An adequate immunologic response may not be obtained if given concomitantly to persons receiving immunosuppressive therapy). Products include:
Gengraf Capsules 457
Neoral Soft Gelatin Capsules 2380
Neoral Oral Solution 2380
Sandimmune 2388

Muromonab-CD3 (An adequate immunologic response may not be obtained if given concomitantly to persons receiving immunosuppressive therapy). Products include:
Orthoclone OKT3 Sterile Solution ... 2498

Mycophenolate Mofetil (An adequate immunologic response may not be obtained if given concomitantly to persons receiving immunosuppressive therapy). Products include:
CellCept Capsules 2951
CellCept Oral Suspension 2951
CellCept Tablets 2951

Sirolimus (An adequate immunologic response may not be obtained if given concomitantly to persons receiving immunosuppressive therapy). Products include:
Rapamune Oral Solution and Tablets 3584

Tacrolimus (An adequate immunologic response may not be obtained if given concomitantly to persons receiving immunosuppressive therapy). Products include:
Prograf 1393
Protopic Ointment 1397

ISCAR MALI INJECTION
(Homeopathic Formulations) 3456
See Iscar Mali Special Injection

ISCAR MALI SPECIAL INJECTION
(Homeopathic Formulations) 3456

Immune modulating drugs, unspecified (Concurrent use requires careful dosing, frequent monitoring of immune function parameters).
No products indexed under this heading.

ISCAR PINI INJECTION
(Homeopathic Formulations) 3456
See Iscar Mali Special Injection

ISCAR QUERCUS INJECTION
(Homeopathic Formulations) 3456
See Iscar Mali Special Injection

ISCAR QUERCUS SPECIAL INJECTION
(Homeopathic Formulations) 3456
See Iscar Mali Special Injection

ISMO TABLETS
(Isosorbide Mononitrate) 3524
May interact with calcium channel blockers, vasodilators, and certain other agents. Compounds in these categories include:

Amlodipine Besylate (Potential for marked symptomatic orthostatic hypotension). Products include:
Lotrel Capsules 2370
Norvasc Tablets 2704

Bepridil Hydrochloride (Potential for marked symptomatic orthostatic hypotension). Products include:
Vascor Tablets 2602

Diazoxide (Additive vasodilating effects).
No products indexed under this heading.

Diltiazem Hydrochloride (Potential for marked symptomatic orthostatic hypotension). Products include:
Cardizem Injectable 1018
Cardizem Lyo-Ject Syringe 1018
Cardizem Monovial 1018
Cardizem CD Capsules 1016
Tiazac Capsules 1378

Epoprostenol Sodium (Additive vasodilating effects). Products include:
Flolan for Injection 1528

Felodipine (Potential for marked symptomatic orthostatic hypotension). Products include:
Lexxel Tablets 608
Plendil Extended-Release Tablets ... 623

Hydralazine Hydrochloride (Additive vasodilating effects).
No products indexed under this heading.

Isradipine (Potential for marked symptomatic orthostatic hypotension). Products include:
DynaCirc Capsules 2921
DynaCirc CR Tablets 2923

Mibefradil Dihydrochloride (Potential for marked symptomatic orthostatic hypotension).
No products indexed under this heading.

Minoxidil (Additive vasodilating effects). Products include:
Rogaine Extra Strength for Men Topical Solution .... ▣ 721
Rogaine for Women Topical Solution .... ▣ 721

Nicardipine Hydrochloride (Potential for marked symptomatic orthostatic hypotension). Products include:
Cardene I.V. 3485

Nifedipine (Potential for marked symptomatic orthostatic hypotension). Products include:
Adalat CC Tablets 877
Procardia Capsules 2708
Procardia XL Extended Release Tablets 2710

Nimodipine (Potential for marked symptomatic orthostatic hypotension). Products include:
Nimotop Capsules 904

Nisoldipine (Potential for marked symptomatic orthostatic hypotension). Products include:
Sular Tablets 688

Sildenafil Citrate (Amplification of the vasodilatory effects of isosorbide mononitrate by sildenafil can result in severe hypotension; the time course and dose dependency of this interaction have not been studied). Products include:
Viagra Tablets 2732

Verapamil Hydrochloride (Potential for marked symptomatic orthostatic hypotension). Products include:
Covera-HS Tablets 3199
Isoptin SR Tablets 467
Tarka Tablets 508
Verelan Capsules 3184
Verelan PM Capsules 3186

Food Interactions

Alcohol (Additive vasodilating effects).

ISOPTIN SR TABLETS
(Verapamil Hydrochloride) 467
May interact with ACE inhibitors, alpha adrenergic blockers, antihypertensives, beta blockers, diuretics, cardiac glycosides, inhalant anesthetics, lithium preparations, neuromuscular blocking agents, quinidine, vasodilators, theophylline, and certain other agents. Compounds in these categories include:

Acebutolol Hydrochloride (Co-administration with beta-adrenergic blockers has resulted in excessive bradycardia and AV block, including complete heart block when combination has been used for the treatment of hypertension). Products include:
Sectral Capsules 3589

Amiloride Hydrochloride (Additive effect on lowering blood pressure). Products include:

Midamor Tablets 2136
Moduretic Tablets 2138

Aminophylline (Inhibition of theophylline clearance and increased plasma levels of theophylline).
No products indexed under this heading.

Amlodipine Besylate (Additive effect on lowering blood pressure). Products include:
Lotrel Capsules 2370
Norvasc Tablets 2704

Atenolol (Co-administration with beta-adrenergic blockers has resulted in excessive bradycardia and AV block, including complete heart block when combination has been used for the treatment of hypertension; potential for a variable effect on atenolol clearance). Products include:
Tenoretic Tablets 690
Tenormin I.V. Injection 692

Atracurium Besylate (Verapamil may potentiate the activity of neuromuscular blocking agents).
No products indexed under this heading.

Benazepril Hydrochloride (Additive effect on lowering blood pressure). Products include:
Lotensin Tablets 2365
Lotensin HCT Tablets 2367
Lotrel Capsules 2370

Bendroflumethiazide (Additive effect on lowering blood pressure). Products include:
Corzide 40/5 Tablets 2247
Corzide 80/5 Tablets 2247

Betaxolol Hydrochloride (Co-administration with beta-adrenergic blockers has resulted in excessive bradycardia and AV block, including complete heart block when combination has been used for the treatment of hypertension). Products include:
Betoptic S Ophthalmic Suspension 537

Bisoprolol Fumarate (Co-administration with beta-adrenergic blockers has resulted in excessive bradycardia and AV block, including complete heart block when combination has been used for the treatment of hypertension). Products include:
Zebeta Tablets 1885
Ziac Tablets 1887

Bumetanide (Additive effect on lowering blood pressure).
No products indexed under this heading.

Candesartan Cilexetil (Additive effect on lowering blood pressure). Products include:
Atacand Tablets 595
Atacand HCT Tablets 597

Captopril (Additive effect on lowering blood pressure). Products include:
Captopril Tablets 2281

Carbamazepine (Increased carbamazepine concentrations; potential for diplopia, headache, ataxia, or dizziness). Products include:
Carbatrol Capsules 3234
Tegretol/Tegretol-XR 2404

Carteolol Hydrochloride (Co-administration with beta-adrenergic blockers has resulted in excessive bradycardia and AV block, including complete heart block when combination has been used for the treatment of hypertension). Products include:
Carteolol Hydrochloride Ophthalmic Solution USP, 1% ⊙258
Ocupress Ophthalmic Solution, 1% Sterile ⊙303

Chlorothiazide (Additive effect on lowering blood pressure). Products include:
Aldoclor Tablets 2035
Diuril Oral 2087

Chlorothiazide Sodium (Additive effect on lowering blood pressure). Products include:
Diuril Sodium Intravenous 2086

Chlorthalidone (Additive effect on lowering blood pressure). Products include:
Clorpres Tablets 1002
Combipres Tablets 1040
Tenoretic Tablets 690

Cimetidine (Possible reduced verapamil clearance). Products include:
Tagamet HB 200 Suspension ▣762
Tagamet HB 200 Tablets ▣761
Tagamet Tablets 1644

Cimetidine Hydrochloride (Possible reduced verapamil clearance). Products include:
Tagamet 1644

Cisatracurium Besylate (Verapamil may potentiate the activity of neuromuscular blocking agents).
No products indexed under this heading.

Clonidine (Additive effect on lowering blood pressure). Products include:
Catapres-TTS 1038

Clonidine Hydrochloride (Additive effect on lowering blood pressure). Products include:
Catapres Tablets 1037
Clorpres Tablets 1002
Combipres Tablets 1040
Duraclon Injection 3057

Cyclosporine (Increased serum levels of cyclosporin). Products include:
Gengraf Capsules 457
Neoral Soft Gelatin Capsules 2380
Neoral Oral Solution 2380
Sandimmune 2388

Deserpidine (Additive effect on lowering blood pressure).
No products indexed under this heading.

Desflurane (Potential for excessive cardiovascular depression). Products include:
Suprane Liquid for Inhalation 874

Deslanoside (Chronic verapamil treatment can increase serum digoxin levels and this can result in digitalis toxicity).
No products indexed under this heading.

Diazoxide (Additive effect on lowering blood pressure).
No products indexed under this heading.

Digitoxin (Chronic verapamil treatment can increase serum digoxin levels and this can result in digitalis toxicity).
No products indexed under this heading.

Digoxin (Chronic verapamil treatment can increase serum digoxin levels and this can result in digitalis toxicity). Products include:
Digitek Tablets 1003
Lanoxicaps Capsules 1574
Lanoxin Injection 1581
Lanoxin Tablets 1587
Lanoxin Elixir Pediatric 1578
Lanoxin Injection Pediatric 1584

Diltiazem Hydrochloride (Additive effect on lowering blood pressure). Products include:
Cardizem Injectable 1018
Cardizem Lyo-Ject Syringe 1018
Cardizem Monovial 1018
Cardizem CD Capsules 1016
Tiazac Capsules 1378

Disopyramide Phosphate (Should not be administered within 48 hours before or 24 hours after verapamil administration).
No products indexed under this heading.

Doxacurium Chloride (Verapamil may potentiate the activity of neuromuscular blocking agents).
No products indexed under this heading.

Doxazosin Mesylate (May result in a reduction in blood pressure that is excessive in some patients). Products include:
Cardura Tablets 2668

Dyphylline (Inhibition of theophylline clearance and increased plasma levels of theophylline). Products include:
Lufyllin Tablets 3347
Lufyllin-400 Tablets 3347
Lufyllin-GG Elixir 3348
Lufyllin-GG Tablets 3348

Enalapril Maleate (Additive effect on lowering blood pressure). Products include:
Lexxel Tablets 608
Vaseretic Tablets 2204
Vasotec Tablets 2210

Enalaprilat (Additive effect on lowering blood pressure). Products include:
Enalaprilat Injection 863
Vasotec I.V. Injection 2207

Enflurane (Potential for excessive cardiovascular depression).
No products indexed under this heading.

Epoprostenol Sodium (Additive effect on lowering blood pressure). Products include:
Flolan for Injection 1528

Eprosartan Mesylate (Additive effect on lowering blood pressure). Products include:
Teveten Tablets 3327

Esmolol Hydrochloride (Co-administration with beta-adrenergic blockers has resulted in excessive bradycardia and AV block, including complete heart block when combination has been used for the treatment of hypertension). Products include:
Brevibloc Injection 858

Ethacrynic Acid (Additive effect on lowering blood pressure). Products include:
Edecrin Tablets 2091

Felodipine (Additive effect on lowering blood pressure). Products include:
Lexxel Tablets 608
Plendil Extended-Release Tablets 623

Flecainide Acetate (Additive effects on myocardial contractility, AV conduction, and repolarization; additive negative inotropic effect). Products include:
Tambocor Tablets 1990

Fosinopril Sodium (Additive effect on lowering blood pressure). Products include:
Monopril Tablets 1091
Monopril HCT 1094

Furosemide (Additive effect on lowering blood pressure). Products include:
Furosemide Tablets 2284

Guanabenz Acetate (Additive effect on lowering blood pressure).
No products indexed under this heading.

Guanethidine Monosulfate (Additive effect on lowering blood pressure).
No products indexed under this heading.

Halothane (Potential for excessive cardiovascular depression). Products include:
Fluothane Inhalation 3508

Hydralazine Hydrochloride (Additive effect on lowering blood pressure).
No products indexed under this heading.

Hydrochlorothiazide (Additive effect on lowering blood pressure). Products include:
Accuretic Tablets 2614
Aldoril Tablets 2039
Atacand HCT Tablets 597
Avalide Tablets 1070
Diovan HCT Tablets 2338
Dyazide Capsules 1515
HydroDIURIL Tablets 2108
Hyzaar 2109
Inderide Tablets 3517
Inderide LA Long-Acting Capsules 3519
Lotensin HCT Tablets 2367
Maxzide 1008
Micardis HCT Tablets 1051
Microzide Capsules 3414
Moduretic Tablets 2138
Monopril HCT 1094
Prinzide Tablets 2168
Timolide Tablets 2187
Uniretic Tablets 3178
Vaseretic Tablets 2204
Zestoretic Tablets 695
Ziac Tablets 1887

Hydroflumethiazide (Additive effect on lowering blood pressure). Products include:
Diucardin Tablets 3494

Indapamide (Additive effect on lowering blood pressure). Products include:
Indapamide Tablets 2286

Irbesartan (Additive effect on lowering blood pressure). Products include:
Avalide Tablets 1070
Avapro Tablets 1074
Avapro Tablets 3076

Isoflurane (Potential for excessive cardiovascular depression).
No products indexed under this heading.

Isradipine (Additive effect on lowering blood pressure). Products include:
DynaCirc Capsules 2921
DynaCirc CR Tablets 2923

Labetalol Hydrochloride (Co-administration with beta-adrenergic blockers has resulted in excessive bradycardia and AV block, including complete heart block when combination has been used for the treatment of hypertension). Products include:
Normodyne Injection 3135
Normodyne Tablets 3137

Levobunolol Hydrochloride (Co-administration with beta-adrenergic blockers has resulted in excessive bradycardia and AV block, including complete heart block when combination has been used for the treatment of hypertension). Products include:
Betagan ⊙228

Lisinopril (Additive effect on lowering blood pressure). Products include:
Prinivil Tablets 2164
Prinzide Tablets 2168
Zestoretic Tablets 695
Zestril Tablets 698

Lithium Carbonate (May result in lowering of serum lithium levels and increased sensitivity to the effects of lithium). Products include:
Eskalith 1527
Lithium Carbonate 3061
Lithobid Slow-Release Tablets 3255

Lithium Citrate (May result in lowering of serum lithium levels and increased sensitivity to the effects of lithium). Products include:
Lithium Citrate Syrup 3061

Losartan Potassium (Additive effect on lowering blood pressure). Products include:
Cozaar Tablets 2067
Hyzaar 2109

Mecamylamine Hydrochloride (Additive effect on lowering blood pressure). Products include:
Inversine Tablets 1850

Methoxyflurane (Potential for excessive cardiovascular depression).
No products indexed under this heading.

Methyclothiazide (Additive effect on lowering blood pressure).
No products indexed under this heading.

Methyldopa (Additive effect on lowering blood pressure). Products include:
- Aldoclor Tablets ... 2035
- Aldomet Tablets ... 2037
- Aldoril Tablets ... 2039

Methyldopate Hydrochloride (Additive effect on lowering blood pressure).
- No products indexed under this heading.

Metipranolol Hydrochloride (Co-administration with beta-adrenergic blockers has resulted in excessive bradycardia and AV block, including complete heart block when combination has been used for the treatment of hypertension).
- No products indexed under this heading.

Metocurine Iodide (Verapamil may potentiate the activity of neuromuscular blocking agents).
- No products indexed under this heading.

Metolazone (Additive effect on lowering blood pressure). Products include:
- Mykrox Tablets ... 1168
- Zaroxolyn Tablets ... 1177

Metoprolol Succinate (Co-administration with beta-adrenergic blockers has resulted in excessive bradycardia and AV block, including complete heart block when combination has been used for the treatment of hypertension; potential for decreased metoprolol clearance). Products include:
- Toprol-XL Tablets ... 651

Metoprolol Tartrate (Co-administration with beta-adrenergic blockers has resulted in excessive bradycardia and AV block, including complete heart block when combination has been used for the treatment of hypertension; potential for decreased metoprolol clearance).
- No products indexed under this heading.

Metyrosine (Additive effect on lowering blood pressure). Products include:
- Demser Capsules ... 2085

Mibefradil Dihydrochloride (Additive effect on lowering blood pressure).
- No products indexed under this heading.

Minoxidil (Additive effect on lowering blood pressure). Products include:
- Rogaine Extra Strength for Men Topical Solution ... ▣721
- Rogaine for Women Topical Solution ... ▣721

Mivacurium Chloride (Verapamil may potentiate the activity of neuromuscular blocking agents).
- No products indexed under this heading.

Moexipril Hydrochloride (Additive effect on lowering blood pressure). Products include:
- Uniretic Tablets ... 3178
- Univasc Tablets ... 3181

Nadolol (Co-administration with beta-adrenergic blockers has resulted in excessive bradycardia and AV block, including complete heart block when combination has been used for the treatment of hypertension). Products include:
- Corgard Tablets ... 2245
- Corzide 40/5 Tablets ... 2247
- Corzide 80/5 Tablets ... 2247
- Nadolol Tablets ... 2288

Nicardipine Hydrochloride (Additive effect on lowering blood pressure). Products include:
- Cardene I.V. ... 3485

Nifedipine (Additive effect on lowering blood pressure). Products include:
- Adalat CC Tablets ... 877
- Procardia Capsules ... 2708
- Procardia XL Extended Release Tablets ... 2710

Nisoldipine (Additive effect on lowering blood pressure). Products include:
- Sular Tablets ... 688

Nitroglycerin (Additive effect on lowering blood pressure). Products include:
- Nitro-Dur Transdermal Infusion System ... 3134
- Nitro-Dur Transdermal Infusion System ... 1834
- Nitrolingual Pumpspray ... 1355
- Nitrostat Tablets ... 2658

Pancuronium Bromide (Verapamil may potentiate the activity of neuromuscular blocking agents).
- No products indexed under this heading.

Penbutolol Sulfate (Co-administration with beta-adrenergic blockers has resulted in excessive bradycardia and AV block, including complete heart block when combination has been used for the treatment of hypertension).
- No products indexed under this heading.

Perindopril Erbumine (Additive effect on lowering blood pressure). Products include:
- Aceon Tablets (2 mg, 4 mg, 8 mg) ... 3249

Phenobarbital (Increases verapamil clearance). Products include:
- Arco-Lase Plus Tablets ... 592
- Donnatal ... 2929
- Donnatal Extentabs ... 2930

Phenoxybenzamine Hydrochloride (Additive effect on lowering blood pressure). Products include:
- Dibenzyline Capsules ... 3457

Phentolamine Mesylate (Additive effect on lowering blood pressure).
- No products indexed under this heading.

Pindolol (Co-administration with beta-adrenergic blockers has resulted in excessive bradycardia and AV block, including complete heart block when combination has been used for the treatment of hypertension).
- No products indexed under this heading.

Polythiazide (Additive effect on lowering blood pressure). Products include:
- Minizide Capsules ... 2700
- Renese Tablets ... 2712

Prazosin Hydrochloride (May result in a reduction in blood pressure that is excessive in some patients). Products include:
- Minipress Capsules ... 2699
- Minizide Capsules ... 2700

Propranolol Hydrochloride (Co-administration with beta-adrenergic blockers has resulted in excessive bradycardia and AV block, including complete heart block when combination has been used for the treatment of hypertension; potential for decreased propranolol clearance). Products include:
- Inderal ... 3513
- Inderal LA Long-Acting Capsules ... 3516
- Inderide Tablets ... 3517
- Inderide LA Long-Acting Capsules ... 3519

Quinapril Hydrochloride (Additive effect on lowering blood pressure). Products include:
- Accupril Tablets ... 2611
- Accuretic Tablets ... 2614

Quinidine Gluconate (Co-administration in patients with hypertrophic cardiomyopathy has resulted in significant hypotension; verapamil significantly counteracted the effects of quinidine on AV conduction and there has been a report of increased quinidine levels during combined therapy). Products include:
- Quinaglute Dura-Tabs Tablets ... 978

Quinidine Polygalacturonate (Co-administration in patients with hypertrophic cardiomyopathy has resulted in significant hypotension; verapamil significantly counteracted the effects of quinidine on AV conduction and there has been a report of increased quinidine levels during combined therapy).
- No products indexed under this heading.

Quinidine Sulfate (Co-administration in patients with hypertrophic cardiomyopathy has resulted in significant hypotension; verapamil significantly counteracted the effects of quinidine on AV conduction and there has been a report of increased quinidine levels during combined therapy). Products include:
- Quinidex Extentabs ... 2933

Ramipril (Additive effect on lowering blood pressure). Products include:
- Altace Capsules ... 2233

Rapacuronium Bromide (Verapamil may potentiate the activity of neuromuscular blocking agents).
- No products indexed under this heading.

Rauwolfia serpentina (Additive effect on lowering blood pressure).
- No products indexed under this heading.

Rescinnamine (Additive effect on lowering blood pressure).
- No products indexed under this heading.

Reserpine (Additive effect on lowering blood pressure).
- No products indexed under this heading.

Rifampin (Reduces oral verapamil bioavailability). Products include:
- Rifadin ... 765
- Rifamate Capsules ... 767
- Rifater Tablets ... 769

Rocuronium Bromide (Verapamil may potentiate the activity of neuromuscular blocking agents). Products include:
- Zemuron Injection ... 2491

Sodium Nitroprusside (Additive effect on lowering blood pressure).
- No products indexed under this heading.

Sotalol Hydrochloride (Co-administration with beta-adrenergic blockers has resulted in excessive bradycardia and AV block, including complete heart block when combination has been used for the treatment of hypertension). Products include:
- Betapace Tablets ... 950
- Betapace AF Tablets ... 954

Spirapril Hydrochloride (Additive effect on lowering blood pressure).
- No products indexed under this heading.

Spironolactone (Additive effect on lowering blood pressure).
- No products indexed under this heading.

Succinylcholine Chloride (Verapamil may potentiate the activity of neuromuscular blocking agents). Products include:
- Anectine Injection ... 1476

Telmisartan (Additive effect on lowering blood pressure). Products include:
- Micardis Tablets ... 1049
- Micardis HCT Tablets ... 1051

Terazosin Hydrochloride (May result in a reduction in blood pressure that is excessive in some patients). Products include:
- Hytrin Capsules ... 464

Theophylline (Inhibition of theophylline clearance and increased plasma levels of theophylline). Products include:
- Aerolate ... 1361
- Theo-Dur Extended-Release Tablets ... 1835
- Uni-Dur Extended-Release Tablets .. 1841
- Uniphyl 400 mg and 600 mg Tablets ... 2903

Theophylline Calcium Salicylate (Inhibition of theophylline clearance and increased plasma levels of theophylline).
- No products indexed under this heading.

Theophylline Sodium Glycinate (Inhibition of theophylline clearance and increased plasma levels of theophylline).
- No products indexed under this heading.

Timolol Hemihydrate (Asymptomatic bradycardia with wandering atrial pacemaker has been observed with ophthalmic timolol and oral verapamil). Products include:
- Betimol Ophthalmic Solution ... ⊙324

Timolol Maleate (Asymptomatic bradycardia with wandering atrial pacemaker has been observed with ophthalmic timolol and oral verapamil; co-administration with beta-adrenergic blockers has resulted in excessive bradycardia and AV block, including complete heart block when combination has been used for the treatment of hypertension). Products include:
- Blocadren Tablets ... 2046
- Cosopt Sterile Ophthalmic Solution ... 2065
- Timolide Tablets ... 2187
- Timolol GFS ... ⊙266
- Timoptic in Ocudose ... 2192
- Timoptic Sterile Ophthalmic Solution ... 2190
- Timoptic-XE Sterile Ophthalmic Gel Forming Solution ... 2194

Torsemide (Additive effect on lowering blood pressure). Products include:
- Demadex Tablets and Injection ... 2965

Trandolapril (Additive effect on lowering blood pressure). Products include:
- Mavik Tablets ... 478
- Tarka Tablets ... 508

Triamterene (Additive effect on lowering blood pressure). Products include:
- Dyazide Capsules ... 1515
- Dyrenium Capsules ... 3458
- Maxzide ... 1008

Trimethaphan Camsylate (Additive effect on lowering blood pressure).
- No products indexed under this heading.

Tubocurarine Chloride (Verapamil may potentiate the activity of neuromuscular blocking agents).
- No products indexed under this heading.

Valsartan (Additive effect on lowering blood pressure). Products include:
- Diovan Capsules ... 2337
- Diovan HCT Tablets ... 2338

Vecuronium Bromide (Verapamil prolongs recovery from the neuromuscular blockade; may potentiate the activity of neuromuscular blocking agents). Products include:
- Norcuron for Injection ... 2478

Food Interactions

Alcohol (Verapamil has been found to significantly inhibit alcohol elimination resulting in elevated blood alcohol concentrations that may prolong the intoxicating effect of alcohol).

Food, unspecified (Produces decreased bioavailability (AUC) but a narrower peak to trough ratio).

ISOPTO CARBACHOL OPHTHALMIC SOLUTION

(Carbachol) ... ⊙215

None cited in PDR database.

ISOPTO CARPINE OPHTHALMIC SOLUTION
(Pilocarpine Hydrochloride) .... ⊙215
None cited in PDR database.

ISORDIL SUBLINGUAL TABLETS
(Isosorbide Dinitrate) 3525
See Isordil Titradose Tablets

ISORDIL TITRADOSE TABLETS
(Isosorbide Dinitrate) 3526
May interact with vasodilators and certain other agents. Compounds in these categories include:

Diazoxide (The vasodilating effects of isosorbide dinitrate may be additive with those of other vasodilators).
No products indexed under this heading.

Epoprostenol Sodium (The vasodilating effects of isosorbide dinitrate may be additive with those of other vasodilators). Products include:
Flolan for Injection 1528

Hydralazine Hydrochloride (The vasodilating effects of isosorbide dinitrate may be additive with those of other vasodilators).
No products indexed under this heading.

Minoxidil (The vasodilating effects of isosorbide dinitrate may be additive with those of other vasodilators). Products include:
Rogaine Extra Strength for Men Topical Solution .... ■721
Rogaine for Women Topical Solution .... ■721

Sildenafil Citrate (Amplification of the vasodilatory effects of isosorbide dinitrate by sildenafil can result in severe hypotension; the time course and dose dependency of this interaction have not been studied). Products include:
Viagra Tablets 2732

Food Interactions

Alcohol (Alcohol exhibits additive vasodilating effects).

IVEEGAM EN
(Globulin, Immune (Human)) 849
May interact with:

Measles, Mumps & Rubella Virus Vaccine, Live (Antibodies in immune globulin preparations may interfere with the responses by pediatric patients to live viral vaccines). Products include:
M-M-R II 2118

JE-VAX VACCINE
(Japanese Encephalitis Vaccine Inactivated) 811
None cited in PDR database.

KADIAN CAPSULES
(Morphine Sulfate) 1335
May interact with central nervous system depressants, diuretics, general anesthetics, hypnotics and sedatives, monoamine oxidase inhibitors, mixed agonist/antagonist opioid analgesics, neuromuscular blocking agents, phenothiazines, and tranquilizers. Compounds in these categories include:

Alfentanil Hydrochloride (Co-administration may increase the risk of respiratory depression, hypotension and profound sedation and coma; when such combined therapy is contemplated, the initial dose of one or both agents should be reduced by at least 50%).
No products indexed under this heading.

Alprazolam (Co-administration may increase the risk of respiratory depression, hypotension and profound sedation and coma; when such combined therapy is contemplated, the initial dose of one or both agents should be reduced by at least 50%). Products include:
Xanax Tablets 2865

Amiloride Hydrochloride (Morphine can reduce the efficacy of diuretics by inducing the release of antidiuretic hormone and by causing spasm of the sphincter of the bladder leading to acute retention of urine). Products include:
Midamor Tablets 2136
Moduretic Tablets 2138

Aprobarbital (Co-administration may increase the risk of respiratory depression, hypotension and profound sedation and coma; when such combined therapy is contemplated, the initial dose of one or both agents should be reduced by at least 50%).
No products indexed under this heading.

Atracurium Besylate (Morphine may enhance the neuromuscular blocking action of skeletal relaxants and produce an increased degree of respiratory depression).
No products indexed under this heading.

Bendroflumethiazide (Morphine can reduce the efficacy of diuretics by inducing the release of antidiuretic hormone and by causing spasm of the sphincter of the bladder leading to acute retention of urine). Products include:
Corzide 40/5 Tablets 2247
Corzide 80/5 Tablets 2247

Bumetanide (Morphine can reduce the efficacy of diuretics by inducing the release of antidiuretic hormone and by causing spasm of the sphincter of the bladder leading to acute retention of urine).
No products indexed under this heading.

Buprenorphine Hydrochloride (May reduce the analgesic effect and/or precipitate withdrawal symptoms). Products include:
Buprenex Injectable 2918

Buspirone Hydrochloride (Co-administration may increase the risk of respiratory depression, hypotension and profound sedation and coma; when such combined therapy is contemplated, the initial dose of one or both agents should be reduced by at least 50%).
No products indexed under this heading.

Butabarbital (Co-administration may increase the risk of respiratory depression, hypotension and profound sedation and coma; when such combined therapy is contemplated, the initial dose of one or both agents should be reduced by at least 50%).
No products indexed under this heading.

Butalbital (Co-administration may increase the risk of respiratory depression, hypotension and profound sedation and coma; when such combined therapy is contemplated, the initial dose of one or both agents should be reduced by at least 50%). Products include:
Phrenilin 578
Sedapap Tablets 50 mg/650 mg ... 2225

Butorphanol Tartrate (May reduce the analgesic effect and/or precipitate withdrawal symptoms). Products include:
Stadol NS Nasal Spray 1108

Chlordiazepoxide (Co-administration may increase the risk of respiratory depression, hypotension and profound sedation and coma; when such combined therapy is contemplated, the initial dose of one or both agents should be reduced by at least 50%). Products include:
Limbitrol 1738

Chlordiazepoxide Hydrochloride (Co-administration may increase the risk of respiratory depression, hypotension and profound sedation and coma; when such combined therapy is contemplated, the initial dose of one or both agents should be reduced by at least 50%). Products include:
Librium Capsules 1736
Librium for Injection 1737

Chlorothiazide (Morphine can reduce the efficacy of diuretics by inducing the release of antidiuretic hormone and by causing spasm of the the sphincter of the bladder leading to acute retention of urine). Products include:
Aldoclor Tablets 2035
Diuril Oral 2087

Chlorothiazide Sodium (Morphine can reduce the efficacy of diuretics by inducing the release of antidiuretic hormone and by causing spasm of the sphincter of the bladder leading to acute retention of urine). Products include:
Diuril Sodium Intravenous 2086

Chlorpromazine (Co-administration may increase the risk of respiratory depression, hypotension and profound sedation and coma; when such combined therapy is contemplated, the initial dose of one or both agents should be reduced by at least 50%). Products include:
Thorazine Suppositories 1656

Chlorpromazine Hydrochloride (Co-administration may increase the risk of respiratory depression, hypotension and profound sedation and coma; when such combined therapy is contemplated, the initial dose of one or both agents should be reduced by at least 50%). Products include:
Thorazine 1656

Chlorprothixene (Co-administration may increase the risk of respiratory depression, hypotension and profound sedation and coma; when such combined therapy is contemplated, the initial dose of one or both agents should be reduced by at least 50%).
No products indexed under this heading.

Chlorprothixene Hydrochloride (Co-administration may increase the risk of respiratory depression, hypotension and profound sedation and coma; when such combined therapy is contemplated, the initial dose of one or both agents should be reduced by at least 50%).
No products indexed under this heading.

Chlorprothixene Lactate (Co-administration may increase the risk of respiratory depression, hypotension and profound sedation and coma; when such combined therapy is contemplated, the initial dose of one or both agents should be reduced by at least 50%).
No products indexed under this heading.

Chlorthalidone (Morphine can reduce the efficacy of diuretics by inducing the release of antidiuretic hormone and by causing spasm of the sphincter of the bladder leading to acute retention of urine). Products include:
Clorpres Tablets 1002
Combipres Tablets 1040
Tenoretic Tablets 690

Cimetidine (Co-administration has resulted in an isolated report of confusion and severe respiratory depression). Products include:
Tagamet HB 200 Suspension .... ■762
Tagamet HB 200 Tablets .... ■761
Tagamet Tablets 1644

Cimetidine Hydrochloride (Co-administration has resulted in an isolated report of confusion and severe respiratory depression). Products include:
Tagamet 1644

Cisatracurium Besylate (Morphine may enhance the neuromuscular blocking action of skeletal relaxants and produce an increased degree of respiratory depression).
No products indexed under this heading.

Clorazepate Dipotassium (Co-administration may increase the risk of respiratory depression, hypotension and profound sedation and coma; when such combined therapy is contemplated, the initial dose of one or both agents should be reduced by at least 50%). Products include:
Tranxene 511

Clozapine (Co-administration may increase the risk of respiratory depression, hypotension and profound sedation and coma; when such combined therapy is contemplated, the initial dose of one or both agents should be reduced by at least 50%). Products include:
Clozaril Tablets 2319

Codeine Phosphate (Co-administration may increase the risk of respiratory depression, hypotension and profound sedation and coma; when such combined therapy is contemplated, the initial dose of one or both agents should be reduced by at least 50%). Products include:
Phenergan with Codeine Syrup 3557
Phenergan VC with Codeine Syrup .. 3561
Robitussin A-C Syrup 2942
Robitussin-DAC Syrup 2942
Ryna-C Liquid .... ■768
Soma Compound w/Codeine Tablets 3355
Tussi-Organidin NR Liquid 3350
Tussi-Organidin-S NR Liquid 3350
Tylenol with Codeine 2595

Desflurane (Co-administration may increase the risk of respiratory depression, hypotension and profound sedation and coma; when such combined therapy is contemplated, the initial dose of one or both agents should be reduced by at least 50%). Products include:
Suprane Liquid for Inhalation 874

Dezocine (Co-administration may increase the risk of respiratory depression, hypotension and profound sedation and coma; when such combined therapy is contemplated, the initial dose of one or both agents should be reduced by at least 50%).
No products indexed under this heading.

Diazepam (Co-administration may increase the risk of respiratory depression, hypotension and profound sedation and coma; when such combined therapy is contemplated, the initial dose of one or both agents should be reduced by at least 50%). Products include:
Valium Injectable 3026
Valium Tablets 3047

Doxacurium Chloride (Morphine may enhance the neuromuscular blocking action of skeletal relaxants and produce an increased degree of respiratory depression).
No products indexed under this heading.

Droperidol (Co-administration may increase the risk of respiratory depression, hypotension and profound sedation and coma; when such combined therapy is contemplated, the initial dose of one or both

agents should be reduced by at least 50%).

No products indexed under this heading.

Enflurane (Co-administration may increase the risk of respiratory depression, hypotension and profound sedation and coma; when such combined therapy is contemplated, the initial dose of one or both agents should be reduced by at least 50%).

No products indexed under this heading.

Estazolam (Co-administration may increase the risk of respiratory depression, hypotension and profound sedation and coma; when such combined therapy is contemplated, the initial dose of one or both agents should be reduced by at least 50%). Products include:

ProSom Tablets 500

Ethacrynic Acid (Morphine can reduce the efficacy of diuretics by inducing the release of antidiuretic hormone and by causing spasm of the sphincter of the bladder leading to acute retention of urine). Products include:

Edecrin Tablets 2091

Ethchlorvynol (Co-administration may increase the risk of respiratory depression, hypotension and profound sedation and coma; when such combined therapy is contemplated, the initial dose of one or both agents should be reduced by at least 50%).

No products indexed under this heading.

Ethinamate (Co-administration may increase the risk of respiratory depression, hypotension and profound sedation and coma; when such combined therapy is contemplated, the initial dose of one or both agents should be reduced by at least 50%).

No products indexed under this heading.

Fentanyl (Co-administration may increase the risk of respiratory depression, hypotension and profound sedation and coma; when such combined therapy is contemplated, the initial dose of one or both agents should be reduced by at least 50%). Products include:

Duragesic Transdermal System 1786

Fentanyl Citrate (Co-administration may increase the risk of respiratory depression, hypotension and profound sedation and coma; when such combined therapy is contemplated, the initial dose of one or both agents should be reduced by at least 50%). Products include:

Actiq 1184

Fluphenazine Decanoate (Co-administration may increase the risk of respiratory depression, hypotension and profound sedation and coma; when such combined therapy is contemplated, the initial dose of one or both agents should be reduced by at least 50%).

No products indexed under this heading.

Fluphenazine Enanthate (Co-administration may increase the risk of respiratory depression, hypotension and profound sedation and coma; when such combined therapy is contemplated, the initial dose of one or both agents should be reduced by at least 50%).

No products indexed under this heading.

Fluphenazine Hydrochloride (Co-administration may increase the risk of respiratory depression, hypotension and profound sedation and coma; when such combined therapy is contemplated, the initial dose of one or both agents should be reduced by at least 50%).

No products indexed under this heading.

Flurazepam Hydrochloride (Co-administration may increase the risk of respiratory depression, hypotension and profound sedation and coma; when such combined therapy is contemplated, the initial dose of one or both agents should be reduced by at least 50%).

No products indexed under this heading.

Furosemide (Morphine can reduce the efficacy of diuretics by inducing the release of antidiuretic hormone and by causing spasm of the sphincter of the bladder leading to acute retention of urine). Products include:

Furosemide Tablets 2284

Glutethimide (Co-administration may increase the risk of respiratory depression, hypotension and profound sedation and coma; when such combined therapy is contemplated, the initial dose of one or both agents should be reduced by at least 50%).

No products indexed under this heading.

Haloperidol (Co-administration may increase the risk of respiratory depression, hypotension and profound sedation and coma; when such combined therapy is contemplated, the initial dose of one or both agents should be reduced by at least 50%). Products include:

Haldol Injection, Tablets and Concentrate 2533

Haloperidol Decanoate (Co-administration may increase the risk of respiratory depression, hypotension and profound sedation and coma; when such combined therapy is contemplated, the initial dose of one or both agents should be reduced by at least 50%). Products include:

Haldol Decanoate 2535

Hydrochlorothiazide (Morphine can reduce the efficacy of diuretics by inducing the release of antidiuretic hormone and by causing spasm of the sphincter of the bladder leading to acute retention of urine). Products include:

Accuretic Tablets 2614
Aldoril Tablets 2039
Atacand HCT Tablets 597
Avalide Tablets 1070
Diovan HCT Tablets 2338
Dyazide Capsules 1515
HydroDIURIL Tablets 2108
Hyzaar 2109
Inderide Tablets 3517
Inderide LA Long-Acting Capsules 3519
Lotensin HCT Tablets 2367
Maxzide 1008
Micardis HCT Tablets 1051
Microzide Capsules 3414
Moduretic Tablets 2138
Monopril HCT 1094
Prinzide Tablets 2168
Timolide Tablets 2187
Uniretic Tablets 3178
Vaseretic Tablets 2204
Zestoretic Tablets 695
Ziac Tablets 1887

Hydrocodone Bitartrate (Co-administration may increase the risk of respiratory depression, hypotension and profound sedation and coma; when such combined therapy is contemplated, the initial dose of one or both agents should be reduced by at least 50%). Products include:

Hycodan 1316
Hycomine Compound Tablets 1317
Hycotuss Expectorant Syrup 1318
Lortab 3319
Lortab Elixir 3317
Maxidone Tablets CIII 3399
Norco 5/325 Tablets CIII 3424
Norco 7.5/325 Tablets CIII 3425
Norco 10/325 Tablets CIII 3427
Norco 10/325 Tablets CIII 3425
Vicodin Tablets 516
Vicodin ES Tablets 517
Vicodin HP Tablets 518
Vicodin Tuss Expectorant 519
Vicoprofen Tablets 520
Zydone Tablets 1330

Hydrocodone Polistirex (Co-administration may increase the risk of respiratory depression, hypotension and profound sedation and coma; when such combined therapy is contemplated, the initial dose of one or both agents should be reduced by at least 50%). Products include:

Tussionex Pennkinetic Extended-Release Suspension 1174

Hydroflumethiazide (Morphine can reduce the efficacy of diuretics by inducing the release of antidiuretic hormone and by causing spasm of the sphincter of the bladder leading to acute retention of urine). Products include:

Diucardin Tablets 3494

Hydromorphone Hydrochloride (Co-administration may increase the risk of respiratory depression, hypotension and profound sedation and coma; when such combined therapy is contemplated, the initial dose of one or both agents should be reduced by at least 50%). Products include:

Dilaudid 441
Dilaudid Oral Liquid 445
Dilaudid Powder 441
Dilaudid Rectal Suppositories 441
Dilaudid Tablets 441
Dilaudid Tablets - 8 mg 445
Dilaudid-HP 443

Hydroxyzine Hydrochloride (Co-administration may increase the risk of respiratory depression, hypotension and profound sedation and coma; when such combined therapy is contemplated, the initial dose of one or both agents should be reduced by at least 50%). Products include:

Atarax Tablets & Syrup 2667
Vistaril Intramuscular Solution 2738

Indapamide (Morphine can reduce the efficacy of diuretics by inducing the release of antidiuretic hormone and by causing spasm of the sphincter of the bladder leading to acute retention of urine). Products include:

Indapamide Tablets 2286

Isocarboxazid (MAO inhibitors have been reported to intensify the effects of opioids causing anxiety, confusion and significant depression of respiration or coma; concurrent and/or sequential use is not recommended).

No products indexed under this heading.

Isoflurane (Co-administration may increase the risk of respiratory depression, hypotension and profound sedation and coma; when such combined therapy is contemplated, the initial dose of one or both agents should be reduced by at least 50%).

No products indexed under this heading.

Ketamine Hydrochloride (Co-administration may increase the risk of respiratory depression, hypotension and profound sedation and coma; when such combined therapy is contemplated, the initial dose of one or both agents should be reduced by at least 50%).

No products indexed under this heading.

Levomethadyl Acetate Hydrochloride (Co-administration may increase the risk of respiratory depression, hypotension and profound sedation and coma; when such combined therapy is contemplated, the initial dose of one or both agents should be reduced by at least 50%). Products include:

No products indexed under this heading.

Levorphanol Tartrate (Co-administration may increase the risk of respiratory depression, hypotension and profound sedation and coma; when such combined therapy is contemplated, the initial dose of one or both agents should be reduced by at least 50%). Products include:

Levo-Dromoran 1734
Levorphanol Tartrate Tablets 3059

Lorazepam (Co-administration may increase the risk of respiratory depression, hypotension and profound sedation and coma; when such combined therapy is contemplated, the initial dose of one or both agents should be reduced by at least 50%). Products include:

Ativan Injection 3478
Ativan Tablets 3482

Loxapine Hydrochloride (Co-administration may increase the risk of respiratory depression, hypotension and profound sedation and coma; when such combined therapy is contemplated, the initial dose of one or both agents should be reduced by at least 50%).

No products indexed under this heading.

Loxapine Succinate (Co-administration may increase the risk of respiratory depression, hypotension and profound sedation and coma; when such combined therapy is contemplated, the initial dose of one or both agents should be reduced by at least 50%). Products include:

Loxitane Capsules 3398

Meperidine Hydrochloride (Co-administration may increase the risk of respiratory depression, hypotension and profound sedation and coma; when such combined therapy is contemplated, the initial dose of one or both agents should be reduced by at least 50%). Products include:

Demerol 3079
Mepergan Injection 3539

Mephobarbital (Co-administration may increase the risk of respiratory depression, hypotension and profound sedation and coma; when such combined therapy is contemplated, the initial dose of one or both agents should be reduced by at least 50%).

No products indexed under this heading.

Meprobamate (Co-administration may increase the risk of respiratory depression, hypotension and profound sedation and coma; when such combined therapy is contemplated, the initial dose of one or both agents should be reduced by at least 50%). Products include:

Miltown Tablets 3349

Mesoridazine Besylate (Co-administration may increase the risk of respiratory depression, hypotension and profound sedation and coma; when such combined therapy is contemplated, the initial dose of one or both agents should be reduced by at least 50%). Products include:

Serentil 1057

Methadone Hydrochloride (Co-administration may increase the risk of respiratory depression, hypotension and profound sedation and coma; when such combined therapy is contemplated, the initial dose of one or both agents should be reduced by at least 50%). Products include:

Dolophine Hydrochloride Tablets 3056

Methohexital Sodium (Co-administration may increase the risk of respiratory depression, hypotension and profound sedation and coma; when such combined therapy is contemplated, the initial dose of one or both agents should be reduced by at least 50%). Products include:

Brevital Sodium for Injection, USP .. 1815

Methotrimeprazine (Co-administration may increase the risk of respiratory depression, hypotension and profound sedation and coma; when such combined therapy is contemplated, the initial dose of one or both agents should be reduced by at least 50%).

No products indexed under this heading.

Methoxyflurane (Co-administration may increase the risk of respiratory depression, hypotension and profound sedation and coma; when such combined therapy is contemplated, the initial dose of one or both agents should be reduced by at least 50%).

No products indexed under this heading.

Methyclothiazide (Morphine can reduce the efficacy of diuretics by inducing the release of antidiuretic hormone and by causing spasm of the sphincter of the bladder leading to acute retention of urine).

No products indexed under this heading.

Metocurine Iodide (Morphine may enhance the neuromuscular blocking action of skeletal relaxants and produce an increased degree of respiratory depression).

No products indexed under this heading.

Metolazone (Morphine can reduce the efficacy of diuretics by inducing the release of antidiuretic hormone and by causing spasm of the sphincter of the bladder leading to acute retention of urine). Products include:

Mykrox Tablets 1168
Zaroxolyn Tablets 1177

Midazolam Hydrochloride (Co-administration may increase the risk of respiratory depression, hypotension and profound sedation and coma; when such combined therapy is contemplated, the initial dose of one or both agents should be reduced by at least 50%). Products include:

Versed Injection 3027
Versed Syrup 3033

Mivacurium Chloride (Morphine may enhance the neuromuscular blocking action of skeletal relaxants and produce an increased degree of respiratory depression).

No products indexed under this heading.

Moclobemide (MAO inhibitors have been reported to intensify the effects of opioids causing anxiety, confusion and significant depression of respiration or coma; concurrent and/or sequential use is not recommended).

No products indexed under this heading.

Molindone Hydrochloride (Co-administration may increase the risk of respiratory depression, hypotension and profound sedation and coma; when such combined therapy is contemplated, the initial dose of one or both agents should be reduced by at least 50%). Products include:

Moban 1320

Nalbuphine Hydrochloride (May reduce the analgesic effect and/or precipitate withdrawal symptoms). Products include:

Nubain Injection 1323

Olanzapine (Co-administration may increase the risk of respiratory depression, hypotension and profound sedation and coma; when such combined therapy is contemplated, the initial dose of one or both agents should be reduced by at least 50%). Products include:

Zyprexa Tablets 1973
Zyprexa ZYDIS Orally Disintegrating Tablets 1973

Oxazepam (Co-administration may increase the risk of respiratory depression, hypotension and profound sedation and coma; when such combined therapy is contemplated, the initial dose of one or both agents should be reduced by at least 50%).

No products indexed under this heading.

Oxycodone Hydrochloride (Co-administration may increase the risk of respiratory depression, hypotension and profound sedation and coma; when such combined therapy is contemplated, the initial dose of one or both agents should be reduced by at least 50%). Products include:

OxyContin Tablets 2912
OxyFast Oral Concentrate Solution . 2916
OxyIR Capsules 2916
Percocet Tablets 1326
Percodan Tablets 1327
Percolone Tablets 1327
Roxicodone 3067
Tylox Capsules 2597

Pancuronium Bromide (Morphine may enhance the neuromuscular blocking action of skeletal relaxants and produce an increased degree of respiratory depression).

No products indexed under this heading.

Pargyline Hydrochloride (MAO inhibitors have been reported to intensify the effects of opioids causing anxiety, confusion and significant depression of respiration or coma; concurrent and/or sequential use is not recommended).

No products indexed under this heading.

Pentazocine Hydrochloride (May reduce the analgesic effect and/or precipitate withdrawal symptoms). Products include:

Talacen Caplets 3089
Talwin Nx Tablets 3090

Pentazocine Lactate (May reduce the analgesic effect and/or precipitate withdrawal symptoms).

No products indexed under this heading.

Pentobarbital Sodium (Co-administration may increase the risk of respiratory depression, hypotension and profound sedation and coma; when such combined therapy is contemplated, the initial dose of one or both agents should be reduced by at least 50%). Products include:

Nembutal Sodium Solution 485

Perphenazine (Co-administration may increase the risk of respiratory depression, hypotension and profound sedation and coma; when such combined therapy is contemplated, the initial dose of one or both agents should be reduced by at least 50%). Products include:

Etrafon 3115
Trilafon 3160

Phenelzine Sulfate (MAO inhibitors have been reported to intensify the effects of opioids causing anxiety, confusion and significant depression of respiration or coma; concurrent and/or sequential use is not recommended). Products include:

Nardil Tablets 2653

Phenobarbital (Co-administration may increase the risk of respiratory depression, hypotension and profound sedation and coma; when such combined therapy is contemplated, the initial dose of one or both agents should be reduced by at least 50%). Products include:

Arco-Lase Plus Tablets 592
Donnatal 2929
Donnatal Extentabs 2930

Polythiazide (Morphine can reduce the efficacy of diuretics by inducing the release of antidiuretic hormone and by causing spasm of the sphincter of the bladder leading to acute retention of urine). Products include:

Minizide Capsules 2700
Renese Tablets 2712

Prazepam (Co-administration may increase the risk of respiratory depression, hypotension and profound sedation and coma; when such combined therapy is contemplated, the initial dose of one or both agents should be reduced by at least 50%).

No products indexed under this heading.

Procarbazine Hydrochloride (MAO inhibitors have been reported to intensify the effects of opioids causing anxiety, confusion and significant depression of respiration or coma; concurrent and/or sequential use is not recommended). Products include:

Matulane Capsules 3246

Prochlorperazine (Co-administration may increase the risk of respiratory depression, hypotension and profound sedation and coma; when such combined therapy is contemplated, the initial dose of one or both agents should be reduced by at least 50%). Products include:

Compazine 1505

Promethazine Hydrochloride (Co-administration may increase the risk of respiratory depression, hypotension and profound sedation and coma; when such combined therapy is contemplated, the initial dose of one or both agents should be reduced by at least 50%). Products include:

Mepergan Injection 3539
Phenergan Injection 3553
Phenergan 3556
Phenergan Syrup 3554
Phenergan with Codeine Syrup 3557
Phenergan with Dextromethorphan Syrup 3559
Phenergan VC Syrup 3560
Phenergan VC with Codeine Syrup .. 3561

Propofol (Co-administration may increase the risk of respiratory depression, hypotension and profound sedation and coma; when such combined therapy is contemplated, the initial dose of one or both agents should be reduced by at least 50%). Products include:

Diprivan Injectable Emulsion 667

Propoxyphene Hydrochloride (Co-administration may increase the risk of respiratory depression, hypotension and profound sedation and coma; when such combined therapy is contemplated, the initial dose of one or both agents should be reduced by at least 50%). Products include:

Darvon Pulvules 1909
Darvon Compound-65 Pulvules 1910

Propoxyphene Napsylate (Co-administration may increase the risk of respiratory depression, hypotension and profound sedation and coma; when such combined therapy is contemplated, the initial dose of one or both agents should be reduced by at least 50%). Products include:

Darvon-N/Darvocet-N 1907
Darvon-N Tablets 1912

Quazepam (Co-administration may increase the risk of respiratory depression, hypotension and profound sedation and coma; when such combined therapy is contemplated, the initial dose of one or both agents should be reduced by at least 50%).

No products indexed under this heading.

Quetiapine Fumarate (Co-administration may increase the risk of respiratory depression, hypotension and profound sedation and coma; when such combined therapy is contemplated, the initial dose of one or both agents should be reduced by at least 50%). Products include:

Seroquel Tablets 684

Rapacuronium Bromide (Morphine may enhance the neuromuscular blocking action of skeletal relaxants and produce an increased degree of respiratory depression).

No products indexed under this heading.

Remifentanil Hydrochloride (Co-administration may increase the risk of respiratory depression, hypotension and profound sedation and coma; when such combined therapy is contemplated, the initial dose of one or both agents should be reduced by at least 50%).

No products indexed under this heading.

Risperidone (Co-administration may increase the risk of respiratory depression, hypotension and profound sedation and coma; when such combined therapy is contemplated, the initial dose of one or both agents should be reduced by at least 50%). Products include:

Risperdal 1796

Rocuronium Bromide (Morphine may enhance the neuromuscular blocking action of skeletal relaxants and produce an increased degree of respiratory depression). Products include:

Zemuron Injection 2491

Secobarbital Sodium (Co-administration may increase the risk of respiratory depression, hypotension and profound sedation and coma; when such combined therapy is contemplated, the initial dose of one or both agents should be reduced by at least 50%).

No products indexed under this heading.

Selegiline Hydrochloride (MAO inhibitors have been reported to intensify the effects of opioids causing anxiety, confusion and significant depression of respiration or coma; concurrent and/or sequential use is not recommended). Products include:

Eldepryl Capsules 3266

Sevoflurane (Co-administration may increase the risk of respiratory depression, hypotension and profound sedation and coma; when such combined therapy is contemplated, the initial dose of one or both agents should be reduced by at least 50%).

No products indexed under this heading.

Spironolactone (Morphine can reduce the efficacy of diuretics by inducing the release of antidiuretic hormone and by causing spasm of the sphincter of the bladder leading to acute retention of urine).

No products indexed under this heading.

Succinylcholine Chloride (Morphine may enhance the neuromuscular blocking action of skeletal relaxants and produce an increased degree of respiratory depression). Products include:

Anectine Injection 1476

Sufentanil Citrate (Co-administration may increase the risk of respiratory depression, hypotension and profound sedation and coma; when such combined therapy is contemplated, the initial dose of one or both agents should be reduced by at least 50%).
No products indexed under this heading.

Temazepam (Co-administration may increase the risk of respiratory depression, hypotension and profound sedation and coma; when such combined therapy is contemplated, the initial dose of one or both agents should be reduced by at least 50%).
No products indexed under this heading.

Thiamylal Sodium (Co-administration may increase the risk of respiratory depression, hypotension and profound sedation and coma; when such combined therapy is contemplated, the initial dose of one or both agents should be reduced by at least 50%).
No products indexed under this heading.

Thioridazine Hydrochloride (Co-administration may increase the risk of respiratory depression, hypotension and profound sedation and coma; when such combined therapy is contemplated, the initial dose of one or both agents should be reduced by at least 50%). Products include:
Thioridazine Hydrochloride Tablets 2289

Thiothixene (Co-administration may increase the risk of respiratory depression, hypotension and profound sedation and coma; when such combined therapy is contemplated, the initial dose of one or both agents should be reduced by at least 50%). Products include:
Navane Capsules 2701
Thiothixene Capsules 2290

Torsemide (Morphine can reduce the efficacy of diuretics by inducing the release of antidiuretic hormone and by causing spasm of the sphincter of the bladder leading to acute retention of urine). Products include:
Demadex Tablets and Injection 2965

Tranylcypromine Sulfate (MAO inhibitors have been reported to intensify the effects of opioids causing anxiety, confusion and significant depression of respiration or coma; concurrent and/or sequential use is not recommended). Products include:
Parnate Tablets 1607

Triamterene (Morphine can reduce the efficacy of diuretics by inducing the release of antidiuretic hormone and by causing spasm of the sphincter of the bladder leading to acute retention of urine). Products include:
Dyazide Capsules 1515
Dyrenium Capsules 3458
Maxzide 1008

Triazolam (Co-administration may increase the risk of respiratory depression, hypotension and profound sedation and coma; when such combined therapy is contemplated, the initial dose of one or both agents should be reduced by at least 50%). Products include:
Halcion Tablets 2823

Trifluoperazine Hydrochloride (Co-administration may increase the risk of respiratory depression, hypotension and profound sedation and coma; when such combined therapy is contemplated, the initial dose of one or both agents should be reduced by at least 50%). Products include:
Stelazine 1640

Vecuronium Bromide (Morphine may enhance the neuromuscular blocking action of skeletal relaxants and produce an increased degree of respiratory depression). Products include:
Norcuron for Injection 2478

Zaleplon (Co-administration may increase the risk of respiratory depression, hypotension and profound sedation and coma; when such combined therapy is contemplated, the initial dose of one or both agents should be reduced by at least 50%). Products include:
Sonata Capsules 3591

Ziprasidone Hydrochloride (Co-administration may increase the risk of respiratory depression, hypotension and profound sedation and coma; when such combined therapy is contemplated, the initial dose of one or both agents should be reduced by at least 50%). Products include:
Geodon Capsules 2688

Zolpidem Tartrate (Co-administration may increase the risk of respiratory depression, hypotension and profound sedation and coma; when such combined therapy is contemplated, the initial dose of one or both agents should be reduced by at least 50%). Products include:
Ambien Tablets 3191

Food Interactions

Alcohol (Co-administration may increase the risk of respiratory depression, hypotension and profound sedation and coma).

Food, unspecified (Slows the rate of absorption of Kadian, the extent of absorption is not affected and Kadian can be administered without regard to meals; the pellets in Kadian should not be dissolved).

KALETRA CAPSULES

(Lopinavir, Ritonavir) 471
May interact with dexamethasone, dihydrofolate reductase inhibitors, ergot-containing drugs, phenytoin, quinidine, and certain other agents. Compounds in these categories include:

Abacavir Sulfate (Kaletra induces glucuronidation; therefore, Kaletra has the potential to reduce abacavir plasma concentrations; the clinical significance is unknown). Products include:
Trizivir Tablets 1669
Ziagen 1692

Amiodarone Hydrochloride (Co-administration can result in increased amiodarone plasma concentrations). Products include:
Cordarone Intravenous 3491
Cordarone Tablets 3487
Pacerone Tablets 3331

Amprenavir (Co-administration results in increased amprenavir plasma concentrations, decreased Cmax and increased Cmin). Products include:
Agenerase Capsules 1454
Agenerase Oral Solution 1459

Astemizole (Kaletra is an in vitro inhibitor of the CYP450 3A and inhibits CYP2D6 to a lesser extent; co-administration with drugs that are highly dependent on these isoforms for clearance and for which elevated plasma concentrations are associated with serious and/or life threatening events, such as astemizole, is contraindicated).
No products indexed under this heading.

Atorvastatin Calcium (Co-administration with HMG-CoA reductase inhibitors that are metabolized by the CYP3A pathway, such as atorvastatin, increases the risk of myopathy including rhabdomyolysis; caution is recommended). Products include:
Lipitor Tablets 2639
Lipitor Tablets 2696

Atovaquone (Co-administration can result in decreased atovaquone plasma concentrations; clinical significance is unknown; however, increase in atovaquone doses may be needed). Products include:
Malarone 1596
Mepron Suspension 1598

Bepridil Hydrochloride (Co-administration can result in increased bepridil plasma concentrations). Products include:
Vascor Tablets 2602

Carbamazepine (Co-administration can result in decreased lopinavir plasma concentrations; Kaletra may be less effective due to decreased lopinavir plasma concentrations). Products include:
Carbatrol Capsules 3234
Tegretol/Tegretol-XR 2404

Cerivastatin Sodium (Co-administration with HMG-CoA reductase inhibitors that are metabolized by the CYP3A pathway, such as cerivastatin, increases the risk of myopathy including rhabdomyolysis; caution is recommended). Products include:
Baycol Tablets 883

Cisapride (Kaletra is an in vitro inhibitor of the CYP450 3A and inhibits CYP2D6 to a lesser extent; co-administration with drugs that are highly dependent on these isoforms for clearance and for which elevated plasma concentrations are associated with serious and/or life threatening events, such as cisapride, is contraindicated).
No products indexed under this heading.

Clarithromycin (Co-administration can result in increased clarithromycin plasma concentrations; for patients with renal impairment, the dosage may need to be adjusted). Products include:
Biaxin/Biaxin XL 403
PREVPAC 3298

Cyclosporine (Co-administration results in increased plasma concentrations of immunosuppressants). Products include:
Gengraf Capsules 457
Neoral Soft Gelatin Capsules 2380
Neoral Oral Solution 2380
Sandimmune 2388

Delavirdine Mesylate (Co-administration has a potential to increase lopinavir plasma concentrations). Products include:
Rescriptor Tablets 526

Dexamethasone (Co-administration can result in decreased lopinavir plasma concentrations; Kaletra may be less effective due to decreased lopinavir plasma concentrations in patients taking these agents concomitantly). Products include:
Decadron Elixir 2078
Decadron Tablets 2079
TobraDex Ophthalmic Ointment 542
TobraDex Ophthalmic Suspension 541

Dexamethasone Acetate (Co-administration can result in decreased lopinavir plasma concentrations; Kaletra may be less effective due to decreased lopinavir plasma concentrations in patients taking these agents concomitantly).
No products indexed under this heading.

Dexamethasone Sodium Phosphate (Co-administration can result in decreased lopinavir plasma concentrations; Kaletra may be less effective due to decreased lopinavir plasma concentrations in patients taking these agents concomitantly). Products include:
Decadron Phosphate Injection 2081
Decadron Phosphate Sterile Ophthalmic Ointment 2083
Decadron Phosphate Sterile Ophthalmic Solution 2084
NeoDecadron Sterile Ophthalmic Solution 2144

Didanosine (Simultaneous administration is not recommended; it is recommended that didanosine be administered on an empty stomach; therefore, didanosine should be given one hour before or two hours after Kaletra). Products include:
Videx 1138
Videx EC Capsules 1143

Dihydroergotamine Mesylate (Kaletra is an in vitro inhibitor of the CYP450 3A and inhibits CYP2D6 to a lesser extent; co-administration with drugs that are highly dependent on these isoforms for clearance and for which elevated plasma concentrations are associated with serious and/or life-threatening events, such as ergot derivatives, is contraindicated). Products include:
D.H.E. 45 Injection 2334
Migranal Nasal Spray 2376

Disulfiram (Kaletra oral solution contains alcohol, which can produce disulfiram-like reactions when co-administered with disulfiram). Products include:
Antabuse Tablets 2444
Antabuse Tablets 3474

Efavirenz (Co-administration with efavirenz has a potential to decrease plasma concentrations of protease inhibitors by inducing the activity of CYP3A). Products include:
Sustiva Capsules 1258

Ergonovine Maleate (Kaletra is an in vitro inhibitor of the CYP450 3A and inhibits CYP2D6 to a lesser extent; co-administration with drugs that are highly dependent on these isoforms for clearance and for which elevated plasma concentrations are associated with serious and/or life-threatening events, such as ergot derivatives, is contraindicated).
No products indexed under this heading.

Ergotamine Tartrate (Kaletra is an in vitro inhibitor of the CYP450 3A and inhibits CYP2D6 to a lesser extent; co-administration with drugs that are highly dependent on these isoforms for clearance and for which elevated plasma concentrations are associated with serious and/or life-threatening events, such as ergot derivatives, is contraindicated).
No products indexed under this heading.

Ethinyl Estradiol (Co-administration results in decreased plasma concentrations of ethinyl estradiol; alternative or additional contraceptive measures should be used when estrogen-based oral contraceptive and Kaletra are co-administered). Products include:
Alesse-21 Tablets 3468
Alesse-28 Tablets 3473
Brevicon 28-Day Tablets 3380
Cyclessa Tablets 2450
Desogen Tablets 2458
Estinyl Tablets 3112
Estrostep 2627
femhrt Tablets 2635
Levlen 962
Levlite 21 Tablets 962
Levlite 28 Tablets 962
Levora Tablets 3389
Loestrin 21 Tablets 2642
Loestrin Fe Tablets 2642
Lo/Ovral Tablets 3532
Lo/Ovral-28 Tablets 3538
Low-Ogestrel-28 Tablets 3392
Microgestin Fe 1.5/30 Tablets 3407
Microgestin Fe 1/20 Tablets 3400
Mircette Tablets 2470

Modicon 2563
Necon 3415
Nordette-28 Tablets 2257
Norinyl 1 +35 28-Day Tablets 3380
Ogestrel 0.5/50-28 Tablets 3428
Ortho-Cept 21 Tablets 2546
Ortho-Cept 28 Tablets 2546
Ortho-Cyclen/Ortho Tri-Cyclen 2573
Ortho-Novum 2563
Ovcon 3364
Ovral Tablets 3551
Ovral-28 Tablets 3552
Tri-Levlen 962
Tri-Norinyl-28 Tablets 3433
Triphasil-21 Tablets 3600
Triphasil-28 Tablets 3605
Trivora Tablets 3439
Yasmin 28 Tablets 980
Zovia 3449

Flecainide Acetate (Kaletra is an in vitro inhibitor of the CYP450 3A and inhibits CYP2D6 to a lesser extent; co-administration with drugs that are highly dependent on these isoforms for clearance and for which elevated plasma concentrations are associated with serious and/or life threatening events, such as flecainide, is contraindicated). Products include:
Tambocor Tablets 1990

Fosphenytoin Sodium (Co-administration can result in decreased lopinavir plasma concentrations; Kaletra may be less effective due to decreased lopinavir plasma concentrations). Products include:
Cerebyx Injection 2619

Hypericum (Co-administration is expected to substantially decrease protease inhibitor concentrations and may result in sub-optimal levels of lopinavir and lead to loss of virologic response and possible resistance to lopinavir or to the class of protease inhibitors; concomitant use is not recommended). Products include:
Brite-Life Caplets .... ▣795
Centrum St. John's Wort Softgels .... ▣853
Metabolic Nutrition System .... ▣798
Movana Tablets .... ▣832
One-A-Day Tension & Mood Softgels .... ▣808
ReSource Wellness StayCalm Caplets .... ▣826
Satiete Tablets .... ▣846

Indinavir Sulfate (Co-administration results in increased indinavir plasma concentrations, decreased Cmax and increased Cmin). Products include:
Crixivan Capsules 2070

Itraconazole (Co-administration can result in increased itraconazole plasma concentrations; high doses of itraconazole (>200 mg/day) are not recommended). Products include:
Sporanox Capsules 1800
Sporanox Injection 1804
Sporanox Injection 2509
Sporanox Oral Solution 1808
Sporanox Oral Solution 2512

Ketoconazole (Co-administration can result in increased ketoconazole plasma concentrations; high doses of ketoconazole (>200 mg/day) are not recommended). Products include:
Nizoral 2% Cream 3620
Nizoral A-D Shampoo 2008
Nizoral 2% Shampoo 2007
Nizoral Tablets 1791

Lidocaine Hydrochloride (Co-administration with systemic lidocaine can result in increased lidocaine plasma concentrations). Products include:
Bactine First Aid Liquid .... ▣611
Xylocaine Injections 653

Lovastatin (Co-administration of Kaletra and lovastatin may increase the risk of myopathy, including rhabdomyolysis; concomitant use is not recommended). Products include:
Mevacor Tablets 2132

Methadone Hydrochloride (Co-administration results in decreased plasma concentrations of methadone; dosage of methadone may need to be increased when co-administered). Products include:
Dolophine Hydrochloride Tablets 3056

Methotrexate Sodium (Co-administration results in increased plasma concentrations of dihydropyridine calcium channel blockers).
No products indexed under this heading.

Methylergonovine Maleate (Kaletra is an in vitro inhibitor of the CYP450 3A and inhibits CYP2D6 to a lesser extent; co-administration with drugs that are highly dependent on these isoforms for clearance and for which elevated plasma concentrations are associated with serious and/or life-threatening events, such as ergot derivatives, is contraindicated).
No products indexed under this heading.

Methysergide Maleate (Kaletra is an in vitro inhibitor of the CYP450 3A and inhibits CYP2D6 to a lesser extent; co-administration with drugs that are highly dependent on these isoforms for clearance and for which elevated plasma concentrations are associated with serious and/or life-threatening events, such as ergot derivatives, is contraindicated).
No products indexed under this heading.

Metronidazole (Kaletra oral solution contains alcohol, which can produce disulfiram-like reactions when co-administered with disulfiram or other drugs that produce this reaction, such as metronidazole). Products include:
MetroCream 1404
MetroGel 1405
MetroGel-Vaginal Gel 1986
MetroLotion 1405
Noritate Cream 1224

Metronidazole Hydrochloride (Kaletra oral solution contains alcohol, which can produce disulfiram-like reactions when co-administered with disulfiram or other drugs that produce this reaction, such as metronidazole).
No products indexed under this heading.

Midazolam Hydrochloride (Kaletra is an in vitro inhibitor of the CYP450 3A and inhibits CYP2D6 to a lesser extent; co-administration with drugs that are highly dependent on these isoforms for clearance and for which elevated plasma concentrations are associated with serious and/or life threatening events, such as midazolam, is contraindicated). Products include:
Versed Injection 3027
Versed Syrup 3033

Nevirapine (Co-administration with nevirapine has a potential to decrease plasma concentrations of protease inhibitors by inducing the activity of CYP3A). Products include:
Viramune Oral Suspension 1060
Viramune Tablets 1060

Phenobarbital (Co-administration can result in decreased lopinavir plasma concentrations; Kaletra may be less effective due to decreased lopinavir plasma concentrations). Products include:
Arco-Lase Plus Tablets 592
Donnatal 2929
Donnatal Extentabs 2930

Phenytoin (Co-administration can result in decreased lopinavir plasma concentrations; Kaletra may be less effective due to decreased lopinavir plasma concentrations). Products include:
Dilantin Infatabs 2624
Dilantin-125 Oral Suspension 2625

Phenytoin Sodium (Co-administration can result in decreased lopinavir plasma concentrations; Kaletra may be less effective due to decreased lopinavir plasma concentrations). Products include:
Dilantin Kapseals 2622

Pimozide (Kaletra is an in vitro inhibitor of the CYP450 3A and inhibits CYP2D6 to a lesser extent; co-administration with drugs that are highly dependent on these isoforms for clearance and for which elevated plasma concentrations are associated with serious and/or life threatening events, such as pimozide, is contraindicated). Products include:
Orap Tablets 1407

Propafenone Hydrochloride (Kaletra is an in vitro inhibitor of the CYP450 3A and inhibits CYP2D6 to a lesser extent; co-administration with drugs that are highly dependent on these isoforms for clearance and for which elevated plasma concentrations are associated with serious and/or life threatening events, such as propafenone, is contraindicated). Products include:
Rythmol Tablets – 150 mg, 225 mg, 300 mg 502

Quinidine Gluconate (Co-administration can result in increased quinidine plasma concentrations). Products include:
Quinaglute Dura-Tabs Tablets 978

Quinidine Polygalacturonate (Co-administration can result in increased quinidine plasma concentrations).
No products indexed under this heading.

Quinidine Sulfate (Co-administration can result in increased quinidine plasma concentrations). Products include:
Quinidex Extentabs 2933

Rapamycin (Co-administration results in increased plasma concentrations of immunosuppressants).
No products indexed under this heading.

Rifabutin (Co-administration can result in increased rifabutin and rifabutin metabolite plasma concentrations; dosage reduction of rifabutin by at least 75% of the usual dose of 300 mg/day is recommended; increased monitoring for adverse reactions is warranted). Products include:
Mycobutin Capsules 2838

Rifampin (Co-administration may lead to loss of virologic response and possible resistance to Kaletra; concomitant use should be avoided). Products include:
Rifadin 765
Rifamate Capsules 767
Rifater Tablets 769

Ritonavir (Co-administration results in increased lopinavir plasma concentrations; appropriate doses of additional ritonavir in combination with Kaletra with safety and efficacy have not been established).

Saquinavir (Co-administration results in increased saquinavir plasma concentrations, decreased Cmax and increased Cmin). Products include:
Fortovase Capsules 2970

Saquinavir Mesylate (Co-administration results in increased saquinavir plasma concentrations, decreased Cmax and increased Cmin). Products include:
Invirase Capsules 2979

Sildenafil Citrate (Co-administration is expected to substantially increase sildenafil concentrations and may result in an increase in sildenafil-associated adverse events including hypotension, syncope, visual changes and prolonged erection). Products include:
Viagra Tablets 2732

Simvastatin (Co-administration of Kaletra and simvastatin may increase the risk of myopathy, including rhabdomyolysis; concomitant use is not recommended). Products include:
Zocor Tablets 2219

Tacrolimus (Co-administration results in increased plasma concentrations of immunosuppressants). Products include:
Prograf 1393
Protopic Ointment 1397

Terfenadine (Kaletra is an in vitro inhibitor of the CYP450 3A and inhibits CYP2D6 to a lesser extent; co-administration with drugs that are highly dependent on these isoforms for clearance and for which elevated plasma concentrations are associated with serious and/or life threatening events, such as terfenadine, is contraindicated).
No products indexed under this heading.

Triazolam (Kaletra is an in vitro inhibitor of the CYP450 3A and inhibits CYP2D6 to a lesser extent; co-administration with drugs that are highly dependent on these isoforms for clearance and for which elevated plasma concentrations are associated with serious and/or life threatening events, such as triazolam, is contraindicated). Products include:
Halcion Tablets 2823

Trimethoprim (Co-administration results in increased plasma concentrations of dihydropyridine calcium channel blockers). Products include:
Bactrim 2949
Septra Suspension 2265
Septra Tablets 2265
Septra DS Tablets 2265

Trimetrexate Glucuronate (Co-administration results in increased plasma concentrations of dihydropyridine calcium channel blockers).
No products indexed under this heading.

Warfarin Sodium (Co-administration can affect concentrations of warfarin; it is recommended that INR be monitored). Products include:
Coumadin for Injection 1243
Coumadin Tablets 1243
Warfarin Sodium Tablets, USP 3302

Zidovudine (Kaletra induces glucuronidation; therefore, Kaletra has the potential to reduce zidovudine plasma concentrations; the clinical significance is unknown). Products include:
Combivir Tablets 1502
Retrovir 1625
Retrovir IV Infusion 1629
Trizivir Tablets 1669

Food Interactions

Food, unspecified (Co-administration with moderate fat meal was associated with a mean increase in AUC and Cmax; to enhance bioavailability Kaletra should be taken with food).

KALETRA ORAL SOLUTION

(Lopinavir, Ritonavir) 471
See Kaletra Capsules

K-DUR MICROBURST RELEASE SYSTEM ER TABLETS

(Potassium Chloride) 1832
May interact with ACE inhibitors, anticholinergics, potassium sparing diuretics, and certain other agents. Compounds in these categories include:

Amiloride Hydrochloride (Co-administration of these agents can

produce severe hyperkalemia; concurrent use is not recommended). Products include:

Midamor Tablets ... 2136
Moduretic Tablets ... 2138

Atropine Sulfate (Concurrent use with anticholinergic drugs or other agents with anticholinergic properties at sufficient doses to exert anticholinergic effects is contraindicated). Products include:

Donnatal ... 2929
Donnatal Extentabs ... 2930
Motofen Tablets ... 577
Prosed/DS Tablets ... 3268
Urised Tablets ... 2876

Belladonna Alkaloids (Concurrent use with anticholinergic drugs or other agents with anticholinergic properties at sufficient doses to exert anticholinergic effects is contraindicated). Products include:

Hyland's Teething Tablets ... ◼766
Urimax Tablets ... 1769

Benazepril Hydrochloride (Potential for increased potassium retention). Products include:

Lotensin Tablets ... 2365
Lotensin HCT Tablets ... 2367
Lotrel Capsules ... 2370

Benztropine Mesylate (Concurrent use with anticholinergic drugs or other agents with anticholinergic properties at sufficient doses to exert anticholinergic effects is contraindicated). Products include:

Cogentin ... 2055

Biperiden Hydrochloride (Concurrent use with anticholinergic drugs or other agents with anticholinergic properties at sufficient doses to exert anticholinergic effects is contraindicated). Products include:

Akineton ... 402

Captopril (Potential for increased potassium retention). Products include:

Captopril Tablets ... 2281

Clidinium Bromide (Concurrent use with anticholinergic drugs or other agents with anticholinergic properties at sufficient doses to exert anticholinergic effects is contraindicated).

No products indexed under this heading.

Dicyclomine Hydrochloride (Concurrent use with anticholinergic drugs or other agents with anticholinergic properties at sufficient doses to exert anticholinergic effects is contraindicated).

No products indexed under this heading.

Enalapril Maleate (Potential for increased potassium retention). Products include:

Lexxel Tablets ... 608
Vaseretic Tablets ... 2204
Vasotec Tablets ... 2210

Enalaprilat (Potential for increased potassium retention). Products include:

Enalaprilat Injection ... 863
Vasotec I.V. Injection ... 2207

Fosinopril Sodium (Potential for increased potassium retention). Products include:

Monopril Tablets ... 1091
Monopril HCT ... 1094

Glycopyrrolate (Concurrent use with anticholinergic drugs or other agents with anticholinergic properties at sufficient doses to exert anticholinergic effects is contraindicated). Products include:

Robinul Forte Tablets ... 1358
Robinul Injectable ... 2940
Robinul Tablets ... 1358

Hyoscyamine (Concurrent use with anticholinergic drugs or other agents with anticholinergic properties at sufficient doses to exert anticholinergic effects is contraindicated). Products include:

Urised Tablets ... 2876

Hyoscyamine Sulfate (Concurrent use with anticholinergic drugs or other agents with anticholinergic properties at sufficient doses to exert anticholinergic effects is contraindicated). Products include:

Arco-Lase Plus Tablets ... 592
Donnatal ... 2929
Donnatal Extentabs ... 2930
Levsin/Levsinex/Levbid ... 3172
NuLev Orally Disintegrating Tablets ... 3176
Prosed/DS Tablets ... 3268
Urimax Tablets ... 1769

Ipratropium Bromide (Concurrent use with anticholinergic drugs or other agents with anticholinergic properties at sufficient doses to exert anticholinergic effects is contraindicated). Products include:

Atrovent Inhalation Aerosol ... 1030
Atrovent Inhalation Solution ... 1031
Atrovent Nasal Spray 0.03% ... 1032
Atrovent Nasal Spray 0.06% ... 1033
Combivent Inhalation Aerosol ... 1041
DuoNeb Inhalation Solution ... 1233

Lisinopril (Potential for increased potassium retention). Products include:

Prinivil Tablets ... 2164
Prinzide Tablets ... 2168
Zestoretic Tablets ... 695
Zestril Tablets ... 698

Mepenzolate Bromide (Concurrent use with anticholinergic drugs or other agents with anticholinergic properties at sufficient doses to exert anticholinergic effects is contraindicated).

No products indexed under this heading.

Moexipril Hydrochloride (Potential for increased potassium retention). Products include:

Uniretic Tablets ... 3178
Univasc Tablets ... 3181

Oxybutynin Chloride (Concurrent use with anticholinergic drugs or other agents with anticholinergic properties at sufficient doses to exert anticholinergic effects is contraindicated). Products include:

Ditropan XL Extended Release Tablets ... 564

Perindopril Erbumine (Potential for increased potassium retention). Products include:

Aceon Tablets (2 mg, 4 mg, 8 mg) ... 3249

Procyclidine Hydrochloride (Concurrent use with anticholinergic drugs or other agents with anticholinergic properties at sufficient doses to exert anticholinergic effects is contraindicated).

No products indexed under this heading.

Propantheline Bromide (Concurrent use with anticholinergic drugs or other agents with anticholinergic properties at sufficient doses to exert anticholinergic effects is contraindicated).

No products indexed under this heading.

Quinapril Hydrochloride (Potential for increased potassium retention). Products include:

Accupril Tablets ... 2611
Accuretic Tablets ... 2614

Ramipril (Potential for increased potassium retention). Products include:

Altace Capsules ... 2233

Scopolamine (Concurrent use with anticholinergic drugs or other agents with anticholinergic properties at sufficient doses to exert anticholinergic effects is contraindicated). Products include:

Transderm Scōp Transdermal Therapeutic System ... 2302

Scopolamine Hydrobromide (Concurrent use with anticholinergic drugs or other agents with anticholinergic properties at sufficient doses to exert anticholinergic effects is contraindicated). Products include:

Donnatal ... 2929
Donnatal Extentabs ... 2930

Spirapril Hydrochloride (Potential for increased potassium retention).

No products indexed under this heading.

Spironolactone (Co-administration of these agents can produce severe hyperkalemia; concurrent use is not recommended).

No products indexed under this heading.

Tolterodine Tartrate (Concurrent use with anticholinergic drugs or other agents with anticholinergic properties at sufficient doses to exert anticholinergic effects is contraindicated). Products include:

Detrol Tablets ... 3623
Detrol LA Capsules ... 2801

Trandolapril (Potential for increased potassium retention). Products include:

Mavik Tablets ... 478
Tarka Tablets ... 508

Triamterene (Co-administration of these agents can produce severe hyperkalemia; concurrent use is not recommended). Products include:

Dyazide Capsules ... 1515
Dyrenium Capsules ... 3458
Maxzide ... 1008

Tridihexethyl Chloride (Concurrent use with anticholinergic drugs or other agents with anticholinergic properties at sufficient doses to exert anticholinergic effects is contraindicated).

No products indexed under this heading.

Trihexyphenidyl Hydrochloride (Concurrent use with anticholinergic drugs or other agents with anticholinergic properties at sufficient doses to exert anticholinergic effects is contraindicated). Products include:

Artane ... 1855

KEFLEX ORAL SUSPENSION

(Cephalexin) ... 1237

See Keflex Pulvules

KEFLEX PULVULES

(Cephalexin) ... 1237

May interact with:

Probenecid (The renal excretion of cephalexin is inhibited by probenecid).

No products indexed under this heading.

KEFUROX VIALS, ADD-VANTAGE

(Cefuroxime Sodium) ... 1948

May interact with aminoglycosides and diuretics. Compounds in these categories include:

Amikacin Sulfate (Co-administration of cephalosporins with aminoglycosides has resulted in nephrotoxicity).

No products indexed under this heading.

Amiloride Hydrochloride (Co-administration of cephalosporins with potent diuretics may result in possible adverse effects on kidney function). Products include:

Midamor Tablets ... 2136
Moduretic Tablets ... 2138

Bendroflumethiazide (Co-administration of cephalosporins with potent diuretics may result in possible adverse effects on kidney function). Products include:

Corzide 40/5 Tablets ... 2247
Corzide 80/5 Tablets ... 2247

Bumetanide (Co-administration of cephalosporins with potent diuretics may result in possible adverse effects on kidney function).

No products indexed under this heading.

Chlorothiazide (Co-administration of cephalosporins with potent diuretics may result in possible adverse effects on kidney function). Products include:

Aldoclor Tablets ... 2035
Diuril Oral ... 2087

Chlorothiazide Sodium (Co-administration of cephalosporins with potent diuretics may result in possible adverse effects on kidney function). Products include:

Diuril Sodium Intravenous ... 2086

Chlorthalidone (Co-administration of cephalosporins with potent diuretics may result in possible adverse effects on kidney function). Products include:

Clorpres Tablets ... 1002
Combipres Tablets ... 1040
Tenoretic Tablets ... 690

Ethacrynic Acid (Co-administration of cephalosporins with potent diuretics may result in possible adverse effects on kidney function). Products include:

Edecrin Tablets ... 2091

Furosemide (Co-administration of cephalosporins with potent diuretics may result in possible adverse effects on kidney function). Products include:

Furosemide Tablets ... 2284

Gentamicin Sulfate (Co-administration of cephalosporins with aminoglycosides has resulted in nephrotoxicity). Products include:

Genoptic Ophthalmic Ointment ... ⊙239
Genoptic Sterile Ophthalmic Solution ... ⊙239
Pred-G Ophthalmic Suspension ... ⊙247
Pred-G Sterile Ophthalmic Ointment ... ⊙248

Hydrochlorothiazide (Co-administration of cephalosporins with potent diuretics may result in possible adverse effects on kidney function). Products include:

Accuretic Tablets ... 2614
Aldoril Tablets ... 2039
Atacand HCT Tablets ... 597
Avalide Tablets ... 1070
Diovan HCT Tablets ... 2338
Dyazide Capsules ... 1515
HydroDIURIL Tablets ... 2108
Hyzaar ... 2109
Inderide Tablets ... 3517
Inderide LA Long-Acting Capsules ... 3519
Lotensin HCT Tablets ... 2367
Maxzide ... 1008
Micardis HCT Tablets ... 1051
Microzide Capsules ... 3414
Moduretic Tablets ... 2138
Monopril HCT ... 1094
Prinzide Tablets ... 2168
Timolide Tablets ... 2187
Uniretic Tablets ... 3178
Vaseretic Tablets ... 2204
Zestoretic Tablets ... 695
Ziac Tablets ... 1887

Hydroflumethiazide (Co-administration of cephalosporins with potent diuretics may result in possible adverse effects on kidney function). Products include:

Diucardin Tablets ... 3494

Indapamide (Co-administration of cephalosporins with potent diuretics may result in possible adverse effects on kidney function). Products include:

Indapamide Tablets ... 2286

Kanamycin Sulfate (Co-administration of cephalosporins with aminoglycosides has resulted in nephrotoxicity).

No products indexed under this heading.

Methyclothiazide (Co-administration of cephalosporins with potent diuretics may result in possible adverse effects on kidney

function).
No products indexed under this heading.

Metolazone (Co-administration of cephalosporins with potent diuretics may result in possible adverse effects on kidney function). Products include:
- Mykrox Tablets ... 1168
- Zaroxolyn Tablets ... 1177

Polythiazide (Co-administration of cephalosporins with potent diuretics may result in possible adverse effects on kidney function). Products include:
- Minizide Capsules ... 2700
- Renese Tablets ... 2712

Spironolactone (Co-administration of cephalosporins with potent diuretics may result in possible adverse effects on kidney function).
No products indexed under this heading.

Streptomycin Sulfate (Co-administration of cephalosporins with aminoglycosides has resulted in nephrotoxicity). Products include:
- Streptomycin Sulfate Injection ... 2714

Tobramycin (Co-administration of cephalosporins with aminoglycosides has resulted in nephrotoxicity). Products include:
- TOBI Solution for Inhalation ... 1206
- TobraDex Ophthalmic Ointment ... 542
- TobraDex Ophthalmic Suspension ... 541
- Tobrex Ophthalmic Ointment ... ⊙220
- Tobrex Ophthalmic Solution ... ⊙221

Tobramycin Sulfate (Co-administration of cephalosporins with aminoglycosides has resulted in nephrotoxicity). Products include:
- Nebcin Vials, Hyporets & ADD-Vantage ... 1955

Torsemide (Co-administration of cephalosporins with potent diuretics may result in possible adverse effects on kidney function). Products include:
- Demadex Tablets and Injection ... 2965

Triamterene (Co-administration of cephalosporins with potent diuretics may result in possible adverse effects on kidney function). Products include:
- Dyazide Capsules ... 1515
- Dyrenium Capsules ... 3458
- Maxzide ... 1008

KEFZOL VIALS, ADD-VANTAGE

(Cefazolin Sodium) ... 1951
May interact with:

Probenecid (May decrease renal tubular secretion of cephalosporins resulting in increased and more prolonged cephalosporin blood levels).
No products indexed under this heading.

KEPPRA TABLETS

(Levetiracetam) ... 3314
May interact with:

Probenecid (Co-administration has resulted in double Cmax of the metabolite, ucb L057, while the fraction of the drug excreted unchanged in the urine; renal clearance of ucb L057 in the presence of probenecid decreased 60%).
No products indexed under this heading.

Food Interactions

Food, unspecified (Decreases Cmax by 20% and delays Tmax by 1.5 hours, does not affect the extent of absorption).

KLARON LOTION 10%

(Sulfacetamide Sodium) ... 1224
None cited in PDR database.

KLONOPIN TABLETS

(Clonazepam) ... 2983
May interact with central nervous system depressants, anticonvulsants, monoamine oxidase inhibitors, phenytoin, tricyclic antidepressants, and certain other agents. Compounds in these categories include:

Alfentanil Hydrochloride (Potentiates CNS-depressant action).
No products indexed under this heading.

Alprazolam (Potentiates CNS-depressant action). Products include:
- Xanax Tablets ... 2865

Amitriptyline Hydrochloride (Potentiates CNS-depressant action). Products include:
- Etrafon ... 3115
- Limbitrol ... 1738

Amoxapine (Potentiates CNS-depressant action).
No products indexed under this heading.

Aprobarbital (Potentiates CNS-depressant action).
No products indexed under this heading.

Buprenorphine Hydrochloride (Potentiates CNS-depressant action). Products include:
- Buprenex Injectable ... 2918

Buspirone Hydrochloride (Potentiates CNS-depressant action).
No products indexed under this heading.

Butabarbital (Potentiates CNS-depressant action).
No products indexed under this heading.

Butalbital (Potentiates CNS-depressant action). Products include:
- Phrenilin ... 578
- Sedapap Tablets 50 mg/650 mg ... 2225

Carbamazepine (Induces clonazepam metabolism causing an approximately 30% decrease in plasma clonazepam levels). Products include:
- Carbatrol Capsules ... 3234
- Tegretol/Tegretol-XR ... 2404

Chlordiazepoxide (Potentiates CNS-depressant action). Products include:
- Limbitrol ... 1738

Chlordiazepoxide Hydrochloride (Potentiates CNS-depressant action). Products include:
- Librium Capsules ... 1736
- Librium for Injection ... 1737

Chlorpromazine (Potentiates CNS-depressant action). Products include:
- Thorazine Suppositories ... 1656

Chlorpromazine Hydrochloride (Potentiates CNS-depressant action). Products include:
- Thorazine ... 1656

Chlorprothixene (Potentiates CNS-depressant action).
No products indexed under this heading.

Chlorprothixene Hydrochloride (Potentiates CNS-depressant action).
No products indexed under this heading.

Chlorprothixene Lactate (Potentiates CNS-depressant action).
No products indexed under this heading.

Clomipramine Hydrochloride (Potentiates CNS-depressant action).
No products indexed under this heading.

Clorazepate Dipotassium (Potentiates CNS-depressant action). Products include:
- Tranxene ... 511

Clozapine (Potentiates CNS-depressant action). Products include:
- Clozaril Tablets ... 2319

Codeine Phosphate (Potentiates CNS-depressant action). Products include:
- Phenergan with Codeine Syrup ... 3557
- Phenergan VC with Codeine Syrup ... 3561
- Robitussin A-C Syrup ... 2942
- Robitussin-DAC Syrup ... 2942
- Ryna-C Liquid ... ■768
- Soma Compound w/Codeine Tablets ... 3355
- Tussi-Organidin NR Liquid ... 3350
- Tussi-Organidin-S NR Liquid ... 3350
- Tylenol with Codeine ... 2595

Desflurane (Potentiates CNS-depressant action). Products include:
- Suprane Liquid for Inhalation ... 874

Desipramine Hydrochloride (Potentiates CNS-depressant action). Products include:
- Norpramin Tablets ... 755

Dezocine (Potentiates CNS-depressant action).
No products indexed under this heading.

Diazepam (Potentiates CNS-depressant action). Products include:
- Valium Injectable ... 3026
- Valium Tablets ... 3047

Divalproex Sodium (Potentiates CNS-depressant action). Products include:
- Depakote Sprinkle Capsules ... 426
- Depakote Tablets ... 430
- Depakote ER Tablets ... 436

Doxepin Hydrochloride (Potentiates CNS-depressant action). Products include:
- Sinequan ... 2713

Droperidol (Potentiates CNS-depressant action).
No products indexed under this heading.

Enflurane (Potentiates CNS-depressant action).
No products indexed under this heading.

Estazolam (Potentiates CNS-depressant action). Products include:
- ProSom Tablets ... 500

Ethchlorvynol (Potentiates CNS-depressant action).
No products indexed under this heading.

Ethinamate (Potentiates CNS-depressant action).
No products indexed under this heading.

Ethosuximide (Potentiates CNS-depressant action). Products include:
- Zarontin Capsules ... 2659
- Zarontin Syrup ... 2660

Ethotoin (Potentiates CNS-depressant action).
No products indexed under this heading.

Felbamate (Potentiates CNS-depressant action). Products include:
- Felbatol ... 3343

Fentanyl (Potentiates CNS-depressant action). Products include:
- Duragesic Transdermal System ... 1786

Fentanyl Citrate (Potentiates CNS-depressant action). Products include:
- Actiq ... 1184

Fluphenazine Decanoate (Potentiates CNS-depressant action).
No products indexed under this heading.

Fluphenazine Enanthate (Potentiates CNS-depressant action).
No products indexed under this heading.

Fluphenazine Hydrochloride (Potentiates CNS-depressant action).
No products indexed under this heading.

Flurazepam Hydrochloride (Potentiates CNS-depressant action).
No products indexed under this heading.

Fosphenytoin Sodium (Induces clonazepam metabolism causing an approximately 30% decrease in plasma clonazepam levels). Products include:
- Cerebyx Injection ... 2619

Glutethimide (Potentiates CNS-depressant action).
No products indexed under this heading.

Haloperidol (Potentiates CNS-depressant action). Products include:
- Haldol Injection, Tablets and Concentrate ... 2533

Haloperidol Decanoate (Potentiates CNS-depressant action). Products include:
- Haldol Decanoate ... 2535

Hydrocodone Bitartrate (Potentiates CNS-depressant action). Products include:
- Hycodan ... 1316
- Hycomine Compound Tablets ... 1317
- Hycotuss Expectorant Syrup ... 1318
- Lortab ... 3319
- Lortab Elixir ... 3317
- Maxidone Tablets CIII ... 3399
- Norco 5/325 Tablets CIII ... 3424
- Norco 7.5/325 Tablets CIII ... 3425
- Norco 10/325 Tablets CIII ... 3427
- Norco 10/325 Tablets CIII ... 3425
- Vicodin Tablets ... 516
- Vicodin ES Tablets ... 517
- Vicodin HP Tablets ... 518
- Vicodin Tuss Expectorant ... 519
- Vicoprofen Tablets ... 520
- Zydone Tablets ... 1330

Hydrocodone Polistirex (Potentiates CNS-depressant action). Products include:
- Tussionex Pennkinetic Extended-Release Suspension ... 1174

Hydromorphone Hydrochloride (Potentiates CNS-depressant action). Products include:
- Dilaudid ... 441
- Dilaudid Oral Liquid ... 445
- Dilaudid Powder ... 441
- Dilaudid Rectal Suppositories ... 441
- Dilaudid Tablets ... 441
- Dilaudid Tablets - 8 mg ... 445
- Dilaudid-HP ... 443

Hydroxyzine Hydrochloride (Potentiates CNS-depressant action). Products include:
- Atarax Tablets & Syrup ... 2667
- Vistaril Intramuscular Solution ... 2738

Imipramine Hydrochloride (Potentiates CNS-depressant action).
No products indexed under this heading.

Imipramine Pamoate (Potentiates CNS-depressant action).
No products indexed under this heading.

Isocarboxazid (Potentiates CNS-depressant action).
No products indexed under this heading.

Isoflurane (Potentiates CNS-depressant action).
No products indexed under this heading.

Itraconazole (Co-administration with CYP450 3A inhibitors should be undertaken with caution). Products include:
- Sporanox Capsules ... 1800
- Sporanox Injection ... 1804
- Sporanox Injection ... 2509
- Sporanox Oral Solution ... 1808
- Sporanox Oral Solution ... 2512

Ketamine Hydrochloride (Potentiates CNS-depressant action).
No products indexed under this heading.

Ketoconazole (Co-administration with CYP450 3A inhibitors should be undertaken with caution). Products include:
- Nizoral 2% Cream ... 3620

Nizoral A-D Shampoo 2008
Nizoral 2% Shampoo 2007
Nizoral Tablets 1791

Lamotrigine (Potentiates CNS-depressant action). Products include:
Lamictal 1567

Levetiracetam (Potentiates CNS-depressant action). Products include:
Keppra Tablets 3314

Levomethadyl Acetate Hydrochloride (Potentiates CNS-depressant action).
No products indexed under this heading.

Levorphanol Tartrate (Potentiates CNS-depressant action). Products include:
Levo-Dromoran 1734
Levorphanol Tartrate Tablets 3059

Lorazepam (Potentiates CNS-depressant action). Products include:
Ativan Injection 3478
Ativan Tablets 3482

Loxapine Hydrochloride (Potentiates CNS-depressant action).
No products indexed under this heading.

Loxapine Succinate (Potentiates CNS-depressant action). Products include:
Loxitane Capsules 3398

Maprotiline Hydrochloride (Potentiates CNS-depressant action).
No products indexed under this heading.

Meperidine Hydrochloride (Potentiates CNS-depressant action). Products include:
Demerol 3079
Mepergan Injection 3539

Mephenytoin (Potentiates CNS-depressant action).
No products indexed under this heading.

Mephobarbital (Potentiates CNS-depressant action).
No products indexed under this heading.

Meprobamate (Potentiates CNS-depressant action). Products include:
Miltown Tablets 3349

Mesoridazine Besylate (Potentiates CNS-depressant action). Products include:
Serentil 1057

Methadone Hydrochloride (Potentiates CNS-depressant action). Products include:
Dolophine Hydrochloride Tablets 3056

Methohexital Sodium (Potentiates CNS-depressant action). Products include:
Brevital Sodium for Injection, USP .. 1815

Methotrimeprazine (Potentiates CNS-depressant action).
No products indexed under this heading.

Methoxyflurane (Potentiates CNS-depressant action).
No products indexed under this heading.

Methsuximide (Potentiates CNS-depressant action). Products include:
Celontin Capsules 2618

Midazolam Hydrochloride (Potentiates CNS-depressant action). Products include:
Versed Injection 3027
Versed Syrup 3033

Moclobemide (Potentiates CNS-depressant action).
No products indexed under this heading.

Molindone Hydrochloride (Potentiates CNS-depressant action). Products include:
Moban 1320

Morphine Sulfate (Potentiates CNS-depressant action). Products include:
Astramorph/PF Injection, USP (Preservative-Free).................... 594
Duramorph Injection 1312
Infumorph 200 and Infumorph 500 Sterile Solutions.................... 1314
Kadian Capsules 1335
MS Contin Tablets 2896
MSIR 2898
Oramorph SR Tablets 3062
Roxanol 3066

Nortriptyline Hydrochloride (Potentiates CNS-depressant action).
No products indexed under this heading.

Olanzapine (Potentiates CNS-depressant action). Products include:
Zyprexa Tablets 1973
Zyprexa ZYDIS Orally Disintegrating Tablets.................... 1973

Oxazepam (Potentiates CNS-depressant action).
No products indexed under this heading.

Oxcarbazepine (Potentiates CNS-depressant action). Products include:
Trileptal Oral Suspension 2407
Trileptal Tablets 2407

Oxycodone Hydrochloride (Potentiates CNS-depressant action). Products include:
OxyContin Tablets 2912
OxyFast Oral Concentrate Solution . 2916
OxyIR Capsules 2916
Percocet Tablets 1326
Percodan Tablets 1327
Percolone Tablets 1327
Roxicodone 3067
Tylox Capsules 2597

Paramethadione (Potentiates CNS-depressant action).
No products indexed under this heading.

Pargyline Hydrochloride (Potentiates CNS-depressant action).
No products indexed under this heading.

Pentobarbital Sodium (Potentiates CNS-depressant action). Products include:
Nembutal Sodium Solution 485

Perphenazine (Potentiates CNS-depressant action). Products include:
Etrafon 3115
Trilafon 3160

Phenacemide (Potentiates CNS-depressant action).
No products indexed under this heading.

Phenelzine Sulfate (Potentiates CNS-depressant action). Products include:
Nardil Tablets 2653

Phenobarbital (Induces clonazepam metabolism causing an approximately 30% decrease in plasma clonazepam levels; CNS depressant action may be potentiated). Products include:
Arco-Lase Plus Tablets 592
Donnatal 2929
Donnatal Extentabs 2930

Phensuximide (Potentiates CNS-depressant action).
No products indexed under this heading.

Phenytoin (Induces clonazepam metabolism causing an approximately 30% decrease in plasma clonazepam levels). Products include:
Dilantin Infatabs 2624
Dilantin-125 Oral Suspension 2625

Phenytoin Sodium (Induces clonazepam metabolism causing an approximately 30% decrease in plasma clonazepam levels). Products include:
Dilantin Kapseals 2622

Prazepam (Potentiates CNS-depressant action).
No products indexed under this heading.

Primidone (Potentiates CNS-depressant action).
No products indexed under this heading.

Procarbazine Hydrochloride (Potentiates CNS-depressant action). Products include:
Matulane Capsules 3246

Prochlorperazine (Potentiates CNS-depressant action). Products include:
Compazine 1505

Promethazine Hydrochloride (Potentiates CNS-depressant action). Products include:
Mepergan Injection 3539
Phenergan Injection 3553
Phenergan 3556
Phenergan Syrup 3554
Phenergan with Codeine Syrup 3557
Phenergan with Dextromethorphan Syrup 3559
Phenergan VC Syrup 3560
Phenergan VC with Codeine Syrup .. 3561

Propofol (Potentiates CNS-depressant action). Products include:
Diprivan Injectable Emulsion 667

Propoxyphene Hydrochloride (Potentiates CNS-depressant action). Products include:
Darvon Pulvules 1909
Darvon Compound-65 Pulvules 1910

Propoxyphene Napsylate (Potentiates CNS-depressant action). Products include:
Darvon-N/Darvocet-N 1907
Darvon-N Tablets 1912

Protriptyline Hydrochloride (Potentiates CNS-depressant action). Products include:
Vivactil Tablets 2446
Vivactil Tablets 2217

Quazepam (Potentiates CNS-depressant action).
No products indexed under this heading.

Quetiapine Fumarate (Potentiates CNS-depressant action). Products include:
Seroquel Tablets 684

Remifentanil Hydrochloride (Potentiates CNS-depressant action).
No products indexed under this heading.

Risperidone (Potentiates CNS-depressant action). Products include:
Risperdal 1796

Secobarbital Sodium (Potentiates CNS-depressant action).
No products indexed under this heading.

Selegiline Hydrochloride (Potentiates CNS-depressant action). Products include:
Eldepryl Capsules 3266

Sevoflurane (Potentiates CNS-depressant action).
No products indexed under this heading.

Sufentanil Citrate (Potentiates CNS-depressant action).
No products indexed under this heading.

Temazepam (Potentiates CNS-depressant action).
No products indexed under this heading.

Thiamylal Sodium (Potentiates CNS-depressant action).
No products indexed under this heading.

Thioridazine Hydrochloride (Potentiates CNS-depressant action). Products include:
Thioridazine Hydrochloride Tablets.................... 2289

Thiothixene (Potentiates CNS-depressant action). Products include:
Navane Capsules 2701
Thiothixene Capsules 2290

Tiagabine Hydrochloride (Potentiates CNS-depressant action). Products include:
Gabitril Tablets 1189

Topiramate (Potentiates CNS-depressant action). Products include:
Topamax Sprinkle Capsules 2590
Topamax Tablets 2590

Tranylcypromine Sulfate (Potentiates CNS-depressant action). Products include:
Parnate Tablets 1607

Triazolam (Potentiates CNS-depressant action). Products include:
Halcion Tablets 2823

Trifluoperazine Hydrochloride (Potentiates CNS-depressant action). Products include:
Stelazine 1640

Trimethadione (Potentiates CNS-depressant action).
No products indexed under this heading.

Trimipramine Maleate (Potentiates CNS-depressant action). Products include:
Surmontil Capsules 3595

Valproate Sodium (Potentiates CNS-depressant action). Products include:
Depacon Injection 416

Valproic Acid (Potentiates CNS-depressant action). Products include:
Depakene 421

Zaleplon (Potentiates CNS-depressant action). Products include:
Sonata Capsules 3591

Ziprasidone Hydrochloride (Potentiates CNS-depressant action). Products include:
Geodon Capsules 2688

Zolpidem Tartrate (Potentiates CNS-depressant action). Products include:
Ambien Tablets 3191

Zonisamide (Potentiates CNS-depressant action). Products include:
Zonegran Capsules 1307

Food Interactions

Alcohol (Potentiates CNS-depressant action).

KLOR-CON M20/ KLOR-CON M10 TABLETS

(Potassium Chloride) 3329
May interact with ACE inhibitors, anticholinergics, potassium preparations, potassium sparing diuretics, and certain other agents. Compounds in these categories include:

Amiloride Hydrochloride (Coadministration of these agents can produce severe hyperkalemia; concurrent use is not recommended). Products include:
Midamor Tablets 2136
Moduretic Tablets 2138

Atropine Sulfate (Concurrent use with anticholinergic drugs or other agents with anticholinergic properties at sufficient doses to exert anticholinergic effects is contraindicated). Products include:
Donnatal 2929
Donnatal Extentabs 2930
Motofen Tablets 577
Prosed/DS Tablets 3268
Urised Tablets 2876

Belladonna Alkaloids (Concurrent use with anticholinergic drugs or other agents with anticholinergic

IMPORTANT NOTE: Always consult each drug listing in the patient's regimen for possible interactions.

properties at sufficient doses to exert anticholinergic effects is contraindicated). Products include:
Hyland's Teething Tablets .... ▭766
Urimax Tablets 1769

Benazepril Hydrochloride (Potential for increased potassium retention). Products include:
Lotensin Tablets 2365
Lotensin HCT Tablets 2367
Lotrel Capsules 2370

Benztropine Mesylate (Concurrent use with anticholinergic drugs or other agents with anticholinergic properties at sufficient doses to exert anticholinergic effects is contraindicated). Products include:
Cogentin 2055

Biperiden Hydrochloride (Concurrent use with anticholinergic drugs or other agents with anticholinergic properties at sufficient doses to exert anticholinergic effects is contraindicated). Products include:
Akineton 402

Captopril (Potential for increased potassium retention). Products include:
Captopril Tablets 2281

Clidinium Bromide (Concurrent use with anticholinergic drugs or other agents with anticholinergic properties at sufficient doses to exert anticholinergic effects is contraindicated).
No products indexed under this heading.

Dicyclomine Hydrochloride (Concurrent use with anticholinergic drugs or other agents with anticholinergic properties at sufficient doses to exert anticholinergic effects is contraindicated).
No products indexed under this heading.

Enalapril Maleate (Potential for increased potassium retention). Products include:
Lexxel Tablets 608
Vaseretic Tablets 2204
Vasotec Tablets 2210

Enalaprilat (Potential for increased potassium retention). Products include:
Enalaprilat Injection 863
Vasotec I.V. Injection 2207

Fosinopril Sodium (Potential for increased potassium retention). Products include:
Monopril Tablets 1091
Monopril HCT 1094

Glycopyrrolate (Concurrent use with anticholinergic drugs or other agents with anticholinergic properties at sufficient doses to exert anticholinergic effects is contraindicated). Products include:
Robinul Forte Tablets 1358
Robinul Injectable 2940
Robinul Tablets 1358

Hyoscyamine (Concurrent use with anticholinergic drugs or other agents with anticholinergic properties at sufficient doses to exert anticholinergic effects is contraindicated). Products include:
Urised Tablets 2876

Hyoscyamine Sulfate (Concurrent use with anticholinergic drugs or other agents with anticholinergic properties at sufficient doses to exert anticholinergic effects is contraindicated). Products include:
Arco-Lase Plus Tablets 592
Donnatal 2929
Donnatal Extentabs 2930
Levsin/Levsinex/Levbid 3172
NuLev Orally Disintegrating Tablets 3176
Prosed/DS Tablets 3268
Urimax Tablets 1769

Ipratropium Bromide (Concurrent use with anticholinergic drugs or other agents with anticholinergic properties at sufficient doses to exert anticholinergic effects is contraindicated). Products include:
Atrovent Inhalation Aerosol 1030
Atrovent Inhalation Solution 1031
Atrovent Nasal Spray 0.03% 1032
Atrovent Nasal Spray 0.06% 1033
Combivent Inhalation Aerosol 1041
DuoNeb Inhalation Solution 1233

Lisinopril (Potential for increased potassium retention). Products include:
Prinivil Tablets 2164
Prinzide Tablets 2168
Zestoretic Tablets 695
Zestril Tablets 698

Mepenzolate Bromide (Concurrent use with anticholinergic drugs or other agents with anticholinergic properties at sufficient doses to exert anticholinergic effects is contraindicated).
No products indexed under this heading.

Moexipril Hydrochloride (Potential for increased potassium retention). Products include:
Uniretic Tablets 3178
Univasc Tablets 3181

Oxybutynin Chloride (Concurrent use with anticholinergic drugs or other agents with anticholinergic properties at sufficient doses to exert anticholinergic effects is contraindicated). Products include:
Ditropan XL Extended Release Tablets 564

Perindopril Erbumine (Potential for increased potassium retention). Products include:
Aceon Tablets (2 mg, 4 mg, 8 mg) 3249

Potassium Acid Phosphate (Co-administration of these agents can produce severe hyperkalemia; concurrent use is not recommended). Products include:
K-Phos Original (Sodium Free) Tablets 947

Potassium Bicarbonate (Co-administration of these agents can produce severe hyperkalemia; concurrent use is not recommended).
No products indexed under this heading.

Potassium Citrate (Co-administration of these agents can produce severe hyperkalemia; concurrent use is not recommended). Products include:
Urocit-K Tablets 2232

Potassium Gluconate (Co-administration of these agents can produce severe hyperkalemia; concurrent use is not recommended).
No products indexed under this heading.

Potassium Phosphate (Co administration of these agents can produce severe hyperkalemia; concurrent use is not recommended). Products include:
K-Phos Neutral Tablets 946

Procyclidine Hydrochloride (Concurrent use with anticholinergic drugs or other agents with anticholinergic properties at sufficient doses to exert anticholinergic effects is contraindicated).
No products indexed under this heading.

Propantheline Bromide (Concurrent use with anticholinergic drugs or other agents with anticholinergic properties at sufficient doses to exert anticholinergic effects is contraindicated).
No products indexed under this heading.

Quinapril Hydrochloride (Potential for increased potassium retention). Products include:
Accupril Tablets 2611
Accuretic Tablets 2614

Ramipril (Potential for increased potassium retention). Products include:
Altace Capsules 2233

Scopolamine (Concurrent use with anticholinergic drugs or other agents with anticholinergic properties at sufficient doses to exert anticholinergic effects is contraindicated). Products include:
Transderm Scōp Transdermal Therapeutic System 2302

Scopolamine Hydrobromide (Concurrent use with anticholinergic drugs or other agents with anticholinergic properties at sufficient doses to exert anticholinergic effects is contraindicated). Products include:
Donnatal 2929
Donnatal Extentabs 2930

Spirapril Hydrochloride (Potential for increased potassium retention).
No products indexed under this heading.

Spironolactone (Co-administration of these agents can produce severe hyperkalemia; concurrent use is not recommended).
No products indexed under this heading.

Tolterodine Tartrate (Concurrent use with anticholinergic drugs or other agents with anticholinergic properties at sufficient doses to exert anticholinergic effects is contraindicated). Products include:
Detrol Tablets 3623
Detrol LA Capsules 2801

Trandolapril (Potential for increased potassium retention). Products include:
Mavik Tablets 478
Tarka Tablets 508

Triamterene (Co-administration of these agents can produce severe hyperkalemia; concurrent use is not recommended). Products include:
Dyazide Capsules 1515
Dyrenium Capsules 3458
Maxzide 1008

Tridihexethyl Chloride (Concurrent use with anticholinergic drugs or other agents with anticholinergic properties at sufficient doses to exert anticholinergic effects is contraindicated).
No products indexed under this heading.

Trihexyphenidyl Hydrochloride (Concurrent use with anticholinergic drugs or other agents with anticholinergic properties at sufficient doses to exert anticholinergic effects is contraindicated). Products include:
Artane 1855

K-LOR POWDER PACKETS
(Potassium Chloride) 469
May interact with ACE inhibitors and potassium sparing diuretics. Compounds in these categories include:

Amiloride Hydrochloride (Co-administration of these agents can produce severe hyperkalemia; concurrent use is not recommended). Products include:
Midamor Tablets 2136
Moduretic Tablets 2138

Benazepril Hydrochloride (Potential for hyperkalemia). Products include:
Lotensin Tablets 2365
Lotensin HCT Tablets 2367
Lotrel Capsules 2370

Captopril (Potential for hyperkalemia). Products include:
Captopril Tablets 2281

Enalapril Maleate (Potential for hyperkalemia). Products include:
Lexxel Tablets 608
Vaseretic Tablets 2204
Vasotec Tablets 2210

Enalaprilat (Potential for hyperkalemia). Products include:
Enalaprilat Injection 863
Vasotec I.V. Injection 2207

Fosinopril Sodium (Potential for hyperkalemia). Products include:
Monopril Tablets 1091
Monopril HCT 1094

Lisinopril (Potential for hyperkalemia). Products include:
Prinivil Tablets 2164
Prinzide Tablets 2168
Zestoretic Tablets 695
Zestril Tablets 698

Moexipril Hydrochloride (Potential for hyperkalemia). Products include:
Uniretic Tablets 3178
Univasc Tablets 3181

Perindopril Erbumine (Potential for hyperkalemia). Products include:
Aceon Tablets (2 mg, 4 mg, 8 mg) 3249

Quinapril Hydrochloride (Potential for hyperkalemia). Products include:
Accupril Tablets 2611
Accuretic Tablets 2614

Ramipril (Potential for hyperkalemia). Products include:
Altace Capsules 2233

Spirapril Hydrochloride (Potential for hyperkalemia).
No products indexed under this heading.

Spironolactone (Co-administration of these agents can produce severe hyperkalemia; concurrent use is not recommended).
No products indexed under this heading.

Trandolapril (Potential for hyperkalemia). Products include:
Mavik Tablets 478
Tarka Tablets 508

Triamterene (Co-administration of these agents can produce severe hyperkalemia; concurrent use is not recommended). Products include:
Dyazide Capsules 1515
Dyrenium Capsules 3458
Maxzide 1008

KOĀTE-DVI
(Antihemophilic Factor (Human)) 931
None cited in PDR database.

KOĀTE-HP
(Antihemophilic Factor (Human)) 932
None cited in PDR database.

KOGENATE
(Antihemophilic Factor (Recombinant)) 934
None cited in PDR database.

KOGENATE FS
(Antihemophilic Factor (Recombinant)) 936
None cited in PDR database.

KONŸNE 80
(Factor IX Complex) 937
None cited in PDR database.

K-PHOS NEUTRAL TABLETS
(Potassium Phosphate, Sodium Phosphate) 946
May interact with antacids containing aluminum, calcium and magnesium, calcium preparations, potassium preparations, potassium sparing diuretics, and certain other agents. Compounds in these categories include:

ACTH (Concurrent use with corticotropin may result in hypernatremia).
No products indexed under this heading.

Aluminum Carbonate (Co-administration with antacids may bind the phosphate and prevent its absorption).
No products indexed under this heading.

Aluminum Hydroxide (Co-administration with antacids may bind the phosphate and prevent its absorption). Products include:
Amphojel Suspension (Mint Flavor) ... 789
Gaviscon Extra Strength Liquid ... 751
Gaviscon Extra Strength Tablets ... 751
Gaviscon Regular Strength Liquid . 751
Gaviscon Regular Strength Tablets ... 750
Maalox Antacid/Anti-Gas Oral Suspension ... 673
Maalox Max Maximum Strength Antacid/Anti-Gas Liquid ... 2300
Maalox Regular Strength Antacid/Antigas Liquid ... 2300
Mylanta ... 1813
Vanquish Caplets ... 617

Amiloride Hydrochloride (Concurrent use with potassium-sparing diuretics may cause hyperkalemia). Products include:
Midamor Tablets ... 2136
Moduretic Tablets ... 2138

Calcium Carbonate (Concurrent use with calcium-containing preparations may antagonize the effects of phosphates in the treatment of hypercalcemia). Products include:
Aspirin Regimen Bayer 81 mg Caplets with Calcium ... 607
Extra Strength Bayer Plus Caplets ... 610
Caltrate 600 Tablets ... 814
Caltrate 600 PLUS ... 815
Caltrate 600 + D Tablets ... 814
Caltrate 600 + Soy Tablets ... 814
D-Cal Chewable Caplets ... 794
Florical Capsules and Tablets ... 2223
Quick Dissolve Maalox Max Maximum Strength Antacid/Antigas Tablets ... 2301
Quick Dissolve Maalox Regular Strength Antacid Tablets ... 2301
Marblen Suspension ... 633
Monocal Tablets ... 2223
Mylanta Fast-Acting ... 1813
Mylanta Calci Tabs ... 636
One-A-Day Bedtime & Rest Tablets ... 805
One-A-Day Calcium Plus Chewable Tablets ... 805
Os-Cal Chewable Tablets ... 838
Pepcid Complete Chewable Tablets ... 1815
ReSource Wellness CalciWise Soft Chews ... 824
Rolaids Tablets ... 706
Extra Strength Rolaids Tablets ... 706
Slow-Mag Tablets ... 835
Titralac ... 640
3M Titralac Plus Antacid Tablets ... 640
Tums ... 763

Calcium Chloride (Concurrent use with calcium-containing preparations may antagonize the effects of phosphates in the treatment of hypercalcemia).
No products indexed under this heading.

Calcium Citrate (Concurrent use with calcium-containing preparations may antagonize the effects of phosphates in the treatment of hypercalcemia). Products include:
Active Calcium Tablets ... 3335
Citracal Liquitab Tablets ... 823
Citracal Tablets ... 2231
Citracal Caplets + D ... 823

Calcium Glubionate (Concurrent use with calcium-containing preparations may antagonize the effects of phosphates in the treatment of hypercalcemia).
No products indexed under this heading.

Deserpidine (Concurrent use with antihypertensives, such as rauwolfia alkaloids, may result in hypernatremia).
No products indexed under this heading.

Diazoxide (Concurrent use with antihypertensives, such as diazoxide, may result in hypernatremia).
No products indexed under this heading.

Fludrocortisone Acetate (Concurrent use with mineralocorticoids may result in hypernatremia). Products include:
Florinef Acetate Tablets ... 2250

Guanethidine Monosulfate (Concurrent use with antihypertensives, such as guanethidine, may result in hypernatremia).
No products indexed under this heading.

Hydralazine Hydrochloride (Concurrent use with antihypertensives, such as hydralazine, may result in hypernatremia).
No products indexed under this heading.

Magaldrate (Co-administration with antacids may bind the phosphate and prevent its absorption).
No products indexed under this heading.

Magnesium Hydroxide (Co-administration with antacids may bind the phosphate and prevent its absorption). Products include:
Ex•Lax Milk of Magnesia Liquid ... 670
Maalox Antacid/Anti-Gas Oral Suspension ... 673
Maalox Max Maximum Strength Antacid/Anti-Gas Liquid ... 2300
Maalox Regular Strength Antacid/Antigas Liquid ... 2300
Mylanta Fast-Acting ... 1813
Mylanta ... 1813
Pepcid Complete Chewable Tablets ... 1815
Phillips' Chewable Tablets ... 615
Phillips' Milk of Magnesia Liquid (Original, Cherry, & Mint) ... 616
Rolaids Tablets ... 706
Extra Strength Rolaids Tablets ... 706
Vanquish Caplets ... 617

Magnesium Oxide (Co-administration with antacids may bind the phosphate and prevent its absorption). Products include:
Beelith Tablets ... 946
Mag-Ox 400 Tablets ... 1024
Uro-Mag Capsules ... 1024

Methyldopa (Concurrent use with antihypertensives, such as methyldopa, may result in hypernatremia). Products include:
Aldoclor Tablets ... 2035
Aldomet Tablets ... 2037
Aldoril Tablets ... 2039

Potassium Acid Phosphate (Concurrent use with potassium-containing medications may cause hyperkalemia). Products include:
K-Phos Original (Sodium Free) Tablets ... 947

Potassium Bicarbonate (Concurrent use with potassium-containing medications may cause hyperkalemia).
No products indexed under this heading.

Potassium Chloride (Concurrent use with potassium-containing medications may cause hyperkalemia). Products include:
Chlor-3 ... 1361
Colyte with Flavor Packs for Oral Solution ... 3170
GoLYTELY and Pineapple Flavor GoLYTELY for Oral Solution ... 1068
K-Dur Microburst Release System ER Tablets ... 1832
Klor-Con M20/Klor-Con M10 Tablets ... 3329
K-Lor Powder Packets ... 469
K-Tab Filmtab Tablets ... 470
Micro-K ... 3311
NuLYTELY, Cherry Flavor, Lemon-Lime Flavor, and Orange Flavor NuLYTELY for Oral Solution ... 1068
Rum-K ... 1363

Potassium Citrate (Concurrent use with potassium-containing medications may cause hyperkalemia). Products include:
Urocit-K Tablets ... 2232

Potassium Gluconate (Concurrent use with potassium-containing medications may cause hyperkalemia).
No products indexed under this heading.

Rauwolfia serpentina (Concurrent use with antihypertensives, such as rauwolfia alkaloids, may result in hypernatremia).
No products indexed under this heading.

Rescinnamine (Concurrent use with antihypertensives, such as rauwolfia alkaloids, may result in hypernatremia).
No products indexed under this heading.

Reserpine (Concurrent use with antihypertensives, such as rauwolfia alkaloids, may result in hypernatremia).
No products indexed under this heading.

Spironolactone (Concurrent use with potassium-sparing diuretics may cause hyperkalemia).
No products indexed under this heading.

Triamterene (Concurrent use with potassium-sparing diuretics may cause hyperkalemia). Products include:
Dyazide Capsules ... 1515
Dyrenium Capsules ... 3458
Maxzide ... 1008

Vitamin D (Concurrent use with vitamin D may antagonize the effects of phosphates in the treatment of hypercalcemia). Products include:
Active Calcium Tablets ... 3335
Caltrate 600 PLUS ... 815
Caltrate 600 + D Tablets ... 814
Centrum Focused Formulas Bone Health Tablets ... 815
Citracal Caplets + D ... 823
D-Cal Chewable Caplets ... 794
One-A-Day Calcium Plus Chewable Tablets ... 805
Os-Cal 250 + D Tablets ... 838
Os-Cal 500 + D Tablets ... 839

K-PHOS ORIGINAL (SODIUM FREE) TABLETS

(Potassium Acid Phosphate) ... 947
May interact with antacids, potassium preparations, potassium sparing diuretics, salicylates, and certain other agents. Compounds in these categories include:

Aluminum Carbonate (May bind phosphate and prevent its absorption).
No products indexed under this heading.

Aluminum Hydroxide (May bind phosphate and prevent its absorption). Products include:
Amphojel Suspension (Mint Flavor) ... 789
Gaviscon Extra Strength Liquid ... 751
Gaviscon Extra Strength Tablets ... 751
Gaviscon Regular Strength Liquid . 751
Gaviscon Regular Strength Tablets ... 750
Maalox Antacid/Anti-Gas Oral Suspension ... 673
Maalox Max Maximum Strength Antacid/Anti-Gas Liquid ... 2300
Maalox Regular Strength Antacid/Antigas Liquid ... 2300
Mylanta ... 1813
Vanquish Caplets ... 617

Amiloride Hydrochloride (Hyperkalemia). Products include:
Midamor Tablets ... 2136
Moduretic Tablets ... 2138

Aspirin (Increased serum salicylate levels; possible toxicity). Products include:
Aggrenox Capsules ... 1026
Alka-Seltzer ... 603
Alka-Seltzer Lemon Lime Antacid and Pain Reliever Effervescent Tablets ... 603
Alka-Seltzer Extra Strength Antacid and Pain Reliever Effervescent Tablets ... 603
Alka-Seltzer PM Effervescent Tablets ... 605
Genuine Bayer Tablets, Caplets and Gelcaps ... 606
Extra Strength Bayer Caplets and Gelcaps ... 610
Aspirin Regimen Bayer Children's Chewable Tablets (Orange or Cherry Flavored) ... 607
Bayer, Aspirin Regimen ... 606
Aspirin Regimen Bayer 81 mg Caplets with Calcium ... 607
Genuine Bayer Professional Labeling (Aspirin Regimen Bayer) ... 608
Extra Strength Bayer Arthritis Caplets ... 610
Extra Strength Bayer Plus Caplets ... 610
Extra Strength Bayer PM Caplets .. 611
BC Powder ... 619
BC Allergy Sinus Cold Powder ... 619
Arthritis Strength BC Powder ... 619
BC Sinus Cold Powder ... 619
Darvon Compound-65 Pulvules ... 1910
Ecotrin Enteric Coated Aspirin Low, Regular and Maximum Strength Tablets ... 1715
Excedrin Extra-Strength Tablets, Caplets, and Geltabs ... 629
Excedrin Migraine ... 1070
Goody's Body Pain Formula Powder ... 620
Goody's Extra Strength Headache Powder ... 620
Goody's Extra Strength Pain Relief Tablets ... 620
Percodan Tablets ... 1327
Robaxisal Tablets ... 2939
Soma Compound Tablets ... 3354
Soma Compound w/Codeine Tablets ... 3355
Vanquish Caplets ... 617

Choline Magnesium Trisalicylate (Increased serum salicylate levels; possible toxicity). Products include:
Trilisate ... 2901

Diflunisal (Increased serum salicylate levels; possible toxicity). Products include:
Dolobid Tablets ... 2088

Magaldrate (May bind phosphate and prevent its absorption).
No products indexed under this heading.

Magnesium Hydroxide (May bind phosphate and prevent its absorption). Products include:
Ex•Lax Milk of Magnesia Liquid ... 670
Maalox Antacid/Anti-Gas Oral Suspension ... 673
Maalox Max Maximum Strength Antacid/Anti-Gas Liquid ... 2300
Maalox Regular Strength Antacid/Antigas Liquid ... 2300
Mylanta Fast-Acting ... 1813
Mylanta ... 1813
Pepcid Complete Chewable Tablets ... 1815
Phillips' Chewable Tablets ... 615
Phillips' Milk of Magnesia Liquid (Original, Cherry, & Mint) ... 616
Rolaids Tablets ... 706
Extra Strength Rolaids Tablets ... 706
Vanquish Caplets ... 617

Magnesium Oxide (May bind phosphate and prevent its absorption). Products include:
Beelith Tablets ... 946
Mag-Ox 400 Tablets ... 1024
Uro-Mag Capsules ... 1024

Magnesium Salicylate (Increased serum salicylate levels; possible toxicity). Products include:
Momentum Backache Relief Extra Strength Caplets ... 666

Potassium Bicarbonate (Potential for hyperkalemia).
No products indexed under this heading.

Potassium Chloride (Potential for hyperkalemia). Products include:
Chlor-3 ... 1361
Colyte with Flavor Packs for Oral Solution ... 3170
GoLYTELY and Pineapple Flavor GoLYTELY for Oral Solution ... 1068
K-Dur Microburst Release System ER Tablets ... 1832
Klor-Con M20/Klor-Con M10 Tablets ... 3329
K-Lor Powder Packets ... 469
K-Tab Filmtab Tablets ... 470
Micro-K ... 3311

IMPORTANT NOTE: Always consult each drug listing in the patient's regimen for possible interactions.

NuLYTELY, Cherry Flavor, Lemon-Lime Flavor, and Orange Flavor NuLYTELY for Oral Solution ... 1068
Rum-K ... 1363

Potassium Citrate (Potential for hyperkalemia). Products include:
Urocit-K Tablets ... 2232

Potassium Gluconate (Potential for hyperkalemia).
No products indexed under this heading.

Potassium Phosphate (Potential for hyperkalemia). Products include:
K-Phos Neutral Tablets ... 946

Salsalate (Increased serum salicylate levels; possible toxicity).
No products indexed under this heading.

Sodium Bicarbonate (May bind phosphate and prevent its absorption). Products include:
Alka-Seltzer ... ▣603
Alka-Seltzer Lemon Lime Antacid and Pain Reliever Effervescent Tablets ... ▣603
Alka-Seltzer Extra Strength Antacid and Pain Reliever Effervescent Tablets ... ▣603
Alka-Seltzer Heartburn Relief Tablets ... ▣604
Ceo-Two Evacuant Suppository ... ▣618
Colyte with Flavor Packs for Oral Solution ... 3170
GoLYTELY and Pineapple Flavor GoLYTELY for Oral Solution ... 1068
NuLYTELY, Cherry Flavor, Lemon-Lime Flavor, and Orange Flavor NuLYTELY for Oral Solution ... 1068

Spironolactone (Hyperkalemia).
No products indexed under this heading.

Triamterene (Hyperkalemia). Products include:
Dyazide Capsules ... 1515
Dyrenium Capsules ... 3458
Maxzide ... 1008

KRISTALOSE FOR ORAL SOLUTION

(Lactulose) ... 1007
May interact with nonabsorbable antacids. Compounds in these categories include:

Aluminum Carbonate (Results of preliminary studies suggests that nonabsorbable antacids given concurrently with lactulose may inhibit the desired lactulose-induced drop in colonic pH).
No products indexed under this heading.

Aluminum Hydroxide (Results of preliminary studies suggests that nonabsorbable antacids given concurrently with lactulose may inhibit the desired lactulose-induced drop in colonic pH). Products include:
Amphojel Suspension (Mint Flavor) ... ▣789
Gaviscon Extra Strength Liquid ... ▣751
Gaviscon Extra Strength Tablets ... ▣751
Gaviscon Regular Strength Liquid ... ▣751
Gaviscon Regular Strength Tablets ... ▣750
Maalox Antacid/Anti-Gas Oral Suspension ... ▣673
Maalox Max Maximum Strength Antacid/Anti-Gas Liquid ... 2300
Maalox Regular Strength Antacid/Antigas Liquid ... 2300
Mylanta ... 1813
Vanquish Caplets ... ▣617

Calcium Carbonate (Results of preliminary studies suggests that nonabsorbable antacids given concurrently with lactulose may inhibit the desired lactulose-induced drop in colonic pH). Products include:
Aspirin Regimen Bayer 81 mg Caplets with Calcium ... ▣607
Extra Strength Bayer Plus Caplets ... ▣610
Caltrate 600 Tablets ... ▣814
Caltrate 600 PLUS ... ▣815
Caltrate 600 + D Tablets ... ▣814
Caltrate 600 + Soy Tablets ... ▣814
D-Cal Chewable Caplets ... ▣794
Florical Capsules and Tablets ... 2223
Quick Dissolve Maalox Max Maximum Strength Antacid/Antigas Tablets ... 2301
Quick Dissolve Maalox Regular Strength Antacid Tablets ... 2301
Marblen Suspension ... ▣633
Monocal Tablets ... 2223
Mylanta Fast-Acting ... 1813
Mylanta Calci Tabs ... ▣636
One-A-Day Bedtime & Rest Tablets ... ▣805
One-A-Day Calcium Plus Chewable Tablets ... ▣805
Os-Cal Chewable Tablets ... ▣838
Pepcid Complete Chewable Tablets ... 1815
ReSource Wellness CalciWise Soft Chews ... ▣824
Rolaids Tablets ... ▣706
Extra Strength Rolaids Tablets ... ▣706
Slow-Mag Tablets ... ▣835
Titralac ... ▣640
3M Titralac Plus Antacid Tablets ... ▣640
Tums ... ▣763

Magnesium Carbonate (Results of preliminary studies suggests that nonabsorbable antacids given concurrently with lactulose may inhibit the desired lactulose-induced drop in colonic pH). Products include:
Gaviscon Extra Strength Liquid ... ▣751
Gaviscon Extra Strength Tablets ... ▣751
Gaviscon Regular Strength Liquid ... ▣751
Marblen Suspension ... ▣633
One-A-Day Calcium Plus Chewable Tablets ... ▣805

Magnesium Hydroxide (Results of preliminary studies suggests that nonabsorbable antacids given concurrently with lactulose may inhibit the desired lactulose-induced drop in colonic pH). Products include:
Ex•Lax Milk of Magnesia Liquid ... ▣670
Maalox Antacid/Anti-Gas Oral Suspension ... ▣673
Maalox Max Maximum Strength Antacid/Anti-Gas Liquid ... 2300
Maalox Regular Strength Antacid/Antigas Liquid ... 2300
Mylanta Fast-Acting ... 1813
Mylanta ... 1813
Pepcid Complete Chewable Tablets ... 1815
Phillips' Chewable Tablets ... ▣615
Phillips' Milk of Magnesia Liquid (Original, Cherry, & Mint) ... ▣616
Rolaids Tablets ... ▣706
Extra Strength Rolaids Tablets ... ▣706
Vanquish Caplets ... ▣617

KRONOFED-A KRONOCAPS

(Chlorpheniramine Maleate, Pseudoephedrine Hydrochloride) ... 1341
None cited in PDR database.

KRONOFED-A-JR. KRONOCAPS

(Chlorpheniramine Maleate, Pseudoephedrine Hydrochloride) ... 1341
None cited in PDR database.

K-TAB FILMTAB TABLETS

(Potassium Chloride) ... 470
May interact with ACE inhibitors, anticholinergics, and potassium sparing diuretics. Compounds in these categories include:

Amiloride Hydrochloride (Potential for severe hyperkalemia). Products include:
Midamor Tablets ... 2136
Moduretic Tablets ... 2138

Atropine Sulfate (Anticholinergic drugs can be cause for delay or arrest in tablet passage through the gastrointestinal tract; concomitant administration of drugs capable of decreasing GI motility should be avoided). Products include:
Donnatal ... 2929
Donnatal Extentabs ... 2930
Motofen Tablets ... 577
Prosed/DS Tablets ... 3268
Urised Tablets ... 2876

Belladonna Alkaloids (Anticholinergic drugs can be cause for delay or arrest in tablet passage through the gastrointestinal tract; concomitant administration of drugs capable of decreasing GI motility should be avoided). Products include:
Hyland's Teething Tablets ... ▣766
Urimax Tablets ... 1769

Benazepril Hydrochloride (Concomitant therapy may result in hyperkalemia; close monitoring is advised). Products include:
Lotensin Tablets ... 2365
Lotensin HCT Tablets ... 2367
Lotrel Capsules ... 2370

Benztropine Mesylate (Anticholinergic drugs can be cause for delay or arrest in tablet passage through the gastrointestinal tract; concomitant administration of drugs capable of decreasing GI motility should be avoided). Products include:
Cogentin ... 2055

Biperiden Hydrochloride (Anticholinergic drugs can be cause for delay or arrest in tablet passage through the gastrointestinal tract; concomitant administration of drugs capable of decreasing GI motility should be avoided). Products include:
Akineton ... 402

Captopril (Concomitant therapy may result in hyperkalemia; close monitoring is advised). Products include:
Captopril Tablets ... 2281

Clidinium Bromide (Anticholinergic drugs can be cause for delay or arrest in tablet passage through the gastrointestinal tract; concomitant administration of drugs capable of decreasing GI motility should be avoided).
No products indexed under this heading.

Dicyclomine Hydrochloride (Anticholinergic drugs can be cause for delay or arrest in tablet passage through the gastrointestinal tract; concomitant administration of drugs capable of decreasing GI motility should be avoided).
No products indexed under this heading.

Enalapril Maleate (Concomitant therapy may result in hyperkalemia; close monitoring is advised). Products include:
Lexxel Tablets ... 608
Vaseretic Tablets ... 2204
Vasotec Tablets ... 2210

Enalaprilat (Concomitant therapy may result in hyperkalemia; close monitoring is advised). Products include:
Enalaprilat Injection ... 863
Vasotec I.V. Injection ... 2207

Fosinopril Sodium (Concomitant therapy may result in hyperkalemia; close monitoring is advised). Products include:
Monopril Tablets ... 1091
Monopril HCT ... 1094

Glycopyrrolate (Anticholinergic drugs can be cause for delay or arrest in tablet passage through the gastrointestinal tract; concomitant administration of drugs capable of decreasing GI motility should be avoided). Products include:
Robinul Forte Tablets ... 1358
Robinul Injectable ... 2940
Robinul Tablets ... 1358

Hyoscyamine (Anticholinergic drugs can be cause for delay or arrest in tablet passage through the gastrointestinal tract; concomitant administration of drugs capable of decreasing GI motility should be avoided). Products include:
Urised Tablets ... 2876

Hyoscyamine Sulfate (Anticholinergic drugs can be cause for delay or arrest in tablet passage through the gastrointestinal tract; concomitant administration of drugs capable of decreasing GI motility should be avoided). Products include:
Arco-Lase Plus Tablets ... 592
Donnatal ... 2929
Donnatal Extentabs ... 2930
Levsin/Levsinex/Levbid ... 3172
NuLev Orally Disintegrating Tablets ... 3176
Prosed/DS Tablets ... 3268
Urimax Tablets ... 1769

Ipratropium Bromide (Anticholinergic drugs can be cause for delay or arrest in tablet passage through the gastrointestinal tract; concomitant administration of drugs capable of decreasing GI motility should be avoided). Products include:
Atrovent Inhalation Aerosol ... 1030
Atrovent Inhalation Solution ... 1031
Atrovent Nasal Spray 0.03% ... 1032
Atrovent Nasal Spray 0.06% ... 1033
Combivent Inhalation Aerosol ... 1041
DuoNeb Inhalation Solution ... 1233

Lisinopril (Concomitant therapy may result in hyperkalemia; close monitoring is advised). Products include:
Prinivil Tablets ... 2164
Prinzide Tablets ... 2168
Zestoretic Tablets ... 695
Zestril Tablets ... 698

Mepenzolate Bromide (Anticholinergic drugs can be cause for delay or arrest in tablet passage through the gastrointestinal tract; concomitant administration of drugs capable of decreasing GI motility should be avoided).
No products indexed under this heading.

Moexipril Hydrochloride (Concomitant therapy may result in hyperkalemia; close monitoring is advised). Products include:
Uniretic Tablets ... 3178
Univasc Tablets ... 3181

Oxybutynin Chloride (Anticholinergic drugs can be cause for delay or arrest in tablet passage through the gastrointestinal tract; concomitant administration of drugs capable of decreasing GI motility should be avoided). Products include:
Ditropan XL Extended Release Tablets ... 564

Perindopril Erbumine (Concomitant therapy may result in hyperkalemia; close monitoring is advised). Products include:
Aceon Tablets (2 mg, 4 mg, 8 mg) ... 3249

Procyclidine Hydrochloride (Anticholinergic drugs can be cause for delay or arrest in tablet passage through the gastrointestinal tract; concomitant administration of drugs capable of decreasing GI motility should be avoided).
No products indexed under this heading.

Propantheline Bromide (Anticholinergic drugs can be cause for delay or arrest in tablet passage through the gastrointestinal tract; concomitant administration of drugs capable of decreasing GI motility should be avoided).
No products indexed under this heading.

Quinapril Hydrochloride (Concomitant therapy may result in hyperkalemia; close monitoring is advised). Products include:
Accupril Tablets ... 2611
Accuretic Tablets ... 2614

Ramipril (Concomitant therapy may result in hyperkalemia; close monitoring is advised). Products include:
Altace Capsules ... 2233

Scopolamine (Anticholinergic drugs can be cause for delay or arrest in tablet passage through the gastrointestinal tract; concomitant administration of drugs capable of decreasing GI motility should be avoided). Products include:

Transderm Scōp Transdermal Therapeutic System 2302

Scopolamine Hydrobromide (Anticholinergic drugs can be cause for delay or arrest in tablet passage through the gastrointestinal tract; concomitant administration of drugs capable of decreasing GI motility should be avoided). Products include:
- Donnatal 2929
- Donnatal Extentabs 2930

Spirapril Hydrochloride (Concomitant therapy may result in hyperkalemia; close monitoring is advised).
No products indexed under this heading.

Spironolactone (Potential for severe hyperkalemia).
No products indexed under this heading.

Tolterodine Tartrate (Anticholinergic drugs can be cause for delay or arrest in tablet passage through the gastrointestinal tract; concomitant administration of drugs capable of decreasing GI motility should be avoided). Products include:
- Detrol Tablets 3623
- Detrol LA Capsules 2801

Trandolapril (Concomitant therapy may result in hyperkalemia; close monitoring is advised). Products include:
- Mavik Tablets 478
- Tarka Tablets 508

Triamterene (Potential for severe hyperkalemia). Products include:
- Dyazide Capsules 1515
- Dyrenium Capsules 3458
- Maxzide 1008

Tridihexethyl Chloride (Anticholinergic drugs can be cause for delay or arrest in tablet passage through the gastrointestinal tract; concomitant administration of drugs capable of decreasing GI motility should be avoided).
No products indexed under this heading.

Trihexyphenidyl Hydrochloride (Anticholinergic drugs can be cause for delay or arrest in tablet passage through the gastrointestinal tract; concomitant administration of drugs capable of decreasing GI motility should be avoided). Products include:
- Artane 1855

KYTRIL INJECTION
(Granisetron Hydrochloride) 2986
See Kytril Tablets

KYTRIL TABLETS
(Granisetron Hydrochloride) 2988
May interact with drugs affecting hepatic drug metabolizing enzyme systems and certain other agents. Compounds in these categories include:

Carbamazepine (May change the clearance and, hence the half-life of granisetron). Products include:
- Carbatrol Capsules 3234
- Tegretol/Tegretol-XR 2404

Cimetidine (May change the clearance and, hence the half-life of granisetron). Products include:
- Tagamet HB 200 Suspension 762
- Tagamet HB 200 Tablets 761
- Tagamet Tablets 1644

Cimetidine Hydrochloride (May change the clearance and, hence the half-life of granisetron). Products include:
- Tagamet 1644

Fosphenytoin Sodium (May change the clearance and, hence the half-life of granisetron). Products include:
- Cerebyx Injection 2619

Phenobarbital (May change the clearance and, hence the half-life of granisetron). Products include:
- Arco-Lase Plus Tablets 592
- Donnatal 2929
- Donnatal Extentabs 2930

Phenytoin (May change the clearance and, hence the half-life of granisetron). Products include:
- Dilantin Infatabs 2624
- Dilantin-125 Oral Suspension 2625

Phenytoin Sodium (May change the clearance and, hence the half-life of granisetron). Products include:
- Dilantin Kapseals 2622

Food Interactions

Food, unspecified (When oral granisetron was administered with food, AUC was decreased by 5% and Cmax increased by 30% in non-fasted individuals).

LAC-HYDRIN CREAM
(Ammonium Lactate) 1118
None cited in PDR database.

LAC-HYDRIN LOTION
(Ammonium Lactate) 1119
None cited in PDR database.

LACRISERT STERILE OPHTHALMIC INSERT
(Hydroxypropyl Cellulose) 2117
None cited in PDR database.

LACTAID EXTRA STRENGTH CAPLETS
(Lactase (beta-d-Galactosidase)) 2002
None cited in PDR database.

LACTAID ORIGINAL STRENGTH CAPLETS
(Lactase (beta-d-Galactosidase)) 2002
None cited in PDR database.

LACTAID ULTRA CAPLETS AND CHEWABLE TABLETS
(Lactase (beta-d-Galactosidase)) 2002
None cited in PDR database.

LAMICTAL TABLETS
(Lamotrigine) 1567
May interact with dihydrofolate reductase inhibitors, phenytoin, valproate, and certain other agents. Compounds in these categories include:

Carbamazepine (Potential for higher incidence of dizziness, diplopia, ataxia, and blurred vision; decreases lamotrigine steady-state concentrations by approximately 40%). Products include:
- Carbatrol Capsules 3234
- Tegretol/Tegretol-XR 2404

Divalproex Sodium (Co-administration in healthy volunteers resulted in decreased trough steady-state VPA concentrations; the addition of VPA increases lamotrigine steady-state concentrations in normal volunteers by slightly more than two-fold). Products include:
- Depakote Sprinkle Capsules 426
- Depakote Tablets 430
- Depakote ER Tablets 436

Fosphenytoin Sodium (Decreases lamotrigine steady-state concentrations by approximately 45% to 54%; lamotrigine has no appreciable effect on steady-state phenytoin plasma concentration). Products include:
- Cerebyx Injection 2619

Methotrexate Sodium (Lamotrigine is an inhibitor of dihydrofolate reductase; prescribers should be aware of this action when used concurrently with agents which inhibit folate metabolism).
No products indexed under this heading.

Phenobarbital (Decreases lamotrigine steady-state concentrations by approximately 40%). Products include:
- Arco-Lase Plus Tablets 592
- Donnatal 2929
- Donnatal Extentabs 2930

Phenytoin (Decreases lamotrigine steady-state concentrations by approximately 45% to 54%; lamotrigine has no appreciable effect on steady-state phenytoin plasma concentration). Products include:
- Dilantin Infatabs 2624
- Dilantin-125 Oral Suspension 2625

Phenytoin Sodium (Decreases lamotrigine steady-state concentrations by approximately 45% to 54%; lamotrigine has no appreciable effect on steady-state phenytoin plasma concentration). Products include:
- Dilantin Kapseals 2622

Primidone (Decreases lamotrigine steady-state concentrations by approximately 40%).
No products indexed under this heading.

Trimethoprim (Lamotrigine is an inhibitor of dihydrofolate reductase; prescribers should be aware of this action when used concurrently with agents which inhibit folate metabolism). Products include:
- Bactrim 2949
- Septra Suspension 2265
- Septra Tablets 2265
- Septra DS Tablets 2265

Trimetrexate Glucuronate (Lamotrigine is an inhibitor of dihydrofolate reductase; prescribers should be aware of this action when used concurrently with agents which inhibit folate metabolism).
No products indexed under this heading.

Valproate Sodium (Co-administration in healthy volunteers resulted in decreased trough steady-state VPA concentrations; the addition of VPA increases lamotrigine steady-state concentrations in normal volunteers by slightly more than two-fold). Products include:
- Depacon Injection 416

Valproic Acid (Co-administration in healthy volunteers resulted in decreased trough steady-state VPA concentrations; the addition of VPA increases lamotrigine steady-state concentrations in normal volunteers by slightly more than two-fold). Products include:
- Depakene 421

LAMICTAL CHEWABLE DISPERSIBLE TABLETS
(Lamotrigine) 1567
See Lamictal Tablets

LAMISIL TABLETS
(Terbinafine Hydrochloride) 2360
May interact with beta blockers, selective serotonin reuptake inhibitors, tricyclic antidepressants, and certain other agents. Compounds in these categories include:

Acebutolol Hydrochloride (In vitro studies show that terbinafine inhibits CYP2D6 mediated metabolism; this may be of clinical relevance for compounds predominantly metabolized by this enzyme, such as beta blockers, if they have a narrow therapeutic window). Products include:
- Sectral Capsules 3589

Amitriptyline Hydrochloride (In vitro studies show that terbinafine inhibits CYP2D6 mediated metabolism; this may be of clinical relevance for compounds predominantly metabolized by this enzyme, such as tricyclic antidepressants, if they have a narrow therapeutic window). Products include:
- Etrafon 3115
- Limbitrol 1738

Amoxapine (In vitro studies show that terbinafine inhibits CYP2D6 mediated metabolism; this may be of clinical relevance for compounds predominantly metabolized by this enzyme, such as tricyclic antidepressants, if they have a narrow therapeutic window).
No products indexed under this heading.

Atenolol (In vitro studies show that terbinafine inhibits CYP2D6 mediated metabolism; this may be of clinical relevance for compounds predominantly metabolized by this enzyme, such as beta blockers, if they have a narrow therapeutic window). Products include:
- Tenoretic Tablets 690
- Tenormin I.V. Injection 692

Betaxolol Hydrochloride (In vitro studies show that terbinafine inhibits CYP2D6 mediated metabolism; this may be of clinical relevance for compounds predominantly metabolized by this enzyme, such as beta blockers, if they have a narrow therapeutic window). Products include:
- Betoptic S Ophthalmic Suspension 537

Bisoprolol Fumarate (In vitro studies show that terbinafine inhibits CYP2D6 mediated metabolism; this may be of clinical relevance for compounds predominantly metabolized by this enzyme, such as beta blockers, if they have a narrow therapeutic window). Products include:
- Zebeta Tablets 1885
- Ziac Tablets 1887

Caffeine (Terbinafine decreases the clearance of intravenously administered caffeine by 19%). Products include:
- BC Powder 619
- Arthritis Strength BC Powder 619
- Darvon Compound-65 Pulvules 1910
- Aspirin Free Excedrin Caplets and Geltabs 628
- Excedrin Extra-Strength Tablets, Caplets, and Geltabs 629
- Excedrin Migraine 1070
- Goody's Extra Strength Headache Powder 620
- Goody's Extra Strength Pain Relief Tablets 620
- Hycomine Compound Tablets 1317
- Maximum Strength Midol Menstrual Caplets and Gelcaps 612
- Vanquish Caplets 617
- Vivarin 763

Caffeine Citrate (Terbinafine decreases the clearance of intravenously administered caffeine by 19%). Products include:
- Cafcit 1035

Carteolol Hydrochloride (In vitro studies show that terbinafine inhibits CYP2D6 mediated metabolism; this may be of clinical relevance for compounds predominantly metabolized by this enzyme, such as beta blockers, if they have a narrow therapeutic window). Products include:
- Carteolol Hydrochloride Ophthalmic Solution USP, 1% .... ⊙ 258
- Ocupress Ophthalmic Solution, 1% Sterile .... ⊙ 303

Cimetidine (Terbinafine clearance is decreased 33% by cimetidine, a CYP450 enzyme inhibitor). Products include:
- Tagamet HB 200 Suspension 762
- Tagamet HB 200 Tablets 761
- Tagamet Tablets 1644

Cimetidine Hydrochloride (Terbinafine clearance is decreased 33% by cimetidine, CYP450 enzyme). Products include:
- Tagamet 1644

Citalopram Hydrobromide (In vitro studies show that terbinafine inhibits CYP2D6 mediated metabolism; this may be of clinical relevance for compounds predominantly metabolized by this enzyme, such as SSRIs, if they have a narrow therapeutic window). Products include:
- Celexa 1365

IMPORTANT NOTE: Always consult each drug listing in the patient's regimen for possible interactions.

Clomipramine Hydrochloride (In vitro studies show that terbinafine inhibits CYP2D6 mediated metabolism; this may be of clinical relevance for compounds predominantly metabolized by this enzyme, such as tricyclic antidepressants, if they have a narrow therapeutic window).
No products indexed under this heading.

Cyclosporine (Terbinafine increases the clearance of cyclosporine by 15%; terbinafine clearance is unaffected by cyclosporine). Products include:
Gengraf Capsules 457
Neoral Soft Gelatin Capsules 2380
Neoral Oral Solution 2380
Sandimmune 2388

Desipramine Hydrochloride (In vitro studies show that terbinafine inhibits CYP2D6 mediated metabolism; this may be of clinical relevance for compounds predominantly metabolized by this enzyme, such as tricyclic antidepressants, if they have a narrow therapeutic window). Products include:
Norpramin Tablets 755

Doxepin Hydrochloride (In vitro studies show that terbinafine inhibits CYP2D6 mediated metabolism; this may be of clinical relevance for compounds predominantly metabolized by this enzyme, such as tricyclic antidepressants, if they have a narrow therapeutic window). Products include:
Sinequan 2713

Esmolol Hydrochloride (In vitro studies show that terbinafine inhibits CYP2D6 mediated metabolism; this may be of clinical relevance for compounds predominantly metabolized by this enzyme, such as beta blockers, if they have a narrow therapeutic window). Products include:
Brevibloc Injection 858

Fluoxetine Hydrochloride (In vitro studies show that terbinafine inhibits CYP2D6 mediated metabolism; this may be of clinical relevance for compounds predominantly metabolized by this enzyme, such as SSRIs, if they have a narrow therapeutic window). Products include:
Prozac Pulvules, Liquid, and Weekly Capsules 1238
Sarafem Pulvules 1962

Fluvoxamine Maleate (In vitro studies show that terbinafine inhibits CYP2D6 mediated metabolism; this may be of clinical relevance for compounds predominantly metabolized by this enzyme, such as SSRIs, if they have a narrow therapeutic window). Products include:
Luvox Tablets (25, 50, 100 mg) 3256

Imipramine Hydrochloride (In vitro studies show that terbinafine inhibits CYP2D6 mediated metabolism; this may be of clinical relevance for compounds predominantly metabolized by this enzyme, such as tricyclic antidepressants, if they have a narrow therapeutic window).
No products indexed under this heading.

Imipramine Pamoate (In vitro studies show that terbinafine inhibits CYP2D6 mediated metabolism; this may be of clinical relevance for compounds predominantly metabolized by this enzyme, such as tricyclic antidepressants, if they have a narrow therapeutic window).
No products indexed under this heading.

Labetalol Hydrochloride (In vitro studies show that terbinafine inhibits CYP2D6 mediated metabolism; this may be of clinical relevance for compounds predominantly metabolized by this enzyme, such as beta blockers, if they have a narrow therapeutic window). Products include:
Normodyne Injection 3135
Normodyne Tablets 3137

Levobunolol Hydrochloride (In vitro studies show that terbinafine inhibits CYP2D6 mediated metabolism; this may be of clinical relevance for compounds predominantly metabolized by this enzyme, such as beta blockers, if they have a narrow therapeutic window). Products include:
Betagan .... ⊙ 228

Maprotiline Hydrochloride (In vitro studies show that terbinafine inhibits CYP2D6 mediated metabolism; this may be of clinical relevance for compounds predominantly metabolized by this enzyme, such as tricyclic antidepressants, if they have a narrow therapeutic window).
No products indexed under this heading.

Metipranolol Hydrochloride (In vitro studies show that terbinafine inhibits CYP2D6 mediated metabolism; this may be of clinical relevance for compounds predominantly metabolized by this enzyme, such as beta blockers, if they have a narrow therapeutic window).
No products indexed under this heading.

Metoprolol Succinate (In vitro studies show that terbinafine inhibits CYP2D6 mediated metabolism; this may be of clinical relevance for compounds predominantly metabolized by this enzyme, such as beta blockers, if they have a narrow therapeutic window). Products include:
Toprol-XL Tablets 651

Metoprolol Tartrate (In vitro studies show that terbinafine inhibits CYP2D6 mediated metabolism; this may be of clinical relevance for compounds predominantly metabolized by this enzyme, such as beta blockers, if they have a narrow therapeutic window).
No products indexed under this heading.

Nadolol (In vitro studies show that terbinafine inhibits CYP2D6 mediated metabolism; this may be of clinical relevance for compounds predominantly metabolized by this enzyme, such as beta blockers, if they have a narrow therapeutic window). Products include:
Corgard Tablets 2245
Corzide 40/5 Tablets 2247
Corzide 80/5 Tablets 2247
Nadolol Tablets 2288

Nortriptyline Hydrochloride (In vitro studies show that terbinafine inhibits CYP2D6 mediated metabolism; this may be of clinical relevance for compounds predominantly metabolized by this enzyme, such as tricyclic antidepressants, if they have a narrow therapeutic window).
No products indexed under this heading.

Paroxetine Hydrochloride (In vitro studies show that terbinafine inhibits CYP2D6 mediated metabolism; this may be of clinical relevance for compounds predominantly metabolized by this enzyme, such as SSRIs, if they have a narrow therapeutic window). Products include:
Paxil 1609

Penbutolol Sulfate (In vitro studies show that terbinafine inhibits CYP2D6 mediated metabolism; this may be of clinical relevance for compounds predominantly metabolized by this enzyme, such as beta blockers, if they have a narrow therapeutic window).
No products indexed under this heading.

Pindolol (In vitro studies show that terbinafine inhibits CYP2D6 mediated metabolism; this may be of clinical relevance for compounds predominantly metabolized by this enzyme, such as beta blockers, if they have a narrow therapeutic window).
No products indexed under this heading.

Propranolol Hydrochloride (In vitro studies show that terbinafine inhibits CYP2D6 mediated metabolism; this may be of clinical relevance for compounds predominantly metabolized by this enzyme, such as beta blockers, if they have a narrow therapeutic window). Products include:
Inderal 3513
Inderal LA Long-Acting Capsules 3516
Inderide Tablets 3517
Inderide LA Long-Acting Capsules 3519

Protriptyline Hydrochloride (In vitro studies show that terbinafine inhibits CYP2D6 mediated metabolism; this may be of clinical relevance for compounds predominantly metabolized by this enzyme, such as tricyclic antidepressants, if they have a narrow therapeutic window). Products include:
Vivactil Tablets 2446
Vivactil Tablets 2217

Rifampin (Terbinafine clearance is increased 100% by rifampin, a CYP450 enzyme inducer). Products include:
Rifadin 765
Rifamate Capsules 767
Rifater Tablets 769

Selegiline Hydrochloride (In vitro studies show that terbinafine inhibits CYP2D6 mediated metabolism; this may be of clinical relevance for compounds predominantly metabolized by this enzyme, such as type B MAO inhibitor, if they have a narrow therapeutic window). Products include:
Eldepryl Capsules 3266

Sertraline Hydrochloride (In vitro studies show that terbinafine inhibits CYP2D6 mediated metabolism; this may be of clinical relevance for compounds predominantly metabolized by this enzyme, such as SSRIs, if they have a narrow therapeutic window). Products include:
Zoloft 2751

Sotalol Hydrochloride (In vitro studies show that terbinafine inhibits CYP2D6 mediated metabolism; this may be of clinical relevance for compounds predominantly metabolized by this enzyme, such as beta blockers, if they have a narrow therapeutic window). Products include:
Betapace Tablets 950
Betapace AF Tablets 954

Terfenadine (Terbinafine clearance is decreased 16% by terfenadine).
No products indexed under this heading.

Timolol Hemihydrate (In vitro studies show that terbinafine inhibits CYP2D6 mediated metabolism; this may be of clinical relevance for compounds predominantly metabolized by this enzyme, such as beta blockers, if they have a narrow therapeutic window). Products include:
Betimol Ophthalmic Solution .... ⊙ 324

Timolol Maleate (In vitro studies show that terbinafine inhibits CYP2D6 mediated metabolism; this may be of clinical relevance for compounds predominantly metabolized by this enzyme, such as beta blockers, if they have a narrow therapeutic window). Products include:
Blocadren Tablets 2046
Cosopt Sterile Ophthalmic Solution 2065
Timolide Tablets 2187
Timolol GFS .... ⊙ 266
Timoptic in Ocudose 2192
Timoptic Sterile Ophthalmic Solution 2190
Timoptic-XE Sterile Ophthalmic Gel Forming Solution 2194

Trimipramine Maleate (In vitro studies show that terbinafine inhibits CYP2D6 mediated metabolism; this may be of clinical relevance for compounds predominantly metabolized by this enzyme, such as tricyclic antidepressants, if they have a narrow therapeutic window). Products include:
Surmontil Capsules 3595

Warfarin Sodium (Co-administration has resulted in altered prothrombin time (prolongation and reduction)). Products include:
Coumadin for Injection 1243
Coumadin Tablets 1243
Warfarin Sodium Tablets, USP 3302

Food Interactions

Food, unspecified (Co-administration has resulted in an increase in the AUC of terbinafine of less than 20%).

LAMISIL AT CREAM

(Terbinafine Hydrochloride) .... ▣ 672
None cited in PDR database.

LAMISIL AT SOLUTION

(Terbinafine Hydrochloride) .... ▣ 672
None cited in PDR database.

LANOXICAPS CAPSULES

(Digoxin) 1574
See Lanoxin Tablets

LANOXIN INJECTION

(Digoxin) 1581
See Lanoxin Tablets

LANOXIN TABLETS

(Digoxin) 1587
May interact with antacids, beta blockers, calcium channel blockers, corticosteroids, erythromycin, macrolide antibiotics, potassium-depleting diuretics, quinidine, sympathomimetics, tetracyclines, thyroid preparations, and certain other agents. Compounds in these categories include:

Acebutolol Hydrochloride (Concomitant use of digoxin and beta-andrenergic blockers may result in the additive effects on AV node conduction). Products include:
Sectral Capsules 3589

Albuterol (Concomitant use of digoxin and sympathomimetics increases the risk of cardiac arrhythmias). Products include:
Proventil Inhalation Aerosol 3142
Ventolin Inhalation Aerosol and Refill 1679

Albuterol Sulfate (Concomitant use of digoxin and sympathomimetics increases the risk of cardiac arrhythmias). Products include:
AccuNeb Inhalation Solution 1230
Combivent Inhalation Aerosol 1041
DuoNeb Inhalation Solution 1233
Proventil Inhalation Solution 0.083% 3146
Proventil Repetabs Tablets 3148
Proventil Solution for Inhalation 0.5% 3144
Proventil HFA Inhalation Aerosol 3150
Ventolin HFA Inhalation Aerosol 3618
Volmax Extended-Release Tablets 2276

Alprazolam (Raises the serum digoxin concentration due to reduction in clearance and/or volume of distribution of the drug, with the implication that digitalis intoxication may result). Products include:
Xanax Tablets 2865

Aluminum Carbonate (Antacids may interfere with intestinal digoxin absorption, resulting in unexpectedly low serum concentrations; antacids may cause hypokalemia or hypomagnesemia and co-administration can cause digitalis toxicity).
No products indexed under this heading.

Aluminum Hydroxide (Antacids may interfere with intestinal digoxin absorption, resulting in unexpectedly low serum concentrations; antacids may cause hypokalemia or hypomagnesemia and co-administration can cause digitalis toxicity). Products include:
- Amphojel Suspension (Mint Flavor) ▣789
- Gaviscon Extra Strength Liquid ▣751
- Gaviscon Extra Strength Tablets ▣751
- Gaviscon Regular Strength Liquid ▣751
- Gaviscon Regular Strength Tablets ▣750
- Maalox Antacid/Anti-Gas Oral Suspension ▣673
- Maalox Max Maximum Strength Antacid/Anti-Gas Liquid 2300
- Maalox Regular Strength Antacid/Antigas Liquid 2300
- Mylanta 1813
- Vanquish Caplets ▣617

Amiodarone Hydrochloride (Raises the serum digoxin concentration due to reduction in clearance and/or volume of distribution of the drug, with the implication that digitalis intoxication may result). Products include:
- Cordarone Intravenous 3491
- Cordarone Tablets 3487
- Pacerone Tablets 3331

Amlodipine Besylate (Concomitant use of digoxin and calcium channel blockers may result in the additive effects on AV node conduction). Products include:
- Lotrel Capsules 2370
- Norvasc Tablets 2704

Amphotericin B (Can cause hypokalemia or hypomagnesemia and potassium or magnesium depletion can sensitize the myocardium to digoxin resulting in digitails toxicity). Products include:
- Abelcet Injection 1273
- AmBisome for Injection 1383
- Amphotec 1774

Anticancer Drugs, unspecified (May interfere with intestinal digoxin absorption, resulting in unexpectedly low serum concentrations).

Atenolol (Concomitant use of digoxin and beta-andrenergic blockers may result in the additive effects on AV node conduction). Products include:
- Tenoretic Tablets 690
- Tenormin I.V. Injection 692

Azithromycin Dihydrate (Macrolide antibiotics may possibly increase digoxin absorption in patients who inactivate digoxin by bacterial metabolism in the lower intestine, so that digitalis intoxication may result). Products include:
- Zithromax 2743
- Zithromax for IV Infusion 2748
- Zithromax for Oral Suspension, 300 mg, 600 mg, 900 mg, 1200 mg 2739
- Zithromax Tablets, 250 mg 2739

Bendroflumethiazide (Potassium-depleting diuretics can cause hypokalemia and co-administration can result in digitalis toxicity). Products include:
- Corzide 40/5 Tablets 2247
- Corzide 80/5 Tablets 2247

Bepridil Hydrochloride (Concomitant use of digoxin and calcium channel blockers may result in the additive effects on AV node conduction). Products include:
- Vascor Tablets 2602

Betamethasone Acetate (Corticosteroids can cause hypokalemia or hypomagnesemia and potassium or magnesium depletion can sensitize the myocardium to digoxin resulting in digitalis toxicity). Products include:
- Celestone Soluspan Injectable Suspension 3097

Betamethasone Sodium Phosphate (Corticosteroids can cause hypokalemia or hypomagnesemia and potassium or magnesium depletion can sensitize the myocardium to digoxin resulting in digitalis toxicity). Products include:
- Celestone Soluspan Injectable Suspension 3097

Betaxolol Hydrochloride (Concomitant use of digoxin and beta-andrenergic blockers may result in the additive effects on AV node conduction). Products include:
- Betoptic S Ophthalmic Suspension 537

Bisoprolol Fumarate (Concomitant use of digoxin and beta-andrenergic blockers may result in the additive effects on AV node conduction). Products include:
- Zebeta Tablets 1885
- Ziac Tablets 1887

Bumetanide (Potassium-depleting diuretics can cause hypokalemia and co-administration can result in digitalis toxicity).
No products indexed under this heading.

Calcium, intravenous (Co-administration with calcium, particularly if administered rapidly by the intravenous route may produce serious arrhythmias in digitalized patients).
No products indexed under this heading.

Carteolol Hydrochloride (Concomitant use of digoxin and beta-andrenergic blockers may result in the additive effects on AV node conduction). Products include:
- Carteolol Hydrochloride Ophthalmic Solution USP, 1% ⊙258
- Ocupress Ophthalmic Solution, 1% Sterile ⊙303

Chlorothiazide (Potassium-depleting diuretics can cause hypokalemia and co-administration can result in digitalis toxicity). Products include:
- Aldoclor Tablets 2035
- Diuril Oral 2087

Chlorothiazide Sodium (Potassium-depleting diuretics can cause hypokalemia and co-administration can result in digitalis toxicity). Products include:
- Diuril Sodium Intravenous 2086

Cholestyramine (May interfere with intestinal digoxin absorption, resulting in unexpectedly low serum concentrations).
No products indexed under this heading.

Clarithromycin (May increase digoxin absorption in patients who inactivate digoxin by bacterial metabolism in the lower intestine, so that digitalis intoxication may result). Products include:
- Biaxin/Biaxin XL 403
- PREVPAC 3298

Cortisone Acetate (Corticosteroids can cause hypokalemia or hypomagnesemia and potassium or magnesium depletion can sensitize the myocardium to digoxin resulting in digitalis toxicity). Products include:
- Cortone Acetate Injectable Suspension 2059
- Cortone Acetate Tablets 2061

Demeclocycline Hydrochloride (May increase digoxin absorption in patients who inactivate digoxin by bacterial metabolism in the lower intestine, so that digitalis intoxication may result). Products include:
- Declomycin Tablets 1855

Dexamethasone (Corticosteroids can cause hypokalemia or hypomagnesemia and potassium or magnesium depletion can sensitize the myocardium to digoxin resulting in digitalis toxicity). Products include:
- Decadron Elixir 2078
- Decadron Tablets 2079
- TobraDex Ophthalmic Ointment 542
- TobraDex Ophthalmic Suspension 541

Dexamethasone Acetate (Corticosteroids can cause hypokalemia or hypomagnesemia and potassium or magnesium depletion can sensitize the myocardium to digoxin resulting in digitalis toxicity).
No products indexed under this heading.

Dexamethasone Sodium Phosphate (Corticosteroids can cause hypokalemia or hypomagnesemia and potassium or magnesium depletion can sensitize the myocardium to digoxin resulting in digitalis toxicity). Products include:
- Decadron Phosphate Injection 2081
- Decadron Phosphate Sterile Ophthalmic Ointment 2083
- Decadron Phosphate Sterile Ophthalmic Solution 2084
- NeoDecadron Sterile Ophthalmic Solution 2144

Diltiazem Hydrochloride (Concomitant use of digoxin and calcium channel blockers may result in the additive effects on AV node conduction). Products include:
- Cardizem Injectable 1018
- Cardizem Lyo-Ject Syringe 1018
- Cardizem Monovial 1018
- Cardizem CD Capsules 1016
- Tiazac Capsules 1378

Diphenoxylate Hydrochloride (Decreases gut motility and may increase digoxin absorption).
No products indexed under this heading.

Dirithromycin (Macrolide antibiotics may possibly increase digoxin absorption in patients who inactivate digoxin by bacterial metabolism in the lower intestine, so that digitalis intoxication may result). Products include:
- Dynabac Tablets 2269

Dobutamine Hydrochloride (Concomitant use of digoxin and sympathomimetics increases the risk of cardiac arrhythmias). Products include:
- Dobutrex Solution Vials 1914

Dopamine Hydrochloride (Concomitant use of digoxin and sympathomimetics increases the risk of cardiac arrhythmias).
No products indexed under this heading.

Doxycycline Calcium (May increase digoxin absorption in patients who inactivate digoxin by bacterial metabolism in the lower intestine, so that digitalis intoxication may result). Products include:
- Vibramycin Calcium Oral Suspension Syrup 2735

Doxycycline Hyclate (May increase digoxin absorption in patients who inactivate digoxin by bacterial metabolism in the lower intestine, so that digitalis intoxication may result). Products include:
- Doryx Coated Pellet Filled Capsules 3357
- Periostat Tablets 1208
- Vibramycin Hyclate Capsules 2735
- Vibramycin Hyclate Intravenous 2737
- Vibra-Tabs Film Coated Tablets 2735

Doxycycline Monohydrate (May increase digoxin absorption in patients who inactivate digoxin by bacterial metabolism in the lower intestine, so that digitalis intoxication may result). Products include:
- Monodox Capsules 2442
- Vibramycin Monohydrate for Oral Suspension 2735

Ephedrine Hydrochloride (Concomitant use of digoxin and sympathomimetics increases the risk of cardiac arrhythmias). Products include:
- Primatene Tablets ▣780

Ephedrine Sulfate (Concomitant use of digoxin and sympathomimetics increases the risk of cardiac arrhythmias).
No products indexed under this heading.

Ephedrine Tannate (Concomitant use of digoxin and sympathomimetics increases the risk of cardiac arrhythmias). Products include:
- Rynatuss Pediatric Suspension 3353
- Rynatuss Tablets 3353

Epinephrine (Concomitant use of digoxin and sympathomimetics increases the risk of cardiac arrhythmias). Products include:
- Epifrin Sterile Ophthalmic Solution ⊙235
- EpiPen 1236
- Primatene Mist ▣779
- Xylocaine with Epinephrine Injection 653

Epinephrine Bitartrate (Concomitant use of digoxin and sympathomimetics increases the risk of cardiac arrhythmias). Products include:
- Sensorcaine 643

Epinephrine Hydrochloride (Concomitant use of digoxin and sympathomimetics increases the risk of cardiac arrhythmias).
No products indexed under this heading.

Erythromycin (May increase digoxin absorption in patients who inactivate digoxin by bacterial metabolism in the lower intestine, so that digitalis intoxication may result). Products include:
- Emgel 2% Topical Gel 1285
- Ery-Tab Tablets 448
- Erythromycin Base Filmtab Tablets 454
- Erythromycin Delayed-Release Capsules, USP 455
- PCE Dispertab Tablets 498

Erythromycin Estolate (May increase digoxin absorption in patients who inactivate digoxin by bacterial metabolism in the lower intestine, so that digitalis intoxication may result).
No products indexed under this heading.

Erythromycin Ethylsuccinate (May increase digoxin absorption in patients who inactivate digoxin by bacterial metabolism in the lower intestine, so that digitalis intoxication may result). Products include:
- E.E.S. 450
- EryPed 446
- Pediazole Suspension 3050

Erythromycin Gluceptate (May increase digoxin absorption in patients who inactivate digoxin by bacterial metabolism in the lower intestine, so that digitalis intoxication may result).
No products indexed under this heading.

Erythromycin Stearate (May increase digoxin absorption in patients who inactivate digoxin by bacterial metabolism in the lower intestine, so that digitalis intoxication may result). Products include:
- Erythrocin Stearate Filmtab Tablets 452

Esmolol Hydrochloride (Concomitant use of digoxin and beta-andrenergic blockers may result in the additive effects on AV node conduction). Products include:
- Brevibloc Injection 858

Ethacrynic Acid (Potassium-depleting diuretics can cause hypokalemia and co-administration can result in digitalis toxicity). Products include:
- Edecrin Tablets 2091

Felodipine (Concomitant use of digoxin and calcium channel blockers may result in the additive effects on AV node conduction). Products include:
- Lexxel Tablets 608
- Plendil Extended-Release Tablets 623

Fludrocortisone Acetate (Corticosteroids can cause hypokalemia

IMPORTANT NOTE: Always consult each drug listing in the patient's regimen for possible interactions.

or hypomagnesemia and potassium or magnesium depletion can sensitize the myocardium to digoxin resulting in digitalis toxicity). Products include:

Florinef Acetate Tablets 2250

Furosemide (Potassium-depleting diuretics can cause hypokalemia and co-administration can result in digitalis toxicity). Products include:

Furosemide Tablets 2284

Hydrochlorothiazide (Potassium-depleting diuretics can cause hypokalemia and co-administration can result in digitalis toxicity). Products include:

Accuretic Tablets 2614
Aldoril Tablets 2039
Atacand HCT Tablets 597
Avalide Tablets 1070
Diovan HCT Tablets 2338
Dyazide Capsules 1515
HydroDIURIL Tablets 2108
Hyzaar 2109
Inderide Tablets 3517
Inderide LA Long-Acting Capsules .. 3519
Lotensin HCT Tablets 2367
Maxzide 1008
Micardis HCT Tablets 1051
Microzide Capsules 3414
Moduretic Tablets 2138
Monopril HCT 1094
Prinzide Tablets 2168
Timolide Tablets 2187
Uniretic Tablets 3178
Vaseretic Tablets 2204
Zestoretic Tablets 695
Ziac Tablets 1887

Hydrocortisone (Corticosteroids can cause hypokalemia or hypomagnesemia and potassium or magnesium depletion can sensitize the myocardium to digoxin resulting in digitalis toxicity). Products include:

Anusol-HC Cream 2.5% 2237
Cipro HC Otic Suspension 540
Cortaid Intensive Therapy Cream .▣717
Cortaid Maximum Strength Cream ....▣717
Cortisporin Ophthalmic Suspension Sterile ....⊙297
Cortizone•5 ....▣699
Cortizone•10 ....▣699
Cortizone•10 Plus Creme ....▣700
Cortizone for Kids Creme ....▣699
Hydrocortone Tablets 2106
Massengill Medicated Soft Cloth Towelette ....▣753
VōSoL HC Otic Solution 3356

Hydrocortisone Acetate (Corticosteroids can cause hypokalemia or hypomagnesemia and potassium or magnesium depletion can sensitize the myocardium to digoxin resulting in digitalis toxicity). Products include:

Analpram-HC 1338
Anusol HC-1 Hydrocortisone Anti-Itch Cream ....▣689
Anusol-HC Suppositories 2238
Cortaid ....▣717
Cortifoam Rectal Foam 3170
Cortisporin-TC Otic Suspension 2246
Hydrocortone Acetate Injectable Suspension 2103
Pramosone 1343
Proctocort Suppositories 2264
ProctoFoam-HC 3177
Terra-Cortril Ophthalmic Suspension 2716

Hydrocortisone Sodium Phosphate (Corticosteroids can cause hypokalemia or hypomagnesemia and potassium or magnesium depletion can sensitize the myocardium to digoxin resulting in digitalis toxicity). Products include:

Hydrocortone Phosphate Injection, Sterile 2105

Hydrocortisone Sodium Succinate (Corticosteroids can cause hypokalemia or hypomagnesemia and potassium or magnesium depletion can sensitize the myocardium to digoxin resulting in digitalis toxicity).

No products indexed under this heading.

Hydroflumethiazide (Potassium-depleting diuretics can cause hypokalemia and co-administration can result in digitalis toxicity). Products include:

Diucardin Tablets 3494

Indomethacin (Raises the serum digoxin concentration due to reduction in clearance and/or volume of distribution of the drug, with the implication that digitalis intoxication may result). Products include:

Indocin 2112

Indomethacin Sodium Trihydrate (Raises the serum digoxin concentration due to reduction in clearance and/or volume of distribution of the drug, with the implication that digitalis intoxication may result). Products include:

Indocin I.V. 2115

Isoproterenol Hydrochloride (Concomitant use of digoxin and sympathomimetics increases the risk of cardiac arrhythmias).

No products indexed under this heading.

Isoproterenol Sulfate (Concomitant use of digoxin and sympathomimetics increases the risk of cardiac arrhythmias).

No products indexed under this heading.

Isradipine (Concomitant use of digoxin and calcium channel blockers may result in the additive effects on AV node conduction). Products include:

DynaCirc Capsules 2921
DynaCirc CR Tablets 2923

Itraconazole (Raises the serum digoxin concentration due to reduction in clearance and/or volume of distribution of the drug, with the implication that digitalis intoxication may result). Products include:

Sporanox Capsules 1800
Sporanox Injection 1804
Sporanox Injection 2509
Sporanox Oral Solution 1808
Sporanox Oral Solution 2512

Kaolin (May interfere with intestinal digoxin absorption, resulting in unexpectedly low serum concentrations).

No products indexed under this heading.

Labetalol Hydrochloride (Concomitant use of digoxin and beta-andrenergic blockers may result in the additive effects on AV node conduction). Products include:

Normodyne Injection 3135
Normodyne Tablets 3137

Levalbuterol Hydrochloride (Concomitant use of digoxin and sympathomimetics increases the risk of cardiac arrhythmias). Products include:

Xopenex Inhalation Solution 3207

Levobunolol Hydrochloride (Concomitant use of digoxin and beta-andrenergic blockers may result in the additive effects on AV node conduction). Products include:

Betagan ....⊙228

Levothyroxine Sodium (Thyroid administration to a digitalized, hypothyroid patient may increase the dose requirement of digoxin). Products include:

Levothroid Tablets 1373
Levoxyl Tablets 1819
Synthroid 505
Unithroid Tablets 3445

Liothyronine Sodium (Thyroid administration to a digitalized, hypothyroid patient may increase the dose requirement of digoxin). Products include:

Cytomel Tablets 1817
Triostat Injection 1825

Liotrix (Thyroid administration to a digitalized, hypothyroid patient may increase the dose requirement of digoxin).

No products indexed under this heading.

Magaldrate (Antacids may interfere with intestinal digoxin absorption, resulting in unexpectedly low serum concentrations; antacids may cause hypokalemia or hypomagnesemia and co-administration can cause digitalis toxicity).

No products indexed under this heading.

Magnesium Hydroxide (Antacids may interfere with intestinal digoxin absorption, resulting in unexpectedly low serum concentrations; antacids may cause hypokalemia or hypomagnesemia and co-administration can cause digitalis toxicity). Products include:

Ex•Lax Milk of Magnesia Liquid ....▣670
Maalox Antacid/Anti-Gas Oral Suspension ....▣673
Maalox Max Maximum Strength Antacid/Anti-Gas Liquid 2300
Maalox Regular Strength Antacid/Antigas Liquid 2300
Mylanta Fast-Acting 1813
Mylanta 1813
Pepcid Complete Chewable Tablets 1815
Phillips' Chewable Tablets ....▣615
Phillips' Milk of Magnesia Liquid (Original, Cherry, & Mint) ....▣616
Rolaids Tablets ....▣706
Extra Strength Rolaids Tablets ......▣706
Vanquish Caplets ....▣617

Magnesium Oxide (Antacids may interfere with intestinal digoxin absorption, resulting in unexpectedly low serum concentrations; antacids may cause hypokalemia or hypomagnesemia and co-administration can cause digitalis toxicity). Products include:

Beelith Tablets 946
Mag-Ox 400 Tablets 1024
Uro-Mag Capsules 1024

Metaproterenol Sulfate (Concomitant use of digoxin and sympathomimetics increases the risk of cardiac arrhythmias). Products include:

Alupent 1029

Metaraminol Bitartrate (Concomitant use of digoxin and sympathomimetics increases the risk of cardiac arrhythmias). Products include:

Aramine Injection 2043

Methacycline Hydrochloride (May increase digoxin absorption in patients who inactivate digoxin by bacterial metabolism in the lower intestine, so that digitalis intoxication may result).

No products indexed under this heading.

Methoxamine Hydrochloride (Concomitant use of digoxin and sympathomimetics increases the risk of cardiac arrhythmias).

No products indexed under this heading.

Methyclothiazide (Potassium-depleting diuretics can cause hypokalemia and co-administration can result in digitalis toxicity).

No products indexed under this heading.

Methylprednisolone Acetate (Corticosteroids can cause hypokalemia or hypomagnesemia and potassium or magnesium depletion can sensitize the myocardium to digoxin resulting in digitalis toxicity). Products include:

Depo-Medrol Injectable Suspension 2795

Methylprednisolone Sodium Succinate (Corticosteroids can cause hypokalemia or hypomagnesemia and potassium or magnesium depletion can sensitize the myocardium to digoxin resulting in digitalis toxicity). Products include:

Solu-Medrol Sterile Powder 2855

Metipranolol Hydrochloride (Concomitant use of digoxin and beta-andrenergic blockers may result in the additive effects on AV node conduction).

No products indexed under this heading.

Metoclopramide Hydrochloride (May interfere with intestinal digoxin absorption, resulting in unexpectedly low serum concentrations). Products include:

Reglan 2935

Metoprolol Succinate (Concomitant use of digoxin and beta-andrenergic blockers may result in the additive effects on AV node conduction). Products include:

Toprol-XL Tablets 651

Metoprolol Tartrate (Concomitant use of digoxin and beta-andrenergic blockers may result in the additive effects on AV node conduction).

No products indexed under this heading.

Mibefradil Dihydrochloride (Concomitant use of digoxin and calcium channel blockers may result in the additive effects on AV node conduction).

No products indexed under this heading.

Minocycline Hydrochloride (May increase digoxin absorption in patients who inactivate digoxin by bacterial metabolism in the lower intestine, so that digitalis intoxication may result). Products include:

Dynacin Capsules 2019
Minocin Intravenous 1862
Minocin Oral Suspension 1865
Minocin Pellet-Filled Capsules 1863

Nadolol (Concomitant use of digoxin and beta-andrenergic blockers may result in the additive effects on AV node conduction). Products include:

Corgard Tablets 2245
Corzide 40/5 Tablets 2247
Corzide 80/5 Tablets 2247
Nadolol Tablets 2288

Neomycin, oral (May interfere with intestinal digoxin absorption, resulting in unexpectedly low serum concentrations).

No products indexed under this heading.

Nicardipine Hydrochloride (Concomitant use of digoxin and calcium channel blockers may result in the additive effects on AV node conduction). Products include:

Cardene I.V. 3485

Nifedipine (Concomitant use of digoxin and calcium channel blockers may result in the additive effects on AV node conduction). Products include:

Adalat CC Tablets 877
Procardia Capsules 2708
Procardia XL Extended Release Tablets 2710

Nimodipine (Concomitant use of digoxin and calcium channel blockers may result in the additive effects on AV node conduction). Products include:

Nimotop Capsules 904

Nisoldipine (Concomitant use of digoxin and calcium channel blockers may result in the additive effects on AV node conduction). Products include:

Sular Tablets 688

Norepinephrine Bitartrate (Concomitant use of digoxin and sympathomimetics increases the risk of cardiac arrhythmias).

No products indexed under this heading.

Oxytetracycline Hydrochloride (May increase digoxin absorption in patients who inactivate digoxin by bacterial metabolism in the lower intestine, so that digitalis intoxication may result). Products include:

Terra-Cortril Ophthalmic Suspension 2716
Urobiotic-250 Capsules 2731

Pectin (May interfere with intestinal digoxin absorption, resulting in unexpectedly low serum concentrations). Products include:
- Celestial Seasonings Soothers Throat Drops ■ 685
- Halls Plus Cough Drops ■ 686

Penbutolol Sulfate (Concomitant use of digoxin and beta-andrenergic blockers may result in the additive effects on AV node conduction).
- No products indexed under this heading.

Penicillamine (Co-administration has resulted in inconsistent reports regarding the effects of penicillamine on serum digoxin concentration). Products include:
- Cuprimine Capsules 2075
- Depen Titratable Tablets 3341

Phenylephrine Bitartrate (Concomitant use of digoxin and sympathomimetics increases the risk of cardiac arrhythmias).
- No products indexed under this heading.

Phenylephrine Hydrochloride (Concomitant use of digoxin and sympathomimetics increases the risk of cardiac arrhythmias). Products include:
- Afrin Nasal Decongestant Children's Pump Mist ■ 734
- Extendryl 1361
- Hycomine Compound Tablets 1317
- Neo-Synephrine ■ 614
- Phenergan VC Syrup 3560
- Phenergan VC with Codeine Syrup 3561
- Preparation H Cream ■ 778
- Preparation H Cooling Gel ■ 778
- Preparation H ■ 778
- Vicks Sinex Nasal Spray and Ultra Fine Mist ■ 729

Phenylephrine Tannate (Concomitant use of digoxin and sympathomimetics increases the risk of cardiac arrhythmias). Products include:
- Ryna-12 S Suspension 3351
- Reformulated Rynatan Pediatric Suspension 3352
- Rynatuss Pediatric Suspension 3353
- Rynatuss Tablets 3353

Phenylpropanolamine Hydrochloride (Concomitant use of digoxin and sympathomimetics increases the risk of cardiac arrhythmias).
- No products indexed under this heading.

Pindolol (Concomitant use of digoxin and beta-andrenergic blockers may result in the additive effects on AV node conduction).
- No products indexed under this heading.

Pirbuterol Acetate (Concomitant use of digoxin and sympathomimetics increases the risk of cardiac arrhythmias). Products include:
- Maxair Autohaler 1981
- Maxair Inhaler 1984

Polythiazide (Potassium-depleting diuretics can cause hypokalemia and co-administration can result in digitalis toxicity). Products include:
- Minizide Capsules 2700
- Renese Tablets 2712

Prednisolone Acetate (Corticosteroids can cause hypokalemia or hypomagnesemia and potassium or magnesium depletion can sensitize the myocardium to digoxin resulting in digitalis toxicity). Products include:
- Blephamide Ophthalmic Ointment 547
- Blephamide Ophthalmic Suspension 548
- Poly-Pred Liquifilm Ophthalmic Suspension ⊙ 245
- Pred Forte Ophthalmic Suspension ⊙ 246
- Pred Mild Sterile Ophthalmic Suspension ⊙ 249
- Pred-G Ophthalmic Suspension ⊙ 247
- Pred-G Sterile Ophthalmic Ointment ⊙ 248

Prednisolone Sodium Phosphate (Corticosteroids can cause hypokalemia or hypomagnesemia and potassium or magnesium depletion can sensitize the myocardium to digoxin resulting in digitalis toxicity). Products include:
- Pediapred Oral Solution 1170

Prednisolone Tebutate (Corticosteroids can cause hypokalemia or hypomagnesemia and potassium or magnesium depletion can sensitize the myocardium to digoxin resulting in digitalis toxicity).
- No products indexed under this heading.

Prednisone (Corticosteroids can cause hypokalemia or hypomagnesemia and potassium or magnesium depletion can sensitize the myocardium to digoxin resulting in digitalis toxicity). Products include:
- Prednisone 3064

Propafenone Hydrochloride (Raises the serum digoxin concentration due to reduction in clearance and/or volume of distribution of the drug, with the implication that digitalis intoxication may result). Products include:
- Rythmol Tablets – 150 mg, 225 mg, 300 mg 502

Propantheline Bromide (Decreases gut motility and may increase digoxin absorption).
- No products indexed under this heading.

Propranolol Hydrochloride (Concomitant use of digoxin and beta-andrenergic blockers may result in the additive effects on AV node conduction). Products include:
- Inderal 3513
- Inderal LA Long-Acting Capsules 3516
- Inderide Tablets 3517
- Inderide LA Long Acting Capsules 3519

Pseudoephedrine Hydrochloride (Concomitant use of digoxin and sympathomimetics increases the risk of cardiac arrhythmias). Products include:
- Actifed Cold & Allergy Tablets ■ 688
- Actifed Cold & Sinus Caplets and Tablets ■ 688
- Advil Cold and Sinus Caplets ■ 771
- Advil Cold and Sinus Tablets ■ 771
- Advil Flu & Body Ache Caplets ■ 772
- Aleve Cold & Sinus Caplets ■ 603
- Alka-Seltzer Plus Liqui-Gels ■ 604
- Alka-Seltzer Plus Cold & Flu Medicine Liqui-Gels ■ 604
- Alka-Seltzer Plus Cold & Sinus Medicine Liqui-Gels ■ 604
- Allegra-D Extended-Release Tablets 714
- BC Cold Powder ■ 619
- Benadryl Allergy/Cold Tablets ■ 691
- Benadryl Allergy/Congestion Tablets ■ 692
- Benadryl Allergy & Sinus Liquid ■ 693
- Benadryl Allergy & Sinus Fastmelt Tablets ■ 693
- Benadryl Allergy Sinus Headache Caplets & Gelcaps ■ 693
- Benadryl Severe Allergy & Sinus Headache Caplets ■ 694
- Benadryl Children's Allergy/Cold Fastmelt Tablets ■ 692
- Benylin Multi-Symptom Liquid ■ 697
- Bromfed Capsules (Extended-Release) 2269
- Bromfed-PD Capsules (Extended-Release) 2269
- Children's Cēpacol Sore Throat ■ 788
- Comtrex Acute Head Cold & Sinus Pressure Relief Tablets ■ 627
- Comtrex Deep Chest Cold & Congestion Relief Softgels ■ 627
- Comtrex Flu Therapy & Fever Relief Daytime Caplets ■ 628
- Comtrex Flu Therapy & Fever Relief Nighttime Tablets ■ 628
- Comtrex Maximum Strength Multi-Symptom Cold & Cough Relief Tablets and Caplets ■ 626
- Contac Non-Drowsy 12 Hour Cold Caplets ■ 745
- Contac Non-Drowsy Timed Release 12 Hour Cold Caplets ■ 746
- Contac Severe Cold and Flu Caplets Maximum Strength ■ 746
- Contac Severe Cold and Flu Caplets Non-Drowsy ■ 746
- Dimetapp Elixir ■ 777
- Dimetapp Cold and Fever Suspension ■ 775
- Dimetapp DM Cold & Cough Elixir ■ 775
- Dimetapp Nighttime Flu Liquid ■ 776
- Dimetapp Non-Drowsy Flu Syrup ■ 777
- Dimetapp Infant Drops Decongestant ■ 775
- Dimetapp Infant Drops Decongestant Plus Cough ■ 776
- Guaifed 2272
- Kronofed-A 1341
- Children's Motrin Cold Oral Suspension 2007
- Motrin Sinus Headache Caplets 2005
- PediaCare Cough-Cold Liquid ■ 719
- PediaCare Infants' Drops Decongestant ■ 719
- PediaCare Infants' Drops Decongestant Plus Cough ■ 719
- PediaCare NightRest Cough-Cold Liquid ■ 719
- Robitussin Cold Caplets Cold & Congestion ■ 780
- Robitussin Cold Softgels Cold & Congestion ■ 780
- Robitussin Cold Caplets Multi-Symptom Cold & Flu ■ 781
- Robitussin Cold Softgels Multi-Symptom Cold & Flu ■ 781
- Robitussin Cold Softgels Severe Congestion ■ 782
- Robitussin Cough & Cold Infant Drops ■ 782
- Robitussin Maximum Strength Cough & Cold Liquid ■ 785
- Robitussin Pediatric Cough & Cold Formula Liquid ■ 785
- Robitussin Multi Symptom Honey Flu Liquid ■ 785
- Robitussin Nighttime Honey Flu Liquid ■ 786
- Robitussin-CF Liquid ■ 783
- Robitussin-DAC Syrup 2942
- Robitussin-PE Liquid ■ 782
- Ryna ■ 768
- Semprex-D Capsules 1172
- Singlet Caplets ■ 761
- Sinutab Non-Drying Liquid Caps ■ 706
- Sinutab Sinus Allergy Medication, Maximum Strength Formula, Tablets & Caplets ■ 707
- Sinutab Sinus Medication, Maximum Strength Without Drowsiness Formula, Tablets & Caplets ■ 707
- Sudafed 12 Hour Tablets ■ 708
- Sudafed 24 Hour Tablets ■ 708
- Children's Sudafed Cold & Cough Liquid ■ 709
- Children's Sudafed Nasal Decongestant Chewables ■ 711
- Children's Sudafed Nasal Decongestant Liquid Medication ■ 711
- Sudafed Cold & Allergy Tablets ■ 708
- Sudafed Cold & Cough Liquid Caps ■ 709
- Sudafed Cold & Sinus Liquid Caps ■ 710
- Sudafed Nasal Decongestant Tablets ■ 710
- Sudafed Non-Drying Sinus Liquid Caps ■ 712
- Sudafed Severe Cold ■ 711
- Sudafed Sinus Headache Caplets ■ 712
- Sudafed Sinus Headache Tablets ■ 712
- Tavist Sinus Non-Drowsy Coated Caplets ■ 676
- TheraFlu Regular Strength Cold & Cough Night Time Hot Liquid ■ 676
- TheraFlu Regular Strength Cold & Sore Throat Night Time Hot Liquid ■ 676
- TheraFlu Maximum Strength Flu & Congestion Non-Drowsy Hot Liquid ■ 677
- TheraFlu Maximum Strength Flu & Cough Night Time Hot Liquid ■ 678
- TheraFlu Maximum Strength Flu & Sore Throat Night Time Hot Liquid ■ 677
- TheraFlu Maximum Strength Severe Cold & Congestion Night Time Caplets ■ 678
- TheraFlu Maximum Strength Severe Cold & Congestion Night Time Hot Liquid ■ 678
- TheraFlu Maximum Strength Severe Cold & Congestion Non-Drowsy ■ 679
- Triaminic Allergy Congestion Liquid ■ 680
- Triaminic Chest Congestion Liquid ■ 680
- Triaminic Cold & Allergy Liquid ■ 681
- Triaminic Cold & Allergy Softchews ■ 683
- Triaminic Cold & Cough Liquid ■ 681
- Triaminic Cold & Cough Softchews ■ 683
- Triaminic Cold & Night Time Cough Liquid ■ 681
- Triaminic Cold, Cough & Fever Liquid ■ 681
- Triaminic Cough Liquid ■ 682
- Triaminic Cough & Congestion Liquid ■ 682
- Triaminic Cough & Sore Throat Liquid ■ 682
- Triaminic Cough & Sore Throat Softchews ■ 684
- Children's Tylenol Allergy-D Liquid 2014
- Children's Tylenol Cold Suspension Liquid and Chewable Tablets 2015
- Children's Tylenol Cold Plus Cough Suspension Liquid and Chewable Tablets 2015
- Children's Tylenol Flu Suspension Liquid 2015
- Children's Tylenol Sinus Suspension Liquid 2017
- Infants' Tylenol Cold Decongestant and Fever Reducer Concentrated Drops 2015
- Infants' Tylenol Cold Decongestant and Fever Reducer Concentrated Drops Plus Cough 2015
- Tylenol Allergy Sinus 2010
- Multi-Symptom Tylenol Cold Complete Formula Caplets 2010
- Multi-Symptom Tylenol Cold Non-Drowsy Caplets and Gelcaps 2010
- Multi-Symptom Tylenol Cold Severe Congestion Non-Drowsy Caplets 2011
- Maximum Strength Tylenol Flu NightTime Gelcaps 2011
- Maximum Strength Tylenol Flu NightTime Liquid 2011
- Maximum Strength Tylenol Flu Non-Drowsy Gelcaps 2011
- Maximum Strength Tylenol Sinus NightTime Caplets 2012
- Maximum Strength Tylenol Sinus Non-Drowsy Geltabs, Gelcaps, Caplets, and Tablets 2012
- Vicks 44D Cough & Head Congestion Relief Liquid ■ 724
- Vicks 44M Cough, Cold & Flu Relief Liquid ■ 725
- Pediatric Vicks 44m Cough & Cold Relief ■ 728
- Vicks DayQuil LiquiCaps/Liquid Multi-Symptom Cold/Flu Relief ■ 727
- Children's Vicks NyQuil Cold/Cough Relief ■ 726
- Vicks NyQuil LiquiCaps/Liquid Multi-Symptom Cold/Flu Relief, Original and Cherry Flavors ■ 727
- Zephrex Tablets 3091
- Zephrex LA Tablets 3092
- Zyrtec-D 12 Hour Extended Relief Tablets 2758

Pseudoephedrine Sulfate (Concomitant use of digoxin and sympathomimetics increases the risk of cardiac arrhythmias). Products include:
- Chlor-Trimeton Allergy/Decongestant Tablets ■ 736
- Claritin-D 12 Hour Extended Release Tablets 3102
- Claritin-D 24 Hour Extended Release Tablets 3104
- Coricidin 'D' Cold, Flu & Sinus Tablets ■ 737
- Drixoral Allergy/Sinus Extended-Release Tablets ■ 741
- Drixoral Cold & Allergy Sustained-Action Tablets ■ 740
- Drixoral Cold & Flu Extended-Release Tablets ■ 740
- Drixoral Nasal Decongestant Long-Acting Non-Drowsy Tablets ■ 740
- Rynatan Tablets 3351

Quinidine Gluconate (Raises the serum digoxin concentration due to reduction in clearance and/or volume of distribution of the drug, with the implication that digitalis intoxication may result). Products include:
- Quinaglute Dura-Tabs Tablets 978

Quinidine Polygalacturonate (Raises the serum digoxin concentration due to reduction in clearance and/or volume of distribution of the drug, with the implication that digita-

IMPORTANT NOTE: Always consult each drug listing in the patient's regimen for possible interactions.

lis intoxication may result).
No products indexed under this heading.

Quinidine Sulfate (Raises the serum digoxin concentration due to reduction in clearance and/or volume of distribution of the drug, with the implication that digitalis intoxication may result). Products include:
Quinidex Extentabs 2933

Quinine (Co-administration has resulted in inconsistent reports regarding the effects of quinine on serum digoxin concentration).
No products indexed under this heading.

Rifampin (May decrease serum digoxin concentration, especially in patients with renal dysfunction, by increasing the non-renal clearance of digoxin). Products include:
Rifadin 765
Rifamate Capsules 767
Rifater Tablets 769

Salmeterol Xinafoate (Concomitant use of digoxin and sympathomimetics increases the risk of cardiac arrhythmias). Products include:
Advair Diskus 100/50 1448
Advair Diskus 250/50 1448
Advair Diskus 500/50 1448
Serevent Diskus 1637
Serevent Inhalation Aerosol 1633

Sodium Bicarbonate (Antacids may interfere with intestinal digoxin absorption, resulting in unexpectedly low serum concentrations; antacids may cause hypokalemia and hypomagnesemia and co-administration can cause digitalis toxicity). Products include:
Alka-Seltzer .... ▣603
Alka-Seltzer Lemon Lime Antacid and Pain Reliever Effervescent Tablets .... ▣603
Alka-Seltzer Extra Strength Antacid and Pain Reliever Effervescent Tablets .... ▣603
Alka-Seltzer Heartburn Relief Tablets .... ▣604
Ceo-Two Evacuant Suppository .... ▣618
Colyte with Flavor Packs for Oral Solution 3170
GoLYTELY and Pineapple Flavor GoLYTELY for Oral Solution 1068
NuLYTELY, Cherry Flavor, Lemon-Lime Flavor, and Orange Flavor NuLYTELY for Oral Solution 1068

Sotalol Hydrochloride (Concomitant use of digoxin and beta-andrenergic blockers may result in the additive effects on AV node conduction). Products include:
Betapace Tablets 950
Betapace AF Tablets 954

Spironolactone (Raises the serum digoxin concentration due to reduction in clearance and/or volume of distribution of the drug, with the implication that digitalis intoxication may result).
No products indexed under this heading.

Succinylcholine Chloride (May cause a sudden extrusion of potassium from muscle cells, and may thereby cause arrhythmias in digitalized patients). Products include:
Anectine Injection 1476

Sulfasalazine (May interfere with intestinal digoxin absorption, resulting in unexpectedly low serum concentrations). Products include:
Azulfidine EN-tabs Tablets 2775

Terbutaline Sulfate (Concomitant use of digoxin and sympathomimetics increases the risk of cardiac arrhythmias). Products include:
Brethine Ampuls 2314
Brethine Tablets 2313

Tetracycline Hydrochloride (May increase digoxin absorption in patients who inactivate digoxin by bacterial metabolism in the lower intestine, so that digitalis intoxication may result).
No products indexed under this heading.

Thyroglobulin (Thyroid administration to a digitalized, hypothyroid patient may increase the dose requirement of digoxin).
No products indexed under this heading.

Thyroid (Thyroid administration to a digitalized, hypothyroid patient may increase the dose requirement of digoxin).
No products indexed under this heading.

Thyroxine (Thyroid administration to a digitalized, hypothyroid patient may increase the dose requirement of digoxin).
No products indexed under this heading.

Thyroxine Sodium (Thyroid administration to a digitalized, hypothyroid patient may increase the dose requirement of digoxin).
No products indexed under this heading.

Timolol Hemihydrate (Concomitant use of digoxin and beta-andrenergic blockers may result in the additive effects on AV node conduction). Products include:
Betimol Ophthalmic Solution .... ⊙324

Timolol Maleate (Concomitant use of digoxin and beta-andrenergic blockers may result in the additive effects on AV node conduction). Products include:
Blocadren Tablets 2046
Cosopt Sterile Ophthalmic Solution 2065
Timolide Tablets 2187
Timolol GFS .... ⊙266
Timoptic in Ocudose 2192
Timoptic Sterile Ophthalmic Solution 2190
Timoptic-XE Sterile Ophthalmic Gel Forming Solution 2194

Torsemide (Potassium-depleting diuretics can cause hypokalemia and co-administration can result in digitalis toxicity). Products include:
Demadex Tablets and Injection 2965

Triamcinolone (Corticosteroids can cause hypokalemia or hypomagnesemia and potassium or magnesium depletion can sensitize the myocardium to digoxin resulting in digitalis toxicity).
No products indexed under this heading.

Triamcinolone Acetonide (Corticosteroids can cause hypokalemia or hypomagnesemia and potassium or magnesium depletion can sensitize the myocardium to digoxin resulting in digitalis toxicity). Products include:
Azmacort Inhalation Aerosol 728
Nasacort Nasal Inhaler 750
Nasacort AQ Nasal Spray 752
Tri-Nasal Spray 2274

Triamcinolone Diacetate (Corticosteroids can cause hypokalemia or hypomagnesemia and potassium or magnesium depletion can sensitize the myocardium to digoxin resulting in digitalis toxicity).
No products indexed under this heading.

Triamcinolone Hexacetonide (Corticosteroids can cause hypokalemia or hypomagnesemia and potassium or magnesium depletion can sensitize the myocardium to digoxin resulting in digitalis toxicity).
No products indexed under this heading.

Troleandomycin (Macrolide antibiotics may possibly increase digoxin absorption in patients who inactivate digoxin by bacterial metabolism in the lower intestine, so that digitalis intoxication may result). Products include:
Tao Capsules 2716

Verapamil Hydrochloride (Raises the serum digoxin concentration due to reduction in clearance and/or volume of distribution of the drug, with the implication that digitalis intoxication may result). Products include:
Covera-HS Tablets 3199
Isoptin SR Tablets 467
Tarka Tablets 508
Verelan Capsules 3184
Verelan PM Capsules 3186

Food Interactions

Meal, high in bran fiber (The amount of digoxin from an oral dose may be reduced).

Meal, unspecified (Slows the rate of absorption).

LANOXIN ELIXIR PEDIATRIC
(Digoxin) 1578
See Lanoxin Tablets

LANOXIN INJECTION PEDIATRIC
(Digoxin) 1584
See Lanoxin Tablets

LANTUS INJECTION
(Insulin glargine) 742
May interact with ACE inhibitors, beta blockers, corticosteroids, diuretics, fibrates, oral hypoglycemic agents, lithium preparations, monoamine oxidase inhibitors, oral contraceptives, phenothiazines, salicylates, sympathomimetics, thyroid preparations, and certain other agents. Compounds in these categories include:

Acarbose (May increase the blood-glucose-lowering effect and susceptibility to hypoglycemia). Products include:
Precose Tablets 906

Acebutolol Hydrochloride (Beta-blockers may either potentiate or weaken the blood-glucose-lowering effect of insulin; signs of hypoglycemia may be reduced or absent with co-administration). Products include:
Sectral Capsules 3589

Albuterol (Sympathomimetic agents may reduce the blood-glucose-lowering effect of insulin). Products include:
Proventil Inhalation Aerosol 3142
Ventolin Inhalation Aerosol and Refill 1679

Albuterol Sulfate (Sympathomimetic agents may reduce the blood-glucose-lowering effect of insulin). Products include:
AccuNeb Inhalation Solution 1230
Combivent Inhalation Aerosol 1041
DuoNeb Inhalation Solution 1233
Proventil Inhalation Solution 0.083% 3146
Proventil Repetabs Tablets 3148
Proventil Solution for Inhalation 0.5% 3144
Proventil HFA Inhalation Aerosol 3150
Ventolin HFA Inhalation Aerosol 3618
Volmax Extended-Release Tablets 2276

Amiloride Hydrochloride (Diuretics may reduce the blood-glucose-lowering effect of insulin). Products include:
Midamor Tablets 2136
Moduretic Tablets 2138

Aspirin (May increase the blood-glucose-lowering effect and susceptibility to hypoglycemia). Products include:
Aggrenox Capsules 1026
Alka-Seltzer .... ▣603
Alka-Seltzer Lemon Lime Antacid and Pain Reliever Effervescent Tablets .... ▣603
Alka-Seltzer Extra Strength Antacid and Pain Reliever Effervescent Tablets .... ▣603
Alka-Seltzer PM Effervescent Tablets .... ▣605
Genuine Bayer Tablets, Caplets and Gelcaps .... ▣606
Extra Strength Bayer Caplets and Gelcaps .... ▣610
Aspirin Regimen Bayer Children's Chewable Tablets (Orange or Cherry Flavored) .... ▣607
Bayer, Aspirin Regimen .... ▣606
Aspirin Regimen Bayer 81 mg Caplets with Calcium .... ▣607
Genuine Bayer Professional Labeling (Aspirin Regimen Bayer) .... ▣608
Extra Strength Bayer Arthritis Caplets .... ▣610
Extra Strength Bayer Plus Caplets .... ▣610
Extra Strength Bayer PM Caplets .... ▣611
BC Powder .... ▣619
BC Allergy Sinus Cold Powder .... ▣619
Arthritis Strength BC Powder .... ▣619
BC Sinus Cold Powder .... ▣619
Darvon Compound-65 Pulvules 1910
Ecotrin Enteric Coated Aspirin Low, Regular and Maximum Strength Tablets 1715
Excedrin Extra-Strength Tablets, Caplets, and Geltabs .... ▣629
Excedrin Migraine 1070
Goody's Body Pain Formula Powder .... ▣620
Goody's Extra Strength Headache Powder .... ▣620
Goody's Extra Strength Pain Relief Tablets .... ▣620
Percodan Tablets 1327
Robaxisal Tablets 2939
Soma Compound Tablets 3354
Soma Compound w/Codeine Tablets 3355
Vanquish Caplets .... ▣617

Atenolol (Beta-blockers may either potentiate or weaken the blood-glucose-lowering effect of insulin; signs of hypoglycemia may be reduced or absent with co-administration). Products include:
Tenoretic Tablets 690
Tenormin I.V. Injection 692

Benazepril Hydrochloride (May increase the blood-glucose-lowering effect and susceptibility to hypoglycemia). Products include:
Lotensin Tablets 2365
Lotensin HCT Tablets 2367
Lotrel Capsules 2370

Bendroflumethiazide (Diuretics may reduce the blood-glucose-lowering effect of insulin). Products include:
Corzide 40/5 Tablets 2247
Corzide 80/5 Tablets 2247

Betamethasone Acetate (Co-administration with corticosteroids may reduce the blood-glucose-lowering effect of insulin). Products include:
Celestone Soluspan Injectable Suspension 3097

Betamethasone Sodium Phosphate (Co-administration with corticosteroids may reduce the blood-glucose-lowering effect of insulin). Products include:
Celestone Soluspan Injectable Suspension 3097

Betaxolol Hydrochloride (Beta-blockers may either potentiate or weaken the blood-glucose-lowering effect of insulin; signs of hypoglycemia may be reduced or absent with co-administration). Products include:
Betoptic S Ophthalmic Suspension 537

Bisoprolol Fumarate (Beta-blockers may either potentiate or weaken the blood-glucose-lowering effect of insulin; signs of hypoglycemia may be reduced or absent with co-administration). Products include:
Zebeta Tablets 1885
Ziac Tablets 1887

Bumetanide (Diuretics may reduce the blood-glucose-lowering effect of insulin).
No products indexed under this heading.

Captopril (May increase the blood-glucose-lowering effect and susceptibility to hypoglycemia). Products include:

Captopril Tablets 2281

Carteolol Hydrochloride (Beta-blockers may either potentiate or weaken the blood-glucose-lowering effect of insulin; signs of hypoglycemia may be reduced or absent with co-administration). Products include:
- Carteolol Hydrochloride Ophthalmic Solution USP, 1% .... ⊙258
- Ocupress Ophthalmic Solution, 1% Sterile .... ⊙303

Chlorothiazide (Diuretics may reduce the blood-glucose-lowering effect of insulin). Products include:
- Aldoclor Tablets 2035
- Diuril Oral 2087

Chlorothiazide Sodium (Diuretics may reduce the blood-glucose-lowering effect of insulin). Products include:
- Diuril Sodium Intravenous 2086

Chlorpromazine (Phenothiazine derivatives may reduce the blood-glucose-lowering effect of insulin). Products include:
- Thorazine Suppositories 1656

Chlorpromazine Hydrochloride (Phenothiazine derivatives may reduce the blood-glucose-lowering effect of insulin). Products include:
- Thorazine 1656

Chlorpropamide (May increase the blood-glucose-lowering effect and susceptibility to hypoglycemia). Products include:
- Diabinese Tablets 2680

Chlorthalidone (Diuretics may reduce the blood-glucose-lowering effect of insulin). Products include:
- Clorpres Tablets 1002
- Combipres Tablets 1040
- Tenoretic Tablets 690

Choline Magnesium Trisalicylate (May increase the blood-glucose-lowering effect and susceptibility to hypoglycemia). Products include:
- Trilisate 2901

Clofibrate (May increase the blood-glucose-lowering effect and susceptibility to hypoglycemia). Products include:
- Atromid-S Capsules 3483

Clonidine (Signs of hypoglycemia may be reduced or absent with co-administration). Products include:
- Catapres-TTS 1038

Clonidine Hydrochloride (Signs of hypoglycemia may be reduced or absent with co-administration). Products include:
- Catapres Tablets 1037
- Clorpres Tablets 1002
- Combipres Tablets 1040
- Duraclon Injection 3057

Cortisone Acetate (Co-administration with corticosteroids may reduce the blood-glucose-lowering effect of insulin). Products include:
- Cortone Acetate Injectable Suspension 2059
- Cortone Acetate Tablets 2061

Danazol (May reduce the blood-glucose-lowering effect of insulin).
- No products indexed under this heading.

Desogestrel (Oral contraceptives may reduce the blood-glucose-lowering effect of insulin). Products include:
- Cyclessa Tablets 2450
- Desogen Tablets 2458
- Mircette Tablets 2470
- Ortho-Cept 21 Tablets 2546
- Ortho-Cept 28 Tablets 2546

Dexamethasone (Co-administration with corticosteroids may reduce the blood-glucose-lowering effect of insulin). Products include:
- Decadron Elixir 2078
- Decadron Tablets 2079
- TobraDex Ophthalmic Ointment 542
- TobraDex Ophthalmic Suspension 541

Dexamethasone Acetate (Co-administration with corticosteroids may reduce the blood-glucose-lowering effect of insulin).
- No products indexed under this heading.

Dexamethasone Sodium Phosphate (Co-administration with corticosteroids may reduce the blood-glucose-lowering effect of insulin). Products include:
- Decadron Phosphate Injection 2081
- Decadron Phosphate Sterile Ophthalmic Ointment 2083
- Decadron Phosphate Sterile Ophthalmic Solution 2084
- NeoDecadron Sterile Ophthalmic Solution 2144

Diflunisal (May increase the blood-glucose-lowering effect and susceptibility to hypoglycemia). Products include:
- Dolobid Tablets 2088

Disopyramide Phosphate (May increase the blood-glucose-lowering effect and susceptibility to hypoglycemia).
- No products indexed under this heading.

Dobutamine Hydrochloride (Sympathomimetic agents may reduce the blood-glucose-lowering effect of insulin). Products include:
- Dobutrex Solution Vials 1914

Dopamine Hydrochloride (Sympathomimetic agents may reduce the blood-glucose-lowering effect of insulin).
- No products indexed under this heading.

Enalapril Maleate (May increase the blood-glucose-lowering effect and susceptibility to hypoglycemia). Products include:
- Lexxel Tablets 608
- Vaseretic Tablets 2204
- Vasotec Tablets 2210

Enalaprilat (May increase the blood-glucose-lowering effect and susceptibility to hypoglycemia). Products include:
- Enalaprilat Injection 863
- Vasotec I.V. Injection 2207

Ephedrine Hydrochloride (Sympathomimetic agents may reduce the blood-glucose-lowering effect of insulin). Products include:
- Primatene Tablets .... ▣780

Ephedrine Sulfate (Sympathomimetic agents may reduce the blood-glucose-lowering effect of insulin).
- No products indexed under this heading.

Ephedrine Tannate (Sympathomimetic agents may reduce the blood-glucose-lowering effect of insulin). Products include:
- Rynatuss Pediatric Suspension 3353
- Rynatuss Tablets 3353

Epinephrine (Sympathomimetic agents may reduce the blood-glucose-lowering effect of insulin). Products include:
- Epifrin Sterile Ophthalmic Solution .... ⊙235
- EpiPen 1236
- Primatene Mist .... ▣779
- Xylocaine with Epinephrine Injection 653

Epinephrine Bitartrate (Sympathomimetic agents may reduce the blood-glucose-lowering effect of insulin). Products include:
- Sensorcaine 643

Epinephrine Hydrochloride (Sympathomimetic agents may reduce the blood-glucose-lowering effect of insulin).
- No products indexed under this heading.

Esmolol Hydrochloride (Beta-blockers may either potentiate or weaken the blood-glucose-lowering effect of insulin; signs of hypoglycemia may be reduced or absent with co-administration). Products include:
- Brevibloc Injection 858

Ethacrynic Acid (Diuretics may reduce the blood-glucose-lowering effect of insulin). Products include:
- Edecrin Tablets 2091

Ethinyl Estradiol (Oral contraceptives may reduce the blood-glucose-lowering effect of insulin). Products include:
- Alesse-21 Tablets 3468
- Alesse-28 Tablets 3473
- Brevicon 28-Day Tablets 3380
- Cyclessa Tablets 2450
- Desogen Tablets 2458
- Estinyl Tablets 3112
- Estrostep 2627
- femhrt Tablets 2635
- Levlen 962
- Levlite 21 Tablets 962
- Levlite 28 Tablets 962
- Levora Tablets 3389
- Loestrin 21 Tablets 2642
- Loestrin Fe Tablets 2642
- Lo/Ovral Tablets 3532
- Lo/Ovral-28 Tablets 3538
- Low-Ogestrel-28 Tablets 3392
- Microgestin Fe 1.5/30 Tablets 3407
- Microgestin Fe 1/20 Tablets 3400
- Mircette Tablets 2470
- Modicon 2563
- Necon 3415
- Nordette-28 Tablets 2257
- Norinyl 1 +35 28-Day Tablets 3380
- Ogestrel 0.5/50-28 Tablets 3428
- Ortho-Cept 21 Tablets 2546
- Ortho-Cept 28 Tablets 2546
- Ortho-Cyclen/Ortho Tri-Cyclen 2573
- Ortho-Novum 2563
- Ovcon 3364
- Ovral Tablets 3551
- Ovral-28 Tablets 3552
- Tri-Levlen 962
- Tri-Norinyl-28 Tablets 3433
- Triphasil-21 Tablets 3600
- Triphasil-28 Tablets 3605
- Trivora Tablets 3439
- Yasmin 28 Tablets 980
- Zovia 3449

Ethynodiol Diacetate (Oral contraceptives may reduce the blood-glucose-lowering effect of insulin). Products include:
- Zovia 3449

Fenofibrate (May increase the blood-glucose-lowering effect and susceptibility to hypoglycemia). Products include:
- Tricor Capsules, Micronized 513

Fludrocortisone Acetate (Co-administration with corticosteroids may reduce the blood-glucose-lowering effect of insulin). Products include:
- Florinef Acetate Tablets 2250

Fluoxetine Hydrochloride (May increase the blood-glucose-lowering effect and susceptibility to hypoglycemia). Products include:
- Prozac Pulvules, Liquid, and Weekly Capsules 1238
- Sarafem Pulvules 1962

Fluphenazine Decanoate (Phenothiazine derivatives may reduce the blood-glucose-lowering effect of insulin).
- No products indexed under this heading.

Fluphenazine Enanthate (Phenothiazine derivatives may reduce the blood-glucose-lowering effect of insulin).
- No products indexed under this heading.

Fluphenazine Hydrochloride (Phenothiazine derivatives may reduce the blood-glucose-lowering effect of insulin).
- No products indexed under this heading.

Fosinopril Sodium (May increase the blood-glucose-lowering effect and susceptibility to hypoglycemia). Products include:
- Monopril Tablets 1091
- Monopril HCT 1094

Furosemide (Diuretics may reduce the blood-glucose-lowering effect of insulin). Products include:
- Furosemide Tablets 2284

Gemfibrozil (May increase the blood-glucose-lowering effect and susceptibility to hypoglycemia). Products include:
- Lopid Tablets 2650

Glimepiride (May increase the blood-glucose-lowering effect and susceptibility to hypoglycemia). Products include:
- Amaryl Tablets 717

Glipizide (May increase the blood-glucose-lowering effect and susceptibility to hypoglycemia). Products include:
- Glucotrol Tablets 2692
- Glucotrol XL Extended Release Tablets 2693

Glyburide (May increase the blood-glucose-lowering effect and susceptibility to hypoglycemia). Products include:
- DiaBeta Tablets 741
- Glucovance Tablets 1086

Guanethidine Monosulfate (Signs of hypoglycemia may be reduced or absent with co-administration).
- No products indexed under this heading.

Hydrochlorothiazide (Diuretics may reduce the blood-glucose-lowering effect of insulin). Products include:
- Accuretic Tablets 2614
- Aldoril Tablets 2039
- Atacand HCT Tablets 597
- Avalide Tablets 1070
- Diovan HCT Tablets 2338
- Dyazide Capsules 1515
- HydroDIURIL Tablets 2108
- Hyzaar 2109
- Inderide Tablets 3517
- Inderide LA Long-Acting Capsules 3519
- Lotensin HCT Tablets 2367
- Maxzide 1008
- Micardis HCT Tablets 1051
- Microzide Capsules 3414
- Moduretic Tablets 2138
- Monopril HCT 1094
- Prinzide Tablets 2168
- Timolide Tablets 2187
- Uniretic Tablets 3178
- Vaseretic Tablets 2204
- Zestoretic Tablets 695
- Ziac Tablets 1887

Hydrocortisone (Co-administration with corticosteroids may reduce the blood-glucose-lowering effect of insulin). Products include:
- Anusol-HC Cream 2.5% 2237
- Cipro HC Otic Suspension 540
- Cortaid Intensive Therapy Cream .... ▣717
- Cortaid Maximum Strength Cream .... ▣717
- Cortisporin Ophthalmic Suspension Sterile .... ⊙297
- Cortizone•5 .... ▣699
- Cortizone•10 .... ▣699
- Cortizone•10 Plus Creme .... ▣700
- Cortizone for Kids Creme .... ▣699
- Hydrocortone Tablets 2106
- Massengill Medicated Soft Cloth Towelette .... ▣753
- VōSoL HC Otic Solution 3356

Hydrocortisone Acetate (Co-administration with corticosteroids may reduce the blood-glucose-lowering effect of insulin). Products include:
- Analpram-HC 1338
- Anusol HC-1 Hydrocortisone Anti-Itch Cream .... ▣689
- Anusol-HC Suppositories 2238
- Cortaid .... ▣717
- Cortifoam Rectal Foam 3170
- Cortisporin-TC Otic Suspension 2246
- Hydrocortone Acetate Injectable Suspension 2103
- Pramosone 1343
- Proctocort Suppositories 2264
- ProctoFoam-HC 3177
- Terra-Cortril Ophthalmic Suspension 2716

Hydrocortisone Sodium Phosphate (Co-administration with corticosteroids may reduce the blood-glucose-lowering effect of insulin). Products include:
- Hydrocortone Phosphate Injection, Sterile 2105

IMPORTANT NOTE: Always consult each drug listing in the patient's regimen for possible interactions.

Hydrocortisone Sodium Succinate (Co-administration with corticosteroids may reduce the blood-glucose-lowering effect of insulin).
No products indexed under this heading.

Hydroflumethiazide (Diuretics may reduce the blood-glucose-lowering effect of insulin). Products include:
Diucardin Tablets 3494

Indapamide (Diuretics may reduce the blood-glucose-lowering effect of insulin). Products include:
Indapamide Tablets 2286

Isocarboxazid (May increase the blood-glucose-lowering effect and susceptibility to hypoglycemia).
No products indexed under this heading.

Isoniazid (May reduce the blood-glucose-lowering effect of insulin). Products include:
Rifamate Capsules 767
Rifater Tablets 769

Isoproterenol Hydrochloride (Sympathomimetic agents may reduce the blood-glucose-lowering effect of insulin).
No products indexed under this heading.

Isoproterenol Sulfate (Sympathomimetic agents may reduce the blood-glucose-lowering effect of insulin).
No products indexed under this heading.

Labetalol Hydrochloride (Beta-blockers may either potentiate or weaken the blood-glucose-lowering effect of insulin; signs of hypoglycemia may be reduced or absent with co-administration). Products include:
Normodyne Injection 3135
Normodyne Tablets 3137

Levalbuterol Hydrochloride (Sympathomimetic agents may reduce the blood-glucose-lowering effect of insulin). Products include:
Xopenex Inhalation Solution 3207

Levobunolol Hydrochloride (Beta-blockers may either potentiate or weaken the blood-glucose-lowering effect of insulin; signs of hypoglycemia may be reduced or absent with co-administration). Products include:
Betagan .... ⊙228

Levonorgestrel (Oral contraceptives may reduce the blood-glucose-lowering effect of insulin). Products include:
Alesse-21 Tablets 3468
Alesse-28 Tablets 3473
Levlen 962
Levlite 21 Tablets 962
Levlite 28 Tablets 962
Levora Tablets 3389
Mirena Intrauterine System 974
Nordette-28 Tablets 2257
Norplant System 3543
Tri-Levlen 962
Triphasil-21 Tablets 3600
Triphasil-28 Tablets 3605
Trivora Tablets 3439

Levothyroxine Sodium (May reduce the blood-glucose-lowering effect of insulin). Products include:
Levothroid Tablets 1373
Levoxyl Tablets 1819
Synthroid 505
Unithroid Tablets 3445

Liothyronine Sodium (May reduce the blood-glucose-lowering effect of insulin). Products include:
Cytomel Tablets 1817
Triostat Injection 1825

Liotrix (May reduce the blood-glucose-lowering effect of insulin).
No products indexed under this heading.

Lisinopril (May increase the blood-glucose-lowering effect and susceptibility to hypoglycemia). Products include:
Prinivil Tablets 2164
Prinzide Tablets 2168
Zestoretic Tablets 695
Zestril Tablets 698

Lithium Carbonate (May either potentiate or weaken the blood-glucose-lowering effect of insulin). Products include:
Eskalith 1527
Lithium Carbonate 3061
Lithobid Slow-Release Tablets 3255

Lithium Citrate (May either potentiate or weaken the blood-glucose-lowering effect of insulin). Products include:
Lithium Citrate Syrup 3061

Magnesium Salicylate (May increase the blood-glucose-lowering effect and susceptibility to hypoglycemia). Products include:
Momentum Backache Relief Extra Strength Caplets.......... ▣666

Mesoridazine Besylate (Phenothiazine derivatives may reduce the blood-glucose-lowering effect of insulin). Products include:
Serentil 1057

Mestranol (Oral contraceptives may reduce the blood-glucose-lowering effect of insulin). Products include:
Necon 1/50 Tablets 3415
Norinyl 1 + 50 28-Day Tablets 3380
Ortho-Novum 1/50□28 Tablets 2556

Metaproterenol Sulfate (Sympathomimetic agents may reduce the blood-glucose-lowering effect of insulin). Products include:
Alupent 1029

Metaraminol Bitartrate (Sympathomimetic agents may reduce the blood-glucose-lowering effect of insulin). Products include:
Aramine Injection 2043

Metformin Hydrochloride (May increase the blood-glucose-lowering effect and susceptibility to hypoglycemia). Products include:
Glucophage Tablets 1080
Glucophage XR Tablets 1080
Glucovance Tablets 1086

Methotrimeprazine (Phenothiazine derivatives may reduce the blood-glucose-lowering effect of insulin).
No products indexed under this heading.

Methoxamine Hydrochloride (Sympathomimetic agents may reduce the blood-glucose-lowering effect of insulin).
No products indexed under this heading.

Methyclothiazide (Diuretics may reduce the blood-glucose-lowering effect of insulin).
No products indexed under this heading.

Methylprednisolone Acetate (Co-administration with corticosteroids may reduce the blood-glucose-lowering effect of insulin). Products include:
Depo-Medrol Injectable Suspension 2795

Methylprednisolone Sodium Succinate (Co-administration with corticosteroids may reduce the blood-glucose-lowering effect of insulin). Products include:
Solu-Medrol Sterile Powder 2855

Metipranolol Hydrochloride (Beta-blockers may either potentiate or weaken the blood-glucose-lowering effect of insulin; signs of hypoglycemia may be reduced or absent with co-administration).
No products indexed under this heading.

Metolazone (Diuretics may reduce the blood-glucose-lowering effect of insulin). Products include:
Mykrox Tablets 1168
Zaroxolyn Tablets 1177

Metoprolol Succinate (Beta-blockers may either potentiate or weaken the blood-glucose-lowering effect of insulin; signs of hypoglycemia may be reduced or absent with co-administration). Products include:
Toprol-XL Tablets 651

Metoprolol Tartrate (Beta-blockers may either potentiate or weaken the blood-glucose-lowering effect of insulin; signs of hypoglycemia may be reduced or absent with co-administration).
No products indexed under this heading.

Miglitol (May increase the blood-glucose-lowering effect and susceptibility to hypoglycemia). Products include:
Glyset Tablets 2821

Moclobemide (May increase the blood-glucose-lowering effect and susceptibility to hypoglycemia).
No products indexed under this heading.

Moexipril Hydrochloride (May increase the blood-glucose-lowering effect and susceptibility to hypoglycemia). Products include:
Uniretic Tablets 3178
Univasc Tablets 3181

Nadolol (Beta-blockers may either potentiate or weaken the blood-glucose-lowering effect of insulin; signs of hypoglycemia may be reduced or absent with co-administration). Products include:
Corgard Tablets 2245
Corzide 40/5 Tablets 2247
Corzide 80/5 Tablets 2247
Nadolol Tablets 2288

Norepinephrine Bitartrate (Sympathomimetic agents may reduce the blood-glucose-lowering effect of insulin).
No products indexed under this heading.

Norethindrone (Oral contraceptives may reduce the blood-glucose-lowering effect of insulin). Products include:
Brevicon 28-Day Tablets 3380
Micronor Tablets 2543
Modicon 2563
Necon 3415
Norinyl 1 +35 28-Day Tablets 3380
Norinyl 1 + 50 28-Day Tablets 3380
Nor-QD Tablets 3423
Ortho-Novum 2563
Ortho-Novum 1/50□28 Tablets 2556
Ovcon 3364
Tri-Norinyl-28 Tablets 3433

Norethynodrel (Oral contraceptives may reduce the blood-glucose-lowering effect of insulin).
No products indexed under this heading.

Norgestimate (Oral contraceptives may reduce the blood-glucose-lowering effect of insulin). Products include:
Ortho-Cyclen/Ortho Tri-Cyclen 2573
Ortho-Prefest Tablets 2570

Norgestrel (Oral contraceptives may reduce the blood-glucose-lowering effect of insulin). Products include:
Lo/Ovral Tablets 3532
Lo/Ovral-28 Tablets 3538
Low-Ogestrel-28 Tablets 3392
Ogestrel 0.5/50-28 Tablets 3428
Ovral Tablets 3551
Ovral-28 Tablets 3552
Ovrette Tablets 3552

Octreotide Acetate (May increase the blood-glucose-lowering effect and susceptibility to hypoglycemia). Products include:
Sandostatin LAR Depot 2395

Pargyline Hydrochloride (May increase the blood-glucose-lowering effect and susceptibility to hypoglycemia).
No products indexed under this heading.

Penbutolol Sulfate (Beta-blockers may either potentiate or weaken the blood-glucose-lowering effect of insulin; signs of hypoglycemia may be reduced or absent with co-administration).
No products indexed under this heading.

Pentamidine Isethionate (May cause hypoglycemia, which may sometimes be followed by hyperglycemia).
No products indexed under this heading.

Perindopril Erbumine (May increase the blood-glucose-lowering effect and susceptibility to hypoglycemia). Products include:
Aceon Tablets (2 mg, 4 mg, 8 mg) 3249

Perphenazine (Phenothiazine derivatives may reduce the blood-glucose-lowering effect of insulin). Products include:
Etrafon 3115
Trilafon 3160

Phenelzine Sulfate (May increase the blood-glucose-lowering effect and susceptibility to hypoglycemia). Products include:
Nardil Tablets 2653

Phenylephrine Bitartrate (Sympathomimetic agents may reduce the blood-glucose-lowering effect of insulin).
No products indexed under this heading.

Phenylephrine Hydrochloride (Sympathomimetic agents may reduce the blood-glucose-lowering effect of insulin). Products include:
Afrin Nasal Decongestant Children's Pump Mist .... ▣734
Extendryl 1361
Hycomine Compound Tablets 1317
Neo-Synephrine .... ▣614
Phenergan VC Syrup 3560
Phenergan VC with Codeine Syrup 3561
Preparation H Cream .... ▣778
Preparation H Cooling Gel .... ▣778
Preparation H .... ▣778
Vicks Sinex Nasal Spray and Ultra Fine Mist .... ▣729

Phenylephrine Tannate (Sympathomimetic agents may reduce the blood-glucose-lowering effect of insulin). Products include:
Ryna-12 S Suspension 3351
Reformulated Rynatan Pediatric Suspension 3352
Rynatuss Pediatric Suspension 3353
Rynatuss Tablets 3353

Phenylpropanolamine Hydrochloride (Sympathomimetic agents may reduce the blood-glucose-lowering effect of insulin).
No products indexed under this heading.

Pindolol (Beta-blockers may either potentiate or weaken the blood-glucose-lowering effect of insulin; signs of hypoglycemia may be reduced or absent with co-administration).
No products indexed under this heading.

Pioglitazone Hydrochloride (May increase the blood-glucose-lowering effect and susceptibility to hypoglycemia). Products include:
Actos Tablets 3275

Pirbuterol Acetate (Sympathomimetic agents may reduce the blood-glucose-lowering effect of insulin). Products include:
Maxair Autohaler 1981
Maxair Inhaler 1984

Polythiazide (Diuretics may reduce the blood-glucose-lowering effect of insulin). Products include:
Minizide Capsules 2700
Renese Tablets 2712

Prednisolone Acetate (Co-administration with corticosteroids may reduce the blood-glucose-lowering effect of insulin). Products include:
Blephamide Ophthalmic Ointment 547
Blephamide Ophthalmic Suspension 548

Poly-Pred Liquifilm Ophthalmic Suspension .... ⊙245
Pred Forte Ophthalmic Suspension .... ⊙246
Pred Mild Sterile Ophthalmic Suspension .... ⊙249
Pred-G Ophthalmic Suspension .... ⊙247
Pred-G Sterile Ophthalmic Ointment .... ⊙248

Prednisolone Sodium Phosphate (Co-administration with corticosteroids may reduce the blood-glucose-lowering effect of insulin). Products include:
Pediapred Oral Solution 1170

Prednisolone Tebutate (Co-administration with corticosteroids may reduce the blood-glucose-lowering effect of insulin).
No products indexed under this heading.

Prednisone (Co-administration with corticosteroids may reduce the blood-glucose-lowering effect of insulin). Products include:
Prednisone 3064

Procarbazine Hydrochloride (May increase the blood-glucose-lowering effect and susceptibility to hypoglycemia). Products include:
Matulane Capsules 3246

Prochlorperazine (Phenothiazine derivatives may reduce the blood-glucose-lowering effect of insulin). Products include:
Compazine 1505

Promethazine Hydrochloride (Phenothiazine derivatives may reduce the blood-glucose-lowering effect of insulin). Products include:
Mepergan Injection 3539
Phenergan Injection 3553
Phenergan 3556
Phenergan Syrup 3554
Phenergan with Codeine Syrup 3557
Phenergan with Dextromethorphan Syrup 3559
Phenergan VC Syrup 3560
Phenergan VC with Codeine Syrup 3561

Propoxyphene Hydrochloride (May increase the blood-glucose-lowering effect and susceptibility to hypoglycemia). Products include:
Darvon Pulvules 1909
Darvon Compound-65 Pulvules 1910

Propoxyphene Napsylate (May increase the blood-glucose-lowering effect and susceptibility to hypoglycemia). Products include:
Darvon-N/Darvocet-N 1907
Darvon-N Tablets 1912

Propranolol Hydrochloride (Beta-blockers may either potentiate or weaken the blood-glucose-lowering effect of insulin; signs of hypoglycemia may be reduced or absent with co-administration). Products include:
Inderal 3513
Inderal LA Long-Acting Capsules 3516
Inderide Tablets 3517
Inderide LA Long-Acting Capsules 3519

Pseudoephedrine Hydrochloride (Sympathomimetic agents may reduce the blood-glucose-lowering effect of insulin). Products include:
Actifed Cold & Allergy Tablets .... ▣688
Actifed Cold & Sinus Caplets and Tablets .... ▣688
Advil Cold and Sinus Caplets .... ▣771
Advil Cold and Sinus Tablets .... ▣771
Advil Flu & Body Ache Caplets .... ▣772
Aleve Cold & Sinus Caplets .... ▣603
Alka-Seltzer Plus Liqui-Gels .... ▣604
Alka-Seltzer Plus Cold & Flu Medicine Liqui-Gels .... ▣604
Alka-Seltzer Plus Cold & Sinus Medicine Liqui-Gels .... ▣604
Allegra-D Extended-Release Tablets 714
BC Cold Powder .... ▣619
Benadryl Allergy/Cold Tablets .... ▣691
Benadryl Allergy/Congestion Tablets .... ▣692
Benadryl Allergy & Sinus Liquid .... ▣693
Benadryl Allergy & Sinus Fastmelt Tablets .... ▣693
Benadryl Allergy Sinus Headache Caplets & Gelcaps .... ▣693
Benadryl Severe Allergy & Sinus Headache Caplets .... ▣694
Benadryl Children's Allergy/Cold Fastmelt Tablets .... ▣692
Benylin Multi-Symptom Liquid .... ▣697
Bromfed Capsules (Extended-Release) 2269
Bromfed-PD Capsules (Extended-Release) 2269
Children's Cēpacol Sore Throat .... ▣788
Comtrex Acute Head Cold & Sinus Pressure Relief Tablets .... ▣627
Comtrex Deep Chest Cold & Congestion Relief Softgels .... ▣627
Comtrex Flu Therapy & Fever Relief Daytime Caplets .... ▣628
Comtrex Flu Therapy & Fever Relief Nighttime Tablets .... ▣628
Comtrex Maximum Strength Multi-Symptom Cold & Cough Relief Tablets and Caplets .... ▣626
Contac Non-Drowsy 12 Hour Cold Caplets .... ▣745
Contac Non-Drowsy Timed Release 12 Hour Cold Caplets .... ▣746
Contac Severe Cold and Flu Caplets Maximum Strength .... ▣746
Contac Severe Cold and Flu Caplets Non-Drowsy .... ▣746
Dimetapp Elixir .... ▣777
Dimetapp Cold and Fever Suspension .... ▣775
Dimetapp DM Cold & Cough Elixir .... ▣775
Dimetapp Nighttime Flu Liquid .... ▣776
Dimetapp Non-Drowsy Flu Syrup .... ▣777
Dimetapp Infant Drops Decongestant .... ▣775
Dimetapp Infant Drops Decongestant Plus Cough .... ▣776
Guaifed 2272
Kronofed-A 1341
Children's Motrin Cold Oral Suspension 2007
Motrin Sinus Headache Caplets 2005
PediaCare Cough-Cold Liquid .... ▣719
PediaCare Infants' Drops Decongestant .... ▣719
PediaCare Infants' Drops Decongestant Plus Cough .... ▣719
PediaCare NightRest Cough-Cold Liquid .... ▣719
Robitussin Cold Caplets Cold & Congestion .... ▣780
Robitussin Cold Softgels Cold & Congestion .... ▣780
Robitussin Cold Caplets Multi-Symptom Cold & Flu .... ▣781
Robitussin Cold Softgels Multi-Symptom Cold & Flu .... ▣781
Robitussin Cold Softgels Severe Congestion .... ▣782
Robitussin Cough & Cold Infant Drops .... ▣782
Robitussin Maximum Strength Cough & Cold Liquid .... ▣785
Robitussin Pediatric Cough & Cold Formula Liquid .... ▣785
Robitussin Multi Symptom Honey Flu Liquid .... ▣785
Robitussin Nighttime Honey Flu Liquid .... ▣786
Robitussin-CF Liquid .... ▣783
Robitussin-DAC Syrup 2942
Robitussin-PE Liquid .... ▣782
Ryna .... ▣768
Semprex-D Capsules 1172
Singlet Caplets .... ▣761
Sinutab Non-Drying Liquid Caps .... ▣706
Sinutab Sinus Allergy Medication, Maximum Strength Formula, Tablets & Caplets .... ▣707
Sinutab Sinus Medication, Maximum Strength Without Drowsiness Formula, Tablets & Caplets .... ▣707
Sudafed 12 Hour Tablets .... ▣708
Sudafed 24 Hour Tablets .... ▣708
Children's Sudafed Cold & Cough Liquid .... ▣709
Children's Sudafed Nasal Decongestant Chewables .... ▣711
Children's Sudafed Nasal Decongestant Liquid Medication .... ▣711
Sudafed Cold & Allergy Tablets .... ▣708
Sudafed Cold & Cough Liquid Caps .... ▣709
Sudafed Cold & Sinus Liquid Caps .... ▣710
Sudafed Nasal Decongestant Tablets .... ▣710
Sudafed Non-Drying Sinus Liquid Caps .... ▣712
Sudafed Severe Cold .... ▣711
Sudafed Sinus Headache Caplets .... ▣712
Sudafed Sinus Headache Tablets .... ▣712
Tavist Sinus Non-Drowsy Coated Caplets .... ▣676
TheraFlu Regular Strength Cold & Cough Night Time Hot Liquid .... ▣676
TheraFlu Regular Strength Cold & Sore Throat Night Time Hot Liquid .... ▣676
TheraFlu Maximum Strength Flu & Congestion Non-Drowsy Hot Liquid .... ▣677
TheraFlu Maximum Strength Flu & Cough Night Time Hot Liquid .... ▣678
TheraFlu Maximum Strength Flu & Sore Throat Night Time Hot Liquid .... ▣677
TheraFlu Maximum Strength Severe Cold & Congestion Night Time Caplets .... ▣678
TheraFlu Maximum Strength Severe Cold & Congestion Night Time Hot Liquid .... ▣678
TheraFlu Maximum Strength Severe Cold & Congestion Non-Drowsy .... ▣679
Triaminic Allergy Congestion Liquid .... ▣680
Triaminic Chest Congestion Liquid .... ▣680
Triaminic Cold & Allergy Liquid .... ▣681
Triaminic Cold & Allergy Softchews .... ▣683
Triaminic Cold & Cough Liquid .... ▣681
Triaminic Cold & Cough Softchews .... ▣683
Triaminic Cold & Night Time Cough Liquid .... ▣681
Triaminic Cold, Cough & Fever Liquid .... ▣681
Triaminic Cough Liquid .... ▣682
Triaminic Cough & Congestion Liquid .... ▣682
Triaminic Cough & Sore Throat Liquid .... ▣682
Triaminic Cough & Sore Throat Softchews .... ▣684
Children's Tylenol Allergy-D Liquid 2014
Children's Tylenol Cold Suspension Liquid and Chewable Tablets 2015
Children's Tylenol Cold Plus Cough Suspension Liquid and Chewable Tablets 2015
Children's Tylenol Flu Suspension Liquid 2015
Children's Tylenol Sinus Suspension Liquid 2017
Infants' Tylenol Cold Decongestant and Fever Reducer Concentrated Drops 2015
Infants' Tylenol Cold Decongestant and Fever Reducer Concentrated Drops Plus Cough 2015
Tylenol Allergy Sinus 2010
Multi-Symptom Tylenol Cold Complete Formula Caplets 2010
Multi-Symptom Tylenol Cold Non-Drowsy Caplets and Gelcaps 2010
Multi-Symptom Tylenol Cold Severe Congestion Non-Drowsy Caplets 2011
Maximum Strength Tylenol Flu NightTime Gelcaps 2011
Maximum Strength Tylenol Flu NightTime Liquid 2011
Maximum Strength Tylenol Flu Non-Drowsy Gelcaps 2011
Maximum Strength Tylenol Sinus NightTime Caplets 2012
Maximum Strength Tylenol Sinus Non-Drowsy Geltabs, Gelcaps, Caplets, and Tablets 2012
Vicks 44D Cough & Head Congestion Relief Liquid .... ▣724
Vicks 44M Cough, Cold & Flu Relief Liquid .... ▣725
Pediatric Vicks 44m Cough & Cold Relief .... ▣728
Vicks DayQuil LiquiCaps/Liquid Multi-Symptom Cold/Flu Relief .... ▣727
Children's Vicks NyQuil Cold/Cough Relief .... ▣726
Vicks NyQuil LiquiCaps/Liquid Multi-Symptom Cold/Flu Relief, Original and Cherry Flavors .... ▣727
Zephrex Tablets 3091
Zephrex LA Tablets 3092
Zyrtec-D 12 Hour Extended Relief Tablets 2758

Pseudoephedrine Sulfate (Sympathomimetic agents may reduce the blood-glucose-lowering effect of insulin). Products include:
Chlor-Trimeton Allergy/Decongestant Tablets .... ▣736
Claritin-D 12 Hour Extended Release Tablets 3102
Claritin-D 24 Hour Extended Release Tablets 3104
Coricidin 'D' Cold, Flu & Sinus Tablets .... ▣737
Drixoral Allergy/Sinus Extended-Release Tablets .... ▣741
Drixoral Cold & Allergy Sustained-Action Tablets .... ▣740
Drixoral Cold & Flu Extended-Release Tablets .... ▣740
Drixoral Nasal Decongestant Long-Acting Non-Drowsy Tablets .... ▣740
Rynatan Tablets 3351

Quinapril Hydrochloride (May increase the blood-glucose-lowering effect and susceptibility to hypoglycemia). Products include:
Accupril Tablets 2611
Accuretic Tablets 2614

Ramipril (May increase the blood-glucose-lowering effect and susceptibility to hypoglycemia). Products include:
Altace Capsules 2233

Repaglinide (May increase the blood-glucose-lowering effect and susceptibility to hypoglycemia). Products include:
Prandin Tablets (0.5, 1, and 2 mg) 2432

Reserpine (Signs of hypoglycemia may be reduced or absent with co-administration).
No products indexed under this heading.

Rosiglitazone Maleate (May increase the blood-glucose-lowering effect and susceptibility to hypoglycemia). Products include:
Avandia Tablets 1490

Salmeterol Xinafoate (Sympathomimetic agents may reduce the blood-glucose-lowering effect of insulin). Products include:
Advair Diskus 100/50 1448
Advair Diskus 250/50 1448
Advair Diskus 500/50 1448
Serevent Diskus 1637
Serevent Inhalation Aerosol 1633

Salsalate (May increase the blood-glucose-lowering effect and susceptibility to hypoglycemia).
No products indexed under this heading.

Selegiline Hydrochloride (May increase the blood-glucose-lowering effect and susceptibility to hypoglycemia). Products include:
Eldepryl Capsules 3266

Somatropin (May reduce the blood-glucose-lowering effect of insulin). Products include:
Genotropin Lyophilized Powder 2818
Humatrope Vials and Cartridges 1930
Norditropin Cartridges 2420
Norditropin for Injection 2419
Nutropin AQ Injection 1420
Nutropin Depot for Injectable Suspension 1423
Nutropin for Injection 1417
Saizen for Injection 3225
Serostim for Injection 3229

Sotalol Hydrochloride (Beta-blockers may either potentiate or weaken the blood-glucose-lowering effect of insulin; signs of hypoglycemia may be reduced or absent with co-administration). Products include:
Betapace Tablets 950
Betapace AF Tablets 954

Spirapril Hydrochloride (May increase the blood-glucose-lowering effect and susceptibility to hypoglycemia).
No products indexed under this heading.

Spironolactone (Diuretics may reduce the blood-glucose-lowering effect of insulin).
No products indexed under this heading.

Sulfamethoxazole (Co-administration with sulfonamide antibiotics may increase the blood-

glucose-lowering effect and susceptibility to hypoglycemia). Products include:

Bactrim ... 2949
Septra Suspension ... 2265
Septra Tablets ... 2265
Septra DS Tablets ... 2265

Sulfisoxazole Acetyl (Co-administration with sulfonamide antibiotics may increase the blood-glucose-lowering effect and susceptibility to hypoglycemia). Products include:

Pediazole Suspension ... 3050

Terbutaline Sulfate (Sympathomimetic agents may reduce the blood-glucose-lowering effect of insulin). Products include:

Brethine Ampuls ... 2314
Brethine Tablets ... 2313

Thioridazine Hydrochloride (Phenothiazine derivatives may reduce the blood-glucose-lowering effect of insulin). Products include:

Thioridazine Hydrochloride Tablets ... 2289

Thyroglobulin (May reduce the blood-glucose-lowering effect of insulin).
No products indexed under this heading.

Thyroid (May reduce the blood-glucose-lowering effect of insulin).
No products indexed under this heading.

Thyroxine (May reduce the blood-glucose-lowering effect of insulin).
No products indexed under this heading.

Thyroxine Sodium (May reduce the blood-glucose-lowering effect of insulin).
No products indexed under this heading.

Timolol Hemihydrate (Beta-blockers may either potentiate or weaken the blood-glucose-lowering effect of insulin; signs of hypoglycemia may be reduced or absent with co-administration). Products include:

Betimol Ophthalmic Solution ... ⊙ 324

Timolol Maleate (Beta-blockers may either potentiate or weaken the blood-glucose-lowering effect of insulin; signs of hypoglycemia may be reduced or absent with co-administration). Products include:

Blocadren Tablets ... 2046
Cosopt Sterile Ophthalmic Solution ... 2065
Timolide Tablets ... 2187
Timolol GFS ... ⊙ 266
Timoptic in Ocudose ... 2192
Timoptic Sterile Ophthalmic Solution ... 2190
Timoptic-XE Sterile Ophthalmic Gel Forming Solution ... 2194

Tolazamide (May increase the blood glucose-lowering effect and susceptibility to hypoglycemia).
No products indexed under this heading.

Tolbutamide (May increase the blood-glucose-lowering effect and susceptibility to hypoglycemia).
No products indexed under this heading.

Torsemide (Diuretics may reduce the blood-glucose-lowering effect of insulin). Products include:

Demadex Tablets and Injection ... 2965

Trandolapril (May increase the blood-glucose-lowering effect and susceptibility to hypoglycemia). Products include:

Mavik Tablets ... 478
Tarka Tablets ... 508

Tranylcypromine Sulfate (May increase the blood-glucose-lowering effect and susceptibility to hypoglycemia). Products include:

Parnate Tablets ... 1607

Triamcinolone (Co-administration with corticosteroids may reduce the blood-glucose-lowering effect of insulin).
No products indexed under this heading.

Triamcinolone Acetonide (Co-administration with corticosteroids may reduce the blood-glucose-lowering effect of insulin). Products include:

Azmacort Inhalation Aerosol ... 728
Nasacort Nasal Inhaler ... 750
Nasacort AQ Nasal Spray ... 752
Tri-Nasal Spray ... 2274

Triamcinolone Diacetate (Co-administration with corticosteroids may reduce the blood-glucose-lowering effect of insulin).
No products indexed under this heading.

Triamcinolone Hexacetonide (Co-administration with corticosteroids may reduce the blood-glucose-lowering effect of insulin).
No products indexed under this heading.

Triamterene (Diuretics may reduce the blood-glucose-lowering effect of insulin). Products include:

Dyazide Capsules ... 1515
Dyrenium Capsules ... 3458
Maxzide ... 1008

Trifluoperazine Hydrochloride (Phenothiazine derivatives may reduce the blood-glucose-lowering effect of insulin). Products include:

Stelazine ... 1640

Troglitazone (May increase the blood-glucose-lowering effect and susceptibility to hypoglycemia).
No products indexed under this heading.

Food Interactions

Alcohol (May either potentiate or weaken the blood-glucose-lowering effect of insulin).

LARIAM TABLETS

(Mefloquine Hydrochloride) ... 2989

May interact with antiarrhythmics, beta blockers, calcium channel blockers, anticonvulsants, phenothiazines, quinidine, tricyclic antidepressants, and certain other agents. Compounds in these categories include:

Acebutolol Hydrochloride (There is a theoretical possibility that co-administration of other drugs known to alter cardiac conduction, such as beta blockers, might also contribute to a prolongation of the QTc interval). Products include:

Sectral Capsules ... 3589

Adenosine (There is a theoretical possibility that co-administration of other drugs known to alter cardiac conduction, such as antiarrhythmic agents, might also contribute to a prolongation of the QTc interval). Products include:

Adenocard Injection ... 1380
Adenoscan ... 1381

Amiodarone Hydrochloride (There is a theoretical possibility that co-administration of other drugs known to alter cardiac conduction, such as antiarrhythmic agents, might also contribute to a prolongation of the QTc interval). Products include:

Cordarone Intravenous ... 3491
Cordarone Tablets ... 3487
Pacerone Tablets ... 3331

Amitriptyline Hydrochloride (There is a theoretical possibility that co-administration of other drugs known to alter cardiac conduction, such as tricyclic antidepressants, might also contribute to a prolongation of the QTc interval). Products include:

Etrafon ... 3115
Limbitrol ... 1738

Amlodipine Besylate (There is a theoretical possibility that co-administration of other drugs known to alter cardiac conduction, such as calcium channel blockers, might also contribute to a prolongation of the QTc interval). Products include:

Lotrel Capsules ... 2370
Norvasc Tablets ... 2704

Amoxapine (There is a theoretical possibility that co-administration of other drugs known to alter cardiac conduction, such as tricyclic antidepressants, might also contribute to a prolongation of the QTc interval).
No products indexed under this heading.

Astemizole (There is a theoretical possibility that co-administration of other drugs known to alter cardiac conduction, such as antihistamine astemizole, might also contribute to a prolongation of the QTc interval).
No products indexed under this heading.

Atenolol (There is a theoretical possibility that co-administration of other drugs known to alter cardiac conduction, such as beta blockers, might also contribute to a prolongation of the QTc interval). Products include:

Tenoretic Tablets ... 690
Tenormin I.V. Injection ... 692

Bepridil Hydrochloride (There is a theoretical possibility that co-administration of other drugs known to alter cardiac conduction, such as calcium channel blockers, might also contribute to a prolongation of the QTc interval). Products include:

Vascor Tablets ... 2602

Betaxolol Hydrochloride (There is a theoretical possibility that co-administration of other drugs known to alter cardiac conduction, such as beta blockers, might also contribute to a prolongation of the QTc interval). Products include:

Betoptic S Ophthalmic Suspension ... 537

Bisoprolol Fumarate (There is a theoretical possibility that co-administration of other drugs known to alter cardiac conduction, such as beta blockers, might also contribute to a prolongation of the QTc interval). Products include:

Zebeta Tablets ... 1885
Ziac Tablets ... 1887

Bretylium Tosylate (There is a theoretical possibility that co-administration of other drugs known to alter cardiac conduction, such as antiarrhythmic agents, might also contribute to a prolongation of the QTc interval).
No products indexed under this heading.

Carbamazepine (Co-administration may reduce seizure control by lowering the plasma levels of anticonvulsant; dosage of anticonvulsant may need to be adjusted). Products include:

Carbatrol Capsules ... 3234
Tegretol/Tegretol-XR ... 2404

Carteolol Hydrochloride (There is a theoretical possibility that co-administration of other drugs known to alter cardiac conduction, such as beta blockers, might also contribute to a prolongation of the QTc interval). Products include:

Carteolol Hydrochloride Ophthalmic Solution USP, 1% ... ⊙ 258
Ocupress Ophthalmic Solution, 1% Sterile ... ⊙ 303

Chloroquine Hydrochloride (Co-administration may produce electrocardiographic abnormalities and increase the risk of convulsions; if these drugs are to be used in the initial treatment of severe malaria, mefloquine administration should be delayed at least 12 hours after the last dose).
No products indexed under this heading.

Chloroquine Phosphate (Co-administration may produce electrocardiographic abnormalities and increase the risk of convulsions; if these drugs are to be used in the initial treatment of severe malaria, mefloquine administration should be delayed at least 12 hours after the last dose). Products include:

Aralen Tablets ... 3075

Chlorpromazine (There is a theoretical possibility that co-administration of other drugs known to alter cardiac conduction, such as phenothiazines, might also contribute to a prolongation of the QTc interval). Products include:

Thorazine Suppositories ... 1656

Chlorpromazine Hydrochloride (There is a theoretical possibility that co-administration of other drugs known to alter cardiac conduction, such as phenothiazines, might also contribute to a prolongation of the QTc interval). Products include:

Thorazine ... 1656

Clomipramine Hydrochloride (There is a theoretical possibility that co-administration of other drugs known to alter cardiac conduction, such as tricyclic antidepressants, might also contribute to a prolongation of the QTc interval).
No products indexed under this heading.

Desipramine Hydrochloride (There is a theoretical possibility that co-administration of other drugs known to alter cardiac conduction, such as tricyclic antidepressants, might also contribute to a prolongation of the QTc interval). Products include:

Norpramin Tablets ... 755

Diltiazem Hydrochloride (There is a theoretical possibility that co-administration of other drugs known to alter cardiac conduction, such as calcium channel blockers, might also contribute to a prolongation of the QTc interval). Products include:

Cardizem Injectable ... 1018
Cardizem Lyo-Ject Syringe ... 1018
Cardizem Monovial ... 1018
Cardizem CD Capsules ... 1016
Tiazac Capsules ... 1378

Disopyramide Phosphate (There is a theoretical possibility that co-administration of other drugs known to alter cardiac conduction, such as antiarrhythmic agents, might also contribute to a prolongation of the QTc interval).
No products indexed under this heading.

Divalproex Sodium (Co-administration may reduce seizure control by lowering the plasma levels of anticonvulsant; dosage of anticonvulsant may need to be adjusted). Products include:

Depakote Sprinkle Capsules ... 426
Depakote Tablets ... 430
Depakote ER Tablets ... 436

Dofetilide (There is a theoretical possibility that co-administration of other drugs known to alter cardiac conduction, such as antiarrhythmic agents, might also contribute to a prolongation of the QTc interval). Products include:

Tikosyn Capsules ... 2717

Doxepin Hydrochloride (There is a theoretical possibility that co-administration of other drugs known to alter cardiac conduction, such as tricyclic antidepressants, might also contribute to a prolongation of the QTc interval). Products include:

Sinequan ... 2713

Esmolol Hydrochloride (There is a theoretical possibility that co-administration of other drugs known to alter cardiac conduction, such as

beta blockers, might also contribute to a prolongation of the QTc interval). Products include:

Brevibloc Injection 858

Ethosuximide (Co-administration may reduce seizure control by lowering the plasma levels of anticonvulsant; dosage of anticonvulsant may need to be adjusted). Products include:

Zarontin Capsules 2659
Zarontin Syrup 2660

Ethotoin (Co-administration may reduce seizure control by lowering the plasma levels of anticonvulsant; dosage of anticonvulsant may need to be adjusted).

No products indexed under this heading.

Felbamate (Co-administration may reduce seizure control by lowering the plasma levels of anticonvulsant; dosage of anticonvulsant may need to be adjusted). Products include:

Felbatol 3343

Felodipine (There is a theoretical possibility that co-administration of other drugs known to alter cardiac conduction, such as calcium channel blockers, might also contribute to a prolongation of the QTc interval). Products include:

Lexxel Tablets 608
Plendil Extended-Release Tablets ... 623

Flecainide Acetate (There is a theoretical possibility that co-administration of other drugs known to alter cardiac conduction, such as antiarrhythmic agents, might also contribute to a prolongation of the QTc interval). Products include:

Tambocor Tablets 1990

Fluphenazine Decanoate (There is a theoretical possibility that co-administration of other drugs known to alter cardiac conduction, such as phenothiazines, might also contribute to a prolongation of the QTc interval).

No products indexed under this heading.

Fluphenazine Enanthate (There is a theoretical possibility that co-administration of other drugs known to alter cardiac conduction, such as phenothiazines, might also contribute to a prolongation of the QTc interval).

No products indexed under this heading.

Fluphenazine Hydrochloride (There is a theoretical possibility that co-administration of other drugs known to alter cardiac conduction, such as phenothiazines, might also contribute to a prolongation of the QTc interval).

No products indexed under this heading.

Fosphenytoin Sodium (Co-administration may reduce seizure control by lowering the plasma levels of anticonvulsant; dosage of anticonvulsant may need to be adjusted). Products include:

Cerebyx Injection 2619

Halofantrine (Administration of halofantrine subsequent to mefloquine suggests a significant, potentially fatal, prolongation of the QTc interval of ECG; halofantrine must not be given simultaneously with or subsequent to mefloquine).

No products indexed under this heading.

Imipramine Hydrochloride (There is a theoretical possibility that co-administration of other drugs known to alter cardiac conduction, such as tricyclic antidepressants, might also contribute to a prolongation of the QTc interval).

No products indexed under this heading.

Imipramine Pamoate (There is a theoretical possibility that co-administration of other drugs known to alter cardiac conduction, such as tricyclic antidepressants, might also contribute to a prolongation of the QTc interval).

No products indexed under this heading.

Isradipine (There is a theoretical possibility that co-administration of other drugs known to alter cardiac conduction, such as calcium channel blockers, might also contribute to a prolongation of the QTc interval). Products include:

DynaCirc Capsules 2921
DynaCirc CR Tablets 2923

Labetalol Hydrochloride (There is a theoretical possibility that co-administration of other drugs known to alter cardiac conduction, such as beta blockers, might also contribute to a prolongation of the QTc interval). Products include:

Normodyne Injection 3135
Normodyne Tablets 3137

Lamotrigine (Co-administration may reduce seizure control by lowering the plasma levels of anticonvulsant; dosage of anticonvulsant may need to be adjusted). Products include:

Lamictal 1567

Levetiracetam (Co-administration may reduce seizure control by lowering the plasma levels of anticonvulsant; dosage of anticonvulsant may need to be adjusted). Products include:

Keppra Tablets 3314

Levobunolol Hydrochloride (There is a theoretical possibility that co-administration of other drugs known to alter cardiac conduction, such as beta blockers, might also contribute to a prolongation of the QTc interval). Products include:

Betagan .... ⊙ 228

Lidocaine Hydrochloride (There is a theoretical possibility that co-administration of other drugs known to alter cardiac conduction, such as antiarrhythmic agents, might also contribute to a prolongation of the QTc interval). Products include:

Bactine First Aid Liquid .... ▣ 611
Xylocaine Injections 653

Maprotiline Hydrochloride (There is a theoretical possibility that co-administration of other drugs known to alter cardiac conduction, such as tricyclic antidepressants, might also contribute to a prolongation of the QTc interval).

No products indexed under this heading.

Mephenytoin (Co-administration may reduce seizure control by lowering the plasma levels of anticonvulsant; dosage of anticonvulsant may need to be adjusted).

No products indexed under this heading.

Mesoridazine Besylate (There is a theoretical possibility that co-administration of other drugs known to alter cardiac conduction, such as phenothiazines, might also contribute to a prolongation of the QTc interval). Products include:

Serentil 1057

Methotrimeprazine (There is a theoretical possibility that co-administration of other drugs known to alter cardiac conduction, such as phenothiazines, might also contribute to a prolongation of the QTc interval).

No products indexed under this heading.

Methsuximide (Co-administration may reduce seizure control by lowering the plasma levels of anticonvulsant; dosage of anticonvulsant may need to be adjusted). Products include:

Celontin Capsules 2618

Metipranolol Hydrochloride (There is a theoretical possibility that co-administration of other drugs known to alter cardiac conduction, such as beta blockers, might also contribute to a prolongation of the QTc interval).

No products indexed under this heading.

Metoprolol Succinate (There is a theoretical possibility that co-administration of other drugs known to alter cardiac conduction, such as beta blockers, might also contribute to a prolongation of the QTc interval). Products include:

Toprol-XL Tablets 651

Metoprolol Tartrate (There is a theoretical possibility that co-administration of other drugs known to alter cardiac conduction, such as beta blockers, might also contribute to a prolongation of the QTc interval).

No products indexed under this heading.

Mexiletine Hydrochloride (There is a theoretical possibility that co-administration of other drugs known to alter cardiac conduction, such as antiarrhythmic agents, might also contribute to a prolongation of the QTc interval). Products include:

Mexitil Capsules 1047

Mibefradil Dihydrochloride (There is a theoretical possibility that co-administration of other drugs known to alter cardiac conduction, such as calcium channel blockers, might also contribute to a prolongation of the QTc interval).

No products indexed under this heading.

Moricizine Hydrochloride (There is a theoretical possibility that co-administration of other drugs known to alter cardiac conduction, such as antiarrhythmic agents, might also contribute to a prolongation of the QTc interval).

No products indexed under this heading.

Nadolol (There is a theoretical possibility that co-administration of other drugs known to alter cardiac conduction, such as beta blockers, might also contribute to a prolongation of the QTc interval). Products include:

Corgard Tablets 2245
Corzide 40/5 Tablets 2247
Corzide 80/5 Tablets 2247
Nadolol Tablets 2288

Nicardipine Hydrochloride (There is a theoretical possibility that co-administration of other drugs known to alter cardiac conduction, such as calcium channel blockers, might also contribute to a prolongation of the QTc interval). Products include:

Cardene I.V. 3485

Nifedipine (There is a theoretical possibility that co-administration of other drugs known to alter cardiac conduction, such as calcium channel blockers, might also contribute to a prolongation of the QTc interval). Products include:

Adalat CC Tablets 877
Procardia Capsules 2708
Procardia XL Extended Release Tablets 2710

Nimodipine (There is a theoretical possibility that co-administration of other drugs known to alter cardiac conduction, such as calcium channel blockers, might also contribute to a prolongation of the QTc interval). Products include:

Nimotop Capsules 904

Nisoldipine (There is a theoretical possibility that co-administration of other drugs known to alter cardiac conduction, such as calcium channel blockers, might also contribute to a prolongation of the QTc interval). Products include:

Sular Tablets 688

Nortriptyline Hydrochloride (There is a theoretical possibility that co-administration of other drugs known to alter cardiac conduction, such as tricyclic antidepressants, might also contribute to a prolongation of the QTc interval).

No products indexed under this heading.

Oxcarbazepine (Co-administration may reduce seizure control by lowering the plasma levels of anticonvulsant; dosage of anticonvulsant may need to be adjusted). Products include:

Trileptal Oral Suspension 2407
Trileptal Tablets 2407

Paramethadione (Co-administration may reduce seizure control by lowering the plasma levels of anticonvulsant; dosage of anticonvulsant may need to be adjusted).

No products indexed under this heading.

Penbutolol Sulfate (There is a theoretical possibility that co-administration of other drugs known to alter cardiac conduction, such as beta blockers, might also contribute to a prolongation of the QTc interval).

No products indexed under this heading.

Perphenazine (There is a theoretical possibility that co-administration of other drugs known to alter cardiac conduction, such as phenothiazines, might also contribute to a prolongation of the QTc interval). Products include:

Etrafon 3115
Trilafon 3160

Phenacemide (Co-administration may reduce seizure control by lowering the plasma levels of anticonvulsant; dosage of anticonvulsant may need to be adjusted).

No products indexed under this heading.

Phenobarbital (Co-administration may reduce seizure control by lowering the plasma levels of anticonvulsant; dosage of anticonvulsant may need to be adjusted). Products include:

Arco-Lase Plus Tablets 592
Donnatal 2929
Donnatal Extentabs 2930

Phensuximide (Co-administration may reduce seizure control by lowering the plasma levels of anticonvulsant; dosage of anticonvulsant may need to be adjusted).

No products indexed under this heading.

Phenytoin (Co-administration may reduce seizure control by lowering the plasma levels of anticonvulsant; dosage of anticonvulsant may need to be adjusted). Products include:

Dilantin Infatabs 2624
Dilantin-125 Oral Suspension 2625

Phenytoin Sodium (Co-administration may reduce seizure control by lowering the plasma levels of anticonvulsant; dosage of anticonvulsant may need to be adjusted). Products include:

Dilantin Kapseals 2622

Pindolol (There is a theoretical possibility that co-administration of other drugs known to alter cardiac conduction, such as beta blockers, might also contribute to a prolongation of the QTc interval).

No products indexed under this heading.

Primidone (Co-administration may reduce seizure control by lowering the plasma levels of anticonvulsant;

dosage of anticonvulsant may need to be adjusted).
No products indexed under this heading.

Procainamide Hydrochloride (There is a theoretical possibility that co-administration of other drugs known to alter cardiac conduction, such as antiarrhythmic agents, might also contribute to a prolongation of the QTc interval). Products include:
Procanbid Extended-Release Tablets 2262

Prochlorperazine (There is a theoretical possibility that co-administration of other drugs known to alter cardiac conduction, such as phenothiazines, might also contribute to a prolongation of the QTc interval). Products include:
Compazine 1505

Promethazine Hydrochloride (There is a theoretical possibility that co-administration of other drugs known to alter cardiac conduction, such as phenothiazines, might also contribute to a prolongation of the QTc interval). Products include:
Mepergan Injection 3539
Phenergan Injection 3553
Phenergan 3556
Phenergan Syrup 3554
Phenergan with Codeine Syrup 3557
Phenergan with Dextromethorphan Syrup 3559
Phenergan VC Syrup 3560
Phenergan VC with Codeine Syrup 3561

Propafenone Hydrochloride (There is a theoretical possibility that co-administration of other drugs known to alter cardiac conduction, such as antiarrhythmic agents, might also contribute to a prolongation of the QTc interval). Products include:
Rythmol Tablets – 150 mg, 225 mg, 300 mg 502

Propranolol Hydrochloride (Co-administration has resulted in one report of cardiopulmonary arrest, with full recovery, in a patient; there is a theoretical possibility that co-administration of other drugs known to alter cardiac conduction, such as beta blockers, might also contribute to a prolongation of the QTc interval). Products include:
Inderal 3513
Inderal LA Long-Acting Capsules 3516
Inderide Tablets 3517
Inderide LA Long-Acting Capsules 3519

Protriptyline Hydrochloride (There is a theoretical possibility that co-administration of other drugs known to alter cardiac conduction, such as tricyclic antidepressants, might also contribute to a prolongation of the QTc interval). Products include:
Vivactil Tablets 2446
Vivactil Tablets 2217

Quinidine Gluconate (Co-administration may produce electrocardiographic abnormalities and increase the risk of convulsions; if these drugs are to be used in the initial treatment of severe malaria, mefloquine administration should be delayed at least 12 hours after the last dose). Products include:
Quinaglute Dura-Tabs Tablets 978

Quinidine Polygalacturonate (Co-administration may produce electrocardiographic abnormalities and increase the risk of convulsions; if these drugs are to be used in the initial treatment of severe malaria, mefloquine administration should be delayed at least 12 hours after the last dose).
No products indexed under this heading.

Quinidine Sulfate (Co-administration may produce electrocardiographic abnormalities and increase the risk of convulsions; if these drugs are to be used in the initial treatment of severe malaria, mefloquine administration should be delayed at least 12 hours after the last dose). Products include:
Quinidex Extentabs 2933

Quinine Sulfate (Co-administration may produce electrocardiographic abnormalities and increase the risk of convulsions; if these drugs are to be used in the initial treatment of severe malaria, mefloquine administration should be delayed at least 12 hours after the last dose).
No products indexed under this heading.

Sotalol Hydrochloride (There is a theoretical possibility that co-administration of other drugs known to alter cardiac conduction, such as beta blockers, might also contribute to a prolongation of the QTc interval). Products include:
Betapace Tablets 950
Betapace AF Tablets 954

Terfenadine (There is a theoretical possibility the the co-administration of other drugs known to alter cardiac conduction, such as antihistamine terfenadine, might also contribute to a prolongation of the QTc interval).
No products indexed under this heading.

Thioridazine Hydrochloride (There is a theoretical possibility that co-administration of other drugs known to alter cardiac conduction, such as phenothiazines, might also contribute to a prolongation of the QTc interval). Products include:
Thioridazine Hydrochloride Tablets 2289

Tiagabine Hydrochloride (Co-administration may reduce seizure control by lowering the plasma levels of anticonvulsant; dosage of anticonvulsant may need to be adjusted). Products include:
Gabitril Tablets 1189

Timolol Hemihydrate (There is a theoretical possibility that co-administration of other drugs known to alter cardiac conduction, such as beta blockers, might also contribute to a prolongation of the QTc interval). Products include:
Betimol Ophthalmic Solution .... ⊙ 324

Timolol Maleate (There is a theoretical possibility that co-administration of other drugs known to alter cardiac conduction, such as beta blockers, might also contribute to a prolongation of the QTc interval). Products include:
Blocadren Tablets 2046
Cosopt Sterile Ophthalmic Solution 2065
Timolide Tablets 2187
Timolol GFS .... ⊙ 266
Timoptic in Ocudose 2192
Timoptic Sterile Ophthalmic Solution 2190
Timoptic-XE Sterile Ophthalmic Gel Forming Solution 2194

Tocainide Hydrochloride (There is a theoretical possibility that co-administration of other drugs known to alter cardiac conduction, such as antiarrhythmic agents, might also contribute to a prolongation of the QTc interval). Products include:
Tonocard Tablets 649

Topiramate (Co-administration may reduce seizure control by lowering the plasma levels of anticonvulsant; dosage of anticonvulsant may need to be adjusted). Products include:
Topamax Sprinkle Capsules 2590
Topamax Tablets 2590

Trifluoperazine Hydrochloride (There is a theoretical possibility that co-administration of other drugs known to alter cardiac conduction, such as phenothiazines, might also contribute to a prolongation of the QTc interval). Products include:
Stelazine 1640

Trimethadione (Co-administration may reduce seizure control by lowering the plasma levels of anticonvulsant; dosage of anticonvulsant may need to be adjusted).
No products indexed under this heading.

Trimipramine Maleate (There is a theoretical possibility that co-administration of other drugs known to alter cardiac conduction, such as tricyclic antidepressants, might also contribute to a prolongation of the QTc interval). Products include:
Surmontil Capsules 3595

Typhoid Vaccine Live Oral TY21a (Attenuation of immunization cannot be excluded when co-administered). Products include:
Vivotif Berna 997

Valproate Sodium (Co-administration may reduce seizure control by lowering the plasma levels of anticonvulsant; dosage of anticonvulsant may need to be adjusted). Products include:
Depacon Injection 416

Valproic Acid (Co-administration may reduce seizure control by lowering the plasma levels of anticonvulsant; dosage of anticonvulsant may need to be adjusted). Products include:
Depakene 421

Verapamil Hydrochloride (There is a theoretical possibility that co-administration of other drugs known to alter cardiac conduction, such as calcium channel blockers, might also contribute to a prolongation of the QTc interval). Products include:
Covera-HS Tablets 3199
Isoptin SR Tablets 467
Tarka Tablets 508
Verelan Capsules 3184
Verelan PM Capsules 3186

Zonisamide (Co-administration may reduce seizure control by lowering the plasma levels of anticonvulsant; dosage of anticonvulsant may need to be adjusted). Products include:
Zonegran Capsules 1307

LESCOL CAPSULES

(Fluvastatin Sodium) 2361
May interact with erythromycin, fibrates, and certain other agents. Compounds in these categories include:

Cholestyramine (Administration of fluvastatin with, or up to 4 hours after cholestyramine results in significant reductions in AUC and Cmax of fluvastatin, however, use of fluvastatin 4 hours after resin results in clinically significant additive effect).
No products indexed under this heading.

Cimetidine (Co-administration results in a significant increase in the fluvastatin Cmax and AUC and a decrease in plasma clearance). Products include:
Tagamet HB 200 Suspension .... ▣ 762
Tagamet HB 200 Tablets .... ▣ 761
Tagamet Tablets 1644

Cimetidine Hydrochloride (Co-administration results in a significant increase in the fluvastatin Cmax and AUC and a decrease in plasma clearance). Products include:
Tagamet 1644

Clofibrate (Myopathy has occasionally been associated with fibrates; combined use should generally be avoided). Products include:
Atromid-S Capsules 3483

Cyclosporine (The risk of myopathy and/or rhabdomyolysis during treatment with HMG-CoA reductase inhibitor has been reported to be increased with concurrent cyclosporine; caution should be exercised). Products include:
Gengraf Capsules 457
Neoral Soft Gelatin Capsules 2380
Neoral Oral Solution 2380
Sandimmune 2388

Diclofenac Potassium (Co-administration increases the mean Cmax and AUC of diclofenac by 60% and 25% respectively). Products include:
Cataflam Tablets 2315

Diclofenac Sodium (Co-administration increases the mean Cmax and AUC of diclofenac by 60% and 25% respectively). Products include:
Arthrotec Tablets 3195
Voltaren Ophthalmic Sterile Ophthalmic Solution .... ⊙ 312
Voltaren Tablets 2315
Voltaren-XR Tablets 2315

Digoxin (Co-administration in patients on chronic digoxin may result in a small increase in digoxin Cmax (11%) and urinary clearance). Products include:
Digitek Tablets 1003
Lanoxicaps Capsules 1574
Lanoxin Injection 1581
Lanoxin Tablets 1587
Lanoxin Elixir Pediatric 1578
Lanoxin Injection Pediatric 1584

Erythromycin (The risk of myopathy and/or rhabdomyolysis during treatment with HMG-CoA reductase inhibitor has been reported to be increased with concurrent erythromycin; caution should be exercised). Products include:
Emgel 2% Topical Gel 1285
Ery-Tab Tablets 448
Erythromycin Base Filmtab Tablets 454
Erythromycin Delayed-Release Capsules, USP 455
PCE Dispertab Tablets 498

Erythromycin Estolate (The risk of myopathy and/or rhabdomyolysis during treatment with HMG-CoA reductase inhibitor has been reported to be increased with concurrent erythromycin; caution should be exercised).
No products indexed under this heading.

Erythromycin Ethylsuccinate (The risk of myopathy and/or rhabdomyolysis during treatment with HMG-CoA reductase inhibitor has been reported to be increased with concurrent erythromycin; caution should be exercised). Products include:
E.E.S. 450
EryPed 446
Pediazole Suspension 3050

Erythromycin Gluceptate (The risk of myopathy and/or rhabdomyolysis during treatment with HMG-CoA reductase inhibitor has been reported to be increased with concurrent erythromycin; caution should be exercised).
No products indexed under this heading.

Erythromycin Stearate (The risk of myopathy and/or rhabdomyolysis during treatment with HMG-CoA reductase inhibitor has been reported to be increased with concurrent erythromycin; caution should be exercised). Products include:
Erythrocin Stearate Filmtab Tablets 452

Fenofibrate (Myopathy has occasionally been associated with fibrates; combined use should generally be avoided). Products include:
Tricor Capsules, Micronized 513

Gemfibrozil (The risk of myopathy and/or rhabdomyolysis during treatment with HMG-CoA reductase inhibitor has been reported to be increased with concurrent gemfibrozil; combined use should generally be avoided). Products include:
Lopid Tablets 2650

Glyburide (Co-administration results in increased mean Cmax, AUC, and

t1/2 of glyburide approximately 50%, 69% and 121% respectively; glyburide increased the mean Cmax and AUC of fluvastatin by 44% and 51% respectively). Products include:

DiaBeta Tablets **741**
Glucovance Tablets **1086**

Ketoconazole (Caution should be exercised if used concurrently with drugs that may decrease the levels of endogenous steroid hormones; increase potential for endocrine dysfunction). Products include:

Nizoral 2% Cream **3620**
Nizoral A-D Shampoo **2008**
Nizoral 2% Shampoo **2007**
Nizoral Tablets **1791**

Nicotinic Acid (The risk of myopathy and/or rhabdomyolysis during treatment with HMG-CoA reductase inhibitor has been reported to be increased with concurrent niacin; caution should be exercised).

No products indexed under this heading.

Omeprazole (Co-administration results in a significant increase in the fluvastatin Cmax and AUC and a decrease in plasma clearance). Products include:

Prilosec Delayed-Release Capsules **628**

Ranitidine Hydrochloride (Co-administration results in a significant increase in the fluvastatin Cmax and AUC and a decrease in plasma clearance). Products include:

Zantac **1690**
Zantac Injection **1688**
Zantac 75 Tablets .... ⊡ **717**

Rifampin (Co-administration in patients pretreated with rifampin results in significant reduction in Cmax (59%) and AUC (51%) with a large increase (95%) in plasma clearance). Products include:

Rifadin **765**
Rifamate Capsules **767**
Rifater Tablets **769**

Spironolactone (Caution should be exercised if used concurrently with drugs that may decrease the levels of endogenous steroid hormones; increase potential for endocrine dysfunction).

No products indexed under this heading.

Warfarin Sodium (Bleeding and/or increased prothrombin time has been reported with other HMG-CoA reductase inhibitors when used concurrently; no interactions at therapeutic concentrations have been demonstrated with fluvastatin and warfarin). Products include:

Coumadin for Injection **1243**
Coumadin Tablets **1243**
Warfarin Sodium Tablets, USP **3302**

Food Interactions

Food, unspecified (Administration of regular formulation of fluvastatin with food reduces the rate but not the extent of absorption; administration with evening meal results in a two-fold decrease in Cmax and more than a two-fold increase in tmax as compared to administration 4 hours after the evening meal; administration of Lescol XL with a high fat meal delayed the absorption and increased the bioavailability by 50%).

LESCOL CAPSULES

(Fluvastatin Sodium) **2925**
May interact with erythromycin, fibrates, and certain other agents. Compounds in these categories include:

Cholestyramine (Administration of fluvastatin with, or up to 4 hours after cholestyramine results in significant reductions in AUC and Cmax of fluvastatin, however, use of fluvastatin 4 hours after resin results in clinically significant additive effect).

No products indexed under this heading.

Cimetidine (Co-administration results in a significant increase in the fluvastatin Cmax and AUC and a decrease in plasma clearance). Products include:

Tagamet HB 200 Suspension .... ⊡ **762**
Tagamet HB 200 Tablets .... ⊡ **761**
Tagamet Tablets **1644**

Cimetidine Hydrochloride (Co-administration results in a significant increase in the fluvastatin Cmax and AUC and a decrease in plasma clearance). Products include:

Tagamet **1644**

Clofibrate (Myopathy has occasionally been associated with fibrates; combined use should generally be avoided). Products include:

Atromid-S Capsules **3483**

Cyclosporine (The risk of myopathy and/or rhabdomyolysis during treatment with HMG-CoA reductase inhibitor has been reported to be increased with concurrent cyclosporine; caution should be exercised). Products include:

Gengraf Capsules **457**
Neoral Soft Gelatin Capsules **2380**
Neoral Oral Solution **2380**
Sandimmune **2388**

Diclofenac Potassium (Co-administration increases the mean Cmax and AUC of diclofenac by 60% and 25% respectively). Products include:

Cataflam Tablets **2315**

Diclofenac Sodium (Co-administration increases the mean Cmax and AUC of diclofenac by 60% and 25% respectively). Products include:

Arthrotec Tablets **3195**
Voltaren Ophthalmic Sterile Ophthalmic Solution .... ⊙ **312**
Voltaren Tablets **2315**
Voltaren-XR Tablets **2315**

Digoxin (Co-administration in patients on chronic digoxin may result in a small increase in digoxin Cmax (11%) and urinary clearance). Products include:

Digitek Tablets **1003**
Lanoxicaps Capsules **1574**
Lanoxin Injection **1581**
Lanoxin Tablets **1587**
Lanoxin Elixir Pediatric **1578**
Lanoxin Injection Pediatric **1584**

Erythromycin (The risk of myopathy and/or rhabdomyolysis during treatment with HMG-CoA reductase inhibitor has been reported to be increased with concurrent erythromycin; caution should be exercised). Products include:

Emgel 2% Topical Gel **1285**
Ery-Tab Tablets **448**
Erythromycin Base Filmtab Tablets .. **454**
Erythromycin Delayed-Release Capsules, USP **455**
PCE Dispertab Tablets **498**

Erythromycin Estolate (The risk of myopathy and/or rhabdomyolysis during treatment with HMG-CoA reductase inhibitor has been reported to be increased with concurrent erythromycin; caution should be exercised).

No products indexed under this heading.

Erythromycin Ethylsuccinate (The risk of myopathy and/or rhabdomyolysis during treatment with HMG-CoA reductase inhibitor has been reported to be increased with concurrent erythromycin; caution should be exercised). Products include:

E.E.S. **450**
EryPed **446**
Pediazole Suspension **3050**

Erythromycin Gluceptate (The risk of myopathy and/or rhabdomyolysis during treatment with HMG-CoA reductase inhibitor has been reported to be increased with concurrent erythromycin; caution should be exercised).

No products indexed under this heading.

Erythromycin Stearate (The risk of myopathy and/or rhabdomyolysis during treatment with HMG-CoA reductase inhibitor has been reported to be increased with concurrent erythromycin; caution should be exercised). Products include:

Erythrocin Stearate Filmtab Tablets **452**

Fenofibrate (Myopathy has occasionally been associated with fibrates; combined use should generally be avoided). Products include:

Tricor Capsules, Micronized **513**

Gemfibrozil (The risk of myopathy and/or rhabdomyolysis during treatment with HMG-CoA reductase inhibitor has been reported to be increased with concurrent gemfibrozil; combined use should generally be avoided). Products include:

Lopid Tablets **2650**

Glyburide (Co-administration results in increased mean Cmax, AUC, and t1/2 of glyburide approximately 50%, 69% and 121% respectively; glyburide increased the mean Cmax and AUC of fluvastatin by 44% and 51% respectively). Products include:

DiaBeta Tablets **741**
Glucovance Tablets **1086**

Ketoconazole (Caution should be exercised if used concurrently with drugs that may decrease the levels of endogenous steroid hormones; increase potential for endocrine dysfunction). Products include:

Nizoral 2% Cream **3620**
Nizoral A-D Shampoo **2008**
Nizoral 2% Shampoo **2007**
Nizoral Tablets **1791**

Nicotinic Acid (The risk of myopathy and/or rhabdomyolysis during treatment with HMG-CoA reductase inhibitor has been reported to be increased with concurrent niacin; caution should be exercised).

No products indexed under this heading.

Omeprazole (Co-administration results in a significant increase in the fluvastatin Cmax and AUC and a decrease in plasma clearance). Products include:

Prilosec Delayed-Release Capsules **628**

Ranitidine Hydrochloride (Co-administration results in a significant increase in the fluvastatin Cmax and AUC and a decrease in plasma clearance). Products include:

Zantac **1690**
Zantac Injection **1688**
Zantac 75 Tablets .... ⊡ **717**

Rifampin (Co-administration in patients pretreated with rifampin results in significant reduction in Cmax (59%) and AUC (51%) with a large increase (95%) in plasma clearance). Products include:

Rifadin **765**
Rifamate Capsules **767**
Rifater Tablets **769**

Spironolactone (Caution should be exercised if used concurrently with drugs that may decrease the levels of endogenous steroid hormones; increase potential for endocrine dysfunction).

No products indexed under this heading.

Warfarin Sodium (Bleeding and/or increased prothrombin time has been reported with other HMG-CoA reductase inhibitors when used concurrently; no interactions at therapeutic concentrations have been demonstrated with fluvastatin and warfarin). Products include:

Coumadin for Injection **1243**
Coumadin Tablets **1243**
Warfarin Sodium Tablets, USP **3302**

Food Interactions

Food, unspecified (Administration of regular formulation of fluvastatin with food reduces the rate but not the extent of absorption; administration with evening meal results in a two-fold decrease in Cmax and more than a two-fold increase in tmax as compared to administration 4 hours after the evening meal; administration of Lescol XL with a high fat meal delayed the absorption and increased the bioavailability by 50%).

LESCOL XL TABLETS

(Fluvastatin Sodium) **2925**
See Lescol Capsules

LESCOL XL TABLETS

(Fluvastatin Sodium) **2361**
See Lescol Capsules

LEUKERAN TABLETS

(Chlorambucil) **1591**
None cited in PDR database.

LEUKINE

(Sargramostim) **1755**
May interact with cytotoxic drugs and drugs with myeloproliferative effects. Compounds in these categories include:

Betamethasone Acetate (May potentiate the myeloproliferative effect). Products include:

Celestone Soluspan Injectable Suspension **3097**

Betamethasone Sodium Phosphate (May potentiate the myeloproliferative effect). Products include:

Celestone Soluspan Injectable Suspension **3097**

Bleomycin Sulfate (Coadministration within 24 hours preceding or following chemotherapy is not recommended because of potential sensitivity of rapidly dividing hematopoietic progenitor cells to cytotoxic therapy).

No products indexed under this heading.

Cortisone Acetate (May potentiate the myeloproliferative effect). Products include:

Cortone Acetate Injectable Suspension **2059**
Cortone Acetate Tablets **2061**

Cyclophosphamide (Coadministration within 24 hours preceding or following chemotherapy is not recommended because of potential sensitivity of rapidly dividing hematopoietic progenitor cells to cytotoxic therapy).

No products indexed under this heading.

Daunorubicin Hydrochloride (Coadministration within 24 hours preceding or following chemotherapy is not recommended because of potential sensitivity of rapidly dividing hematopoietic progenitor cells to cytotoxic therapy). Products include:

Cerubidine for Injection **947**

Dexamethasone (May potentiate the myeloproliferative effect). Products include:

Decadron Elixir **2078**
Decadron Tablets **2079**
TobraDex Ophthalmic Ointment **542**
TobraDex Ophthalmic Suspension **541**

Dexamethasone Acetate (May potentiate the myeloproliferative effect).

No products indexed under this heading.

Dexamethasone Sodium Phosphate (May potentiate the myeloproliferative effect). Products include:

Decadron Phosphate Injection **2081**
Decadron Phosphate Sterile Ophthalmic Ointment **2083**

Decadron Phosphate Sterile Ophthalmic Solution ... 2084
NeoDecadron Sterile Ophthalmic Solution ... 2144

Doxorubicin Hydrochloride (Coadministration within 24 hours preceding or following chemotherapy is not recommended because of potential sensitivity of rapidly dividing hematopoietic progenitor cells to cytotoxic therapy). Products include:
Adriamycin PFS/RDF Injection ... 2767
Doxil Injection ... 566

Epirubicin Hydrochloride (Coadministration within 24 hours preceding or following chemotherapy is not recommended because of potential sensitivity of rapidly dividing hematopoietic progenitor cells to cytotoxic therapy). Products include:
Ellence Injection ... 2806

Fluorouracil (Coadministration within 24 hours preceding or following chemotherapy is not recommended because of potential sensitivity of rapidly dividing hematopoietic progenitor cells to cytotoxic therapy). Products include:
Carac Cream ... 1222
Efudex ... 1733
Fluoroplex ... 552

Hydrocortisone (May potentiate the myeloproliferative effect). Products include:
Anusol-HC Cream 2.5% ... 2237
Cipro HC Otic Suspension ... 540
Cortaid Intensive Therapy Cream ... ▣717
Cortaid Maximum Strength Cream ... ▣717
Cortisporin Ophthalmic Suspension Sterile ... ⊙297
Cortizone•5 ... ▣699
Cortizone•10 ... ▣699
Cortizone•10 Plus Creme ... ▣700
Cortizone for Kids Creme ... ▣699
Hydrocortone Tablets ... 2106
Massengill Medicated Soft Cloth Towelette ... ▣753
VōSoL HC Otic Solution ... 3356

Hydrocortisone Acetate (May potentiate the myeloproliferative effect). Products include:
Analpram-HC ... 1338
Anusol HC-1 Hydrocortisone Anti-Itch Cream ... ▣689
Anusol-HC Suppositories ... 2238
Cortaid ... ▣717
Cortifoam Rectal Foam ... 3170
Cortisporin-TC Otic Suspension ... 2246
Hydrocortone Acetate Injectable Suspension ... 2103
Pramosone ... 1343
Proctocort Suppositories ... 2264
ProctoFoam-HC ... 3177
Terra-Cortril Ophthalmic Suspension ... 2716

Hydrocortisone Sodium Phosphate (May potentiate the myeloproliferative effect). Products include:
Hydrocortone Phosphate Injection, Sterile ... 2105

Hydrocortisone Sodium Succinate (May potentiate the myeloproliferative effect).
No products indexed under this heading.

Hydroxyurea (Coadministration within 24 hours preceding or following chemotherapy is not recommended because of potential sensitivity of rapidly dividing hematopoietic progenitor cells to cytotoxic therapy). Products include:
Mylocel Tablets ... 2227

Lithium Carbonate (May potentiate the myeloproliferative effect). Products include:
Eskalith ... 1527
Lithium Carbonate ... 3061
Lithobid Slow-Release Tablets ... 3255

Lithium Citrate (May potentiate the myeloproliferative effect). Products include:
Lithium Citrate Syrup ... 3061

Methotrexate Sodium (Coadministration within 24 hours preceding or following chemotherapy is not recommended because of potential sensitivity of rapidly dividing hematopoietic progenitor cells to cytotoxic therapy).
No products indexed under this heading.

Methylprednisolone Acetate (May potentiate the myeloproliferative effect). Products include:
Depo-Medrol Injectable Suspension ... 2795

Methylprednisolone Sodium Succinate (May potentiate the myeloproliferative effect). Products include:
Solu-Medrol Sterile Powder ... 2855

Mitotane (Coadministration within 24 hours preceding or following chemotherapy is not recommended because of potential sensitivity of rapidly dividing hematopoietic progenitor cells to cytotoxic therapy).
No products indexed under this heading.

Mitoxantrone Hydrochloride (Coadministration within 24 hours preceding or following chemotherapy is not recommended because of potential sensitivity of rapidly dividing hematopoietic progenitor cells to cytotoxic therapy). Products include:
Novantrone for Injection ... 1760

Prednisolone Acetate (May potentiate the myeloproliferative effect). Products include:
Blephamide Ophthalmic Ointment ... 547
Blephamide Ophthalmic Suspension ... 548
Poly-Pred Liquifilm Ophthalmic Suspension ... ⊙245
Pred Forte Ophthalmic Suspension ... ⊙246
Pred Mild Sterile Ophthalmic Suspension ... ⊙249
Pred-G Ophthalmic Suspension ... ⊙247
Pred-G Sterile Ophthalmic Ointment ... ⊙248

Prednisolone Sodium Phosphate (May potentiate the myeloproliferative effect). Products include:
Pediapred Oral Solution ... 1170

Prednisolone Tebutate (May potentiate the myeloproliferative effect).
No products indexed under this heading.

Prednisone (May potentiate the myeloproliferative effect). Products include:
Prednisone ... 3064

Procarbazine Hydrochloride (Coadministration within 24 hours preceding or following chemotherapy is not recommended because of potential sensitivity of rapidly dividing hematopoietic progenitor cells to cytotoxic therapy). Products include:
Matulane Capsules ... 3246

Tamoxifen Citrate (Coadministration within 24 hours preceding or following chemotherapy is not recommended because of potential sensitivity of rapidly dividing hematopoietic progenitor cells to cytotoxic therapy). Products include:
Nolvadex Tablets ... 678

Triamcinolone (May potentiate the myeloproliferative effect).
No products indexed under this heading.

Triamcinolone Acetonide (May potentiate the myeloproliferative effect). Products include:
Azmacort Inhalation Aerosol ... 728
Nasacort Nasal Inhaler ... 750
Nasacort AQ Nasal Spray ... 752
Tri-Nasal Spray ... 2274

Triamcinolone Diacetate (May potentiate the myeloproliferative effect).
No products indexed under this heading.

Triamcinolone Hexacetonide (May potentiate the myeloproliferative effect).
No products indexed under this heading.

Vincristine Sulfate (Coadministration within 24 hours preceding or following chemotherapy is not recommended because of potential sensitivity of rapidly dividing hematopoietic progenitor cells to cytotoxic therapy).
No products indexed under this heading.

LEUSTATIN INJECTION

(Cladribine) ... 2495
May interact with:

Bone Marrow Depressants, unspecified (Caution should be exercised if co-administered with other drugs known to cause myelosuppression).

LEVAQUIN INJECTION

(Levofloxacin) ... 2537
See Levaquin Tablets

LEVAQUIN TABLETS

(Levofloxacin) ... 2537
May interact with antacids containing aluminum, calcium and magnesium, oral hypoglycemic agents, iron containing oral preparations, non-steroidal anti-inflammatory agents, theophylline, and certain other agents. Compounds in these categories include:

Acarbose (Disturbances of blood glucose, including hyper- and hypoglycemia, have been reported in patients treated concomitantly with quinolones and an antidiabetic agent; careful monitoring of blood glucose levels is recommended). Products include:
Precose Tablets ... 906

Aluminum Carbonate (Antacids containing aluminum or magnesium may interfere with the gastrointestinal absorption of levofloxacin resulting in systemic levels considerably lower than desired; these agents should be taken at least 2 hours before or after levofloxacin administration).
No products indexed under this heading.

Aluminum Hydroxide (Antacids containing aluminum or magnesium may interfere with the gastrointestinal absorption of levofloxacin resulting in systemic levels considerably lower than desired; these agents should be taken at least 2 hours before or after levofloxacin administration). Products include:
Amphojel Suspension (Mint Flavor) ... ▣789
Gaviscon Extra Strength Liquid ... ▣751
Gaviscon Extra Strength Tablets ... ▣751
Gaviscon Regular Strength Liquid ... ▣751
Gaviscon Regular Strength Tablets ... ▣750
Maalox Antacid/Anti-Gas Oral Suspension ... ▣673
Maalox Max Maximum Strength Antacid/Anti-Gas Liquid ... 2300
Maalox Regular Strength Antacid/Antigas Liquid ... 2300
Mylanta ... 1813
Vanquish Caplets ... ▣617

Aminophylline (Co-administration of other quinolones with theophylline has resulted in prolonged elimination half-life, elevated serum theophylline levels, and increased risk of theophylline related toxicity; no significant effect of levofloxacin on theophylline pharmacokinetic parameters has been detected, however, caution should be exercised).
No products indexed under this heading.

Celecoxib (Co-administration may increase the risk of CNS stimulation and convulsive seizures). Products include:
Celebrex Capsules ... 2676
Celebrex Capsules ... 2780

Chlorpropamide (Disturbances of blood glucose, including hyper- and hypoglycemia, have been reported in patients treated concomitantly with quinolones and an antidiabetic agent; careful monitoring of blood glucose levels is recommended). Products include:
Diabinese Tablets ... 2680

Cimetidine (Co-administration has resulted in higher levofloxacin AUC and t1/2, while CL/F and CLr were lower during concomitant treatment with cimetidine). Products include:
Tagamet HB 200 Suspension ... ▣762
Tagamet HB 200 Tablets ... ▣761
Tagamet Tablets ... 1644

Cimetidine Hydrochloride (Co-administration has resulted in higher levofloxacin AUC and t1/2, while CL/F and CLr were lower during concomitant treatment with cimetidine). Products include:
Tagamet ... 1644

Cyclosporine (Levofloxacin Cmax and Ke were slightly lower while Tmax and t1/2 were slightly longer in the presence of cyclosporine; these differences, however, are not clinically significant, therefore, no dosage adjustment is required). Products include:
Gengraf Capsules ... 457
Neoral Soft Gelatin Capsules ... 2380
Neoral Oral Solution ... 2380
Sandimmune ... 2388

Diclofenac Potassium (Co-administration may increase the risk of CNS stimulation and convulsive seizures). Products include:
Cataflam Tablets ... 2315

Diclofenac Sodium (Co-administration may increase the risk of CNS stimulation and convulsive seizures). Products include:
Arthrotec Tablets ... 3195
Voltaren Ophthalmic Sterile Ophthalmic Solution ... ⊙312
Voltaren Tablets ... 2315
Voltaren-XR Tablets ... 2315

Didanosine (Antacids contained in Videx chewable/buffered tablets or pediatric powder for oral solution may substantially interfere with the gastrointestinal absorption of levofloxacin, resulting in systemic levels considerably lower than desired). Products include:
Videx ... 1138
Videx EC Capsules ... 1143

Dyphylline (Co-administration of other quinolones with theophylline has resulted in prolonged elimination half-life, elevated serum theophylline levels, and increased risk of theophylline related toxicity; no significant effect of levofloxacin on theophylline pharmacokinetic parameters has been detected, however, caution should be exercised). Products include:
Lufyllin Tablets ... 3347
Lufyllin-400 Tablets ... 3347
Lufyllin-GG Elixir ... 3348
Lufyllin-GG Tablets ... 3348

Etodolac (Co-administration may increase the risk of CNS stimulation and convulsive seizures). Products include:
Lodine ... 3528
Lodine XL Extended-Release Tablets ... 3530

Fenoprofen Calcium (Co-administration may increase the risk of CNS stimulation and convulsive seizures).
No products indexed under this heading.

Ferrous Fumarate (Iron-containing preparations may interfere with the gastrointestinal absorption of levofloxacin resulting in systemic levels considerably lower than desired; these agents should be taken at

least 2 hours before or after levofloxacin administration). Products include:
- New Formulation Chromagen OB Capsules 3094
- Loestrin Fe Tablets 2642
- NataChew Tablets 3364

Ferrous Gluconate (Iron-containing preparations may interfere with the gastrointestinal absorption of levofloxacin resulting in systemic levels considerably lower than desired; these agents should be taken at least 2 hours before or after levofloxacin administration). Products include:
- Fergon Iron Tablets 802

Ferrous Sulfate (Iron-containing preparations may interfere with the gastrointestinal absorption of levofloxacin resulting in systemic levels considerably lower than desired; these agents should be taken at least 2 hours before or after levofloxacin administration). Products include:
- Feosol Tablets 1717
- Slow Fe Tablets 827
- Slow Fe with Folic Acid Tablets 828

Flurbiprofen (Co-administration may increase the risk of CNS stimulation and convulsive seizures).
No products indexed under this heading.

Glimepiride (Disturbances of blood glucose, including hyper- and hypoglycemia, have been reported in patients treated concomitantly with quinolones and an antidiabetic agent; careful monitoring of blood glucose levels is recommended). Products include:
- Amaryl Tablets 717

Glipizide (Disturbances of blood glucose, including hyper- and hypoglycemia, have been reported in patients treated concomitantly with quinolones and an antidiabetic agent; careful monitoring of blood glucose levels is recommended). Products include:
- Glucotrol Tablets 2692
- Glucotrol XL Extended Release Tablets 2693

Glyburide (Disturbances of blood glucose, including hyper- and hypoglycemia, have been reported in patients treated concomitantly with quinolones and an antidiabetic agent; careful monitoring of blood glucose levels is recommended). Products include:
- DiaBeta Tablets 741
- Glucovance Tablets 1086

Ibuprofen (Co-administration may increase the risk of CNS stimulation and convulsive seizures). Products include:
- Advil 771
- Children's Advil Oral Suspension 773
- Children's Advil Chewable Tablets 773
- Advil Cold and Sinus Caplets 771
- Advil Cold and Sinus Tablets 771
- Advil Flu & Body Ache Caplets 772
- Infants' Advil Drops 773
- Junior Strength Advil Tablets 773
- Junior Strength Advil Chewable Tablets 773
- Advil Migraine Liquigels 772
- Children's Motrin Oral Suspension and Chewable Tablets 2006
- Children's Motrin Cold Oral Suspension 2007
- Children's Motrin Oral Suspension 643
- Motrin Suspension, Oral Drops, Chewable Tablets, and Caplets 2002
- Infants' Motrin Concentrated Drops 2006
- Junior Strength Motrin Caplets and Chewable Tablets 2006
- Motrin IB Tablets, Caplets, and Gelcaps 2002
- Motrin Migraine Pain Caplets 2005
- Motrin Sinus Headache Caplets 2005
- Vicoprofen Tablets 520

Indomethacin (Co-administration may increase the risk of CNS stimulation and convulsive seizures). Products include:
- Indocin 2112

Indomethacin Sodium Trihydrate (Co-administration may increase the risk of CNS stimulation and convulsive seizures). Products include:
- Indocin I.V. 2115

Iron (Iron-containing preparations may interfere with the gastrointestinal absorption of levofloxacin resulting in systemic levels considerably lower than desired; these agents should be taken at least 2 hours before or after levofloxacin administration).
No products indexed under this heading.

Ketoprofen (Co-administration may increase the risk of CNS stimulation and convulsive seizures). Products include:
- Orudis Capsules 3548
- Orudis KT Tablets 778
- Oruvail Capsules 3548

Ketorolac Tromethamine (Co-administration may increase the risk of CNS stimulation and convulsive seizures). Products include:
- Acular Ophthalmic Solution 544
- Acular PF Ophthalmic Solution 544
- Toradol 3018

Magaldrate (Antacids containing aluminum or magnesium may interfere with the gastrointestinal absorption of levofloxacin resulting in systemic levels considerably lower than desired; these agents should be taken at least 2 hours before or after levofloxacin administration).
No products indexed under this heading.

Magnesium Hydroxide (Antacids containing aluminum or magnesium may interfere with the gastrointestinal absorption of levofloxacin resulting in systemic levels considerably lower than desired; these agents should be taken at least 2 hours before or after levofloxacin administration). Products include:
- Ex•Lax Milk of Magnesia Liquid 670
- Maalox Antacid/Anti-Gas Oral Suspension 673
- Maalox Max Maximum Strength Antacid/Anti-Gas Liquid 2300
- Maalox Regular Strength Antacid/Antigas Liquid 2300
- Mylanta Fast-Acting 1813
- Mylanta 1813
- Pepcid Complete Chewable Tablets 1815
- Phillips' Chewable Tablets 615
- Phillips' Milk of Magnesia Liquid (Original, Cherry, & Mint) 616
- Rolaids Tablets 706
- Extra Strength Rolaids Tablets 706
- Vanquish Caplets 617

Magnesium Oxide (Antacids containing aluminum or magnesium may interfere with the gastrointestinal absorption of levofloxacin resulting in systemic levels considerably lower than desired; these agents should be taken at least 2 hours before or after levofloxacin administration). Products include:
- Beelith Tablets 946
- Mag-Ox 400 Tablets 1024
- Uro-Mag Capsules 1024

Meclofenamate Sodium (Co-administration may increase the risk of CNS stimulation and convulsive seizures).
No products indexed under this heading.

Mefenamic Acid (Co-administration may increase the risk of CNS stimulation and convulsive seizures). Products include:
- Ponstel Capsules 1356

Meloxicam (Co-administration may increase the risk of CNS stimulation and convulsive seizures). Products include:
- Mobic Tablets 1054

Metformin Hydrochloride (Disturbances of blood glucose, including hyper- and hypoglycemia, have been reported in patients treated concomitantly with quinolones and an antidiabetic agent; careful monitoring of blood glucose levels is recommended). Products include:
- Glucophage Tablets 1080
- Glucophage XR Tablets 1080
- Glucovance Tablets 1086

Miglitol (Disturbances of blood glucose, including hyper- and hypoglycemia, have been reported in patients treated concomitantly with quinolones and an antidiabetic agent; careful monitoring of blood glucose levels is recommended). Products include:
- Glyset Tablets 2821

Nabumetone (Co-administration may increase the risk of CNS stimulation and convulsive seizures). Products include:
- Relafen Tablets 1617

Naproxen (Co-administration may increase the risk of CNS stimulation and convulsive seizures). Products include:
- EC-Naprosyn Delayed-Release Tablets 2967
- Naprosyn Suspension 2967
- Naprosyn Tablets 2967

Naproxen Sodium (Co-administration may increase the risk of CNS stimulation and convulsive seizures). Products include:
- Aleve Tablets, Caplets and Gelcaps 602
- Aleve Cold & Sinus Caplets 603
- Anaprox Tablets 2967
- Anaprox DS Tablets 2967
- Naprelan Tablets 1293

Oxaprozin (Co-administration may increase the risk of CNS stimulation and convulsive seizures).
No products indexed under this heading.

Phenylbutazone (Co-administration may increase the risk of CNS stimulation and convulsive seizures).
No products indexed under this heading.

Pioglitazone Hydrochloride (Disturbances of blood glucose, including hyper- and hypoglycemia, have been reported in patients treated concomitantly with quinolones and an antidiabetic agent; careful monitoring of blood glucose levels is recommended). Products include:
- Actos Tablets 3275

Piroxicam (Co-administration may increase the risk of CNS stimulation and convulsive seizures). Products include:
- Feldene Capsules 2685

Polysaccharide-Iron Complex (Iron-containing preparations may interfere with the gastrointestinal absorption of levofloxacin resulting in systemic levels considerably lower than desired; these agents should be taken at least 2 hours before or after levofloxacin administration). Products include:
- Niferex 3176
- Niferex-150 Capsules 3176
- Nu-Iron 150 Capsules 2224

Probenecid (Co-administration has resulted in higher levofloxacin AUC and t1/2, while CL/F and CLr were lower during concomitant treatment with probenecid).
No products indexed under this heading.

Repaglinide (Disturbances of blood glucose, including hyper- and hypoglycemia, have been reported in patients treated concomitantly with quinolones and an antidiabetic agent; careful monitoring of blood glucose levels is recommended). Products include:
- Prandin Tablets (0.5, 1, and 2 mg) 2432

Rofecoxib (Co-administration may increase the risk of CNS stimulation and convulsive seizures). Products include:
- Vioxx 2213

Rosiglitazone Maleate (Disturbances of blood glucose, including hyper- and hypoglycemia, have been reported in patients treated concomitantly with quinolones and an antidiabetic agent; careful monitoring of blood glucose levels is recommended). Products include:
- Avandia Tablets 1490

Sucralfate (May interfere with the gastrointestinal absorption of levofloxacin resulting in systemic levels considerably lower than desired; sucralfate should be taken at least 2 hours before or after levofloxacin administration). Products include:
- Carafate Suspension 731
- Carafate Tablets 730

Sulindac (Co-administration may increase the risk of CNS stimulation and convulsive seizures). Products include:
- Clinoril Tablets 2053

Theophylline (Co-administration of other quinolones with theophylline has resulted in prolonged elimination half-life, elevated serum theophylline levels, and increased risk of theophylline related toxicity; no significant effect of levofloxacin on theophylline pharmacokinetic parameters has been detected, however, caution should be exercised). Products include:
- Aerolate 1361
- Theo-Dur Extended-Release Tablets 1835
- Uni-Dur Extended-Release Tablets 1841
- Uniphyl 400 mg and 600 mg Tablets 2903

Theophylline Calcium Salicylate (Co-administration of other quinolones with theophylline has resulted in prolonged elimination half-life, elevated serum theophylline levels, and increased risk of theophylline related toxicity; no significant effect of levofloxacin on theophylline pharmacokinetic parameters has been detected, however, caution should be exercised).
No products indexed under this heading.

Theophylline Sodium Glycinate (Co-administration of other quinolones with theophylline has resulted in prolonged elimination half-life, elevated serum theophylline levels, and increased risk of theophylline related toxicity; no significant effect of levofloxacin on theophylline pharmacokinetic parameters has been detected, however, caution should be exercised).
No products indexed under this heading.

Tolazamide (Disturbances of blood glucose, including hyper- and hypoglycemia, have been reported in patients treated concomitantly with quinolones and an antidiabetic agent; careful monitoring of blood glucose levels is recommended).
No products indexed under this heading.

Tolbutamide (Disturbances of blood glucose, including hyper- and hypoglycemia, have been reported in patients treated concomitantly with quinolones and an antidiabetic agent; careful monitoring of blood glucose levels is recommended).
No products indexed under this heading.

Tolmetin Sodium (Co-administration may increase the risk of CNS stimulation and convulsive seizures). Products include:

Tolectin 2589

Troglitazone (Disturbances of blood glucose, including hyper- and hypoglycemia, have been reported in patients treated concomitantly with quinolones and an antidiabetic agent; careful monitoring of blood glucose levels is recommended).

No products indexed under this heading.

Warfarin Sodium (Co-administration of other quinolones with warfarin has resulted in enhanced effects of warfarin; no significant effect of levofloxacin on warfarin pharmacokinetic parameters has been detected in clinical studies, however, caution should be exercised and coagulation test should be closely monitored). Products include:

Coumadin for Injection 1243
Coumadin Tablets 1243
Warfarin Sodium Tablets, USP 3302

Food Interactions

Food, unspecified (Co-administration slightly prolongs the time to peak concentration by approximately 1 hour and slightly decreases the peak concentration by approximately 14%; levofloxacin can be administered without regard to food).

LEVBID EXTENDED-RELEASE TABLETS

(Hyoscyamine Sulfate) 3172
See Levsin Drops

LEVLEN 21 TABLETS

(Ethinyl Estradiol, Levonorgestrel) 962
See Levlite 21 Tablets

LEVLEN 28 TABLETS

(Ethinyl Estradiol, Levonorgestrel) 962
See Levlite 21 Tablets

LEVLITE 21 TABLETS

(Ethinyl Estradiol, Levonorgestrel) 962
May interact with barbiturates, cholinergic agents, phenytoin, tetracyclines, theophylline, and certain other agents. Compounds in these categories include:

Aminophylline (Ethinyl estradiol may interfere with the metabolism of theophylline by inhibiting hepatic microsomal enzymes thereby increasing theophylline concentrations).

No products indexed under this heading.

Ampicillin (Co-administration of estrogens with certain antibiotics, such as ampicillin, may decrease the enterohepatic circulation and may reduce ethinyl estradiol concentrations; potential for reduced efficacy and increased incidence of breakthrough bleeding and menstrual irregularities).

No products indexed under this heading.

Ampicillin Sodium (Co-administration of estrogens with certain antibiotics, such as ampicillin, may decrease the enterohepatic circulation and may reduce ethinyl estradiol concentrations; potential for reduced efficacy and increased incidence of breakthrough bleeding and menstrual irregularities). Products include:

Unasyn for Injection 2728

Aprobarbital (Co-administration with hepatic microsomal enzyme inducers, such as barbiturates, can decrease ethinyl estradiol concentrations; potential for reduced efficacy and increased incidence of breakthrough bleeding and menstrual irregularities).

No products indexed under this heading.

Bethanechol Chloride (Diarrhea may increase gastrointestinal motility and reduce hormone absorption; co-administration with drugs which reduce gut transit time, such as cholinergic agents, may reduce hormone concentrations in the blood). Products include:

Urecholine 2198
Urecholine Tablets 2445

Butabarbital (Co-administration with hepatic microsomal enzyme inducers, such as barbiturates, can decrease ethinyl estradiol concentrations; potential for reduced efficacy and increased incidence of breakthrough bleeding and menstrual irregularities).

No products indexed under this heading.

Butalbital (Co-administration with hepatic microsomal enzyme inducers, such as barbiturates, can decrease ethinyl estradiol concentrations; potential for reduced efficacy and increased incidence of breakthrough bleeding and menstrual irregularities). Products include:

Phrenilin 578
Sedapap Tablets 50 mg/650 mg 2225

Cevimeline Hydrochloride (Diarrhea may increase gastrointestinal motility and reduce hormone absorption; co-administration with drugs which reduce gut transit time, such as cholinergic agents, may reduce hormone concentrations in the blood). Products include:

Evoxac Capsules 1217

Cisapride (Diarrhea may increase gastrointestinal motility and reduce hormone absorption; co-administration with drugs which reduce gut transit time, such as prokinetic agents, may reduce hormone concentrations in the blood).

No products indexed under this heading.

Cyclosporine (Ethinyl estradiol may interfere with the metabolism of cyclosporine by inhibiting hepatic microsomal enzymes thereby increasing cyclosporine concentrations). Products include:

Gengraf Capsules 457
Neoral Soft Gelatin Capsules 2380
Neoral Oral Solution 2380
Sandimmune 2388

Demeclocycline Hydrochloride (Co-administration of estrogens with certain antibiotics, such as tetracyclines, may decrease the enterohepatic circulation and may reduce ethinyl estradiol concentrations; potential for reduced efficacy and increased incidence of breakthrough bleeding and menstrual irregularities). Products include:

Declomycin Tablets 1855

Donepezil Hydrochloride (Diarrhea may increase gastrointestinal motility and reduce hormone absorption; co-administration with drugs which reduce gut transit time, such as cholinergic agents, may reduce hormone concentrations in the blood). Products include:

Aricept Tablets 1270
Aricept Tablets 2665

Doxycycline Calcium (Co-administration of estrogens with certain antibiotics, such as tetracyclines, may decrease the enterohepatic circulation and may reduce ethinyl estradiol concentrations; potential for reduced efficacy and increased incidence of breakthrough bleeding and menstrual irregularities). Products include:

Vibramycin Calcium Oral Suspension Syrup 2735

Doxycycline Hyclate (Co-administration of estrogens with certain antibiotics, such as tetracyclines, may decrease the enterohepatic circulation and may reduce ethinyl estradiol concentrations; potential for reduced efficacy and increased incidence of breakthrough bleeding and menstrual irregularities). Products include:

Doryx Coated Pellet Filled Capsules 3357
Periostat Tablets 1208
Vibramycin Hyclate Capsules 2735
Vibramycin Hyclate Intravenous 2737
Vibra-Tabs Film Coated Tablets 2735

Doxycycline Monohydrate (Co-administration of estrogens with certain antibiotics, such as tetracyclines, may decrease the enterohepatic circulation and may reduce ethinyl estradiol concentrations; potential for reduced efficacy and increased incidence of breakthrough bleeding and menstrual irregularities). Products include:

Monodox Capsules 2442
Vibramycin Monohydrate for Oral Suspension 2735

Dyphylline (Ethinyl estradiol may interfere with the metabolism of theophylline by inhibiting hepatic microsomal enzymes thereby increasing theophylline concentrations). Products include:

Lufyllin Tablets 3347
Lufyllin-400 Tablets 3347
Lufyllin-GG Elixir 3348
Lufyllin-GG Tablets 3348

Edrophonium Chloride (Diarrhea may increase gastrointestinal motility and reduce hormone absorption; co-administration with drugs which reduce gut transit time, such as cholinergic agents, may reduce hormone concentrations in the blood). Products include:

Tensilon Injectable 1745

Fosphenytoin Sodium (Co-administration with hepatic microsomal enzyme inducers, such as phenytoin, can decrease ethinyl estradiol concentrations; potential for reduced efficacy and increased incidence of breakthrough bleeding and menstrual irregularities). Products include:

Cerebyx Injection 2619

Galantamine Hydrobromide (Diarrhea may increase gastrointestinal motility and reduce hormone absorption; co-administration with drugs which reduce gut transit time, such as cholinergic agents, may reduce hormone concentrations in the blood). Products include:

Reminyl Oral Solution 1792
Reminyl Tablets 1792

Griseofulvin (Co-administration with hepatic microsomal enzyme inducers, such as griseofulvin, can decrease ethinyl estradiol concentrations; potential for reduced efficacy and increased incidence of breakthrough bleeding and menstrual irregularities). Products include:

Grifulvin V Tablets Microsize and Oral Suspension Microsize 2518
Gris-PEG Tablets 2661

Mephobarbital (Co-administration with hepatic microsomal enzyme inducers, such as barbiturates, can decrease ethinyl estradiol concentrations; potential for reduced efficacy and increased incidence of breakthrough bleeding and menstrual irregularities).

No products indexed under this heading.

Methacycline Hydrochloride (Co-administration of estrogens with certain antibiotics, such as tetracyclines, may decrease the enterohepatic circulation and may reduce ethinyl estradiol concentrations; potential for reduced efficacy and increased incidence of breakthrough bleeding and menstrual irregularities).

No products indexed under this heading.

Metoclopramide Hydrochloride (Diarrhea may increase gastrointestinal motility and reduce hormone absorption; co-administration with drugs which reduce gut transit time, such as prokinetic agents, may reduce hormone concentrations in the blood). Products include:

Reglan 2935

Minocycline Hydrochloride (Co-administration of estrogens with certain antibiotics, such as tetracyclines, may decrease the enterohepatic circulation and may reduce ethinyl estradiol concentrations; potential for reduced efficacy and increased incidence of breakthrough bleeding and menstrual irregularities). Products include:

Dynacin Capsules 2019
Minocin Intravenous 1862
Minocin Oral Suspension 1865
Minocin Pellet-Filled Capsules 1863

Neostigmine Bromide (Diarrhea may increase gastrointestinal motility and reduce hormone absorption; co-administration with drugs which reduce gut transit time, such as cholinergic agents, may reduce hormone concentrations in the blood). Products include:

Prostigmin Tablets 1744

Neostigmine Methylsulfate (Diarrhea may increase gastrointestinal motility and reduce hormone absorption; co-administration with drugs which reduce gut transit time, such as cholinergic agents, may reduce hormone concentrations in the blood). Products include:

Prostigmin Injectable 1744

Oxytetracycline Hydrochloride (Co-administration of estrogens with certain antibiotics, such as tetracyclines, may decrease the enterohepatic circulation and may reduce ethinyl estradiol concentrations; potential for reduced efficacy and increased incidence of breakthrough bleeding and menstrual irregularities). Products include:

Terra-Cortril Ophthalmic Suspension 2716
Urobiotic-250 Capsules 2731

Pentobarbital Sodium (Co-administration with hepatic microsomal enzyme inducers, such as barbiturates, can decrease ethinyl estradiol concentrations; potential for reduced efficacy and increased incidence of breakthrough bleeding and menstrual irregularities). Products include:

Nembutal Sodium Solution 485

Phenobarbital (Co-administration with hepatic microsomal enzyme inducers, such as barbiturates, can decrease ethinyl estradiol concentrations; potential for reduced efficacy and increased incidence of breakthrough bleeding and menstrual irregularities). Products include:

Arco-Lase Plus Tablets 592
Donnatal 2929
Donnatal Extentabs 2930

Phenylbutazone (Co-administration with hepatic microsomal enzyme inducers, such as phenylbutazone, can decrease ethinyl estradiol concentrations; potential for reduced efficacy and increased incidence of breakthrough bleeding and menstrual irregularities).

No products indexed under this heading.

Phenytoin (Co-administration with hepatic microsomal enzyme inducers, such as phenytoin, can decrease ethinyl estradiol concentrations; potential for reduced efficacy

and increased incidence of breakthrough bleeding and menstrual irregularities). Products include:
- Dilantin Infatabs 2624
- Dilantin-125 Oral Suspension 2625

Phenytoin Sodium (Co-administration with hepatic microsomal enzyme inducers, such as phenytoin, can decrease ethinyl estradiol concentrations; potential for reduced efficacy and increased incidence of breakthrough bleeding and menstrual irregularities). Products include:
- Dilantin Kapseals 2622

Pyridostigmine Bromide (Diarrhea may increase gastrointestinal motility and reduce hormone absorption; co-administration with drugs which reduce gut transit time, such as cholinergic agents, may reduce hormone concentrations in the blood). Products include:
- Mestinon 1740

Rifampin (Co-administration with hepatic microsomal enzyme inducers, such as rifampin, can decrease ethinyl estradiol concentrations; this interaction has been associated with reduced efficacy and increased incidence of breakthrough bleeding and menstrual irregularities). Products include:
- Rifadin 765
- Rifamate Capsules 767
- Rifater Tablets 769

Rivastigmine Tartrate (Diarrhea may increase gastrointestinal motility and reduce hormone absorption; co-administration with drugs which reduce gut transit time, such as cholinergic agents, may reduce hormone concentrations in the blood). Products include:
- Exelon Capsules 2342
- Exelon Oral Solution 2345

Secobarbital Sodium (Co-administration with hepatic microsomal enzyme inducers, such as barbiturates, can decrease ethinyl estradiol concentrations; potential for reduced efficacy and increased incidence of breakthrough bleeding and menstrual irregularities).
No products indexed under this heading.

Tacrine Hydrochloride (Diarrhea may increase gastrointestinal motility and reduce hormone absorption; co-administration with drugs which reduce gut transit time, such as cholinergic agents, may reduce hormone concentrations in the blood). Products include:
- Cognex Capsules 1351

Tetracycline Hydrochloride (Co-administration of estrogens with certain antibiotics, such as tetracyclines, may decrease the enterohepatic circulation and may reduce ethinyl estradiol concentrations; potential for reduced efficacy and increased incidence of breakthrough bleeding and menstrual irregularities).
No products indexed under this heading.

Theophylline (Ethinyl estradiol may interfere with the metabolism of theophylline by inhibiting hepatic microsomal enzymes thereby increasing theophylline concentrations). Products include:
- Aerolate 1361
- Theo-Dur Extended-Release Tablets 1835
- Uni-Dur Extended-Release Tablets 1841
- Uniphyl 400 mg and 600 mg Tablets 2903

Theophylline Calcium Salicylate (Ethinyl estradiol may interfere with the metabolism of theophylline by inhibiting hepatic microsomal enzymes thereby increasing theophylline concentrations).
No products indexed under this heading.

Theophylline Sodium Glycinate (Ethinyl estradiol may interfere with the metabolism of theophylline by inhibiting hepatic microsomal enzymes thereby increasing theophylline concentrations).
No products indexed under this heading.

Thiamylal Sodium (Co-administration with hepatic microsomal enzyme inducers, such as barbiturates, can decrease ethinyl estradiol concentrations; potential for reduced efficacy and increased incidence of breakthrough bleeding and menstrual irregularities).
No products indexed under this heading.

Vitamin C (Sulfation of ethinyl estradiol occurs in gastrointestinal wall, therefore, drugs which interfere with the sulfation in the GI wall, such as ascorbic acid, may increase ethinyl estradiol bioavailabilty). Products include:
- Beta-C Tablets .... ▣811
- C-Grams Caplets .... ▣795
- Halls Defense Drops .... ▣687
- Peridin-C Tablets .... ▣618

LEVLITE 28 TABLETS

(Ethinyl Estradiol, Levonorgestrel) 962
See Levlite 21 Tablets

LEVO-DROMORAN INJECTABLE

(Levorphanol Tartrate) 1734
May interact with antihistamines, barbiturates, central nervous system depressants, general anesthetics, hypnotics and sedatives, monoamine oxidase inhibitors, mixed agonist/antagonist opioid analgesics, narcotic analgesics, phenothiazines, skeletal muscle relaxants, tranquilizers, tricyclic antidepressants, and certain other agents. Compounds in these categories include:

Acrivastine (Concurrent use may result in additive central nervous system depressant effects, including respiratory depression, hypotension, profound sedation and coma). Products include:
- Semprex-D Capsules 1172

Alfentanil Hydrochloride (Concurrent use may result in additive central nervous system depressant effects, including respiratory depression, hypotension, profound sedation and coma).
No products indexed under this heading.

Alprazolam (Concurrent use may result in additive central nervous system depressant effects, including respiratory depression, hypotension, profound sedation and coma). Products include:
- Xanax Tablets 2865

Amitriptyline Hydrochloride (Concurrent use may result in additive central nervous system depressant effects, including respiratory depression, hypotension, profound sedation and coma). Products include:
- Etrafon 3115
- Limbitrol 1738

Amoxapine (Concurrent use may result in additive central nervous system depressant effects, including respiratory depression, hypotension, profound sedation and coma).
No products indexed under this heading.

Aprobarbital (Concurrent use may result in additive central nervous system depressant effects, including respiratory depression, hypotension, profound sedation and coma).
No products indexed under this heading.

Astemizole (Concurrent use may result in additive central nervous system depressant effects, including respiratory depression, hypotension, profound sedation and coma).
No products indexed under this heading.

Azatadine Maleate (Concurrent use may result in additive central nervous system depressant effects, including respiratory depression, hypotension, profound sedation and coma). Products include:
- Rynatan Tablets 3351

Baclofen (Concurrent use may result in additive central nervous system depressant effects, including respiratory depression, hypotension, profound sedation and coma).
No products indexed under this heading.

Bromodiphenhydramine Hydrochloride (Concurrent use may result in additive central nervous system depressant effects, including respiratory depression, hypotension, profound sedation and coma).
No products indexed under this heading.

Brompheniramine Maleate (Concurrent use may result in additive central nervous system depressant effects, including respiratory depression, hypotension, profound sedation and coma). Products include:
- Bromfed Capsules (Extended-Release) 2269
- Bromfed-PD Capsules (Extended-Release) 2269
- Comtrex Acute Head Cold & Sinus Pressure Relief Tablets .... ▣627
- Dimetapp Elixir .... ▣777
- Dimetapp Cold and Fever Suspension .... ▣775
- Dimetapp DM Cold & Cough Elixir .... ▣775
- Dimetapp Nighttime Flu Liquid .... ▣776

Buprenorphine Hydrochloride (In patients on pure opioid agonist therapy, mixed agonist/antagonist analgesics may precipitate withdrawal symptoms). Products include:
- Buprenex Injectable 2918

Buspirone Hydrochloride (Concurrent use may result in additive central nervous system depressant effects, including respiratory depression, hypotension, profound sedation and coma).
No products indexed under this heading.

Butabarbital (Concurrent use may result in additive central nervous system depressant effects, including respiratory depression, hypotension, profound sedation and coma).
No products indexed under this heading.

Butalbital (Concurrent use may result in additive central nervous system depressant effects, including respiratory depression, hypotension, profound sedation and coma). Products include:
- Phrenilin 578
- Sedapap Tablets 50 mg/650 mg 2225

Butorphanol Tartrate (In patients on pure opioid agonist therapy, mixed agonist/antagonist analgesics may precipitate withdrawal symptoms). Products include:
- Stadol NS Nasal Spray 1108

Carisoprodol (Concurrent use may result in additive central nervous system depressant effects, including respiratory depression, hypotension, profound sedation and coma). Products include:
- Soma Tablets 3353
- Soma Compound Tablets 3354
- Soma Compound w/Codeine Tablets 3355

Cetirizine Hydrochloride (Concurrent use may result in additive central nervous system depressant effects, including respiratory depression, hypotension, profound sedation and coma). Products include:
- Zyrtec 2756
- Zyrtec-D 12 Hour Extended Relief Tablets 2758

Chlordiazepoxide (Concurrent use may result in additive central nervous system depressant effects, including respiratory depression, hypotension, profound sedation and coma). Products include:
- Limbitrol 1738

Chlordiazepoxide Hydrochloride (Concurrent use may result in additive central nervous system depressant effects, including respiratory depression, hypotension, profound sedation and coma). Products include:
- Librium Capsules 1736
- Librium for Injection 1737

Chlorpheniramine Maleate (Concurrent use may result in additive central nervous system depressant effects, including respiratory depression, hypotension, profound sedation and coma). Products include:
- Actifed Cold & Sinus Caplets and Tablets .... ▣688
- Alka-Seltzer Plus Liqui-Gels .... ▣604
- BC Allergy Sinus Cold Powder .... ▣619
- Chlor-Trimeton Allergy Tablets .... ▣735
- Chlor-Trimeton Allergy/Decongestant Tablets .... ▣736
- Comtrex Flu Therapy & Fever Relief Nighttime Tablets .... ▣628
- Comtrex Maximum Strength Multi-Symptom Cold & Cough Relief Tablets and Caplets .... ▣626
- Contac Severe Cold and Flu Caplets Maximum Strength .... ▣746
- Coricidin 'D' Cold, Flu & Sinus Tablets .... ▣737
- Coricidin/Coricidin D .... ▣738
- Coricidin HBP Maximum Strength Flu Tablets .... ▣738
- Extendryl 1361
- Hycomine Compound Tablets 1317
- Kronofed-A 1341
- PediaCare Cough-Cold Liquid .... ▣719
- PediaCare NightRest Cough-Cold Liquid .... ▣719
- Robitussin Nighttime Honey Flu Liquid .... ▣786
- Ryna .... ▣768
- Singlet Caplets .... ▣761
- Sinutab Sinus Allergy Medication, Maximum Strength Formula, Tablets & Caplets .... ▣707
- Sudafed Cold & Allergy Tablets .... ▣708
- TheraFlu Regular Strength Cold & Cough Night Time Hot Liquid .... ▣676
- TheraFlu Regular Strength Cold & Sore Throat Night Time Hot Liquid .... ▣676
- TheraFlu Maximum Strength Flu & Cough Night Time Hot Liquid .... ▣678
- TheraFlu Maximum Strength Flu & Sore Throat Night Time Hot Liquid .... ▣677
- TheraFlu Maximum Strength Severe Cold & Congestion Night Time Caplets .... ▣678
- TheraFlu Maximum Strength Severe Cold & Congestion Night Time Hot Liquid .... ▣678
- Triaminic Cold & Allergy Liquid .... ▣681
- Triaminic Cold & Allergy Softchews .... ▣683
- Triaminic Cold & Cough Liquid .... ▣681
- Triaminic Cold & Cough Softchews .... ▣683
- Triaminic Cold & Night Time Cough Liquid .... ▣681
- Triaminic Cold, Cough & Fever Liquid .... ▣681
- Children's Tylenol Cold Suspension Liquid and Chewable Tablets 2015
- Children's Tylenol Cold Plus Cough Suspension Liquid and Chewable Tablets 2015
- Children's Tylenol Flu Suspension Liquid 2015
- Maximum Strength Tylenol Allergy Sinus Caplets, Gelcaps, and Geltabs 2010
- Multi-Symptom Tylenol Cold Complete Formula Caplets 2010
- Vicks 44M Cough, Cold & Flu Relief Liquid .... ▣725
- Pediatric Vicks 44m Cough & Cold Relief .... ▣728

IMPORTANT NOTE: Always consult each drug listing in the patient's regimen for possible interactions.

Children's Vicks NyQuil
Cold/Cough Relief ▣726

Chlorpheniramine Polistirex (Concurrent use may result in additive central nervous system depressant effects, including respiratory depression, hypotension, profound sedation and coma). Products include:

Tussionex Pennkinetic
Extended-Release Suspension 1174

Chlorpheniramine Tannate (Concurrent use may result in additive central nervous system depressant effects, including respiratory depression, hypotension, profound sedation and coma). Products include:

Reformulated Rynatan Pediatric
Suspension 3352
Rynatuss Pediatric Suspension 3353
Rynatuss Tablets 3353
Tussi-12 S Suspension 3356
Tussi-12 Tablets 3356

Chlorpromazine (Concurrent use may result in additive central nervous system depressant effects, including respiratory depression, hypotension, profound sedation and coma). Products include:

Thorazine Suppositories 1656

Chlorpromazine Hydrochloride (Concurrent use may result in additive central nervous system depressant effects, including respiratory depression, hypotension, profound sedation and coma). Products include:

Thorazine 1656

Chlorprothixene (Concurrent use may result in additive central nervous system depressant effects, including respiratory depression, hypotension, profound sedation and coma).

No products indexed under this heading.

Chlorprothixene Hydrochloride (Concurrent use may result in additive central nervous system depressant effects, including respiratory depression, hypotension, profound sedation and coma).

No products indexed under this heading.

Chlorprothixene Lactate (Concurrent use may result in additive central nervous system depressant effects, including respiratory depression, hypotension, profound sedation and coma).

No products indexed under this heading.

Chlorzoxazone (Concurrent use may result in additive central nervous system depressant effects, including respiratory depression, hypotension, profound sedation and coma). Products include:

Parafon Forte DSC Caplets 2582

Clemastine Fumarate (Concurrent use may result in additive central nervous system depressant effects, including respiratory depression, hypotension, profound sedation and coma). Products include:

Tavist 12 Hour Allergy Tablets ▣676

Clomipramine Hydrochloride (Concurrent use may result in additive central nervous system depressant effects, including respiratory depression, hypotension, profound sedation and coma).

No products indexed under this heading.

Clorazepate Dipotassium (Concurrent use may result in additive central nervous system depressant effects, including respiratory depression, hypotension, profound sedation and coma). Products include:

Tranxene 511

Clozapine (Concurrent use may result in additive central nervous system depressant effects, including respiratory depression, hypotension, profound sedation and coma). Products include:

Clozaril Tablets 2319

Codeine Phosphate (Concurrent use may result in additive central nervous system depressant effects, including respiratory depression, hypotension, profound sedation and coma). Products include:

Phenergan with Codeine Syrup 3557
Phenergan VC with Codeine Syrup 3561
Robitussin A-C Syrup 2942
Robitussin-DAC Syrup 2942
Ryna-C Liquid ▣768
Soma Compound w/Codeine
Tablets 3355
Tussi-Organidin NR Liquid 3350
Tussi-Organidin-S NR Liquid 3350
Tylenol with Codeine 2595

Cyclobenzaprine Hydrochloride (Concurrent use may result in additive central nervous system depressant effects, including respiratory depression, hypotension, profound sedation and coma). Products include:

Flexeril Tablets 572
Flexeril Tablets 2094

Cyproheptadine Hydrochloride (Concurrent use may result in additive central nervous system depressant effects, including respiratory depression, hypotension, profound sedation and coma). Products include:

Periactin Tablets 2155

Dantrolene Sodium (Concurrent use may result in additive central nervous system depressant effects, including respiratory depression, hypotension, profound sedation and coma). Products include:

Dantrium Capsules 2885
Dantrium Intravenous 2886

Desflurane (Concurrent use may result in additive central nervous system depressant effects, including respiratory depression, hypotension, profound sedation and coma). Products include:

Suprane Liquid for Inhalation 874

Desipramine Hydrochloride (Concurrent use may result in additive central nervous system depressant effects, including respiratory depression, hypotension, profound sedation and coma). Products include:

Norpramin Tablets 755

Dexchlorpheniramine Maleate (Concurrent use may result in additive central nervous system depressant effects, including respiratory depression, hypotension, profound sedation and coma).

No products indexed under this heading.

Dezocine (In patients on pure opioid agonist therapy, mixed agonist/antagonist analgesics may precipitate withdrawal symptoms).

No products indexed under this heading.

Diazepam (Concurrent use may result in additive central nervous system depressant effects, including respiratory depression, hypotension, profound sedation and coma). Products include:

Valium Injectable 3026
Valium Tablets 3047

Diphenhydramine Citrate (Concurrent use may result in additive central nervous system depressant effects, including respiratory depression, hypotension, profound sedation and coma). Products include:

Alka-Seltzer PM Effervescent
Tablets ▣605
Benadryl Allergy & Sinus Fastmelt
Tablets ▣693
Benadryl Children's Allergy/Cold
Fastmelt Tablets ▣692
Excedrin PM Tablets, Caplets,
and Geltabs ▣631
Goody's PM Powder ▣621

Diphenhydramine Hydrochloride (Concurrent use may result in additive central nervous system depressant effects, including respiratory depression, hypotension, profound sedation and coma). Products include:

Extra Strength Bayer PM
Caplets ▣611
Benadryl Allergy Chewables ▣689
Benadryl Allergy ▣691
Benadryl Allergy Liquid ▣690
Benadryl Allergy/Cold Tablets ▣691
Benadryl Allergy/Congestion
Tablets ▣692
Benadryl Allergy & Sinus Liquid ▣693
Benadryl Allergy Sinus Headache
Caplets & Gelcaps ▣693
Benadryl Severe Allergy & Sinus
Headache Caplets ▣694
Benadryl Dye-Free Allergy Liquid ▣690
Benadryl Dye-Free Allergy
Liqui-Gels Softgels ▣690
Benadryl Itch Relief Stick Extra
Strength ▣695
Benadryl Cream ▣695
Benadryl Gel ▣695
Benadryl Spray ▣696
Benadryl Parenteral 2617
Coricidin HBP Night-Time Cold &
Flu Tablets ▣738
Nytol QuickCaps Caplets ▣622
Maximum Strength Nytol
QuickGels Softgels ▣621
Extra Strength Percogesic
Aspirin-Free Coated Caplets ▣665
Simply Sleep Caplets 2008
Sominex Original Formula Tablets ▣761
Children's Tylenol Allergy-D Liquid 2014
Maximum Strength Tylenol Allergy
Sinus NightTime Caplets 2010
Tylenol Severe Allergy Caplets 2010
Maximum Strength Tylenol Flu
NightTime Gelcaps 2011
Extra Strength Tylenol PM Caplets,
Geltabs, and Gelcaps 2012
Unisom Maximum Strength
SleepGels ▣713

Diphenylpyraline Hydrochloride (Concurrent use may result in additive central nervous system depressant effects, including respiratory depression, hypotension, profound sedation and coma).

No products indexed under this heading.

Doxepin Hydrochloride (Concurrent use may result in additive central nervous system depressant effects, including respiratory depression, hypotension, profound sedation and coma). Products include:

Sinequan 2713

Droperidol (Concurrent use may result in additive central nervous system depressant effects, including respiratory depression, hypotension, profound sedation and coma).

No products indexed under this heading.

Enflurane (Concurrent use may result in additive central nervous system depressant effects, including respiratory depression, hypotension, profound sedation and coma).

No products indexed under this heading.

Estazolam (Concurrent use may result in additive central nervous system depressant effects, including respiratory depression, hypotension, profound sedation and coma). Products include:

ProSom Tablets 500

Ethchlorvynol (Concurrent use may result in additive central nervous system depressant effects, including respiratory depression, hypotension, profound sedation and coma).

No products indexed under this heading.

Ethinamate (Concurrent use may result in additive central nervous system depressant effects, including respiratory depression, hypotension, profound sedation and coma).

No products indexed under this heading.

Fentanyl (Concurrent use may result in additive central nervous system depressant effects, including respiratory depression, hypotension, profound sedation and coma). Products include:

Duragesic Transdermal System 1786

Fentanyl Citrate (Concurrent use may result in additive central nervous system depressant effects, including respiratory depression, hypotension, profound sedation and coma). Products include:

Actiq 1184

Fexofenadine Hydrochloride (Concurrent use may result in additive central nervous system depressant effects, including respiratory depression, hypotension, profound sedation and coma). Products include:

Allegra 712
Allegra-D Extended-Release
Tablets 714

Fluphenazine Decanoate (Concurrent use may result in additive central nervous system depressant effects, including respiratory depression, hypotension, profound sedation and coma).

No products indexed under this heading.

Fluphenazine Enanthate (Concurrent use may result in additive central nervous system depressant effects, including respiratory depression, hypotension, profound sedation and coma).

No products indexed under this heading.

Fluphenazine Hydrochloride (Concurrent use may result in additive central nervous system depressant effects, including respiratory depression, hypotension, profound sedation and coma).

No products indexed under this heading.

Flurazepam Hydrochloride (Concurrent use may result in additive central nervous system depressant effects, including respiratory depression, hypotension, profound sedation and coma).

No products indexed under this heading.

Glutethimide (Concurrent use may result in additive central nervous system depressant effects, including respiratory depression, hypotension, profound sedation and coma).

No products indexed under this heading.

Haloperidol (Concurrent use may result in additive central nervous system depressant effects, including respiratory depression, hypotension, profound sedation and coma). Products include:

Haldol Injection, Tablets and
Concentrate 2533

Haloperidol Decanoate (Concurrent use may result in additive central nervous system depressant effects, including respiratory depression, hypotension, profound sedation and coma). Products include:

Haldol Decanoate 2535

Hydrocodone Bitartrate (Concurrent use may result in additive central nervous system depressant effects, including respiratory depression, hypotension, profound sedation and coma). Products include:

Hycodan 1316
Hycomine Compound Tablets 1317
Hycotuss Expectorant Syrup 1318
Lortab 3319
Lortab Elixir 3317
Maxidone Tablets CIII 3399
Norco 5/325 Tablets CIII 3424
Norco 7.5/325 Tablets CIII 3425
Norco 10/325 Tablets CIII 3427
Norco 10/325 Tablets CIII 3425
Vicodin Tablets 516
Vicodin ES Tablets 517

Vicodin HP Tablets 518
Vicodin Tuss Expectorant 519
Vicoprofen Tablets 520
Zydone Tablets 1330

Hydrocodone Polistirex (Concurrent use may result in additive central nervous system depressant effects, including respiratory depression, hypotension, profound sedation and coma). Products include:
Tussionex Pennkinetic Extended-Release Suspension 1174

Hydromorphone Hydrochloride (Concurrent use may result in additive central nervous system depressant effects, including respiratory depression, hypotension, profound sedation and coma). Products include:
Dilaudid 441
Dilaudid Oral Liquid 445
Dilaudid Powder 441
Dilaudid Rectal Suppositories 441
Dilaudid Tablets 441
Dilaudid Tablets - 8 mg 445
Dilaudid-HP 443

Hydroxyzine Hydrochloride (Concurrent use may result in additive central nervous system depressant effects, including respiratory depression, hypotension, profound sedation and coma). Products include:
Atarax Tablets & Syrup 2667
Vistaril Intramuscular Solution 2738

Imipramine Hydrochloride (Concurrent use may result in additive central nervous system depressant effects, including respiratory depression, hypotension, profound sedation and coma).
No products indexed under this heading.

Imipramine Pamoate (Concurrent use may result in additive central nervous system depressant effects, including respiratory depression, hypotension, profound sedation and coma).
No products indexed under this heading.

Isocarboxazid (Although no interaction between MAO inhibitors and levorphanol has been observed, concurrent use is not recommended).
No products indexed under this heading.

Isoflurane (Concurrent use may result in additive central nervous system depressant effects, including respiratory depression, hypotension, profound sedation and coma).
No products indexed under this heading.

Ketamine Hydrochloride (Concurrent use may result in additive central nervous system depressant effects, including respiratory depression, hypotension, profound sedation and coma).
No products indexed under this heading.

Levomethadyl Acetate Hydrochloride (Concurrent use may result in additive central nervous system depressant effects, including respiratory depression, hypotension, profound sedation and coma).
No products indexed under this heading.

Loratadine (Concurrent use may result in additive central nervous system depressant effects, including respiratory depression, hypotension, profound sedation and coma). Products include:
Claritin 3100
Claritin-D 12 Hour Extended Release Tablets 3102
Claritin-D 24 Hour Extended Release Tablets 3104

Lorazepam (Concurrent use may result in additive central nervous system depressant effects, including respiratory depression, hypotension, profound sedation and coma). Products include:
Ativan Injection 3478
Ativan Tablets 3482

Loxapine Hydrochloride (Concurrent use may result in additive central nervous system depressant effects, including respiratory depression, hypotension, profound sedation and coma).
No products indexed under this heading.

Loxapine Succinate (Concurrent use may result in additive central nervous system depressant effects, including respiratory depression, hypotension, profound sedation and coma). Products include:
Loxitane Capsules 3398

Maprotiline Hydrochloride (Concurrent use may result in additive central nervous system depressant effects, including respiratory depression, hypotension, profound sedation and coma).
No products indexed under this heading.

Meperidine Hydrochloride (Concurrent use may result in additive central nervous system depressant effects, including respiratory depression, hypotension, profound sedation and coma). Products include:
Demerol 3079
Mepergan Injection 3539

Mephobarbital (Concurrent use may result in additive central nervous system depressant effects, including respiratory depression, hypotension, profound sedation and coma).
No products indexed under this heading.

Meprobamate (Concurrent use may result in additive central nervous system depressant effects, including respiratory depression, hypotension, profound sedation and coma). Products include:
Miltown Tablets 3349

Mesoridazine Besylate (Concurrent use may result in additive central nervous system depressant effects, including respiratory depression, hypotension, profound sedation and coma). Products include:
Serentil 1057

Metaxalone (Concurrent use may result in additive central nervous system depressant effects, including respiratory depression, hypotension, profound sedation and coma). Products include:
Skelaxin Tablets 1301

Methadone Hydrochloride (Concurrent use may result in additive central nervous system depressant effects, including respiratory depression, hypotension, profound sedation and coma). Products include:
Dolophine Hydrochloride Tablets 3056

Methdilazine Hydrochloride (Concurrent use may result in additive central nervous system depressant effects, including respiratory depression, hypotension, profound sedation and coma).
No products indexed under this heading.

Methocarbamol (Concurrent use may result in additive central nervous system depressant effects, including respiratory depression, hypotension, profound sedation and coma). Products include:
Robaxin Injectable 2938
Robaxin Tablets 2939
Robaxisal Tablets 2939

Methohexital Sodium (Concurrent use may result in additive central nervous system depressant effects, including respiratory depression, hypotension, profound sedation and coma). Products include:
Brevital Sodium for Injection, USP .. 1815

Methotrimeprazine (Concurrent use may result in additive central nervous system depressant effects, including respiratory depression, hypotension, profound sedation and coma).
No products indexed under this heading.

Methoxyflurane (Concurrent use may result in additive central nervous system depressant effects, including respiratory depression, hypotension, profound sedation and coma).
No products indexed under this heading.

Midazolam Hydrochloride (Concurrent use may result in additive central nervous system depressant effects, including respiratory depression, hypotension, profound sedation and coma). Products include:
Versed Injection 3027
Versed Syrup 3033

Moclobemide (Although no interaction between MAO inhibitors and levorphanol has been observed, concurrent use is not recommended).
No products indexed under this heading.

Molindone Hydrochloride (Concurrent use may result in additive central nervous system depressant effects, including respiratory depression, hypotension, profound sedation and coma). Products include:
Moban 1320

Morphine Sulfate (Concurrent use may result in additive central nervous system depressant effects, including respiratory depression, hypotension, profound sedation and coma). Products include:
Astramorph/PF Injection, USP (Preservative-Free)........................ 594
Duramorph Injection 1312
Infumorph 200 and Infumorph 500 Sterile Solutions........................... 1314
Kadian Capsules 1335
MS Contin Tablets 2896
MSIR 2898
Oramorph SR Tablets 3062
Roxanol 3066

Nalbuphine Hydrochloride (In patients on pure opioid agonist therapy, mixed agonist/antagonist analgesics may precipitate withdrawal symptoms). Products include:
Nubain Injection 1323

Nortriptyline Hydrochloride (Concurrent use may result in additive central nervous system depressant effects, including respiratory depression, hypotension, profound sedation and coma).
No products indexed under this heading.

Olanzapine (Concurrent use may result in additive central nervous system depressant effects, including respiratory depression, hypotension, profound sedation and coma). Products include:
Zyprexa Tablets 1973
Zyprexa ZYDIS Orally Disintegrating Tablets.................. 1973

Orphenadrine Citrate (Concurrent use may result in additive central nervous system depressant effects, including respiratory depression, hypotension, profound sedation and coma). Products include:
Norflex 1987

Oxazepam (Concurrent use may result in additive central nervous system depressant effects, including respiratory depression, hypotension, profound sedation and coma).
No products indexed under this heading.

Oxycodone Hydrochloride (Concurrent use may result in additive central nervous system depressant effects, including respiratory depression, hypotension, profound sedation and coma). Products include:
OxyContin Tablets 2912
OxyFast Oral Concentrate Solution . 2916
OxyIR Capsules 2916
Percocet Tablets 1326
Percodan Tablets 1327
Percolone Tablets 1327
Roxicodone 3067
Tylox Capsules 2597

Pargyline Hydrochloride (Although no interaction between MAO inhibitors and levorphanol has been observed, concurrent use is not recommended).
No products indexed under this heading.

Pentazocine Hydrochloride (In patients on pure opioid agonist therapy, mixed agonist/antagonist analgesics may precipitate withdrawal symptoms). Products include:
Talacen Caplets 3089
Talwin Nx Tablets 3090

Pentazocine Lactate (In patients on pure opioid agonist therapy, mixed agonist/antagonist analgesics may precipitate withdrawal symptoms).
No products indexed under this heading.

Pentobarbital Sodium (Concurrent use may result in additive central nervous system depressant effects, including respiratory depression, hypotension, profound sedation and coma). Products include:
Nembutal Sodium Solution 485

Perphenazine (Concurrent use may result in additive central nervous system depressant effects, including respiratory depression, hypotension, profound sedation and coma). Products include:
Etrafon 3115
Trilafon 3160

Phenelzine Sulfate (Although no interaction between MAO inhibitors and levorphanol has been observed, concurrent use is not recommended). Products include:
Nardil Tablets 2653

Phenobarbital (Concurrent use may result in additive central nervous system depressant effects, including respiratory depression, hypotension, profound sedation and coma). Products include:
Arco-Lase Plus Tablets 592
Donnatal 2929
Donnatal Extentabs 2930

Prazepam (Concurrent use may result in additive central nervous system depressant effects, including respiratory depression, hypotension, profound sedation and coma).
No products indexed under this heading.

Procarbazine Hydrochloride (Although no interaction between MAO inhibitors and levorphanol has been observed, concurrent use is not recommended). Products include:
Matulane Capsules 3246

Prochlorperazine (Concurrent use may result in additive central nervous system depressant effects, including respiratory depression, hypotension, profound sedation and coma). Products include:
Compazine 1505

Promethazine Hydrochloride (Concurrent use may result in additive central nervous system depressant effects, including respiratory depression, hypotension, profound sedation and coma). Products include:
Mepergan Injection 3539
Phenergan Injection 3553
Phenergan 3556
Phenergan Syrup 3554
Phenergan with Codeine Syrup 3557
Phenergan with Dextromethorphan Syrup 3559
Phenergan VC Syrup 3560
Phenergan VC with Codeine Syrup .. 3561

Propofol (Concurrent use may result in additive central nervous

system depressant effects, including respiratory depression, hypotension, profound sedation and coma). Products include:

Diprivan Injectable Emulsion 667

Propoxyphene Hydrochloride (Concurrent use may result in additive central nervous system depressant effects, including respiratory depression, hypotension, profound sedation and coma). Products include:

Darvon Pulvules 1909
Darvon Compound-65 Pulvules 1910

Propoxyphene Napsylate (Concurrent use may result in additive central nervous system depressant effects, including respiratory depression, hypotension, profound sedation and coma). Products include:

Darvon-N/Darvocet-N 1907
Darvon-N Tablets 1912

Protriptyline Hydrochloride (Concurrent use may result in additive central nervous system depressant effects, including respiratory depression, hypotension, profound sedation and coma). Products include:

Vivactil Tablets 2446
Vivactil Tablets 2217

Pyrilamine Maleate (Concurrent use may result in additive central nervous system depressant effects, including respiratory depression, hypotension, profound sedation and coma). Products include:

Maximum Strength Midol Menstrual Caplets and Gelcaps.................................. ▣612
Maximum Strength Midol PMS Caplets and Gelcaps................. ▣613

Pyrilamine Tannate (Concurrent use may result in additive central nervous system depressant effects, including respiratory depression, hypotension, profound sedation and coma). Products include:

Ryna-12 S Suspension 3351

Quazepam (Concurrent use may result in additive central nervous system depressant effects, including respiratory depression, hypotension, profound sedation and coma).

No products indexed under this heading.

Quetiapine Fumarate (Concurrent use may result in additive central nervous system depressant effects, including respiratory depression, hypotension, profound sedation and coma). Products include:

Seroquel Tablets 684

Remifentanil Hydrochloride (Concurrent use may result in additive central nervous system depressant effects, including respiratory depression, hypotension, profound sedation and coma).

No products indexed under this heading.

Risperidone (Concurrent use may result in additive central nervous system depressant effects, including respiratory depression, hypotension, profound sedation and coma). Products include:

Risperdal 1796

Secobarbital Sodium (Concurrent use may result in additive central nervous system depressant effects, including respiratory depression, hypotension, profound sedation and coma).

No products indexed under this heading.

Selegiline Hydrochloride (Although no interaction between MAO inhibitors and levorphanol has been observed, concurrent use is not recommended). Products include:

Eldepryl Capsules 3266

Sevoflurane (Concurrent use may result in additive central nervous system depressant effects, including respiratory depression, hypotension, profound sedation and coma).

No products indexed under this heading.

Sufentanil Citrate (Concurrent use may result in additive central nervous system depressant effects, including respiratory depression, hypotension, profound sedation and coma).

No products indexed under this heading.

Temazepam (Concurrent use may result in additive central nervous system depressant effects, including respiratory depression, hypotension, profound sedation and coma).

No products indexed under this heading.

Terfenadine (Concurrent use may result in additive central nervous system depressant effects, including respiratory depression, hypotension, profound sedation and coma).

No products indexed under this heading.

Thiamylal Sodium (Concurrent use may result in additive central nervous system depressant effects, including respiratory depression, hypotension, profound sedation and coma).

No products indexed under this heading.

Thioridazine Hydrochloride (Concurrent use may result in additive central nervous system depressant effects, including respiratory depression, hypotension, profound sedation and coma). Products include:

Thioridazine Hydrochloride Tablets.. 2289

Thiothixene (Concurrent use may result in additive central nervous system depressant effects, including respiratory depression, hypotension, profound sedation and coma). Products include:

Navane Capsules 2701
Thiothixene Capsules 2290

Tranylcypromine Sulfate (Although no interaction between MAO inhibitors and levorphanol has been observed, concurrent use is not recommended). Products include:

Parnate Tablets 1607

Triazolam (Concurrent use may result in additive central nervous system depressant effects, including respiratory depression, hypotension, profound sedation and coma). Products include:

Halcion Tablets 2823

Trifluoperazine Hydrochloride (Concurrent use may result in additive central nervous system depressant effects, including respiratory depression, hypotension, profound sedation and coma). Products include:

Stelazine 1640

Trimeprazine Tartrate (Concurrent use may result in additive central nervous system depressant effects, including respiratory depression, hypotension, profound sedation and coma).

No products indexed under this heading.

Trimipramine Maleate (Concurrent use may result in additive central nervous system depressant effects, including respiratory depression, hypotension, profound sedation and coma). Products include:

Surmontil Capsules 3595

Tripelennamine Hydrochloride (Concurrent use may result in additive central nervous system depressant effects, including respiratory depression, hypotension, profound sedation and coma).

No products indexed under this heading.

Triprolidine Hydrochloride (Concurrent use may result in additive central nervous system depressant effects, including respiratory depression, hypotension, profound sedation and coma). Products include:

Actifed Cold & Allergy Tablets .... ▣688

Zaleplon (Concurrent use may result in additive central nervous system depressant effects, including respiratory depression, hypotension, profound sedation and coma). Products include:

Sonata Capsules 3591

Ziprasidone Hydrochloride (Concurrent use may result in additive central nervous system depressant effects, including respiratory depression, hypotension, profound sedation and coma). Products include:

Geodon Capsules 2688

Zolpidem Tartrate (Concurrent use may result in additive central nervous system depressant effects, including respiratory depression, hypotension, profound sedation and coma). Products include:

Ambien Tablets 3191

Food Interactions

Alcohol (Concurrent use may result in additive central nervous system depressant effects, including respiratory depression, hypotension, profound sedation and coma).

LEVO-DROMORAN TABLETS

(Levorphanol Tartrate) 1734

See Levo-Dromoran Injectable

LEVORA TABLETS

(Ethinyl Estradiol, Levonorgestrel) 3389

May interact with barbiturates, phenytoin, tetracyclines, and certain other agents. Compounds in these categories include:

Ampicillin (Potential for reduced efficacy and increased incidence of breakthrough bleeding and menstrual irregularities with concomitant use).

No products indexed under this heading.

Ampicillin Sodium (Potential for reduced efficacy and increased incidence of breakthrough bleeding and menstrual irregularities with concomitant use). Products include:

Unasyn for Injection 2728

Aprobarbital (Potential for reduced efficacy and increased incidence of breakthrough bleeding and menstrual irregularities with concomitant use).

No products indexed under this heading.

Butabarbital (Potential for reduced efficacy and increased incidence of breakthrough bleeding and menstrual irregularities with concomitant use).

No products indexed under this heading.

Butalbital (Potential for reduced efficacy and increased incidence of breakthrough bleeding and menstrual irregularities with concomitant use). Products include:

Phrenilin 578
Sedapap Tablets 50 mg/650 mg ... 2225

Demeclocycline Hydrochloride (Potential for reduced efficacy and increased incidence of breakthrough bleeding and menstrual irregularities with concomitant use). Products include:

Declomycin Tablets 1855

Doxycycline Calcium (Potential for reduced efficacy and increased incidence of breakthrough bleeding and menstrual irregularities with concomitant use). Products include:

Vibramycin Calcium Oral Suspension Syrup 2735

Doxycycline Hyclate (Potential for reduced efficacy and increased incidence of breakthrough bleeding and menstrual irregularities with concomitant use). Products include:

Doryx Coated Pellet Filled Capsules.. 3357
Periostat Tablets 1208
Vibramycin Hyclate Capsules 2735
Vibramycin Hyclate Intravenous 2737
Vibra-Tabs Film Coated Tablets 2735

Doxycycline Monohydrate (Potential for reduced efficacy and increased incidence of breakthrough bleeding and menstrual irregularities with concomitant use). Products include:

Monodox Capsules 2442
Vibramycin Monohydrate for Oral Suspension 2735

Fosphenytoin Sodium (Potential for reduced efficacy and increased incidence of breakthrough bleeding and menstrual irregularities with concomitant use). Products include:

Cerebyx Injection 2619

Griseofulvin (Potential for reduced efficacy and increased incidence of breakthrough bleeding and menstrual irregularities with concomitant use). Products include:

Grifulvin V Tablets Microsize and Oral Suspension Microsize 2518
Gris-PEG Tablets 2661

Mephobarbital (Potential for reduced efficacy and increased incidence of breakthrough bleeding and menstrual irregularities with concomitant use).

No products indexed under this heading.

Methacycline Hydrochloride (Potential for reduced efficacy and increased incidence of breakthrough bleeding and menstrual irregularities with concomitant use).

No products indexed under this heading.

Minocycline Hydrochloride (Potential for reduced efficacy and increased incidence of breakthrough bleeding and menstrual irregularities with concomitant use). Products include:

Dynacin Capsules 2019
Minocin Intravenous 1862
Minocin Oral Suspension 1865
Minocin Pellet-Filled Capsules 1863

Oxytetracycline Hydrochloride (Potential for reduced efficacy and increased incidence of breakthrough bleeding and menstrual irregularities with concomitant use). Products include:

Terra-Cortril Ophthalmic Suspension 2716
Urobiotic-250 Capsules 2731

Pentobarbital Sodium (Potential for reduced efficacy and increased incidence of breakthrough bleeding and menstrual irregularities with concomitant use). Products include:

Nembutal Sodium Solution 485

Phenobarbital (Potential for reduced efficacy and increased incidence of breakthrough bleeding and menstrual irregularities with concomitant use). Products include:

Arco-Lase Plus Tablets 592
Donnatal 2929
Donnatal Extentabs 2930

Phenylbutazone (Potential for reduced efficacy and increased incidence of breakthrough bleeding and menstrual irregularities with concomitant use).

No products indexed under this heading.

Phenytoin (Potential for reduced efficacy and increased incidence of breakthrough bleeding and menstrual irregularities with concomitant use). Products include:

Dilantin Infatabs 2624

Dilantin-125 Oral Suspension 2625

Phenytoin Sodium (Potential for reduced efficacy and increased incidence of breakthrough bleeding and menstrual irregularities with concomitant use). Products include:

Dilantin Kapseals 2622

Rifampin (Co-administration has been associated with reduced efficacy and increased incidence of breakthrough bleeding and menstrual irregularities). Products include:

Rifadin 765
Rifamate Capsules 767
Rifater Tablets 769

Secobarbital Sodium (Potential for reduced efficacy and increased incidence of breakthrough bleeding and menstrual irregularities with concomitant use).

No products indexed under this heading.

Tetracycline Hydrochloride (Potential for reduced efficacy and increased incidence of breakthrough bleeding and menstrual irregularities with concomitant use).

No products indexed under this heading.

Thiamylal Sodium (Potential for reduced efficacy and increased incidence of breakthrough bleeding and menstrual irregularities with concomitant use).

No products indexed under this heading.

LEVORPHANOL TARTRATE TABLETS

(Levorphanol Tartrate) 3059

May interact with antihistamines, central nervous system depressants, monoamine oxidase inhibitors, and certain other agents. Compounds in these categories include:

Acrivastine (Concurrent use may result in additive CNS depressant effects). Products include:

Semprex-D Capsules 1172

Alfentanil Hydrochloride (Concurrent use may result in additive CNS depressant effects).

No products indexed under this heading.

Alprazolam (Concurrent use may result in additive CNS depressant effects). Products include:

Xanax Tablets 2865

Aprobarbital (Concurrent use may result in additive CNS depressant effects).

No products indexed under this heading.

Astemizole (Concurrent use may result in additive CNS depressant effects).

No products indexed under this heading.

Azatadine Maleate (Concurrent use may result in additive CNS depressant effects). Products include:

Rynatan Tablets 3351

Bromodiphenhydramine Hydrochloride (Concurrent use may result in additive CNS depressant effects).

No products indexed under this heading.

Brompheniramine Maleate (Concurrent use may result in additive CNS depressant effects). Products include:

Bromfed Capsules (Extended-Release) 2269
Bromfed-PD Capsules (Extended-Release) 2269
Comtrex Acute Head Cold & Sinus Pressure Relief Tablets .... ▣627
Dimetapp Elixir .... ▣777
Dimetapp Cold and Fever Suspension .... ▣775
Dimetapp DM Cold & Cough Elixir .... ▣775
Dimetapp Nighttime Flu Liquid .... ▣776

Buprenorphine Hydrochloride (Concurrent use may result in additive CNS depressant effects). Products include:

Buprenex Injectable 2918

Buspirone Hydrochloride (Concurrent use may result in additive CNS depressant effects).

No products indexed under this heading.

Butabarbital (Concurrent use may result in additive CNS depressant effects).

No products indexed under this heading.

Butalbital (Concurrent use may result in additive CNS depressant effects). Products include:

Phrenilin 578
Sedapap Tablets 50 mg/650 mg ... 2225

Cetirizine Hydrochloride (Concurrent use may result in additive CNS depressant effects). Products include:

Zyrtec 2756
Zyrtec-D 12 Hour Extended Relief Tablets 2758

Chlordiazepoxide (Concurrent use may result in additive CNS depressant effects). Products include:

Limbitrol 1738

Chlordiazepoxide Hydrochloride (Concurrent use may result in additive CNS depressant effects). Products include:

Librium Capsules 1736
Librium for Injection 1737

Chlorpheniramine Maleate (Concurrent use may result in additive CNS depressant effects). Products include:

Actifed Cold & Sinus Caplets and Tablets .... ▣688
Alka-Seltzer Plus Liqui-Gels .... ▣604
BC Allergy Sinus Cold Powder .... ▣619
Chlor-Trimeton Allergy Tablets .... ▣735
Chlor-Trimeton Allergy/Decongestant Tablets .... ▣736
Comtrex Flu Therapy & Fever Relief Nighttime Tablets .... ▣628
Comtrex Maximum Strength Multi-Symptom Cold & Cough Relief Tablets and Caplets .... ▣626
Contac Severe Cold and Flu Caplets Maximum Strength .... ▣746
Coricidin 'D' Cold, Flu & Sinus Tablets .... ▣737
Coricidin/Coricidin D .... ▣738
Coricidin HBP Maximum Strength Flu Tablets .... ▣738
Extendryl 1361
Hycomine Compound Tablets 1317
Kronofed-A 1341
PediaCare Cough-Cold Liquid .... ▣719
PediaCare NightRest Cough-Cold Liquid .... ▣719
Robitussin Nighttime Honey Flu Liquid .... ▣786
Ryna .... ▣768
Singlet Caplets .... ▣761
Sinutab Sinus Allergy Medication, Maximum Strength Formula, Tablets & Caplets .... ▣707
Sudafed Cold & Allergy Tablets .... ▣708
TheraFlu Regular Strength Cold & Cough Night Time Hot Liquid .... ▣676
TheraFlu Regular Strength Cold & Sore Throat Night Time Hot Liquid .... ▣676
TheraFlu Maximum Strength Flu & Cough Night Time Hot Liquid .... ▣678
TheraFlu Maximum Strength Flu & Sore Throat Night Time Hot Liquid .... ▣677
TheraFlu Maximum Strength Severe Cold & Congestion Night Time Caplets .... ▣678
TheraFlu Maximum Strength Severe Cold & Congestion Night Time Hot Liquid .... ▣678
Triaminic Cold & Allergy Liquid .... ▣681
Triaminic Cold & Allergy Softchews .... ▣683
Triaminic Cold & Cough Liquid .... ▣681
Triaminic Cold & Cough Softchews .... ▣683
Triaminic Cold & Night Time Cough Liquid .... ▣681
Triaminic Cold, Cough & Fever Liquid .... ▣681
Children's Tylenol Cold Suspension Liquid and Chewable Tablets 2015
Children's Tylenol Cold Plus Cough Suspension Liquid and Chewable Tablets 2015
Children's Tylenol Flu Suspension Liquid 2015
Maximum Strength Tylenol Allergy Sinus Caplets, Gelcaps, and Geltabs 2010
Multi-Symptom Tylenol Cold Complete Formula Caplets 2010
Vicks 44M Cough, Cold & Flu Relief Liquid .... ▣725
Pediatric Vicks 44m Cough & Cold Relief .... ▣728
Children's Vicks NyQuil Cold/Cough Relief .... ▣726

Chlorpheniramine Polistirex (Concurrent use may result in additive CNS depressant effects). Products include:

Tussionex Pennkinetic Extended-Release Suspension 1174

Chlorpheniramine Tannate (Concurrent use may result in additive CNS depressant effects). Products include:

Reformulated Rynatan Pediatric Suspension 3352
Rynatuss Pediatric Suspension 3353
Rynatuss Tablets 3353
Tussi-12 S Suspension 3356
Tussi-12 Tablets 3356

Chlorpromazine (Concurrent use may result in additive CNS depressant effects). Products include:

Thorazine Suppositories 1656

Chlorpromazine Hydrochloride (Concurrent use may result in additive CNS depressant effects). Products include:

Thorazine 1656

Chlorprothixene (Concurrent use may result in additive CNS depressant effects).

No products indexed under this heading.

Chlorprothixene Hydrochloride (Concurrent use may result in additive CNS depressant effects).

No products indexed under this heading.

Chlorprothixene Lactate (Concurrent use may result in additive CNS depressant effects).

No products indexed under this heading.

Clemastine Fumarate (Concurrent use may result in additive CNS depressant effects). Products include:

Tavist 12 Hour Allergy Tablets .... ▣676

Clorazepate Dipotassium (Concurrent use may result in additive CNS depressant effects). Products include:

Tranxene 511

Clozapine (Concurrent use may result in additive CNS depressant effects). Products include:

Clozaril Tablets 2319

Codeine Phosphate (Concurrent use may result in additive CNS depressant effects). Products include:

Phenergan with Codeine Syrup 3557
Phenergan VC with Codeine Syrup 3561
Robitussin A-C Syrup 2942
Robitussin-DAC Syrup 2942
Ryna-C Liquid .... ▣768
Soma Compound w/Codeine Tablets 3355
Tussi-Organidin NR Liquid 3350
Tussi-Organidin-S NR Liquid 3350
Tylenol with Codeine 2595

Cyproheptadine Hydrochloride (Concurrent use may result in additive CNS depressant effects). Products include:

Periactin Tablets 2155

Desflurane (Concurrent use may result in additive CNS depressant effects). Products include:

Suprane Liquid for Inhalation 874

Dexchlorpheniramine Maleate (Concurrent use may result in additive CNS depressant effects).

No products indexed under this heading.

Dezocine (Concurrent use may result in additive CNS depressant effects).

No products indexed under this heading.

Diazepam (Concurrent use may result in additive CNS depressant effects). Products include:

Valium Injectable 3026
Valium Tablets 3047

Diphenhydramine Citrate (Concurrent use may result in additive CNS depressant effects). Products include:

Alka-Seltzer PM Effervescent Tablets .... ▣605
Benadryl Allergy & Sinus Fastmelt Tablets .... ▣693
Benadryl Children's Allergy/Cold Fastmelt Tablets .... ▣692
Excedrin PM Tablets, Caplets, and Geltabs .... ▣631
Goody's PM Powder .... ▣621

Diphenhydramine Hydrochloride (Concurrent use may result in additive CNS depressant effects). Products include:

Extra Strength Bayer PM Caplets .... ▣611
Benadryl Allergy Chewables .... ▣689
Benadryl Allergy .... ▣691
Benadryl Allergy Liquid .... ▣690
Benadryl Allergy/Cold Tablets .... ▣691
Benadryl Allergy/Congestion Tablets .... ▣692
Benadryl Allergy & Sinus Liquid .... ▣693
Benadryl Allergy Sinus Headache Caplets & Gelcaps .... ▣693
Benadryl Severe Allergy & Sinus Headache Caplets .... ▣694
Benadryl Dye-Free Allergy Liquid .... ▣690
Benadryl Dye-Free Allergy Liqui-Gels Softgels .... ▣690
Benadryl Itch Relief Stick Extra Strength .... ▣695
Benadryl Cream .... ▣695
Benadryl Gel .... ▣695
Benadryl Spray .... ▣696
Benadryl Parenteral 2617
Coricidin HBP Night-Time Cold & Flu Tablets .... ▣738
Nytol QuickCaps Caplets .... ▣622
Maximum Strength Nytol QuickGels Softgels .... ▣621
Extra Strength Percogesic Aspirin-Free Coated Caplets .... ▣665
Simply Sleep Caplets 2008
Sominex Original Formula Tablets .... ▣761
Children's Tylenol Allergy-D Liquid 2014
Maximum Strength Tylenol Allergy Sinus NightTime Caplets 2010
Tylenol Severe Allergy Caplets 2010
Maximum Strength Tylenol Flu NightTime Gelcaps 2011
Extra Strength Tylenol PM Caplets, Geltabs, and Gelcaps 2012
Unisom Maximum Strength SleepGels .... ▣713

Diphenylpyraline Hydrochloride (Concurrent use may result in additive CNS depressant effects).

No products indexed under this heading.

Droperidol (Concurrent use may result in additive CNS depressant effects).

No products indexed under this heading.

Enflurane (Concurrent use may result in additive CNS depressant effects).

No products indexed under this heading.

Estazolam (Concurrent use may result in additive CNS depressant effects). Products include:

ProSom Tablets 500

Ethchlorvynol (Concurrent use may result in additive CNS depressant effects).

No products indexed under this heading.

Ethinamate (Concurrent use may result in additive CNS depressant

effects).
No products indexed under this heading.

Fentanyl (Concurrent use may result in additive CNS depressant effects). Products include:
- Duragesic Transdermal System 1786

Fentanyl Citrate (Concurrent use may result in additive CNS depressant effects). Products include:
- Actiq 1184

Fexofenadine Hydrochloride (Concurrent use may result in additive CNS depressant effects). Products include:
- Allegra 712
- Allegra-D Extended-Release Tablets 714

Fluphenazine Decanoate (Concurrent use may result in additive CNS depressant effects).
No products indexed under this heading.

Fluphenazine Enanthate (Concurrent use may result in additive CNS depressant effects).
No products indexed under this heading.

Fluphenazine Hydrochloride (Concurrent use may result in additive CNS depressant effects).
No products indexed under this heading.

Flurazepam Hydrochloride (Concurrent use may result in additive CNS depressant effects).
No products indexed under this heading.

Glutethimide (Concurrent use may result in additive CNS depressant effects).
No products indexed under this heading.

Haloperidol (Concurrent use may result in additive CNS depressant effects). Products include:
- Haldol Injection, Tablets and Concentrate 2533

Haloperidol Decanoate (Concurrent use may result in additive CNS depressant effects). Products include:
- Haldol Decanoate 2535

Hydrocodone Bitartrate (Concurrent use may result in additive CNS depressant effects). Products include:
- Hycodan 1316
- Hycomine Compound Tablets 1317
- Hycotuss Expectorant Syrup 1318
- Lortab 3319
- Lortab Elixir 3317
- Maxidone Tablets CIII 3399
- Norco 5/325 Tablets CIII 3424
- Norco 7.5/325 Tablets CIII 3425
- Norco 10/325 Tablets CIII 3427
- Norco 10/325 Tablets CIII 3425
- Vicodin Tablets 516
- Vicodin ES Tablets 517
- Vicodin HP Tablets 518
- Vicodin Tuss Expectorant 519
- Vicoprofen Tablets 520
- Zydone Tablets 1330

Hydrocodone Polistirex (Concurrent use may result in additive CNS depressant effects). Products include:
- Tussionex Pennkinetic Extended-Release Suspension 1174

Hydromorphone Hydrochloride (Concurrent use may result in additive CNS depressant effects). Products include:
- Dilaudid 441
- Dilaudid Oral Liquid 445
- Dilaudid Powder 441
- Dilaudid Rectal Suppositories 441
- Dilaudid Tablets 441
- Dilaudid Tablets - 8 mg 445
- Dilaudid-HP 443

Hydroxyzine Hydrochloride (Concurrent use may result in additive CNS depressant effects). Products include:
- Atarax Tablets & Syrup 2667
- Vistaril Intramuscular Solution 2738

Isocarboxazid (Although no interaction between MAO inhibitors and levorphanol has been observed, other narcotic analgesics have produced severe interactions with co-administered MAO inhibitor; concurrent use is not recommended).
No products indexed under this heading.

Isoflurane (Concurrent use may result in additive CNS depressant effects).
No products indexed under this heading.

Ketamine Hydrochloride (Concurrent use may result in additive CNS depressant effects).
No products indexed under this heading.

Levomethadyl Acetate Hydrochloride (Concurrent use may result in additive CNS depressant effects).
No products indexed under this heading.

Loratadine (Concurrent use may result in additive CNS depressant effects). Products include:
- Claritin 3100
- Claritin-D 12 Hour Extended Release Tablets 3102
- Claritin-D 24 Hour Extended Release Tablets 3104

Lorazepam (Concurrent use may result in additive CNS depressant effects). Products include:
- Ativan Injection 3478
- Ativan Tablets 3482

Loxapine Hydrochloride (Concurrent use may result in additive CNS depressant effects).
No products indexed under this heading.

Loxapine Succinate (Concurrent use may result in additive CNS depressant effects). Products include:
- Loxitane Capsules 3398

Meperidine Hydrochloride (Concurrent use may result in additive CNS depressant effects). Products include:
- Demerol 3079
- Mepergan Injection 3539

Mephobarbital (Concurrent use may result in additive CNS depressant effects).
No products indexed under this heading.

Meprobamate (Concurrent use may result in additive CNS depressant effects). Products include:
- Miltown Tablets 3349

Mesoridazine Besylate (Concurrent use may result in additive CNS depressant effects). Products include:
- Serentil 1057

Methadone Hydrochloride (Concurrent use may result in additive CNS depressant effects). Products include:
- Dolophine Hydrochloride Tablets 3056

Methdilazine Hydrochloride (Concurrent use may result in additive CNS depressant effects).
No products indexed under this heading.

Methohexital Sodium (Concurrent use may result in additive CNS depressant effects). Products include:
- Brevital Sodium for Injection, USP 1815

Methotrimeprazine (Concurrent use may result in additive CNS depressant effects).
No products indexed under this heading.

Methoxyflurane (Concurrent use may result in additive CNS depressant effects).
No products indexed under this heading.

Midazolam Hydrochloride (Concurrent use may result in additive CNS depressant effects). Products include:
- Versed Injection 3027
- Versed Syrup 3033

Moclobemide (Although no interaction between MAO inhibitors and levorphanol has been observed, other narcotic analgesics have produced severe interactions with co-administered MAO inhibitor; concurrent use is not recommended).
No products indexed under this heading.

Molindone Hydrochloride (Concurrent use may result in additive CNS depressant effects). Products include:
- Moban 1320

Morphine Sulfate (Concurrent use may result in additive CNS depressant effects). Products include:
- Astramorph/PF Injection, USP (Preservative-Free) 594
- Duramorph Injection 1312
- Infumorph 200 and Infumorph 500 Sterile Solutions 1314
- Kadian Capsules 1335
- MS Contin Tablets 2896
- MSIR 2898
- Oramorph SR Tablets 3062
- Roxanol 3066

Olanzapine (Concurrent use may result in additive CNS depressant effects). Products include:
- Zyprexa Tablets 1973
- Zyprexa ZYDIS Orally Disintegrating Tablets 1973

Oxazepam (Concurrent use may result in additive CNS depressant effects).
No products indexed under this heading.

Oxycodone Hydrochloride (Concurrent use may result in additive CNS depressant effects). Products include:
- OxyContin Tablets 2912
- OxyFast Oral Concentrate Solution 2916
- OxyIR Capsules 2916
- Percocet Tablets 1326
- Percodan Tablets 1327
- Percolone Tablets 1327
- Roxicodone 3067
- Tylox Capsules 2597

Pargyline Hydrochloride (Although no interaction between MAO inhibitors and levorphanol has been observed, other narcotic analgesics have produced severe interactions with co-administered MAO inhibitor; concurrent use is not recommended).
No products indexed under this heading.

Pentobarbital Sodium (Concurrent use may result in additive CNS depressant effects). Products include:
- Nembutal Sodium Solution 485

Perphenazine (Concurrent use may result in additive CNS depressant effects). Products include:
- Etrafon 3115
- Trilafon 3160

Phenelzine Sulfate (Although no interaction between MAO inhibitors and levorphanol has been observed, other narcotic analgesics have produced severe interactions with co-administered MAO inhibitor; concurrent use is not recommended). Products include:
- Nardil Tablets 2653

Phenobarbital (Concurrent use may result in additive CNS depressant effects). Products include:
- Arco-Lase Plus Tablets 592
- Donnatal 2929
- Donnatal Extentabs 2930

Prazepam (Concurrent use may result in additive CNS depressant effects).
No products indexed under this heading.

Procarbazine Hydrochloride (Although no interaction between MAO inhibitors and levorphanol has been observed, other narcotic analgesics have produced severe interactions with co-administered MAO inhibitor; concurrent use is not recommended). Products include:
- Matulane Capsules 3246

Prochlorperazine (Concurrent use may result in additive CNS depressant effects). Products include:
- Compazine 1505

Promethazine Hydrochloride (Concurrent use may result in additive CNS depressant effects). Products include:
- Mepergan Injection 3539
- Phenergan Injection 3553
- Phenergan 3556
- Phenergan Syrup 3554
- Phenergan with Codeine Syrup 3557
- Phenergan with Dextromethorphan Syrup 3559
- Phenergan VC Syrup 3560
- Phenergan VC with Codeine Syrup 3561

Propofol (Concurrent use may result in additive CNS depressant effects). Products include:
- Diprivan Injectable Emulsion 667

Propoxyphene Hydrochloride (Concurrent use may result in additive CNS depressant effects). Products include:
- Darvon Pulvules 1909
- Darvon Compound-65 Pulvules 1910

Propoxyphene Napsylate (Concurrent use may result in additive CNS depressant effects). Products include:
- Darvon-N/Darvocet-N 1907
- Darvon-N Tablets 1912

Pyrilamine Maleate (Concurrent use may result in additive CNS depressant effects). Products include:
- Maximum Strength Midol Menstrual Caplets and Gelcaps ..... ▣612
- Maximum Strength Midol PMS Caplets and Gelcaps ..... ▣613

Pyrilamine Tannate (Concurrent use may result in additive CNS depressant effects). Products include:
- Ryna-12 S Suspension 3351

Quazepam (Concurrent use may result in additive CNS depressant effects).
No products indexed under this heading.

Quetiapine Fumarate (Concurrent use may result in additive CNS depressant effects). Products include:
- Seroquel Tablets 684

Remifentanil Hydrochloride (Concurrent use may result in additive CNS depressant effects).
No products indexed under this heading.

Risperidone (Concurrent use may result in additive CNS depressant effects). Products include:
- Risperdal 1796

Secobarbital Sodium (Concurrent use may result in additive CNS depressant effects).
No products indexed under this heading.

Selegiline Hydrochloride (Although no interaction between MAO inhibitors and levorphanol has been observed, other narcotic analgesics have produced severe interactions with co-administered MAO inhibitor; concurrent use is not recommended). Products include:
- Eldepryl Capsules 3266

Sevoflurane (Concurrent use may result in additive CNS depressant effects).
No products indexed under this heading.

Sufentanil Citrate (Concurrent use may result in additive CNS depressant effects).
No products indexed under this heading.

Temazepam (Concurrent use may result in additive CNS depressant effects).
No products indexed under this heading.

Terfenadine (Concurrent use may result in additive CNS depressant effects).
No products indexed under this heading.

Thiamylal Sodium (Concurrent use may result in additive CNS depressant effects).
No products indexed under this heading.

Thioridazine Hydrochloride (Concurrent use may result in additive CNS depressant effects). Products include:
Thioridazine Hydrochloride Tablets 2289

Thiothixene (Concurrent use may result in additive CNS depressant effects). Products include:
Navane Capsules 2701
Thiothixene Capsules 2290

Tranylcypromine Sulfate (Although no interaction between MAO inhibitors and levorphanol has been observed, other narcotic analgesics have produced severe interactions with co-administered MAO inhibitor; concurrent use is not recommended). Products include:
Parnate Tablets 1607

Triazolam (Concurrent use may result in additive CNS depressant effects). Products include:
Halcion Tablets 2823

Trifluoperazine Hydrochloride (Concurrent use may result in additive CNS depressant effects). Products include:
Stelazine 1640

Trimeprazine Tartrate (Concurrent use may result in additive CNS depressant effects).
No products indexed under this heading.

Tripelennamine Hydrochloride (Concurrent use may result in additive CNS depressant effects).
No products indexed under this heading.

Triprolidine Hydrochloride (Concurrent use may result in additive CNS depressant effects). Products include:
Actifed Cold & Allergy Tablets 688

Zaleplon (Concurrent use may result in additive CNS depressant effects). Products include:
Sonata Capsules 3591

Ziprasidone Hydrochloride (Concurrent use may result in additive CNS depressant effects). Products include:
Geodon Capsules 2688

Zolpidem Tartrate (Concurrent use may result in additive CNS depressant effects). Products include:
Ambien Tablets 3191

Food Interactions

Alcohol (Concurrent use may result in additive CNS depressant effects).

LEVOTHROID TABLETS

(Levothyroxine Sodium) 1373
May interact with oral anticoagulants, estrogens, oral hypoglycemic agents, insulin, oral contraceptives, and certain other agents. Compounds in these categories include:

Acarbose (Dosage of hypoglycemic agent may need to be adjusted). Products include:
Precose Tablets 906

Chlorotrianisene (Estrogens tend to increase serum thyroxine-binding globulin; patients with non-functioning thyroid may need to adjust thyroid dosage).
No products indexed under this heading.

Chlorpropamide (Dosage of hypoglycemic agent may need to be adjusted). Products include:
Diabinese Tablets 2680

Cholestyramine (Binds both T_4 and T_3 in the intestine, thus impairing absorption of thyroid hormone; four to five hours should elapse between administration of cholestyramine and thyroid hormone).
No products indexed under this heading.

Colestipol Hydrochloride (Binds both T_4 and T_3 in the intestine, thus impairing absorption of thyroid hormone; four to five hours should elapse between administration of cholestyramine and thyroid hormone). Products include:
Colestid Tablets 2791

Desogestrel (Estrogens tend to increase serum thyroxine-binding globulin; patients with non-functioning thyroid may need to adjust thyroid dosage). Products include:
Cyclessa Tablets 2450
Desogen Tablets 2458
Mircette Tablets 2470
Ortho-Cept 21 Tablets 2546
Ortho-Cept 28 Tablets 2546

Dicumarol (Anticoagulant effects may be potentiated; dosage adjustment should be made).
No products indexed under this heading.

Dienestrol (Estrogens tend to increase serum thyroxine-binding globulin; patients with non-functioning thyroid may need to adjust thyroid dosage). Products include:
Ortho Dienestrol Cream 2554

Diethylstilbestrol (Estrogens tend to increase serum thyroxine-binding globulin; patients with non-functioning thyroid may need to adjust thyroid dosage).
No products indexed under this heading.

Epinephrine Hydrochloride (Enhanced coronary insufficiency).
No products indexed under this heading.

Estradiol (Estrogens tend to increase serum thyroxine-binding globulin; patients with non-functioning thyroid may need to adjust thyroid dosage). Products include:
Activella Tablets 2764
Alora Transdermal System 3372
Climara Transdermal System 958
CombiPatch Transdermal System 2323
Esclim Transdermal System 3460
Estrace Vaginal Cream 3358
Estrace Tablets 3361
Estring Vaginal Ring 2811
Ortho-Prefest Tablets 2570
Vagifem Tablets 2857
Vivelle Transdermal System 2412
Vivelle-Dot Transdermal System 2416

Estrogens, Conjugated (Estrogens tend to increase serum thyroxine-binding globulin; patients with non-functioning thyroid may need to adjust thyroid dosage). Products include:
Premarin Intravenous 3563
Premarin Tablets 3566
Premarin Vaginal Cream 3570
Premphase Tablets 3572
Prempro Tablets 3572

Estrogens, Esterified (Estrogens tend to increase serum thyroxine-binding globulin; patients with non-functioning thyroid may need to adjust thyroid dosage). Products include:
Estratest 3252
Menest Tablets 2254

Estropipate (Estrogens tend to increase serum thyroxine-binding globulin; patients with non-functioning thyroid may need to adjust thyroid dosage). Products include:
Ogen Tablets 2846
Ortho-Est Tablets 3464

Ethinyl Estradiol (Estrogens tend to increase serum thyroxine-binding globulin; patients with non-functioning thyroid may need to adjust thyroid dosage). Products include:
Alesse-21 Tablets 3468
Alesse-28 Tablets 3473
Brevicon 28-Day Tablets 3380
Cyclessa Tablets 2450
Desogen Tablets 2458
Estinyl Tablets 3112
Estrostep 2627
femhrt Tablets 2635
Levlen 962
Levlite 21 Tablets 962
Levlite 28 Tablets 962
Levora Tablets 3389
Loestrin 21 Tablets 2642
Loestrin Fe Tablets 2642
Lo/Ovral Tablets 3532
Lo/Ovral-28 Tablets 3538
Low-Ogestrel-28 Tablets 3392
Microgestin Fe 1.5/30 Tablets 3407
Microgestin Fe 1/20 Tablets 3400
Mircette Tablets 2470
Modicon 2563
Necon 3415
Nordette-28 Tablets 2257
Norinyl 1 +35 28-Day Tablets 3380
Ogestrel 0.5/50-28 Tablets 3428
Ortho-Cept 21 Tablets 2546
Ortho-Cept 28 Tablets 2546
Ortho-Cyclen/Ortho Tri-Cyclen 2573
Ortho-Novum 2563
Ovcon 3364
Ovral Tablets 3551
Ovral-28 Tablets 3552
Tri-Levlen 962
Tri-Norinyl-28 Tablets 3433
Triphasil-21 Tablets 3600
Triphasil-28 Tablets 3605
Trivora Tablets 3439
Yasmin 28 Tablets 980
Zovia 3449

Ethynodiol Diacetate (Estrogens tend to increase serum thyroxine-binding globulin; patients with non-functioning thyroid may need to adjust thyroid dosage). Products include:
Zovia 3449

Glimepiride (Dosage of hypoglycemic agent may need to be adjusted). Products include:
Amaryl Tablets 717

Glipizide (Dosage of hypoglycemic agent may need to be adjusted). Products include:
Glucotrol Tablets 2692
Glucotrol XL Extended Release Tablets 2693

Glyburide (Dosage of hypoglycemic agent may need to be adjusted). Products include:
DiaBeta Tablets 741
Glucovance Tablets 1086

Insulin, Human, Zinc Suspension (Dosage of insulin may need to be adjusted). Products include:
Humulin L, 100 Units 1937
Humulin U, 100 Units 1943
Novolin L Human Insulin 10 ml Vials 2422

Insulin, Human NPH (Dosage of insulin may need to be adjusted). Products include:
Humulin N, 100 Units 1939
Humulin N NPH Pen 1940
Novolin N Human Insulin 10 ml Vials 2422
Novolin N PenFill 2423
Novolin N Prefilled Syringe Disposable Insulin Delivery System 2425

Insulin, Human Regular (Dosage of insulin may need to be adjusted). Products include:
Humulin R Regular (U-500) 1943
Humulin R, 100 Units 1941
Novolin R Human Insulin 10 ml Vials 2423
Novolin R PenFill 2423
Novolin R Prefilled Syringe Disposable Insulin Delivery System 2425
Velosulin BR Human Insulin 10 ml Vials 2435

Insulin, Human Regular and Human NPH Mixture (Dosage of insulin may need to be adjusted). Products include:
Humulin 50/50, 100 Units 1934
Humulin 70/30, 100 Units 1935
Humulin 70/30 Pen 1936
Novolin 70/30 Human Insulin 10 ml Vials 2421
Novolin 70/30 PenFill 2423
Novolin 70/30 Prefilled Disposable Insulin Delivery System 2425

Insulin, NPH (Dosage of insulin may need to be adjusted). Products include:
Iletin II, NPH (Pork), 100 Units 1946

Insulin, Regular (Dosage of insulin may need to be adjusted). Products include:
Iletin II, Regular (Pork), 100 Units 1947

Insulin, Zinc Crystals (Dosage of insulin may need to be adjusted).
No products indexed under this heading.

Insulin, Zinc Suspension (Dosage of insulin may need to be adjusted). Products include:
Iletin II, Lente (Pork), 100 Units 1945

Insulin Aspart, Human Regular (Dosage of insulin may need to be adjusted).
No products indexed under this heading.

Insulin glargine (Dosage of insulin may need to be adjusted). Products include:
Lantus Injection 742

Insulin Lispro, Human (Dosage of insulin may need to be adjusted). Products include:
Humalog 1926
Humalog Mix 75/25 Pen 1928

Insulin Lispro Protamine, Human (Dosage of insulin may need to be adjusted). Products include:
Humalog Mix 75/25 Pen 1928

Levonorgestrel (Estrogens tend to increase serum thyroxine-binding globulin; patients with non-functioning thyroid may need to adjust thyroid dosage). Products include:
Alesse-21 Tablets 3468
Alesse-28 Tablets 3473
Levlen 962
Levlite 21 Tablets 962
Levlite 28 Tablets 962
Levora Tablets 3389
Mirena Intrauterine System 974
Nordette-28 Tablets 2257
Norplant System 3543
Tri-Levlen 962
Triphasil-21 Tablets 3600
Triphasil-28 Tablets 3605
Trivora Tablets 3439

Mestranol (Estrogens tend to increase serum thyroxine-binding globulin; patients with non-functioning thyroid may need to adjust thyroid dosage). Products include:
Necon 1/50 Tablets 3415
Norinyl 1 + 50 28-Day Tablets 3380
Ortho-Novum 1/50□28 Tablets 2556

Metformin Hydrochloride (Dosage of hypoglycemic agent may need to be adjusted). Products include:
Glucophage Tablets 1080
Glucophage XR Tablets 1080
Glucovance Tablets 1086

Miglitol (Dosage of hypoglycemic agent may need to be adjusted). Products include:
Glyset Tablets 2821

Norethindrone (Estrogens tend to increase serum thyroxine-binding globulin; patients with non-

IMPORTANT NOTE: Always consult each drug listing in the patient's regimen for possible interactions.

functioning thyroid may need to adjust thyroid dosage). Products include:

- Brevicon 28-Day Tablets 3380
- Micronor Tablets 2543
- Modicon 2563
- Necon 3415
- Norinyl 1 +35 28-Day Tablets 3380
- Norinyl 1 + 50 28-Day Tablets 3380
- Nor-QD Tablets 3423
- Ortho-Novum 2563
- Ortho-Novum 1/50▣28 Tablets 2556
- Ovcon 3364
- Tri-Norinyl-28 Tablets 3433

Norethynodrel (Estrogens tend to increase serum thyroxine-binding globulin; patients with non-functioning thyroid may need to adjust thyroid dosage).

No products indexed under this heading.

Norgestimate (Estrogens tend to increase serum thyroxine-binding globulin; patients with non-functioning thyroid may need to adjust thyroid dosage). Products include:

- Ortho-Cyclen/Ortho Tri-Cyclen 2573
- Ortho-Prefest Tablets 2570

Norgestrel (Estrogens tend to increase serum thyroxine-binding globulin; patients with non-functioning thyroid may need to adjust thyroid dosage). Products include:

- Lo/Ovral Tablets 3532
- Lo/Ovral-28 Tablets 3538
- Low-Ogestrel-28 Tablets 3392
- Ogestrel 0.5/50-28 Tablets 3428
- Ovral Tablets 3551
- Ovral-28 Tablets 3552
- Ovrette Tablets 3552

Pioglitazone Hydrochloride (Dosage of hypoglycemic agent may need to be adjusted). Products include:

- Actos Tablets 3275

Polyestradiol Phosphate (Estrogens tend to increase serum thyroxine-binding globulin; patients with non-functioning thyroid may need to adjust thyroid dosage).

No products indexed under this heading.

Quinestrol (Estrogens tend to increase serum thyroxine-binding globulin; patients with non-functioning thyroid may need to adjust thyroid dosage).

No products indexed under this heading.

Repaglinide (Dosage of hypoglycemic agent may need to be adjusted). Products include:

- Prandin Tablets (0.5, 1, and 2 mg) 2432

Rosiglitazone Maleate (Dosage of hypoglycemic agent may need to be adjusted). Products include:

- Avandia Tablets 1490

Tolazamide (Dosage of hypoglycemic agent may need to be adjusted).

No products indexed under this heading.

Tolbutamide (Dosage of hypoglycemic agent may need to be adjusted).

No products indexed under this heading.

Troglitazone (Dosage of hypoglycemic agent may need to be adjusted).

No products indexed under this heading.

Warfarin Sodium (Anticoagulant effects may be potentiated; dosage adjustment should be made). Products include:

- Coumadin for Injection 1243
- Coumadin Tablets 1243
- Warfarin Sodium Tablets, USP 3302

LEVOXYL TABLETS

(Levothyroxine Sodium) 1819

May interact with androgens, antacids containing aluminum, calcium and magnesium, beta blockers, oral anticoagulants, dopamine agonists, estrogens, glucocorticoids, cardiac glycosides, hydantoin anticonvulsants, oral hypoglycemic agents, insulin, lithium preparations, phenytoin, radiographic iodinated contrast media, salicylates, sympathomimetics, thiazides, tricyclic antidepressants, and theophylline. Compounds in these categories include:

Acarbose (Addition of levothyroxine to antidiabetic therapy may result in increased antidiabetic agent requirements). Products include:

- Precose Tablets 906

Acebutolol Hydrochloride (Co-administration with beta-blockers may decrease T_4 5'-deiodinase activity; action of beta-blocker may be impaired when the hypothyroid patient is converted to euthyroid). Products include:

- Sectral Capsules 3589

Albuterol (Co-administration of sympathomimetic agents may increase the effects of sympathomimetics or thyroid hormone; thyroid hormones may increase risk of coronary insufficiency when sympathomimetic agents are administered to patients with coronary disease). Products include:

- Proventil Inhalation Aerosol 3142
- Ventolin Inhalation Aerosol and Refill 1679

Albuterol Sulfate (Co-administration of sympathomimetic agents may increase the effects of sympathomimetics or thyroid hormone; thyroid hormones may increase risk of coronary insufficiency when sympathomimetic agents are administered to patients with coronary disease). Products include:

- AccuNeb Inhalation Solution 1230
- Combivent Inhalation Aerosol 1041
- DuoNeb Inhalation Solution 1233
- Proventil Inhalation Solution 0.083% 3146
- Proventil Repetabs Tablets 3148
- Proventil Solution for Inhalation 0.5% 3144
- Proventil HFA Inhalation Aerosol 3150
- Ventolin HFA Inhalation Aerosol 3618
- Volmax Extended-Release Tablets .. 2276

Aldesleukin (Co-administration has been associated with transient painless thyroiditis in 20% of patients). Products include:

- Proleukin for Injection 1199

Aluminum Carbonate (Co-administration with antacids may reduce the efficacy of levothyroxine by binding and delaying or preventing absorption, potentially resulting in hypothyroidism; administer levothyroxine at least 4 hours apart from these agents).

No products indexed under this heading.

Aluminum Hydroxide (Co-administration with antacids may reduce the efficacy of levothyroxine by binding and delaying or preventing absorption, potentially resulting in hypothyroidism; administer levothyroxine at least 4 hours apart from these agents). Products include:

- Amphojel Suspension (Mint Flavor) .... ▣789
- Gaviscon Extra Strength Liquid ..... ▣751
- Gaviscon Extra Strength Tablets ... ▣751
- Gaviscon Regular Strength Liquid . ▣751
- Gaviscon Regular Strength Tablets .... ▣750
- Maalox Antacid/Anti-Gas Oral Suspension .... ▣673
- Maalox Max Maximum Strength Antacid/Anti-Gas Liquid 2300
- Maalox Regular Strength Antacid/Antigas Liquid 2300
- Mylanta 1813
- Vanquish Caplets .... ▣617

Aminoglutethimide (May decrease thyroid hormone secretion, which may result in hypothyrodism).

No products indexed under this heading.

Aminophylline (Decreased theophylline clearance may occur in hypothyroid patients; clearance returns to normal when euthyroid state is achieved).

No products indexed under this heading.

p-Aminosalicylic Acid (Co-administration has been associated with thyroid hormone and/or TSH level alterations by various mechanisms).

No products indexed under this heading.

Amiodarone Hydrochloride (May decrease thyroid hormone secretion, which may result in hypothyrodism; amiodarone is slowly excreted, producing more prolonged hypothyroidism; amiodarone may induce hyperthyroidism by causing thyroiditis). Products include:

- Cordarone Intravenous 3491
- Cordarone Tablets 3487
- Pacerone Tablets 3331

Amitriptyline Hydrochloride (Co-administration may increase the therapeutic and toxic effects of both drugs possibly due to increased receptor sensitivity to catecholamines; toxic effects may include increased risk of arrhythmias and CNS stimulation; onset of tricyclics may be accelerated). Products include:

- Etrafon 3115
- Limbitrol 1738

Amoxapine (Co-administration may increase the therapeutic and toxic effects of both drugs possibly due to increased receptor sensitivity to catecholamines; toxic effects may include increased risk of arrhythmias and CNS stimulation; onset of tricyclics may be accelerated).

No products indexed under this heading.

Asparaginase (Co-administration may result in decreased serum TBG concentration). Products include:

- Elspar for Injection 2092

Aspirin (Co-administration with salicylates at greater than 2 gm inhibit binding of T_4 and T_3 to TBG and transthyrelin; an initial increase in serum FT_4 is followed by return of FT_4 to normal levels with sustained therapeutic salicylate concentrations, although total T_4 levels may decrease by as much as 30%). Products include:

- Aggrenox Capsules 1026
- Alka-Seltzer .... ▣603
- Alka-Seltzer Lemon Lime Antacid and Pain Reliever Effervescent Tablets .... ▣603
- Alka-Seltzer Extra Strength Antacid and Pain Reliever Effervescent Tablets .... ▣603
- Alka-Seltzer PM Effervescent Tablets .... ▣605
- Genuine Bayer Tablets, Caplets and Gelcaps .... ▣606
- Extra Strength Bayer Caplets and Gelcaps .... ▣610
- Aspirin Regimen Bayer Children's Chewable Tablets (Orange or Cherry Flavored) .... ▣607
- Bayer, Aspirin Regimen .... ▣606
- Aspirin Regimen Bayer 81 mg Caplets with Calcium .... ▣607
- Genuine Bayer Professional Labeling (Aspirin Regimen Bayer) .... ▣608
- Extra Strength Bayer Arthritis Caplets .... ▣610
- Extra Strength Bayer Plus Caplets .... ▣610
- Extra Strength Bayer PM Caplets .. ▣611
- BC Powder .... ▣619
- BC Allergy Sinus Cold Powder ...... ▣619
- Arthritis Strength BC Powder .... ▣619
- BC Sinus Cold Powder .... ▣619
- Darvon Compound-65 Pulvules 1910
- Ecotrin Enteric Coated Aspirin Low, Regular and Maximum Strength Tablets 1715
- Excedrin Extra-Strength Tablets, Caplets, and Geltabs .... ▣629
- Excedrin Migraine 1070
- Goody's Body Pain Formula Powder .... ▣620
- Goody's Extra Strength Headache Powder .... ▣620
- Goody's Extra Strength Pain Relief Tablets .... ▣620
- Percodan Tablets 1327
- Robaxisal Tablets 2939
- Soma Compound Tablets 3354
- Soma Compound w/Codeine Tablets 3355
- Vanquish Caplets .... ▣617

Atenolol (Co-administration with beta-blockers may decrease T_4 5'-deiodinase activity; action of beta-blocker may be impaired when the hypothyroid patient is converted to euthyroid). Products include:

- Tenoretic Tablets 690
- Tenormin I.V. Injection 692

Bendroflumethiazide (Co-administration has been associated with thyroid hormone and/or TSH level alterations by various mechanisms). Products include:

- Corzide 40/5 Tablets 2247
- Corzide 80/5 Tablets 2247

Betamethasone Acetate (Co-administration with glucocorticoids may result in a transient reduction in TSH secretion; the reduction is not sustained, therefore, hypothyroidism does not occur; glucocorticoids may decrease serum TBG concentration). Products include:

- Celestone Soluspan Injectable Suspension 3097

Betamethasone Sodium Phosphate (Co-administration with glucocorticoids may result in a transient reduction in TSH secretion; the reduction is not sustained, therefore, hypothyroidism does not occur; glucocorticoids may decrease serum TBG concentration). Products include:

- Celestone Soluspan Injectable Suspension 3097

Betaxolol Hydrochloride (Co-administration with beta-blockers may decrease T_4 5'-deiodinase activity; action of beta-blocker may be impaired when the hypothyroid patient is converted to euthyroid). Products include:

- Betoptic S Ophthalmic Suspension 537

Bisoprolol Fumarate (Co-administration with beta-blockers may decrease T_4 5'-deiodinase activity; action of beta-blocker may be impaired when the hypothyroid patient is converted to euthyroid). Products include:

- Zebeta Tablets 1885
- Ziac Tablets 1887

Bromocriptine Mesylate (Co-administration with dopamine agonists may result in a transient reduction in TSH secretion; the reduction is not sustained, therefore, hypothyroidism does not occur).

No products indexed under this heading.

Calcium Carbonate (Co-administration with calcium carbonate may form insoluble chelate with levothyroxine, which may result in hypothyroidism; administer levothyroxine at least 4 hours apart from these agents). Products include:

- Aspirin Regimen Bayer 81 mg Caplets with Calcium .... ▣607
- Extra Strength Bayer Plus Caplets .... ▣610
- Caltrate 600 Tablets .... ▣814
- Caltrate 600 PLUS .... ▣815
- Caltrate 600 + D Tablets .... ▣814
- Caltrate 600 + Soy Tablets .... ▣814
- D-Cal Chewable Caplets .... ▣794
- Florical Capsules and Tablets 2223

Quick Dissolve Maalox Max Maximum Strength Antacid/Antigas Tablets 2301
Quick Dissolve Maalox Regular Strength Antacid Tablets 2301
Marblen Suspension .... ■633
Monocal Tablets 2223
Mylanta Fast-Acting 1813
Mylanta Calci Tabs .... ■636
One-A-Day Bedtime & Rest Tablets .... ■805
One-A-Day Calcium Plus Chewable Tablets .... ■805
Os-Cal Chewable Tablets .... ■838
Pepcid Complete Chewable Tablets 1815
ReSource Wellness CalciWise Soft Chews .... ■824
Rolaids Tablets .... ■706
Extra Strength Rolaids Tablets .... ■706
Slow-Mag Tablets .... ■835
Titralac .... ■640
3M Titralac Plus Antacid Tablets .... ■640
Tums .... ■763

Carbamazepine (Co-administration may increase hepatic metabolism, which may result in hypothyroidism, resulting in increased levothyroxine requirements; carbamazepine reduces serum protein binding of levothyroxine, and total- and free-T_4 may be reduced by 20% to 40%, but most patients have normal serum TSH levels and are clinically euthyroid). Products include:
Carbatrol Capsules 3234
Tegretol/Tegretol-XR 2404

Carteolol Hydrochloride (Co-administration with beta-blockers may decrease T_4 5'-deiodinase activity; action of beta-blocker may be impaired when the hypothyroid patient is converted to euthyroid). Products include:
Carteolol Hydrochloride Ophthalmic Solution USP, 1% .... ⊙258
Ocupress Ophthalmic Solution, 1% Sterile .... ⊙303

Chloral Hydrate (Co-administration has been associated with thyroid hormone and/or TSH level alterations by various mechanisms).
No products indexed under this heading.

Chlorothiazide (Co-administration has been associated with thyroid hormone and/or TSH level alterations by various mechanisms). Products include:
Aldoclor Tablets 2035
Diuril Oral 2087

Chlorothiazide Sodium (Co-administration has been associated with thyroid hormone and/or TSH level alterations by various mechanisms). Products include:
Diuril Sodium Intravenous 2086

Chlorotrianisene (Co-administration with oral estrogens may result in increased serum TBG concentrations).
No products indexed under this heading.

Chlorpropamide (Addition of levothyroxine to antidiabetic therapy may result in increased antidiabetic agent requirements). Products include:
Diabinese Tablets 2680

Cholestyramine (Co-administration may result in decreased T_4 absorption, which may result in hypothyroidism; administer levothyroxine at least 4 hours apart from these agents).
No products indexed under this heading.

Choline Magnesium Trisalicylate (Co-administration with salicylates at greater than 2 gm inhibit binding of T_4 and T_3 to TBG and transthyrelin; an initial increase in serum FT_4 is followed by return of FT_4 to normal levels with sustained therapeutic salicylate concentrations, although total T_4 levels may decrease by as much as 30%). Products include:
Trilisate 2901

Clofibrate (Co-administration may result in increased serum TBG concentrations). Products include:
Atromid-S Capsules 3483

Clomipramine Hydrochloride (Co-administration may increase the therapeutic and toxic effects of both drugs possibly due to increased receptor sensitivity to catecholamines; toxic effects may include increased risk of arrhythmias and CNS stimulation; onset of tricyclics may be accelerated).
No products indexed under this heading.

Colestipol Hydrochloride (Co-administration may result in decreased T_4 absorption, which may result in hypothyroidism; administer levothyroxine at least 4 hours apart from these agents). Products include:
Colestid Tablets 2791

Cortisone Acetate (Co-administration with glucocorticoids may result in a transient reduction in TSH secretion; the reduction is not sustained, therefore, hypothyroidism does not occur; glucocorticoids may decrease serum TBG concentration). Products include:
Cortone Acetate Injectable Suspension 2059
Cortone Acetate Tablets 2061

Desipramine Hydrochloride (Co-administration may increase the therapeutic and toxic effects of both drugs possibly due to increased receptor sensitivity to catecholamines; toxic effects may include increased risk of arrhythmias and CNS stimulation; onset of tricyclics may be accelerated). Products include:
Norpramin Tablets 755

Deslanoside (Co-administration may result in reduced serum digitalis glycosides in hyperthyroidism or when the hypothyroid patient is converted to euthyroid state; therapeutic effect of digitalis glycoside may be reduced).
No products indexed under this heading.

Dexamethasone (Co-administration with glucocorticoids may result in a transient reduction in TSH secretion; the reduction is not sustained, therefore, hypothyroidism does not occur; glucocorticoids may decrease serum TBG concentration). Products include:
Decadron Elixir 2078
Decadron Tablets 2079
TobraDex Ophthalmic Ointment 542
TobraDex Ophthalmic Suspension .. 541

Dexamethasone Acetate (Co-administration with glucocorticoids may result in a transient reduction in TSH secretion; the reduction is not sustained, therefore, hypothyroidism does not occur; glucocorticoids may decrease serum TBG concentration).
No products indexed under this heading.

Dexamethasone Sodium Phosphate (Co-administration with glucocorticoids may result in a transient reduction in TSH secretion; the reduction is not sustained, therefore, hypothyroidism does not occur; glucocorticoids may decrease serum TBG concentration). Products include:
Decadron Phosphate Injection 2081
Decadron Phosphate Sterile Ophthalmic Ointment 2083
Decadron Phosphate Sterile Ophthalmic Solution 2084
NeoDecadron Sterile Ophthalmic Solution 2144

Diatrizoate Meglumine (May decrease thyroid hormone secretion, which may result in hypothyroidism; the fetus, elderly, and euthyroid patients with underlying thyroid disease are among those individuals who are susceptible to iodine-induced hypothyroidism; oral cholecytographic agents slowly excreted, producing more prolonged hypothyroidism; iodide drugs that contain pharmacologic amounts of iodide may cause hypothyroidism in euthyroid patients with Grave's disease previously treated with thyroid autonomy; hyperthyroidism may develop over several weeks and may persist for several months after therapy discontinuation).
No products indexed under this heading.

Diatrizoate Sodium (May decrease thyroid hormone secretion, which may result in hypothyroidism; the fetus, elderly, and euthyroid patients with underlying thyroid disease are among those individuals who are susceptible to iodine-induced hypothyroidism; oral cholecytographic agents slowly excreted, producing more prolonged hypothyroidism; iodide drugs that contain pharmacologic amounts of iodide may cause hypothyroidism in euthyroid patients with Grave's disease previously treated with thyroid autonomy; hyperthyroidism may develop over several weeks and may persist for several months after therapy discontinuation).
No products indexed under this heading.

Diazepam (Co-administration has been associated with thyroid hormone and/or TSH level alterations by various mechanisms). Products include:
Valium Injectable 3026
Valium Tablets 3047

Dicumarol (Thyroid hormones appear to increase the catabolism of vitamin K-dependent clotting factors, thereby increasing the anticoagulant activity of oral anticoagulants).
No products indexed under this heading.

Dienestrol (Co-administration with oral estrogens may result in increased serum TBG concentrations). Products include:
Ortho Dienestrol Cream 2554

Diethylstilbestrol (Co-administration with oral estrogens may result in increased serum TBG concentrations).
No products indexed under this heading.

Diflunisal (Co-administration with salicylates at greater than 2 gm inhibit binding of T_4 and T_3 to TBG and transthyrelin; an initial increase in serum FT_4 is followed by return of FT_4 to normal levels with sustained therapeutic salicylate concentrations, although total T_4 levels may decrease by as much as 30%). Products include:
Dolobid Tablets 2088

Digitoxin (Co-administration may result in reduced serum digitalis glycosides in hyperthyroidism or when the hypothyroid patient is converted to euthyroid state; therapeutic effect of digitalis glycoside may be reduced).
No products indexed under this heading.

Digoxin (Co-administration may result in reduced serum digitalis glycosides in hyperthyroidism or when the hypothyroid patient is converted to euthyroid state; therapeutic effect of digitalis glycoside may be reduced). Products include:
Digitek Tablets 1003
Lanoxicaps Capsules 1574
Lanoxin Injection 1581
Lanoxin Tablets 1587
Lanoxin Elixir Pediatric 1578
Lanoxin Injection Pediatric 1584

Dobutamine Hydrochloride (Co-administration of sympathomimetic agents may increase the effects of sympathomimetics or thyroid hormone; thyroid hormones may increase risk of coronary insufficiency when sympathomimetic agents are administered to patients with coronary disease). Products include:
Dobutrex Solution Vials 1914

Dopamine Hydrochloride (Co-administration with dopamine may result in a transient reduction in TSH secretion; the reduction is not sustained, therefore, hypothyroidism does not occur).
No products indexed under this heading.

Doxepin Hydrochloride (Co-administration may increase the therapeutic and toxic effects of both drugs possibly due to increased receptor sensitivity to catecholamines; toxic effects may include increased risk of arrhythmias and CNS stimulation; onset of tricyclics may be accelerated). Products include:
Sinequan 2713

Dyphylline (Decreased theophylline clearance may occur in hypothyroid patients; clearance returns to normal when euthyroid state is achieved). Products include:
Lufyllin Tablets 3347
Lufyllin-400 Tablets 3347
Lufyllin-GG Elixir 3348
Lufyllin-GG Tablets 3348

Ephedrine Hydrochloride (Co-administration of sympathomimetic agents may increase the effects of sympathomimetics or thyroid hormone; thyroid hormones may increase risk of coronary insufficiency when sympathomimetic agents are administered to patients with coronary disease). Products include:
Primatene Tablets .... ■780

Ephedrine Sulfate (Co-administration of sympathomimetic agents may increase the effects of sympathomimetics or thyroid hormone; thyroid hormones may increase risk of coronary insufficiency when sympathomimetic agents are administered to patients with coronary disease).
No products indexed under this heading.

Ephedrine Tannate (Co-administration of sympathomimetic agents may increase the effects of sympathomimetics or thyroid hormone; thyroid hormones may increase risk of coronary insufficiency when sympathomimetic agents are administered to patients with coronary disease). Products include:
Rynatuss Pediatric Suspension 3353
Rynatuss Tablets 3353

Epinephrine (Co-administration of sympathomimetic agents may increase the effects of sympathomimetics or thyroid hormone; thyroid hormones may increase risk of coronary insufficiency when sympathomimetic agents are administered to patients with coronary disease). Products include:
Epifrin Sterile Ophthalmic Solution .... ⊙235
EpiPen 1236
Primatene Mist .... ■779
Xylocaine with Epinephrine Injection 653

Epinephrine Bitartrate (Co-administration of sympathomimetic agents may increase the effects of sympathomimetics or thyroid hormone; thyroid hormones may increase risk of coronary insufficiency when sympathomimetic agents are administered to patients with coronary disease). Products include:
Sensorcaine 643

Epinephrine Hydrochloride (Co-administration of sympathomimetic agents may increase the effects of sympathomimetics or thyroid hormone; thyroid hormones may increase risk of coronary insufficiency when sympathomimetic agents are administered to patients with coronary disease).
No products indexed under this heading.

Esmolol Hydrochloride (Co-administration with beta-blockers may decrease T_4 5'-deiodinase activity; action of beta-blocker may be impaired when the hypothyroid patient is converted to euthyroid). Products include:
Brevibloc Injection 858

Estradiol (Co-administration with oral estrogens may result in increased serum TBG concentrations). Products include:
Activella Tablets 2764
Alora Transdermal System 3372
Climara Transdermal System 958
CombiPatch Transdermal System .. 2323
Esclim Transdermal System 3460
Estrace Vaginal Cream 3358
Estrace Tablets 3361
Estring Vaginal Ring 2811
Ortho-Prefest Tablets 2570
Vagifem Tablets 2857
Vivelle Transdermal System 2412
Vivelle-Dot Transdermal System 2416

Estrogens, Conjugated (Co-administration with oral estrogens may result in increased serum TBG concentrations). Products include:
Premarin Intravenous 3563
Premarin Tablets 3566
Premarin Vaginal Cream 3570
Premphase Tablets 3572
Prempro Tablets 3572

Estrogens, Esterified (Co-administration with oral estrogens may result in increased serum TBG concentrations). Products include:
Estratest 3252
Menest Tablets 2254

Estropipate (Co-administration with oral estrogens may result in increased serum TBG concentrations). Products include:
Ogen Tablets 2846
Ortho-Est Tablets 3464

Ethinyl Estradiol (Co-administration with estrogen containing oral contraceptives may result in increased serum TBG concentrations). Products include:
Alesse-21 Tablets 3468
Alesse-28 Tablets 3473
Brevicon 28-Day Tablets 3380
Cyclessa Tablets 2450
Desogen Tablets 2458
Estinyl Tablets 3112
Estrostep 2627
femhrt Tablets 2635
Levlen 962
Levlite 21 Tablets 962
Levlite 28 Tablets 962
Levora Tablets 3389
Loestrin 21 Tablets 2642
Loestrin Fe Tablets 2642
Lo/Ovral Tablets 3532
Lo/Ovral-28 Tablets 3538
Low-Ogestrel-28 Tablets 3392
Microgestin Fe 1.5/30 Tablets 3407
Microgestin Fe 1/20 Tablets 3400
Mircette Tablets 2470
Modicon 2563
Necon 3415
Nordette-28 Tablets 2257
Norinyl 1 +35 28-Day Tablets 3380
Ogestrel 0.5/50-28 Tablets 3428
Ortho-Cept 21 Tablets 2546
Ortho-Cept 28 Tablets 2546
Ortho-Cyclen/Ortho Tri-Cyclen 2573
Ortho-Novum 2563
Ovcon 3364
Ovral Tablets 3551
Ovral-28 Tablets 3552
Tri-Levlen 962
Tri-Norinyl-28 Tablets 3433
Triphasil-21 Tablets 3600
Triphasil-28 Tablets 3605
Trivora Tablets 3439
Yasmin 28 Tablets 980
Zovia 3449

Ethiodized Oil (May decrease thyroid hormone secretion, which may result in hypothyrodism; the fetus, elderly, and euthyroid patients with underlying thyroid disease are among those individuals who are susceptible to iodine-induced hypothyroidism; oral cholecytographic agents slowly excreted, producing more prolonged hypothyroidism; iodide drugs that contain pharmacologic amounts of iodide may cause hypothyroidism in euthyroid patients with Grave's disease previously treated with thyroid autonomy; hyperthyroidism may develop over several weeks and may persist for several months after therapy discontinuation). Products include:
Ethiodol Injection 3095

Ethionamide (Co-administration has been associated with thyroid hormone and/or TSH level alterations by various mechanisms). Products include:
Trecator-SC Tablets 3598

Ethotoin (Hydantoins may cause protein-binding site displacement; co-administration results in an initial transient increase in FT_4; continued administration results in a decrease in serum T_4 and normal FT_4 and TSH concentrations and, therefore, patients are clinically euthyroid).
No products indexed under this heading.

Ferrous Sulfate (Co-administration may result in decreased T_4 absorption, which may result in hypothyroidism; ferrous sulfate may form a ferric-thyroxine complex; administer levothyroxine at least 4 hours apart from these agents). Products include:
Feosol Tablets 1717
Slow Fe Tablets .... ▣827
Slow Fe with Folic Acid Tablets ..... ▣828

Fiber Supplement (Concurrent use of dietary fiber may bind and decrease the absorption of levothyroxine sodium from GI tract).
No products indexed under this heading.

Fludrocortisone Acetate (Co-administration with glucocorticoids may result in a transient reduction in TSH secretion; the reduction is not sustained, therefore, hypothyroidism does not occur; glucocorticoids may decrease serum TBG concentration). Products include:
Florinef Acetate Tablets 2250

Fluorouracil (Co-administration with 5-FU may result in increased serum TBG concentrations). Products include:
Carac Cream 1222
Efudex 1733
Fluoroplex 552

Fluoxymesterone (Co-administration with androgens/anabolic steroids may result in decreased serum TBG concentration).
No products indexed under this heading.

Fosphenytoin Sodium (Hydantoins may cause protein-binding site displacement; co-administration results in an initial transient increase in FT_4; co-administration may increase hepatic metabolism, which may result in hypothyroidism, resulting in increased levothyroxine requirements; phenytoin reduces serum protein binding of levothyroxine, and total- and free-T_4 may be reduced by 20% to 40%, but most patients have normal serum TSH levels and are clinically euthyroid). Products include:
Cerebyx Injection 2619

Furosemide (May cause protein-binding site displacement at greater than 80 mg IV; co-administration results in an initial transient increase in FT_4; continued administration results in a decrease in serum T_4 and normal FT_4 and TSH concentrations and, therefore, patients are clinically euthyroid). Products include:
Furosemide Tablets 2284

Gadopentetate Dimeglumine (May decrease thyroid hormone secretion, which may result in hypothyrodism; the fetus, elderly, and euthyroid patients with underlying thyroid disease are among those individuals who are susceptible to iodine-induced hypothyroidism; oral cholecytographic agents slowly excreted, producing more prolonged hypothyroidism; iodide drugs that contain pharmacologic amounts of iodide may cause hypothyroidism in euthyroid patients with Grave's disease previously treated with thyroid autonomy; hyperthyroidism may develop over several weeks and may persist for several months after therapy discontinuation).
No products indexed under this heading.

Glimepiride (Addition of levothyroxine to antidiabetic therapy may result in increased antidiabetic agent requirements). Products include:
Amaryl Tablets 717

Glipizide (Addition of levothyroxine to antidiabetic therapy may result in increased antidiabetic agent requirements). Products include:
Glucotrol Tablets 2692
Glucotrol XL Extended Release Tablets 2693

Glyburide (Addition of levothyroxine to antidiabetic therapy may result in increased antidiabetic agent requirements). Products include:
DiaBeta Tablets 741
Glucovance Tablets 1086

Heparin Sodium (May cause protein-binding site displacement; co-administration results in an initial transient increase in FT_4; continued administration results in a decrease in serum T_4 and normal FT_4 and TSH concentrations and, therefore, patients are clinically euthyroid). Products include:
Heparin Lock Flush Solution 3509
Heparin Sodium Injection 3511

Heroin (Co-administration may result in increased serum TBG concentrations).
No products indexed under this heading.

Hydrochlorothiazide (Co-administration has been associated with thyroid hormone and/or TSH level alterations by various mechanisms). Products include:
Accuretic Tablets 2614
Aldoril Tablets 2039
Atacand HCT Tablets 597
Avalide Tablets 1070
Diovan HCT Tablets 2338
Dyazide Capsules 1515
HydroDIURIL Tablets 2108
Hyzaar 2109
Inderide Tablets 3517
Inderide LA Long-Acting Capsules .. 3519
Lotensin HCT Tablets 2367
Maxzide 1008
Micardis HCT Tablets 1051
Microzide Capsules 3414
Moduretic Tablets 2138
Monopril HCT 1094
Prinzide Tablets 2168
Timolide Tablets 2187
Uniretic Tablets 3178
Vaseretic Tablets 2204
Zestoretic Tablets 695
Ziac Tablets 1887

Hydrocortisone (Co-administration with glucocorticoids may result in a transient reduction in TSH secretion; the reduction is not sustained, therefore, hypothyroidism does not occur; glucocorticoids may decrease serum TBG concentration). Products include:
Anusol-HC Cream 2.5% 2237
Cipro HC Otic Suspension 540
Cortaid Intensive Therapy Cream .. ▣717
Cortaid Maximum Strength Cream .... ▣717
Cortisporin Ophthalmic Suspension Sterile .... ⊙297
Cortizone•5 .... ▣699
Cortizone•10 .... ▣699
Cortizone•10 Plus Creme .... ▣700
Cortizone for Kids Creme .... ▣699
Hydrocortone Tablets 2106
Massengill Medicated Soft Cloth Towelette .... ▣753
VōSoL HC Otic Solution 3356

Hydrocortisone Acetate (Co-administration with glucocorticoids may result in a transient reduction in TSH secretion; the reduction is not sustained, therefore, hypothyroidism does not occur; glucocorticoids may decrease serum TBG concentration). Products include:
Analpram-HC 1338
Anusol HC-1 Hydrocortisone Anti-Itch Cream .... ▣689
Anusol-HC Suppositories 2238
Cortaid .... ▣717
Cortifoam Rectal Foam 3170
Cortisporin-TC Otic Suspension 2246
Hydrocortone Acetate Injectable Suspension 2103
Pramosone 1343
Proctocort Suppositories 2264
ProctoFoam-HC 3177
Terra-Cortril Ophthalmic Suspension 2716

Hydrocortisone Sodium Phosphate (Co-administration with glucocorticoids may result in a transient reduction in TSH secretion; the reduction is not sustained, therefore, hypothyroidism does not occur; glucocorticoids may decrease serum TBG concentration). Products include:
Hydrocortone Phosphate Injection, Sterile 2105

Hydrocortisone Sodium Succinate (Co-administration with glucocorticoids may result in a transient reduction in TSH secretion; the reduction is not sustained, therefore, hypothyroidism does not occur; glucocorticoids may decrease serum TBG concentration).
No products indexed under this heading.

Hydroflumethiazide (Co-administration has been associated with thyroid hormone and/or TSH level alterations by various mechanisms). Products include:
Diucardin Tablets 3494

Imipramine Hydrochloride (Co-administration may increase the therapeutic and toxic effects of both drugs possibly due to increased receptor sensitivity to catecholamines; toxic effects may include increased risk of arrhythmias and CNS stimulation; onset of tricyclics may be accelerated).
No products indexed under this heading.

Imipramine Pamoate (Co-administration may increase the therapeutic and toxic effects of both drugs possibly due to increased receptor sensitivity to catecholamines; toxic effects may include increased risk of arrhythmias and CNS stimulation; onset of tricyclics may be accelerated).
No products indexed under this heading.

Infant Formula (Concurrent use of soybean flour may bind and decrease the absorption of levothyroxine sodium from GI tract).

Insulin, Human, Zinc Suspension (Addition of levothyroxine to insulin therapy may result in increased insulin requirements). Products include:

Humulin L, 100 Units 1937
Humulin U, 100 Units 1943
Novolin L Human Insulin 10 ml Vials..................................... 2422

Insulin, Human NPH (Addition of levothyroxine to insulin therapy may result in increased insulin requirements). Products include:
Humulin N, 100 Units 1939
Humulin N NPH Pen 1940
Novolin N Human Insulin 10 ml Vials..................................... 2422
Novolin N PenFill 2423
Novolin N Prefilled Syringe Disposable Insulin Delivery System 2425

Insulin, Human Regular (Addition of levothyroxine to insulin therapy may result in increased insulin requirements). Products include:
Humulin R Regular (U-500) 1943
Humulin R, 100 Units 1941
Novolin R Human Insulin 10 ml Vials..................................... 2423
Novolin R PenFill 2423
Novolin R Prefilled Syringe Disposable Insulin Delivery System 2425
Velosulin BR Human Insulin 10 ml Vials..................................... 2435

Insulin, Human Regular and Human NPH Mixture (Addition of levothyroxine to insulin therapy may result in increased insulin requirements). Products include:
Humulin 50/50, 100 Units 1934
Humulin 70/30, 100 Units 1935
Humulin 70/30 Pen 1936
Novolin 70/30 Human Insulin 10 ml Vials 2421
Novolin 70/30 PenFill 2423
Novolin 70/30 Prefilled Disposable Insulin Delivery System 2425

Insulin, NPH (Addition of levothyroxine to insulin therapy may result in increased insulin requirements). Products include:
Iletin II, NPH (Pork), 100 Units 1946

Insulin, Regular (Addition of levothyroxine to insulin therapy may result in increased insulin requirements). Products include:
Iletin II, Regular (Pork), 100 Units ... 1947

Insulin, Zinc Crystals (Addition of levothyroxine to insulin therapy may result in increased insulin requirements).
No products indexed under this heading.

Insulin, Zinc Suspension (Addition of levothyroxine to insulin therapy may result in increased insulin requirements). Products include:
Iletin II, Lente (Pork), 100 Units 1945

Insulin Aspart, Human Regular (Addition of levothyroxine to insulin therapy may result in increased insulin requirements).
No products indexed under this heading.

Insulin glargine (Addition of levothyroxine to insulin therapy may result in increased insulin requirements). Products include:
Lantus Injection 742

Insulin Lispro, Human (Addition of levothyroxine to insulin therapy may result in increased insulin requirements). Products include:
Humalog 1926
Humalog Mix 75/25 Pen 1928

Insulin Lispro Protamine, Human (Addition of levothyroxine to insulin therapy may result in increased insulin requirements). Products include:
Humalog Mix 75/25 Pen 1928

Interferon alfa-2A, Recombinant (Co-administration with interferon alpha has been associated with the development of antithyroid microsomal antibodies in 20% of patients and some have transient hypothyroidism, hyperthyroidism, or both; patients who have antithyroid antibodies before treatment are at higher risk for thyroid dysfunction). Products include:
Roferon-A Injection 2996

Interferon alfa-2B, Recombinant (Co-administration with interferon alpha has been associated with the development of antithyroid microsomal antibodies in 20% of patients and some have transient hypothyroidism, hyperthyroidism, or both; patients who have antithyroid antibodies before treatment are at higher risk for thyroid dysfunction). Products include:
Intron A for Injection 3120
Rebetron Combination Therapy 3153

Interferon alfa-N3 (Human Leukocyte Derived) (Co-administration with interferon alpha has been associated with the development of antithyroid microsomal antibodies in 20% of patients and some have transient hypothyroidism, hyperthyroidism, or both; patients who have antithyroid antibodies before treatment are at higher risk for thyroid dysfunction). Products include:
Alferon N Injection 1770

Iodamide Meglumine (May decrease thyroid hormone secretion, which may result in hypothyrodism; the fetus, elderly, and euthyroid patients with underlying thyroid disease are among those individuals who are susceptible to iodine-induced hypothyroidism; oral cholecytographic agents slowly excreted, producing more prolonged hypothyroidism; iodide drugs that contain pharmacologic amounts of iodide may cause hypothyroidism in euthyroid patients with Grave's disease previously treated with thyroid autonomy; hyperthyroidism may develop over several weeks and may persist for several months after therapy discontinuation).
No products indexed under this heading.

Iohexol (May decrease thyroid hormone secretion, which may result in hypothyrodism; the fetus, elderly, and euthyroid patients with underlying thyroid disease are among those individuals who are susceptible to iodine-induced hypothyroidism; oral cholecytographic agents slowly excreted, producing more prolonged hypothyroidism; iodide drugs that contain pharmacologic amounts of iodide may cause hypothyroidism in euthyroid patients with Grave's disease previously treated with thyroid autonomy; hyperthyroidism may develop over several weeks and may persist for several months after therapy discontinuation).
No products indexed under this heading.

Iopamidol (May decrease thyroid hormone secretion, which may result in hypothyrodism; the fetus, elderly, and euthyroid patients with underlying thyroid disease are among those individuals who are susceptible to iodine-induced hypothyroidism; oral cholecytographic agents slowly excreted, producing more prolonged hypothyroidism; iodide drugs that contain pharmacologic amounts of iodide may cause hypothyroidism in euthyroid patients with Grave's disease previously treated with thyroid autonomy; hyperthyroidism may develop over several weeks and may persist for several months after therapy discontinuation).
No products indexed under this heading.

Iopanoic Acid (May decrease thyroid hormone secretion, which may result in hypothyrodism; the fetus, elderly, and euthyroid patients with underlying thyroid disease are among those individuals who are susceptible to iodine-induced hypothyroidism; oral cholecytographic agents slowly excreted, producing more prolonged hypothyroidism; iodide drugs that contain pharmacologic amounts of iodide may cause hypothyroidism in euthyroid patients with Grave's disease previously treated with thyroid autonomy; hyperthyroidism may develop over several weeks and may persist for several months after therapy discontinuation).
No products indexed under this heading.

Iothalamate Meglumine (May decrease thyroid hormone secretion, which may result in hypothyrodism; the fetus, elderly, and euthyroid patients with underlying thyroid disease are among those individuals who are susceptible to iodine-induced hypothyroidism; oral cholecytographic agents slowly excreted, producing more prolonged hypothyroidism; iodide drugs that contain pharmacologic amounts of iodide may cause hypothyroidism in euthyroid patients with Grave's disease previously treated with thyroid autonomy; hyperthyroidism may develop over several weeks and may persist for several months after therapy discontinuation).
No products indexed under this heading.

Ioxaglate Meglumine (May decrease thyroid hormone secretion, which may result in hypothyrodism; the fetus, elderly, and euthyroid patients with underlying thyroid disease are among those individuals who are susceptible to iodine-induced hypothyroidism; oral cholecytographic agents slowly excreted, producing more prolonged hypothyroidism; iodide drugs that contain pharmacologic amounts of iodide may cause hypothyroidism in euthyroid patients with Grave's disease previously treated with thyroid autonomy; hyperthyroidism may develop over several weeks and may persist for several months after therapy discontinuation).
No products indexed under this heading.

Ioxaglate Sodium (May decrease thyroid hormone secretion, which may result in hypothyrodism; the fetus, elderly, and euthyroid patients with underlying thyroid disease are among those individuals who are susceptible to iodine-induced hypothyroidism; oral cholecytographic agents slowly excreted, producing more prolonged hypothyroidism; iodide drugs that contain pharmacologic amounts of iodide may cause hypothyroidism in euthyroid patients with Grave's disease previously treated with thyroid autonomy; hyperthyroidism may develop over several weeks and may persist for several months after therapy discontinuation).
No products indexed under this heading.

Isoproterenol Hydrochloride (Co-administration of sympathomimetic agents may increase the effects of sympathomimetics or thyroid hormone; thyroid hormones may increase risk of coronary insufficiency when sympathomimetic agents are administered to patients with coronary disease).
No products indexed under this heading.

Isoproterenol Sulfate (Co-administration of sympathomimetic agents may increase the effects of sympathomimetics or thyroid hormone; thyroid hormones may increase risk of coronary insufficiency when sympathomimetic agents are administered to patients with coronary disease).
No products indexed under this heading.

Ketamine Hydrochloride (Co-administration may produce marked hypertension and tachycardia).
No products indexed under this heading.

Labetalol Hydrochloride (Co-administration with beta-blockers may decrease T_4 5'-deiodinase activity; action of beta-blocker may be impaired when the hypothyroid patient is converted to euthyroid). Products include:
Normodyne Injection 3135
Normodyne Tablets 3137

Levalbuterol Hydrochloride (Co-administration of sympathomimetic agents may increase the effects of sympathomimetics or thyroid hormone; thyroid hormones may increase risk of coronary insufficiency when sympathomimetic agents are administered to patients with coronary disease). Products include:
Xopenex Inhalation Solution 3207

Levobunolol Hydrochloride (Co-administration with beta-blockers may decrease T_4 5'-deiodinase activity; action of beta-blocker may be impaired when the hypothyroid patient is converted to euthyroid). Products include:
Betagan .... ⊙ 228

Lithium Carbonate (May decrease thyroid hormone secretion, which may result in hypothyrodism; long-term lithium therapy can result in goiter in up to 50% of patients, and either subclinical or overt hypothyroidism, each in up to 20% of patients). Products include:
Eskalith 1527
Lithium Carbonate 3061
Lithobid Slow-Release Tablets 3255

Lithium Citrate (May decrease thyroid hormone secretion, which may result in hypothyrodism; long-term lithium therapy can result in goiter in up to 50% of patients, and either subclinical or overt hypothyroidism, each in up to 20% of patients). Products include:
Lithium Citrate Syrup 3061

Lovastatin (Co-administration has been associated with thyroid hormone and/or TSH level alterations by various mechanisms). Products include:
Mevacor Tablets 2132

Magaldrate (Co-administration with antacids may reduce the efficacy of levothyroxine by binding and delaying or preventing absorption, potentially resulting in hypothyroidism; administer levothyroxine at least 4 hours apart from these agents).
No products indexed under this heading.

Magnesium Hydroxide (Co-administration with antacids may reduce the efficacy of levothyroxine by binding and delaying or preventing absorption, potentially resulting in hypothyroidism; administer levothyroxine at least 4 hours apart from these agents). Products include:
Ex•Lax Milk of Magnesia Liquid .... ◘670
Maalox Antacid/Anti-Gas Oral Suspension...................................... ◘673
Maalox Max Maximum Strength Antacid/Anti-Gas Liquid 2300
Maalox Regular Strength Antacid/Antigas Liquid 2300
Mylanta Fast-Acting 1813
Mylanta 1813
Pepcid Complete Chewable Tablets.. 1815
Phillips' Chewable Tablets .... ◘615
Phillips' Milk of Magnesia Liquid (Original, Cherry, & Mint)........... ◘616
Rolaids Tablets .... ◘706
Extra Strength Rolaids Tablets ...... ◘706
Vanquish Caplets .... ◘617

Magnesium Oxide (Co-administration with antacids may reduce the efficacy of levothyroxine by binding and delaying or prevent-

ing absorption, potentially resulting in hypothyroidism; administer levothyroxine at least 4 hours apart from these agents). Products include:
- Beelith Tablets ... 946
- Mag-Ox 400 Tablets ... 1024
- Uro-Mag Capsules ... 1024

Magnesium Salicylate (Co-administration with salicylates at greater than 2 gm inhibit binding of T_4 and T_3 to TBG and transthyrelin; an initial increase in serum FT_4 is followed by return of FT_4 to normal levels with sustained therapeutic salicylate concentrations, although total T_4 levels may decrease by as much as 30%). Products include:
- Momentum Backache Relief Extra Strength Caplets ... ▣666

Maprotiline Hydrochloride (Co-administration may increase the therapeutic and toxic effects of both drugs possibly due to increased receptor sensitivity to catecholamines; toxic effects may include increased risk of arrhythmias and CNS stimulation; onset of tricyclics may be accelerated).
No products indexed under this heading.

Meclofenamate Sodium (Co-administration with fenamate NSAID may result in decreased serum TBG concentration).
No products indexed under this heading.

Mefenamic Acid (Co-administration with fenamate NSAID may result in decreased serum TBG concentration). Products include:
- Ponstel Capsules ... 1356

Mephenytoin (Hydantoins may cause protein-binding site displacement; co-administration results in an initial transient increase in FT_4; continued administration results in a decrease in serum T_4 and normal FT_4 and TSH concentrations and, therefore, patients are clinically euthyroid).
No products indexed under this heading.

Mercaptopurine (Co-administration has been associated with thyroid hormone and/or TSH level alterations by various mechanisms). Products include:
- Purinethol Tablets ... 1615

Mestranol (Co-administration with estrogen containing oral contraceptives may result in increased serum TBG concentrations). Products include:
- Necon 1/50 Tablets ... 3415
- Norinyl 1 + 50 28-Day Tablets ... 3380
- Ortho-Novum 1/50□28 Tablets ... 2556

Metaproterenol Sulfate (Co-administration of sympathomimetic agents may increase the effects of sympathomimetics or thyroid hormone; thyroid hormones may increase risk of coronary insufficiency when sympathomimetic agents are administered to patients with coronary disease). Products include:
- Alupent ... 1029

Metaraminol Bitartrate (Co-administration of sympathomimetic agents may increase the effects of sympathomimetics or thyroid hormone; thyroid hormones may increase risk of coronary insufficiency when sympathomimetic agents are administered to patients with coronary disease). Products include:
- Aramine Injection ... 2043

Metformin Hydrochloride (Addition of levothyroxine to antidiabetic therapy may result in increased antidiabetic agent requirements). Products include:
- Glucophage Tablets ... 1080
- Glucophage XR Tablets ... 1080
- Glucovance Tablets ... 1086

Methadone Hydrochloride (Co-administration may result in increased serum TBG concentrations). Products include:
- Dolophine Hydrochloride Tablets ... 3056

Methimazole (May decrease thyroid hormone secretion, which may result in hypothyrodism).
No products indexed under this heading.

Methoxamine Hydrochloride (Co-administration of sympathomimetic agents may increase the effects of sympathomimetics or thyroid hormone; thyroid hormones may increase risk of coronary insufficiency when sympathomimetic agents are administered to patients with coronary disease).
No products indexed under this heading.

Methyclothiazide (Co-administration has been associated with thyroid hormone and/or TSH level alterations by various mechanisms).
No products indexed under this heading.

Methylprednisolone Acetate (Co-administration with glucocorticoids may result in a transient reduction in TSH secretion; the reduction is not sustained, therefore, hypothyroidism does not occur; glucocorticoids may decrease serum TBG concentration). Products include:
- Depo-Medrol Injectable Suspension ... 2795

Methylprednisolone Sodium Succinate (Co-administration with glucocorticoids may result in a transient reduction in TSH secretion; the reduction is not sustained, therefore, hypothyroidism does not occur; glucocorticoids may decrease serum TBG concentration). Products include:
- Solu-Medrol Sterile Powder ... 2855

Methyltestosterone (Co-administration with androgens/anabolic steroids may result in decreased serum TBG concentration). Products include:
- Android Capsules, 10 mg ... 1731
- Estratest ... 3252
- Testred Capsules, 10 mg ... 1746

Metipranolol Hydrochloride (Co-administration with beta-blockers may decrease T_4 5'-deiodinase activity; action of beta-blocker may be impaired when the hypothyroid patient is converted to euthyroid).
No products indexed under this heading.

Metoclopramide Hydrochloride (Co-administration has been associated with thyroid hormone and/or TSH level alterations by various mechanisms). Products include:
- Reglan ... 2935

Metoprolol Succinate (Co-administration with beta-blockers may decrease T_4 5'-deiodinase activity; action of beta-blocker may be impaired when the hypothyroid patient is converted to euthyroid). Products include:
- Toprol-XL Tablets ... 651

Metoprolol Tartrate (Co-administration with beta-blockers may decrease T_4 5'-deiodinase activity; action of beta-blocker may be impaired when the hypothyroid patient is converted to euthyroid).
No products indexed under this heading.

Miglitol (Addition of levothyroxine to antidiabetic therapy may result in increased antidiabetic agent requirements). Products include:
- Glyset Tablets ... 2821

Mitotane (Co-administration may result in increased serum TBG concentrations).
No products indexed under this heading.

Nadolol (Co-administration with beta-blockers may decrease T_4 5'-deiodinase activity; action of beta-blocker may be impaired when the hypothyroid patient is converted to euthyroid). Products include:
- Corgard Tablets ... 2245
- Corzide 40/5 Tablets ... 2247
- Corzide 80/5 Tablets ... 2247
- Nadolol Tablets ... 2288

Niacin (Co-administration with slow-release nicotinic acid may result in decreased serum TBG concentration). Products include:
- Niaspan Extended-Release Tablets ... 1846
- Nicotinex Elixir ... ▣633

Norepinephrine Bitartrate (Co-administration of sympathomimetic agents may increase the effects of sympathomimetics or thyroid hormone; thyroid hormones may increase risk of coronary insufficiency when sympathomimetic agents are administered to patients with coronary disease).
No products indexed under this heading.

Nortriptyline Hydrochloride (Co-administration may increase the therapeutic and toxic effects of both drugs possibly due to increased receptor sensitivity to catecholamines; toxic effects may include increased risk of arrhythmias and CNS stimulation; onset of tricyclics may be accelerated).
No products indexed under this heading.

Octreotide Acetate (Co-administration with octreotide may result in a transient reduction in TSH secretion; the reduction is not sustained, therefore, hypothyroidism does not occur). Products include:
- Sandostatin LAR Depot ... 2395

Oxandrolone (Co-administration with androgens/anabolic steroids may result in decreased serum TBG concentration). Products include:
- Oxandrin Tablets ... 1153

Oxymetholone (Co-administration with androgens/anabolic steroids may result in decreased serum TBG concentration). Products include:
- Anadrol-50 Tablets ... 3321

Penbutolol Sulfate (Co-administration with beta-blockers may decrease T_4 5'-deiodinase activity; action of beta-blocker may be impaired when the hypothyroid patient is converted to euthyroid).
No products indexed under this heading.

Pergolide Mesylate (Co-administration with dopamine agonists may result in a transient reduction in TSH secretion; the reduction is not sustained, therefore, hypothyroidism does not occur). Products include:
- Permax Tablets ... 1299

Perphenazine (Co-administration has been associated with thyroid hormone and/or TSH level alterations by various mechanisms). Products include:
- Etrafon ... 3115
- Trilafon ... 3160

Phenobarbital (Co-administration may increase hepatic metabolism, which may result in hypothyroidism, resulting in increased levothyroxine requirements). Products include:
- Arco-Lase Plus Tablets ... 592
- Donnatal ... 2929
- Donnatal Extentabs ... 2930

Phenylbutazone (Co-administration may cause protein-binding site displacement).
No products indexed under this heading.

Phenylephrine Bitartrate (Co-administration of sympathomimetic agents may increase the effects of sympathomimetics or thyroid hormone; thyroid hormones may increase risk of coronary insufficiency when sympathomimetic agents are administered to patients with coronary disease).
No products indexed under this heading.

Phenylephrine Hydrochloride (Co-administration of sympathomimetic agents may increase the effects of sympathomimetics or thyroid hormone; thyroid hormones may increase risk of coronary insufficiency when sympathomimetic agents are administered to patients with coronary disease). Products include:
- Afrin Nasal Decongestant Children's Pump Mist ... ▣734
- Extendryl ... 1361
- Hycomine Compound Tablets ... 1317
- Neo-Synephrine ... ▣614
- Phenergan VC Syrup ... 3560
- Phenergan VC with Codeine Syrup .. 3561
- Preparation H Cream ... ▣778
- Preparation H Cooling Gel ... ▣778
- Preparation H ... ▣778
- Vicks Sinex Nasal Spray and Ultra Fine Mist ... ▣729

Phenylephrine Tannate (Co-administration of sympathomimetic agents may increase the effects of sympathomimetics or thyroid hormone; thyroid hormones may increase risk of coronary insufficiency when sympathomimetic agents are administered to patients with coronary disease). Products include:
- Ryna-12 S Suspension ... 3351
- Reformulated Rynatan Pediatric Suspension ... 3352
- Rynatuss Pediatric Suspension ... 3353
- Rynatuss Tablets ... 3353

Phenylpropanolamine Hydrochloride (Co-administration of sympathomimetic agents may increase the effects of sympathomimetics or thyroid hormone; thyroid hormones may increase risk of coronary insufficiency when sympathomimetic agents are administered to patients with coronary disease).
No products indexed under this heading.

Phenytoin (Hydantoins may cause protein-binding site displacement; co-administration results in an initial transient increase in FT_4; co-administration may increase hepatic metabolism, which may result in hypothyroidism, resulting in increased levothyroxine requirements; phenytoin reduces serum protein binding of levothyroxine, and total- and free-T_4 may be reduced by 20% to 40%, but most patients have normal serum TSH levels and are clinicly euthyroid). Products include:
- Dilantin Infatabs ... 2624
- Dilantin-125 Oral Suspension ... 2625

Phenytoin Sodium (Hydantoins may cause protein-binding site displacement; co-administration results in an initial transient increase in FT_4; co-administration may increase hepatic metabolism, which may result in hypothyroidism, resulting in increased levothyroxine requirements; phenytoin reduces serum protein binding of levothyroxine, and total- and free-T_4 may be reduced by 20% to 40%, but most patients have normal serum TSH levels and are clinicly euthyroid). Products include:
- Dilantin Kapseals ... 2622

Pindolol (Co-administration with beta-blockers may decrease T_4 5'-deiodinase activity; action of beta-blocker may be impaired when the hypothyroid patient is converted to

euthyroid).
No products indexed under this heading.

Pioglitazone Hydrochloride (Addition of levothyroxine to antidiabetic therapy may result in increased antidiabetic agent requirements). Products include:
Actos Tablets 3275

Pirbuterol Acetate (Co-administration of sympathomimetic agents may increase the effects of sympathomimetics or thyroid hormone; thyroid hormones may increase risk of coronary insufficiency when sympathomimetic agents are administered to patients with coronary disease). Products include:
Maxair Autohaler 1981
Maxair Inhaler 1984

Polyestradiol Phosphate (Co-administration with oral estrogens may result in increased serum TBG concentrations).
No products indexed under this heading.

Polythiazide (Co-administration has been associated with thyroid hormone and/or TSH level alterations by various mechanisms). Products include:
Minizide Capsules 2700
Renese Tablets 2712

Potassium Iodide (May decrease thyroid hormone secretion, which may result in hypothyrodism; iodide drugs that contain pharmacologic amounts of iodide may cause hypothyroidism in euthyroid patients with Grave's disease previously treated with thyroid autonomy; hyperthyroidism may develop over several weeks and may persist for several months after therapy discontinuation). Products include:
Pima Syrup 1362

Pramipexole Dihydrochloride (Co-administration with dopamine agonists may result in a transient reduction in TSH secretion; the reduction is not sustained, therefore, hypothyroidism does not occur). Products include:
Mirapex Tablets 2834

Prednisolone Acetate (Co-administration with glucocorticoids may result in a transient reduction in TSH secretion; the reduction is not sustained, therefore, hypothyroidism does not occur; glucocorticoids may decrease serum TBG concentration). Products include:
Blephamide Ophthalmic Ointment 547
Blephamide Ophthalmic Suspension 548
Poly-Pred Liquifilm Ophthalmic Suspension .... ⊙245
Pred Forte Ophthalmic Suspension .... ⊙246
Pred Mild Sterile Ophthalmic Suspension .... ⊙249
Pred-G Ophthalmic Suspension .... ⊙247
Pred-G Sterile Ophthalmic Ointment .... ⊙248

Prednisolone Sodium Phosphate (Co-administration with glucocorticoids may result in a transient reduction in TSH secretion; the reduction is not sustained, therefore, hypothyroidism does not occur; glucocorticoids may decrease serum TBG concentration). Products include:
Pediapred Oral Solution 1170

Prednisolone Tebutate (Co-administration with glucocorticoids may result in a transient reduction in TSH secretion; the reduction is not sustained, therefore, hypothyroidism does not occur; glucocorticoids may decrease serum TBG concentration).
No products indexed under this heading.

Prednisone (Co-administration with glucocorticoids may result in a transient reduction in TSH secretion; the reduction is not sustained, therefore, hypothyroidism does not occur; glucocorticoids may decrease serum TBG concentration). Products include:
Prednisone 3064

Propranolol Hydrochloride (Co-administration with beta-blockers may decrease T_4 5'-deiodinase activity; in patients treated with large doses of propranolol, greater than 160 mg/day, T_3 and T_4 levels change slightly, TSH levels remain normal, and patients are clinically euthyroid; action of beta-blocker may be impaired when the hypothyroid patient is converted to euthyroid). Products include:
Inderal 3513
Inderal LA Long-Acting Capsules 3516
Inderide Tablets 3517
Inderide LA Long-Acting Capsules 3519

Propylthiouracil (May decrease thyroid hormone secretion, which may result in hypothyrodism).
No products indexed under this heading.

Protriptyline Hydrochloride (Co-administration may increase the therapeutic and toxic effects of both drugs possibly due to increased receptor sensitivity to catecholamines; toxic effects may include increased risk of arrhythmias and CNS stimulation; onset of tricyclics may be accelerated). Products include:
Vivactil Tablets 2446
Vivactil Tablets 2217

Pseudoephedrine Hydrochloride (Co-administration of sympathomimetic agents may increase the effects of sympathomimetics or thyroid hormone; thyroid hormones may increase risk of coronary insufficiency when sympathomimetic agents are administered to patients with coronary disease). Products include:
Actifed Cold & Allergy Tablets .... ▣688
Actifed Cold & Sinus Caplets and Tablets .... ▣688
Advil Cold and Sinus Caplets .... ▣771
Advil Cold and Sinus Tablets .... ▣771
Advil Flu & Body Ache Caplets .... ▣772
Aleve Cold & Sinus Caplets .... ▣603
Alka-Seltzer Plus Liqui-Gels .... ▣604
Alka-Seltzer Plus Cold & Flu Medicine Liqui-Gels .... ▣604
Alka-Seltzer Plus Cold & Sinus Medicine Liqui-Gels .... ▣604
Allegra-D Extended-Release Tablets 714
BC Cold Powder .... ▣619
Benadryl Allergy/Cold Tablets .... ▣691
Benadryl Allergy/Congestion Tablets .... ▣692
Benadryl Allergy & Sinus Liquid .... ▣693
Benadryl Allergy & Sinus Fastmelt Tablets .... ▣693
Benadryl Allergy Sinus Headache Caplets & Gelcaps .... ▣693
Benadryl Severe Allergy & Sinus Headache Caplets .... ▣694
Benadryl Children's Allergy/Cold Fastmelt Tablets .... ▣692
Benylin Multi-Symptom Liquid .... ▣697
Bromfed Capsules (Extended-Release) 2269
Bromfed-PD Capsules (Extended-Release) 2269
Children's Cēpacol Sore Throat .... ▣788
Comtrex Acute Head Cold & Sinus Pressure Relief Tablets .... ▣627
Comtrex Deep Chest Cold & Congestion Relief Softgels .... ▣627
Comtrex Flu Therapy & Fever Relief Daytime Caplets .... ▣628
Comtrex Flu Therapy & Fever Relief Nighttime Tablets .... ▣628
Comtrex Maximum Strength Multi-Symptom Cold & Cough Relief Tablets and Caplets .... ▣626
Contac Non-Drowsy 12 Hour Cold Caplets .... ▣745
Contac Non-Drowsy Timed Release 12 Hour Cold Caplets .... ▣746
Contac Severe Cold and Flu Caplets Maximum Strength .... ▣746
Contac Severe Cold and Flu Caplets Non-Drowsy .... ▣746
Dimetapp Elixir .... ▣777
Dimetapp Cold and Fever Suspension .... ▣775
Dimetapp DM Cold & Cough Elixir .... ▣775
Dimetapp Nighttime Flu Liquid .... ▣776
Dimetapp Non-Drowsy Flu Syrup .... ▣777
Dimetapp Infant Drops Decongestant .... ▣775
Dimetapp Infant Drops Decongestant Plus Cough .... ▣776
Guaifed 2272
Kronofed-A 1341
Children's Motrin Cold Oral Suspension 2007
Motrin Sinus Headache Caplets 2005
PediaCare Cough-Cold Liquid .... ▣719
PediaCare Infants' Drops Decongestant .... ▣719
PediaCare Infants' Drops Decongestant Plus Cough .... ▣719
PediaCare NightRest Cough-Cold Liquid .... ▣719
Robitussin Cold Caplets Cold & Congestion .... ▣780
Robitussin Cold Softgels Cold & Congestion .... ▣780
Robitussin Cold Caplets Multi-Symptom Cold & Flu .... ▣781
Robitussin Cold Softgels Multi-Symptom Cold & Flu .... ▣781
Robitussin Cold Softgels Severe Congestion .... ▣782
Robitussin Cough & Cold Infant Drops .... ▣782
Robitussin Maximum Strength Cough & Cold Liquid .... ▣785
Robitussin Pediatric Cough & Cold Formula Liquid .... ▣785
Robitussin Multi Symptom Honey Flu Liquid .... ▣785
Robitussin Nighttime Honey Flu Liquid .... ▣786
Robitussin-CF Liquid .... ▣783
Robitussin-DAC Syrup 2942
Robitussin-PE Liquid .... ▣782
Ryna .... ▣768
Semprex-D Capsules 1172
Singlet Caplets .... ▣761
Sinutab Non-Drying Liquid Caps .... ▣706
Sinutab Sinus Allergy Medication, Maximum Strength Formula, Tablets & Caplets .... ▣707
Sinutab Sinus Medication, Maximum Strength Without Drowsiness Formula, Tablets & Caplets .... ▣707
Sudafed 12 Hour Tablets .... ▣708
Sudafed 24 Hour Tablets .... ▣708
Children's Sudafed Cold & Cough Liquid .... ▣709
Children's Sudafed Nasal Decongestant Chewables .... ▣711
Children's Sudafed Nasal Decongestant Liquid Medication .... ▣711
Sudafed Cold & Allergy Tablets .... ▣708
Sudafed Cold & Cough Liquid Caps .... ▣709
Sudafed Cold & Sinus Liquid Caps .... ▣710
Sudafed Nasal Decongestant Tablets .... ▣710
Sudafed Non-Drying Sinus Liquid Caps .... ▣712
Sudafed Severe Cold .... ▣711
Sudafed Sinus Headache Caplets .... ▣712
Sudafed Sinus Headache Tablets .... ▣712
Tavist Sinus Non-Drowsy Coated Caplets .... ▣676
TheraFlu Regular Strength Cold & Cough Night Time Hot Liquid .... ▣676
TheraFlu Regular Strength Cold & Sore Throat Night Time Hot Liquid .... ▣676
TheraFlu Maximum Strength Flu & Congestion Non-Drowsy Hot Liquid .... ▣677
TheraFlu Maximum Strength Flu & Cough Night Time Hot Liquid .... ▣678
TheraFlu Maximum Strength Flu & Sore Throat Night Time Hot Liquid .... ▣677
TheraFlu Maximum Strength Severe Cold & Congestion Night Time Caplets .... ▣678
TheraFlu Maximum Strength Severe Cold & Congestion Night Time Hot Liquid .... ▣678
TheraFlu Maximum Strength Severe Cold & Congestion Non-Drowsy .... ▣679
Triaminic Allergy Congestion Liquid .... ▣680
Triaminic Chest Congestion Liquid .... ▣680
Triaminic Cold & Allergy Liquid .... ▣681
Triaminic Cold & Allergy Softchews .... ▣683
Triaminic Cold & Cough Liquid .... ▣681
Triaminic Cold & Cough Softchews .... ▣683
Triaminic Cold & Night Time Cough Liquid .... ▣681
Triaminic Cold, Cough & Fever Liquid .... ▣681
Triaminic Cough Liquid .... ▣682
Triaminic Cough & Congestion Liquid .... ▣682
Triaminic Cough & Sore Throat Liquid .... ▣682
Triaminic Cough & Sore Throat Softchews .... ▣684
Children's Tylenol Allergy-D Liquid 2014
Children's Tylenol Cold Suspension Liquid and Chewable Tablets 2015
Children's Tylenol Cold Plus Cough Suspension Liquid and Chewable Tablets 2015
Children's Tylenol Flu Suspension Liquid 2015
Children's Tylenol Sinus Suspension Liquid 2017
Infants' Tylenol Cold Decongestant and Fever Reducer Concentrated Drops 2015
Infants' Tylenol Cold Decongestant and Fever Reducer Concentrated Drops Plus Cough 2015
Tylenol Allergy Sinus 2010
Multi-Symptom Tylenol Cold Complete Formula Caplets 2010
Multi-Symptom Tylenol Cold Non-Drowsy Caplets and Gelcaps 2010
Multi-Symptom Tylenol Cold Severe Congestion Non-Drowsy Caplets 2011
Maximum Strength Tylenol Flu NightTime Gelcaps 2011
Maximum Strength Tylenol Flu NightTime Liquid 2011
Maximum Strength Tylenol Flu Non-Drowsy Gelcaps 2011
Maximum Strength Tylenol Sinus NightTime Caplets 2012
Maximum Strength Tylenol Sinus Non-Drowsy Geltabs, Gelcaps, Caplets, and Tablets 2012
Vicks 44D Cough & Head Congestion Relief Liquid .... ▣724
Vicks 44M Cough, Cold & Flu Relief Liquid .... ▣725
Pediatric Vicks 44m Cough & Cold Relief .... ▣728
Vicks DayQuil LiquiCaps/Liquid Multi-Symptom Cold/Flu Relief .... ▣727
Children's Vicks NyQuil Cold/Cough Relief .... ▣726
Vicks NyQuil LiquiCaps/Liquid Multi-Symptom Cold/Flu Relief, Original and Cherry Flavors .... ▣727
Zephrex Tablets 3091
Zephrex LA Tablets 3092
Zyrtec-D 12 Hour Extended Relief Tablets 2758

Pseudoephedrine Sulfate (Co-administration of sympathomimetic agents may increase the effects of sympathomimetics or thyroid hormone; thyroid hormones may increase risk of coronary insufficiency when sympathomimetic agents are administered to patients with coronary disease). Products include:
Chlor-Trimeton Allergy/Decongestant Tablets .... ▣736
Claritin-D 12 Hour Extended Release Tablets 3102
Claritin-D 24 Hour Extended Release Tablets 3104
Coricidin 'D' Cold, Flu & Sinus Tablets .... ▣737
Drixoral Allergy/Sinus Extended-Release Tablets .... ▣741
Drixoral Cold & Allergy Sustained-Action Tablets .... ▣740
Drixoral Cold & Flu Extended-Release Tablets .... ▣740
Drixoral Nasal Decongestant Long-Acting Non-Drowsy Tablets .... ▣740
Rynatan Tablets 3351

Quinestrol (Co-administration with oral estrogens may result in increased serum TBG concentrations).
No products indexed under this heading.

Repaglinide (Addition of levothyroxine to antidiabetic therapy may result in increased antidiabetic agent requirements). Products include:
- Prandin Tablets (0.5, 1, and 2 mg) ... **2432**

Resorcinol (Co-administration of excessive topical use of resorcinol has been associated with thyroid hormone and/or TSH level alterations by various mechanisms).
No products indexed under this heading.

Rifampin (Co-administration may increase hepatic metabolism, which may result in hypothyroidism, resulting in increased levothyroxine requirements). Products include:
- Rifadin ... **765**
- Rifamate Capsules ... **767**
- Rifater Tablets ... **769**

Ropinirole Hydrochloride (Co-administration with dopamine agonists may result in a transient reduction in TSH secretion; the reduction is not sustained, therefore, hypothyroidism does not occur). Products include:
- Requip Tablets ... **1621**

Rosiglitazone Maleate (Addition of levothyroxine to antidiabetic therapy may result in increased antidiabetic agent requirements). Products include:
- Avandia Tablets ... **1490**

Salmeterol Xinafoate (Co-administration of sympathomimetic agents may increase the effects of sympathomimetics or thyroid hormone; thyroid hormones may increase risk of coronary insufficiency when sympathomimetic agents are administered to patients with coronary disease). Products include:
- Advair Diskus 100/50 ... **1448**
- Advair Diskus 250/50 ... **1448**
- Advair Diskus 500/50 ... **1448**
- Serevent Diskus ... **1637**
- Serevent Inhalation Aerosol ... **1633**

Salsalate (Co-administration with salicylates at greater than 2 gm inhibit binding of T_4 and T_3 to TBG and transthyrelin; an initial increase in serum FT_4 is followed by return of FT_4 to normal levels with sustained therapeutic salicylate concentrations, although total T_4 levels may decrease by as much as 30%).
No products indexed under this heading.

Sertraline Hydrochloride (Co-administration of sertraline in patients stabilized on levothyroxine may result in increased levothyroxine requirements). Products include:
- Zoloft ... **2751**

Sodium Nitroprusside (Co-administration has been associated with thyroid hormone and/or TSH level alterations by various mechanisms).
No products indexed under this heading.

Sodium Polystyrene Sulfonate (Co-administration may result in decreased T_4 absorption, which may result in hypothyroidism; administer levothyroxine at least 4 hours apart from these agents).
No products indexed under this heading.

Somatrem (Excessive use of thyroid hormone with growth hormones may accelerate epiphyseal closure; however, untreated hypothyroidism may interfere with growth response to growth hormone).
No products indexed under this heading.

Somatropin (Excessive use of thyroid hormone with growth hormones may accelerate epiphyseal closure; however, untreated hypothyroidism may interfere with growth response to growth hormone). Products include:
- Genotropin Lyophilized Powder ... **2818**
- Humatrope Vials and Cartridges ... **1930**
- Norditropin Cartridges ... **2420**
- Norditropin for Injection ... **2419**
- Nutropin AQ Injection ... **1420**
- Nutropin Depot for Injectable Suspension ... **1423**
- Nutropin for Injection ... **1417**
- Saizen for Injection ... **3225**
- Serostim for Injection ... **3229**

Sotalol Hydrochloride (Co-administration with beta-blockers may decrease T_4 5'-deiodinase activity; action of beta-blocker may be impaired when the hypothyroid patient is converted to euthyroid). Products include:
- Betapace Tablets ... **950**
- Betapace AF Tablets ... **954**

Soybean Preparations (Concurrent use of soybean flour may bind and decrease the absorption of levothyroxine sodium from GI tract).
No products indexed under this heading.

Stanozolol (Co-administration with androgens/anabolic steroids may result in decreased serum TBG concentration).
No products indexed under this heading.

Sucralfate (Co-administration may result in decreased T_4 absorption, which may result in hypothyroidism; administer levothyroxine at least 4 hours apart from these agents). Products include:
- Carafate Suspension ... **731**
- Carafate Tablets ... **730**

Sulfamethoxazole (May decrease thyroid hormone secretion, which may result in hypothyrodism). Products include:
- Bactrim ... **2949**
- Septra Suspension ... **2265**
- Septra Tablets ... **2265**
- Septra DS Tablets ... **2265**

Sulfisoxazole Acetyl (May decrease thyroid hormone secretion, which may result in hypothyrodism). Products include:
- Pediazole Suspension ... **3050**

Tamoxifen Citrate (Co-administration may result in increased serum TBG concentrations). Products include:
- Nolvadex Tablets ... **678**

Terbutaline Sulfate (Co-administration of sympathomimetic agents may increase the effects of sympathomimetics or thyroid hormone; thyroid hormones may increase risk of coronary insufficiency when sympathomimetic agents are administered to patients with coronary disease). Products include:
- Brethine Ampuls ... **2314**
- Brethine Tablets ... **2313**

Theophylline (Decreased theophylline clearance may occur in hypothyroid patients; clearance returns to normal when euthyroid state is achieved). Products include:
- Aerolate ... **1361**
- Theo-Dur Extended-Release Tablets ... **1835**
- Uni-Dur Extended-Release Tablets .. **1841**
- Uniphyl 400 mg and 600 mg Tablets ... **2903**

Theophylline Calcium Salicylate (Decreased theophylline clearance may occur in hypothyroid patients; clearance returns to normal when euthyroid state is achieved).
No products indexed under this heading.

Theophylline Sodium Glycinate (Decreased theophylline clearance may occur in hypothyroid patients; clearance returns to normal when euthyroid state is achieved).
No products indexed under this heading.

Timolol Hemihydrate (Co-administration with beta-blockers may decrease T_4 5'-deiodinase activity; action of beta-blocker may be impaired when the hypothyroid patient is converted to euthyroid). Products include:
- Betimol Ophthalmic Solution ... ⊙**324**

Timolol Maleate (Co-administration with beta-blockers may decrease T_4 5'-deiodinase activity; action of beta-blocker may be impaired when the hypothyroid patient is converted to euthyroid). Products include:
- Blocadren Tablets ... **2046**
- Cosopt Sterile Ophthalmic Solution ... **2065**
- Timolide Tablets ... **2187**
- Timolol GFS ... ⊙**266**
- Timoptic in Ocudose ... **2192**
- Timoptic Sterile Ophthalmic Solution ... **2190**
- Timoptic-XE Sterile Ophthalmic Gel Forming Solution ... **2194**

Tolazamide (Addition of levothyroxine to antidiabetic therapy may result in increased antidiabetic agent requirements).
No products indexed under this heading.

Tolbutamide (May decrease thyroid hormone secretion, which may result in hypothyrodism).
No products indexed under this heading.

Triamcinolone (Co-administration with glucocorticoids may result in a transient reduction in TSH secretion; the reduction is not sustained, therefore, hypothyroidism does not occur; glucocorticoids may decrease serum TBG concentration).
No products indexed under this heading.

Triamcinolone Acetonide (Co-administration with glucocorticoids may result in a transient reduction in TSH secretion; the reduction is not sustained, therefore, hypothyroidism does not occur; glucocorticoids may decrease serum TBG concentration). Products include:
- Azmacort Inhalation Aerosol ... **728**
- Nasacort Nasal Inhaler ... **750**
- Nasacort AQ Nasal Spray ... **752**
- Tri-Nasal Spray ... **2274**

Triamcinolone Diacetate (Co-administration with glucocorticoids may result in a transient reduction in TSH secretion; the reduction is not sustained, therefore, hypothyroidism does not occur; glucocorticoids may decrease serum TBG concentration).
No products indexed under this heading.

Triamcinolone Hexacetonide (Co-administration with glucocorticoids may result in a transient reduction in TSH secretion; the reduction is not sustained, therefore, hypothyroidism does not occur; glucocorticoids may decrease serum TBG concentration).
No products indexed under this heading.

Trimipramine Maleate (Co-administration may increase the therapeutic and toxic effects of both drugs possibly due to increased receptor sensitivity to catecholamines; toxic effects may include increased risk of arrhythmias and CNS stimulation; onset of tricyclics may be accelerated). Products include:
- Surmontil Capsules ... **3595**

Troglitazone (Addition of levothyroxine to antidiabetic therapy may result in increased antidiabetic agent requirements).
No products indexed under this heading.

Tyropanoate Sodium (May decrease thyroid hormone secretion, which may result in hypothyrodism; the fetus, elderly, and euthyroid patients with underlying thyroid disease are among those individuals who are susceptible to iodine-induced hypothyroidism; oral cholecytographic agents slowly excreted, producing more prolonged hypothyroidism; iodide drugs that contain pharmacologic amounts of iodide may cause hypothyroidism in euthyroid patients with Grave's disease previously treated with thyroid autonomy; hyperthyroidism may develop over several weeks and may persist for several months after therapy discontinuation).
No products indexed under this heading.

Warfarin Sodium (Thyroid hormones appear to increase the catabolism of vitamin K-dependent clotting factors, thereby increasing the anticoagulant activity of oral anticoagulants). Products include:
- Coumadin for Injection ... **1243**
- Coumadin Tablets ... **1243**
- Warfarin Sodium Tablets, USP ... **3302**

Food Interactions

Cotton seed meal (Concurrent use of cotton seed meal may bind and decrease the absorption of levothyroxine sodium from GI tract).
No products indexed under this heading.

Dietary Fiber (Concurrent use of dietary fiber may bind and decrease the absorption of levothyroxine sodium from GI tract).

Soybean Formula, Children's (Concurrent use of soybean flour may bind and decrease the absorption of levothyroxine sodium from GI tract).

Walnuts (Concurrent use of walnuts may bind and decrease the absorption of levothyroxine sodium from GI tract).
No products indexed under this heading.

LEVSIN DROPS

(Hyoscyamine Sulfate) ... **3172**

May interact with antacids, antihistamines, antimuscarinic drugs, monoamine oxidase inhibitors, phenothiazines, tricyclic antidepressants, and certain other agents. Compounds in these categories include:

Acrivastine (Additive adverse effects). Products include:
- Semprex-D Capsules ... **1172**

Aluminum Carbonate (Interferes with absorption of Levsin).
No products indexed under this heading.

Aluminum Hydroxide (Interferes with absorption of Levsin). Products include:
- Amphojel Suspension (Mint Flavor) ... ▣**789**
- Gaviscon Extra Strength Liquid ... ▣**751**
- Gaviscon Extra Strength Tablets ... ▣**751**
- Gaviscon Regular Strength Liquid . ▣**751**
- Gaviscon Regular Strength Tablets ... ▣**750**
- Maalox Antacid/Anti-Gas Oral Suspension ... ▣**673**
- Maalox Max Maximum Strength Antacid/Anti-Gas Liquid ... **2300**
- Maalox Regular Strength Antacid/Antigas Liquid ... **2300**
- Mylanta ... **1813**
- Vanquish Caplets ... ▣**617**

Amantadine Hydrochloride (Additive adverse effects). Products include:
- Symmetrel ... **1328**

Amitriptyline Hydrochloride (Additive adverse effects). Products include:
- Etrafon ... **3115**
- Limbitrol ... **1738**

Amoxapine (Additive adverse effects).
No products indexed under this heading.

Astemizole (Additive adverse effects).
No products indexed under this heading.

Atropine Sulfate (Additive adverse effects). Products include:
Donnatal 2929
Donnatal Extentabs 2930
Motofen Tablets 577
Prosed/DS Tablets 3268
Urised Tablets 2876

Azatadine Maleate (Additive adverse effects). Products include:
Rynatan Tablets 3351

Belladonna Alkaloids (Additive adverse effects). Products include:
Hyland's Teething Tablets 766
Urimax Tablets 1769

Bromodiphenhydramine Hydrochloride (Additive adverse effects).
No products indexed under this heading.

Brompheniramine Maleate (Additive adverse effects). Products include:
Bromfed Capsules (Extended-Release) 2269
Bromfed-PD Capsules (Extended-Release) 2269
Comtrex Acute Head Cold & Sinus Pressure Relief Tablets 627
Dimetapp Elixir 777
Dimetapp Cold and Fever Suspension 775
Dimetapp DM Cold & Cough Elixir 775
Dimetapp Nighttime Flu Liquid 776

Cetirizine Hydrochloride (Additive adverse effects). Products include:
Zyrtec 2756
Zyrtec-D 12 Hour Extended Relief Tablets 2758

Chlorpheniramine Maleate (Additive adverse effects). Products include:
Actifed Cold & Sinus Caplets and Tablets 688
Alka-Seltzer Plus Liqui-Gels 604
BC Allergy Sinus Cold Powder 619
Chlor-Trimeton Allergy Tablets 735
Chlor-Trimeton Allergy/Decongestant Tablets 736
Comtrex Flu Therapy & Fever Relief Nighttime Tablets 628
Comtrex Maximum Strength Multi-Symptom Cold & Cough Relief Tablets and Caplets 626
Contac Severe Cold and Flu Caplets Maximum Strength 746
Coricidin 'D' Cold, Flu & Sinus Tablets 737
Coricidin/Coricidin D 738
Coricidin HBP Maximum Strength Flu Tablets 738
Extendryl 1361
Hycomine Compound Tablets 1317
Kronofed-A 1341
PediaCare Cough-Cold Liquid 719
PediaCare NightRest Cough-Cold Liquid 719
Robitussin Nighttime Honey Flu Liquid 786
Ryna 768
Singlet Caplets 761
Sinutab Sinus Allergy Medication, Maximum Strength Formula, Tablets & Caplets 707
Sudafed Cold & Allergy Tablets 708
TheraFlu Regular Strength Cold & Cough Night Time Hot Liquid 676
TheraFlu Regular Strength Cold & Sore Throat Night Time Hot Liquid 676
TheraFlu Maximum Strength Flu & Cough Night Time Hot Liquid 678
TheraFlu Maximum Strength Flu & Sore Throat Night Time Hot Liquid 677
TheraFlu Maximum Strength Severe Cold & Congestion Night Time Caplets 678
TheraFlu Maximum Strength Severe Cold & Congestion Night Time Hot Liquid 678
Triaminic Cold & Allergy Liquid 681
Triaminic Cold & Allergy Softchews 683
Triaminic Cold & Cough Liquid 681
Triaminic Cold & Cough Softchews 683
Triaminic Cold & Night Time Cough Liquid 681
Triaminic Cold, Cough & Fever Liquid 681
Children's Tylenol Cold Suspension Liquid and Chewable Tablets 2015
Children's Tylenol Cold Plus Cough Suspension Liquid and Chewable Tablets 2015
Children's Tylenol Flu Suspension Liquid 2015
Maximum Strength Tylenol Allergy Sinus Caplets, Gelcaps, and Geltabs 2010
Multi-Symptom Tylenol Cold Complete Formula Caplets 2010
Vicks 44M Cough, Cold & Flu Relief Liquid 725
Pediatric Vicks 44m Cough & Cold Relief 728
Children's Vicks NyQuil Cold/Cough Relief 726

Chlorpheniramine Polistirex (Additive adverse effects). Products include:
Tussionex Pennkinetic Extended-Release Suspension 1174

Chlorpheniramine Tannate (Additive adverse effects). Products include:
Reformulated Rynatan Pediatric Suspension 3352
Rynatuss Pediatric Suspension 3353
Rynatuss Tablets 3353
Tussi-12 S Suspension 3356
Tussi-12 Tablets 3356

Chlorpromazine (Additive adverse effects). Products include:
Thorazine Suppositories 1656

Chlorpromazine Hydrochloride (Additive adverse effects). Products include:
Thorazine 1656

Clemastine Fumarate (Additive adverse effects). Products include:
Tavist 12 Hour Allergy Tablets 676

Clidinium Bromide (Additive adverse effects).
No products indexed under this heading.

Clomipramine Hydrochloride (Additive adverse effects).
No products indexed under this heading.

Cyproheptadine Hydrochloride (Additive adverse effects). Products include:
Periactin Tablets 2155

Desipramine Hydrochloride (Additive adverse effects). Products include:
Norpramin Tablets 755

Dexchlorpheniramine Maleate (Additive adverse effects).
No products indexed under this heading.

Dicyclomine Hydrochloride (Additive adverse effects).
No products indexed under this heading.

Diphenhydramine Citrate (Additive adverse effects). Products include:
Alka-Seltzer PM Effervescent Tablets 605
Benadryl Allergy & Sinus Fastmelt Tablets 693
Benadryl Children's Allergy/Cold Fastmelt Tablets 692
Excedrin PM Tablets, Caplets, and Geltabs 631
Goody's PM Powder 621

Diphenhydramine Hydrochloride (Additive adverse effects). Products include:
Extra Strength Bayer PM Caplets 611
Benadryl Allergy Chewables 689
Benadryl Allergy 691
Benadryl Allergy Liquid 690
Benadryl Allergy/Cold Tablets 691
Benadryl Allergy/Congestion Tablets 692
Benadryl Allergy & Sinus Liquid 693
Benadryl Allergy Sinus Headache Caplets & Gelcaps 693
Benadryl Severe Allergy & Sinus Headache Caplets 694
Benadryl Dye-Free Allergy Liquid 690
Benadryl Dye-Free Allergy Liqui-Gels Softgels 690
Benadryl Itch Relief Stick Extra Strength 695
Benadryl Cream 695
Benadryl Gel 695
Benadryl Spray 696
Benadryl Parenteral 2617
Coricidin HBP Night-Time Cold & Flu Tablets 738
Nytol QuickCaps Caplets 622
Maximum Strength Nytol QuickGels Softgels 621
Extra Strength Percogesic Aspirin-Free Coated Caplets 665
Simply Sleep Caplets 2008
Sominex Original Formula Tablets 761
Children's Tylenol Allergy-D Liquid 2014
Maximum Strength Tylenol Allergy Sinus NightTime Caplets 2010
Tylenol Severe Allergy Caplets 2010
Maximum Strength Tylenol Flu NightTime Gelcaps 2011
Extra Strength Tylenol PM Caplets, Geltabs, and Gelcaps 2012
Unisom Maximum Strength SleepGels 713

Diphenylpyraline Hydrochloride (Additive adverse effects).
No products indexed under this heading.

Doxepin Hydrochloride (Additive adverse effects). Products include:
Sinequan 2713

Fexofenadine Hydrochloride (Additive adverse effects). Products include:
Allegra 712
Allegra-D Extended-Release Tablets 714

Fluphenazine Decanoate (Additive adverse effects).
No products indexed under this heading.

Fluphenazine Enanthate (Additive adverse effects).
No products indexed under this heading.

Fluphenazine Hydrochloride (Additive adverse effects).
No products indexed under this heading.

Glycopyrrolate (Additive adverse effects). Products include:
Robinul Forte Tablets 1358
Robinul Injectable 2940
Robinul Tablets 1358

Haloperidol (Additive adverse effects). Products include:
Haldol Injection, Tablets and Concentrate 2533

Haloperidol Decanoate (Additive adverse effects). Products include:
Haldol Decanoate 2535

Hyoscyamine (Additive adverse effects). Products include:
Urised Tablets 2876

Imipramine Hydrochloride (Additive adverse effects).
No products indexed under this heading.

Imipramine Pamoate (Additive adverse effects).
No products indexed under this heading.

Ipratropium Bromide (Additive adverse effects). Products include:
Atrovent Inhalation Aerosol 1030
Atrovent Inhalation Solution 1031
Atrovent Nasal Spray 0.03% 1032
Atrovent Nasal Spray 0.06% 1033
Combivent Inhalation Aerosol 1041
DuoNeb Inhalation Solution 1233

Isocarboxazid (Additive adverse effects).
No products indexed under this heading.

Loratadine (Additive adverse effects). Products include:
Claritin 3100
Claritin-D 12 Hour Extended Release Tablets 3102
Claritin-D 24 Hour Extended Release Tablets 3104

Magaldrate (Interferes with absorption of Levsin).
No products indexed under this heading.

Magnesium Hydroxide (Interferes with absorption of Levsin). Products include:
Ex•Lax Milk of Magnesia Liquid 670
Maalox Antacid/Anti-Gas Oral Suspension 673
Maalox Max Maximum Strength Antacid/Anti-Gas Liquid 2300
Maalox Regular Strength Antacid/Antigas Liquid 2300
Mylanta Fast-Acting 1813
Mylanta 1813
Pepcid Complete Chewable Tablets 1815
Phillips' Chewable Tablets 615
Phillips' Milk of Magnesia Liquid (Original, Cherry, & Mint) 616
Rolaids Tablets 706
Extra Strength Rolaids Tablets 706
Vanquish Caplets 617

Magnesium Oxide (Interferes with absorption of Levsin). Products include:
Beelith Tablets 946
Mag-Ox 400 Tablets 1024
Uro-Mag Capsules 1024

Maprotiline Hydrochloride (Additive adverse effects).
No products indexed under this heading.

Mepenzolate Bromide (Additive adverse effects).
No products indexed under this heading.

Mesoridazine Besylate (Additive adverse effects). Products include:
Serentil 1057

Methdilazine Hydrochloride (Additive adverse effects).
No products indexed under this heading.

Methotrimeprazine (Additive adverse effects).
No products indexed under this heading.

Moclobemide (Additive adverse effects).
No products indexed under this heading.

Nortriptyline Hydrochloride (Additive adverse effects).
No products indexed under this heading.

Oxyphenonium Bromide (Additive adverse effects).
No products indexed under this heading.

Pargyline Hydrochloride (Additive adverse effects).
No products indexed under this heading.

Perphenazine (Additive adverse effects). Products include:
Etrafon 3115
Trilafon 3160

Phenelzine Sulfate (Additive adverse effects). Products include:
Nardil Tablets 2653

Procarbazine Hydrochloride (Additive adverse effects). Products include:
Matulane Capsules 3246

Prochlorperazine (Additive adverse effects). Products include:
Compazine 1505

Promethazine Hydrochloride (Additive adverse effects). Products include:
Mepergan Injection 3539
Phenergan Injection 3553
Phenergan 3556
Phenergan Syrup 3554
Phenergan with Codeine Syrup 3557
Phenergan with Dextromethorphan Syrup 3559
Phenergan VC Syrup 3560
Phenergan VC with Codeine Syrup 3561

Propantheline Bromide (Additive adverse effects).
No products indexed under this heading.

IMPORTANT NOTE: Always consult each drug listing in the patient's regimen for possible interactions.

Protriptyline Hydrochloride (Additive adverse effects). Products include:
- Vivactil Tablets 2446
- Vivactil Tablets 2217

Pyrilamine Maleate (Additive adverse effects). Products include:
- Maximum Strength Midol Menstrual Caplets and Gelcaps ..... ■612
- Maximum Strength Midol PMS Caplets and Gelcaps ..... ■613

Pyrilamine Tannate (Additive adverse effects). Products include:
- Ryna-12 S Suspension 3351

Scopolamine (Additive adverse effects). Products include:
- Transderm Scōp Transdermal Therapeutic System 2302

Scopolamine Hydrobromide (Additive adverse effects). Products include:
- Donnatal 2929
- Donnatal Extentabs 2930

Selegiline Hydrochloride (Additive adverse effects). Products include:
- Eldepryl Capsules 3266

Sodium Bicarbonate (Interferes with absorption of Levsin). Products include:
- Alka-Seltzer ..... ■603
- Alka-Seltzer Lemon Lime Antacid and Pain Reliever Effervescent Tablets ..... ■603
- Alka-Seltzer Extra Strength Antacid and Pain Reliever Effervescent Tablets ..... ■603
- Alka-Seltzer Heartburn Relief Tablets ..... ■604
- Ceo-Two Evacuant Suppository ..... ■618
- Colyte with Flavor Packs for Oral Solution 3170
- GoLYTELY and Pineapple Flavor GoLYTELY for Oral Solution 1068
- NuLYTELY, Cherry Flavor, Lemon-Lime Flavor, and Orange Flavor NuLYTELY for Oral Solution 1068

Terfenadine (Additive adverse effects).
No products indexed under this heading.

Thioridazine Hydrochloride (Additive adverse effects). Products include:
- Thioridazine Hydrochloride Tablets 2289

Tolterodine Tartrate (Additive adverse effects). Products include:
- Detrol Tablets 3623
- Detrol LA Capsules 2801

Tranylcypromine Sulfate (Additive adverse effects). Products include:
- Parnate Tablets 1607

Tridihexethyl Chloride (Additive adverse effects).
No products indexed under this heading.

Trifluoperazine Hydrochloride (Additive adverse effects). Products include:
- Stelazine 1640

Trimeprazine Tartrate (Additive adverse effects).
No products indexed under this heading.

Trimipramine Maleate (Additive adverse effects). Products include:
- Surmontil Capsules 3595

Tripelennamine Hydrochloride (Additive adverse effects).
No products indexed under this heading.

Triprolidine Hydrochloride (Additive adverse effects). Products include:
- Actifed Cold & Allergy Tablets ..... ■688

LEVSIN ELIXIR
(Hyoscyamine Sulfate) 3172
See Levsin Drops

LEVSIN INJECTION
(Hyoscyamine Sulfate) 3172
See Levsin Drops

LEVSIN TABLETS
(Hyoscyamine Sulfate) 3172
See Levsin Drops

LEVSIN/SL TABLETS
(Hyoscyamine Sulfate) 3172
See Levsin Drops

LEVSINEX TIMECAPS
(Hyoscyamine Sulfate) 3172
See Levsin Drops

LEVULAN KERASTICK
(Aminolevulinic Acid Hydrochloride) 971

May interact with phenothiazines, sulfonamides, sulfonylureas, tetracyclines, thiazides, and certain other agents. Compounds in these categories include:

Bendroflumethiazide (Co-administration with other photosensitizing agents, such as thiazide diuretics, might increase photosensitivity reactions of actinic ketoses treated with aminolevulinic acid HCL). Products include:
- Corzide 40/5 Tablets 2247
- Corzide 80/5 Tablets 2247

Chlorothiazide (Co-administration with other photosensitizing agents, such as thiazide diuretics, might increase photosensitivity reactions of actinic ketoses treated with aminolevulinic acid HCL). Products include:
- Aldoclor Tablets 2035
- Diuril Oral 2087

Chlorothiazide Sodium (Co-administration with other photosensitizing agents, such as thiazide diuretics, might increase photosensitivity reactions of actinic ketoses treated with aminolevulinic acid HCL). Products include:
- Diuril Sodium Intravenous 2086

Chlorpromazine (Co-administration with other photosensitizing agents, such as phenothiazines, might increase photosensitivity reactions of actinic ketoses treated with aminolevulinic acid HCL). Products include:
- Thorazine Suppositories 1656

Chlorpromazine Hydrochloride (Co-administration with other photosensitizing agents, such as phenothiazines, might increase photosensitivity reactions of actinic ketoses treated with aminolevulinic acid HCL). Products include:
- Thorazine 1656

Chlorpropamide (Co-administration with other photosensitizing agents, such as sulfonylureas, might increase photosensitivity reactions of actinic ketoses treated with aminolevulinic acid HCL). Products include:
- Diabinese Tablets 2680

Demeclocycline Hydrochloride (Co-administration with other photosensitizing agents, such as tetracyclines, might increase photosensitivity reactions of actinic ketoses treated with aminolevulinic acid HCL). Products include:
- Declomycin Tablets 1855

Doxycycline Calcium (Co-administration with other photosensitizing agents, such as tetracyclines, might increase photosensitivity reactions of actinic ketoses treated with aminolevulinic acid HCL). Products include:
- Vibramycin Calcium Oral Suspension Syrup 2735

Doxycycline Hyclate (Co-administration with other photosensitizing agents, such as tetracyclines, might increase photosensitivity reactions of actinic ketoses treated with aminolevulinic acid HCL). Products include:
- Doryx Coated Pellet Filled Capsules 3357
- Periostat Tablets 1208
- Vibramycin Hyclate Capsules 2735
- Vibramycin Hyclate Intravenous 2737
- Vibra-Tabs Film Coated Tablets 2735

Doxycycline Monohydrate (Co-administration with other photosensitizing agents, such as tetracyclines, might increase photosensitivity reactions of actinic ketoses treated with aminolevulinic acid HCL). Products include:
- Monodox Capsules 2442
- Vibramycin Monohydrate for Oral Suspension 2735

Fluphenazine Decanoate (Co-administration with other photosensitizing agents, such as phenothiazines, might increase photosensitivity reactions of actinic ketoses treated with aminolevulinic acid HCL).
No products indexed under this heading.

Fluphenazine Enanthate (Co-administration with other photosensitizing agents, such as phenothiazines, might increase photosensitivity reactions of actinic ketoses treated with aminolevulinic acid HCL).
No products indexed under this heading.

Fluphenazine Hydrochloride (Co-administration with other photosensitizing agents, such as phenothiazines, might increase photosensitivity reactions of actinic ketoses treated with aminolevulinic acid HCL).
No products indexed under this heading.

Glimepiride (Co-administration with other photosensitizing agents, such as sulfonylureas, might increase photosensitivity reactions of actinic ketoses treated with aminolevulinic acid HCL). Products include:
- Amaryl Tablets 717

Glipizide (Co-administration with other photosensitizing agents, such as sulfonylureas, might increase photosensitivity reactions of actinic ketoses treated with aminolevulinic acid HCL). Products include:
- Glucotrol Tablets 2692
- Glucotrol XL Extended Release Tablets 2693

Glyburide (Co-administration with other photosensitizing agents, such as sulfonylureas, might increase photosensitivity reactions of actinic ketoses treated with aminolevulinic acid HCL). Products include:
- DiaBeta Tablets 741
- Glucovance Tablets 1086

Griseofulvin (Co-administration with other photosensitizing agents, such as griseofulvin, might increase photosensitivity reactions of actinic ketoses treated with aminolevulinic acid HCL). Products include:
- Grifulvin V Tablets Microsize and Oral Suspension Microsize 2518
- Gris-PEG Tablets 2661

Hydrochlorothiazide (Co-administration with other photosensitizing agents, such as thiazide diuretics, might increase photosensitivity reactions of actinic ketoses treated with aminolevulinic acid HCL). Products include:
- Accuretic Tablets 2614
- Aldoril Tablets 2039
- Atacand HCT Tablets 597
- Avalide Tablets 1070
- Diovan HCT Tablets 2338
- Dyazide Capsules 1515
- HydroDIURIL Tablets 2108
- Hyzaar 2109
- Inderide Tablets 3517
- Inderide LA Long-Acting Capsules 3519
- Lotensin HCT Tablets 2367
- Maxzide 1008
- Micardis HCT Tablets 1051
- Microzide Capsules 3414
- Moduretic Tablets 2138
- Monopril HCT 1094
- Prinzide Tablets 2168
- Timolide Tablets 2187
- Uniretic Tablets 3178
- Vaseretic Tablets 2204
- Zestoretic Tablets 695
- Ziac Tablets 1887

Hydroflumethiazide (Co-administration with other photosensitizing agents, such as thiazide diuretics, might increase photosensitivity reactions of actinic ketoses treated with aminolevulinic acid HCL). Products include:
- Diucardin Tablets 3494

Mesoridazine Besylate (Co-administration with other photosensitizing agents, such as phenothiazines, might increase photosensitivity reactions of actinic ketoses treated with aminolevulinic acid HCL). Products include:
- Serentil 1057

Methacycline Hydrochloride (Co-administration with other photosensitizing agents, such as tetracyclines, might increase photosensitivity reactions of actinic ketoses treated with aminolevulinic acid HCL).
No products indexed under this heading.

Methotrimeprazine (Co-administration with other photosensitizing agents, such as phenothiazines, might increase photosensitivity reactions of actinic ketoses treated with aminolevulinic acid HCL).
No products indexed under this heading.

Methyclothiazide (Co-administration with other photosensitizing agents, such as thiazide diuretics, might increase photosensitivity reactions of actinic ketoses treated with aminolevulinic acid HCL).
No products indexed under this heading.

Minocycline Hydrochloride (Co-administration with other photosensitizing agents, such as tetracyclines, might increase photosensitivity reactions of actinic ketoses treated with aminolevulinic acid HCL). Products include:
- Dynacin Capsules 2019
- Minocin Intravenous 1862
- Minocin Oral Suspension 1865
- Minocin Pellet-Filled Capsules 1863

Oxytetracycline Hydrochloride (Co-administration with other photosensitizing agents, such as tetracyclines, might increase photosensitivity reactions of actinic ketoses treated with aminolevulinic acid HCL). Products include:
- Terra-Cortril Ophthalmic Suspension 2716
- Urobiotic-250 Capsules 2731

Perphenazine (Co-administration with other photosensitizing agents, such as phenothiazines, might increase photosensitivity reactions of actinic ketoses treated with aminolevulinic acid HCL). Products include:
- Etrafon 3115
- Trilafon 3160

Polythiazide (Co-administration with other photosensitizing agents, such as thiazide diuretics, might increase photosensitivity reactions of actinic ketoses treated with aminolevulinic acid HCL). Products include:
- Minizide Capsules 2700
- Renese Tablets 2712

Prochlorperazine (Co-administration with other photosensitizing agents, such as phenothiazines, might increase photosensitivity reactions of actinic ketoses treated with aminolevulinic acid HCL). Products include:
- Compazine 1505

Promethazine Hydrochloride (Co-administration with other photosensitizing agents, such as phenothiazines, might increase photosensitivity reactions of actinic ketoses treated with aminolevulinic acid HCL). Products include:

- Mepergan Injection 3539
- Phenergan Injection 3553
- Phenergan 3556
- Phenergan Syrup 3554
- Phenergan with Codeine Syrup 3557
- Phenergan with Dextromethorphan Syrup 3559
- Phenergan VC Syrup 3560
- Phenergan VC with Codeine Syrup .. 3561

Sulfacytine (Co-administration with other photosensitizing agents, such as sulfonamides, might increase photosensitivity reactions of actinic ketoses treated with aminolevulinic acid HCL).

No products indexed under this heading.

Sulfamethizole (Co-administration with other photosensitizing agents, such as sulfonamides, might increase photosensitivity reactions of actinic ketoses treated with aminolevulinic acid HCL). Products include:

- Urobiotic-250 Capsules 2731

Sulfamethoxazole (Co-administration with other photosensitizing agents, such as sulfonamides, might increase photosensitivity reactions of actinic ketoses treated with aminolevulinic acid HCL). Products include:

- Bactrim 2949
- Septra Suspension 2265
- Septra Tablets 2265
- Septra DS Tablets 2265

Sulfasalazine (Co-administration with other photosensitizing agents, such as sulfonamides, might increase photosensitivity reactions of actinic ketoses treated with aminolevulinic acid HCL). Products include:

- Azulfidine EN-tabs Tablets 2775

Sulfinpyrazone (Co-administration with other photosensitizing agents, such as sulfonamides, might increase photosensitivity reactions of actinic ketoses treated with aminolevulinic acid HCL).

No products indexed under this heading.

Sulfisoxazole (Co-administration with other photosensitizing agents, such as sulfonamides, might increase photosensitivity reactions of actinic ketoses treated with aminolevulinic acid HCL).

No products indexed under this heading.

Sulfisoxazole Acetyl (Co-administration with other photosensitizing agents, such as sulfonamides, might increase photosensitivity reactions of actinic ketoses treated with aminolevulinic acid HCL). Products include:

- Pediazole Suspension 3050

Sulfisoxazole Diolamine (Co-administration with other photosensitizing agents, such as sulfonamides, might increase photosensitivity reactions of actinic ketoses treated with aminolevulinic acid HCL).

No products indexed under this heading.

Tetracycline Hydrochloride (Co-administration with other photosensitizing agents, such as tetracyclines, might increase photosensitivity reactions of actinic ketoses treated with aminolevulinic acid HCL).

No products indexed under this heading.

Thioridazine Hydrochloride (Co-administration with other photosensitizing agents, such as phenothiazines, might increase photosensitivity reactions of actinic ketoses treated with aminolevulinic acid HCL). Products include:

- Thioridazine Hydrochloride Tablets 2289

Tolazamide (Co-administration with other photosensitizing agents, such as sulfonylureas, might increase photosensitivity reactions of actinic ketoses treated with aminolevulinic acid HCL).

No products indexed under this heading.

Tolbutamide (Co-administration with other photosensitizing agents, such as sulfonylureas, might increase photosensitivity reactions of actinic ketoses treated with aminolevulinic acid HCL).

No products indexed under this heading.

Trifluoperazine Hydrochloride (Co-administration with other photosensitizing agents, such as phenothiazines, might increase photosensitivity reactions of actinic ketoses treated with aminolevulinic acid HCL). Products include:

- Stelazine 1640

LEXXEL TABLETS

(Enalapril Maleate, Felodipine) 608

May interact with diuretics, anticonvulsants, erythromycin, lithium preparations, non-steroidal anti-inflammatory agents, potassium preparations, potassium sparing diuretics, agents causing renin release, and certain other agents. Compounds in these categories include:

Amiloride Hydrochloride (Co-administration with potassium-sparing diuretics may lead to significant increase in serum potassium). Products include:

- Midamor Tablets 2136
- Moduretic Tablets 2138

Bendroflumethiazide (The antihypertensive effect of enalapril is augmented by agents that cause renin release; potential for excessive hypotension). Products include:

- Corzide 40/5 Tablets 2247
- Corzide 80/5 Tablets 2247

Bumetanide (Co-administration in patients on diuretics, especially those in whom diuretic therapy was recently instituted, may experience an excessive hypotension after initiation of therapy with enalapril).

No products indexed under this heading.

Carbamazepine (Maximum plasma concentrations of felodipine can be considerably lower in epileptic patients on long-term anticonvulsant therapy). Products include:

- Carbatrol Capsules 3234
- Tegretol/Tegretol-XR 2404

Celecoxib (Co-administration of enalapril in some patients with compromised renal function who are being treated with non-steroidal anti-inflammatory drugs may result in a further deterioration of renal function; these effects are usually reversible). Products include:

- Celebrex Capsules 2676
- Celebrex Capsules 2780

Chlorothiazide (The antihypertensive effect of enalapril is augmented by agents that cause renin release; potential for excessive hypotension). Products include:

- Aldoclor Tablets 2035
- Diuril Oral 2087

Chlorothiazide Sodium (The antihypertensive effect of enalapril is augmented by agents that cause renin release; potential for excessive hypotension). Products include:

- Diuril Sodium Intravenous 2086

Chlorthalidone (Co-administration in patients on diuretics, especially those in whom diuretic therapy was recently instituted, may experience an excessive hypotension after initiation of therapy with enalapril). Products include:

- Clorpres Tablets 1002
- Combipres Tablets 1040
- Tenoretic Tablets 690

Cimetidine (Co-administration has resulted in an approximately 50% increase in the AUC and Cmax of felodipine; clinically significant interaction may occur in some hypertensive patients). Products include:

- Tagamet HB 200 Suspension 762
- Tagamet HB 200 Tablets 761
- Tagamet Tablets 1644

Cimetidine Hydrochloride (Co-administration has resulted in an approximately 50% increase in the AUC and Cmax of felodipine; clinically significant interaction may occur in some hypertensive patients). Products include:

- Tagamet 1644

Diclofenac Potassium (Co-administration of enalapril in some patients with compromised renal function who are being treated with non-steroidal anti-inflammatory drugs may result in a further deterioration of renal function; these effects are usually reversible). Products include:

- Cataflam Tablets 2315

Diclofenac Sodium (Co-administration of enalapril in some patients with compromised renal function who are being treated with non-steroidal anti-inflammatory drugs may result in a further deterioration of renal function; these effects are usually reversible). Products include:

- Arthrotec Tablets 3195
- Voltaren Ophthalmic Sterile Ophthalmic Solution .... ⊙ 312
- Voltaren Tablets 2315
- Voltaren-XR Tablets 2315

Divalproex Sodium (Maximum plasma concentrations of felodipine can be considerably lower in epileptic patients on long-term anticonvulsant therapy). Products include:

- Depakote Sprinkle Capsules 426
- Depakote Tablets 430
- Depakote ER Tablets 436

Erythromycin (Co-administration of felodipine with erythromycin has resulted in approximately 2.5-fold increase in the AUC and Cmax, but no prolongation in the half-life of felodipine). Products include:

- Emgel 2% Topical Gel 1285
- Ery-Tab Tablets 448
- Erythromycin Base Filmtab Tablets .. 454
- Erythromycin Delayed-Release Capsules, USP 455
- PCE Dispertab Tablets 498

Erythromycin Estolate (Co-administration of felodipine with erythromycin has resulted in approximately 2.5-fold increase in the AUC and Cmax, but no prolongation in the half-life of felodipine).

No products indexed under this heading.

Erythromycin Ethylsuccinate (Co-administration of felodipine with erythromycin has resulted in approximately 2.5-fold increase in the AUC and Cmax, but no prolongation in the half-life of felodipine). Products include:

- E.E.S. 450
- EryPed 446
- Pediazole Suspension 3050

Erythromycin Gluceptate (Co-administration of felodipine with erythromycin has resulted in approximately 2.5-fold increase in the AUC and Cmax, but no prolongation in the half-life of felodipine).

No products indexed under this heading.

Erythromycin Stearate (Co-administration of felodipine with erythromycin has resulted in approximately 2.5-fold increase in the AUC and Cmax, but no prolongation in the half-life of felodipine). Products include:

- Erythrocin Stearate Filmtab Tablets 452

Ethacrynic Acid (Co-administration in patients on diuretics, especially those in whom diuretic therapy was recently instituted, may experience an excessive hypotension after initiation of therapy with enalapril). Products include:

- Edecrin Tablets 2091

Ethosuximide (Maximum plasma concentrations of felodipine can be considerably lower in epileptic patients on long-term anticonvulsant therapy). Products include:

- Zarontin Capsules 2659
- Zarontin Syrup 2660

Ethotoin (Maximum plasma concentrations of felodipine can be considerably lower in epileptic patients on long-term anticonvulsant therapy).

No products indexed under this heading.

Etodolac (Co-administration of enalapril in some patients with compromised renal function who are being treated with non-steroidal anti-inflammatory drugs may result in a further deterioration of renal function; these effects are usually reversible). Products include:

- Lodine 3528
- Lodine XL Extended-Release Tablets 3530

Felbamate (Maximum plasma concentrations of felodipine can be considerably lower in epileptic patients on long-term anticonvulsant therapy). Products include:

- Felbatol 3343

Fenoprofen Calcium (Co-administration of enalapril in some patients with compromised renal function who are being treated with non-steroidal anti-inflammatory drugs may result in a further deterioration of renal function; these effects are usually reversible).

No products indexed under this heading.

Flurbiprofen (Co-administration of enalapril in some patients with compromised renal function who are being treated with non-steroidal anti-inflammatory drugs may result in a further deterioration of renal function; these effects are usually reversible).

No products indexed under this heading.

Fosphenytoin Sodium (Maximum plasma concentrations of felodipine can be considerably lower in epileptic patients on long-term anticonvulsant therapy). Products include:

- Cerebyx Injection 2619

Furosemide (Co-administration in patients on diuretics, especially those in whom diuretic therapy was recently instituted, may experience an excessive hypotension after initiation of therapy with enalapril). Products include:

- Furosemide Tablets 2284

Hydrochlorothiazide (The antihypertensive effect of enalapril is augmented by agents that cause renin release; potential for excessive hypotension). Products include:

- Accuretic Tablets 2614
- Aldoril Tablets 2039
- Atacand HCT Tablets 597
- Avalide Tablets 1070
- Diovan HCT Tablets 2338
- Dyazide Capsules 1515
- HydroDIURIL Tablets 2108
- Hyzaar 2109
- Inderide Tablets 3517
- Inderide LA Long-Acting Capsules .. 3519
- Lotensin HCT Tablets 2367
- Maxzide 1008
- Micardis HCT Tablets 1051
- Microzide Capsules 3414

Moduretic Tablets 2138
Monopril HCT 1094
Prinzide Tablets 2168
Timolide Tablets 2187
Uniretic Tablets 3178
Vaseretic Tablets 2204
Zestoretic Tablets 695
Ziac Tablets 1887

Hydroflumethiazide (The antihypertensive effect of enalapril is augmented by agents that cause renin release; potential for excessive hypotension). Products include:
Diucardin Tablets 3494

Ibuprofen (Co-administration of enalapril in some patients with compromised renal function who are being treated with non-steroidal anti-inflammatory drugs may result in a further deterioration of renal function; these effects are usually reversible). Products include:
Advil .... ▣ 771
Children's Advil Oral Suspension ... ▣ 773
Children's Advil Chewable Tablets . ▣ 773
Advil Cold and Sinus Caplets .... ▣ 771
Advil Cold and Sinus Tablets .... ▣ 771
Advil Flu & Body Ache Caplets .... ▣ 772
Infants' Advil Drops .... ▣ 773
Junior Strength Advil Tablets .... ▣ 773
Junior Strength Advil Chewable Tablets .... ▣ 773
Advil Migraine Liquigels .... ▣ 772
Children's Motrin Oral Suspension and Chewable Tablets 2006
Children's Motrin Cold Oral Suspension 2007
Children's Motrin Oral Suspension .... ▣ 643
Motrin Suspension, Oral Drops, Chewable Tablets, and Caplets 2002
Infants' Motrin Concentrated Drops 2006
Junior Strength Motrin Caplets and Chewable Tablets 2006
Motrin IB Tablets, Caplets, and Gelcaps 2002
Motrin Migraine Pain Caplets 2005
Motrin Sinus Headache Caplets 2005
Vicoprofen Tablets 520

Indapamide (Co-administration in patients on diuretics, especially those in whom diuretic therapy was recently instituted, may experience an excessive hypotension after initiation of therapy with enalapril). Products include:
Indapamide Tablets 2286

Indomethacin (Co-administration of enalapril in some patients with compromised renal function who are being treated with non-steroidal anti-inflammatory drugs may result in a further deterioration of renal function; these effects are usually reversible). Products include:
Indocin 2112

Indomethacin Sodium Trihydrate (Co-administration of enalapril in some patients with compromised renal function who are being treated with non-steroidal anti-inflammatory drugs may result in a further deterioration of renal function; these effects are usually reversible). Products include:
Indocin I.V. 2115

Itraconazole (Felodipine is metabolized by CYP3A4; co-administration of CYP3A4 inhibitors, such as itraconazole, with another extended release formulation of felodipine has resulted in approximately 8-fold increase in the AUC, more than 6-fold increase in the Cmax, and 2-fold prolongation in the half-life of felodpine). Products include:
Sporanox Capsules 1800
Sporanox Injection 1804
Sporanox Injection 2509
Sporanox Oral Solution 1808
Sporanox Oral Solution 2512

Ketoconazole (Felodipine is metabolized by CYP3A4; co-administration of CYP3A4 inhibitors, such as ketoconazole, with felodipine may lead to several-fold increases in the plasma levels of felodipine). Products include:
Nizoral 2% Cream 3620
Nizoral A-D Shampoo 2008
Nizoral 2% Shampoo 2007
Nizoral Tablets 1791

Ketoprofen (Co-administration of enalapril in some patients with compromised renal function who are being treated with non-steroidal anti-inflammatory drugs may result in a further deterioration of renal function; these effects are usually reversible). Products include:
Orudis Capsules 3548
Orudis KT Tablets .... ▣ 778
Oruvail Capsules 3548

Ketorolac Tromethamine (Co-administration of enalapril in some patients with compromised renal function who are being treated with non-steroidal anti-inflammatory drugs may result in a further deterioration of renal function; these effects are usually reversible). Products include:
Acular Ophthalmic Solution 544
Acular PF Ophthalmic Solution 544
Toradol 3018

Lamotrigine (Maximum plasma concentrations of felodipine can be considerably lower in epileptic patients on long-term anticonvulsant therapy). Products include:
Lamictal 1567

Levetiracetam (Maximum plasma concentrations of felodipine can be considerably lower in epileptic patients on long-term anticonvulsant therapy). Products include:
Keppra Tablets 3314

Lithium Carbonate (Co-administration can lead to lithium toxicity; frequent monitoring of serum lithium levels is recommended). Products include:
Eskalith 1527
Lithium Carbonate 3061
Lithobid Slow-Release Tablets 3255

Lithium Citrate (Co-administration can lead to lithium toxicity; frequent monitoring of serum lithium levels is recommended). Products include:
Lithium Citrate Syrup 3061

Meclofenamate Sodium (Co-administration of enalapril in some patients with compromised renal function who are being treated with non-steroidal anti-inflammatory drugs may result in a further deterioration of renal function; these effects are usually reversible).
No products indexed under this heading.

Mefenamic Acid (Co-administration of enalapril in some patients with compromised renal function who are being treated with non-steroidal anti-inflammatory drugs may result in a further deterioration of renal function; these effects are usually reversible). Products include:
Ponstel Capsules 1356

Meloxicam (Co-administration of enalapril in some patients with compromised renal function who are being treated with non-steroidal anti-inflammatory drugs may result in a further deterioration of renal function; these effects are usually reversible). Products include:
Mobic Tablets 1054

Mephenytoin (Maximum plasma concentrations of felodipine can be considerably lower in epileptic patients on long-term anticonvulsant therapy).
No products indexed under this heading.

Methsuximide (Maximum plasma concentrations of felodipine can be considerably lower in epileptic patients on long-term anticonvulsant therapy). Products include:
Celontin Capsules 2618

Methyclothiazide (The antihypertensive effect of enalapril is augmented by agents that cause renin release; potential for excessive hypotension).
No products indexed under this heading.

Metolazone (Co-administration in patients on diuretics, especially those in whom diuretic therapy was recently instituted, may experience an excessive hypotension after initiation of therapy with enalapril). Products include:
Mykrox Tablets 1168
Zaroxolyn Tablets 1177

Metoprolol Succinate (Co-administration has resulted in an increase in the AUC (31%) and Cmax (38%) of metoprolol). Products include:
Toprol-XL Tablets 651

Metoprolol Tartrate (Co-administration has resulted in an increase in the AUC (31%) and Cmax (38%) of metoprolol).
No products indexed under this heading.

Nabumetone (Co-administration of enalapril in some patients with compromised renal function who are being treated with non-steroidal anti-inflammatory drugs may result in a further deterioration of renal function; these effects are usually reversible). Products include:
Relafen Tablets 1617

Naproxen (Co-administration of enalapril in some patients with compromised renal function who are being treated with non-steroidal anti-inflammatory drugs may result in a further deterioration of renal function; these effects are usually reversible). Products include:
EC-Naprosyn Delayed-Release Tablets 2967
Naprosyn Suspension 2967
Naprosyn Tablets 2967

Naproxen Sodium (Co-administration of enalapril in some patients with compromised renal function who are being treated with non-steroidal anti-inflammatory drugs may result in a further deterioration of renal function; these effects are usually reversible). Products include:
Aleve Tablets, Caplets and Gelcaps .... ▣ 602
Aleve Cold & Sinus Caplets .... ▣ 603
Anaprox Tablets 2967
Anaprox DS Tablets 2967
Naprelan Tablets 1293

Oxaprozin (Co-administration of enalapril in some patients with compromised renal function who are being treated with non-steroidal anti-inflammatory drugs may result in a further deterioration of renal function; these effects are usually reversible).
No products indexed under this heading.

Oxcarbazepine (Maximum plasma concentrations of felodipine can be considerably lower in epileptic patients on long-term anticonvulsant therapy). Products include:
Trileptal Oral Suspension 2407
Trileptal Tablets 2407

Paramethadione (Maximum plasma concentrations of felodipine can be considerably lower in epileptic patients on long-term anticonvulsant therapy).
No products indexed under this heading.

Phenacemide (Maximum plasma concentrations of felodipine can be considerably lower in epileptic patients on long-term anticonvulsant therapy).
No products indexed under this heading.

Phenobarbital (Maximum plasma concentrations of felodipine can be considerably lower in epileptic patients on long-term anticonvulsant therapy). Products include:
Arco-Lase Plus Tablets 592
Donnatal 2929
Donnatal Extentabs 2930

Phensuximide (Maximum plasma concentrations of felodipine can be considerably lower in epileptic patients on long-term anticonvulsant therapy).
No products indexed under this heading.

Phenylbutazone (Co-administration of enalapril in some patients with compromised renal function who are being treated with non-steroidal anti-inflammatory drugs may result in a further deterioration of renal function; these effects are usually reversible).
No products indexed under this heading.

Phenytoin (Maximum plasma concentrations of felodipine can be considerably lower in epileptic patients on long-term anticonvulsant therapy). Products include:
Dilantin Infatabs 2624
Dilantin-125 Oral Suspension 2625

Phenytoin Sodium (Maximum plasma concentrations of felodipine can be considerably lower in epileptic patients on long-term anticonvulsant therapy). Products include:
Dilantin Kapseals 2622

Piroxicam (Co-administration of enalapril in some patients with compromised renal function who are being treated with non-steroidal anti-inflammatory drugs may result in a further deterioration of renal function; these effects are usually reversible). Products include:
Feldene Capsules 2685

Polythiazide (The antihypertensive effect of enalapril is augmented by agents that cause renin release; potential for excessive hypotension). Products include:
Minizide Capsules 2700
Renese Tablets 2712

Potassium Acid Phosphate (Co-administration may lead to significant increase in serum potassium). Products include:
K-Phos Original (Sodium Free) Tablets 947

Potassium Bicarbonate (Co-administration may lead to significant increase in serum potassium).
No products indexed under this heading.

Potassium Chloride (Co-administration may lead to significant increase in serum potassium). Products include:
Chlor-3 1361
Colyte with Flavor Packs for Oral Solution 3170
GoLYTELY and Pineapple Flavor GoLYTELY for Oral Solution 1068
K-Dur Microburst Release System ER Tablets 1832
Klor-Con M20/Klor-Con M10 Tablets 3329
K-Lor Powder Packets 469
K-Tab Filmtab Tablets 470
Micro-K 3311
NuLYTELY, Cherry Flavor, Lemon-Lime Flavor, and Orange Flavor NuLYTELY for Oral Solution 1068
Rum-K 1363

Potassium Citrate (Co-administration may lead to significant increase in serum potassium). Products include:
Urocit-K Tablets 2232

Potassium Gluconate (Co-administration may lead to significant increase in serum potassium).
No products indexed under this heading.

Potassium Phosphate (Co-administration may lead to significant increase in serum potassium). Products include:
K-Phos Neutral Tablets 946

Primidone (Maximum plasma concentrations of felodipine can be considerably lower in epileptic patients on long-term anticonvulsant therapy).
No products indexed under this heading.

Rofecoxib (Co-administration of enalapril in some patients with compromised renal function who are being treated with non-steroidal anti-inflammatory drugs may result in a further deterioration of renal function; these effects are usually reversible). Products include:
Vioxx 2213

Spironolactone (Co-administration with potassium-sparing diuretics may lead to significant increase in serum potassium).
No products indexed under this heading.

Sulindac (Co-administration of enalapril in some patients with compromised renal function who are being treated with non-steroidal anti-inflammatory drugs may result in a further deterioration of renal function; these effects are usually reversible). Products include:
Clinoril Tablets 2053

Tiagabine Hydrochloride (Maximum plasma concentrations of felodipine can be considerably lower in epileptic patients on long-term anticonvulsant therapy). Products include:
Gabitril Tablets 1189

Tolmetin Sodium (Co-administration of enalapril in some patients with compromised renal function who are being treated with non-steroidal anti-inflammatory drugs may result in a further deterioration of renal function; these effects are usually reversible). Products include:
Tolectin 2589

Topiramate (Maximum plasma concentrations of felodipine can be considerably lower in epileptic patients on long-term anticonvulsant therapy). Products include:
Topamax Sprinkle Capsules 2590
Topamax Tablets 2590

Torsemide (Co-administration in patients on diuretics, especially those in whom diuretic therapy was recently instituted, may experience an excessive hypotension after initiation of therapy with enalapril). Products include:
Demadex Tablets and Injection 2965

Triamterene (Co-administration with potassium-sparing diuretics may lead to significant increase in serum potassium). Products include:
Dyazide Capsules 1515
Dyrenium Capsules 3458
Maxzide 1008

Trimethadione (Maximum plasma concentrations of felodipine can be considerably lower in epileptic patients on long-term anticonvulsant therapy).
No products indexed under this heading.

Valproate Sodium (Maximum plasma concentrations of felodipine can be considerably lower in epileptic patients on long-term anticonvulsant therapy). Products include:
Depacon Injection 416

Valproic Acid (Maximum plasma concentrations of felodipine can be considerably lower in epileptic patients on long-term anticonvulsant therapy). Products include:
Depakene 421

Zonisamide (Maximum plasma concentrations of felodipine can be considerably lower in epileptic patients on long-term anticonvulsant therapy). Products include:
Zonegran Capsules 1307

Food Interactions

Food, unspecified (When Lexxel is taken with food (a substantial meal of 650 Kcal or greater), some of the pharmacokinetics of its components are changed; Lexxel should be regularly taken either without food or with a light meal).

Grapefruit Juice (Felodipine is metabolized by CYP3A4; co-administration of CYP3A4 inhibitors, such as grapefruit juice has resulted in more than 2-fold increase in the AUC and Cmax).

LIBRIUM CAPSULES

(Chlordiazepoxide Hydrochloride) 1736
May interact with central nervous system depressants, oral anticoagulants, monoamine oxidase inhibitors, phenothiazines, and certain other agents. Compounds in these categories include:

Alfentanil Hydrochloride (Potential for additive effects).
No products indexed under this heading.

Alprazolam (Potential for additive effects). Products include:
Xanax Tablets 2865

Aprobarbital (Potential for additive effects).
No products indexed under this heading.

Buprenorphine Hydrochloride (Potential for additive effects). Products include:
Buprenex Injectable 2918

Buspirone Hydrochloride (Potential for additive effects).
No products indexed under this heading.

Butabarbital (Potential for additive effects).
No products indexed under this heading.

Butalbital (Potential for additive effects). Products include:
Phrenilin 578
Sedapap Tablets 50 mg/650 mg 2225

Chlordiazepoxide (Potential for additive effects). Products include:
Limbitrol 1738

Chlorpromazine (Concomitant use should be avoided due to the possibility of potentiation). Products include:
Thorazine Suppositories 1656

Chlorpromazine Hydrochloride (Concomitant use should be avoided due to the possibility of potentiation). Products include:
Thorazine 1656

Chlorprothixene (Potential for additive effects).
No products indexed under this heading.

Chlorprothixene Hydrochloride (Potential for additive effects).
No products indexed under this heading.

Chlorprothixene Lactate (Potential for additive effects).
No products indexed under this heading.

Clorazepate Dipotassium (Potential for additive effects). Products include:
Tranxene 511

Clozapine (Potential for additive effects). Products include:
Clozaril Tablets 2319

Codeine Phosphate (Potential for additive effects). Products include:
Phenergan with Codeine Syrup 3557
Phenergan VC with Codeine Syrup 3561
Robitussin A-C Syrup 2942
Robitussin-DAC Syrup 2942
Ryna-C Liquid 768
Soma Compound w/Codeine Tablets 3355
Tussi-Organidin NR Liquid 3350
Tussi-Organidin-S NR Liquid 3350
Tylenol with Codeine 2595

Desflurane (Potential for additive effects). Products include:
Suprane Liquid for Inhalation 874

Dezocine (Potential for additive effects).
No products indexed under this heading.

Diazepam (Potential for additive effects). Products include:
Valium Injectable 3026
Valium Tablets 3047

Dicumarol (Variable effects on blood coagulation have been reported very rarely with concomitant use).
No products indexed under this heading.

Droperidol (Potential for additive effects).
No products indexed under this heading.

Enflurane (Potential for additive effects).
No products indexed under this heading.

Estazolam (Potential for additive effects). Products include:
ProSom Tablets 500

Ethchlorvynol (Potential for additive effects).
No products indexed under this heading.

Ethinamate (Potential for additive effects).
No products indexed under this heading.

Fentanyl (Potential for additive effects). Products include:
Duragesic Transdermal System 1786

Fentanyl Citrate (Potential for additive effects). Products include:
Actiq 1184

Fluphenazine Decanoate (Concomitant use should be avoided due to the possibility of potentiation).
No products indexed under this heading.

Fluphenazine Enanthate (Concomitant use should be avoided due to the possibility of potentiation).
No products indexed under this heading.

Fluphenazine Hydrochloride (Concomitant use should be avoided due to the possibility of potentiation).
No products indexed under this heading.

Flurazepam Hydrochloride (Potential for additive effects).
No products indexed under this heading.

Glutethimide (Potential for additive effects).
No products indexed under this heading.

Haloperidol (Potential for additive effects). Products include:
Haldol Injection, Tablets and Concentrate 2533

Haloperidol Decanoate (Potential for additive effects). Products include:
Haldol Decanoate 2535

Hydrocodone Bitartrate (Potential for additive effects). Products include:
Hycodan 1316
Hycomine Compound Tablets 1317
Hycotuss Expectorant Syrup 1318
Lortab 3319
Lortab Elixir 3317
Maxidone Tablets CIII 3399
Norco 5/325 Tablets CIII 3424
Norco 7.5/325 Tablets CIII 3425
Norco 10/325 Tablets CIII 3427
Norco 10/325 Tablets CIII 3425
Vicodin Tablets 516
Vicodin ES Tablets 517
Vicodin HP Tablets 518
Vicodin Tuss Expectorant 519
Vicoprofen Tablets 520
Zydone Tablets 1330

Hydrocodone Polistirex (Potential for additive effects). Products include:
Tussionex Pennkinetic Extended-Release Suspension 1174

Hydromorphone Hydrochloride (Potential for additive effects). Products include:
Dilaudid 441
Dilaudid Oral Liquid 445
Dilaudid Powder 441
Dilaudid Rectal Suppositories 441
Dilaudid Tablets 441
Dilaudid Tablets - 8 mg 445
Dilaudid-HP 443

Hydroxyzine Hydrochloride (Potential for additive effects). Products include:
Atarax Tablets & Syrup 2667
Vistaril Intramuscular Solution 2738

Isocarboxazid (Concomitant use should be avoided due to the possibility of potentiation).
No products indexed under this heading.

Isoflurane (Potential for additive effects).
No products indexed under this heading.

Ketamine Hydrochloride (Potential for additive effects).
No products indexed under this heading.

Levomethadyl Acetate Hydrochloride (Potential for additive effects).
No products indexed under this heading.

Levorphanol Tartrate (Potential for additive effects). Products include:
Levo-Dromoran 1734
Levorphanol Tartrate Tablets 3059

Lorazepam (Potential for additive effects). Products include:
Ativan Injection 3478
Ativan Tablets 3482

Loxapine Hydrochloride (Potential for additive effects).
No products indexed under this heading.

Loxapine Succinate (Potential for additive effects). Products include:
Loxitane Capsules 3398

Meperidine Hydrochloride (Potential for additive effects). Products include:
Demerol 3079
Mepergan Injection 3539

Mephobarbital (Potential for additive effects).
No products indexed under this heading.

Meprobamate (Potential for additive effects). Products include:
Miltown Tablets 3349

Mesoridazine Besylate (Concomitant use should be avoided due to the possibility of potentiation). Products include:
Serentil 1057

Methadone Hydrochloride (Potential for additive effects). Products include:
Dolophine Hydrochloride Tablets 3056

Methohexital Sodium (Potential for additive effects). Products include:
Brevital Sodium for Injection, USP 1815

Methotrimeprazine (Concomitant use should be avoided due to the possibility of potentiation).
No products indexed under this heading.

Methoxyflurane (Potential for additive effects).
No products indexed under this heading.

Midazolam Hydrochloride (Potential for additive effects). Products include:
Versed Injection 3027
Versed Syrup 3033

Moclobemide (Concomitant use should be avoided due to the possi-

IMPORTANT NOTE: Always consult each drug listing in the patient's regimen for possible interactions.

bility of potentiation).
No products indexed under this heading.

Molindone Hydrochloride (Potential for additive effects). Products include:
Moban ... 1320

Morphine Sulfate (Potential for additive effects). Products include:
Astramorph/PF Injection, USP (Preservative-Free) ... 594
Duramorph Injection ... 1312
Infumorph 200 and Infumorph 500 Sterile Solutions ... 1314
Kadian Capsules ... 1335
MS Contin Tablets ... 2896
MSIR ... 2898
Oramorph SR Tablets ... 3062
Roxanol ... 3066

Olanzapine (Potential for additive effects). Products include:
Zyprexa Tablets ... 1973
Zyprexa ZYDIS Orally Disintegrating Tablets ... 1973

Oxazepam (Potential for additive effects).
No products indexed under this heading.

Oxycodone Hydrochloride (Potential for additive effects). Products include:
OxyContin Tablets ... 2912
OxyFast Oral Concentrate Solution . 2916
OxyIR Capsules ... 2916
Percocet Tablets ... 1326
Percodan Tablets ... 1327
Percolone Tablets ... 1327
Roxicodone ... 3067
Tylox Capsules ... 2597

Pargyline Hydrochloride (Concomitant use should be avoided due to the possibility of potentiation).
No products indexed under this heading.

Pentobarbital Sodium (Potential for additive effects). Products include:
Nembutal Sodium Solution ... 485

Perphenazine (Concomitant use should be avoided due to the possibility of potentiation). Products include:
Etrafon ... 3115
Trilafon ... 3160

Phenelzine Sulfate (Concomitant use should be avoided due to the possibility of potentiation). Products include:
Nardil Tablets ... 2653

Phenobarbital (Potential for additive effects). Products include:
Arco-Lase Plus Tablets ... 592
Donnatal ... 2929
Donnatal Extentabs ... 2930

Prazepam (Potential for additive effects).
No products indexed under this heading.

Procarbazine Hydrochloride (Concomitant use should be avoided due to the possibility of potentiation). Products include:
Matulane Capsules ... 3246

Prochlorperazine (Concomitant use should be avoided due to the possibility of potentiation). Products include:
Compazine ... 1505

Promethazine Hydrochloride (Concomitant use should be avoided due to the possibility of potentiation). Products include:
Mepergan Injection ... 3539
Phenergan Injection ... 3553
Phenergan ... 3556
Phenergan Syrup ... 3554
Phenergan with Codeine Syrup ... 3557
Phenergan with Dextromethorphan Syrup ... 3559
Phenergan VC Syrup ... 3560
Phenergan VC with Codeine Syrup .. 3561

Propofol (Potential for additive effects). Products include:
Diprivan Injectable Emulsion ... 667

Propoxyphene Hydrochloride (Potential for additive effects). Products include:
Darvon Pulvules ... 1909
Darvon Compound-65 Pulvules ... 1910

Propoxyphene Napsylate (Potential for additive effects). Products include:
Darvon-N/Darvocet-N ... 1907
Darvon-N Tablets ... 1912

Quazepam (Potential for additive effects).
No products indexed under this heading.

Quetiapine Fumarate (Potential for additive effects). Products include:
Seroquel Tablets ... 684

Remifentanil Hydrochloride (Potential for additive effects).
No products indexed under this heading.

Risperidone (Potential for additive effects). Products include:
Risperdal ... 1796

Secobarbital Sodium (Potential for additive effects).
No products indexed under this heading.

Selegiline Hydrochloride (Concomitant use should be avoided due to the possibility of potentiation). Products include:
Eldepryl Capsules ... 3266

Sevoflurane (Potential for additive effects).
No products indexed under this heading.

Sufentanil Citrate (Potential for additive effects).
No products indexed under this heading.

Temazepam (Potential for additive effects).
No products indexed under this heading.

Thiamylal Sodium (Potential for additive effects).
No products indexed under this heading.

Thioridazine Hydrochloride (Concomitant use should be avoided due to the possibility of potentiation). Products include:
Thioridazine Hydrochloride Tablets ... 2289

Thiothixene (Potential for additive effects). Products include:
Navane Capsules ... 2701
Thiothixene Capsules ... 2290

Tranylcypromine Sulfate (Concomitant use should be avoided due to the possibility of potentiation). Products include:
Parnate Tablets ... 1607

Triazolam (Potential for additive effects). Products include:
Halcion Tablets ... 2823

Trifluoperazine Hydrochloride (Concomitant use should be avoided due to the possibility of potentiation). Products include:
Stelazine ... 1640

Warfarin Sodium (Variable effects on blood coagulation have been reported very rarely with concomitant use). Products include:
Coumadin for Injection ... 1243
Coumadin Tablets ... 1243
Warfarin Sodium Tablets, USP ... 3302

Zaleplon (Potential for additive effects). Products include:
Sonata Capsules ... 3591

Ziprasidone Hydrochloride (Potential for additive effects). Products include:
Geodon Capsules ... 2688

Zolpidem Tartrate (Potential for additive effects). Products include:
Ambien Tablets ... 3191

Food Interactions

Alcohol (Potential for additive effects).

LIBRIUM FOR INJECTION
(Chlordiazepoxide Hydrochloride) ... 1737
See Librium Capsules

LIDEX CREAM
(Fluocinonide) ... 2020
None cited in PDR database.

LIDEX GEL
(Fluocinonide) ... 2020
None cited in PDR database.

LIDEX OINTMENT
(Fluocinonide) ... 2020
None cited in PDR database.

LIDEX TOPICAL SOLUTION
(Fluocinonide) ... 2020
None cited in PDR database.

LIDEX-E CREAM
(Fluocinonide) ... 2020
None cited in PDR database.

LIDODERM PATCH
(Lidocaine) ... 1319
May interact with:

Mexiletine Hydrochloride (Co-administration in patients receiving Class-1 antiarrhythmic drugs, such as mexiletine, may result in additive toxic effects). Products include:
Mexitil Capsules ... 1047

Tocainide Hydrochloride (Co-administration in patients receiving Class-1 antiarrhythmic drugs, such as tocainide, may result in additive toxic effects). Products include:
Tonocard Tablets ... 649

LIMBITROL TABLETS
(Amitriptyline Hydrochloride, Chlordiazepoxide) ... 1738
May interact with anticholinergics, central nervous system depressants, antidepressant drugs, monoamine oxidase inhibitors, phenothiazines, quinidine, thyroid preparations, and certain other agents. Compounds in these categories include:

Alfentanil Hydrochloride (Co-administration may produce additive effects resulting in harmful level of sedation and CNS depression).
No products indexed under this heading.

Alprazolam (Co-administration may produce additive effects resulting in harmful level of sedation and CNS depression). Products include:
Xanax Tablets ... 2865

Amoxapine (May inhibit the activity of cytochrome P450 2D6 isoenzyme and are substrates for P450 2D6 and may make normal metabolizers resemble poor metabolizers resulting in higher than expected plasma levels of tricyclic antidepressants).
No products indexed under this heading.

Aprobarbital (Co-administration may produce additive effects resulting in harmful level of sedation and CNS depression).
No products indexed under this heading.

Atropine Sulfate (Severe constipation may result with concurrent use of tricyclic antidepressants and anticholinergic drugs). Products include:
Donnatal ... 2929
Donnatal Extentabs ... 2930
Motofen Tablets ... 577
Prosed/DS Tablets ... 3268
Urised Tablets ... 2876

Belladonna Alkaloids (Severe constipation may result with concurrent use of tricyclic antidepressants and anticholinergic drugs). Products include:
Hyland's Teething Tablets ... ▣766
Urimax Tablets ... 1769

Benztropine Mesylate (Severe constipation may result with concurrent use of tricyclic antidepressants and anticholinergic drugs). Products include:
Cogentin ... 2055

Biperiden Hydrochloride (Severe constipation may result with concurrent use of tricyclic antidepressants and anticholinergic drugs). Products include:
Akineton ... 402

Buprenorphine Hydrochloride (Co-administration may produce additive effects resulting in harmful level of sedation and CNS depression). Products include:
Buprenex Injectable ... 2918

Bupropion Hydrochloride (May inhibit the activity of cytochrome P450 2D6 isoenzyme and are substrates for P450 2D6 and may make normal metabolizers resemble poor metabolizers resulting in higher than expected plasma levels of tricyclic antidepressants). Products include:
Wellbutrin Tablets ... 1680
Wellbutrin SR Sustained-Release Tablets ... 1684
Zyban Sustained-Release Tablets ... 1710

Buspirone Hydrochloride (Co-administration may produce additive effects resulting in harmful level of sedation and CNS depression).
No products indexed under this heading.

Butabarbital (Co-administration may produce additive effects resulting in harmful level of sedation and CNS depression).
No products indexed under this heading.

Butalbital (Co-administration may produce additive effects resulting in harmful level of sedation and CNS depression). Products include:
Phrenilin ... 578
Sedapap Tablets 50 mg/650 mg ... 2225

Chlordiazepoxide Hydrochloride (Co-administration may produce additive effects resulting in harmful level of sedation and CNS depression). Products include:
Librium Capsules ... 1736
Librium for Injection ... 1737

Chlorpromazine (May inhibit the activity of cytochrome P450 2D6 isoenzyme and are substrates for P450 2D6 and may make normal metabolizers resemble poor metabolizers resulting in higher than expected plasma levels of tricyclic antidepressants; co-administration may produce additive effects resulting in harmful level of sedation and CNS depression). Products include:
Thorazine Suppositories ... 1656

Chlorpromazine Hydrochloride (May inhibit the activity of cytochrome P450 2D6 isoenzyme and are substrates for P450 2D6 and may make normal metabolizers resemble poor metabolizers resulting in higher than expected plasma levels of tricyclic antidepressants; co-administration may produce additive effects resulting in harmful level of sedation and CNS depression). Products include:
Thorazine ... 1656

Chlorprothixene (Co-administration may produce additive effects resulting in harmful level of sedation and CNS depression).
No products indexed under this heading.

Chlorprothixene Hydrochloride (Co-administration may produce additive effects resulting in harmful level of sedation and CNS depression).
No products indexed under this heading.

Chlorprothixene Lactate (Co-administration may produce additive

effects resulting in harmful level of sedation and CNS depression).
No products indexed under this heading.

Cimetidine (Cimetidine is reported to reduce hepatic metabolism of certain tricyclic antidepressants and benzodiazepines, thereby delaying elimination and increasing steady-state concentrations of these drugs). Products include:
Tagamet HB 200 Suspension 762
Tagamet HB 200 Tablets 761
Tagamet Tablets 1644

Cimetidine Hydrochloride (Cimetidine is reported to reduce hepatic metabolism of certain tricyclic antidepressants and benzodiazepines, thereby delaying elimination and increasing steady-state concentrations of these drugs). Products include:
Tagamet 1644

Citalopram Hydrobromide (May inhibit the activity of cytochrome P450 2D6 isoenzyme and are substrates for P450 2D6 and may make normal metabolizers resemble poor metabolizers resulting in higher than expected plasma levels of tricyclic antidepressants). Products include:
Celexa 1365

Clidinium Bromide (Severe constipation may result with concurrent use of tricyclic antidepressants and anticholinergic drugs).
No products indexed under this heading.

Clonidine (Amitriptyline may block the antihypertensive effects). Products include:
Catapres-TTS 1038

Clonidine Hydrochloride (Amitriptyline may block the antihypertensive effects). Products include:
Catapres Tablets 1037
Clorpres Tablets 1002
Combipres Tablets 1040
Duraclon Injection 3057

Clorazepate Dipotassium (Co-administration may produce additive effects resulting in harmful level of sedation and CNS depression). Products include:
Tranxene 511

Clozapine (Co-administration may produce additive effects resulting in harmful level of sedation and CNS depression). Products include:
Clozaril Tablets 2319

Codeine Phosphate (Co-administration may produce additive effects resulting in harmful level of sedation and CNS depression). Products include:
Phenergan with Codeine Syrup 3557
Phenergan VC with Codeine Syrup .. 3561
Robitussin A-C Syrup 2942
Robitussin-DAC Syrup 2942
Ryna-C Liquid 768
Soma Compound w/Codeine Tablets 3355
Tussi-Organidin NR Liquid 3350
Tussi-Organidin-S NR Liquid 3350
Tylenol with Codeine 2595

Desflurane (Co-administration may produce additive effects resulting in harmful level of sedation and CNS depression). Products include:
Suprane Liquid for Inhalation 874

Desipramine Hydrochloride (May inhibit the activity of cytochrome P450 2D6 isoenzyme and are substrates for P450 2D6 and may make normal metabolizers resemble poor metabolizers resulting in higher than expected plasma levels of tricyclic antidepressants). Products include:
Norpramin Tablets 755

Dezocine (Co-administration may produce additive effects resulting in harmful level of sedation and CNS depression).
No products indexed under this heading.

Diazepam (Co-administration may produce additive effects resulting in harmful level of sedation and CNS depression). Products include:
Valium Injectable 3026
Valium Tablets 3047

Dicyclomine Hydrochloride (Severe constipation may result with concurrent use of tricyclic antidepressants and anticholinergic drugs).
No products indexed under this heading.

Doxepin Hydrochloride (May inhibit the activity of cytochrome P450 2D6 isoenzyme and are substrates for P450 2D6 and may make normal metabolizers resemble poor metabolizers resulting in higher than expected plasma levels of tricyclic antidepressants). Products include:
Sinequan 2713

Droperidol (Co-administration may produce additive effects resulting in harmful level of sedation and CNS depression).
No products indexed under this heading.

Enflurane (Co-administration may produce additive effects resulting in harmful level of sedation and CNS depression).
No products indexed under this heading.

Estazolam (Co-administration may produce additive effects resulting in harmful level of sedation and CNS depression). Products include:
ProSom Tablets 500

Ethchlorvynol (Co-administration may produce additive effects resulting in harmful level of sedation and CNS depression).
No products indexed under this heading.

Ethinamate (Co-administration may produce additive effects resulting in harmful level of sedation and CNS depression).
No products indexed under this heading.

Fentanyl (Co-administration may produce additive effects resulting in harmful level of sedation and CNS depression). Products include:
Duragesic Transdermal System 1786

Fentanyl Citrate (Co-administration may produce additive effects resulting in harmful level of sedation and CNS depression). Products include:
Actiq 1184

Flecainide Acetate (May inhibit the activity of cytochrome P450 2D6 isoenzyme and are substrates for P450 2D6 and may make normal metabolizers resemble poor metabolizers resulting in higher than expected plasma levels of tricyclic antidepressants). Products include:
Tambocor Tablets 1990

Fluoxetine Hydrochloride (Selective serotonin reuptake inhibitors, such as fluoxetine, may have variable extent of inhibition of P450 2D6; potential for higher than expected plasma levels of tricyclic antidepressants; due to long half-life of fluoxetine, at least 5 weeks should elapse before initiating TCA treatment in a patient being withdrawn from fluoxetine). Products include:
Prozac Pulvules, Liquid, and Weekly Capsules 1238
Sarafem Pulvules 1962

Fluphenazine Decanoate (May inhibit the activity of cytochrome P450 2D6 isoenzyme and are substrates for P450 2D6 and may make normal metabolizers resemble poor metabolizers resulting in higher than expected plasma levels of tricyclic antidepressants; co-administration may produce additive effects resulting in harmful level of sedation and CNS depression).
No products indexed under this heading.

Fluphenazine Enanthate (May inhibit the activity of cytochrome P450 2D6 isoenzyme and are substrates for P450 2D6 and may make normal metabolizers resemble poor metabolizers resulting in higher than expected plasma levels of tricyclic antidepressants; co-administration may produce additive effects resulting in harmful level of sedation and CNS depression).
No products indexed under this heading.

Fluphenazine Hydrochloride (May inhibit the activity of cytochrome P450 2D6 isoenzyme and are substrates for P450 2D6 and may make normal metabolizers resemble poor metabolizers resulting in higher than expected plasma levels of tricyclic antidepressants; co-administration may produce additive effects resulting in harmful level of sedation and CNS depression).
No products indexed under this heading.

Flurazepam Hydrochloride (Co-administration may produce additive effects resulting in harmful level of sedation and CNS depression).
No products indexed under this heading.

Glutethimide (Co-administration may produce additive effects resulting in harmful level of sedation and CNS depression).
No products indexed under this heading.

Glycopyrrolate (Severe constipation may result with concurrent use of tricyclic antidepressants and anticholinergic drugs). Products include:
Robinul Forte Tablets 1358
Robinul Injectable 2940
Robinul Tablets 1358

Guanadrel Sulfate (Amitriptyline may block the antihypertensive effects).
No products indexed under this heading.

Guanethidine Monosulfate (Amitriptyline may block the antihypertensive effects).
No products indexed under this heading.

Haloperidol (Co-administration may produce additive effects resulting in harmful level of sedation and CNS depression). Products include:
Haldol Injection, Tablets and Concentrate 2533

Haloperidol Decanoate (Co-administration may produce additive effects resulting in harmful level of sedation and CNS depression). Products include:
Haldol Decanoate 2535

Hydrocodone Bitartrate (Co-administration may produce additive effects resulting in harmful level of sedation and CNS depression). Products include:
Hycodan 1316
Hycomine Compound Tablets 1317
Hycotuss Expectorant Syrup 1318
Lortab 3319
Lortab Elixir 3317
Maxidone Tablets CIII 3399
Norco 5/325 Tablets CIII 3424
Norco 7.5/325 Tablets CIII 3425
Norco 10/325 Tablets CIII 3427
Norco 10/325 Tablets CIII 3425
Vicodin Tablets 516
Vicodin ES Tablets 517
Vicodin HP Tablets 518
Vicodin Tuss Expectorant 519
Vicoprofen Tablets 520
Zydone Tablets 1330

Hydrocodone Polistirex (Co-administration may produce additive effects resulting in harmful level of sedation and CNS depression). Products include:
Tussionex Pennkinetic Extended-Release Suspension 1174

Hydromorphone Hydrochloride (Co-administration may produce additive effects resulting in harmful level of sedation and CNS depression). Products include:
Dilaudid 441
Dilaudid Oral Liquid 445
Dilaudid Powder 441
Dilaudid Rectal Suppositories 441
Dilaudid Tablets 441
Dilaudid Tablets - 8 mg 445
Dilaudid-HP 443

Hydroxyzine Hydrochloride (Co-administration may produce additive effects resulting in harmful level of sedation and CNS depression). Products include:
Atarax Tablets & Syrup 2667
Vistaril Intramuscular Solution 2738

Hyoscyamine (Severe constipation may result with concurrent use of tricyclic antidepressants and anticholinergic drugs). Products include:
Urised Tablets 2876

Hyoscyamine Sulfate (Severe constipation may result with concurrent use of tricyclic antidepressants and anticholinergic drugs). Products include:
Arco-Lase Plus Tablets 592
Donnatal 2929
Donnatal Extentabs 2930
Levsin/Levsinex/Levbid 3172
NuLev Orally Disintegrating Tablets 3176
Prosed/DS Tablets 3268
Urimax Tablets 1769

Imipramine Hydrochloride (May inhibit the activity of cytochrome P450 2D6 isoenzyme and are substrates for P450 2D6 and may make normal metabolizers resemble poor metabolizers resulting in higher than expected plasma levels of tricyclic antidepressants).
No products indexed under this heading.

Imipramine Pamoate (May inhibit the activity of cytochrome P450 2D6 isoenzyme and are substrates for P450 2D6 and may make normal metabolizers resemble poor metabolizers resulting in higher than expected plasma levels of tricyclic antidepressants).
No products indexed under this heading.

Ipratropium Bromide (Severe constipation may result with concurrent use of tricyclic antidepressants and anticholinergic drugs). Products include:
Atrovent Inhalation Aerosol 1030
Atrovent Inhalation Solution 1031
Atrovent Nasal Spray 0.03% 1032
Atrovent Nasal Spray 0.06% 1033
Combivent Inhalation Aerosol 1041
DuoNeb Inhalation Solution 1233

Isocarboxazid (Co-administration of tricyclic antidepressants and MAO inhibitor has produced hyperpyretic crises, severe convulsions, and deaths; concurrent and/or sequential use is contraindicated).
No products indexed under this heading.

Isoflurane (Co-administration may produce additive effects resulting in harmful level of sedation and CNS depression).
No products indexed under this heading.

Ketamine Hydrochloride (Co-administration may produce additive effects resulting in harmful level of sedation and CNS depression).
No products indexed under this heading.

Levomethadyl Acetate Hydrochloride (Co-administration may produce additive effects resulting in harmful level of sedation and CNS

depression).
No products indexed under this heading.

Levorphanol Tartrate (Co-administration may produce additive effects resulting in harmful level of sedation and CNS depression). Products include:
Levo-Dromoran 1734
Levorphanol Tartrate Tablets 3059

Levothyroxine Sodium (Close supervision is required when Limbitrol is given to patients on thyroid medications). Products include:
Levothroid Tablets 1373
Levoxyl Tablets 1819
Synthroid 505
Unithroid Tablets 3445

Liothyronine Sodium (Close supervision is required when Limbitrol is given to patients on thyroid medications). Products include:
Cytomel Tablets 1817
Triostat Injection 1825

Liotrix (Close supervision is required when Limbitrol is given to patients on thyroid medications).
No products indexed under this heading.

Lorazepam (Co-administration may produce additive effects resulting in harmful level of sedation and CNS depression). Products include:
Ativan Injection 3478
Ativan Tablets 3482

Loxapine Hydrochloride (Co-administration may produce additive effects resulting in harmful level of sedation and CNS depression).
No products indexed under this heading.

Loxapine Succinate (Co-administration may produce additive effects resulting in harmful level of sedation and CNS depression). Products include:
Loxitane Capsules 3398

Maprotiline Hydrochloride (May inhibit the activity of cytochrome P450 2D6 isoenzyme and are substrates for P450 2D6 and may make normal metabolizers resemble poor metabolizers resulting in higher than expected plasma levels of tricyclic antidepressants).
No products indexed under this heading.

Mepenzolate Bromide (Severe constipation may result with concurrent use of tricyclic antidepressants and anticholinergic drugs).
No products indexed under this heading.

Meperidine Hydrochloride (Co-administration may produce additive effects resulting in harmful level of sedation and CNS depression). Products include:
Demerol 3079
Mepergan Injection 3539

Mephobarbital (Co-administration may produce additive effects resulting in harmful level of sedation and CNS depression).
No products indexed under this heading.

Meprobamate (Co-administration may produce additive effects resulting in harmful level of sedation and CNS depression). Products include:
Miltown Tablets 3349

Mesoridazine Besylate (May inhibit the activity of cytochrome P450 2D6 isoenzyme and are substrates for P450 2D6 and may make normal metabolizers resemble poor metabolizers resulting in higher than expected plasma levels of tricyclic antidepressants; co-administration may produce additive effects resulting in harmful level of sedation and CNS depression). Products include:
Serentil 1057

Methadone Hydrochloride (Co-administration may produce additive effects resulting in harmful level of sedation and CNS depression). Products include:
Dolophine Hydrochloride Tablets 3056

Methohexital Sodium (Co-administration may produce additive effects resulting in harmful level of sedation and CNS depression). Products include:
Brevital Sodium for Injection, USP .. 1815

Methotrimeprazine (May inhibit the activity of cytochrome P450 2D6 isoenzyme and are substrates for P450 2D6 and may make normal metabolizers resemble poor metabolizers resulting in higher than expected plasma levels of tricyclic antidepressants; co-administration may produce additive effects resulting in harmful level of sedation and CNS depression).
No products indexed under this heading.

Methoxyflurane (Co-administration may produce additive effects resulting in harmful level of sedation and CNS depression).
No products indexed under this heading.

Midazolam Hydrochloride (Co-administration may produce additive effects resulting in harmful level of sedation and CNS depression). Products include:
Versed Injection 3027
Versed Syrup 3033

Mirtazapine (May inhibit the activity of cytochrome P450 2D6 isoenzyme and are substrates for P450 2D6 and may make normal metabolizers resemble poor metabolizers resulting in higher than expected plasma levels of tricyclic antidepressants). Products include:
Remeron Tablets 2483
Remeron SolTab Tablets 2486

Moclobemide (Co-administration of tricyclic antidepressants and MAO inhibitor has produced hyperpyretic crises, severe convulsions, and deaths; concurrent and/or sequential use is contrainidicated).
No products indexed under this heading.

Molindone Hydrochloride (Co-administration may produce additive effects resulting in harmful level of sedation and CNS depression). Products include:
Moban 1320

Morphine Sulfate (Co-administration may produce additive effects resulting in harmful level of sedation and CNS depression). Products include:
Astramorph/PF Injection, USP (Preservative-Free) 594
Duramorph Injection 1312
Infumorph 200 and Infumorph 500 Sterile Solutions 1314
Kadian Capsules 1335
MS Contin Tablets 2896
MSIR 2898
Oramorph SR Tablets 3062
Roxanol 3066

Nefazodone Hydrochloride (May inhibit the activity of cytochrome P450 2D6 isoenzyme and are substrates for P450 2D6 and may make normal metabolizers resemble poor metabolizers resulting in higher than expected plasma levels of tricyclic antidepressants). Products include:
Serzone Tablets 1104

Nortriptyline Hydrochloride (May inhibit the activity of cytochrome P450 2D6 isoenzyme and are substrates for P450 2D6 and may make normal metabolizers resemble poor metabolizers resulting in higher than expected plasma levels of tricyclic antidepressants).
No products indexed under this heading.

Olanzapine (Co-administration may produce additive effects resulting in harmful level of sedation and CNS depression). Products include:
Zyprexa Tablets 1973
Zyprexa ZYDIS Orally Disintegrating Tablets 1973

Oxazepam (Co-administration may produce additive effects resulting in harmful level of sedation and CNS depression).
No products indexed under this heading.

Oxybutynin Chloride (Severe constipation may result with concurrent use of tricyclic antidepressants and anticholinergic drugs). Products include:
Ditropan XL Extended Release Tablets 564

Oxycodone Hydrochloride (Co-administration may produce additive effects resulting in harmful level of sedation and CNS depression). Products include:
OxyContin Tablets 2912
OxyFast Oral Concentrate Solution . 2916
OxyIR Capsules 2916
Percocet Tablets 1326
Percodan Tablets 1327
Percolone Tablets 1327
Roxicodone 3067
Tylox Capsules 2597

Pargyline Hydrochloride (Co-administration of tricyclic antidepressants and MAO inhibitor has produced hyperpyretic crises, severe convulsions, and deaths; concurrent and/or sequential use is contrainidicated).
No products indexed under this heading.

Paroxetine Hydrochloride (Selective serotonin reuptake inhibitors, such as paroxetine, may have variable extent of inhibition of P450 2D6; potential for higher than expected plasma levels of tricyclic antidepressants). Products include:
Paxil 1609

Pentobarbital Sodium (Co-administration may produce additive effects resulting in harmful level of sedation and CNS depression). Products include:
Nembutal Sodium Solution 485

Perphenazine (May inhibit the activity of cytochrome P450 2D6 isoenzyme and are substrates for P450 2D6 and may make normal metabolizers resemble poor metabolizers resulting in higher than expected plasma levels of tricyclic antidepressants; co-administration may produce additive effects resulting in harmful level of sedation and CNS depression). Products include:
Etrafon 3115
Trilafon 3160

Phenelzine Sulfate (Co-administration of tricyclic antidepressants and MAO inhibitor has produced hyperpyretic crises, severe convulsions, and deaths; concurrent and/or sequential use is contrainidicated). Products include:
Nardil Tablets 2653

Phenobarbital (Co-administration may produce additive effects resulting in harmful level of sedation and CNS depression). Products include:
Arco-Lase Plus Tablets 592
Donnatal 2929
Donnatal Extentabs 2930

Prazepam (Co-administration may produce additive effects resulting in harmful level of sedation and CNS depression).
No products indexed under this heading.

Procarbazine Hydrochloride (Co-administration of tricyclic antidepressants and MAO inhibitor has produced hyperpyretic crises, severe convulsions, and deaths; concurrent and/or sequential use is contrainidicated). Products include:
Matulane Capsules 3246

Prochlorperazine (May inhibit the activity of cytochrome P450 2D6 isoenzyme and are substrates for P450 2D6 and may make normal metabolizers resemble poor metabolizers resulting in higher than expected plasma levels of tricyclic antidepressants; co-administration may produce additive effects resulting in harmful level of sedation and CNS depression). Products include:
Compazine 1505

Procyclidine Hydrochloride (Severe constipation may result with concurrent use of tricyclic antidepressants and anticholinergic drugs).
No products indexed under this heading.

Promethazine Hydrochloride (May inhibit the activity of cytochrome P450 2D6 isoenzyme and are substrates for P450 2D6 and may make normal metabolizers resemble poor metabolizers resulting in higher than expected plasma levels of tricyclic antidepressants; co-administration may produce additive effects resulting in harmful level of sedation and CNS depression). Products include:
Mepergan Injection 3539
Phenergan Injection 3553
Phenergan 3556
Phenergan Syrup 3554
Phenergan with Codeine Syrup 3557
Phenergan with Dextromethorphan Syrup 3559
Phenergan VC Syrup 3560
Phenergan VC with Codeine Syrup .. 3561

Propafenone Hydrochloride (May inhibit the activity of cytochrome P450 2D6 isoenzyme and are substrates for P450 2D6 and may make normal metabolizers resemble poor metabolizers resulting in higher than expected plasma levels of tricyclic antidepressants). Products include:
Rythmol Tablets – 150 mg, 225 mg, 300 mg 502

Propantheline Bromide (Severe constipation may result with concurrent use of tricyclic antidepressants and anticholinergic drugs).
No products indexed under this heading.

Propofol (Co-administration may produce additive effects resulting in harmful level of sedation and CNS depression). Products include:
Diprivan Injectable Emulsion 667

Propoxyphene Hydrochloride (Co-administration may produce additive effects resulting in harmful level of sedation and CNS depression). Products include:
Darvon Pulvules 1909
Darvon Compound-65 Pulvules 1910

Propoxyphene Napsylate (Co-administration may produce additive effects resulting in harmful level of sedation and CNS depression). Products include:
Darvon-N/Darvocet-N 1907
Darvon-N Tablets 1912

Protriptyline Hydrochloride (May inhibit the activity of cytochrome P450 2D6 isoenzyme and are substrates for P450 2D6 and may make normal metabolizers resemble poor metabolizers resulting in higher than expected plasma levels of tricyclic antidepressants). Products include:
Vivactil Tablets 2446
Vivactil Tablets 2217

Quazepam (Co-administration may produce additive effects resulting in harmful level of sedation and CNS depression).
No products indexed under this heading.

Quetiapine Fumarate (Co-administration may produce additive

effects resulting in harmful level of sedation and CNS depression). Products include:
Seroquel Tablets 684

Quinidine Gluconate (May inhibit the activity of cytochrome P450 2D6 isoenzyme and may make normal metabolizers resemble poor metabolizers resulting in higher than expected plasma levels of tricyclic antidepressants). Products include:
Quinaglute Dura-Tabs Tablets 978

Quinidine Polygalacturonate (May inhibit the activity of cytochrome P450 2D6 isoenzyme and may make normal metabolizers resemble poor metabolizers resulting in higher than expected plasma levels of tricyclic antidepressants).
No products indexed under this heading.

Quinidine Sulfate (May inhibit the activity of cytochrome P450 2D6 isoenzyme and may make normal metabolizers resemble poor metabolizers resulting in higher than expected plasma levels of tricyclic antidepressants). Products include:
Quinidex Extentabs 2933

Remifentanil Hydrochloride (Co-administration may produce additive effects resulting in harmful level of sedation and CNS depression).
No products indexed under this heading.

Risperidone (Co-administration may produce additive effects resulting in harmful level of sedation and CNS depression). Products include:
Risperdal 1796

Scopolamine (Severe constipation may result with concurrent use of tricyclic antidepressants and anticholinergic drugs). Products include:
Transderm Scōp Transdermal Therapeutic System 2302

Scopolamine Hydrobromide (Severe constipation may result with concurrent use of tricyclic antidepressants and anticholinergic drugs). Products include:
Donnatal 2929
Donnatal Extentabs 2930

Secobarbital Sodium (Co-administration may produce additive effects resulting in harmful level of sedation and CNS depression).
No products indexed under this heading.

Selegiline Hydrochloride (Co-administration of tricyclic antidepressants and MAO inhibitor has produced hyperpyretic crises, severe convulsions, and deaths; concurrent and/or sequential use is contraindicated). Products include:
Eldepryl Capsules 3266

Sertraline Hydrochloride (Selective serotonin reuptake inhibitors, such as sertraline, may have variable extent of inhibition of P450 2D6; potential for higher than expected plasma levels of tricyclic antidepressants). Products include:
Zoloft 2751

Sevoflurane (Co-administration may produce additive effects resulting in harmful level of sedation and CNS depression).
No products indexed under this heading.

Sufentanil Citrate (Co-administration may produce additive effects resulting in harmful level of sedation and CNS depression).
No products indexed under this heading.

Temazepam (Co-administration may produce additive effects resulting in harmful level of sedation and CNS depression).
No products indexed under this heading.

Thiamylal Sodium (Co-administration may produce additive effects resulting in harmful level of sedation and CNS depression).
No products indexed under this heading.

Thioridazine Hydrochloride (May inhibit the activity of cytochrome P450 2D6 isoenzyme and are substrates for P450 2D6 and may make normal metabolizers resemble poor metabolizers resulting in higher than expected plasma levels of tricyclic antidepressants; co-administration may produce additive effects resulting in harmful level of sedation and CNS depression). Products include:
Thioridazine Hydrochloride Tablets 2289

Thiothixene (Co-administration may produce additive effects resulting in harmful level of sedation and CNS depression). Products include:
Navane Capsules 2701
Thiothixene Capsules 2290

Thyroglobulin (Close supervision is required when Limbitrol is given to patients on thyroid medications).
No products indexed under this heading.

Thyroid (Close supervision is required when Limbitrol is given to patients on thyroid medications).
No products indexed under this heading.

Thyroxine (Close supervision is required when Limbitrol is given to patients on thyroid medications).
No products indexed under this heading.

Thyroxine Sodium (Close supervision is required when Limbitrol is given to patients on thyroid medications).
No products indexed under this heading.

Tolterodine Tartrate (Severe constipation may result with concurrent use of tricyclic antidepressants and anticholinergic drugs). Products include:
Detrol Tablets 3623
Detrol LA Capsules 2801

Tranylcypromine Sulfate (Co-administration of tricyclic antidepressants and MAO inhibitor has produced hyperpyretic crises, severe convulsions, and deaths; concurrent and/or sequential use is contraindicated). Products include:
Parnate Tablets 1607

Trazodone Hydrochloride (May inhibit the activity of cytochrome P450 2D6 isoenzyme and are substrates for P450 2D6 and may make normal metabolizers resemble poor metabolizers resulting in higher than expected plasma levels of tricyclic antidepressants).
No products indexed under this heading.

Triazolam (Co-administration may produce additive effects resulting in harmful level of sedation and CNS depression). Products include:
Halcion Tablets 2823

Tridihexethyl Chloride (Severe constipation may result with concurrent use of tricyclic antidepressants and anticholinergic drugs).
No products indexed under this heading.

Trifluoperazine Hydrochloride (May inhibit the activity of cytochrome P450 2D6 isoenzyme and are substrates for P450 2D6 and may make normal metabolizers resemble poor metabolizers resulting in higher than expected plasma levels of tricyclic antidepressants; co-administration may produce additive effects resulting in harmful level of sedation and CNS depression). Products include:
Stelazine 1640

Trihexyphenidyl Hydrochloride (Severe constipation may result with concurrent use of tricyclic antidepressants and anticholinergic drugs). Products include:
Artane 1855

Trimipramine Maleate (May inhibit the activity of cytochrome P450 2D6 isoenzyme and are substrates for P450 2D6 and may make normal metabolizers resemble poor metabolizers resulting in higher than expected plasma levels of tricyclic antidepressants). Products include:
Surmontil Capsules 3595

Venlafaxine Hydrochloride (May inhibit the activity of cytochrome P450 2D6 isoenzyme and are substrates for P450 2D6 and may make normal metabolizers resemble poor metabolizers resulting in higher than expected plasma levels of tricyclic antidepressants). Products include:
Effexor Tablets 3495
Effexor XR Capsules 3499

Zaleplon (Co-administration may produce additive effects resulting in harmful level of sedation and CNS depression). Products include:
Sonata Capsules 3591

Ziprasidone Hydrochloride (Co-administration may produce additive effects resulting in harmful level of sedation and CNS depression). Products include:
Geodon Capsules 2688

Zolpidem Tartrate (Co-administration may produce additive effects resulting in harmful level of sedation and CNS depression). Products include:
Ambien Tablets 3191

Food Interactions

Alcohol (Concurrent use may produce additive effects resulting in harmful level of sedation and CNS depression).

LIMBITROL DS TABLETS

(Amitriptyline Hydrochloride, Chlordiazepoxide)............................ 1738
See Limbitrol Tablets

LINDANE LOTION USP 1%

(Lindane) 559
May interact with:

Oils, unspecified (May enhance absorption; avoid concurrent use).

LINDANE SHAMPOO USP 1%

(Lindane) 560
May interact with:

Oils, unspecified (May enhance absorption; avoid concurrent use).

LIPITOR TABLETS

(Atorvastatin Calcium) 2696
May interact with azole antifungals, erythromycin, fibrates, and certain other agents. Compounds in these categories include:

Aluminum Hydroxide (Co-administration with aluminum hydroxide/magnesium hydroxide antacid has resulted in decreased atorvastatin plasma concentrations by 35%; LDL-C reduction was unaltered). Products include:
Amphojel Suspension (Mint Flavor)... 789
Gaviscon Extra Strength Liquid 751
Gaviscon Extra Strength Tablets 751
Gaviscon Regular Strength Liquid . 751
Gaviscon Regular Strength Tablets 750
Maalox Antacid/Anti-Gas Oral Suspension.. 673
Maalox Max Maximum Strength Antacid/Anti-Gas Liquid 2300
Maalox Regular Strength Antacid/Antigas Liquid 2300
Mylanta 1813
Vanquish Caplets 617

Clofibrate (Co-administration with fibric acid derivatives increases the risk of myopathy). Products include:
Atromid-S Capsules 3483

Clotrimazole (Co-administration with azole antifungals increases the risk of myopathy). Products include:
Gyne-Lotrimin 3, 3-Day Cream 741
Lotrimin AF Cream, Lotion, Solution, and Jock Itch Cream.... 742
Lotrimin 3128
Lotrisone 3129
Mycelex Troche 573
Mycelex-7 Combination-Pack Vaginal Inserts & External Vulvar Cream.................................. 614
Mycelex-7 Vaginal Cream 614
Mycelex-7 Vaginal Cream with 7 Disposable Applicators.................. 614

Colestipol Hydrochloride (Co-administration has resulted in decreased atorvastatin plasma concentrations by 25%, however, LDL-C reduction was greater when these drugs were given together than when either drug was given alone). Products include:
Colestid Tablets 2791

Cyclosporine (Co-administration increases the risk of myopathy). Products include:
Gengraf Capsules 457
Neoral Soft Gelatin Capsules......... 2380
Neoral Oral Solution 2380
Sandimmune 2388

Digoxin (Co-administration has resulted in increased steady-state digoxin plasma concentrations by 20%). Products include:
Digitek Tablets 1003
Lanoxicaps Capsules 1574
Lanoxin Injection 1581
Lanoxin Tablets 1587
Lanoxin Elixir Pediatric 1578
Lanoxin Injection Pediatric 1584

Erythromycin (Co-administration increases the risk of myopathy; plasma concentrations of atorvastatin has increased by 40% when co-administered with erythromycin, a known inhibitor of cytochrome P4503A4). Products include:
Emgel 2% Topical Gel 1285
Ery-Tab Tablets 448
Erythromycin Base Filmtab Tablets . 454
Erythromycin Delayed-Release Capsules, USP.............................. 455
PCE Dispertab Tablets 498

Erythromycin Estolate (Co-administration increases the risk of myopathy; plasma concentrations of atorvastatin has increased by 40% when co-administered with erythromycin, a known inhibitor of cytochrome P4503A4).
No products indexed under this heading.

Erythromycin Ethylsuccinate (Co-administration increases the risk of myopathy; plasma concentrations of atorvastatin has increased by 40% when co-administered with erythromycin, a known inhibitor of cytochrome P4503A4). Products include:
E.E.S. 450
EryPed 446
Pediazole Suspension 3050

Erythromycin Gluceptate (Co-administration increases the risk of myopathy; plasma concentrations of atorvastatin has increased by 40% when co-administered with erythromycin, a known inhibitor of cytochrome P4503A4).
No products indexed under this heading.

Erythromycin Stearate (Co-administration increases the risk of myopathy; plasma concentrations of atorvastatin has increased by 40% when co-administered with erythromycin, a known inhibitor of cytochrome P4503A4). Products include:
Erythrocin Stearate Filmtab Tablets 452

Ethinyl Estradiol (Co-administration with an oral contraceptive has increased AUC values for norethindrone and ethinyl estradiol by 30% and 20%). Products include:
Alesse-21 Tablets 3468

Alesse-28 Tablets ... 3473
Brevicon 28-Day Tablets ... 3380
Cyclessa Tablets ... 2450
Desogen Tablets ... 2458
Estinyl Tablets ... 3112
Estrostep ... 2627
femhrt Tablets ... 2635
Levlen ... 962
Levlite 21 Tablets ... 962
Levlite 28 Tablets ... 962
Levora Tablets ... 3389
Loestrin 21 Tablets ... 2642
Loestrin Fe Tablets ... 2642
Lo/Ovral Tablets ... 3532
Lo/Ovral-28 Tablets ... 3538
Low-Ogestrel-28 Tablets ... 3392
Microgestin Fe 1.5/30 Tablets ... 3407
Microgestin Fe 1/20 Tablets ... 3400
Mircette Tablets ... 2470
Modicon ... 2563
Necon ... 3415
Nordette-28 Tablets ... 2257
Norinyl 1 +35 28-Day Tablets ... 3380
Ogestrel 0.5/50-28 Tablets ... 3428
Ortho-Cept 21 Tablets ... 2546
Ortho-Cept 28 Tablets ... 2546
Ortho-Cyclen/Ortho Tri-Cyclen ... 2573
Ortho-Novum ... 2563
Ovcon ... 3364
Ovral Tablets ... 3551
Ovral-28 Tablets ... 3552
Tri-Levlen ... 962
Tri-Norinyl-28 Tablets ... 3433
Triphasil-21 Tablets ... 3600
Triphasil-28 Tablets ... 3605
Trivora Tablets ... 3439
Yasmin 28 Tablets ... 980
Zovia ... 3449

Fenofibrate (Co-administration with fibric acid derivatives increases the risk of myopathy). Products include:
Tricor Capsules, Micronized ... 513

Fluconazole (Co-administration with azole antifungals increases the risk of myopathy). Products include:
Diflucan Tablets, Injection, and Oral Suspension ... 2681

Gemfibrozil (Co-administration with fibric acid derivatives increases the risk of myopathy). Products include:
Lopid Tablets ... 2650

Itraconazole (Co-administration with azole antifungals increases the risk of myopathy). Products include:
Sporanox Capsules ... 1800
Sporanox Injection ... 1804
Sporanox Injection ... 2509
Sporanox Oral Solution ... 1808
Sporanox Oral Solution ... 2512

Ketoconazole (Co-administration with azole antifungals increases the risk of myopathy). Products include:
Nizoral 2% Cream ... 3620
Nizoral A-D Shampoo ... 2008
Nizoral 2% Shampoo ... 2007
Nizoral Tablets ... 1791

Miconazole (Co-administration with azole antifungals increases the risk of myopathy).
No products indexed under this heading.

Niacin (Co-administration increases the risk of myopathy). Products include:
Niaspan Extended-Release Tablets ... 1846
Nicotinex Elixir ... ■633

Norethindrone (Co-administration with an oral contraceptive has increased AUC values for norethindrone and ethinyl estradiol by 30% and 20%). Products include:
Brevicon 28-Day Tablets ... 3380
Micronor Tablets ... 2543
Modicon ... 2563
Necon ... 3415
Norinyl 1 +35 28-Day Tablets ... 3380
Norinyl 1 + 50 28-Day Tablets ... 3380
Nor-QD Tablets ... 3423
Ortho-Novum ... 2563
Ortho-Novum 1/50□28 Tablets ... 2556
Ovcon ... 3364
Tri-Norinyl-28 Tablets ... 3433

Oxiconazole Nitrate (Co-administration with azole antifungals increases the risk of myopathy). Products include:
Oxistat ... 1298

Terconazole (Co-administration with azole antifungals increases the risk of myopathy). Products include:
Terazol 3 Vaginal Cream ... 2587
Terazol 3 Vaginal Suppositories ... 2587
Terazol 7 Vaginal Cream ... 2587

LIPITOR TABLETS

(Atorvastatin Calcium) ... 2639
May interact with azole antifungals, erythromycin, fibrates, and certain other agents. Compounds in these categories include:

Aluminum Hydroxide (Co-administration with aluminum hydroxide/magnesium hydroxide antacid has resulted in decreased atorvastatin plasma concentrations by 35%; LDL-C reduction was unaltered). Products include:
Amphojel Suspension (Mint Flavor) ... ■789
Gaviscon Extra Strength Liquid ... ■751
Gaviscon Extra Strength Tablets ... ■751
Gaviscon Regular Strength Liquid ... ■751
Gaviscon Regular Strength Tablets ... ■750
Maalox Antacid/Anti-Gas Oral Suspension ... ■673
Maalox Max Maximum Strength Antacid/Anti-Gas Liquid ... 2300
Maalox Regular Strength Antacid/Antigas Liquid ... 2300
Mylanta ... 1813
Vanquish Caplets ... ■617

Clofibrate (Co-administration with fibric acid derivatives increases the risk of myopathy). Products include:
Atromid-S Capsules ... 3483

Clotrimazole (Co-administration with azole antifungals increases the risk of myopathy). Products include:
Gyne-Lotrimin 3, 3-Day Cream ... ■741
Lotrimin AF Cream, Lotion, Solution, and Jock Itch Cream ... ■742
Lotrimin ... 3128
Lotrisone ... 3129
Mycelex Troche ... 573
Mycelex-7 Combination-Pack Vaginal Inserts & External Vulvar Cream ... ■614
Mycelex-7 Vaginal Cream ... ■614
Mycelex-7 Vaginal Cream with 7 Disposable Applicators ... ■614

Colestipol Hydrochloride (Co-administration has resulted in decreased atorvastatin plasma concentrations by 25%, however, LDL-C reduction was greater when these drugs were given together than when either drug was given alone). Products include:
Colestid Tablets ... 2791

Cyclosporine (Co-administration increases the risk of myopathy). Products include:
Gengraf Capsules ... 457
Neoral Soft Gelatin Capsules ... 2380
Neoral Oral Solution ... 2380
Sandimmune ... 2388

Digoxin (Co-administration has resulted in increased steady-state digoxin plasma concentrations by 20%). Products include:
Digitek Tablets ... 1003
Lanoxicaps Capsules ... 1574
Lanoxin Injection ... 1581
Lanoxin Tablets ... 1587
Lanoxin Elixir Pediatric ... 1578
Lanoxin Injection Pediatric ... 1584

Erythromycin (Co-administration increases the risk of myopathy; plasma concentrations of atorvastatin has increased by 40% when co-administered with erythromycin, a known inhibitor of cytochrome P4503A4). Products include:
Emgel 2% Topical Gel ... 1285
Ery-Tab Tablets ... 448
Erythromycin Base Filmtab Tablets ... 454
Erythromycin Delayed-Release Capsules, USP ... 455
PCE Dispertab Tablets ... 498

Erythromycin Estolate (Co-administration increases the risk of myopathy; plasma concentrations of atorvastatin has increased by 40% when co-administered with erythromycin, a known inhibitor of cytochrome P4503A4).
No products indexed under this heading.

Erythromycin Ethylsuccinate (Co-administration increases the risk of myopathy; plasma concentrations of atorvastatin has increased by 40% when co-administered with erythromycin, a known inhibitor of cytochrome P4503A4). Products include:
E.E.S. ... 450
EryPed ... 446
Pediazole Suspension ... 3050

Erythromycin Gluceptate (Co-administration increases the risk of myopathy; plasma concentrations of atorvastatin has increased by 40% when co-administered with erythromycin, a known inhibitor of cytochrome P4503A4).
No products indexed under this heading.

Erythromycin Stearate (Co-administration increases the risk of myopathy; plasma concentrations of atorvastatin has increased by 40% when co-administered with erythromycin, a known inhibitor of cytochrome P4503A4). Products include:
Erythrocin Stearate Filmtab Tablets ... 452

Ethinyl Estradiol (Co-administration with an oral contraceptive has increased AUC values for norethindrone and ethinyl estradiol by 30% and 20%). Products include:
Alesse-21 Tablets ... 3468
Alesse-28 Tablets ... 3473
Brevicon 28-Day Tablets ... 3380
Cyclessa Tablets ... 2450
Desogen Tablets ... 2458
Estinyl Tablets ... 3112
Estrostep ... 2627
femhrt Tablets ... 2635
Levlen ... 962
Levlite 21 Tablets ... 962
Levlite 28 Tablets ... 962
Levora Tablets ... 3389
Loestrin 21 Tablets ... 2642
Loestrin Fe Tablets ... 2642
Lo/Ovral Tablets ... 3532
Lo/Ovral-28 Tablets ... 3538
Low-Ogestrel-28 Tablets ... 3392
Microgestin Fe 1.5/30 Tablets ... 3407
Microgestin Fe 1/20 Tablets ... 3400
Mircette Tablets ... 2470
Modicon ... 2563
Necon ... 3415
Nordette-28 Tablets ... 2257
Norinyl 1 +35 28-Day Tablets ... 3380
Ogestrel 0.5/50-28 Tablets ... 3428
Ortho-Cept 21 Tablets ... 2546
Ortho-Cept 28 Tablets ... 2546
Ortho-Cyclen/Ortho Tri-Cyclen ... 2573
Ortho-Novum ... 2563
Ovcon ... 3364
Ovral Tablets ... 3551
Ovral-28 Tablets ... 3552
Tri-Levlen ... 962
Tri-Norinyl-28 Tablets ... 3433
Triphasil-21 Tablets ... 3600
Triphasil-28 Tablets ... 3605
Trivora Tablets ... 3439
Yasmin 28 Tablets ... 980
Zovia ... 3449

Fenofibrate (Co-administration with fibric acid derivatives increases the risk of myopathy). Products include:
Tricor Capsules, Micronized ... 513

Fluconazole (Co-administration with azole antifungals increases the risk of myopathy). Products include:
Diflucan Tablets, Injection, and Oral Suspension ... 2681

Gemfibrozil (Co-administration with fibric acid derivatives increases the risk of myopathy). Products include:
Lopid Tablets ... 2650

Itraconazole (Co-administration with azole antifungals increases the risk of myopathy). Products include:
Sporanox Capsules ... 1800
Sporanox Injection ... 1804
Sporanox Injection ... 2509
Sporanox Oral Solution ... 1808
Sporanox Oral Solution ... 2512

Ketoconazole (Co-administration with azole antifungals increases the risk of myopathy). Products include:
Nizoral 2% Cream ... 3620
Nizoral A-D Shampoo ... 2008
Nizoral 2% Shampoo ... 2007
Nizoral Tablets ... 1791

Miconazole (Co-administration with azole antifungals increases the risk of myopathy).
No products indexed under this heading.

Niacin (Co-administration increases the risk of myopathy). Products include:
Niaspan Extended-Release Tablets ... 1846
Nicotinex Elixir ... ■633

Norethindrone (Co-administration with an oral contraceptive has increased AUC values for norethindrone and ethinyl estradiol by 30% and 20%). Products include:
Brevicon 28-Day Tablets ... 3380
Micronor Tablets ... 2543
Modicon ... 2563
Necon ... 3415
Norinyl 1 +35 28-Day Tablets ... 3380
Norinyl 1 + 50 28-Day Tablets ... 3380
Nor-QD Tablets ... 3423
Ortho-Novum ... 2563
Ortho-Novum 1/50□28 Tablets ... 2556
Ovcon ... 3364
Tri-Norinyl-28 Tablets ... 3433

Oxiconazole Nitrate (Co-administration with azole antifungals increases the risk of myopathy). Products include:
Oxistat ... 1298

Terconazole (Co-administration with azole antifungals increases the risk of myopathy). Products include:
Terazol 3 Vaginal Cream ... 2587
Terazol 3 Vaginal Suppositories ... 2587
Terazol 7 Vaginal Cream ... 2587

LIPOFLAVONOID CAPLETS

(Bioflavonoids, Vitamins, Multiple) ... ■828
None cited in PDR database.

LISTERINE MOUTHRINSE

(Eucalyptol, Menthol, Methyl Salicylate) ... ■702
None cited in PDR database.

COOL MINT LISTERINE MOUTHRINSE

(Eucalyptol, Menthol, Methyl Salicylate, Thymol) ... ■702
None cited in PDR database.

FRESHBURST LISTERINE MOUTHRINSE

(Eucalyptol, Menthol, Methyl Salicylate, Thymol) ... ■702
None cited in PDR database.

TARTAR CONTROL LISTERINE MOUTHRINSE

(Eucalyptol, Menthol, Methyl Salicylate) ... ■702
None cited in PDR database.

LISTERMINT ALCOHOL-FREE MOUTHRINSE

(Sodium Fluoride) ... ■703
None cited in PDR database.

LITHIUM CARBONATE CAPSULES

(Lithium Carbonate) ... 3061
May interact with ACE inhibitors, diuretics, antipsychotic agents, neuromuscular blocking agents, non-steroidal anti-inflammatory agents, and certain other agents. Compounds in these categories include:

Amiloride Hydrochloride (Co-administration results in reduced

renal clearance of lithium and increased serum lithium levels with risk of lithium toxicity). Products include:
- Midamor Tablets 2136
- Moduretic Tablets 2138

Atracurium Besylate (Lithium may prolong the effects of neuromuscular blocking agents).
- No products indexed under this heading.

Benazepril Hydrochloride (Co-administration results in reduced renal clearance of lithium and increased serum lithium levels with risk of lithium toxicity). Products include:
- Lotensin Tablets 2365
- Lotensin HCT Tablets 2367
- Lotrel Capsules 2370

Bendroflumethiazide (Co-administration results in reduced renal clearance of lithium and increased serum lithium levels with risk of lithium toxicity). Products include:
- Corzide 40/5 Tablets 2247
- Corzide 80/5 Tablets 2247

Bumetanide (Co-administration results in reduced renal clearance of lithium and increased serum lithium levels with risk of lithium toxicity).
- No products indexed under this heading.

Captopril (Co-administration results in reduced renal clearance of lithium and increased serum lithium levels with risk of lithium toxicity). Products include:
- Captopril Tablets 2281

Celecoxib (Potential for increased plasma lithium levels). Products include:
- Celebrex Capsules 2676
- Celebrex Capsules 2780

Chlorothiazide (Co-administration results in reduced renal clearance of lithium and increased serum lithium levels with risk of lithium toxicity). Products include:
- Aldoclor Tablets 2035
- Diuril Oral 2087

Chlorothiazide Sodium (Co-administration results in reduced renal clearance of lithium and increased serum lithium levels with risk of lithium toxicity). Products include:
- Diuril Sodium Intravenous 2086

Chlorpromazine (Potential for encephalopathic syndrome). Products include:
- Thorazine Suppositories 1656

Chlorpromazine Hydrochloride (Potential for encephalopathic syndrome). Products include:
- Thorazine 1656

Chlorprothixene (Potential for encephalopathic syndrome).
- No products indexed under this heading.

Chlorprothixene Hydrochloride (Potential for encephalopathic syndrome).
- No products indexed under this heading.

Chlorthalidone (Co-administration results in reduced renal clearance of lithium and increased serum lithium levels with risk of lithium toxicity). Products include:
- Clorpres Tablets 1002
- Combipres Tablets 1040
- Tenoretic Tablets 690

Cisatracurium Besylate (Lithium may prolong the effects of neuromuscular blocking agents).
- No products indexed under this heading.

Clozapine (Potential for encephalopathic syndrome). Products include:
- Clozaril Tablets 2319

Diclofenac Potassium (Potential for increased plasma lithium levels). Products include:
- Cataflam Tablets 2315

Diclofenac Sodium (Potential for increased plasma lithium levels). Products include:
- Arthrotec Tablets 3195
- Voltaren Ophthalmic Sterile Ophthalmic Solution .... ⊙312
- Voltaren Tablets 2315
- Voltaren-XR Tablets 2315

Doxacurium Chloride (Lithium may prolong the effects of neuromuscular blocking agents).
- No products indexed under this heading.

Enalapril Maleate (Co-administration results in reduced renal clearance of lithium and increased serum lithium levels with risk of lithium toxicity). Products include:
- Lexxel Tablets 608
- Vaseretic Tablets 2204
- Vasotec Tablets 2210

Enalaprilat (Co-administration results in reduced renal clearance of lithium and increased serum lithium levels with risk of lithium toxicity). Products include:
- Enalaprilat Injection 863
- Vasotec I.V. Injection 2207

Ethacrynic Acid (Co-administration results in reduced renal clearance of lithium and increased serum lithium levels with risk of lithium toxicity). Products include:
- Edecrin Tablets 2091

Etodolac (Potential for increased plasma lithium levels). Products include:
- Lodine 3528
- Lodine XL Extended-Release Tablets 3530

Fenoprofen Calcium (Potential for increased plasma lithium levels).
- No products indexed under this heading.

Fluphenazine Decanoate (Potential for encephalopathic syndrome).
- No products indexed under this heading.

Fluphenazine Enanthate (Potential for encephalopathic syndrome).
- No products indexed under this heading.

Fluphenazine Hydrochloride (Potential for encephalopathic syndrome).
- No products indexed under this heading.

Flurbiprofen (Potential for increased plasma lithium levels).
- No products indexed under this heading.

Fosinopril Sodium (Co-administration results in reduced renal clearance of lithium and increased serum lithium levels with risk of lithium toxicity). Products include:
- Monopril Tablets 1091
- Monopril HCT 1094

Furosemide (Co-administration results in reduced renal clearance of lithium and increased serum lithium levels with risk of lithium toxicity). Products include:
- Furosemide Tablets 2284

Haloperidol (Co-administration has resulted in an encephalopathic syndrome characterized by weakness, lethargy, confusion, extrapyramidal symptoms, and others followed by irreversible brain damage). Products include:
- Haldol Injection, Tablets and Concentrate 2533

Haloperidol Decanoate (Co-administration has resulted in an encephalopathic syndrome characterized by weakness, lethargy, confusion, extrapyramidal symptoms, and others followed by irreversible brain damage). Products include:
- Haldol Decanoate 2535

Hydrochlorothiazide (Co-administration results in reduced renal clearance of lithium and increased serum lithium levels with risk of lithium toxicity). Products include:
- Accuretic Tablets 2614
- Aldoril Tablets 2039
- Atacand HCT Tablets 597
- Avalide Tablets 1070
- Diovan HCT Tablets 2338
- Dyazide Capsules 1515
- HydroDIURIL Tablets 2108
- Hyzaar 2109
- Inderide Tablets 3517
- Inderide LA Long-Acting Capsules .. 3519
- Lotensin HCT Tablets 2367
- Maxzide 1008
- Micardis HCT Tablets 1051
- Microzide Capsules 3414
- Moduretic Tablets 2138
- Monopril HCT 1094
- Prinzide Tablets 2168
- Timolide Tablets 2187
- Uniretic Tablets 3178
- Vaseretic Tablets 2204
- Zestoretic Tablets 695
- Ziac Tablets 1887

Hydroflumethiazide (Co-administration results in reduced renal clearance of lithium and increased serum lithium levels with risk of lithium toxicity). Products include:
- Diucardin Tablets 3494

Ibuprofen (Potential for increased plasma lithium levels). Products include:
- Advil .... ■771
- Children's Advil Oral Suspension ... ■773
- Children's Advil Chewable Tablets . ■773
- Advil Cold and Sinus Caplets .... ■771
- Advil Cold and Sinus Tablets .... ■771
- Advil Flu & Body Ache Caplets .... ■772
- Infants' Advil Drops .... ■773
- Junior Strength Advil Tablets .... ■773
- Junior Strength Advil Chewable Tablets .... ■773
- Advil Migraine Liquigels .... ■772
- Children's Motrin Oral Suspension and Chewable Tablets 2006
- Children's Motrin Cold Oral Suspension 2007
- Children's Motrin Oral Suspension .... ■643
- Motrin Suspension, Oral Drops, Chewable Tablets, and Caplets 2002
- Infants' Motrin Concentrated Drops 2006
- Junior Strength Motrin Caplets and Chewable Tablets 2006
- Motrin IB Tablets, Caplets, and Gelcaps 2002
- Motrin Migraine Pain Caplets 2005
- Motrin Sinus Headache Caplets 2005
- Vicoprofen Tablets 520

Indapamide (Co-administration results in reduced renal clearance of lithium and increased serum lithium levels with risk of lithium toxicity). Products include:
- Indapamide Tablets 2286

Indomethacin (Significant increases in steady state plasma lithium levels). Products include:
- Indocin 2112

Indomethacin Sodium Trihydrate (Potential for increased plasma lithium levels). Products include:
- Indocin I.V. 2115

Ketoprofen (Potential for increased plasma lithium levels). Products include:
- Orudis Capsules 3548
- Orudis KT Tablets .... ■778
- Oruvail Capsules 3548

Ketorolac Tromethamine (Potential for increased plasma lithium levels). Products include:
- Acular Ophthalmic Solution 544
- Acular PF Ophthalmic Solution 544
- Toradol 3018

Lisinopril (Co-administration results in reduced renal clearance of lithium and increased serum lithium levels with risk of lithium toxicity). Products include:
- Prinivil Tablets 2164
- Prinzide Tablets 2168
- Zestoretic Tablets 695
- Zestril Tablets 698

Lithium Citrate (Potential for encephalopathic syndrome). Products include:
- Lithium Citrate Syrup 3061

Loxapine Hydrochloride (Potential for encephalopathic syndrome).
- No products indexed under this heading.

Loxapine Succinate (Potential for encephalopathic syndrome). Products include:
- Loxitane Capsules 3398

Meclofenamate Sodium (Potential for increased plasma lithium levels).
- No products indexed under this heading.

Mefenamic Acid (Potential for increased plasma lithium levels). Products include:
- Ponstel Capsules 1356

Meloxicam (Potential for increased plasma lithium levels). Products include:
- Mobic Tablets 1054

Mesoridazine Besylate (Potential for encephalopathic syndrome). Products include:
- Serentil 1057

Methotrimeprazine (Potential for encephalopathic syndrome).
- No products indexed under this heading.

Methyclothiazide (Co-administration results in reduced renal clearance of lithium and increased serum lithium levels with risk of lithium toxicity).
- No products indexed under this heading.

Metocurine Iodide (Lithium may prolong the effects of neuromuscular blocking agents).
- No products indexed under this heading.

Metolazone (Co-administration results in reduced renal clearance of lithium and increased serum lithium levels with risk of lithium toxicity). Products include:
- Mykrox Tablets 1168
- Zaroxolyn Tablets 1177

Mivacurium Chloride (Lithium may prolong the effects of neuromuscular blocking agents).
- No products indexed under this heading.

Moexipril Hydrochloride (Co-administration results in reduced renal clearance of lithium and increased serum lithium levels with risk of lithium toxicity). Products include:
- Uniretic Tablets 3178
- Univasc Tablets 3181

Molindone Hydrochloride (Potential for encephalopathic syndrome). Products include:
- Moban 1320

Nabumetone (Potential for increased plasma lithium levels). Products include:
- Relafen Tablets 1617

Naproxen (Potential for increased plasma lithium levels). Products include:
- EC-Naprosyn Delayed-Release Tablets 2967
- Naprosyn Suspension 2967
- Naprosyn Tablets 2967

Naproxen Sodium (Potential for increased plasma lithium levels). Products include:
- Aleve Tablets, Caplets and Gelcaps .... ■602
- Aleve Cold & Sinus Caplets .... ■603
- Anaprox Tablets 2967
- Anaprox DS Tablets 2967
- Naprelan Tablets 1293

Olanzapine (Potential for encephalopathic syndrome). Products include:
- Zyprexa Tablets 1973

IMPORTANT NOTE: Always consult each drug listing in the patient's regimen for possible interactions.

Zyprexa ZYDIS Orally Disintegrating Tablets ... 1973

Oxaprozin (Potential for increased plasma lithium levels).
No products indexed under this heading.

Pancuronium Bromide (Lithium may prolong the effects of neuromuscular blocking agents).
No products indexed under this heading.

Perindopril Erbumine (Co-administration results in reduced renal clearance of lithium and increased serum lithium levels with risk of lithium toxicity). Products include:
Aceon Tablets (2 mg, 4 mg, 8 mg) ... 3249

Perphenazine (Potential for encephalopathic syndrome). Products include:
Etrafon ... 3115
Trilafon ... 3160

Phenylbutazone (Potential for increased plasma lithium levels).
No products indexed under this heading.

Pimozide (Potential for encephalopathic syndrome). Products include:
Orap Tablets ... 1407

Piroxicam (Significant increases in steady state plasma lithium levels). Products include:
Feldene Capsules ... 2685

Polythiazide (Co-administration results in reduced renal clearance of lithium and increased serum lithium levels with risk of lithium toxicity). Products include:
Minizide Capsules ... 2700
Renese Tablets ... 2712

Prochlorperazine (Potential for encephalopathic syndrome). Products include:
Compazine ... 1505

Promethazine Hydrochloride (Potential for encephalopathic syndrome). Products include:
Mepergan Injection ... 3539
Phenergan Injection ... 3553
Phenergan ... 3556
Phenergan Syrup ... 3554
Phenergan with Codeine Syrup ... 3557
Phenergan with Dextromethorphan Syrup ... 3559
Phenergan VC Syrup ... 3560
Phenergan VC with Codeine Syrup ... 3561

Quetiapine Fumarate (Potential for encephalopathic syndrome). Products include:
Seroquel Tablets ... 684

Quinapril Hydrochloride (Co-administration results in reduced renal clearance of lithium and increased serum lithium levels with risk of lithium toxicity). Products include:
Accupril Tablets ... 2611
Accuretic Tablets ... 2614

Ramipril (Co-administration results in reduced renal clearance of lithium and increased serum lithium levels with risk of lithium toxicity). Products include:
Altace Capsules ... 2233

Rapacuronium Bromide (Lithium may prolong the effects of neuromuscular blocking agents).
No products indexed under this heading.

Risperidone (Potential for encephalopathic syndrome). Products include:
Risperdal ... 1796

Rocuronium Bromide (Lithium may prolong the effects of neuromuscular blocking agents). Products include:
Zemuron Injection ... 2491

Rofecoxib (Potential for increased plasma lithium levels). Products include:
Vioxx ... 2213

Spirapril Hydrochloride (Co-administration results in reduced renal clearance of lithium and increased serum lithium levels with risk of lithium toxicity).
No products indexed under this heading.

Spironolactone (Co-administration results in reduced renal clearance of lithium and increased serum lithium levels with risk of lithium toxicity).
No products indexed under this heading.

Succinylcholine Chloride (Lithium may prolong the effects of neuromuscular blocking agents). Products include:
Anectine Injection ... 1476

Sulindac (Potential for increased plasma lithium levels). Products include:
Clinoril Tablets ... 2053

Thioridazine Hydrochloride (Potential for encephalopathic syndrome). Products include:
Thioridazine Hydrochloride Tablets ... 2289

Thiothixene (Potential for encephalopathic syndrome). Products include:
Navane Capsules ... 2701
Thiothixene Capsules ... 2290

Tolmetin Sodium (Potential for increased plasma lithium levels). Products include:
Tolectin ... 2589

Torsemide (Co-administration results in reduced renal clearance of lithium and increased serum lithium levels with risk of lithium toxicity). Products include:
Demadex Tablets and Injection ... 2965

Trandolapril (Co-administration results in reduced renal clearance of lithium and increased serum lithium levels with risk of lithium toxicity). Products include:
Mavik Tablets ... 478
Tarka Tablets ... 508

Triamterene (Co-administration results in reduced renal clearance of lithium and increased serum lithium levels with risk of lithium toxicity). Products include:
Dyazide Capsules ... 1515
Dyrenium Capsules ... 3458
Maxzide ... 1008

Trifluoperazine Hydrochloride (Potential for encephalopathic syndrome). Products include:
Stelazine ... 1640

Vecuronium Bromide (Lithium may prolong the effects of neuromuscular blocking agents). Products include:
Norcuron for Injection ... 2478

Ziprasidone Hydrochloride (Potential for encephalopathic syndrome). Products include:
Geodon Capsules ... 2688

LITHIUM CARBONATE TABLETS

(Lithium Carbonate) ... 3061
See Lithium Carbonate Capsules

LITHIUM CITRATE SYRUP

(Lithium Citrate) ... 3061
See Lithium Carbonate Capsules

LITHOBID SLOW-RELEASE TABLETS

(Lithium Carbonate) ... 3255
May interact with ACE inhibitors, calcium channel blockers, diuretics, antipsychotic agents, neuromuscular blocking agents, non-steroidal anti-inflammatory agents, theophylline, and certain other agents. Compounds in these categories include:

Acetazolamide (Lowers serum lithium concentrations by increasing urinary lithium excretions). Products include:
Diamox Sequels Sustained Release Capsules ... ⊙270
Diamox Tablets ... ⊙269

Acetazolamide Sodium (Lowers serum lithium concentrations by increasing urinary lithium excretions). Products include:
Diamox Intravenous ... ⊙269

Amiloride Hydrochloride (Sodium loss from diuretics may reduce the renal clearance of lithium resulting in increased serum lithium concentrations with the risk of lithium toxicity; concomitant use should be avoided, if used concurrently, lithium dosage may need to be decreased and more frequent monitoring of lithium serum concentrations is recommended). Products include:
Midamor Tablets ... 2136
Moduretic Tablets ... 2138

Aminophylline (Lowers serum lithium concentrations by increasing urinary lithium excretions).
No products indexed under this heading.

Amlodipine Besylate (Concurrent use may increase the risk of neurotoxicity in the form of ataxia, tremors, nausea, vomiting, diarrhea, and/or tinnitus). Products include:
Lotrel Capsules ... 2370
Norvasc Tablets ... 2704

Atracurium Besylate (Prolonged effects of neuromuscular blocking agents).
No products indexed under this heading.

Benazepril Hydrochloride (ACE inhibitors may reduce the renal clearance of lithium resulting in increased serum lithium concentrations with the risk of lithium toxicity; concomitant use should be avoided, if used concurrently, lithium dosage may need to be decreased and more frequent monitoring of lithium serum concentrations is recommended). Products include:
Lotensin Tablets ... 2365
Lotensin HCT Tablets ... 2367
Lotrel Capsules ... 2370

Bendroflumethiazide (Sodium loss from diuretics may reduce the renal clearance of lithium resulting in increased serum lithium concentrations with the risk of lithium toxicity; concomitant use should be avoided, if used concurrently, lithium dosage may need to be decreased and more frequent monitoring of lithium serum concentrations is recommended). Products include:
Corzide 40/5 Tablets ... 2247
Corzide 80/5 Tablets ... 2247

Bepridil Hydrochloride (Concurrent use may increase the risk of neurotoxicity in the form of ataxia, tremors, nausea, vomiting, diarrhea, and/or tinnitus). Products include:
Vascor Tablets ... 2602

Bumetanide (Sodium loss from diuretics may reduce the renal clearance of lithium resulting in increased serum lithium concentrations with the risk of lithium toxicity; concomitant use should be avoided, if used concurrently, lithium dosage may need to be decreased and more frequent monitoring of lithium serum concentrations is recommended).
No products indexed under this heading.

Captopril (ACE inhibitors may reduce the renal clearance of lithium resulting in increased serum lithium concentrations with the risk of lithium toxicity; concomitant use should be avoided, if used concurrently, lithium dosage may need to be decreased and more frequent monitoring of lithium serum concentrations is recommended). Products include:
Captopril Tablets ... 2281

Carbamazepine (Increased risk of neurotoxic side effects). Products include:
Carbatrol Capsules ... 3234
Tegretol/Tegretol-XR ... 2404

Celecoxib (Potential for increased steady-state plasma lithium levels resulting in lithium toxicity). Products include:
Celebrex Capsules ... 2676
Celebrex Capsules ... 2780

Chlorothiazide (Sodium loss from diuretics may reduce the renal clearance of lithium resulting in increased serum lithium concentrations with the risk of lithium toxicity; concomitant use should be avoided, if used concurrently, lithium dosage may need to be decreased and more frequent monitoring of lithium serum concentrations is recommended). Products include:
Aldoclor Tablets ... 2035
Diuril Oral ... 2087

Chlorothiazide Sodium (Sodium loss from diuretics may reduce the renal clearance of lithium resulting in increased serum lithium concentrations with the risk of lithium toxicity; concomitant use should be avoided, if used concurrently, lithium dosage may need to be decreased and more frequent monitoring of lithium serum concentrations is recommended). Products include:
Diuril Sodium Intravenous ... 2086

Chlorpromazine (Possible haloperidol-type interaction has been extended to other antipsychotics). Products include:
Thorazine Suppositories ... 1656

Chlorpromazine Hydrochloride (Possible haloperidol-type interaction has been extended to other antipsychotics). Products include:
Thorazine ... 1656

Chlorprothixene (Possible haloperidol-type interaction has been extended to other antipsychotics).
No products indexed under this heading.

Chlorprothixene Hydrochloride (Possible haloperidol-type interaction has been extended to other antipsychotics).
No products indexed under this heading.

Chlorthalidone (Sodium loss from diuretics may reduce the renal clearance of lithium resulting in increased serum lithium concentrations with the risk of lithium toxicity; concomitant use should be avoided, if used concurrently, lithium dosage may need to be decreased and more frequent monitoring of lithium serum concentrations is recommended). Products include:
Clorpres Tablets ... 1002
Combipres Tablets ... 1040
Tenoretic Tablets ... 690

Cisatracurium Besylate (Prolonged effects of neuromuscular blocking agents).
No products indexed under this heading.

Clozapine (Possible haloperidol-type interaction has been extended to other antipsychotics). Products include:
Clozaril Tablets ... 2319

Decamethonium (Prolonged effects of neuromuscular blocking agents).
No products indexed under this heading.

Diclofenac Potassium (Potential for increased steady-state plasma lithium levels resulting in lithium toxicity). Products include:
Cataflam Tablets ... 2315

Diclofenac Sodium (Potential for increased steady-state plasma lithium levels resulting in lithium toxicity). Products include:
Arthrotec Tablets ... 3195

Voltaren Ophthalmic Sterile Ophthalmic Solution .... ⊙ 312
Voltaren Tablets 2315
Voltaren-XR Tablets 2315

Diltiazem Hydrochloride (Concurrent use may increase the risk of neurotoxicity in the form of ataxia, tremors, nausea, vomiting, diarrhea, and/or tinnitus). Products include:
Cardizem Injectable 1018
Cardizem Lyo-Ject Syringe 1018
Cardizem Monovial 1018
Cardizem CD Capsules 1016
Tiazac Capsules 1378

Doxacurium Chloride (Prolonged effects of neuromuscular blocking agents).
No products indexed under this heading.

Dyphylline (Lowers serum lithium concentrations by increasing urinary lithium excretions). Products include:
Lufyllin Tablets 3347
Lufyllin-400 Tablets 3347
Lufyllin-GG Elixir 3348
Lufyllin-GG Tablets 3348

Enalapril Maleate (ACE inhibitors may reduce the renal clearance of lithium resulting in increased serum lithium concentrations with the risk of lithium toxicity; concomitant use should be avoided, if used concurrently, lithium dosage may need to be decreased and more frequent monitoring of lithium serum concentrations is recommended). Products include:
Lexxel Tablets 608
Vaseretic Tablets 2204
Vasotec Tablets 2210

Enalaprilat (ACE inhibitors may reduce the renal clearance of lithium resulting in increased serum lithium concentrations with the risk of lithium toxicity; concomitant use should be avoided, if used concurrently, lithium dosage may need to be decreased and more frequent monitoring of lithium serum concentrations is recommended). Products include:
Enalaprilat Injection 863
Vasotec I.V. Injection 2207

Ethacrynic Acid (Sodium loss from diuretics may reduce the renal clearance of lithium resulting in increased serum lithium concentrations with the risk of lithium toxicity; concomitant use should be avoided, if used concurrently, lithium dosage may need to be decreased and more frequent monitoring of lithium serum concentrations is recommended). Products include:
Edecrin Tablets 2091

Etodolac (Potential for increased steady-state plasma lithium levels resulting in lithium toxicity). Products include:
Lodine 3528
Lodine XL Extended-Release Tablets 3530

Felodipine (Concurrent use may increase the risk of neurotoxicity in the form of ataxia, tremors, nausea, vomiting, diarrhea, and/or tinnitus). Products include:
Lexxel Tablets 608
Plendil Extended-Release Tablets 623

Fenoprofen Calcium (Potential for increased steady-state plasma lithium levels resulting in lithium toxicity).
No products indexed under this heading.

Fluoxetine Hydrochloride (Coadministration has resulted in both increased and decreased serum lithium concentrations). Products include:
Prozac Pulvules, Liquid, and Weekly Capsules 1238
Sarafem Pulvules 1962

Fluphenazine Decanoate (Possible haloperidol-type interaction has been extended to other antipsychotics).
No products indexed under this heading.

Fluphenazine Enanthate (Possible haloperidol-type interaction has been extended to other antipsychotics).
No products indexed under this heading.

Fluphenazine Hydrochloride (Possible haloperidol-type interaction has been extended to other antipsychotics).
No products indexed under this heading.

Flurbiprofen (Potential for increased steady-state plasma lithium levels resulting in lithium toxicity).
No products indexed under this heading.

Fosinopril Sodium (ACE inhibitors may reduce the renal clearance of lithium resulting in increased serum lithium concentrations with the risk of lithium toxicity; concomitant use should be avoided, if used concurrently, lithium dosage may need to be decreased and more frequent monitoring of lithium serum concentrations is recommended). Products include:
Monopril Tablets 1091
Monopril HCT 1094

Furosemide (Sodium loss from diuretics may reduce the renal clearance of lithium resulting in increased serum lithium concentrations with the risk of lithium toxicity; concomitant use should be avoided, if used concurrently, lithium dosage may need to be decreased and more frequent monitoring of lithium serum concentrations is recommended). Products include:
Furosemide Tablets 2284

Haloperidol (Concomitant use may lead to encephalopathic syndrome followed by irreversible brain damage). Products include:
Haldol Injection, Tablets and Concentrate 2533

Haloperidol Decanoate (Concomitant use may lead to encephalopathic syndrome followed by irreversible brain damage). Products include:
Haldol Decanoate 2535

Hydrochlorothiazide (Sodium loss from diuretics may reduce the renal clearance of lithium resulting in increased serum lithium concentrations with the risk of lithium toxicity; concomitant use should be avoided, if used concurrently, lithium dosage may need to be decreased and more frequent monitoring of lithium serum concentrations is recommended). Products include:
Accuretic Tablets 2614
Aldoril Tablets 2039
Atacand HCT Tablets 597
Avalide Tablets 1070
Diovan HCT Tablets 2338
Dyazide Capsules 1515
HydroDIURIL Tablets 2108
Hyzaar 2109
Inderide Tablets 3517
Inderide LA Long-Acting Capsules 3519
Lotensin HCT Tablets 2367
Maxzide 1008
Micardis HCT Tablets 1051
Microzide Capsules 3414
Moduretic Tablets 2138
Monopril HCT 1094
Prinzide Tablets 2168
Timolide Tablets 2187
Uniretic Tablets 3178
Vaseretic Tablets 2204
Zestoretic Tablets 695
Ziac Tablets 1887

Hydroflumethiazide (Sodium loss from diuretics may reduce the renal clearance of lithium resulting in increased serum lithium concentrations with the risk of lithium toxicity; concomitant use should be avoided, if used concurrently, lithium dosage may need to be decreased and more frequent monitoring of lithium serum concentrations is recommended). Products include:
Diucardin Tablets 3494

Ibuprofen (Potential for increased steady-state plasma lithium levels resulting in lithium toxicity). Products include:
Advil 771
Children's Advil Oral Suspension 773
Children's Advil Chewable Tablets 773
Advil Cold and Sinus Caplets 771
Advil Cold and Sinus Tablets 771
Advil Flu & Body Ache Caplets 772
Infants' Advil Drops 773
Junior Strength Advil Tablets 773
Junior Strength Advil Chewable Tablets 773
Advil Migraine Liquigels 772
Children's Motrin Oral Suspension and Chewable Tablets 2006
Children's Motrin Cold Oral Suspension 2007
Children's Motrin Oral Suspension 643
Motrin Suspension, Oral Drops, Chewable Tablets, and Caplets 2002
Infants' Motrin Concentrated Drops 2006
Junior Strength Motrin Caplets and Chewable Tablets 2006
Motrin IB Tablets, Caplets, and Gelcaps 2002
Motrin Migraine Pain Caplets 2005
Motrin Sinus Headache Caplets 2005
Vicoprofen Tablets 520

Indapamide (Sodium loss from diuretics may reduce the renal clearance of lithium resulting in increased serum lithium concentrations with the risk of lithium toxicity; concomitant use should be avoided, if used concurrently, lithium dosage may need to be decreased and more frequent monitoring of lithium serum concentrations is recommended). Products include:
Indapamide Tablets 2286

Indomethacin (Potential for increased steady-state plasma lithium levels resulting in lithium toxicity). Products include:
Indocin 2112

Indomethacin Sodium Trihydrate (Potential for increased steady-state plasma lithium levels resulting in lithium toxicity). Products include:
Indocin I.V. 2115

Isradipine (Concurrent use may increase the risk of neurotoxicity in the form of ataxia, tremors, nausea, vomiting, diarrhea, and/or tinnitus). Products include:
DynaCirc Capsules 2921
DynaCirc CR Tablets 2923

Ketoprofen (Potential for increased steady-state plasma lithium levels resulting in lithium toxicity). Products include:
Orudis Capsules 3548
Orudis KT Tablets 778
Oruvail Capsules 3548

Ketorolac Tromethamine (Potential for increased steady-state plasma lithium levels resulting in lithium toxicity). Products include:
Acular Ophthalmic Solution 544
Acular PF Ophthalmic Solution 544
Toradol 3018

Lisinopril (ACE inhibitors may reduce the renal clearance of lithium resulting in increased serum lithium concentrations with the risk of lithium toxicity; concomitant use should be avoided, if used concurrently, lithium dosage may need to be decreased and more frequent monitoring of lithium serum concentrations is recommended). Products include:
Prinivil Tablets 2164
Prinzide Tablets 2168
Zestoretic Tablets 695
Zestril Tablets 698

Lithium Citrate (Possible haloperidol-type interaction has been extended to other antipsychotics). Products include:
Lithium Citrate Syrup 3061

Loxapine Hydrochloride (Possible haloperidol-type interaction has been extended to other antipsychotics).
No products indexed under this heading.

Loxapine Succinate (Possible haloperidol-type interaction has been extended to other antipsychotics). Products include:
Loxitane Capsules 3398

Meclofenamate Sodium (Potential for increased steady-state plasma lithium levels resulting in lithium toxicity).
No products indexed under this heading.

Mefenamic Acid (Potential for increased steady-state plasma lithium levels resulting in lithium toxicity). Products include:
Ponstel Capsules 1356

Meloxicam (Potential for increased steady-state plasma lithium levels resulting in lithium toxicity). Products include:
Mobic Tablets 1054

Mesoridazine Besylate (Possible haloperidol-type interaction has been extended to other antipsychotics). Products include:
Serentil 1057

Methotrimeprazine (Possible haloperidol-type interaction has been extended to other antipsychotics).
No products indexed under this heading.

Methyclothiazide (Sodium loss from diuretics may reduce the renal clearance of lithium resulting in increased serum lithium concentrations with the risk of lithium toxicity; concomitant use should be avoided, if used concurrently, lithium dosage may need to be decreased and more frequent monitoring of lithium serum concentrations is recommended).
No products indexed under this heading.

Metocurine Iodide (Prolonged effects of neuromuscular blocking agents).
No products indexed under this heading.

Metolazone (Sodium loss from diuretics may reduce the renal clearance of lithium resulting in increased serum lithium concentrations with the risk of lithium toxicity; concomitant use should be avoided, if used concurrently, lithium dosage may need to be decreased and more frequent monitoring of lithium serum concentrations is recommended). Products include:
Mykrox Tablets 1168
Zaroxolyn Tablets 1177

Metronidazole (Concurrent use may provoke lithium toxicity due to reduced renal clearance). Products include:
MetroCream 1404
MetroGel 1405
MetroGel-Vaginal Gel 1986
MetroLotion 1405
Noritate Cream 1224

Metronidazole Sodium (Concurrent use may provoke lithium due to reduced renal clearance).
No products indexed under this heading.

Mibefradil Dihydrochloride (Concurrent use may increase the risk of neurotoxicity in the form of ataxia, tremors, nausea, vomiting, diarrhea, and/or tinnitus).
No products indexed under this heading.

Mivacurium Chloride (Prolonged effects of neuromuscular blocking

agents).
No products indexed under this heading.

Moexipril Hydrochloride (ACE inhibitors may reduce the renal clearance of lithium resulting in increased serum lithium concentrations with the risk of lithium toxicity; concomitant use should be avoided, if used concurrently, lithium dosage may need to be decreased and more frequent monitoring of lithium serum concentrations is recommended). Products include:
Uniretic Tablets ... 3178
Univasc Tablets ... 3181

Molindone Hydrochloride (Possible haloperidol-type interaction has been extended to other antipsychotics). Products include:
Moban ... 1320

Nabumetone (Potential for increased steady-state plasma lithium levels resulting in lithium toxicity). Products include:
Relafen Tablets ... 1617

Naproxen (Potential for increased steady-state plasma lithium levels resulting in lithium toxicity). Products include:
EC-Naprosyn Delayed-Release Tablets ... 2967
Naprosyn Suspension ... 2967
Naprosyn Tablets ... 2967

Naproxen Sodium (Potential for increased steady-state plasma lithium levels resulting in lithium toxicity). Products include:
Aleve Tablets, Caplets and Gelcaps ... ▣602
Aleve Cold & Sinus Caplets ... ▣603
Anaprox Tablets ... 2967
Anaprox DS Tablets ... 2967
Naprelan Tablets ... 1293

Nicardipine Hydrochloride (Concurrent use may increase the risk of neurotoxicity in the form of ataxia, tremors, nausea, vomiting, diarrhea, and/or tinnitus). Products include:
Cardene I.V. ... 3485

Nifedipine (Concurrent use may increase the risk of neurotoxicity in the form of ataxia, tremors, nausea, vomiting, diarrhea, and/or tinnitus). Products include:
Adalat CC Tablets ... 877
Procardia Capsules ... 2708
Procardia XL Extended Release Tablets ... 2710

Nimodipine (Concurrent use may increase the risk of neurotoxicity in the form of ataxia, tremors, nausea, vomiting, diarrhea, and/or tinnitus). Products include:
Nimotop Capsules ... 904

Nisoldipine (Concurrent use may increase the risk of neurotoxicity in the form of ataxia, tremors, nausea, vomiting, diarrhea, and/or tinnitus). Products include:
Sular Tablets ... 688

Olanzapine (Possible haloperidol-type interaction has been extended to other antipsychotics). Products include:
Zyprexa Tablets ... 1973
Zyprexa ZYDIS Orally Disintegrating Tablets ... 1973

Oxaprozin (Potential for increased steady-state plasma lithium levels resulting in lithium toxicity).
No products indexed under this heading.

Pancuronium Bromide (Prolonged effects of neuromuscular blocking agents).
No products indexed under this heading.

Perindopril Erbumine (ACE inhibitors may reduce the renal clearance of lithium resulting in increased serum lithium concentrations with the risk of lithium toxicity; concomitant use should be avoided, if used concurrently, lithium dosage may need to be decreased and more frequent monitoring of lithium serum concentrations is recommended). Products include:
Aceon Tablets (2 mg, 4 mg, 8 mg) ... 3249

Perphenazine (Possible haloperidol-type interaction has been extended to other antipsychotics). Products include:
Etrafon ... 3115
Trilafon ... 3160

Phenylbutazone (Potential for increased steady-state plasma lithium levels resulting in lithium toxicity).
No products indexed under this heading.

Pimozide (Possible haloperidol-type interaction has been extended to other antipsychotics). Products include:
Orap Tablets ... 1407

Piroxicam (Potential for increased steady-state plasma lithium levels resulting in lithium toxicity). Products include:
Feldene Capsules ... 2685

Polythiazide (Sodium loss from diuretics may reduce the renal clearance of lithium resulting in increased serum lithium concentrations with the risk of lithium toxicity; concomitant use should be avoided, if used concurrently, lithium dosage may need to be decreased and more frequent monitoring of lithium serum concentrations is recommended). Products include:
Minizide Capsules ... 2700
Renese Tablets ... 2712

Potassium Iodide (Concomitant extended use of iodide preparation may produce hypothyroidism). Products include:
Pima Syrup ... 1362

Prochlorperazine (Possible haloperidol-type interaction has been extended to other antipsychotics). Products include:
Compazine ... 1505

Promethazine Hydrochloride (Possible haloperidol-type interaction has been extended to other antipsychotics). Products include:
Mepergan Injection ... 3539
Phenergan Injection ... 3553
Phenergan ... 3556
Phenergan Syrup ... 3554
Phenergan with Codeine Syrup ... 3557
Phenergan with Dextromethorphan Syrup ... 3559
Phenergan VC Syrup ... 3560
Phenergan VC with Codeine Syrup ... 3561

Quetiapine Fumarate (Possible haloperidol-type interaction has been extended to other antipsychotics). Products include:
Seroquel Tablets ... 684

Quinapril Hydrochloride (ACE inhibitors may reduce the renal clearance of lithium resulting in increased serum lithium concentrations with the risk of lithium toxicity; concomitant use should be avoided, if used concurrently, lithium dosage may need to be decreased and more frequent monitoring of lithium serum concentrations is recommended). Products include:
Accupril Tablets ... 2611
Accuretic Tablets ... 2614

Ramipril (ACE inhibitors may reduce the renal clearance of lithium resulting in increased serum lithium concentrations with the risk of lithium toxicity; concomitant use should be avoided, if used concurrently, lithium dosage may need to be decreased and more frequent monitoring of lithium serum concentrations is recommended). Products include:
Altace Capsules ... 2233

Rapacuronium Bromide (Prolonged effects of neuromuscular blocking agents).
No products indexed under this heading.

Risperidone (Possible haloperidol-type interaction has been extended to other antipsychotics). Products include:
Risperdal ... 1796

Rocuronium Bromide (Prolonged effects of neuromuscular blocking agents). Products include:
Zemuron Injection ... 2491

Rofecoxib (Potential for increased steady-state plasma lithium levels resulting in lithium toxicity). Products include:
Vioxx ... 2213

Sodium Bicarbonate (Lowers serum lithium concentrations by increasing urinary lithium excretions). Products include:
Alka-Seltzer ... ▣603
Alka-Seltzer Lemon Lime Antacid and Pain Reliever Effervescent Tablets ... ▣603
Alka-Seltzer Extra Strength Antacid and Pain Reliever Effervescent Tablets ... ▣603
Alka-Seltzer Heartburn Relief Tablets ... ▣604
Ceo-Two Evacuant Suppository ... ▣618
Colyte with Flavor Packs for Oral Solution ... 3170
GoLYTELY and Pineapple Flavor GoLYTELY for Oral Solution ... 1068
NuLYTELY, Cherry Flavor, Lemon-Lime Flavor, and Orange Flavor NuLYTELY for Oral Solution ... 1068

Spirapril Hydrochloride (ACE inhibitors may reduce the renal clearance of lithium resulting in increased serum lithium concentrations with the risk of lithium toxicity; concomitant use should be avoided, if used concurrently, lithium dosage may need to be decreased and more frequent monitoring of lithium serum concentrations is recommended).
No products indexed under this heading.

Spironolactone (Sodium loss from diuretics may reduce the renal clearance of lithium resulting in increased serum lithium concentrations with the risk of lithium toxicity; concomitant use should be avoided, if used concurrently, lithium dosage may need to be decreased and more frequent monitoring of lithium serum concentrations is recommended).
No products indexed under this heading.

Succinylcholine Chloride (Prolonged effects of neuromuscular blocking agents). Products include:
Anectine Injection ... 1476

Sulindac (Potential for increased steady-state plasma lithium levels resulting in lithium toxicity). Products include:
Clinoril Tablets ... 2053

Theophylline (Lowers serum lithium concentrations by increasing urinary lithium excretions). Products include:
Aerolate ... 1361
Theo-Dur Extended-Release Tablets ... 1835
Uni-Dur Extended-Release Tablets ... 1841
Uniphyl 400 mg and 600 mg Tablets ... 2903

Theophylline Calcium Salicylate (Lowers serum lithium concentrations by increasing urinary lithium excretions).
No products indexed under this heading.

Theophylline Sodium Glycinate (Lowers serum lithium concentrations by increasing urinary lithium excretions).
No products indexed under this heading.

Thioridazine Hydrochloride (Possible haloperidol-type interaction has been extended to other antipsychotics). Products include:
Thioridazine Hydrochloride Tablets ... 2289

Thiothixene (Possible haloperidol-type interaction has been extended to other antipsychotics). Products include:
Navane Capsules ... 2701
Thiothixene Capsules ... 2290

Tolmetin Sodium (Potential for increased steady-state plasma lithium levels resulting in lithium toxicity). Products include:
Tolectin ... 2589

Torsemide (Sodium loss from diuretics may reduce the renal clearance of lithium resulting in increased serum lithium concentrations with the risk of lithium toxicity; concomitant use should be avoided, if used concurrently, lithium dosage may need to be decreased and more frequent monitoring of lithium serum concentrations is recommended). Products include:
Demadex Tablets and Injection ... 2965

Trandolapril (ACE inhibitors may reduce the renal clearance of lithium resulting in increased serum lithium concentrations with the risk of lithium toxicity; concomitant use should be avoided, if used concurrently, lithium dosage may need to be decreased and more frequent monitoring of lithium serum concentrations is recommended). Products include:
Mavik Tablets ... 478
Tarka Tablets ... 508

Triamterene (Sodium loss from diuretics may reduce the renal clearance of lithium resulting in increased serum lithium concentrations with the risk of lithium toxicity; concomitant use should be avoided, if used concurrently, lithium dosage may need to be decreased and more frequent monitoring of lithium serum concentrations is recommended). Products include:
Dyazide Capsules ... 1515
Dyrenium Capsules ... 3458
Maxzide ... 1008

Trifluoperazine Hydrochloride (Possible haloperidol-type interaction has been extended to other antipsychotics). Products include:
Stelazine ... 1640

Vecuronium Bromide (Prolonged effects of neuromuscular blocking agents). Products include:
Norcuron for Injection ... 2478

Verapamil Hydrochloride (Concurrent use may increase the risk of neurotoxicity in the form of ataxia, tremors, nausea, vomiting, diarrhea, and/or tinnitus). Products include:
Covera-HS Tablets ... 3199
Isoptin SR Tablets ... 467
Tarka Tablets ... 508
Verelan Capsules ... 3184
Verelan PM Capsules ... 3186

Ziprasidone Hydrochloride (Possible haloperidol-type interaction has been extended to other antipsychotics). Products include:
Geodon Capsules ... 2688

LIVOSTIN
(Levocabastine Hydrochloride) ... ⊙305
None cited in PDR database.

LOCOID CREAM
(Hydrocortisone Butyrate) ... 1341
None cited in PDR database.

LOCOID LIPOCREAM CREAM
(Hydrocortisone Butyrate) ... 1342
None cited in PDR database.

LOCOID OINTMENT
(Hydrocortisone Butyrate) ... 1341
None cited in PDR database.

LOCOID TOPICAL SOLUTION
(Hydrocortisone Butyrate) ... 1341
None cited in PDR database.

LODINE CAPSULES

(Etodolac) 3528
See Lodine XL Extended-Release Tablets

LODINE TABLETS

(Etodolac) 3528
See Lodine XL Extended-Release Tablets

LODINE XL EXTENDED-RELEASE TABLETS

(Etodolac) 3530
May interact with ACE inhibitors, oral anticoagulants, lithium preparations, thiazides, and certain other agents. Compounds in these categories include:

Aluminum Carbonate (Co-administration with antacids has no apparent effect on the extent of absorption, however, antacids can decrease the peak concentration reached by 15% to 20%).
No products indexed under this heading.

Aluminum Hydroxide (Co-administration with antacids has no apparent effect on the extent of absorption, however, antacids can decrease the peak concentration reached by 15% to 20%). Products include:
- Amphojel Suspension (Mint Flavor) 789
- Gaviscon Extra Strength Liquid 751
- Gaviscon Extra Strength Tablets 751
- Gaviscon Regular Strength Liquid 751
- Gaviscon Regular Strength Tablets 750
- Maalox Antacid/Anti-Gas Oral Suspension 673
- Maalox Max Maximum Strength Antacid/Anti-Gas Liquid 2300
- Maalox Regular Strength Antacid/Antigas Liquid 2300
- Mylanta 1813
- Vanquish Caplets 617

Aspirin (Co-administration reduces protein binding, although the clearance of free etodolac is not altered; concurrent use is not recommended because of potential for increased adverse effects). Products include:
- Aggrenox Capsules 1026
- Alka-Seltzer 603
- Alka-Seltzer Lemon Lime Antacid and Pain Reliever Effervescent Tablets 603
- Alka-Seltzer Extra Strength Antacid and Pain Reliever Effervescent Tablets 603
- Alka-Seltzer PM Effervescent Tablets 605
- Genuine Bayer Tablets, Caplets and Gelcaps 606
- Extra Strength Bayer Caplets and Gelcaps 610
- Aspirin Regimen Bayer Children's Chewable Tablets (Orange or Cherry Flavored) 607
- Bayer, Aspirin Regimen 606
- Aspirin Regimen Bayer 81 mg Caplets with Calcium 607
- Genuine Bayer Professional Labeling (Aspirin Regimen Bayer) 608
- Extra Strength Bayer Arthritis Caplets 610
- Extra Strength Bayer Plus Caplets 610
- Extra Strength Bayer PM Caplets 611
- BC Powder 619
- BC Allergy Sinus Cold Powder 619
- Arthritis Strength BC Powder 619
- BC Sinus Cold Powder 619
- Darvon Compound-65 Pulvules 1910
- Ecotrin Enteric Coated Aspirin Low, Regular and Maximum Strength Tablets 1715
- Excedrin Extra-Strength Tablets, Caplets, and Geltabs 629
- Excedrin Migraine 1070
- Goody's Body Pain Formula Powder 620
- Goody's Extra Strength Headache Powder 620
- Goody's Extra Strength Pain Relief Tablets 620
- Percodan Tablets 1327
- Robaxisal Tablets 2939
- Soma Compound Tablets 3354
- Soma Compound w/Codeine Tablets 3355
- Vanquish Caplets 617

Benazepril Hydrochloride (NSAIDs may diminish the antihypertensive effect of ACE inhibitors). Products include:
- Lotensin Tablets 2365
- Lotensin HCT Tablets 2367
- Lotrel Capsules 2370

Bendroflumethiazide (Etodolac can reduce the natriuretic effect of thiazide diuretics due to inhibition of renal prostaglandin synthesis). Products include:
- Corzide 40/5 Tablets 2247
- Corzide 80/5 Tablets 2247

Captopril (NSAIDs may diminish the antihypertensive effect of ACE inhibitors). Products include:
- Captopril Tablets 2281

Chlorothiazide (Etodolac can reduce the natriuretic effect of thiazide diuretics due to inhibition of renal prostaglandin synthesis). Products include:
- Aldoclor Tablets 2035
- Diuril Oral 2087

Chlorothiazide Sodium (Etodolac can reduce the natriuretic effect of thiazide diuretics due to inhibition of renal prostaglandin synthesis). Products include:
- Diuril Sodium Intravenous 2086

Cyclosporine (Etodolac, like other NSAIDs, may cause changes in the elimination of cyclosporine; nephrotoxicity associated with cyclosporine may also be enhanced). Products include:
- Gengraf Capsules 457
- Neoral Soft Gelatin Capsules 2380
- Neoral Oral Solution 2380
- Sandimmune 2388

Dicumarol (NSAIDs inhibit platelet aggregation and have been shown to prolong bleeding time in some patients; concurrent use with anticoagulants may adversely affect platelet function).
No products indexed under this heading.

Digoxin (Etodolac, like other NSAIDs, may cause changes in the elimination of digoxin through its effects on renal prostaglandins, leading to elevated serum levels of digoxin and increased toxicity). Products include:
- Digitek Tablets 1003
- Lanoxicaps Capsules 1574
- Lanoxin Injection 1581
- Lanoxin Tablets 1587
- Lanoxin Elixir Pediatric 1578
- Lanoxin Injection Pediatric 1584

Enalapril Maleate (NSAIDs may diminish the antihypertensive effect of ACE inhibitors). Products include:
- Lexxel Tablets 608
- Vaseretic Tablets 2204
- Vasotec Tablets 2210

Enalaprilat (NSAIDs may diminish the antihypertensive effect of ACE inhibitors). Products include:
- Enalaprilat Injection 863
- Vasotec I.V. Injection 2207

Fosinopril Sodium (NSAIDs may diminish the antihypertensive effect of ACE inhibitors). Products include:
- Monopril Tablets 1091
- Monopril HCT 1094

Furosemide (Etodolac can reduce the natriuretic effect of furosemide diuretics due to inhibition of renal prostaglandin synthesis). Products include:
- Furosemide Tablets 2284

Hydrochlorothiazide (Etodolac can reduce the natriuretic effect of thiazide diuretics due to inhibition of renal prostaglandin synthesis). Products include:
- Accuretic Tablets 2614
- Aldoril Tablets 2039
- Atacand HCT Tablets 597
- Avalide Tablets 1070
- Diovan HCT Tablets 2338
- Dyazide Capsules 1515
- HydroDIURIL Tablets 2108
- Hyzaar 2109
- Inderide Tablets 3517
- Inderide LA Long-Acting Capsules 3519
- Lotensin HCT Tablets 2367
- Maxzide 1008
- Micardis HCT Tablets 1051
- Microzide Capsules 3414
- Moduretic Tablets 2138
- Monopril HCT 1094
- Prinzide Tablets 2168
- Timolide Tablets 2187
- Uniretic Tablets 3178
- Vaseretic Tablets 2204
- Zestoretic Tablets 695
- Ziac Tablets 1887

Hydroflumethiazide (Etodolac can reduce the natriuretic effect of thiazide diuretics due to inhibition of renal prostaglandin synthesis). Products include:
- Diucardin Tablets 3494

Lisinopril (NSAIDs may diminish the antihypertensive effect of ACE inhibitors). Products include:
- Prinivil Tablets 2164
- Prinzide Tablets 2168
- Zestoretic Tablets 695
- Zestril Tablets 698

Lithium Carbonate (NSAIDs have produced an elevation of plasma lithium levels and a reduction in renal lithium clearance due to inhibition of renal prostaglandin synthesis). Products include:
- Eskalith 1527
- Lithium Carbonate 3061
- Lithobid Slow-Release Tablets 3255

Lithium Citrate (NSAIDs have produced an elevation of plasma lithium levels and a reduction in renal lithium clearance due to inhibition of renal prostaglandin synthesis). Products include:
- Lithium Citrate Syrup 3061

Magnesium Hydroxide (Co-administration with antacids has no apparent effect on the extent of absorption, however, antacids can decrease the peak concentration reached by 15% to 20%). Products include:
- Ex•Lax Milk of Magnesia Liquid 670
- Maalox Antacid/Anti-Gas Oral Suspension 673
- Maalox Max Maximum Strength Antacid/Anti-Gas Liquid 2300
- Maalox Regular Strength Antacid/Antigas Liquid 2300
- Mylanta Fast-Acting 1813
- Mylanta 1813
- Pepcid Complete Chewable Tablets 1815
- Phillips' Chewable Tablets 615
- Phillips' Milk of Magnesia Liquid (Original, Cherry, & Mint) 616
- Rolaids Tablets 706
- Extra Strength Rolaids Tablets 706
- Vanquish Caplets 617

Magnesium Oxide (Co-administration with antacids has no apparent effect on the extent of absorption, however, antacids can decrease the peak concentration reached by 15% to 20%). Products include:
- Beelith Tablets 946
- Mag-Ox 400 Tablets 1024
- Uro-Mag Capsules 1024

Methotrexate Sodium (Etodolac, like other NSAIDs, may cause changes in the elimination of methotrexate through its effects on renal prostaglandins, leading to elevated serum levels of methotrexate and increased toxicity).
No products indexed under this heading.

Methyclothiazide (Etodolac can reduce the natriuretic effect of thiazide diuretics due to inhibition of renal prostaglandin synthesis).
No products indexed under this heading.

Moexipril Hydrochloride (NSAIDs may diminish the antihypertensive effect of ACE inhibitors). Products include:
- Uniretic Tablets 3178
- Univasc Tablets 3181

Perindopril Erbumine (NSAIDs may diminish the antihypertensive effect of ACE inhibitors). Products include:
- Aceon Tablets (2 mg, 4 mg, 8 mg) 3249

Phenylbutazone (Co-administration causes an increase (by about 80%) in the free fraction of etodolac; concomitant use is not recommended).
No products indexed under this heading.

Polythiazide (Etodolac can reduce the natriuretic effect of thiazide diuretics due to inhibition of renal prostaglandin synthesis). Products include:
- Minizide Capsules 2700
- Renese Tablets 2712

Quinapril Hydrochloride (NSAIDs may diminish the antihypertensive effect of ACE inhibitors). Products include:
- Accupril Tablets 2611
- Accuretic Tablets 2614

Ramipril (NSAIDs may diminish the antihypertensive effect of ACE inhibitors). Products include:
- Altace Capsules 2233

Spirapril Hydrochloride (NSAIDs may diminish the antihypertensive effect of ACE inhibitors).
No products indexed under this heading.

Trandolapril (NSAIDs may diminish the antihypertensive effect of ACE inhibitors). Products include:
- Mavik Tablets 478
- Tarka Tablets 508

Warfarin Sodium (Co-administration results in synergistic bleeding; there have been few spontaneous reports or prolonged prothrombin times with or without bleeding). Products include:
- Coumadin for Injection 1243
- Coumadin Tablets 1243
- Warfarin Sodium Tablets, USP 3302

Food Interactions

Food, unspecified (Food significantly increased Cmax (54%) following 600 mg dose).

LODOSYN TABLETS

(Carbidopa) 1251
May interact with antihypertensives, dopamine D2 antagonists, iron containing oral preparations, nonselective MAO inhibitors, phenytoin, tricyclic antidepressants, and certain other agents. Compounds in these categories include:

Acebutolol Hydrochloride (Co-administration with some antihypertensive agents has resulted in symptomatic postural hypotension). Products include:
- Sectral Capsules 3589

Amitriptyline Hydrochloride (Co-administration of tricyclic antidepressants and carbidopa-levodopa preparations has resulted in rare reports of adverse reactions; including hypertension and dyskinesia). Products include:
- Etrafon 3115
- Limbitrol 1738

Amlodipine Besylate (Co-administration with some antihypertensive agents has resulted in symptomatic postural hypotension). Products include:
- Lotrel Capsules 2370
- Norvasc Tablets 2704

Amoxapine (Co-administration of tricyclic antidepressants and carbidopa-levodopa preparations has resulted in rare reports of

adverse reactions; including hypertension and dyskinesia).
No products indexed under this heading.

Atenolol (Co-administration with some antihypertensive agents has resulted in symptomatic postural hypotension). Products include:
Tenoretic Tablets **690**
Tenormin I.V. Injection **692**

Benazepril Hydrochloride (Co-administration with some antihypertensive agents has resulted in symptomatic postural hypotension).
Products include:
Lotensin Tablets **2365**
Lotensin HCT Tablets **2367**
Lotrel Capsules **2370**

Bendroflumethiazide (Co-administration with some antihypertensive agents has resulted in symptomatic postural hypotension).
Products include:
Corzide 40/5 Tablets **2247**
Corzide 80/5 Tablets **2247**

Betaxolol Hydrochloride (Co-administration with some antihypertensive agents has resulted in symptomatic postural hypotension).
Products include:
Betoptic S Ophthalmic Suspension **537**

Bisoprolol Fumarate (Co-administration with some antihypertensive agents has resulted in symptomatic postural hypotension).
Products include:
Zebeta Tablets **1885**
Ziac Tablets **1887**

Candesartan Cilexetil (Co-administration with some antihypertensive agents has resulted in symptomatic postural hypotension).
Products include:
Atacand Tablets **595**
Atacand HCT Tablets **597**

Captopril (Co-administration with some antihypertensive agents has resulted in symptomatic postural hypotension). Products include:
Captopril Tablets **2281**

Carteolol Hydrochloride (Co-administration with some antihypertensive agents has resulted in symptomatic postural hypotension).
Products include:
Carteolol Hydrochloride Ophthalmic Solution USP, 1% .... ⊙**258**
Ocupress Ophthalmic Solution, 1% Sterile .... ⊙**303**

Chlorothiazide (Co-administration with some antihypertensive agents has resulted in symptomatic postural hypotension). Products include:
Aldoclor Tablets **2035**
Diuril Oral **2087**

Chlorothiazide Sodium (Co-administration with some antihypertensive agents has resulted in symptomatic postural hypotension).
Products include:
Diuril Sodium Intravenous **2086**

Chlorpromazine (Co-administration with dopamine D2 receptor antagonists may reduce the therapeutic effects of levodopa). Products include:
Thorazine Suppositories **1656**

Chlorpromazine Hydrochloride (Co-administration with dopamine D2 receptor antagonists may reduce the therapeutic effects of levodopa).
Products include:
Thorazine **1656**

Chlorprothixene (Co-administration with dopamine D2 receptor antagonists may reduce the therapeutic effects of levodopa).
No products indexed under this heading.

Chlorprothixene Hydrochloride (Co-administration with dopamine D2 receptor antagonists may reduce the therapeutic effects of levodopa).
No products indexed under this heading.

Chlorthalidone (Co-administration with some antihypertensive agents has resulted in symptomatic postural hypotension). Products include:
Clorpres Tablets **1002**
Combipres Tablets **1040**
Tenoretic Tablets **690**

Clomipramine Hydrochloride (Co-administration of tricyclic antidepressants and carbidopa-levodopa preparations has resulted in rare reports of adverse reactions; including hypertension and dyskinesia).
No products indexed under this heading.

Clonidine (Co-administration with some antihypertensive agents has resulted in symptomatic postural hypotension). Products include:
Catapres-TTS **1038**

Clonidine Hydrochloride (Co-administration with some antihypertensive agents has resulted in symptomatic postural hypotension).
Products include:
Catapres Tablets **1037**
Clorpres Tablets **1002**
Combipres Tablets **1040**
Duraclon Injection **3057**

Deserpidine (Co-administration with some antihypertensive agents has resulted in symptomatic postural hypotension).
No products indexed under this heading.

Desipramine Hydrochloride (Co-administration of tricyclic antidepressants and carbidopa-levodopa preparations has resulted in rare reports of adverse reactions; including hypertension and dyskinesia).
Products include:
Norpramin Tablets **755**

Diazoxide (Co-administration with some antihypertensive agents has resulted in symptomatic postural hypotension).
No products indexed under this heading.

Diltiazem Hydrochloride (Co-administration with some antihypertensive agents has resulted in symptomatic postural hypotension).
Products include:
Cardizem Injectable **1018**
Cardizem Lyo-Ject Syringe **1018**
Cardizem Monovial **1018**
Cardizem CD Capsules **1016**
Tiazac Capsules **1378**

Doxazosin Mesylate (Co-administration with some antihypertensive agents has resulted in symptomatic postural hypotension).
Products include:
Cardura Tablets **2668**

Doxepin Hydrochloride (Co-administration of tricyclic antidepressants and carbidopa-levodopa preparations has resulted in rare reports of adverse reactions; including hypertension and dyskinesia).
Products include:
Sinequan **2713**

Enalapril Maleate (Co-administration with some antihypertensive agents has resulted in symptomatic postural hypotension).
Products include:
Lexxel Tablets **608**
Vaseretic Tablets **2204**
Vasotec Tablets **2210**

Enalaprilat (Co-administration with some antihypertensive agents has resulted in symptomatic postural hypotension). Products include:
Enalaprilat Injection **863**
Vasotec I.V. Injection **2207**

Eprosartan Mesylate (Co-administration with some antihypertensive agents has resulted in symptomatic postural hypotension).
Products include:
Teveten Tablets **3327**

Esmolol Hydrochloride (Co-administration with some antihypertensive agents has resulted in symptomatic postural hypotension).
Products include:
Brevibloc Injection **858**

Felodipine (Co-administration with some antihypertensive agents has resulted in symptomatic postural hypotension). Products include:
Lexxel Tablets **608**
Plendil Extended-Release Tablets **623**

Ferrous Fumarate (Iron salts may reduce the bioavailability of carbidopa-levodopa; the clinical significance is unclear). Products include:
New Formulation Chromagen OB Capsules **3094**
Loestrin Fe Tablets **2642**
NataChew Tablets **3364**

Ferrous Gluconate (Iron salts may reduce the bioavailability of carbidopa-levodopa; the clinical significance is unclear). Products include:
Fergon Iron Tablets .... ▣**802**

Ferrous Sulfate (Iron salts may reduce the bioavailability of carbidopa-levodopa; the clinical significance is unclear). Products include:
Feosol Tablets **1717**
Slow Fe Tablets .... ▣**827**
Slow Fe with Folic Acid Tablets .... ▣**828**

Fluphenazine Decanoate (Co-administration with dopamine D2 receptor antagonists may reduce the therapeutic effects of levodopa).
No products indexed under this heading.

Fluphenazine Enanthate (Co-administration with dopamine D2 receptor antagonists may reduce the therapeutic effects of levodopa).
No products indexed under this heading.

Fluphenazine Hydrochloride (Co-administration with dopamine D2 receptor antagonists may reduce the therapeutic effects of levodopa).
No products indexed under this heading.

Fosinopril Sodium (Co-administration with some antihypertensive agents has resulted in symptomatic postural hypotension).
Products include:
Monopril Tablets **1091**
Monopril HCT **1094**

Fosphenytoin Sodium (The beneficial effects of levodopa in Parkinson's disease have been reported to be reversed by phenytoin). Products include:
Cerebyx Injection **2619**

Furosemide (Co-administration with some antihypertensive agents has resulted in symptomatic postural hypotension). Products include:
Furosemide Tablets **2284**

Guanabenz Acetate (Co-administration with some antihypertensive agents has resulted in symptomatic postural hypotension).
No products indexed under this heading.

Guanethidine Monosulfate (Co-administration with some antihypertensive agents has resulted in symptomatic postural hypotension).
No products indexed under this heading.

Haloperidol (Co-administration with dopamine D2 receptor antagonists may reduce the therapeutic effects of levodopa). Products include:
Haldol Injection, Tablets and Concentrate **2533**

Haloperidol Decanoate (Co-administration with dopamine D2 receptor antagonists may reduce the therapeutic effects of levodopa).
Products include:
Haldol Decanoate **2535**

Hydralazine Hydrochloride (Co-administration with some antihypertensive agents has resulted in symptomatic postural hypotension).
No products indexed under this heading.

Hydrochlorothiazide (Co-administration with some antihypertensive agents has resulted in symptomatic postural hypotension).
Products include:
Accuretic Tablets **2614**
Aldoril Tablets **2039**
Atacand HCT Tablets **597**
Avalide Tablets **1070**
Diovan HCT Tablets **2338**
Dyazide Capsules **1515**
HydroDIURIL Tablets **2108**
Hyzaar **2109**
Inderide Tablets **3517**
Inderide LA Long-Acting Capsules **3519**
Lotensin HCT Tablets **2367**
Maxzide **1008**
Micardis HCT Tablets **1051**
Microzide Capsules **3414**
Moduretic Tablets **2138**
Monopril HCT **1094**
Prinzide Tablets **2168**
Timolide Tablets **2187**
Uniretic Tablets **3178**
Vaseretic Tablets **2204**
Zestoretic Tablets **695**
Ziac Tablets **1887**

Hydroflumethiazide (Co-administration with some antihypertensive agents has resulted in symptomatic postural hypotension).
Products include:
Diucardin Tablets **3494**

Imipramine Hydrochloride (Co-administration of tricyclic antidepressants and carbidopa-levodopa preparations has resulted in rare reports of adverse reactions; including hypertension and dyskinesia).
No products indexed under this heading.

Imipramine Pamoate (Co-administration of tricyclic antidepressants and carbidopa-levodopa preparations has resulted in rare reports of adverse reactions; including hypertension and dyskinesia).
No products indexed under this heading.

Indapamide (Co-administration with some antihypertensive agents has resulted in symptomatic postural hypotension). Products include:
Indapamide Tablets **2286**

Irbesartan (Co-administration with some antihypertensive agents has resulted in symptomatic postural hypotension). Products include:
Avalide Tablets **1070**
Avapro Tablets **1074**
Avapro Tablets **3076**

Iron (Iron salts may reduce the bioavailability of carbidopa-levodopa; the clinical significance is unclear).
No products indexed under this heading.

Isocarboxazid (Concurrent and/or sequential use of levodopa or carbidopa-levodopa with nonselective MAO inhibitors is contraindicated).
No products indexed under this heading.

Isradipine (Co-administration with some antihypertensive agents has resulted in symptomatic postural hypotension). Products include:
DynaCirc Capsules **2921**
DynaCirc CR Tablets **2923**

Labetalol Hydrochloride (Co-administration with some antihypertensive agents has resulted in symptomatic postural hypotension).
Products include:
Normodyne Injection **3135**
Normodyne Tablets **3137**

Lisinopril (Co-administration with some antihypertensive agents has resulted in symptomatic postural hypotension). Products include:
Prinivil Tablets 2164
Prinzide Tablets 2168
Zestoretic Tablets 695
Zestril Tablets 698

Losartan Potassium (Co-administration with some antihypertensive agents has resulted in symptomatic postural hypotension). Products include:
Cozaar Tablets 2067
Hyzaar 2109

Loxapine Hydrochloride (Co-administration with dopamine D2 receptor antagonists may reduce the therapeutic effects of levodopa).
No products indexed under this heading.

Loxapine Succinate (Co-administration with dopamine D2 receptor antagonists may reduce the therapeutic effects of levodopa). Products include:
Loxitane Capsules 3398

Maprotiline Hydrochloride (Co-administration of tricyclic antidepressants and carbidopa-levodopa preparations has resulted in rare reports of adverse reactions; including hypertension and dyskinesia).
No products indexed under this heading.

Mecamylamine Hydrochloride (Co-administration with some antihypertensive agents has resulted in symptomatic postural hypotension). Products include:
Inversine Tablets 1850

Mesoridazine Besylate (Co-administration with dopamine D2 receptor antagonists may reduce the therapeutic effects of levodopa). Products include:
Serentil 1057

Methotrimeprazine (Co-administration with dopamine D2 receptor antagonists may reduce the therapeutic effects of levodopa).
No products indexed under this heading.

Methyclothiazide (Co-administration with some antihypertensive agents has resulted in symptomatic postural hypotension).
No products indexed under this heading.

Methyldopa (Co-administration with some antihypertensive agents has resulted in symptomatic postural hypotension). Products include:
Aldoclor Tablets 2035
Aldomet Tablets 2037
Aldoril Tablets 2039

Methyldopate Hydrochloride (Co-administration with some antihypertensive agents has resulted in symptomatic postural hypotension).
No products indexed under this heading.

Metoclopramide Hydrochloride (Co-administration with dopamine D2 receptor antagonists may reduce the therapeutic effects of levodopa). Products include:
Reglan 2935

Metolazone (Co-administration with some antihypertensive agents has resulted in symptomatic postural hypotension). Products include:
Mykrox Tablets 1168
Zaroxolyn Tablets 1177

Metoprolol Succinate (Co-administration with some antihypertensive agents has resulted in symptomatic postural hypotension). Products include:
Toprol-XL Tablets 651

Metoprolol Tartrate (Co-administration with some antihypertensive agents has resulted in symptomatic postural hypotension).
No products indexed under this heading.

Metyrosine (Co-administration with some antihypertensive agents has resulted in symptomatic postural hypotension). Products include:
Demser Capsules 2085

Mibefradil Dihydrochloride (Co-administration with some antihypertensive agents has resulted in symptomatic postural hypotension).
No products indexed under this heading.

Minoxidil (Co-administration with some antihypertensive agents has resulted in symptomatic postural hypotension). Products include:
Rogaine Extra Strength for Men Topical Solution .... ■721
Rogaine for Women Topical Solution .... ■721

Moexipril Hydrochloride (Co-administration with some antihypertensive agents has resulted in symptomatic postural hypotension). Products include:
Uniretic Tablets 3178
Univasc Tablets 3181

Molindone Hydrochloride (Co-administration with dopamine D2 receptor antagonists may reduce the therapeutic effects of levodopa). Products include:
Moban 1320

Nadolol (Co-administration with some antihypertensive agents has resulted in symptomatic postural hypotension). Products include:
Corgard Tablets 2245
Corzide 40/5 Tablets 2247
Corzide 80/5 Tablets 2247
Nadolol Tablets 2288

Nicardipine Hydrochloride (Co-administration with some antihypertensive agents has resulted in symptomatic postural hypotension). Products include:
Cardene I.V. 3485

Nifedipine (Co-administration with some antihypertensive agents has resulted in symptomatic postural hypotension). Products include:
Adalat CC Tablets 877
Procardia Capsules 2708
Procardia XL Extended Release Tablets 2710

Nisoldipine (Co-administration with some antihypertensive agents has resulted in symptomatic postural hypotension). Products include:
Sular Tablets 688

Nitroglycerin (Co-administration with some antihypertensive agents has resulted in symptomatic postural hypotension). Products include:
Nitro-Dur Transdermal Infusion System 3134
Nitro-Dur Transdermal Infusion System 1834
Nitrolingual Pumpspray 1355
Nitrostat Tablets 2658

Nortriptyline Hydrochloride (Co-administration of tricyclic antidepressants and carbidopa-levodopa preparations has resulted in rare reports of adverse reactions; including hypertension and dyskinesia).
No products indexed under this heading.

Papaverine Hydrochloride (The beneficial effects of levodopa in Parkinson's disease have been reported to be reversed by papaverine).
No products indexed under this heading.

Pargyline Hydrochloride (Concurrent and/or sequential use of levodopa or carbidopa-levodopa with nonselective MAO inhibitors is contraindicated).
No products indexed under this heading.

Penbutolol Sulfate (Co-administration with some antihypertensive agents has resulted in symptomatic postural hypotension).
No products indexed under this heading.

Perindopril Erbumine (Co-administration with some antihypertensive agents has resulted in symptomatic postural hypotension). Products include:
Aceon Tablets (2 mg, 4 mg, 8 mg) 3249

Perphenazine (Co-administration with dopamine D2 receptor antagonists may reduce the therapeutic effects of levodopa). Products include:
Etrafon 3115
Trilafon 3160

Phenelzine Sulfate (Concurrent and/or sequential use of levodopa or carbidopa-levodopa with nonselective MAO inhibitors is contraindicated). Products include:
Nardil Tablets 2653

Phenoxybenzamine Hydrochloride (Co-administration with some antihypertensive agents has resulted in symptomatic postural hypotension). Products include:
Dibenzyline Capsules 3457

Phentolamine Mesylate (Co-administration with some antihypertensive agents has resulted in symptomatic postural hypotension).
No products indexed under this heading.

Phenytoin (The beneficial effects of levodopa in Parkinson's disease have been reported to be reversed by phenytoin). Products include:
Dilantin Infatabs 2624
Dilantin-125 Oral Suspension 2625

Phenytoin Sodium (The beneficial effects of levodopa in Parkinson's disease have been reported to be reversed by phenytoin). Products include:
Dilantin Kapseals 2622

Pindolol (Co-administration with some antihypertensive agents has resulted in symptomatic postural hypotension).
No products indexed under this heading.

Polysaccharide-Iron Complex (Iron salts may reduce the bioavailability of carbidopa-levodopa; the clinical significance is unclear). Products include:
Niferex 3176
Niferex-150 Capsules 3176
Nu-Iron 150 Capsules 2224

Polythiazide (Co-administration with some antihypertensive agents has resulted in symptomatic postural hypotension). Products include:
Minizide Capsules 2700
Renese Tablets 2712

Prazosin Hydrochloride (Co-administration with some antihypertensive agents has resulted in symptomatic postural hypotension). Products include:
Minipress Capsules 2699
Minizide Capsules 2700

Procarbazine Hydrochloride (Concurrent and/or sequential use of levodopa or carbidopa-levodopa with nonselective MAO inhibitors is contraindicated). Products include:
Matulane Capsules 3246

Prochlorperazine (Co-administration with dopamine D2 receptor antagonists may reduce the therapeutic effects of levodopa). Products include:
Compazine 1505

Promethazine Hydrochloride (Co-administration with dopamine D2 receptor antagonists may reduce the therapeutic effects of levodopa). Products include:
Mepergan Injection 3539
Phenergan Injection 3553
Phenergan 3556
Phenergan Syrup 3554
Phenergan with Codeine Syrup 3557
Phenergan with Dextromethorphan Syrup 3559
Phenergan VC Syrup 3560
Phenergan VC with Codeine Syrup .. 3561

Propranolol Hydrochloride (Co-administration with some antihypertensive agents has resulted in symptomatic postural hypotension). Products include:
Inderal 3513
Inderal LA Long-Acting Capsules 3516
Inderide Tablets 3517
Inderide LA Long-Acting Capsules .. 3519

Protriptyline Hydrochloride (Co-administration of tricyclic antidepressants and carbidopa-levodopa preparations has resulted in rare reports of adverse reactions; including hypertension and dyskinesia). Products include:
Vivactil Tablets 2446
Vivactil Tablets 2217

Quetiapine Fumarate (Co-administration with dopamine D2 receptor antagonists may reduce the therapeutic effects of levodopa). Products include:
Seroquel Tablets 684

Quinapril Hydrochloride (Co-administration with some antihypertensive agents has resulted in symptomatic postural hypotension). Products include:
Accupril Tablets 2611
Accuretic Tablets 2614

Ramipril (Co-administration with some antihypertensive agents has resulted in symptomatic postural hypotension). Products include:
Altace Capsules 2233

Rauwolfia serpentina (Co-administration with some antihypertensive agents has resulted in symptomatic postural hypotension).
No products indexed under this heading.

Rescinnamine (Co-administration with some antihypertensive agents has resulted in symptomatic postural hypotension).
No products indexed under this heading.

Reserpine (Co-administration with some antihypertensive agents has resulted in symptomatic postural hypotension).
No products indexed under this heading.

Risperidone (Co-administration with dopamine D2 receptor antagonists may reduce the therapeutic effects of levodopa). Products include:
Risperdal 1796

Selegiline Hydrochloride (Concomitant therapy with selegiline and carbidopa-levodopa may be associated with severe orthostatic hypotension not attributable to carbidopa-levodopa alone). Products include:
Eldepryl Capsules 3266

Sodium Nitroprusside (Co-administration with some antihypertensive agents has resulted in symptomatic postural hypotension).
No products indexed under this heading.

Sotalol Hydrochloride (Co-administration with some antihypertensive agents has resulted in symptomatic postural hypotension). Products include:
Betapace Tablets 950
Betapace AF Tablets 954

Spirapril Hydrochloride (Co-administration with some antihypertensive agents has resulted in symptomatic postural hypotension).
No products indexed under this heading.

Telmisartan (Co-administration with some antihypertensive agents has resulted in symptomatic postural hypotension). Products include:

Micardis Tablets 1049
Micardis HCT Tablets 1051

Terazosin Hydrochloride (Co-administration with some antihypertensive agents has resulted in symptomatic postural hypotension). Products include:
Hytrin Capsules 464

Thioridazine Hydrochloride (Co-administration with dopamine D2 receptor antagonists may reduce the therapeutic effects of levodopa). Products include:
Thioridazine Hydrochloride Tablets 2289

Thiothixene (Co-administration with dopamine D2 receptor antagonists may reduce the therapeutic effects of levodopa). Products include:
Navane Capsules 2701
Thiothixene Capsules 2290

Timolol Maleate (Co-administration with some antihypertensive agents has resulted in symptomatic postural hypotension). Products include:
Blocadren Tablets 2046
Cosopt Sterile Ophthalmic Solution 2065
Timolide Tablets 2187
Timolol GFS ⊙266
Timoptic in Ocudose 2192
Timoptic Sterile Ophthalmic Solution 2190
Timoptic-XE Sterile Ophthalmic Gel Forming Solution 2194

Torsemide (Co-administration with some antihypertensive agents has resulted in symptomatic postural hypotension). Products include:
Demadex Tablets and Injection 2965

Trandolapril (Co-administration with some antihypertensive agents has resulted in symptomatic postural hypotension). Products include:
Mavik Tablets 478
Tarka Tablets 508

Tranylcypromine Sulfate (Concurrent and/or sequential use of levodopa or carbidopa-levodopa with nonselective MAO inhibitors is contraindicated). Products include:
Parnate Tablets 1607

Trifluoperazine Hydrochloride (Co-administration with dopamine D2 receptor antagonists may reduce the therapeutic effects of levodopa). Products include:
Stelazine 1640

Trimethaphan Camsylate (Co-administration with some antihypertensive agents has resulted in symptomatic postural hypotension).
No products indexed under this heading.

Trimipramine Maleate (Co-administration of tricyclic antidepressants and carbidopa-levodopa preparations has resulted in rare reports of adverse reactions; including hypertension and dyskinesia). Products include:
Surmontil Capsules 3595

Valsartan (Co-administration with some antihypertensive agents has resulted in symptomatic postural hypotension). Products include:
Diovan Capsules 2337
Diovan HCT Tablets 2338

Verapamil Hydrochloride (Co-administration with some antihypertensive agents has resulted in symptomatic postural hypotension). Products include:
Covera-HS Tablets 3199
Isoptin SR Tablets 467
Tarka Tablets 508
Verelan Capsules 3184
Verelan PM Capsules 3186

LOESTRIN 21 TABLETS

(Ethinyl Estradiol, Norethindrone Acetate) 2642

May interact with methylprednisolone, phenytoin, prednisolone, tetracyclines, theophylline, and certain other agents. Compounds in these categories include:

Acetaminophen (May increase plasma ethinyl estradiol concentrations, possibly by inhibition of conjugation; oral contraceptives may induce the conjugation of other compounds, such as acetaminophen, resulting in decreased plasma concentrations of acetaminophen). Products include:
Actifed Cold & Sinus Caplets and Tablets ■688
Alka-Seltzer Plus Liqui-Gels ■604
Alka-Seltzer Plus Cold & Flu Medicine Liqui-Gels ■604
Alka-Seltzer Plus Cold & Sinus Medicine Liqui-Gels ■604
Benadryl Allergy/Cold Tablets ■691
Benadryl Allergy Sinus Headache Caplets & Gelcaps ■693
Benadryl Severe Allergy & Sinus Headache Caplets ■694
Children's Cēpacol Sore Throat ■788
Comtrex Acute Head Cold & Sinus Pressure Relief Tablets ■627
Comtrex Deep Chest Cold & Congestion Relief Softgels ■627
Comtrex Flu Therapy & Fever Relief Daytime Caplets ■628
Comtrex Flu Therapy & Fever Relief Nighttime Tablets ■628
Comtrex Maximum Strength Multi-Symptom Cold & Cough Relief Tablets and Caplets ■626
Contac Severe Cold and Flu Caplets Maximum Strength ■746
Contac Severe Cold and Flu Caplets Non-Drowsy ■746
Coricidin 'D' Cold, Flu & Sinus Tablets ■737
Coricidin HBP Cold & Flu Tablets ■738
Coricidin HBP Maximum Strength Flu Tablets ■738
Coricidin HBP Night-Time Cold & Flu Tablets ■738
Darvon-N/Darvocet-N 1907
Dimetapp Cold and Fever Suspension ■775
Dimetapp Nighttime Flu Liquid ■776
Dimetapp Non-Drowsy Flu Syrup ■777
Drixoral Allergy/Sinus Extended-Release Tablets ■741
Drixoral Cold & Flu Extended-Release Tablets ■740
Aspirin Free Excedrin Caplets and Geltabs ■628
Excedrin Extra-Strength Tablets, Caplets, and Geltabs ■629
Excedrin Migraine 1070
Excedrin PM Tablets, Caplets, and Geltabs ■631
Goody's Body Pain Formula Powder ■620
Goody's Extra Strength Headache Powder ■620
Goody's Extra Strength Pain Relief Tablets ■620
Goody's PM Powder ■621
Hycomine Compound Tablets 1317
Lortab 3319
Lortab Elixir 3317
Maxidone Tablets CIII 3399
Maximum Strength Midol Menstrual Caplets and Gelcaps ■612
Maximum Strength Midol PMS Caplets and Gelcaps ■613
Maximum Strength Midol Teen Caplets ■612
Midrin Capsules 3464
Norco 5/325 Tablets CIII 3424
Norco 7.5/325 Tablets CIII 3425
Norco 10/325 Tablets CIII 3427
Norco 10/325 Tablets CIII 3425
Percocet Tablets 1326
Percogesic Aspirin-Free Coated Tablets ■667
Extra Strength Percogesic Aspirin-Free Coated Caplets ■665
Phrenilin 578
Robitussin Cold Caplets Multi-Symptom Cold & Flu ■781
Robitussin Cold Softgels Multi-Symptom Cold & Flu ■781
Robitussin Multi Symptom Honey Flu Liquid ■785
Robitussin Nighttime Honey Flu Liquid ■786
Sedapap Tablets 50 mg/650 mg 2225
Singlet Caplets ■761
Sinutab Sinus Allergy Medication, Maximum Strength Formula, Tablets & Caplets ■707
Sinutab Sinus Medication, Maximum Strength Without Drowsiness Formula, Tablets & Caplets ■707
Sudafed Cold & Cough Liquid Caps ■709
Sudafed Cold & Sinus Liquid Caps ■710
Sudafed Severe Cold ■711
Sudafed Sinus Headache Caplets ■712
Sudafed Sinus Headache Tablets ■712
Tavist Sinus Non-Drowsy Coated Caplets ■676
TheraFlu Regular Strength Cold & Cough Night Time Hot Liquid ■676
TheraFlu Regular Strength Cold & Sore Throat Night Time Hot Liquid ■676
TheraFlu Maximum Strength Flu & Congestion Non-Drowsy Hot Liquid ■677
TheraFlu Maximum Strength Flu & Cough Night Time Hot Liquid ■678
TheraFlu Maximum Strength Flu & Sore Throat Night Time Hot Liquid ■677
TheraFlu Maximum Strength Severe Cold & Congestion Night Time Caplets ■678
TheraFlu Maximum Strength Severe Cold & Congestion Night Time Hot Liquid ■678
TheraFlu Maximum Strength Severe Cold & Congestion Non-Drowsy ■679
Triaminic Cold, Cough & Fever Liquid ■681
Triaminic Cough & Sore Throat Liquid ■682
Triaminic Cough & Sore Throat Softchews ■684
Tylenol, Children's 2014
Children's Tylenol Allergy-D Liquid 2014
Children's Tylenol Cold Suspension Liquid and Chewable Tablets 2015
Children's Tylenol Cold Plus Cough Suspension Liquid and Chewable Tablets 2015
Children's Tylenol Flu Suspension Liquid 2015
Children's Tylenol Sinus Suspension Liquid 2017
Infants' Tylenol Cold Decongestant and Fever Reducer Concentrated Drops 2015
Infants' Tylenol Cold Decongestant and Fever Reducer Concentrated Drops Plus Cough 2015
Junior Strength Tylenol Soft Chews Chewable Tablets 2014
Tylenol 2009
Tylenol Allergy Sinus 2010
Tylenol Severe Allergy Caplets 2010
Multi-Symptom Tylenol Cold Complete Formula Caplets 2010
Multi-Symptom Tylenol Cold Non-Drowsy Caplets and Gelcaps 2010
Multi-Symptom Tylenol Cold Severe Congestion Non-Drowsy Caplets 2011
Maximum Strength Tylenol Flu NightTime Gelcaps 2011
Maximum Strength Tylenol Flu NightTime Liquid 2011
Maximum Strength Tylenol Flu Non-Drowsy Gelcaps 2011
Extra Strength Tylenol PM Caplets, Geltabs, and Gelcaps 2012
Maximum Strength Tylenol Sinus NightTime Caplets 2012
Maximum Strength Tylenol Sinus Non-Drowsy Geltabs, Gelcaps, Caplets, and Tablets 2012
Maximum Strength Tylenol Sore Throat Adult Liquid 2013
Tylenol with Codeine 2595
Women's Tylenol Menstrual Relief Caplets 2013
Tylox Capsules 2597
Ultracet Tablets 2597
Vanquish Caplets ■617
Vicks 44M Cough, Cold & Flu Relief Liquid ■725
Vicks DayQuil LiquiCaps/Liquid Multi-Symptom Cold/Flu Relief ■727
Vicks NyQuil LiquiCaps/Liquid Multi-Symptom Cold/Flu Relief, Original and Cherry Flavors ■727
Vicodin Tablets 516
Vicodin ES Tablets 517
Vicodin HP Tablets 518
Zydone Tablets 1330

Aminophylline (Co-administration of oral contraceptives containing ethinyl estradiol may inhibit metabolism of theophylline resulting in increased plasma concentrations of theophylline).
No products indexed under this heading.

Ampicillin (Pregnancy while taking oral contraceptives has been reported when oral contraceptives were administered with ampicillin; clinical pharmacokinetic studies have not demonstrated any consistent effect of antibiotics on plasma concentrations of synthetic steroids).
No products indexed under this heading.

Ampicillin Sodium (Pregnancy while taking oral contraceptives has been reported when oral contraceptives were administered with ampicillin; clinical pharmacokinetic studies have not demonstrated any consistent effect of antibiotics on plasma concentrations of synthetic steroids). Products include:
Unasyn for Injection 2728

Atorvastatin Calcium (Co-administration has resulted in increased AUC values for norethindrone and ethinyl estradiol by approximately 30% and 20% respectively). Products include:
Lipitor Tablets 2639
Lipitor Tablets 2696

Carbamazepine (Anticonvulsants such as carbamazepine have been shown to increase the metabolism of ethinyl estradiol and/or norethindrone which could result in a reduction in contraceptive effectiveness). Products include:
Carbatrol Capsules 3234
Tegretol/Tegretol-XR 2404

Clofibrate (Co-administration of oral contraceptives has resulted in increased clearance of clofibric acid). Products include:
Atromid-S Capsules 3483

Cyclosporine (Co-administration of oral contraceptives containing ethinyl estradiol may inhibit metabolism of cyclosporine resulting in increased plasma concentrations of cyclosporine). Products include:
Gengraf Capsules 457
Neoral Soft Gelatin Capsules 2380
Neoral Oral Solution 2380
Sandimmune 2388

Demeclocycline Hydrochloride (Pregnancy while taking oral contraceptives has been reported when oral contraceptives were administered with tetracyclines; clinical pharmacokinetic studies have not demonstrated any consistent effect of antibiotics on plasma concentrations of synthetic steroids). Products include:
Declomycin Tablets 1855

Doxycycline Calcium (Pregnancy while taking oral contraceptives has been reported when oral contraceptives were administered with tetracyclines; clinical pharmacokinetic studies have not demonstrated any consistent effect of antibiotics on plasma concentrations of synthetic steroids). Products include:
Vibramycin Calcium Oral Suspension Syrup 2735

Doxycycline Hyclate (Pregnancy while taking oral contraceptives has been reported when oral contraceptives were administered with tetracyclines; clinical pharmacokinetic studies have not demonstrated any consistent effect of antibiotics on plasma concentrations of synthetic steroids). Products include:
Doryx Coated Pellet Filled Capsules 3357
Periostat Tablets 1208
Vibramycin Hyclate Capsules 2735
Vibramycin Hyclate Intravenous 2737
Vibra-Tabs Film Coated Tablets 2735

Doxycycline Monohydrate (Pregnancy while taking oral contraceptives has been reported when oral contraceptives were administered with tetracyclines; clinical pharmacokinetic studies have not demonstrated any consistent effect of antibiot-

ics on plasma concentrations of synthetic steroids). Products include:
- Monodox Capsules 2442
- Vibramycin Monohydrate for Oral Suspension 2735

Dyphylline (Co-administration of oral contraceptives containing ethinyl estradiol may inhibit metabolism of theophylline resulting in increased plasma concentrations of theophylline). Products include:
- Lufyllin Tablets 3347
- Lufyllin-400 Tablets 3347
- Lufyllin-GG Elixir 3348
- Lufyllin-GG Tablets 3348

Fosphenytoin Sodium (Anticonvulsants such as phenytoin have been shown to increase the metabolism of ethinyl estradiol and/or norethindrone which could result in a reduction in contraceptive effectiveness). Products include:
- Cerebyx Injection 2619

Griseofulvin (Pregnancy while taking oral contraceptives has been reported when oral contraceptives were administered with griseofulvin; clinical pharmacokinetic studies have not demonstrated any consistent effect of antibiotics on plasma concentrations of synthetic steroids). Products include:
- Grifulvin V Tablets Microsize and Oral Suspension Microsize 2518
- Gris-PEG Tablets 2661

Methacycline Hydrochloride (Pregnancy while taking oral contraceptives has been reported when oral contraceptives were administered with tetracyclines; clinical pharmacokinetic studies have not demonstrated any consistent effect of antibiotics on plasma concentrations of synthetic steroids).
No products indexed under this heading.

Methylprednisolone (Co-administration of oral contraceptives containing ethinyl estradiol may inhibit metabolism of prednisolone resulting in increased plasma concentrations of prednisolone).
No products indexed under this heading.

Methylprednisolone Acetate (Co-administration of oral contraceptives containing ethinyl estradiol may inhibit metabolism of prednisolone resulting in increased plasma concentrations of prednisolone). Products include:
- Depo-Medrol Injectable Suspension 2795

Methylprednisolone Sodium Succinate (Co-administration of oral contraceptives containing ethinyl estradiol may inhibit metabolism of prednisolone resulting in increased plasma concentrations of prednisolone). Products include:
- Solu-Medrol Sterile Powder 2855

Minocycline Hydrochloride (Pregnancy while taking oral contraceptives has been reported when oral contraceptives were administered with tetracyclines; clinical pharmacokinetic studies have not demonstrated any consistent effect of antibiotics on plasma concentrations of synthetic steroids). Products include:
- Dynacin Capsules 2019
- Minocin Intravenous 1862
- Minocin Oral Suspension 1865
- Minocin Pellet-Filled Capsules 1863

Morphine Sulfate (Co-administration of oral contraceptives has resulted in increased clearance of morphine). Products include:
- Astramorph/PF Injection, USP (Preservative-Free) 594
- Duramorph Injection 1312
- Infumorph 200 and Infumorph 500 Sterile Solutions 1314
- Kadian Capsules 1335
- MS Contin Tablets 2896
- MSIR 2898
- Oramorph SR Tablets 3062
- Roxanol 3066

Oxytetracycline Hydrochloride (Pregnancy while taking oral contraceptives has been reported when oral contraceptives were administered with tetracyclines; clinical pharmacokinetic studies have not demonstrated any consistent effect of antibiotics on plasma concentrations of synthetic steroids). Products include:
- Terra-Cortril Ophthalmic Suspension 2716
- Urobiotic-250 Capsules 2731

Phenobarbital (Anticonvulsants such as phenobarbital have been shown to increase the metabolism of ethinyl estradiol and/or norethindrone which could result in a reduction in contraceptive effectiveness). Products include:
- Arco-Lase Plus Tablets 592
- Donnatal 2929
- Donnatal Extentabs 2930

Phenylbutazone (Co-administration has resulted in a reduction in contraceptive effectiveness and increased incidence of breakthrough bleeding).
No products indexed under this heading.

Phenytoin (Anticonvulsants such as phenytoin have been shown to increase the metabolism of ethinyl estradiol and/or norethindrone which could result in a reduction in contraceptive effectiveness). Products include:
- Dilantin Infatabs 2624
- Dilantin-125 Oral Suspension 2625

Phenytoin Sodium (Anticonvulsants such as phenytoin have been shown to increase the metabolism of ethinyl estradiol and/or norethindrone which could result in a reduction in contraceptive effectiveness). Products include:
- Dilantin Kapseals 2622

Prednisolone (Co-administration of oral contraceptives containing ethinyl estradiol may inhibit metabolism of prednisolone resulting in increased plasma concentrations of prednisolone). Products include:
- Prelone Syrup 2273

Prednisolone Acetate (Co-administration of oral contraceptives containing ethinyl estradiol may inhibit metabolism of prednisolone resulting in increased plasma concentrations of prednisolone). Products include:
- Blephamide Ophthalmic Ointment .. 547
- Blephamide Ophthalmic Suspension 548
- Poly-Pred Liquifilm Ophthalmic Suspension .... ⊙245
- Pred Forte Ophthalmic Suspension .... ⊙246
- Pred Mild Sterile Ophthalmic Suspension .... ⊙249
- Pred-G Ophthalmic Suspension .... ⊙247
- Pred-G Sterile Ophthalmic Ointment .... ⊙248

Prednisolone Sodium Phosphate (Co-administration of oral contraceptives containing ethinyl estradiol may inhibit metabolism of prednisolone resulting in increased plasma concentrations of prednisolone). Products include:
- Pediapred Oral Solution 1170

Prednisolone Tebutate (Co-administration of oral contraceptives containing ethinyl estradiol may inhibit metabolism of prednisolone resulting in increased plasma concentrations of prednisolone).
No products indexed under this heading.

Rifampin (Metabolism of both norethindrone and ethinyl estradiol is increased by rifampin; co-administration has resulted in a reduction of contraceptive effectiveness and increased incidence of breakthrough bleeding and menstrual irregularities). Products include:
- Rifadin 765
- Rifamate Capsules 767
- Rifater Tablets 769

Salicylic Acid (Co-administration of oral contraceptives has resulted in increased clearance of salicylic acid). Products include:
- Clear Away Gel with Aloe Wart Remover System 736
- Clear Away Liquid Wart Remover System 736
- Clear Away One Step Wart Remover 737
- Clear Away One Step Wart Remover for Kids 737
- Clear Away One Step Plantar Wart Remover 737
- Compound W One Step Pads for Kids 664
- Compound W One Step Plantar Pads 664
- Compound W One Step Wart Remover Pads 664
- Compound W Wart Remover Gel 665
- Compound W Wart Remover Liquid 665
- Wart-Off Liquid 716

Temazepam (Co-administration of oral contraceptives has resulted in increased clearance of temazepam).
No products indexed under this heading.

Tetracycline Hydrochloride (Pregnancy while taking oral contraceptives has been reported when oral contraceptives were administered with tetracyclines; clinical pharmacokinetic studies have not demonstrated any consistent effect of antibiotics on plasma concentrations of synthetic steroids).
No products indexed under this heading.

Theophylline (Co-administration of oral contraceptives containing ethinyl estradiol may inhibit metabolism of theophylline resulting in increased plasma concentrations of theophylline). Products include:
- Aerolate 1361
- Theo-Dur Extended-Release Tablets 1835
- Uni-Dur Extended-Release Tablets .. 1841
- Uniphyl 400 mg and 600 mg Tablets 2903

Theophylline Calcium Salicylate (Co-administration of oral contraceptives containing ethinyl estradiol may inhibit metabolism of theophylline resulting in increased plasma concentrations of theophylline).
No products indexed under this heading.

Theophylline Sodium Glycinate (Co-administration of oral contraceptives containing ethinyl estradiol may inhibit metabolism of theophylline resulting in increased plasma concentrations of theophylline).
No products indexed under this heading.

Troglitazone (Co-administration has reduced the plasma concentrations of both norethindrone and ethinyl estradiol by approximately 30%, which could result in a reduction in contraceptive effectiveness).
No products indexed under this heading.

Vitamin C (May increase plasma ethinyl estradiol concentrations, possibly by inhibition of conjugation). Products include:
- Beta-C Tablets 811
- C-Grams Caplets 795
- Halls Defense Drops 687
- Peridin-C Tablets 618

LOESTRIN FE TABLETS

(Ethinyl Estradiol, Ferrous Fumarate, Norethindrone Acetate) 2642

See Loestrin 21 Tablets

LO/OVRAL TABLETS

(Ethinyl Estradiol, Norgestrel) 3532

May interact with barbiturates, phenytoin, tetracyclines, and certain other agents. Compounds in these categories include:

Ampicillin (Co-administration with ampicillin may result in reduced efficacy and increased incidence of breakthrough bleeding and menstrual irregularities).
No products indexed under this heading.

Ampicillin Sodium (Co-administration with ampicillin may result in reduced efficacy and increased incidence of breakthrough bleeding and menstrual irregularities). Products include:
- Unasyn for Injection 2728

Aprobarbital (Co-administration with barbiturates may result in reduced efficacy and increased incidence of breakthrough bleeding and menstrual irregularities).
No products indexed under this heading.

Butabarbital (Co-administration with barbiturates may result in reduced efficacy and increased incidence of breakthrough bleeding and menstrual irregularities).
No products indexed under this heading.

Butalbital (Co-administration with barbiturates may result in reduced efficacy and increased incidence of breakthrough bleeding and menstrual irregularities). Products include:
- Phrenilin 578
- Sedapap Tablets 50 mg/650 mg ... 2225

Demeclocycline Hydrochloride (Co-administration with tetracyclines may result in reduced efficacy and increased incidence of breakthrough bleeding and menstrual irregularities). Products include:
- Declomycin Tablets 1855

Doxycycline Calcium (Co-administration with tetracyclines may result in reduced efficacy and increased incidence of breakthrough bleeding and menstrual irregularities). Products include:
- Vibramycin Calcium Oral Suspension Syrup 2735

Doxycycline Hyclate (Co-administration with tetracyclines may result in reduced efficacy and increased incidence of breakthrough bleeding and menstrual irregularities). Products include:
- Doryx Coated Pellet Filled Capsules 3357
- Periostat Tablets 1208
- Vibramycin Hyclate Capsules 2735
- Vibramycin Hyclate Intravenous 2737
- Vibra-Tabs Film Coated Tablets 2735

Doxycycline Monohydrate (Co-administration with tetracyclines may result in reduced efficacy and increased incidence of breakthrough bleeding and menstrual irregularities). Products include:
- Monodox Capsules 2442
- Vibramycin Monohydrate for Oral Suspension 2735

Fosphenytoin Sodium (Co-administration with phenytoin may result in reduced efficacy and increased incidence of breakthrough bleeding and menstrual irregularities). Products include:
- Cerebyx Injection 2619

Griseofulvin (Co-administration with griseofulvin may result in reduced efficacy and increased incidence of breakthrough bleeding and menstrual irregularities). Products include:
- Grifulvin V Tablets Microsize and Oral Suspension Microsize 2518
- Gris-PEG Tablets 2661

Mephobarbital (Co-administration with barbiturates may result in reduced efficacy and increased inci-

dence of breakthrough bleeding and menstrual irregularities).
No products indexed under this heading.

Methacycline Hydrochloride (Co-administration with tetracyclines may result in reduced efficacy and increased incidence of breakthrough bleeding and menstrual irregularities).
No products indexed under this heading.

Minocycline Hydrochloride (Co-administration with tetracyclines may result in reduced efficacy and increased incidence of breakthrough bleeding and menstrual irregularities). Products include:
Dynacin Capsules 2019
Minocin Intravenous 1862
Minocin Oral Suspension 1865
Minocin Pellet-Filled Capsules 1863

Oxytetracycline Hydrochloride (Co-administration with tetracyclines may result in reduced efficacy and increased incidence of breakthrough bleeding and menstrual irregularities). Products include:
Terra-Cortril Ophthalmic Suspension 2716
Urobiotic-250 Capsules 2731

Pentobarbital Sodium (Co-administration with barbiturates may result in reduced efficacy and increased incidence of breakthrough bleeding and menstrual irregularities). Products include:
Nembutal Sodium Solution 485

Phenobarbital (Co-administration with barbiturates may result in reduced efficacy and increased incidence of breakthrough bleeding and menstrual irregularities). Products include:
Arco-Lase Plus Tablets 592
Donnatal 2929
Donnatal Extentabs 2930

Phenylbutazone (Co-administration with phenylbutazone may result in reduced efficacy and increased incidence of breakthrough bleeding and menstrual irregularities).
No products indexed under this heading.

Phenytoin (Co-administration with phenytoin may result in reduced efficacy and increased incidence of breakthrough bleeding and menstrual irregularities). Products include:
Dilantin Infatabs 2624
Dilantin-125 Oral Suspension 2625

Phenytoin Sodium (Co-administration with phenytoin may result in reduced efficacy and increased incidence of breakthrough bleeding and menstrual irregularities). Products include:
Dilantin Kapseals 2622

Rifampin (Co-administration reduces efficacy and increased incidence of breakthrough bleeding and menstrual irregularities). Products include:
Rifadin 765
Rifamate Capsules 767
Rifater Tablets 769

Secobarbital Sodium (Co-administration with barbiturates may result in reduced efficacy and increased incidence of breakthrough bleeding and menstrual irregularities).
No products indexed under this heading.

Tetracycline Hydrochloride (Co-administration with tetracyclines may result in reduced efficacy and increased incidence of breakthrough bleeding and menstrual irregularities).
No products indexed under this heading.

Thiamylal Sodium (Co-administration with barbiturates may result in reduced efficacy and increased incidence of breakthrough bleeding and menstrual irregularities).
No products indexed under this heading.

Troleandomycin (Co-administration may increase the risk of intrahepatic cholestasis). Products include:
Tao Capsules 2716

LO/OVRAL-28 TABLETS

(Ethinyl Estradiol, Norgestrel) 3538
See Lo/Ovral Tablets

LOPID TABLETS

(Gemfibrozil) 2650
May interact with oral anticoagulants, HMG-CoA reductase inhibitors, and certain other agents. Compounds in these categories include:

Atorvastatin Calcium (The risk of myopathy and rhabdomyolysis is increased with combined gemfibrozil and HMG-CoA reductase inhibitor therapy; myopathy rhabdomyolysis with or without acute renal failure has been reported as early as 3 weeks after initiation of combined therapy; there is no assurance that periodic monitoring of creatine kinase will prevent the occurrence of severe myopathy and kidney damage). Products include:
Lipitor Tablets 2639
Lipitor Tablets 2696

Cerivastatin Sodium (Co-administration is contraindicated because of an observed marked increased risk of myopathy and rhabdomyolysis). Products include:
Baycol Tablets 883

Dicumarol (The dosage of the anticoagulant should be reduced to maintain the prothrombin time at the desired level to prevent bleeding complications).
No products indexed under this heading.

Fluvastatin Sodium (The risk of myopathy and rhabdomyolysis is increased with combined gemfibrozil and HMG-CoA reductase inhibitor therapy; myopathy rhabdomyolysis with or without acute renal failure has been reported as early as 3 weeks after initiation of combined therapy; there is no assurance that periodic monitoring of creatine kinase will prevent the occurrence of severe myopathy and kidney damage). Products include:
Lescol Capsules 2361
Lescol 2925
Lescol XL Tablets 2361

Lovastatin (The risk of myopathy and rhabdomyolysis is increased with combined gemfibrozil and HMG-CoA reductase inhibitor therapy; myopathy rhabdomyolysis with or without acute renal failure has been reported as early as 3 weeks after initiation of combined therapy; there is no assurance that periodic monitoring of creatine kinase will prevent the occurrence of severe myopathy and kidney damage). Products include:
Mevacor Tablets 2132

Pravastatin Sodium (The risk of myopathy and rhabdomyolysis is increased with combined gemfibrozil and HMG-CoA reductase inhibitor therapy; myopathy rhabdomyolysis with or without acute renal failure has been reported as early as 3 weeks after initiation of combined therapy; there is no assurance that periodic monitoring of creatine kinase will prevent the occurrence of severe myopathy and kidney damage). Products include:
Pravachol Tablets 1099

Simvastatin (The risk of myopathy and rhabdomyolysis is increased with combined gemfibrozil and HMG-CoA reductase inhibitor therapy; myopathy rhabdomyolysis with or without acute renal failure has been reported as early as 3 weeks after initiation of combined therapy; there is no assurance that periodic monitoring of creatine kinase will prevent the occurrence of severe myopathy and kidney damage). Products include:
Zocor Tablets 2219

Warfarin Sodium (The dosage of the anticoagulant should be reduced to maintain the prothrombin time at the desired level to prevent bleeding complications). Products include:
Coumadin for Injection 1243
Coumadin Tablets 1243
Warfarin Sodium Tablets, USP 3302

Food Interactions

Food, unspecified (Gemfibrozil pharmacokinetics are affected by the timing of meals relative to dosing; the rate and extent of absorption of gemfibrozil were significantly increased when administered 0.5 hours before meals; AUC is decreased when it is after meals).

LOPROX CREAM

(Ciclopirox Olamine) 2021
None cited in PDR database.

LOPROX GEL

(Ciclopirox) 2022
None cited in PDR database.

LOPROX LOTION

(Ciclopirox Olamine) 2021
None cited in PDR database.

LORABID SUSPENSION AND PULVULES

(Loracarbef) 2251
May interact with:

Probenecid (Inhibits renal excretion resulting in an approximately 80% increase in the AUC for loracarbef).
No products indexed under this heading.

Food Interactions

Food, unspecified (Delays the peak plasma concentration with no change in the total absorption).

LORTAB 2.5/500 TABLETS

(Acetaminophen, Hydrocodone Bitartrate) 3319
See Lortab 10/500 Tablets

LORTAB 5/500 TABLETS

(Acetaminophen, Hydrocodone Bitartrate) 3319
See Lortab 10/500 Tablets

LORTAB 7.5/500 TABLETS

(Acetaminophen, Hydrocodone Bitartrate) 3319
See Lortab 10/500 Tablets

LORTAB 10/500 TABLETS

(Acetaminophen, Hydrocodone Bitartrate) 3319
May interact with antihistamines, central nervous system depressants, monoamine oxidase inhibitors, narcotic analgesics, tranquilizers, and tricyclic antidepressants. Compounds in these categories include:

Acrivastine (Co-administration may exhibit additive CNS-depression). Products include:
Semprex-D Capsules 1172

Alfentanil Hydrochloride (Co-administration may exhibit additive CNS-depression).
No products indexed under this heading.

Alprazolam (Co-administration may exhibit additive CNS-depression). Products include:
Xanax Tablets 2865

Amitriptyline Hydrochloride (Co-administration may increase the effect of either the antidepressant or hydrocodone). Products include:
Etrafon 3115
Limbitrol 1738

Amoxapine (Co-administration may increase the effect of either the antidepressant or hydrocodone).
No products indexed under this heading.

Aprobarbital (Co-administration may exhibit additive CNS-depression).
No products indexed under this heading.

Astemizole (Co-administration may exhibit additive CNS-depression).
No products indexed under this heading.

Azatadine Maleate (Co-administration may exhibit additive CNS-depression). Products include:
Rynatan Tablets 3351

Bromodiphenhydramine Hydrochloride (Co-administration may exhibit additive CNS-depression).
No products indexed under this heading.

Brompheniramine Maleate (Co-administration may exhibit additive CNS-depression). Products include:
Bromfed Capsules (Extended-Release) 2269
Bromfed-PD Capsules (Extended-Release) 2269
Comtrex Acute Head Cold & Sinus Pressure Relief Tablets .... ▣627
Dimetapp Elixir .... ▣777
Dimetapp Cold and Fever Suspension .... ▣775
Dimetapp DM Cold & Cough Elixir .... ▣775
Dimetapp Nighttime Flu Liquid .... ▣776

Buprenorphine Hydrochloride (Co-administration may exhibit additive CNS-depression). Products include:
Buprenex Injectable 2918

Buspirone Hydrochloride (Co-administration may exhibit additive CNS-depression).
No products indexed under this heading.

Butabarbital (Co-administration may exhibit additive CNS-depression).
No products indexed under this heading.

Butalbital (Co-administration may exhibit additive CNS-depression). Products include:
Phrenilin 578
Sedapap Tablets 50 mg/650 mg 2225

Cetirizine Hydrochloride (Co-administration may exhibit additive CNS-depression). Products include:
Zyrtec 2756
Zyrtec-D 12 Hour Extended Relief Tablets 2758

Chlordiazepoxide (Co-administration may exhibit additive CNS-depression). Products include:
Limbitrol 1738

Chlordiazepoxide Hydrochloride (Co-administration may exhibit additive CNS-depression). Products include:
Librium Capsules 1736
Librium for Injection 1737

Chlorpheniramine Maleate (Co-administration may exhibit additive CNS-depression). Products include:
Actifed Cold & Sinus Caplets and Tablets .... ▣688
Alka-Seltzer Plus Liqui-Gels .... ▣604
BC Allergy Sinus Cold Powder .... ▣619
Chlor-Trimeton Allergy Tablets .... ▣735
Chlor-Trimeton Allergy/Decongestant Tablets .... ▣736
Comtrex Flu Therapy & Fever Relief Nighttime Tablets .... ▣628
Comtrex Maximum Strength Multi-Symptom Cold & Cough Relief Tablets and Caplets .... ▣626
Contac Severe Cold and Flu Caplets Maximum Strength .... ▣746

Coricidin 'D' Cold, Flu & Sinus Tablets ■737
Coricidin/Coricidin D ■738
Coricidin HBP Maximum Strength Flu Tablets ■738
Extendryl 1361
Hycomine Compound Tablets 1317
Kronofed-A 1341
PediaCare Cough-Cold Liquid ■719
PediaCare NightRest Cough-Cold Liquid ■719
Robitussin Nighttime Honey Flu Liquid ■786
Ryna ■768
Singlet Caplets ■761
Sinutab Sinus Allergy Medication, Maximum Strength Formula, Tablets & Caplets ■707
Sudafed Cold & Allergy Tablets ■708
TheraFlu Regular Strength Cold & Cough Night Time Hot Liquid ■676
TheraFlu Regular Strength Cold & Sore Throat Night Time Hot Liquid ■676
TheraFlu Maximum Strength Flu & Cough Night Time Hot Liquid ■678
TheraFlu Maximum Strength Flu & Sore Throat Night Time Hot Liquid ■677
TheraFlu Maximum Strength Severe Cold & Congestion Night Time Caplets ■678
TheraFlu Maximum Strength Severe Cold & Congestion Night Time Hot Liquid ■678
Triaminic Cold & Allergy Liquid ■681
Triaminic Cold & Allergy Softchews ■683
Triaminic Cold & Cough Liquid ■681
Triaminic Cold & Cough Softchews ■683
Triaminic Cold & Night Time Cough Liquid ■681
Triaminic Cold, Cough & Fever Liquid ■681
Children's Tylenol Cold Suspension Liquid and Chewable Tablets 2015
Children's Tylenol Cold Plus Cough Suspension Liquid and Chewable Tablets 2015
Children's Tylenol Flu Suspension Liquid 2015
Maximum Strength Tylenol Allergy Sinus Caplets, Gelcaps, and Geltabs 2010
Multi-Symptom Tylenol Cold Complete Formula Caplets 2010
Vicks 44M Cough, Cold & Flu Relief Liquid ■725
Pediatric Vicks 44m Cough & Cold Relief ■728
Children's Vicks NyQuil Cold/Cough Relief ■726

Chlorpheniramine Polistirex (Co-administration may exhibit additive CNS-depression). Products include:
Tussionex Pennkinetic Extended-Release Suspension 1174

Chlorpheniramine Tannate (Co-administration may exhibit additive CNS-depression). Products include:
Reformulated Rynatan Pediatric Suspension 3352
Rynatuss Pediatric Suspension 3353
Rynatuss Tablets 3353
Tussi-12 S Suspension 3356
Tussi-12 Tablets 3356

Chlorpromazine (Co-administration may exhibit additive CNS-depression). Products include:
Thorazine Suppositories 1656

Chlorpromazine Hydrochloride (Co-administration may exhibit additive CNS-depression). Products include:
Thorazine 1656

Chlorprothixene (Co-administration may exhibit additive CNS-depression).
No products indexed under this heading.

Chlorprothixene Hydrochloride (Co-administration may exhibit additive CNS-depression).
No products indexed under this heading.

Chlorprothixene Lactate (Co-administration may exhibit additive CNS-depression).
No products indexed under this heading.

Clemastine Fumarate (Co-administration may exhibit additive CNS-depression). Products include:
Tavist 12 Hour Allergy Tablets ■676

Clomipramine Hydrochloride (Co-administration may increase the effect of either the antidepressant or hydrocodone).
No products indexed under this heading.

Clorazepate Dipotassium (Co-administration may exhibit additive CNS-depression). Products include:
Tranxene 511

Clozapine (Co-administration may exhibit additive CNS-depression). Products include:
Clozaril Tablets 2319

Codeine Phosphate (Co-administration may exhibit additive CNS-depression). Products include:
Phenergan with Codeine Syrup 3557
Phenergan VC with Codeine Syrup 3561
Robitussin A-C Syrup 2942
Robitussin-DAC Syrup 2942
Ryna-C Liquid ■768
Soma Compound w/Codeine Tablets 3355
Tussi-Organidin NR Liquid 3350
Tussi-Organidin-S NR Liquid 3350
Tylenol with Codeine 2595

Cyproheptadine Hydrochloride (Co-administration may exhibit additive CNS-depression). Products include:
Periactin Tablets 2155

Desflurane (Co-administration may exhibit additive CNS-depression). Products include:
Suprane Liquid for Inhalation 874

Desipramine Hydrochloride (Co-administration may increase the effect of either the antidepressant or hydrocodone). Products include:
Norpramin Tablets 755

Dexchlorpheniramine Maleate (Co-administration may exhibit additive CNS-depression).
No products indexed under this heading.

Dezocine (Co-administration may exhibit additive CNS-depression).
No products indexed under this heading.

Diazepam (Co-administration may exhibit additive CNS-depression). Products include:
Valium Injectable 3026
Valium Tablets 3047

Diphenhydramine Citrate (Co-administration may exhibit additive CNS-depression). Products include:
Alka-Seltzer PM Effervescent Tablets ■605
Benadryl Allergy & Sinus Fastmelt Tablets ■693
Benadryl Children's Allergy/Cold Fastmelt Tablets ■692
Excedrin PM Tablets, Caplets, and Geltabs ■631
Goody's PM Powder ■621

Diphenhydramine Hydrochloride (Co-administration may exhibit additive CNS-depression). Products include:
Extra Strength Bayer PM Caplets ■611
Benadryl Allergy Chewables ■689
Benadryl Allergy ■691
Benadryl Allergy Liquid ■690
Benadryl Allergy/Cold Tablets ■691
Benadryl Allergy/Congestion Tablets ■692
Benadryl Allergy & Sinus Liquid ■693
Benadryl Allergy Sinus Headache Caplets & Gelcaps ■693
Benadryl Severe Allergy & Sinus Headache Caplets ■694
Benadryl Dye-Free Allergy Liquid ■690
Benadryl Dye-Free Allergy Liqui-Gels Softgels ■690
Benadryl Itch Relief Stick Extra Strength ■695
Benadryl Cream ■695
Benadryl Gel ■695
Benadryl Spray ■696
Benadryl Parenteral 2617
Coricidin HBP Night-Time Cold & Flu Tablets ■738
Nytol QuickCaps Caplets ■622
Maximum Strength Nytol QuickGels Softgels ■621
Extra Strength Percogesic Aspirin-Free Coated Caplets ■665
Simply Sleep Caplets 2008
Sominex Original Formula Tablets ■761
Children's Tylenol Allergy-D Liquid 2014
Maximum Strength Tylenol Allergy Sinus NightTime Caplets 2010
Tylenol Severe Allergy Caplets 2010
Maximum Strength Tylenol Flu NightTime Gelcaps 2011
Extra Strength Tylenol PM Caplets, Geltabs, and Gelcaps 2012
Unisom Maximum Strength SleepGels ■713

Diphenylpyraline Hydrochloride (Co-administration may exhibit additive CNS-depression).
No products indexed under this heading.

Doxepin Hydrochloride (Co-administration may increase the effect of either the antidepressant or hydrocodone). Products include:
Sinequan 2713

Droperidol (Co-administration may exhibit additive CNS-depression).
No products indexed under this heading.

Enflurane (Co-administration may exhibit additive CNS-depression).
No products indexed under this heading.

Estazolam (Co-administration may exhibit additive CNS-depression). Products include:
ProSom Tablets 500

Ethchlorvynol (Co-administration may exhibit additive CNS-depression).
No products indexed under this heading.

Ethinamate (Co-administration may exhibit additive CNS-depression).
No products indexed under this heading.

Fentanyl (Co-administration may exhibit additive CNS-depression). Products include:
Duragesic Transdermal System 1786

Fentanyl Citrate (Co-administration may exhibit additive CNS-depression). Products include:
Actiq 1184

Fexofenadine Hydrochloride (Co-administration may exhibit additive CNS-depression). Products include:
Allegra 712
Allegra-D Extended-Release Tablets 714

Fluphenazine Decanoate (Co-administration may exhibit additive CNS-depression).
No products indexed under this heading.

Fluphenazine Enanthate (Co-administration may exhibit additive CNS-depression).
No products indexed under this heading.

Fluphenazine Hydrochloride (Co-administration may exhibit additive CNS-depression).
No products indexed under this heading.

Flurazepam Hydrochloride (Co-administration may exhibit additive CNS-depression).
No products indexed under this heading.

Glutethimide (Co-administration may exhibit additive CNS-depression).
No products indexed under this heading.

Haloperidol (Co-administration may exhibit additive CNS-depression). Products include:
Haldol Injection, Tablets and Concentrate 2533

Haloperidol Decanoate (Co-administration may exhibit additive CNS-depression). Products include:
Haldol Decanoate 2535

Hydrocodone Polistirex (Co-administration may exhibit additive CNS-depression). Products include:
Tussionex Pennkinetic Extended-Release Suspension 1174

Hydromorphone Hydrochloride (Co-administration may exhibit additive CNS depression). Products include:
Dilaudid 441
Dilaudid Oral Liquid 445
Dilaudid Powder 441
Dilaudid Rectal Suppositories 441
Dilaudid Tablets 441
Dilaudid Tablets - 8 mg 445
Dilaudid-HP 443

Hydroxyzine Hydrochloride (Co-administration may exhibit additive CNS-depression). Products include:
Atarax Tablets & Syrup 2667
Vistaril Intramuscular Solution 2738

Imipramine Hydrochloride (Co-administration may increase the effect of either the antidepressant or hydrocodone).
No products indexed under this heading.

Imipramine Pamoate (Co-administration may increase the effect of either the antidepressant or hydrocodone).
No products indexed under this heading.

Isocarboxazid (Co-administration may increase the effect of either the MAO inhibitor or hydrocodone).
No products indexed under this heading.

Isoflurane (Co-administration may exhibit additive CNS-depression).
No products indexed under this heading.

Ketamine Hydrochloride (Co-administration may exhibit additive CNS-depression).
No products indexed under this heading.

Levomethadyl Acetate Hydrochloride (Co-administration may exhibit additive CNS-depression).
No products indexed under this heading.

Levorphanol Tartrate (Co-administration may exhibit additive CNS-depression). Products include:
Levo-Dromoran 1734
Levorphanol Tartrate Tablets 3059

Loratadine (Co-administration may exhibit additive CNS-depression). Products include:
Claritin 3100
Claritin-D 12 Hour Extended Release Tablets 3102
Claritin-D 24 Hour Extended Release Tablets 3104

Lorazepam (Co-administration may exhibit additive CNS-depression). Products include:
Ativan Injection 3478
Ativan Tablets 3482

Loxapine Hydrochloride (Co-administration may exhibit additive CNS-depression).
No products indexed under this heading.

Loxapine Succinate (Co-administration may exhibit additive CNS-depression). Products include:
Loxitane Capsules 3398

Maprotiline Hydrochloride (Co-administration may increase the effect of either the antidepressant or hydrocodone).
No products indexed under this heading.

Meperidine Hydrochloride (Co-administration may exhibit additive CNS-depression). Products include:
Demerol 3079
Mepergan Injection 3539

IMPORTANT NOTE: Always consult each drug listing in the patient's regimen for possible interactions.

Mephobarbital (Co-administration may exhibit additive CNS-depression).
No products indexed under this heading.

Meprobamate (Co-administration may exhibit additive CNS-depression). Products include:
Miltown Tablets ... 3349

Mesoridazine Besylate (Co-administration may exhibit additive CNS-depression). Products include:
Serentil ... 1057

Methadone Hydrochloride (Co-administration may exhibit additive CNS-depression). Products include:
Dolophine Hydrochloride Tablets ... 3056

Methdilazine Hydrochloride (Co-administration may exhibit additive CNS-depression).
No products indexed under this heading.

Methohexital Sodium (Co-administration may exhibit additive CNS-depression). Products include:
Brevital Sodium for Injection, USP .. 1815

Methotrimeprazine (Co-administration may exhibit additive CNS-depression).
No products indexed under this heading.

Methoxyflurane (Co-administration may exhibit additive CNS-depression).
No products indexed under this heading.

Midazolam Hydrochloride (Co-administration may exhibit additive CNS-depression). Products include:
Versed Injection ... 3027
Versed Syrup ... 3033

Moclobemide (Co-administration may increase the effect of either the MAO inhibitor or hydrocodone).
No products indexed under this heading.

Molindone Hydrochloride (Co-administration may exhibit additive CNS-depression). Products include:
Moban ... 1320

Morphine Sulfate (Co-administration may exhibit additive CNS-depression). Products include:
Astramorph/PF Injection, USP (Preservative-Free) ... 594
Duramorph Injection ... 1312
Infumorph 200 and Infumorph 500 Sterile Solutions ... 1314
Kadian Capsules ... 1335
MS Contin Tablets ... 2896
MSIR ... 2898
Oramorph SR Tablets ... 3062
Roxanol ... 3066

Nortriptyline Hydrochloride (Co-administration may increase the effect of either the antidepressant or hydrocodone).
No products indexed under this heading.

Olanzapine (Co-administration may exhibit additive CNS-depression). Products include:
Zyprexa Tablets ... 1973
Zyprexa ZYDIS Orally Disintegrating Tablets ... 1973

Oxazepam (Co-administration may exhibit additive CNS-depression).
No products indexed under this heading.

Oxycodone Hydrochloride (Co-administration may exhibit additive CNS-depression). Products include:
OxyContin Tablets ... 2912
OxyFast Oral Concentrate Solution . 2916
OxyIR Capsules ... 2916
Percocet Tablets ... 1326
Percodan Tablets ... 1327
Percolone Tablets ... 1327
Roxicodone ... 3067
Tylox Capsules ... 2597

Pargyline Hydrochloride (Co-administration may increase the effect of either the MAO inhibitor or hydrocodone).
No products indexed under this heading.

Pentobarbital Sodium (Co-administration may exhibit additive CNS-depression). Products include:
Nembutal Sodium Solution ... 485

Perphenazine (Co-administration may exhibit additive CNS-depression). Products include:
Etrafon ... 3115
Trilafon ... 3160

Phenelzine Sulfate (Co-administration may increase the effect of either the MAO inhibitor or hydrocodone). Products include:
Nardil Tablets ... 2653

Phenobarbital (Co-administration may exhibit additive CNS-depression). Products include:
Arco-Lase Plus Tablets ... 592
Donnatal ... 2929
Donnatal Extentabs ... 2930

Prazepam (Co-administration may exhibit additive CNS-depression).
No products indexed under this heading.

Procarbazine Hydrochloride (Co-administration may increase the effect of either the MAO inhibitor or hydrocodone). Products include:
Matulane Capsules ... 3246

Prochlorperazine (Co-administration may exhibit additive CNS-depression). Products include:
Compazine ... 1505

Promethazine Hydrochloride (Co-administration may exhibit additive CNS-depression). Products include:
Mepergan Injection ... 3539
Phenergan Injection ... 3553
Phenergan ... 3556
Phenergan Syrup ... 3554
Phenergan with Codeine Syrup ... 3557
Phenergan with Dextromethorphan Syrup ... 3559
Phenergan VC Syrup ... 3560
Phenergan VC with Codeine Syrup .. 3561

Propofol (Co-administration may exhibit additive CNS-depression). Products include:
Diprivan Injectable Emulsion ... 667

Propoxyphene Hydrochloride (Co-administration may exhibit additive CNS-depression). Products include:
Darvon Pulvules ... 1909
Darvon Compound-65 Pulvules ... 1910

Propoxyphene Napsylate (Co-administration may exhibit additive CNS-depression). Products include:
Darvon-N/Darvocet-N ... 1907
Darvon-N Tablets ... 1912

Protriptyline Hydrochloride (Co-administration may increase the effect of either the antidepressant or hydrocodone). Products include:
Vivactil Tablets ... 2446
Vivactil Tablets ... 2217

Pyrilamine Maleate (Co-administration may exhibit additive CNS-depression). Products include:
Maximum Strength Midol Menstrual Caplets and Gelcaps ... ▣612
Maximum Strength Midol PMS Caplets and Gelcaps ... ▣613

Pyrilamine Tannate (Co-administration may exhibit additive CNS-depression). Products include:
Ryna-12 S Suspension ... 3351

Quazepam (Co-administration may exhibit additive CNS-depression).
No products indexed under this heading.

Quetiapine Fumarate (Co-administration may exhibit additive CNS-depression). Products include:
Seroquel Tablets ... 684

Remifentanil Hydrochloride (Co-administration may exhibit additive CNS-depression).
No products indexed under this heading.

Risperidone (Co-administration may exhibit additive CNS-depression). Products include:
Risperdal ... 1796

Secobarbital Sodium (Co-administration may exhibit additive CNS-depression).
No products indexed under this heading.

Selegiline Hydrochloride (Co-administration may increase the effect of either the MAO inhibitor or hydrocodone). Products include:
Eldepryl Capsules ... 3266

Sevoflurane (Co-administration may exhibit additive CNS-depression).
No products indexed under this heading.

Sufentanil Citrate (Co-administration may exhibit additive CNS-depression).
No products indexed under this heading.

Temazepam (Co-administration may exhibit additive CNS-depression).
No products indexed under this heading.

Terfenadine (Co-administration may exhibit additive CNS-depression).
No products indexed under this heading.

Thiamylal Sodium (Co-administration may exhibit additive CNS-depression).
No products indexed under this heading.

Thioridazine Hydrochloride (Co-administration may exhibit additive CNS-depression). Products include:
Thioridazine Hydrochloride Tablets ... 2289

Thiothixene (Co-administration may exhibit additive CNS-depression). Products include:
Navane Capsules ... 2701
Thiothixene Capsules ... 2290

Tranylcypromine Sulfate (Co-administration may increase the effect of either the MAO inhibitor or hydrocodone). Products include:
Parnate Tablets ... 1607

Triazolam (Co-administration may exhibit additive CNS-depression). Products include:
Halcion Tablets ... 2823

Trifluoperazine Hydrochloride (Co-administration may exhibit additive CNS-depression). Products include:
Stelazine ... 1640

Trimeprazine Tartrate (Co-administration may exhibit additive CNS-depression).
No products indexed under this heading.

Trimipramine Maleate (Co-administration may increase the effect of either the antidepressant or hydrocodone). Products include:
Surmontil Capsules ... 3595

Tripelennamine Hydrochloride (Co-administration may exhibit additive CNS-depression).
No products indexed under this heading.

Triprolidine Hydrochloride (Co-administration may exhibit additive CNS-depression). Products include:
Actifed Cold & Allergy Tablets ... ▣688

Zaleplon (Co-administration may exhibit additive CNS-depression). Products include:
Sonata Capsules ... 3591

Ziprasidone Hydrochloride (Co-administration may exhibit additive CNS-depression). Products include:
Geodon Capsules ... 2688

Zolpidem Tartrate (Co-administration may exhibit additive CNS-depression). Products include:
Ambien Tablets ... 3191

Food Interactions

Alcohol (Co-administration may exhibit additive CNS-depression; concurrent use should be avoided).

LORTAB ELIXIR
(Acetaminophen, Hydrocodone Bitartrate) ... 3317
See Lortab 10/500 Tablets

LOTEMAX STERILE OPHTHALMIC SUSPENSION 0.5%
(Loteprednol Etabonate) ... ⊙261
None cited in PDR database.

LOTENSIN TABLETS
(Benazepril Hydrochloride) ... 2365
May interact with diuretics, lithium preparations, potassium preparations, and potassium sparing diuretics. Compounds in these categories include:

Amiloride Hydrochloride (Co-administration with potassium-sparing diuretics can increase the risk of hyperkalemia). Products include:
Midamor Tablets ... 2136
Moduretic Tablets ... 2138

Bendroflumethiazide (Patients on diuretics, especially those in whom diuretic therapy was recently instituted, may occasionally experience an excessive reduction in blood pressure). Products include:
Corzide 40/5 Tablets ... 2247
Corzide 80/5 Tablets ... 2247

Bumetanide (Patients on diuretics, especially those in whom diuretic therapy was recently instituted, may occasionally experience an excessive reduction in blood pressure).
No products indexed under this heading.

Chlorothiazide (Patients on diuretics, especially those in whom diuretic therapy was recently instituted, may occasionally experience an excessive reduction in blood pressure). Products include:
Aldoclor Tablets ... 2035
Diuril Oral ... 2087

Chlorothiazide Sodium (Patients on diuretics, especially those in whom diuretic therapy was recently instituted, may occasionally experience an excessive reduction in blood pressure). Products include:
Diuril Sodium Intravenous ... 2086

Chlorthalidone (Patients on diuretics, especially those in whom diuretic therapy was recently instituted, may occasionally experience an excessive reduction in blood pressure). Products include:
Clorpres Tablets ... 1002
Combipres Tablets ... 1040
Tenoretic Tablets ... 690

Ethacrynic Acid (Patients on diuretics, especially those in whom diuretic therapy was recently instituted, may occasionally experience an excessive reduction in blood pressure). Products include:
Edecrin Tablets ... 2091

Furosemide (Patients on diuretics, especially those in whom diuretic therapy was recently instituted, may occasionally experience an excessive reduction in blood pressure). Products include:
Furosemide Tablets ... 2284

Hydrochlorothiazide (Patients on diuretics, especially those in whom diuretic therapy was recently instituted, may occasionally experience an excessive reduction in blood pressure). Products include:
Accuretic Tablets ... 2614
Aldoril Tablets ... 2039
Atacand HCT Tablets ... 597
Avalide Tablets ... 1070
Diovan HCT Tablets ... 2338

Dyazide Capsules 1515
HydroDIURIL Tablets 2108
Hyzaar 2109
Inderide Tablets 3517
Inderide LA Long-Acting Capsules 3519
Lotensin HCT Tablets 2367
Maxzide 1008
Micardis HCT Tablets 1051
Microzide Capsules 3414
Moduretic Tablets 2138
Monopril HCT 1094
Prinzide Tablets 2168
Timolide Tablets 2187
Uniretic Tablets 3178
Vaseretic Tablets 2204
Zestoretic Tablets 695
Ziac Tablets 1887

Hydroflumethiazide (Patients on diuretics, especially those in whom diuretic therapy was recently instituted, may occasionally experience an excessive reduction in blood pressure). Products include:
Diucardin Tablets 3494

Indapamide (Patients on diuretics, especially those in whom diuretic therapy was recently instituted, may occasionally experience an excessive reduction in blood pressure). Products include:
Indapamide Tablets 2286

Lithium Carbonate (Co-administration with lithium results in increased serum lithium levels and symptoms of lithium toxicity). Products include:
Eskalith 1527
Lithium Carbonate 3061
Lithobid Slow-Release Tablets 3255

Lithium Citrate (Co-administration with lithium results in increased serum lithium levels and symptoms of lithium toxicity). Products include:
Lithium Citrate Syrup 3061

Methyclothiazide (Patients on diuretics, especially those in whom diuretic therapy was recently instituted, may occasionally experience an excessive reduction in blood pressure).
No products indexed under this heading.

Metolazone (Patients on diuretics, especially those in whom diuretic therapy was recently instituted, may occasionally experience an excessive reduction in blood pressure). Products include:
Mykrox Tablets 1168
Zaroxolyn Tablets 1177

Polythiazide (Patients on diuretics, especially those in whom diuretic therapy was recently instituted, may occasionally experience an excessive reduction in blood pressure). Products include:
Minizide Capsules 2700
Renese Tablets 2712

Potassium Acid Phosphate (Co-administration with potassium supplements can increase the risk of hyperkalemia). Products include:
K-Phos Original (Sodium Free) Tablets 947

Potassium Bicarbonate (Co-administration with potassium supplements can increase the risk of hyperkalemia).
No products indexed under this heading.

Potassium Chloride (Co-administration with potassium supplements can increase the risk of hyperkalemia). Products include:
Chlor-3 1361
Colyte with Flavor Packs for Oral Solution 3170
GoLYTELY and Pineapple Flavor GoLYTELY for Oral Solution 1068
K-Dur Microburst Release System ER Tablets 1832
Klor-Con M20/Klor-Con M10 Tablets 3329
K-Lor Powder Packets 469
K-Tab Filmtab Tablets 470
Micro-K 3311
NuLYTELY, Cherry Flavor, Lemon-Lime Flavor, and Orange Flavor NuLYTELY for Oral Solution 1068
Rum-K 1363

Potassium Citrate (Co-administration with potassium supplements can increase the risk of hyperkalemia). Products include:
Urocit-K Tablets 2232

Potassium Gluconate (Co-administration with potassium supplements can increase the risk of hyperkalemia).
No products indexed under this heading.

Potassium Phosphate (Co-administration with potassium supplements can increase the risk of hyperkalemia). Products include:
K-Phos Neutral Tablets 946

Spironolactone (Co-administration with potassium-sparing diuretics can increase the risk of hyperkalemia).
No products indexed under this heading.

Torsemide (Patients on diuretics, especially those in whom diuretic therapy was recently instituted, may occasionally experience an excessive reduction in blood pressure). Products include:
Demadex Tablets and Injection 2965

Triamterene (Co-administration with potassium-sparing diuretics can increase the risk of hyperkalemia). Products include:
Dyazide Capsules 1515
Dyrenium Capsules 3458
Maxzide 1008

LOTENSIN HCT TABLETS

(Benazepril Hydrochloride, Hydrochlorothiazide) 2367

May interact with barbiturates, insulin, lithium preparations, narcotic analgesics, non-steroidal anti-inflammatory agents, potassium preparations, potassium sparing diuretics, and certain other agents. Compounds in these categories include:

Alfentanil Hydrochloride (Orthostatic hypotension produced by thiazides may be potentiated by narcotics).
No products indexed under this heading.

Amiloride Hydrochloride (Co-administration with potassium-sparing diuretics can increase the risk of hyperkalemia). Products include:
Midamor Tablets 2136
Moduretic Tablets 2138

Aprobarbital (Orthostatic hypotension produced by thiazides may be potentiated by barbiturates).
No products indexed under this heading.

Buprenorphine Hydrochloride (Orthostatic hypotension produced by thiazides may be potentiated by narcotics). Products include:
Buprenex Injectable 2918

Butabarbital (Orthostatic hypotension produced by thiazides may be potentiated by barbiturates).
No products indexed under this heading.

Butalbital (Orthostatic hypotension produced by thiazides may be potentiated by barbiturates). Products include:
Phrenilin 578
Sedapap Tablets 50 mg/650 mg 2225

Celecoxib (The diuretic, natriuretic, and antihypertensive effects of thiazide diuretics may be reduced by concurrent administration of non-steroidal anti-inflammatory agents). Products include:
Celebrex Capsules 2676
Celebrex Capsules 2780

Cholestyramine (Absorption of hydrochlorothiazide is impaired in the presence of anionic exchange resins; cholestyramine resins bind the hydrochlorothiazide and reduce its absorption from GI tract by up to 85%).
No products indexed under this heading.

Codeine Phosphate (Orthostatic hypotension produced by thiazides may be potentiated by narcotics). Products include:
Phenergan with Codeine Syrup 3557
Phenergan VC with Codeine Syrup 3561
Robitussin A-C Syrup 2942
Robitussin-DAC Syrup 2942
Ryna-C Liquid 768
Soma Compound w/Codeine Tablets 3355
Tussi-Organidin NR Liquid 3350
Tussi-Organidin-S NR Liquid 3350
Tylenol with Codeine 2595

Colestipol Hydrochloride (Absorption of hydrochlorothiazide is impaired in the presence of anionic exchange resins; colestipol resins bind the hydrochlorothiazide and reduce its absorption from GI tract by up to 43%). Products include:
Colestid Tablets 2791

Dezocine (Orthostatic hypotension produced by thiazides may be potentiated by narcotics).
No products indexed under this heading.

Diclofenac Potassium (The diuretic, natriuretic, and antihypertensive effects of thiazide diuretics may be reduced by concurrent administration of non-steroidal anti-inflammatory agents). Products include:
Cataflam Tablets 2315

Diclofenac Sodium (The diuretic, natriuretic, and antihypertensive effects of thiazide diuretics may be reduced by concurrent administration of non-steroidal anti-inflammatory agents). Products include:
Arthrotec Tablets 3195
Voltaren Ophthalmic Sterile Ophthalmic Solution ⊙312
Voltaren Tablets 2315
Voltaren-XR Tablets 2315

Etodolac (The diuretic, natriuretic, and antihypertensive effects of thiazide diuretics may be reduced by concurrent administration of non-steroidal anti-inflammatory agents). Products include:
Lodine 3528
Lodine XL Extended-Release Tablets 3530

Fenoprofen Calcium (The diuretic, natriuretic, and antihypertensive effects of thiazide diuretics may be reduced by concurrent administration of non-steroidal anti-inflammatory agents).
No products indexed under this heading.

Fentanyl (Orthostatic hypotension produced by thiazides may be potentiated by narcotics). Products include:
Duragesic Transdermal System 1786

Fentanyl Citrate (Orthostatic hypotension produced by thiazides may be potentiated by narcotics). Products include:
Actiq 1184

Flurbiprofen (The diuretic, natriuretic, and antihypertensive effects of thiazide diuretics may be reduced by concurrent administration of non-steroidal anti-inflammatory agents).
No products indexed under this heading.

Hydrocodone Bitartrate (Orthostatic hypotension produced by thiazides may be potentiated by narcotics). Products include:
Hycodan 1316
Hycomine Compound Tablets 1317
Hycotuss Expectorant Syrup 1318
Lortab 3319
Lortab Elixir 3317
Maxidone Tablets CIII 3399
Norco 5/325 Tablets CIII 3424
Norco 7.5/325 Tablets CIII 3425
Norco 10/325 Tablets CIII 3427
Norco 10/325 Tablets CIII 3425
Vicodin Tablets 516
Vicodin ES Tablets 517
Vicodin HP Tablets 518
Vicodin Tuss Expectorant 519
Vicoprofen Tablets 520
Zydone Tablets 1330

Hydrocodone Polistirex (Orthostatic hypotension produced by thiazides may be potentiated by narcotics). Products include:
Tussionex Pennkinetic Extended-Release Suspension 1174

Hydromorphone Hydrochloride (Orthostatic hypotension produced by thiazides may be potentiated by narcotics). Products include:
Dilaudid 441
Dilaudid Oral Liquid 445
Dilaudid Powder 441
Dilaudid Rectal Suppositories 441
Dilaudid Tablets 441
Dilaudid Tablets - 8 mg 445
Dilaudid-HP 443

Ibuprofen (The diuretic, natriuretic, and antihypertensive effects of thiazide diuretics may be reduced by concurrent administration of non-steroidal anti-inflammatory agents). Products include:
Advil 771
Children's Advil Oral Suspension 773
Children's Advil Chewable Tablets 773
Advil Cold and Sinus Caplets 771
Advil Cold and Sinus Tablets 771
Advil Flu & Body Ache Caplets 772
Infants' Advil Drops 773
Junior Strength Advil Tablets 773
Junior Strength Advil Chewable Tablets 773
Advil Migraine Liquigels 772
Children's Motrin Oral Suspension and Chewable Tablets 2006
Children's Motrin Cold Oral Suspension 2007
Children's Motrin Oral Suspension 643
Motrin Suspension, Oral Drops, Chewable Tablets, and Caplets 2002
Infants' Motrin Concentrated Drops 2006
Junior Strength Motrin Caplets and Chewable Tablets 2006
Motrin IB Tablets, Caplets, and Gelcaps 2002
Motrin Migraine Pain Caplets 2005
Motrin Sinus Headache Caplets 2005
Vicoprofen Tablets 520

Indomethacin (The diuretic, natriuretic, and antihypertensive effects of thiazide diuretics may be reduced by concurrent administration of non-steroidal anti-inflammatory agents). Products include:
Indocin 2112

Indomethacin Sodium Trihydrate (The diuretic, natriuretic, and antihypertensive effects of thiazide diuretics may be reduced by concurrent administration of non-steroidal anti-inflammatory agents). Products include:
Indocin I.V. 2115

Insulin, Human, Zinc Suspension (Hydrochlorothiazide causes hyperglycemia and tends to reduce glucose tolerance; insulin requirements may be increased, decreased, or unchanged). Products include:
Humulin L, 100 Units 1937
Humulin U, 100 Units 1943
Novolin L Human Insulin 10 ml Vials 2422

Insulin, Human NPH (Hydrochlorothiazide causes hyperglycemia and tends to reduce glucose tolerance; insulin requirements may be increased, decreased, or unchanged). Products include:
Humulin N, 100 Units 1939
Humulin N NPH Pen 1940
Novolin N Human Insulin 10 ml Vials 2422
Novolin N PenFill 2423
Novolin N Prefilled Syringe Disposable Insulin Delivery System 2425

Insulin, Human Regular (Hydrochlorothiazide causes hyperglycemia and tends to reduce glucose tolerance; insulin requirements may be increased, decreased, or unchanged). Products include:
- Humulin R Regular (U-500) 1943
- Humulin R, 100 Units 1941
- Novolin R Human Insulin 10 ml Vials 2423
- Novolin R PenFill 2423
- Novolin R Prefilled Syringe Disposable Insulin Delivery System 2425
- Velosulin BR Human Insulin 10 ml Vials 2435

Insulin, Human Regular and Human NPH Mixture (Hydrochlorothiazide causes hyperglycemia and tends to reduce glucose tolerance; insulin requirements may be increased, decreased, or unchanged). Products include:
- Humulin 50/50, 100 Units 1934
- Humulin 70/30, 100 Units 1935
- Humulin 70/30 Pen 1936
- Novolin 70/30 Human Insulin 10 ml Vials 2421
- Novolin 70/30 PenFill 2423
- Novolin 70/30 Prefilled Disposable Insulin Delivery System 2425

Insulin, NPH (Hydrochlorothiazide causes hyperglycemia and tends to reduce glucose tolerance; insulin requirements may be increased, decreased, or unchanged). Products include:
- Iletin II, NPH (Pork), 100 Units 1946

Insulin, Regular (Hydrochlorothiazide causes hyperglycemia and tends to reduce glucose tolerance; insulin requirements may be increased, decreased, or unchanged). Products include:
- Iletin II, Regular (Pork), 100 Units ... 1947

Insulin, Zinc Crystals (Hydrochlorothiazide causes hyperglycemia and tends to reduce glucose tolerance; insulin requirements may be increased, decreased, or unchanged).
No products indexed under this heading.

Insulin, Zinc Suspension (Hydrochlorothiazide causes hyperglycemia and tends to reduce glucose tolerance; insulin requirements may be increased, decreased, or unchanged). Products include:
- Iletin II, Lente (Pork), 100 Units 1945

Insulin Aspart, Human Regular (Hydrochlorothiazide causes hyperglycemia and tends to reduce glucose tolerance; insulin requirements may be increased, decreased, or unchanged).
No products indexed under this heading.

Insulin glargine (Hydrochlorothiazide causes hyperglycemia and tends to reduce glucose tolerance; insulin requirements may be increased, decreased, or unchanged). Products include:
- Lantus Injection 742

Insulin Lispro, Human (Hydrochlorothiazide causes hyperglycemia and tends to reduce glucose tolerance; insulin requirements may be increased, decreased, or unchanged). Products include:
- Humalog 1926
- Humalog Mix 75/25 Pen 1928

Insulin Lispro Protamine, Human (Hydrochlorothiazide causes hyperglycemia and tends to reduce glucose tolerance; insulin requirements may be increased, decreased, or unchanged). Products include:
- Humalog Mix 75/25 Pen 1928

Ketoprofen (The diuretic, natriuretic, and antihypertensive effects of thiazide diuretics may be reduced by concurrent administration of non-steroidal anti-inflammatory agents). Products include:
- Orudis Capsules 3548
- Orudis KT Tablets .... ▣778
- Oruvail Capsules 3548

Ketorolac Tromethamine (The diuretic, natriuretic, and antihypertensive effects of thiazide diuretics may be reduced by concurrent administration of non-steroidal anti-inflammatory agents). Products include:
- Acular Ophthalmic Solution 544
- Acular PF Ophthalmic Solution 544
- Toradol 3018

Levorphanol Tartrate (Orthostatic hypotension produced by thiazides may be potentiated by narcotics). Products include:
- Levo-Dromoran 1734
- Levorphanol Tartrate Tablets 3059

Lithium Carbonate (Co-administration with lithium results in increased serum lithium levels; renal clearance of lithium is reduced by thiazides; increased risk of lithium toxicity). Products include:
- Eskalith 1527
- Lithium Carbonate 3061
- Lithobid Slow-Release Tablets 3255

Lithium Citrate (Co-administration with lithium results in increased serum lithium levels; renal clearance of lithium is reduced by thiazides; increased risk of lithium toxicity). Products include:
- Lithium Citrate Syrup 3061

Meclofenamate Sodium (The diuretic, natriuretic, and antihypertensive effects of thiazide diuretics may be reduced by concurrent administration of non-steroidal anti-inflammatory agents).
No products indexed under this heading.

Mefenamic Acid (The diuretic, natriuretic, and antihypertensive effects of thiazide diuretics may be reduced by concurrent administration of non-steroidal anti-inflammatory agents). Products include:
- Ponstel Capsules 1356

Meloxicam (The diuretic, natriuretic, and antihypertensive effects of thiazide diuretics may be reduced by concurrent administration of non-steroidal anti-inflammatory agents). Products include:
- Mobic Tablets 1054

Meperidine Hydrochloride (Orthostatic hypotension produced by thiazides may be potentiated by narcotics). Products include:
- Demerol 3079
- Mepergan Injection 3539

Mephobarbital (Orthostatic hypotension produced by thiazides may be potentiated by barbiturates).
No products indexed under this heading.

Methadone Hydrochloride (Orthostatic hypotension produced by thiazides may be potentiated by narcotics). Products include:
- Dolophine Hydrochloride Tablets 3056

Morphine Sulfate (Orthostatic hypotension produced by thiazides may be potentiated by narcotics). Products include:
- Astramorph/PF Injection, USP (Preservative-Free) 594
- Duramorph Injection 1312
- Infumorph 200 and Infumorph 500 Sterile Solutions 1314
- Kadian Capsules 1335
- MS Contin Tablets 2896
- MSIR 2898
- Oramorph SR Tablets 3062
- Roxanol 3066

Nabumetone (The diuretic, natriuretic, and antihypertensive effects of thiazide diuretics may be reduced by concurrent administration of non-steroidal anti-inflammatory agents). Products include:
- Relafen Tablets 1617

Naproxen (The diuretic, natriuretic, and antihypertensive effects of thiazide diuretics may be reduced by concurrent administration of non-steroidal anti-inflammatory agents). Products include:
- EC-Naprosyn Delayed-Release Tablets 2967
- Naprosyn Suspension 2967
- Naprosyn Tablets 2967

Naproxen Sodium (The diuretic, natriuretic, and antihypertensive effects of thiazide diuretics may be reduced by concurrent administration of non-steroidal anti-inflammatory agents). Products include:
- Aleve Tablets, Caplets and Gelcaps .... ▣602
- Aleve Cold & Sinus Caplets .... ▣603
- Anaprox Tablets 2967
- Anaprox DS Tablets 2967
- Naprelan Tablets 1293

Norepinephrine Hydrochloride (Thiazides may decrease arterial responsiveness to norepinephrine).
No products indexed under this heading.

Oxaprozin (The diuretic, natriuretic, and antihypertensive effects of thiazide diuretics may be reduced by concurrent administration of non-steroidal anti-inflammatory agents).
No products indexed under this heading.

Oxycodone Hydrochloride (Orthostatic hypotension produced by thiazides may be potentiated by narcotics). Products include:
- OxyContin Tablets 2912
- OxyFast Oral Concentrate Solution 2916
- OxyIR Capsules 2916
- Percocet Tablets 1326
- Percodan Tablets 1327
- Percolone Tablets 1327
- Roxicodone 3067
- Tylox Capsules 2597

Pentobarbital Sodium (Orthostatic hypotension produced by thiazides may be potentiated by barbiturates). Products include:
- Nembutal Sodium Solution 485

Phenobarbital (Orthostatic hypotension produced by thiazides may be potentiated by barbiturates). Products include:
- Arco-Lase Plus Tablets 592
- Donnatal 2929
- Donnatal Extentabs 2930

Phenylbutazone (The diuretic, natriuretic, and antihypertensive effects of thiazide diuretics may be reduced by concurrent administration of non-steroidal anti-inflammatory agents).
No products indexed under this heading.

Piroxicam (The diuretic, natriuretic, and antihypertensive effects of thiazide diuretics may be reduced by concurrent administration of non-steroidal anti-inflammatory agents). Products include:
- Feldene Capsules 2685

Potassium Acid Phosphate (Co-administration with potassium supplements can increase the risk of hyperkalemia). Products include:
- K-Phos Original (Sodium Free) Tablets 947

Potassium Bicarbonate (Co-administration with potassium supplements can increase the risk of hyperkalemia).
No products indexed under this heading.

Potassium Chloride (Co-administration with potassium supplements can increase the risk of hyperkalemia). Products include:
- Chlor-3 1361
- Colyte with Flavor Packs for Oral Solution 3170
- GoLYTELY and Pineapple Flavor GoLYTELY for Oral Solution 1068
- K-Dur Microburst Release System ER Tablets 1832
- Klor-Con M20/Klor-Con M10 Tablets 3329
- K-Lor Powder Packets 469
- K-Tab Filmtab Tablets 470
- Micro-K 3311
- NuLYTELY, Cherry Flavor, Lemon-Lime Flavor, and Orange Flavor NuLYTELY for Oral Solution 1068
- Rum-K 1363

Potassium Citrate (Co-administration with potassium supplements can increase the risk of hyperkalemia). Products include:
- Urocit-K Tablets 2232

Potassium Gluconate (Co-administration with potassium supplements can increase the risk of hyperkalemia).
No products indexed under this heading.

Potassium Phosphate (Co-administration with potassium supplements can increase the risk of hyperkalemia). Products include:
- K-Phos Neutral Tablets 946

Propoxyphene Hydrochloride (Orthostatic hypotension produced by thiazides may be potentiated by narcotics). Products include:
- Darvon Pulvules 1909
- Darvon Compound-65 Pulvules 1910

Propoxyphene Napsylate (Orthostatic hypotension produced by thiazides may be potentiated by narcotics). Products include:
- Darvon-N/Darvocet-N 1907
- Darvon-N Tablets 1912

Remifentanil Hydrochloride (Orthostatic hypotension produced by thiazides may be potentiated by narcotics).
No products indexed under this heading.

Rofecoxib (The diuretic, natriuretic, and antihypertensive effects of thiazide diuretics may be reduced by concurrent administration of non-steroidal anti-inflammatory agents). Products include:
- Vioxx 2213

Secobarbital Sodium (Orthostatic hypotension produced by thiazides may be potentiated by barbiturates).
No products indexed under this heading.

Spironolactone (Co-administration with potassium-sparing diuretics can increase the risk of hyperkalemia).
No products indexed under this heading.

Sufentanil Citrate (Orthostatic hypotension produced by thiazides may be potentiated by narcotics).
No products indexed under this heading.

Sulindac (The diuretic, natriuretic, and antihypertensive effects of thiazide diuretics may be reduced by concurrent administration of non-steroidal anti-inflammatory agents). Products include:
- Clinoril Tablets 2053

Thiamylal Sodium (Orthostatic hypotension produced by thiazides may be potentiated by barbiturates).
No products indexed under this heading.

Tolmetin Sodium (The diuretic, natriuretic, and antihypertensive effects of thiazide diuretics may be reduced by concurrent administration of non-steroidal anti-inflammatory agents). Products include:
- Tolectin 2589

Triamterene (Co-administration with potassium-sparing diuretics can increase the risk of hyperkalemia). Products include:
- Dyazide Capsules 1515
- Dyrenium Capsules 3458
- Maxzide 1008

Tubocurarine Chloride (Thiazides may increase the responsiveness to tubocurarine).
No products indexed under this heading.

Food Interactions

Alcohol (Orthostatic hypotension produced by thiazides may be potentiated by alcohol).

LOTREL CAPSULES

(Amlodipine Besylate, Benazepril Hydrochloride)........................ 2370

May interact with diuretics, lithium preparations, potassium preparations, and potassium sparing diuretics. Compounds in these categories include:

Amiloride Hydrochloride (Potential for the increased risk of hyperkalemia; patients on diuretics, especially those in whom diuretic therapy was recently instituted, may experience an excessive reduction in blood pressure). Products include:
- Midamor Tablets 2136
- Moduretic Tablets 2138

Bendroflumethiazide (Patients on diuretics, especially those in whom diuretic therapy was recently instituted, may experience an excessive reduction in blood pressure). Products include:
- Corzide 40/5 Tablets 2247
- Corzide 80/5 Tablets 2247

Bumetanide (Patients on diuretics, especially those in whom diuretic therapy was recently instituted, may experience an excessive reduction in blood pressure).
No products indexed under this heading.

Chlorothiazide (Patients on diuretics, especially those in whom diuretic therapy was recently instituted, may experience an excessive reduction in blood pressure). Products include:
- Aldoclor Tablets 2035
- Diuril Oral 2087

Chlorothiazide Sodium (Patients on diuretics, especially those in whom diuretic therapy was recently instituted, may experience an excessive reduction in blood pressure). Products include:
- Diuril Sodium Intravenous 2086

Chlorthalidone (Patients on diuretics, especially those in whom diuretic therapy was recently instituted, may experience an excessive reduction in blood pressure). Products include:
- Clorpres Tablets 1002
- Combipres Tablets 1040
- Tenoretic Tablets 690

Ethacrynic Acid (Patients on diuretics, especially those in whom diuretic therapy was recently instituted, may experience an excessive reduction in blood pressure). Products include:
- Edecrin Tablets 2091

Furosemide (Patients on diuretics, especially those in whom diuretic therapy was recently instituted, may experience an excessive reduction in blood pressure). Products include:
- Furosemide Tablets 2284

Hydrochlorothiazide (Patients on diuretics, especially those in whom diuretic therapy was recently instituted, may experience an excessive reduction in blood pressure). Products include:
- Accuretic Tablets 2614
- Aldoril Tablets 2039
- Atacand HCT Tablets 597
- Avalide Tablets 1070
- Diovan HCT Tablets 2338
- Dyazide Capsules 1515
- HydroDIURIL Tablets 2108
- Hyzaar 2109
- Inderide Tablets 3517
- Inderide LA Long-Acting Capsules .. 3519
- Lotensin HCT Tablets 2367
- Maxzide 1008
- Micardis HCT Tablets 1051
- Microzide Capsules 3414
- Moduretic Tablets 2138
- Monopril HCT 1094
- Prinzide Tablets 2168
- Timolide Tablets 2187
- Uniretic Tablets 3178
- Vaseretic Tablets 2204
- Zestoretic Tablets 695
- Ziac Tablets 1887

Hydroflumethiazide (Patients on diuretics, especially those in whom diuretic therapy was recently instituted, may experience an excessive reduction in blood pressure). Products include:
- Diucardin Tablets 3494

Indapamide (Patients on diuretics, especially those in whom diuretic therapy was recently instituted, may experience an excessive reduction in blood pressure). Products include:
- Indapamide Tablets 2286

Lithium Carbonate (Potential for increased serum lithium levels and symptoms of lithium toxicity). Products include:
- Eskalith 1527
- Lithium Carbonate 3061
- Lithobid Slow-Release Tablets 3255

Lithium Citrate (Potential for increased serum lithium levels and symptoms of lithium toxicity). Products include:
- Lithium Citrate Syrup 3061

Methyclothiazide (Patients on diuretics, especially those in whom diuretic therapy was recently instituted, may experience an excessive reduction in blood pressure).
No products indexed under this heading.

Metolazone (Patients on diuretics, especially those in whom diuretic therapy was recently instituted, may experience an excessive reduction in blood pressure). Products include:
- Mykrox Tablets 1168
- Zaroxolyn Tablets 1177

Polythiazide (Patients on diuretics, especially those in whom diuretic therapy was recently instituted, may experience an excessive reduction in blood pressure). Products include:
- Minizide Capsules 2700
- Renese Tablets 2712

Potassium Acid Phosphate (Potential for the increased risk of hyperkalemia). Products include:
- K-Phos Original (Sodium Free) Tablets 947

Potassium Bicarbonate (Potential for the increased risk of hyperkalemia).
No products indexed under this heading.

Potassium Chloride (Potential for the increased risk of hyperkalemia). Products include:
- Chlor-3 1361
- Colyte with Flavor Packs for Oral Solution 3170
- GoLYTELY and Pineapple Flavor GoLYTELY for Oral Solution 1068
- K-Dur Microburst Release System ER Tablets 1832
- Klor-Con M20/Klor-Con M10 Tablets 3329
- K-Lor Powder Packets 469
- K-Tab Filmtab Tablets 470
- Micro-K 3311
- NuLYTELY, Cherry Flavor, Lemon-Lime Flavor, and Orange Flavor NuLYTELY for Oral Solution 1068
- Rum-K 1363

Potassium Citrate (Potential for the increased risk of hyperkalemia). Products include:
- Urocit-K Tablets 2232

Potassium Gluconate (Potential for the increased risk of hyperkalemia).
No products indexed under this heading.

Potassium Phosphate (Potential for the increased risk of hyperkalemia). Products include:
- K-Phos Neutral Tablets 946

Spironolactone (Potential for the increased risk of hyperkalemia; patients on diuretics, especially those in whom diuretic therapy was recently instituted, may experience an excessive reduction in blood pressure).
No products indexed under this heading.

Torsemide (Patients on diuretics, especially those in whom diuretic therapy was recently instituted, may experience an excessive reduction in blood pressure). Products include:
- Demadex Tablets and Injection 2965

Triamterene (Potential for the increased risk of hyperkalemia; patients on diuretics, especially those in whom diuretic therapy was recently instituted, may experience an excessive reduction in blood pressure). Products include:
- Dyazide Capsules 1515
- Dyrenium Capsules 3458
- Maxzide 1008

LOTRIMIN AF CREAM, LOTION, SOLUTION, AND JOCK ITCH CREAM

(Clotrimazole) .... ▣742

None cited in PDR database.

LOTRIMIN AF SPRAY POWDER, SPRAY LIQUID, SPRAY DEODORANT POWDER, SHAKER POWDER AND JOCK ITCH SPRAY POWDER

(Miconazole Nitrate) .... ▣742

None cited in PDR database.

LOTRIMIN CREAM 1%

(Clotrimazole) 3128

None cited in PDR database.

LOTRIMIN LOTION 1%

(Clotrimazole) 3128

None cited in PDR database.

LOTRIMIN TOPICAL SOLUTION 1%

(Clotrimazole) 3128

None cited in PDR database.

LOTRISONE CREAM

(Betamethasone Dipropionate, Clotrimazole) 3129

None cited in PDR database.

LOTRISONE LOTION

(Betamethasone Dipropionate, Clotrimazole) 3129

None cited in PDR database.

LOVENOX INJECTION

(Enoxaparin) 746

May interact with anticoagulants, non-steroidal anti-inflammatory agents, salicylates, and certain other agents. Compounds in these categories include:

Ardeparin Sodium (Agents which may enhance the risk of hemorrhage, such as other anticoagulants, should be discontinued prior to initiation of Lovenox therapy; the risk of developing epidural or spinal hematoma which can result in long-term or permanent paralysis is increased by the concomitant use of drugs affecting hemostasis).
No products indexed under this heading.

Aspirin (Agents which may enhance the risk of hemorrhage, such as platelet inhibitors, should be discontinued prior to initiation of Lovenox therapy; the risk of developing epidural or spinal hematoma which can result in long-term or permanent paralysis is increased by the concomitant use of drugs affecting hemostasis). Products include:
- Aggrenox Capsules 1026
- Alka-Seltzer .... ▣603
- Alka-Seltzer Lemon Lime Antacid and Pain Reliever Effervescent Tablets .... ▣603
- Alka-Seltzer Extra Strength Antacid and Pain Reliever Effervescent Tablets .... ▣603
- Alka-Seltzer PM Effervescent Tablets .... ▣605
- Genuine Bayer Tablets, Caplets and Gelcaps .... ▣606
- Extra Strength Bayer Caplets and Gelcaps .... ▣610
- Aspirin Regimen Bayer Children's Chewable Tablets (Orange or Cherry Flavored) .... ▣607
- Bayer, Aspirin Regimen .... ▣606
- Aspirin Regimen Bayer 81 mg Caplets with Calcium .... ▣607
- Genuine Bayer Professional Labeling (Aspirin Regimen Bayer) .... ▣608
- Extra Strength Bayer Arthritis Caplets .... ▣610
- Extra Strength Bayer Plus Caplets .... ▣610
- Extra Strength Bayer PM Caplets . ▣611
- BC Powder .... ▣619
- BC Allergy Sinus Cold Powder .... ▣619
- Arthritis Strength BC Powder .... ▣619
- BC Sinus Cold Powder .... ▣619
- Darvon Compound-65 Pulvules 1910
- Ecotrin Enteric Coated Aspirin Low, Regular and Maximum Strength Tablets 1715
- Excedrin Extra-Strength Tablets, Caplets, and Geltabs .... ▣629
- Excedrin Migraine 1070
- Goody's Body Pain Formula Powder .... ▣620
- Goody's Extra Strength Headache Powder .... ▣620
- Goody's Extra Strength Pain Relief Tablets .... ▣620
- Percodan Tablets 1327
- Robaxisal Tablets 2939
- Soma Compound Tablets 3354
- Soma Compound w/Codeine Tablets 3355
- Vanquish Caplets .... ▣617

Celecoxib (Agents which may enhance the risk of hemorrhage, such as platelet inhibitors, should be discontinued prior to initiation of Lovenox therapy; the risk of developing epidural or spinal hematoma which can result in long-term or permanent paralysis is increased by the concomitant use of drugs affecting hemostasis). Products include:
- Celebrex Capsules 2676
- Celebrex Capsules 2780

Choline Magnesium Trisalicylate (Agents which may enhance the risk of hemorrhage, such as platelet inhibitors, should be discontinued prior to initiation of Lovenox therapy; the risk of developing epidural or spinal hematoma which can result in long-term or permanent paralysis is increased by the concomitant use of drugs affecting hemostasis). Products include:
- Trilisate 2901

Clopidogrel Bisulfate (Agents which may enhance the risk of hemorrhage, such as platelet aggregation inhibitors, should be discontinued prior to initiation of Lovenox therapy; the risk of developing epidural or spinal hematoma which can result in long-term or permanent paralysis is increased by the concomitant use of drugs affecting hemostasis). Products include:
- Plavix Tablets 1097
- Plavix Tablets 3084

Dalteparin Sodium (Agents which may enhance the risk of hemorrhage, such as other anticoagulants, should be discontinued prior to initiation of Lovenox therapy; the risk of developing epidural or spinal hematoma which can result in long-term or permanent paralysis is increased by the concomitant use of drugs affecting hemostasis). Products include:
- Fragmin Injection 2814

Danaparoid Sodium (Agents which may enhance the risk of hemorrhage, such as other anticoagulants, should be discontinued prior to initia-

tion of Lovenox therapy; the risk of developing epidural or spinal hematoma which can result in long-term or permanent paralysis is increased by the concomitant use of drugs affecting hemostasis). Products include:

Orgaran Injection 2480

Diclofenac Potassium (Agents which may enhance the risk of hemorrhage, such as platelet inhibitors, should be discontinued prior to initiation of Lovenox therapy; the risk of developing epidural or spinal hematoma which can result in long-term or permanent paralysis is increased by the concomitant use of drugs affecting hemostasis). Products include:

Cataflam Tablets 2315

Diclofenac Sodium (Agents which may enhance the risk of hemorrhage, such as platelet inhibitors, should be discontinued prior to initiation of Lovenox therapy; the risk of developing epidural or spinal hematoma which can result in long-term or permanent paralysis is increased by the concomitant use of drugs affecting hemostasis). Products include:

Arthrotec Tablets 3195
Voltaren Ophthalmic Sterile Ophthalmic Solution .... ⊙312
Voltaren Tablets 2315
Voltaren-XR Tablets 2315

Dicumarol (Agents which may enhance the risk of hemorrhage, such as other anticoagulants, should be discontinued prior to initiation of Lovenox therapy; the risk of developing epidural or spinal hematoma which can result in long-term or permanent paralysis is increased by the concomitant use of drugs affecting hemostasis).

No products indexed under this heading.

Diflunisal (Agents which may enhance the risk of hemorrhage, such as platelet inhibitors, should be discontinued prior to initiation of Lovenox therapy; the risk of developing epidural or spinal hematoma which can result in long-term or permanent paralysis is increased by the concomitant use of drugs affecting hemostasis). Products include:

Dolobid Tablets 2088

Dipyridamole (Agents which may enhance the risk of hemorrhage, such as dipyridamole, should be discontinued prior to initiation of Lovenox therapy). Products include:

Aggrenox Capsules 1026
Persantine Tablets 1057

Eptifibatide (Agents which may enhance the risk of hemorrhage, such as platelet aggregation inhibitors, should be discontinued prior to initiation of Lovenox therapy; the risk of developing epidural or spinal hematoma which can result in long-term or permanent paralysis is increased by the concomitant use of drugs affecting hemostasis). Products include:

Integrilin Injection 1213
Integrilin Injection 1828

Etodolac (Agents which may enhance the risk of hemorrhage, such as platelet inhibitors, should be discontinued prior to initiation of Lovenox therapy; the risk of developing epidural or spinal hematoma which can result in long-term or permanent paralysis is increased by the concomitant use of drugs affecting hemostasis). Products include:

Lodine 3528
Lodine XL Extended-Release Tablets 3530

Fenoprofen Calcium (Agents which may enhance the risk of hemorrhage, such as platelet inhibitors, should be discontinued prior to initiation of Lovenox therapy; the risk of developing epidural or spinal hematoma which can result in long-term or permanent paralysis is increased by the concomitant use of drugs affecting hemostasis).

No products indexed under this heading.

Flurbiprofen (Agents which may enhance the risk of hemorrhage, such as platelet inhibitors, should be discontinued prior to initiation of Lovenox therapy; the risk of developing epidural or spinal hematoma which can result in long-term or permanent paralysis is increased by the concomitant use of drugs affecting hemostasis).

No products indexed under this heading.

Heparin Sodium (Agents which may enhance the risk of hemorrhage, such as other anticoagulants, should be discontinued prior to initiation of Lovenox therapy; the risk of developing epidural or spinal hematoma which can result in long-term or permanent paralysis is increased by the concomitant use of drugs affecting hemostasis). Products include:

Heparin Lock Flush Solution 3509
Heparin Sodium Injection 3511

Ibuprofen (Agents which may enhance the risk of hemorrhage, such as platelet inhibitors, should be discontinued prior to initiation of Lovenox therapy; the risk of developing epidural or spinal hematoma which can result in long-term or permanent paralysis is increased by the concomitant use of drugs affecting hemostasis). Products include:

Advil .... ▣771
Children's Advil Oral Suspension .... ▣773
Children's Advil Chewable Tablets .... ▣773
Advil Cold and Sinus Caplets .... ▣771
Advil Cold and Sinus Tablets .... ▣771
Advil Flu & Body Ache Caplets .... ▣772
Infants' Advil Drops .... ▣773
Junior Strength Advil Tablets .... ▣773
Junior Strength Advil Chewable Tablets .... ▣773
Advil Migraine Liquigels .... ▣772
Children's Motrin Oral Suspension and Chewable Tablets 2006
Children's Motrin Cold Oral Suspension 2007
Children's Motrin Oral Suspension .... ▣643
Motrin Suspension, Oral Drops, Chewable Tablets, and Caplets 2002
Infants' Motrin Concentrated Drops 2006
Junior Strength Motrin Caplets and Chewable Tablets 2006
Motrin IB Tablets, Caplets, and Gelcaps 2002
Motrin Migraine Pain Caplets 2005
Motrin Sinus Headache Caplets 2005
Vicoprofen Tablets 520

Indomethacin (Agents which may enhance the risk of hemorrhage, such as platelet inhibitors, should be discontinued prior to initiation of Lovenox therapy; the risk of developing epidural or spinal hematoma which can result in long-term or permanent paralysis is increased by the concomitant use of drugs affecting hemostasis). Products include:

Indocin 2112

Indomethacin Sodium Trihydrate (Agents which may enhance the risk of hemorrhage, such as platelet inhibitors, should be discontinued prior to initiation of Lovenox therapy; the risk of developing epidural or spinal hematoma which can result in long-term or permanent paralysis is increased by the concomitant use of drugs affecting hemostasis). Products include:

Indocin I.V. 2115

Ketoprofen (Agents which may enhance the risk of hemorrhage, such as platelet inhibitors, should be discontinued prior to initiation of Lovenox therapy; the risk of developing epidural or spinal hematoma which can result in long-term or permanent paralysis is increased by the concomitant use of drugs affecting hemostasis). Products include:

Orudis Capsules 3548
Orudis KT Tablets .... ▣778
Oruvail Capsules 3548

Ketorolac Tromethamine (Agents which may enhance the risk of hemorrhage, such as platelet inhibitors, should be discontinued prior to initiation of Lovenox therapy; the risk of developing epidural or spinal hematoma which can result in long-term or permanent paralysis is increased by the concomitant use of drugs affecting hemostasis). Products include:

Acular Ophthalmic Solution 544
Acular PF Ophthalmic Solution 544
Toradol 3018

Magnesium Salicylate (Agents which may enhance the risk of hemorrhage, such as platelet inhibitors, should be discontinued prior to initiation of Lovenox therapy; the risk of developing epidural or spinal hematoma which can result in long-term or permanent paralysis is increased by the concomitant use of drugs affecting hemostasis). Products include:

Momentum Backache Relief Extra Strength Caplets .... ▣666

Meclofenamate Sodium (Agents which may enhance the risk of hemorrhage, such as platelet inhibitors, should be discontinued prior to initiation of Lovenox therapy; the risk of developing epidural or spinal hematoma which can result in long-term or permanent paralysis is increased by the concomitant use of drugs affecting hemostasis).

No products indexed under this heading.

Mefenamic Acid (Agents which may enhance the risk of hemorrhage, such as platelet inhibitors, should be discontinued prior to initiation of Lovenox therapy; the risk of developing epidural or spinal hematoma which can result in long-term or permanent paralysis is increased by the concomitant use of drugs affecting hemostasis). Products include:

Ponstel Capsules 1356

Meloxicam (Agents which may enhance the risk of hemorrhage, such as platelet inhibitors, should be discontinued prior to initiation of Lovenox therapy; the risk of developing epidural or spinal hematoma which can result in long-term or permanent paralysis is increased by the concomitant use of drugs affecting hemostasis). Products include:

Mobic Tablets 1054

Nabumetone (Agents which may enhance the risk of hemorrhage, such as platelet inhibitors, should be discontinued prior to initiation of Lovenox therapy; the risk of developing epidural or spinal hematoma which can result in long-term or permanent paralysis is increased by the concomitant use of drugs affecting hemostasis). Products include:

Relafen Tablets 1617

Naproxen (Agents which may enhance the risk of hemorrhage, such as platelet inhibitors, should be discontinued prior to initiation of Lovenox therapy; the risk of developing epidural or spinal hematoma which can result in long-term or permanent paralysis is increased by the concomitant use of drugs affecting hemostasis). Products include:

EC-Naprosyn Delayed-Release Tablets 2967
Naprosyn Suspension 2967
Naprosyn Tablets 2967

Naproxen Sodium (Agents which may enhance the risk of hemorrhage, such as platelet inhibitors, should be discontinued prior to initiation of Lovenox therapy; the risk of developing epidural or spinal hematoma which can result in long-term or permanent paralysis is increased by the concomitant use of drugs affecting hemostasis). Products include:

Aleve Tablets, Caplets and Gelcaps .... ▣602
Aleve Cold & Sinus Caplets .... ▣603
Anaprox Tablets 2967
Anaprox DS Tablets 2967
Naprelan Tablets 1293

Oxaprozin (Agents which may enhance the risk of hemorrhage, such as platelet inhibitors, should be discontinued prior to initiation of Lovenox therapy; the risk of developing epidural or spinal hematoma which can result in long-term or permanent paralysis is increased by the concomitant use of drugs affecting hemostasis).

No products indexed under this heading.

Phenylbutazone (Agents which may enhance the risk of hemorrhage, such as platelet inhibitors, should be discontinued prior to initiation of Lovenox therapy; the risk of developing epidural or spinal hematoma which can result in long-term or permanent paralysis is increased by the concomitant use of drugs affecting hemostasis).

No products indexed under this heading.

Piroxicam (Agents which may enhance the risk of hemorrhage, such as platelet inhibitors, should be discontinued prior to initiation of Lovenox therapy; the risk of developing epidural or spinal hematoma which can result in long-term or permanent paralysis is increased by the concomitant use of drugs affecting hemostasis). Products include:

Feldene Capsules 2685

Rofecoxib (Agents which may enhance the risk of hemorrhage, such as platelet inhibitors, should be discontinued prior to initiation of Lovenox therapy; the risk of developing epidural or spinal hematoma which can result in long-term or permanent paralysis is increased by the concomitant use of drugs affecting hemostasis). Products include:

Vioxx 2213

Salsalate (Agents which may enhance the risk of hemorrhage, such as platelet inhibitors, should be discontinued prior to initiation of Lovenox therapy; the risk of developing epidural or spinal hematoma which can result in long-term or permanent paralysis is increased by the concomitant use of drugs affecting hemostasis).

No products indexed under this heading.

Sulfinpyrazone (Agents which may enhance the risk of hemorrhage, such as sulfinpyrazone, should be discontinued prior to initiation of Lovenox therapy).

No products indexed under this heading.

Sulindac (Agents which may enhance the risk of hemorrhage, such as platelet inhibitors, should be discontinued prior to initiation of Lovenox therapy; the risk of developing epidural or spinal hematoma which can result in long-term or permanent paralysis is increased by the concomitant use of drugs affecting hemostasis). Products include:

Clinoril Tablets 2053

Tinzaparin sodium (Agents which may enhance the risk of hemorrhage, such as other anticoagulants, should be discontinued prior to initiation of Lovenox therapy; the risk of developing epidural or spinal hematoma which can result in long-term or permanent paralysis is increased by the concomitant use of drugs affecting hemostasis). Products include:

Innohep Injection ... 1248

Tirofiban Hydrochloride (Agents which may enhance the risk of hemorrhage, such as platelet aggregation inhibitors, should be discontinued prior to initiation of Lovenox therapy; the risk of developing epidural or spinal hematoma which can result in long-term or permanent paralysis is increased by the concomitant use of drugs affecting hemostasis). Products include:
Aggrastat ... 2031

Tolmetin Sodium (Agents which may enhance the risk of hemorrhage, such as platelet inhibitors, should be discontinued prior to initiation of Lovenox therapy; the risk of developing epidural or spinal hematoma which can result in long-term or permanent paralysis is increased by the concomitant use of drugs affecting hemostasis). Products include:
Tolectin ... 2589

Warfarin Sodium (Agents which may enhance the risk of hemorrhage, such as other anticoagulants, should be discontinued prior to initiation of Lovenox therapy; the risk of developing epidural or spinal hematoma which can result in long-term or permanent paralysis is increased by the concomitant use of drugs affecting hemostasis). Products include:
Coumadin for Injection ... 1243
Coumadin Tablets ... 1243
Warfarin Sodium Tablets, USP ... 3302

LOW-OGESTREL-28 TABLETS

(Ethinyl Estradiol, Norgestrel) ... 3392
May interact with barbiturates and certain other agents. Compounds in these categories include:

Ampicillin Sodium (Reduced efficacy; increased incidence of breakthrough bleeding). Products include:
Unasyn for Injection ... 2728

Aprobarbital (Reduced efficacy; increased incidence of breakthrough bleeding).
No products indexed under this heading.

Butabarbital (Reduced efficacy; increased incidence of breakthrough bleeding).
No products indexed under this heading.

Butalbital (Reduced efficacy; increased incidence of breakthrough bleeding). Products include:
Phrenilin ... 578
Sedapap Tablets 50 mg/650 mg ... 2225

Mephobarbital (Reduced efficacy; increased incidence of breakthrough bleeding).
No products indexed under this heading.

Oxytetracycline (Reduced efficacy; increased incidence of breakthrough bleeding).
No products indexed under this heading.

Oxytetracycline Hydrochloride (Reduced efficacy; increased incidence of breakthrough bleeding). Products include:
Terra-Cortril Ophthalmic Suspension ... 2716
Urobiotic-250 Capsules ... 2731

Pentobarbital Sodium (Reduced efficacy; increased incidence of breakthrough bleeding). Products include:
Nembutal Sodium Solution ... 485

Phenobarbital (Reduced efficacy; increased incidence of breakthrough bleeding). Products include:
Arco-Lase Plus Tablets ... 592
Donnatal ... 2929
Donnatal Extentabs ... 2930

Phenylbutazone (Reduced efficacy; increased incidence of breakthrough bleeding).
No products indexed under this heading.

Phenytoin Sodium (Reduced efficacy; increased incidence of breakthrough bleeding). Products include:
Dilantin Kapseals ... 2622

Rifampin (Reduced efficacy; increased incidence of breakthrough bleeding). Products include:
Rifadin ... 765
Rifamate Capsules ... 767
Rifater Tablets ... 769

Secobarbital Sodium (Reduced efficacy; increased incidence of breakthrough bleeding).
No products indexed under this heading.

Tetracycline Hydrochloride (Reduced efficacy; increased incidence of breakthrough bleeding).
No products indexed under this heading.

Thiamylal Sodium (Reduced efficacy; increased incidence of breakthrough bleeding).
No products indexed under this heading.

LOXITANE CAPSULES

(Loxapine Succinate) ... 3398
May interact with barbiturates, central nervous system depressants, narcotic analgesics, and certain other agents. Compounds in these categories include:

Alfentanil Hydrochloride (Loxapine may impair mental and/or physical abilities; concomitant use may result in additive effects; loxapine is contraindicated in severe narcotic-induced depressed state).
No products indexed under this heading.

Alprazolam (Loxapine may impair mental and/or physical abilities; concomitant use may result in additive effects). Products include:
Xanax Tablets ... 2865

Aprobarbital (Loxapine may impair mental and/or physical abilities; concomitant use may result in additive effects; loxapine is contraindicated in severe barbiturate-induced depressed state).
No products indexed under this heading.

Buprenorphine Hydrochloride (Loxapine may impair mental and/or physical abilities; concomitant use may result in additive effects; loxapine is contraindicated in severe narcotic-induced depressed state). Products include:
Buprenex Injectable ... 2918

Buspirone Hydrochloride (Loxapine may impair mental and/or physical abilities; concomitant use may result in additive effects).
No products indexed under this heading.

Butabarbital (Loxapine may impair mental and/or physical abilities; concomitant use may result in additive effects; loxapine is contraindicated in severe barbiturate-induced depressed state).
No products indexed under this heading.

Butalbital (Loxapine may impair mental and/or physical abilities; concomitant use may result in additive effects; loxapine is contraindicated in severe barbiturate-induced depressed state). Products include:
Phrenilin ... 578
Sedapap Tablets 50 mg/650 mg ... 2225

Chlordiazepoxide (Loxapine may impair mental and/or physical abilities; concomitant use may result in additive effects). Products include:
Limbitrol ... 1738

Chlordiazepoxide Hydrochloride (Loxapine may impair mental and/or physical abilities; concomitant use may result in additive effects). Products include:
Librium Capsules ... 1736
Librium for Injection ... 1737

Chlorpromazine (Loxapine may impair mental and/or physical abilities; concomitant use may result in additive effects). Products include:
Thorazine Suppositories ... 1656

Chlorpromazine Hydrochloride (Loxapine may impair mental and/or physical abilities; concomitant use may result in additive effects). Products include:
Thorazine ... 1656

Chlorprothixene (Loxapine may impair mental and/or physical abilities; concomitant use may result in additive effects).
No products indexed under this heading.

Chlorprothixene Hydrochloride (Loxapine may impair mental and/or physical abilities; concomitant use may result in additive effects).
No products indexed under this heading.

Chlorprothixene Lactate (Loxapine may impair mental and/or physical abilities; concomitant use may result in additive effects).
No products indexed under this heading.

Clorazepate Dipotassium (Loxapine may impair mental and/or physical abilities; concomitant use may result in additive effects). Products include:
Tranxene ... 511

Clozapine (Loxapine may impair mental and/or physical abilities; concomitant use may result in additive effects). Products include:
Clozaril Tablets ... 2319

Codeine Phosphate (Loxapine may impair mental and/or physical abilities; concomitant use may result in additive effects; loxapine is contraindicated in severe narcotic-induced depressed state). Products include:
Phenergan with Codeine Syrup ... 3557
Phenergan VC with Codeine Syrup ... 3561
Robitussin A-C Syrup ... 2942
Robitussin-DAC Syrup ... 2942
Ryna-C Liquid ... 768
Soma Compound w/Codeine Tablets ... 3355
Tussi-Organidin NR Liquid ... 3350
Tussi-Organidin-S NR Liquid ... 3350
Tylenol with Codeine ... 2595

Desflurane (Loxapine may impair mental and/or physical abilities; concomitant use may result in additive effects). Products include:
Suprane Liquid for Inhalation ... 874

Dezocine (Loxapine may impair mental and/or physical abilities; concomitant use may result in additive effects; loxapine is contraindicated in severe narcotic-induced depressed state).
No products indexed under this heading.

Diazepam (Loxapine may impair mental and/or physical abilities; concomitant use may result in additive effects). Products include:
Valium Injectable ... 3026
Valium Tablets ... 3047

Droperidol (Loxapine may impair mental and/or physical abilities; concomitant use may result in additive effects).
No products indexed under this heading.

Enflurane (Loxapine may impair mental and/or physical abilities; concomitant use may result in additive effects).
No products indexed under this heading.

Estazolam (Loxapine may impair mental and/or physical abilities; concomitant use may result in additive effects). Products include:
ProSom Tablets ... 500

Ethchlorvynol (Loxapine may impair mental and/or physical abilities; concomitant use may result in additive effects).
No products indexed under this heading.

Ethinamate (Loxapine may impair mental and/or physical abilities; concomitant use may result in additive effects).
No products indexed under this heading.

Fentanyl (Loxapine may impair mental and/or physical abilities; concomitant use may result in additive effects; loxapine is contraindicated in severe narcotic-induced depressed state). Products include:
Duragesic Transdermal System ... 1786

Fentanyl Citrate (Loxapine may impair mental and/or physical abilities; concomitant use may result in additive effects; loxapine is contraindicated in severe narcotic-induced depressed state). Products include:
Actiq ... 1184

Fluphenazine Decanoate (Loxapine may impair mental and/or physical abilities; concomitant use may result in additive effects).
No products indexed under this heading.

Fluphenazine Enanthate (Loxapine may impair mental and/or physical abilities; concomitant use may result in additive effects).
No products indexed under this heading.

Fluphenazine Hydrochloride (Loxapine may impair mental and/or physical abilities; concomitant use may result in additive effects).
No products indexed under this heading.

Flurazepam Hydrochloride (Loxapine may impair mental and/or physical abilities; concomitant use may result in additive effects).
No products indexed under this heading.

Glutethimide (Loxapine may impair mental and/or physical abilities; concomitant use may result in additive effects).
No products indexed under this heading.

Haloperidol (Loxapine may impair mental and/or physical abilities; concomitant use may result in additive effects). Products include:
Haldol Injection, Tablets and Concentrate ... 2533

Haloperidol Decanoate (Loxapine may impair mental and/or physical abilities; concomitant use may result in additive effects). Products include:
Haldol Decanoate ... 2535

Hydrocodone Bitartrate (Loxapine may impair mental and/or physical abilities; concomitant use may result in additive effects; loxapine is contraindicated in severe narcotic-induced depressed state). Products include:
Hycodan ... 1316
Hycomine Compound Tablets ... 1317
Hycotuss Expectorant Syrup ... 1318
Lortab ... 3319
Lortab Elixir ... 3317
Maxidone Tablets CIII ... 3399
Norco 5/325 Tablets CIII ... 3424
Norco 7.5/325 Tablets CIII ... 3425
Norco 10/325 Tablets CIII ... 3427
Norco 10/325 Tablets CIII ... 3425
Vicodin Tablets ... 516
Vicodin ES Tablets ... 517
Vicodin HP Tablets ... 518
Vicodin Tuss Expectorant ... 519
Vicoprofen Tablets ... 520
Zydone Tablets ... 1330

Hydrocodone Polistirex (Loxapine may impair mental and/or physical abilities; concomitant use may result in additive effects; loxapine is contraindicated in severe narcotic-induced depressed state). Products include:
- Tussionex Pennkinetic Extended-Release Suspension 1174

Hydromorphone Hydrochloride (Loxapine may impair mental and/or physical abilities; concomitant use may result in additive effects; loxapine is contraindicated in severe narcotic-induced depressed state). Products include:
- Dilaudid 441
- Dilaudid Oral Liquid 445
- Dilaudid Powder 441
- Dilaudid Rectal Suppositories 441
- Dilaudid Tablets 441
- Dilaudid Tablets - 8 mg 445
- Dilaudid-HP 443

Hydroxyzine Hydrochloride (Loxapine may impair mental and/or physical abilities; concomitant use may result in additive effects). Products include:
- Atarax Tablets & Syrup 2667
- Vistaril Intramuscular Solution 2738

Isoflurane (Loxapine may impair mental and/or physical abilities; concomitant use may result in additive effects).
No products indexed under this heading.

Ketamine Hydrochloride (Loxapine may impair mental and/or physical abilities; concomitant use may result in additive effects).
No products indexed under this heading.

Levomethadyl Acetate Hydrochloride (Loxapine may impair mental and/or physical abilities; concomitant use may result in additive effects).
No products indexed under this heading.

Levorphanol Tartrate (Loxapine may impair mental and/or physical abilities; concomitant use may result in additive effects; loxapine is contraindicated in severe narcotic-induced depressed state). Products include:
- Levo-Dromoran 1734
- Levorphanol Tartrate Tablets 3059

Lorazepam (Co-administration has resulted in rare reports of significant respiratory depression, stupor and/or hypotension). Products include:
- Ativan Injection 3478
- Ativan Tablets 3482

Loxapine Hydrochloride (Loxapine may impair mental and/or physical abilities; concomitant use may result in additive effects).
No products indexed under this heading.

Meperidine Hydrochloride (Loxapine may impair mental and/or physical abilities; concomitant use may result in additive effects; loxapine is contraindicated in severe narcotic-induced depressed state). Products include:
- Demerol 3079
- Mepergan Injection 3539

Mephobarbital (Loxapine may impair mental and/or physical abilities; concomitant use may result in additive effects; loxapine is contraindicated in severe barbiturate-induced depressed state).
No products indexed under this heading.

Meprobamate (Loxapine may impair mental and/or physical abilities; concomitant use may result in additive effects). Products include:
- Miltown Tablets 3349

Mesoridazine Besylate (Loxapine may impair mental and/or physical abilities; concomitant use may result in additive effects). Products include:
- Serentil 1057

Methadone Hydrochloride (Loxapine may impair mental and/or physical abilities; concomitant use may result in additive effects; loxapine is contraindicated in severe narcotic-induced depressed state). Products include:
- Dolophine Hydrochloride Tablets 3056

Methohexital Sodium (Loxapine may impair mental and/or physical abilities; concomitant use may result in additive effects). Products include:
- Brevital Sodium for Injection, USP .. 1815

Methotrimeprazine (Loxapine may impair mental and/or physical abilities; concomitant use may result in additive effects).
No products indexed under this heading.

Methoxyflurane (Loxapine may impair mental and/or physical abilities; concomitant use may result in additive effects).
No products indexed under this heading.

Midazolam Hydrochloride (Loxapine may impair mental and/or physical abilities; concomitant use may result in additive effects). Products include:
- Versed Injection 3027
- Versed Syrup 3033

Molindone Hydrochloride (Loxapine may impair mental and/or physical abilities; concomitant use may result in additive effects). Products include:
- Moban 1320

Morphine Sulfate (Loxapine may impair mental and/or physical abilities; concomitant use may result in additive effects; loxapine is contraindicated in severe narcotic-induced depressed state). Products include:
- Astramorph/PF Injection, USP (Preservative-Free) 594
- Duramorph Injection 1312
- Infumorph 200 and Infumorph 500 Sterile Solutions 1314
- Kadian Capsules 1335
- MS Contin Tablets 2896
- MSIR 2898
- Oramorph SR Tablets 3062
- Roxanol 3066

Olanzapine (Loxapine may impair mental and/or physical abilities; concomitant use may result in additive effects). Products include:
- Zyprexa Tablets 1973
- Zyprexa ZYDIS Orally Disintegrating Tablets 1973

Oxazepam (Loxapine may impair mental and/or physical abilities; concomitant use may result in additive effects).
No products indexed under this heading.

Oxycodone Hydrochloride (Loxapine may impair mental and/or physical abilities; concomitant use may result in additive effects; loxapine is contraindicated in severe narcotic-induced depressed state). Products include:
- OxyContin Tablets 2912
- OxyFast Oral Concentrate Solution . 2916
- OxyIR Capsules 2916
- Percocet Tablets 1326
- Percodan Tablets 1327
- Percolone Tablets 1327
- Roxicodone 3067
- Tylox Capsules 2597

Pentobarbital Sodium (Loxapine may impair mental and/or physical abilities; concomitant use may result in additive effects; loxapine is contraindicated in severe barbiturate-induced depressed state). Products include:
- Nembutal Sodium Solution 485

Perphenazine (Loxapine may impair mental and/or physical abilities; concomitant use may result in additive effects). Products include:
- Etrafon 3115
- Trilafon 3160

Phenobarbital (Loxapine may impair mental and/or physical abilities; concomitant use may result in additive effects; loxapine is contraindicated in severe barbiturate-induced depressed state). Products include:
- Arco-Lase Plus Tablets 592
- Donnatal 2929
- Donnatal Extentabs 2930

Prazepam (Loxapine may impair mental and/or physical abilities; concomitant use may result in additive effects).
No products indexed under this heading.

Prochlorperazine (Loxapine may impair mental and/or physical abilities; concomitant use may result in additive effects). Products include:
- Compazine 1505

Promethazine Hydrochloride (Loxapine may impair mental and/or physical abilities; concomitant use may result in additive effects). Products include:
- Mepergan Injection 3539
- Phenergan Injection 3553
- Phenergan 3556
- Phenergan Syrup 3554
- Phenergan with Codeine Syrup 3557
- Phenergan with Dextromethorphan Syrup 3559
- Phenergan VC Syrup 3560
- Phenergan VC with Codeine Syrup .. 3561

Propofol (Loxapine may impair mental and/or physical abilities; concomitant use may result in additive effects). Products include:
- Diprivan Injectable Emulsion 667

Propoxyphene Hydrochloride (Loxapine may impair mental and/or physical abilities; concomitant use may result in additive effects; loxapine is contraindicated in severe narcotic-induced depressed state). Products include:
- Darvon Pulvules 1909
- Darvon Compound-65 Pulvules 1910

Propoxyphene Napsylate (Loxapine may impair mental and/or physical abilities; concomitant use may result in additive effects; loxapine is contraindicated in severe narcotic-induced depressed state). Products include:
- Darvon-N/Darvocet-N 1907
- Darvon-N Tablets 1912

Quazepam (Loxapine may impair mental and/or physical abilities; concomitant use may result in additive effects).
No products indexed under this heading.

Quetiapine Fumarate (Loxapine may impair mental and/or physical abilities; concomitant use may result in additive effects). Products include:
- Seroquel Tablets 684

Remifentanil Hydrochloride (Loxapine may impair mental and/or physical abilities; concomitant use may result in additive effects; loxapine is contraindicated in severe narcotic-induced depressed state).
No products indexed under this heading.

Risperidone (Loxapine may impair mental and/or physical abilities; concomitant use may result in additive effects). Products include:
- Risperdal 1796

Secobarbital Sodium (Loxapine may impair mental and/or physical abilities; concomitant use may result in additive effects; loxapine is contraindicated in severe barbiturate-induced depressed state).
No products indexed under this heading.

Sevoflurane (Loxapine may impair mental and/or physical abilities; concomitant use may result in additive effects).
No products indexed under this heading.

Sufentanil Citrate (Loxapine may impair mental and/or physical abilities; concomitant use may result in additive effects; loxapine is contraindicated in severe narcotic-induced depressed state).
No products indexed under this heading.

Temazepam (Loxapine may impair mental and/or physical abilities; concomitant use may result in additive effects).
No products indexed under this heading.

Thiamylal Sodium (Loxapine may impair mental and/or physical abilities; concomitant use may result in additive effects; loxapine is contraindicated in severe barbiturate-induced depressed state).
No products indexed under this heading.

Thioridazine Hydrochloride (Loxapine may impair mental and/or physical abilities; concomitant use may result in additive effects). Products include:
- Thioridazine Hydrochloride Tablets 2289

Thiothixene (Loxapine may impair mental and/or physical abilities; concomitant use may result in additive effects). Products include:
- Navane Capsules 2701
- Thiothixene Capsules 2290

Triazolam (Loxapine may impair mental and/or physical abilities; concomitant use may result in additive effects). Products include:
- Halcion Tablets 2823

Trifluoperazine Hydrochloride (Loxapine may impair mental and/or physical abilities; concomitant use may result in additive effects). Products include:
- Stelazine 1640

Zaleplon (Loxapine may impair mental and/or physical abilities; concomitant use may result in additive effects). Products include:
- Sonata Capsules 3591

Ziprasidone Hydrochloride (Loxapine may impair mental and/or physical abilities; concomitant use may result in additive effects). Products include:
- Geodon Capsules 2688

Zolpidem Tartrate (Loxapine may impair mental and/or physical abilities; concomitant use may result in additive effects). Products include:
- Ambien Tablets 3191

Food Interactions

Alcohol (Loxapine may impair mental and/or physical abilities; concomitant use may result in additive effects; loxapine is contraindicated in severe alcohol-induced depressed state).

LUBRIDERM ADVANCED THERAPY CREAMY LOTION

(Cetyl Alcohol, Glycerin, Mineral Oil) ..... ▣703
None cited in PDR database.

LUBRIDERM DAILY UV LOTION

(Octyl Methoxycinnamate, Octyl Salicylate, Oxybenzone) ..... ▣703
None cited in PDR database.

LUBRIDERM SERIOUSLY SENSITIVE LOTION

(Glycerin, Mineral Oil, Petrolatum) ..... ▣703
None cited in PDR database.

LUBRIDERM SKIN THERAPY MOISTURIZING LOTION
(Lanolin, Mineral Oil, Petrolatum) .... ■703
None cited in PDR database.

LUFYLLIN TABLETS
(Dyphylline) 3347
May interact with sympathomimetic bronchodilators and certain other agents. Compounds in these categories include:

Albuterol (Co-administration with sympathomimetic bronchodilators has been reported to produce synergism). Products include:
Proventil Inhalation Aerosol 3142
Ventolin Inhalation Aerosol and Refill.. 1679

Albuterol Sulfate (Co-administration with sympathomimetic bronchodilators has been reported to produce synergism). Products include:
AccuNeb Inhalation Solution 1230
Combivent Inhalation Aerosol 1041
DuoNeb Inhalation Solution 1233
Proventil Inhalation Solution 0.083% 3146
Proventil Repetabs Tablets 3148
Proventil Solution for Inhalation 0.5% 3144
Proventil HFA Inhalation Aerosol 3150
Ventolin HFA Inhalation Aerosol 3618
Volmax Extended-Release Tablets .. 2276

Bitolterol Mesylate (Co-administration with sympathomimetic bronchodilators has been reported to produce synergism).
No products indexed under this heading.

Ephedrine Hydrochloride (Co-administration with sympathomimetic bronchodilators has been reported to produce synergism). Products include:
Primatene Tablets .... ■780

Ephedrine Sulfate (Co-administration with sympathomimetic bronchodilators has been reported to produce synergism).
No products indexed under this heading.

Ephedrine Tannate (Co-administration with sympathomimetic bronchodilators has been reported to produce synergism). Products include:
Rynatuss Pediatric Suspension 3353
Rynatuss Tablets 3353

Epinephrine (Co-administration with sympathomimetic bronchodilators has been reported to produce synergism). Products include:
Epifrin Sterile Ophthalmic Solution .... ⊙235
EpiPen 1236
Primatene Mist .... ■779
Xylocaine with Epinephrine Injection 653

Epinephrine Hydrochloride (Co-administration with sympathomimetic bronchodilators has been reported to produce synergism).
No products indexed under this heading.

Isoetharine (Co-administration with sympathomimetic bronchodilators has been reported to produce synergism).
No products indexed under this heading.

Isoproterenol Hydrochloride (Co-administration with sympathomimetic bronchodilators has been reported to produce synergism).
No products indexed under this heading.

Isoproterenol Sulfate (Co-administration with sympathomimetic bronchodilators has been reported to produce synergism).
No products indexed under this heading.

Levalbuterol Hydrochloride (Co-administration with sympathomimetic bronchodilators has been reported to produce synergism). Products include:
Xopenex Inhalation Solution 3207

Metaproterenol Sulfate (Co-administration with sympathomimetic bronchodilators has been reported to produce synergism). Products include:
Alupent 1029

Pirbuterol Acetate (Co-administration with sympathomimetic bronchodilators has been reported to produce synergism). Products include:
Maxair Autohaler 1981
Maxair Inhaler 1984

Probenecid (Concurrent use with probenecid, which competes for tubular secretion, has shown to increase plasma half-life of dyphylline).
No products indexed under this heading.

Salmeterol Xinafoate (Co-administration with sympathomimetic bronchodilators has been reported to produce synergism). Products include:
Advair Diskus 100/50 1448
Advair Diskus 250/50 1448
Advair Diskus 500/50 1448
Serevent Diskus 1637
Serevent Inhalation Aerosol 1633

Terbutaline Sulfate (Co-administration with sympathomimetic bronchodilators has been reported to produce synergism). Products include:
Brethine Ampuls 2314
Brethine Tablets 2313

LUFYLLIN-400 TABLETS
(Dyphylline) 3347
See Lufyllin Tablets

LUFYLLIN-GG ELIXIR
(Dyphylline, Guaifenesin) 3348
See Lufyllin-GG Tablets

LUFYLLIN-GG TABLETS
(Dyphylline, Guaifenesin) 3348
May interact with sympathomimetic bronchodilators and certain other agents. Compounds in these categories include:

Albuterol (Co-administration with sympathomimetic bronchodilators has been reported to produce synergism). Products include:
Proventil Inhalation Aerosol 3142
Ventolin Inhalation Aerosol and Refill 1679

Albuterol Sulfate (Co-administration with sympathomimetic bronchodilators has been reported to produce synergism). Products include:
AccuNeb Inhalation Solution 1230
Combivent Inhalation Aerosol 1041
DuoNeb Inhalation Solution 1233
Proventil Inhalation Solution 0.083% 3146
Proventil Repetabs Tablets 3148
Proventil Solution for Inhalation 0.5% 3144
Proventil HFA Inhalation Aerosol 3150
Ventolin HFA Inhalation Aerosol 3618
Volmax Extended-Release Tablets .. 2276

Bitolterol Mesylate (Co-administration with sympathomimetic bronchodilators has been reported to produce synergism).
No products indexed under this heading.

Ephedrine Hydrochloride (Co-administration with sympathomimetic bronchodilators has been reported to produce synergism). Products include:
Primatene Tablets .... ■780

Ephedrine Sulfate (Co-administration with sympathomimetic bronchodilators has been reported to produce synergism).
No products indexed under this heading.

Ephedrine Tannate (Co-administration with sympathomimetic bronchodilators has been reported to produce synergism). Products include:
Rynatuss Pediatric Suspension 3353
Rynatuss Tablets 3353

Epinephrine (Co-administration with sympathomimetic bronchodilators has been reported to produce synergism). Products include:
Epifrin Sterile Ophthalmic Solution .... ⊙235
EpiPen 1236
Primatene Mist .... ■779
Xylocaine with Epinephrine Injection 653

Epinephrine Hydrochloride (Co-administration with sympathomimetic bronchodilators has been reported to produce synergism).
No products indexed under this heading.

Isoetharine (Co-administration with sympathomimetic bronchodilators has been reported to produce synergism).
No products indexed under this heading.

Isoproterenol Hydrochloride (Co-administration with sympathomimetic bronchodilators has been reported to produce synergism).
No products indexed under this heading.

Isoproterenol Sulfate (Co-administration with sympathomimetic bronchodilators has been reported to produce synergism).
No products indexed under this heading.

Levalbuterol Hydrochloride (Co-administration with sympathomimetic bronchodilators has been reported to produce synergism). Products include:
Xopenex Inhalation Solution 3207

Metaproterenol Sulfate (Co-administration with sympathomimetic bronchodilators has been reported to produce synergism). Products include:
Alupent 1029

Pirbuterol Acetate (Co-administration with sympathomimetic bronchodilators has been reported to produce synergism). Products include:
Maxair Autohaler 1981
Maxair Inhaler 1984

Probenecid (Concurrent use with probenecid, which competes for tubular secretion, has shown to increase plasma half-life of dyphylline).
No products indexed under this heading.

Salmeterol Xinafoate (Co-administration with sympathomimetic bronchodilators has been reported to produce synergism). Products include:
Advair Diskus 100/50 1448
Advair Diskus 250/50 1448
Advair Diskus 500/50 1448
Serevent Diskus 1637
Serevent Inhalation Aerosol 1633

Terbutaline Sulfate (Co-administration with sympathomimetic bronchodilators has been reported to produce synergism). Products include:
Brethine Ampuls 2314
Brethine Tablets 2313

LUMIGAN OPHTHALMIC SOLUTION
(Bimatoprost) 553
None cited in PDR database.

LUNELLE MONTHLY INJECTION
(Estradiol Cypionate, Medroxyprogesterone Acetate) 2827
May interact with phenytoin, prednisolone, tetracyclines, theophylline, and certain other agents. Compounds in these categories include:

Acetaminophen (May increase plasma concentrations of synthetic estrogens, possibly by inhibition of conjugation; oral contraceptives may induce the conjugation of other compounds and decreases the plasma concentrations of acetaminophen). Products include:
Actifed Cold & Sinus Caplets and Tablets .... ■688
Alka-Seltzer Plus Liqui-Gels .... ■604
Alka-Seltzer Plus Cold & Flu Medicine Liqui-Gels .... ■604
Alka-Seltzer Plus Cold & Sinus Medicine Liqui-Gels .... ■604
Benadryl Allergy/Cold Tablets .... ■691
Benadryl Allergy Sinus Headache Caplets & Gelcaps .... ■693
Benadryl Severe Allergy & Sinus Headache Caplets .... ■694
Children's Cēpacol Sore Throat .... ■788
Comtrex Acute Head Cold & Sinus Pressure Relief Tablets ..... ■627
Comtrex Deep Chest Cold & Congestion Relief Softgels .... ■627
Comtrex Flu Therapy & Fever Relief Daytime Caplets .... ■628
Comtrex Flu Therapy & Fever Relief Nighttime Tablets .... ■628
Comtrex Maximum Strength Multi-Symptom Cold & Cough Relief Tablets and Caplets .... ■626
Contac Severe Cold and Flu Caplets Maximum Strength .... ■746
Contac Severe Cold and Flu Caplets Non-Drowsy .... ■746
Coricidin 'D' Cold, Flu & Sinus Tablets .... ■737
Coricidin HBP Cold & Flu Tablets .. ■738
Coricidin HBP Maximum Strength Flu Tablets .... ■738
Coricidin HBP Night-Time Cold & Flu Tablets .... ■738
Darvon-N/Darvocet-N 1907
Dimetapp Cold and Fever Suspension .... ■775
Dimetapp Nighttime Flu Liquid ...... ■776
Dimetapp Non-Drowsy Flu Syrup .. ■777
Drixoral Allergy/Sinus Extended-Release Tablets .... ■741
Drixoral Cold & Flu Extended-Release Tablets .... ■740
Aspirin Free Excedrin Caplets and Geltabs .... ■628
Excedrin Extra-Strength Tablets, Caplets, and Geltabs .... ■629
Excedrin Migraine 1070
Excedrin PM Tablets, Caplets, and Geltabs .... ■631
Goody's Body Pain Formula Powder .... ■620
Goody's Extra Strength Headache Powder .... ■620
Goody's Extra Strength Pain Relief Tablets .... ■620
Goody's PM Powder .... ■621
Hycomine Compound Tablets 1317
Lortab 3319
Lortab Elixir 3317
Maxidone Tablets CIII 3399
Maximum Strength Midol Menstrual Caplets and Gelcaps .. ■612
Maximum Strength Midol PMS Caplets and Gelcaps .... ■613
Maximum Strength Midol Teen Caplets .... ■612
Midrin Capsules 3464
Norco 5/325 Tablets CIII 3424
Norco 7.5/325 Tablets CIII 3425
Norco 10/325 Tablets CIII 3427
Norco 10/325 Tablets CIII 3425
Percocet Tablets 1326
Percogesic Aspirin-Free Coated Tablets .... ■667
Extra Strength Percogesic Aspirin-Free Coated Caplets ...... ■665
Phrenilin 578
Robitussin Cold Caplets Multi-Symptom Cold & Flu .... ■781
Robitussin Cold Softgels Multi-Symptom Cold & Flu .... ■781
Robitussin Multi Symptom Honey Flu Liquid .... ■785
Robitussin Nighttime Honey Flu Liquid .... ■786
Sedapap Tablets 50 mg/650 mg ... 2225

Singlet Caplets ▣ 761
Sinutab Sinus Allergy Medication, Maximum Strength Formula, Tablets & Caplets ▣ 707
Sinutab Sinus Medication, Maximum Strength Without Drowsiness Formula, Tablets & Caplets ▣ 707
Sudafed Cold & Cough Liquid Caps ▣ 709
Sudafed Cold & Sinus Liquid Caps ▣ 710
Sudafed Severe Cold ▣ 711
Sudafed Sinus Headache Caplets ▣ 712
Sudafed Sinus Headache Tablets ▣ 712
Tavist Sinus Non-Drowsy Coated Caplets ▣ 676
TheraFlu Regular Strength Cold & Cough Night Time Hot Liquid ▣ 676
TheraFlu Regular Strength Cold & Sore Throat Night Time Hot Liquid ▣ 676
TheraFlu Maximum Strength Flu & Congestion Non-Drowsy Hot Liquid ▣ 677
TheraFlu Maximum Strength Flu & Cough Night Time Hot Liquid ▣ 678
TheraFlu Maximum Strength Flu & Sore Throat Night Time Hot Liquid ▣ 677
TheraFlu Maximum Strength Severe Cold & Congestion Night Time Caplets ▣ 678
TheraFlu Maximum Strength Severe Cold & Congestion Night Time Hot Liquid ▣ 678
TheraFlu Maximum Strength Severe Cold & Congestion Non-Drowsy ▣ 679
Triaminic Cold, Cough & Fever Liquid ▣ 681
Triaminic Cough & Sore Throat Liquid ▣ 682
Triaminic Cough & Sore Throat Softchews ▣ 684
Tylenol, Children's 2014
Children's Tylenol Allergy-D Liquid 2014
Children's Tylenol Cold Suspension Liquid and Chewable Tablets 2015
Children's Tylenol Cold Plus Cough Suspension Liquid and Chewable Tablets 2015
Children's Tylenol Flu Suspension Liquid 2015
Children's Tylenol Sinus Suspension Liquid 2017
Infants' Tylenol Cold Decongestant and Fever Reducer Concentrated Drops 2015
Infants' Tylenol Cold Decongestant and Fever Reducer Concentrated Drops Plus Cough 2015
Junior Strength Tylenol Soft Chews Chewable Tablets 2014
Tylenol 2009
Tylenol Allergy Sinus 2010
Tylenol Severe Allergy Caplets 2010
Multi-Symptom Tylenol Cold Complete Formula Caplets 2010
Multi-Symptom Tylenol Cold Non-Drowsy Caplets and Gelcaps 2010
Multi-Symptom Tylenol Cold Severe Congestion Non-Drowsy Caplets 2011
Maximum Strength Tylenol Flu NightTime Gelcaps 2011
Maximum Strength Tylenol Flu NightTime Liquid 2011
Maximum Strength Tylenol Flu Non-Drowsy Gelcaps 2011
Extra Strength Tylenol PM Caplets, Geltabs, and Gelcaps 2012
Maximum Strength Tylenol Sinus NightTime Caplets 2012
Maximum Strength Tylenol Sinus Non-Drowsy Geltabs, Gelcaps, Caplets, and Tablets 2012
Maximum Strength Tylenol Sore Throat Adult Liquid 2013
Tylenol with Codeine 2595
Women's Tylenol Menstrual Relief Caplets 2013
Tylox Capsules 2597
Ultracet Tablets 2597
Vanquish Caplets ▣ 617
Vicks 44M Cough, Cold & Flu Relief Liquid ▣ 725
Vicks DayQuil LiquiCaps/Liquid Multi-Symptom Cold/Flu Relief ▣ 727
Vicks NyQuil LiquiCaps/Liquid Multi-Symptom Cold/Flu Relief, Original and Cherry Flavors ▣ 727
Vicodin Tablets 516
Vicodin ES Tablets 517
Vicodin HP Tablets 518
Zydone Tablets 1330

Aminoglutethimide (May decrease the serum concentration of medroxyprogesterone acetate (MPA); possibility of decreased efficacy with concurrent use).
No products indexed under this heading.

Aminophylline (Combined hormonal contraceptives containing some synthetic estrogens, e.g., ethinyl estradiol, may inhibit the metabolism of theophylline).
No products indexed under this heading.

Ampicillin (Pregnancy while taking oral contraceptives has been reported when the oral contraceptives were administered with antimicrobials, such as ampicillin).
No products indexed under this heading.

Ampicillin Sodium (Pregnancy while taking oral contraceptives has been reported when the oral contraceptives were administered with antimicrobials, such as ampicillin). Products include:
Unasyn for Injection 2728

Carbamazepine (Anticonvulsants, such as carbamazepine, have been shown to increase the metabolism of some synthetic estrogens and progestins, which could result in a reduction of contraceptive effectiveness). Products include:
Carbatrol Capsules 3234
Tegretol/Tegretol-XR 2404

Clofibrate (Increased clearance of clofibric acid has been noted when co-administered with oral contraceptives). Products include:
Atromid-S Capsules 3483

Cyclosporine (Combined hormonal contraceptives containing some synthetic estrogens, e.g., ethinyl estradiol, may inhibit the metabolism of cyclosporine). Products include:
Gengraf Capsules 457
Neoral Soft Gelatin Capsules 2380
Neoral Oral Solution 2380
Sandimmune 2388

Demeclocycline Hydrochloride (Pregnancy while taking oral contraceptives has been reported when the oral contraceptives were administered with antimicrobials, such as tetracyclines). Products include:
Declomycin Tablets 1855

Doxycycline Calcium (Pregnancy while taking oral contraceptives has been reported when the oral contraceptives were administered with antimicrobials, such as tetracyclines). Products include:
Vibramycin Calcium Oral Suspension Syrup 2735

Doxycycline Hyclate (Pregnancy while taking oral contraceptives has been reported when the oral contraceptives were administered with antimicrobials, such as tetracyclines). Products include:
Doryx Coated Pellet Filled Capsules 3357
Periostat Tablets 1208
Vibramycin Hyclate Capsules 2735
Vibramycin Hyclate Intravenous 2737
Vibra-Tabs Film Coated Tablets 2735

Doxycycline Monohydrate (Pregnancy while taking oral contraceptives has been reported when the oral contraceptives were administered with antimicrobials, such as tetracyclines). Products include:
Monodox Capsules 2442
Vibramycin Monohydrate for Oral Suspension 2735

Dyphylline (Combined hormonal contraceptives containing some synthetic estrogens, e.g., ethinyl estradiol, may inhibit the metabolism of theophylline). Products include:
Lufyllin Tablets 3347
Lufyllin-400 Tablets 3347
Lufyllin-GG Elixir 3348
Lufyllin-GG Tablets 3348

Fosphenytoin Sodium (Anticonvulsants, such as phenytoin, have been shown to increase the metabolism of some synthetic estrogens and progestins, which could result in a reduction of contraceptive effectiveness). Products include:
Cerebyx Injection 2619

Griseofulvin (Pregnancy while taking oral contraceptives has been reported when the oral contraceptives were administered with antimicrobials, such as griseofulvin). Products include:
Grifulvin V Tablets Microsize and Oral Suspension Microsize 2518
Gris-PEG Tablets 2661

Hypericum (Herbal products containing St. John's Wort may induce hepatic enzymes (CYP450) and glycoprotein transporter and may reduce the effectiveness of contraceptive steroids; may result in breakthrough bleeding). Products include:
Brite-Life Caplets ▣ 795
Centrum St. John's Wort Softgels ▣ 853
Metabolic Nutrition System ▣ 798
Movana Tablets ▣ 832
One-A-Day Tension & Mood Softgels ▣ 808
ReSource Wellness StayCalm Caplets ▣ 826
Satiete Tablets ▣ 846

Methacycline Hydrochloride (Pregnancy while taking oral contraceptives has been reported when the oral contraceptives were administered with antimicrobials, such as tetracyclines).
No products indexed under this heading.

Minocycline Hydrochloride (Pregnancy while taking oral contraceptives has been reported when the oral contraceptives were administered with antimicrobials, such as tetracyclines). Products include:
Dynacin Capsules 2019
Minocin Intravenous 1862
Minocin Oral Suspension 1865
Minocin Pellet-Filled Capsules 1863

Morphine Sulfate (Increased clearance of morphine has been noted when co-administered with oral contraceptives). Products include:
Astramorph/PF Injection, USP (Preservative-Free) 594
Duramorph Injection 1312
Infumorph 200 and Infumorph 500 Sterile Solutions 1314
Kadian Capsules 1335
MS Contin Tablets 2896
MSIR 2898
Oramorph SR Tablets 3062
Roxanol 3066

Oxytetracycline Hydrochloride (Pregnancy while taking oral contraceptives has been reported when the oral contraceptives were administered with antimicrobials, such as tetracyclines). Products include:
Terra-Cortril Ophthalmic Suspension 2716
Urobiotic-250 Capsules 2731

Phenobarbital (Anticonvulsants, such as phenobarbital, have been shown to increase the metabolism of some synthetic estrogens and progestins, which could result in a reduction of contraceptive effectiveness). Products include:
Arco-Lase Plus Tablets 592
Donnatal 2929
Donnatal Extentabs 2930

Phenylbutazone (A reduction in contraceptive effectiveness and an increased incidence of menstrual irregularities has been suggested with concomitant phenylbutazone).
No products indexed under this heading.

Phenytoin (Anticonvulsants, such as phenytoin, have been shown to increase the metabolism of some synthetic estrogens and progestins, which could result in a reduction of contraceptive effectiveness). Products include:
Dilantin Infatabs 2624
Dilantin-125 Oral Suspension 2625

Phenytoin Sodium (Anticonvulsants, such as phenytoin, have been shown to increase the metabolism of some synthetic estrogens and progestins, which could result in a reduction of contraceptive effectiveness). Products include:
Dilantin Kapseals 2622

Prednisolone (Combined hormonal contraceptives containing some synthetic estrogens, e.g., ethinyl estradiol, may inhibit the metabolism of prednisolone). Products include:
Prelone Syrup 2273

Prednisolone Acetate (Combined hormonal contraceptives containing some synthetic estrogens, e.g., ethinyl estradiol, may inhibit the metabolism of prednisolone). Products include:
Blephamide Ophthalmic Ointment 547
Blephamide Ophthalmic Suspension 548
Poly-Pred Liquifilm Ophthalmic Suspension ⊙ 245
Pred Forte Ophthalmic Suspension ⊙ 246
Pred Mild Sterile Ophthalmic Suspension ⊙ 249
Pred-G Ophthalmic Suspension ⊙ 247
Pred-G Sterile Ophthalmic Ointment ⊙ 248

Prednisolone Sodium Phosphate (Combined hormonal contraceptives containing some synthetic estrogens, e.g., ethinyl estradiol, may inhibit the metabolism of prednisolone). Products include:
Pediapred Oral Solution 1170

Prednisolone Tebutate (Combined hormonal contraceptives containing some synthetic estrogens, e.g., ethinyl estradiol, may inhibit the metabolism of prednisolone).
No products indexed under this heading.

Rifampin (Metabolism of some synthetic estrogens, e.g., ethinyl estradiol, and progestins, e.g., norethindrone is increased by rifampin; a reduction in contraceptive effectiveness and an increase in menstrual irregularities have been associated with concomitant use of rifampin). Products include:
Rifadin 765
Rifamate Capsules 767
Rifater Tablets 769

Salicylic Acid (Increased clearance of salicylic acid has been noted when co-administered with oral contraceptives). Products include:
Clear Away Gel with Aloe Wart Remover System ▣ 736
Clear Away Liquid Wart Remover System ▣ 736
Clear Away One Step Wart Remover ▣ 737
Clear Away One Step Wart Remover for Kids ▣ 737
Clear Away One Step Plantar Wart Remover ▣ 737
Compound W One Step Pads for Kids ▣ 664
Compound W One Step Plantar Pads ▣ 664
Compound W One Step Wart Remover Pads ▣ 664
Compound W Wart Remover Gel ▣ 665
Compound W Wart Remover Liquid ▣ 665
Wart-Off Liquid ▣ 716

Temazepam (Increased clearance of temazepam has been noted when co-administered with oral contraceptives).
No products indexed under this heading.

Tetracycline Hydrochloride (Pregnancy while taking oral contraceptives has been reported when the oral contraceptives were administered with antimicrobials, such as

tetracyclines).
No products indexed under this heading.

Theophylline (Combined hormonal contraceptives containing some synthetic estrogens, e.g., ethinyl estradiol, may inhibit the metabolism of theophylline). Products include:
Aerolate 1361
Theo-Dur Extended-Release Tablets 1835
Uni-Dur Extended-Release Tablets .. 1841
Uniphyl 400 mg and 600 mg Tablets 2903

Theophylline Calcium Salicylate (Combined hormonal contraceptives containing some synthetic estrogens, e.g., ethinyl estradiol, may inhibit the metabolism of theophylline).
No products indexed under this heading.

Theophylline Sodium Glycinate (Combined hormonal contraceptives containing some synthetic estrogens, e.g., ethinyl estradiol, may inhibit the metabolism of theophylline).
No products indexed under this heading.

Vitamin C (May increase plasma concentrations of synthetic estrogens, possibly by inhibition of conjugation). Products include:
Beta-C Tablets 811
C-Grams Caplets 795
Halls Defense Drops 687
Peridin-C Tablets 618

LUPRON DEPOT 3.75 MG
(Leuprolide Acetate) 3281
None cited in PDR database.

LUPRON DEPOT 7.5 MG
(Leuprolide Acetate) 3284
None cited in PDR database.

LUPRON DEPOT--3 MONTH 11.25 MG
(Leuprolide Acetate) 3285
None cited in PDR database.

LUPRON DEPOT--3 MONTH 22.5 MG
(Leuprolide Acetate) 3288
None cited in PDR database.

LUPRON DEPOT--4 MONTH 30 MG
(Leuprolide Acetate) 3289
None cited in PDR database.

LUPRON DEPOT-PED 7.5 MG, 11.25 MG AND 15 MG
(Leuprolide Acetate) 3291
None cited in PDR database.

LUPRON INJECTION
(Leuprolide Acetate) 3279
None cited in PDR database.

LUPRON INJECTION PEDIATRIC
(Leuprolide Acetate) 3280
None cited in PDR database.

LUSTRA CREAM
(Hydroquinone) 2023
None cited in PDR database.

LUSTRA-AF CREAM
(Hydroquinone) 2023
None cited in PDR database.

LUVOX TABLETS (25, 50, 100 MG)
(Fluvoxamine Maleate) 3256
May interact with benzodiazepines metabolised by glucuronidation, benzodiazepines metabolised by hepatic oxidation, lithium preparations, monoamine oxidase inhibitors, phenytoin, quinidine, theophylline, and certain other agents. Compounds in these categories include:

Alprazolam (Co-administration may result in reduced alprazolam clearance, pharmacokinetic parameters (AUC, Cmax, T1/2) and steady-state plasma concentrations of alprazolam are twice those observed when alprazolam was used alone). Products include:
Xanax Tablets 2865

Aminophylline (Decreased clearance of theophylline by approximately 3-fold; dose of theophylline should be reduced to one-third of the usual daily dose).
No products indexed under this heading.

Amitriptyline Hydrochloride (Co-administration has resulted in significant increases in plasma tricyclic antidepressant levels). Products include:
Etrafon 3115
Limbitrol 1738

Astemizole (Fluvoxamine may be a potent inhibitor of P450IIIA4, co-administration may lead to the potential for QT prolongation and torsade de pointes-type ventricular tachycardia; concurrent use is contraindicated).
No products indexed under this heading.

Carbamazepine (Elevated plasma carbamazepine levels and symptoms of toxicity). Products include:
Carbatrol Capsules 3234
Tegretol/Tegretol-XR 2404

Chlordiazepoxide (Potential for reduced clearance of benzodiazepines metabolized by hepatic oxidation). Products include:
Limbitrol 1738

Chlordiazepoxide Hydrochloride (Potential for reduced clearance of benzodiazepines metabolized by hepatic oxidation). Products include:
Librium Capsules 1736
Librium for Injection 1737

Cisapride (Fluvoxamine may be a potent inhibitor of P450IIIA4, co-administration may lead to the potential for QT prolongation and torsade de pointes-type ventricular tachycardia; concurrent use is contraindicated).
No products indexed under this heading.

Clomipramine Hydrochloride (Co-administration has resulted in significant increases in plasma tricyclic antidepressant levels).
No products indexed under this heading.

Clozapine (Co-administration has resulted in elevated serum levels of clozapine; the risk of clozapine-related seizures and orthostatic hypotension may be increased). Products include:
Clozaril Tablets 2319

Diazepam (Reduced clearance of both diazepam and its active metabolite; co-administration is not advisable). Products include:
Valium Injectable 3026
Valium Tablets 3047

Diltiazem Hydrochloride (Co-administration has resulted in bradycardia). Products include:
Cardizem Injectable 1018
Cardizem Lyo-Ject Syringe 1018
Cardizem Monovial 1018
Cardizem CD Capsules 1016
Tiazac Capsules 1378

Dyphylline (Decreased clearance of theophylline by approximately 3-fold; dose of theophylline should be reduced to one-third of the usual daily dose). Products include:
Lufyllin Tablets 3347
Lufyllin-400 Tablets 3347
Lufyllin-GG Elixir 3348
Lufyllin-GG Tablets 3348

Estazolam (Potential for reduced clearance of benzodiazepines metabolized by hepatic oxidation). Products include:
ProSom Tablets 500

Flurazepam Hydrochloride (Potential for reduced clearance of benzodiazepines metabolized by hepatic oxidation).
No products indexed under this heading.

Fosphenytoin Sodium (A clinically significant fluvoxamine interaction is possible with drugs having a narrow therapeutic ratio, such as phenytoin). Products include:
Cerebyx Injection 2619

Halazepam (Potential for reduced clearance of benzodiazepines metabolized by hepatic oxidation).
No products indexed under this heading.

Imipramine Hydrochloride (Co-administration has resulted in significant increases in plasma tricyclic antidepressant levels).
No products indexed under this heading.

Isocarboxazid (Co-administration of another serotonin reuptake inhibitor and MAO inhibitors has resulted in serious, sometimes fatal, reactions including hyperthermia, rigidity, extreme agitation, delirium, and coma; concurrent and/or sequential use of Luvox and an MAOI is not recommended).
No products indexed under this heading.

Ketoconazole (Caution is advised if used concurrently with inhibitor of P450IIIA4, such as ketoconazole). Products include:
Nizoral 2% Cream 3620
Nizoral A-D Shampoo 2008
Nizoral 2% Shampoo 2007
Nizoral Tablets 1791

Lithium Carbonate (Co-administration has resulted in seizures; lithium may enhance the serotonergic effects of fluvoxamine). Products include:
Eskalith 1527
Lithium Carbonate 3061
Lithobid Slow-Release Tablets 3255

Lithium Citrate (Co-administration has resulted in seizures; lithium may enhance the serotonergic effects of fluvoxamine). Products include:
Lithium Citrate Syrup 3061

Lorazepam (Possible substantial decrements in cognitive functioning; the clearance of benzodiazepines metabolized by glucuronidation is unlikely to be affected). Products include:
Ativan Injection 3478
Ativan Tablets 3482

Methadone Hydrochloride (Significantly increased methadone (plasma level:dose) ratios). Products include:
Dolophine Hydrochloride Tablets 3056

Metoprolol Succinate (Co-administration has resulted in one case of bradycardia and hypotension and a second case of orthostatic hypotension). Products include:
Toprol-XL Tablets 651

Metoprolol Tartrate (Co-administration has resulted in one case of bradycardia and hypotension and a second case of orthostatic hypotension).
No products indexed under this heading.

Midazolam Hydrochloride (Potential for reduced clearance of benzodiazepines metabolized by hepatic oxidation). Products include:
Versed Injection 3027
Versed Syrup 3033

Moclobemide (Co-administration of another serotonin reuptake inhibitor and MAO inhibitors has resulted in serious, sometimes fatal, reactions including hyperthermia, rigidity, extreme agitation, delirium, and coma; concurrent and/or sequential use of Luvox and an MAOI is not recommended).
No products indexed under this heading.

Oxazepam (The clearance of benzodiazepines metabolized by glucuronidation is unlikely to be affected).
No products indexed under this heading.

Pargyline Hydrochloride (Co-administration of another serotonin reuptake inhibitor and MAO inhibitors has resulted in serious, sometimes fatal, reactions including hyperthermia, rigidity, extreme agitation, delirium, and coma; concurrent and/or sequential use of Luvox and an MAOI is not recommended).
No products indexed under this heading.

Phenelzine Sulfate (Co-administration of another serotonin reuptake inhibitor and MAO inhibitors has resulted in serious, sometimes fatal, reactions including hyperthermia, rigidity, extreme agitation, delirium, and coma; concurrent and/or sequential use of Luvox and an MAOI is not recommended). Products include:
Nardil Tablets 2653

Phenytoin (A clinically significant fluvoxamine interaction is possible with drugs having a narrow therapeutic ratio, such as phenytoin). Products include:
Dilantin Infatabs 2624
Dilantin-125 Oral Suspension 2625

Phenytoin Sodium (A clinically significant fluvoxamine interaction is possible with drugs having a narrow therapeutic ratio, such as phenytoin). Products include:
Dilantin Kapseals 2622

Pimozide (Fluvoxamine may be a potent inhibitor of CYP4503A4; co-administration may lead to the potential for QT prolongation and torsade de pointes-type ventricular tachycardia; concurrent use is contraindicated). Products include:
Orap Tablets 1407

Procarbazine Hydrochloride (Co-administration of another serotonin reuptake inhibitor and MAO inhibitors has resulted in serious, sometimes fatal, reactions including hyperthermia, rigidity, extreme agitation, delirium, and coma; concurrent and/or sequential use of Luvox and an MAOI is not recommended). Products include:
Matulane Capsules 3246

Propranolol Hydrochloride (Potential for five-fold increase in minimum propranolol plasma concentrations; slight potentiation of the propranolol-induced reduction in heart rate and reduction in the exercise diastolic pressure). Products include:
Inderal 3513
Inderal LA Long-Acting Capsules 3516
Inderide Tablets 3517
Inderide LA Long-Acting Capsules .. 3519

Quazepam (Potential for reduced clearance of benzodiazepines metabolized by hepatic oxidation).
No products indexed under this heading.

Quinidine Gluconate (Fluvoxamine is metabolized, at least in part, by P450IID6 isoenzyme; caution is indicated in patients receiving known inhibitor, such as quinidine, of this isoenzyme). Products include:
Quinaglute Dura-Tabs Tablets 978

Quinidine Polygalacturonate (Fluvoxamine is metabolized, at least in part, by P450IID6 isoenzyme; caution is indicated in patients receiving known inhibitor, such as quinidine, of this isoenzyme).
No products indexed under this heading.

Quinidine Sulfate (Fluvoxamine is metabolized, at least in part, by P450IID6 isoenzyme; caution is indicated in patients receiving known inhibitor, such as quinidine, of this isoenzyme). Products include:
Quinidex Extentabs 2933

Selegiline Hydrochloride (Co-administration of another serotonin reuptake inhibitor and MAO inhibitors has resulted in serious, sometimes fatal, reactions including hyperthermia, rigidity, extreme agitation, delirium, and coma; concurrent and/or sequential use of Luvox and an MAOI is not recommended). Products include:
Eldepryl Capsules 3266

Sumatriptan (Co-administration of SSRI with sumatriptan has resulted in rare reports of weakness, hyperreflexia, and incoordination). Products include:
Imitrex Nasal Spray 1554

Sumatriptan Succinate (Co-administration of SSRI with sumatriptan has resulted in rare reports of weakness, hyperrflexia, and incoordination). Products include:
Imitrex Injection 1549
Imitrex Tablets 1558

Temazepam (The clearance of benzodiazepines metabolized by glucuronidation is unlikely to be affected).
No products indexed under this heading.

Terfenadine (Fluvoxamine may be a potent inhibitor of P450IIIA4, co-administration may lead to the potential for QT prolongation and torsade de pointes-type ventricular tachycardia; concurrent use is contraindicated).
No products indexed under this heading.

Theophylline (Decreased clearance of theophylline by approximately 3-fold; dose of theophylline should be reduced to one-third of the usual daily dose). Products include:
Aerolate 1361
Theo-Dur Extended-Release Tablets 1835
Uni-Dur Extended-Release Tablets .. 1841
Uniphyl 400 mg and 600 mg Tablets 2903

Theophylline Calcium Salicylate (Decreased clearance of theophylline by approximately 3-fold; dose of theophylline should be reduced to one-third of the usual daily dose).
No products indexed under this heading.

Theophylline Sodium Glycinate (Decreased clearance of theophylline by approximately 3-fold; dose of theophylline should be reduced to one-third of the usual daily dose).
No products indexed under this heading.

Thioridazine Hydrochloride (Co-administration has resulted in three-fold elevation in plasma levels of thioridazine and its active metabolites; because thioridazine administration produces a dose-related prolongation of the QTc interval, which is associated with serious ventricularrhythmias, such as torsade de pointes-type arrhythmias, and sudden death; concurrent use is contraindicated). Products include:
Thioridazine Hydrochloride Tablets 2289

Tranylcypromine Sulfate (Co-administration of another serotonin reuptake inhibitor and MAO inhibitors has resulted in serious, sometimes fatal, reactions including hyperthermia, rigidity, extreme agitation, delirium, and coma; concurrent and/or sequential use of Luvox and an MAOI is not recommended). Products include:
Parnate Tablets 1607

Triazolam (The clearance of benzodiazepines metabolized by glucuronidation is unlikely to be affected). Products include:
Halcion Tablets 2823

L-Tryptophan (Enhances serotogenic effects; potential for severe vomiting).
No products indexed under this heading.

Warfarin Sodium (Co-administration has resulted in increased warfarin plasma concentrations by 98% and prothrombin time prolongation). Products include:
Coumadin for Injection 1243
Coumadin Tablets 1243
Warfarin Sodium Tablets, USP 3302

Food Interactions

Alcohol (Concurrent use should be avoided).

LUXIQ FOAM

(Betamethasone Valerate) 1210
None cited in PDR database.

LYMERIX VACCINE

(Lyme Disease Vaccine (Recombinant OspA)) 1592
May interact with anticoagulants. Compounds in these categories include:

Ardeparin Sodium (As with other intramuscular injections, LYMErix should not be given to individuals on anticoagulant therapy).
No products indexed under this heading.

Dalteparin Sodium (As with other intramuscular injections, LYMErix should not be given to individuals on anticoagulant therapy). Products include:
Fragmin Injection 2814

Danaparoid Sodium (As with other intramuscular injections, LYMErix should not be given to individuals on anticoagulant therapy). Products include:
Orgaran Injection 2480

Dicumarol (As with other intramuscular injections, LYMErix should not be given to individuals on anticoagulant therapy).
No products indexed under this heading.

Enoxaparin (As with other intramuscular injections, LYMErix should not be given to individuals on anticoagulant therapy). Products include:
Lovenox Injection 746

Heparin Sodium (As with other intramuscular injections, LYMErix should not be given to individuals on anticoagulant therapy). Products include:
Heparin Lock Flush Solution 3509
Heparin Sodium Injection 3511

Tinzaparin sodium (As with other intramuscular injections, LYMErix should not be given to individuals on anticoagulant therapy). Products include:
Innohep Injection 1248

Warfarin Sodium (As with other intramuscular injections, LYMErix should not be given to individuals on anticoagulant therapy). Products include:
Coumadin for Injection 1243
Coumadin Tablets 1243
Warfarin Sodium Tablets, USP 3302

MAALOX ANTACID/ ANTI-GAS ORAL SUSPENSION

(Aluminum Hydroxide, Magnesium Hydroxide, Simethicone) .... ▣673
May interact with:

Prescription Drugs, unspecified (Antacids may interact with certain unspecified prescription drugs).

MAALOX MAX MAXIMUM STRENGTH ANTACID/ ANTI-GAS LIQUID

(Aluminum Hydroxide, Magnesium Hydroxide, Simethicone) 2300
May interact with:

Prescription Drugs, unspecified (Antacids may interfere with certain unspecified prescription drugs; resulting effect not specified).

MAALOX REGULAR STRENGTH ANTACID/ ANTIGAS LIQUID

(Aluminum Hydroxide, Magnesium Hydroxide) 2300
May interact with:

Prescription Drugs, unspecified (Antacids may interact with certain unspecified prescription drugs).

QUICK DISSOLVE MAALOX MAX MAXIMUM STRENGTH ANTACID/ ANTIGAS TABLETS

(Calcium Carbonate) 2301
See Quick Dissolve Maalox Regular Strength Antacid Tablets

QUICK DISSOLVE MAALOX REGULAR STRENGTH ANTACID TABLETS

(Calcium Carbonate) 2301
May interact with:

Drugs, Oral, unspecified (Antacids may interact with certain unspecified prescription drugs).

QUICK DISSOLVE MAALOX MAX MAXIMUM STRENGTH ANTACID/ ANTIGAS CHEWABLE TABLETS

(Calcium Carbonate, Simethicone) .... ▣674

MACROBID CAPSULES

(Nitrofurantoin Monohydrate) 2889
May interact with:

Magnesium Trisilicate (Co-administration with antacids containing magnesium trisilicate reduces both the rate and extent of absorption). Products include:
Gaviscon Regular Strength Tablets .... ▣750

Probenecid (Inhibition of renal tubular secretion of nitrofurantoin; increases toxicity and could lessen its efficacy as a urinary tract antibacterial).
No products indexed under this heading.

Sulfinpyrazone (Inhibition of renal tubular secretion of nitrofurantoin; increases toxicity and could lessen its efficacy as a urinary tract antibacterial).
No products indexed under this heading.

Food Interactions

Food, unspecified (Increases bioavailability by approximately 40%).

MACRODANTIN CAPSULES

(Nitrofurantoin) 2891
May interact with:

Magnesium Trisilicate (Co-administration with antacids containing magnesium trisilicate reduces both the rate and extent of absorption). Products include:
Gaviscon Regular Strength Tablets .... ▣750

Probenecid (Inhibition of renal tubular secretion of nitrofurantoin increases toxicity and could lessen its efficacy as a urinary tract antibacterial).
No products indexed under this heading.

Sulfinpyrazone (Inhibition of renal tubular secretion of nitrofurantoin increases toxicity and could lessen its efficacy as a urinary tract antibacterial).
No products indexed under this heading.

Food Interactions

Food, unspecified (Increases bioavailability of Macrodantin).

MACRO-MINERAL COMPLEX CAPLETS

(Herbals with Vitamins & Minerals) .... ▣797
None cited in PDR database.

MAGONATE NATAL LIQUID

(Magnesium Gluconate) 1362
None cited in PDR database.

MAGONATE TABLETS AND LIQUID

(Magnesium Gluconate) 1362
None cited in PDR database.

MAG-OX 400 TABLETS

(Magnesium Oxide) 1024
May interact with:

Prescription Drugs, unspecified (Antacids may interact with certain prescription drugs; concurrent use should not be undertaken without prior consultation with healthcare professional).

MALARONE TABLETS

(Atovaquone, Proguanil Hydrochloride) 1596
May interact with tetracyclines. Compounds in these categories include:

Demeclocycline Hydrochloride (Co-administration with tetracycline has been associated with approximately a 40% reduction in plasma concentrations of atovaquone). Products include:
Declomycin Tablets 1855

Doxycycline Calcium (Co-administration with tetracycline has been associated with approximately a 40% reduction in plasma concentrations of atovaquone). Products include:
Vibramycin Calcium Oral Suspension Syrup 2735

Doxycycline Hyclate (Co-administration with tetracycline has been associated with approximately a 40% reduction in plasma concentrations of atovaquone). Products include:
Doryx Coated Pellet Filled Capsules 3357
Periostat Tablets 1208
Vibramycin Hyclate Capsules 2735
Vibramycin Hyclate Intravenous 2737
Vibra-Tabs Film Coated Tablets 2735

Doxycycline Monohydrate (Co-administration with tetracycline has been associated with approximately a 40% reduction in plasma concentrations of atovaquone). Products include:
Monodox Capsules 2442
Vibramycin Monohydrate for Oral Suspension 2735

Methacycline Hydrochloride (Co-administration with tetracycline has been associated with approximately a 40% reduction in plasma concentrations of atovaquone).
No products indexed under this heading.

Metoclopramide Hydrochloride (May reduce the bioavailability of atovaquone and should be used only if other antiemetics are not available). Products include:
- Reglan 2935

Minocycline Hydrochloride (Co-administration with tetracycline has been associated with approximately a 40% reduction in plasma concentrations of atovaquone). Products include:
- Dynacin Capsules 2019
- Minocin Intravenous 1862
- Minocin Oral Suspension 1865
- Minocin Pellet-Filled Capsules 1863

Oxytetracycline Hydrochloride (Co-administration with tetracycline has been associated with approximately a 40% reduction in plasma concentrations of atovaquone). Products include:
- Terra-Cortril Ophthalmic Suspension 2716
- Urobiotic-250 Capsules 2731

Rifabutin (Co-administration of rifabutin is known to reduce atovaquone levels by approximately 34%; concomitant therapy is not recommended). Products include:
- Mycobutin Capsules 2838

Rifampin (Co-administration of rifampin is known to reduce atovaquone levels by approximately 50%; concomitant therapy is not recommended). Products include:
- Rifadin 765
- Rifamate Capsules 767
- Rifater Tablets 769

Tetracycline Hydrochloride (Co-administration with tetracycline has been associated with approximately a 40% reduction in plasma concentrations of atovaquone).
No products indexed under this heading.

Food Interactions

Food, unspecified (Dietary fat intake with atovaquone increases the rate and extent of absorption; Malarone should be taken with food or milky drink).

MALARONE PEDIATRIC TABLETS
(Atovaquone, Proguanil Hydrochloride) 1596
See Malarone Tablets

MALTSUPEX POWDER, LIQUID, TABLETS
(Malt Soup Extract) .... ■767
None cited in PDR database.

MANDOL VIALS
(Cefamandole Nafate) 1953
May interact with aminoglycosides and certain other agents. Compounds in these categories include:

Amikacin Sulfate (Nephrotoxicity).
No products indexed under this heading.

Gentamicin Sulfate (Nephrotoxicity). Products include:
- Genoptic Ophthalmic Ointment .... ⊙239
- Genoptic Sterile Ophthalmic Solution .... ⊙239
- Pred-G Ophthalmic Suspension .... ⊙247
- Pred-G Sterile Ophthalmic Ointment .... ⊙248

Kanamycin Sulfate (Nephrotoxicity).
No products indexed under this heading.

Probenecid (Slows tubular excretion and doubles the peak serum levels).
No products indexed under this heading.

Streptomycin Sulfate (Nephrotoxicity). Products include:
- Streptomycin Sulfate Injection 2714

Tobramycin (Nephrotoxicity). Products include:
- TOBI Solution for Inhalation 1206
- TobraDex Ophthalmic Ointment 542
- TobraDex Ophthalmic Suspension 541
- Tobrex Ophthalmic Ointment .... ⊙220
- Tobrex Ophthalmic Solution .... ⊙221

Tobramycin Sulfate (Nephrotoxicity). Products include:
- Nebcin Vials, Hyporets & ADD-Vantage 1955

Food Interactions

Alcohol (Concurrent ingestion of ethanol may result in nausea, vomiting, vasomotor instability with hypotension and peripheral vasodilation).

MARBLEN SUSPENSION
(Calcium Carbonate, Magnesium Carbonate) .... ■633
May interact with:

Prescription Drugs, unspecified (Antacids may interact with certain unspecified prescription drugs; consult your physician).

MARINOL CAPSULES
(Dronabinol) 3325
May interact with anticholinergics, antihistamines, barbiturates, benzodiazepines, central nervous system depressants, lithium preparations, narcotic analgesics, sympathomimetics, tricyclic antidepressants, theophylline, and certain other agents. Compounds in these categories include:

Acrivastine (Co-administration results in additive CNS depression or super-additive tachycardia and drowsiness). Products include:
- Semprex-D Capsules 1172

Albuterol (Co-administration with sympathomimetics may result in additive hypertension, tachycardia, and possibly cardiotoxicity). Products include:
- Proventil Inhalation Aerosol 3142
- Ventolin Inhalation Aerosol and Refill 1679

Albuterol Sulfate (Co-administration with sympathomimetics may result in additive hypertension, tachycardia, and possibly cardiotoxicity). Products include:
- AccuNeb Inhalation Solution 1230
- Combivent Inhalation Aerosol 1041
- DuoNeb Inhalation Solution 1233
- Proventil Inhalation Solution 0.083% 3146
- Proventil Repetabs Tablets 3148
- Proventil Solution for Inhalation 0.5% 3144
- Proventil HFA Inhalation Aerosol 3150
- Ventolin HFA Inhalation Aerosol 3618
- Volmax Extended-Release Tablets 2276

Alfentanil Hydrochloride (Co-administration results in additive drowsiness and CNS depression).
No products indexed under this heading.

Alprazolam (Co-administration results in additive drowsiness and CNS depression). Products include:
- Xanax Tablets 2865

Aminophylline (Increased theophylline metabolism has resulted with smoking marijuana).
No products indexed under this heading.

Amitriptyline Hydrochloride (Co-administration results in additive tachycardia, hypertension, and drowsiness). Products include:
- Etrafon 3115
- Limbitrol 1738

Amoxapine (Co-administration results in additive tachycardia, hypertension, and drowsiness).
No products indexed under this heading.

Amphetamine Sulfate (Co-administration with amphetamine may result in additive hypertension, tachycardia, and possibly cardiotoxicity). Products include:
- Adderall Tablets 3231
- Adderall XR Capsules

Aprobarbital (Co-administration results in decreased clearance of barbiturates via competitive inhibition of metabolism; additive drowsiness and CNS depression).
No products indexed under this heading.

Astemizole (Co-administration results in additive CNS depression or super-additive tachycardia and drowsiness).
No products indexed under this heading.

Atropine Sulfate (Co-administration with anticholinergic agents may result in additive or super-additive tachycardia and drowsiness). Products include:
- Donnatal 2929
- Donnatal Extentabs 2930
- Motofen Tablets 577
- Prosed/DS Tablets 3268
- Urised Tablets 2876

Azatadine Maleate (Co-administration results in additive CNS depression or super-additive tachycardia and drowsiness). Products include:
- Rynatan Tablets 3351

Belladonna Alkaloids (Co-administration with anticholinergic agents may result in additive or super-additive tachycardia and drowsiness). Products include:
- Hyland's Teething Tablets .... ■766
- Urimax Tablets 1769

Benztropine Mesylate (Co-administration with anticholinergic agents may result in additive or super-additive tachycardia and drowsiness). Products include:
- Cogentin 2055

Biperiden Hydrochloride (Co-administration with anticholinergic agents may result in additive or super-additive tachycardia and drowsiness). Products include:
- Akineton 402

Bromodiphenhydramine Hydrochloride (Co-administration results in additive CNS depression or super-additive tachycardia and drowsiness).
No products indexed under this heading.

Brompheniramine Maleate (Co-administration results in additive CNS depression or super-additive tachycardia and drowsiness). Products include:
- Bromfed Capsules (Extended-Release) 2269
- Bromfed-PD Capsules (Extended-Release) 2269
- Comtrex Acute Head Cold & Sinus Pressure Relief Tablets .... ■627
- Dimetapp Elixir .... ■777
- Dimetapp Cold and Fever Suspension .... ■775
- Dimetapp DM Cold & Cough Elixir .... ■775
- Dimetapp Nighttime Flu Liquid .... ■776

Buprenorphine Hydrochloride (Co-administration results in additive drowsiness and CNS depression). Products include:
- Buprenex Injectable 2918

Buspirone Hydrochloride (Co-administration results in additive drowsiness and CNS depression).
No products indexed under this heading.

Butabarbital (Co-administration results in decreased clearance of barbiturates via competitive inhibition of metabolism; additive drowsiness and CNS depression).
No products indexed under this heading.

Butalbital (Co-administration results in decreased clearance of barbiturates via competitive inhibition of metabolism; additive drowsiness and CNS depression). Products include:
- Phrenilin 578
- Sedapap Tablets 50 mg/650 mg 2225

Carisoprodol (Co-administration with muscle relaxants may result in additive drowsiness and CNS depression). Products include:
- Soma Tablets 3353
- Soma Compound Tablets 3354
- Soma Compound w/Codeine Tablets 3355

Cetirizine Hydrochloride (Co-administration results in additive CNS depression or super-additive tachycardia and drowsiness). Products include:
- Zyrtec 2756
- Zyrtec-D 12 Hour Extended Relief Tablets 2758

Chlordiazepoxide (Co-administration results in additive drowsiness and CNS depression). Products include:
- Limbitrol 1738

Chlordiazepoxide Hydrochloride (Co-administration results in additive drowsiness and CNS depression). Products include:
- Librium Capsules 1736
- Librium for Injection 1737

Chlorpheniramine Maleate (Co-administration results in additive CNS depression or super-additive tachycardia and drowsiness). Products include:
- Actifed Cold & Sinus Caplets and Tablets .... ■688
- Alka-Seltzer Plus Liqui-Gels .... ■604
- BC Allergy Sinus Cold Powder .... ■619
- Chlor-Trimeton Allergy Tablets .... ■735
- Chlor-Trimeton Allergy/Decongestant Tablets .... ■736
- Comtrex Flu Therapy & Fever Relief Nighttime Tablets .... ■628
- Comtrex Maximum Strength Multi-Symptom Cold & Cough Relief Tablets and Caplets .... ■626
- Contac Severe Cold and Flu Caplets Maximum Strength .... ■746
- Coricidin 'D' Cold, Flu & Sinus Tablets .... ■737
- Coricidin/Coricidin D .... ■738
- Coricidin HBP Maximum Strength Flu Tablets .... ■738
- Extendryl 1361
- Hycomine Compound Tablets 1317
- Kronofed-A 1341
- PediaCare Cough-Cold Liquid .... ■719
- PediaCare NightRest Cough-Cold Liquid .... ■719
- Robitussin Nighttime Honey Flu Liquid .... ■786
- Ryna .... ■768
- Singlet Caplets .... ■761
- Sinutab Sinus Allergy Medication, Maximum Strength Formula, Tablets & Caplets .... ■707
- Sudafed Cold & Allergy Tablets .... ■708
- TheraFlu Regular Strength Cold & Cough Night Time Hot Liquid .... ■676
- TheraFlu Regular Strength Cold & Sore Throat Night Time Hot Liquid .... ■676
- TheraFlu Maximum Strength Flu & Cough Night Time Hot Liquid .... ■678
- TheraFlu Maximum Strength Flu & Sore Throat Night Time Hot Liquid .... ■677
- TheraFlu Maximum Strength Severe Cold & Congestion Night Time Caplets .... ■678
- TheraFlu Maximum Strength Severe Cold & Congestion Night Time Hot Liquid .... ■678
- Triaminic Cold & Allergy Liquid .... ■681
- Triaminic Cold & Allergy Softchews .... ■683
- Triaminic Cold & Cough Liquid .... ■681
- Triaminic Cold & Cough Softchews .... ■683
- Triaminic Cold & Night Time Cough Liquid .... ■681
- Triaminic Cold, Cough & Fever Liquid .... ■681
- Children's Tylenol Cold Suspension Liquid and Chewable Tablets 2015
- Children's Tylenol Cold Plus Cough Suspension Liquid and Chewable Tablets 2015
- Children's Tylenol Flu Suspension Liquid 2015
- Maximum Strength Tylenol Allergy Sinus Caplets, Gelcaps, and Geltabs 2010

Multi-Symptom Tylenol Cold Complete Formula Caplets.......... 2010
Vicks 44M Cough, Cold & Flu Relief Liquid.............................. ▣725
Pediatric Vicks 44m Cough & Cold Relief................................ ▣728
Children's Vicks NyQuil Cold/Cough Relief.............................. ▣726

Chlorpheniramine Polistirex (Co-administration results in additive CNS depression or super-additive tachycardia and drowsiness). Products include:
Tussionex Pennkinetic Extended-Release Suspension..... 1174

Chlorpheniramine Tannate (Co-administration results in additive CNS depression or super-additive tachycardia and drowsiness). Products include:
Reformulated Rynatan Pediatric Suspension.............................. 3352
Rynatuss Pediatric Suspension...... 3353
Rynatuss Tablets.............................. 3353
Tussi-12 S Suspension.................. 3356
Tussi-12 Tablets.............................. 3356

Chlorpromazine (Co-administration results in additive drowsiness and CNS depression). Products include:
Thorazine Suppositories................ 1656

Chlorpromazine Hydrochloride (Co-administration results in additive drowsiness and CNS depression). Products include:
Thorazine.. 1656

Chlorprothixene (Co-administration results in additive drowsiness and CNS depression).
No products indexed under this heading.

Chlorprothixene Hydrochloride (Co-administration results in additive drowsiness and CNS depression).
No products indexed under this heading.

Chlorprothixene Lactate (Co-administration results in additive drowsiness and CNS depression).
No products indexed under this heading.

Chlorzoxazone (Co-administration with muscle relaxants may result in additive drowsiness and CNS depression). Products include:
Parafon Forte DSC Caplets............ 2582

Clemastine Fumarate (Co-administration results in additive CNS depression or super-additive tachycardia and drowsiness). Products include:
Tavist 12 Hour Allergy Tablets....... ▣676

Clidinium Bromide (Co-administration with anticholinergic agents may result in additive or super-additive tachycardia and drowsiness).
No products indexed under this heading.

Clomipramine Hydrochloride (Co-administration results in additive tachycardia, hypertension, and drowsiness).
No products indexed under this heading.

Clorazepate Dipotassium (Co-administration results in additive drowsiness and CNS depression). Products include:
Tranxene.. 511

Clozapine (Co-administration results in additive drowsiness and CNS depression). Products include:
Clozaril Tablets.............................. 2319

Cocaine Hydrochloride (Co-administration with cocaine may result in additive hypertension, tachycardia, and possibly cardiotoxicity).
No products indexed under this heading.

Codeine Phosphate (Co-administration results in additive drowsiness and CNS depression). Products include:
Phenergan with Codeine Syrup....... 3557
Phenergan VC with Codeine Syrup.. 3561
Robitussin A-C Syrup...................... 2942
Robitussin-DAC Syrup.................... 2942
Ryna-C Liquid.................................. ▣768
Soma Compound w/Codeine Tablets.. 3355
Tussi-Organidin NR Liquid.............. 3350
Tussi-Organidin-S NR Liquid.......... 3350
Tylenol with Codeine...................... 2595

Cyclobenzaprine Hydrochloride (Co-administration with muscle relaxants may result in additive drowsiness and CNS depression). Products include:
Flexeril Tablets................................ 572
Flexeril Tablets................................ 2094

Cyproheptadine Hydrochloride (Co-administration results in additive CNS depression or super-additive tachycardia and drowsiness). Products include:
Periactin Tablets.............................. 2155

Desflurane (Co-administration results in additive drowsiness and CNS depression). Products include:
Suprane Liquid for Inhalation.......... 874

Desipramine Hydrochloride (Co-administration results in additive tachycardia, hypertension, and drowsiness). Products include:
Norpramin Tablets............................ 755

Dexchlorpheniramine Maleate (Co-administration results in additive CNS depression or super-additive tachycardia and drowsiness).
No products indexed under this heading.

Dextroamphetamine Sulfate (Co-administration with amphetamine may result in additive hypertension, tachycardia, and possibly cardiotoxicity). Products include:
Adderall Tablets.............................. 3231
Adderall XR Capsules......................
Dexedrine.. 1512
DextroStat Tablets.......................... 3236

Dezocine (Co-administration results in additive drowsiness and CNS depression).
No products indexed under this heading.

Diazepam (Co-administration results in additive drowsiness and CNS depression). Products include:
Valium Injectable............................ 3026
Valium Tablets.................................. 3047

Dicyclomine Hydrochloride (Co-administration with anticholinergic agents may result in additive or super-additive tachycardia and drowsiness).
No products indexed under this heading.

Diphenhydramine Citrate (Co-administration results in additive CNS depression or super-additive tachycardia and drowsiness). Products include:
Alka-Seltzer PM Effervescent Tablets.. ▣605
Benadryl Allergy & Sinus Fastmelt Tablets.. ▣693
Benadryl Children's Allergy/Cold Fastmelt Tablets.......................... ▣692
Excedrin PM Tablets, Caplets, and Geltabs.................................. ▣631
Goody's PM Powder........................ ▣621

Diphenhydramine Hydrochloride (Co-administration results in additive CNS depression or super-additive tachycardia and drowsiness). Products include:
Extra Strength Bayer PM Caplets.. ▣611
Benadryl Allergy Chewables............ ▣689
Benadryl Allergy.............................. ▣691
Benadryl Allergy Liquid.................. ▣690
Benadryl Allergy/Cold Tablets........ ▣691
Benadryl Allergy/Congestion Tablets.. ▣692
Benadryl Allergy & Sinus Liquid...... ▣693
Benadryl Allergy Sinus Headache Caplets & Gelcaps........................ ▣693
Benadryl Severe Allergy & Sinus Headache Caplets........................ ▣694
Benadryl Dye-Free Allergy Liquid... ▣690
Benadryl Dye-Free Allergy Liqui-Gels Softgels............................ ▣690
Benadryl Itch Relief Stick Extra Strength.. ▣695
Benadryl Cream................................ ▣695
Benadryl Gel.................................... ▣695
Benadryl Spray................................ ▣696
Benadryl Parenteral........................ 2617
Coricidin HBP Night-Time Cold & Flu Tablets.................................... ▣738
Nytol QuickCaps Caplets................ ▣622
Maximum Strength Nytol QuickGels Softgels.......................... ▣621
Extra Strength Percogesic Aspirin-Free Coated Caplets......... ▣665
Simply Sleep Caplets...................... 2008
Sominex Original Formula Tablets.. ▣761
Children's Tylenol Allergy-D Liquid... 2014
Maximum Strength Tylenol Allergy Sinus NightTime Caplets.............. 2010
Tylenol Severe Allergy Caplets........ 2010
Maximum Strength Tylenol Flu NightTime Gelcaps........................ 2011
Extra Strength Tylenol PM Caplets, Geltabs, and Gelcaps.................... 2012
Unisom Maximum Strength SleepGels.. ▣713

Diphenylpyraline Hydrochloride (Co-administration results in additive CNS depression or super-additive tachycardia and drowsiness).
No products indexed under this heading.

Disulfiram (Co-administration of disulfiram in a patient who smoked marijuana has resulted in a reversible hypomanic reaction). Products include:
Antabuse Tablets............................ 2444
Antabuse Tablets............................ 3474

Dobutamine Hydrochloride (Co-administration with sympathomimetics may result in additive hypertension, tachycardia, and possibly cardiotoxicity). Products include:
Dobutrex Solution Vials.................. 1914

Dopamine Hydrochloride (Co-administration with sympathomimetics may result in additive hypertension, tachycardia, and possibly cardiotoxicity).
No products indexed under this heading.

Doxepin Hydrochloride (Co-administration results in additive tachycardia, hypertension, and drowsiness). Products include:
Sinequan.. 2713

Droperidol (Co-administration results in additive drowsiness and CNS depression).
No products indexed under this heading.

Dyphylline (Increased theophylline metabolism has resulted with smoking marijuana). Products include:
Lufyllin Tablets.............................. 3347
Lufyllin-400 Tablets........................ 3347
Lufyllin-GG Elixir............................ 3348
Lufyllin-GG Tablets.......................... 3348

Enflurane (Co-administration results in additive drowsiness and CNS depression).
No products indexed under this heading.

Ephedrine Hydrochloride (Co-administration with sympathomimetics may result in additive hypertension, tachycardia, and possibly cardiotoxicity). Products include:
Primatene Tablets............................ ▣780

Ephedrine Sulfate (Co-administration with sympathomimetics may result in additive hypertension, tachycardia, and possibly cardiotoxicity).
No products indexed under this heading.

Ephedrine Tannate (Co-administration with sympathomimetics may result in additive hypertension, tachycardia, and possibly cardiotoxicity). Products include:
Rynatuss Pediatric Suspension...... 3353
Rynatuss Tablets.............................. 3353

Epinephrine (Co-administration with sympathomimetics may result in additive hypertension, tachycardia, and possibly cardiotoxicity). Products include:
Epifrin Sterile Ophthalmic Solution.. ⊙235
EpiPen.. 1236
Primatene Mist.................................. ▣779
Xylocaine with Epinephrine Injection.. 653

Epinephrine Bitartrate (Co-administration with sympathomimetics may result in additive hypertension, tachycardia, and possibly cardiotoxicity). Products include:
Sensorcaine...................................... 643

Epinephrine Hydrochloride (Co-administration with sympathomimetics may result in additive hypertension, tachycardia, and possibly cardiotoxicity).
No products indexed under this heading.

Estazolam (Co-administration results in additive drowsiness and CNS depression). Products include:
ProSom Tablets................................ 500

Ethchlorvynol (Co-administration results in additive drowsiness and CNS depression).
No products indexed under this heading.

Ethinamate (Co-administration results in additive drowsiness and CNS depression).
No products indexed under this heading.

Fentanyl (Co-administration results in additive drowsiness and CNS depression). Products include:
Duragesic Transdermal System...... 1786

Fentanyl Citrate (Co-administration results in additive drowsiness and CNS depression). Products include:
Actiq.. 1184

Fexofenadine Hydrochloride (Co-administration results in additive CNS depression or super-additive tachycardia and drowsiness). Products include:
Allegra.. 712
Allegra-D Extended-Release Tablets.. 714

Fluoxetine Hydrochloride (Co-administration of fluoxetine in a patient who smoked marijuana has resulted in a hypomanic reaction). Products include:
Prozac Pulvules, Liquid, and Weekly Capsules.............................. 1238
Sarafem Pulvules.............................. 1962

Fluphenazine Decanoate (Co-administration results in additive drowsiness and CNS depression).
No products indexed under this heading.

Fluphenazine Enanthate (Co-administration results in additive drowsiness and CNS depression).
No products indexed under this heading.

Fluphenazine Hydrochloride (Co-administration results in additive drowsiness and CNS depression).
No products indexed under this heading.

Flurazepam Hydrochloride (Co-administration results in additive drowsiness and CNS depression).
No products indexed under this heading.

Glutethimide (Co-administration results in additive drowsiness and CNS depression).
No products indexed under this heading.

Glycopyrrolate (Co-administration with anticholinergic agents may result in additive or super-additive tachycardia and drowsiness). Products include:
Robinul Forte Tablets...................... 1358
Robinul Injectable............................ 2940
Robinul Tablets................................ 1358

Halazepam (Co-administration results in additive drowsiness and

CNS depression).
No products indexed under this heading.

Haloperidol (Co-administration results in additive drowsiness and CNS depression). Products include:
Haldol Injection, Tablets and Concentrate 2533

Haloperidol Decanoate (Co-administration results in additive drowsiness and CNS depression). Products include:
Haldol Decanoate 2535

Hydrocodone Bitartrate (Co-administration results in additive drowsiness and CNS depression). Products include:
Hycodan 1316
Hycomine Compound Tablets 1317
Hycotuss Expectorant Syrup 1318
Lortab 3319
Lortab Elixir 3317
Maxidone Tablets CIII 3399
Norco 5/325 Tablets CIII 3424
Norco 7.5/325 Tablets CIII 3425
Norco 10/325 Tablets CIII 3427
Norco 10/325 Tablets CIII 3425
Vicodin Tablets 516
Vicodin ES Tablets 517
Vicodin HP Tablets 518
Vicodin Tuss Expectorant 519
Vicoprofen Tablets 520
Zydone Tablets 1330

Hydrocodone Polistirex (Co-administration results in additive drowsiness and CNS depression). Products include:
Tussionex Pennkinetic Extended-Release Suspension 1174

Hydromorphone Hydrochloride (Co-administration results in additive drowsiness and CNS depression). Products include:
Dilaudid 441
Dilaudid Oral Liquid 445
Dilaudid Powder 441
Dilaudid Rectal Suppositories 441
Dilaudid Tablets 441
Dilaudid Tablets - 8 mg 445
Dilaudid-HP 443

Hydroxyzine Hydrochloride (Co-administration results in additive drowsiness and CNS depression). Products include:
Atarax Tablets & Syrup 2667
Vistaril Intramuscular Solution 2738

Hyoscyamine (Co-administration with anticholinergic agents may result in additive or super-additive tachycardia and drowsiness). Products include:
Urised Tablets 2876

Hyoscyamine Sulfate (Co-administration with anticholinergic agents may result in additive or super-additive tachycardia and drowsiness). Products include:
Arco-Lase Plus Tablets 592
Donnatal 2929
Donnatal Extentabs 2930
Levsin/Levsinex/Levbid 3172
NuLev Orally Disintegrating Tablets 3176
Prosed/DS Tablets 3268
Urimax Tablets 1769

Imipramine Hydrochloride (Co-administration results in additive tachycardia, hypertension, and drowsiness).
No products indexed under this heading.

Imipramine Pamoate (Co-administration results in additive tachycardia, hypertension, and drowsiness).
No products indexed under this heading.

Ipratropium Bromide (Co-administration with anticholinergic agents may result in additive or super-additive tachycardia and drowsiness). Products include:
Atrovent Inhalation Aerosol 1030
Atrovent Inhalation Solution 1031
Atrovent Nasal Spray 0.03% 1032
Atrovent Nasal Spray 0.06% 1033
Combivent Inhalation Aerosol 1041
DuoNeb Inhalation Solution 1233

Isoflurane (Co-administration results in additive drowsiness and CNS depression).
No products indexed under this heading.

Isoproterenol Hydrochloride (Co-administration with sympathomimetics may result in additive hypertension, tachycardia, and possibly cardiotoxicity).
No products indexed under this heading.

Isoproterenol Sulfate (Co-administration with sympathomimetics may result in additive hypertension, tachycardia, and possibly cardiotoxicity).
No products indexed under this heading.

Ketamine Hydrochloride (Co-administration results in additive drowsiness and CNS depression).
No products indexed under this heading.

Levalbuterol Hydrochloride (Co-administration with sympathomimetics may result in additive hypertension, tachycardia, and possibly cardiotoxicity). Products include:
Xopenex Inhalation Solution 3207

Levomethadyl Acetate Hydrochloride (Co-administration results in additive drowsiness and CNS depression).
No products indexed under this heading.

Levorphanol Tartrate (Co-administration results in additive drowsiness and CNS depression). Products include:
Levo-Dromoran 1734
Levorphanol Tartrate Tablets 3059

Lithium Carbonate (Co-administration results in additive drowsiness and CNS depression). Products include:
Eskalith 1527
Lithium Carbonate 3061
Lithobid Slow-Release Tablets 3255

Lithium Citrate (Co-administration results in additive drowsiness and CNS depression). Products include:
Lithium Citrate Syrup 3061

Loratadine (Co-administration results in additive CNS depression or super-additive tachycardia and drowsiness). Products include:
Claritin 3100
Claritin-D 12 Hour Extended Release Tablets 3102
Claritin-D 24 Hour Extended Release Tablets 3104

Lorazepam (Co-administration results in additive drowsiness and CNS depression). Products include:
Ativan Injection 3478
Ativan Tablets 3482

Loxapine Hydrochloride (Co-administration results in additive drowsiness and CNS depression).
No products indexed under this heading.

Loxapine Succinate (Co-administration results in additive drowsiness and CNS depression). Products include:
Loxitane Capsules 3398

Maprotiline Hydrochloride (Co-administration results in additive tachycardia, hypertension, and drowsiness).
No products indexed under this heading.

Mepenzolate Bromide (Co-administration with anticholinergic agents may result in additive or super-additive tachycardia and drowsiness).
No products indexed under this heading.

Meperidine Hydrochloride (Co-administration results in additive drowsiness and CNS depression). Products include:
Demerol 3079
Mepergan Injection 3539

Mephobarbital (Co-administration results in decreased clearance of barbiturates via competitive inhibition of metabolism; additive drowsiness and CNS depression).
No products indexed under this heading.

Meprobamate (Co-administration results in additive drowsiness and CNS depression). Products include:
Miltown Tablets 3349

Mesoridazine Besylate (Co-administration results in additive drowsiness and CNS depression). Products include:
Serentil 1057

Metaproterenol Sulfate (Co-administration with sympathomimetics may result in additive hypertension, tachycardia, and possibly cardiotoxicity). Products include:
Alupent 1029

Metaraminol Bitartrate (Co-administration with sympathomimetics may result in additive hypertension, tachycardia, and possibly cardiotoxicity). Products include:
Aramine Injection 2043

Methadone Hydrochloride (Co-administration results in additive drowsiness and CNS depression). Products include:
Dolophine Hydrochloride Tablets 3056

Methamphetamine Hydrochloride (Co-administration with amphetamine may result in additive hypertension, tachycardia, and possibly cardiotoxicity). Products include:
Desoxyn Tablets 440

Methdilazine Hydrochloride (Co-administration results in additive CNS depression or super-additive tachycardia and drowsiness).
No products indexed under this heading.

Methocarbamol (Co-administration with muscle relaxants may result in additive drowsiness and CNS depression). Products include:
Robaxin Injectable 2938
Robaxin Tablets 2939
Robaxisal Tablets 2939

Methohexital Sodium (Co-administration results in additive drowsiness and CNS depression). Products include:
Brevital Sodium for Injection, USP 1815

Methotrimeprazine (Co-administration results in additive drowsiness and CNS depression).
No products indexed under this heading.

Methoxamine Hydrochloride (Co-administration with sympathomimetics may result in additive hypertension, tachycardia, and possibly cardiotoxicity).
No products indexed under this heading.

Methoxyflurane (Co-administration results in additive drowsiness and CNS depression).
No products indexed under this heading.

Midazolam Hydrochloride (Co-administration results in additive drowsiness and CNS depression). Products include:
Versed Injection 3027
Versed Syrup 3033

Molindone Hydrochloride (Co-administration results in additive drowsiness and CNS depression). Products include:
Moban 1320

Morphine Sulfate (Co-administration results in additive drowsiness and CNS depression). Products include:
Astramorph/PF Injection, USP (Preservative-Free) 594
Duramorph Injection 1312
Infumorph 200 and Infumorph 500 Sterile Solutions 1314
Kadian Capsules 1335
MS Contin Tablets 2896
MSIR 2898
Oramorph SR Tablets 3062
Roxanol 3066

Norepinephrine Bitartrate (Co-administration with sympathomimetics may result in additive hypertension, tachycardia, and possibly cardiotoxicity).
No products indexed under this heading.

Nortriptyline Hydrochloride (Co-administration results in additive tachycardia, hypertension, and drowsiness).
No products indexed under this heading.

Olanzapine (Co-administration results in additive drowsiness and CNS depression). Products include:
Zyprexa Tablets 1973
Zyprexa ZYDIS Orally Disintegrating Tablets 1973

Orphenadrine Citrate (Co-administration with muscle relaxants may result in additive drowsiness and CNS depression). Products include:
Norflex 1987

Oxazepam (Co-administration results in additive drowsiness and CNS depression).
No products indexed under this heading.

Oxybutynin Chloride (Co-administration with anticholinergic agents may result in additive or super-additive tachycardia and drowsiness). Products include:
Ditropan XL Extended Release Tablets 564

Oxycodone Hydrochloride (Co-administration results in additive drowsiness and CNS depression). Products include:
OxyContin Tablets 2912
OxyFast Oral Concentrate Solution 2916
OxyIR Capsules 2916
Percocet Tablets 1326
Percodan Tablets 1327
Percolone Tablets 1327
Roxicodone 3067
Tylox Capsules 2597

Pentobarbital Sodium (Co-administration results in decreased clearance of barbiturates via competitive inhibition of metabolism; additive drowsiness and CNS depression). Products include:
Nembutal Sodium Solution 485

Perphenazine (Co-administration results in additive drowsiness and CNS depression). Products include:
Etrafon 3115
Trilafon 3160

Phenobarbital (Co-administration results in decreased clearance of barbiturates via competitive inhibition of metabolism; additive drowsiness and CNS depression). Products include:
Arco-Lase Plus Tablets 592
Donnatal 2929
Donnatal Extentabs 2930

Phenylephrine Bitartrate (Co-administration with sympathomimetics may result in additive hypertension, tachycardia, and possibly cardiotoxicity).
No products indexed under this heading.

Phenylephrine Hydrochloride (Co-administration with sympathomimetics may result in additive hypertension, tachycardia, and possibly cardiotoxicity). Products include:
Afrin Nasal Decongestant Children's Pump Mist 734
Extendryl 1361
Hycomine Compound Tablets 1317
Neo-Synephrine 614
Phenergan VC Syrup 3560
Phenergan VC with Codeine Syrup 3561
Preparation H Cream 778

Preparation H Cooling Gel ... 778
Preparation H ... 778
Vicks Sinex Nasal Spray and Ultra Fine Mist ... 729

Phenylephrine Tannate (Co-administration with sympathomimetics may result in additive hypertension, tachycardia, and possibly cardiotoxicity). Products include:
Ryna-12 S Suspension ... 3351
Reformulated Rynatan Pediatric Suspension ... 3352
Rynatuss Pediatric Suspension ... 3353
Rynatuss Tablets ... 3353

Phenylpropanolamine Hydrochloride (Co-administration with sympathomimetics may result in additive hypertension, tachycardia, and possibly cardiotoxicity).
No products indexed under this heading.

Pirbuterol Acetate (Co-administration with sympathomimetics may result in additive hypertension, tachycardia, and possibly cardiotoxicity). Products include:
Maxair Autohaler ... 1981
Maxair Inhaler ... 1984

Prazepam (Co-administration results in additive drowsiness and CNS depression).
No products indexed under this heading.

Prochlorperazine (Co-administration results in additive drowsiness and CNS depression). Products include:
Compazine ... 1505

Procyclidine Hydrochloride (Co-administration with anticholinergic agents may result in additive or super-additive tachycardia and drowsiness).
No products indexed under this heading.

Promethazine Hydrochloride (Co-administration results in additive drowsiness and CNS depression). Products include:
Mepergan Injection ... 3539
Phenergan Injection ... 3553
Phenergan ... 3556
Phenergan Syrup ... 3554
Phenergan with Codeine Syrup ... 3557
Phenergan with Dextromethorphan Syrup ... 3559
Phenergan VC Syrup ... 3560
Phenergan VC with Codeine Syrup ... 3561

Propantheline Bromide (Co-administration with anticholinergic agents may result in additive or super-additive tachycardia and drowsiness).
No products indexed under this heading.

Propofol (Co-administration results in additive drowsiness and CNS depression). Products include:
Diprivan Injectable Emulsion ... 667

Propoxyphene Hydrochloride (Co-administration results in additive drowsiness and CNS depression). Products include:
Darvon Pulvules ... 1909
Darvon Compound-65 Pulvules ... 1910

Propoxyphene Napsylate (Co-administration results in additive drowsiness and CNS depression). Products include:
Darvon-N/Darvocet-N ... 1907
Darvon-N Tablets ... 1912

Protriptyline Hydrochloride (Co-administration results in additive tachycardia, hypertension, and drowsiness). Products include:
Vivactil Tablets ... 2446
Vivactil Tablets ... 2217

Pseudoephedrine Hydrochloride (Co-administration with sympathomimetics may result in additive hypertension, tachycardia, and possibly cardiotoxicity). Products include:
Actifed Cold & Allergy Tablets ... 688
Actifed Cold & Sinus Caplets and Tablets ... 688
Advil Cold and Sinus Caplets ... 771
Advil Cold and Sinus Tablets ... 771
Advil Flu & Body Ache Caplets ... 772
Aleve Cold & Sinus Caplets ... 603
Alka-Seltzer Plus Liqui-Gels ... 604
Alka-Seltzer Plus Cold & Flu Medicine Liqui-Gels ... 604
Alka-Seltzer Plus Cold & Sinus Medicine Liqui-Gels ... 604
Allegra-D Extended-Release Tablets ... 714
BC Cold Powder ... 619
Benadryl Allergy/Cold Tablets ... 691
Benadryl Allergy/Congestion Tablets ... 692
Benadryl Allergy & Sinus Liquid ... 693
Benadryl Allergy & Sinus Fastmelt Tablets ... 693
Benadryl Allergy Sinus Headache Caplets & Gelcaps ... 693
Benadryl Severe Allergy & Sinus Headache Caplets ... 694
Benadryl Children's Allergy/Cold Fastmelt Tablets ... 692
Benylin Multi-Symptom Liquid ... 697
Bromfed Capsules (Extended-Release) ... 2269
Bromfed-PD Capsules (Extended-Release) ... 2269
Children's Cēpacol Sore Throat ... 788
Comtrex Acute Head Cold & Sinus Pressure Relief Tablets ... 627
Comtrex Deep Chest Cold & Congestion Relief Softgels ... 627
Comtrex Flu Therapy & Fever Relief Daytime Caplets ... 628
Comtrex Flu Therapy & Fever Relief Nighttime Tablets ... 628
Comtrex Maximum Strength Multi-Symptom Cold & Cough Relief Tablets and Caplets ... 626
Contac Non-Drowsy 12 Hour Cold Caplets ... 745
Contac Non-Drowsy Timed Release 12 Hour Cold Caplets ... 746
Contac Severe Cold and Flu Caplets Maximum Strength ... 746
Contac Severe Cold and Flu Caplets Non-Drowsy ... 746
Dimetapp Elixir ... 777
Dimetapp Cold and Fever Suspension ... 775
Dimetapp DM Cold & Cough Elixir ... 775
Dimetapp Nighttime Flu Liquid ... 776
Dimetapp Non-Drowsy Flu Syrup ... 777
Dimetapp Infant Drops Decongestant ... 775
Dimetapp Infant Drops Decongestant Plus Cough ... 776
Guaifed ... 2272
Kronofed-A ... 1341
Children's Motrin Cold Oral Suspension ... 2007
Motrin Sinus Headache Caplets ... 2005
PediaCare Cough-Cold Liquid ... 719
PediaCare Infants' Drops Decongestant ... 719
PediaCare Infants' Drops Decongestant Plus Cough ... 719
PediaCare NightRest Cough-Cold Liquid ... 719
Robitussin Cold Caplets Cold & Congestion ... 780
Robitussin Cold Softgels Cold & Congestion ... 780
Robitussin Cold Caplets Multi-Symptom Cold & Flu ... 781
Robitussin Cold Softgels Multi-Symptom Cold & Flu ... 781
Robitussin Cold Softgels Severe Congestion ... 782
Robitussin Cough & Cold Infant Drops ... 782
Robitussin Maximum Strength Cough & Cold Liquid ... 785
Robitussin Pediatric Cough & Cold Formula Liquid ... 785
Robitussin Multi Symptom Honey Flu Liquid ... 785
Robitussin Nighttime Honey Flu Liquid ... 786
Robitussin-CF Liquid ... 783
Robitussin-DAC Syrup ... 2942
Robitussin-PE Liquid ... 782
Ryna ... 768
Semprex-D Capsules ... 1172
Singlet Caplets ... 761
Sinutab Non-Drying Liquid Caps ... 706
Sinutab Sinus Allergy Medication, Maximum Strength Formula, Tablets & Caplets ... 707
Sinutab Sinus Medication, Maximum Strength Without Drowsiness Formula, Tablets & Caplets ... 707
Sudafed 12 Hour Tablets ... 708
Sudafed 24 Hour Tablets ... 708
Children's Sudafed Cold & Cough Liquid ... 709
Children's Sudafed Nasal Decongestant Chewables ... 711
Children's Sudafed Nasal Decongestant Liquid Medication ... 711
Sudafed Cold & Allergy Tablets ... 708
Sudafed Cold & Cough Liquid Caps ... 709
Sudafed Cold & Sinus Liquid Caps ... 710
Sudafed Nasal Decongestant Tablets ... 710
Sudafed Non-Drying Sinus Liquid Caps ... 712
Sudafed Severe Cold ... 711
Sudafed Sinus Headache Caplets ... 712
Sudafed Sinus Headache Tablets ... 712
Tavist Sinus Non-Drowsy Coated Caplets ... 676
TheraFlu Regular Strength Cold & Cough Night Time Hot Liquid ... 676
TheraFlu Regular Strength Cold & Sore Throat Night Time Hot Liquid ... 676
TheraFlu Maximum Strength Flu & Congestion Non-Drowsy Hot Liquid ... 677
TheraFlu Maximum Strength Flu & Cough Night Time Hot Liquid ... 678
TheraFlu Maximum Strength Flu & Sore Throat Night Time Hot Liquid ... 677
TheraFlu Maximum Strength Severe Cold & Congestion Night Time Caplets ... 678
TheraFlu Maximum Strength Severe Cold & Congestion Night Time Hot Liquid ... 678
TheraFlu Maximum Strength Severe Cold & Congestion Non-Drowsy ... 679
Triaminic Allergy Congestion Liquid ... 680
Triaminic Chest Congestion Liquid ... 680
Triaminic Cold & Allergy Liquid ... 681
Triaminic Cold & Allergy Softchews ... 683
Triaminic Cold & Cough Liquid ... 681
Triaminic Cold & Cough Softchews ... 683
Triaminic Cold & Night Time Cough Liquid ... 681
Triaminic Cold, Cough & Fever Liquid ... 681
Triaminic Cough Liquid ... 682
Triaminic Cough & Congestion Liquid ... 682
Triaminic Cough & Sore Throat Liquid ... 682
Triaminic Cough & Sore Throat Softchews ... 684
Children's Tylenol Allergy-D Liquid ... 2014
Children's Tylenol Cold Suspension Liquid and Chewable Tablets ... 2015
Children's Tylenol Cold Plus Cough Suspension Liquid and Chewable Tablets ... 2015
Children's Tylenol Flu Suspension Liquid ... 2015
Children's Tylenol Sinus Suspension Liquid ... 2017
Infants' Tylenol Cold Decongestant and Fever Reducer Concentrated Drops ... 2015
Infants' Tylenol Cold Decongestant and Fever Reducer Concentrated Drops Plus Cough ... 2015
Tylenol Allergy Sinus ... 2010
Multi-Symptom Tylenol Cold Complete Formula Caplets ... 2010
Multi-Symptom Tylenol Cold Non-Drowsy Caplets and Gelcaps ... 2010
Multi-Symptom Tylenol Cold Severe Congestion Non-Drowsy Caplets ... 2011
Maximum Strength Tylenol Flu NightTime Gelcaps ... 2011
Maximum Strength Tylenol Flu NightTime Liquid ... 2011
Maximum Strength Tylenol Flu Non-Drowsy Gelcaps ... 2011
Maximum Strength Tylenol Sinus NightTime Caplets ... 2012
Maximum Strength Tylenol Sinus Non-Drowsy Geltabs, Gelcaps, Caplets, and Tablets ... 2012
Vicks 44D Cough & Head Congestion Relief Liquid ... 724
Vicks 44M Cough, Cold & Flu Relief Liquid ... 725
Pediatric Vicks 44m Cough & Cold Relief ... 728
Vicks DayQuil LiquiCaps/Liquid Multi-Symptom Cold/Flu Relief ... 727
Children's Vicks NyQuil Cold/Cough Relief ... 726
Vicks NyQuil LiquiCaps/Liquid Multi-Symptom Cold/Flu Relief, Original and Cherry Flavors ... 727
Zephrex Tablets ... 3091
Zephrex LA Tablets ... 3092
Zyrtec-D 12 Hour Extended Relief Tablets ... 2758

Pseudoephedrine Sulfate (Co-administration with sympathomimetics may result in additive hypertension, tachycardia, and possibly cardiotoxicity). Products include:
Chlor-Trimeton Allergy/Decongestant Tablets ... 736
Claritin-D 12 Hour Extended Release Tablets ... 3102
Claritin-D 24 Hour Extended Release Tablets ... 3104
Coricidin 'D' Cold, Flu & Sinus Tablets ... 737
Drixoral Allergy/Sinus Extended-Release Tablets ... 741
Drixoral Cold & Allergy Sustained-Action Tablets ... 740
Drixoral Cold & Flu Extended-Release Tablets ... 740
Drixoral Nasal Decongestant Long-Acting Non-Drowsy Tablets ... 740
Rynatan Tablets ... 3351

Pyrilamine Maleate (Co-administration results in additive CNS depression or super-additive tachycardia and drowsiness). Products include:
Maximum Strength Midol Menstrual Caplets and Gelcaps ... 612
Maximum Strength Midol PMS Caplets and Gelcaps ... 613

Pyrilamine Tannate (Co-administration results in additive CNS depression or super-additive tachycardia and drowsiness). Products include:
Ryna-12 S Suspension ... 3351

Quazepam (Co-administration results in additive drowsiness and CNS depression).
No products indexed under this heading.

Quetiapine Fumarate (Co-administration results in additive drowsiness and CNS depression). Products include:
Seroquel Tablets ... 684

Remifentanil Hydrochloride (Co-administration results in additive drowsiness and CNS depression).
No products indexed under this heading.

Risperidone (Co-administration results in additive drowsiness and CNS depression). Products include:
Risperdal ... 1796

Salmeterol Xinafoate (Co-administration with sympathomimetics may result in additive hypertension, tachycardia, and possibly cardiotoxicity). Products include:
Advair Diskus 100/50 ... 1448
Advair Diskus 250/50 ... 1448
Advair Diskus 500/50 ... 1448
Serevent Diskus ... 1637
Serevent Inhalation Aerosol ... 1633

Scopolamine (Co-administration with anticholinergic agents may result in additive or super-additive tachycardia and drowsiness). Products include:
Transderm Scōp Transdermal Therapeutic System ... 2302

Scopolamine Hydrobromide (Co-administration with anticholinergic agents may result in additive or super-additive tachycardia and drowsiness). Products include:
Donnatal ... 2929
Donnatal Extentabs ... 2930

Secobarbital Sodium (Co-administration results in decreased clearance of barbiturates via competitive inhibition of metabolism; additive drowsiness and CNS

depression).
No products indexed under this heading.

Sevoflurane (Co-administration results in additive drowsiness and CNS depression).
No products indexed under this heading.

Sufentanil Citrate (Co-administration results in additive drowsiness and CNS depression).
No products indexed under this heading.

Temazepam (Co-administration results in additive drowsiness and CNS depression).
No products indexed under this heading.

Terbutaline Sulfate (Co-administration with sympathomimetics may result in additive hypertension, tachycardia, and possibly cardiotoxicity). Products include:
Brethine Ampuls 2314
Brethine Tablets 2313

Terfenadine (Co-administration results in additive CNS depression or super-additive tachycardia and drowsiness).
No products indexed under this heading.

Theophylline (Increased theophylline metabolism has resulted with smoking marijuana). Products include:
Aerolate 1361
Theo-Dur Extended-Release Tablets 1835
Uni-Dur Extended-Release Tablets .. 1841
Uniphyl 400 mg and 600 mg Tablets 2903

Theophylline Calcium Salicylate (Increased theophylline metabolism has resulted with smoking marijuana).
No products indexed under this heading.

Theophylline Sodium Glycinate (Increased theophylline metabolism has resulted with smoking marijuana).
No products indexed under this heading.

Thiamylal Sodium (Co-administration results in decreased clearance of barbiturates via competitive inhibition of metabolism; additive drowsiness and CNS depression).
No products indexed under this heading.

Thioridazine Hydrochloride (Co-administration results in additive drowsiness and CNS depression). Products include:
Thioridazine Hydrochloride Tablets 2289

Thiothixene (Co-administration results in additive drowsiness and CNS depression). Products include:
Navane Capsules 2701
Thiothixene Capsules 2290

Tolterodine Tartrate (Co-administration with anticholinergic agents may result in additive or super-additive tachycardia and drowsiness). Products include:
Detrol Tablets 3623
Detrol LA Capsules 2801

Triazolam (Co-administration results in additive drowsiness and CNS depression). Products include:
Halcion Tablets 2823

Tridihexethyl Chloride (Co-administration with anticholinergic agents may result in additive or super-additive tachycardia and drowsiness).
No products indexed under this heading.

Trifluoperazine Hydrochloride (Co-administration results in additive drowsiness and CNS depression). Products include:
Stelazine 1640

Trihexyphenidyl Hydrochloride (Co-administration with anticholinergic agents may result in additive or super-additive tachycardia and drowsiness). Products include:
Artane 1855

Trimeprazine Tartrate (Co-administration results in additive CNS depression or super-additive tachycardia and drowsiness).
No products indexed under this heading.

Trimipramine Maleate (Co-administration results in additive tachycardia, hypertension, and drowsiness). Products include:
Surmontil Capsules 3595

Tripelennamine Hydrochloride (Co-administration results in additive CNS depression or super-additive tachycardia and drowsiness).
No products indexed under this heading.

Triprolidine Hydrochloride (Co-administration results in additive CNS depression or super-additive tachycardia and drowsiness). Products include:
Actifed Cold & Allergy Tablets 688

Zaleplon (Co-administration results in additive drowsiness and CNS depression). Products include:
Sonata Capsules 3591

Ziprasidone Hydrochloride (Co-administration results in additive drowsiness and CNS depression). Products include:
Geodon Capsules 2688

Zolpidem Tartrate (Co-administration results in additive drowsiness and CNS depression). Products include:
Ambien Tablets 3191

Food Interactions

Alcohol (Co-administration results in additive drowsiness and CNS depression).

MARLYN FORMULA 50 CAPSULES
(Amino Acid Preparations, Vitamin B_6) 1997
None cited in PDR database.

MASS APPEAL TABLETS
(Amino Acid Preparations) 845
None cited in PDR database.

MASSENGILL FEMININE CLEANSING WASH
(Cleanser) 753
None cited in PDR database.

MASSENGILL DISPOSABLE DOUCHES
(Vinegar) 752
None cited in PDR database.

MASSENGILL BABY POWDER SCENT SOFT CLOTH TOWELETTE
(Lactic Acid, Potassium Sorbate, Sodium Lactate) 753
None cited in PDR database.

MASSENGILL MEDICATED DISPOSABLE DOUCHE
(Povidone Iodine) 753
None cited in PDR database.

MASSENGILL MEDICATED SOFT CLOTH TOWELETTE
(Hydrocortisone) 753
None cited in PDR database.

MATERNA TABLETS
(Vitamins, Prenatal, Vitamins with Minerals) 1862
None cited in PDR database.

MATULANE CAPSULES
(Procarbazine Hydrochloride) 3246
May interact with antihistamines, antihypertensives, barbiturates, narcotic analgesics, phenothiazines, sympathomimetics, tricyclic antidepressants, and certain other agents. Compounds in these categories include:

Acebutolol Hydrochloride (To minimize CNS depression and possible potentiation, hypotensive agents should be used with caution). Products include:
Sectral Capsules 3589

Acrivastine (Potential for increased CNS depression and possible potentiation). Products include:
Semprex-D Capsules 1172

Albuterol (Procarbazine exhibits some MAO inhibitory activity; concurrent use should be avoided). Products include:
Proventil Inhalation Aerosol 3142
Ventolin Inhalation Aerosol and Refill 1679

Albuterol Sulfate (Procarbazine exhibits some MAO inhibitory activity; concurrent use should be avoided). Products include:
AccuNeb Inhalation Solution 1230
Combivent Inhalation Aerosol 1041
DuoNeb Inhalation Solution 1233
Proventil Inhalation Solution 0.083% 3146
Proventil Repetabs Tablets 3148
Proventil Solution for Inhalation 0.5% 3144
Proventil HFA Inhalation Aerosol 3150
Ventolin HFA Inhalation Aerosol 3618
Volmax Extended-Release Tablets .. 2276

Alfentanil Hydrochloride (Potential for increased CNS depression and possible potentiation).
No products indexed under this heading.

Amitriptyline Hydrochloride (Procarbazine exhibits some MAO inhibitory activity; concurrent use should be avoided). Products include:
Etrafon 3115
Limbitrol 1738

Amlodipine Besylate (To minimize CNS depression and possible potentiation, hypotensive agents should be used with caution). Products include:
Lotrel Capsules 2370
Norvasc Tablets 2704

Amoxapine (Procarbazine exhibits some MAO inhibitory activity; concurrent use should be avoided).
No products indexed under this heading.

Aprobarbital (Potential for increased CNS depression and possible potentiation).
No products indexed under this heading.

Astemizole (Potential for increased CNS depression and possible potentiation).
No products indexed under this heading.

Atenolol (To minimize CNS depression and possible potentiation, hypotensive agents should be used with caution). Products include:
Tenoretic Tablets 690
Tenormin I.V. Injection 692

Azatadine Maleate (Potential for increased CNS depression and possible potentiation). Products include:
Rynatan Tablets 3351

Benazepril Hydrochloride (To minimize CNS depression and possible potentiation, hypotensive agents should be used with caution). Products include:
Lotensin Tablets 2365
Lotensin HCT Tablets 2367
Lotrel Capsules 2370

Bendroflumethiazide (To minimize CNS depression and possible potentiation, hypotensive agents should be used with caution). Products include:
Corzide 40/5 Tablets 2247
Corzide 80/5 Tablets 2247

Betaxolol Hydrochloride (To minimize CNS depression and possible potentiation, hypotensive agents should be used with caution). Products include:
Betoptic S Ophthalmic Suspension 537

Bisoprolol Fumarate (To minimize CNS depression and possible potentiation, hypotensive agents should be used with caution). Products include:
Zebeta Tablets 1885
Ziac Tablets 1887

Bromodiphenhydramine Hydrochloride (Potential for increased CNS depression and possible potentiation).
No products indexed under this heading.

Brompheniramine Maleate (Potential for increased CNS depression and possible potentiation). Products include:
Bromfed Capsules (Extended-Release) 2269
Bromfed-PD Capsules (Extended-Release) 2269
Comtrex Acute Head Cold & Sinus Pressure Relief Tablets 627
Dimetapp Elixir 777
Dimetapp Cold and Fever Suspension 775
Dimetapp DM Cold & Cough Elixir . 775
Dimetapp Nighttime Flu Liquid 776

Buprenorphine Hydrochloride (Potential for increased CNS depression and possible potentiation). Products include:
Buprenex Injectable 2918

Butabarbital (Potential for increased CNS depression and possible potentiation).
No products indexed under this heading.

Butalbital (Potential for increased CNS depression and possible potentiation). Products include:
Phrenilin 578
Sedapap Tablets 50 mg/650 mg ... 2225

Candesartan Cilexetil (To minimize CNS depression and possible potentiation, hypotensive agents should be used with caution). Products include:
Atacand Tablets 595
Atacand HCT Tablets 597

Captopril (To minimize CNS depression and possible potentiation, hypotensive agents should be used with caution). Products include:
Captopril Tablets 2281

Carteolol Hydrochloride (To minimize CNS depression and possible potentiation, hypotensive agents should be used with caution). Products include:
Carteolol Hydrochloride Ophthalmic Solution USP, 1% ...... ⊙258
Ocupress Ophthalmic Solution, 1% Sterile .... ⊙303

Cetirizine Hydrochloride (Potential for increased CNS depression and possible potentiation). Products include:
Zyrtec 2756
Zyrtec-D 12 Hour Extended Relief Tablets 2758

Chlorothiazide (To minimize CNS depression and possible potentiation, hypotensive agents should be used with caution). Products include:
Aldoclor Tablets 2035
Diuril Oral 2087

Chlorothiazide Sodium (To minimize CNS depression and possible potentiation, hypotensive agents should be used with caution). Products include:
Diuril Sodium Intravenous 2086

IMPORTANT NOTE: Always consult each drug listing in the patient's regimen for possible interactions.

Chlorpheniramine Maleate (Potential for increased CNS depression and possible potentiation). Products include:
- Actifed Cold & Sinus Caplets and Tablets .... ▣688
- Alka-Seltzer Plus Liqui-Gels .... ▣604
- BC Allergy Sinus Cold Powder .... ▣619
- Chlor-Trimeton Allergy Tablets .... ▣735
- Chlor-Trimeton Allergy/Decongestant Tablets .... ▣736
- Comtrex Flu Therapy & Fever Relief Nighttime Tablets .... ▣628
- Comtrex Maximum Strength Multi-Symptom Cold & Cough Relief Tablets and Caplets .... ▣626
- Contac Severe Cold and Flu Caplets Maximum Strength .... ▣746
- Coricidin 'D' Cold, Flu & Sinus Tablets .... ▣737
- Coricidin/Coricidin D .... ▣738
- Coricidin HBP Maximum Strength Flu Tablets .... ▣738
- Extendryl 1361
- Hycomine Compound Tablets 1317
- Kronofed-A 1341
- PediaCare Cough-Cold Liquid .... ▣719
- PediaCare NightRest Cough-Cold Liquid .... ▣719
- Robitussin Nighttime Honey Flu Liquid .... ▣786
- Ryna .... ▣768
- Singlet Caplets .... ▣761
- Sinutab Sinus Allergy Medication, Maximum Strength Formula, Tablets & Caplets .... ▣707
- Sudafed Cold & Allergy Tablets .... ▣708
- TheraFlu Regular Strength Cold & Cough Night Time Hot Liquid .... ▣676
- TheraFlu Regular Strength Cold & Sore Throat Night Time Hot Liquid .... ▣676
- TheraFlu Maximum Strength Flu & Cough Night Time Hot Liquid .... ▣678
- TheraFlu Maximum Strength Flu & Sore Throat Night Time Hot Liquid .... ▣677
- TheraFlu Maximum Strength Severe Cold & Congestion Night Time Caplets .... ▣678
- TheraFlu Maximum Strength Severe Cold & Congestion Night Time Hot Liquid .... ▣678
- Triaminic Cold & Allergy Liquid .... ▣681
- Triaminic Cold & Allergy Softchews .... ▣683
- Triaminic Cold & Cough Liquid .... ▣681
- Triaminic Cold & Cough Softchews .... ▣683
- Triaminic Cold & Night Time Cough Liquid .... ▣681
- Triaminic Cold, Cough & Fever Liquid .... ▣681
- Children's Tylenol Cold Suspension Liquid and Chewable Tablets 2015
- Children's Tylenol Cold Plus Cough Suspension Liquid and Chewable Tablets 2015
- Children's Tylenol Flu Suspension Liquid 2015
- Maximum Strength Tylenol Allergy Sinus Caplets, Gelcaps, and Geltabs 2010
- Multi-Symptom Tylenol Cold Complete Formula Caplets 2010
- Vicks 44M Cough, Cold & Flu Relief Liquid .... ▣725
- Pediatric Vicks 44m Cough & Cold Relief .... ▣728
- Children's Vicks NyQuil Cold/Cough Relief .... ▣726

Chlorpheniramine Polistirex (Potential for increased CNS depression and possible potentiation). Products include:
- Tussionex Pennkinetic Extended-Release Suspension 1174

Chlorpheniramine Tannate (Potential for increased CNS depression and possible potentiation). Products include:
- Reformulated Rynatan Pediatric Suspension 3352
- Rynatuss Pediatric Suspension 3353
- Rynatuss Tablets 3353
- Tussi-12 S Suspension 3356
- Tussi-12 Tablets 3356

Chlorpromazine (Potential for increased CNS depression and possible potentiation). Products include:
- Thorazine Suppositories 1656

Chlorpromazine Hydrochloride (Potential for increased CNS depression and possible potentiation). Products include:
- Thorazine 1656

Chlorthalidone (To minimize CNS depression and possible potentiation, hypotensive agents should be used with caution). Products include:
- Clorpres Tablets 1002
- Combipres Tablets 1040
- Tenoretic Tablets 690

Clemastine Fumarate (Potential for increased CNS depression and possible potentiation). Products include:
- Tavist 12 Hour Allergy Tablets .... ▣676

Clomipramine Hydrochloride (Procarbazine exhibits some MAO inhibitory activity; concurrent use should be avoided).
- No products indexed under this heading.

Clonidine (To minimize CNS depression and possible potentiation, hypotensive agents should be used with caution). Products include:
- Catapres-TTS 1038

Clonidine Hydrochloride (To minimize CNS depression and possible potentiation, hypotensive agents should be used with caution). Products include:
- Catapres Tablets 1037
- Clorpres Tablets 1002
- Combipres Tablets 1040
- Duraclon Injection 3057

Codeine Phosphate (Potential for increased CNS depression and possible potentiation). Products include:
- Phenergan with Codeine Syrup 3557
- Phenergan VC with Codeine Syrup 3561
- Robitussin A-C Syrup 2942
- Robitussin-DAC Syrup 2942
- Ryna-C Liquid .... ▣768
- Soma Compound w/Codeine Tablets 3355
- Tussi-Organidin NR Liquid 3350
- Tussi-Organidin-S NR Liquid 3350
- Tylenol with Codeine 2595

Cyproheptadine Hydrochloride (Potential for increased CNS depression and possible potentiation). Products include:
- Periactin Tablets 2155

Deserpidine (To minimize CNS depression and possible potentiation, hypotensive agents should be used with caution).
- No products indexed under this heading.

Desipramine Hydrochloride (Procarbazine exhibits some MAO inhibitory activity; concurrent use should be avoided). Products include:
- Norpramin Tablets 755

Dexchlorpheniramine Maleate (Potential for increased CNS depression and possible potentiation).
- No products indexed under this heading.

Dezocine (Potential for increased CNS depression and possible potentiation).
- No products indexed under this heading.

Diazoxide (To minimize CNS depression and possible potentiation, hypotensive agents should be used with caution).
- No products indexed under this heading.

Diltiazem Hydrochloride (To minimize CNS depression and possible potentiation, hypotensive agents should be used with caution). Products include:
- Cardizem Injectable 1018
- Cardizem Lyo-Ject Syringe 1018
- Cardizem Monovial 1018
- Cardizem CD Capsules 1016
- Tiazac Capsules 1378

Diphenhydramine Citrate (Potential for increased CNS depression and possible potentiation). Products include:
- Alka-Seltzer PM Effervescent Tablets .... ▣605
- Benadryl Allergy & Sinus Fastmelt Tablets .... ▣693
- Benadryl Children's Allergy/Cold Fastmelt Tablets .... ▣692
- Excedrin PM Tablets, Caplets, and Geltabs .... ▣631
- Goody's PM Powder .... ▣621

Diphenhydramine Hydrochloride (Potential for increased CNS depression and possible potentiation). Products include:
- Extra Strength Bayer PM Caplets .... ▣611
- Benadryl Allergy Chewables .... ▣689
- Benadryl Allergy .... ▣691
- Benadryl Allergy Liquid .... ▣690
- Benadryl Allergy/Cold Tablets .... ▣691
- Benadryl Allergy/Congestion Tablets .... ▣692
- Benadryl Allergy & Sinus Liquid .... ▣693
- Benadryl Allergy Sinus Headache Caplets & Gelcaps .... ▣693
- Benadryl Severe Allergy & Sinus Headache Caplets .... ▣694
- Benadryl Dye-Free Allergy Liquid .... ▣690
- Benadryl Dye-Free Allergy Liqui-Gels Softgels .... ▣690
- Benadryl Itch Relief Stick Extra Strength .... ▣695
- Benadryl Cream .... ▣695
- Benadryl Gel .... ▣695
- Benadryl Spray .... ▣696
- Benadryl Parenteral 2617
- Coricidin HBP Night-Time Cold & Flu Tablets .... ▣738
- Nytol QuickCaps Caplets .... ▣622
- Maximum Strength Nytol QuickGels Softgels .... ▣621
- Extra Strength Percogesic Aspirin-Free Coated Caplets .... ▣665
- Simply Sleep Caplets 2008
- Sominex Original Formula Tablets .... ▣761
- Children's Tylenol Allergy-D Liquid 2014
- Maximum Strength Tylenol Allergy Sinus NightTime Caplets 2010
- Tylenol Severe Allergy Caplets 2010
- Maximum Strength Tylenol Flu NightTime Gelcaps 2011
- Extra Strength Tylenol PM Caplets, Geltabs, and Gelcaps 2012
- Unisom Maximum Strength SleepGels .... ▣713

Diphenylpyraline Hydrochloride (Potential for increased CNS depression and possible potentiation).
- No products indexed under this heading.

Dobutamine Hydrochloride (Procarbazine exhibits some MAO inhibitory activity; concurrent use should be avoided). Products include:
- Dobutrex Solution Vials 1914

Dopamine Hydrochloride (Procarbazine exhibits some MAO inhibitory activity; concurrent use should be avoided).
- No products indexed under this heading.

Doxazosin Mesylate (To minimize CNS depression and possible potentiation, hypotensive agents should be used with caution). Products include:
- Cardura Tablets 2668

Doxepin Hydrochloride (Procarbazine exhibits some MAO inhibitory activity; concurrent use should be avoided). Products include:
- Sinequan 2713

Enalapril Maleate (To minimize CNS depression and possible potentiation, hypotensive agents should be used with caution). Products include:
- Lexxel Tablets 608
- Vaseretic Tablets 2204
- Vasotec Tablets 2210

Enalaprilat (To minimize CNS depression and possible potentiation, hypotensive agents should be used with caution). Products include:
- Enalaprilat Injection 863
- Vasotec I.V. Injection 2207

Ephedrine Hydrochloride (Procarbazine exhibits some MAO inhibitory activity; concurrent use should be avoided). Products include:
- Primatene Tablets .... ▣780

Ephedrine Sulfate (Procarbazine exhibits some MAO inhibitory activity; concurrent use should be avoided).
- No products indexed under this heading.

Ephedrine Tannate (Procarbazine exhibits some MAO inhibitory activity; concurrent use should be avoided). Products include:
- Rynatuss Pediatric Suspension 3353
- Rynatuss Tablets 3353

Epinephrine (Procarbazine exhibits some MAO inhibitory activity; concurrent use should be avoided). Products include:
- Epifrin Sterile Ophthalmic Solution .... ⊙235
- EpiPen 1236
- Primatene Mist .... ▣779
- Xylocaine with Epinephrine Injection 653

Epinephrine Bitartrate (Procarbazine exhibits some MAO inhibitory activity; concurrent use should be avoided). Products include:
- Sensorcaine 643

Epinephrine Hydrochloride (Procarbazine exhibits some MAO inhibitory activity; concurrent use should be avoided).
- No products indexed under this heading.

Eprosartan Mesylate (To minimize CNS depression and possible potentiation, hypotensive agents should be used with caution). Products include:
- Teveten Tablets 3327

Esmolol Hydrochloride (To minimize CNS depression and possible potentiation, hypotensive agents should be used with caution). Products include:
- Brevibloc Injection 858

Felodipine (To minimize CNS depression and possible potentiation, hypotensive agents should be used with caution). Products include:
- Lexxel Tablets 608
- Plendil Extended-Release Tablets 623

Fentanyl (Potential for increased CNS depression and possible potentiation). Products include:
- Duragesic Transdermal System 1786

Fentanyl Citrate (Potential for increased CNS depression and possible potentiation). Products include:
- Actiq 1184

Fexofenadine Hydrochloride (Potential for increased CNS depression and possible potentiation). Products include:
- Allegra 712
- Allegra-D Extended-Release Tablets 714

Fluphenazine Decanoate (Potential for increased CNS depression and possible potentiation).
- No products indexed under this heading.

Fluphenazine Enanthate (Potential for increased CNS depression and possible potentiation).
- No products indexed under this heading.

Fluphenazine Hydrochloride (Potential for increased CNS depression and possible potentiation).
- No products indexed under this heading.

Fosinopril Sodium (To minimize CNS depression and possible potentiation, hypotensive agents should be used with caution). Products include:
- Monopril Tablets 1091
- Monopril HCT 1094

Furosemide (To minimize CNS depression and possible potentia-

tion, hypotensive agents should be used with caution). Products include:
Furosemide Tablets 2284

Guanabenz Acetate (To minimize CNS depression and possible potentiation, hypotensive agents should be used with caution).
No products indexed under this heading.

Guanethidine Monosulfate (To minimize CNS depression and possible potentiation, hypotensive agents should be used with caution).
No products indexed under this heading.

Hydralazine Hydrochloride (To minimize CNS depression and possible potentiation, hypotensive agents should be used with caution).
No products indexed under this heading.

Hydrochlorothiazide (To minimize CNS depression and possible potentiation, hypotensive agents should be used with caution). Products include:
Accuretic Tablets 2614
Aldoril Tablets 2039
Atacand HCT Tablets 597
Avalide Tablets 1070
Diovan HCT Tablets 2338
Dyazide Capsules 1515
HydroDIURIL Tablets 2108
Hyzaar 2109
Inderide Tablets 3517
Inderide LA Long-Acting Capsules 3519
Lotensin HCT Tablets 2367
Maxzide 1008
Micardis HCT Tablets 1051
Microzide Capsules 3414
Moduretic Tablets 2138
Monopril HCT 1094
Prinzide Tablets 2168
Timolide Tablets 2187
Uniretic Tablets 3178
Vaseretic Tablets 2204
Zestoretic Tablets 695
Ziac Tablets 1887

Hydrocodone Bitartrate (Potential for increased CNS depression and possible potentiation). Products include:
Hycodan 1316
Hycomine Compound Tablets 1317
Hycotuss Expectorant Syrup 1318
Lortab 3319
Lortab Elixir 3317
Maxidone Tablets CIII 3399
Norco 5/325 Tablets CIII 3424
Norco 7.5/325 Tablets CIII 3425
Norco 10/325 Tablets CIII 3427
Norco 10/325 Tablets CIII 3425
Vicodin Tablets 516
Vicodin ES Tablets 517
Vicodin HP Tablets 518
Vicodin Tuss Expectorant 519
Vicoprofen Tablets 520
Zydone Tablets 1330

Hydrocodone Polistirex (Potential for increased CNS depression and possible potentiation). Products include:
Tussionex Pennkinetic Extended-Release Suspension 1174

Hydroflumethiazide (To minimize CNS depression and possible potentiation, hypotensive agents should be used with caution). Products include:
Diucardin Tablets 3494

Hydromorphone Hydrochloride (Potential for increased CNS depression and possible potentiation). Products include:
Dilaudid 441
Dilaudid Oral Liquid 445
Dilaudid Powder 441
Dilaudid Rectal Suppositories 441
Dilaudid Tablets 441
Dilaudid Tablets - 8 mg 445
Dilaudid-HP 443

Imipramine Hydrochloride (Procarbazine exhibits some MAO inhibitory activity; concurrent use should be avoided).
No products indexed under this heading.

Imipramine Pamoate (Procarbazine exhibits some MAO inhibitory activity; concurrent use should be avoided).
No products indexed under this heading.

Indapamide (To minimize CNS depression and possible potentiation, hypotensive agents should be used with caution). Products include:
Indapamide Tablets 2286

Irbesartan (To minimize CNS depression and possible potentiation, hypotensive agents should be used with caution). Products include:
Avalide Tablets 1070
Avapro Tablets 1074
Avapro Tablets 3076

Isoproterenol Hydrochloride (Procarbazine exhibits some MAO inhibitory activity; concurrent use should be avoided).
No products indexed under this heading.

Isoproterenol Sulfate (Procarbazine exhibits some MAO inhibitory activity; concurrent use should be avoided).
No products indexed under this heading.

Isradipine (To minimize CNS depression and possible potentiation, hypotensive agents should be used with caution). Products include:
DynaCirc Capsules 2921
DynaCirc CR Tablets 2923

Labetalol Hydrochloride (To minimize CNS depression and possible potentiation, hypotensive agents should be used with caution). Products include:
Normodyne Injection 3135
Normodyne Tablets 3137

Levalbuterol Hydrochloride (Procarbazine exhibits some MAO inhibitory activity; concurrent use should be avoided). Products include:
Xopenex Inhalation Solution 3207

Levorphanol Tartrate (Potential for increased CNS depression and possible potentiation). Products include:
Levo-Dromoran 1734
Levorphanol Tartrate Tablets 3059

Lisinopril (To minimize CNS depression and possible potentiation, hypotensive agents should be used with caution). Products include:
Prinivil Tablets 2164
Prinzide Tablets 2168
Zestoretic Tablets 695
Zestril Tablets 698

Loratadine (Potential for increased CNS depression and possible potentiation). Products include:
Claritin 3100
Claritin-D 12 Hour Extended Release Tablets 3102
Claritin-D 24 Hour Extended Release Tablets 3104

Losartan Potassium (To minimize CNS depression and possible potentiation, hypotensive agents should be used with caution). Products include:
Cozaar Tablets 2067
Hyzaar 2109

Maprotiline Hydrochloride (Procarbazine exhibits some MAO inhibitory activity; concurrent use should be avoided).
No products indexed under this heading.

Mecamylamine Hydrochloride (To minimize CNS depression and possible potentiation, hypotensive agents should be used with caution). Products include:
Inversine Tablets 1850

Meperidine Hydrochloride (Potential for increased CNS depression and possible potentiation). Products include:
Demerol 3079
Mepergan Injection 3539

Mephobarbital (Potential for increased CNS depression and possible potentiation).
No products indexed under this heading.

Mesoridazine Besylate (Potential for increased CNS depression and possible potentiation). Products include:
Serentil 1057

Metaproterenol Sulfate (Procarbazine exhibits some MAO inhibitory activity; concurrent use should be avoided). Products include:
Alupent 1029

Metaraminol Bitartrate (Procarbazine exhibits some MAO inhibitory activity; concurrent use should be avoided). Products include:
Aramine Injection 2043

Methadone Hydrochloride (Potential for increased CNS depression and possible potentiation). Products include:
Dolophine Hydrochloride Tablets 3056

Methdilazine Hydrochloride (Potential for increased CNS depression and possible potentiation).
No products indexed under this heading.

Methotrimeprazine (Potential for increased CNS depression and possible potentiation).
No products indexed under this heading.

Methoxamine Hydrochloride (Procarbazine exhibits some MAO inhibitory activity; concurrent use should be avoided).
No products indexed under this heading.

Methyclothiazide (To minimize CNS depression and possible potentiation, hypotensive agents should be used with caution).
No products indexed under this heading.

Methyldopa (To minimize CNS depression and possible potentiation, hypotensive agents should be used with caution). Products include:
Aldoclor Tablets 2035
Aldomet Tablets 2037
Aldoril Tablets 2039

Methyldopate Hydrochloride (To minimize CNS depression and possible potentiation, hypotensive agents should be used with caution).
No products indexed under this heading.

Metolazone (To minimize CNS depression and possible potentiation, hypotensive agents should be used with caution). Products include:
Mykrox Tablets 1168
Zaroxolyn Tablets 1177

Metoprolol Succinate (To minimize CNS depression and possible potentiation, hypotensive agents should be used with caution). Products include:
Toprol-XL Tablets 651

Metoprolol Tartrate (To minimize CNS depression and possible potentiation, hypotensive agents should be used with caution).
No products indexed under this heading.

Metyrosine (To minimize CNS depression and possible potentiation, hypotensive agents should be used with caution). Products include:
Demser Capsules 2085

Mibefradil Dihydrochloride (To minimize CNS depression and possible potentiation, hypotensive agents should be used with caution).
No products indexed under this heading.

Minoxidil (To minimize CNS depression and possible potentiation, hypotensive agents should be used with caution). Products include:
Rogaine Extra Strength for Men Topical Solution .... ▣721
Rogaine for Women Topical Solution .... ▣721

Moexipril Hydrochloride (To minimize CNS depression and possible potentiation, hypotensive agents should be used with caution). Products include:
Uniretic Tablets 3178
Univasc Tablets 3181

Morphine Sulfate (Potential for increased CNS depression and possible potentiation). Products include:
Astramorph/PF Injection, USP (Preservative-Free) 594
Duramorph Injection 1312
Infumorph 200 and Infumorph 500 Sterile Solutions 1314
Kadian Capsules 1335
MS Contin Tablets 2896
MSIR 2898
Oramorph SR Tablets 3062
Roxanol 3066

Nadolol (To minimize CNS depression and possible potentiation, hypotensive agents should be used with caution). Products include:
Corgard Tablets 2245
Corzide 40/5 Tablets 2247
Corzide 80/5 Tablets 2247
Nadolol Tablets 2288

Nicardipine Hydrochloride (To minimize CNS depression and possible potentiation, hypotensive agents should be used with caution). Products include:
Cardene I.V. 3485

Nifedipine (To minimize CNS depression and possible potentiation, hypotensive agents should be used with caution). Products include:
Adalat CC Tablets 877
Procardia Capsules 2708
Procardia XL Extended Release Tablets 2710

Nisoldipine (To minimize CNS depression and possible potentiation, hypotensive agents should be used with caution). Products include:
Sular Tablets 688

Nitroglycerin (To minimize CNS depression and possible potentiation, hypotensive agents should be used with caution). Products include:
Nitro-Dur Transdermal Infusion System 3134
Nitro-Dur Transdermal Infusion System 1834
Nitrolingual Pumpspray 1355
Nitrostat Tablets 2658

Norepinephrine Bitartrate (Procarbazine exhibits some MAO inhibitory activity; concurrent use should be avoided).
No products indexed under this heading.

Nortriptyline Hydrochloride (Procarbazine exhibits some MAO inhibitory activity; concurrent use should be avoided).
No products indexed under this heading.

Oxycodone Hydrochloride (Potential for increased CNS depression and possible potentiation). Products include:
OxyContin Tablets 2912
OxyFast Oral Concentrate Solution 2916
OxyIR Capsules 2916
Percocet Tablets 1326
Percodan Tablets 1327
Percolone Tablets 1327
Roxicodone 3067
Tylox Capsules 2597

Penbutolol Sulfate (To minimize CNS depression and possible potentiation, hypotensive agents should be used with caution).
No products indexed under this heading.

Pentobarbital Sodium (Potential for increased CNS depression and possible potentiation). Products include:
Nembutal Sodium Solution 485

IMPORTANT NOTE: Always consult each drug listing in the patient's regimen for possible interactions.

Perindopril Erbumine (To minimize CNS depression and possible potentiation, hypotensive agents should be used with caution). Products include:
- Aceon Tablets (2 mg, 4 mg, 8 mg) ... 3249

Perphenazine (Potential for increased CNS depression and possible potentiation). Products include:
- Etrafon ... 3115
- Trilafon ... 3160

Phenobarbital (Potential for increased CNS depression and possible potentiation). Products include:
- Arco-Lase Plus Tablets ... 592
- Donnatal ... 2929
- Donnatal Extentabs ... 2930

Phenoxybenzamine Hydrochloride (To minimize CNS depression and possible potentiation, hypotensive agents should be used with caution). Products include:
- Dibenzyline Capsules ... 3457

Phentolamine Mesylate (To minimize CNS depression and possible potentiation, hypotensive agents should be used with caution).
- No products indexed under this heading.

Phenylephrine Bitartrate (Procarbazine exhibits some MAO inhibitory activity; concurrent use should be avoided).
- No products indexed under this heading.

Phenylephrine Hydrochloride (Procarbazine exhibits some MAO inhibitory activity; concurrent use should be avoided). Products include:
- Afrin Nasal Decongestant Children's Pump Mist ... ▣734
- Extendryl ... 1361
- Hycomine Compound Tablets ... 1317
- Neo-Synephrine ... ▣614
- Phenergan VC Syrup ... 3560
- Phenergan VC with Codeine Syrup . 3561
- Preparation H Cream ... ▣778
- Preparation H Cooling Gel ... ▣778
- Preparation H ... ▣778
- Vicks Sinex Nasal Spray and Ultra Fine Mist ... ▣729

Phenylephrine Tannate (Procarbazine exhibits some MAO inhibitory activity; concurrent use should be avoided). Products include:
- Ryna-12 S Suspension ... 3351
- Reformulated Rynatan Pediatric Suspension ... 3352
- Rynatuss Pediatric Suspension ... 3353
- Rynatuss Tablets ... 3353

Phenylpropanolamine Hydrochloride (Procarbazine exhibits some MAO inhibitory activity; concurrent use should be avoided).
- No products indexed under this heading.

Pindolol (To minimize CNS depression and possible potentiation, hypotensive agents should be used with caution).
- No products indexed under this heading.

Pirbuterol Acetate (Procarbazine exhibits some MAO inhibitory activity; concurrent use should be avoided). Products include:
- Maxair Autohaler ... 1981
- Maxair Inhaler ... 1984

Polythiazide (To minimize CNS depression and possible potentiation, hypotensive agents should be used with caution). Products include:
- Minizide Capsules ... 2700
- Renese Tablets ... 2712

Prazosin Hydrochloride (To minimize CNS depression and possible potentiation, hypotensive agents should be used with caution). Products include:
- Minipress Capsules ... 2699
- Minizide Capsules ... 2700

Prochlorperazine (Potential for increased CNS depression and possible potentiation). Products include:
- Compazine ... 1505

Promethazine Hydrochloride (Potential for increased CNS depression and possible potentiation). Products include:
- Mepergan Injection ... 3539
- Phenergan Injection ... 3553
- Phenergan ... 3556
- Phenergan Syrup ... 3554
- Phenergan with Codeine Syrup ... 3557
- Phenergan with Dextromethorphan Syrup ... 3559
- Phenergan VC Syrup ... 3560
- Phenergan VC with Codeine Syrup .. 3561

Propoxyphene Hydrochloride (Potential for increased CNS depression and possible potentiation). Products include:
- Darvon Pulvules ... 1909
- Darvon Compound-65 Pulvules ... 1910

Propoxyphene Napsylate (Potential for increased CNS depression and possible potentiation). Products include:
- Darvon-N/Darvocet-N ... 1907
- Darvon-N Tablets ... 1912

Propranolol Hydrochloride (To minimize CNS depression and possible potentiation, hypotensive agents should be used with caution). Products include:
- Inderal ... 3513
- Inderal LA Long-Acting Capsules ... 3516
- Inderide Tablets ... 3517
- Inderide LA Long-Acting Capsules . 3519

Protriptyline Hydrochloride (Procarbazine exhibits some MAO inhibitory activity; concurrent use should be avoided). Products include:
- Vivactil Tablets ... 2446
- Vivactil Tablets ... 2217

Pseudoephedrine Hydrochloride (Procarbazine exhibits some MAO inhibitory activity; concurrent use should be avoided). Products include:
- Actifed Cold & Allergy Tablets ... ▣688
- Actifed Cold & Sinus Caplets and Tablets ... ▣688
- Advil Cold and Sinus Caplets ... ▣771
- Advil Cold and Sinus Tablets ... ▣771
- Advil Flu & Body Ache Caplets ... ▣772
- Aleve Cold & Sinus Caplets ... ▣603
- Alka-Seltzer Plus Liqui-Gels ... ▣604
- Alka-Seltzer Plus Cold & Flu Medicine Liqui-Gels ... ▣604
- Alka-Seltzer Plus Cold & Sinus Medicine Liqui-Gels ... ▣604
- Allegra-D Extended-Release Tablets ... 714
- BC Cold Powder ... ▣619
- Benadryl Allergy/Cold Tablets ... ▣691
- Benadryl Allergy/Congestion Tablets ... ▣692
- Benadryl Allergy & Sinus Liquid ... ▣693
- Benadryl Allergy & Sinus Fastmelt Tablets ... ▣693
- Benadryl Allergy Sinus Headache Caplets & Gelcaps ... ▣693
- Benadryl Severe Allergy & Sinus Headache Caplets ... ▣694
- Benadryl Children's Allergy/Cold Fastmelt Tablets ... ▣692
- Benylin Multi-Symptom Liquid ... ▣697
- Bromfed Capsules (Extended-Release) ... 2269
- Bromfed-PD Capsules (Extended-Release) ... 2269
- Children's Cēpacol Sore Throat ... ▣788
- Comtrex Acute Head Cold & Sinus Pressure Relief Tablets ... ▣627
- Comtrex Deep Chest Cold & Congestion Relief Softgels ... ▣627
- Comtrex Flu Therapy & Fever Relief Daytime Caplets ... ▣628
- Comtrex Flu Therapy & Fever Relief Nighttime Tablets ... ▣628
- Comtrex Maximum Strength Multi-Symptom Cold & Cough Relief Tablets and Caplets ... ▣626
- Contac Non-Drowsy 12 Hour Cold Caplets ... ▣745
- Contac Non-Drowsy Timed Release 12 Hour Cold Caplets ... ▣746
- Contac Severe Cold and Flu Caplets Maximum Strength ... ▣746
- Contac Severe Cold and Flu Caplets Non-Drowsy ... ▣746
- Dimetapp Elixir ... ▣777
- Dimetapp Cold and Fever Suspension ... ▣775
- Dimetapp DM Cold & Cough Elixir . ▣775
- Dimetapp Nighttime Flu Liquid ... ▣776
- Dimetapp Non-Drowsy Flu Syrup ... ▣777
- Dimetapp Infant Drops Decongestant ... ▣775
- Dimetapp Infant Drops Decongestant Plus Cough ... ▣776
- Guaifed ... 2272
- Kronofed-A ... 1341
- Children's Motrin Cold Oral Suspension ... 2007
- Motrin Sinus Headache Caplets ... 2005
- PediaCare Cough-Cold Liquid ... ▣719
- PediaCare Infants' Drops Decongestant ... ▣719
- PediaCare Infants' Drops Decongestant Plus Cough ... ▣719
- PediaCare NightRest Cough-Cold Liquid ... ▣719
- Robitussin Cold Caplets Cold & Congestion ... ▣780
- Robitussin Cold Softgels Cold & Congestion ... ▣780
- Robitussin Cold Caplets Multi-Symptom Cold & Flu ... ▣781
- Robitussin Cold Softgels Multi-Symptom Cold & Flu ... ▣781
- Robitussin Cold Softgels Severe Congestion ... ▣782
- Robitussin Cough & Cold Infant Drops ... ▣782
- Robitussin Maximum Strength Cough & Cold Liquid ... ▣785
- Robitussin Pediatric Cough & Cold Formula Liquid ... ▣785
- Robitussin Multi Symptom Honey Flu Liquid ... ▣785
- Robitussin Nighttime Honey Flu Liquid ... ▣786
- Robitussin-CF Liquid ... ▣783
- Robitussin-DAC Syrup ... 2942
- Robitussin-PE Liquid ... ▣782
- Ryna ... ▣768
- Semprex-D Capsules ... 1172
- Singlet Caplets ... ▣761
- Sinutab Non-Drying Liquid Caps ... ▣706
- Sinutab Sinus Allergy Medication, Maximum Strength Formula, Tablets & Caplets ... ▣707
- Sinutab Sinus Medication, Maximum Strength Without Drowsiness Formula, Tablets & Caplets ... ▣707
- Sudafed 12 Hour Tablets ... ▣708
- Sudafed 24 Hour Tablets ... ▣708
- Children's Sudafed Cold & Cough Liquid ... ▣709
- Children's Sudafed Nasal Decongestant Chewables ... ▣711
- Children's Sudafed Nasal Decongestant Liquid Medication ... ▣711
- Sudafed Cold & Allergy Tablets ... ▣708
- Sudafed Cold & Cough Liquid Caps ... ▣709
- Sudafed Cold & Sinus Liquid Caps ... ▣710
- Sudafed Nasal Decongestant Tablets ... ▣710
- Sudafed Non-Drying Sinus Liquid Caps ... ▣712
- Sudafed Severe Cold ... ▣711
- Sudafed Sinus Headache Caplets ... ▣712
- Sudafed Sinus Headache Tablets ... ▣712
- Tavist Sinus Non-Drowsy Coated Caplets ... ▣676
- TheraFlu Regular Strength Cold & Cough Night Time Hot Liquid ... ▣676
- TheraFlu Regular Strength Cold & Sore Throat Night Time Hot Liquid ... ▣676
- TheraFlu Maximum Strength Flu & Congestion Non-Drowsy Hot Liquid ... ▣677
- TheraFlu Maximum Strength Flu & Cough Night Time Hot Liquid .. ▣678
- TheraFlu Maximum Strength Flu & Sore Throat Night Time Hot Liquid ... ▣677
- TheraFlu Maximum Strength Severe Cold & Congestion Night Time Caplets ... ▣678
- TheraFlu Maximum Strength Severe Cold & Congestion Night Time Hot Liquid ... ▣678
- TheraFlu Maximum Strength Severe Cold & Congestion Non-Drowsy ... ▣679
- Triaminic Allergy Congestion Liquid ... ▣680
- Triaminic Chest Congestion Liquid ... ▣680
- Triaminic Cold & Allergy Liquid ... ▣681
- Triaminic Cold & Allergy Softchews ... ▣683
- Triaminic Cold & Cough Liquid ... ▣681
- Triaminic Cold & Cough Softchews ... ▣683
- Triaminic Cold & Night Time Cough Liquid ... ▣681
- Triaminic Cold, Cough & Fever Liquid ... ▣681
- Triaminic Cough Liquid ... ▣682
- Triaminic Cough & Congestion Liquid ... ▣682
- Triaminic Cough & Sore Throat Liquid ... ▣682
- Triaminic Cough & Sore Throat Softchews ... ▣684
- Children's Tylenol Allergy-D Liquid ... 2014
- Children's Tylenol Cold Suspension Liquid and Chewable Tablets ... 2015
- Children's Tylenol Cold Plus Cough Suspension Liquid and Chewable Tablets ... 2015
- Children's Tylenol Flu Suspension Liquid ... 2015
- Children's Tylenol Sinus Suspension Liquid ... 2017
- Infants' Tylenol Cold Decongestant and Fever Reducer Concentrated Drops ... 2015
- Infants' Tylenol Cold Decongestant and Fever Reducer Concentrated Drops Plus Cough .. 2015
- Tylenol Allergy Sinus ... 2010
- Multi-Symptom Tylenol Cold Complete Formula Caplets ... 2010
- Multi-Symptom Tylenol Cold Non-Drowsy Caplets and Gelcaps ... 2010
- Multi-Symptom Tylenol Cold Severe Congestion Non-Drowsy Caplets ... 2011
- Maximum Strength Tylenol Flu NightTime Gelcaps ... 2011
- Maximum Strength Tylenol Flu NightTime Liquid ... 2011
- Maximum Strength Tylenol Flu Non-Drowsy Gelcaps ... 2011
- Maximum Strength Tylenol Sinus NightTime Caplets ... 2012
- Maximum Strength Tylenol Sinus Non-Drowsy Geltabs, Gelcaps, Caplets, and Tablets ... 2012
- Vicks 44D Cough & Head Congestion Relief Liquid ... ▣724
- Vicks 44M Cough, Cold & Flu Relief Liquid ... ▣725
- Pediatric Vicks 44m Cough & Cold Relief ... ▣728
- Vicks DayQuil LiquiCaps/Liquid Multi-Symptom Cold/Flu Relief ... ▣727
- Children's Vicks NyQuil Cold/Cough Relief ... ▣726
- Vicks NyQuil LiquiCaps/Liquid Multi-Symptom Cold/Flu Relief, Original and Cherry Flavors ... ▣727
- Zephrex Tablets ... 3091
- Zephrex LA Tablets ... 3092
- Zyrtec-D 12 Hour Extended Relief Tablets ... 2758

Pseudoephedrine Sulfate (Procarbazine exhibits some MAO inhibitory activity; concurrent use should be avoided). Products include:
- Chlor-Trimeton Allergy/Decongestant Tablets ... ▣736
- Claritin-D 12 Hour Extended Release Tablets ... 3102
- Claritin-D 24 Hour Extended Release Tablets ... 3104
- Coricidin 'D' Cold, Flu & Sinus Tablets ... ▣737
- Drixoral Allergy/Sinus Extended-Release Tablets ... ▣741
- Drixoral Cold & Allergy Sustained-Action Tablets ... ▣740
- Drixoral Cold & Flu Extended-Release Tablets ... ▣740
- Drixoral Nasal Decongestant Long-Acting Non-Drowsy Tablets ... ▣740
- Rynatan Tablets ... 3351

Pyrilamine Maleate (Potential for increased CNS depression and possible potentiation). Products include:
- Maximum Strength Midol Menstrual Caplets and Gelcaps ... ▣612
- Maximum Strength Midol PMS Caplets and Gelcaps ... ▣613

Pyrilamine Tannate (Potential for increased CNS depression and possible potentiation). Products include:
- Ryna-12 S Suspension ... 3351

Quinapril Hydrochloride (To minimize CNS depression and possible potentiation, hypotensive agents should be used with caution). Products include:
- Accupril Tablets ... 2611

Accuretic Tablets 2614

Ramipril (To minimize CNS depression and possible potentiation, hypotensive agents should be used with caution). Products include:

Altace Capsules 2233

Rauwolfia serpentina (To minimize CNS depression and possible potentiation, hypotensive agents should be used with caution).

No products indexed under this heading.

Remifentanil Hydrochloride (Potential for increased CNS depression and possible potentiation).

No products indexed under this heading.

Rescinnamine (To minimize CNS depression and possible potentiation, hypotensive agents should be used with caution).

No products indexed under this heading.

Reserpine (To minimize CNS depression and possible potentiation, hypotensive agents should be used with caution).

No products indexed under this heading.

Salmeterol Xinafoate (Procarbazine exhibits some MAO inhibitory activity; concurrent use should be avoided). Products include:

Advair Diskus 100/50 1448
Advair Diskus 250/50 1448
Advair Diskus 500/50 1448
Serevent Diskus 1637
Serevent Inhalation Aerosol 1633

Secobarbital Sodium (Potential for increased CNS depression and possible potentiation).

No products indexed under this heading.

Sodium Nitroprusside (To minimize CNS depression and possible potentiation, hypotensive agents should be used with caution).

No products indexed under this heading.

Sotalol Hydrochloride (To minimize CNS depression and possible potentiation, hypotensive agents should be used with caution). Products include:

Betapace Tablets 950
Betapace AF Tablets 954

Spirapril Hydrochloride (To minimize CNS depression and possible potentiation, hypotensive agents should be used with caution).

No products indexed under this heading.

Sufentanil Citrate (Potential for increased CNS depression and possible potentiation).

No products indexed under this heading.

Telmisartan (To minimize CNS depression and possible potentiation, hypotensive agents should be used with caution). Products include:

Micardis Tablets 1049
Micardis HCT Tablets 1051

Terazosin Hydrochloride (To minimize CNS depression and possible potentiation, hypotensive agents should be used with caution). Products include:

Hytrin Capsules 464

Terbutaline Sulfate (Procarbazine exhibits some MAO inhibitory activity; concurrent use should be avoided). Products include:

Brethine Ampuls 2314
Brethine Tablets 2313

Terfenadine (Potential for increased CNS depression and possible potentiation).

No products indexed under this heading.

Thiamylal Sodium (Potential for increased CNS depression and possible potentiation).

No products indexed under this heading.

Thioridazine Hydrochloride (Potential for increased CNS depression and possible potentiation). Products include:

Thioridazine Hydrochloride Tablets 2289

Timolol Maleate (To minimize CNS depression and possible potentiation, hypotensive agents should be used with caution). Products include:

Blocadren Tablets 2046
Cosopt Sterile Ophthalmic Solution 2065
Timolide Tablets 2187
Timolol GFS .... ⊙266
Timoptic in Ocudose 2192
Timoptic Sterile Ophthalmic Solution 2190
Timoptic-XE Sterile Ophthalmic Gel Forming Solution 2194

Torsemide (To minimize CNS depression and possible potentiation, hypotensive agents should be used with caution). Products include:

Demadex Tablets and Injection 2965

Trandolapril (To minimize CNS depression and possible potentiation, hypotensive agents should be used with caution). Products include:

Mavik Tablets 478
Tarka Tablets 508

Trifluoperazine Hydrochloride (Potential for increased CNS depression and possible potentiation). Products include:

Stelazine 1640

Trimeprazine Tartrate (Potential for increased CNS depression and possible potentiation).

No products indexed under this heading.

Trimethaphan Camsylate (To minimize CNS depression and possible potentiation, hypotensive agents should be used with caution).

No products indexed under this heading.

Trimipramine Maleate (Procarbazine exhibits some MAO inhibitory activity; concurrent use should be avoided). Products include:

Surmontil Capsules 3595

Tripelennamine Hydrochloride (Potential for increased CNS depression and possible potentiation).

No products indexed under this heading.

Triprolidine Hydrochloride (Potential for increased CNS depression and possible potentiation). Products include:

Actifed Cold & Allergy Tablets .... ▣688

Valsartan (To minimize CNS depression and possible potentiation, hypotensive agents should be used with caution). Products include:

Diovan Capsules 2337
Diovan HCT Tablets 2338

Verapamil Hydrochloride (To minimize CNS depression and possible potentiation, hypotensive agents should be used with caution). Products include:

Covera-HS Tablets 3199
Isoptin SR Tablets 467
Tarka Tablets 508
Verelan Capsules 3184
Verelan PM Capsules 3186

Food Interactions

Alcohol (Concurrent use may produce an Antabuse-like reaction; concomitant use should be avoided).

Bananas (Procarbazine exhibits some MAO inhibitory activity: concurrent use should be avoided).

Cheese, aged (Procarbazine exhibits some MAO inhibitory activity: concurrent use should be avoided).

Food with high concentration of tyramine (Procarbazine exhibits some MAO inhibitory activity: concurrent use should be avoided).

Wine, unspecified (Procarbazine exhibits some MAO inhibitory activity: concurrent use should be avoided).

Yogurt (Procarbazine exhibits some MAO inhibitory activity: concurrent use should be avoided).

MAVIK TABLETS

(Trandolapril) 478

May interact with diuretics, lithium preparations, potassium preparations, potassium sparing diuretics, and certain other agents. Compounds in these categories include:

Amiloride Hydrochloride (Co-administration increases the risk of hyperkalemia; patients on diuretics, especially those on recently instituted diuretic therapy, may experience an excessive reduction in blood pressure after initiation of therapy with trandolapril). Products include:

Midamor Tablets 2136
Moduretic Tablets 2138

Bendroflumethiazide (Patients on diuretics, especially those on recently instituted diuretic therapy, may experience an excessive reduction in blood pressure after initiation of therapy with trandolapril). Products include:

Corzide 40/5 Tablets 2247
Corzide 80/5 Tablets 2247

Bumetanide (Patients on diuretics, especially those on recently instituted diuretic therapy, may experience an excessive reduction in blood pressure after initiation of therapy with trandolapril).

No products indexed under this heading.

Chlorothiazide (Patients on diuretics, especially those on recently instituted diuretic therapy, may experience an excessive reduction in blood pressure after initiation of therapy with trandolapril). Products include:

Aldoclor Tablets 2035
Diuril Oral 2087

Chlorothiazide Sodium (Patients on diuretics, especially those on recently instituted diuretic therapy, may experience an excessive reduction in blood pressure after initiation of therapy with trandolapril). Products include:

Diuril Sodium Intravenous 2086

Chlorthalidone (Patients on diuretics, especially those on recently instituted diuretic therapy, may experience an excessive reduction in blood pressure after initiation of therapy with trandolapril). Products include:

Clorpres Tablets 1002
Combipres Tablets 1040
Tenoretic Tablets 690

Cimetidine (Co-administration has led to an increase of about 44% in Cmax for trandolapril with no effect on ACE inhibition). Products include:

Tagamet HB 200 Suspension .... ▣762
Tagamet HB 200 Tablets .... ▣761
Tagamet Tablets 1644

Cimetidine Hydrochloride (Co-administration has led to an increase of about 44% in Cmax for trandolapril with no effect on ACE inhibition). Products include:

Tagamet 1644

Ethacrynic Acid (Patients on diuretics, especially those on recently instituted diuretic therapy, may experience an excessive reduction in blood pressure after initiation of therapy with trandolapril). Products include:

Edecrin Tablets 2091

Furosemide (Co-administration has led to an increase of about 25% in the renal clearance of trandolapril with no effect on ACE inhibition; patients on diuretics, especially those on recently instituted diuretic therapy, may experience an excessive reduction in bloodpressure after initiation of therapy with trandolapril). Products include:

Furosemide Tablets 2284

Hydrochlorothiazide (Patients on diuretics, especially those on recently instituted diuretic therapy, may experience an excessive reduction in blood pressure after initiation of therapy with trandolapril). Products include:

Accuretic Tablets 2614
Aldoril Tablets 2039
Atacand HCT Tablets 597
Avalide Tablets 1070
Diovan HCT Tablets 2338
Dyazide Capsules 1515
HydroDIURIL Tablets 2108
Hyzaar 2109
Inderide Tablets 3517
Inderide LA Long-Acting Capsules 3519
Lotensin HCT Tablets 2367
Maxzide 1008
Micardis HCT Tablets 1051
Microzide Capsules 3414
Moduretic Tablets 2138
Monopril HCT 1094
Prinzide Tablets 2168
Timolide Tablets 2187
Uniretic Tablets 3178
Vaseretic Tablets 2204
Zestoretic Tablets 695
Ziac Tablets 1887

Hydroflumethiazide (Patients on diuretics, especially those on recently instituted diuretic therapy, may experience an excessive reduction in blood pressure after initiation of therapy with trandolapril). Products include:

Diucardin Tablets 3494

Indapamide (Patients on diuretics, especially those on recently instituted diuretic therapy, may experience an excessive reduction in blood pressure after initiation of therapy with trandolapril). Products include:

Indapamide Tablets 2286

Lithium Carbonate (Co-administration of ACE inhibitors and lithium has resulted in increased serum lithium levels and symptoms of lithium toxicity). Products include:

Eskalith 1527
Lithium Carbonate 3061
Lithobid Slow-Release Tablets 3255

Lithium Citrate (Co-administration of ACE inhibitors and lithium has resulted in increased serum lithium levels and symptoms of lithium toxicity). Products include:

Lithium Citrate Syrup 3061

Methyclothiazide (Patients on diuretics, especially those on recently instituted diuretic therapy, may experience an excessive reduction in blood pressure after initiation of therapy with trandolapril).

No products indexed under this heading.

Metolazone (Patients on diuretics, especially those on recently instituted diuretic therapy, may experience an excessive reduction in blood pressure after initiation of therapy with trandolapril). Products include:

Mykrox Tablets 1168
Zaroxolyn Tablets 1177

Polythiazide (Patients on diuretics, especially those on recently instituted diuretic therapy, may experience an excessive reduction in blood pressure after initiation of therapy with trandolapril). Products include:

Minizide Capsules 2700
Renese Tablets 2712

Potassium Acid Phosphate (Co-administration increases the risk of hyperkalemia). Products include:

K-Phos Original (Sodium Free) Tablets 947

Potassium Bicarbonate (Co-administration increases the risk of hyperkalemia).

No products indexed under this heading.

Potassium Chloride (Co-administration increases the risk of hyperkalemia). Products include:
- Chlor-3 1361
- Colyte with Flavor Packs for Oral Solution.......... 3170
- GoLYTELY and Pineapple Flavor GoLYTELY for Oral Solution.......... 1068
- K-Dur Microburst Release System ER Tablets.......... 1832
- Klor-Con M20/Klor-Con M10 Tablets.......... 3329
- K-Lor Powder Packets 469
- K-Tab Filmtab Tablets 470
- Micro-K 3311
- NuLYTELY, Cherry Flavor, Lemon-Lime Flavor, and Orange Flavor NuLYTELY for Oral Solution.......... 1068
- Rum-K 1363

Potassium Citrate (Co-administration increases the risk of hyperkalemia). Products include:
- Urocit-K Tablets 2232

Potassium Gluconate (Co-administration increases the risk of hyperkalemia).
No products indexed under this heading.

Potassium Phosphate (Co-administration increases the risk of hyperkalemia). Products include:
- K-Phos Neutral Tablets 946

Spironolactone (Co-administration increases the risk of hyperkalemia; patients on diuretics, especially those on recently instituted diuretic therapy, may experience an excessive reduction in blood pressure after initiation of therapy with trandolapril).
No products indexed under this heading.

Torsemide (Patients on diuretics, especially those on recently instituted diuretic therapy, may experience an excessive reduction in blood pressure after initiation of therapy with trandolapril). Products include:
- Demadex Tablets and Injection 2965

Triamterene (Co-administration increases the risk of hyperkalemia; patients on diuretics, especially those on recently instituted diuretic therapy, may experience an excessive reduction in blood pressure after initiation of therapy with trandolapril). Products include:
- Dyazide Capsules 1515
- Dyrenium Capsules 3458
- Maxzide 1008

Food Interactions

Food, unspecified (Slows absorption of trandolapril but does not affect AUC or Cmax).

MAXAIR AUTOHALER

(Pirbuterol Acetate) 1981

May interact with beta blockers, monoamine oxidase inhibitors, potassium-depleting diuretics, sympathomimetic aerosol bronchodilators, and tricyclic antidepressants. Compounds in these categories include:

Acebutolol Hydrochloride (Co-administration with beta adrenergic receptor blocking agents blocks the pulmonary effect of pirbuterol and may produce severe bronchospasm in asthmatic patients). Products include:
- Sectral Capsules 3589

Albuterol (Potential for additive effects). Products include:
- Proventil Inhalation Aerosol 3142
- Ventolin Inhalation Aerosol and Refill.......... 1679

Amitriptyline Hydrochloride (Concurrent and/or sequential use with tricyclic antidepressants can result in the potentiation of pirbuterol's action on the vascular system). Products include:
- Etrafon 3115
- Limbitrol 1738

Amoxapine (Concurrent and/or sequential use with tricyclic antidepressants can result in the potentiation of pirbuterol's action on the vascular system).
No products indexed under this heading.

Atenolol (Co-administration with beta adrenergic receptor blocking agents blocks the pulmonary effect of pirbuterol and may produce severe bronchospasm in asthmatic patients). Products include:
- Tenoretic Tablets 690
- Tenormin I.V. Injection 692

Bendroflumethiazide (The ECG changes and/or hypokalemia that may result from administration of non-potassium sparing diuretics can be acutely worsened by beta-agonists; clinical significance is not known). Products include:
- Corzide 40/5 Tablets 2247
- Corzide 80/5 Tablets 2247

Betaxolol Hydrochloride (Co-administration with beta adrenergic receptor blocking agents blocks the pulmonary effect of pirbuterol and may produce severe bronchospasm in asthmatic patients). Products include:
- Betoptic S Ophthalmic Suspension 537

Bisoprolol Fumarate (Co-administration with beta adrenergic receptor blocking agents blocks the pulmonary effect of pirbuterol and may produce severe bronchospasm in asthmatic patients). Products include:
- Zebeta Tablets 1885
- Ziac Tablets 1887

Bitolterol Mesylate (Potential for additive effects).
No products indexed under this heading.

Bumetanide (The ECG changes and/or hypokalemia that may result from administration of non-potassium sparing diuretics can be acutely worsened by beta-agonists; clinical significance is not known).
No products indexed under this heading.

Carteolol Hydrochloride (Co-administration with beta adrenergic receptor blocking agents blocks the pulmonary effect of pirbuterol and may produce severe bronchospasm in asthmatic patients). Products include:
- Carteolol Hydrochloride Ophthalmic Solution USP, 1% .... ⊙258
- Ocupress Ophthalmic Solution, 1% Sterile .... ⊙303

Chlorothiazide (The ECG changes and/or hypokalemia that may result from administration of non-potassium sparing diuretics can be acutely worsened by beta-agonists; clinical significance is not known). Products include:
- Aldoclor Tablets 2035
- Diuril Oral 2087

Chlorothiazide Sodium (The ECG changes and/or hypokalemia that may result from administration of non-potassium sparing diuretics can be acutely worsened by beta-agonists; clinical significance is not known). Products include:
- Diuril Sodium Intravenous 2086

Clomipramine Hydrochloride (Concurrent and/or sequential use with tricyclic antidepressants can result in the potentiation of pirbuterol's action on the vascular system).
No products indexed under this heading.

Desipramine Hydrochloride (Concurrent and/or sequential use with tricyclic antidepressants can result in the potentiation of pirbuterol's action on the vascular system). Products include:
- Norpramin Tablets 755

Doxepin Hydrochloride (Concurrent and/or sequential use with tricyclic antidepressants can result in the potentiation of pirbuterol's action on the vascular system). Products include:
- Sinequan 2713

Esmolol Hydrochloride (Co-administration with beta adrenergic receptor blocking agents blocks the pulmonary effect of pirbuterol and may produce severe bronchospasm in asthmatic patients). Products include:
- Brevibloc Injection 858

Ethacrynic Acid (The ECG changes and/or hypokalemia that may result from administration of non-potassium sparing diuretics can be acutely worsened by beta-agonists; clinical significance is not known). Products include:
- Edecrin Tablets 2091

Furosemide (The ECG changes and/or hypokalemia that may result from administration of non-potassium sparing diuretics can be acutely worsened by beta-agonists; clinical significance is not known). Products include:
- Furosemide Tablets 2284

Hydrochlorothiazide (The ECG changes and/or hypokalemia that may result from administration of non-potassium sparing diuretics can be acutely worsened by beta-agonists; clinical significance is not known). Products include:
- Accuretic Tablets 2614
- Aldoril Tablets 2039
- Atacand HCT Tablets 597
- Avalide Tablets 1070
- Diovan HCT Tablets 2338
- Dyazide Capsules 1515
- HydroDIURIL Tablets 2108
- Hyzaar 2109
- Inderide Tablets 3517
- Inderide LA Long-Acting Capsules 3519
- Lotensin HCT Tablets 2367
- Maxzide 1008
- Micardis HCT Tablets 1051
- Microzide Capsules 3414
- Moduretic Tablets 2138
- Monopril HCT 1094
- Prinzide Tablets 2168
- Timolide Tablets 2187
- Uniretic Tablets 3178
- Vaseretic Tablets 2204
- Zestoretic Tablets 695
- Ziac Tablets 1887

Hydroflumethiazide (The ECG changes and/or hypokalemia that may result from administration of non-potassium sparing diuretics can be acutely worsened by beta-agonists; clinical significance is not known). Products include:
- Diucardin Tablets 3494

Imipramine Hydrochloride (Concurrent and/or sequential use with tricyclic antidepressants can result in the potentiation of pirbuterol's action on the vascular system).
No products indexed under this heading.

Imipramine Pamoate (Concurrent and/or sequential use with tricyclic antidepressants can result in the potentiation of pirbuterol's action on the vascular system).
No products indexed under this heading.

Isocarboxazid (Concurrent and/or sequential use with MAO inhibitors can result in the potentiation of pirbuterol's action on the vascular system).
No products indexed under this heading.

Isoetharine (Potential for additive effects).
No products indexed under this heading.

Isoproterenol Hydrochloride (Potential for additive effects).
No products indexed under this heading.

Labetalol Hydrochloride (Co-administration with beta adrenergic receptor blocking agents blocks the pulmonary effect of pirbuterol and may produce severe bronchospasm in asthmatic patients). Products include:
- Normodyne Injection 3135
- Normodyne Tablets 3137

Levalbuterol Hydrochloride (Potential for additive effects). Products include:
- Xopenex Inhalation Solution 3207

Levobunolol Hydrochloride (Co-administration with beta adrenergic receptor blocking agents blocks the pulmonary effect of pirbuterol and may produce severe bronchospasm in asthmatic patients). Products include:
- Betagan .... ⊙228

Maprotiline Hydrochloride (Concurrent and/or sequential use with tricyclic antidepressants can result in the potentiation of pirbuterol's action on the vascular system).
No products indexed under this heading.

Metaproterenol Sulfate (Potential for additive effects). Products include:
- Alupent 1029

Methyclothiazide (The ECG changes and/or hypokalemia that may result from administration of non-potassium sparing diuretics can be acutely worsened by beta-agonists; clinical significance is not known).
No products indexed under this heading.

Metipranolol Hydrochloride (Co-administration with beta adrenergic receptor blocking agents blocks the pulmonary effect of pirbuterol and may produce severe bronchospasm in asthmatic patients).
No products indexed under this heading.

Metoprolol Succinate (Co-administration with beta adrenergic receptor blocking agents blocks the pulmonary effect of pirbuterol and may produce severe bronchospasm in asthmatic patients). Products include:
- Toprol-XL Tablets 651

Metoprolol Tartrate (Co-administration with beta adrenergic receptor blocking agents blocks the pulmonary effect of pirbuterol and may produce severe bronchospasm in asthmatic patients).
No products indexed under this heading.

Moclobemide (Concurrent and/or sequential use with MAO inhibitors can result in the potentiation of pirbuterol's action on the vascular system).
No products indexed under this heading.

Nadolol (Co-administration with beta adrenergic receptor blocking agents blocks the pulmonary effect of pirbuterol and may produce severe bronchospasm in asthmatic patients). Products include:
- Corgard Tablets 2245
- Corzide 40/5 Tablets 2247
- Corzide 80/5 Tablets 2247
- Nadolol Tablets 2288

Nortriptyline Hydrochloride (Concurrent and/or sequential use with tricyclic antidepressants can result in the potentiation of pirbuterol's action on the vascular system).
No products indexed under this heading.

Pargyline Hydrochloride (Concurrent and/or sequential use with MAO

inhibitors can result in the potentiation of pirbuterol's action on the vascular system).
No products indexed under this heading.

Penbutolol Sulfate (Co-administration with beta adrenergic receptor blocking agents blocks the pulmonary effect of pirbuterol and may produce severe bronchospasm in asthmatic patients).
No products indexed under this heading.

Phenelzine Sulfate (Concurrent and/or sequential use with MAO inhibitors can result in the potentiation of pirbuterol's action on the vascular system). Products include:
Nardil Tablets 2653

Pindolol (Co-administration with beta adrenergic receptor blocking agents blocks the pulmonary effect of pirbuterol and may produce severe bronchospasm in asthmatic patients).
No products indexed under this heading.

Polythiazide (The ECG changes and/or hypokalemia that may result from administration of non-potassium sparing diuretics can be acutely worsened by beta-agonists; clinical significance is not known). Products include:
Minizide Capsules 2700
Renese Tablets 2712

Procarbazine Hydrochloride (Concurrent and/or sequential use with MAO inhibitors can result in the potentiation of pirbuterol's action on the vascular system). Products include:
Matulane Capsules 3246

Propranolol Hydrochloride (Co-administration with beta adrenergic receptor blocking agents blocks the pulmonary effect of pirbuterol and may produce severe bronchospasm in asthmatic patients). Products include:
Inderal 3513
Inderal LA Long-Acting Capsules 3516
Inderide Tablets 3517
Inderide LA Long-Acting Capsules .. 3519

Protriptyline Hydrochloride (Concurrent and/or sequential use with tricyclic antidepressants can result in the potentiation of pirbuterol's action on the vascular system). Products include:
Vivactil Tablets 2446
Vivactil Tablets 2217

Salmeterol Xinafoate (Potential for additive effects). Products include:
Advair Diskus 100/50 1448
Advair Diskus 250/50 1448
Advair Diskus 500/50 1448
Serevent Diskus 1637
Serevent Inhalation Aerosol 1633

Selegiline Hydrochloride (Concurrent and/or sequential use with MAO inhibitors can result in the potentiation of pirbuterol's action on the vascular system). Products include:
Eldepryl Capsules 3266

Sotalol Hydrochloride (Co-administration with beta adrenergic receptor blocking agents blocks the pulmonary effect of pirbuterol and may produce severe bronchospasm in asthmatic patients). Products include:
Betapace Tablets 950
Betapace AF Tablets 954

Terbutaline Sulfate (Potential for additive effects). Products include:
Brethine Ampuls 2314
Brethine Tablets 2313

Timolol Hemihydrate (Co-administration with beta adrenergic receptor blocking agents blocks the pulmonary effect of pirbuterol and may produce severe bronchospasm in asthmatic patients). Products include:
Betimol Ophthalmic Solution .... ⊙324

Timolol Maleate (Co-administration with beta adrenergic receptor blocking agents blocks the pulmonary effect of pirbuterol and may produce severe bronchospasm in asthmatic patients). Products include:
Blocadren Tablets 2046
Cosopt Sterile Ophthalmic Solution 2065
Timolide Tablets 2187
Timolol GFS .... ⊙266
Timoptic in Ocudose 2192
Timoptic Sterile Ophthalmic Solution 2190
Timoptic-XE Sterile Ophthalmic Gel Forming Solution 2194

Torsemide (The ECG changes and/or hypokalemia that may result from administration of non-potassium sparing diuretics can be acutely worsened by beta-agonists; clinical significance is not known). Products include:
Demadex Tablets and Injection 2965

Tranylcypromine Sulfate (Concurrent and/or sequential use with MAO inhibitors can result in the potentiation of pirbuterol's action on the vascular system). Products include:
Parnate Tablets 1607

Trimipramine Maleate (Concurrent and/or sequential use with tricyclic antidepressants can result in the potentiation of pirbuterol's action on the vascular system). Products include:
Surmontil Capsules 3595

MAXAIR INHALER

(Pirbuterol Acetate) 1984
May interact with beta blockers, monoamine oxidase inhibitors, potassium-depleting diuretics, sympathomimetic bronchodilators, and tricyclic antidepressants. Compounds in these categories include:

Acebutolol Hydrochloride (Beta blockers not only block the pulmonary effect of beta-agonists but may produce severe bronchospasm in asthmatic patients). Products include:
Sectral Capsules 3589

Albuterol (Potential for additive effects). Products include:
Proventil Inhalation Aerosol 3142
Ventolin Inhalation Aerosol and Refill 1679

Albuterol Sulfate (Potential for additive effects). Products include:
AccuNeb Inhalation Solution 1230
Combivent Inhalation Aerosol 1041
DuoNeb Inhalation Solution 1233
Proventil Inhalation Solution 0.083% 3146
Proventil Repetabs Tablets 3148
Proventil Solution for Inhalation 0.5% 3144
Proventil HFA Inhalation Aerosol 3150
Ventolin HFA Inhalation Aerosol 3618
Volmax Extended-Release Tablets .. 2276

Amitriptyline Hydrochloride (Co-administration may potentiate the action of pirbuterol on the vascular system; concurrent and/or sequential use should be undertaken with extreme caution). Products include:
Etrafon 3115
Limbitrol 1738

Amoxapine (Co-administration may potentiate the action of pirbuterol on the vascular system; concurrent and/or sequential use should be undertaken with extreme caution).
No products indexed under this heading.

Atenolol (Beta blockers not only block the pulmonary effect of beta-agonists but may produce severe bronchospasm in asthmatic patients). Products include:
Tenoretic Tablets 690
Tenormin I.V. Injection 692

Bendroflumethiazide (The ECG changes and/or hypokalemia that may result from the administration of non-potassium sparing diuretics can be acutely worsened by the beta agonists). Products include:
Corzide 40/5 Tablets 2247
Corzide 80/5 Tablets 2247

Betaxolol Hydrochloride (Beta blockers not only block the pulmonary effect of beta-agonists but may produce severe bronchospasm in asthmatic patients). Products include:
Betoptic S Ophthalmic Suspension 537

Bisoprolol Fumarate (Beta blockers not only block the pulmonary effect of beta-agonists but may produce severe bronchospasm in asthmatic patients). Products include:
Zebeta Tablets 1885
Ziac Tablets 1887

Bitolterol Mesylate (Potential for additive effects).
No products indexed under this heading.

Bumetanide (The ECG changes and/or hypokalemia that may result from the administration of non-potassium sparing diuretics can be acutely worsened by the beta agonists).
No products indexed under this heading.

Carteolol Hydrochloride (Beta blockers not only block the pulmonary effect of beta-agonists but may produce severe bronchospasm in asthmatic patients). Products include:
Carteolol Hydrochloride Ophthalmic Solution USP, 1% ..... ⊙258
Ocupress Ophthalmic Solution, 1% Sterile .... ⊙303

Chlorothiazide (The ECG changes and/or hypokalemia that may result from the administration of non-potassium sparing diuretics can be acutely worsened by the beta agonists). Products include:
Aldoclor Tablets 2035
Diuril Oral 2087

Chlorothiazide Sodium (The ECG changes and/or hypokalemia that may result from the administration of non-potassium sparing diuretics can be acutely worsened by the beta agonists). Products include:
Diuril Sodium Intravenous 2086

Clomipramine Hydrochloride (Co-administration may potentiate the action of pirbuterol on the vascular system; concurrent and/or sequential use should be undertaken with extreme caution).
No products indexed under this heading.

Desipramine Hydrochloride (Co-administration may potentiate the action of pirbuterol on the vascular system; concurrent and/or sequential use should be undertaken with extreme caution). Products include:
Norpramin Tablets 755

Doxepin Hydrochloride (Co-administration may potentiate the action of pirbuterol on the vascular system; concurrent and/or sequential use should be undertaken with extreme caution). Products include:
Sinequan 2713

Ephedrine Hydrochloride (Potential for additive effects). Products include:
Primatene Tablets 780

Ephedrine Sulfate (Potential for additive effects).
No products indexed under this heading.

Ephedrine Tannate (Potential for additive effects). Products include:
Rynatuss Pediatric Suspension 3353
Rynatuss Tablets 3353

Epinephrine (Potential for additive effects). Products include:
Epifrin Sterile Ophthalmic Solution .... ⊙235
EpiPen 1236
Primatene Mist 779
Xylocaine with Epinephrine Injection 653

Epinephrine Hydrochloride (Potential for additive effects).
No products indexed under this heading.

Esmolol Hydrochloride (Beta blockers not only block the pulmonary effect of beta-agonists but may produce severe bronchospasm in asthmatic patients). Products include:
Brevibloc Injection 858

Ethacrynic Acid (The ECG changes and/or hypokalemia that may result from the administration of non-potassium sparing diuretics can be acutely worsened by the beta agonists). Products include:
Edecrin Tablets 2091

Furosemide (The ECG changes and/or hypokalemia that may result from the administration of non-potassium sparing diuretics can be acutely worsened by the beta agonists). Products include:
Furosemide Tablets 2284

Hydrochlorothiazide (The ECG changes and/or hypokalemia that may result from the administration of non-potassium sparing diuretics can be acutely worsened by the beta agonists). Products include:
Accuretic Tablets 2614
Aldoril Tablets 2039
Atacand HCT Tablets 597
Avalide Tablets 1070
Diovan HCT Tablets 2338
Dyazide Capsules 1515
HydroDIURIL Tablets 2108
Hyzaar 2109
Inderide Tablets 3517
Inderide LA Long-Acting Capsules .. 3519
Lotensin HCT Tablets 2367
Maxzide 1008
Micardis HCT Tablets 1051
Microzide Capsules 3414
Moduretic Tablets 2138
Monopril HCT 1094
Prinzide Tablets 2168
Timolide Tablets 2187
Uniretic Tablets 3178
Vaseretic Tablets 2204
Zestoretic Tablets 695
Ziac Tablets 1887

Hydroflumethiazide (The ECG changes and/or hypokalemia that may result from the administration of non-potassium sparing diuretics can be acutely worsened by the beta agonists). Products include:
Diucardin Tablets 3494

Imipramine Hydrochloride (Co-administration may potentiate the action of pirbuterol on the vascular system; concurrent and/or sequential use should be undertaken with extreme caution).
No products indexed under this heading.

Imipramine Pamoate (Co-administration may potentiate the action of pirbuterol on the vascular system; concurrent and/or sequential use should be undertaken with extreme caution).
No products indexed under this heading.

Isocarboxazid (Co-administration may potentiate the action of pirbuterol on the vascular system; concurrent and/or sequential use should be undertaken with extreme caution).
No products indexed under this heading.

Isoetharine (Potential for additive effects).
No products indexed under this heading.

Isoproterenol Hydrochloride (Potential for additive effects).
No products indexed under this heading.

Isoproterenol Sulfate (Potential for additive effects).
No products indexed under this heading.

Labetalol Hydrochloride (Beta blockers not only block the pulmonary effect of beta-agonists but may produce severe bronchospasm in asthmatic patients). Products include:
Normodyne Injection 3135
Normodyne Tablets 3137

Levalbuterol Hydrochloride (Potential for additive effects). Products include:
Xopenex Inhalation Solution 3207

Levobunolol Hydrochloride (Beta blockers not only block the pulmonary effect of beta-agonists but may produce severe bronchospasm in asthmatic patients). Products include:
Betagan .... ⊙228

Maprotiline Hydrochloride (Co-administration may potentiate the action of pirbuterol on the vascular system; concurrent and/or sequential use should be undertaken with extreme caution).
No products indexed under this heading.

Metaproterenol Sulfate (Potential for additive effects). Products include:
Alupent 1029

Methyclothiazide (The ECG changes and/or hypokalemia that may result from the administration of non-potassium sparing diuretics can be acutely worsened by the beta agonists).
No products indexed under this heading.

Metipranolol Hydrochloride (Beta blockers not only block the pulmonary effect of beta-agonists but may produce severe bronchospasm in asthmatic patients).
No products indexed under this heading.

Metoprolol Succinate (Beta blockers not only block the pulmonary effect of beta-agonists but may produce severe bronchospasm in asthmatic patients). Products include:
Toprol-XL Tablets 651

Metoprolol Tartrate (Beta blockers not only block the pulmonary effect of beta-agonists but may produce severe bronchospasm in asthmatic patients).
No products indexed under this heading.

Moclobemide (Co-administration may potentiate the action of pirbuterol on the vascular system; concurrent and/or sequential use should be undertaken with extreme caution).
No products indexed under this heading.

Nadolol (Beta blockers not only block the pulmonary effect of beta-agonists but may produce severe bronchospasm in asthmatic patients). Products include:
Corgard Tablets 2245
Corzide 40/5 Tablets 2247
Corzide 80/5 Tablets 2247
Nadolol Tablets 2288

Nortriptyline Hydrochloride (Co-administration may potentiate the action of pirbuterol on the vascular system; concurrent and/or sequential use should be undertaken with extreme caution).
No products indexed under this heading.

Pargyline Hydrochloride (Co-administration may potentiate the action of pirbuterol on the vascular system; concurrent and/or sequential use should be undertaken with extreme caution).
No products indexed under this heading.

Penbutolol Sulfate (Beta blockers not only block the pulmonary effect of beta-agonists but may produce severe bronchospasm in asthmatic patients).
No products indexed under this heading.

Phenelzine Sulfate (Co-administration may potentiate the action of pirbuterol on the vascular system; concurrent and/or sequential use should be undertaken with extreme caution). Products include:
Nardil Tablets 2653

Pindolol (Beta blockers not only block the pulmonary effect of beta-agonists but may produce severe bronchospasm in asthmatic patients).
No products indexed under this heading.

Polythiazide (The ECG changes and/or hypokalemia that may result from the administration of non-potassium sparing diuretics can be acutely worsened by the beta agonists). Products include:
Minizide Capsules 2700
Renese Tablets 2712

Procarbazine Hydrochloride (Co-administration may potentiate the action of pirbuterol on the vascular system; concurrent and/or sequential use should be undertaken with extreme caution). Products include:
Matulane Capsules 3246

Propranolol Hydrochloride (Beta blockers not only block the pulmonary effect of beta-agonists but may produce severe bronchospasm in asthmatic patients). Products include:
Inderal 3513
Inderal LA Long-Acting Capsules 3516
Inderide Tablets 3517
Inderide LA Long-Acting Capsules .. 3519

Protriptyline Hydrochloride (Co-administration may potentiate the action of pirbuterol on the vascular system; concurrent and/or sequential use should be undertaken with extreme caution). Products include:
Vivactil Tablets 2446
Vivactil Tablets 2217

Salmeterol Xinafoate (Potential for additive effects). Products include:
Advair Diskus 100/50 1448
Advair Diskus 250/50 1448
Advair Diskus 500/50 1448
Serevent Diskus 1637
Serevent Inhalation Aerosol 1633

Selegiline Hydrochloride (Co-administration may potentiate the action of pirbuterol on the vascular system; concurrent and/or sequential use should be undertaken with extreme caution). Products include:
Eldepryl Capsules 3266

Sotalol Hydrochloride (Beta blockers not only block the pulmonary effect of beta-agonists but may produce severe bronchospasm in asthmatic patients). Products include:
Betapace Tablets 950
Betapace AF Tablets 954

Terbutaline Sulfate (Potential for additive effects). Products include:
Brethine Ampuls 2314
Brethine Tablets 2313

Timolol Hemihydrate (Beta blockers not only block the pulmonary effect of beta-agonists but may produce severe bronchospasm in asthmatic patients). Products include:
Betimol Ophthalmic Solution .... ⊙324

Timolol Maleate (Beta blockers not only block the pulmonary effect of beta-agonists but may produce severe bronchospasm in asthmatic patients). Products include:
Blocadren Tablets 2046
Cosopt Sterile Ophthalmic Solution 2065
Timolide Tablets 2187
Timolol GFS .... ⊙266
Timoptic in Ocudose 2192
Timoptic Sterile Ophthalmic Solution 2190
Timoptic-XE Sterile Ophthalmic Gel Forming Solution 2194

Torsemide (The ECG changes and/or hypokalemia that may result from the administration of non-potassium sparing diuretics can be acutely worsened by the beta agonists). Products include:
Demadex Tablets and Injection 2965

Tranylcypromine Sulfate (Co-administration may potentiate the action of pirbuterol on the vascular system; concurrent and/or sequential use should be undertaken with extreme caution). Products include:
Parnate Tablets 1607

Trimipramine Maleate (Co-administration may potentiate the action of pirbuterol on the vascular system; concurrent and/or sequential use should be undertaken with extreme caution). Products include:
Surmontil Capsules 3595

MAXALT TABLETS

(Rizatriptan Benzoate) 2120
May interact with 5HT1-receptor agonists, ergot-containing drugs, monoamine oxidase inhibitors, selective serotonin reuptake inhibitors, and certain other agents. Compounds in these categories include:

Citalopram Hydrobromide (Co-administration of 5-HT1 agonists with selective serotonin reuptake inhibitors (SSRIs) has resulted, rarely, in hyperreflexia, weakness, and incoordination). Products include:
Celexa 1365

Dihydroergotamine Mesylate (Ergot-containing drugs have been reported to cause prolonged vasospastic reactions; because there is a theoretical basis that these effects may be additive, use of ergot-type agents and rizatriptan within 24 hours is contraindicated). Products include:
D.H.E. 45 Injection 2334
Migranal Nasal Spray 2376

Ergonovine Maleate (Ergot-containing drugs have been reported to cause prolonged vasospastic reactions; because there is a theoretical basis that these effects may be additive, use of ergot-type agents and rizatriptan within 24 hours is contraindicated).
No products indexed under this heading.

Ergotamine Tartrate (Ergot-containing drugs have been reported to cause prolonged vasospastic reactions; because there is a theoretical basis that these effects may be additive, use of ergot-type agents and rizatriptan within 24 hours is contraindicated).
No products indexed under this heading.

Fluoxetine Hydrochloride (Co-administration of 5-HT1 agonists with selective serotonin reuptake inhibitors (SSRIs) has resulted, rarely, in hyperreflexia, weakness, and incoordination). Products include:
Prozac Pulvules, Liquid, and Weekly Capsules 1238
Sarafem Pulvules 1962

Fluvoxamine Maleate (Co-administration of 5-HT1 agonists with selective serotonin reuptake inhibitors (SSRIs) has resulted, rarely, in hyperreflexia, weakness, and incoordination). Products include:
Luvox Tablets (25, 50, 100 mg) 3256

Isocarboxazid (Plasma concentrations of rizatriptan may be increased by MAO inhibitors; concurrent and/or sequential use is contraindicated).
No products indexed under this heading.

Methylergonovine Maleate (Ergot-containing drugs have been reported to cause prolonged vasospastic reactions; because there is a theoretical basis that these effects may be additive, use of ergot-type agents and rizatriptan within 24 hours is contraindicated).
No products indexed under this heading.

Methysergide Maleate (Ergot-containing drugs have been reported to cause prolonged vasospastic reactions; because there is a theoretical basis that these effects may be additive, use of ergot-type agents and rizatriptan within 24 hours is contraindicated).
No products indexed under this heading.

Moclobemide (Concomitant therapy with the selective, reversible MAO-A inhibitor, moclobemide, has resulted in increased systemic exposure of rizatriptan and its metabolite; concurrent and/or sequential use is contraindicated).
No products indexed under this heading.

Naratriptan Hydrochloride (Co-administration with other 5-HT1 agonists within 24 hours of each other is contraindicated because the vasospastic effects may be additive). Products include:
Amerge Tablets 1467

Pargyline Hydrochloride (Plasma concentrations of rizatriptan may be increased by MAO inhibitors; concurrent and/or sequential use is contraindicated).
No products indexed under this heading.

Paroxetine Hydrochloride (Co-administration of 5-HT1 agonists with selective serotonin reuptake inhibitors (SSRIs) has resulted, rarely, in hyperreflexia, weakness, and incoordination; no pharmacokinetic interaction was observed with a single dose study). Products include:
Paxil 1609

Phenelzine Sulfate (Plasma concentrations of rizatriptan may be increased by MAO inhibitors; concurrent and/or sequential use is contraindicated). Products include:
Nardil Tablets 2653

Procarbazine Hydrochloride (Plasma concentrations of rizatriptan may be increased by MAO inhibitors; concurrent and/or sequential use is contraindicated). Products include:
Matulane Capsules 3246

Propranolol Hydrochloride (Co-administration has resulted in an increase in mean plasma AUC for rizatriptan by 70%). Products include:
Inderal 3513
Inderal LA Long-Acting Capsules 3516
Inderide Tablets 3517
Inderide LA Long-Acting Capsules .. 3519

Selegiline Hydrochloride (Plasma concentrations of rizatriptan may be increased by MAO inhibitors; concurrent and/or sequential use is contraindicated). Products include:
Eldepryl Capsules 3266

Sertraline Hydrochloride (Co-administration of 5-HT1 agonists with selective serotonin reuptake inhibitors (SSRIs) has resulted, rarely, in hyperreflexia, weakness, and incoordination). Products include:
Zoloft 2751

Sumatriptan (Co-administration with other 5-HT1 agonists within 24

hours of each other is contraindicated because the vasospastic effects may be additive). Products include:

Imitrex Nasal Spray 1554

Sumatriptan Succinate (Co-administration with other 5-HT1 agonists within 24 hours of each other is contraindicated because the vasospastic effects may be additive). Products include:

Imitrex Injection 1549
Imitrex Tablets 1558

Tranylcypromine Sulfate (Plasma concentrations of rizatriptan may be increased by MAO inhibitors; concurrent and/or sequential use is contraindicated). Products include:

Parnate Tablets 1607

Zolmitriptan (Co-administration with other 5-HT1 agonists within 24 hours of each other is contraindicated because the vasospastic effects may be additive). Products include:

Zomig Tablets 708
Zomig-ZMT Tablets 708

Food Interactions

Food, unspecified (Delays the time to reach peak concentration by an hour; no significant effect on the bioavailability).

MAXALT-MLT ORALLY DISINTEGRATING TABLETS

(Rizatriptan Benzoate) 2120
See Maxalt Tablets

MAXIDONE TABLETS CIII

(Acetaminophen, Hydrocodone Bitartrate) 3399

May interact with antihistamines, central nervous system depressants, hypnotics and sedatives, monoamine oxidase inhibitors, antipsychotic agents, tricyclic antidepressants, and certain other agents. Compounds in these categories include:

Acrivastine (Co-administration may exhibit an additive CNS depression). Products include:

Semprex-D Capsules 1172

Alfentanil Hydrochloride (Co-administration may exhibit an additive CNS depression).

No products indexed under this heading.

Alprazolam (Co-administration may exhibit an additive CNS depression). Products include:

Xanax Tablets 2865

Amitriptyline Hydrochloride (Co-administration with tricyclic antidepressant may increase the effect of either hydrocodone or tricyclic antidepressant). Products include:

Etrafon 3115
Limbitrol 1738

Amoxapine (Co-administration with tricyclic antidepressant may increase the effect of either hydrocodone or tricyclic antidepressant).

No products indexed under this heading.

Aprobarbital (Co-administration may exhibit an additive CNS depression).

No products indexed under this heading.

Astemizole (Co-administration may exhibit an additive CNS depression).

No products indexed under this heading.

Azatadine Maleate (Co-administration may exhibit an additive CNS depression). Products include:

Rynatan Tablets 3351

Bromodiphenhydramine Hydrochloride (Co-administration may exhibit an additive CNS depression).

No products indexed under this heading.

Brompheniramine Maleate (Co-administration may exhibit an additive CNS depression). Products include:

Bromfed Capsules (Extended-Release) 2269
Bromfed-PD Capsules (Extended-Release) 2269
Comtrex Acute Head Cold & Sinus Pressure Relief Tablets 627
Dimetapp Elixir 777
Dimetapp Cold and Fever Suspension 775
Dimetapp DM Cold & Cough Elixir 775
Dimetapp Nighttime Flu Liquid 776

Buprenorphine Hydrochloride (Co-administration may exhibit an additive CNS depression). Products include:

Buprenex Injectable 2918

Buspirone Hydrochloride (Co-administration may exhibit an additive CNS depression).

No products indexed under this heading.

Butabarbital (Co-administration may exhibit an additive CNS depression).

No products indexed under this heading.

Butalbital (Co-administration may exhibit an additive CNS depression). Products include:

Phrenilin 578
Sedapap Tablets 50 mg/650 mg ... 2225

Cetirizine Hydrochloride (Co-administration may exhibit an additive CNS depression). Products include:

Zyrtec 2756
Zyrtec-D 12 Hour Extended Relief Tablets 2758

Chlordiazepoxide (Co-administration may exhibit an additive CNS depression). Products include:

Limbitrol 1738

Chlordiazepoxide Hydrochloride (Co-administration may exhibit an additive CNS depression). Products include:

Librium Capsules 1736
Librium for Injection 1737

Chlorpheniramine Maleate (Co-administration may exhibit an additive CNS depression). Products include:

Actifed Cold & Sinus Caplets and Tablets 688
Alka-Seltzer Plus Liqui-Gels 604
BC Allergy Sinus Cold Powder 619
Chlor-Trimeton Allergy Tablets 735
Chlor-Trimeton Allergy/Decongestant Tablets 736
Comtrex Flu Therapy & Fever Relief Nighttime Tablets 628
Comtrex Maximum Strength Multi-Symptom Cold & Cough Relief Tablets and Caplets 626
Contac Severe Cold and Flu Caplets Maximum Strength 746
Coricidin 'D' Cold, Flu & Sinus Tablets 737
Coricidin/Coricidin D 738
Coricidin HBP Maximum Strength Flu Tablets 738
Extendryl 1361
Hycomine Compound Tablets 1317
Kronofed-A 1341
PediaCare Cough-Cold Liquid 719
PediaCare NightRest Cough-Cold Liquid 719
Robitussin Nighttime Honey Flu Liquid 786
Ryna 768
Singlet Caplets 761
Sinutab Sinus Allergy Medication, Maximum Strength Formula, Tablets & Caplets 707
Sudafed Cold & Allergy Tablets 708
TheraFlu Regular Strength Cold & Cough Night Time Hot Liquid 676
TheraFlu Regular Strength Cold & Sore Throat Night Time Hot Liquid 676
TheraFlu Maximum Strength Flu & Cough Night Time Hot Liquid .. 678
TheraFlu Maximum Strength Flu & Sore Throat Night Time Hot Liquid 677
TheraFlu Maximum Strength Severe Cold & Congestion Night Time Caplets 678
TheraFlu Maximum Strength Severe Cold & Congestion Night Time Hot Liquid 678
Triaminic Cold & Allergy Liquid 681
Triaminic Cold & Allergy Softchews 683
Triaminic Cold & Cough Liquid 681
Triaminic Cold & Cough Softchews 683
Triaminic Cold & Night Time Cough Liquid 681
Triaminic Cold, Cough & Fever Liquid 681
Children's Tylenol Cold Suspension Liquid and Chewable Tablets 2015
Children's Tylenol Cold Plus Cough Suspension Liquid and Chewable Tablets 2015
Children's Tylenol Flu Suspension Liquid 2015
Maximum Strength Tylenol Allergy Sinus Caplets, Gelcaps, and Geltabs 2010
Multi-Symptom Tylenol Cold Complete Formula Caplets 2010
Vicks 44M Cough, Cold & Flu Relief Liquid 725
Pediatric Vicks 44m Cough & Cold Relief 728
Children's Vicks NyQuil Cold/Cough Relief 726

Chlorpheniramine Polistirex (Co-administration may exhibit an additive CNS depression). Products include:

Tussionex Pennkinetic Extended-Release Suspension 1174

Chlorpheniramine Tannate (Co-administration may exhibit an additive CNS depression). Products include:

Reformulated Rynatan Pediatric Suspension 3352
Rynatuss Pediatric Suspension 3353
Rynatuss Tablets 3353
Tussi-12 S Suspension 3356
Tussi-12 Tablets 3356

Chlorpromazine (Co-administration may exhibit an additive CNS depression). Products include:

Thorazine Suppositories 1656

Chlorpromazine Hydrochloride (Co-administration may exhibit an additive CNS depression). Products include:

Thorazine 1656

Chlorprothixene (Co-administration may exhibit an additive CNS depression).

No products indexed under this heading.

Chlorprothixene Hydrochloride (Co-administration may exhibit an additive CNS depression).

No products indexed under this heading.

Chlorprothixene Lactate (Co-administration may exhibit an additive CNS depression).

No products indexed under this heading.

Clemastine Fumarate (Co-administration may exhibit an additive CNS depression). Products include:

Tavist 12 Hour Allergy Tablets 676

Clomipramine Hydrochloride (Co-administration with tricyclic antidepressant may increase the effect of either hydrocodone or tricyclic antidepressant).

No products indexed under this heading.

Clorazepate Dipotassium (Co-administration may exhibit an additive CNS depression). Products include:

Tranxene 511

Clozapine (Co-administration may exhibit an additive CNS depression). Products include:

Clozaril Tablets 2319

Codeine Phosphate (Co-administration may exhibit an additive CNS depression). Products include:

Phenergan with Codeine Syrup 3557
Phenergan VC with Codeine Syrup .. 3561
Robitussin A-C Syrup 2942
Robitussin-DAC Syrup 2942
Ryna-C Liquid 768
Soma Compound w/Codeine Tablets 3355
Tussi-Organidin NR Liquid 3350
Tussi-Organidin-S NR Liquid 3350
Tylenol with Codeine 2595

Cyproheptadine Hydrochloride (Co-administration may exhibit an additive CNS depression). Products include:

Periactin Tablets 2155

Desflurane (Co-administration may exhibit an additive CNS depression). Products include:

Suprane Liquid for Inhalation 874

Desipramine Hydrochloride (Co-administration with tricyclic antidepressant may increase the effect of either hydrocodone or tricyclic antidepressant). Products include:

Norpramin Tablets 755

Dexchlorpheniramine Maleate (Co-administration may exhibit an additive CNS depression).

No products indexed under this heading.

Dezocine (Co-administration may exhibit an additive CNS depression).

No products indexed under this heading.

Diazepam (Co-administration may exhibit an additive CNS depression). Products include:

Valium Injectable 3026
Valium Tablets 3047

Diphenhydramine Citrate (Co-administration may exhibit an additive CNS depression). Products include:

Alka-Seltzer PM Effervescent Tablets 605
Benadryl Allergy & Sinus Fastmelt Tablets 693
Benadryl Children's Allergy/Cold Fastmelt Tablets 692
Excedrin PM Tablets, Caplets, and Geltabs 631
Goody's PM Powder 621

Diphenhydramine Hydrochloride (Co-administration may exhibit an additive CNS depression). Products include:

Extra Strength Bayer PM Caplets 611
Benadryl Allergy Chewables 689
Benadryl Allergy 691
Benadryl Allergy Liquid 690
Benadryl Allergy/Cold Tablets 691
Benadryl Allergy/Congestion Tablets 692
Benadryl Allergy & Sinus Liquid 693
Benadryl Allergy Sinus Headache Caplets & Gelcaps 693
Benadryl Severe Allergy & Sinus Headache Caplets 694
Benadryl Dye-Free Allergy Liquid ... 690
Benadryl Dye-Free Allergy Liqui-Gels Softgels 690
Benadryl Itch Relief Stick Extra Strength 695
Benadryl Cream 695
Benadryl Gel 695
Benadryl Spray 696
Benadryl Parenteral 2617
Coricidin HBP Night-Time Cold & Flu Tablets 738
Nytol QuickCaps Caplets 622
Maximum Strength Nytol QuickGels Softgels 621
Extra Strength Percogesic Aspirin-Free Coated Caplets 665
Simply Sleep Caplets 2008
Sominex Original Formula Tablets . 761
Children's Tylenol Allergy-D Liquid ... 2014
Maximum Strength Tylenol Allergy Sinus NightTime Caplets 2010
Tylenol Severe Allergy Caplets 2010
Maximum Strength Tylenol Flu NightTime Gelcaps 2011
Extra Strength Tylenol PM Caplets, Geltabs, and Gelcaps 2012

Unisom Maximum Strength SleepGels .... ▣713

Diphenylpyraline Hydrochloride (Co-administration may exhibit an additive CNS depression).
No products indexed under this heading.

Doxepin Hydrochloride (Co-administration with tricyclic antidepressant may increase the effect of either hydrocodone or tricyclic antidepressant). Products include:
Sinequan 2713

Droperidol (Co-administration may exhibit an additive CNS depression).
No products indexed under this heading.

Enflurane (Co-administration may exhibit an additive CNS depression).
No products indexed under this heading.

Estazolam (Co-administration may exhibit an additive CNS depression). Products include:
ProSom Tablets 500

Ethchlorvynol (Co-administration may exhibit an additive CNS depression).
No products indexed under this heading.

Ethinamate (Co-administration may exhibit an additive CNS depression).
No products indexed under this heading.

Fentanyl (Co-administration may exhibit an additive CNS depression). Products include:
Duragesic Transdermal System 1786

Fentanyl Citrate (Co-administration may exhibit an additive CNS depression). Products include:
Actiq 1184

Fexofenadine Hydrochloride (Co-administration may exhibit an additive CNS depression). Products include:
Allegra 712
Allegra-D Extended-Release Tablets 714

Fluphenazine Decanoate (Co-administration may exhibit an additive CNS depression).
No products indexed under this heading.

Fluphenazine Enanthate (Co-administration may exhibit an additive CNS depression).
No products indexed under this heading.

Fluphenazine Hydrochloride (Co-administration may exhibit an additive CNS depression).
No products indexed under this heading.

Flurazepam Hydrochloride (Co-administration may exhibit an additive CNS depression).
No products indexed under this heading.

Glutethimide (Co-administration may exhibit an additive CNS depression).
No products indexed under this heading.

Haloperidol (Co-administration may exhibit an additive CNS depression). Products include:
Haldol Injection, Tablets and Concentrate 2533

Haloperidol Decanoate (Co-administration may exhibit an additive CNS depression). Products include:
Haldol Decanoate 2535

Hydrocodone Polistirex (Co-administration may exhibit an additive CNS depression). Products include:
Tussionex Pennkinetic Extended-Release Suspension 1174

Hydromorphone Hydrochloride (Co-administration may exhibit an additive CNS depression). Products include:
Dilaudid 441
Dilaudid Oral Liquid 445
Dilaudid Powder 441
Dilaudid Rectal Suppositories 441
Dilaudid Tablets 441
Dilaudid Tablets - 8 mg 445
Dilaudid-HP 443

Hydroxyzine Hydrochloride (Co-administration may exhibit an additive CNS depression). Products include:
Atarax Tablets & Syrup 2667
Vistaril Intramuscular Solution 2738

Imipramine Hydrochloride (Co-administration with tricyclic antidepressant may increase the effect of either hydrocodone or tricyclic antidepressant).
No products indexed under this heading.

Imipramine Pamoate (Co-administration with tricyclic antidepressant may increase the effect of either hydrocodone or tricyclic antidepressant).
No products indexed under this heading.

Isocarboxazid (Co-administration with MAO inhibitors may increase the effect of either hydrocodone or MAO inhibitor).
No products indexed under this heading.

Isoflurane (Co-administration may exhibit an additive CNS depression).
No products indexed under this heading.

Ketamine Hydrochloride (Co-administration may exhibit an additive CNS depression).
No products indexed under this heading.

Levomethadyl Acetate Hydrochloride (Co-administration may exhibit an additive CNS depression).
No products indexed under this heading.

Levorphanol Tartrate (Co-administration may exhibit an additive CNS depression). Products include:
Levo-Dromoran 1734
Levorphanol Tartrate Tablets 3059

Lithium Carbonate (Co-administration may exhibit an additive CNS depression). Products include:
Eskalith 1527
Lithium Carbonate 3061
Lithobid Slow-Release Tablets 3255

Lithium Citrate (Co-administration may exhibit an additive CNS depression). Products include:
Lithium Citrate Syrup 3061

Loratadine (Co-administration may exhibit an additive CNS depression). Products include:
Claritin 3100
Claritin-D 12 Hour Extended Release Tablets 3102
Claritin-D 24 Hour Extended Release Tablets 3104

Lorazepam (Co-administration may exhibit an additive CNS depression). Products include:
Ativan Injection 3478
Ativan Tablets 3482

Loxapine Hydrochloride (Co-administration may exhibit an additive CNS depression).
No products indexed under this heading.

Loxapine Succinate (Co-administration may exhibit an additive CNS depression). Products include:
Loxitane Capsules 3398

Maprotiline Hydrochloride (Co-administration with tricyclic antidepressant may increase the effect of either hydrocodone or tricyclic antidepressant).
No products indexed under this heading.

Meperidine Hydrochloride (Co-administration may exhibit an additive CNS depression). Products include:
Demerol 3079
Mepergan Injection 3539

Mephobarbital (Co-administration may exhibit an additive CNS depression).
No products indexed under this heading.

Meprobamate (Co-administration may exhibit an additive CNS depression). Products include:
Miltown Tablets 3349

Mesoridazine Besylate (Co-administration may exhibit an additive CNS depression). Products include:
Serentil 1057

Methadone Hydrochloride (Co-administration may exhibit an additive CNS depression). Products include:
Dolophine Hydrochloride Tablets 3056

Methdilazine Hydrochloride (Co-administration may exhibit an additive CNS depression).
No products indexed under this heading.

Methohexital Sodium (Co-administration may exhibit an additive CNS depression). Products include:
Brevital Sodium for Injection, USP 1815

Methotrimeprazine (Co-administration may exhibit an additive CNS depression).
No products indexed under this heading.

Methoxyflurane (Co-administration may exhibit an additive CNS depression).
No products indexed under this heading.

Midazolam Hydrochloride (Co-administration may exhibit an additive CNS depression). Products include:
Versed Injection 3027
Versed Syrup 3033

Moclobemide (Co-administration with MAO inhibitors may increase the effect of either hydrocodone or MAO inhibitor).
No products indexed under this heading.

Molindone Hydrochloride (Co-administration may exhibit an additive CNS depression). Products include:
Moban 1320

Morphine Sulfate (Co-administration may exhibit an additive CNS depression). Products include:
Astramorph/PF Injection, USP (Preservative-Free) 594
Duramorph Injection 1312
Infumorph 200 and Infumorph 500 Sterile Solutions 1314
Kadian Capsules 1335
MS Contin Tablets 2896
MSIR 2898
Oramorph SR Tablets 3062
Roxanol 3066

Nortriptyline Hydrochloride (Co-administration with tricyclic antidepressant may increase the effect of either hydrocodone or tricyclic antidepressant).
No products indexed under this heading.

Olanzapine (Co-administration may exhibit an additive CNS depression). Products include:
Zyprexa Tablets 1973
Zyprexa ZYDIS Orally Disintegrating Tablets 1973

Oxazepam (Co-administration may exhibit an additive CNS depression).
No products indexed under this heading.

Oxycodone Hydrochloride (Co-administration may exhibit an additive CNS depression). Products include:
OxyContin Tablets 2912
OxyFast Oral Concentrate Solution 2916
OxyIR Capsules 2916
Percocet Tablets 1326
Percodan Tablets 1327
Percolone Tablets 1327
Roxicodone 3067
Tylox Capsules 2597

Pargyline Hydrochloride (Co-administration with MAO inhibitors may increase the effect of either hydrocodone or MAO inhibitor).
No products indexed under this heading.

Pentobarbital Sodium (Co-administration may exhibit an additive CNS depression). Products include:
Nembutal Sodium Solution 485

Perphenazine (Co-administration may exhibit an additive CNS depression). Products include:
Etrafon 3115
Trilafon 3160

Phenelzine Sulfate (Co-administration with MAO inhibitors may increase the effect of either hydrocodone or MAO inhibitor). Products include:
Nardil Tablets 2653

Phenobarbital (Co-administration may exhibit an additive CNS depression). Products include:
Arco-Lase Plus Tablets 592
Donnatal 2929
Donnatal Extentabs 2930

Pimozide (Co-administration may exhibit an additive CNS depression). Products include:
Orap Tablets 1407

Prazepam (Co-administration may exhibit an additive CNS depression).
No products indexed under this heading.

Procarbazine Hydrochloride (Co-administration with MAO inhibitors may increase the effect of either hydrocodone or MAO inhibitor). Products include:
Matulane Capsules 3246

Prochlorperazine (Co-administration may exhibit an additive CNS depression). Products include:
Compazine 1505

Promethazine Hydrochloride (Co-administration may exhibit an additive CNS depression). Products include:
Mepergan Injection 3539
Phenergan Injection 3553
Phenergan 3556
Phenergan Syrup 3554
Phenergan with Codeine Syrup 3557
Phenergan with Dextromethorphan Syrup 3559
Phenergan VC Syrup 3560
Phenergan VC with Codeine Syrup 3561

Propofol (Co-administration may exhibit an additive CNS depression). Products include:
Diprivan Injectable Emulsion 667

Propoxyphene Hydrochloride (Co-administration may exhibit an additive CNS depression). Products include:
Darvon Pulvules 1909
Darvon Compound-65 Pulvules 1910

Propoxyphene Napsylate (Co-administration may exhibit an additive CNS depression). Products include:
Darvon-N/Darvocet-N 1907
Darvon-N Tablets 1912

Protriptyline Hydrochloride (Co-administration with tricyclic antidepressant may increase the effect of either hydrocodone or tricyclic antidepressant). Products include:
Vivactil Tablets 2446
Vivactil Tablets 2217

Pyrilamine Maleate (Co-administration may exhibit an additive CNS depression). Products include:
- Maximum Strength Midol Menstrual Caplets and Gelcaps .... ⊡612
- Maximum Strength Midol PMS Caplets and Gelcaps .... ⊡613

Pyrilamine Tannate (Co-administration may exhibit an additive CNS depression). Products include:
- Ryna-12 S Suspension 3351

Quazepam (Co-administration may exhibit an additive CNS depression).
- No products indexed under this heading.

Quetiapine Fumarate (Co-administration may exhibit an additive CNS depression). Products include:
- Seroquel Tablets 684

Remifentanil Hydrochloride (Co-administration may exhibit an additive CNS depression).
- No products indexed under this heading.

Risperidone (Co-administration may exhibit an additive CNS depression). Products include:
- Risperdal 1796

Secobarbital Sodium (Co-administration may exhibit an additive CNS depression).
- No products indexed under this heading.

Selegiline Hydrochloride (Co-administration with MAO inhibitors may increase the effect of either hydrocodone or MAO inhibitor). Products include:
- Eldepryl Capsules 3266

Sevoflurane (Co-administration may exhibit an additive CNS depression).
- No products indexed under this heading.

Sufentanil Citrate (Co-administration may exhibit an additive CNS depression).
- No products indexed under this heading.

Temazepam (Co-administration may exhibit an additive CNS depression).
- No products indexed under this heading.

Terfenadine (Co-administration may exhibit an additive CNS depression).
- No products indexed under this heading.

Thiamylal Sodium (Co-administration may exhibit an additive CNS depression).
- No products indexed under this heading.

Thioridazine Hydrochloride (Co-administration may exhibit an additive CNS depression). Products include:
- Thioridazine Hydrochloride Tablets 2289

Thiothixene (Co-administration may exhibit an additive CNS depression). Products include:
- Navane Capsules 2701
- Thiothixene Capsules 2290

Tranylcypromine Sulfate (Co-administration with MAO inhibitors may increase the effect of either hydrocodone or MAO inhibitor). Products include:
- Parnate Tablets 1607

Triazolam (Co-administration may exhibit an additive CNS depression). Products include:
- Halcion Tablets 2823

Trifluoperazine Hydrochloride (Co-administration may exhibit an additive CNS depression). Products include:
- Stelazine 1640

Trimeprazine Tartrate (Co-administration may exhibit an additive CNS depression).
- No products indexed under this heading.

Trimipramine Maleate (Co-administration with tricyclic antidepressant may increase the effect of either hydrocodone or tricyclic antidepressant). Products include:
- Surmontil Capsules 3595

Tripelennamine Hydrochloride (Co-administration may exhibit an additive CNS depression).
- No products indexed under this heading.

Triprolidine Hydrochloride (Co-administration may exhibit an additive CNS depression). Products include:
- Actifed Cold & Allergy Tablets .... ⊡688

Zaleplon (Co-administration may exhibit an additive CNS depression). Products include:
- Sonata Capsules 3591

Ziprasidone Hydrochloride (Co-administration may exhibit an additive CNS depression). Products include:
- Geodon Capsules 2688

Zolpidem Tartrate (Co-administration may exhibit an additive CNS depression). Products include:
- Ambien Tablets 3191

Food Interactions

Alcohol (Co-administration may exhibit an additive CNS depression).

MAXIPIME FOR INJECTION
(Cefepime Hydrochloride) 1285
May interact with aminoglycosides and certain other agents. Compounds in these categories include:

Amikacin Sulfate (Co-administration increases the potential for nephrotoxicity and ototoxicity of aminoglycoside antibiotics).
- No products indexed under this heading.

Furosemide (Co-administration with furosemide and other cephalosporins has resulted in nephrotoxicity). Products include:
- Furosemide Tablets 2284

Gentamicin Sulfate (Co-administration increases the potential for nephrotoxicity and ototoxicity of aminoglycoside antibiotics). Products include:
- Genoptic Ophthalmic Ointment .... ⊙239
- Genoptic Sterile Ophthalmic Solution .... ⊙239
- Pred-G Ophthalmic Suspension .... ⊙247
- Pred-G Sterile Ophthalmic Ointment .... ⊙248

Kanamycin Sulfate (Co-administration increases the potential for nephrotoxicity and ototoxicity of aminoglycoside antibiotics).
- No products indexed under this heading.

Streptomycin Sulfate (Co-administration increases the potential for nephrotoxicity and ototoxicity of aminoglycoside antibiotics). Products include:
- Streptomycin Sulfate Injection 2714

Tobramycin (Co-administration increases the potential for nephrotoxicity and ototoxicity of aminoglycoside antibiotics). Products include:
- TOBI Solution for Inhalation 1206
- TobraDex Ophthalmic Ointment 542
- TobraDex Ophthalmic Suspension 541
- Tobrex Ophthalmic Ointment .... ⊙220
- Tobrex Ophthalmic Solution .... ⊙221

Tobramycin Sulfate (Co-administration increases the potential for nephrotoxicity and ototoxicity of aminoglycoside antibiotics). Products include:
- Nebcin Vials, Hyporets & ADD-Vantage 1955

MAXZIDE TABLETS
(Hydrochlorothiazide, Triamterene) 1008
May interact with ACE inhibitors, antihypertensives, barbiturates, cardiac glycosides, insulin, lithium preparations, narcotic analgesics, non-steroidal anti-inflammatory agents, potassium preparations, potassium sparing diuretics, and certain other agents. Compounds in these categories include:

Acebutolol Hydrochloride (Potential for additive or augmentative effect). Products include:
- Sectral Capsules 3589

Alfentanil Hydrochloride (May aggravate orthostatic hypotension).
- No products indexed under this heading.

Amiloride Hydrochloride (Increased risk of hyperkalemia; co-administration with other potassium-conserving agents is contraindicated). Products include:
- Midamor Tablets 2136
- Moduretic Tablets 2138

Amlodipine Besylate (Potential for additive or augmentative effect). Products include:
- Lotrel Capsules 2370
- Norvasc Tablets 2704

Aprobarbital (May aggravate orthostatic hypotension).
- No products indexed under this heading.

Atenolol (Potential for additive or augmentative effect). Products include:
- Tenoretic Tablets 690
- Tenormin I.V. Injection 692

Benazepril Hydrochloride (Co-administration of potassium-sparing agents with ACE inhibitors greatly increases the risk of hyperkalemia; concurrent use should be undertaken with extreme caution). Products include:
- Lotensin Tablets 2365
- Lotensin HCT Tablets 2367
- Lotrel Capsules 2370

Bendroflumethiazide (Potential for additive or augmentative effect). Products include:
- Corzide 40/5 Tablets 2247
- Corzide 80/5 Tablets 2247

Betaxolol Hydrochloride (Potential for additive or augmentative effect). Products include:
- Betoptic S Ophthalmic Suspension 537

Bisoprolol Fumarate (Potential for additive or augmentative effect). Products include:
- Zebeta Tablets 1885
- Ziac Tablets 1887

Buprenorphine Hydrochloride (May aggravate orthostatic hypotension). Products include:
- Buprenex Injectable 2918

Butabarbital (May aggravate orthostatic hypotension).
- No products indexed under this heading.

Butalbital (May aggravate orthostatic hypotension). Products include:
- Phrenilin 578
- Sedapap Tablets 50 mg/650 mg 2225

Candesartan Cilexetil (Potential for additive or augmentative effect). Products include:
- Atacand Tablets 595
- Atacand HCT Tablets 597

Captopril (Co-administration of potassium-sparing agents with ACE inhibitors greatly increases the risk of hyperkalemia; concurrent use should be undertaken with extreme caution). Products include:
- Captopril Tablets 2281

Carteolol Hydrochloride (Potential for additive or augmentative effect). Products include:
- Carteolol Hydrochloride Ophthalmic Solution USP, 1% .... ⊙258
- Ocupress Ophthalmic Solution, 1% Sterile .... ⊙303

Celecoxib (Potential for acute renal failure). Products include:
- Celebrex Capsules 2676
- Celebrex Capsules 2780

Chlorothiazide (Potential for additive or augmentative effect). Products include:
- Aldoclor Tablets 2035
- Diuril Oral 2087

Chlorothiazide Sodium (Potential for additive or augmentative effect). Products include:
- Diuril Sodium Intravenous 2086

Chlorthalidone (Potential for additive or augmentative effect). Products include:
- Clorpres Tablets 1002
- Combipres Tablets 1040
- Tenoretic Tablets 690

Clonidine (Potential for additive or augmentative effect). Products include:
- Catapres-TTS 1038

Clonidine Hydrochloride (Potential for additive or augmentative effect). Products include:
- Catapres Tablets 1037
- Clorpres Tablets 1002
- Combipres Tablets 1040
- Duraclon Injection 3057

Codeine Phosphate (May aggravate orthostatic hypotension). Products include:
- Phenergan with Codeine Syrup 3557
- Phenergan VC with Codeine Syrup 3561
- Robitussin A-C Syrup 2942
- Robitussin-DAC Syrup 2942
- Ryna-C Liquid .... ⊡768
- Soma Compound w/Codeine Tablets 3355
- Tussi-Organidin NR Liquid 3350
- Tussi-Organidin-S NR Liquid 3350
- Tylenol with Codeine 2595

Deserpidine (Potential for additive or augmentative effect).
- No products indexed under this heading.

Deslanoside (Potential for digitalis toxicity due to hypokalemia).
- No products indexed under this heading.

Dezocine (May aggravate orthostatic hypotension).
- No products indexed under this heading.

Diazoxide (Potential for additive or augmentative effect).
- No products indexed under this heading.

Diclofenac Potassium (Potential for acute renal failure). Products include:
- Cataflam Tablets 2315

Diclofenac Sodium (Potential for acute renal failure). Products include:
- Arthrotec Tablets 3195
- Voltaren Ophthalmic Sterile Ophthalmic Solution .... ⊙312
- Voltaren Tablets 2315
- Voltaren-XR Tablets 2315

Digitoxin (Potential for digitalis toxicity due to hypokalemia).
- No products indexed under this heading.

Digoxin (Potential for digitalis toxicity due to hypokalemia). Products include:
- Digitek Tablets 1003
- Lanoxicaps Capsules 1574
- Lanoxin Injection 1581
- Lanoxin Tablets 1587
- Lanoxin Elixir Pediatric 1578
- Lanoxin Injection Pediatric 1584

Diltiazem Hydrochloride (Potential for additive or augmentative effect). Products include:
- Cardizem Injectable 1018
- Cardizem Lyo-Ject Syringe 1018

Cardizem Monovial 1018
Cardizem CD Capsules 1016
Tiazac Capsules 1378

Doxazosin Mesylate (Potential for additive or augmentative effect). Products include:
Cardura Tablets 2668

Enalapril Maleate (Co-administration of potassium-sparing agents with ACE inhibitors greatly increases the risk of hyperkalemia; concurrent use should be undertaken with extreme caution). Products include:
Lexxel Tablets 608
Vaseretic Tablets 2204
Vasotec Tablets 2210

Enalaprilat (Co-administration of potassium-sparing agents with ACE inhibitors greatly increases the risk of hyperkalemia; concurrent use should be undertaken with extreme caution). Products include:
Enalaprilat Injection 863
Vasotec I.V. Injection 2207

Eprosartan Mesylate (Potential for additive or augmentative effect). Products include:
Teveten Tablets 3327

Esmolol Hydrochloride (Potential for additive or augmentative effect). Products include:
Brevibloc Injection 858

Etodolac (Potential for acute renal failure). Products include:
Lodine 3528
Lodine XL Extended-Release Tablets 3530

Felodipine (Potential for additive or augmentative effect). Products include:
Lexxel Tablets 608
Plendil Extended-Release Tablets ... 623

Fenoprofen Calcium (Potential for acute renal failure).
No products indexed under this heading.

Fentanyl (May aggravate orthostatic hypotension). Products include:
Duragesic Transdermal System 1786

Fentanyl Citrate (May aggravate orthostatic hypotension). Products include:
Actiq 1184

Flurbiprofen (Potential for acute renal failure).
No products indexed under this heading.

Fosinopril Sodium (Co-administration of potassium-sparing agents with ACE inhibitors greatly increases the risk of hyperkalemia; concurrent use should be undertaken with extreme caution). Products include:
Monopril Tablets 1091
Monopril HCT 1094

Furosemide (Potential for additive or augmentative effect). Products include:
Furosemide Tablets 2284

Guanabenz Acetate (Potential for additive or augmentative effect).
No products indexed under this heading.

Guanethidine Monosulfate (Potential for additive or augmentative effect).
No products indexed under this heading.

Hydralazine Hydrochloride (Potential for additive or augmentative effect).
No products indexed under this heading.

Hydrocodone Bitartrate (May aggravate orthostatic hypotension). Products include:
Hycodan 1316
Hycomine Compound Tablets 1317
Hycotuss Expectorant Syrup 1318
Lortab 3319
Lortab Elixir 3317
Maxidone Tablets CIII 3399
Norco 5/325 Tablets CIII 3424
Norco 7.5/325 Tablets CIII 3425
Norco 10/325 Tablets CIII 3427
Norco 10/325 Tablets CIII 3425
Vicodin Tablets 516
Vicodin ES Tablets 517
Vicodin HP Tablets 518
Vicodin Tuss Expectorant 519
Vicoprofen Tablets 520
Zydone Tablets 1330

Hydrocodone Polistirex (May aggravate orthostatic hypotension). Products include:
Tussionex Pennkinetic Extended-Release Suspension 1174

Hydroflumethiazide (Potential for additive or augmentative effect). Products include:
Diucardin Tablets 3494

Hydromorphone Hydrochloride (May aggravate orthostatic hypotension). Products include:
Dilaudid 441
Dilaudid Oral Liquid 445
Dilaudid Powder 441
Dilaudid Rectal Suppositories 441
Dilaudid Tablets 441
Dilaudid Tablets - 8 mg 445
Dilaudid-HP 443

Ibuprofen (Potential for acute renal failure). Products include:
Advil .... ▣771
Children's Advil Oral Suspension ... ▣773
Children's Advil Chewable Tablets ... ▣773
Advil Cold and Sinus Caplets .... ▣771
Advil Cold and Sinus Tablets .... ▣771
Advil Flu & Body Ache Caplets ...... ▣772
Infants' Advil Drops .... ▣773
Junior Strength Advil Tablets .... ▣773
Junior Strength Advil Chewable Tablets .... ▣773
Advil Migraine Liquigels .... ▣772
Children's Motrin Oral Suspension and Chewable Tablets 2006
Children's Motrin Cold Oral Suspension 2007
Children's Motrin Oral Suspension .... ▣643
Motrin Suspension, Oral Drops, Chewable Tablets, and Caplets 2002
Infants' Motrin Concentrated Drops 2006
Junior Strength Motrin Caplets and Chewable Tablets 2006
Motrin IB Tablets, Caplets, and Gelcaps 2002
Motrin Migraine Pain Caplets 2005
Motrin Sinus Headache Caplets 2005
Vicoprofen Tablets 520

Indapamide (Potential for additive or augmentative effect). Products include:
Indapamide Tablets 2286

Indomethacin (Potential for acute renal failure). Products include:
Indocin 2112

Indomethacin Sodium Trihydrate (Potential for acute renal failure). Products include:
Indocin I.V. 2115

Insulin, Human, Zinc Suspension (Insulin requirements in diabetics may be altered). Products include:
Humulin L, 100 Units 1937
Humulin U, 100 Units 1943
Novolin L Human Insulin 10 ml Vials 2422

Insulin, Human NPH (Insulin requirements in diabetics may be altered). Products include:
Humulin N, 100 Units 1939
Humulin N NPH Pen 1940
Novolin N Human Insulin 10 ml Vials 2422
Novolin N PenFill 2423
Novolin N Prefilled Syringe Disposable Insulin Delivery System 2425

Insulin, Human Regular (Insulin requirements in diabetics may be altered). Products include:
Humulin R Regular (U-500) 1943
Humulin R, 100 Units 1941
Novolin R Human Insulin 10 ml Vials 2423
Novolin R PenFill 2423
Novolin R Prefilled Syringe Disposable Insulin Delivery System 2425
Velosulin BR Human Insulin 10 ml Vials 2435

Insulin, Human Regular and Human NPH Mixture (Insulin requirements in diabetics may be altered). Products include:
Humulin 50/50, 100 Units 1934
Humulin 70/30, 100 Units 1935
Humulin 70/30 Pen 1936
Novolin 70/30 Human Insulin 10 ml Vials 2421
Novolin 70/30 PenFill 2423
Novolin 70/30 Prefilled Disposable Insulin Delivery System 2425

Insulin, NPH (Insulin requirements in diabetics may be altered). Products include:
Iletin II, NPH (Pork), 100 Units 1946

Insulin, Regular (Insulin requirements in diabetics may be altered). Products include:
Iletin II, Regular (Pork), 100 Units ... 1947

Insulin, Zinc Crystals (Insulin requirements in diabetics may be altered).
No products indexed under this heading.

Insulin, Zinc Suspension (Insulin requirements in diabetics may be altered). Products include:
Iletin II, Lente (Pork), 100 Units 1945

Insulin Aspart, Human Regular (Insulin requirements in diabetics may be altered).
No products indexed under this heading.

Insulin glargine (Insulin requirements in diabetics may be altered). Products include:
Lantus Injection 742

Insulin Lispro, Human (Insulin requirements in diabetics may be altered). Products include:
Humalog 1926
Humalog Mix 75/25 Pen 1928

Insulin Lispro Protamine, Human (Insulin requirements in diabetics may be altered). Products include:
Humalog Mix 75/25 Pen 1928

Irbesartan (Potential for additive or augmentative effect). Products include:
Avalide Tablets 1070
Avapro Tablets 1074
Avapro Tablets 3076

Isradipine (Potential for additive or augmentative effect). Products include:
DynaCirc Capsules 2921
DynaCirc CR Tablets 2923

Ketoprofen (Potential for acute renal failure). Products include:
Orudis Capsules 3548
Orudis KT Tablets .... ▣778
Oruvail Capsules 3548

Ketorolac Tromethamine (Potential for acute renal failure). Products include:
Acular Ophthalmic Solution 544
Acular PF Ophthalmic Solution 544
Toradol 3018

Labetalol Hydrochloride (Potential for additive or augmentative effect). Products include:
Normodyne Injection 3135
Normodyne Tablets 3137

Levorphanol Tartrate (May aggravate orthostatic hypotension). Products include:
Levo-Dromoran 1734
Levorphanol Tartrate Tablets 3059

Lisinopril (Co-administration of potassium-sparing agents with ACE inhibitors greatly increases the risk of hyperkalemia; concurrent use should be undertaken with extreme caution). Products include:
Prinivil Tablets 2164
Prinzide Tablets 2168
Zestoretic Tablets 695
Zestril Tablets 698

Lithium Carbonate (Diuretics tend to reduce lithium renal clearance and add a high risk of lithium toxicity). Products include:
Eskalith 1527
Lithium Carbonate 3061
Lithobid Slow-Release Tablets 3255

Lithium Citrate (Diuretics tend to reduce lithium renal clearance and add a high risk of lithium toxicity). Products include:
Lithium Citrate Syrup 3061

Losartan Potassium (Potential for additive or augmentative effect). Products include:
Cozaar Tablets 2067
Hyzaar 2109

Mecamylamine Hydrochloride (Potential for additive or augmentative effect). Products include:
Inversine Tablets 1850

Meclofenamate Sodium (Potential for acute renal failure).
No products indexed under this heading.

Mefenamic Acid (Potential for acute renal failure). Products include:
Ponstel Capsules 1356

Meloxicam (Potential for acute renal failure). Products include:
Mobic Tablets 1054

Meperidine Hydrochloride (May aggravate orthostatic hypotension). Products include:
Demerol 3079
Mepergan Injection 3539

Mephobarbital (May aggravate orthostatic hypotension).
No products indexed under this heading.

Methadone Hydrochloride (May aggravate orthostatic hypotension). Products include:
Dolophine Hydrochloride Tablets 3056

Methyclothiazide (Potential for additive or augmentative effect).
No products indexed under this heading.

Methyldopa (Potential for additive or augmentative effect). Products include:
Aldoclor Tablets 2035
Aldomet Tablets 2037
Aldoril Tablets 2039

Methyldopate Hydrochloride (Potential for additive or augmentative effect).
No products indexed under this heading.

Metolazone (Potential for additive or augmentative effect). Products include:
Mykrox Tablets 1168
Zaroxolyn Tablets 1177

Metoprolol Succinate (Potential for additive or augmentative effect). Products include:
Toprol-XL Tablets 651

Metoprolol Tartrate (Potential for additive or augmentative effect).
No products indexed under this heading.

Metyrosine (Potential for additive or augmentative effect). Products include:
Demser Capsules 2085

Mibefradil Dihydrochloride (Potential for additive or augmentative effect).
No products indexed under this heading.

Minoxidil (Potential for additive or augmentative effect). Products include:
Rogaine Extra Strength for Men Topical Solution .... ▣721
Rogaine for Women Topical Solution .... ▣721

Moexipril Hydrochloride (Co-administration of potassium-sparing agents with ACE inhibitors greatly increases the risk of hyperkalemia; concurrent use should be undertaken with extreme caution). Products include:
Uniretic Tablets 3178
Univasc Tablets 3181

Morphine Sulfate (May aggravate orthostatic hypotension). Products include:
- Astramorph/PF Injection, USP (Preservative-Free) 594
- Duramorph Injection 1312
- Infumorph 200 and Infumorph 500 Sterile Solutions 1314
- Kadian Capsules 1335
- MS Contin Tablets 2896
- MSIR 2898
- Oramorph SR Tablets 3062
- Roxanol 3066

Nabumetone (Potential for acute renal failure). Products include:
- Relafen Tablets 1617

Nadolol (Potential for additive or augmentative effect). Products include:
- Corgard Tablets 2245
- Corzide 40/5 Tablets 2247
- Corzide 80/5 Tablets 2247
- Nadolol Tablets 2288

Naproxen (Potential for acute renal failure). Products include:
- EC-Naprosyn Delayed-Release Tablets 2967
- Naprosyn Suspension 2967
- Naprosyn Tablets 2967

Naproxen Sodium (Potential for acute renal failure). Products include:
- Aleve Tablets, Caplets and Gelcaps 602
- Aleve Cold & Sinus Caplets 603
- Anaprox Tablets 2967
- Anaprox DS Tablets 2967
- Naprelan Tablets 1293

Nicardipine Hydrochloride (Potential for additive or augmentative effect). Products include:
- Cardene I.V. 3485

Nifedipine (Potential for additive or augmentative effect). Products include:
- Adalat CC Tablets 877
- Procardia Capsules 2708
- Procardia XL Extended Release Tablets 2710

Nisoldipine (Potential for additive or augmentative effect). Products include:
- Sular Tablets 688

Nitroglycerin (Potential for additive or augmentative effect). Products include:
- Nitro-Dur Transdermal Infusion System 3134
- Nitro-Dur Transdermal Infusion System 1834
- Nitrolingual Pumpspray 1355
- Nitrostat Tablets 2658

Oxaprozin (Potential for acute renal failure).
No products indexed under this heading.

Oxycodone Hydrochloride (May aggravate orthostatic hypotension). Products include:
- OxyContin Tablets 2912
- OxyFast Oral Concentrate Solution 2916
- OxyIR Capsules 2916
- Percocet Tablets 1326
- Percodan Tablets 1327
- Percolone Tablets 1327
- Roxicodone 3067
- Tylox Capsules 2597

Penbutolol Sulfate (Potential for additive or augmentative effect).
No products indexed under this heading.

Pentobarbital Sodium (May aggravate orthostatic hypotension). Products include:
- Nembutal Sodium Solution 485

Perindopril Erbumine (Co-administration of potassium-sparing agents with ACE inhibitors greatly increases the risk of hyperkalemia; concurrent use should be undertaken with extreme caution). Products include:
- Aceon Tablets (2 mg, 4 mg, 8 mg) 3249

Phenobarbital (May aggravate orthostatic hypotension). Products include:
- Arco-Lase Plus Tablets 592
- Donnatal 2929
- Donnatal Extentabs 2930

Phenoxybenzamine Hydrochloride (Potential for additive or augmentative effect). Products include:
- Dibenzyline Capsules 3457

Phentolamine Mesylate (Potential for additive or augmentative effect).
No products indexed under this heading.

Phenylbutazone (Potential for acute renal failure).
No products indexed under this heading.

Pindolol (Potential for additive or augmentative effect).
No products indexed under this heading.

Piroxicam (Potential for acute renal failure). Products include:
- Feldene Capsules 2685

Polythiazide (Potential for additive or augmentative effect). Products include:
- Minizide Capsules 2700
- Renese Tablets 2712

Potassium Acid Phosphate (Concomitant administration is contraindicated). Products include:
- K-Phos Original (Sodium Free) Tablets 947

Potassium Bicarbonate (Concomitant administration is contraindicated).
No products indexed under this heading.

Potassium Chloride (Concomitant administration is contraindicated). Products include:
- Chlor-3 1361
- Colyte with Flavor Packs for Oral Solution 3170
- GoLYTELY and Pineapple Flavor GoLYTELY for Oral Solution 1068
- K-Dur Microburst Release System ER Tablets 1832
- Klor-Con M20/Klor-Con M10 Tablets 3329
- K-Lor Powder Packets 469
- K-Tab Filmtab Tablets 470
- Micro-K 3311
- NuLYTELY, Cherry Flavor, Lemon-Lime Flavor, and Orange Flavor NuLYTELY for Oral Solution 1068
- Rum-K 1363

Potassium Citrate (Concomitant administration is contraindicated). Products include:
- Urocit-K Tablets 2232

Potassium Gluconate (Concomitant administration is contraindicated).
No products indexed under this heading.

Potassium Phosphate (Concomitant administration is contraindicated). Products include:
- K-Phos Neutral Tablets 946

Prazosin Hydrochloride (Potential for additive or augmentative effect). Products include:
- Minipress Capsules 2699
- Minizide Capsules 2700

Propoxyphene Hydrochloride (May aggravate orthostatic hypotension). Products include:
- Darvon Pulvules 1909
- Darvon Compound-65 Pulvules 1910

Propoxyphene Napsylate (May aggravate orthostatic hypotension). Products include:
- Darvon-N/Darvocet-N 1907
- Darvon-N Tablets 1912

Propranolol Hydrochloride (Potential for additive or augmentative effect). Products include:
- Inderal 3513
- Inderal LA Long-Acting Capsules 3516
- Inderide Tablets 3517
- Inderide LA Long-Acting Capsules 3519

Quinapril Hydrochloride (Co-administration of potassium-sparing agents with ACE inhibitors greatly increases the risk of hyperkalemia; concurrent use should be undertaken with extreme caution). Products include:
- Accupril Tablets 2611
- Accuretic Tablets 2614

Ramipril (Co-administration of potassium-sparing agents with ACE inhibitors greatly increases the risk of hyperkalemia; concurrent use should be undertaken with extreme caution). Products include:
- Altace Capsules 2233

Rauwolfia serpentina (Potential for additive or augmentative effect).
No products indexed under this heading.

Remifentanil Hydrochloride (May aggravate orthostatic hypotension).
No products indexed under this heading.

Rescinnamine (Potential for additive or augmentative effect).
No products indexed under this heading.

Reserpine (Potential for additive or augmentative effect).
No products indexed under this heading.

Rofecoxib (Potential for acute renal failure). Products include:
- Vioxx 2213

Secobarbital Sodium (May aggravate orthostatic hypotension).
No products indexed under this heading.

Sodium Nitroprusside (Potential for additive or augmentative effect).
No products indexed under this heading.

Sotalol Hydrochloride (Potential for additive or augmentative effect). Products include:
- Betapace Tablets 950
- Betapace AF Tablets 954

Spirapril Hydrochloride (Co-administration of potassium-sparing agents with ACE inhibitors greatly increases the risk of hyperkalemia; concurrent use should be undertaken with extreme caution).
No products indexed under this heading.

Spironolactone (Increased risk of hyperkalemia; co-administration with other potassium-conserving agents is contraindicated).
No products indexed under this heading.

Sufentanil Citrate (May aggravate orthostatic hypotension).
No products indexed under this heading.

Sulindac (Potential for acute renal failure). Products include:
- Clinoril Tablets 2053

Telmisartan (Potential for additive or augmentative effect). Products include:
- Micardis Tablets 1049
- Micardis HCT Tablets 1051

Terazosin Hydrochloride (Potential for additive or augmentative effect). Products include:
- Hytrin Capsules 464

Thiamylal Sodium (May aggravate orthostatic hypotension).
No products indexed under this heading.

Timolol Maleate (Potential for additive or augmentative effect). Products include:
- Blocadren Tablets 2046
- Cosopt Sterile Ophthalmic Solution 2065
- Timolide Tablets 2187
- Timolol GFS .... ⊙266
- Timoptic in Ocudose 2192
- Timoptic Sterile Ophthalmic Solution 2190
- Timoptic-XE Sterile Ophthalmic Gel Forming Solution 2194

Tolmetin Sodium (Potential for acute renal failure). Products include:
- Tolectin 2589

Torsemide (Potential for additive or augmentative effect). Products include:
- Demadex Tablets and Injection 2965

Trandolapril (Co-administration of potassium-sparing agents with ACE inhibitors greatly increases the risk of hyperkalemia; concurrent use should be undertaken with extreme caution). Products include:
- Mavik Tablets 478
- Tarka Tablets 508

Trimethaphan Camsylate (Potential for additive or augmentative effect).
No products indexed under this heading.

Valsartan (Potential for additive or augmentative effect). Products include:
- Diovan Capsules 2337
- Diovan HCT Tablets 2338

Verapamil Hydrochloride (Potential for additive or augmentative effect). Products include:
- Covera-HS Tablets 3199
- Isoptin SR Tablets 467
- Tarka Tablets 508
- Verelan Capsules 3184
- Verelan PM Capsules 3186

Food Interactions

Alcohol (May aggravate orthostatic hypotension).

Diet, potassium-rich (Concurrent use is contraindicated).

MAXZIDE-25 MG TABLETS
(Hydrochlorothiazide, Triamterene) 1008
See Maxzide Tablets

MAY-VITA ELIXIR
(Vitamins with Minerals) 2224
None cited in PDR database.

MDR FITNESS TABS FOR MEN AND WOMEN
(Vitamins with Minerals) 2018
None cited in PDR database.

MEFOXIN FOR INJECTION
(Cefoxitin Sodium) 2124
May interact with aminoglycosides and certain other agents. Compounds in these categories include:

Amikacin Sulfate (Increased nephrotoxicity).
No products indexed under this heading.

Gentamicin Sulfate (Increased nephrotoxicity). Products include:
- Genoptic Ophthalmic Ointment .... ⊙239
- Genoptic Sterile Ophthalmic Solution .... ⊙239
- Pred-G Ophthalmic Suspension .... ⊙247
- Pred-G Sterile Ophthalmic Ointment .... ⊙248

Kanamycin Sulfate (Increased nephrotoxicity).
No products indexed under this heading.

Probenecid (Slows tubular excretion and produces higher serum levels of cefoxitin).
No products indexed under this heading.

Streptomycin Sulfate (Increased nephrotoxicity). Products include:
- Streptomycin Sulfate Injection 2714

Tobramycin (Increased nephrotoxicity). Products include:
- TOBI Solution for Inhalation 1206
- TobraDex Ophthalmic Ointment 542
- TobraDex Ophthalmic Suspension 541
- Tobrex Ophthalmic Ointment .... ⊙220
- Tobrex Ophthalmic Solution .... ⊙221

Tobramycin Sulfate (Increased nephrotoxicity). Products include:
- Nebcin Vials, Hyporets & ADD-Vantage 1955

MEFOXIN PREMIXED INTRAVENOUS SOLUTION
(Cefoxitin Sodium) 2127
May interact with aminoglycosides and certain other agents. Compounds in these categories include:

Amikacin Sulfate (Increased nephrotoxicity).
No products indexed under this heading.

Gentamicin Sulfate (Increased nephrotoxicity). Products include:
Genoptic Ophthalmic Ointment ...... ⊙239
Genoptic Sterile Ophthalmic Solution .... ⊙239
Pred-G Ophthalmic Suspension ..... ⊙247
Pred-G Sterile Ophthalmic Ointment .... ⊙248

Kanamycin Sulfate (Increased nephrotoxicity).
No products indexed under this heading.

Probenecid (Higher serum levels of cefoxitin).
No products indexed under this heading.

Streptomycin Sulfate (Increased nephrotoxicity). Products include:
Streptomycin Sulfate Injection 2714

Tobramycin (Increased nephrotoxicity). Products include:
TOBI Solution for Inhalation 1206
TobraDex Ophthalmic Ointment 542
TobraDex Ophthalmic Suspension .. 541
Tobrex Ophthalmic Ointment .... ⊙220
Tobrex Ophthalmic Solution .... ⊙221

Tobramycin Sulfate (Increased nephrotoxicity). Products include:
Nebcin Vials, Hyporets & ADD-Vantage 1955

MEGA ANTIOXIDANT TABLETS
(Vitamins, Multiple) 3335
None cited in PDR database.

MEGA-B TABLETS
(Vitamin B Complex) 592
None cited in PDR database.

MEGACE ORAL SUSPENSION
(Megestrol Acetate) 1124
May interact with insulin. Compounds in these categories include:

Insulin, Human, Zinc Suspension (Exacerbation of pre-existing diabetes with increased insulin requirements have been reported in association with the use of Megace).
Products include:
Humulin L, 100 Units 1937
Humulin U, 100 Units 1943
Novolin L Human Insulin 10 ml Vials 2422

Insulin, Human NPH (Exacerbation of pre-existing diabetes with increased insulin requirements have been reported in association with the use of Megace). Products include:
Humulin N, 100 Units 1939
Humulin N NPH Pen 1940
Novolin N Human Insulin 10 ml Vials 2422
Novolin N PenFill 2423
Novolin N Prefilled Syringe Disposable Insulin Delivery System 2425

Insulin, Human Regular (Exacerbation of pre-existing diabetes with increased insulin requirements have been reported in association with the use of Megace). Products include:
Humulin R Regular (U-500) 1943
Humulin R, 100 Units 1941
Novolin R Human Insulin 10 ml Vials 2423
Novolin R PenFill 2423
Novolin R Prefilled Syringe Disposable Insulin Delivery System 2425
Velosulin BR Human Insulin 10 ml Vials 2435

Insulin, Human Regular and Human NPH Mixture (Exacerbation of pre-existing diabetes with increased insulin requirements have been reported in association with the use of Megace). Products include:
Humulin 50/50, 100 Units 1934
Humulin 70/30, 100 Units 1935
Humulin 70/30 Pen 1936
Novolin 70/30 Human Insulin 10 ml Vials 2421
Novolin 70/30 PenFill 2423
Novolin 70/30 Prefilled Disposable Insulin Delivery System 2425

Insulin, NPH (Exacerbation of pre-existing diabetes with increased insulin requirements have been reported in association with the use of Megace). Products include:
Iletin II, NPH (Pork), 100 Units 1946

Insulin, Regular (Exacerbation of pre-existing diabetes with increased insulin requirements have been reported in association with the use of Megace). Products include:
Iletin II, Regular (Pork), 100 Units ... 1947

Insulin, Zinc Crystals (Exacerbation of pre-existing diabetes with increased insulin requirements have been reported in association with the use of Megace).
No products indexed under this heading.

Insulin, Zinc Suspension (Exacerbation of pre-existing diabetes with increased insulin requirements have been reported in association with the use of Megace). Products include:
Iletin II, Lente (Pork), 100 Units 1945

Insulin Aspart, Human Regular (Exacerbation of pre-existing diabetes with increased insulin requirements have been reported in association with the use of Megace).
No products indexed under this heading.

Insulin glargine (Exacerbation of pre-existing diabetes with increased insulin requirements have been reported in association with the use of Megace). Products include:
Lantus Injection 742

Insulin Lispro, Human (Exacerbation of pre-existing diabetes with increased insulin requirements have been reported in association with the use of Megace). Products include:
Humalog 1926
Humalog Mix 75/25 Pen 1928

Insulin Lispro Protamine, Human (Exacerbation of pre-existing diabetes with increased insulin requirements have been reported in association with the use of Megace).
Products include:
Humalog Mix 75/25 Pen 1928

MEGADOSE TABLETS
(Vitamins with Minerals) 593
None cited in PDR database.

MELANEX TOPICAL SOLUTION
(Hydroquinone) 2300
May interact with:

Hydrogen Peroxide (May result in transient dark staining of skin areas so treated).
No products indexed under this heading.

MENEST TABLETS
(Estrogens, Esterified) 2254
None cited in PDR database.

MENOMUNE-A/C/Y/W-135 VACCINE
(Meningococcal Polysaccharide Vaccine) 813
May interact with immunosuppressive agents. Compounds in these categories include:

Azathioprine (Co-administration with immunosuppressive therapy may not result in adequate immunologic response).
No products indexed under this heading.

Basiliximab (Co-administration with immunosuppressive therapy may not result in adequate immunologic response). Products include:
Simulect for Injection 2399

Cyclosporine (Co-administration with immunosuppressive therapy may not result in adequate immunologic response). Products include:
Gengraf Capsules 457
Neoral Soft Gelatin Capsules 2380
Neoral Oral Solution 2380
Sandimmune 2388

Muromonab-CD3 (Co-administration with immunosuppressive therapy may not result in adequate immunologic response).
Products include:
Orthoclone OKT3 Sterile Solution ... 2498

Mycophenolate Mofetil (Co-administration with immunosuppressive therapy may not result in adequate immunologic response).
Products include:
CellCept Capsules 2951
CellCept Oral Suspension 2951
CellCept Tablets 2951

Sirolimus (Co-administration with immunosuppressive therapy may not result in adequate immunologic response). Products include:
Rapamune Oral Solution and Tablets 3584

Tacrolimus (Co-administration with immunosuppressive therapy may not result in adequate immunologic response). Products include:
Prograf 1393
Protopic Ointment 1397

MENTAX CREAM
(Butenafine Hydrochloride) 1009
None cited in PDR database.

MEPERGAN INJECTION
(Meperidine Hydrochloride, Promethazine Hydrochloride)............ 3539
May interact with barbiturates, central nervous system depressants, general anesthetics, hypnotics and sedatives, monoamine oxidase inhibitors, narcotic analgesics, phenothiazines, tranquilizers, tricyclic antidepressants, and certain other agents. Compounds in these categories include:

Alfentanil Hydrochloride (Respiratory depression, hypotension, profound sedation or coma).
No products indexed under this heading.

Alprazolam (Respiratory depression, hypotension, profound sedation or coma). Products include:
Xanax Tablets 2865

Amitriptyline Hydrochloride (Respiratory depression, hypotension, profound sedation or coma).
Products include:
Etrafon 3115
Limbitrol 1738

Amoxapine (Respiratory depression, hypotension, profound sedation or coma).
No products indexed under this heading.

Aprobarbital (Respiratory depression, hypotension, profound sedation or coma).
No products indexed under this heading.

Buprenorphine Hydrochloride (Respiratory depression, hypotension, profound sedation or coma).
Products include:
Buprenex Injectable 2918

Buspirone Hydrochloride (Respiratory depression, hypotension, profound sedation or coma).
No products indexed under this heading.

Butabarbital (Respiratory depression, hypotension, profound sedation or coma).
No products indexed under this heading.

Butalbital (Respiratory depression, hypotension, profound sedation or coma). Products include:
Phrenilin 578
Sedapap Tablets 50 mg/650 mg ... 2225

Chlordiazepoxide (Respiratory depression, hypotension, profound sedation or coma). Products include:
Limbitrol 1738

Chlordiazepoxide Hydrochloride (Respiratory depression, hypotension, profound sedation or coma).
Products include:
Librium Capsules 1736
Librium for Injection 1737

Chlorpromazine (Respiratory depression, hypotension, profound sedation or coma). Products include:
Thorazine Suppositories 1656

Chlorpromazine Hydrochloride (Respiratory depression, hypotension, profound sedation or coma).
Products include:
Thorazine 1656

Chlorprothixene (Respiratory depression, hypotension, profound sedation or coma).
No products indexed under this heading.

Chlorprothixene Hydrochloride (Respiratory depression, hypotension, profound sedation or coma).
No products indexed under this heading.

Chlorprothixene Lactate (Respiratory depression, hypotension, profound sedation or coma).
No products indexed under this heading.

Clomipramine Hydrochloride (Respiratory depression, hypotension, profound sedation or coma).
No products indexed under this heading.

Clorazepate Dipotassium (Respiratory depression, hypotension, profound sedation or coma). Products include:
Tranxene 511

Clozapine (Respiratory depression, hypotension, profound sedation or coma). Products include:
Clozaril Tablets 2319

Codeine Phosphate (Respiratory depression, hypotension, profound sedation or coma). Products include:
Phenergan with Codeine Syrup 3557
Phenergan VC with Codeine Syrup .. 3561
Robitussin A-C Syrup 2942
Robitussin-DAC Syrup 2942
Ryna-C Liquid .... ▣768
Soma Compound w/Codeine Tablets 3355
Tussi-Organidin NR Liquid 3350
Tussi-Organidin-S NR Liquid 3350
Tylenol with Codeine 2595

Desflurane (Respiratory depression, hypotension, profound sedation or coma). Products include:
Suprane Liquid for Inhalation 874

Desipramine Hydrochloride (Respiratory depression, hypotension, profound sedation or coma).
Products include:
Norpramin Tablets 755

Dezocine (Respiratory depression, hypotension, profound sedation or coma).
No products indexed under this heading.

Diazepam (Respiratory depression, hypotension, profound sedation or coma). Products include:
Valium Injectable 3026
Valium Tablets 3047

Doxepin Hydrochloride (Respiratory depression, hypotension, profound sedation or coma). Products include:

Sinequan 2713
Droperidol (Respiratory depression, hypotension, profound sedation or coma).
No products indexed under this heading.
Enflurane (Respiratory depression, hypotension, profound sedation or coma).
No products indexed under this heading.
Estazolam (Respiratory depression, hypotension, profound sedation or coma). Products include:
ProSom Tablets 500
Ethchlorvynol (Respiratory depression, hypotension, profound sedation or coma).
No products indexed under this heading.
Ethinamate (Respiratory depression, hypotension, profound sedation or coma).
No products indexed under this heading.
Fentanyl (Respiratory depression, hypotension, profound sedation or coma). Products include:
Duragesic Transdermal System 1786
Fentanyl Citrate (Respiratory depression, hypotension, profound sedation or coma). Products include:
Actiq 1184
Fluphenazine Decanoate (Respiratory depression, hypotension, profound sedation or coma).
No products indexed under this heading.
Fluphenazine Enanthate (Respiratory depression, hypotension, profound sedation or coma).
No products indexed under this heading.
Fluphenazine Hydrochloride (Respiratory depression, hypotension, profound sedation or coma).
No products indexed under this heading.
Flurazepam Hydrochloride (Respiratory depression, hypotension, profound sedation or coma).
No products indexed under this heading.
Glutethimide (Respiratory depression, hypotension, profound sedation or coma).
No products indexed under this heading.
Haloperidol (Respiratory depression, hypotension, profound sedation or coma). Products include:
Haldol Injection, Tablets and Concentrate 2533
Haloperidol Decanoate (Respiratory depression, hypotension, profound sedation or coma). Products include:
Haldol Decanoate 2535
Hydrocodone Bitartrate (Respiratory depression, hypotension, profound sedation or coma). Products include:
Hycodan 1316
Hycomine Compound Tablets 1317
Hycotuss Expectorant Syrup 1318
Lortab 3319
Lortab Elixir 3317
Maxidone Tablets CIII 3399
Norco 5/325 Tablets CIII 3424
Norco 7.5/325 Tablets CIII 3425
Norco 10/325 Tablets CIII 3427
Norco 10/325 Tablets CIII 3425
Vicodin Tablets 516
Vicodin ES Tablets 517
Vicodin HP Tablets 518
Vicodin Tuss Expectorant 519
Vicoprofen Tablets 520
Zydone Tablets 1330
Hydrocodone Polistirex (Respiratory depression, hypotension, profound sedation or coma). Products include:
Tussionex Pennkinetic Extended-Release Suspension 1174
Hydromorphone Hydrochloride (Respiratory depression, hypotension, profound sedation or coma). Products include:
Dilaudid 441
Dilaudid Oral Liquid 445
Dilaudid Powder 441
Dilaudid Rectal Suppositories 441
Dilaudid Tablets 441
Dilaudid Tablets - 8 mg 445
Dilaudid-HP 443
Hydroxyzine Hydrochloride (Respiratory depression, hypotension, profound sedation or coma). Products include:
Atarax Tablets & Syrup 2667
Vistaril Intramuscular Solution 2738
Imipramine Hydrochloride (Respiratory depression, hypotension, profound sedation or coma).
No products indexed under this heading.
Imipramine Pamoate (Respiratory depression, hypotension, profound sedation or coma).
No products indexed under this heading.
Isocarboxazid (Concurrent administration is contraindicated).
No products indexed under this heading.
Isoflurane (Respiratory depression, hypotension, profound sedation or coma).
No products indexed under this heading.
Ketamine Hydrochloride (Respiratory depression, hypotension, profound sedation or coma).
No products indexed under this heading.
Levomethadyl Acetate Hydrochloride (Respiratory depression, hypotension, profound sedation or coma).
No products indexed under this heading.
Levorphanol Tartrate (Respiratory depression, hypotension, profound sedation or coma). Products include:
Levo-Dromoran 1734
Levorphanol Tartrate Tablets 3059
Lorazepam (Respiratory depression, hypotension, profound sedation or coma). Products include:
Ativan Injection 3478
Ativan Tablets 3482
Loxapine Hydrochloride (Respiratory depression, hypotension, profound sedation or coma).
No products indexed under this heading.
Loxapine Succinate (Respiratory depression, hypotension, profound sedation or coma). Products include:
Loxitane Capsules 3398
Maprotiline Hydrochloride (Respiratory depression, hypotension, profound sedation or coma).
No products indexed under this heading.
Mephobarbital (Respiratory depression, hypotension, profound sedation or coma).
No products indexed under this heading.
Meprobamate (Respiratory depression, hypotension, profound sedation or coma). Products include:
Miltown Tablets 3349
Mesoridazine Besylate (Respiratory depression, hypotension, profound sedation or coma). Products include:
Serentil 1057
Methadone Hydrochloride (Respiratory depression, hypotension, profound sedation or coma). Products include:
Dolophine Hydrochloride Tablets 3056
Methohexital Sodium (Respiratory depression, hypotension, profound sedation or coma). Products include:
Brevital Sodium for Injection, USP 1815
Methotrimeprazine (Respiratory depression, hypotension, profound sedation or coma).
No products indexed under this heading.
Methoxyflurane (Respiratory depression, hypotension, profound sedation or coma).
No products indexed under this heading.
Midazolam Hydrochloride (Respiratory depression, hypotension, profound sedation or coma). Products include:
Versed Injection 3027
Versed Syrup 3033
Moclobemide (Concurrent administration is contraindicated).
No products indexed under this heading.
Molindone Hydrochloride (Respiratory depression, hypotension, profound sedation or coma). Products include:
Moban 1320
Morphine Sulfate (Respiratory depression, hypotension, profound sedation or coma). Products include:
Astramorph/PF Injection, USP (Preservative-Free) 594
Duramorph Injection 1312
Infumorph 200 and Infumorph 500 Sterile Solutions 1314
Kadian Capsules 1335
MS Contin Tablets 2896
MSIR 2898
Oramorph SR Tablets 3062
Roxanol 3066
Nortriptyline Hydrochloride (Respiratory depression, hypotension, profound sedation or coma).
No products indexed under this heading.
Olanzapine (Respiratory depression, hypotension, profound sedation or coma). Products include:
Zyprexa Tablets 1973
Zyprexa ZYDIS Orally Disintegrating Tablets 1973
Oxazepam (Respiratory depression, hypotension, profound sedation or coma).
No products indexed under this heading.
Oxycodone Hydrochloride (Respiratory depression, hypotension, profound sedation or coma). Products include:
OxyContin Tablets 2912
OxyFast Oral Concentrate Solution 2916
OxyIR Capsules 2916
Percocet Tablets 1326
Percodan Tablets 1327
Percolone Tablets 1327
Roxicodone 3067
Tylox Capsules 2597
Pargyline Hydrochloride (Concurrent administration is contraindicated).
No products indexed under this heading.
Pentobarbital Sodium (Respiratory depression, hypotension, profound sedation or coma). Products include:
Nembutal Sodium Solution 485
Perphenazine (Respiratory depression, hypotension, profound sedation or coma). Products include:
Etrafon 3115
Trilafon 3160
Phenelzine Sulfate (Concurrent administration is contraindicated). Products include:
Nardil Tablets 2653
Phenobarbital (Respiratory depression, hypotension, profound sedation or coma). Products include:
Arco-Lase Plus Tablets 592
Donnatal 2929
Donnatal Extentabs 2930
Prazepam (Respiratory depression, hypotension, profound sedation or coma).
No products indexed under this heading.
Procarbazine Hydrochloride (Concurrent administration is contraindicated). Products include:
Matulane Capsules 3246
Prochlorperazine (Respiratory depression, hypotension, profound sedation or coma). Products include:
Compazine 1505
Propofol (Respiratory depression, hypotension, profound sedation or coma). Products include:
Diprivan Injectable Emulsion 667
Propoxyphene Hydrochloride (Respiratory depression, hypotension, profound sedation or coma). Products include:
Darvon Pulvules 1909
Darvon Compound-65 Pulvules 1910
Propoxyphene Napsylate (Respiratory depression, hypotension, profound sedation or coma). Products include:
Darvon-N/Darvocet-N 1907
Darvon-N Tablets 1912
Protriptyline Hydrochloride (Respiratory depression, hypotension, profound sedation or coma). Products include:
Vivactil Tablets 2446
Vivactil Tablets 2217
Quazepam (Respiratory depression, hypotension, profound sedation or coma).
No products indexed under this heading.
Quetiapine Fumarate (Respiratory depression, hypotension, profound sedation or coma). Products include:
Seroquel Tablets 684
Remifentanil Hydrochloride (Respiratory depression, hypotension, profound sedation or coma).
No products indexed under this heading.
Risperidone (Respiratory depression, hypotension, profound sedation or coma). Products include:
Risperdal 1796
Secobarbital Sodium (Respiratory depression, hypotension, profound sedation or coma).
No products indexed under this heading.
Selegiline Hydrochloride (Concurrent administration is contraindicated). Products include:
Eldepryl Capsules 3266
Sevoflurane (Respiratory depression, hypotension, profound sedation or coma).
No products indexed under this heading.
Sufentanil Citrate (Respiratory depression, hypotension, profound sedation or coma).
No products indexed under this heading.
Temazepam (Respiratory depression, hypotension, profound sedation or coma).
No products indexed under this heading.
Thiamylal Sodium (Respiratory depression, hypotension, profound sedation or coma).
No products indexed under this heading.
Thioridazine Hydrochloride (Respiratory depression, hypotension, profound sedation or coma). Products include:
Thioridazine Hydrochloride Tablets 2289
Thiothixene (Respiratory depression, hypotension, profound sedation or coma). Products include:
Navane Capsules 2701
Thiothixene Capsules 2290
Tranylcypromine Sulfate (Concurrent administration is contraindicated). Products include:
Parnate Tablets 1607

IMPORTANT NOTE: Always consult each drug listing in the patient's regimen for possible interactions.

Triazolam (Respiratory depression, hypotension, profound sedation or coma). Products include:
- Halcion Tablets 2823

Trifluoperazine Hydrochloride (Respiratory depression, hypotension, profound sedation or coma). Products include:
- Stelazine 1640

Trimipramine Maleate (Respiratory depression, hypotension, profound sedation or coma). Products include:
- Surmontil Capsules 3595

Zaleplon (Respiratory depression, hypotension, profound sedation or coma). Products include:
- Sonata Capsules 3591

Ziprasidone Hydrochloride (Respiratory depression, hypotension, profound sedation or coma). Products include:
- Geodon Capsules 2688

Zolpidem Tartrate (Respiratory depression, hypotension, profound sedation or coma). Products include:
- Ambien Tablets 3191

Food Interactions

Alcohol (Respiratory depression, hypotension, profound sedation or coma).

MEPHYTON TABLETS

(Vitamin K_1) 2129

None cited in PDR database.

MEPRON SUSPENSION

(Atovaquone) 1598

May interact with highly protein bound drugs (selected) and certain other agents. Compounds in these categories include:

Amiodarone Hydrochloride (Atovaquone is highly bound to plasma protein (greater than 99.9%); caution is advised when co-administered with other highly protein bound drugs with narrow therapeutic indices). Products include:
- Cordarone Intravenous 3491
- Cordarone Tablets 3487
- Pacerone Tablets 3331

Amitriptyline Hydrochloride (Atovaquone is highly bound to plasma protein (greater than 99.9%); caution is advised when co-administered with other highly protein bound drugs with narrow therapeutic indices). Products include:
- Etrafon 3115
- Limbitrol 1738

Cefonicid Sodium (Atovaquone is highly bound to plasma protein (greater than 99.9%); caution is advised when co-administered with other highly protein bound drugs with narrow therapeutic indices).

No products indexed under this heading.

Celecoxib (Atovaquone is highly bound to plasma protein (greater than 99.9%); caution is advised when co-administered with other highly protein bound drugs with narrow therapeutic indices). Products include:
- Celebrex Capsules 2676
- Celebrex Capsules 2780

Chlordiazepoxide (Atovaquone is highly bound to plasma protein (greater than 99.9%); caution is advised when co-administered with other highly protein bound drugs with narrow therapeutic indices). Products include:
- Limbitrol 1738

Chlordiazepoxide Hydrochloride (Atovaquone is highly bound to plasma protein (greater than 99.9%); caution is advised when co-administered with other highly protein bound drugs with narrow therapeutic indices). Products include:
- Librium Capsules 1736
- Librium for Injection 1737

Chlorpromazine (Atovaquone is highly bound to plasma protein (greater than 99.9%); caution is advised when co-administered with other highly protein bound drugs with narrow therapeutic indices). Products include:
- Thorazine Suppositories 1656

Chlorpromazine Hydrochloride (Atovaquone is highly bound to plasma protein (greater than 99.9%); caution is advised when co-administered with other highly protein bound drugs with narrow therapeutic indices). Products include:
- Thorazine 1656

Clomipramine Hydrochloride (Atovaquone is highly bound to plasma protein (greater than 99.9%); caution is advised when co-administered with other highly protein bound drugs with narrow therapeutic indices).

No products indexed under this heading.

Clozapine (Atovaquone is highly bound to plasma protein (greater than 99.9%); caution is advised when co-administered with other highly protein bound drugs with narrow therapeutic indices). Products include:
- Clozaril Tablets 2319

Cyclosporine (Atovaquone is highly bound to plasma protein (greater than 99.9%); caution is advised when co-administered with other highly protein bound drugs with narrow therapeutic indices). Products include:
- Gengraf Capsules 457
- Neoral Soft Gelatin Capsules 2380
- Neoral Oral Solution 2380
- Sandimmune 2388

Diazepam (Atovaquone is highly bound to plasma protein (greater than 99.9%); caution is advised when co-administered with other highly protein bound drugs with narrow therapeutic indices). Products include:
- Valium Injectable 3026
- Valium Tablets 3047

Diclofenac Potassium (Atovaquone is highly bound to plasma protein (greater than 99.9%); caution is advised when co-administered with other highly protein bound drugs with narrow therapeutic indices). Products include:
- Cataflam Tablets 2315

Diclofenac Sodium (Atovaquone is highly bound to plasma protein (greater than 99.9%); caution is advised when co-administered with other highly protein bound drugs with narrow therapeutic indices). Products include:
- Arthrotec Tablets 3195
- Voltaren Ophthalmic Sterile Ophthalmic Solution .... ⊙ 312
- Voltaren Tablets 2315
- Voltaren-XR Tablets 2315

Dipyridamole (Atovaquone is highly bound to plasma protein (greater than 99.9%); caution is advised when co-administered with other highly protein bound drugs with narrow therapeutic indices). Products include:
- Aggrenox Capsules 1026
- Persantine Tablets 1057

Fenoprofen Calcium (Atovaquone is highly bound to plasma protein (greater than 99.9%); caution is advised when co-administered with other highly protein bound drugs with narrow therapeutic indices).

No products indexed under this heading.

Flurazepam Hydrochloride (Atovaquone is highly bound to plasma protein (greater than 99.9%); caution is advised when co-administered with other highly protein bound drugs with narrow therapeutic indices).

No products indexed under this heading.

Flurbiprofen (Atovaquone is highly bound to plasma protein (greater than 99.9%); caution is advised when co-administered with other highly protein bound drugs with narrow therapeutic indices).

No products indexed under this heading.

Glipizide (Atovaquone is highly bound to plasma protein (greater than 99.9%); caution is advised when co-administered with other highly protein bound drugs with narrow therapeutic indices). Products include:
- Glucotrol Tablets 2692
- Glucotrol XL Extended Release Tablets 2693

Ibuprofen (Atovaquone is highly bound to plasma protein (greater than 99.9%); caution is advised when co-administered with other highly protein bound drugs with narrow therapeutic indices). Products include:
- Advil .... ▣ 771
- Children's Advil Oral Suspension .... ▣ 773
- Children's Advil Chewable Tablets .... ▣ 773
- Advil Cold and Sinus Caplets .... ▣ 771
- Advil Cold and Sinus Tablets .... ▣ 771
- Advil Flu & Body Ache Caplets .... ▣ 772
- Infants' Advil Drops .... ▣ 773
- Junior Strength Advil Tablets .... ▣ 773
- Junior Strength Advil Chewable Tablets .... ▣ 773
- Advil Migraine Liquigels .... ▣ 772
- Children's Motrin Oral Suspension and Chewable Tablets 2006
- Children's Motrin Cold Oral Suspension 2007
- Children's Motrin Oral Suspension .... ▣ 643
- Motrin Suspension, Oral Drops, Chewable Tablets, and Caplets 2002
- Infants' Motrin Concentrated Drops 2006
- Junior Strength Motrin Caplets and Chewable Tablets 2006
- Motrin IB Tablets, Caplets, and Gelcaps 2002
- Motrin Migraine Pain Caplets 2005
- Motrin Sinus Headache Caplets 2005
- Vicoprofen Tablets 520

Imipramine Hydrochloride (Atovaquone is highly bound to plasma protein (greater than 99.9%); caution is advised when co-administered with other highly protein bound drugs with narrow therapeutic indices).

No products indexed under this heading.

Imipramine Pamoate (Atovaquone is highly bound to plasma protein (greater than 99.9%); caution is advised when co-administered with other highly protein bound drugs with narrow therapeutic indices).

No products indexed under this heading.

Indomethacin (Atovaquone is highly bound to plasma protein (greater than 99.9%); caution is advised when co-administered with other highly protein bound drugs with narrow therapeutic indices). Products include:
- Indocin 2112

Indomethacin Sodium Trihydrate (Atovaquone is highly bound to plasma protein (greater than 99.9%); caution is advised when co-administered with other highly protein bound drugs with narrow therapeutic indices). Products include:
- Indocin I.V. 2115

Ketoprofen (Atovaquone is highly bound to plasma protein (greater than 99.9%); caution is advised when co-administered with other highly protein bound drugs with narrow therapeutic indices). Products include:
- Orudis Capsules 3548
- Orudis KT Tablets .... ▣ 778
- Oruvail Capsules 3548

Ketorolac Tromethamine (Atovaquone is highly bound to plasma protein (greater than 99.9%); caution is advised when co-administered with other highly protein bound drugs with narrow therapeutic indices). Products include:
- Acular Ophthalmic Solution 544
- Acular PF Ophthalmic Solution 544
- Toradol 3018

Meclofenamate Sodium (Atovaquone is highly bound to plasma protein (greater than 99.9%); caution is advised when co-administered with other highly protein bound drugs with narrow therapeutic indices).

No products indexed under this heading.

Mefenamic Acid (Atovaquone is highly bound to plasma protein (greater than 99.9%); caution is advised when co-administered with other highly protein bound drugs with narrow therapeutic indices). Products include:
- Ponstel Capsules 1356

Midazolam Hydrochloride (Atovaquone is highly bound to plasma protein (greater than 99.9%); caution is advised when co-administered with other highly protein bound drugs with narrow therapeutic indices). Products include:
- Versed Injection 3027
- Versed Syrup 3033

Naproxen (Atovaquone is highly bound to plasma protein (greater than 99.9%); caution is advised when co-administered with other highly protein bound drugs with narrow therapeutic indices). Products include:
- EC-Naprosyn Delayed-Release Tablets 2967
- Naprosyn Suspension 2967
- Naprosyn Tablets 2967

Naproxen Sodium (Atovaquone is highly bound to plasma protein (greater than 99.9%); caution is advised when co-administered with other highly protein bound drugs with narrow therapeutic indices). Products include:
- Aleve Tablets, Caplets and Gelcaps .... ▣ 602
- Aleve Cold & Sinus Caplets .... ▣ 603
- Anaprox Tablets 2967
- Anaprox DS Tablets 2967
- Naprelan Tablets 1293

Nortriptyline Hydrochloride (Atovaquone is highly bound to plasma protein (greater than 99.9%); caution is advised when co-administered with other highly protein bound drugs with narrow therapeutic indices).

No products indexed under this heading.

Oxaprozin (Atovaquone is highly bound to plasma protein (greater than 99.9%); caution is advised when co-administered with other highly protein bound drugs with narrow therapeutic indices).

No products indexed under this heading.

Oxazepam (Atovaquone is highly bound to plasma protein (greater than 99.9%); caution is advised when co-administered with other highly protein bound drugs with narrow therapeutic indices).

No products indexed under this heading.

Phenylbutazone (Atovaquone is highly bound to plasma protein (greater than 99.9%); caution is advised when co-administered with other highly protein bound drugs

with narrow therapeutic indices).
No products indexed under this heading.

Piroxicam (Atovaquone is highly bound to plasma protein (greater than 99.9%); caution is advised when co-administered with other highly protein bound drugs with narrow therapeutic indices). Products include:
Feldene Capsules ... 2685

Propranolol Hydrochloride (Atovaquone is highly bound to plasma protein (greater than 99.9%); caution is advised when co-administered with other highly protein bound drugs with narrow therapeutic indices). Products include:
Inderal ... 3513
Inderal LA Long-Acting Capsules ... 3516
Inderide Tablets ... 3517
Inderide LA Long-Acting Capsules .. 3519

Rifabutin (Due to structural similarity to rifampin, rifabutin may decrease average steady-state plasma atovaquone concentration). Products include:
Mycobutin Capsules ... 2838

Rifampin (Co-administration with oral rifampin in HIV-infected individuals may result in a 52% ±13% decrease in the average steady-state plasma atovaquone concentration and a 37% ±42% increase in the average steady-state plasma rifampin concentration). Products include:
Rifadin ... 765
Rifamate Capsules ... 767
Rifater Tablets ... 769

Sulfamethoxazole (Co-administration with TMP-SMX may result in slight decrease in average steady-state concentrations of TMP-SMX; this effect is minor and would not expect to produce clinically significant events). Products include:
Bactrim ... 2949
Septra Suspension ... 2265
Septra Tablets ... 2265
Septra DS Tablets ... 2265

Sulindac (Atovaquone is highly bound to plasma protein (greater than 99.9%); caution is advised when co-administered with other highly protein bound drugs with narrow therapeutic indices). Products include:
Clinoril Tablets ... 2053

Temazepam (Atovaquone is highly bound to plasma protein (greater than 99.9%); caution is advised when co-administered with other highly protein bound drugs with narrow therapeutic indices).
No products indexed under this heading.

Tolbutamide (Atovaquone is highly bound to plasma protein (greater than 99.9%); caution is advised when co-administered with other highly protein bound drugs with narrow therapeutic indices).
No products indexed under this heading.

Tolmetin Sodium (Atovaquone is highly bound to plasma protein (greater than 99.9%); caution is advised when co-administered with other highly protein bound drugs with narrow therapeutic indices). Products include:
Tolectin ... 2589

Trimethoprim (Co-administration with TMP-SMX may result in slight decrease in average steady-state concentrations of TMP-SMX; this effect is minor and would not expect to produce clinically significant events). Products include:
Bactrim ... 2949
Septra Suspension ... 2265
Septra Tablets ... 2265
Septra DS Tablets ... 2265

Trimipramine Maleate (Atovaquone is highly bound to plasma protein (greater than 99.9%); caution is advised when co-administered with other highly protein bound drugs with narrow therapeutic indices). Products include:
Surmontil Capsules ... 3595

Warfarin Sodium (Atovaquone is highly bound to plasma protein (greater than 99.9%); caution is advised when co-administered with other highly protein bound drugs with narrow therapeutic indices). Products include:
Coumadin for Injection ... 1243
Coumadin Tablets ... 1243
Warfarin Sodium Tablets, USP ... 3302

Zidovudine (Atovaquone tablets have shown to decrease zidovudine apparent oral clearance leading to an increase in plasma zidovudine AUC; this effect is minor and would not expect to produce clinically significant events). Products include:
Combivir Tablets ... 1502
Retrovir ... 1625
Retrovir IV Infusion ... 1629
Trizivir Tablets ... 1669

Food Interactions

Food, unspecified (Food enhances absorption by approximately two-fold).

MERIDIA CAPSULES

(Sibutramine Hydrochloride Monohydrate) ... 481
May interact with anorexiants, erythromycin, lithium preparations, monoamine oxidase inhibitors, serotonergic agents, and certain other agents. Compounds in these categories include:

Amphetamine Resins (Concurrent use with other centrally acting appetite suppressant drugs is contraindicated).
No products indexed under this heading.

Benzphetamine Hydrochloride (Concurrent use with other centrally acting appetite suppressant drugs is contraindicated).
No products indexed under this heading.

Cimetidine (Co-administration has resulted in small increases in combined (M1 and M2 metabolites) plasma Cmax and AUC; these differences are unlikely to be of clinical significance). Products include:
Tagamet HB 200 Suspension ... 762
Tagamet HB 200 Tablets ... 761
Tagamet Tablets ... 1644

Cimetidine Hydrochloride (Co-administration has resulted in small increases in combined (M1 and M2 metabolites) plasma Cmax and AUC; these differences are unlikely to be of clinical significance). Products include:
Tagamet ... 1644

Citalopram Hydrobromide (Sibutramine inhibits serotonin reuptake and serotonin syndrome, a rare, but serious constellation of symptoms, has been reported with the concomitant use of two SSRIs; concurrent use should be avoided). Products include:
Celexa ... 1365

Dexfenfluramine Hydrochloride (Concurrent use with other centrally acting appetite suppressant drugs is contraindicated).
No products indexed under this heading.

Dextroamphetamine Sulfate (Concurrent use with other centrally acting appetite suppressant drugs is contraindicated). Products include:
Adderall Tablets ... 3231
Adderall XR Capsules ...
Dexedrine ... 1512
DextroStat Tablets ... 3236

Dextromethorphan Hydrobromide (Sibutramine inhibits serotonin reuptake and combination of SSRIs and dextromethorphan has resulted in serious, sometimes fatal, reactions, serotonin syndrome). Products include:
Alka-Seltzer Plus Liqui-Gels ... 604
Alka-Seltzer Plus Cold & Flu Medicine Liqui-Gels ... 604
Benylin Adult Formula Cough Suppressant Liquid ... 696
Benylin Cough Suppressant/Expectorant Liquid ... 697
Benylin Multi-Symptom Liquid ... 697
Benylin Pediatric Cough Suppressant Liquid ... 698
Comtrex Deep Chest Cold & Congestion Relief Softgels ... 627
Comtrex Maximum Strength Multi-Symptom Cold & Cough Relief Tablets and Caplets ... 626
Contac Severe Cold and Flu Caplets Maximum Strength ... 746
Contac Severe Cold and Flu Caplets Non-Drowsy ... 746
Coricidin HBP Cough & Cold Tablets ... 738
Coricidin HBP Maximum Strength Flu Tablets ... 738
Dimetapp DM Cold & Cough Elixir ... 775
Dimetapp Nighttime Flu Liquid ... 776
Dimetapp Non-Drowsy Flu Syrup ... 777
Dimetapp Infant Drops Decongestant Plus Cough ... 776
PediaCare Cough-Cold Liquid ... 719
PediaCare Infants' Drops Decongestant Plus Cough ... 719
PediaCare NightRest Cough-Cold Liquid ... 719
Phenergan with Dextromethorphan Syrup ... 3559
Robitussin Cold Caplets Cold & Congestion ... 780
Robitussin Cold Softgels Cold & Congestion ... 780
Robitussin Cold Caplets Multi-Symptom Cold & Flu ... 781
Robitussin Cold Softgels Multi-Symptom Cold & Flu ... 781
Robitussin Cough & Cold Infant Drops ... 782
Robitussin Maximum Strength Cough & Cold Liquid ... 785
Robitussin Pediatric Cough & Cold Formula Liquid ... 785
Robitussin Maximum Strength Cough Suppressant Liquid ... 784
Robitussin Pediatric Cough Suppressant Liquid ... 784
Robitussin Multi Symptom Honey Flu Liquid ... 785
Robitussin Nighttime Honey Flu Liquid ... 786
Robitussin-CF Liquid ... 783
Robitussin DM Infant Drops ... 783
Robitussin-DM Liquid ... 783
Children's Sudafed Cold & Cough Liquid ... 709
Sudafed Cold & Cough Liquid Caps ... 709
Sudafed Severe Cold ... 711
TheraFlu Regular Strength Cold & Cough Night Time Hot Liquid ... 676
TheraFlu Maximum Strength Flu & Congestion Non-Drowsy Hot Liquid ... 677
TheraFlu Maximum Strength Flu & Cough Night Time Hot Liquid ... 678
TheraFlu Maximum Strength Severe Cold & Congestion Night Time Caplets ... 678
TheraFlu Maximum Strength Severe Cold & Congestion Night Time Hot Liquid ... 678
TheraFlu Maximum Strength Severe Cold & Congestion Non-Drowsy ... 679
Triaminic Cold & Cough Liquid ... 681
Triaminic Cold & Cough Softchews ... 683
Triaminic Cold & Night Time Cough Liquid ... 681
Triaminic Cold, Cough & Fever Liquid ... 681
Triaminic Cough Liquid ... 682
Triaminic Cough Softchews ... 684
Triaminic Cough & Congestion Liquid ... 682
Triaminic Cough & Sore Throat Liquid ... 682
Triaminic Cough & Sore Throat Softchews ... 684
Tussi-Organidin DM NR Liquid ... 3350
Tussi-Organidin DM-S NR Liquid ... 3350
Children's Tylenol Cold Plus Cough Suspension Liquid and Chewable Tablets ... 2015
Children's Tylenol Flu Suspension Liquid ... 2015
Infants' Tylenol Cold Decongestant and Fever Reducer Concentrated Drops Plus Cough .. 2015
Multi-Symptom Tylenol Cold Complete Formula Caplets ... 2010
Multi-Symptom Tylenol Cold Non-Drowsy Caplets and Gelcaps ... 2010
Multi-Symptom Tylenol Cold Severe Congestion Non-Drowsy Caplets ... 2011
Maximum Strength Tylenol Flu NightTime Liquid ... 2011
Maximum Strength Tylenol Flu Non-Drowsy Gelcaps ... 2011
Vicks 44 Cough Relief Liquid ... 724
Vicks 44D Cough & Head Congestion Relief Liquid ... 724
Vicks 44E Cough & Chest Congestion Relief Liquid ... 725
Pediatric Vicks 44e Cough & Chest Congestion Relief Liquid ... 728
Vicks 44M Cough, Cold & Flu Relief Liquid ... 725
Pediatric Vicks 44m Cough & Cold Relief ... 728
Vicks DayQuil LiquiCaps/Liquid Multi-Symptom Cold/Flu Relief ... 727
Children's Vicks NyQuil Cold/Cough Relief ... 726
Vicks NyQuil LiquiCaps/Liquid Multi-Symptom Cold/Flu Relief, Original and Cherry Flavors ... 727

Dextromethorphan Polistirex (Sibutramine inhibits serotonin reuptake and combination of SSRIs and dextromethorphan has resulted in serious, sometimes fatal, reactions, serotonin syndrome). Products include:
Delsym Extended-Release Suspension ... 664

Diethylpropion Hydrochloride (Concurrent use with other centrally acting appetite suppressant drugs is contraindicated).
No products indexed under this heading.

Dihydroergotamine Mesylate (Sibutramine inhibits serotonin reuptake and combination of SSRIs and agents for migraine, such as dihydroergotamine, has resulted in serious, sometimes fatal, reactions, serotonin syndrome). Products include:
D.H.E. 45 Injection ... 2334
Migranal Nasal Spray ... 2376

Erythromycin (Co-administration has resulted in a small increase in the AUC and a small reduction in Cmax of sibutramine metabolites). Products include:
Emgel 2% Topical Gel ... 1285
Ery-Tab Tablets ... 448
Erythromycin Base Filmtab Tablets . 454
Erythromycin Delayed-Release Capsules, USP ... 455
PCE Dispertab Tablets ... 498

Erythromycin Estolate (Co-administration has resulted in a small increase in the AUC and a small reduction in Cmax of sibutramine metabolites).
No products indexed under this heading.

Erythromycin Ethylsuccinate (Co-administration has resulted in a small increase in the AUC and a small reduction in Cmax of sibutramine metabolites). Products include:
E.E.S. ... 450
EryPed ... 446
Pediazole Suspension ... 3050

Erythromycin Gluceptate (Co-administration has resulted in a small increase in the AUC and a small reduction in Cmax of sibutramine metabolites).
No products indexed under this heading.

Erythromycin Stearate (Co-administration has resulted in a small

increase in the AUC and a small reduction in Cmax of sibutramine metabolites). Products include:
Erythrocin Stearate Filmtab Tablets 452

Fenfluramine Hydrochloride (Concurrent use with other centrally acting appetite suppressant drugs is contraindicated).
No products indexed under this heading.

Fentanyl (Sibutramine inhibits serotonin reuptake and combination of SSRIs and certain opioids, such as fentanyl, has resulted in serious, sometimes fatal, reactions, serotonin syndrome). Products include:
Duragesic Transdermal System 1786

Fentanyl Citrate (Sibutramine inhibits serotonin reuptake and combination of SSRIs and certain opioids, such as fentanyl, has resulted in serious, sometimes fatal, reactions, serotonin syndrome). Products include:
Actiq 1184

Fluoxetine Hydrochloride (Sibutramine inhibits serotonin reuptake and serotonin syndrome, a rare, but serious constellation of symptoms, has been reported with the concomitant use of two SSRIs; concurrent use should be avoided). Products include:
Prozac Pulvules, Liquid, and Weekly Capsules 1238
Sarafem Pulvules 1962

Fluvoxamine Maleate (Sibutramine inhibits serotonin reuptake and serotonin syndrome, a rare, but serious constellation of symptoms, has been reported with the concomitant use of two SSRIs; concurrent use should be avoided). Products include:
Luvox Tablets (25, 50, 100 mg) 3256

Isocarboxazid (Concurrent and/or sequential use with MAO inhibitors is contraindicated; sibutramine inhibits serotonin reuptake and combination of MAO inhibitor and serotonergic agents has resulted in serious, sometimes fatal, reactions, serotonin syndrome).
No products indexed under this heading.

Ketoconazole (Co-administration has resulted in a moderate increase in AUC and Cmax of sibutramine). Products include:
Nizoral 2% Cream 3620
Nizoral A-D Shampoo 2008
Nizoral 2% Shampoo 2007
Nizoral Tablets 1791

Lithium Carbonate (Sibutramine inhibits serotonin reuptake and combination of SSRIs and lithium has resulted in serious, sometimes fatal, reactions, serotonin syndrome). Products include:
Eskalith 1527
Lithium Carbonate 3061
Lithobid Slow-Release Tablets 3255

Lithium Citrate (Sibutramine inhibits serotonin reuptake and combination of SSRIs and lithium has resulted in serious, sometimes fatal, reactions, serotonin syndrome). Products include:
Lithium Citrate Syrup 3061

Mazindol (Concurrent use with other centrally acting appetite suppressant drugs is contraindicated).
No products indexed under this heading.

Meperidine Hydrochloride (Sibutramine inhibits serotonin reuptake and combination of SSRIs and certain opioids, such as meperidine, has resulted in serious, sometimes fatal, reactions, serotonin syndrome). Products include:
Demerol 3079
Mepergan Injection 3539

Methamphetamine Hydrochloride (Concurrent use with other centrally acting appetite suppressant drugs is contraindicated). Products include:
Desoxyn Tablets 440

Moclobemide (Concurrent and/or sequential use with MAO inhibitors is contraindicated; sibutramine inhibits serotonin reuptake and combination of MAO inhibitor and serotonergic agents has resulted in serious, sometimes fatal, reactions, serotonin syndrome).
No products indexed under this heading.

Pargyline Hydrochloride (Concurrent and/or sequential use with MAO inhibitors is contraindicated; sibutramine inhibits serotonin reuptake and combination of MAO inhibitor and serotonergic agents has resulted in serious, sometimes fatal, reactions, serotonin syndrome).
No products indexed under this heading.

Paroxetine Hydrochloride (Sibutramine inhibits serotonin reuptake and serotonin syndrome, a rare, but serious constellation of symptoms, has been reported with the concomitant use of two SSRIs; concurrent use should be avoided). Products include:
Paxil 1609

Pentazocine Hydrochloride (Sibutramine inhibits serotonin reuptake and combination of SSRIs and pentazocine has resulted in serious, sometimes fatal, reactions, serotonin syndrome). Products include:
Talacen Caplets 3089
Talwin Nx Tablets 3090

Phendimetrazine Tartrate (Concurrent use with other centrally acting appetite suppressant drugs is contraindicated). Products include:
Bontril Slow-Release Capsules 576

Phenelzine Sulfate (Concurrent and/or sequential use with MAO inhibitors is contraindicated; sibutramine inhibits serotonin reuptake and combination of MAO inhibitor and serotonergic agents has resulted in serious, sometimes fatal, reactions, serotonin syndrome). Products include:
Nardil Tablets 2653

Phenmetrazine Hydrochloride (Concurrent use with other centrally acting appetite suppressant drugs is contraindicated).
No products indexed under this heading.

Phentermine Hydrochloride (Concurrent use with other centrally acting appetite suppressant drugs is contraindicated). Products include:
Adipex-P 1406

Phentermine Resin (Concurrent use with other centrally acting appetite suppressant drugs is contraindicated). Products include:
Ionamin Capsules 1163

Phenylephrine Hydrochloride (Sibutramine substantially raises blood in some patients and concomitant use of sibutramine and drugs that raise blood pressure and/or heart rate, such as decongestants, requires caution). Products include:
Afrin Nasal Decongestant Children's Pump Mist .... ▣734
Extendryl 1361
Hycomine Compound Tablets 1317
Neo-Synephrine .... ▣614
Phenergan VC Syrup 3560
Phenergan VC with Codeine Syrup . 3561
Preparation H Cream .... ▣778
Preparation H Cooling Gel .... ▣778
Preparation H .... ▣778
Vicks Sinex Nasal Spray and Ultra Fine Mist .... ▣729

Phenylephrine Tannate (Sibutramine substantially raises blood in some patients and concomitant use of sibutramine and drugs that raise blood pressure and/or heart rate, such as decongestants, requires caution). Products include:
Ryna-12 S Suspension 3351
Reformulated Rynatan Pediatric Suspension 3352
Rynatuss Pediatric Suspension 3353
Rynatuss Tablets 3353

Phenylpropanolamine Hydrochloride (Sibutramine substantially raises blood in some patients and concomitant use of sibutramine and drugs that raise blood pressure and/or heart rate, such as decongestants, requires caution).
No products indexed under this heading.

Procarbazine Hydrochloride (Concurrent and/or sequential use with MAO inhibitors is contraindicated; sibutramine inhibits serotonin reuptake and combination of MAO inhibitor and serotonergic agents has resulted in serious, sometimes fatal, reactions, serotonin syndrome). Products include:
Matulane Capsules 3246

Pseudoephedrine Hydrochloride (Sibutramine substantially raises blood in some patients and concomitant use of sibutramine and drugs that raise blood pressure and/or heart rate, such as decongestants, requires caution). Products include:
Actifed Cold & Allergy Tablets .... ▣688
Actifed Cold & Sinus Caplets and Tablets .... ▣688
Advil Cold and Sinus Caplets .... ▣771
Advil Cold and Sinus Tablets .... ▣771
Advil Flu & Body Ache Caplets .... ▣772
Aleve Cold & Sinus Caplets .... ▣603
Alka-Seltzer Plus Liqui-Gels .... ▣604
Alka-Seltzer Plus Cold & Flu Medicine Liqui-Gels .... ▣604
Alka-Seltzer Plus Cold & Sinus Medicine Liqui-Gels .... ▣604
Allegra-D Extended-Release Tablets 714
BC Cold Powder .... ▣619
Benadryl Allergy/Cold Tablets .... ▣691
Benadryl Allergy/Congestion Tablets .... ▣692
Benadryl Allergy & Sinus Liquid .... ▣693
Benadryl Allergy & Sinus Fastmelt Tablets .... ▣693
Benadryl Allergy Sinus Headache Caplets & Gelcaps .... ▣693
Benadryl Severe Allergy & Sinus Headache Caplets .... ▣694
Benadryl Children's Allergy/Cold Fastmelt Tablets .... ▣692
Benylin Multi-Symptom Liquid .... ▣697
Bromfed Capsules (Extended-Release) 2269
Bromfed-PD Capsules (Extended-Release) 2269
Children's Cēpacol Sore Throat .... ▣788
Comtrex Acute Head Cold & Sinus Pressure Relief Tablets .... ▣627
Comtrex Deep Chest Cold & Congestion Relief Softgels .... ▣627
Comtrex Flu Therapy & Fever Relief Daytime Caplets .... ▣628
Comtrex Flu Therapy & Fever Relief Nighttime Tablets .... ▣628
Comtrex Maximum Strength Multi-Symptom Cold & Cough Relief Tablets and Caplets .... ▣626
Contac Non-Drowsy 12 Hour Cold Caplets .... ▣745
Contac Non-Drowsy Timed Release 12 Hour Cold Caplets .... ▣746
Contac Severe Cold and Flu Caplets Maximum Strength .... ▣746
Contac Severe Cold and Flu Caplets Non-Drowsy .... ▣746
Dimetapp Elixir .... ▣777
Dimetapp Cold and Fever Suspension .... ▣775
Dimetapp DM Cold & Cough Elixir .... ▣775
Dimetapp Nighttime Flu Liquid .... ▣776
Dimetapp Non-Drowsy Flu Syrup .... ▣777
Dimetapp Infant Drops Decongestant .... ▣775
Dimetapp Infant Drops Decongestant Plus Cough .... ▣776
Guaifed 2272
Kronofed-A 1341
Children's Motrin Cold Oral Suspension 2007
Motrin Sinus Headache Caplets 2005
PediaCare Cough-Cold Liquid .... ▣719
PediaCare Infants' Drops Decongestant .... ▣719
PediaCare Infants' Drops Decongestant Plus Cough .... ▣719
PediaCare NightRest Cough-Cold Liquid .... ▣719
Robitussin Cold Caplets Cold & Congestion .... ▣780
Robitussin Cold Softgels Cold & Congestion .... ▣780
Robitussin Cold Caplets Multi-Symptom Cold & Flu .... ▣781
Robitussin Cold Softgels Multi-Symptom Cold & Flu .... ▣781
Robitussin Cold Softgels Severe Congestion .... ▣782
Robitussin Cough & Cold Infant Drops .... ▣782
Robitussin Maximum Strength Cough & Cold Liquid .... ▣785
Robitussin Pediatric Cough & Cold Formula Liquid .... ▣785
Robitussin Multi Symptom Honey Flu Liquid .... ▣785
Robitussin Nighttime Honey Flu Liquid .... ▣786
Robitussin-CF Liquid .... ▣783
Robitussin-DAC Syrup 2942
Robitussin-PE Liquid .... ▣782
Ryna .... ▣768
Semprex-D Capsules 1172
Singlet Caplets .... ▣761
Sinutab Non-Drying Liquid Caps .... ▣706
Sinutab Sinus Allergy Medication, Maximum Strength Formula, Tablets & Caplets .... ▣707
Sinutab Sinus Medication, Maximum Strength Without Drowsiness Formula, Tablets & Caplets .... ▣707
Sudafed 12 Hour Tablets .... ▣708
Sudafed 24 Hour Tablets .... ▣708
Children's Sudafed Cold & Cough Liquid .... ▣709
Children's Sudafed Nasal Decongestant Chewables .... ▣711
Children's Sudafed Nasal Decongestant Liquid Medication .... ▣711
Sudafed Cold & Allergy Tablets .... ▣708
Sudafed Cold & Cough Liquid Caps .... ▣709
Sudafed Cold & Sinus Liquid Caps .... ▣710
Sudafed Nasal Decongestant Tablets .... ▣710
Sudafed Non-Drying Sinus Liquid Caps .... ▣712
Sudafed Severe Cold .... ▣711
Sudafed Sinus Headache Caplets .... ▣712
Sudafed Sinus Headache Tablets .... ▣712
Tavist Sinus Non-Drowsy Coated Caplets .... ▣676
TheraFlu Regular Strength Cold & Cough Night Time Hot Liquid .... ▣676
TheraFlu Regular Strength Cold & Sore Throat Night Time Hot Liquid .... ▣676
TheraFlu Maximum Strength Flu & Congestion Non-Drowsy Hot Liquid .... ▣677
TheraFlu Maximum Strength Flu & Cough Night Time Hot Liquid .... ▣678
TheraFlu Maximum Strength Flu & Sore Throat Night Time Hot Liquid .... ▣677
TheraFlu Maximum Strength Severe Cold & Congestion Night Time Caplets .... ▣678
TheraFlu Maximum Strength Severe Cold & Congestion Night Time Hot Liquid .... ▣678
TheraFlu Maximum Strength Severe Cold & Congestion Non-Drowsy .... ▣679
Triaminic Allergy Congestion Liquid .... ▣680
Triaminic Chest Congestion Liquid .... ▣680
Triaminic Cold & Allergy Liquid .... ▣681
Triaminic Cold & Allergy Softchews .... ▣683
Triaminic Cold & Cough Liquid .... ▣681
Triaminic Cold & Cough Softchews .... ▣683
Triaminic Cold & Night Time Cough Liquid .... ▣681
Triaminic Cold, Cough & Fever Liquid .... ▣681
Triaminic Cough Liquid .... ▣682
Triaminic Cough & Congestion Liquid .... ▣682
Triaminic Cough & Sore Throat Liquid .... ▣682
Triaminic Cough & Sore Throat Softchews .... ▣684
Children's Tylenol Allergy-D Liquid ... 2014

Children's Tylenol Cold Suspension Liquid and Chewable Tablets ... 2015
Children's Tylenol Cold Plus Cough Suspension Liquid and Chewable Tablets ... 2015
Children's Tylenol Flu Suspension Liquid ... 2015
Children's Tylenol Sinus Suspension Liquid ... 2017
Infants' Tylenol Cold Decongestant and Fever Reducer Concentrated Drops ... 2015
Infants' Tylenol Cold Decongestant and Fever Reducer Concentrated Drops Plus Cough .. 2015
Tylenol Allergy Sinus ... 2010
Multi-Symptom Tylenol Cold Complete Formula Caplets ... 2010
Multi-Symptom Tylenol Cold Non-Drowsy Caplets and Gelcaps ... 2010
Multi-Symptom Tylenol Cold Severe Congestion Non-Drowsy Caplets ... 2011
Maximum Strength Tylenol Flu NightTime Gelcaps ... 2011
Maximum Strength Tylenol Flu NightTime Liquid ... 2011
Maximum Strength Tylenol Flu Non-Drowsy Gelcaps ... 2011
Maximum Strength Tylenol Sinus NightTime Caplets ... 2012
Maximum Strength Tylenol Sinus Non-Drowsy Geltabs, Gelcaps, Caplets, and Tablets ... 2012
Vicks 44D Cough & Head Congestion Relief Liquid ... 724
Vicks 44M Cough, Cold & Flu Relief Liquid ... 725
Pediatric Vicks 44m Cough & Cold Relief ... 728
Vicks DayQuil LiquiCaps/Liquid Multi-Symptom Cold/Flu Relief ... 727
Children's Vicks NyQuil Cold/Cough Relief ... 726
Vicks NyQuil LiquiCaps/Liquid Multi-Symptom Cold/Flu Relief, Original and Cherry Flavors ... 727
Zephrex Tablets ... 3091
Zephrex LA Tablets ... 3092
Zyrtec-D 12 Hour Extended Relief Tablets ... 2758

Pseudoephedrine Sulfate (Sibutramine substantially raises blood in some patients and concomitant use of sibutramine and drugs that raise blood pressure and/or heart rate, such as decongestants, requires caution). Products include:
Chlor-Trimeton Allergy/Decongestant Tablets ... 736
Claritin-D 12 Hour Extended Release Tablets ... 3102
Claritin-D 24 Hour Extended Release Tablets ... 3104
Coricidin 'D' Cold, Flu & Sinus Tablets ... 737
Drixoral Allergy/Sinus Extended-Release Tablets ... 741
Drixoral Cold & Allergy Sustained-Action Tablets ... 740
Drixoral Cold & Flu Extended-Release Tablets ... 740
Drixoral Nasal Decongestant Long-Acting Non-Drowsy Tablets ... 740
Rynatan Tablets ... 3351

Selegiline Hydrochloride (Concurrent and/or sequential use with MAO inhibitors is contraindicated; sibutramine inhibits serotonin reuptake and combination of MAO inhibitor and serotonergic agents has resulted in serious, sometimes fatal, reactions, serotonin syndrome). Products include:
Eldepryl Capsules ... 3266

Sertraline Hydrochloride (Sibutramine inhibits serotonin reuptake and serotonin syndrome, a rare, but serious constellation of symptoms, has been reported with the concomitant use of two SSRIs; concurrent use should be avoided). Products include:
Zoloft ... 2751

Sumatriptan (Sibutramine inhibits serotonin reuptake and combination of SSRIs and agents for migraine, such as sumatriptan, has resulted in serious, sometimes fatal, reactions, serotonin syndrome). Products include:
Imitrex Nasal Spray ... 1554

Sumatriptan Succinate (Sibutramine inhibits serotonin reuptake and combination of SSRIs and agents for migraine, such as sumatriptan, has resulted in serious, sometimes fatal, reactions, serotonin syndrome). Products include:
Imitrex Injection ... 1549
Imitrex Tablets ... 1558

Tranylcypromine Sulfate (Concurrent and/or sequential use with MAO inhibitors is contraindicated; sibutramine inhibits serotonin reuptake and combination of MAO inhibitor and serotonergic agents has resulted in serious, sometimes fatal, reactions, serotonin syndrome). Products include:
Parnate Tablets ... 1607

L-Tryptophan (Sibutramine inhibits serotonin reuptake and combination of SSRIs and tryptophan has resulted in serious, sometimes fatal, reactions, serotonin syndrome).
No products indexed under this heading.

Venlafaxine Hydrochloride (Sibutramine inhibits serotonin reuptake and serotonin syndrome, a rare, but serious constellation of symptoms, has been reported with the concomitant use of two SSRIs; concurrent use should be avoided). Products include:
Effexor Tablets ... 3495
Effexor XR Capsules ... 3499

Food Interactions

Alcohol (Concurrent use has not resulted in psychomotor reactions of clinical significance, however, concomitant use with excessive alcohol is not recommended).

Food, unspecified (Co-administration with a standard breakfast has resulted in reduced peak M1 and M2 amine concentrations and delayed the time to peak by approximately three hours; the AUCs of M1 and M2 were not significantly altered).

MERREM I.V.

(Meropenem) ... 673
May interact with:

Probenecid (Competes with meropenem for active tubular secretion and thus inhibits the renal excretion of meropenem; statistically significant increases in the elimination half-life and the extent of systemic exposure has been reported; co-administration is not recommended).
No products indexed under this heading.

MERUVAX II

(Rubella Virus Vaccine Live) ... 2130
May interact with immunosuppressive agents. Compounds in these categories include:

Azathioprine (Concurrent immunosuppressive therapy is contraindicated).
No products indexed under this heading.

Basiliximab (Concurrent immunosuppressive therapy is contraindicated). Products include:
Simulect for Injection ... 2399

Cyclosporine (Concurrent immunosuppressive therapy is contraindicated). Products include:
Gengraf Capsules ... 457
Neoral Soft Gelatin Capsules ... 2380
Neoral Oral Solution ... 2380
Sandimmune ... 2388

Muromonab-CD3 (Concurrent immunosuppressive therapy is contraindicated). Products include:
Orthoclone OKT3 Sterile Solution ... 2498

Mycophenolate Mofetil (Concurrent immunosuppressive therapy is contraindicated). Products include:
CellCept Capsules ... 2951
CellCept Oral Suspension ... 2951
CellCept Tablets ... 2951

Sirolimus (Concurrent immunosuppressive therapy is contraindicated). Products include:
Rapamune Oral Solution and Tablets ... 3584

Tacrolimus (Concurrent immunosuppressive therapy is contraindicated). Products include:
Prograf ... 1393
Protopic Ointment ... 1397

MESTINON SYRUP

(Pyridostigmine Bromide) ... 1740
None cited in PDR database.

MESTINON TABLETS

(Pyridostigmine Bromide) ... 1740
None cited in PDR database.

MESTINON TIMESPAN TABLETS

(Pyridostigmine Bromide) ... 1740
None cited in PDR database.

METABOLIC NUTRITION SYSTEM

(Ephedra, Ginseng, Herbals with Vitamins & Minerals, Hypericum) ... 798
None cited in PDR database.

METADATE CD CAPSULES

(Methylphenidate Hydrochloride) ... 1164
May interact with oral anticoagulants, monoamine oxidase inhibitors, phenytoin, selective serotonin reuptake inhibitors, tricyclic antidepressants, vasopressors, and certain other agents. Compounds in these categories include:

Amitriptyline Hydrochloride (Methylphenidate may inhibit the metabolism of tricyclic antidepressants; downward dosage adjustment of tricyclic antidepressants may be required). Products include:
Etrafon ... 3115
Limbitrol ... 1738

Amoxapine (Methylphenidate may inhibit the metabolism of tricyclic antidepressants; downward dosage adjustment of tricyclic antidepressants may be required).
No products indexed under this heading.

Citalopram Hydrobromide (Methylphenidate may inhibit the metabolism of selective serotonin reuptake inhibitors; downward dosage adjustment of SSRI may be required). Products include:
Celexa ... 1365

Clomipramine Hydrochloride (Methylphenidate may inhibit the metabolism of tricyclic antidepressants; downward dosage adjustment of tricyclic antidepressants may be required).
No products indexed under this heading.

Clonidine (Co-administration has resulted in serious adverse events; the safety of this combination has not been systemically established). Products include:
Catapres-TTS ... 1038

Clonidine Hydrochloride (Co-administration has resulted in serious adverse events; the safety of this combination has not been systemically established). Products include:
Catapres Tablets ... 1037
Clorpres Tablets ... 1002
Combipres Tablets ... 1040
Duraclon Injection ... 3057

Desipramine Hydrochloride (Methylphenidate may inhibit the metabolism of tricyclic antidepressants; downward dosage adjustment of tricyclic antidepressants may be required). Products include:
Norpramin Tablets ... 755

Dicumarol (Methylphenidate may inhibit the metabolism of coumarin anticoagulants; downward dosage adjustment of anticoagulants may be required).
No products indexed under this heading.

Dopamine Hydrochloride (Methylphenidate causes rise in blood pressure; co-administration with other pressor agents should be undertaken with caution).
No products indexed under this heading.

Doxepin Hydrochloride (Methylphenidate may inhibit the metabolism of tricyclic antidepressants; downward dosage adjustment of tricyclic antidepressants may be required). Products include:
Sinequan ... 2713

Epinephrine Bitartrate (Methylphenidate causes rise in blood pressure; co-administration with other pressor agents should be undertaken with caution). Products include:
Sensorcaine ... 643

Epinephrine Hydrochloride (Methylphenidate causes rise in blood pressure; co-administration with other pressor agents should be undertaken with caution).
No products indexed under this heading.

Fluoxetine Hydrochloride (Methylphenidate may inhibit the metabolism of selective serotonin reuptake inhibitors; downward dosage adjustment of SSRI may be required). Products include:
Prozac Pulvules, Liquid, and Weekly Capsules ... 1238
Sarafem Pulvules ... 1962

Fluvoxamine Maleate (Methylphenidate may inhibit the metabolism of selective serotonin reuptake inhibitors; downward dosage adjustment of SSRI may be required). Products include:
Luvox Tablets (25, 50, 100 mg) ... 3256

Fosphenytoin Sodium (Methylphenidate may inhibit the metabolism of anticonvulsants, such as phenytoin; additionally methylphenidate may lower the convulsive threshold in patients with prior history of seizures). Products include:
Cerebyx Injection ... 2619

Guanethidine Monosulfate (Methylphenidate may decrease the hypotensive effect of guanethidine).
No products indexed under this heading.

Imipramine Hydrochloride (Methylphenidate may inhibit the metabolism of tricyclic antidepressants; downward dosage adjustment of tricyclic antidepressants may be required).
No products indexed under this heading.

Imipramine Pamoate (Methylphenidate may inhibit the metabolism of tricyclic antidepressants; downward dosage adjustment of tricyclic antidepressants may be required).
No products indexed under this heading.

Isocarboxazid (Co-administration can result in hypertensive crises; concurrent and/or sequential use with MAO inhibitors is contraindicated).
No products indexed under this heading.

Maprotiline Hydrochloride (Methylphenidate may inhibit the metabolism of tricyclic antidepressants; downward dosage adjustment of

tricyclic antidepressants may be required).
No products indexed under this heading.

Metaraminol Bitartrate (Methylphenidate causes rise in blood pressure; co-administration with other pressor agents should be undertaken with caution). Products include:
Aramine Injection 2043

Methoxamine Hydrochloride (Methylphenidate causes rise in blood pressure; co-administration with other pressor agents should be undertaken with caution).
No products indexed under this heading.

Moclobemide (Co-administration can result in hypertensive crises; concurrent and/or sequential use with MAO inhibitors is contraindicated).
No products indexed under this heading.

Norepinephrine Bitartrate (Methylphenidate causes rise in blood pressure; co-administration with other pressor agents should be undertaken with caution).
No products indexed under this heading.

Nortriptyline Hydrochloride (Methylphenidate may inhibit the metabolism of tricyclic antidepressants; downward dosage adjustment of tricyclic antidepressants may be required).
No products indexed under this heading.

Pargyline Hydrochloride (Co-administration can result in hypertensive crises; concurrent and/or sequential use with MAO inhibitors is contraindicated).
No products indexed under this heading.

Paroxetine Hydrochloride (Methylphenidate may inhibit the metabolism of selective serotonin reuptake inhibitors; downward dosage adjustment of SSRI may be required). Products include:
Paxil 1609

Phenelzine Sulfate (Co-administration can result in hypertensive crises; concurrent and/or sequential use with MAO inhibitors is contraindicated). Products include:
Nardil Tablets 2653

Phenobarbital (Methylphenidate may inhibit the metabolism of anticonvulsants, such as phenobarbital; additionally methylphenidate may lower the convulsive threshold in patients with prior history of seizures). Products include:
Arco-Lase Plus Tablets 592
Donnatal 2929
Donnatal Extentabs 2930

Phenylephrine Hydrochloride (Methylphenidate causes rise in blood pressure; co-administration with other pressor agents should be undertaken with caution). Products include:
Afrin Nasal Decongestant Children's Pump Mist .... ▣734
Extendryl 1361
Hycomine Compound Tablets 1317
Neo-Synephrine .... ▣614
Phenergan VC Syrup 3560
Phenergan VC with Codeine Syrup 3561
Preparation H Cream .... ▣778
Preparation H Cooling Gel .... ▣778
Preparation H .... ▣778
Vicks Sinex Nasal Spray and Ultra Fine Mist .... ▣729

Phenytoin (Methylphenidate may inhibit the metabolism of anticonvulsants, such as phenytoin; additionally methylphenidate may lower the convulsive threshold in patients with prior history of seizures). Products include:
Dilantin Infatabs 2624
Dilantin-125 Oral Suspension 2625

Phenytoin Sodium (Methylphenidate may inhibit the metabolism of anticonvulsants, such as phenytoin; additionally methylphenidate may lower the convulsive threshold in patients with prior history of seizures). Products include:
Dilantin Kapseals 2622

Primidone (Methylphenidate may inhibit the metabolism of anticonvulsants, such as primidone; additionally methylphenidate may lower the convulsive threshold in patients with prior history of seizures).
No products indexed under this heading.

Procarbazine Hydrochloride (Co-administration can result in hypertensive crises; concurrent and/or sequential use with MAO inhibitors is contraindicated). Products include:
Matulane Capsules 3246

Protriptyline Hydrochloride (Methylphenidate may inhibit the metabolism of tricyclic antidepressants; downward dosage adjustment of tricyclic antidepressants may be required). Products include:
Vivactil Tablets 2446
Vivactil Tablets 2217

Selegiline Hydrochloride (Co-administration can result in hypertensive crises; concurrent and/or sequential use with MAO inhibitors is contraindicated). Products include:
Eldepryl Capsules 3266

Sertraline Hydrochloride (Methylphenidate may inhibit the metabolism of selective serotonin reuptake inhibitors; downward dosage adjustment of SSRI may be required). Products include:
Zoloft 2751

Tranylcypromine Sulfate (Co-administration can result in hypertensive crises; concurrent and/or sequential use with MAO inhibitors is contraindicated). Products include:
Parnate Tablets 1607

Trimipramine Maleate (Methylphenidate may inhibit the metabolism of tricyclic antidepressants; downward dosage adjustment of tricyclic antidepressants may be required). Products include:
Surmontil Capsules 3595

Venlafaxine Hydrochloride (Co-administration in a patient on methylphenidate for 18 months has resulted in neuroleptic malignant syndrome within 45 minutes of ingesting his first dose of venlafaxine). Products include:
Effexor Tablets 3495
Effexor XR Capsules 3499

Warfarin Sodium (Methylphenidate may inhibit the metabolism of coumarin anticoagulants; downward dosage adjustment of anticoagulants may be required). Products include:
Coumadin for Injection 1243
Coumadin Tablets 1243
Warfarin Sodium Tablets, USP 3302

METADATE ER TABLETS
(Methylphenidate Hydrochloride) 1167
See Metadate CD Capsules

METAMUCIL DIETARY FIBER SUPPLEMENT
(Psyllium Preparations) .... ▣834
None cited in PDR database.

METAMUCIL ORIGINAL TEXTURE POWDER, ORANGE FLAVOR
(Psyllium Preparations) 2877
None cited in PDR database.

METAMUCIL ORIGINAL TEXTURE POWDER, REGULAR FLAVOR
(Psyllium Preparations) 2877
None cited in PDR database.

METAMUCIL SMOOTH TEXTURE POWDER, ORANGE FLAVOR
(Psyllium Preparations) 2877
None cited in PDR database.

METAMUCIL SMOOTH TEXTURE POWDER, SUGAR-FREE, ORANGE FLAVOR
(Psyllium Preparations) 2877
None cited in PDR database.

METAMUCIL SMOOTH TEXTURE POWDER, SUGAR-FREE, REGULAR FLAVOR
(Psyllium Preparations) 2877
None cited in PDR database.

METAMUCIL WAFERS, APPLE CRISP AND CINNAMON SPICE FLAVORS
(Psyllium Preparations) 2877
None cited in PDR database.

METHYLIN TABLETS
(Methylphenidate Hydrochloride) 1995
May interact with oral anticoagulants, anticonvulsants, monoamine oxidase inhibitors, vasopressors, and certain other agents. Compounds in these categories include:

Carbamazepine (Menthylphenidate may lower the convulsive threshold in patients with prior history of seizures; safe concomitant use of anticonvulsants and Methylin has not been established). Products include:
Carbatrol Capsules 3234
Tegretol/Tegretol-XR 2404

Clomipramine Hydrochloride (Menthylphenidate may inhibit the metabolism of clomipramine; downward dosage adjustment of clomipramine may be required).
No products indexed under this heading.

Desipramine Hydrochloride (Menthylphenidate may inhibit the metabolism of desipramine; downward dosage adjustment of desipramine may be required). Products include:
Norpramin Tablets 755

Dicumarol (Menthylphenidate may inhibit the metabolism of coumarin anticoagulants; downward dosage adjustment of anticoagulants may be required).
No products indexed under this heading.

Divalproex Sodium (Menthylphenidate may lower the convulsive threshold in patients with prior history of seizures; safe concomitant use of anticonvulsants and Methylin has not been established). Products include:
Depakote Sprinkle Capsules 426
Depakote Tablets 430
Depakote ER Tablets 436

Dopamine Hydrochloride (Menthylphenidate causes rise in blood pressure; co-administration with other pressor agents should be undertaken with caution).
No products indexed under this heading.

Epinephrine Bitartrate (Menthylphenidate causes rise in blood pressure; co-administration with other pressor agents should be undertaken with caution). Products include:
Sensorcaine 643

Epinephrine Hydrochloride (Menthylphenidate causes rise in blood pressure; co-administration with other pressor agents should be undertaken with caution).
No products indexed under this heading.

Ethosuximide (Menthylphenidate may lower the convulsive threshold in patients with prior history of seizures; safe concomitant use of anticonvulsants and Methylin has not been established). Products include:
Zarontin Capsules 2659
Zarontin Syrup 2660

Ethotoin (Menthylphenidate may lower the convulsive threshold in patients with prior history of seizures; safe concomitant use of anticonvulsants and Methylin has not been established).
No products indexed under this heading.

Felbamate (Menthylphenidate may lower the convulsive threshold in patients with prior history of seizures; safe concomitant use of anticonvulsants and Methylin has not been established). Products include:
Felbatol 3343

Fosphenytoin Sodium (Menthylphenidate may lower the convulsive threshold in patients with prior history of seizures; safe concomitant use of anticonvulsants and Methylin has not been established). Products include:
Cerebyx Injection 2619

Imipramine Hydrochloride (Menthylphenidate may inhibit the metabolism of imipramine; downward dosage adjustment of imipramine may be required).
No products indexed under this heading.

Imipramine Pamoate (Menthylphenidate may inhibit the metabolism of imipramine; downward dosage adjustment of imipramine may be required).
No products indexed under this heading.

Isocarboxazid (Menthylphenidate causes rise in blood pressure; co-administration with MAOI should be undertaken with caution).
No products indexed under this heading.

Lamotrigine (Menthylphenidate may lower the convulsive threshold in patients with prior history of seizures; safe concomitant use of anticonvulsants and Methylin has not been established). Products include:
Lamictal 1567

Levetiracetam (Menthylphenidate may lower the convulsive threshold in patients with prior history of seizures; safe concomitant use of anticonvulsants and Methylin has not been established). Products include:
Keppra Tablets 3314

Mephenytoin (Menthylphenidate may lower the convulsive threshold in patients with prior history of seizures; safe concomitant use of anticonvulsants and Methylin has not been established).
No products indexed under this heading.

Metaraminol Bitartrate (Menthylphenidate causes rise in blood pressure; co-administration with other pressor agents should be undertaken with caution). Products include:
Aramine Injection 2043

Methoxamine Hydrochloride (Menthylphenidate causes rise in blood pressure; co-administration with other pressor agents should be undertaken with caution).
No products indexed under this heading.

Methsuximide (Menthylphenidate may lower the convulsive threshold in patients with prior history of seizures; safe concomitant use of anti-

convulsants and Methylin has not been established). Products include:
Celontin Capsules 2618

Moclobemide (Menthylphenidate causes rise in blood pressure; co-administration with MAOI should be undertaken with caution).
No products indexed under this heading.

Norepinephrine Bitartrate (Menthylphenidate causes rise in blood pressure; co-administration with other pressor agents should be undertaken with caution).
No products indexed under this heading.

Oxcarbazepine (Menthylphenidate may lower the convulsive threshold in patients with prior history of seizures; safe concomitant use of anticonvulsants and Methylin has not been established). Products include:
Trileptal Oral Suspension 2407
Trileptal Tablets 2407

Paramethadione (Menthylphenidate may lower the convulsive threshold in patients with prior history of seizures; safe concomitant use of anticonvulsants and Methylin has not been established).
No products indexed under this heading.

Pargyline Hydrochloride (Menthylphenidate causes rise in blood pressure; co-administration with MAOI should be undertaken with caution).
No products indexed under this heading.

Phenacemide (Menthylphenidate may lower the convulsive threshold in patients with prior history of seizures; safe concomitant use of anticonvulsants and Methylin has not been established).
No products indexed under this heading.

Phenelzine Sulfate (Menthylphenidate causes rise in blood pressure; co-administration with MAOI should be undertaken with caution).
Products include:
Nardil Tablets 2653

Phenobarbital (Menthylphenidate may inhibit the metabolism of phenobarbital; downward dosage adjustment of phenobarbital may be required; menthylphenidate may lower the convulsive threshold in patients with prior history of seizures; safe concomitant use of anticonvulsants and Methylin has not been established). Products include:
Arco-Lase Plus Tablets 592
Donnatal 2929
Donnatal Extentabs 2930

Phensuximide (Menthylphenidate may lower the convulsive threshold in patients with prior history of seizures; safe concomitant use of anticonvulsants and Methylin has not been established).
No products indexed under this heading.

Phenylbutazone (Menthylphenidate may inhibit the metabolism of phenylbutazone; downward dosage adjustment of phenylbutazone may be required).
No products indexed under this heading.

Phenylephrine Hydrochloride (Menthylphenidate causes rise in blood pressure; co-administration with other pressor agents should be undertaken with caution). Products include:
Afrin Nasal Decongestant Children's Pump Mist 734
Extendryl 1361
Hycomine Compound Tablets 1317
Neo-Synephrine 614
Phenergan VC Syrup 3560
Phenergan VC with Codeine Syrup 3561
Preparation H Cream 778
Preparation H Cooling Gel 778
Preparation H 778
Vicks Sinex Nasal Spray and Ultra Fine Mist 729

Phenytoin (Menthylphenidate may lower the convulsive threshold in patients with prior history of seizures; safe concomitant use of anticonvulsants and Methylin has not been established). Products include:
Dilantin Infatabs 2624
Dilantin-125 Oral Suspension 2625

Phenytoin Sodium (Menthylphenidate may lower the convulsive threshold in patients with prior history of seizures; safe concomitant use of anticonvulsants and Methylin has not been established). Products include:
Dilantin Kapseals 2622

Primidone (Menthylphenidate may inhibit the metabolism of primidone; downward dosage adjustment of primidone may be required; menthylphenidate may lower the convulsive threshold in patients with prior history of seizures; safe concomitant use of anticonvulsants and Methylin has not been established).
No products indexed under this heading.

Procarbazine Hydrochloride (Menthylphenidate causes rise in blood pressure; co-administration with MAOI should be undertaken with caution). Products include:
Matulane Capsules 3246

Selegiline Hydrochloride (Menthylphenidate causes rise in blood pressure; co-administration with MAOI should be undertaken with caution). Products include:
Eldepryl Capsules 3266

Tiagabine Hydrochloride (Menthylphenidate may lower the convulsive threshold in patients with prior history of seizures; safe concomitant use of anticonvulsants and Methylin has not been established). Products include:
Gabitril Tablets 1189

Topiramate (Menthylphenidate may lower the convulsive threshold in patients with prior history of seizures; safe concomitant use of anticonvulsants and Methylin has not been established). Products include:
Topamax Sprinkle Capsules 2590
Topamax Tablets 2590

Tranylcypromine Sulfate (Menthylphenidate causes rise in blood pressure; co-administration with MAOI should be undertaken with caution). Products include:
Parnate Tablets 1607

Trimethadione (Menthylphenidate may lower the convulsive threshold in patients with prior history of seizures; safe concomitant use of anticonvulsants and Methylin has not been established).
No products indexed under this heading.

Valproate Sodium (Menthylphenidate may lower the convulsive threshold in patients with prior history of seizures; safe concomitant use of anticonvulsants and Methylin has not been established). Products include:
Depacon Injection 416

Valproic Acid (Menthylphenidate may lower the convulsive threshold in patients with prior history of seizures; safe concomitant use of anticonvulsants and Methylin has not been established). Products include:
Depakene 421

Venlafaxine Hydrochloride (Co-administration in a patient on menthylphenidate for 18 months has resulted in neuroleptic malignant syndrome within 45 minutes of ingesting his first dose of venlafaxine). Products include:
Effexor Tablets 3495
Effexor XR Capsules 3499

Warfarin Sodium (Menthylphenidate may inhibit the metabolism of coumarin anticoagulants; downward dosage adjustment of anticoagulants may be required). Products include:
Coumadin for Injection 1243
Coumadin Tablets 1243
Warfarin Sodium Tablets, USP 3302

Zonisamide (Menthylphenidate may lower the convulsive threshold in patients with prior history of seizures; safe concomitant use of anticonvulsants and Methylin has not been established). Products include:
Zonegran Capsules 1307

METHYLIN ER TABLETS
(Methylphenidate Hydrochloride) 1995
See Methylin Tablets

METROCREAM
(Metronidazole) 1404
May interact with oral anticoagulants. Compounds in these categories include:

Dicumarol (Oral metronidazole potentiates the anticoagulant effect resulting in a prolongation of prothrombin time; the effect of topical metronidazole on prothrombin time is not known).
No products indexed under this heading.

Warfarin Sodium (Oral metronidazole potentiates the anticoagulant effect resulting in a prolongation of prothrombin time; the effect of topical metronidazole on prothrombin time is not known). Products include:
Coumadin for Injection 1243
Coumadin Tablets 1243
Warfarin Sodium Tablets, USP 3302

METROGEL
(Metronidazole) 1405
May interact with oral anticoagulants. Compounds in these categories include:

Dicumarol (Prolonged prothrombin time and potentiation of oral anticoagulant with systemic metronidazole; the effect of topical metronidazole on prothrombin is unknown).
No products indexed under this heading.

Warfarin Sodium (Prolonged prothrombin time and potentiation of oral anticoagulant with systemic metronidazole; the effect of topical metronidazole on prothrombin is unknown). Products include:
Coumadin for Injection 1243
Coumadin Tablets 1243
Warfarin Sodium Tablets, USP 3302

METROGEL-VAGINAL GEL
(Metronidazole) 1986
May interact with oral anticoagulants and certain other agents. Compounds in these categories include:

Dicumarol (Oral metronidazole potentiates the anticoagulant effect of warfarin).
No products indexed under this heading.

Disulfiram (Psychotic reactions to oral metronidazole have been reported in alcoholics who are using metronidazole and disulfiram concurrently). Products include:
Antabuse Tablets 2444
Antabuse Tablets 3474

Warfarin Sodium (Oral metronidazole potentiates the anticoagulant effect of warfarin). Products include:
Coumadin for Injection 1243
Coumadin Tablets 1243
Warfarin Sodium Tablets, USP 3302

Food Interactions

Alcohol (Possibility of a disulfiram-like reaction).

METROLOTION
(Metronidazole) 1405
See MetroCream

MEVACOR TABLETS
(Lovastatin) 2132
May interact with azole antifungals, oral anticoagulants, erythromycin, fibrates, protease inhibitors, and certain other agents. Compounds in these categories include:

Amprenavir (The risk of myopathy appears to be increased by high levels of HMG-CoA reductase inhibitory activity in plasma; lovastatin is metabolized by CYP3A4 isoenzyme, certain agents, such as HIV protease inhibitors, share this metabolic pathway and can raise the plasma levels of lovastatin and may increase the risk of myopathy). Products include:
Agenerase Capsules 1454
Agenerase Oral Solution 1459

Clarithromycin (The risk of myopathy appears to be increased by high levels of HMG-CoA reductase inhibitory activity in plasma; lovastatin is metabolized by CYP3A4 isoenzyme, certain agents, such as macrolide antibiotics clarithromycin, share this metabolic pathway and can raise the plasma levels of lovastatin and may increase the risk of myopathy). Products include:
Biaxin/Biaxin XL 403
PREVPAC 3298

Clofibrate (The incidence and severity of myopathy are increased by co-administration of HMG-CoA reductase inhibitors with drugs that cause myopathy when given alone, such as fibrates; combined use should be avoided; if used concurrently, the dose of lovastatin should generally not exceed 20 mg). Products include:
Atromid-S Capsules 3483

Clotrimazole (The risk of myopathy appears to be increased by high levels of HMG-CoA reductase inhibitory activity in plasma; lovastatin is metabolized by CYP3A4 isoenzyme, certain agents, such as azole antifungals, share this metabolic pathway and can raise the plasma levels of lovastatin and may increase the risk of myopathy). Products include:
Gyne-Lotrimin 3, 3-Day Cream 741
Lotrimin AF Cream, Lotion, Solution, and Jock Itch Cream 742
Lotrimin 3128
Lotrisone 3129
Mycelex Troche 573
Mycelex-7 Combination-Pack Vaginal Inserts & External Vulvar Cream 614
Mycelex-7 Vaginal Cream 614
Mycelex-7 Vaginal Cream with 7 Disposable Applicators 614

Cyclosporine (The risk of myopathy appears to be increased by high levels of HMG-CoA reductase inhibitory activity in plasma; lovastatin is metabolized by CYP3A4 isoenzyme, certain agents, such as cyclosporine, share this metabolic pathway and can raise the plasma levels of lovastatin and may increase the risk of myopathy; the dose of lovastatin should generally not exceed 20 mg if used concomitantly). Products include:
Gengraf Capsules 457
Neoral Soft Gelatin Capsules 2380
Neoral Oral Solution 2380
Sandimmune 2388

Dicumarol (Co-administration has resulted in bleeding and/or prothrombin time in few patients).
No products indexed under this heading.

Erythromycin (The risk of myopathy appears to be increased by high levels of HMG-CoA reductase inhibitory activity in plasma; lovastatin is metabolized by CYP3A4 isoenzyme,

certain agents, such as macrolide antibiotics erythromycin, share this metabolic pathway and can raise the plasma levels of lovastatin and may increase the risk of myopathy). Products include:

Emgel 2% Topical Gel 1285
Ery-Tab Tablets 448
Erythromycin Base Filmtab Tablets . 454
Erythromycin Delayed-Release Capsules, USP 455
PCE Dispertab Tablets 498

Erythromycin Estolate (The risk of myopathy appears to be increased by high levels of HMG-CoA reductase inhibitory activity in plasma; lovastatin is metabolized by CYP3A4 isoenzyme, certain agents, such as macrolide antibiotics erythromycin, share this metabolic pathway and can raise the plasma levels of lovastatin and may increase the risk of myopathy).

No products indexed under this heading.

Erythromycin Ethylsuccinate (The risk of myopathy appears to be increased by high levels of HMG-CoA reductase inhibitory activity in plasma; lovastatin is metabolized by CYP3A4 isoenzyme, certain agents, such as macrolide antibiotics erythromycin, share this metabolic pathway and can raise the plasma levels of lovastatin and may increase the risk of myopathy). Products include:

E.E.S. 450
EryPed 446
Pediazole Suspension 3050

Erythromycin Gluceptate (The risk of myopathy appears to be increased by high levels of HMG-CoA reductase inhibitory activity in plasma; lovastatin is metabolized by CYP3A4 isoenzyme, certain agents, such as macrolide antibiotics erythromycin, share this metabolic pathway and can raise the plasma levels of lovastatin and may increase the risk of myopathy).

No products indexed under this heading.

Erythromycin Stearate (The risk of myopathy appears to be increased by high levels of HMG-CoA reductase inhibitory activity in plasma; lovastatin is metabolized by CYP3A4 isoenzyme, certain agents, such as macrolide antibiotics erythromycin, share this metabolic pathway and can raise the plasma levels of lovastatin and may increase the risk of myopathy). Products include:

Erythrocin Stearate Filmtab Tablets 452

Fenofibrate (The incidence and severity of myopathy are increased by co-administration of HMG-CoA reductase inhibitors with drugs that cause myopathy when given alone, such as fibrates; combined use should be avoided; if used concurrently, the dose of lovastatin should generally not exceed 20 mg). Products include:

Tricor Capsules, Micronized 513

Fluconazole (The risk of myopathy appears to be increased by high levels of HMG-CoA reductase inhibitory activity in plasma; lovastatin is metabolized by CYP3A4 isoenzyme, certain agents, such as azole antifungals, share this metabolic pathway and can raise the plasma levels of lovastatin and may increase the risk of myopathy). Products include:

Diflucan Tablets, Injection, and Oral Suspension 2681

Gemfibrozil (The incidence and severity of myopathy are increased by co-administration of HMG-CoA reductase inhibitors with drugs that cause myopathy when given alone, such as fibrates; combined use should be avoided; if used concurrently, the dose of lovastatin should generally not exceed 20 mg). Products include:

Lopid Tablets 2650

Indinavir Sulfate (The risk of myopathy appears to be increased by high levels of HMG-CoA reductase inhibitory activity in plasma; lovastatin is metabolized by CYP3A4 isoenzyme, certain agents, such as HIV protease inhibitors, share this metabolic pathway and can raise the plasma levels of lovastatin and may increase the risk of myopathy). Products include:

Crixivan Capsules 2070

Itraconazole (The risk of myopathy appears to be increased by high levels of HMG-CoA reductase inhibitory activity in plasma; lovastatin is metabolized by CYP3A4 isoenzyme, certain agents, such as itraconazole, share this metabolic pathway and can raise the plasma levels of lovastatin and may increase the risk of myopathy). Products include:

Sporanox Capsules 1800
Sporanox Injection 1804
Sporanox Injection 2509
Sporanox Oral Solution 1808
Sporanox Oral Solution 2512

Ketoconazole (The risk of myopathy appears to be increased by high levels of HMG-CoA reductase inhibitory activity in plasma; lovastatin is metabolized by CYP3A4 isoenzyme, certain agents, such as ketoconazole, share this metabolic pathway and can raise the plasma levels of lovastatin and may increase the risk of myopathy). Products include:

Nizoral 2% Cream 3620
Nizoral A-D Shampoo 2008
Nizoral 2% Shampoo 2007
Nizoral Tablets 1791

Lopinavir (The risk of myopathy appears to be increased by high levels of HMG-CoA reductase inhibitory activity in plasma; lovastatin is metabolized by CYP3A4 isoenzyme, certain agents, such as HIV protease inhibitors, share this metabolic pathway and can raise the plasma levels of lovastatin and may increase the risk of myopathy). Products include:

Kaletra Capsules 471
Kaletra Oral Solution 471

Miconazole (The risk of myopathy appears to be increased by high levels of HMG-CoA reductase inhibitory activity in plasma; lovastatin is metabolized by CYP3A4 isoenzyme, certain agents, such as azole antifungals, share this metabolic pathway and can raise the plasma levels of lovastatin and may increase the risk of myopathy).

No products indexed under this heading.

Nefazodone Hydrochloride (The risk of myopathy appears to be increased by high levels of HMG-CoA reductase inhibitory activity in plasma; lovastatin is metabolized by CYP3A4 isoenzyme, certain agents, such as antidepressant nefazodone, share this metabolic pathway and can raise the plasma levels of lovastatin and may increase the risk of myopathy). Products include:

Serzone Tablets 1104

Nelfinavir Mesylate (The risk of myopathy appears to be increased by high levels of HMG-CoA reductase inhibitory activity in plasma; lovastatin is metabolized by CYP3A4 isoenzyme, certain agents, such as HIV protease inhibitors, share this metabolic pathway and can raise the plasma levels of lovastatin and may increase the risk of myopathy). Products include:

Viracept 532

Niacin (The incidence and severity of myopathy are increased by co-administration of HMG-CoA reductase inhibitors with drugs that cause myopathy when given alone, such as lipid-lowering doses of niacin; combined use should be avoided; if used concurrently, the dose of lovastatin should generally not exceed 20 mg). Products include:

Niaspan Extended-Release Tablets 1846
Nicotinex Elixir .... ■633

Oxiconazole Nitrate (The risk of myopathy appears to be increased by high levels of HMG-CoA reductase inhibitory activity in plasma; lovastatin is metabolized by CYP3A4 isoenzyme, certain agents, such as azole antifungals, share this metabolic pathway and can raise the plasma levels of lovastatin and may increase the risk of myopathy). Products include:

Oxistat 1298

Ritonavir (The risk of myopathy appears to be increased by high levels of HMG-CoA reductase inhibitory activity in plasma; lovastatin is metabolized by CYP3A4 isoenzyme, certain agents, such as HIV protease inhibitors, share this metabolic pathway and can raise the plasma levels of lovastatin and may increase the risk of myopathy). Products include:

Kaletra Capsules 471
Kaletra Oral Solution 471
Norvir Capsules 487
Norvir Oral Solution 487

Saquinavir (The risk of myopathy appears to be increased by high levels of HMG-CoA reductase inhibitory activity in plasma; lovastatin is metabolized by CYP3A4 isoenzyme, certain agents, such as HIV protease inhibitors, share this metabolic pathway and can raise the plasma levels of lovastatin and may increase the risk of myopathy). Products include:

Fortovase Capsules 2970

Saquinavir Mesylate (The risk of myopathy appears to be increased by high levels of HMG-CoA reductase inhibitory activity in plasma; lovastatin is metabolized by CYP3A4 isoenzyme, certain agents, such as HIV protease inhibitors, share this metabolic pathway and can raise the plasma levels of lovastatin and may increase the risk of myopathy). Products include:

Invirase Capsules 2979

Terconazole (The risk of myopathy appears to be increased by high levels of HMG-CoA reductase inhibitory activity in plasma; lovastatin is metabolized by CYP3A4 isoenzyme, certain agents, such as azole antifungals, share this metabolic pathway and can raise the plasma levels of lovastatin and may increase the risk of myopathy). Products include:

Terazol 3 Vaginal Cream 2587
Terazol 3 Vaginal Suppositories 2587
Terazol 7 Vaginal Cream 2587

Verapamil Hydrochloride (Co-administration may increase the risk of myopathy; although the data are insufficient for lovastatin). Products include:

Covera-HS Tablets 3199
Isoptin SR Tablets 467
Tarka Tablets 508
Verelan Capsules 3184
Verelan PM Capsules 3186

Warfarin Sodium (Co-administration has resulted in bleeding and/or prothrombin time in few patients). Products include:

Coumadin for Injection 1243
Coumadin Tablets 1243
Warfarin Sodium Tablets, USP 3302

Food Interactions

Alcohol (Lovastatin should be used with caution in patients who have consumed substantial quantity of alcohol and have a past history of liver disease; active liver disease and unexplained elevation in transaminase are contraindications to the use of lovastatin).

Grapefruit Juice (Lovastatin is a substrate for CYP4503A4 and grapefruit juice contains one or more components that inhibit CYP3A4; co-administration with grapefruit juice can increase the plasma concentrations of lovastatin and its B-hydroxyacid metabolite; large quantity of grapefruit juice (> 1 quart daily) significantly increase the serum concentrations and should be avoided).

Meal, unspecified (When lovastatin was given under fasting conditions, plasma concentrations of total inhibitors were on average about two-thirds those found when lovastatin was administered immediately after a standard meal).

MEXITIL CAPSULES

(Mexiletine Hydrochloride) 1047

May interact with narcotic analgesics, phenytoin, theophylline, and certain other agents. Compounds in these categories include:

Alfentanil Hydrochloride (Narcotics have been reported to slow the absorption of mexiletine).

No products indexed under this heading.

Aluminum Hydroxide (Magnesium-aluminum hydroxide has been reported to slow the absorption of mexiletine). Products include:

Amphojel Suspension (Mint Flavor) .... ■789
Gaviscon Extra Strength Liquid .... ■751
Gaviscon Extra Strength Tablets .... ■751
Gaviscon Regular Strength Liquid .... ■751
Gaviscon Regular Strength Tablets .... ■750
Maalox Antacid/Anti-Gas Oral Suspension .... ■673
Maalox Max Maximum Strength Antacid/Anti-Gas Liquid 2300
Maalox Regular Strength Antacid/Antigas Liquid 2300
Mylanta 1813
Vanquish Caplets .... ■617

Aminophylline (Co-administration may lead to increased plasma theophylline levels).

No products indexed under this heading.

Atropine Sulfate (Atropine has been reported to slow the absorption of mexiletine). Products include:

Donnatal 2929
Donnatal Extentabs 2930
Motofen Tablets 577
Prosed/DS Tablets 3268
Urised Tablets 2876

Buprenorphine Hydrochloride (Narcotics have been reported to slow the absorption of mexiletine). Products include:

Buprenex Injectable 2918

Caffeine (Co-administration leads to a decrease in caffeine clearance). Products include:

BC Powder .... ■619
Arthritis Strength BC Powder .... ■619
Darvon Compound-65 Pulvules 1910
Aspirin Free Excedrin Caplets and Geltabs .... ■628
Excedrin Extra-Strength Tablets, Caplets, and Geltabs .... ■629
Excedrin Migraine 1070
Goody's Extra Strength Headache Powder .... ■620
Goody's Extra Strength Pain Relief Tablets .... ■620
Hycomine Compound Tablets 1317
Maximum Strength Midol Menstrual Caplets and Gelcaps .... ■612
Vanquish Caplets .... ■617
Vivarin .... ■763

Cimetidine (Co-administration has been reported to increase, decrease, or leave unchanged mexiletine plasma levels). Products include:

Tagamet HB 200 Suspension .... ■762
Tagamet HB 200 Tablets .... ■761
Tagamet Tablets 1644

Cimetidine Hydrochloride (Co-administration has been reported to increase, decrease, or leave unchanged mexiletine plasma levels). Products include:

Tagamet 1644

Codeine Phosphate (Narcotics have been reported to slow the absorption of mexiletine). Products include:
- Phenergan with Codeine Syrup 3557
- Phenergan VC with Codeine Syrup .. 3561
- Robitussin A-C Syrup 2942
- Robitussin-DAC Syrup 2942
- Ryna-C Liquid 768
- Soma Compound w/Codeine Tablets 3355
- Tussi-Organidin NR Liquid 3350
- Tussi-Organidin-S NR Liquid 3350
- Tylenol with Codeine 2595

Dezocine (Narcotics have been reported to slow the absorption of mexiletine).
- No products indexed under this heading.

Digoxin (Mexiletine does not alter serum digoxin levels, but magnesium-aluminum hydroxide, when used to treat gastrointestinal symptoms due to mexiletine, has been reported to lower serum digoxin levels). Products include:
- Digitek Tablets 1003
- Lanoxicaps Capsules 1574
- Lanoxin Injection 1581
- Lanoxin Tablets 1587
- Lanoxin Elixir Pediatric 1578
- Lanoxin Injection Pediatric 1584

Dyphylline (Co-administration may lead to increased plasma theophylline levels). Products include:
- Lufyllin Tablets 3347
- Lufyllin-400 Tablets 3347
- Lufyllin-GG Elixir 3348
- Lufyllin-GG Tablets 3348

Fentanyl (Narcotics have been reported to slow the absorption of mexiletine). Products include:
- Duragesic Transdermal System 1786

Fentanyl Citrate (Narcotics have been reported to slow the absorption of mexiletine). Products include:
- Actiq 1184

Fosphenytoin Sodium (Co-administration with hepatic enzyme inducers, such as phenytoin, has been reported to lower mexiletine plasma levels). Products include:
- Cerebyx Injection 2619

Hydrocodone Bitartrate (Narcotics have been reported to slow the absorption of mexiletine). Products include:
- Hycodan 1316
- Hycomine Compound Tablets 1317
- Hycotuss Expectorant Syrup 1318
- Lortab 3319
- Lortab Elixir 3317
- Maxidone Tablets CIII 3399
- Norco 5/325 Tablets CIII 3424
- Norco 7.5/325 Tablets CIII 3425
- Norco 10/325 Tablets CIII 3427
- Norco 10/325 Tablets CIII 3425
- Vicodin Tablets 516
- Vicodin ES Tablets 517
- Vicodin HP Tablets 518
- Vicodin Tuss Expectorant 519
- Vicoprofen Tablets 520
- Zydone Tablets 1330

Hydrocodone Polistirex (Narcotics have been reported to slow the absorption of mexiletine). Products include:
- Tussionex Pennkinetic Extended-Release Suspension 1174

Hydromorphone Hydrochloride (Narcotics have been reported to slow the absorption of mexiletine). Products include:
- Dilaudid 441
- Dilaudid Oral Liquid 445
- Dilaudid Powder 441
- Dilaudid Rectal Suppositories 441
- Dilaudid Tablets 441
- Dilaudid Tablets - 8 mg 445
- Dilaudid-HP 443

Levorphanol Tartrate (Narcotics have been reported to slow the absorption of mexiletine). Products include:
- Levo-Dromoran 1734
- Levorphanol Tartrate Tablets 3059

Magnesium Hydroxide (Magnesium-aluminum hydroxide has been reported to slow the absorption of mexiletine). Products include:
- Ex•Lax Milk of Magnesia Liquid 670
- Maalox Antacid/Anti-Gas Oral Suspension 673
- Maalox Max Maximum Strength Antacid/Anti-Gas Liquid 2300
- Maalox Regular Strength Antacid/Antigas Liquid 2300
- Mylanta Fast-Acting 1813
- Mylanta 1813
- Pepcid Complete Chewable Tablets 1815
- Phillips' Chewable Tablets 615
- Phillips' Milk of Magnesia Liquid (Original, Cherry, & Mint) 616
- Rolaids Tablets 706
- Extra Strength Rolaids Tablets 706
- Vanquish Caplets 617

Meperidine Hydrochloride (Narcotics have been reported to slow the absorption of mexiletine). Products include:
- Demerol 3079
- Mepergan Injection 3539

Methadone Hydrochloride (Narcotics have been reported to slow the absorption of mexiletine). Products include:
- Dolophine Hydrochloride Tablets 3056

Metoclopramide Hydrochloride (Co-administration has been reported to accelerate absorption). Products include:
- Reglan 2935

Morphine Sulfate (Narcotics have been reported to slow the absorption of mexiletine). Products include:
- Astramorph/PF Injection, USP (Preservative-Free) 594
- Duramorph Injection 1312
- Infumorph 200 and Infumorph 500 Sterile Solutions 1314
- Kadian Capsules 1335
- MS Contin Tablets 2896
- MSIR 2898
- Oramorph SR Tablets 3062
- Roxanol 3066

Oxycodone Hydrochloride (Narcotics have been reported to slow the absorption of mexiletine). Products include:
- OxyContin Tablets 2912
- OxyFast Oral Concentrate Solution 2916
- OxyIR Capsules 2916
- Percocet Tablets 1326
- Percodan Tablets 1327
- Percolone Tablets 1327
- Roxicodone 3067
- Tylox Capsules 2597

Phenobarbital (Co-administration with hepatic enzyme inducers, such as phenobarbital, has been reported to lower mexiletine plasma levels). Products include:
- Arco-Lase Plus Tablets 592
- Donnatal 2929
- Donnatal Extentabs 2930

Phenytoin (Co-administration with hepatic enzyme inducers, such as phenytoin, has been reported to lower mexiletine plasma levels). Products include:
- Dilantin Infatabs 2624
- Dilantin-125 Oral Suspension 2625

Phenytoin Sodium (Co-administration with hepatic enzyme inducers, such as phenytoin, has been reported to lower mexiletine plasma levels). Products include:
- Dilantin Kapseals 2622

Propoxyphene Hydrochloride (Narcotics have been reported to slow the absorption of mexiletine). Products include:
- Darvon Pulvules 1909
- Darvon Compound-65 Pulvules 1910

Propoxyphene Napsylate (Narcotics have been reported to slow the absorption of mexiletine). Products include:
- Darvon-N/Darvocet-N 1907
- Darvon-N Tablets 1912

Remifentanil Hydrochloride (Narcotics have been reported to slow the absorption of mexiletine).
- No products indexed under this heading.

Rifampin (Co-administration with hepatic enzyme inducers, such as rifampin, has been reported to lower mexiletine plasma levels). Products include:
- Rifadin 765
- Rifamate Capsules 767
- Rifater Tablets 769

Sufentanil Citrate (Narcotics have been reported to slow the absorption of mexiletine).
- No products indexed under this heading.

Theophylline (Co-administration may lead to increased plasma theophylline levels). Products include:
- Aerolate 1361
- Theo-Dur Extended-Release Tablets 1835
- Uni-Dur Extended-Release Tablets 1841
- Uniphyl 400 mg and 600 mg Tablets 2903

Theophylline Calcium Salicylate (Co-administration may lead to increased plasma theophylline levels).
- No products indexed under this heading.

Theophylline Sodium Glycinate (Co-administration may lead to increased plasma theophylline levels).
- No products indexed under this heading.

MEYENBERG GOAT MILK
(Goat Milk) 823
None cited in PDR database.

MIACALCIN INJECTION
(Calcitonin-Salmon) 2373
None cited in PDR database.

MIACALCIN NASAL SPRAY
(Calcitonin-Salmon) 2375
May interact with:

Etidronate Disodium (Diphosphonate) (Prior diphosphonate use may reduce the anti-resorptive response to calcitonin-salmon nasal spray).
- No products indexed under this heading.

Pamidronate Disodium (Prior diphosphonate use may reduce the anti-resorptive response to calcitonin-salmon nasal spray). Products include:
- Aredia for Injection 2309

MICARDIS TABLETS
(Telmisartan) 1049
May interact with:

Digoxin (Co-administration has resulted in median increases in digoxin peak plasma concentration (49%) and in trough concentration (20%); digoxin levels should be monitored when initiating, adjusting, and discontinuing telmisartan to avoid possible over- or under- digitalization). Products include:
- Digitek Tablets 1003
- Lanoxicaps Capsules 1574
- Lanoxin Injection 1581
- Lanoxin Tablets 1587
- Lanoxin Elixir Pediatric 1578
- Lanoxin Injection Pediatric 1584

Warfarin Sodium (Co-administration has resulted in slight decrease in the mean warfarin trough plasma concentration; this decrease did not result in a change in INR). Products include:
- Coumadin for Injection 1243
- Coumadin Tablets 1243
- Warfarin Sodium Tablets, USP 3302

Food Interactions

Food, unspecified (Slightly reduces the bioavailability of telmisartan; Micardis tablets may be administered with or without food).

MICARDIS HCT TABLETS
(Hydrochlorothiazide, Telmisartan) 1051
May interact with certain other agents. Compounds in these categories include:

Acarbose (Thiazide diuretics may cause hyperglycemia; dosage adjustment of oral hypoglycemia agents may be required). Products include:
- Precose Tablets 906

Acebutolol Hydrochloride (Co-administration with other antihypertensive agents may result in additive effect or potentiation). Products include:
- Sectral Capsules 3589

ACTH (Intensifies electrolyte depletion, particularly hypokalemia).
- No products indexed under this heading.

Alfentanil Hydrochloride (Potentiation of orthostatic hypotension).
- No products indexed under this heading.

Amlodipine Besylate (Co-administration with other antihypertensive agents may result in additive effect or potentiation). Products include:
- Lotrel Capsules 2370
- Norvasc Tablets 2704

Aprobarbital (Potentiation of orthostatic hypotension).
- No products indexed under this heading.

Atenolol (Co-administration with other antihypertensive agents may result in additive effect or potentiation). Products include:
- Tenoretic Tablets 690
- Tenormin I.V. Injection 692

Atracurium Besylate (Possible increased responsiveness to the muscle relaxants).
- No products indexed under this heading.

Benazepril Hydrochloride (Co-administration with other antihypertensive agents may result in additive effect or potentiation). Products include:
- Lotensin Tablets 2365
- Lotensin HCT Tablets 2367
- Lotrel Capsules 2370

Bendroflumethiazide (Co-administration with other antihypertensive agents may result in additive effect or potentiation). Products include:
- Corzide 40/5 Tablets 2247
- Corzide 80/5 Tablets 2247

Betamethasone Acetate (Corticosteroids intensify electrolyte depletion, particularly hypokalemia). Products include:
- Celestone Soluspan Injectable Suspension 3097

Betamethasone Sodium Phosphate (Corticosteroids intensify electrolyte depletion, particularly hypokalemia). Products include:
- Celestone Soluspan Injectable Suspension 3097

Betaxolol Hydrochloride (Co-administration with other antihypertensive agents may result in additive effect or potentiation). Products include:
- Betoptic S Ophthalmic Suspension 537

Bisoprolol Fumarate (Co-administration with other antihypertensive agents may result in additive effect or potentiation). Products include:
- Zebeta Tablets 1885
- Ziac Tablets 1887

Buprenorphine Hydrochloride (Potentiation of orthostatic hypotension). Products include:
- Buprenex Injectable 2918

Butabarbital (Potentiation of orthostatic hypotension).
No products indexed under this heading.

Butalbital (Potentiation of orthostatic hypotension). Products include:
Phrenilin 578
Sedapap Tablets 50 mg/650 mg 2225

Candesartan Cilexetil (Co-administration with other antihypertensive agents may result in additive effect or potentiation). Products include:
Atacand Tablets 595
Atacand HCT Tablets 597

Captopril (Co-administration with other antihypertensive agents may result in additive effect or potentiation). Products include:
Captopril Tablets 2281

Carteolol Hydrochloride (Co-administration with other antihypertensive agents may result in additive effect or potentiation). Products include:
Carteolol Hydrochloride Ophthalmic Solution USP, 1% .... ⊙258
Ocupress Ophthalmic Solution, 1% Sterile .... ⊙303

Celecoxib (Co-administration in some patients can result in reduced diuretic, natriuretic, and antihypertensive effects). Products include:
Celebrex Capsules 2676
Celebrex Capsules 2780

Chlorothiazide (Co-administration with other antihypertensive agents may result in additive effect or potentiation). Products include:
Aldoclor Tablets 2035
Diuril Oral 2087

Chlorothiazide Sodium (Co-administration with other antihypertensive agents may result in additive effect or potentiation). Products include:
Diuril Sodium Intravenous 2086

Chlorpropamide (Thiazide diuretics may cause hyperglycemia; dosage adjustment of oral hypoglycemia agents may be required). Products include:
Diabinese Tablets 2680

Chlorthalidone (Co-administration with other antihypertensive agents may result in additive effect or potentiation). Products include:
Clorpres Tablets 1002
Combipres Tablets 1040
Tenoretic Tablets 690

Cholestyramine (Absorption of hydrochlorothiazide is impaired in the presence of anionic exchange resins; cholestyramine binds the hydrochlorothiazide from the GI tract by up to 85%).
No products indexed under this heading.

Cisatracurium Besylate (Possible increased responsiveness to the muscle relaxants).
No products indexed under this heading.

Clonidine (Co-administration with other antihypertensive agents may result in additive effect or potentiation). Products include:
Catapres-TTS 1038

Clonidine Hydrochloride (Co-administration with other antihypertensive agents may result in additive effect or potentiation). Products include:
Catapres Tablets 1037
Clorpres Tablets 1002
Combipres Tablets 1040
Duraclon Injection 3057

Codeine Phosphate (Potentiation of orthostatic hypotension). Products include:
Phenergan with Codeine Syrup 3557
Phenergan VC with Codeine Syrup 3561
Robitussin A-C Syrup 2942
Robitussin-DAC Syrup 2942
Ryna-C Liquid .... ▣768
Soma Compound w/Codeine Tablets 3355
Tussi-Organidin NR Liquid 3350
Tussi-Organidin-S NR Liquid 3350
Tylenol with Codeine 2595

Colestipol Hydrochloride (Absorption of hydrochlorothiazide is impaired in the presence of anionic exchange resins; colestipol binds the hydroclorothiazide from the GI tract by up to 43%). Products include:
Colestid Tablets 2791

Cortisone Acetate (Corticosteroids intensify electrolyte depletion, particularly hypokalemia). Products include:
Cortone Acetate Injectable Suspension 2059
Cortone Acetate Tablets 2061

Deserpidine (Co-administration with other antihypertensive agents may result in additive effect or potentiation).
No products indexed under this heading.

Dexamethasone (Corticosteroids intensify electrolyte depletion, particularly hypokalemia). Products include:
Decadron Elixir 2078
Decadron Tablets 2079
TobraDex Ophthalmic Ointment 542
TobraDex Ophthalmic Suspension 541

Dexamethasone Acetate (Corticosteroids intensify electrolyte depletion, particularly hypokalemia).
No products indexed under this heading.

Dexamethasone Sodium Phosphate (Corticosteroids intensify electrolyte depletion, particularly hypokalemia). Products include:
Decadron Phosphate Injection 2081
Decadron Phosphate Sterile Ophthalmic Ointment 2083
Decadron Phosphate Sterile Ophthalmic Solution 2084
NeoDecadron Sterile Ophthalmic Solution 2144

Dezocine (Potentiation of orthostatic hypotension).
No products indexed under this heading.

Diazoxide (Co-administration with other antihypertensive agents may result in additive effect or potentiation).
No products indexed under this heading.

Diclofenac Potassium (Co-administration in some patients can result in reduced diuretic, natriuretic, and antihypertensive effects). Products include:
Cataflam Tablets 2315

Diclofenac Sodium (Co-administration in some patients can result in reduced diuretic, natriuretic, and antihypertensive effects). Products include:
Arthrotec Tablets 3195
Voltaren Ophthalmic Sterile Ophthalmic Solution .... ⊙312
Voltaren Tablets 2315
Voltaren-XR Tablets 2315

Digoxin (Co-administration has resulted in median increases in digoxin peak plasma concentration (49%) and in trough concentration (20%); digoxin levels should be monitored when initiating, adjusting, and discontinuing telmisartan to avoid possible over- or under-digitalization; thiazide-induced hypokalemia exaggerate or sensitize the response of the heart to the toxic effects of digitalis, i.e., increased ventricular irritability). Products include:
Digitek Tablets 1003
Lanoxicaps Capsules 1574
Lanoxin Injection 1581
Lanoxin Tablets 1587
Lanoxin Elixir Pediatric 1578
Lanoxin Injection Pediatric 1584

Diltiazem Hydrochloride (Co-administration with other antihypertensive agents may result in additive effect or potentiation). Products include:
Cardizem Injectable 1018
Cardizem Lyo-Ject Syringe 1018
Cardizem Monovial 1018
Cardizem CD Capsules 1016
Tiazac Capsules 1378

Doxazosin Mesylate (Co-administration with other antihypertensive agents may result in additive effect or potentiation). Products include:
Cardura Tablets 2668

Enalapril Maleate (Co-administration with other antihypertensive agents may result in additive effect or potentiation). Products include:
Lexxel Tablets 608
Vaseretic Tablets 2204
Vasotec Tablets 2210

Enalaprilat (Co-administration with other antihypertensive agents may result in additive effect or potentiation). Products include:
Enalaprilat Injection 863
Vasotec I.V. Injection 2207

Eprosartan Mesylate (Co-administration with other antihypertensive agents may result in additive effect or potentiation). Products include:
Teveten Tablets 3327

Esmolol Hydrochloride (Co-administration with other antihypertensive agents may result in additive effect or potentiation). Products include:
Brevibloc Injection 858

Etodolac (Co-administration in some patients can result in reduced diuretic, natriuretic, and antihypertensive effects). Products include:
Lodine 3528
Lodine XL Extended-Release Tablets 3530

Felodipine (Co-administration with other antihypertensive agents may result in additive effect or potentiation). Products include:
Lexxel Tablets 608
Plendil Extended-Release Tablets 623

Fenoprofen Calcium (Co-administration in some patients can result in reduced diuretic, natriuretic, and antihypertensive effects).
No products indexed under this heading.

Fentanyl (Potentiation of orthostatic hypotension). Products include:
Duragesic Transdermal System 1786

Fentanyl Citrate (Potentiation of orthostatic hypotension). Products include:
Actiq 1184

Fludrocortisone Acetate (Corticosteroids intensify electrolyte depletion, particularly hypokalemia). Products include:
Florinef Acetate Tablets 2250

Flurbiprofen (Co-administration in some patients can result in reduced diuretic, natriuretic, and antihypertensive effects).
No products indexed under this heading.

Fosinopril Sodium (Co-administration with other antihypertensive agents may result in additive effect or potentiation). Products include:
Monopril Tablets 1091
Monopril HCT 1094

Furosemide (Co-administration with other antihypertensive agents may result in additive effect or potentiation). Products include:
Furosemide Tablets 2284

Glimepiride (Thiazide diuretics may cause hyperglycemia; dosage adjustment of oral hypoglycemia agents may be required). Products include:
Amaryl Tablets 717

Glipizide (Thiazide diuretics may cause hyperglycemia; dosage adjustment of oral hypoglycemia agents may be required). Products include:
Glucotrol Tablets 2692
Glucotrol XL Extended Release Tablets 2693

Glyburide (Thiazide diuretics may cause hyperglycemia; dosage adjustment of oral hypoglycemia agents may be required). Products include:
DiaBeta Tablets 741
Glucovance Tablets 1086

Guanabenz Acetate (Co-administration with other antihypertensive agents may result in additive effect or potentiation).
No products indexed under this heading.

Guanethidine Monosulfate (Co-administration with other antihypertensive agents may result in additive effect or potentiation).
No products indexed under this heading.

Hydralazine Hydrochloride (Co-administration with other antihypertensive agents may result in additive effect or potentiation).
No products indexed under this heading.

Hydrocodone Bitartrate (Potentiation of orthostatic hypotension). Products include:
Hycodan 1316
Hycomine Compound Tablets 1317
Hycotuss Expectorant Syrup 1318
Lortab 3319
Lortab Elixir 3317
Maxidone Tablets CIII 3399
Norco 5/325 Tablets CIII 3424
Norco 7.5/325 Tablets CIII 3425
Norco 10/325 Tablets CIII 3427
Norco 10/325 Tablets CIII 3425
Vicodin Tablets 516
Vicodin ES Tablets 517
Vicodin HP Tablets 518
Vicodin Tuss Expectorant 519
Vicoprofen Tablets 520
Zydone Tablets 1330

Hydrocodone Polistirex (Potentiation of orthostatic hypotension). Products include:
Tussionex Pennkinetic Extended-Release Suspension 1174

Hydrocortisone (Corticosteroids intensify electrolyte depletion, particularly hypokalemia). Products include:
Anusol-HC Cream 2.5% 2237
Cipro HC Otic Suspension 540
Cortaid Intensive Therapy Cream .... ▣717
Cortaid Maximum Strength Cream .... ▣717
Cortisporin Ophthalmic Suspension Sterile .... ⊙297
Cortizone•5 .... ▣699
Cortizone•10 .... ▣699
Cortizone•10 Plus Creme .... ▣700
Cortizone for Kids Creme .... ▣699
Hydrocortone Tablets 2106
Massengill Medicated Soft Cloth Towelette .... ▣753
VōSoL HC Otic Solution 3356

Hydrocortisone Acetate (Corticosteroids intensify electrolyte depletion, particularly hypokalemia). Products include:
Analpram-HC 1338
Anusol HC-1 Hydrocortisone Anti-Itch Cream .... ▣689
Anusol-HC Suppositories 2238
Cortaid .... ▣717
Cortifoam Rectal Foam 3170
Cortisporin-TC Otic Suspension 2246
Hydrocortone Acetate Injectable Suspension 2103
Pramosone 1343
Proctocort Suppositories 2264
ProctoFoam-HC 3177
Terra-Cortril Ophthalmic Suspension 2716

Hydrocortisone Sodium Phosphate (Corticosteroids intensify electrolyte depletion, particularly hypokalemia). Products include:
Hydrocortone Phosphate Injection, Sterile 2105

Hydrocortisone Sodium Succinate (Corticosteroids intensify electrolyte depletion, particularly hypokalemia).
No products indexed under this heading.

Hydroflumethiazide (Co-administration with other antihypertensive agents may result in additive effect or potentiation). Products include:
Diucardin Tablets 3494

Hydromorphone Hydrochloride (Potentiation of orthostatic hypotension). Products include:
Dilaudid 441
Dilaudid Oral Liquid 445
Dilaudid Powder 441
Dilaudid Rectal Suppositories 441
Dilaudid Tablets 441
Dilaudid Tablets - 8 mg 445
Dilaudid-HP 443

Ibuprofen (Co-administration in some patients can result in reduced diuretic, natriuretic, and antihypertensive effects). Products include:
Advil 771
Children's Advil Oral Suspension 773
Children's Advil Chewable Tablets 773
Advil Cold and Sinus Caplets 771
Advil Cold and Sinus Tablets 771
Advil Flu & Body Ache Caplets 772
Infants' Advil Drops 773
Junior Strength Advil Tablets 773
Junior Strength Advil Chewable Tablets 773
Advil Migraine Liquigels 772
Children's Motrin Oral Suspension and Chewable Tablets 2006
Children's Motrin Cold Oral Suspension 2007
Children's Motrin Oral Suspension 643
Motrin Suspension, Oral Drops, Chewable Tablets, and Caplets 2002
Infants' Motrin Concentrated Drops 2006
Junior Strength Motrin Caplets and Chewable Tablets 2006
Motrin IB Tablets, Caplets, and Gelcaps 2002
Motrin Migraine Pain Caplets 2005
Motrin Sinus Headache Caplets 2005
Vicoprofen Tablets 520

Indapamide (Co-administration with other antihypertensive agents may result in additive effect or potentiation). Products include:
Indapamide Tablets 2286

Indomethacin (Co-administration in some patients can result in reduced diuretic, natriuretic, and antihypertensive effects). Products include:
Indocin 2112

Indomethacin Sodium Trihydrate (Co-administration in some patients can result in reduced diuretic, natriuretic, and antihypertensive effects). Products include:
Indocin I.V. 2115

Insulin, Human, Zinc Suspension (Thiazide diuretics may cause hyperglycemia; dosage adjustment of insulin may be required). Products include:
Humulin L, 100 Units 1937
Humulin U, 100 Units 1943
Novolin L Human Insulin 10 ml Vials 2422

Insulin, Human NPH (Thiazide diuretics may cause hyperglycemia; dosage adjustment of insulin may be required). Products include:
Humulin N, 100 Units 1939
Humulin N NPH Pen 1940
Novolin N Human Insulin 10 ml Vials 2422
Novolin N PenFill 2423
Novolin N Prefilled Syringe Disposable Insulin Delivery System 2425

Insulin, Human Regular (Thiazide diuretics may cause hyperglycemia; dosage adjustment of insulin may be required). Products include:
Humulin R Regular (U-500) 1943
Humulin R, 100 Units 1941
Novolin R Human Insulin 10 ml Vials 2423
Novolin R PenFill 2423
Novolin R Prefilled Syringe Disposable Insulin Delivery System 2425
Velosulin BR Human Insulin 10 ml Vials 2435

Insulin, Human Regular and Human NPH Mixture (Thiazide diuretics may cause hyperglycemia; dosage adjustment of insulin may be required). Products include:
Humulin 50/50, 100 Units 1934
Humulin 70/30, 100 Units 1935
Humulin 70/30 Pen 1936
Novolin 70/30 Human Insulin 10 ml Vials 2421
Novolin 70/30 PenFill 2423
Novolin 70/30 Prefilled Disposable Insulin Delivery System 2425

Insulin, NPH (Thiazide diuretics may cause hyperglycemia; dosage adjustment of insulin may be required). Products include:
Iletin II, NPH (Pork), 100 Units 1946

Insulin, Regular (Thiazide diuretics may cause hyperglycemia; dosage adjustment of insulin may be required). Products include:
Iletin II, Regular (Pork), 100 Units 1947

Insulin, Zinc Crystals (Thiazide diuretics may cause hyperglycemia; dosage adjustment of insulin may be required).
No products indexed under this heading.

Insulin, Zinc Suspension (Thiazide diuretics may cause hyperglycemia; dosage adjustment of insulin may be required). Products include:
Iletin II, Lente (Pork), 100 Units 1945

Insulin Aspart, Human Regular (Thiazide diuretics may cause hyperglycemia; dosage adjustment of insulin may be required).
No products indexed under this heading.

Insulin glargine (Thiazide diuretics may cause hyperglycemia; dosage adjustment of insulin may be required). Products include:
Lantus Injection 742

Insulin Lispro, Human (Thiazide diuretics may cause hyperglycemia; dosage adjustment of insulin may be required). Products include:
Humalog 1926
Humalog Mix 75/25 Pen 1928

Insulin Lispro Protamine, Human (Thiazide diuretics may cause hyperglycemia; dosage adjustment of insulin may be required). Products include:
Humalog Mix 75/25 Pen 1928

Irbesartan (Co-administration with other antihypertensive agents may result in additive effect or potentiation). Products include:
Avalide Tablets 1070
Avapro Tablets 1074
Avapro Tablets 3076

Isradipine (Co-administration with other antihypertensive agents may result in additive effect or potentiation). Products include:
DynaCirc Capsules 2921
DynaCirc CR Tablets 2923

Ketoprofen (Co-administration in some patients can result in reduced diuretic, natriuretic, and antihypertensive effects). Products include:
Orudis Capsules 3548
Orudis KT Tablets 778
Oruvail Capsules 3548

Ketorolac Tromethamine (Co-administration in some patients can result in reduced diuretic, natriuretic, and antihypertensive effects). Products include:
Acular Ophthalmic Solution 544
Acular PF Ophthalmic Solution 544
Toradol 3018

Labetalol Hydrochloride (Co-administration with other antihypertensive agents may result in additive effect or potentiation). Products include:
Normodyne Injection 3135
Normodyne Tablets 3137

Levorphanol Tartrate (Potentiation of orthostatic hypotension). Products include:
Levo-Dromoran 1734
Levorphanol Tartrate Tablets 3059

Lisinopril (Co-administration with other antihypertensive agents may result in additive effect or potentiation). Products include:
Prinivil Tablets 2164
Prinzide Tablets 2168
Zestoretic Tablets 695
Zestril Tablets 698

Lithium Carbonate (Diuretics reduce the renal clearance of lithium and add a high risk of lithium toxicity; concurrent use should be avoided). Products include:
Eskalith 1527
Lithium Carbonate 3061
Lithobid Slow-Release Tablets 3255

Lithium Citrate (Diuretics reduce the renal clearance of lithium and add a high risk of lithium toxicity; concurrent use should be avoided). Products include:
Lithium Citrate Syrup 3061

Losartan Potassium (Co-administration with other antihypertensive agents may result in additive effect or potentiation). Products include:
Cozaar Tablets 2067
Hyzaar 2109

Mecamylamine Hydrochloride (Co-administration with other antihypertensive agents may result in additive effect or potentiation). Products include:
Inversine Tablets 1850

Meclofenamate Sodium (Co-administration in some patients can result in reduced diuretic, natriuretic, and antihypertensive effects).
No products indexed under this heading.

Mefenamic Acid (Co-administration in some patients can result in reduced diuretic, natriuretic, and antihypertensive effects). Products include:
Ponstel Capsules 1356

Meloxicam (Co-administration in some patients can result in reduced diuretic, natriuretic, and antihypertensive effects). Products include:
Mobic Tablets 1054

Meperidine Hydrochloride (Potentiation of orthostatic hypotension). Products include:
Demerol 3079
Mepergan Injection 3539

Mephobarbital (Potentiation of orthostatic hypotension).
No products indexed under this heading.

Metformin Hydrochloride (Thiazide diuretics may cause hyperglycemia; dosage adjustment of oral hypoglycemia agents may be required). Products include:
Glucophage Tablets 1080
Glucophage XR Tablets 1080
Glucovance Tablets 1086

Methadone Hydrochloride (Potentiation of orthostatic hypotension). Products include:
Dolophine Hydrochloride Tablets 3056

Methyclothiazide (Co-administration with other antihypertensive agents may result in additive effect or potentiation).
No products indexed under this heading.

Methyldopa (Co-administration with other antihypertensive agents may result in additive effect or potentiation). Products include:
Aldoclor Tablets 2035
Aldomet Tablets 2037
Aldoril Tablets 2039

Methyldopate Hydrochloride (Co-administration with other antihypertensive agents may result in additive effect or potentiation).
No products indexed under this heading.

Methylprednisolone Acetate (Corticosteroids intensify electrolyte depletion, particularly hypokalemia). Products include:
Depo-Medrol Injectable Suspension 2795

Methylprednisolone Sodium Succinate (Corticosteroids intensify electrolyte depletion, particularly hypokalemia). Products include:
Solu-Medrol Sterile Powder 2855

Metocurine Iodide (Possible increased responsiveness to the muscle relaxants).
No products indexed under this heading.

Metolazone (Co-administration with other antihypertensive agents may result in additive effect or potentiation). Products include:
Mykrox Tablets 1168
Zaroxolyn Tablets 1177

Metoprolol Succinate (Co-administration with other antihypertensive agents may result in additive effect or potentiation). Products include:
Toprol-XL Tablets 651

Metoprolol Tartrate (Co-administration with other antihypertensive agents may result in additive effect or potentiation).
No products indexed under this heading.

Metyrosine (Co-administration with other antihypertensive agents may result in additive effect or potentiation). Products include:
Demser Capsules 2085

Mibefradil Dihydrochloride (Co-administration with other antihypertensive agents may result in additive effect or potentiation).
No products indexed under this heading.

Miglitol (Thiazide diuretics may cause hyperglycemia; dosage adjustment of oral hypoglycemia agents may be required). Products include:
Glyset Tablets 2821

Minoxidil (Co-administration with other antihypertensive agents may result in additive effect or potentiation). Products include:
Rogaine Extra Strength for Men Topical Solution 721
Rogaine for Women Topical Solution 721

Mivacurium Chloride (Possible increased responsiveness to the muscle relaxants).
No products indexed under this heading.

Moexipril Hydrochloride (Co-administration with other antihypertensive agents may result in additive effect or potentiation). Products include:
Uniretic Tablets 3178
Univasc Tablets 3181

Morphine Sulfate (Potentiation of orthostatic hypotension). Products include:
Astramorph/PF Injection, USP (Preservative-Free) 594
Duramorph Injection 1312
Infumorph 200 and Infumorph 500 Sterile Solutions 1314
Kadian Capsules 1335
MS Contin Tablets 2896
MSIR 2898
Oramorph SR Tablets 3062
Roxanol 3066

Nabumetone (Co-administration in some patients can result in reduced diuretic, natriuretic, and antihypertensive effects). Products include:
Relafen Tablets 1617

IMPORTANT NOTE: Always consult each drug listing in the patient's regimen for possible interactions.

Nadolol (Co-administration with other antihypertensive agents may result in additive effect or potentiation). Products include:
- Corgard Tablets 2245
- Corzide 40/5 Tablets 2247
- Corzide 80/5 Tablets 2247
- Nadolol Tablets 2288

Naproxen (Co-administration in some patients can result in reduced diuretic, natriuretic, and antihypertensive effects). Products include:
- EC-Naprosyn Delayed-Release Tablets 2967
- Naprosyn Suspension 2967
- Naprosyn Tablets 2967

Naproxen Sodium (Co-administration in some patients can result in reduced diuretic, natriuretic, and antihypertensive effects). Products include:
- Aleve Tablets, Caplets and Gelcaps .... ■602
- Aleve Cold & Sinus Caplets .... ■603
- Anaprox Tablets 2967
- Anaprox DS Tablets 2967
- Naprelan Tablets 1293

Nicardipine Hydrochloride (Co-administration with other antihypertensive agents may result in additive effect or potentiation). Products include:
- Cardene I.V. 3485

Nifedipine (Co-administration with other antihypertensive agents may result in additive effect or potentiation). Products include:
- Adalat CC Tablets 877
- Procardia Capsules 2708
- Procardia XL Extended Release Tablets 2710

Nisoldipine (Co-administration with other antihypertensive agents may result in additive effect or potentiation). Products include:
- Sular Tablets 688

Nitroglycerin (Co-administration with other antihypertensive agents may result in additive effect or potentiation). Products include:
- Nitro-Dur Transdermal Infusion System 3134
- Nitro-Dur Transdermal Infusion System 1834
- Nitrolingual Pumpspray 1355
- Nitrostat Tablets 2658

Norepinephrine Bitartrate (Possible decreased response to pressure amines).
- No products indexed under this heading.

Oxaprozin (Co-administration in some patients can result in reduced diuretic, natriuretic, and antihypertensive effects).
- No products indexed under this heading.

Oxycodone Hydrochloride (Potentiation of orthostatic hypotension). Products include:
- OxyContin Tablets 2912
- OxyFast Oral Concentrate Solution 2916
- OxyIR Capsules 2916
- Percocet Tablets 1326
- Percodan Tablets 1327
- Percolone Tablets 1327
- Roxicodone 3067
- Tylox Capsules 2597

Pancuronium Bromide (Possible increased responsiveness to the muscle relaxants).
- No products indexed under this heading.

Penbutolol Sulfate (Co-administration with other antihypertensive agents may result in additive effect or potentiation).
- No products indexed under this heading.

Pentobarbital Sodium (Potentiation of orthostatic hypotension). Products include:
- Nembutal Sodium Solution 485

Perindopril Erbumine (Co-administration with other antihypertensive agents may result in additive effect or potentiation). Products include:
- Aceon Tablets (2 mg, 4 mg, 8 mg) 3249

Phenobarbital (Potentiation of orthostatic hypotension). Products include:
- Arco-Lase Plus Tablets 592
- Donnatal 2929
- Donnatal Extentabs 2930

Phenoxybenzamine Hydrochloride (Co-administration with other antihypertensive agents may result in additive effect or potentiation). Products include:
- Dibenzyline Capsules 3457

Phentolamine Mesylate (Co-administration with other antihypertensive agents may result in additive effect or potentiation).
- No products indexed under this heading.

Phenylbutazone (Co-administration in some patients can result in reduced diuretic, natriuretic, and antihypertensive effects).
- No products indexed under this heading.

Pindolol (Co-administration with other antihypertensive agents may result in additive effect or potentiation).
- No products indexed under this heading.

Pioglitazone Hydrochloride (Thiazide diuretics may cause hyperglycemia; dosage adjustment of oral hypoglycemia agents may be required). Products include:
- Actos Tablets 3275

Piroxicam (Co-administration in some patients can result in reduced diuretic, natriuretic, and antihypertensive effects). Products include:
- Feldene Capsules 2685

Polythiazide (Co-administration with other antihypertensive agents may result in additive effect or potentiation). Products include:
- Minizide Capsules 2700
- Renese Tablets 2712

Potassium Acid Phosphate (Concurrent use of potassium supplements or salt substitute is not recommended). Products include:
- K-Phos Original (Sodium Free) Tablets 947

Potassium Bicarbonate (Concurrent use of potassium supplements or salt substitute is not recommended).
- No products indexed under this heading.

Potassium Chloride (Concurrent use of potassium supplements or salt substitute is not recommended). Products include:
- Chlor-3 1361
- Colyte with Flavor Packs for Oral Solution 3170
- GoLYTELY and Pineapple Flavor GoLYTELY for Oral Solution 1068
- K-Dur Microburst Release System ER Tablets 1832
- Klor-Con M20/Klor-Con M10 Tablets 3329
- K-Lor Powder Packets 469
- K-Tab Filmtab Tablets 470
- Micro-K 3311
- NuLYTELY, Cherry Flavor, Lemon-Lime Flavor, and Orange Flavor NuLYTELY for Oral Solution 1068
- Rum-K 1363

Potassium Citrate (Concurrent use of potassium supplements or salt substitute is not recommended). Products include:
- Urocit-K Tablets 2232

Potassium Gluconate (Concurrent use of potassium supplements or salt substitute is not recommended).
- No products indexed under this heading.

Potassium Phosphate (Concurrent use of potassium supplements or salt substitute is not recommended). Products include:
- K-Phos Neutral Tablets 946

Prazosin Hydrochloride (Co-administration with other antihypertensive agents may result in additive effect or potentiation). Products include:
- Minipress Capsules 2699
- Minizide Capsules 2700

Prednisolone Acetate (Corticosteroids intensify electrolyte depletion, particularly hypokalemia). Products include:
- Blephamide Ophthalmic Ointment 547
- Blephamide Ophthalmic Suspension 548
- Poly-Pred Liquifilm Ophthalmic Suspension .... ⊙245
- Pred Forte Ophthalmic Suspension .... ⊙246
- Pred Mild Sterile Ophthalmic Suspension .... ⊙249
- Pred-G Ophthalmic Suspension .... ⊙247
- Pred-G Sterile Ophthalmic Ointment .... ⊙248

Prednisolone Sodium Phosphate (Corticosteroids intensify electrolyte depletion, particularly hypokalemia). Products include:
- Pediapred Oral Solution 1170

Prednisolone Tebutate (Corticosteroids intensify electrolyte depletion, particularly hypokalemia).
- No products indexed under this heading.

Prednisone (Corticosteroids intensify electrolyte depletion, particularly hypokalemia). Products include:
- Prednisone 3064

Propoxyphene Hydrochloride (Potentiation of orthostatic hypotension). Products include:
- Darvon Pulvules 1909
- Darvon Compound-65 Pulvules 1910

Propoxyphene Napsylate (Potentiation of orthostatic hypotension). Products include:
- Darvon-N/Darvocet-N 1907
- Darvon-N Tablets 1912

Propranolol Hydrochloride (Co-administration with other antihypertensive agents may result in additive effect or potentiation). Products include:
- Inderal 3513
- Inderal LA Long-Acting Capsules 3516
- Inderide Tablets 3517
- Inderide LA Long-Acting Capsules 3519

Quinapril Hydrochloride (Co-administration with other antihypertensive agents may result in additive effect or potentiation). Products include:
- Accupril Tablets 2611
- Accuretic Tablets 2614

Ramipril (Co-administration with other antihypertensive agents may result in additive effect or potentiation). Products include:
- Altace Capsules 2233

Rapacuronium Bromide (Possible increased responsiveness to the muscle relaxants).
- No products indexed under this heading.

Rauwolfia serpentina (Co-administration with other antihypertensive agents may result in additive effect or potentiation).
- No products indexed under this heading.

Remifentanil Hydrochloride (Potentiation of orthostatic hypotension).
- No products indexed under this heading.

Repaglinide (Thiazide diuretics may cause hyperglycemia; dosage adjustment of oral hypoglycemia agents may be required). Products include:
- Prandin Tablets (0.5, 1, and 2 mg) 2432

Rescinnamine (Co-administration with other antihypertensive agents may result in additive effect or potentiation).
- No products indexed under this heading.

Reserpine (Co-administration with other antihypertensive agents may result in additive effect or potentiation).
- No products indexed under this heading.

Rocuronium Bromide (Possible increased responsiveness to the muscle relaxants). Products include:
- Zemuron Injection 2491

Rofecoxib (Co-administration in some patients can result in reduced diuretic, natriuretic, and antihypertensive effects). Products include:
- Vioxx 2213

Rosiglitazone Maleate (Thiazide diuretics may cause hyperglycemia; dosage adjustment of oral hypoglycemia agents may be required). Products include:
- Avandia Tablets 1490

Secobarbital Sodium (Potentiation of orthostatic hypotension).
- No products indexed under this heading.

Sodium Nitroprusside (Co-administration with other antihypertensive agents may result in additive effect or potentiation).
- No products indexed under this heading.

Sotalol Hydrochloride (Co-administration with other antihypertensive agents may result in additive effect or potentiation). Products include:
- Betapace Tablets 950
- Betapace AF Tablets 954

Spirapril Hydrochloride (Co-administration with other antihypertensive agents may result in additive effect or potentiation).
- No products indexed under this heading.

Sufentanil Citrate (Potentiation of orthostatic hypotension).
- No products indexed under this heading.

Sulindac (Co-administration in some patients can result in reduced diuretic, natriuretic, and antihypertensive effects). Products include:
- Clinoril Tablets 2053

Terazosin Hydrochloride (Co-administration with other antihypertensive agents may result in additive effect or potentiation). Products include:
- Hytrin Capsules 464

Thiamylal Sodium (Potentiation of orthostatic hypotension).
- No products indexed under this heading.

Timolol Maleate (Co-administration with other antihypertensive agents may result in additive effect or potentiation). Products include:
- Blocadren Tablets 2046
- Cosopt Sterile Ophthalmic Solution 2065
- Timolide Tablets 2187
- Timolol GFS .... ⊙266
- Timoptic in Ocudose 2192
- Timoptic Sterile Ophthalmic Solution 2190
- Timoptic-XE Sterile Ophthalmic Gel Forming Solution 2194

Tolazamide (Thiazide diuretics may cause hyperglycemia; dosage adjustment of oral hypoglycemia agents may be required).
- No products indexed under this heading.

Tolbutamide (Thiazide diuretics may cause hyperglycemia; dosage adjustment of oral hypoglycemia agents may be required).
- No products indexed under this heading.

Tolmetin Sodium (Co-administration in some patients can result in reduced diuretic, natriuretic, and antihypertensive effects). Products include:
- Tolectin 2589

Torsemide (Co-administration with other antihypertensive agents may result in additive effect or potentiation). Products include:
- Demadex Tablets and Injection 2965

Trandolapril (Co-administration with other antihypertensive agents may result in additive effect or potentiation). Products include:
- Mavik Tablets 478
- Tarka Tablets 508

Triamcinolone (Corticosteroids intensify electrolyte depletion, particularly hypokalemia).
- No products indexed under this heading.

Triamcinolone Acetonide (Corticosteroids intensify electrolyte depletion, particularly hypokalemia). Products include:
- Azmacort Inhalation Aerosol 728
- Nasacort Nasal Inhaler 750
- Nasacort AQ Nasal Spray 752
- Tri-Nasal Spray 2274

Triamcinolone Diacetate (Corticosteroids intensify electrolyte depletion, particularly hypokalemia).
- No products indexed under this heading.

Triamcinolone Hexacetonide (Corticosteroids intensify electrolyte depletion, particularly hypokalemia).
- No products indexed under this heading.

Trimethaphan Camsylate (Co-administration with other antihypertensive agents may result in additive effect or potentiation).
- No products indexed under this heading.

Troglitazone (Thiazide diuretics may cause hyperglycemia; dosage adjustment of oral hypoglycemia agents may be required).
- No products indexed under this heading.

Valsartan (Co-administration with other antihypertensive agents may result in additive effect or potentiation). Products include:
- Diovan Capsules 2337
- Diovan HCT Tablets 2338

Vecuronium Bromide (Possible increased responsiveness to the muscle relaxants). Products include:
- Norcuron for Injection 2478

Verapamil Hydrochloride (Co-administration with other antihypertensive agents may result in additive effect or potentiation). Products include:
- Covera-HS Tablets 3199
- Isoptin SR Tablets 467
- Tarka Tablets 508
- Verelan Capsules 3184
- Verelan PM Capsules 3186

Warfarin Sodium (Co-administration has resulted in slight decrease in the mean warfarin trough plasma concentration; this decrease did not result in a change in INR). Products include:
- Coumadin for Injection 1243
- Coumadin Tablets 1243
- Warfarin Sodium Tablets, USP 3302

Food Interactions

Alcohol (Potentiation of orthostatic hypotension).

Food, unspecified (Slightly reduces the bioavailability of telmisartan with reduction in AUC of about 6%).

MICRHOGAM INJECTION

(Rh_o (D) Immune Globulin (Human)) 2524

None cited in PDR database.

MICRO-K EXTENCAPS

(Potassium Chloride) 3311

May interact with ACE inhibitors, anticholinergics, and potassium sparing diuretics. Compounds in these categories include:

Amiloride Hydrochloride (Hypokalemia should not be treated by the co-administration of potassium salts and a potassium sparing diuretic, since the simultaneous administration of these agents can produce severe hyperkalemia). Products include:
- Midamor Tablets 2136
- Moduretic Tablets 2138

Atropine Sulfate (Anticholinergic drugs can be cause for delay or arrest in tablet passage through the gastrointestinal tract; concomitant administration of drugs capable of decreasing GI motility should be avoided). Products include:
- Donnatal 2929
- Donnatal Extentabs 2930
- Motofen Tablets 577
- Prosed/DS Tablets 3268
- Urised Tablets 2876

Belladonna Alkaloids (Anticholinergic drugs can be cause for delay or arrest in tablet passage through the gastrointestinal tract; concomitant administration of drugs capable of decreasing GI motility should be avoided). Products include:
- Hyland's Teething Tablets 766
- Urimax Tablets 1769

Benazepril Hydrochloride (ACE inhibitors can produce some potassium retention and co-administration of potassium supplements with ACE inhibitors can increase the risk of hyperkalemia). Products include:
- Lotensin Tablets 2365
- Lotensin HCT Tablets 2367
- Lotrel Capsules 2370

Benztropine Mesylate (Anticholinergic drugs can be cause for delay or arrest in tablet passage through the gastrointestinal tract; concomitant administration of drugs capable of decreasing GI motility should be avoided). Products include:
- Cogentin 2055

Biperiden Hydrochloride (Anticholinergic drugs can be cause for delay or arrest in tablet passage through the gastrointestinal tract; concomitant administration of drugs capable of decreasing GI motility should be avoided). Products include:
- Akineton 402

Captopril (ACE inhibitors can produce some potassium retention and co-administration of potassium supplements with ACE inhibitors can increase the risk of hyperkalemia). Products include:
- Captopril Tablets 2281

Clidinium Bromide (Anticholinergic drugs can be cause for delay or arrest in tablet passage through the gastrointestinal tract; concomitant administration of drugs capable of decreasing GI motility should be avoided).
- No products indexed under this heading.

Dicyclomine Hydrochloride (Anticholinergic drugs can be cause for delay or arrest in tablet passage through the gastrointestinal tract; concomitant administration of drugs capable of decreasing GI motility should be avoided).
- No products indexed under this heading.

Enalapril Maleate (ACE inhibitors can produce some potassium retention and co-administration of potassium supplements with ACE inhibitors can increase the risk of hyperkalemia). Products include:
- Lexxel Tablets 608
- Vaseretic Tablets 2204
- Vasotec Tablets 2210

Enalaprilat (ACE inhibitors can produce some potassium retention and co-administration of potassium supplements with ACE inhibitors can increase the risk of hyperkalemia). Products include:
- Enalaprilat Injection 863
- Vasotec I.V. Injection 2207

Fosinopril Sodium (ACE inhibitors can produce some potassium retention and co-administration of potassium supplements with ACE inhibitors can increase the risk of hyperkalemia). Products include:
- Monopril Tablets 1091
- Monopril HCT 1094

Glycopyrrolate (Anticholinergic drugs can be cause for delay or arrest in tablet passage through the gastrointestinal tract; concomitant administration of drugs capable of decreasing GI motility should be avoided). Products include:
- Robinul Forte Tablets 1358
- Robinul Injectable 2940
- Robinul Tablets 1358

Hyoscyamine (Anticholinergic drugs can be cause for delay or arrest in tablet passage through the gastrointestinal tract; concomitant administration of drugs capable of decreasing GI motility should be avoided). Products include:
- Urised Tablets 2876

Hyoscyamine Sulfate (Anticholinergic drugs can be cause for delay or arrest in tablet passage through the gastrointestinal tract; concomitant administration of drugs capable of decreasing GI motility should be avoided). Products include:
- Arco-Lase Plus Tablets 592
- Donnatal 2929
- Donnatal Extentabs 2930
- Levsin/Levsinex/Levbid 3172
- NuLev Orally Disintegrating Tablets 3176
- Prosed/DS Tablets 3268
- Urimax Tablets 1769

Ipratropium Bromide (Anticholinergic drugs can be cause for delay or arrest in tablet passage through the gastrointestinal tract; concomitant administration of drugs capable of decreasing GI motility should be avoided). Products include:
- Atrovent Inhalation Aerosol 1030
- Atrovent Inhalation Solution 1031
- Atrovent Nasal Spray 0.03% 1032
- Atrovent Nasal Spray 0.06% 1033
- Combivent Inhalation Aerosol 1041
- DuoNeb Inhalation Solution 1233

Lisinopril (ACE inhibitors can produce some potassium retention and co-administration of potassium supplements with ACE inhibitors can increase the risk of hyperkalemia). Products include:
- Prinivil Tablets 2164
- Prinzide Tablets 2168
- Zestoretic Tablets 695
- Zestril Tablets 698

Mepenzolate Bromide (Anticholinergic drugs can be cause for delay or arrest in tablet passage through the gastrointestinal tract; concomitant administration of drugs capable of decreasing GI motility should be avoided).
- No products indexed under this heading.

Moexipril Hydrochloride (ACE inhibitors can produce some potassium retention and co-administration of potassium supplements with ACE inhibitors can increase the risk of hyperkalemia). Products include:
- Uniretic Tablets 3178
- Univasc Tablets 3181

Oxybutynin Chloride (Anticholinergic drugs can be cause for delay or arrest in tablet passage through the gastrointestinal tract; concomitant administration of drugs capable of decreasing GI motility should be avoided). Products include:
- Ditropan XL Extended Release Tablets 564

Perindopril Erbumine (ACE inhibitors can produce some potassium retention and co-administration of potassium supplements with ACE inhibitors can increase the risk of hyperkalemia). Products include:
- Aceon Tablets (2 mg, 4 mg, 8 mg) 3249

Procyclidine Hydrochloride (Anticholinergic drugs can be cause for delay or arrest in tablet passage through the gastrointestinal tract; concomitant administration of drugs capable of decreasing GI motility should be avoided).
- No products indexed under this heading.

Propantheline Bromide (Anticholinergic drugs can be cause for delay or arrest in tablet passage through the gastrointestinal tract; concomitant administration of drugs capable of decreasing GI motility should be avoided).
- No products indexed under this heading.

Quinapril Hydrochloride (ACE inhibitors can produce some potassium retention and co-administration of potassium supplements with ACE inhibitors can increase the risk of hyperkalemia). Products include:
- Accupril Tablets 2611
- Accuretic Tablets 2614

Ramipril (ACE inhibitors can produce some potassium retention and co-administration of potassium supplements with ACE inhibitors can increase the risk of hyperkalemia). Products include:
- Altace Capsules 2233

Scopolamine (Anticholinergic drugs can be cause for delay or arrest in tablet passage through the gastrointestinal tract; concomitant administration of drugs capable of decreasing GI motility should be avoided). Products include:
- Transderm Scōp Transdermal Therapeutic System 2302

Scopolamine Hydrobromide (Anticholinergic drugs can be cause for delay or arrest in tablet passage through the gastrointestinal tract; concomitant administration of drugs capable of decreasing GI motility should be avoided). Products include:
- Donnatal 2929
- Donnatal Extentabs 2930

Spirapril Hydrochloride (ACE inhibitors can produce some potassium retention and co-administration of potassium supplements with ACE inhibitors can increase the risk of hyperkalemia).
- No products indexed under this heading.

Spironolactone (Hypokalemia should not be treated by the co-administration of potassium salts and a potassium sparing diuretic, since the simultaneous administration of these agents can produce severe hyperkalemia).
- No products indexed under this heading.

Tolterodine Tartrate (Anticholinergic drugs can be cause for delay or arrest in tablet passage through the gastrointestinal tract; concomitant administration of drugs capable of decreasing GI motility should be avoided). Products include:
- Detrol Tablets 3623
- Detrol LA Capsules 2801

Trandolapril (ACE inhibitors can produce some potassium retention and co-administration of potassium supplements with ACE inhibitors can increase the risk of hyperkalemia). Products include:
- Mavik Tablets 478

Tarka Tablets 508

Triamterene (Hypokalemia should not be treated by the co-administration of potassium salts and a potassium sparing diuretic, since the simultaneous administration of these agents can produce severe hyperkalemia). Products include:

Dyazide Capsules 1515
Dyrenium Capsules 3458
Maxzide 1008

Tridihexethyl Chloride (Anticholinergic drugs can be cause for delay or arrest in tablet passage through the gastrointestinal tract; concomitant administration of drugs capable of decreasing GI motility should be avoided).

No products indexed under this heading.

Trihexyphenidyl Hydrochloride (Anticholinergic drugs can be cause for delay or arrest in tablet passage through the gastrointestinal tract; concomitant administration of drugs capable of decreasing GI motility should be avoided). Products include:

Artane 1855

MICRO-K 10 EXTENCAPS

(Potassium Chloride) 3311
See Micro-K Extencaps

MICROGESTIN FE 1.5/30 TABLETS

(Ethinyl Estradiol, Norethindrone Acetate) 3407
See Microgestin Fe 1/20 Tablets

MICROGESTIN FE 1/20 TABLETS

(Ethinyl Estradiol, Norethindrone Acetate) 3400

May interact with phenytoin, prednisolone, theophylline, and certain other agents. Compounds in these categories include:

Acetaminophen (May increase AUC and/or plasma concentrations of ethinyl estradiol; co-administration may decrease plasma concentrations of acetaminophen). Products include:

Actifed Cold & Sinus Caplets and Tablets .... ▣ 688
Alka-Seltzer Plus Liqui-Gels .... ▣ 604
Alka-Seltzer Plus Cold & Flu Medicine Liqui-Gels .... ▣ 604
Alka-Seltzer Plus Cold & Sinus Medicine Liqui-Gels .... ▣ 604
Benadryl Allergy/Cold Tablets .... ▣ 691
Benadryl Allergy Sinus Headache Caplets & Gelcaps .... ▣ 693
Benadryl Severe Allergy & Sinus Headache Caplets .... ▣ 694
Children's Cēpacol Sore Throat .... ▣ 788
Comtrex Acute Head Cold & Sinus Pressure Relief Tablets ..... ▣ 627
Comtrex Deep Chest Cold & Congestion Relief Softgels .... ▣ 627
Comtrex Flu Therapy & Fever Relief Daytime Caplets .... ▣ 628
Comtrex Flu Therapy & Fever Relief Nighttime Tablets .... ▣ 628
Comtrex Maximum Strength Multi-Symptom Cold & Cough Relief Tablets and Caplets .... ▣ 626
Contac Severe Cold and Flu Caplets Maximum Strength .... ▣ 746
Contac Severe Cold and Flu Caplets Non-Drowsy .... ▣ 746
Coricidin 'D' Cold, Flu & Sinus Tablets .... ▣ 737
Coricidin HBP Cold & Flu Tablets .. ▣ 738
Coricidin HBP Maximum Strength Flu Tablets .... ▣ 738
Coricidin HBP Night-Time Cold & Flu Tablets .... ▣ 738
Darvon-N/Darvocet-N 1907
Dimetapp Cold and Fever Suspension .... ▣ 775
Dimetapp Nighttime Flu Liquid ...... ▣ 776
Dimetapp Non-Drowsy Flu Syrup .. ▣ 777
Drixoral Allergy/Sinus Extended-Release Tablets .... ▣ 741
Drixoral Cold & Flu Extended-Release Tablets .... ▣ 740
Aspirin Free Excedrin Caplets and Geltabs .... ▣ 628
Excedrin Extra-Strength Tablets, Caplets, and Geltabs .... ▣ 629
Excedrin Migraine 1070
Excedrin PM Tablets, Caplets, and Geltabs .... ▣ 631
Goody's Body Pain Formula Powder .... ▣ 620
Goody's Extra Strength Headache Powder .... ▣ 620
Goody's Extra Strength Pain Relief Tablets .... ▣ 620
Goody's PM Powder .... ▣ 621
Hycomine Compound Tablets 1317
Lortab 3319
Lortab Elixir 3317
Maxidone Tablets CIII 3399
Maximum Strength Midol Menstrual Caplets and Gelcaps.. ▣ 612
Maximum Strength Midol PMS Caplets and Gelcaps .... ▣ 613
Maximum Strength Midol Teen Caplets .... ▣ 612
Midrin Capsules 3464
Norco 5/325 Tablets CIII 3424
Norco 7.5/325 Tablets CIII 3425
Norco 10/325 Tablets CIII 3427
Norco 10/325 Tablets CIII 3425
Percocet Tablets 1326
Percogesic Aspirin-Free Coated Tablets .... ▣ 667
Extra Strength Percogesic Aspirin-Free Coated Caplets .... ▣ 665
Phrenilin 578
Robitussin Cold Caplets Multi-Symptom Cold & Flu .... ▣ 781
Robitussin Cold Softgels Multi-Symptom Cold & Flu .... ▣ 781
Robitussin Multi Symptom Honey Flu Liquid .... ▣ 785
Robitussin Nighttime Honey Flu Liquid .... ▣ 786
Sedapap Tablets 50 mg/650 mg 2225
Singlet Caplets .... ▣ 761
Sinutab Sinus Allergy Medication, Maximum Strength Formula, Tablets & Caplets .... ▣ 707
Sinutab Sinus Medication, Maximum Strength Without Drowsiness Formula, Tablets & Caplets .... ▣ 707
Sudafed Cold & Cough Liquid Caps .... ▣ 709
Sudafed Cold & Sinus Liquid Caps .... ▣ 710
Sudafed Severe Cold .... ▣ 711
Sudafed Sinus Headache Caplets .. ▣ 712
Sudafed Sinus Headache Tablets .. ▣ 712
Tavist Sinus Non-Drowsy Coated Caplets .... ▣ 676
TheraFlu Regular Strength Cold & Cough Night Time Hot Liquid ..... ▣ 676
TheraFlu Regular Strength Cold & Sore Throat Night Time Hot Liquid .... ▣ 676
TheraFlu Maximum Strength Flu & Congestion Non-Drowsy Hot Liquid .... ▣ 677
TheraFlu Maximum Strength Flu & Cough Night Time Hot Liquid .. ▣ 678
TheraFlu Maximum Strength Flu & Sore Throat Night Time Hot Liquid .... ▣ 677
TheraFlu Maximum Strength Severe Cold & Congestion Night Time Caplets .... ▣ 678
TheraFlu Maximum Strength Severe Cold & Congestion Night Time Hot Liquid .... ▣ 678
TheraFlu Maximum Strength Severe Cold & Congestion Non-Drowsy .... ▣ 679
Triaminic Cold, Cough & Fever Liquid .... ▣ 681
Triaminic Cough & Sore Throat Liquid .... ▣ 682
Triaminic Cough & Sore Throat Softchews .... ▣ 684
Tylenol, Children's 2014
Children's Tylenol Allergy-D Liquid .. 2014
Children's Tylenol Cold Suspension Liquid and Chewable Tablets 2015
Children's Tylenol Cold Plus Cough Suspension Liquid and Chewable Tablets 2015
Children's Tylenol Flu Suspension Liquid 2015
Children's Tylenol Sinus Suspension Liquid 2017
Infants' Tylenol Cold Decongestant and Fever Reducer Concentrated Drops 2015
Infants' Tylenol Cold Decongestant and Fever Reducer Concentrated Drops Plus Cough .. 2015
Junior Strength Tylenol Soft Chews Chewable Tablets 2014
Tylenol 2009
Tylenol Allergy Sinus 2010
Tylenol Severe Allergy Caplets 2010
Multi-Symptom Tylenol Cold Complete Formula Caplets 2010
Multi-Symptom Tylenol Cold Non-Drowsy Caplets and Gelcaps 2010
Multi-Symptom Tylenol Cold Severe Congestion Non-Drowsy Caplets 2011
Maximum Strength Tylenol Flu NightTime Gelcaps 2011
Maximum Strength Tylenol Flu NightTime Liquid 2011
Maximum Strength Tylenol Flu Non-Drowsy Gelcaps 2011
Extra Strength Tylenol PM Caplets, Geltabs, and Gelcaps 2012
Maximum Strength Tylenol Sinus NightTime Caplets 2012
Maximum Strength Tylenol Sinus Non-Drowsy Geltabs, Gelcaps, Caplets, and Tablets 2012
Maximum Strength Tylenol Sore Throat Adult Liquid 2013
Tylenol with Codeine 2595
Women's Tylenol Menstrual Relief Caplets 2013
Tylox Capsules 2597
Ultracet Tablets 2597
Vanquish Caplets .... ▣ 617
Vicks 44M Cough, Cold & Flu Relief Liquid .... ▣ 725
Vicks DayQuil LiquiCaps/Liquid Multi-Symptom Cold/Flu Relief ... ▣ 727
Vicks NyQuil LiquiCaps/Liquid Multi-Symptom Cold/Flu Relief, Original and Cherry Flavors .... ▣ 727
Vicodin Tablets 516
Vicodin ES Tablets 517
Vicodin HP Tablets 518
Zydone Tablets 1330

Aminophylline (Co-administration of products containing ethinyl estradiol may inhibit the metabolism of other compounds, such as theophylline, resulting in increased plasma concentrations of theophylline).

No products indexed under this heading.

Atorvastatin Calcium (Co-administration of atorvastatin and an oral contraceptive increased AUC values for ethinyl estradiol and norethindrone by approximately 20% and 30% respectively). Products include:

Lipitor Tablets 2639
Lipitor Tablets 2696

Carbamazepine (Co-administration with carbamazepine results in increased metabolism of ethinyl estradiol and/or norethindrone that could result in a reduction of contraceptive effectiveness). Products include:

Carbatrol Capsules 3234
Tegretol/Tegretol-XR 2404

Clofibrate (Co-administration of products containing ethinyl estradiol may increase clearance of clofibric acid). Products include:

Atromid-S Capsules 3483

Cyclosporine (Co-administration of products containing ethinyl estradiol may inhibit the metabolism of other compounds, such as cyclosporine, resulting in increased plasma concentrations of cyclosporine). Products include:

Gengraf Capsules 457
Neoral Soft Gelatin Capsules 2380
Neoral Oral Solution 2380
Sandimmune 2388

Dyphylline (Co-administration of products containing ethinyl estradiol may inhibit the metabolism of other compounds, such as theophylline, resulting in increased plasma concentrations of theophylline). Products include:

Lufyllin Tablets 3347
Lufyllin-400 Tablets 3347
Lufyllin-GG Elixir 3348
Lufyllin-GG Tablets 3348

Fosphenytoin Sodium (Co-administration with phenytoin results in increased metabolism of ethinyl estradiol and/or norethindrone that could result in a reduction of contraceptive effectiveness). Products include:

Cerebyx Injection 2619

Morphine Sulfate (Co-administration of products containing ethinyl estradiol may increase clearance of morphine). Products include:

Astramorph/PF Injection, USP (Preservative-Free) 594
Duramorph Injection 1312
Infumorph 200 and Infumorph 500 Sterile Solutions 1314
Kadian Capsules 1335
MS Contin Tablets 2896
MSIR 2898
Oramorph SR Tablets 3062
Roxanol 3066

Phenobarbital (Co-administration with phenobarbital results in increased metabolism of ethinyl estradiol and/or norethindrone that could result in a reduction of contraceptive effectiveness). Products include:

Arco-Lase Plus Tablets 592
Donnatal 2929
Donnatal Extentabs 2930

Phenylbutazone (Co-administration has resulted in a reduction in contraceptive effectiveness and increased incidence of breakthrough bleeding).

No products indexed under this heading.

Phenytoin (Co-administration with phenytoin results in increased metabolism of ethinyl estradiol and/or norethindrone that could result in a reduction of contraceptive effectiveness). Products include:

Dilantin Infatabs 2624
Dilantin-125 Oral Suspension 2625

Phenytoin Sodium (Co-administration with phenytoin results in increased metabolism of ethinyl estradiol and/or norethindrone that could result in a reduction of contraceptive effectiveness). Products include:

Dilantin Kapseals 2622

Prednisolone (Co-administration of products containing ethinyl estradiol may inhibit the metabolism of other compounds, such as prednisolone, resulting in increased plasma concentrations of prednisolone). Products include:

Prelone Syrup 2273

Prednisolone Acetate (Co-administration of products containing ethinyl estradiol may inhibit the metabolism of other compounds, such as prednisolone, resulting in increased plasma concentrations of prednisolone). Products include:

Blephamide Ophthalmic Ointment .. 547
Blephamide Ophthalmic Suspension 548
Poly-Pred Liquifilm Ophthalmic Suspension .... ⊙ 245
Pred Forte Ophthalmic Suspension .... ⊙ 246
Pred Mild Sterile Ophthalmic Suspension .... ⊙ 249
Pred-G Ophthalmic Suspension ..... ⊙ 247
Pred-G Sterile Ophthalmic Ointment .... ⊙ 248

Prednisolone Sodium Phosphate (Co-administration of products containing ethinyl estradiol may inhibit the metabolism of other compounds, such as prednisolone, resulting in increased plasma concentrations of prednisolone). Products include:

Pediapred Oral Solution 1170

Prednisolone Tebutate (Co-administration of products containing ethinyl estradiol may inhibit the metabolism of other compounds, such as prednisolone, resulting in increased plasma concentrations of prednisolone).

No products indexed under this heading.

Rifampin (Co-administration with rifampin results in increased metabolism of ethinyl estradiol and norethindrone; a reduction in contraceptive effectiveness and increased incidence of breakthrough bleeding and menstrual irregularities has been associated with concomitant use of rifampin). Products include:
Rifadin 765
Rifamate Capsules 767
Rifater Tablets 769

Salicylic Acid (Co-administration of products containing ethinyl estradiol may increase clearance of salicylic acid). Products include:
Clear Away Gel with Aloe Wart Remover System 736
Clear Away Liquid Wart Remover System 736
Clear Away One Step Wart Remover 737
Clear Away One Step Wart Remover for Kids 737
Clear Away One Step Plantar Wart Remover 737
Compound W One Step Pads for Kids 664
Compound W One Step Plantar Pads 664
Compound W One Step Wart Remover Pads 664
Compound W Wart Remover Gel 665
Compound W Wart Remover Liquid 665
Wart-Off Liquid 716

Temazepam (Co-administration of products containing ethinyl estradiol may increase clearance of temazepam).
No products indexed under this heading.

Theophylline (Co-administration of products containing ethinyl estradiol may inhibit the metabolism of other compounds, such as theophylline, resulting in increased plasma concentrations of theophylline). Products include:
Aerolate 1361
Theo-Dur Extended-Release Tablets 1835
Uni-Dur Extended-Release Tablets .. 1841
Uniphyl 400 mg and 600 mg Tablets 2903

Theophylline Calcium Salicylate (Co-administration of products containing ethinyl estradiol may inhibit the metabolism of other compounds, such as theophylline, resulting in increased plasma concentrations of theophylline).
No products indexed under this heading.

Theophylline Sodium Glycinate (Co-administration of products containing ethinyl estradiol may inhibit the metabolism of other compounds, such as theophylline, resulting in increased plasma concentrations of theophylline).
No products indexed under this heading.

Troglitazone (Co-administration of troglitazone with an oral contraceptive containing ethinyl estradiol and norethindrone reduces the plasma concentrations of both by 30% which could result in a reduction of contraceptive effectiveness).
No products indexed under this heading.

Vitamin C (May increase AUC and/or plasma concentrations of ethinyl estradiol). Products include:
Beta-C Tablets 811
C-Grams Caplets 795
Halls Defense Drops 687
Peridin-C Tablets 618

MICRONOR TABLETS

(Norethindrone) 2543
May interact with barbiturates, phenytoin, and certain other agents. Compounds in these categories include:

Aprobarbital (The effectiveness of progestin-only oral contraceptives is reduced by hepatic enzyme-inducing agents such as barbiturates).
No products indexed under this heading.

Butabarbital (The effectiveness of progestin-only oral contraceptives is reduced by hepatic enzyme-inducing agents such as barbiturates).
No products indexed under this heading.

Butalbital (The effectiveness of progestin-only oral contraceptives is reduced by hepatic enzyme-inducing agents such as barbiturates). Products include:
Phrenilin 578
Sedapap Tablets 50 mg/650 mg ... 2225

Carbamazepine (The effectiveness of progestin-only oral contraceptives is reduced by hepatic enzyme-inducing agents such as carbamazepine). Products include:
Carbatrol Capsules 3234
Tegretol/Tegretol-XR 2404

Fosphenytoin Sodium (The effectiveness of progestin-only oral contraceptives is reduced by hepatic enzyme-inducing agents such as phenytoin). Products include:
Cerebyx Injection 2619

Mephobarbital (The effectiveness of progestin-only oral contraceptives is reduced by hepatic enzyme-inducing agents such as barbiturates).
No products indexed under this heading.

Pentobarbital Sodium (The effectiveness of progestin-only oral contraceptives is reduced by hepatic enzyme-inducing agents such as barbiturates). Products include:
Nembutal Sodium Solution 485

Phenobarbital (The effectiveness of progestin-only oral contraceptives is reduced by hepatic enzyme-inducing agents such as barbiturates). Products include:
Arco-Lase Plus Tablets 592
Donnatal 2929
Donnatal Extentabs 2930

Phenytoin (The effectiveness of progestin-only oral contraceptives is reduced by hepatic enzyme-inducing agents such as phenytoin). Products include:
Dilantin Infatabs 2624
Dilantin-125 Oral Suspension 2625

Phenytoin Sodium (The effectiveness of progestin-only oral contraceptives is reduced by hepatic enzyme-inducing agents such as phenytoin). Products include:
Dilantin Kapseals 2622

Rifampin (The effectiveness of progestin-only oral contraceptives is reduced by hepatic enzyme-inducing agents such as rifampin). Products include:
Rifadin 765
Rifamate Capsules 767
Rifater Tablets 769

Secobarbital Sodium (The effectiveness of progestin-only oral contraceptives is reduced by hepatic enzyme-inducing agents such as barbiturates).
No products indexed under this heading.

Thiamylal Sodium (The effectiveness of progestin-only oral contraceptives is reduced by hepatic enzyme-inducing agents such as barbiturates).
No products indexed under this heading.

MICROZIDE CAPSULES

(Hydrochlorothiazide) 3414
May interact with antihypertensives, barbiturates, corticosteroids, cardiac glycosides, oral hypoglycemic agents, insulin, lithium preparations, narcotic analgesics, nondepolarizing neuromuscular blocking agents, non-steroidal anti-inflammatory agents, and certain other agents. Compounds in these categories include:

Acarbose (Thiazides may cause hyperglycemia; dosage adjustment of oral hypoglycemic agent may be required). Products include:
Precose Tablets 906

Acebutolol Hydrochloride (Co-administration with other antihypertensive agents may result in additive effect or potentiation). Products include:
Sectral Capsules 3589

ACTH (Co-administration with adrenocorticotropin hormone may result in intensified electrolyte depletion, particularly hypokalemia).
No products indexed under this heading.

Alfentanil Hydrochloride (May potentiate orthostatic hypotension).
No products indexed under this heading.

Amlodipine Besylate (Co-administration with other antihypertensive agents may result in additive effect or potentiation). Products include:
Lotrel Capsules 2370
Norvasc Tablets 2704

Aprobarbital (May potentiate orthostatic hypotension).
No products indexed under this heading.

Atenolol (Co-administration with other antihypertensive agents may result in additive effect or potentiation). Products include:
Tenoretic Tablets 690
Tenormin I.V. Injection 692

Atracurium Besylate (Possible increased responsiveness to the muscle relaxant).
No products indexed under this heading.

Benazepril Hydrochloride (Co-administration with other antihypertensive agents may result in additive effect or potentiation). Products include:
Lotensin Tablets 2365
Lotensin HCT Tablets 2367
Lotrel Capsules 2370

Bendroflumethiazide (Co-administration with other antihypertensive agents may result in additive effect or potentiation). Products include:
Corzide 40/5 Tablets 2247
Corzide 80/5 Tablets 2247

Betamethasone Acetate (Co-administration with corticosteroids may result in intensified electrolyte depletion, particularly hypokalemia). Products include:
Celestone Soluspan Injectable Suspension 3097

Betamethasone Sodium Phosphate (Co-administration with corticosteroids may result in intensified electrolyte depletion, particularly hypokalemia). Products include:
Celestone Soluspan Injectable Suspension 3097

Betaxolol Hydrochloride (Co-administration with other antihypertensive agents may result in additive effect or potentiation). Products include:
Betoptic S Ophthalmic Suspension 537

Bisoprolol Fumarate (Co-administration with other antihypertensive agents may result in additive effect or potentiation). Products include:
Zebeta Tablets 1885
Ziac Tablets 1887

Buprenorphine Hydrochloride (May potentiate orthostatic hypotension). Products include:
Buprenex Injectable 2918

Butabarbital (May potentiate orthostatic hypotension).
No products indexed under this heading.

Butalbital (May potentiate orthostatic hypotension). Products include:
Phrenilin 578
Sedapap Tablets 50 mg/650 mg ... 2225

Candesartan Cilexetil (Co-administration with other antihypertensive agents may result in additive effect or potentiation). Products include:
Atacand Tablets 595
Atacand HCT Tablets 597

Captopril (Co-administration with other antihypertensive agents may result in additive effect or potentiation). Products include:
Captopril Tablets 2281

Carteolol Hydrochloride (Co-administration with other antihypertensive agents may result in additive effect or potentiation). Products include:
Carteolol Hydrochloride Ophthalmic Solution USP, 1% .... ⊙258
Ocupress Ophthalmic Solution, 1% Sterile .... ⊙303

Celecoxib (Co-administration with non-steroidal anti-inflammatory drugs can result in reduced diuretic, natriuretic, and antihypertensive effects). Products include:
Celebrex Capsules 2676
Celebrex Capsules 2780

Chlorothiazide (Co-administration with other antihypertensive agents may result in additive effect or potentiation). Products include:
Aldoclor Tablets 2035
Diuril Oral 2087

Chlorothiazide Sodium (Co-administration with other antihypertensive agents may result in additive effect or potentiation). Products include:
Diuril Sodium Intravenous 2086

Chlorpropamide (Thiazides may cause hyperglycemia; dosage adjustment of oral hypoglycemic agent may be required). Products include:
Diabinese Tablets 2680

Chlorthalidone (Co-administration with other antihypertensive agents may result in additive effect or potentiation). Products include:
Clorpres Tablets 1002
Combipres Tablets 1040
Tenoretic Tablets 690

Cholestyramine (Binds hydrochlorothiazide and reduces its absorption from gastrointestinal tract by up to 85%).
No products indexed under this heading.

Cisatracurium Besylate (Possible increased responsiveness to the muscle relaxant).
No products indexed under this heading.

Clonidine (Co-administration with other antihypertensive agents may result in additive effect or potentiation). Products include:
Catapres-TTS 1038

Clonidine Hydrochloride (Co-administration with other antihypertensive agents may result in additive effect or potentiation). Products include:
Catapres Tablets 1037
Clorpres Tablets 1002
Combipres Tablets 1040
Duraclon Injection 3057

Codeine Phosphate (May potentiate orthostatic hypotension). Products include:
Phenergan with Codeine Syrup 3557
Phenergan VC with Codeine Syrup . 3561
Robitussin A-C Syrup 2942
Robitussin-DAC Syrup 2942
Ryna-C Liquid 768
Soma Compound w/Codeine Tablets 3355
Tussi-Organidin NR Liquid 3350
Tussi-Organidin-S NR Liquid 3350
Tylenol with Codeine 2595

Colestipol Hydrochloride (Binds hydrochlorothiazide and reduces its absorption from gastrointestinal tract by up to 43%). Products include:
Colestid Tablets 2791

IMPORTANT NOTE: Always consult each drug listing in the patient's regimen for possible interactions.

Cortisone Acetate (Co-administration with corticosteroids may result in intensified electrolyte depletion, particularly hypokalemia). Products include:
- Cortone Acetate Injectable Suspension 2059
- Cortone Acetate Tablets 2061

Deserpidine (Co-administration with other antihypertensive agents may result in additive effect or potentiation).
- No products indexed under this heading.

Deslanoside (Thiazide-induced hypokalemia can sensitize or exaggerate the response of the heart to the toxic effects of digitalis).
- No products indexed under this heading.

Dexamethasone (Co-administration with corticosteroids may result in intensified electrolyte depletion, particularly hypokalemia). Products include:
- Decadron Elixir 2078
- Decadron Tablets 2079
- TobraDex Ophthalmic Ointment 542
- TobraDex Ophthalmic Suspension 541

Dexamethasone Acetate (Co-administration with corticosteroids may result in intensified electrolyte depletion, particularly hypokalemia).
- No products indexed under this heading.

Dexamethasone Sodium Phosphate (Co-administration with corticosteroids may result in intensified electrolyte depletion, particularly hypokalemia). Products include:
- Decadron Phosphate Injection 2081
- Decadron Phosphate Sterile Ophthalmic Ointment 2083
- Decadron Phosphate Sterile Ophthalmic Solution 2084
- NeoDecadron Sterile Ophthalmic Solution 2144

Dezocine (May potentiate orthostatic hypotension).
- No products indexed under this heading.

Diazoxide (Co-administration with other antihypertensive agents may result in additive effect or potentiation).
- No products indexed under this heading.

Diclofenac Potassium (Co-administration with non-steroidal anti-inflammatory drugs can result in reduced diuretic, natriuretic, and antihypertensive effects). Products include:
- Cataflam Tablets 2315

Diclofenac Sodium (Co-administration with non-steroidal anti-inflammatory drugs can result in reduced diuretic, natriuretic, and antihypertensive effects). Products include:
- Arthrotec Tablets 3195
- Voltaren Ophthalmic Sterile Ophthalmic Solution ..... ⊙ 312
- Voltaren Tablets 2315
- Voltaren-XR Tablets 2315

Digitoxin (Thiazide-induced hypokalemia can sensitize or exaggerate the response of the heart to the toxic effects of digitalis).
- No products indexed under this heading.

Digoxin (Thiazide-induced hypokalemia can sensitize or exaggerate the response of the heart to the toxic effects of digitalis). Products include:
- Digitek Tablets 1003
- Lanoxicaps Capsules 1574
- Lanoxin Injection 1581
- Lanoxin Tablets 1587
- Lanoxin Elixir Pediatric 1578
- Lanoxin Injection Pediatric 1584

Diltiazem Hydrochloride (Co-administration with other antihypertensive agents may result in additive effect or potentiation). Products include:
- Cardizem Injectable 1018
- Cardizem Lyo-Ject Syringe 1018
- Cardizem Monovial 1018
- Cardizem CD Capsules 1016
- Tiazac Capsules 1378

Doxazosin Mesylate (Co-administration with other antihypertensive agents may result in additive effect or potentiation). Products include:
- Cardura Tablets 2668

Enalapril Maleate (Co-administration with other antihypertensive agents may result in additive effect or potentiation). Products include:
- Lexxel Tablets 608
- Vaseretic Tablets 2204
- Vasotec Tablets 2210

Enalaprilat (Co-administration with other antihypertensive agents may result in additive effect or potentiation). Products include:
- Enalaprilat Injection 863
- Vasotec I.V. Injection 2207

Eprosartan Mesylate (Co-administration with other antihypertensive agents may result in additive effect or potentiation). Products include:
- Teveten Tablets 3327

Esmolol Hydrochloride (Co-administration with other antihypertensive agents may result in additive effect or potentiation). Products include:
- Brevibloc Injection 858

Etodolac (Co-administration with non-steroidal anti-inflammatory drugs can result in reduced diuretic, natriuretic, and antihypertensive effects). Products include:
- Lodine 3528
- Lodine XL Extended-Release Tablets 3530

Felodipine (Co-administration with other antihypertensive agents may result in additive effect or potentiation). Products include:
- Lexxel Tablets 608
- Plendil Extended-Release Tablets 623

Fenoprofen Calcium (Co-administration with non-steroidal anti-inflammatory drugs can result in reduced diuretic, natriuretic, and antihypertensive effects).
- No products indexed under this heading.

Fentanyl (May potentiate orthostatic hypotension). Products include:
- Duragesic Transdermal System 1786

Fentanyl Citrate (May potentiate orthostatic hypotension). Products include:
- Actiq 1184

Fludrocortisone Acetate (Co-administration with corticosteroids may result in intensified electrolyte depletion, particularly hypokalemia). Products include:
- Florinef Acetate Tablets 2250

Flurbiprofen (Co-administration with non-steroidal anti-inflammatory drugs can result in reduced diuretic, natriuretic, and antihypertensive effects).
- No products indexed under this heading.

Fosinopril Sodium (Co-administration with other antihypertensive agents may result in additive effect or potentiation). Products include:
- Monopril Tablets 1091
- Monopril HCT 1094

Furosemide (Co-administration with other antihypertensive agents may result in additive effect or potentiation). Products include:
- Furosemide Tablets 2284

Glimepiride (Thiazides may cause hyperglycemia; dosage adjustment of oral hypoglycemic agent may be required). Products include:
- Amaryl Tablets 717

Glipizide (Thiazides may cause hyperglycemia; dosage adjustment of oral hypoglycemic agent may be required). Products include:
- Glucotrol Tablets 2692
- Glucotrol XL Extended Release Tablets 2693

Glyburide (Thiazides may cause hyperglycemia; dosage adjustment of oral hypoglycemic agent may be required). Products include:
- DiaBeta Tablets 741
- Glucovance Tablets 1086

Guanabenz Acetate (Co-administration with other antihypertensive agents may result in additive effect or potentiation).
- No products indexed under this heading.

Guanethidine Monosulfate (Co-administration with other antihypertensive agents may result in additive effect or potentiation).
- No products indexed under this heading.

Hydralazine Hydrochloride (Co-administration with other antihypertensive agents may result in additive effect or potentiation).
- No products indexed under this heading.

Hydrochlorothiazide (Co-administration with other antihypertensive agents may result in additive effect or potentiation). Products include:
- Accuretic Tablets 2614
- Aldoril Tablets 2039
- Atacand HCT Tablets 597
- Avalide Tablets 1070
- Diovan HCT Tablets 2338
- Dyazide Capsules 1515
- HydroDIURIL Tablets 2108
- Hyzaar 2109
- Inderide Tablets 3517
- Inderide LA Long-Acting Capsules 3519
- Lotensin HCT Tablets 2367
- Maxzide 1008
- Micardis HCT Tablets 1051
- Microzide Capsules 3414
- Moduretic Tablets 2138
- Monopril HCT 1094
- Prinzide Tablets 2168
- Timolide Tablets 2187
- Uniretic Tablets 3178
- Vaseretic Tablets 2204
- Zestoretic Tablets 695
- Ziac Tablets 1887

Hydrocodone Bitartrate (May potentiate orthostatic hypotension). Products include:
- Hycodan 1316
- Hycomine Compound Tablets 1317
- Hycotuss Expectorant Syrup 1318
- Lortab 3319
- Lortab Elixir 3317
- Maxidone Tablets CIII 3399
- Norco 5/325 Tablets CIII 3424
- Norco 7.5/325 Tablets CIII 3425
- Norco 10/325 Tablets CIII 3427
- Norco 10/325 Tablets CIII 3425
- Vicodin Tablets 516
- Vicodin ES Tablets 517
- Vicodin HP Tablets 518
- Vicodin Tuss Expectorant 519
- Vicoprofen Tablets 520
- Zydone Tablets 1330

Hydrocodone Polistirex (May potentiate orthostatic hypotension). Products include:
- Tussionex Pennkinetic Extended-Release Suspension 1174

Hydrocortisone (Co-administration with corticosteroids may result in intensified electrolyte depletion, particularly hypokalemia). Products include:
- Anusol-HC Cream 2.5% 2237
- Cipro HC Otic Suspension 540
- Cortaid Intensive Therapy Cream ..... ■ 717
- Cortaid Maximum Strength Cream ..... ■ 717
- Cortisporin Ophthalmic Suspension Sterile ..... ⊙ 297
- Cortizone•5 ..... ■ 699
- Cortizone•10 ..... ■ 699
- Cortizone•10 Plus Creme ..... ■ 700
- Cortizone for Kids Creme ..... ■ 699
- Hydrocortone Tablets 2106
- Massengill Medicated Soft Cloth Towelette ..... ■ 753
- VōSoL HC Otic Solution 3356

Hydrocortisone Acetate (Co-administration with corticosteroids may result in intensified electrolyte depletion, particularly hypokalemia). Products include:
- Analpram-HC 1338
- Anusol HC-1 Hydrocortisone Anti-Itch Cream ..... ■ 689
- Anusol-HC Suppositories 2238
- Cortaid ..... ■ 717
- Cortifoam Rectal Foam 3170
- Cortisporin-TC Otic Suspension 2246
- Hydrocortone Acetate Injectable Suspension 2103
- Pramosone 1343
- Proctocort Suppositories 2264
- ProctoFoam-HC 3177
- Terra-Cortril Ophthalmic Suspension 2716

Hydrocortisone Sodium Phosphate (Co-administration with corticosteroids may result in intensified electrolyte depletion, particularly hypokalemia). Products include:
- Hydrocortone Phosphate Injection, Sterile 2105

Hydrocortisone Sodium Succinate (Co-administration with corticosteroids may result in intensified electrolyte depletion, particularly hypokalemia).
- No products indexed under this heading.

Hydroflumethiazide (Co-administration with other antihypertensive agents may result in additive effect or potentiation). Products include:
- Diucardin Tablets 3494

Hydromorphone Hydrochloride (May potentiate orthostatic hypotension). Products include:
- Dilaudid 441
- Dilaudid Oral Liquid 445
- Dilaudid Powder 441
- Dilaudid Rectal Suppositories 441
- Dilaudid Tablets 441
- Dilaudid Tablets - 8 mg 445
- Dilaudid-HP 443

Ibuprofen (Co-administration with non-steroidal anti-inflammatory drugs can result in reduced diuretic, natriuretic, and antihypertensive effects). Products include:
- Advil ..... ■ 771
- Children's Advil Oral Suspension ..... ■ 773
- Children's Advil Chewable Tablets ..... ■ 773
- Advil Cold and Sinus Caplets ..... ■ 771
- Advil Cold and Sinus Tablets ..... ■ 771
- Advil Flu & Body Ache Caplets ..... ■ 772
- Infants' Advil Drops ..... ■ 773
- Junior Strength Advil Tablets ..... ■ 773
- Junior Strength Advil Chewable Tablets ..... ■ 773
- Advil Migraine Liquigels ..... ■ 772
- Children's Motrin Oral Suspension and Chewable Tablets 2006
- Children's Motrin Cold Oral Suspension 2007
- Children's Motrin Oral Suspension ..... ■ 643
- Motrin Suspension, Oral Drops, Chewable Tablets, and Caplets 2002
- Infants' Motrin Concentrated Drops 2006
- Junior Strength Motrin Caplets and Chewable Tablets 2006
- Motrin IB Tablets, Caplets, and Gelcaps 2002
- Motrin Migraine Pain Caplets 2005
- Motrin Sinus Headache Caplets 2005
- Vicoprofen Tablets 520

Indapamide (Co-administration with other antihypertensive agents may result in additive effect or potentiation). Products include:
- Indapamide Tablets 2286

Indomethacin (Co-administration with non-steroidal anti-inflammatory

drugs can result in reduced diuretic, natriuretic, and antihypertensive effects). Products include:
- Indocin 2112

Indomethacin Sodium Trihydrate (Co-administration with non-steroidal anti-inflammatory drugs can result in reduced diuretic, natriuretic, and antihypertensive effects). Products include:
- Indocin I.V. 2115

Insulin, Human, Zinc Suspension (Thiazides may cause hyperglycemia; insulin dosage adjustment may be required). Products include:
- Humulin L, 100 Units 1937
- Humulin U, 100 Units 1943
- Novolin L Human Insulin 10 ml Vials 2422

Insulin, Human NPH (Thiazides may cause hyperglycemia; insulin dosage adjustment may be required). Products include:
- Humulin N, 100 Units 1939
- Humulin N NPH Pen 1940
- Novolin N Human Insulin 10 ml Vials 2422
- Novolin N PenFill 2423
- Novolin N Prefilled Syringe Disposable Insulin Delivery System 2425

Insulin, Human Regular (Thiazides may cause hyperglycemia; insulin dosage adjustment may be required). Products include:
- Humulin R Regular (U-500) 1943
- Humulin R, 100 Units 1941
- Novolin R Human Insulin 10 ml Vials 2423
- Novolin R PenFill 2423
- Novolin R Prefilled Syringe Disposable Insulin Delivery System 2425
- Velosulin BR Human Insulin 10 ml Vials 2435

Insulin, Human Regular and Human NPH Mixture (Thiazides may cause hyperglycemia; insulin dosage adjustment may be required). Products include:
- Humulin 50/50, 100 Units 1934
- Humulin 70/30, 100 Units 1935
- Humulin 70/30 Pen 1936
- Novolin 70/30 Human Insulin 10 ml Vials 2421
- Novolin 70/30 PenFill 2423
- Novolin 70/30 Prefilled Disposable Insulin Delivery System 2425

Insulin, NPH (Thiazides may cause hyperglycemia; insulin dosage adjustment may be required). Products include:
- Iletin II, NPH (Pork), 100 Units 1946

Insulin, Regular (Thiazides may cause hyperglycemia; insulin dosage adjustment may be required). Products include:
- Iletin II, Regular (Pork), 100 Units ... 1947

Insulin, Zinc Crystals (Thiazides may cause hyperglycemia; insulin dosage adjustment may be required).
- No products indexed under this heading.

Insulin, Zinc Suspension (Thiazides may cause hyperglycemia; insulin dosage adjustment may be required). Products include:
- Iletin II, Lente (Pork), 100 Units 1945

Insulin Aspart, Human Regular (Thiazides may cause hyperglycemia; insulin dosage adjustment may be required).
- No products indexed under this heading.

Insulin glargine (Thiazides may cause hyperglycemia; insulin dosage adjustment may be required). Products include:
- Lantus Injection 742

Insulin Lispro, Human (Thiazides may cause hyperglycemia; insulin dosage adjustment may be required). Products include:
- Humalog 1926
- Humalog Mix 75/25 Pen 1928

Insulin Lispro Protamine, Human (Thiazides may cause hyperglycemia; insulin dosage adjustment may be required). Products include:
- Humalog Mix 75/25 Pen 1928

Irbesartan (Co-administration with other antihypertensive agents may result in additive effect or potentiation). Products include:
- Avalide Tablets 1070
- Avapro Tablets 1074
- Avapro Tablets 3076

Isradipine (Co-administration with other antihypertensive agents may result in additive effect or potentiation). Products include:
- DynaCirc Capsules 2921
- DynaCirc CR Tablets 2923

Ketoprofen (Co-administration with non-steroidal anti-inflammatory drugs can result in reduced diuretic, natriuretic, and antihypertensive effects). Products include:
- Orudis Capsules 3548
- Orudis KT Tablets 778
- Oruvail Capsules 3548

Ketorolac Tromethamine (Co-administration with non-steroidal anti-inflammatory drugs can result in reduced diuretic, natriuretic, and antihypertensive effects). Products include:
- Acular Ophthalmic Solution 544
- Acular PF Ophthalmic Solution 544
- Toradol 3018

Labetalol Hydrochloride (Co-administration with other antihypertensive agents may result in additive effect or potentiation). Products include:
- Normodyne Injection 3135
- Normodyne Tablets 3137

Levorphanol Tartrate (May potentiate orthostatic hypotension). Products include:
- Levo-Dromoran 1734
- Levorphanol Tartrate Tablets 3059

Lisinopril (Co-administration with other antihypertensive agents may result in additive effect or potentiation). Products include:
- Prinivil Tablets 2164
- Prinzide Tablets 2168
- Zestoretic Tablets 695
- Zestril Tablets 698

Lithium Carbonate (Diuretics reduce the renal clearance of lithium and greatly increase the risk of lithium toxicity). Products include:
- Eskalith 1527
- Lithium Carbonate 3061
- Lithobid Slow-Release Tablets 3255

Lithium Citrate (Diuretics reduce the renal clearance of lithium and greatly increase the risk of lithium toxicity). Products include:
- Lithium Citrate Syrup 3061

Losartan Potassium (Co-administration with other antihypertensive agents may result in additive effect or potentiation). Products include:
- Cozaar Tablets 2067
- Hyzaar 2109

Mecamylamine Hydrochloride (Co-administration with other antihypertensive agents may result in additive effect or potentiation). Products include:
- Inversine Tablets 1850

Meclofenamate Sodium (Co-administration with non-steroidal anti-inflammatory drugs can result in reduced diuretic, natriuretic, and antihypertensive effects).
- No products indexed under this heading.

Mefenamic Acid (Co-administration with non-steroidal anti-inflammatory drugs can result in reduced diuretic, natriuretic, and antihypertensive effects). Products include:
- Ponstel Capsules 1356

Meloxicam (Co-administration with non-steroidal anti-inflammatory drugs can result in reduced diuretic, natriuretic, and antihypertensive effects). Products include:
- Mobic Tablets 1054

Meperidine Hydrochloride (May potentiate orthostatic hypotension). Products include:
- Demerol 3079
- Mepergan Injection 3539

Mephobarbital (May potentiate orthostatic hypotension).
- No products indexed under this heading.

Metformin Hydrochloride (Thiazides may cause hyperglycemia; dosage adjustment of oral hypoglycemic agent may be required). Products include:
- Glucophage Tablets 1080
- Glucophage XR Tablets 1080
- Glucovance Tablets 1086

Methadone Hydrochloride (May potentiate orthostatic hypotension). Products include:
- Dolophine Hydrochloride Tablets 3056

Methyclothiazide (Co-administration with other antihypertensive agents may result in additive effect or potentiation).
- No products indexed under this heading.

Methyldopa (Co-administration with other antihypertensive agents may result in additive effect or potentiation). Products include:
- Aldoclor Tablets 2035
- Aldomet Tablets 2037
- Aldoril Tablets 2039

Methyldopate Hydrochloride (Co-administration with other antihypertensive agents may result in additive effect or potentiation).
- No products indexed under this heading.

Methylprednisolone Acetate (Co-administration with corticosteroids may result in intensified electrolyte depletion, particularly hypokalemia). Products include:
- Depo-Medrol Injectable Suspension 2795

Methylprednisolone Sodium Succinate (Co-administration with corticosteroids may result in intensified electrolyte depletion, particularly hypokalemia). Products include:
- Solu-Medrol Sterile Powder 2855

Metocurine Iodide (Possible increased responsiveness to the muscle relaxant).
- No products indexed under this heading.

Metolazone (Co-administration with other antihypertensive agents may result in additive effect or potentiation). Products include:
- Mykrox Tablets 1168
- Zaroxolyn Tablets 1177

Metoprolol Succinate (Co-administration with other antihypertensive agents may result in additive effect or potentiation). Products include:
- Toprol-XL Tablets 651

Metoprolol Tartrate (Co-administration with other antihypertensive agents may result in additive effect or potentiation).
- No products indexed under this heading.

Metyrosine (Co-administration with other antihypertensive agents may result in additive effect or potentiation). Products include:
- Demser Capsules 2085

Mibefradil Dihydrochloride (Co-administration with other antihypertensive agents may result in additive effect or potentiation).
- No products indexed under this heading.

Miglitol (Thiazides may cause hyperglycemia; dosage adjustment of oral hypoglycemic agent may be required). Products include:
- Glyset Tablets 2821

Minoxidil (Co-administration with other antihypertensive agents may result in additive effect or potentiation). Products include:
- Rogaine Extra Strength for Men Topical Solution 721
- Rogaine for Women Topical Solution 721

Mivacurium Chloride (Possible increased responsiveness to the muscle relaxant).
- No products indexed under this heading.

Moexipril Hydrochloride (Co-administration with other antihypertensive agents may result in additive effect or potentiation). Products include:
- Uniretic Tablets 3178
- Univasc Tablets 3181

Morphine Sulfate (May potentiate orthostatic hypotension). Products include:
- Astramorph/PF Injection, USP (Preservative-Free) 594
- Duramorph Injection 1312
- Infumorph 200 and Infumorph 500 Sterile Solutions 1314
- Kadian Capsules 1335
- MS Contin Tablets 2896
- MSIR 2898
- Oramorph SR Tablets 3062
- Roxanol 3066

Nabumetone (Co-administration with non-steroidal anti-inflammatory drugs can result in reduced diuretic, natriuretic, and antihypertensive effects). Products include:
- Relafen Tablets 1617

Nadolol (Co-administration with other antihypertensive agents may result in additive effect or potentiation). Products include:
- Corgard Tablets 2245
- Corzide 40/5 Tablets 2247
- Corzide 80/5 Tablets 2247
- Nadolol Tablets 2288

Naproxen (Co-administration with non-steroidal anti-inflammatory drugs can result in reduced diuretic, natriuretic, and antihypertensive effects). Products include:
- EC-Naprosyn Delayed-Release Tablets 2967
- Naprosyn Suspension 2967
- Naprosyn Tablets 2967

Naproxen Sodium (Co-administration with non-steroidal anti-inflammatory drugs can result in reduced diuretic, natriuretic, and antihypertensive effects). Products include:
- Aleve Tablets, Caplets and Gelcaps 602
- Aleve Cold & Sinus Caplets 603
- Anaprox Tablets 2967
- Anaprox DS Tablets 2967
- Naprelan Tablets 1293

Nicardipine Hydrochloride (Co-administration with other antihypertensive agents may result in additive effect or potentiation). Products include:
- Cardene I.V. 3485

Nifedipine (Co-administration with other antihypertensive agents may result in additive effect or potentiation). Products include:
- Adalat CC Tablets 877
- Procardia Capsules 2708
- Procardia XL Extended Release Tablets 2710

Nisoldipine (Co-administration with other antihypertensive agents may result in additive effect or potentiation). Products include:
- Sular Tablets 688

Nitroglycerin (Co-administration with other antihypertensive agents may result in additive effect or potentiation). Products include:
- Nitro-Dur Transdermal Infusion System 3134
- Nitro-Dur Transdermal Infusion System 1834
- Nitrolingual Pumpspray 1355

Nitrostat Tablets 2658

Norepinephrine Bitartrate (Co-administration may result in possible decreased response to pressor amines).
No products indexed under this heading.

Oxaprozin (Co-administration with non-steroidal anti-inflammatory drugs can result in reduced diuretic, natriuretic, and antihypertensive effects).
No products indexed under this heading.

Oxycodone Hydrochloride (May potentiate orthostatic hypotension). Products include:
OxyContin Tablets 2912
OxyFast Oral Concentrate Solution . 2916
OxyIR Capsules 2916
Percocet Tablets 1326
Percodan Tablets 1327
Percolone Tablets 1327
Roxicodone 3067
Tylox Capsules 2597

Pancuronium Bromide (Possible increased responsiveness to the muscle relaxant).
No products indexed under this heading.

Penbutolol Sulfate (Co-administration with other antihypertensive agents may result in additive effect or potentiation).
No products indexed under this heading.

Pentobarbital Sodium (May potentiate orthostatic hypotension). Products include:
Nembutal Sodium Solution 485

Perindopril Erbumine (Co-administration with other antihypertensive agents may result in additive effect or potentiation). Products include:
Aceon Tablets (2 mg, 4 mg, 8 mg) 3249

Phenobarbital (May potentiate orthostatic hypotension). Products include:
Arco-Lase Plus Tablets 592
Donnatal 2929
Donnatal Extentabs 2930

Phenoxybenzamine Hydrochloride (Co-administration with other antihypertensive agents may result in additive effect or potentiation). Products include:
Dibenzyline Capsules 3457

Phentolamine Mesylate (Co-administration with other antihypertensive agents may result in additive effect or potentiation).
No products indexed under this heading.

Phenylbutazone (Co-administration with non-steroidal anti-inflammatory drugs can result in reduced diuretic, natriuretic, and antihypertensive effects).
No products indexed under this heading.

Pindolol (Co-administration with other antihypertensive agents may result in additive effect or potentiation).
No products indexed under this heading.

Pioglitazone Hydrochloride (Thiazides may cause hyperglycemia; dosage adjustment of oral hypoglycemic agent may be required). Products include:
Actos Tablets 3275

Piroxicam (Co-administration with non-steroidal anti-inflammatory drugs can result in reduced diuretic, natriuretic, and antihypertensive effects). Products include:
Feldene Capsules 2685

Polythiazide (Co-administration with other antihypertensive agents may result in additive effect or potentiation). Products include:
Minizide Capsules 2700
Renese Tablets 2712

Prazosin Hydrochloride (Co-administration with other antihypertensive agents may result in additive effect or potentiation). Products include:
Minipress Capsules 2699
Minizide Capsules 2700

Prednisolone Acetate (Co-administration with corticosteroids may result in intensified electrolyte depletion, particularly hypokalemia). Products include:
Blephamide Ophthalmic Ointment ... 547
Blephamide Ophthalmic Suspension 548
Poly-Pred Liquifilm Ophthalmic Suspension .... ⊙245
Pred Forte Ophthalmic Suspension .... ⊙246
Pred Mild Sterile Ophthalmic Suspension .... ⊙249
Pred-G Ophthalmic Suspension ..... ⊙247
Pred-G Sterile Ophthalmic Ointment .... ⊙248

Prednisolone Sodium Phosphate (Co-administration with corticosteroids may result in intensified electrolyte depletion, particularly hypokalemia). Products include:
Pediapred Oral Solution 1170

Prednisolone Tebutate (Co-administration with corticosteroids may result in intensified electrolyte depletion, particularly hypokalemia).
No products indexed under this heading.

Prednisone (Co-administration with corticosteroids may result in intensified electrolyte depletion, particularly hypokalemia). Products include:
Prednisone 3064

Propoxyphene Hydrochloride (May potentiate orthostatic hypotension). Products include:
Darvon Pulvules 1909
Darvon Compound-65 Pulvules 1910

Propoxyphene Napsylate (May potentiate orthostatic hypotension). Products include:
Darvon-N/Darvocet-N 1907
Darvon-N Tablets 1912

Propranolol Hydrochloride (Co-administration with other antihypertensive agents may result in additive effect or potentiation). Products include:
Inderal 3513
Inderal LA Long-Acting Capsules 3516
Inderide Tablets 3517
Inderide LA Long-Acting Capsules .. 3519

Quinapril Hydrochloride (Co-administration with other antihypertensive agents may result in additive effect or potentiation). Products include:
Accupril Tablets 2611
Accuretic Tablets 2614

Ramipril (Co-administration with other antihypertensive agents may result in additive effect or potentiation). Products include:
Altace Capsules 2233

Rapacuronium Bromide (Possible increased responsiveness to the muscle relaxant).
No products indexed under this heading.

Rauwolfia serpentina (Co-administration with other antihypertensive agents may result in additive effect or potentiation).
No products indexed under this heading.

Remifentanil Hydrochloride (May potentiate orthostatic hypotension).
No products indexed under this heading.

Repaglinide (Thiazides may cause hyperglycemia; dosage adjustment of oral hypoglycemic agent may be required). Products include:
Prandin Tablets (0.5, 1, and 2 mg) 2432

Rescinnamine (Co-administration with other antihypertensive agents may result in additive effect or potentiation).
No products indexed under this heading.

Reserpine (Co-administration with other antihypertensive agents may result in additive effect or potentiation).
No products indexed under this heading.

Rocuronium Bromide (Possible increased responsiveness to the muscle relaxant). Products include:
Zemuron Injection 2491

Rofecoxib (Co-administration with non-steroidal anti-inflammatory drugs can result in reduced diuretic, natriuretic, and antihypertensive effects). Products include:
Vioxx 2213

Rosiglitazone Maleate (Thiazides may cause hyperglycemia; dosage adjustment of oral hypoglycemic agent may be required). Products include:
Avandia Tablets 1490

Secobarbital Sodium (May potentiate orthostatic hypotension).
No products indexed under this heading.

Sodium Nitroprusside (Co-administration with other antihypertensive agents may result in additive effect or potentiation).
No products indexed under this heading.

Sotalol Hydrochloride (Co-administration with other antihypertensive agents may result in additive effect or potentiation). Products include:
Betapace Tablets 950
Betapace AF Tablets 954

Spirapril Hydrochloride (Co-administration with other antihypertensive agents may result in additive effect or potentiation).
No products indexed under this heading.

Sufentanil Citrate (May potentiate orthostatic hypotension).
No products indexed under this heading.

Sulindac (Co-administration with non-steroidal anti-inflammatory drugs can result in reduced diuretic, natriuretic, and antihypertensive effects). Products include:
Clinoril Tablets 2053

Telmisartan (Co-administration with other antihypertensive agents may result in additive effect or potentiation). Products include:
Micardis Tablets 1049
Micardis HCT Tablets 1051

Terazosin Hydrochloride (Co-administration with other antihypertensive agents may result in additive effect or potentiation). Products include:
Hytrin Capsules 464

Thiamylal Sodium (May potentiate orthostatic hypotension).
No products indexed under this heading.

Timolol Maleate (Co-administration with other antihypertensive agents may result in additive effect or potentiation). Products include:
Blocadren Tablets 2046
Cosopt Sterile Ophthalmic Solution 2065
Timolide Tablets 2187
Timolol GFS .... ⊙266
Timoptic in Ocudose 2192
Timoptic Sterile Ophthalmic Solution 2190
Timoptic-XE Sterile Ophthalmic Gel Forming Solution 2194

Tolazamide (Thiazides may cause hyperglycemia; dosage adjustment of oral hypoglycemic agent may be required).
No products indexed under this heading.

Tolbutamide (Thiazides may cause hyperglycemia; dosage adjustment of oral hypoglycemic agent may be required).
No products indexed under this heading.

Tolmetin Sodium (Co-administration with non-steroidal anti-inflammatory drugs can result in reduced diuretic, natriuretic, and antihypertensive effects). Products include:
Tolectin 2589

Torsemide (Co-administration with other antihypertensive agents may result in additive effect or potentiation). Products include:
Demadex Tablets and Injection 2965

Trandolapril (Co-administration with other antihypertensive agents may result in additive effect or potentiation). Products include:
Mavik Tablets 478
Tarka Tablets 508

Triamcinolone (Co-administration with corticosteroids may result in intensified electrolyte depletion, particularly hypokalemia).
No products indexed under this heading.

Triamcinolone Acetonide (Co-administration with corticosteroids may result in intensified electrolyte depletion, particularly hypokalemia). Products include:
Azmacort Inhalation Aerosol 728
Nasacort Nasal Inhaler 750
Nasacort AQ Nasal Spray 752
Tri-Nasal Spray 2274

Triamcinolone Diacetate (Co-administration with corticosteroids may result in intensified electrolyte depletion, particularly hypokalemia).
No products indexed under this heading.

Triamcinolone Hexacetonide (Co-administration with corticosteroids may result in intensified electrolyte depletion, particularly hypokalemia).
No products indexed under this heading.

Trimethaphan Camsylate (Co-administration with other antihypertensive agents may result in additive effect or potentiation).
No products indexed under this heading.

Troglitazone (Thiazides may cause hyperglycemia; dosage adjustment of oral hypoglycemic agent may be required).
No products indexed under this heading.

Tubocurarine Chloride (Possible increased responsiveness to the muscle relaxant).
No products indexed under this heading.

Valsartan (Co-administration with other antihypertensive agents may result in additive effect or potentiation). Products include:
Diovan Capsules 2337
Diovan HCT Tablets 2338

Vecuronium Bromide (Possible increased responsiveness to the muscle relaxant). Products include:
Norcuron for Injection 2478

Verapamil Hydrochloride (Co-administration with other antihypertensive agents may result in additive effect or potentiation). Products include:
Covera-HS Tablets 3199
Isoptin SR Tablets 467
Tarka Tablets 508
Verelan Capsules 3184
Verelan PM Capsules 3186

Food Interactions

Alcohol (May potentiate orthostatic hypotension).

MIDAMOR TABLETS

(Amiloride Hydrochloride) 2136

May interact with ACE inhibitors, diuretics, lithium preparations, non-steroidal anti-inflammatory agents, potassium preparations, potassium sparing diuretics, and certain other agents. Compounds in these categories include:

Benazepril Hydrochloride (Increased risk of hyperkalemia). Products include:
- Lotensin Tablets 2365
- Lotensin HCT Tablets 2367
- Lotrel Capsules 2370

Bendroflumethiazide (Hyponatremia; hypochloremia; increases in BUN levels). Products include:
- Corzide 40/5 Tablets 2247
- Corzide 80/5 Tablets 2247

Bumetanide (Hyponatremia; hypochloremia; increases in BUN levels).
- No products indexed under this heading.

Captopril (Increased risk of hyperkalemia). Products include:
- Captopril Tablets 2281

Celecoxib (Reduced diuretic, natriuretic, and antihypertensive effects of Midamor). Products include:
- Celebrex Capsules 2676
- Celebrex Capsules 2780

Chlorothiazide (Hyponatremia; hypochloremia; increases in BUN levels). Products include:
- Aldoclor Tablets 2035
- Diuril Oral 2087

Chlorothiazide Sodium (Hyponatremia; hypochloremia; increases in BUN levels). Products include:
- Diuril Sodium Intravenous 2086

Chlorthalidone (Hyponatremia; hypochloremia; increases in BUN levels). Products include:
- Clorpres Tablets 1002
- Combipres Tablets 1040
- Tenoretic Tablets 690

Diclofenac Potassium (Reduced diuretic, natriuretic, and antihypertensive effects of Midamor). Products include:
- Cataflam Tablets 2315

Diclofenac Sodium (Reduced diuretic, natriuretic, and antihypertensive effects of Midamor). Products include:
- Arthrotec Tablets 3195
- Voltaren Ophthalmic Sterile Ophthalmic Solution .... ⊙312
- Voltaren Tablets 2315
- Voltaren-XR Tablets 2315

Enalapril Maleate (Increased risk of hyperkalemia). Products include:
- Lexxel Tablets 608
- Vaseretic Tablets 2204
- Vasotec Tablets 2210

Enalaprilat (Increased risk of hyperkalemia). Products include:
- Enalaprilat Injection 863
- Vasotec I.V. Injection 2207

Ethacrynic Acid (Hyponatremia; hypochloremia; increases in BUN levels). Products include:
- Edecrin Tablets 2091

Etodolac (Reduced diuretic, natriuretic, and antihypertensive effects of Midamor). Products include:
- Lodine 3528
- Lodine XL Extended-Release Tablets 3530

Fenoprofen Calcium (Reduced diuretic, natriuretic, and antihypertensive effects of Midamor).
- No products indexed under this heading.

Flurbiprofen (Reduced diuretic, natriuretic, and antihypertensive effects of Midamor).
- No products indexed under this heading.

Fosinopril Sodium (Increased risk of hyperkalemia). Products include:
- Monopril Tablets 1091
- Monopril HCT 1094

Furosemide (Hyponatremia; hypochloremia; increases in BUN levels). Products include:
- Furosemide Tablets 2284

Hydrochlorothiazide (Hyponatremia; hypochloremia; increases in BUN levels). Products include:
- Accuretic Tablets 2614
- Aldoril Tablets 2039
- Atacand HCT Tablets 597
- Avalide Tablets 1070
- Diovan HCT Tablets 2338
- Dyazide Capsules 1515
- HydroDIURIL Tablets 2108
- Hyzaar 2109
- Inderide Tablets 3517
- Inderide LA Long-Acting Capsules 3519
- Lotensin HCT Tablets 2367
- Maxzide 1008
- Micardis HCT Tablets 1051
- Microzide Capsules 3414
- Moduretic Tablets 2138
- Monopril HCT 1094
- Prinzide Tablets 2168
- Timolide Tablets 2187
- Uniretic Tablets 3178
- Vaseretic Tablets 2204
- Zestoretic Tablets 695
- Ziac Tablets 1887

Hydroflumethiazide (Hyponatremia; hypochloremia; increases in BUN levels). Products include:
- Diucardin Tablets 3494

Ibuprofen (Reduced diuretic, natriuretic, and antihypertensive effects of Midamor). Products include:
- Advil .... ▣771
- Children's Advil Oral Suspension .... ▣773
- Children's Advil Chewable Tablets .... ▣773
- Advil Cold and Sinus Caplets .... ▣771
- Advil Cold and Sinus Tablets .... ▣771
- Advil Flu & Body Ache Caplets .... ▣772
- Infants' Advil Drops .... ▣773
- Junior Strength Advil Tablets .... ▣773
- Junior Strength Advil Chewable Tablets .... ▣773
- Advil Migraine Liquigels .... ▣772
- Children's Motrin Oral Suspension and Chewable Tablets 2006
- Children's Motrin Cold Oral Suspension 2007
- Children's Motrin Oral Suspension .... ▣643
- Motrin Suspension, Oral Drops, Chewable Tablets, and Caplets 2002
- Infants' Motrin Concentrated Drops 2006
- Junior Strength Motrin Caplets and Chewable Tablets 2006
- Motrin IB Tablets, Caplets, and Gelcaps 2002
- Motrin Migraine Pain Caplets 2005
- Motrin Sinus Headache Caplets 2005
- Vicoprofen Tablets 520

Indapamide (Hyponatremia; hypochloremia; increases in BUN levels). Products include:
- Indapamide Tablets 2286

Indomethacin (Reduced diuretic, natriuretic, and antihypertensive effects of Midamor; increased serum potassium levels of both drugs). Products include:
- Indocin 2112

Indomethacin Sodium Trihydrate (Reduced diuretic, natriuretic, and antihypertensive effects of Midamor; increased serum potassium levels of both drugs). Products include:
- Indocin I.V. 2115

Ketoprofen (Reduced diuretic, natriuretic, and antihypertensive effects of Midamor). Products include:
- Orudis Capsules 3548
- Orudis KT Tablets .... ▣778
- Oruvail Capsules 3548

Ketorolac Tromethamine (Reduced diuretic, natriuretic, and antihypertensive effects of Midamor). Products include:
- Acular Ophthalmic Solution 544
- Acular PF Ophthalmic Solution 544
- Toradol 3018

Lisinopril (Increased risk of hyperkalemia). Products include:
- Prinivil Tablets 2164
- Prinzide Tablets 2168
- Zestoretic Tablets 695
- Zestril Tablets 698

Lithium Carbonate (High risk of lithium toxicity). Products include:
- Eskalith 1527
- Lithium Carbonate 3061
- Lithobid Slow-Release Tablets 3255

Lithium Citrate (High risk of lithium toxicity). Products include:
- Lithium Citrate Syrup 3061

Meclofenamate Sodium (Reduced diuretic, natriuretic, and antihypertensive effects of Midamor).
- No products indexed under this heading.

Mefenamic Acid (Reduced diuretic, natriuretic, and antihypertensive effects of Midamor). Products include:
- Ponstel Capsules 1356

Meloxicam (Reduced diuretic, natriuretic, and antihypertensive effects of Midamor). Products include:
- Mobic Tablets 1054

Methyclothiazide (Hyponatremia; hypochloremia; increases in BUN levels).
- No products indexed under this heading.

Metolazone (Hyponatremia; hypochloremia; increases in BUN levels). Products include:
- Mykrox Tablets 1168
- Zaroxolyn Tablets 1177

Moexipril Hydrochloride (Increased risk of hyperkalemia). Products include:
- Uniretic Tablets 3178
- Univasc Tablets 3181

Nabumetone (Reduced diuretic, natriuretic, and antihypertensive effects of Midamor). Products include:
- Relafen Tablets 1617

Naproxen (Reduced diuretic, natriuretic, and antihypertensive effects of Midamor). Products include:
- EC-Naprosyn Delayed-Release Tablets 2967
- Naprosyn Suspension 2967
- Naprosyn Tablets 2967

Naproxen Sodium (Reduced diuretic, natriuretic, and antihypertensive effects of Midamor). Products include:
- Aleve Tablets, Caplets and Gelcaps .... ▣602
- Aleve Cold & Sinus Caplets .... ▣603
- Anaprox Tablets 2967
- Anaprox DS Tablets 2967
- Naprelan Tablets 1293

Oxaprozin (Reduced diuretic, natriuretic, and antihypertensive effects of Midamor).
- No products indexed under this heading.

Perindopril Erbumine (Increased risk of hyperkalemia). Products include:
- Aceon Tablets (2 mg, 4 mg, 8 mg) 3249

Phenylbutazone (Reduced diuretic, natriuretic, and antihypertensive effects of Midamor).
- No products indexed under this heading.

Piroxicam (Reduced diuretic, natriuretic, and antihypertensive effects of Midamor). Products include:
- Feldene Capsules 2685

Polythiazide (Hyponatremia; hypochloremia; increases in BUN levels). Products include:
- Minizide Capsules 2700
- Renese Tablets 2712

Potassium Acid Phosphate (Concomitant therapy is contraindicated). Products include:
- K-Phos Original (Sodium Free) Tablets 947

Potassium Bicarbonate (Concomitant therapy is contraindicated).
- No products indexed under this heading.

Potassium Chloride (Concomitant therapy is contraindicated). Products include:
- Chlor-3 1361
- Colyte with Flavor Packs for Oral Solution 3170
- GoLYTELY and Pineapple Flavor GoLYTELY for Oral Solution 1068
- K-Dur Microburst Release System ER Tablets 1832
- Klor-Con M20/Klor-Con M10 Tablets 3329
- K-Lor Powder Packets 469
- K-Tab Filmtab Tablets 470
- Micro-K 3311
- NuLYTELY, Cherry Flavor, Lemon-Lime Flavor, and Orange Flavor NuLYTELY for Oral Solution 1068
- Rum-K 1363

Potassium Citrate (Concomitant therapy is contraindicated). Products include:
- Urocit-K Tablets 2232

Potassium Gluconate (Concomitant therapy is contraindicated).
- No products indexed under this heading.

Potassium Phosphate (Concomitant therapy is contraindicated). Products include:
- K-Phos Neutral Tablets 946

Quinapril Hydrochloride (Increased risk of hyperkalemia). Products include:
- Accupril Tablets 2611
- Accuretic Tablets 2614

Ramipril (Increased risk of hyperkalemia). Products include:
- Altace Capsules 2233

Rofecoxib (Reduced diuretic, natriuretic, and antihypertensive effects of Midamor). Products include:
- Vioxx 2213

Spirapril Hydrochloride (Increased risk of hyperkalemia).
- No products indexed under this heading.

Spironolactone (Do not administer concomitantly; rapid increases in serum potassium).
- No products indexed under this heading.

Sulindac (Reduced diuretic, natriuretic, and antihypertensive effects of Midamor). Products include:
- Clinoril Tablets 2053

Tolmetin Sodium (Reduced diuretic, natriuretic, and antihypertensive effects of Midamor). Products include:
- Tolectin 2589

Torsemide (Hyponatremia; hypochloremia; increases in BUN levels). Products include:
- Demadex Tablets and Injection 2965

Trandolapril (Increased risk of hyperkalemia). Products include:
- Mavik Tablets 478
- Tarka Tablets 508

Triamterene (Do not administer concomitantly; rapid increases in serum potassium). Products include:
- Dyazide Capsules 1515
- Dyrenium Capsules 3458
- Maxzide 1008

Food Interactions

Diet, potassium-rich (Potential for rapid increases in serum potassium levels).

MAXIMUM STRENGTH MIDOL MENSTRUAL CAPLETS AND GELCAPS

(Acetaminophen, Caffeine, Pyrilamine Maleate) .... ▣612

May interact with hypnotics and sedatives, tranquilizers, and certain other agents. Compounds in these categories include:

Alprazolam (May increase drowsiness). Products include:
- Xanax Tablets 2865

Buspirone Hydrochloride (May increase drowsiness).
No products indexed under this heading.

Caffeine-containing medications (Concomitant use may cause nervousness, irritability, sleeplessness, and occasionally, rapid heartbeat).

Chlordiazepoxide (May increase drowsiness). Products include:
Limbitrol ... 1738

Chlordiazepoxide Hydrochloride (May increase drowsiness). Products include:
Librium Capsules ... 1736
Librium for Injection ... 1737

Chlorpromazine (May increase drowsiness). Products include:
Thorazine Suppositories ... 1656

Chlorpromazine Hydrochloride (May increase drowsiness). Products include:
Thorazine ... 1656

Chlorprothixene (May increase drowsiness).
No products indexed under this heading.

Chlorprothixene Hydrochloride (May increase drowsiness).
No products indexed under this heading.

Clorazepate Dipotassium (May increase drowsiness). Products include:
Tranxene ... 511

Diazepam (May increase drowsiness). Products include:
Valium Injectable ... 3026
Valium Tablets ... 3047

Droperidol (May increase drowsiness).
No products indexed under this heading.

Estazolam (May increase drowsiness). Products include:
ProSom Tablets ... 500

Ethchlorvynol (May increase drowsiness).
No products indexed under this heading.

Ethinamate (May increase drowsiness).
No products indexed under this heading.

Fluphenazine Decanoate (May increase drowsiness).
No products indexed under this heading.

Fluphenazine Enanthate (May increase drowsiness).
No products indexed under this heading.

Fluphenazine Hydrochloride (May increase drowsiness).
No products indexed under this heading.

Flurazepam Hydrochloride (May increase drowsiness).
No products indexed under this heading.

Glutethimide (May increase drowsiness).
No products indexed under this heading.

Haloperidol (May increase drowsiness). Products include:
Haldol Injection, Tablets and Concentrate ... 2533

Haloperidol Decanoate (May increase drowsiness). Products include:
Haldol Decanoate ... 2535

Hydroxyzine Hydrochloride (May increase drowsiness). Products include:
Atarax Tablets & Syrup ... 2667
Vistaril Intramuscular Solution ... 2738

Lorazepam (May increase drowsiness). Products include:
Ativan Injection ... 3478
Ativan Tablets ... 3482

Loxapine Hydrochloride (May increase drowsiness).
No products indexed under this heading.

Loxapine Succinate (May increase drowsiness). Products include:
Loxitane Capsules ... 3398

Meprobamate (May increase drowsiness). Products include:
Miltown Tablets ... 3349

Mesoridazine Besylate (May increase drowsiness). Products include:
Serentil ... 1057

Midazolam Hydrochloride (May increase drowsiness). Products include:
Versed Injection ... 3027
Versed Syrup ... 3033

Molindone Hydrochloride (May increase drowsiness). Products include:
Moban ... 1320

Oxazepam (May increase drowsiness).
No products indexed under this heading.

Perphenazine (May increase drowsiness). Products include:
Etrafon ... 3115
Trilafon ... 3160

Prazepam (May increase drowsiness).
No products indexed under this heading.

Prochlorperazine (May increase drowsiness). Products include:
Compazine ... 1505

Promethazine Hydrochloride (May increase drowsiness). Products include:
Mepergan Injection ... 3539
Phenergan Injection ... 3553
Phenergan ... 3556
Phenergan Syrup ... 3554
Phenergan with Codeine Syrup ... 3557
Phenergan with Dextromethorphan Syrup ... 3559
Phenergan VC Syrup ... 3560
Phenergan VC with Codeine Syrup ... 3561

Propofol (May increase drowsiness). Products include:
Diprivan Injectable Emulsion ... 667

Quazepam (May increase drowsiness).
No products indexed under this heading.

Secobarbital Sodium (May increase drowsiness).
No products indexed under this heading.

Temazepam (May increase drowsiness).
No products indexed under this heading.

Thioridazine Hydrochloride (May increase drowsiness). Products include:
Thioridazine Hydrochloride Tablets ... 2289

Thiothixene (May increase drowsiness). Products include:
Navane Capsules ... 2701
Thiothixene Capsules ... 2290

Triazolam (May increase drowsiness). Products include:
Halcion Tablets ... 2823

Trifluoperazine Hydrochloride (May increase drowsiness). Products include:
Stelazine ... 1640

Zaleplon (May increase drowsiness). Products include:
Sonata Capsules ... 3591

Zolpidem Tartrate (May increase drowsiness). Products include:
Ambien Tablets ... 3191

Food Interactions

Alcohol (Chronic heavy alcohol users, 3 or more drinks per day, should consult their physicians for advice on when and how they should take pain relievers/fever reducers including acetaminophen; increases drowsiness effect).

Beverages, caffeine-containing (Concomitant use may cause nervousness, irritability, sleeplessness, and occasionally, rapid heartbeat).

Food, caffeine-containing (Concomitant use may cause nervousness, irritability, sleeplessness, and occasionally, rapid heartbeat).

MAXIMUM STRENGTH MIDOL PMS CAPLETS AND GELCAPS

(Acetaminophen, Pamabrom, Pyrilamine Maleate) ... ▭613
May interact with hypnotics and sedatives, tranquilizers, and certain other agents. Compounds in these categories include:

Alprazolam (May increase drowsiness). Products include:
Xanax Tablets ... 2865

Buspirone Hydrochloride (May increase drowsiness).
No products indexed under this heading.

Chlordiazepoxide (May increase drowsiness). Products include:
Limbitrol ... 1738

Chlordiazepoxide Hydrochloride (May increase drowsiness). Products include:
Librium Capsules ... 1736
Librium for Injection ... 1737

Chlorpromazine (May increase drowsiness). Products include:
Thorazine Suppositories ... 1656

Chlorpromazine Hydrochloride (May increase drowsiness). Products include:
Thorazine ... 1656

Chlorprothixene (May increase drowsiness).
No products indexed under this heading.

Chlorprothixene Hydrochloride (May increase drowsiness).
No products indexed under this heading.

Clorazepate Dipotassium (May increase drowsiness). Products include:
Tranxene ... 511

Diazepam (May increase drowsiness). Products include:
Valium Injectable ... 3026
Valium Tablets ... 3047

Droperidol (May increase drowsiness).
No products indexed under this heading.

Estazolam (May increase drowsiness). Products include:
ProSom Tablets ... 500

Ethchlorvynol (May increase drowsiness).
No products indexed under this heading.

Ethinamate (May increase drowsiness).
No products indexed under this heading.

Fluphenazine Decanoate (May increase drowsiness).
No products indexed under this heading.

Fluphenazine Enanthate (May increase drowsiness).
No products indexed under this heading.

Fluphenazine Hydrochloride (May increase drowsiness).
No products indexed under this heading.

Flurazepam Hydrochloride (May increase drowsiness).
No products indexed under this heading.

Glutethimide (May increase drowsiness).
No products indexed under this heading.

Haloperidol (May increase drowsiness). Products include:
Haldol Injection, Tablets and Concentrate ... 2533

Haloperidol Decanoate (May increase drowsiness). Products include:
Haldol Decanoate ... 2535

Hydroxyzine Hydrochloride (May increase drowsiness). Products include:
Atarax Tablets & Syrup ... 2667
Vistaril Intramuscular Solution ... 2738

Lorazepam (May increase drowsiness). Products include:
Ativan Injection ... 3478
Ativan Tablets ... 3482

Loxapine Hydrochloride (May increase drowsiness).
No products indexed under this heading.

Loxapine Succinate (May increase drowsiness). Products include:
Loxitane Capsules ... 3398

Meprobamate (May increase drowsiness). Products include:
Miltown Tablets ... 3349

Mesoridazine Besylate (May increase drowsiness). Products include:
Serentil ... 1057

Midazolam Hydrochloride (May increase drowsiness). Products include:
Versed Injection ... 3027
Versed Syrup ... 3033

Molindone Hydrochloride (May increase drowsiness). Products include:
Moban ... 1320

Oxazepam (May increase drowsiness).
No products indexed under this heading.

Perphenazine (May increase drowsiness). Products include:
Etrafon ... 3115
Trilafon ... 3160

Prazepam (May increase drowsiness).
No products indexed under this heading.

Prochlorperazine (May increase drowsiness). Products include:
Compazine ... 1505

Promethazine Hydrochloride (May increase drowsiness). Products include:
Mepergan Injection ... 3539
Phenergan Injection ... 3553
Phenergan ... 3556
Phenergan Syrup ... 3554
Phenergan with Codeine Syrup ... 3557
Phenergan with Dextromethorphan Syrup ... 3559
Phenergan VC Syrup ... 3560
Phenergan VC with Codeine Syrup ... 3561

Propofol (May increase drowsiness). Products include:
Diprivan Injectable Emulsion ... 667

Quazepam (May increase drowsiness).
No products indexed under this heading.

Secobarbital Sodium (May increase drowsiness).
No products indexed under this heading.

Temazepam (May increase drowsiness).
No products indexed under this heading.

Thioridazine Hydrochloride (May increase drowsiness). Products include:
Thioridazine Hydrochloride Tablets ... 2289

Thiothixene (May increase drowsiness). Products include:
Navane Capsules ... 2701

Thiothixene Capsules 2290

Triazolam (May increase drowsiness). Products include:
Halcion Tablets 2823

Trifluoperazine Hydrochloride (May increase drowsiness). Products include:
Stelazine 1640

Zaleplon (May increase drowsiness). Products include:
Sonata Capsules 3591

Zolpidem Tartrate (May increase drowsiness). Products include:
Ambien Tablets 3191

Food Interactions

Alcohol (Chronic heavy alcohol users, 3 or more drinks per day, should consult their physicians for advice on when and how they should take pain relievers/fever reducers including acetaminophen; increases drowsiness effect).

MAXIMUM STRENGTH MIDOL TEEN CAPLETS

(Acetaminophen, Pamabrom) .... ▣612
May interact with:

Food Interactions

Alcohol (Chronic heavy alcohol users, 3 or more drinks per day, should consult their physicians for advice on when and how they should take pain relievers/fever reducers including acetaminophen; increases drowsiness effect).

MIDRIN CAPSULES

(Acetaminophen, Dichloralphenazone, Isometheptene Mucate).................... 3464
May interact with monoamine oxidase inhibitors. Compounds in these categories include:

Isocarboxazid (Concurrent therapy contraindicated).
No products indexed under this heading.

Moclobemide (Concurrent therapy contraindicated).
No products indexed under this heading.

Pargyline Hydrochloride (Concurrent therapy contraindicated).
No products indexed under this heading.

Phenelzine Sulfate (Concurrent therapy contraindicated). Products include:
Nardil Tablets 2653

Procarbazine Hydrochloride (Concurrent therapy contraindicated). Products include:
Matulane Capsules 3246

Selegiline Hydrochloride (Concurrent therapy contraindicated). Products include:
Eldepryl Capsules 3266

Tranylcypromine Sulfate (Concurrent therapy contraindicated). Products include:
Parnate Tablets 1607

MIGRANAL NASAL SPRAY

(Dihydroergotamine Mesylate) 2376
May interact with 5HT1-receptor agonists, macrolide antibiotics, vasopressors, and certain other agents. Compounds in these categories include:

Azithromycin Dihydrate (Co-administration of ergot alkaloids with macrolide antibiotics has resulted in increased plasma levels of unchanged alkaloids and peripheral vasoconstriction; vasospastic reactions have been reported with concurrent use at therapeutic doses). Products include:
Zithromax 2743
Zithromax for IV Infusion 2748
Zithromax for Oral Suspension, 300 mg, 600 mg, 900 mg, 1200 mg.................... 2739
Zithromax Tablets, 250 mg 2739

Clarithromycin (Co-administration of ergot alkaloids with macrolide antibiotics has resulted in increased plasma levels of unchanged alkaloids and peripheral vasoconstriction; vasospastic reactions have been reported with concurrent use at therapeutic doses). Products include:
Biaxin/Biaxin XL 403
PREVPAC 3298

Dirithromycin (Co-administration of ergot alkaloids with macrolide antibiotics has resulted in increased plasma levels of unchanged alkaloids and peripheral vasoconstriction; vasospastic reactions have been reported with concurrent use at therapeutic doses). Products include:
Dynabac Tablets 2269

Dopamine Hydrochloride (Concurrent use with peripheral and central vasoconstrictors is not recommended because the combination may result in additive or synergistic elevation of blood pressure).
No products indexed under this heading.

Epinephrine Bitartrate (Concurrent use with peripheral and central vasoconstrictors is not recommended because the combination may result in additive or synergistic elevation of blood pressure). Products include:
Sensorcaine 643

Epinephrine Hydrochloride (Concurrent use with peripheral and central vasoconstrictors is not recommended because the combination may result in additive or synergistic elevation of blood pressure).
No products indexed under this heading.

Erythromycin (Co-administration of ergot alkaloids with macrolide antibiotics has resulted in increased plasma levels of unchanged alkaloids and peripheral vasoconstriction; vasospastic reactions have been reported with concurrent use at therapeutic doses). Products include:
Emgel 2% Topical Gel 1285
Ery-Tab Tablets 448
Erythromycin Base Filmtab Tablets 454
Erythromycin Delayed-Release Capsules, USP 455
PCE Dispertab Tablets 498

Erythromycin Estolate (Co-administration of ergot alkaloids with macrolide antibiotics has resulted in increased plasma levels of unchanged alkaloids and peripheral vasoconstriction; vasospastic reactions have been reported with concurrent use at therapeutic doses).
No products indexed under this heading.

Erythromycin Ethylsuccinate (Co-administration of ergot alkaloids with macrolide antibiotics has resulted in increased plasma levels of unchanged alkaloids and peripheral vasoconstriction; vasospastic reactions have been reported with concurrent use at therapeutic doses). Products include:
E.E.S. 450
EryPed 446
Pediazole Suspension 3050

Erythromycin Gluceptate (Co-administration of ergot alkaloids with macrolide antibiotics has resulted in increased plasma levels of unchanged alkaloids and peripheral vasoconstriction; vasospastic reactions have been reported with concurrent use at therapeutic doses).
No products indexed under this heading.

Erythromycin Stearate (Co-administration of ergot alkaloids with macrolide antibiotics has resulted in increased plasma levels of unchanged alkaloids and peripheral vasoconstriction; vasospastic reactions have been reported with concurrent use at therapeutic doses). Products include:
Erythrocin Stearate Filmtab Tablets 452

Metaraminol Bitartrate (Concurrent use with peripheral and central vasoconstrictors is not recommended because the combination may result in additive or synergistic elevation of blood pressure). Products include:
Aramine Injection 2043

Methoxamine Hydrochloride (Concurrent use with peripheral and central vasoconstrictors is not recommended because the combination may result in additive or synergistic elevation of blood pressure).
No products indexed under this heading.

Naratriptan Hydrochloride (Concurrent use of 5-HT1 agonists and ergot-containing or ergot-type medications should not be undertaken within 24 hours of each other). Products include:
Amerge Tablets 1467

Nicotine (May provoke vasoconstriction in some patients, predisposing to a greater ischemic response to ergot). Products include:
Nicoderm CQ Patch 1717
Nicotrol Inhaler 2840
Nicotrol Nasal Spray 2843
Nicotrol Patch 2840

Nicotine Polacrilex (May provoke vasoconstriction in some patients, predisposing to a greater ischemic response to ergot). Products include:
Nicorette Gum 1720

Norepinephrine Bitartrate (Concurrent use with peripheral and central vasoconstrictors is not recommended because the combination may result in additive or synergistic elevation of blood pressure).
No products indexed under this heading.

Phenylephrine Hydrochloride (Concurrent use with peripheral and central vasoconstrictors is not recommended because the combination may result in additive or synergistic elevation of blood pressure). Products include:
Afrin Nasal Decongestant Children's Pump Mist .... ▣734
Extendryl 1361
Hycomine Compound Tablets 1317
Neo-Synephrine .... ▣614
Phenergan VC Syrup 3560
Phenergan VC with Codeine Syrup 3561
Preparation H Cream .... ▣778
Preparation H Cooling Gel .... ▣778
Preparation H .... ▣778
Vicks Sinex Nasal Spray and Ultra Fine Mist .... ▣729

Propranolol Hydrochloride (May potentiate the vasoconstrictive action of ergotamine by blocking the vasodilating property of epinephrine). Products include:
Inderal 3513
Inderal LA Long-Acting Capsules 3516
Inderide Tablets 3517
Inderide LA Long-Acting Capsules 3519

Rizatriptan Benzoate (Concurrent use of 5-HT1 agonists and ergot-containing or ergot-type medications should not be undertaken within 24 hours of each other). Products include:
Maxalt Tablets 2120
Maxalt-MLT Orally Disintegrating Tablets 2120

Sumatriptan (Co-administration could lead to additive coronary artery vasospasm effect; concurrent use should not be undertaken within 24 hours of each other). Products include:
Imitrex Nasal Spray 1554

Sumatriptan Succinate (Co-administration could lead to additive coronary artery vasospasm effect; concurrent use should not be undertaken within 24 hours of each other). Products include:
Imitrex Injection 1549
Imitrex Tablets 1558

Troleandomycin (Co-administration of ergot alkaloids with macrolide antibiotics has resulted in increased plasma levels of unchanged alkaloids and peripheral vasoconstriction; vasospastic reactions have been reported with concurrent use at therapeutic doses). Products include:
Tao Capsules 2716

Zolmitriptan (Concurrent use of 5-HT1 agonists and ergot-containing or ergot-type medications should not be undertaken within 24 hours of each other). Products include:
Zomig Tablets 708
Zomig-ZMT Tablets 708

MILTOWN TABLETS

(Meprobamate) 3349
May interact with central nervous system depressants and certain other agents. Compounds in these categories include:

Alfentanil Hydrochloride (Simultaneous use can lead to additive CNS depressant effects).
No products indexed under this heading.

Alprazolam (Simultaneous use can lead to additive CNS depressant effects). Products include:
Xanax Tablets 2865

Aprobarbital (Simultaneous use can lead to additive CNS depressant effects).
No products indexed under this heading.

Buprenorphine Hydrochloride (Simultaneous use can lead to additive CNS depressant effects). Products include:
Buprenex Injectable 2918

Buspirone Hydrochloride (Simultaneous use can lead to additive CNS depressant effects).
No products indexed under this heading.

Butabarbital (Simultaneous use can lead to additive CNS depressant effects).
No products indexed under this heading.

Butalbital (Simultaneous use can lead to additive CNS depressant effects). Products include:
Phrenilin 578
Sedapap Tablets 50 mg/650 mg 2225

Chlordiazepoxide (Simultaneous use can lead to additive CNS depressant effects). Products include:
Limbitrol 1738

Chlordiazepoxide Hydrochloride (Simultaneous use can lead to additive CNS depressant effects). Products include:
Librium Capsules 1736
Librium for Injection 1737

Chlorpromazine (Simultaneous use can lead to additive CNS depressant effects). Products include:
Thorazine Suppositories 1656

Chlorpromazine Hydrochloride (Simultaneous use can lead to additive CNS depressant effects). Products include:
Thorazine 1656

Chlorprothixene (Simultaneous use can lead to additive CNS depressant effects).
No products indexed under this heading.

Chlorprothixene Hydrochloride (Simultaneous use can lead to additive CNS depressant effects).
No products indexed under this heading.

Chlorprothixene Lactate (Simultaneous use can lead to additive CNS depressant effects).
No products indexed under this heading.

Clorazepate Dipotassium (Simultaneous use can lead to additive CNS depressant effects). Products include:
Tranxene 511

Clozapine (Simultaneous use can lead to additive CNS depressant effects). Products include:
Clozaril Tablets 2319

Codeine Phosphate (Simultaneous use can lead to additive CNS depressant effects). Products include:
Phenergan with Codeine Syrup 3557
Phenergan VC with Codeine Syrup .. 3561
Robitussin A-C Syrup 2942
Robitussin-DAC Syrup 2942
Ryna-C Liquid ..... ▣768
Soma Compound w/Codeine Tablets 3355
Tussi-Organidin NR Liquid 3350
Tussi-Organidin-S NR Liquid 3350
Tylenol with Codeine 2595

Desflurane (Simultaneous use can lead to additive CNS depressant effects). Products include:
Suprane Liquid for Inhalation 874

Dezocine (Simultaneous use can lead to additive CNS depressant effects).
No products indexed under this heading.

Diazepam (Simultaneous use can lead to additive CNS depressant effects). Products include:
Valium Injectable 3026
Valium Tablets 3047

Droperidol (Simultaneous use can lead to additive CNS depressant effects).
No products indexed under this heading.

Enflurane (Simultaneous use can lead to additive CNS depressant effects).
No products indexed under this heading.

Estazolam (Simultaneous use can lead to additive CNS depressant effects). Products include:
ProSom Tablets 500

Ethchlorvynol (Simultaneous use can lead to additive CNS depressant effects).
No products indexed under this heading.

Ethinamate (Simultaneous use can lead to additive CNS depressant effects).
No products indexed under this heading.

Fentanyl (Simultaneous use can lead to additive CNS depressant effects). Products include:
Duragesic Transdermal System 1786

Fentanyl Citrate (Simultaneous use can lead to additive CNS depressant effects). Products include:
Actiq 1184

Fluphenazine Decanoate (Simultaneous use can lead to additive CNS depressant effects).
No products indexed under this heading.

Fluphenazine Enanthate (Simultaneous use can lead to additive CNS depressant effects).
No products indexed under this heading.

Fluphenazine Hydrochloride (Simultaneous use can lead to additive CNS depressant effects).
No products indexed under this heading.

Flurazepam Hydrochloride (Simultaneous use can lead to additive CNS depressant effects).
No products indexed under this heading.

Glutethimide (Simultaneous use can lead to additive CNS depressant effects).
No products indexed under this heading.

Haloperidol (Simultaneous use can lead to additive CNS depressant effects). Products include:
Haldol Injection, Tablets and Concentrate 2533

Haloperidol Decanoate (Simultaneous use can lead to additive CNS depressant effects). Products include:
Haldol Decanoate 2535

Hydrocodone Bitartrate (Simultaneous use can lead to additive CNS depressant effects). Products include:
Hycodan 1316
Hycomine Compound Tablets 1317
Hycotuss Expectorant Syrup 1318
Lortab 3319
Lortab Elixir 3317
Maxidone Tablets CIII 3399
Norco 5/325 Tablets CIII 3424
Norco 7.5/325 Tablets CIII 3425
Norco 10/325 Tablets CIII 3427
Norco 10/325 Tablets CIII 3425
Vicodin Tablets 516
Vicodin ES Tablets 517
Vicodin HP Tablets 518
Vicodin Tuss Expectorant 519
Vicoprofen Tablets 520
Zydone Tablets 1330

Hydrocodone Polistirex (Simultaneous use can lead to additive CNS depressant effects). Products include:
Tussionex Pennkinetic Extended-Release Suspension 1174

Hydromorphone Hydrochloride (Simultaneous use can lead to additive CNS depressant effects). Products include:
Dilaudid 441
Dilaudid Oral Liquid 445
Dilaudid Powder 441
Dilaudid Rectal Suppositories 441
Dilaudid Tablets 441
Dilaudid Tablets - 8 mg 445
Dilaudid-HP 443

Hydroxyzine Hydrochloride (Simultaneous use can lead to additive CNS depressant effects). Products include:
Atarax Tablets & Syrup 2667
Vistaril Intramuscular Solution 2738

Isoflurane (Simultaneous use can lead to additive CNS depressant effects).
No products indexed under this heading.

Ketamine Hydrochloride (Simultaneous use can lead to additive CNS depressant effects).
No products indexed under this heading.

Levomethadyl Acetate Hydrochloride (Simultaneous use can lead to additive CNS depressant effects).
No products indexed under this heading.

Levorphanol Tartrate (Simultaneous use can lead to additive CNS depressant effects). Products include:
Levo-Dromoran 1734
Levorphanol Tartrate Tablets 3059

Lorazepam (Simultaneous use can lead to additive CNS depressant effects). Products include:
Ativan Injection 3478
Ativan Tablets 3482

Loxapine Hydrochloride (Simultaneous use can lead to additive CNS depressant effects).
No products indexed under this heading.

Loxapine Succinate (Simultaneous use can lead to additive CNS depressant effects). Products include:
Loxitane Capsules 3398

Meperidine Hydrochloride (Simultaneous use can lead to additive CNS depressant effects). Products include:
Demerol 3079
Mepergan Injection 3539

Mephobarbital (Simultaneous use can lead to additive CNS depressant effects).
No products indexed under this heading.

Mesoridazine Besylate (Simultaneous use can lead to additive CNS depressant effects). Products include:
Serentil 1057

Methadone Hydrochloride (Simultaneous use can lead to additive CNS depressant effects). Products include:
Dolophine Hydrochloride Tablets 3056

Methohexital Sodium (Simultaneous use can lead to additive CNS depressant effects). Products include:
Brevital Sodium for Injection, USP .. 1815

Methotrimeprazine (Simultaneous use can lead to additive CNS depressant effects).
No products indexed under this heading.

Methoxyflurane (Simultaneous use can lead to additive CNS depressant effects).
No products indexed under this heading.

Midazolam Hydrochloride (Simultaneous use can lead to additive CNS depressant effects). Products include:
Versed Injection 3027
Versed Syrup 3033

Molindone Hydrochloride (Simultaneous use can lead to additive CNS depressant effects). Products include:
Moban 1320

Morphine Sulfate (Simultaneous use can lead to additive CNS depressant effects). Products include:
Astramorph/PF Injection, USP (Preservative-Free) 594
Duramorph Injection 1312
Infumorph 200 and Infumorph 500 Sterile Solutions 1314
Kadian Capsules 1335
MS Contin Tablets 2896
MSIR 2898
Oramorph SR Tablets 3062
Roxanol 3066

Olanzapine (Simultaneous use can lead to additive CNS depressant effects). Products include:
Zyprexa Tablets 1973
Zyprexa ZYDIS Orally Disintegrating Tablets 1973

Oxazepam (Simultaneous use can lead to additive CNS depressant effects).
No products indexed under this heading.

Oxycodone Hydrochloride (Simultaneous use can lead to additive CNS depressant effects). Products include:
OxyContin Tablets 2912
OxyFast Oral Concentrate Solution . 2916
OxyIR Capsules 2916
Percocet Tablets 1326
Percodan Tablets 1327
Percolone Tablets 1327
Roxicodone 3067
Tylox Capsules 2597

Pentobarbital Sodium (Simultaneous use can lead to additive CNS depressant effects). Products include:
Nembutal Sodium Solution 485

Perphenazine (Simultaneous use can lead to additive CNS depressant effects). Products include:
Etrafon 3115
Trilafon 3160

Phenobarbital (Simultaneous use can lead to additive CNS depressant effects). Products include:
Arco-Lase Plus Tablets 592
Donnatal 2929
Donnatal Extentabs 2930

Prazepam (Simultaneous use can lead to additive CNS depressant effects).
No products indexed under this heading.

Prochlorperazine (Simultaneous use can lead to additive CNS depressant effects). Products include:
Compazine 1505

Promethazine Hydrochloride (Simultaneous use can lead to additive CNS depressant effects). Products include:
Mepergan Injection 3539
Phenergan Injection 3553
Phenergan 3556
Phenergan Syrup 3554
Phenergan with Codeine Syrup 3557
Phenergan with Dextromethorphan Syrup 3559
Phenergan VC Syrup 3560
Phenergan VC with Codeine Syrup .. 3561

Propofol (Simultaneous use can lead to additive CNS depressant effects). Products include:
Diprivan Injectable Emulsion 667

Propoxyphene Hydrochloride (Simultaneous use can lead to additive CNS depressant effects). Products include:
Darvon Pulvules 1909
Darvon Compound-65 Pulvules 1910

Propoxyphene Napsylate (Simultaneous use can lead to additive CNS depressant effects). Products include:
Darvon-N/Darvocet-N 1907
Darvon-N Tablets 1912

Quazepam (Simultaneous use can lead to additive CNS depressant effects).
No products indexed under this heading.

Quetiapine Fumarate (Simultaneous use can lead to additive CNS depressant effects). Products include:
Seroquel Tablets 684

Remifentanil Hydrochloride (Simultaneous use can lead to additive CNS depressant effects).
No products indexed under this heading.

Risperidone (Simultaneous use can lead to additive CNS depressant effects). Products include:
Risperdal 1796

Secobarbital Sodium (Simultaneous use can lead to additive CNS depressant effects).
No products indexed under this heading.

Sevoflurane (Simultaneous use can lead to additive CNS depressant effects).
No products indexed under this heading.

Sufentanil Citrate (Simultaneous use can lead to additive CNS depressant effects).
No products indexed under this heading.

Temazepam (Simultaneous use can lead to additive CNS depressant effects).
No products indexed under this heading.

Thiamylal Sodium (Simultaneous use can lead to additive CNS depressant effects).
No products indexed under this heading.

Thioridazine Hydrochloride (Simultaneous use can lead to additive CNS depressant effects). Products include:
Thioridazine Hydrochloride Tablets 2289

Thiothixene (Simultaneous use can lead to additive CNS depressant effects). Products include:

Navane Capsules 2701
Thiothixene Capsules 2290

Triazolam (Simultaneous use can lead to additive CNS depressant effects). Products include:
Halcion Tablets 2823

Trifluoperazine Hydrochloride (Simultaneous use can lead to additive CNS depressant effects). Products include:
Stelazine 1640

Zaleplon (Simultaneous use can lead to additive CNS depressant effects). Products include:
Sonata Capsules 3591

Ziprasidone Hydrochloride (Simultaneous use can lead to additive CNS depressant effects). Products include:
Geodon Capsules 2688

Zolpidem Tartrate (Simultaneous use can lead to additive CNS depressant effects). Products include:
Ambien Tablets 3191

Food Interactions

Alcohol (Simultaneous use can lead to additive CNS depressant effects).

MINIPRESS CAPSULES
(Prazosin Hydrochloride) 2699
May interact with antihypertensives, beta blockers, and diuretics. Compounds in these categories include:

Acebutolol Hydrochloride (Potential for additive hypotensive effect; hypotension may develop with concurrent use of beta blockers). Products include:
Sectral Capsules 3589

Amiloride Hydrochloride (Potential for additive hypotensive effect). Products include:
Midamor Tablets 2136
Moduretic Tablets 2138

Amlodipine Besylate (Potential for additive hypotensive effect). Products include:
Lotrel Capsules 2370
Norvasc Tablets 2704

Atenolol (Potential for additive hypotensive effect; hypotension may develop with concurrent use of beta blockers). Products include:
Tenoretic Tablets 690
Tenormin I.V. Injection 692

Benazepril Hydrochloride (Potential for additive hypotensive effect). Products include:
Lotensin Tablets 2365
Lotensin HCT Tablets 2367
Lotrel Capsules 2370

Bendroflumethiazide (Potential for additive hypotensive effect). Products include:
Corzide 40/5 Tablets 2247
Corzide 80/5 Tablets 2247

Betaxolol Hydrochloride (Potential for additive hypotensive effect; hypotension may develop with concurrent use of beta blockers). Products include:
Betoptic S Ophthalmic Suspension 537

Bisoprolol Fumarate (Potential for additive hypotensive effect; hypotension may develop with concurrent use of beta blockers). Products include:
Zebeta Tablets 1885
Ziac Tablets 1887

Bumetanide (Potential for additive hypotensive effect).
No products indexed under this heading.

Candesartan Cilexetil (Potential for additive hypotensive effect). Products include:
Atacand Tablets 595
Atacand HCT Tablets 597

Captopril (Potential for additive hypotensive effect). Products include:
Captopril Tablets 2281

Carteolol Hydrochloride (Potential for additive hypotensive effect; hypotension may develop with concurrent use of beta blockers). Products include:
Carteolol Hydrochloride Ophthalmic Solution USP, 1% .... ⊙ 258
Ocupress Ophthalmic Solution, 1% Sterile .... ⊙ 303

Chlorothiazide (Potential for additive hypotensive effect). Products include:
Aldoclor Tablets 2035
Diuril Oral 2087

Chlorothiazide Sodium (Potential for additive hypotensive effect). Products include:
Diuril Sodium Intravenous 2086

Chlorthalidone (Potential for additive hypotensive effect). Products include:
Clorpres Tablets 1002
Combipres Tablets 1040
Tenoretic Tablets 690

Clonidine (Potential for additive hypotensive effect). Products include:
Catapres-TTS 1038

Clonidine Hydrochloride (Potential for additive hypotensive effect). Products include:
Catapres Tablets 1037
Clorpres Tablets 1002
Combipres Tablets 1040
Duraclon Injection 3057

Deserpidine (Potential for additive hypotensive effect).
No products indexed under this heading.

Diazoxide (Potential for additive hypotensive effect).
No products indexed under this heading.

Diltiazem Hydrochloride (Potential for additive hypotensive effect). Products include:
Cardizem Injectable 1018
Cardizem Lyo-Ject Syringe 1018
Cardizem Monovial 1018
Cardizem CD Capsules 1016
Tiazac Capsules 1378

Doxazosin Mesylate (Potential for additive hypotensive effect). Products include:
Cardura Tablets 2668

Enalapril Maleate (Potential for additive hypotensive effect). Products include:
Lexxel Tablets 608
Vaseretic Tablets 2204
Vasotec Tablets 2210

Enalaprilat (Potential for additive hypotensive effect). Products include:
Enalaprilat Injection 863
Vasotec I.V. Injection 2207

Eprosartan Mesylate (Potential for additive hypotensive effect). Products include:
Teveten Tablets 3327

Esmolol Hydrochloride (Potential for additive hypotensive effect; hypotension may develop with concurrent use of beta blockers). Products include:
Brevibloc Injection 858

Ethacrynic Acid (Potential for additive hypotensive effect). Products include:
Edecrin Tablets 2091

Felodipine (Potential for additive hypotensive effect). Products include:
Lexxel Tablets 608
Plendil Extended-Release Tablets 623

Fosinopril Sodium (Potential for additive hypotensive effect). Products include:
Monopril Tablets 1091
Monopril HCT 1094

Furosemide (Potential for additive hypotensive effect). Products include:
Furosemide Tablets 2284

Guanabenz Acetate (Potential for additive hypotensive effect).
No products indexed under this heading.

Guanethidine Monosulfate (Potential for additive hypotensive effect).
No products indexed under this heading.

Hydralazine Hydrochloride (Potential for additive hypotensive effect).
No products indexed under this heading.

Hydrochlorothiazide (Potential for additive hypotensive effect). Products include:
Accuretic Tablets 2614
Aldoril Tablets 2039
Atacand HCT Tablets 597
Avalide Tablets 1070
Diovan HCT Tablets 2338
Dyazide Capsules 1515
HydroDIURIL Tablets 2108
Hyzaar 2109
Inderide Tablets 3517
Inderide LA Long-Acting Capsules 3519
Lotensin HCT Tablets 2367
Maxzide 1008
Micardis HCT Tablets 1051
Microzide Capsules 3414
Moduretic Tablets 2138
Monopril HCT 1094
Prinzide Tablets 2168
Timolide Tablets 2187
Uniretic Tablets 3178
Vaseretic Tablets 2204
Zestoretic Tablets 695
Ziac Tablets 1887

Hydroflumethiazide (Potential for additive hypotensive effect). Products include:
Diucardin Tablets 3494

Indapamide (Potential for additive hypotensive effect). Products include:
Indapamide Tablets 2286

Irbesartan (Potential for additive hypotensive effect). Products include:
Avalide Tablets 1070
Avapro Tablets 1074
Avapro Tablets 3076

Isradipine (Potential for additive hypotensive effect). Products include:
DynaCirc Capsules 2921
DynaCirc CR Tablets 2923

Labetalol Hydrochloride (Potential for additive hypotensive effect; hypotension may develop with concurrent use of beta blockers). Products include:
Normodyne Injection 3135
Normodyne Tablets 3137

Levobunolol Hydrochloride (Potential for additive hypotensive effect; hypotension may develop with concurrent use of beta blockers). Products include:
Betagan .... ⊙ 228

Lisinopril (Potential for additive hypotensive effect). Products include:
Prinivil Tablets 2164
Prinzide Tablets 2168
Zestoretic Tablets 695
Zestril Tablets 698

Losartan Potassium (Potential for additive hypotensive effect). Products include:
Cozaar Tablets 2067
Hyzaar 2109

Mecamylamine Hydrochloride (Potential for additive hypotensive effect). Products include:
Inversine Tablets 1850

Methyclothiazide (Potential for additive hypotensive effect).
No products indexed under this heading.

Methyldopa (Potential for additive hypotensive effect). Products include:
Aldoclor Tablets 2035
Aldomet Tablets 2037
Aldoril Tablets 2039

Methyldopate Hydrochloride (Potential for additive hypotensive effect).
No products indexed under this heading.

Metipranolol Hydrochloride (Potential for additive hypotensive effect; hypotension may develop with concurrent use of beta blockers).
No products indexed under this heading.

Metolazone (Potential for additive hypotensive effect). Products include:
Mykrox Tablets 1168
Zaroxolyn Tablets 1177

Metoprolol Succinate (Potential for additive hypotensive effect; hypotension may develop with concurrent use of beta blockers). Products include:
Toprol-XL Tablets 651

Metoprolol Tartrate (Potential for additive hypotensive effect; hypotension may develop with concurrent use of beta blockers).
No products indexed under this heading.

Metyrosine (Potential for additive hypotensive effect). Products include:
Demser Capsules 2085

Mibefradil Dihydrochloride (Potential for additive hypotensive effect).
No products indexed under this heading.

Minoxidil (Potential for additive hypotensive effect). Products include:
Rogaine Extra Strength for Men Topical Solution .... ▣ 721
Rogaine for Women Topical Solution .... ▣ 721

Moexipril Hydrochloride (Potential for additive hypotensive effect). Products include:
Uniretic Tablets 3178
Univasc Tablets 3181

Nadolol (Potential for additive hypotensive effect; hypotension may develop with concurrent use of beta blockers). Products include:
Corgard Tablets 2245
Corzide 40/5 Tablets 2247
Corzide 80/5 Tablets 2247
Nadolol Tablets 2288

Nicardipine Hydrochloride (Potential for additive hypotensive effect). Products include:
Cardene I.V. 3485

Nifedipine (Potential for additive hypotensive effect). Products include:
Adalat CC Tablets 877
Procardia Capsules 2708
Procardia XL Extended Release Tablets 2710

Nisoldipine (Potential for additive hypotensive effect). Products include:
Sular Tablets 688

Nitroglycerin (Potential for additive hypotensive effect). Products include:
Nitro-Dur Transdermal Infusion System 3134
Nitro-Dur Transdermal Infusion System 1834
Nitrolingual Pumpspray 1355
Nitrostat Tablets 2658

Penbutolol Sulfate (Potential for additive hypotensive effect; hypotension may develop with concurrent use of beta blockers).
No products indexed under this heading.

Perindopril Erbumine (Potential for additive hypotensive effect). Products include:
Aceon Tablets (2 mg, 4 mg, 8 mg) 3249

IMPORTANT NOTE: Always consult each drug listing in the patient's regimen for possible interactions.

Phenoxybenzamine Hydrochloride (Potential for additive hypotensive effect). Products include:
Dibenzyline Capsules ... 3457

Phentolamine Mesylate (Potential for additive hypotensive effect).
No products indexed under this heading.

Pindolol (Potential for additive hypotensive effect; hypotension may develop with concurrent use of beta blockers).
No products indexed under this heading.

Polythiazide (Potential for additive hypotensive effect). Products include:
Minizide Capsules ... 2700
Renese Tablets ... 2712

Propranolol Hydrochloride (Potential for additive hypotensive effect; hypotension may develop with concurrent use of beta blockers). Products include:
Inderal ... 3513
Inderal LA Long-Acting Capsules ... 3516
Inderide Tablets ... 3517
Inderide LA Long-Acting Capsules ... 3519

Quinapril Hydrochloride (Potential for additive hypotensive effect). Products include:
Accupril Tablets ... 2611
Accuretic Tablets ... 2614

Ramipril (Potential for additive hypotensive effect). Products include:
Altace Capsules ... 2233

Rauwolfia serpentina (Potential for additive hypotensive effect).
No products indexed under this heading.

Rescinnamine (Potential for additive hypotensive effect).
No products indexed under this heading.

Reserpine (Potential for additive hypotensive effect).
No products indexed under this heading.

Sodium Nitroprusside (Potential for additive hypotensive effect).
No products indexed under this heading.

Sotalol Hydrochloride (Potential for additive hypotensive effect; hypotension may develop with concurrent use of beta blockers). Products include:
Betapace Tablets ... 950
Betapace AF Tablets ... 954

Spirapril Hydrochloride (Potential for additive hypotensive effect).
No products indexed under this heading.

Spironolactone (Potential for additive hypotensive effect).
No products indexed under this heading.

Telmisartan (Potential for additive hypotensive effect). Products include:
Micardis Tablets ... 1049
Micardis HCT Tablets ... 1051

Terazosin Hydrochloride (Potential for additive hypotensive effect). Products include:
Hytrin Capsules ... 464

Timolol Hemihydrate (Potential for additive hypotensive effect; hypotension may develop with concurrent use of beta blockers). Products include:
Betimol Ophthalmic Solution ... ⊙ 324

Timolol Maleate (Potential for additive hypotensive effect; hypotension may develop with concurrent use of beta blockers). Products include:
Blocadren Tablets ... 2046
Cosopt Sterile Ophthalmic Solution ... 2065
Timolide Tablets ... 2187
Timolol GFS ... ⊙ 266
Timoptic in Ocudose ... 2192
Timoptic Sterile Ophthalmic Solution ... 2190
Timoptic-XE Sterile Ophthalmic Gel Forming Solution ... 2194

Torsemide (Potential for additive hypotensive effect). Products include:
Demadex Tablets and Injection ... 2965

Trandolapril (Potential for additive hypotensive effect). Products include:
Mavik Tablets ... 478
Tarka Tablets ... 508

Triamterene (Potential for additive hypotensive effect). Products include:
Dyazide Capsules ... 1515
Dyrenium Capsules ... 3458
Maxzide ... 1008

Trimethaphan Camsylate (Potential for additive hypotensive effect).
No products indexed under this heading.

Valsartan (Potential for additive hypotensive effect). Products include:
Diovan Capsules ... 2337
Diovan HCT Tablets ... 2338

Verapamil Hydrochloride (Potential for additive hypotensive effect). Products include:
Covera-HS Tablets ... 3199
Isoptin SR Tablets ... 467
Tarka Tablets ... 508
Verelan Capsules ... 3184
Verelan PM Capsules ... 3186

MINIZIDE CAPSULES

(Polythiazide, Prazosin Hydrochloride) ... 2700
May interact with antihypertensives, barbiturates, corticosteroids, cardiac glycosides, insulin, narcotic analgesics, and certain other agents. Compounds in these categories include:

Acebutolol Hydrochloride (Co-administration may result in additive or potentiative action of other antihypertensives). Products include:
Sectral Capsules ... 3589

ACTH (Concomitant use with ACTH may increase the risk of developing hypokalemia).
No products indexed under this heading.

Alfentanil Hydrochloride (Co-administration may aggravate orthostatic hypotension).
No products indexed under this heading.

Amlodipine Besylate (Co-administration may result in additive or potentiative action of other antihypertensives). Products include:
Lotrel Capsules ... 2370
Norvasc Tablets ... 2704

Aprobarbital (Co-administration may aggravate orthostatic hypotension).
No products indexed under this heading.

Atenolol (Co-administration may result in additive or potentiative action of other antihypertensives). Products include:
Tenoretic Tablets ... 690
Tenormin I.V. Injection ... 692

Benazepril Hydrochloride (Co-administration may result in additive or potentiative action of other antihypertensives). Products include:
Lotensin Tablets ... 2365
Lotensin HCT Tablets ... 2367
Lotrel Capsules ... 2370

Bendroflumethiazide (Co-administration may result in additive or potentiative action of other antihypertensives). Products include:
Corzide 40/5 Tablets ... 2247
Corzide 80/5 Tablets ... 2247

Betamethasone Acetate (Concomitant use with corticosteroids may increase the risk of developing hypokalemia). Products include:
Celestone Soluspan Injectable Suspension ... 3097

Betamethasone Sodium Phosphate (Concomitant use with corticosteroids may increase the risk of developing hypokalemia). Products include:
Celestone Soluspan Injectable Suspension ... 3097

Betaxolol Hydrochloride (Co-administration may result in additive or potentiative action of other antihypertensives). Products include:
Betoptic S Ophthalmic Suspension ... 537

Bisoprolol Fumarate (Co-administration may result in additive or potentiative action of other antihypertensives). Products include:
Zebeta Tablets ... 1885
Ziac Tablets ... 1887

Buprenorphine Hydrochloride (Co-administration may aggravate orthostatic hypotension). Products include:
Buprenex Injectable ... 2918

Butabarbital (Co-administration may aggravate orthostatic hypotension).
No products indexed under this heading.

Butalbital (Co-administration may aggravate orthostatic hypotension). Products include:
Phrenilin ... 578
Sedapap Tablets 50 mg/650 mg ... 2225

Candesartan Cilexetil (Co-administration may result in additive or potentiative action of other antihypertensives). Products include:
Atacand Tablets ... 595
Atacand HCT Tablets ... 597

Captopril (Co-administration may result in additive or potentiative action of other antihypertensives). Products include:
Captopril Tablets ... 2281

Carteolol Hydrochloride (Co-administration may result in additive or potentiative action of other antihypertensives). Products include:
Carteolol Hydrochloride Ophthalmic Solution USP, 1% ... ⊙ 258
Ocupress Ophthalmic Solution, 1% Sterile ... ⊙ 303

Chlorothiazide (Co-administration may result in additive or potentiative action of other antihypertensives). Products include:
Aldoclor Tablets ... 2035
Diuril Oral ... 2087

Chlorothiazide Sodium (Co-administration may result in additive or potentiative action of other antihypertensives). Products include:
Diuril Sodium Intravenous ... 2086

Chlorthalidone (Co-administration may result in additive or potentiative action of other antihypertensives). Products include:
Clorpres Tablets ... 1002
Combipres Tablets ... 1040
Tenoretic Tablets ... 690

Clonidine (Co-administration may result in additive or potentiative action of other antihypertensives). Products include:
Catapres-TTS ... 1038

Clonidine Hydrochloride (Co-administration may result in additive or potentiative action of other antihypertensives). Products include:
Catapres Tablets ... 1037
Clorpres Tablets ... 1002
Combipres Tablets ... 1040
Duraclon Injection ... 3057

Codeine Phosphate (Co-administration may aggravate orthostatic hypotension). Products include:
Phenergan with Codeine Syrup ... 3557
Phenergan VC with Codeine Syrup ... 3561
Robitussin A-C Syrup ... 2942
Robitussin-DAC Syrup ... 2942
Ryna-C Liquid ... ■□ 768
Soma Compound w/Codeine Tablets ... 3355
Tussi-Organidin NR Liquid ... 3350
Tussi-Organidin-S NR Liquid ... 3350
Tylenol with Codeine ... 2595

Cortisone Acetate (Concomitant use with corticosteroids may increase the risk of developing hypokalemia). Products include:
Cortone Acetate Injectable Suspension ... 2059
Cortone Acetate Tablets ... 2061

Deserpidine (Co-administration may result in additive or potentiative action of other antihypertensives).
No products indexed under this heading.

Deslanoside (Co-administration with digitalis may exaggerate the metabolic effects of hypokalemia, especially with reference to myocardial activity).
No products indexed under this heading.

Dexamethasone (Concomitant use with corticosteroids may increase the risk of developing hypokalemia). Products include:
Decadron Elixir ... 2078
Decadron Tablets ... 2079
TobraDex Ophthalmic Ointment ... 542
TobraDex Ophthalmic Suspension ... 541

Dexamethasone Acetate (Concomitant use with corticosteroids may increase the risk of developing hypokalemia).
No products indexed under this heading.

Dexamethasone Sodium Phosphate (Concomitant use with corticosteroids may increase the risk of developing hypokalemia). Products include:
Decadron Phosphate Injection ... 2081
Decadron Phosphate Sterile Ophthalmic Ointment ... 2083
Decadron Phosphate Sterile Ophthalmic Solution ... 2084
NeoDecadron Sterile Ophthalmic Solution ... 2144

Dezocine (Co-administration may aggravate orthostatic hypotension).
No products indexed under this heading.

Diazoxide (Co-administration may result in additive or potentiative action of other antihypertensives).
No products indexed under this heading.

Digitoxin (Co-administration with digitalis may exaggerate the metabolic effects of hypokalemia, especially with reference to myocardial activity).
No products indexed under this heading.

Digoxin (Co-administration with digitalis may exaggerate the metabolic effects of hypokalemia, especially with reference to myocardial activity). Products include:
Digitek Tablets ... 1003
Lanoxicaps Capsules ... 1574
Lanoxin Injection ... 1581
Lanoxin Tablets ... 1587
Lanoxin Elixir Pediatric ... 1578
Lanoxin Injection Pediatric ... 1584

Diltiazem Hydrochloride (Co-administration may result in additive or potentiative action of other antihypertensives). Products include:
Cardizem Injectable ... 1018
Cardizem Lyo-Ject Syringe ... 1018
Cardizem Monovial ... 1018
Cardizem CD Capsules ... 1016
Tiazac Capsules ... 1378

Doxazosin Mesylate (Co-administration may result in additive or potentiative action of other antihypertensives). Products include:
Cardura Tablets ... 2668

Enalapril Maleate (Co-administration may result in additive or potentiative action of other antihypertensives). Products include:
Lexxel Tablets ... 608

Vaseretic Tablets 2204
Vasotec Tablets 2210

Enalaprilat (Co-administration may result in additive or potentiative action of other antihypertensives). Products include:
Enalaprilat Injection 863
Vasotec I.V. Injection 2207

Eprosartan Mesylate (Co-administration may result in additive or potentiative action of other antihypertensives). Products include:
Teveten Tablets 3327

Esmolol Hydrochloride (Co-administration may result in additive or potentiative action of other antihypertensives). Products include:
Brevibloc Injection 858

Felodipine (Co-administration may result in additive or potentiative action of other antihypertensives). Products include:
Lexxel Tablets 608
Plendil Extended-Release Tablets 623

Fentanyl (Co-administration may aggravate orthostatic hypotension). Products include:
Duragesic Transdermal System 1786

Fentanyl Citrate (Co-administration may aggravate orthostatic hypotension). Products include:
Actiq 1184

Fludrocortisone Acetate (Concomitant use with corticosteroids may increase the risk of developing hypokalemia). Products include:
Florinef Acetate Tablets 2250

Fosinopril Sodium (Co-administration may result in additive or potentiative action of other antihypertensives). Products include:
Monopril Tablets 1091
Monopril HCT 1094

Furosemide (Co-administration may result in additive or potentiative action of other antihypertensives). Products include:
Furosemide Tablets 2284

Guanabenz Acetate (Co-administration may result in additive or potentiative action of other antihypertensives).
No products indexed under this heading.

Guanethidine Monosulfate (Co-administration may result in additive or potentiative action of other antihypertensives).
No products indexed under this heading.

Hydralazine Hydrochloride (Co-administration may result in additive or potentiative action of other antihypertensives).
No products indexed under this heading.

Hydrochlorothiazide (Co-administration may result in additive or potentiative action of other antihypertensives). Products include:
Accuretic Tablets 2614
Aldoril Tablets 2039
Atacand HCT Tablets 597
Avalide Tablets 1070
Diovan HCT Tablets 2338
Dyazide Capsules 1515
HydroDIURIL Tablets 2108
Hyzaar 2109
Inderide Tablets 3517
Inderide LA Long-Acting Capsules 3519
Lotensin HCT Tablets 2367
Maxzide 1008
Micardis HCT Tablets 1051
Microzide Capsules 3414
Moduretic Tablets 2138
Monopril HCT 1094
Prinzide Tablets 2168
Timolide Tablets 2187
Uniretic Tablets 3178
Vaseretic Tablets 2204
Zestoretic Tablets 695
Ziac Tablets 1887

Hydrocodone Bitartrate (Co-administration may aggravate orthostatic hypotension). Products include:
Hycodan 1316
Hycomine Compound Tablets 1317
Hycotuss Expectorant Syrup 1318
Lortab 3319
Lortab Elixir 3317
Maxidone Tablets CIII 3399
Norco 5/325 Tablets CIII 3424
Norco 7.5/325 Tablets CIII 3425
Norco 10/325 Tablets CIII 3427
Norco 10/325 Tablets CIII 3425
Vicodin Tablets 516
Vicodin ES Tablets 517
Vicodin HP Tablets 518
Vicodin Tuss Expectorant 519
Vicoprofen Tablets 520
Zydone Tablets 1330

Hydrocodone Polistirex (Co-administration may aggravate orthostatic hypotension). Products include:
Tussionex Pennkinetic Extended-Release Suspension 1174

Hydrocortisone (Concomitant use with corticosteroids may increase the risk of developing hypokalemia). Products include:
Anusol-HC Cream 2.5% 2237
Cipro HC Otic Suspension 540
Cortaid Intensive Therapy Cream 717
Cortaid Maximum Strength Cream 717
Cortisporin Ophthalmic Suspension Sterile ⊙297
Cortizone•5 699
Cortizone•10 699
Cortizone•10 Plus Creme 700
Cortizone for Kids Creme 699
Hydrocortone Tablets 2106
Massengill Medicated Soft Cloth Towelette 753
VōSoL HC Otic Solution 3356

Hydrocortisone Acetate (Concomitant use with corticosteroids may increase the risk of developing hypokalemia). Products include:
Analpram-HC 1338
Anusol HC-1 Hydrocortisone Anti-Itch Cream 689
Anusol-HC Suppositories 2238
Cortaid 717
Cortifoam Rectal Foam 3170
Cortisporin-TC Otic Suspension 2246
Hydrocortone Acetate Injectable Suspension 2103
Pramosone 1343
Proctocort Suppositories 2264
ProctoFoam-HC 3177
Terra-Cortril Ophthalmic Suspension 2716

Hydrocortisone Sodium Phosphate (Concomitant use with corticosteroids may increase the risk of developing hypokalemia). Products include:
Hydrocortone Phosphate Injection, Sterile 2105

Hydrocortisone Sodium Succinate (Concomitant use with corticosteroids may increase the risk of developing hypokalemia).
No products indexed under this heading.

Hydroflumethiazide (Co-administration may result in additive or potentiative action of other antihypertensives). Products include:
Diucardin Tablets 3494

Hydromorphone Hydrochloride (Co-administration may aggravate orthostatic hypotension). Products include:
Dilaudid 441
Dilaudid Oral Liquid 445
Dilaudid Powder 441
Dilaudid Rectal Suppositories 441
Dilaudid Tablets 441
Dilaudid Tablets - 8 mg 445
Dilaudid-HP 443

Indapamide (Co-administration may result in additive or potentiative action of other antihypertensives). Products include:
Indapamide Tablets 2286

Insulin, Human, Zinc Suspension (Hyperglycemia is a side effect of thiazides, insulin dosage may need to be altered). Products include:
Humulin L, 100 Units 1937
Humulin U, 100 Units 1943
Novolin L Human Insulin 10 ml Vials 2422

Insulin, Human NPH (Hyperglycemia is a side effect of thiazides, insulin dosage may need to be altered). Products include:
Humulin N, 100 Units 1939
Humulin N NPH Pen 1940
Novolin N Human Insulin 10 ml Vials 2422
Novolin N PenFill 2423
Novolin N Prefilled Syringe Disposable Insulin Delivery System 2425

Insulin, Human Regular (Hyperglycemia is a side effect of thiazides, insulin dosage may need to be altered). Products include:
Humulin R Regular (U-500) 1943
Humulin R, 100 Units 1941
Novolin R Human Insulin 10 ml Vials 2423
Novolin R PenFill 2423
Novolin R Prefilled Syringe Disposable Insulin Delivery System 2425
Velosulin BR Human Insulin 10 ml Vials 2435

Insulin, Human Regular and Human NPH Mixture (Hyperglycemia is a side effect of thiazides, insulin dosage may need to be altered). Products include:
Humulin 50/50, 100 Units 1934
Humulin 70/30, 100 Units 1935
Humulin 70/30 Pen 1936
Novolin 70/30 Human Insulin 10 ml Vials 2421
Novolin 70/30 PenFill 2423
Novolin 70/30 Prefilled Disposable Insulin Delivery System 2425

Insulin, NPH (Hyperglycemia is a side effect of thiazides, insulin dosage may need to be altered). Products include:
Iletin II, NPH (Pork), 100 Units 1946

Insulin, Regular (Hyperglycemia is a side effect of thiazides, insulin dosage may need to be altered). Products include:
Iletin II, Regular (Pork), 100 Units 1947

Insulin, Zinc Crystals (Hyperglycemia is a side effect of thiazides, insulin dosage may need to be altered).
No products indexed under this heading.

Insulin, Zinc Suspension (Hyperglycemia is a side effect of thiazides, insulin dosage may need to be altered). Products include:
Iletin II, Lente (Pork), 100 Units 1945

Insulin Aspart, Human Regular (Hyperglycemia is a side effect of thiazides, insulin dosage may need to be altered).
No products indexed under this heading.

Insulin glargine (Hyperglycemia is a side effect of thiazides, insulin dosage may need to be altered). Products include:
Lantus Injection 742

Insulin Lispro, Human (Hyperglycemia is a side effect of thiazides, insulin dosage may need to be altered). Products include:
Humalog 1926
Humalog Mix 75/25 Pen 1928

Insulin Lispro Protamine, Human (Hyperglycemia is a side effect of thiazides, insulin dosage may need to be altered). Products include:
Humalog Mix 75/25 Pen 1928

Irbesartan (Co-administration may result in additive or potentiative action of other antihypertensives). Products include:
Avalide Tablets 1070
Avapro Tablets 1074
Avapro Tablets 3076

Isradipine (Co-administration may result in additive or potentiative action of other antihypertensives). Products include:
DynaCirc Capsules 2921
DynaCirc CR Tablets 2923

Labetalol Hydrochloride (Co-administration may result in additive or potentiative action of other antihypertensives). Products include:
Normodyne Injection 3135
Normodyne Tablets 3137

Levorphanol Tartrate (Co-administration may aggravate orthostatic hypotension). Products include:
Levo-Dromoran 1734
Levorphanol Tartrate Tablets 3059

Lisinopril (Co-administration may result in additive or potentiative action of other antihypertensives). Products include:
Prinivil Tablets 2164
Prinzide Tablets 2168
Zestoretic Tablets 695
Zestril Tablets 698

Losartan Potassium (Co-administration may result in additive or potentiative action of other antihypertensives). Products include:
Cozaar Tablets 2067
Hyzaar 2109

Mecamylamine Hydrochloride (Co-administration may result in additive or potentiative action of other antihypertensives). Products include:
Inversine Tablets 1850

Meperidine Hydrochloride (Co-administration may aggravate orthostatic hypotension). Products include:
Demerol 3079
Mepergan Injection 3539

Mephobarbital (Co-administration may aggravate orthostatic hypotension).
No products indexed under this heading.

Methadone Hydrochloride (Co-administration may aggravate orthostatic hypotension). Products include:
Dolophine Hydrochloride Tablets 3056

Methyclothiazide (Co-administration may result in additive or potentiative action of other antihypertensives).
No products indexed under this heading.

Methyldopa (Co-administration may result in additive or potentiative action of other antihypertensives). Products include:
Aldoclor Tablets 2035
Aldomet Tablets 2037
Aldoril Tablets 2039

Methyldopate Hydrochloride (Co-administration may result in additive or potentiative action of other antihypertensives).
No products indexed under this heading.

Methylprednisolone Acetate (Concomitant use with corticosteroids may increase the risk of developing hypokalemia). Products include:
Depo-Medrol Injectable Suspension 2795

Methylprednisolone Sodium Succinate (Concomitant use with corticosteroids may increase the risk of developing hypokalemia). Products include:
Solu-Medrol Sterile Powder 2855

Metolazone (Co-administration may result in additive or potentiative action of other antihypertensives). Products include:
Mykrox Tablets 1168
Zaroxolyn Tablets 1177

Metoprolol Succinate (Co-administration may result in additive or potentiative action of other antihypertensives). Products include:
Toprol-XL Tablets 651

Metoprolol Tartrate (Co-administration may result in additive or potentiative action of other antihy-

IMPORTANT NOTE: Always consult each drug listing in the patient's regimen for possible interactions.

pertensives).
No products indexed under this heading.

Metyrosine (Co-administration may result in additive or potentiative action of other antihypertensives). Products include:
Demser Capsules 2085

Mibefradil Dihydrochloride (Co-administration may result in additive or potentiative action of other antihypertensives).
No products indexed under this heading.

Minoxidil (Co-administration may result in additive or potentiative action of other antihypertensives). Products include:
Rogaine Extra Strength for Men Topical Solution .... ▣721
Rogaine for Women Topical Solution .... ▣721

Moexipril Hydrochloride (Co-administration may result in additive or potentiative action of other antihypertensives). Products include:
Uniretic Tablets 3178
Univasc Tablets 3181

Morphine Sulfate (Co-administration may aggravate orthostatic hypotension). Products include:
Astramorph/PF Injection, USP (Preservative-Free) 594
Duramorph Injection 1312
Infumorph 200 and Infumorph 500 Sterile Solutions 1314
Kadian Capsules 1335
MS Contin Tablets 2896
MSIR 2898
Oramorph SR Tablets 3062
Roxanol 3066

Nadolol (Co-administration may result in additive or potentiative action of other antihypertensives). Products include:
Corgard Tablets 2245
Corzide 40/5 Tablets 2247
Corzide 80/5 Tablets 2247
Nadolol Tablets 2288

Nicardipine Hydrochloride (Co-administration may result in additive or potentiative action of other antihypertensives). Products include:
Cardene I.V. 3485

Nifedipine (Co-administration may result in additive or potentiative action of other antihypertensives). Products include:
Adalat CC Tablets 877
Procardia Capsules 2708
Procardia XL Extended Release Tablets 2710

Nisoldipine (Co-administration may result in additive or potentiative action of other antihypertensives). Products include:
Sular Tablets 688

Nitroglycerin (Co-administration may result in additive or potentiative action of other antihypertensives). Products include:
Nitro-Dur Transdermal Infusion System 3134
Nitro-Dur Transdermal Infusion System 1834
Nitrolingual Pumpspray 1355
Nitrostat Tablets 2658

Norepinephrine Bitartrate (Thiazides may decrease the arterial responsiveness to norepinephrine).
No products indexed under this heading.

Oxycodone Hydrochloride (Co-administration may aggravate orthostatic hypotension). Products include:
OxyContin Tablets 2912
OxyFast Oral Concentrate Solution 2916
OxyIR Capsules 2916
Percocet Tablets 1326
Percodan Tablets 1327
Percolone Tablets 1327
Roxicodone 3067
Tylox Capsules 2597

Penbutolol Sulfate (Co-administration may result in additive or potentiative action of other antihypertensives).
No products indexed under this heading.

Pentobarbital Sodium (Co-administration may aggravate orthostatic hypotension). Products include:
Nembutal Sodium Solution 485

Perindopril Erbumine (Co-administration may result in additive or potentiative action of other antihypertensives). Products include:
Aceon Tablets (2 mg, 4 mg, 8 mg) 3249

Phenobarbital (Co-administration may aggravate orthostatic hypotension). Products include:
Arco-Lase Plus Tablets 592
Donnatal 2929
Donnatal Extentabs 2930

Phenoxybenzamine Hydrochloride (Co-administration may result in additive or potentiative action of other antihypertensives). Products include:
Dibenzyline Capsules 3457

Phentolamine Mesylate (Co-administration may result in additive or potentiative action of other antihypertensives).
No products indexed under this heading.

Pindolol (Co-administration may result in additive or potentiative action of other antihypertensives).
No products indexed under this heading.

Prednisolone Acetate (Concomitant use with corticosteroids may increase the risk of developing hypokalemia). Products include:
Blephamide Ophthalmic Ointment 547
Blephamide Ophthalmic Suspension 548
Poly-Pred Liquifilm Ophthalmic Suspension .... ⊙245
Pred Forte Ophthalmic Suspension .... ⊙246
Pred Mild Sterile Ophthalmic Suspension .... ⊙249
Pred-G Ophthalmic Suspension .... ⊙247
Pred-G Sterile Ophthalmic Ointment .... ⊙248

Prednisolone Sodium Phosphate (Concomitant use with corticosteroids may increase the risk of developing hypokalemia). Products include:
Pediapred Oral Solution 1170

Prednisolone Tebutate (Concomitant use with corticosteroids may increase the risk of developing hypokalemia).
No products indexed under this heading.

Prednisone (Concomitant use with corticosteroids may increase the risk of developing hypokalemia). Products include:
Prednisone 3064

Propoxyphene Hydrochloride (Co-administration may aggravate orthostatic hypotension). Products include:
Darvon Pulvules 1909
Darvon Compound-65 Pulvules 1910

Propoxyphene Napsylate (Co-administration may aggravate orthostatic hypotension). Products include:
Darvon-N/Darvocet-N 1907
Darvon-N Tablets 1912

Propranolol Hydrochloride (Co-administration may result in additive or potentiative action of other antihypertensives). Products include:
Inderal 3513
Inderal LA Long-Acting Capsules 3516
Inderide Tablets 3517
Inderide LA Long-Acting Capsules 3519

Quinapril Hydrochloride (Co-administration may result in additive or potentiative action of other antihypertensives). Products include:
Accupril Tablets 2611
Accuretic Tablets 2614

Ramipril (Co-administration may result in additive or potentiative action of other antihypertensives). Products include:
Altace Capsules 2233

Rauwolfia serpentina (Co-administration may result in additive or potentiative action of other antihypertensives).
No products indexed under this heading.

Remifentanil Hydrochloride (Co-administration may aggravate orthostatic hypotension).
No products indexed under this heading.

Rescinnamine (Co-administration may result in additive or potentiative action of other antihypertensives).
No products indexed under this heading.

Reserpine (Co-administration may result in additive or potentiative action of other antihypertensives).
No products indexed under this heading.

Secobarbital Sodium (Co-administration may aggravate orthostatic hypotension).
No products indexed under this heading.

Sodium Nitroprusside (Co-administration may result in additive or potentiative action of other antihypertensives).
No products indexed under this heading.

Sotalol Hydrochloride (Co-administration may result in additive or potentiative action of other antihypertensives). Products include:
Betapace Tablets 950
Betapace AF Tablets 954

Spirapril Hydrochloride (Co-administration may result in additive or potentiative action of other antihypertensives).
No products indexed under this heading.

Sufentanil Citrate (Co-administration may aggravate orthostatic hypotension).
No products indexed under this heading.

Telmisartan (Co-administration may result in additive or potentiative action of other antihypertensives). Products include:
Micardis Tablets 1049
Micardis HCT Tablets 1051

Terazosin Hydrochloride (Co-administration may result in additive or potentiative action of other antihypertensives). Products include:
Hytrin Capsules 464

Thiamylal Sodium (Co-administration may aggravate orthostatic hypotension).
No products indexed under this heading.

Timolol Maleate (Co-administration may result in additive or potentiative action of other antihypertensives). Products include:
Blocadren Tablets 2046
Cosopt Sterile Ophthalmic Solution 2065
Timolide Tablets 2187
Timolol GFS .... ⊙266
Timoptic in Ocudose 2192
Timoptic Sterile Ophthalmic Solution 2190
Timoptic-XE Sterile Ophthalmic Gel Forming Solution 2194

Torsemide (Co-administration may result in additive or potentiative action of other antihypertensives). Products include:
Demadex Tablets and Injection 2965

Trandolapril (Co-administration may result in additive or potentiative action of other antihypertensives). Products include:
Mavik Tablets 478
Tarka Tablets 508

Triamcinolone (Concomitant use with corticosteroids may increase the risk of developing hypokalemia).
No products indexed under this heading.

Triamcinolone Acetonide (Concomitant use with corticosteroids may increase the risk of developing hypokalemia). Products include:
Azmacort Inhalation Aerosol 728
Nasacort Nasal Inhaler 750
Nasacort AQ Nasal Spray 752
Tri-Nasal Spray 2274

Triamcinolone Diacetate (Concomitant use with corticosteroids may increase the risk of developing hypokalemia).
No products indexed under this heading.

Triamcinolone Hexacetonide (Concomitant use with corticosteroids may increase the risk of developing hypokalemia).
No products indexed under this heading.

Trimethaphan Camsylate (Co-administration may result in additive or potentiative action of other antihypertensives).
No products indexed under this heading.

Tubocurarine Chloride (Thiazides may increase the responsiveness to tubocurarine).
No products indexed under this heading.

Valsartan (Co-administration may result in additive or potentiative action of other antihypertensives). Products include:
Diovan Capsules 2337
Diovan HCT Tablets 2338

Verapamil Hydrochloride (Co-administration may result in additive or potentiative action of other antihypertensives). Products include:
Covera-HS Tablets 3199
Isoptin SR Tablets 467
Tarka Tablets 508
Verelan Capsules 3184
Verelan PM Capsules 3186

Food Interactions

Alcohol (Concurrent use may aggravate orthostatic hypotension).

MINOCIN INTRAVENOUS
(Minocycline Hydrochloride) 1862
May interact with anticoagulants, oral contraceptives, penicillins, and certain other agents. Compounds in these categories include:

Amoxicillin Trihydrate (Interference with bactericidal action of penicillins; avoid concurrent use).

Ampicillin (Interference with bactericidal action of penicillins; avoid concurrent use).
No products indexed under this heading.

Ampicillin Sodium (Interference with bactericidal action of penicillins; avoid concurrent use). Products include:
Unasyn for Injection 2728

Ampicillin Trihydrate (Interference with bactericidal action of penicillins; avoid concurrent use).
No products indexed under this heading.

Ardeparin Sodium (Depressed plasma prothrombin activity).
No products indexed under this heading.

Azlocillin Sodium (Interference with bactericidal action of penicillins; avoid concurrent use).
No products indexed under this heading.

Bacampicillin Hydrochloride (Interference with bactericidal action

of penicillins; avoid concurrent use).
No products indexed under this heading.

Carbenicillin Disodium (Interference with bactericidal action of penicillins; avoid concurrent use).
No products indexed under this heading.

Carbenicillin Indanyl Sodium (Interference with bactericidal action of penicillins; avoid concurrent use). Products include:
Geocillin Tablets ... 2687

Dalteparin Sodium (Depressed plasma prothrombin activity). Products include:
Fragmin Injection ... 2814

Danaparoid Sodium (Depressed plasma prothrombin activity). Products include:
Orgaran Injection ... 2480

Desogestrel (Reduced efficacy and increased incidence of breakthrough bleeding). Products include:
Cyclessa Tablets ... 2450
Desogen Tablets ... 2458
Mircette Tablets ... 2470
Ortho-Cept 21 Tablets ... 2546
Ortho-Cept 28 Tablets ... 2546

Dicloxacillin Sodium (Interference with bactericidal action of penicillins; avoid concurrent use).
No products indexed under this heading.

Dicumarol (Depressed plasma prothrombin activity).
No products indexed under this heading.

Enoxaparin (Depressed plasma prothrombin activity). Products include:
Lovenox Injection ... 746

Ethinyl Estradiol (Reduced efficacy and increased incidence of breakthrough bleeding). Products include:
Alesse-21 Tablets ... 3468
Alesse-28 Tablets ... 3473
Brevicon 28-Day Tablets ... 3380
Cyclessa Tablets ... 2450
Desogen Tablets ... 2458
Estinyl Tablets ... 3112
Estrostep ... 2627
femhrt Tablets ... 2635
Levlen ... 962
Levlite 21 Tablets ... 962
Levlite 28 Tablets ... 962
Levora Tablets ... 3389
Loestrin 21 Tablets ... 2642
Loestrin Fe Tablets ... 2642
Lo/Ovral Tablets ... 3532
Lo/Ovral-28 Tablets ... 3538
Low-Ogestrel-28 Tablets ... 3392
Microgestin Fe 1.5/30 Tablets ... 3407
Microgestin Fe 1/20 Tablets ... 3400
Mircette Tablets ... 2470
Modicon ... 2563
Necon ... 3415
Nordette-28 Tablets ... 2257
Norinyl 1 +35 28-Day Tablets ... 3380
Ogestrel 0.5/50-28 Tablets ... 3428
Ortho-Cept 21 Tablets ... 2546
Ortho-Cept 28 Tablets ... 2546
Ortho-Cyclen/Ortho Tri-Cyclen ... 2573
Ortho-Novum ... 2563
Ovcon ... 3364
Ovral Tablets ... 3551
Ovral-28 Tablets ... 3552
Tri-Levlen ... 962
Tri-Norinyl-28 Tablets ... 3433
Triphasil-21 Tablets ... 3600
Triphasil-28 Tablets ... 3605
Trivora Tablets ... 3439
Yasmin 28 Tablets ... 980
Zovia ... 3449

Ethynodiol Diacetate (Reduced efficacy and increased incidence of breakthrough bleeding). Products include:
Zovia ... 3449

Heparin Sodium (Depressed plasma prothrombin activity). Products include:
Heparin Lock Flush Solution ... 3509
Heparin Sodium Injection ... 3511

Levonorgestrel (Reduced efficacy and increased incidence of breakthrough bleeding). Products include:
Alesse-21 Tablets ... 3468
Alesse-28 Tablets ... 3473
Levlen ... 962
Levlite 21 Tablets ... 962
Levlite 28 Tablets ... 962
Levora Tablets ... 3389
Mirena Intrauterine System ... 974
Nordette-28 Tablets ... 2257
Norplant System ... 3543
Tri-Levlen ... 962
Triphasil-21 Tablets ... 3600
Triphasil-28 Tablets ... 3605
Trivora Tablets ... 3439

Mestranol (Reduced efficacy and increased incidence of breakthrough bleeding). Products include:
Necon 1/50 Tablets ... 3415
Norinyl 1 + 50 28-Day Tablets ... 3380
Ortho-Novum 1/50□28 Tablets ... 2556

Mezlocillin Sodium (Interference with bactericidal action of penicillins; avoid concurrent use).
No products indexed under this heading.

Nafcillin Sodium (Interference with bactericidal action of penicillins; avoid concurrent use).
No products indexed under this heading.

Norethindrone (Reduced efficacy and increased incidence of breakthrough bleeding). Products include:
Brevicon 28-Day Tablets ... 3380
Micronor Tablets ... 2543
Modicon ... 2563
Necon ... 3415
Norinyl 1 +35 28-Day Tablets ... 3380
Norinyl 1 + 50 28-Day Tablets ... 3380
Nor-QD Tablets ... 3423
Ortho-Novum ... 2563
Ortho-Novum 1/50□28 Tablets ... 2556
Ovcon ... 3364
Tri-Norinyl-28 Tablets ... 3433

Norethynodrel (Reduced efficacy and increased incidence of breakthrough bleeding).
No products indexed under this heading.

Norgestimate (Reduced efficacy and increased incidence of breakthrough bleeding). Products include:
Ortho-Cyclen/Ortho Tri-Cyclen ... 2573
Ortho-Prefest Tablets ... 2570

Norgestrel (Reduced efficacy and increased incidence of breakthrough bleeding). Products include:
Lo/Ovral Tablets ... 3532
Lo/Ovral-28 Tablets ... 3538
Low-Ogestrel-28 Tablets ... 3392
Ogestrel 0.5/50-28 Tablets ... 3428
Ovral Tablets ... 3551
Ovral-28 Tablets ... 3552
Ovrette Tablets ... 3552

Penicillin G Benzathine (Interference with bactericidal action of penicillins; avoid concurrent use). Products include:
Bicillin C-R 900/300 Injection ... 2240
Bicillin C-R Injection ... 2238
Bicillin L-A Injection ... 2242
Permapen Isoject ... 2706

Penicillin G Potassium (Interference with bactericidal action of penicillins; avoid concurrent use). Products include:
Pfizerpen for Injection ... 2707

Penicillin G Procaine (Interference with bactericidal action of penicillins; avoid concurrent use). Products include:
Bicillin C-R 900/300 Injection ... 2240
Bicillin C-R Injection ... 2238

Penicillin G Sodium (Interference with bactericidal action of penicillins; avoid concurrent use).
No products indexed under this heading.

Penicillin V Potassium (Interference with bactericidal action of penicillins; avoid concurrent use).
No products indexed under this heading.

Ticarcillin Disodium (Interference with bactericidal action of penicillins; avoid concurrent use). Products include:
Timentin Injection- ADD-Vantage Vial ... 1661
Timentin Injection-Galaxy Container ... 1664
Timentin Injection-Pharmacy Bulk Package ... 1666
Timentin for Intravenous Administration ... 1658

Tinzaparin sodium (Depressed plasma prothrombin activity). Products include:
Innohep Injection ... 1248

Warfarin Sodium (Depressed plasma prothrombin activity). Products include:
Coumadin for Injection ... 1243
Coumadin Tablets ... 1243
Warfarin Sodium Tablets, USP ... 3302

MINOCIN ORAL SUSPENSION

(Minocycline Hydrochloride) ... 1865
May interact with antacids containing aluminum, calcium and magnesium, anticoagulants, oral contraceptives, penicillins, and certain other agents. Compounds in these categories include:

Aluminum Carbonate (Absorption of tetracyclines is impaired).
No products indexed under this heading.

Aluminum Hydroxide (Absorption of tetracyclines is impaired). Products include:
Amphojel Suspension (Mint Flavor) ... ▣789
Gaviscon Extra Strength Liquid ... ▣751
Gaviscon Extra Strength Tablets ... ▣751
Gaviscon Regular Strength Liquid . ▣751
Gaviscon Regular Strength Tablets ... ▣750
Maalox Antacid/Anti-Gas Oral Suspension ... ▣673
Maalox Max Maximum Strength Antacid/Anti-Gas Liquid ... 2300
Maalox Regular Strength Antacid/Antigas Liquid ... 2300
Mylanta ... 1813
Vanquish Caplets ... ▣617

Amoxicillin Trihydrate (Interference with bactericidal action of penicillin; avoid concurrent use).

Ampicillin (Interference with bactericidal action of penicillin; avoid concurrent use).
No products indexed under this heading.

Ampicillin Sodium (Interference with bactericidal action of penicillin; avoid concurrent use). Products include:
Unasyn for Injection ... 2728

Ampicillin Trihydrate (Interference with bactericidal action of penicillin; avoid concurrent use).
No products indexed under this heading.

Ardeparin Sodium (Depressed plasma prothrombin activity; may require downward adjustment of the anticoagulant dosage).
No products indexed under this heading.

Azlocillin Sodium (Interference with bactericidal action of penicillin; avoid concurrent use).
No products indexed under this heading.

Bacampicillin Hydrochloride (Interference with bactericidal action of penicillin; avoid concurrent use).
No products indexed under this heading.

Carbenicillin Disodium (Interference with bactericidal action of penicillin; avoid concurrent use).
No products indexed under this heading.

Carbenicillin Indanyl Sodium (Interference with bactericidal action of penicillin; avoid concurrent use). Products include:
Geocillin Tablets ... 2687

Dalteparin Sodium (Depressed plasma prothrombin activity; may require downward adjustment of the anticoagulant dosage). Products include:
Fragmin Injection ... 2814

Danaparoid Sodium (Depressed plasma prothrombin activity; may require downward adjustment of the anticoagulant dosage). Products include:
Orgaran Injection ... 2480

Desogestrel (Concurrent use may render oral contraceptives less effective; potential for breakthrough bleeding). Products include:
Cyclessa Tablets ... 2450
Desogen Tablets ... 2458
Mircette Tablets ... 2470
Ortho-Cept 21 Tablets ... 2546
Ortho-Cept 28 Tablets ... 2546

Dicloxacillin Sodium (Interference with bactericidal action of penicillin; avoid concurrent use).
No products indexed under this heading.

Dicumarol (Depressed plasma prothrombin activity; may require downward adjustment of the anticoagulant dosage).
No products indexed under this heading.

Enoxaparin (Depressed plasma prothrombin activity; may require downward adjustment of the anticoagulant dosage). Products include:
Lovenox Injection ... 746

Ethinyl Estradiol (Concurrent use may render oral contraceptives less effective; potential for breakthrough bleeding). Products include:
Alesse-21 Tablets ... 3468
Alesse-28 Tablets ... 3473
Brevicon 28-Day Tablets ... 3380
Cyclessa Tablets ... 2450
Desogen Tablets ... 2458
Estinyl Tablets ... 3112
Estrostep ... 2627
femhrt Tablets ... 2635
Levlen ... 962
Levlite 21 Tablets ... 962
Levlite 28 Tablets ... 962
Levora Tablets ... 3389
Loestrin 21 Tablets ... 2642
Loestrin Fe Tablets ... 2642
Lo/Ovral Tablets ... 3532
Lo/Ovral-28 Tablets ... 3538
Low-Ogestrel-28 Tablets ... 3392
Microgestin Fe 1.5/30 Tablets ... 3407
Microgestin Fe 1/20 Tablets ... 3400
Mircette Tablets ... 2470
Modicon ... 2563
Necon ... 3415
Nordette-28 Tablets ... 2257
Norinyl 1 +35 28-Day Tablets ... 3380
Ogestrel 0.5/50-28 Tablets ... 3428
Ortho-Cept 21 Tablets ... 2546
Ortho-Cept 28 Tablets ... 2546
Ortho-Cyclen/Ortho Tri-Cyclen ... 2573
Ortho-Novum ... 2563
Ovcon ... 3364
Ovral Tablets ... 3551
Ovral-28 Tablets ... 3552
Tri-Levlen ... 962
Tri-Norinyl-28 Tablets ... 3433
Triphasil-21 Tablets ... 3600
Triphasil-28 Tablets ... 3605
Trivora Tablets ... 3439
Yasmin 28 Tablets ... 980
Zovia ... 3449

Ethynodiol Diacetate (Concurrent use may render oral contraceptives less effective; potential for breakthrough bleeding). Products include:
Zovia ... 3449

Ferrous Fumarate (Absorption of tetracyclines is impaired). Products include:
New Formulation Chromagen OB Capsules ... 3094
Loestrin Fe Tablets ... 2642
NataChew Tablets ... 3364

Ferrous Gluconate (Absorption of tetracyclines is impaired). Products include:
Fergon Iron Tablets ... ▣802

Ferrous Sulfate (Absorption of tetracyclines is impaired). Products include:
Feosol Tablets ... 1717

Slow Fe Tablets .... ▣827
Slow Fe with Folic Acid Tablets ..... ▣828

Heparin Sodium (Depressed plasma prothrombin activity; may require downward adjustment of the anticoagulant dosage). Products include:
Heparin Lock Flush Solution 3509
Heparin Sodium Injection 3511

Levonorgestrel (Concurrent use may render oral contraceptives less effective; potential for breakthrough bleeding). Products include:
Alesse-21 Tablets 3468
Alesse-28 Tablets 3473
Levlen 962
Levlite 21 Tablets 962
Levlite 28 Tablets 962
Levora Tablets 3389
Mirena Intrauterine System 974
Nordette-28 Tablets 2257
Norplant System 3543
Tri-Levlen 962
Triphasil-21 Tablets 3600
Triphasil-28 Tablets 3605
Trivora Tablets 3439

Magaldrate (Absorption of tetracyclines is impaired).
No products indexed under this heading.

Magnesium Hydroxide (Absorption of tetracyclines is impaired). Products include:
Ex•Lax Milk of Magnesia Liquid .... ▣670
Maalox Antacid/Anti-Gas Oral Suspension .... ▣673
Maalox Max Maximum Strength Antacid/Anti-Gas Liquid 2300
Maalox Regular Strength Antacid/Antigas Liquid 2300
Mylanta Fast-Acting 1813
Mylanta 1813
Pepcid Complete Chewable Tablets 1815
Phillips' Chewable Tablets .... ▣615
Phillips' Milk of Magnesia Liquid (Original, Cherry, & Mint)........... ▣616
Rolaids Tablets .... ▣706
Extra Strength Rolaids Tablets ...... ▣706
Vanquish Caplets .... ▣617

Magnesium Oxide (Absorption of tetracyclines is impaired). Products include:
Beelith Tablets 946
Mag-Ox 400 Tablets 1024
Uro-Mag Capsules 1024

Mestranol (Concurrent use may render oral contraceptives less effective; potential for breakthrough bleeding). Products include:
Necon 1/50 Tablets 3415
Norinyl 1 + 50 28-Day Tablets 3380
Ortho-Novum 1/50▫28 Tablets 2556

Mezlocillin Sodium (Interference with bactericidal action of penicillin; avoid concurrent use).
No products indexed under this heading.

Nafcillin Sodium (Interference with bactericidal action of penicillin; avoid concurrent use).
No products indexed under this heading.

Norethindrone (Concurrent use may render oral contraceptives less effective; potential for breakthrough bleeding). Products include:
Brevicon 28-Day Tablets 3380
Micronor Tablets 2543
Modicon 2563
Necon 3415
Norinyl 1 +35 28-Day Tablets 3380
Norinyl 1 + 50 28-Day Tablets 3380
Nor-QD Tablets 3423
Ortho-Novum 2563
Ortho-Novum 1/50▫28 Tablets 2556
Ovcon 3364
Tri-Norinyl-28 Tablets 3433

Norethynodrel (Concurrent use may render oral contraceptives less effective; potential for breakthrough bleeding).
No products indexed under this heading.

Norgestimate (Concurrent use may render oral contraceptives less effective; potential for breakthrough bleeding). Products include:
Ortho-Cyclen/Ortho Tri-Cyclen 2573
Ortho-Prefest Tablets 2570

Norgestrel (Concurrent use may render oral contraceptives less effective; potential for breakthrough bleeding). Products include:
Lo/Ovral Tablets 3532
Lo/Ovral-28 Tablets 3538
Low-Ogestrel-28 Tablets 3392
Ogestrel 0.5/50-28 Tablets 3428
Ovral Tablets 3551
Ovral-28 Tablets 3552
Ovrette Tablets 3552

Penicillin G Benzathine (Interference with bactericidal action of penicillin; avoid concurrent use). Products include:
Bicillin C-R 900/300 Injection 2240
Bicillin C-R Injection 2238
Bicillin L-A Injection 2242
Permapen Isoject 2706

Penicillin G Potassium (Interference with bactericidal action of penicillin; avoid concurrent use). Products include:
Pfizerpen for Injection 2707

Penicillin G Procaine (Interference with bactericidal action of penicillin; avoid concurrent use). Products include:
Bicillin C-R 900/300 Injection 2240
Bicillin C-R Injection 2238

Penicillin G Sodium (Interference with bactericidal action of penicillin; avoid concurrent use).
No products indexed under this heading.

Penicillin V Potassium (Interference with bactericidal action of penicillin; avoid concurrent use).
No products indexed under this heading.

Ticarcillin Disodium (Interference with bactericidal action of penicillin; avoid concurrent use). Products include:
Timentin Injection- ADD-Vantage Vial 1661
Timentin Injection-Galaxy Container 1664
Timentin Injection-Pharmacy Bulk Package 1666
Timentin for Intravenous Administration 1658

Tinzaparin sodium (Depressed plasma prothrombin activity; may require downward adjustment of the anticoagulant dosage). Products include:
Innohep Injection 1248

Warfarin Sodium (Depressed plasma prothrombin activity; may require downward adjustment of the anticoagulant dosage). Products include:
Coumadin for Injection 1243
Coumadin Tablets 1243
Warfarin Sodium Tablets, USP 3302

MINOCIN PELLET-FILLED CAPSULES

(Minocycline Hydrochloride) 1863
May interact with antacids containing aluminum, calcium and magnesium, anticoagulants, iron containing oral preparations, oral contraceptives, penicillins, and certain other agents. Compounds in these categories include:

Aluminum Carbonate (Absorption of tetracyclines is impaired).
No products indexed under this heading.

Aluminum Hydroxide (Absorption of tetracyclines is impaired). Products include:
Amphojel Suspension (Mint Flavor) .... ▣789
Gaviscon Extra Strength Liquid ..... ▣751
Gaviscon Extra Strength Tablets ... ▣751
Gaviscon Regular Strength Liquid . ▣751
Gaviscon Regular Strength Tablets .... ▣750
Maalox Antacid/Anti-Gas Oral Suspension .... ▣673
Maalox Max Maximum Strength Antacid/Anti-Gas Liquid 2300
Maalox Regular Strength Antacid/Antigas Liquid 2300
Mylanta 1813
Vanquish Caplets .... ▣617

Amoxicillin Trihydrate (Interference with bactericidal action of penicillin; avoid concurrent use).

Ampicillin (Interference with bactericidal action of penicillin; avoid concurrent use).
No products indexed under this heading.

Ampicillin Sodium (Interference with bactericidal action of penicillin; avoid concurrent use). Products include:
Unasyn for Injection 2728

Ampicillin Trihydrate (Interference with bactericidal action of penicillin; avoid concurrent use).
No products indexed under this heading.

Ardeparin Sodium (Depressed plasma prothrombin activity; may require downward adjustment of the anticoagulant dosage).
No products indexed under this heading.

Azlocillin Sodium (Interference with bactericidal action of penicillin; avoid concurrent use).
No products indexed under this heading.

Bacampicillin Hydrochloride (Interference with bactericidal action of penicillin; avoid concurrent use).
No products indexed under this heading.

Carbenicillin Disodium (Interference with bactericidal action of penicillin; avoid concurrent use).
No products indexed under this heading.

Carbenicillin Indanyl Sodium (Interference with bactericidal action of penicillin; avoid concurrent use). Products include:
Geocillin Tablets 2687

Dalteparin Sodium (Depressed plasma prothrombin activity; may require downward adjustment of the anticoagulant dosage). Products include:
Fragmin Injection 2814

Danaparoid Sodium (Depressed plasma prothrombin activity; may require downward adjustment of the anticoagulant dosage). Products include:
Orgaran Injection 2480

Desogestrel (Concurrent use may render oral contraceptives less effective; potential for breakthrough bleeding). Products include:
Cyclessa Tablets 2450
Desogen Tablets 2458
Mircette Tablets 2470
Ortho-Cept 21 Tablets 2546
Ortho-Cept 28 Tablets 2546

Dicloxacillin Sodium (Interference with bactericidal action of penicillin; avoid concurrent use).
No products indexed under this heading.

Dicumarol (Depressed plasma prothrombin activity; may require downward adjustment of the anticoagulant dosage).
No products indexed under this heading.

Enoxaparin (Depressed plasma prothrombin activity; may require downward adjustment of the anticoagulant dosage). Products include:
Lovenox Injection 746

Ethinyl Estradiol (Concurrent use may render oral contraceptives less effective; potential for breakthrough bleeding). Products include:
Alesse-21 Tablets 3468
Alesse-28 Tablets 3473
Brevicon 28-Day Tablets 3380
Cyclessa Tablets 2450
Desogen Tablets 2458
Estinyl Tablets 3112
Estrostep 2627
femhrt Tablets 2635
Levlen 962
Levlite 21 Tablets 962
Levlite 28 Tablets 962
Levora Tablets 3389
Loestrin 21 Tablets 2642
Loestrin Fe Tablets 2642
Lo/Ovral Tablets 3532
Lo/Ovral-28 Tablets 3538
Low-Ogestrel-28 Tablets 3392
Microgestin Fe 1.5/30 Tablets 3407
Microgestin Fe 1/20 Tablets 3400
Mircette Tablets 2470
Modicon 2563
Necon 3415
Nordette-28 Tablets 2257
Norinyl 1 +35 28-Day Tablets 3380
Ogestrel 0.5/50-28 Tablets 3428
Ortho-Cept 21 Tablets 2546
Ortho-Cept 28 Tablets 2546
Ortho-Cyclen/Ortho Tri-Cyclen 2573
Ortho-Novum 2563
Ovcon 3364
Ovral Tablets 3551
Ovral-28 Tablets 3552
Tri-Levlen 962
Tri-Norinyl-28 Tablets 3433
Triphasil-21 Tablets 3600
Triphasil-28 Tablets 3605
Trivora Tablets 3439
Yasmin 28 Tablets 980
Zovia 3449

Ethynodiol Diacetate (Concurrent use may render oral contraceptives less effective; potential for breakthrough bleeding). Products include:
Zovia 3449

Ferrous Fumarate (Absorption of tetracyclines is impaired). Products include:
New Formulation Chromagen OB Capsules 3094
Loestrin Fe Tablets 2642
NataChew Tablets 3364

Ferrous Gluconate (Absorption of tetracyclines is impaired). Products include:
Fergon Iron Tablets .... ▣802

Ferrous Sulfate (Absorption of tetracyclines is impaired). Products include:
Feosol Tablets 1717
Slow Fe Tablets .... ▣827
Slow Fe with Folic Acid Tablets ..... ▣828

Heparin Sodium (Depressed plasma prothrombin activity; may require downward adjustment of the anticoagulant dosage). Products include:
Heparin Lock Flush Solution 3509
Heparin Sodium Injection 3511

Iron (Absorption of tetracyclines is impaired).
No products indexed under this heading.

Levonorgestrel (Concurrent use may render oral contraceptives less effective; potential for breakthrough bleeding). Products include:
Alesse-21 Tablets 3468
Alesse-28 Tablets 3473
Levlen 962
Levlite 21 Tablets 962
Levlite 28 Tablets 962
Levora Tablets 3389
Mirena Intrauterine System 974
Nordette-28 Tablets 2257
Norplant System 3543
Tri-Levlen 962
Triphasil-21 Tablets 3600
Triphasil-28 Tablets 3605
Trivora Tablets 3439

Magaldrate (Absorption of tetracyclines is impaired).
No products indexed under this heading.

Magnesium Hydroxide (Absorption of tetracyclines is impaired). Products include:
Ex•Lax Milk of Magnesia Liquid .... ▣670
Maalox Antacid/Anti-Gas Oral Suspension .... ▣673
Maalox Max Maximum Strength Antacid/Anti-Gas Liquid 2300
Maalox Regular Strength Antacid/Antigas Liquid 2300
Mylanta Fast-Acting 1813
Mylanta 1813
Pepcid Complete Chewable Tablets 1815

Phillips' Chewable Tablets .... ▣615
Phillips' Milk of Magnesia Liquid (Original, Cherry, & Mint)........... ▣616
Rolaids Tablets .... ▣706
Extra Strength Rolaids Tablets ...... ▣706
Vanquish Caplets .... ▣617

Magnesium Oxide (Absorption of tetracyclines is impaired). Products include:
Beelith Tablets 946
Mag-Ox 400 Tablets 1024
Uro-Mag Capsules 1024

Mestranol (Concurrent use may render oral contraceptives less effective; potential for breakthrough bleeding). Products include:
Necon 1/50 Tablets 3415
Norinyl 1 + 50 28-Day Tablets 3380
Ortho-Novum 1/50□28 Tablets 2556

Methoxyflurane (Potential for fatal renal toxicity).
No products indexed under this heading.

Mezlocillin Sodium (Interference with bactericidal action of penicillin; avoid concurrent use).
No products indexed under this heading.

Nafcillin Sodium (Interference with bactericidal action of penicillin; avoid concurrent use).
No products indexed under this heading.

Norethindrone (Concurrent use may render oral contraceptives less effective; potential for breakthrough bleeding). Products include:
Brevicon 28-Day Tablets 3380
Micronor Tablets 2543
Modicon 2563
Necon 3415
Norinyl 1 +35 28-Day Tablets 3380
Norinyl 1 + 50 28-Day Tablets 3380
Nor-QD Tablets 3423
Ortho-Novum 2563
Ortho-Novum 1/50□28 Tablets 2556
Ovcon 3364
Tri-Norinyl-28 Tablets 3433

Norethynodrel (Concurrent use may render oral contraceptives less effective; potential for breakthrough bleeding).
No products indexed under this heading.

Norgestimate (Concurrent use may render oral contraceptives less effective; potential for breakthrough bleeding). Products include:
Ortho-Cyclen/Ortho Tri-Cyclen 2573
Ortho-Prefest Tablets 2570

Norgestrel (Concurrent use may render oral contraceptives less effective; potential for breakthrough bleeding). Products include:
Lo/Ovral Tablets 3532
Lo/Ovral-28 Tablets 3538
Low-Ogestrel-28 Tablets 3392
Ogestrel 0.5/50-28 Tablets 3428
Ovral Tablets 3551
Ovral-28 Tablets 3552
Ovrette Tablets 3552

Penicillin G Benzathine (Interference with bactericidal action of penicillin; avoid concurrent use). Products include:
Bicillin C-R 900/300 Injection 2240
Bicillin C-R Injection 2238
Bicillin L-A Injection 2242
Permapen Isoject 2706

Penicillin G Potassium (Interference with bactericidal action of penicillin; avoid concurrent use). Products include:
Pfizerpen for Injection 2707

Penicillin G Procaine (Interference with bactericidal action of penicillin; avoid concurrent use). Products include:
Bicillin C-R 900/300 Injection 2240
Bicillin C-R Injection 2238

Penicillin G Sodium (Interference with bactericidal action of penicillin; avoid concurrent use).
No products indexed under this heading.

Penicillin V Potassium (Interference with bactericidal action of penicillin; avoid concurrent use).
No products indexed under this heading.

Polysaccharide-Iron Complex (Absorption of tetracyclines is impaired). Products include:
Niferex 3176
Niferex-150 Capsules 3176
Nu-Iron 150 Capsules 2224

Ticarcillin Disodium (Interference with bactericidal action of penicillin; avoid concurrent use). Products include:
Timentin Injection- ADD-Vantage Vial 1661
Timentin Injection-Galaxy Container 1664
Timentin Injection-Pharmacy Bulk Package 1666
Timentin for Intravenous Administration 1658

Tinzaparin sodium (Depressed plasma prothrombin activity; may require downward adjustment of the anticoagulant dosage). Products include:
Innohep Injection 1248

Warfarin Sodium (Depressed plasma prothrombin activity; may require downward adjustment of the anticoagulant dosage). Products include:
Coumadin for Injection 1243
Coumadin Tablets 1243
Warfarin Sodium Tablets, USP 3302

Food Interactions

Dairy products (The peak plasma concentrations were slightly decreased (11.2%) and delayed by 1 hour).

Meal with dairy products (The peak plasma concentrations were slightly decreased (11.2%) and delayed by 1 hour).

MINTEZOL SUSPENSION
(Thiabendazole) 2137
See Mintezol Chewable Tablets

MINTEZOL CHEWABLE TABLETS
(Thiabendazole) 2137
May interact with theophylline. Compounds in these categories include:

Aminophylline (Thiabendazole may compete with theophylline for sites of metabolism in the liver, thus elevating the serum levels of theophylline to toxic levels; monitor theophylline blood levels).
No products indexed under this heading.

Dyphylline (Thiabendazole may compete with theophylline for sites of metabolism in the liver, thus elevating the serum levels of theophylline to toxic levels; monitor theophylline blood levels). Products include:
Lufyllin Tablets 3347
Lufyllin-400 Tablets 3347
Lufyllin-GG Elixir 3348
Lufyllin-GG Tablets 3348

Theophylline (Thiabendazole may compete with theophylline for sites of metabolism in the liver, thus elevating the serum levels of theophylline to toxic levels; monitor theophylline blood levels). Products include:
Aerolate 1361
Theo-Dur Extended-Release Tablets 1835
Uni-Dur Extended-Release Tablets .. 1841
Uniphyl 400 mg and 600 mg Tablets 2903

Theophylline Calcium Salicylate (Thiabendazole may compete with theophylline for sites of metabolism in the liver, thus elevating the serum levels of theophylline to toxic levels; monitor theophylline blood levels).
No products indexed under this heading.

Theophylline Sodium Glycinate (Thiabendazole may compete with theophylline for sites of metabolism in the liver, thus elevating the serum levels of theophylline to toxic levels; monitor theophylline blood levels).
No products indexed under this heading.

MIOCHOL-E SYSTEM PAK
(Acetylcholine Chloride) .... ⊙305
See Miochol-E with Steri-Tags

MIOCHOL-E WITH STERI-TAGS
(Acetylcholine Chloride) .... ⊙305
May interact with topical nonsteroidal anti-inflammatory agents. Compounds in these categories include:

Diclofenac Sodium (Acetylcholine and carbachol have been ineffective when used in patients with topical nonsteroidal anti-inflammatory agents). Products include:
Arthrotec Tablets 3195
Voltaren Ophthalmic Sterile Ophthalmic Solution .... ⊙312
Voltaren Tablets 2315
Voltaren-XR Tablets 2315

Flurbiprofen Sodium (Acetylcholine and carbachol have been ineffective when used in patients with topical nonsteroidal anti-inflammatory agents). Products include:
Ocufen Ophthalmic Solution .... ⊙242

Suprofen (Acetylcholine and carbachol have been ineffective when used in patients with topical nonsteroidal anti-inflammatory agents).
No products indexed under this heading.

MIRALAX POWDER FOR ORAL SOLUTION
(Polyethylene Glycol) 1069
None cited in PDR database.

MIRAPEX TABLETS
(Pramipexole Dihydrochloride) 2834
May interact with central nervous system depressants, dopamine D2 antagonists, quinidine, and certain other agents. Compounds in these categories include:

Alfentanil Hydrochloride (Pramipexole may cause somnolence and because of possible additive sedative effect, caution should be exercised if used concurrently with CNS depressants).
No products indexed under this heading.

Alprazolam (Pramipexole may cause somnolence and because of possible additive sedative effect, caution should be exercised if used concurrently with CNS depressants). Products include:
Xanax Tablets 2865

Aprobarbital (Pramipexole may cause somnolence and because of possible additive sedative effect, caution should be exercised if used concurrently with CNS depressants).
No products indexed under this heading.

Buprenorphine Hydrochloride (Pramipexole may cause somnolence and because of possible additive sedative effect, caution should be exercised if used concurrently with CNS depressants). Products include:
Buprenex Injectable 2918

Buspirone Hydrochloride (Pramipexole may cause somnolence and because of possible additive sedative effect, caution should be exercised if used concurrently with CNS depressants).
No products indexed under this heading.

Butabarbital (Pramipexole may cause somnolence and because of possible additive sedative effect, caution should be exercised if used concurrently with CNS depressants).
No products indexed under this heading.

Butalbital (Pramipexole may cause somnolence and because of possible additive sedative effect, caution should be exercised if used concurrently with CNS depressants). Products include:
Phrenilin 578
Sedapap Tablets 50 mg/650 mg ... 2225

Chlordiazepoxide (Pramipexole may cause somnolence and because of possible additive sedative effect, caution should be exercised if used concurrently with CNS depressants). Products include:
Limbitrol 1738

Chlordiazepoxide Hydrochloride (Pramipexole may cause somnolence and because of possible additive sedative effect, caution should be exercised if used concurrently with CNS depressants). Products include:
Librium Capsules 1736
Librium for Injection 1737

Chlorpromazine (Co-administration with domamine antagonists may diminish the effectiveness of pramipexole). Products include:
Thorazine Suppositories 1656

Chlorpromazine Hydrochloride (Co-administration with domamine antagonists may diminish the effectiveness of pramipexole). Products include:
Thorazine 1656

Chlorprothixene (Co-administration with domamine antagonists may diminish the effectiveness of pramipexole).
No products indexed under this heading.

Chlorprothixene Hydrochloride (Co-administration with domamine antagonists may diminish the effectiveness of pramipexole).
No products indexed under this heading.

Chlorprothixene Lactate (Pramipexole may cause somnolence and because of possible additive sedative effect, caution should be exercised if used concurrently with CNS depressants).
No products indexed under this heading.

Cimetidine (Co-administration with cimetidine, a known inhibitor of renal tubular secretion of organic acids via anionic transport, has caused a 50% increase in pramipexole AUC and a 40% increase in half-life). Products include:
Tagamet HB 200 Suspension .... ▣762
Tagamet HB 200 Tablets .... ▣761
Tagamet Tablets 1644

Cimetidine Hydrochloride (Co-administration with cimetidine, a known inhibitor of renal tubular secretion of organic acids via anionic transport, has caused a 50% increase in pramipexole AUC and a 40% increase in half-life). Products include:
Tagamet 1644

Clorazepate Dipotassium (Pramipexole may cause somnolence and because of possible additive sedative effect, caution should be exercised if used concurrently with CNS depressants). Products include:
Tranxene 511

Clozapine (Pramipexole may cause somnolence and because of possible additive sedative effect, caution should be exercised if used concurrently with CNS depressants). Products include:
Clozaril Tablets 2319

Codeine Phosphate (Pramipexole may cause somnolence and because of possible additive sedative effect,

caution should be exercised if used concurrently with CNS depressants). Products include:

Phenergan with Codeine Syrup 3557
Phenergan VC with Codeine Syrup .. 3561
Robitussin A-C Syrup 2942
Robitussin-DAC Syrup 2942
Ryna-C Liquid .... ▭ 768
Soma Compound w/Codeine Tablets 3355
Tussi-Organidin NR Liquid 3350
Tussi-Organidin-S NR Liquid 3350
Tylenol with Codeine 2595

Desflurane (Pramipexole may cause somnolence and because of possible additive sedative effect, caution should be exercised if used concurrently with CNS depressants). Products include:

Suprane Liquid for Inhalation 874

Dezocine (Pramipexole may cause somnolence and because of possible additive sedative effect, caution should be exercised if used concurrently with CNS depressants).

No products indexed under this heading.

Diazepam (Pramipexole may cause somnolence and because of possible additive sedative effect, caution should be exercised if used concurrently with CNS depressants). Products include:

Valium Injectable 3026
Valium Tablets 3047

Diltiazem Hydrochloride (Co-administration of drugs that are secreted by the cationic transport system, e.g., diltiazem, decrease the oral clearance of pramipexole by about 20%). Products include:

Cardizem Injectable 1018
Cardizem Lyo-Ject Syringe 1018
Cardizem Monovial 1018
Cardizem CD Capsules 1016
Tiazac Capsules 1378

Droperidol (Pramipexole may cause somnolence and because of possible additive sedative effect, caution should be exercised if used concurrently with CNS depressants).

No products indexed under this heading.

Enflurane (Pramipexole may cause somnolence and because of possible additive sedative effect, caution should be exercised if used concurrently with CNS depressants).

No products indexed under this heading.

Estazolam (Pramipexole may cause somnolence and because of possible additive sedative effect, caution should be exercised if used concurrently with CNS depressants). Products include:

ProSom Tablets 500

Ethchlorvynol (Pramipexole may cause somnolence and because of possible additive sedative effect, caution should be exercised if used concurrently with CNS depressants).

No products indexed under this heading.

Ethinamate (Pramipexole may cause somnolence and because of possible additive sedative effect, caution should be exercised if used concurrently with CNS depressants).

No products indexed under this heading.

Fentanyl (Pramipexole may cause somnolence and because of possible additive sedative effect, caution should be exercised if used concurrently with CNS depressants). Products include:

Duragesic Transdermal System 1786

Fentanyl Citrate (Pramipexole may cause somnolence and because of possible additive sedative effect, caution should be exercised if used concurrently with CNS depressants). Products include:

Actiq 1184

Fluphenazine Decanoate (Co-administration with domamine antagonists may diminish the effectiveness of pramipexole).

No products indexed under this heading.

Fluphenazine Enanthate (Co-administration with domamine antagonists may diminish the effectiveness of pramipexole).

No products indexed under this heading.

Fluphenazine Hydrochloride (Co-administration with domamine antagonists may diminish the effectiveness of pramipexole).

No products indexed under this heading.

Flurazepam Hydrochloride (Pramipexole may cause somnolence and because of possible additive sedative effect, caution should be exercised if used concurrently with CNS depressants).

No products indexed under this heading.

Glutethimide (Pramipexole may cause somnolence and because of possible additive sedative effect, caution should be exercised if used concurrently with CNS depressants).

No products indexed under this heading.

Haloperidol (Co-administration with domamine antagonists may diminish the effectiveness of pramipexole). Products include:

Haldol Injection, Tablets and Concentrate 2533

Haloperidol Decanoate (Co-administration with domamine antagonists may diminish the effectiveness of pramipexole). Products include:

Haldol Decanoate 2535

Hydrocodone Bitartrate (Pramipexole may cause somnolence and because of possible additive sedative effect, caution should be exercised if used concurrently with CNS depressants). Products include:

Hycodan 1316
Hycomine Compound Tablets 1317
Hycotuss Expectorant Syrup 1318
Lortab 3319
Lortab Elixir 3317
Maxidone Tablets CIII 3399
Norco 5/325 Tablets CIII 3424
Norco 7.5/325 Tablets CIII 3425
Norco 10/325 Tablets CIII 3427
Norco 10/325 Tablets CIII 3425
Vicodin Tablets 516
Vicodin ES Tablets 517
Vicodin HP Tablets 518
Vicodin Tuss Expectorant 519
Vicoprofen Tablets 520
Zydone Tablets 1330

Hydrocodone Polistirex (Pramipexole may cause somnolence and because of possible additive sedative effect, caution should be exercised if used concurrently with CNS depressants). Products include:

Tussionex Pennkinetic Extended-Release Suspension 1174

Hydromorphone Hydrochloride (Pramipexole may cause somnolence and because of possible additive sedative effect, caution should be exercised if used concurrently with CNS depressants). Products include:

Dilaudid 441
Dilaudid Oral Liquid 445
Dilaudid Powder 441
Dilaudid Rectal Suppositories 441
Dilaudid Tablets 441
Dilaudid Tablets - 8 mg 445
Dilaudid-HP 443

Hydroxyzine Hydrochloride (Pramipexole may cause somnolence and because of possible additive sedative effect, caution should be exercised if used concurrently with CNS depressants). Products include:

Atarax Tablets & Syrup 2667
Vistaril Intramuscular Solution 2738

Isoflurane (Pramipexole may cause somnolence and because of possible additive sedative effect, caution should be exercised if used concurrently with CNS depressants).

No products indexed under this heading.

Ketamine Hydrochloride (Pramipexole may cause somnolence and because of possible additive sedative effect, caution should be exercised if used concurrently with CNS depressants).

No products indexed under this heading.

Levodopa (Pramipexole may potentiate the dopaminergic side effects of levodopa and may cause or exacerbate pre-existing dyskinesia; pramipexole may cause an increase in levodopa Cmax by about 40% and a decrease in Tmax from 2.5 to 0.6 hours). Products include:

Sinemet Tablets 1253
Sinemet CR Tablets 1255

Levomethadyl Acetate Hydrochloride (Pramipexole may cause somnolence and because of possible additive sedative effect, caution should be exercised if used concurrently with CNS depressants).

No products indexed under this heading.

Levorphanol Tartrate (Pramipexole may cause somnolence and because of possible additive sedative effect, caution should be exercised if used concurrently with CNS depressants). Products include:

Levo-Dromoran 1734
Levorphanol Tartrate Tablets 3059

Lorazepam (Pramipexole may cause somnolence and because of possible additive sedative effect, caution should be exercised if used concurrently with CNS depressants). Products include:

Ativan Injection 3478
Ativan Tablets 3482

Loxapine Hydrochloride (Co-administration with domamine antagonists may diminish the effectiveness of pramipexole).

No products indexed under this heading.

Loxapine Succinate (Co-administration with domamine antagonists may diminish the effectiveness of pramipexole). Products include:

Loxitane Capsules 3398

Meperidine Hydrochloride (Pramipexole may cause somnolence and because of possible additive sedative effect, caution should be exercised if used concurrently with CNS depressants). Products include:

Demerol 3079
Mepergan Injection 3539

Mephobarbital (Pramipexole may cause somnolence and because of possible additive sedative effect, caution should be exercised if used concurrently with CNS depressants).

No products indexed under this heading.

Meprobamate (Pramipexole may cause somnolence and because of possible additive sedative effect, caution should be exercised if used concurrently with CNS depressants). Products include:

Miltown Tablets 3349

Mesoridazine Besylate (Co-administration with domamine antagonists may diminish the effectiveness of pramipexole). Products include:

Serentil 1057

Methadone Hydrochloride (Pramipexole may cause somnolence and because of possible additive sedative effect, caution should be exercised if used concurrently with CNS depressants). Products include:

Dolophine Hydrochloride Tablets 3056

Methohexital Sodium (Pramipexole may cause somnolence and because of possible additive sedative effect, caution should be exercised if used concurrently with CNS depressants). Products include:

Brevital Sodium for Injection, USP .. 1815

Methotrimeprazine (Co-administration with domamine antagonists may diminish the effectiveness of pramipexole).

No products indexed under this heading.

Methoxyflurane (Pramipexole may cause somnolence and because of possible additive sedative effect, caution should be exercised if used concurrently with CNS depressants).

No products indexed under this heading.

Metoclopramide Hydrochloride (Co-administration with domamine antagonists may diminish the effectiveness of pramipexole). Products include:

Reglan 2935

Midazolam Hydrochloride (Pramipexole may cause somnolence and because of possible additive sedative effect, caution should be exercised if used concurrently with CNS depressants). Products include:

Versed Injection 3027
Versed Syrup 3033

Molindone Hydrochloride (Co-administration with domamine antagonists may diminish the effectiveness of pramipexole). Products include:

Moban 1320

Morphine Sulfate (Pramipexole may cause somnolence and because of possible additive sedative effect, caution should be exercised if used concurrently with CNS depressants). Products include:

Astramorph/PF Injection, USP (Preservative-Free) 594
Duramorph Injection 1312
Infumorph 200 and Infumorph 500 Sterile Solutions 1314
Kadian Capsules 1335
MS Contin Tablets 2896
MSIR 2898
Oramorph SR Tablets 3062
Roxanol 3066

Olanzapine (Pramipexole may cause somnolence and because of possible additive sedative effect, caution should be exercised if used concurrently with CNS depressants). Products include:

Zyprexa Tablets 1973
Zyprexa ZYDIS Orally Disintegrating Tablets 1973

Oxazepam (Pramipexole may cause somnolence and because of possible additive sedative effect, caution should be exercised if used concurrently with CNS depressants).

No products indexed under this heading.

Oxycodone Hydrochloride (Pramipexole may cause somnolence and because of possible additive sedative effect, caution should be exercised if used concurrently with CNS depressants). Products include:

OxyContin Tablets 2912
OxyFast Oral Concentrate Solution . 2916
OxyIR Capsules 2916
Percocet Tablets 1326
Percodan Tablets 1327
Percolone Tablets 1327
Roxicodone 3067
Tylox Capsules 2597

Pentobarbital Sodium (Pramipexole may cause somnolence and because of possible additive seda-

tive effect, caution should be exercised if used concurrently with CNS depressants). Products include:

Nembutal Sodium Solution 485

Perphenazine (Co-administration with domamine antagonists may diminish the effectiveness of pramipexole). Products include:

Etrafon 3115
Trilafon 3160

Phenobarbital (Pramipexole may cause somnolence and because of possible additive sedative effect, caution should be exercised if used concurrently with CNS depressants). Products include:

Arco-Lase Plus Tablets 592
Donnatal 2929
Donnatal Extentabs 2930

Prazepam (Pramipexole may cause somnolence and because of possible additive sedative effect, caution should be exercised if used concurrently with CNS depressants).

No products indexed under this heading.

Prochlorperazine (Co-administration with domamine antagonists may diminish the effectiveness of pramipexole). Products include:

Compazine 1505

Promethazine Hydrochloride (Co-administration with domamine antagonists may diminish the effectiveness of pramipexole). Products include:

Mepergan Injection 3539
Phenergan Injection 3553
Phenergan 3556
Phenergan Syrup 3554
Phenergan with Codeine Syrup 3557
Phenergan with Dextromethorphan Syrup 3559
Phenergan VC Syrup 3560
Phenergan VC with Codeine Syrup 3561

Propofol (Pramipexole may cause somnolence and because of possible additive sedative effect, caution should be exercised if used concurrently with CNS depressants). Products include:

Diprivan Injectable Emulsion 667

Propoxyphene Hydrochloride (Pramipexole may cause somnolence and because of possible additive sedative effect, caution should be exercised if used concurrently with CNS depressants). Products include:

Darvon Pulvules 1909
Darvon Compound-65 Pulvules 1910

Propoxyphene Napsylate (Pramipexole may cause somnolence and because of possible additive sedative effect, caution should be exercised if used concurrently with CNS depressants). Products include:

Darvon-N/Darvocet-N 1907
Darvon-N Tablets 1912

Quazepam (Pramipexole may cause somnolence and because of possible additive sedative effect, caution should be exercised if used concurrently with CNS depressants).

No products indexed under this heading.

Quetiapine Fumarate (Co-administration with domamine antagonists may diminish the effectiveness of pramipexole). Products include:

Seroquel Tablets 684

Quinidine Gluconate (Co-administration of drugs that are secreted by the cationic transport system, e.g., quinidine, decrease the oral clearance of pramipexole by about 20%). Products include:

Quinaglute Dura-Tabs Tablets 978

Quinidine Polygalacturonate (Co-administration of drugs that are secreted by the cationic transport system, e.g., quinidine, decrease the oral clearance of pramipexole by about 20%).

No products indexed under this heading.

Quinidine Sulfate (Co-administration of drugs that are secreted by the cationic transport system, e.g., quinidine, decrease the oral clearance of pramipexole by about 20%). Products include:

Quinidex Extentabs 2933

Quinine Sulfate (Co-administration of drugs that are secreted by the cationic transport system, e.g., quinine, decrease the oral clearance of pramipexole by about 20%).

No products indexed under this heading.

Ranitidine Hydrochloride (Co-administration of drugs that are secreted by the cationic transport system, e.g., ranitidine, decrease the oral clearance of pramipexole by about 20%). Products include:

Zantac 1690
Zantac Injection 1688
Zantac 75 Tablets 717

Remifentanil Hydrochloride (Pramipexole may cause somnolence and because of possible additive sedative effect, caution should be exercised if used concurrently with CNS depressants).

No products indexed under this heading.

Risperidone (Co-administration with domamine antagonists may diminish the effectiveness of pramipexole). Products include:

Risperdal 1796

Secobarbital Sodium (Pramipexole may cause somnolence and because of possible additive sedative effect, caution should be exercised if used concurrently with CNS depressants).

No products indexed under this heading.

Sevoflurane (Pramipexole may cause somnolence and because of possible additive sedative effect, caution should be exercised if used concurrently with CNS depressants).

No products indexed under this heading.

Sufentanil Citrate (Pramipexole may cause somnolence and because of possible additive sedative effect, caution should be exercised if used concurrently with CNS depressants).

No products indexed under this heading.

Temazepam (Pramipexole may cause somnolence and because of possible additive sedative effect, caution should be exercised if used concurrently with CNS depressants).

No products indexed under this heading.

Thiamylal Sodium (Pramipexole may cause somnolence and because of possible additive sedative effect, caution should be exercised if used concurrently with CNS depressants).

No products indexed under this heading.

Thioridazine Hydrochloride (Co-administration with domamine antagonists may diminish the effectiveness of pramipexole). Products include:

Thioridazine Hydrochloride Tablets 2289

Thiothixene (Co-administration with domamine antagonists may diminish the effectiveness of pramipexole). Products include:

Navane Capsules 2701
Thiothixene Capsules 2290

Triamterene (Co-administration of drugs that are secreted by the cationic transport system, e.g., triamterene, decrease the oral clearance of pramipexole by about 20%). Products include:

Dyazide Capsules 1515
Dyrenium Capsules 3458
Maxzide 1008

Triazolam (Pramipexole may cause somnolence and because of possible additive sedative effect, caution should be exercised if used concurrently with CNS depressants). Products include:

Halcion Tablets 2823

Trifluoperazine Hydrochloride (Co-administration with domamine antagonists may diminish the effectiveness of pramipexole). Products include:

Stelazine 1640

Verapamil Hydrochloride (Co-administration of drugs that are secreted by the cationic transport system, e.g., verapamil, decrease the oral clearance of pramipexole by about 20%). Products include:

Covera-HS Tablets 3199
Isoptin SR Tablets 467
Tarka Tablets 508
Verelan Capsules 3184
Verelan PM Capsules 3186

Zaleplon (Pramipexole may cause somnolence and because of possible additive sedative effect, caution should be exercised if used concurrently with CNS depressants). Products include:

Sonata Capsules 3591

Ziprasidone Hydrochloride (Pramipexole may cause somnolence and because of possible additive sedative effect, caution should be exercised if used concurrently with CNS depressants). Products include:

Geodon Capsules 2688

Zolpidem Tartrate (Pramipexole may cause somnolence and because of possible additive sedative effect, caution should be exercised if used concurrently with CNS depressants). Products include:

Ambien Tablets 3191

Food Interactions

Food, unspecified (Food does not affect the extent of pramipexole absorption, although the time of maximum plasma concentration is increased by about 1 hour when the drug is taken with a meal).

MIRCETTE TABLETS

(Desogestrel, Ethinyl Estradiol) 2470

May interact with barbiturates, phenytoin, tetracyclines, and certain other agents. Compounds in these categories include:

Ampicillin (Potential for reduced efficacy and increased incidence of breakthrough bleeding and menstrual irregularities with concomitant use).

No products indexed under this heading.

Ampicillin Sodium (Potential for reduced efficacy and increased incidence of breakthrough bleeding and menstrual irregularities with concomitant use). Products include:

Unasyn for Injection 2728

Aprobarbital (Potential for reduced efficacy and increased incidence of breakthrough bleeding and menstrual irregularities with concomitant use).

No products indexed under this heading.

Butabarbital (Potential for reduced efficacy and increased incidence of breakthrough bleeding and menstrual irregularities with concomitant use).

No products indexed under this heading.

Butalbital (Potential for reduced efficacy and increased incidence of breakthrough bleeding and menstrual irregularities with concomitant use). Products include:

Phrenilin 578
Sedapap Tablets 50 mg/650 mg 2225

Demeclocycline Hydrochloride (Potential for reduced efficacy and increased incidence of breakthrough bleeding and menstrual irregularities with concomitant use). Products include:

Declomycin Tablets 1855

Doxycycline Calcium (Potential for reduced efficacy and increased incidence of breakthrough bleeding and menstrual irregularities with concomitant use). Products include:

Vibramycin Calcium Oral Suspension Syrup 2735

Doxycycline Hyclate (Potential for reduced efficacy and increased incidence of breakthrough bleeding and menstrual irregularities with concomitant use). Products include:

Doryx Coated Pellet Filled Capsules 3357
Periostat Tablets 1208
Vibramycin Hyclate Capsules 2735
Vibramycin Hyclate Intravenous 2737
Vibra-Tabs Film Coated Tablets 2735

Doxycycline Monohydrate (Potential for reduced efficacy and increased incidence of breakthrough bleeding and menstrual irregularities with concomitant use). Products include:

Monodox Capsules 2442
Vibramycin Monohydrate for Oral Suspension 2735

Fosphenytoin Sodium (Potential for reduced efficacy and increased incidence of breakthrough bleeding and menstrual irregularities with concomitant use). Products include:

Cerebyx Injection 2619

Griseofulvin (Potential for reduced efficacy and increased incidence of breakthrough bleeding and menstrual irregularities with concomitant use). Products include:

Grifulvin V Tablets Microsize and Oral Suspension Microsize 2518
Gris-PEG Tablets 2661

Mephobarbital (Potential for reduced efficacy and increased incidence of breakthrough bleeding and menstrual irregularities with concomitant use).

No products indexed under this heading.

Methacycline Hydrochloride (Potential for reduced efficacy and increased incidence of breakthrough bleeding and menstrual irregularities with concomitant use).

No products indexed under this heading.

Minocycline Hydrochloride (Potential for reduced efficacy and increased incidence of breakthrough bleeding and menstrual irregularities with concomitant use). Products include:

Dynacin Capsules 2019
Minocin Intravenous 1862
Minocin Oral Suspension 1865
Minocin Pellet-Filled Capsules 1863

Oxytetracycline Hydrochloride (Potential for reduced efficacy and increased incidence of breakthrough bleeding and menstrual irregularities with concomitant use). Products include:

Terra-Cortril Ophthalmic Suspension 2716
Urobiotic-250 Capsules 2731

Pentobarbital Sodium (Potential for reduced efficacy and increased incidence of breakthrough bleeding and menstrual irregularities with concomitant use). Products include:

Nembutal Sodium Solution 485

Phenobarbital (Potential for reduced efficacy and increased incidence of breakthrough bleeding and menstrual irregularities with concomitant use). Products include:

Arco-Lase Plus Tablets 592
Donnatal 2929
Donnatal Extentabs 2930

Phenylbutazone (Potential for reduced efficacy and increased incidence of breakthrough bleeding and

menstrual irregularities with concomitant use).
No products indexed under this heading.

Phenytoin (Potential for reduced efficacy and increased incidence of breakthrough bleeding and menstrual irregularities with concomitant use). Products include:
- Dilantin Infatabs 2624
- Dilantin-125 Oral Suspension 2625

Phenytoin Sodium (Potential for reduced efficacy and increased incidence of breakthrough bleeding and menstrual irregularities with concomitant use). Products include:
- Dilantin Kapseals 2622

Rifampin (Co-administration has been associated with reduced efficacy and increased incidence of breakthrough bleeding and menstrual irregularities). Products include:
- Rifadin 765
- Rifamate Capsules 767
- Rifater Tablets 769

Secobarbital Sodium (Potential for reduced efficacy and increased incidence of breakthrough bleeding and menstrual irregularities with concomitant use).
No products indexed under this heading.

Tetracycline Hydrochloride (Potential for reduced efficacy and increased incidence of breakthrough bleeding and menstrual irregularities with concomitant use).
No products indexed under this heading.

Thiamylal Sodium (Potential for reduced efficacy and increased incidence of breakthrough bleeding and menstrual irregularities with concomitant use).
No products indexed under this heading.

MIRENA INTRAUTERINE SYSTEM

(Levonorgestrel) 974

May interact with phenytoin and certain other agents. Compounds in these categories include:

Carbamazepine (Co-administration with drugs that induce liver enzymes may impair the effect of hormonal contraceptives). Products include:
- Carbatrol Capsules 3234
- Tegretol/Tegretol-XR 2404

Fosphenytoin Sodium (Co-administration with drugs that induce liver enzymes may impair the effect of hormonal contraceptives). Products include:
- Cerebyx Injection 2619

Phenytoin (Co-administration with drugs that induce liver enzymes may impair the effect of hormonal contraceptives). Products include:
- Dilantin Infatabs 2624
- Dilantin-125 Oral Suspension 2625

Phenytoin Sodium (Co-administration with drugs that induce liver enzymes may impair the effect of hormonal contraceptives). Products include:
- Dilantin Kapseals 2622

Rifampin (Co-administration with drugs that induce liver enzymes may impair the effect of hormonal contraceptives). Products include:
- Rifadin 765
- Rifamate Capsules 767
- Rifater Tablets 769

MITHRACIN FOR INTRAVENOUS USE

(Plicamycin) 903

None cited in PDR database.

MITROLAN CHEWABLE TABLETS

(Calcium Polycarbophil) .... ▣789

May interact with tetracyclines. Compounds in these categories include:

Demeclocycline Hydrochloride (Mitrolan releases free calcium after ingestion, which may impair oral absorption of tetracycline). Products include:
- Declomycin Tablets 1855

Doxycycline Calcium (Mitrolan releases free calcium after ingestion, which may impair oral absorption of tetracycline). Products include:
- Vibramycin Calcium Oral Suspension Syrup 2735

Doxycycline Hyclate (Mitrolan releases free calcium after ingestion, which may impair oral absorption of tetracycline). Products include:
- Doryx Coated Pellet Filled Capsules 3357
- Periostat Tablets 1208
- Vibramycin Hyclate Capsules 2735
- Vibramycin Hyclate Intravenous 2737
- Vibra-Tabs Film Coated Tablets 2735

Doxycycline Monohydrate (Mitrolan releases free calcium after ingestion, which may impair oral absorption of tetracycline). Products include:
- Monodox Capsules 2442
- Vibramycin Monohydrate for Oral Suspension 2735

Methacycline Hydrochloride (Mitrolan releases free calcium after ingestion, which may impair oral absorption of tetracycline).
No products indexed under this heading.

Minocycline Hydrochloride (Mitrolan releases free calcium after ingestion, which may impair oral absorption of tetracycline). Products include:
- Dynacin Capsules 2019
- Minocin Intravenous 1862
- Minocin Oral Suspension 1865
- Minocin Pellet-Filled Capsules 1863

Oxytetracycline Hydrochloride (Mitrolan releases free calcium after ingestion, which may impair oral absorption of tetracycline). Products include:
- Terra-Cortril Ophthalmic Suspension 2716
- Urobiotic-250 Capsules 2731

Tetracycline Hydrochloride (Mitrolan releases free calcium after ingestion, which may impair oral absorption of tetracycline).
No products indexed under this heading.

M-M-R II

(Measles, Mumps & Rubella Virus Vaccine, Live) 2118

May interact with immunosuppressive agents. Compounds in these categories include:

Azathioprine (Concurrent administration with immunosuppressant is contraindicated).
No products indexed under this heading.

Basiliximab (Concurrent administration with immunosuppressant is contraindicated). Products include:
- Simulect for Injection 2399

Cyclosporine (Concurrent administration with immunosuppressant is contraindicated). Products include:
- Gengraf Capsules 457
- Neoral Soft Gelatin Capsules 2380
- Neoral Oral Solution 2380
- Sandimmune 2388

Muromonab-CD3 (Concurrent administration with immunosuppressant is contraindicated). Products include:
- Orthoclone OKT3 Sterile Solution 2498

Mycophenolate Mofetil (Concurrent administration with immunosuppressant is contraindicated). Products include:
- CellCept Capsules 2951
- CellCept Oral Suspension 2951
- CellCept Tablets 2951

Sirolimus (Concurrent administration with immunosuppressant is contraindicated). Products include:
- Rapamune Oral Solution and Tablets 3584

Tacrolimus (Concurrent administration with immunosuppressant is contraindicated). Products include:
- Prograf 1393
- Protopic Ointment 1397

MOBAN ORAL CONCENTRATE

(Molindone Hydrochloride) 1320

See Moban Tablets

MOBAN TABLETS

(Molindone Hydrochloride) 1320

May interact with tetracyclines and certain other agents. Compounds in these categories include:

Demeclocycline Hydrochloride (Calcium sulfate present as an excipient may interfere with the absorption of oral tetracyclines). Products include:
- Declomycin Tablets 1855

Doxycycline Calcium (Calcium sulfate present as an excipient may interfere with the absorption of oral tetracyclines). Products include:
- Vibramycin Calcium Oral Suspension Syrup 2735

Doxycycline Hyclate (Calcium sulfate present as an excipient may interfere with the absorption of oral tetracyclines). Products include:
- Doryx Coated Pellet Filled Capsules 3357
- Periostat Tablets 1208
- Vibramycin Hyclate Capsules 2735
- Vibramycin Hyclate Intravenous 2737
- Vibra-Tabs Film Coated Tablets 2735

Doxycycline Monohydrate (Calcium sulfate present as an excipient may interfere with the absorption of oral tetracyclines). Products include:
- Monodox Capsules 2442
- Vibramycin Monohydrate for Oral Suspension 2735

Methacycline Hydrochloride (Calcium sulfate present as an excipient may interfere with the absorption of oral tetracyclines).
No products indexed under this heading.

Minocycline Hydrochloride (Calcium sulfate present as an excipient may interfere with the absorption of oral tetracyclines). Products include:
- Dynacin Capsules 2019
- Minocin Intravenous 1862
- Minocin Oral Suspension 1865
- Minocin Pellet-Filled Capsules 1863

Oxytetracycline Hydrochloride (Calcium sulfate present as an excipient may interfere with the absorption of oral tetracyclines). Products include:
- Terra-Cortril Ophthalmic Suspension 2716
- Urobiotic-250 Capsules 2731

Phenytoin Sodium (Calcium sulfate present as an excipient may interfere with the absorption of oral phenytoin sodium). Products include:
- Dilantin Kapseals 2622

Tetracycline Hydrochloride (Calcium sulfate present as an excipient may interfere with the absorption of oral tetracyclines).
No products indexed under this heading.

MOBIC TABLETS

(Meloxicam) 1054

May interact with ACE inhibitors, lithium preparations, thiazides, and certain other agents. Compounds in these categories include:

Aspirin (Co-administration of aspirin to healthy volunteers tended to increase the AUC and Cmax of meloxicam; the clinical significance of this interaction is not known; concurrent use may result in an increased rate of GI ulceration or other complications). Products include:
- Aggrenox Capsules 1026
- Alka-Seltzer .... ▣603
- Alka-Seltzer Lemon Lime Antacid and Pain Reliever Effervescent Tablets .... ▣603
- Alka-Seltzer Extra Strength Antacid and Pain Reliever Effervescent Tablets .... ▣603
- Alka-Seltzer PM Effervescent Tablets .... ▣605
- Genuine Bayer Tablets, Caplets and Gelcaps .... ▣606
- Extra Strength Bayer Caplets and Gelcaps .... ▣610
- Aspirin Regimen Bayer Children's Chewable Tablets (Orange or Cherry Flavored) .... ▣607
- Bayer, Aspirin Regimen .... ▣606
- Aspirin Regimen Bayer 81 mg Caplets with Calcium .... ▣607
- Genuine Bayer Professional Labeling (Aspirin Regimen Bayer) .... ▣608
- Extra Strength Bayer Arthritis Caplets .... ▣610
- Extra Strength Bayer Plus Caplets .... ▣610
- Extra Strength Bayer PM Caplets .... ▣611
- BC Powder .... ▣619
- BC Allergy Sinus Cold Powder .... ▣619
- Arthritis Strength BC Powder .... ▣619
- BC Sinus Cold Powder .... ▣619
- Darvon Compound-65 Pulvules 1910
- Ecotrin Enteric Coated Aspirin Low, Regular and Maximum Strength Tablets 1715
- Excedrin Extra-Strength Tablets, Caplets, and Geltabs .... ▣629
- Excedrin Migraine 1070
- Goody's Body Pain Formula Powder .... ▣620
- Goody's Extra Strength Headache Powder .... ▣620
- Goody's Extra Strength Pain Relief Tablets .... ▣620
- Percodan Tablets 1327
- Robaxisal Tablets 2939
- Soma Compound Tablets 3354
- Soma Compound w/Codeine Tablets 3355
- Vanquish Caplets .... ▣617

Benazepril Hydrochloride (Co-administration of NSAIDs with ACE inhibitors may diminish the antihypertensive effects of ACE inhibitors). Products include:
- Lotensin Tablets 2365
- Lotensin HCT Tablets 2367
- Lotrel Capsules 2370

Bendroflumethiazide (NSAIDs can reduce the natriuretic effect of thiazide diuretics in some patients). Products include:
- Corzide 40/5 Tablets 2247
- Corzide 80/5 Tablets 2247

Captopril (Co-administration of NSAIDs with ACE inhibitors may diminish the antihypertensive effects of ACE inhibitors). Products include:
- Captopril Tablets 2281

Chlorothiazide (NSAIDs can reduce the natriuretic effect of thiazide diuretics in some patients). Products include:
- Aldoclor Tablets 2035
- Diuril Oral 2087

Chlorothiazide Sodium (NSAIDs can reduce the natriuretic effect of thiazide diuretics in some patients). Products include:
- Diuril Sodium Intravenous 2086

Cholestyramine (Pretreatment for four days with cholestyramine significantly increased clearance of meloxicam by 50% resulting in a decrease

in t1/2 from 19.2 hours to 12.5 hours, and a 35% reduction in AUC; the clinical significance of this interaction is not known).
No products indexed under this heading.

Enalapril Maleate (Co-administration of NSAIDs with ACE inhibitors may diminish the antihypertensive effects of ACE inhibitors). Products include:
Lexxel Tablets ... 608
Vaseretic Tablets ... 2204
Vasotec Tablets ... 2210

Enalaprilat (Co-administration of NSAIDs with ACE inhibitors may diminish the antihypertensive effects of ACE inhibitors). Products include:
Enalaprilat Injection ... 863
Vasotec I.V. Injection ... 2207

Fosinopril Sodium (Co-administration of NSAIDs with ACE inhibitors may diminish the antihypertensive effects of ACE inhibitors). Products include:
Monopril Tablets ... 1091
Monopril HCT ... 1094

Furosemide (NSAIDs can reduce the natriuretic effect of furosemide in some patients; in clinical studies, pharmacokinetics and pharmacodynamics of furosemide were not affected by multiple doses of meloxicam). Products include:
Furosemide Tablets ... 2284

Hydrochlorothiazide (NSAIDs can reduce the natriuretic effect of thiazide diuretics in some patients). Products include:
Accuretic Tablets ... 2614
Aldoril Tablets ... 2039
Atacand HCT Tablets ... 597
Avalide Tablets ... 1070
Diovan HCT Tablets ... 2338
Dyazide Capsules ... 1515
HydroDIURIL Tablets ... 2108
Hyzaar ... 2109
Inderide Tablets ... 3517
Inderide LA Long-Acting Capsules ... 3519
Lotensin HCT Tablets ... 2367
Maxzide ... 1008
Micardis HCT Tablets ... 1051
Microzide Capsules ... 3414
Moduretic Tablets ... 2138
Monopril HCT ... 1094
Prinzide Tablets ... 2168
Timolide Tablets ... 2187
Uniretic Tablets ... 3178
Vaseretic Tablets ... 2204
Zestoretic Tablets ... 695
Ziac Tablets ... 1887

Hydroflumethiazide (NSAIDs can reduce the natriuretic effect of thiazide diuretics in some patients). Products include:
Diucardin Tablets ... 3494

Lisinopril (Co-administration of NSAIDs with ACE inhibitors may diminish the antihypertensive effects of ACE inhibitors). Products include:
Prinivil Tablets ... 2164
Prinzide Tablets ... 2168
Zestoretic Tablets ... 695
Zestril Tablets ... 698

Lithium Carbonate (NSAIDs can produce an elevation of plasma lithium levels and a reduction in renal lithium clearance; co-administration in healthy subjects has resulted in increased lithium concentration and AUC). Products include:
Eskalith ... 1527
Lithium Carbonate ... 3061
Lithobid Slow-Release Tablets ... 3255

Lithium Citrate (NSAIDs can produce an elevation of plasma lithium levels and a reduction in renal lithium clearance; co-administration in healthy subjects has resulted in increased lithium concentration and AUC). Products include:
Lithium Citrate Syrup ... 3061

Methyclothiazide (NSAIDs can reduce the natriuretic effect of thiazide diuretics in some patients).
No products indexed under this heading.

Moexipril Hydrochloride (Co-administration of NSAIDs with ACE inhibitors may diminish the antihypertensive effects of ACE inhibitors). Products include:
Uniretic Tablets ... 3178
Univasc Tablets ... 3181

Perindopril Erbumine (Co-administration of NSAIDs with ACE inhibitors may diminish the antihypertensive effects of ACE inhibitors). Products include:
Aceon Tablets (2 mg, 4 mg, 8 mg) ... 3249

Polythiazide (NSAIDs can reduce the natriuretic effect of thiazide diuretics in some patients). Products include:
Minizide Capsules ... 2700
Renese Tablets ... 2712

Quinapril Hydrochloride (Co-administration of NSAIDs with ACE inhibitors may diminish the antihypertensive effects of ACE inhibitors). Products include:
Accupril Tablets ... 2611
Accuretic Tablets ... 2614

Ramipril (Co-administration of NSAIDs with ACE inhibitors may diminish the antihypertensive effects of ACE inhibitors). Products include:
Altace Capsules ... 2233

Spirapril Hydrochloride (Co-administration of NSAIDs with ACE inhibitors may diminish the antihypertensive effects of ACE inhibitors).
No products indexed under this heading.

Trandolapril (Co-administration of NSAIDs with ACE inhibitors may diminish the antihypertensive effects of ACE inhibitors). Products include:
Mavik Tablets ... 478
Tarka Tablets ... 508

Warfarin Sodium (Potential for increased risk of bleeding). Products include:
Coumadin for Injection ... 1243
Coumadin Tablets ... 1243
Warfarin Sodium Tablets, USP ... 3302

Food Interactions

Food, unspecified (Co-administration with a high fat breakfast did not affect extent of absorption of meloxicam capsules but led to 22% higher Cmax values; mean Cmax values were achieved between 5 to 6 hours; Mobic tablets can be administered without regard to timing of meals).

MODICON 21 TABLETS

(Ethinyl Estradiol, Norethindrone) ... 2563
See Ortho-Novum 7/7/7▢21 Tablets

MODICON 28 TABLETS

(Ethinyl Estradiol, Norethindrone) ... 2563
See Ortho-Novum 7/7/7▢21 Tablets

MODURETIC TABLETS

(Amiloride Hydrochloride, Hydrochlorothiazide) ... 2138
May interact with ACE inhibitors, antihypertensives, barbiturates, bile acid sequestering agents, corticosteroids, cardiac glycosides, oral hypoglycemic agents, insulin, lithium preparations, narcotic analgesics, non-steroidal anti-inflammatory agents, potassium preparations, and certain other agents. Compounds in these categories include:

Acarbose (Dosage adjustment of the antidiabetic drug may be required). Products include:
Precose Tablets ... 906

Acebutolol Hydrochloride (Potentiated or additive action). Products include:
Sectral Capsules ... 3589

ACTH (Hypokalemia).
No products indexed under this heading.

Alfentanil Hydrochloride (Potentiation of orthostatic hypotension).
No products indexed under this heading.

Amlodipine Besylate (Potentiated or additive action). Products include:
Lotrel Capsules ... 2370
Norvasc Tablets ... 2704

Aprobarbital (Potentiation of orthostatic hypotension).
No products indexed under this heading.

Atenolol (Potentiated or additive action). Products include:
Tenoretic Tablets ... 690
Tenormin I.V. Injection ... 692

Benazepril Hydrochloride (Potentiated or additive action; increased risk of hyperkalemia). Products include:
Lotensin Tablets ... 2365
Lotensin HCT Tablets ... 2367
Lotrel Capsules ... 2370

Bendroflumethiazide (Potentiated or additive action). Products include:
Corzide 40/5 Tablets ... 2247
Corzide 80/5 Tablets ... 2247

Betamethasone Acetate (Hypokalemia). Products include:
Celestone Soluspan Injectable Suspension ... 3097

Betamethasone Sodium Phosphate (Hypokalemia). Products include:
Celestone Soluspan Injectable Suspension ... 3097

Betaxolol Hydrochloride (Potentiated or additive action). Products include:
Betoptic S Ophthalmic Suspension ... 537

Bisoprolol Fumarate (Potentiated or additive action). Products include:
Zebeta Tablets ... 1885
Ziac Tablets ... 1887

Buprenorphine Hydrochloride (Potentiation of orthostatic hypotension). Products include:
Buprenex Injectable ... 2918

Butabarbital (Potentiation of orthostatic hypotension).
No products indexed under this heading.

Butalbital (Potentiation of orthostatic hypotension). Products include:
Phrenilin ... 578
Sedapap Tablets 50 mg/650 mg ... 2225

Candesartan Cilexetil (Potentiated or additive action). Products include:
Atacand Tablets ... 595
Atacand HCT Tablets ... 597

Captopril (Potentiated or additive action; increased risk of hyperkalemia). Products include:
Captopril Tablets ... 2281

Carteolol Hydrochloride (Potentiated or additive action). Products include:
Carteolol Hydrochloride Ophthalmic Solution USP, 1% ... ⊙258
Ocupress Ophthalmic Solution, 1% Sterile ... ⊙303

Celecoxib (Reduced diuretic, natriuretic, and antihypertensive effects of Moduretic). Products include:
Celebrex Capsules ... 2676
Celebrex Capsules ... 2780

Chlorothiazide (Potentiated or additive action). Products include:
Aldoclor Tablets ... 2035
Diuril Oral ... 2087

Chlorothiazide Sodium (Potentiated or additive action). Products include:
Diuril Sodium Intravenous ... 2086

Chlorpropamide (Dosage adjustment of the antidiabetic drug may be required). Products include:
Diabinese Tablets ... 2680

Chlorthalidone (Potentiated or additive effects). Products include:
Clorpres Tablets ... 1002
Combipres Tablets ... 1040

Tenoretic Tablets ... 690

Cholestyramine (Cholestyramine resin has potential of binding hydrochlorothiazide and reducing its absorption from the GI tract by up to 85%).
No products indexed under this heading.

Clonidine (Potentiated or additive action). Products include:
Catapres-TTS ... 1038

Clonidine Hydrochloride (Potentiated or additive action). Products include:
Catapres Tablets ... 1037
Clorpres Tablets ... 1002
Combipres Tablets ... 1040
Duraclon Injection ... 3057

Codeine Phosphate (Potentiation of orthostatic hypotension). Products include:
Phenergan with Codeine Syrup ... 3557
Phenergan VC with Codeine Syrup ... 3561
Robitussin A-C Syrup ... 2942
Robitussin-DAC Syrup ... 2942
Ryna-C Liquid ... ◘768
Soma Compound w/Codeine Tablets ... 3355
Tussi-Organidin NR Liquid ... 3350
Tussi-Organidin-S NR Liquid ... 3350
Tylenol with Codeine ... 2595

Colestipol Hydrochloride (Colestipol resin has potential of binding hydrochlorothiazide and reducing its absorption from the GI tract by up to 43%). Products include:
Colestid Tablets ... 2791

Cortisone Acetate (Hypokalemia). Products include:
Cortone Acetate Injectable Suspension ... 2059
Cortone Acetate Tablets ... 2061

Deserpidine (Potentiated or additive action).
No products indexed under this heading.

Deslanoside (Potential for exaggerated response of the heart to the toxic effects of digitalis).
No products indexed under this heading.

Dexamethasone (Hypokalemia). Products include:
Decadron Elixir ... 2078
Decadron Tablets ... 2079
TobraDex Ophthalmic Ointment ... 542
TobraDex Ophthalmic Suspension ... 541

Dexamethasone Acetate (Hypokalemia).
No products indexed under this heading.

Dexamethasone Sodium Phosphate (Hypokalemia). Products include:
Decadron Phosphate Injection ... 2081
Decadron Phosphate Sterile Ophthalmic Ointment ... 2083
Decadron Phosphate Sterile Ophthalmic Solution ... 2084
NeoDecadron Sterile Ophthalmic Solution ... 2144

Dezocine (Potentiation of orthostatic hypotension).
No products indexed under this heading.

Diazoxide (Potentiated or additive action).
No products indexed under this heading.

Diclofenac Potassium (Reduced diuretic, natriuretic, and antihypertensive effects of Moduretic). Products include:
Cataflam Tablets ... 2315

Diclofenac Sodium (Reduced diuretic, natriuretic, and antihypertensive effects of Moduretic). Products include:
Arthrotec Tablets ... 3195
Voltaren Ophthalmic Sterile Ophthalmic Solution ... ⊙312
Voltaren Tablets ... 2315
Voltaren-XR Tablets ... 2315

Digitoxin (Potential for exaggerated response of the heart to the toxic

IMPORTANT NOTE: Always consult each drug listing in the patient's regimen for possible interactions.

effects of digitalis).
No products indexed under this heading.

Digoxin (Potential for exaggerated response of the heart to the toxic effects of digitalis). Products include:
- Digitek Tablets ... 1003
- Lanoxicaps Capsules ... 1574
- Lanoxin Injection ... 1581
- Lanoxin Tablets ... 1587
- Lanoxin Elixir Pediatric ... 1578
- Lanoxin Injection Pediatric ... 1584

Diltiazem Hydrochloride (Potentiated or additive action). Products include:
- Cardizem Injectable ... 1018
- Cardizem Lyo-Ject Syringe ... 1018
- Cardizem Monovial ... 1018
- Cardizem CD Capsules ... 1016
- Tiazac Capsules ... 1378

Doxazosin Mesylate (Potentiated or additive action). Products include:
- Cardura Tablets ... 2668

Enalapril Maleate (Potentiated or additive action; increased risk of hyperkalemia). Products include:
- Lexxel Tablets ... 608
- Vaseretic Tablets ... 2204
- Vasotec Tablets ... 2210

Enalaprilat (Potentiated or additive action; increased risk of hyperkalemia). Products include:
- Enalaprilat Injection ... 863
- Vasotec I.V. Injection ... 2207

Eprosartan Mesylate (Potentiated or additive action). Products include:
- Teveten Tablets ... 3327

Esmolol Hydrochloride (Potentiated or additive action). Products include:
- Brevibloc Injection ... 858

Etodolac (Reduced diuretic, natriuretic, and antihypertensive effects of Moduretic). Products include:
- Lodine ... 3528
- Lodine XL Extended-Release Tablets ... 3530

Felodipine (Potentiated or additive action). Products include:
- Lexxel Tablets ... 608
- Plendil Extended-Release Tablets ... 623

Fenoprofen Calcium (Reduced diuretic, natriuretic, and antihypertensive effects of Moduretic).
No products indexed under this heading.

Fentanyl (Potentiation of orthostatic hypotension). Products include:
- Duragesic Transdermal System ... 1786

Fentanyl Citrate (Potentiation of orthostatic hypotension). Products include:
- Actiq ... 1184

Fludrocortisone Acetate (Hypokalemia). Products include:
- Florinef Acetate Tablets ... 2250

Flurbiprofen (Reduced diuretic, natriuretic, and antihypertensive effects of Moduretic).
No products indexed under this heading.

Fosinopril Sodium (Potentiated or additive action; increased risk of hyperkalemia). Products include:
- Monopril Tablets ... 1091
- Monopril HCT ... 1094

Furosemide (Potentiated or additive action). Products include:
- Furosemide Tablets ... 2284

Glimepiride (Dosage adjustment of the antidiabetic drug may be required). Products include:
- Amaryl Tablets ... 717

Glipizide (Dosage adjustment of the antidiabetic drug may be required). Products include:
- Glucotrol Tablets ... 2692
- Glucotrol XL Extended Release Tablets ... 2693

Glyburide (Dosage adjustment of the antidiabetic drug may be required). Products include:
- DiaBeta Tablets ... 741
- Glucovance Tablets ... 1086

Guanabenz Acetate (Potentiated or additive action).
No products indexed under this heading.

Guanethidine Monosulfate (Potentiated or additive action).
No products indexed under this heading.

Hydralazine Hydrochloride (Potentiated or additive effects).
No products indexed under this heading.

Hydrocodone Bitartrate (Potentiation of orthostatic hypotension). Products include:
- Hycodan ... 1316
- Hycomine Compound Tablets ... 1317
- Hycotuss Expectorant Syrup ... 1318
- Lortab ... 3319
- Lortab Elixir ... 3317
- Maxidone Tablets CIII ... 3399
- Norco 5/325 Tablets CIII ... 3424
- Norco 7.5/325 Tablets CIII ... 3425
- Norco 10/325 Tablets CIII ... 3427
- Norco 10/325 Tablets CIII ... 3425
- Vicodin Tablets ... 516
- Vicodin ES Tablets ... 517
- Vicodin HP Tablets ... 518
- Vicodin Tuss Expectorant ... 519
- Vicoprofen Tablets ... 520
- Zydone Tablets ... 1330

Hydrocodone Polistirex (Potentiation of orthostatic hypotension). Products include:
- Tussionex Pennkinetic Extended-Release Suspension ... 1174

Hydrocortisone (Hypokalemia). Products include:
- Anusol-HC Cream 2.5% ... 2237
- Cipro HC Otic Suspension ... 540
- Cortaid Intensive Therapy Cream ... ⊡717
- Cortaid Maximum Strength Cream ... ⊡717
- Cortisporin Ophthalmic Suspension Sterile ... ⊙297
- Cortizone•5 ... ⊡699
- Cortizone•10 ... ⊡699
- Cortizone•10 Plus Creme ... ⊡700
- Cortizone for Kids Creme ... ⊡699
- Hydrocortone Tablets ... 2106
- Massengill Medicated Soft Cloth Towelette ... ⊡753
- VōSoL HC Otic Solution ... 3356

Hydrocortisone Acetate (Hypokalemia). Products include:
- Analpram-HC ... 1338
- Anusol HC-1 Hydrocortisone Anti-Itch Cream ... ⊡689
- Anusol-HC Suppositories ... 2238
- Cortaid ... ⊡717
- Cortifoam Rectal Foam ... 3170
- Cortisporin-TC Otic Suspension ... 2246
- Hydrocortone Acetate Injectable Suspension ... 2103
- Pramosone ... 1343
- Proctocort Suppositories ... 2264
- ProctoFoam-HC ... 3177
- Terra-Cortril Ophthalmic Suspension ... 2716

Hydrocortisone Sodium Phosphate (Hypokalemia). Products include:
- Hydrocortone Phosphate Injection, Sterile ... 2105

Hydrocortisone Sodium Succinate (Hypokalemia).
No products indexed under this heading.

Hydroflumethiazide (Potentiated or additive action). Products include:
- Diucardin Tablets ... 3494

Hydromorphone Hydrochloride (Potentiation of orthostatic hypotension). Products include:
- Dilaudid ... 441
- Dilaudid Oral Liquid ... 445
- Dilaudid Powder ... 441
- Dilaudid Rectal Suppositories ... 441
- Dilaudid Tablets ... 441
- Dilaudid Tablets - 8 mg ... 445
- Dilaudid-HP ... 443

Ibuprofen (Reduced diuretic, natriuretic, and antihypertensive effects of Moduretic). Products include:
- Advil ... ⊡771
- Children's Advil Oral Suspension ... ⊡773
- Children's Advil Chewable Tablets ... ⊡773
- Advil Cold and Sinus Caplets ... ⊡771
- Advil Cold and Sinus Tablets ... ⊡771
- Advil Flu & Body Ache Caplets ... ⊡772
- Infants' Advil Drops ... ⊡773
- Junior Strength Advil Tablets ... ⊡773
- Junior Strength Advil Chewable Tablets ... ⊡773
- Advil Migraine Liquigels ... ⊡772
- Children's Motrin Oral Suspension and Chewable Tablets ... 2006
- Children's Motrin Cold Oral Suspension ... 2007
- Children's Motrin Oral Suspension ... ⊡643
- Motrin Suspension, Oral Drops, Chewable Tablets, and Caplets ... 2002
- Infants' Motrin Concentrated Drops ... 2006
- Junior Strength Motrin Caplets and Chewable Tablets ... 2006
- Motrin IB Tablets, Caplets, and Gelcaps ... 2002
- Motrin Migraine Pain Caplets ... 2005
- Motrin Sinus Headache Caplets ... 2005
- Vicoprofen Tablets ... 520

Indapamide (Potentiated or additive action). Products include:
- Indapamide Tablets ... 2286

Indomethacin (Reduced diuretic, natriuretic, and antihypertensive effects of Moduretic; increased serum potassium levels of both drugs). Products include:
- Indocin ... 2112

Indomethacin Sodium Trihydrate (Reduced diuretic, natriuretic, and antihypertensive effects of Moduretic; increased serum potassium levels of both drugs). Products include:
- Indocin I.V. ... 2115

Insulin, Human, Zinc Suspension (Altered insulin requirements). Products include:
- Humulin L, 100 Units ... 1937
- Humulin U, 100 Units ... 1943
- Novolin L Human Insulin 10 ml Vials ... 2422

Insulin, Human NPH (Altered insulin requirements). Products include:
- Humulin N, 100 Units ... 1939
- Humulin N NPH Pen ... 1940
- Novolin N Human Insulin 10 ml Vials ... 2422
- Novolin N PenFill ... 2423
- Novolin N Prefilled Syringe Disposable Insulin Delivery System ... 2425

Insulin, Human Regular (Altered insulin requirements). Products include:
- Humulin R Regular (U-500) ... 1943
- Humulin R, 100 Units ... 1941
- Novolin R Human Insulin 10 ml Vials ... 2423
- Novolin R PenFill ... 2423
- Novolin R Prefilled Syringe Disposable Insulin Delivery System ... 2425
- Velosulin BR Human Insulin 10 ml Vials ... 2435

Insulin, Human Regular and Human NPH Mixture (Altered insulin requirements). Products include:
- Humulin 50/50, 100 Units ... 1934
- Humulin 70/30, 100 Units ... 1935
- Humulin 70/30 Pen ... 1936
- Novolin 70/30 Human Insulin 10 ml Vials ... 2421
- Novolin 70/30 PenFill ... 2423
- Novolin 70/30 Prefilled Disposable Insulin Delivery System ... 2425

Insulin, NPH (Altered insulin requirements). Products include:
- Iletin II, NPH (Pork), 100 Units ... 1946

Insulin, Regular (Altered insulin requirements). Products include:
- Iletin II, Regular (Pork), 100 Units ... 1947

Insulin, Zinc Crystals (Altered insulin requirements).
No products indexed under this heading.

Insulin, Zinc Suspension (Altered insulin requirements). Products include:
- Iletin II, Lente (Pork), 100 Units ... 1945

Insulin Aspart, Human Regular (Altered insulin requirements).
No products indexed under this heading.

Insulin glargine (Altered insulin requirements). Products include:
- Lantus Injection ... 742

Insulin Lispro, Human (Altered insulin requirements). Products include:
- Humalog ... 1926
- Humalog Mix 75/25 Pen ... 1928

Insulin Lispro Protamine, Human (Altered insulin requirements). Products include:
- Humalog Mix 75/25 Pen ... 1928

Irbesartan (Potentiated or additive action). Products include:
- Avalide Tablets ... 1070
- Avapro Tablets ... 1074
- Avapro Tablets ... 3076

Isradipine (Potentiated or additive action). Products include:
- DynaCirc Capsules ... 2921
- DynaCirc CR Tablets ... 2923

Ketoprofen (Reduced diuretic, natriuretic, and antihypertensive effects of Moduretic). Products include:
- Orudis Capsules ... 3548
- Orudis KT Tablets ... ⊡778
- Oruvail Capsules ... 3548

Ketorolac Tromethamine (Reduced diuretic, natriuretic, and antihypertensive effects of Moduretic). Products include:
- Acular Ophthalmic Solution ... 544
- Acular PF Ophthalmic Solution ... 544
- Toradol ... 3018

Labetalol Hydrochloride (Potentiated or additive action). Products include:
- Normodyne Injection ... 3135
- Normodyne Tablets ... 3137

Levorphanol Tartrate (Potentiation of orthostatic hypotension). Products include:
- Levo-Dromoran ... 1734
- Levorphanol Tartrate Tablets ... 3059

Lisinopril (Potentiated or additive action; increased risk of hyperkalemia). Products include:
- Prinivil Tablets ... 2164
- Prinzide Tablets ... 2168
- Zestoretic Tablets ... 695
- Zestril Tablets ... 698

Lithium Carbonate (High risk of lithium toxicity). Products include:
- Eskalith ... 1527
- Lithium Carbonate ... 3061
- Lithobid Slow-Release Tablets ... 3255

Lithium Citrate (High risk of lithium toxicity). Products include:
- Lithium Citrate Syrup ... 3061

Losartan Potassium (Potentiated or additive action). Products include:
- Cozaar Tablets ... 2067
- Hyzaar ... 2109

Mecamylamine Hydrochloride (Potentiated or additive action). Products include:
- Inversine Tablets ... 1850

Meclofenamate Sodium (Reduced diuretic, natriuretic, and antihypertensive effects of Moduretic).
No products indexed under this heading.

Mefenamic Acid (Reduced diuretic, natriuretic, and antihypertensive effects of Moduretic). Products include:
- Ponstel Capsules ... 1356

Meloxicam (Reduced diuretic, natriuretic, and antihypertensive effects of Moduretic). Products include:
- Mobic Tablets ... 1054

Meperidine Hydrochloride (Potentiation of orthostatic hypotension). Products include:
- Demerol ... 3079
- Mepergan Injection ... 3539

Mephobarbital (Potentiation of orthostatic hypotension).
No products indexed under this heading.

Metformin Hydrochloride (Dosage adjustment of the antidiabetic drug may be required). Products include:

Glucophage Tablets 1080
Glucophage XR Tablets 1080
Glucovance Tablets 1086

Methadone Hydrochloride (Potentiation of orthostatic hypotension). Products include:
Dolophine Hydrochloride Tablets 3056

Methyclothiazide (Potentiated or additive action).
No products indexed under this heading.

Methyldopa (Potentiated or additive action). Products include:
Aldoclor Tablets 2035
Aldomet Tablets 2037
Aldoril Tablets 2039

Methyldopate Hydrochloride (Potentiated or additive action).
No products indexed under this heading.

Methylprednisolone Acetate (Hypokalemia). Products include:
Depo-Medrol Injectable Suspension 2795

Methylprednisolone Sodium Succinate (Hypokalemia). Products include:
Solu-Medrol Sterile Powder 2855

Metolazone (Potentiated or additive action). Products include:
Mykrox Tablets 1168
Zaroxolyn Tablets 1177

Metoprolol Succinate (Potentiated or additive action). Products include:
Toprol-XL Tablets 651

Metoprolol Tartrate (Potentiated or additive action).
No products indexed under this heading.

Metyrosine (Potentiated or additive action). Products include:
Demser Capsules 2085

Mibefradil Dihydrochloride (Potentiated or additive action).
No products indexed under this heading.

Miglitol (Dosage adjustment of the antidiabetic drug may be required). Products include:
Glyset Tablets 2821

Minoxidil (Potentiated or additive action). Products include:
Rogaine Extra Strength for Men Topical Solution .... ◙ 721
Rogaine for Women Topical Solution .... ◙ 721

Moexipril Hydrochloride (Potentiated or additive action; increased risk of hyperkalemia). Products include:
Uniretic Tablets 3178
Univasc Tablets 3181

Morphine Sulfate (Potentiation of orthostatic hypotension). Products include:
Astramorph/PF Injection, USP (Preservative-Free) 594
Duramorph Injection 1312
Infumorph 200 and Infumorph 500 Sterile Solutions 1314
Kadian Capsules 1335
MS Contin Tablets 2896
MSIR 2898
Oramorph SR Tablets 3062
Roxanol 3066

Nabumetone (Reduced diuretic, natriuretic, and antihypertensive effects of Moduretic). Products include:
Relafen Tablets 1617

Nadolol (Potentiated or additive action). Products include:
Corgard Tablets 2245
Corzide 40/5 Tablets 2247
Corzide 80/5 Tablets 2247
Nadolol Tablets 2288

Naproxen (Reduced diuretic, natriuretic, and antihypertensive effects of Moduretic). Products include:
EC-Naprosyn Delayed-Release Tablets 2967
Naprosyn Suspension 2967
Naprosyn Tablets 2967

Naproxen Sodium (Reduced diuretic, natriuretic, and antihypertensive effects of Moduretic). Products include:
Aleve Tablets, Caplets and Gelcaps .... ◙ 602
Aleve Cold & Sinus Caplets .... ◙ 603
Anaprox Tablets 2967
Anaprox DS Tablets 2967
Naprelan Tablets 1293

Nicardipine Hydrochloride (Potentiated or additive action). Products include:
Cardene I.V. 3485

Nifedipine (Potentiated or additive action). Products include:
Adalat CC Tablets 877
Procardia Capsules 2708
Procardia XL Extended Release Tablets 2710

Nisoldipine (Potentiated or additive action). Products include:
Sular Tablets 688

Nitroglycerin (Potentiated or additive action). Products include:
Nitro-Dur Transdermal Infusion System 3134
Nitro-Dur Transdermal Infusion System 1834
Nitrolingual Pumpspray 1355
Nitrostat Tablets 2658

Norepinephrine Bitartrate (Possible decreased response to pressor amines).
No products indexed under this heading.

Oxaprozin (Reduced diuretic, natriuretic, and antihypertensive effects of Moduretic).
No products indexed under this heading.

Oxycodone Hydrochloride (Potentiation of orthostatic hypotension). Products include:
OxyContin Tablets 2912
OxyFast Oral Concentrate Solution 2916
OxyIR Capsules 2916
Percocet Tablets 1326
Percodan Tablets 1327
Percolone Tablets 1327
Roxicodone 3067
Tylox Capsules 2597

Penbutolol Sulfate (Potentiated or additive action).
No products indexed under this heading.

Pentobarbital Sodium (Potentiation of orthostatic hypotension). Products include:
Nembutal Sodium Solution 485

Perindopril Erbumine (Potentiated or additive action; increased risk of hyperkalemia). Products include:
Aceon Tablets (2 mg, 4 mg, 8 mg) 3249

Phenobarbital (Potentiation of orthostatic hypotension). Products include:
Arco-Lase Plus Tablets 592
Donnatal 2929
Donnatal Extentabs 2930

Phenoxybenzamine Hydrochloride (Potentiated or additive action). Products include:
Dibenzyline Capsules 3457

Phentolamine Mesylate (Potentiated or additive action).
No products indexed under this heading.

Phenylbutazone (Reduced diuretic, natriuretic, and antihypertensive effects of Moduretic).
No products indexed under this heading.

Pindolol (Potentiated or additive action).
No products indexed under this heading.

Pioglitazone Hydrochloride (Dosage adjustment of the antidiabetic drug may be required). Products include:
Actos Tablets 3275

Piroxicam (Reduced diuretic, natriuretic, and antihypertensive effects of Moduretic). Products include:
Feldene Capsules 2685

Polythiazide (Potentiated or additive action). Products include:
Minizide Capsules 2700
Renese Tablets 2712

Potassium Acid Phosphate (Potential for rapid increase in serum potassium levels). Products include:
K-Phos Original (Sodium Free) Tablets 947

Potassium Bicarbonate (Potential for rapid increase in serum potassium levels).
No products indexed under this heading.

Potassium Chloride (Potential for rapid increase in serum potassium levels). Products include:
Chlor-3 1361
Colyte with Flavor Packs for Oral Solution 3170
GoLYTELY and Pineapple Flavor GoLYTELY for Oral Solution 1068
K-Dur Microburst Release System ER Tablets 1832
Klor-Con M20/Klor-Con M10 Tablets 3329
K-Lor Powder Packets 469
K-Tab Filmtab Tablets 470
Micro-K 3311
NuLYTELY, Cherry Flavor, Lemon-Lime Flavor, and Orange Flavor NuLYTELY for Oral Solution 1068
Rum-K 1363

Potassium Citrate (Potential for rapid increase in serum potassium levels). Products include:
Urocit-K Tablets 2232

Potassium Gluconate (Potential for rapid increase in serum potassium levels).
No products indexed under this heading.

Potassium Phosphate (Potential for rapid increase in serum potassium levels). Products include:
K-Phos Neutral Tablets 946

Prazosin Hydrochloride (Potentiated or additive action). Products include:
Minipress Capsules 2699
Minizide Capsules 2700

Prednisolone Acetate (Hypokalemia). Products include:
Blephamide Ophthalmic Ointment 547
Blephamide Ophthalmic Suspension 548
Poly-Pred Liquifilm Ophthalmic Suspension .... ⊙ 245
Pred Forte Ophthalmic Suspension .... ⊙ 246
Pred Mild Sterile Ophthalmic Suspension .... ⊙ 249
Pred-G Ophthalmic Suspension .... ⊙ 247
Pred-G Sterile Ophthalmic Ointment .... ⊙ 248

Prednisolone Sodium Phosphate (Hypokalemia). Products include:
Pediapred Oral Solution 1170

Prednisolone Tebutate (Hypokalemia).
No products indexed under this heading.

Prednisone (Hypokalemia). Products include:
Prednisone 3064

Propoxyphene Hydrochloride (Potentiation of orthostatic hypotension). Products include:
Darvon Pulvules 1909
Darvon Compound-65 Pulvules 1910

Propoxyphene Napsylate (Potentiation of orthostatic hypotension). Products include:
Darvon-N/Darvocet-N 1907
Darvon-N Tablets 1912

Propranolol Hydrochloride (Potentiated or additive action). Products include:
Inderal 3513
Inderal LA Long-Acting Capsules 3516
Inderide Tablets 3517
Inderide LA Long-Acting Capsules 3519

Quinapril Hydrochloride (Potentiated or additive action; increased risk of hyperkalemia). Products include:
Accupril Tablets 2611
Accuretic Tablets 2614

Ramipril (Potentiated or additive action; increased risk of hyperkalemia). Products include:
Altace Capsules 2233

Rauwolfia serpentina (Potentiated or additive action).
No products indexed under this heading.

Remifentanil Hydrochloride (Potentiation of orthostatic hypotension).
No products indexed under this heading.

Repaglinide (Dosage adjustment of the antidiabetic drug may be required). Products include:
Prandin Tablets (0.5, 1, and 2 mg) 2432

Rescinnamine (Potentiated or additive action).
No products indexed under this heading.

Reserpine (Potentiated or additive action).
No products indexed under this heading.

Rofecoxib (Reduced diuretic, natriuretic, and antihypertensive effects of Moduretic). Products include:
Vioxx 2213

Rosiglitazone Maleate (Dosage adjustment of the antidiabetic drug may be required). Products include:
Avandia Tablets 1490

Secobarbital Sodium (Potentiation of orthostatic hypotension).
No products indexed under this heading.

Sodium Nitroprusside (Potentiated or additive action).
No products indexed under this heading.

Sotalol Hydrochloride (Potentiated or additive action). Products include:
Betapace Tablets 950
Betapace AF Tablets 954

Spirapril Hydrochloride (Potentiated or additive action; increased risk of hyperkalemia).
No products indexed under this heading.

Spironolactone (Potential for rapid increase in serum potassium levels).
No products indexed under this heading.

Sufentanil Citrate (Potentiation of orthostatic hypotension).
No products indexed under this heading.

Sulindac (Reduced diuretic, natriuretic, and antihypertensive effects of Moduretic). Products include:
Clinoril Tablets 2053

Telmisartan (Potentiated or additive action). Products include:
Micardis Tablets 1049
Micardis HCT Tablets 1051

Terazosin Hydrochloride (Potentiated or additive action). Products include:
Hytrin Capsules 464

Thiamylal Sodium (Potentiation of orthostatic hypotension).
No products indexed under this heading.

Timolol Maleate (Potentiated or additive action). Products include:
Blocadren Tablets 2046
Cosopt Sterile Ophthalmic Solution 2065
Timolide Tablets 2187
Timolol GFS .... ⊙ 266
Timoptic in Ocudose 2192
Timoptic Sterile Ophthalmic Solution 2190
Timoptic-XE Sterile Ophthalmic Gel Forming Solution 2194

Tolazamide (Dosage adjustment of the antidiabetic drug may be required).
No products indexed under this heading.

Tolbutamide (Dosage adjustment of the antidiabetic drug may be required).
No products indexed under this heading.

Tolmetin Sodium (Reduced diuretic, natriuretic, and antihypertensive effects of Moduretic). Products include:
- Tolectin 2589

Torsemide (Potentiated or additive action; increased risk of hyperkalemia). Products include:
- Demadex Tablets and Injection 2965

Trandolapril (Potentiated or additive action; increased risk of hyperkalemia). Products include:
- Mavik Tablets 478
- Tarka Tablets 508

Triamcinolone (Hypokalemia).
No products indexed under this heading.

Triamcinolone Acetonide (Hypokalemia). Products include:
- Azmacort Inhalation Aerosol 728
- Nasacort Nasal Inhaler 750
- Nasacort AQ Nasal Spray 752
- Tri-Nasal Spray 2274

Triamcinolone Diacetate (Hypokalemia).
No products indexed under this heading.

Triamcinolone Hexacetonide (Hypokalemia).
No products indexed under this heading.

Triamterene (Potential for rapid increase in serum potassium levels). Products include:
- Dyazide Capsules 1515
- Dyrenium Capsules 3458
- Maxzide 1008

Trimethaphan Camsylate (Potentiated or additive action).
No products indexed under this heading.

Troglitazone (Dosage adjustment of the antidiabetic drug may be required).
No products indexed under this heading.

Tubocurarine Chloride (Increased responsiveness to tubocurarine).
No products indexed under this heading.

Valsartan (Potentiated or additive action). Products include:
- Diovan Capsules 2337
- Diovan HCT Tablets 2338

Verapamil Hydrochloride (Potentiated or additive action). Products include:
- Covera-HS Tablets 3199
- Isoptin SR Tablets 467
- Tarka Tablets 508
- Verelan Capsules 3184
- Verelan PM Capsules 3186

Food Interactions

Alcohol (Potentiation of orthostatic hypotension).

Diet, potassium-rich (Potential for rapid increases in serum potassium levels).

MOISTURE EYES EYE DROPS
(Glycerin, Propylene Glycol) .... ⊙252
None cited in PDR database.

MOISTURE EYES PRESERVATIVE FREE EYE DROPS
(Propylene Glycol) .... ⊙253
None cited in PDR database.

MOISTURE EYES PM PRESERVATIVE FREE EYE OINTMENT
(Mineral Oil, Petrolatum, White) .... ⊙253
None cited in PDR database.

MOMENTUM BACKACHE RELIEF EXTRA STRENGTH CAPLETS
(Magnesium Salicylate) .... ◘666
May interact with oral anticoagulants, oral hypoglycemic agents, and certain other agents. Compounds in these categories include:

Acarbose (Concurrent use with antidiabetic agents should be avoided). Products include:
- Precose Tablets 906

Antiarthritic Drugs, unspecified (Concurrent use with certain unspecified arthritis drugs should be avoided).

Chlorpropamide (Concurrent use with antidiabetic agents should be avoided). Products include:
- Diabinese Tablets 2680

Dicumarol (Concurrent use with anticoagulant agents should be avoided).
No products indexed under this heading.

Glimepiride (Concurrent use with antidiabetic agents should be avoided). Products include:
- Amaryl Tablets 717

Glipizide (Concurrent use with antidiabetic agents should be avoided). Products include:
- Glucotrol Tablets 2692
- Glucotrol XL Extended Release Tablets 2693

Glyburide (Concurrent use with antidiabetic agents should be avoided). Products include:
- DiaBeta Tablets 741
- Glucovance Tablets 1086

Metformin Hydrochloride (Concurrent use with antidiabetic agents should be avoided). Products include:
- Glucophage Tablets 1080
- Glucophage XR Tablets 1080
- Glucovance Tablets 1086

Miglitol (Concurrent use with antidiabetic agents should be avoided). Products include:
- Glyset Tablets 2821

Pioglitazone Hydrochloride (Concurrent use with antidiabetic agents should be avoided). Products include:
- Actos Tablets 3275

Probenecid (Concurrent use with drugs for gout, such as probenecid, should be avoided).
No products indexed under this heading.

Repaglinide (Concurrent use with antidiabetic agents should be avoided). Products include:
- Prandin Tablets (0.5, 1, and 2 mg) 2432

Rosiglitazone Maleate (Concurrent use with antidiabetic agents should be avoided). Products include:
- Avandia Tablets 1490

Sulfinpyrazone (Concurrent use with drugs for gout, such as sulfinpyrazone, should be avoided).
No products indexed under this heading.

Tolazamide (Concurrent use with antidiabetic agents should be avoided).
No products indexed under this heading.

Tolbutamide (Concurrent use with antidiabetic agents should be avoided).
No products indexed under this heading.

Troglitazone (Concurrent use with antidiabetic agents should be avoided).
No products indexed under this heading.

Warfarin Sodium (Concurrent use with anticoagulant agents should be avoided). Products include:
- Coumadin for Injection 1243
- Coumadin Tablets 1243
- Warfarin Sodium Tablets, USP 3302

Food Interactions

Alcohol (Chronic heavy alcohol users, 3 or more drinks per day, should consult their physician for advice on when and how they should take pain relievers/fever reducers including salicylates).

MONOCAL TABLETS
(Calcium Carbonate, Sodium Monofluorophosphate) 2223
None cited in PDR database.

MONOCLATE-P CONCENTRATE
(Antihemophilic Factor (Human)) 793
None cited in PDR database.

MONODOX CAPSULES
(Doxycycline Monohydrate) 2442
May interact with antacids containing aluminum, calcium and magnesium, barbiturates, oral anticoagulants, oral contraceptives, penicillins, phenytoin, and certain other agents. Compounds in these categories include:

Aluminum Carbonate (Absorption of tetracyclines is impaired).
No products indexed under this heading.

Aluminum Hydroxide (Absorption of tetracyclines is impaired). Products include:
- Amphojel Suspension (Mint Flavor) .... ◘789
- Gaviscon Extra Strength Liquid .... ◘751
- Gaviscon Extra Strength Tablets .... ◘751
- Gaviscon Regular Strength Liquid .... ◘751
- Gaviscon Regular Strength Tablets .... ◘750
- Maalox Antacid/Anti-Gas Oral Suspension .... ◘673
- Maalox Max Maximum Strength Antacid/Anti-Gas Liquid 2300
- Maalox Regular Strength Antacid/Antigas Liquid 2300
- Mylanta 1813
- Vanquish Caplets .... ◘617

Amoxicillin Trihydrate (Interference with penicillins' bactericidal action).

Ampicillin (Interference with penicillins' bactericidal action).
No products indexed under this heading.

Ampicillin Sodium (Interference with penicillins' bactericidal action). Products include:
- Unasyn for Injection 2728

Ampicillin Trihydrate (Interference with penicillins' bactericidal action).
No products indexed under this heading.

Aprobarbital (Decreases the half-life of doxycycline).
No products indexed under this heading.

Azlocillin Sodium (Interference with penicillins' bactericidal action).
No products indexed under this heading.

Bacampicillin Hydrochloride (Interference with penicillins' bactericidal action).
No products indexed under this heading.

Butabarbital (Decreases the half-life of doxycycline).
No products indexed under this heading.

Butalbital (Decreases the half-life of doxycycline). Products include:
- Phrenilin 578
- Sedapap Tablets 50 mg/650 mg 2225

Carbamazepine (Decreases the half-life of doxycycline). Products include:
- Carbatrol Capsules 3234
- Tegretol/Tegretol-XR 2404

Carbenicillin Disodium (Interference with penicillins' bactericidal action).
No products indexed under this heading.

Carbenicillin Indanyl Sodium (Interference with penicillins' bactericidal action). Products include:
- Geocillin Tablets 2687

Desogestrel (Concurrent use may render oral contraceptives less effective). Products include:
- Cyclessa Tablets 2450
- Desogen Tablets 2458
- Mircette Tablets 2470
- Ortho-Cept 21 Tablets 2546
- Ortho-Cept 28 Tablets 2546

Dicloxacillin Sodium (Interference with penicillins' bactericidal action).
No products indexed under this heading.

Dicumarol (Depressed plasma prothrombin activity).
No products indexed under this heading.

Ethinyl Estradiol (Concurrent use may render oral contraceptives less effective). Products include:
- Alesse-21 Tablets 3468
- Alesse-28 Tablets 3473
- Brevicon 28-Day Tablets 3380
- Cyclessa Tablets 2450
- Desogen Tablets 2458
- Estinyl Tablets 3112
- Estrostep 2627
- femhrt Tablets 2635
- Levlen 962
- Levlite 21 Tablets 962
- Levlite 28 Tablets 962
- Levora Tablets 3389
- Loestrin 21 Tablets 2642
- Loestrin Fe Tablets 2642
- Lo/Ovral Tablets 3532
- Lo/Ovral-28 Tablets 3538
- Low-Ogestrel-28 Tablets 3392
- Microgestin Fe 1.5/30 Tablets 3407
- Microgestin Fe 1/20 Tablets 3400
- Mircette Tablets 2470
- Modicon 2563
- Necon 3415
- Nordette-28 Tablets 2257
- Norinyl 1 +35 28-Day Tablets 3380
- Ogestrel 0.5/50-28 Tablets 3428
- Ortho-Cept 21 Tablets 2546
- Ortho-Cept 28 Tablets 2546
- Ortho-Cyclen/Ortho Tri-Cyclen 2573
- Ortho-Novum 2563
- Ovcon 3364
- Ovral Tablets 3551
- Ovral-28 Tablets 3552
- Tri-Levlen 962
- Tri-Norinyl-28 Tablets 3433
- Triphasil-21 Tablets 3600
- Triphasil-28 Tablets 3605
- Trivora Tablets 3439
- Yasmin 28 Tablets 980
- Zovia 3449

Ethynodiol Diacetate (Concurrent use may render oral contraceptives less effective). Products include:
- Zovia 3449

Fosphenytoin Sodium (Decreases the half-life of doxycycline). Products include:
- Cerebyx Injection 2619

Levonorgestrel (Concurrent use may render oral contraceptives less effective). Products include:
- Alesse-21 Tablets 3468
- Alesse-28 Tablets 3473
- Levlen 962
- Levlite 21 Tablets 962
- Levlite 28 Tablets 962
- Levora Tablets 3389
- Mirena Intrauterine System 974
- Nordette-28 Tablets 2257
- Norplant System 3543
- Tri-Levlen 962
- Triphasil-21 Tablets 3600
- Triphasil-28 Tablets 3605
- Trivora Tablets 3439

Magaldrate (Absorption of tetracyclines is impaired).
No products indexed under this heading.

Magnesium Hydroxide (Absorption of tetracyclines is impaired). Products include:
Ex•Lax Milk of Magnesia Liquid ... ▣670
Maalox Antacid/Anti-Gas Oral Suspension ... ▣673
Maalox Max Maximum Strength Antacid/Anti-Gas Liquid ... 2300
Maalox Regular Strength Antacid/Antigas Liquid ... 2300
Mylanta Fast-Acting ... 1813
Mylanta ... 1813
Pepcid Complete Chewable Tablets ... 1815
Phillips' Chewable Tablets ... ▣615
Phillips' Milk of Magnesia Liquid (Original, Cherry, & Mint) ... ▣616
Rolaids Tablets ... ▣706
Extra Strength Rolaids Tablets ... ▣706
Vanquish Caplets ... ▣617

Magnesium Oxide (Absorption of tetracyclines is impaired). Products include:
Beelith Tablets ... 946
Mag-Ox 400 Tablets ... 1024
Uro-Mag Capsules ... 1024

Mephobarbital (Decreases the half-life of doxycycline).
No products indexed under this heading.

Mestranol (Concurrent use may render oral contraceptives less effective). Products include:
Necon 1/50 Tablets ... 3415
Norinyl 1 + 50 28-Day Tablets ... 3380
Ortho-Novum 1/50□28 Tablets ... 2556

Methoxyflurane (Potential for fatal renal toxicity).
No products indexed under this heading.

Mezlocillin Sodium (Interference with penicillins' bactericidal action).
No products indexed under this heading.

Nafcillin Sodium (Interference with penicillins' bactericidal action).
No products indexed under this heading.

Norethindrone (Concurrent use may render oral contraceptives less effective). Products include:
Brevicon 28-Day Tablets ... 3380
Micronor Tablets ... 2543
Modicon ... 2563
Necon ... 3415
Norinyl 1 +35 28-Day Tablets ... 3380
Norinyl 1 + 50 28-Day Tablets ... 3380
Nor-QD Tablets ... 3423
Ortho-Novum ... 2563
Ortho-Novum 1/50□28 Tablets ... 2556
Ovcon ... 3364
Tri-Norinyl-28 Tablets ... 3433

Norethynodrel (Concurrent use may render oral contraceptives less effective).
No products indexed under this heading.

Norgestimate (Concurrent use may render oral contraceptives less effective). Products include:
Ortho-Cyclen/Ortho Tri-Cyclen ... 2573
Ortho-Prefest Tablets ... 2570

Norgestrel (Concurrent use may render oral contraceptives less effective). Products include:
Lo/Ovral Tablets ... 3532
Lo/Ovral-28 Tablets ... 3538
Low-Ogestrel-28 Tablets ... 3392
Ogestrel 0.5/50-28 Tablets ... 3428
Ovral Tablets ... 3551
Ovral-28 Tablets ... 3552
Ovrette Tablets ... 3552

Penicillin G Benzathine (Interference with penicillins' bactericidal action). Products include:
Bicillin C-R 900/300 Injection ... 2240
Bicillin C-R Injection ... 2238
Bicillin L-A Injection ... 2242
Permapen Isoject ... 2706

Penicillin G Potassium (Interference with penicillins' bactericidal action). Products include:
Pfizerpen for Injection ... 2707

Penicillin G Procaine (Interference with penicillins' bactericidal action). Products include:
Bicillin C-R 900/300 Injection ... 2240
Bicillin C-R Injection ... 2238

Penicillin G Sodium (Interference with penicillins' bactericidal action).
No products indexed under this heading.

Penicillin V Potassium (Interference with penicillins' bactericidal action).
No products indexed under this heading.

Pentobarbital Sodium (Decreases the half-life of doxycycline). Products include:
Nembutal Sodium Solution ... 485

Phenobarbital (Decreases the half-life of doxycycline). Products include:
Arco-Lase Plus Tablets ... 592
Donnatal ... 2929
Donnatal Extentabs ... 2930

Phenytoin (Decreases the half-life of doxycycline). Products include:
Dilantin Infatabs ... 2624
Dilantin-125 Oral Suspension ... 2625

Phenytoin Sodium (Decreases the half-life of doxycycline). Products include:
Dilantin Kapseals ... 2622

Secobarbital Sodium (Decreases the half-life of doxycycline).
No products indexed under this heading.

Thiamylal Sodium (Decreases the half-life of doxycycline).
No products indexed under this heading.

Ticarcillin Disodium (Interference with penicillins' bactericidal action). Products include:
Timentin Injection- ADD-Vantage Vial ... 1661
Timentin Injection-Galaxy Container ... 1664
Timentin Injection-Pharmacy Bulk Package ... 1666
Timentin for Intravenous Administration ... 1658

Warfarin Sodium (Depressed plasma prothrombin activity). Products include:
Coumadin for Injection ... 1243
Coumadin Tablets ... 1243
Warfarin Sodium Tablets, USP ... 3302

MONONINE CONCENTRATE
(Factor IX (Human)) ... 794
None cited in PDR database.

MONOPRIL TABLETS
(Fosinopril Sodium) ... 1091
May interact with diuretics, lithium preparations, potassium preparations, potassium sparing diuretics, and certain other agents. Compounds in these categories include:

Aluminum Hydroxide (Co-administration with an antacid containing aluminum hydroxide, magnesium hydroxide, and simethicone has resulted in reduced serum levels and urinary excretion of fosinoprilat; dosing should be separated by two hours). Products include:
Amphojel Suspension (Mint Flavor) ... ▣789
Gaviscon Extra Strength Liquid ... ▣751
Gaviscon Extra Strength Tablets ... ▣751
Gaviscon Regular Strength Liquid ... ▣751
Gaviscon Regular Strength Tablets ... ▣750
Maalox Antacid/Anti-Gas Oral Suspension ... ▣673
Maalox Max Maximum Strength Antacid/Anti-Gas Liquid ... 2300
Maalox Regular Strength Antacid/Antigas Liquid ... 2300
Mylanta ... 1813
Vanquish Caplets ... ▣617

Amiloride Hydrochloride (Fosinopril attenuates diuretic-induced potassium loss; concomitant use can lead to hyperkalemia; frequent monitoring of serum potassium is recommended if used concurrently; co-administration can result in excessive hypotension). Products include:
Midamor Tablets ... 2136
Moduretic Tablets ... 2138

Bendroflumethiazide (Co-administration of fosinopril in patients on diuretics, especially those in who diuretic therapy was recently instituted, may occasionally experience excessive hypotension; antihypertensive effects of fosinopril are augmented by antihypertensive agents that cause renin release). Products include:
Corzide 40/5 Tablets ... 2247
Corzide 80/5 Tablets ... 2247

Bumetanide (Co-administration of fosinopril in patients on diuretics, especially those in who diuretic therapy was recently instituted, may occasionally experience excessive hypotension; antihypertensive effects of fosinopril are augmented by antihypertensive agents that cause renin release).
No products indexed under this heading.

Chlorothiazide (Co-administration of fosinopril in patients on diuretics, especially those in who diuretic therapy was recently instituted, may occasionally experience excessive hypotension; antihypertensive effects of fosinopril are augmented by antihypertensive agents that cause renin release). Products include:
Aldoclor Tablets ... 2035
Diuril Oral ... 2087

Chlorothiazide Sodium (Co-administration of fosinopril in patients on diuretics, especially those in who diuretic therapy was recently instituted, may occasionally experience excessive hypotension; antihypertensive effects of fosinopril are augmented by antihypertensive agents that cause renin release). Products include:
Diuril Sodium Intravenous ... 2086

Chlorthalidone (Co-administration of fosinopril in patients on diuretics, especially those in who diuretic therapy was recently instituted, may occasionally experience excessive hypotension; antihypertensive effects of fosinopril are augmented by antihypertensive agents that cause renin release). Products include:
Clorpres Tablets ... 1002
Combipres Tablets ... 1040
Tenoretic Tablets ... 690

Ethacrynic Acid (Co-administration of fosinopril in patients on diuretics, especially those in who diuretic therapy was recently instituted, may occasionally experience excessive hypotension; antihypertensive effects of fosinopril are augmented by antihypertensive agents that cause renin release). Products include:
Edecrin Tablets ... 2091

Furosemide (Co-administration of fosinopril in patients on diuretics, especially those in who diuretic therapy was recently instituted, may occasionally experience excessive hypotension; antihypertensive effects of fosinopril are augmented by antihypertensive agents that cause renin release). Products include:
Furosemide Tablets ... 2284

Hydrochlorothiazide (Co-administration of fosinopril in patients on diuretics, especially those in who diuretic therapy was recently instituted, may occasionally experience excessive hypotension; antihypertensive effects of fosinopril are augmented by antihypertensive agents that cause renin release). Products include:
Accuretic Tablets ... 2614
Aldoril Tablets ... 2039
Atacand HCT Tablets ... 597
Avalide Tablets ... 1070
Diovan HCT Tablets ... 2338
Dyazide Capsules ... 1515
HydroDIURIL Tablets ... 2108
Hyzaar ... 2109
Inderide Tablets ... 3517
Inderide LA Long-Acting Capsules ... 3519
Lotensin HCT Tablets ... 2367
Maxzide ... 1008
Micardis HCT Tablets ... 1051
Microzide Capsules ... 3414
Moduretic Tablets ... 2138
Monopril HCT ... 1094
Prinzide Tablets ... 2168
Timolide Tablets ... 2187
Uniretic Tablets ... 3178
Vaseretic Tablets ... 2204
Zestoretic Tablets ... 695
Ziac Tablets ... 1887

Hydroflumethiazide (Co-administration of fosinopril in patients on diuretics, especially those in who diuretic therapy was recently instituted, may occasionally experience excessive hypotension; antihypertensive effects of fosinopril are augmented by antihypertensive agents that cause renin release). Products include:
Diucardin Tablets ... 3494

Indapamide (Co-administration of fosinopril in patients on diuretics, especially those in who diuretic therapy was recently instituted, may occasionally experience excessive hypotension; antihypertensive effects of fosinopril are augmented by antihypertensive agents that cause renin release). Products include:
Indapamide Tablets ... 2286

Lithium Carbonate (Co-administration of lithium with drugs that cause elimination of sodium, including ACE inhibitors, can lead to lithium toxicity). Products include:
Eskalith ... 1527
Lithium Carbonate ... 3061
Lithobid Slow-Release Tablets ... 3255

Lithium Citrate (Co-administration of lithium with drugs that cause elimination of sodium, including ACE inhibitors, can lead to lithium toxicity). Products include:
Lithium Citrate Syrup ... 3061

Magnesium Hydroxide (Co-administration with an antacid containing aluminum hydroxide, magnesium hydroxide, and simethicone has resulted in reduced serum levels and urinary excretion of fosinoprilat; dosing should be separated by two hours). Products include:
Ex•Lax Milk of Magnesia Liquid ... ▣670
Maalox Antacid/Anti-Gas Oral Suspension ... ▣673
Maalox Max Maximum Strength Antacid/Anti-Gas Liquid ... 2300
Maalox Regular Strength Antacid/Antigas Liquid ... 2300
Mylanta Fast-Acting ... 1813
Mylanta ... 1813
Pepcid Complete Chewable Tablets ... 1815
Phillips' Chewable Tablets ... ▣615
Phillips' Milk of Magnesia Liquid (Original, Cherry, & Mint) ... ▣616
Rolaids Tablets ... ▣706
Extra Strength Rolaids Tablets ... ▣706
Vanquish Caplets ... ▣617

Methyclothiazide (Co-administration of fosinopril in patients on diuretics, especially those in who diuretic therapy was recently instituted, may occasionally experience excessive hypotension; antihypertensive effects of fosinopril are augmented by antihypertensive agents that cause renin release).
No products indexed under this heading.

Metolazone (Co-administration of fosinopril in patients on diuretics, especially those in who diuretic therapy was recently instituted, may occasionally experience excessive

IMPORTANT NOTE: Always consult each drug listing in the patient's regimen for possible interactions.

hypotension; antihypertensive effects of fosinopril are augmented by antihypertensive agents that cause renin release). Products include:

Mykrox Tablets 1168
Zaroxolyn Tablets 1177

Polythiazide (Co-administration of fosinopril in patients on diuretics, especially those in who diuretic therapy was recently instituted, may occasionally experience excessive hypotension; antihypertensive effects of fosinopril are augmented by antihypertensive agents that cause renin release). Products include:

Minizide Capsules 2700
Renese Tablets 2712

Potassium Acid Phosphate (Concomitant use of potassium-containing salt substitute or potassium supplements can lead to hyperkalemia; frequent monitoring of serum potassium is recommended if used concurrently). Products include:

K-Phos Original (Sodium Free) Tablets 947

Potassium Bicarbonate (Concomitant use of potassium-containing salt substitute or potassium supplements can lead to hyperkalemia; frequent monitoring of serum potassium is recommended if used concurrently).

No products indexed under this heading.

Potassium Chloride (Concomitant use of potassium-containing salt substitute or potassium supplements can lead to hyperkalemia; frequent monitoring of serum potassium is recommended if used concurrently). Products include:

Chlor-3 1361
Colyte with Flavor Packs for Oral Solution 3170
GoLYTELY and Pineapple Flavor GoLYTELY for Oral Solution 1068
K-Dur Microburst Release System ER Tablets 1832
Klor-Con M20/Klor-Con M10 Tablets 3329
K-Lor Powder Packets 469
K-Tab Filmtab Tablets 470
Micro-K 3311
NuLYTELY, Cherry Flavor, Lemon-Lime Flavor, and Orange Flavor NuLYTELY for Oral Solution 1068
Rum-K 1363

Potassium Citrate (Concomitant use of potassium-containing salt substitute or potassium supplements can lead to hyperkalemia; frequent monitoring of serum potassium is recommended if used concurrently). Products include:

Urocit-K Tablets 2232

Potassium Gluconate (Concomitant use of potassium-containing salt substitute or potassium supplements can lead to hyperkalemia; frequent monitoring of serum potassium is recommended if used concurrently).

No products indexed under this heading.

Potassium Phosphate (Concomitant use of potassium-containing salt substitute or potassium supplements can lead to hyperkalemia; frequent monitoring of serum potassium is recommended if used concurrently). Products include:

K-Phos Neutral Tablets 946

Spironolactone (Fosinopril attenuates diuretic-induced potassium loss; concomitant use can lead to hyperkalemia; frequent monitoring of serum potassium is recommended if used concurrently; co-administration can result in excessive hypotension).

No products indexed under this heading.

Torsemide (Co-administration of fosinopril in patients on diuretics, especially those in who diuretic therapy was recently instituted, may occasionally experience excessive hypotension; antihypertensive effects of fosinopril are augmented by antihypertensive agents that cause renin release). Products include:

Demadex Tablets and Injection 2965

Triamterene (Fosinopril attenuates diuretic-induced potassium loss; concomitant use can lead to hyperkalemia; frequent monitoring of serum potassium is recommended if used concurrently; co-administration can result in excessive hypotension). Products include:

Dyazide Capsules 1515
Dyrenium Capsules 3458
Maxzide 1008

Food Interactions

Food, unspecified (Rate of absorption may be slowed by the presence of food in the GI tract; the extent of absorption is not affected).

MONOPRIL HCT 10/12.5 TABLETS

(Fosinopril Sodium, Hydrochlorothiazide) 1094

May interact with antacids containing aluminum, calcium and magnesium, insulin, lithium preparations, methenamine, non-steroidal anti-inflammatory agents, potassium preparations, potassium sparing diuretics, and certain other agents. Compounds in these categories include:

Aluminum Carbonate (Co-administration with antacids may impair absorption of fosinopril; if concomitant use of these agents is indicated, dosing should be separated by 2 hours).

No products indexed under this heading.

Aluminum Hydroxide (Co-administration with antacids may impair absorption of fosinopril; if concomitant use of these agents is indicated, dosing should be separated by 2 hours). Products include:

Amphojel Suspension (Mint Flavor) .... ■789
Gaviscon Extra Strength Liquid .... ■751
Gaviscon Extra Strength Tablets .... ■751
Gaviscon Regular Strength Liquid .... ■751
Gaviscon Regular Strength Tablets .... ■750
Maalox Antacid/Anti-Gas Oral Suspension .... ■673
Maalox Max Maximum Strength Antacid/Anti-Gas Liquid 2300
Maalox Regular Strength Antacid/Antigas Liquid 2300
Mylanta 1813
Vanquish Caplets .... ■617

Amiloride Hydrochloride (Co-administration can increase the risk of hyperlipidemia). Products include:

Midamor Tablets 2136
Moduretic Tablets 2138

Celecoxib (The diuretic, natriuretic, and antihypertensive effects of thiazide diuretics may be reduced by co-administration with NSAID's). Products include:

Celebrex Capsules 2676
Celebrex Capsules 2780

Cholestyramine (Absorption of hydrochlorothiazide is impaired in the presence of anionic exchange resins; reduced absorption of hydrochlorothiazide by 85%).

No products indexed under this heading.

Colestipol Hydrochloride (Absorption of hydrochlorothiazide is impaired in the presence of anionic exchange resins; reduced absorption of hydrochlorothiazide by 43%). Products include:

Colestid Tablets 2791

Diclofenac Potassium (The diuretic, natriuretic, and antihypertensive effects of thiazide diuretics may be reduced by co-administration with NSAID's). Products include:

Cataflam Tablets 2315

Diclofenac Sodium (The diuretic, natriuretic, and antihypertensive effects of thiazide diuretics may be reduced by co-administration with NSAID's). Products include:

Arthrotec Tablets 3195
Voltaren Ophthalmic Sterile Ophthalmic Solution .... ⊙312
Voltaren Tablets 2315
Voltaren-XR Tablets 2315

Etodolac (The diuretic, natriuretic, and antihypertensive effects of thiazide diuretics may be reduced by co-administration with NSAID's). Products include:

Lodine 3528
Lodine XL Extended-Release Tablets 3530

Fenoprofen Calcium (The diuretic, natriuretic, and antihypertensive effects of thiazide diuretics may be reduced by co-administration with NSAID's).

No products indexed under this heading.

Flurbiprofen (The diuretic, natriuretic, and antihypertensive effects of thiazide diuretics may be reduced by co-administration with NSAID's).

No products indexed under this heading.

Ibuprofen (The diuretic, natriuretic, and antihypertensive effects of thiazide diuretics may be reduced by co-administration with NSAID's). Products include:

Advil .... ■771
Children's Advil Oral Suspension .... ■773
Children's Advil Chewable Tablets .... ■773
Advil Cold and Sinus Caplets .... ■771
Advil Cold and Sinus Tablets .... ■771
Advil Flu & Body Ache Caplets .... ■772
Infants' Advil Drops .... ■773
Junior Strength Advil Tablets .... ■773
Junior Strength Advil Chewable Tablets .... ■773
Advil Migraine Liquigels .... ■772
Children's Motrin Oral Suspension and Chewable Tablets 2006
Children's Motrin Cold Oral Suspension 2007
Children's Motrin Oral Suspension .... ■643
Motrin Suspension, Oral Drops, Chewable Tablets, and Caplets 2002
Infants' Motrin Concentrated Drops 2006
Junior Strength Motrin Caplets and Chewable Tablets 2006
Motrin IB Tablets, Caplets, and Gelcaps 2002
Motrin Migraine Pain Caplets 2005
Motrin Sinus Headache Caplets 2005
Vicoprofen Tablets 520

Indomethacin (The diuretic, natriuretic, and antihypertensive effects of thiazide diuretics may be reduced by co-administration with NSAID's). Products include:

Indocin 2112

Indomethacin Sodium Trihydrate (The diuretic, natriuretic, and antihypertensive effects of thiazide diuretics may be reduced by co-administration with NSAID's). Products include:

Indocin I.V. 2115

Insulin, Human, Zinc Suspension (Thiazide diuretics tend to reduce glucose tolerance, therefore, insulin requirements in diabetic patients may be increased, decreased, or unchanged). Products include:

Humulin L, 100 Units 1937
Humulin U, 100 Units 1943
Novolin L Human Insulin 10 ml Vials 2422

Insulin, Human NPH (Thiazide diuretics tend to reduce glucose tolerance, therefore, insulin requirements in diabetic patients may be increased, decreased, or unchanged). Products include:

Humulin N, 100 Units 1939
Humulin N NPH Pen 1940
Novolin N Human Insulin 10 ml Vials 2422
Novolin N PenFill 2423
Novolin N Prefilled Syringe Disposable Insulin Delivery System 2425

Insulin, Human Regular (Thiazide diuretics tend to reduce glucose tolerance, therefore, insulin requirements in diabetic patients may be increased, decreased, or unchanged). Products include:

Humulin R Regular (U-500) 1943
Humulin R, 100 Units 1941
Novolin R Human Insulin 10 ml Vials 2423
Novolin R PenFill 2423
Novolin R Prefilled Syringe Disposable Insulin Delivery System 2425
Velosulin BR Human Insulin 10 ml Vials 2435

Insulin, Human Regular and Human NPH Mixture (Thiazide diuretics tend to reduce glucose tolerance, therefore, insulin requirements in diabetic patients may be increased, decreased, or unchanged). Products include:

Humulin 50/50, 100 Units 1934
Humulin 70/30, 100 Units 1935
Humulin 70/30 Pen 1936
Novolin 70/30 Human Insulin 10 ml Vials 2421
Novolin 70/30 PenFill 2423
Novolin 70/30 Prefilled Disposable Insulin Delivery System 2425

Insulin, NPH (Thiazide diuretics tend to reduce glucose tolerance, therefore, insulin requirements in diabetic patients may be increased, decreased, or unchanged). Products include:

Iletin II, NPH (Pork), 100 Units 1946

Insulin, Regular (Thiazide diuretics tend to reduce glucose tolerance, therefore, insulin requirements in diabetic patients may be increased, decreased, or unchanged). Products include:

Iletin II, Regular (Pork), 100 Units 1947

Insulin, Zinc Crystals (Thiazide diuretics tend to reduce glucose tolerance, therefore, insulin requirements in diabetic patients may be increased, decreased, or unchanged).

No products indexed under this heading.

Insulin, Zinc Suspension (Thiazide diuretics tend to reduce glucose tolerance, therefore, insulin requirements in diabetic patients may be increased, decreased, or unchanged). Products include:

Iletin II, Lente (Pork), 100 Units 1945

Insulin Aspart, Human Regular (Thiazide diuretics tend to reduce glucose tolerance, therefore, insulin requirements in diabetic patients may be increased, decreased, or unchanged).

No products indexed under this heading.

Insulin glargine (Thiazide diuretics tend to reduce glucose tolerance, therefore, insulin requirements in diabetic patients may be increased, decreased, or unchanged). Products include:

Lantus Injection 742

Insulin Lispro, Human (Thiazide diuretics tend to reduce glucose tolerance, therefore, insulin requirements in diabetic patients may be increased, decreased, or unchanged). Products include:

Humalog 1926
Humalog Mix 75/25 Pen 1928

Insulin Lispro Protamine, Human (Thiazide diuretics tend to reduce glucose tolerance, therefore, insulin requirements in diabetic patients may be increased, decreased, or unchanged). Products include:

Humalog Mix 75/25 Pen 1928

Ketoprofen (The diuretic, natriuretic, and antihypertensive effects of thiazide diuretics may be reduced by co-administration with NSAID's). Products include:
Orudis Capsules 3548
Orudis KT Tablets 778
Oruvail Capsules 3548

Ketorolac Tromethamine (The diuretic, natriuretic, and antihypertensive effects of thiazide diuretics may be reduced by co-administration with NSAID's). Products include:
Acular Ophthalmic Solution 544
Acular PF Ophthalmic Solution 544
Toradol 3018

Lithium Carbonate (Increased serum lithium levels and symptoms of lithium toxicity; renal clearance of lithium is reduced by thiazides, therefore the risk is raised further). Products include:
Eskalith 1527
Lithium Carbonate 3061
Lithobid Slow-Release Tablets 3255

Lithium Citrate (Increased serum lithium levels and symptoms of lithium toxicity; renal clearance of lithium is reduced by thiazides, therefore the risk is raised further). Products include:
Lithium Citrate Syrup 3061

Magaldrate (Co-administration with antacids may impair absorption of fosinopril; if concomitant use of these agents is indicated, dosing should be separated by 2 hours).
No products indexed under this heading.

Magnesium Hydroxide (Co-administration with antacids may impair absorption of fosinopril; if concomitant use of these agents is indicated, dosing should be separated by 2 hours). Products include:
Ex•Lax Milk of Magnesia Liquid 670
Maalox Antacid/Anti-Gas Oral Suspension 673
Maalox Max Maximum Strength Antacid/Anti-Gas Liquid 2300
Maalox Regular Strength Antacid/Antigas Liquid 2300
Mylanta Fast-Acting 1813
Mylanta 1813
Pepcid Complete Chewable Tablets 1815
Phillips' Chewable Tablets 615
Phillips' Milk of Magnesia Liquid (Original, Cherry, & Mint) 616
Rolaids Tablets 706
Extra Strength Rolaids Tablets 706
Vanquish Caplets 617

Magnesium Oxide (Co-administration with antacids may impair absorption of fosinopril; if concomitant use of these agents is indicated, dosing should be separated by 2 hours). Products include:
Beelith Tablets 946
Mag-Ox 400 Tablets 1024
Uro-Mag Capsules 1024

Meclofenamate Sodium (The diuretic, natriuretic, and antihypertensive effects of thiazide diuretics may be reduced by co-administration with NSAID's).
No products indexed under this heading.

Mefenamic Acid (The diuretic, natriuretic, and antihypertensive effects of thiazide diuretics may be reduced by co-administration with NSAID's). Products include:
Ponstel Capsules 1356

Meloxicam (The diuretic, natriuretic, and antihypertensive effects of thiazide diuretics may be reduced by co-administration with NSAID's). Products include:
Mobic Tablets 1054

Methenamine (Hydrochlorothiazide alkalinizes urine, therefore, may reduce the effectiveness of methenamine). Products include:
Prosed/DS Tablets 3268
Urimax Tablets 1769
Urised Tablets 2876

Methenamine Hippurate (Hydrochlorothiazide alkalinizes urine, therefore, may reduce the effectiveness of methenamine).
No products indexed under this heading.

Methenamine Mandelate (Hydrochlorothiazide alkalinizes urine, therefore, may reduce the effectiveness of methenamine). Products include:
Uroqid-Acid No. 2 Tablets 947

Nabumetone (The diuretic, natriuretic, and antihypertensive effects of thiazide diuretics may be reduced by co-administration with NSAID's). Products include:
Relafen Tablets 1617

Naproxen (The diuretic, natriuretic, and antihypertensive effects of thiazide diuretics may be reduced by co-administration with NSAID's). Products include:
EC-Naprosyn Delayed-Release Tablets 2967
Naprosyn Suspension 2967
Naprosyn Tablets 2967

Naproxen Sodium (The diuretic, natriuretic, and antihypertensive effects of thiazide diuretics may be reduced by co-administration with NSAID's). Products include:
Aleve Tablets, Caplets and Gelcaps 602
Aleve Cold & Sinus Caplets 603
Anaprox Tablets 2967
Anaprox DS Tablets 2967
Naprelan Tablets 1293

Norepinephrine Hydrochloride (Thiazides may decrease arterial responsiveness to norepinephrine).
No products indexed under this heading.

Oxaprozin (The diuretic, natriuretic, and antihypertensive effects of thiazide diuretics may be reduced by co-administration with NSAID's).
No products indexed under this heading.

Phenylbutazone (The diuretic, natriuretic, and antihypertensive effects of thiazide diuretics may be reduced by co-administration with NSAID's).
No products indexed under this heading.

Piroxicam (The diuretic, natriuretic, and antihypertensive effects of thiazide diuretics may be reduced by co-administration with NSAID's). Products include:
Feldene Capsules 2685

Potassium Acid Phosphate (Co-administration with potassium supplements can increase the risk of hyperlipidemia). Products include:
K-Phos Original (Sodium Free) Tablets 947

Potassium Bicarbonate (Co-administration with potassium supplements can increase the risk of hyperlipidemia).
No products indexed under this heading.

Potassium Chloride (Co-administration with potassium supplements can increase the risk of hyperlipidemia). Products include:
Chlor-3 1361
Colyte with Flavor Packs for Oral Solution 3170
GoLYTELY and Pineapple Flavor GoLYTELY for Oral Solution 1068
K-Dur Microburst Release System ER Tablets 1832
Klor-Con M20/Klor-Con M10 Tablets 3329
K-Lor Powder Packets 469
K-Tab Filmtab Tablets 470
Micro-K 3311
NuLYTELY, Cherry Flavor, Lemon-Lime Flavor, and Orange Flavor NuLYTELY for Oral Solution 1068
Rum-K 1363

Potassium Citrate (Co-administration with potassium supplements can increase the risk of hyperlipidemia). Products include:
Urocit-K Tablets 2232

Potassium Gluconate (Co-administration with potassium supplements can increase the risk of hyperlipidemia).
No products indexed under this heading.

Potassium Phosphate (Co-administration with potassium supplements can increase the risk of hyperlipidemia). Products include:
K-Phos Neutral Tablets 946

Rofecoxib (The diuretic, natriuretic, and antihypertensive effects of thiazide diuretics may be reduced by co-administration with NSAID's). Products include:
Vioxx 2213

Spironolactone (Co-administration can increase the risk of hyperlipidemia).
No products indexed under this heading.

Sulindac (The diuretic, natriuretic, and antihypertensive effects of thiazide diuretics may be reduced by co-administration with NSAID's). Products include:
Clinoril Tablets 2053

Tolmetin Sodium (The diuretic, natriuretic, and antihypertensive effects of thiazide diuretics may be reduced by co-administration with NSAID's). Products include:
Tolectin 2589

Triamterene (Co-administration can increase the risk of hyperlipidemia). Products include:
Dyazide Capsules 1515
Dyrenium Capsules 3458
Maxzide 1008

Tubocurarine Chloride (Thiazides may increase the responsiveness to tubocurarine).
No products indexed under this heading.

MONOPRIL HCT 20/12.5 TABLETS

(Fosinopril Sodium, Hydrochlorothiazide) 1094
See Monopril HCT 10/12.5 Tablets

MONUROL SACHET

(Fosfomycin Tromethamine) 1375
May interact with:

Cisapride (Increases gastrointestinal motility and may lower the serum concentration and urinary excretion of fosfomycin).
No products indexed under this heading.

Metoclopramide Hydrochloride (Lowers the serum concentration and urinary excretion of fosfomycin). Products include:
Reglan 2935

Food Interactions

Food, unspecified (The oral bioavailability of fosfomycin is reduced to 30% under fed conditions compared to 37% under fasting condition; Monurol can be taken with or without food).

MOISTURE EYES PROTECT AND PRESERVATIVE-FREE MOISTURE EYES PROTECT

(Dextran 70, Hydroxypropyl Methylcellulose) .... ⊙253
None cited in PDR database.

MOTOFEN TABLETS

(Atropine Sulfate, Difenoxin Hydrochloride) 577
May interact with barbiturates, monoamine oxidase inhibitors, narcotic analgesics, tranquilizers, and certain other agents. Compounds in these categories include:

Alfentanil Hydrochloride (Effects potentiated).
No products indexed under this heading.

Alprazolam (Effects potentiated). Products include:
Xanax Tablets 2865

Aprobarbital (Effects potentiated).
No products indexed under this heading.

Buprenorphine Hydrochloride (Effects potentiated). Products include:
Buprenex Injectable 2918

Buspirone Hydrochloride (Effects potentiated).
No products indexed under this heading.

Butabarbital (Effects potentiated).
No products indexed under this heading.

Butalbital (Effects potentiated). Products include:
Phrenilin 578
Sedapap Tablets 50 mg/650 mg 2225

Chlordiazepoxide (Effects potentiated). Products include:
Limbitrol 1738

Chlordiazepoxide Hydrochloride (Effects potentiated). Products include:
Librium Capsules 1736
Librium for Injection 1737

Chlorpromazine (Effects potentiated). Products include:
Thorazine Suppositories 1656

Chlorpromazine Hydrochloride (Effects potentiated). Products include:
Thorazine 1656

Chlorprothixene (Effects potentiated).
No products indexed under this heading.

Chlorprothixene Hydrochloride (Effects potentiated).
No products indexed under this heading.

Clorazepate Dipotassium (Effects potentiated). Products include:
Tranxene 511

Codeine Phosphate (Effects potentiated). Products include:
Phenergan with Codeine Syrup 3557
Phenergan VC with Codeine Syrup 3561
Robitussin A-C Syrup 2942
Robitussin-DAC Syrup 2942
Ryna-C Liquid 768
Soma Compound w/Codeine Tablets 3355
Tussi-Organidin NR Liquid 3350
Tussi-Organidin-S NR Liquid 3350
Tylenol with Codeine 2595

Dezocine (Effects potentiated).
No products indexed under this heading.

Diazepam (Effects potentiated). Products include:
Valium Injectable 3026
Valium Tablets 3047

Droperidol (Effects potentiated).
No products indexed under this heading.

Fentanyl (Effects potentiated). Products include:
Duragesic Transdermal System 1786

Fentanyl Citrate (Effects potentiated). Products include:
Actiq 1184

Fluphenazine Decanoate (Effects potentiated).
No products indexed under this heading.

Fluphenazine Enanthate (Effects potentiated).
No products indexed under this heading.

Fluphenazine Hydrochloride (Effects potentiated).
No products indexed under this heading.

Haloperidol (Effects potentiated). Products include:
Haldol Injection, Tablets and Concentrate ... 2533

Haloperidol Decanoate (Effects potentiated). Products include:
Haldol Decanoate ... 2535

Hydrocodone Bitartrate (Effects potentiated). Products include:
Hycodan ... 1316
Hycomine Compound Tablets ... 1317
Hycotuss Expectorant Syrup ... 1318
Lortab ... 3319
Lortab Elixir ... 3317
Maxidone Tablets CIII ... 3399
Norco 5/325 Tablets CIII ... 3424
Norco 7.5/325 Tablets CIII ... 3425
Norco 10/325 Tablets CIII ... 3427
Norco 10/325 Tablets CIII ... 3425
Vicodin Tablets ... 516
Vicodin ES Tablets ... 517
Vicodin HP Tablets ... 518
Vicodin Tuss Expectorant ... 519
Vicoprofen Tablets ... 520
Zydone Tablets ... 1330

Hydrocodone Polistirex (Effects potentiated). Products include:
Tussionex Pennkinetic Extended-Release Suspension ... 1174

Hydromorphone Hydrochloride (Effects potentiated). Products include:
Dilaudid ... 441
Dilaudid Oral Liquid ... 445
Dilaudid Powder ... 441
Dilaudid Rectal Suppositories ... 441
Dilaudid Tablets ... 441
Dilaudid Tablets - 8 mg ... 445
Dilaudid-HP ... 443

Hydroxyzine Hydrochloride (Effects potentiated). Products include:
Atarax Tablets & Syrup ... 2667
Vistaril Intramuscular Solution ... 2738

Isocarboxazid (Concurrent use may precipitate hypertensive crisis).
No products indexed under this heading.

Levorphanol Tartrate (Effects potentiated). Products include:
Levo-Dromoran ... 1734
Levorphanol Tartrate Tablets ... 3059

Lorazepam (Effects potentiated). Products include:
Ativan Injection ... 3478
Ativan Tablets ... 3482

Loxapine Hydrochloride (Effects potentiated).
No products indexed under this heading.

Loxapine Succinate (Effects potentiated). Products include:
Loxitane Capsules ... 3398

Meperidine Hydrochloride (Effects potentiated). Products include:
Demerol ... 3079
Mepergan Injection ... 3539

Mephobarbital (Effects potentiated).
No products indexed under this heading.

Meprobamate (Effects potentiated). Products include:
Miltown Tablets ... 3349

Mesoridazine Besylate (Effects potentiated). Products include:
Serentil ... 1057

Methadone Hydrochloride (Effects potentiated). Products include:
Dolophine Hydrochloride Tablets ... 3056

Moclobemide (Concurrent use may precipitate hypertensive crisis).
No products indexed under this heading.

Molindone Hydrochloride (Effects potentiated). Products include:
Moban ... 1320

Morphine Sulfate (Effects potentiated). Products include:
Astramorph/PF Injection, USP (Preservative-Free) ... 594
Duramorph Injection ... 1312
Infumorph 200 and Infumorph 500 Sterile Solutions ... 1314
Kadian Capsules ... 1335
MS Contin Tablets ... 2896
MSIR ... 2898
Oramorph SR Tablets ... 3062
Roxanol ... 3066

Oxazepam (Effects potentiated).
No products indexed under this heading.

Oxycodone Hydrochloride (Effects potentiated). Products include:
OxyContin Tablets ... 2912
OxyFast Oral Concentrate Solution ... 2916
OxyIR Capsules ... 2916
Percocet Tablets ... 1326
Percodan Tablets ... 1327
Percolone Tablets ... 1327
Roxicodone ... 3067
Tylox Capsules ... 2597

Pargyline Hydrochloride (Concurrent use may precipitate hypertensive crisis).
No products indexed under this heading.

Pentobarbital Sodium (Effects potentiated). Products include:
Nembutal Sodium Solution ... 485

Perphenazine (Effects potentiated). Products include:
Etrafon ... 3115
Trilafon ... 3160

Phenelzine Sulfate (Concurrent use may precipitate hypertensive crisis). Products include:
Nardil Tablets ... 2653

Phenobarbital (Effects potentiated). Products include:
Arco-Lase Plus Tablets ... 592
Donnatal ... 2929
Donnatal Extentabs ... 2930

Prazepam (Effects potentiated).
No products indexed under this heading.

Procarbazine Hydrochloride (Concurrent use may precipitate hypertensive crisis). Products include:
Matulane Capsules ... 3246

Prochlorperazine (Effects potentiated). Products include:
Compazine ... 1505

Promethazine Hydrochloride (Effects potentiated). Products include:
Mepergan Injection ... 3539
Phenergan Injection ... 3553
Phenergan ... 3556
Phenergan Syrup ... 3554
Phenergan with Codeine Syrup ... 3557
Phenergan with Dextromethorphan Syrup ... 3559
Phenergan VC Syrup ... 3560
Phenergan VC with Codeine Syrup ... 3561

Propoxyphene Hydrochloride (Effects potentiated). Products include:
Darvon Pulvules ... 1909
Darvon Compound-65 Pulvules ... 1910

Propoxyphene Napsylate (Effects potentiated). Products include:
Darvon-N/Darvocet-N ... 1907
Darvon-N Tablets ... 1912

Remifentanil Hydrochloride (Effects potentiated).
No products indexed under this heading.

Secobarbital Sodium (Effects potentiated).
No products indexed under this heading.

Selegiline Hydrochloride (Concurrent use may precipitate hypertensive crisis). Products include:
Eldepryl Capsules ... 3266

Sufentanil Citrate (Effects potentiated).
No products indexed under this heading.

Thiamylal Sodium (Effects potentiated).
No products indexed under this heading.

Thioridazine Hydrochloride (Effects potentiated). Products include:
Thioridazine Hydrochloride Tablets ... 2289

Thiothixene (Effects potentiated). Products include:
Navane Capsules ... 2701
Thiothixene Capsules ... 2290

Tranylcypromine Sulfate (Concurrent use may precipitate hypertensive crisis). Products include:
Parnate Tablets ... 1607

Trifluoperazine Hydrochloride (Effects potentiated). Products include:
Stelazine ... 1640

Food Interactions

Alcohol (Effects potentiated).

CHILDREN'S MOTRIN ORAL SUSPENSION AND CHEWABLE TABLETS
(Ibuprofen) ... 2006
None cited in PDR database.

CHILDREN'S MOTRIN COLD ORAL SUSPENSION
(Ibuprofen, Pseudoephedrine Hydrochloride) ... 2007
See Motrin Sinus Headache Caplets

CHILDREN'S MOTRIN ORAL SUSPENSION
(Ibuprofen) ... ■643
None cited in PDR database.

CHILDREN'S MOTRIN COLD ORAL SUSPENSION
(Ibuprofen, Pseudoephedrine Hydrochloride) ... ■645
May interact with monoamine oxidase inhibitors. Compounds in these categories include:

Isocarboxazid (Concurrent and/or sequential use with MAO inhibitors is not recommended).
No products indexed under this heading.

Moclobemide (Concurrent and/or sequential use with MAO inhibitors is not recommended).
No products indexed under this heading.

Pargyline Hydrochloride (Concurrent and/or sequential use with MAO inhibitors is not recommended).
No products indexed under this heading.

Phenelzine Sulfate (Concurrent and/or sequential use with MAO inhibitors is not recommended). Products include:
Nardil Tablets ... 2653

Procarbazine Hydrochloride (Concurrent and/or sequential use with MAO inhibitors is not recommended). Products include:
Matulane Capsules ... 3246

Selegiline Hydrochloride (Concurrent and/or sequential use with MAO inhibitors is not recommended). Products include:
Eldepryl Capsules ... 3266

Tranylcypromine Sulfate (Concurrent and/or sequential use with MAO inhibitors is not recommended). Products include:
Parnate Tablets ... 1607

MOTRIN SUSPENSION, ORAL DROPS, CHEWABLE TABLETS, AND CAPLETS
(Ibuprofen) ... 2002
May interact with ACE inhibitors, oral anticoagulants, lithium preparations, thiazides, and certain other agents. Compounds in these categories include:

Aspirin (Yields a net decrease in anti-inflammatory activity with lowered blood levels of non-aspirin drug in animal studies). Products include:
Aggrenox Capsules ... 1026
Alka-Seltzer ... ■603
Alka-Seltzer Lemon Lime Antacid and Pain Reliever Effervescent Tablets ... ■603
Alka-Seltzer Extra Strength Antacid and Pain Reliever Effervescent Tablets ... ■603
Alka-Seltzer PM Effervescent Tablets ... ■605
Genuine Bayer Tablets, Caplets and Gelcaps ... ■606
Extra Strength Bayer Caplets and Gelcaps ... ■610
Aspirin Regimen Bayer Children's Chewable Tablets (Orange or Cherry Flavored) ... ■607
Bayer, Aspirin Regimen ... ■606
Aspirin Regimen Bayer 81 mg Caplets with Calcium ... ■607
Genuine Bayer Professional Labeling (Aspirin Regimen Bayer) ... ■608
Extra Strength Bayer Arthritis Caplets ... ■610
Extra Strength Bayer Plus Caplets ... ■610
Extra Strength Bayer PM Caplets ... ■611
BC Powder ... ■619
BC Allergy Sinus Cold Powder ... ■619
Arthritis Strength BC Powder ... ■619
BC Sinus Cold Powder ... ■619
Darvon Compound-65 Pulvules ... 1910
Ecotrin Enteric Coated Aspirin Low, Regular and Maximum Strength Tablets ... 1715
Excedrin Extra-Strength Tablets, Caplets, and Geltabs ... ■629
Excedrin Migraine ... 1070
Goody's Body Pain Formula Powder ... ■620
Goody's Extra Strength Headache Powder ... ■620
Goody's Extra Strength Pain Relief Tablets ... ■620
Percodan Tablets ... 1327
Robaxisal Tablets ... 2939
Soma Compound Tablets ... 3354
Soma Compound w/Codeine Tablets ... 3355
Vanquish Caplets ... ■617

Benazepril Hydrochloride (Ibuprofen may diminish the antihypertensive effect). Products include:
Lotensin Tablets ... 2365
Lotensin HCT Tablets ... 2367
Lotrel Capsules ... 2370

Bendroflumethiazide (Ibuprofen can reduce the natriuretic effect of thiazide diuretics in some patients). Products include:
Corzide 40/5 Tablets ... 2247
Corzide 80/5 Tablets ... 2247

Captopril (Ibuprofen may diminish the antihypertensive effect). Products include:
Captopril Tablets ... 2281

Chlorothiazide (Ibuprofen can reduce the natriuretic effect of thiazide diuretics in some patients). Products include:
Aldoclor Tablets ... 2035
Diuril Oral ... 2087

Chlorothiazide Sodium (Ibuprofen can reduce the natriuretic effect of thiazide diuretics in some patients). Products include:
Diuril Sodium Intravenous ... 2086

Dicumarol (Concurrent use may result in bleeding).
No products indexed under this heading.

Enalapril Maleate (Ibuprofen may diminish the antihypertensive effect). Products include:
Lexxel Tablets ... 608
Vaseretic Tablets ... 2204

Vasotec Tablets 2210

Enalaprilat (Ibuprofen may diminish the antihypertensive effect). Products include:

Enalaprilat Injection 863
Vasotec I.V. Injection 2207

Fosinopril Sodium (Ibuprofen may diminish the antihypertensive effect). Products include:

Monopril Tablets 1091
Monopril HCT 1094

Furosemide (Ibuprofen can reduce the natriurectic effect furosemide). Products include:

Furosemide Tablets 2284

Hydrochlorothiazide (Ibuprofen can reduce the natriuretic effect of thiazide diuretics in some patients). Products include:

Accuretic Tablets 2614
Aldoril Tablets 2039
Atacand HCT Tablets 597
Avalide Tablets 1070
Diovan HCT Tablets 2338
Dyazide Capsules 1515
HydroDIURIL Tablets 2108
Hyzaar 2109
Inderide Tablets 3517
Inderide LA Long-Acting Capsules 3519
Lotensin HCT Tablets 2367
Maxzide 1008
Micardis HCT Tablets 1051
Microzide Capsules 3414
Moduretic Tablets 2138
Monopril HCT 1094
Prinzide Tablets 2168
Timolide Tablets 2187
Uniretic Tablets 3178
Vaseretic Tablets 2204
Zestoretic Tablets 695
Ziac Tablets 1887

Hydroflumethiazide (Ibuprofen can reduce the natriuretic effect of thiazide diuretics in some patients). Products include:

Diucardin Tablets 3494

Lisinopril (Ibuprofen may diminish the antihypertensive effect). Products include:

Prinivil Tablets 2164
Prinzide Tablets 2168
Zestoretic Tablets 695
Zestril Tablets 698

Lithium Carbonate (Ibuprofen can produce an elevation of plasma lithium levels and a reduction in renal lithium clearance). Products include:

Eskalith 1527
Lithium Carbonate 3061
Lithobid Slow-Release Tablets 3255

Lithium Citrate (Ibuprofen can produce an elevation of plasma lithium levels and a reduction in renal lithium clearance). Products include:

Lithium Citrate Syrup 3061

Methotrexate Sodium (Potential for enhanced methotrexate toxicity possibly resulting from competitively inhibiting methotrexate accumulation).

No products indexed under this heading.

Methyclothiazide (Ibuprofen can reduce the natriuretic effect of thiazide diuretics in some patients).

No products indexed under this heading.

Moexipril Hydrochloride (Ibuprofen may diminish the antihypertensive effect). Products include:

Uniretic Tablets 3178
Univasc Tablets 3181

Perindopril Erbumine (Ibuprofen may diminish the antihypertensive effect). Products include:

Aceon Tablets (2 mg, 4 mg, 8 mg) 3249

Polythiazide (Ibuprofen can reduce the natriuretic effect of thiazide diuretics in some patients). Products include:

Minizide Capsules 2700
Renese Tablets 2712

Quinapril Hydrochloride (Ibuprofen may diminish the antihypertensive effect). Products include:

Accupril Tablets 2611
Accuretic Tablets 2614

Ramipril (Ibuprofen may diminish the antihypertensive effect). Products include:

Altace Capsules 2233

Spirapril Hydrochloride (Ibuprofen may diminish the antihypertensive effect).

No products indexed under this heading.

Trandolapril (Ibuprofen may diminish the antihypertensive effect). Products include:

Mavik Tablets 478
Tarka Tablets 508

Warfarin Sodium (Concurrent use may result in bleeding). Products include:

Coumadin for Injection 1243
Coumadin Tablets 1243
Warfarin Sodium Tablets, USP 3302

Food Interactions

Food, unspecified (Food affects the rate but not the extent of absorption; Tmax is delayed by approximately 30 to 60 minutes and peak levels are reduced by approximately 30 to 50%).

INFANTS' MOTRIN CONCENTRATED DROPS

(Ibuprofen) 2006
None cited in PDR database.

JUNIOR STRENGTH MOTRIN CAPLETS AND CHEWABLE TABLETS

(Ibuprofen) 2006
None cited in PDR database.

MOTRIN IB TABLETS, CAPLETS, AND GELCAPS

(Ibuprofen) 2002
May interact with:

Acetaminophen (Concurrent administration should not be undertaken without physician's direction). Products include:

Actifed Cold & Sinus Caplets and Tablets 688
Alka-Seltzer Plus Liqui-Gels 604
Alka-Seltzer Plus Cold & Flu Medicine Liqui-Gels 604
Alka-Seltzer Plus Cold & Sinus Medicine Liqui-Gels 604
Benadryl Allergy/Cold Tablets 691
Benadryl Allergy Sinus Headache Caplets & Gelcaps 693
Benadryl Severe Allergy & Sinus Headache Caplets 694
Children's Cēpacol Sore Throat 788
Comtrex Acute Head Cold & Sinus Pressure Relief Tablets 627
Comtrex Deep Chest Cold & Congestion Relief Softgels 627
Comtrex Flu Therapy & Fever Relief Daytime Caplets 628
Comtrex Flu Therapy & Fever Relief Nighttime Tablets 628
Comtrex Maximum Strength Multi-Symptom Cold & Cough Relief Tablets and Caplets 626
Contac Severe Cold and Flu Caplets Maximum Strength 746
Contac Severe Cold and Flu Caplets Non-Drowsy 746
Coricidin 'D' Cold, Flu & Sinus Tablets 737
Coricidin HBP Cold & Flu Tablets 738
Coricidin HBP Maximum Strength Flu Tablets 738
Coricidin HBP Night-Time Cold & Flu Tablets 738
Darvon-N/Darvocet-N 1907
Dimetapp Cold and Fever Suspension 775
Dimetapp Nighttime Flu Liquid 776
Dimetapp Non-Drowsy Flu Syrup 777
Drixoral Allergy/Sinus Extended-Release Tablets 741
Drixoral Cold & Flu Extended-Release Tablets 740
Aspirin Free Excedrin Caplets and Geltabs 628
Excedrin Extra-Strength Tablets, Caplets, and Geltabs 629
Excedrin Migraine 1070
Excedrin PM Tablets, Caplets, and Geltabs 631
Goody's Body Pain Formula Powder 620
Goody's Extra Strength Headache Powder 620
Goody's Extra Strength Pain Relief Tablets 620
Goody's PM Powder 621
Hycomine Compound Tablets 1317
Lortab 3319
Lortab Elixir 3317
Maxidone Tablets CIII 3399
Maximum Strength Midol Menstrual Caplets and Gelcaps 612
Maximum Strength Midol PMS Caplets and Gelcaps 613
Maximum Strength Midol Teen Caplets 612
Midrin Capsules 3464
Norco 5/325 Tablets CIII 3424
Norco 7.5/325 Tablets CIII 3425
Norco 10/325 Tablets CIII 3427
Norco 10/325 Tablets CIII 3425
Percocet Tablets 1326
Percogesic Aspirin-Free Coated Tablets 667
Extra Strength Percogesic Aspirin-Free Coated Caplets 665
Phrenilin 578
Robitussin Cold Caplets Multi-Symptom Cold & Flu 781
Robitussin Cold Softgels Multi-Symptom Cold & Flu 781
Robitussin Multi Symptom Honey Flu Liquid 785
Robitussin Nighttime Honey Flu Liquid 786
Sedapap Tablets 50 mg/650 mg 2225
Singlet Caplets 761
Sinutab Sinus Allergy Medication, Maximum Strength Formula, Tablets & Caplets 707
Sinutab Sinus Medication, Maximum Strength Without Drowsiness Formula, Tablets & Caplets 707
Sudafed Cold & Cough Liquid Caps 709
Sudafed Cold & Sinus Liquid Caps 710
Sudafed Severe Cold 711
Sudafed Sinus Headache Caplets 712
Sudafed Sinus Headache Tablets 712
Tavist Sinus Non-Drowsy Coated Caplets 676
TheraFlu Regular Strength Cold & Cough Night Time Hot Liquid 676
TheraFlu Regular Strength Cold & Sore Throat Night Time Hot Liquid 676
TheraFlu Maximum Strength Flu & Congestion Non-Drowsy Hot Liquid 677
TheraFlu Maximum Strength Flu & Cough Night Time Hot Liquid 678
TheraFlu Maximum Strength Flu & Sore Throat Night Time Hot Liquid 677
TheraFlu Maximum Strength Severe Cold & Congestion Night Time Caplets 678
TheraFlu Maximum Strength Severe Cold & Congestion Night Time Hot Liquid 678
TheraFlu Maximum Strength Severe Cold & Congestion Non-Drowsy 679
Triaminic Cold, Cough & Fever Liquid 681
Triaminic Cough & Sore Throat Liquid 682
Triaminic Cough & Sore Throat Softchews 684
Tylenol, Children's 2014
Children's Tylenol Allergy-D Liquid 2014
Children's Tylenol Cold Suspension Liquid and Chewable Tablets 2015
Children's Tylenol Cold Plus Cough Suspension Liquid and Chewable Tablets 2015
Children's Tylenol Flu Suspension Liquid 2015
Children's Tylenol Sinus Suspension Liquid 2017
Infants' Tylenol Cold Decongestant and Fever Reducer Concentrated Drops 2015
Infants' Tylenol Cold Decongestant and Fever Reducer Concentrated Drops Plus Cough 2015
Junior Strength Tylenol Soft Chews Chewable Tablets 2014
Tylenol 2009
Tylenol Allergy Sinus 2010
Tylenol Severe Allergy Caplets 2010
Multi-Symptom Tylenol Cold Complete Formula Caplets 2010
Multi-Symptom Tylenol Cold Non-Drowsy Caplets and Gelcaps 2010
Multi-Symptom Tylenol Cold Severe Congestion Non-Drowsy Caplets 2011
Maximum Strength Tylenol Flu NightTime Gelcaps 2011
Maximum Strength Tylenol Flu NightTime Liquid 2011
Maximum Strength Tylenol Flu Non-Drowsy Gelcaps 2011
Extra Strength Tylenol PM Caplets, Geltabs, and Gelcaps 2012
Maximum Strength Tylenol Sinus NightTime Caplets 2012
Maximum Strength Tylenol Sinus Non-Drowsy Geltabs, Gelcaps, Caplets, and Tablets 2012
Maximum Strength Tylenol Sore Throat Adult Liquid 2013
Tylenol with Codeine 2595
Women's Tylenol Menstrual Relief Caplets 2013
Tylox Capsules 2597
Ultracet Tablets 2597
Vanquish Caplets 617
Vicks 44M Cough, Cold & Flu Relief Liquid 725
Vicks DayQuil LiquiCaps/Liquid Multi-Symptom Cold/Flu Relief 727
Vicks NyQuil LiquiCaps/Liquid Multi-Symptom Cold/Flu Relief, Original and Cherry Flavors 727
Vicodin Tablets 516
Vicodin ES Tablets 517
Vicodin HP Tablets 518
Zydone Tablets 1330

Aspirin (Concurrent administration should not be undertaken without physician's direction). Products include:

Aggrenox Capsules 1026
Alka-Seltzer 603
Alka-Seltzer Lemon Lime Antacid and Pain Reliever Effervescent Tablets 603
Alka-Seltzer Extra Strength Antacid and Pain Reliever Effervescent Tablets 603
Alka-Seltzer PM Effervescent Tablets 605
Genuine Bayer Tablets, Caplets and Gelcaps 606
Extra Strength Bayer Caplets and Gelcaps 610
Aspirin Regimen Bayer Children's Chewable Tablets (Orange or Cherry Flavored) 607
Bayer, Aspirin Regimen 606
Aspirin Regimen Bayer 81 mg Caplets with Calcium 607
Genuine Bayer Professional Labeling (Aspirin Regimen Bayer) 608
Extra Strength Bayer Arthritis Caplets 610
Extra Strength Bayer Plus Caplets 610
Extra Strength Bayer PM Caplets 611
BC Powder 619
BC Allergy Sinus Cold Powder 619
Arthritis Strength BC Powder 619
BC Sinus Cold Powder 619
Darvon Compound-65 Pulvules 1910
Ecotrin Enteric Coated Aspirin Low, Regular and Maximum Strength Tablets 1715
Excedrin Extra-Strength Tablets, Caplets, and Geltabs 629
Excedrin Migraine 1070
Goody's Body Pain Formula Powder 620
Goody's Extra Strength Headache Powder 620
Goody's Extra Strength Pain Relief Tablets 620
Percodan Tablets 1327
Robaxisal Tablets 2939
Soma Compound Tablets 3354
Soma Compound w/Codeine Tablets 3355
Vanquish Caplets 617

Food Interactions

Alcohol (Chronic heavy alcohol users, 3 or more drinks per day, should consult their physicians for advice on when and how they should take pain relievers/fever reducers including ibuprofen).

MOTRIN MIGRAINE PAIN CAPLETS

(Ibuprofen) 2005

IMPORTANT NOTE: Always consult each drug listing in the patient's regimen for possible interactions.

Food Interactions

Alcohol (Chronic heavy alcohol users, 3 or more drinks per day, should consult their physicians for advice on when and how they should take pain relievers, including ibuprofen).

MOTRIN SINUS HEADACHE CAPLETS

(Ibuprofen, Pseudoephedrine Hydrochloride)....... 2005

May interact with monoamine oxidase inhibitors and certain other agents. Compounds in these categories include:

Isocarboxazid (Concurrent and/or sequential use with MAO inhibitors is not recommended).
No products indexed under this heading.

Moclobemide (Concurrent and/or sequential use with MAO inhibitors is not recommended).
No products indexed under this heading.

Pargyline Hydrochloride (Concurrent and/or sequential use with MAO inhibitors is not recommended).
No products indexed under this heading.

Phenelzine Sulfate (Concurrent and/or sequential use with MAO inhibitors is not recommended). Products include:
Nardil Tablets 2653

Procarbazine Hydrochloride (Concurrent and/or sequential use with MAO inhibitors is not recommended). Products include:
Matulane Capsules 3246

Selegiline Hydrochloride (Concurrent and/or sequential use with MAO inhibitors is not recommended). Products include:
Eldepryl Capsules 3266

Tranylcypromine Sulfate (Concurrent and/or sequential use with MAO inhibitors is not recommended). Products include:
Parnate Tablets 1607

Food Interactions

Alcohol (Chronic heavy alcohol users, three or more drinks per day, should consult their physicians for advice on when and how they should take pain relievers/fever reducers including ibuprofen).

MOVANA TABLETS

(Hypericum) .... ▣832

May interact with oral contraceptives and certain other agents. Compounds in these categories include:

Desogestrel (Co-administration of St. John's Wort and oral contraceptives in some women has resulted in irregular menstrual cycles). Products include:
Cyclessa Tablets 2450
Desogen Tablets 2458
Mircette Tablets 2470
Ortho-Cept 21 Tablets 2546
Ortho-Cept 28 Tablets 2546

Ethinyl Estradiol (Co-administration of St. John's Wort and oral contraceptives in some women has resulted in irregular menstrual cycles). Products include:
Alesse-21 Tablets 3468
Alesse-28 Tablets 3473
Brevicon 28-Day Tablets 3380
Cyclessa Tablets 2450
Desogen Tablets 2458
Estinyl Tablets 3112
Estrostep 2627
femhrt Tablets 2635
Levlen 962
Levlite 21 Tablets 962
Levlite 28 Tablets 962
Levora Tablets 3389
Loestrin 21 Tablets 2642
Loestrin Fe Tablets 2642
Lo/Ovral Tablets 3532
Lo/Ovral-28 Tablets 3538
Low-Ogestrel-28 Tablets 3392
Microgestin Fe 1.5/30 Tablets 3407
Microgestin Fe 1/20 Tablets 3400
Mircette Tablets 2470
Modicon 2563
Necon 3415
Nordette-28 Tablets 2257
Norinyl 1 +35 28-Day Tablets 3380
Ogestrel 0.5/50-28 Tablets 3428
Ortho-Cept 21 Tablets 2546
Ortho-Cept 28 Tablets 2546
Ortho-Cyclen/Ortho Tri-Cyclen 2573
Ortho-Novum 2563
Ovcon 3364
Ovral Tablets 3551
Ovral-28 Tablets 3552
Tri-Levlen 962
Tri-Norinyl-28 Tablets 3433
Triphasil-21 Tablets 3600
Triphasil-28 Tablets 3605
Trivora Tablets 3439
Yasmin 28 Tablets 980
Zovia 3449

Ethynodiol Diacetate (Co-administration of St. John's Wort and oral contraceptives in some women has resulted in irregular menstrual cycles). Products include:
Zovia 3449

Levonorgestrel (Co-administration of St. John's Wort and oral contraceptives in some women has resulted in irregular menstrual cycles). Products include:
Alesse-21 Tablets 3468
Alesse-28 Tablets 3473
Levlen 962
Levlite 21 Tablets 962
Levlite 28 Tablets 962
Levora Tablets 3389
Mirena Intrauterine System 974
Nordette-28 Tablets 2257
Norplant System 3543
Tri-Levlen 962
Triphasil-21 Tablets 3600
Triphasil-28 Tablets 3605
Trivora Tablets 3439

Mestranol (Co-administration of St. John's Wort and oral contraceptives in some women has resulted in irregular menstrual cycles). Products include:
Necon 1/50 Tablets 3415
Norinyl 1 + 50 28-Day Tablets 3380
Ortho-Novum 1/50▫28 Tablets 2556

Norethindrone (Co-administration of St. John's Wort and oral contraceptives in some women has resulted in irregular menstrual cycles). Products include:
Brevicon 28-Day Tablets 3380
Micronor Tablets 2543
Modicon 2563
Necon 3415
Norinyl 1 +35 28-Day Tablets 3380
Norinyl 1 + 50 28-Day Tablets 3380
Nor-QD Tablets 3423
Ortho-Novum 2563
Ortho-Novum 1/50▫28 Tablets 2556
Ovcon 3364
Tri-Norinyl-28 Tablets 3433

Norethynodrel (Co-administration of St. John's Wort and oral contraceptives in some women has resulted in irregular menstrual cycles).
No products indexed under this heading.

Norgestimate (Co-administration of St. John's Wort and oral contraceptives in some women has resulted in irregular menstrual cycles). Products include:
Ortho-Cyclen/Ortho Tri-Cyclen 2573
Ortho-Prefest Tablets 2570

Norgestrel (Co-administration of St. John's Wort and oral contraceptives in some women has resulted in irregular menstrual cycles). Products include:
Lo/Ovral Tablets 3532
Lo/Ovral-28 Tablets 3538
Low-Ogestrel-28 Tablets 3392
Ogestrel 0.5/50-28 Tablets 3428
Ovral Tablets 3551
Ovral-28 Tablets 3552
Ovrette Tablets 3552

Warfarin Sodium (St. John's Wort may reduce the effect of oral anticoagulant). Products include:
Coumadin for Injection 1243
Coumadin Tablets 1243
Warfarin Sodium Tablets, USP 3302

MS CONTIN TABLETS

(Morphine Sulfate) 2896

May interact with central nervous system depressants, general anesthetics, hypnotics and sedatives, mixed agonist/antagonist opioid analgesics, neuromuscular blocking agents, phenothiazines, tranquilizers, and certain other agents. Compounds in these categories include:

Alfentanil Hydrochloride (Profound sedation; coma; severe hypotension; respiratory depression).
No products indexed under this heading.

Alprazolam (Profound sedation; coma; severe hypotension; respiratory depression). Products include:
Xanax Tablets 2865

Aprobarbital (Profound sedation; coma; severe hypotension; respiratory depression).
No products indexed under this heading.

Atracurium Besylate (Increased respiratory depression).
No products indexed under this heading.

Buprenorphine Hydrochloride (Mixed agonist/antagonist analgesics may reduce the analgesic effect or may precipitate withdrawal symptoms). Products include:
Buprenex Injectable 2918

Buspirone Hydrochloride (Profound sedation; coma; severe hypotension; respiratory depression).
No products indexed under this heading.

Butabarbital (Profound sedation; coma; severe hypotension; respiratory depression).
No products indexed under this heading.

Butalbital (Profound sedation; coma; severe hypotension; respiratory depression). Products include:
Phrenilin 578
Sedapap Tablets 50 mg/650 mg 2225

Butorphanol Tartrate (Mixed agonist/antagonist analgesics may reduce the analgesic effect or may precipitate withdrawal symptoms). Products include:
Stadol NS Nasal Spray 1108

Chlordiazepoxide (Profound sedation; coma; severe hypotension; respiratory depression). Products include:
Limbitrol 1738

Chlordiazepoxide Hydrochloride (Profound sedation; coma; severe hypotension; respiratory depression). Products include:
Librium Capsules 1736
Librium for Injection 1737

Chlorpromazine (Profound sedation; coma; severe hypotension; respiratory depression). Products include:
Thorazine Suppositories 1656

Chlorpromazine Hydrochloride (Profound sedation; coma; severe hypotension; respiratory depression). Products include:
Thorazine 1656

Chlorprothixene (Profound sedation; coma; severe hypotension; respiratory depression).
No products indexed under this heading.

Chlorprothixene Hydrochloride (Profound sedation; coma; severe hypotension; respiratory depression).
No products indexed under this heading.

Chlorprothixene Lactate (Profound sedation; coma; severe hypotension; respiratory depression).
No products indexed under this heading.

Cisatracurium Besylate (Increased respiratory depression).
No products indexed under this heading.

Clorazepate Dipotassium (Profound sedation; coma; severe hypotension; respiratory depression). Products include:
Tranxene 511

Clozapine (Profound sedation; coma; severe hypotension; respiratory depression). Products include:
Clozaril Tablets 2319

Codeine Phosphate (Profound sedation; coma; severe hypotension; respiratory depression). Products include:
Phenergan with Codeine Syrup 3557
Phenergan VC with Codeine Syrup 3561
Robitussin A-C Syrup 2942
Robitussin-DAC Syrup 2942
Ryna-C Liquid .... ▣768
Soma Compound w/Codeine Tablets 3355
Tussi-Organidin NR Liquid 3350
Tussi-Organidin-S NR Liquid 3350
Tylenol with Codeine 2595

Desflurane (Profound sedation; coma; severe hypotension; respiratory depression). Products include:
Suprane Liquid for Inhalation 874

Dezocine (Profound sedation; coma; severe hypotension; respiratory depression).
No products indexed under this heading.

Diazepam (Profound sedation; coma; severe hypotension; respiratory depression). Products include:
Valium Injectable 3026
Valium Tablets 3047

Doxacurium Chloride (Increased respiratory depression).
No products indexed under this heading.

Droperidol (Profound sedation; coma; severe hypotension; respiratory depression).
No products indexed under this heading.

Enflurane (Profound sedation; coma; severe hypotension; respiratory depression).
No products indexed under this heading.

Estazolam (Profound sedation; coma; severe hypotension; respiratory depression). Products include:
ProSom Tablets 500

Ethchlorvynol (Profound sedation; coma; severe hypotension; respiratory depression).
No products indexed under this heading.

Ethinamate (Profound sedation; coma; severe hypotension; respiratory depression).
No products indexed under this heading.

Fentanyl (Profound sedation; coma; severe hypotension; respiratory depression). Products include:
Duragesic Transdermal System 1786

Fentanyl Citrate (Profound sedation; coma; severe hypotension; respiratory depression). Products include:
Actiq 1184

Fluphenazine Decanoate (Profound sedation; coma; severe hypotension; respiratory depression).
No products indexed under this heading.

Fluphenazine Enanthate (Profound sedation; coma; severe hypotension; respiratory depression).
No products indexed under this heading.

Fluphenazine Hydrochloride (Profound sedation; coma; severe hypotension; respiratory

depression).
No products indexed under this heading.

Flurazepam Hydrochloride (Profound sedation; coma; severe hypotension; respiratory depression).
No products indexed under this heading.

Glutethimide (Profound sedation; coma; severe hypotension; respiratory depression).
No products indexed under this heading.

Haloperidol (Profound sedation; coma; severe hypotension; respiratory depression). Products include:
Haldol Injection, Tablets and Concentrate 2533

Haloperidol Decanoate (Profound sedation; coma; severe hypotension; respiratory depression). Products include:
Haldol Decanoate 2535

Hydrocodone Bitartrate (Profound sedation; coma; severe hypotension; respiratory depression). Products include:
Hycodan 1316
Hycomine Compound Tablets 1317
Hycotuss Expectorant Syrup 1318
Lortab 3319
Lortab Elixir 3317
Maxidone Tablets CIII 3399
Norco 5/325 Tablets CIII 3424
Norco 7.5/325 Tablets CIII 3425
Norco 10/325 Tablets CIII 3427
Norco 10/325 Tablets CIII 3425
Vicodin Tablets 516
Vicodin ES Tablets 517
Vicodin HP Tablets 518
Vicodin Tuss Expectorant 519
Vicoprofen Tablets 520
Zydone Tablets 1330

Hydrocodone Polistirex (Profound sedation; coma; severe hypotension; respiratory depression). Products include:
Tussionex Pennkinetic Extended-Release Suspension 1174

Hydromorphone Hydrochloride (Profound sedation; coma; severe hypotension; respiratory depression). Products include:
Dilaudid 441
Dilaudid Oral Liquid 445
Dilaudid Powder 441
Dilaudid Rectal Suppositories 441
Dilaudid Tablets 441
Dilaudid Tablets - 8 mg 445
Dilaudid-HP 443

Hydroxyzine Hydrochloride (Profound sedation; coma; severe hypotension; respiratory depression). Products include:
Atarax Tablets & Syrup 2667
Vistaril Intramuscular Solution 2738

Isoflurane (Profound sedation; coma; severe hypotension; respiratory depression).
No products indexed under this heading.

Ketamine Hydrochloride (Profound sedation; coma; severe hypotension; respiratory depression).
No products indexed under this heading.

Levomethadyl Acetate Hydrochloride (Profound sedation; coma; severe hypotension; respiratory depression).
No products indexed under this heading.

Levorphanol Tartrate (Profound sedation; coma; severe hypotension; respiratory depression). Products include:
Levo-Dromoran 1734
Levorphanol Tartrate Tablets 3059

Lorazepam (Profound sedation; coma; severe hypotension; respiratory depression). Products include:
Ativan Injection 3478
Ativan Tablets 3482

Loxapine Hydrochloride (Profound sedation; coma; severe hypotension; respiratory depression).
No products indexed under this heading.

Loxapine Succinate (Profound sedation; coma; severe hypotension; respiratory depression). Products include:
Loxitane Capsules 3398

Meperidine Hydrochloride (Profound sedation; coma; severe hypotension; respiratory depression). Products include:
Demerol 3079
Mepergan Injection 3539

Mephobarbital (Profound sedation; coma; severe hypotension; respiratory depression).
No products indexed under this heading.

Meprobamate (Profound sedation; coma; severe hypotension; respiratory depression). Products include:
Miltown Tablets 3349

Mesoridazine Besylate (Profound sedation; coma; severe hypotension; respiratory depression). Products include:
Serentil 1057

Methadone Hydrochloride (Profound sedation; coma; severe hypotension; respiratory depression). Products include:
Dolophine Hydrochloride Tablets 3056

Methohexital Sodium (Profound sedation; coma; severe hypotension; respiratory depression). Products include:
Brevital Sodium for Injection, USP 1815

Methotrimeprazine (Profound sedation; coma; severe hypotension; respiratory depression).
No products indexed under this heading.

Methoxyflurane (Profound sedation; coma; severe hypotension; respiratory depression).
No products indexed under this heading.

Metocurine Iodide (Increased respiratory depression).
No products indexed under this heading.

Midazolam Hydrochloride (Profound sedation; coma; severe hypotension; respiratory depression). Products include:
Versed Injection 3027
Versed Syrup 3033

Mivacurium Chloride (Increased respiratory depression).
No products indexed under this heading.

Molindone Hydrochloride (Profound sedation; coma; severe hypotension; respiratory depression). Products include:
Moban 1320

Nalbuphine Hydrochloride (Mixed agonist/antagonist analgesics may reduce the analgesic effect or may precipitate withdrawal symptoms). Products include:
Nubain Injection 1323

Olanzapine (Profound sedation; coma; severe hypotension; respiratory depression). Products include:
Zyprexa Tablets 1973
Zyprexa ZYDIS Orally Disintegrating Tablets 1973

Oxazepam (Profound sedation; coma; severe hypotension; respiratory depression).
No products indexed under this heading.

Oxycodone Hydrochloride (Profound sedation; coma; severe hypotension; respiratory depression). Products include:
OxyContin Tablets 2912
OxyFast Oral Concentrate Solution 2916
OxyIR Capsules 2916
Percocet Tablets 1326
Percodan Tablets 1327
Percolone Tablets 1327
Roxicodone 3067
Tylox Capsules 2597

Pancuronium Bromide (Increased respiratory depression).
No products indexed under this heading.

Pentazocine Hydrochloride (Mixed agonist/antagonist analgesics may reduce the analgesic effect or may precipitate withdrawal symptoms). Products include:
Talacen Caplets 3089
Talwin Nx Tablets 3090

Pentazocine Lactate (Mixed agonist/antagonist analgesics may reduce the analgesic effect or may precipitate withdrawal symptoms).
No products indexed under this heading.

Pentobarbital Sodium (Profound sedation; coma; severe hypotension; respiratory depression). Products include:
Nembutal Sodium Solution 485

Perphenazine (Profound sedation; coma; severe hypotension; respiratory depression). Products include:
Etrafon 3115
Trilafon 3160

Phenobarbital (Profound sedation; coma; severe hypotension; respiratory depression). Products include:
Arco-Lase Plus Tablets 592
Donnatal 2929
Donnatal Extentabs 2930

Prazepam (Profound sedation; coma; severe hypotension; respiratory depression).
No products indexed under this heading.

Prochlorperazine (Profound sedation; coma; severe hypotension; respiratory depression). Products include:
Compazine 1505

Promethazine Hydrochloride (Profound sedation; coma; severe hypotension; respiratory depression). Products include:
Mepergan Injection 3539
Phenergan Injection 3553
Phenergan 3556
Phenergan Syrup 3554
Phenergan with Codeine Syrup 3557
Phenergan with Dextromethorphan Syrup 3559
Phenergan VC Syrup 3560
Phenergan VC with Codeine Syrup 3561

Propofol (Profound sedation; coma; severe hypotension; respiratory depression). Products include:
Diprivan Injectable Emulsion 667

Propoxyphene Hydrochloride (Profound sedation; coma; severe hypotension; respiratory depression). Products include:
Darvon Pulvules 1909
Darvon Compound-65 Pulvules 1910

Propoxyphene Napsylate (Profound sedation; coma; severe hypotension; respiratory depression). Products include:
Darvon-N/Darvocet-N 1907
Darvon-N Tablets 1912

Quazepam (Profound sedation; coma; severe hypotension; respiratory depression).
No products indexed under this heading.

Quetiapine Fumarate (Profound sedation; coma; severe hypotension; respiratory depression). Products include:
Seroquel Tablets 684

Rapacuronium Bromide (Increased respiratory depression).
No products indexed under this heading.

Remifentanil Hydrochloride (Profound sedation; coma; severe hypotension; respiratory depression).
No products indexed under this heading.

Risperidone (Profound sedation; coma; severe hypotension; respiratory depression). Products include:
Risperdal 1796

Rocuronium Bromide (Increased respiratory depression). Products include:
Zemuron Injection 2491

Secobarbital Sodium (Profound sedation; coma; severe hypotension; respiratory depression).
No products indexed under this heading.

Sevoflurane (Profound sedation; coma; severe hypotension; respiratory depression).
No products indexed under this heading.

Succinylcholine Chloride (Increased respiratory depression). Products include:
Anectine Injection 1476

Sufentanil Citrate (Profound sedation; coma; severe hypotension; respiratory depression).
No products indexed under this heading.

Temazepam (Profound sedation; coma; severe hypotension; respiratory depression).
No products indexed under this heading.

Thiamylal Sodium (Profound sedation; coma; severe hypotension; respiratory depression).
No products indexed under this heading.

Thioridazine Hydrochloride (Profound sedation; coma; severe hypotension; respiratory depression). Products include:
Thioridazine Hydrochloride Tablets 2289

Thiothixene (Profound sedation; coma; severe hypotension; respiratory depression). Products include:
Navane Capsules 2701
Thiothixene Capsules 2290

Triazolam (Profound sedation; coma; severe hypotension; respiratory depression). Products include:
Halcion Tablets 2823

Trifluoperazine Hydrochloride (Profound sedation; coma; severe hypotension; respiratory depression). Products include:
Stelazine 1640

Vecuronium Bromide (Increased respiratory depression). Products include:
Norcuron for Injection 2478

Zaleplon (Profound sedation; coma; severe hypotension; respiratory depression). Products include:
Sonata Capsules 3591

Ziprasidone Hydrochloride (Profound sedation; coma; severe hypotension; respiratory depression). Products include:
Geodon Capsules 2688

Zolpidem Tartrate (Profound sedation; coma; severe hypotension; respiratory depression). Products include:
Ambien Tablets 3191

Food Interactions

Alcohol (Respiratory depression, hypotension and profound sedation or coma may result).

MSIR ORAL CAPSULES

(Morphine Sulfate) 2898

See MSIR Oral Solution

MSIR ORAL SOLUTION

(Morphine Sulfate) 2898

May interact with central nervous system depressants, general anesthetics, hypnotics and sedatives, muscle relaxants, phenothiazines, tranquilizers, and certain other agents. Compounds in these categories include:

Alfentanil Hydrochloride (Additive depressant effects; potential for respiratory depression, hypotension and profound sedation or coma; the dose of one or both agents should be reduced).
No products indexed under this heading.

Alprazolam (Additive depressant effects; potential for respiratory depression, hypotension and profound sedation or coma; the dose of one or both agents should be reduced). Products include:
Xanax Tablets 2865

Aprobarbital (Additive depressant effects; potential for respiratory depression, hypotension and profound sedation or coma; the dose of one or both agents should be reduced).
No products indexed under this heading.

Atracurium Besylate (Increased respiratory depression).
No products indexed under this heading.

Baclofen (Increased respiratory depression).
No products indexed under this heading.

Buprenorphine Hydrochloride (Additive depressant effects; potential for respiratory depression, hypotension and profound sedation or coma; the dose of one or both agents should be reduced). Products include:
Buprenex Injectable 2918

Buspirone Hydrochloride (Additive depressant effects; potential for respiratory depression, hypotension and profound sedation or coma; the dose of one or both agents should be reduced).
No products indexed under this heading.

Butabarbital (Additive depressant effects; potential for respiratory depression, hypotension and profound sedation or coma; the dose of one or both agents should be reduced).
No products indexed under this heading.

Butalbital (Additive depressant effects; potential for respiratory depression, hypotension and profound sedation or coma; the dose of one or both agents should be reduced). Products include:
Phrenilin 578
Sedapap Tablets 50 mg/650 mg 2225

Carisoprodol (Increased respiratory depression). Products include:
Soma Tablets 3353
Soma Compound Tablets 3354
Soma Compound w/Codeine Tablets 3355

Chlordiazepoxide (Additive depressant effects; potential for respiratory depression, hypotension and profound sedation or coma; the dose of one or both agents should be reduced). Products include:
Limbitrol 1738

Chlordiazepoxide Hydrochloride (Additive depressant effects; potential for respiratory depression, hypotension and profound sedation or coma; the dose of one or both agents should be reduced). Products include:
Librium Capsules 1736
Librium for Injection 1737

Chlorpromazine (Additive depressant effects; potential for respiratory depression, hypotension and profound sedation or coma; the dose of one or both agents should be reduced). Products include:
Thorazine Suppositories 1656

Chlorpromazine Hydrochloride (Additive depressant effects; potential for respiratory depression, hypotension and profound sedation or coma; the dose of one or both agents should be reduced). Products include:
Thorazine 1656

Chlorprothixene (Additive depressant effects; potential for respiratory depression, hypotension and profound sedation or coma; the dose of one or both agents should be reduced).
No products indexed under this heading.

Chlorprothixene Hydrochloride (Additive depressant effects; potential for respiratory depression, hypotension and profound sedation or coma; the dose of one or both agents should be reduced).
No products indexed under this heading.

Chlorprothixene Lactate (Additive depressant effects; potential for respiratory depression, hypotension and profound sedation or coma; the dose of one or both agents should be reduced).
No products indexed under this heading.

Chlorzoxazone (Increased respiratory depression). Products include:
Parafon Forte DSC Caplets 2582

Cisatracurium Besylate (Increased respiratory depression).
No products indexed under this heading.

Clorazepate Dipotassium (Additive depressant effects; potential for respiratory depression, hypotension and profound sedation or coma; the dose of one or both agents should be reduced). Products include:
Tranxene 511

Clozapine (Additive depressant effects; potential for respiratory depression, hypotension and profound sedation or coma; the dose of one or both agents should be reduced). Products include:
Clozaril Tablets 2319

Codeine Phosphate (Additive depressant effects; potential for respiratory depression, hypotension and profound sedation or coma; the dose of one or both agents should be reduced). Products include:
Phenergan with Codeine Syrup 3557
Phenergan VC with Codeine Syrup .. 3561
Robitussin A-C Syrup 2942
Robitussin-DAC Syrup 2942
Ryna-C Liquid .... ■ 768
Soma Compound w/Codeine Tablets 3355
Tussi-Organidin NR Liquid 3350
Tussi-Organidin-S NR Liquid 3350
Tylenol with Codeine 2595

Cyclobenzaprine Hydrochloride (Increased respiratory depression). Products include:
Flexeril Tablets 572
Flexeril Tablets 2094

Dantrolene Sodium (Increased respiratory depression). Products include:
Dantrium Capsules 2885
Dantrium Intravenous 2886

Desflurane (Additive depressant effects; potential for respiratory depression, hypotension and profound sedation or coma; the dose of one or both agents should be reduced). Products include:
Suprane Liquid for Inhalation 874

Dezocine (Additive depressant effects; potential for respiratory depression, hypotension and profound sedation or coma; the dose of one or both agents should be reduced).
No products indexed under this heading.

Diazepam (Additive depressant effects; potential for respiratory depression, hypotension and profound sedation or coma; the dose of one or both agents should be reduced). Products include:
Valium Injectable 3026
Valium Tablets 3047

Doxacurium Chloride (Increased respiratory depression).
No products indexed under this heading.

Droperidol (Additive depressant effects; potential for respiratory depression, hypotension and profound sedation or coma; the dose of one or both agents should be reduced).
No products indexed under this heading.

Enflurane (Additive depressant effects; potential for respiratory depression, hypotension and profound sedation or coma; the dose of one or both agents should be reduced).
No products indexed under this heading.

Estazolam (Additive depressant effects; potential for respiratory depression, hypotension and profound sedation or coma; the dose of one or both agents should be reduced). Products include:
ProSom Tablets 500

Ethchlorvynol (Additive depressant effects; potential for respiratory depression, hypotension and profound sedation or coma; the dose of one or both agents should be reduced).
No products indexed under this heading.

Ethinamate (Additive depressant effects; potential for respiratory depression, hypotension and profound sedation or coma; the dose of one or both agents should be reduced).
No products indexed under this heading.

Fentanyl (Additive depressant effects; potential for respiratory depression, hypotension and profound sedation or coma; the dose of one or both agents should be reduced). Products include:
Duragesic Transdermal System 1786

Fentanyl Citrate (Additive depressant effects; potential for respiratory depression, hypotension and profound sedation or coma; the dose of one or both agents should be reduced). Products include:
Actiq 1184

Fluphenazine Decanoate (Additive depressant effects; potential for respiratory depression, hypotension and profound sedation or coma; the dose of one or both agents should be reduced).
No products indexed under this heading.

Fluphenazine Enanthate (Additive depressant effects; potential for respiratory depression, hypotension and profound sedation or coma; the dose of one or both agents should be reduced).
No products indexed under this heading.

Fluphenazine Hydrochloride (Additive depressant effects; potential for respiratory depression, hypotension and profound sedation or coma; the dose of one or both agents should be reduced).
No products indexed under this heading.

Flurazepam Hydrochloride (Additive depressant effects; potential for respiratory depression, hypotension and profound sedation or coma; the dose of one or both agents should be reduced).
No products indexed under this heading.

Glutethimide (Additive depressant effects; potential for respiratory depression, hypotension and profound sedation or coma; the dose of one or both agents should be reduced).
No products indexed under this heading.

Haloperidol (Additive depressant effects; potential for respiratory depression, hypotension and profound sedation or coma; the dose of one or both agents should be reduced). Products include:
Haldol Injection, Tablets and Concentrate 2533

Haloperidol Decanoate (Additive depressant effects; potential for respiratory depression, hypotension and profound sedation or coma; the dose of one or both agents should be reduced). Products include:
Haldol Decanoate 2535

Hydrocodone Bitartrate (Additive depressant effects; potential for respiratory depression, hypotension and profound sedation or coma; the dose of one or both agents should be reduced). Products include:
Hycodan 1316
Hycomine Compound Tablets 1317
Hycotuss Expectorant Syrup 1318
Lortab 3319
Lortab Elixir 3317
Maxidone Tablets CIII 3399
Norco 5/325 Tablets CIII 3424
Norco 7.5/325 Tablets CIII 3425
Norco 10/325 Tablets CIII 3427
Norco 10/325 Tablets CIII 3425
Vicodin Tablets 516
Vicodin ES Tablets 517
Vicodin HP Tablets 518
Vicodin Tuss Expectorant 519
Vicoprofen Tablets 520
Zydone Tablets 1330

Hydrocodone Polistirex (Additive depressant effects; potential for respiratory depression, hypotension and profound sedation or coma; the dose of one or both agents should be reduced). Products include:
Tussionex Pennkinetic Extended-Release Suspension..... 1174

Hydromorphone Hydrochloride (Additive depressant effects; potential for respiratory depression, hypotension and profound sedation or coma; the dose of one or both agents should be reduced). Products include:
Dilaudid 441
Dilaudid Oral Liquid 445
Dilaudid Powder 441
Dilaudid Rectal Suppositories 441
Dilaudid Tablets 441
Dilaudid Tablets - 8 mg 445
Dilaudid-HP 443

Hydroxyzine Hydrochloride (Additive depressant effects; potential for respiratory depression, hypotension and profound sedation or coma; the dose of one or both agents should be reduced). Products include:
Atarax Tablets & Syrup 2667
Vistaril Intramuscular Solution 2738

Isoflurane (Additive depressant effects; potential for respiratory depression, hypotension and profound sedation or coma; the dose of one or both agents should be reduced).
No products indexed under this heading.

Ketamine Hydrochloride (Additive depressant effects; potential for res-

piratory depression, hypotension and profound sedation or coma; the dose of one or both agents should be reduced).
No products indexed under this heading.

Levomethadyl Acetate Hydrochloride (Additive depressant effects; potential for respiratory depression, hypotension and profound sedation or coma; the dose of one or both agents should be reduced).
No products indexed under this heading.

Levorphanol Tartrate (Additive depressant effects; potential for respiratory depression, hypotension and profound sedation or coma; the dose of one or both agents should be reduced). Products include:
Levo-Dromoran 1734
Levorphanol Tartrate Tablets 3059

Lorazepam (Additive depressant effects; potential for respiratory depression, hypotension and profound sedation or coma; the dose of one or both agents should be reduced). Products include:
Ativan Injection 3478
Ativan Tablets 3482

Loxapine Hydrochloride (Additive depressant effects; potential for respiratory depression, hypotension and profound sedation or coma; the dose of one or both agents should be reduced).
No products indexed under this heading.

Loxapine Succinate (Additive depressant effects; potential for respiratory depression, hypotension and profound sedation or coma; the dose of one or both agents should be reduced). Products include:
Loxitane Capsules 3398

Meperidine Hydrochloride (Additive depressant effects; potential for respiratory depression, hypotension and profound sedation or coma; the dose of one or both agents should be reduced). Products include:
Demerol 3079
Mepergan Injection 3539

Mephobarbital (Additive depressant effects; potential for respiratory depression, hypotension and profound sedation or coma; the dose of one or both agents should be reduced).
No products indexed under this heading.

Meprobamate (Additive depressant effects; potential for respiratory depression, hypotension and profound sedation or coma; the dose of one or both agents should be reduced). Products include:
Miltown Tablets 3349

Mesoridazine Besylate (Additive depressant effects; potential for respiratory depression, hypotension and profound sedation or coma; the dose of one or both agents should be reduced). Products include:
Serentil 1057

Metaxalone (Increased respiratory depression). Products include:
Skelaxin Tablets 1301

Methadone Hydrochloride (Additive depressant effects; potential for respiratory depression, hypotension and profound sedation or coma; the dose of one or both agents should be reduced). Products include:
Dolophine Hydrochloride Tablets 3056

Methocarbamol (Increased respiratory depression). Products include:
Robaxin Injectable 2938
Robaxin Tablets 2939
Robaxisal Tablets 2939

Methohexital Sodium (Additive depressant effects; potential for respiratory depression, hypotension and profound sedation or coma; the dose of one or both agents should be reduced). Products include:
Brevital Sodium for Injection, USP 1815

Methotrimeprazine (Additive depressant effects; potential for respiratory depression, hypotension and profound sedation or coma; the dose of one or both agents should be reduced).
No products indexed under this heading.

Methoxyflurane (Additive depressant effects; potential for respiratory depression, hypotension and profound sedation or coma; the dose of one or both agents should be reduced).
No products indexed under this heading.

Metocurine Iodide (Increased respiratory depression).
No products indexed under this heading.

Midazolam Hydrochloride (Additive depressant effects; potential for respiratory depression, hypotension and profound sedation or coma; the dose of one or both agents should be reduced). Products include:
Versed Injection 3027
Versed Syrup 3033

Mivacurium Chloride (Increased respiratory depression).
No products indexed under this heading.

Molindone Hydrochloride (Additive depressant effects; potential for respiratory depression, hypotension and profound sedation or coma; the dose of one or both agents should be reduced). Products include:
Moban 1320

Olanzapine (Additive depressant effects; potential for respiratory depression, hypotension and profound sedation or coma; the dose of one or both agents should be reduced). Products include:
Zyprexa Tablets 1973
Zyprexa ZYDIS Orally Disintegrating Tablets 1973

Orphenadrine Citrate (Increased respiratory depression). Products include:
Norflex 1987

Oxazepam (Additive depressant effects; potential for respiratory depression, hypotension and profound sedation or coma; the dose of one or both agents should be reduced).
No products indexed under this heading.

Oxycodone Hydrochloride (Additive depressant effects; potential for respiratory depression, hypotension and profound sedation or coma; the dose of one or both agents should be reduced). Products include:
OxyContin Tablets 2912
OxyFast Oral Concentrate Solution 2916
OxyIR Capsules 2916
Percocet Tablets 1326
Percodan Tablets 1327
Percolone Tablets 1327
Roxicodone 3067
Tylox Capsules 2597

Pancuronium Bromide (Increased respiratory depression).
No products indexed under this heading.

Pentazocine Hydrochloride (Reduced analgesic effect; precipitation of withdrawal). Products include:
Talacen Caplets 3089
Talwin Nx Tablets 3090

Pentazocine Lactate (Reduced analgesic effect; precipitation of withdrawal).
No products indexed under this heading.

Pentobarbital Sodium (Additive depressant effects; potential for respiratory depression, hypotension and profound sedation or coma; the dose of one or both agents should be reduced). Products include:
Nembutal Sodium Solution 485

Perphenazine (Additive depressant effects; potential for respiratory depression, hypotension and profound sedation or coma; the dose of one or both agents should be reduced). Products include:
Etrafon 3115
Trilafon 3160

Phenobarbital (Additive depressant effects; potential for respiratory depression, hypotension and profound sedation or coma; the dose of one or both agents should be reduced). Products include:
Arco-Lase Plus Tablets 592
Donnatal 2929
Donnatal Extentabs 2930

Prazepam (Additive depressant effects; potential for respiratory depression, hypotension and profound sedation or coma; the dose of one or both agents should be reduced).
No products indexed under this heading.

Prochlorperazine (Additive depressant effects; potential for respiratory depression, hypotension and profound sedation or coma; the dose of one or both agents should be reduced). Products include:
Compazine 1505

Promethazine Hydrochloride (Additive depressant effects; potential for respiratory depression, hypotension and profound sedation or coma; the dose of one or both agents should be reduced). Products include:
Mepergan Injection 3539
Phenergan Injection 3553
Phenergan 3556
Phenergan Syrup 3554
Phenergan with Codeine Syrup 3557
Phenergan with Dextromethorphan Syrup 3559
Phenergan VC Syrup 3560
Phenergan VC with Codeine Syrup 3561

Propofol (Additive depressant effects; potential for respiratory depression, hypotension and profound sedation or coma; the dose of one or both agents should be reduced). Products include:
Diprivan Injectable Emulsion 667

Propoxyphene Hydrochloride (Additive depressant effects; potential for respiratory depression, hypotension and profound sedation or coma; the dose of one or both agents should be reduced). Products include:
Darvon Pulvules 1909
Darvon Compound-65 Pulvules 1910

Propoxyphene Napsylate (Additive depressant effects; potential for respiratory depression, hypotension and profound sedation or coma; the dose of one or both agents should be reduced). Products include:
Darvon-N/Darvocet-N 1907
Darvon-N Tablets 1912

Quazepam (Additive depressant effects; potential for respiratory depression, hypotension and profound sedation or coma; the dose of one or both agents should be reduced).
No products indexed under this heading.

Quetiapine Fumarate (Additive depressant effects; potential for respiratory depression, hypotension and profound sedation or coma; the dose of one or both agents should be reduced). Products include:
Seroquel Tablets 684

Rapacuronium Bromide (Increased respiratory depression).
No products indexed under this heading.

Remifentanil Hydrochloride (Additive depressant effects; potential for respiratory depression, hypotension and profound sedation or coma; the dose of one or both agents should be reduced).
No products indexed under this heading.

Risperidone (Additive depressant effects; potential for respiratory depression, hypotension and profound sedation or coma; the dose of one or both agents should be reduced). Products include:
Risperdal 1796

Rocuronium Bromide (Increased respiratory depression). Products include:
Zemuron Injection 2491

Secobarbital Sodium (Additive depressant effects; potential for respiratory depression, hypotension and profound sedation or coma; the dose of one or both agents should be reduced).
No products indexed under this heading.

Sevoflurane (Additive depressant effects; potential for respiratory depression, hypotension and profound sedation or coma; the dose of one or both agents should be reduced).
No products indexed under this heading.

Succinylcholine Chloride (Increased respiratory depression). Products include:
Anectine Injection 1476

Sufentanil Citrate (Additive depressant effects; potential for respiratory depression, hypotension and profound sedation or coma; the dose of one or both agents should be reduced).
No products indexed under this heading.

Temazepam (Additive depressant effects; potential for respiratory depression, hypotension and profound sedation or coma; the dose of one or both agents should be reduced).
No products indexed under this heading.

Thiamylal Sodium (Additive depressant effects; potential for respiratory depression, hypotension and profound sedation or coma; the dose of one or both agents should be reduced).
No products indexed under this heading.

Thioridazine Hydrochloride (Additive depressant effects; potential for respiratory depression, hypotension and profound sedation or coma; the dose of one or both agents should be reduced). Products include:
Thioridazine Hydrochloride Tablets 2289

Thiothixene (Additive depressant effects; potential for respiratory depression, hypotension and profound sedation or coma; the dose of one or both agents should be reduced). Products include:
Navane Capsules 2701
Thiothixene Capsules 2290

Triazolam (Additive depressant effects; potential for respiratory depression, hypotension and profound sedation or coma; the dose of one or both agents should be reduced). Products include:
Halcion Tablets 2823

Trifluoperazine Hydrochloride (Additive depressant effects; potential for respiratory depression, hypotension and profound sedation or coma; the dose of one or both agents should be reduced). Products include:
Stelazine 1640

Vecuronium Bromide (Increased respiratory depression). Products include:
Norcuron for Injection 2478

Zaleplon (Additive depressant effects; potential for respiratory depression, hypotension and profound sedation or coma; the dose of one or both agents should be reduced). Products include:
Sonata Capsules 3591

Ziprasidone Hydrochloride (Additive depressant effects; potential for respiratory depression, hypotension and profound sedation or coma; the dose of one or both agents should be reduced). Products include:
Geodon Capsules 2688

Zolpidem Tartrate (Additive depressant effects; potential for respiratory depression, hypotension and profound sedation or coma; the dose of one or both agents should be reduced). Products include:
Ambien Tablets 3191

Food Interactions

Alcohol (Additive depressant effects; potential for respiratory depression, hypotension and profound sedation or coma).

MSIR ORAL SOLUTION CONCENTRATE
(Morphine Sulfate) 2898
See MSIR Oral Solution

MSIR ORAL TABLETS
(Morphine Sulfate) 2898
See MSIR Oral Solution

MUMPSVAX
(Mumps Virus Vaccine, Live) 2141
May interact with immunosuppressive agents. Compounds in these categories include:

Azathioprine (Concurrent immunosuppressive therapy is contraindicated).
No products indexed under this heading.

Basiliximab (Concurrent immunosuppressive therapy is contraindicated). Products include:
Simulect for Injection 2399

Cyclosporine (Concurrent immunosuppressive therapy is contraindicated). Products include:
Gengraf Capsules 457
Neoral Soft Gelatin Capsules 2380
Neoral Oral Solution 2380
Sandimmune 2388

Muromonab-CD3 (Concurrent immunosuppressive therapy is contraindicated). Products include:
Orthoclone OKT3 Sterile Solution 2498

Mycophenolate Mofetil (Concurrent immunosuppressive therapy is contraindicated). Products include:
CellCept Capsules 2951
CellCept Oral Suspension 2951
CellCept Tablets 2951

Sirolimus (Concurrent immunosuppressive therapy is contraindicated). Products include:
Rapamune Oral Solution and Tablets 3584

Tacrolimus (Concurrent immunosuppressive therapy is contraindicated). Products include:
Prograf 1393
Protopic Ointment 1397

MURINE TEARS LUBRICANT EYE DROPS
(Polyvinyl Alcohol, Povidone) .... ⊙323
None cited in PDR database.

MURINE TEARS PLUS LUBRICANT REDNESS RELIEVER EYE DROPS
(Polyvinyl Alcohol, Povidone, Tetrahydrozoline Hydrochloride)....... ⊙323
None cited in PDR database.

MURO 128 STERILE OPHTHALMIC OINTMENT
(Sodium Chloride) .... ⊙262
None cited in PDR database.

MURO 128 STERILE OPHTHALMIC SOLUTION 2% AND 5%
(Sodium Chloride) .... ⊙262
None cited in PDR database.

MUSE URETHRAL SUPPOSITORY
(Alprostadil) 3335
May interact with anticoagulants and certain other agents. Compounds in these categories include:

Ardeparin Sodium (Patients on anticoagulant therapy may be at higher risk of bleeding when treated with MUSE).
No products indexed under this heading.

Dalteparin Sodium (Patients on anticoagulant therapy may be at higher risk of bleeding when treated with MUSE). Products include:
Fragmin Injection 2814

Danaparoid Sodium (Patients on anticoagulant therapy may be at higher risk of bleeding when treated with MUSE). Products include:
Orgaran Injection 2480

Dicumarol (Patients on anticoagulant therapy may be at higher risk of bleeding when treated with MUSE).
No products indexed under this heading.

Drugs that Attenuate Erectile Dysfunction (Co-administration may influence the response to MUSE).
No products indexed under this heading.

Enoxaparin (Patients on anticoagulant therapy may be at higher risk of bleeding when treated with MUSE). Products include:
Lovenox Injection 746

Heparin Sodium (Patients on anticoagulant therapy may be at higher risk of bleeding when treated with MUSE). Products include:
Heparin Lock Flush Solution 3509
Heparin Sodium Injection 3511

Tinzaparin sodium (Patients on anticoagulant therapy may be at higher risk of bleeding when treated with MUSE). Products include:
Innohep Injection 1248

Warfarin Sodium (Patients on anticoagulant therapy may be at higher risk of bleeding when treated with MUSE). Products include:
Coumadin for Injection 1243
Coumadin Tablets 1243
Warfarin Sodium Tablets, USP 3302

MUSTARGEN FOR INJECTION
(Mechlorethamine Hydrochloride) 2142
May interact with antineoplastics. Compounds in these categories include:

Altretamine (Hematopoiesis may be further compromised in patients who have been previously treated with chemotherapeutic agents). Products include:
Hexalen Capsules 2226

Anastrozole (Hematopoiesis may be further compromised in patients who have been previously treated with chemotherapeutic agents). Products include:
Arimidex Tablets 659

Asparaginase (Hematopoiesis may be further compromised in patients who have been previously treated with chemotherapeutic agents). Products include:
Elspar for Injection 2092

Bicalutamide (Hematopoiesis may be further compromised in patients who have been previously treated with chemotherapeutic agents). Products include:
Casodex Tablets 662

Bleomycin Sulfate (Hematopoiesis may be further compromised in patients who have been previously treated with chemotherapeutic agents).
No products indexed under this heading.

Busulfan (Hematopoiesis may be further compromised in patients who have been previously treated with chemotherapeutic agents). Products include:
Myleran Tablets 1603

Carboplatin (Hematopoiesis may be further compromised in patients who have been previously treated with chemotherapeutic agents). Products include:
Paraplatin for Injection 1126

Carmustine (BCNU) (Hematopoiesis may be further compromised in patients who have been previously treated with chemotherapeutic agents). Products include:
Gliadel Wafer 1723

Chlorambucil (Hematopoiesis may be further compromised in patients who have been previously treated with chemotherapeutic agents). Products include:
Leukeran Tablets 1591

Cisplatin (Hematopoiesis may be further compromised in patients who have been previously treated with chemotherapeutic agents).
No products indexed under this heading.

Cyclophosphamide (Hematopoiesis may be further compromised in patients who have been previously treated with chemotherapeutic agents).
No products indexed under this heading.

Dacarbazine (Hematopoiesis may be further compromised in patients who have been previously treated with chemotherapeutic agents). Products include:
DTIC-Dome 902

Daunorubicin Citrate (Hematopoiesis may be further compromised in patients who have been previously treated with chemotherapeutic agents). Products include:
DaunoXome Injection 1442

Daunorubicin Hydrochloride (Hematopoiesis may be further compromised in patients who have been previously treated with chemotherapeutic agents). Products include:
Cerubidine for Injection 947

Denileukin Diftitox (Hematopoiesis may be further compromised in patients who have been previously treated with chemotherapeutic agents).
No products indexed under this heading.

Docetaxel (Hematopoiesis may be further compromised in patients who have been previously treated with chemotherapeutic agents). Products include:
Taxotere for Injection Concentrate 778

Doxorubicin Hydrochloride (Hematopoiesis may be further compromised in patients who have been previously treated with chemotherapeutic agents). Products include:
Adriamycin PFS/RDF Injection 2767
Doxil Injection 566

Epirubicin Hydrochloride (Hematopoiesis may be further compromised in patients who have been previously treated with chemotherapeutic agents). Products include:
Ellence Injection 2806

Estramustine Phosphate Sodium (Hematopoiesis may be further compromised in patients who have been previously treated with chemotherapeutic agents). Products include:
Emcyt Capsules 2810

Etoposide (Hematopoiesis may be further compromised in patients who have been previously treated with chemotherapeutic agents).
No products indexed under this heading.

Exemestane (Hematopoiesis may be further compromised in patients who have been previously treated with chemotherapeutic agents). Products include:
Aromasin Tablets 2769

Floxuridine (Hematopoiesis may be further compromised in patients who have been previously treated with chemotherapeutic agents). Products include:
Sterile FUDR 2974

Fluorouracil (Hematopoiesis may be further compromised in patients who have been previously treated with chemotherapeutic agents). Products include:
Carac Cream 1222
Efudex 1733
Fluoroplex 552

Flutamide (Hematopoiesis may be further compromised in patients who have been previously treated with chemotherapeutic agents). Products include:
Eulexin Capsules 3118

Gemcitabine Hydrochloride (Hematopoiesis may be further compromised in patients who have been previously treated with chemotherapeutic agents). Products include:
Gemzar for Injection 1919

Hydroxyurea (Hematopoiesis may be further compromised in patients who have been previously treated with chemotherapeutic agents). Products include:
Mylocel Tablets 2227

Idarubicin Hydrochloride (Hematopoiesis may be further compromised in patients who have been previously treated with chemotherapeutic agents). Products include:
Idamycin PFS Injection 2825

Ifosfamide (Hematopoiesis may be further compromised in patients who have been previously treated with chemotherapeutic agents). Products include:
Ifex for Injection 1123

Interferon alfa-2A, Recombinant (Hematopoiesis may be further compromised in patients who have been previously treated with chemotherapeutic agents). Products include:
Roferon-A Injection 2996

Interferon alfa-2B, Recombinant (Hematopoiesis may be further compromised in patients who have been previously treated with chemotherapeutic agents). Products include:
Intron A for Injection 3120
Rebetron Combination Therapy 3153

Irinotecan Hydrochloride (Hematopoiesis may be further compromised in patients who have been previously treated with chemotherapeutic agents).
No products indexed under this heading.

Levamisole Hydrochloride (Hematopoiesis may be further compromised in patients who have been previously treated with chemotherapeutic agents). Products include:
Ergamisol Tablets 1789

Lomustine (CCNU) (Hematopoiesis may be further compromised in patients who have been previously treated with chemotherapeutic agents).
No products indexed under this heading.

Megestrol Acetate (Hematopoiesis may be further compromised in patients who have been previously treated with chemotherapeutic agents). Products include:
Megace Oral Suspension 1124

Melphalan (Hematopoiesis may be further compromised in patients who have been previously treated with chemotherapeutic agents). Products include:
Alkeran Tablets 1466

Mercaptopurine (Hematopoiesis may be further compromised in patients who have been previously treated with chemotherapeutic agents). Products include:
Purinethol Tablets 1615

Methotrexate Sodium (Hematopoiesis may be further compromised in patients who have been previously treated with chemotherapeutic agents).
No products indexed under this heading.

Mitomycin (Mitomycin-C) (Hematopoiesis may be further compromised in patients who have been previously treated with chemotherapeutic agents).
No products indexed under this heading.

Mitotane (Hematopoiesis may be further compromised in patients who have been previously treated with chemotherapeutic agents).
No products indexed under this heading.

Mitoxantrone Hydrochloride (Hematopoiesis may be further compromised in patients who have been previously treated with chemotherapeutic agents). Products include:
Novantrone for Injection 1760

Paclitaxel (Hematopoiesis may be further compromised in patients who have been previously treated with chemotherapeutic agents). Products include:
Taxol Injection 1129

Procarbazine Hydrochloride (Hematopoiesis may be further compromised in patients who have been previously treated with chemotherapeutic agents). Products include:
Matulane Capsules 3246

Streptozocin (Hematopoiesis may be further compromised in patients who have been previously treated with chemotherapeutic agents).
No products indexed under this heading.

Tamoxifen Citrate (Hematopoiesis may be further compromised in patients who have been previously treated with chemotherapeutic agents). Products include:
Nolvadex Tablets 678

Teniposide (Hematopoiesis may be further compromised in patients who have been previously treated with chemotherapeutic agents).
No products indexed under this heading.

Thioguanine (Hematopoiesis may be further compromised in patients who have been previously treated with chemotherapeutic agents). Products include:
Tabloid Tablets 1642

Thiotepa (Hematopoiesis may be further compromised in patients who have been previously treated with chemotherapeutic agents). Products include:
Thioplex for Injection 1765

Topotecan Hydrochloride (Hematopoiesis may be further compromised in patients who have been previously treated with chemotherapeutic agents). Products include:
Hycamtin for Injection 1546

Toremifene Citrate (Hematopoiesis may be further compromised in patients who have been previously treated with chemotherapeutic agents). Products include:
Fareston Tablets 3237

Valrubicin (Hematopoiesis may be further compromised in patients who have been previously treated with chemotherapeutic agents). Products include:
Valstar Sterile Solution for Intravesical Instillation 1175

Vincristine Sulfate (Hematopoiesis may be further compromised in patients who have been previously treated with chemotherapeutic agents).
No products indexed under this heading.

Vinorelbine Tartrate (Hematopoiesis may be further compromised in patients who have been previously treated with chemotherapeutic agents). Products include:
Navelbine Injection 1604

MYAMBUTOL TABLETS
(Ethambutol Hydrochloride) 1290
None cited in PDR database.

MYCELEX-3 VAGINAL CREAM WITH 3 DISPOSABLE APPLICATORS
(Butoconazole Nitrate) .... ▣613
None cited in PDR database.

MYCELEX-3 VAGINAL CREAM IN 3 PRE-FILLED APPLICATORS
(Butoconazole Nitrate) .... ▣613
None cited in PDR database.

MYCELEX TROCHE
(Clotrimazole) 573
None cited in PDR database.

MYCELEX-7 COMBINATION-PACK VAGINAL INSERTS & EXTERNAL VULVAR CREAM
(Clotrimazole) .... ▣614
None cited in PDR database.

MYCELEX-7 VAGINAL CREAM
(Clotrimazole) .... ▣614
None cited in PDR database.

MYCELEX-7 VAGINAL CREAM WITH 7 DISPOSABLE APPLICATORS
(Clotrimazole) .... ▣614
None cited in PDR database.

MYCOBUTIN CAPSULES
(Rifabutin) 2838
May interact with barbiturates, beta blockers, corticosteroids, oral anticoagulants, anticonvulsants, cardiac glycosides, macrolide antibiotics, narcotic analgesics, oral contraceptives, progestins, sulfonylureas, theophylline, and certain other agents. Compounds in these categories include:

Acebutolol Hydrochloride (Potential for decreased effects of concurrently administered beta-adrenergic blockers). Products include:
Sectral Capsules 3589

Alfentanil Hydrochloride (Potential for reduced activity of narcotics through liver enzyme-inducing properties).
No products indexed under this heading.

Aminophylline (Potential for decreased effects of concurrently administered theophylline).
No products indexed under this heading.

Analgesics, unspecified (Potential for reduced activity of analgesics through liver enzyme-inducing properties).

Aprobarbital (Potential for decreased effects of concurrently administered barbiturates).
No products indexed under this heading.

Atenolol (Potential for decreased effects of concurrently administered beta-adrenergic blockers). Products include:
Tenoretic Tablets 690
Tenormin I.V. Injection 692

Azithromycin Dihydrate (Concomitant administration with higher doses of rifabutin results in higher incidence of uveitis). Products include:
Zithromax 2743
Zithromax for IV Infusion 2748
Zithromax for Oral Suspension, 300 mg, 600 mg, 900 mg, 1200 mg 2739
Zithromax Tablets, 250 mg 2739

Betamethasone Acetate (Potential for reduced activity of corticosteroids through liver enzyme-inducing properties). Products include:
Celestone Soluspan Injectable Suspension 3097

Betamethasone Sodium Phosphate (Potential for reduced activity of corticosteroids through liver enzyme-inducing properties). Products include:
Celestone Soluspan Injectable Suspension 3097

Betaxolol Hydrochloride (Potential for decreased effects of concurrently administered beta-adrenergic blockers). Products include:
Betoptic S Ophthalmic Suspension 537

Bisoprolol Fumarate (Potential for decreased effects of concurrently administered beta-adrenergic blockers). Products include:
Zebeta Tablets 1885
Ziac Tablets 1887

Buprenorphine Hydrochloride (Potential for reduced activity of narcotics through liver enzyme-inducing properties). Products include:
Buprenex Injectable 2918

Butabarbital (Potential for decreased effects of concurrently administered barbiturates).
No products indexed under this heading.

Butalbital (Potential for decreased effects of concurrently administered barbiturates). Products include:
Phrenilin 578
Sedapap Tablets 50 mg/650 mg 2225

Carbamazepine (Potential for decreased effects of concurrently administered anticonvulsants). Products include:
Carbatrol Capsules 3234
Tegretol/Tegretol-XR 2404

Carteolol Hydrochloride (Potential for decreased effects of concurrently administered beta-adrenergic blockers). Products include:
Carteolol Hydrochloride Ophthalmic Solution USP, 1% .... ⊙258
Ocupress Ophthalmic Solution, 1% Sterile .... ⊙303

Chloramphenicol (Potential for decreased effects of concurrently administered chloramphenicol). Products include:
Chloromycetin Ophthalmic Ointment, 1% .... ⊙296
Chloromycetin Ophthalmic Solution .... ⊙297
Chloroptic Sterile Ophthalmic Ointment .... ⊙234
Chloroptic Sterile Ophthalmic Solution .... ⊙235

Chloramphenicol Palmitate (Potential for decreased effects of concurrently administered chloramphenicol).
No products indexed under this heading.

Chloramphenicol Sodium Succinate (Potential for decreased effects of concurrently administered chloramphenicol).
No products indexed under this heading.

Chlorpropamide (Potential for reduced activity of oral sulfonylureas through liver enzyme-inducing properties). Products include:
Diabinese Tablets 2680

Clarithromycin (Concomitant administration with higher doses of rifabutin results in higher incidence of uveitis). Products include:
Biaxin/Biaxin XL 403
PREVPAC 3298

Clofibrate (Potential for decreased effects of concurrently administered clofibrate). Products include:
Atromid-S Capsules 3483

Clonazepam (Potential for decreased effects of concurrently administered anticonvulsants). Products include:
Klonopin Tablets 2983

Codeine Phosphate (Potential for reduced activity of narcotics through liver enzyme-inducing properties). Products include:
Phenergan with Codeine Syrup 3557
Phenergan VC with Codeine Syrup 3561
Robitussin A-C Syrup 2942
Robitussin-DAC Syrup 2942
Ryna-C Liquid .... ▣768
Soma Compound w/Codeine Tablets 3355
Tussi-Organidin NR Liquid 3350
Tussi-Organidin-S NR Liquid 3350
Tylenol with Codeine 2595

Cortisone Acetate (Potential for reduced activity of corticosteroids through liver enzyme-inducing properties). Products include:
Cortone Acetate Injectable Suspension 2059
Cortone Acetate Tablets 2061

Cyclosporine (Potential for reduced activity of cyclosporine through liver enzyme-inducing properties). Products include:
Gengraf Capsules 457
Neoral Soft Gelatin Capsules 2380
Neoral Oral Solution 2380
Sandimmune 2388

Dapsone (Potential for reduced activity of dapsone through liver enzyme-inducing properties). Products include:
Dapsone Tablets USP 1780

Deslanoside (Potential for reduced activity of cardiac glycoside agents through liver enzyme-inducing properties).
No products indexed under this heading.

Desogestrel (Potential for decreased effects of concurrently administered progestins). Products include:
Cyclessa Tablets 2450
Desogen Tablets 2458
Mircette Tablets 2470
Ortho-Cept 21 Tablets 2546
Ortho-Cept 28 Tablets 2546

Dexamethasone (Potential for reduced activity of corticosteroids through liver enzyme-inducing properties). Products include:
Decadron Elixir 2078
Decadron Tablets 2079
TobraDex Ophthalmic Ointment 542
TobraDex Ophthalmic Suspension 541

Dexamethasone Acetate (Potential for reduced activity of corticosteroids through liver enzyme-inducing properties).
No products indexed under this heading.

Dexamethasone Sodium Phosphate (Potential for reduced activity of corticosteroids through liver enzyme-inducing properties). Products include:
- Decadron Phosphate Injection 2081
- Decadron Phosphate Sterile Ophthalmic Ointment.................. 2083
- Decadron Phosphate Sterile Ophthalmic Solution 2084
- NeoDecadron Sterile Ophthalmic Solution.................................. 2144

Dezocine (Potential for reduced activity of narcotics through liver enzyme-inducing properties).
No products indexed under this heading.

Diazepam (Potential for decreased effects of concurrently administered diazepam). Products include:
- Valium Injectable 3026
- Valium Tablets 3047

Dicumarol (Potential for reduced activity of anticoagulants through liver enzyme-inducing properties).
No products indexed under this heading.

Digitoxin (Potential for reduced activity of cardiac glycoside agents through liver enzyme-inducing properties).
No products indexed under this heading.

Digoxin (Potential for reduced activity of cardiac glycoside agents through liver enzyme-inducing properties). Products include:
- Digitek Tablets 1003
- Lanoxicaps Capsules 1574
- Lanoxin Injection 1581
- Lanoxin Tablets 1587
- Lanoxin Elixir Pediatric 1578
- Lanoxin Injection Pediatric 1584

Dirithromycin (Concomitant administration with higher doses of rifabutin results in higher incidence of uveitis). Products include:
- Dynabac Tablets 2269

Disopyramide Phosphate (Potential for decreased effects of concurrently administered mexiletine).
No products indexed under this heading.

Divalproex Sodium (Potential for decreased effects of concurrently administered anticonvulsants). Products include:
- Depakote Sprinkle Capsules 426
- Depakote Tablets 430
- Depakote ER Tablets 436

Dyphylline (Potential for decreased effects of concurrently administered theophylline). Products include:
- Lufyllin Tablets 3347
- Lufyllin-400 Tablets 3347
- Lufyllin-GG Elixir 3348
- Lufyllin-GG Tablets 3348

Erythromycin (Concomitant administration with higher doses of rifabutin results in higher incidence of uveitis). Products include:
- Emgel 2% Topical Gel 1285
- Ery-Tab Tablets 448
- Erythromycin Base Filmtab Tablets . 454
- Erythromycin Delayed-Release Capsules, USP 455
- PCE Dispertab Tablets 498

Erythromycin Estolate (Concomitant administration with higher doses of rifabutin results in higher incidence of uveitis).
No products indexed under this heading.

Erythromycin Ethylsuccinate (Concomitant administration with higher doses of rifabutin results in higher incidence of uveitis). Products include:
- E.E.S. 450
- EryPed 446
- Pediazole Suspension 3050

Erythromycin Gluceptate (Concomitant administration with higher doses of rifabutin results in higher incidence of uveitis).
No products indexed under this heading.

Erythromycin Stearate (Concomitant administration with higher doses of rifabutin results in higher incidence of uveitis). Products include:
- Erythrocin Stearate Filmtab Tablets 452

Esmolol Hydrochloride (Potential for decreased effects of concurrently administered beta-adrenergic blockers). Products include:
- Brevibloc Injection 858

Ethinyl Estradiol (Potential for reduced activity of oral contraceptives through liver enzyme-inducing properties). Products include:
- Alesse-21 Tablets 3468
- Alesse-28 Tablets 3473
- Brevicon 28-Day Tablets 3380
- Cyclessa Tablets 2450
- Desogen Tablets 2458
- Estinyl Tablets 3112
- Estrostep 2627
- femhrt Tablets 2635
- Levlen 962
- Levlite 21 Tablets 962
- Levlite 28 Tablets 962
- Levora Tablets 3389
- Loestrin 21 Tablets 2642
- Loestrin Fe Tablets 2642
- Lo/Ovral Tablets 3532
- Lo/Ovral-28 Tablets 3538
- Low-Ogestrel-28 Tablets 3392
- Microgestin Fe 1.5/30 Tablets 3407
- Microgestin Fe 1/20 Tablets 3400
- Mircette Tablets 2470
- Modicon 2563
- Necon 3415
- Nordette-28 Tablets 2257
- Norinyl 1 +35 28-Day Tablets 3380
- Ogestrel 0.5/50-28 Tablets 3428
- Ortho-Cept 21 Tablets 2546
- Ortho-Cept 28 Tablets 2546
- Ortho-Cyclen/Ortho Tri-Cyclen 2573
- Ortho-Novum 2563
- Ovcon 3364
- Ovral Tablets 3551
- Ovral-28 Tablets 3552
- Tri-Levlen 962
- Tri-Norinyl-28 Tablets 3433
- Triphasil-21 Tablets 3600
- Triphasil-28 Tablets 3605
- Trivora Tablets 3439
- Yasmin 28 Tablets 980
- Zovia 3449

Ethosuximide (Potential for decreased effects of concurrently administered anticonvulsants). Products include:
- Zarontin Capsules 2659
- Zarontin Syrup 2660

Ethotoin (Potential for decreased effects of concurrently administered anticonvulsants).
No products indexed under this heading.

Ethynodiol Diacetate (Potential for reduced activity of oral contraceptives through liver enzyme-inducing properties). Products include:
- Zovia 3449

Felbamate (Potential for decreased effects of concurrently administered anticonvulsants). Products include:
- Felbatol 3343

Fentanyl (Potential for reduced activity of narcotics through liver enzyme-inducing properties). Products include:
- Duragesic Transdermal System 1786

Fentanyl Citrate (Potential for reduced activity of narcotics through liver enzyme-inducing properties). Products include:
- Actiq 1184

Fluconazole (Concomitant administration with higher doses of rifabutin results in higher incidence of uveitis). Products include:
- Diflucan Tablets, Injection, and Oral Suspension 2681

Fludrocortisone Acetate (Potential for reduced activity of corticosteroids through liver enzyme-inducing properties). Products include:
- Florinef Acetate Tablets 2250

Fosphenytoin Sodium (Potential for decreased effects of concurrently administered anticonvulsants). Products include:
- Cerebyx Injection 2619

Glimepiride (Potential for reduced activity of oral sulfonylureas through liver enzyme-inducing properties). Products include:
- Amaryl Tablets 717

Glipizide (Potential for reduced activity of oral sulfonylureas through liver enzyme-inducing properties). Products include:
- Glucotrol Tablets 2692
- Glucotrol XL Extended Release Tablets 2693

Glyburide (Potential for reduced activity of oral sulfonylureas through liver enzyme-inducing properties). Products include:
- DiaBeta Tablets 741
- Glucovance Tablets 1086

Hydrocodone Bitartrate (Potential for reduced activity of narcotics through liver enzyme-inducing properties). Products include:
- Hycodan 1316
- Hycomine Compound Tablets 1317
- Hycotuss Expectorant Syrup 1318
- Lortab 3319
- Lortab Elixir 3317
- Maxidone Tablets CIII 3399
- Norco 5/325 Tablets CIII 3424
- Norco 7.5/325 Tablets CIII 3425
- Norco 10/325 Tablets CIII 3427
- Norco 10/325 Tablets CIII 3425
- Vicodin Tablets 516
- Vicodin ES Tablets 517
- Vicodin HP Tablets 518
- Vicodin Tuss Expectorant 519
- Vicoprofen Tablets 520
- Zydone Tablets 1330

Hydrocodone Polistirex (Potential for reduced activity of narcotics through liver enzyme-inducing properties). Products include:
- Tussionex Pennkinetic Extended-Release Suspension 1174

Hydrocortisone (Potential for reduced activity of corticosteroids through liver enzyme-inducing properties). Products include:
- Anusol-HC Cream 2.5% 2237
- Cipro HC Otic Suspension 540
- Cortaid Intensive Therapy Cream . ▣717
- Cortaid Maximum Strength Cream .... ▣717
- Cortisporin Ophthalmic Suspension Sterile .... ⊙297
- Cortizone•5 .... ▣699
- Cortizone•10 .... ▣699
- Cortizone•10 Plus Creme .... ▣700
- Cortizone for Kids Creme .... ▣699
- Hydrocortone Tablets 2106
- Massengill Medicated Soft Cloth Towelette .... ▣753
- VōSoL HC Otic Solution 3356

Hydrocortisone Acetate (Potential for reduced activity of corticosteroids through liver enzyme-inducing properties). Products include:
- Analpram-HC 1338
- Anusol HC-1 Hydrocortisone Anti-Itch Cream .... ▣689
- Anusol-HC Suppositories 2238
- Cortaid .... ▣717
- Cortifoam Rectal Foam 3170
- Cortisporin-TC Otic Suspension 2246
- Hydrocortone Acetate Injectable Suspension 2103
- Pramosone 1343
- Proctocort Suppositories 2264
- ProctoFoam-HC 3177
- Terra-Cortril Ophthalmic Suspension 2716

Hydrocortisone Sodium Phosphate (Potential for reduced activity of corticosteroids through liver enzyme-inducing properties). Products include:
- Hydrocortone Phosphate Injection, Sterile 2105

Hydrocortisone Sodium Succinate (Potential for reduced activity of corticosteroids through liver enzyme-inducing properties).
No products indexed under this heading.

Hydromorphone Hydrochloride (Potential for reduced activity of narcotics through liver enzyme-inducing properties). Products include:
- Dilaudid 441
- Dilaudid Oral Liquid 445
- Dilaudid Powder 441
- Dilaudid Rectal Suppositories 441
- Dilaudid Tablets 441
- Dilaudid Tablets - 8 mg 445
- Dilaudid-HP 443

Ketoconazole (Potential for decreased effects of concurrently administered ketoconazole). Products include:
- Nizoral 2% Cream 3620
- Nizoral A-D Shampoo 2008
- Nizoral 2% Shampoo 2007
- Nizoral Tablets 1791

Labetalol Hydrochloride (Potential for decreased effects of concurrently administered beta-adrenergic blockers). Products include:
- Normodyne Injection 3135
- Normodyne Tablets 3137

Lamotrigine (Potential for decreased effects of concurrently administered anticonvulsants). Products include:
- Lamictal 1567

Levetiracetam (Potential for decreased effects of concurrently administered anticonvulsants). Products include:
- Keppra Tablets 3314

Levobunolol Hydrochloride (Potential for decreased effects of concurrently administered beta-adrenergic blockers). Products include:
- Betagan .... ⊙228

Levonorgestrel (Potential for reduced activity of oral contraceptives through liver enzyme-inducing properties). Products include:
- Alesse-21 Tablets 3468
- Alesse-28 Tablets 3473
- Levlen 962
- Levlite 21 Tablets 962
- Levlite 28 Tablets 962
- Levora Tablets 3389
- Mirena Intrauterine System 974
- Nordette-28 Tablets 2257
- Norplant System 3543
- Tri-Levlen 962
- Triphasil-21 Tablets 3600
- Triphasil-28 Tablets 3605
- Trivora Tablets 3439

Levorphanol Tartrate (Potential for reduced activity of narcotics through liver enzyme-inducing properties). Products include:
- Levo-Dromoran 1734
- Levorphanol Tartrate Tablets 3059

Medroxyprogesterone Acetate (Potential for decreased effects of concurrently administered progestins). Products include:
- Depo-Provera Contraceptive Injection 2798
- Lunelle Monthly Injection 2827
- Premphase Tablets 3572
- Prempro Tablets 3572
- Provera Tablets 2853

Megestrol Acetate (Potential for decreased effects of concurrently administered progestins). Products include:
- Megace Oral Suspension 1124

Meperidine Hydrochloride (Potential for reduced activity of narcotics through liver enzyme-inducing properties). Products include:
- Demerol 3079
- Mepergan Injection 3539

Mephenytoin (Potential for decreased effects of concurrently administered anticonvulsants).
No products indexed under this heading.

Mephobarbital (Potential for decreased effects of concurrently administered barbiturates).
No products indexed under this heading.

Mestranol (Potential for reduced activity of oral contraceptives through liver enzyme-inducing properties). Products include:
Necon 1/50 Tablets ... 3415
Norinyl 1 + 50 28-Day Tablets ... 3380
Ortho-Novum 1/50□28 Tablets ... 2556

Methadone Hydrochloride (Potential for reduced activity of methadone-and narcotics through liver enzyme inducing properties). Products include:
Dolophine Hydrochloride Tablets ... 3056

Methsuximide (Potential for decreased effects of concurrently administered anticonvulsants). Products include:
Celontin Capsules ... 2618

Methylprednisolone Acetate (Potential for reduced activity of corticosteroids through liver enzyme-inducing properties). Products include:
Depo-Medrol Injectable Suspension ... 2795

Methylprednisolone Sodium Succinate (Potential for reduced activity of corticosteroids through liver enzyme-inducing properties). Products include:
Solu-Medrol Sterile Powder ... 2855

Metipranolol Hydrochloride (Potential for decreased effects of concurrently administered beta-adrenergic blockers).
No products indexed under this heading.

Metoprolol Succinate (Potential for decreased effects of concurrently administered beta-adrenergic blockers). Products include:
Toprol-XL Tablets ... 651

Metoprolol Tartrate (Potential for decreased effects of concurrently administered beta-adrenergic blockers).
No products indexed under this heading.

Morphine Sulfate (Potential for reduced activity of narcotics through liver enzyme-inducing properties). Products include:
Astramorph/PF Injection, USP (Preservative-Free) ... 594
Duramorph Injection ... 1312
Infumorph 200 and Infumorph 500 Sterile Solutions ... 1314
Kadian Capsules ... 1335
MS Contin Tablets ... 2896
MSIR ... 2898
Oramorph SR Tablets ... 3062
Roxanol ... 3066

Nadolol (Potential for decreased effects of concurrently administered beta-adrenergic blockers). Products include:
Corgard Tablets ... 2245
Corzide 40/5 Tablets ... 2247
Corzide 80/5 Tablets ... 2247
Nadolol Tablets ... 2288

Norethindrone (Potential for reduced activity of oral contraceptives through liver enzyme-inducing properties). Products include:
Brevicon 28-Day Tablets ... 3380
Micronor Tablets ... 2543
Modicon ... 2563
Necon ... 3415
Norinyl 1 +35 28-Day Tablets ... 3380
Norinyl 1 + 50 28-Day Tablets ... 3380
Nor-QD Tablets ... 3423
Ortho-Novum ... 2563
Ortho-Novum 1/50□28 Tablets ... 2556
Ovcon ... 3364
Tri-Norinyl-28 Tablets ... 3433

Norethynodrel (Potential for reduced activity of oral contraceptives through liver enzyme-inducing properties).
No products indexed under this heading.

Norgestimate (Potential for decreased effects of concurrently administered progestins). Products include:
Ortho-Cyclen/Ortho Tri-Cyclen ... 2573
Ortho-Prefest Tablets ... 2570

Norgestrel (Potential for reduced activity of oral contraceptives through liver enzyme-inducing properties). Products include:
Lo/Ovral Tablets ... 3532
Lo/Ovral-28 Tablets ... 3538
Low-Ogestrel-28 Tablets ... 3392
Ogestrel 0.5/50-28 Tablets ... 3428
Ovral Tablets ... 3551
Ovral-28 Tablets ... 3552
Ovrette Tablets ... 3552

Oxcarbazepine (Potential for decreased effects of concurrently administered anticonvulsants). Products include:
Trileptal Oral Suspension ... 2407
Trileptal Tablets ... 2407

Oxycodone Hydrochloride (Potential for reduced activity of narcotics through liver enzyme-inducing properties). Products include:
OxyContin Tablets ... 2912
OxyFast Oral Concentrate Solution ... 2916
OxyIR Capsules ... 2916
Percocet Tablets ... 1326
Percodan Tablets ... 1327
Percolone Tablets ... 1327
Roxicodone ... 3067
Tylox Capsules ... 2597

Paramethadione (Potential for decreased effects of concurrently administered anticonvulsants).
No products indexed under this heading.

Penbutolol Sulfate (Potential for decreased effects of concurrently administered beta-adrenergic blockers).
No products indexed under this heading.

Pentobarbital Sodium (Potential for decreased effects of concurrently administered barbiturates). Products include:
Nembutal Sodium Solution ... 485

Phenacemide (Potential for decreased effects of concurrently administered anticonvulsants).
No products indexed under this heading.

Phenobarbital (Potential for decreased effects of concurrently administered anticonvulsants and barbiturates). Products include:
Arco-Lase Plus Tablets ... 592
Donnatal ... 2929
Donnatal Extentabs ... 2930

Phensuximide (Potential for decreased effects of concurrently administered anticonvulsants).
No products indexed under this heading.

Phenytoin (Potential for decreased effects of concurrently administered anticonvulsants). Products include:
Dilantin Infatabs ... 2624
Dilantin-125 Oral Suspension ... 2625

Phenytoin Sodium (Potential for decreased effects of concurrently administered anticonvulsants). Products include:
Dilantin Kapseals ... 2622

Pindolol (Potential for decreased effects of concurrently administered beta-adrenergic blockers).
No products indexed under this heading.

Prednisolone Acetate (Potential for reduced activity of corticosteroids through liver enzyme-inducing properties). Products include:
Blephamide Ophthalmic Ointment ... 547
Blephamide Ophthalmic Suspension ... 548
Poly-Pred Liquifilm Ophthalmic Suspension ... ⊙ 245
Pred Forte Ophthalmic Suspension ... ⊙ 246
Pred Mild Sterile Ophthalmic Suspension ... ⊙ 249
Pred-G Ophthalmic Suspension ... ⊙ 247
Pred-G Sterile Ophthalmic Ointment ... ⊙ 248

Prednisolone Sodium Phosphate (Potential for reduced activity of corticosteroids through liver enzyme-inducing properties). Products include:
Pediapred Oral Solution ... 1170

Prednisolone Tebutate (Potential for reduced activity of corticosteroids through liver enzyme-inducing properties).
No products indexed under this heading.

Prednisone (Potential for reduced activity of corticosteroids through liver enzyme-inducing properties). Products include:
Prednisone ... 3064

Primidone (Potential for decreased effects of concurrently administered anticonvulsants).
No products indexed under this heading.

Propoxyphene Hydrochloride (Potential for reduced activity of narcotics through liver enzyme-inducing properties). Products include:
Darvon Pulvules ... 1909
Darvon Compound-65 Pulvules ... 1910

Propoxyphene Napsylate (Potential for reduced activity of narcotics through liver enzyme-inducing properties). Products include:
Darvon-N/Darvocet-N ... 1907
Darvon-N Tablets ... 1912

Propranolol Hydrochloride (Potential for decreased effects of concurrently administered beta-adrenergic blockers). Products include:
Inderal ... 3513
Inderal LA Long-Acting Capsules ... 3516
Inderide Tablets ... 3517
Inderide LA Long-Acting Capsules ... 3519

Quinidine Gluconate (Potential for reduced activity of quinidine through liver enzyme-inducing properties). Products include:
Quinaglute Dura-Tabs Tablets ... 978

Quinidine Polygalacturonate (Potential for reduced activity of quinidine through liver enzyme-inducing properties).
No products indexed under this heading.

Quinidine Sulfate (Potential for reduced activity of quinidine through liver enzyme-inducing properties). Products include:
Quinidex Extentabs ... 2933

Remifentanil Hydrochloride (Potential for reduced activity of narcotics through liver enzyme-inducing properties).
No products indexed under this heading.

Secobarbital Sodium (Potential for decreased effects of concurrently administered barbiturates).
No products indexed under this heading.

Sotalol Hydrochloride (Potential for decreased effects of concurrently administered beta-adrenergic blockers). Products include:
Betapace Tablets ... 950
Betapace AF Tablets ... 954

Sufentanil Citrate (Potential for reduced activity of narcotics through liver enzyme-inducing properties).
No products indexed under this heading.

Theophylline (Potential for decreased effects of concurrently administered theophylline). Products include:
Aerolate ... 1361
Theo-Dur Extended-Release Tablets ... 1835
Uni-Dur Extended-Release Tablets ... 1841
Uniphyl 400 mg and 600 mg Tablets ... 2903

Theophylline Calcium Salicylate (Potential for decreased effects of concurrently administered theophylline).
No products indexed under this heading.

Theophylline Sodium Glycinate (Potential for decreased effects of concurrently administered theophylline).
No products indexed under this heading.

Thiamylal Sodium (Potential for decreased effects of concurrently administered barbiturates).
No products indexed under this heading.

Tiagabine Hydrochloride (Potential for decreased effects of concurrently administered anticonvulsants). Products include:
Gabitril Tablets ... 1189

Timolol Hemihydrate (Potential for decreased effects of concurrently administered beta-adrenergic blockers). Products include:
Betimol Ophthalmic Solution ... ⊙ 324

Timolol Maleate (Potential for decreased effects of concurrently administered beta-adrenergic blockers). Products include:
Blocadren Tablets ... 2046
Cosopt Sterile Ophthalmic Solution ... 2065
Timolide Tablets ... 2187
Timolol GFS ... ⊙ 266
Timoptic in Ocudose ... 2192
Timoptic Sterile Ophthalmic Solution ... 2190
Timoptic-XE Sterile Ophthalmic Gel Forming Solution ... 2194

Tolazamide (Potential for reduced activity of oral sulfonylureas through liver enzyme-inducing properties).
No products indexed under this heading.

Tolbutamide (Potential for reduced activity of oral sulfonylureas through liver enzyme-inducing properties).
No products indexed under this heading.

Topiramate (Potential for decreased effects of concurrently administered anticonvulsants). Products include:
Topamax Sprinkle Capsules ... 2590
Topamax Tablets ... 2590

Triamcinolone (Potential for reduced activity of corticosteroids through liver enzyme-inducing properties).
No products indexed under this heading.

Triamcinolone Acetonide (Potential for reduced activity of corticosteroids through liver enzyme-inducing properties). Products include:
Azmacort Inhalation Aerosol ... 728
Nasacort Nasal Inhaler ... 750
Nasacort AQ Nasal Spray ... 752
Tri-Nasal Spray ... 2274

Triamcinolone Diacetate (Potential for reduced activity of corticosteroids through liver enzyme-inducing properties).
No products indexed under this heading.

Triamcinolone Hexacetonide (Potential for reduced activity of corticosteroids through liver enzyme-inducing properties).
No products indexed under this heading.

Trimethadione (Potential for decreased effects of concurrently administered anticonvulsants).
No products indexed under this heading.

Troleandomycin (Concomitant administration with higher doses of rifabutin results in higher incidence of uveitis). Products include:
Tao Capsules ... 2716

Valproate Sodium (Potential for decreased effects of concurrently administered anticonvulsants). Products include:
Depacon Injection ... 416

IMPORTANT NOTE: Always consult each drug listing in the patient's regimen for possible interactions.

Valproic Acid (Potential for decreased effects of concurrently administered anticonvulsants). Products include:
- Depakene ... 421

Verapamil Hydrochloride (Potential for decreased effects of concurrently administered verapamil). Products include:
- Covera-HS Tablets ... 3199
- Isoptin SR Tablets ... 467
- Tarka Tablets ... 508
- Verelan Capsules ... 3184
- Verelan PM Capsules ... 3186

Warfarin Sodium (Potential for reduced activity of anticoagulants through liver enzyme-inducing properties). Products include:
- Coumadin for Injection ... 1243
- Coumadin Tablets ... 1243
- Warfarin Sodium Tablets, USP ... 3302

Zidovudine (Reduced steady-state plasma levels of zidovudine after repeated Mycobutin dosing). Products include:
- Combivir Tablets ... 1502
- Retrovir ... 1625
- Retrovir IV Infusion ... 1629
- Trizivir Tablets ... 1669

Zonisamide (Potential for decreased effects of concurrently administered anticonvulsants). Products include:
- Zonegran Capsules ... 1307

Food Interactions

Diet, high-lipid (High-fat meals slow the rate without influencing the extent of absorption from the capsule dosage form).

MYKROX TABLETS

(Metolazone) ... 1168

May interact with antihypertensives, barbiturates, corticosteroids, cardiac glycosides, oral hypoglycemic agents, insulin, lithium preparations, loop diuretics, narcotic analgesics, non-steroidal anti-inflammatory agents, salicylates, and certain other agents. Compounds in these categories include:

Acarbose (Blood glucose concentrations may be raised by metolazone in diabetics). Products include:
- Precose Tablets ... 906

Acebutolol Hydrochloride (Orthostatic hypotension may occur with concurrent therapy). Products include:
- Sectral Capsules ... 3589

ACTH (Potential for increased hypokalemia).
- No products indexed under this heading.

Alfentanil Hydrochloride (Potentiates orthostatic hypotensive effects).
- No products indexed under this heading.

Amlodipine Besylate (Orthostatic hypotension may occur with concurrent therapy). Products include:
- Lotrel Capsules ... 2370
- Norvasc Tablets ... 2704

Aprobarbital (Potentiates orthostatic hypotensive effects).
- No products indexed under this heading.

Aspirin (Antihypertensive effects of Mykrox may be decreased). Products include:
- Aggrenox Capsules ... 1026
- Alka-Seltzer ... ▣603
- Alka-Seltzer Lemon Lime Antacid and Pain Reliever Effervescent Tablets ... ▣603
- Alka-Seltzer Extra Strength Antacid and Pain Reliever Effervescent Tablets ... ▣603
- Alka-Seltzer PM Effervescent Tablets ... ▣605
- Genuine Bayer Tablets, Caplets and Gelcaps ... ▣606
- Extra Strength Bayer Caplets and Gelcaps ... ▣610
- Aspirin Regimen Bayer Children's Chewable Tablets (Orange or Cherry Flavored) ... ▣607
- Bayer, Aspirin Regimen ... ▣606
- Aspirin Regimen Bayer 81 mg Caplets with Calcium ... ▣607
- Genuine Bayer Professional Labeling (Aspirin Regimen Bayer) ... ▣608
- Extra Strength Bayer Arthritis Caplets ... ▣610
- Extra Strength Bayer Plus Caplets ... ▣610
- Extra Strength Bayer PM Caplets ... ▣611
- BC Powder ... ▣619
- BC Allergy Sinus Cold Powder ... ▣619
- Arthritis Strength BC Powder ... ▣619
- BC Sinus Cold Powder ... ▣619
- Darvon Compound-65 Pulvules ... 1910
- Ecotrin Enteric Coated Aspirin Low, Regular and Maximum Strength Tablets ... 1715
- Excedrin Extra-Strength Tablets, Caplets, and Geltabs ... ▣629
- Excedrin Migraine ... 1070
- Goody's Body Pain Formula Powder ... ▣620
- Goody's Extra Strength Headache Powder ... ▣620
- Goody's Extra Strength Pain Relief Tablets ... ▣620
- Percodan Tablets ... 1327
- Robaxisal Tablets ... 2939
- Soma Compound Tablets ... 3354
- Soma Compound w/Codeine Tablets ... 3355
- Vanquish Caplets ... ▣617

Atenolol (Orthostatic hypotension may occur with concurrent therapy). Products include:
- Tenoretic Tablets ... 690
- Tenormin I.V. Injection ... 692

Benazepril Hydrochloride (Orthostatic hypotension may occur with concurrent therapy). Products include:
- Lotensin Tablets ... 2365
- Lotensin HCT Tablets ... 2367
- Lotrel Capsules ... 2370

Bendroflumethiazide (Orthostatic hypotension may occur with concurrent therapy). Products include:
- Corzide 40/5 Tablets ... 2247
- Corzide 80/5 Tablets ... 2247

Betamethasone Acetate (Potential for increased hypokalemia). Products include:
- Celestone Soluspan Injectable Suspension ... 3097

Betamethasone Sodium Phosphate (Potential for increased hypokalemia). Products include:
- Celestone Soluspan Injectable Suspension ... 3097

Betaxolol Hydrochloride (Orthostatic hypotension may occur with concurrent therapy). Products include:
- Betoptic S Ophthalmic Suspension ... 537

Bisoprolol Fumarate (Orthostatic hypotension may occur with concurrent therapy). Products include:
- Zebeta Tablets ... 1885
- Ziac Tablets ... 1887

Bumetanide (Large or prolonged losses of fluids and electrolytes may result).
- No products indexed under this heading.

Buprenorphine Hydrochloride (Potentiates orthostatic hypotensive effects). Products include:
- Buprenex Injectable ... 2918

Butabarbital (Potentiates orthostatic hypotensive effects).
- No products indexed under this heading.

Butalbital (Potentiates orthostatic hypotensive effects). Products include:
- Phrenilin ... 578
- Sedapap Tablets 50 mg/650 mg ... 2225

Candesartan Cilexetil (Orthostatic hypotension may occur with concurrent therapy). Products include:
- Atacand Tablets ... 595
- Atacand HCT Tablets ... 597

Captopril (Orthostatic hypotension may occur with concurrent therapy). Products include:
- Captopril Tablets ... 2281

Carteolol Hydrochloride (Orthostatic hypotension may occur with concurrent therapy). Products include:
- Carteolol Hydrochloride Ophthalmic Solution USP, 1% ... ⊙258
- Ocupress Ophthalmic Solution, 1% Sterile ... ⊙303

Celecoxib (Antihypertensive effects of Mykrox may be decreased). Products include:
- Celebrex Capsules ... 2676
- Celebrex Capsules ... 2780

Chlorothiazide (Orthostatic hypotension may occur with concurrent therapy). Products include:
- Aldoclor Tablets ... 2035
- Diuril Oral ... 2087

Chlorothiazide Sodium (Orthostatic hypotension may occur with concurrent therapy). Products include:
- Diuril Sodium Intravenous ... 2086

Chlorpropamide (Blood glucose concentrations may be raised by metolazone in diabetics). Products include:
- Diabinese Tablets ... 2680

Chlorthalidone (Orthostatic hypotension may occur with concurrent therapy). Products include:
- Clorpres Tablets ... 1002
- Combipres Tablets ... 1040
- Tenoretic Tablets ... 690

Choline Magnesium Trisalicylate (Antihypertensive effects of Mykrox may be decreased). Products include:
- Trilisate ... 2901

Clonidine (Orthostatic hypotension may occur with concurrent therapy). Products include:
- Catapres-TTS ... 1038

Clonidine Hydrochloride (Orthostatic hypotension may occur with concurrent therapy). Products include:
- Catapres Tablets ... 1037
- Clorpres Tablets ... 1002
- Combipres Tablets ... 1040
- Duraclon Injection ... 3057

Codeine Phosphate (Potentiates orthostatic hypotensive effects). Products include:
- Phenergan with Codeine Syrup ... 3557
- Phenergan VC with Codeine Syrup ... 3561
- Robitussin A-C Syrup ... 2942
- Robitussin-DAC Syrup ... 2942
- Ryna-C Liquid ... ▣768
- Soma Compound w/Codeine Tablets ... 3355
- Tussi-Organidin NR Liquid ... 3350
- Tussi-Organidin-S NR Liquid ... 3350
- Tylenol with Codeine ... 2595

Cortisone Acetate (Potential for increased hypokalemia). Products include:
- Cortone Acetate Injectable Suspension ... 2059
- Cortone Acetate Tablets ... 2061

Deserpidine (Orthostatic hypotension may occur with concurrent therapy).
- No products indexed under this heading.

Deslanoside (Hypokalemia increases sensitivity of the myocardium to digitalis toxicity).
- No products indexed under this heading.

Dexamethasone (Potential for increased hypokalemia). Products include:
- Decadron Elixir ... 2078
- Decadron Tablets ... 2079
- TobraDex Ophthalmic Ointment ... 542
- TobraDex Ophthalmic Suspension ... 541

Dexamethasone Acetate (Potential for increased hypokalemia).
- No products indexed under this heading.

Dexamethasone Sodium Phosphate (Potential for increased hypokalemia). Products include:
- Decadron Phosphate Injection ... 2081
- Decadron Phosphate Sterile Ophthalmic Ointment ... 2083
- Decadron Phosphate Sterile Ophthalmic Solution ... 2084
- NeoDecadron Sterile Ophthalmic Solution ... 2144

Dezocine (Potentiates orthostatic hypotensive effects).
- No products indexed under this heading.

Diazoxide (Orthostatic hypotension may occur with concurrent therapy).
- No products indexed under this heading.

Diclofenac Potassium (Antihypertensive effects of Mykrox may be decreased). Products include:
- Cataflam Tablets ... 2315

Diclofenac Sodium (Antihypertensive effects of Mykrox may be decreased). Products include:
- Arthrotec Tablets ... 3195
- Voltaren Ophthalmic Sterile Ophthalmic Solution ... ⊙312
- Voltaren Tablets ... 2315
- Voltaren-XR Tablets ... 2315

Dicumarol (May affect the hypoprothrombinemic response to anticoagulants; dosage adjustments may be necessary).
- No products indexed under this heading.

Diflunisal (Antihypertensive effects of Mykrox may be decreased). Products include:
- Dolobid Tablets ... 2088

Digitoxin (Hypokalemia increases sensitivity of the myocardium to digitalis toxicity).
- No products indexed under this heading.

Digoxin (Hypokalemia increases sensitivity of the myocardium to digitalis toxicity). Products include:
- Digitek Tablets ... 1003
- Lanoxicaps Capsules ... 1574
- Lanoxin Injection ... 1581
- Lanoxin Tablets ... 1587
- Lanoxin Elixir Pediatric ... 1578
- Lanoxin Injection Pediatric ... 1584

Diltiazem Hydrochloride (Orthostatic hypotension may occur with concurrent therapy). Products include:
- Cardizem Injectable ... 1018
- Cardizem Lyo-Ject Syringe ... 1018
- Cardizem Monovial ... 1018
- Cardizem CD Capsules ... 1016
- Tiazac Capsules ... 1378

Doxazosin Mesylate (Orthostatic hypotension may occur with concurrent therapy). Products include:
- Cardura Tablets ... 2668

Enalapril Maleate (Orthostatic hypotension may occur with concurrent therapy). Products include:
- Lexxel Tablets ... 608
- Vaseretic Tablets ... 2204
- Vasotec Tablets ... 2210

Enalaprilat (Orthostatic hypotension may occur with concurrent therapy). Products include:
- Enalaprilat Injection ... 863
- Vasotec I.V. Injection ... 2207

Eprosartan Mesylate (Orthostatic hypotension may occur with concurrent therapy). Products include:
- Teveten Tablets ... 3327

Esmolol Hydrochloride (Orthostatic hypotension may occur with concurrent therapy). Products include:
- Brevibloc Injection ... 858

Ethacrynic Acid (Large or prolonged losses of fluids and electrolytes may result). Products include:
- Edecrin Tablets ... 2091

Etodolac (Antihypertensive effects of Mykrox may be decreased). Products include:
- Lodine ... 3528

Lodine XL Extended-Release Tablets 3530

Felodipine (Orthostatic hypotension may occur with concurrent therapy). Products include:
Lexxel Tablets 608
Plendil Extended-Release Tablets 623

Fenoprofen Calcium (Antihypertensive effects of Mykrox may be decreased).
No products indexed under this heading.

Fentanyl (Potentiates orthostatic hypotensive effects). Products include:
Duragesic Transdermal System 1786

Fentanyl Citrate (Potentiates orthostatic hypotensive effects). Products include:
Actiq 1184

Fludrocortisone Acetate (Potential for increased hypokalemia). Products include:
Florinef Acetate Tablets 2250

Flurbiprofen (Antihypertensive effects of Mykrox may be decreased).
No products indexed under this heading.

Fosinopril Sodium (Orthostatic hypotension may occur with concurrent therapy). Products include:
Monopril Tablets 1091
Monopril HCT 1094

Furosemide (Large or prolonged losses of fluids and electrolytes may result; orthostatic hypotension may occur with concurrent therapy). Products include:
Furosemide Tablets 2284

Glimepiride (Blood glucose concentrations may be raised by metolazone in diabetics). Products include:
Amaryl Tablets 717

Glipizide (Blood glucose concentrations may be raised by metolazone in diabetics). Products include:
Glucotrol Tablets 2692
Glucotrol XL Extended Release Tablets 2693

Glyburide (Blood glucose concentrations may be raised by metolazone in diabetics). Products include:
DiaBeta Tablets 741
Glucovance Tablets 1086

Guanabenz Acetate (Orthostatic hypotension may occur with concurrent therapy).
No products indexed under this heading.

Guanethidine Monosulfate (Orthostatic hypotension may occur with concurrent therapy).
No products indexed under this heading.

Hydralazine Hydrochloride (Orthostatic hypotension may occur with concurrent therapy).
No products indexed under this heading.

Hydrochlorothiazide (Orthostatic hypotension may occur with concurrent therapy). Products include:
Accuretic Tablets 2614
Aldoril Tablets 2039
Atacand HCT Tablets 597
Avalide Tablets 1070
Diovan HCT Tablets 2338
Dyazide Capsules 1515
HydroDIURIL Tablets 2108
Hyzaar 2109
Inderide Tablets 3517
Inderide LA Long-Acting Capsules 3519
Lotensin HCT Tablets 2367
Maxzide 1008
Micardis HCT Tablets 1051
Microzide Capsules 3414
Moduretic Tablets 2138
Monopril HCT 1094
Prinzide Tablets 2168
Timolide Tablets 2187
Uniretic Tablets 3178
Vaseretic Tablets 2204
Zestoretic Tablets 695
Ziac Tablets 1887

Hydrocodone Bitartrate (Potentiates orthostatic hypotensive effects). Products include:
Hycodan 1316
Hycomine Compound Tablets 1317
Hycotuss Expectorant Syrup 1318
Lortab 3319
Lortab Elixir 3317
Maxidone Tablets CIII 3399
Norco 5/325 Tablets CIII 3424
Norco 7.5/325 Tablets CIII 3425
Norco 10/325 Tablets CIII 3427
Norco 10/325 Tablets CIII 3425
Vicodin Tablets 516
Vicodin ES Tablets 517
Vicodin HP Tablets 518
Vicodin Tuss Expectorant 519
Vicoprofen Tablets 520
Zydone Tablets 1330

Hydrocodone Polistirex (Potentiates orthostatic hypotensive effects). Products include:
Tussionex Pennkinetic Extended-Release Suspension 1174

Hydrocortisone (Potential for increased hypokalemia). Products include:
Anusol-HC Cream 2.5% 2237
Cipro HC Otic Suspension 540
Cortaid Intensive Therapy Cream 717
Cortaid Maximum Strength Cream 717
Cortisporin Ophthalmic Suspension Sterile 297
Cortizone•5 699
Cortizone•10 699
Cortizone•10 Plus Creme 700
Cortizone for Kids Creme 699
Hydrocortone Tablets 2106
Massengill Medicated Soft Cloth Towelette 753
VōSoL HC Otic Solution 3356

Hydrocortisone Acetate (Potential for increased hypokalemia). Products include:
Analpram-HC 1338
Anusol HC-1 Hydrocortisone Anti-Itch Cream 689
Anusol-HC Suppositories 2238
Cortaid 717
Cortifoam Rectal Foam 3170
Cortisporin-TC Otic Suspension 2246
Hydrocortone Acetate Injectable Suspension 2103
Pramosone 1343
Proctocort Suppositories 2264
ProctoFoam-HC 3177
Terra-Cortril Ophthalmic Suspension 2716

Hydrocortisone Sodium Phosphate (Potential for increased hypokalemia). Products include:
Hydrocortone Phosphate Injection, Sterile 2105

Hydrocortisone Sodium Succinate (Potential for increased hypokalemia).
No products indexed under this heading.

Hydroflumethiazide (Orthostatic hypotension may occur with concurrent therapy). Products include:
Diucardin Tablets 3494

Hydromorphone Hydrochloride (Potentiates orthostatic hypotensive effects). Products include:
Dilaudid 441
Dilaudid Oral Liquid 445
Dilaudid Powder 441
Dilaudid Rectal Suppositories 441
Dilaudid Tablets 441
Dilaudid Tablets - 8 mg 445
Dilaudid-HP 443

Ibuprofen (Antihypertensive effects of Mykrox may be decreased). Products include:
Advil 771
Children's Advil Oral Suspension 773
Children's Advil Chewable Tablets 773
Advil Cold and Sinus Caplets 771
Advil Cold and Sinus Tablets 771
Advil Flu & Body Ache Caplets 772
Infants' Advil Drops 773
Junior Strength Advil Tablets 773
Junior Strength Advil Chewable Tablets 773
Advil Migraine Liquigels 772
Children's Motrin Oral Suspension and Chewable Tablets 2006
Children's Motrin Cold Oral Suspension 2007
Children's Motrin Oral Suspension 643
Motrin Suspension, Oral Drops, Chewable Tablets, and Caplets 2002
Infants' Motrin Concentrated Drops 2006
Junior Strength Motrin Caplets and Chewable Tablets 2006
Motrin IB Tablets, Caplets, and Gelcaps 2002
Motrin Migraine Pain Caplets 2005
Motrin Sinus Headache Caplets 2005
Vicoprofen Tablets 520

Indapamide (Orthostatic hypotension may occur with concurrent therapy). Products include:
Indapamide Tablets 2286

Indomethacin (Antihypertensive effects of Mykrox may be decreased). Products include:
Indocin 2112

Indomethacin Sodium Trihydrate (Antihypertensive effects of Mykrox may be decreased). Products include:
Indocin I.V. 2115

Insulin, Human, Zinc Suspension (Blood glucose concentrations may be raised by metolazone in diabetics). Products include:
Humulin L, 100 Units 1937
Humulin U, 100 Units 1943
Novolin L Human Insulin 10 ml Vials 2422

Insulin, Human NPH (Blood glucose concentrations may be raised by metolazone in diabetics). Products include:
Humulin N, 100 Units 1939
Humulin N NPH Pen 1940
Novolin N Human Insulin 10 ml Vials 2422
Novolin N PenFill 2423
Novolin N Prefilled Syringe Disposable Insulin Delivery System 2425

Insulin, Human Regular (Blood glucose concentrations may be raised by metolazone in diabetics). Products include:
Humulin R Regular (U-500) 1943
Humulin R, 100 Units 1941
Novolin R Human Insulin 10 ml Vials 2423
Novolin R PenFill 2423
Novolin R Prefilled Syringe Disposable Insulin Delivery System 2425
Velosulin BR Human Insulin 10 ml Vials 2435

Insulin, Human Regular and Human NPH Mixture (Blood glucose concentrations may be raised by metolazone in diabetics). Products include:
Humulin 50/50, 100 Units 1934
Humulin 70/30, 100 Units 1935
Humulin 70/30 Pen 1936
Novolin 70/30 Human Insulin 10 ml Vials 2421
Novolin 70/30 PenFill 2423
Novolin 70/30 Prefilled Disposable Insulin Delivery System 2425

Insulin, NPH (Blood glucose concentrations may be raised by metolazone in diabetics). Products include:
Iletin II, NPH (Pork), 100 Units 1946

Insulin, Regular (Blood glucose concentrations may be raised by metolazone in diabetics). Products include:
Iletin II, Regular (Pork), 100 Units 1947

Insulin, Zinc Crystals (Blood glucose concentrations may be raised by metolazone in diabetics).
No products indexed under this heading.

Insulin, Zinc Suspension (Blood glucose concentrations may be raised by metolazone in diabetics). Products include:
Iletin II, Lente (Pork), 100 Units 1945

Insulin Aspart, Human Regular (Blood glucose concentrations may be raised by metolazone in diabetics).
No products indexed under this heading.

Insulin glargine (Blood glucose concentrations may be raised by metolazone in diabetics). Products include:
Lantus Injection 742

Insulin Lispro, Human (Blood glucose concentrations may be raised by metolazone in diabetics). Products include:
Humalog 1926
Humalog Mix 75/25 Pen 1928

Insulin Lispro Protamine, Human (Blood glucose concentrations may be raised by metolazone in diabetics). Products include:
Humalog Mix 75/25 Pen 1928

Irbesartan (Orthostatic hypotension may occur with concurrent therapy). Products include:
Avalide Tablets 1070
Avapro Tablets 1074
Avapro Tablets 3076

Isradipine (Orthostatic hypotension may occur with concurrent therapy). Products include:
DynaCirc Capsules 2921
DynaCirc CR Tablets 2923

Ketoprofen (Antihypertensive effects of Mykrox may be decreased). Products include:
Orudis Capsules 3548
Orudis KT Tablets 778
Oruvail Capsules 3548

Ketorolac Tromethamine (Antihypertensive effects of Mykrox may be decreased). Products include:
Acular Ophthalmic Solution 544
Acular PF Ophthalmic Solution 544
Toradol 3018

Labetalol Hydrochloride (Orthostatic hypotension may occur with concurrent therapy). Products include:
Normodyne Injection 3135
Normodyne Tablets 3137

Levorphanol Tartrate (Potentiates orthostatic hypotensive effects). Products include:
Levo-Dromoran 1734
Levorphanol Tartrate Tablets 3059

Lisinopril (Orthostatic hypotension may occur with concurrent therapy). Products include:
Prinivil Tablets 2164
Prinzide Tablets 2168
Zestoretic Tablets 695
Zestril Tablets 698

Lithium Carbonate (Reduced renal clearance of lithium; high risk of lithium toxicity). Products include:
Eskalith 1527
Lithium Carbonate 3061
Lithobid Slow-Release Tablets 3255

Lithium Citrate (Reduced renal clearance of lithium; high risk of lithium toxicity). Products include:
Lithium Citrate Syrup 3061

Losartan Potassium (Orthostatic hypotension may occur with concurrent therapy). Products include:
Cozaar Tablets 2067
Hyzaar 2109

Magnesium Salicylate (Antihypertensive effects of Mykrox may be decreased). Products include:
Momentum Backache Relief Extra Strength Caplets 666

Mecamylamine Hydrochloride (Orthostatic hypotension may occur with concurrent therapy). Products include:
Inversine Tablets 1850

Meclofenamate Sodium (Antihypertensive effects of Mykrox may be decreased).
No products indexed under this heading.

Mefenamic Acid (Antihypertensive effects of Mykrox may be decreased). Products include:
Ponstel Capsules 1356

IMPORTANT NOTE: Always consult each drug listing in the patient's regimen for possible interactions.

Meloxicam (Antihypertensive effects of Mykrox may be decreased). Products include:
Mobic Tablets 1054

Meperidine Hydrochloride (Potentiates orthostatic hypotensive effects). Products include:
Demerol 3079
Mepergan Injection 3539

Mephobarbital (Potentiates orthostatic hypotensive effects).
No products indexed under this heading.

Metformin Hydrochloride (Blood glucose concentrations may be raised by metolazone in diabetics). Products include:
Glucophage Tablets 1080
Glucophage XR Tablets 1080
Glucovance Tablets 1086

Methadone Hydrochloride (Potentiates orthostatic hypotensive effects). Products include:
Dolophine Hydrochloride Tablets 3056

Methenamine (Efficacy of methenamine may be decreased). Products include:
Prosed/DS Tablets 3268
Urimax Tablets 1769
Urised Tablets 2876

Methenamine Hippurate (Efficacy of methenamine may be decreased).
No products indexed under this heading.

Methenamine Mandelate (Efficacy of methenamine may be decreased). Products include:
Uroqid-Acid No. 2 Tablets 947

Methyclothiazide (Orthostatic hypotension may occur with concurrent therapy).
No products indexed under this heading.

Methyldopa (Orthostatic hypotension may occur with concurrent therapy). Products include:
Aldoclor Tablets 2035
Aldomet Tablets 2037
Aldoril Tablets 2039

Methyldopate Hydrochloride (Orthostatic hypotension may occur with concurrent therapy).
No products indexed under this heading.

Methylprednisolone Acetate (Potential for increased hypokalemia). Products include:
Depo-Medrol Injectable Suspension 2795

Methylprednisolone Sodium Succinate (Potential for increased hypokalemia). Products include:
Solu-Medrol Sterile Powder 2855

Metoprolol Succinate (Orthostatic hypotension may occur with concurrent therapy). Products include:
Toprol-XL Tablets 651

Metoprolol Tartrate (Orthostatic hypotension may occur with concurrent therapy).
No products indexed under this heading.

Metyrosine (Orthostatic hypotension may occur with concurrent therapy). Products include:
Demser Capsules 2085

Mibefradil Dihydrochloride (Orthostatic hypotension may occur with concurrent therapy).
No products indexed under this heading.

Miglitol (Blood glucose concentrations may be raised by metolazone in diabetics). Products include:
Glyset Tablets 2821

Minoxidil (Orthostatic hypotension may occur with concurrent therapy). Products include:
Rogaine Extra Strength for Men Topical Solution .... ▣721
Rogaine for Women Topical Solution .... ▣721

Moexipril Hydrochloride (Orthostatic hypotension may occur with concurrent therapy). Products include:
Uniretic Tablets 3178
Univasc Tablets 3181

Morphine Sulfate (Potentiates orthostatic hypotensive effects). Products include:
Astramorph/PF Injection, USP (Preservative-Free) 594
Duramorph Injection 1312
Infumorph 200 and Infumorph 500 Sterile Solutions 1314
Kadian Capsules 1335
MS Contin Tablets 2896
MSIR 2898
Oramorph SR Tablets 3062
Roxanol 3066

Nabumetone (Antihypertensive effects of Mykrox may be decreased). Products include:
Relafen Tablets 1617

Nadolol (Orthostatic hypotension may occur with concurrent therapy). Products include:
Corgard Tablets 2245
Corzide 40/5 Tablets 2247
Corzide 80/5 Tablets 2247
Nadolol Tablets 2288

Naproxen (Antihypertensive effects of Mykrox may be decreased). Products include:
EC-Naprosyn Delayed-Release Tablets 2967
Naprosyn Suspension 2967
Naprosyn Tablets 2967

Naproxen Sodium (Antihypertensive effects of Mykrox may be decreased). Products include:
Aleve Tablets, Caplets and Gelcaps .... ▣602
Aleve Cold & Sinus Caplets .... ▣603
Anaprox Tablets 2967
Anaprox DS Tablets 2967
Naprelan Tablets 1293

Nicardipine Hydrochloride (Orthostatic hypotension may occur with concurrent therapy). Products include:
Cardene I.V. 3485

Nifedipine (Orthostatic hypotension may occur with concurrent therapy). Products include:
Adalat CC Tablets 877
Procardia Capsules 2708
Procardia XL Extended Release Tablets 2710

Nisoldipine (Orthostatic hypotension may occur with concurrent therapy). Products include:
Sular Tablets 688

Nitroglycerin (Orthostatic hypotension may occur with concurrent therapy). Products include:
Nitro-Dur Transdermal Infusion System 3134
Nitro-Dur Transdermal Infusion System 1834
Nitrolingual Pumpspray 1355
Nitrostat Tablets 2658

Norepinephrine Bitartrate (Arterial responsiveness to norepinephrine may be decreased).
No products indexed under this heading.

Oxaprozin (Antihypertensive effects of Mykrox may be decreased).
No products indexed under this heading.

Oxycodone Hydrochloride (Potentiates orthostatic hypotensive effects). Products include:
OxyContin Tablets 2912
OxyFast Oral Concentrate Solution 2916
OxyIR Capsules 2916
Percocet Tablets 1326
Percodan Tablets 1327
Percolone Tablets 1327
Roxicodone 3067
Tylox Capsules 2597

Penbutolol Sulfate (Orthostatic hypotension may occur with concurrent therapy).
No products indexed under this heading.

Pentobarbital Sodium (Potentiates orthostatic hypotensive effects). Products include:
Nembutal Sodium Solution 485

Perindopril Erbumine (Orthostatic hypotension may occur with concurrent therapy). Products include:
Aceon Tablets (2 mg, 4 mg, 8 mg) 3249

Phenobarbital (Potentiates orthostatic hypotensive effects). Products include:
Arco-Lase Plus Tablets 592
Donnatal 2929
Donnatal Extentabs 2930

Phenoxybenzamine Hydrochloride (Orthostatic hypotension may occur with concurrent therapy). Products include:
Dibenzyline Capsules 3457

Phentolamine Mesylate (Orthostatic hypotension may occur with concurrent therapy).
No products indexed under this heading.

Phenylbutazone (Antihypertensive effects of Mykrox may be decreased).
No products indexed under this heading.

Pindolol (Orthostatic hypotension may occur with concurrent therapy).
No products indexed under this heading.

Pioglitazone Hydrochloride (Blood glucose concentrations may be raised by metolazone in diabetics). Products include:
Actos Tablets 3275

Piroxicam (Antihypertensive effects of Mykrox may be decreased). Products include:
Feldene Capsules 2685

Polythiazide (Orthostatic hypotension may occur with concurrent therapy). Products include:
Minizide Capsules 2700
Renese Tablets 2712

Prazosin Hydrochloride (Orthostatic hypotension may occur with concurrent therapy). Products include:
Minipress Capsules 2699
Minizide Capsules 2700

Prednisolone Acetate (Potential for increased hypokalemia). Products include:
Blephamide Ophthalmic Ointment 547
Blephamide Ophthalmic Suspension 548
Poly-Pred Liquifilm Ophthalmic Suspension .... ⊙245
Pred Forte Ophthalmic Suspension .... ⊙246
Pred Mild Sterile Ophthalmic Suspension .... ⊙249
Pred-G Ophthalmic Suspension .... ⊙247
Pred-G Sterile Ophthalmic Ointment .... ⊙248

Prednisolone Sodium Phosphate (Potential for increased hypokalemia). Products include:
Pediapred Oral Solution 1170

Prednisolone Tebutate (Potential for increased hypokalemia).
No products indexed under this heading.

Prednisone (Potential for increased hypokalemia). Products include:
Prednisone 3064

Propoxyphene Hydrochloride (Potentiates orthostatic hypotensive effects). Products include:
Darvon Pulvules 1909
Darvon Compound-65 Pulvules 1910

Propoxyphene Napsylate (Potentiates orthostatic hypotensive effects). Products include:
Darvon-N/Darvocet-N 1907
Darvon-N Tablets 1912

Propranolol Hydrochloride (Orthostatic hypotension may occur with concurrent therapy). Products include:
Inderal 3513
Inderal LA Long-Acting Capsules 3516
Inderide Tablets 3517
Inderide LA Long-Acting Capsules 3519

Quinapril Hydrochloride (Orthostatic hypotension may occur with concurrent therapy). Products include:
Accupril Tablets 2611
Accuretic Tablets 2614

Ramipril (Orthostatic hypotension may occur with concurrent therapy). Products include:
Altace Capsules 2233

Rauwolfia serpentina (Orthostatic hypotension may occur with concurrent therapy).
No products indexed under this heading.

Remifentanil Hydrochloride (Potentiates orthostatic hypotensive effects).
No products indexed under this heading.

Repaglinide (Blood glucose concentrations may be raised by metolazone in diabetics). Products include:
Prandin Tablets (0.5, 1, and 2 mg) 2432

Rescinnamine (Orthostatic hypotension may occur with concurrent therapy).
No products indexed under this heading.

Reserpine (Orthostatic hypotension may occur with concurrent therapy).
No products indexed under this heading.

Rofecoxib (Antihypertensive effects of Mykrox may be decreased). Products include:
Vioxx 2213

Rosiglitazone Maleate (Blood glucose concentrations may be raised by metolazone in diabetics). Products include:
Avandia Tablets 1490

Salsalate (Antihypertensive effects of Mykrox may be decreased).
No products indexed under this heading.

Secobarbital Sodium (Potentiates orthostatic hypotensive effects).
No products indexed under this heading.

Sodium Nitroprusside (Orthostatic hypotension may occur with concurrent therapy).
No products indexed under this heading.

Sotalol Hydrochloride (Orthostatic hypotension may occur with concurrent therapy). Products include:
Betapace Tablets 950
Betapace AF Tablets 954

Spirapril Hydrochloride (Orthostatic hypotension may occur with concurrent therapy).
No products indexed under this heading.

Sufentanil Citrate (Potentiates orthostatic hypotensive effects).
No products indexed under this heading.

Sulindac (Antihypertensive effects of Mykrox may be decreased). Products include:
Clinoril Tablets 2053

Telmisartan (Orthostatic hypotension may occur with concurrent therapy). Products include:
Micardis Tablets 1049
Micardis HCT Tablets 1051

Terazosin Hydrochloride (Orthostatic hypotension may occur with concurrent therapy). Products include:
Hytrin Capsules 464

Thiamylal Sodium (Potentiates orthostatic hypotensive effects).
No products indexed under this heading.

Timolol Maleate (Orthostatic hypotension may occur with concurrent therapy). Products include:

Blocadren Tablets 2046
Cosopt Sterile Ophthalmic Solution.. 2065
Timolide Tablets 2187
Timolol GFS .... ⊙ 266
Timoptic in Ocudose 2192
Timoptic Sterile Ophthalmic Solution.. 2190
Timoptic-XE Sterile Ophthalmic Gel Forming Solution.................. 2194

Tolazamide (Blood glucose concentrations may be raised by metolazone in diabetics).

No products indexed under this heading.

Tolbutamide (Blood glucose concentrations may be raised by metolazone in diabetics).

No products indexed under this heading.

Tolmetin Sodium (Antihypertensive effects of Mykrox may be decreased). Products include:

Tolectin 2589

Torsemide (Orthostatic hypotension may occur with concurrent therapy). Products include:

Demadex Tablets and Injection 2965

Trandolapril (Orthostatic hypotension may occur with concurrent therapy). Products include:

Mavik Tablets 478
Tarka Tablets 508

Triamcinolone (Potential for increased hypokalemia).

No products indexed under this heading.

Triamcinolone Acetonide (Potential for increased hypokalemia). Products include:

Azmacort Inhalation Aerosol 728
Nasacort Nasal Inhaler 750
Nasacort AQ Nasal Spray 752
Tri-Nasal Spray 2274

Triamcinolone Diacetate (Potential for increased hypokalemia).

No products indexed under this heading.

Triamcinolone Hexacetonide (Potential for increased hypokalemia).

No products indexed under this heading.

Trimethaphan Camsylate (Orthostatic hypotension may occur with concurrent therapy).

No products indexed under this heading.

Troglitazone (Blood glucose concentrations may be raised by metolazone in diabetics).

No products indexed under this heading.

Tubocurarine Chloride (Neuromuscular blocking effects of curariform drugs may be enhanced).

No products indexed under this heading.

Valsartan (Orthostatic hypotension may occur with concurrent therapy). Products include:

Diovan Capsules 2337
Diovan HCT Tablets 2338

Verapamil Hydrochloride (Orthostatic hypotension may occur with concurrent therapy). Products include:

Covera-HS Tablets 3199
Isoptin SR Tablets 467
Tarka Tablets 508
Verelan Capsules 3184
Verelan PM Capsules 3186

Warfarin Sodium (May affect the hypoprothrombinemic response to anticoagulants; dosage adjustments may be necessary). Products include:

Coumadin for Injection 1243
Coumadin Tablets 1243
Warfarin Sodium Tablets, USP 3302

Food Interactions

Alcohol (Potentiates orthostatic hypotensive effects).

FAST-ACTING MYLANTA ANTACID GELCAPS
(Calcium Carbonate, Magnesium Hydroxide).. 1813
May interact with:

Prescription Drugs, unspecified (Resultant effects of concurrent use not specified).

FAST-ACTING MYLANTA LIQUID ANTACID
(Aluminum Hydroxide, Magnesium Hydroxide, Simethicone).................. 1813
May interact with:

Prescription Drugs, unspecified (Antacids interact with certain prescription drugs; physician's consultation is required if used concurrently).

EXTRA STRENGTH FAST-ACTING MYLANTA LIQUID
(Aluminum Hydroxide, Magnesium Hydroxide, Simethicone).................. 1813
See Fast-Acting Mylanta Liquid Antacid

FAST-ACTING MYLANTA ULTRA TABS
(Calcium Carbonate, Magnesium Hydroxide).. 1813
See Fast-Acting Mylanta Antacid Gelcaps

MAXIMUM STRENGTH MYLANTA GAS RELIEF SOFTGELS
(Simethicone) 1814
None cited in PDR database.

MYLANTA GAS RELIEF TABLETS
(Simethicone) 1814
None cited in PDR database.

MAXIMUM STRENGTH MYLANTA GAS RELIEF TABLETS
(Simethicone) 1814
None cited in PDR database.

EXTRA STRENGTH MYLANTA CALCI TABS TABLETS
(Calcium Carbonate) 636
May interact with:

Prescription Drugs, unspecified (Antacids may interact with certain prescription drugs; consultation with physician or pharmacist is required before using these drugs concurrently).

ULTRA MYLANTA CALCI TABS TABLETS
(Calcium Carbonate) 636
None cited in PDR database.

MYLERAN TABLETS
(Busulfan) 1603
May interact with antineoplastics, cytotoxic drugs, and certain other agents. Compounds in these categories include:

Altretamine (Potential for rare life-threatening hepatic veno-occlusive disease). Products include:

Hexalen Capsules 2226

Anastrozole (Potential for rare life-threatening hepatic veno-occlusive disease). Products include:

Arimidex Tablets 659

Asparaginase (Potential for rare life-threatening hepatic veno-occlusive disease). Products include:

Elspar for Injection 2092

Bicalutamide (Potential for rare life-threatening hepatic veno-occlusive disease). Products include:

Casodex Tablets 662

Bleomycin Sulfate (Busulfan-induced pulmonary toxicity may be additive to the effects produced by other cytotoxic agents).

No products indexed under this heading.

Bone Marrow Depressants, unspecified (Additive myelosuppression).

Carboplatin (Potential for rare life-threatening hepatic veno-occlusive disease). Products include:

Paraplatin for Injection 1126

Carmustine (BCNU) (Potential for rare life-threatening hepatic veno-occlusive disease). Products include:

Gliadel Wafer 1723

Chlorambucil (Potential for rare life-threatening hepatic veno-occlusive disease). Products include:

Leukeran Tablets 1591

Cisplatin (Potential for rare life-threatening hepatic veno-occlusive disease).

No products indexed under this heading.

Cyclophosphamide (Potential for rare life-threatening hepatic veno-occlusive disease; potential for cardiac temponade).

No products indexed under this heading.

Dacarbazine (Potential for rare life-threatening hepatic veno-occlusive disease). Products include:

DTIC-Dome 902

Daunorubicin Citrate (Potential for rare life-threatening hepatic veno-occlusive disease). Products include:

DaunoXome Injection 1442

Daunorubicin Hydrochloride (Busulfan-induced pulmonary toxicity may be additive to the effects produced by other cytotoxic agents). Products include:

Cerubidine for Injection 947

Denileukin Diftitox (Potential for rare life-threatening hepatic veno-occlusive disease).

No products indexed under this heading.

Docetaxel (Potential for rare life-threatening hepatic veno-occlusive disease). Products include:

Taxotere for Injection Concentrate 778

Doxorubicin Hydrochloride (Busulfan-induced pulmonary toxicity may be additive to the effects produced by other cytotoxic agents). Products include:

Adriamycin PFS/RDF Injection 2767
Doxil Injection 566

Epirubicin Hydrochloride (Busulfan-induced pulmonary toxicity may be additive to the effects produced by other cytotoxic agents). Products include:

Ellence Injection 2806

Estramustine Phosphate Sodium (Potential for rare life-threatening hepatic veno-occlusive disease). Products include:

Emcyt Capsules 2810

Etoposide (Potential for rare life-threatening hepatic veno-occlusive disease).

No products indexed under this heading.

Exemestane (Potential for rare life-threatening hepatic veno-occlusive disease). Products include:

Aromasin Tablets 2769

Floxuridine (Potential for rare life-threatening hepatic veno-occlusive disease). Products include:

Sterile FUDR 2974

Fluorouracil (Busulfan-induced pulmonary toxicity may be additive to the effects produced by other cytotoxic agents). Products include:

Carac Cream 1222
Efudex 1733
Fluoroplex 552

Flutamide (Potential for rare life-threatening hepatic veno-occlusive disease). Products include:

Eulexin Capsules 3118

Gemcitabine Hydrochloride (Potential for rare life-threatening hepatic veno-occlusive disease). Products include:

Gemzar for Injection 1919

Hydroxyurea (Busulfan-induced pulmonary toxicity may be additive to the effects produced by other cytotoxic agents). Products include:

Mylocel Tablets 2227

Idarubicin Hydrochloride (Potential for rare life-threatening hepatic veno-occlusive disease). Products include:

Idamycin PFS Injection 2825

Ifosfamide (Potential for rare life-threatening hepatic veno-occlusive disease). Products include:

Ifex for Injection 1123

Interferon alfa-2A, Recombinant (Potential for rare life-threatening hepatic veno-occlusive disease). Products include:

Roferon-A Injection 2996

Interferon alfa-2B, Recombinant (Potential for rare life-threatening hepatic veno-occlusive disease). Products include:

Intron A for Injection 3120
Rebetron Combination Therapy 3153

Irinotecan Hydrochloride (Potential for rare life-threatening hepatic veno-occlusive disease).

No products indexed under this heading.

Itraconazole (Co-administration may result in increased busulfan toxicity). Products include:

Sporanox Capsules 1800
Sporanox Injection 1804
Sporanox Injection 2509
Sporanox Oral Solution 1808
Sporanox Oral Solution 2512

Levamisole Hydrochloride (Potential for rare life-threatening hepatic veno-occlusive disease). Products include:

Ergamisol Tablets 1789

Lomustine (CCNU) (Potential for rare life-threatening hepatic veno-occlusive disease).

No products indexed under this heading.

Mechlorethamine Hydrochloride (Potential for rare life-threatening hepatic veno-occlusive disease). Products include:

Mustargen for Injection 2142

Megestrol Acetate (Potential for rare life-threatening hepatic veno-occlusive disease). Products include:

Megace Oral Suspension 1124

Melphalan (Potential for rare life-threatening hepatic veno-occlusive disease). Products include:

Alkeran Tablets 1466

Mercaptopurine (Potential for rare life-threatening hepatic veno-occlusive disease). Products include:

Purinethol Tablets 1615

Methotrexate Sodium (Busulfan-induced pulmonary toxicity may be additive to the effects produced by other cytotoxic agents).

No products indexed under this heading.

Mitomycin (Mitomycin-C) (Potential for rare life-threatening hepatic veno-occlusive disease).

No products indexed under this heading.

Mitotane (Busulfan-induced pulmonary toxicity may be additive to the effects produced by other cytotoxic agents).

No products indexed under this heading.

IMPORTANT NOTE: Always consult each drug listing in the patient's regimen for possible interactions.

Mitoxantrone Hydrochloride (Busulfan-induced pulmonary toxicity may be additive to the effects produced by other cytotoxic agents). Products include:
Novantrone for Injection 1760

Paclitaxel (Potential for rare life-threatening hepatic veno-occlusive disease). Products include:
Taxol Injection 1129

Procarbazine Hydrochloride (Busulfan-induced pulmonary toxicity may be additive to the effects produced by other cytotoxic agents). Products include:
Matulane Capsules 3246

Streptozocin (Potential for rare life-threatening hepatic veno-occlusive disease).
No products indexed under this heading.

Tamoxifen Citrate (Busulfan-induced pulmonary toxicity may be additive to the effects produced by other cytotoxic agents). Products include:
Nolvadex Tablets 678

Teniposide (Potential for rare life-threatening hepatic veno-occlusive disease).
No products indexed under this heading.

Thioguanine (Potential for esophageal varices associated with abnormal liver function tests; potential for rare life-threatening hepatic veno-occulsive disease). Products include:
Tabloid Tablets 1642

Thiotepa (Potential for rare life-threatening hepatic veno-occlusive disease). Products include:
Thioplex for Injection 1765

Topotecan Hydrochloride (Potential for rare life-threatening hepatic veno-occlusive disease). Products include:
Hycamtin for Injection 1546

Toremifene Citrate (Potential for rare life-threatening hepatic veno-occlusive disease). Products include:
Fareston Tablets 3237

Valrubicin (Potential for rare life-threatening hepatic veno-occlusive disease). Products include:
Valstar Sterile Solution for Intravesical Instillation 1175

Vincristine Sulfate (Busulfan-induced pulmonary toxicity may be additive to the effects produced by other cytotoxic agents).
No products indexed under this heading.

Vinorelbine Tartrate (Potential for rare life-threatening hepatic veno-occlusive disease). Products include:
Navelbine Injection 1604

MYLICON INFANTS' DROPS
(Simethicone) 1813
None cited in PDR database.

INFANTS' MYLICON DROPS
(Simethicone) ....■634

MYLOCEL TABLETS
(Hydroxyurea) 2227
May interact with:

Bone Marrow Suppressants, unspecified (Concurrent use with other myelosuppressive agents may increase the likelihood of bone marrow depression).

MYLOTARG FOR INJECTION
(Gemtuzumab ozogamicin) 3540
None cited in PDR database.

MYOBLOC INJECTABLE SOLUTION
(Botulinum Toxin Type B) 1291
May interact with aminoglycosides, neuromuscular blocking agents, and certain other agents. Compounds in these categories include:

Amikacin Sulfate (Co-administration with aminoglycosides may potentiate the effect of the toxin).
No products indexed under this heading.

Atracurium Besylate (Co-administration with neuromuscular blocking agents may potentiate the effect of the toxin).
No products indexed under this heading.

Cisatracurium Besylate (Co-administration with neuromuscular blocking agents may potentiate the effect of the toxin).
No products indexed under this heading.

Doxacurium Chloride (Co-administration with neuromuscular blocking agents may potentiate the effect of the toxin).
No products indexed under this heading.

Gentamicin Sulfate (Co-administration with aminoglycosides may potentiate the effect of the toxin). Products include:
Genoptic Ophthalmic Ointment .....⊙239
Genoptic Sterile Ophthalmic Solution ....⊙239
Pred-G Ophthalmic Suspension .....⊙247
Pred-G Sterile Ophthalmic Ointment ....⊙248

Kanamycin Sulfate (Co-administration with aminoglycosides may potentiate the effect of the toxin).
No products indexed under this heading.

Metocurine Iodide (Co-administration with neuromuscular blocking agents may potentiate the effect of the toxin).
No products indexed under this heading.

Mivacurium Chloride (Co-administration with neuromuscular blocking agents may potentiate the effect of the toxin).
No products indexed under this heading.

Pancuronium Bromide (Co-administration with neuromuscular blocking agents may potentiate the effect of the toxin).
No products indexed under this heading.

Rapacuronium Bromide (Co-administration with neuromuscular blocking agents may potentiate the effect of the toxin).
No products indexed under this heading.

Rocuronium Bromide (Co-administration with neuromuscular blocking agents may potentiate the effect of the toxin). Products include:
Zemuron Injection 2491

Streptomycin Sulfate (Co-administration with aminoglycosides may potentiate the effect of the toxin). Products include:
Streptomycin Sulfate Injection 2714

Succinylcholine Chloride (Co-administration with neuromuscular blocking agents may potentiate the effect of the toxin). Products include:
Anectine Injection 1476

Tobramycin (Co-administration with aminoglycosides may potentiate the effect of the toxin). Products include:
TOBI Solution for Inhalation 1206
TobraDex Ophthalmic Ointment 542
TobraDex Ophthalmic Suspension .. 541
Tobrex Ophthalmic Ointment ....⊙220
Tobrex Ophthalmic Solution ....⊙221

Tobramycin Sulfate (Co-administration with aminoglycosides may potentiate the effect of the toxin). Products include:
Nebcin Vials, Hyporets & ADD-Vantage 1955

Tubocurarine Chloride (Co-administration with curare-like compounds may potentiate the effect of the toxin).
No products indexed under this heading.

Vecuronium Bromide (Co-administration with neuromuscular blocking agents may potentiate the effect of the toxin). Products include:
Norcuron for Injection 2478

NABI-HB
(Hepatitis B Immune Globulin (Human)).. 2295
May interact with:

Mumps Virus Vaccine, Live (H-Big may interfere with the immune response to vaccination, therefore, vaccination with live virus vaccine should be deferred until approximately 3 months). Products include:
Mumpsvax 2141

Rubella & Mumps Virus Vaccine Live (H-Big may interfere with the immune response to vaccination, therefore, vaccination with live virus vaccine should be deferred until approximately 3 months).
No products indexed under this heading.

Rubella Virus Vaccine Live (H-Big may interfere with the immune response to vaccination, therefore, vaccination with live virus vaccine should be deferred until approximately 3 months). Products include:
Meruvax II 2130

NADOLOL TABLETS
(Nadolol) 2288
May interact with general anesthetics, oral hypoglycemic agents, insulin, and certain other agents. Compounds in these categories include:

Acarbose (Beta-adrenergic blockade may prevent the appearance of premonitory signs and symptoms, such as tachycardia and blood pressure changes, of acute hypoglycemia; beta-blockade also reduces the release of insulin in response to hyperglycemia; adjust dosage of oral antidiabetic drugs). Products include:
Precose Tablets 906

Chlorpropamide (Beta-adrenergic blockade may prevent the appearance of premonitory signs and symptoms, such as tachycardia and blood pressure changes, of acute hypoglycemia; beta-blockade also reduces the release of insulin in response to hyperglycemia; adjust dosage of oral antidiabetic drugs). Products include:
Diabinese Tablets 2680

Enflurane (Co-administration may result in exaggeration of the hypotension induced by general anesthetics).
No products indexed under this heading.

Epinephrine (Patients with a history of severe anaphylactic reaction to variety of allergens may be more reactive to repeated challenge; potential for unresponsiveness to the usual dose of epinephrine). Products include:
Epifrin Sterile Ophthalmic Solution ....⊙235
EpiPen 1236
Primatene Mist ....■779
Xylocaine with Epinephrine Injection 653

Epinephrine Hydrochloride (Patients with a history of severe anaphylactic reaction to variety of allergens may be more reactive to repeated challenge; potential for unresponsiveness to the usual dose of epinephrine).
No products indexed under this heading.

Glimepiride (Beta-adrenergic blockade may prevent the appearance of premonitory signs and symptoms, such as tachycardia and blood pressure changes, of acute hypoglycemia; beta-blockade also reduces the release of insulin in response to hyperglycemia; adjust dosage of oral antidiabetic drugs). Products include:
Amaryl Tablets 717

Glipizide (Beta-adrenergic blockade may prevent the appearance of premonitory signs and symptoms, such as tachycardia and blood pressure changes, of acute hypoglycemia; beta-blockade also reduces the release of insulin in response to hyperglycemia; adjust dosage of oral antidiabetic drugs). Products include:
Glucotrol Tablets 2692
Glucotrol XL Extended Release Tablets 2693

Glyburide (Beta-adrenergic blockade may prevent the appearance of premonitory signs and symptoms, such as tachycardia and blood pressure changes, of acute hypoglycemia; beta-blockade also reduces the release of insulin in response to hyperglycemia; adjust dosage of oral antidiabetic drugs). Products include:
DiaBeta Tablets 741
Glucovance Tablets 1086

Insulin, Human, Zinc Suspension (Beta-adrenergic blockade may prevent the appearance of premonitory signs and symptoms, such as tachycardia and blood pressure changes, of acute hypoglycemia; beta-blockade also reduces the release of insulin in response to hyperglycemia; adjust dosage of insulin). Products include:
Humulin L, 100 Units 1937
Humulin U, 100 Units 1943
Novolin L Human Insulin 10 ml Vials 2422

Insulin, Human NPH (Beta-adrenergic blockade may prevent the appearance of premonitory signs and symptoms, such as tachycardia and blood pressure changes, of acute hypoglycemia; beta-blockade also reduces the release of insulin in response to hyperglycemia; adjust dosage of insulin). Products include:
Humulin N, 100 Units 1939
Humulin N NPH Pen 1940
Novolin N Human Insulin 10 ml Vials 2422
Novolin N PenFill 2423
Novolin N Prefilled Syringe Disposable Insulin Delivery System 2425

Insulin, Human Regular (Beta-adrenergic blockade may prevent the appearance of premonitory signs and symptoms, such as tachycardia and blood pressure changes, of acute hypoglycemia; beta-blockade also reduces the release of insulin in response to hyperglycemia; adjust dosage of insulin). Products include:
Humulin R Regular (U-500) 1943
Humulin R, 100 Units 1941
Novolin R Human Insulin 10 ml Vials 2423
Novolin R PenFill 2423
Novolin R Prefilled Syringe Disposable Insulin Delivery System 2425
Velosulin BR Human Insulin 10 ml Vials 2435

Insulin, Human Regular and Human NPH Mixture (Beta-adrenergic blockade may prevent the appearance of premonitory signs and symptoms, such as tachycardia

and blood pressure changes, of acute hypoglycemia; beta-blockade also reduces the release of insulin in response to hyperglycemia; adjust dosage of insulin). Products include:

- Humulin 50/50, 100 Units 1934
- Humulin 70/30, 100 Units 1935
- Humulin 70/30 Pen 1936
- Novolin 70/30 Human Insulin 10 ml Vials 2421
- Novolin 70/30 PenFill 2423
- Novolin 70/30 Prefilled Disposable Insulin Delivery System 2425

Insulin, NPH (Beta-adrenergic blockade may prevent the appearance of premonitory signs and symptoms, such as tachycardia and blood pressure changes, of acute hypoglycemia; beta-blockade also reduces the release of insulin in response to hyperglycemia; adjust dosage of insulin). Products include:

- Iletin II, NPH (Pork), 100 Units 1946

Insulin, Regular (Beta-adrenergic blockade may prevent the appearance of premonitory signs and symptoms, such as tachycardia and blood pressure changes, of acute hypoglycemia; beta-blockade also reduces the release of insulin in response to hyperglycemia; adjust dosage of insulin). Products include:

- Iletin II, Regular (Pork), 100 Units ... 1947

Insulin, Zinc Crystals (Beta-adrenergic blockade may prevent the appearance of premonitory signs and symptoms, such as tachycardia and blood pressure changes, of acute hypoglycemia; beta-blockade also reduces the release of insulin in response to hyperglycemia; adjust dosage of insulin).

No products indexed under this heading.

Insulin, Zinc Suspension (Beta-adrenergic blockade may prevent the appearance of premonitory signs and symptoms, such as tachycardia and blood pressure changes, of acute hypoglycemia; beta-blockade also reduces the release of insulin in response to hyperglycemia; adjust dosage of insulin). Products include:

- Iletin II, Lente (Pork), 100 Units 1945

Insulin Aspart, Human Regular (Beta-adrenergic blockade may prevent the appearance of premonitory signs and symptoms, such as tachycardia and blood pressure changes, of acute hypoglycemia; beta-blockade also reduces the release of insulin in response to hyperglycemia; adjust dosage of insulin).

No products indexed under this heading.

Insulin glargine (Beta-adrenergic blockade may prevent the appearance of premonitory signs and symptoms, such as tachycardia and blood pressure changes, of acute hypoglycemia; beta-blockade also reduces the release of insulin in response to hyperglycemia; adjust dosage of insulin). Products include:

- Lantus Injection 742

Insulin Lispro, Human (Beta-adrenergic blockade may prevent the appearance of premonitory signs and symptoms, such as tachycardia and blood pressure changes, of acute hypoglycemia; beta-blockade also reduces the release of insulin in response to hyperglycemia; adjust dosage of insulin). Products include:

- Humalog 1926
- Humalog Mix 75/25 Pen 1928

Insulin Lispro Protamine, Human (Beta-adrenergic blockade may prevent the appearance of premonitory signs and symptoms, such as tachycardia and blood pressure changes, of acute hypoglycemia; beta-blockade also reduces the release of insulin in response to hyperglycemia; adjust dosage of insulin). Products include:

- Humalog Mix 75/25 Pen 1928

Isoflurane (Co-administration may result in exaggeration of the hypotension induced by general anesthetics).

No products indexed under this heading.

Ketamine Hydrochloride (Co-administration may result in exaggeration of the hypotension induced by general anesthetics).

No products indexed under this heading.

Metformin Hydrochloride (Beta-adrenergic blockade may prevent the appearance of premonitory signs and symptoms, such as tachycardia and blood pressure changes, of acute hypoglycemia; beta-blockade also reduces the release of insulin in response to hyperglycemia; adjust dosage of oral antidiabetic drugs). Products include:

- Glucophage Tablets 1080
- Glucophage XR Tablets 1080
- Glucovance Tablets 1086

Methohexital Sodium (Co-administration may result in exaggeration of the hypotension induced by general anesthetics). Products include:

- Brevital Sodium for Injection, USP .. 1815

Methoxyflurane (Co-administration may result in exaggeration of the hypotension induced by general anesthetics).

No products indexed under this heading.

Miglitol (Beta-adrenergic blockade may prevent the appearance of premonitory signs and symptoms, such as tachycardia and blood pressure changes, of acute hypoglycemia; beta-blockade also reduces the release of insulin in response to hyperglycemia; adjust dosage of oral antidiabetic drugs). Products include:

- Glyset Tablets 2821

Pioglitazone Hydrochloride (Beta-adrenergic blockade may prevent the appearance of premonitory signs and symptoms, such as tachycardia and blood pressure changes, of acute hypoglycemia; beta-blockade also reduces the release of insulin in response to hyperglycemia; adjust dosage of oral antidiabetic drugs). Products include:

- Actos Tablets 3275

Propofol (Co-administration may result in exaggeration of the hypotension induced by general anesthetics). Products include:

- Diprivan Injectable Emulsion 667

Repaglinide (Beta-adrenergic blockade may prevent the appearance of premonitory signs and symptoms, such as tachycardia and blood pressure changes, of acute hypoglycemia; beta-blockade also reduces the release of insulin in response to hyperglycemia; adjust dosage of oral antidiabetic drugs). Products include:

- Prandin Tablets (0.5, 1, and 2 mg) 2432

Reserpine (Potential for additive effects resulting in hypotension and/or excessive bradycardia (vertigo, syncope, postural hypotension)).

No products indexed under this heading.

Rosiglitazone Maleate (Beta-adrenergic blockade may prevent the appearance of premonitory signs and symptoms, such as tachycardia and blood pressure changes, of acute hypoglycemia; beta-blockade also reduces the release of insulin in response to hyperglycemia; adjust dosage of oral antidiabetic drugs). Products include:

- Avandia Tablets 1490

Sevoflurane (Co-administration may result in exaggeration of the hypotension induced by general anesthetics).

No products indexed under this heading.

Tolazamide (Beta-adrenergic blockade may prevent the appearance of premonitory signs and symptoms, such as tachycardia and blood pressure changes, of acute hypoglycemia; beta-blockade also reduces the release of insulin in response to hyperglycemia; adjust dosage of oral antidiabetic drugs).

No products indexed under this heading.

Tolbutamide (Beta-adrenergic blockade may prevent the appearance of premonitory signs and symptoms, such as tachycardia and blood pressure changes, of acute hypoglycemia; beta-blockade also reduces the release of insulin in response to hyperglycemia; adjust dosage of oral antidiabetic drugs).

No products indexed under this heading.

Troglitazone (Beta-adrenergic blockade may prevent the appearance of premonitory signs and symptoms, such as tachycardia and blood pressure changes, of acute hypoglycemia; beta-blockade also reduces the release of insulin in response to hyperglycemia; adjust dosage of oral antidiabetic drugs).

No products indexed under this heading.

NAFTIN CREAM

(Naftifine Hydrochloride) 2224
None cited in PDR database.

NAFTIN GEL

(Naftifine Hydrochloride) 2224
None cited in PDR database.

NAPHCON-A OPHTHALMIC SOLUTION

(Naphazoline Hydrochloride, Pheniramine Maleate) 540
None cited in PDR database.

NAPRELAN TABLETS

(Naproxen Sodium) 1293

May interact with ACE inhibitors, beta blockers, oral anticoagulants, hydantoin anticonvulsants, lithium preparations, sulfonamides, sulfonylureas, and certain other agents. Compounds in these categories include:

Acebutolol Hydrochloride (Reduced antihypertensive effect of beta blockers). Products include:

- Sectral Capsules 3589

Aspirin (Naproxen is displaced from its binding sites during concomitant use of aspirin resulting in lower plasma concentrations and peak plasma levels). Products include:

- Aggrenox Capsules 1026
- Alka-Seltzer .... ▣603
- Alka-Seltzer Lemon Lime Antacid and Pain Reliever Effervescent Tablets .... ▣603
- Alka-Seltzer Extra Strength Antacid and Pain Reliever Effervescent Tablets .... ▣603
- Alka-Seltzer PM Effervescent Tablets .... ▣605
- Genuine Bayer Tablets, Caplets and Gelcaps .... ▣606
- Extra Strength Bayer Caplets and Gelcaps .... ▣610
- Aspirin Regimen Bayer Children's Chewable Tablets (Orange or Cherry Flavored) .... ▣607
- Bayer, Aspirin Regimen .... ▣606
- Aspirin Regimen Bayer 81 mg Caplets with Calcium .... ▣607
- Genuine Bayer Professional Labeling (Aspirin Regimen Bayer) .... ▣608
- Extra Strength Bayer Arthritis Caplets .... ▣610
- Extra Strength Bayer Plus Caplets .... ▣610
- Extra Strength Bayer PM Caplets .. ▣611
- BC Powder .... ▣619
- BC Allergy Sinus Cold Powder ...... ▣619
- Arthritis Strength BC Powder .... ▣619
- BC Sinus Cold Powder .... ▣619
- Darvon Compound-65 Pulvules 1910
- Ecotrin Enteric Coated Aspirin Low, Regular and Maximum Strength Tablets 1715
- Excedrin Extra-Strength Tablets, Caplets, and Geltabs .... ▣629
- Excedrin Migraine 1070
- Goody's Body Pain Formula Powder .... ▣620
- Goody's Extra Strength Headache Powder .... ▣620
- Goody's Extra Strength Pain Relief Tablets .... ▣620
- Percodan Tablets 1327
- Robaxisal Tablets 2939
- Soma Compound Tablets 3354
- Soma Compound w/Codeine Tablets 3355
- Vanquish Caplets .... ▣617

Atenolol (Reduced antihypertensive effect of beta blockers). Products include:

- Tenoretic Tablets 690
- Tenormin I.V. Injection 692

Benazepril Hydrochloride (Co-administration may potentiate renal disease states). Products include:

- Lotensin Tablets 2365
- Lotensin HCT Tablets 2367
- Lotrel Capsules 2370

Bendroflumethiazide (Potential for sulfonamide toxicity). Products include:

- Corzide 40/5 Tablets 2247
- Corzide 80/5 Tablets 2247

Betaxolol Hydrochloride (Reduced antihypertensive effect of beta blockers). Products include:

- Betoptic S Ophthalmic Suspension 537

Bisoprolol Fumarate (Reduced antihypertensive effect of beta blockers). Products include:

- Zebeta Tablets 1885
- Ziac Tablets 1887

Captopril (Co-administration may potentiate renal disease states). Products include:

- Captopril Tablets 2281

Carteolol Hydrochloride (Reduced antihypertensive effect of beta blockers). Products include:

- Carteolol Hydrochloride Ophthalmic Solution USP, 1% ..... ⊙258
- Ocupress Ophthalmic Solution, 1% Sterile .... ⊙303

Chlorothiazide (Potential for sulfonamide toxicity). Products include:

- Aldoclor Tablets 2035
- Diuril Oral 2087

Chlorothiazide Sodium (Potential for sulfonamide toxicity). Products include:

- Diuril Sodium Intravenous 2086

Chlorpropamide (Potential for sulfonylurea toxicity). Products include:

- Diabinese Tablets 2680

Dicumarol (Naproxen may decrease platelet aggregation and prolong bleeding time; caution is advised if co-administered).

No products indexed under this heading.

Enalapril Maleate (Co-administration may potentiate renal disease states). Products include:

- Lexxel Tablets 608
- Vaseretic Tablets 2204
- Vasotec Tablets 2210

Enalaprilat (Co-administration may potentiate renal disease states). Products include:

- Enalaprilat Injection 863
- Vasotec I.V. Injection 2207

Esmolol Hydrochloride (Reduced antihypertensive effect of beta blockers). Products include:

- Brevibloc Injection 858

Ethotoin (Potential for hydantoin toxicity).
No products indexed under this heading.

Fosinopril Sodium (Co-administration may potentiate renal disease states). Products include:
- Monopril Tablets ... 1091
- Monopril HCT ... 1094

Fosphenytoin Sodium (Potential for hydantoin toxicity). Products include:
- Cerebyx Injection ... 2619

Furosemide (Potential for inhibition of natriuretic effect of furosemide). Products include:
- Furosemide Tablets ... 2284

Glimepiride (Potential for sulfonylurea toxicity). Products include:
- Amaryl Tablets ... 717

Glipizide (Potential for sulfonylurea toxicity). Products include:
- Glucotrol Tablets ... 2692
- Glucotrol XL Extended Release Tablets ... 2693

Glyburide (Potential for sulfonylurea toxicity). Products include:
- DiaBeta Tablets ... 741
- Glucovance Tablets ... 1086

Hydrochlorothiazide (Potential for sulfonamide toxicity). Products include:
- Accuretic Tablets ... 2614
- Aldoril Tablets ... 2039
- Atacand HCT Tablets ... 597
- Avalide Tablets ... 1070
- Diovan HCT Tablets ... 2338
- Dyazide Capsules ... 1515
- HydroDIURIL Tablets ... 2108
- Hyzaar ... 2109
- Inderide Tablets ... 3517
- Inderide LA Long-Acting Capsules .. 3519
- Lotensin HCT Tablets ... 2367
- Maxzide ... 1008
- Micardis HCT Tablets ... 1051
- Microzide Capsules ... 3414
- Moduretic Tablets ... 2138
- Monopril HCT ... 1094
- Prinzide Tablets ... 2168
- Timolide Tablets ... 2187
- Uniretic Tablets ... 3178
- Vaseretic Tablets ... 2204
- Zestoretic Tablets ... 695
- Ziac Tablets ... 1887

Hydroflumethiazide (Potential for sulfonamide toxicity). Products include:
- Diucardin Tablets ... 3494

Labetalol Hydrochloride (Reduced antihypertensive effect of beta blockers). Products include:
- Normodyne Injection ... 3135
- Normodyne Tablets ... 3137

Levobunolol Hydrochloride (Reduced antihypertensive effect of beta blockers). Products include:
- Betagan ... ⊙228

Lisinopril (Co-administration may potentiate renal disease states). Products include:
- Prinivil Tablets ... 2164
- Prinzide Tablets ... 2168
- Zestoretic Tablets ... 695
- Zestril Tablets ... 698

Lithium Carbonate (Inhibition of lithium renal clearance leading to increase in plasma lithium concentrations). Products include:
- Eskalith ... 1527
- Lithium Carbonate ... 3061
- Lithobid Slow-Release Tablets ... 3255

Lithium Citrate (Inhibition of lithium renal clearance leading to increase in plasma lithium concentrations). Products include:
- Lithium Citrate Syrup ... 3061

Mephenytoin (Potential for hydantoin toxicity).
No products indexed under this heading.

Methotrexate Sodium (Potential for reduced tubular secretion of methotrexate and possible increased methotrexate toxicity as shown in animal model; caution is recommended).
No products indexed under this heading.

Methyclothiazide (Potential for sulfohamide toxicity).
No products indexed under this heading.

Metipranolol Hydrochloride (Reduced antihypertensive effect of beta blockers).
No products indexed under this heading.

Metoprolol Succinate (Reduced antihypertensive effect of beta blockers). Products include:
- Toprol-XL Tablets ... 651

Metoprolol Tartrate (Reduced antihypertensive effect of beta blockers).
No products indexed under this heading.

Moexipril Hydrochloride (Co-administration may potentiate renal disease states). Products include:
- Uniretic Tablets ... 3178
- Univasc Tablets ... 3181

Nadolol (Reduced antihypertensive effect of beta blockers). Products include:
- Corgard Tablets ... 2245
- Corzide 40/5 Tablets ... 2247
- Corzide 80/5 Tablets ... 2247
- Nadolol Tablets ... 2288

Naproxen (Concurrent use of Naprelan with other naproxen products should be avoided since they all circulate in the plasma as the naproxen anion). Products include:
- EC-Naprosyn Delayed-Release Tablets ... 2967
- Naprosyn Suspension ... 2967
- Naprosyn Tablets ... 2967

Penbutolol Sulfate (Reduced antihypertensive effect of beta blockers).
No products indexed under this heading.

Perindopril Erbumine (Co-administration may potentiate renal disease states). Products include:
- Aceon Tablets (2 mg, 4 mg, 8 mg) ... 3249

Phenytoin (Potential for hydantoin toxicity). Products include:
- Dilantin Infatabs ... 2624
- Dilantin-125 Oral Suspension ... 2625

Phenytoin Sodium (Potential for hydantoin toxicity). Products include:
- Dilantin Kapseals ... 2622

Pindolol (Reduced antihypertensive effect of beta blockers).
No products indexed under this heading.

Polythiazide (Potential for sulfonamide toxicity). Products include:
- Minizide Capsules ... 2700
- Renese Tablets ... 2712

Probenecid (Probenecid given concurrently increases naproxen anion plasma levels and extends its plasma half-life significantly).
No products indexed under this heading.

Propranolol Hydrochloride (Reduced antihypertensive effect of beta blockers). Products include:
- Inderal ... 3513
- Inderal LA Long-Acting Capsules ... 3516
- Inderide Tablets ... 3517
- Inderide LA Long-Acting Capsules .. 3519

Quinapril Hydrochloride (Co-administration may potentiate renal disease states). Products include:
- Accupril Tablets ... 2611
- Accuretic Tablets ... 2614

Ramipril (Co-administration may potentiate renal disease states). Products include:
- Altace Capsules ... 2233

Sotalol Hydrochloride (Reduced antihypertensive effect of beta blockers). Products include:
- Betapace Tablets ... 950
- Betapace AF Tablets ... 954

Spirapril Hydrochloride (Co-administration may potentiate renal disease states).
No products indexed under this heading.

Sulfacytine (Potential for sulfonamide toxicity).

Sulfamethizole (Potential for sulfonamide toxicity). Products include:
- Urobiotic-250 Capsules ... 2731

Sulfamethoxazole (Potential for sulfonamide toxicity). Products include:
- Bactrim ... 2949
- Septra Suspension ... 2265
- Septra Tablets ... 2265
- Septra DS Tablets ... 2265

Sulfasalazine (Potential for sulfonamide toxicity). Products include:
- Azulfidine EN-tabs Tablets ... 2775

Sulfinpyrazone (Potential for sulfonamide toxicity).
No products indexed under this heading.

Sulfisoxazole (Potential for sulfonamide toxicity).
No products indexed under this heading.

Sulfisoxazole Acetyl (Potential for sulfonamide toxicity). Products include:
- Pediazole Suspension ... 3050

Sulfisoxazole Diolamine (Potential for sulfonamide toxicity).
No products indexed under this heading.

Timolol Hemihydrate (Reduced antihypertensive effect of beta blockers). Products include:
- Betimol Ophthalmic Solution ... ⊙324

Timolol Maleate (Reduced antihypertensive effect of beta blockers). Products include:
- Blocadren Tablets ... 2046
- Cosopt Sterile Ophthalmic Solution ... 2065
- Timolide Tablets ... 2187
- Timolol GFS ... ⊙266
- Timoptic in Ocudose ... 2192
- Timoptic Sterile Ophthalmic Solution ... 2190
- Timoptic-XE Sterile Ophthalmic Gel Forming Solution ... 2194

Tolazamide (Potential for sulfonylurea toxicity).
No products indexed under this heading.

Tolbutamide (Potential for sulfonylurea toxicity).
No products indexed under this heading.

Trandolapril (Co-administration may potentiate renal disease states). Products include:
- Mavik Tablets ... 478
- Tarka Tablets ... 508

Warfarin Sodium (Naproxen may decrease platelet aggregation and prolong bleeding time; caution is advised if co-administered). Products include:
- Coumadin for Injection ... 1243
- Coumadin Tablets ... 1243
- Warfarin Sodium Tablets, USP ... 3302

Food Interactions

Food, unspecified (Food causes a slight decrease in the rate of naproxen absorption following Naprelan administration).

NAPROSYN SUSPENSION

(Naproxen) ... 2967
See EC-Naprosyn Delayed-Release Tablets

NAPROSYN TABLETS

(Naproxen) ... 2967
See EC-Naprosyn Delayed-Release Tablets

NARCAN INJECTION

(Naloxone Hydrochloride) ... 1322
May interact with:

Cardiotoxic drugs, unspecified (Narcan should be used with caution in patients who have received potentially cardiotoxic drugs).

NARDIL TABLETS

(Phenelzine Sulfate) ... 2653
May interact with alpha adrenergic stimulants, anorexiants, antihypertensives, barbiturates, beta blockers, catecholamine depleting drugs, antidepressant drugs, dibenzazepines, monoamine oxidase inhibitors, narcotic analgesics, phenylpropanolamine containing anorectics, serotoninergic agents, sympathomimetics, thiazides, tricyclic antidepressants, and certain other agents. Compounds in these categories include:

Acebutolol Hydrochloride (Exaggerated hypotensive effects). Products include:
- Sectral Capsules ... 3589

Albuterol (Potentiation of sympathomimetic agents and related compounds resulting in hypertensive crises; concurrent use is contraindicated). Products include:
- Proventil Inhalation Aerosol ... 3142
- Ventolin Inhalation Aerosol and Refill ... 1679

Albuterol Sulfate (Potentiation of sympathomimetic agents and related compounds resulting in hypertensive crises; concurrent use is contraindicated). Products include:
- AccuNeb Inhalation Solution ... 1230
- Combivent Inhalation Aerosol ... 1041
- DuoNeb Inhalation Solution ... 1233
- Proventil Inhalation Solution 0.083% ... 3146
- Proventil Repetabs Tablets ... 3148
- Proventil Solution for Inhalation 0.5% ... 3144
- Proventil HFA Inhalation Aerosol ... 3150
- Ventolin HFA Inhalation Aerosol ... 3618
- Volmax Extended-Release Tablets .. 2276

Alfentanil Hydrochloride (Contraindication warning for meperidine is extended to other narcotics).
No products indexed under this heading.

Amitriptyline Hydrochloride (Concurrent or in rapid succession administration is contraindicated). Products include:
- Etrafon ... 3115
- Limbitrol ... 1738

Amlodipine Besylate (Exaggerated hypotensive effects). Products include:
- Lotrel Capsules ... 2370
- Norvasc Tablets ... 2704

Amoxapine (Concurrent or in rapid succession administration is contraindicated).
No products indexed under this heading.

Amphetamine Resins (Potentiation of sympathomimetic agents and related compounds resulting in hypertensive crises; concurrent use is contraindicated).
No products indexed under this heading.

Amphetamine Sulfate (Potentiation of sympathomimetic agents and related compounds resulting in hypertensive crises; concurrent use is contraindicated). Products include:
- Adderall Tablets ... 3231
- Adderall XR Capsules ...

Aprobarbital (Potential for increased hypnosis).
No products indexed under this heading.

Atenolol (Exaggerated hypotensive effects). Products include:
- Tenoretic Tablets ... 690
- Tenormin I.V. Injection ... 692

Benazepril Hydrochloride (Exaggerated hypotensive effects). Products include:
- Lotensin Tablets ... 2365
- Lotensin HCT Tablets ... 2367
- Lotrel Capsules ... 2370

Bendroflumethiazide (Exaggerated hypotensive effects). Products include:

Corzide 40/5 Tablets 2247
Corzide 80/5 Tablets 2247

Benzphetamine Hydrochloride (Concurrent administration is not recommended).
No products indexed under this heading.

Betaxolol Hydrochloride (Exaggerated hypotensive effects). Products include:
Betoptic S Ophthalmic Suspension 537

Bisoprolol Fumarate (Exaggerated hypotensive effects). Products include:
Zebeta Tablets 1885
Ziac Tablets 1887

Buprenorphine Hydrochloride (Contraindication warning for meperidine is extended to other narcotics). Products include:
Buprenex Injectable 2918

Bupropion Hydrochloride (Concurrent administration is contraindicated; at least 14 days should elapse between discontinuation of an MAOI inhibitor and initiation of treatment with bupropion hydrochloride). Products include:
Wellbutrin Tablets 1680
Wellbutrin SR Sustained-Release Tablets 1684
Zyban Sustained-Release Tablets 1710

Buspirone Hydrochloride (Elevated blood pressure; concurrent therapy is contraindicated).
No products indexed under this heading.

Butabarbital (Potential for increased hypnosis).
No products indexed under this heading.

Butalbital (Potential for increased hypnosis). Products include:
Phrenilin 578
Sedapap Tablets 50 mg/650 mg 2225

Caffeine-containing medications (Concurrent use with excessive caffeine intake should be avoided).

Candesartan Cilexetil (Exaggerated hypotensive effects). Products include:
Atacand Tablets 595
Atacand HCT Tablets 597

Captopril (Exaggerated hypotensive effects). Products include:
Captopril Tablets 2281

Carbamazepine (Concurrent or in rapid succession administration is contraindicated). Products include:
Carbatrol Capsules 3234
Tegretol/Tegretol-XR 2404

Carteolol Hydrochloride (Exaggerated hypotensive effects). Products include:
Carteolol Hydrochloride Ophthalmic Solution USP, 1% .... ⊙258
Ocupress Ophthalmic Solution, 1% Sterile .... ⊙303

Chlorothiazide (Exaggerated hypotensive effects). Products include:
Aldoclor Tablets 2035
Diuril Oral 2087

Chlorothiazide Sodium (Exaggerated hypotensive effects). Products include:
Diuril Sodium Intravenous 2086

Chlorthalidone (Exaggerated hypotensive effects). Products include:
Clorpres Tablets 1002
Combipres Tablets 1040
Tenoretic Tablets 690

Citalopram Hydrobromide (Concurrent or in rapid succession administration is contraindicated). Products include:
Celexa 1365

Clomipramine Hydrochloride (Concurrent or in rapid succession administration is contraindicated).
No products indexed under this heading.

Clonidine (Exaggerated hypotensive effects). Products include:
Catapres-TTS 1038

Clonidine Hydrochloride (Exaggerated hypotensive effects). Products include:
Catapres Tablets 1037
Clorpres Tablets 1002
Combipres Tablets 1040
Duraclon Injection 3057

Clozapine (Concurrent or in rapid succession administration is contraindicated). Products include:
Clozaril Tablets 2319

Cocaine Hydrochloride (Potentiation of sympathomimetic agents and related compounds resulting in hypertensive crises; concurrent use is contraindicated).
No products indexed under this heading.

Codeine Phosphate (Contraindication warning for meperidine is extended to other narcotics). Products include:
Phenergan with Codeine Syrup 3557
Phenergan VC with Codeine Syrup 3561
Robitussin A-C Syrup 2942
Robitussin-DAC Syrup 2942
Ryna-C Liquid 768
Soma Compound w/Codeine Tablets 3355
Tussi-Organidin NR Liquid 3350
Tussi-Organidin-S NR Liquid 3350
Tylenol with Codeine 2595

Cyclobenzaprine Hydrochloride (Possibility of unspecified adverse drug interaction; concurrent or in rapid succession administration should be avoided). Products include:
Flexeril Tablets 572
Flexeril Tablets 2094

Deserpidine (Exaggerated hypotensive effects; exercise caution).
No products indexed under this heading.

Desipramine Hydrochloride (Concurrent or in rapid succession administration is contraindicated). Products include:
Norpramin Tablets 755

Dexfenfluramine Hydrochloride (Co-administration with serotoninergic drugs has resulted in serious reactions, including hyperthermia, rigidity, myoclonic movements and death; concurrent and/or sequential use is contraindicated).
No products indexed under this heading.

Dextroamphetamine (Hypertensive crises; concurrent administration is not recommended).
No products indexed under this heading.

Dextroamphetamine Sulfate (Hypertensive crises; concurrent administration is not recommended). Products include:
Adderall Tablets 3231
Adderall XR Capsules ....
Dexedrine 1512
DextroStat Tablets 3236

Dextromethorphan Hydrobromide (Concurrent administration is not recommended; may cause drowsiness and bizarre behavior). Products include:
Alka-Seltzer Plus Liqui-Gels 604
Alka-Seltzer Plus Cold & Flu Medicine Liqui-Gels 604
Benylin Adult Formula Cough Suppressant Liquid 696
Benylin Cough Suppressant/Expectorant Liquid 697
Benylin Multi-Symptom Liquid 697
Benylin Pediatric Cough Suppressant Liquid 698
Comtrex Deep Chest Cold & Congestion Relief Softgels 627
Comtrex Maximum Strength Multi-Symptom Cold & Cough Relief Tablets and Caplets 626
Contac Severe Cold and Flu Caplets Maximum Strength 746
Contac Severe Cold and Flu Caplets Non-Drowsy 746
Coricidin HBP Cough & Cold Tablets 738
Coricidin HBP Maximum Strength Flu Tablets 738
Dimetapp DM Cold & Cough Elixir 775
Dimetapp Nighttime Flu Liquid 776
Dimetapp Non-Drowsy Flu Syrup 777
Dimetapp Infant Drops Decongestant Plus Cough 776
PediaCare Cough-Cold Liquid 719
PediaCare Infants' Drops Decongestant Plus Cough 719
PediaCare NightRest Cough-Cold Liquid 719
Phenergan with Dextromethorphan Syrup 3559
Robitussin Cold Caplets Cold & Congestion 780
Robitussin Cold Softgels Cold & Congestion 780
Robitussin Cold Caplets Multi-Symptom Cold & Flu 781
Robitussin Cold Softgels Multi-Symptom Cold & Flu 781
Robitussin Cough & Cold Infant Drops 782
Robitussin Maximum Strength Cough & Cold Liquid 785
Robitussin Pediatric Cough & Cold Formula Liquid 785
Robitussin Maximum Strength Cough Suppressant Liquid 784
Robitussin Pediatric Cough Suppressant Liquid 784
Robitussin Multi Symptom Honey Flu Liquid 785
Robitussin Nighttime Honey Flu Liquid 786
Robitussin-CF Liquid 783
Robitussin DM Infant Drops 783
Robitussin-DM Liquid 783
Children's Sudafed Cold & Cough Liquid 709
Sudafed Cold & Cough Liquid Caps 709
Sudafed Severe Cold 711
TheraFlu Regular Strength Cold & Cough Night Time Hot Liquid 676
TheraFlu Maximum Strength Flu & Congestion Non-Drowsy Hot Liquid 677
TheraFlu Maximum Strength Flu & Cough Night Time Hot Liquid 678
TheraFlu Maximum Strength Severe Cold & Congestion Night Time Caplets 678
TheraFlu Maximum Strength Severe Cold & Congestion Night Time Hot Liquid 678
TheraFlu Maximum Strength Severe Cold & Congestion Non-Drowsy 679
Triaminic Cold & Cough Liquid 681
Triaminic Cold & Cough Softchews 683
Triaminic Cold & Night Time Cough Liquid 681
Triaminic Cold, Cough & Fever Liquid 681
Triaminic Cough Liquid 682
Triaminic Cough Softchews 684
Triaminic Cough & Congestion Liquid 682
Triaminic Cough & Sore Throat Liquid 682
Triaminic Cough & Sore Throat Softchews 684
Tussi-Organidin DM NR Liquid 3350
Tussi-Organidin DM-S NR Liquid 3350
Children's Tylenol Cold Plus Cough Suspension Liquid and Chewable Tablets 2015
Children's Tylenol Flu Suspension Liquid 2015
Infants' Tylenol Cold Decongestant and Fever Reducer Concentrated Drops Plus Cough 2015
Multi-Symptom Tylenol Cold Complete Formula Caplets 2010
Multi-Symptom Tylenol Cold Non-Drowsy Caplets and Gelcaps 2010
Multi-Symptom Tylenol Cold Severe Congestion Non-Drowsy Caplets 2011
Maximum Strength Tylenol Flu NightTime Liquid 2011
Maximum Strength Tylenol Flu Non-Drowsy Gelcaps 2011
Vicks 44 Cough Relief Liquid 724
Vicks 44D Cough & Head Congestion Relief Liquid 724
Vicks 44E Cough & Chest Congestion Relief Liquid 725
Pediatric Vicks 44e Cough & Chest Congestion Relief Liquid 728
Vicks 44M Cough, Cold & Flu Relief Liquid 725
Pediatric Vicks 44m Cough & Cold Relief 728
Vicks DayQuil LiquiCaps/Liquid Multi-Symptom Cold/Flu Relief 727
Children's Vicks NyQuil Cold/Cough Relief 726
Vicks NyQuil LiquiCaps/Liquid Multi-Symptom Cold/Flu Relief, Original and Cherry Flavors 727

Dextromethorphan Polistirex (Concurrent administration is not recommended; may cause drowsiness and bizarre behavior). Products include:
Delsym Extended-Release Suspension 664

Dezocine (Contraindication warning for meperidine is extended to other narcotics).
No products indexed under this heading.

Diazoxide (Exaggerated hypotensive effects).
No products indexed under this heading.

Diethylpropion Hydrochloride (Concurrent administration is not recommended).
No products indexed under this heading.

Diltiazem Hydrochloride (Exaggerated hypotensive effects). Products include:
Cardizem Injectable 1018
Cardizem Lyo-Ject Syringe 1018
Cardizem Monovial 1018
Cardizem CD Capsules 1016
Tiazac Capsules 1378

Dobutamine Hydrochloride (Potentiation of sympathomimetic agents and related compounds resulting in hypertensive crises; concurrent use is contraindicated). Products include:
Dobutrex Solution Vials 1914

Dopamine Hydrochloride (Potentiation of sympathomimetic agents and related compounds resulting in hypertensive crises; concurrent use is contraindicated).
No products indexed under this heading.

Doxazosin Mesylate (Exaggerated hypotensive effects). Products include:
Cardura Tablets 2668

Doxepin Hydrochloride (Concurrent or in rapid succession administration is contraindicated). Products include:
Sinequan 2713

Enalapril Maleate (Exaggerated hypotensive effects). Products include:
Lexxel Tablets 608
Vaseretic Tablets 2204
Vasotec Tablets 2210

Enalaprilat (Exaggerated hypotensive effects). Products include:
Enalaprilat Injection 863
Vasotec I.V. Injection 2207

Ephedrine Hydrochloride (Potentiation of sympathomimetic agents and related compounds resulting in hypertensive crises; concurrent use is contraindicated). Products include:
Primatene Tablets 780

Ephedrine Sulfate (Potentiation of sympathomimetic agents and related compounds resulting in hypertensive crises; concurrent use is contraindicated).
No products indexed under this heading.

Ephedrine Tannate (Potentiation of sympathomimetic agents and related compounds resulting in hypertensive crises; concurrent use is contraindicated). Products include:
Rynatuss Pediatric Suspension 3353
Rynatuss Tablets 3353

Epinephrine (Potentiation of sympathomimetic agents and related compounds resulting in hypertensive crises; concurrent use is contraindicated). Products include:
Epifrin Sterile Ophthalmic Solution ⊙235
EpiPen 1236
Primatene Mist ▣779
Xylocaine with Epinephrine Injection 653

Epinephrine Bitartrate (Potentiation of sympathomimetic agents and related compounds resulting in hypertensive crises; concurrent use is contraindicated). Products include:
Sensorcaine 643

Epinephrine Hydrochloride (Potentiation of sympathomimetic agents and related compounds resulting in hypertensive crises; concurrent use is contraindicated).
No products indexed under this heading.

Eprosartan Mesylate (Exaggerated hypotensive effects). Products include:
Teveten Tablets 3327

Esmolol Hydrochloride (Exaggerated hypotensive effects). Products include:
Brevibloc Injection 858

Felodipine (Exaggerated hypotensive effects). Products include:
Lexxel Tablets 608
Plendil Extended-Release Tablets 623

Fenfluramine Hydrochloride (Concurrent administration is not recommended).
No products indexed under this heading.

Fentanyl (Contraindication warning for meperidine is extended to other narcotics). Products include:
Duragesic Transdermal System 1786

Fentanyl Citrate (Contraindication warning for meperidine is extended to other narcotics). Products include:
Actiq 1184

Fluoxetine Hydrochloride (Coadministration with serotoninergic drugs has resulted in serious reactions, including hyperthermia, rigidity, myoclonic movements and death; concurrent and/or sequential use is contraindicated). Products include:
Prozac Pulvules, Liquid, and Weekly Capsules 1238
Sarafem Pulvules 1962

Fluvoxamine Maleate (Coadministration with serotoninergic drugs has resulted in serious reactions, including hyperthermia, rigidity, myoclonic movements and death; concurrent and/or sequential use is contraindicated). Products include:
Luvox Tablets (25, 50, 100 mg) 3256

Fosinopril Sodium (Exaggerated hypotensive effects). Products include:
Monopril Tablets 1091
Monopril HCT 1094

Furazolidone (Hypertensive crises; at least 10 days should elapse between discontinuation of Nardil and institution of another MAOI).
No products indexed under this heading.

Furosemide (Exaggerated hypotensive effects). Products include:
Furosemide Tablets 2284

Guanabenz Acetate (Exaggerated hypotensive effects).
No products indexed under this heading.

Guanethidine Monosulfate (Exaggerated hypotensive effects; contraindication).
No products indexed under this heading.

Hexobarbital (Potential for increased hypnosis).

Hydralazine Hydrochloride (Exaggerated hypotensive effects).
No products indexed under this heading.

Hydrochlorothiazide (Exaggerated hypotensive effects). Products include:
Accuretic Tablets 2614
Aldoril Tablets 2039
Atacand HCT Tablets 597
Avalide Tablets 1070
Diovan HCT Tablets 2338
Dyazide Capsules 1515
HydroDIURIL Tablets 2108
Hyzaar 2109
Inderide Tablets 3517
Inderide LA Long-Acting Capsules 3519
Lotensin HCT Tablets 2367
Maxzide 1008
Micardis HCT Tablets 1051
Microzide Capsules 3414
Moduretic Tablets 2138
Monopril HCT 1094
Prinzide Tablets 2168
Timolide Tablets 2187
Uniretic Tablets 3178
Vaseretic Tablets 2204
Zestoretic Tablets 695
Ziac Tablets 1887

Hydrocodone Bitartrate (Contraindication warning for meperidine is extended to other narcotics). Products include:
Hycodan 1316
Hycomine Compound Tablets 1317
Hycotuss Expectorant Syrup 1318
Lortab 3319
Lortab Elixir 3317
Maxidone Tablets CIII 3399
Norco 5/325 Tablets CIII 3424
Norco 7.5/325 Tablets CIII 3425
Norco 10/325 Tablets CIII 3427
Norco 10/325 Tablets CIII 3425
Vicodin Tablets 516
Vicodin ES Tablets 517
Vicodin HP Tablets 518
Vicodin Tuss Expectorant 519
Vicoprofen Tablets 520
Zydone Tablets 1330

Hydrocodone Polistirex (Contraindication warning for meperidine is extended to other narcotics). Products include:
Tussionex Pennkinetic Extended-Release Suspension 1174

Hydroflumethiazide (Exaggerated hypotensive effects). Products include:
Diucardin Tablets 3494

Hydromorphone Hydrochloride (Contraindication warning for meperidine is extended to other narcotics). Products include:
Dilaudid 441
Dilaudid Oral Liquid 445
Dilaudid Powder 441
Dilaudid Rectal Suppositories 441
Dilaudid Tablets 441
Dilaudid Tablets - 8 mg 445
Dilaudid-HP 443

Imipramine Hydrochloride (Concurrent or in rapid succession administration is contraindicated).
No products indexed under this heading.

Imipramine Pamoate (Concurrent or in rapid succession administration is contraindicated).
No products indexed under this heading.

Indapamide (Exaggerated hypotensive effects). Products include:
Indapamide Tablets 2286

Irbesartan (Exaggerated hypotensive effects). Products include:
Avalide Tablets 1070
Avapro Tablets 1074
Avapro Tablets 3076

Isocarboxazid (Hypertensive crises; at least 10 days should elapse between discontinuation of Nardil and institution of another MAOI).
No products indexed under this heading.

Isoproterenol Hydrochloride (Potentiation of sympathomimetic agents and related compounds resulting in hypertensive crises; concurrent use is contraindicated).
No products indexed under this heading.

Isoproterenol Sulfate (Potentiation of sympathomimetic agents and related compounds resulting in hypertensive crises; concurrent use is contraindicated).
No products indexed under this heading.

Isradipine (Exaggerated hypotensive effects). Products include:
DynaCirc Capsules 2921
DynaCirc CR Tablets 2923

Labetalol Hydrochloride (Exaggerated hypotensive effects). Products include:
Normodyne Injection 3135
Normodyne Tablets 3137

Levalbuterol Hydrochloride (Potentiation of sympathomimetic agents and related compounds resulting in hypertensive crises; concurrent use is contraindicated). Products include:
Xopenex Inhalation Solution 3207

Levodopa (Potentiation of sympathomimetic agents and related compounds, including levodopa, resulting in hypertensive crises; concurrent use is contraindicated). Products include:
Sinemet Tablets 1253
Sinemet CR Tablets 1255

Levorphanol Tartrate (Contraindication warning for meperidine is extended to other narcotics). Products include:
Levo-Dromoran 1734
Levorphanol Tartrate Tablets 3059

Lisinopril (Exaggerated hypotensive effects). Products include:
Prinivil Tablets 2164
Prinzide Tablets 2168
Zestoretic Tablets 695
Zestril Tablets 698

Losartan Potassium (Exaggerated hypotensive effects). Products include:
Cozaar Tablets 2067
Hyzaar 2109

Maprotiline Hydrochloride (Concurrent or in rapid succession administration is contraindicated).
No products indexed under this heading.

Mazindol (Concurrent administration is not recommended).
No products indexed under this heading.

Mecamylamine Hydrochloride (Exaggerated hypotensive effects). Products include:
Inversine Tablets 1850

Meperidine Hydrochloride (Coadministration with a single dose of meperidine has resulted in excitation, seizures, delirium, hyperpyrexia, circulatory collapse, coma, and death; concurrent use is contraindicated). Products include:
Demerol 3079
Mepergan Injection 3539

Mephobarbital (Potential for increased hypnosis).
No products indexed under this heading.

Metaproterenol Sulfate (Potentiation of sympathomimetic agents and related compounds resulting in hypertensive crises; concurrent use is contraindicated). Products include:
Alupent 1029

Metaraminol Bitartrate (Potentiation of sympathomimetic agents and related compounds resulting in hypertensive crises; concurrent use is contraindicated). Products include:
Aramine Injection 2043

Methadone Hydrochloride (Contraindication warning for meperidine is extended to other narcotics). Products include:
Dolophine Hydrochloride Tablets 3056

Methamphetamine Hydrochloride (Concurrent administration is not recommended). Products include:
Desoxyn Tablets 440

Methoxamine Hydrochloride (Potentiation of sympathomimetic agents and related compounds resulting in hypertensive crises; concurrent use is contraindicated).
No products indexed under this heading.

Methyclothiazide (Exaggerated hypotensive effects).
No products indexed under this heading.

Methyldopa (Potentiation of sympathomimetic agents and related compounds, including methyldopa, resulting in hypertensive crises; concurrent use is contraindicated). Products include:
Aldoclor Tablets 2035
Aldomet Tablets 2037
Aldoril Tablets 2039

Methyldopate Hydrochloride (Potentiation of sympathomimetic agents and related compounds, including methyldopa, resulting in hypertensive crises; concurrent use is contraindicated).
No products indexed under this heading.

Methylphenidate Hydrochloride (Potentiation of sympathomimetic agents and related compounds resulting in hypertensive crises; concurrent use is contraindicated). Products include:
Concerta Extended-Release Tablets 1998
Concerta Tablets 561
Metadate CD Capsules 1164
Metadate ER Tablets 1167
Methylin Tablets 1995
Methylin ER Tablets 1995
Ritalin 2387

Metipranolol Hydrochloride (Exaggerated hypotensive effects).
No products indexed under this heading.

Metolazone (Exaggerated hypotensive effects). Products include:
Mykrox Tablets 1168
Zaroxolyn Tablets 1177

Metoprolol Succinate (Exaggerated hypotensive effects). Products include:
Toprol-XL Tablets 651

Metoprolol Tartrate (Exaggerated hypotensive effects).
No products indexed under this heading.

Metyrosine (Exaggerated hypotensive effects). Products include:
Demser Capsules 2085

Mibefradil Dihydrochloride (Exaggerated hypotensive effects).
No products indexed under this heading.

Minoxidil (Exaggerated hypotensive effects). Products include:
Rogaine Extra Strength for Men Topical Solution ▣721
Rogaine for Women Topical Solution ▣721

Mirtazapine (Concurrent or in rapid succession administration is contraindicated). Products include:
Remeron Tablets 2483
Remeron SolTab Tablets 2486

Moclobemide (Hypertensive crises; at least 10 days should elapse between discontinuation of Nardil and institution of another MAOI).
No products indexed under this heading.

Moexipril Hydrochloride (Exaggerated hypotensive effects). Products include:
Uniretic Tablets 3178
Univasc Tablets 3181

Morphine Sulfate (Contraindication warning for meperidine is extended to other narcotics). Products include:
- Astramorph/PF Injection, USP (Preservative-Free) ... 594
- Duramorph Injection ... 1312
- Infumorph 200 and Infumorph 500 Sterile Solutions ... 1314
- Kadian Capsules ... 1335
- MS Contin Tablets ... 2896
- MSIR ... 2898
- Oramorph SR Tablets ... 3062
- Roxanol ... 3066

Nadolol (Exaggerated hypotensive effects). Products include:
- Corgard Tablets ... 2245
- Corzide 40/5 Tablets ... 2247
- Corzide 80/5 Tablets ... 2247
- Nadolol Tablets ... 2288

Naphazoline Hydrochloride (Contraindicated). Products include:
- Albalon Ophthalmic Solution ... ⊙ 225
- All Clear Eye Drops ... ⊙ 252
- All Clear AR Eye Drops ... ⊙ 252
- Clear Eyes ACR Astringent/Lubricant Eye Redness Reliever ... ⊙ 322
- Clear Eyes Lubricant Eye Redness Reliever ... ⊙ 322
- Naphcon-A Ophthalmic Solution ... 540
- Opcon-A Eye Drops ... ⊙ 253
- Vasocon-A Eye Drops ... ⊙ 307
- Visine-A Eye Allergy Relief Eye Drops ... ⊙ 314
- Visine-A Eye Drops ... ▣ 714

Nefazodone Hydrochloride (Concurrent or in rapid succession administration is contraindicated). Products include:
- Serzone Tablets ... 1104

Nicardipine Hydrochloride (Exaggerated hypotensive effects). Products include:
- Cardene I.V. ... 3485

Nifedipine (Exaggerated hypotensive effects). Products include:
- Adalat CC Tablets ... 877
- Procardia Capsules ... 2708
- Procardia XL Extended Release Tablets ... 2710

Nisoldipine (Exaggerated hypotensive effects). Products include:
- Sular Tablets ... 688

Nitroglycerin (Exaggerated hypotensive effects). Products include:
- Nitro-Dur Transdermal Infusion System ... 3134
- Nitro-Dur Transdermal Infusion System ... 1834
- Nitrolingual Pumpspray ... 1355
- Nitrostat Tablets ... 2658

Norepinephrine Bitartrate (Potentiation of sympathomimetic agents and related compounds resulting in hypertensive crises; concurrent use is contraindicated).
- No products indexed under this heading.

Nortriptyline Hydrochloride (Hypertensive crises; concurrent or in rapid succession administration is contraindicated).
- No products indexed under this heading.

Oxycodone Hydrochloride (Contraindication warning for meperidine is extended to other narcotics). Products include:
- OxyContin Tablets ... 2912
- OxyFast Oral Concentrate Solution ... 2916
- OxyIR Capsules ... 2916
- Percocet Tablets ... 1326
- Percodan Tablets ... 1327
- Percolone Tablets ... 1327
- Roxicodone ... 3067
- Tylox Capsules ... 2597

Oxymetazoline Hydrochloride (Contraindicated). Products include:
- Afrin ... ▣ 733
- Afrin No Drip Original Nasal Spray ... ▣ 735
- Afrin No Drip Extra Moisturizing Nasal Spray ... ▣ 735
- Afrin No Drip Severe Congestion Nasal Spray ... ▣ 735
- Afrin No Drip Sinus Nasal Spray ... ▣ 735
- Afrin Original Pump Mist ... ▣ 733
- Neo-Synephrine 12 Hour ... ▣ 615
- Vicks Sinex 12-Hour Nasal Spray and Ultra Fine Mist ... ▣ 729
- Visine L.R. Long Lasting Eye Drops ... ⊙ 315

Pargyline Hydrochloride (Hypertensive crises; at least 10 days should elapse between discontinuation of Nardil and institution of another MAOI).
- No products indexed under this heading.

Paroxetine Hydrochloride (Coadministration with serotoninergic drugs has resulted in serious reactions, including hyperthermia, rigidity, myoclonic movements and death; concurrent and/or sequential use is contraindicated). Products include:
- Paxil ... 1609

Penbutolol Sulfate (Exaggerated hypotensive effects).
- No products indexed under this heading.

Pentobarbital Sodium (Potential for increased hypnosis). Products include:
- Nembutal Sodium Solution ... 485

Perindopril Erbumine (Exaggerated hypotensive effects). Products include:
- Aceon Tablets (2 mg, 4 mg, 8 mg) ... 3249

Phendimetrazine Tartrate (Concurrent administration is not recommended). Products include:
- Bontril Slow-Release Capsules ... 576

Phenmetrazine Hydrochloride (Concurrent administration is not recommended).
- No products indexed under this heading.

Phenobarbital (Potential for increased hypnosis). Products include:
- Arco-Lase Plus Tablets ... 592
- Donnatal ... 2929
- Donnatal Extentabs ... 2930

Phenoxybenzamine Hydrochloride (Exaggerated hypotensive effects). Products include:
- Dibenzyline Capsules ... 3457

Phentolamine Mesylate (Exaggerated hypotensive effects).
- No products indexed under this heading.

D-Phenylalanine (Potentiation of sympathomimetic agents and related compounds resulting in hypertensive crises; concurrent use is contraindicated).

L-Phenylalanine (Potentiation of sympathomimetic agents and related compounds resulting in hypertensive crises; concurrent use is contraindicated).

Phenylephrine Bitartrate (Potentiation of sympathomimetic agents and related compounds resulting in hypertensive crises; concurrent use is contraindicated).
- No products indexed under this heading.

Phenylephrine Hydrochloride (Potentiation of sympathomimetic agents and related compounds resulting in hypertensive crises; concurrent use is contraindicated). Products include:
- Afrin Nasal Decongestant Children's Pump Mist ... ▣ 734
- Extendryl ... 1361
- Hycomine Compound Tablets ... 1317
- Neo-Synephrine ... ▣ 614
- Phenergan VC Syrup ... 3560
- Phenergan VC with Codeine Syrup ... 3561
- Preparation H Cream ... ▣ 778
- Preparation H Cooling Gel ... ▣ 778
- Preparation H ... ▣ 778
- Vicks Sinex Nasal Spray and Ultra Fine Mist ... ▣ 729

Phenylephrine Tannate (Potentiation of sympathomimetic agents and related compounds resulting in hypertensive crises; concurrent use is contraindicated). Products include:
- Ryna-12 S Suspension ... 3351
- Reformulated Rynatan Pediatric Suspension ... 3352
- Rynatuss Pediatric Suspension ... 3353
- Rynatuss Tablets ... 3353

Phenylpropanolamine Containing Anorectics (Concurrent administration is not recommended).
- No products indexed under this heading.

Phenylpropanolamine Hydrochloride (Potentiation of sympathomimetic agents and related compounds resulting in hypertensive crises; concurrent use is contraindicated).
- No products indexed under this heading.

Pindolol (Exaggerated hypotensive effects).
- No products indexed under this heading.

Pirbuterol Acetate (Potentiation of sympathomimetic agents and related compounds resulting in hypertensive crises; concurrent use is contraindicated). Products include:
- Maxair Autohaler ... 1981
- Maxair Inhaler ... 1984

Polythiazide (Exaggerated hypotensive effects). Products include:
- Minizide Capsules ... 2700
- Renese Tablets ... 2712

Prazosin Hydrochloride (Exaggerated hypotensive effects). Products include:
- Minipress Capsules ... 2699
- Minizide Capsules ... 2700

Procarbazine Hydrochloride (Hypertensive crises; at least 10 days should elapse between discontinuation of Nardil and institution of another MAOI). Products include:
- Matulane Capsules ... 3246

Propoxyphene Hydrochloride (Contraindication warning for meperidine is extended to other narcotics). Products include:
- Darvon Pulvules ... 1909
- Darvon Compound-65 Pulvules ... 1910

Propoxyphene Napsylate (Contraindication warning for meperidine is extended to other narcotics). Products include:
- Darvon-N/Darvocet-N ... 1907
- Darvon-N Tablets ... 1912

Propranolol Hydrochloride (Exaggerated hypotensive effects). Products include:
- Inderal ... 3513
- Inderal LA Long-Acting Capsules ... 3516
- Inderide Tablets ... 3517
- Inderide LA Long-Acting Capsules ... 3519

Protriptyline Hydrochloride (Concurrent or in rapid succession administration is contraindicated). Products include:
- Vivactil Tablets ... 2446
- Vivactil Tablets ... 2217

Pseudoephedrine Hydrochloride (Potentiation of sympathomimetic agents and related compounds resulting in hypertensive crises; concurrent use is contraindicated). Products include:
- Actifed Cold & Allergy Tablets ... ▣ 688
- Actifed Cold & Sinus Caplets and Tablets ... ▣ 688
- Advil Cold and Sinus Caplets ... ▣ 771
- Advil Cold and Sinus Tablets ... ▣ 771
- Advil Flu & Body Ache Caplets ... ▣ 772
- Aleve Cold & Sinus Caplets ... ▣ 603
- Alka-Seltzer Plus Liqui-Gels ... ▣ 604
- Alka-Seltzer Plus Cold & Flu Medicine Liqui-Gels ... ▣ 604
- Alka-Seltzer Plus Cold & Sinus Medicine Liqui-Gels ... ▣ 604
- Allegra-D Extended-Release Tablets ... 714
- BC Cold Powder ... ▣ 619
- Benadryl Allergy/Cold Tablets ... ▣ 691
- Benadryl Allergy/Congestion Tablets ... ▣ 692
- Benadryl Allergy & Sinus Liquid ... ▣ 693
- Benadryl Allergy & Sinus Fastmelt Tablets ... ▣ 693
- Benadryl Allergy Sinus Headache Caplets & Gelcaps ... ▣ 693
- Benadryl Severe Allergy & Sinus Headache Caplets ... ▣ 694
- Benadryl Children's Allergy/Cold Fastmelt Tablets ... ▣ 692
- Benylin Multi-Symptom Liquid ... ▣ 697
- Bromfed Capsules (Extended-Release) ... 2269
- Bromfed-PD Capsules (Extended-Release) ... 2269
- Children's Cēpacol Sore Throat ... ▣ 788
- Comtrex Acute Head Cold & Sinus Pressure Relief Tablets ... ▣ 627
- Comtrex Deep Chest Cold & Congestion Relief Softgels ... ▣ 627
- Comtrex Flu Therapy & Fever Relief Daytime Caplets ... ▣ 628
- Comtrex Flu Therapy & Fever Relief Nighttime Tablets ... ▣ 628
- Comtrex Maximum Strength Multi-Symptom Cold & Cough Relief Tablets and Caplets ... ▣ 626
- Contac Non-Drowsy 12 Hour Cold Caplets ... ▣ 745
- Contac Non-Drowsy Timed Release 12 Hour Cold Caplets ... ▣ 746
- Contac Severe Cold and Flu Caplets Maximum Strength ... ▣ 746
- Contac Severe Cold and Flu Caplets Non-Drowsy ... ▣ 746
- Dimetapp Elixir ... ▣ 777
- Dimetapp Cold and Fever Suspension ... ▣ 775
- Dimetapp DM Cold & Cough Elixir ... ▣ 775
- Dimetapp Nighttime Flu Liquid ... ▣ 776
- Dimetapp Non-Drowsy Flu Syrup ... ▣ 777
- Dimetapp Infant Drops Decongestant ... ▣ 775
- Dimetapp Infant Drops Decongestant Plus Cough ... ▣ 776
- Guaifed ... 2272
- Kronofed-A ... 1341
- Children's Motrin Cold Oral Suspension ... 2007
- Motrin Sinus Headache Caplets ... 2005
- PediaCare Cough-Cold Liquid ... ▣ 719
- PediaCare Infants' Drops Decongestant ... ▣ 719
- PediaCare Infants' Drops Decongestant Plus Cough ... ▣ 719
- PediaCare NightRest Cough-Cold Liquid ... ▣ 719
- Robitussin Cold Caplets Cold & Congestion ... ▣ 780
- Robitussin Cold Softgels Cold & Congestion ... ▣ 780
- Robitussin Cold Caplets Multi-Symptom Cold & Flu ... ▣ 781
- Robitussin Cold Softgels Multi-Symptom Cold & Flu ... ▣ 781
- Robitussin Cold Softgels Severe Congestion ... ▣ 782
- Robitussin Cough & Cold Infant Drops ... ▣ 782
- Robitussin Maximum Strength Cough & Cold Liquid ... ▣ 785
- Robitussin Pediatric Cough & Cold Formula Liquid ... ▣ 785
- Robitussin Multi Symptom Honey Flu Liquid ... ▣ 785
- Robitussin Nighttime Honey Flu Liquid ... ▣ 786
- Robitussin-CF Liquid ... ▣ 783
- Robitussin-DAC Syrup ... 2942
- Robitussin-PE Liquid ... ▣ 782
- Ryna ... ▣ 768
- Semprex-D Capsules ... 1172
- Singlet Caplets ... ▣ 761
- Sinutab Non-Drying Liquid Caps ... ▣ 706
- Sinutab Sinus Allergy Medication, Maximum Strength Formula, Tablets & Caplets ... ▣ 707
- Sinutab Sinus Medication, Maximum Strength Without Drowsiness Formula, Tablets & Caplets ... ▣ 707
- Sudafed 12 Hour Tablets ... ▣ 708
- Sudafed 24 Hour Tablets ... ▣ 708
- Children's Sudafed Cold & Cough Liquid ... ▣ 709
- Children's Sudafed Nasal Decongestant Chewables ... ▣ 711
- Children's Sudafed Nasal Decongestant Liquid Medication ... ▣ 711
- Sudafed Cold & Allergy Tablets ... ▣ 708
- Sudafed Cold & Cough Liquid Caps ... ▣ 709
- Sudafed Cold & Sinus Liquid Caps ... ▣ 710
- Sudafed Nasal Decongestant Tablets ... ▣ 710
- Sudafed Non-Drying Sinus Liquid Caps ... ▣ 712
- Sudafed Severe Cold ... ▣ 711
- Sudafed Sinus Headache Caplets ... ▣ 712

Sudafed Sinus Headache Tablets .. ▣712
Tavist Sinus Non-Drowsy Coated Caplets ▣676
TheraFlu Regular Strength Cold & Cough Night Time Hot Liquid ▣676
TheraFlu Regular Strength Cold & Sore Throat Night Time Hot Liquid ▣676
TheraFlu Maximum Strength Flu & Congestion Non-Drowsy Hot Liquid ▣677
TheraFlu Maximum Strength Flu & Cough Night Time Hot Liquid ▣678
TheraFlu Maximum Strength Flu & Sore Throat Night Time Hot Liquid ▣677
TheraFlu Maximum Strength Severe Cold & Congestion Night Time Caplets ▣678
TheraFlu Maximum Strength Severe Cold & Congestion Night Time Hot Liquid ▣678
TheraFlu Maximum Strength Severe Cold & Congestion Non-Drowsy ▣679
Triaminic Allergy Congestion Liquid ▣680
Triaminic Chest Congestion Liquid ▣680
Triaminic Cold & Allergy Liquid ▣681
Triaminic Cold & Allergy Softchews ▣683
Triaminic Cold & Cough Liquid ▣681
Triaminic Cold & Cough Softchews ▣683
Triaminic Cold & Night Time Cough Liquid ▣681
Triaminic Cold, Cough & Fever Liquid ▣681
Triaminic Cough Liquid ▣682
Triaminic Cough & Congestion Liquid ▣682
Triaminic Cough & Sore Throat Liquid ▣682
Triaminic Cough & Sore Throat Softchews ▣684
Children's Tylenol Allergy-D Liquid ... 2014
Children's Tylenol Cold Suspension Liquid and Chewable Tablets 2015
Children's Tylenol Cold Plus Cough Suspension Liquid and Chewable Tablets 2015
Children's Tylenol Flu Suspension Liquid 2015
Children's Tylenol Sinus Suspension Liquid 2017
Infants' Tylenol Cold Decongestant and Fever Reducer Concentrated Drops 2015
Infants' Tylenol Cold Decongestant and Fever Reducer Concentrated Drops Plus Cough .. 2015
Tylenol Allergy Sinus 2010
Multi-Symptom Tylenol Cold Complete Formula Caplets 2010
Multi-Symptom Tylenol Cold Non-Drowsy Caplets and Gelcaps 2010
Multi-Symptom Tylenol Cold Severe Congestion Non-Drowsy Caplets 2011
Maximum Strength Tylenol Flu NightTime Gelcaps 2011
Maximum Strength Tylenol Flu NightTime Liquid 2011
Maximum Strength Tylenol Flu Non-Drowsy Gelcaps 2011
Maximum Strength Tylenol Sinus NightTime Caplets 2012
Maximum Strength Tylenol Sinus Non-Drowsy Geltabs, Gelcaps, Caplets, and Tablets 2012
Vicks 44D Cough & Head Congestion Relief Liquid ▣724
Vicks 44M Cough, Cold & Flu Relief Liquid ▣725
Pediatric Vicks 44m Cough & Cold Relief ▣728
Vicks DayQuil LiquiCaps/Liquid Multi-Symptom Cold/Flu Relief ... ▣727
Children's Vicks NyQuil Cold/Cough Relief ▣726
Vicks NyQuil LiquiCaps/Liquid Multi-Symptom Cold/Flu Relief, Original and Cherry Flavors ▣727
Zephrex Tablets 3091
Zephrex LA Tablets 3092
Zyrtec-D 12 Hour Extended Relief Tablets 2758

Pseudoephedrine Sulfate (Potentiation of sympathomimetic agents and related compounds resulting in hypertensive crises; concurrent use is contraindicated). Products include:
Chlor-Trimeton Allergy/Decongestant Tablets ▣736
Claritin-D 12 Hour Extended Release Tablets 3102
Claritin-D 24 Hour Extended Release Tablets 3104
Coricidin 'D' Cold, Flu & Sinus Tablets ▣737
Drixoral Allergy/Sinus Extended-Release Tablets ▣741
Drixoral Cold & Allergy Sustained-Action Tablets ▣740
Drixoral Cold & Flu Extended-Release Tablets ▣740
Drixoral Nasal Decongestant Long-Acting Non-Drowsy Tablets ▣740
Rynatan Tablets 3351

Quinapril Hydrochloride (Exaggerated hypotensive effects). Products include:
Accupril Tablets 2611
Accuretic Tablets 2614

Ramipril (Exaggerated hypotensive effects). Products include:
Altace Capsules 2233

Rauwolfia serpentina (Exaggerated hypotensive effects; exercise caution).
No products indexed under this heading.

Remifentanil Hydrochloride (Contraindication warning for meperidine is extended to other narcotics).
No products indexed under this heading.

Rescinnamine (Exaggerated hypotensive effects; exercise caution).
No products indexed under this heading.

Reserpine (Exaggerated hypotensive effects; exercise caution).
No products indexed under this heading.

Salmeterol Xinafoate (Potentiation of sympathomimetic agents and related compounds resulting in hypertensive crises; concurrent use is contraindicated). Products include:
Advair Diskus 100/50 1448
Advair Diskus 250/50 1448
Advair Diskus 500/50 1448
Serevent Diskus 1637
Serevent Inhalation Aerosol 1633

Secobarbital Sodium (Potential for increased hypnosis).
No products indexed under this heading.

Selegiline Hydrochloride (Hypertensive crises; at least 10 days should elapse between discontinuation of Nardil and institution of another MAOI). Products include:
Eldepryl Capsules 3266

Sertraline Hydrochloride (Concurrent or in rapid succession administration is contraindicated). Products include:
Zoloft 2751

Sibutramine Hydrochloride Monohydrate (Concurrent administration is not recommended). Products include:
Meridia Capsules 481

Sodium Nitroprusside (Exaggerated hypotensive effects).
No products indexed under this heading.

Sotalol Hydrochloride (Exaggerated hypotensive effects). Products include:
Betapace Tablets 950
Betapace AF Tablets 954

Spirapril Hydrochloride (Exaggerated hypotensive effects).
No products indexed under this heading.

Sufentanil Citrate (Contraindication warning for meperidine is extended to other narcotics).
No products indexed under this heading.

Telmisartan (Exaggerated hypotensive effects). Products include:
Micardis Tablets 1049
Micardis HCT Tablets 1051

Terazosin Hydrochloride (Exaggerated hypotensive effects). Products include:
Hytrin Capsules 464

Terbutaline Sulfate (Potentiation of sympathomimetic agents and related compounds resulting in hypertensive crises; concurrent use is contraindicated). Products include:
Brethine Ampuls 2314
Brethine Tablets 2313

Tetrahydrozoline Hydrochloride (Contraindicated). Products include:
Murine Tears Plus Lubricant Redness Reliever Eye Drops ⊙323
Visine Original Eye Drops ⊙315
Visine A.C. Seasonal Relief From Pollen & Dust Eye Drops ⊙314
Advanced Relief Visine Eye Drops . ⊙313

Thiamylal Sodium (Potential for increased hypnosis).
No products indexed under this heading.

Timolol Hemihydrate (Exaggerated hypotensive effects). Products include:
Betimol Ophthalmic Solution ⊙324

Timolol Maleate (Exaggerated hypotensive effects). Products include:
Blocadren Tablets 2046
Cosopt Sterile Ophthalmic Solution 2065
Timolide Tablets 2187
Timolol GFS ⊙266
Timoptic in Ocudose 2192
Timoptic Sterile Ophthalmic Solution 2190
Timoptic-XE Sterile Ophthalmic Gel Forming Solution 2194

Torsemide (Exaggerated hypotensive effects). Products include:
Demadex Tablets and Injection 2965

Trandolapril (Exaggerated hypotensive effects). Products include:
Mavik Tablets 478
Tarka Tablets 508

Tranylcypromine Sulfate (Hypertensive crises; at least 10 days should elapse between discontinuation of Nardil and institution of another MAOI). Products include:
Parnate Tablets 1607

Trazodone Hydrochloride (Concurrent or in rapid succession administration is contraindicated).
No products indexed under this heading.

Trimethaphan Camsylate (Exaggerated hypotensive effects).
No products indexed under this heading.

Trimipramine Maleate (Concurrent or in rapid succession administration is contraindicated). Products include:
Surmontil Capsules 3595

L-Tryptophan (Potentiation of sympathomimetic agents and related compounds, including tryptophan, resulting in hypertensive crises; concurrent use is contraindicated).
No products indexed under this heading.

Tyramine (Concurrent use should be avoided).
No products indexed under this heading.

L-Tyrosine (Potentiation of sympathomimetic agents and related compounds, including tyrosine, resulting in hypertensive crises; concurrent use is contraindicated).
No products indexed under this heading.

Valsartan (Exaggerated hypotensive effects). Products include:
Diovan Capsules 2337
Diovan HCT Tablets 2338

Venlafaxine Hydrochloride (Co-administration with serotoninergic drugs has resulted in serious reactions, including hyperthermia, rigidity, myoclonic movements and death; concurrent and/or sequential use is contraindicated). Products include:
Effexor Tablets 3495
Effexor XR Capsules 3499

Verapamil Hydrochloride (Exaggerated hypotensive effects). Products include:
Covera-HS Tablets 3199
Isoptin SR Tablets 467
Tarka Tablets 508
Verelan Capsules 3184
Verelan PM Capsules 3186

Food Interactions

Alcohol (Concurrent use should be avoided).

Beans, broad (Concurrent and/or sequential intake must be avoided).

Beans, Fava (Concurrent and/or sequential intake must be avoided).

Beer, alcohol-free (Concurrent and/or sequential intake must be avoided).

Beer, reduced-alcohol (Concurrent and/or sequential intake must be avoided).

Beer, unspecified (Concurrent and/or sequential intake must be avoided).

Beverages, caffeine-containing (Excessive caffeine intake should be avoided).

Bologna, Lebanon (Concurrent and/or sequential intake must be avoided).

Cheese, aged (Concurrent and/or sequential intake must be avoided).

Cheese, unspecified (Concurrent and/or sequential intake must be avoided).

Chocolate (Concurrent and/or sequential intake must be avoided).

Fish, smoked (Concurrent and/or sequential intake must be avoided).

Food with high concentration of dopamine (Concurrent and/or sequential intake must be avoided).

Food with high concentration of tyramine (Concurrent and/or sequential intake must be avoided).

Herring, pickled (Concurrent and/or sequential intake must be avoided).

Liver (Concurrent and/or sequential intake must be avoided).

Meat, unspecified (Concurrent and/or sequential intake must be avoided).

Meat extracts (Concurrent and/or sequential intake must be avoided).

Pepperoni (Concurrent and/or sequential intake must be avoided).

Salami, Genoa (Concurrent and/or sequential intake must be avoided).

Salami, Hard (Concurrent and/or sequential intake must be avoided).

Sauerkraut (Concurrent and/or sequential intake must be avoided).

Sausage, Dry (Concurrent and/or sequential intake must be avoided).

Wine, unspecified (Concurrent and/or sequential intake must be avoided).

Wine products (Concurrent and/or sequential intake must be avoided).

Yeast, Brewer's (Concurrent and/or sequential intake must be avoided).

Yeast Extract (Concurrent and/or sequential intake must be avoided).

Yogurt (Concurrent and/or sequential intake must be avoided).

NAROPIN INJECTION

(Ropivacaine Hydrochloride) 612
May interact with local anesthetics, theophylline, and certain other agents. Compounds in these categories include:

Aminophylline (Co-administration with drugs known to be metabolized by CYP1A2 via competitive inhibition, such as theophylline, may result in an interaction; caution is advised if used concurrently).
No products indexed under this heading.

Bupivacaine Hydrochloride (Co-administration with other local anesthetics or agents structurally related to amide-type local anesthetics may result in additive toxic effects). Products include:
- Sensorcaine 643
- Sensorcaine-MPF Injection 643

Chloroprocaine Hydrochloride (Co-administration with other local anesthetics or agents structurally related to amide-type local anesthetics may result in additive toxic effects). Products include:
- Nesacaine/Nesacaine MPF 617

Dyphylline (Co-administration with drugs known to be metabolized by CYP1A2 via competitive inhibition, such as theophylline, may result in an interaction; caution is advised if used concurrently). Products include:
- Lufyllin Tablets 3347
- Lufyllin-400 Tablets 3347
- Lufyllin-GG Elixir 3348
- Lufyllin-GG Tablets 3348

Etidocaine Hydrochloride (Co-administration with other local anesthetics or agents structurally related to amide-type local anesthetics may result in additive toxic effects). Products include:
- Duranest Injections 600

Fluvoxamine Maleate (Co-administration with fluvoxamine, a selective and potent inhibitor of CYP1A2, has resulted in reduced plasma clearance by 70% leading to increased ropivacaine plasma levels). Products include:
- Luvox Tablets (25, 50, 100 mg) 3256

Imipramine Hydrochloride (Co-administration with drugs known to be metabolized by CYP1A2 via competitive inhibition, such as imipramine, may result in an interaction; caution is advised if used concurrently).
No products indexed under this heading.

Imipramine Pamoate (Co-administration with drugs known to be metabolized by CYP1A2 via competitive inhibition, such as imipramine, may result in an interaction; caution is advised if used concurrently).
No products indexed under this heading.

Ketoconazole (Co-administration has resulted in a 15% reduction in *in vivo* plasma clearance of ropivacaine). Products include:
- Nizoral 2% Cream 3620
- Nizoral A-D Shampoo 2008
- Nizoral 2% Shampoo 2007
- Nizoral Tablets 1791

Levobupivacaine Hydrochloride (Co-administration with other local anesthetics or agents structurally related to amide-type local anesthetics may result in additive toxic effects). Products include:
- Chirocaine Injection 2909

Lidocaine Hydrochloride (Co-administration with other local anesthetics or agents structurally related to amide-type local anesthetics may result in additive toxic effects). Products include:
- Bactine First Aid Liquid 611
- Xylocaine Injections 653

Mepivacaine Hydrochloride (Co-administration with other local anesthetics or agents structurally related to amide-type local anesthetics may result in additive toxic effects). Products include:
- Polocaine Injection, USP 625
- Polocaine-MPF Injection, USP 625

Procaine Hydrochloride (Co-administration with other local anesthetics or agents structurally related to amide-type local anesthetics may result in additive toxic effects).
No products indexed under this heading.

Tetracaine Hydrochloride (Co-administration with other local anesthetics or agents structurally related to amide-type local anesthetics may result in additive toxic effects). Products include:
- Cēpacol Viractin Cold Sore and Fever Blister Treatment, Gel........ 788
- Cetacaine Topical Anesthetic 1196

Theophylline (Co-administration with drugs known to be metabolized by CYP1A2 via competitive inhibition, such as theophylline, may result in an interaction; caution is advised if used concurrently). Products include:
- Aerolate 1361
- Theo-Dur Extended-Release Tablets 1835
- Uni-Dur Extended-Release Tablets .. 1841
- Uniphyl 400 mg and 600 mg Tablets 2903

Theophylline Calcium Salicylate (Co-administration with drugs known to be metabolized by CYP1A2 via competitive inhibition, such as theophylline, may result in an interaction; caution is advised if used concurrently).
No products indexed under this heading.

Theophylline Sodium Glycinate (Co-administration with drugs known to be metabolized by CYP1A2 via competitive inhibition, such as theophylline, may result in an interaction; caution is advised if used concurrently).
No products indexed under this heading.

Verapamil Hydrochloride (*In vitro* studies indicate that cytochrome P450 IA is involved in the formation of 3-hydroxy ropivacaine, the major metabolite; co-administration with other agents which are potent inhibitors of this enzyme, such as verapamil, may potentially interact with Naropin). Products include:
- Covera-HS Tablets 3199
- Isoptin SR Tablets 467
- Tarka Tablets 508
- Verelan Capsules 3184
- Verelan PM Capsules 3186

NASACORT NASAL INHALER
(Triamcinolone Acetonide) 750
May interact with:

Prednisone (Concomitant use with alternate-day systemic prednisone could increase the likelihood of hypothalamic-pituitary-adrenal (HPA) suppression). Products include:
- Prednisone 3064

NASACORT AQ NASAL SPRAY
(Triamcinolone Acetonide) 752
None cited in PDR database.

NASALCROM NASAL SPRAY
(Cromolyn Sodium) 719
None cited in PDR database.

NASALIDE NASAL SPRAY
(Flunisolide) 1295
None cited in PDR database.

NASAREL NASAL SOLUTION 0.025%
(Flunisolide) 1296
None cited in PDR database.

NASCOBAL GEL
(Vitamin B_{12}) 3174
May interact with:

Bone Marrow Suppressants, unspecified (Blunted or impeded therapeutic response to vitamin B_{12} may be due to co-administration of drugs with bone marrow suppressant properties).

Chloramphenicol Sodium Succinate (Blunted or impeded therapeutic response to vitamin B_{12} may be due to co-administration of drugs with bone marrow suppressant properties, such as chloramphenicol).
No products indexed under this heading.

Food Interactions

Food, unspecified (Hot foods may cause nasal secretions and a resulting loss of medication; therefore, patients should be told to administer Nascobal at least one hour before or one hour after ingestion of hot foods or liquids).

NASONEX NASAL SPRAY
(Mometasone Furoate Monohydrate) 3131
None cited in PDR database.

NATACHEW TABLETS
(Ferrous Fumarate, Vitamins, Prenatal, Vitamins with Iron) 3364
None cited in PDR database.

NATACYN ANTIFUNGAL OPHTHALMIC SUSPENSION
(Natamycin) .... ⊙216
None cited in PDR database.

NATRECOR FOR INJECTION
(Nesiritide) 3189
None cited in PDR database.

NATRU-VENT NASAL SPRAY, ADULT STRENGTH
(Xylometazoline Hydrochloride) 624
None cited in PDR database.

NATRU-VENT NASAL SPRAY, PEDIATRIC STRENGTH
(Xylometazoline Hydrochloride) 625
None cited in PDR database.

NATRU-VENT SALINE NASAL SPRAY
(Sodium Chloride) 625
None cited in PDR database.

NATURAL AROUSAL CREAM
(L-Arginine) 840
None cited in PDR database.

NATURAL SENSATION CREAM
(L-Arginine) 841
None cited in PDR database.

NATURE'S OWN PAIN EXPELLER CREAM
(L-Arginine, Capsaicin) 841
None cited in PDR database.

NATURE'S REMEDY TABLETS
(Sennosides) 621
None cited in PDR database.

NAVANE CAPSULES
(Thiothixene) 2701
May interact with anticholinergics, central nervous system depressants, and certain other agents. Compounds in these categories include:

Alfentanil Hydrochloride (Co-administration may result in possible additive effects which may include hypotension; careful dosage adjustment is indicated when used concurrently).
No products indexed under this heading.

Alprazolam (Co-administration may result in possible additive effects which may include hypotension; careful dosage adjustment is indicated when used concurrently). Products include:
- Xanax Tablets 2865

Aprobarbital (Co-administration may result in possible additive effects which may include hypotension; careful dosage adjustment is indicated when used concurrently).
No products indexed under this heading.

Atropine Sulfate (Thiothixene possesses weak anticholinergic properties; concurrent use requires caution because of increased atropine-like effect). Products include:
- Donnatal 2929
- Donnatal Extentabs 2930
- Motofen Tablets 577
- Prosed/DS Tablets 3268
- Urised Tablets 2876

Belladonna Alkaloids (Thiothixene possesses weak anticholinergic properties; concurrent use requires caution because of increased atropine-like effect). Products include:
- Hyland's Teething Tablets 766
- Urimax Tablets 1769

Benztropine Mesylate (Thiothixene possesses weak anticholinergic properties; concurrent use requires caution because of increased atropine-like effect). Products include:
- Cogentin 2055

Biperiden Hydrochloride (Thiothixene possesses weak anticholinergic properties; concurrent use requires caution because of increased atropine-like effect). Products include:
- Akineton 402

Buprenorphine Hydrochloride (Co-administration may result in possible additive effects which may include hypotension; careful dosage adjustment is indicated when used concurrently). Products include:
- Buprenex Injectable 2918

Buspirone Hydrochloride (Co-administration may result in possible additive effects which may include hypotension; careful dosage adjustment is indicated when used concurrently).
No products indexed under this heading.

Butabarbital (Co-administration may result in possible additive effects which may include hypotension; careful dosage adjustment is indicated when used concurrently).
No products indexed under this heading.

Butalbital (Co-administration may result in possible additive effects which may include hypotension; careful dosage adjustment is indicated when used concurrently). Products include:
- Phrenilin 578
- Sedapap Tablets 50 mg/650 mg ... 2225

Chlordiazepoxide (Co-administration may result in possible additive effects which may include hypotension; careful dosage adjustment is indicated when used concurrently). Products include:
- Limbitrol 1738

Chlordiazepoxide Hydrochloride (Co-administration may result in possible additive effects which may include hypotension; careful dosage adjustment is indicated when used concurrently). Products include:
- Librium Capsules 1736
- Librium for Injection 1737

Chlorpromazine (Co-administration may result in possible additive effects which may include hypotension; careful dosage adjustment is indicated when used concurrently). Products include:
- Thorazine Suppositories 1656

Chlorpromazine Hydrochloride (Co-administration may result in possible additive effects which may include hypotension; careful dosage adjustment is indicated when used concurrently). Products include:
- Thorazine 1656

Chlorprothixene (Co-administration may result in possible additive effects which may include hypotension; careful dosage adjustment is indicated when used concurrently).
No products indexed under this heading.

Chlorprothixene Hydrochloride (Co-administration may result in possible additive effects which may include hypotension; careful dosage adjustment is indicated when used concurrently).
No products indexed under this heading.

Chlorprothixene Lactate (Co-administration may result in possible additive effects which may include hypotension; careful dosage adjustment is indicated when used concurrently).
No products indexed under this heading.

Clidinium Bromide (Thiothixene possesses weak anticholinergic properties; concurrent use requires caution because of increased atropine-like effect).
No products indexed under this heading.

Clorazepate Dipotassium (Co-administration may result in possible additive effects which may include hypotension; careful dosage adjustment is indicated when used concurrently). Products include:
- Tranxene 511

Clozapine (Co-administration may result in possible additive effects which may include hypotension; careful dosage adjustment is indicated when used concurrently). Products include:
- Clozaril Tablets 2319

Codeine Phosphate (Co-administration may result in possible additive effects which may include hypotension; careful dosage adjustment is indicated when used concurrently). Products include:
- Phenergan with Codeine Syrup 3557
- Phenergan VC with Codeine Syrup .. 3561
- Robitussin A-C Syrup 2942
- Robitussin-DAC Syrup 2942
- Ryna-C Liquid .... ▣768
- Soma Compound w/Codeine Tablets 3355
- Tussi-Organidin NR Liquid 3350
- Tussi-Organidin-S NR Liquid 3350
- Tylenol with Codeine 2595

Desflurane (Co-administration may result in possible additive effects which may include hypotension; careful dosage adjustment is indicated when used concurrently). Products include:
- Suprane Liquid for Inhalation 874

Dezocine (Co-administration may result in possible additive effects which may include hypotension; careful dosage adjustment is indicated when used concurrently).
No products indexed under this heading.

Diazepam (Co-administration may result in possible additive effects which may include hypotension; careful dosage adjustment is indicated when used concurrently). Products include:
- Valium Injectable 3026
- Valium Tablets 3047

Dicyclomine Hydrochloride (Thiothixene possesses weak anticholinergic properties; concurrent use requires caution because of increased atropine-like effect).
No products indexed under this heading.

Droperidol (Co-administration may result in possible additive effects which may include hypotension; careful dosage adjustment is indicated when used concurrently).
No products indexed under this heading.

Enflurane (Co-administration may result in possible additive effects which may include hypotension; careful dosage adjustment is indicated when used concurrently).
No products indexed under this heading.

Estazolam (Co-administration may result in possible additive effects which may include hypotension; careful dosage adjustment is indicated when used concurrently). Products include:
- ProSom Tablets 500

Ethchlorvynol (Co-administration may result in possible additive effects which may include hypotension; careful dosage adjustment is indicated when used concurrently).
No products indexed under this heading.

Ethinamate (Co-administration may result in possible additive effects which may include hypotension; careful dosage adjustment is indicated when used concurrently).
No products indexed under this heading.

Fentanyl (Co-administration may result in possible additive effects which may include hypotension; careful dosage adjustment is indicated when used concurrently). Products include:
- Duragesic Transdermal System 1786

Fentanyl Citrate (Co-administration may result in possible additive effects which may include hypotension; careful dosage adjustment is indicated when used concurrently). Products include:
- Actiq 1184

Fluphenazine Decanoate (Co-administration may result in possible additive effects which may include hypotension; careful dosage adjustment is indicated when used concurrently).
No products indexed under this heading.

Fluphenazine Enanthate (Co-administration may result in possible additive effects which may include hypotension; careful dosage adjustment is indicated when used concurrently).
No products indexed under this heading.

Fluphenazine Hydrochloride (Co-administration may result in possible additive effects which may include hypotension; careful dosage adjustment is indicated when used concurrently).
No products indexed under this heading.

Flurazepam Hydrochloride (Co-administration may result in possible additive effects which may include hypotension; careful dosage adjustment is indicated when used concurrently).
No products indexed under this heading.

Glutethimide (Co-administration may result in possible additive effects which may include hypotension; careful dosage adjustment is indicated when used concurrently).
No products indexed under this heading.

Glycopyrrolate (Thiothixene possesses weak anticholinergic properties; concurrent use requires caution because of increased atropine-like effect). Products include:
- Robinul Forte Tablets 1358
- Robinul Injectable 2940
- Robinul Tablets 1358

Haloperidol (Co-administration may result in possible additive effects which may include hypotension; careful dosage adjustment is indicated when used concurrently). Products include:
- Haldol Injection, Tablets and Concentrate 2533

Haloperidol Decanoate (Co-administration may result in possible additive effects which may include hypotension; careful dosage adjustment is indicated when used concurrently). Products include:
- Haldol Decanoate 2535

Hydrocodone Bitartrate (Co-administration may result in possible additive effects which may include hypotension; careful dosage adjustment is indicated when used concurrently). Products include:
- Hycodan 1316
- Hycomine Compound Tablets 1317
- Hycotuss Expectorant Syrup 1318
- Lortab 3319
- Lortab Elixir 3317
- Maxidone Tablets CIII 3399
- Norco 5/325 Tablets CIII 3424
- Norco 7.5/325 Tablets CIII 3425
- Norco 10/325 Tablets CIII 3427
- Norco 10/325 Tablets CIII 3425
- Vicodin Tablets 516
- Vicodin ES Tablets 517
- Vicodin HP Tablets 518
- Vicodin Tuss Expectorant 519
- Vicoprofen Tablets 520
- Zydone Tablets 1330

Hydrocodone Polistirex (Co-administration may result in possible additive effects which may include hypotension; careful dosage adjustment is indicated when used concurrently). Products include:
- Tussionex Pennkinetic Extended-Release Suspension 1174

Hydromorphone Hydrochloride (Co-administration may result in possible additive effects which may include hypotension; careful dosage adjustment is indicated when used concurrently). Products include:
- Dilaudid 441
- Dilaudid Oral Liquid 445
- Dilaudid Powder 441
- Dilaudid Rectal Suppositories 441
- Dilaudid Tablets 441
- Dilaudid Tablets - 8 mg 445
- Dilaudid-HP 443

Hydroxyzine Hydrochloride (Co-administration may result in possible additive effects which may include hypotension; careful dosage adjustment is indicated when used concurrently). Products include:
- Atarax Tablets & Syrup 2667
- Vistaril Intramuscular Solution 2738

Hyoscyamine (Thiothixene possesses weak anticholinergic properties; concurrent use requires caution because of increased atropine-like effect). Products include:
- Urised Tablets 2876

Hyoscyamine Sulfate (Thiothixene possesses weak anticholinergic properties; concurrent use requires caution because of increased atropine-like effect). Products include:
- Arco-Lase Plus Tablets 592
- Donnatal 2929
- Donnatal Extentabs 2930
- Levsin/Levsinex/Levbid 3172
- NuLev Orally Disintegrating Tablets 3176
- Prosed/DS Tablets 3268
- Urimax Tablets 1769

Ipratropium Bromide (Thiothixene possesses weak anticholinergic properties; concurrent use requires caution because of increased atropine-like effect). Products include:
- Atrovent Inhalation Aerosol 1030
- Atrovent Inhalation Solution 1031
- Atrovent Nasal Spray 0.03% 1032
- Atrovent Nasal Spray 0.06% 1033
- Combivent Inhalation Aerosol 1041
- DuoNeb Inhalation Solution 1233

Isoflurane (Co-administration may result in possible additive effects which may include hypotension; careful dosage adjustment is indicated when used concurrently).
No products indexed under this heading.

Ketamine Hydrochloride (Co-administration may result in possible additive effects which may include hypotension; careful dosage adjustment is indicated when used concurrently).
No products indexed under this heading.

Levomethadyl Acetate Hydrochloride (Co-administration may result in possible additive effects which may include hypotension; careful dosage adjustment is indicated when used concurrently).
No products indexed under this heading.

Levorphanol Tartrate (Co-administration may result in possible additive effects which may include hypotension; careful dosage adjustment is indicated when used concurrently). Products include:
- Levo-Dromoran 1734
- Levorphanol Tartrate Tablets 3059

Lorazepam (Co-administration may result in possible additive effects which may include hypotension; careful dosage adjustment is indicated when used concurrently). Products include:
- Ativan Injection 3478
- Ativan Tablets 3482

Loxapine Hydrochloride (Co-administration may result in possible additive effects which may include hypotension; careful dosage adjustment is indicated when used concurrently).
No products indexed under this heading.

Loxapine Succinate (Co-administration may result in possible additive effects which may include hypotension; careful dosage adjustment is indicated when used concurrently). Products include:
- Loxitane Capsules 3398

Mepenzolate Bromide (Thiothixene possesses weak anticholinergic properties; concurrent use requires caution because of increased atropine-like effect).
No products indexed under this heading.

Meperidine Hydrochloride (Co-administration may result in possible additive effects which may include hypotension; careful dosage adjustment is indicated when used concurrently). Products include:
- Demerol 3079
- Mepergan Injection 3539

Mephobarbital (Thiothixene potentiates the action of barbiturates, however, the dosage of anticonvulsant barbiturates should not be reduced since thiothixene is capable of precipitating convulsion).
No products indexed under this heading.

Meprobamate (Co-administration may result in possible additive effects which may include hypotension; careful dosage adjustment is indicated when used concurrently). Products include:

Miltown Tablets 3349

Mesoridazine Besylate (Co-administration may result in possible additive effects which may include hypotension; careful dosage adjustment is indicated when used concurrently). Products include:

Serentil 1057

Methadone Hydrochloride (Co-administration may result in possible additive effects which may include hypotension; careful dosage adjustment is indicated when used concurrently). Products include:

Dolophine Hydrochloride Tablets 3056

Methohexital Sodium (Co-administration may result in possible additive effects which may include hypotension; careful dosage adjustment is indicated when used concurrently). Products include:

Brevital Sodium for Injection, USP .. 1815

Methotrimeprazine (Co-administration may result in possible additive effects which may include hypotension; careful dosage adjustment is indicated when used concurrently).

No products indexed under this heading.

Methoxyflurane (Co-administration may result in possible additive effects which may include hypotension; careful dosage adjustment is indicated when used concurrently).

No products indexed under this heading.

Midazolam Hydrochloride (Co-administration may result in possible additive effects which may include hypotension; careful dosage adjustment is indicated when used concurrently). Products include:

Versed Injection 3027
Versed Syrup 3033

Molindone Hydrochloride (Co-administration may result in possible additive effects which may include hypotension; careful dosage adjustment is indicated when used concurrently). Products include:

Moban 1320

Morphine Sulfate (Co-administration may result in possible additive effects which may include hypotension; careful dosage adjustment is indicated when used concurrently). Products include:

Astramorph/PF Injection, USP (Preservative-Free)........................ 594
Duramorph Injection 1312
Infumorph 200 and Infumorph 500 Sterile Solutions............................ 1314
Kadian Capsules 1335
MS Contin Tablets 2896
MSIR 2898
Oramorph SR Tablets 3062
Roxanol 3066

Olanzapine (Co-administration may result in possible additive effects which may include hypotension; careful dosage adjustment is indicated when used concurrently). Products include:

Zyprexa Tablets 1973
Zyprexa ZYDIS Orally Disintegrating Tablets.................. 1973

Oxazepam (Co-administration may result in possible additive effects which may include hypotension; careful dosage adjustment is indicated when used concurrently).

No products indexed under this heading.

Oxybutynin Chloride (Thiothixene possesses weak anticholinergic properties; concurrent use requires caution because of increased atropine-like effect). Products include:

Ditropan XL Extended Release Tablets.. 564

Oxycodone Hydrochloride (Co-administration may result in possible additive effects which may include hypotension; careful dosage adjustment is indicated when used concurrently). Products include:

OxyContin Tablets 2912
OxyFast Oral Concentrate Solution . 2916
OxyIR Capsules 2916
Percocet Tablets 1326
Percodan Tablets 1327
Percolone Tablets 1327
Roxicodone 3067
Tylox Capsules 2597

Pentobarbital Sodium (Co-administration may result in possible additive effects which may include hypotension; careful dosage adjustment is indicated when used concurrently). Products include:

Nembutal Sodium Solution 485

Perphenazine (Co-administration may result in possible additive effects which may include hypotension; careful dosage adjustment is indicated when used concurrently). Products include:

Etrafon 3115
Trilafon 3160

Phenobarbital (Thiothixene potentiates the action of barbiturates, however, the dosage of anticonvulsant barbiturates should not be reduced since thiothixene is capable of precipitating convulsion). Products include:

Arco-Lase Plus Tablets 592
Donnatal 2929
Donnatal Extentabs 2930

Prazepam (Co-administration may result in possible additive effects which may include hypotension; careful dosage adjustment is indicated when used concurrently).

No products indexed under this heading.

Prochlorperazine (Co-administration may result in possible additive effects which may include hypotension; careful dosage adjustment is indicated when used concurrently). Products include:

Compazine 1505

Procyclidine Hydrochloride (Thiothixene possesses weak anticholinergic properties; concurrent use requires caution because of increased atropine-like effect).

No products indexed under this heading.

Promethazine Hydrochloride (Co-administration may result in possible additive effects which may include hypotension; careful dosage adjustment is indicated when used concurrently). Products include:

Mepergan Injection 3539
Phenergan Injection 3553
Phenergan 3556
Phenergan Syrup 3554
Phenergan with Codeine Syrup 3557
Phenergan with Dextromethorphan Syrup 3559
Phenergan VC Syrup 3560
Phenergan VC with Codeine Syrup .. 3561

Propantheline Bromide (Thiothixene possesses weak anticholinergic properties; concurrent use requires caution because of increased atropine-like effect).

No products indexed under this heading.

Propofol (Co-administration may result in possible additive effects which may include hypotension; careful dosage adjustment is indicated when used concurrently). Products include:

Diprivan Injectable Emulsion 667

Propoxyphene Hydrochloride (Co-administration may result in possible additive effects which may include hypotension; careful dosage adjustment is indicated when used concurrently). Products include:

Darvon Pulvules 1909
Darvon Compound-65 Pulvules 1910

Propoxyphene Napsylate (Co-administration may result in possible additive effects which may include hypotension; careful dosage adjustment is indicated when used concurrently). Products include:

Darvon-N/Darvocet-N 1907
Darvon-N Tablets 1912

Quazepam (Co-administration may result in possible additive effects which may include hypotension; careful dosage adjustment is indicated when used concurrently).

No products indexed under this heading.

Quetiapine Fumarate (Co-administration may result in possible additive effects which may include hypotension; careful dosage adjustment is indicated when used concurrently). Products include:

Seroquel Tablets 684

Remifentanil Hydrochloride (Co-administration may result in possible additive effects which may include hypotension; careful dosage adjustment is indicated when used concurrently).

No products indexed under this heading.

Risperidone (Co-administration may result in possible additive effects which may include hypotension; careful dosage adjustment is indicated when used concurrently). Products include:

Risperdal 1796

Scopolamine (Thiothixene possesses weak anticholinergic properties; concurrent use requires caution because of increased atropine-like effect). Products include:

Transderm Scōp Transdermal Therapeutic System.......................... 2302

Scopolamine Hydrobromide (Thiothixene possesses weak anticholinergic properties; concurrent use requires caution because of increased atropine-like effect). Products include:

Donnatal 2929
Donnatal Extentabs 2930

Secobarbital Sodium (Co-administration may result in possible additive effects which may include hypotension; careful dosage adjustment is indicated when used concurrently).

No products indexed under this heading.

Sevoflurane (Co-administration may result in possible additive effects which may include hypotension; careful dosage adjustment is indicated when used concurrently).

No products indexed under this heading.

Sufentanil Citrate (Co-administration may result in possible additive effects which may include hypotension; careful dosage adjustment is indicated when used concurrently).

No products indexed under this heading.

Temazepam (Co-administration may result in possible additive effects which may include hypotension; careful dosage adjustment is indicated when used concurrently).

No products indexed under this heading.

Thiamylal Sodium (Co-administration may result in possible additive effects which may include hypotension; careful dosage adjustment is indicated when used concurrently).

No products indexed under this heading.

Thioridazine Hydrochloride (Co-administration may result in possible additive effects which may include hypotension; careful dosage adjustment is indicated when used concurrently). Products include:

Thioridazine Hydrochloride Tablets 2289

Tolterodine Tartrate (Thiothixene possesses weak anticholinergic properties; concurrent use requires caution because of increased atropine-like effect). Products include:

Detrol Tablets 3623
Detrol LA Capsules 2801

Triazolam (Co-administration may result in possible additive effects which may include hypotension; careful dosage adjustment is indicated when used concurrently). Products include:

Halcion Tablets 2823

Tridihexethyl Chloride (Thiothixene possesses weak anticholinergic properties; concurrent use requires caution because of increased atropine-like effect).

No products indexed under this heading.

Trifluoperazine Hydrochloride (Co-administration may result in possible additive effects which may include hypotension; careful dosage adjustment is indicated when used concurrently). Products include:

Stelazine 1640

Trihexyphenidyl Hydrochloride (Thiothixene possesses weak anticholinergic properties; concurrent use requires caution because of increased atropine-like effect). Products include:

Artane 1855

Zaleplon (Co-administration may result in possible additive effects which may include hypotension; careful dosage adjustment is indicated when used concurrently). Products include:

Sonata Capsules 3591

Ziprasidone Hydrochloride (Co-administration may result in possible additive effects which may include hypotension; careful dosage adjustment is indicated when used concurrently). Products include:

Geodon Capsules 2688

Zolpidem Tartrate (Co-administration may result in possible additive effects which may include hypotension; careful dosage adjustment is indicated when used concurrently). Products include:

Ambien Tablets 3191

Food Interactions

Alcohol (Possible additive effects which may include hypotension).

NAVANE CONCENTRATE

(Thiothixene Hydrochloride) 2701
See Navane Capsules

NAVANE INTRAMUSCULAR

(Thiothixene Hydrochloride) 2703
See Navane Capsules

NAVELBINE INJECTION

(Vinorelbine Tartrate) 1604

May interact with CYP450 3A4 isoenzyme inhibitors (selected) and certain other agents. Compounds in these categories include:

Amiodarone Hydrochloride (Co-administration of vinorelbine with an inhibitor of CYP3A metabolic pathway may cause an earlier onset and/or an increased severity of side effects). Products include:

Cordarone Intravenous 3491
Cordarone Tablets 3487
Pacerone Tablets 3331

Amprenavir (Co-administration of vinorelbine with an inhibitor of CYP3A metabolic pathway may cause an earlier onset and/or an increased severity of side effects). Products include:

Agenerase Capsules 1454
Agenerase Oral Solution 1459

Cimetidine (Co-administration of vinorelbine with an inhibitor of CYP3A

metabolic pathway may cause an earlier onset and/or an increased severity of side effects). Products include:
- Tagamet HB 200 Suspension .... ▣762
- Tagamet HB 200 Tablets .... ▣761
- Tagamet Tablets 1644

Cimetidine Hydrochloride (Co-administration of vinorelbine with an inhibitor of CYP3A metabolic pathway may cause an earlier onset and/or an increased severity of side effects). Products include:
- Tagamet 1644

Cisplatin (Potential for higher incidence of granulocytopenia with vinorelbine used in combination with cisplatin; vestibular and auditory deficits have been observed with combination therapy).
No products indexed under this heading.

Clarithromycin (Co-administration of vinorelbine with an inhibitor of CYP3A metabolic pathway may cause an earlier onset and/or an increased severity of side effects). Products include:
- Biaxin/Biaxin XL 403
- PREVPAC 3298

Erythromycin (Co-administration of vinorelbine with an inhibitor of CYP3A metabolic pathway may cause an earlier onset and/or an increased severity of side effects). Products include:
- Emgel 2% Topical Gel 1285
- Ery-Tab Tablets 448
- Erythromycin Base Filmtab Tablets . 454
- Erythromycin Delayed-Release Capsules, USP 455
- PCE Dispertab Tablets 498

Erythromycin Estolate (Co-administration of vinorelbine with an inhibitor of CYP3A metabolic pathway may cause an earlier onset and/or an increased severity of side effects).
No products indexed under this heading.

Erythromycin Ethylsuccinate (Co-administration of vinorelbine with an inhibitor of CYP3A metabolic pathway may cause an earlier onset and/or an increased severity of side effects). Products include:
- E.E.S. 450
- EryPed 446
- Pediazole Suspension 3050

Erythromycin Gluceptate (Co-administration of vinorelbine with an inhibitor of CYP3A metabolic pathway may cause an earlier onset and/or an increased severity of side effects).
No products indexed under this heading.

Erythromycin Stearate (Co-administration of vinorelbine with an inhibitor of CYP3A metabolic pathway may cause an earlier onset and/or an increased severity of side effects). Products include:
- Erythrocin Stearate Filmtab Tablets 452

Fluconazole (Co-administration of vinorelbine with an inhibitor of CYP3A metabolic pathway may cause an earlier onset and/or an increased severity of side effects). Products include:
- Diflucan Tablets, Injection, and Oral Suspension 2681

Fluvoxamine Maleate (Co-administration of vinorelbine with an inhibitor of CYP3A metabolic pathway may cause an earlier onset and/or an increased severity of side effects). Products include:
- Luvox Tablets (25, 50, 100 mg) 3256

Indinavir Sulfate (Co-administration of vinorelbine with an inhibitor of CYP3A metabolic pathway may cause an earlier onset and/or an increased severity of side effects). Products include:
- Crixivan Capsules 2070

Itraconazole (Co-administration of vinorelbine with an inhibitor of CYP3A metabolic pathway may cause an earlier onset and/or an increased severity of side effects). Products include:
- Sporanox Capsules 1800
- Sporanox Injection 1804
- Sporanox Injection 2509
- Sporanox Oral Solution 1808
- Sporanox Oral Solution 2512

Ketoconazole (Co-administration of vinorelbine with an inhibitor of CYP3A metabolic pathway may cause an earlier onset and/or an increased severity of side effects). Products include:
- Nizoral 2% Cream 3620
- Nizoral A-D Shampoo 2008
- Nizoral 2% Shampoo 2007
- Nizoral Tablets 1791

Mitomycin (Mitomycin-C) (Acute pulmonary reactions have been reported with vinorelbine and other vinca alkaloids used in conjunction with mitomycin).
No products indexed under this heading.

Nefazodone Hydrochloride (Co-administration of vinorelbine with an inhibitor of CYP3A metabolic pathway may cause an earlier onset and/or an increased severity of side effects). Products include:
- Serzone Tablets 1104

Nelfinavir Mesylate (Co-administration of vinorelbine with an inhibitor of CYP3A metabolic pathway may cause an earlier onset and/or an increased severity of side effects). Products include:
- Viracept 532

Paclitaxel (Patients on concomitant and/or sequential administration should be monitored for signs and symptoms of neuropathy). Products include:
- Taxol Injection 1129

Ritonavir (Co-administration of vinorelbine with an inhibitor of CYP3A metabolic pathway may cause an earlier onset and/or an increased severity of side effects). Products include:
- Kaletra Capsules 471
- Kaletra Oral Solution 471
- Norvir Capsules 487
- Norvir Oral Solution 487

Saquinavir (Co-administration of vinorelbine with an inhibitor of CYP3A metabolic pathway may cause an earlier onset and/or an increased severity of side effects). Products include:
- Fortovase Capsules 2970

Saquinavir Mesylate (Co-administration of vinorelbine with an inhibitor of CYP3A metabolic pathway may cause an earlier onset and/or an increased severity of side effects). Products include:
- Invirase Capsules 2979

Troleandomycin (Co-administration of vinorelbine with an inhibitor of CYP3A metabolic pathway may cause an earlier onset and/or an increased severity of side effects). Products include:
- Tao Capsules 2716

NEBCIN VIALS, HYPORETS & ADD-VANTAGE

(Tobramycin Sulfate) 1955

May interact with aminoglycosides, cephalosporins, and certain other agents. Compounds in these categories include:

Amikacin Sulfate (Tobramycin has an inherent potential for causing nephrotoxicity and ototoxicity; concurrent and sequential use should be avoided).
No products indexed under this heading.

Cefaclor (Co-administration has resulted in an increased incidence of nephrotoxicity). Products include:
- Ceclor CD Tablets 1279
- Ceclor 1905

Cefadroxil (Co-administration has resulted in an increased incidence of nephrotoxicity). Products include:
- Duricef 1079

Cefamandole Nafate (Co-administration has resulted in an increased incidence of nephrotoxicity). Products include:
- Mandol Vials 1953

Cefazolin Sodium (Co-administration has resulted in an increased incidence of nephrotoxicity). Products include:
- Ancef for Injection 1474
- Ancef Injection 1474
- Kefzol Vials, ADD-Vantage 1951

Cefdinir (Co-administration has resulted in an increased incidence of nephrotoxicity). Products include:
- Omnicef 493

Cefepime Hydrochloride (Co-administration has resulted in an increased incidence of nephrotoxicity). Products include:
- Maxipime for Injection 1285

Cefixime (Co-administration has resulted in an increased incidence of nephrotoxicity). Products include:
- Suprax 1877

Cefmetazole Sodium (Co-administration has resulted in an increased incidence of nephrotoxicity).
No products indexed under this heading.

Cefonicid Sodium (Co-administration has resulted in an increased incidence of nephrotoxicity).
No products indexed under this heading.

Cefoperazone Sodium (Co-administration has resulted in an increased incidence of nephrotoxicity). Products include:
- Cefobid Pharmacy Bulk Package - Not for Direct Infusion 2673

Ceforanide (Co-administration has resulted in an increased incidence of nephrotoxicity).
No products indexed under this heading.

Cefotaxime Sodium (Co-administration has resulted in an increased incidence of nephrotoxicity). Products include:
- Claforan Injection 732

Cefotetan (Co-administration has resulted in an increased incidence of nephrotoxicity). Products include:
- Cefotan 664

Cefoxitin Sodium (Co-administration has resulted in an increased incidence of nephrotoxicity). Products include:
- Mefoxin for Injection 2124
- Mefoxin Premixed Intravenous Solution 2127

Cefpodoxime Proxetil (Co-administration has resulted in an increased incidence of nephrotoxicity). Products include:
- Vantin Tablets and Oral Suspension 2860

Cefprozil (Co-administration has resulted in an increased incidence of nephrotoxicity). Products include:
- Cefzil 1076

Ceftazidime (Co-administration has resulted in an increased incidence of nephrotoxicity). Products include:
- Ceptaz for Injection 1499
- Fortaz for Injection 1541
- Tazicef for Injection 1647
- Tazicef Pharmacy Bulk Package 1653
- Tazidime Vials, Faspak & ADD-Vantage 1966

Ceftizoxime Sodium (Co-administration has resulted in an increased incidence of nephrotoxicity). Products include:
- Cefizox for Intramuscular or Intravenous Use 1390

Ceftriaxone Sodium (Co-administration has resulted in an increased incidence of nephrotoxicity). Products include:
- Rocephin Injectable Vials, ADD-Vantage, Galaxy, Bulk........... 2993

Cefuroxime Axetil (Co-administration has resulted in an increased incidence of nephrotoxicity). Products include:
- Ceftin 1898

Cefuroxime Sodium (Co-administration has resulted in an increased incidence of nephrotoxicity). Products include:
- Kefurox Vials, ADD-Vantage 1948

Cephalexin (Co-administration has resulted in an increased incidence of nephrotoxicity). Products include:
- Keflex 1237

Cephaloridine (Tobramycin has an inherent potential for causing nephrotoxicity and ototoxicity; concurrent and sequential use should be avoided).

Cephalothin Sodium (Co-administration has resulted in an increased incidence of nephrotoxicity).

Cephapirin Sodium (Co-administration has resulted in an increased incidence of nephrotoxicity).
No products indexed under this heading.

Cephradine (Co-administration has resulted in an increased incidence of nephrotoxicity).
No products indexed under this heading.

Cisplatin (Tobramycin has an inherent potential for causing nephrotoxicity and ototoxicity; concurrent and sequential use should be avoided).
No products indexed under this heading.

Colistin Sulfate (Tobramycin has an inherent potential for causing nephrotoxicity and ototoxicity; concurrent and sequential use should be avoided). Products include:
- Cortisporin-TC Otic Suspension 2246

Ethacrynic Acid (Co-administration should be avoided; ethacrynic acid enhances aminoglycoside toxicity by altering antibiotic concentrations in serum and tissue; increased potential for ototoxicity). Products include:
- Edecrin Tablets 2091

Furosemide (Co-administration should be avoided; furosemide enhances aminoglycoside toxicity by altering antibiotic concentrations in serum and tissue; increased potential for ototoxicity). Products include:
- Furosemide Tablets 2284

Gentamicin Sulfate (Tobramycin has an inherent potential for causing nephrotoxicity and ototoxicity; concurrent and sequential use should be avoided). Products include:
- Genoptic Ophthalmic Ointment ..... ⊙239
- Genoptic Sterile Ophthalmic Solution .... ⊙239
- Pred-G Ophthalmic Suspension ..... ⊙247
- Pred-G Sterile Ophthalmic Ointment .... ⊙248

Kanamycin Sulfate (Tobramycin has an inherent potential for causing nephrotoxicity and ototoxicity; concurrent and sequential use should be avoided).
No products indexed under this heading.

Loracarbef (Co-administration has resulted in an increased incidence of nephrotoxicity). Products include:
- Lorabid Suspension and Pulvules ... 2251

Neomycin Sulfate (Tobramycin has an inherent potential for causing nephrotoxicity and ototoxicity; concurrent and sequential use should be avoided). Products include:
- Cortisporin Ophthalmic Suspension Sterile .... ⊙297
- Cortisporin-TC Otic Suspension 2246
- NeoDecadron Sterile Ophthalmic Solution 2144
- Neosporin G.U. Irrigant Sterile 2256
- Neosporin Ophthalmic Ointment Sterile .... ⊙299
- Neosporin Ophthalmic Solution Sterile .... ⊙300
- Poly-Pred Liquifilm Ophthalmic Suspension .... ⊙245

Paromomycin Sulfate (Tobramycin has an inherent potential for causing nephrotoxicity and ototoxicity; concurrent and sequential use should be avoided).
No products indexed under this heading.

Polymyxin B Sulfate (Tobramycin has an inherent potential for causing nephrotoxicity and ototoxicity; concurrent and sequential use should be avoided). Products include:
- Betadine Brand First Aid Antibiotics & Moisturizer Ointment 2894
- Betadine Brand Plus First Aid Antibiotics & Pain Reliever Ointment 2894
- Cortisporin Ophthalmic Suspension Sterile .... ⊙297
- Neosporin G.U. Irrigant Sterile 2256
- Neosporin Ointment .... ◙704
- Neosporin Ophthalmic Ointment Sterile .... ⊙299
- Neosporin Ophthalmic Solution Sterile .... ⊙300
- Neosporin + Pain Relief Maximum Strength Cream .... ◙704
- Neosporin + Pain Relief Maximum Strength Ointment .... ◙704
- Poly-Pred Liquifilm Ophthalmic Suspension .... ⊙245
- Polysporin Ointment .... ◙706
- Polysporin Ophthalmic Ointment Sterile .... ⊙301
- Polysporin Powder .... ◙706
- Polytrim Ophthalmic Solution 556

Streptomycin Sulfate (Tobramycin has an inherent potential for causing nephrotoxicity and ototoxicity; concurrent and sequential use should be avoided). Products include:
- Streptomycin Sulfate Injection 2714

Tobramycin (Tobramycin has an inherent potential for causing nephrotoxicity and ototoxicity; concurrent and sequential use should be avoided). Products include:
- TOBI Solution for Inhalation 1206
- TobraDex Ophthalmic Ointment 542
- TobraDex Ophthalmic Suspension 541
- Tobrex Ophthalmic Ointment .... ⊙220
- Tobrex Ophthalmic Solution .... ⊙221

Vancomycin Hydrochloride (Tobramycin has an inherent potential for causing nephrotoxicity and ototoxicity; concurrent and sequential use should be avoided). Products include:
- Vancocin HCl Capsules & Pulvules 1972
- Vancocin HCl Oral Solution 1971
- Vancocin HCl, Vials & ADD-Vantage 1970

Viomycin (Tobramycin has an inherent potential for causing nephrotoxicity and ototoxicity; concurrent and sequential use should be avoided).

NECON 0.5/35 TABLETS
(Ethinyl Estradiol, Norethindrone) 3415
See Necon 1/35 Tablets

NECON 1/50 TABLETS
(Mestranol, Norethindrone) 3415
See Necon 1/35 Tablets

NECON 1/35 TABLETS
(Ethinyl Estradiol, Norethindrone) 3415
May interact with barbiturates, phenytoin, tetracyclines, and certain other agents. Compounds in these categories include:

Ampicillin (Potential for reduced efficacy and increased incidence of breakthrough bleeding and menstrual irregularities with concomnitant use).
No products indexed under this heading.

Ampicillin Sodium (Potential for reduced efficacy and increased incidence of breakthrough bleeding and menstrual irregularities with concomnitant use). Products include:
- Unasyn for Injection 2728

Aprobarbital (Potential for reduced efficacy and increased incidence of breakthrough bleeding and menstrual irregularities with concomitant use).
No products indexed under this heading.

Butabarbital (Potential for reduced efficacy and increased incidence of breakthrough bleeding and menstrual irregularities with concomitant use).
No products indexed under this heading.

Butalbital (Potential for reduced efficacy and increased incidence of breakthrough bleeding and menstrual irregularities with concomitant use). Products include:
- Phrenilin 578
- Sedapap Tablets 50 mg/650 mg 2225

Demeclocycline Hydrochloride (Potential for reduced efficacy and increased incidence of breakthrough bleeding and menstrual irregularities with concomitant use). Products include:
- Declomycin Tablets 1855

Doxycycline Calcium (Potential for reduced efficacy and increased incidence of breakthrough bleeding and menstrual irregularities with concomitant use). Products include:
- Vibramycin Calcium Oral Suspension Syrup 2735

Doxycycline Hyclate (Potential for reduced efficacy and increased incidence of breakthrough bleeding and menstrual irregularities with concomitant use). Products include:
- Doryx Coated Pellet Filled Capsules 3357
- Periostat Tablets 1208
- Vibramycin Hyclate Capsules 2735
- Vibramycin Hyclate Intravenous 2737
- Vibra-Tabs Film Coated Tablets 2735

Doxycycline Monohydrate (Potential for reduced efficacy and increased incidence of breakthrough bleeding and menstrual irregularities with concomitant use). Products include:
- Monodox Capsules 2442
- Vibramycin Monohydrate for Oral Suspension 2735

Fosphenytoin Sodium (Potential for reduced efficacy and increased incidence of breakthrough bleeding and menstrual irregularities with concomitant use). Products include:
- Cerebyx Injection 2619

Griseofulvin (Potential for reduced efficacy and increased incidence of breakthrough bleeding and menstrual irregularities with concomnitant use). Products include:
- Grifulvin V Tablets Microsize and Oral Suspension Microsize 2518
- Gris-PEG Tablets 2661

Mephobarbital (Potential for reduced efficacy and increased incidence of breakthrough bleeding and menstrual irregularities with concomitant use).
No products indexed under this heading.

Methacycline Hydrochloride (Potential for reduced efficacy and increased incidence of breakthrough bleeding and menstrual irregularities with concomitant use).
No products indexed under this heading.

Minocycline Hydrochloride (Potential for reduced efficacy and increased incidence of breakthrough bleeding and menstrual irregularities with concomitant use). Products include:
- Dynacin Capsules 2019
- Minocin Intravenous 1862
- Minocin Oral Suspension 1865
- Minocin Pellet-Filled Capsules 1863

Oxytetracycline Hydrochloride (Potential for reduced efficacy and increased incidence of breakthrough bleeding and menstrual irregularities with concomitant use). Products include:
- Terra-Cortril Ophthalmic Suspension 2716
- Urobiotic-250 Capsules 2731

Pentobarbital Sodium (Potential for reduced efficacy and increased incidence of breakthrough bleeding and menstrual irregularities with concomitant use). Products include:
- Nembutal Sodium Solution 485

Phenobarbital (Potential for reduced efficacy and increased incidence of breakthrough bleeding and menstrual irregularities with concomitant use). Products include:
- Arco-Lase Plus Tablets 592
- Donnatal 2929
- Donnatal Extentabs 2930

Phenylbutazone (Potential for reduced efficacy and increased incidence of breakthrough bleeding and menstrual irregularities with concomitant use).
No products indexed under this heading.

Phenytoin (Potential for reduced efficacy and increased incidence of breakthrough bleeding and menstrual irregularities with concomitant use). Products include:
- Dilantin Infatabs 2624
- Dilantin-125 Oral Suspension 2625

Phenytoin Sodium (Potential for reduced efficacy and increased incidence of breakthrough bleeding and menstrual irregularities with concomitant use). Products include:
- Dilantin Kapseals 2622

Rifampin (Co-administration has been associated with reduced efficacy and increased incidence of breakthrough bleeding and menstrual irregularities). Products include:
- Rifadin 765
- Rifamate Capsules 767
- Rifater Tablets 769

Secobarbital Sodium (Potential for reduced efficacy and increased incidence of breakthrough bleeding and menstrual irregularities with concomitant use).
No products indexed under this heading.

Tetracycline Hydrochloride (Potential for reduced efficacy and increased incidence of breakthrough bleeding and menstrual irregularities with concomitant use).
No products indexed under this heading.

Thiamylal Sodium (Potential for reduced efficacy and increased incidence of breakthrough bleeding and menstrual irregularities with concomitant use).
No products indexed under this heading.

NECON 10/11 TABLETS
(Ethinyl Estradiol, Norethindrone) 3415
See Necon 1/35 Tablets

NEMBUTAL SODIUM SOLUTION
(Pentobarbital Sodium) 485
May interact with central nervous system depressants, corticosteroids, oral anticoagulants, doxycycline, estrogens, monoamine oxidase inhibitors, oral contraceptives, phenytoin, and certain other agents. Compounds in these categories include:

Alfentanil Hydrochloride (Concomitant use of other CNS depressants may produce additive depressant effects).
No products indexed under this heading.

Alprazolam (Concomitant use of other CNS depressants may produce additive depressant effects). Products include:
- Xanax Tablets 2865

Aprobarbital (Concomitant use of other CNS depressants may produce additive depressant effects).
No products indexed under this heading.

Betamethasone Acetate (Barbiturates appear to enhance the metabolism of exogenous corticosteroids probably through the induction of hepatic microsomal enzymes). Products include:
- Celestone Soluspan Injectable Suspension 3097

Betamethasone Sodium Phosphate (Barbiturates appear to enhance the metabolism of exogenous corticosteroids probably through the induction of hepatic microsomal enzymes). Products include:
- Celestone Soluspan Injectable Suspension 3097

Buprenorphine Hydrochloride (Concomitant use of other CNS depressants may produce additive depressant effects). Products include:
- Buprenex Injectable 2918

Buspirone Hydrochloride (Concomitant use of other CNS depressants may produce additive depressant effects).
No products indexed under this heading.

Butabarbital (Concomitant use of other CNS depressants may produce additive depressant effects).
No products indexed under this heading.

Butalbital (Concomitant use of other CNS depressants may produce additive depressant effects). Products include:
- Phrenilin 578
- Sedapap Tablets 50 mg/650 mg 2225

Chlordiazepoxide (Concomitant use of other CNS depressants may produce additive depressant effects). Products include:
- Limbitrol 1738

Chlordiazepoxide Hydrochloride (Concomitant use of other CNS depressants may produce additive depressant effects). Products include:
- Librium Capsules 1736
- Librium for Injection 1737

Chlorotrianisene (Pretreatment with or co-administration of phenobarbital may decrease the effect of estrogen by increasing its metabolism; application of this data to other barbiturates appears valid).
No products indexed under this heading.

Chlorpromazine (Concomitant use of other CNS depressants may produce additive depressant effects). Products include:
- Thorazine Suppositories 1656

Chlorpromazine Hydrochloride (Concomitant use of other CNS depressants may produce additive depressant effects). Products include:
- Thorazine 1656

Chlorprothixene (Concomitant use of other CNS depressants may produce additive depressant effects).
No products indexed under this heading.

Chlorprothixene Hydrochloride (Concomitant use of other CNS depressants may produce additive

depressant effects).
No products indexed under this heading.

Chlorprothixene Lactate (Concomitant use of other CNS depressants may produce additive depressant effects).
No products indexed under this heading.

Clorazepate Dipotassium (Concomitant use of other CNS depressants may produce additive depressant effects). Products include:
Tranxene 511

Clozapine (Concomitant use of other CNS depressants may produce additive depressant effects). Products include:
Clozaril Tablets 2319

Codeine Phosphate (Concomitant use of other CNS depressants may produce additive depressant effects). Products include:
Phenergan with Codeine Syrup 3557
Phenergan VC with Codeine Syrup .. 3561
Robitussin A-C Syrup 2942
Robitussin-DAC Syrup 2942
Ryna-C Liquid .... ▣768
Soma Compound w/Codeine Tablets 3355
Tussi-Organidin NR Liquid 3350
Tussi-Organidin-S NR Liquid 3350
Tylenol with Codeine 2595

Cortisone Acetate (Barbiturates appear to enhance the metabolism of exogenous corticosteroids probably through the induction of hepatic microsomal enzymes). Products include:
Cortone Acetate Injectable Suspension 2059
Cortone Acetate Tablets 2061

Desflurane (Concomitant use of other CNS depressants may produce additive depressant effects). Products include:
Suprane Liquid for Inhalation 874

Desogestrel (Pretreatment with or co-administration of phenobarbital may decrease the effect of estrogen by increasing its metabolism; application of this data to other barbiturates appears valid; higher incidence of pregnancy in patients on co-administration). Products include:
Cyclessa Tablets 2450
Desogen Tablets 2458
Mircette Tablets 2470
Ortho-Cept 21 Tablets 2546
Ortho-Cept 28 Tablets 2546

Dexamethasone (Barbiturates appear to enhance the metabolism of exogenous corticosteroids probably through the induction of hepatic microsomal enzymes). Products include:
Decadron Elixir 2078
Decadron Tablets 2079
TobraDex Ophthalmic Ointment 542
TobraDex Ophthalmic Suspension .. 541

Dexamethasone Acetate (Barbiturates appear to enhance the metabolism of exogenous corticosteroids probably through the induction of hepatic microsomal enzymes).
No products indexed under this heading.

Dexamethasone Sodium Phosphate (Barbiturates appear to enhance the metabolism of exogenous corticosteroids probably through the induction of hepatic microsomal enzymes). Products include:
Decadron Phosphate Injection 2081
Decadron Phosphate Sterile Ophthalmic Ointment 2083
Decadron Phosphate Sterile Ophthalmic Solution 2084
NeoDecadron Sterile Ophthalmic Solution 2144

Dezocine (Concomitant use of other CNS depressants may produce additive depressant effects).
No products indexed under this heading.

Diazepam (Concomitant use of other CNS depressants may produce additive depressant effects). Products include:
Valium Injectable 3026
Valium Tablets 3047

Dicumarol (Barbiturates can induce hepatic microsomal enzymes resulting in increased metabolism and decreased anticoagulant response of oral anticoagulants).
No products indexed under this heading.

Dienestrol (Pretreatment with or co-administration of phenobarbital may decrease the effect of estrogen by increasing its metabolism; application of this data to other barbiturates appears valid). Products include:
Ortho Dienestrol Cream 2554

Diethylstilbestrol (Pretreatment with or co-administration of phenobarbital may decrease the effect of estrogen by increasing its metabolism; application of this data to other barbiturates appears valid).
No products indexed under this heading.

Divalproex Sodium (Valproate appears to decrease barbiturate metabolism). Products include:
Depakote Sprinkle Capsules 426
Depakote Tablets 430
Depakote ER Tablets 436

Doxycycline Calcium (Phenobarbital has been shown to shorten the half-life of doxycycline for as long as 2 weeks after barbiturate therapy is discontinued; application of this data to other barbiturates appears valid). Products include:
Vibramycin Calcium Oral Suspension Syrup 2735

Doxycycline Hyclate (Phenobarbital has been shown to shorten the half-life of doxycycline for as long as 2 weeks after barbiturate therapy is discontinued; application of this data to other barbiturates appears valid). Products include:
Doryx Coated Pellet Filled Capsules 3357
Periostat Tablets 1208
Vibramycin Hyclate Capsules 2735
Vibramycin Hyclate Intravenous 2737
Vibra-Tabs Film Coated Tablets 2735

Doxycycline Monohydrate (Phenobarbital has been shown to shorten the half-life of doxycycline for as long as 2 weeks after barbiturate therapy is discontinued; application of this data to other barbiturates appears valid). Products include:
Monodox Capsules 2442
Vibramycin Monohydrate for Oral Suspension 2735

Droperidol (Concomitant use of other CNS depressants may produce additive depressant effects).
No products indexed under this heading.

Enflurane (Concomitant use of other CNS depressants may produce additive depressant effects).
No products indexed under this heading.

Estazolam (Concomitant use of other CNS depressants may produce additive depressant effects). Products include:
ProSom Tablets 500

Estradiol (Pretreatment with or co-administration of phenobarbital may decrease the effect of estrogen by increasing its metabolism; application of this data to other barbiturates appears valid). Products include:
Activella Tablets 2764
Alora Transdermal System 3372
Climara Transdermal System 958
CombiPatch Transdermal System .. 2323
Esclim Transdermal System 3460
Estrace Vaginal Cream 3358
Estrace Tablets 3361
Estring Vaginal Ring 2811
Ortho-Prefest Tablets 2570
Vagifem Tablets 2857
Vivelle Transdermal System 2412
Vivelle-Dot Transdermal System 2416

Estrogens, Conjugated (Pretreatment with or co-administration of phenobarbital may decrease the effect of estrogen by increasing its metabolism; application of this data to other barbiturates appears valid). Products include:
Premarin Intravenous 3563
Premarin Tablets 3566
Premarin Vaginal Cream 3570
Premphase Tablets 3572
Prempro Tablets 3572

Estrogens, Esterified (Pretreatment with or co-administration of phenobarbital may decrease the effect of estrogen by increasing its metabolism; application of this data to other barbiturates appears valid). Products include:
Estratest 3252
Menest Tablets 2254

Estropipate (Pretreatment with or co-administration of phenobarbital may decrease the effect of estrogen by increasing its metabolism; application of this data to other barbiturates appears valid). Products include:
Ogen Tablets 2846
Ortho-Est Tablets 3464

Ethchlorvynol (Concomitant use of other CNS depressants may produce additive depressant effects).
No products indexed under this heading.

Ethinamate (Concomitant use of other CNS depressants may produce additive depressant effects).
No products indexed under this heading.

Ethinyl Estradiol (Pretreatment with or co-administration of phenobarbital may decrease the effect of estrogen by increasing its metabolism; application of this data to other barbiturates appears valid; higher incidence of pregnancy in patients on co-administration). Products include:
Alesse-21 Tablets 3468
Alesse-28 Tablets 3473
Brevicon 28-Day Tablets 3380
Cyclessa Tablets 2450
Desogen Tablets 2458
Estinyl Tablets 3112
Estrostep 2627
femhrt Tablets 2635
Levlen 962
Levlite 21 Tablets 962
Levlite 28 Tablets 962
Levora Tablets 3389
Loestrin 21 Tablets 2642
Loestrin Fe Tablets 2642
Lo/Ovral Tablets 3532
Lo/Ovral-28 Tablets 3538
Low-Ogestrel-28 Tablets 3392
Microgestin Fe 1.5/30 Tablets 3407
Microgestin Fe 1/20 Tablets 3400
Mircette Tablets 2470
Modicon 2563
Necon 3415
Nordette-28 Tablets 2257
Norinyl 1 +35 28-Day Tablets 3380
Ogestrel 0.5/50-28 Tablets 3428
Ortho-Cept 21 Tablets 2546
Ortho-Cept 28 Tablets 2546
Ortho-Cyclen/Ortho Tri-Cyclen 2573
Ortho-Novum 2563
Ovcon 3364
Ovral Tablets 3551
Ovral-28 Tablets 3552
Tri-Levlen 962
Tri-Norinyl-28 Tablets 3433
Triphasil-21 Tablets 3600
Triphasil-28 Tablets 3605
Trivora Tablets 3439
Yasmin 28 Tablets 980
Zovia 3449

Ethynodiol Diacetate (Pretreatment with or co-administration of phenobarbital may decrease the effect of estrogen by increasing its metabolism; application of this data to other barbiturates appears valid; higher incidence of pregnancy in patients on co-administration). Products include:
Zovia 3449

Fentanyl (Concomitant use of other CNS depressants may produce additive depressant effects). Products include:
Duragesic Transdermal System 1786

Fentanyl Citrate (Concomitant use of other CNS depressants may produce additive depressant effects). Products include:
Actiq 1184

Fludrocortisone Acetate (Barbiturates appear to enhance the metabolism of exogenous corticosteroids probably through the induction of hepatic microsomal enzymes). Products include:
Florinef Acetate Tablets 2250

Fluphenazine Decanoate (Concomitant use of other CNS depressants may produce additive depressant effects).
No products indexed under this heading.

Fluphenazine Enanthate (Concomitant use of other CNS depressants may produce additive depressant effects).
No products indexed under this heading.

Fluphenazine Hydrochloride (Concomitant use of other CNS depressants may produce additive depressant effects).
No products indexed under this heading.

Flurazepam Hydrochloride (Concomitant use of other CNS depressants may produce additive depressant effects).
No products indexed under this heading.

Fosphenytoin Sodium (The effect of barbiturates on the metabolism of phenytoin appears to be variable). Products include:
Cerebyx Injection 2619

Furazolidone (Co-administration with MAO inhibitors prolongs the effects of barbiturates probably because the metabolism of the barbiturate is inhibited).
No products indexed under this heading.

Glutethimide (Concomitant use of other CNS depressants may produce additive depressant effects).
No products indexed under this heading.

Griseofulvin (Phenobarbital appears to interfere with the absorption of orally administered griseofulvin, thus decreasing its blood level; application of this data to other barbiturates appears valid). Products include:
Grifulvin V Tablets Microsize and Oral Suspension Microsize 2518
Gris-PEG Tablets 2661

Haloperidol (Concomitant use of other CNS depressants may produce additive depressant effects). Products include:
Haldol Injection, Tablets and Concentrate 2533

Haloperidol Decanoate (Concomitant use of other CNS depressants may produce additive depressant effects). Products include:
Haldol Decanoate 2535

Hydrocodone Bitartrate (Concomitant use of other CNS depressants may produce additive depressant effects). Products include:
Hycodan 1316
Hycomine Compound Tablets 1317
Hycotuss Expectorant Syrup 1318
Lortab 3319
Lortab Elixir 3317
Maxidone Tablets CIII 3399
Norco 5/325 Tablets CIII 3424
Norco 7.5/325 Tablets CIII 3425

Norco 10/325 Tablets CIII 3427
Norco 10/325 Tablets CIII 3425
Vicodin Tablets 516
Vicodin ES Tablets 517
Vicodin HP Tablets 518
Vicodin Tuss Expectorant 519
Vicoprofen Tablets 520
Zydone Tablets 1330

Hydrocodone Polistirex (Concomitant use of other CNS depressants may produce additive depressant effects). Products include:
Tussionex Pennkinetic Extended-Release Suspension 1174

Hydrocortisone (Barbiturates appear to enhance the metabolism of exogenous corticosteroids probably through the induction of hepatic microsomal enzymes). Products include:
Anusol-HC Cream 2.5% 2237
Cipro HC Otic Suspension 540
Cortaid Intensive Therapy Cream 717
Cortaid Maximum Strength Cream 717
Cortisporin Ophthalmic Suspension Sterile ⊙297
Cortizone•5 699
Cortizone•10 699
Cortizone•10 Plus Creme 700
Cortizone for Kids Creme 699
Hydrocortone Tablets 2106
Massengill Medicated Soft Cloth Towelette 753
VōSoL HC Otic Solution 3356

Hydrocortisone Acetate (Barbiturates appear to enhance the metabolism of exogenous corticosteroids probably through the induction of hepatic microsomal enzymes). Products include:
Analpram-HC 1338
Anusol HC-1 Hydrocortisone Anti-Itch Cream 689
Anusol-HC Suppositories 2238
Cortaid 717
Cortifoam Rectal Foam 3170
Cortisporin-TC Otic Suspension 2246
Hydrocortone Acetate Injectable Suspension 2103
Pramosone 1343
Proctocort Suppositories 2264
ProctoFoam-HC 3177
Terra-Cortril Ophthalmic Suspension 2716

Hydrocortisone Sodium Phosphate (Barbiturates appear to enhance the metabolism of exogenous corticosteroids probably through the induction of hepatic microsomal enzymes). Products include:
Hydrocortone Phosphate Injection, Sterile 2105

Hydrocortisone Sodium Succinate (Barbiturates appear to enhance the metabolism of exogenous corticosteroids probably through the induction of hepatic microsomal enzymes).
No products indexed under this heading.

Hydromorphone Hydrochloride (Concomitant use of other CNS depressants may produce additive depressant effects). Products include:
Dilaudid 441
Dilaudid Oral Liquid 445
Dilaudid Powder 441
Dilaudid Rectal Suppositories 441
Dilaudid Tablets 441
Dilaudid Tablets - 8 mg 445
Dilaudid-HP 443

Hydroxyzine Hydrochloride (Concomitant use of other CNS depressants may produce additive depressant effects). Products include:
Atarax Tablets & Syrup 2667
Vistaril Intramuscular Solution 2738

Isocarboxazid (Co-administration with MAO inhibitors prolongs the effects of barbiturates probably because the metabolism of the barbiturate is inhibited).
No products indexed under this heading.

Isoflurane (Concomitant use of other CNS depressants may produce additive depressant effects).
No products indexed under this heading.

Ketamine Hydrochloride (Concomitant use of other CNS depressants may produce additive depressant effects).
No products indexed under this heading.

Levomethadyl Acetate Hydrochloride (Concomitant use of other CNS depressants may produce additive depressant effects).
No products indexed under this heading.

Levonorgestrel (Pretreatment with or co-administration of phenobarbital may decrease the effect of estrogen by increasing its metabolism; application of this data to other barbiturates appears valid; higher incidence of pregnancy in patients on co-administration). Products include:
Alesse-21 Tablets 3468
Alesse-28 Tablets 3473
Levlen 962
Levlite 21 Tablets 962
Levlite 28 Tablets 962
Levora Tablets 3389
Mirena Intrauterine System 974
Nordette-28 Tablets 2257
Norplant System 3543
Tri-Levlen 962
Triphasil-21 Tablets 3600
Triphasil-28 Tablets 3605
Trivora Tablets 3439

Levorphanol Tartrate (Concomitant use of other CNS depressants may produce additive depressant effects). Products include:
Levo-Dromoran 1734
Levorphanol Tartrate Tablets 3059

Lorazepam (Concomitant use of other CNS depressants may produce additive depressant effects). Products include:
Ativan Injection 3478
Ativan Tablets 3482

Loxapine Hydrochloride (Concomitant use of other CNS depressants may produce additive depressant effects).
No products indexed under this heading.

Loxapine Succinate (Concomitant use of other CNS depressants may produce additive depressant effects). Products include:
Loxitane Capsules 3398

Meperidine Hydrochloride (Concomitant use of other CNS depressants may produce additive depressant effects). Products include:
Demerol 3079
Mepergan Injection 3539

Mephobarbital (Concomitant use of other CNS depressants may produce additive depressant effects).
No products indexed under this heading.

Meprobamate (Concomitant use of other CNS depressants may produce additive depressant effects). Products include:
Miltown Tablets 3349

Mesoridazine Besylate (Concomitant use of other CNS depressants may produce additive depressant effects). Products include:
Serentil 1057

Mestranol (Pretreatment with or co-administration of phenobarbital may decrease the effect of estrogen by increasing its metabolism; application of this data to other barbiturates appears valid; higher incidence of pregnancy in patients on co-administration). Products include:
Necon 1/50 Tablets 3415
Norinyl 1 + 50 28-Day Tablets 3380
Ortho-Novum 1/50□28 Tablets 2556

Methadone Hydrochloride (Concomitant use of other CNS depressants may produce additive depressant effects). Products include:
Dolophine Hydrochloride Tablets 3056

Methohexital Sodium (Concomitant use of other CNS depressants may produce additive depressant effects). Products include:
Brevital Sodium for Injection, USP 1815

Methotrimeprazine (Concomitant use of other CNS depressants may produce additive depressant effects).
No products indexed under this heading.

Methoxyflurane (Concomitant use of other CNS depressants may produce additive depressant effects).
No products indexed under this heading.

Methylprednisolone Acetate (Barbiturates appear to enhance the metabolism of exogenous corticosteroids probably through the induction of hepatic microsomal enzymes). Products include:
Depo-Medrol Injectable Suspension 2795

Methylprednisolone Sodium Succinate (Barbiturates appear to enhance the metabolism of exogenous corticosteroids probably through the induction of hepatic microsomal enzymes). Products include:
Solu-Medrol Sterile Powder 2855

Midazolam Hydrochloride (Concomitant use of other CNS depressants may produce additive depressant effects). Products include:
Versed Injection 3027
Versed Syrup 3033

Moclobemide (Co-administration with MAO inhibitors prolongs the effects of barbiturates probably because the metabolism of the barbiturate is inhibited).
No products indexed under this heading.

Molindone Hydrochloride (Concomitant use of other CNS depressants may produce additive depressant effects). Products include:
Moban 1320

Morphine Sulfate (Concomitant use of other CNS depressants may produce additive depressant effects). Products include:
Astramorph/PF Injection, USP (Preservative-Free) 594
Duramorph Injection 1312
Infumorph 200 and Infumorph 500 Sterile Solutions 1314
Kadian Capsules 1335
MS Contin Tablets 2896
MSIR 2898
Oramorph SR Tablets 3062
Roxanol 3066

Norethindrone (Pretreatment with or co-administration of phenobarbital may decrease the effect of estrogen by increasing its metabolism; application of this data to other barbiturates appears valid; higher incidence of pregnancy in patients on co-administration). Products include:
Brevicon 28-Day Tablets 3380
Micronor Tablets 2543
Modicon 2563
Necon 3415
Norinyl 1 +35 28-Day Tablets 3380
Norinyl 1 + 50 28-Day Tablets 3380
Nor-QD Tablets 3423
Ortho-Novum 2563
Ortho-Novum 1/50□28 Tablets 2556
Ovcon 3364
Tri-Norinyl-28 Tablets 3433

Norethynodrel (Pretreatment with or co-administration of phenobarbital may decrease the effect of estrogen by increasing its metabolism; application of this data to other barbiturates appears valid; higher incidence of pregnancy in patients on co-administration).
No products indexed under this heading.

Norgestimate (Pretreatment with or co-administration of phenobarbital may decrease the effect of estrogen by increasing its metabolism; application of this data to other barbiturates appears valid; higher incidence of pregnancy in patients on co-administration). Products include:
Ortho-Cyclen/Ortho Tri-Cyclen 2573
Ortho-Prefest Tablets 2570

Norgestrel (Pretreatment with or co-administration of phenobarbital may decrease the effect of estrogen by increasing its metabolism; application of this data to other barbiturates appears valid; higher incidence of pregnancy in patients on co-administration). Products include:
Lo/Ovral Tablets 3532
Lo/Ovral-28 Tablets 3538
Low-Ogestrel-28 Tablets 3392
Ogestrel 0.5/50-28 Tablets 3428
Ovral Tablets 3551
Ovral-28 Tablets 3552
Ovrette Tablets 3552

Olanzapine (Concomitant use of other CNS depressants may produce additive depressant effects). Products include:
Zyprexa Tablets 1973
Zyprexa ZYDIS Orally Disintegrating Tablets 1973

Oxazepam (Concomitant use of other CNS depressants may produce additive depressant effects).
No products indexed under this heading.

Oxycodone Hydrochloride (Concomitant use of other CNS depressants may produce additive depressant effects). Products include:
OxyContin Tablets 2912
OxyFast Oral Concentrate Solution 2916
OxyIR Capsules 2916
Percocet Tablets 1326
Percodan Tablets 1327
Percolone Tablets 1327
Roxicodone 3067
Tylox Capsules 2597

Pargyline Hydrochloride (Co-administration with MAO inhibitors prolongs the effects of barbiturates probably because the metabolism of the barbiturate is inhibited).
No products indexed under this heading.

Perphenazine (Concomitant use of other CNS depressants may produce additive depressant effects). Products include:
Etrafon 3115
Trilafon 3160

Phenelzine Sulfate (Co-administration with MAO inhibitors prolongs the effects of barbiturates probably because the metabolism of the barbiturate is inhibited). Products include:
Nardil Tablets 2653

Phenobarbital (Concomitant use of other CNS depressants may produce additive depressant effects). Products include:
Arco-Lase Plus Tablets 592
Donnatal 2929
Donnatal Extentabs 2930

Phenytoin (The effect of barbiturates on the metabolism of phenytoin appears to be variable). Products include:
Dilantin Infatabs 2624
Dilantin-125 Oral Suspension 2625

Phenytoin Sodium (The effect of barbiturates on the metabolism of phenytoin appears to be variable). Products include:
Dilantin Kapseals 2622

Polyestradiol Phosphate (Pretreatment with or co-administration of phenobarbital may decrease the effect of estrogen by increasing its metabolism; application of this data to other barbiturates appears valid).
No products indexed under this heading.

Prazepam (Concomitant use of other CNS depressants may pro-

IMPORTANT NOTE: Always consult each drug listing in the patient's regimen for possible interactions.

duce additive depressant effects).
No products indexed under this heading.

Prednisolone Acetate (Barbiturates appear to enhance the metabolism of exogenous corticosteroids probably through the induction of hepatic microsomal enzymes).
Products include:
- Blephamide Ophthalmic Ointment.... **547**
- Blephamide Ophthalmic Suspension.... **548**
- Poly-Pred Liquifilm Ophthalmic Suspension.... ⊙**245**
- Pred Forte Ophthalmic Suspension.... ⊙**246**
- Pred Mild Sterile Ophthalmic Suspension.... ⊙**249**
- Pred-G Ophthalmic Suspension.... ⊙**247**
- Pred-G Sterile Ophthalmic Ointment.... ⊙**248**

Prednisolone Sodium Phosphate (Barbiturates appear to enhance the metabolism of exogenous corticosteroids probably through the induction of hepatic microsomal enzymes). Products include:
- Pediapred Oral Solution.... **1170**

Prednisolone Tebutate (Barbiturates appear to enhance the metabolism of exogenous corticosteroids probably through the induction of hepatic microsomal enzymes).
No products indexed under this heading.

Prednisone (Barbiturates appear to enhance the metabolism of exogenous corticosteroids probably through the induction of hepatic microsomal enzymes). Products include:
- Prednisone.... **3064**

Procarbazine Hydrochloride (Co-administration with MAO inhibitors prolongs the effects of barbiturates probably because the metabolism of the barbiturate is inhibited). Products include:
- Matulane Capsules.... **3246**

Prochlorperazine (Concomitant use of other CNS depressants may produce additive depressant effects). Products include:
- Compazine.... **1505**

Promethazine Hydrochloride (Concomitant use of other CNS depressants may produce additive depressant effects). Products include:
- Mepergan Injection.... **3539**
- Phenergan Injection.... **3553**
- Phenergan.... **3556**
- Phenergan Syrup.... **3554**
- Phenergan with Codeine Syrup.... **3557**
- Phenergan with Dextromethorphan Syrup.... **3559**
- Phenergan VC Syrup.... **3560**
- Phenergan VC with Codeine Syrup.. **3561**

Propofol (Concomitant use of other CNS depressants may produce additive depressant effects). Products include:
- Diprivan Injectable Emulsion.... **667**

Propoxyphene Hydrochloride (Concomitant use of other CNS depressants may produce additive depressant effects). Products include:
- Darvon Pulvules.... **1909**
- Darvon Compound-65 Pulvules.... **1910**

Propoxyphene Napsylate (Concomitant use of other CNS depressants may produce additive depressant effects). Products include:
- Darvon-N/Darvocet-N.... **1907**
- Darvon-N Tablets.... **1912**

Quazepam (Concomitant use of other CNS depressants may produce additive depressant effects).
No products indexed under this heading.

Quetiapine Fumarate (Concomitant use of other CNS depressants may produce additive depressant effects). Products include:
- Seroquel Tablets.... **684**

Quinestrol (Pretreatment with or co-administration of phenobarbital may decrease the effect of estrogen by increasing its metabolism; application of this data to other barbiturates appears valid).
No products indexed under this heading.

Remifentanil Hydrochloride (Concomitant use of other CNS depressants may produce additive depressant effects).
No products indexed under this heading.

Risperidone (Concomitant use of other CNS depressants may produce additive depressant effects). Products include:
- Risperdal.... **1796**

Secobarbital Sodium (Concomitant use of other CNS depressants may produce additive depressant effects).
No products indexed under this heading.

Selegiline Hydrochloride (Co-administration with MAO inhibitors prolongs the effects of barbiturates probably because the metabolism of the barbiturate is inhibited). Products include:
- Eldepryl Capsules.... **3266**

Sevoflurane (Concomitant use of other CNS depressants may produce additive depressant effects).
No products indexed under this heading.

Sufentanil Citrate (Concomitant use of other CNS depressants may produce additive depressant effects).
No products indexed under this heading.

Temazepam (Concomitant use of other CNS depressants may produce additive depressant effects).
No products indexed under this heading.

Thiamylal Sodium (Concomitant use of other CNS depressants may produce additive depressant effects).
No products indexed under this heading.

Thioridazine Hydrochloride (Concomitant use of other CNS depressants may produce additive depressant effects). Products include:
- Thioridazine Hydrochloride Tablets.... **2289**

Thiothixene (Concomitant use of other CNS depressants may produce additive depressant effects). Products include:
- Navane Capsules.... **2701**
- Thiothixene Capsules.... **2290**

Tranylcypromine Sulfate (Co-administration with MAO inhibitors prolongs the effects of barbiturates probably because the metabolism of the barbiturate is inhibited). Products include:
- Parnate Tablets.... **1607**

Triamcinolone (Barbiturates appear to enhance the metabolism of exogenous corticosteroids probably through the induction of hepatic microsomal enzymes).
No products indexed under this heading.

Triamcinolone Acetonide (Barbiturates appear to enhance the metabolism of exogenous corticosteroids probably through the induction of hepatic microsomal enzymes). Products include:
- Azmacort Inhalation Aerosol.... **728**
- Nasacort Nasal Inhaler.... **750**
- Nasacort AQ Nasal Spray.... **752**
- Tri-Nasal Spray.... **2274**

Triamcinolone Diacetate (Barbiturates appear to enhance the metabolism of exogenous corticosteroids probably through the induction of hepatic microsomal enzymes).
No products indexed under this heading.

Triamcinolone Hexacetonide (Barbiturates appear to enhance the metabolism of exogenous corticosteroids probably through the induction of hepatic microsomal enzymes).
No products indexed under this heading.

Triazolam (Concomitant use of other CNS depressants may produce additive depressant effects). Products include:
- Halcion Tablets.... **2823**

Trifluoperazine Hydrochloride (Concomitant use of other CNS depressants may produce additive depressant effects). Products include:
- Stelazine.... **1640**

Valproate Sodium (Valproate appears to decrease barbiturate metabolism). Products include:
- Depacon Injection.... **416**

Valproic Acid (Appears to decrease barbiturate metabolism). Products include:
- Depakene.... **421**

Warfarin Sodium (Barbiturates can induce hepatic microsomal enzymes resulting in increased metabolism and decreased anticoagulant response of oral anticoagulants). Products include:
- Coumadin for Injection.... **1243**
- Coumadin Tablets.... **1243**
- Warfarin Sodium Tablets, USP.... **3302**

Zaleplon (Concomitant use of other CNS depressants may produce additive depressant effects). Products include:
- Sonata Capsules.... **3591**

Ziprasidone Hydrochloride (Concomitant use of other CNS depressants may produce additive depressant effects). Products include:
- Geodon Capsules.... **2688**

Zolpidem Tartrate (Concomitant use of other CNS depressants may produce additive depressant effects). Products include:
- Ambien Tablets.... **3191**

Food Interactions

Alcohol (Concomitant use of other CNS depressants may produce additive depressant effects).

NEODECADRON STERILE OPHTHALMIC SOLUTION

(Dexamethasone Sodium Phosphate, Neomycin Sulfate).... **2144**
None cited in PDR database.

NEORAL SOFT GELATIN CAPSULES

(Cyclosporine).... **2380**
May interact with erythromycin, nonsteroidal anti-inflammatory agents, protease inhibitors, potassium sparing diuretics, and certain other agents. Compounds in these categories include:

Allopurinol (Increases cyclosporine concentrations).
No products indexed under this heading.

Amiloride Hydrochloride (Cyclosporine may cause hyperkalemia; concurrent use should be avoided). Products include:
- Midamor Tablets.... **2136**
- Moduretic Tablets.... **2138**

Amiodarone Hydrochloride (Increases cyclosporine concentrations). Products include:
- Cordarone Intravenous.... **3491**
- Cordarone Tablets.... **3487**
- Pacerone Tablets.... **3331**

Amphotericin B (May potentiate renal dysfunction). Products include:
- Abelcet Injection.... **1273**
- AmBisome for Injection.... **1383**
- Amphotec.... **1774**

Amprenavir (The HIV protease inhibitors are known to inhibit cytochrome P450IIIA and increase the concentration of drugs metabolized by this enzyme system; agents that inhibit this enzyme could decrease metabolism and increase cyclosporine concentrations; this interaction has not been studied, however, care should be exercised). Products include:
- Agenerase Capsules.... **1454**
- Agenerase Oral Solution.... **1459**

Azapropazon (May potentiate renal dysfunction).

Azathioprine (May potentiate renal dysfunction).
No products indexed under this heading.

Bromocriptine Mesylate (Increases cyclosporine concentrations).
No products indexed under this heading.

Carbamazepine (Decreases cyclosporine concentrations). Products include:
- Carbatrol Capsules.... **3234**
- Tegretol/Tegretol-XR.... **2404**

Celecoxib (Co-administration with NSAID's particularly in the setting of dehydration, may potentiate renal dysfunction). Products include:
- Celebrex Capsules.... **2676**
- Celebrex Capsules.... **2780**

Cimetidine (May potentiate renal dysfunction). Products include:
- Tagamet HB 200 Suspension.... ▣**762**
- Tagamet HB 200 Tablets.... ▣**761**
- Tagamet Tablets.... **1644**

Cimetidine Hydrochloride (May potentiate renal dysfunction). Products include:
- Tagamet.... **1644**

Clarithromycin (Increases cyclosporine concentrations). Products include:
- Biaxin/Biaxin XL.... **403**
- PREVPAC.... **3298**

Colchicine (Co-administration results in increased cyclosporine concentrations and potentiation of renal dysfunction).
No products indexed under this heading.

Dalfopristin (Co-administration with substrate that inhibit CYP450 3A such as dalfopristin, could decrease metabolism and increase cyclosporine concentrations). Products include:
- Synercid I.V.... **775**

Danazol (Increases cyclosporine concentrations).
No products indexed under this heading.

Diclofenac Potassium (Co-administration has been associated with approximate doubling of diclofenac blood levels and occasional reports of reversible decreases in renal function; possible potentiation of renal dysfunction; the dose of diclofenac should be in the lower end of the therapeutic range). Products include:
- Cataflam Tablets.... **2315**

Diclofenac Sodium (Co-administration has been associated with approximate doubling of diclofenac blood levels and occasional reports of reversible decreases in renal function; possible potentiation of renal dysfunction; the dose of diclofenac should be in the lower end of the therapeutic range). Products include:
- Arthrotec Tablets.... **3195**
- Voltaren Ophthalmic Sterile Ophthalmic Solution.... ⊙**312**
- Voltaren Tablets.... **2315**
- Voltaren-XR Tablets.... **2315**

Digoxin (Reduced clearance of digoxin; decrease in the apparent volume of distribution of digoxin; severe digoxin toxicity can occur). Products include:
- Digitek Tablets 1003
- Lanoxicaps Capsules 1574
- Lanoxin Injection 1581
- Lanoxin Tablets 1587
- Lanoxin Elixir Pediatric 1578
- Lanoxin Injection Pediatric 1584

Diltiazem Hydrochloride (Increases cyclosporine concentrations). Products include:
- Cardizem Injectable 1018
- Cardizem Lyo-Ject Syringe 1018
- Cardizem Monovial 1018
- Cardizem CD Capsules 1016
- Tiazac Capsules 1378

Erythromycin (Co-administration with substrate that inhibit CYP450 3A, such as erythromycin, could decrease metabolism and increase cyclosporine concentrations). Products include:
- Emgel 2% Topical Gel 1285
- Ery-Tab Tablets 448
- Erythromycin Base Filmtab Tablets . 454
- Erythromycin Delayed-Release Capsules, USP 455
- PCE Dispertab Tablets 498

Erythromycin Estolate (Co-administration with substrate that inhibit CYP450 3A, such as erythromycin, could decrease metabolism and increase cyclosporine concentrations).
No products indexed under this heading.

Erythromycin Ethylsuccinate (Co-administration with substrate that inhibit CYP450 3A, such as erythromycin, could decrease metabolism and increase cyclosporine concentrations). Products include:
- E.E.S. 450
- EryPed 446
- Pediazole Suspension 3050

Erythromycin Gluceptate (Co-administration with substrate that inhibit CYP450 3A, such as erythromycin, could decrease metabolism and increase cyclosporine concentrations).
No products indexed under this heading.

Erythromycin Stearate (Co-administration with substrate that inhibit CYP450 3A, such as erythromycin, could decrease metabolism and increase cyclosporine concentrations). Products include:
- Erythrocin Stearate Filmtab Tablets 452

Etodolac (Co-administration with NSAID's particularly in the setting of dehydration, may potentiate renal dysfunction). Products include:
- Lodine 3528
- Lodine XL Extended-Release Tablets 3530

Fenoprofen Calcium (Co-administration with NSAID's particularly in the setting of dehydration, may potentiate renal dysfunction).
No products indexed under this heading.

Fluconazole (Increases cyclosporine concentrations). Products include:
- Diflucan Tablets, Injection, and Oral Suspension 2681

Flurbiprofen (Co-administration with NSAID's particularly in the setting of dehydration, may potentiate renal dysfunction).
No products indexed under this heading.

Gentamicin Sulfate (May potentiate renal dysfunction). Products include:
- Genoptic Ophthalmic Ointment .... ⊙239
- Genoptic Sterile Ophthalmic Solution .... ⊙239
- Pred-G Ophthalmic Suspension .... ⊙247
- Pred-G Sterile Ophthalmic Ointment .... ⊙248

Hypericum (Co-administration has been reported to produce a marked reduction in blood cyclosporine concentrations, resulting in subtherapeutic levels, rejection of transplanted organs, and graft loss). Products include:
- Brite-Life Caplets .... ▣795
- Centrum St. John's Wort Softgels . ▣853
- Metabolic Nutrition System .... ▣798
- Movana Tablets .... ▣832
- One-A-Day Tension & Mood Softgels .... ▣808
- ReSource Wellness StayCalm Caplets .... ▣826
- Satiete Tablets .... ▣846

Ibuprofen (Co-administration with NSAID's particularly in the setting of dehydration, may potentiate renal dysfunction). Products include:
- Advil .... ▣771
- Children's Advil Oral Suspension ... ▣773
- Children's Advil Chewable Tablets . ▣773
- Advil Cold and Sinus Caplets .... ▣771
- Advil Cold and Sinus Tablets .... ▣771
- Advil Flu & Body Ache Caplets .... ▣772
- Infants' Advil Drops .... ▣773
- Junior Strength Advil Tablets .... ▣773
- Junior Strength Advil Chewable Tablets .... ▣773
- Advil Migraine Liquigels .... ▣772
- Children's Motrin Oral Suspension and Chewable Tablets 2006
- Children's Motrin Cold Oral Suspension 2007
- Children's Motrin Oral Suspension .... ▣643
- Motrin Suspension, Oral Drops, Chewable Tablets, and Caplets 2002
- Infants' Motrin Concentrated Drops 2006
- Junior Strength Motrin Caplets and Chewable Tablets 2006
- Motrin IB Tablets, Caplets, and Gelcaps 2002
- Motrin Migraine Pain Caplets 2005
- Motrin Sinus Headache Caplets 2005
- Vicoprofen Tablets 520

Indinavir Sulfate (The HIV protease inhibitors are known to inhibit cytochrome P450IIIA and increase the concentration of drugs metabolized by this enzyme system; agents that inhibit this enzyme could decrease metabolism and increase cyclosporine concentrations; this interaction has not been studied, however, care should be exercised). Products include:
- Crixivan Capsules 2070

Indomethacin (Co-administration with NSAID's particularly in the setting of dehydration, may potentiate renal dysfunction). Products include:
- Indocin 2112

Indomethacin Sodium Trihydrate (Co-administration with NSAID's particularly in the setting of dehydration, may potentiate renal dysfunction). Products include:
- Indocin I.V. 2115

Itraconazole (Increases cyclosporine concentrations). Products include:
- Sporanox Capsules 1800
- Sporanox Injection 1804
- Sporanox Injection 2509
- Sporanox Oral Solution 1808
- Sporanox Oral Solution 2512

Ketoconazole (May potentiate renal dysfunction; co-administration with substrate that inhibit CYP450 3A, such as ketoconazole, could decrease metabolism and increase cyclosporine concentrations). Products include:
- Nizoral 2% Cream 3620
- Nizoral A-D Shampoo 2008
- Nizoral 2% Shampoo 2007
- Nizoral Tablets 1791

Ketoprofen (Co-administration with NSAID's particularly in the setting of dehydration, may potentiate renal dysfunction). Products include:
- Orudis Capsules 3548
- Orudis KT Tablets .... ▣778
- Oruvail Capsules 3548

Ketorolac Tromethamine (Co-administration with NSAID's particularly in the setting of dehydration, may potentiate renal dysfunction). Products include:
- Acular Ophthalmic Solution 544
- Acular PF Ophthalmic Solution 544
- Toradol 3018

Lopinavir (The HIV protease inhibitors are known to inhibit cytochrome P450IIIA and increase the concentration of drugs metabolized by this enzyme system; agents that inhibit this enzyme could decrease metabolism and increase cyclosporine concentrations; this interaction has not been studied, however, care should be exercised). Products include:
- Kaletra Capsules 471
- Kaletra Oral Solution 471

Lovastatin (Reduced clearance of lovastatin; potential for mycositis). Products include:
- Mevacor Tablets 2132

Meclofenamate Sodium (Co-administration with NSAID's particularly in the setting of dehydration, may potentiate renal dysfunction).
No products indexed under this heading.

Mefenamic Acid (Co-administration with NSAID's particularly in the setting of dehydration, may potentiate renal dysfunction). Products include:
- Ponstel Capsules 1356

Meloxicam (Co-administration with NSAID's particularly in the setting of dehydration, may potentiate renal dysfunction). Products include:
- Mobic Tablets 1054

Melphalan (May potentiate renal dysfunction). Products include:
- Alkeran Tablets 1466

Methotrexate Sodium (Increased risk of developing skin malignancies in psoriasis patients with concurrent use; in rheumatoid arthritis patients, methotrexate concentrations (AUCs) were increased approximately 30% and concentrations (AUCs) were increased approximately 80%; the clinical significance is unknown).
No products indexed under this heading.

Metoclopramide Hydrochloride (Increases cyclosporine concentrations). Products include:
- Reglan 2935

Muromonab-CD3 (Psoriasis patients receiving other immunosuppressive agents, such as muromonab-CD3, should not receive concurrent cyclosporine because of the possibility of excessive immunosuppression). Products include:
- Orthoclone OKT3 Sterile Solution ... 2498

Mycophenolate Mofetil (Psoriasis patients receiving other immunosuppressive agents, such as mycophenolate mofetil, should not receive concurrent cyclosporine because of the possibility of excessive immunosuppression). Products include:
- CellCept Capsules 2951
- CellCept Oral Suspension 2951
- CellCept Tablets 2951

Nabumetone (Co-administration with NSAID's particularly in the setting of dehydration, may potentiate renal dysfunction). Products include:
- Relafen Tablets 1617

Nafcillin Sodium (Decreases cyclosporine concentrations).
No products indexed under this heading.

Naproxen (Concomitant use is associated with additive decreases in renal function with possible potentiation of renal dysfunction). Products include:
- EC-Naprosyn Delayed-Release Tablets 2967
- Naprosyn Suspension 2967
- Naprosyn Tablets 2967

Naproxen Sodium (Concomitant use is associated with additive decreases in renal function with possible potentiation of renal dysfunction). Products include:
- Aleve Tablets, Caplets and Gelcaps .... ▣602
- Aleve Cold & Sinus Caplets .... ▣603
- Anaprox Tablets 2967
- Anaprox DS Tablets 2967
- Naprelan Tablets 1293

Nelfinavir Mesylate (The HIV protease inhibitors are known to inhibit cytochrome P450IIIA and increase the concentration of drugs metabolized by this enzyme system; agents that inhibit this enzyme could decrease metabolism and increase cyclosporine concentrations; this interaction has not been studied, however, care should be exercised). Products include:
- Viracept 532

Nephrotoxic Drugs (Potential for increased nephrotoxicity; careful monitoring of renal function is required).

Nicardipine Hydrochloride (Increases cyclosporine concentrations). Products include:
- Cardene I.V. 3485

Nifedipine (Potential for frequent gingival hyperplasia). Products include:
- Adalat CC Tablets 877
- Procardia Capsules 2708
- Procardia XL Extended Release Tablets 2710

Octreotide Acetate (Decreases cyclosporine concentrations). Products include:
- Sandostatin LAR Depot 2395

Orlistat (Co-administration can result in decreased absorption of cyclosporine; concomitant use should be avoided). Products include:
- Xenical Capsules 3043

Oxaprozin (Co-administration with NSAID's particularly in the setting of dehydration, may potentiate renal dysfunction).
No products indexed under this heading.

Phenobarbital (Decreases cyclosporine concentrations). Products include:
- Arco-Lase Plus Tablets 592
- Donnatal 2929
- Donnatal Extentabs 2930

Phenylbutazone (Co-administration with NSAID's particularly in the setting of dehydration, may potentiate renal dysfunction).
No products indexed under this heading.

Piroxicam (Co-administration with NSAID's particularly in the setting of dehydration, may potentiate renal dysfunction). Products include:
- Feldene Capsules 2685

Quinupristin (Co-administration with substrate that inhibit CYP450 3A, such as quinupristine, could decrease metabolism and increase cyclosporine concentrations). Products include:
- Synercid I.V. 775

Ranitidine Hydrochloride (May potentiate renal dysfunction). Products include:
- Zantac 1690
- Zantac Injection 1688
- Zantac 75 Tablets .... ▣717

Rifabutin (Substances that are inducers of cytochrome P450 activity could increase metabolism and decrease cyclosporine concentrations; rifabutin is known to increase the metabolism of other drugs metabolized by the cytochrome P450; this interaction has not been studied, however, care should be exercised). Products include:
- Mycobutin Capsules 2838

IMPORTANT NOTE: Always consult each drug listing in the patient's regimen for possible interactions.

Rifampin (Decreases cyclosporine concentrations). Products include:
- Rifadin ... 765
- Rifamate Capsules ... 767
- Rifater Tablets ... 769

Ritonavir (The HIV protease inhibitors are known to inhibit cytochrome P450IIIA and increase the concentration of drugs metabolized by this enzyme system; agents that inhibit this enzyme could decrease metabolism and increase cyclosporine concentrations; this interaction has not been studied, however, care should be exercised). Products include:
- Kaletra Capsules ... 471
- Kaletra Oral Solution ... 471
- Norvir Capsules ... 487
- Norvir Oral Solution ... 487

Rofecoxib (Co-administration with NSAID's particularly in the setting of dehydration, may potentiate renal dysfunction). Products include:
- Vioxx ... 2213

Saquinavir (The HIV protease inhibitors are known to inhibit cytochrome P450IIIA and increase the concentration of drugs metabolized by this enzyme system; agents that inhibit this enzyme could decrease metabolism and increase cyclosporine concentrations; this interaction has not been studied, however, care should be exercised). Products include:
- Fortovase Capsules ... 2970

Saquinavir Mesylate (The HIV protease inhibitors are known to inhibit cytochrome P450IIIA and increase the concentration of drugs metabolized by this enzyme system; agents that inhibit this enzyme could decrease metabolism and increase cyclosporine concentrations; this interaction has not been studied, however, care should be exercised). Products include:
- Invirase Capsules ... 2979

Spironolactone (Cyclosporine may cause hyperkalemia; concurrent use should be avoided).
No products indexed under this heading.

Sulfamethoxazole (Co-administration with trimethoprim/sulfamethoxazole may potentiate renal dysfunction). Products include:
- Bactrim ... 2949
- Septra Suspension ... 2265
- Septra Tablets ... 2265
- Septra DS Tablets ... 2265

Sulindac (Concomitant use is associated with additive decreases in renal function with possible potentiation of renal dysfunction). Products include:
- Clinoril Tablets ... 2053

Tacrolimus (May potentiate renal dysfunction). Products include:
- Prograf ... 1393
- Protopic Ointment ... 1397

Ticlopidine Hydrochloride (Decreases cyclosporine concentrations). Products include:
- Ticlid Tablets ... 3015

Tobramycin (May potentiate renal dysfunction). Products include:
- TOBI Solution for Inhalation ... 1206
- TobraDex Ophthalmic Ointment ... 542
- TobraDex Ophthalmic Suspension .. 541
- Tobrex Ophthalmic Ointment ... ⊙220
- Tobrex Ophthalmic Solution ... ⊙221

Tobramycin Sulfate (May potentiate renal dysfunction). Products include:
- Nebcin Vials, Hyporets & ADD-Vantage ... 1955

Tolmetin Sodium (Co-administration with NSAID's particularly in the setting of dehydration, may potentiate renal dysfunction). Products include:
- Tolectin ... 2589

Triamterene (Cyclosporine may cause hyperkalemia; concurrent use should be avoided). Products include:
- Dyazide Capsules ... 1515
- Dyrenium Capsules ... 3458
- Maxzide ... 1008

Trimethoprim (Co-administration with trimethoprim/sulfamethoxazole may potentiate renal dysfunction). Products include:
- Bactrim ... 2949
- Septra Suspension ... 2265
- Septra Tablets ... 2265
- Septra DS Tablets ... 2265

Vaccines (Live) (Vaccination may be less effective).
No products indexed under this heading.

Vancomycin Hydrochloride (May potentiate renal dysfunction). Products include:
- Vancocin HCl Capsules & Pulvules .. 1972
- Vancocin HCl Oral Solution ... 1971
- Vancocin HCl, Vials & ADD-Vantage ... 1970

Verapamil Hydrochloride (Increases cyclosporine concentrations). Products include:
- Covera-HS Tablets ... 3199
- Isoptin SR Tablets ... 467
- Tarka Tablets ... 508
- Verelan Capsules ... 3184
- Verelan PM Capsules ... 3186

Food Interactions

Diet, high-lipid (A high fat meal consumed within one-half hour before Neoral administration decreased the AUC by 13% and Cmax by 33%).

Food, unspecified (Administration of food with Neoral decreases the AUC and Cmax).

Grapefruit (Affects the metabolism of cyclosporine and should be avoided).

Grapefruit Juice (Affects the metabolism of cyclosporine and should be avoided).

NEORAL ORAL SOLUTION
(Cyclosporine) ... 2380
See Neoral Soft Gelatin Capsules

NEOSPORIN G.U. IRRIGANT STERILE
(Neomycin Sulfate, Polymyxin B Sulfate) ... 2256
None cited in PDR database.

NEOSPORIN OINTMENT
(Bacitracin Zinc, Neomycin, Polymyxin B Sulfate) ... ■704
None cited in PDR database.

NEOSPORIN OPHTHALMIC OINTMENT STERILE
(Bacitracin Zinc, Neomycin Sulfate, Polymyxin B Sulfate) ... ⊙299
None cited in PDR database.

NEOSPORIN OPHTHALMIC SOLUTION STERILE
(Gramicidin, Neomycin Sulfate, Polymyxin B Sulfate) ... ⊙300
None cited in PDR database.

NEOSPORIN + PAIN RELIEF MAXIMUM STRENGTH CREAM
(Neomycin, Polymyxin B Sulfate, Pramoxine Hydrochloride) ... ■704
None cited in PDR database.

NEOSPORIN + PAIN RELIEF MAXIMUM STRENGTH OINTMENT
(Bacitracin Zinc, Neomycin, Polymyxin B Sulfate, Pramoxine Hydrochloride) ... ■704
None cited in PDR database.

NEO-SYNEPHRINE NASAL DROPS, REGULAR AND EXTRA STRENGTH
(Phenylephrine Hydrochloride) ... ■614
None cited in PDR database.

NEO-SYNEPHRINE NASAL SPRAYS, MILD, REGULAR AND EXTRA STRENGTH
(Phenylephrine Hydrochloride) ... ■614
None cited in PDR database.

NEO-SYNEPHRINE 12 HOUR NASAL SPRAY
(Oxymetazoline Hydrochloride) ... ■615
None cited in PDR database.

NEO-SYNEPHRINE 12 HOUR EXTRA MOISTURIZING NASAL SPRAY
(Oxymetazoline Hydrochloride) ... ■615
None cited in PDR database.

NEPHROCAPS
(Vitamins, Multiple) ... 1362
None cited in PDR database.

NEPTAZANE TABLETS
(Methazolamide) ... ⊙271
May interact with corticosteroids and certain other agents. Compounds in these categories include:

Aspirin (Concomitant use of high-dose aspirin and carbonic anhydrase inhibitors may produce anorexia, tachypnea, lethargy, coma, and death). Products include:
- Aggrenox Capsules ... 1026
- Alka-Seltzer ... ■603
- Alka-Seltzer Lemon Lime Antacid and Pain Reliever Effervescent Tablets ... ■603
- Alka-Seltzer Extra Strength Antacid and Pain Reliever Effervescent Tablets ... ■603
- Alka-Seltzer PM Effervescent Tablets ... ■605
- Genuine Bayer Tablets, Caplets and Gelcaps ... ■606
- Extra Strength Bayer Caplets and Gelcaps ... ■610
- Aspirin Regimen Bayer Children's Chewable Tablets (Orange or Cherry Flavored) ... ■607
- Bayer, Aspirin Regimen ... ■606
- Aspirin Regimen Bayer 81 mg Caplets with Calcium ... ■607
- Genuine Bayer Professional Labeling (Aspirin Regimen Bayer) ... ■608
- Extra Strength Bayer Arthritis Caplets ... ■610
- Extra Strength Bayer Plus Caplets ... ■610
- Extra Strength Bayer PM Caplets .. ■611
- BC Powder ... ■619
- BC Allergy Sinus Cold Powder ... ■619
- Arthritis Strength BC Powder ... ■619
- BC Sinus Cold Powder ... ■619
- Darvon Compound-65 Pulvules ... 1910
- Ecotrin Enteric Coated Aspirin Low, Regular and Maximum Strength Tablets ... 1715
- Excedrin Extra-Strength Tablets, Caplets, and Geltabs ... ■629
- Excedrin Migraine ... 1070
- Goody's Body Pain Formula Powder ... ■620
- Goody's Extra Strength Headache Powder ... ■620
- Goody's Extra Strength Pain Relief Tablets ... ■620
- Percodan Tablets ... 1327
- Robaxisal Tablets ... 2939
- Soma Compound Tablets ... 3354
- Soma Compound w/Codeine Tablets ... 3355
- Vanquish Caplets ... ■617

Betamethasone Acetate (Potential for developing hypokalemia). Products include:
- Celestone Soluspan Injectable Suspension ... 3097

Betamethasone Sodium Phosphate (Potential for developing hypokalemia). Products include:
- Celestone Soluspan Injectable Suspension ... 3097

Cortisone Acetate (Potential for developing hypokalemia). Products include:
- Cortone Acetate Injectable Suspension ... 2059
- Cortone Acetate Tablets ... 2061

Dexamethasone (Potential for developing hypokalemia). Products include:
- Decadron Elixir ... 2078
- Decadron Tablets ... 2079
- TobraDex Ophthalmic Ointment ... 542
- TobraDex Ophthalmic Suspension .. 541

Dexamethasone Acetate (Potential for developing hypokalemia).
No products indexed under this heading.

Dexamethasone Sodium Phosphate (Potential for developing hypokalemia). Products include:
- Decadron Phosphate Injection ... 2081
- Decadron Phosphate Sterile Ophthalmic Ointment ... 2083
- Decadron Phosphate Sterile Ophthalmic Solution ... 2084
- NeoDecadron Sterile Ophthalmic Solution ... 2144

Fludrocortisone Acetate (Potential for developing hypokalemia). Products include:
- Florinef Acetate Tablets ... 2250

Hydrocortisone (Potential for developing hypokalemia). Products include:
- Anusol-HC Cream 2.5% ... 2237
- Cipro HC Otic Suspension ... 540
- Cortaid Intensive Therapy Cream .. ■717
- Cortaid Maximum Strength Cream ... ■717
- Cortisporin Ophthalmic Suspension Sterile ... ⊙297
- Cortizone•5 ... ■699
- Cortizone•10 ... ■699
- Cortizone•10 Plus Creme ... ■700
- Cortizone for Kids Creme ... ■699
- Hydrocortone Tablets ... 2106
- Massengill Medicated Soft Cloth Towelette ... ■753
- VōSoL HC Otic Solution ... 3356

Hydrocortisone Acetate (Potential for developing hypokalemia). Products include:
- Analpram-HC ... 1338
- Anusol HC-1 Hydrocortisone Anti-Itch Cream ... ■689
- Anusol-HC Suppositories ... 2238
- Cortaid ... ■717
- Cortifoam Rectal Foam ... 3170
- Cortisporin-TC Otic Suspension ... 2246
- Hydrocortone Acetate Injectable Suspension ... 2103
- Pramosone ... 1343
- Proctocort Suppositories ... 2264
- ProctoFoam-HC ... 3177
- Terra-Cortril Ophthalmic Suspension ... 2716

Hydrocortisone Sodium Phosphate (Potential for developing hypokalemia). Products include:
- Hydrocortone Phosphate Injection, Sterile ... 2105

Hydrocortisone Sodium Succinate (Potential for developing hypokalemia).
No products indexed under this heading.

Methylprednisolone Acetate (Potential for developing hypokalemia). Products include:
- Depo-Medrol Injectable Suspension ... 2795

Methylprednisolone Sodium Succinate (Potential for developing hypokalemia). Products include:
- Solu-Medrol Sterile Powder ... 2855

Prednisolone Acetate (Potential for developing hypokalemia). Products include:
- Blephamide Ophthalmic Ointment ... 547
- Blephamide Ophthalmic Suspension ... 548
- Poly-Pred Liquifilm Ophthalmic Suspension ... ⊙245
- Pred Forte Ophthalmic Suspension ... ⊙246
- Pred Mild Sterile Ophthalmic Suspension ... ⊙249
- Pred-G Ophthalmic Suspension ... ⊙247
- Pred-G Sterile Ophthalmic Ointment ... ⊙248

Prednisolone Sodium Phosphate (Potential for developing hypokalemia). Products include:
- Pediapred Oral Solution ... 1170

Prednisolone Tebutate (Potential for developing hypokalemia).
No products indexed under this heading.

Prednisone (Potential for developing hypokalemia). Products include:

Prednisone 3064

Triamcinolone (Potential for developing hypokalemia).
No products indexed under this heading.

Triamcinolone Acetonide (Potential for developing hypokalemia). Products include:
Azmacort Inhalation Aerosol 728
Nasacort Nasal Inhaler 750
Nasacort AQ Nasal Spray 752
Tri-Nasal Spray 2274

Triamcinolone Diacetate (Potential for developing hypokalemia).
No products indexed under this heading.

Triamcinolone Hexacetonide (Potential for developing hypokalemia).
No products indexed under this heading.

NESACAINE INJECTION

(Chloroprocaine Hydrochloride) 617
May interact with ergot-type oxytocic drugs, monoamine oxidase inhibitors, phenothiazines, tricyclic antidepressants, and certain other agents. Compounds in these categories include:

Amitriptyline Hydrochloride (Co-administration of local anesthetic solutions containing epinephrine may produce severe, prolonged hypotension or hypertension; concurrent use should be avoided). Products include:
Etrafon 3115
Limbitrol 1738

Amoxapine (Co-administration of local anesthetic solutions containing epinephrine may produce severe, prolonged hypotension or hypertension; concurrent use should be avoided).
No products indexed under this heading.

Chlorpromazine (Co-administration of local anesthetic solutions containing epinephrine may produce severe, prolonged hypotension or hypertension; concurrent use should be avoided). Products include:
Thorazine Suppositories 1656

Chlorpromazine Hydrochloride (Co-administration of local anesthetic solutions containing epinephrine may produce severe, prolonged hypotension or hypertension; concurrent use should be avoided). Products include:
Thorazine 1656

Clomipramine Hydrochloride (Co-administration of local anesthetic solutions containing epinephrine may produce severe, prolonged hypotension or hypertension; concurrent use should be avoided).
No products indexed under this heading.

Desipramine Hydrochloride (Co-administration of local anesthetic solutions containing epinephrine may produce severe, prolonged hypotension or hypertension; concurrent use should be avoided). Products include:
Norpramin Tablets 755

Doxepin Hydrochloride (Co-administration of local anesthetic solutions containing epinephrine may produce severe, prolonged hypotension or hypertension; concurrent use should be avoided). Products include:
Sinequan 2713

Fluphenazine Decanoate (Co-administration of local anesthetic solutions containing epinephrine may produce severe, prolonged hypotension or hypertension; concurrent use should be avoided).
No products indexed under this heading.

Fluphenazine Enanthate (Co-administration of local anesthetic solutions containing epinephrine may produce severe, prolonged hypotension or hypertension; concurrent use should be avoided).
No products indexed under this heading.

Fluphenazine Hydrochloride (Co-administration of local anesthetic solutions containing epinephrine may produce severe, prolonged hypotension or hypertension; concurrent use should be avoided).
No products indexed under this heading.

Imipramine Hydrochloride (Co-administration of local anesthetic solutions containing epinephrine may produce severe, prolonged hypotension or hypertension; concurrent use should be avoided).
No products indexed under this heading.

Imipramine Pamoate (Co-administration of local anesthetic solutions containing epinephrine may produce severe, prolonged hypotension or hypertension; concurrent use should be avoided).
No products indexed under this heading.

Isocarboxazid (Co-administration of local anesthetic solutions containing epinephrine may produce severe, prolonged hypotension or hypertension; concurrent use should be avoided).
No products indexed under this heading.

Maprotiline Hydrochloride (Co-administration of local anesthetic solutions containing epinephrine may produce severe, prolonged hypotension or hypertension; concurrent use should be avoided).
No products indexed under this heading.

Mesoridazine Besylate (Co-administration of local anesthetic solutions containing epinephrine may produce severe, prolonged hypotension or hypertension; concurrent use should be avoided). Products include:
Serentil 1057

Methotrimeprazine (Co-administration of local anesthetic solutions containing epinephrine may produce severe, prolonged hypotension or hypertension; concurrent use should be avoided).
No products indexed under this heading.

Methylergonovine Maleate (Co-administration of vasopressors (for the treatment of hypotension related to obstetrical blocks) and ergot-type oxytocic drugs may cause severe, persistant hypertension or cerebrovascular accidents).
No products indexed under this heading.

Moclobemide (Co-administration of local anesthetic solutions containing epinephrine may produce severe, prolonged hypotension or hypertension; concurrent use should be avoided).
No products indexed under this heading.

Nortriptyline Hydrochloride (Co-administration of local anesthetic solutions containing epinephrine may produce severe, prolonged hypotension or hypertension; concurrent use should be avoided).
No products indexed under this heading.

Pargyline Hydrochloride (Co-administration of local anesthetic solutions containing epinephrine may produce severe, prolonged hypotension or hypertension; concurrent use should be avoided).
No products indexed under this heading.

Perphenazine (Co-administration of local anesthetic solutions containing epinephrine may produce severe, prolonged hypotension or hypertension; concurrent use should be avoided). Products include:
Etrafon 3115
Trilafon 3160

Phenelzine Sulfate (Co-administration of local anesthetic solutions containing epinephrine may produce severe, prolonged hypotension or hypertension; concurrent use should be avoided). Products include:
Nardil Tablets 2653

Procarbazine Hydrochloride (Co-administration of local anesthetic solutions containing epinephrine may produce severe, prolonged hypotension or hypertension; concurrent use should be avoided). Products include:
Matulane Capsules 3246

Prochlorperazine (Co-administration of local anesthetic solutions containing epinephrine may produce severe, prolonged hypotension or hypertension; concurrent use should be avoided). Products include:
Compazine 1505

Promethazine Hydrochloride (Co-administration of local anesthetic solutions containing epinephrine may produce severe, prolonged hypotension or hypertension; concurrent use should be avoided). Products include:
Mepergan Injection 3539
Phenergan Injection 3553
Phenergan 3556
Phenergan Syrup 3554
Phenergan with Codeine Syrup 3557
Phenergan with Dextromethorphan Syrup 3559
Phenergan VC Syrup 3560
Phenergan VC with Codeine Syrup 3561

Protriptyline Hydrochloride (Co-administration of local anesthetic solutions containing epinephrine may produce severe, prolonged hypotension or hypertension; concurrent use should be avoided). Products include:
Vivactil Tablets 2446
Vivactil Tablets 2217

Selegiline Hydrochloride (Co-administration of local anesthetic solutions containing epinephrine may produce severe, prolonged hypotension or hypertension; concurrent use should be avoided). Products include:
Eldepryl Capsules 3266

Sulfamethizole (The para-aminobenzoic acid metabolite of chloroprocaine inhibits the action of sulfonamides; concurrent use should be avoided). Products include:
Urobiotic-250 Capsules 2731

Sulfamethoxazole (The para-aminobenzoic acid metabolite of chloroprocaine inhibits the action of sulfonamides; concurrent use should be avoided). Products include:
Bactrim 2949
Septra Suspension 2265
Septra Tablets 2265
Septra DS Tablets 2265

Sulfisoxazole (The para-aminobenzoic acid metabolite of chloroprocaine inhibits the action of sulfonamides; concurrent use should be avoided).
No products indexed under this heading.

Thioridazine Hydrochloride (Co-administration of local anesthetic solutions containing epinephrine may produce severe, prolonged hypotension or hypertension; concurrent use should be avoided). Products include:
Thioridazine Hydrochloride Tablets 2289

Tranylcypromine Sulfate (Co-administration of local anesthetic solutions containing epinephrine may produce severe, prolonged hypotension or hypertension; concurrent use should be avoided). Products include:
Parnate Tablets 1607

Trifluoperazine Hydrochloride (Co-administration of local anesthetic solutions containing epinephrine may produce severe, prolonged hypotension or hypertension; concurrent use should be avoided). Products include:
Stelazine 1640

Trimipramine Maleate (Co-administration of local anesthetic solutions containing epinephrine may produce severe, prolonged hypotension or hypertension; concurrent use should be avoided). Products include:
Surmontil Capsules 3595

NESACAINE-MPF INJECTION

(Chloroprocaine Hydrochloride) 617
See Nesacaine Injection

NESTABS RX TABLETS

(Vitamins, Prenatal, Vitamins with Minerals) 1351
None cited in PDR database.

NEUMEGA FOR INJECTION

(Oprelvekin) 1434
None cited in PDR database.

NEUPOGEN FOR INJECTION

(Filgrastim) 587
May interact with drugs which potentiate the release of neutrophils. Compounds in these categories include:

Lithium Carbonate (Concurrent use should be undertaken with caution since lithium potentiates the release of neutrophils). Products include:
Eskalith 1527
Lithium Carbonate 3061
Lithobid Slow-Release Tablets 3255

Lithium Citrate (Concurrent use should be undertaken with caution since lithium potentiates the release of neutrophils). Products include:
Lithium Citrate Syrup 3061

NEURONTIN CAPSULES

(Gabapentin) 2655
May interact with:

Aluminum Hydroxide (Coadministration reduces bioavailability of gabapentin by 20%; gabapentin should be taken at least 2 hours following antacid containing aluminum hydroxide and magnesium hydroxide). Products include:
Amphojel Suspension (Mint Flavor) 789
Gaviscon Extra Strength Liquid 751
Gaviscon Extra Strength Tablets 751
Gaviscon Regular Strength Liquid 751
Gaviscon Regular Strength Tablets 750
Maalox Antacid/Anti-Gas Oral Suspension 673
Maalox Max Maximum Strength Antacid/Anti-Gas Liquid 2300
Maalox Regular Strength Antacid/Antigas Liquid 2300
Mylanta 1813
Vanquish Caplets 617

Cimetidine (Alters renal clearance of gabapentin and creatinine; this

IMPORTANT NOTE: Always consult each drug listing in the patient's regimen for possible interactions.

small decrease in excretion of gabapentin is not expected to be of clinical importance). Products include:
Tagamet HB 200 Suspension .... ▣762
Tagamet HB 200 Tablets .... ▣761
Tagamet Tablets 1644

Cimetidine Hydrochloride (Alters renal clearance of gabapentin and creatinine; this small decrease in excretion of gabapentin is not expected to be of clinical importance). Products include:
Tagamet 1644

Magnesium Hydroxide (Coadministration reduces bioavailability of gabapentin by 20%; gabapentin should be taken at least 2 hours following antacid containing aluminum hydroxide and magnesium hydroxide). Products include:
Ex•Lax Milk of Magnesia Liquid .... ▣670
Maalox Antacid/Anti-Gas Oral Suspension .... ▣673
Maalox Max Maximum Strength Antacid/Anti-Gas Liquid 2300
Maalox Regular Strength Antacid/Antigas Liquid 2300
Mylanta Fast-Acting 1813
Mylanta 1813
Pepcid Complete Chewable Tablets 1815
Phillips' Chewable Tablets .... ▣615
Phillips' Milk of Magnesia Liquid (Original, Cherry, & Mint) .... ▣616
Rolaids Tablets .... ▣706
Extra Strength Rolaids Tablets ...... ▣706
Vanquish Caplets .... ▣617

Norethindrone (The Cmax of norethindrone was 13% higher when it was coadministered with gabapentin; this interaction is not expected to be of clinical importance). Products include:
Brevicon 28-Day Tablets 3380
Micronor Tablets 2543
Modicon 2563
Necon 3415
Norinyl 1 +35 28-Day Tablets 3380
Norinyl 1 + 50 28-Day Tablets 3380
Nor-QD Tablets 3423
Ortho-Novum 2563
Ortho-Novum 1/50□28 Tablets 2556
Ovcon 3364
Tri-Norinyl-28 Tablets 3433

Norethindrone Acetate (The Cmax of norethindrone was 13% higher when it was coadministered with gabapentin; this interaction is not expected to be of clinical importance). Products include:
Activella Tablets 2764
Aygestin Tablets 1333
CombiPatch Transdermal System .. 2323
Estrostep 2627
femhrt Tablets 2635
Loestrin 21 Tablets 2642
Loestrin Fe Tablets 2642
Microgestin Fe 1.5/30 Tablets 3407
Microgestin Fe 1/20 Tablets 3400

NEURONTIN ORAL SOLUTION
(Gabapentin) 2655
See Neurontin Capsules

NEURONTIN TABLETS
(Gabapentin) 2655
See Neurontin Capsules

NEW SKIN LIQUID BANDAGE
(Pyroxylin) .... ▣667
None cited in PDR database.

NEXIUM DELAYED-RELEASE CAPSULES
(Esomeprazole Magnesium) 619
May interact with iron containing oral preparations and certain other agents. Compounds in these categories include:

Amoxicillin (Co-administration of esomeprazole, clarithromycin, and amoxicillin has resulted in increase in the plasma levels of esomeprazole and 14-hydroxyxclarithromycin; the observed increase in esomeprazole exposure during co-administration with clarithromycin and amoxicillin is not expected to produce safety concerns). Products include:
Amoxil Chewable Tablets 1471
Amoxil for Oral Suspension 1471
Amoxil 1471
Augmentin Chewable Tablets 1482
Augmentin Powder for Oral Suspension 1482
Augmentin Tablets 1485
Augmentin ES-600 Powder for Oral Suspension 1487
PREVPAC 3298

Amoxicillin Trihydrate (Co-administration of esomeprazole, clarithromycin, and amoxicillin has resulted in increase in the plasma levels of esomeprazole and 14-hydroxyxclarithromycin; the observed increase in esomeprazole exposure during co-administration with clarithromycin and amoxicillin is not expected to produce safety concerns).

Clarithromycin (Co-administration of esomeprazole, clarithromycin, and amoxicillin has resulted in increase in the plasma levels of esomeprazole and 14-hydroxyxclarithromycin; the observed increase in esomeprazole exposure during co-administration with clarithromycin and amoxicillin is not expected to produce safety concerns). Products include:
Biaxin/Biaxin XL 403
PREVPAC 3298

Diazepam (Esomeprazole may interfere with CYP2C19, the major metabolizing enzyme; co-administration of esomeprazole and diazepam, a CYP2C19 substrate, resulted in a 45% decrease in clearance of diazepam; increased plasma levels of diazepam were observed 12 hours after dosing and onwards; however, at that time the plasma levels of diazepam were below the therapeutic interval, and this interaction is unlikely to be of clinical relevance). Products include:
Valium Injectable 3026
Valium Tablets 3047

Digoxin (Esomeprazole inhibits gastric acid secretion; therefore, esomeprazole may interfere with the absorption of drugs where gastric pH is an important determinant of bioavailability, such as digoxin). Products include:
Digitek Tablets 1003
Lanoxicaps Capsules 1574
Lanoxin Injection 1581
Lanoxin Tablets 1587
Lanoxin Elixir Pediatric 1578
Lanoxin Injection Pediatric 1584

Ferrous Fumarate (Esomeprazole inhibits gastric acid secretion; therefore, esomeprazole may interfere with the absorption of drugs where gastric pH is an important determinant of bioavailability, such as oral iron salts). Products include:
New Formulation Chromagen OB Capsules 3094
Loestrin Fe Tablets 2642
NataChew Tablets 3364

Ferrous Gluconate (Esomeprazole inhibits gastric acid secretion; therefore, esomeprazole may interfere with the absorption of drugs where gastric pH is an important determinant of bioavailability, such as oral iron salts). Products include:
Fergon Iron Tablets .... ▣802

Ferrous Sulfate (Esomeprazole inhibits gastric acid secretion; therefore, esomeprazole may interfere with the absorption of drugs where gastric pH is an important determinant of bioavailability, such as oral iron salts). Products include:
Feosol Tablets 1717
Slow Fe Tablets .... ▣827
Slow Fe with Folic Acid Tablets ..... ▣828

Iron (Esomeprazole inhibits gastric acid secretion; therefore, esomeprazole may interfere with the absorption of drugs where gastric pH is an important determinant of bioavailability, such as oral iron salts).
No products indexed under this heading.

Ketoconazole (Esomeprazole inhibits gastric acid secretion; therefore, esomeprazole may interfere with the absorption of drugs where gastric pH is an important determinant of bioavailability, such as ketoconazole). Products include:
Nizoral 2% Cream 3620
Nizoral A-D Shampoo 2008
Nizoral 2% Shampoo 2007
Nizoral Tablets 1791

Pimozide (Co-administration of clarithromycin-esomeprazole combination with pimozide is contraindicated; concurrent use of clarithromycin and/or erythromycin with pimozide has resulted in cardiac arrhythmias including QT prolongation, ventricular tachycardia, ventricular fibrillations and torsade de pointes). Products include:
Orap Tablets 1407

Polysaccharide-Iron Complex (Esomeprazole inhibits gastric acid secretion; therefore, esomeprazole may interfere with the absorption of drugs where gastric pH is an important determinant of bioavailability, such as oral iron salts). Products include:
Niferex 3176
Niferex-150 Capsules 3176
Nu-Iron 150 Capsules 2224

NIASPAN EXTENDED-RELEASE TABLETS
(Niacin) 1846
May interact with beta blockers, calcium channel blockers, oral anticoagulants, HMG-CoA reductase inhibitors, nitrates and nitrites, and certain other agents. Compounds in these categories include:

Acebutolol Hydrochloride (Co-administration with vasoactive drugs, such as adrenergic blocking agents, may result in postural hypotension, particularly in patients with unstable angina or acute phase of myocardial infarction). Products include:
Sectral Capsules 3589

Amlodipine Besylate (Co-administration with vasoactive drugs, such as calcium channel blocker, may result in postural hypotension, particularly in patients with unstable angina or acute phase of myocardial infarction). Products include:
Lotrel Capsules 2370
Norvasc Tablets 2704

Amyl Nitrite (Co-administration with vasoactive drugs, such as nitrates, may result in postural hypotension, particularly in patients with unstable angina or acute phase of myocardial infarction).
No products indexed under this heading.

Aspirin (Concomitant aspirin may decrease the metabolic clearance of nicotinic acid; the clinical relevance of this finding is unclear). Products include:
Aggrenox Capsules 1026
Alka-Seltzer .... ▣603
Alka-Seltzer Lemon Lime Antacid and Pain Reliever Effervescent Tablets .... ▣603
Alka-Seltzer Extra Strength Antacid and Pain Reliever Effervescent Tablets .... ▣603
Alka-Seltzer PM Effervescent Tablets .... ▣605
Genuine Bayer Tablets, Caplets and Gelcaps .... ▣606
Extra Strength Bayer Caplets and Gelcaps .... ▣610
Aspirin Regimen Bayer Children's Chewable Tablets (Orange or Cherry Flavored) .... ▣607
Bayer, Aspirin Regimen .... ▣606
Aspirin Regimen Bayer 81 mg Caplets with Calcium .... ▣607
Genuine Bayer Professional Labeling (Aspirin Regimen Bayer) .... ▣608
Extra Strength Bayer Arthritis Caplets .... ▣610
Extra Strength Bayer Plus Caplets .... ▣610
Extra Strength Bayer PM Caplets .. ▣611
BC Powder .... ▣619
BC Allergy Sinus Cold Powder ...... ▣619
Arthritis Strength BC Powder .... ▣619
BC Sinus Cold Powder .... ▣619
Darvon Compound-65 Pulvules 1910
Ecotrin Enteric Coated Aspirin Low, Regular and Maximum Strength Tablets 1715
Excedrin Extra-Strength Tablets, Caplets, and Geltabs .... ▣629
Excedrin Migraine 1070
Goody's Body Pain Formula Powder .... ▣620
Goody's Extra Strength Headache Powder .... ▣620
Goody's Extra Strength Pain Relief Tablets .... ▣620
Percodan Tablets 1327
Robaxisal Tablets 2939
Soma Compound Tablets 3354
Soma Compound w/Codeine Tablets 3355
Vanquish Caplets .... ▣617

Atenolol (Co-administration with vasoactive drugs, such as adrenergic blocking agents, may result in postural hypotension, particularly in patients with unstable angina or acute phase of myocardial infarction). Products include:
Tenoretic Tablets 690
Tenormin I.V. Injection 692

Atorvastatin Calcium (Co-administration of lipid-altering doses ($\geq$ 1 g/day) of niacin and HMG-CoA reductase inhibitors has resulted in rare cases of rhabdomyolysis). Products include:
Lipitor Tablets 2639
Lipitor Tablets 2696

Bepridil Hydrochloride (Co-administration with vasoactive drugs, such as calcium channel blocker, may result in postural hypotension, particularly in patients with unstable angina or acute phase of myocardial infarction). Products include:
Vascor Tablets 2602

Betaxolol Hydrochloride (Co-administration with vasoactive drugs, such as adrenergic blocking agents, may result in postural hypotension, particularly in patients with unstable angina or acute phase of myocardial infarction). Products include:
Betoptic S Ophthalmic Suspension 537

Bisoprolol Fumarate (Co-administration with vasoactive drugs, such as adrenergic blocking agents, may result in postural hypotension, particularly in patients with unstable angina or acute phase of myocardial infarction). Products include:
Zebeta Tablets 1885
Ziac Tablets 1887

Carteolol Hydrochloride (Co-administration with vasoactive drugs, such as adrenergic blocking agents, may result in postural hypotension, particularly in patients with unstable angina or acute phase of myocardial infarction). Products include:
Carteolol Hydrochloride Ophthalmic Solution USP, 1% ..... ⊙258
Ocupress Ophthalmic Solution, 1% Sterile .... ⊙303

Cerivastatin Sodium (Co-administration of lipid-altering doses ($\geq$ 1 g/day) of niacin and HMG-CoA

reductase inhibitors has resulted in rare cases of rhabdomyolysis). Products include:
- Baycol Tablets 883

Cholestyramine (*In vitro* study resulted in approximately 10% to 30% of available niacin bound to cholestyramine; 4 to 6 hours or greater should elapse between ingestion of bile acid-binding resins and the administration of Niaspan).
No products indexed under this heading.

Colestipol Hydrochloride (*In vitro* study resulted in approximately 90% of available niacin bound to colestipol; 4 to 6 hours or greater should elapse between ingestion of bile acid-binding resins and the administration of Niaspan). Products include:
- Colestid Tablets 2791

Dicumarol (Niacin prolongs prothrombin time; caution should be exercised when used concurrently).
No products indexed under this heading.

Diltiazem Hydrochloride (Co-administration with vasoactive drugs, such as calcium channel blocker, may result in postural hypotension, particularly in patients with unstable angina or acute phase of myocardial infarction). Products include:
- Cardizem Injectable 1018
- Cardizem Lyo-Ject Syringe 1018
- Cardizem Monovial 1018
- Cardizem CD Capsules 1016
- Tiazac Capsules 1378

Erythrityl Tetranitrate (Co-administration with vasoactive drugs, such as nitrates, may result in postural hypotension, particularly in patients with unstable angina or acute phase of myocardial infarction).
No products indexed under this heading.

Esmolol Hydrochloride (Co-administration with vasoactive drugs, such as adrenergic blocking agents, may result in postural hypotension, particularly in patients with unstable angina or acute phase of myocardial infarction). Products include:
- Brevibloc Injection 858

Felodipine (Co-administration with vasoactive drugs, such as calcium channel blocker, may result in postural hypotension, particularly in patients with unstable angina or acute phase of myocardial infarction). Products include:
- Lexxel Tablets 608
- Plendil Extended-Release Tablets ... 623

Fluvastatin Sodium (Co-administration of lipid-altering doses ($\geq$ 1 g/day) of niacin and HMG-CoA reductase inhibitors has resulted in rare cases of rhabdomyolysis). Products include:
- Lescol Capsules 2361
- Lescol 2925
- Lescol XL Tablets 2361

Isosorbide Dinitrate (Co-administration with vasoactive drugs, such as nitrates, may result in postural hypotension, particularly in patients with unstable angina or acute phase of myocardial infarction). Products include:
- Isordil Sublingual Tablets 3525
- Isordil Titradose Tablets 3526

Isosorbide Mononitrate (Co-administration with vasoactive drugs, such as nitrates, may result in postural hypotension, particularly in patients with unstable angina or acute phase of myocardial infarction). Products include:
- Imdur Tablets 1826
- Ismo Tablets 3524

Isradipine (Co-administration with vasoactive drugs, such as calcium channel blocker, may result in postural hypotension, particularly in patients with unstable angina or acute phase of myocardial infarction). Products include:
- DynaCirc Capsules 2921
- DynaCirc CR Tablets 2923

Labetalol Hydrochloride (Co-administration with vasoactive drugs, such as adrenergic blocking agents, may result in postural hypotension, particularly in patients with unstable angina or acute phase of myocardial infarction). Products include:
- Normodyne Injection 3135
- Normodyne Tablets 3137

Levobunolol Hydrochloride (Co-administration with vasoactive drugs, such as adrenergic blocking agents, may result in postural hypotension, particularly in patients with unstable angina or acute phase of myocardial infarction). Products include:
- Betagan .... ⊙ 228

Lovastatin (Co-administration of lipid-altering doses ($\geq$ 1 g/day) of niacin and HMG-CoA reductase inhibitors has resulted in rare cases of rhabdomyolysis). Products include:
- Mevacor Tablets 2132

Mecamylamine Hydrochloride (Niacin may potentiate the effects of ganglionic blocking agents, such as mecamylamine, resulting in postural hypotension). Products include:
- Inversine Tablets 1850

Metipranolol Hydrochloride (Co-administration with vasoactive drugs, such as adrenergic blocking agents, may result in postural hypotension, particularly in patients with unstable angina or acute phase of myocardial infarction).
No products indexed under this heading.

Metoprolol Succinate (Co-administration with vasoactive drugs, such as adrenergic blocking agents, may result in postural hypotension, particularly in patients with unstable angina or acute phase of myocardial infarction). Products include:
- Toprol-XL Tablets 651

Metoprolol Tartrate (Co-administration with vasoactive drugs, such as adrenergic blocking agents, may result in postural hypotension, particularly in patients with unstable angina or acute phase of myocardial infarction).
No products indexed under this heading.

Mibefradil Dihydrochloride (Co-administration with vasoactive drugs, such as calcium channel blocker, may result in postural hypotension, particularly in patients with unstable angina or acute phase of myocardial infarction).
No products indexed under this heading.

Nadolol (Co-administration with vasoactive drugs, such as adrenergic blocking agents, may result in postural hypotension, particularly in patients with unstable angina or acute phase of myocardial infarction). Products include:
- Corgard Tablets 2245
- Corzide 40/5 Tablets 2247
- Corzide 80/5 Tablets 2247
- Nadolol Tablets 2288

Nicardipine Hydrochloride (Co-administration with vasoactive drugs, such as calcium channel blocker, may result in postural hypotension, particularly in patients with unstable angina or acute phase of myocardial infarction). Products include:
- Cardene I.V. 3485

Nicotinamide (May potentiate the adverse effects of Niaspan). Products include:
- Nicomide Tablets 3247

Nifedipine (Co-administration with vasoactive drugs, such as calcium channel blocker, may result in postural hypotension, particularly in patients with unstable angina or acute phase of myocardial infarction). Products include:
- Adalat CC Tablets 877
- Procardia Capsules 2708
- Procardia XL Extended Release Tablets 2710

Nimodipine (Co-administration with vasoactive drugs, such as calcium channel blocker, may result in postural hypotension, particularly in patients with unstable angina or acute phase of myocardial infarction). Products include:
- Nimotop Capsules 904

Nisoldipine (Co-administration with vasoactive drugs, such as calcium channel blocker, may result in postural hypotension, particularly in patients with unstable angina or acute phase of myocardial infarction). Products include:
- Sular Tablets 688

Nitroglycerin (Co-administration with vasoactive drugs, such as nitrates, may result in postural hypotension, particularly in patients with unstable angina or acute phase of myocardial infarction). Products include:
- Nitro-Dur Transdermal Infusion System 3134
- Nitro-Dur Transdermal Infusion System 1834
- Nitrolingual Pumpspray 1355
- Nitrostat Tablets 2658

Penbutolol Sulfate (Co-administration with vasoactive drugs, such as adrenergic blocking agents, may result in postural hypotension, particularly in patients with unstable angina or acute phase of myocardial infarction).
No products indexed under this heading.

Pentaerythritol Tetranitrate (Co-administration with vasoactive drugs, such as nitrates, may result in postural hypotension, particularly in patients with unstable angina or acute phase of myocardial infarction).
No products indexed under this heading.

Pindolol (Co-administration with vasoactive drugs, such as adrenergic blocking agents, may result in postural hypotension, particularly in patients with unstable angina or acute phase of myocardial infarction).
No products indexed under this heading.

Pravastatin Sodium (Co-administration of lipid-altering doses ($\geq$ 1 g/day) of niacin and HMG-CoA reductase inhibitors has resulted in rare cases of rhabdomyolysis). Products include:
- Pravachol Tablets 1099

Propranolol Hydrochloride (Co-administration with vasoactive drugs, such as adrenergic blocking agents, may result in postural hypotension, particularly in patients with unstable angina or acute phase of myocardial infarction). Products include:
- Inderal 3513
- Inderal LA Long-Acting Capsules 3516
- Inderide Tablets 3517
- Inderide LA Long-Acting Capsules .. 3519

Simvastatin (Co-administration of lipid-altering doses ($\geq$ 1 g/day) of niacin and HMG-CoA reductase inhibitors has resulted in rare cases of rhabdomyolysis). Products include:
- Zocor Tablets 2219

Sotalol Hydrochloride (Co-administration with vasoactive drugs, such as adrenergic blocking agents, may result in postural hypotension, particularly in patients with unstable angina or acute phase of myocardial infarction). Products include:
- Betapace Tablets 950
- Betapace AF Tablets 954

Timolol Hemihydrate (Co-administration with vasoactive drugs, such as adrenergic blocking agents, may result in postural hypotension, particularly in patients with unstable angina or acute phase of myocardial infarction). Products include:
- Betimol Ophthalmic Solution .... ⊙ 324

Timolol Maleate (Co-administration with vasoactive drugs, such as adrenergic blocking agents, may result in postural hypotension, particularly in patients with unstable angina or acute phase of myocardial infarction). Products include:
- Blocadren Tablets 2046
- Cosopt Sterile Ophthalmic Solution 2065
- Timolide Tablets 2187
- Timolol GFS .... ⊙ 266
- Timoptic in Ocudose 2192
- Timoptic Sterile Ophthalmic Solution 2190
- Timoptic-XE Sterile Ophthalmic Gel Forming Solution 2194

Verapamil Hydrochloride (Co-administration with vasoactive drugs, such as calcium channel blocker, may result in postural hypotension, particularly in patients with unstable angina or acute phase of myocardial infarction). Products include:
- Covera-HS Tablets 3199
- Isoptin SR Tablets 467
- Tarka Tablets 508
- Verelan Capsules 3184
- Verelan PM Capsules 3186

Warfarin Sodium (Niacin prolongs prothrombin time; caution should be exercised when used concurrently). Products include:
- Coumadin for Injection 1243
- Coumadin Tablets 1243
- Warfarin Sodium Tablets, USP 3302

Food Interactions

Alcohol (Concomitant alcohol may increase the side effects of flushing and pruritus and should be avoided around the time of Niaspan ingestion).

Drinks, hot, unspecified (Concomitant hot drinks may increase the side effects of flushing and pruritus and should be avoided around the time of Niaspan ingestion).

NICODERM CQ PATCH

(Nicotine) 1717
See Nicorette Gum

NICOMIDE TABLETS

(Folic Acid, Nicotinamide, Zinc Oxide) 3247

May interact with fluoroquinolone antibiotics, tetracyclines, and certain other agents. Compounds in these categories include:

Alatrofloxacin Mesylate (Decreased absorption of oral quinolones). Products include:
- Trovan I.V. 2722

Carbamazepine (Reduced clearance of carbamazepine). Products include:
- Carbatrol Capsules 3234
- Tegretol/Tegretol-XR 2404

Ciprofloxacin (Decreased absorption of oral quinolones). Products include:
- Cipro I.V. 893
- Cipro I.V. Pharmacy Bulk Package .. 897
- Cipro Oral Suspension 887

Ciprofloxacin Hydrochloride (Decreased absorption of oral quinolones). Products include:

Ciloxan 538
Cipro HC Otic Suspension 540
Cipro Tablets 887

Demeclocycline Hydrochloride (Decreased absorption of oral tetracyclines). Products include:
Declomycin Tablets 1855

Doxycycline Calcium (Decreased absorption of oral tetracyclines). Products include:
Vibramycin Calcium Oral Suspension Syrup 2735

Doxycycline Hyclate (Decreased absorption of oral tetracyclines). Products include:
Doryx Coated Pellet Filled Capsules 3357
Periostat Tablets 1208
Vibramycin Hyclate Capsules 2735
Vibramycin Hyclate Intravenous 2737
Vibra-Tabs Film Coated Tablets 2735

Doxycycline Monohydrate (Decreased absorption of oral tetracyclines). Products include:
Monodox Capsules 2442
Vibramycin Monohydrate for Oral Suspension 2735

Enoxacin (Decreased absorption of oral quinolones).
No products indexed under this heading.

Grepafloxacin Hydrochloride (Decreased absorption of oral quinolones).
No products indexed under this heading.

Lomefloxacin Hydrochloride (Decreased absorption of oral quinolones).
No products indexed under this heading.

Methacycline Hydrochloride (Decreased absorption of oral tetracyclines).
No products indexed under this heading.

Minocycline Hydrochloride (Decreased absorption of oral tetracyclines). Products include:
Dynacin Capsules 2019
Minocin Intravenous 1862
Minocin Oral Suspension 1865
Minocin Pellet-Filled Capsules 1863

Moxifloxacin Hydrochloride (Decreased absorption of oral quinolones). Products include:
Avelox Tablets 879

Norfloxacin (Decreased absorption of oral quinolones). Products include:
Chibroxin Sterile Ophthalmic Solution 2051
Noroxin Tablets 2145

Ofloxacin (Decreased absorption of oral quinolones). Products include:
Floxin I.V. 2526
Floxin Otic Solution 1219
Floxin Tablets 2529
Ocuflox Ophthalmic Solution 554

Oxytetracycline Hydrochloride (Decreased absorption of oral tetracyclines). Products include:
Terra-Cortril Ophthalmic Suspension 2716
Urobiotic-250 Capsules 2731

Primidone (Reduced clearance of primidone).
No products indexed under this heading.

Tetracycline Hydrochloride (Decreased absorption of oral tetracyclines).
No products indexed under this heading.

Trovafloxacin Mesylate (Decreased absorption of oral quinolones). Products include:
Trovan Tablets 2722

NICORETTE GUM

(Nicotine Polacrilex) 1720
May interact with asthma medications and antidepressant drugs. Compounds in these categories include:

Albuterol (Concurrent use with asthma medications should be undertaken under physician's supervision). Products include:
Proventil Inhalation Aerosol 3142
Ventolin Inhalation Aerosol and Refill 1679

Albuterol Sulfate (Concurrent use with asthma medications should be undertaken under physician's supervision). Products include:
AccuNeb Inhalation Solution 1230
Combivent Inhalation Aerosol 1041
DuoNeb Inhalation Solution 1233
Proventil Inhalation Solution 0.083% 3146
Proventil Repetabs Tablets 3148
Proventil Solution for Inhalation 0.5% 3144
Proventil HFA Inhalation Aerosol 3150
Ventolin HFA Inhalation Aerosol 3618
Volmax Extended-Release Tablets 2276

Amitriptyline Hydrochloride (Concurrent use with antidepressant should be undertaken under physician's supervision). Products include:
Etrafon 3115
Limbitrol 1738

Amoxapine (Concurrent use with antidepressant should be undertaken under physician's supervision).
No products indexed under this heading.

Bitolterol Mesylate (Concurrent use with asthma medications should be undertaken under physician's supervision).
No products indexed under this heading.

Bupropion Hydrochloride (Concurrent use with antidepressant should be undertaken under physician's supervision). Products include:
Wellbutrin Tablets 1680
Wellbutrin SR Sustained-Release Tablets 1684
Zyban Sustained-Release Tablets 1710

Citalopram Hydrobromide (Concurrent use with antidepressant should be undertaken under physician's supervision). Products include:
Celexa 1365

Desipramine Hydrochloride (Concurrent use with antidepressant should be undertaken under physician's supervision). Products include:
Norpramin Tablets 755

Doxepin Hydrochloride (Concurrent use with antidepressant should be undertaken under physician's supervision). Products include:
Sinequan 2713

Ephedrine Hydrochloride (Concurrent use with asthma medications should be undertaken under physician's supervision). Products include:
Primatene Tablets .... ▣780

Ephedrine Sulfate (Concurrent use with asthma medications should be undertaken under physician's supervision).
No products indexed under this heading.

Ephedrine Tannate (Concurrent use with asthma medications should be undertaken under physician's supervision). Products include:
Rynatuss Pediatric Suspension 3353
Rynatuss Tablets 3353

Epinephrine (Concurrent use with asthma medications should be undertaken under physician's supervision). Products include:
Epifrin Sterile Ophthalmic Solution .... ⊙235
EpiPen 1236
Primatene Mist .... ▣779
Xylocaine with Epinephrine Injection 653

Epinephrine Bitartrate (Concurrent use with asthma medications should be undertaken under physician's supervision). Products include:
Sensorcaine 643

Epinephrine Hydrochloride (Concurrent use with asthma medications should be undertaken under physician's supervision).
No products indexed under this heading.

Fluoxetine Hydrochloride (Concurrent use with antidepressant should be undertaken under physician's supervision). Products include:
Prozac Pulvules, Liquid, and Weekly Capsules 1238
Sarafem Pulvules 1962

Imipramine Hydrochloride (Concurrent use with antidepressant should be undertaken under physician's supervision).
No products indexed under this heading.

Imipramine Pamoate (Concurrent use with antidepressant should be undertaken under physician's supervision).
No products indexed under this heading.

Isocarboxazid (Concurrent use with antidepressant should be undertaken under physician's supervision).
No products indexed under this heading.

Isoetharine (Concurrent use with asthma medications should be undertaken under physician's supervision).
No products indexed under this heading.

Isoproterenol Hydrochloride (Concurrent use with asthma medications should be undertaken under physician's supervision).
No products indexed under this heading.

Isoproterenol Sulfate (Concurrent use with asthma medications should be undertaken under physician's supervision).
No products indexed under this heading.

Levalbuterol Hydrochloride (Concurrent use with asthma medications should be undertaken under physician's supervision). Products include:
Xopenex Inhalation Solution 3207

Maprotiline Hydrochloride (Concurrent use with antidepressant should be undertaken under physician's supervision).
No products indexed under this heading.

Metaproterenol Sulfate (Concurrent use with asthma medications should be undertaken under physician's supervision). Products include:
Alupent 1029

Mirtazapine (Concurrent use with antidepressant should be undertaken under physician's supervision). Products include:
Remeron Tablets 2483
Remeron SolTab Tablets 2486

Nefazodone Hydrochloride (Concurrent use with antidepressant should be undertaken under physician's supervision). Products include:
Serzone Tablets 1104

Nortriptyline Hydrochloride (Concurrent use with antidepressant should be undertaken under physician's supervision).
No products indexed under this heading.

Paroxetine Hydrochloride (Concurrent use with antidepressant should be undertaken under physician's supervision). Products include:
Paxil 1609

Phenelzine Sulfate (Concurrent use with antidepressant should be undertaken under physician's supervision). Products include:
Nardil Tablets 2653

Pirbuterol Acetate (Concurrent use with asthma medications should be undertaken under physician's supervision). Products include:
Maxair Autohaler 1981
Maxair Inhaler 1984

Protriptyline Hydrochloride (Concurrent use with antidepressant should be undertaken under physician's supervision). Products include:
Vivactil Tablets 2446
Vivactil Tablets 2217

Salmeterol Xinafoate (Concurrent use with asthma medications should be undertaken under physician's supervision). Products include:
Advair Diskus 100/50 1448
Advair Diskus 250/50 1448
Advair Diskus 500/50 1448
Serevent Diskus 1637
Serevent Inhalation Aerosol 1633

Sertraline Hydrochloride (Concurrent use with antidepressant should be undertaken under physician's supervision). Products include:
Zoloft 2751

Terbutaline Sulfate (Concurrent use with asthma medications should be undertaken under physician's supervision). Products include:
Brethine Ampuls 2314
Brethine Tablets 2313

Tranylcypromine Sulfate (Concurrent use with antidepressant should be undertaken under physician's supervision). Products include:
Parnate Tablets 1607

Trazodone Hydrochloride (Concurrent use with antidepressant should be undertaken under physician's supervision).
No products indexed under this heading.

Trimipramine Maleate (Concurrent use with antidepressant should be undertaken under physician's supervision). Products include:
Surmontil Capsules 3595

Venlafaxine Hydrochloride (Concurrent use with antidepressant should be undertaken under physician's supervision). Products include:
Effexor Tablets 3495
Effexor XR Capsules 3499

NICOTINEX ELIXIR

(Niacin) .... ▣633
None cited in PDR database.

NICOTROL INHALER

(Nicotine) 2840
May interact with tricyclic antidepressants and theophylline. Compounds in these categories include:

Aminophylline (Physiological changes resulting from smoking cessation, with or without nicotine replacement, may alter the pharmacokinetics of concomitant drugs such as theophylline).
No products indexed under this heading.

Amitriptyline Hydrochloride (Physiological changes resulting from smoking cessation, with or without nicotine replacement, may alter the pharmacokinetics of concomitant drugs such as tricyclic antidepressants). Products include:
Etrafon 3115
Limbitrol 1738

Amoxapine (Physiological changes resulting from smoking cessation, with or without nicotine replacement, may alter the pharmacokinetics of concomitant drugs such as tricyclic antidepressants).
No products indexed under this heading.

Clomipramine Hydrochloride (Physiological changes resulting from smoking cessation, with or without nicotine replacement, may alter the pharmacokinetics of concomitant drugs such as tricyclic antidepressants).
No products indexed under this heading.

Desipramine Hydrochloride (Physiological changes resulting from smoking cessation, with or without nicotine replacement, may alter the pharmacokinetics of concomitant drugs such as tricyclic antidepressants). Products include:
Norpramin Tablets 755

Doxepin Hydrochloride (Physiological changes resulting from smoking cessation, with or without nicotine replacement, may alter the pharmacokinetics of concomitant drugs such as tricyclic antidepressants). Products include:
Sinequan 2713

Dyphylline (Physiological changes resulting from smoking cessation, with or without nicotine replacement, may alter the pharmacokinetics of concomitant drugs such as theophylline). Products include:
Lufyllin Tablets 3347
Lufyllin-400 Tablets 3347
Lufyllin-GG Elixir 3348
Lufyllin-GG Tablets 3348

Imipramine Hydrochloride (Physiological changes resulting from smoking cessation, with or without nicotine replacement, may alter the pharmacokinetics of concomitant drugs such as tricyclic antidepressants).
No products indexed under this heading.

Imipramine Pamoate (Physiological changes resulting from smoking cessation, with or without nicotine replacement, may alter the pharmacokinetics of concomitant drugs such as tricyclic antidepressants).
No products indexed under this heading.

Maprotiline Hydrochloride (Physiological changes resulting from smoking cessation, with or without nicotine replacement, may alter the pharmacokinetics of concomitant drugs such as tricyclic antidepressants).
No products indexed under this heading.

Nortriptyline Hydrochloride (Physiological changes resulting from smoking cessation, with or without nicotine replacement, may alter the pharmacokinetics of concomitant drugs such as tricyclic antidepressants).
No products indexed under this heading.

Protriptyline Hydrochloride (Physiological changes resulting from smoking cessation, with or without nicotine replacement, may alter the pharmacokinetics of concomitant drugs such as tricyclic antidepressants). Products include:
Vivactil Tablets 2446
Vivactil Tablets 2217

Theophylline (Physiological changes resulting from smoking cessation, with or without nicotine replacement, may alter the pharmacokinetics of concomitant drugs such as theophylline). Products include:
Aerolate 1361
Theo-Dur Extended-Release Tablets 1835
Uni-Dur Extended-Release Tablets .. 1841
Uniphyl 400 mg and 600 mg Tablets 2903

Theophylline Calcium Salicylate (Physiological changes resulting from smoking cessation, with or without nicotine replacement, may alter the pharmacokinetics of concomitant drugs such as theophylline).
No products indexed under this heading.

Theophylline Sodium Glycinate (Physiological changes resulting from smoking cessation, with or without nicotine replacement, may alter the pharmacokinetics of concomitant drugs such as theophylline).
No products indexed under this heading.

Trimipramine Maleate (Physiological changes resulting from smoking cessation, with or without nicotine replacement, may alter the pharmacokinetics of concomitant drugs such as tricyclic antidepressants). Products include:
Surmontil Capsules 3595

NICOTROL NASAL SPRAY

(Nicotine) 2843
May interact with beta blockers, insulin, sympathomimetics, theophylline, and certain other agents. Compounds in these categories include:

Acebutolol Hydrochloride (Deinduction of hepatic enzyme on smoking cessation; may require a decrease in dose at cessation of smoking). Products include:
Sectral Capsules 3589

Acetaminophen (Deinduction of hepatic enzyme on smoking cessation; may require a decrease in dose at cessation of smoking). Products include:
Actifed Cold & Sinus Caplets and Tablets 688
Alka-Seltzer Plus Liqui-Gels 604
Alka-Seltzer Plus Cold & Flu Medicine Liqui-Gels 604
Alka-Seltzer Plus Cold & Sinus Medicine Liqui-Gels 604
Benadryl Allergy/Cold Tablets 691
Benadryl Allergy Sinus Headache Caplets & Gelcaps 693
Benadryl Severe Allergy & Sinus Headache Caplets 694
Children's Cēpacol Sore Throat 788
Comtrex Acute Head Cold & Sinus Pressure Relief Tablets 627
Comtrex Deep Chest Cold & Congestion Relief Softgels 627
Comtrex Flu Therapy & Fever Relief Daytime Caplets 628
Comtrex Flu Therapy & Fever Relief Nighttime Tablets 628
Comtrex Maximum Strength Multi-Symptom Cold & Cough Relief Tablets and Caplets 626
Contac Severe Cold and Flu Caplets Maximum Strength 746
Contac Severe Cold and Flu Caplets Non-Drowsy 746
Coricidin 'D' Cold, Flu & Sinus Tablets 737
Coricidin HBP Cold & Flu Tablets .. 738
Coricidin HBP Maximum Strength Flu Tablets 738
Coricidin HBP Night-Time Cold & Flu Tablets 738
Darvon-N/Darvocet-N 1907
Dimetapp Cold and Fever Suspension 775
Dimetapp Nighttime Flu Liquid 776
Dimetapp Non-Drowsy Flu Syrup .. 777
Drixoral Allergy/Sinus Extended-Release Tablets 741
Drixoral Cold & Flu Extended-Release Tablets 740
Aspirin Free Excedrin Caplets and Geltabs 628
Excedrin Extra-Strength Tablets, Caplets, and Geltabs 629
Excedrin Migraine 1070
Excedrin PM Tablets, Caplets, and Geltabs 631
Goody's Body Pain Formula Powder 620
Goody's Extra Strength Headache Powder 620
Goody's Extra Strength Pain Relief Tablets 620
Goody's PM Powder 621
Hycomine Compound Tablets 1317
Lortab 3319
Lortab Elixir 3317
Maxidone Tablets CIII 3399
Maximum Strength Midol Menstrual Caplets and Gelcaps .. 612
Maximum Strength Midol PMS Caplets and Gelcaps 613
Maximum Strength Midol Teen Caplets 612
Midrin Capsules 3464
Norco 5/325 Tablets CIII 3424
Norco 7.5/325 Tablets CIII 3425
Norco 10/325 Tablets CIII 3427
Norco 10/325 Tablets CIII 3425
Percocet Tablets 1326
Percogesic Aspirin-Free Coated Tablets 667
Extra Strength Percogesic Aspirin-Free Coated Caplets 665
Phrenilin 578
Robitussin Cold Caplets Multi-Symptom Cold & Flu 781
Robitussin Cold Softgels Multi-Symptom Cold & Flu 781
Robitussin Multi Symptom Honey Flu Liquid 785
Robitussin Nighttime Honey Flu Liquid 786
Sedapap Tablets 50 mg/650 mg ... 2225
Singlet Caplets 761
Sinutab Sinus Allergy Medication, Maximum Strength Formula, Tablets & Caplets 707
Sinutab Sinus Medication, Maximum Strength Without Drowsiness Formula, Tablets & Caplets 707
Sudafed Cold & Cough Liquid Caps 709
Sudafed Cold & Sinus Liquid Caps 710
Sudafed Severe Cold 711
Sudafed Sinus Headache Caplets .. 712
Sudafed Sinus Headache Tablets .. 712
Tavist Sinus Non-Drowsy Coated Caplets 676
TheraFlu Regular Strength Cold & Cough Night Time Hot Liquid 676
TheraFlu Regular Strength Cold & Sore Throat Night Time Hot Liquid 676
TheraFlu Maximum Strength Flu & Congestion Non-Drowsy Hot Liquid 677
TheraFlu Maximum Strength Flu & Cough Night Time Hot Liquid .. 678
TheraFlu Maximum Strength Flu & Sore Throat Night Time Hot Liquid 677
TheraFlu Maximum Strength Severe Cold & Congestion Night Time Caplets 678
TheraFlu Maximum Strength Severe Cold & Congestion Night Time Hot Liquid 678
TheraFlu Maximum Strength Severe Cold & Congestion Non-Drowsy 679
Triaminic Cold, Cough & Fever Liquid 681
Triaminic Cough & Sore Throat Liquid 682
Triaminic Cough & Sore Throat Softchews 684
Tylenol, Children's 2014
Children's Tylenol Allergy-D Liquid ... 2014
Children's Tylenol Cold Suspension Liquid and Chewable Tablets 2015
Children's Tylenol Cold Plus Cough Suspension Liquid and Chewable Tablets 2015
Children's Tylenol Flu Suspension Liquid 2015
Children's Tylenol Sinus Suspension Liquid 2017
Infants' Tylenol Cold Decongestant and Fever Reducer Concentrated Drops 2015
Infants' Tylenol Cold Decongestant and Fever Reducer Concentrated Drops Plus Cough .. 2015
Junior Strength Tylenol Soft Chews Chewable Tablets 2014
Tylenol 2009
Tylenol Allergy Sinus 2010
Tylenol Severe Allergy Caplets 2010
Multi-Symptom Tylenol Cold Complete Formula Caplets 2010
Multi-Symptom Tylenol Cold Non-Drowsy Caplets and Gelcaps 2010
Multi-Symptom Tylenol Cold Severe Congestion Non-Drowsy Caplets 2011
Maximum Strength Tylenol Flu NightTime Gelcaps 2011
Maximum Strength Tylenol Flu NightTime Liquid 2011
Maximum Strength Tylenol Flu Non-Drowsy Gelcaps 2011
Extra Strength Tylenol PM Caplets, Geltabs, and Gelcaps 2012
Maximum Strength Tylenol Sinus NightTime Caplets 2012
Maximum Strength Tylenol Sinus Non-Drowsy Geltabs, Gelcaps, Caplets, and Tablets 2012
Maximum Strength Tylenol Sore Throat Adult Liquid 2013
Tylenol with Codeine 2595
Women's Tylenol Menstrual Relief Caplets 2013
Tylox Capsules 2597
Ultracet Tablets 2597
Vanquish Caplets 617
Vicks 44M Cough, Cold & Flu Relief Liquid 725
Vicks DayQuil LiquiCaps/Liquid Multi-Symptom Cold/Flu Relief ... 727
Vicks NyQuil LiquiCaps/Liquid Multi-Symptom Cold/Flu Relief, Original and Cherry Flavors 727
Vicodin Tablets 516
Vicodin ES Tablets 517
Vicodin HP Tablets 518
Zydone Tablets 1330

Albuterol (Decrease in circulating catecholamines with smoking cessation; may require an increase in dose at cessation of smoking). Products include:
Proventil Inhalation Aerosol 3142
Ventolin Inhalation Aerosol and Refill 1679

Albuterol Sulfate (Decrease in circulating catecholamines with smoking cessation; may require an increase in dose at cessation of smoking). Products include:
AccuNeb Inhalation Solution 1230
Combivent Inhalation Aerosol 1041
DuoNeb Inhalation Solution 1233
Proventil Inhalation Solution 0.083% 3146
Proventil Repetabs Tablets 3148
Proventil Solution for Inhalation 0.5% 3144
Proventil HFA Inhalation Aerosol 3150
Ventolin HFA Inhalation Aerosol 3618
Volmax Extended-Release Tablets .. 2276

Aminophylline (Deinduction of hepatic enzyme on smoking cessation; may require a decrease in dose at cessation of smoking).
No products indexed under this heading.

Atenolol (Deinduction of hepatic enzyme on smoking cessation; may require a decrease in dose at cessation of smoking). Products include:
Tenoretic Tablets 690
Tenormin I.V. Injection 692

Betaxolol Hydrochloride (Deinduction of hepatic enzyme on smoking cessation; may require a decrease in dose at cessation of smoking). Products include:
Betoptic S Ophthalmic Suspension 537

Bisoprolol Fumarate (Deinduction of hepatic enzyme on smoking cessation; may require a decrease in dose at cessation of smoking). Products include:
Zebeta Tablets 1885
Ziac Tablets 1887

Caffeine (Deinduction of hepatic enzyme on smoking cessation; may require a decrease in dose at cessation of smoking). Products include:
BC Powder 619
Arthritis Strength BC Powder 619
Darvon Compound-65 Pulvules 1910
Aspirin Free Excedrin Caplets and Geltabs 628
Excedrin Extra-Strength Tablets, Caplets, and Geltabs 629
Excedrin Migraine 1070
Goody's Extra Strength Headache Powder 620
Goody's Extra Strength Pain Relief Tablets 620
Hycomine Compound Tablets 1317
Maximum Strength Midol Menstrual Caplets and Gelcaps .. 612
Vanquish Caplets 617
Vivarin 763

Carteolol Hydrochloride (Deinduction of hepatic enzyme on smok-

IMPORTANT NOTE: Always consult each drug listing in the patient's regimen for possible interactions.

ing cessation; may require a decrease in dose at cessation of smoking). Products include:
- Carteolol Hydrochloride Ophthalmic Solution USP, 1% ..... ⊙258
- Ocupress Ophthalmic Solution, 1% Sterile ..... ⊙303

Dobutamine Hydrochloride (Decrease in circulating catecholamines with smoking cessation; may require an increase in dose at cessation of smoking). Products include:
- Dobutrex Solution Vials 1914

Dopamine Hydrochloride (Decrease in circulating catecholamines with smoking cessation; may require an increase in dose at cessation of smoking).
- No products indexed under this heading.

Dyphylline (Deinduction of hepatic enzyme on smoking cessation; may require a decrease in dose at cessation of smoking). Products include:
- Lufyllin Tablets 3347
- Lufyllin-400 Tablets 3347
- Lufyllin-GG Elixir 3348
- Lufyllin-GG Tablets 3348

Ephedrine Hydrochloride (Decrease in circulating catecholamines with smoking cessation; may require an increase in dose at cessation of smoking). Products include:
- Primatene Tablets ..... ▣780

Ephedrine Sulfate (Decrease in circulating catecholamines with smoking cessation; may require an increase in dose at cessation of smoking).
- No products indexed under this heading.

Ephedrine Tannate (Decrease in circulating catecholamines with smoking cessation; may require an increase in dose at cessation of smoking). Products include:
- Rynatuss Pediatric Suspension 3353
- Rynatuss Tablets 3353

Epinephrine (Decrease in circulating catecholamines with smoking cessation; may require an increase in dose at cessation of smoking). Products include:
- Epifrin Sterile Ophthalmic Solution ..... ⊙235
- EpiPen 1236
- Primatene Mist ..... ▣779
- Xylocaine with Epinephrine Injection 653

Epinephrine Bitartrate (Decrease in circulating catecholamines with smoking cessation; may require an increase in dose at cessation of smoking). Products include:
- Sensorcaine 643

Epinephrine Hydrochloride (Decrease in circulating catecholamines with smoking cessation; may require an increase in dose at cessation of smoking).
- No products indexed under this heading.

Esmolol Hydrochloride (Deinduction of hepatic enzyme on smoking cessation; may require a decrease in dose at cessation of smoking). Products include:
- Brevibloc Injection 858

Imipramine Hydrochloride (Deinduction of hepatic enzyme on smoking cessation; may require a decrease in dose at cessation of smoking).
- No products indexed under this heading.

Imipramine Pamoate (Deinduction of hepatic enzyme on smoking cessation; may require a decrease in dose at cessation of smoking).
- No products indexed under this heading.

Insulin, Human, Zinc Suspension (Increase of subcutaneous insulin absorption with smoking cessation; may require a decrease in dose at cessation of smoking). Products include:
- Humulin L, 100 Units 1937
- Humulin U, 100 Units 1943
- Novolin L Human Insulin 10 ml Vials 2422

Insulin, Human NPH (Increase of subcutaneous insulin absorption with smoking cessation; may require a decrease in dose at cessation of smoking). Products include:
- Humulin N, 100 Units 1939
- Humulin N NPH Pen 1940
- Novolin N Human Insulin 10 ml Vials 2422
- Novolin N PenFill 2423
- Novolin N Prefilled Syringe Disposable Insulin Delivery System 2425

Insulin, Human Regular (Increase of subcutaneous insulin absorption with smoking cessation; may require a decrease in dose at cessation of smoking). Products include:
- Humulin R Regular (U-500) 1943
- Humulin R, 100 Units 1941
- Novolin R Human Insulin 10 ml Vials 2423
- Novolin R PenFill 2423
- Novolin R Prefilled Syringe Disposable Insulin Delivery System 2425
- Velosulin BR Human Insulin 10 ml Vials 2435

Insulin, Human Regular and Human NPH Mixture (Increase of subcutaneous insulin absorption with smoking cessation; may require a decrease in dose at cessation of smoking). Products include:
- Humulin 50/50, 100 Units 1934
- Humulin 70/30, 100 Units 1935
- Humulin 70/30 Pen 1936
- Novolin 70/30 Human Insulin 10 ml Vials 2421
- Novolin 70/30 PenFill 2423
- Novolin 70/30 Prefilled Disposable Insulin Delivery System 2425

Insulin, NPH (Increase of subcutaneous insulin absorption with smoking cessation; may require a decrease in dose at cessation of smoking). Products include:
- Iletin II, NPH (Pork), 100 Units 1946

Insulin, Regular (Increase of subcutaneous insulin absorption with smoking cessation; may require a decrease in dose at cessation of smoking). Products include:
- Iletin II, Regular (Pork), 100 Units 1947

Insulin, Zinc Crystals (Increase of subcutaneous insulin absorption with smoking cessation; may require a decrease in dose at cessation of smoking).
- No products indexed under this heading.

Insulin, Zinc Suspension (Increase of subcutaneous insulin absorption with smoking cessation; may require a decrease in dose at cessation of smoking). Products include:
- Iletin II, Lente (Pork), 100 Units 1945

Insulin Aspart, Human Regular (Increase of subcutaneous insulin absorption with smoking cessation; may require a decrease in dose at cessation of smoking).
- No products indexed under this heading.

Insulin glargine (Increase of subcutaneous insulin absorption with smoking cessation; may require a decrease in dose at cessation of smoking). Products include:
- Lantus Injection 742

Insulin Lispro, Human (Increase of subcutaneous insulin absorption with smoking cessation; may require a decrease in dose at cessation of smoking). Products include:
- Humalog 1926
- Humalog Mix 75/25 Pen 1928

Insulin Lispro Protamine, Human (Increase of subcutaneous insulin absorption with smoking cessation; may require a decrease in dose at cessation of smoking). Products include:
- Humalog Mix 75/25 Pen 1928

Isoproterenol Hydrochloride (Decrease in circulating catecholamines with smoking cessation; may require an increase in dose at cessation of smoking).
- No products indexed under this heading.

Isoproterenol Sulfate (Decrease in circulating catecholamines with smoking cessation; may require an increase in dose at cessation of smoking).
- No products indexed under this heading.

Labetalol Hydrochloride (Decrease in circulating catecholamines with smoking cessation; may require a decrease in dose at cessation of smoking). Products include:
- Normodyne Injection 3135
- Normodyne Tablets 3137

Levalbuterol Hydrochloride (Decrease in circulating catecholamines with smoking cessation; may require an increase in dose at cessation of smoking). Products include:
- Xopenex Inhalation Solution 3207

Levobunolol Hydrochloride (Deinduction of hepatic enzyme on smoking cessation; may require a decrease in dose at cessation of smoking). Products include:
- Betagan ..... ⊙228

Metaproterenol Sulfate (Decrease in circulating catecholamines with smoking cessation; may require an increase in dose at cessation of smoking). Products include:
- Alupent 1029

Metaraminol Bitartrate (Decrease in circulating catecholamines with smoking cessation; may require an increase in dose at cessation of smoking). Products include:
- Aramine Injection 2043

Methoxamine Hydrochloride (Decrease in circulating catecholamines with smoking cessation; may require an increase in dose at cessation of smoking).
- No products indexed under this heading.

Metipranolol Hydrochloride (Deinduction of hepatic enzyme on smoking cessation; may require a decrease in dose at cessation of smoking).
- No products indexed under this heading.

Metoprolol Succinate (Deinduction of hepatic enzyme on smoking cessation; may require a decrease in dose at cessation of smoking). Products include:
- Toprol-XL Tablets 651

Metoprolol Tartrate (Deinduction of hepatic enzyme on smoking cessation; may require a decrease in dose at cessation of smoking).
- No products indexed under this heading.

Nadolol (Deinduction of hepatic enzyme on smoking cessation; may require a decrease in dose at cessation of smoking). Products include:
- Corgard Tablets 2245
- Corzide 40/5 Tablets 2247
- Corzide 80/5 Tablets 2247
- Nadolol Tablets 2288

Norepinephrine Bitartrate (Decrease in circulating catecholamines with smoking cessation; may require an increase in dose at cessation of smoking).
- No products indexed under this heading.

Oxazepam (Deinduction of hepatic enzyme on smoking cessation; may require a decrease in dose at cessation of smoking).
- No products indexed under this heading.

Penbutolol Sulfate (Deinduction of hepatic enzyme on smoking cessation; may require a decrease in dose at cessation of smoking).
- No products indexed under this heading.

Pentazocine Hydrochloride (Deinduction of hepatic enzyme on smoking cessation; may require a decrease in dose at cessation of smoking). Products include:
- Talacen Caplets 3089
- Talwin Nx Tablets 3090

Pentazocine Lactate (Deinduction of hepatic enzyme on smoking cessation; may require a decrease in dose at cessation of smoking).
- No products indexed under this heading.

Phenylephrine Bitartrate (Decrease in circulating catecholamines with smoking cessation; may require an increase in dose at cessation of smoking).
- No products indexed under this heading.

Phenylephrine Hydrochloride (Decrease in circulating catecholamines with smoking cessation; may require an increase in dose at cessation of smoking). Products include:
- Afrin Nasal Decongestant Children's Pump Mist ..... ▣734
- Extendryl 1361
- Hycomine Compound Tablets 1317
- Neo-Synephrine ..... ▣614
- Phenergan VC Syrup 3560
- Phenergan VC with Codeine Syrup 3561
- Preparation H Cream ..... ▣778
- Preparation H Cooling Gel ..... ▣778
- Preparation H ..... ▣778
- Vicks Sinex Nasal Spray and Ultra Fine Mist ..... ▣729

Phenylephrine Tannate (Decrease in circulating catecholamines with smoking cessation; may require an increase in dose at cessation of smoking). Products include:
- Ryna-12 S Suspension 3351
- Reformulated Rynatan Pediatric Suspension 3352
- Rynatuss Pediatric Suspension 3353
- Rynatuss Tablets 3353

Phenylpropanolamine Hydrochloride (Decrease in circulating catecholamines with smoking cessation; may require an increase in dose at cessation of smoking).
- No products indexed under this heading.

Pindolol (Deinduction of hepatic enzyme on smoking cessation; may require a decrease in dose at cessation of smoking).
- No products indexed under this heading.

Pirbuterol Acetate (Decrease in circulating catecholamines with smoking cessation; may require an increase in dose at cessation of smoking). Products include:
- Maxair Autohaler 1981
- Maxair Inhaler 1984

Prazosin Hydrochloride (Decrease in circulating catecholamines with smoking cessation; may require a decrease in dose at cessation of smoking). Products include:
- Minipress Capsules 2699
- Minizide Capsules 2700

Propranolol Hydrochloride (Deinduction of hepatic enzyme on smoking cessation; may require a decrease in dose at cessation of smoking). Products include:
- Inderal 3513
- Inderal LA Long-Acting Capsules 3516
- Inderide Tablets 3517
- Inderide LA Long-Acting Capsules 3519

Pseudoephedrine Hydrochloride (Decrease in circulating catechola-

mines with smoking cessation; may require an increase in dose at cessation of smoking). Products include:
Actifed Cold & Allergy Tablets 688
Actifed Cold & Sinus Caplets and Tablets 688
Advil Cold and Sinus Caplets 771
Advil Cold and Sinus Tablets 771
Advil Flu & Body Ache Caplets 772
Aleve Cold & Sinus Caplets 603
Alka-Seltzer Plus Liqui-Gels 604
Alka-Seltzer Plus Cold & Flu Medicine Liqui-Gels 604
Alka-Seltzer Plus Cold & Sinus Medicine Liqui-Gels 604
Allegra-D Extended-Release Tablets 714
BC Cold Powder 619
Benadryl Allergy/Cold Tablets 691
Benadryl Allergy/Congestion Tablets 692
Benadryl Allergy & Sinus Liquid 693
Benadryl Allergy & Sinus Fastmelt Tablets 693
Benadryl Allergy Sinus Headache Caplets & Gelcaps 693
Benadryl Severe Allergy & Sinus Headache Caplets 694
Benadryl Children's Allergy/Cold Fastmelt Tablets 692
Benylin Multi-Symptom Liquid 697
Bromfed Capsules (Extended-Release) 2269
Bromfed-PD Capsules (Extended-Release) 2269
Children's Cēpacol Sore Throat 788
Comtrex Acute Head Cold & Sinus Pressure Relief Tablets 627
Comtrex Deep Chest Cold & Congestion Relief Softgels 627
Comtrex Flu Therapy & Fever Relief Daytime Caplets 628
Comtrex Flu Therapy & Fever Relief Nighttime Tablets 628
Comtrex Maximum Strength Multi-Symptom Cold & Cough Relief Tablets and Caplets 626
Contac Non-Drowsy 12 Hour Cold Caplets 745
Contac Non-Drowsy Timed Release 12 Hour Cold Caplets 746
Contac Severe Cold and Flu Caplets Maximum Strength 746
Contac Severe Cold and Flu Caplets Non-Drowsy 746
Dimetapp Elixir 777
Dimetapp Cold and Fever Suspension 775
Dimetapp DM Cold & Cough Elixir 775
Dimetapp Nighttime Flu Liquid 776
Dimetapp Non-Drowsy Flu Syrup 777
Dimetapp Infant Drops Decongestant 775
Dimetapp Infant Drops Decongestant Plus Cough 776
Guaifed 2272
Kronofed-A 1341
Children's Motrin Cold Oral Suspension 2007
Motrin Sinus Headache Caplets 2005
PediaCare Cough-Cold Liquid 719
PediaCare Infants' Drops Decongestant 719
PediaCare Infants' Drops Decongestant Plus Cough 719
PediaCare NightRest Cough-Cold Liquid 719
Robitussin Cold Caplets Cold & Congestion 780
Robitussin Cold Softgels Cold & Congestion 780
Robitussin Cold Caplets Multi-Symptom Cold & Flu 781
Robitussin Cold Softgels Multi-Symptom Cold & Flu 781
Robitussin Cold Softgels Severe Congestion 782
Robitussin Cough & Cold Infant Drops 782
Robitussin Maximum Strength Cough & Cold Liquid 785
Robitussin Pediatric Cough & Cold Formula Liquid 785
Robitussin Multi Symptom Honey Flu Liquid 785
Robitussin Nighttime Honey Flu Liquid 786
Robitussin-CF Liquid 783
Robitussin-DAC Syrup 2942
Robitussin-PE Liquid 782
Ryna 768
Semprex-D Capsules 1172
Singlet Caplets 761
Sinutab Non-Drying Liquid Caps 706
Sinutab Sinus Allergy Medication, Maximum Strength Formula, Tablets & Caplets 707
Sinutab Sinus Medication, Maximum Strength Without Drowsiness Formula, Tablets & Caplets 707
Sudafed 12 Hour Tablets 708
Sudafed 24 Hour Tablets 708
Children's Sudafed Cold & Cough Liquid 709
Children's Sudafed Nasal Decongestant Chewables 711
Children's Sudafed Nasal Decongestant Liquid Medication 711
Sudafed Cold & Allergy Tablets 708
Sudafed Cold & Cough Liquid Caps 709
Sudafed Cold & Sinus Liquid Caps 710
Sudafed Nasal Decongestant Tablets 710
Sudafed Non-Drying Sinus Liquid Caps 712
Sudafed Severe Cold 711
Sudafed Sinus Headache Caplets 712
Sudafed Sinus Headache Tablets 712
Tavist Sinus Non-Drowsy Coated Caplets 676
TheraFlu Regular Strength Cold & Cough Night Time Hot Liquid 676
TheraFlu Regular Strength Cold & Sore Throat Night Time Hot Liquid 676
TheraFlu Maximum Strength Flu & Congestion Non-Drowsy Hot Liquid 677
TheraFlu Maximum Strength Flu & Cough Night Time Hot Liquid 678
TheraFlu Maximum Strength Flu & Sore Throat Night Time Hot Liquid 677
TheraFlu Maximum Strength Severe Cold & Congestion Night Time Caplets 678
TheraFlu Maximum Strength Severe Cold & Congestion Night Time Hot Liquid 678
TheraFlu Maximum Strength Severe Cold & Congestion Non-Drowsy 679
Triaminic Allergy Congestion Liquid 680
Triaminic Chest Congestion Liquid 680
Triaminic Cold & Allergy Liquid 681
Triaminic Cold & Allergy Softchews 683
Triaminic Cold & Cough Liquid 681
Triaminic Cold & Cough Softchews 683
Triaminic Cold & Night Time Cough Liquid 681
Triaminic Cold, Cough & Fever Liquid 681
Triaminic Cough Liquid 682
Triaminic Cough & Congestion Liquid 682
Triaminic Cough & Sore Throat Liquid 682
Triaminic Cough & Sore Throat Softchews 684
Children's Tylenol Allergy-D Liquid 2014
Children's Tylenol Cold Suspension Liquid and Chewable Tablets 2015
Children's Tylenol Cold Plus Cough Suspension Liquid and Chewable Tablets 2015
Children's Tylenol Flu Suspension Liquid 2015
Children's Tylenol Sinus Suspension Liquid 2017
Infants' Tylenol Cold Decongestant and Fever Reducer Concentrated Drops 2015
Infants' Tylenol Cold Decongestant and Fever Reducer Concentrated Drops Plus Cough 2015
Tylenol Allergy Sinus 2010
Multi-Symptom Tylenol Cold Complete Formula Caplets 2010
Multi-Symptom Tylenol Cold Non-Drowsy Caplets and Gelcaps 2010
Multi-Symptom Tylenol Cold Severe Congestion Non-Drowsy Caplets 2011
Maximum Strength Tylenol Flu NightTime Gelcaps 2011
Maximum Strength Tylenol Flu NightTime Liquid 2011
Maximum Strength Tylenol Flu Non-Drowsy Gelcaps 2011
Maximum Strength Tylenol Sinus NightTime Caplets 2012
Maximum Strength Tylenol Sinus Non-Drowsy Geltabs, Gelcaps, Caplets, and Tablets 2012
Vicks 44D Cough & Head Congestion Relief Liquid 724
Vicks 44M Cough, Cold & Flu Relief Liquid 725
Pediatric Vicks 44m Cough & Cold Relief 728
Vicks DayQuil LiquiCaps/Liquid Multi-Symptom Cold/Flu Relief 727
Children's Vicks NyQuil Cold/Cough Relief 726
Vicks NyQuil LiquiCaps/Liquid Multi-Symptom Cold/Flu Relief, Original and Cherry Flavors 727
Zephrex Tablets 3091
Zephrex LA Tablets 3092
Zyrtec-D 12 Hour Extended Relief Tablets 2758

Pseudoephedrine Sulfate (Decrease in circulating catecholamines with smoking cessation; may require an increase in dose at cessation of smoking). Products include:
Chlor-Trimeton Allergy/Decongestant Tablets 736
Claritin-D 12 Hour Extended Release Tablets 3102
Claritin-D 24 Hour Extended Release Tablets 3104
Coricidin 'D' Cold, Flu & Sinus Tablets 737
Drixoral Allergy/Sinus Extended-Release Tablets 741
Drixoral Cold & Allergy Sustained-Action Tablets 740
Drixoral Cold & Flu Extended-Release Tablets 740
Drixoral Nasal Decongestant Long-Acting Non-Drowsy Tablets 740
Rynatan Tablets 3351

Salmeterol Xinafoate (Decrease in circulating catecholamines with smoking cessation; may require an increase in dose at cessation of smoking). Products include:
Advair Diskus 100/50 1448
Advair Diskus 250/50 1448
Advair Diskus 500/50 1448
Serevent Diskus 1637
Serevent Inhalation Aerosol 1633

Sotalol Hydrochloride (Deinduction of hepatic enzyme on smoking cessation; may require a decrease in dose at cessation of smoking). Products include:
Betapace Tablets 950
Betapace AF Tablets 954

Terbutaline Sulfate (Decrease in circulating catecholamines with smoking cessation; may require an increase in dose at cessation of smoking). Products include:
Brethine Ampuls 2314
Brethine Tablets 2313

Theophylline (Deinduction of hepatic enzyme on smoking cessation; may require a decrease in dose at cessation of smoking). Products include:
Aerolate 1361
Theo-Dur Extended-Release Tablets 1835
Uni-Dur Extended-Release Tablets 1841
Uniphyl 400 mg and 600 mg Tablets 2903

Theophylline Calcium Salicylate (Deinduction of hepatic enzyme on smoking cessation; may require a decrease in dose at cessation of smoking).
No products indexed under this heading.

Theophylline Sodium Glycinate (Deinduction of hepatic enzyme on smoking cessation; may require a decrease in dose at cessation of smoking).
No products indexed under this heading.

Timolol Hemihydrate (Deinduction of hepatic enzyme on smoking cessation; may require a decrease in dose at cessation of smoking). Products include:
Betimol Ophthalmic Solution .... ⊙ 324

Timolol Maleate (Deinduction of hepatic enzyme on smoking cessation; may require a decrease in dose at cessation of smoking). Products include:
Blocadren Tablets 2046
Cosopt Sterile Ophthalmic Solution 2065
Timolide Tablets 2187
Timolol GFS .... ⊙ 266
Timoptic in Ocudose 2192
Timoptic Sterile Ophthalmic Solution 2190
Timoptic-XE Sterile Ophthalmic Gel Forming Solution 2194

Xylometazoline Hydrochloride (The extent of absorption and peak plasma concentration is slightly reduced in patients with common cold/rhinitis; time to peak concentration is prolonged with the use of xylometazoline). Products include:
Natru-Vent Nasal Spray, Adult Strength 624
Natru-Vent Nasal Spray, Pediatric Strength 625

NICOTROL PATCH
(Nicotine) 2840
None cited in PDR database.

NIFEREX ELIXIR
(Polysaccharide-Iron Complex) 3176
None cited in PDR database.

NIFEREX TABLETS
(Polysaccharide-Iron Complex) 3176
None cited in PDR database.

NIFEREX-150 CAPSULES
(Polysaccharide-Iron Complex) 3176
None cited in PDR database.

NILANDRON TABLETS
(Nilutamide) 753
May interact with phenytoin, vitamin K antagonists, theophylline, and certain other agents. Compounds in these categories include:

Aminophylline (Co-administration of nilutamide with theophylline may result in delayed elimination and increase in its serum half-life leading to a toxic level).
No products indexed under this heading.

Dicumarol (Co-administration of nilutamide with vitamin K antagonists may result in delayed elimination and increases in their serum half-life leading to a toxic level).
No products indexed under this heading.

Dyphylline (Co-administration of nilutamide with theophylline may result in delayed elimination and increase in its serum half-life leading to a toxic level). Products include:
Lufyllin Tablets 3347
Lufyllin-400 Tablets 3347
Lufyllin-GG Elixir 3348
Lufyllin-GG Tablets 3348

Fosphenytoin Sodium (Co-administration of nilutamide with phenytoin may result in delayed elimination and increase in its serum half-life leading to a toxic level). Products include:
Cerebyx Injection 2619

Phenytoin (Co-administration of nilutamide with phenytoin may result in delayed elimination and increase in its serum half-life leading to a toxic level). Products include:
Dilantin Infatabs 2624
Dilantin-125 Oral Suspension 2625

Phenytoin Sodium (Co-administration of nilutamide with phenytoin may result in delayed elimination and increase in its serum half-life leading to a toxic level). Products include:
Dilantin Kapseals 2622

Theophylline (Co-administration of nilutamide with theophylline may result in delayed elimination and increase in its serum half-life leading to a toxic level). Products include:

Aerolate 1361
Theo-Dur Extended-Release Tablets 1835
Uni-Dur Extended-Release Tablets .. 1841
Uniphyl 400 mg and 600 mg Tablets 2903

Theophylline Calcium Salicylate (Co-administration of nilutamide with theophylline may result in delayed elimination and increase in its serum half-life leading to a toxic level).
No products indexed under this heading.

Theophylline Sodium Glycinate (Co-administration of nilutamide with theophylline may result in delayed elimination and increase in its serum half-life leading to a toxic level).
No products indexed under this heading.

Warfarin Sodium (Co-administration of nilutamide with vitamin K antagonists may result in delayed elimination and increases in their serum half-life leading to a toxic level). Products include:
Coumadin for Injection 1243
Coumadin Tablets 1243
Warfarin Sodium Tablets, USP 3302

Food Interactions

Alcohol (Because of possibility of an intolerance to alcohol (facial flushes, malaise, hypotension) following ingestion of Nilandron, it is recommended that intake of alcohol be avoided by patients who experience this reaction).

NIMOTOP CAPSULES

(Nimodipine) 904
May interact with antihypertensives, calcium channel blockers, and certain other agents. Compounds in these categories include:

Acebutolol Hydrochloride (Concomitant administration results in intensified effect). Products include:
Sectral Capsules 3589

Amlodipine Besylate (Possibility of enhanced cardiovascular action). Products include:
Lotrel Capsules 2370
Norvasc Tablets 2704

Atenolol (Concomitant administration results in intensified effect). Products include:
Tenoretic Tablets 690
Tenormin I.V. Injection 692

Benazepril Hydrochloride (Concomitant administration results in intensified effect). Products include:
Lotensin Tablets 2365
Lotensin HCT Tablets 2367
Lotrel Capsules 2370

Bendroflumethiazide (Concomitant administration results in intensified effect). Products include:
Corzide 40/5 Tablets 2247
Corzide 80/5 Tablets 2247

Bepridil Hydrochloride (Possibility of enhanced cardiovascular action). Products include:
Vascor Tablets 2602

Betaxolol Hydrochloride (Concomitant administration results in intensified effect). Products include:
Betoptic S Ophthalmic Suspension 537

Bisoprolol Fumarate (Concomitant administration results in intensified effect). Products include:
Zebeta Tablets 1885
Ziac Tablets 1887

Candesartan Cilexetil (Concomitant administration results in intensified effect). Products include:
Atacand Tablets 595
Atacand HCT Tablets 597

Captopril (Concomitant administration results in intensified effect). Products include:
Captopril Tablets 2281

Carteolol Hydrochloride (Concomitant administration results in intensified effect). Products include:
Carteolol Hydrochloride Ophthalmic Solution USP, 1% .... ⊙258
Ocupress Ophthalmic Solution, 1% Sterile .... ⊙303

Chlorothiazide (Concomitant administration results in intensified effect). Products include:
Aldoclor Tablets 2035
Diuril Oral 2087

Chlorothiazide Sodium (Concomitant administration results in intensified effect). Products include:
Diuril Sodium Intravenous 2086

Chlorthalidone (Concomitant administration results in intensified effect). Products include:
Clorpres Tablets 1002
Combipres Tablets 1040
Tenoretic Tablets 690

Cimetidine (May increase peak nimodipine plasma concentrations and AUC). Products include:
Tagamet HB 200 Suspension .... ▣762
Tagamet HB 200 Tablets .... ▣761
Tagamet Tablets 1644

Cimetidine Hydrochloride (May increase peak nimodipine plasma concentrations and AUC). Products include:
Tagamet 1644

Clonidine (Concomitant administration results in intensified effect). Products include:
Catapres-TTS 1038

Clonidine Hydrochloride (Concomitant administration results in intensified effect). Products include:
Catapres Tablets 1037
Clorpres Tablets 1002
Combipres Tablets 1040
Duraclon Injection 3057

Deserpidine (Concomitant administration results in intensified effect).
No products indexed under this heading.

Diazoxide (Concomitant administration results in intensified effect).
No products indexed under this heading.

Diltiazem Hydrochloride (Possibility of enhanced cardiovascular action). Products include:
Cardizem Injectable 1018
Cardizem Lyo-Ject Syringe 1018
Cardizem Monovial 1018
Cardizem CD Capsules 1016
Tiazac Capsules 1378

Doxazosin Mesylate (Concomitant administration results in intensified effect). Products include:
Cardura Tablets 2668

Enalapril Maleate (Concomitant administration results in intensified effect). Products include:
Lexxel Tablets 608
Vaseretic Tablets 2204
Vasotec Tablets 2210

Enalaprilat (Concomitant administration results in intensified effect). Products include:
Enalaprilat Injection 863
Vasotec I.V. Injection 2207

Eprosartan Mesylate (Concomitant administration results in intensified effect). Products include:
Teveten Tablets 3327

Esmolol Hydrochloride (Concomitant administration results in intensified effect). Products include:
Brevibloc Injection 858

Felodipine (Possibility of enhanced cardiovascular action). Products include:
Lexxel Tablets 608
Plendil Extended-Release Tablets ... 623

Fosinopril Sodium (Concomitant administration results in intensified effect). Products include:
Monopril Tablets 1091
Monopril HCT 1094

Furosemide (Concomitant administration results in intensified effect). Products include:
Furosemide Tablets 2284

Guanabenz Acetate (Concomitant administration results in intensified effect).
No products indexed under this heading.

Guanethidine Monosulfate (Concomitant administration results in intensified effect).
No products indexed under this heading.

Hydralazine Hydrochloride (Concomitant administration results in intensified effect).
No products indexed under this heading.

Hydrochlorothiazide (Concomitant administration results in intensified effect). Products include:
Accuretic Tablets 2614
Aldoril Tablets 2039
Atacand HCT Tablets 597
Avalide Tablets 1070
Diovan HCT Tablets 2338
Dyazide Capsules 1515
HydroDIURIL Tablets 2108
Hyzaar 2109
Inderide Tablets 3517
Inderide LA Long-Acting Capsules .. 3519
Lotensin HCT Tablets 2367
Maxzide 1008
Micardis HCT Tablets 1051
Microzide Capsules 3414
Moduretic Tablets 2138
Monopril HCT 1094
Prinzide Tablets 2168
Timolide Tablets 2187
Uniretic Tablets 3178
Vaseretic Tablets 2204
Zestoretic Tablets 695
Ziac Tablets 1887

Hydroflumethiazide (Concomitant administration results in intensified effect). Products include:
Diucardin Tablets 3494

Indapamide (Concomitant administration results in intensified effect). Products include:
Indapamide Tablets 2286

Irbesartan (Concomitant administration results in intensified effect). Products include:
Avalide Tablets 1070
Avapro Tablets 1074
Avapro Tablets 3076

Isradipine (Possibility of enhanced cardiovascular action). Products include:
DynaCirc Capsules 2921
DynaCirc CR Tablets 2923

Labetalol Hydrochloride (Concomitant administration results in intensified effect). Products include:
Normodyne Injection 3135
Normodyne Tablets 3137

Lisinopril (Concomitant administration results in intensified effect). Products include:
Prinivil Tablets 2164
Prinzide Tablets 2168
Zestoretic Tablets 695
Zestril Tablets 698

Losartan Potassium (Concomitant administration results in intensified effect). Products include:
Cozaar Tablets 2067
Hyzaar 2109

Mecamylamine Hydrochloride (Concomitant administration results in intensified effect). Products include:
Inversine Tablets 1850

Methyclothiazide (Concomitant administration results in intensified effect).
No products indexed under this heading.

Methyldopa (Concomitant administration results in intensified effect). Products include:
Aldoclor Tablets 2035
Aldomet Tablets 2037
Aldoril Tablets 2039

Methyldopate Hydrochloride (Concomitant administration results in intensified effect).
No products indexed under this heading.

Metolazone (Concomitant administration results in intensified effect). Products include:
Mykrox Tablets 1168
Zaroxolyn Tablets 1177

Metoprolol Succinate (Concomitant administration results in intensified effect). Products include:
Toprol-XL Tablets 651

Metoprolol Tartrate (Concomitant administration results in intensified effect).
No products indexed under this heading.

Metyrosine (Concomitant administration results in intensified effect). Products include:
Demser Capsules 2085

Mibefradil Dihydrochloride (Possibility of enhanced cardiovascular action).
No products indexed under this heading.

Minoxidil (Concomitant administration results in intensified effect). Products include:
Rogaine Extra Strength for Men Topical Solution .... ▣721
Rogaine for Women Topical Solution .... ▣721

Moexipril Hydrochloride (Concomitant administration results in intensified effect). Products include:
Uniretic Tablets 3178
Univasc Tablets 3181

Nadolol (Concomitant administration results in intensified effect). Products include:
Corgard Tablets 2245
Corzide 40/5 Tablets 2247
Corzide 80/5 Tablets 2247
Nadolol Tablets 2288

Nicardipine Hydrochloride (Possibility of enhanced cardiovascular action). Products include:
Cardene I.V. 3485

Nifedipine (Possibility of enhanced cardiovascular action). Products include:
Adalat CC Tablets 877
Procardia Capsules 2708
Procardia XL Extended Release Tablets 2710

Nisoldipine (Possibility of enhanced cardiovascular action). Products include:
Sular Tablets 688

Nitroglycerin (Concomitant administration results in intensified effect). Products include:
Nitro-Dur Transdermal Infusion System 3134
Nitro-Dur Transdermal Infusion System 1834
Nitrolingual Pumpspray 1355
Nitrostat Tablets 2658

Penbutolol Sulfate (Concomitant administration results in intensified effect).
No products indexed under this heading.

Perindopril Erbumine (Concomitant administration results in intensified effect). Products include:
Aceon Tablets (2 mg, 4 mg, 8 mg) 3249

Phenoxybenzamine Hydrochloride (Concomitant administration results in intensified effect). Products include:
Dibenzyline Capsules 3457

Phentolamine Mesylate (Concomitant administration results in intensified effect).
No products indexed under this heading.

Phenytoin (Potential for phenytoin toxicity). Products include:
Dilantin Infatabs 2624
Dilantin-125 Oral Suspension 2625

Phenytoin Sodium (Potential for phenytoin toxicity). Products include:

Dilantin Kapseals 2622

Pindolol (Concomitant administration results in intensified effect).
No products indexed under this heading.

Polythiazide (Concomitant administration results in intensified effect). Products include:
Minizide Capsules 2700
Renese Tablets 2712

Prazosin Hydrochloride (Concomitant administration results in intensified effect). Products include:
Minipress Capsules 2699
Minizide Capsules 2700

Propranolol Hydrochloride (Concomitant administration results in intensified effect). Products include:
Inderal 3513
Inderal LA Long-Acting Capsules 3516
Inderide Tablets 3517
Inderide LA Long-Acting Capsules .. 3519

Quinapril Hydrochloride (Concomitant administration results in intensified effect). Products include:
Accupril Tablets 2611
Accuretic Tablets 2614

Ramipril (Concomitant administration results in intensified effect). Products include:
Altace Capsules 2233

Rauwolfia serpentina (Concomitant administration results in intensified effect).
No products indexed under this heading.

Rescinnamine (Concomitant administration results in intensified effect).
No products indexed under this heading.

Reserpine (Concomitant administration results in intensified effect).
No products indexed under this heading.

Sodium Nitroprusside (Concomitant administration results in intensified effect).
No products indexed under this heading.

Sotalol Hydrochloride (Concomitant administration results in intensified effect). Products include:
Betapace Tablets 950
Betapace AF Tablets 954

Spirapril Hydrochloride (Concomitant administration results in intensified effect).
No products indexed under this heading.

Telmisartan (Concomitant administration results in intensified effect). Products include:
Micardis Tablets 1049
Micardis HCT Tablets 1051

Terazosin Hydrochloride (Concomitant administration results in intensified effect). Products include:
Hytrin Capsules 464

Timolol Maleate (Concomitant administration results in intensified effect). Products include:
Blocadren Tablets 2046
Cosopt Sterile Ophthalmic Solution 2065
Timolide Tablets 2187
Timolol GFS .... ⊙266
Timoptic in Ocudose 2192
Timoptic Sterile Ophthalmic Solution 2190
Timoptic-XE Sterile Ophthalmic Gel Forming Solution 2194

Torsemide (Concomitant administration results in intensified effect). Products include:
Demadex Tablets and Injection 2965

Trandolapril (Concomitant administration results in intensified effect). Products include:
Mavik Tablets 478
Tarka Tablets 508

Trimethaphan Camsylate (Concomitant administration results in intensified effect).
No products indexed under this heading.

Valsartan (Concomitant administration results in intensified effect). Products include:
Diovan Capsules 2337
Diovan HCT Tablets 2338

Verapamil Hydrochloride (Possibility of enhanced cardiovascular action). Products include:
Covera-HS Tablets 3199
Isoptin SR Tablets 467
Tarka Tablets 508
Verelan Capsules 3184
Verelan PM Capsules 3186

Food Interactions

Meal, unspecified (Administration of nimodipine capsules following a standard breakfast resulted in 68% lower peak plasma concentration and 38% lower bioavailability).

NIPENT FOR INJECTION
(Pentostatin) 3272
May interact with:

Allopurinol (Both drugs are associated with skin rashes; concomitant therapy in one patient has resulted in a fatal hypersensitivity vasculitis).
No products indexed under this heading.

Carmustine (BCNU) (Co-administration with high dose cyclophosphamide, carmustine, and etoposide has resulted in a report of acute pulmonary edema, hypotension, and death). Products include:
Gliadel Wafer 1723

Cyclophosphamide (Co-administration with high dose cyclophosphamide, carmustine, and etoposide has resulted in a report of acute pulmonary edema, hypotension, and death).
No products indexed under this heading.

Etoposide (Co-administration with high dose cyclophosphamide, carmustine, and etoposide has resulted in a report of acute pulmonary edema, hypotension, and death).
No products indexed under this heading.

Fludarabine Phosphate (Increased risk of fatal pulmonary toxicity; combined use is not recommended). Products include:
Fludara for Injection 995

Vidarabine (Enhanced effects of vidarabine and may result in increased adverse reactions associated with each drug).
No products indexed under this heading.

NITRO-DUR TRANSDERMAL INFUSION SYSTEM
(Nitroglycerin) 3134
May interact with calcium channel blockers, vasodilators, and certain other agents. Compounds in these categories include:

Amlodipine Besylate (Vasodilating effects of nitroglycerin may be additive with those of other vasodilators). Products include:
Lotrel Capsules 2370
Norvasc Tablets 2704

Bepridil Hydrochloride (Vasodilating effects of nitroglycerin may be additive with those of other vasodilators). Products include:
Vascor Tablets 2602

Diazoxide (Vasodilating effects of nitroglycerin may be additive with those of other vasodilators).
No products indexed under this heading.

Diltiazem Hydrochloride (Vasodilating effects of nitroglycerin may be additive with those of other vasodilators). Products include:
Cardizem Injectable 1018
Cardizem Lyo-Ject Syringe 1018
Cardizem Monovial 1018
Cardizem CD Capsules 1016
Tiazac Capsules 1378

Epoprostenol Sodium (Vasodilating effects of nitroglycerin may be additive with those of other vasodilators). Products include:
Flolan for Injection 1528

Felodipine (Vasodilating effects of nitroglycerin may be additive with those of other vasodilators). Products include:
Lexxel Tablets 608
Plendil Extended-Release Tablets ... 623

Hydralazine Hydrochloride (Vasodilating effects of nitroglycerin may be additive with those of other vasodilators).
No products indexed under this heading.

Isradipine (Vasodilating effects of nitroglycerin may be additive with those of other vasodilators). Products include:
DynaCirc Capsules 2921
DynaCirc CR Tablets 2923

Mibefradil Dihydrochloride (Vasodilating effects of nitroglycerin may be additive with those of other vasodilators).
No products indexed under this heading.

Minoxidil (Vasodilating effects of nitroglycerin may be additive with those of other vasodilators). Products include:
Rogaine Extra Strength for Men Topical Solution 721
Rogaine for Women Topical Solution 721

Nicardipine Hydrochloride (Vasodilating effects of nitroglycerin may be additive with those of other vasodilators). Products include:
Cardene I.V. 3485

Nifedipine (Vasodilating effects of nitroglycerin may be additive with those of other vasodilators). Products include:
Adalat CC Tablets 877
Procardia Capsules 2708
Procardia XL Extended Release Tablets 2710

Nimodipine (Vasodilating effects of nitroglycerin may be additive with those of other vasodilators). Products include:
Nimotop Capsules 904

Nisoldipine (Vasodilating effects of nitroglycerin may be additive with those of other vasodilators). Products include:
Sular Tablets 688

Sildenafil Citrate (Amplification of the vasodilatory effects of the nitroglycerin patch by sildenafil can result in severe hypotension). Products include:
Viagra Tablets 2732

Verapamil Hydrochloride (Vasodilating effects of nitroglycerin may be additive with those of other vasodilators). Products include:
Covera-HS Tablets 3199
Isoptin SR Tablets 467
Tarka Tablets 508
Verelan Capsules 3184
Verelan PM Capsules 3186

Food Interactions

Alcohol (Enhances sensitivity to the hypotensive effects).

NITRO-DUR TRANSDERMAL INFUSION SYSTEM
(Nitroglycerin) 1834
May interact with calcium channel blockers, vasodilators, and certain other agents. Compounds in these categories include:

Amlodipine Besylate (Vasodilating effects of nitroglycerin may be additive with those of other vasodilators). Products include:
Lotrel Capsules 2370
Norvasc Tablets 2704

Bepridil Hydrochloride (Vasodilating effects of nitroglycerin may be additive with those of other vasodilators). Products include:
Vascor Tablets 2602

Diazoxide (Vasodilating effects of nitroglycerin may be additive with those of other vasodilators).
No products indexed under this heading.

Diltiazem Hydrochloride (Vasodilating effects of nitroglycerin may be additive with those of other vasodilators). Products include:
Cardizem Injectable 1018
Cardizem Lyo-Ject Syringe 1018
Cardizem Monovial 1018
Cardizem CD Capsules 1016
Tiazac Capsules 1378

Epoprostenol Sodium (Vasodilating effects of nitroglycerin may be additive with those of other vasodilators). Products include:
Flolan for Injection 1528

Felodipine (Vasodilating effects of nitroglycerin may be additive with those of other vasodilators). Products include:
Lexxel Tablets 608
Plendil Extended-Release Tablets ... 623

Hydralazine Hydrochloride (Vasodilating effects of nitroglycerin may be additive with those of other vasodilators).
No products indexed under this heading.

Isradipine (Vasodilating effects of nitroglycerin may be additive with those of other vasodilators). Products include:
DynaCirc Capsules 2921
DynaCirc CR Tablets 2923

Mibefradil Dihydrochloride (Vasodilating effects of nitroglycerin may be additive with those of other vasodilators).
No products indexed under this heading.

Minoxidil (Vasodilating effects of nitroglycerin may be additive with those of other vasodilators). Products include:
Rogaine Extra Strength for Men Topical Solution 721
Rogaine for Women Topical Solution 721

Nicardipine Hydrochloride (Vasodilating effects of nitroglycerin may be additive with those of other vasodilators). Products include:
Cardene I.V. 3485

Nifedipine (Vasodilating effects of nitroglycerin may be additive with those of other vasodilators). Products include:
Adalat CC Tablets 877
Procardia Capsules 2708
Procardia XL Extended Release Tablets 2710

Nimodipine (Vasodilating effects of nitroglycerin may be additive with those of other vasodilators). Products include:
Nimotop Capsules 904

Nisoldipine (Vasodilating effects of nitroglycerin may be additive with those of other vasodilators). Products include:
Sular Tablets 688

Sildenafil Citrate (Amplification of the vasodilatory effects of the nitroglycerin patch by sildenafil can result in severe hypotension). Products include:
Viagra Tablets 2732

Verapamil Hydrochloride (Vasodilating effects of nitroglycerin may be additive with those of other vasodilators). Products include:
Covera-HS Tablets 3199
Isoptin SR Tablets 467
Tarka Tablets 508
Verelan Capsules 3184

Verelan PM Capsules 3186

Food Interactions

Alcohol (Enhances sensitivity to the hypotensive effects).

NITROLINGUAL PUMPSPRAY

(Nitroglycerin) 1355

May interact with calcium channel blockers and certain other agents. Compounds in these categories include:

Amlodipine Besylate (Marked symptomatic orthostatic hypotension). Products include:

- Lotrel Capsules 2370
- Norvasc Tablets 2704

Bepridil Hydrochloride (Marked symptomatic orthostatic hypotension). Products include:

- Vascor Tablets 2602

Diltiazem Hydrochloride (Marked symptomatic orthostatic hypotension). Products include:

- Cardizem Injectable 1018
- Cardizem Lyo-Ject Syringe 1018
- Cardizem Monovial 1018
- Cardizem CD Capsules 1016
- Tiazac Capsules 1378

Drugs Depending On Vascular Smooth Muscle (Decreased or increased effect).

No products indexed under this heading.

Felodipine (Marked symptomatic orthostatic hypotension). Products include:

- Lexxel Tablets 608
- Plendil Extended-Release Tablets ... 623

Isradipine (Marked symptomatic orthostatic hypotension). Products include:

- DynaCirc Capsules 2921
- DynaCirc CR Tablets 2923

Mibefradil Dihydrochloride (Marked symptomatic orthostatic hypotension).

No products indexed under this heading.

Nicardipine Hydrochloride (Marked symptomatic orthostatic hypotension). Products include:

- Cardene I.V. 3485

Nifedipine (Marked symptomatic orthostatic hypotension). Products include:

- Adalat CC Tablets 877
- Procardia Capsules 2708
- Procardia XL Extended Release Tablets 2710

Nimodipine (Marked symptomatic orthostatic hypotension). Products include:

- Nimotop Capsules 904

Nisoldipine (Marked symptomatic orthostatic hypotension). Products include:

- Sular Tablets 688

Sildenafil Citrate (Amplification of the vasodilatory effects of nitroglycerine by sildenafil can result in severe hypotension; the time course and dose dependency of this interaction have not been studied; concurrent use is contraindicated). Products include:

- Viagra Tablets 2732

Verapamil Hydrochloride (Marked symptomatic orthostatic hypotension). Products include:

- Covera-HS Tablets 3199
- Isoptin SR Tablets 467
- Tarka Tablets 508
- Verelan Capsules 3184
- Verelan PM Capsules 3186

Food Interactions

Alcohol (Enhanced sensitivity to hypotensive effects).

NITROSTAT TABLETS

(Nitroglycerin) 2658

May interact with anticholinergics, antihypertensives, beta blockers, calcium channel blockers, phenothiazines, and tricyclic antidepressants. Compounds in these categories include:

Acebutolol Hydrochloride (Co-administration of nitrates with beta-blockers may result in possible additive hypotensive effects). Products include:

- Sectral Capsules 3589

Alteplase, Recombinant (Intravenous nitroglycerin decreases the thrombolytic effect of alteplase). Products include:

- Activase I.V. 1410
- Cathflo Activase 3611

Amitriptyline Hydrochloride (Tricyclic antidepressants may cause dry mouth and diminished salivary secretions; this may make dissolution of sublingual nitroglycerin difficult; increasing salivation with chewing gum or artificial saliva products may prove useful in aiding dissolutionof sublingual nitroglycerin). Products include:

- Etrafon 3115
- Limbitrol 1738

Amlodipine Besylate (Co-administration of organic nitrates with calcium channel blockers has resulted in marked orthostatic hypotension). Products include:

- Lotrel Capsules 2370
- Norvasc Tablets 2704

Amoxapine (Tricyclic antidepressants may cause dry mouth and diminished salivary secretions; this may make dissolution of sublingual nitroglycerin difficult; increasing salivation with chewing gum or artificial saliva products may prove useful in aiding dissolutionof sublingual nitroglycerin).

No products indexed under this heading.

Aspirin (Co-administration with aspirin enhances the vasodilatory and hemodynamic effects of nitroglycerin). Products include:

- Aggrenox Capsules 1026
- Alka-Seltzer .... ▣603
- Alka-Seltzer Lemon Lime Antacid and Pain Reliever Effervescent Tablets .... ▣603
- Alka-Seltzer Extra Strength Antacid and Pain Reliever Effervescent Tablets .... ▣603
- Alka-Seltzer PM Effervescent Tablets .... ▣605
- Genuine Bayer Tablets, Caplets and Gelcaps .... ▣606
- Extra Strength Bayer Caplets and Gelcaps .... ▣610
- Aspirin Regimen Bayer Children's Chewable Tablets (Orange or Cherry Flavored) .... ▣607
- Bayer, Aspirin Regimen .... ▣606
- Aspirin Regimen Bayer 81 mg Caplets with Calcium .... ▣607
- Genuine Bayer Professional Labeling (Aspirin Regimen Bayer) .... ▣608
- Extra Strength Bayer Arthritis Caplets .... ▣610
- Extra Strength Bayer Plus Caplets .... ▣610
- Extra Strength Bayer PM Caplets .. ▣611
- BC Powder .... ▣619
- BC Allergy Sinus Cold Powder ...... ▣619
- Arthritis Strength BC Powder .... ▣619
- BC Sinus Cold Powder .... ▣619
- Darvon Compound-65 Pulvules 1910
- Ecotrin Enteric Coated Aspirin Low, Regular and Maximum Strength Tablets 1715
- Excedrin Extra-Strength Tablets, Caplets, and Geltabs .... ▣629
- Excedrin Migraine 1070
- Goody's Body Pain Formula Powder .... ▣620
- Goody's Extra Strength Headache Powder .... ▣620
- Goody's Extra Strength Pain Relief Tablets .... ▣620
- Percodan Tablets 1327
- Robaxisal Tablets 2939
- Soma Compound Tablets 3354
- Soma Compound w/Codeine Tablets 3355
- Vanquish Caplets .... ▣617

Atenolol (Co-administration of nitrates with beta-blockers may result in possible additive hypotensive effects). Products include:

- Tenoretic Tablets 690
- Tenormin I.V. Injection 692

Atropine Sulfate (Anticholinergic drugs may cause dry mouth and diminished salivary secretions; this may make dissolution of sublingual nitroglycerin difficult; increasing salivation with chewing gum or artificial saliva products may prove useful in aiding dissolution of sublingual nitroglycerin). Products include:

- Donnatal 2929
- Donnatal Extentabs 2930
- Motofen Tablets 577
- Prosed/DS Tablets 3268
- Urised Tablets 2876

Belladonna Alkaloids (Anticholinergic drugs may cause dry mouth and diminished salivary secretions; this may make dissolution of sublingual nitroglycerin difficult; increasing salivation with chewing gum or artificial saliva products may prove useful in aiding dissolution of sublingual nitroglycerin). Products include:

- Hyland's Teething Tablets .... ▣766
- Urimax Tablets 1769

Benazepril Hydrochloride (Co-administration of nitrates with other antihypertensive agents may result in possible additive hypotensive effects). Products include:

- Lotensin Tablets 2365
- Lotensin HCT Tablets 2367
- Lotrel Capsules 2370

Bendroflumethiazide (Co-administration of nitrates with other antihypertensive agents may result in possible additive hypotensive effects). Products include:

- Corzide 40/5 Tablets 2247
- Corzide 80/5 Tablets 2247

Benztropine Mesylate (Anticholinergic drugs may cause dry mouth and diminished salivary secretions; this may make dissolution of sublingual nitroglycerin difficult; increasing salivation with chewing gum or artificial saliva products may prove useful in aiding dissolution of sublingual nitroglycerin). Products include:

- Cogentin 2055

Bepridil Hydrochloride (Co-administration of organic nitrates with calcium channel blockers has resulted in marked orthostatic hypotension). Products include:

- Vascor Tablets 2602

Betaxolol Hydrochloride (Co-administration of nitrates with beta-blockers may result in possible additive hypotensive effects). Products include:

- Betoptic S Ophthalmic Suspension 537

Biperiden Hydrochloride (Anticholinergic drugs may cause dry mouth and diminished salivary secretions; this may make dissolution of sublingual nitroglycerin difficult; increasing salivation with chewing gum or artificial saliva products may prove useful in aiding dissolution of sublingual nitroglycerin). Products include:

- Akineton 402

Bisoprolol Fumarate (Co-administration of nitrates with beta-blockers may result in possible additive hypotensive effects). Products include:

- Zebeta Tablets 1885
- Ziac Tablets 1887

Candesartan Cilexetil (Co-administration of nitrates with other antihypertensive agents may result in possible additive hypotensive effects). Products include:

- Atacand Tablets 595
- Atacand HCT Tablets 597

Captopril (Co-administration of nitrates with other antihypertensive agents may result in possible additive hypotensive effects). Products include:

- Captopril Tablets 2281

Carteolol Hydrochloride (Co-administration of nitrates with beta-blockers may result in possible additive hypotensive effects). Products include:

- Carteolol Hydrochloride Ophthalmic Solution USP, 1% ..... ⊙258
- Ocupress Ophthalmic Solution, 1% Sterile .... ⊙303

Chlorothiazide (Co-administration of nitrates with other antihypertensive agents may result in possible additive hypotensive effects). Products include:

- Aldoclor Tablets 2035
- Diuril Oral 2087

Chlorothiazide Sodium (Co-administration of nitrates with other antihypertensive agents may result in possible additive hypotensive effects). Products include:

- Diuril Sodium Intravenous 2086

Chlorpromazine (Co-administration of nitrates with phenothiazines may result in possible additive hypotensive effects). Products include:

- Thorazine Suppositories 1656

Chlorpromazine Hydrochloride (Co-administration of nitrates with phenothiazines may result in possible additive hypotensive effects). Products include:

- Thorazine 1656

Chlorthalidone (Co-administration of nitrates with other antihypertensive agents may result in possible additive hypotensive effects). Products include:

- Clorpres Tablets 1002
- Combipres Tablets 1040
- Tenoretic Tablets 690

Clidinium Bromide (Anticholinergic drugs may cause dry mouth and diminished salivary secretions; this may make dissolution of sublingual nitroglycerin difficult; increasing salivation with chewing gum or artificial saliva products may prove useful in aiding dissolution of sublingual nitroglycerin).

No products indexed under this heading.

Clomipramine Hydrochloride (Tricyclic antidepressants may cause dry mouth and diminished salivary secretions; this may make dissolution of sublingual nitroglycerin difficult; increasing salivation with chewing gum or artificial saliva products may prove useful in aiding dissolutionof sublingual nitroglycerin).

No products indexed under this heading.

Clonidine (Co-administration of nitrates with other antihypertensive agents may result in possible additive hypotensive effects). Products include:

- Catapres-TTS 1038

Clonidine Hydrochloride (Co-administration of nitrates with other antihypertensive agents may result in possible additive hypotensive effects). Products include:

- Catapres Tablets 1037
- Clorpres Tablets 1002
- Combipres Tablets 1040
- Duraclon Injection 3057

Deserpidine (Co-administration of nitrates with other antihypertensive agents may result in possible additive hypotensive effects).

No products indexed under this heading.

Desipramine Hydrochloride (Tricyclic antidepressants may cause dry mouth and diminished salivary

secretions; this may make dissolution of sublingual nitroglycerin difficult; increasing salivation with chewing gum or artificial saliva products may prove useful in aiding dissolutionof sublingual nitroglycerin). Products include:

Norpramin Tablets 755

Diazoxide (Co-administration of nitrates with other antihypertensive agents may result in possible additive hypotensive effects).

No products indexed under this heading.

Dicyclomine Hydrochloride (Anticholinergic drugs may cause dry mouth and diminished salivary secretions; this may make dissolution of sublingual nitroglycerin difficult; increasing salivation with chewing gum or artificial saliva products may prove useful in aiding dissolution of sublingual nitroglycerin).

No products indexed under this heading.

Dihydroergotamine Mesylate (Oral administration of nitroglycerin markedly decreases the first-pass metabolism of dihydroergotamine and subsequently increases its oral bioavailability; ergotamine is known to precipitate angina pectoris, therefore, patients receiving sublingual nitroglycerin should avoid ergotamine and related drugs). Products include:

D.H.E. 45 Injection 2334
Migranal Nasal Spray 2376

Diltiazem Hydrochloride (Co-administration of organic nitrates with calcium channel blockers has resulted in marked orthostatic hypotension). Products include:

Cardizem Injectable 1018
Cardizem Lyo-Ject Syringe 1018
Cardizem Monovial 1018
Cardizem CD Capsules 1016
Tiazac Capsules 1378

Doxazosin Mesylate (Co-administration of nitrates with other antihypertensive agents may result in possible additive hypotensive effects). Products include:

Cardura Tablets 2668

Doxepin Hydrochloride (Tricyclic antidepressants may cause dry mouth and diminished salivary secretions; this may make dissolution of sublingual nitroglycerin difficult; increasing salivation with chewing gum or artificial saliva products may prove useful in aiding dissolutionof sublingual nitroglycerin). Products include:

Sinequan 2713

Enalapril Maleate (Co-administration of nitrates with other antihypertensive agents may result in possible additive hypotensive effects). Products include:

Lexxel Tablets 608
Vaseretic Tablets 2204
Vasotec Tablets 2210

Enalaprilat (Co-administration of nitrates with other antihypertensive agents may result in possible additive hypotensive effects). Products include:

Enalaprilat Injection 863
Vasotec I.V. Injection 2207

Eprosartan Mesylate (Co-administration of nitrates with other antihypertensive agents may result in possible additive hypotensive effects). Products include:

Teveten Tablets 3327

Ergotamine Tartrate (Oral administration of nitroglycerin markedly decreases the first-pass metabolism of dihydroergotamine and subsequently increases its oral bioavailability; ergotamine is known to precipitate angina pectoris, therefore, patients receiving sublingual nitroglycerin should avoid ergotamine and related drugs).

No products indexed under this heading.

Esmolol Hydrochloride (Co-administration of nitrates with beta-blockers may result in possible additive hypotensive effects). Products include:

Brevibloc Injection 858

Felodipine (Co-administration of organic nitrates with calcium channel blockers has resulted in marked orthostatic hypotension). Products include:

Lexxel Tablets 608
Plendil Extended-Release Tablets ... 623

Fluphenazine Decanoate (Co-administration of nitrates with phenothiazines may result in possible additive hypotensive effects).

No products indexed under this heading.

Fluphenazine Enanthate (Co-administration of nitrates with phenothiazines may result in possible additive hypotensive effects).

No products indexed under this heading.

Fluphenazine Hydrochloride (Co-administration of nitrates with phenothiazines may result in possible additive hypotensive effects).

No products indexed under this heading.

Fosinopril Sodium (Co-administration of nitrates with other antihypertensive agents may result in possible additive hypotensive effects). Products include:

Monopril Tablets 1091
Monopril HCT 1094

Furosemide (Co-administration of nitrates with other antihypertensive agents may result in possible additive hypotensive effects). Products include:

Furosemide Tablets 2284

Glycopyrrolate (Anticholinergic drugs may cause dry mouth and diminished salivary secretions; this may make dissolution of sublingual nitroglycerin difficult; increasing salivation with chewing gum or artificial saliva products may prove useful in aiding dissolution of sublingual nitroglycerin). Products include:

Robinul Forte Tablets 1358
Robinul Injectable 2940
Robinul Tablets 1358

Guanabenz Acetate (Co-administration of nitrates with other antihypertensive agents may result in possible additive hypotensive effects).

No products indexed under this heading.

Guanethidine Monosulfate (Co-administration of nitrates with other antihypertensive agents may result in possible additive hypotensive effects).

No products indexed under this heading.

Heparin Sodium (Intravenous nitroglycerin reduces the anticoagulant effect of heparin and activated partial thromboplastin times should be monitored). Products include:

Heparin Lock Flush Solution 3509
Heparin Sodium Injection 3511

Hydralazine Hydrochloride (Co-administration of nitrates with other antihypertensive agents may result in possible additive hypotensive effects).

No products indexed under this heading.

Hydrochlorothiazide (Co-administration of nitrates with other antihypertensive agents may result in possible additive hypotensive effects). Products include:

Accuretic Tablets 2614
Aldoril Tablets 2039
Atacand HCT Tablets 597
Avalide Tablets 1070
Diovan HCT Tablets 2338
Dyazide Capsules 1515
HydroDIURIL Tablets 2108
Hyzaar 2109
Inderide Tablets 3517
Inderide LA Long-Acting Capsules .. 3519
Lotensin HCT Tablets 2367
Maxzide 1008
Micardis HCT Tablets 1051
Microzide Capsules 3414
Moduretic Tablets 2138
Monopril HCT 1094
Prinzide Tablets 2168
Timolide Tablets 2187
Uniretic Tablets 3178
Vaseretic Tablets 2204
Zestoretic Tablets 695
Ziac Tablets 1887

Hydroflumethiazide (Co-administration of nitrates with other antihypertensive agents may result in possible additive hypotensive effects). Products include:

Diucardin Tablets 3494

Hyoscyamine (Anticholinergic drugs may cause dry mouth and diminished salivary secretions; this may make dissolution of sublingual nitroglycerin difficult; increasing salivation with chewing gum or artificial saliva products may prove useful in aiding dissolution of sublingual nitroglycerin). Products include:

Urised Tablets 2876

Hyoscyamine Sulfate (Anticholinergic drugs may cause dry mouth and diminished salivary secretions; this may make dissolution of sublingual nitroglycerin difficult; increasing salivation with chewing gum or artificial saliva products may prove useful in aiding dissolution of sublingual nitroglycerin). Products include:

Arco-Lase Plus Tablets 592
Donnatal 2929
Donnatal Extentabs 2930
Levsin/Levsinex/Levbid 3172
NuLev Orally Disintegrating Tablets 3176
Prosed/DS Tablets 3268
Urimax Tablets 1769

Imipramine Hydrochloride (Tricyclic antidepressants may cause dry mouth and diminished salivary secretions; this may make dissolution of sublingual nitroglycerin difficult; increasing salivation with chewing gum or artificial saliva products may prove useful in aiding dissolutionof sublingual nitroglycerin).

No products indexed under this heading.

Imipramine Pamoate (Tricyclic antidepressants may cause dry mouth and diminished salivary secretions; this may make dissolution of sublingual nitroglycerin difficult; increasing salivation with chewing gum or artificial saliva products may prove useful in aiding dissolutionof sublingual nitroglycerin).

No products indexed under this heading.

Indapamide (Co-administration of nitrates with other antihypertensive agents may result in possible additive hypotensive effects). Products include:

Indapamide Tablets 2286

Ipratropium Bromide (Anticholinergic drugs may cause dry mouth and diminished salivary secretions; this may make dissolution of sublingual nitroglycerin difficult; increasing salivation with chewing gum or artificial saliva products may prove useful in aiding dissolution of sublingual nitroglycerin). Products include:

Atrovent Inhalation Aerosol 1030
Atrovent Inhalation Solution 1031
Atrovent Nasal Spray 0.03% 1032
Atrovent Nasal Spray 0.06% 1033
Combivent Inhalation Aerosol 1041
DuoNeb Inhalation Solution 1233

Irbesartan (Co-administration of nitrates with other antihypertensive agents may result in possible additive hypotensive effects). Products include:

Avalide Tablets 1070
Avapro Tablets 1074
Avapro Tablets 3076

Isosorbide Dinitrate (A decrease in therapeutic effect of sublingual nitroglycerin may result from use of long-acting nitrates). Products include:

Isordil Sublingual Tablets 3525
Isordil Titradose Tablets 3526

Isosorbide Mononitrate (A decrease in therapeutic effect of sublingual nitroglycerin may result from use of long-acting nitrates). Products include:

Imdur Tablets 1826
Ismo Tablets 3524

Isradipine (Co-administration of organic nitrates with calcium channel blockers has resulted in marked orthostatic hypotension). Products include:

DynaCirc Capsules 2921
DynaCirc CR Tablets 2923

Labetalol Hydrochloride (Co-administration of nitrates with beta-blockers may result in possible additive hypotensive effects). Products include:

Normodyne Injection 3135
Normodyne Tablets 3137

Levobunolol Hydrochloride (Co-administration of nitrates with beta-blockers may result in possible additive hypotensive effects). Products include:

Betagan .... ⊙ 228

Lisinopril (Co-administration of nitrates with other antihypertensive agents may result in possible additive hypotensive effects). Products include:

Prinivil Tablets 2164
Prinzide Tablets 2168
Zestoretic Tablets 695
Zestril Tablets 698

Losartan Potassium (Co-administration of nitrates with other antihypertensive agents may result in possible additive hypotensive effects). Products include:

Cozaar Tablets 2067
Hyzaar 2109

Maprotiline Hydrochloride (Tricyclic antidepressants may cause dry mouth and diminished salivary secretions; this may make dissolution of sublingual nitroglycerin difficult; increasing salivation with chewing gum or artificial saliva products may prove useful in aiding dissolutionof sublingual nitroglycerin).

No products indexed under this heading.

Mecamylamine Hydrochloride (Co-administration of nitrates with other antihypertensive agents may result in possible additive hypotensive effects). Products include:

Inversine Tablets 1850

Mepenzolate Bromide (Anticholinergic drugs may cause dry mouth and diminished salivary secretions; this may make dissolution of sublingual nitroglycerin difficult; increasing salivation with chewing gum or artificial saliva products may prove useful in aiding dissolution of sublingual nitroglycerin).

No products indexed under this heading.

Mesoridazine Besylate (Co-administration of nitrates with phenothiazines may result in possible additive hypotensive effects). Products include:

Serentil 1057

Methotrimeprazine (Co-administration of nitrates with phenothiazines may result in possible additive hypotensive effects).

No products indexed under this heading.

Methyclothiazide (Co-administration of nitrates with other antihypertensive agents may result in possible additive hypotensive effects).
No products indexed under this heading.

Methyldopa (Co-administration of nitrates with other antihypertensive agents may result in possible additive hypotensive effects). Products include:
Aldoclor Tablets **2035**
Aldomet Tablets **2037**
Aldoril Tablets **2039**

Methyldopate Hydrochloride (Co-administration of nitrates with other antihypertensive agents may result in possible additive hypotensive effects).
No products indexed under this heading.

Metipranolol Hydrochloride (Co-administration of nitrates with beta-blockers may result in possible additive hypotensive effects).
No products indexed under this heading.

Metolazone (Co-administration of nitrates with other antihypertensive agents may result in possible additive hypotensive effects). Products include:
Mykrox Tablets **1168**
Zaroxolyn Tablets **1177**

Metoprolol Succinate (Co-administration of nitrates with beta-blockers may result in possible additive hypotensive effects). Products include:
Toprol-XL Tablets **651**

Metoprolol Tartrate (Co-administration of nitrates with beta-blockers may result in possible additive hypotensive effects).
No products indexed under this heading.

Metyrosine (Co-administration of nitrates with other antihypertensive agents may result in possible additive hypotensive effects). Products include:
Demser Capsules **2085**

Mibefradil Dihydrochloride (Co-administration of organic nitrates with calcium channel blockers has resulted in marked orthostatic hypotension).
No products indexed under this heading.

Minoxidil (Co-administration of nitrates with other antihypertensive agents may result in possible additive hypotensive effects). Products include:
Rogaine Extra Strength for Men Topical Solution .... ■□**721**
Rogaine for Women Topical Solution .... ■□**721**

Moexipril Hydrochloride (Co-administration of nitrates with other antihypertensive agents may result in possible additive hypotensive effects). Products include:
Uniretic Tablets **3178**
Univasc Tablets **3181**

Nadolol (Co-administration of nitrates with beta-blockers may result in possible additive hypotensive effects). Products include:
Corgard Tablets **2245**
Corzide 40/5 Tablets **2247**
Corzide 80/5 Tablets **2247**
Nadolol Tablets **2288**

Nicardipine Hydrochloride (Co-administration of organic nitrates with calcium channel blockers has resulted in marked orthostatic hypotension). Products include:
Cardene I.V. **3485**

Nifedipine (Co-administration of organic nitrates with calcium channel blockers has resulted in marked orthostatic hypotension). Products include:
Adalat CC Tablets **877**
Procardia Capsules **2708**
Procardia XL Extended Release Tablets **2710**

Nimodipine (Co-administration of organic nitrates with calcium channel blockers has resulted in marked orthostatic hypotension). Products include:
Nimotop Capsules **904**

Nisoldipine (Co-administration of organic nitrates with calcium channel blockers has resulted in marked orthostatic hypotension). Products include:
Sular Tablets **688**

Nitroglycerin, long-acting formulations (A decrease in the therapeutic effects of sublingual nitroglycerin may result from use of long-acting nitrates).

Nortriptyline Hydrochloride (Tricyclic antidepressants may cause dry mouth and diminished salivary secretions; this may make dissolution of sublingual nitroglycerin difficult; increasing salivation with chewing gum or artificial saliva products may prove useful in aiding dissolutionof sublingual nitroglycerin).
No products indexed under this heading.

Oxybutynin Chloride (Anticholinergic drugs may cause dry mouth and diminished salivary secretions; this may make dissolution of sublingual nitroglycerin difficult; increasing salivation with chewing gum or artificial saliva products may prove useful in aiding dissolution of sublingual nitroglycerin). Products include:
Ditropan XL Extended Release Tablets **564**

Penbutolol Sulfate (Co-administration of nitrates with beta-blockers may result in possible additive hypotensive effects).
No products indexed under this heading.

Perindopril Erbumine (Co-administration of nitrates with other antihypertensive agents may result in possible additive hypotensive effects). Products include:
Aceon Tablets (2 mg, 4 mg, 8 mg) **3249**

Perphenazine (Co-administration of nitrates with phenothiazines may result in possible additive hypotensive effects). Products include:
Etrafon **3115**
Trilafon **3160**

Phenoxybenzamine Hydrochloride (Co-administration of nitrates with other antihypertensive agents may result in possible additive hypotensive effects). Products include:
Dibenzyline Capsules **3457**

Phentolamine Mesylate (Co-administration of nitrates with other antihypertensive agents may result in possible additive hypotensive effects).
No products indexed under this heading.

Pindolol (Co-administration of nitrates with beta-blockers may result in possible additive hypotensive effects).
No products indexed under this heading.

Polythiazide (Co-administration of nitrates with other antihypertensive agents may result in possible additive hypotensive effects). Products include:
Minizide Capsules **2700**
Renese Tablets **2712**

Prazosin Hydrochloride (Co-administration of nitrates with other antihypertensive agents may result in possible additive hypotensive effects). Products include:
Minipress Capsules **2699**
Minizide Capsules **2700**

Prochlorperazine (Co-administration of nitrates with phenothiazines may result in possible additive hypotensive effects). Products include:
Compazine **1505**

Procyclidine Hydrochloride (Anticholinergic drugs may cause dry mouth and diminished salivary secretions; this may make dissolution of sublingual nitroglycerin difficult; increasing salivation with chewing gum or artificial saliva products may prove useful in aiding dissolution of sublingual nitroglycerin).
No products indexed under this heading.

Promethazine Hydrochloride (Co-administration of nitrates with phenothiazines may result in possible additive hypotensive effects). Products include:
Mepergan Injection **3539**
Phenergan Injection **3553**
Phenergan **3556**
Phenergan Syrup **3554**
Phenergan with Codeine Syrup **3557**
Phenergan with Dextromethorphan Syrup **3559**
Phenergan VC Syrup **3560**
Phenergan VC with Codeine Syrup .. **3561**

Propantheline Bromide (Anticholinergic drugs may cause dry mouth and diminished salivary secretions; this may make dissolution of sublingual nitroglycerin difficult; increasing salivation with chewing gum or artificial saliva products may prove useful in aiding dissolution of sublingual nitroglycerin).
No products indexed under this heading.

Propranolol Hydrochloride (Co-administration of nitrates with beta-blockers may result in possible additive hypotensive effects). Products include:
Inderal **3513**
Inderal LA Long-Acting Capsules **3516**
Inderide Tablets **3517**
Inderide LA Long-Acting Capsules .. **3519**

Protriptyline Hydrochloride (Tricyclic antidepressants may cause dry mouth and diminished salivary secretions; this may make dissolution of sublingual nitroglycerin difficult; increasing salivation with chewing gum or artificial saliva products may prove useful in aiding dissolutionof sublingual nitroglycerin). Products include:
Vivactil Tablets **2446**
Vivactil Tablets **2217**

Quinapril Hydrochloride (Co-administration of nitrates with other antihypertensive agents may result in possible additive hypotensive effects). Products include:
Accupril Tablets **2611**
Accuretic Tablets **2614**

Ramipril (Co-administration of nitrates with other antihypertensive agents may result in possible additive hypotensive effects). Products include:
Altace Capsules **2233**

Rauwolfia serpentina (Co-administration of nitrates with other antihypertensive agents may result in possible additive hypotensive effects).
No products indexed under this heading.

Rescinnamine (Co-administration of nitrates with other antihypertensive agents may result in possible additive hypotensive effects).
No products indexed under this heading.

Reserpine (Co-administration of nitrates with other antihypertensive agents may result in possible additive hypotensive effects).
No products indexed under this heading.

Scopolamine (Anticholinergic drugs may cause dry mouth and diminished salivary secretions; this may make dissolution of sublingual nitroglycerin difficult; increasing salivation with chewing gum or artificial saliva products may prove useful in aiding dissolution of sublingual nitroglycerin). Products include:
Transderm Scōp Transdermal Therapeutic System **2302**

Scopolamine Hydrobromide (Anticholinergic drugs may cause dry mouth and diminished salivary secretions; this may make dissolution of sublingual nitroglycerin difficult; increasing salivation with chewing gum or artificial saliva products may prove useful in aiding dissolution of sublingual nitroglycerin). Products include:
Donnatal **2929**
Donnatal Extentabs **2930**

Sildenafil Citrate (Co-administration of organic nitrates with sildenafil has been shown to potentiate the hypotensive effects of organic nitrates; concurrent use is contraindicated). Products include:
Viagra Tablets **2732**

Sodium Nitroprusside (Co-administration of nitrates with other antihypertensive agents may result in possible additive hypotensive effects).
No products indexed under this heading.

Sotalol Hydrochloride (Co-administration of nitrates with beta-blockers may result in possible additive hypotensive effects). Products include:
Betapace Tablets **950**
Betapace AF Tablets **954**

Spirapril Hydrochloride (Co-administration of nitrates with other antihypertensive agents may result in possible additive hypotensive effects).
No products indexed under this heading.

Telmisartan (Co-administration of nitrates with other antihypertensive agents may result in possible additive hypotensive effects). Products include:
Micardis Tablets **1049**
Micardis HCT Tablets **1051**

Terazosin Hydrochloride (Co-administration of nitrates with other antihypertensive agents may result in possible additive hypotensive effects). Products include:
Hytrin Capsules **464**

Thioridazine Hydrochloride (Co-administration of nitrates with phenothiazines may result in possible additive hypotensive effects). Products include:
Thioridazine Hydrochloride Tablets **2289**

Timolol Hemihydrate (Co-administration of nitrates with beta-blockers may result in possible additive hypotensive effects). Products include:
Betimol Ophthalmic Solution .... ⊙**324**

Timolol Maleate (Co-administration of nitrates with beta-blockers may result in possible additive hypotensive effects). Products include:
Blocadren Tablets **2046**
Cosopt Sterile Ophthalmic Solution **2065**
Timolide Tablets **2187**
Timolol GFS .... ⊙**266**
Timoptic in Ocudose **2192**
Timoptic Sterile Ophthalmic Solution **2190**
Timoptic-XE Sterile Ophthalmic Gel Forming Solution **2194**

Tolterodine Tartrate (Anticholinergic drugs may cause dry mouth and diminished salivary secretions; this may make dissolution of sublingual nitroglycerin difficult; increasing

salivation with chewing gum or artificial saliva products may prove useful in aiding dissolution of sublingual nitroglycerin). Products include:

Detrol Tablets ... 3623
Detrol LA Capsules ... 2801

Torsemide (Co-administration of nitrates with other antihypertensive agents may result in possible additive hypotensive effects). Products include:

Demadex Tablets and Injection ... 2965

Trandolapril (Co-administration of nitrates with other antihypertensive agents may result in possible additive hypotensive effects). Products include:

Mavik Tablets ... 478
Tarka Tablets ... 508

Tridihexethyl Chloride (Anticholinergic drugs may cause dry mouth and diminished salivary secretions; this may make dissolution of sublingual nitroglycerin difficult; increasing salivation with chewing gum or artificial saliva products may prove useful in aiding dissolution of sublingual nitroglycerin).

No products indexed under this heading.

Trifluoperazine Hydrochloride (Co-administration of nitrates with phenothiazines may result in possible additive hypotensive effects). Products include:

Stelazine ... 1640

Trihexyphenidyl Hydrochloride (Anticholinergic drugs may cause dry mouth and diminished salivary secretions; this may make dissolution of sublingual nitroglycerin difficult; increasing salivation with chewing gum or artificial saliva products may prove useful in aiding dissolution of sublingual nitroglycerin). Products include:

Artane ... 1855

Trimethaphan Camsylate (Co-administration of nitrates with other antihypertensive agents may result in possible additive hypotensive effects).

No products indexed under this heading.

Trimipramine Maleate (Tricyclic antidepressants may cause dry mouth and diminished salivary secretions; this may make dissolution of sublingual nitroglycerin difficult; increasing salivation with chewing gum or artificial saliva products may prove useful in aiding dissolution of sublingual nitroglycerin). Products include:

Surmontil Capsules ... 3595

Valsartan (Co-administration of nitrates with other antihypertensive agents may result in possible additive hypotensive effects). Products include:

Diovan Capsules ... 2337
Diovan HCT Tablets ... 2338

Verapamil Hydrochloride (Co-administration of organic nitrates with calcium channel blockers has resulted in marked orthostatic hypotension). Products include:

Covera-HS Tablets ... 3199
Isoptin SR Tablets ... 467
Tarka Tablets ... 508
Verelan Capsules ... 3184
Verelan PM Capsules ... 3186

Food Interactions

Alcohol (Concomitant use may cause hypotension).

NIX CREME RINSE

(Permethrin) ... 704
None cited in PDR database.

NIZORAL 2% CREAM

(Ketoconazole) ... 3620
None cited in PDR database.

NIZORAL A-D SHAMPOO

(Ketoconazole) ... 2008
None cited in PDR database.

NIZORAL 2% SHAMPOO

(Ketoconazole) ... 2007
None cited in PDR database.

NIZORAL TABLETS

(Ketoconazole) ... 1791
May interact with antacids, anticholinergics, oral anticoagulants, histamine H_2-receptor antagonists, oral hypoglycemic agents, and certain other agents. Compounds in these categories include:

Acarbose (Possibility of severe hypoglycemia cannot be ruled out). Products include:

Precose Tablets ... 906

Aluminum Carbonate (Nizoral requires acidity for dissolution, antacids should be given at least two hours after Nizoral administration).

No products indexed under this heading.

Aluminum Hydroxide (Nizoral requires acidity for dissolution, antacids should be given at least two hours after Nizoral administration). Products include:

Amphojel Suspension (Mint Flavor) ... 789
Gaviscon Extra Strength Liquid ... 751
Gaviscon Extra Strength Tablets ... 751
Gaviscon Regular Strength Liquid ... 751
Gaviscon Regular Strength Tablets ... 750
Maalox Antacid/Anti-Gas Oral Suspension ... 673
Maalox Max Maximum Strength Antacid/Anti-Gas Liquid ... 2300
Maalox Regular Strength Antacid/Antigas Liquid ... 2300
Mylanta ... 1813
Vanquish Caplets ... 617

Astemizole (Co-administration is contraindicated; elevated plasma levels of astemizole resulting in prolonged QT intervals).

No products indexed under this heading.

Atropine Sulfate (Nizoral requires acidity for dissolution, these drugs should be given at least two hours after Nizoral administration). Products include:

Donnatal ... 2929
Donnatal Extentabs ... 2930
Motofen Tablets ... 577
Prosed/DS Tablets ... 3268
Urised Tablets ... 2876

Belladonna Alkaloids (Nizoral requires acidity for dissolution, these drugs should be given at least two hours after Nizoral administration). Products include:

Hyland's Teething Tablets ... 766
Urimax Tablets ... 1769

Benztropine Mesylate (Nizoral requires acidity for dissolution, these drugs should be given at least two hours after Nizoral administration). Products include:

Cogentin ... 2055

Biperiden Hydrochloride (Nizoral requires acidity for dissolution, these drugs should be given at least two hours after Nizoral administration). Products include:

Akineton ... 402

Chlorpropamide (Possibility of severe hypoglycemia cannot be ruled out). Products include:

Diabinese Tablets ... 2680

Cimetidine (Nizoral requires acidity for dissolution, these drugs should be given at least two hours after Nizoral administration). Products include:

Tagamet HB 200 Suspension ... 762
Tagamet HB 200 Tablets ... 761
Tagamet Tablets ... 1644

Cimetidine Hydrochloride (Nizoral requires acidity for dissolution, these drugs should be given at least two hours after Nizoral administration). Products include:

Tagamet ... 1644

Cisapride (Co-administration has resulted in serious cardiovascular adverse events including ventricular tachycardia, ventricular fibrillation and torsade de pointes; concurrent use is contraindicated).

No products indexed under this heading.

Clidinium Bromide (Nizoral requires acidity for dissolution, these drugs should be given at least two hours after Nizoral administration).

No products indexed under this heading.

Cyclosporine (Co-administration may alter the metabolism of cyclosporine resulting in increased plasma concentration of cyclosporine). Products include:

Gengraf Capsules ... 457
Neoral Soft Gelatin Capsules ... 2380
Neoral Oral Solution ... 2380
Sandimmune ... 2388

Dicumarol (Anticoagulant effect enhanced).

No products indexed under this heading.

Dicyclomine Hydrochloride (Nizoral requires acidity for dissolution, these drugs should be given at least two hours after Nizoral administration).

No products indexed under this heading.

Digoxin (Rare cases of elevated plasma concentrations of digoxin; monitor digoxin concentration). Products include:

Digitek Tablets ... 1003
Lanoxicaps Capsules ... 1574
Lanoxin Injection ... 1581
Lanoxin Tablets ... 1587
Lanoxin Elixir Pediatric ... 1578
Lanoxin Injection Pediatric ... 1584

Famotidine (Nizoral requires acidity for dissolution, these drugs should be given at least two hours after Nizoral administration). Products include:

Famotidine Injection ... 866
Pepcid AC ... 1814
Pepcid Complete Chewable Tablets ... 1815
Pepcid Injection ... 2153
Pepcid for Oral Suspension ... 2150
Pepcid RPD Orally Disintegrating Tablets ... 2150
Pepcid Tablets ... 2150

Fosphenytoin Sodium (Co-administration may alter metabolism of one or both of the drugs). Products include:

Cerebyx Injection ... 2619

Glimepiride (Possibility of severe hypoglycemia cannot be ruled out). Products include:

Amaryl Tablets ... 717

Glipizide (Possibility of severe hypoglycemia cannot be ruled out). Products include:

Glucotrol Tablets ... 2692
Glucotrol XL Extended Release Tablets ... 2693

Glyburide (Possibility of severe hypoglycemia cannot be ruled out). Products include:

DiaBeta Tablets ... 741
Glucovance Tablets ... 1086

Glycopyrrolate (Nizoral requires acidity for dissolution, these drugs should be given at least two hours after Nizoral administration). Products include:

Robinul Forte Tablets ... 1358
Robinul Injectable ... 2940
Robinul Tablets ... 1358

Hyoscyamine (Nizoral requires acidity for dissolution, these drugs should be given at least two hours after Nizoral administration). Products include:

Urised Tablets ... 2876

Hyoscyamine Sulfate (Nizoral requires acidity for dissolution, these drugs should be given at least two hours after Nizoral administration). Products include:

Arco-Lase Plus Tablets ... 592
Donnatal ... 2929
Donnatal Extentabs ... 2930
Levsin/Levsinex/Levbid ... 3172
NuLev Orally Disintegrating Tablets ... 3176
Prosed/DS Tablets ... 3268
Urimax Tablets ... 1769

Ipratropium Bromide (Nizoral requires acidity for dissolution, these drugs should be given at least two hours after Nizoral administration). Products include:

Atrovent Inhalation Aerosol ... 1030
Atrovent Inhalation Solution ... 1031
Atrovent Nasal Spray 0.03% ... 1032
Atrovent Nasal Spray 0.06% ... 1033
Combivent Inhalation Aerosol ... 1041
DuoNeb Inhalation Solution ... 1233

Isoniazid (Affects ketoconazole concentrations adversely). Products include:

Rifamate Capsules ... 767
Rifater Tablets ... 769

Loratadine (AUC and Cmax of loratadine averaged 302% and 251% respectively following coadministration; no cardiac changes were noted). Products include:

Claritin ... 3100
Claritin-D 12 Hour Extended Release Tablets ... 3102
Claritin-D 24 Hour Extended Release Tablets ... 3104

Magaldrate (Nizoral requires acidity for dissolution, antacids should be given at least two hours after Nizoral administration).

No products indexed under this heading.

Magnesium Hydroxide (Nizoral requires acidity for dissolution, antacids should be given at least two hours after Nizoral administration). Products include:

Ex•Lax Milk of Magnesia Liquid ... 670
Maalox Antacid/Anti-Gas Oral Suspension ... 673
Maalox Max Maximum Strength Antacid/Anti-Gas Liquid ... 2300
Maalox Regular Strength Antacid/Antigas Liquid ... 2300
Mylanta Fast-Acting ... 1813
Mylanta ... 1813
Pepcid Complete Chewable Tablets ... 1815
Phillips' Chewable Tablets ... 615
Phillips' Milk of Magnesia Liquid (Original, Cherry, & Mint) ... 616
Rolaids Tablets ... 706
Extra Strength Rolaids Tablets ... 706
Vanquish Caplets ... 617

Magnesium Oxide (Nizoral requires acidity for dissolution, antacids should be given at least two hours after Nizoral administration). Products include:

Beelith Tablets ... 946
Mag-Ox 400 Tablets ... 1024
Uro-Mag Capsules ... 1024

Mepenzolate Bromide (Nizoral requires acidity for dissolution, these drugs should be given at least two hours after Nizoral administration).

No products indexed under this heading.

Metformin Hydrochloride (Possibility of severe hypoglycemia cannot be ruled out). Products include:

Glucophage Tablets ... 1080
Glucophage XR Tablets ... 1080
Glucovance Tablets ... 1086

Methylprednisolone (Co-administration may alter the metabolism of methylprednisolone resulting in increased plasma concentration; dosage of methylprednisolone may have to be adjusted).

No products indexed under this heading.

Methylprednisolone Acetate (Co-administration may alter the metabolism of methylprednisolone resulting in increased plasma concentration;

dosage of methylprednisolone may have to be adjusted). Products include:
Depo-Medrol Injectable Suspension 2795

Methylprednisolone Sodium Succinate (Co-administration may alter the metabolism of methylprednisolone resulting in increased plasma concentration; dosage of methylprednisolone may have to be adjusted). Products include:
Solu-Medrol Sterile Powder 2855

Midazolam Hydrochloride (Co-administration with oral midazolam has resulted in elevated plasma concentration of midazolam resulting in prolonged hypnotic and sedative effects; concurrent oral use should be avoided). Products include:
Versed Injection 3027
Versed Syrup 3033

Miglitol (Possibility of severe hypoglycemia cannot be ruled out). Products include:
Glyset Tablets 2821

Nizatidine (Nizoral requires acidity for dissolution, these drugs should be given at least two hours after Nizoral administration). Products include:
Axid Pulvules 1903
Axid Pulvules 2919

Oxybutynin Chloride (Nizoral requires acidity for dissolution, these drugs should be given at least two hours after Nizoral administration). Products include:
Ditropan XL Extended Release Tablets 564

Phenytoin (Co-administration may alter metabolism of one or both of the drugs). Products include:
Dilantin Infatabs 2624
Dilantin-125 Oral Suspension 2625

Phenytoin Sodium (Co-administration may alter metabolism of one or both of the drugs). Products include:
Dilantin Kapseals 2622

Pioglitazone Hydrochloride (Possibility of severe hypoglycemia cannot be ruled out). Products include:
Actos Tablets 3275

Procyclidine Hydrochloride (Nizoral requires acidity for dissolution, these drugs should be given at least two hours after Nizoral administration).
No products indexed under this heading.

Propantheline Bromide (Nizoral requires acidity for dissolution, these drugs should be given at least two hours after Nizoral administration).
No products indexed under this heading.

Ranitidine Bismuth Citrate (Nizoral requires acidity for dissolution, these drugs should be given at least two hours after Nizoral administration).
No products indexed under this heading.

Ranitidine Hydrochloride (Nizoral requires acidity for dissolution, these drugs should be given at least two hours after Nizoral administration). Products include:
Zantac 1690
Zantac Injection 1688
Zantac 75 Tablets .... ■717

Repaglinide (Possibility of severe hypoglycemia cannot be ruled out). Products include:
Prandin Tablets (0.5, 1, and 2 mg) 2432

Rifampin (Reduces blood levels of ketoconazole). Products include:
Rifadin 765
Rifamate Capsules 767
Rifater Tablets 769

Rosiglitazone Maleate (Possibility of severe hypoglycemia cannot be ruled out). Products include:
Avandia Tablets 1490

Scopolamine (Nizoral requires acidity for dissolution, these drugs should be given at least two hours after Nizoral administration). Products include:
Transderm Scōp Transdermal Therapeutic System 2302

Scopolamine Hydrobromide (Nizoral requires acidity for dissolution, these drugs should be given at least two hours after Nizoral administration). Products include:
Donnatal 2929
Donnatal Extentabs 2930

Sodium Bicarbonate (Nizoral requires acidity for dissolution, antacids should be given at least two hours after Nizoral administration). Products include:
Alka-Seltzer .... ■603
Alka-Seltzer Lemon Lime Antacid and Pain Reliever Effervescent Tablets .... ■603
Alka-Seltzer Extra Strength Antacid and Pain Reliever Effervescent Tablets .... ■603
Alka-Seltzer Heartburn Relief Tablets .... ■604
Ceo-Two Evacuant Suppository .... ■618
Colyte with Flavor Packs for Oral Solution 3170
GoLYTELY and Pineapple Flavor GoLYTELY for Oral Solution 1068
NuLYTELY, Cherry Flavor, Lemon-Lime Flavor, and Orange Flavor NuLYTELY for Oral Solution 1068

Tacrolimus (Co-administration may alter the metabolism of tacrolimus resulting in increased plasma concentration; dosage of tacrolimus may have to be adjusted). Products include:
Prograf 1393
Protopic Ointment 1397

Terfenadine (Co-administration has resulted in rare cases of serious cardiovascular adverse events including death, ventricular tachycardia, and torsade de pointes due to increased terfenadine concentrations caused by ketoconazole tablets; concurrent use is contraindicated).
No products indexed under this heading.

Tolazamide (Possibility of severe hypoglycemia cannot be ruled out).
No products indexed under this heading.

Tolbutamide (Possibility of severe hypoglycemia cannot be ruled out).
No products indexed under this heading.

Tolterodine Tartrate (Nizoral requires acidity for dissolution, these drugs should be given at least two hours after Nizoral administration). Products include:
Detrol Tablets 3623
Detrol LA Capsules 2801

Triazolam (Co-administration has resulted in elevated plasma concentration of triazolam resulting in prolonged hypnotic and sedative effects; concurrent use with oral triazolam is contraindicated). Products include:
Halcion Tablets 2823

Tridihexethyl Chloride (Nizoral requires acidity for dissolution, these drugs should be given at least two hours after Nizoral administration).
No products indexed under this heading.

Trihexyphenidyl Hydrochloride (Nizoral requires acidity for dissolution, these drugs should be given at least two hours after Nizoral administration). Products include:
Artane 1855

Troglitazone (Possibility of severe hypoglycemia cannot be ruled out).
No products indexed under this heading.

Warfarin Sodium (Anticoagulant effect enhanced). Products include:
Coumadin for Injection 1243
Coumadin Tablets 1243
Warfarin Sodium Tablets, USP 3302

Food Interactions

Alcohol (Potential for disulfiram-like reaction to alcohol resulting in flushing, rash, peripheral edema, nausea and headache).

NOLVADEX TABLETS

(Tamoxifen Citrate) 678
May interact with oral anticoagulants, cytotoxic drugs, and certain other agents. Compounds in these categories include:

Bleomycin Sulfate (Increased incidence of thromboembolic events when cytotoxic agents are combined with Nolvadex).
No products indexed under this heading.

Bromocriptine Mesylate (Concomitant therapy has been shown to elevate serum tamoxifen and N-desmethyl-tamoxifen).
No products indexed under this heading.

Cyclophosphamide (Increased incidence of thromboembolic events when cytotoxic agents are combined with Nolvadex).
No products indexed under this heading.

Daunorubicin Hydrochloride (Increased incidence of thromboembolic events when cytotoxic agents are combined with Nolvadex). Products include:
Cerubidine for Injection 947

Dicumarol (Increased anticoagulant effect; monitor patient's prothrombin time).
No products indexed under this heading.

Doxorubicin Hydrochloride (Increased incidence of thromboembolic events when cytotoxic agents are combined with Nolvadex). Products include:
Adriamycin PFS/RDF Injection 2767
Doxil Injection 566

Epirubicin Hydrochloride (Increased incidence of thromboembolic events when cytotoxic agents are combined with Nolvadex). Products include:
Ellence Injection 2806

Fluorouracil (Increased incidence of thromboembolic events when cytotoxic agents are combined with Nolvadex). Products include:
Carac Cream 1222
Efudex 1733
Fluoroplex 552

Hydroxyurea (Increased incidence of thromboembolic events when cytotoxic agents are combined with Nolvadex). Products include:
Mylocel Tablets 2227

Methotrexate Sodium (Increased incidence of thromboembolic events when cytotoxic agents are combined with Nolvadex).
No products indexed under this heading.

Mitotane (Increased incidence of thromboembolic events when cytotoxic agents are combined with Nolvadex).
No products indexed under this heading.

Mitoxantrone Hydrochloride (Increased incidence of thromboembolic events when cytotoxic agents are combined with Nolvadex). Products include:
Novantrone for Injection 1760

Phenobarbital (Concomitant therapy in one patient resulted in lower steady state serum level of tamoxifen). Products include:
Arco-Lase Plus Tablets 592
Donnatal 2929
Donnatal Extentabs 2930

Procarbazine Hydrochloride (Increased incidence of thromboembolic events when cytotoxic agents are combined with Nolvadex). Products include:
Matulane Capsules 3246

Vincristine Sulfate (Increased incidence of thromboembolic events when cytotoxic agents are combined with Nolvadex).
No products indexed under this heading.

Warfarin Sodium (Increased anticoagulant effect; monitor patient's prothrombin time). Products include:
Coumadin for Injection 1243
Coumadin Tablets 1243
Warfarin Sodium Tablets, USP 3302

NORCO 5/325 TABLETS CIII

(Acetaminophen, Hydrocodone Bitartrate) 3424
See Norco 7.5/325 Tablets CIII

NORCO 7.5/325 TABLETS CIII

(Acetaminophen, Hydrocodone Bitartrate) 3425
May interact with antihistamines, central nervous system depressants, monoamine oxidase inhibitors, narcotic analgesics, antipsychotic agents, tricyclic antidepressants, and certain other agents. Compounds in these categories include:

Acrivastine (Co-administration may exhibit an additive CNS depression). Products include:
Semprex-D Capsules 1172

Alfentanil Hydrochloride (Co-administration may exhibit an additive CNS depression).
No products indexed under this heading.

Alprazolam (Co-administration may exhibit an additive CNS depression). Products include:
Xanax Tablets 2865

Amitriptyline Hydrochloride (Co-administration with tricyclic antidepressant may increase the effect of either hydrocodone or tricyclic antidepressant). Products include:
Etrafon 3115
Limbitrol 1738

Amoxapine (Co-administration with tricyclic antidepressant may increase the effect of either hydrocodone or tricyclic antidepressant).
No products indexed under this heading.

Aprobarbital (Co-administration may exhibit an additive CNS depression).
No products indexed under this heading.

Astemizole (Co-administration may exhibit an additive CNS depression).
No products indexed under this heading.

Azatadine Maleate (Co-administration may exhibit an additive CNS depression). Products include:
Rynatan Tablets 3351

Bromodiphenhydramine Hydrochloride (Co-administration may exhibit an additive CNS depression).
No products indexed under this heading.

Brompheniramine Maleate (Co-administration may exhibit an additive CNS depression). Products include:
Bromfed Capsules (Extended-Release) 2269
Bromfed-PD Capsules (Extended-Release) 2269
Comtrex Acute Head Cold & Sinus Pressure Relief Tablets .... ■627

Dimetapp Elixir .... ■777
Dimetapp Cold and Fever Suspension .... ■775
Dimetapp DM Cold & Cough Elixir . ■775
Dimetapp Nighttime Flu Liquid ...... ■776

Buprenorphine Hydrochloride (Co-administration may exhibit an additive CNS depression). Products include:
Buprenex Injectable 2918

Buspirone Hydrochloride (Co-administration may exhibit an additive CNS depression).
No products indexed under this heading.

Butabarbital (Co-administration may exhibit an additive CNS depression).
No products indexed under this heading.

Butalbital (Co-administration may exhibit an additive CNS depression). Products include:
Phrenilin 578
Sedapap Tablets 50 mg/650 mg 2225

Cetirizine Hydrochloride (Co-administration may exhibit an additive CNS depression). Products include:
Zyrtec 2756
Zyrtec-D 12 Hour Extended Relief Tablets 2758

Chlordiazepoxide (Co-administration may exhibit an additive CNS depression). Products include:
Limbitrol 1738

Chlordiazepoxide Hydrochloride (Co-administration may exhibit an additive CNS depression). Products include:
Librium Capsules 1736
Librium for Injection 1737

Chlorpheniramine Maleate (Co-administration may exhibit an additive CNS depression). Products include:
Actifed Cold & Sinus Caplets and Tablets .... ■688
Alka-Seltzer Plus Liqui-Gels .... ■604
BC Allergy Sinus Cold Powder .... ■619
Chlor-Trimeton Allergy Tablets ...... ■735
Chlor-Trimeton Allergy/Decongestant Tablets .... ■736
Comtrex Flu Therapy & Fever Relief Nighttime Tablets .... ■628
Comtrex Maximum Strength Multi-Symptom Cold & Cough Relief Tablets and Caplets .... ■626
Contac Severe Cold and Flu Caplets Maximum Strength .... ■746
Coricidin 'D' Cold, Flu & Sinus Tablets .... ■737
Coricidin/Coricidin D .... ■738
Coricidin HBP Maximum Strength Flu Tablets .... ■738
Extendryl 1361
Hycomine Compound Tablets 1317
Kronofed-A 1341
PediaCare Cough-Cold Liquid .... ■719
PediaCare NightRest Cough-Cold Liquid .... ■719
Robitussin Nighttime Honey Flu Liquid .... ■786
Ryna .... ■768
Singlet Caplets .... ■761
Sinutab Sinus Allergy Medication, Maximum Strength Formula, Tablets & Caplets .... ■707
Sudafed Cold & Allergy Tablets .... ■708
TheraFlu Regular Strength Cold & Cough Night Time Hot Liquid...... ■676
TheraFlu Regular Strength Cold & Sore Throat Night Time Hot Liquid .... ■676
TheraFlu Maximum Strength Flu & Cough Night Time Hot Liquid .. ■678
TheraFlu Maximum Strength Flu & Sore Throat Night Time Hot Liquid .... ■677
TheraFlu Maximum Strength Severe Cold & Congestion Night Time Caplets .... ■678
TheraFlu Maximum Strength Severe Cold & Congestion Night Time Hot Liquid .... ■678
Triaminic Cold & Allergy Liquid .... ■681
Triaminic Cold & Allergy Softchews .... ■683
Triaminic Cold & Cough Liquid ...... ■681
Triaminic Cold & Cough Softchews .... ■683
Triaminic Cold & Night Time Cough Liquid .... ■681
Triaminic Cold, Cough & Fever Liquid .... ■681
Children's Tylenol Cold Suspension Liquid and Chewable Tablets 2015
Children's Tylenol Cold Plus Cough Suspension Liquid and Chewable Tablets 2015
Children's Tylenol Flu Suspension Liquid 2015
Maximum Strength Tylenol Allergy Sinus Caplets, Gelcaps, and Geltabs 2010
Multi-Symptom Tylenol Cold Complete Formula Caplets 2010
Vicks 44M Cough, Cold & Flu Relief Liquid .... ■725
Pediatric Vicks 44m Cough & Cold Relief .... ■728
Children's Vicks NyQuil Cold/Cough Relief .... ■726

Chlorpheniramine Polistirex (Co-administration may exhibit an additive CNS depression). Products include:
Tussionex Pennkinetic Extended-Release Suspension..... 1174

Chlorpheniramine Tannate (Co-administration may exhibit an additive CNS depression). Products include:
Reformulated Rynatan Pediatric Suspension 3352
Rynatuss Pediatric Suspension 3353
Rynatuss Tablets 3353
Tussi-12 S Suspension 3356
Tussi-12 Tablets 3356

Chlorpromazine (Co-administration may exhibit an additive CNS depression). Products include:
Thorazine Suppositories 1656

Chlorpromazine Hydrochloride (Co-administration may exhibit an additive CNS depression). Products include:
Thorazine 1656

Chlorprothixene (Co-administration may exhibit an additive CNS depression).
No products indexed under this heading.

Chlorprothixene Hydrochloride (Co-administration may exhibit an additive CNS depression).
No products indexed under this heading.

Chlorprothixene Lactate (Co-administration may exhibit an additive CNS depression).
No products indexed under this heading.

Clemastine Fumarate (Co-administration may exhibit an additive CNS depression). Products include:
Tavist 12 Hour Allergy Tablets ...... ■676

Clomipramine Hydrochloride (Co-administration with tricyclic antidepressant may increase the effect of either hydrocodone or tricyclic antidepressant).
No products indexed under this heading.

Clorazepate Dipotassium (Co-administration may exhibit an additive CNS depression). Products include:
Tranxene 511

Clozapine (Co-administration may exhibit an additive CNS depression). Products include:
Clozaril Tablets 2319

Codeine Phosphate (Co-administration may exhibit an additive CNS depression). Products include:
Phenergan with Codeine Syrup 3557
Phenergan VC with Codeine Syrup .. 3561
Robitussin A-C Syrup 2942
Robitussin-DAC Syrup 2942
Ryna-C Liquid .... ■768
Soma Compound w/Codeine Tablets 3355
Tussi-Organidin NR Liquid 3350
Tussi-Organidin-S NR Liquid 3350
Tylenol with Codeine 2595

Cyproheptadine Hydrochloride (Co-administration may exhibit an additive CNS depression). Products include:
Periactin Tablets 2155

Desflurane (Co-administration may exhibit an additive CNS depression). Products include:
Suprane Liquid for Inhalation 874

Desipramine Hydrochloride (Co-administration with tricyclic antidepressant may increase the effect of either hydrocodone or tricyclic antidepressant). Products include:
Norpramin Tablets 755

Dexchlorpheniramine Maleate (Co-administration may exhibit an additive CNS depression).
No products indexed under this heading.

Dezocine (Co-administration may exhibit an additive CNS depression).
No products indexed under this heading.

Diazepam (Co-administration may exhibit an additive CNS depression). Products include:
Valium Injectable 3026
Valium Tablets 3047

Diphenhydramine Citrate (Co-administration may exhibit an additive CNS depression). Products include:
Alka-Seltzer PM Effervescent Tablets .... ■605
Benadryl Allergy & Sinus Fastmelt Tablets .... ■693
Benadryl Children's Allergy/Cold Fastmelt Tablets .... ■692
Excedrin PM Tablets, Caplets, and Geltabs .... ■631
Goody's PM Powder .... ■621

Diphenhydramine Hydrochloride (Co-administration may exhibit an additive CNS depression). Products include:
Extra Strength Bayer PM Caplets .... ■611
Benadryl Allergy Chewables .... ■689
Benadryl Allergy .... ■691
Benadryl Allergy Liquid .... ■690
Benadryl Allergy/Cold Tablets .... ■691
Benadryl Allergy/Congestion Tablets .... ■692
Benadryl Allergy & Sinus Liquid ..... ■693
Benadryl Allergy Sinus Headache Caplets & Gelcaps .... ■693
Benadryl Severe Allergy & Sinus Headache Caplets .... ■694
Benadryl Dye-Free Allergy Liquid .... ■690
Benadryl Dye-Free Allergy Liqui-Gels Softgels .... ■690
Benadryl Itch Relief Stick Extra Strength .... ■695
Benadryl Cream .... ■695
Benadryl Gel .... ■695
Benadryl Spray .... ■696
Benadryl Parenteral 2617
Coricidin HBP Night-Time Cold & Flu Tablets .... ■738
Nytol QuickCaps Caplets .... ■622
Maximum Strength Nytol QuickGels Softgels .... ■621
Extra Strength Percogesic Aspirin-Free Coated Caplets .... ■665
Simply Sleep Caplets 2008
Sominex Original Formula Tablets . ■761
Children's Tylenol Allergy-D Liquid ... 2014
Maximum Strength Tylenol Allergy Sinus NightTime Caplets 2010
Tylenol Severe Allergy Caplets 2010
Maximum Strength Tylenol Flu NightTime Gelcaps 2011
Extra Strength Tylenol PM Caplets, Geltabs, and Gelcaps 2012
Unisom Maximum Strength SleepGels .... ■713

Diphenylpyraline Hydrochloride (Co-administration may exhibit an additive CNS depression).
No products indexed under this heading.

Doxepin Hydrochloride (Co-administration with tricyclic antidepressant may increase the effect of either hydrocodone or tricyclic antidepressant). Products include:
Sinequan 2713

Droperidol (Co-administration may exhibit an additive CNS depression).
No products indexed under this heading.

Enflurane (Co-administration may exhibit an additive CNS depression).
No products indexed under this heading.

Estazolam (Co-administration may exhibit an additive CNS depression). Products include:
ProSom Tablets 500

Ethchlorvynol (Co-administration may exhibit an additive CNS depression).
No products indexed under this heading.

Ethinamate (Co-administration may exhibit an additive CNS depression).
No products indexed under this heading.

Fentanyl (Co-administration may exhibit an additive CNS depression). Products include:
Duragesic Transdermal System 1786

Fentanyl Citrate (Co-administration may exhibit an additive CNS depression). Products include:
Actiq 1184

Fexofenadine Hydrochloride (Co-administration may exhibit an additive CNS depression). Products include:
Allegra 712
Allegra-D Extended-Release Tablets 714

Fluphenazine Decanoate (Co-administration may exhibit an additive CNS depression).
No products indexed under this heading.

Fluphenazine Enanthate (Co-administration may exhibit an additive CNS depression).
No products indexed under this heading.

Fluphenazine Hydrochloride (Co-administration may exhibit an additive CNS depression).
No products indexed under this heading.

Flurazepam Hydrochloride (Co-administration may exhibit an additive CNS depression).
No products indexed under this heading.

Glutethimide (Co-administration may exhibit an additive CNS depression).
No products indexed under this heading.

Haloperidol (Co-administration may exhibit an additive CNS depression). Products include:
Haldol Injection, Tablets and Concentrate 2533

Haloperidol Decanoate (Co-administration may exhibit an additive CNS depression). Products include:
Haldol Decanoate 2535

Hydrocodone Polistirex (Co-administration may exhibit an additive CNS depression). Products include:
Tussionex Pennkinetic Extended-Release Suspension 1174

Hydromorphone Hydrochloride (Co-administration may exhibit an additive CNS depression). Products include:
Dilaudid 441
Dilaudid Oral Liquid 445
Dilaudid Powder 441
Dilaudid Rectal Suppositories 441
Dilaudid Tablets 441
Dilaudid Tablets - 8 mg 445
Dilaudid-HP 443

Hydroxyzine Hydrochloride (Co-administration may exhibit an additive CNS depression). Products include:
Atarax Tablets & Syrup 2667

Vistaril Intramuscular Solution 2738

Imipramine Hydrochloride (Co-administration with tricyclic antidepressant may increase the effect of either hydrocodone or tricyclic antidepressant).
No products indexed under this heading.

Imipramine Pamoate (Co-administration with tricyclic antidepressant may increase the effect of either hydrocodone or tricyclic antidepressant).
No products indexed under this heading.

Isocarboxazid (Co-administration with an MAO inhibitor may increase the effect of either hydrocodone or MAO inhibitor).
No products indexed under this heading.

Isoflurane (Co-administration may exhibit an additive CNS depression).
No products indexed under this heading.

Ketamine Hydrochloride (Co-administration may exhibit an additive CNS depression).
No products indexed under this heading.

Levomethadyl Acetate Hydrochloride (Co-administration may exhibit an additive CNS depression).
No products indexed under this heading.

Levorphanol Tartrate (Co-administration may exhibit an additive CNS depression). Products include:
Levo-Dromoran 1734
Levorphanol Tartrate Tablets 3059

Lithium Carbonate (Co-administration may exhibit an additive CNS depression). Products include:
Eskalith 1527
Lithium Carbonate 3061
Lithobid Slow-Release Tablets 3255

Lithium Citrate (Co-administration may exhibit an additive CNS depression). Products include:
Lithium Citrate Syrup 3061

Loratadine (Co-administration may exhibit an additive CNS depression). Products include:
Claritin 3100
Claritin-D 12 Hour Extended Release Tablets 3102
Claritin-D 24 Hour Extended Release Tablets 3104

Lorazepam (Co-administration may exhibit an additive CNS depression). Products include:
Ativan Injection 3478
Ativan Tablets 3482

Loxapine Hydrochloride (Co-administration may exhibit an additive CNS depression).
No products indexed under this heading.

Loxapine Succinate (Co-administration may exhibit an additive CNS depression). Products include:
Loxitane Capsules 3398

Maprotiline Hydrochloride (Co-administration with tricyclic antidepressant may increase the effect of either hydrocodone or tricyclic antidepressant).
No products indexed under this heading.

Meperidine Hydrochloride (Co-administration may exhibit an additive CNS depression). Products include:
Demerol 3079
Mepergan Injection 3539

Mephobarbital (Co-administration may exhibit an additive CNS depression).
No products indexed under this heading.

Meprobamate (Co-administration may exhibit an additive CNS depression). Products include:
Miltown Tablets 3349

Mesoridazine Besylate (Co-administration may exhibit an additive CNS depression). Products include:
Serentil 1057

Methadone Hydrochloride (Co-administration may exhibit an additive CNS depression). Products include:
Dolophine Hydrochloride Tablets 3056

Methdilazine Hydrochloride (Co-administration may exhibit an additive CNS depression).
No products indexed under this heading.

Methohexital Sodium (Co-administration may exhibit an additive CNS depression). Products include:
Brevital Sodium for Injection, USP .. 1815

Methotrimeprazine (Co-administration may exhibit an additive CNS depression).
No products indexed under this heading.

Methoxyflurane (Co-administration may exhibit an additive CNS depression).
No products indexed under this heading.

Midazolam Hydrochloride (Co-administration may exhibit an additive CNS depression). Products include:
Versed Injection 3027
Versed Syrup 3033

Moclobemide (Co-administration with an MAO inhibitor may increase the effect of either hydrocodone or MAO inhibitor).
No products indexed under this heading.

Molindone Hydrochloride (Co-administration may exhibit an additive CNS depression). Products include:
Moban 1320

Morphine Sulfate (Co-administration may exhibit an additive CNS depression). Products include:
Astramorph/PF Injection, USP (Preservative-Free)...................... 594
Duramorph Injection 1312
Infumorph 200 and Infumorph 500 Sterile Solutions......................... 1314
Kadian Capsules 1335
MS Contin Tablets 2896
MSIR 2898
Oramorph SR Tablets 3062
Roxanol 3066

Nortriptyline Hydrochloride (Co-administration with tricyclic antidepressant may increase the effect of either hydrocodone or tricyclic antidepressant).
No products indexed under this heading.

Olanzapine (Co-administration may exhibit an additive CNS depression). Products include:
Zyprexa Tablets 1973
Zyprexa ZYDIS Orally Disintegrating Tablets................. 1973

Oxazepam (Co-administration may exhibit an additive CNS depression).
No products indexed under this heading.

Oxycodone Hydrochloride (Co-administration may exhibit an additive CNS depression). Products include:
OxyContin Tablets 2912
OxyFast Oral Concentrate Solution . 2916
OxyIR Capsules 2916
Percocet Tablets 1326
Percodan Tablets 1327
Percolone Tablets 1327
Roxicodone 3067
Tylox Capsules 2597

Pargyline Hydrochloride (Co-administration with an MAO inhibitor may increase the effect of either hydrocodone or MAO inhibitor).
No products indexed under this heading.

Pentobarbital Sodium (Co-administration may exhibit an additive CNS depression). Products include:
Nembutal Sodium Solution 485

Perphenazine (Co-administration may exhibit an additive CNS depression). Products include:
Etrafon 3115
Trilafon 3160

Phenelzine Sulfate (Co-administration with an MAO inhibitor may increase the effect of either hydrocodone or MAO inhibitor). Products include:
Nardil Tablets 2653

Phenobarbital (Co-administration may exhibit an additive CNS depression). Products include:
Arco-Lase Plus Tablets 592
Donnatal 2929
Donnatal Extentabs 2930

Pimozide (Co-administration may exhibit an additive CNS depression). Products include:
Orap Tablets 1407

Prazepam (Co-administration may exhibit an additive CNS depression).
No products indexed under this heading.

Procarbazine Hydrochloride (Co-administration with an MAO inhibitor may increase the effect of either hydrocodone or MAO inhibitor). Products include:
Matulane Capsules 3246

Prochlorperazine (Co-administration may exhibit an additive CNS depression). Products include:
Compazine 1505

Promethazine Hydrochloride (Co-administration may exhibit an additive CNS depression). Products include:
Mepergan Injection 3539
Phenergan Injection 3553
Phenergan 3556
Phenergan Syrup 3554
Phenergan with Codeine Syrup 3557
Phenergan with Dextromethorphan Syrup 3559
Phenergan VC Syrup 3560
Phenergan VC with Codeine Syrup .. 3561

Propofol (Co-administration may exhibit an additive CNS depression). Products include:
Diprivan Injectable Emulsion 667

Propoxyphene Hydrochloride (Co-administration may exhibit an additive CNS depression). Products include:
Darvon Pulvules 1909
Darvon Compound-65 Pulvules 1910

Propoxyphene Napsylate (Co-administration may exhibit an additive CNS depression). Products include:
Darvon-N/Darvocet-N 1907
Darvon-N Tablets 1912

Protriptyline Hydrochloride (Co-administration with tricyclic antidepressant may increase the effect of either hydrocodone or tricyclic antidepressant). Products include:
Vivactil Tablets 2446
Vivactil Tablets 2217

Pyrilamine Maleate (Co-administration may exhibit an additive CNS depression). Products include:
Maximum Strength Midol Menstrual Caplets and Gelcaps...................................... ▭612
Maximum Strength Midol PMS Caplets and Gelcaps................. ▭613

Pyrilamine Tannate (Co-administration may exhibit an additive CNS depression). Products include:
Ryna-12 S Suspension 3351

Quazepam (Co-administration may exhibit an additive CNS depression).
No products indexed under this heading.

Quetiapine Fumarate (Co-administration may exhibit an additive CNS depression). Products include:
Seroquel Tablets 684

Remifentanil Hydrochloride (Co-administration may exhibit an additive CNS depression).
No products indexed under this heading.

Risperidone (Co-administration may exhibit an additive CNS depression). Products include:
Risperdal 1796

Secobarbital Sodium (Co-administration may exhibit an additive CNS depression).
No products indexed under this heading.

Selegiline Hydrochloride (Co-administration with an MAO inhibitor may increase the effect of either hydrocodone or MAO inhibitor). Products include:
Eldepryl Capsules 3266

Sevoflurane (Co-administration may exhibit an additive CNS depression).
No products indexed under this heading.

Sufentanil Citrate (Co-administration may exhibit an additive CNS depression).
No products indexed under this heading.

Temazepam (Co-administration may exhibit an additive CNS depression).
No products indexed under this heading.

Terfenadine (Co-administration may exhibit an additive CNS depression).
No products indexed under this heading.

Thiamylal Sodium (Co-administration may exhibit an additive CNS depression).
No products indexed under this heading.

Thioridazine Hydrochloride (Co-administration may exhibit an additive CNS depression). Products include:
Thioridazine Hydrochloride Tablets....................................... 2289

Thiothixene (Co-administration may exhibit an additive CNS depression). Products include:
Navane Capsules 2701
Thiothixene Capsules 2290

Tranylcypromine Sulfate (Co-administration with an MAO inhibitor may increase the effect of either hydrocodone or MAO inhibitor). Products include:
Parnate Tablets 1607

Triazolam (Co-administration may exhibit an additive CNS depression). Products include:
Halcion Tablets 2823

Trifluoperazine Hydrochloride (Co-administration may exhibit an additive CNS depression). Products include:
Stelazine 1640

Trimeprazine Tartrate (Co-administration may exhibit an additive CNS depression).
No products indexed under this heading.

Trimipramine Maleate (Co-administration with tricyclic antidepressant may increase the effect of either hydrocodone or tricyclic antidepressant). Products include:
Surmontil Capsules 3595

Tripelennamine Hydrochloride (Co-administration may exhibit an

additive CNS depression).
No products indexed under this heading.

Triprolidine Hydrochloride (Co-administration may exhibit an additive CNS depression). Products include:
Actifed Cold & Allergy Tablets .... ▣688

Zaleplon (Co-administration may exhibit an additive CNS depression). Products include:
Sonata Capsules 3591

Ziprasidone Hydrochloride (Co-administration may exhibit an additive CNS depression). Products include:
Geodon Capsules 2688

Zolpidem Tartrate (Co-administration may exhibit an additive CNS depression). Products include:
Ambien Tablets 3191

Food Interactions

Alcohol (Concurrent use results in additive CNS depression; alcohol intake should be avoided).

NORCO 10/325 TABLETS CIII

(Acetaminophen, Hydrocodone Bitartrate) 3425
See Norco 7.5/325 Tablets CIII

NORCO 10/325 TABLETS CIII

(Acetaminophen, Hydrocodone Bitartrate) 3427
See Norco 7.5/325 Tablets CIII

NORCURON FOR INJECTION

(Vecuronium Bromide) 2478
May interact with aminoglycosides, inhalant anesthetics, nondepolarizing neuromuscular blocking agents, tetracyclines, and certain other agents. Compounds in these categories include:

Amikacin Sulfate (Possible prolongation of neuromuscular blockade).
No products indexed under this heading.

Atracurium Besylate (Additive effect).
No products indexed under this heading.

Bacitracin (Possible prolongation of neuromuscular blockade).
No products indexed under this heading.

Cisatracurium Besylate (Additive effect).
No products indexed under this heading.

Colistimethate Sodium (Possible prolongation of neuromuscular blockade). Products include:
Coly-Mycin M Parenteral 2243

Colistin Sulfate (Possible prolongation of neuromuscular blockade). Products include:
Cortisporin-TC Otic Suspension 2246

Demeclocycline Hydrochloride (Possible prolongation of neuromuscular blockade). Products include:
Declomycin Tablets 1855

Desflurane (Pronounced enhancement of neuromuscular blockade). Products include:
Suprane Liquid for Inhalation 874

Doxycycline Calcium (Possible prolongation of neuromuscular blockade). Products include:
Vibramycin Calcium Oral Suspension Syrup 2735

Doxycycline Hyclate (Possible prolongation of neuromuscular blockade). Products include:
Doryx Coated Pellet Filled Capsules 3357
Periostat Tablets 1208
Vibramycin Hyclate Capsules 2735
Vibramycin Hyclate Intravenous 2737
Vibra-Tabs Film Coated Tablets 2735

Doxycycline Monohydrate (Possible prolongation of neuromuscular blockade). Products include:
Monodox Capsules 2442
Vibramycin Monohydrate for Oral Suspension 2735

Enflurane (Pronounced enhancement of neuromuscular blockade).
No products indexed under this heading.

Gentamicin Sulfate (Possible prolongation of neuromuscular blockade). Products include:
Genoptic Ophthalmic Ointment ...... ⊙239
Genoptic Sterile Ophthalmic Solution .... ⊙239
Pred-G Ophthalmic Suspension ..... ⊙247
Pred-G Sterile Ophthalmic Ointment .... ⊙248

Halothane (Pronounced enhancement of neuromuscular blockade). Products include:
Fluothane Inhalation 3508

Isoflurane (Pronounced enhancement of neuromuscular blockade).
No products indexed under this heading.

Kanamycin Sulfate (Possible prolongation of neuromuscular blockade).
No products indexed under this heading.

Magnesium Sulfate Injection (May enhance the neuromuscular blockade).

Methacycline Hydrochloride (Possible prolongation of neuromuscular blockade).
No products indexed under this heading.

Methoxyflurane (Pronounced enhancement of neuromuscular blockade).
No products indexed under this heading.

Metocurine Iodide (Additive effect).
No products indexed under this heading.

Minocycline Hydrochloride (Possible prolongation of neuromuscular blockade). Products include:
Dynacin Capsules 2019
Minocin Intravenous 1862
Minocin Oral Suspension 1865
Minocin Pellet-Filled Capsules 1863

Mivacurium Chloride (Additive effect).
No products indexed under this heading.

Neomycin, oral (Possible prolongation of neuromuscular blockade).

Oxytetracycline (Possible prolongation of neuromuscular blockade).
No products indexed under this heading.

Oxytetracycline Hydrochloride (Possible prolongation of neuromuscular blockade). Products include:
Terra-Cortril Ophthalmic Suspension 2716
Urobiotic-250 Capsules 2731

Pancuronium Bromide (Additive effect).
No products indexed under this heading.

Polymyxin B Sulfate (Possible prolongation of neuromuscular blockade). Products include:
Betadine Brand First Aid Antibiotics & Moisturizer Ointment 2894
Betadine Brand Plus First Aid Antibiotics & Pain Reliever Ointment 2894
Cortisporin Ophthalmic Suspension Sterile .... ⊙297
Neosporin G.U. Irrigant Sterile 2256
Neosporin Ointment .... ▣704
Neosporin Ophthalmic Ointment Sterile .... ⊙299
Neosporin Ophthalmic Solution Sterile .... ⊙300
Neosporin + Pain Relief Maximum Strength Cream .... ▣704
Neosporin + Pain Relief Maximum Strength Ointment .... ▣704
Poly-Pred Liquifilm Ophthalmic Suspension .... ⊙245
Polysporin Ointment .... ▣706
Polysporin Ophthalmic Ointment Sterile .... ⊙301
Polysporin Powder .... ▣706
Polytrim Ophthalmic Solution 556

Quinidine Gluconate (Possible recurrent paralysis). Products include:
Quinaglute Dura-Tabs Tablets 978

Quinidine Polygalacturonate (Possible recurrent paralysis).
No products indexed under this heading.

Quinidine Sulfate (Possible recurrent paralysis). Products include:
Quinidex Extentabs 2933

Rapacuronium Bromide (Additive effect).
No products indexed under this heading.

Rocuronium Bromide (Additive effect). Products include:
Zemuron Injection 2491

Streptomycin Sulfate (Possible prolongation of neuromuscular blockade). Products include:
Streptomycin Sulfate Injection 2714

Succinylcholine Chloride (Prior administration may enhance neuromuscular blocking effect and duration of action of Norcuron). Products include:
Anectine Injection 1476

Tetracycline Hydrochloride (Possible prolongation of neuromuscular blockade).
No products indexed under this heading.

Tobramycin (Possible prolongation of neuromuscular blockade). Products include:
TOBI Solution for Inhalation 1206
TobraDex Ophthalmic Ointment 542
TobraDex Ophthalmic Suspension .. 541
Tobrex Ophthalmic Ointment .... ⊙220
Tobrex Ophthalmic Solution .... ⊙221

Tobramycin Sulfate (Possible prolongation of neuromuscular blockade). Products include:
Nebcin Vials, Hyporets & ADD-Vantage 1955

NORDETTE-28 TABLETS

(Ethinyl Estradiol, Levonorgestrel) 2257
May interact with barbiturates and certain other agents. Compounds in these categories include:

Ampicillin Sodium (Reduced efficacy; increased incidence of breakthrough bleeding). Products include:
Unasyn for Injection 2728

Aprobarbital (Reduced efficacy; increased incidence of breakthrough bleeding).
No products indexed under this heading.

Butabarbital (Reduced efficacy; increased incidence of breakthrough bleeding).
No products indexed under this heading.

Butalbital (Reduced efficacy; increased incidence of breakthrough bleeding). Products include:
Phrenilin 578
Sedapap Tablets 50 mg/650 mg ... 2225

Mephobarbital (Reduced efficacy; increased incidence of breakthrough bleeding).
No products indexed under this heading.

Oxytetracycline (Reduced efficacy; increased incidence of breakthrough bleeding).
No products indexed under this heading.

Oxytetracycline Hydrochloride (Reduced efficacy; increased incidence of breakthrough bleeding). Products include:
Terra-Cortril Ophthalmic Suspension 2716
Urobiotic-250 Capsules 2731

Pentobarbital Sodium (Reduced efficacy; increased incidence of breakthrough bleeding). Products include:
Nembutal Sodium Solution 485

Phenobarbital (Reduced efficacy; increased incidence of breakthrough bleeding). Products include:
Arco-Lase Plus Tablets 592
Donnatal 2929
Donnatal Extentabs 2930

Phenylbutazone (Reduced efficacy; increased incidence of breakthrough bleeding).
No products indexed under this heading.

Phenytoin Sodium (Reduced efficacy; increased incidence of breakthrough bleeding). Products include:
Dilantin Kapseals 2622

Rifampin (Reduced efficacy; increased incidence of breakthrough bleeding). Products include:
Rifadin 765
Rifamate Capsules 767
Rifater Tablets 769

Secobarbital Sodium (Reduced efficacy; increased incidence of breakthrough bleeding).
No products indexed under this heading.

Tetracycline Hydrochloride (Reduced efficacy; increased incidence of breakthrough bleeding).
No products indexed under this heading.

Thiamylal Sodium (Reduced efficacy; increased incidence of breakthrough bleeding).
No products indexed under this heading.

NORDITROPIN CARTRIDGES

(Somatropin) 2420
See Norditropin for Injection

NORDITROPIN FOR INJECTION

(Somatropin) 2419
May interact with corticosteroids. Compounds in these categories include:

Betamethasone Acetate (Concomitant glucocorticoid therapy may inhibit the growth promoting effect of somatropin). Products include:
Celestone Soluspan Injectable Suspension 3097

Betamethasone Sodium Phosphate (Concomitant glucocorticoid therapy may inhibit the growth promoting effect of somatropin). Products include:
Celestone Soluspan Injectable Suspension 3097

Cortisone Acetate (Concomitant glucocorticoid therapy may inhibit the growth promoting effect of somatropin). Products include:
Cortone Acetate Injectable Suspension 2059
Cortone Acetate Tablets 2061

Dexamethasone (Concomitant glucocorticoid therapy may inhibit the growth promoting effect of somatropin). Products include:
Decadron Elixir 2078
Decadron Tablets 2079
TobraDex Ophthalmic Ointment 542
TobraDex Ophthalmic Suspension .. 541

Dexamethasone Acetate (Concomitant glucocorticoid therapy may inhibit the growth promoting effect

of somatropin).
No products indexed under this heading.

Dexamethasone Sodium Phosphate (Concomitant glucocorticoid therapy may inhibit the growth promoting effect of somatropin). Products include:
Decadron Phosphate Injection 2081
Decadron Phosphate Sterile Ophthalmic Ointment........................ 2083
Decadron Phosphate Sterile Ophthalmic Solution 2084
NeoDecadron Sterile Ophthalmic Solution..................................... 2144

Fludrocortisone Acetate (Concomitant glucocorticoid therapy may inhibit the growth promoting effect of somatropin). Products include:
Florinef Acetate Tablets 2250

Hydrocortisone (Concomitant glucocorticoid therapy may inhibit the growth promoting effect of somatropin). Products include:
Anusol-HC Cream 2.5% 2237
Cipro HC Otic Suspension 540
Cortaid Intensive Therapy Cream . ▣717
Cortaid Maximum Strength Cream ....▣717
Cortisporin Ophthalmic Suspension Sterile ....⊙297
Cortizone•5 ....▣699
Cortizone•10 ....▣699
Cortizone•10 Plus Creme ....▣700
Cortizone for Kids Creme ....▣699
Hydrocortone Tablets 2106
Massengill Medicated Soft Cloth Towelette ....▣753
VōSoL HC Otic Solution 3356

Hydrocortisone Acetate (Concomitant glucocorticoid therapy may inhibit the growth promoting effect of somatropin). Products include:
Analpram-HC 1338
Anusol HC-1 Hydrocortisone Anti-Itch Cream ....▣689
Anusol-HC Suppositories 2238
Cortaid ....▣717
Cortifoam Rectal Foam 3170
Cortisporin-TC Otic Suspension 2246
Hydrocortone Acetate Injectable Suspension 2103
Pramosone 1343
Proctocort Suppositories 2264
ProctoFoam-HC 3177
Terra-Cortril Ophthalmic Suspension 2716

Hydrocortisone Sodium Phosphate (Concomitant glucocorticoid therapy may inhibit the growth promoting effect of somatropin). Products include:
Hydrocortone Phosphate Injection, Sterile 2105

Hydrocortisone Sodium Succinate (Concomitant glucocorticoid therapy may inhibit the growth promoting effect of somatropin).
No products indexed under this heading.

Methylprednisolone Acetate (Concomitant glucocorticoid therapy may inhibit the growth promoting effect of somatropin). Products include:
Depo-Medrol Injectable Suspension 2795

Methylprednisolone Sodium Succinate (Concomitant glucocorticoid therapy may inhibit the growth promoting effect of somatropin). Products include:
Solu-Medrol Sterile Powder 2855

Prednisolone Acetate (Concomitant glucocorticoid therapy may inhibit the growth promoting effect of somatropin). Products include:
Blephamide Ophthalmic Ointment .. 547
Blephamide Ophthalmic Suspension 548
Poly-Pred Liquifilm Ophthalmic Suspension ....⊙245
Pred Forte Ophthalmic Suspension ....⊙246
Pred Mild Sterile Ophthalmic Suspension ....⊙249
Pred-G Ophthalmic Suspension .....⊙247
Pred-G Sterile Ophthalmic Ointment ....⊙248

Prednisolone Sodium Phosphate (Concomitant glucocorticoid therapy may inhibit the growth promoting effect of somatropin). Products include:
Pediapred Oral Solution 1170

Prednisolone Tebutate (Concomitant glucocorticoid therapy may inhibit the growth promoting effect of somatropin).
No products indexed under this heading.

Prednisone (Concomitant glucocorticoid therapy may inhibit the growth promoting effect of somatropin). Products include:
Prednisone 3064

Triamcinolone (Concomitant glucocorticoid therapy may inhibit the growth promoting effect of somatropin).
No products indexed under this heading.

Triamcinolone Acetonide (Concomitant glucocorticoid therapy may inhibit the growth promoting effect of somatropin). Products include:
Azmacort Inhalation Aerosol 728
Nasacort Nasal Inhaler 750
Nasacort AQ Nasal Spray 752
Tri-Nasal Spray 2274

Triamcinolone Diacetate (Concomitant glucocorticoid therapy may inhibit the growth promoting effect of somatropin).
No products indexed under this heading.

Triamcinolone Hexacetonide (Concomitant glucocorticoid therapy may inhibit the growth promoting effect of somatropin).
No products indexed under this heading.

NORFLEX EXTENDED-RELEASE TABLETS
(Orphenadrine Citrate) 1987
May interact with:

Propoxyphene Hydrochloride (Concomitant use results in confusion, anxiety and tremors). Products include:
Darvon Pulvules 1909
Darvon Compound-65 Pulvules 1910

Propoxyphene Napsylate (Concomitant use results in confusion, anxiety and tremors). Products include:
Darvon-N/Darvocet-N 1907
Darvon-N Tablets 1912

NORFLEX INJECTION
(Orphenadrine Citrate) 1987
See Norflex Extended-Release Tablets

NORINYL 1 +35 28-DAY TABLETS
(Ethinyl Estradiol, Norethindrone) 3380
See Brevicon 28-Day Tablets

NORINYL 1 + 50 28-DAY TABLETS
(Mestranol, Norethindrone) 3380
See Brevicon 28-Day Tablets

NORITATE CREAM
(Metronidazole) 1224
May interact with oral anticoagulants. Compounds in these categories include:

Dicumarol (Oral metronidazole has been reported to potentiate the anticoagulant effect of coumarin and warfarin resulting in a prolongation of prothrombin time; this interaction should be kept in mind if Noritate is used concurrently with oral coagulants).
No products indexed under this heading.

Warfarin Sodium (Oral metronidazole has been reported to potentiate the anticoagulant effect of coumarin and warfarin resulting in a prolongation of prothrombin time; this interaction should be kept in mind if Noritate is used concurrently with oral coagulants). Products include:
Coumadin for Injection 1243
Coumadin Tablets 1243
Warfarin Sodium Tablets, USP 3302

NORMODYNE INJECTION
(Labetalol Hydrochloride) 3135
See Normodyne Tablets

NORMODYNE TABLETS
(Labetalol Hydrochloride) 3137
May interact with diphenylalkylamine-type calcium antagonists, oral hypoglycemic agents, insulin, sympathomimetic bronchodilators, tricyclic antidepressants, and certain other agents. Compounds in these categories include:

Acarbose (Beta blockade may prevent the appearance of premonitory signs and symptoms of acute hypoglycemia; additionally, beta blockade reduces the release of insulin in response to hyperglycemia; it may be necessary to adjust the dosage of antidiabetic drugs). Products include:
Precose Tablets 906

Albuterol (Beta-blocker can blunt the bronchodilator effect of beta-receptor agonists in patients with bronchospasm; greater than normal anti-asthmatic dose of beta-agonist may be required). Products include:
Proventil Inhalation Aerosol 3142
Ventolin Inhalation Aerosol and Refill 1679

Albuterol Sulfate (Beta-blocker can blunt the bronchodilator effect of beta-receptor agonists in patients with bronchospasm; greater than normal anti-asthmatic dose of beta-agonist may be required). Products include:
AccuNeb Inhalation Solution 1230
Combivent Inhalation Aerosol 1041
DuoNeb Inhalation Solution 1233
Proventil Inhalation Solution 0.083% 3146
Proventil Repetabs Tablets 3148
Proventil Solution for Inhalation 0.5% 3144
Proventil HFA Inhalation Aerosol 3150
Ventolin HFA Inhalation Aerosol 3618
Volmax Extended-Release Tablets ..2276

Amitriptyline Hydrochloride (Potential for tremor). Products include:
Etrafon 3115
Limbitrol 1738

Amoxapine (Potential for tremor).
No products indexed under this heading

Bitolterol Mesylate (Beta-blocker can blunt the bronchodilator effect of beta-receptor agonists in patients with bronchospasm; greater than normal anti-asthmatic dose of beta-agonist may be required).
No products indexed under this heading.

Chlorpropamide (Beta blockade may prevent the appearance of premonitory signs and symptoms of acute hypoglycemia; additionally, beta blockade reduces the release of insulin in response to hyperglycemia; it may be necessary to adjust the dosage of antidiabetic drugs). Products include:
Diabinese Tablets 2680

Cimetidine (Increases bioavailability of labetalol). Products include:
Tagamet HB 200 Suspension ....▣762
Tagamet HB 200 Tablets ....▣761
Tagamet Tablets 1644

Cimetidine Hydrochloride (Increases bioavailability of labetalol). Products include:
Tagamet 1644

Clomipramine Hydrochloride (Potential for tremor).
No products indexed under this heading.

Desipramine Hydrochloride (Potential for tremor). Products include:
Norpramin Tablets 755

Doxepin Hydrochloride (Potential for tremor). Products include:
Sinequan 2713

Ephedrine Hydrochloride (Beta-blocker can blunt the bronchodilator effect of beta-receptor agonists in patients with bronchospasm; greater than normal anti-asthmatic dose of beta-agonist may be required). Products include:
Primatene Tablets ....▣780

Ephedrine Sulfate (Beta-blocker can blunt the bronchodilator effect of beta-receptor agonists in patients with bronchospasm; greater than normal anti-asthmatic dose of beta-agonist may be required).
No products indexed under this heading.

Ephedrine Tannate (Beta-blocker can blunt the bronchodilator effect of beta-receptor agonists in patients with bronchospasm; greater than normal anti-asthmatic dose of beta-agonist may be required). Products include:
Rynatuss Pediatric Suspension 3353
Rynatuss Tablets 3353

Epinephrine (Potential for unresponsiveness to the usual dose of epinephrine to treat allergic reaction). Products include:
Epifrin Sterile Ophthalmic Solution ....⊙235
EpiPen 1236
Primatene Mist ....▣779
Xylocaine with Epinephrine Injection 653

Epinephrine Hydrochloride (Potential for unresponsiveness to the usual dose of epinephrine to treat allergic reaction).
No products indexed under this heading.

Glimepiride (Beta blockade may prevent the appearance of premonitory signs and symptoms of acute hypoglycemia; additionally, beta blockade reduces the release of insulin in response to hyperglycemia; it may be necessary to adjust the dosage of antidiabetic drugs). Products include:
Amaryl Tablets 717

Glipizide (Beta blockade may prevent the appearance of premonitory signs and symptoms of acute hypoglycemia; additionally, beta blockade reduces the release of insulin in response to hyperglycemia; it may be necessary to adjust the dosage of antidiabetic drugs). Products include:
Glucotrol Tablets 2692
Glucotrol XL Extended Release Tablets 2693

Glyburide (Beta blockade may prevent the appearance of premonitory signs and symptoms of acute hypoglycemia; additionally, beta blockade reduces the release of insulin in response to hyperglycemia; it may be necessary to adjust the dosage of antidiabetic drugs). Products include:
DiaBeta Tablets 741
Glucovance Tablets 1086

Halothane (Synergism has been reported between labetalol I.V. and halothane anesthesia; potential increased hypotensive effect, reduction in cardiac output and increased in central venous pressure). Products include:
Fluothane Inhalation 3508

Imipramine Hydrochloride (Potential for tremor).
No products indexed under this heading.

Imipramine Pamoate (Potential for tremor).
No products indexed under this heading.

Insulin, Human, Zinc Suspension (Beta blockade may prevent the appearance of premonitory signs and symptoms of acute hypoglycemia; additionally, beta blockade reduces the release of insulin in response to hyperglycemia; it may be necessary to adjust the dosage of insulin). Products include:
Humulin L, 100 Units **1937**
Humulin U, 100 Units **1943**
Novolin L Human Insulin 10 ml Vials **2422**

Insulin, Human NPH (Beta blockade may prevent the appearance of premonitory signs and symptoms of acute hypoglycemia; additionally, beta blockade reduces the release of insulin in response to hyperglycemia; it may be necessary to adjust the dosage of insulin). Products include:
Humulin N, 100 Units **1939**
Humulin N NPH Pen **1940**
Novolin N Human Insulin 10 ml Vials **2422**
Novolin N PenFill **2423**
Novolin N Prefilled Syringe Disposable Insulin Delivery System **2425**

Insulin, Human Regular (Beta blockade may prevent the appearance of premonitory signs and symptoms of acute hypoglycemia; additionally, beta blockade reduces the release of insulin in response to hyperglycemia; it may be necessary to adjust the dosage of insulin). Products include:
Humulin R Regular (U-500) **1943**
Humulin R, 100 Units **1941**
Novolin R Human Insulin 10 ml Vials **2423**
Novolin R PenFill **2423**
Novolin R Prefilled Syringe Disposable Insulin Delivery System **2425**
Velosulin BR Human Insulin 10 ml Vials **2435**

Insulin, Human Regular and Human NPH Mixture (Beta blockade may prevent the appearance of premonitory signs and symptoms of acute hypoglycemia; additionally, beta blockade reduces the release of insulin in response to hyperglycemia; it may be necessary to adjust the dosage of insulin). Products include:
Humulin 50/50, 100 Units **1934**
Humulin 70/30, 100 Units **1935**
Humulin 70/30 Pen **1936**
Novolin 70/30 Human Insulin 10 ml Vials **2421**
Novolin 70/30 PenFill **2423**
Novolin 70/30 Prefilled Disposable Insulin Delivery System **2425**

Insulin, NPH (Beta blockade may prevent the appearance of premonitory signs and symptoms of acute hypoglycemia; additionally, beta blockade reduces the release of insulin in response to hyperglycemia; it may be necessary to adjust the dosage of insulin). Products include:
Iletin II, NPH (Pork), 100 Units **1946**

Insulin, Regular (Beta blockade may prevent the appearance of premonitory signs and symptoms of acute hypoglycemia; additionally, beta blockade reduces the release of insulin in response to hyperglycemia; it may be necessary to adjust the dosage of insulin). Products include:
Iletin II, Regular (Pork), 100 Units ... **1947**

Insulin, Zinc Crystals (Beta blockade may prevent the appearance of premonitory signs and symptoms of acute hypoglycemia; additionally, beta blockade reduces the release of insulin in response to hyperglycemia; it may be necessary to adjust the dosage of insulin).
No products indexed under this heading.

Insulin, Zinc Suspension (Beta blockade may prevent the appearance of premonitory signs and symptoms of acute hypoglycemia; additionally, beta blockade reduces the release of insulin in response to hyperglycemia; it may be necessary to adjust the dosage of insulin). Products include:
Iletin II, Lente (Pork), 100 Units **1945**

Insulin Aspart, Human Regular (Beta blockade may prevent the appearance of premonitory signs and symptoms of acute hypoglycemia; additionally, beta blockade reduces the release of insulin in response to hyperglycemia; it may be necessary to adjust the dosage of insulin).
No products indexed under this heading.

Insulin glargine (Beta blockade may prevent the appearance of premonitory signs and symptoms of acute hypoglycemia; additionally, beta blockade reduces the release of insulin in response to hyperglycemia; it may be necessary to adjust the dosage of insulin). Products include:
Lantus Injection **742**

Insulin Lispro, Human (Beta blockade may prevent the appearance of premonitory signs and symptoms of acute hypoglycemia; additionally, beta blockade reduces the release of insulin in response to hyperglycemia; it may be necessary to adjust the dosage of insulin). Products include:
Humalog **1926**
Humalog Mix 75/25 Pen **1928**

Insulin Lispro Protamine, Human (Beta blockade may prevent the appearance of premonitory signs and symptoms of acute hypoglycemia; additionally, beta blockade reduces the release of insulin in response to hyperglycemia; it may be necessary to adjust the dosage of insulin). Products include:
Humalog Mix 75/25 Pen **1928**

Isoetharine (Beta-blocker can blunt the bronchodilator effect of beta-receptor agonists in patients with bronchospasm; greater than normal anti-asthmatic dose of beta-agonist may be required).
No products indexed under this heading.

Isoproterenol Hydrochloride (Beta-blocker can blunt the bronchodilator effect of beta-receptor agonists in patients with bronchospasm; greater than normal anti-asthmatic dose of beta-agonist may be required).
No products indexed under this heading.

Isoproterenol Sulfate (Beta-blocker can blunt the bronchodilator effect of beta-receptor agonists in patients with bronchospasm; greater than normal anti-asthmatic dose of beta-agonist may be required).
No products indexed under this heading.

Levalbuterol Hydrochloride (Beta-blocker can blunt the bronchodilator effect of beta-receptor agonists in patients with bronchospasm; greater than normal anti-asthmatic dose of beta-agonist may be required). Products include:
Xopenex Inhalation Solution **3207**

Maprotiline Hydrochloride (Potential for tremor).
No products indexed under this heading.

Metaproterenol Sulfate (Beta-blocker can blunt the bronchodilator effect of beta-receptor agonists in patients with bronchospasm; greater than normal anti-asthmatic dose of beta-agonist may be required). Products include:
Alupent **1029**

Metformin Hydrochloride (Beta blockade may prevent the appearance of premonitory signs and symptoms of acute hypoglycemia; additionally, beta blockade reduces the release of insulin in response to hyperglycemia; it may be necessary to adjust the dosage of antidiabetic drugs). Products include:
Glucophage Tablets **1080**
Glucophage XR Tablets **1080**
Glucovance Tablets **1086**

Miglitol (Beta blockade may prevent the appearance of premonitory signs and symptoms of acute hypoglycemia; additionally, beta blockade reduces the release of insulin in response to hyperglycemia; it may be necessary to adjust the dosage of antidiabetic drugs). Products include:
Glyset Tablets **2821**

Nitroglycerin (Reflex tachycardia produced by nitroglycerin blunted). Products include:
Nitro-Dur Transdermal Infusion System **3134**
Nitro-Dur Transdermal Infusion System **1834**
Nitrolingual Pumpspray **1355**
Nitrostat Tablets **2658**

Nortriptyline Hydrochloride (Potential for tremor).
No products indexed under this heading.

Pioglitazone Hydrochloride (Beta blockade may prevent the appearance of premonitory signs and symptoms of acute hypoglycemia; additionally, beta blockade reduces the release of insulin in response to hyperglycemia; it may be necessary to adjust the dosage of antidiabetic drugs). Products include:
Actos Tablets **3275**

Pirbuterol Acetate (Beta-blocker can blunt the bronchodilator effect of beta-receptor agonists in patients with bronchospasm; greater than normal anti-asthmatic dose of beta-agonist may be required). Products include:
Maxair Autohaler **1981**
Maxair Inhaler **1984**

Protriptyline Hydrochloride (Potential for tremor). Products include:
Vivactil Tablets **2446**
Vivactil Tablets **2217**

Repaglinide (Beta blockade may prevent the appearance of premonitory signs and symptoms of acute hypoglycemia; additionally, beta blockade reduces the release of insulin in response to hyperglycemia; it may be necessary to adjust the dosage of antidiabetic drugs). Products include:
Prandin Tablets (0.5, 1, and 2 mg) **2432**

Rosiglitazone Maleate (Beta blockade may prevent the appearance of premonitory signs and symptoms of acute hypoglycemia; additionally, beta blockade reduces the release of insulin in response to hyperglycemia; it may be necessary to adjust the dosage of antidiabetic drugs). Products include:
Avandia Tablets **1490**

Salmeterol Xinafoate (Beta-blocker can blunt the bronchodilator effect of beta-receptor agonists in patients with bronchospasm; greater than normal anti-asthmatic dose of beta-agonist may be required). Products include:
Advair Diskus 100/50 .... **1448**
Advair Diskus 250/50 .... **1448**
Advair Diskus 500/50 .... **1448**
Serevent Diskus **1637**
Serevent Inhalation Aerosol **1633**

Terbutaline Sulfate (Beta-blocker can blunt the bronchodilator effect of beta-receptor agonists in patients with bronchospasm; greater than normal anti-asthmatic dose of beta-agonist may be required). Products include:
Brethine Ampuls **2314**
Brethine Tablets **2313**

Tolazamide (Beta blockade may prevent the appearance of premonitory signs and symptoms of acute hypoglycemia; additionally, beta blockade reduces the release of insulin in response to hyperglycemia; it may be necessary to adjust the dosage of antidiabetic drugs).
No products indexed under this heading.

Tolbutamide (Beta blockade may prevent the appearance of premonitory signs and symptoms of acute hypoglycemia; additionally, beta blockade reduces the release of insulin in response to hyperglycemia; it may be necessary to adjust the dosage of antidiabetic drugs).
No products indexed under this heading.

Trimipramine Maleate (Potential for tremor). Products include:
Surmontil Capsules **3595**

Troglitazone (Beta blockade may prevent the appearance of premonitory signs and symptoms of acute hypoglycemia; additionally, beta blockade reduces the release of insulin in response to hyperglycemia; it may be necessary to adjust the dosage of antidiabetic drugs).
No products indexed under this heading.

Verapamil Hydrochloride (Care should be taken if coadministered; effects of concomitant use not specified). Products include:
Covera-HS Tablets **3199**
Isoptin SR Tablets **467**
Tarka Tablets **508**
Verelan Capsules **3184**
Verelan PM Capsules **3186**

NOROXIN TABLETS

(Norfloxacin) **2145**

May interact with antacids containing aluminum, calcium and magnesium, oral anticoagulants, iron containing oral preparations, theophylline, and certain other agents. Compounds in these categories include:

Aluminum Carbonate (May interfere with absorption resulting in lower serum and urine levels of norfloxacin; antacids should not be administered concomitantly with, or within 2 hours of, the administration of norfloxacin).
No products indexed under this heading.

Aluminum Hydroxide (May interfere with absorption resulting in lower serum and urine levels of norfloxacin; antacids should not be administered concomitantly with, or within 2 hours of, the administration of norfloxacin). Products include:
Amphojel Suspension (Mint Flavor) .... ■ **789**
Gaviscon Extra Strength Liquid ..... ■ **751**
Gaviscon Extra Strength Tablets ... ■ **751**
Gaviscon Regular Strength Liquid . ■ **751**
Gaviscon Regular Strength Tablets .... ■ **750**
Maalox Antacid/Anti-Gas Oral Suspension .... ■ **673**
Maalox Max Maximum Strength Antacid/Anti-Gas Liquid **2300**

Maalox Regular Strength Antacid/Antigas Liquid 2300
Mylanta 1813
Vanquish Caplets .... ▣617

Aminophylline (Co-administration of quinolone with theophylline has resulted in elevated plasma levels of theophylline resulting in theophylline-related side effects).
No products indexed under this heading.

Caffeine (Some quinolones have been shown to interfere with the metabolism of caffeine leading to reduced clearance of caffeine and a prolongation of its plasma half-life). Products include:
BC Powder .... ▣619
Arthritis Strength BC Powder .... ▣619
Darvon Compound-65 Pulvules 1910
Aspirin Free Excedrin Caplets and Geltabs .... ▣628
Excedrin Extra-Strength Tablets, Caplets, and Geltabs .... ▣629
Excedrin Migraine 1070
Goody's Extra Strength Headache Powder .... ▣620
Goody's Extra Strength Pain Relief Tablets .... ▣620
Hycomine Compound Tablets 1317
Maximum Strength Midol Menstrual Caplets and Gelcaps .... ▣612
Vanquish Caplets .... ▣617
Vivarin .... ▣763

Cyclosporine (Co-administration has resulted in elevated serum levels of cyclosporine). Products include:
Gengraf Capsules 457
Neoral Soft Gelatin Capsules 2380
Neoral Oral Solution 2380
Sandimmune 2388

Dicumarol (Co-administration may enhance the effects of oral anticoagulants).
No products indexed under this heading.

Didanosine (Co-administration with Videx, didanosine chewable/buffered tablets or the pediatric powder for oral solution may interfere with the absorption resulting in lower serum and urine levels of norfloxacin; this combination should not be administered concomitantly or within 2 hours of administration of norfloxacin). Products include:
Videx 1138
Videx EC Capsules 1143

Dyphylline (Co-administration of quinolone with theophylline has resulted in elevated plasma levels of theophylline resulting in theophylline-related side effects). Products include:
Lufyllin Tablets 3347
Lufyllin-400 Tablets 3347
Lufyllin-GG Elixir 3348
Lufyllin-GG Tablets 3348

Ferrous Fumarate (May interfere with absorption resulting in lower serum and urine levels of norfloxacin; iron containing products should not be administered concomitantly with, or within 2 hours of, the administration of norfloxacin). Products include:
New Formulation Chromagen OB Capsules 3094
Loestrin Fe Tablets 2642
NataChew Tablets 3364

Ferrous Gluconate (May interfere with absorption resulting in lower serum and urine levels of norfloxacin; iron containing products should not be administered concomitantly with, or within 2 hours of, the administration of norfloxacin). Products include:
Fergon Iron Tablets .... ▣802

Ferrous Sulfate (May interfere with absorption resulting in lower serum and urine levels of norfloxacin; iron containing products should not be administered concomitantly with, or within 2 hours of, the administration of norfloxacin). Products include:
Feosol Tablets 1717
Slow Fe Tablets .... ▣827
Slow Fe with Folic Acid Tablets .... ▣828

Iron (May interfere with absorption resulting in lower serum and urine levels of norfloxacin; iron containing products should not be administered concomitantly with, or within 2 hours of, the administration of norfloxacin).
No products indexed under this heading.

Magaldrate (May interfere with absorption resulting in lower serum and urine levels of norfloxacin; antacids should not be administered concomitantly with, or within 2 hours of, the administration of norfloxacin).
No products indexed under this heading.

Magnesium Hydroxide (May interfere with absorption resulting in lower serum and urine levels of norfloxacin; antacids should not be administered concomitantly with, or within 2 hours of, the administration of norfloxacin). Products include:
Ex•Lax Milk of Magnesia Liquid .... ▣670
Maalox Antacid/Anti-Gas Oral Suspension .... ▣673
Maalox Max Maximum Strength Antacid/Anti-Gas Liquid 2300
Maalox Regular Strength Antacid/Antigas Liquid 2300
Mylanta Fast-Acting 1813
Mylanta 1813
Pepcid Complete Chewable Tablets 1815
Phillips' Chewable Tablets .... ▣615
Phillips' Milk of Magnesia Liquid (Original, Cherry, & Mint) .... ▣616
Rolaids Tablets .... ▣706
Extra Strength Rolaids Tablets .... ▣706
Vanquish Caplets .... ▣617

Magnesium Oxide (May interfere with absorption resulting in lower serum and urine levels of norfloxacin; antacids should not be administered concomitantly with, or within 2 hours of, the administration of norfloxacin). Products include:
Beelith Tablets 946
Mag-Ox 400 Tablets 1024
Uro-Mag Capsules 1024

Nitrofurantoin (Nitrofurantoin may antagonize the antibacterial effect of norfloxacin in the urinary tract; concurrent use is not recommended). Products include:
Macrodantin Capsules 2891

Polysaccharide-Iron Complex (May interfere with absorption resulting in lower serum and urine levels of norfloxacin; iron containing products should not be administered concomitantly with, or within 2 hours of, the administration of norfloxacin). Products include:
Niferex 3176
Niferex-150 Capsules 3176
Nu-Iron 150 Capsules 2224

Probenecid (Co-administration with probenecid has resulted in diminished urinary excretion).
No products indexed under this heading.

Sucralfate (May interfere with absorption resulting in lower serum and urine levels of norfloxacin; sucralfate should not be administered concomitantly with, or within 2 hours of, the administration of norfloxacin). Products include:
Carafate Suspension 731
Carafate Tablets 730

Theophylline (Co-administration of quinolone with theophylline has resulted in elevated plasma levels of theophylline resulting in theophylline-related side effects). Products include:
Aerolate 1361
Theo-Dur Extended-Release Tablets 1835
Uni-Dur Extended-Release Tablets 1841
Uniphyl 400 mg and 600 mg Tablets 2903

Theophylline Calcium Salicylate (Co-administration of quinolone with theophylline has resulted in elevated plasma levels of theophylline resulting in theophylline-related side effects).
No products indexed under this heading.

Theophylline Sodium Glycinate (Co-administration of quinolone with theophylline has resulted in elevated plasma levels of theophylline resulting in theophylline-related side effects).
No products indexed under this heading.

Warfarin Sodium (Co-administration may enhance the effects of oral anticoagulants). Products include:
Coumadin for Injection 1243
Coumadin Tablets 1243
Warfarin Sodium Tablets, USP 3302

Zinc Sulfate (May interfere with absorption resulting in lower serum and urine levels of norfloxacin; zinc containing oral products should not be administered concomitantly with, or within 2 hours of, the administration of norfloxacin). Products include:
Clear Eyes ACR Astringent/Lubricant Eye Redness Reliever .... ⊙322
Visine A.C. Seasonal Relief From Pollen & Dust Eye Drops .... ⊙314

Food Interactions

Dairy products (Avoid simultaneous ingestion; administer norfloxacin at least one hour before or two hours after ingestion of milk and/or other dairy products).

Food, unspecified (Co-administration may decrease the absorption of norfloxacin; administer at least one hour before or two hours after a meal).

NORPLANT SYSTEM

(Levonorgestrel) 3543
May interact with phenytoin and certain other agents. Compounds in these categories include:

Carbamazepine (Co-administration with carbamazepine may increase the metabolism of levonorgestrel through induction of microsomal liver enzyme; potential for reduced efficacy of contraceptive that may result in pregnancy; alternative method of contraception should be considered). Products include:
Carbatrol Capsules 3234
Tegretol/Tegretol-XR 2404

Fosphenytoin Sodium (Co-administration with phenytoin may increase the metabolism of levonorgestrel through induction of microsomal liver enzyme; potential for reduced efficacy of contraceptive that may result in pregnancy; alternative method of contraception should be considered). Products include:
Cerebyx Injection 2619

Phenytoin (Co-administration with phenytoin may increase the metabolism of levonorgestrel through induction of microsomal liver enzyme; potential for reduced efficacy of contraceptive that may result in pregnancy; alternative method of contraception should be considered). Products include:
Dilantin Infatabs 2624
Dilantin-125 Oral Suspension 2625

Phenytoin Sodium (Co-administration with phenytoin may increase the metabolism of levonorgestrel through induction of microsomal liver enzyme; potential for reduced efficacy of contraceptive that may result in pregnancy; alternative method of contraception should be considered). Products include:
Dilantin Kapseals 2622

Rifampin (Co-administration with rifampin may increase the metabolism of levonorgestrel through induction of microsomal liver enzyme; potential for reduced efficacy of contraceptive that may result in pregnancy; alternative method of contraception should be considered). Products include:
Rifadin 765
Rifamate Capsules 767
Rifater Tablets 769

NORPRAMIN TABLETS

(Desipramine Hydrochloride) 755
May interact with anticholinergics, barbiturates, antidepressant drugs, hypnotics and sedatives, monoamine oxidase inhibitors, phenothiazines, quinidine, sympathomimetics, thyroid preparations, tranquilizers, and certain other agents. Compounds in these categories include:

Albuterol (Tricyclic antidepressants may potentiate the effects of sympathomimetics; close supervision and careful adjustment of dosage are required). Products include:
Proventil Inhalation Aerosol 3142
Ventolin Inhalation Aerosol and Refill 1679

Albuterol Sulfate (Tricyclic antidepressants may potentiate the effects of sympathomimetics; close supervision and careful adjustment of dosage are required). Products include:
AccuNeb Inhalation Solution 1230
Combivent Inhalation Aerosol 1041
DuoNeb Inhalation Solution 1233
Proventil Inhalation Solution 0.083% 3146
Proventil Repetabs Tablets 3148
Proventil Solution for Inhalation 0.5% 3144
Proventil HFA Inhalation Aerosol 3150
Ventolin HFA Inhalation Aerosol 3618
Volmax Extended-Release Tablets 2276

Alprazolam (Co-administration with major tranquilizers may produce additive sedative and anticholinergic effects). Products include:
Xanax Tablets 2865

Amitriptyline Hydrochloride (Co-administration with substrates for P450 2D6, such as many other antidepressants, may make normal metabolizers resemble poor metabolizers resulting in higher than expected plasma levels of tricyclic antidepressants). Products include:
Etrafon 3115
Limbitrol 1738

Amoxapine (Co-administration with substrates for P450 2D6, such as many other antidepressants, may make normal metabolizers resemble poor metabolizers resulting in higher than expected plasma levels of tricyclic antidepressants).
No products indexed under this heading.

Aprobarbital (Barbiturates induce liver enzyme activity and thereby reduce tricyclic antidepressant plasma levels; co-administration may produce additive sedative effects).
No products indexed under this heading.

Atropine Sulfate (Co-administration results in additive anticholinergic effects; close supervision and careful adjustment of dosage are required). Products include:
Donnatal 2929
Donnatal Extentabs 2930
Motofen Tablets 577
Prosed/DS Tablets 3268
Urised Tablets 2876

Belladonna Alkaloids (Co-administration results in additive anticholinergic effects; close supervision and careful adjustment of dosage are required). Products include:
Hyland's Teething Tablets .... ▣766
Urimax Tablets 1769

Benztropine Mesylate (Co-administration results in additive anticholinergic effects; close supervi-

sion and careful adjustment of dosage are required). Products include:
Cogentin 2055

Biperiden Hydrochloride (Co-administration results in additive anticholinergic effects; close supervision and careful adjustment of dosage are required). Products include:
Akineton 402

Bupropion Hydrochloride (Co-administration with substrates for P450 2D6, such as many other antidepressants, may make normal metabolizers resemble poor metabolizers resulting in higher than expected plasma levels of tricyclic antidepressants). Products include:
Wellbutrin Tablets 1680
Wellbutrin SR Sustained-Release Tablets 1684
Zyban Sustained-Release Tablets 1710

Buspirone Hydrochloride (Co-administration with tranquilizers may produce additive sedative effects).
No products indexed under this heading.

Butabarbital (Barbiturates induce liver enzyme activity and thereby reduce tricyclic antidepressant plasma levels; co-administration may produce additive sedative effects).
No products indexed under this heading.

Butalbital (Barbiturates induce liver enzyme activity and thereby reduce tricyclic antidepressant plasma levels; co-administration may produce additive sedative effects). Products include:
Phrenilin 578
Sedapap Tablets 50 mg/650 mg 2225

Chlordiazepoxide (Co-administration with major tranquilizers may produce additive sedative and anticholinergic effects).
Products include:
Limbitrol 1738

Chlordiazepoxide Hydrochloride (Co-administration with major tranquilizers may produce additive sedative and anticholinergic effects).
Products include:
Librium Capsules 1736
Librium for Injection 1737

Chlorpromazine (Phenothiazines are substrates for P450 2D6 and co-administration may make normal metabolizers resemble poor metabolizers resulting in higher than expected plasma levels of tricyclic antidepressants; co-administration with major tranquilizers may produce additive sedative and anticholinergic effects). Products include:
Thorazine Suppositories 1656

Chlorpromazine Hydrochloride (Phenothiazines are substrates for P450 2D6 and co-administration may make normal metabolizers resemble poor metabolizers resulting in higher than expected plasma levels of tricyclic antidepressants; co-administration with major tranquilizers may produce additive sedative and anticholinergic effects).
Products include:
Thorazine 1656

Chlorprothixene (Co-administration with major tranquilizers may produce additive sedative and anticholinergic effects).
No products indexed under this heading.

Chlorprothixene Hydrochloride (Co-administration with major tranquilizers may produce additive sedative and anticholinergic effects).
No products indexed under this heading.

Cimetidine (Concurrent administration can produce clinically significant increase in the plasma concentrations of the tricyclic antidepressants through competition for the same metabolic enzyme systems; decreases in plasma levels of the TCA have been reported upon discontinuation of cimetidine, which may result in the loss of the therapeutic efficacy of TCA). Products include:
Tagamet HB 200 Suspension .... ◻762
Tagamet HB 200 Tablets .... ◻761
Tagamet Tablets 1644

Cimetidine Hydrochloride (Concurrent administration can produce clinically significant increase in the plasma concentrations of the tricyclic antidepressants through competition for the same metabolic enzyme systems; decreases in plasma levels of the TCA have been reported upon discontinuation of cimetidine, which may result in the loss of the therapeutic efficacy of TCA). Products include:
Tagamet 1644

Citalopram Hydrobromide (Co-administration with substrates for P450 2D6, such as many other antidepressants, may make normal metabolizers resemble poor metabolizers resulting in higher than expected plasma levels of tricyclic antidepressants). Products include:
Celexa 1365

Clidinium Bromide (Co-administration results in additive anticholinergic effects; close supervision and careful adjustment of dosage are required).
No products indexed under this heading.

Clonidine (Desipramine may block the antihypertensive effects).
Products include:
Catapres-TTS 1038

Clonidine Hydrochloride (Desipramine may block the antihypertensive effects). Products include:
Catapres Tablets 1037
Clorpres Tablets 1002
Combipres Tablets 1040
Duraclon Injection 3057

Clorazepate Dipotassium (Co-administration with major tranquilizers may produce additive sedative and anticholinergic effects).
Products include:
Tranxene 511

Diazepam (Co-administration with major tranquilizers may produce additive sedative and anticholinergic effects). Products include:
Valium Injectable 3026
Valium Tablets 3047

Dicyclomine Hydrochloride (Co-administration results in additive anticholinergic effects; close supervision and careful adjustment of dosage are required).
No products indexed under this heading.

Dobutamine Hydrochloride (Tricyclic antidepressants may potentiate the effects of sympathomimetics; close supervision and careful adjustment of dosage are required).
Products include:
Dobutrex Solution Vials 1914

Dopamine Hydrochloride (Tricyclic antidepressants may potentiate the effects of sympathomimetics; close supervision and careful adjustment of dosage are required).
No products indexed under this heading.

Doxepin Hydrochloride (Co-administration with substrates for P450 2D6, such as many other antidepressants, may make normal metabolizers resemble poor metabolizers resulting in higher than expected plasma levels of tricyclic antidepressants). Products include:
Sinequan 2713

Droperidol (Co-administration with major tranquilizers may produce additive sedative and anticholinergic effects).
No products indexed under this heading.

Ephedrine Hydrochloride (Tricyclic antidepressants may potentiate the effects of sympathomimetics; close supervision and careful adjustment of dosage are required).
Products include:
Primatene Tablets .... ◻780

Ephedrine Sulfate (Tricyclic antidepressants may potentiate the effects of sympathomimetics; close supervision and careful adjustment of dosage are required).
No products indexed under this heading.

Ephedrine Tannate (Tricyclic antidepressants may potentiate the effects of sympathomimetics; close supervision and careful adjustment of dosage are required). Products include:
Rynatuss Pediatric Suspension 3353
Rynatuss Tablets 3353

Epinephrine (Tricyclic antidepressants may potentiate the effects of sympathomimetics; close supervision and careful adjustment of dosage are required). Products include:
Epifrin Sterile Ophthalmic Solution .... ⊙235
EpiPen 1236
Primatene Mist .... ◻779
Xylocaine with Epinephrine Injection 653

Epinephrine Bitartrate (Tricyclic antidepressants may potentiate the effects of sympathomimetics; close supervision and careful adjustment of dosage are required). Products include:
Sensorcaine 643

Epinephrine Hydrochloride (Tricyclic antidepressants may potentiate the effects of sympathomimetics; close supervision and careful adjustment of dosage are required).
No products indexed under this heading.

Estazolam (Co-administration may produce additive sedative effects).
Products include:
ProSom Tablets 500

Ethchlorvynol (Co-administration may produce additive sedative effects).
No products indexed under this heading.

Ethinamate (Co-administration may produce additive sedative effects).
No products indexed under this heading.

Flecainide Acetate (Co-administration with substrates for P450 2D6, such as flecainide, may make normal metabolizers resemble poor metabolizers resulting in higher than expected plasma levels of tricyclic antidepressants). Products include:
Tambocor Tablets 1990

Fluoxetine Hydrochloride (Selective serotonin reuptake inhibitors, such as fluoxetine, may have variable extent of inhibition of P450 2D6; potential for higher than expected plasma levels of tricyclic antidepressants; due to long half-life of fluoxetine, at least 5 weeks should elapse before initiating TCA treatment in a patient being withdrawn from fluoxetine). Products include:
Prozac Pulvules, Liquid, and Weekly Capsules 1238
Sarafem Pulvules 1962

Fluphenazine Decanoate (Phenothiazines are substrates for P450 2D6 and co-administration may make normal metabolizers resemble poor metabolizers resulting in higher than expected plasma levels of tricyclic antidepressants; co-administration with major tranquilizers may produce additive sedative and anticholinergic effects).
No products indexed under this heading.

Fluphenazine Enanthate (Phenothiazines are substrates for P450 2D6 and co-administration may make normal metabolizers resemble poor metabolizers resulting in higher than expected plasma levels of tricyclic antidepressants; co-administration with major tranquilizers may produce additive sedative and anticholinergic effects).
No products indexed under this heading.

Fluphenazine Hydrochloride (Phenothiazines are substrates for P450 2D6 and co-administration may make normal metabolizers resemble poor metabolizers resulting in higher than expected plasma levels of tricyclic antidepressants; co-administration with major tranquilizers may produce additive sedative and anticholinergic effects).
No products indexed under this heading.

Flurazepam Hydrochloride (Co-administration may produce additive sedative effects).
No products indexed under this heading.

Glutethimide (Co-administration may produce additive sedative effects).
No products indexed under this heading.

Glycopyrrolate (Co-administration results in additive anticholinergic effects; close supervision and careful adjustment of dosage are required). Products include:
Robinul Forte Tablets 1358
Robinul Injectable 2940
Robinul Tablets 1358

Guanadrel Sulfate (Desipramine may block the antihypertensive effects).
No products indexed under this heading.

Guanethidine Monosulfate (Desipramine may block the antihypertensive effects).
No products indexed under this heading.

Haloperidol (Co-administration with major tranquilizers may produce additive sedative and anticholinergic effects). Products include:
Haldol Injection, Tablets and Concentrate 2533

Haloperidol Decanoate (Co-administration with major tranquilizers may produce additive sedative and anticholinergic effects).
Products include:
Haldol Decanoate 2535

Hydroxyzine Hydrochloride (Co-administration with major tranquilizers may produce additive sedative and anticholinergic effects).
Products include:
Atarax Tablets & Syrup 2667
Vistaril Intramuscular Solution 2738

Hyoscyamine (Co-administration results in additive anticholinergic effects; close supervision and careful adjustment of dosage are required). Products include:
Urised Tablets 2876

Hyoscyamine Sulfate (Co-administration results in additive anticholinergic effects; close supervision and careful adjustment of dosage are required). Products include:
Arco-Lase Plus Tablets 592
Donnatal 2929
Donnatal Extentabs 2930
Levsin/Levsinex/Levbid 3172
NuLev Orally Disintegrating Tablets 3176
Prosed/DS Tablets 3268

IMPORTANT NOTE: Always consult each drug listing in the patient's regimen for possible interactions.

Urimax Tablets 1769

Imipramine Hydrochloride (Co-administration with substrates for P450 2D6, such as many other antidepressants, may make normal metabolizers resemble poor metabolizers resulting in higher than expected plasma levels of tricyclic antidepressants).
No products indexed under this heading.

Imipramine Pamoate (Co-administration with substrates for P450 2D6, such as many other antidepressants, may make normal metabolizers resemble poor metabolizers resulting in higher than expected plasma levels of tricyclic antidepressants).
No products indexed under this heading.

Ipratropium Bromide (Co-administration results in additive anticholinergic effects; close supervision and careful adjustment of dosage are required). Products include:
Atrovent Inhalation Aerosol 1030
Atrovent Inhalation Solution 1031
Atrovent Nasal Spray 0.03% 1032
Atrovent Nasal Spray 0.06% 1033
Combivent Inhalation Aerosol 1041
DuoNeb Inhalation Solution 1233

Isocarboxazid (Co-administration of tricyclic antidepressants and MAO inhibitor has produced hyperpyretic crises, severe convulsions, and deaths; concurrent and/or sequential use is contraindicated).
No products indexed under this heading.

Isoproterenol Hydrochloride (Tricyclic antidepressants may potentiate the effects of sympathomimetics; close supervision and careful adjustment of dosage are required).
No products indexed under this heading.

Isoproterenol Sulfate (Tricyclic antidepressants may potentiate the effects of sympathomimetics; close supervision and careful adjustment of dosage are required).
No products indexed under this heading.

Levalbuterol Hydrochloride (Tricyclic antidepressants may potentiate the effects of sympathomimetics; close supervision and careful adjustment of dosage are required). Products include:
Xopenex Inhalation Solution 3207

Levothyroxine Sodium (Co-administration with thyroid medications may increase the possibility of cardiovascular toxicity, including arrhythmias). Products include:
Levothroid Tablets 1373
Levoxyl Tablets 1819
Synthroid 505
Unithroid Tablets 3445

Liothyronine Sodium (Co-administration with thyroid medications may increase the possibility of cardiovascular toxicity, including arrhythmias). Products include:
Cytomel Tablets 1817
Triostat Injection 1825

Liotrix (Co-administration with thyroid medications may increase the possibility of cardiovascular toxicity, including arrhythmias).
No products indexed under this heading.

Lorazepam (Co-administration with tranquilizers may produce additive sedative and anticholinergic effects). Products include:
Ativan Injection 3478
Ativan Tablets 3482

Loxapine Hydrochloride (Co-administration with major tranquilizers may produce additive sedative and anticholinergic effects).
No products indexed under this heading.

Loxapine Succinate (Co-administration with major tranquilizers may produce additive sedative and anticholinergic effects). Products include:
Loxitane Capsules 3398

Maprotiline Hydrochloride (Co-administration with substrates for P450 2D6, such as many other antidepressants, may make normal metabolizers resemble poor metabolizers resulting in higher than expected plasma levels of tricyclic antidepressants).
No products indexed under this heading.

Mepenzolate Bromide (Co-administration results in additive anticholinergic effects; close supervision and careful adjustment of dosage are required).
No products indexed under this heading.

Mephobarbital (Barbiturates induce liver enzyme activity and thereby reduce tricyclic antidepressant plasma levels; co-administration may produce additive sedative effects).
No products indexed under this heading.

Meprobamate (Co-administration with major tranquilizers may produce additive sedative effects). Products include:
Miltown Tablets 3349

Mesoridazine Besylate (Phenothiazines are substrates for P450 2D6 and co-administration may make normal metabolizers resemble poor metabolizers resulting in higher than expected plasma levels of tricyclic antidepressants; co-administration with major tranquilizers may produce additive sedative and anticholinergic effects). Products include:
Serentil 1057

Metaproterenol Sulfate (Tricyclic antidepressants may potentiate the effects of sympathomimetics; close supervision and careful adjustment of dosage are required). Products include:
Alupent 1029

Metaraminol Bitartrate (Tricyclic antidepressants may potentiate the effects of sympathomimetics; close supervision and careful adjustment of dosage are required). Products include:
Aramine Injection 2043

Methotrimeprazine (Phenothiazines are substrates for P450 2D6 and co-administration may make normal metabolizers resemble poor metabolizers resulting in higher than expected plasma levels of tricyclic antidepressants; co-administration with major tranquilizers may produce additive sedative and anticholinergic effects).
No products indexed under this heading.

Methoxamine Hydrochloride (Tricyclic antidepressants may potentiate the effects of sympathomimetics; close supervision and careful adjustment of dosage are required).
No products indexed under this heading.

Midazolam Hydrochloride (Co-administration may produce additive sedative effects). Products include:
Versed Injection 3027
Versed Syrup 3033

Mirtazapine (Co-administration with substrates for P450 2D6, such as many other antidepressants, may make normal metabolizers resemble poor metabolizers resulting in higher than expected plasma levels of tricyclic antidepressants). Products include:
Remeron Tablets 2483
Remeron SolTab Tablets 2486

Moclobemide (Co-administration of tricyclic antidepressants and MAO inhibitor has produced hyperpyretic crises, severe convulsions, and deaths; concurrent and/or sequential use is contraindicated).
No products indexed under this heading.

Molindone Hydrochloride (Co-administration with major tranquilizers may produce additive sedative and anticholinergic effects). Products include:
Moban 1320

Nefazodone Hydrochloride (Co-administration with substrates for P450 2D6, such as many other antidepressants, may make normal metabolizers resemble poor metabolizers resulting in higher than expected plasma levels of tricyclic antidepressants). Products include:
Serzone Tablets 1104

Norepinephrine Bitartrate (Tricyclic antidepressants may potentiate the effects of sympathomimetics; close supervision and careful adjustment of dosage are required).
No products indexed under this heading.

Nortriptyline Hydrochloride (Co-administration with substrates for P450 2D6, such as many other antidepressants, may make normal metabolizers resemble poor metabolizers resulting in higher than expected plasma levels of tricyclic antidepressants).
No products indexed under this heading.

Oxazepam (Co-administration with major tranquilizers may produce additive sedative effects).
No products indexed under this heading.

Oxybutynin Chloride (Co-administration results in additive anticholinergic effects; close supervision and careful adjustment of dosage are required). Products include:
Ditropan XL Extended Release Tablets 564

Pargyline Hydrochloride (Co-administration of tricyclic antidepressants and MAO inhibitor has produced hyperpyretic crises, severe convulsions, and deaths; concurrent and/or sequential use is contraindicated).
No products indexed under this heading.

Paroxetine Hydrochloride (Selective serotonin reuptake inhibitors, such as paroxetine, may have variable extent of inhibition of P450 2D6; potential for higher than expected plasma levels of tricyclic antidepressants). Products include:
Paxil 1609

Pentobarbital Sodium (Barbiturates induce liver enzyme activity and thereby reduce tricyclic antidepressant plasma levels; co-administration may produce additive sedative effects). Products include:
Nembutal Sodium Solution 485

Perphenazine (Phenothiazines are substrates for P450 2D6 and co-administration may make normal metabolizers resemble poor metabolizers resulting in higher than expected plasma levels of tricyclic antidepressants; co-administration with major tranquilizers may produce additive sedative and anticholinergic effects). Products include:
Etrafon 3115
Trilafon 3160

Phenelzine Sulfate (Co-administration of tricyclic antidepressants and MAO inhibitor has produced hyperpyretic crises, severe convulsions, and deaths; concurrent and/or sequential use is contraindicated). Products include:
Nardil Tablets 2653

Phenobarbital (Barbiturates induce liver enzyme activity and thereby reduce tricyclic antidepressant plasma levels; co-administration may produce additive sedative effects). Products include:
Arco-Lase Plus Tablets 592
Donnatal 2929
Donnatal Extentabs 2930

Phenylephrine Bitartrate (Tricyclic antidepressants may potentiate the effects of sympathomimetics; close supervision and careful adjustment of dosage are required).
No products indexed under this heading.

Phenylephrine Hydrochloride (Tricyclic antidepressants may potentiate the effects of sympathomimetics; close supervision and careful adjustment of dosage are required). Products include:
Afrin Nasal Decongestant Children's Pump Mist .... ▣734
Extendryl 1361
Hycomine Compound Tablets 1317
Neo-Synephrine .... ▣614
Phenergan VC Syrup 3560
Phenergan VC with Codeine Syrup . 3561
Preparation H Cream .... ▣778
Preparation H Cooling Gel .... ▣778
Preparation H .... ▣778
Vicks Sinex Nasal Spray and Ultra Fine Mist .... ▣729

Phenylephrine Tannate (Tricyclic antidepressants may potentiate the effects of sympathomimetics; close supervision and careful adjustment of dosage are required). Products include:
Ryna-12 S Suspension 3351
Reformulated Rynatan Pediatric Suspension 3352
Rynatuss Pediatric Suspension 3353
Rynatuss Tablets 3353

Phenylpropanolamine Hydrochloride (Tricyclic antidepressants may potentiate the effects of sympathomimetics; close supervision and careful adjustment of dosage are required).
No products indexed under this heading.

Pirbuterol Acetate (Tricyclic antidepressants may potentiate the effects of sympathomimetics; close supervision and careful adjustment of dosage are required). Products include:
Maxair Autohaler 1981
Maxair Inhaler 1984

Prazepam (Co-administration with major tranquilizers may produce additive sedative effects).
No products indexed under this heading.

Procarbazine Hydrochloride (Co-administration of tricyclic antidepressants and MAO inhibitor has produced hyperpyretic crises, severe convulsions, and deaths; concurrent and/or sequential use is contraindicated). Products include:
Matulane Capsules 3246

Prochlorperazine (Phenothiazines are substrates for P450 2D6 and co-administration may make normal metabolizers resemble poor metabolizers resulting in higher than expected plasma levels of tricyclic antidepressants; co-administration with major tranquilizers may produce additive sedative and anticholinergic effects). Products include:
Compazine 1505

Procyclidine Hydrochloride (Co-administration results in additive anticholinergic effects; close supervi-

sion and careful adjustment of dosage are required).
No products indexed under this heading.

Promethazine Hydrochloride (Phenothiazines are substrates for P450 2D6 and co-administration may make normal metabolizers resemble poor metabolizers resulting in higher than expected plasma levels of tricyclic antidepressants; co-administration with major tranquilizers may produce additive sedative and anticholinergic effects). Products include:
- Mepergan Injection ... 3539
- Phenergan Injection ... 3553
- Phenergan ... 3556
- Phenergan Syrup ... 3554
- Phenergan with Codeine Syrup ... 3557
- Phenergan with Dextromethorphan Syrup ... 3559
- Phenergan VC Syrup ... 3560
- Phenergan VC with Codeine Syrup . 3561

Propafenone Hydrochloride (Co-administration with substrates for P450 2D6, such as propafenone, may make normal metabolizers resemble poor metabolizers resulting in higher than expected plasma levels of tricyclic antidepressants). Products include:
- Rythmol Tablets – 150 mg, 225 mg, 300 mg ... 502

Propantheline Bromide (Co-administration results in additive anticholinergic effects; close supervision and careful adjustment of dosage are required).
No products indexed under this heading.

Propofol (Co-administration may produce additive sedative effects). Products include:
- Diprivan Injectable Emulsion ... 667

Protriptyline Hydrochloride (Co-administration with substrates for P450 2D6, such as many other antidepressants, may make normal metabolizers resemble poor metabolizers resulting in higher than expected plasma levels of tricyclic antidepressants). Products include:
- Vivactil Tablets ... 2446
- Vivactil Tablets ... 2217

Pseudoephedrine Hydrochloride (Tricyclic antidepressants may potentiate the effects of sympathomimetics; close supervision and careful adjustment of dosage are required). Products include:
- Actifed Cold & Allergy Tablets ... 688
- Actifed Cold & Sinus Caplets and Tablets ... 688
- Advil Cold and Sinus Caplets ... 771
- Advil Cold and Sinus Tablets ... 771
- Advil Flu & Body Ache Caplets ... 772
- Aleve Cold & Sinus Caplets ... 603
- Alka-Seltzer Plus Liqui-Gels ... 604
- Alka-Seltzer Plus Cold & Flu Medicine Liqui-Gels ... 604
- Alka-Seltzer Plus Cold & Sinus Medicine Liqui-Gels ... 604
- Allegra-D Extended-Release Tablets ... 714
- BC Cold Powder ... 619
- Benadryl Allergy/Cold Tablets ... 691
- Benadryl Allergy/Congestion Tablets ... 692
- Benadryl Allergy & Sinus Liquid ... 693
- Benadryl Allergy & Sinus Fastmelt Tablets ... 693
- Benadryl Allergy Sinus Headache Caplets & Gelcaps ... 693
- Benadryl Severe Allergy & Sinus Headache Caplets ... 694
- Benadryl Children's Allergy/Cold Fastmelt Tablets ... 692
- Benylin Multi-Symptom Liquid ... 697
- Bromfed Capsules (Extended-Release) ... 2269
- Bromfed-PD Capsules (Extended-Release) ... 2269
- Children's Cēpacol Sore Throat ... 788
- Comtrex Acute Head Cold & Sinus Pressure Relief Tablets ... 627
- Comtrex Deep Chest Cold & Congestion Relief Softgels ... 627
- Comtrex Flu Therapy & Fever Relief Daytime Caplets ... 628
- Comtrex Flu Therapy & Fever Relief Nighttime Tablets ... 628
- Comtrex Maximum Strength Multi-Symptom Cold & Cough Relief Tablets and Caplets ... 626
- Contac Non-Drowsy 12 Hour Cold Caplets ... 745
- Contac Non-Drowsy Timed Release 12 Hour Cold Caplets ... 746
- Contac Severe Cold and Flu Caplets Maximum Strength ... 746
- Contac Severe Cold and Flu Caplets Non-Drowsy ... 746
- Dimetapp Elixir ... 777
- Dimetapp Cold and Fever Suspension ... 775
- Dimetapp DM Cold & Cough Elixir . 775
- Dimetapp Nighttime Flu Liquid ... 776
- Dimetapp Non-Drowsy Flu Syrup ... 777
- Dimetapp Infant Drops Decongestant ... 775
- Dimetapp Infant Drops Decongestant Plus Cough ... 776
- Guaifed ... 2272
- Kronofed-A ... 1341
- Children's Motrin Cold Oral Suspension ... 2007
- Motrin Sinus Headache Caplets ... 2005
- PediaCare Cough-Cold Liquid ... 719
- PediaCare Infants' Drops Decongestant ... 719
- PediaCare Infants' Drops Decongestant Plus Cough ... 719
- PediaCare NightRest Cough-Cold Liquid ... 719
- Robitussin Cold Caplets Cold & Congestion ... 780
- Robitussin Cold Softgels Cold & Congestion ... 780
- Robitussin Cold Caplets Multi-Symptom Cold & Flu ... 781
- Robitussin Cold Softgels Multi-Symptom Cold & Flu ... 781
- Robitussin Cold Softgels Severe Congestion ... 782
- Robitussin Cough & Cold Infant Drops ... 782
- Robitussin Maximum Strength Cough & Cold Liquid ... 785
- Robitussin Pediatric Cough & Cold Formula Liquid ... 785
- Robitussin Multi Symptom Honey Flu Liquid ... 785
- Robitussin Nighttime Honey Flu Liquid ... 786
- Robitussin-CF Liquid ... 783
- Robitussin-DAC Syrup ... 2942
- Robitussin-PE Liquid ... 782
- Ryna ... 768
- Semprex-D Capsules ... 1172
- Singlet Caplets ... 761
- Sinutab Non-Drying Liquid Caps ... 706
- Sinutab Sinus Allergy Medication, Maximum Strength Formula, Tablets & Caplets ... 707
- Sinutab Sinus Medication, Maximum Strength Without Drowsiness Formula, Tablets & Caplets ... 707
- Sudafed 12 Hour Tablets ... 708
- Sudafed 24 Hour Tablets ... 708
- Children's Sudafed Cold & Cough Liquid ... 709
- Children's Sudafed Nasal Decongestant Chewables ... 711
- Children's Sudafed Nasal Decongestant Liquid Medication ... 711
- Sudafed Cold & Allergy Tablets ... 708
- Sudafed Cold & Cough Liquid Caps ... 709
- Sudafed Cold & Sinus Liquid Caps ... 710
- Sudafed Nasal Decongestant Tablets ... 710
- Sudafed Non-Drying Sinus Liquid Caps ... 712
- Sudafed Severe Cold ... 711
- Sudafed Sinus Headache Caplets ... 712
- Sudafed Sinus Headache Tablets . 712
- Tavist Sinus Non-Drowsy Coated Caplets ... 676
- TheraFlu Regular Strength Cold & Cough Night Time Hot Liquid ... 676
- TheraFlu Regular Strength Cold & Sore Throat Night Time Hot Liquid ... 676
- TheraFlu Maximum Strength Flu & Congestion Non-Drowsy Hot Liquid ... 677
- TheraFlu Maximum Strength Flu & Cough Night Time Hot Liquid .. 678
- TheraFlu Maximum Strength Flu & Sore Throat Night Time Hot Liquid ... 677
- TheraFlu Maximum Strength Severe Cold & Congestion Night Time Caplets ... 678
- TheraFlu Maximum Strength Severe Cold & Congestion Night Time Hot Liquid ... 678
- TheraFlu Maximum Strength Severe Cold & Congestion Non-Drowsy ... 679
- Triaminic Allergy Congestion Liquid ... 680
- Triaminic Chest Congestion Liquid ... 680
- Triaminic Cold & Allergy Liquid ... 681
- Triaminic Cold & Allergy Softchews ... 683
- Triaminic Cold & Cough Liquid ... 681
- Triaminic Cold & Cough Softchews ... 683
- Triaminic Cold & Night Time Cough Liquid ... 681
- Triaminic Cold, Cough & Fever Liquid ... 681
- Triaminic Cough Liquid ... 682
- Triaminic Cough & Congestion Liquid ... 682
- Triaminic Cough & Sore Throat Liquid ... 682
- Triaminic Cough & Sore Throat Softchews ... 684
- Children's Tylenol Allergy-D Liquid ... 2014
- Children's Tylenol Cold Suspension Liquid and Chewable Tablets ... 2015
- Children's Tylenol Cold Plus Cough Suspension Liquid and Chewable Tablets ... 2015
- Children's Tylenol Flu Suspension Liquid ... 2015
- Children's Tylenol Sinus Suspension Liquid ... 2017
- Infants' Tylenol Cold Decongestant and Fever Reducer Concentrated Drops ... 2015
- Infants' Tylenol Cold Decongestant and Fever Reducer Concentrated Drops Plus Cough .. 2015
- Tylenol Allergy Sinus ... 2010
- Multi-Symptom Tylenol Cold Complete Formula Caplets ... 2010
- Multi-Symptom Tylenol Cold Non-Drowsy Caplets and Gelcaps ... 2010
- Multi-Symptom Tylenol Cold Severe Congestion Non-Drowsy Caplets ... 2011
- Maximum Strength Tylenol Flu NightTime Gelcaps ... 2011
- Maximum Strength Tylenol Flu NightTime Liquid ... 2011
- Maximum Strength Tylenol Flu Non-Drowsy Gelcaps ... 2011
- Maximum Strength Tylenol Sinus NightTime Caplets ... 2012
- Maximum Strength Tylenol Sinus Non-Drowsy Geltabs, Gelcaps, Caplets, and Tablets ... 2012
- Vicks 44D Cough & Head Congestion Relief Liquid ... 724
- Vicks 44M Cough, Cold & Flu Relief Liquid ... 725
- Pediatric Vicks 44m Cough & Cold Relief ... 728
- Vicks DayQuil LiquiCaps/Liquid Multi-Symptom Cold/Flu Relief ... 727
- Children's Vicks NyQuil Cold/Cough Relief ... 726
- Vicks NyQuil LiquiCaps/Liquid Multi-Symptom Cold/Flu Relief, Original and Cherry Flavors ... 727
- Zephrex Tablets ... 3091
- Zephrex LA Tablets ... 3092
- Zyrtec-D 12 Hour Extended Relief Tablets ... 2758

Pseudoephedrine Sulfate (Tricyclic antidepressants may potentiate the effects of sympathomimetics; close supervision and careful adjustment of dosage are required). Products include:
- Chlor-Trimeton Allergy/Decongestant Tablets ... 736
- Claritin-D 12 Hour Extended Release Tablets ... 3102
- Claritin-D 24 Hour Extended Release Tablets ... 3104
- Coricidin 'D' Cold, Flu & Sinus Tablets ... 737
- Drixoral Allergy/Sinus Extended-Release Tablets ... 741
- Drixoral Cold & Allergy Sustained-Action Tablets ... 740
- Drixoral Cold & Flu Extended-Release Tablets ... 740
- Drixoral Nasal Decongestant Long-Acting Non-Drowsy Tablets ... 740
- Rynatan Tablets ... 3351

Quazepam (Co-administration may produce additive sedative effects).
No products indexed under this heading.

Quinidine Gluconate (May inhibit the activity of cytochrome P450 2D6 isoenzyme and may make normal metabolizers resemble poor metabolizers resulting in higher than expected plasma levels of tricyclic antidepressants). Products include:
- Quinaglute Dura-Tabs Tablets ... 978

Quinidine Polygalacturonate (May inhibit the activity of cytochrome P450 2D6 isoenzyme and may make normal metabolizers resemble poor metabolizers resulting in higher than expected plasma levels of tricyclic antidepressants).
No products indexed under this heading.

Quinidine Sulfate (May inhibit the activity of cytochrome P450 2D6 isoenzyme and may make normal metabolizers resemble poor metabolizers resulting in higher than expected plasma levels of tricyclic antidepressants). Products include:
- Quinidex Extentabs ... 2933

Salmeterol Xinafoate (Tricyclic antidepressants may potentiate the effects of sympathomimetics; close supervision and careful adjustment of dosage are required). Products include:
- Advair Diskus 100/50 ... 1448
- Advair Diskus 250/50 ... 1448
- Advair Diskus 500/50 ... 1448
- Serevent Diskus ... 1637
- Serevent Inhalation Aerosol ... 1633

Scopolamine (Co-administration results in additive anticholinergic effects; close supervision and careful adjustment of dosage are required). Products include:
- Transderm Scōp Transdermal Therapeutic System ... 2302

Scopolamine Hydrobromide (Co-administration results in additive anticholinergic effects; close supervision and careful adjustment of dosage are required). Products include:
- Donnatal ... 2929
- Donnatal Extentabs ... 2930

Secobarbital Sodium (Barbiturates induce liver enzyme activity and thereby reduce tricyclic antidepressant plasma levels; co-administration may produce additive sedative effects).
No products indexed under this heading.

Selegiline Hydrochloride (Co-administration of tricyclic antidepressants and MAO inhibitor has produced hyperpyretic crises, severe convulsions, and deaths; concurrent and/or sequential use is contraindicated). Products include:
- Eldepryl Capsules ... 3266

Sertraline Hydrochloride (Selective serotonin reuptake inhibitors, such as sertraline, may have variable extent of inhibition of P450 2D6; potential for higher than expected plasma levels of tricyclic antidepressants). Products include:
- Zoloft ... 2751

Temazepam (Co-administration may produce additive sedative effects).
No products indexed under this heading.

Terbutaline Sulfate (Tricyclic antidepressants may potentiate the effects of sympathomimetics; close supervision and careful adjustment of dosage are required). Products include:
- Brethine Ampuls ... 2314

IMPORTANT NOTE: Always consult each drug listing in the patient's regimen for possible interactions.

Brethine Tablets 2313

Thiamylal Sodium (Barbiturates induce liver enzyme activity and thereby reduce tricyclic antidepressant plasma levels; co-administration may produce additive sedative effects).

No products indexed under this heading.

Thioridazine Hydrochloride (Phenothiazines are substrates for P450 2D6 and co-administration may make normal metabolizers resemble poor metabolizers resulting in higher than expected plasma levels of tricyclic antidepressants; co-administration with major tranquilizers may produce additive sedative and anticholinergic effects). Products include:

Thioridazine Hydrochloride Tablets 2289

Thiothixene (Co-administration with major tranquilizers may produce additive sedative and anticholinergic effects). Products include:

Navane Capsules 2701
Thiothixene Capsules 2290

Thyroglobulin (Co-administration with thyroid medications may increase the possibility of cardiovascular toxicity, including arrhythmias).

No products indexed under this heading.

Thyroid (Co-administration with thyroid medications may increase the possibility of cardiovascular toxicity, including arrhythmias).

No products indexed under this heading.

Thyroxine (Co-administration with thyroid medications may increase the possibility of cardiovascular toxicity, including arrhythmias).

No products indexed under this heading.

Thyroxine Sodium (Co-administration with thyroid medications may increase the possibility of cardiovascular toxicity, including arrhythmias).

No products indexed under this heading.

Tolterodine Tartrate (Co-administration results in additive anticholinergic effects; close supervision and careful adjustment of dosage are required). Products include:

Detrol Tablets 3623
Detrol LA Capsules 2801

Tranylcypromine Sulfate (Co-administration of tricyclic antidepressants and MAO inhibitor has produced hyperpyretic crises, severe convulsions, and deaths; concurrent and/or sequential use is contraindicated). Products include:

Parnate Tablets 1607

Trazodone Hydrochloride (Co-administration with substrates for P450 2D6, such as many other antidepressants, may make normal metabolizers resemble poor metabolizers resulting in higher than expected plasma levels of tricyclic antidepressants).

No products indexed under this heading.

Triazolam (Co-administration may produce additive sedative effects). Products include:

Halcion Tablets 2823

Tridihexethyl Chloride (Co-administration results in additive anticholinergic effects; close supervision and careful adjustment of dosage are required).

No products indexed under this heading.

Trifluoperazine Hydrochloride (Phenothiazines are substrates for P450 2D6 and co-administration may make normal metabolizers resemble poor metabolizers resulting in higher than expected plasma levels of tricyclic antidepressants; co-administration with major tranquilizers may produce additive sedative and anticholinergic effects). Products include:

Stelazine 1640

Trihexyphenidyl Hydrochloride (Co-administration results in additive anticholinergic effects; close supervision and careful adjustment of dosage are required). Products include:

Artane 1855

Trimipramine Maleate (Co-administration with substrates for P450 2D6, such as many other antidepressants, may make normal metabolizers resemble poor metabolizers resulting in higher than expected plasma levels of tricyclic antidepressants). Products include:

Surmontil Capsules 3595

Venlafaxine Hydrochloride (Co-administration with substrates for P450 2D6, such as many other antidepressants, may make normal metabolizers resemble poor metabolizers resulting in higher than expected plasma levels of tricyclic antidepressants). Products include:

Effexor Tablets 3495
Effexor XR Capsules 3499

Zaleplon (Co-administration may produce additive sedative effects). Products include:

Sonata Capsules 3591

Zolpidem Tartrate (Co-administration may produce additive sedative effects). Products include:

Ambien Tablets 3191

Food Interactions

Alcohol (Concurrent use results in exaggerated response to alcohol; alcohol induces liver enzyme activity and thereby reduces tricyclic antidepressant plasma levels).

NOR-QD TABLETS

(Norethindrone) 3423

May interact with barbiturates, phenytoin, and certain other agents. Compounds in these categories include:

Aprobarbital (The effectiveness of progestin-only pills is reduced by hepatic enzyme-inducing drugs such as barbiturates).

No products indexed under this heading.

Butabarbital (The effectiveness of progestin-only pills is reduced by hepatic enzyme-inducing drugs such as barbiturates).

No products indexed under this heading.

Butalbital (The effectiveness of progestin-only pills is reduced by hepatic enzyme-inducing drugs such as barbiturates). Products include:

Phrenilin 578
Sedapap Tablets 50 mg/650 mg ... 2225

Carbamazepine (The effectiveness of progestin-only pills is reduced by hepatic enzyme-inducing drugs such as carbamazepine). Products include:

Carbatrol Capsules 3234
Tegretol/Tegretol-XR 2404

Fosphenytoin Sodium (The effectiveness of progestin-only pills is reduced by hepatic enzyme-inducing drugs such as phenytoin). Products include:

Cerebyx Injection 2619

Mephobarbital (The effectiveness of progestin-only pills is reduced by hepatic enzyme-inducing drugs such as barbiturates).

No products indexed under this heading.

Pentobarbital Sodium (The effectiveness of progestin-only pills is reduced by hepatic enzyme-inducing drugs such as barbiturates). Products include:

Nembutal Sodium Solution 485

Phenobarbital (The effectiveness of progestin-only pills is reduced by hepatic enzyme-inducing drugs such as barbiturates). Products include:

Arco-Lase Plus Tablets 592
Donnatal 2929
Donnatal Extentabs 2930

Phenytoin (The effectiveness of progestin-only pills is reduced by hepatic enzyme-inducing drugs such as phenytoin). Products include:

Dilantin Infatabs 2624
Dilantin-125 Oral Suspension 2625

Phenytoin Sodium (The effectiveness of progestin-only pills is reduced by hepatic enzyme-inducing drugs such as phenytoin). Products include:

Dilantin Kapseals 2622

Rifampin (The effectiveness of progestin-only pills is reduced by hepatic enzyme-inducing drugs such as rifampin). Products include:

Rifadin 765
Rifamate Capsules 767
Rifater Tablets 769

Secobarbital Sodium (The effectiveness of progestin-only pills is reduced by hepatic enzyme-inducing drugs such as barbiturates).

No products indexed under this heading.

Thiamylal Sodium (The effectiveness of progestin-only pills is reduced by hepatic enzyme-inducing drugs such as barbiturates).

No products indexed under this heading.

NORVASC TABLETS

(Amlodipine Besylate) 2704

None cited in PDR database.

NORVIR CAPSULES

(Ritonavir) 487

May interact with beta blockers, agents which increase cytochrome P4503A activity, dexamethasone, erythromycin, HMG-CoA reductase inhibitors, oral hypoglycemic agents, highly metabolized sedatives and hypnotics, insulin, phenytoin, selective serotonin reuptake inhibitors, tricyclic antidepressants, valproate, theophylline, and certain other agents. Compounds in these categories include:

Acarbose (New onset diabetes mellitus, exacerbation of pre-existing diabetes, and hyperglycemia have been reported with protease inhibitors; dosage adjustment of oral hypoglycemic agents may be required). Products include:

Precose Tablets 906

Acebutolol Hydrochloride (Co-administration with beta blockers has resulted in cardiac and neurologic events). Products include:

Sectral Capsules 3589

Albendazole (Co-administration results in a possible increase in AUC of albendazole; dosage adjustments may be required). Products include:

Albenza Tablets 1463

Alfentanil Hydrochloride (Co-administration results in a large increase (> 3x) in AUC of alfentanil; dosage adjustments may be required).

No products indexed under this heading.

Alprazolam (Co-administration is likely to produce large increases in highly metabolized sedatives and hypnotics resulting in extreme sedation and respiratory depression; concurrent use is contraindicated). Products include:

Xanax Tablets 2865

Aminophylline (Co-administration results in the reduction of the average AUC of theophylline; increased dosage of theophylline may be required).

No products indexed under this heading.

Amitriptyline Hydrochloride (Co-administration may result in increased tricyclic antidepressant's plasma concentrations; dose decrease of tricyclics may be needed). Products include:

Etrafon 3115
Limbitrol 1738

Amoxapine (Co-administration may result in increased tricyclic antidepressant's plasma concentrations; dose decrease of tricyclics may be needed).

No products indexed under this heading.

Atenolol (Co-administration with beta blockers has resulted in cardiac and neurologic events). Products include:

Tenoretic Tablets 690
Tenormin I.V. Injection 692

Atorvastatin Calcium (Co-administration results in increased plasma concentrations of HMG-CoA reductase inhibitors; the risk of myopathy including rhabdomyolysis may be increased). Products include:

Lipitor Tablets 2639
Lipitor Tablets 2696

Atovaquone (Co-administration may result in decreased atovaquone plasma concentrations; dose increase of atovaquone may be needed). Products include:

Malarone 1596
Mepron Suspension 1598

Betaxolol Hydrochloride (Co-administration results in a possible increase in AUC of betaxolol; dosage adjustments may be required). Products include:

Betoptic S Ophthalmic Suspension 537

Bisoprolol Fumarate (Co-administration with beta blockers has resulted in cardiac and neurologic events). Products include:

Zebeta Tablets 1885
Ziac Tablets 1887

Bromocriptine Mesylate (Co-administration results in a large increase (> 3x) in AUC of bromocriptine; dosage adjustments may be required).

No products indexed under this heading.

Bupropion Hydrochloride (Co-administration may result in increased bupropion plasma concentrations; dose decrease of bupropion may be needed). Products include:

Wellbutrin Tablets 1680
Wellbutrin SR Sustained-Release Tablets 1684
Zyban Sustained-Release Tablets 1710

Carbamazepine (Co-administration may result in increased carbamazepine plasma concentrations; dose decrease of carbamazepine may be needed). Products include:

Carbatrol Capsules 3234
Tegretol/Tegretol-XR 2404

Carteolol Hydrochloride (Co-administration with beta blockers has resulted in cardiac and neurologic events). Products include:

Carteolol Hydrochloride Ophthalmic Solution USP, 1% ..... ⊙ 258
Ocupress Ophthalmic Solution, 1% Sterile .... ⊙ 303

Cerivastatin Sodium (Co-administration results in increased plasma concentrations of HMG-CoA reductase inhibitors; the risk of myopathy including rhabdomyolysis may be increased). Products include:

Baycol Tablets 883

Chloroquine Hydrochloride (Co-administration results in a possible

increase in AUC of chloroquine; dosage adjustments may be required).
No products indexed under this heading.

Chloroquine Phosphate (Co-administration results in a possible increase in AUC of chloroquine; dosage adjustments may be required). Products include:
Aralen Tablets 3075

Chlorpromazine (Co-administration results in a moderate increase (1.5 to 3x) in AUC of chlorpromazine; dosage adjustments may be required). Products include:
Thorazine Suppositories 1656

Chlorpromazine Hydrochloride (Co-administration results in a moderate increase (1.5 to 3x) in AUC of chlorpromazine; dosage adjustments may be required). Products include:
Thorazine 1656

Chlorpropamide (New onset diabetes mellitus, exacerbation of pre-existing diabetes, and hyperglycemia have been reported with protease inhibitors; dosage adjustment of oral hypoglycemic agents may be required). Products include:
Diabinese Tablets 2680

Cisapride (Ritonavir is expected to produce a large increase in the plasma cisapride concentrations; cisapride has recognized risk to induce serious cardiac arrhythmias; co-administration is contraindicated).
No products indexed under this heading.

Citalopram Hydrobromide (Co-administration may result in increased selective serotonin reuptake inhibitors' plasma concentrations; dose decrease of SSRIs may be needed). Products include:
Celexa 1365

Clofibrate (Ritonavir may increase the activity of glucuronosyltransferase; co-administration results in a decrease in AUC of clofibrate; dosage adjustments may be required). Products include:
Atromid-S Capsules 3483

Clomipramine Hydrochloride (Co-administration may result in increased tricyclic antidepressant's plasma concentrations; dose decrease of tricyclics may be needed).
No products indexed under this heading.

Clonazepam (Co-administration may result in increased clonazepam plasma concentrations; dose decrease of clonazepam may be needed). Products include:
Klonopin Tablets 2983

Clorazepate Dipotassium (Co-administration may result in increased clorazepate plasma concentrations; dose decrease of clorazepate may be needed). Products include:
Tranxene 511

Clozapine (Ritonavir is expected to produce a large increase in the plasma clozapine concentrations; clozapine has recognized risk to induce hematologic abnormalities; co-administration is contraindicated). Products include:
Clozaril Tablets 2319

Codeine Phosphate (Ritonavir may increase the activity of glucuronosyltransferase; co-administration results in possible decrease in AUC of codeine; possible need for dosage alterations of codeine). Products include:
Phenergan with Codeine Syrup 3557
Phenergan VC with Codeine Syrup 3561
Robitussin A-C Syrup 2942
Robitussin-DAC Syrup 2942
Ryna-C Liquid 768
Soma Compound w/Codeine Tablets 3355
Tussi-Organidin NR Liquid 3350
Tussi-Organidin-S NR Liquid 3350
Tylenol with Codeine 2595

Cyclophosphamide (An increase in the AUC of cyclophosphamide, activated by CYP, may correspond to a decrease in the AUC of the active metabolite(s) and a possible decrease in efficacy of cyclophosphamide).
No products indexed under this heading.

Cyclosporine (Co-administration may result in increased cyclosporine plasma concentrations; dose decrease of cyclosporine may be needed). Products include:
Gengraf Capsules 457
Neoral Soft Gelatin Capsules 2380
Neoral Oral Solution 2380
Sandimmune 2388

Daunorubicin Hydrochloride (Co-administration results in a possible increase in AUC of daunorubicin; dosage adjustments may be required). Products include:
Cerubidine for Injection 947

Desipramine Hydrochloride (Co-administration results in a 145% mean increase in the AUC of desipramine; dosage reduction of desipramine should be considered). Products include:
Norpramin Tablets 755

Dexamethasone (Co-administration results in a large increase (> 3x) in AUC of dexamethasone; dosage adjustments may be required; potential for increase in the clearance of ritonavir resulting in decreased ritonavir plasma concentrations). Products include:
Decadron Elixir 2078
Decadron Tablets 2079
TobraDex Ophthalmic Ointment 542
TobraDex Ophthalmic Suspension 541

Dexamethasone Acetate (Co-administration results in a large increase (> 3x) in AUC of dexamethasone; dosage adjustments may be required; potential for increase in the clearance of ritonavir resulting in decreased ritonavir plasma concentrations).
No products indexed under this heading.

Dexamethasone Phosphate (Co-administration results in a large increase (> 3x) in AUC of dexamethasone; dosage adjustments may be required; potential for increase in the clearance of ritonavir resulting in decreased ritonavir plasma concentrations).
No products indexed under this heading.

Dexamethasone Sodium Phosphate (Co-administration results in a large increase (> 3x) in AUC of dexamethasone; dosage adjustments may be required; potential for increase in the clearance of ritonavir resulting in decreased ritonavir plasma concentrations). Products include:
Decadron Phosphate Injection 2081
Decadron Phosphate Sterile Ophthalmic Ointment 2083
Decadron Phosphate Sterile Ophthalmic Solution 2084
NeoDecadron Sterile Ophthalmic Solution 2144

Dexfenfluramine Hydrochloride (Co-administration results in a moderate (1.5 to 3x) increase in AUC of dexfenfluramine; dosage adjustments may be required).
No products indexed under this heading.

Diazepam (Co-administration may result in increased diazepam plasma concentrations; dose decrease of diazepam may be needed). Products include:
Valium Injectable 3026
Valium Tablets 3047

Diclofenac Potassium (Co-administration results in a moderate (1.5 to 3x) increase or decrease in AUC of diclofenac). Products include:
Cataflam Tablets 2315

Diclofenac Sodium (Co-administration results in a moderate (1.5 to 3x) increase or decrease in AUC of diclofenac). Products include:
Arthrotec Tablets 3195
Voltaren Ophthalmic Sterile Ophthalmic Solution .... ⊙312
Voltaren Tablets 2315
Voltaren-XR Tablets 2315

Didanosine (Co-administration results in a decreased AUC of didanosine by 13%; dosing of these two drugs should be separated by 2.5 hours to avoid formulation incompatability). Products include:
Videx 1138
Videx EC Capsules 1143

Diltiazem Hydrochloride (Co-administration may result in increased diltiazem plasma concentrations; dose decrease of diltiazem may be needed). Products include:
Cardizem Injectable 1018
Cardizem Lyo-Ject Syringe 1018
Cardizem Monovial 1018
Cardizem CD Capsules 1016
Tiazac Capsules 1378

Diphenoxylate Hydrochloride (Ritonavir may increase the activity of glucuronosyltransferase; co-administration results in a decrease in AUC of diphenoxylate; dosage adjustments may be required).
No products indexed under this heading.

Disopyramide Phosphate (Co-administration may result in increased disopyramide plasma concentrations; cardiac and neurologic events have been reported with co-administration).
No products indexed under this heading.

Disulfiram (Potential for disulfiram-like reactions due to the presence of ethanol in the ritonavir formulations). Products include:
Antabuse Tablets 2444
Antabuse Tablets 3474

Divalproex Sodium (Co-administration may result in decreased valproate plasma concentrations; dose increase of valproate may be needed). Products include:
Depakote Sprinkle Capsules 426
Depakote Tablets 430
Depakote ER Tablets 436

Doxazosin Mesylate (Co-administration results in a possible increase in AUC of doxazosin; dosage adjustments may be required). Products include:
Cardura Tablets 2668

Doxepin Hydrochloride (Co-administration results in a possible increase in the AUC of doxepin; dosage adjustment of doxepine may be required). Products include:
Sinequan 2713

Doxorubicin Hydrochloride (Co-administration results in a possible increase in AUC of doxorubicin; dosage adjustments may be required). Products include:
Adriamycin PFS/RDF Injection 2767
Doxil Injection 566

Dronabinol (Co-administration may result in increased dronabinol plasma concentrations; dose decrease of dronabinol may be needed). Products include:
Marinol Capsules 3325

Dyphylline (Co-administration results in the reduction of the average AUC of theophylline; increased dosage of theophylline may be required). Products include:
Lufyllin Tablets 3347
Lufyllin-400 Tablets 3347
Lufyllin-GG Elixir 3348
Lufyllin-GG Tablets 3348

Encainide Hydrochloride (Ritonavir is expected to produce a large increase in the plasma concentrations of encainide; concurrent use is contraindicated).
No products indexed under this heading.

Ergonovine Maleate (Co-administration may result in a possible increase in concentrations of ergonovine, in general, concurrent use with ergot alkaloid preparations is contraindicated).
No products indexed under this heading.

Erythromycin (Co-administration results in a large increase (> 3x) in AUC of erythromycin; dosage adjustments may be required). Products include:
Emgel 2% Topical Gel 1285
Ery-Tab Tablets 448
Erythromycin Base Filmtab Tablets 454
Erythromycin Delayed-Release Capsules, USP 455
PCE Dispertab Tablets 498

Erythromycin Estolate (Co-administration results in a large increase (> 3x) in AUC of erythromycin; dosage adjustments may be required).
No products indexed under this heading.

Erythromycin Ethylsuccinate (Co-administration results in a large increase (> 3x) in AUC of erythromycin; dosage adjustments may be required). Products include:
E.E.S. 450
EryPed 446
Pediazole Suspension 3050

Erythromycin Gluceptate (Co-administration results in a large increase (> 3x) in AUC of erythromycin; dosage adjustments may be required).
No products indexed under this heading.

Erythromycin Stearate (Co-administration results in a large increase (> 3x) in AUC of erythromycin; dosage adjustments may be required). Products include:
Erythrocin Stearate Filmtab Tablets 452

Esmolol Hydrochloride (Co-administration with beta blockers has resulted in cardiac and neurologic events). Products include:
Brevibloc Injection 858

Estazolam (Co-administration may result in increased estazolam plasma concentrations; dose decrease of estazolam may be needed). Products include:
ProSom Tablets 500

Ethinyl Estradiol (Co-administration results in the reduction in the mean AUC of ethinyl estradiol, a component of oral contraceptives; dosage increase or alternate contraceptive measures should be considered). Products include:
Alesse-21 Tablets 3468
Alesse-28 Tablets 3473
Brevicon 28-Day Tablets 3380
Cyclessa Tablets 2450
Desogen Tablets 2458
Estinyl Tablets 3112
Estrostep 2627
femhrt Tablets 2635
Levlen 962
Levlite 21 Tablets 962
Levlite 28 Tablets 962
Levora Tablets 3389
Loestrin 21 Tablets 2642
Loestrin Fe Tablets 2642
Lo/Ovral Tablets 3532
Lo/Ovral-28 Tablets 3538
Low-Ogestrel-28 Tablets 3392
Microgestin Fe 1.5/30 Tablets 3407
Microgestin Fe 1/20 Tablets 3400

IMPORTANT NOTE: Always consult each drug listing in the patient's regimen for possible interactions.

Mircette Tablets 2470
Modicon 2563
Necon 3415
Nordette-28 Tablets 2257
Norinyl 1 +35 28-Day Tablets 3380
Ogestrel 0.5/50-28 Tablets 3428
Ortho-Cept 21 Tablets 2546
Ortho-Cept 28 Tablets 2546
Ortho-Cyclen/Ortho Tri-Cyclen 2573
Ortho-Novum 2563
Ovcon 3364
Ovral Tablets 3551
Ovral-28 Tablets 3552
Tri-Levlen 962
Tri-Norinyl-28 Tablets 3433
Triphasil-21 Tablets 3600
Triphasil-28 Tablets 3605
Trivora Tablets 3439
Yasmin 28 Tablets 980
Zovia 3449

Ethosuximide (Co-administration may result in increased ethosuximide plasma concentrations; dose decrease of ethosuximide may be needed). Products include:
Zarontin Capsules 2659
Zarontin Syrup 2660

Etoposide (Co-administration results in a large increase (> 3x) in AUC of etoposide; dosage adjustments may be required).
No products indexed under this heading.

Fentanyl (Co-administration results in a large increase (> 3x) in AUC of fentanyl; dosage adjustments may be required). Products include:
Duragesic Transdermal System 1786

Fentanyl Citrate (Co-administration results in a large increase (> 3x) in AUC of fentanyl; dosage adjustments may be required). Products include:
Actiq 1184

Fluconazole (Co-administration has resulted in an increase in AUC and Cmax of ritonavir by 12% and 15% respectively). Products include:
Diflucan Tablets, Injection, and Oral Suspension 2681

Fluoxetine Hydrochloride (Cardiac and neurologic events have been reported when ritonavir has been co-administered with fluoxetine). Products include:
Prozac Pulvules, Liquid, and Weekly Capsules 1238
Sarafem Pulvules 1962

Flurazepam Hydrochloride (Co-administration may result in increased flurazepam plasma concentrations; dose decrease of flurazepam may be needed).
No products indexed under this heading.

Flurbiprofen (Co-administration results in a moderate (1.5 to 3x) increase or decrease in AUC of flurbiprofen).
No products indexed under this heading.

Fluvastatin Sodium (Co-administration results in a possible increase in AUC of fluvastatin; dosage adjustments may be required). Products include:
Lescol Capsules 2361
Lescol 2925
Lescol XL Tablets 2361

Fluvoxamine Maleate (Co-administration may result in increased selective serotonin reuptake inhibitors' plasma concentrations; dose decrease of SSRIs may be needed). Products include:
Luvox Tablets (25, 50, 100 mg) 3256

Fosphenytoin Sodium (Co-administration results in a moderate increase or decrease in AUC of phenytoin; dosage adjustments may be required; potential for increase in the clearance of ritonavir resulting in decreased ritonavir plasma concentrations). Products include:
Cerebyx Injection 2619

Gemfibrozil (Co-administration results in a possible increase in AUC of gemfibrozil; dosage adjustments may be required). Products include:
Lopid Tablets 2650

Glimepiride (Co-administration results in a moderate increase or decrease in AUC of glimepiride; dosage adjustments may be required). Products include:
Amaryl Tablets 717

Glipizide (Co-administration results in a moderate increase or decrease in AUC of glipizide; dosage adjustments may be required). Products include:
Glucotrol Tablets 2692
Glucotrol XL Extended Release Tablets 2693

Glyburide (Co-administration results in a moderate increase or decrease in AUC of glyburide; dosage adjustments may be required). Products include:
DiaBeta Tablets 741
Glucovance Tablets 1086

Haloperidol (Co-administration results in a moderate increase (1.5 to 3x) in AUC of haloperidol; dosage adjustments may be required). Products include:
Haldol Injection, Tablets and Concentrate 2533

Haloperidol Decanoate (Co-administration results in a moderate increase (1.5 to 3x) in AUC of haloperidol; dosage adjustments may be required). Products include:
Haldol Decanoate 2535

Hydrocodone Bitartrate (Co-administration results in a moderate increase (1.5 to 3x) in AUC of hydrocodone; dosage adjustments may be required). Products include:
Hycodan 1316
Hycomine Compound Tablets 1317
Hycotuss Expectorant Syrup 1318
Lortab 3319
Lortab Elixir 3317
Maxidone Tablets CIII 3399
Norco 5/325 Tablets CIII 3424
Norco 7.5/325 Tablets CIII 3425
Norco 10/325 Tablets CIII 3427
Norco 10/325 Tablets CIII 3425
Vicodin Tablets 516
Vicodin ES Tablets 517
Vicodin HP Tablets 518
Vicodin Tuss Expectorant 519
Vicoprofen Tablets 520
Zydone Tablets 1330

Hydromorphone Hydrochloride (Ritonavir may increase the activity of glucuronosyltransferase; co-administration results in possible decrease in AUC of hydromorphone; possible need for dosage alterations of hydromorphone). Products include:
Dilaudid 441
Dilaudid Oral Liquid 445
Dilaudid Powder 441
Dilaudid Rectal Suppositories 441
Dilaudid Tablets 441
Dilaudid Tablets - 8 mg 445
Dilaudid-HP 443

Hypericum (Co-administration is expected to substantially decrease protease inhibitor concentrations and may result in sub-optimal levels of Norvir and lead to loss of virologic response and possible resistance to Norvir; concomitant use of Norvir and St. John's Wort or products containing St. John's Wort is not recommended). Products include:
Brite-Life Caplets ▣795
Centrum St. John's Wort Softgels ▣853
Metabolic Nutrition System ▣798
Movana Tablets ▣832
One-A-Day Tension & Mood Softgels ▣808
ReSource Wellness StayCalm Caplets ▣826
Satiete Tablets ▣846

Ibuprofen (Co-administration results in a moderate (1.5 to 3x) increase or decrease in AUC of ibuprofen). Products include:
Advil ▣771
Children's Advil Oral Suspension ▣773
Children's Advil Chewable Tablets ▣773
Advil Cold and Sinus Caplets ▣771
Advil Cold and Sinus Tablets ▣771
Advil Flu & Body Ache Caplets ▣772
Infants' Advil Drops ▣773
Junior Strength Advil Tablets ▣773
Junior Strength Advil Chewable Tablets ▣773
Advil Migraine Liquigels ▣772
Children's Motrin Oral Suspension and Chewable Tablets 2006
Children's Motrin Cold Oral Suspension 2007
Children's Motrin Oral Suspension ▣643
Motrin Suspension, Oral Drops, Chewable Tablets, and Caplets 2002
Infants' Motrin Concentrated Drops 2006
Junior Strength Motrin Caplets and Chewable Tablets 2006
Motrin IB Tablets, Caplets, and Gelcaps 2002
Motrin Migraine Pain Caplets 2005
Motrin Sinus Headache Caplets 2005
Vicoprofen Tablets 520

Ifosfamide (An increase in the AUC of ifosfamide, activated by CYP, may correspond to a decrease in the AUC of the active metabolite(s) and a possible decrease in efficacy of ifosfamide). Products include:
Ifex for Injection 1123

Imipramine Hydrochloride (Co-administration may result in increased tricyclic antidepressant's plasma concentrations; dose decrease of tricyclics may be needed).
No products indexed under this heading.

Imipramine Pamoate (Co-administration may result in increased tricyclic antidepressant's plasma concentrations; dose decrease of tricyclics may be needed).
No products indexed under this heading.

Indinavir Sulfate (Co-administration results in increased indinavir concentration; appropriate doses for this combination with respect to efficacy and safety have not been established). Products include:
Crixivan Capsules 2070

Indomethacin (Co-administration results in a moderate (1.5 to 3x) increase or decrease in AUC of indomethacin). Products include:
Indocin 2112

Insulin, Human, Zinc Suspension (New onset diabetes mellitus, exacerbation of pre-existing diabetes, and hyperglycemia have been reported with protease inhibitors; dosage adjustment of insulin may be required). Products include:
Humulin L, 100 Units 1937
Humulin U, 100 Units 1943
Novolin L Human Insulin 10 ml Vials 2422

Insulin, Human NPH (New onset diabetes mellitus, exacerbation of pre-existing diabetes, and hyperglycemia have been reported with protease inhibitors; dosage adjustment of insulin may be required). Products include:
Humulin N, 100 Units 1939
Humulin N NPH Pen 1940
Novolin N Human Insulin 10 ml Vials 2422
Novolin N PenFill 2423
Novolin N Prefilled Syringe Disposable Insulin Delivery System 2425

Insulin, Human Regular (New onset diabetes mellitus, exacerbation of pre-existing diabetes, and hyperglycemia have been reported with protease inhibitors; dosage adjustment of insulin may be required). Products include:
Humulin R Regular (U-500) 1943
Humulin R, 100 Units 1941
Novolin R Human Insulin 10 ml Vials 2423
Novolin R PenFill 2423
Novolin R Prefilled Syringe Disposable Insulin Delivery System 2425
Velosulin BR Human Insulin 10 ml Vials 2435

Insulin, Human Regular and Human NPH Mixture (New onset diabetes mellitus, exacerbation of pre-existing diabetes, and hyperglycemia have been reported with protease inhibitors; dosage adjustment of insulin may be required). Products include:
Humulin 50/50, 100 Units 1934
Humulin 70/30, 100 Units 1935
Humulin 70/30 Pen 1936
Novolin 70/30 Human Insulin 10 ml Vials 2421
Novolin 70/30 PenFill 2423
Novolin 70/30 Prefilled Disposable Insulin Delivery System 2425

Insulin, NPH (New onset diabetes mellitus, exacerbation of pre-existing diabetes, and hyperglycemia have been reported with protease inhibitors; dosage adjustment of insulin may be required). Products include:
Iletin II, NPH (Pork), 100 Units 1946

Insulin, Regular (New onset diabetes mellitus, exacerbation of pre-existing diabetes, and hyperglycemia have been reported with protease inhibitors; dosage adjustment of insulin may be required). Products include:
Iletin II, Regular (Pork), 100 Units 1947

Insulin, Zinc Crystals (New onset diabetes mellitus, exacerbation of pre-existing diabetes, and hyperglycemia have been reported with protease inhibitors; dosage adjustment of insulin may be required).
No products indexed under this heading.

Insulin, Zinc Suspension (New onset diabetes mellitus, exacerbation of pre-existing diabetes, and hyperglycemia have been reported with protease inhibitors; dosage adjustment of insulin may be required). Products include:
Iletin II, Lente (Pork), 100 Units 1945

Insulin Aspart, Human Regular (New onset diabetes mellitus, exacerbation of pre-existing diabetes, and hyperglycemia have been reported with protease inhibitors; dosage adjustment of insulin may be required).
No products indexed under this heading.

Insulin glargine (New onset diabetes mellitus, exacerbation of pre-existing diabetes, and hyperglycemia have been reported with protease inhibitors; dosage adjustment of insulin may be required). Products include:
Lantus Injection 742

Insulin Lispro, Human (New onset diabetes mellitus, exacerbation of pre-existing diabetes, and hyperglycemia have been reported with protease inhibitors; dosage adjustment of insulin may be required). Products include:
Humalog 1926
Humalog Mix 75/25 Pen 1928

Insulin Lispro Protamine, Human (New onset diabetes mellitus, exacerbation of pre-existing diabetes, and hyperglycemia have been reported with protease inhibitors; dosage adjustment of insulin may be required). Products include:
Humalog Mix 75/25 Pen 1928

Itraconazole (Co-administration results in a possible increase in AUC of itraconazole; dosage adjustments may be required). Products include:
Sporanox Capsules 1800
Sporanox Injection 1804
Sporanox Injection 2509
Sporanox Oral Solution 1808
Sporanox Oral Solution 2512

Ketoconazole (Co-administration results in increased ketoconazole concentration; high doses of ketoconazole (>200 mg/day) are not recommended). Products include:
- Nizoral 2% Cream 3620
- Nizoral A-D Shampoo 2008
- Nizoral 2% Shampoo 2007
- Nizoral Tablets 1791

Ketoprofen (Ritonavir may increase the activity of glucuronosyltransferase; co-administration results in possible decrease in AUC of ketoprofen; possible need for dosage alterations of ketoprofen). Products include:
- Orudis Capsules 3548
- Orudis KT Tablets 778
- Oruvail Capsules 3548

Ketorolac Tromethamine (Ritonavir may increase the activity of glucuronosyltransferase; co-administration results in possible decrease in AUC of ketorolac; possible need for dosage alterations of ketorolac). Products include:
- Acular Ophthalmic Solution 544
- Acular PF Ophthalmic Solution 544
- Toradol 3018

Labetalol Hydrochloride (Co-administration with beta blockers has resulted in cardiac and neurologic events). Products include:
- Normodyne Injection 3135
- Normodyne Tablets 3137

Lamotrigine (Co-administration may result in decreased lamotrigine plasma concentrations; dose increase of lamotrigine may be needed). Products include:
- Lamictal 1567

Lansoprazole (Co-administration results in a moderate increase or decrease in AUC of lansoprazole; dosage adjustments may be required). Products include:
- Prevacid Delayed-Release Capsules 3292
- PREVPAC 3298

Levobunolol Hydrochloride (Co-administration with beta blockers has resulted in cardiac and neurologic events). Products include:
- Betagan 228

Lidocaine Hydrochloride (Co-administration results in an increase in plasma concentrations of lidocaine; dosage adjustments may be required). Products include:
- Bactine First Aid Liquid 611
- Xylocaine Injections 653

Loperamide Hydrochloride (Co-administration results in a decrease in AUC of loperamide). Products include:
- Imodium A-D Liquid and Caplets 2001
- Imodium Advanced Caplets and Chewable Tablets 2001

Loratadine (Ritonavir is expected to produce a large increase (> 3x) in the plasma concentrations of loratadine; dosage adjustments may be required). Products include:
- Claritin 3100
- Claritin-D 12 Hour Extended Release Tablets 3102
- Claritin-D 24 Hour Extended Release Tablets 3104

Lorazepam (Ritonavir may increase the activity of glucuronosyltransferase; co-administration results in a decrease in AUC of lorazepam; dosage adjustments may be required). Products include:
- Ativan Injection 3478
- Ativan Tablets 3482

Losartan Potassium (Co-administration results in a moderate increase or decrease in AUC of losartan; dosage adjustments may be required). Products include:
- Cozaar Tablets 2067
- Hyzaar 2109

Lovastatin (Co-administration results in increased plasma concentrations of lovastatin; the risk of myopathy including rhabdomyolysis may be increased; concomitant use is not recommended). Products include:
- Mevacor Tablets 2132

Maprotiline Hydrochloride (Co-administration may result in increased tricyclic antidepressant's plasma concentrations; dose decrease of tricyclics may be needed).

No products indexed under this heading.

Meperidine Hydrochloride (Co-administration results in decreased meperidine concentration and increased normeperidine concentration; dosage increase and long-term use of meperidine with ritonavir are not recommended due to the increased concentrations of the metabolite normeperidine which has both analgesic activity and CNS stimulant activity such as seizures). Products include:
- Demerol 3079
- Mepergan Injection 3539

Metformin Hydrochloride (New onset diabetes mellitus, exacerbation of pre-existing diabetes, and hyperglycemia have been reported with protease inhibitors; dosage adjustment of oral hypoglycemic agents may be required). Products include:
- Glucophage Tablets 1080
- Glucophage XR Tablets 1080
- Glucovance Tablets 1086

Methadone Hydrochloride (Co-administration results in decreased methadone concentration; dosage increase of methadone may be considered). Products include:
- Dolophine Hydrochloride Tablets 3056

Methamphetamine Hydrochloride (Co-administration may result in increased methamphetamine plasma concentrations; dose decrease of methamphetamine may be needed). Products include:
- Desoxyn Tablets 440

Methylphenidate Hydrochloride (Co-administration results in a possible increase in AUC of methylphenidate; dosage adjustments may be required). Products include:
- Concerta Extended-Release Tablets 1998
- Concerta Tablets 561
- Metadate CD Capsules 1164
- Metadate ER Tablets 1167
- Methylin Tablets 1995
- Methylin ER Tablets 1995
- Ritalin 2387

Metipranolol Hydrochloride (Co-administration with beta blockers has resulted in cardiac and neurologic events).

No products indexed under this heading.

Metoclopramide Hydrochloride (Ritonavir may increase the activity of glucuronosyltransferase; co-administration results in a decrease in AUC of metoclopramide; dosage adjustments may be required). Products include:
- Reglan 2935

Metoprolol Succinate (Co-administration may result in increased metoprolol plasma concentrations; cardiac and neurologic events have been reported with co-administration). Products include:
- Toprol-XL Tablets 651

Metoprolol Tartrate (Co-administration may result in increased metoprolol plasma concentrations; cardiac and neurologic events have been reported with co-administration).

No products indexed under this heading.

Metronidazole (Potential for disulfiram-like reactions due to the presence of ethanol in the ritonavir formulations). Products include:
- MetroCream 1404
- MetroGel 1405
- MetroGel-Vaginal Gel 1986
- MetroLotion 1405
- Noritate Cream 1224

Metronidazole Hydrochloride (Potential for disulfiram-like reactions due to the presence of ethanol in the ritonavir formulations).

No products indexed under this heading.

Mexiletine Hydrochloride (Co-administration may result in increased mexiletine plasma concentrations; cardiac and neurologic events have been reported with co-administration). Products include:
- Mexitil Capsules 1047

Miconazole (Co-administration results in a possible increase in AUC of miconazole; dosage adjustments may be required).

No products indexed under this heading.

Miconazole Nitrate (Co-administration results in a possible increase in AUC of miconazole; dosage adjustments may be required). Products include:
- Desenex 668
- Desenex Jock Itch Spray Powder 668
- Lotrimin AF Spray Powder, Spray Liquid, Spray Deodorant Powder, Shaker Powder and Jock Itch Spray Powder 742

Midazolam Hydrochloride (Co-administration is likely to produce large increases in highly metabolized sedatives and hypnotics resulting in extreme sedation and respiratory depression; concurrent use is contraindicated). Products include:
- Versed Injection 3027
- Versed Syrup 3033

Miglitol (New onset diabetes mellitus, exacerbation of pre-existing diabetes, and hyperglycemia have been reported with protease inhibitors; dosage adjustment of oral hypoglycemic agents may be required). Products include:
- Glyset Tablets 2821

Morphine Sulfate (Ritonavir may increase the activity of glucuronosyltransferase; co-administration results in possible decrease in AUC of morphine; possible need for dosage alterations of morphine). Products include:
- Astramorph/PF Injection, USP (Preservative-Free) 594
- Duramorph Injection 1312
- Infumorph 200 and Infumorph 500 Sterile Solutions 1314
- Kadian Capsules 1335
- MS Contin Tablets 2896
- MSIR 2898
- Oramorph SR Tablets 3062
- Roxanol 3066

Nadolol (Co-administration with beta blockers has resulted in cardiac and neurologic events). Products include:
- Corgard Tablets 2245
- Corzide 40/5 Tablets 2247
- Corzide 80/5 Tablets 2247
- Nadolol Tablets 2288

Naproxen (Ritonavir may increase the activity of glucuronosyltransferase; co-administration results in possible decrease in AUC of naproxen; possible need for dosage alterations of naproxen). Products include:
- EC-Naprosyn Delayed-Release Tablets 2967
- Naprosyn Suspension 2967
- Naprosyn Tablets 2967

Naproxen Sodium (Ritonavir may increase the activity of glucuronosyltransferase; co-administration results in possible decrease in AUC of naproxen; possible need for dosage alterations of naproxen). Products include:
- Aleve Tablets, Caplets and Gelcaps 602
- Aleve Cold & Sinus Caplets 603
- Anaprox Tablets 2967
- Anaprox DS Tablets 2967
- Naprelan Tablets 1293

Nefazodone Hydrochloride (Co-administration may result in increased nefazodone plasma concentrations; cardiac and neurologic events have been reported with co-administration). Products include:
- Serzone Tablets 1104

Nevirapine (Co-administration may result in a possible increase in concentrations of nevirapine). Products include:
- Viramune Oral Suspension 1060
- Viramune Tablets 1060

Nifedipine (Co-administration may result in increased nifedipine plasma concentrations; dose decrease of nifedipine may be needed). Products include:
- Adalat CC Tablets 877
- Procardia Capsules 2708
- Procardia XL Extended Release Tablets 2710

Nitrendipine (Co-administration results in a large increase (> 3x) in AUC of nitrendipine; dosage adjustments may be required).

No products indexed under this heading.

Nortriptyline Hydrochloride (Co-administration may result in increased tricyclic antidepressant's plasma concentrations; dose decrease of tricyclics may be needed).

No products indexed under this heading.

Omeprazole (Co-administration results in a moderate increase or decrease in AUC of omeprazole; dosage adjustments may be required). Products include:
- Prilosec Delayed-Release Capsules 628

Ondansetron Hydrochloride (Co-administration results in a large increase (> 3x) in AUC of ondansetron; dosage adjustments may be required). Products include:
- Zofran Injection 1698
- Zofran 1703

Oxazepam (Ritonavir may increase the activity of glucuronosyltransferase; co-administration results in a decrease in AUC of oxazepam; dosage adjustments may be required).

No products indexed under this heading.

Oxycodone Hydrochloride (Co-administration results in a moderate increase (1.5 to 3x) in AUC of oxycodone; dosage adjustments may be required). Products include:
- OxyContin Tablets 2912
- OxyFast Oral Concentrate Solution 2916
- OxyIR Capsules 2916
- Percocet Tablets 1326
- Percodan Tablets 1327
- Percolone Tablets 1327
- Roxicodone 3067
- Tylox Capsules 2597

Paclitaxel (Co-administration results in a large increase (> 3x) in AUC of paclitaxel; dosage adjustments may be required). Products include:
- Taxol Injection 1129

Paroxetine Hydrochloride (Co-administration results in a moderate increase (1.5 to 3x) in AUC of paroxetine; dosage adjustments may be required). Products include:
- Paxil 1609

Penbutolol Sulfate (Co-administration results in a possible increase in AUC of penbutolol; dosage adjustments may be required).

No products indexed under this heading.

Pentoxifylline (Co-administration results in a possible increase in AUC of pentoxifylline; dosage adjustments may be required). Products include:
- Trental Tablets 784

Perphenazine (Co-administration may result in increased perphenazine plasma concentrations; dose decrease of perphenazine may be needed). Products include:
- Etrafon 3115
- Trilafon 3160

Phenobarbital (Co-administration results in a possible increase in AUC of phenobarbital; dosage adjustments may be required; potential for increase in the clearance of ritonavir resulting in decreased ritonavir plasma concentrations). Products include:
- Arco-Lase Plus Tablets 592
- Donnatal 2929
- Donnatal Extentabs 2930

Phenytoin (Co-administration results in a moderate increase or decrease in AUC of phenytoin; dosage adjustments may be required; potential for increase in the clearance of ritonavir resulting in decreased ritonavir plasma concentrations). Products include:
- Dilantin Infatabs 2624
- Dilantin-125 Oral Suspension 2625

Phenytoin Sodium (Co-administration results in a moderate increase or decrease in AUC of phenytoin; dosage adjustments may be required; potential for increase in the clearance of ritonavir resulting in decreased ritonavir plasma concentrations). Products include:
- Dilantin Kapseals 2622

Pimozide (Co-administration is expected to produce large increases in the plasma concentrations of pimozide; co-administration is contraindicated). Products include:
- Orap Tablets 1407

Pindolol (Co-administration results in a possible increase in AUC of pindolol; dosage adjustments may be required).
- No products indexed under this heading.

Pioglitazone Hydrochloride (New onset diabetes mellitus, exacerbation of pre-existing diabetes, and hyperglycemia have been reported with protease inhibitors; dosage adjustment of oral hypoglycemic agents may be required). Products include:
- Actos Tablets 3275

Piroxicam (Ritonavir is expected to produce a large increase in the plasma concentrations of piroxicam; concurrent use is contraindicated). Products include:
- Feldene Capsules 2685

Pravastatin Sodium (Co-administration results in a large increase (> 3x) in AUC of pravastatin; dosage adjustments may be required). Products include:
- Pravachol Tablets 1099

Prazosin Hydrochloride (Co-administration results in a possible increase in AUC of prazosin; dosage adjustments may be required). Products include:
- Minipress Capsules 2699
- Minizide Capsules 2700

Prednisone (Co-administration may result in increased prednisone plasma concentrations; dose decrease of prednisone may be needed). Products include:
- Prednisone 3064

Primaquine Phosphate (Co-administration results in a possible increase in AUC of primaquine; dosage adjustments may be required).
- No products indexed under this heading.

Prochlorperazine (Co-administration results in a possible increase in AUC of prochlorperazine; dosage adjustments may be required). Products include:
- Compazine 1505

Proguanil (Co-administration results in a moderate increase or decrease in AUC of proguanil; dosage adjustments may be required).
- No products indexed under this heading.

Promethazine Hydrochloride (Co-administration results in a possible increase in AUC of promethazine; dosage adjustments may be required). Products include:
- Mepergan Injection 3539
- Phenergan Injection 3553
- Phenergan 3556
- Phenergan Syrup 3554
- Phenergan with Codeine Syrup 3557
- Phenergan with Dextromethorphan Syrup 3559
- Phenergan VC Syrup 3560
- Phenergan VC with Codeine Syrup .. 3561

Propofol (Ritonavir may increase the activity of glucuronosyltransferase; co-administration results in a decrease in AUC of propofol; dosage adjustments may be required). Products include:
- Diprivan Injectable Emulsion 667

Propoxyphene Hydrochloride (Ritonavir is expected to produce an increase in the plasma concentrations of propoxyphene). Products include:
- Darvon Pulvules 1909
- Darvon Compound-65 Pulvules 1910

Propoxyphene Napsylate (Ritonavir is expected to produce an increase in the plasma concentrations of propoxyphene). Products include:
- Darvon-N/Darvocet-N 1907
- Darvon-N Tablets 1912

Propranolol Hydrochloride (Co-administration results in a moderate increase (1.5 to 3x) in AUC of propanolol; dosage adjustments may be required). Products include:
- Inderal 3513
- Inderal LA Long-Acting Capsules 3516
- Inderide Tablets 3517
- Inderide LA Long-Acting Capsules .. 3519

Protriptyline Hydrochloride (Co-administration may result in increased tricyclic antidepressant's plasma concentrations; dose decrease of tricyclics may be needed). Products include:
- Vivactil Tablets 2446
- Vivactil Tablets 2217

Pyrimethamine (Co-administration results in a possible increase in AUC of pyrimethamine; dosage adjustments may be required). Products include:
- Daraprim Tablets 1511

Quinidine Gluconate (Ritonavir is expected to produce a large increase in the plasma concentrations of quinidine; concurrent use is contraindicated). Products include:
- Quinaglute Dura-Tabs Tablets 978

Quinidine Polygalacturonate (Ritonavir is expected to produce a large increase in the plasma concentration of quinidine; concurrent use is contraindicated).
- No products indexed under this heading.

Quinidine Sulfate (Ritonavir is expected to produce a large increase in the plasma concentrations of quinidine; concurrent use is contraindicated). Products include:
- Quinidex Extentabs 2933

Quinine Sulfate (Co-administration may result in increased quinine plasma concentrations; dose decrease of quinine may be needed).
- No products indexed under this heading.

Repaglinide (New onset diabetes mellitus, exacerbation of pre-existing diabetes, and hyperglycemia have been reported with protease inhibitors; dosage adjustment of oral hypoglycemic agents may be required). Products include:
- Prandin Tablets (0.5, 1, and 2 mg) 2432

Rifabutin (Co-administration results in increased rifabutin and rifabutin metabolite concentration; dosage reduction of rifabutin by at least three-quarters of the usual dose of 300 mg/day is recommended). Products include:
- Mycobutin Capsules 2838

Rifampin (Co-administration results in decreased ritonavir concentration). Products include:
- Rifadin 765
- Rifamate Capsules 767
- Rifater Tablets 769

Rifapentine (Potential for increase in the clearance of ritonavir resulting in decreased ritonavir plasma concentrations). Products include:
- Priftin Tablets 758

Risperidone (Co-administration may result in increased risperidone plasma concentrations; dose decrease of risperidone may be needed). Products include:
- Risperdal 1796

Rosiglitazone Maleate (New onset diabetes mellitus, exacerbation of pre-existing diabetes, and hyperglycemia have been reported with protease inhibitors; dosage adjustment of oral hypoglycemic agents may be required). Products include:
- Avandia Tablets 1490

Saquinavir (Ritonavir extensively inhibits the metabolism of saquinavir resulting in greatly increased saquinavir plasma concentrations). Products include:
- Fortovase Capsules 2970

Saquinavir Mesylate (Ritonavir extensively inhibits the metabolism of saquinavir resulting in greatly increased saquinavir plasma concentrations). Products include:
- Invirase Capsules 2979

Sertraline Hydrochloride (Co-administration results in a large increase (> 3x) in AUC of sertraline; dosage adjustments may be required). Products include:
- Zoloft 2751

Sildenafil Citrate (Co-administration is expected to substantially increase sildenafil concentrations, 11-fold increase in AUC, and may result in an increase in sildenafil-associated adverse events, including hypotension, syncope, visual changes, and prolonged erection; sildenafil should not exceed a maximum dose of 25 mg in a 48-hour period in patients receiving concomitant therapy). Products include:
- Viagra Tablets 2732

Simvastatin (Co-administration results in increased plasma concentrations of simvastatin; the risk of myopathy including rhabdomyolysis may be increased; concomitant use is not recommended). Products include:
- Zocor Tablets 2219

Sotalol Hydrochloride (Co-administration with beta blockers has resulted in cardiac and neurologic events). Products include:
- Betapace Tablets 950
- Betapace AF Tablets 954

Sulfamethoxazole (Co-administration with a combination tablet containing sulfamethoxazole and trimethoprim has resulted in decreased AUC of sulfamethoxazole by 20% and no change in AUC). Products include:
- Bactrim 2949
- Septra Suspension 2265
- Septra Tablets 2265
- Septra DS Tablets 2265

Tacrolimus (Co-administration may result in increased tacrolimus plasma concentrations; dose decrease of tacrolimus may be needed). Products include:
- Prograf 1393
- Protopic Ointment 1397

Tamoxifen Citrate (Co-administration results in a large increase (> 3x) in AUC of tamoxifen; dosage adjustments may be required). Products include:
- Nolvadex Tablets 678

Temazepam (Ritonavir may increase the activity of glucuronosyltransferase; co-administration results in a decrease in AUC of temazepam; dosage adjustments may be required).
- No products indexed under this heading.

Terazosin Hydrochloride (Co-administration results in a possible increase in AUC of terazosin; dosage adjustments may be required). Products include:
- Hytrin Capsules 464

Theophylline (Co-administration results in the reduction of the average AUC of theophylline; increased dosage of theophylline may be required). Products include:
- Aerolate 1361
- Theo-Dur Extended-Release Tablets 1835
- Uni-Dur Extended-Release Tablets .. 1841
- Uniphyl 400 mg and 600 mg Tablets 2903

Theophylline Calcium Salicylate (Co-administration results in the reduction of the average AUC of theophylline; increased dosage of theophylline may be required).
- No products indexed under this heading.

Theophylline Sodium Glycinate (Co-administration results in the reduction of the average AUC of theophylline; increased dosage of theophylline may be required).
- No products indexed under this heading.

Thioridazine Hydrochloride (Co-administration may result in increased thioridazine plasma concentrations; dose decrease of thioridazine may be needed). Products include:
- Thioridazine Hydrochloride Tablets 2289

Timolol Hemihydrate (Co-administration may result in increased timolol plasma concentrations; cardiac and neurologic events have been reported with co-administration). Products include:
- Betimol Ophthalmic Solution .... ⊙ 324

Timolol Maleate (Co-administration may result in increased timolol plasma concentrations; cardiac and neurologic events have been reported with co-administration). Products include:
- Blocadren Tablets 2046
- Cosopt Sterile Ophthalmic Solution 2065
- Timolide Tablets 2187
- Timolol GFS .... ⊙ 266
- Timoptic in Ocudose 2192
- Timoptic Sterile Ophthalmic Solution 2190
- Timoptic-XE Sterile Ophthalmic Gel Forming Solution 2194

Tocainide Hydrochloride (Co-administration results in a possible increase in AUC of tocainide; dosage adjustments may be required). Products include:
- Tonocard Tablets 649

Tolazamide (New onset diabetes mellitus, exacerbation of pre-existing diabetes, and hyperglycemia have

been reported with protease inhibitors; dosage adjustment of oral hypoglycemic agents may be required).
No products indexed under this heading.

Tolbutamide (Co-administration results in a moderate increase or decrease in AUC of tolbutamide; dosage adjustments may be required).
No products indexed under this heading.

Tramadol Hydrochloride (Co-administration results in an increase in AUC of tramadol; dosage adjustments may be required). Products include:
Ultracet Tablets 2597
Ultram Tablets 2600

Trazodone Hydrochloride (Co-administration results in a large increase (> 3x) in AUC of trazodone; dosage adjustments may be required).
No products indexed under this heading.

Triazolam (Co-administration is likely to produce large increases in highly metabolized sedatives and hypnotics resulting in extreme sedation and respiratory depression; concurrent use is contraindicated). Products include:
Halcion Tablets 2823

Trimethoprim (Co-administration with a combination tablet containing sulfamethoxazole and trimethoprim has resulted in increased AUC of trimethoprim by 20% and no change in AUC). Products include:
Bactrim 2949
Septra Suspension 2265
Septra Tablets 2265
Septra DS Tablets 2265

Trimipramine Maleate (Co-administration may result in increased tricyclic antidepressant's plasma concentrations; dose decrease of tricyclics may be needed). Products include:
Surmontil Capsules 3595

Troglitazone (New onset diabetes mellitus, exacerbation of pre-existing diabetes, and hyperglycemia have been reported with protease inhibitors; dosage adjustment of oral hypoglycemic agents may be required).
No products indexed under this heading.

Valproate Sodium (Co-administration may result in decreased valproate plasma concentrations; dose increase of valproate may be needed). Products include:
Depacon Injection 416

Valproic Acid (Co-administration may result in decreased valproate plasma concentrations; dose increase of valproate may be needed). Products include:
Depakene 421

Venlafaxine Hydrochloride (Co-administration results in a moderate increase (1.5 to 3x) in AUC of venlafaxine; dosage adjustments may be required). Products include:
Effexor Tablets 3495
Effexor XR Capsules 3499

Verapamil Hydrochloride (Co-administration may result in increased verapamil plasma concentrations; dose decrease of verapamil may be needed). Products include:
Covera-HS Tablets 3199
Isoptin SR Tablets 467
Tarka Tablets 508
Verelan Capsules 3184
Verelan PM Capsules 3186

Vinblastine Sulfate (Co-administration results in a large increase (> 3x) in AUC of vinblastine; dosage adjustments may be required).
No products indexed under this heading.

Vincristine Sulfate (Co-administration results in a large increase (> 3x) in AUC of vincristine; dosage adjustments may be required).
No products indexed under this heading.

Warfarin Sodium (Co-administration may result in decreased warfarin plasma concentrations; dose increase of warfarin may be needed). Products include:
Coumadin for Injection 1243
Coumadin Tablets 1243
Warfarin Sodium Tablets, USP 3302

Zidovudine (Co-administration has resulted in decreased AUC and Cmax of zidovudine by 25% and 27% respectively and no change in ritonavir AUC and/or Cmax). Products include:
Combivir Tablets 1502
Retrovir 1625
Retrovir IV Infusion 1629
Trizivir Tablets 1669

Zolpidem Tartrate (Co-administration may result in increased zolpidem plasma concentrations; dose decrease of zolpidem may be needed). Products include:
Ambien Tablets 3191

Food Interactions

Meal, unspecified (Relative to fasting conditions, the extent of absorption of ritonavir from capsule formulation was 15% higher when administered with a meal; decreased peak ritonavir concentrations when oral solution was given under non-fasting condition).

NORVIR ORAL SOLUTION
(Ritonavir) 487
See Norvir Capsules

NOVANTRONE FOR INJECTION
(Mitoxantrone Hydrochloride) 1760
May interact with:

Daunorubicin Citrate (Increased risk of cardiac effects in patients previously treated with daunorubicin). Products include:
DaunoXome Injection 1442

Daunorubicin Hydrochloride (Increased risk of cardiac effects in patients previously treated with daunorubicin). Products include:
Cerubidine for Injection 947

Doxorubicin Hydrochloride (Increased risk of cardiac effects in patients previously treated with doxorubicin). Products include:
Adriamycin PFS/RDF Injection 2767
Doxil Injection 566

NOVAREL FOR INJECTION
(Chorionic Gonadotropin) 1347
None cited in PDR database.

NOVOLIN 70/30 HUMAN INSULIN 10 ML VIALS
(Insulin, Human Regular and Human NPH Mixture) 2421
None cited in PDR database.

NOVOLIN 70/30 PENFILL 1.5 ML CARTRIDGES
(Insulin, Human Regular and Human NPH Mixture) 2423
None cited in PDR database.

NOVOLIN 70/30 PENFILL 3 ML CARTRIDGES
(Insulin, Human Regular and Human NPH Mixture) 2423
None cited in PDR database.

NOVOLIN 70/30 PREFILLED DISPOSABLE INSULIN DELIVERY SYSTEM
(Insulin, Human Regular and Human NPH Mixture) 2425
None cited in PDR database.

NOVOLIN L HUMAN INSULIN 10 ML VIALS
(Insulin, Human, Zinc Suspension) 2422
None cited in PDR database.

NOVOLIN N HUMAN INSULIN 10 ML VIALS
(Insulin, Human NPH) 2422
None cited in PDR database.

NOVOLIN N PENFILL 1.5 ML CARTRIDGES
(Insulin, Human NPH) 2423
None cited in PDR database.

NOVOLIN N PENFILL 3 ML CARTRIDGES
(Insulin, Human NPH) 2423
None cited in PDR database.

NOVOLIN N PREFILLED SYRINGE DISPOSABLE INSULIN DELIVERY SYSTEM
(Insulin, Human NPH) 2425
None cited in PDR database.

NOVOLIN R HUMAN INSULIN 10 ML VIALS
(Insulin, Human Regular) 2423
None cited in PDR database.

NOVOLIN R PENFILL 1.5 ML CARTRIDGES
(Insulin, Human Regular) 2423
None cited in PDR database.

NOVOLIN R PENFILL 3 ML CARTRIDGES
(Insulin, Human Regular) 2423
None cited in PDR database.

NOVOLIN R PREFILLED SYRINGE DISPOSABLE INSULIN DELIVERY SYSTEM
(Insulin, Human Regular) 2425
None cited in PDR database.

NOVOSEVEN
(Antihemophilic Factor (Recombinant)) 2430
None cited in PDR database.

NUBAIN INJECTION
(Nalbuphine Hydrochloride) 1323
May interact with anesthetics, central nervous system depressants, general anesthetics, hypnotics and sedatives, narcotic analgesics, phenothiazines, tranquilizers, and certain other agents. Compounds in these categories include:

Alfentanil Hydrochloride (Additive CNS depression).
No products indexed under this heading.

Alprazolam (Additive CNS depression). Products include:
Xanax Tablets 2865

Aprobarbital (Additive CNS depression).
No products indexed under this heading.

Buprenorphine Hydrochloride (Additive CNS depression). Products include:
Buprenex Injectable 2918

Buspirone Hydrochloride (Additive CNS depression).
No products indexed under this heading.

Butabarbital (Additive CNS depression).
No products indexed under this heading.

Butalbital (Additive CNS depression). Products include:
Phrenilin 578
Sedapap Tablets 50 mg/650 mg 2225

Chlordiazepoxide (Additive CNS depression). Products include:
Limbitrol 1738

Chlordiazepoxide Hydrochloride (Additive CNS depression). Products include:
Librium Capsules 1736
Librium for Injection 1737

Chlorpromazine (Additive CNS depression). Products include:
Thorazine Suppositories 1656

Chlorpromazine Hydrochloride (Additive CNS depression). Products include:
Thorazine 1656

Chlorprothixene (Additive CNS depression).
No products indexed under this heading.

Chlorprothixene Hydrochloride (Additive CNS depression).
No products indexed under this heading.

Chlorprothixene Lactate (Additive CNS depression).
No products indexed under this heading.

Clorazepate Dipotassium (Additive CNS depression). Products include:
Tranxene 511

Clozapine (Additive CNS depression). Products include:
Clozaril Tablets 2319

Codeine Phosphate (Additive CNS depression). Products include:
Phenergan with Codeine Syrup 3557
Phenergan VC with Codeine Syrup .. 3561
Robitussin A-C Syrup 2942
Robitussin-DAC Syrup 2942
Ryna-C Liquid 768
Soma Compound w/Codeine Tablets 3355
Tussi-Organidin NR Liquid 3350
Tussi-Organidin-S NR Liquid 3350
Tylenol with Codeine 2595

Desflurane (Additive CNS depression). Products include:
Suprane Liquid for Inhalation 874

Dezocine (Additive CNS depression).
No products indexed under this heading.

Diazepam (Additive CNS depression). Products include:
Valium Injectable 3026
Valium Tablets 3047

Droperidol (Additive CNS depression).
No products indexed under this heading.

Enflurane (Additive CNS depression).
No products indexed under this heading.

Estazolam (Additive CNS depression). Products include:
ProSom Tablets 500

Ethchlorvynol (Additive CNS depression).
No products indexed under this heading.

Ethinamate (Additive CNS depression).
No products indexed under this heading.

Fentanyl (Additive CNS depression). Products include:
Duragesic Transdermal System 1786

Fentanyl Citrate (Additive CNS depression). Products include:
Actiq 1184

Fluphenazine Decanoate (Additive CNS depression).
No products indexed under this heading.

Fluphenazine Enanthate (Additive CNS depression).
No products indexed under this heading.

Fluphenazine Hydrochloride (Additive CNS depression).
No products indexed under this heading.

Flurazepam Hydrochloride (Additive CNS depression).
No products indexed under this heading.

Glutethimide (Additive CNS depression).
No products indexed under this heading.

Haloperidol (Additive CNS depression). Products include:
Haldol Injection, Tablets and Concentrate 2533

Haloperidol Decanoate (Additive CNS depression). Products include:
Haldol Decanoate 2535

Halothane (Additive CNS depression). Products include:
Fluothane Inhalation 3508

Hydrocodone Bitartrate (Additive CNS depression). Products include:
Hycodan 1316
Hycomine Compound Tablets 1317
Hycotuss Expectorant Syrup 1318
Lortab 3319
Lortab Elixir 3317
Maxidone Tablets CIII 3399
Norco 5/325 Tablets CIII 3424
Norco 7.5/325 Tablets CIII 3425
Norco 10/325 Tablets CIII 3427
Norco 10/325 Tablets CIII 3425
Vicodin Tablets 516
Vicodin ES Tablets 517
Vicodin HP Tablets 518
Vicodin Tuss Expectorant 519
Vicoprofen Tablets 520
Zydone Tablets 1330

Hydrocodone Polistirex (Additive CNS depression). Products include:
Tussionex Pennkinetic Extended-Release Suspension 1174

Hydromorphone Hydrochloride (Additive CNS depression). Products include:
Dilaudid 441
Dilaudid Oral Liquid 445
Dilaudid Powder 441
Dilaudid Rectal Suppositories 441
Dilaudid Tablets 441
Dilaudid Tablets - 8 mg 445
Dilaudid-HP 443

Hydroxyzine Hydrochloride (Additive CNS depression). Products include:
Atarax Tablets & Syrup 2667
Vistaril Intramuscular Solution 2738

Isoflurane (Additive CNS depression).
No products indexed under this heading.

Ketamine Hydrochloride (Additive CNS depression).
No products indexed under this heading.

Levomethadyl Acetate Hydrochloride (Additive CNS depression).
No products indexed under this heading.

Levorphanol Tartrate (Additive CNS depression). Products include:
Levo-Dromoran 1734
Levorphanol Tartrate Tablets 3059

Lorazepam (Additive CNS depression). Products include:
Ativan Injection 3478
Ativan Tablets 3482

Loxapine Hydrochloride (Additive CNS depression).
No products indexed under this heading.

Loxapine Succinate (Additive CNS depression). Products include:
Loxitane Capsules 3398

Meperidine Hydrochloride (Additive CNS depression). Products include:
Demerol 3079
Mepergan Injection 3539

Mephobarbital (Additive CNS depression).
No products indexed under this heading.

Meprobamate (Additive CNS depression). Products include:
Miltown Tablets 3349

Mesoridazine Besylate (Additive CNS depression). Products include:
Serentil 1057

Methadone Hydrochloride (Additive CNS depression). Products include:
Dolophine Hydrochloride Tablets 3056

Methohexital Sodium (Additive CNS depression). Products include:
Brevital Sodium for Injection, USP 1815

Methotrimeprazine (Additive CNS depression).
No products indexed under this heading.

Methoxyflurane (Additive CNS depression).
No products indexed under this heading.

Midazolam Hydrochloride (Additive CNS depression). Products include:
Versed Injection 3027
Versed Syrup 3033

Molindone Hydrochloride (Additive CNS depression). Products include:
Moban 1320

Morphine Sulfate (Additive CNS depression). Products include:
Astramorph/PF Injection, USP (Preservative-Free) 594
Duramorph Injection 1312
Infumorph 200 and Infumorph 500 Sterile Solutions 1314
Kadian Capsules 1335
MS Contin Tablets 2896
MSIR 2898
Oramorph SR Tablets 3062
Roxanol 3066

Olanzapine (Additive CNS depression). Products include:
Zyprexa Tablets 1973
Zyprexa ZYDIS Orally Disintegrating Tablets 1973

Oxazepam (Additive CNS depression).
No products indexed under this heading.

Oxycodone Hydrochloride (Additive CNS depression). Products include:
OxyContin Tablets 2912
OxyFast Oral Concentrate Solution 2916
OxyIR Capsules 2916
Percocet Tablets 1326
Percodan Tablets 1327
Percolone Tablets 1327
Roxicodone 3067
Tylox Capsules 2597

Pentobarbital Sodium (Additive CNS depression). Products include:
Nembutal Sodium Solution 485

Perphenazine (Additive CNS depression). Products include:
Etrafon 3115
Trilafon 3160

Phenobarbital (Additive CNS depression). Products include:
Arco-Lase Plus Tablets 592
Donnatal 2929
Donnatal Extentabs 2930

Prazepam (Additive CNS depression).
No products indexed under this heading.

Prochlorperazine (Additive CNS depression). Products include:
Compazine 1505

Promethazine Hydrochloride (Additive CNS depression). Products include:
Mepergan Injection 3539
Phenergan Injection 3553
Phenergan 3556
Phenergan Syrup 3554
Phenergan with Codeine Syrup 3557
Phenergan with Dextromethorphan Syrup 3559
Phenergan VC Syrup 3560
Phenergan VC with Codeine Syrup 3561

Propofol (Additive CNS depression). Products include:
Diprivan Injectable Emulsion 667

Propoxyphene Hydrochloride (Additive CNS depression). Products include:
Darvon Pulvules 1909
Darvon Compound-65 Pulvules 1910

Propoxyphene Napsylate (Additive CNS depression). Products include:
Darvon-N/Darvocet-N 1907
Darvon-N Tablets 1912

Quazepam (Additive CNS depression).
No products indexed under this heading.

Quetiapine Fumarate (Additive CNS depression). Products include:
Seroquel Tablets 684

Remifentanil Hydrochloride (Additive CNS depression).
No products indexed under this heading.

Risperidone (Additive CNS depression). Products include:
Risperdal 1796

Secobarbital Sodium (Additive CNS depression).
No products indexed under this heading.

Sevoflurane (Additive CNS depression).
No products indexed under this heading.

Sufentanil Citrate (Additive CNS depression).
No products indexed under this heading.

Temazepam (Additive CNS depression).
No products indexed under this heading.

Thiamylal Sodium (Additive CNS depression).
No products indexed under this heading.

Thioridazine Hydrochloride (Additive CNS depression). Products include:
Thioridazine Hydrochloride Tablets 2289

Thiothixene (Additive CNS depression). Products include:
Navane Capsules 2701
Thiothixene Capsules 2290

Triazolam (Additive CNS depression). Products include:
Halcion Tablets 2823

Trifluoperazine Hydrochloride (Additive CNS depression). Products include:
Stelazine 1640

Zaleplon (Additive CNS depression). Products include:
Sonata Capsules 3591

Ziprasidone Hydrochloride (Additive CNS depression). Products include:
Geodon Capsules 2688

Zolpidem Tartrate (Additive CNS depression). Products include:
Ambien Tablets 3191

Food Interactions

Alcohol (Additive CNS depression).

NU-IRON 150 CAPSULES
(Polysaccharide-Iron Complex) 2224
None cited in PDR database.

NULEV ORALLY DISINTEGRATING TABLETS
(Hyoscyamine Sulfate) 3176
May interact with antacids, antihistamines, antimuscarinic drugs, monoamine oxidase inhibitors, phenothiazines, tricyclic antidepressants, and certain other agents. Compounds in these categories include:

Acrivastine (Co-administration with certain antihistamines may result in additive adverse effects resulting from cholinergic blockade). Products include:
Semprex-D Capsules 1172

Aluminum Carbonate (Co-administration with antacids may interfere with the absorption of hyoscyamine; administer NuLev before meals and antacids after meals).
No products indexed under this heading.

Aluminum Hydroxide (Co-administration with antacids may interfere with the absorption of hyoscyamine; administer NuLev before meals and antacids after meals). Products include:
Amphojel Suspension (Mint Flavor) .... ▣789
Gaviscon Extra Strength Liquid .... ▣751
Gaviscon Extra Strength Tablets .... ▣751
Gaviscon Regular Strength Liquid .... ▣751
Gaviscon Regular Strength Tablets .... ▣750
Maalox Antacid/Anti-Gas Oral Suspension .... ▣673
Maalox Max Maximum Strength Antacid/Anti-Gas Liquid 2300
Maalox Regular Strength Antacid/Antigas Liquid 2300
Mylanta 1813
Vanquish Caplets .... ▣617

Amantadine Hydrochloride (Co-administration may result in additive adverse effects resulting from cholinergic blockade). Products include:
Symmetrel 1328

Amitriptyline Hydrochloride (Co-administration with tricyclic antidepressants may result in additive adverse effects resulting from cholinergic blockade). Products include:
Etrafon 3115
Limbitrol 1738

Amoxapine (Co-administration with tricyclic antidepressants may result in additive adverse effects resulting from cholinergic blockade).
No products indexed under this heading.

Astemizole (Co-administration with certain antihistamines may result in additive adverse effects resulting from cholinergic blockade).
No products indexed under this heading.

Atropine Sulfate (Co-administration with certain antimuscarinic drugs may result in additive adverse effects resulting from cholinergic blockade). Products include:
Donnatal 2929
Donnatal Extentabs 2930
Motofen Tablets 577
Prosed/DS Tablets 3268
Urised Tablets 2876

Azatadine Maleate (Co-administration with certain antihistamines may result in additive adverse effects resulting from cholinergic blockade). Products include:
Rynatan Tablets 3351

Belladonna Alkaloids (Co-administration with certain antimuscarinic drugs may result in additive adverse effects resulting from cholinergic blockade). Products include:
Hyland's Teething Tablets .... ▣766
Urimax Tablets 1769

Bromodiphenhydramine Hydrochloride (Co-administration with certain antihistamines may result in additive adverse effects resulting from cholinergic blockade).
No products indexed under this heading.

Brompheniramine Maleate (Co-administration with certain antihistamines may result in additive adverse effects resulting from cholinergic blockade). Products include:
Bromfed Capsules (Extended-Release) 2269
Bromfed-PD Capsules (Extended-Release) 2269
Comtrex Acute Head Cold & Sinus Pressure Relief Tablets .... ▣627

Dimetapp Elixir 777
Dimetapp Cold and Fever Suspension........ 775
Dimetapp DM Cold & Cough Elixir . 775
Dimetapp Nighttime Flu Liquid 776

Cetirizine Hydrochloride (Co-administration with certain antihistamines may result in additive adverse effects resulting from cholinergic blockade). Products include:
Zyrtec 2756
Zyrtec-D 12 Hour Extended Relief Tablets........ 2758

Chlorpheniramine Maleate (Co-administration with certain antihistamines may result in additive adverse effects resulting from cholinergic blockade). Products include:
Actifed Cold & Sinus Caplets and Tablets........ 688
Alka-Seltzer Plus Liqui-Gels 604
BC Allergy Sinus Cold Powder 619
Chlor-Trimeton Allergy Tablets 735
Chlor-Trimeton Allergy/Decongestant Tablets 736
Comtrex Flu Therapy & Fever Relief Nighttime Tablets 628
Comtrex Maximum Strength Multi-Symptom Cold & Cough Relief Tablets and Caplets 626
Contac Severe Cold and Flu Caplets Maximum Strength 746
Coricidin 'D' Cold, Flu & Sinus Tablets 737
Coricidin/Coricidin D 738
Coricidin HBP Maximum Strength Flu Tablets 738
Extendryl 1361
Hycomine Compound Tablets 1317
Kronofed-A 1341
PediaCare Cough-Cold Liquid 719
PediaCare NightRest Cough-Cold Liquid 719
Robitussin Nighttime Honey Flu Liquid 786
Ryna 768
Singlet Caplets 761
Sinutab Sinus Allergy Medication, Maximum Strength Formula, Tablets & Caplets 707
Sudafed Cold & Allergy Tablets 708
TheraFlu Regular Strength Cold & Cough Night Time Hot Liquid 676
TheraFlu Regular Strength Cold & Sore Throat Night Time Hot Liquid 676
TheraFlu Maximum Strength Flu & Cough Night Time Hot Liquid .. 678
TheraFlu Maximum Strength Flu & Sore Throat Night Time Hot Liquid 677
TheraFlu Maximum Strength Severe Cold & Congestion Night Time Caplets 678
TheraFlu Maximum Strength Severe Cold & Congestion Night Time Hot Liquid 678
Triaminic Cold & Allergy Liquid 681
Triaminic Cold & Allergy Softchews 683
Triaminic Cold & Cough Liquid 681
Triaminic Cold & Cough Softchews 683
Triaminic Cold & Night Time Cough Liquid 681
Triaminic Cold, Cough & Fever Liquid 681
Children's Tylenol Cold Suspension Liquid and Chewable Tablets 2015
Children's Tylenol Cold Plus Cough Suspension Liquid and Chewable Tablets 2015
Children's Tylenol Flu Suspension Liquid 2015
Maximum Strength Tylenol Allergy Sinus Caplets, Gelcaps, and Geltabs 2010
Multi-Symptom Tylenol Cold Complete Formula Caplets 2010
Vicks 44M Cough, Cold & Flu Relief Liquid 725
Pediatric Vicks 44m Cough & Cold Relief 728
Children's Vicks NyQuil Cold/Cough Relief 726

Chlorpheniramine Polistirex (Co-administration with certain antihistamines may result in additive adverse effects resulting from cholinergic blockade). Products include:
Tussionex Pennkinetic Extended-Release Suspension 1174

Chlorpheniramine Tannate (Co-administration with certain antihistamines may result in additive adverse effects resulting from cholinergic blockade). Products include:
Reformulated Rynatan Pediatric Suspension 3352
Rynatuss Pediatric Suspension 3353
Rynatuss Tablets 3353
Tussi-12 S Suspension 3356
Tussi-12 Tablets 3356

Chlorpromazine (Co-administration with phenothiazines may result in additive adverse effects resulting from cholinergic blockade). Products include:
Thorazine Suppositories 1656

Chlorpromazine Hydrochloride (Co-administration with phenothiazines may result in additive adverse effects resulting from cholinergic blockade). Products include:
Thorazine 1656

Clemastine Fumarate (Co-administration with certain antihistamines may result in additive adverse effects resulting from cholinergic blockade). Products include:
Tavist 12 Hour Allergy Tablets 676

Clidinium Bromide (Co-administration with certain antimuscarinic drugs may result in additive adverse effects resulting from cholinergic blockade).
No products indexed under this heading.

Clomipramine Hydrochloride (Co-administration with tricyclic antidepressants may result in additive adverse effects resulting from cholinergic blockade).
No products indexed under this heading.

Cyproheptadine Hydrochloride (Co-administration with certain antihistamines may result in additive adverse effects resulting from cholinergic blockade). Products include:
Periactin Tablets 2155

Desipramine Hydrochloride (Co-administration with tricyclic antidepressants may result in additive adverse effects resulting from cholinergic blockade). Products include:
Norpramin Tablets 755

Dexchlorpheniramine Maleate (Co-administration with certain antihistamines may result in additive adverse effects resulting from cholinergic blockade).
No products indexed under this heading.

Dicyclomine Hydrochloride (Co-administration with certain antimuscarinic drugs may result in additive adverse effects resulting from cholinergic blockade).
No products indexed under this heading.

Diphenhydramine Citrate (Co-administration with certain antihistamines may result in additive adverse effects resulting from cholinergic blockade). Products include:
Alka-Seltzer PM Effervescent Tablets 605
Benadryl Allergy & Sinus Fastmelt Tablets 693
Benadryl Children's Allergy/Cold Fastmelt Tablets 692
Excedrin PM Tablets, Caplets, and Geltabs 631
Goody's PM Powder 621

Diphenhydramine Hydrochloride (Co-administration with certain antihistamines may result in additive adverse effects resulting from cholinergic blockade). Products include:
Extra Strength Bayer PM Caplets 611
Benadryl Allergy Chewables 689
Benadryl Allergy 691
Benadryl Allergy Liquid 690
Benadryl Allergy/Cold Tablets 691
Benadryl Allergy/Congestion Tablets 692
Benadryl Allergy & Sinus Liquid 693
Benadryl Allergy Sinus Headache Caplets & Gelcaps........ 693
Benadryl Severe Allergy & Sinus Headache Caplets 694
Benadryl Dye-Free Allergy Liquid ... 690
Benadryl Dye-Free Allergy Liqui-Gels Softgels........ 690
Benadryl Itch Relief Stick Extra Strength........ 695
Benadryl Cream 695
Benadryl Gel 695
Benadryl Spray 696
Benadryl Parenteral 2617
Coricidin HBP Night-Time Cold & Flu Tablets........ 738
Nytol QuickCaps Caplets 622
Maximum Strength Nytol QuickGels Softgels........ 621
Extra Strength Percogesic Aspirin-Free Coated Caplets........ 665
Simply Sleep Caplets 2008
Sominex Original Formula Tablets . 761
Children's Tylenol Allergy-D Liquid ... 2014
Maximum Strength Tylenol Allergy Sinus NightTime Caplets 2010
Tylenol Severe Allergy Caplets 2010
Maximum Strength Tylenol Flu NightTime Gelcaps 2011
Extra Strength Tylenol PM Caplets, Geltabs, and Gelcaps 2012
Unisom Maximum Strength SleepGels 713

Diphenylpyraline Hydrochloride (Co-administration with certain antihistamines may result in additive adverse effects resulting from cholinergic blockade).
No products indexed under this heading.

Doxepin Hydrochloride (Co-administration with tricyclic antidepressants may result in additive adverse effects resulting from cholinergic blockade). Products include:
Sinequan 2713

Fexofenadine Hydrochloride (Co-administration with certain antihistamines may result in additive adverse effects resulting from cholinergic blockade). Products include:
Allegra 712
Allegra-D Extended-Release Tablets 714

Fluphenazine Decanoate (Co-administration with phenothiazines may result in additive adverse effects resulting from cholinergic blockade).
No products indexed under this heading.

Fluphenazine Enanthate (Co-administration with phenothiazines may result in additive adverse effects resulting from cholinergic blockade).
No products indexed under this heading.

Fluphenazine Hydrochloride (Co-administration with phenothiazines may result in additive adverse effects resulting from cholinergic blockade).
No products indexed under this heading.

Glycopyrrolate (Co-administration with certain antimuscarinic drugs may result in additive adverse effects resulting from cholinergic blockade). Products include:
Robinul Forte Tablets 1358
Robinul Injectable 2940
Robinul Tablets 1358

Haloperidol (Co-administration may result in additive adverse effects resulting from cholinergic blockade). Products include:
Haldol Injection, Tablets and Concentrate 2533

Haloperidol Decanoate (Co-administration may result in additive adverse effects resulting from cholinergic blockade). Products include:
Haldol Decanoate 2535

Hyoscyamine (Co-administration with certain antimuscarinic drugs may result in additive adverse effects resulting from cholinergic blockade). Products include:
Urised Tablets 2876

Imipramine Hydrochloride (Co-administration with tricyclic antidepressants may result in additive adverse effects resulting from cholinergic blockade).
No products indexed under this heading.

Imipramine Pamoate (Co-administration with tricyclic antidepressants may result in additive adverse effects resulting from cholinergic blockade).
No products indexed under this heading.

Ipratropium Bromide (Co-administration with certain antimuscarinic drugs may result in additive adverse effects resulting from cholinergic blockade). Products include:
Atrovent Inhalation Aerosol 1030
Atrovent Inhalation Solution 1031
Atrovent Nasal Spray 0.03% 1032
Atrovent Nasal Spray 0.06% 1033
Combivent Inhalation Aerosol 1041
DuoNeb Inhalation Solution 1233

Isocarboxazid (Co-administration with MAO inhibitors may result in additive adverse effects resulting from cholinergic blockade).
No products indexed under this heading.

Loratadine (Co-administration with certain antihistamines may result in additive adverse effects resulting from cholinergic blockade). Products include:
Claritin 3100
Claritin-D 12 Hour Extended Release Tablets 3102
Claritin-D 24 Hour Extended Release Tablets 3104

Magaldrate (Co-administration with antacids may interfere with the absorption of hyoscyamine; administer NuLev before meals and antacids after meals).
No products indexed under this heading.

Magnesium Hydroxide (Co-administration with antacids may interfere with the absorption of hyoscyamine; administer NuLev before meals and antacids after meals). Products include:
Ex•Lax Milk of Magnesia Liquid 670
Maalox Antacid/Anti-Gas Oral Suspension 673
Maalox Max Maximum Strength Antacid/Anti-Gas Liquid 2300
Maalox Regular Strength Antacid/Antigas Liquid 2300
Mylanta Fast-Acting 1813
Mylanta 1813
Pepcid Complete Chewable Tablets 1815
Phillips' Chewable Tablets 615
Phillips' Milk of Magnesia Liquid (Original, Cherry, & Mint) 616
Rolaids Tablets 706
Extra Strength Rolaids Tablets 706
Vanquish Caplets 617

Magnesium Oxide (Co-administration with antacids may interfere with the absorption of hyoscyamine; administer NuLev before meals and antacids after meals). Products include:
Beelith Tablets 946
Mag-Ox 400 Tablets 1024
Uro-Mag Capsules 1024

Maprotiline Hydrochloride (Co-administration with tricyclic antidepressants may result in additive adverse effects resulting from cholinergic blockade).
No products indexed under this heading.

Mepenzolate Bromide (Co-administration with certain antimuscarinic drugs may result in additive adverse effects resulting from cholinergic blockade).
No products indexed under this heading.

Mesoridazine Besylate (Co-administration with phenothiazines

may result in additive adverse effects resulting from cholinergic blockade). Products include:
Serentil 1057

Methdilazine Hydrochloride (Co-administration with certain antihistamines may result in additive adverse effects resulting from cholinergic blockade).
No products indexed under this heading.

Methotrimeprazine (Co-administration with phenothiazines may result in additive adverse effects resulting from cholinergic blockade).
No products indexed under this heading.

Moclobemide (Co-administration with MAO inhibitors may result in additive adverse effects resulting from cholinergic blockade).
No products indexed under this heading.

Nortriptyline Hydrochloride (Co-administration with tricyclic antidepressants may result in additive adverse effects resulting from cholinergic blockade).
No products indexed under this heading.

Oxyphenonium Bromide (Co-administration with certain antimuscarinic drugs may result in additive adverse effects resulting from cholinergic blockade).
No products indexed under this heading.

Pargyline Hydrochloride (Co-administration with MAO inhibitors may result in additive adverse effects resulting from cholinergic blockade).
No products indexed under this heading.

Perphenazine (Co-administration with phenothiazines may result in additive adverse effects resulting from cholinergic blockade). Products include:
Etrafon 3115
Trilafon 3160

Phenelzine Sulfate (Co-administration with MAO inhibitors may result in additive adverse effects resulting from cholinergic blockade). Products include:
Nardil Tablets 2653

Procarbazine Hydrochloride (Co-administration with MAO inhibitors may result in additive adverse effects resulting from cholinergic blockade). Products include:
Matulane Capsules 3246

Prochlorperazine (Co-administration with phenothiazines may result in additive adverse effects resulting from cholinergic blockade). Products include:
Compazine 1505

Promethazine Hydrochloride (Co-administration with phenothiazines may result in additive adverse effects resulting from cholinergic blockade). Products include:
Mepergan Injection 3539
Phenergan Injection 3553
Phenergan 3556
Phenergan Syrup 3554
Phenergan with Codeine Syrup 3557
Phenergan with Dextromethorphan Syrup 3559
Phenergan VC Syrup 3560
Phenergan VC with Codeine Syrup .. 3561

Propantheline Bromide (Co-administration with certain antimuscarinic drugs may result in additive adverse effects resulting from cholinergic blockade).
No products indexed under this heading.

Protriptyline Hydrochloride (Co-administration with tricyclic antidepressants may result in additive adverse effects resulting from cholinergic blockade). Products include:
Vivactil Tablets 2446
Vivactil Tablets 2217

Pyrilamine Maleate (Co-administration with certain antihistamines may result in additive adverse effects resulting from cholinergic blockade). Products include:
Maximum Strength Midol Menstrual Caplets and Gelcaps .... ▣612
Maximum Strength Midol PMS Caplets and Gelcaps .... ▣613

Pyrilamine Tannate (Co-administration with certain antihistamines may result in additive adverse effects resulting from cholinergic blockade). Products include:
Ryna-12 S Suspension 3351

Scopolamine (Co-administration with certain antimuscarinic drugs may result in additive adverse effects resulting from cholinergic blockade). Products include:
Transderm Scōp Transdermal Therapeutic System 2302

Scopolamine Hydrobromide (Co-administration with certain antimuscarinic drugs may result in additive adverse effects resulting from cholinergic blockade). Products include:
Donnatal 2929
Donnatal Extentabs 2930

Selegiline Hydrochloride (Co-administration with MAO inhibitors may result in additive adverse effects resulting from cholinergic blockade). Products include:
Eldepryl Capsules 3266

Sodium Bicarbonate (Co-administration with antacids may interfere with the absorption of hyoscyamine; administer NuLev before meals and antacids after meals). Products include:
Alka-Seltzer .... ▣603
Alka-Seltzer Lemon Lime Antacid and Pain Reliever Effervescent Tablets .... ▣603
Alka-Seltzer Extra Strength Antacid and Pain Reliever Effervescent Tablets .... ▣603
Alka-Seltzer Heartburn Relief Tablets .... ▣604
Ceo-Two Evacuant Suppository .... ▣618
Colyte with Flavor Packs for Oral Solution 3170
GoLYTELY and Pineapple Flavor GoLYTELY for Oral Solution 1068
NuLYTELY, Cherry Flavor, Lemon-Lime Flavor, and Orange Flavor NuLYTELY for Oral Solution 1068

Terfenadine (Co-administration with certain antihistamines may result in additive adverse effects resulting from cholinergic blockade).
No products indexed under this heading.

Thioridazine Hydrochloride (Co-administration with phenothiazines may result in additive adverse effects resulting from cholinergic blockade). Products include:
Thioridazine Hydrochloride Tablets 2289

Tolterodine Tartrate (Co-administration with certain antimuscarinic drugs may result in additive adverse effects resulting from cholinergic blockade). Products include:
Detrol Tablets 3623
Detrol LA Capsules 2801

Tranylcypromine Sulfate (Co-administration with MAO inhibitors may result in additive adverse effects resulting from cholinergic blockade). Products include:
Parnate Tablets 1607

Tridihexethyl Chloride (Co-administration with certain antimuscarinic drugs may result in additive adverse effects resulting from cholinergic blockade).
No products indexed under this heading.

Trifluoperazine Hydrochloride (Co-administration with phenothiazines may result in additive adverse effects resulting from cholinergic blockade). Products include:
Stelazine 1640

Trimeprazine Tartrate (Co-administration with certain antihistamines may result in additive adverse effects resulting from cholinergic blockade).
No products indexed under this heading.

Trimipramine Maleate (Co-administration with tricyclic antidepressants may result in additive adverse effects resulting from cholinergic blockade). Products include:
Surmontil Capsules 3595

Tripelennamine Hydrochloride (Co-administration with certain antihistamines may result in additive adverse effects resulting from cholinergic blockade).
No products indexed under this heading.

Triprolidine Hydrochloride (Co-administration with certain antihistamines may result in additive adverse effects resulting from cholinergic blockade). Products include:
Actifed Cold & Allergy Tablets .... ▣688

NULYTELY, CHERRY FLAVOR, LEMON-LIME FLAVOR, AND ORANGE FLAVOR NULYTELY FOR ORAL SOLUTION

(Polyethylene Glycol, Potassium Chloride, Sodium Bicarbonate, Sodium Chloride) 1068
May interact with:

Oral Medications, unspecified (Oral medications may not be absorbed if given within one hour).

Food Interactions

Food, unspecified (Solid food should not be given for at least two hours before the solution is given).

NUMORPHAN INJECTION

(Oxymorphone Hydrochloride) 1324
May interact with anticholinergics, central nervous system depressants, general anesthetics, hypnotics and sedatives, monoamine oxidase inhibitors, narcotic analgesics, phenothiazines, tranquilizers, tricyclic antidepressants, and certain other agents. Compounds in these categories include:

Alfentanil Hydrochloride (Concomitant use may produce additive CNS depressant effects).
No products indexed under this heading.

Alprazolam (Concomitant use may produce additive CNS depressant effects). Products include:
Xanax Tablets 2865

Amitriptyline Hydrochloride (Concomitant use may produce additive CNS depressant effects). Products include:
Etrafon 3115
Limbitrol 1738

Amoxapine (Concomitant use may produce additive CNS depressant effects).
No products indexed under this heading.

Aprobarbital (Concomitant use may produce additive CNS depressant effects).
No products indexed under this heading.

Atropine Sulfate (Co-administration of anticholinergics and opioid analgesics may result in increased risk of urinary retention and/or severe constipation and paralytic ileus). Products include:
Donnatal 2929
Donnatal Extentabs 2930
Motofen Tablets 577
Prosed/DS Tablets 3268
Urised Tablets 2876

Belladonna Alkaloids (Co-administration of anticholinergics and opioid analgesics may result in increased risk of urinary retention and/or severe constipation and paralytic ileus). Products include:
Hyland's Teething Tablets .... ▣766
Urimax Tablets 1769

Benztropine Mesylate (Co-administration of anticholinergics and opioid analgesics may result in increased risk of urinary retention and/or severe constipation and paralytic ileus). Products include:
Cogentin 2055

Biperiden Hydrochloride (Co-administration of anticholinergics and opioid analgesics may result in increased risk of urinary retention and/or severe constipation and paralytic ileus). Products include:
Akineton 402

Buprenorphine Hydrochloride (Concomitant use may produce additive CNS depressant effects). Products include:
Buprenex Injectable 2918

Buspirone Hydrochloride (Concomitant use may produce additive CNS depressant effects).
No products indexed under this heading.

Butabarbital (Concomitant use may produce additive CNS depressant effects).
No products indexed under this heading.

Butalbital (Concomitant use may produce additive CNS depressant effects). Products include:
Phrenilin 578
Sedapap Tablets 50 mg/650 mg ... 2225

Chlordiazepoxide (Concomitant use may produce additive CNS depressant effects). Products include:
Limbitrol 1738

Chlordiazepoxide Hydrochloride (Concomitant use may produce additive CNS depressant effects). Products include:
Librium Capsules 1736
Librium for Injection 1737

Chlorpromazine (Concomitant use may produce additive CNS depressant effects). Products include:
Thorazine Suppositories 1656

Chlorpromazine Hydrochloride (Concomitant use may produce additive CNS depressant effects). Products include:
Thorazine 1656

Chlorprothixene (Concomitant use may produce additive CNS depressant effects).
No products indexed under this heading.

Chlorprothixene Hydrochloride (Concomitant use may produce additive CNS depressant effects).
No products indexed under this heading.

Chlorprothixene Lactate (Concomitant use may produce additive CNS depressant effects).
No products indexed under this heading.

Cimetidine (Co-administration of cimetidine and opioid analgesics has resulted in confusion, disorientation, respiratory depression, apnea, and seizures; no clear-cut cause and effect relationship was established). Products include:
Tagamet HB 200 Suspension .... ▣762
Tagamet HB 200 Tablets .... ▣761
Tagamet Tablets 1644

Cimetidine Hydrochloride (Co-administration of cimetidine and opioid analgesics has resulted in confusion, disorientation, respiratory

depression, apnea, and seizures; no clear-cut cause and effect relationship was established). Products include:
Tagamet ... 1644

Clidinium Bromide (Co-administration of anticholinergics and opioid analgesics may result in increased risk of urinary retention and/or severe constipation and paralytic ileus).
No products indexed under this heading.

Clomipramine Hydrochloride (Concomitant use may produce additive CNS depressant effects).
No products indexed under this heading.

Clorazepate Dipotassium (Concomitant use may produce additive CNS depressant effects). Products include:
Tranxene ... 511

Clozapine (Concomitant use may produce additive CNS depressant effects). Products include:
Clozaril Tablets ... 2319

Codeine Phosphate (Concomitant use may produce additive CNS depressant effects). Products include:
Phenergan with Codeine Syrup ... 3557
Phenergan VC with Codeine Syrup ... 3561
Robitussin A-C Syrup ... 2942
Robitussin-DAC Syrup ... 2942
Ryna-C Liquid ... 768
Soma Compound w/Codeine Tablets ... 3355
Tussi-Organidin NR Liquid ... 3350
Tussi-Organidin-S NR Liquid ... 3350
Tylenol with Codeine ... 2595

Desflurane (Concomitant use may produce additive CNS depressant effects). Products include:
Suprane Liquid for Inhalation ... 874

Desipramine Hydrochloride (Concomitant use may produce additive CNS depressant effects). Products include:
Norpramin Tablets ... 755

Dezocine (Concomitant use may produce additive CNS depressant effects).
No products indexed under this heading.

Diazepam (Concomitant use may produce additive CNS depressant effects). Products include:
Valium Injectable ... 3026
Valium Tablets ... 3047

Dicyclomine Hydrochloride (Co-administration of anticholinergics and opioid analgesics may result in increased risk of urinary retention and/or severe constipation and paralytic ileus).
No products indexed under this heading.

Doxepin Hydrochloride (Concomitant use may produce additive CNS depressant effects). Products include:
Sinequan ... 2713

Droperidol (Concomitant use may produce additive CNS depressant effects).
No products indexed under this heading.

Enflurane (Concomitant use may produce additive CNS depressant effects).
No products indexed under this heading.

Estazolam (Concomitant use may produce additive CNS depressant effects). Products include:
ProSom Tablets ... 500

Ethchlorvynol (Concomitant use may produce additive CNS depressant effects).
No products indexed under this heading.

Ethinamate (Concomitant use may produce additive CNS depressant effects).
No products indexed under this heading.

Fentanyl (Concomitant use may produce additive CNS depressant effects). Products include:
Duragesic Transdermal System ... 1786

Fentanyl Citrate (Concomitant use may produce additive CNS depressant effects). Products include:
Actiq ... 1184

Fluphenazine Decanoate (Concomitant use may produce additive CNS depressant effects).
No products indexed under this heading.

Fluphenazine Enanthate (Concomitant use may produce additive CNS depressant effects).
No products indexed under this heading.

Fluphenazine Hydrochloride (Concomitant use may produce additive CNS depressant effects).
No products indexed under this heading.

Flurazepam Hydrochloride (Concomitant use may produce additive CNS depressant effects).
No products indexed under this heading.

Glutethimide (Concomitant use may produce additive CNS depressant effects).
No products indexed under this heading.

Glycopyrrolate (Co-administration of anticholinergics and opiod analgesics may result in increased risk of urinary retention and/or severe constipation and paralytic ileus). Products include:
Robinul Forte Tablets ... 1358
Robinul Injectable ... 2940
Robinul Tablets ... 1358

Haloperidol (Concomitant use may produce additive CNS depressant effects). Products include:
Haldol Injection, Tablets and Concentrate ... 2533

Haloperidol Decanoate (Concomitant use may produce additive CNS depressant effects). Products include:
Haldol Decanoate ... 2535

Hydrocodone Bitartrate (Concomitant use may produce additive CNS depressant effects). Products include:
Hycodan ... 1316
Hycomine Compound Tablets ... 1317
Hycotuss Expectorant Syrup ... 1318
Lortab ... 3319
Lortab Elixir ... 3317
Maxidone Tablets CIII ... 3399
Norco 5/325 Tablets CIII ... 3424
Norco 7.5/325 Tablets CIII ... 3425
Norco 10/325 Tablets CIII ... 3427
Norco 10/325 Tablets CIII ... 3425
Vicodin Tablets ... 516
Vicodin ES Tablets ... 517
Vicodin HP Tablets ... 518
Vicodin Tuss Expectorant ... 519
Vicoprofen Tablets ... 520
Zydone Tablets ... 1330

Hydrocodone Polistirex (Concomitant use may produce additive CNS depressant effects). Products include:
Tussionex Pennkinetic Extended-Release Suspension ... 1174

Hydromorphone Hydrochloride (Concomitant use may produce additive CNS depressant effects). Products include:
Dilaudid ... 441
Dilaudid Oral Liquid ... 445
Dilaudid Powder ... 441
Dilaudid Rectal Suppositories ... 441
Dilaudid Tablets ... 441
Dilaudid Tablets - 8 mg ... 445
Dilaudid-HP ... 443

Hydroxyzine Hydrochloride (Concomitant use may produce additive CNS depressant effects). Products include:
Atarax Tablets & Syrup ... 2667
Vistaril Intramuscular Solution ... 2738

Hyoscyamine (Co-administration of anticholinergics and opiod analgesics may result in increased risk of urinary retention and/or severe constipation and paralytic ileus). Products include:
Urised Tablets ... 2876

Hyoscyamine Sulfate (Co-administration of anticholinergics and opioid analgesics may result in increased risk of urinary retention and/or severe constipation and paralytic ileus). Products include:
Arco-Lase Plus Tablets ... 592
Donnatal ... 2929
Donnatal Extentabs ... 2930
Levsin/Levsinex/Levbid ... 3172
NuLev Orally Disintegrating Tablets ... 3176
Prosed/DS Tablets ... 3268
Urimax Tablets ... 1769

Imipramine Hydrochloride (Concomitant use may produce additive CNS depressant effects).
No products indexed under this heading.

Imipramine Pamoate (Concomitant use may produce additive CNS depressant effects).
No products indexed under this heading.

Ipratropium Bromide (Co-administration of anticholinergics and opioid analgesics may result in increased risk of urinary retention and/or severe constipation and paralytic ileus). Products include:
Atrovent Inhalation Aerosol ... 1030
Atrovent Inhalation Solution ... 1031
Atrovent Nasal Spray 0.03% ... 1032
Atrovent Nasal Spray 0.06% ... 1033
Combivent Inhalation Aerosol ... 1041
DuoNeb Inhalation Solution ... 1233

Isocarboxazid (Concomitant use may produce additive CNS depressant effects).
No products indexed under this heading.

Isoflurane (Concomitant use may produce additive CNS depressant effects).
No products indexed under this heading.

Ketamine Hydrochloride (Concomitant use may produce additive CNS depressant effects).
No products indexed under this heading.

Levomethadyl Acetate Hydrochloride (Concomitant use may produce additive CNS depressant effects).
No products indexed under this heading.

Levorphanol Tartrate (Concomitant use may produce additive CNS depressant effects). Products include:
Levo-Dromoran ... 1734
Levorphanol Tartrate Tablets ... 3059

Lorazepam (Concomitant use may produce additive CNS depressant effects). Products include:
Ativan Injection ... 3478
Ativan Tablets ... 3482

Loxapine Hydrochloride (Concomitant use may produce additive CNS depressant effects).
No products indexed under this heading.

Loxapine Succinate (Concomitant use may produce additive CNS depressant effects). Products include:
Loxitane Capsules ... 3398

Maprotiline Hydrochloride (Concomitant use may produce additive CNS depressant effects).
No products indexed under this heading.

Mepenzolate Bromide (Co-administration of anticholinergics and opioid analgesics may result in increased risk of urinary retention and/or severe constipation and paralytic ileus).
No products indexed under this heading.

Meperidine Hydrochloride (Concomitant use may produce additive CNS depressant effects). Products include:
Demerol ... 3079
Mepergan Injection ... 3539

Mephobarbital (Concomitant use may produce additive CNS depressant effects).
No products indexed under this heading.

Meprobamate (Concomitant use may produce additive CNS depressant effects). Products include:
Miltown Tablets ... 3349

Mesoridazine Besylate (Concomitant use may produce additive CNS depressant effects). Products include:
Serentil ... 1057

Methadone Hydrochloride (Concomitant use may produce additive CNS depressant effects). Products include:
Dolophine Hydrochloride Tablets ... 3056

Methohexital Sodium (Concomitant use may produce additive CNS depressant effects). Products include:
Brevital Sodium for Injection, USP ... 1815

Methotrimeprazine (Concomitant use may produce additive CNS depressant effects).
No products indexed under this heading.

Methoxyflurane (Concomitant use may produce additive CNS depressant effects).
No products indexed under this heading.

Midazolam Hydrochloride (Concomitant use may produce additive CNS depressant effects). Products include:
Versed Injection ... 3027
Versed Syrup ... 3033

Moclobemide (Concomitant use may produce additive CNS depressant effects).
No products indexed under this heading.

Molindone Hydrochloride (Concomitant use may produce additive CNS depressant effects). Products include:
Moban ... 1320

Morphine Sulfate (Concomitant use may produce additive CNS depressant effects). Products include:
Astramorph/PF Injection, USP (Preservative-Free) ... 594
Duramorph Injection ... 1312
Infumorph 200 and Infumorph 500 Sterile Solutions ... 1314
Kadian Capsules ... 1335
MS Contin Tablets ... 2896
MSIR ... 2898
Oramorph SR Tablets ... 3062
Roxanol ... 3066

Nortriptyline Hydrochloride (Concomitant use may produce additive CNS depressant effects).
No products indexed under this heading.

Olanzapine (Concomitant use may produce additive CNS depressant effects). Products include:
Zyprexa Tablets ... 1973
Zyprexa ZYDIS Orally Disintegrating Tablets ... 1973

Oxazepam (Concomitant use may produce additive CNS depressant effects).
No products indexed under this heading.

Oxybutynin Chloride (Co-administration of anticholinergics and opioid analgesics may result in

IMPORTANT NOTE: Always consult each drug listing in the patient's regimen for possible interactions.

increased risk of urinary retention and/or severe constipation and paralytic ileus). Products include:
Ditropan XL Extended Release Tablets 564

Oxycodone Hydrochloride (Concomitant use may produce additive CNS depressant effects). Products include:
OxyContin Tablets 2912
OxyFast Oral Concentrate Solution . 2916
OxyIR Capsules 2916
Percocet Tablets 1326
Percodan Tablets 1327
Percolone Tablets 1327
Roxicodone 3067
Tylox Capsules 2597

Pargyline Hydrochloride (Concomitant use may produce additive CNS depressant effects).
No products indexed under this heading.

Pentobarbital Sodium (Concomitant use may produce additive CNS depressant effects). Products include:
Nembutal Sodium Solution 485

Perphenazine (Concomitant use may produce additive CNS depressant effects). Products include:
Etrafon 3115
Trilafon 3160

Phenelzine Sulfate (Concomitant use may produce additive CNS depressant effects). Products include:
Nardil Tablets 2653

Phenobarbital (Concomitant use may produce additive CNS depressant effects). Products include:
Arco-Lase Plus Tablets 592
Donnatal 2929
Donnatal Extentabs 2930

Prazepam (Concomitant use may produce additive CNS depressant effects).
No products indexed under this heading.

Procarbazine Hydrochloride (Concomitant use may produce additive CNS depressant effects). Products include:
Matulane Capsules 3246

Prochlorperazine (Concomitant use may produce additive CNS depressant effects). Products include:
Compazine 1505

Procyclidine Hydrochloride (Co-administration of anticholinergics and opiod analgesics may result in increased risk of urinary retention and/or severe constipation and paralytic ileus).
No products indexed under this heading.

Promethazine Hydrochloride (Concomitant use may produce additive CNS depressant effects). Products include:
Mepergan Injection 3539
Phenergan Injection 3553
Phenergan 3556
Phenergan Syrup 3554
Phenergan with Codeine Syrup 3557
Phenergan with Dextromethorphan Syrup 3559
Phenergan VC Syrup 3560
Phenergan VC with Codeine Syrup .. 3561

Propantheline Bromide (Co-administration of anticholinergics and opiod analgesics may result in increased risk of urinary retention and/or severe constipation and paralytic ileus).
No products indexed under this heading.

Propofol (Co-administration has resulted in increased incidence of bradycardia; concomitant use may produce additive CNS depressant effects). Products include:
Diprivan Injectable Emulsion 667

Propoxyphene Hydrochloride (Concomitant use may produce additive CNS depressant effects). Products include:
Darvon Pulvules 1909
Darvon Compound-65 Pulvules 1910

Propoxyphene Napsylate (Concomitant use may produce additive CNS depressant effects). Products include:
Darvon-N/Darvocet-N 1907
Darvon-N Tablets 1912

Protriptyline Hydrochloride (Concomitant use may produce additive CNS depressant effects). Products include:
Vivactil Tablets 2446
Vivactil Tablets 2217

Quazepam (Concomitant use may produce additive CNS depressant effects).
No products indexed under this heading.

Quetiapine Fumarate (Concomitant use may produce additive CNS depressant effects). Products include:
Seroquel Tablets 684

Remifentanil Hydrochloride (Concomitant use may produce additive CNS depressant effects).
No products indexed under this heading.

Risperidone (Concomitant use may produce additive CNS depressant effects). Products include:
Risperdal 1796

Scopolamine (Co-administration of anticholinergics and opiod analgesics may result in increased risk of urinary retention and/or severe constipation and paralytic ileus). Products include:
Transderm Scōp Transdermal Therapeutic System 2302

Scopolamine Hydrobromide (Co-administration of anticholinergics and opiod analgesics may result in increased risk of urinary retention and/or severe constipation and paralytic ileus). Products include:
Donnatal 2929
Donnatal Extentabs 2930

Secobarbital Sodium (Concomitant use may produce additive CNS depressant effects).
No products indexed under this heading.

Selegiline Hydrochloride (Concomitant use may produce additive CNS depressant effects). Products include:
Eldepryl Capsules 3266

Sevoflurane (Concomitant use may produce additive CNS depressant effects).
No products indexed under this heading.

Sufentanil Citrate (Concomitant use may produce additive CNS depressant effects).
No products indexed under this heading.

Temazepam (Concomitant use may produce additive CNS depressant effects).
No products indexed under this heading.

Thiamylal Sodium (Concomitant use may produce additive CNS depressant effects).
No products indexed under this heading.

Thioridazine Hydrochloride (Concomitant use may produce additive CNS depressant effects). Products include:
Thioridazine Hydrochloride Tablets 2289

Thiothixene (Concomitant use may produce additive CNS depressant effects). Products include:
Navane Capsules 2701
Thiothixene Capsules 2290

Tolterodine Tartrate (Co-administration of anticholinergics and opiod analgesics may result in increased risk of urinary retention and/or severe constipation and paralytic ileus). Products include:
Detrol Tablets 3623
Detrol LA Capsules 2801

Tranylcypromine Sulfate (Concomitant use may produce additive CNS depressant effects). Products include:
Parnate Tablets 1607

Triazolam (Concomitant use may produce additive CNS depressant effects). Products include:
Halcion Tablets 2823

Tridihexethyl Chloride (Co-administration of anticholinergics and opiod analgesics may result in increased risk of urinary retention and/or severe constipation and paralytic ileus).
No products indexed under this heading.

Trifluoperazine Hydrochloride (Concomitant use may produce additive CNS depressant effects). Products include:
Stelazine 1640

Trihexyphenidyl Hydrochloride (Co-administration of anticholinergics and opiod analgesics may result in increased risk of urinary retention and/or severe constipation and paralytic ileus). Products include:
Artane 1855

Trimipramine Maleate (Concomitant use may produce additive CNS depressant effects). Products include:
Surmontil Capsules 3595

Zaleplon (Concomitant use may produce additive CNS depressant effects). Products include:
Sonata Capsules 3591

Ziprasidone Hydrochloride (Concomitant use may produce additive CNS depressant effects). Products include:
Geodon Capsules 2688

Zolpidem Tartrate (Concomitant use may produce additive CNS depressant effects). Products include:
Ambien Tablets 3191

Food Interactions

Alcohol (Concomitant use may produce additive CNS depressant effects).

NUMORPHAN SUPPOSITORIES

(Oxymorphone Hydrochloride) 1324
See Numorphan Injection

NUTR-E-SOL LIQUID

(Vitamin E) 526
None cited in PDR database.

NUTROPIN AQ INJECTION

(Somatropin) 1420
See Nutropin for Injection

NUTROPIN DEPOT FOR INJECTABLE SUSPENSION

(Somatropin) 1423
See Nutropin for Injection

NUTROPIN FOR INJECTION

(Somatropin) 1417
May interact with corticosteroids, phenytoin, and certain other agents. Compounds in these categories include:

Betamethasone Acetate (Excessive glucocorticoid therapy will inhibit the growth-promoting effect of human growth hormone). Products include:
Celestone Soluspan Injectable Suspension 3097

Betamethasone Sodium Phosphate (Excessive glucocorticoid therapy will inhibit the growth-promoting effect of human growth hormone). Products include:
Celestone Soluspan Injectable Suspension 3097

Carbamazepine (Limited published data suggests that growth hormone treatment increased CYP450 mediated antipyrine clearance in man, therefore, growth hormone administration may alter the clearance of compounds known to be metabolized by CYP450 liver enzymes, such as anticonvulsants like carbamazepine). Products include:
Carbatrol Capsules 3234
Tegretol/Tegretol-XR 2404

Cortisone Acetate (Excessive glucocorticoid therapy will inhibit the growth-promoting effect of human growth hormone). Products include:
Cortone Acetate Injectable Suspension 2059
Cortone Acetate Tablets 2061

Cyclosporine (Limited published data suggests that growth hormone treatment increases CYP450 mediated antipyrine clearance in man, therefore, growth hormone administration may alter the clearance of compounds known to be metabolized by CYP450 liver enzymes, such as cyclosporine). Products include:
Gengraf Capsules 457
Neoral Soft Gelatin Capsules 2380
Neoral Oral Solution 2380
Sandimmune 2388

Dexamethasone (Excessive glucocorticoid therapy will inhibit the growth-promoting effect of human growth hormone). Products include:
Decadron Elixir 2078
Decadron Tablets 2079
TobraDex Ophthalmic Ointment 542
TobraDex Ophthalmic Suspension .. 541

Dexamethasone Acetate (Excessive glucocorticoid therapy will inhibit the growth-promoting effect of human growth hormone).
No products indexed under this heading.

Dexamethasone Sodium Phosphate (Excessive glucocorticoid therapy will inhibit the growth-promoting effect of human growth hormone). Products include:
Decadron Phosphate Injection 2081
Decadron Phosphate Sterile Ophthalmic Ointment 2083
Decadron Phosphate Sterile Ophthalmic Solution 2084
NeoDecadron Sterile Ophthalmic Solution 2144

Fludrocortisone Acetate (Excessive glucocorticoid therapy will inhibit the growth-promoting effect of human growth hormone). Products include:
Florinef Acetate Tablets 2250

Fosphenytoin Sodium (Limited published data suggests that growth hormone treatment increases CYP450 mediated antipyrine clearance in man, therefore, growth hormone administration may alter the clearance of compounds known to be metabolized by CYP450 liver enzymes, such as anticonvulsants like phenytoin). Products include:
Cerebyx Injection 2619

Hydrocortisone (Excessive glucocorticoid therapy will inhibit the growth-promoting effect of human growth hormone). Products include:
Anusol-HC Cream 2.5% 2237
Cipro HC Otic Suspension 540
Cortaid Intensive Therapy Cream .. ■ 717
Cortaid Maximum Strength Cream .... ■ 717
Cortisporin Ophthalmic Suspension Sterile .... ⊙ 297
Cortizone•5 .... ■ 699
Cortizone•10 .... ■ 699

Cortizone•10 Plus Creme .... ▣700
Cortizone for Kids Creme .... ▣699
Hydrocortone Tablets 2106
Massengill Medicated Soft Cloth Towelette .... ▣753
VōSoL HC Otic Solution 3356

Hydrocortisone Acetate (Excessive glucocorticoid therapy will inhibit the growth-promoting effect of human growth hormone). Products include:
Analpram-HC 1338
Anusol HC-1 Hydrocortisone Anti-Itch Cream .... ▣689
Anusol-HC Suppositories 2238
Cortaid .... ▣717
Cortifoam Rectal Foam 3170
Cortisporin-TC Otic Suspension 2246
Hydrocortone Acetate Injectable Suspension 2103
Pramosone 1343
Proctocort Suppositories 2264
ProctoFoam-HC 3177
Terra-Cortril Ophthalmic Suspension 2716

Hydrocortisone Sodium Phosphate (Excessive glucocorticoid therapy will inhibit the growth-promoting effect of human growth hormone). Products include:
Hydrocortone Phosphate Injection, Sterile 2105

Hydrocortisone Sodium Succinate (Excessive glucocorticoid therapy will inhibit the growth-promoting effect of human growth hormone).
No products indexed under this heading.

Methylprednisolone Acetate (Excessive glucocorticoid therapy will inhibit the growth-promoting effect of human growth hormone). Products include:
Depo-Medrol Injectable Suspension 2795

Methylprednisolone Sodium Succinate (Excessive glucocorticoid therapy will inhibit the growth-promoting effect of human growth hormone). Products include:
Solu-Medrol Sterile Powder 2855

Phenytoin (Limited published data suggests that growth hormone treatment increases CYP450 mediated antipyrine clearance in man, therefore, growth hormone administration may alter the clearance of compounds known to be metabolized by CYP450 liver enzymes, such as anticonvulsants like phenytoin). Products include:
Dilantin Infatabs 2624
Dilantin-125 Oral Suspension 2625

Phenytoin Sodium (Limited published data suggests that growth hormone treatment increases CYP450 mediated antipyrine clearance in man, therefore, growth hormone administration may alter the clearance of compounds known to be metabolized by CYP450 liver enzymes, such as anticonvulsants like phenytoin). Products include:
Dilantin Kapseals 2622

Prednisolone Acetate (Excessive glucocorticoid therapy will inhibit the growth-promoting effect of human growth hormone). Products include:
Blephamide Ophthalmic Ointment .. 547
Blephamide Ophthalmic Suspension 548
Poly-Pred Liquifilm Ophthalmic Suspension .... ⊙245
Pred Forte Ophthalmic Suspension .... ⊙246
Pred Mild Sterile Ophthalmic Suspension .... ⊙249
Pred-G Ophthalmic Suspension ...... ⊙247
Pred-G Sterile Ophthalmic Ointment .... ⊙248

Prednisolone Sodium Phosphate (Excessive glucocorticoid therapy will inhibit the growth-promoting effect of human growth hormone). Products include:
Pediapred Oral Solution 1170

Prednisolone Tebutate (Excessive glucocorticoid therapy will inhibit the growth-promoting effect of human growth hormone).
No products indexed under this heading.

Prednisone (Excessive glucocorticoid therapy will inhibit the growth-promoting effect of human growth hormone). Products include:
Prednisone 3064

Triamcinolone (Excessive glucocorticoid therapy will inhibit the growth-promoting effect of human growth hormone).
No products indexed under this heading.

Triamcinolone Acetonide (Excessive glucocorticoid therapy will inhibit the growth-promoting effect of human growth hormone). Products include:
Azmacort Inhalation Aerosol 728
Nasacort Nasal Inhaler 750
Nasacort AQ Nasal Spray 752
Tri-Nasal Spray 2274

Triamcinolone Diacetate (Excessive glucocorticoid therapy will inhibit the growth-promoting effect of human growth hormone).
No products indexed under this heading.

Triamcinolone Hexacetonide (Excessive glucocorticoid therapy will inhibit the growth-promoting effect of human growth hormone).
No products indexed under this heading.

NYSTATIN VAGINAL TABLETS, USP

(Nystatin) 2445
None cited in PDR database.

NYSTOP TOPICAL POWDER USP

(Nystatin) 2608
None cited in PDR database.

NYTOL NATURAL TABLETS

(Aconite, Ignatius Beans) .... ▣622
May interact with hypnotics and sedatives, tranquilizers, and certain other agents. Compounds in these categories include:

Alprazolam (Concurrent use should be avoided unless directed by a physician). Products include:
Xanax Tablets 2865

Buspirone Hydrochloride (Concurrent use should be avoided unless directed by a physician).
No products indexed under this heading.

Chlordiazepoxide (Concurrent use should be avoided unless directed by a physician). Products include:
Limbitrol 1738

Chlordiazepoxide Hydrochloride (Concurrent use should be avoided unless directed by a physician). Products include:
Librium Capsules 1736
Librium for Injection 1737

Chlorpromazine (Concurrent use should be avoided unless directed by a physician). Products include:
Thorazine Suppositories 1656

Chlorpromazine Hydrochloride (Concurrent use should be avoided unless directed by a physician). Products include:
Thorazine 1656

Chlorprothixene (Concurrent use should be avoided unless directed by a physician).
No products indexed under this heading.

Chlorprothixene Hydrochloride (Concurrent use should be avoided unless directed by a physician).
No products indexed under this heading.

Clorazepate Dipotassium (Concurrent use should be avoided unless directed by a physician). Products include:
Tranxene 511

Diazepam (Concurrent use should be avoided unless directed by a physician). Products include:
Valium Injectable 3026
Valium Tablets 3047

Droperidol (Concurrent use should be avoided unless directed by a physician).
No products indexed under this heading.

Estazolam (Concurrent use should be avoided unless directed by a physician). Products include:
ProSom Tablets 500

Ethchlorvynol (Concurrent use should be avoided unless directed by a physician).
No products indexed under this heading.

Ethinamate (Concurrent use should be avoided unless directed by a physician).
No products indexed under this heading.

Fluphenazine Decanoate (Concurrent use should be avoided unless directed by a physician).
No products indexed under this heading.

Fluphenazine Enanthate (Concurrent use should be avoided unless directed by a physician).
No products indexed under this heading.

Fluphenazine Hydrochloride (Concurrent use should be avoided unless directed by a physician).
No products indexed under this heading.

Flurazepam Hydrochloride (Concurrent use should be avoided unless directed by a physician).
No products indexed under this heading.

Glutethimide (Concurrent use should be avoided unless directed by a physician).
No products indexed under this heading.

Haloperidol (Concurrent use should be avoided unless directed by a physician). Products include:
Haldol Injection, Tablets and Concentrate 2533

Haloperidol Decanoate (Concurrent use should be avoided unless directed by a physician). Products include:
Haldol Decanoate 2535

Hydroxyzine Hydrochloride (Concurrent use should be avoided unless directed by a physician). Products include:
Atarax Tablets & Syrup 2667
Vistaril Intramuscular Solution 2738

Lorazepam (Concurrent use should be avoided unless directed by a physician). Products include:
Ativan Injection 3478
Ativan Tablets 3482

Loxapine Hydrochloride (Concurrent use should be avoided unless directed by a physician).
No products indexed under this heading.

Loxapine Succinate (Concurrent use should be avoided unless directed by a physician). Products include:
Loxitane Capsules 3398

Meprobamate (Concurrent use should be avoided unless directed by a physician). Products include:
Miltown Tablets 3349

Mesoridazine Besylate (Concurrent use should be avoided unless directed by a physician). Products include:
Serentil 1057

Midazolam Hydrochloride (Concurrent use should be avoided unless directed by a physician). Products include:
Versed Injection 3027
Versed Syrup 3033

Molindone Hydrochloride (Concurrent use should be avoided unless directed by a physician). Products include:
Moban 1320

Oxazepam (Concurrent use should be avoided unless directed by a physician).
No products indexed under this heading.

Perphenazine (Concurrent use should be avoided unless directed by a physician). Products include:
Etrafon 3115
Trilafon 3160

Prazepam (Concurrent use should be avoided unless directed by a physician).
No products indexed under this heading.

Prochlorperazine (Concurrent use should be avoided unless directed by a physician). Products include:
Compazine 1505

Promethazine Hydrochloride (Concurrent use should be avoided unless directed by a physician). Products include:
Mepergan Injection 3539
Phenergan Injection 3553
Phenergan 3556
Phenergan Syrup 3554
Phenergan with Codeine Syrup 3557
Phenergan with Dextromethorphan Syrup 3559
Phenergan VC Syrup 3560
Phenergan VC with Codeine Syrup . 3561

Propofol (Concurrent use should be avoided unless directed by a physician). Products include:
Diprivan Injectable Emulsion 667

Quazepam (Concurrent use should be avoided unless directed by a physician).
No products indexed under this heading.

Secobarbital Sodium (Concurrent use should be avoided unless directed by a physician).
No products indexed under this heading.

Temazepam (Concurrent use should be avoided unless directed by a physician).
No products indexed under this heading.

Thioridazine Hydrochloride (Concurrent use should be avoided unless directed by a physician). Products include:
Thioridazine Hydrochloride Tablets 2289

Thiothixene (Concurrent use should be avoided unless directed by a physician). Products include:
Navane Capsules 2701
Thiothixene Capsules 2290

Triazolam (Concurrent use should be avoided unless directed by a physician). Products include:
Halcion Tablets 2823

Trifluoperazine Hydrochloride (Concurrent use should be avoided unless directed by a physician). Products include:
Stelazine 1640

Zaleplon (Concurrent use should be avoided unless directed by a physician). Products include:
Sonata Capsules 3591

Zolpidem Tartrate (Concurrent use should be avoided unless directed by a physician). Products include:
Ambien Tablets 3191

Food Interactions

Alcohol (Concurrent use should be avoided while taking this product).

NYTOL QUICKCAPS CAPLETS
(Diphenhydramine Hydrochloride) .... ▣622
See Maximum Strength Nytol QuickGels Softgels

MAXIMUM STRENGTH NYTOL QUICKGELS SOFTGELS
(Diphenhydramine Hydrochloride) .... ▣621
May interact with central nervous system depressants, monoamine oxidase inhibitors, and certain other agents. Compounds in these categories include:

Alfentanil Hydrochloride (Concurrent use with CNS depressant will heighten the depressant effect of Nytol).
No products indexed under this heading.

Alprazolam (Concurrent use with CNS depressant will heighten the depressant effect of Nytol). Products include:
Xanax Tablets 2865

Aprobarbital (Concurrent use with CNS depressant will heighten the depressant effect of Nytol).
No products indexed under this heading.

Buprenorphine Hydrochloride (Concurrent use with CNS depressant will heighten the depressant effect of Nytol). Products include:
Buprenex Injectable 2918

Buspirone Hydrochloride (Concurrent use with CNS depressant will heighten the depressant effect of Nytol).
No products indexed under this heading.

Butabarbital (Concurrent use with CNS depressant will heighten the depressant effect of Nytol).
No products indexed under this heading.

Butalbital (Concurrent use with CNS depressant will heighten the depressant effect of Nytol). Products include:
Phrenilin 578
Sedapap Tablets 50 mg/650 mg 2225

Chlordiazepoxide (Concurrent use with CNS depressant will heighten the depressant effect of Nytol). Products include:
Limbitrol 1738

Chlordiazepoxide Hydrochloride (Concurrent use with CNS depressant will heighten the depressant effect of Nytol). Products include:
Librium Capsules 1736
Librium for Injection 1737

Chlorpromazine (Concurrent use with CNS depressant will heighten the depressant effect of Nytol). Products include:
Thorazine Suppositories 1656

Chlorpromazine Hydrochloride (Concurrent use with CNS depressant will heighten the depressant effect of Nytol). Products include:
Thorazine 1656

Chlorprothixene (Concurrent use with CNS depressant will heighten the depressant effect of Nytol).
No products indexed under this heading.

Chlorprothixene Hydrochloride (Concurrent use with CNS depressant will heighten the depressant effect of Nytol).
No products indexed under this heading.

Chlorprothixene Lactate (Concurrent use with CNS depressant will heighten the depressant effect of Nytol).
No products indexed under this heading.

Clorazepate Dipotassium (Concurrent use with CNS depressant will heighten the depressant effect of Nytol). Products include:
Tranxene 511

Clozapine (Concurrent use with CNS depressant will heighten the depressant effect of Nytol). Products include:
Clozaril Tablets 2319

Codeine Phosphate (Concurrent use with CNS depressant will heighten the depressant effect of Nytol). Products include:
Phenergan with Codeine Syrup 3557
Phenergan VC with Codeine Syrup 3561
Robitussin A-C Syrup 2942
Robitussin-DAC Syrup 2942
Ryna-C Liquid .... ▣768
Soma Compound w/Codeine Tablets 3355
Tussi-Organidin NR Liquid 3350
Tussi-Organidin-S NR Liquid 3350
Tylenol with Codeine 2595

Desflurane (Concurrent use with CNS depressant will heighten the depressant effect of Nytol). Products include:
Suprane Liquid for Inhalation 874

Dezocine (Concurrent use with CNS depressant will heighten the depressant effect of Nytol).
No products indexed under this heading.

Diazepam (Concurrent use with CNS depressant will heighten the depressant effect of Nytol). Products include:
Valium Injectable 3026
Valium Tablets 3047

Droperidol (Concurrent use with CNS depressant will heighten the depressant effect of Nytol).
No products indexed under this heading.

Enflurane (Concurrent use with CNS depressant will heighten the depressant effect of Nytol).
No products indexed under this heading.

Estazolam (Concurrent use with CNS depressant will heighten the depressant effect of Nytol). Products include:
ProSom Tablets 500

Ethchlorvynol (Concurrent use with CNS depressant will heighten the depressant effect of Nytol).
No products indexed under this heading.

Ethinamate (Concurrent use with CNS depressant will heighten the depressant effect of Nytol).
No products indexed under this heading.

Fentanyl (Concurrent use with CNS depressant will heighten the depressant effect of Nytol). Products include:
Duragesic Transdermal System 1786

Fentanyl Citrate (Concurrent use with CNS depressant will heighten the depressant effect of Nytol). Products include:
Actiq 1184

Fluphenazine Decanoate (Concurrent use with CNS depressant will heighten the depressant effect of Nytol).
No products indexed under this heading.

Fluphenazine Enanthate (Concurrent use with CNS depressant will heighten the depressant effect of Nytol).
No products indexed under this heading.

Fluphenazine Hydrochloride (Concurrent use with CNS depressant will heighten the depressant effect of Nytol).
No products indexed under this heading.

Flurazepam Hydrochloride (Concurrent use with CNS depressant will heighten the depressant effect of Nytol).
No products indexed under this heading.

Glutethimide (Concurrent use with CNS depressant will heighten the depressant effect of Nytol).
No products indexed under this heading.

Haloperidol (Concurrent use with CNS depressant will heighten the depressant effect of Nytol). Products include:
Haldol Injection, Tablets and Concentrate 2533

Haloperidol Decanoate (Concurrent use with CNS depressant will heighten the depressant effect of Nytol). Products include:
Haldol Decanoate 2535

Hydrocodone Bitartrate (Concurrent use with CNS depressant will heighten the depressant effect of Nytol). Products include:
Hycodan 1316
Hycomine Compound Tablets 1317
Hycotuss Expectorant Syrup 1318
Lortab 3319
Lortab Elixir 3317
Maxidone Tablets CIII 3399
Norco 5/325 Tablets CIII 3424
Norco 7.5/325 Tablets CIII 3425
Norco 10/325 Tablets CIII 3427
Norco 10/325 Tablets CIII 3425
Vicodin Tablets 516
Vicodin ES Tablets 517
Vicodin HP Tablets 518
Vicodin Tuss Expectorant 519
Vicoprofen Tablets 520
Zydone Tablets 1330

Hydrocodone Polistirex (Concurrent use with CNS depressant will heighten the depressant effect of Nytol). Products include:
Tussionex Pennkinetic Extended-Release Suspension 1174

Hydromorphone Hydrochloride (Concurrent use with CNS depressant will heighten the depressant effect of Nytol). Products include:
Dilaudid 441
Dilaudid Oral Liquid 445
Dilaudid Powder 441
Dilaudid Rectal Suppositories 441
Dilaudid Tablets 441
Dilaudid Tablets - 8 mg 445
Dilaudid-HP 443

Hydroxyzine Hydrochloride (Concurrent use with CNS depressant will heighten the depressant effect of Nytol). Products include:
Atarax Tablets & Syrup 2667
Vistaril Intramuscular Solution 2738

Isocarboxazid (Concurrent use with MAO inhibitor will prolong and intensify the anticholinergic effects of antihistamines).
No products indexed under this heading.

Isoflurane (Concurrent use with CNS depressant will heighten the depressant effect of Nytol).
No products indexed under this heading.

Ketamine Hydrochloride (Concurrent use with CNS depressant will heighten the depressant effect of Nytol).
No products indexed under this heading.

Levomethadyl Acetate Hydrochloride (Concurrent use with CNS depressant will heighten the depressant effect of Nytol).
No products indexed under this heading.

Levorphanol Tartrate (Concurrent use with CNS depressant will heighten the depressant effect of Nytol). Products include:
Levo-Dromoran 1734
Levorphanol Tartrate Tablets 3059

Lorazepam (Concurrent use with CNS depressant will heighten the depressant effect of Nytol). Products include:
Ativan Injection 3478
Ativan Tablets 3482

Loxapine Hydrochloride (Concurrent use with CNS depressant will heighten the depressant effect of Nytol).
No products indexed under this heading.

Loxapine Succinate (Concurrent use with CNS depressant will heighten the depressant effect of Nytol). Products include:
Loxitane Capsules 3398

Meperidine Hydrochloride (Concurrent use with CNS depressant will heighten the depressant effect of Nytol). Products include:
Demerol 3079
Mepergan Injection 3539

Mephobarbital (Concurrent use with CNS depressant will heighten the depressant effect of Nytol).
No products indexed under this heading.

Meprobamate (Concurrent use with CNS depressant will heighten the depressant effect of Nytol). Products include:
Miltown Tablets 3349

Mesoridazine Besylate (Concurrent use with CNS depressant will heighten the depressant effect of Nytol). Products include:
Serentil 1057

Methadone Hydrochloride (Concurrent use with CNS depressant will heighten the depressant effect of Nytol). Products include:
Dolophine Hydrochloride Tablets 3056

Methohexital Sodium (Concurrent use with CNS depressant will heighten the depressant effect of Nytol). Products include:
Brevital Sodium for Injection, USP 1815

Methotrimeprazine (Concurrent use with CNS depressant will heighten the depressant effect of Nytol).
No products indexed under this heading.

Methoxyflurane (Concurrent use with CNS depressant will heighten the depressant effect of Nytol).
No products indexed under this heading.

Midazolam Hydrochloride (Concurrent use with CNS depressant will heighten the depressant effect of Nytol). Products include:
Versed Injection 3027
Versed Syrup 3033

Moclobemide (Concurrent use with MAO inhibitor will prolong and intensify the anticholinergic effects of antihistamines).
No products indexed under this heading.

Molindone Hydrochloride (Concurrent use with CNS depressant will heighten the depressant effect of Nytol). Products include:
Moban 1320

Morphine Sulfate (Concurrent use with CNS depressant will heighten the depressant effect of Nytol). Products include:
Astramorph/PF Injection, USP (Preservative-Free) 594
Duramorph Injection 1312
Infumorph 200 and Infumorph 500 Sterile Solutions 1314
Kadian Capsules 1335
MS Contin Tablets 2896
MSIR 2898
Oramorph SR Tablets 3062
Roxanol 3066

Olanzapine (Concurrent use with CNS depressant will heighten the depressant effect of Nytol). Products include:
Zyprexa Tablets 1973

Zyprexa ZYDIS Orally Disintegrating Tablets ... 1973

Oxazepam (Concurrent use with CNS depressant will heighten the depressant effect of Nytol).
No products indexed under this heading.

Oxycodone Hydrochloride (Concurrent use with CNS depressant will heighten the depressant effect of Nytol). Products include:
OxyContin Tablets ... 2912
OxyFast Oral Concentrate Solution . 2916
OxyIR Capsules ... 2916
Percocet Tablets ... 1326
Percodan Tablets ... 1327
Percolone Tablets ... 1327
Roxicodone ... 3067
Tylox Capsules ... 2597

Pargyline Hydrochloride (Concurrent use with MAO inhibitor will prolong and intensify the anticholinergic effects of antihistamines).
No products indexed under this heading.

Pentobarbital Sodium (Concurrent use with CNS depressant will heighten the depressant effect of Nytol). Products include:
Nembutal Sodium Solution ... 485

Perphenazine (Concurrent use with CNS depressant will heighten the depressant effect of Nytol). Products include:
Etrafon ... 3115
Trilafon ... 3160

Phenelzine Sulfate (Concurrent use with MAO inhibitor will prolong and intensify the anticholinergic effects of antihistamines). Products include:
Nardil Tablets ... 2653

Phenobarbital (Concurrent use with CNS depressant will heighten the depressant effect of Nytol). Products include:
Arco-Lase Plus Tablets ... 592
Donnatal ... 2929
Donnatal Extentabs ... 2930

Prazepam (Concurrent use with CNS depressant will heighten the depressant effect of Nytol).
No products indexed under this heading.

Procarbazine Hydrochloride (Concurrent use with MAO inhibitor will prolong and intensify the anticholinergic effects of antihistamines). Products include:
Matulane Capsules ... 3246

Prochlorperazine (Concurrent use with CNS depressant will heighten the depressant effect of Nytol). Products include:
Compazine ... 1505

Promethazine Hydrochloride (Concurrent use with CNS depressant will heighten the depressant effect of Nytol). Products include:
Mepergan Injection ... 3539
Phenergan Injection ... 3553
Phenergan ... 3556
Phenergan Syrup ... 3554
Phenergan with Codeine Syrup ... 3557
Phenergan with Dextromethorphan Syrup ... 3559
Phenergan VC Syrup ... 3560
Phenergan VC with Codeine Syrup .. 3561

Propofol (Concurrent use with CNS depressant will heighten the depressant effect of Nytol). Products include:
Diprivan Injectable Emulsion ... 667

Propoxyphene Hydrochloride (Concurrent use with CNS depressant will heighten the depressant effect of Nytol). Products include:
Darvon Pulvules ... 1909
Darvon Compound-65 Pulvules ... 1910

Propoxyphene Napsylate (Concurrent use with CNS depressant will heighten the depressant effect of Nytol). Products include:
Darvon-N/Darvocet-N ... 1907
Darvon-N Tablets ... 1912

Quazepam (Concurrent use with CNS depressant will heighten the depressant effect of Nytol).
No products indexed under this heading.

Quetiapine Fumarate (Concurrent use with CNS depressant will heighten the depressant effect of Nytol). Products include:
Seroquel Tablets ... 684

Remifentanil Hydrochloride (Concurrent use with CNS depressant will heighten the depressant effect of Nytol).
No products indexed under this heading.

Risperidone (Concurrent use with CNS depressant will heighten the depressant effect of Nytol). Products include:
Risperdal ... 1796

Secobarbital Sodium (Concurrent use with CNS depressant will heighten the depressant effect of Nytol).
No products indexed under this heading.

Selegiline Hydrochloride (Concurrent use with MAO inhibitor will prolong and intensify the anticholinergic effects of antihistamines). Products include:
Eldepryl Capsules ... 3266

Sevoflurane (Concurrent use with CNS depressant will heighten the depressant effect of Nytol).
No products indexed under this heading.

Sufentanil Citrate (Concurrent use with CNS depressant will heighten the depressant effect of Nytol).
No products indexed under this heading.

Temazepam (Concurrent use with CNS depressant will heighten the depressant effect of Nytol).
No products indexed under this heading.

Thiamylal Sodium (Concurrent use with CNS depressant will heighten the depressant effect of Nytol).
No products indexed under this heading.

Thioridazine Hydrochloride (Concurrent use with CNS depressant will heighten the depressant effect of Nytol). Products include:
Thioridazine Hydrochloride Tablets ... 2289

Thiothixene (Concurrent use with CNS depressant will heighten the depressant effect of Nytol). Products include:
Navane Capsules ... 2701
Thiothixene Capsules ... 2290

Tranylcypromine Sulfate (Concurrent use with MAO inhibitor will prolong and intensify the anticholinergic effects of antihistamines). Products include:
Parnate Tablets ... 1607

Triazolam (Concurrent use with CNS depressant will heighten the depressant effect of Nytol). Products include:
Halcion Tablets ... 2823

Trifluoperazine Hydrochloride (Concurrent use with CNS depressant will heighten the depressant effect of Nytol). Products include:
Stelazine ... 1640

Zaleplon (Concurrent use with CNS depressant will heighten the depressant effect of Nytol). Products include:
Sonata Capsules ... 3591

Ziprasidone Hydrochloride (Concurrent use with CNS depressant will heighten the depressant effect of Nytol). Products include:
Geodon Capsules ... 2688

Zolpidem Tartrate (Concurrent use with CNS depressant will heighten the depressant effect of Nytol). Products include:
Ambien Tablets ... 3191

Food Interactions

Alcohol (Concurrent use will heighten the depressant effect of Nytol; avoid alcoholic beverages while taking this product).

OBEGYN PRENATAL SUPPLEMENT

(Vitamins, Prenatal) ... 1362
None cited in PDR database.

OCEAN NASAL MIST

(Sodium Chloride) ... ⊡633
None cited in PDR database.

OCUCOAT

(Hydroxypropyl Methylcellulose) ... ⊙330
None cited in PDR database.

OCUFEN OPHTHALMIC SOLUTION

(Flurbiprofen Sodium) ... ⊙242
May interact with:

Acetylcholine Chloride (There have been reports that acetylcholine chloride is ineffective when used in patients treated with ophthalmic flurbiprofen). Products include:
Miochol-E System Pak ... ⊙305
Miochol-E with Steri-Tags ... ⊙305

Carbachol (There have been reports that carbachol is ineffective when used in patients treated with ophthalmic flurbiprofen). Products include:
Isopto Carbachol Ophthalmic Solution ... ⊙215

OCUFLOX OPHTHALMIC SOLUTION

(Ofloxacin) ... 554
May interact with oral anticoagulants, theophylline, and certain other agents. Compounds in these categories include:

Aminophylline (Systemic administration of quinolone has shown to elevate plasma theophylline levels; specific drug interactions studies have not been conducted with the ofloxacin ophthalmic solution).
No products indexed under this heading.

Caffeine-containing medications (Systemic administration of quinolone has shown to interfere with the metabolism of caffeine; specific drug interactions studies have not been conducted with the ofloxacin ophthalmic solution).

Cyclosporine (Systemic administration of quinolone has been associated with transient elevations in serum creatinine; specific drug interactions studies have not been conducted with the ofloxacin ophthalmic solution). Products include:
Gengraf Capsules ... 457
Neoral Soft Gelatin Capsules ... 2380
Neoral Oral Solution ... 2380
Sandimmune ... 2388

Dicumarol (Systemic administration of quinolone has shown to enhance the effects of oral anticoagulants; specific drug interactions studies have not been conducted with the ofloxacin ophthalmic solution).
No products indexed under this heading.

Dyphylline (Systemic administration of quinolone has shown to elevate plasma theophylline levels; specific drug interactions studies have not been conducted with the ofloxacin ophthalmic solution). Products include:
Lufyllin Tablets ... 3347
Lufyllin-400 Tablets ... 3347
Lufyllin-GG Elixir ... 3348
Lufyllin-GG Tablets ... 3348

Theophylline (Systemic administration of quinolone has shown to elevate plasma theophylline levels; specific drug interactions studies have not been conducted with the ofloxacin ophthalmic solution). Products include:
Aerolate ... 1361
Theo-Dur Extended-Release Tablets ... 1835
Uni-Dur Extended-Release Tablets .. 1841
Uniphyl 400 mg and 600 mg Tablets ... 2903

Theophylline Calcium Salicylate (Systemic administration of quinolone has shown to elevate plasma theophylline levels; specific drug interactions studies have not been conducted with the ofloxacin ophthalmic solution).
No products indexed under this heading.

Theophylline Sodium Glycinate (Systemic administration of quinolone has shown to elevate plasma theophylline levels; specific drug interactions studies have not been conducted with the ofloxacin ophthalmic solution).
No products indexed under this heading.

Warfarin Sodium (Systemic administration of quinolone has shown to enhance the effects of oral anticoagulants; specific drug interactions studies have not been conducted with the ofloxacin ophthalmic solution). Products include:
Coumadin for Injection ... 1243
Coumadin Tablets ... 1243
Warfarin Sodium Tablets, USP ... 3302

OCUPRESS OPHTHALMIC SOLUTION, 1% STERILE

(Carteolol Hydrochloride) ... ⊙303
May interact with beta blockers and catecholamine depleting drugs. Compounds in these categories include:

Acebutolol Hydrochloride (Potential for additive effects). Products include:
Sectral Capsules ... 3589

Atenolol (Potential for additive effects). Products include:
Tenoretic Tablets ... 690
Tenormin I.V. Injection ... 692

Betaxolol Hydrochloride (Potential for additive effects). Products include:
Betoptic S Ophthalmic Suspension ... 537

Bisoprolol Fumarate (Potential for additive effects). Products include:
Zebeta Tablets ... 1885
Ziac Tablets ... 1887

Deserpidine (Possible additive effects and the production of hypotension and/or marked bradycardia).
No products indexed under this heading.

Esmolol Hydrochloride (Potential for additive effects). Products include:
Brevibloc Injection ... 858

Guanethidine Monosulfate (Possible additive effects and the production of hypotension and/or marked bradycardia).
No products indexed under this heading.

Labetalol Hydrochloride (Potential for additive effects). Products include:
Normodyne Injection ... 3135
Normodyne Tablets ... 3137

Levobunolol Hydrochloride (Potential for additive effects). Products include:
Betagan ... ⊙228

Metipranolol Hydrochloride (Potential for additive effects).
No products indexed under this heading.

Metoprolol Succinate (Potential for additive effects). Products include:
Toprol-XL Tablets 651

Metoprolol Tartrate (Potential for additive effects).
No products indexed under this heading.

Nadolol (Potential for additive effects). Products include:
Corgard Tablets 2245
Corzide 40/5 Tablets 2247
Corzide 80/5 Tablets 2247
Nadolol Tablets 2288

Penbutolol Sulfate (Potential for additive effects).
No products indexed under this heading.

Pindolol (Potential for additive effects).
No products indexed under this heading.

Propranolol Hydrochloride (Potential for additive effects). Products include:
Inderal 3513
Inderal LA Long-Acting Capsules 3516
Inderide Tablets 3517
Inderide LA Long-Acting Capsules .. 3519

Rauwolfia serpentina (Possible additive effects and the production of hypotension and/or marked bradycardia).
No products indexed under this heading.

Rescinnamine (Possible additive effects and the production of hypotension and/or marked bradycardia).
No products indexed under this heading.

Reserpine (Possible additive effects and the production of hypotension and/or marked bradycardia).
No products indexed under this heading.

Sotalol Hydrochloride (Potential for additive effects). Products include:
Betapace Tablets 950
Betapace AF Tablets 954

Timolol Hemihydrate (Potential for additive effects). Products include:
Betimol Ophthalmic Solution .... ⊙324

Timolol Maleate (Potential for additive effects). Products include:
Blocadren Tablets 2046
Cosopt Sterile Ophthalmic Solution 2065
Timolide Tablets 2187
Timolol GFS .... ⊙266
Timoptic in Ocudose 2192
Timoptic Sterile Ophthalmic Solution 2190
Timoptic-XE Sterile Ophthalmic Gel Forming Solution 2194

OCUVITE LUTEIN VITAMIN AND MINERAL SUPPLEMENT
(Vitamins with Minerals) .... ⊙263
None cited in PDR database.

OCUVITE VITAMIN AND MINERAL SUPPLEMENT
(Vitamins with Minerals) .... ⊙263
None cited in PDR database.

OCUVITE EXTRA VITAMIN AND MINERAL SUPPLEMENT
(Vitamins with Minerals) .... ⊙263
None cited in PDR database.

OGEN TABLETS
(Estropipate) 2846
May interact with:

Medroxyprogesterone Acetate (Possible adverse effects on lipoprotein metabolism; impairment of glucose tolerance and possible enhancement of mitotic activity in breast epithelial tissues). Products include:
Depo-Provera Contraceptive Injection 2798
Lunelle Monthly Injection 2827
Premphase Tablets 3572
Prempro Tablets 3572
Provera Tablets 2853

OGESTREL 0.5/50-28 TABLETS
(Ethinyl Estradiol, Norgestrel) 3428
See Low-Ogestrel-28 Tablets

OLUX FOAM
(Clobetasol Propionate) 1211
None cited in PDR database.

OMNICEF CAPSULES
(Cefdinir) 493
May interact with antacids containing aluminum, calcium and magnesium, iron containing oral preparations, and certain other agents. Compounds in these categories include:

Aluminum Carbonate (Antacids (aluminum- or magnesium-containing) interfere with the absorption of cefdinir; Omnicef should be taken at least 2 hours before or after the antacids).
No products indexed under this heading.

Aluminum Hydroxide (Antacids (aluminum- or magnesium-containing) interfere with the absorption of cefdinir; Omnicef should be taken at least 2 hours before or after the antacids). Products include:
Amphojel Suspension (Mint Flavor) .... ▣789
Gaviscon Extra Strength Liquid ..... ▣751
Gaviscon Extra Strength Tablets ... ▣751
Gaviscon Regular Strength Liquid . ▣751
Gaviscon Regular Strength Tablets .... ▣750
Maalox Antacid/Anti-Gas Oral Suspension .... ▣673
Maalox Max Maximum Strength Antacid/Anti-Gas Liquid 2300
Maalox Regular Strength Antacid/Antigas Liquid 2300
Mylanta 1813
Vanquish Caplets .... ▣617

Ferrous Fumarate (Iron supplements, including multivitamins that contain iron, interfere with the absorption of cefdinir; Omnicef should be taken at least 2 hours before or after the administration of iron-containing products). Products include:
New Formulation Chromagen OB Capsules 3094
Loestrin Fe Tablets 2642
NataChew Tablets 3364

Ferrous Gluconate (Iron supplements, including multivitamins that contain iron, interfere with the absorption of cefdinir; Omnicef should be taken at least 2 hours before or after the administration of iron-containing products). Products include:
Fergon Iron Tablets .... ▣802

Ferrous Sulfate (Iron supplements, including multivitamins that contain iron, interfere with the absorption of cefdinir; Omnicef should be taken at least 2 hours before or after the administration of iron-containing products). Products include:
Feosol Tablets 1717
Slow Fe Tablets .... ▣827
Slow Fe with Folic Acid Tablets ..... ▣828

Iron (Iron supplements, including multivitamins that contain iron, interfere with the absorption of cefdinir; Omnicef should be taken at least 2 hours before or after the administration of iron-containing products).
No products indexed under this heading.

Magaldrate (Antacids (aluminum- or magnesium-containing) interfere with the absorption of cefdinir; Omnicef should be taken at least 2 hours before or after the antacids).
No products indexed under this heading.

Magnesium Hydroxide (Antacids (aluminum- or magnesium-containing) interfere with the absorption of cefdinir; Omnicef should be taken at least 2 hours before or after the antacids). Products include:
Ex•Lax Milk of Magnesia Liquid .... ▣670
Maalox Antacid/Anti-Gas Oral Suspension .... ▣673
Maalox Max Maximum Strength Antacid/Anti-Gas Liquid 2300
Maalox Regular Strength Antacid/Antigas Liquid 2300
Mylanta Fast-Acting 1813
Mylanta 1813
Pepcid Complete Chewable Tablets 1815
Phillips' Chewable Tablets .... ▣615
Phillips' Milk of Magnesia Liquid (Original, Cherry, & Mint) .... ▣616
Rolaids Tablets .... ▣706
Extra Strength Rolaids Tablets ...... ▣706
Vanquish Caplets .... ▣617

Magnesium Oxide (Antacids (aluminum- or magnesium-containing) interfere with the absorption of cefdinir; Omnicef should be taken at least 2 hours before or after the antacids). Products include:
Beelith Tablets 946
Mag-Ox 400 Tablets 1024
Uro-Mag Capsules 1024

Polysaccharide-Iron Complex (Iron supplements, including multivitamins that contain iron, interfere with the absorption of cefdinir; Omnicef should be taken at least 2 hours before or after the administration of iron-containing products). Products include:
Niferex 3176
Niferex-150 Capsules 3176
Nu-Iron 150 Capsules 2224

Probenecid (Inhibits renal excretion of cefdinir, resulting in an approximate doubling in AUC, a 54% increase in peak cefdinir plasma levels, and a 50% prolongation in the apparent elimination).
No products indexed under this heading.

Food Interactions

Food, unspecified (Although Cmax and AUC of cefdinir absorption from capsules are reduced by 16% and 10% respectively, when given with a high-fat meal, the magnitude of these reduction is not likely to clinically significant, therefore, cefdinir may be taken without regard to food).

OMNICEF FOR ORAL SUSPENSION
(Cefdinir) 493
See Omnicef Capsules

ONCASPAR
(Pegaspargase) 756
May interact with antineoplastics, anticoagulants, non-steroidal anti-inflammatory agents, highly protein bound drugs (selected), and certain other agents. Compounds in these categories include:

Altretamine (Potential for unspecified unfavorable interactions). Products include:
Hexalen Capsules 2226

Amiodarone Hydrochloride (Depletion of serum proteins by pegaspargase may increase the toxicity of other drugs which are protein bound). Products include:
Cordarone Intravenous 3491
Cordarone Tablets 3487
Pacerone Tablets 3331

Amitriptyline Hydrochloride (Depletion of serum proteins by pegaspargase may increase the toxicity of other drugs which are protein bound). Products include:
Etrafon 3115
Limbitrol 1738

Anastrozole (Potential for unspecified unfavorable interactions). Products include:
Arimidex Tablets 659

Ardeparin Sodium (Increased risk of bleeding and/or thrombosis).
No products indexed under this heading.

Asparaginase (Potential for unspecified unfavorable interactions). Products include:
Elspar for Injection 2092

Aspirin (Increased risk of bleeding and/or thrombosis). Products include:
Aggrenox Capsules 1026
Alka-Seltzer .... ▣603
Alka-Seltzer Lemon Lime Antacid and Pain Reliever Effervescent Tablets .... ▣603
Alka-Seltzer Extra Strength Antacid and Pain Reliever Effervescent Tablets .... ▣603
Alka-Seltzer PM Effervescent Tablets .... ▣605
Genuine Bayer Tablets, Caplets and Gelcaps .... ▣606
Extra Strength Bayer Caplets and Gelcaps .... ▣610
Aspirin Regimen Bayer Children's Chewable Tablets (Orange or Cherry Flavored) .... ▣607
Bayer, Aspirin Regimen .... ▣606
Aspirin Regimen Bayer 81 mg Caplets with Calcium .... ▣607
Genuine Bayer Professional Labeling (Aspirin Regimen Bayer) .... ▣608
Extra Strength Bayer Arthritis Caplets .... ▣610
Extra Strength Bayer Plus Caplets .... ▣610
Extra Strength Bayer PM Caplets .. ▣611
BC Powder .... ▣619
BC Allergy Sinus Cold Powder .... ▣619
Arthritis Strength BC Powder .... ▣619
BC Sinus Cold Powder .... ▣619
Darvon Compound-65 Pulvules 1910
Ecotrin Enteric Coated Aspirin Low, Regular and Maximum Strength Tablets 1715
Excedrin Extra-Strength Tablets, Caplets, and Geltabs .... ▣629
Excedrin Migraine 1070
Goody's Body Pain Formula Powder .... ▣620
Goody's Extra Strength Headache Powder .... ▣620
Goody's Extra Strength Pain Relief Tablets .... ▣620
Percodan Tablets 1327
Robaxisal Tablets 2939
Soma Compound Tablets 3354
Soma Compound w/Codeine Tablets 3355
Vanquish Caplets .... ▣617

Atovaquone (Depletion of serum proteins by pegaspargase may increase the toxicity of other drugs which are protein bound). Products include:
Malarone 1596
Mepron Suspension 1598

Bicalutamide (Potential for unspecified unfavorable interactions). Products include:
Casodex Tablets 662

Bleomycin Sulfate (Potential for unspecified unfavorable interactions).
No products indexed under this heading.

Busulfan (Potential for unspecified unfavorable interactions). Products include:
Myleran Tablets 1603

Carboplatin (Potential for unspecified unfavorable interactions). Products include:
Paraplatin for Injection 1126

Carmustine (BCNU) (Potential for unspecified unfavorable interactions). Products include:
Gliadel Wafer 1723

Cefonicid Sodium (Depletion of serum proteins by pegaspargase may increase the toxicity of other drugs which are protein bound).
No products indexed under this heading.

Celecoxib (Increased risk of bleeding and/or thrombosis). Products include:
Celebrex Capsules 2676
Celebrex Capsules 2780

Chlorambucil (Potential for unspecified unfavorable interactions). Products include:
Leukeran Tablets 1591

Chlordiazepoxide (Depletion of serum proteins by pegaspargase may increase the toxicity of other drugs which are protein bound). Products include:
Limbitrol 1738

Chlordiazepoxide Hydrochloride (Depletion of serum proteins by pegaspargase may increase the toxicity of other drugs which are protein bound). Products include:
Librium Capsules 1736
Librium for Injection 1737

Chlorpromazine (Depletion of serum proteins by pegaspargase may increase the toxicity of other drugs which are protein bound). Products include:
Thorazine Suppositories 1656

Chlorpromazine Hydrochloride (Depletion of serum proteins by pegaspargase may increase the toxicity of other drugs which are protein bound). Products include:
Thorazine 1656

Cisplatin (Potential for unspecified unfavorable interactions).
No products indexed under this heading.

Clomipramine Hydrochloride (Depletion of serum proteins by pegaspargase may increase the toxicity of other drugs which are protein bound).
No products indexed under this heading.

Clozapine (Depletion of serum proteins by pegaspargase may increase the toxicity of other drugs which are protein bound). Products include:
Clozaril Tablets 2319

Cyclophosphamide (Potential for unspecified unfavorable interactions).
No products indexed under this heading.

Cyclosporine (Depletion of serum proteins by pegaspargase may increase the toxicity of other drugs which are protein bound). Products include:
Gengraf Capsules 457
Neoral Soft Gelatin Capsules 2380
Neoral Oral Solution 2380
Sandimmune 2388

Dacarbazine (Potential for unspecified unfavorable interactions). Products include:
DTIC-Dome 902

Dalteparin Sodium (Increased risk of bleeding and/or thrombosis). Products include:
Fragmin Injection 2814

Danaparoid Sodium (Increased risk of bleeding and/or thrombosis). Products include:
Orgaran Injection 2480

Daunorubicin Citrate (Potential for unspecified unfavorable interactions). Products include:
DaunoXome Injection 1442

Daunorubicin Hydrochloride (Potential for unspecified unfavorable interactions). Products include:
Cerubidine for Injection 947

Denileukin Diftitox (Potential for unspecified unfavorable interactions).
No products indexed under this heading.

Diazepam (Depletion of serum proteins by pegaspargase may increase the toxicity of other drugs which are protein bound). Products include:
Valium Injectable 3026
Valium Tablets 3047

Diclofenac Potassium (Depletion of serum proteins by pegaspargase may increase the toxicity of other drugs which are protein bound; increased risk of bleeding and/or thrombosis). Products include:
Cataflam Tablets 2315

Diclofenac Sodium (Depletion of serum proteins by pegaspargase may increase the toxicity of other drugs which are protein bound; increased risk of bleeding and/or thrombosis). Products include:
Arthrotec Tablets 3195
Voltaren Ophthalmic Sterile Ophthalmic Solution .... ⊙ 312
Voltaren Tablets 2315
Voltaren-XR Tablets 2315

Dicumarol (Increased risk of bleeding and/or thrombosis).
No products indexed under this heading.

Dipyridamole (Depletion of serum proteins by pegaspargase may increase the toxicity of other drugs which are protein bound). Products include:
Aggrenox Capsules 1026
Persantine Tablets 1057

Docetaxel (Potential for unspecified unfavorable interactions). Products include:
Taxotere for Injection Concentrate 778

Doxorubicin Hydrochloride (Potential for unspecified unfavorable interactions). Products include:
Adriamycin PFS/RDF Injection 2767
Doxil Injection 566

Enoxaparin (Increased risk of bleeding and/or thrombosis). Products include:
Lovenox Injection 746

Epirubicin Hydrochloride (Potential for unspecified unfavorable interactions). Products include:
Ellence Injection 2806

Estramustine Phosphate Sodium (Potential for unspecified unfavorable interactions). Products include:
Emcyt Capsules 2810

Etodolac (Increased risk of bleeding and/or thrombosis). Products include:
Lodine 3528
Lodine XL Extended-Release Tablets 3530

Etoposide (Potential for unspecified unfavorable interactions).
No products indexed under this heading.

Exemestane (Potential for unspecified unfavorable interactions). Products include:
Aromasin Tablets 2769

Fenoprofen Calcium (Depletion of serum proteins by pegaspargase may increase the toxicity of other drugs which are protein bound; increased risk of bleeding and/or thrombosis).
No products indexed under this heading.

Floxuridine (Potential for unspecified unfavorable interactions). Products include:
Sterile FUDR 2974

Fluorouracil (Potential for unspecified unfavorable interactions). Products include:
Carac Cream 1222
Efudex 1733
Fluoroplex 552

Flurazepam Hydrochloride (Depletion of serum proteins by pegaspargase may increase the toxicity of other drugs which are protein bound).
No products indexed under this heading.

Flurbiprofen (Depletion of serum proteins by pegaspargase may increase the toxicity of other drugs which are protein bound; increased risk of bleeding and/or thrombosis).
No products indexed under this heading.

Flutamide (Potential for unspecified unfavorable interactions). Products include:
Eulexin Capsules 3118

Gemcitabine Hydrochloride (Potential for unspecified unfavorable interactions). Products include:
Gemzar for Injection 1919

Glipizide (Depletion of serum proteins by pegaspargase may increase the toxicity of other drugs which are protein bound). Products include:
Glucotrol Tablets 2692
Glucotrol XL Extended Release Tablets 2693

Heparin Sodium (Increased risk of bleeding and/or thrombosis). Products include:
Heparin Lock Flush Solution 3509
Heparin Sodium Injection 3511

Hydroxyurea (Potential for unspecified unfavorable interactions). Products include:
Mylocel Tablets 2227

Ibuprofen (Depletion of serum proteins by pegaspargase may increase the toxicity of other drugs which are protein bound; increased risk of bleeding and/or thrombosis). Products include:
Advil .... ▣771
Children's Advil Oral Suspension .... ▣773
Children's Advil Chewable Tablets .... ▣773
Advil Cold and Sinus Caplets .... ▣771
Advil Cold and Sinus Tablets .... ▣771
Advil Flu & Body Ache Caplets .... ▣772
Infants' Advil Drops .... ▣773
Junior Strength Advil Tablets .... ▣773
Junior Strength Advil Chewable Tablets .... ▣773
Advil Migraine Liquigels .... ▣772
Children's Motrin Oral Suspension and Chewable Tablets 2006
Children's Motrin Cold Oral Suspension 2007
Children's Motrin Oral Suspension .... ▣643
Motrin Suspension, Oral Drops, Chewable Tablets, and Caplets 2002
Infants' Motrin Concentrated Drops 2006
Junior Strength Motrin Caplets and Chewable Tablets 2006
Motrin IB Tablets, Caplets, and Gelcaps 2002
Motrin Migraine Pain Caplets 2005
Motrin Sinus Headache Caplets 2005
Vicoprofen Tablets 520

Idarubicin Hydrochloride (Potential for unspecified unfavorable interactions). Products include:
Idamycin PFS Injection 2825

Ifosfamide (Potential for unspecified unfavorable interactions). Products include:
Ifex for Injection 1123

Imipramine Hydrochloride (Depletion of serum proteins by pegaspargase may increase the toxicity of other drugs which are protein bound).
No products indexed under this heading.

Imipramine Pamoate (Depletion of serum proteins by pegaspargase may increase the toxicity of other drugs which are protein bound).
No products indexed under this heading.

Indomethacin (Depletion of serum proteins by pegaspargase may increase the toxicity of other drugs which are protein bound; increased risk of bleeding and/or thrombosis). Products include:
Indocin 2112

Indomethacin Sodium Trihydrate (Depletion of serum proteins by pegaspargase may increase the toxicity of other drugs which are protein bound; increased risk of bleeding and/or thrombosis). Products include:
Indocin I.V. 2115

Interferon alfa-2A, Recombinant (Potential for unspecified unfavorable interactions). Products include:
Roferon-A Injection 2996

Interferon alfa-2B, Recombinant (Potential for unspecified unfavorable interactions). Products include:
Intron A for Injection 3120
Rebetron Combination Therapy 3153

Irinotecan Hydrochloride (Potential for unspecified unfavorable interactions).
No products indexed under this heading.

Ketoprofen (Depletion of serum proteins by pegaspargase may increase the toxicity of other drugs which are protein bound; increased risk of bleeding and/or thrombosis). Products include:
Orudis Capsules 3548
Orudis KT Tablets .... ▣778
Oruvail Capsules 3548

Ketorolac Tromethamine (Depletion of serum proteins by pegaspargase may increase the toxicity of other drugs which are protein bound; increased risk of bleeding and/or thrombosis). Products include:
Acular Ophthalmic Solution 544
Acular PF Ophthalmic Solution 544
Toradol 3018

Levamisole Hydrochloride (Potential for unspecified unfavorable interactions). Products include:
Ergamisol Tablets 1789

Lomustine (CCNU) (Potential for unspecified unfavorable interactions).
No products indexed under this heading.

Mechlorethamine Hydrochloride (Potential for unspecified unfavorable interactions). Products include:
Mustargen for Injection 2142

Meclofenamate Sodium (Depletion of serum proteins by pegaspargase may increase the toxicity of other drugs which are protein bound; increased risk of bleeding and/or thrombosis).
No products indexed under this heading.

Mefenamic Acid (Depletion of serum proteins by pegaspargase may increase the toxicity of other drugs which are protein bound; increased risk of bleeding and/or thrombosis). Products include:
Ponstel Capsules 1356

Megestrol Acetate (Potential for unspecified unfavorable interactions). Products include:
Megace Oral Suspension 1124

Meloxicam (Increased risk of bleeding and/or thrombosis). Products include:
Mobic Tablets 1054

Melphalan (Potential for unspecified unfavorable interactions). Products include:
Alkeran Tablets 1466

Mercaptopurine (Potential for unspecified unfavorable interactions). Products include:
Purinethol Tablets 1615

Methotrexate Sodium (Pegaspargase inhibits protein synthesis and cell replication and thus interferes with the action of methotrexate which requires cell replication for its lethal effect; potential for unspecified unfavorable interactions).
No products indexed under this heading.

Midazolam Hydrochloride (Depletion of serum proteins by pegaspargase may increase the toxicity of other drugs which are protein bound). Products include:
Versed Injection 3027
Versed Syrup 3033

Mitomycin (Mitomycin-C) (Potential for unspecified unfavorable interactions).
No products indexed under this heading.

Mitotane (Potential for unspecified unfavorable interactions).
No products indexed under this heading.

Mitoxantrone Hydrochloride (Potential for unspecified unfavorable interactions). Products include:
Novantrone for Injection 1760

Nabumetone (Increased risk of bleeding and/or thrombosis). Products include:
Relafen Tablets 1617

Naproxen (Depletion of serum proteins by pegaspargase may increase the toxicity of other drugs which are protein bound; increased risk of bleeding and/or thrombosis). Products include:
EC-Naprosyn Delayed-Release Tablets 2967
Naprosyn Suspension 2967
Naprosyn Tablets 2967

Naproxen Sodium (Depletion of serum proteins by pegaspargase may increase the toxicity of other drugs which are protein bound; increased risk of bleeding and/or thrombosis). Products include:
Aleve Tablets, Caplets and Gelcaps ....▣ 602
Aleve Cold & Sinus Caplets ....▣ 603
Anaprox Tablets 2967
Anaprox DS Tablets 2967
Naprelan Tablets 1293

Nortriptyline Hydrochloride (Depletion of serum proteins by pegaspargase may increase the toxicity of other drugs which are protein bound).
No products indexed under this heading.

Oxaprozin (Depletion of serum proteins by pegaspargase may increase the toxicity of other drugs which are protein bound; increased risk of bleeding and/or thrombosis).
No products indexed under this heading.

Oxazepam (Depletion of serum proteins by pegaspargase may increase the toxicity of other drugs which are protein bound).
No products indexed under this heading.

Paclitaxel (Potential for unspecified unfavorable interactions). Products include:
Taxol Injection 1129

Phenylbutazone (Depletion of serum proteins by pegaspargase may increase the toxicity of other drugs which are protein bound; increased risk of bleeding and/or thrombosis).
No products indexed under this heading.

Piroxicam (Depletion of serum proteins by pegaspargase may increase the toxicity of other drugs which are protein bound; increased risk of bleeding and/or thrombosis). Products include:
Feldene Capsules 2685

Procarbazine Hydrochloride (Potential for unspecified unfavorable interactions). Products include:
Matulane Capsules 3246

Propranolol Hydrochloride (Depletion of serum proteins by pegaspargase may increase the toxicity of other drugs which are protein bound). Products include:
Inderal 3513
Inderal LA Long-Acting Capsules 3516
Inderide Tablets 3517
Inderide LA Long-Acting Capsules .. 3519

Rofecoxib (Increased risk of bleeding and/or thrombosis). Products include:
Vioxx 2213

Streptozocin (Potential for unspecified unfavorable interactions).
No products indexed under this heading.

Sulindac (Depletion of serum proteins by pegaspargase may increase the toxicity of other drugs which are protein bound; increased risk of bleeding and/or thrombosis). Products include:
Clinoril Tablets 2053

Tamoxifen Citrate (Potential for unspecified unfavorable interactions). Products include:
Nolvadex Tablets 678

Temazepam (Depletion of serum proteins by pegaspargase may increase the toxicity of other drugs which are protein bound).
No products indexed under this heading.

Teniposide (Potential for unspecified unfavorable interactions).
No products indexed under this heading.

Thioguanine (Potential for unspecified unfavorable interactions). Products include:
Tabloid Tablets 1642

Thiotepa (Potential for unspecified unfavorable interactions). Products include:
Thioplex for Injection 1765

Tinzaparin sodium (Increased risk of bleeding and/or thrombosis). Products include:
Innohep Injection 1248

Tolbutamide (Depletion of serum proteins by pegaspargase may increase the toxicity of other drugs which are protein bound).
No products indexed under this heading.

Tolmetin Sodium (Depletion of serum proteins by pegaspargase may increase the toxicity of other drugs which are protein bound; increased risk of bleeding and/or thrombosis). Products include:
Tolectin 2589

Topotecan Hydrochloride (Potential for unspecified unfavorable interactions). Products include:
Hycamtin for Injection 1546

Toremifene Citrate (Potential for unspecified unfavorable interactions). Products include:
Fareston Tablets 3237

Trimipramine Maleate (Depletion of serum proteins by pegaspargase may increase the toxicity of other drugs which are protein bound). Products include:
Surmontil Capsules 3595

Valrubicin (Potential for unspecified unfavorable interactions). Products include:
Valstar Sterile Solution for Intravesical Instillation 1175

Vincristine Sulfate (Potential for unspecified unfavorable interactions).
No products indexed under this heading.

Vinorelbine Tartrate (Potential for unspecified unfavorable interactions). Products include:
Navelbine Injection 1604

Warfarin Sodium (Depletion of serum proteins by pegaspargase may increase the toxicity of other drugs which are protein bound; increased risk of bleeding and/or thrombosis). Products include:
Coumadin for Injection 1243
Coumadin Tablets 1243
Warfarin Sodium Tablets, USP 3302

ONE-A-DAY ANTIOXIDANT SOFTGELS

(Vitamins with Minerals) .... ▣ 805
None cited in PDR database.

ONE-A-DAY BEDTIME & REST TABLETS

(Calcium Carbonate, Herbals with Minerals, Kava-Kava, Valeriana officinalis)......................... ▣ 805
May interact with hypnotics and sedatives, tranquilizers, and certain other agents. Compounds in these categories include:

Alprazolam (Kava-Kava and Valerian Root may potentiate the effect of sedatives and tranquilizers). Products include:
Xanax Tablets 2865

Buspirone Hydrochloride (Kava-Kava and Valerian Root may potentiate the effect of sedatives and tranquilizers).
No products indexed under this heading.

Chlordiazepoxide (Kava-Kava and Valerian Root may potentiate the effect of sedatives and tranquilizers). Products include:
Limbitrol 1738

Chlordiazepoxide Hydrochloride (Kava-Kava and Valerian Root may potentiate the effect of sedatives and tranquilizers). Products include:
Librium Capsules 1736
Librium for Injection 1737

Chlorpromazine (Kava-Kava and Valerian Root may potentiate the effect of sedatives and tranquilizers). Products include:
Thorazine Suppositories 1656

Chlorpromazine Hydrochloride (Kava-Kava and Valerian Root may potentiate the effect of sedatives and tranquilizers). Products include:
Thorazine 1656

Chlorprothixene (Kava-Kava and Valerian Root may potentiate the effect of sedatives and tranquilizers).
No products indexed under this heading.

Chlorprothixene Hydrochloride (Kava-Kava and Valerian Root may potentiate the effect of sedatives and tranquilizers).
No products indexed under this heading.

Clorazepate Dipotassium (Kava-Kava and Valerian Root may potentiate the effect of sedatives and tranquilizers). Products include:
Tranxene 511

Diazepam (Kava-Kava and Valerian Root may potentiate the effect of sedatives and tranquilizers). Products include:
Valium Injectable 3026
Valium Tablets 3047

Droperidol (Kava-Kava and Valerian Root may potentiate the effect of sedatives and tranquilizers).
No products indexed under this heading.

Estazolam (Kava-Kava and Valerian Root may potentiate the effect of sedatives and tranquilizers). Products include:
ProSom Tablets 500

Ethchlorvynol (Kava-Kava and Valerian Root may potentiate the effect of sedatives and tranquilizers).
No products indexed under this heading.

Ethinamate (Kava-Kava and Valerian Root may potentiate the effect of sedatives and tranquilizers).
No products indexed under this heading.

Fluphenazine Decanoate (Kava-Kava and Valerian Root may potentiate the effect of sedatives and tranquilizers).
No products indexed under this heading.

Fluphenazine Enanthate (Kava-Kava and Valerian Root may potentiate the effect of sedatives and tranquilizers).
No products indexed under this heading.

Fluphenazine Hydrochloride (Kava-Kava and Valerian Root may potentiate the effect of sedatives and tranquilizers).
No products indexed under this heading.

Flurazepam Hydrochloride (Kava-Kava and Valerian Root may potentiate the effect of sedatives and tranquilizers).
No products indexed under this heading.

Glutethimide (Kava-Kava and Valerian Root may potentiate the effect of sedatives and tranquilizers).
No products indexed under this heading.

Haloperidol (Kava-Kava and Valerian Root may potentiate the effect of sedatives and tranquilizers). Products include:
Haldol Injection, Tablets and Concentrate 2533

Haloperidol Decanoate (Kava-Kava and Valerian Root may potentiate the effect of sedatives and tranquilizers). Products include:
Haldol Decanoate 2535

Hydroxyzine Hydrochloride (Kava-Kava and Valerian Root may potentiate the effect of sedatives and tranquilizers). Products include:
Atarax Tablets & Syrup 2667
Vistaril Intramuscular Solution 2738

Lorazepam (Kava-Kava and Valerian Root may potentiate the effect of sedatives and tranquilizers). Products include:
Ativan Injection 3478
Ativan Tablets 3482

Loxapine Hydrochloride (Kava-Kava and Valerian Root may potentiate the effect of sedatives and tranquilizers).
No products indexed under this heading.

Loxapine Succinate (Kava-Kava and Valerian Root may potentiate the effect of sedatives and tranquilizers). Products include:
Loxitane Capsules 3398

Meprobamate (Kava-Kava and Valerian Root may potentiate the effect of sedatives and tranquilizers). Products include:
Miltown Tablets 3349

Mesoridazine Besylate (Kava-Kava and Valerian Root may potentiate the effect of sedatives and tranquilizers). Products include:
Serentil 1057

Midazolam Hydrochloride (Kava-Kava and Valerian Root may potentiate the effect of sedatives and tranquilizers). Products include:
Versed Injection 3027
Versed Syrup 3033

Molindone Hydrochloride (Kava-Kava and Valerian Root may potentiate the effect of sedatives and tranquilizers). Products include:
Moban 1320

Oxazepam (Kava-Kava and Valerian Root may potentiate the effect of sedatives and tranquilizers).
No products indexed under this heading.

Perphenazine (Kava-Kava and Valerian Root may potentiate the effect of sedatives and tranquilizers). Products include:
Etrafon 3115
Trilafon 3160

Prazepam (Kava-Kava and Valerian Root may potentiate the effect of

sedatives and tranquilizers).
No products indexed under this heading.

Prochlorperazine (Kava-Kava and Valerian Root may potentiate the effect of sedatives and tranquilizers). Products include:
Compazine 1505

Promethazine Hydrochloride (Kava-Kava and Valerian Root may potentiate the effect of sedatives and tranquilizers). Products include:
Mepergan Injection 3539
Phenergan Injection 3553
Phenergan 3556
Phenergan Syrup 3554
Phenergan with Codeine Syrup 3557
Phenergan with Dextromethorphan Syrup 3559
Phenergan VC Syrup 3560
Phenergan VC with Codeine Syrup .. 3561

Propofol (Kava-Kava and Valerian Root may potentiate the effect of sedatives and tranquilizers). Products include:
Diprivan Injectable Emulsion 667

Quazepam (Kava-Kava and Valerian Root may potentiate the effect of sedatives and tranquilizers).
No products indexed under this heading.

Secobarbital Sodium (Kava-Kava and Valerian Root may potentiate the effect of sedatives and tranquilizers).
No products indexed under this heading.

Temazepam (Kava-Kava and Valerian Root may potentiate the effect of sedatives and tranquilizers).
No products indexed under this heading.

Thioridazine Hydrochloride (Kava-Kava and Valerian Root may potentiate the effect of sedatives and tranquilizers). Products include:
Thioridazine Hydrochloride Tablets 2289

Thiothixene (Kava-Kava and Valerian Root may potentiate the effect of sedatives and tranquilizers). Products include:
Navane Capsules 2701
Thiothixene Capsules 2290

Triazolam (Kava-Kava and Valerian Root may potentiate the effect of sedatives and tranquilizers). Products include:
Halcion Tablets 2823

Trifluoperazine Hydrochloride (Kava-Kava and Valerian Root may potentiate the effect of sedatives and tranquilizers). Products include:
Stelazine 1640

Zaleplon (Kava-Kava and Valerian Root may potentiate the effect of sedatives and tranquilizers). Products include:
Sonata Capsules 3591

Zolpidem Tartrate (Kava-Kava and Valerian Root may potentiate the effect of sedatives and tranquilizers). Products include:
Ambien Tablets 3191

Food Interactions

Alcohol (Kava-Kava and Valerian Root may potentiate the effect of alcohol).

ONE-A-DAY CALCIUM PLUS CHEWABLE TABLETS
(Calcium Carbonate, Magnesium Carbonate, Vitamin D) 805
None cited in PDR database.

ONE-A-DAY CHOLESTEROL HEALTH TABLETS
(Allium sativum, Herbals with Vitamins, Vitamin E) 805
None cited in PDR database.

ONE-A-DAY ENERGY FORMULA TABLETS
(Chromium Picolinate, Ginseng, Vitamin B Complex) 806
May interact with:

Antihypertensive agents, unspecified (Concurrent use with medication for high blood pressure requires consultation with a health care professional).

ONE-A-DAY ESSENTIAL TABLETS
(Vitamins with Minerals) 806
None cited in PDR database.

ONE-A-DAY 50 PLUS TABLETS
(Vitamins with Minerals) 804
None cited in PDR database.

ONE-A-DAY GARLIC SOFTGELS
(Garlic Oil) 806
None cited in PDR database.

ONE-A-DAY JOINT HEALTH TABLETS
(Glucosamine Sulfate, Herbals with Vitamins) 806
None cited in PDR database.

ONE-A-DAY KIDS COMPLETE TABLETS
(Vitamins with Minerals) 806
None cited in PDR database.

ONE-A-DAY MAXIMUM TABLETS
(Vitamins with Minerals) 807
None cited in PDR database.

ONE-A-DAY MEMORY & CONCENTRATION TABLETS
(Choline, Ginkgo biloba, Vitamin B_{12}, Vitamin B_6) 807
May interact with oral anticoagulants. Compounds in these categories include:

Dicumarol (Concurrent use with anticoagulants is not recommended).
No products indexed under this heading.

Warfarin Sodium (Concurrent use with anticoagulants is not recommended). Products include:
Coumadin for Injection 1243
Coumadin Tablets 1243
Warfarin Sodium Tablets, USP 3302

ONE-A-DAY MENOPAUSE HEALTH TABLETS
(Black Cohosh, Lecithin, Vitamin E) 808
May interact with:

Antihypertensive agents, unspecified (Concurrent use with medication for high blood pressure requires consultation with a health care professional).

ONE-A-DAY MEN'S TABLETS
(Vitamins with Minerals) 808
None cited in PDR database.

ONE-A-DAY PROSTATE HEALTH SOFTGELS
(Pumpkin, Serenoa repens, Zinc) 808
None cited in PDR database.

ONE-A-DAY TENSION & MOOD SOFTGELS
(Hypericum, Kava-Kava, Vitamin B Complex With Vitamin C) 808
May interact with hypnotics and sedatives, monoamine oxidase inhibitors, tranquilizers, and certain other agents. Compounds in these categories include:

Alprazolam (May increase drowsiness effect). Products include:
Xanax Tablets 2865

Buspirone Hydrochloride (May increase drowsiness effect).
No products indexed under this heading.

Chlordiazepoxide (May increase drowsiness effect). Products include:
Limbitrol 1738

Chlordiazepoxide Hydrochloride (May increase drowsiness effect). Products include:
Librium Capsules 1736
Librium for Injection 1737

Chlorpromazine (May increase drowsiness effect). Products include:
Thorazine Suppositories 1656

Chlorpromazine Hydrochloride (May increase drowsiness effect). Products include:
Thorazine 1656

Chlorprothixene (May increase drowsiness effect).
No products indexed under this heading.

Chlorprothixene Hydrochloride (May increase drowsiness effect).
No products indexed under this heading.

Clorazepate Dipotassium (May increase drowsiness effect). Products include:
Tranxene 511

Diazepam (May increase drowsiness effect). Products include:
Valium Injectable 3026
Valium Tablets 3047

Droperidol (May increase drowsiness effect).
No products indexed under this heading.

Estazolam (May increase drowsiness effect). Products include:
ProSom Tablets 500

Ethchlorvynol (May increase drowsiness effect).
No products indexed under this heading.

Ethinamate (May increase drowsiness effect).
No products indexed under this heading.

Fluphenazine Decanoate (May increase drowsiness effect).
No products indexed under this heading.

Fluphenazine Enanthate (May increase drowsiness effect).
No products indexed under this heading.

Fluphenazine Hydrochloride (May increase drowsiness effect).
No products indexed under this heading.

Flurazepam Hydrochloride (May increase drowsiness effect).
No products indexed under this heading.

Glutethimide (May increase drowsiness effect).
No products indexed under this heading.

Haloperidol (May increase drowsiness effect). Products include:
Haldol Injection, Tablets and Concentrate 2533

Haloperidol Decanoate (May increase drowsiness effect). Products include:
Haldol Decanoate 2535

Hydroxyzine Hydrochloride (May increase drowsiness effect). Products include:
Atarax Tablets & Syrup 2667
Vistaril Intramuscular Solution 2738

Isocarboxazid (Concurrent and/or sequential use with MAO inhibitors is not recommended).
No products indexed under this heading.

Lorazepam (May increase drowsiness effect). Products include:
Ativan Injection 3478
Ativan Tablets 3482

Loxapine Hydrochloride (May increase drowsiness effect).
No products indexed under this heading.

Loxapine Succinate (May increase drowsiness effect). Products include:
Loxitane Capsules 3398

Meprobamate (May increase drowsiness effect). Products include:
Miltown Tablets 3349

Mesoridazine Besylate (May increase drowsiness effect). Products include:
Serentil 1057

Midazolam Hydrochloride (May increase drowsiness effect). Products include:
Versed Injection 3027
Versed Syrup 3033

Moclobemide (Concurrent and/or sequential use with MAO inhibitors is not recommended).
No products indexed under this heading.

Molindone Hydrochloride (May increase drowsiness effect). Products include:
Moban 1320

Oxazepam (May increase drowsiness effect).
No products indexed under this heading.

Pargyline Hydrochloride (Concurrent and/or sequential use with MAO inhibitors is not recommended).
No products indexed under this heading.

Perphenazine (May increase drowsiness effect). Products include:
Etrafon 3115
Trilafon 3160

Phenelzine Sulfate (Concurrent and/or sequential use with MAO inhibitors is not recommended). Products include:
Nardil Tablets 2653

Prazepam (May increase drowsiness effect).
No products indexed under this heading.

Procarbazine Hydrochloride (Concurrent and/or sequential use with MAO inhibitors is not recommended). Products include:
Matulane Capsules 3246

Prochlorperazine (May increase drowsiness effect). Products include:
Compazine 1505

Promethazine Hydrochloride (May increase drowsiness effect). Products include:
Mepergan Injection 3539
Phenergan Injection 3553
Phenergan 3556
Phenergan Syrup 3554
Phenergan with Codeine Syrup 3557
Phenergan with Dextromethorphan Syrup 3559
Phenergan VC Syrup 3560
Phenergan VC with Codeine Syrup . 3561

Propofol (May increase drowsiness effect). Products include:
Diprivan Injectable Emulsion 667

Quazepam (May increase drowsiness effect).
No products indexed under this heading.

Secobarbital Sodium (May increase drowsiness effect).
No products indexed under this heading.

Selegiline Hydrochloride (Concurrent and/or sequential use with MAO inhibitors is not recommended). Products include:
Eldepryl Capsules 3266

Temazepam (May increase drowsiness effect).
No products indexed under this heading.

Thioridazine Hydrochloride (May increase drowsiness effect). Products include:
- Thioridazine Hydrochloride Tablets 2289

Thiothixene (May increase drowsiness effect). Products include:
- Navane Capsules 2701
- Thiothixene Capsules 2290

Tranylcypromine Sulfate (Concurrent and/or sequential use with MAO inhibitors is not recommended). Products include:
- Parnate Tablets 1607

Triazolam (May increase drowsiness effect). Products include:
- Halcion Tablets 2823

Trifluoperazine Hydrochloride (May increase drowsiness effect). Products include:
- Stelazine 1640

Zaleplon (May increase drowsiness effect). Products include:
- Sonata Capsules 3591

Zolpidem Tartrate (May increase drowsiness effect). Products include:
- Ambien Tablets 3191

Food Interactions

Alcohol (May increase drowsiness effect; avoid alcoholic beverages).

ONE-A-DAY WOMEN'S TABLETS

(Vitamins with Minerals) .... ▣ 809

None cited in PDR database.

OPCON-A EYE DROPS

(Naphazoline Hydrochloride, Pheniramine Maleate) .... ⊙ 253

None cited in PDR database.

OPHTHETIC OPHTHALMIC SOLUTION

(Proparacaine Hydrochloride) .... ⊙ 244

None cited in PDR database.

OPTICROM OPHTHALMIC SOLUTION

(Cromolyn Sodium) 555

None cited in PDR database.

OPTIPRANOLOL METIPRANOLOL OPHTHALMIC SOLUTION 0.3%

(Metipranolol) .... ⊙ 263

May interact with adrenergic augmenting psychotropics, beta blockers, calcium channel blockers, cardiac glycosides, and certain other agents. Compounds in these categories include:

Acebutolol Hydrochloride (Co-administration with oral beta blockers may result in additive effects or systemic beta blockade). Products include:
- Sectral Capsules 3589

Amlodipine Besylate (Co-administration with oral or intravenous calcium channel antagonists may result in possible precipitation of left ventricular failure and hypotension). Products include:
- Lotrel Capsules 2370
- Norvasc Tablets 2704

Atenolol (Co-administration with oral beta blockers may result in additive effects or systemic beta blockade). Products include:
- Tenoretic Tablets 690
- Tenormin I.V. Injection 692

Bepridil Hydrochloride (Co-administration with oral or intravenous calcium channel antagonists may result in possible precipitation of left ventricular failure and hypotension). Products include:
- Vascor Tablets 2602

Betaxolol Hydrochloride (Co-administration with oral beta blockers may result in additive effects or systemic beta blockade). Products include:
- Betoptic S Ophthalmic Suspension 537

Bisoprolol Fumarate (Co-administration with oral beta blockers may result in additive effects or systemic beta blockade). Products include:
- Zebeta Tablets 1885
- Ziac Tablets 1887

Carteolol Hydrochloride (Co-administration with oral beta blockers may result in additive effects or systemic beta blockade). Products include:
- Carteolol Hydrochloride Ophthalmic Solution USP, 1% .... ⊙ 258
- Ocupress Ophthalmic Solution, 1% Sterile .... ⊙ 303

Deserpidine (Possible additive effects and production of hypotension and/or bradycardia when beta blocker is concurrently used with catecholamine-depleting drugs).
No products indexed under this heading.

Deslanoside (Concomitant use of beta blockers with digitalis and calcium channel blockers may result in additive effects in prolonging atrioventricular conduction time).
No products indexed under this heading.

Digitoxin (Concomitant use of beta blockers with digitalis and calcium channel blockers may result in additive effects in prolonging atrioventricular conduction time).
No products indexed under this heading.

Digoxin (Concomitant use of beta blockers with digitalis and calcium channel blockers may result in additive effects in prolonging atrioventricular conduction time). Products include:
- Digitek Tablets 1003
- Lanoxicaps Capsules 1574
- Lanoxin Injection 1581
- Lanoxin Tablets 1587
- Lanoxin Elixir Pediatric 1578
- Lanoxin Injection Pediatric 1584

Diltiazem Hydrochloride (Co-administration with oral or intravenous calcium channel antagonists may result in possible precipitation of left ventricular failure and hypotension). Products include:
- Cardizem Injectable 1018
- Cardizem Lyo-Ject Syringe 1018
- Cardizem Monovial 1018
- Cardizem CD Capsules 1016
- Tiazac Capsules 1378

Epinephrine (Concurrent use in patients with history of atopy or severe anaphylactic reaction to allergens may be unresponsive to the usual doses of epinephrine used to treat anaphylactic reaction). Products include:
- Epifrin Sterile Ophthalmic Solution .... ⊙ 235
- EpiPen 1236
- Primatene Mist .... ▣ 779
- Xylocaine with Epinephrine Injection 653

Epinephrine Hydrochloride (Concurrent use in patients with history of atopy or severe anaphylactic reaction to allergens may be unresponsive to the usual doses of epinephrine used to treat anaphylactic reaction).
No products indexed under this heading.

Esmolol Hydrochloride (Co-administration with oral beta blockers may result in additive effects or systemic beta blockade). Products include:
- Brevibloc Injection 858

Felodipine (Co-administration with oral or intravenous calcium channel antagonists may result in possible precipitation of left ventricular failure and hypotension). Products include:
- Lexxel Tablets 608
- Plendil Extended-Release Tablets 623

Isocarboxazid (Exercise caution when used concurrently with adrenergic psychotropic drugs).
No products indexed under this heading.

Isradipine (Co-administration with oral or intravenous calcium channel antagonists may result in possible precipitation of left ventricular failure and hypotension). Products include:
- DynaCirc Capsules 2921
- DynaCirc CR Tablets 2923

Labetalol Hydrochloride (Co-administration with oral beta blockers may result in additive effects or systemic beta blockade). Products include:
- Normodyne Injection 3135
- Normodyne Tablets 3137

Levobunolol Hydrochloride (Co-administration with oral beta blockers may result in additive effects or systemic beta blockade). Products include:
- Betagan .... ⊙ 228

Metoprolol Succinate (Co-administration with oral beta blockers may result in additive effects or systemic beta blockade). Products include:
- Toprol-XL Tablets 651

Metoprolol Tartrate (Co-administration with oral beta blockers may result in additive effects or systemic beta blockade).
No products indexed under this heading.

Mibefradil Dihydrochloride (Co-administration with oral or intravenous calcium channel antagonists may result in possible precipitation of left ventricular failure and hypotension).
No products indexed under this heading.

Nadolol (Co-administration with oral beta blockers may result in additive effects or systemic beta blockade). Products include:
- Corgard Tablets 2245
- Corzide 40/5 Tablets 2247
- Corzide 80/5 Tablets 2247
- Nadolol Tablets 2288

Nicardipine Hydrochloride (Co-administration with oral or intravenous calcium channel antagonists may result in possible precipitation of left ventricular failure and hypotension). Products include:
- Cardene I.V. 3485

Nifedipine (Co-administration with oral or intravenous calcium channel antagonists may result in possible precipitation of left ventricular failure and hypotension). Products include:
- Adalat CC Tablets 877
- Procardia Capsules 2708
- Procardia XL Extended Release Tablets 2710

Nimodipine (Co-administration with oral or intravenous calcium channel antagonists may result in possible precipitation of left ventricular failure and hypotension). Products include:
- Nimotop Capsules 904

Nisoldipine (Co-administration with oral or intravenous calcium channel antagonists may result in possible precipitation of left ventricular failure and hypotension). Products include:
- Sular Tablets 688

Pargyline Hydrochloride (Exercise caution when used concurrently with adrenergic psychotropic drugs).
No products indexed under this heading.

Penbutolol Sulfate (Co-administration with oral beta blockers may result in additive effects or systemic beta blockade).
No products indexed under this heading.

Phenelzine Sulfate (Exercise caution when used concurrently with adrenergic psychotropic drugs). Products include:
- Nardil Tablets 2653

Pindolol (Co-administration with oral beta blockers may result in additive effects or systemic beta blockade).
No products indexed under this heading.

Propranolol Hydrochloride (Co-administration with oral beta blockers may result in additive effects or systemic beta blockade). Products include:
- Inderal 3513
- Inderal LA Long-Acting Capsules 3516
- Inderide Tablets 3517
- Inderide LA Long-Acting Capsules 3519

Rauwolfia serpentina (Possible additive effects and production of hypotension and/or bradycardia when beta blocker is concurrently used with catecholamine-depleting drugs).
No products indexed under this heading.

Rescinnamine (Possible additive effects and production of hypotension and/or bradycardia when beta blocker is concurrently used with catecholamine-depleting drugs).
No products indexed under this heading.

Reserpine (Possible additive effects and production of hypotension and/or bradycardia when beta blocker is concurrently used with catecholamine-depleting drugs).
No products indexed under this heading.

Sotalol Hydrochloride (Co-administration with oral beta blockers may result in additive effects or systemic beta blockade). Products include:
- Betapace Tablets 950
- Betapace AF Tablets 954

Timolol Hemihydrate (Co-administration with oral beta blockers may result in additive effects or systemic beta blockade). Products include:
- Betimol Ophthalmic Solution .... ⊙ 324

Timolol Maleate (Co-administration with oral beta blockers may result in additive effects or systemic beta blockade). Products include:
- Blocadren Tablets 2046
- Cosopt Sterile Ophthalmic Solution 2065
- Timolide Tablets 2187
- Timolol GFS .... ⊙ 266
- Timoptic in Ocudose 2192
- Timoptic Sterile Ophthalmic Solution 2190
- Timoptic-XE Sterile Ophthalmic Gel Forming Solution 2194

Tranylcypromine Sulfate (Exercise caution when used concurrently with adrenergic psychotropic drugs). Products include:
- Parnate Tablets 1607

Verapamil Hydrochloride (Co-administration with oral or intravenous calcium channel antagonists may result in possible precipitation of left ventricular failure and hypotension). Products include:
- Covera-HS Tablets 3199
- Isoptin SR Tablets 467
- Tarka Tablets 508
- Verelan Capsules 3184
- Verelan PM Capsules 3186

OPTIVAR OPHTHALMIC SOLUTION

(Azelastine Hydrochloride) 2273

None cited in PDR database.

ORAMORPH SR TABLETS

(Morphine Sulfate) 3062

May interact with antihistamines, central nervous system depressants, hypnotics and sedatives, psychotropics, and certain other agents. Compounds in these categories include:

Acrivastine (CNS depressant effects are potentiated). Products include:
- Semprex-D Capsules 1172

Alfentanil Hydrochloride (CNS depressant effects are potentiated).
- No products indexed under this heading.

Alprazolam (CNS depressant effects are potentiated). Products include:
- Xanax Tablets 2865

Amitriptyline Hydrochloride (CNS depressant effects are potentiated). Products include:
- Etrafon 3115
- Limbitrol 1738

Amoxapine (CNS depressant effects are potentiated).
- No products indexed under this heading.

Aprobarbital (CNS depressant effects are potentiated).
- No products indexed under this heading.

Astemizole (CNS depressant effects are potentiated).
- No products indexed under this heading.

Azatadine Maleate (CNS depressant effects are potentiated). Products include:
- Rynatan Tablets 3351

Bromodiphenhydramine Hydrochloride (CNS depressant effects are potentiated).
- No products indexed under this heading.

Brompheniramine Maleate (CNS depressant effects are potentiated). Products include:
- Bromfed Capsules (Extended-Release) 2269
- Bromfed-PD Capsules (Extended-Release) 2269
- Comtrex Acute Head Cold & Sinus Pressure Relief Tablets 627
- Dimetapp Elixir 777
- Dimetapp Cold and Fever Suspension 775
- Dimetapp DM Cold & Cough Elixir 775
- Dimetapp Nighttime Flu Liquid 776

Buprenorphine Hydrochloride (CNS depressant effects are potentiated; may alter analgesic effect or may precipitate withdrawal symptoms). Products include:
- Buprenex Injectable 2918

Buspirone Hydrochloride (CNS depressant effects are potentiated).
- No products indexed under this heading.

Butabarbital (CNS depressant effects are potentiated).
- No products indexed under this heading.

Butalbital (CNS depressant effects are potentiated). Products include:
- Phrenilin 578
- Sedapap Tablets 50 mg/650 mg 2225

Butorphanol Tartrate (May alter analgesic effect or may precipitate withdrawal symptoms). Products include:
- Stadol NS Nasal Spray 1108

Cetirizine Hydrochloride (CNS depressant effects are potentiated). Products include:
- Zyrtec 2756
- Zyrtec-D 12 Hour Extended Relief Tablets 2758

Chlordiazepoxide (CNS depressant effects are potentiated). Products include:
- Limbitrol 1738

Chlordiazepoxide Hydrochloride (CNS depressant effects are potentiated). Products include:
- Librium Capsules 1736
- Librium for Injection 1737

Chlorpheniramine Maleate (CNS depressant effects are potentiated). Products include:
- Actifed Cold & Sinus Caplets and Tablets 688
- Alka-Seltzer Plus Liqui-Gels 604
- BC Allergy Sinus Cold Powder 619
- Chlor-Trimeton Allergy Tablets 735
- Chlor-Trimeton Allergy/Decongestant Tablets 736
- Comtrex Flu Therapy & Fever Relief Nighttime Tablets 628
- Comtrex Maximum Strength Multi-Symptom Cold & Cough Relief Tablets and Caplets 626
- Contac Severe Cold and Flu Caplets Maximum Strength 746
- Coricidin 'D' Cold, Flu & Sinus Tablets 737
- Coricidin/Coricidin D 738
- Coricidin HBP Maximum Strength Flu Tablets 738
- Extendryl 1361
- Hycomine Compound Tablets 1317
- Kronofed-A 1341
- PediaCare Cough-Cold Liquid 719
- PediaCare NightRest Cough-Cold Liquid 719
- Robitussin Nighttime Honey Flu Liquid 786
- Ryna 768
- Singlet Caplets 761
- Sinutab Sinus Allergy Medication, Maximum Strength Formula, Tablets & Caplets 707
- Sudafed Cold & Allergy Tablets 708
- TheraFlu Regular Strength Cold & Cough Night Time Hot Liquid 676
- TheraFlu Regular Strength Cold & Sore Throat Night Time Hot Liquid 676
- TheraFlu Maximum Strength Flu & Cough Night Time Hot Liquid 678
- TheraFlu Maximum Strength Flu & Sore Throat Night Time Hot Liquid 677
- TheraFlu Maximum Strength Severe Cold & Congestion Night Time Caplets 678
- TheraFlu Maximum Strength Severe Cold & Congestion Night Time Hot Liquid 678
- Triaminic Cold & Allergy Liquid 681
- Triaminic Cold & Allergy Softchews 683
- Triaminic Cold & Cough Liquid 681
- Triaminic Cold & Cough Softchews 683
- Triaminic Cold & Night Time Cough Liquid 681
- Triaminic Cold, Cough & Fever Liquid 681
- Children's Tylenol Cold Suspension Liquid and Chewable Tablets 2015
- Children's Tylenol Cold Plus Cough Suspension Liquid and Chewable Tablets 2015
- Children's Tylenol Flu Suspension Liquid 2015
- Maximum Strength Tylenol Allergy Sinus Caplets, Gelcaps, and Geltabs 2010
- Multi-Symptom Tylenol Cold Complete Formula Caplets 2010
- Vicks 44M Cough, Cold & Flu Relief Liquid 725
- Pediatric Vicks 44m Cough & Cold Relief 728
- Children's Vicks NyQuil Cold/Cough Relief 726

Chlorpheniramine Polistirex (CNS depressant effects are potentiated). Products include:
- Tussionex Pennkinetic Extended-Release Suspension 1174

Chlorpheniramine Tannate (CNS depressant effects are potentiated). Products include:
- Reformulated Rynatan Pediatric Suspension 3352
- Rynatuss Pediatric Suspension 3353
- Rynatuss Tablets 3353
- Tussi-12 S Suspension 3356
- Tussi-12 Tablets 3356

Chlorpromazine (CNS depressant effects are potentiated). Products include:
- Thorazine Suppositories 1656

Chlorpromazine Hydrochloride (CNS depressant effects are potentiated). Products include:
- Thorazine 1656

Chlorprothixene (CNS depressant effects are potentiated).
- No products indexed under this heading.

Chlorprothixene Hydrochloride (CNS depressant effects are potentiated).
- No products indexed under this heading.

Chlorprothixene Lactate (CNS depressant effects are potentiated).
- No products indexed under this heading.

Clemastine Fumarate (CNS depressant effects are potentiated). Products include:
- Tavist 12 Hour Allergy Tablets 676

Clorazepate Dipotassium (CNS depressant effects are potentiated). Products include:
- Tranxene 511

Clozapine (CNS depressant effects are potentiated). Products include:
- Clozaril Tablets 2319

Codeine Phosphate (CNS depressant effects are potentiated). Products include:
- Phenergan with Codeine Syrup 3557
- Phenergan VC with Codeine Syrup 3561
- Robitussin A-C Syrup 2942
- Robitussin-DAC Syrup 2942
- Ryna-C Liquid 768
- Soma Compound w/Codeine Tablets 3355
- Tussi-Organidin NR Liquid 3350
- Tussi-Organidin-S NR Liquid 3350
- Tylenol with Codeine 2595

Cyproheptadine Hydrochloride (CNS depressant effects are potentiated). Products include:
- Periactin Tablets 2155

Desflurane (CNS depressant effects are potentiated). Products include:
- Suprane Liquid for Inhalation 874

Desipramine Hydrochloride (CNS depressant effects are potentiated). Products include:
- Norpramin Tablets 755

Dexchlorpheniramine Maleate (CNS depressant effects are potentiated).
- No products indexed under this heading.

Dezocine (CNS depressant effects are potentiated).
- No products indexed under this heading.

Diazepam (CNS depressant effects are potentiated). Products include:
- Valium Injectable 3026
- Valium Tablets 3047

Diphenhydramine Citrate (CNS depressant effects are potentiated). Products include:
- Alka-Seltzer PM Effervescent Tablets 605
- Benadryl Allergy & Sinus Fastmelt Tablets 693
- Benadryl Children's Allergy/Cold Fastmelt Tablets 692
- Excedrin PM Tablets, Caplets, and Geltabs 631
- Goody's PM Powder 621

Diphenhydramine Hydrochloride (CNS depressant effects are potentiated). Products include:
- Extra Strength Bayer PM Caplets 611
- Benadryl Allergy Chewables 689
- Benadryl Allergy 691
- Benadryl Allergy Liquid 690
- Benadryl Allergy/Cold Tablets 691
- Benadryl Allergy/Congestion Tablets 692
- Benadryl Allergy & Sinus Liquid 693
- Benadryl Allergy Sinus Headache Caplets & Gelcaps 693
- Benadryl Severe Allergy & Sinus Headache Caplets 694
- Benadryl Dye-Free Allergy Liquid 690
- Benadryl Dye-Free Allergy Liqui-Gels Softgels 690
- Benadryl Itch Relief Stick Extra Strength 695
- Benadryl Cream 695
- Benadryl Gel 695
- Benadryl Spray 696
- Benadryl Parenteral 2617
- Coricidin HBP Night-Time Cold & Flu Tablets 738
- Nytol QuickCaps Caplets 622
- Maximum Strength Nytol QuickGels Softgels 621
- Extra Strength Percogesic Aspirin-Free Coated Caplets 665
- Simply Sleep Caplets 2008
- Sominex Original Formula Tablets 761
- Children's Tylenol Allergy-D Liquid 2014
- Maximum Strength Tylenol Allergy Sinus NightTime Caplets 2010
- Tylenol Severe Allergy Caplets 2010
- Maximum Strength Tylenol Flu NightTime Gelcaps 2011
- Extra Strength Tylenol PM Caplets, Geltabs, and Gelcaps 2012
- Unisom Maximum Strength SleepGels 713

Diphenylpyraline Hydrochloride (CNS depressant effects are potentiated).
- No products indexed under this heading.

Doxepin Hydrochloride (CNS depressant effects are potentiated). Products include:
- Sinequan 2713

Droperidol (CNS depressant effects are potentiated).
- No products indexed under this heading.

Enflurane (CNS depressant effects are potentiated).
- No products indexed under this heading.

Estazolam (CNS depressant effects are potentiated). Products include:
- ProSom Tablets 500

Ethchlorvynol (CNS depressant effects are potentiated).
- No products indexed under this heading.

Ethinamate (CNS depressant effects are potentiated).
- No products indexed under this heading.

Fentanyl (CNS depressant effects are potentiated). Products include:
- Duragesic Transdermal System 1786

Fentanyl Citrate (CNS depressant effects are potentiated). Products include:
- Actiq 1184

Fexofenadine Hydrochloride (CNS depressant effects are potentiated). Products include:
- Allegra 712
- Allegra-D Extended-Release Tablets 714

Fluphenazine Decanoate (CNS depressant effects are potentiated).
- No products indexed under this heading.

Fluphenazine Enanthate (CNS depressant effects are potentiated).
- No products indexed under this heading.

Fluphenazine Hydrochloride (CNS depressant effects are potentiated).
- No products indexed under this heading.

Flurazepam Hydrochloride (CNS depressant effects are potentiated).
- No products indexed under this heading.

Glutethimide (CNS depressant effects are potentiated).
- No products indexed under this heading.

Haloperidol (CNS depressant effects are potentiated). Products include:
- Haldol Injection, Tablets and Concentrate 2533

Haloperidol Decanoate (CNS depressant effects are potentiated). Products include:

Haldol Decanoate 2535

Hydrocodone Bitartrate (CNS depressant effects are potentiated). Products include:
Hycodan 1316
Hycomine Compound Tablets 1317
Hycotuss Expectorant Syrup 1318
Lortab 3319
Lortab Elixir 3317
Maxidone Tablets CIII 3399
Norco 5/325 Tablets CIII 3424
Norco 7.5/325 Tablets CIII 3425
Norco 10/325 Tablets CIII 3427
Norco 10/325 Tablets CIII 3425
Vicodin Tablets 516
Vicodin ES Tablets 517
Vicodin HP Tablets 518
Vicodin Tuss Expectorant 519
Vicoprofen Tablets 520
Zydone Tablets 1330

Hydrocodone Polistirex (CNS depressant effects are potentiated). Products include:
Tussionex Pennkinetic Extended-Release Suspension 1174

Hydromorphone Hydrochloride (CNS depressant effects are potentiated). Products include:
Dilaudid 441
Dilaudid Oral Liquid 445
Dilaudid Powder 441
Dilaudid Rectal Suppositories 441
Dilaudid Tablets 441
Dilaudid Tablets - 8 mg 445
Dilaudid-HP 443

Hydroxyzine Hydrochloride (CNS depressant effects are potentiated). Products include:
Atarax Tablets & Syrup 2667
Vistaril Intramuscular Solution 2738

Imipramine Hydrochloride (CNS depressant effects are potentiated).
No products indexed under this heading.

Imipramine Pamoate (CNS depressant effects are potentiated).
No products indexed under this heading.

Isocarboxazid (CNS depressant effects are potentiated).
No products indexed under this heading.

Isoflurane (CNS depressant effects are potentiated).
No products indexed under this heading.

Ketamine Hydrochloride (CNS depressant effects are potentiated).
No products indexed under this heading.

Levomethadyl Acetate Hydrochloride (CNS depressant effects are potentiated).
No products indexed under this heading.

Levorphanol Tartrate (CNS depressant effects are potentiated). Products include:
Levo-Dromoran 1734
Levorphanol Tartrate Tablets 3059

Lithium Carbonate (CNS depressant effects are potentiated). Products include:
Eskalith 1527
Lithium Carbonate 3061
Lithobid Slow-Release Tablets 3255

Lithium Citrate (CNS depressant effects are potentiated). Products include:
Lithium Citrate Syrup 3061

Loratadine (CNS depressant effects are potentiated). Products include:
Claritin 3100
Claritin-D 12 Hour Extended Release Tablets 3102
Claritin-D 24 Hour Extended Release Tablets 3104

Lorazepam (CNS depressant effects are potentiated). Products include:
Ativan Injection 3478
Ativan Tablets 3482

Loxapine Hydrochloride (CNS depressant effects are potentiated).
No products indexed under this heading.

Loxapine Succinate (CNS depressant effects are potentiated). Products include:
Loxitane Capsules 3398

Maprotiline Hydrochloride (CNS depressant effects are potentiated).
No products indexed under this heading.

Meperidine Hydrochloride (CNS depressant effects are potentiated). Products include:
Demerol 3079
Mepergan Injection 3539

Mephobarbital (CNS depressant effects are potentiated).
No products indexed under this heading.

Meprobamate (CNS depressant effects are potentiated). Products include:
Miltown Tablets 3349

Mesoridazine Besylate (CNS depressant effects are potentiated). Products include:
Serentil 1057

Methadone Hydrochloride (CNS depressant effects are potentiated). Products include:
Dolophine Hydrochloride Tablets 3056

Methdilazine Hydrochloride (CNS depressant effects are potentiated).
No products indexed under this heading.

Methohexital Sodium (CNS depressant effects are potentiated). Products include:
Brevital Sodium for Injection, USP 1815

Methotrimeprazine (CNS depressant effects are potentiated).
No products indexed under this heading.

Methoxyflurane (CNS depressant effects are potentiated).
No products indexed under this heading.

Midazolam Hydrochloride (CNS depressant effects are potentiated). Products include:
Versed Injection 3027
Versed Syrup 3033

Molindone Hydrochloride (CNS depressant effects are potentiated). Products include:
Moban 1320

Nalbuphine Hydrochloride (May alter analgesic effect or may precipitate withdrawal symptoms). Products include:
Nubain Injection 1323

Nortriptyline Hydrochloride (CNS depressant effects are potentiated).
No products indexed under this heading.

Olanzapine (CNS depressant effects are potentiated). Products include:
Zyprexa Tablets 1973
Zyprexa ZYDIS Orally Disintegrating Tablets 1973

Oxazepam (CNS depressant effects are potentiated).
No products indexed under this heading.

Oxycodone Hydrochloride (CNS depressant effects are potentiated). Products include:
OxyContin Tablets 2912
OxyFast Oral Concentrate Solution 2916
OxyIR Capsules 2916
Percocet Tablets 1326
Percodan Tablets 1327
Percolone Tablets 1327
Roxicodone 3067
Tylox Capsules 2597

Pentazocine Hydrochloride (May alter analgesic effect or may precipitate withdrawal symptoms). Products include:
Talacen Caplets 3089
Talwin Nx Tablets 3090

Pentazocine Lactate (May alter analgesic effect or may precipitate withdrawal symptoms).
No products indexed under this heading.

Pentobarbital Sodium (CNS depressant effects are potentiated). Products include:
Nembutal Sodium Solution 485

Perphenazine (CNS depressant effects are potentiated). Products include:
Etrafon 3115
Trilafon 3160

Phenelzine Sulfate (CNS depressant effects are potentiated). Products include:
Nardil Tablets 2653

Phenobarbital (CNS depressant effects are potentiated). Products include:
Arco-Lase Plus Tablets 592
Donnatal 2929
Donnatal Extentabs 2930

Prazepam (CNS depressant effects are potentiated).
No products indexed under this heading.

Prochlorperazine (CNS depressant effects are potentiated). Products include:
Compazine 1505

Promethazine Hydrochloride (CNS depressant effects are potentiated). Products include:
Mepergan Injection 3539
Phenergan Injection 3553
Phenergan 3556
Phenergan Syrup 3554
Phenergan with Codeine Syrup 3557
Phenergan with Dextromethorphan Syrup 3559
Phenergan VC Syrup 3560
Phenergan VC with Codeine Syrup 3561

Propofol (CNS depressant effects are potentiated). Products include:
Diprivan Injectable Emulsion 667

Propoxyphene Hydrochloride (CNS depressant effects are potentiated). Products include:
Darvon Pulvules 1909
Darvon Compound-65 Pulvules 1910

Propoxyphene Napsylate (CNS depressant effects are potentiated). Products include:
Darvon-N/Darvocet-N 1907
Darvon-N Tablets 1912

Protriptyline Hydrochloride (CNS depressant effects are potentiated). Products include:
Vivactil Tablets 2446
Vivactil Tablets 2217

Pyrilamine Maleate (CNS depressant effects are potentiated). Products include:
Maximum Strength Midol Menstrual Caplets and Gelcaps .... ▣612
Maximum Strength Midol PMS Caplets and Gelcaps .... ▣613

Pyrilamine Tannate (CNS depressant effects are potentiated). Products include:
Ryna-12 S Suspension 3351

Quazepam (CNS depressant effects are potentiated).
No products indexed under this heading.

Quetiapine Fumarate (CNS depressant effects are potentiated). Products include:
Seroquel Tablets 684

Remifentanil Hydrochloride (CNS depressant effects are potentiated).
No products indexed under this heading.

Risperidone (CNS depressant effects are potentiated). Products include:
Risperdal 1796

Secobarbital Sodium (CNS depressant effects are potentiated).
No products indexed under this heading.

Sevoflurane (CNS depressant effects are potentiated).
No products indexed under this heading.

Sufentanil Citrate (CNS depressant effects are potentiated).
No products indexed under this heading.

Temazepam (CNS depressant effects are potentiated).
No products indexed under this heading.

Terfenadine (CNS depressant effects are potentiated).
No products indexed under this heading.

Thiamylal Sodium (CNS depressant effects are potentiated).
No products indexed under this heading.

Thioridazine Hydrochloride (CNS depressant effects are potentiated). Products include:
Thioridazine Hydrochloride Tablets 2289

Thiothixene (CNS depressant effects are potentiated). Products include:
Navane Capsules 2701
Thiothixene Capsules 2290

Tranylcypromine Sulfate (CNS depressant effects are potentiated). Products include:
Parnate Tablets 1607

Triazolam (CNS depressant effects are potentiated). Products include:
Halcion Tablets 2823

Trifluoperazine Hydrochloride (CNS depressant effects are potentiated). Products include:
Stelazine 1640

Trimeprazine Tartrate (CNS depressant effects are potentiated).
No products indexed under this heading.

Trimipramine Maleate (CNS depressant effects are potentiated). Products include:
Surmontil Capsules 3595

Tripelennamine Hydrochloride (CNS depressant effects are potentiated).
No products indexed under this heading.

Triprolidine Hydrochloride (CNS depressant effects are potentiated). Products include:
Actifed Cold & Allergy Tablets .... ▣688

Zaleplon (CNS depressant effects are potentiated). Products include:
Sonata Capsules 3591

Ziprasidone Hydrochloride (CNS depressant effects are potentiated). Products include:
Geodon Capsules 2688

Zolpidem Tartrate (CNS depressant effects are potentiated). Products include:
Ambien Tablets 3191

Food Interactions

Alcohol (CNS depressant effects are potentiated).

ORAP TABLETS

(Pimozide) 1407

May interact with central nervous system depressants, macrolide antibiotics, protease inhibitors, drugs that prolong the QT interval, and certain other agents. Compounds in these categories include:

Alfentanil Hydrochloride (Pimozide may be capable of potentiating CNS depressants).
No products indexed under this heading.

Alprazolam (Pimozide may be capable of potentiating CNS depressants). Products include:
Xanax Tablets 2865

Amiodarone Hydrochloride (Coadministration with other drugs

which prolong the QT interval may result in additive effect on the QT interval). Products include:
Cordarone Intravenous 3491
Cordarone Tablets 3487
Pacerone Tablets 3331

Amitriptyline Hydrochloride (Co-administration with other drugs which prolong the QT interval may result in additive effect on the QT interval). Products include:
Etrafon 3115
Limbitrol 1738

Amoxapine (Co-administration with other drugs which prolong the QT interval may result in additive effect on the QT interval).
No products indexed under this heading.

Amphetamine Sulfate (Pimozide should not be used in patients taking drugs that themselves cause motor and phonic tics; such as amphetamine). Products include:
Adderall Tablets 3231
Adderall XR Capsules

Amprenavir (Protease inhibitor drugs are inhibitors of CYP3A and thus could potentially impede pimozide metabolism; co-administration is contraindicated). Products include:
Agenerase Capsules 1454
Agenerase Oral Solution 1459

Aprobarbital (Pimozide may be capable of potentiating CNS depressants).
No products indexed under this heading.

Astemizole (Co-administration with other drugs which prolong the QT interval may result in additive effect on the QT interval).
No products indexed under this heading.

Azithromycin Dihydrate (Macrolide antibiotics are inhibitors of CYP3A and thus could potentially impede pimozide metabolism; ventricular arrhythmias have been rarely associated with the use of macrolide antibiotics in patients with prolonged QT intervals, as might be produced by pimozide; co-administration is contraindicated). Products include:
Zithromax 2743
Zithromax for IV Infusion 2748
Zithromax for Oral Suspension, 300 mg, 600 mg, 900 mg, 1200 mg 2739
Zithromax Tablets, 250 mg 2739

Bretylium Tosylate (Co-administration with other drugs which prolong the QT interval may result in additive effect on the QT interval).
No products indexed under this heading.

Buprenorphine Hydrochloride (Pimozide may be capable of potentiating CNS depressants). Products include:
Buprenex Injectable 2918

Buspirone Hydrochloride (Pimozide may be capable of potentiating CNS depressants).
No products indexed under this heading.

Butabarbital (Pimozide may be capable of potentiating CNS depressants).
No products indexed under this heading.

Butalbital (Pimozide may be capable of potentiating CNS depressants). Products include:
Phrenilin 578
Sedapap Tablets 50 mg/650 mg 2225

Chlordiazepoxide (Pimozide may be capable of potentiating CNS depressants). Products include:
Limbitrol 1738

Chlordiazepoxide Hydrochloride (Pimozide may be capable of potentiating CNS depressants). Products include:
Librium Capsules 1736
Librium for Injection 1737

Chlorpromazine (Co-administration with other drugs which prolong the QT interval may result in additive effect on the QT interval). Products include:
Thorazine Suppositories 1656

Chlorpromazine Hydrochloride (Co-administration with other drugs which prolong the QT interval may result in additive effect on the QT interval). Products include:
Thorazine 1656

Chlorprothixene (Pimozide may be capable of potentiating CNS depressants).
No products indexed under this heading.

Chlorprothixene Hydrochloride (Pimozide may be capable of potentiating CNS depressants).
No products indexed under this heading.

Chlorprothixene Lactate (Pimozide may be capable of potentiating CNS depressants).
No products indexed under this heading.

Clarithromycin (Marcolide antibiotics are inhibitors of CYP3A and thus could potentially impede pimozide metabolism; ventricular arrhythmias have been rarely associated with the use of macrolide antibiotics in patients with prolonged QT intervals, as might be produced by pimozide; two sudden deaths have been reported when clarithromycin was added to ongoing pimozide therapy; co-administration is contraindicated). Products include:
Biaxin/Biaxin XL 403
PREVPAC 3298

Clomipramine Hydrochloride (Co-administration with other drugs which prolong the QT interval may result in additive effect on the QT interval).
No products indexed under this heading.

Clorazepate Dipotassium (Pimozide may be capable of potentiating CNS depressants). Products include:
Tranxene 511

Clozapine (Pimozide may be capable of potentiating CNS depressants). Products include:
Clozaril Tablets 2319

Codeine Phosphate (Pimozide may be capable of potentiating CNS depressants). Products include:
Phenergan with Codeine Syrup 3557
Phenergan VC with Codeine Syrup 3561
Robitussin A-C Syrup 2942
Robitussin-DAC Syrup 2942
Ryna-C Liquid 768
Soma Compound w/Codeine Tablets 3355
Tussi-Organidin NR Liquid 3350
Tussi-Organidin-S NR Liquid 3350
Tylenol with Codeine 2595

Desflurane (Pimozide may be capable of potentiating CNS depressants). Products include:
Suprane Liquid for Inhalation 874

Desipramine Hydrochloride (Co-administration with other drugs which prolong the QT interval may result in additive effect on the QT interval). Products include:
Norpramin Tablets 755

Dextroamphetamine Sulfate (Pimozide should not be used in patients taking drugs that themselves cause motor and phonic tics; such as amphetamine). Products include:
Adderall Tablets 3231
Adderall XR Capsules
Dexedrine 1512
DextroStat Tablets 3236

Dezocine (Pimozide may be capable of potentiating CNS depressants).
No products indexed under this heading.

Diazepam (Pimozide may be capable of potentiating CNS depressants). Products include:
Valium Injectable 3026
Valium Tablets 3047

Dirithromycin (Macrolide antibiotics are inhibitors of CYP3A and thus could potentially impede pimozide metabolism; ventricular arrhythmias have been rarely associated with the use of macrolide antibiotics in patients with prolonged QT intervals, as might be produced by pimozide; co-administration is contraindicated). Products include:
Dynabac Tablets 2269

Disopyramide Phosphate (Co-administration with other drugs which prolong the QT interval may result in additive effect on the QT interval).
No products indexed under this heading.

Dofetilide (Co-administration with other drugs which prolong the QT interval may result in additive effect on the QT interval). Products include:
Tikosyn Capsules 2717

Doxepin Hydrochloride (Co-administration with other drugs which prolong the QT interval may result in additive effect on the QT interval). Products include:
Sinequan 2713

Droperidol (Pimozide may be capable of potentiating CNS depressants).
No products indexed under this heading.

Enflurane (Pimozide may be capable of potentiating CNS depressants).
No products indexed under this heading.

Erythromycin (Macrolide antibiotics are inhibitors of CYP3A and thus could potentially impede pimozide metabolism; ventricular arrhythmias have been rarely associated with the use of macrolide antibiotics in patients with prolonged QT intervals, as might be produced by pimozide; co-administration is contraindicated). Products include:
Emgel 2% Topical Gel 1285
Ery-Tab Tablets 448
Erythromycin Base Filmtab Tablets 454
Erythromycin Delayed-Release Capsules, USP 455
PCE Dispertab Tablets 498

Erythromycin Estolate (Macrolide antibiotics are inhibitors of CYP3A and thus could potentially impede pimozide metabolism; ventricular arrhythmias have been rarely associated with the use of macrolide antibiotics in patients with prolonged QT intervals, as might be produced by pimozide; co-administration is contraindicated).
No products indexed under this heading.

Erythromycin Ethylsuccinate (Macrolide antibiotics are inhibitors of CYP3A and thus could potentially impede pimozide metabolism; ventricular arrhythmias have been rarely associated with the use of macrolide antibiotics in patients with prolonged QT intervals, as might be produced by pimozide; co-administration is contraindicated). Products include:
E.E.S. 450
EryPed 446
Pediazole Suspension 3050

Erythromycin Gluceptate (Macrolide antibiotics are inhibitors of CYP3A and thus could potentially impede pimozide metabolism; ventricular arrhythmias have been rarely associated with the use of macrolide antibiotics in patients with prolonged QT intervals, as might be produced by pimozide; co-administration is contraindicated).
No products indexed under this heading.

Erythromycin Stearate (Macrolide antibiotics are inhibitors of CYP3A and thus could potentially impede pimozide metabolism; ventricular arrhythmias have been rarely associated with the use of macrolide antibiotics in patients with prolonged QT intervals, as might be produced by pimozide; co-administration is contraindicated). Products include:
Erythrocin Stearate Filmtab Tablets 452

Estazolam (Pimozide may be capable of potentiating CNS depressants). Products include:
ProSom Tablets 500

Ethchlorvynol (Pimozide may be capable of potentiating CNS depressants).
No products indexed under this heading.

Ethinamate (Pimozide may be capable of potentiating CNS depressants).
No products indexed under this heading.

Fentanyl (Pimozide may be capable of potentiating CNS depressants). Products include:
Duragesic Transdermal System 1786

Fentanyl Citrate (Pimozide may be capable of potentiating CNS depressants). Products include:
Actiq 1184

Flecainide Acetate (Co-administration with other drugs which prolong the QT interval may result in additive effect on the QT interval). Products include:
Tambocor Tablets 1990

Fluoxetine Hydrochloride (Co-administration has resulted in a single case report of possible additive effects of pimozide and fluoxetine leading to bradycardia). Products include:
Prozac Pulvules, Liquid, and Weekly Capsules 1238
Sarafem Pulvules 1962

Fluphenazine Decanoate (Co-administration with other drugs which prolong the QT interval may result in additive effect on the QT interval).
No products indexed under this heading.

Fluphenazine Enanthate (Co-administration with other drugs which prolong the QT interval may result in additive effect on the QT interval).
No products indexed under this heading.

Fluphenazine Hydrochloride (Co-administration with other drugs which prolong the QT interval may result in additive effect on the QT interval).
No products indexed under this heading.

Flurazepam Hydrochloride (Pimozide may be capable of potentiating CNS depressants).
No products indexed under this heading.

Glutethimide (Pimozide may be capable of potentiating CNS depressants).
No products indexed under this heading.

Haloperidol (Pimozide may be capable of potentiating CNS depressants). Products include:
Haldol Injection, Tablets and Concentrate 2533

Haloperidol Decanoate (Pimozide may be capable of potentiating CNS depressants). Products include:
Haldol Decanoate 2535

Hydrocodone Bitartrate (Pimozide may be capable of potentiating CNS depressants). Products include:
Hycodan 1316
Hycomine Compound Tablets 1317
Hycotuss Expectorant Syrup 1318
Lortab 3319
Lortab Elixir 3317
Maxidone Tablets CIII 3399
Norco 5/325 Tablets CIII 3424
Norco 7.5/325 Tablets CIII 3425
Norco 10/325 Tablets CIII 3427
Norco 10/325 Tablets CIII 3425
Vicodin Tablets 516
Vicodin ES Tablets 517
Vicodin HP Tablets 518
Vicodin Tuss Expectorant 519
Vicoprofen Tablets 520
Zydone Tablets 1330

Hydrocodone Polistirex (Pimozide may be capable of potentiating CNS depressants). Products include:
Tussionex Pennkinetic Extended-Release Suspension 1174

Hydromorphone Hydrochloride (Pimozide may be capable of potentiating CNS depressants). Products include:
Dilaudid 441
Dilaudid Oral Liquid 445
Dilaudid Powder 441
Dilaudid Rectal Suppositories 441
Dilaudid Tablets 441
Dilaudid Tablets - 8 mg 445
Dilaudid-HP 443

Hydroxyzine Hydrochloride (Pimozide may be capable of potentiating CNS depressants). Products include:
Atarax Tablets & Syrup 2667
Vistaril Intramuscular Solution 2738

Imipramine Hydrochloride (Co-administration with other drugs which prolong the QT interval may result in additive effect on the QT interval).
No products indexed under this heading.

Imipramine Pamoate (Co-administration with other drugs which prolong the QT interval may result in additive effect on the QT interval).
No products indexed under this heading.

Indinavir Sulfate (Protease inhibitor drugs are inhibitors of CYP3A and thus could potentially impede pimozide metabolism; co-administration is contraindicated). Products include:
Crixivan Capsules 2070

Isoflurane (Pimozide may be capable of potentiating CNS depressants).
No products indexed under this heading.

Itraconazole (Azole antifungals are inhibitors of CYP3A and thus could potentially impede pimozide metabolism; co-administration is contraindicated). Products include:
Sporanox Capsules 1800
Sporanox Injection 1804
Sporanox Injection 2509
Sporanox Oral Solution 1808
Sporanox Oral Solution 2512

Ketamine Hydrochloride (Pimozide may be capable of potentiating CNS depressants).
No products indexed under this heading.

Ketoconazole (Azole antifungals are inhibitors of CYP3A and thus could potentially impede pimozide metabolism; co-administration is contraindicated). Products include:
Nizoral 2% Cream 3620
Nizoral A-D Shampoo 2008
Nizoral 2% Shampoo 2007
Nizoral Tablets 1791

Levomethadyl Acetate Hydrochloride (Pimozide may be capable of potentiating CNS depressants).
No products indexed under this heading.

Levorphanol Tartrate (Pimozide may be capable of potentiating CNS depressants). Products include:
Levo-Dromoran 1734
Levorphanol Tartrate Tablets 3059

Lidocaine Hydrochloride (Co-administration with other drugs which prolong the QT interval may result in additive effect on the QT interval). Products include:
Bactine First Aid Liquid .... ▣611
Xylocaine Injections 653

Lopinavir (Protease inhibitor drugs are inhibitors of CYP3A and thus could potentially impede pimozide metabolism; co-administration is contraindicated). Products include:
Kaletra Capsules 471
Kaletra Oral Solution 471

Lorazepam (Pimozide may be capable of potentiating CNS depressants). Products include:
Ativan Injection 3478
Ativan Tablets 3482

Loxapine Hydrochloride (Pimozide may be capable of potentiating CNS depressants).
No products indexed under this heading.

Loxapine Succinate (Pimozide may be capable of potentiating CNS depressants). Products include:
Loxitane Capsules 3398

Maprotiline Hydrochloride (Co-administration with other drugs which prolong the QT interval may result in additive effect on the QT interval).
No products indexed under this heading.

Meperidine Hydrochloride (Pimozide may be capable of potentiating CNS depressants). Products include:
Demerol 3079
Mepergan Injection 3539

Mephobarbital (Pimozide may be capable of potentiating CNS depressants).
No products indexed under this heading.

Meprobamate (Pimozide may be capable of potentiating CNS depressants). Products include:
Miltown Tablets 3349

Mesoridazine Besylate (Co-administration with other drugs which prolong the QT interval may result in additive effect on the QT interval). Products include:
Serentil 1057

Methadone Hydrochloride (Pimozide may be capable of potentiating CNS depressants). Products include:
Dolophine Hydrochloride Tablets 3056

Methamphetamine Hydrochloride (Pimozide should not be used in patients taking drugs that themselves cause motor and phonic tics; such as amphetamine). Products include:
Desoxyn Tablets 440

Methohexital Sodium (Pimozide may be capable of potentiating CNS depressants). Products include:
Brevital Sodium for Injection, USP .. 1815

Methotrimeprazine (Pimozide may be capable of potentiating CNS depressants).
No products indexed under this heading.

Methoxyflurane (Pimozide may be capable of potentiating CNS depressants).
No products indexed under this heading.

Methylphenidate Hydrochloride (Pimozide should not be used in patients taking drugs that themselves cause motor and phonic tics; such as methylphenidate). Products include:
Concerta Extended-Release Tablets 1998
Concerta Tablets 561
Metadate CD Capsules 1164
Metadate ER Tablets 1167
Methylin Tablets 1995
Methylin ER Tablets 1995
Ritalin 2387

Mexiletine Hydrochloride (Co-administration with other drugs which prolong the QT interval may result in additive effect on the QT interval). Products include:
Mexitil Capsules 1047

Midazolam Hydrochloride (Pimozide may be capable of potentiating CNS depressants). Products include:
Versed Injection 3027
Versed Syrup 3033

Molindone Hydrochloride (Pimozide may be capable of potentiating CNS depressants). Products include:
Moban 1320

Morphine Sulfate (Pimozide may be capable of potentiating CNS depressants). Products include:
Astramorph/PF Injection, USP (Preservative-Free) 594
Duramorph Injection 1312
Infumorph 200 and Infumorph 500 Sterile Solutions 1314
Kadian Capsules 1335
MS Contin Tablets 2896
MSIR 2898
Oramorph SR Tablets 3062
Roxanol 3066

Nefazodone Hydrochloride (Pimozide is metabolized by CYP3A; co-administration with potent inhibitors of this enzyme system, such as nefazodone, could potentially impede pimozide metabolism; concurrent use is contraindicated). Products include:
Serzone Tablets 1104

Nelfinavir Mesylate (Protease inhibitor drugs are inhibitors of CYP3A and thus could potentially impede pimozide metabolism; co-administration is contraindicated). Products include:
Viracept 532

Nortriptyline Hydrochloride (Co-administration with other drugs which prolong the QT interval may result in additive effect on the QT interval).
No products indexed under this heading.

Olanzapine (Pimozide may be capable of potentiating CNS depressants). Products include:
Zyprexa Tablets 1973
Zyprexa ZYDIS Orally Disintegrating Tablets 1973

Oxazepam (Pimozide may be capable of potentiating CNS depressants).
No products indexed under this heading.

Oxycodone Hydrochloride (Pimozide may be capable of potentiating CNS depressants). Products include:
OxyContin Tablets 2912
OxyFast Oral Concentrate Solution . 2916
OxyIR Capsules 2916
Percocet Tablets 1326
Percodan Tablets 1327
Percolone Tablets 1327
Roxicodone 3067
Tylox Capsules 2597

Pemoline (Pimozide should not be used in patients taking drugs that themselves cause motor and phonic tics; such as pemoline). Products include:
Cylert Tablets 415

Pentobarbital Sodium (Pimozide may be capable of potentiating CNS depressants). Products include:
Nembutal Sodium Solution 485

Perphenazine (Co-administration with other drugs which prolong the QT interval may result in additive effect on the QT interval). Products include:
Etrafon 3115
Trilafon 3160

Phenobarbital (Pimozide may be capable of potentiating CNS depressants). Products include:
Arco-Lase Plus Tablets 592
Donnatal 2929
Donnatal Extentabs 2930

Prazepam (Pimozide may be capable of potentiating CNS depressants).
No products indexed under this heading.

Procainamide Hydrochloride (Co-administration with other drugs which prolong the QT interval may result in additive effect on the QT interval). Products include:
Procanbid Extended-Release Tablets 2262

Prochlorperazine (Co-administration with other drugs which prolong the QT interval may result in additive effect on the QT interval). Products include:
Compazine 1505

Promethazine Hydrochloride (Co-administration with other drugs which prolong the QT interval may result in additive effect on the QT interval). Products include:
Mepergan Injection 3539
Phenergan Injection 3553
Phenergan 3556
Phenergan Syrup 3554
Phenergan with Codeine Syrup 3557
Phenergan with Dextromethorphan Syrup 3559
Phenergan VC Syrup 3560
Phenergan VC with Codeine Syrup .. 3561

Propafenone Hydrochloride (Co-administration with other drugs which prolong the QT interval may result in additive effect on the QT interval). Products include:
Rythmol Tablets – 150 mg, 225 mg, 300 mg 502

Propofol (Pimozide may be capable of potentiating CNS depressants). Products include:
Diprivan Injectable Emulsion 667

Propoxyphene Hydrochloride (Pimozide may be capable of potentiating CNS depressants). Products include:
Darvon Pulvules 1909
Darvon Compound-65 Pulvules 1910

Propoxyphene Napsylate (Pimozide may be capable of potentiating CNS depressants). Products include:
Darvon-N/Darvocet-N 1907
Darvon-N Tablets 1912

Protriptyline Hydrochloride (Co-administration with other drugs which prolong the QT interval may result in additive effect on the QT interval). Products include:
Vivactil Tablets 2446
Vivactil Tablets 2217

Quazepam (Pimozide may be capable of potentiating CNS depressants).
No products indexed under this heading.

Quetiapine Fumarate (Pimozide may be capable of potentiating CNS depressants). Products include:
Seroquel Tablets 684

Quinidine Gluconate (Co-administration with other drugs which prolong the QT interval may result in additive effect on the QT interval). Products include:
Quinaglute Dura-Tabs Tablets 978

Quinidine Polygalacturonate (Co-administration with other drugs which prolong the QT interval may result in additive effect on the QT

interval).
No products indexed under this heading.

Quinidine Sulfate (Co-administration with other drugs which prolong the QT interval may result in additive effect on the QT interval). Products include:
Quinidex Extentabs 2933

Remifentanil Hydrochloride (Pimozide may be capable of potentiating CNS depressants).
No products indexed under this heading.

Risperidone (Pimozide may be capable of potentiating CNS depressants). Products include:
Risperdal 1796

Ritonavir (Protease inhibitor drugs are inhibitors of CYP3A and thus could potentially impede pimozide metabolism; co-administration is contraindicated). Products include:
Kaletra Capsules 471
Kaletra Oral Solution 471
Norvir Capsules 487
Norvir Oral Solution 487

Saquinavir (Protease inhibitor drugs are inhibitors of CYP3A and thus could potentially impede pimozide metabolism; co-administration is contraindicated). Products include:
Fortovase Capsules 2970

Saquinavir Mesylate (Protease inhibitor drugs are inhibitors of CYP3A and thus could potentially impede pimozide metabolism; co-administration is contraindicated). Products include:
Invirase Capsules 2979

Secobarbital Sodium (Pimozide may be capable of potentiating CNS depressants).
No products indexed under this heading.

Sevoflurane (Pimozide may be capable of potentiating CNS depressants).
No products indexed under this heading.

Sufentanil Citrate (Pimozide may be capable of potentiating CNS depressants).
No products indexed under this heading.

Temazepam (Pimozide may be capable of potentiating CNS depressants).
No products indexed under this heading.

Terfenadine (Co-administration with other drugs which prolong the QT interval may result in additive effect on the QT interval).
No products indexed under this heading.

Thiamylal Sodium (Pimozide may be capable of potentiating CNS depressants).
No products indexed under this heading.

Thioridazine Hydrochloride (Co-administration with other drugs which prolong the QT interval may result in additive effect on the QT interval). Products include:
Thioridazine Hydrochloride Tablets 2289

Thiothixene (Pimozide may be capable of potentiating CNS depressants). Products include:
Navane Capsules 2701
Thiothixene Capsules 2290

Tocainide Hydrochloride (Co-administration with other drugs which prolong the QT interval may result in additive effect on the QT interval). Products include:
Tonocard Tablets 649

Triazolam (Pimozide may be capable of potentiating CNS depressants). Products include:
Halcion Tablets 2823

Trifluoperazine Hydrochloride (Co-administration with other drugs which prolong the QT interval may result in additive effect on the QT interval). Products include:
Stelazine 1640

Trimipramine Maleate (Co-administration with other drugs which prolong the QT interval may result in additive effect on the QT interval). Products include:
Surmontil Capsules 3595

Troleandomycin (Macrolide antibiotics are inhibitors of CYP3A and thus could potentially impede pimozide metabolism; ventricular arrhythmias have been rarely associated with the use of macrolide antibiotics in patients with prolonged QT intervals, as might be produced by pimozide; co-administration is contraindicated). Products include:
Tao Capsules 2716

Zaleplon (Pimozide may be capable of potentiating CNS depressants). Products include:
Sonata Capsules 3591

Zileuton (Pimozide is metabolized by CYP3A; co-administration with inhibitors of this enzyme system, such as zileuton, could potentially impede pimozide metabolism; concurrent use should be avoided). Products include:
Zyflo Filmtab Tablets 524

Ziprasidone Hydrochloride (Co-administration with other drugs which prolong the QT interval may result in additive effect on the QT interval). Products include:
Geodon Capsules 2688

Zolpidem Tartrate (Pimozide may be capable of potentiating CNS depressants). Products include:
Ambien Tablets 3191

Food Interactions

Alcohol (Pimozide may be capable of potentiating CNS depressants, including alcohol).

ORGANIDIN NR LIQUID

(Guaifenesin) 3350
See Tussi-Organidin DM NR Liquid

ORGANIDIN NR TABLETS

(Guaifenesin) 3350
None cited in PDR database.

ORGARAN INJECTION

(Danaparoid Sodium) 2480
May interact with anticoagulants, non-steroidal anti-inflammatory agents, salicylates, and certain other agents. Compounds in these categories include:

Ardeparin Sodium (Co-administration of danaparoid during neuraxial anesthesia with other drugs affecting hemostasis, such as anticoagulants, may increase the risk of developing an epidural or spinal hematoma which can result in long-term or permanent paralysis; concurrent use in other situations may induce or augment bleeding).
No products indexed under this heading.

Aspirin (Co-administration of danaparoid during neuraxial anesthesia with other drugs affecting hemostasis, such as salicylates, may increase the risk of developing an epidural or spinal hematoma which can result in long-term or permanent paralysis; concurrent use in other situations may induce or augment bleeding). Products include:
Aggrenox Capsules 1026
Alka-Seltzer .... ■603
Alka-Seltzer Lemon Lime Antacid and Pain Reliever Effervescent Tablets .... ■603
Alka-Seltzer Extra Strength Antacid and Pain Reliever Effervescent Tablets .... ■603
Alka-Seltzer PM Effervescent Tablets .... ■605
Genuine Bayer Tablets, Caplets and Gelcaps .... ■606
Extra Strength Bayer Caplets and Gelcaps .... ■610
Aspirin Regimen Bayer Children's Chewable Tablets (Orange or Cherry Flavored) .... ■607
Bayer, Aspirin Regimen .... ■606
Aspirin Regimen Bayer 81 mg Caplets with Calcium .... ■607
Genuine Bayer Professional Labeling (Aspirin Regimen Bayer) .... ■608
Extra Strength Bayer Arthritis Caplets .... ■610
Extra Strength Bayer Plus Caplets .... ■610
Extra Strength Bayer PM Caplets .. ■611
BC Powder .... ■619
BC Allergy Sinus Cold Powder .... ■619
Arthritis Strength BC Powder .... ■619
BC Sinus Cold Powder .... ■619
Darvon Compound-65 Pulvules 1910
Ecotrin Enteric Coated Aspirin Low, Regular and Maximum Strength Tablets 1715
Excedrin Extra-Strength Tablets, Caplets, and Geltabs .... ■629
Excedrin Migraine 1070
Goody's Body Pain Formula Powder .... ■620
Goody's Extra Strength Headache Powder .... ■620
Goody's Extra Strength Pain Relief Tablets .... ■620
Percodan Tablets 1327
Robaxisal Tablets 2939
Soma Compound Tablets 3354
Soma Compound w/Codeine Tablets 3355
Vanquish Caplets .... ■617

Celecoxib (Co-administration of danaparoid during neuraxial anesthesia with other drugs affecting hemostasis, such as non-steroidal anti-inflammatory agents, may increase the risk of developing an epidural or spinal hematoma which can result in long-term or permanent paralysis; concurrent use in other situations may induce or augment bleeding). Products include:
Celebrex Capsules 2676
Celebrex Capsules 2780

Choline Magnesium Trisalicylate (Co-administration of danaparoid during neuraxial anesthesia with other drugs affecting hemostasis, such as salicylates, may increase the risk of developing an epidural or spinal hematoma which can result in long-term or permanent paralysis; concurrent use in other situations may induce or augment bleeding). Products include:
Trilisate 2901

Clopidogrel Bisulfate (Co-administration of danaparoid during neuraxial anesthesia with other drugs affecting hemostasis, such as platelet inhibitors, may increase the risk of developing an epidural or spinal hematoma which can result in long-term or permanent paralysis; concurrent use in other situations may induce or augment bleeding). Products include:
Plavix Tablets 1097
Plavix Tablets 3084

Dalteparin Sodium (Co-administration of danaparoid during neuraxial anesthesia with other drugs affecting hemostasis, such as anticoagulants, may increase the risk of developing an epidural or spinal hematoma which can result in long-term or permanent paralysis; concurrent use in other situations may induce or augment bleeding). Products include:
Fragmin Injection 2814

Diclofenac Potassium (Co-administration of danaparoid during neuraxial anesthesia with other drugs affecting hemostasis, such as non-steroidal anti-inflammatory agents, may increase the risk of developing an epidural or spinal hematoma which can result in long-term or permanent paralysis; concurrent use in other situations may induce or augment bleeding). Products include:
Cataflam Tablets 2315

Diclofenac Sodium (Co-administration of danaparoid during neuraxial anesthesia with other drugs affecting hemostasis, such as non-steroidal anti-inflammatory agents, may increase the risk of developing an epidural or spinal hematoma which can result in long-term or permanent paralysis; concurrent use in other situations may induce or augment bleeding). Products include:
Arthrotec Tablets 3195
Voltaren Ophthalmic Sterile Ophthalmic Solution .... ⊙312
Voltaren Tablets 2315
Voltaren-XR Tablets 2315

Dicumarol (Co-administration of danaparoid during neuraxial anesthesia with other drugs affecting hemostasis, such as anticoagulants, may increase the risk of developing an epidural or spinal hematoma which can result in long-term or permanent paralysis; concurrent use in other situations may induce or augment bleeding).
No products indexed under this heading.

Diflunisal (Co-administration of danaparoid during neuraxial anesthesia with other drugs affecting hemostasis, such as salicylates, may increase the risk of developing an epidural or spinal hematoma which can result in long-term or permanent paralysis; concurrent use in other situations may induce or augment bleeding). Products include:
Dolobid Tablets 2088

Dipyridamole (Co-administration of danaparoid during neuraxial anesthesia with other drugs affecting hemostasis, such as platelet inhibitors, may increase the risk of developing an epidural or spinal hematoma which can result in long-term or permanent paralysis; concurrent use in other situations may induce or augment bleeding). Products include:
Aggrenox Capsules 1026
Persantine Tablets 1057

Enoxaparin (Co-administration of danaparoid during neuraxial anesthesia with other drugs affecting hemostasis, such as anticoagulants, may increase the risk of developing an epidural or spinal hematoma which can result in long-term or permanent paralysis; concurrent use in other situations may induce or augment bleeding). Products include:
Lovenox Injection 746

Etodolac (Co-administration of danaparoid during neuraxial anesthesia with other drugs affecting hemostasis, such as non-steroidal anti-inflammatory agents, may increase the risk of developing an epidural or spinal hematoma which can result in long-term or permanent paralysis; concurrent use in other situations may induce or augment bleeding). Products include:
Lodine 3528
Lodine XL Extended-Release Tablets 3530

Fenoprofen Calcium (Co-administration of danaparoid during neuraxial anesthesia with other drugs affecting hemostasis, such as non-steroidal anti-inflammatory agents, may increase the risk of developing an epidural or spinal hematoma which can result in long-term or permanent paralysis; concurrent use in other situations may

induce or augment bleeding).
No products indexed under this heading.

Flurbiprofen (Co-administration of danaparoid during neuraxial anesthesia with other drugs affecting hemostasis, such as non-steroidal anti-inflammatory agents, may increase the risk of developing an epidural or spinal hematoma which can result in long-term or permanent paralysis; concurrent use in other situations may induce or augment bleeding).
No products indexed under this heading.

Heparin Sodium (Co-administration of danaparoid during neuraxial anesthesia with other drugs affecting hemostasis, such as anticoagulants, may increase the risk of developing an epidural or spinal hematoma which can result in long-term or permanent paralysis; concurrent use in other situations may induce or augment bleeding). Products include:
Heparin Lock Flush Solution 3509
Heparin Sodium Injection 3511

Ibuprofen (Co-administration of danaparoid during neuraxial anesthesia with other drugs affecting hemostasis, such as non-steroidal anti-inflammatory agents, may increase the risk of developing an epidural or spinal hematoma which can result in long-term or permanent paralysis; concurrent use in other situations may induce or augment bleeding). Products include:
Advil .... ▣771
Children's Advil Oral Suspension ... ▣773
Children's Advil Chewable Tablets . ▣773
Advil Cold and Sinus Caplets .... ▣771
Advil Cold and Sinus Tablets .... ▣771
Advil Flu & Body Ache Caplets ...... ▣772
Infants' Advil Drops .... ▣773
Junior Strength Advil Tablets .... ▣773
Junior Strength Advil Chewable Tablets .... ▣773
Advil Migraine Liquigels .... ▣772
Children's Motrin Oral Suspension and Chewable Tablets 2006
Children's Motrin Cold Oral Suspension 2007
Children's Motrin Oral Suspension .... ▣643
Motrin Suspension, Oral Drops, Chewable Tablets, and Caplets 2002
Infants' Motrin Concentrated Drops 2006
Junior Strength Motrin Caplets and Chewable Tablets 2006
Motrin IB Tablets, Caplets, and Gelcaps 2002
Motrin Migraine Pain Caplets 2005
Motrin Sinus Headache Caplets 2005
Vicoprofen Tablets 520

Indomethacin (Co-administration of danaparoid during neuraxial anesthesia with other drugs affecting hemostasis, such as non-steroidal anti-inflammatory agents, may increase the risk of developing an epidural or spinal hematoma which can result in long-term or permanent paralysis; concurrent use in other situations may induce or augment bleeding). Products include:
Indocin 2112

Indomethacin Sodium Trihydrate (Co-administration of danaparoid during neuraxial anesthesia with other drugs affecting hemostasis, such as non-steroidal anti-inflammatory agents, may increase the risk of developing an epidural or spinal hematoma which can result in long-term or permanent paralysis; concurrent use in other situations may induce or augment bleeding). Products include:
Indocin I.V. 2115

Ketoprofen (Co-administration of danaparoid during neuraxial anesthesia with other drugs affecting hemostasis, such as non-steroidal anti-inflammatory agents, may increase the risk of developing an epidural or spinal hematoma which can result in long-term or permanent paralysis; concurrent use in other situations may induce or augment bleeding).
Products include:
Orudis Capsules 3548
Orudis KT Tablets .... ▣778
Oruvail Capsules 3548

Ketorolac Tromethamine (Co-administration of danaparoid during neuraxial anesthesia with other drugs affecting hemostasis, such as non-steroidal anti-inflammatory agents, may increase the risk of developing an epidural or spinal hematoma which can result in long-term or permanent paralysis; concurrent use in other situations may induce or augment bleeding).
Products include:
Acular Ophthalmic Solution 544
Acular PF Ophthalmic Solution 544
Toradol 3018

Magnesium Salicylate (Co-administration of danaparoid during neuraxial anesthesia with other drugs affecting hemostasis, such as salicylates, may increase the risk of developing an epidural or spinal hematoma which can result in long-term or permanent paralysis; concurrent use in other situations may induce or augment bleeding).
Products include:
Momentum Backache Relief Extra Strength Caplets .... ▣666

Meclofenamate Sodium (Co-administration of danaparoid during neuraxial anesthesia with other drugs affecting hemostasis, such as non-steroidal anti-inflammatory agents, may increase the risk of developing an epidural or spinal hematoma which can result in long-term or permanent paralysis; concurrent use in other situations may induce or augment bleeding).
No products indexed under this heading.

Mefenamic Acid (Co-administration of danaparoid during neuraxial anesthesia with other drugs affecting hemostasis, such as non-steroidal anti-inflammatory agents, may increase the risk of developing an epidural or spinal hematoma which can result in long-term or permanent paralysis; concurrent use in other situations may induce or augment bleeding).
Products include:
Ponstel Capsules 1356

Meloxicam (Co-administration of danaparoid during neuraxial anesthesia with other drugs affecting hemostasis, such as non-steroidal anti-inflammatory agents, may increase the risk of developing an epidural or spinal hematoma which can result in long-term or permanent paralysis; concurrent use in other situations may induce or augment bleeding).
Products include:
Mobic Tablets 1054

Nabumetone (Co-administration of danaparoid during neuraxial anesthesia with other drugs affecting hemostasis, such as non-steroidal anti-inflammatory agents, may increase the risk of developing an epidural or spinal hematoma which can result in long-term or permanent paralysis; concurrent use in other situations may induce or augment bleeding).
Products include:
Relafen Tablets 1617

Naproxen (Co-administration of danaparoid during neuraxial anesthesia with other drugs affecting hemostasis, such as non-steroidal anti-inflammatory agents, may increase the risk of developing an epidural or spinal hematoma which can result in long-term or permanent paralysis; concurrent use in other situations may induce or augment bleeding).
Products include:
EC-Naprosyn Delayed-Release Tablets 2967
Naprosyn Suspension 2967
Naprosyn Tablets 2967

Naproxen Sodium (Co-administration of danaparoid during neuraxial anesthesia with other drugs affecting hemostasis, such as non-steroidal anti-inflammatory agents, may increase the risk of developing an epidural or spinal hematoma which can result in long-term or permanent paralysis; concurrent use in other situations may induce or augment bleeding).
Products include:
Aleve Tablets, Caplets and Gelcaps .... ▣602
Aleve Cold & Sinus Caplets .... ▣603
Anaprox Tablets 2967
Anaprox DS Tablets 2967
Naprelan Tablets 1293

Oxaprozin (Co-administration of danaparoid during neuraxial anesthesia with other drugs affecting hemostasis, such as non-steroidal anti-inflammatory agents, may increase the risk of developing an epidural or spinal hematoma which can result in long-term or permanent paralysis; concurrent use in other situations may induce or augment bleeding).
No products indexed under this heading.

Phenylbutazone (Co-administration of danaparoid during neuraxial anesthesia with other drugs affecting hemostasis, such as non-steroidal anti-inflammatory agents, may increase the risk of developing an epidural or spinal hematoma which can result in long-term or permanent paralysis; concurrent use in other situations may induce or augment bleeding).
No products indexed under this heading.

Piroxicam (Co-administration of danaparoid during neuraxial anesthesia with other drugs affecting hemostasis, such as non-steroidal anti-inflammatory agents, may increase the risk of developing an epidural or spinal hematoma which can result in long-term or permanent paralysis; concurrent use in other situations may induce or augment bleeding).
Products include:
Feldene Capsules 2685

Rofecoxib (Co-administration of danaparoid during neuraxial anesthesia with other drugs affecting hemostasis, such as non-steroidal anti-inflammatory agents, may increase the risk of developing an epidural or spinal hematoma which can result in long-term or permanent paralysis; concurrent use in other situations may induce or augment bleeding).
Products include:
Vioxx 2213

Salsalate (Co-administration of danaparoid during neuraxial anesthesia with other drugs affecting hemostasis, such as salicylates, may increase the risk of developing an epidural or spinal hematoma which can result in long-term or permanent paralysis; concurrent use in other situations may induce or augment bleeding).
No products indexed under this heading.

Sulindac (Co-administration of danaparoid during neuraxial anesthesia with other drugs affecting hemostasis, such as non-steroidal anti-inflammatory agents, may increase the risk of developing an epidural or spinal hematoma which can result in long-term or permanent paralysis; concurrent use in other situations may induce or augment bleeding).
Products include:
Clinoril Tablets 2053

Tinzaparin sodium (Co-administration of danaparoid during neuraxial anesthesia with other drugs affecting hemostasis, such as anticoagulants, may increase the risk of developing an epidural or spinal hematoma which can result in long-term or permanent paralysis; concurrent use in other situations may induce or augment bleeding).
Products include:
Innohep Injection 1248

Tolmetin Sodium (Co-administration of danaparoid during neuraxial anesthesia with other drugs affecting hemostasis, such as non-steroidal anti-inflammatory agents, may increase the risk of developing an epidural or spinal hematoma which can result in long-term or permanent paralysis; concurrent use in other situations may induce or augment bleeding).
Products include:
Tolectin 2589

Warfarin Sodium (Co-administration of danaparoid during neuraxial anesthesia with other drugs affecting hemostasis, such as anticoagulants, may increase the risk of developing an epidural or spinal hematoma which can result in long-term or permanent paralysis; concurrent use in other situations may induce or augment bleeding).
Products include:
Coumadin for Injection 1243
Coumadin Tablets 1243
Warfarin Sodium Tablets, USP 3302

ORTHO DIAPHRAGM KITS -- ALL-FLEX ARCING SPRING; ORTHO COIL SPRING

(Diaphragm) 2552
None cited in PDR database.

ORTHO DIENESTROL CREAM

(Dienestrol) 2554
None cited in PDR database.

ORTHO-CEPT 21 TABLETS

(Desogestrel, Ethinyl Estradiol) 2546
May interact with barbiturates, tetracyclines, and certain other agents. Compounds in these categories include:

Ampicillin (Potential for reduced efficacy and increased incidence of breakthrough bleeding and menstrual irregularities with concomitant use).
No products indexed under this heading.

Ampicillin Sodium (Potential for reduced efficacy and increased incidence of breakthrough bleeding and menstrual irregularities with concomitant use). Products include:
Unasyn for Injection 2728

Aprobarbital (Potential for reduced efficacy and increased incidence of breakthrough bleeding and menstrual irregularities with concomitant use).
No products indexed under this heading.

Butabarbital (Potential for reduced efficacy and increased incidence of breakthrough bleeding and menstrual irregularities with concomitant use).
No products indexed under this heading.

Butalbital (Potential for reduced efficacy and increased incidence of breakthrough bleeding and menstrual irregularities with concomitant use). Products include:
Phrenilin 578
Sedapap Tablets 50 mg/650 mg ... 2225

Carbamazepine (Potential for reduced efficacy and increased inci-

dence of breakthrough bleeding and menstrual irregularities with concomitant use). Products include:

Carbatrol Capsules 3234
Tegretol/Tegretol-XR 2404

Demeclocycline Hydrochloride (Potential for reduced efficacy and increased incidence of breakthrough bleeding and menstrual irregularities with concomitant use). Products include:

Declomycin Tablets 1855

Doxycycline Calcium (Potential for reduced efficacy and increased incidence of breakthrough bleeding and menstrual irregularities with concomitant use). Products include:

Vibramycin Calcium Oral Suspension Syrup 2735

Doxycycline Hyclate (Potential for reduced efficacy and increased incidence of breakthrough bleeding and menstrual irregularities with concomitant use). Products include:

Doryx Coated Pellet Filled Capsules 3357
Periostat Tablets 1208
Vibramycin Hyclate Capsules 2735
Vibramycin Hyclate Intravenous 2737
Vibra-Tabs Film Coated Tablets 2735

Doxycycline Monohydrate (Potential for reduced efficacy and increased incidence of breakthrough bleeding and menstrual irregularities with concomitant use). Products include:

Monodox Capsules 2442
Vibramycin Monohydrate for Oral Suspension 2735

Fosphenytoin Sodium (Potential for reduced efficacy and increased incidence of breakthrough bleeding and menstrual irregularities with concomitant use). Products include:

Cerebyx Injection 2619

Griseofulvin (Potential for reduced efficacy and increased incidence of breakthrough bleeding and menstrual irregularities with concomitant use). Products include:

Grifulvin V Tablets Microsize and Oral Suspension Microsize 2518
Gris-PEG Tablets 2661

Hypericum (Co-administration of hormonal contraceptives and St. John's Wort has resulted in breakthrough bleeding). Products include:

Brite-Life Caplets .... ▣795
Centrum St. John's Wort Softgels .... ▣853
Metabolic Nutrition System .... ▣798
Movana Tablets .... ▣832
One-A-Day Tension & Mood Softgels .... ▣808
ReSource Wellness StayCalm Caplets .... ▣826
Satiete Tablets .... ▣846

Mephobarbital (Potential for reduced efficacy and increased incidence of breakthrough bleeding and menstrual irregularities with concomitant use).

No products indexed under this heading.

Methacycline Hydrochloride (Potential for reduced efficacy and increased incidence of breakthrough bleeding and menstrual irregularities with concomitant use).

No products indexed under this heading.

Minocycline Hydrochloride (Potential for reduced efficacy and increased incidence of breakthrough bleeding and menstrual irregularities with concomitant use). Products include:

Dynacin Capsules 2019
Minocin Intravenous 1862
Minocin Oral Suspension 1865
Minocin Pellet-Filled Capsules 1863

Oxytetracycline Hydrochloride (Potential for reduced efficacy and increased incidence of breakthrough bleeding and menstrual irregularities with concomitant use). Products include:

Terra-Cortril Ophthalmic Suspension 2716
Urobiotic-250 Capsules 2731

Pentobarbital Sodium (Potential for reduced efficacy and increased incidence of breakthrough bleeding and menstrual irregularities with concomitant use). Products include:

Nembutal Sodium Solution 485

Phenobarbital (Potential for reduced efficacy and increased incidence of breakthrough bleeding and menstrual irregularities with concomitant use). Products include:

Arco-Lase Plus Tablets 592
Donnatal 2929
Donnatal Extentabs 2930

Phenylbutazone (Potential for reduced efficacy and increased incidence of breakthrough bleeding and menstrual irregularities with concomitant use).

No products indexed under this heading.

Phenytoin (Potential for reduced efficacy and increased incidence of breakthrough bleeding and menstrual irregularities with concomitant use). Products include:

Dilantin Infatabs 2624
Dilantin-125 Oral Suspension 2625

Phenytoin Sodium (Potential for reduced efficacy and increased incidence of breakthrough bleeding and menstrual irregularities with concomitant use). Products include:

Dilantin Kapseals 2622

Rifampin (Co-administration has been associated with reduced efficacy and increased incidence of breakthrough bleeding and menstrual irregularities). Products include:

Rifadin 765
Rifamate Capsules 767
Rifater Tablets 769

Secobarbital Sodium (Potential for reduced efficacy and increased incidence of breakthrough bleeding and menstrual irregularities with concomitant use).

No products indexed under this heading.

Tetracycline Hydrochloride (Potential for reduced efficacy and increased incidence of breakthrough bleeding and menstrual irregularities with concomitant use).

No products indexed under this heading.

Thiamylal Sodium (Potential for reduced efficacy and increased incidence of breakthrough bleeding and menstrual irregularities with concomitant use).

No products indexed under this heading.

Topiramate (Potential for reduced efficacy and increased incidence of breakthrough bleeding and menstrual irregularities with concomitant use). Products include:

Topamax Sprinkle Capsules 2590
Topamax Tablets 2590

ORTHO-CEPT 28 TABLETS

(Desogestrel, Ethinyl Estradiol) 2546

See Ortho-Cept 21 Tablets

ORTHOCLONE OKT3 STERILE SOLUTION

(Muromonab-CD3) 2498

May interact with corticosteroids and certain other agents. Compounds in these categories include:

Azathioprine (Infection or malignancies have been reported with azathioprine alone and in conjunction with muromonab-CD3).

No products indexed under this heading.

Betamethasone Acetate (Psychosis and infection have been reported in patients treated with corticosteroids alone and in conjunction with muromonab-CD3). Products include:

Celestone Soluspan Injectable Suspension 3097

Betamethasone Sodium Phosphate (Psychosis and infection have been reported in patients treated with corticosteroids alone and in conjunction with muromonab-CD3). Products include:

Celestone Soluspan Injectable Suspension 3097

Cortisone Acetate (Psychosis and infection have been reported in patients treated with corticosteroids alone and in conjunction with muromonab-CD3). Products include:

Cortone Acetate Injectable Suspension 2059
Cortone Acetate Tablets 2061

Cyclosporine (Seizures, encephalopathy, infections, malignancies, and thrombotic events have been reported in patients receiving cyclosporine alone and in conjunction with muromonab-CD3). Products include:

Gengraf Capsules 457
Neoral Soft Gelatin Capsules 2380
Neoral Oral Solution 2380
Sandimmune 2388

Dexamethasone (Psychosis and infection have been reported in patients treated with corticosteroids alone and in conjunction with muromonab-CD3). Products include:

Decadron Elixir 2078
Decadron Tablets 2079
TobraDex Ophthalmic Ointment 542
TobraDex Ophthalmic Suspension 541

Dexamethasone Acetate (Psychosis and infection have been reported in patients treated with corticosteroids alone and in conjunction with muromonab-CD3).

No products indexed under this heading.

Dexamethasone Sodium Phosphate (Psychosis and infection have been reported in patients treated with corticosteroids alone and in conjunction with muromonab-CD3). Products include:

Decadron Phosphate Injection 2081
Decadron Phosphate Sterile Ophthalmic Ointment 2083
Decadron Phosphate Sterile Ophthalmic Solution 2084
NeoDecadron Sterile Ophthalmic Solution 2144

Fludrocortisone Acetate (Psychosis and infection have been reported in patients treated with corticosteroids alone and in conjunction with muromonab-CD3). Products include:

Florinef Acetate Tablets 2250

Hydrocortisone (Psychosis and infection have been reported in patients treated with corticosteroids alone and in conjunction with muromonab-CD3). Products include:

Anusol-HC Cream 2.5% 2237
Cipro HC Otic Suspension 540
Cortaid Intensive Therapy Cream .... ▣717
Cortaid Maximum Strength Cream .... ▣717
Cortisporin Ophthalmic Suspension Sterile .... ⊙297
Cortizone•5 .... ▣699
Cortizone•10 .... ▣699
Cortizone•10 Plus Creme .... ▣700
Cortizone for Kids Creme .... ▣699
Hydrocortone Tablets 2106
Massengill Medicated Soft Cloth Towelette .... ▣753
VōSoL HC Otic Solution 3356

Hydrocortisone Acetate (Psychosis and infection have been reported in patients treated with corticosteroids alone and in conjunction with muromonab-CD3). Products include:

Analpram-HC 1338
Anusol HC-1 Hydrocortisone Anti-Itch Cream .... ▣689
Anusol-HC Suppositories 2238
Cortaid .... ▣717
Cortifoam Rectal Foam 3170
Cortisporin-TC Otic Suspension 2246
Hydrocortone Acetate Injectable Suspension 2103
Pramosone 1343
Proctocort Suppositories 2264
ProctoFoam-HC 3177
Terra-Cortril Ophthalmic Suspension 2716

Hydrocortisone Sodium Phosphate (Psychosis and infection have been reported in patients treated with corticosteroids alone and in conjunction with muromonab-CD3). Products include:

Hydrocortone Phosphate Injection, Sterile 2105

Hydrocortisone Sodium Succinate (Psychosis and infection have been reported in patients treated with corticosteroids alone and in conjunction with muromonab-CD3).

No products indexed under this heading.

Indomethacin (Encephalopathy and other CNS effects have been reported in patients treated with indomethacin alone and in conjunction with muromonab-CD3). Products include:

Indocin 2112

Indomethacin Sodium Trihydrate (Encephalopathy and other CNS effects have been reported in patients treated with indomethacin alone and in conjunction with muromonab-CD3). Products include:

Indocin I.V. 2115

Methylprednisolone Acetate (Psychosis and infection have been reported in patients treated with corticosteroids alone and in conjunction with muromonab-CD3). Products include:

Depo-Medrol Injectable Suspension 2795

Methylprednisolone Sodium Succinate (Psychosis and infection have been reported in patients treated with corticosteroids alone and in conjunction with muromonab-CD3). Products include:

Solu-Medrol Sterile Powder 2855

Prednisolone Acetate (Psychosis and infection have been reported in patients treated with corticosteroids alone and in conjunction with muromonab-CD3). Products include:

Blephamide Ophthalmic Ointment 547
Blephamide Ophthalmic Suspension 548
Poly-Pred Liquifilm Ophthalmic Suspension .... ⊙245
Pred Forte Ophthalmic Suspension .... ⊙246
Pred Mild Sterile Ophthalmic Suspension .... ⊙249
Pred-G Ophthalmic Suspension .... ⊙247
Pred-G Sterile Ophthalmic Ointment .... ⊙248

Prednisolone Sodium Phosphate (Psychosis and infection have been reported in patients treated with corticosteroids alone and in conjunction with muromonab-CD3). Products include:

Pediapred Oral Solution 1170

Prednisolone Tebutate (Psychosis and infection have been reported in patients treated with corticosteroids alone and in conjunction with muromonab-CD3).

No products indexed under this heading.

Prednisone (Psychosis and infection have been reported in patients treated with corticosteroids alone and in conjunction with muromonab-CD3). Products include:

Prednisone 3064

Triamcinolone (Psychosis and infection have been reported in patients treated with corticosteroids alone and in conjunction with muromonab-CD3).

No products indexed under this heading.

Triamcinolone Acetonide (Psychosis and infection have been

reported in patients treated with corticosteroids alone and in conjunction with muromonab-CD3). Products include:

Azmacort Inhalation Aerosol 728
Nasacort Nasal Inhaler 750
Nasacort AQ Nasal Spray 752
Tri-Nasal Spray 2274

Triamcinolone Diacetate (Psychosis and infection have been reported in patients treated with corticosteroids alone and in conjunction with muromonab-CD3).

No products indexed under this heading.

Triamcinolone Hexacetonide (Psychosis and infection have been reported in patients treated with corticosteroids alone and in conjunction with muromonab-CD3).

No products indexed under this heading.

ORTHO-CYCLEN 21 TABLETS

(Ethinyl Estradiol, Norgestimate) 2573

May interact with barbiturates, phenytoin, tetracyclines, and certain other agents. Compounds in these categories include:

Ampicillin (Potential for reduced efficacy and increased incidence of breakthrough bleeding and menstrual irregularities with concomitant use).

No products indexed under this heading.

Ampicillin Sodium (Potential for reduced efficacy and increased incidence of breakthrough bleeding and menstrual irregularities with concomitant use). Products include:

Unasyn for Injection 2728

Aprobarbital (Potential for reduced efficacy and increased incidence of breakthrough bleeding and menstrual irregularities with concomitant use).

No products indexed under this heading.

Butabarbital (Potential for reduced efficacy and increased incidence of breakthrough bleeding and menstrual irregularities with concomitant use).

No products indexed under this heading.

Butalbital (Potential for reduced efficacy and increased incidence of breakthrough bleeding and menstrual irregularities with concomitant use). Products include:

Phrenilin 578
Sedapap Tablets 50 mg/650 mg ... 2225

Carbamazepine (Potential for reduced efficacy and increased incidence of breakthrough bleeding and menstrual irregularities with concomitant use). Products include:

Carbatrol Capsules 3234
Tegretol/Tegretol-XR 2404

Demeclocycline Hydrochloride (Potential for reduced efficacy and increased incidence of breakthrough bleeding and menstrual irregularities with concomitant use). Products include:

Declomycin Tablets 1855

Doxycycline Calcium (Potential for reduced efficacy and increased incidence of breakthrough bleeding and menstrual irregularities with concomitant use). Products include:

Vibramycin Calcium Oral Suspension Syrup 2735

Doxycycline Hyclate (Potential for reduced efficacy and increased incidence of breakthrough bleeding and menstrual irregularities with concomitant use). Products include:

Doryx Coated Pellet Filled Capsules 3357
Periostat Tablets 1208
Vibramycin Hyclate Capsules 2735
Vibramycin Hyclate Intravenous 2737
Vibra-Tabs Film Coated Tablets 2735

Doxycycline Monohydrate (Potential for reduced efficacy and increased incidence of breakthrough bleeding and menstrual irregularities with concomitant use). Products include:

Monodox Capsules 2442
Vibramycin Monohydrate for Oral Suspension 2735

Fosphenytoin Sodium (Potential for reduced efficacy and increased incidence of breakthrough bleeding and menstrual irregularities with concomitant use). Products include:

Cerebyx Injection 2619

Griseofulvin (Potential for reduced efficacy and increased incidence of breakthrough bleeding and menstrual irregularities with concomitant use). Products include:

Grifulvin V Tablets Microsize and Oral Suspension Microsize 2518
Gris-PEG Tablets 2661

Hypericum (Co-administration of hormonal contraceptives and St. John's Wort containing herbal supplements has resulted in breakthrough bleeding shortly after starting St. John's Wort and pregnancies have been reported with concomitant therapy in some patients). Products include:

Brite-Life Caplets .... ▣795
Centrum St. John's Wort Softgels . ▣853
Metabolic Nutrition System .... ▣798
Movana Tablets .... ▣832
One-A-Day Tension & Mood Softgels .... ▣808
ReSource Wellness StayCalm Caplets .... ▣826
Satiete Tablets .... ▣846

Mephobarbital (Potential for reduced efficacy and increased incidence of breakthrough bleeding and menstrual irregularities with concomitant use).

No products indexed under this heading.

Methacycline Hydrochloride (Potential for reduced efficacy and increased incidence of breakthrough bleeding and menstrual irregularities with concomitant use).

No products indexed under this heading.

Minocycline Hydrochloride (Potential for reduced efficacy and increased incidence of breakthrough bleeding and menstrual irregularities with concomitant use). Products include:

Dynacin Capsules 2019
Minocin Intravenous 1862
Minocin Oral Suspension 1865
Minocin Pellet-Filled Capsules 1863

Oxytetracycline Hydrochloride (Potential for reduced efficacy and increased incidence of breakthrough bleeding and menstrual irregularities with concomitant use). Products include:

Terra-Cortril Ophthalmic Suspension 2716
Urobiotic-250 Capsules 2731

Pentobarbital Sodium (Potential for reduced efficacy and increased incidence of breakthrough bleeding and menstrual irregularities with concomitant use). Products include:

Nembutal Sodium Solution 485

Phenobarbital (Potential for reduced efficacy and increased incidence of breakthrough bleeding and menstrual irregularities with concomitant use). Products include:

Arco-Lase Plus Tablets 592
Donnatal 2929
Donnatal Extentabs 2930

Phenylbutazone (Potential for reduced efficacy and increased incidence of breakthrough bleeding and menstrual irregularities with concomitant use).

No products indexed under this heading.

Phenytoin (Potential for reduced efficacy and increased incidence of breakthrough bleeding and menstrual irregularities with concomitant use). Products include:

Dilantin Infatabs 2624
Dilantin-125 Oral Suspension 2625

Phenytoin Sodium (Potential for reduced efficacy and increased incidence of breakthrough bleeding and menstrual irregularities with concomitant use). Products include:

Dilantin Kapseals 2622

Rifampin (Co-administration has been associated with reduced efficacy and increased incidence of breakthrough bleeding and menstrual irregularities). Products include:

Rifadin 765
Rifamate Capsules 767
Rifater Tablets 769

Secobarbital Sodium (Potential for reduced efficacy and increased incidence of breakthrough bleeding and menstrual irregularities with concomitant use).

No products indexed under this heading.

Tetracycline Hydrochloride (Potential for reduced efficacy and increased incidence of breakthrough bleeding and menstrual irregularities with concomitant use).

No products indexed under this heading.

Thiamylal Sodium (Potential for reduced efficacy and increased incidence of breakthrough bleeding and menstrual irregularities with concomitant use).

No products indexed under this heading.

Topiramate (Co-administration may result in reduced efficacy and increased incidence of breakthrough bleeding and menstrual irregularities). Products include:

Topamax Sprinkle Capsules 2590
Topamax Tablets 2590

ORTHO-CYCLEN 28 TABLETS

(Ethinyl Estradiol, Norgestimate) 2573

See Ortho-Cyclen 21 Tablets

ORTHO-EST TABLETS

(Estropipate) 3464

May interact with progestins. Compounds in these categories include:

Desogestrel (Potential risk of adverse effects on carbohydrate and lipid metabolism; the choice of progestin and dosage may be important in minimizing these adverse effects). Products include:

Cyclessa Tablets 2450
Desogen Tablets 2458
Mircette Tablets 2470
Ortho-Cept 21 Tablets 2546
Ortho-Cept 28 Tablets 2546

Medroxyprogesterone Acetate (Potential risk of adverse effects on carbohydrate and lipid metabolism; the choice of progestin and dosage may be important in minimizing these adverse effects). Products include:

Depo-Provera Contraceptive Injection 2798
Lunelle Monthly Injection 2827
Premphase Tablets 3572
Prempro Tablets 3572
Provera Tablets 2853

Megestrol Acetate (Potential risk of adverse effects on carbohydrate and lipid metabolism; the choice of progestin and dosage may be important in minimizing these adverse effects). Products include:

Megace Oral Suspension 1124

Norgestimate (Potential risk of adverse effects on carbohydrate and lipid metabolism; the choice of progestin and dosage may be important in minimizing these adverse effects). Products include:

Ortho-Cyclen/Ortho Tri-Cyclen 2573
Ortho-Prefest Tablets 2570

ORTHO-NOVUM 1/35□21 TABLETS

(Ethinyl Estradiol, Norethindrone) 2563

See Ortho-Novum 7/7/7□21 Tablets

ORTHO-NOVUM 1/35□28 TABLETS

(Ethinyl Estradiol, Norethindrone) 2563

See Ortho-Novum 7/7/7□21 Tablets

ORTHO-NOVUM 1/50□28 TABLETS

(Mestranol, Norethindrone) 2556

See Ortho-Novum 7/7/7□21 Tablets

ORTHO-NOVUM 7/7/7□21 TABLETS

(Ethinyl Estradiol, Norethindrone) 2563

May interact with barbiturates, phenytoin, tetracyclines, and certain other agents. Compounds in these categories include:

Ampicillin (Potential for reduced efficacy and increased incidence of breakthrough bleeding and menstrual irregularities with concomitant use).

No products indexed under this heading.

Ampicillin Sodium (Potential for reduced efficacy and increased incidence of breakthrough bleeding and menstrual irregularities with concomitant use). Products include:

Unasyn for Injection 2728

Aprobarbital (Potential for reduced efficacy and increased incidence of breakthrough bleeding and menstrual irregularities with concomitant use).

No products indexed under this heading.

Butabarbital (Potential for reduced efficacy and increased incidence of breakthrough bleeding and menstrual irregularities with concomitant use).

No products indexed under this heading.

Butalbital (Potential for reduced efficacy and increased incidence of breakthrough bleeding and menstrual irregularities with concomitant use). Products include:

Phrenilin 578
Sedapap Tablets 50 mg/650 mg ... 2225

Demeclocycline Hydrochloride (Potential for reduced efficacy and increased incidence of breakthrough bleeding and menstrual irregularities with concomitant use). Products include:

Declomycin Tablets 1855

Doxycycline Calcium (Potential for reduced efficacy and increased incidence of breakthrough bleeding and menstrual irregularities with concomitant use). Products include:

Vibramycin Calcium Oral Suspension Syrup 2735

Doxycycline Hyclate (Potential for reduced efficacy and increased incidence of breakthrough bleeding and menstrual irregularities with concomitant use). Products include:

Doryx Coated Pellet Filled Capsules 3357
Periostat Tablets 1208
Vibramycin Hyclate Capsules 2735
Vibramycin Hyclate Intravenous 2737
Vibra-Tabs Film Coated Tablets 2735

Doxycycline Monohydrate (Potential for reduced efficacy and increased incidence of breakthrough bleeding and menstrual irregularities with concomitant use). Products include:

Monodox Capsules 2442

Vibramycin Monohydrate for Oral Suspension 2735

Fosphenytoin Sodium (Potential for reduced efficacy and increased incidence of breakthrough bleeding and menstrual irregularities with concomitant use). Products include:

Cerebyx Injection 2619

Griseofulvin (Potential for reduced efficacy and increased incidence of breakthrough bleeding and menstrual irregularities with concomitant use). Products include:

Grifulvin V Tablets Microsize and Oral Suspension Microsize 2518
Gris-PEG Tablets 2661

Hypericum (Co-administration of hormonal contraceptives and St. John's Wort containing herbal supplements has resulted in breakthrough bleeding shortly after starting St. John's Wort and pregnancies have been reported with concomitant therapy in some patients). Products include:

Brite-Life Caplets .... ▣795
Centrum St. John's Wort Softgels .... ▣853
Metabolic Nutrition System .... ▣798
Movana Tablets .... ▣832
One-A-Day Tension & Mood Softgels .... ▣808
ReSource Wellness StayCalm Caplets .... ▣826
Satiete Tablets .... ▣846

Mephobarbital (Potential for reduced efficacy and increased incidence of breakthrough bleeding and menstrual irregularities with concomitant use).

No products indexed under this heading.

Methacycline Hydrochloride (Potential for reduced efficacy and increased incidence of breakthrough bleeding and menstrual irregularities with concomitant use).

No products indexed under this heading.

Minocycline Hydrochloride (Potential for reduced efficacy and increased incidence of breakthrough bleeding and menstrual irregularities with concomitant use). Products include:

Dynacin Capsules 2019
Minocin Intravenous 1862
Minocin Oral Suspension 1865
Minocin Pellet-Filled Capsules 1863

Oxytetracycline Hydrochloride (Potential for reduced efficacy and increased incidence of breakthrough bleeding and menstrual irregularities with concomitant use). Products include:

Terra-Cortril Ophthalmic Suspension 2716
Urobiotic-250 Capsules 2731

Pentobarbital Sodium (Potential for reduced efficacy and increased incidence of breakthrough bleeding and menstrual irregularities with concomitant use). Products include:

Nembutal Sodium Solution 485

Phenobarbital (Potential for reduced efficacy and increased incidence of breakthrough bleeding and menstrual irregularities with concomitant use). Products include:

Arco-Lase Plus Tablets 592
Donnatal 2929
Donnatal Extentabs 2930

Phenylbutazone (Potential for reduced efficacy and increased incidence of breakthrough bleeding and menstrual irregularities with concomitant use).

No products indexed under this heading.

Phenytoin (Potential for reduced efficacy and increased incidence of breakthrough bleeding and menstrual irregularities with concomitant use). Products include:

Dilantin Infatabs 2624
Dilantin-125 Oral Suspension 2625

Phenytoin Sodium (Potential for reduced efficacy and increased incidence of breakthrough bleeding and menstrual irregularities with concomitant use). Products include:

Dilantin Kapseals 2622

Rifampin (Co-administration has been associated with reduced efficacy and increased incidence of breakthrough bleeding and menstrual irregularities). Products include:

Rifadin 765
Rifamate Capsules 767
Rifater Tablets 769

Secobarbital Sodium (Potential for reduced efficacy and increased incidence of breakthrough bleeding and menstrual irregularities with concomitant use).

No products indexed under this heading.

Tetracycline Hydrochloride (Potential for reduced efficacy and increased incidence of breakthrough bleeding and menstrual irregularities with concomitant use).

No products indexed under this heading.

Thiamylal Sodium (Potential for reduced efficacy and increased incidence of breakthrough bleeding and menstrual irregularities with concomitant use).

No products indexed under this heading.

Topiramate (Co-administration may result in reduced efficacy and increased incidence of breakthrough bleeding and menstrual irregularities). Products include:

Topamax Sprinkle Capsules 2590
Topamax Tablets 2590

ORTHO-NOVUM 7/7/7□28 TABLETS

(Ethinyl Estradiol, Norethindrone) 2563
See Ortho-Novum 7/7/7□21 Tablets

ORTHO-NOVUM 10/11□21 TABLETS

(Ethinyl Estradiol, Norethindrone) 2563
See Ortho-Novum 7/7/7□21 Tablets

ORTHO-NOVUM 10/11□28 TABLETS

(Ethinyl Estradiol, Norethindrone) 2563
See Ortho-Novum 7/7/7□21 Tablets

ORTHO-PREFEST TABLETS

(Estradiol, Norgestimate) 2570
May interact with:

Food Interactions

Food, unspecified (Co-administration with a high fat meal results in increased Cmax values for estrone and estrone sulfate; Cmax values 17- deacetylnorgestimate were decreased; the AUC values for these analytes were not significantly affected by food).

ORTHO TRI-CYCLEN 21 TABLETS

(Ethinyl Estradiol, Norgestimate) 2573
See Ortho-Cyclen 21 Tablets

ORTHO TRI-CYCLEN 28 TABLETS

(Ethinyl Estradiol, Norgestimate) 2573
See Ortho-Cyclen 21 Tablets

ORUDIS CAPSULES

(Ketoprofen) 3548
May interact with diuretics, lithium preparations, and certain other agents. Compounds in these categories include:

Amiloride Hydrochloride (Reduced urinary potassium and chloride excretion). Products include:

Midamor Tablets 2136
Moduretic Tablets 2138

Aspirin (Decreased protein-binding and increased plasma clearance of ketoprofen). Products include:

Aggrenox Capsules 1026
Alka-Seltzer .... ▣603
Alka-Seltzer Lemon Lime Antacid and Pain Reliever Effervescent Tablets .... ▣603
Alka-Seltzer Extra Strength Antacid and Pain Reliever Effervescent Tablets .... ▣603
Alka-Seltzer PM Effervescent Tablets .... ▣605
Genuine Bayer Tablets, Caplets and Gelcaps .... ▣606
Extra Strength Bayer Caplets and Gelcaps .... ▣610
Aspirin Regimen Bayer Children's Chewable Tablets (Orange or Cherry Flavored) .... ▣607
Bayer, Aspirin Regimen .... ▣606
Aspirin Regimen Bayer 81 mg Caplets with Calcium .... ▣607
Genuine Bayer Professional Labeling (Aspirin Regimen Bayer) .... ▣608
Extra Strength Bayer Arthritis Caplets .... ▣610
Extra Strength Bayer Plus Caplets .... ▣610
Extra Strength Bayer PM Caplets .... ▣611
BC Powder .... ▣619
BC Allergy Sinus Cold Powder .... ▣619
Arthritis Strength BC Powder .... ▣619
BC Sinus Cold Powder .... ▣619
Darvon Compound-65 Pulvules 1910
Ecotrin Enteric Coated Aspirin Low, Regular and Maximum Strength Tablets 1715
Excedrin Extra-Strength Tablets, Caplets, and Geltabs .... ▣629
Excedrin Migraine 1070
Goody's Body Pain Formula Powder .... ▣620
Goody's Extra Strength Headache Powder .... ▣620
Goody's Extra Strength Pain Relief Tablets .... ▣620
Percodan Tablets 1327
Robaxisal Tablets 2939
Soma Compound Tablets 3354
Soma Compound w/Codeine Tablets 3355
Vanquish Caplets .... ▣617

Bendroflumethiazide (Reduced urinary potassium and chloride excretion). Products include:

Corzide 40/5 Tablets 2247
Corzide 80/5 Tablets 2247

Bumetanide (Reduced urinary potassium and chloride excretion).

No products indexed under this heading.

Chlorothiazide (Reduced urinary potassium and chloride excretion). Products include:

Aldoclor Tablets 2035
Diuril Oral 2087

Chlorothiazide Sodium (Reduced urinary potassium and chloride excretion). Products include:

Diuril Sodium Intravenous 2086

Chlorthalidone (Reduced urinary potassium and chloride excretion). Products include:

Clorpres Tablets 1002
Combipres Tablets 1040
Tenoretic Tablets 690

Ethacrynic Acid (Reduced urinary potassium and chloride excretion). Products include:

Edecrin Tablets 2091

Furosemide (Reduced urinary potassium and chloride excretion). Products include:

Furosemide Tablets 2284

Hydrochlorothiazide (Reduced urinary potassium and chloride excretion). Products include:

Accuretic Tablets 2614
Aldoril Tablets 2039
Atacand HCT Tablets 597
Avalide Tablets 1070
Diovan HCT Tablets 2338
Dyazide Capsules 1515
HydroDIURIL Tablets 2108
Hyzaar 2109
Inderide Tablets 3517
Inderide LA Long-Acting Capsules 3519
Lotensin HCT Tablets 2367
Maxzide 1008
Micardis HCT Tablets 1051
Microzide Capsules 3414
Moduretic Tablets 2138
Monopril HCT 1094
Prinzide Tablets 2168
Timolide Tablets 2187
Uniretic Tablets 3178
Vaseretic Tablets 2204
Zestoretic Tablets 695
Ziac Tablets 1887

Hydroflumethiazide (Reduced urinary potassium and chloride excretion). Products include:

Diucardin Tablets 3494

Indapamide (Reduced urinary potassium and chloride excretion). Products include:

Indapamide Tablets 2286

Lithium Carbonate (Increased steady-state plasma lithium levels). Products include:

Eskalith 1527
Lithium Carbonate 3061
Lithobid Slow-Release Tablets 3255

Lithium Citrate (Increased steady-state plasma lithium levels). Products include:

Lithium Citrate Syrup 3061

Methotrexate Sodium (Increased toxicity; avoid coadministration).

No products indexed under this heading.

Methyclothiazide (Reduced urinary potassium and chloride excretion).

No products indexed under this heading.

Metolazone (Reduced urinary potassium and chloride excretion). Products include:

Mykrox Tablets 1168
Zaroxolyn Tablets 1177

Polythiazide (Reduced urinary potassium and chloride excretion). Products include:

Minizide Capsules 2700
Renese Tablets 2712

Probenecid (Decreased protein-binding and increased plasma clearance of ketoprofen).

No products indexed under this heading.

Spironolactone (Reduced urinary potassium and chloride excretion).

No products indexed under this heading.

Torsemide (Reduced urinary potassium and chloride excretion). Products include:

Demadex Tablets and Injection 2965

Triamterene (Reduced urinary potassium and chloride excretion). Products include:

Dyazide Capsules 1515
Dyrenium Capsules 3458
Maxzide 1008

Warfarin Sodium (Concurrent therapy requires close monitoring of patients on both drugs). Products include:

Coumadin for Injection 1243
Coumadin Tablets 1243
Warfarin Sodium Tablets, USP 3302

Food Interactions

Food, unspecified (Slows rate of absorption resulting in delayed and reduced peak concentrations).

ORUDIS KT TABLETS

(Ketoprofen) .... ▣778
May interact with:

Food Interactions

Alcohol (Patients consuming three or more alcohol-containing drinks should consult their doctor for advice on when and how they should take Orudis KT).

ORUVAIL CAPSULES

(Ketoprofen) 3548
See Orudis Capsules

OS-CAL CHEWABLE TABLETS

(Calcium Carbonate) .... ▣838
None cited in PDR database.

OS-CAL 250 + D TABLETS

(Calcium, Vitamin D) .... ▣838
None cited in PDR database.

IMPORTANT NOTE: Always consult each drug listing in the patient's regimen for possible interactions.

OS-CAL 500 TABLETS
(Calcium) .... ▣839
None cited in PDR database.

OS-CAL 500 + D TABLETS
(Calcium, Vitamin D) .... ▣839
None cited in PDR database.

OSCILLOCOCCINUM PELLETS
(Anas Barbariae Hepatis et Cordis Extractum)........................... ▣625
None cited in PDR database.

OVCON 35 TABLETS
(Ethinyl Estradiol, Norethindrone) 3364
May interact with barbiturates, phenytoin, tetracyclines, and certain other agents. Compounds in these categories include:

Ampicillin (Potential for reduced efficacy and increased incidence of breakthrough bleeding and menstrual irregularities with concomitant use).
No products indexed under this heading.

Ampicillin Sodium (Potential for reduced efficacy and increased incidence of breakthrough bleeding and menstrual irregularities with concomitant use). Products include:
Unasyn for Injection 2728

Aprobarbital (Potential for reduced efficacy and increased incidence of breakthrough bleeding and menstrual irregularities with concomitant use).
No products indexed under this heading.

Butabarbital (Potential for reduced efficacy and increased incidence of breakthrough bleeding and menstrual irregularities with concomitant use).
No products indexed under this heading.

Butalbital (Potential for reduced efficacy and increased incidence of breakthrough bleeding and menstrual irregularities with concomitant use). Products include:
Phrenilin 578
Sedapap Tablets 50 mg/650 mg 2225

Demeclocycline Hydrochloride (Potential for reduced efficacy and increased incidence of breakthrough bleeding and menstrual irregularities with concomitant use). Products include:
Declomycin Tablets 1855

Doxycycline Calcium (Potential for reduced efficacy and increased incidence of breakthrough bleeding and menstrual irregularities with concomitant use). Products include:
Vibramycin Calcium Oral Suspension Syrup 2735

Doxycycline Hyclate (Potential for reduced efficacy and increased incidence of breakthrough bleeding and menstrual irregularities with concomitant use). Products include:
Doryx Coated Pellet Filled Capsules 3357
Periostat Tablets 1208
Vibramycin Hyclate Capsules 2735
Vibramycin Hyclate Intravenous 2737
Vibra-Tabs Film Coated Tablets 2735

Doxycycline Monohydrate (Potential for reduced efficacy and increased incidence of breakthrough bleeding and menstrual irregularities with concomitant use). Products include:
Monodox Capsules 2442
Vibramycin Monohydrate for Oral Suspension 2735

Fosphenytoin Sodium (Potential for reduced efficacy and increased incidence of breakthrough bleeding and menstrual irregularities with concomitant use). Products include:
Cerebyx Injection 2619

Griseofulvin (Potential for reduced efficacy and increased incidence of breakthrough bleeding and menstrual irregularities with concomitant use). Products include:
Grifulvin V Tablets Microsize and Oral Suspension Microsize 2518
Gris-PEG Tablets 2661

Mephobarbital (Potential for reduced efficacy and increased incidence of breakthrough bleeding and menstrual irregularities with concomitant use).
No products indexed under this heading.

Methacycline Hydrochloride (Potential for reduced efficacy and increased incidence of breakthrough bleeding and menstrual irregularities with concomitant use).
No products indexed under this heading.

Minocycline Hydrochloride (Potential for reduced efficacy and increased incidence of breakthrough bleeding and menstrual irregularities with concomitant use). Products include:
Dynacin Capsules 2019
Minocin Intravenous 1862
Minocin Oral Suspension 1865
Minocin Pellet-Filled Capsules 1863

Oxytetracycline Hydrochloride (Potential for reduced efficacy and increased incidence of breakthrough bleeding and menstrual irregularities with concomitant use). Products include:
Terra-Cortril Ophthalmic Suspension 2716
Urobiotic-250 Capsules 2731

Pentobarbital Sodium (Potential for reduced efficacy and increased incidence of breakthrough bleeding and menstrual irregularities with concomitant use). Products include:
Nembutal Sodium Solution 485

Phenobarbital (Potential for reduced efficacy and increased incidence of breakthrough bleeding and menstrual irregularities with concomitant use). Products include:
Arco-Lase Plus Tablets 592
Donnatal 2929
Donnatal Extentabs 2930

Phenylbutazone (Potential for reduced efficacy and increased incidence of breakthrough bleeding and menstrual irregularities with concomitant use).
No products indexed under this heading.

Phenytoin (Potential for reduced efficacy and increased incidence of breakthrough bleeding and menstrual irregularities with concomitant use). Products include:
Dilantin Infatabs 2624
Dilantin 125 Oral Suspension 2625

Phenytoin Sodium (Potential for reduced efficacy and increased incidence of breakthrough bleeding and menstrual irregularities with concomitant use). Products include:
Dilantin Kapseals 2622

Rifampin (Co-administration has been associated with reduced efficacy and increased incidence of breakthrough bleeding and menstrual irregularities). Products include:
Rifadin 765
Rifamate Capsules 767
Rifater Tablets 769

Secobarbital Sodium (Potential for reduced efficacy and increased incidence of breakthrough bleeding and menstrual irregularities with concomitant use).
No products indexed under this heading.

Tetracycline Hydrochloride (Potential for reduced efficacy and increased incidence of breakthrough bleeding and menstrual irregularities with concomitant use).
No products indexed under this heading.

Thiamylal Sodium (Potential for reduced efficacy and increased incidence of breakthrough bleeding and menstrual irregularities with concomitant use).
No products indexed under this heading.

OVCON 50 TABLETS
(Ethinyl Estradiol, Norethindrone) 3364
See Ovcon 35 Tablets

OVIDE LOTION
(Malathion) 2023
None cited in PDR database.

OVIDREL FOR INJECTION
(Choriogonadotropin Alfa) 3220
None cited in PDR database.

OVRAL TABLETS
(Ethinyl Estradiol, Norgestrel) 3551
See Lo/Ovral Tablets

OVRAL-28 TABLETS
(Ethinyl Estradiol, Norgestrel) 3552
See Lo/Ovral Tablets

OVRETTE TABLETS
(Norgestrel) 3552
See Lo/Ovral Tablets

OXANDRIN TABLETS
(Oxandrolone) 1153
May interact with corticosteroids, oral anticoagulants, oral hypoglycemic agents, and certain other agents. Compounds in these categories include:

Acarbose (Oxandrolone may inhibit the metabolism of oral hypoglycemic agents). Products include:
Precose Tablets 906

ACTH (In patients with edema, co-administration with ACTH may increase the edema).
No products indexed under this heading.

Betamethasone Acetate (In patients with edema, co-administration with adrenal cortical steroids may increase the edema). Products include:
Celestone Soluspan Injectable Suspension 3097

Betamethasone Sodium Phosphate (In patients with edema, co-administration with adrenal cortical steroids may increase the edema). Products include:
Celestone Soluspan Injectable Suspension 3097

Chlorpropamide (Oxandrolone may inhibit the metabolism of oral hypoglycemic agents). Products include:
Diabinese Tablets 2680

Cortisone Acetate (In patients with edema, co-administration with adrenal cortical steroids may increase the edema). Products include:
Cortone Acetate Injectable Suspension 2059
Cortone Acetate Tablets 2061

Dexamethasone (In patients with edema, co-administration with adrenal cortical steroids may increase the edema). Products include:
Decadron Elixir 2078
Decadron Tablets 2079
TobraDex Ophthalmic Ointment 542
TobraDex Ophthalmic Suspension .. 541

Dexamethasone Acetate (In patients with edema, co-administration with adrenal cortical steroids may increase the edema).
No products indexed under this heading.

Dexamethasone Sodium Phosphate (In patients with edema, co-administration with adrenal cortical steroids may increase the edema). Products include:
Decadron Phosphate Injection 2081
Decadron Phosphate Sterile Ophthalmic Ointment 2083
Decadron Phosphate Sterile Ophthalmic Solution 2084
NeoDecadron Sterile Ophthalmic Solution... 2144

Dicumarol (Anabolic steroids may increase the sensitivity to oral anticoagulants; dosage of the anticoagulants may have to be decreased in order to maintain desired prothrombin time).
No products indexed under this heading.

Fludrocortisone Acetate (In patients with edema, co-administration with adrenal cortical steroids may increase the edema). Products include:
Florinef Acetate Tablets 2250

Glimepiride (Oxandrolone may inhibit the metabolism of oral hypoglycemic agents). Products include:
Amaryl Tablets 717

Glipizide (Oxandrolone may inhibit the metabolism of oral hypoglycemic agents). Products include:
Glucotrol Tablets 2692
Glucotrol XL Extended Release Tablets 2693

Glyburide (Oxandrolone may inhibit the metabolism of oral hypoglycemic agents). Products include:
DiaBeta Tablets 741
Glucovance Tablets 1086

Hydrocortisone (In patients with edema, co-administration with adrenal cortical steroids may increase the edema). Products include:
Anusol-HC Cream 2.5% 2237
Cipro HC Otic Suspension 540
Cortaid Intensive Therapy Cream . ▣717
Cortaid Maximum Strength Cream .... ▣717
Cortisporin Ophthalmic Suspension Sterile .... ⊙297
Cortizone•5 .... ▣699
Cortizone•10 .... ▣699
Cortizone•10 Plus Creme .... ▣700
Cortizone for Kids Creme .... ▣699
Hydrocortone Tablets 2106
Massengill Medicated Soft Cloth Towelette .... ▣753
VōSoL HC Otic Solution 3356

Hydrocortisone Acetate (In patients with edema, co-administration with adrenal cortical steroids may increase the edema). Products include:
Analpram-HC 1338
Anusol HC-1 Hydrocortisone Anti-Itch Cream .... ▣689
Anusol-HC Suppositories 2238
Cortaid .... ▣717
Cortifoam Rectal Foam 3170
Cortisporin-TC Otic Suspension 2246
Hydrocortone Acetate Injectable Suspension 2103
Pramosone 1343
Proctocort Suppositories 2264
ProctoFoam-HC 3177
Terra-Cortril Ophthalmic Suspension 2716

Hydrocortisone Sodium Phosphate (In patients with edema, co-administration with adrenal cortical steroids may increase the edema). Products include:
Hydrocortone Phosphate Injection, Sterile 2105

Hydrocortisone Sodium Succinate (In patients with edema, co-administration with adrenal cortical steroids may increase the edema).
No products indexed under this heading.

Metformin Hydrochloride (Oxandrolone may inhibit the metabolism of oral hypoglycemic agents). Products include:
Glucophage Tablets 1080
Glucophage XR Tablets 1080
Glucovance Tablets 1086

Methylprednisolone Acetate (In patients with edema, co-administration with adrenal cortical steroids may increase the edema). Products include:
Depo-Medrol Injectable Suspension 2795

Methylprednisolone Sodium Succinate (In patients with edema, co-administration with adrenal cortical steroids may increase the edema). Products include:
Solu-Medrol Sterile Powder 2855

Miglitol (Oxandrolone may inhibit the metabolism of oral hypoglycemic agents). Products include:
Glyset Tablets 2821

Pioglitazone Hydrochloride (Oxandrolone may inhibit the metabolism of oral hypoglycemic agents). Products include:
Actos Tablets 3275

Prednisolone Acetate (In patients with edema, co-administration with adrenal cortical steroids may increase the edema). Products include:
Blephamide Ophthalmic Ointment 547
Blephamide Ophthalmic Suspension 548
Poly-Pred Liquifilm Ophthalmic Suspension .... ⊙245
Pred Forte Ophthalmic Suspension .... ⊙246
Pred Mild Sterile Ophthalmic Suspension .... ⊙249
Pred-G Ophthalmic Suspension .... ⊙247
Pred-G Sterile Ophthalmic Ointment .... ⊙248

Prednisolone Sodium Phosphate (In patients with edema, co-administration with adrenal cortical steroids may increase the edema). Products include:
Pediapred Oral Solution 1170

Prednisolone Tebutate (In patients with edema, co-administration with adrenal cortical steroids may increase the edema).
No products indexed under this heading.

Prednisone (In patients with edema, co-administration with adrenal cortical steroids may increase the edema). Products include:
Prednisone 3064

Repaglinide (Oxandrolone may inhibit the metabolism of oral hypoglycemic agents). Products include:
Prandin Tablets (0.5, 1, and 2 mg) 2432

Rosiglitazone Maleate (Oxandrolone may inhibit the metabolism of oral hypoglycemic agents). Products include:
Avandia Tablets 1490

Tolazamide (Oxandrolone may inhibit the metabolism of oral hypoglycemic agents).
No products indexed under this heading.

Tolbutamide (Oxandrolone may inhibit the metabolism of oral hypoglycemic agents).
No products indexed under this heading.

Triamcinolone (In patients with edema, co-administration with adrenal cortical steroids may increase the edema).
No products indexed under this heading.

Triamcinolone Acetonide (In patients with edema, co-administration with adrenal cortical steroids may increase the edema). Products include:
Azmacort Inhalation Aerosol 728
Nasacort Nasal Inhaler 750
Nasacort AQ Nasal Spray 752
Tri-Nasal Spray 2274

Triamcinolone Diacetate (In patients with edema, co-administration with adrenal cortical steroids may increase the edema).
No products indexed under this heading.

Triamcinolone Hexacetonide (In patients with edema, co-administration with adrenal cortical steroids may increase the edema).
No products indexed under this heading.

Troglitazone (Oxandrolone may inhibit the metabolism of oral hypoglycemic agents).
No products indexed under this heading.

Warfarin Sodium (Anabolic steroids may increase the sensitivity to oral anticoagulants; dosage of the anticoagulants may have to be decreased in order to maintain desired prothrombin time). Products include:
Coumadin for Injection 1243
Coumadin Tablets 1243
Warfarin Sodium Tablets, USP 3302

OXISTAT CREAM
(Oxiconazole Nitrate) 1298
None cited in PDR database.

OXISTAT LOTION
(Oxiconazole Nitrate) 1298
None cited in PDR database.

OXSORALEN LOTION 1%
(Methoxsalen) 1740
May interact with phenothiazines, sulfonamides, tetracyclines, thiazides, and certain other agents. Compounds in these categories include:

Anthralin (Possible photosensitivity effects). Products include:
Psoriatec Cream 3247

Bendroflumethiazide (Possible photosensitivity effects). Products include:
Corzide 40/5 Tablets 2247
Corzide 80/5 Tablets 2247

Chlorothiazide (Possible photosensitivity effects). Products include:
Aldoclor Tablets 2035
Diuril Oral 2087

Chlorothiazide Sodium (Possible photosensitivity effects). Products include:
Diuril Sodium Intravenous 2086

Chlorpromazine (Possible photosensitivity effects). Products include:
Thorazine Suppositories 1656

Chlorpromazine Hydrochloride (Possible photosensitivity effects). Products include:
Thorazine 1656

Chlorpropamide (Possible photosensitivity effects). Products include:
Diabinese Tablets 2680

Coal Tar (Possible photosensitivity effects). Products include:
Tegrin Dandruff Shampoo - Extra Conditioning 623
Tegrin Dandruff Shampoo - Fresh Herbal 624
Tegrin Skin Cream 624

Demeclocycline Hydrochloride (Possible photosensitivity effects). Products include:
Declomycin Tablets 1855

Doxycycline Calcium (Possible photosensitivity effects). Products include:
Vibramycin Calcium Oral Suspension Syrup 2735

Doxycycline Hyclate (Possible photosensitivity effects). Products include:
Doryx Coated Pellet Filled Capsules 3357
Periostat Tablets 1208
Vibramycin Hyclate Capsules 2735
Vibramycin Hyclate Intravenous 2737
Vibra-Tabs Film Coated Tablets 2735

Doxycycline Monohydrate (Possible photosensitivity effects). Products include:
Monodox Capsules 2442
Vibramycin Monohydrate for Oral Suspension 2735

Fluphenazine Decanoate (Possible photosensitivity effects).
No products indexed under this heading.

Fluphenazine Enanthate (Possible photosensitivity effects).
No products indexed under this heading.

Fluphenazine Hydrochloride (Possible photosensitivity effects).
No products indexed under this heading.

Glipizide (Possible photosensitivity effects). Products include:
Glucotrol Tablets 2692
Glucotrol XL Extended Release Tablets 2693

Glyburide (Possible photosensitivity effects). Products include:
DiaBeta Tablets 741
Glucovance Tablets 1086

Griseofulvin (Possible photosensitivity effects). Products include:
Grifulvin V Tablets Microsize and Oral Suspension Microsize 2518
Gris-PEG Tablets 2661

Hydrochlorothiazide (Possible photosensitivity effects). Products include:
Accuretic Tablets 2614
Aldoril Tablets 2039
Atacand HCT Tablets 597
Avalide Tablets 1070
Diovan HCT Tablets 2338
Dyazide Capsules 1515
HydroDIURIL Tablets 2108
Hyzaar 2109
Inderide Tablets 3517
Inderide LA Long-Acting Capsules 3519
Lotensin HCT Tablets 2367
Maxzide 1008
Micardis HCT Tablets 1051
Microzide Capsules 3414
Moduretic Tablets 2138
Monopril HCT 1094
Prinzide Tablets 2168
Timolide Tablets 2187
Uniretic Tablets 3178
Vaseretic Tablets 2204
Zestoretic Tablets 695
Ziac Tablets 1887

Hydroflumethiazide (Possible photosensitivity effects). Products include:
Diucardin Tablets 3494

Mesoridazine Besylate (Possible photosensitivity effects). Products include:
Serentil 1057

Methacycline Hydrochloride (Possible photosensitivity effects).
No products indexed under this heading.

Methotrimeprazine (Possible photosensitivity effects).
No products indexed under this heading.

Methyclothiazide (Possible photosensitivity effects).
No products indexed under this heading.

Methylene Blue (Possible photosensitivity effects). Products include:
Prosed/DS Tablets 3268
Urimax Tablets 1769
Urised Tablets 2876

Minocycline Hydrochloride (Possible photosensitivity effects). Products include:
Dynacin Capsules 2019
Minocin Intravenous 1862
Minocin Oral Suspension 1865
Minocin Pellet-Filled Capsules 1863

Nalidixic Acid (Possible photosensitivity effects).
No products indexed under this heading.

Oxytetracycline (Possible photosensitivity effects).
No products indexed under this heading.

Oxytetracycline Hydrochloride (Possible photosensitivity effects). Products include:
Terra-Cortril Ophthalmic Suspension 2716
Urobiotic-250 Capsules 2731

Perphenazine (Possible photosensitivity effects). Products include:
Etrafon 3115
Trilafon 3160

Polythiazide (Possible photosensitivity effects). Products include:
Minizide Capsules 2700
Renese Tablets 2712

Prochlorperazine (Possible photosensitivity effects). Products include:
Compazine 1505

Promethazine Hydrochloride (Possible photosensitivity effects). Products include:
Mepergan Injection 3539
Phenergan Injection 3553
Phenergan 3556
Phenergan Syrup 3554
Phenergan with Codeine Syrup 3557
Phenergan with Dextromethorphan Syrup 3559
Phenergan VC Syrup 3560
Phenergan VC with Codeine Syrup 3561

Sulfacytine (Possible photosensitivity effects).

Sulfamethizole (Possible photosensitivity effects). Products include:
Urobiotic-250 Capsules 2731

Sulfamethoxazole (Possible photosensitivity effects). Products include:
Bactrim 2949
Septra Suspension 2265
Septra Tablets 2265
Septra DS Tablets 2265

Sulfasalazine (Possible photosensitivity effects). Products include:
Azulfidine EN-tabs Tablets 2775

Sulfinpyrazone (Possible photosensitivity effects).
No products indexed under this heading.

Sulfisoxazole (Possible photosensitivity effects).
No products indexed under this heading.

Sulfisoxazole Acetyl (Possible photosensitivity effects). Products include:
Pediazole Suspension 3050

Sulfisoxazole Diolamine (Possible photosensitivity effects).
No products indexed under this heading.

Tetracycline Hydrochloride (Possible photosensitivity effects).
No products indexed under this heading.

Thioridazine Hydrochloride (Possible photosensitivity effects). Products include:
Thioridazine Hydrochloride Tablets 2289

Tolazamide (Possible photosensitivity effects).
No products indexed under this heading.

Tolbutamide (Possible photosensitivity effects).
No products indexed under this heading.

Trifluoperazine Hydrochloride (Possible photosensitivity effects). Products include:
Stelazine 1640

OXSORALEN-ULTRA CAPSULES
(Methoxsalen) 1741
May interact with phenothiazines, sulfonamides, tetracyclines, thiazides, and certain other agents. Compounds in these categories include:

Anthralin (Possible photosensitivity effects). Products include:
Psoriatec Cream 3247

Bendroflumethiazide (Possible photosensitivity effects). Products include:
Corzide 40/5 Tablets 2247
Corzide 80/5 Tablets 2247

IMPORTANT NOTE: Always consult each drug listing in the patient's regimen for possible interactions.

Chlorothiazide (Possible photosensitivity effects). Products include:
Aldoclor Tablets 2035
Diuril Oral 2087

Chlorothiazide Sodium (Possible photosensitivity effects). Products include:
Diuril Sodium Intravenous 2086

Chlorpromazine (Possible photosensitivity effects). Products include:
Thorazine Suppositories 1656

Chlorpromazine Hydrochloride (Possible photosensitivity effects). Products include:
Thorazine 1656

Chlorpropamide (Possible photosensitivity effects). Products include:
Diabinese Tablets 2680

Coal Tar (Possible photosensitivity effects). Products include:
Tegrin Dandruff Shampoo - Extra Conditioning .... ▣623
Tegrin Dandruff Shampoo - Fresh Herbal .... ▣624
Tegrin Skin Cream .... ▣624

Demeclocycline Hydrochloride (Possible photosensitivity effects). Products include:
Declomycin Tablets 1855

Doxycycline Calcium (Possible photosensitivity effects). Products include:
Vibramycin Calcium Oral Suspension Syrup 2735

Doxycycline Hyclate (Possible photosensitivity effects). Products include:
Doryx Coated Pellet Filled Capsules 3357
Periostat Tablets 1208
Vibramycin Hyclate Capsules 2735
Vibramycin Hyclate Intravenous 2737
Vibra-Tabs Film Coated Tablets 2735

Doxycycline Monohydrate (Possible photosensitivity effects). Products include:
Monodox Capsules 2442
Vibramycin Monohydrate for Oral Suspension 2735

Fluphenazine Decanoate (Possible photosensitivity effects).
No products indexed under this heading.

Fluphenazine Enanthate (Possible photosensitivity effects).
No products indexed under this heading.

Fluphenazine Hydrochloride (Possible photosensitivity effects).
No products indexed under this heading.

Glipizide (Possible photosensitivity effects). Products include:
Glucotrol Tablets 2692
Glucotrol XL Extended Release Tablets 2693

Glyburide (Possible photosensitivity effects). Products include:
DiaBeta Tablets 741
Glucovance Tablets 1086

Griseofulvin (Possible photosensitivity effects). Products include:
Grifulvin V Tablets Microsize and Oral Suspension Microsize 2518
Gris-PEG Tablets 2661

Hydrochlorothiazide (Possible photosensitivity effects). Products include:
Accuretic Tablets 2614
Aldoril Tablets 2039
Atacand HCT Tablets 597
Avalide Tablets 1070
Diovan HCT Tablets 2338
Dyazide Capsules 1515
HydroDIURIL Tablets 2108
Hyzaar 2109
Inderide Tablets 3517
Inderide LA Long-Acting Capsules 3519
Lotensin HCT Tablets 2367
Maxzide 1008
Micardis HCT Tablets 1051
Microzide Capsules 3414
Moduretic Tablets 2138
Monopril HCT 1094
Prinzide Tablets 2168
Timolide Tablets 2187
Uniretic Tablets 3178
Vaseretic Tablets 2204
Zestoretic Tablets 695
Ziac Tablets 1887

Hydroflumethiazide (Possible photosensitivity effects). Products include:
Diucardin Tablets 3494

Mesoridazine Besylate (Possible photosensitivity effects). Products include:
Serentil 1057

Methacycline Hydrochloride (Possible photosensitivity effects).
No products indexed under this heading.

Methotrimeprazine (Possible photosensitivity effects).
No products indexed under this heading.

Methyclothiazide (Possible photosensitivity effects).
No products indexed under this heading.

Methylene Blue (Possible photosensitivity effects). Products include:
Prosed/DS Tablets 3268
Urimax Tablets 1769
Urised Tablets 2876

Minocycline Hydrochloride (Possible photosensitivity effects). Products include:
Dynacin Capsules 2019
Minocin Intravenous 1862
Minocin Oral Suspension 1865
Minocin Pellet-Filled Capsules 1863

Nalidixic Acid (Possible photosensitivity effects).
No products indexed under this heading.

Oxytetracycline (Possible photosensitivity effects).
No products indexed under this heading.

Oxytetracycline Hydrochloride (Possible photosensitivity effects). Products include:
Terra-Cortril Ophthalmic Suspension 2716
Urobiotic-250 Capsules 2731

Perphenazine (Possible photosensitivity effects). Products include:
Etrafon 3115
Trilafon 3160

Polythiazide (Possible photosensitivity effects). Products include:
Minizide Capsules 2700
Renese Tablets 2712

Prochlorperazine (Possible photosensitivity effects). Products include:
Compazine 1505

Promethazine Hydrochloride (Possible photosensitivity effects). Products include:
Mepergan Injection 3539
Phenergan Injection 3553
Phenergan 3556
Phenergan Syrup 3554
Phenergan with Codeine Syrup 3557
Phenergan with Dextromethorphan Syrup 3559
Phenergan VC Syrup 3560
Phenergan VC with Codeine Syrup 3561

Sulfacytine (Possible photosensitivity effects).
No products indexed under this heading.

Sulfamethizole (Possible photosensitivity effects). Products include:
Urobiotic-250 Capsules 2731

Sulfamethoxazole (Possible photosensitivity effects). Products include:
Bactrim 2949
Septra Suspension 2265
Septra Tablets 2265
Septra DS Tablets 2265

Sulfasalazine (Possible photosensitivity effects). Products include:
Azulfidine EN-tabs Tablets 2775

Sulfinpyrazone (Possible photosensitivity effects).
No products indexed under this heading.

Sulfisoxazole (Possible photosensitivity effects).
No products indexed under this heading.

Sulfisoxazole Acetyl (Possible photosensitivity effects). Products include:
Pediazole Suspension 3050

Sulfisoxazole Diolamine (Possible photosensitivity effects).
No products indexed under this heading.

Tetracycline Hydrochloride (Possible photosensitivity effects).
No products indexed under this heading.

Thioridazine Hydrochloride (Possible photosensitivity effects). Products include:
Thioridazine Hydrochloride Tablets 2289

Tolazamide (Possible photosensitivity effects).
No products indexed under this heading.

Tolbutamide (Possible photosensitivity effects).
No products indexed under this heading.

Trifluoperazine Hydrochloride (Possible photosensitivity effects). Products include:
Stelazine 1640

OXYCONTIN TABLETS

(Oxycodone Hydrochloride) 2912

May interact with central nervous system depressants, general anesthetics, hypnotics and sedatives, mixed agonist/antagonist opioid analgesics, phenothiazines, tranquilizers, and certain other agents. Compounds in these categories include:

Alfentanil Hydrochloride (Concurrent use with the usual dose of OxyContin may result in respiratory depression, profound sedation or coma; reduced dosage (1/3 to 1/2 of the usual dosage) may be necessary).
No products indexed under this heading.

Alprazolam (Concurrent use with the usual dose of OxyContin may result in respiratory depression, profound sedation or coma; reduced dosage (1/3 to 1/2 of the usual dosage) may be necessary). Products include:
Xanax Tablets 2865

Aprobarbital (Concurrent use with the usual dose of OxyContin may result in respiratory depression, profound sedation or coma; reduced dosage (1/3 to 1/2 of the usual dosage) may be necessary).
No products indexed under this heading.

Buprenorphine Hydrochloride (Mixed agonist/antagonist analgesics may reduce the analgesic effect of oxycodone and/or may precipitate withdrawal symptoms). Products include:
Buprenex Injectable 2918

Buspirone Hydrochloride (Concurrent use with the usual dose of OxyContin may result in respiratory depression, profound sedation or coma; reduced dosage (1/3 to 1/2 of the usual dosage) may be necessary).
No products indexed under this heading.

Butabarbital (Concurrent use with the usual dose of OxyContin may result in respiratory depression, profound sedation or coma; reduced dosage (1/3 to 1/2 of the usual dosage) may be necessary).
No products indexed under this heading.

Butalbital (Concurrent use with the usual dose of OxyContin may result in respiratory depression, profound sedation or coma; reduced dosage (1/3 to 1/2 of the usual dosage) may be necessary). Products include:
Phrenilin 578
Sedapap Tablets 50 mg/650 mg 2225

Butorphanol Tartrate (Mixed agonist/antagonist analgesics may reduce the analgesic effect of oxycodone and/or may precipitate withdrawal symptoms). Products include:
Stadol NS Nasal Spray 1108

Chlordiazepoxide (Concurrent use with the usual dose of OxyContin may result in respiratory depression, profound sedation or coma; reduced dosage (1/3 to 1/2 of the usual dosage) may be necessary). Products include:
Limbitrol 1738

Chlordiazepoxide Hydrochloride (Concurrent use with the usual dose of OxyContin may result in respiratory depression, profound sedation or coma; reduced dosage (1/3 to 1/2 of the usual dosage) may be necessary). Products include:
Librium Capsules 1736
Librium for Injection 1737

Chlorpromazine (Concurrent use with the usual dose of OxyContin may result in respiratory depression, profound sedation or coma; reduced dosage (1/3 to 1/2 of the usual dosage) may be necessary). Products include:
Thorazine Suppositories 1656

Chlorpromazine Hydrochloride (Concurrent use with the usual dose of OxyContin may result in respiratory depression, profound sedation or coma; reduced dosage (1/3 to 1/2 of the usual dosage) may be necessary). Products include:
Thorazine 1656

Chlorprothixene (Concurrent use with the usual dose of OxyContin may result in respiratory depression, profound sedation or coma; reduced dosage (1/3 to 1/2 of the usual dosage) may be necessary).
No products indexed under this heading.

Chlorprothixene Hydrochloride (Concurrent use with the usual dose of OxyContin may result in respiratory depression, profound sedation or coma; reduced dosage (1/3 to 1/2 of the usual dosage) may be necessary).
No products indexed under this heading.

Chlorprothixene Lactate (Concurrent use with the usual dose of OxyContin may result in respiratory depression, profound sedation or coma; reduced dosage (1/3 to 1/2 of the usual dosage) may be necessary).
No products indexed under this heading.

Clorazepate Dipotassium (Concurrent use with the usual dose of OxyContin may result in respiratory depression, profound sedation or coma; reduced dosage (1/3 to 1/2 of the usual dosage) may be necessary). Products include:
Tranxene 511

Clozapine (Concurrent use with the usual dose of OxyContin may result in respiratory depression, profound sedation or coma; reduced dosage (1/3 to 1/2 of the usual dosage) may be necessary). Products include:
Clozaril Tablets 2319

Codeine Phosphate (Concurrent use with the usual dose of OxyContin may result in respiratory depression, profound sedation or coma; reduced dosage (1/3 to 1/2 of the usual dosage) may be necessary). Products include:
Phenergan with Codeine Syrup 3557
Phenergan VC with Codeine Syrup 3561

Robitussin A-C Syrup 2942
Robitussin-DAC Syrup 2942
Ryna-C Liquid 768
Soma Compound w/Codeine Tablets 3355
Tussi-Organidin NR Liquid 3350
Tussi-Organidin-S NR Liquid 3350
Tylenol with Codeine 2595

Desflurane (Concurrent use with the usual dose of OxyContin may result in respiratory depression, profound sedation or coma; reduced dosage (1/3 to 1/2 of the usual dosage) may be necessary). Products include:
Suprane Liquid for Inhalation 874

Dezocine (Concurrent use with the usual dose of OxyContin may result in respiratory depression, profound sedation or coma; reduced dosage (1/3 to 1/2 of the usual dosage) may be necessary).
No products indexed under this heading.

Diazepam (Concurrent use with the usual dose of OxyContin may result in respiratory depression, profound sedation or coma; reduced dosage (1/3 to 1/2 of the usual dosage) may be necessary). Products include:
Valium Injectable 3026
Valium Tablets 3047

Droperidol (Concurrent use with the usual dose of OxyContin may result in respiratory depression, profound sedation or coma; reduced dosage (1/3 to 1/2 of the usual dosage) may be necessary).
No products indexed under this heading.

Enflurane (Concurrent use with the usual dose of OxyContin may result in respiratory depression, profound sedation or coma; reduced dosage (1/3 to 1/2 of the usual dosage) may be necessary).
No products indexed under this heading.

Estazolam (Concurrent use with the usual dose of OxyContin may result in respiratory depression, profound sedation or coma; reduced dosage (1/3 to 1/2 of the usual dosage) may be necessary). Products include:
ProSom Tablets 500

Ethchlorvynol (Concurrent use with the usual dose of OxyContin may result in respiratory depression, profound sedation or coma; reduced dosage (1/3 to 1/2 of the usual dosage) may be necessary).
No products indexed under this heading.

Ethinamate (Concurrent use with the usual dose of OxyContin may result in respiratory depression, profound sedation or coma; reduced dosage (1/3 to 1/2 of the usual dosage) may be necessary).
No products indexed under this heading.

Fentanyl (Concurrent use with the usual dose of OxyContin may result in respiratory depression, profound sedation or coma; reduced dosage (1/3 to 1/2 of the usual dosage) may be necessary). Products include:
Duragesic Transdermal System 1786

Fentanyl Citrate (Concurrent use with the usual dose of OxyContin may result in respiratory depression, profound sedation or coma; reduced dosage (1/3 to 1/2 of the usual dosage) may be necessary). Products include:
Actiq 1184

Fluphenazine Decanoate (Concurrent use with the usual dose of OxyContin may result in respiratory depression, profound sedation or coma; reduced dosage (1/3 to 1/2 of the usual dosage) may be necessary).
No products indexed under this heading.

Fluphenazine Enanthate (Concurrent use with the usual dose of OxyContin may result in respiratory depression, profound sedation or coma; reduced dosage (1/3 to 1/2 of the usual dosage) may be necessary).
No products indexed under this heading.

Fluphenazine Hydrochloride (Concurrent use with the usual dose of OxyContin may result in respiratory depression, profound sedation or coma; reduced dosage (1/3 to 1/2 of the usual dosage) may be necessary).
No products indexed under this heading.

Flurazepam Hydrochloride (Concurrent use with the usual dose of OxyContin may result in respiratory depression, profound sedation or coma; reduced dosage (1/3 to 1/2 of the usual dosage) may be necessary).
No products indexed under this heading.

Glutethimide (Concurrent use with the usual dose of OxyContin may result in respiratory depression, profound sedation or coma; reduced dosage (1/3 to 1/2 of the usual dosage) may be necessary).
No products indexed under this heading.

Haloperidol (Concurrent use with the usual dose of OxyContin may result in respiratory depression, profound sedation or coma; reduced dosage (1/3 to 1/2 of the usual dosage) may be necessary). Products include:
Haldol Injection, Tablets and Concentrate 2533

Haloperidol Decanoate (Concurrent use with the usual dose of OxyContin may result in respiratory depression, profound sedation or coma; reduced dosage (1/3 to 1/2 of the usual dosage) may be necessary). Products include:
Haldol Decanoate 2535

Hydrocodone Bitartrate (Concurrent use with the usual dose of OxyContin may result in respiratory depression, profound sedation or coma; reduced dosage (1/3 to 1/2 of the usual dosage) may be necessary). Products include:
Hycodan 1316
Hycomine Compound Tablets 1317
Hycotuss Expectorant Syrup 1318
Lortab 3319
Lortab Elixir 3317
Maxidone Tablets CIII 3399
Norco 5/325 Tablets CIII 3424
Norco 7.5/325 Tablets CIII 3425
Norco 10/325 Tablets CIII 3427
Norco 10/325 Tablets CIII 3425
Vicodin Tablets 516
Vicodin ES Tablets 517
Vicodin HP Tablets 518
Vicodin Tuss Expectorant 519
Vicoprofen Tablets 520
Zydone Tablets 1330

Hydrocodone Polistirex (Concurrent use with the usual dose of OxyContin may result in respiratory depression, profound sedation or coma; reduced dosage (1/3 to 1/2 of the usual dosage) may be necessary). Products include:
Tussionex Pennkinetic Extended-Release Suspension 1174

Hydromorphone Hydrochloride (Concurrent use with the usual dose of OxyContin may result in respiratory depression, profound sedation or coma; reduced dosage (1/3 to 1/2 of the usual dosage) may be necessary). Products include:
Dilaudid 441
Dilaudid Oral Liquid 445
Dilaudid Powder 441
Dilaudid Rectal Suppositories 441
Dilaudid Tablets 441
Dilaudid Tablets - 8 mg 445
Dilaudid-HP 443

Hydroxyzine Hydrochloride (Concurrent use with the usual dose of OxyContin may result in respiratory depression, profound sedation or coma; reduced dosage (1/3 to 1/2 of the usual dosage) may be necessary). Products include:
Atarax Tablets & Syrup 2667
Vistaril Intramuscular Solution 2738

Isoflurane (Concurrent use with the usual dose of OxyContin may result in respiratory depression, profound sedation or coma; reduced dosage (1/3 to 1/2 of the usual dosage) may be necessary).
No products indexed under this heading.

Ketamine Hydrochloride (Concurrent use with the usual dose of OxyContin may result in respiratory depression, profound sedation or coma; reduced dosage (1/3 to 1/2 of the usual dosage) may be necessary).
No products indexed under this heading.

Levomethadyl Acetate Hydrochloride (Concurrent use with the usual dose of OxyContin may result in respiratory depression, profound sedation or coma; reduced dosage (1/3 to 1/2 of the usual dosage) may be necessary).
No products indexed under this heading.

Levorphanol Tartrate (Concurrent use with the usual dose of OxyContin may result in respiratory depression, profound sedation or coma; reduced dosage (1/3 to 1/2 of the usual dosage) may be necessary). Products include:
Levo-Dromoran 1734
Levorphanol Tartrate Tablets 3059

Lorazepam (Concurrent use with the usual dose of OxyContin may result in respiratory depression, profound sedation or coma; reduced dosage (1/3 to 1/2 of the usual dosage) may be necessary). Products include:
Ativan Injection 3478
Ativan Tablets 3482

Loxapine Hydrochloride (Concurrent use with the usual dose of OxyContin may result in respiratory depression, profound sedation or coma; reduced dosage (1/3 to 1/2 of the usual dosage) may be necessary).
No products indexed under this heading.

Loxapine Succinate (Concurrent use with the usual dose of OxyContin may result in respiratory depression, profound sedation or coma; reduced dosage (1/3 to 1/2 of the usual dosage) may be necessary). Products include:
Loxitane Capsules 3398

Meperidine Hydrochloride (Concurrent use with the usual dose of OxyContin may result in respiratory depression, profound sedation or coma; reduced dosage (1/3 to 1/2 of the usual dosage) may be necessary). Products include:
Demerol 3079
Mepergan Injection 3539

Mephobarbital (Concurrent use with the usual dose of OxyContin may result in respiratory depression, profound sedation or coma; reduced dosage (1/3 to 1/2 of the usual dosage) may be necessary).
No products indexed under this heading.

Meprobamate (Concurrent use with the usual dose of OxyContin may result in respiratory depression, profound sedation or coma; reduced dosage (1/3 to 1/2 of the usual dosage) may be necessary). Products include:
Miltown Tablets 3349

Mesoridazine Besylate (Concurrent use with the usual dose of OxyContin may result in respiratory depression, profound sedation or coma; reduced dosage (1/3 to 1/2 of the usual dosage) may be necessary). Products include:
Serentil 1057

Methadone Hydrochloride (Concurrent use with the usual dose of OxyContin may result in respiratory depression, profound sedation or coma; reduced dosage (1/3 to 1/2 of the usual dosage) may be necessary). Products include:
Dolophine Hydrochloride Tablets 3056

Methohexital Sodium (Concurrent use with the usual dose of OxyContin may result in respiratory depression, profound sedation or coma; reduced dosage (1/3 to 1/2 of the usual dosage) may be necessary). Products include:
Brevital Sodium for Injection, USP .. 1815

Methotrimeprazine (Concurrent use with the usual dose of OxyContin may result in respiratory depression, profound sedation or coma; reduced dosage (1/3 to 1/2 of the usual dosage) may be necessary).
No products indexed under this heading.

Methoxyflurane (Concurrent use with the usual dose of OxyContin may result in respiratory depression, profound sedation or coma; reduced dosage (1/3 to 1/2 of the usual dosage) may be necessary).
No products indexed under this heading.

Midazolam Hydrochloride (Concurrent use with the usual dose of OxyContin may result in respiratory depression, profound sedation or coma; reduced dosage (1/3 to 1/2 of the usual dosage) may be necessary). Products include:
Versed Injection 3027
Versed Syrup 3033

Molindone Hydrochloride (Concurrent use with the usual dose of OxyContin may result in respiratory depression, profound sedation or coma; reduced dosage (1/3 to 1/2 of the usual dosage) may be necessary). Products include:
Moban 1320

Morphine Sulfate (Concurrent use with the usual dose of OxyContin may result in respiratory depression, profound sedation or coma; reduced dosage (1/3 to 1/2 of the usual dosage) may be necessary). Products include:
Astramorph/PF Injection, USP (Preservative-Free) 594
Duramorph Injection 1312
Infumorph 200 and Infumorph 500 Sterile Solutions 1314
Kadian Capsules 1335
MS Contin Tablets 2896
MSIR 2898
Oramorph SR Tablets 3062
Roxanol 3066

Nalbuphine Hydrochloride (Mixed agonist/antagonist analgesics may reduce the analgesic effect of oxycodone and/or may precipitate withdrawal symptoms). Products include:
Nubain Injection 1323

Olanzapine (Concurrent use with the usual dose of OxyContin may result in respiratory depression, profound sedation or coma; reduced dosage (1/3 to 1/2 of the usual dosage) may be necessary). Products include:
Zyprexa Tablets 1973
Zyprexa ZYDIS Orally Disintegrating Tablets 1973

Oxazepam (Concurrent use with the usual dose of OxyContin may result in respiratory depression, profound sedation or coma; reduced dosage (1/3 to 1/2 of the usual dosage) may be necessary).
No products indexed under this heading.

Pentazocine Hydrochloride (Mixed agonist/antagonist analgesics may reduce the analgesic effect of oxycodone and/or may precipitate withdrawal symptoms). Products include:
Talacen Caplets 3089
Talwin Nx Tablets 3090

Pentazocine Lactate (Mixed agonist/antagonist analgesics may reduce the analgesic effect of oxycodone and/or may precipitate withdrawal symptoms).
No products indexed under this heading.

Pentobarbital Sodium (Concurrent use with the usual dose of OxyContin may result in respiratory depression, profound sedation or coma; reduced dosage (1/3 to 1/2 of the usual dosage) may be necessary). Products include:
Nembutal Sodium Solution 485

Perphenazine (Concurrent use with the usual dose of OxyContin may result in respiratory depression, profound sedation or coma; reduced dosage (1/3 to 1/2 of the usual dosage) may be necessary). Products include:
Etrafon 3115
Trilafon 3160

Phenobarbital (Concurrent use with the usual dose of OxyContin may result in respiratory depression, profound sedation or coma; reduced dosage (1/3 to 1/2 of the usual dosage) may be necessary). Products include:
Arco-Lase Plus Tablets 592
Donnatal 2929
Donnatal Extentabs 2930

Prazepam (Concurrent use with the usual dose of OxyContin may result in respiratory depression, profound sedation or coma; reduced dosage (1/3 to 1/2 of the usual dosage) may be necessary).
No products indexed under this heading.

Prochlorperazine (Concurrent use with the usual dose of OxyContin may result in respiratory depression, profound sedation or coma; reduced dosage (1/3 to 1/2 of the usual dosage) may be necessary). Products include:
Compazine 1505

Promethazine Hydrochloride (Concurrent use with the usual dose of OxyContin may result in respiratory depression, profound sedation or coma; reduced dosage (1/3 to 1/2 of the usual dosage) may be necessary). Products include:
Mepergan Injection 3539
Phenergan Injection 3553
Phenergan 3556
Phenergan Syrup 3554
Phenergan with Codeine Syrup 3557
Phenergan with Dextromethorphan Syrup 3559
Phenergan VC Syrup 3560
Phenergan VC with Codeine Syrup .. 3561

Propofol (Concurrent use with the usual dose of OxyContin may result in respiratory depression, profound sedation or coma; reduced dosage (1/3 to 1/2 of the usual dosage) may be necessary). Products include:
Diprivan Injectable Emulsion 667

Propoxyphene Hydrochloride (Concurrent use with the usual dose of OxyContin may result in respiratory depression, profound sedation or coma; reduced dosage (1/3 to 1/2 of the usual dosage) may be necessary). Products include:
Darvon Pulvules 1909
Darvon Compound-65 Pulvules 1910

Propoxyphene Napsylate (Concurrent use with the usual dose of OxyContin may result in respiratory depression, profound sedation or coma; reduced dosage (1/3 to 1/2 of the usual dosage) may be necessary). Products include:
Darvon-N/Darvocet-N 1907
Darvon-N Tablets 1912

Quazepam (Concurrent use with the usual dose of OxyContin may result in respiratory depression, profound sedation or coma; reduced dosage (1/3 to 1/2 of the usual dosage) may be necessary).
No products indexed under this heading.

Quetiapine Fumarate (Concurrent use with the usual dose of OxyContin may result in respiratory depression, profound sedation or coma; reduced dosage (1/3 to 1/2 of the usual dosage) may be necessary). Products include:
Seroquel Tablets 684

Remifentanil Hydrochloride (Concurrent use with the usual dose of OxyContin may result in respiratory depression, profound sedation or coma; reduced dosage (1/3 to 1/2 of the usual dosage) may be necessary).
No products indexed under this heading.

Risperidone (Concurrent use with the usual dose of OxyContin may result in respiratory depression, profound sedation or coma; reduced dosage (1/3 to 1/2 of the usual dosage) may be necessary). Products include:
Risperdal 1796

Secobarbital Sodium (Concurrent use with the usual dose of OxyContin may result in respiratory depression, profound sedation or coma; reduced dosage (1/3 to 1/2 of the usual dosage) may be necessary).
No products indexed under this heading.

Sevoflurane (Concurrent use with the usual dose of OxyContin may result in respiratory depression, profound sedation or coma; reduced dosage (1/3 to 1/2 of the usual dosage) may be necessary).
No products indexed under this heading.

Sufentanil Citrate (Concurrent use with the usual dose of OxyContin may result in respiratory depression, profound sedation or coma; reduced dosage (1/3 to 1/2 of the usual dosage) may be necessary).
No products indexed under this heading.

Temazepam (Concurrent use with the usual dose of OxyContin may result in respiratory depression, profound sedation or coma; reduced dosage (1/3 to 1/2 of the usual dosage) may be necessary).
No products indexed under this heading.

Thiamylal Sodium (Concurrent use with the usual dose of OxyContin may result in respiratory depression, profound sedation or coma; reduced dosage (1/3 to 1/2 of the usual dosage) may be necessary).
No products indexed under this heading.

Thioridazine Hydrochloride (Concurrent use with the usual dose of OxyContin may result in respiratory depression, profound sedation or coma; reduced dosage (1/3 to 1/2 of the usual dosage) may be necessary). Products include:
Thioridazine Hydrochloride Tablets 2289

Thiothixene (Concurrent use with the usual dose of OxyContin may result in respiratory depression, profound sedation or coma; reduced dosage (1/3 to 1/2 of the usual dosage) may be necessary). Products include:
Navane Capsules 2701
Thiothixene Capsules 2290

Triazolam (Concurrent use with the usual dose of OxyContin may result in respiratory depression, profound sedation or coma; reduced dosage (1/3 to 1/2 of the usual dosage) may be necessary). Products include:
Halcion Tablets 2823

Trifluoperazine Hydrochloride (Concurrent use with the usual dose of OxyContin may result in respiratory depression, profound sedation or coma; reduced dosage (1/3 to 1/2 of the usual dosage) may be necessary). Products include:
Stelazine 1640

Zaleplon (Concurrent use with the usual dose of OxyContin may result in respiratory depression, profound sedation or coma; reduced dosage (1/3 to 1/2 of the usual dosage) may be necessary). Products include:
Sonata Capsules 3591

Ziprasidone Hydrochloride (Concurrent use with the usual dose of OxyContin may result in respiratory depression, profound sedation or coma; reduced dosage (1/3 to 1/2 of the usual dosage) may be necessary). Products include:
Geodon Capsules 2688

Zolpidem Tartrate (Concurrent use with the usual dose of OxyContin may result in respiratory depression, profound sedation or coma; reduced dosage (1/3 to 1/2 of the usual dosage) may be necessary). Products include:
Ambien Tablets 3191

Food Interactions

Alcohol (Concurrent use with the usual dose of OxyContin may result in respiratory depression, profound sedation or coma).

OXYFAST ORAL CONCENTRATE SOLUTION

(Oxycodone Hydrochloride) 2916
See OxyIR Capsules

OXYIR CAPSULES

(Oxycodone Hydrochloride) 2916
May interact with central nervous system depressants, general anesthetics, hypnotics and sedatives, mixed agonist/antagonist opioid analgesics, narcotic analgesics, phenothiazines, tranquilizers, and certain other agents. Compounds in these categories include:

Alfentanil Hydrochloride (Concomitant use may exhibit an additive CNS depression).
No products indexed under this heading.

Alprazolam (Concomitant use may exhibit an additive CNS depression). Products include:
Xanax Tablets 2865

Aprobarbital (Concomitant use may exhibit an additive CNS depression).
No products indexed under this heading.

Buprenorphine Hydrochloride (Co-administration with mixed agonist/antagonist analgesics may reduce the analgesic effect of oxycodone and/or may precipitate withdrawal symptoms). Products include:
Buprenex Injectable 2918

Buspirone Hydrochloride (Concomitant use may exhibit an additive CNS depression).
No products indexed under this heading.

Butabarbital (Concomitant use may exhibit an additive CNS depression).
No products indexed under this heading.

Butalbital (Concomitant use may exhibit an additive CNS depression). Products include:
Phrenilin 578
Sedapap Tablets 50 mg/650 mg ... 2225

Butorphanol Tartrate (Co-administration with mixed agonist/antagonist analgesics may reduce the analgesic effect of oxycodone and/or may precipitate withdrawal symptoms). Products include:
Stadol NS Nasal Spray 1108

Chlordiazepoxide (Concomitant use may exhibit an additive CNS depression). Products include:
Limbitrol 1738

Chlordiazepoxide Hydrochloride (Concomitant use may exhibit an additive CNS depression). Products include:
Librium Capsules 1736
Librium for Injection 1737

Chlorpromazine (Concomitant use may exhibit an additive CNS depression). Products include:
Thorazine Suppositories 1656

Chlorpromazine Hydrochloride (Concomitant use may exhibit an additive CNS depression). Products include:
Thorazine 1656

Chlorprothixene (Concomitant use may exhibit an additive CNS depression).
No products indexed under this heading.

Chlorprothixene Hydrochloride (Concomitant use may exhibit an additive CNS depression).
No products indexed under this heading.

Chlorprothixene Lactate (Concomitant use may exhibit an additive CNS depression).
No products indexed under this heading.

Clorazepate Dipotassium (Concomitant use may exhibit an additive CNS depression). Products include:
Tranxene 511

Clozapine (Concomitant use may exhibit an additive CNS depression). Products include:
Clozaril Tablets 2319

Codeine Phosphate (Concomitant use may exhibit an additive CNS depression). Products include:
Phenergan with Codeine Syrup 3557
Phenergan VC with Codeine Syrup .. 3561
Robitussin A-C Syrup 2942
Robitussin-DAC Syrup 2942
Ryna-C Liquid .... ▣768
Soma Compound w/Codeine Tablets 3355
Tussi-Organidin NR Liquid 3350
Tussi-Organidin-S NR Liquid 3350
Tylenol with Codeine 2595

Desflurane (Concomitant use may exhibit an additive CNS depression). Products include:
Suprane Liquid for Inhalation 874

Dezocine (Concomitant use may exhibit an additive CNS depression).
No products indexed under this heading.

Diazepam (Concomitant use may exhibit an additive CNS depression). Products include:
Valium Injectable 3026
Valium Tablets 3047

Droperidol (Concomitant use may exhibit an additive CNS depression).
No products indexed under this heading.

Enflurane (Concomitant use may exhibit an additive CNS depression).
No products indexed under this heading.

Estazolam (Concomitant use may exhibit an additive CNS depression). Products include:
ProSom Tablets 500

Ethchlorvynol (Concomitant use may exhibit an additive CNS depression).
No products indexed under this heading.

Ethinamate (Concomitant use may exhibit an additive CNS depression).
No products indexed under this heading.

Fentanyl (Concomitant use may exhibit an additive CNS depression). Products include:
Duragesic Transdermal System 1786

Fentanyl Citrate (Concomitant use may exhibit an additive CNS depression). Products include:
Actiq 1184

Fluphenazine Decanoate (Concomitant use may exhibit an additive CNS depression).
No products indexed under this heading.

Fluphenazine Enanthate (Concomitant use may exhibit an additive CNS depression).
No products indexed under this heading.

Fluphenazine Hydrochloride (Concomitant use may exhibit an additive CNS depression).
No products indexed under this heading.

Flurazepam Hydrochloride (Concomitant use may exhibit an additive CNS depression).
No products indexed under this heading.

Glutethimide (Concomitant use may exhibit an additive CNS depression).
No products indexed under this heading.

Haloperidol (Concomitant use may exhibit an additive CNS depression). Products include:
Haldol Injection, Tablets and Concentrate 2533

Haloperidol Decanoate (Concomitant use may exhibit an additive CNS depression). Products include:
Haldol Decanoate 2535

Hydrocodone Bitartrate (Concomitant use may exhibit an additive CNS depression). Products include:
Hycodan 1316
Hycomine Compound Tablets 1317
Hycotuss Expectorant Syrup 1318
Lortab 3319
Lortab Elixir 3317
Maxidone Tablets CIII 3399
Norco 5/325 Tablets CIII 3424
Norco 7.5/325 Tablets CIII 3425
Norco 10/325 Tablets CIII 3427
Norco 10/325 Tablets CIII 3425
Vicodin Tablets 516
Vicodin ES Tablets 517
Vicodin HP Tablets 518
Vicodin Tuss Expectorant 519
Vicoprofen Tablets 520
Zydone Tablets 1330

Hydrocodone Polistirex (Concomitant use may exhibit an additive CNS depression). Products include:
Tussionex Pennkinetic Extended-Release Suspension 1174

Hydromorphone Hydrochloride (Concomitant use may exhibit an additive CNS depression). Products include:
Dilaudid 441
Dilaudid Oral Liquid 445
Dilaudid Powder 441
Dilaudid Rectal Suppositories 441
Dilaudid Tablets 441
Dilaudid Tablets - 8 mg 445
Dilaudid-HP 443

Hydroxyzine Hydrochloride (Concomitant use may exhibit an additive CNS depression). Products include:
Atarax Tablets & Syrup 2667
Vistaril Intramuscular Solution 2738

Isoflurane (Concomitant use may exhibit an additive CNS depression).
No products indexed under this heading.

Ketamine Hydrochloride (Concomitant use may exhibit an additive CNS depression).
No products indexed under this heading.

Levomethadyl Acetate Hydrochloride (Concomitant use may exhibit an additive CNS depression).
No products indexed under this heading.

Levorphanol Tartrate (Concomitant use may exhibit an additive CNS depression). Products include:
Levo-Dromoran 1734
Levorphanol Tartrate Tablets 3059

Lorazepam (Concomitant use may exhibit an additive CNS depression). Products include:
Ativan Injection 3478
Ativan Tablets 3482

Loxapine Hydrochloride (Concomitant use may exhibit an additive CNS depression).
No products indexed under this heading.

Loxapine Succinate (Concomitant use may exhibit an additive CNS depression). Products include:
Loxitane Capsules 3398

Meperidine Hydrochloride (Concomitant use may exhibit an additive CNS depression). Products include:
Demerol 3079
Mepergan Injection 3539

Mephobarbital (Concomitant use may exhibit an additive CNS depression).
No products indexed under this heading.

Meprobamate (Concomitant use may exhibit an additive CNS depression). Products include:
Miltown Tablets 3349

Mesoridazine Besylate (Concomitant use may exhibit an additive CNS depression). Products include:
Serentil 1057

Methadone Hydrochloride (Concomitant use may exhibit an additive CNS depression). Products include:
Dolophine Hydrochloride Tablets 3056

Methohexital Sodium (Concomitant use may exhibit an additive CNS depression). Products include:
Brevital Sodium for Injection, USP 1815

Methotrimeprazine (Concomitant use may exhibit an additive CNS depression).
No products indexed under this heading.

Methoxyflurane (Concomitant use may exhibit an additive CNS depression).
No products indexed under this heading.

Midazolam Hydrochloride (Concomitant use may exhibit an additive CNS depression). Products include:
Versed Injection 3027
Versed Syrup 3033

Molindone Hydrochloride (Concomitant use may exhibit an additive CNS depression). Products include:
Moban 1320

Morphine Sulfate (Concomitant use may exhibit an additive CNS depression). Products include:
Astramorph/PF Injection, USP (Preservative-Free) 594
Duramorph Injection 1312
Infumorph 200 and Infumorph 500 Sterile Solutions 1314
Kadian Capsules 1335
MS Contin Tablets 2896
MSIR 2898
Oramorph SR Tablets 3062
Roxanol 3066

Nalbuphine Hydrochloride (Coadministration with mixed agonist/antagonist analgesics may reduce the analgesic effect of oxycodone and/or may precipitate withdrawal symptoms). Products include:
Nubain Injection 1323

Olanzapine (Concomitant use may exhibit an additive CNS depression). Products include:
Zyprexa Tablets 1973
Zyprexa ZYDIS Orally Disintegrating Tablets 1973

Oxazepam (Concomitant use may exhibit an additive CNS depression).
No products indexed under this heading.

Pentazocine Hydrochloride (Coadministration with mixed agonist/antagonist analgesics may reduce the analgesic effect of oxycodone and/or may precipitate withdrawal symptoms). Products include:
Talacen Caplets 3089
Talwin Nx Tablets 3090

Pentazocine Lactate (Coadministration with mixed agonist/antagonist analgesics may reduce the analgesic effect of oxycodone and/or may precipitate withdrawal symptoms).
No products indexed under this heading.

Pentobarbital Sodium (Concomitant use may exhibit an additive CNS depression). Products include:
Nembutal Sodium Solution 485

Perphenazine (Concomitant use may exhibit an additive CNS depression). Products include:
Etrafon 3115
Trilafon 3160

Phenobarbital (Concomitant use may exhibit an additive CNS depression). Products include:
Arco-Lase Plus Tablets 592
Donnatal 2929
Donnatal Extentabs 2930

Prazepam (Concomitant use may exhibit an additive CNS depression).
No products indexed under this heading.

Prochlorperazine (Concomitant use may exhibit an additive CNS depression). Products include:
Compazine 1505

Promethazine Hydrochloride (Concomitant use may exhibit an additive CNS depression). Products include:
Mepergan Injection 3539
Phenergan Injection 3553
Phenergan 3556
Phenergan Syrup 3554
Phenergan with Codeine Syrup 3557
Phenergan with Dextromethorphan Syrup 3559
Phenergan VC Syrup 3560
Phenergan VC with Codeine Syrup 3561

Propofol (Concomitant use may exhibit an additive CNS depression). Products include:
Diprivan Injectable Emulsion 667

Propoxyphene Hydrochloride (Concomitant use may exhibit an additive CNS depression). Products include:
Darvon Pulvules 1909
Darvon Compound-65 Pulvules 1910

Propoxyphene Napsylate (Concomitant use may exhibit an additive CNS depression). Products include:
Darvon-N/Darvocet-N 1907
Darvon-N Tablets 1912

Quazepam (Concomitant use may exhibit an additive CNS depression).
No products indexed under this heading.

Quetiapine Fumarate (Concomitant use may exhibit an additive CNS depression). Products include:
Seroquel Tablets 684

Remifentanil Hydrochloride (Concomitant use may exhibit an additive CNS depression).
No products indexed under this heading.

Risperidone (Concomitant use may exhibit an additive CNS depression). Products include:
Risperdal 1796

Secobarbital Sodium (Concomitant use may exhibit an additive CNS depression).
No products indexed under this heading.

Sevoflurane (Concomitant use may exhibit an additive CNS depression).
No products indexed under this heading.

Sufentanil Citrate (Concomitant use may exhibit an additive CNS depression).
No products indexed under this heading.

Temazepam (Concomitant use may exhibit an additive CNS depression).
No products indexed under this heading.

Thiamylal Sodium (Concomitant use may exhibit an additive CNS depression).
No products indexed under this heading.

Thioridazine Hydrochloride (Concomitant use may exhibit an additive CNS depression). Products include:
Thioridazine Hydrochloride Tablets 2289

Thiothixene (Concomitant use may exhibit an additive CNS depression). Products include:
Navane Capsules 2701
Thiothixene Capsules 2290

Triazolam (Concomitant use may exhibit an additive CNS depression). Products include:
Halcion Tablets 2823

Trifluoperazine Hydrochloride (Concomitant use may exhibit an additive CNS depression). Products include:
Stelazine 1640

Zaleplon (Concomitant use may exhibit an additive CNS depression). Products include:
Sonata Capsules 3591

Ziprasidone Hydrochloride (Concomitant use may exhibit an additive CNS depression). Products include:
Geodon Capsules 2688

Zolpidem Tartrate (Concomitant use may exhibit an additive CNS depression). Products include:
Ambien Tablets 3191

Food Interactions

Alcohol (Concomitant use may exhibit an additive CNS depression).

PACERONE TABLETS

(Amiodarone Hydrochloride) 3331
May interact with beta blockers, calcium channel blockers, oral anticoagulants, cardiac glycosides, phenytoin, quinidine, and certain other agents. Compounds in these categories include:

Acebutolol Hydrochloride (Possible potentiation of bradycardia, sinus arrest, and AV block when co-administered with beta-blocking agents). Products include:
Sectral Capsules 3589

Amlodipine Besylate (Possible potentiation of bradycardia, sinus arrest, and AV block when co-administered with calcium antagonists). Products include:
Lotrel Capsules 2370
Norvasc Tablets 2704

Atenolol (Possible potentiation of bradycardia, sinus arrest, and AV block when co-administered with beta-blocking agents). Products include:
Tenoretic Tablets 690
Tenormin I.V. Injection 692

Bepridil Hydrochloride (Possible potentiation of bradycardia, sinus

arrest, and AV block when co-administered with calcium antagonists). Products include:
Vascor Tablets 2602

Betaxolol Hydrochloride (Possible potentiation of bradycardia, sinus arrest, and AV block when co-administered with beta-blocking agents). Products include:
Betoptic S Ophthalmic Suspension.............................. 537

Bisoprolol Fumarate (Possible potentiation of bradycardia, sinus arrest, and AV block when co-administered with beta-blocking agents). Products include:
Zebeta Tablets 1885
Ziac Tablets 1887

Carteolol Hydrochloride (Possible potentiation of bradycardia, sinus arrest, and AV block when co-administered with beta-blocking agents). Products include:
Carteolol Hydrochloride Ophthalmic Solution USP, 1% ..... ⊙258
Ocupress Ophthalmic Solution, 1% Sterile .... ⊙303

Cyclosporine (Co-administration has been reported to produce persistently elevated plasma concentrations of cyclosporine resulting in elevated creatinine, despite reduction in dose of cyclosporine). Products include:
Gengraf Capsules 457
Neoral Soft Gelatin Capsules 2380
Neoral Oral Solution 2380
Sandimmune 2388

Deslanoside (Co-administration of amiodarone to patients receiving digitalis therapy regularly results in an increase in the serum digoxin concentration that may reach toxic levels with resultant toxicity).
No products indexed under this heading.

Dicumarol (Co-administration results in potentiation of warfarin-type anticoagulant response and can result in serious bleeding).
No products indexed under this heading.

Digitoxin (Co-administration of amiodarone to patients receiving digitalis therapy regularly results in an increase in the serum digoxin concentration that may reach toxic levels with resultant toxicity).
No products indexed under this heading.

Digoxin (Co-administration of amiodarone to patients receiving digitalis therapy regularly results in an increase in the serum digoxin concentration that may reach toxic levels with resultant toxicity). Products include:
Digitek Tablets 1003
Lanoxicaps Capsules 1574
Lanoxin Injection 1581
Lanoxin Tablets 1587
Lanoxin Elixir Pediatric 1578
Lanoxin Injection Pediatric 1584

Diltiazem Hydrochloride (Possible potentiation of bradycardia, sinus arrest, and AV block when co-administered with calcium antagonists). Products include:
Cardizem Injectable 1018
Cardizem Lyo-Ject Syringe 1018
Cardizem Monovial 1018
Cardizem CD Capsules 1016
Tiazac Capsules 1378

Esmolol Hydrochloride (Possible potentiation of bradycardia, sinus arrest, and AV block when co-administered with beta-blocking agents). Products include:
Brevibloc Injection 858

Felodipine (Possible potentiation of bradycardia, sinus arrest, and AV block when co-administered with calcium antagonists). Products include:
Lexxel Tablets 608
Plendil Extended-Release Tablets ... 623

Fosphenytoin Sodium (Co-administration has resulted in increased steady-state levels of phenytoin). Products include:
Cerebyx Injection 2619

Isradipine (Possible potentiation of bradycardia, sinus arrest, and AV block when co-administered with calcium antagonists). Products include:
DynaCirc Capsules 2921
DynaCirc CR Tablets 2923

Labetalol Hydrochloride (Possible potentiation of bradycardia, sinus arrest, and AV block when co-administered with beta-blocking agents). Products include:
Normodyne Injection 3135
Normodyne Tablets 3137

Levobunolol Hydrochloride (Possible potentiation of bradycardia, sinus arrest, and AV block when co-administered with beta-blocking agents). Products include:
Betagan .... ⊙228

Metipranolol Hydrochloride (Possible potentiation of bradycardia, sinus arrest, and AV block when co-administered with beta-blocking agents).
No products indexed under this heading.

Metoprolol Succinate (Possible potentiation of bradycardia, sinus arrest, and AV block when co-administered with beta-blocking agents). Products include:
Toprol-XL Tablets 651

Metoprolol Tartrate (Possible potentiation of bradycardia, sinus arrest, and AV block when co-administered with beta-blocking agents).
No products indexed under this heading.

Mibefradil Dihydrochloride (Possible potentiation of bradycardia, sinus arrest, and AV block when co-administered with calcium antagonists).
No products indexed under this heading.

Nadolol (Possible potentiation of bradycardia, sinus arrest, and AV block when co-administered with beta-blocking agents). Products include:
Corgard Tablets 2245
Corzide 40/5 Tablets 2247
Corzide 80/5 Tablets 2247
Nadolol Tablets 2288

Nicardipine Hydrochloride (Possible potentiation of bradycardia, sinus arrest, and AV block when co-administered with calcium antagonists). Products include:
Cardene I.V. 3485

Nifedipine (Possible potentiation of bradycardia, sinus arrest, and AV block when co-administered with calcium antagonists). Products include:
Adalat CC Tablets 877
Procardia Capsules 2708
Procardia XL Extended Release Tablets 2710

Nimodipine (Possible potentiation of bradycardia, sinus arrest, and AV block when co-administered with calcium antagonists). Products include:
Nimotop Capsules 904

Nisoldipine (Possible potentiation of bradycardia, sinus arrest, and AV block when co-administered with calcium antagonists). Products include:
Sular Tablets 688

Penbutolol Sulfate (Possible potentiation of bradycardia, sinus arrest, and AV block when co-administered with beta-blocking agents).
No products indexed under this heading.

Phenytoin (Co-administration has resulted in increased steady-state levels of phenytoin). Products include:
Dilantin Infatabs 2624
Dilantin-125 Oral Suspension 2625

Phenytoin Sodium (Co-administration has resulted in increased steady-state levels of phenytoin). Products include:
Dilantin Kapseals 2622

Pindolol (Possible potentiation of bradycardia, sinus arrest, and AV block when co-administered with beta-blocking agents).
No products indexed under this heading.

Procainamide Hydrochloride (Co-administration has resulted in increased plasma concentration by 55% and NAPA concentration by 33%; dose of procainamide should be reduced by 13%). Products include:
Procanbid Extended-Release Tablets 2262

Propranolol Hydrochloride (Possible potentiation of bradycardia, sinus arrest, and AV block when co-administered with beta-blocking agents). Products include:
Inderal 3513
Inderal LA Long-Acting Capsules 3516
Inderide Tablets 3517
Inderide LA Long-Acting Capsules .. 3519

Quinidine Gluconate (Co-administration has resulted in increased serum concentration by 33%; dose of quinidine should be reduced by 1/3 to 1/2). Products include:
Quinaglute Dura-Tabs Tablets 978

Quinidine Polygalacturonate (Co-administration has resulted in increased serum concentration by 33%; dose of quinidine should be reduced by 1/3 to 1/2).
No products indexed under this heading.

Quinidine Sulfate (Co-administration has resulted in increased serum concentration by 33%; dose of quinidine should be reduced by 1/3 to 1/2). Products include:
Quinidex Extentabs 2933

Sotalol Hydrochloride (Possible potentiation of bradycardia, sinus arrest, and AV block when co-administered with beta-blocking agents). Products include:
Betapace Tablets 950
Betapace AF Tablets 954

Timolol Hemihydrate (Possible potentiation of bradycardia, sinus arrest, and AV block when co-administered with beta-blocking agents). Products include:
Betimol Ophthalmic Solution .... ⊙324

Timolol Maleate (Possible potentiation of bradycardia, sinus arrest, and AV block when co-administered with beta-blocking agents). Products include:
Blocadren Tablets 2046
Cosopt Sterile Ophthalmic Solution 2065
Timolide Tablets 2187
Timolol GFS .... ⊙266
Timoptic in Ocudose 2192
Timoptic Sterile Ophthalmic Solution 2190
Timoptic-XE Sterile Ophthalmic Gel Forming Solution 2194

Verapamil Hydrochloride (Possible potentiation of bradycardia, sinus arrest, and AV block when co-administered with calcium antagonists). Products include:
Covera-HS Tablets 3199
Isoptin SR Tablets 467
Tarka Tablets 508
Verelan Capsules 3184
Verelan PM Capsules 3186

Warfarin Sodium (Co-administration results in potentiation of warfarin-type anticoagulant response resulting in increased prothrombin time by 100%; dose of warfarin should be reduced by 1/3 to 1/2). Products include:
Coumadin for Injection 1243
Coumadin Tablets 1243
Warfarin Sodium Tablets, USP 3302

PANAFIL OINTMENT
(Chlorophyllin Copper Complex Sodium, Papain, Urea).............................. 1726
May interact with:

Heavy metal salts, unspecified (Papain may be inactivated by the salts of heavy metals).

Hydrogen Peroxide (May inactivate papain).
No products indexed under this heading.

PANCREASE CAPSULES
(Pancrelipase) 2580
None cited in PDR database.

PANCREASE MT CAPSULES
(Pancrelipase) 2581
None cited in PDR database.

PANHEMATIN FOR INJECTION
(Hemin) 497
May interact with barbiturates, oral anticoagulants, and estrogens. Compounds in these categories include:

Aprobarbital (Hemin inhibits the enzyme delta-aminolevulinic acid synthetase; concurrent use with drugs that increase the activity of delta-aminolevulinic acid synthetase, such as barbiturates, should be avoided).
No products indexed under this heading.

Butabarbital (Hemin inhibits the enzyme delta-aminolevulinic acid synthetase; concurrent use with drugs that increase the activity of delta-aminolevulinic acid synthetase, such as barbiturates, should be avoided).
No products indexed under this heading.

Butalbital (Hemin inhibits the enzyme delta-aminolevulinic acid synthetase; concurrent use with drugs that increase the activity of delta-aminolevulinic acid synthetase, such as barbiturates, should be avoided). Products include:
Phrenilin 578
Sedapap Tablets 50 mg/650 mg ... 2225

Chlorotrianisene (Hemin inhibits the enzyme delta-aminolevulinic acid synthetase; concurrent use with drugs that increase the activity of delta-aminolevulinic acid synthetase, such as estrogens, should be avoided).
No products indexed under this heading.

Dicumarol (Hemin exhibits transient, mild anticoagulant effects, therefore, concurrent anticoagulant therapy should be avoided).
No products indexed under this heading.

Dienestrol (Hemin inhibits the enzyme delta-aminolevulinic acid synthetase; concurrent use with drugs that increase the activity of delta-aminolevulinic acid synthetase, such as estrogens, should be avoided). Products include:
Ortho Dienestrol Cream 2554

Diethylstilbestrol (Hemin inhibits the enzyme delta-aminolevulinic acid synthetase; concurrent use with drugs that increase the activity of delta-aminolevulinic acid synthetase, such as estrogens, should be

avoided).
No products indexed under this heading.

Estradiol (Hemin inhibits the enzyme delta-aminolevulinic acid synthetase; concurrent use with drugs that increase the activity of delta-aminolevulinic acid synthetase, such as estrogens, should be avoided). Products include:
Activella Tablets 2764
Alora Transdermal System 3372
Climara Transdermal System 958
CombiPatch Transdermal System 2323
Esclim Transdermal System 3460
Estrace Vaginal Cream 3358
Estrace Tablets 3361
Estring Vaginal Ring 2811
Ortho-Prefest Tablets 2570
Vagifem Tablets 2857
Vivelle Transdermal System 2412
Vivelle-Dot Transdermal System 2416

Estrogens, Conjugated (Hemin inhibits the enzyme delta-aminolevulinic acid synthetase; concurrent use with drugs that increase the activity of delta-aminolevulinic acid synthetase, such as estrogens, should be avoided). Products include:
Premarin Intravenous 3563
Premarin Tablets 3566
Premarin Vaginal Cream 3570
Premphase Tablets 3572
Prempro Tablets 3572

Estrogens, Esterified (Hemin inhibits the enzyme delta-aminolevulinic acid synthetase; concurrent use with drugs that increase the activity of delta-aminolevulinic acid synthetase, such as estrogens, should be avoided). Products include:
Estratest 3252
Menest Tablets 2254

Estropipate (Hemin inhibits the enzyme delta-aminolevulinic acid synthetase; concurrent use with drugs that increase the activity of delta-aminolevulinic acid synthetase, such as estrogens, should be avoided). Products include:
Ogen Tablets 2846
Ortho-Est Tablets 3464

Ethinyl Estradiol (Hemin inhibits the enzyme delta-aminolevulinic acid synthetase; concurrent use with drugs that increase the activity of delta-aminolevulinic acid synthetase, such as estrogens, should be avoided). Products include:
Alesse-21 Tablets 3468
Alesse-28 Tablets 3473
Brevicon 28-Day Tablets 3380
Cyclessa Tablets 2450
Desogen Tablets 2458
Estinyl Tablets 3112
Estrostep 2627
femhrt Tablets 2635
Levlen 962
Levlite 21 Tablets 962
Levlite 28 Tablets 962
Levora Tablets 3389
Loestrin 21 Tablets 2642
Loestrin Fe Tablets 2642
Lo/Ovral Tablets 3532
Lo/Ovral-28 Tablets 3538
Low-Ogestrel-28 Tablets 3392
Microgestin Fe 1.5/30 Tablets 3407
Microgestin Fe 1/20 Tablets 3400
Mircette Tablets 2470
Modicon 2563
Necon 3415
Nordette-28 Tablets 2257
Norinyl 1 +35 28-Day Tablets 3380
Ogestrel 0.5/50-28 Tablets 3428
Ortho-Cept 21 Tablets 2546
Ortho-Cept 28 Tablets 2546
Ortho-Cyclen/Ortho Tri-Cyclen 2573
Ortho-Novum 2563
Ovcon 3364
Ovral Tablets 3551
Ovral-28 Tablets 3552
Tri-Levlen 962
Tri-Norinyl-28 Tablets 3433
Triphasil-21 Tablets 3600
Triphasil-28 Tablets 3605
Trivora Tablets 3439
Yasmin 28 Tablets 980
Zovia 3449

Mephobarbital (Hemin inhibits the enzyme delta-aminolevulinic acid synthetase; concurrent use with drugs that increase the activity of delta-aminolevulinic acid synthetase, such as barbiturates, should be avoided).
No products indexed under this heading.

Pentobarbital Sodium (Hemin inhibits the enzyme delta-aminolevulinic acid synthetase; concurrent use with drugs that increase the activity of delta-aminolevulinic acid synthetase, such as barbiturates, should be avoided). Products include:
Nembutal Sodium Solution 485

Phenobarbital (Hemin inhibits the enzyme delta-aminolevulinic acid synthetase; concurrent use with drugs that increase the activity of delta-aminolevulinic acid synthetase, such as barbiturates, should be avoided). Products include:
Arco-Lase Plus Tablets 592
Donnatal 2929
Donnatal Extentabs 2930

Polyestradiol Phosphate (Hemin inhibits the enzyme delta-aminolevulinic acid synthetase; concurrent use with drugs that increase the activity of delta-aminolevulinic acid synthetase, such as estrogens, should be avoided).
No products indexed under this heading.

Quinestrol (Hemin inhibits the enzyme delta-aminolevulinic acid synthetase; concurrent use with drugs that increase the activity of delta-aminolevulinic acid synthetase, such as estrogens, should be avoided).
No products indexed under this heading.

Secobarbital Sodium (Hemin inhibits the enzyme delta-aminolevulinic acid synthetase; concurrent use with drugs that increase the activity of delta-aminolevulinic acid synthetase, such as barbiturates, should be avoided).
No products indexed under this heading.

Thiamylal Sodium (Hemin inhibits the enzyme delta-aminolevulinic acid synthetase; concurrent use with drugs that increase the activity of delta-aminolevulinic acid synthetase, such as barbiturates, should be avoided).
No products indexed under this heading.

Warfarin Sodium (Hemin exhibits transient, mild anticoagulant effects, therefore, concurrent anticoagulant therapy should be avoided). Products include:
Coumadin for Injection 1243
Coumadin Tablets 1243
Warfarin Sodium Tablets, USP 3302

PARAFON FORTE DSC CAPLETS

(Chlorzoxazone) 2582
May interact with central nervous system depressants and certain other agents. Compounds in these categories include:

Alfentanil Hydrochloride (May produce additive effect).
No products indexed under this heading.

Alprazolam (May produce additive effect). Products include:
Xanax Tablets 2865

Aprobarbital (May produce additive effect).
No products indexed under this heading.

Buprenorphine Hydrochloride (May produce additive effect). Products include:
Buprenex Injectable 2918

Buspirone Hydrochloride (May produce additive effect).
No products indexed under this heading.

Butabarbital (May produce additive effect).
No products indexed under this heading.

Butalbital (May produce additive effect). Products include:
Phrenilin 578
Sedapap Tablets 50 mg/650 mg 2225

Chlordiazepoxide (May produce additive effect). Products include:
Limbitrol 1738

Chlordiazepoxide Hydrochloride (May produce additive effect). Products include:
Librium Capsules 1736
Librium for Injection 1737

Chlorpromazine (May produce additive effect). Products include:
Thorazine Suppositories 1656

Chlorpromazine Hydrochloride (May produce additive effect). Products include:
Thorazine 1656

Chlorprothixene (May produce additive effect).
No products indexed under this heading.

Chlorprothixene Hydrochloride (May produce additive effect).
No products indexed under this heading.

Chlorprothixene Lactate (May produce additive effect).
No products indexed under this heading.

Clorazepate Dipotassium (May produce additive effect). Products include:
Tranxene 511

Clozapine (May produce additive effect). Products include:
Clozaril Tablets 2319

Codeine Phosphate (May produce additive effect). Products include:
Phenergan with Codeine Syrup 3557
Phenergan VC with Codeine Syrup 3561
Robitussin A-C Syrup 2942
Robitussin-DAC Syrup 2942
Ryna-C Liquid 768
Soma Compound w/Codeine Tablets 3355
Tussi-Organidin NR Liquid 3350
Tussi-Organidin-S NR Liquid 3350
Tylenol with Codeine 2595

Desflurane (May produce additive effect). Products include:
Suprane Liquid for Inhalation 874

Dezocine (May produce additive effect).
No products indexed under this heading.

Diazepam (May produce additive effect). Products include:
Valium Injectable 3026
Valium Tablets 3047

Droperidol (May produce additive effect).
No products indexed under this heading.

Enflurane (May produce additive effect).
No products indexed under this heading.

Estazolam (May produce additive effect). Products include:
ProSom Tablets 500

Ethchlorvynol (May produce additive effect).
No products indexed under this heading.

Ethinamate (May produce additive effect).
No products indexed under this heading.

Fentanyl (May produce additive effect). Products include:
Duragesic Transdermal System 1786

Fentanyl Citrate (May produce additive effect). Products include:
Actiq 1184

Fluphenazine Decanoate (May produce additive effect).
No products indexed under this heading.

Fluphenazine Enanthate (May produce additive effect).
No products indexed under this heading.

Fluphenazine Hydrochloride (May produce additive effect).
No products indexed under this heading.

Flurazepam Hydrochloride (May produce additive effect).
No products indexed under this heading.

Glutethimide (May produce additive effect).
No products indexed under this heading.

Haloperidol (May produce additive effect). Products include:
Haldol Injection, Tablets and Concentrate 2533

Haloperidol Decanoate (May produce additive effect). Products include:
Haldol Decanoate 2535

Hydrocodone Bitartrate (May produce additive effect). Products include:
Hycodan 1316
Hycomine Compound Tablets 1317
Hycotuss Expectorant Syrup 1318
Lortab 3319
Lortab Elixir 3317
Maxidone Tablets CIII 3399
Norco 5/325 Tablets CIII 3424
Norco 7.5/325 Tablets CIII 3425
Norco 10/325 Tablets CIII 3427
Norco 10/325 Tablets CIII 3425
Vicodin Tablets 516
Vicodin ES Tablets 517
Vicodin HP Tablets 518
Vicodin Tuss Expectorant 519
Vicoprofen Tablets 520
Zydone Tablets 1330

Hydrocodone Polistirex (May produce additive effect). Products include:
Tussionex Pennkinetic Extended-Release Suspension 1174

Hydromorphone Hydrochloride (May produce additive effect). Products include:
Dilaudid 441
Dilaudid Oral Liquid 445
Dilaudid Powder 441
Dilaudid Rectal Suppositories 441
Dilaudid Tablets 441
Dilaudid Tablets - 8 mg 445
Dilaudid-HP 443

Hydroxyzine Hydrochloride (May produce additive effect). Products include:
Atarax Tablets & Syrup 2667
Vistaril Intramuscular Solution 2738

Isoflurane (May produce additive effect).
No products indexed under this heading.

Ketamine Hydrochloride (May produce additive effect).
No products indexed under this heading.

Levomethadyl Acetate Hydrochloride (May produce additive effect).
No products indexed under this heading.

Levorphanol Tartrate (May produce additive effect). Products include:
Levo-Dromoran 1734
Levorphanol Tartrate Tablets 3059

Lorazepam (May produce additive effect). Products include:
Ativan Injection 3478
Ativan Tablets 3482

Loxapine Hydrochloride (May produce additive effect).
No products indexed under this heading.

IMPORTANT NOTE: Always consult each drug listing in the patient's regimen for possible interactions.

Loxapine Succinate (May produce additive effect). Products include:
Loxitane Capsules 3398

Meperidine Hydrochloride (May produce additive effect). Products include:
Demerol 3079
Mepergan Injection 3539

Mephobarbital (May produce additive effect).
No products indexed under this heading.

Meprobamate (May produce additive effect). Products include:
Miltown Tablets 3349

Mesoridazine Besylate (May produce additive effect). Products include:
Serentil 1057

Methadone Hydrochloride (May produce additive effect). Products include:
Dolophine Hydrochloride Tablets 3056

Methohexital Sodium (May produce additive effect). Products include:
Brevital Sodium for Injection, USP .. 1815

Methotrimeprazine (May produce additive effect).
No products indexed under this heading.

Methoxyflurane (May produce additive effect).
No products indexed under this heading.

Midazolam Hydrochloride (May produce additive effect). Products include:
Versed Injection 3027
Versed Syrup 3033

Molindone Hydrochloride (May produce additive effect). Products include:
Moban 1320

Morphine Sulfate (May produce additive effect). Products include:
Astramorph/PF Injection, USP (Preservative-Free) 594
Duramorph Injection 1312
Infumorph 200 and Infumorph 500 Sterile Solutions 1314
Kadian Capsules 1335
MS Contin Tablets 2896
MSIR 2898
Oramorph SR Tablets 3062
Roxanol 3066

Olanzapine (May produce additive effect). Products include:
Zyprexa Tablets 1973
Zyprexa ZYDIS Orally Disintegrating Tablets 1973

Oxazepam (May produce additive effect).
No products indexed under this heading.

Oxycodone Hydrochloride (May produce additive effect). Products include:
OxyContin Tablets 2912
OxyFast Oral Concentrate Solution . 2916
OxyIR Capsules 2916
Percocet Tablets 1326
Percodan Tablets 1327
Percolone Tablets 1327
Roxicodone 3067
Tylox Capsules 2597

Pentobarbital Sodium (May produce additive effect). Products include:
Nembutal Sodium Solution 485

Perphenazine (May produce additive effect). Products include:
Etrafon 3115
Trilafon 3160

Phenobarbital (May produce additive effect). Products include:
Arco-Lase Plus Tablets 592
Donnatal 2929
Donnatal Extentabs 2930

Prazepam (May produce additive effect).
No products indexed under this heading.

Prochlorperazine (May produce additive effect). Products include:
Compazine 1505

Promethazine Hydrochloride (May produce additive effect). Products include:
Mepergan Injection 3539
Phenergan Injection 3553
Phenergan 3556
Phenergan Syrup 3554
Phenergan with Codeine Syrup 3557
Phenergan with Dextromethorphan Syrup 3559
Phenergan VC Syrup 3560
Phenergan VC with Codeine Syrup .. 3561

Propofol (May produce additive effect). Products include:
Diprivan Injectable Emulsion 667

Propoxyphene Hydrochloride (May produce additive effect). Products include:
Darvon Pulvules 1909
Darvon Compound-65 Pulvules 1910

Propoxyphene Napsylate (May produce additive effect). Products include:
Darvon-N/Darvocet-N 1907
Darvon-N Tablets 1912

Quazepam (May produce additive effect).
No products indexed under this heading.

Quetiapine Fumarate (May produce additive effect). Products include:
Seroquel Tablets 684

Remifentanil Hydrochloride (May produce additive effect).
No products indexed under this heading.

Risperidone (May produce additive effect). Products include:
Risperdal 1796

Secobarbital Sodium (May produce additive effect).
No products indexed under this heading.

Sevoflurane (May produce additive effect).
No products indexed under this heading.

Sufentanil Citrate (May produce additive effect).
No products indexed under this heading.

Temazepam (May produce additive effect).
No products indexed under this heading.

Thiamylal Sodium (May produce additive effect).
No products indexed under this heading.

Thioridazine Hydrochloride (May produce additive effect). Products include:
Thioridazine Hydrochloride Tablets 2289

Thiothixene (May produce additive effect). Products include:
Navane Capsules 2701
Thiothixene Capsules 2290

Triazolam (May produce additive effect). Products include:
Halcion Tablets 2823

Trifluoperazine Hydrochloride (May produce additive effect). Products include:
Stelazine 1640

Zaleplon (May produce additive effect). Products include:
Sonata Capsules 3591

Ziprasidone Hydrochloride (May produce additive effect). Products include:
Geodon Capsules 2688

Zolpidem Tartrate (May produce additive effect). Products include:
Ambien Tablets 3191

Food Interactions

Alcohol (May produce additive effect).

PARAGARD T 380A INTRAUTERINE COPPER CONTRACEPTIVE
(Copper, Intrauterine) 2582
None cited in PDR database.

PARAPLATIN FOR INJECTION
(Carboplatin) 1126
May interact with aminoglycosides and certain other agents. Compounds in these categories include:

Amikacin Sulfate (Concomitant treatment has resulted in increased renal and/or audiologic toxicity).
No products indexed under this heading.

Gentamicin Sulfate (Concomitant treatment has resulted in increased renal and/or audiologic toxicity). Products include:
Genoptic Ophthalmic Ointment ..... ⊙239
Genoptic Sterile Ophthalmic Solution ..... ⊙239
Pred-G Ophthalmic Suspension ..... ⊙247
Pred-G Sterile Ophthalmic Ointment ..... ⊙248

Kanamycin Sulfate (Concomitant treatment has resulted in increased renal and/or audiologic toxicity).
No products indexed under this heading.

Nephrotoxic Drugs (Renal effects may be potentiated).
No products indexed under this heading.

Streptomycin Sulfate (Concomitant treatment has resulted in increased renal and/or audiologic toxicity). Products include:
Streptomycin Sulfate Injection 2714

Tobramycin (Concomitant treatment has resulted in increased renal and/or audiologic toxicity). Products include:
TOBI Solution for Inhalation 1206
TobraDex Ophthalmic Ointment 542
TobraDex Ophthalmic Suspension 541
Tobrex Ophthalmic Ointment ..... ⊙220
Tobrex Ophthalmic Solution ..... ⊙221

Tobramycin Sulfate (Concomitant treatment has resulted in increased renal and/or audiologic toxicity). Products include:
Nebcin Vials, Hyporets & ADD-Vantage 1955

PARNATE TABLETS
(Tranylcypromine Sulfate) 1607
May interact with alpha adrenergic stimulants, amphetamines, anesthetics, anorexiants, antihistamines, antihypertensives, anticholinergic-type antiparkinsonism drugs, dibenzazepines, diuretics, oral hypoglycemic agents, hypnotics and sedatives, insulin, monoamine oxidase inhibitors, narcotic analgesics, phenothiazines, selective serotonin reuptake inhibitors, sympathomimetics, tricyclic antidepressants, and certain other agents. Compounds in these categories include:

Acarbose (Some MAO inhibitors have contributed to hypoglycemic episodes in diabetic patients receiving oral hypoglycemic agents). Products include:
Precose Tablets 906

Acebutolol Hydrochloride (Concurrent use with hypotensive agents is contraindicated; a marked potentiating effect on these classes of drugs has been reported). Products include:
Sectral Capsules 3589

Acrivastine (Concurrent use is contraindicated). Products include:
Semprex-D Capsules 1172

Albuterol (Concurrent and/or sequential use is contraindicated; combination therapy may precipitate hypertension, headache and related symptoms). Products include:
Proventil Inhalation Aerosol 3142
Ventolin Inhalation Aerosol and Refill 1679

Albuterol Sulfate (Concurrent and/or sequential use is contraindicated; combination therapy may precipitate hypertension, headache and related symptoms). Products include:
AccuNeb Inhalation Solution 1230
Combivent Inhalation Aerosol 1041
DuoNeb Inhalation Solution 1233
Proventil Inhalation Solution 0.083% 3146
Proventil Repetabs Tablets 3148
Proventil Solution for Inhalation 0.5% 3144
Proventil HFA Inhalation Aerosol 3150
Ventolin HFA Inhalation Aerosol 3618
Volmax Extended-Release Tablets .. 2276

Alfentanil Hydrochloride (Concurrent use is contraindicated; a marked potentiating effect on these classes of drugs has been reported).
No products indexed under this heading.

Amiloride Hydrochloride (Concurrent use with hypotensive agents is contraindicated; a marked potentiating effect on these classes of drugs has been reported). Products include:
Midamor Tablets 2136
Moduretic Tablets 2138

Amitriptyline Hydrochloride (Concurrent use with tricyclic antidepressants may result in hypertensive crises or severe convulsive seizures; concurrent and/or sequential use is contraindicated). Products include:
Etrafon 3115
Limbitrol 1738

Amlodipine Besylate (Concurrent use with hypotensive agents is contraindicated; a marked potentiating effect on these classes of drugs has been reported). Products include:
Lotrel Capsules 2370
Norvasc Tablets 2704

Amoxapine (Concurrent use with tricyclic antidepressants may result in hypertensive crises or severe convulsive seizures; concurrent and/or sequential use is contraindicated).
No products indexed under this heading.

Amphetamine Resins (Concurrent and/or sequential use is contraindicated).
No products indexed under this heading.

Amphetamine Sulfate (Concurrent and/or sequential use is contraindicated). Products include:
Adderall Tablets 3231
Adderall XR Capsules .....

Astemizole (Concurrent use is contraindicated).
No products indexed under this heading.

Atenolol (Concurrent use with hypotensive agents is contraindicated; a marked potentiating effect on these classes of drugs has been reported). Products include:
Tenoretic Tablets 690
Tenormin I.V. Injection 692

Azatadine Maleate (Concurrent use is contraindicated). Products include:
Rynatan Tablets 3351

Benazepril Hydrochloride (Concurrent use with hypotensive agents is contraindicated; a marked potentiating effect on these classes of drugs has been reported). Products include:
Lotensin Tablets 2365
Lotensin HCT Tablets 2367
Lotrel Capsules 2370

Bendroflumethiazide (Concurrent use with hypotensive agents is contraindicated; a marked potentiating effect on these classes of drugs has been reported). Products include:
Corzide 40/5 Tablets 2247
Corzide 80/5 Tablets 2247

Benzphetamine Hydrochloride (Concurrent and/or sequential use is

contraindicated).
No products indexed under this heading.

Benztropine Mesylate (Anti-Parkinsonism drugs should be used with caution in patients receiving Parnate since severe reactions have been reported). Products include:
Cogentin 2055

Betaxolol Hydrochloride (Concurrent use with hypotensive agents is contraindicated; a marked potentiating effect on these classes of drugs has been reported). Products include:
Betoptic S Ophthalmic Suspension 537

Biperiden Hydrochloride (Anti-Parkinsonism drugs should be used with caution in patients receiving Parnate since severe reactions have been reported). Products include:
Akineton 402

Bisoprolol Fumarate (Concurrent use with hypotensive agents is contraindicated; a marked potentiating effect on these classes of drugs has been reported). Products include:
Zebeta Tablets 1885
Ziac Tablets 1887

Bromodiphenhydramine Hydrochloride (Concurrent use is contraindicated).
No products indexed under this heading.

Brompheniramine Maleate (Concurrent use is contraindicated). Products include:
Bromfed Capsules (Extended-Release) 2269
Bromfed-PD Capsules (Extended-Release) 2269
Comtrex Acute Head Cold & Sinus Pressure Relief Tablets 627
Dimetapp Elixir 777
Dimetapp Cold and Fever Suspension 775
Dimetapp DM Cold & Cough Elixir 775
Dimetapp Nighttime Flu Liquid 776

Bumetanide (Concurrent use with hypotensive agents is contraindicated; a marked potentiating effect on these classes of drugs has been reported).
No products indexed under this heading.

Buprenorphine Hydrochloride (Concurrent use is contraindicated; a marked potentiating effect on these classes of drugs has been reported). Products include:
Buprenex Injectable 2918

Bupropion Hydrochloride (Concurrent use is contraindicated; at least 14 days should elapse between discontinuation of an MAO inhibitor and initiation of treatment with bupropion). Products include:
Wellbutrin Tablets 1680
Wellbutrin SR Sustained-Release Tablets 1684
Zyban Sustained-Release Tablets 1710

Buspirone Hydrochloride (Concurrent use of buspirone and MAO inhibitor has resulted in several cases of hypertension; concurrent use is contraindicated; at least 10 days should elapse between the discontinuation of Parnate and the institution of buspirone).
No products indexed under this heading.

Caffeine (Excessive use of caffeine in any form is contraindicated). Products include:
BC Powder 619
Arthritis Strength BC Powder 619
Darvon Compound-65 Pulvules 1910
Aspirin Free Excedrin Caplets and Geltabs 628
Excedrin Extra-Strength Tablets, Caplets, and Geltabs 629
Excedrin Migraine 1070
Goody's Extra Strength Headache Powder 620
Goody's Extra Strength Pain Relief Tablets 620
Hycomine Compound Tablets 1317
Maximum Strength Midol Menstrual Caplets and Gelcaps 612
Vanquish Caplets 617
Vivarin 763

Candesartan Cilexetil (Concurrent use with hypotensive agents is contraindicated; a marked potentiating effect on these classes of drugs has been reported). Products include:
Atacand Tablets 595
Atacand HCT Tablets 597

Captopril (Concurrent use with hypotensive agents is contraindicated; a marked potentiating effect on these classes of drugs has been reported). Products include:
Captopril Tablets 2281

Carbamazepine (Concurrent use with dibenzazepine-related entities may result in hypertensive crises or severe convulsive seizures; concurrent and/or sequential use is contraindicated). Products include:
Carbatrol Capsules 3234
Tegretol/Tegretol-XR 2404

Carteolol Hydrochloride (Concurrent use with hypotensive agents is contraindicated; a marked potentiating effect on these classes of drugs has been reported). Products include:
Carteolol Hydrochloride Ophthalmic Solution USP, 1% .... ⊙ 258
Ocupress Ophthalmic Solution, 1% Sterile .... ⊙ 303

Cetirizine Hydrochloride (Concurrent use is contraindicated). Products include:
Zyrtec 2756
Zyrtec-D 12 Hour Extended Relief Tablets 2758

Chlorothiazide (Concurrent use with hypotensive agents is contraindicated; a marked potentiating effect on these classes of drugs has been reported). Products include:
Aldoclor Tablets 2035
Diuril Oral 2087

Chlorothiazide Sodium (Concurrent use with hypotensive agents is contraindicated; a marked potentiating effect on these classes of drugs has been reported). Products include:
Diuril Sodium Intravenous 2086

Chlorpheniramine Maleate (Concurrent use is contraindicated). Products include:
Actifed Cold & Sinus Caplets and Tablets 688
Alka-Seltzer Plus Liqui-Gels 604
BC Allergy Sinus Cold Powder 619
Chlor-Trimeton Allergy Tablets 735
Chlor-Trimeton Allergy/Decongestant Tablets 736
Comtrex Flu Therapy & Fever Relief Nighttime Tablets 628
Comtrex Maximum Strength Multi-Symptom Cold & Cough Relief Tablets and Caplets 626
Contac Severe Cold and Flu Caplets Maximum Strength 746
Coricidin 'D' Cold, Flu & Sinus Tablets 737
Coricidin/Coricidin D 738
Coricidin HBP Maximum Strength Flu Tablets 738
Extendryl 1361
Hycomine Compound Tablets 1317
Kronofed-A 1341
PediaCare Cough-Cold Liquid 719
PediaCare NightRest Cough-Cold Liquid 719
Robitussin Nighttime Honey Flu Liquid 786
Ryna 768
Singlet Caplets 761
Sinutab Sinus Allergy Medication, Maximum Strength Formula, Tablets & Caplets 707
Sudafed Cold & Allergy Tablets 708
TheraFlu Regular Strength Cold & Cough Night Time Hot Liquid 676
TheraFlu Regular Strength Cold & Sore Throat Night Time Hot Liquid 676
TheraFlu Maximum Strength Flu & Cough Night Time Hot Liquid 678
TheraFlu Maximum Strength Flu & Sore Throat Night Time Hot Liquid 677
TheraFlu Maximum Strength Severe Cold & Congestion Night Time Caplets 678
TheraFlu Maximum Strength Severe Cold & Congestion Night Time Hot Liquid 678
Triaminic Cold & Allergy Liquid 681
Triaminic Cold & Allergy Softchews 683
Triaminic Cold & Cough Liquid 681
Triaminic Cold & Cough Softchews 683
Triaminic Cold & Night Time Cough Liquid 681
Triaminic Cold, Cough & Fever Liquid 681
Children's Tylenol Cold Suspension Liquid and Chewable Tablets 2015
Children's Tylenol Cold Plus Cough Suspension Liquid and Chewable Tablets 2015
Children's Tylenol Flu Suspension Liquid 2015
Maximum Strength Tylenol Allergy Sinus Caplets, Gelcaps, and Geltabs 2010
Multi-Symptom Tylenol Cold Complete Formula Caplets 2010
Vicks 44M Cough, Cold & Flu Relief Liquid 725
Pediatric Vicks 44m Cough & Cold Relief 728
Children's Vicks NyQuil Cold/Cough Relief 726

Chlorpheniramine Polistirex (Concurrent use is contraindicated). Products include:
Tussionex Pennkinetic Extended-Release Suspension 1174

Chlorpheniramine Tannate (Concurrent use is contraindicated). Products include:
Reformulated Rynatan Pediatric Suspension 3352
Rynatuss Pediatric Suspension 3353
Rynatuss Tablets 3353
Tussi-12 S Suspension 3356
Tussi-12 Tablets 3356

Chlorpromazine (Possibility of additive hypotensive effects). Products include:
Thorazine Suppositories 1656

Chlorpromazine Hydrochloride (Possibility of additive hypotensive effects). Products include:
Thorazine 1656

Chlorpropamide (Some MAO inhibitors have contributed to hypoglycemic episodes in diabetic patients receiving oral hypoglycemic agents). Products include:
Diabinese Tablets 2680

Chlorthalidone (Concurrent use with hypotensive agents is contraindicated; a marked potentiating effect on these classes of drugs has been reported). Products include:
Clorpres Tablets 1002
Combipres Tablets 1040
Tenoretic Tablets 690

Citalopram Hydrobromide (Concurrent and/or sequential use is contraindicated; potential for serious, sometimes fatal, reactions including hyperthermia, rigidity, myoclonus, and other toxicities). Products include:
Celexa 1365

Clemastine Fumarate (Concurrent use is contraindicated). Products include:
Tavist 12 Hour Allergy Tablets 676

Clomipramine Hydrochloride (Concurrent use with tricyclic antidepressants may result in hypertensive crises or severe convulsive seizures; concurrent and/or sequential use is contraindicated).
No products indexed under this heading.

Clonidine (Concurrent use with hypotensive agents is contraindicated; a marked potentiating effect on these classes of drugs has been reported). Products include:
Catapres-TTS 1038

Clonidine Hydrochloride (Concurrent use with hypotensive agents is contraindicated; a marked potentiating effect on these classes of drugs has been reported). Products include:
Catapres Tablets 1037
Clorpres Tablets 1002
Combipres Tablets 1040
Duraclon Injection 3057

Clozapine (Concurrent use with dibenzazepine-related entities may result in hypertensive crises or severe convulsive seizures; concurrent and/or sequential use is contraindicated). Products include:
Clozaril Tablets 2319

Cocaine Hydrochloride (Concurrent use is contraindicated).
No products indexed under this heading.

Codeine Phosphate (Concurrent use is contraindicated; a marked potentiating effect on these classes of drugs has been reported). Products include:
Phenergan with Codeine Syrup 3557
Phenergan VC with Codeine Syrup 3561
Robitussin A-C Syrup 2942
Robitussin-DAC Syrup 2942
Ryna-C Liquid 768
Soma Compound w/Codeine Tablets 3355
Tussi-Organidin NR Liquid 3350
Tussi-Organidin-S NR Liquid 3350
Tylenol with Codeine 2595

Cyclobenzaprine Hydrochloride (Concurrent use with dibenzazepine-related entities may result in hypertensive crises or severe convulsive seizures; concurrent and/or sequential use is contraindicated). Products include:
Flexeril Tablets 572
Flexeril Tablets 2094

Cyproheptadine Hydrochloride (Concurrent use is contraindicated). Products include:
Periactin Tablets 2155

Deserpidine (Concurrent use with hypotensive agents is contraindicated; a marked potentiating effect on these classes of drugs has been reported).
No products indexed under this heading.

Desipramine Hydrochloride (Concurrent use with tricyclic antidepressants may result in hypertensive crises or severe convulsive seizures; concurrent and/or sequential use is contraindicated). Products include:
Norpramin Tablets 755

Dexchlorpheniramine Maleate (Concurrent use is contraindicated).
No products indexed under this heading.

Dexfenfluramine Hydrochloride (Co-administration with dexfenfluramine, a serotonin releaser and reuptake inhibitor, is contraindicated).
No products indexed under this heading.

Dextroamphetamine Sulfate (Concurrent and/or sequential use is contraindicated). Products include:
Adderall Tablets 3231
Adderall XR Capsules
Dexedrine 1512
DextroStat Tablets 3236

Dextromethorphan Hydrobromide (The combination of dextromethorphan and MAO inhibitors have been reported to cause brief episodes of psychosis or bizzare behavior; concurrent use is contraindicated). Products include:
Alka-Seltzer Plus Liqui-Gels 604
Alka-Seltzer Plus Cold & Flu Medicine Liqui-Gels 604
Benylin Adult Formula Cough Suppressant Liquid 696

Benylin Cough Suppressant/Expectorant Liquid .... ▣697
Benylin Multi-Symptom Liquid .... ▣697
Benylin Pediatric Cough Suppressant Liquid .... ▣698
Comtrex Deep Chest Cold & Congestion Relief Softgels .... ▣627
Comtrex Maximum Strength Multi-Symptom Cold & Cough Relief Tablets and Caplets .... ▣626
Contac Severe Cold and Flu Caplets Maximum Strength .... ▣746
Contac Severe Cold and Flu Caplets Non-Drowsy .... ▣746
Coricidin HBP Cough & Cold Tablets .... ▣738
Coricidin HBP Maximum Strength Flu Tablets .... ▣738
Dimetapp DM Cold & Cough Elixir .... ▣775
Dimetapp Nighttime Flu Liquid .... ▣776
Dimetapp Non-Drowsy Flu Syrup .... ▣777
Dimetapp Infant Drops Decongestant Plus Cough .... ▣776
PediaCare Cough-Cold Liquid .... ▣719
PediaCare Infants' Drops Decongestant Plus Cough .... ▣719
PediaCare NightRest Cough-Cold Liquid .... ▣719
Phenergan with Dextromethorphan Syrup 3559
Robitussin Cold Caplets Cold & Congestion .... ▣780
Robitussin Cold Softgels Cold & Congestion .... ▣780
Robitussin Cold Caplets Multi-Symptom Cold & Flu .... ▣781
Robitussin Cold Softgels Multi-Symptom Cold & Flu .... ▣781
Robitussin Cough & Cold Infant Drops .... ▣782
Robitussin Maximum Strength Cough & Cold Liquid .... ▣785
Robitussin Pediatric Cough & Cold Formula Liquid .... ▣785
Robitussin Maximum Strength Cough Suppressant Liquid .... ▣784
Robitussin Pediatric Cough Suppressant Liquid .... ▣784
Robitussin Multi Symptom Honey Flu Liquid .... ▣785
Robitussin Nighttime Honey Flu Liquid .... ▣786
Robitussin-CF Liquid .... ▣783
Robitussin DM Infant Drops .... ▣783
Robitussin-DM Liquid .... ▣783
Children's Sudafed Cold & Cough Liquid .... ▣709
Sudafed Cold & Cough Liquid Caps .... ▣709
Sudafed Severe Cold .... ▣711
TheraFlu Regular Strength Cold & Cough Night Time Hot Liquid .... ▣676
TheraFlu Maximum Strength Flu & Congestion Non-Drowsy Hot Liquid .... ▣677
TheraFlu Maximum Strength Flu & Cough Night Time Hot Liquid .... ▣678
TheraFlu Maximum Strength Severe Cold & Congestion Night Time Caplets .... ▣678
TheraFlu Maximum Strength Severe Cold & Congestion Night Time Hot Liquid .... ▣678
TheraFlu Maximum Strength Severe Cold & Congestion Non-Drowsy .... ▣679
Triaminic Cold & Cough Liquid .... ▣681
Triaminic Cold & Cough Softchews .... ▣683
Triaminic Cold & Night Time Cough Liquid .... ▣681
Triaminic Cold, Cough & Fever Liquid .... ▣681
Triaminic Cough Liquid .... ▣682
Triaminic Cough Softchews .... ▣684
Triaminic Cough & Congestion Liquid .... ▣682
Triaminic Cough & Sore Throat Liquid .... ▣682
Triaminic Cough & Sore Throat Softchews .... ▣684
Tussi-Organidin DM NR Liquid 3350
Tussi-Organidin DM-S NR Liquid 3350
Children's Tylenol Cold Plus Cough Suspension Liquid and Chewable Tablets 2015
Children's Tylenol Flu Suspension Liquid 2015
Infants' Tylenol Cold Decongestant and Fever Reducer Concentrated Drops Plus Cough 2015
Multi-Symptom Tylenol Cold Complete Formula Caplets 2010
Multi-Symptom Tylenol Cold Non-Drowsy Caplets and Gelcaps 2010
Multi-Symptom Tylenol Cold Severe Congestion Non-Drowsy Caplets 2011
Maximum Strength Tylenol Flu NightTime Liquid 2011
Maximum Strength Tylenol Flu Non-Drowsy Gelcaps 2011
Vicks 44 Cough Relief Liquid .... ▣724
Vicks 44D Cough & Head Congestion Relief Liquid .... ▣724
Vicks 44E Cough & Chest Congestion Relief Liquid .... ▣725
Pediatric Vicks 44e Cough & Chest Congestion Relief Liquid .... ▣728
Vicks 44M Cough, Cold & Flu Relief Liquid .... ▣725
Pediatric Vicks 44m Cough & Cold Relief .... ▣728
Vicks DayQuil LiquiCaps/Liquid Multi-Symptom Cold/Flu Relief .... ▣727
Children's Vicks NyQuil Cold/Cough Relief .... ▣726
Vicks NyQuil LiquiCaps/Liquid Multi-Symptom Cold/Flu Relief, Original and Cherry Flavors .... ▣727

Dextromethorphan Polistirex (The combination of dextromethorphan and MAO inhibitors have been reported to cause brief episodes of psychosis or bizzare behavior; concurrent use is contraindicated). Products include:
Delsym Extended-Release Suspension .... ▣664

Dezocine (Concurrent use is contraindicated; a marked potentiating effect on these classes of drugs has been reported).
No products indexed under this heading.

Diazoxide (Concurrent use with hypotensive agents is contraindicated; a marked potentiating effect on these classes of drugs has been reported).
No products indexed under this heading.

Diethylpropion Hydrochloride (Concurrent and/or sequential use is contraindicated).
No products indexed under this heading.

Diltiazem Hydrochloride (Concurrent use with hypotensive agents is contraindicated; a marked potentiating effect on these classes of drugs has been reported). Products include:
Cardizem Injectable 1018
Cardizem Lyo-Ject Syringe 1018
Cardizem Monovial 1018
Cardizem CD Capsules 1016
Tiazac Capsules 1378

Diphenhydramine Citrate (Concurrent use is contraindicated). Products include:
Alka-Seltzer PM Effervescent Tablets .... ▣605
Benadryl Allergy & Sinus Fastmelt Tablets .... ▣693
Benadryl Children's Allergy/Cold Fastmelt Tablets .... ▣692
Excedrin PM Tablets, Caplets, and Geltabs .... ▣631
Goody's PM Powder .... ▣621

Diphenhydramine Hydrochloride (Concurrent use is contraindicated). Products include:
Extra Strength Bayer PM Caplets .... ▣611
Benadryl Allergy Chewables .... ▣689
Benadryl Allergy .... ▣691
Benadryl Allergy Liquid .... ▣690
Benadryl Allergy/Cold Tablets .... ▣691
Benadryl Allergy/Congestion Tablets .... ▣692
Benadryl Allergy & Sinus Liquid .... ▣693
Benadryl Allergy Sinus Headache Caplets & Gelcaps .... ▣693
Benadryl Severe Allergy & Sinus Headache Caplets .... ▣694
Benadryl Dye-Free Allergy Liquid .... ▣690
Benadryl Dye-Free Allergy Liqui-Gels Softgels .... ▣690
Benadryl Itch Relief Stick Extra Strength .... ▣695
Benadryl Cream .... ▣695
Benadryl Gel .... ▣695
Benadryl Spray .... ▣696
Benadryl Parenteral 2617
Coricidin HBP Night-Time Cold & Flu Tablets .... ▣738
Nytol QuickCaps Caplets .... ▣622
Maximum Strength Nytol QuickGels Softgels .... ▣621
Extra Strength Percogesic Aspirin-Free Coated Caplets .... ▣665
Simply Sleep Caplets 2008
Sominex Original Formula Tablets .... ▣761
Children's Tylenol Allergy-D Liquid 2014
Maximum Strength Tylenol Allergy Sinus NightTime Caplets 2010
Tylenol Severe Allergy Caplets 2010
Maximum Strength Tylenol Flu NightTime Gelcaps 2011
Extra Strength Tylenol PM Caplets, Geltabs, and Gelcaps 2012
Unisom Maximum Strength SleepGels .... ▣713

Diphenylpyraline Hydrochloride (Concurrent use is contraindicated).
No products indexed under this heading.

Disulfiram (Concurrent use requires caution; co-administration in animal models has resulted in severe toxicity including convulsions and death). Products include:
Antabuse Tablets 2444
Antabuse Tablets 3474

Dobutamine Hydrochloride (Concurrent and/or sequential use is contraindicated; combination therapy may precipitate hypertension, headache and related symptoms). Products include:
Dobutrex Solution Vials 1914

Dopamine Hydrochloride (Concurrent and/or sequential use is contraindicated; combination therapy may precipitate hypertension, headache and related symptoms).
No products indexed under this heading.

Doxazosin Mesylate (Concurrent use with hypotensive agents is contraindicated; a marked potentiating effect on these classes of drugs has been reported). Products include:
Cardura Tablets 2668

Doxepin Hydrochloride (Concurrent use with tricyclic antidepressants may result in hypertensive crises or severe convulsive seizures; concurrent and/or sequential use is contraindicated). Products include:
Sinequan 2713

Enalapril Maleate (Concurrent use with hypotensive agents is contraindicated; a marked potentiating effect on these classes of drugs has been reported). Products include:
Lexxel Tablets 608
Vaseretic Tablets 2204
Vasotec Tablets 2210

Enalaprilat (Concurrent use with hypotensive agents is contraindicated; a marked potentiating effect on these classes of drugs has been reported). Products include:
Enalaprilat Injection 863
Vasotec I.V. Injection 2207

Enflurane (Concurrent use is contraindicated).
No products indexed under this heading.

Ephedrine Hydrochloride (Concurrent and/or sequential use is contraindicated; combination therapy may precipitate hypertension, headache and related symptoms). Products include:
Primatene Tablets .... ▣780

Ephedrine Sulfate (Concurrent and/or sequential use is contraindicated; combination therapy may precipitate hypertension, headache and related symptoms).
No products indexed under this heading.

Ephedrine Tannate (Concurrent and/or sequential use is contraindicated; combination therapy may precipitate hypertension, headache and related symptoms). Products include:
Rynatuss Pediatric Suspension 3353
Rynatuss Tablets 3353

Epinephrine (Concurrent and/or sequential use is contraindicated; combination therapy may precipitate hypertension, headache and related symptoms). Products include:
Epifrin Sterile Ophthalmic Solution .... ⊙235
EpiPen 1236
Primatene Mist .... ▣779
Xylocaine with Epinephrine Injection 653

Epinephrine Bitartrate (Concurrent and/or sequential use is contraindicated; combination therapy may precipitate hypertension, headache and related symptoms). Products include:
Sensorcaine 643

Epinephrine Hydrochloride (Concurrent and/or sequential use is contraindicated; combination therapy may precipitate hypertension, headache and related symptoms).
No products indexed under this heading.

Eprosartan Mesylate (Concurrent use with hypotensive agents is contraindicated; a marked potentiating effect on these classes of drugs has been reported). Products include:
Teveten Tablets 3327

Esmolol Hydrochloride (Concurrent use with hypotensive agents is contraindicated; a marked potentiating effect on these classes of drugs has been reported). Products include:
Brevibloc Injection 858

Estazolam (Concurrent use is contraindicated). Products include:
ProSom Tablets 500

Ethacrynic Acid (Concurrent use with hypotensive agents is contraindicated; a marked potentiating effect on these classes of drugs has been reported). Products include:
Edecrin Tablets 2091

Ethchlorvynol (Concurrent use is contraindicated).
No products indexed under this heading.

Ethinamate (Concurrent use is contraindicated).
No products indexed under this heading.

Felodipine (Concurrent use with hypotensive agents is contraindicated; a marked potentiating effect on these classes of drugs has been reported). Products include:
Lexxel Tablets 608
Plendil Extended-Release Tablets 623

Fenfluramine Hydrochloride (Concurrent and/or sequential use is contraindicated).
No products indexed under this heading.

Fentanyl (Concurrent use is contraindicated; a marked potentiating effect on these classes of drugs has been reported). Products include:
Duragesic Transdermal System 1786

Fentanyl Citrate (Concurrent use is contraindicated; a marked potentiating effect on these classes of drugs has been reported). Products include:
Actiq 1184

Fexofenadine Hydrochloride (Concurrent use is contraindicated). Products include:
Allegra 712
Allegra-D Extended-Release Tablets 714

Fluoxetine Hydrochloride (Concurrent use has resulted in serious, sometimes fatal, reactions including hyperthermia, rigidity, myoclonus, autonomic instability with possible rapid fluctuations of vital signs and mental status; concurrent use is contraindicated; at least 5 weeks should

be allowed after stopping fluoxetine before starting an MAO inhibitor). Products include:
Prozac Pulvules, Liquid, and Weekly Capsules 1238
Sarafem Pulvules 1962

Fluphenazine Decanoate (Possibility of additive hypotensive effects).
No products indexed under this heading.

Fluphenazine Enanthate (Possibility of additive hypotensive effects).
No products indexed under this heading.

Fluphenazine Hydrochloride (Possibility of additive hypotensive effects).
No products indexed under this heading.

Flurazepam Hydrochloride (Concurrent use is contraindicated).
No products indexed under this heading.

Fluvoxamine Maleate (Concurrent and/or sequential use is contraindicated; potential for serious, sometimes fatal, reactions including hyperthermia, rigidity, myoclonus, and other toxicities). Products include:
Luvox Tablets (25, 50, 100 mg) 3256

Fosinopril Sodium (Concurrent use with hypotensive agents is contraindicated; a marked potentiating effect on these classes of drugs has been reported). Products include:
Monopril Tablets 1091
Monopril HCT 1094

Furosemide (Concurrent use with hypotensive agents is contraindicated; a marked potentiating effect on these classes of drugs has been reported). Products include:
Furosemide Tablets 2284

Glimepiride (Some MAO inhibitors have contributed to hypoglycemic episodes in diabetic patients receiving oral hypoglycemic agents). Products include:
Amaryl Tablets 717

Glipizide (Some MAO inhibitors have contributed to hypoglycemic episodes in diabetic patients receiving oral hypoglycemic agents). Products include:
Glucotrol Tablets 2692
Glucotrol XL Extended Release Tablets 2693

Glutethimide (Concurrent use is contraindicated).
No products indexed under this heading.

Glyburide (Some MAO inhibitors have contributed to hypoglycemic episodes in diabetic patients receiving oral hypoglycemic agents). Products include:
DiaBeta Tablets 741
Glucovance Tablets 1086

Guanabenz Acetate (Concurrent use with hypotensive agents is contraindicated; a marked potentiating effect on these classes of drugs has been reported).
No products indexed under this heading.

Guanethidine Monosulfate (Concurrent and/or sequential use is contraindicated; combination therapy may precipitate hypertension, headache and related symptoms).
No products indexed under this heading.

Halothane (Concurrent use is contraindicated). Products include:
Fluothane Inhalation 3508

Hydralazine Hydrochloride (Concurrent use with hypotensive agents is contraindicated; a marked potentiating effect on these classes of drugs has been reported).
No products indexed under this heading.

Hydrochlorothiazide (Concurrent use with hypotensive agents is contraindicated; a marked potentiating effect on these classes of drugs has been reported). Products include:
Accuretic Tablets 2614
Aldoril Tablets 2039
Atacand HCT Tablets 597
Avalide Tablets 1070
Diovan HCT Tablets 2338
Dyazide Capsules 1515
HydroDIURIL Tablets 2108
Hyzaar 2109
Inderide Tablets 3517
Inderide LA Long-Acting Capsules 3519
Lotensin HCT Tablets 2367
Maxzide 1008
Micardis HCT Tablets 1051
Microzide Capsules 3414
Moduretic Tablets 2138
Monopril HCT 1094
Prinzide Tablets 2168
Timolide Tablets 2187
Uniretic Tablets 3178
Vaseretic Tablets 2204
Zestoretic Tablets 695
Ziac Tablets 1887

Hydrocodone Bitartrate (Concurrent use is contraindicated; a marked potentiating effect on these classes of drugs has been reported). Products include:
Hycodan 1316
Hycomine Compound Tablets 1317
Hycotuss Expectorant Syrup 1318
Lortab 3319
Lortab Elixir 3317
Maxidone Tablets CIII 3399
Norco 5/325 Tablets CIII 3424
Norco 7.5/325 Tablets CIII 3425
Norco 10/325 Tablets CIII 3427
Norco 10/325 Tablets CIII 3425
Vicodin Tablets 516
Vicodin ES Tablets 517
Vicodin HP Tablets 518
Vicodin Tuss Expectorant 519
Vicoprofen Tablets 520
Zydone Tablets 1330

Hydrocodone Polistirex (Concurrent use is contraindicated; a marked potentiating effect on these classes of drugs has been reported). Products include:
Tussionex Pennkinetic Extended-Release Suspension 1174

Hydroflumethiazide (Concurrent use with hypotensive agents is contraindicated; a marked potentiating effect on these classes of drugs has been reported). Products include:
Diucardin Tablets 3494

Hydromorphone Hydrochloride (Concurrent use is contraindicated; a marked potentiating effect on these classes of drugs has been reported). Products include:
Dilaudid 441
Dilaudid Oral Liquid 445
Dilaudid Powder 441
Dilaudid Rectal Suppositories 441
Dilaudid Tablets 441
Dilaudid Tablets - 8 mg 445
Dilaudid-HP 443

Imipramine Hydrochloride (Concurrent use with tricyclic antidepressants may result in hypertensive crises or severe convulsive seizures; concurrent and/or sequential use is contraindicated).
No products indexed under this heading.

Imipramine Pamoate (Concurrent use with tricyclic antidepressants may result in hypertensive crises or severe convulsive seizures; concurrent and/or sequential use is contraindicated).
No products indexed under this heading.

Indapamide (Concurrent use with hypotensive agents is contraindicated; a marked potentiating effect on these classes of drugs has been reported). Products include:
Indapamide Tablets 2286

Insulin, Human, Zinc Suspension (Some MAO inhibitors have contributed to hypoglycemic episodes in diabetic patients receiving insulin). Products include:
Humulin L, 100 Units 1937
Humulin U, 100 Units 1943
Novolin L Human Insulin 10 ml Vials 2422

Insulin, Human NPH (Some MAO inhibitors have contributed to hypoglycemic episodes in diabetic patients receiving insulin). Products include:
Humulin N, 100 Units 1939
Humulin N NPH Pen 1940
Novolin N Human Insulin 10 ml Vials 2422
Novolin N PenFill 2423
Novolin N Prefilled Syringe Disposable Insulin Delivery System 2425

Insulin, Human Regular (Some MAO inhibitors have contributed to hypoglycemic episodes in diabetic patients receiving insulin). Products include:
Humulin R Regular (U-500) 1943
Humulin R, 100 Units 1941
Novolin R Human Insulin 10 ml Vials 2423
Novolin R PenFill 2423
Novolin R Prefilled Syringe Disposable Insulin Delivery System 2425
Velosulin BR Human Insulin 10 ml Vials 2435

Insulin, Human Regular and Human NPH Mixture (Some MAO inhibitors have contributed to hypoglycemic episodes in diabetic patients receiving insulin). Products include:
Humulin 50/50, 100 Units 1934
Humulin 70/30, 100 Units 1935
Humulin 70/30 Pen 1936
Novolin 70/30 Human Insulin 10 ml Vials 2421
Novolin 70/30 PenFill 2423
Novolin 70/30 Prefilled Disposable Insulin Delivery System 2425

Insulin, NPH (Some MAO inhibitors have contributed to hypoglycemic episodes in diabetic patients receiving insulin). Products include:
Iletin II, NPH (Pork), 100 Units 1946

Insulin, Regular (Some MAO inhibitors have contributed to hypoglycemic episodes in diabetic patients receiving insulin). Products include:
Iletin II, Regular (Pork), 100 Units 1947

Insulin, Zinc Crystals (Some MAO inhibitors have contributed to hypoglycemic episodes in diabetic patients receiving insulin).
No products indexed under this heading.

Insulin, Zinc Suspension (Some MAO inhibitors have contributed to hypoglycemic episodes in diabetic patients receiving insulin). Products include:
Iletin II, Lente (Pork), 100 Units 1945

Insulin Aspart, Human Regular (Some MAO inhibitors have contributed to hypoglycemic episodes in diabetic patients receiving insulin).
No products indexed under this heading.

Insulin glargine (Some MAO inhibitors have contributed to hypoglycemic episodes in diabetic patients receiving insulin). Products include:
Lantus Injection 742

Insulin Lispro, Human (Some MAO inhibitors have contributed to hypoglycemic episodes in diabetic patients receiving insulin). Products include:
Humalog 1926
Humalog Mix 75/25 Pen 1928

Insulin Lispro Protamine, Human (Some MAO inhibitors have contributed to hypoglycemic episodes in diabetic patients receiving insulin). Products include:
Humalog Mix 75/25 Pen 1928

Irbesartan (Concurrent use with hypotensive agents is contraindicated; a marked potentiating effect on these classes of drugs has been reported). Products include:
Avalide Tablets 1070
Avapro Tablets 1074
Avapro Tablets 3076

Isocarboxazid (Concurrent use with another MAO inhibitor may result in hypertensive crises or severe convulsive seizures; concurrent and/or sequential use is contraindicated).
No products indexed under this heading.

Isoflurane (Concurrent use is contraindicated).
No products indexed under this heading.

Isoproterenol Hydrochloride (Concurrent and/or sequential use is contraindicated; combination therapy may precipitate hypertension, headache and related symptoms).
No products indexed under this heading.

Isoproterenol Sulfate (Concurrent and/or sequential use is contraindicated; combination therapy may precipitate hypertension, headache and related symptoms).
No products indexed under this heading.

Isradipine (Concurrent use with hypotensive agents is contraindicated; a marked potentiating effect on these classes of drugs has been reported). Products include:
DynaCirc Capsules 2921
DynaCirc CR Tablets 2923

Ketamine Hydrochloride (Concurrent use is contraindicated).
No products indexed under this heading.

Labetalol Hydrochloride (Concurrent use with hypotensive agents is contraindicated; a marked potentiating effect on these classes of drugs has been reported). Products include:
Normodyne Injection 3135
Normodyne Tablets 3137

Levalbuterol Hydrochloride (Concurrent and/or sequential use is contraindicated; combination therapy may precipitate hypertension, headache and related symptoms). Products include:
Xopenex Inhalation Solution 3207

Levodopa (Concurrent and/or sequential use is contraindicated; combination therapy may precipitate hypertension, headache and related symptoms). Products include:
Sinemet Tablets 1253
Sinemet CR Tablets 1255

Levorphanol Tartrate (Concurrent use is contraindicated; a marked potentiating effect on these classes of drugs has been reported). Products include:
Levo-Dromoran 1734
Levorphanol Tartrate Tablets 3059

Lisinopril (Concurrent use with hypotensive agents is contraindicated; a marked potentiating effect on these classes of drugs has been reported). Products include:
Prinivil Tablets 2164
Prinzide Tablets 2168
Zestoretic Tablets 695
Zestril Tablets 698

Loratadine (Concurrent use is contraindicated). Products include:
Claritin 3100
Claritin-D 12 Hour Extended Release Tablets 3102
Claritin-D 24 Hour Extended Release Tablets 3104

Lorazepam (Concurrent use is contraindicated). Products include:
Ativan Injection 3478
Ativan Tablets 3482

Losartan Potassium (Concurrent use with hypotensive agents is contraindicated; a marked potentiating effect on these classes of drugs has been reported). Products include:
Cozaar Tablets 2067
Hyzaar 2109

Maprotiline Hydrochloride (Concurrent use with tricyclic antidepressants may result in hypertensive crises or severe convulsive seizures; concurrent and/or sequential use is contraindicated).
No products indexed under this heading.

Mazindol (Concurrent and/or sequential use is contraindicated).
No products indexed under this heading.

Mecamylamine Hydrochloride (Concurrent use with hypotensive agents is contraindicated; a marked potentiating effect on these classes of drugs has been reported). Products include:
Inversine Tablets 1850

Meperidine Hydrochloride (Concomitant use or within 2 or 3 weeks following MAOI therapy is contraindicated; serious reactions including coma, severe hypertension or hypotension, convulsion, severe respiratory depression, malignant hyperplexia, excitation, peripheral vascular collapse, and death have been reported with combined use). Products include:
Demerol 3079
Mepergan Injection 3539

Mesoridazine Besylate (Possibility of additive hypotensive effects). Products include:
Serentil 1057

Metaproterenol Sulfate (Concurrent and/or sequential use is contraindicated; combination therapy may precipitate hypertension, headache and related symptoms). Products include:
Alupent 1029

Metaraminol Bitartrate (Concurrent and/or sequential use is contraindicated; combination therapy may precipitate hypertension, headache and related symptoms). Products include:
Aramine Injection 2043

Metformin Hydrochloride (Some MAO inhibitors have contributed to hypoglycemic episodes in diabetic patients receiving oral hypoglycemic agents). Products include:
Glucophage Tablets 1080
Glucophage XR Tablets 1080
Glucovance Tablets 1086

Methadone Hydrochloride (Concurrent use is contraindicated; a marked potentiating effect on these classes of drugs has been reported). Products include:
Dolophine Hydrochloride Tablets 3056

Methamphetamine Hydrochloride (Concurrent and/or sequential use is contraindicated). Products include:
Desoxyn Tablets 440

Methdilazine Hydrochloride (Concurrent use is contraindicated).
No products indexed under this heading.

Methohexital Sodium (Concurrent use is contraindicated). Products include:
Brevital Sodium for Injection, USP .. 1815

Methotrimeprazine (Possibility of additive hypotensive effects).
No products indexed under this heading.

Methoxamine Hydrochloride (Concurrent and/or sequential use is contraindicated; combination therapy may precipitate hypertension, headache and related symptoms).
No products indexed under this heading.

Methyclothiazide (Concurrent use with hypotensive agents is contraindicated; a marked potentiating effect on these classes of drugs has been reported).
No products indexed under this heading.

Methyldopa (Concurrent and/or sequential use is contraindicated; combination therapy may precipitate hypertension, headache and related symptoms). Products include:
Aldoclor Tablets 2035
Aldomet Tablets 2037
Aldoril Tablets 2039

Methyldopate Hydrochloride (Concurrent and/or sequential use is contraindicated; combination therapy may precipitate hypertension, headache and related symptoms).
No products indexed under this heading.

Metolazone (Concurrent use with hypotensive agents is contraindicated; a marked potentiating effect on these classes of drugs has been reported). Products include:
Mykrox Tablets 1168
Zaroxolyn Tablets 1177

Metoprolol Succinate (Concurrent use with hypotensive agents is contraindicated; a marked potentiating effect on these classes of drugs has been reported). Products include:
Toprol-XL Tablets 651

Metoprolol Tartrate (Concurrent use with hypotensive agents is contraindicated; a marked potentiating effect on these classes of drugs has been reported).
No products indexed under this heading.

Metrizamide (Concurrent use with drugs which lower seizure threshold, including MAO inhibitors, should not be used with metrizamide).
No products indexed under this heading.

Metyrosine (Concurrent use with hypotensive agents is contraindicated; a marked potentiating effect on these classes of drugs has been reported). Products include:
Demser Capsules 2085

Mibefradil Dihydrochloride (Concurrent use with hypotensive agents is contraindicated; a marked potentiating effect on these classes of drugs has been reported).
No products indexed under this heading.

Midazolam Hydrochloride (Concurrent use is contraindicated). Products include:
Versed Injection 3027
Versed Syrup 3033

Miglitol (Some MAO inhibitors have contributed to hypoglycemic episodes in diabetic patients receiving oral hypoglycemic agents). Products include:
Glyset Tablets 2821

Minoxidil (Concurrent use with hypotensive agents is contraindicated; a marked potentiating effect on these classes of drugs has been reported). Products include:
Rogaine Extra Strength for Men Topical Solution .... ■721
Rogaine for Women Topical Solution .... ■721

Moclobemide (Concurrent use with another MAO inhibitor may result in hypertensive crises or severe convulsive seizures; concurrent and/or sequential use is contraindicated).
No products indexed under this heading.

Moexipril Hydrochloride (Concurrent use with hypotensive agents is contraindicated; a marked potentiating effect on these classes of drugs has been reported). Products include:
Uniretic Tablets 3178
Univasc Tablets 3181

Morphine Sulfate (Concurrent use is contraindicated; a marked potentiating effect on these classes of drugs has been reported). Products include:
Astramorph/PF Injection, USP (Preservative-Free) 594
Duramorph Injection 1312
Infumorph 200 and Infumorph 500 Sterile Solutions 1314
Kadian Capsules 1335
MS Contin Tablets 2896
MSIR 2898
Oramorph SR Tablets 3062
Roxanol 3066

Nadolol (Concurrent use with hypotensive agents is contraindicated; a marked potentiating effect on these classes of drugs has been reported). Products include:
Corgard Tablets 2245
Corzide 40/5 Tablets 2247
Corzide 80/5 Tablets 2247
Nadolol Tablets 2288

Naphazoline Hydrochloride (Concurrent and/or sequential use is contraindicated; combination therapy may precipitate hypertension, headache and related symptoms). Products include:
Albalon Ophthalmic Solution .... ⊙225
All Clear Eye Drops .... ⊙252
All Clear AR Eye Drops .... ⊙252
Clear Eyes ACR Astringent/Lubricant Eye Redness Reliever .... ⊙322
Clear Eyes Lubricant Eye Redness Reliever .... ⊙322
Naphcon-A Ophthalmic Solution 540
Opcon-A Eye Drops .... ⊙253
Vasocon-A Eye Drops .... ⊙307
Visine-A Eye Allergy Relief Eye Drops .... ⊙314
Visine-A Eye Drops .... ■714

Nicardipine Hydrochloride (Concurrent use with hypotensive agents is contraindicated; a marked potentiating effect on these classes of drugs has been reported). Products include:
Cardene I.V. 3485

Nifedipine (Concurrent use with hypotensive agents is contraindicated; a marked potentiating effect on these classes of drugs has been reported). Products include:
Adalat CC Tablets 877
Procardia Capsules 2708
Procardia XL Extended Release Tablets 2710

Nisoldipine (Concurrent use with hypotensive agents is contraindicated; a marked potentiating effect on these classes of drugs has been reported). Products include:
Sular Tablets 688

Nitroglycerin (Concurrent use with hypotensive agents is contraindicated; a marked potentiating effect on these classes of drugs has been reported). Products include:
Nitro-Dur Transdermal Infusion System 3134
Nitro-Dur Transdermal Infusion System 1834
Nitrolingual Pumpspray 1355
Nitrostat Tablets 2658

Norepinephrine Bitartrate (Concurrent and/or sequential use is contraindicated; combination therapy may precipitate hypertension, headache and related symptoms).
No products indexed under this heading.

Nortriptyline Hydrochloride (Concurrent use with tricyclic antidepressants may result in hypertensive crises or severe convulsive seizures; concurrent and/or sequential use is contraindicated).
No products indexed under this heading.

Oxycodone Hydrochloride (Concurrent use is contraindicated; a marked potentiating effect on these classes of drugs has been reported). Products include:
OxyContin Tablets 2912
OxyFast Oral Concentrate Solution . 2916
OxyIR Capsules 2916
Percocet Tablets 1326
Percodan Tablets 1327
Percolone Tablets 1327
Roxicodone 3067
Tylox Capsules 2597

Oxymetazoline Hydrochloride (Concurrent and/or sequential use is contraindicated; combination therapy may precipitate hypertension, headache and related symptoms). Products include:
Afrin .... ■733
Afrin No Drip Original Nasal Spray .... ■735
Afrin No Drip Extra Moisturizing Nasal Spray .... ■735
Afrin No Drip Severe Congestion Nasal Spray .... ■735
Afrin No Drip Sinus Nasal Spray ... ■735
Afrin Original Pump Mist .... ■733
Neo-Synephrine 12 Hour .... ■615
Vicks Sinex 12-Hour Nasal Spray and Ultra Fine Mist .... ■729
Visine L.R. Long Lasting Eye Drops .... ⊙315

Pargyline Hydrochloride (Concurrent use with another MAO inhibitor may result in hypertensive crises or severe convulsive seizures; concurrent and/or sequential use is contraindicated).
No products indexed under this heading.

Paroxetine Hydrochloride (Concurrent and/or sequential use is contraindicated; potential for serious, sometimes fatal, reactions including hyperthermia, rigidity, myoclonus, and other toxicities; at least 2 weeks should be allowed after stopping paroxetine before starting an MAO inhibitor). Products include:
Paxil 1609

Penbutolol Sulfate (Concurrent use with hypotensive agents is contraindicated; a marked potentiating effect on these classes of drugs has been reported).
No products indexed under this heading.

Perindopril Erbumine (Concurrent use with hypotensive agents is contraindicated; a marked potentiating effect on these classes of drugs has been reported). Products include:
Aceon Tablets (2 mg, 4 mg, 8 mg) 3249

Perphenazine (Possibility of additive hypotensive effects). Products include:
Etrafon 3115
Trilafon 3160

Phendimetrazine Tartrate (Concurrent and/or sequential use is contraindicated). Products include:
Bontril Slow-Release Capsules 576

Phenelzine Sulfate (Concurrent use with another MAO inhibitor may result in hypertensive crises or severe convulsive seizures; concurrent and/or sequential use is contraindicated). Products include:
Nardil Tablets 2653

Phenmetrazine Hydrochloride (Concurrent and/or sequential use is contraindicated).
No products indexed under this heading.

Phenoxybenzamine Hydrochloride (Concurrent use with hypotensive agents is contraindicated; a marked potentiating effect on these classes of drugs has been reported). Products include:
Dibenzyline Capsules 3457

Phentolamine Mesylate (Concurrent use with hypotensive agents is contraindicated; a marked potentiat-

ing effect on these classes of drugs has been reported).

No products indexed under this heading.

Phenylephrine Bitartrate (Concurrent and/or sequential use is contraindicated; combination therapy may precipitate hypertension, headache and related symptoms).

No products indexed under this heading.

Phenylephrine Hydrochloride (Concurrent and/or sequential use is contraindicated; combination therapy may precipitate hypertension, headache and related symptoms). Products include:

- Afrin Nasal Decongestant Children's Pump Mist ▣734
- Extendryl 1361
- Hycomine Compound Tablets 1317
- Neo-Synephrine ▣614
- Phenergan VC Syrup 3560
- Phenergan VC with Codeine Syrup 3561
- Preparation H Cream ▣778
- Preparation H Cooling Gel ▣778
- Preparation H ▣778
- Vicks Sinex Nasal Spray and Ultra Fine Mist ▣729

Phenylephrine Tannate (Concurrent and/or sequential use is contraindicated; combination therapy may precipitate hypertension, headache and related symptoms). Products include:

- Ryna-12 S Suspension 3351
- Reformulated Rynatan Pediatric Suspension 3352
- Rynatuss Pediatric Suspension 3353
- Rynatuss Tablets 3353

Phenylpropanolamine Hydrochloride (Concurrent and/or sequential use is contraindicated; combination therapy may precipitate hypertension, headache and related symptoms).

No products indexed under this heading.

Pindolol (Concurrent use with hypotensive agents is contraindicated; a marked potentiating effect on these classes of drugs has been reported).

No products indexed under this heading.

Pioglitazone Hydrochloride (Some MAO inhibitors have contributed to hypoglycemic episodes in diabetic patients receiving oral hypoglycemic agents). Products include:

- Actos Tablets 3275

Pirbuterol Acetate (Concurrent and/or sequential use is contraindicated; combination therapy may precipitate hypertension, headache and related symptoms). Products include:

- Maxair Autohaler 1981
- Maxair Inhaler 1984

Polythiazide (Concurrent use with hypotensive agents is contraindicated; a marked potentiating effect on these classes of drugs has been reported). Products include:

- Minizide Capsules 2700
- Renese Tablets 2712

Prazosin Hydrochloride (Concurrent use with hypotensive agents is contraindicated; a marked potentiating effect on these classes of drugs has been reported). Products include:

- Minipress Capsules 2699
- Minizide Capsules 2700

Procarbazine Hydrochloride (Concurrent use with another MAO inhibitor may result in hypertensive crises or severe convulsive seizures; concurrent and/or sequential use is contraindicated). Products include:

- Matulane Capsules 3246

Prochlorperazine (Possibility of additive hypotensive effects). Products include:

- Compazine 1505

Procyclidine Hydrochloride (Anti-Parkinsonism drugs should be used with caution in patients receiving Parnate since severe reactions have been reported).

No products indexed under this heading.

Promethazine Hydrochloride (Concurrent use is contraindicated). Products include:

- Mepergan Injection 3539
- Phenergan Injection 3553
- Phenergan 3556
- Phenergan Syrup 3554
- Phenergan with Codeine Syrup 3557
- Phenergan with Dextromethorphan Syrup 3559
- Phenergan VC Syrup 3560
- Phenergan VC with Codeine Syrup 3561

Propofol (Concurrent use is contraindicated). Products include:

- Diprivan Injectable Emulsion 667

Propoxyphene Hydrochloride (Concurrent use is contraindicated; a marked potentiating effect on these classes of drugs has been reported). Products include:

- Darvon Pulvules 1909
- Darvon Compound-65 Pulvules 1910

Propoxyphene Napsylate (Concurrent use is contraindicated; a marked potentiating effect on these classes of drugs has been reported). Products include:

- Darvon-N/Darvocet-N 1907
- Darvon-N Tablets 1912

Propranolol Hydrochloride (Concurrent use with hypotensive agents is contraindicated; a marked potentiating effect on these classes of drugs has been reported). Products include:

- Inderal 3513
- Inderal LA Long-Acting Capsules 3516
- Inderide Tablets 3517
- Inderide LA Long-Acting Capsules 3519

Protriptyline Hydrochloride (Concurrent use with tricyclic antidepressants may result in hypertensive crises or severe convulsive seizures; concurrent and/or sequential use is contraindicated). Products include:

- Vivactil Tablets 2446
- Vivactil Tablets 2217

Pseudoephedrine Hydrochloride (Concurrent and/or sequential use is contraindicated; combination therapy may precipitate hypertension, headache and related symptoms). Products include:

- Actifed Cold & Allergy Tablets ▣688
- Actifed Cold & Sinus Caplets and Tablets ▣688
- Advil Cold and Sinus Caplets ▣771
- Advil Cold and Sinus Tablets ▣771
- Advil Flu & Body Ache Caplets ▣772
- Aleve Cold & Sinus Caplets ▣603
- Alka-Seltzer Plus Liqui-Gels ▣604
- Alka-Seltzer Plus Cold & Flu Medicine Liqui-Gels ▣604
- Alka-Seltzer Plus Cold & Sinus Medicine Liqui-Gels ▣604
- Allegra-D Extended-Release Tablets 714
- BC Cold Powder ▣619
- Benadryl Allergy/Cold Tablets ▣691
- Benadryl Allergy/Congestion Tablets ▣692
- Benadryl Allergy & Sinus Liquid ▣693
- Benadryl Allergy & Sinus Fastmelt Tablets ▣693
- Benadryl Allergy Sinus Headache Caplets & Gelcaps ▣693
- Benadryl Severe Allergy & Sinus Headache Caplets ▣694
- Benadryl Children's Allergy/Cold Fastmelt Tablets ▣692
- Benylin Multi-Symptom Liquid ▣697
- Bromfed Capsules (Extended-Release) 2269
- Bromfed-PD Capsules (Extended-Release) 2269
- Children's Cēpacol Sore Throat ▣788
- Comtrex Acute Head Cold & Sinus Pressure Relief Tablets ▣627
- Comtrex Deep Chest Cold & Congestion Relief Softgels ▣627
- Comtrex Flu Therapy & Fever Relief Daytime Caplets ▣628
- Comtrex Flu Therapy & Fever Relief Nighttime Tablets ▣628
- Comtrex Maximum Strength Multi-Symptom Cold & Cough Relief Tablets and Caplets ▣626
- Contac Non-Drowsy 12 Hour Cold Caplets ▣745
- Contac Non-Drowsy Timed Release 12 Hour Cold Caplets ▣746
- Contac Severe Cold and Flu Caplets Maximum Strength ▣746
- Contac Severe Cold and Flu Caplets Non-Drowsy ▣746
- Dimetapp Elixir ▣777
- Dimetapp Cold and Fever Suspension ▣775
- Dimetapp DM Cold & Cough Elixir ▣775
- Dimetapp Nighttime Flu Liquid ▣776
- Dimetapp Non-Drowsy Flu Syrup ▣777
- Dimetapp Infant Drops Decongestant ▣775
- Dimetapp Infant Drops Decongestant Plus Cough ▣776
- Guaifed 2272
- Kronofed-A 1341
- Children's Motrin Cold Oral Suspension 2007
- Motrin Sinus Headache Caplets 2005
- PediaCare Cough-Cold Liquid ▣719
- PediaCare Infants' Drops Decongestant ▣719
- PediaCare Infants' Drops Decongestant Plus Cough ▣719
- PediaCare NightRest Cough-Cold Liquid ▣719
- Robitussin Cold Caplets Cold & Congestion ▣780
- Robitussin Cold Softgels Cold & Congestion ▣780
- Robitussin Cold Caplets Multi-Symptom Cold & Flu ▣781
- Robitussin Cold Softgels Multi-Symptom Cold & Flu ▣781
- Robitussin Cold Softgels Severe Congestion ▣782
- Robitussin Cough & Cold Infant Drops ▣782
- Robitussin Maximum Strength Cough & Cold Liquid ▣785
- Robitussin Pediatric Cough & Cold Formula Liquid ▣785
- Robitussin Multi Symptom Honey Flu Liquid ▣785
- Robitussin Nighttime Honey Flu Liquid ▣786
- Robitussin-CF Liquid ▣783
- Robitussin-DAC Syrup 2942
- Robitussin-PE Liquid ▣782
- Ryna ▣768
- Semprex-D Capsules 1172
- Singlet Caplets ▣761
- Sinutab Non-Drying Liquid Caps ▣706
- Sinutab Sinus Allergy Medication, Maximum Strength Formula, Tablets & Caplets ▣707
- Sinutab Sinus Medication, Maximum Strength Without Drowsiness Formula, Tablets & Caplets ▣707
- Sudafed 12 Hour Tablets ▣708
- Sudafed 24 Hour Tablets ▣708
- Children's Sudafed Cold & Cough Liquid ▣709
- Children's Sudafed Nasal Decongestant Chewables ▣711
- Children's Sudafed Nasal Decongestant Liquid Medication ▣711
- Sudafed Cold & Allergy Tablets ▣708
- Sudafed Cold & Cough Liquid Caps ▣709
- Sudafed Cold & Sinus Liquid Caps ▣710
- Sudafed Nasal Decongestant Tablets ▣710
- Sudafed Non-Drying Sinus Liquid Caps ▣712
- Sudafed Severe Cold ▣711
- Sudafed Sinus Headache Caplets ▣712
- Sudafed Sinus Headache Tablets ▣712
- Tavist Sinus Non-Drowsy Coated Caplets ▣676
- TheraFlu Regular Strength Cold & Cough Night Time Hot Liquid ▣676
- TheraFlu Regular Strength Cold & Sore Throat Night Time Hot Liquid ▣676
- TheraFlu Maximum Strength Flu & Congestion Non-Drowsy Hot Liquid ▣677
- TheraFlu Maximum Strength Flu & Cough Night Time Hot Liquid ▣678
- TheraFlu Maximum Strength Flu & Sore Throat Night Time Hot Liquid ▣677
- TheraFlu Maximum Strength Severe Cold & Congestion Night Time Caplets ▣678
- TheraFlu Maximum Strength Severe Cold & Congestion Night Time Hot Liquid ▣678
- TheraFlu Maximum Strength Severe Cold & Congestion Non-Drowsy ▣679
- Triaminic Allergy Congestion Liquid ▣680
- Triaminic Chest Congestion Liquid ▣680
- Triaminic Cold & Allergy Liquid ▣681
- Triaminic Cold & Allergy Softchews ▣683
- Triaminic Cold & Cough Liquid ▣681
- Triaminic Cold & Cough Softchews ▣683
- Triaminic Cold & Night Time Cough Liquid ▣681
- Triaminic Cold, Cough & Fever Liquid ▣681
- Triaminic Cough Liquid ▣682
- Triaminic Cough & Congestion Liquid ▣682
- Triaminic Cough & Sore Throat Liquid ▣682
- Triaminic Cough & Sore Throat Softchews ▣684
- Children's Tylenol Allergy-D Liquid 2014
- Children's Tylenol Cold Suspension Liquid and Chewable Tablets 2015
- Children's Tylenol Cold Plus Cough Suspension Liquid and Chewable Tablets 2015
- Children's Tylenol Flu Suspension Liquid 2015
- Children's Tylenol Sinus Suspension Liquid 2017
- Infants' Tylenol Cold Decongestant and Fever Reducer Concentrated Drops 2015
- Infants' Tylenol Cold Decongestant and Fever Reducer Concentrated Drops Plus Cough 2015
- Tylenol Allergy Sinus 2010
- Multi-Symptom Tylenol Cold Complete Formula Caplets 2010
- Multi-Symptom Tylenol Cold Non-Drowsy Caplets and Gelcaps 2010
- Multi-Symptom Tylenol Cold Severe Congestion Non-Drowsy Caplets 2011
- Maximum Strength Tylenol Flu NightTime Gelcaps 2011
- Maximum Strength Tylenol Flu NightTime Liquid 2011
- Maximum Strength Tylenol Flu Non-Drowsy Gelcaps 2011
- Maximum Strength Tylenol Sinus NightTime Caplets 2012
- Maximum Strength Tylenol Sinus Non-Drowsy Geltabs, Gelcaps, Caplets, and Tablets 2012
- Vicks 44D Cough & Head Congestion Relief Liquid ▣724
- Vicks 44M Cough, Cold & Flu Relief Liquid ▣725
- Pediatric Vicks 44m Cough & Cold Relief ▣728
- Vicks DayQuil LiquiCaps/Liquid Multi-Symptom Cold/Flu Relief ▣727
- Children's Vicks NyQuil Cold/Cough Relief ▣726
- Vicks NyQuil LiquiCaps/Liquid Multi-Symptom Cold/Flu Relief, Original and Cherry Flavors ▣727
- Zephrex Tablets 3091
- Zephrex LA Tablets 3092
- Zyrtec-D 12 Hour Extended Relief Tablets 2758

Pseudoephedrine Sulfate (Concurrent and/or sequential use is contraindicated; combination therapy may precipitate hypertension, headache and related symptoms). Products include:

- Chlor-Trimeton Allergy/Decongestant Tablets ▣736
- Claritin-D 12 Hour Extended Release Tablets 3102
- Claritin-D 24 Hour Extended Release Tablets 3104
- Coricidin 'D' Cold, Flu & Sinus Tablets ▣737
- Drixoral Allergy/Sinus Extended-Release Tablets ▣741
- Drixoral Cold & Allergy Sustained-Action Tablets ▣740
- Drixoral Cold & Flu Extended-Release Tablets ▣740
- Drixoral Nasal Decongestant Long-Acting Non-Drowsy Tablets ▣740
- Rynatan Tablets 3351

IMPORTANT NOTE: Always consult each drug listing in the patient's regimen for possible interactions.

Pyrilamine Maleate (Concurrent use is contraindicated). Products include:
- Maximum Strength Midol Menstrual Caplets and Gelcaps .... ▣612
- Maximum Strength Midol PMS Caplets and Gelcaps .... ▣613

Pyrilamine Tannate (Concurrent use is contraindicated). Products include:
- Ryna-12 S Suspension 3351

Quazepam (Concurrent use is contraindicated).
No products indexed under this heading.

Quinapril Hydrochloride (Concurrent use with hypotensive agents is contraindicated; a marked potentiating effect on these classes of drugs has been reported). Products include:
- Accupril Tablets 2611
- Accuretic Tablets 2614

Ramipril (Concurrent use with hypotensive agents is contraindicated; a marked potentiating effect on these classes of drugs has been reported). Products include:
- Altace Capsules 2233

Rauwolfia serpentina (Concurrent use with hypotensive agents is contraindicated; a marked potentiating effect on these classes of drugs has been reported).
No products indexed under this heading.

Remifentanil Hydrochloride (Concurrent use is contraindicated; a marked potentiating effect on these classes of drugs has been reported).
No products indexed under this heading.

Repaglinide (Some MAO inhibitors have contributed to hypoglycemic episodes in diabetic patients receiving oral hypoglycemic agents). Products include:
- Prandin Tablets (0.5, 1, and 2 mg) 2432

Rescinnamine (Concurrent use with hypotensive agents is contraindicated; a marked potentiating effect on these classes of drugs has been reported).
No products indexed under this heading.

Reserpine (Concurrent and/or sequential use is contraindicated; combination therapy may precipitate hypertension, headache and related symptoms).
No products indexed under this heading.

Rosiglitazone Maleate (Some MAO inhibitors have contributed to hypoglycemic episodes in diabetic patients receiving oral hypoglycemic agents). Products include:
- Avandia Tablets 1490

Salmeterol Xinafoate (Concurrent and/or sequential use is contraindicated; combination therapy may precipitate hypertension, headache and related symptoms). Products include:
- Advair Diskus 100/50 1448
- Advair Diskus 250/50 1448
- Advair Diskus 500/50 1448
- Serevent Diskus 1637
- Serevent Inhalation Aerosol 1633

Secobarbital Sodium (Concurrent use is contraindicated).
No products indexed under this heading.

Selegiline Hydrochloride (Concurrent use with another MAO inhibitor may result in hypertensive crises or severe convulsive seizures; concurrent and/or sequential use is contraindicated). Products include:
- Eldepryl Capsules 3266

Sertraline Hydrochloride (Concurrent and/or sequential use is contraindicated; potential for serious, sometimes fatal, reactions including hyperthermia, rigidity, myoclonus, and other toxicities; at least 2 weeks should be allowed after stopping sertraline before starting an MAO inhibitor). Products include:
- Zoloft 2751

Sibutramine Hydrochloride Monohydrate (Concurrent and/or sequential use is contraindicated). Products include:
- Meridia Capsules 481

Sodium Nitroprusside (Concurrent use with hypotensive agents is contraindicated; a marked potentiating effect on these classes of drugs has been reported).
No products indexed under this heading.

Sotalol Hydrochloride (Concurrent use with hypotensive agents is contraindicated; a marked potentiating effect on these classes of drugs has been reported). Products include:
- Betapace Tablets 950
- Betapace AF Tablets 954

Spirapril Hydrochloride (Concurrent use with hypotensive agents is contraindicated; a marked potentiating effect on these classes of drugs has been reported).
No products indexed under this heading.

Spironolactone (Concurrent use with hypotensive agents is contraindicated; a marked potentiating effect on these classes of drugs has been reported).
No products indexed under this heading.

Sufentanil Citrate (Concurrent use is contraindicated; a marked potentiating effect on these classes of drugs has been reported).
No products indexed under this heading.

Telmisartan (Concurrent use with hypotensive agents is contraindicated; a marked potentiating effect on these classes of drugs has been reported). Products include:
- Micardis Tablets 1049
- Micardis HCT Tablets 1051

Temazepam (Concurrent use is contraindicated).
No products indexed under this heading.

Terazosin Hydrochloride (Concurrent use with hypotensive agents is contraindicated; a marked potentiating effect on these classes of drugs has been reported). Products include:
- Hytrin Capsules 464

Terbutaline Sulfate (Concurrent and/or sequential use is contraindicated; combination therapy may precipitate hypertension, headache and related symptoms). Products include:
- Brethine Ampuls 2314
- Brethine Tablets 2313

Terfenadine (Concurrent use is contraindicated).
No products indexed under this heading.

Tetrahydrozoline Hydrochloride (Concurrent and/or sequential use is contraindicated; combination therapy may precipitate hypertension, headache and related symptoms). Products include:
- Murine Tears Plus Lubricant Redness Reliever Eye Drops .... ⊙323
- Visine Original Eye Drops .... ⊙315
- Visine A.C. Seasonal Relief From Pollen & Dust Eye Drops .... ⊙314
- Advanced Relief Visine Eye Drops .... ⊙313

Thiamylal Sodium (Concurrent use is contraindicated).
No products indexed under this heading.

Thioridazine Hydrochloride (Possibility of additive hypotensive effects). Products include:
- Thioridazine Hydrochloride Tablets 2289

Timolol Maleate (Concurrent use with hypotensive agents is contraindicated; a marked potentiating effect on these classes of drugs has been reported). Products include:
- Blocadren Tablets 2046
- Cosopt Sterile Ophthalmic Solution 2065
- Timolide Tablets 2187
- Timolol GFS .... ⊙266
- Timoptic in Ocudose 2192
- Timoptic Sterile Ophthalmic Solution 2190
- Timoptic-XE Sterile Ophthalmic Gel Forming Solution 2194

Tolazamide (Some MAO inhibitors have contributed to hypoglycemic episodes in diabetic patients receiving oral hypoglycemic agents).
No products indexed under this heading.

Tolbutamide (Some MAO inhibitors have contributed to hypoglycemic episodes in diabetic patients receiving oral hypoglycemic agents).
No products indexed under this heading.

Torsemide (Concurrent use with hypotensive agents is contraindicated; a marked potentiating effect on these classes of drugs has been reported). Products include:
- Demadex Tablets and Injection 2965

Trandolapril (Concurrent use with hypotensive agents is contraindicated; a marked potentiating effect on these classes of drugs has been reported). Products include:
- Mavik Tablets 478
- Tarka Tablets 508

Triamterene (Concurrent use with hypotensive agents is contraindicated; a marked potentiating effect on these classes of drugs has been reported). Products include:
- Dyazide Capsules 1515
- Dyrenium Capsules 3458
- Maxzide 1008

Triazolam (Concurrent use is contraindicated). Products include:
- Halcion Tablets 2823

Tridihexethyl Chloride (Anti-Parkinsonism drugs should be used with caution in patients receiving Parnate since severe reactions have been reported).
No products indexed under this heading.

Trifluoperazine Hydrochloride (Possibility of additive hypotensive effects). Products include:
- Stelazine 1640

Trihexyphenidyl Hydrochloride (Anti-Parkinsonism drugs should be used with caution in patients receiving Parnate since severe reactions have been reported). Products include:
- Artane 1855

Trimeprazine Tartrate (Concurrent use is contraindicated).
No products indexed under this heading.

Trimethaphan Camsylate (Concurrent use with hypotensive agents is contraindicated; a marked potentiating effect on these classes of drugs has been reported).
No products indexed under this heading.

Trimipramine Maleate (Concurrent use with tricyclic antidepressants may result in hypertensive crises or severe convulsive seizures; concurrent and/or sequential use is contraindicated). Products include:
- Surmontil Capsules 3595

Tripelennamine Hydrochloride (Concurrent use is contraindicated).
No products indexed under this heading.

Triprolidine Hydrochloride (Concurrent use is contraindicated). Products include:
- Actifed Cold & Allergy Tablets .... ▣688

Troglitazone (Some MAO inhibitors have contributed to hypoglycemic episodes in diabetic patients receiving oral hypoglycemic agents).
No products indexed under this heading.

L-Tryptophan (Concurrent and/or sequential use is contraindicated; combination therapy may precipitate hypertension, disorientation, memory impairment, other neurologic and behavioral changes, headache and related symptoms).
No products indexed under this heading.

Tyramine (Concurrent use is contraindicated).
No products indexed under this heading.

Valsartan (Concurrent use with hypotensive agents is contraindicated; a marked potentiating effect on these classes of drugs has been reported). Products include:
- Diovan Capsules 2337
- Diovan HCT Tablets 2338

Verapamil Hydrochloride (Concurrent use with hypotensive agents is contraindicated; a marked potentiating effect on these classes of drugs has been reported). Products include:
- Covera-HS Tablets 3199
- Isoptin SR Tablets 467
- Tarka Tablets 508
- Verelan Capsules 3184
- Verelan PM Capsules 3186

Zaleplon (Concurrent use is contraindicated). Products include:
- Sonata Capsules 3591

Zolpidem Tartrate (Concurrent use is contraindicated). Products include:
- Ambien Tablets 3191

Food Interactions

Alcohol (Concurrent use is contraindicated; a marked potentiating effect on alcohol has been reported).

Anchovies (Potential for hypertensive crisis; concurrent use is contraindicated).

Avocados (Potential for hypertensive crisis; concurrent use is contraindicated).

Bananas (Potential for hypertensive crisis; concurrent use is contraindicated).

Beans, broad (Potential for hypertensive crisis; concurrent use is contraindicated).

Beans, Fava (Potential for hypertensive crisis; concurrent use is contraindicated).

Beer, alcohol-free (Potential for hypertensive crisis; concurrent use is contraindicated).

Beer, unspecified (Potential for hypertensive crisis; concurrent use is contraindicated).

Beverages, caffeine-containing (Potential for hypertensive crisis; concurrent use is contraindicated).

Caviar (Potential for hypertensive crisis; concurrent use is contraindicated).

Cheese, aged (Potential for hypertensive crisis; concurrent use is contraindicated).

Cheese, strong, unpasteurized (Potential for hypertensive crisis; concurrent use is contraindicated).

Cheese, unspecified (Potential for hypertensive crisis; concurrent use is contraindicated).

Chocolate (Potential for hypertensive crisis; concurrent use is contraindicated).

Cream, sour (Potential for hypertensive crisis; concurrent use is contraindicated).

Figs, canned (Potential for hypertensive crisis; concurrent use is contraindicated).

Food with high concentration of tyramine (Potential for hypertensive crisis; concurrent use is contraindicated).

Fruits, dried (Potential for hypertensive crisis; concurrent use is contraindicated).

Fruits, overripe (Potential for hypertensive crisis; concurrent use is contraindicated).

Herring, pickled (Potential for hypertensive crisis; concurrent use is contraindicated).

Liqueurs (Potential for hypertensive crisis; concurrent use is contraindicated).

Liver (Potential for hypertensive crisis; concurrent use is contraindicated).

Meat extracts (Potential for hypertensive crisis; concurrent use is contraindicated).

Meat prepared with tenderizers (Potential for hypertensive crisis; concurrent use is contraindicated).

Prunes (Potential for hypertensive crisis; concurrent use is contraindicated).

Raisins (Potential for hypertensive crisis; concurrent use is contraindicated).

Raspberries (Potential for hypertensive crisis; concurrent use is contraindicated).

Sauerkraut (Potential for hypertensive crisis; concurrent use is contraindicated).

Sherry (Potential for hypertensive crisis; concurrent use is contraindicated).

Soy Sauce (Potential for hypertensive crisis; concurrent use is contraindicated).

Wine, Chianti (Potential for hypertensive crisis; concurrent use is contraindicated).

Yeast Extract (Potential for hypertensive crisis; concurrent use is contraindicated).

Yogurt (Potential for hypertensive crisis; concurrent use is contraindicated).

PASER GRANULES

(Aminosalicylic Acid) 1781
May interact with:

Digoxin (Potential for reduced digoxin levels). Products include:
- Digitek Tablets 1003
- Lanoxicaps Capsules 1574
- Lanoxin Injection 1581
- Lanoxin Tablets 1587
- Lanoxin Elixir Pediatric 1578
- Lanoxin Injection Pediatric 1584

Isoniazid (Concurrent use with a rapidly available form of aminosalicylic acid has been reported to produce a 20% reduction in the acetylation of INH; the lower serum levels produced by delayed release preparation will result in a reduced effect on the acetylation of INH). Products include:
- Rifamate Capsules 767
- Rifater Tablets 769

Rifampin (May block the absorption of rifampin; PASER granules do not contain excipient that blocks the absorption). Products include:
- Rifadin 765
- Rifamate Capsules 767
- Rifater Tablets 769

Vitamin B_{12} (Reduced absorption of vitamin B_{12} with clinically significant erythrocyte abnormalities developing after depletion). Products include:
- Bevitamel Tablets 3459
- Nascobal Gel 3174
- One-A-Day Memory & Concentration Tablets .... ▣807

PATANOL OPHTHALMIC SOLUTION

(Olopatadine Hydrochloride) 540
None cited in PDR database.

PAXIL ORAL SUSPENSION

(Paroxetine Hydrochloride) 1609
See Paxil Tablets

PAXIL TABLETS

(Paroxetine Hydrochloride) 1609
May interact with lithium preparations, monoamine oxidase inhibitors, phenothiazines, phenytoin, quinidine, tricyclic antidepressants, theophylline, and certain other agents. Compounds in these categories include:

Aminophylline (There have been reports of elevated theophylline levels associated with co-administration).
No products indexed under this heading.

Amitriptyline Hydrochloride (Co-administration may result in inhibition of tricyclic antidepressants by paroxetine; monitor plasma concentration of tricyclic antidepressant). Products include:
- Etrafon 3115
- Limbitrol 1738

Amoxapine (Co-administration may result in inhibition of tricyclic antidepressants by paroxetine; monitor plasma concentration of tricyclic antidepressant).
No products indexed under this heading.

Chlorpromazine (Paroxetine may significantly inhibit the activity of cytochrome isoenzyme P450IID6; co-administration should be approached with caution). Products include:
- Thorazine Suppositories 1656

Chlorpromazine Hydrochloride (Paroxetine may significantly inhibit the activity of cytochrome isoenzyme P450IID6; co-administration should be approached with caution). Products include:
- Thorazine 1656

Cimetidine (Co-administration with oral cimetidine has resulted in an increase in steady-state plasma concentrations of paroxetine). Products include:
- Tagamet HB 200 Suspension .... ▣762
- Tagamet HB 200 Tablets .... ▣761
- Tagamet Tablets 1644

Cimetidine Hydrochloride (Co-administration with oral cimetidine has resulted in an increase in steady-state plasma concentrations of paroxetine). Products include:
- Tagamet 1644

Clomipramine Hydrochloride (Co-administration may result in inhibition of tricyclic antidepressants by paroxetine; monitor plasma concentration of tricyclic antidepressant).
No products indexed under this heading.

Desipramine Hydrochloride (Co-administration with desipramine has resulted in an increase in Cmax, AUC and T1/2 by an average of approximately two-, five- and three-fold respectively). Products include:
- Norpramin Tablets 755

Diazepam (Under steady-state conditions, diazepam does not appear to affect paroxetine kinetics, however, paroxetine is highly protein bound to plasma protein; co-administration may result in displacement from binding sites of either drug resulting in increased adverse effects). Products include:
- Valium Injectable 3026
- Valium Tablets 3047

Digoxin (Potential for decrease in mean digoxin AUC). Products include:
- Digitek Tablets 1003
- Lanoxicaps Capsules 1574
- Lanoxin Injection 1581
- Lanoxin Tablets 1587
- Lanoxin Elixir Pediatric 1578
- Lanoxin Injection Pediatric 1584

Doxepin Hydrochloride (Co-administration may result in inhibition of tricyclic antidepressants by paroxetine; monitor plasma concentration of tricyclic antidepressant). Products include:
- Sinequan 2713

Dyphylline (There have been reports of elevated theophylline levels associated with co-administration). Products include:
- Lufyllin Tablets 3347
- Lufyllin-400 Tablets 3347
- Lufyllin-GG Elixir 3348
- Lufyllin-GG Tablets 3348

Fluphenazine Decanoate (Paroxetine may significantly inhibit the activity of cytochrome isoenzyme P450IID6; co-administration should be approached with caution).
No products indexed under this heading.

Fluphenazine Enanthate (Paroxetine may significantly inhibit the activity of cytochrome isoenzyme P450IID6; co-administration should be approached with caution).
No products indexed under this heading.

Fluphenazine Hydrochloride (Paroxetine may significantly inhibit the activity of cytochrome isoenzyme P450IID6; co-administration should be approached with caution).
No products indexed under this heading.

Fosphenytoin Sodium (Co-administration has resulted in reduction of paroxetine AUC and T1/2; potential for elevated phenytoin levels or slight reduction in phenytoin AUC). Products include:
- Cerebyx Injection 2619

Imipramine Hydrochloride (Co-administration may result in inhibition of tricyclic antidepressants by paroxetine; monitor plasma concentration of tricyclic antidepressant).
No products indexed under this heading.

Imipramine Pamoate (Co-administration may result in inhibition of tricyclic antidepressants by paroxetine; monitor plasma concentration of tricyclic antidepressant).
No products indexed under this heading.

Isocarboxazid (Potential for serious and fatal reactions including hyperthermia, rigidity, myoclonus and other serious reactions; concurrent and/or sequential use is contraindicated).
No products indexed under this heading.

Lithium Carbonate (Concurrent administration should be undertaken with caution). Products include:
- Eskalith 1527
- Lithium Carbonate 3061
- Lithobid Slow-Release Tablets 3255

Lithium Citrate (Concurrent administration should be undertaken with caution). Products include:
- Lithium Citrate Syrup 3061

Maprotiline Hydrochloride (Co-administration may result in inhibition of tricyclic antidepressants by paroxetine; monitor plasma concentration of tricyclic antidepressant).
No products indexed under this heading.

Mesoridazine Besylate (Paroxetine may significantly inhibit the activity of cytochrome isoenzyme P450IID6; co-administration should be approached with caution). Products include:
- Serentil 1057

Methotrimeprazine (Paroxetine may significantly inhibit the activity of cytochrome isoenzyme P450IID6; co-administration should be approached with caution).
No products indexed under this heading.

Metoprolol Succinate (There has been a case report of severe hypotension when paroxetine was added to chronic metoprolol treatment). Products include:
- Toprol-XL Tablets 651

Metoprolol Tartrate (There has been a case report of severe hypotension when paroxetine was added to chronic metoprolol treatment).
No products indexed under this heading.

Moclobemide (Potential for serious and fatal reactions including hyperthermia, rigidity, myoclonus and other serious reactions; concurrent and/or sequential use is contraindicated).
No products indexed under this heading.

Nortriptyline Hydrochloride (Co-administration may result in inhibition of tricyclic antidepressants by paroxetine; monitor plasma concentration of tricyclic antidepressant).
No products indexed under this heading.

Pargyline Hydrochloride (Potential for serious and fatal reactions including hyperthermia, rigidity, myoclonus and other serious reactions; concurrent and/or sequential use is contraindicated).
No products indexed under this heading.

Perphenazine (Paroxetine may significantly inhibit the activity of cytochrome isoenzyme P450IID6; co-administration should be approached with caution). Products include:
- Etrafon 3115
- Trilafon 3160

Phenelzine Sulfate (Potential for serious and fatal reactions including hyperthermia, rigidity, myoclonus and other serious reactions; concurrent and/or sequential use is contraindicated). Products include:
- Nardil Tablets 2653

Phenobarbital (Co-administration has resulted in reduction of paroxetine AUC and T1/2). Products include:
- Arco-Lase Plus Tablets 592
- Donnatal 2929
- Donnatal Extentabs 2930

Phenytoin (Co-administration has resulted in reduction of paroxetine AUC and T1/2; potential for elevated phenytoin levels or slight reduction in phenytoin AUC). Products include:
- Dilantin Infatabs 2624
- Dilantin-125 Oral Suspension 2625

Phenytoin Sodium (Co-administration has resulted in reduction of paroxetine AUC and T1/2; potential for elevated phenytoin levels or slight reduction in phenytoin AUC). Products include:
- Dilantin Kapseals 2622

Pimozide (Concomitant use has been associated with extrapyramidal symptoms including dystonia, akathisia, bradykinesia, cogwheel rigidity, hypertonia, and oculogyric crisis). Products include:
- Orap Tablets 1407

Procarbazine Hydrochloride (Potential for serious and fatal reactions including hyperthermia, rigidity, myoclonus and other serious reactions; concurrent and/or sequential use is contraindicated). Products include:
- Matulane Capsules 3246

Prochlorperazine (Paroxetine may significantly inhibit the activity of cytochrome isoenzyme P450IID6; co-administration should be approached with caution). Products include:

Compazine 1505

Procyclidine Hydrochloride (Increased steady-state AUC, Cmax and Cmin values of procyclidine with concurrent use).
No products indexed under this heading.

Promethazine Hydrochloride (Paroxetine may significantly inhibit the activity of cytochrome isoenzyme P450IID6; co-administration should be approached with caution). Products include:
Mepergan Injection 3539
Phenergan Injection 3553
Phenergan 3556
Phenergan Syrup 3554
Phenergan with Codeine Syrup 3557
Phenergan with Dextromethorphan Syrup 3559
Phenergan VC Syrup 3560
Phenergan VC with Codeine Syrup . 3561

Protriptyline Hydrochloride (Co-administration may result in inhibition of tricyclic antidepressants by paroxetine; monitor plasma concentration of tricyclic antidepressant). Products include:
Vivactil Tablets 2446
Vivactil Tablets 2217

Quinidine Gluconate (Paroxetine is metabolized by the cytochrome P450IID6 and co-administration with agents that inhibit this enzyme, such as quinidine, should be undertaken with caution). Products include:
Quinaglute Dura-Tabs Tablets 978

Quinidine Polygalacturonate (Paroxetine is metabolized by the cytochrome P450IID6 and co-administration with agents that inhibit this enzyme, such as quinidine, should be undertaken with caution).
No products indexed under this heading.

Quinidine Sulfate (Paroxetine is metabolized by the cytochrome P450IID6 and co-administration with agents that inhibit this enzyme, such as quinidine, should be undertaken with caution). Products include:
Quinidex Extentabs 2933

Selegiline Hydrochloride (Potential for serious and fatal reactions including hyperthermia, rigidity, myoclonus and other serious reactions; concurrent and/or sequential use is contraindicated). Products include:
Eldepryl Capsules 3266

Sumatriptan (Co-administration of a selective serotonin reuptake inhibitor (SSRI) and sumatriptan has resulted in weakness, hyperreflexia, and incoordination). Products include:
Imitrex Nasal Spray 1554

Sumatriptan Succinate (Co-administration of a selective serotonin reuptake inhibitor (SSRI) and sumatriptan has resulted in weakness, hyperreflexia, and incoordination). Products include:
Imitrex Injection 1549
Imitrex Tablets 1558

Theophylline (There have been reports of elevated theophylline levels associated with co-administration). Products include:
Aerolate 1361
Theo-Dur Extended-Release Tablets 1835
Uni-Dur Extended-Release Tablets .. 1841
Uniphyl 400 mg and 600 mg Tablets 2903

Theophylline Calcium Salicylate (There have been reports of elevated theophylline levels associated with co-administration).
No products indexed under this heading.

Theophylline Sodium Glycinate (There have been reports of elevated theophylline levels associated with co-administration).
No products indexed under this heading.

Thioridazine Hydrochloride (Co-administration of drugs which inhibit CYP450IID6, such as paroxetine will elevate plasma levels of thioridazine; because thioridazine administration produces a dose-related prolongation of the QTc interval, which is associated with serious ventricular arrhythmias, such as torsade de pointes-type arrhythmias, and sudden death; concurrent use is contraindicated). Products include:
Thioridazine Hydrochloride Tablets 2289

Tranylcypromine Sulfate (Potential for serious and fatal reactions including hyperthermia, rigidity, myoclonus and other serious reactions; concurrent and/or sequential use is contraindicated). Products include:
Parnate Tablets 1607

Trifluoperazine Hydrochloride (Paroxetine may significantly inhibit the activity of cytochrome isoenzyme P450IID6; co-administration should be approached with caution). Products include:
Stelazine 1640

Trimipramine Maleate (Co-administration may result in inhibition of tricyclic antidepressants by paroxetine; monitor plasma concentration of tricyclic antidepressant). Products include:
Surmontil Capsules 3595

L-Tryptophan (Potential for headache, nausea, sweating and dizziness; concomitant use is not recommended).
No products indexed under this heading.

Warfarin Sodium (Potential for pharmacodynamic interaction that causes an increased bleeding diathesis in the face of unaltered prothrombin time). Products include:
Coumadin for Injection 1243
Coumadin Tablets 1243
Warfarin Sodium Tablets, USP 3302

Food Interactions

Alcohol (Concurrent use should be avoided).

Food, unspecified (Co-administration with food resulted in slight increase (6%) in AUC, but Cmax was 29% greater, while time to reach plasma concentration decreased from 6.4 hours post-dosing to 4.9 hours).

PCE DISPERTAB TABLETS

(Erythromycin) 498
May interact with oral anticoagulants, phenytoin, valproate, theophylline, and certain other agents. Compounds in these categories include:

Alfentanil Hydrochloride (Concurrent use of erythromycin in patients receiving drugs metabolized by the cytochrome P450 system may be associated with elevation in serum levels of alfentanil).
No products indexed under this heading.

Aminophylline (Co-administration in patients who are receiving high doses of theophylline may be associated with an increase in serum theophylline levels and potential theophylline toxicity).
No products indexed under this heading.

Astemizole (Concurrent use of erythromycin in patients receiving astemizole has been reported to significantly alter the metabolism of astemizole; rare cases of cardiovascular adverse events, including prolonged QT interval, cardiac arrest, torsade de pointes, and other ventricular arrhythmias have been reported; co-administration is contraindicated).
No products indexed under this heading.

Bromocriptine Mesylate (Concurrent use of erythromycin in patients receiving drugs metabolized by the cytochrome P450 system may be associated with elevation in serum levels of bromocriptine).
No products indexed under this heading.

Carbamazepine (Concurrent use of erythromycin in patients receiving drugs metabolized by the cytochrome P450 system may be associated with elevation in serum levels of carbamazepine). Products include:
Carbatrol Capsules 3234
Tegretol/Tegretol-XR 2404

Cisapride (Concurrent use of erythromycin in patients receiving cisapride has been reported to inhibit the metabolism of cisapride; cases of cardiovascular adverse events, including prolonged QT interval, torsade de pointes, ventricular tachycardia, and ventricular fibrillation have been reported; co-administration is contraindicated).
No products indexed under this heading.

Cyclosporine (Concurrent use of erythromycin in patients receiving drugs metabolized by the cytochrome P450 system may be associated with elevation in serum levels of cyclosporine). Products include:
Gengraf Capsules 457
Neoral Soft Gelatin Capsules 2380
Neoral Oral Solution 2380
Sandimmune 2388

Dicumarol (Co-administration has resulted in increased anticoagulant effects).
No products indexed under this heading.

Digoxin (Co-administration has been reported to result in elevated digoxin serum levels). Products include:
Digitek Tablets 1003
Lanoxicaps Capsules 1574
Lanoxin Injection 1581
Lanoxin Tablets 1587
Lanoxin Elixir Pediatric 1578
Lanoxin Injection Pediatric 1584

Dihydroergotamine Mesylate (Co-administration has been associated in some patients with acute ergot toxicity characterized by severe peripheral vasospasm and dysesthesia). Products include:
D.H.E. 45 Injection 2334
Migranal Nasal Spray 2376

Disopyramide Phosphate (Concurrent use of erythromycin in patients receiving drugs metabolized by the cytochrome P450 system may be associated with elevation in serum levels of disopyramide).
No products indexed under this heading.

Divalproex Sodium (Concurrent use of erythromycin in patients receiving drugs metabolized by the cytochrome P450 system may be associated with elevation in serum levels of valproate). Products include:
Depakote Sprinkle Capsules 426
Depakote Tablets 430
Depakote ER Tablets 436

Dyphylline (Co-administration in patients who are receiving high doses of theophylline may be associated with an increase in serum theophylline levels and potential theophylline toxicity). Products include:
Lufyllin Tablets 3347
Lufyllin-400 Tablets 3347
Lufyllin-GG Elixir 3348
Lufyllin-GG Tablets 3348

Ergotamine Tartrate (Co-administration has been associated in some patients with acute ergot toxicity characterized by severe peripheral vasospasm and dysesthesia).
No products indexed under this heading.

Fosphenytoin Sodium (Concurrent use of erythromycin in patients receiving drugs metabolized by the cytochrome P450 system may be associated with elevation in serum levels of phenytoin). Products include:
Cerebyx Injection 2619

Hexobarbital (Concurrent use of erythromycin in patients receiving drugs metabolized by the cytochrome P450 system may be associated with elevation in serum levels of hexobarbital).
No products indexed under this heading.

Lovastatin (Co-administration in seriously ill patients has resulted in rhabdomyolysis with or without renal impairment). Products include:
Mevacor Tablets 2132

Midazolam Hydrochloride (Erythromycin has been reported to decrease the clearance of triazolam and, thus, may increase the pharmacologic effect of the benzodiazepine). Products include:
Versed Injection 3027
Versed Syrup 3033

Phenytoin (Concurrent use of erythromycin in patients receiving drugs metabolized by the cytochrome P450 system may be associated with elevation in serum levels of phenytoin). Products include:
Dilantin Infatabs 2624
Dilantin-125 Oral Suspension 2625

Phenytoin Sodium (Concurrent use of erythromycin in patients receiving drugs metabolized by the cytochrome P450 system may be associated with elevation in serum levels of phenytoin). Products include:
Dilantin Kapseals 2622

Tacrolimus (Concurrent use of erythromycin in patients receiving drugs metabolized by the cytochrome P450 system may be associated with elevation in serum levels of tacrolimus). Products include:
Prograf 1393
Protopic Ointment 1397

Terfenadine (Concurrent use of erythromycin in patients receiving terfenadine has been reported to significantly alter the metabolism of terfenadine; rare cases of cardiovascular adverse events, including prolonged QT interval, cardiac arrest, torsade de pointes, other ventricular arrhythmias, and death have been reported; co-administration is contraindicated).
No products indexed under this heading.

Theophylline (Co-administration in patients who are receiving high doses of theophylline may be associated with an increase in serum theophylline levels and potential theophylline toxicity). Products include:
Aerolate 1361
Theo-Dur Extended-Release Tablets 1835
Uni-Dur Extended-Release Tablets .. 1841
Uniphyl 400 mg and 600 mg Tablets 2903

Theophylline Calcium Salicylate (Co-administration in patients who are receiving high doses of theophylline may be associated with an increase in serum theophylline levels and potential theophylline toxicity).
No products indexed under this heading.

Theophylline Sodium Glycinate (Co-administration in patients who are receiving high doses of theophylline may be associated with an increase in serum theophylline levels

and potential theophylline toxicity).
No products indexed under this heading.

Triazolam (Erythromycin has been reported to decrease the clearance of triazolam and, thus, may increase the pharmacologic effect of the benzodiazepine). Products include:
Halcion Tablets 2823

Valproate Sodium (Concurrent use of erythromycin in patients receiving drugs metabolized by the cytochrome P450 system may be associated with elevation in serum levels of valproate). Products include:
Depacon Injection 416

Valproic Acid (Concurrent use of erythromycin in patients receiving drugs metabolized by the cytochrome P450 system may be associated with elevation in serum levels of valproate). Products include:
Depakene 421

Warfarin Sodium (Co-administration has resulted in increased anticoagulant effects). Products include:
Coumadin for Injection 1243
Coumadin Tablets 1243
Warfarin Sodium Tablets, USP 3302

Food Interactions

Meal, unspecified (Presence of food results in lower blood levels; optimal blood levels are obtained when PCE is given in the fasting state (at least ½ hour and preferably 2 hours before meals)).

PEDIACARE COUGH-COLD LIQUID

(Chlorpheniramine Maleate, Dextromethorphan Hydrobromide, Pseudoephedrine Hydrochloride) .... ■719
See PediaCare NightRest Cough-Cold Liquid

PEDIACARE INFANTS' DROPS DECONGESTANT

(Pseudoephedrine Hydrochloride) .... ■719
See PediaCare NightRest Cough-Cold Liquid

PEDIACARE INFANTS' DROPS DECONGESTANT PLUS COUGH

(Dextromethorphan Hydrobromide, Pseudoephedrine Hydrochloride) .... ■719
See PediaCare NightRest Cough-Cold Liquid

PEDIACARE NIGHTREST COUGH-COLD LIQUID

(Chlorpheniramine Maleate, Dextromethorphan Hydrobromide, Pseudoephedrine Hydrochloride) .... ■719
May interact with hypnotics and sedatives, monoamine oxidase inhibitors, and tranquilizers. Compounds in these categories include:

Alprazolam (Increases the drowsiness effect). Products include:
Xanax Tablets 2865

Buspirone Hydrochloride (Increases the drowsiness effect).
No products indexed under this heading.

Chlordiazepoxide (Increases the drowsiness effect). Products include:
Limbitrol 1738

Chlordiazepoxide Hydrochloride (Increases the drowsiness effect). Products include:
Librium Capsules 1736
Librium for Injection 1737

Chlorpromazine (Increases the drowsiness effect). Products include:
Thorazine Suppositories 1656

Chlorpromazine Hydrochloride (Increases the drowsiness effect). Products include:
Thorazine 1656

Chlorprothixene (Increases the drowsiness effect).
No products indexed under this heading.

Chlorprothixene Hydrochloride (Increases the drowsiness effect).
No products indexed under this heading.

Clorazepate Dipotassium (Increases the drowsiness effect). Products include:
Tranxene 511

Diazepam (Increases the drowsiness effect). Products include:
Valium Injectable 3026
Valium Tablets 3047

Droperidol (Increases the drowsiness effect).
No products indexed under this heading.

Estazolam (Increases the drowsiness effect). Products include:
ProSom Tablets 500

Ethchlorvynol (Increases the drowsiness effect).
No products indexed under this heading.

Ethinamate (Increases the drowsiness effect).
No products indexed under this heading.

Fluphenazine Decanoate (Increases the drowsiness effect).
No products indexed under this heading.

Fluphenazine Enanthate (Increases the drowsiness effect).
No products indexed under this heading.

Fluphenazine Hydrochloride (Increases the drowsiness effect).
No products indexed under this heading.

Flurazepam Hydrochloride (Increases the drowsiness effect).
No products indexed under this heading.

Glutethimide (Increases the drowsiness effect).
No products indexed under this heading.

Haloperidol (Increases the drowsiness effect). Products include:
Haldol Injection, Tablets and Concentrate 2533

Haloperidol Decanoate (Increases the drowsiness effect). Products include:
Haldol Decanoate 2535

Hydroxyzine Hydrochloride (Increases the drowsiness effect). Products include:
Atarax Tablets & Syrup 2667
Vistaril Intramuscular Solution 2738

Isocarboxazid (Concurrent and/or sequential use is not recommended).
No products indexed under this heading.

Lorazepam (Increases the drowsiness effect). Products include:
Ativan Injection 3478
Ativan Tablets 3482

Loxapine Hydrochloride (Increases the drowsiness effect).
No products indexed under this heading.

Loxapine Succinate (Increases the drowsiness effect). Products include:
Loxitane Capsules 3398

Meprobamate (Increases the drowsiness effect). Products include:
Miltown Tablets 3349

Mesoridazine Besylate (Increases the drowsiness effect). Products include:
Serentil 1057

Midazolam Hydrochloride (Increases the drowsiness effect). Products include:
Versed Injection 3027
Versed Syrup 3033

Moclobemide (Concurrent and/or sequential use is not recommended).
No products indexed under this heading.

Molindone Hydrochloride (Increases the drowsiness effect). Products include:
Moban 1320

Oxazepam (Increases the drowsiness effect).
No products indexed under this heading.

Pargyline Hydrochloride (Concurrent and/or sequential use is not recommended).
No products indexed under this heading.

Perphenazine (Increases the drowsiness effect). Products include:
Etrafon 3115
Trilafon 3160

Phenelzine Sulfate (Concurrent and/or sequential use is not recommended). Products include:
Nardil Tablets 2653

Prazepam (Increases the drowsiness effect).
No products indexed under this heading.

Procarbazine Hydrochloride (Concurrent and/or sequential use is not recommended). Products include:
Matulane Capsules 3246

Prochlorperazine (Increases the drowsiness effect). Products include:
Compazine 1505

Promethazine Hydrochloride (Increases the drowsiness effect). Products include:
Mepergan Injection 3539
Phenergan Injection 3553
Phenergan 3556
Phenergan Syrup 3554
Phenergan with Codeine Syrup 3557
Phenergan with Dextromethorphan Syrup 3559
Phenergan VC Syrup 3560
Phenergan VC with Codeine Syrup 3561

Propofol (Increases the drowsiness effect). Products include:
Diprivan Injectable Emulsion 667

Quazepam (Increases the drowsiness effect).
No products indexed under this heading.

Secobarbital Sodium (Increases the drowsiness effect).
No products indexed under this heading.

Selegiline Hydrochloride (Concurrent and/or sequential use is not recommended). Products include:
Eldepryl Capsules 3266

Temazepam (Increases the drowsiness effect).
No products indexed under this heading.

Thioridazine Hydrochloride (Increases the drowsiness effect). Products include:
Thioridazine Hydrochloride Tablets 2289

Thiothixene (Increases the drowsiness effect). Products include:
Navane Capsules 2701
Thiothixene Capsules 2290

Tranylcypromine Sulfate (Concurrent and/or sequential use is not recommended). Products include:
Parnate Tablets 1607

Triazolam (Increases the drowsiness effect). Products include:
Halcion Tablets 2823

Trifluoperazine Hydrochloride (Increases the drowsiness effect). Products include:
Stelazine 1640

Zaleplon (Increases the drowsiness effect). Products include:
Sonata Capsules 3591

Zolpidem Tartrate (Increases the drowsiness effect). Products include:
Ambien Tablets 3191

PEDIALYTE ORAL ELECTROLYTE MAINTENANCE SOLUTION

(Electrolyte Supplement) 3049
None cited in PDR database.

PEDIAPRED ORAL SOLUTION

(Prednisolone Sodium Phosphate) 1170
May interact with barbiturates, oral hypoglycemic agents, insulin, and certain other agents. Compounds in these categories include:

Acarbose (Increased requirement of hypoglycemic agents in diabetes). Products include:
Precose Tablets 906

Aprobarbital (Induces hepatic microsomal drug metabolizing enzyme activity which may result in enhanced metabolism of prednisolone; dosage of prednisolone may need to be increased).
No products indexed under this heading.

Aspirin (Aspirin should be used cautiously in conjunction with corticosteroids in hypoprothrobinemia). Products include:
Aggrenox Capsules 1026
Alka-Seltzer .... ■603
Alka-Seltzer Lemon Lime Antacid and Pain Reliever Effervescent Tablets .... ■603
Alka-Seltzer Extra Strength Antacid and Pain Reliever Effervescent Tablets .... ■603
Alka-Seltzer PM Effervescent Tablets .... ■605
Genuine Bayer Tablets, Caplets and Gelcaps .... ■606
Extra Strength Bayer Caplets and Gelcaps .... ■610
Aspirin Regimen Bayer Children's Chewable Tablets (Orange or Cherry Flavored) .... ■607
Bayer, Aspirin Regimen .... ■606
Aspirin Regimen Bayer 81 mg Caplets with Calcium .... ■607
Genuine Bayer Professional Labeling (Aspirin Regimen Bayer) .... ■608
Extra Strength Bayer Arthritis Caplets .... ■610
Extra Strength Bayer Plus Caplets .... ■610
Extra Strength Bayer PM Caplets .... ■611
BC Powder .... ■619
BC Allergy Sinus Cold Powder .... ■619
Arthritis Strength BC Powder .... ■619
BC Sinus Cold Powder .... ■619
Darvon Compound-65 Pulvules 1910
Ecotrin Enteric Coated Aspirin Low, Regular and Maximum Strength Tablets 1715
Excedrin Extra-Strength Tablets, Caplets, and Geltabs .... ■629
Excedrin Migraine 1070
Goody's Body Pain Formula Powder .... ■620
Goody's Extra Strength Headache Powder .... ■620
Goody's Extra Strength Pain Relief Tablets .... ■620
Percodan Tablets 1327
Robaxisal Tablets 2939
Soma Compound Tablets 3354
Soma Compound w/Codeine Tablets 3355
Vanquish Caplets .... ■617

Butabarbital (Induces hepatic microsomal drug metabolizing enzyme activity which may result in enhanced metabolism of prednisolone; dosage of prednisolone may need to be increased).
No products indexed under this heading.

Butalbital (Induces hepatic microsomal drug metabolizing enzyme activity which may result in enhanced metabolism of prednisolone; dosage of prednisolone may need to be increased). Products include:
Phrenilin 578
Sedapap Tablets 50 mg/650 mg 2225

Chlorpropamide (Increased requirement of hypoglycemic agents in diabetes). Products include:
Diabinese Tablets 2680
Glimepiride (Increased requirement of hypoglycemic agents in diabetes). Products include:
Amaryl Tablets 717
Glipizide (Increased requirement of hypoglycemic agents in diabetes). Products include:
Glucotrol Tablets 2692
Glucotrol XL Extended Release Tablets 2693
Glyburide (Increased requirement of hypoglycemic agents in diabetes). Products include:
DiaBeta Tablets 741
Glucovance Tablets 1086
Insulin, Human, Zinc Suspension (Increased requirement of insulin in diabetes). Products include:
Humulin L, 100 Units 1937
Humulin U, 100 Units 1943
Novolin L Human Insulin 10 ml Vials 2422
Insulin, Human NPH (Increased requirement of insulin in diabetes). Products include:
Humulin N, 100 Units 1939
Humulin N NPH Pen 1940
Novolin N Human Insulin 10 ml Vials 2422
Novolin N PenFill 2423
Novolin N Prefilled Syringe Disposable Insulin Delivery System 2425
Insulin, Human Regular (Increased requirement of insulin in diabetes). Products include:
Humulin R Regular (U-500) 1943
Humulin R, 100 Units 1941
Novolin R Human Insulin 10 ml Vials 2423
Novolin R PenFill 2423
Novolin R Prefilled Syringe Disposable Insulin Delivery System 2425
Velosulin BR Human Insulin 10 ml Vials 2435
Insulin, Human Regular and Human NPH Mixture (Increased requirement of insulin in diabetes). Products include:
Humulin 50/50, 100 Units 1934
Humulin 70/30, 100 Units 1935
Humulin 70/30 Pen 1936
Novolin 70/30 Human Insulin 10 ml Vials 2421
Novolin 70/30 PenFill 2423
Novolin 70/30 Prefilled Disposable Insulin Delivery System 2425
Insulin, NPH (Increased requirement of insulin in diabetes). Products include:
Iletin II, NPH (Pork), 100 Units 1946
Insulin, Regular (Increased requirement of insulin in diabetes). Products include:
Iletin II, Regular (Pork), 100 Units ... 1947
Insulin, Zinc Crystals (Increased requirement of insulin in diabetes).
No products indexed under this heading.
Insulin, Zinc Suspension (Increased requirement of insulin in diabetes). Products include:
Iletin II, Lente (Pork), 100 Units 1945
Insulin Aspart, Human Regular (Increased requirement of insulin in diabetes).
No products indexed under this heading.
Insulin glargine (Increased requirement of insulin in diabetes). Products include:
Lantus Injection 742
Insulin Lispro, Human (Increased requirement of insulin in diabetes). Products include:
Humalog 1926
Humalog Mix 75/25 Pen 1928
Insulin Lispro Protamine, Human (Increased requirement of insulin in diabetes). Products include:
Humalog Mix 75/25 Pen 1928
Mephobarbital (Induces hepatic microsomal drug metabolizing enzyme activity which may result in enhanced metabolism of prednisolone; dosage of prednisolone may need to be increased).
No products indexed under this heading.
Metformin Hydrochloride (Increased requirement of hypoglycemic agents in diabetes). Products include:
Glucophage Tablets 1080
Glucophage XR Tablets 1080
Glucovance Tablets 1086
Miglitol (Increased requirement of hypoglycemic agents in diabetes). Products include:
Glyset Tablets 2821
Pentobarbital Sodium (Induces hepatic microsomal drug metabolizing enzyme activity which may result in enhanced metabolism of prednisolone; dosage of prednisolone may need to be increased). Products include:
Nembutal Sodium Solution 485
Phenobarbital (Induces hepatic microsomal drug metabolizing enzyme activity which may result in enhanced metabolism of prednisolone; dosage of prednisolone may need to be increased). Products include:
Arco-Lase Plus Tablets 592
Donnatal 2929
Donnatal Extentabs 2930
Pioglitazone Hydrochloride (Increased requirement of hypoglycemic agents in diabetes). Products include:
Actos Tablets 3275
Repaglinide (Increased requirement of hypoglycemic agents in diabetes). Products include:
Prandin Tablets (0.5, 1, and 2 mg) 2432
Rosiglitazone Maleate (Increased requirement of hypoglycemic agents in diabetes). Products include:
Avandia Tablets 1490
Secobarbital Sodium (Induces hepatic microsomal drug metabolizing enzyme activity which may result in enhanced metabolism of prednisolone; dosage of prednisolone may need to be increased).
No products indexed under this heading.
Thiamylal Sodium (Induces hepatic microsomal drug metabolizing enzyme activity which may result in enhanced metabolism of prednisolone; dosage of prednisolone may need to be increased).
No products indexed under this heading.
Tolazamide (Increased requirement of hypoglycemic agents in diabetes).
No products indexed under this heading.
Tolbutamide (Increased requirement of hypoglycemic agents in diabetes).
No products indexed under this heading.
Troglitazone (Increased requirement of hypoglycemic agents in diabetes).
No products indexed under this heading.

PEDIASURE ENTERAL FORMULA

(Entereal Nutrition) 3052
None cited in PDR database.

PEDIASURE FORMULA

(Entereal Nutrition) 3052
None cited in PDR database.

PEDIAZOLE SUSPENSION

(Erythromycin Ethylsuccinate, Sulfisoxazole Acetyl) 3050
May interact with oral anticoagulants, sulfonylureas, theophylline, and certain other agents. Compounds in these categories include:

Alfentanil Hydrochloride (Co-administration is associated with elevation in alfentanil serum levels).
No products indexed under this heading.
Aminophylline (Erythromycin use in patients who are receiving high doses of theophylline may be associated with an increase in serum theophylline levels and potential theophylline toxicity).
No products indexed under this heading.
Bromocriptine Mesylate (Co-administration is associated with elevation in bromocriptine serum levels).
No products indexed under this heading.
Carbamazepine (Co-administration is associated with elevation in carbamazepine serum levels). Products include:
Carbatrol Capsules 3234
Tegretol/Tegretol-XR 2404
Chlorpropamide (Sulfisoxazole can potentiate the blood-sugar-lowering activities of sulfonylureas). Products include:
Diabinese Tablets 2680
Cyclosporine (Co-administration is associated with elevation in cyclosporine serum levels). Products include:
Gengraf Capsules 457
Neoral Soft Gelatin Capsules 2380
Neoral Oral Solution 2380
Sandimmune 2388
Dicumarol (Co-administration of erythromycin and oral anticoagulants has resulted in increased anticoagulant effects; sulfisoxazole may prolong the prothrombin time with concurrent use).
No products indexed under this heading.
Digoxin (Co-administration has been reported to result in elevated digoxin serum levels). Products include:
Digitek Tablets 1003
Lanoxicaps Capsules 1574
Lanoxin Injection 1581
Lanoxin Tablets 1587
Lanoxin Elixir Pediatric 1578
Lanoxin Injection Pediatric 1584
Dihydroergotamine Mesylate (Co-administration has been associated with acute ergot toxicity characterized by severe peripheral vasospasm and dysesthesia). Products include:
D.H.E. 45 Injection 2334
Migranal Nasal Spray 2376
Disopyramide Phosphate (Co-administration is associated with elevation in disopyramide serum levels).
No products indexed under this heading.
Dyphylline (Erythromycin use in patients who are receiving high doses of theophylline may be associated with an increase in serum theophylline levels and potential theophylline toxicity). Products include:
Lufyllin Tablets 3347
Lufyllin-400 Tablets 3347
Lufyllin-GG Elixir 3348
Lufyllin-GG Tablets 3348
Ergotamine Tartrate (Co-administration has been associated with acute ergot toxicity characterized by severe peripheral vasospasm and dysesthesia).
No products indexed under this heading.
Fosphenytoin Sodium (Co-administration is associated with elevation in phenytoin serum levels). Products include:
Cerebyx Injection 2619
Glimepiride (Sulfisoxazole can potentiate the blood-sugar-lowering activities of sulfonylureas). Products include:
Amaryl Tablets 717
Glipizide (Sulfisoxazole can potentiate the blood-sugar-lowering activities of sulfonylureas). Products include:
Glucotrol Tablets 2692
Glucotrol XL Extended Release Tablets 2693
Glyburide (Sulfisoxazole can potentiate the blood-sugar-lowering activities of sulfonylureas). Products include:
DiaBeta Tablets 741
Glucovance Tablets 1086
Hexobarbital (Co-administration is associated with elevation in hexobarbital serum levels).
Lovastatin (Co-administration is associated with elevation in lovastatin serum levels; combined therapy has resulted in rhabdomyolysis with or without renal impairment in seriously ill patients; carefully monitor creatine kinase and serum transaminase levels). Products include:
Mevacor Tablets 2132
Methotrexate Sodium (Sulfonamides can displace methotrexate from plasma binding sites, thus increasing free methotrexate concentrations).
No products indexed under this heading.
Midazolam Hydrochloride (Erythromycin has been reported to decrease the clearance of midazolam and thus may increase the pharmacological effect of midazolam). Products include:
Versed Injection 3027
Versed Syrup 3033
Phenytoin (Co-administration is associated with elevation in phenytoin serum levels). Products include:
Dilantin Infatabs 2624
Dilantin-125 Oral Suspension 2625
Phenytoin Sodium (Co-administration is associated with elevation in phenytoin serum levels). Products include:
Dilantin Kapseals 2622
Sodium Thiopental (Sulfisoxazole competes with thiopental for plasma protein binding resulting in a decrease in the amount of thiopental required for anesthesia).
No products indexed under this heading.
Terfenadine (Concomitant use significantly alters the metabolism of terfenadine metabolism; rare cases of serious cardiovascular adverse events, including cardiac arrest, torsades de pointes, other ventricular arrhythmias, and death have been observed; concurrent use is contraindicated).
No products indexed under this heading.
Theophylline (Erythromycin use in patients who are receiving high doses of theophylline may be associated with an increase in serum theophylline levels and potential theophylline toxicity). Products include:
Aerolate 1361
Theo-Dur Extended-Release Tablets 1835
Uni-Dur Extended-Release Tablets .. 1841
Uniphyl 400 mg and 600 mg Tablets 2903
Theophylline Calcium Salicylate (Erythromycin use in patients who are receiving high doses of theophylline may be associated with an increase in serum theophylline levels

and potential theophylline toxicity).
No products indexed under this heading.

Theophylline Sodium Glycinate (Erythromycin use in patients who are receiving high doses of theophylline may be associated with an increase in serum theophylline levels and potential theophylline toxicity).
No products indexed under this heading.

Tolazamide (Sulfisoxazole can potentiate the blood-sugar-lowering activities of sulfonylureas).
No products indexed under this heading.

Tolbutamide (Sulfisoxazole can potentiate the blood-sugar-lowering activities of sulfonylureas).
No products indexed under this heading.

Triazolam (Erythromycin has been reported to decrease the clearance of triazolam and thus may increase the pharmacological effect of triazolam). Products include:
Halcion Tablets 2823

Warfarin Sodium (Co-administration of erythromycin and oral anticoagulants has resulted in increased anticoagulant effects; sulfisoxazole may prolong the prothrombin time with concurrent use). Products include:
Coumadin for Injection 1243
Coumadin Tablets 1243
Warfarin Sodium Tablets, USP 3302

LIQUID PEDVAXHIB
(Haemophilus B Conjugate Vaccine) 2148
None cited in PDR database.

PEG-INTRON POWDER FOR INJECTION
(Peginterferon Alfa-2B) 3140
None cited in PDR database.

PENLAC NAIL LACQUER, TOPICAL SOLUTION
(Ciclopirox) 1225
None cited in PDR database.

PENTASA CAPSULES
(Mesalamine) 3239
None cited in PDR database.

PEPCID AC CHEWABLE TABLETS
(Famotidine) 1814
None cited in PDR database.

PEPCID AC GELCAPS
(Famotidine) 1814
None cited in PDR database.

PEPCID AC TABLETS
(Famotidine) 1814
None cited in PDR database.

PEPCID COMPLETE CHEWABLE TABLETS
(Calcium Carbonate, Famotidine, Magnesium Hydroxide) .... ▣638
May interact with:

Prescription Drugs, unspecified (Antacids contained in Pepcid Complete may interact with certain prescription drugs).

PEPCID COMPLETE CHEWABLE TABLETS
(Calcium Carbonate, Famotidine, Magnesium Hydroxide) 1815
May interact with:

Prescription Drugs, unspecified (Antacids contained in Pepcid Complete may interact with certain prescription drugs).

PEPCID INJECTION
(Famotidine) 2153
None cited in PDR database.

PEPCID INJECTION PREMIXED
(Famotidine) 2153
None cited in PDR database.

PEPCID FOR ORAL SUSPENSION
(Famotidine) 2150
May interact with antacids and certain other agents. Compounds in these categories include:

Aluminum Carbonate (Bioavailability may be slightly decreased by antacids).
No products indexed under this heading.

Aluminum Hydroxide (Bioavailability may be slightly decreased by antacids). Products include:
Amphojel Suspension (Mint Flavor) .... ▣789
Gaviscon Extra Strength Liquid .... ▣751
Gaviscon Extra Strength Tablets .... ▣751
Gaviscon Regular Strength Liquid .... ▣751
Gaviscon Regular Strength Tablets .... ▣750
Maalox Antacid/Anti-Gas Oral Suspension .... ▣673
Maalox Max Maximum Strength Antacid/Anti-Gas Liquid 2300
Maalox Regular Strength Antacid/Antigas Liquid 2300
Mylanta 1813
Vanquish Caplets .... ▣617

Magaldrate (Bioavailability may be slightly decreased by antacids).
No products indexed under this heading.

Magnesium Hydroxide (Bioavailability may be slightly decreased by antacids). Products include:
Ex•Lax Milk of Magnesia Liquid .... ▣670
Maalox Antacid/Anti-Gas Oral Suspension .... ▣673
Maalox Max Maximum Strength Antacid/Anti-Gas Liquid 2300
Maalox Regular Strength Antacid/Antigas Liquid 2300
Mylanta Fast-Acting 1813
Mylanta 1813
Pepcid Complete Chewable Tablets 1815
Phillips' Chewable Tablets .... ▣615
Phillips' Milk of Magnesia Liquid (Original, Cherry, & Mint) .... ▣616
Rolaids Tablets .... ▣706
Extra Strength Rolaids Tablets .... ▣706
Vanquish Caplets .... ▣617

Magnesium Oxide (Bioavailability may be slightly decreased by antacids). Products include:
Beelith Tablets 946
Mag-Ox 400 Tablets 1024
Uro-Mag Capsules 1024

Sodium Bicarbonate (Bioavailability may be slightly decreased by antacids). Products include:
Alka-Seltzer .... ▣603
Alka-Seltzer Lemon Lime Antacid and Pain Reliever Effervescent Tablets .... ▣603
Alka-Seltzer Extra Strength Antacid and Pain Reliever Effervescent Tablets .... ▣603
Alka-Seltzer Heartburn Relief Tablets .... ▣604
Ceo-Two Evacuant Suppository .... ▣618
Colyte with Flavor Packs for Oral Solution 3170
GoLYTELY and Pineapple Flavor GoLYTELY for Oral Solution 1068
NuLYTELY, Cherry Flavor, Lemon-Lime Flavor, and Orange Flavor NuLYTELY for Oral Solution 1068

Food Interactions

Food, unspecified (Bioavailability may be slightly increased by antacids).

PEPCID RPD ORALLY DISINTEGRATING TABLETS
(Famotidine) 2150
See Pepcid for Oral Suspension

PEPCID TABLETS
(Famotidine) 2150
See Pepcid for Oral Suspension

PEPTO-BISMOL MAXIMUM STRENGTH LIQUID
(Bismuth Subsalicylate) 2878
May interact with oral anticoagulants, antigout agents, and oral hypoglycemic agents. Compounds in these categories include:

Acarbose (Use cautiously). Products include:
Precose Tablets 906

Allopurinol (Use cautiously).
No products indexed under this heading.

Chlorpropamide (Use cautiously). Products include:
Diabinese Tablets 2680

Dicumarol (Use cautiously).
No products indexed under this heading.

Glimepiride (Use cautiously). Products include:
Amaryl Tablets 717

Glipizide (Use cautiously). Products include:
Glucotrol Tablets 2692
Glucotrol XL Extended Release Tablets 2693

Glyburide (Use cautiously). Products include:
DiaBeta Tablets 741
Glucovance Tablets 1086

Metformin Hydrochloride (Use cautiously). Products include:
Glucophage Tablets 1080
Glucophage XR Tablets 1080
Glucovance Tablets 1086

Miglitol (Use cautiously). Products include:
Glyset Tablets 2821

Pioglitazone Hydrochloride (Use cautiously). Products include:
Actos Tablets 3275

Probenecid (Use cautiously).
No products indexed under this heading.

Repaglinide (Use cautiously). Products include:
Prandin Tablets (0.5, 1, and 2 mg) 2432

Rosiglitazone Maleate (Use cautiously). Products include:
Avandia Tablets 1490

Sulfinpyrazone (Use cautiously).
No products indexed under this heading.

Tolazamide (Use cautiously).
No products indexed under this heading.

Tolbutamide (Use cautiously).
No products indexed under this heading.

Troglitazone (Use cautiously).
No products indexed under this heading.

Warfarin Sodium (Use cautiously). Products include:
Coumadin for Injection 1243
Coumadin Tablets 1243
Warfarin Sodium Tablets, USP 3302

PEPTO-BISMOL ORIGINAL LIQUID, ORIGINAL AND CHERRY TABLETS AND EASY-TO-SWALLOW CAPLETS
(Bismuth Subsalicylate) 2878
May interact with oral anticoagulants, antigout agents, and oral hypoglycemic agents. Compounds in these categories include:

Acarbose (Use cautiously). Products include:
Precose Tablets 906

Allopurinol (Use cautiously).
No products indexed under this heading.

Chlorpropamide (Use cautiously). Products include:
Diabinese Tablets 2680

Dicumarol (Use cautiously).
No products indexed under this heading.

Glimepiride (Use cautiously). Products include:
Amaryl Tablets 717

Glipizide (Use cautiously). Products include:
Glucotrol Tablets 2692
Glucotrol XL Extended Release Tablets 2693

Glyburide (Use cautiously). Products include:
DiaBeta Tablets 741
Glucovance Tablets 1086

Metformin Hydrochloride (Use cautiously). Products include:
Glucophage Tablets 1080
Glucophage XR Tablets 1080
Glucovance Tablets 1086

Miglitol (Use cautiously). Products include:
Glyset Tablets 2821

Pioglitazone Hydrochloride (Use cautiously). Products include:
Actos Tablets 3275

Probenecid (Use cautiously).
No products indexed under this heading.

Repaglinide (Use cautiously). Products include:
Prandin Tablets (0.5, 1, and 2 mg) 2432

Rosiglitazone Maleate (Use cautiously). Products include:
Avandia Tablets 1490

Sulfinpyrazone (Use cautiously).
No products indexed under this heading.

Tolazamide (Use cautiously).
No products indexed under this heading.

Tolbutamide (Use cautiously).
No products indexed under this heading.

Troglitazone (Use cautiously).
No products indexed under this heading.

Warfarin Sodium (Use cautiously). Products include:
Coumadin for Injection 1243
Coumadin Tablets 1243
Warfarin Sodium Tablets, USP 3302

PERCOCET TABLETS
(Acetaminophen, Oxycodone Hydrochloride) 1326
May interact with anticholinergics, central nervous system depressants, general anesthetics, hypnotics and sedatives, monoamine oxidase inhibitors, narcotic analgesics, phenothiazines, tranquilizers, tricyclic antidepressants, and certain other agents. Compounds in these categories include:

Alfentanil Hydrochloride (Additive CNS depression; dose of one or both agents should be reduced).
No products indexed under this heading.

Alprazolam (Additive CNS depression; dose of one or both agents should be reduced). Products include:
Xanax Tablets 2865

Amitriptyline Hydrochloride (Increased effect of antidepressant or oxycodone). Products include:
Etrafon 3115
Limbitrol 1738

Amoxapine (Increased effect of antidepressant or oxycodone).
No products indexed under this heading.

Aprobarbital (Additive CNS depression; dose of one or both agents should be reduced).
No products indexed under this heading.

Atropine Sulfate (May produce paralytic ileus). Products include:
Donnatal ... 2929
Donnatal Extentabs ... 2930
Motofen Tablets ... 577
Prosed/DS Tablets ... 3268
Urised Tablets ... 2876

Belladonna Alkaloids (May produce paralytic ileus). Products include:
Hyland's Teething Tablets ... ▣766
Urimax Tablets ... 1769

Benztropine Mesylate (May produce paralytic ileus). Products include:
Cogentin ... 2055

Biperiden Hydrochloride (May produce paralytic ileus). Products include:
Akineton ... 402

Buprenorphine Hydrochloride (Additive CNS depression; dose of one or both agents should be reduced). Products include:
Buprenex Injectable ... 2918

Buspirone Hydrochloride (Additive CNS depression; dose of one or both agents should be reduced).
No products indexed under this heading.

Butabarbital (Additive CNS depression; dose of one or both agents should be reduced).
No products indexed under this heading.

Butalbital (Additive CNS depression; dose of one or both agents should be reduced). Products include:
Phrenilin ... 578
Sedapap Tablets 50 mg/650 mg ... 2225

Chlordiazepoxide (Additive CNS depression; dose of one or both agents should be reduced). Products include:
Limbitrol ... 1738

Chlordiazepoxide Hydrochloride (Additive CNS depression; dose of one or both agents should be reduced). Products include:
Librium Capsules ... 1736
Librium for Injection ... 1737

Chlorpromazine (Additive CNS depression; dose of one or both agents should be reduced). Products include:
Thorazine Suppositories ... 1656

Chlorpromazine Hydrochloride (Additive CNS depression; dose of one or both agents should be reduced). Products include:
Thorazine ... 1656

Chlorprothixene (Additive CNS depression; dose of one or both agents should be reduced).
No products indexed under this heading.

Chlorprothixene Hydrochloride (Additive CNS depression; dose of one or both agents should be reduced).
No products indexed under this heading.

Chlorprothixene Lactate (Additive CNS depression; dose of one or both agents should be reduced).
No products indexed under this heading.

Clidinium Bromide (May produce paralytic ileus).
No products indexed under this heading.

Clomipramine Hydrochloride (Increased effect of antidepressant or oxycodone).
No products indexed under this heading.

Clorazepate Dipotassium (Additive CNS depression; dose of one or both agents should be reduced). Products include:
Tranxene ... 511

Clozapine (Additive CNS depression; dose of one or both agents should be reduced). Products include:
Clozaril Tablets ... 2319

Codeine Phosphate (Additive CNS depression; dose of one or both agents should be reduced). Products include:
Phenergan with Codeine Syrup ... 3557
Phenergan VC with Codeine Syrup ... 3561
Robitussin A-C Syrup ... 2942
Robitussin-DAC Syrup ... 2942
Ryna-C Liquid ... ▣768
Soma Compound w/Codeine Tablets ... 3355
Tussi-Organidin NR Liquid ... 3350
Tussi-Organidin-S NR Liquid ... 3350
Tylenol with Codeine ... 2595

Desflurane (Additive CNS depression; dose of one or both agents should be reduced). Products include:
Suprane Liquid for Inhalation ... 874

Desipramine Hydrochloride (Increased effect of antidepressant or oxycodone). Products include:
Norpramin Tablets ... 755

Dezocine (Additive CNS depression; dose of one or both agents should be reduced).
No products indexed under this heading.

Diazepam (Additive CNS depression; dose of one or both agents should be reduced). Products include:
Valium Injectable ... 3026
Valium Tablets ... 3047

Dicyclomine Hydrochloride (May produce paralytic ileus).
No products indexed under this heading.

Doxepin Hydrochloride (Increased effect of antidepressant or oxycodone). Products include:
Sinequan ... 2713

Droperidol (Additive CNS depression; dose of one or both agents should be reduced).
No products indexed under this heading.

Enflurane (Additive CNS depression; dose of one or both agents should be reduced).
No products indexed under this heading.

Estazolam (Additive CNS depression; dose of one or both agents should be reduced). Products include:
ProSom Tablets ... 500

Ethchlorvynol (Additive CNS depression; dose of one or both agents should be reduced).
No products indexed under this heading.

Ethinamate (Additive CNS depression; dose of one or both agents should be reduced).
No products indexed under this heading.

Ethopropazine Hydrochloride (May produce paralytic ileus).
No products indexed under this heading.

Fentanyl (Additive CNS depression; dose of one or both agents should be reduced). Products include:
Duragesic Transdermal System ... 1786

Fentanyl Citrate (Additive CNS depression; dose of one or both agents should be reduced). Products include:
Actiq ... 1184

Fluphenazine Decanoate (Additive CNS depression; dose of one or both agents should be reduced).
No products indexed under this heading.

Fluphenazine Enanthate (Additive CNS depression; dose of one or both agents should be reduced).
No products indexed under this heading.

Fluphenazine Hydrochloride (Additive CNS depression; dose of one or both agents should be reduced).
No products indexed under this heading.

Flurazepam Hydrochloride (Additive CNS depression; dose of one or both agents should be reduced).
No products indexed under this heading.

Glutethimide (Additive CNS depression; dose of one or both agents should be reduced).
No products indexed under this heading.

Glycopyrrolate (May produce paralytic ileus). Products include:
Robinul Forte Tablets ... 1358
Robinul Injectable ... 2940
Robinul Tablets ... 1358

Haloperidol (Additive CNS depression; dose of one or both agents should be reduced). Products include:
Haldol Injection, Tablets and Concentrate ... 2533

Haloperidol Decanoate (Additive CNS depression; dose of one or both agents should be reduced). Products include:
Haldol Decanoate ... 2535

Hydrocodone Bitartrate (Additive CNS depression; dose of one or both agents should be reduced). Products include:
Hycodan ... 1316
Hycomine Compound Tablets ... 1317
Hycotuss Expectorant Syrup ... 1318
Lortab ... 3319
Lortab Elixir ... 3317
Maxidone Tablets CIII ... 3399
Norco 5/325 Tablets CIII ... 3424
Norco 7.5/325 Tablets CIII ... 3425
Norco 10/325 Tablets CIII ... 3427
Norco 10/325 Tablets CIII ... 3425
Vicodin Tablets ... 516
Vicodin ES Tablets ... 517
Vicodin HP Tablets ... 518
Vicodin Tuss Expectorant ... 519
Vicoprofen Tablets ... 520
Zydone Tablets ... 1330

Hydrocodone Polistirex (Additive CNS depression; dose of one or both agents should be reduced). Products include:
Tussionex Pennkinetic Extended-Release Suspension ... 1174

Hydromorphone Hydrochloride (Additive CNS depression; dose of one or both agents should be reduced). Products include:
Dilaudid ... 441
Dilaudid Oral Liquid ... 445
Dilaudid Powder ... 441
Dilaudid Rectal Suppositories ... 441
Dilaudid Tablets ... 441
Dilaudid Tablets - 8 mg ... 445
Dilaudid-HP ... 443

Hydroxyzine Hydrochloride (Additive CNS depression; dose of one or both agents should be reduced). Products include:
Atarax Tablets & Syrup ... 2667
Vistaril Intramuscular Solution ... 2738

Hyoscyamine (May produce paralytic ileus). Products include:
Urised Tablets ... 2876

Hyoscyamine Sulfate (May produce paralytic ileus). Products include:
Arco-Lase Plus Tablets ... 592
Donnatal ... 2929
Donnatal Extentabs ... 2930
Levsin/Levsinex/Levbid ... 3172
NuLev Orally Disintegrating Tablets ... 3176
Prosed/DS Tablets ... 3268
Urimax Tablets ... 1769

Imipramine Hydrochloride (Increased effect of antidepressant or oxycodone).
No products indexed under this heading.

Imipramine Pamoate (Increased effect of antidepressant or oxycodone).
No products indexed under this heading.

Ipratropium Bromide (May produce paralytic ileus). Products include:
Atrovent Inhalation Aerosol ... 1030
Atrovent Inhalation Solution ... 1031
Atrovent Nasal Spray 0.03% ... 1032
Atrovent Nasal Spray 0.06% ... 1033
Combivent Inhalation Aerosol ... 1041
DuoNeb Inhalation Solution ... 1233

Isocarboxazid (Increased effect of either oxycodone or MAO inhibitor).
No products indexed under this heading.

Isoflurane (Additive CNS depression; dose of one or both agents should be reduced).
No products indexed under this heading.

Ketamine Hydrochloride (Additive CNS depression; dose of one or both agents should be reduced).
No products indexed under this heading.

Levomethadyl Acetate Hydrochloride (Additive CNS depression; dose of one or both agents should be reduced).
No products indexed under this heading.

Levorphanol Tartrate (Additive CNS depression; dose of one or both agents should be reduced). Products include:
Levo-Dromoran ... 1734
Levorphanol Tartrate Tablets ... 3059

Lorazepam (Additive CNS depression; dose of one or both agents should be reduced). Products include:
Ativan Injection ... 3478
Ativan Tablets ... 3482

Loxapine Hydrochloride (Additive CNS depression; dose of one or both agents should be reduced).
No products indexed under this heading.

Loxapine Succinate (Additive CNS depression; dose of one or both agents should be reduced). Products include:
Loxitane Capsules ... 3398

Maprotiline Hydrochloride (Increased effect of antidepressant or oxycodone).
No products indexed under this heading.

Mepenzolate Bromide (May produce paralytic ileus).
No products indexed under this heading.

Meperidine Hydrochloride (Additive CNS depression; dose of one or both agents should be reduced). Products include:
Demerol ... 3079
Mepergan Injection ... 3539

Mephobarbital (Additive CNS depression; dose of one or both agents should be reduced).
No products indexed under this heading.

Meprobamate (Additive CNS depression; dose of one or both agents should be reduced). Products include:
Miltown Tablets ... 3349

Mesoridazine Besylate (Additive CNS depression; dose of one or both agents should be reduced). Products include:
Serentil ... 1057

Methadone Hydrochloride (Additive CNS depression; dose of one or both agents should be reduced). Products include:
Dolophine Hydrochloride Tablets ... 3056

Methohexital Sodium (Additive CNS depression; dose of one or both agents should be reduced). Products include:
Brevital Sodium for Injection, USP ... 1815

Methotrimeprazine (Additive CNS depression; dose of one or both agents should be reduced).
No products indexed under this heading.

Methoxyflurane (Additive CNS depression; dose of one or both agents should be reduced).
No products indexed under this heading.

Midazolam Hydrochloride (Additive CNS depression; dose of one or both agents should be reduced). Products include:
- Versed Injection 3027
- Versed Syrup 3033

Moclobemide (Increased effect of either oxycodone or MAO inhibitor).
No products indexed under this heading.

Molindone Hydrochloride (Additive CNS depression; dose of one or both agents should be reduced). Products include:
- Moban 1320

Morphine Sulfate (Additive CNS depression; dose of one or both agents should be reduced). Products include:
- Astramorph/PF Injection, USP (Preservative-Free) 594
- Duramorph Injection 1312
- Infumorph 200 and Infumorph 500 Sterile Solutions 1314
- Kadian Capsules 1335
- MS Contin Tablets 2896
- MSIR 2898
- Oramorph SR Tablets 3062
- Roxanol 3066

Nortriptyline Hydrochloride (Increased effect of antidepressant or oxycodone).
No products indexed under this heading.

Olanzapine (Additive CNS depression; dose of one or both agents should be reduced). Products include:
- Zyprexa Tablets 1973
- Zyprexa ZYDIS Orally Disintegrating Tablets 1973

Oxazepam (Additive CNS depression; dose of one or both agents should be reduced; increased effect of antidepressant).
No products indexed under this heading.

Oxybutynin Chloride (May produce paralytic ileus). Products include:
- Ditropan XL Extended Release Tablets 564

Oxyphenonium Bromide (May produce paralytic ileus).
No products indexed under this heading.

Pargyline Hydrochloride (Increased effect of either oxycodone or MAO inhibitor).
No products indexed under this heading.

Pentobarbital Sodium (Additive CNS depression; dose of one or both agents should be reduced). Products include:
- Nembutal Sodium Solution 485

Perphenazine (Additive CNS depression; dose of one or both agents should be reduced). Products include:
- Etrafon 3115
- Trilafon 3160

Phenelzine Sulfate (Increased effect of either oxycodone or MAO inhibitor). Products include:
- Nardil Tablets 2653

Phenobarbital (Additive CNS depression; dose of one or both agents should be reduced). Products include:
- Arco-Lase Plus Tablets 592
- Donnatal 2929
- Donnatal Extentabs 2930

Prazepam (Additive CNS depression; dose of one or both agents should be reduced).
No products indexed under this heading.

Procarbazine Hydrochloride (Increased effect of either oxycodone or MAO inhibitor). Products include:
- Matulane Capsules 3246

Prochlorperazine (Additive CNS depression; dose of one or both agents should be reduced). Products include:
- Compazine 1505

Procyclidine Hydrochloride (May produce paralytic ileus).
No products indexed under this heading.

Promethazine Hydrochloride (Additive CNS depression; dose of one or both agents should be reduced). Products include:
- Mepergan Injection 3539
- Phenergan Injection 3553
- Phenergan 3556
- Phenergan Syrup 3554
- Phenergan with Codeine Syrup 3557
- Phenergan with Dextromethorphan Syrup 3559
- Phenergan VC Syrup 3560
- Phenergan VC with Codeine Syrup 3561

Propantheline Bromide (May produce paralytic ileus).
No products indexed under this heading.

Propofol (Additive CNS depression; dose of one or both agents should be reduced). Products include:
- Diprivan Injectable Emulsion 667

Propoxyphene Hydrochloride (Additive CNS depression; dose of one or both agents should be reduced). Products include:
- Darvon Pulvules 1909
- Darvon Compound-65 Pulvules 1910

Propoxyphene Napsylate (Additive CNS depression; dose of one or both agents should be reduced). Products include:
- Darvon-N/Darvocet-N 1907
- Darvon-N Tablets 1912

Protriptyline Hydrochloride (Increased effect of antidepressant or oxycodone). Products include:
- Vivactil Tablets 2446
- Vivactil Tablets 2217

Quazepam (Additive CNS depression; dose of one or both agents should be reduced).
No products indexed under this heading.

Quetiapine Fumarate (Additive CNS depression; dose of one or both agents should be reduced). Products include:
- Seroquel Tablets 684

Remifentanil Hydrochloride (Additive CNS depression; dose of one or both agents should be reduced).
No products indexed under this heading.

Risperidone (Additive CNS depression; dose of one or both agents should be reduced). Products include:
- Risperdal 1796

Scopolamine (May produce paralytic ileus). Products include:
- Transderm Scōp Transdermal Therapeutic System 2302

Scopolamine Hydrobromide (May produce paralytic ileus). Products include:
- Donnatal 2929
- Donnatal Extentabs 2930

Secobarbital Sodium (Additive CNS depression; dose of one or both agents should be reduced).
No products indexed under this heading.

Selegiline Hydrochloride (Increased effect of either oxycodone or MAO inhibitor). Products include:
- Eldepryl Capsules 3266

Sevoflurane (Additive CNS depression; dose of one or both agents should be reduced).
No products indexed under this heading.

Sufentanil Citrate (Additive CNS depression; dose of one or both agents should be reduced).
No products indexed under this heading.

Temazepam (Additive CNS depression; dose of one or both agents should be reduced).
No products indexed under this heading.

Thiamylal Sodium (Additive CNS depression; dose of one or both agents should be reduced).
No products indexed under this heading.

Thioridazine Hydrochloride (Additive CNS depression; dose of one or both agents should be reduced). Products include:
- Thioridazine Hydrochloride Tablets 2289

Thiothixene (Additive CNS depression; dose of one or both agents should be reduced). Products include:
- Navane Capsules 2701
- Thiothixene Capsules 2290

Tolterodine Tartrate (May produce paralytic ileus). Products include:
- Detrol Tablets 3623
- Detrol LA Capsules 2801

Tranylcypromine Sulfate (Increased effect of either oxycodone or MAO inhibitor). Products include:
- Parnate Tablets 1607

Triazolam (Additive CNS depression; dose of one or both agents should be reduced). Products include:
- Halcion Tablets 2823

Tridihexethyl Chloride (May produce paralytic ileus).
No products indexed under this heading.

Trifluoperazine Hydrochloride (Additive CNS depression; dose of one or both agents should be reduced). Products include:
- Stelazine 1640

Trihexyphenidyl Hydrochloride (May produce paralytic ileus). Products include:
- Artane 1855

Trimipramine Maleate (Increased effect of antidepressant or oxycodone). Products include:
- Surmontil Capsules 3595

Zaleplon (Additive CNS depression; dose of one or both agents should be reduced). Products include:
- Sonata Capsules 3591

Ziprasidone Hydrochloride (Additive CNS depression; dose of one or both agents should be reduced). Products include:
- Geodon Capsules 2688

Zolpidem Tartrate (Additive CNS depression; dose of one or both agents should be reduced). Products include:
- Ambien Tablets 3191

Food Interactions

Alcohol (Additive CNS depression).

PERCODAN TABLETS

(Aspirin, Oxycodone Hydrochloride, Oxycodone Terephthalate) 1327

May interact with central nervous system depressants, anticoagulants, general anesthetics, hypnotics and sedatives, narcotic analgesics, phenothiazines, tranquilizers, and certain other agents. Compounds in these categories include:

Alfentanil Hydrochloride (Additive CNS depression).
No products indexed under this heading.

Alprazolam (Additive CNS depression). Products include:
- Xanax Tablets 2865

Aprobarbital (Additive CNS depression).
No products indexed under this heading.

Ardeparin Sodium (Enhanced effect of anticoagulant).
No products indexed under this heading.

Buprenorphine Hydrochloride (Additive CNS depression). Products include:
- Buprenex Injectable 2918

Buspirone Hydrochloride (Additive CNS depression).
No products indexed under this heading.

Butabarbital (Additive CNS depression).
No products indexed under this heading.

Butalbital (Additive CNS depression). Products include:
- Phrenilin 578
- Sedapap Tablets 50 mg/650 mg 2225

Chlordiazepoxide (Additive CNS depression). Products include:
- Limbitrol 1738

Chlordiazepoxide Hydrochloride (Additive CNS depression). Products include:
- Librium Capsules 1736
- Librium for Injection 1737

Chlorpromazine (Additive CNS depression). Products include:
- Thorazine Suppositories 1656

Chlorpromazine Hydrochloride (Additive CNS depression). Products include:
- Thorazine 1656

Chlorprothixene (Additive CNS depression).
No products indexed under this heading.

Chlorprothixene Hydrochloride (Additive CNS depression).
No products indexed under this heading.

Chlorprothixene Lactate (Additive CNS depression).
No products indexed under this heading.

Clorazepate Dipotassium (Additive CNS depression). Products include:
- Tranxene 511

Clozapine (Additive CNS depression). Products include:
- Clozaril Tablets 2319

Codeine Phosphate (Additive CNS depression). Products include:
- Phenergan with Codeine Syrup 3557
- Phenergan VC with Codeine Syrup 3561
- Robitussin A-C Syrup 2942
- Robitussin-DAC Syrup 2942
- Ryna-C Liquid 768
- Soma Compound w/Codeine Tablets 3355
- Tussi-Organidin NR Liquid 3350
- Tussi-Organidin-S NR Liquid 3350
- Tylenol with Codeine 2595

Dalteparin Sodium (Enhanced effect of anticoagulant). Products include:
- Fragmin Injection 2814

Danaparoid Sodium (Enhanced effect of anticoagulant). Products include:
- Orgaran Injection 2480

Desflurane (Additive CNS depression). Products include:
- Suprane Liquid for Inhalation 874

Dezocine (Additive CNS depression).
No products indexed under this heading.

Diazepam (Additive CNS depression). Products include:
- Valium Injectable 3026
- Valium Tablets 3047

IMPORTANT NOTE: Always consult each drug listing in the patient's regimen for possible interactions.

Dicumarol (Enhanced effect of anticoagulant).
No products indexed under this heading.

Droperidol (Additive CNS depression).
No products indexed under this heading.

Enflurane (Additive CNS depression).
No products indexed under this heading.

Enoxaparin (Enhanced effect of anticoagulant). Products include:
Lovenox Injection 746

Estazolam (Additive CNS depression). Products include:
ProSom Tablets 500

Ethchlorvynol (Additive CNS depression).
No products indexed under this heading.

Ethinamate (Additive CNS depression).
No products indexed under this heading.

Fentanyl (Additive CNS depression). Products include:
Duragesic Transdermal System 1786

Fentanyl Citrate (Additive CNS depression). Products include:
Actiq 1184

Fluphenazine Decanoate (Additive CNS depression).
No products indexed under this heading.

Fluphenazine Enanthate (Additive CNS depression).
No products indexed under this heading.

Fluphenazine Hydrochloride (Additive CNS depression).
No products indexed under this heading.

Flurazepam Hydrochloride (Additive CNS depression).
No products indexed under this heading.

Glutethimide (Additive CNS depression).
No products indexed under this heading.

Haloperidol (Additive CNS depression). Products include:
Haldol Injection, Tablets and Concentrate 2533

Haloperidol Decanoate (Additive CNS depression). Products include:
Haldol Decanoate 2535

Heparin Sodium (Enhanced effect of anticoagulant). Products include:
Heparin Lock Flush Solution 3509
Heparin Sodium Injection 3511

Hydrocodone Bitartrate (Additive CNS depression). Products include:
Hycodan 1316
Hycomine Compound Tablets 1317
Hycotuss Expectorant Syrup 1318
Lortab 3319
Lortab Elixir 3317
Maxidone Tablets CIII 3399
Norco 5/325 Tablets CIII 3424
Norco 7.5/325 Tablets CIII 3425
Norco 10/325 Tablets CIII 3427
Norco 10/325 Tablets CIII 3425
Vicodin Tablets 516
Vicodin ES Tablets 517
Vicodin HP Tablets 518
Vicodin Tuss Expectorant 519
Vicoprofen Tablets 520
Zydone Tablets 1330

Hydrocodone Polistirex (Additive CNS depression). Products include:
Tussionex Pennkinetic Extended-Release Suspension 1174

Hydromorphone Hydrochloride (Additive CNS depression). Products include:
Dilaudid 441
Dilaudid Oral Liquid 445
Dilaudid Powder 441
Dilaudid Rectal Suppositories 441
Dilaudid Tablets 441
Dilaudid Tablets - 8 mg 445
Dilaudid-HP 443

Hydroxyzine Hydrochloride (Additive CNS depression). Products include:
Atarax Tablets & Syrup 2667
Vistaril Intramuscular Solution 2738

Isoflurane (Additive CNS depression).
No products indexed under this heading.

Ketamine Hydrochloride (Additive CNS depression).
No products indexed under this heading.

Levomethadyl Acetate Hydrochloride (Additive CNS depression).
No products indexed under this heading.

Levorphanol Tartrate (Additive CNS depression). Products include:
Levo-Dromoran 1734
Levorphanol Tartrate Tablets 3059

Lorazepam (Additive CNS depression). Products include:
Ativan Injection 3478
Ativan Tablets 3482

Loxapine Hydrochloride (Additive CNS depression).
No products indexed under this heading.

Loxapine Succinate (Additive CNS depression). Products include:
Loxitane Capsules 3398

Meperidine Hydrochloride (Additive CNS depression). Products include:
Demerol 3079
Mepergan Injection 3539

Mephobarbital (Additive CNS depression).
No products indexed under this heading.

Meprobamate (Additive CNS depression). Products include:
Miltown Tablets 3349

Mesoridazine Besylate (Additive CNS depression). Products include:
Serentil 1057

Methadone Hydrochloride (Additive CNS depression). Products include:
Dolophine Hydrochloride Tablets 3056

Methohexital Sodium (Additive CNS depression). Products include:
Brevital Sodium for Injection, USP 1815

Methotrimeprazine (Additive CNS depression).
No products indexed under this heading.

Methoxyflurane (Additive CNS depression).
No products indexed under this heading.

Midazolam Hydrochloride (Additive CNS depression). Products include:
Versed Injection 3027
Versed Syrup 3033

Molindone Hydrochloride (Additive CNS depression). Products include:
Moban 1320

Morphine Sulfate (Additive CNS depression). Products include:
Astramorph/PF Injection, USP (Preservative-Free) 594
Duramorph Injection 1312
Infumorph 200 and Infumorph 500 Sterile Solutions 1314
Kadian Capsules 1335
MS Contin Tablets 2896
MSIR 2898
Oramorph SR Tablets 3062
Roxanol 3066

Olanzapine (Additive CNS depression). Products include:
Zyprexa Tablets 1973
Zyprexa ZYDIS Orally Disintegrating Tablets 1973

Oxazepam (Additive CNS depression).
No products indexed under this heading.

Pentobarbital Sodium (Additive CNS depression). Products include:
Nembutal Sodium Solution 485

Perphenazine (Additive CNS depression). Products include:
Etrafon 3115
Trilafon 3160

Phenobarbital (Additive CNS depression). Products include:
Arco-Lase Plus Tablets 592
Donnatal 2929
Donnatal Extentabs 2930

Prazepam (Additive CNS depression).
No products indexed under this heading.

Probenecid (Aspirin may inhibit the uricosuric effects).
No products indexed under this heading.

Prochlorperazine (Additive CNS depression). Products include:
Compazine 1505

Promethazine Hydrochloride (Additive CNS depression). Products include:
Mepergan Injection 3539
Phenergan Injection 3553
Phenergan 3556
Phenergan Syrup 3554
Phenergan with Codeine Syrup 3557
Phenergan with Dextromethorphan Syrup 3559
Phenergan VC Syrup 3560
Phenergan VC with Codeine Syrup 3561

Propofol (Additive CNS depression). Products include:
Diprivan Injectable Emulsion 667

Propoxyphene Hydrochloride (Additive CNS depression). Products include:
Darvon Pulvules 1909
Darvon Compound-65 Pulvules 1910

Propoxyphene Napsylate (Additive CNS depression). Products include:
Darvon-N/Darvocet-N 1907
Darvon-N Tablets 1912

Quazepam (Additive CNS depression).
No products indexed under this heading.

Quetiapine Fumarate (Additive CNS depression). Products include:
Seroquel Tablets 684

Remifentanil Hydrochloride (Additive CNS depression).
No products indexed under this heading.

Risperidone (Additive CNS depression). Products include:
Risperdal 1796

Secobarbital Sodium (Additive CNS depression).
No products indexed under this heading.

Sevoflurane (Additive CNS depression).
No products indexed under this heading.

Sufentanil Citrate (Additive CNS depression).
No products indexed under this heading.

Sulfinpyrazone (Aspirin may inhibit the uricosuric effects).
No products indexed under this heading.

Temazepam (Additive CNS depression).
No products indexed under this heading.

Thiamylal Sodium (Additive CNS depression).
No products indexed under this heading.

Thioridazine Hydrochloride (Additive CNS depression). Products include:
Thioridazine Hydrochloride Tablets 2289

Thiothixene (Additive CNS depression). Products include:
Navane Capsules 2701
Thiothixene Capsules 2290

Tinzaparin sodium (Enhanced effect of anticoagulant). Products include:
Innohep Injection 1248

Triazolam (Additive CNS depression). Products include:
Halcion Tablets 2823

Trifluoperazine Hydrochloride (Additive CNS depression). Products include:
Stelazine 1640

Warfarin Sodium (Enhanced effect of anticoagulant). Products include:
Coumadin for Injection 1243
Coumadin Tablets 1243
Warfarin Sodium Tablets, USP 3302

Zaleplon (Additive CNS depression). Products include:
Sonata Capsules 3591

Ziprasidone Hydrochloride (Additive CNS depression). Products include:
Geodon Capsules 2688

Zolpidem Tartrate (Additive CNS depression). Products include:
Ambien Tablets 3191

Food Interactions

Alcohol (Additive CNS depression).

PERCOGESIC ASPIRIN-FREE COATED TABLETS

(Acetaminophen, Phenyltoloxamine Citrate) .... ■667
See Extra Strength Percogesic Aspirin-Free Coated Caplets

EXTRA STRENGTH PERCOGESIC ASPIRIN-FREE COATED CAPLETS

(Acetaminophen, Diphenhydramine Hydrochloride) .... ■665

May interact with hypnotics and sedatives, tranquilizers, and certain other agents. Compounds in these categories include:

Alprazolam (May increase drowsiness effect). Products include:
Xanax Tablets 2865

Buspirone Hydrochloride (May increase drowsiness effect).
No products indexed under this heading.

Chlordiazepoxide (May increase drowsiness effect). Products include:
Limbitrol 1738

Chlordiazepoxide Hydrochloride (May increase drowsiness effect). Products include:
Librium Capsules 1736
Librium for Injection 1737

Chlorpromazine (May increase drowsiness effect). Products include:
Thorazine Suppositories 1656

Chlorpromazine Hydrochloride (May increase drowsiness effect). Products include:
Thorazine 1656

Chlorprothixene (May increase drowsiness effect).
No products indexed under this heading.

Chlorprothixene Hydrochloride (May increase drowsiness effect).
No products indexed under this heading.

Clorazepate Dipotassium (May increase drowsiness effect). Products include:
Tranxene 511

Diazepam (May increase drowsiness effect). Products include:
Valium Injectable 3026
Valium Tablets 3047

Droperidol (May increase drowsiness effect).
No products indexed under this heading.

Estazolam (May increase drowsiness effect). Products include:
ProSom Tablets 500

Ethchlorvynol (May increase drowsiness effect).
No products indexed under this heading.

Ethinamate (May increase drowsiness effect).
No products indexed under this heading.

Fluphenazine Decanoate (May increase drowsiness effect).
No products indexed under this heading.

Fluphenazine Enanthate (May increase drowsiness effect).
No products indexed under this heading.

Fluphenazine Hydrochloride (May increase drowsiness effect).
No products indexed under this heading.

Flurazepam Hydrochloride (May increase drowsiness effect).
No products indexed under this heading.

Glutethimide (May increase drowsiness effect).
No products indexed under this heading.

Haloperidol (May increase drowsiness effect). Products include:
Haldol Injection, Tablets and Concentrate 2533

Haloperidol Decanoate (May increase drowsiness effect). Products include:
Haldol Decanoate 2535

Hydroxyzine Hydrochloride (May increase drowsiness effect). Products include:
Atarax Tablets & Syrup 2667
Vistaril Intramuscular Solution 2738

Lorazepam (May increase drowsiness effect). Products include:
Ativan Injection 3478
Ativan Tablets 3482

Loxapine Hydrochloride (May increase drowsiness effect).
No products indexed under this heading.

Loxapine Succinate (May increase drowsiness effect). Products include:
Loxitane Capsules 3398

Meprobamate (May increase drowsiness effect). Products include:
Miltown Tablets 3349

Mesoridazine Besylate (May increase drowsiness effect). Products include:
Serentil 1057

Midazolam Hydrochloride (May increase drowsiness effect). Products include:
Versed Injection 3027
Versed Syrup 3033

Molindone Hydrochloride (May increase drowsiness effect). Products include:
Moban 1320

Oxazepam (May increase drowsiness effect).
No products indexed under this heading.

Perphenazine (May increase drowsiness effect). Products include:
Etrafon 3115
Trilafon 3160

Prazepam (May increase drowsiness effect).
No products indexed under this heading.

Prochlorperazine (May increase drowsiness effect). Products include:
Compazine 1505

Promethazine Hydrochloride (May increase drowsiness effect). Products include:
Mepergan Injection 3539
Phenergan Injection 3553
Phenergan 3556
Phenergan Syrup 3554
Phenergan with Codeine Syrup 3557
Phenergan with Dextromethorphan Syrup 3559
Phenergan VC Syrup 3560
Phenergan VC with Codeine Syrup 3561

Propofol (May increase drowsiness effect). Products include:
Diprivan Injectable Emulsion 667

Quazepam (May increase drowsiness effect).
No products indexed under this heading.

Secobarbital Sodium (May increase drowsiness effect).
No products indexed under this heading.

Temazepam (May increase drowsiness effect).
No products indexed under this heading.

Thioridazine Hydrochloride (May increase drowsiness effect). Products include:
Thioridazine Hydrochloride Tablets 2289

Thiothixene (May increase drowsiness effect). Products include:
Navane Capsules 2701
Thiothixene Capsules 2290

Triazolam (May increase drowsiness effect). Products include:
Halcion Tablets 2823

Trifluoperazine Hydrochloride (May increase drowsiness effect). Products include:
Stelazine 1640

Zaleplon (May increase drowsiness effect). Products include:
Sonata Capsules 3591

Zolpidem Tartrate (May increase drowsiness effect). Products include:
Ambien Tablets 3191

Food Interactions

Alcohol (Chronic heavy alcohol users, 3 or more drinks per day, should consult their physician for advice on when and how they should take pain relievers/fever reducers including acetaminophen; increases drowsiness effect; avoid alcoholic beverages).

PERCOLONE TABLETS

(Oxycodone Hydrochloride) 1327

May interact with central nervous system depressants, hypnotics and sedatives, narcotic analgesics, phenothiazines, tranquilizers, and certain other agents. Compounds in these categories include:

Alfentanil Hydrochloride (Co-administration may exhibit an additive CNS depression).
No products indexed under this heading.

Alprazolam (Co-administration may exhibit an additive CNS depression). Products include:
Xanax Tablets 2865

Aprobarbital (Co-administration may exhibit an additive CNS depression).
No products indexed under this heading.

Buprenorphine Hydrochloride (Co-administration may exhibit an additive CNS depression). Products include:
Buprenex Injectable 2918

Buspirone Hydrochloride (Co-administration may exhibit an additive CNS depression).
No products indexed under this heading.

Butabarbital (Co-administration may exhibit an additive CNS depression).
No products indexed under this heading.

Butalbital (Co-administration may exhibit an additive CNS depression). Products include:
Phrenilin 578
Sedapap Tablets 50 mg/650 mg 2225

Chlordiazepoxide (Co-administration may exhibit an additive CNS depression). Products include:
Limbitrol 1738

Chlordiazepoxide Hydrochloride (Co-administration may exhibit an additive CNS depression). Products include:
Librium Capsules 1736
Librium for Injection 1737

Chlorpromazine (Co-administration may exhibit an additive CNS depression). Products include:
Thorazine Suppositories 1656

Chlorpromazine Hydrochloride (Co-administration may exhibit an additive CNS depression). Products include:
Thorazine 1656

Chlorprothixene (Co-administration may exhibit an additive CNS depression).
No products indexed under this heading.

Chlorprothixene Hydrochloride (Co-administration may exhibit an additive CNS depression).
No products indexed under this heading.

Chlorprothixene Lactate (Co-administration may exhibit an additive CNS depression).
No products indexed under this heading.

Clorazepate Dipotassium (Co-administration may exhibit an additive CNS depression). Products include:
Tranxene 511

Clozapine (Co-administration may exhibit an additive CNS depression). Products include:
Clozaril Tablets 2319

Codeine Phosphate (Co-administration may exhibit an additive CNS depression). Products include:
Phenergan with Codeine Syrup 3557
Phenergan VC with Codeine Syrup 3561
Robitussin A-C Syrup 2942
Robitussin-DAC Syrup 2942
Ryna-C Liquid 768
Soma Compound w/Codeine Tablets 3355
Tussi-Organidin NR Liquid 3350
Tussi-Organidin-S NR Liquid 3350
Tylenol with Codeine 2595

Desflurane (Co-administration may exhibit an additive CNS depression). Products include:
Suprane Liquid for Inhalation 874

Dezocine (Co-administration may exhibit an additive CNS depression).
No products indexed under this heading.

Diazepam (Co-administration may exhibit an additive CNS depression). Products include:
Valium Injectable 3026
Valium Tablets 3047

Droperidol (Co-administration may exhibit an additive CNS depression).
No products indexed under this heading.

Enflurane (Co-administration may exhibit an additive CNS depression).
No products indexed under this heading.

Estazolam (Co-administration may exhibit an additive CNS depression). Products include:
ProSom Tablets 500

Ethchlorvynol (Co-administration may exhibit an additive CNS depression).
No products indexed under this heading.

Ethinamate (Co-administration may exhibit an additive CNS depression).
No products indexed under this heading.

Fentanyl (Co-administration may exhibit an additive CNS depression). Products include:
Duragesic Transdermal System 1786

Fentanyl Citrate (Co-administration may exhibit an additive CNS depression). Products include:
Actiq 1184

Fluphenazine Decanoate (Co-administration may exhibit an additive CNS depression).
No products indexed under this heading.

Fluphenazine Enanthate (Co-administration may exhibit an additive CNS depression).
No products indexed under this heading.

Fluphenazine Hydrochloride (Co-administration may exhibit an additive CNS depression).
No products indexed under this heading.

Flurazepam Hydrochloride (Co-administration may exhibit an additive CNS depression).
No products indexed under this heading.

Glutethimide (Co-administration may exhibit an additive CNS depression).
No products indexed under this heading.

Haloperidol (Co-administration may exhibit an additive CNS depression). Products include:
Haldol Injection, Tablets and Concentrate 2533

Haloperidol Decanoate (Co-administration may exhibit an additive CNS depression). Products include:
Haldol Decanoate 2535

Hydrocodone Bitartrate (Co-administration may exhibit an additive CNS depression). Products include:
Hycodan 1316
Hycomine Compound Tablets 1317
Hycotuss Expectorant Syrup 1318
Lortab 3319
Lortab Elixir 3317
Maxidone Tablets CIII 3399
Norco 5/325 Tablets CIII 3424
Norco 7.5/325 Tablets CIII 3425
Norco 10/325 Tablets CIII 3427
Norco 10/325 Tablets CIII 3425
Vicodin Tablets 516
Vicodin ES Tablets 517
Vicodin HP Tablets 518
Vicodin Tuss Expectorant 519
Vicoprofen Tablets 520
Zydone Tablets 1330

Hydrocodone Polistirex (Co-administration may exhibit an additive CNS depression). Products include:
Tussionex Pennkinetic Extended-Release Suspension 1174

Hydromorphone Hydrochloride (Co-administration may exhibit an additive CNS depression). Products include:
Dilaudid 441
Dilaudid Oral Liquid 445
Dilaudid Powder 441
Dilaudid Rectal Suppositories 441
Dilaudid Tablets 441
Dilaudid Tablets - 8 mg 445
Dilaudid-HP 443

Hydroxyzine Hydrochloride (Co-administration may exhibit an additive CNS depression). Products include:
Atarax Tablets & Syrup 2667
Vistaril Intramuscular Solution 2738

Isoflurane (Co-administration may exhibit an additive CNS depression).
No products indexed under this heading.

Ketamine Hydrochloride (Co-administration may exhibit an additive CNS depression).
No products indexed under this heading.

Levomethadyl Acetate Hydrochloride (Co-administration may exhibit an additive CNS depression).
No products indexed under this heading.

Levorphanol Tartrate (Co-administration may exhibit an additive CNS depression). Products include:
Levo-Dromoran 1734
Levorphanol Tartrate Tablets 3059

Lorazepam (Co-administration may exhibit an additive CNS depression). Products include:
Ativan Injection 3478
Ativan Tablets 3482

Loxapine Hydrochloride (Co-administration may exhibit an additive CNS depression).
No products indexed under this heading.

Loxapine Succinate (Co-administration may exhibit an additive CNS depression). Products include:
Loxitane Capsules 3398

Meperidine Hydrochloride (Co-administration may exhibit an additive CNS depression). Products include:
Demerol 3079
Mepergan Injection 3539

Mephobarbital (Co-administration may exhibit an additive CNS depression).
No products indexed under this heading.

Meprobamate (Co-administration may exhibit an additive CNS depression). Products include:
Miltown Tablets 3349

Mesoridazine Besylate (Co-administration may exhibit an additive CNS depression). Products include:
Serentil 1057

Methadone Hydrochloride (Co-administration may exhibit an additive CNS depression). Products include:
Dolophine Hydrochloride Tablets 3056

Methohexital Sodium (Co-administration may exhibit an additive CNS depression). Products include:
Brevital Sodium for Injection, USP 1815

Methotrimeprazine (Co-administration may exhibit an additive CNS depression).
No products indexed under this heading.

Methoxyflurane (Co-administration may exhibit an additive CNS depression).
No products indexed under this heading.

Midazolam Hydrochloride (Co-administration may exhibit an additive CNS depression). Products include:
Versed Injection 3027
Versed Syrup 3033

Molindone Hydrochloride (Co-administration may exhibit an additive CNS depression). Products include:
Moban 1320

Morphine Sulfate (Co-administration may exhibit an additive CNS depression). Products include:
Astramorph/PF Injection, USP (Preservative-Free) 594
Duramorph Injection 1312
Infumorph 200 and Infumorph 500 Sterile Solutions 1314
Kadian Capsules 1335
MS Contin Tablets 2896
MSIR 2898
Oramorph SR Tablets 3062
Roxanol 3066

Olanzapine (Co-administration may exhibit an additive CNS depression). Products include:
Zyprexa Tablets 1973
Zyprexa ZYDIS Orally Disintegrating Tablets 1973

Oxazepam (Co-administration may exhibit an additive CNS depression).
No products indexed under this heading.

Pentobarbital Sodium (Co-administration may exhibit an additive CNS depression). Products include:
Nembutal Sodium Solution 485

Perphenazine (Co-administration may exhibit an additive CNS depression). Products include:
Etrafon 3115
Trilafon 3160

Phenobarbital (Co-administration may exhibit an additive CNS depression). Products include:
Arco-Lase Plus Tablets 592
Donnatal 2929
Donnatal Extentabs 2930

Prazepam (Co-administration may exhibit an additive CNS depression).
No products indexed under this heading.

Prochlorperazine (Co-administration may exhibit an additive CNS depression). Products include:
Compazine 1505

Promethazine Hydrochloride (Co-administration may exhibit an additive CNS depression). Products include:
Mepergan Injection 3539
Phenergan Injection 3553
Phenergan 3556
Phenergan Syrup 3554
Phenergan with Codeine Syrup 3557
Phenergan with Dextromethorphan Syrup 3559
Phenergan VC Syrup 3560
Phenergan VC with Codeine Syrup 3561

Propofol (Co-administration may exhibit an additive CNS depression). Products include:
Diprivan Injectable Emulsion 667

Propoxyphene Hydrochloride (Co-administration may exhibit an additive CNS depression). Products include:
Darvon Pulvules 1909
Darvon Compound-65 Pulvules 1910

Propoxyphene Napsylate (Co-administration may exhibit an additive CNS depression). Products include:
Darvon-N/Darvocet-N 1907
Darvon-N Tablets 1912

Quazepam (Co-administration may exhibit an additive CNS depression).
No products indexed under this heading.

Quetiapine Fumarate (Co-administration may exhibit an additive CNS depression). Products include:
Seroquel Tablets 684

Remifentanil Hydrochloride (Co-administration may exhibit an additive CNS depression).
No products indexed under this heading.

Risperidone (Co-administration may exhibit an additive CNS depression). Products include:
Risperdal 1796

Secobarbital Sodium (Co-administration may exhibit an additive CNS depression).
No products indexed under this heading.

Sevoflurane (Co-administration may exhibit an additive CNS depression).
No products indexed under this heading.

Sufentanil Citrate (Co-administration may exhibit an additive CNS depression).
No products indexed under this heading.

Temazepam (Co-administration may exhibit an additive CNS depression).
No products indexed under this heading.

Thiamylal Sodium (Co-administration may exhibit an additive CNS depression).
No products indexed under this heading.

Thioridazine Hydrochloride (Co-administration may exhibit an additive CNS depression). Products include:
Thioridazine Hydrochloride Tablets 2289

Thiothixene (Co-administration may exhibit an additive CNS depression). Products include:
Navane Capsules 2701
Thiothixene Capsules 2290

Triazolam (Co-administration may exhibit an additive CNS depression). Products include:
Halcion Tablets 2823

Trifluoperazine Hydrochloride (Co-administration may exhibit an additive CNS depression). Products include:
Stelazine 1640

Zaleplon (Co-administration may exhibit an additive CNS depression). Products include:
Sonata Capsules 3591

Ziprasidone Hydrochloride (Co-administration may exhibit an additive CNS depression). Products include:
Geodon Capsules 2688

Zolpidem Tartrate (Co-administration may exhibit an additive CNS depression). Products include:
Ambien Tablets 3191

Food Interactions

Alcohol (Concurrent use may exhibit an additive CNS depression).

PERDIEM FIBER THERAPY

(Psyllium Preparations) 2301
None cited in PDR database.

PERDIEM OVERNIGHT RELIEF

(Psyllium Preparations, Senna) 2301
None cited in PDR database.

PERFECT MEAL

(Amino Acid Preparations, Lactobacillus Acidophilus, Vitamins with Minerals) .... ▣798
None cited in PDR database.

PERFORMANCE GOLD CAPLETS

(Ginseng, Golden Root, Whey) .... ▣798
None cited in PDR database.

PERFORMANCE OPTIMIZER SYSTEM

(Amino Acid Preparations, Ginseng, Herbals, Multiple, Herbals with Vitamins & Minerals, Serenoa repens) .... ▣798
None cited in PDR database.

PERGONAL FOR INJECTION

(Menotropins) 3223
None cited in PDR database.

PERIACTIN TABLETS

(Cyproheptadine Hydrochloride) 2155
May interact with central nervous system depressants and monoamine oxidase inhibitors. Compounds in these categories include:

Alfentanil Hydrochloride (Antihistimines may have additive effects with central nervous system depressants).
No products indexed under this heading.

Alprazolam (Antihistimines may have additive effects with central nervous system depressants). Products include:
Xanax Tablets 2865

Aprobarbital (Antihistimines may have additive effects with central nervous system depressants).
No products indexed under this heading.

Buprenorphine Hydrochloride (Antihistimines may have additive effects with central nervous system depressants). Products include:
Buprenex Injectable 2918

Buspirone Hydrochloride (Antihistimines may have additive effects with central nervous system depressants).
No products indexed under this heading.

Butabarbital (Antihistimines may have additive effects with central nervous system depressants).
No products indexed under this heading.

Butalbital (Antihistimines may have additive effects with central nervous system depressants). Products include:
Phrenilin 578
Sedapap Tablets 50 mg/650 mg 2225

Chlordiazepoxide (Antihistimines may have additive effects with central nervous system depressants). Products include:
Limbitrol 1738

Chlordiazepoxide Hydrochloride (Antihistimines may have additive effects with central nervous system depressants). Products include:
Librium Capsules 1736
Librium for Injection 1737

Chlorpromazine (Antihistimines may have additive effects with central nervous system depressants). Products include:
Thorazine Suppositories 1656

Chlorpromazine Hydrochloride (Antihistimines may have additive effects with central nervous system depressants). Products include:
Thorazine 1656

Chlorprothixene (Antihistimines may have additive effects with central nervous system depressants).
No products indexed under this heading.

Chlorprothixene Hydrochloride (Antihistimines may have additive effects with central nervous system depressants).
No products indexed under this heading.

Chlorprothixene Lactate (Antihistimines may have additive effects with central nervous system depressants).
No products indexed under this heading.

Clorazepate Dipotassium (Antihistimines may have additive effects with central nervous system depressants). Products include:
Tranxene 511

Clozapine (Antihistimines may have additive effects with central nervous system depressants). Products include:
Clozaril Tablets 2319

Codeine Phosphate (Antihistimines may have additive effects with central nervous system depressants). Products include:
Phenergan with Codeine Syrup 3557
Phenergan VC with Codeine Syrup 3561
Robitussin A-C Syrup 2942
Robitussin-DAC Syrup 2942
Ryna-C Liquid .... ▣768
Soma Compound w/Codeine Tablets 3355

Tussi-Organidin NR Liquid 3350
Tussi-Organidin-S NR Liquid 3350
Tylenol with Codeine 2595

Desflurane (Antihistimines may have additive effects with central nervous system depressants). Products include:
Suprane Liquid for Inhalation 874

Dezocine (Antihistimines may have additive effects with central nervous system depressants).
No products indexed under this heading.

Diazepam (Antihistimines may have additive effects with central nervous system depressants). Products include:
Valium Injectable 3026
Valium Tablets 3047

Droperidol (Antihistimines may have additive effects with central nervous system depressants).
No products indexed under this heading.

Enflurane (Antihistimines may have additive effects with central nervous system depressants).
No products indexed under this heading.

Estazolam (Antihistimines may have additive effects with central nervous system depressants). Products include:
ProSom Tablets 500

Ethchlorvynol (Antihistimines may have additive effects with central nervous system depressants).
No products indexed under this heading.

Ethinamate (Antihistimines may have additive effects with central nervous system depressants).
No products indexed under this heading.

Fentanyl (Antihistimines may have additive effects with central nervous system depressants). Products include:
Duragesic Transdermal System 1786

Fentanyl Citrate (Antihistimines may have additive effects with central nervous system depressants). Products include:
Actiq 1184

Fluphenazine Decanoate (Antihistimines may have additive effects with central nervous system depressants).
No products indexed under this heading.

Fluphenazine Enanthate (Antihistimines may have additive effects with central nervous system depressants).
No products indexed under this heading.

Fluphenazine Hydrochloride (Antihistimines may have additive effects with central nervous system depressants).
No products indexed under this heading.

Flurazepam Hydrochloride (Antihistimines may have additive effects with central nervous system depressants).
No products indexed under this heading.

Glutethimide (Antihistimines may have additive effects with central nervous system depressants).
No products indexed under this heading.

Haloperidol (Antihistimines may have additive effects with central nervous system depressants). Products include:
Haldol Injection, Tablets and Concentrate 2533

Haloperidol Decanoate (Antihistimines may have additive effects with central nervous system depressants). Products include:
Haldol Decanoate 2535

Hydrocodone Bitartrate (Antihistimines may have additive effects with central nervous system depressants). Products include:
Hycodan 1316
Hycomine Compound Tablets 1317
Hycotuss Expectorant Syrup 1318
Lortab 3319
Lortab Elixir 3317
Maxidone Tablets CIII 3399
Norco 5/325 Tablets CIII 3424
Norco 7.5/325 Tablets CIII 3425
Norco 10/325 Tablets CIII 3427
Norco 10/325 Tablets CIII 3425
Vicodin Tablets 516
Vicodin ES Tablets 517
Vicodin HP Tablets 518
Vicodin Tuss Expectorant 519
Vicoprofen Tablets 520
Zydone Tablets 1330

Hydrocodone Polistirex (Antihistimines may have additive effects with central nervous system depressants). Products include:
Tussionex Pennkinetic Extended-Release Suspension 1174

Hydromorphone Hydrochloride (Antihistimines may have additive effects with central nervous system depressants). Products include:
Dilaudid 441
Dilaudid Oral Liquid 445
Dilaudid Powder 441
Dilaudid Rectal Suppositories 441
Dilaudid Tablets 441
Dilaudid Tablets - 8 mg 445
Dilaudid-HP 443

Hydroxyzine Hydrochloride (Antihistimines may have additive effects with central nervous system depressants). Products include:
Atarax Tablets & Syrup 2667
Vistaril Intramuscular Solution 2738

Isocarboxazid (MAO inhibitors prolong and intensify anticholinergic effects of antihistimines; concurrent use is contraindicated).
No products indexed under this heading.

Isoflurane (Antihistimines may have additive effects with central nervous system depressants).
No products indexed under this heading.

Ketamine Hydrochloride (Antihistimines may have additive effects with central nervous system depressants).
No products indexed under this heading.

Levomethadyl Acetate Hydrochloride (Antihistimines may have additive effects with central nervous system depressants).
No products indexed under this heading.

Levorphanol Tartrate (Antihistimines may have additive effects with central nervous system depressants). Products include:
Levo-Dromoran 1734
Levorphanol Tartrate Tablets 3059

Lorazepam (Antihistimines may have additive effects with central nervous system depressants). Products include:
Ativan Injection 3478
Ativan Tablets 3482

Loxapine Hydrochloride (Antihistimines may have additive effects with central nervous system depressants).
No products indexed under this heading.

Loxapine Succinate (Antihistimines may have additive effects with central nervous system depressants). Products include:
Loxitane Capsules 3398

Meperidine Hydrochloride (Antihistimines may have additive effects with central nervous system depressants). Products include:
Demerol 3079
Mepergan Injection 3539

Mephobarbital (Antihistimines may have additive effects with central nervous system depressants).
No products indexed under this heading.

Meprobamate (Antihistimines may have additive effects with central nervous system depressants). Products include:
Miltown Tablets 3349

Mesoridazine Besylate (Antihistimines may have additive effects with central nervous system depressants). Products include:
Serentil 1057

Methadone Hydrochloride (Antihistimines may have additive effects with central nervous system depressants). Products include:
Dolophine Hydrochloride Tablets 3056

Methohexital Sodium (Antihistimines may have additive effects with central nervous system depressants). Products include:
Brevital Sodium for Injection, USP .. 1815

Methotrimeprazine (Antihistimines may have additive effects with central nervous system depressants).
No products indexed under this heading.

Methoxyflurane (Antihistimines may have additive effects with central nervous system depressants).
No products indexed under this heading.

Midazolam Hydrochloride (Antihistimines may have additive effects with central nervous system depressants). Products include:
Versed Injection 3027
Versed Syrup 3033

Moclobemide (MAO inhibitors prolong and intensify anticholinergic effects of antihistimines; concurrent use is contraindicated).
No products indexed under this heading.

Molindone Hydrochloride (Antihistimines may have additive effects with central nervous system depressants). Products include:
Moban 1320

Morphine Sulfate (Antihistimines may have additive effects with central nervous system depressants). Products include:
Astramorph/PF Injection, USP (Preservative-Free) 594
Duramorph Injection 1312
Infumorph 200 and Infumorph 500 Sterile Solutions 1314
Kadian Capsules 1335
MS Contin Tablets 2896
MSIR 2898
Oramorph SR Tablets 3062
Roxanol 3066

Olanzapine (Antihistimines may have additive effects with central nervous system depressants). Products include:
Zyprexa Tablets 1973
Zyprexa ZYDIS Orally Disintegrating Tablets 1973

Oxazepam (Antihistimines may have additive effects with central nervous system depressants).
No products indexed under this heading.

Oxycodone Hydrochloride (Antihistimines may have additive effects with central nervous system depressants). Products include:
OxyContin Tablets 2912
OxyFast Oral Concentrate Solution . 2916
OxyIR Capsules 2916
Percocet Tablets 1326
Percodan Tablets 1327
Percolone Tablets 1327
Roxicodone 3067
Tylox Capsules 2597

Pargyline Hydrochloride (MAO inhibitors prolong and intensify anticholinergic effects of antihistimines; concurrent use is contraindicated).
No products indexed under this heading.

Pentobarbital Sodium (Antihistimines may have additive effects with central nervous system depressants). Products include:
Nembutal Sodium Solution 485

Perphenazine (Antihistimines may have additive effects with central nervous system depressants). Products include:
Etrafon 3115
Trilafon 3160

Phenelzine Sulfate (MAO inhibitors prolong and intensify anticholinergic effects of antihistimines; concurrent use is contraindicated). Products include:
Nardil Tablets 2653

Phenobarbital (Antihistimines may have additive effects with central nervous system depressants). Products include:
Arco-Lase Plus Tablets 592
Donnatal 2929
Donnatal Extentabs 2930

Prazepam (Antihistimines may have additive effects with central nervous system depressants).
No products indexed under this heading.

Procarbazine Hydrochloride (MAO inhibitors prolong and intensify anticholinergic effects of antihistimines; concurrent use is contraindicated). Products include:
Matulane Capsules 3246

Prochlorperazine (Antihistimines may have additive effects with central nervous system depressants). Products include:
Compazine 1505

Promethazine Hydrochloride (Antihistimines may have additive effects with central nervous system depressants). Products include:
Mepergan Injection 3539
Phenergan Injection 3553
Phenergan 3556
Phenergan Syrup 3554
Phenergan with Codeine Syrup 3557
Phenergan with Dextromethorphan Syrup 3559
Phenergan VC Syrup 3560
Phenergan VC with Codeine Syrup .. 3561

Propofol (Antihistimines may have additive effects with central nervous system depressants). Products include:
Diprivan Injectable Emulsion 667

Propoxyphene Hydrochloride (Antihistimines may have additive effects with central nervous system depressants). Products include:
Darvon Pulvules 1909
Darvon Compound-65 Pulvules 1910

Propoxyphene Napsylate (Antihistimines may have additive effects with central nervous system depressants). Products include:
Darvon-N/Darvocet-N 1907
Darvon-N Tablets 1912

Quazepam (Antihistimines may have additive effects with central nervous system depressants).
No products indexed under this heading.

Quetiapine Fumarate (Antihistimines may have additive effects with central nervous system depressants). Products include:
Seroquel Tablets 684

Remifentanil Hydrochloride (Antihistimines may have additive effects with central nervous system depressants).
No products indexed under this heading.

Risperidone (Antihistimines may have additive effects with central nervous system depressants). Products include:
Risperdal 1796

Secobarbital Sodium (Antihistimines may have additive effects with central nervous system

depressants).
No products indexed under this heading.
Selegiline Hydrochloride (MAO inhibitors prolong and intensify anticholinergic effects of antihistimines; concurrent use is contraindicated). Products include:
Eldepryl Capsules 3266
Sevoflurane (Antihistimines may have additive effects with central nervous system depressants).
No products indexed under this heading.
Sufentanil Citrate (Antihistimines may have additive effects with central nervous system depressants).
No products indexed under this heading.
Temazepam (Antihistimines may have additive effects with central nervous system depressants).
No products indexed under this heading.
Thiamylal Sodium (Antihistimines may have additive effects with central nervous system depressants).
No products indexed under this heading.
Thioridazine Hydrochloride (Antihistimines may have additive effects with central nervous system depressants). Products include:
Thioridazine Hydrochloride Tablets 2289
Thiothixene (Antihistimines may have additive effects with central nervous system depressants). Products include:
Navane Capsules 2701
Thiothixene Capsules 2290
Tranylcypromine Sulfate (MAO inhibitors prolong and intensify anticholinergic effects of antihistimines; concurrent use is contraindicated). Products include:
Parnate Tablets 1607
Triazolam (Antihistimines may have additive effects with central nervous system depressants). Products include:
Halcion Tablets 2823
Trifluoperazine Hydrochloride (Antihistimines may have additive effects with central nervous system depressants). Products include:
Stelazine 1640
Zaleplon (Antihistimines may have additive effects with central nervous system depressants). Products include:
Sonata Capsules 3591
Ziprasidone Hydrochloride (Antihistimines may have additive effects with central nervous system depressants). Products include:
Geodon Capsules 2688
Zolpidem Tartrate (Antihistimines may have additive effects with central nervous system depressants). Products include:
Ambien Tablets 3191

Food Interactions

Alcohol (Antihistimines may have additive effects with alcohol).

PERI-COLACE CAPSULES AND SYRUP
(Casanthranol, Docusate Sodium) 3240
None cited in PDR database.

PERIDIN-C TABLETS
(Bioflavonoids, Hesperidin Complex, Hesperidin Methyl Chalcone, Vitamin C) .... ▣618
None cited in PDR database.

PERIOSTAT TABLETS
(Doxycycline Hyclate) 1208
May interact with antacids containing aluminum, calcium and magnesium, barbiturates, oral anticoagulants, iron containing oral preparations, oral contraceptives, penicillins, phenytoin, and certain other agents. Compounds in these categories include:

Aluminum Carbonate (Absorption of tetracyclines is impaired by antacids containing aluminum, calcium, or magnesium).
No products indexed under this heading.
Aluminum Hydroxide (Absorption of tetracyclines is impaired by antacids containing aluminum, calcium, or magnesium). Products include:
Amphojel Suspension (Mint Flavor) .... ▣789
Gaviscon Extra Strength Liquid .... ▣751
Gaviscon Extra Strength Tablets .... ▣751
Gaviscon Regular Strength Liquid .... ▣751
Gaviscon Regular Strength Tablets .... ▣750
Maalox Antacid/Anti-Gas Oral Suspension .... ▣673
Maalox Max Maximum Strength Antacid/Anti-Gas Liquid 2300
Maalox Regular Strength Antacid/Antigas Liquid 2300
Mylanta 1813
Vanquish Caplets .... ▣617
Amoxicillin Trihydrate (Co-administration of bacteriostatic antibiotics, such as the tetracycline class of antibiotics, may interfere with the bactericidal action of members of the beta lactam antibiotics, such as penicillins; concurrent use should be avoided).
Ampicillin (Co-administration of bacteriostatic antibiotics, such as the tetracycline class of antibiotics, may interfere with the bactericidal action of members of the beta lactam antibiotics, such as penicillins; concurrent use should be avoided).
No products indexed under this heading.
Ampicillin Sodium (Co-administration of bacteriostatic antibiotics, such as the tetracycline class of antibiotics, may interfere with the bactericidal action of members of the beta lactam antibiotics, such as penicillins; concurrent use should be avoided). Products include:
Unasyn for Injection 2728
Ampicillin Trihydrate (Co-administration of bacteriostatic antibiotics, such as the tetracycline class of antibiotics, may interfere with the bactericidal action of members of the beta lactam antibiotics, such as penicillins; concurrent use should be avoided).
No products indexed under this heading.
Aprobarbital (Co-administration with barbiturates decreases the half-life of doxycycline).
No products indexed under this heading.
Azlocillin Sodium (Co-administration of bacteriostatic antibiotics, such as the tetracycline class of antibiotics, may interfere with the bactericidal action of members of the beta lactam antibiotics, such as penicillins; concurrent use should be avoided).
No products indexed under this heading.
Bacampicillin Hydrochloride (Co-administration of bacteriostatic antibiotics, such as the tetracycline class of antibiotics, may interfere with the bactericidal action of members of the beta lactam antibiotics, such as penicillins; concurrent use should be avoided).
No products indexed under this heading.
Bismuth Subsalicylate (Absorption of tetracyclines is impaired by bismuth subsalicylate). Products include:
Pepto-Bismol Maximum Strength Liquid 2878
Pepto-Bismol Original Liquid, Original and Cherry Tablets and Easy-To-Swallow Caplets 2878
Butabarbital (Co-administration with barbiturates decreases the half-life of doxycycline).
No products indexed under this heading.
Butalbital (Co-administration with barbiturates decreases the half-life of doxycycline). Products include:
Phrenilin 578
Sedapap Tablets 50 mg/650 mg 2225
Calcium Carbonate (Absorption of tetracyclines is impaired by antacids containing aluminum, calcium, or magnesium). Products include:
Aspirin Regimen Bayer 81 mg Caplets with Calcium .... ▣607
Extra Strength Bayer Plus Caplets .... ▣610
Caltrate 600 Tablets .... ▣814
Caltrate 600 PLUS .... ▣815
Caltrate 600 + D Tablets .... ▣814
Caltrate 600 + Soy Tablets .... ▣814
D-Cal Chewable Caplets .... ▣794
Florical Capsules and Tablets 2223
Quick Dissolve Maalox Max Maximum Strength Antacid/Antigas Tablets 2301
Quick Dissolve Maalox Regular Strength Antacid Tablets 2301
Marblen Suspension .... ▣633
Monocal Tablets 2223
Mylanta Fast-Acting 1813
Mylanta Calci Tabs .... ▣636
One-A-Day Bedtime & Rest Tablets .... ▣805
One-A-Day Calcium Plus Chewable Tablets .... ▣805
Os-Cal Chewable Tablets .... ▣838
Pepcid Complete Chewable Tablets 1815
ReSource Wellness CalciWise Soft Chews .... ▣824
Rolaids Tablets .... ▣706
Extra Strength Rolaids Tablets .... ▣706
Slow-Mag Tablets .... ▣835
Titralac .... ▣640
3M Titralac Plus Antacid Tablets .... ▣640
Tums .... ▣763
Carbamazepine (Co-administration with carbamazepine decreases the half-life of doxycycline). Products include:
Carbatrol Capsules 3234
Tegretol/Tegretol-XR 2404
Carbenicillin Disodium (Co-administration of bacteriostatic antibiotics, such as the tetracycline class of antibiotics, may interfere with the bactericidal action of members of the beta lactam antibiotics, such as penicillins; concurrent use should be avoided).
No products indexed under this heading.
Carbenicillin Indanyl Sodium (Co-administration of bacteriostatic antibiotics, such as the tetracycline class of antibiotics, may interfere with the bactericidal action of members of the beta lactam antibiotics, such as penicillins; concurrent use should be avoided). Products include:
Geocillin Tablets 2687
Desogestrel (Concurrent use of tetracycline may render oral contraceptives less effective). Products include:
Cyclessa Tablets 2450
Desogen Tablets 2458
Mircette Tablets 2470
Ortho-Cept 21 Tablets 2546
Ortho-Cept 28 Tablets 2546
Dicloxacillin Sodium (Co-administration of bacteriostatic antibiotics, such as the tetracycline class of antibiotics, may interfere with the bactericidal action of members of the beta lactam antibiotics, such as penicillins; concurrent use should be avoided).
No products indexed under this heading.
Dicumarol (Co-administration of tetracyclines with anticoagulants results in depressed prothrombin activity; downward adjustment of anticoagulant may be required).
No products indexed under this heading.
Ethinyl Estradiol (Concurrent use of tetracycline may render oral contraceptives less effective). Products include:
Alesse-21 Tablets 3468
Alesse-28 Tablets 3473
Brevicon 28-Day Tablets 3380
Cyclessa Tablets 2450
Desogen Tablets 2458
Estinyl Tablets 3112
Estrostep 2627
femhrt Tablets 2635
Levlen 962
Levlite 21 Tablets 962
Levlite 28 Tablets 962
Levora Tablets 3389
Loestrin 21 Tablets 2642
Loestrin Fe Tablets 2642
Lo/Ovral Tablets 3532
Lo/Ovral-28 Tablets 3538
Low-Ogestrel-28 Tablets 3392
Microgestin Fe 1.5/30 Tablets 3407
Microgestin Fe 1/20 Tablets 3400
Mircette Tablets 2470
Modicon 2563
Necon 3415
Nordette-28 Tablets 2257
Norinyl 1 +35 28-Day Tablets 3380
Ogestrel 0.5/50-28 Tablets 3428
Ortho-Cept 21 Tablets 2546
Ortho-Cept 28 Tablets 2546
Ortho-Cyclen/Ortho Tri-Cyclen 2573
Ortho-Novum 2563
Ovcon 3364
Ovral Tablets 3551
Ovral-28 Tablets 3552
Tri-Levlen 962
Tri-Norinyl-28 Tablets 3433
Triphasil-21 Tablets 3600
Triphasil-28 Tablets 3605
Trivora Tablets 3439
Yasmin 28 Tablets 980
Zovia 3449
Ethynodiol Diacetate (Concurrent use of tetracycline may render oral contraceptives less effective). Products include:
Zovia 3449
Ferrous Fumarate (Absorption of tetracyclines is impaired by iron-containing preparations). Products include:
New Formulation Chromagen OB Capsules 3094
Loestrin Fe Tablets 2642
NataChew Tablets 3364
Ferrous Gluconate (Absorption of tetracyclines is impaired by iron-containing preparations). Products include:
Fergon Iron Tablets .... ▣802
Ferrous Sulfate (Absorption of tetracyclines is impaired by iron-containing preparations). Products include:
Feosol Tablets 1717
Slow Fe Tablets .... ▣827
Slow Fe with Folic Acid Tablets .... ▣828
Fosphenytoin Sodium (Co-administration with phenytoin decreases the half-life of doxycycline). Products include:
Cerebyx Injection 2619
Iron (Absorption of tetracyclines is impaired by iron-containing preparations).
No products indexed under this heading.
Levonorgestrel (Concurrent use of tetracycline may render oral contraceptives less effective). Products include:
Alesse-21 Tablets 3468
Alesse-28 Tablets 3473
Levlen 962
Levlite 21 Tablets 962
Levlite 28 Tablets 962
Levora Tablets 3389
Mirena Intrauterine System 974
Nordette-28 Tablets 2257
Norplant System 3543
Tri-Levlen 962
Triphasil-21 Tablets 3600
Triphasil-28 Tablets 3605
Trivora Tablets 3439
Magaldrate (Absorption of tetracyclines is impaired by antacids containing aluminum, calcium, or mag-

nesium).
No products indexed under this heading.

Magnesium Hydroxide (Absorption of tetracyclines is impaired by antacids containing aluminum, calcium, or magnesium). Products include:
- Ex•Lax Milk of Magnesia Liquid 670
- Maalox Antacid/Anti-Gas Oral Suspension 673
- Maalox Max Maximum Strength Antacid/Anti-Gas Liquid 2300
- Maalox Regular Strength Antacid/Antigas Liquid 2300
- Mylanta Fast-Acting 1813
- Mylanta 1813
- Pepcid Complete Chewable Tablets 1815
- Phillips' Chewable Tablets 615
- Phillips' Milk of Magnesia Liquid (Original, Cherry, & Mint) 616
- Rolaids Tablets 706
- Extra Strength Rolaids Tablets 706
- Vanquish Caplets 617

Magnesium Oxide (Absorption of tetracyclines is impaired by antacids containing aluminum, calcium, or magnesium). Products include:
- Beelith Tablets 946
- Mag-Ox 400 Tablets 1024
- Uro-Mag Capsules 1024

Mephobarbital (Co-administration with barbiturates decreases the half-life of doxycycline).
No products indexed under this heading.

Mestranol (Concurrent use of tetracycline may render oral contraceptives less effective). Products include:
- Necon 1/50 Tablets 3415
- Norinyl 1 + 50 28-Day Tablets 3380
- Ortho-Novum 1/50□28 Tablets 2556

Methoxyflurane (Concurrent use of tetracycline and methoxyflurane has been reported to result in fatal renal toxicity).
No products indexed under this heading.

Mezlocillin Sodium (Co-administration of bacteriostatic antibiotics, such as the tetracycline class of antibiotics, may interfere with the bactericidal action of members of the beta lactam antibiotics, such as penicillins; concurrent use should be avoided).
No products indexed under this heading.

Nafcillin Sodium (Co-administration of bacteriostatic antibiotics, such as the tetracycline class of antibiotics, may interfere with the bactericidal action of members of the beta lactam antibiotics, such as penicillins; concurrent use should be avoided).
No products indexed under this heading.

Norethindrone (Concurrent use of tetracycline may render oral contraceptives less effective). Products include:
- Brevicon 28-Day Tablets 3380
- Micronor Tablets 2543
- Modicon 2563
- Necon 3415
- Norinyl 1 +35 28-Day Tablets 3380
- Norinyl 1 + 50 28-Day Tablets 3380
- Nor-QD Tablets 3423
- Ortho-Novum 2563
- Ortho-Novum 1/50□28 Tablets 2556
- Ovcon 3364
- Tri-Norinyl-28 Tablets 3433

Norethynodrel (Concurrent use of tetracycline may render oral contraceptives less effective).
No products indexed under this heading.

Norgestimate (Concurrent use of tetracycline may render oral contraceptives less effective). Products include:
- Ortho-Cyclen/Ortho Tri-Cyclen 2573
- Ortho-Prefest Tablets 2570

Norgestrel (Concurrent use of tetracycline may render oral contraceptives less effective). Products include:
- Lo/Ovral Tablets 3532
- Lo/Ovral-28 Tablets 3538
- Low-Ogestrel-28 Tablets 3392
- Ogestrel 0.5/50-28 Tablets 3428
- Ovral Tablets 3551
- Ovral-28 Tablets 3552
- Ovrette Tablets 3552

Penicillin G Benzathine (Co-administration of bacteriostatic antibiotics, such as the tetracycline class of antibiotics, may interfere with the bactericidal action of members of the beta lactam antibiotics, such as penicillins; concurrent use should be avoided). Products include:
- Bicillin C-R 900/300 Injection 2240
- Bicillin C-R Injection 2238
- Bicillin L-A Injection 2242
- Permapen Isoject 2706

Penicillin G Potassium (Co-administration of bacteriostatic antibiotics, such as the tetracycline class of antibiotics, may interfere with the bactericidal action of members of the beta lactam antibiotics, such as penicillins; concurrent use should be avoided). Products include:
- Pfizerpen for Injection 2707

Penicillin G Procaine (Co-administration of bacteriostatic antibiotics, such as the tetracycline class of antibiotics, may interfere with the bactericidal action of members of the beta lactam antibiotics, such as penicillins; concurrent use should be avoided). Products include:
- Bicillin C-R 900/300 Injection 2240
- Bicillin C-R Injection 2238

Penicillin G Sodium (Co-administration of bacteriostatic antibiotics, such as the tetracycline class of antibiotics, may interfere with the bactericidal action of members of the beta lactam antibiotics, such as penicillins; concurrent use should be avoided).
No products indexed under this heading.

Penicillin V Potassium (Co-administration of bacteriostatic antibiotics, such as the tetracycline class of antibiotics, may interfere with the bactericidal action of members of the beta lactam antibiotics, such as penicillins; concurrent use should be avoided).
No products indexed under this heading.

Pentobarbital Sodium (Co-administration with barbiturates decreases the half-life of doxycycline). Products include:
- Nembutal Sodium Solution 485

Phenobarbital (Co-administration with barbiturates decreases the half-life of doxycycline). Products include:
- Arco-Lase Plus Tablets 592
- Donnatal 2929
- Donnatal Extentabs 2930

Phenytoin (Co-administration with phenytoin decreases the half-life of doxycycline). Products include:
- Dilantin Infatabs 2624
- Dilantin-125 Oral Suspension 2625

Phenytoin Sodium (Co-administration with phenytoin decreases the half-life of doxycycline). Products include:
- Dilantin Kapseals 2622

Polysaccharide-Iron Complex (Absorption of tetracyclines is impaired by iron-containing preparations). Products include:
- Niferex 3176
- Niferex-150 Capsules 3176
- Nu-Iron 150 Capsules 2224

Secobarbital Sodium (Co-administration with barbiturates decreases the half-life of doxycycline).
No products indexed under this heading.

Thiamylal Sodium (Co-administration with barbiturates decreases the half-life of doxycycline).
No products indexed under this heading.

Ticarcillin Disodium (Co-administration of bacteriostatic antibiotics, such as the tetracycline class of antibiotics, may interfere with the bactericidal action of members of the beta lactam antibiotics, such as penicillins; concurrent use should be avoided). Products include:
- Timentin Injection- ADD-Vantage Vial 1661
- Timentin Injection-Galaxy Container 1664
- Timentin Injection-Pharmacy Bulk Package 1666
- Timentin for Intravenous Administration 1658

Warfarin Sodium (Co-administration of tetracyclines with anticoagulants results in depressed prothrombin activity; downward adjustment of anticoagulant may be required). Products include:
- Coumadin for Injection 1243
- Coumadin Tablets 1243
- Warfarin Sodium Tablets, USP 3302

PERMAPEN ISOJECT

(Penicillin G Benzathine) 2706
May interact with erythromycin, highly protein bound drugs (selected), tetracyclines, and certain other agents. Compounds in these categories include:

Amiodarone Hydrochloride (Displacement of penicillins from plasma protein binding sites by highly protein bound drugs will elevate the level of free penicillin in the serum). Products include:
- Cordarone Intravenous 3491
- Cordarone Tablets 3487
- Pacerone Tablets 3331

Amitriptyline Hydrochloride (Displacement of penicillins from plasma protein binding sites by highly protein bound drugs will elevate the level of free penicillin in the serum). Products include:
- Etrafon 3115
- Limbitrol 1738

Atovaquone (Displacement of penicillins from plasma protein binding sites by highly protein bound drugs will elevate the level of free penicillin in the serum). Products include:
- Malarone 1596
- Mepron Suspension 1598

Cefonicid Sodium (Displacement of penicillins from plasma protein binding sites by highly protein bound drugs will elevate the level of free penicillin in the serum).
No products indexed under this heading.

Celecoxib (Displacement of penicillins from plasma protein binding sites by highly protein bound drugs will elevate the level of free penicillin in the serum). Products include:
- Celebrex Capsules 2676
- Celebrex Capsules 2780

Chlordiazepoxide (Displacement of penicillins from plasma protein binding sites by highly protein bound drugs will elevate the level of free penicillin in the serum). Products include:
- Limbitrol 1738

Chlordiazepoxide Hydrochloride (Displacement of penicillins from plasma protein binding sites by highly protein bound drugs will elevate the level of free penicillin in the serum). Products include:
- Librium Capsules 1736
- Librium for Injection 1737

Chlorpromazine (Displacement of penicillins from plasma protein binding sites by highly protein bound drugs will elevate the level of free penicillin in the serum). Products include:
- Thorazine Suppositories 1656

Chlorpromazine Hydrochloride (Displacement of penicillins from plasma protein binding sites by highly protein bound drugs will elevate the level of free penicillin in the serum). Products include:
- Thorazine 1656

Clomipramine Hydrochloride (Displacement of penicillins from plasma protein binding sites by highly protein bound drugs will elevate the level of free penicillin in the serum).
No products indexed under this heading.

Clozapine (Displacement of penicillins from plasma protein binding sites by highly protein bound drugs will elevate the level of free penicillin in the serum). Products include:
- Clozaril Tablets 2319

Cyclosporine (Displacement of penicillins from plasma protein binding sites by highly protein bound drugs will elevate the level of free penicillin in the serum). Products include:
- Gengraf Capsules 457
- Neoral Soft Gelatin Capsules 2380
- Neoral Oral Solution 2380
- Sandimmune 2388

Demeclocycline Hydrochloride (Co-administration of bacteriostatic antibiotics, such as tetracycline, may diminish bactericidal effects of penicillins by slowing the rate of bacterial growth). Products include:
- Declomycin Tablets 1855

Diazepam (Displacement of penicillins from plasma protein binding sites by highly protein bound drugs will elevate the level of free penicillin in the serum). Products include:
- Valium Injectable 3026
- Valium Tablets 3047

Diclofenac Potassium (Displacement of penicillins from plasma protein binding sites by highly protein bound drugs will elevate the level of free penicillin in the serum). Products include:
- Cataflam Tablets 2315

Diclofenac Sodium (Displacement of penicillins from plasma protein binding sites by highly protein bound drugs will elevate the level of free penicillin in the serum). Products include:
- Arthrotec Tablets 3195
- Voltaren Ophthalmic Sterile Ophthalmic Solution .... ⊙ 312
- Voltaren Tablets 2315
- Voltaren-XR Tablets 2315

Dipyridamole (Displacement of penicillins from plasma protein binding sites by highly protein bound drugs will elevate the level of free penicillin in the serum). Products include:
- Aggrenox Capsules 1026
- Persantine Tablets 1057

Doxycycline Calcium (Co-administration of bacteriostatic antibiotics, such as tetracycline, may diminish bactericidal effects of penicillins by slowing the rate of bacterial growth). Products include:
- Vibramycin Calcium Oral Suspension Syrup 2735

Doxycycline Hyclate (Co-administration of bacteriostatic antibiotics, such as tetracycline, may diminish bactericidal effects of penicillins by slowing the rate of bacterial growth). Products include:
- Doryx Coated Pellet Filled Capsules 3357
- Periostat Tablets 1208

Vibramycin Hyclate Capsules 2735
Vibramycin Hyclate Intravenous 2737
Vibra-Tabs Film Coated Tablets 2735

Doxycycline Monohydrate (Co-administration of bacteriostatic antibiotics, such as tetracycline, may diminish bactericidal effects of penicillins by slowing the rate of bacterial growth). Products include:
Monodox Capsules 2442
Vibramycin Monohydrate for Oral Suspension 2735

Erythromycin (Co-administration of bacteriostatic antibiotics, such as erythromycin, may diminish bactericidal effects of penicillins by slowing the rate of bacterial growth). Products include:
Emgel 2% Topical Gel 1285
Ery-Tab Tablets 448
Erythromycin Base Filmtab Tablets . 454
Erythromycin Delayed-Release Capsules, USP 455
PCE Dispertab Tablets 498

Erythromycin Estolate (Co-administration of bacteriostatic antibiotics, such as erythromycin, may diminish bactericidal effects of penicillins by slowing the rate of bacterial growth).
No products indexed under this heading.

Erythromycin Ethylsuccinate (Co-administration of bacteriostatic antibiotics, such as erythromycin, may diminish bactericidal effects of penicillins by slowing the rate of bacterial growth). Products include:
E.E.S. 450
EryPed 446
Pediazole Suspension 3050

Erythromycin Gluceptate (Co-administration of bacteriostatic antibiotics, such as erythromycin, may diminish bactericidal effects of penicillins by slowing the rate of bacterial growth).
No products indexed under this heading.

Erythromycin Stearate (Co-administration of bacteriostatic antibiotics, such as erythromycin, may diminish bactericidal effects of penicillins by slowing the rate of bacterial growth). Products include:
Erythrocin Stearate Filmtab Tablets 452

Fenoprofen Calcium (Displacement of penicillins from plasma protein binding sites by highly protein bound drugs will elevate the level of free penicillin in the serum).
No products indexed under this heading.

Flurazepam Hydrochloride (Displacement of penicillins from plasma protein binding sites by highly protein bound drugs will elevate the level of free penicillin in the serum).
No products indexed under this heading.

Flurbiprofen (Displacement of penicillins from plasma protein binding sites by highly protein bound drugs will elevate the level of free penicillin in the serum).
No products indexed under this heading.

Glipizide (Displacement of penicillins from plasma protein binding sites by highly protein bound drugs will elevate the level of free penicillin in the serum). Products include:
Glucotrol Tablets 2692
Glucotrol XL Extended Release Tablets 2693

Ibuprofen (Displacement of penicillins from plasma protein binding sites by highly protein bound drugs will elevate the level of free penicillin in the serum). Products include:
Advil .... ▣771
Children's Advil Oral Suspension ... ▣773
Children's Advil Chewable Tablets . ▣773
Advil Cold and Sinus Caplets .... ▣771
Advil Cold and Sinus Tablets .... ▣771
Advil Flu & Body Ache Caplets ...... ▣772
Infants' Advil Drops .... ▣773
Junior Strength Advil Tablets .... ▣773
Junior Strength Advil Chewable Tablets .... ▣773
Advil Migraine Liquigels .... ▣772
Children's Motrin Oral Suspension and Chewable Tablets.................. 2006
Children's Motrin Cold Oral Suspension 2007
Children's Motrin Oral Suspension................................ ▣643
Motrin Suspension, Oral Drops, Chewable Tablets, and Caplets.... 2002
Infants' Motrin Concentrated Drops.. 2006
Junior Strength Motrin Caplets and Chewable Tablets 2006
Motrin IB Tablets, Caplets, and Gelcaps.................................... 2002
Motrin Migraine Pain Caplets 2005
Motrin Sinus Headache Caplets 2005
Vicoprofen Tablets 520

Imipramine Hydrochloride (Displacement of penicillins from plasma protein binding sites by highly protein bound drugs will elevate the level of free penicillin in the serum).
No products indexed under this heading.

Imipramine Pamoate (Displacement of penicillins from plasma protein binding sites by highly protein bound drugs will elevate the level of free penicillin in the serum).
No products indexed under this heading.

Indomethacin (Displacement of penicillins from plasma protein binding sites by highly protein bound drugs will elevate the level of free penicillin in the serum). Products include:
Indocin 2112

Indomethacin Sodium Trihydrate (Displacement of penicillins from plasma protein binding sites by highly protein bound drugs will elevate the level of free penicillin in the serum). Products include:
Indocin I.V. 2115

Ketoprofen (Displacement of penicillins from plasma protein binding sites by highly protein bound drugs will elevate the level of free penicillin in the serum). Products include:
Orudis Capsules 3548
Orudis KT Tablets .... ▣778
Oruvail Capsules 3548

Ketorolac Tromethamine (Displacement of penicillins from plasma protein binding sites by highly protein bound drugs will elevate the level of free penicillin in the serum). Products include:
Acular Ophthalmic Solution 544
Acular PF Ophthalmic Solution 544
Toradol 3018

Meclofenamate Sodium (Displacement of penicillins from plasma protein binding sites by highly protein bound drugs will elevate the level of free penicillin in the serum).
No products indexed under this heading.

Mefenamic Acid (Displacement of penicillins from plasma protein binding sites by highly protein bound drugs will elevate the level of free penicillin in the serum). Products include:
Ponstel Capsules 1356

Methacycline Hydrochloride (Co-administration of bacteriostatic antibiotics, such as tetracycline, may diminish bactericidal effects of penicillins by slowing the rate of bacterial growth).
No products indexed under this heading.

Midazolam Hydrochloride (Displacement of penicillins from plasma protein binding sites by highly protein bound drugs will elevate the level of free penicillin in the serum). Products include:
Versed Injection 3027
Versed Syrup 3033

Minocycline Hydrochloride (Co-administration of bacteriostatic antibiotics, such as tetracycline, may diminish bactericidal effects of penicillins by slowing the rate of bacterial growth). Products include:
Dynacin Capsules 2019
Minocin Intravenous 1862
Minocin Oral Suspension 1865
Minocin Pellet-Filled Capsules 1863

Naproxen (Displacement of penicillins from plasma protein binding sites by highly protein bound drugs will elevate the level of free penicillin in the serum). Products include:
EC-Naprosyn Delayed-Release Tablets 2967
Naprosyn Suspension 2967
Naprosyn Tablets 2967

Naproxen Sodium (Displacement of penicillins from plasma protein binding sites by highly protein bound drugs will elevate the level of free penicillin in the serum). Products include:
Aleve Tablets, Caplets and Gelcaps.. ▣602
Aleve Cold & Sinus Caplets .... ▣603
Anaprox Tablets 2967
Anaprox DS Tablets 2967
Naprelan Tablets 1293

Nortriptyline Hydrochloride (Displacement of penicillins from plasma protein binding sites by highly protein bound drugs will elevate the level of free penicillin in the serum).
No products indexed under this heading.

Oxaprozin (Displacement of penicillins from plasma protein binding sites by highly protein bound drugs will elevate the level of free penicillin in the serum).
No products indexed under this heading.

Oxazepam (Displacement of penicillins from plasma protein binding sites by highly protein bound drugs will elevate the level of free penicillin in the serum).
No products indexed under this heading.

Oxytetracycline Hydrochloride (Co-administration of bacteriostatic antibiotics, such as tetracycline, may diminish bactericidal effects of penicillins by slowing the rate of bacterial growth). Products include:
Terra-Cortril Ophthalmic Suspension................................ 2716
Urobiotic-250 Capsules 2731

Phenylbutazone (Displacement of penicillins from plasma protein binding sites by highly protein bound drugs will elevate the level of free penicillin in the serum).
No products indexed under this heading.

Piroxicam (Displacement of penicillins from plasma protein binding sites by highly protein bound drugs will elevate the level of free penicillin in the serum). Products include:
Feldene Capsules 2685

Probenecid (Penicillin blood levels may be prolonged by co-administration of probenecid which blocks renal tubular secretion of penicillin).
No products indexed under this heading.

Propranolol Hydrochloride (Displacement of penicillins from plasma protein binding sites by highly protein bound drugs will elevate the level of free penicillin in the serum). Products include:
Inderal 3513
Inderal LA Long-Acting Capsules 3516
Inderide Tablets 3517
Inderide LA Long-Acting Capsules .. 3519

Sulindac (Displacement of penicillins from plasma protein binding sites by highly protein bound drugs will elevate the level of free penicillin in the serum). Products include:
Clinoril Tablets 2053

Temazepam (Displacement of penicillins from plasma protein binding sites by highly protein bound drugs will elevate the level of free penicillin in the serum).
No products indexed under this heading.

Tetracycline Hydrochloride (Co-administration of bacteriostatic antibiotics, such as tetracycline, may diminish bactericidal effects of penicillins by slowing the rate of bacterial growth).
No products indexed under this heading.

Tolbutamide (Displacement of penicillins from plasma protein binding sites by highly protein bound drugs will elevate the level of free penicillin in the serum).
No products indexed under this heading.

Tolmetin Sodium (Displacement of penicillins from plasma protein binding sites by highly protein bound drugs will elevate the level of free penicillin in the serum). Products include:
Tolectin 2589

Trimipramine Maleate (Displacement of penicillins from plasma protein binding sites by highly protein bound drugs will elevate the level of free penicillin in the serum). Products include:
Surmontil Capsules 3595

Warfarin Sodium (Displacement of penicillins from plasma protein binding sites by highly protein bound drugs will elevate the level of free penicillin in the serum). Products include:
Coumadin for Injection 1243
Coumadin Tablets 1243
Warfarin Sodium Tablets, USP 3302

PERMAX TABLETS

(Pergolide Mesylate) 1299
May interact with dopamine antagonists, central nervous system depressants, and certain other agents. Compounds in these categories include:

Alfentanil Hydrochloride (Pergolide may cause somnolence and concurrent use with CNS depressants may result in additive sedative effects).
No products indexed under this heading.

Alprazolam (Pergolide may cause somnolence and concurrent use with CNS depressants may result in additive sedative effects). Products include:
Xanax Tablets 2865

Aprobarbital (Pergolide may cause somnolence and concurrent use with CNS depressants may result in additive sedative effects).
No products indexed under this heading.

Buprenorphine Hydrochloride (Pergolide may cause somnolence and concurrent use with CNS depressants may result in additive sedative effects). Products include:
Buprenex Injectable 2918

Buspirone Hydrochloride (Pergolide may cause somnolence and concurrent use with CNS depressants may result in additive sedative effects).
No products indexed under this heading.

Butabarbital (Pergolide may cause somnolence and concurrent use with CNS depressants may result in addi-

tive sedative effects).
No products indexed under this heading.

Butalbital (Pergolide may cause somnolence and concurrent use with CNS depressants may result in additive sedative effects). Products include:
Phrenilin 578
Sedapap Tablets 50 mg/650 mg ... 2225

Chlordiazepoxide (Pergolide may cause somnolence and concurrent use with CNS depressants may result in additive sedative effects). Products include:
Limbitrol 1738

Chlordiazepoxide Hydrochloride (Pergolide may cause somnolence and concurrent use with CNS depressants may result in additive sedative effects). Products include:
Librium Capsules 1736
Librium for Injection 1737

Chlorpromazine (May diminish the effectiveness of Permax; caution should be exercised if co-administered). Products include:
Thorazine Suppositories 1656

Chlorpromazine Hydrochloride (Concurrent use with dopamine antagonists may diminish the effectiveness of pergolide). Products include:
Thorazine 1656

Chlorprothixene (Pergolide may cause somnolence and concurrent use with CNS depressants may result in additive sedative effects).
No products indexed under this heading.

Chlorprothixene Hydrochloride (Pergolide may cause somnolence and concurrent use with CNS depressants may result in additive sedative effects).
No products indexed under this heading.

Chlorprothixene Lactate (Pergolide may cause somnolence and concurrent use with CNS depressants may result in additive sedative effects).
No products indexed under this heading.

Clorazepate Dipotassium (Pergolide may cause somnolence and concurrent use with CNS depressants may result in additive sedative effects). Products include:
Tranxene 511

Clozapine (Concurrent use with dopamine antagonists may diminish the effectiveness of pergolide). Products include:
Clozaril Tablets 2319

Codeine Phosphate (Pergolide may cause somnolence and concurrent use with CNS depressants may result in additive sedative effects). Products include:
Phenergan with Codeine Syrup 3557
Phenergan VC with Codeine Syrup .. 3561
Robitussin A-C Syrup 2942
Robitussin-DAC Syrup 2942
Ryna-C Liquid 768
Soma Compound w/Codeine Tablets 3355
Tussi-Organidin NR Liquid 3350
Tussi-Organidin-S NR Liquid 3350
Tylenol with Codeine 2595

Desflurane (Pergolide may cause somnolence and concurrent use with CNS depressants may result in additive sedative effects). Products include:
Suprane Liquid for Inhalation 874

Dezocine (Pergolide may cause somnolence and concurrent use with CNS depressants may result in additive sedative effects).
No products indexed under this heading.

Diazepam (Pergolide may cause somnolence and concurrent use with CNS depressants may result in additive sedative effects). Products include:
Valium Injectable 3026
Valium Tablets 3047

Droperidol (Pergolide may cause somnolence and concurrent use with CNS depressants may result in additive sedative effects).
No products indexed under this heading.

Enflurane (Pergolide may cause somnolence and concurrent use with CNS depressants may result in additive sedative effects).
No products indexed under this heading.

Estazolam (Pergolide may cause somnolence and concurrent use with CNS depressants may result in additive sedative effects). Products include:
ProSom Tablets 500

Ethchlorvynol (Pergolide may cause somnolence and concurrent use with CNS depressants may result in additive sedative effects).
No products indexed under this heading.

Ethinamate (Pergolide may cause somnolence and concurrent use with CNS depressants may result in additive sedative effects).
No products indexed under this heading.

Fentanyl (Pergolide may cause somnolence and concurrent use with CNS depressants may result in additive sedative effects). Products include:
Duragesic Transdermal System 1786

Fentanyl Citrate (Pergolide may cause somnolence and concurrent use with CNS depressants may result in additive sedative effects). Products include:
Actiq 1184

Fluphenazine Decanoate (Concurrent use with dopamine antagonists may diminish the effectiveness of pergolide).
No products indexed under this heading.

Fluphenazine Enanthate (Concurrent use with dopamine antagonists may diminish the effectiveness of pergolide).
No products indexed under this heading.

Fluphenazine Hydrochloride (Concurrent use with dopamine antagonists may diminish the effectiveness of pergolide).
No products indexed under this heading.

Flurazepam Hydrochloride (Pergolide may cause somnolence and concurrent use with CNS depressants may result in additive sedative effects).
No products indexed under this heading.

Glutethimide (Pergolide may cause somnolence and concurrent use with CNS depressants may result in additive sedative effects).
No products indexed under this heading.

Haloperidol (Concurrent use with dopamine antagonists may diminish the effectiveness of pergolide). Products include:
Haldol Injection, Tablets and Concentrate 2533

Haloperidol Decanoate (Concurrent use with dopamine antagonists may diminish the effectiveness of pergolide). Products include:
Haldol Decanoate 2535

Hydrocodone Bitartrate (Pergolide may cause somnolence and concurrent use with CNS depressants may result in additive sedative effects). Products include:
Hycodan 1316
Hycomine Compound Tablets 1317
Hycotuss Expectorant Syrup 1318
Lortab 3319
Lortab Elixir 3317
Maxidone Tablets CIII 3399
Norco 5/325 Tablets CIII 3424
Norco 7.5/325 Tablets CIII 3425
Norco 10/325 Tablets CIII 3427
Norco 10/325 Tablets CIII 3425
Vicodin Tablets 516
Vicodin ES Tablets 517
Vicodin HP Tablets 518
Vicodin Tuss Expectorant 519
Vicoprofen Tablets 520
Zydone Tablets 1330

Hydrocodone Polistirex (Pergolide may cause somnolence and concurrent use with CNS depressants may result in additive sedative effects). Products include:
Tussionex Pennkinetic Extended-Release Suspension..... 1174

Hydromorphone Hydrochloride (Pergolide may cause somnolence and concurrent use with CNS depressants may result in additive sedative effects). Products include:
Dilaudid 441
Dilaudid Oral Liquid 445
Dilaudid Powder 441
Dilaudid Rectal Suppositories 441
Dilaudid Tablets 441
Dilaudid Tablets - 8 mg 445
Dilaudid-HP 443

Hydroxyzine Hydrochloride (Pergolide may cause somnolence and concurrent use with CNS depressants may result in additive sedative effects). Products include:
Atarax Tablets & Syrup 2667
Vistaril Intramuscular Solution 2738

Isoflurane (Pergolide may cause somnolence and concurrent use with CNS depressants may result in additive sedative effects).
No products indexed under this heading.

Ketamine Hydrochloride (Pergolide may cause somnolence and concurrent use with CNS depressants may result in additive sedative effects).
No products indexed under this heading.

Levodopa (Concomitant use may cause and/or exacerbate preexisting states of confusion and hallucination). Products include:
Sinemet Tablets 1253
Sinemet CR Tablets 1255

Levomethadyl Acetate Hydrochloride (Pergolide may cause somnolence and concurrent use with CNS depressants may result in additive sedative effects).
No products indexed under this heading.

Levorphanol Tartrate (Pergolide may cause somnolence and concurrent use with CNS depressants may result in additive sedative effects). Products include:
Levo-Dromoran 1734
Levorphanol Tartrate Tablets 3059

Lorazepam (Pergolide may cause somnolence and concurrent use with CNS depressants may result in additive sedative effects). Products include:
Ativan Injection 3478
Ativan Tablets 3482

Loxapine Hydrochloride (Pergolide may cause somnolence and concurrent use with CNS depressants may result in additive sedative effects).
No products indexed under this heading.

Loxapine Succinate (Pergolide may cause somnolence and concurrent use with CNS depressants may result in additive sedative effects). Products include:
Loxitane Capsules 3398

Meperidine Hydrochloride (Pergolide may cause somnolence and concurrent use with CNS depressants may result in additive sedative effects). Products include:
Demerol 3079
Mepergan Injection 3539

Mephobarbital (Pergolide may cause somnolence and concurrent use with CNS depressants may result in additive sedative effects).
No products indexed under this heading.

Meprobamate (Pergolide may cause somnolence and concurrent use with CNS depressants may result in additive sedative effects). Products include:
Miltown Tablets 3349

Mesoridazine Besylate (Concurrent use with dopamine antagonists may diminish the effectiveness of pergolide). Products include:
Serentil 1057

Methadone Hydrochloride (Pergolide may cause somnolence and concurrent use with CNS depressants may result in additive sedative effects). Products include:
Dolophine Hydrochloride Tablets 3056

Methohexital Sodium (Pergolide may cause somnolence and concurrent use with CNS depressants may result in additive sedative effects). Products include:
Brevital Sodium for Injection, USP .. 1815

Methotrimeprazine (Concurrent use with dopamine antagonists may diminish the effectiveness of pergolide).
No products indexed under this heading.

Methoxyflurane (Pergolide may cause somnolence and concurrent use with CNS depressants may result in additive sedative effects).
No products indexed under this heading.

Metoclopramide Hydrochloride (Concurrent use with dopamine antagonists may diminish the effectiveness of pergolide). Products include:
Reglan 2935

Midazolam Hydrochloride (Pergolide may cause somnolence and concurrent use with CNS depressants may result in additive sedative effects). Products include:
Versed Injection 3027
Versed Syrup 3033

Molindone Hydrochloride (Pergolide may cause somnolence and concurrent use with CNS depressants may result in additive sedative effects). Products include:
Moban 1320

Morphine Sulfate (Pergolide may cause somnolence and concurrent use with CNS depressants may result in additive sedative effects). Products include:
Astramorph/PF Injection, USP (Preservative-Free) 594
Duramorph Injection 1312
Infumorph 200 and Infumorph 500 Sterile Solutions 1314
Kadian Capsules 1335
MS Contin Tablets 2896
MSIR 2898
Oramorph SR Tablets 3062
Roxanol 3066

Olanzapine (Concurrent use with dopamine antagonists may diminish the effectiveness of pergolide). Products include:
Zyprexa Tablets 1973
Zyprexa ZYDIS Orally Disintegrating Tablets 1973

Oxazepam (Pergolide may cause somnolence and concurrent use with CNS depressants may result in additive sedative effects).
No products indexed under this heading.

Oxycodone Hydrochloride (Pergolide may cause somnolence and

concurrent use with CNS depressants may result in additive sedative effects). Products include:
- OxyContin Tablets 2912
- OxyFast Oral Concentrate Solution . 2916
- OxyIR Capsules 2916
- Percocet Tablets 1326
- Percodan Tablets 1327
- Percolone Tablets 1327
- Roxicodone 3067
- Tylox Capsules 2597

Pentobarbital Sodium (Pergolide may cause somnolence and concurrent use with CNS depressants may result in additive sedative effects). Products include:
- Nembutal Sodium Solution 485

Perphenazine (Concurrent use with dopamine antagonists may diminish the effectiveness of pergolide). Products include:
- Etrafon 3115
- Trilafon 3160

Phenobarbital (Pergolide may cause somnolence and concurrent use with CNS depressants may result in additive sedative effects). Products include:
- Arco-Lase Plus Tablets 592
- Donnatal 2929
- Donnatal Extentabs 2930

Pimozide (Concurrent use with dopamine antagonists may diminish the effectiveness of pergolide). Products include:
- Orap Tablets 1407

Prazepam (Pergolide may cause somnolence and concurrent use with CNS depressants may result in additive sedative effects).
No products indexed under this heading.

Prochlorperazine (Concurrent use with dopamine antagonists may diminish the effectiveness of pergolide). Products include:
- Compazine 1505

Promethazine Hydrochloride (Concurrent use with dopamine antagonists may diminish the effectiveness of pergolide). Products include:
- Mepergan Injection 3539
- Phenergan Injection 3553
- Phenergan 3556
- Phenergan Syrup 3554
- Phenergan with Codeine Syrup 3557
- Phenergan with Dextromethorphan Syrup 3559
- Phenergan VC Syrup 3560
- Phenergan VC with Codeine Syrup .. 3561

Propofol (Pergolide may cause somnolence and concurrent use with CNS depressants may result in additive sedative effects). Products include:
- Diprivan Injectable Emulsion 667

Propoxyphene Hydrochloride (Pergolide may cause somnolence and concurrent use with CNS depressants may result in additive sedative effects). Products include:
- Darvon Pulvules 1909
- Darvon Compound-65 Pulvules 1910

Propoxyphene Napsylate (Pergolide may cause somnolence and concurrent use with CNS depressants may result in additive sedative effects). Products include:
- Darvon-N/Darvocet-N 1907
- Darvon-N Tablets 1912

Quazepam (Pergolide may cause somnolence and concurrent use with CNS depressants may result in additive sedative effects).
No products indexed under this heading.

Quetiapine Fumarate (Concurrent use with dopamine antagonists may diminish the effectiveness of pergolide). Products include:
- Seroquel Tablets 684

Remifentanil Hydrochloride (Pergolide may cause somnolence and concurrent use with CNS depressants may result in additive sedative effects).
No products indexed under this heading.

Risperidone (Pergolide may cause somnolence and concurrent use with CNS depressants may result in additive sedative effects). Products include:
- Risperdal 1796

Secobarbital Sodium (Pergolide may cause somnolence and concurrent use with CNS depressants may result in additive sedative effects).
No products indexed under this heading.

Sevoflurane (Pergolide may cause somnolence and concurrent use with CNS depressants may result in additive sedative effects).
No products indexed under this heading.

Sufentanil Citrate (Pergolide may cause somnolence and concurrent use with CNS depressants may result in additive sedative effects).
No products indexed under this heading.

Temazepam (Pergolide may cause somnolence and concurrent use with CNS depressants may result in additive sedative effects).
No products indexed under this heading.

Thiamylal Sodium (Pergolide may cause somnolence and concurrent use with CNS depressants may result in additive sedative effects).
No products indexed under this heading.

Thioridazine Hydrochloride (Concurrent use with dopamine antagonists may diminish the effectiveness of pergolide). Products include:
- Thioridazine Hydrochloride Tablets 2289

Thiothixene (May diminish the effectiveness of Permax). Products include:
- Navane Capsules 2701
- Thiothixene Capsules 2290

Triazolam (Pergolide may cause somnolence and concurrent use with CNS depressants may result in additive sedative effects). Products include:
- Halcion Tablets 2823

Trifluoperazine Hydrochloride (Concurrent use with dopamine antagonists may diminish the effectiveness of pergolide). Products include:
- Stelazine 1640

Zaleplon (Pergolide may cause somnolence and concurrent use with CNS depressants may result in additive sedative effects). Products include:
- Sonata Capsules 3591

Ziprasidone Hydrochloride (Pergolide may cause somnolence and concurrent use with CNS depressants may result in additive sedative effects). Products include:
- Geodon Capsules 2688

Zolpidem Tartrate (Pergolide may cause somnolence and concurrent use with CNS depressants may result in additive sedative effects). Products include:
- Ambien Tablets 3191

Food Interactions

Alcohol (Pergolide may cause somnolence and concurrent use with alcohol may result in additive sedative effects).

PERMETHRIN LOTION

(Permethrin) .... ▣602
None cited in PDR database.

PERSANTINE TABLETS

(Dipyridamole) 1057
None cited in PDR database.

PFIZERPEN FOR INJECTION

(Penicillin G Potassium) 2707
May interact with erythromycin, tetracyclines, and certain other agents. Compounds in these categories include:

Demeclocycline Hydrochloride (Co-administration of bacteriostatic antibiotics, such as tetracycline, may diminish the bactericidal effects of penicillins by slowing the rate of bacterial growth). Products include:
- Declomycin Tablets 1855

Doxycycline Calcium (Co-administration of bacteriostatic antibiotics, such as tetracycline, may diminish the bactericidal effects of penicillins by slowing the rate of bacterial growth). Products include:
- Vibramycin Calcium Oral Suspension Syrup 2735

Doxycycline Hyclate (Co-administration of bacteriostatic antibiotics, such as tetracycline, may diminish the bactericidal effects of penicillins by slowing the rate of bacterial growth). Products include:
- Doryx Coated Pellet Filled Capsules 3357
- Periostat Tablets 1208
- Vibramycin Hyclate Capsules 2735
- Vibramycin Hyclate Intravenous 2737
- Vibra-Tabs Film Coated Tablets 2735

Doxycycline Monohydrate (Co-administration of bacteriostatic antibiotics, such as tetracycline, may diminish the bactericidal effects of penicillins by slowing the rate of bacterial growth). Products include:
- Monodox Capsules 2442
- Vibramycin Monohydrate for Oral Suspension 2735

Erythromycin (Co-administration of bacteriostatic antibiotics, such as erythromycin, may diminish the bactericidal effects of penicillins by slowing the rate of bacterial growth). Products include:
- Emgel 2% Topical Gel 1285
- Ery-Tab Tablets 448
- Erythromycin Base Filmtab Tablets . 454
- Erythromycin Delayed-Release Capsules, USP 455
- PCE Dispertab Tablets 498

Erythromycin Estolate (Co-administration of bacteriostatic antibiotics, such as erythromycin, may diminish the bactericidal effects of penicillins by slowing the rate of bacterial growth).
No products indexed under this heading.

Erythromycin Ethylsuccinate (Co-administration of bacteriostatic antibiotics, such as erythromycin, may diminish the bactericidal effects of penicillins by slowing the rate of bacterial growth). Products include:
- E.E.S. 450
- EryPed 446
- Pediazole Suspension 3050

Erythromycin Gluceptate (Co-administration of bacteriostatic antibiotics, such as erythromycin, may diminish the bactericidal effects of penicillins by slowing the rate of bacterial growth).
No products indexed under this heading.

Erythromycin Stearate (Co-administration of bacteriostatic antibiotics, such as erythromycin, may diminish the bactericidal effects of penicillins by slowing the rate of bacterial growth). Products include:
- Erythrocin Stearate Filmtab Tablets 452

Methacycline Hydrochloride (Co-administration of bacteriostatic antibiotics, such as tetracycline, may diminish the bactericidal effects of penicillins by slowing the rate of bacterial growth).
No products indexed under this heading.

Minocycline Hydrochloride (Co-administration of bacteriostatic antibiotics, such as tetracycline, may diminish the bactericidal effects of penicillins by slowing the rate of bacterial growth). Products include:
- Dynacin Capsules 2019
- Minocin Intravenous 1862
- Minocin Oral Suspension 1865
- Minocin Pellet-Filled Capsules 1863

Oxytetracycline Hydrochloride (Co-administration of bacteriostatic antibiotics, such as tetracycline, may diminish the bactericidal effects of penicillins by slowing the rate of bacterial growth). Products include:
- Terra-Cortril Ophthalmic Suspension 2716
- Urobiotic-250 Capsules 2731

Probenecid (Blocks the renal tubular secretion of penicillin and co-administration with probenecid may prolong penicillin blood levels).
No products indexed under this heading.

Tetracycline Hydrochloride (Co-administration of bacteriostatic antibiotics, such as tetracycline, may diminish the bactericidal effects of penicillins by slowing the rate of bacterial growth).
No products indexed under this heading.

PHAZYME-125 MG QUICK DISSOLVE CHEWABLE TABLETS

(Simethicone) .... ▣622
None cited in PDR database.

PHAZYME-180 MG ULTRA STRENGTH SOFTGELS

(Simethicone) .... ▣622
None cited in PDR database.

PHENERGAN INJECTION

(Promethazine Hydrochloride) 3553
May interact with anticholinergics, barbiturates, central nervous system depressants, monoamine oxidase inhibitors, narcotic analgesics, and certain other agents. Compounds in these categories include:

Alfentanil Hydrochloride (Co-administration may increase, prolong, or intensify the sedative action of CNS depressants; the dose of narcotics should be reduced by one-quarter to one-half when given concurrently; excessive amounts of Phenergan relative to narcotic may lead to restlessness and minor hyperactivity in the patient with pain).
No products indexed under this heading.

Alprazolam (Co-administration may increase, prolong, or intensify the sedative action of CNS depressants). Products include:
- Xanax Tablets 2865

Aprobarbital (Co-administration may increase, prolong, or intensify the sedative action of CNS depressants; the dose of barbiturates should be reduced by at least one-half when given concurrently).
No products indexed under this heading.

Atropine Sulfate (Concomitant use of other anticholinergic agents should be undertaken with caution because of possible additive effects). Products include:
- Donnatal 2929
- Donnatal Extentabs 2930
- Motofen Tablets 577
- Prosed/DS Tablets 3268
- Urised Tablets 2876

Belladonna Alkaloids (Concomitant use of other anticholinergic agents should be undertaken with caution because of possible additive effects). Products include:
- Hyland's Teething Tablets .... ▣766
- Urimax Tablets 1769

Benztropine Mesylate (Concomitant use of other anticholinergic agents should be undertaken with caution because of possible additive effects). Products include:
Cogentin 2055

Biperiden Hydrochloride (Concomitant use of other anticholinergic agents should be undertaken with caution because of possible additive effects). Products include:
Akineton 402

Buprenorphine Hydrochloride (Co-administration may increase, prolong, or intensify the sedative action of CNS depressants; the dose of narcotics should be reduced by one-quarter to one-half when given concurrently; excessive amounts of Phenergan relative to narcotic may lead to restlessness and minor hyperactivity in the patient with pain). Products include:
Buprenex Injectable 2918

Buspirone Hydrochloride (Co-administration may increase, prolong, or intensify the sedative action of CNS depressants).
No products indexed under this heading.

Butabarbital (Co-administration may increase, prolong, or intensify the sedative action of CNS depressants; the dose of barbiturates should be reduced by at least one-half when given concurrently).
No products indexed under this heading.

Butalbital (Co-administration may increase, prolong, or intensify the sedative action of CNS depressants; the dose of barbiturates should be reduced by at least one-half when given concurrently). Products include:
Phrenilin 578
Sedapap Tablets 50 mg/650 mg 2225

Chlordiazepoxide (Co-administration may increase, prolong, or intensify the sedative action of CNS depressants). Products include:
Limbitrol 1738

Chlordiazepoxide Hydrochloride (Co-administration may increase, prolong, or intensify the sedative action of CNS depressants). Products include:
Librium Capsules 1736
Librium for Injection 1737

Chlorpromazine (Co-administration may increase, prolong, or intensify the sedative action of CNS depressants). Products include:
Thorazine Suppositories 1656

Chlorpromazine Hydrochloride (Co-administration may increase, prolong, or intensify the sedative action of CNS depressants). Products include:
Thorazine 1656

Chlorprothixene (Co-administration may increase, prolong, or intensify the sedative action of CNS depressants).
No products indexed under this heading.

Chlorprothixene Hydrochloride (Co-administration may increase, prolong, or intensify the sedative action of CNS depressants).
No products indexed under this heading.

Chlorprothixene Lactate (Co-administration may increase, prolong, or intensify the sedative action of CNS depressants).
No products indexed under this heading.

Clidinium Bromide (Concomitant use of other anticholinergic agents should be undertaken with caution because of possible additive effects).
No products indexed under this heading.

Clorazepate Dipotassium (Co-administration may increase, prolong, or intensify the sedative action of CNS depressants). Products include:
Tranxene 511

Clozapine (Co-administration may increase, prolong, or intensify the sedative action of CNS depressants). Products include:
Clozaril Tablets 2319

Codeine Phosphate (Co-administration may increase, prolong, or intensify the sedative action of CNS depressants; the dose of narcotics should be reduced by one-quarter to one-half when given concurrently; excessive amounts of Phenergan relative to narcotic may lead to restlessness and minor hyperactivity in the patient with pain). Products include:
Phenergan with Codeine Syrup 3557
Phenergan VC with Codeine Syrup .. 3561
Robitussin A-C Syrup 2942
Robitussin-DAC Syrup 2942
Ryna-C Liquid .... ⊞768
Soma Compound w/Codeine Tablets 3355
Tussi-Organidin NR Liquid 3350
Tussi-Organidin-S NR Liquid 3350
Tylenol with Codeine 2595

Desflurane (Co-administration may increase, prolong, or intensify the sedative action of CNS depressants). Products include:
Suprane Liquid for Inhalation 874

Dezocine (Co-administration may increase, prolong, or intensify the sedative action of CNS depressants; the dose of narcotics should be reduced by one-quarter to one-half when given concurrently; excessive amounts of Phenergan relative to narcotic may lead to restlessness and minor hyperactivity in the patient with pain).
No products indexed under this heading.

Diazepam (Co-administration may increase, prolong, or intensify the sedative action of CNS depressants). Products include:
Valium Injectable 3026
Valium Tablets 3047

Dicyclomine Hydrochloride (Concomitant use of other anticholinergic agents should be undertaken with caution because of possible additive effects).
No products indexed under this heading.

Droperidol (Co-administration may increase, prolong, or intensify the sedative action of CNS depressants).
No products indexed under this heading.

Enflurane (Co-administration may increase, prolong, or intensify the sedative action of CNS depressants).
No products indexed under this heading.

Epinephrine Hydrochloride (Potential for reversal of the vasopressor effect).
No products indexed under this heading.

Estazolam (Co-administration may increase, prolong, or intensify the sedative action of CNS depressants). Products include:
ProSom Tablets 500

Ethchlorvynol (Co-administration may increase, prolong, or intensify the sedative action of CNS depressants).
No products indexed under this heading.

Ethinamate (Co-administration may increase, prolong, or intensify the sedative action of CNS depressants).
No products indexed under this heading.

Fentanyl (Co-administration may increase, prolong, or intensify the sedative action of CNS depressants; the dose of narcotics should be reduced by one-quarter to one-half when given concurrently; excessive amounts of Phenergan relative to narcotic may lead to restlessness and minor hyperactivity in the patient with pain). Products include:
Duragesic Transdermal System 1786

Fentanyl Citrate (Co-administration may increase, prolong, or intensify the sedative action of CNS depressants; the dose of narcotics should be reduced by one-quarter to one-half when given concurrently; excessive amounts of Phenergan relative to narcotic may lead to restlessness and minor hyperactivity in the patient with pain). Products include:
Actiq 1184

Fluphenazine Decanoate (Co-administration may increase, prolong, or intensify the sedative action of CNS depressants).
No products indexed under this heading.

Fluphenazine Enanthate (Co-administration may increase, prolong, or intensify the sedative action of CNS depressants).
No products indexed under this heading.

Fluphenazine Hydrochloride (Co-administration may increase, prolong, or intensify the sedative action of CNS depressants).
No products indexed under this heading.

Flurazepam Hydrochloride (Co-administration may increase, prolong, or intensify the sedative action of CNS depressants).
No products indexed under this heading.

Glutethimide (Co-administration may increase, prolong, or intensify the sedative action of CNS depressants).
No products indexed under this heading.

Glycopyrrolate (Concomitant use of other anticholinergic agents should be undertaken with caution because of possible additive effects). Products include:
Robinul Forte Tablets 1358
Robinul Injectable 2940
Robinul Tablets 1358

Haloperidol (Co-administration may increase, prolong, or intensify the sedative action of CNS depressants). Products include:
Haldol Injection, Tablets and Concentrate 2533

Haloperidol Decanoate (Co-administration may increase, prolong, or intensify the sedative action of CNS depressants). Products include:
Haldol Decanoate 2535

Hydrocodone Bitartrate (Co-administration may increase, prolong, or intensify the sedative action of CNS depressants; the dose of narcotics should be reduced by one-quarter to one-half when given concurrently; excessive amounts of Phenergan relative to narcotic may lead to restlessness and minor hyperactivity in the patient with pain). Products include:
Hycodan 1316
Hycomine Compound Tablets 1317
Hycotuss Expectorant Syrup 1318
Lortab 3319
Lortab Elixir 3317
Maxidone Tablets CIII 3399
Norco 5/325 Tablets CIII 3424
Norco 7.5/325 Tablets CIII 3425
Norco 10/325 Tablets CIII 3427
Norco 10/325 Tablets CIII 3425
Vicodin Tablets 516
Vicodin ES Tablets 517
Vicodin HP Tablets 518
Vicodin Tuss Expectorant 519
Vicoprofen Tablets 520
Zydone Tablets 1330

Hydrocodone Polistirex (Co-administration may increase, prolong, or intensify the sedative action of CNS depressants; the dose of narcotics should be reduced by one-quarter to one-half when given concurrently; excessive amounts of Phenergan relative to narcotic may lead to restlessness and minor hyperactivity in the patient with pain). Products include:
Tussionex Pennkinetic Extended-Release Suspension 1174

Hydromorphone Hydrochloride (Additive sedative effects). Products include:
Dilaudid 441
Dilaudid Oral Liquid 445
Dilaudid Powder 441
Dilaudid Rectal Suppositories 441
Dilaudid Tablets 441
Dilaudid Tablets - 8 mg 445
Dilaudid-HP 443

Hydroxyzine Hydrochloride (Co-administration may increase, prolong, or intensify the sedative action of CNS depressants). Products include:
Atarax Tablets & Syrup 2667
Vistaril Intramuscular Solution 2738

Hyoscyamine (Concomitant use of other anticholinergic agents should be undertaken with caution because of possible additive effects). Products include:
Urised Tablets 2876

Hyoscyamine Sulfate (Concomitant use of other anticholinergic agents should be undertaken with caution because of possible additive effects). Products include:
Arco-Lase Plus Tablets 592
Donnatal 2929
Donnatal Extentabs 2930
Levsin/Levsinex/Levbid 3172
NuLev Orally Disintegrating Tablets 3176
Prosed/DS Tablets 3268
Urimax Tablets 1769

Ipratropium Bromide (Concomitant use of other anticholinergic agents should be undertaken with caution because of possible additive effects). Products include:
Atrovent Inhalation Aerosol 1030
Atrovent Inhalation Solution 1031
Atrovent Nasal Spray 0.03% 1032
Atrovent Nasal Spray 0.06% 1033
Combivent Inhalation Aerosol 1041
DuoNeb Inhalation Solution 1233

Isocarboxazid (Co-administration of MAO inhibitors with phenothiazines has resulted in increased incidence of extrapyramidal effects; although such a reaction has not been reported with Phenergan, the possibility should be considered).
No products indexed under this heading.

Isoflurane (Co-administration may increase, prolong, or intensify the sedative action of CNS depressants).
No products indexed under this heading.

Ketamine Hydrochloride (Co-administration may increase, prolong, or intensify the sedative action of CNS depressants).
No products indexed under this heading.

Levomethadyl Acetate Hydrochloride (Co-administration may increase, prolong, or intensify the sedative action of CNS depressants).
No products indexed under this heading.

Levorphanol Tartrate (Co-administration may increase, prolong, or intensify the sedative action of CNS depressants; the dose of narcotics should be reduced by one-quarter to one-half when given concurrently; excessive amounts of Phenergan relative to narcotic may lead to restlessness and minor hyperactivity in the patient with pain). Products include:
- Levo-Dromoran 1734
- Levorphanol Tartrate Tablets 3059

Lorazepam (Co-administration may increase, prolong, or intensify the sedative action of CNS depressants). Products include:
- Ativan Injection 3478
- Ativan Tablets 3482

Loxapine Hydrochloride (Co-administration may increase, prolong, or intensify the sedative action of CNS depressants).
No products indexed under this heading.

Loxapine Succinate (Co-administration may increase, prolong, or intensify the sedative action of CNS depressants). Products include:
- Loxitane Capsules 3398

Mepenzolate Bromide (Concomitant use of other anticholinergic agents should be undertaken with caution because of possible additive effects).
No products indexed under this heading.

Meperidine Hydrochloride (Co-administration may increase, prolong, or intensify the sedative action of CNS depressants; the dose of narcotics should be reduced by one-quarter to one-half when given concurrently; excessive amounts of Phenergan relative to narcotic may lead to restlessness and minor hyperactivity in the patient with pain). Products include:
- Demerol 3079
- Mepergan Injection 3539

Mephobarbital (Co-administration may increase, prolong, or intensify the sedative action of CNS depressants; the dose of barbiturates should be reduced by at least one-half when given concurrently).
No products indexed under this heading.

Meprobamate (Co-administration may increase, prolong, or intensify the sedative action of CNS depressants). Products include:
- Miltown Tablets 3349

Mesoridazine Besylate (Co-administration may increase, prolong, or intensify the sedative action of CNS depressants). Products include:
- Serentil 1057

Methadone Hydrochloride (Co-administration may increase, prolong, or intensify the sedative action of CNS depressants; the dose of narcotics should be reduced by one-quarter to one-half when given concurrently; excessive amounts of Phenergan relative to narcotic may lead to restlessness and minor hyperactivity in the patient with pain). Products include:
- Dolophine Hydrochloride Tablets 3056

Methohexital Sodium (Co-administration may increase, prolong, or intensify the sedative action of CNS depressants). Products include:
- Brevital Sodium for Injection, USP .. 1815

Methotrimeprazine (Co-administration may increase, prolong, or intensify the sedative action of CNS depressants).
No products indexed under this heading.

Methoxyflurane (Co-administration may increase, prolong, or intensify the sedative action of CNS depressants).
No products indexed under this heading.

Midazolam Hydrochloride (Co-administration may increase, prolong, or intensify the sedative action of CNS depressants). Products include:
- Versed Injection 3027
- Versed Syrup 3033

Moclobemide (Co-administration of MAO inhibitors with phenothiazines has resulted in increased incidence of extrapyramidal effects; although such a reaction has not been reported with Phenergan, the possibility should be considered).
No products indexed under this heading.

Molindone Hydrochloride (Co-administration may increase, prolong, or intensify the sedative action of CNS depressants). Products include:
- Moban 1320

Morphine Sulfate (Co-administration may increase, prolong, or intensify the sedative action of CNS depressants; the dose of narcotics should be reduced by one-quarter to one-half when given concurrently; excessive amounts of Phenergan relative to narcotic may lead to restlessness and minor hyperactivity in the patient with pain). Products include:
- Astramorph/PF Injection, USP (Preservative-Free) 594
- Duramorph Injection 1312
- Infumorph 200 and Infumorph 500 Sterile Solutions 1314
- Kadian Capsules 1335
- MS Contin Tablets 2896
- MSIR 2898
- Oramorph SR Tablets 3062
- Roxanol 3066

Olanzapine (Co-administration may increase, prolong, or intensify the sedative action of CNS depressants). Products include:
- Zyprexa Tablets 1973
- Zyprexa ZYDIS Orally Disintegrating Tablets 1973

Oxazepam (Co-administration may increase, prolong, or intensify the sedative action of CNS depressants).
No products indexed under this heading.

Oxybutynin Chloride (Concomitant use of other anticholinergic agents should be undertaken with caution because of possible additive effects). Products include:
- Ditropan XL Extended Release Tablets 564

Oxycodone Hydrochloride (Co-administration may increase, prolong, or intensify the sedative action of CNS depressants; the dose of narcotics should be reduced by one-quarter to one-half when given concurrently; excessive amounts of Phenergan relative to narcotic may lead to restlessness and minor hyperactivity in the patient with pain). Products include:
- OxyContin Tablets 2912
- OxyFast Oral Concentrate Solution . 2916
- OxyIR Capsules 2916
- Percocet Tablets 1326
- Percodan Tablets 1327
- Percolone Tablets 1327
- Roxicodone 3067
- Tylox Capsules 2597

Pargyline Hydrochloride (Co-administration of MAO inhibitors with phenothiazines has resulted in increased incidence of extrapyramidal effects; although such a reaction has not been reported with Phenergan, the possibility should be considered).
No products indexed under this heading.

Pentobarbital Sodium (Co-administration may increase, prolong, or intensify the sedative action of CNS depressants; the dose of barbiturates should be reduced by at least one-half when given concurrently). Products include:
- Nembutal Sodium Solution 485

Perphenazine (Co-administration may increase, prolong, or intensify the sedative action of CNS depressants). Products include:
- Etrafon 3115
- Trilafon 3160

Phenelzine Sulfate (Co-administration of MAO inhibitors with phenothiazines has resulted in increased incidence of extrapyramidal effects; although such a reaction has not been reported with Phenergan, the possibility should be considered). Products include:
- Nardil Tablets 2653

Phenobarbital (Co-administration may increase, prolong, or intensify the sedative action of CNS depressants; the dose of barbiturates should be reduced by at least one-half when given concurrently). Products include:
- Arco-Lase Plus Tablets 592
- Donnatal 2929
- Donnatal Extentabs 2930

Prazepam (Co-administration may increase, prolong, or intensify the sedative action of CNS depressants).
No products indexed under this heading.

Procarbazine Hydrochloride (Co-administration of MAO inhibitors with phenothiazines has resulted in increased incidence of extrapyramidal effects; although such a reaction has not been reported with Phenergan, the possibility should be considered). Products include:
- Matulane Capsules 3246

Prochlorperazine (Co-administration may increase, prolong, or intensify the sedative action of CNS depressants). Products include:
- Compazine 1505

Procyclidine Hydrochloride (Concomitant use of other anticholinergic agents should be undertaken with caution because of possible additive effects).
No products indexed under this heading.

Propantheline Bromide (Concomitant use of other anticholinergic agents should be undertaken with caution because of possible additive effects).
No products indexed under this heading.

Propofol (Co-administration may increase, prolong, or intensify the sedative action of CNS depressants). Products include:
- Diprivan Injectable Emulsion 667

Propoxyphene Hydrochloride (Co-administration may increase, prolong, or intensify the sedative action of CNS depressants; the dose of narcotics should be reduced by one-quarter to one-half when given concurrently; excessive amounts of Phenergan relative to narcotic may lead to restlessness and minor hyperactivity in the patient with pain). Products include:
- Darvon Pulvules 1909
- Darvon Compound-65 Pulvules 1910

Propoxyphene Napsylate (Co-administration may increase, prolong, or intensify the sedative action of CNS depressants; the dose of narcotics should be reduced by one-quarter to one-half when given concurrently; excessive amounts of Phenergan relative to narcotic may lead to restlessness and minor hyperactivity in the patient with pain). Products include:
- Darvon-N/Darvocet-N 1907
- Darvon-N Tablets 1912

Quazepam (Co-administration may increase, prolong, or intensify the sedative action of CNS depressants).
No products indexed under this heading.

Quetiapine Fumarate (Co-administration may increase, prolong, or intensify the sedative action of CNS depressants). Products include:
- Seroquel Tablets 684

Remifentanil Hydrochloride (Co-administration may increase, prolong, or intensify the sedative action of CNS depressants; the dose of narcotics should be reduced by one-quarter to one-half when given concurrently; excessive amounts of Phenergan relative to narcotic may lead to restlessness and minor hyperactivity in the patient with pain).
No products indexed under this heading.

Risperidone (Co-administration may increase, prolong, or intensify the sedative action of CNS depressants). Products include:
- Risperdal 1796

Scopolamine (Concomitant use of other anticholinergic agents should be undertaken with caution because of possible additive effects). Products include:
- Transderm Scōp Transdermal Therapeutic System 2302

Scopolamine Hydrobromide (Concomitant use of other anticholinergic agents should be undertaken with caution because of possible additive effects). Products include:
- Donnatal 2929
- Donnatal Extentabs 2930

Secobarbital Sodium (Co-administration may increase, prolong, or intensify the sedative action of CNS depressants; the dose of barbiturates should be reduced by at least one-half when given concurrently).
No products indexed under this heading.

Selegiline Hydrochloride (Co-administration of MAO inhibitors with phenothiazines has resulted in increased incidence of extrapyramidal effects; although such a reaction has not been reported with Phenergan, the possibility should be considered). Products include:
- Eldepryl Capsules 3266

Sevoflurane (Co-administration may increase, prolong, or intensify the sedative action of CNS depressants).
No products indexed under this heading.

Sufentanil Citrate (Co-administration may increase, prolong, or intensify the sedative action of CNS depressants; the dose of narcotics should be reduced by one-quarter to one-half when given concurrently; excessive amounts of Phenergan relative to narcotic may lead to restlessness and minor hyperactivity in the patient with pain).
No products indexed under this heading.

Temazepam (Co-administration may increase, prolong, or intensify the sedative action of CNS depressants).
No products indexed under this heading.

Thiamylal Sodium (Co-administration may increase, prolong, or intensify the sedative action

of CNS depressants; the dose of barbiturates should be reduced by at least one-half when given concurrently).

No products indexed under this heading.

Thioridazine Hydrochloride (Co-administration may increase, prolong, or intensify the sedative action of CNS depressants). Products include:

Thioridazine Hydrochloride Tablets 2289

Thiothixene (Co-administration may increase, prolong, or intensify the sedative action of CNS depressants). Products include:

Navane Capsules 2701
Thiothixene Capsules 2290

Tolterodine Tartrate (Concomitant use of other anticholinergic agents should be undertaken with caution because of possible additive effects). Products include:

Detrol Tablets 3623
Detrol LA Capsules 2801

Tranylcypromine Sulfate (Co-administration of MAO inhibitors with phenothiazines has resulted in increased incidence of extrapyramidal effects; although such a reaction has not been reported with Phenergan, the possibility should be considered). Products include:

Parnate Tablets 1607

Triazolam (Co-administration may increase, prolong, or intensify the sedative action of CNS depressants). Products include:

Halcion Tablets 2823

Tridihexethyl Chloride (Concomitant use of other anticholinergic agents should be undertaken with caution because of possible additive effects).

No products indexed under this heading.

Trifluoperazine Hydrochloride (Co-administration may increase, prolong, or intensify the sedative action of CNS depressants). Products include:

Stelazine 1640

Trihexyphenidyl Hydrochloride (Concomitant use of other anticholinergic agents should be undertaken with caution because of possible additive effects). Products include:

Artane 1855

Zaleplon (Co-administration may increase, prolong, or intensify the sedative action of CNS depressants). Products include:

Sonata Capsules 3591

Ziprasidone Hydrochloride (Co-administration may increase, prolong, or intensify the sedative action of CNS depressants). Products include:

Geodon Capsules 2688

Zolpidem Tartrate (Co-administration may increase, prolong, or intensify the sedative action of CNS depressants). Products include:

Ambien Tablets 3191

Food Interactions

Alcohol (Co-administration may increase, prolong, or intensify the sedative action of CNS depressants, such as alcohol).

PHENERGAN SUPPOSITORIES

(Promethazine Hydrochloride) 3556

May interact with anticholinergics, barbiturates, central nervous system depressants, monoamine oxidase inhibitors, narcotic analgesics, tricyclic antidepressants, and certain other agents. Compounds in these categories include:

Alfentanil Hydrochloride (Promethazine may increase, prolong, or intensify the sedative action of other CNS depressants; when co-administered with narcotics, the dose of narcotics should be reduced by at least one-quarter to one-half; excessive amount of promethazine relative to narcotic may lead to restlessness and motor hyperactivity in the patient with pain).

No products indexed under this heading.

Alprazolam (Promethazine may increase, prolong, or intensify the sedative action of other CNS depressants; concurrent use should be avoided with other CNS depressants or administered in reduced dosage to patient receiving promethazine). Products include:

Xanax Tablets 2865

Amitriptyline Hydrochloride (Promethazine may increase, prolong, or intensify the sedative action of other CNS depressants; concurrent use should be avoided with tricyclic antidepressants or administered in reduced dosage to patient receiving promethazine). Products include:

Etrafon 3115
Limbitrol 1738

Amoxapine (Promethazine may increase, prolong, or intensify the sedative action of other CNS depressants; concurrent use should be avoided with tricyclic antidepressants or administered in reduced dosage to patient receiving promethazine).

No products indexed under this heading.

Aprobarbital (Promethazine may increase, prolong, or intensify the sedative action of other CNS depressants; when co-administered with barbiturates, the dose of barbiturates should be reduced by one-quarter to one-half).

No products indexed under this heading.

Atropine Sulfate (Co-administration with agents with anticholinergic properties should be undertaken with caution). Products include:

Donnatal 2929
Donnatal Extentabs 2930
Motofen Tablets 577
Prosed/DS Tablets 3268
Urised Tablets 2876

Belladonna Alkaloids (Co-administration with agents with anticholinergic properties should be undertaken with caution). Products include:

Hyland's Teething Tablets 766
Urimax Tablets 1769

Benztropine Mesylate (Co-administration with agents with anticholinergic properties should be undertaken with caution). Products include:

Cogentin 2055

Biperiden Hydrochloride (Co-administration with agents with anticholinergic properties should be undertaken with caution). Products include:

Akineton 402

Buprenorphine Hydrochloride (Promethazine may increase, prolong, or intensify the sedative action of other CNS depressants; when co-administered with narcotics, the dose of narcotics should be reduced by at least one-quarter to one-half; excessive amount of promethazine relative to narcotic may lead to restlessness and motor hyperactivity in the patient with pain). Products include:

Buprenex Injectable 2918

Buspirone Hydrochloride (Promethazine may increase, prolong, or intensify the sedative action of other CNS depressants; concurrent use should be avoided with other CNS depressants or administered in reduced dosage to patient receiving promethazine).

No products indexed under this heading.

Butabarbital (Promethazine may increase, prolong, or intensify the sedative action of other CNS depressants; when co-administered with barbiturates, the dose of barbiturates should be reduced by one-quarter to one-half).

No products indexed under this heading.

Butalbital (Promethazine may increase, prolong, or intensify the sedative action of other CNS depressants; when co-administered with barbiturates, the dose of barbiturates should be reduced by one-quarter to one-half). Products include:

Phrenilin 578
Sedapap Tablets 50 mg/650 mg ... 2225

Chlordiazepoxide (Promethazine may increase, prolong, or intensify the sedative action of other CNS depressants; concurrent use should be avoided with other CNS depressants or administered in reduced dosage to patient receiving promethazine). Products include:

Limbitrol 1738

Chlordiazepoxide Hydrochloride (Promethazine may increase, prolong, or intensify the sedative action of other CNS depressants; concurrent use should be avoided with other CNS depressants or administered in reduced dosage to patient receiving promethazine). Products include:

Librium Capsules 1736
Librium for Injection 1737

Chlorpromazine (Promethazine may increase, prolong, or intensify the sedative action of other CNS depressants; concurrent use should be avoided with other CNS depressants or administered in reduced dosage to patient receiving promethazine). Products include:

Thorazine Suppositories 1656

Chlorpromazine Hydrochloride (Promethazine may increase, prolong, or intensify the sedative action of other CNS depressants; concurrent use should be avoided with other CNS depressants or administered in reduced dosage to patient receiving promethazine). Products include:

Thorazine 1656

Chlorprothixene (Promethazine may increase, prolong, or intensify the sedative action of other CNS depressants; concurrent use should be avoided with other CNS depressants or administered in reduced dosage to patient receiving promethazine).

No products indexed under this heading.

Chlorprothixene Hydrochloride (Promethazine may increase, prolong, or intensify the sedative action of other CNS depressants; concurrent use should be avoided with other CNS depressants or administered in reduced dosage to patient receiving promethazine).

No products indexed under this heading.

Chlorprothixene Lactate (Promethazine may increase, prolong, or intensify the sedative action of other CNS depressants; concurrent use should be avoided with other CNS depressants or administered in reduced dosage to patient receiving promethazine).

No products indexed under this heading.

Clidinium Bromide (Co-administration with agents with anticholinergic properties should be undertaken with caution).

No products indexed under this heading.

Clomipramine Hydrochloride (Promethazine may increase, prolong, or intensify the sedative action of other CNS depressants; concurrent use should be avoided with tricyclic antidepressants or administered in reduced dosage to patient receiving promethazine).

No products indexed under this heading.

Clorazepate Dipotassium (Promethazine may increase, prolong, or intensify the sedative action of other CNS depressants; concurrent use should be avoided with other CNS depressants or administered in reduced dosage to patient receiving promethazine). Products include:

Tranxene 511

Clozapine (Promethazine may increase, prolong, or intensify the sedative action of other CNS depressants; concurrent use should be avoided with other CNS depressants or administered in reduced dosage to patient receiving promethazine). Products include:

Clozaril Tablets 2319

Codeine Phosphate (Promethazine may increase, prolong, or intensify the sedative action of other CNS depressants; when co-administered with narcotics, the dose of narcotics should be reduced by at least one-quarter to one-half; excessive amount of promethazine relative to narcotic may lead to restlessness and motor hyperactivity in the patient with pain). Products include:

Phenergan with Codeine Syrup 3557
Phenergan VC with Codeine Syrup .. 3561
Robitussin A-C Syrup 2942
Robitussin-DAC Syrup 2942
Ryna-C Liquid 768
Soma Compound w/Codeine Tablets 3355
Tussi-Organidin NR Liquid 3350
Tussi-Organidin-S NR Liquid 3350
Tylenol with Codeine 2595

Desflurane (Promethazine may increase, prolong, or intensify the sedative action of other CNS depressants; concurrent use should be avoided with other CNS depressants or administered in reduced dosage to patient receiving promethazine). Products include:

Suprane Liquid for Inhalation 874

Desipramine Hydrochloride (Promethazine may increase, prolong, or intensify the sedative action of other CNS depressants; concurrent use should be avoided with tricyclic antidepressants or administered in reduced dosage to patient receiving promethazine). Products include:

Norpramin Tablets 755

Dezocine (Promethazine may increase, prolong, or intensify the sedative action of other CNS depressants; when co-administered with narcotics, the dose of narcotics should be reduced by at least one-quarter to one-half; excessive amount of promethazine relative to narcotic may lead to restlessness and motor hyperactivity in the patient with pain).

No products indexed under this heading.

Diazepam (Promethazine may increase, prolong, or intensify the sedative action of other CNS depressants; concurrent use should be avoided with other CNS depressants or administered in reduced dosage to patient receiving promethazine). Products include:

Valium Injectable 3026
Valium Tablets 3047

Dicyclomine Hydrochloride (Co-administration with agents with anticholinergic properties should be

undertaken with caution).
No products indexed under this heading.

Doxepin Hydrochloride (Promethazine may increase, prolong, or intensify the sedative action of other CNS depressants; concurrent use should be avoided with tricyclic antidepressants or administered in reduced dosage to patient receiving promethazine). Products include:
Sinequan 2713

Droperidol (Promethazine may increase, prolong, or intensify the sedative action of other CNS depressants; concurrent use should be avoided with other CNS depressants or administered in reduced dosage to patient receiving promethazine).
No products indexed under this heading.

Enflurane (Promethazine may increase, prolong, or intensify the sedative action of other CNS depressants; concurrent use should be avoided with other CNS depressants or administered in reduced dosage to patient receiving promethazine).
No products indexed under this heading.

Estazolam (Promethazine may increase, prolong, or intensify the sedative action of other CNS depressants; concurrent use should be avoided with other CNS depressants or administered in reduced dosage to patient receiving promethazine). Products include:
ProSom Tablets 500

Ethchlorvynol (Promethazine may increase, prolong, or intensify the sedative action of other CNS depressants; concurrent use should be avoided with other CNS depressants or administered in reduced dosage to patient receiving promethazine).
No products indexed under this heading.

Ethinamate (Promethazine may increase, prolong, or intensify the sedative action of other CNS depressants; concurrent use should be avoided with other CNS depressants or administered in reduced dosage to patient receiving promethazine).
No products indexed under this heading.

Fentanyl (Promethazine may increase, prolong, or intensify the sedative action of other CNS depressants; when co-administered with narcotics, the dose of narcotics should be reduced by at least one-quarter to one-half; excessive amount of promethazine relative to narcotic may lead to restlessness and motor hyperactivity in the patient with pain). Products include:
Duragesic Transdermal System 1786

Fentanyl Citrate (Promethazine may increase, prolong, or intensify the sedative action of other CNS depressants; when co-administered with narcotics, the dose of narcotics should be reduced by at least one-quarter to one-half; excessive amount of promethazine relative to narcotic may lead to restlessness and motor hyperactivity in the patient with pain). Products include:
Actiq 1184

Fluphenazine Decanoate (Promethazine may increase, prolong, or intensify the sedative action of other CNS depressants; concurrent use should be avoided with other CNS depressants or administered in reduced dosage to patient receiving promethazine).
No products indexed under this heading.

Fluphenazine Enanthate (Promethazine may increase, prolong, or intensify the sedative action of other CNS depressants; concurrent use should be avoided with other CNS depressants or administered in reduced dosage to patient receiving promethazine).
No products indexed under this heading.

Fluphenazine Hydrochloride (Promethazine may increase, prolong, or intensify the sedative action of other CNS depressants; concurrent use should be avoided with other CNS depressants or administered in reduced dosage to patient receiving promethazine).
No products indexed under this heading.

Flurazepam Hydrochloride (Promethazine may increase, prolong, or intensify the sedative action of other CNS depressants; concurrent use should be avoided with other CNS depressants or administered in reduced dosage to patient receiving promethazine).
No products indexed under this heading.

Glutethimide (Promethazine may increase, prolong, or intensify the sedative action of other CNS depressants; concurrent use should be avoided with other CNS depressants or administered in reduced dosage to patient receiving promethazine).
No products indexed under this heading.

Glycopyrrolate (Co-administration with agents with anticholinergic properties should be undertaken with caution). Products include:
Robinul Forte Tablets 1358
Robinul Injectable 2940
Robinul Tablets 1358

Haloperidol (Promethazine may increase, prolong, or intensify the sedative action of other CNS depressants; concurrent use should be avoided with other CNS depressants or administered in reduced dosage to patient receiving promethazine). Products include:
Haldol Injection, Tablets and Concentrate 2533

Haloperidol Decanoate (Promethazine may increase, prolong, or intensify the sedative action of other CNS depressants; concurrent use should be avoided with other CNS depressants or administered in reduced dosage to patient receiving promethazine). Products include:
Haldol Decanoate 2535

Hydrocodone Bitartrate (Promethazine may increase, prolong, or intensify the sedative action of other CNS depressants; when co-administered with narcotics, the dose of narcotics should be reduced by at least one-quarter to one-half; excessive amount of promethazine relative to narcotic may lead to restlessness and motor hyperactivity in the patient with pain). Products include:
Hycodan 1316
Hycomine Compound Tablets 1317
Hycotuss Expectorant Syrup 1318
Lortab 3319
Lortab Elixir 3317
Maxidone Tablets CIII 3399
Norco 5/325 Tablets CIII 3424
Norco 7.5/325 Tablets CIII 3425
Norco 10/325 Tablets CIII 3427
Norco 10/325 Tablets CIII 3425
Vicodin Tablets 516
Vicodin ES Tablets 517
Vicodin HP Tablets 518
Vicodin Tuss Expectorant 519
Vicoprofen Tablets 520
Zydone Tablets 1330

Hydrocodone Polistirex (Promethazine may increase, prolong, or intensify the sedative action of other CNS depressants; when co-administered with narcotics, the dose of narcotics should be reduced by at least one-quarter to one-half; excessive amount of promethazine relative to narcotic may lead to restlessness and motor hyperactivity in the patient with pain). Products include:
Tussionex Pennkinetic Extended-Release Suspension..... 1174

Hydromorphone Hydrochloride (Promethazine may increase, prolong, or intensify the sedative action of other CNS depressants; when co-administered with narcotics, the dose of narcotics should be reduced by at least one-quarter to one-half; excessive amount of promethazine relative to narcotic may lead to restlessness and motor hyperactivity in the patient with pain). Products include:
Dilaudid 441
Dilaudid Oral Liquid 445
Dilaudid Powder 441
Dilaudid Rectal Suppositories 441
Dilaudid Tablets 441
Dilaudid Tablets - 8 mg 445
Dilaudid-HP 443

Hydroxyzine Hydrochloride (Promethazine may increase, prolong, or intensify the sedative action of other CNS depressants; concurrent use should be avoided with other CNS depressants or administered in reduced dosage to patient receiving promethazine). Products include:
Atarax Tablets & Syrup 2667
Vistaril Intramuscular Solution 2738

Hyoscyamine (Co-administration with agents with anticholinergic properties should be undertaken with caution). Products include:
Urised Tablets 2876

Hyoscyamine Sulfate (Co-administration with agents with anticholinergic properties should be undertaken with caution). Products include:
Arco-Lase Plus Tablets 592
Donnatal 2929
Donnatal Extentabs 2930
Levsin/Levsinex/Levbid 3172
NuLev Orally Disintegrating Tablets 3176
Prosed/DS Tablets 3268
Urimax Tablets 1769

Imipramine Hydrochloride (Promethazine may increase, prolong, or intensify the sedative action of other CNS depressants; concurrent use should be avoided with tricyclic antidepressants or administered in reduced dosage to patient receiving promethazine).
No products indexed under this heading.

Imipramine Pamoate (Promethazine may increase, prolong, or intensify the sedative action of other CNS depressants; concurrent use should be avoided with tricyclic antidepressants or administered in reduced dosage to patient receiving promethazine).
No products indexed under this heading.

Ipratropium Bromide (Co-administration with agents with anticholinergic properties should be undertaken with caution). Products include:
Atrovent Inhalation Aerosol 1030
Atrovent Inhalation Solution 1031
Atrovent Nasal Spray 0.03% 1032
Atrovent Nasal Spray 0.06% 1033
Combivent Inhalation Aerosol 1041
DuoNeb Inhalation Solution 1233

Isocarboxazid (Co-administration of phenothiazines with MAO inhibitors may increase the incidence of extrapyramidal effects).
No products indexed under this heading.

Isoflurane (Promethazine may increase, prolong, or intensify the sedative action of other CNS depressants; concurrent use should be avoided with other CNS depressants or administered in reduced dosage to patient receiving promethazine).
No products indexed under this heading.

Ketamine Hydrochloride (Promethazine may increase, prolong, or intensify the sedative action of other CNS depressants; concurrent use should be avoided with other CNS depressants or administered in reduced dosage to patient receiving promethazine).
No products indexed under this heading.

Levomethadyl Acetate Hydrochloride (Promethazine may increase, prolong, or intensify the sedative action of other CNS depressants; concurrent use should be avoided with other CNS depressants or administered in reduced dosage to patient receiving promethazine).
No products indexed under this heading.

Levorphanol Tartrate (Promethazine may increase, prolong, or intensify the sedative action of other CNS depressants; when co-administered with narcotics, the dose of narcotics should be reduced by at least one-quarter to one-half; excessive amount of promethazine relative to narcotic may lead to restlessness and motor hyperactivity in the patient with pain). Products include:
Levo-Dromoran 1734
Levorphanol Tartrate Tablets 3059

Lorazepam (Promethazine may increase, prolong, or intensify the sedative action of other CNS depressants; concurrent use should be avoided with other CNS depressants or administered in reduced dosage to patient receiving promethazine). Products include:
Ativan Injection 3478
Ativan Tablets 3482

Loxapine Hydrochloride (Promethazine may increase, prolong, or intensify the sedative action of other CNS depressants; concurrent use should be avoided with other CNS depressants or administered in reduced dosage to patient receiving promethazine).
No products indexed under this heading.

Loxapine Succinate (Promethazine may increase, prolong, or intensify the sedative action of other CNS depressants; concurrent use should be avoided with other CNS depressants or administered in reduced dosage to patient receiving promethazine). Products include:
Loxitane Capsules 3398

Maprotiline Hydrochloride (Promethazine may increase, prolong, or intensify the sedative action of other CNS depressants; concurrent use should be avoided with tricyclic antidepressants or administered in reduced dosage to patient receiving promethazine).
No products indexed under this heading.

Mepenzolate Bromide (Co-administration with agents with anticholinergic properties should be undertaken with caution).
No products indexed under this heading.

Meperidine Hydrochloride (Promethazine may increase, prolong, or intensify the sedative action of other CNS depressants; when co-administered with narcotics, the dose of narcotics should be reduced by at least one-quarter to one-half; excessive amount of promethazine relative to narcotic may lead to restlessness and motor hyperactivity in the patient with pain). Products include:
Demerol 3079
Mepergan Injection 3539

Mephobarbital (Promethazine may increase, prolong, or intensify the sedative action of other CNS depressants; when co-administered with barbiturates, the dose of barbiturates should be reduced by one-quarter to one-half).
No products indexed under this heading.

Meprobamate (Promethazine may increase, prolong, or intensify the sedative action of other CNS depressants; concurrent use should be avoided with other CNS depressants or administered in reduced dosage to patient receiving promethazine). Products include:
Miltown Tablets ... 3349

Mesoridazine Besylate (Promethazine may increase, prolong, or intensify the sedative action of other CNS depressants; concurrent use should be avoided with other CNS depressants or administered in reduced dosage to patient receiving promethazine). Products include:
Serentil ... 1057

Methadone Hydrochloride (Promethazine may increase, prolong, or intensify the sedative action of other CNS depressants; when co-administered with narcotics, the dose of narcotics should be reduced by at least one-quarter to one-half; excessive amount of promethazine relative to narcotic may lead to restlessness and motor hyperactivity in the patient with pain). Products include:
Dolophine Hydrochloride Tablets ... 3056

Methohexital Sodium (Promethazine may increase, prolong, or intensify the sedative action of other CNS depressants; concurrent use should be avoided with other CNS depressants or administered in reduced dosage to patient receiving promethazine). Products include:
Brevital Sodium for Injection, USP .. 1815

Methotrimeprazine (Promethazine may increase, prolong, or intensify the sedative action of other CNS depressants; concurrent use should be avoided with other CNS depressants or administered in reduced dosage to patient receiving promethazine).
No products indexed under this heading.

Methoxyflurane (Promethazine may increase, prolong, or intensify the sedative action of other CNS depressants; concurrent use should be avoided with other CNS depressants or administered in reduced dosage to patient receiving promethazine).
No products indexed under this heading.

Midazolam Hydrochloride (Promethazine may increase, prolong, or intensify the sedative action of other CNS depressants; concurrent use should be avoided with other CNS depressants or administered in reduced dosage to patient receiving promethazine). Products include:
Versed Injection ... 3027
Versed Syrup ... 3033

Moclobemide (Co-administration of phenothiazines with MAO inhibitors may increase the incidence of extrapyramidal effects).
No products indexed under this heading.

Molindone Hydrochloride (Promethazine may increase, prolong, or intensify the sedative action of other CNS depressants; concurrent use should be avoided with other CNS depressants or administered in reduced dosage to patient receiving promethazine). Products include:
Moban ... 1320

Morphine Sulfate (Promethazine may increase, prolong, or intensify the sedative action of other CNS depressants; when co-administered with narcotics, the dose of narcotics should be reduced by at least one-quarter to one-half; excessive amount of promethazine relative to narcotic may lead to restlessness and motor hyperactivity in the patient with pain). Products include:
Astramorph/PF Injection, USP (Preservative-Free) ... 594
Duramorph Injection ... 1312
Infumorph 200 and Infumorph 500 Sterile Solutions ... 1314
Kadian Capsules ... 1335
MS Contin Tablets ... 2896
MSIR ... 2898
Oramorph SR Tablets ... 3062
Roxanol ... 3066

Nortriptyline Hydrochloride (Promethazine may increase, prolong, or intensify the sedative action of other CNS depressants; concurrent use should be avoided with tricyclic antidepressants or administered in reduced dosage to patient receiving promethazine).
No products indexed under this heading.

Olanzapine (Promethazine may increase, prolong, or intensify the sedative action of other CNS depressants; concurrent use should be avoided with other CNS depressants or administered in reduced dosage to patient receiving promethazine). Products include:
Zyprexa Tablets ... 1973
Zyprexa ZYDIS Orally Disintegrating Tablets ... 1973

Oxazepam (Promethazine may increase, prolong, or intensify the sedative action of other CNS depressants; concurrent use should be avoided with other CNS depressants or administered in reduced dosage to patient receiving promethazine).
No products indexed under this heading.

Oxybutynin Chloride (Co-administration with agents with anticholinergic properties should be undertaken with caution). Products include:
Ditropan XL Extended Release Tablets ... 564

Oxycodone Hydrochloride (Promethazine may increase, prolong, or intensify the sedative action of other CNS depressants; when co-administered with narcotics, the dose of narcotics should be reduced by at least one-quarter to one-half; excessive amount of promethazine relative to narcotic may lead to restlessness and motor hyperactivity in the patient with pain). Products include:
OxyContin Tablets ... 2912
OxyFast Oral Concentrate Solution . 2916
OxyIR Capsules ... 2916
Percocet Tablets ... 1326
Percodan Tablets ... 1327
Percolone Tablets ... 1327
Roxicodone ... 3067
Tylox Capsules ... 2597

Pargyline Hydrochloride (Co-administration of phenothiazines with MAO inhibitors may increase the incidence of extrapyramidal effects).
No products indexed under this heading.

Pentobarbital Sodium (Promethazine may increase, prolong, or intensify the sedative action of other CNS depressants; when co-administered with barbiturates, the dose of barbiturates should be reduced by one-quarter to one-half). Products include:
Nembutal Sodium Solution ... 485

Perphenazine (Promethazine may increase, prolong, or intensify the sedative action of other CNS depressants; concurrent use should be avoided with other CNS depressants or administered in reduced dosage to patient receiving promethazine). Products include:
Etrafon ... 3115
Trilafon ... 3160

Phenelzine Sulfate (Co-administration of phenothiazines with MAO inhibitors may increase the incidence of extrapyramidal effects). Products include:
Nardil Tablets ... 2653

Phenobarbital (Promethazine may increase, prolong, or intensify the sedative action of other CNS depressants; when co-administered with barbiturates, the dose of barbiturates should be reduced by one-quarter to one-half). Products include:
Arco-Lase Plus Tablets ... 592
Donnatal ... 2929
Donnatal Extentabs ... 2930

Prazepam (Promethazine may increase, prolong, or intensify the sedative action of other CNS depressants; concurrent use should be avoided with other CNS depressants or administered in reduced dosage to patient receiving promethazine).
No products indexed under this heading.

Procarbazine Hydrochloride (Co-administration of phenothiazines with MAO inhibitors may increase the incidence of extrapyramidal effects). Products include:
Matulane Capsules ... 3246

Prochlorperazine (Promethazine may increase, prolong, or intensify the sedative action of other CNS depressants; concurrent use should be avoided with other CNS depressants or administered in reduced dosage to patient receiving promethazine). Products include:
Compazine ... 1505

Procyclidine Hydrochloride (Co-administration with agents with anticholinergic properties should be undertaken with caution).
No products indexed under this heading.

Propantheline Bromide (Co-administration with agents with anticholinergic properties should be undertaken with caution).
No products indexed under this heading.

Propofol (Promethazine may increase, prolong, or intensify the sedative action of other CNS depressants; concurrent use should be avoided with other CNS depressants or administered in reduced dosage to patient receiving promethazine). Products include:
Diprivan Injectable Emulsion ... 667

Propoxyphene Hydrochloride (Promethazine may increase, prolong, or intensify the sedative action of other CNS depressants; when co-administered with narcotics, the dose of narcotics should be reduced by at least one-quarter to one-half; excessive amount of promethazine relative to narcotic may lead to restlessness and motor hyperactivity in the patient with pain). Products include:
Darvon Pulvules ... 1909
Darvon Compound-65 Pulvules ... 1910

Propoxyphene Napsylate (Promethazine may increase, prolong, or intensify the sedative action of other CNS depressants; when co-administered with narcotics, the dose of narcotics should be reduced by at least one-quarter to one-half; excessive amount of promethazine relative to narcotic may lead to restlessness and motor hyperactivity in the patient with pain). Products include:
Darvon-N/Darvocet-N ... 1907
Darvon-N Tablets ... 1912

Protriptyline Hydrochloride (Promethazine may increase, prolong, or intensify the sedative action of other CNS depressants; concurrent use should be avoided with tricyclic antidepressants or administered in reduced dosage to patient receiving promethazine). Products include:
Vivactil Tablets ... 2446
Vivactil Tablets ... 2217

Quazepam (Promethazine may increase, prolong, or intensify the sedative action of other CNS depressants; concurrent use should be avoided with other CNS depressants or administered in reduced dosage to patient receiving promethazine).
No products indexed under this heading.

Quetiapine Fumarate (Promethazine may increase, prolong, or intensify the sedative action of other CNS depressants; concurrent use should be avoided with other CNS depressants or administered in reduced dosage to patient receiving promethazine). Products include:
Seroquel Tablets ... 684

Remifentanil Hydrochloride (Promethazine may increase, prolong, or intensify the sedative action of other CNS depressants; when co-administered with narcotics, the dose of narcotics should be reduced by at least one-quarter to one-half; excessive amount of promethazine relative to narcotic may lead to restlessness and motor hyperactivity in the patient with pain).
No products indexed under this heading.

Risperidone (Promethazine may increase, prolong, or intensify the sedative action of other CNS depressants; concurrent use should be avoided with other CNS depressants or administered in reduced dosage to patient receiving promethazine). Products include:
Risperdal ... 1796

Scopolamine (Co-administration with agents with anticholinergic properties should be undertaken with caution). Products include:
Transderm Scōp Transdermal Therapeutic System ... 2302

Scopolamine Hydrobromide (Co-administration with agents with anticholinergic properties should be undertaken with caution). Products include:
Donnatal ... 2929
Donnatal Extentabs ... 2930

Secobarbital Sodium (Promethazine may increase, prolong, or intensify the sedative action of other CNS depressants; when co-administered with barbiturates, the dose of barbiturates should be reduced by one-quarter to one-half).
No products indexed under this heading.

Selegiline Hydrochloride (Co-administration of phenothiazines with MAO inhibitors may increase the incidence of extrapyramidal effects). Products include:
Eldepryl Capsules ... 3266

Sevoflurane (Promethazine may increase, prolong, or intensify the sedative action of other CNS depressants; concurrent use should be avoided with other CNS depressants or administered in reduced dosage to patient receiving promethazine).
No products indexed under this heading.

Sufentanil Citrate (Promethazine may increase, prolong, or intensify the sedative action of other CNS depressants; when co-administered with narcotics, the dose of narcotics should be reduced by at least one-quarter to one-half; excessive

amount of promethazine relative to narcotic may lead to restlessness and motor hyperactivity in the patient with pain).
No products indexed under this heading.

Temazepam (Promethazine may increase, prolong, or intensify the sedative action of other CNS depressants; concurrent use should be avoided with other CNS depressants or administered in reduced dosage to patient receiving promethazine).
No products indexed under this heading.

Thiamylal Sodium (Promethazine may increase, prolong, or intensify the sedative action of other CNS depressants; when co-administered with barbiturates, the dose of barbiturates should be reduced by one-quarter to one-half).
No products indexed under this heading.

Thioridazine Hydrochloride (Promethazine may increase, prolong, or intensify the sedative action of other CNS depressants; concurrent use should be avoided with other CNS depressants or administered in reduced dosage to patient receiving promethazine). Products include:
Thioridazine Hydrochloride Tablets 2289

Thiothixene (Promethazine may increase, prolong, or intensify the sedative action of other CNS depressants; concurrent use should be avoided with other CNS depressants or administered in reduced dosage to patient receiving promethazine). Products include:
Navane Capsules 2701
Thiothixene Capsules 2290

Tolterodine Tartrate (Co-administration with agents with anticholinergic properties should be undertaken with caution). Products include:
Detrol Tablets 3623
Detrol LA Capsules 2801

Tranylcypromine Sulfate (Co-administration of phenothiazines with MAO inhibitors may increase the incidence of extrapyramidal effects). Products include:
Parnate Tablets 1607

Triazolam (Promethazine may increase, prolong, or intensify the sedative action of other CNS depressants; concurrent use should be avoided with other CNS depressants or administered in reduced dosage to patient receiving promethazine). Products include:
Halcion Tablets 2823

Tridihexethyl Chloride (Co-administration with agents with anticholinergic properties should be undertaken with caution).
No products indexed under this heading.

Trifluoperazine Hydrochloride (Promethazine may increase, prolong, or intensify the sedative action of other CNS depressants; concurrent use should be avoided with other CNS depressants or administered in reduced dosage to patient receiving promethazine). Products include:
Stelazine 1640

Trihexyphenidyl Hydrochloride (Co-administration with agents with anticholinergic properties should be undertaken with caution). Products include:
Artane 1855

Trimipramine Maleate (Promethazine may increase, prolong, or intensify the sedative action of other CNS depressants; concurrent use should be avoided with tricyclic antidepressants or administered in reduced dosage to patient receiving promethazine). Products include:
Surmontil Capsules 3595

Zaleplon (Promethazine may increase, prolong, or intensify the sedative action of other CNS depressants; concurrent use should be avoided with other CNS depressants or administered in reduced dosage to patient receiving promethazine). Products include:
Sonata Capsules 3591

Ziprasidone Hydrochloride (Promethazine may increase, prolong, or intensify the sedative action of other CNS depressants; concurrent use should be avoided with other CNS depressants or administered in reduced dosage to patient receiving promethazine). Products include:
Geodon Capsules 2688

Zolpidem Tartrate (Promethazine may increase, prolong, or intensify the sedative action of other CNS depressants; concurrent use should be avoided with other CNS depressants or administered in reduced dosage to patient receiving promethazine). Products include:
Ambien Tablets 3191

Food Interactions

Alcohol (Promethazine may increase, prolong, or intensify the sedative action of other CNS depressants, such as alcohol).

PHENERGAN SYRUP FORTIS

(Promethazine Hydrochloride) 3554
May interact with hypnotics and sedatives, narcotic analgesics, tranquilizers, tricyclic antidepressants, and certain other agents. Compounds in these categories include:

Alfentanil Hydrochloride (Additive sedative effects).
No products indexed under this heading.

Alprazolam (Additive sedative effects). Products include:
Xanax Tablets 2865

Amitriptyline Hydrochloride (Additive sedative effects). Products include:
Etrafon 3115
Limbitrol 1738

Amoxapine (Additive sedative effects).
No products indexed under this heading.

Buprenorphine Hydrochloride (Additive sedative effects). Products include:
Buprenex Injectable 2918

Buspirone Hydrochloride (Additive sedative effects).
No products indexed under this heading.

Chlordiazepoxide (Additive sedative effects). Products include:
Limbitrol 1738

Chlordiazepoxide Hydrochloride (Additive sedative effects). Products include:
Librium Capsules 1736
Librium for Injection 1737

Chlorpromazine (Additive sedative effects). Products include:
Thorazine Suppositories 1656

Chlorpromazine Hydrochloride (Additive sedative effects). Products include:
Thorazine 1656

Chlorprothixene (Additive sedative effects).
No products indexed under this heading.

Chlorprothixene Hydrochloride (Additive sedative effects).
No products indexed under this heading.

Clomipramine Hydrochloride (Additive sedative effects).
No products indexed under this heading.

Clorazepate Dipotassium (Additive sedative effects). Products include:
Tranxene 511

Codeine Phosphate (Additive sedative effects). Products include:
Phenergan with Codeine Syrup 3557
Phenergan VC with Codeine Syrup 3561
Robitussin A-C Syrup 2942
Robitussin-DAC Syrup 2942
Ryna-C Liquid .... ■ 768
Soma Compound w/Codeine Tablets 3355
Tussi-Organidin NR Liquid 3350
Tussi-Organidin-S NR Liquid 3350
Tylenol with Codeine 2595

Desipramine Hydrochloride (Additive sedative effects). Products include:
Norpramin Tablets 755

Dezocine (Additive sedative effects).
No products indexed under this heading.

Diazepam (Additive sedative effects). Products include:
Valium Injectable 3026
Valium Tablets 3047

Doxepin Hydrochloride (Additive sedative effects). Products include:
Sinequan 2713

Droperidol (Additive sedative effects).
No products indexed under this heading.

Estazolam (Additive sedative effects). Products include:
ProSom Tablets 500

Ethchlorvynol (Additive sedative effects).
No products indexed under this heading.

Ethinamate (Additive sedative effects).
No products indexed under this heading.

Fentanyl (Additive sedative effects). Products include:
Duragesic Transdermal System 1786

Fentanyl Citrate (Additive sedative effects). Products include:
Actiq 1184

Fluphenazine Decanoate (Additive sedative effects).
No products indexed under this heading.

Fluphenazine Enanthate (Additive sedative effects).
No products indexed under this heading.

Fluphenazine Hydrochloride (Additive sedative effects).
No products indexed under this heading.

Flurazepam Hydrochloride (Additive sedative effects).
No products indexed under this heading.

Glutethimide (Additive sedative effects).
No products indexed under this heading.

Haloperidol (Additive sedative effects). Products include:
Haldol Injection, Tablets and Concentrate 2533

Haloperidol Decanoate (Additive sedative effects). Products include:
Haldol Decanoate 2535

Hydrocodone Bitartrate (Additive sedative effects). Products include:
Hycodan 1316
Hycomine Compound Tablets 1317
Hycotuss Expectorant Syrup 1318
Lortab 3319
Lortab Elixir 3317
Maxidone Tablets CIII 3399
Norco 5/325 Tablets CIII 3424
Norco 7.5/325 Tablets CIII 3425
Norco 10/325 Tablets CIII 3427
Norco 10/325 Tablets CIII 3425
Vicodin Tablets 516
Vicodin ES Tablets 517
Vicodin HP Tablets 518
Vicodin Tuss Expectorant 519
Vicoprofen Tablets 520
Zydone Tablets 1330

Hydrocodone Polistirex (Additive sedative effects). Products include:
Tussionex Pennkinetic Extended-Release Suspension 1174

Hydromorphone Hydrochloride (Additive sedative effects). Products include:
Dilaudid 441
Dilaudid Oral Liquid 445
Dilaudid Powder 441
Dilaudid Rectal Suppositories 441
Dilaudid Tablets 441
Dilaudid Tablets - 8 mg 445
Dilaudid-HP 443

Hydroxyzine Hydrochloride (Additive sedative effects). Products include:
Atarax Tablets & Syrup 2667
Vistaril Intramuscular Solution 2738

Imipramine Hydrochloride (Additive sedative effects).
No products indexed under this heading.

Imipramine Pamoate (Additive sedative effects).
No products indexed under this heading.

Levorphanol Tartrate (Additive sedative effects). Products include:
Levo-Dromoran 1734
Levorphanol Tartrate Tablets 3059

Lorazepam (Additive sedative effects). Products include:
Ativan Injection 3478
Ativan Tablets 3482

Loxapine Hydrochloride (Additive sedative effects).
No products indexed under this heading.

Loxapine Succinate (Additive sedative effects). Products include:
Loxitane Capsules 3398

Maprotiline Hydrochloride (Additive sedative effects).
No products indexed under this heading.

Meperidine Hydrochloride (Additive sedative effects). Products include:
Demerol 3079
Mepergan Injection 3539

Meprobamate (Additive sedative effects). Products include:
Miltown Tablets 3349

Mesoridazine Besylate (Additive sedative effects). Products include:
Serentil 1057

Methadone Hydrochloride (Additive sedative effects). Products include:
Dolophine Hydrochloride Tablets 3056

Midazolam Hydrochloride (Additive sedative effects). Products include:
Versed Injection 3027
Versed Syrup 3033

Molindone Hydrochloride (Additive sedative effects). Products include:
Moban 1320

Morphine Sulfate (Additive sedative effects). Products include:
Astramorph/PF Injection, USP (Preservative-Free) 594
Duramorph Injection 1312
Infumorph 200 and Infumorph 500 Sterile Solutions 1314
Kadian Capsules 1335
MS Contin Tablets 2896
MSIR 2898
Oramorph SR Tablets 3062
Roxanol 3066

Nortriptyline Hydrochloride (Additive sedative effects).
No products indexed under this heading.

Oxazepam (Additive sedative effects).
No products indexed under this heading.

Oxycodone Hydrochloride (Additive sedative effects). Products include:
OxyContin Tablets ... 2912
OxyFast Oral Concentrate Solution . 2916
OxyIR Capsules ... 2916
Percocet Tablets ... 1326
Percodan Tablets ... 1327
Percolone Tablets ... 1327
Roxicodone ... 3067
Tylox Capsules ... 2597

Perphenazine (Additive sedative effects). Products include:
Etrafon ... 3115
Trilafon ... 3160

Prazepam (Additive sedative effects).
No products indexed under this heading.

Prochlorperazine (Additive sedative effects). Products include:
Compazine ... 1505

Propofol (Additive sedative effects). Products include:
Diprivan Injectable Emulsion ... 667

Propoxyphene Hydrochloride (Additive sedative effects). Products include:
Darvon Pulvules ... 1909
Darvon Compound-65 Pulvules ... 1910

Propoxyphene Napsylate (Additive sedative effects). Products include:
Darvon-N/Darvocet-N ... 1907
Darvon-N Tablets ... 1912

Protriptyline Hydrochloride (Additive sedative effects). Products include:
Vivactil Tablets ... 2446
Vivactil Tablets ... 2217

Quazepam (Additive sedative effects).
No products indexed under this heading.

Remifentanil Hydrochloride (Additive sedative effects).
No products indexed under this heading.

Secobarbital Sodium (Additive sedative effects).
No products indexed under this heading.

Sufentanil Citrate (Additive sedative effects).
No products indexed under this heading.

Temazepam (Additive sedative effects).
No products indexed under this heading.

Thioridazine Hydrochloride (Additive sedative effects). Products include:
Thioridazine Hydrochloride Tablets ... 2289

Thiothixene (Additive sedative effects). Products include:
Navane Capsules ... 2701
Thiothixene Capsules ... 2290

Triazolam (Additive sedative effects). Products include:
Halcion Tablets ... 2823

Trifluoperazine Hydrochloride (Additive sedative effects). Products include:
Stelazine ... 1640

Trimipramine Maleate (Additive sedative effects). Products include:
Surmontil Capsules ... 3595

Zaleplon (Additive sedative effects). Products include:
Sonata Capsules ... 3591

Zolpidem Tartrate (Additive sedative effects). Products include:
Ambien Tablets ... 3191

Food Interactions

Alcohol (Additive sedative effects).

PHENERGAN SYRUP PLAIN

(Promethazine Hydrochloride) ... 3554
See Phenergan Syrup Fortis

PHENERGAN TABLETS

(Promethazine Hydrochloride) ... 3556
See Phenergan Suppositories

PHENERGAN WITH CODEINE SYRUP

(Codeine Phosphate, Promethazine Hydrochloride) ... 3557
May interact with hypnotics and sedatives, monoamine oxidase inhibitors, narcotic analgesics, tranquilizers, tricyclic antidepressants, and certain other agents. Compounds in these categories include:

Alfentanil Hydrochloride (Additive sedative effects).
No products indexed under this heading.

Alprazolam (Additive sedative effects). Products include:
Xanax Tablets ... 2865

Amitriptyline Hydrochloride (Additive sedative effects). Products include:
Etrafon ... 3115
Limbitrol ... 1738

Amoxapine (Additive sedative effects).
No products indexed under this heading.

Buprenorphine Hydrochloride (Additive sedative effects). Products include:
Buprenex Injectable ... 2918

Buspirone Hydrochloride (Additive sedative effects).
No products indexed under this heading.

Chlordiazepoxide (Additive sedative effects). Products include:
Limbitrol ... 1738

Chlordiazepoxide Hydrochloride (Additive sedative effects). Products include:
Librium Capsules ... 1736
Librium for Injection ... 1737

Chlorpromazine (Additive sedative effects). Products include:
Thorazine Suppositories ... 1656

Chlorpromazine Hydrochloride (Additive sedative effects). Products include:
Thorazine ... 1656

Chlorprothixene (Additive sedative effects).
No products indexed under this heading.

Chlorprothixene Hydrochloride (Additive sedative effects).
No products indexed under this heading.

Clomipramine Hydrochloride (Additive sedative effects).
No products indexed under this heading.

Clorazepate Dipotassium (Additive sedative effects). Products include:
Tranxene ... 511

Desipramine Hydrochloride (Additive sedative effects). Products include:
Norpramin Tablets ... 755

Dezocine (Additive sedative effects).
No products indexed under this heading.

Diazepam (Additive sedative effects). Products include:
Valium Injectable ... 3026
Valium Tablets ... 3047

Doxepin Hydrochloride (Additive sedative effects). Products include:
Sinequan ... 2713

Droperidol (Additive sedative effects).
No products indexed under this heading.

Estazolam (Additive sedative effects). Products include:
ProSom Tablets ... 500

Ethchlorvynol (Additive sedative effects).
No products indexed under this heading.

Ethinamate (Additive sedative effects).
No products indexed under this heading.

Fentanyl (Additive sedative effects). Products include:
Duragesic Transdermal System ... 1786

Fentanyl Citrate (Additive sedative effects). Products include:
Actiq ... 1184

Fluphenazine Decanoate (Additive sedative effects).
No products indexed under this heading.

Fluphenazine Enanthate (Additive sedative effects).
No products indexed under this heading.

Fluphenazine Hydrochloride (Additive sedative effects).
No products indexed under this heading.

Flurazepam Hydrochloride (Additive sedative effects).
No products indexed under this heading.

Glutethimide (Additive sedative effects).
No products indexed under this heading.

Haloperidol (Additive sedative effects). Products include:
Haldol Injection, Tablets and Concentrate ... 2533

Haloperidol Decanoate (Additive sedative effects). Products include:
Haldol Decanoate ... 2535

Hydrocodone Bitartrate (Additive sedative effects). Products include:
Hycodan ... 1316
Hycomine Compound Tablets ... 1317
Hycotuss Expectorant Syrup ... 1318
Lortab ... 3319
Lortab Elixir ... 3317
Maxidone Tablets CIII ... 3399
Norco 5/325 Tablets CIII ... 3424
Norco 7.5/325 Tablets CIII ... 3425
Norco 10/325 Tablets CIII ... 3427
Norco 10/325 Tablets CIII ... 3425
Vicodin Tablets ... 516
Vicodin ES Tablets ... 517
Vicodin HP Tablets ... 518
Vicodin Tuss Expectorant ... 519
Vicoprofen Tablets ... 520
Zydone Tablets ... 1330

Hydrocodone Polistirex (Additive sedative effects). Products include:
Tussionex Pennkinetic Extended-Release Suspension ... 1174

Hydromorphone Hydrochloride (Additive sedative effects). Products include:
Dilaudid ... 441
Dilaudid Oral Liquid ... 445
Dilaudid Powder ... 441
Dilaudid Rectal Suppositories ... 441
Dilaudid Tablets ... 441
Dilaudid Tablets - 8 mg ... 445
Dilaudid-HP ... 443

Hydroxyzine Hydrochloride (Additive sedative effects). Products include:
Atarax Tablets & Syrup ... 2667
Vistaril Intramuscular Solution ... 2738

Imipramine Hydrochloride (Additive sedative effects).
No products indexed under this heading.

Imipramine Pamoate (Additive sedative effects).
No products indexed under this heading.

Isocarboxazid (Excessive narcotic effects).
No products indexed under this heading.

Levorphanol Tartrate (Additive sedative effects). Products include:
Levo-Dromoran ... 1734
Levorphanol Tartrate Tablets ... 3059

Lorazepam (Additive sedative effects). Products include:
Ativan Injection ... 3478
Ativan Tablets ... 3482

Loxapine Hydrochloride (Additive sedative effects).
No products indexed under this heading.

Loxapine Succinate (Additive sedative effects). Products include:
Loxitane Capsules ... 3398

Maprotiline Hydrochloride (Additive sedative effects).
No products indexed under this heading.

Meperidine Hydrochloride (Additive sedative effects). Products include:
Demerol ... 3079
Mepergan Injection ... 3539

Meprobamate (Additive sedative effects). Products include:
Miltown Tablets ... 3349

Mesoridazine Besylate (Additive sedative effects). Products include:
Serentil ... 1057

Methadone Hydrochloride (Additive sedative effects). Products include:
Dolophine Hydrochloride Tablets ... 3056

Midazolam Hydrochloride (Additive sedative effects). Products include:
Versed Injection ... 3027
Versed Syrup ... 3033

Moclobemide (Excessive narcotic effects).
No products indexed under this heading.

Molindone Hydrochloride (Additive sedative effects). Products include:
Moban ... 1320

Morphine Sulfate (Additive sedative effects). Products include:
Astramorph/PF Injection, USP (Preservative-Free) ... 594
Duramorph Injection ... 1312
Infumorph 200 and Infumorph 500 Sterile Solutions ... 1314
Kadian Capsules ... 1335
MS Contin Tablets ... 2896
MSIR ... 2898
Oramorph SR Tablets ... 3062
Roxanol ... 3066

Nortriptyline Hydrochloride (Additive sedative effects).
No products indexed under this heading.

Oxazepam (Additive sedative effects).
No products indexed under this heading.

Oxycodone Hydrochloride (Additive sedative effects). Products include:
OxyContin Tablets ... 2912
OxyFast Oral Concentrate Solution . 2916
OxyIR Capsules ... 2916
Percocet Tablets ... 1326
Percodan Tablets ... 1327
Percolone Tablets ... 1327
Roxicodone ... 3067
Tylox Capsules ... 2597

Pargyline Hydrochloride (Excessive narcotic effects).
No products indexed under this heading.

Perphenazine (Additive sedative effects). Products include:
Etrafon ... 3115
Trilafon ... 3160

Phenelzine Sulfate (Excessive narcotic effects). Products include:
Nardil Tablets ... 2653

Prazepam (Additive sedative effects).
No products indexed under this heading.

Procarbazine Hydrochloride (Excessive narcotic effects). Products include:
Matulane Capsules 3246
Prochlorperazine (Additive sedative effects). Products include:
Compazine 1505
Propofol (Additive sedative effects). Products include:
Diprivan Injectable Emulsion 667
Propoxyphene Hydrochloride (Additive sedative effects). Products include:
Darvon Pulvules 1909
Darvon Compound-65 Pulvules 1910
Propoxyphene Napsylate (Additive sedative effects). Products include:
Darvon-N/Darvocet-N 1907
Darvon-N Tablets 1912
Protriptyline Hydrochloride (Additive sedative effects). Products include:
Vivactil Tablets 2446
Vivactil Tablets 2217
Quazepam (Additive sedative effects).
No products indexed under this heading.
Remifentanil Hydrochloride (Additive sedative effects).
No products indexed under this heading.
Secobarbital Sodium (Additive sedative effects).
No products indexed under this heading.
Selegiline Hydrochloride (Excessive narcotic effects). Products include:
Eldepryl Capsules 3266
Sufentanil Citrate (Additive sedative effects).
No products indexed under this heading.
Temazepam (Additive sedative effects).
No products indexed under this heading.
Thioridazine Hydrochloride (Additive sedative effects). Products include:
Thioridazine Hydrochloride Tablets 2289
Thiothixene (Additive sedative effects). Products include:
Navane Capsules 2701
Thiothixene Capsules 2290
Tranylcypromine Sulfate (Excessive narcotic effects). Products include:
Parnate Tablets 1607
Triazolam (Additive sedative effects). Products include:
Halcion Tablets 2823
Trifluoperazine Hydrochloride (Additive sedative effects). Products include:
Stelazine 1640
Trimipramine Maleate (Additive sedative effects). Products include:
Surmontil Capsules 3595
Zaleplon (Additive sedative effects). Products include:
Sonata Capsules 3591
Zolpidem Tartrate (Additive sedative effects). Products include:
Ambien Tablets 3191

Food Interactions

Alcohol (Additive sedative effects).

PHENERGAN WITH DEXTROMETHORPHAN SYRUP
(Dextromethorphan Hydrobromide, Promethazine Hydrochloride) 3559
May interact with hypnotics and sedatives, monoamine oxidase inhibitors, narcotic analgesics, tranquilizers, tricyclic antidepressants, and certain other agents. Compounds in these categories include:

Alfentanil Hydrochloride (Additive sedative effects).
No products indexed under this heading.
Alprazolam (Additive sedative effects). Products include:
Xanax Tablets 2865
Amitriptyline Hydrochloride (Additive sedative effects). Products include:
Etrafon 3115
Limbitrol 1738
Amoxapine (Additive sedative effects).
No products indexed under this heading.
Buprenorphine Hydrochloride (Additive sedative effects). Products include:
Buprenex Injectable 2918
Buspirone Hydrochloride (Additive sedative effects).
No products indexed under this heading.
Chlordiazepoxide (Additive sedative effects). Products include:
Limbitrol 1738
Chlordiazepoxide Hydrochloride (Additive sedative effects). Products include:
Librium Capsules 1736
Librium for Injection 1737
Chlorpromazine (Additive sedative effects). Products include:
Thorazine Suppositories 1656
Chlorpromazine Hydrochloride (Additive sedative effects). Products include:
Thorazine 1656
Chlorprothixene (Additive sedative effects).
No products indexed under this heading.
Chlorprothixene Hydrochloride (Additive sedative effects).
No products indexed under this heading.
Clomipramine Hydrochloride (Additive sedative effects).
No products indexed under this heading.
Clorazepate Dipotassium (Additive sedative effects). Products include:
Tranxene 511
Codeine Phosphate (Additive sedative effects). Products include:
Phenergan with Codeine Syrup 3557
Phenergan VC with Codeine Syrup 3561
Robitussin A-C Syrup 2942
Robitussin-DAC Syrup 2942
Ryna-C Liquid .... ▣ 768
Soma Compound w/Codeine Tablets 3355
Tussi-Organidin NR Liquid 3350
Tussi-Organidin-S NR Liquid 3350
Tylenol with Codeine 2595
Desipramine Hydrochloride (Additive sedative effects). Products include:
Norpramin Tablets 755
Dezocine (Additive sedative effects).
No products indexed under this heading.
Diazepam (Additive sedative effects). Products include:
Valium Injectable 3026
Valium Tablets 3047
Doxepin Hydrochloride (Additive sedative effects). Products include:
Sinequan 2713
Droperidol (Additive sedative effects).
No products indexed under this heading.
Estazolam (Additive sedative effects). Products include:
ProSom Tablets 500
Ethchlorvynol (Additive sedative effects).
No products indexed under this heading.
Ethinamate (Additive sedative effects).
No products indexed under this heading.
Fentanyl (Additive sedative effects). Products include:
Duragesic Transdermal System 1786
Fentanyl Citrate (Additive sedative effects). Products include:
Actiq 1184
Fluphenazine Decanoate (Additive sedative effects).
No products indexed under this heading.
Fluphenazine Enanthate (Additive sedative effects).
No products indexed under this heading.
Fluphenazine Hydrochloride (Additive sedative effects).
No products indexed under this heading.
Flurazepam Hydrochloride (Additive sedative effects).
No products indexed under this heading.
Glutethimide (Additive sedative effects).
No products indexed under this heading.
Haloperidol (Additive sedative effects). Products include:
Haldol Injection, Tablets and Concentrate 2533
Haloperidol Decanoate (Additive sedative effects). Products include:
Haldol Decanoate 2535
Hydrocodone Bitartrate (Additive sedative effects). Products include:
Hycodan 1316
Hycomine Compound Tablets 1317
Hycotuss Expectorant Syrup 1318
Lortab 3319
Lortab Elixir 3317
Maxidone Tablets CIII 3399
Norco 5/325 Tablets CIII 3424
Norco 7.5/325 Tablets CIII 3425
Norco 10/325 Tablets CIII 3427
Norco 10/325 Tablets CIII 3425
Vicodin Tablets 516
Vicodin ES Tablets 517
Vicodin HP Tablets 518
Vicodin Tuss Expectorant 519
Vicoprofen Tablets 520
Zydone Tablets 1330
Hydrocodone Polistirex (Additive sedative effects). Products include:
Tussionex Pennkinetic Extended-Release Suspension 1174
Hydromorphone Hydrochloride (Additive sedative effects). Products include:
Dilaudid 441
Dilaudid Oral Liquid 445
Dilaudid Powder 441
Dilaudid Rectal Suppositories 441
Dilaudid Tablets 441
Dilaudid Tablets - 8 mg 445
Dilaudid-HP 443
Hydroxyzine Hydrochloride (Additive sedative effects). Products include:
Atarax Tablets & Syrup 2667
Vistaril Intramuscular Solution 2738
Imipramine Hydrochloride (Additive sedative effects).
No products indexed under this heading.
Imipramine Pamoate (Additive sedative effects).
No products indexed under this heading.
Isocarboxazid (Co-administration with MAO inhibitors has resulted in hyperpyrexia, hypotension, and death; concomitant use is contraindicated).
No products indexed under this heading.
Levorphanol Tartrate (Additive sedative effects). Products include:
Levo-Dromoran 1734
Levorphanol Tartrate Tablets 3059
Lorazepam (Additive sedative effects). Products include:
Ativan Injection 3478
Ativan Tablets 3482
Loxapine Hydrochloride (Additive sedative effects).
No products indexed under this heading.
Loxapine Succinate (Additive sedative effects). Products include:
Loxitane Capsules 3398
Maprotiline Hydrochloride (Additive sedative effects).
No products indexed under this heading.
Meperidine Hydrochloride (Additive sedative effects). Products include:
Demerol 3079
Mepergan Injection 3539
Meprobamate (Additive sedative effects). Products include:
Miltown Tablets 3349
Mesoridazine Besylate (Additive sedative effects). Products include:
Serentil 1057
Methadone Hydrochloride (Additive sedative effects). Products include:
Dolophine Hydrochloride Tablets 3056
Midazolam Hydrochloride (Additive sedative effects). Products include:
Versed Injection 3027
Versed Syrup 3033
Moclobemide (Co-administration with MAO inhibitors has resulted in hyperpyrexia, hypotension, and death; concomitant use is contraindicated).
No products indexed under this heading.
Molindone Hydrochloride (Additive sedative effects). Products include:
Moban 1320
Morphine Sulfate (Additive sedative effects). Products include:
Astramorph/PF Injection, USP (Preservative-Free) 594
Duramorph Injection 1312
Infumorph 200 and Infumorph 500 Sterile Solutions 1314
Kadian Capsules 1335
MS Contin Tablets 2896
MSIR 2898
Oramorph SR Tablets 3062
Roxanol 3066
Nortriptyline Hydrochloride (Additive sedative effects).
No products indexed under this heading.
Oxazepam (Additive sedative effects).
No products indexed under this heading.
Oxycodone Hydrochloride (Additive sedative effects). Products include:
OxyContin Tablets 2912
OxyFast Oral Concentrate Solution 2916
OxyIR Capsules 2916
Percocet Tablets 1326
Percodan Tablets 1327
Percolone Tablets 1327
Roxicodone 3067
Tylox Capsules 2597
Pargyline Hydrochloride (Co-administration with MAO inhibitors has resulted in hyperpyrexia, hypotension, and death; concomitant use is contraindicated).
No products indexed under this heading.
Perphenazine (Additive sedative effects). Products include:
Etrafon 3115
Trilafon 3160
Phenelzine Sulfate (Co-administration with MAO inhibitors has resulted in hyperpyrexia, hypotension, and death; concomitant use is contraindicated). Products include:
Nardil Tablets 2653
Prazepam (Additive sedative effects).
No products indexed under this heading.

Procarbazine Hydrochloride (Co-administration with MAO inhibitors has resulted in hyperpyrexia, hypotension, and death; concomitant use is contraindicated). Products include:
- Matulane Capsules 3246

Prochlorperazine (Additive sedative effects). Products include:
- Compazine 1505

Propofol (Additive sedative effects). Products include:
- Diprivan Injectable Emulsion 667

Propoxyphene Hydrochloride (Additive sedative effects). Products include:
- Darvon Pulvules 1909
- Darvon Compound-65 Pulvules 1910

Propoxyphene Napsylate (Additive sedative effects). Products include:
- Darvon-N/Darvocet-N 1907
- Darvon-N Tablets 1912

Protriptyline Hydrochloride (Additive sedative effects). Products include:
- Vivactil Tablets 2446
- Vivactil Tablets 2217

Quazepam (Additive sedative effects).
No products indexed under this heading.

Remifentanil Hydrochloride (Additive sedative effects).
No products indexed under this heading.

Secobarbital Sodium (Additive sedative effects).
No products indexed under this heading.

Selegiline Hydrochloride (Co-administration with MAO inhibitors has resulted in hyperpyrexia, hypotension, and death; concomitant use is contraindicated). Products include:
- Eldepryl Capsules 3266

Sufentanil Citrate (Additive sedative effects).
No products indexed under this heading.

Temazepam (Additive sedative effects).
No products indexed under this heading.

Thioridazine Hydrochloride (Additive sedative effects). Products include:
- Thioridazine Hydrochloride Tablets 2289

Thiothixene (Additive sedative effects). Products include:
- Navane Capsules 2701
- Thiothixene Capsules 2290

Tranylcypromine Sulfate (Co-administration with MAO inhibitors has resulted in hyperpyrexia, hypotension, and death; concomitant use is contraindicated). Products include:
- Parnate Tablets 1607

Triazolam (Additive sedative effects). Products include:
- Halcion Tablets 2823

Trifluoperazine Hydrochloride (Additive sedative effects). Products include:
- Stelazine 1640

Trimipramine Maleate (Additive sedative effects). Products include:
- Surmontil Capsules 3595

Zaleplon (Additive sedative effects). Products include:
- Sonata Capsules 3591

Zolpidem Tartrate (Additive sedative effects). Products include:
- Ambien Tablets 3191

Food Interactions

Alcohol (Additive sedative effects).

PHENERGAN VC SYRUP

(Phenylephrine Hydrochloride, Promethazine Hydrochloride) 3560

May interact with alpha adrenergic blockers, beta blockers, hypnotics and sedatives, monoamine oxidase inhibitors, narcotic analgesics, sympathomimetic bronchodilators, sympathomimetics, tranquilizers, tricyclic antidepressants, and certain other agents. Compounds in these categories include:

Acebutolol Hydrochloride (Cardiostimulating effects blocked). Products include:
- Sectral Capsules 3589

Albuterol (Tachycardia or arrhythmias may occur). Products include:
- Proventil Inhalation Aerosol 3142
- Ventolin Inhalation Aerosol and Refill 1679

Albuterol Sulfate (Tachycardia or arrhythmias may occur). Products include:
- AccuNeb Inhalation Solution 1230
- Combivent Inhalation Aerosol 1041
- DuoNeb Inhalation Solution 1233
- Proventil Inhalation Solution 0.083% 3146
- Proventil Repetabs Tablets 3148
- Proventil Solution for Inhalation 0.5% 3144
- Proventil HFA Inhalation Aerosol 3150
- Ventolin HFA Inhalation Aerosol 3618
- Volmax Extended-Release Tablets 2276

Alfentanil Hydrochloride (Additive sedative effects).
No products indexed under this heading.

Alprazolam (Additive sedative effects). Products include:
- Xanax Tablets 2865

Amitriptyline Hydrochloride (Additive sedative effects; increased pressor response). Products include:
- Etrafon 3115
- Limbitrol 1738

Amoxapine (Additive sedative effects; increased pressor response).
No products indexed under this heading.

Amphetamine Aspartate (Synergistic adrenergic response). Products include:
- Adderall Tablets 3231
- Adderall XR Capsules

Amphetamine Resins (Synergistic adrenergic response).
No products indexed under this heading.

Amphetamine Sulfate (Synergistic adrenergic response). Products include:
- Adderall Tablets 3231
- Adderall XR Capsules

Atenolol (Cardiostimulating effects blocked). Products include:
- Tenoretic Tablets 690
- Tenormin I.V. Injection 692

Atropine Sulfate (Enhanced pressor response; reflex bradycardia blocked). Products include:
- Donnatal 2929
- Donnatal Extentabs 2930
- Motofen Tablets 577
- Prosed/DS Tablets 3268
- Urised Tablets 2876

Betaxolol Hydrochloride (Cardiostimulating effects blocked). Products include:
- Betoptic S Ophthalmic Suspension 537

Bisoprolol Fumarate (Cardiostimulating effects blocked). Products include:
- Zebeta Tablets 1885
- Ziac Tablets 1887

Bitolterol Mesylate (Tachycardia or arrhythmias may occur).
No products indexed under this heading.

Buprenorphine Hydrochloride (Additive sedative effects). Products include:
- Buprenex Injectable 2918

Buspirone Hydrochloride (Additive sedative effects).
No products indexed under this heading.

Carteolol Hydrochloride (Cardiostimulating effects blocked). Products include:
- Carteolol Hydrochloride Ophthalmic Solution USP, 1% .... ⊙258
- Ocupress Ophthalmic Solution, 1% Sterile .... ⊙303

Chlordiazepoxide (Additive sedative effects). Products include:
- Limbitrol 1738

Chlordiazepoxide Hydrochloride (Additive sedative effects). Products include:
- Librium Capsules 1736
- Librium for Injection 1737

Chlorpromazine (Additive sedative effects). Products include:
- Thorazine Suppositories 1656

Chlorpromazine Hydrochloride (Additive sedative effects). Products include:
- Thorazine 1656

Chlorprothixene (Additive sedative effects).
No products indexed under this heading.

Chlorprothixene Hydrochloride (Additive sedative effects).
No products indexed under this heading.

Clomipramine Hydrochloride (Additive sedative effects; increased pressor response).
No products indexed under this heading.

Clorazepate Dipotassium (Additive sedative effects). Products include:
- Tranxene 511

Codeine Phosphate (Additive sedative effects). Products include:
- Phenergan with Codeine Syrup 3557
- Phenergan VC with Codeine Syrup 3561
- Robitussin A-C Syrup 2942
- Robitussin-DAC Syrup 2942
- Ryna-C Liquid .... ▣768
- Soma Compound w/Codeine Tablets 3355
- Tussi-Organidin NR Liquid 3350
- Tussi-Organidin-S NR Liquid 3350
- Tylenol with Codeine 2595

Desipramine Hydrochloride (Additive sedative effects; increased pressor response). Products include:
- Norpramin Tablets 755

Dezocine (Additive sedative effects).
No products indexed under this heading.

Diazepam (Additive sedative effects). Products include:
- Valium Injectable 3026
- Valium Tablets 3047

Dobutamine Hydrochloride (Tachycardia or arrhythmias may occur). Products include:
- Dobutrex Solution Vials 1914

Dopamine Hydrochloride (Tachycardia or arrhythmias may occur).
No products indexed under this heading.

Doxazosin Mesylate (Decreased pressor response). Products include:
- Cardura Tablets 2668

Doxepin Hydrochloride (Additive sedative effects; increased pressor response). Products include:
- Sinequan 2713

Droperidol (Additive sedative effects).
No products indexed under this heading.

Ephedrine Hydrochloride (Tachycardia or arrhythmias may occur). Products include:
- Primatene Tablets .... ▣780

Ephedrine Sulfate (Tachycardia or arrhythmias may occur).
No products indexed under this heading.

Ephedrine Tannate (Tachycardia or arrhythmias may occur). Products include:
- Rynatuss Pediatric Suspension 3353
- Rynatuss Tablets 3353

Epinephrine (Tachycardia or arrhythmias may occur). Products include:
- Epifrin Sterile Ophthalmic Solution .... ⊙235
- EpiPen 1236
- Primatene Mist .... ▣779
- Xylocaine with Epinephrine Injection 653

Epinephrine Bitartrate (Tachycardia or arrhythmias may occur). Products include:
- Sensorcaine 643

Epinephrine Hydrochloride (Tachycardia or arrhythmias may occur).
No products indexed under this heading.

Ergotamine Tartrate (Excessive rise in blood pressure).
No products indexed under this heading.

Esmolol Hydrochloride (Cardiostimulating effects blocked). Products include:
- Brevibloc Injection 858

Estazolam (Additive sedative effects). Products include:
- ProSom Tablets 500

Ethchlorvynol (Additive sedative effects).
No products indexed under this heading.

Ethinamate (Additive sedative effects).
No products indexed under this heading.

Fentanyl (Additive sedative effects). Products include:
- Duragesic Transdermal System 1786

Fentanyl Citrate (Additive sedative effects). Products include:
- Actiq 1184

Fluphenazine Decanoate (Additive sedative effects).
No products indexed under this heading.

Fluphenazine Enanthate (Additive sedative effects).
No products indexed under this heading.

Fluphenazine Hydrochloride (Additive sedative effects).
No products indexed under this heading.

Flurazepam Hydrochloride (Additive sedative effects).
No products indexed under this heading.

Glutethimide (Additive sedative effects).
No products indexed under this heading.

Haloperidol (Additive sedative effects). Products include:
- Haldol Injection, Tablets and Concentrate 2533

Haloperidol Decanoate (Additive sedative effects). Products include:
- Haldol Decanoate 2535

Hydrocodone Bitartrate (Additive sedative effects). Products include:
- Hycodan 1316
- Hycomine Compound Tablets 1317
- Hycotuss Expectorant Syrup 1318
- Lortab 3319
- Lortab Elixir 3317
- Maxidone Tablets CIII 3399
- Norco 5/325 Tablets CIII 3424
- Norco 7.5/325 Tablets CIII 3425
- Norco 10/325 Tablets CIII 3427
- Norco 10/325 Tablets CIII 3425
- Vicodin Tablets 516
- Vicodin ES Tablets 517
- Vicodin HP Tablets 518
- Vicodin Tuss Expectorant 519
- Vicoprofen Tablets 520
- Zydone Tablets 1330

Hydrocodone Polistirex (Additive sedative effects). Products include:

Tussionex Pennkinetic Extended-Release Suspension..... 1174

Hydromorphone Hydrochloride (Additive sedative effects). Products include:
Dilaudid 441
Dilaudid Oral Liquid 445
Dilaudid Powder 441
Dilaudid Rectal Suppositories 441
Dilaudid Tablets 441
Dilaudid Tablets - 8 mg 445
Dilaudid-HP 443

Hydroxyzine Hydrochloride (Additive sedative effects). Products include:
Atarax Tablets & Syrup 2667
Vistaril Intramuscular Solution 2738

Imipramine Hydrochloride (Additive sedative effects; increased pressor response).
No products indexed under this heading.

Imipramine Pamoate (Additive sedative effects; increased pressor response).
No products indexed under this heading.

Isocarboxazid (Acute hypertensive crisis; concurrent use is contraindicated).
No products indexed under this heading.

Isoetharine (Tachycardia or arrhythmias may occur).
No products indexed under this heading.

Isoproterenol Hydrochloride (Tachycardia or arrhythmias may occur).
No products indexed under this heading.

Isoproterenol Sulfate (Tachycardia or arrhythmias may occur).
No products indexed under this heading.

Labetalol Hydrochloride (Cardiostimulating effects blocked). Products include:
Normodyne Injection 3135
Normodyne Tablets 3137

Levalbuterol Hydrochloride (Tachycardia or arrhythmias may occur). Products include:
Xopenex Inhalation Solution 3207

Levobunolol Hydrochloride (Cardiostimulating effects blocked). Products include:
Betagan .... ⊙228

Levorphanol Tartrate (Additive sedative effects). Products include:
Levo-Dromoran 1734
Levorphanol Tartrate Tablets 3059

Lorazepam (Additive sedative effects). Products include:
Ativan Injection 3478
Ativan Tablets 3482

Loxapine Hydrochloride (Additive sedative effects).
No products indexed under this heading.

Loxapine Succinate (Additive sedative effects). Products include:
Loxitane Capsules 3398

Maprotiline Hydrochloride (Additive sedative effects; increased pressor response).
No products indexed under this heading.

Meperidine Hydrochloride (Additive sedative effects). Products include:
Demerol 3079
Mepergan Injection 3539

Meprobamate (Additive sedative effects). Products include:
Miltown Tablets 3349

Mesoridazine Besylate (Additive sedative effects). Products include:
Serentil 1057

Metaproterenol Sulfate (Tachycardia or arrhythmias may occur). Products include:
Alupent 1029

Metaraminol Bitartrate (Tachycardia or arrhythmias may occur). Products include:
Aramine Injection 2043

Methadone Hydrochloride (Additive sedative effects). Products include:
Dolophine Hydrochloride Tablets 3056

Methoxamine Hydrochloride (Tachycardia or arrhythmias may occur).
No products indexed under this heading.

Metipranolol Hydrochloride (Cardiostimulating effects blocked).
No products indexed under this heading.

Metoprolol Succinate (Cardiostimulating effects blocked). Products include:
Toprol-XL Tablets 651

Metoprolol Tartrate (Cardiostimulating effects blocked).
No products indexed under this heading.

Midazolam Hydrochloride (Additive sedative effects). Products include:
Versed Injection 3027
Versed Syrup 3033

Moclobemide (Acute hypertensive crisis; concurrent use is contraindicated).
No products indexed under this heading.

Molindone Hydrochloride (Additive sedative effects). Products include:
Moban 1320

Morphine Sulfate (Additive sedative effects). Products include:
Astramorph/PF Injection, USP (Preservative-Free) 594
Duramorph Injection 1312
Infumorph 200 and Infumorph 500 Sterile Solutions 1314
Kadian Capsules 1335
MS Contin Tablets 2896
MSIR 2898
Oramorph SR Tablets 3062
Roxanol 3066

Nadolol (Cardiostimulating effects blocked). Products include:
Corgard Tablets 2245
Corzide 40/5 Tablets 2247
Corzide 80/5 Tablets 2247
Nadolol Tablets 2288

Norepinephrine Bitartrate (Tachycardia or arrhythmias may occur).
No products indexed under this heading.

Nortriptyline Hydrochloride (Additive sedative effects; increased pressor response).
No products indexed under this heading.

Oxazepam (Additive sedative effects).
No products indexed under this heading.

Oxycodone Hydrochloride (Additive sedative effects). Products include:
OxyContin Tablets 2912
OxyFast Oral Concentrate Solution 2916
OxyIR Capsules 2916
Percocet Tablets 1326
Percodan Tablets 1327
Percolone Tablets 1327
Roxicodone 3067
Tylox Capsules 2597

Pargyline Hydrochloride (Acute hypertensive crisis; concurrent use is contraindicated).
No products indexed under this heading.

Penbutolol Sulfate (Cardiostimulating effects blocked).
No products indexed under this heading.

Perphenazine (Additive sedative effects). Products include:
Etrafon 3115
Trilafon 3160

Phenelzine Sulfate (Acute hypertensive crisis; concurrent use is contraindicated). Products include:
Nardil Tablets 2653

Phentolamine Mesylate (Decreased pressor response).
No products indexed under this heading.

Phenylephrine Bitartrate (Tachycardia or arrhythmias may occur).
No products indexed under this heading.

Phenylephrine Tannate (Tachycardia or arrhythmias may occur). Products include:
Ryna-12 S Suspension 3351
Reformulated Rynatan Pediatric Suspension 3352
Rynatuss Pediatric Suspension 3353
Rynatuss Tablets 3353

Phenylpropanolamine Hydrochloride (Tachycardia or arrhythmias may occur).
No products indexed under this heading.

Pindolol (Cardiostimulating effects blocked).
No products indexed under this heading.

Pirbuterol Acetate (Tachycardia or arrhythmias may occur). Products include:
Maxair Autohaler 1981
Maxair Inhaler 1984

Prazepam (Additive sedative effects).
No products indexed under this heading.

Prazosin Hydrochloride (Decreased pressor response). Products include:
Minipress Capsules 2699
Minizide Capsules 2700

Procarbazine Hydrochloride (Acute hypertensive crisis; concurrent use is contraindicated). Products include:
Matulane Capsules 3246

Prochlorperazine (Additive sedative effects). Products include:
Compazine 1505

Propofol (Additive sedative effects). Products include:
Diprivan Injectable Emulsion 667

Propoxyphene Hydrochloride (Additive sedative effects). Products include:
Darvon Pulvules 1909
Darvon Compound-65 Pulvules 1910

Propoxyphene Napsylate (Additive sedative effects). Products include:
Darvon-N/Darvocet-N 1907
Darvon-N Tablets 1912

Propranolol Hydrochloride (Cardiostimulating effects blocked). Products include:
Inderal 3513
Inderal LA Long-Acting Capsules 3516
Inderide Tablets 3517
Inderide LA Long-Acting Capsules .. 3519

Protriptyline Hydrochloride (Additive sedative effects; increased pressor response). Products include:
Vivactil Tablets 2446
Vivactil Tablets 2217

Pseudoephedrine Hydrochloride (Tachycardia or arrhythmias may occur). Products include:
Actifed Cold & Allergy Tablets ....▣688
Actifed Cold & Sinus Caplets and Tablets .... ▣688
Advil Cold and Sinus Caplets ....▣771
Advil Cold and Sinus Tablets ....▣771
Advil Flu & Body Ache Caplets ....▣772
Aleve Cold & Sinus Caplets ....▣603
Alka-Seltzer Plus Liqui-Gels ....▣604
Alka-Seltzer Plus Cold & Flu Medicine Liqui-Gels ....▣604
Alka-Seltzer Plus Cold & Sinus Medicine Liqui-Gels ....▣604
Allegra-D Extended-Release Tablets 714
BC Cold Powder ....▣619
Benadryl Allergy/Cold Tablets ....▣691
Benadryl Allergy/Congestion Tablets ....▣692
Benadryl Allergy & Sinus Liquid ....▣693
Benadryl Allergy & Sinus Fastmelt Tablets ....▣693
Benadryl Allergy Sinus Headache Caplets & Gelcaps ....▣693
Benadryl Severe Allergy & Sinus Headache Caplets ....▣694
Benadryl Children's Allergy/Cold Fastmelt Tablets ....▣692
Benylin Multi-Symptom Liquid ....▣697
Bromfed Capsules (Extended-Release) 2269
Bromfed-PD Capsules (Extended-Release) 2269
Children's Cēpacol Sore Throat ....▣788
Comtrex Acute Head Cold & Sinus Pressure Relief Tablets ....▣627
Comtrex Deep Chest Cold & Congestion Relief Softgels ....▣627
Comtrex Flu Therapy & Fever Relief Daytime Caplets ....▣628
Comtrex Flu Therapy & Fever Relief Nighttime Tablets ....▣628
Comtrex Maximum Strength Multi-Symptom Cold & Cough Relief Tablets and Caplets ....▣626
Contac Non-Drowsy 12 Hour Cold Caplets ....▣745
Contac Non-Drowsy Timed Release 12 Hour Cold Caplets ...▣746
Contac Severe Cold and Flu Caplets Maximum Strength ....▣746
Contac Severe Cold and Flu Caplets Non-Drowsy ....▣746
Dimetapp Elixir ....▣777
Dimetapp Cold and Fever Suspension ....▣775
Dimetapp DM Cold & Cough Elixir .▣775
Dimetapp Nighttime Flu Liquid ....▣776
Dimetapp Non-Drowsy Flu Syrup ..▣777
Dimetapp Infant Drops Decongestant ....▣775
Dimetapp Infant Drops Decongestant Plus Cough ....▣776
Guaifed 2272
Kronofed-A 1341
Children's Motrin Cold Oral Suspension 2007
Motrin Sinus Headache Caplets 2005
PediaCare Cough-Cold Liquid ....▣719
PediaCare Infants' Drops Decongestant ....▣719
PediaCare Infants' Drops Decongestant Plus Cough ....▣719
PediaCare NightRest Cough-Cold Liquid ....▣719
Robitussin Cold Caplets Cold & Congestion ....▣780
Robitussin Cold Softgels Cold & Congestion ....▣780
Robitussin Cold Caplets Multi-Symptom Cold & Flu ....▣781
Robitussin Cold Softgels Multi-Symptom Cold & Flu ....▣781
Robitussin Cold Softgels Severe Congestion ....▣782
Robitussin Cough & Cold Infant Drops ....▣782
Robitussin Maximum Strength Cough & Cold Liquid ....▣785
Robitussin Pediatric Cough & Cold Formula Liquid ....▣785
Robitussin Multi Symptom Honey Flu Liquid ....▣785
Robitussin Nighttime Honey Flu Liquid ....▣786
Robitussin-CF Liquid ....▣783
Robitussin-DAC Syrup 2942
Robitussin-PE Liquid ....▣782
Ryna ....▣768
Semprex-D Capsules 1172
Singlet Caplets ....▣761
Sinutab Non-Drying Liquid Caps ....▣706
Sinutab Sinus Allergy Medication, Maximum Strength Formula, Tablets & Caplets ....▣707
Sinutab Sinus Medication, Maximum Strength Without Drowsiness Formula, Tablets & Caplets ....▣707
Sudafed 12 Hour Tablets ....▣708
Sudafed 24 Hour Tablets ....▣708
Children's Sudafed Cold & Cough Liquid ....▣709
Children's Sudafed Nasal Decongestant Chewables ....▣711
Children's Sudafed Nasal Decongestant Liquid Medication ....▣711
Sudafed Cold & Allergy Tablets ....▣708
Sudafed Cold & Cough Liquid Caps ....▣709
Sudafed Cold & Sinus Liquid Caps ....▣710

Sudafed Nasal Decongestant Tablets 710
Sudafed Non-Drying Sinus Liquid Caps 712
Sudafed Severe Cold 711
Sudafed Sinus Headache Caplets . 712
Sudafed Sinus Headache Tablets .. 712
Tavist Sinus Non-Drowsy Coated Caplets 676
TheraFlu Regular Strength Cold & Cough Night Time Hot Liquid 676
TheraFlu Regular Strength Cold & Sore Throat Night Time Hot Liquid 676
TheraFlu Maximum Strength Flu & Congestion Non-Drowsy Hot Liquid 677
TheraFlu Maximum Strength Flu & Cough Night Time Hot Liquid .. 678
TheraFlu Maximum Strength Flu & Sore Throat Night Time Hot Liquid 677
TheraFlu Maximum Strength Severe Cold & Congestion Night Time Caplets 678
TheraFlu Maximum Strength Severe Cold & Congestion Night Time Hot Liquid 678
TheraFlu Maximum Strength Severe Cold & Congestion Non-Drowsy 679
Triaminic Allergy Congestion Liquid 680
Triaminic Chest Congestion Liquid 680
Triaminic Cold & Allergy Liquid 681
Triaminic Cold & Allergy Softchews 683
Triaminic Cold & Cough Liquid 681
Triaminic Cold & Cough Softchews 683
Triaminic Cold & Night Time Cough Liquid 681
Triaminic Cold, Cough & Fever Liquid 681
Triaminic Cough Liquid 682
Triaminic Cough & Congestion Liquid 682
Triaminic Cough & Sore Throat Liquid 682
Triaminic Cough & Sore Throat Softchews 684
Children's Tylenol Allergy-D Liquid ... 2014
Children's Tylenol Cold Suspension Liquid and Chewable Tablets 2015
Children's Tylenol Cold Plus Cough Suspension Liquid and Chewable Tablets 2015
Children's Tylenol Flu Suspension Liquid 2015
Children's Tylenol Sinus Suspension Liquid 2017
Infants' Tylenol Cold Decongestant and Fever Reducer Concentrated Drops 2015
Infants' Tylenol Cold Decongestant and Fever Reducer Concentrated Drops Plus Cough .. 2015
Tylenol Allergy Sinus 2010
Multi-Symptom Tylenol Cold Complete Formula Caplets 2010
Multi-Symptom Tylenol Cold Non-Drowsy Caplets and Gelcaps 2010
Multi-Symptom Tylenol Cold Severe Congestion Non-Drowsy Caplets 2011
Maximum Strength Tylenol Flu NightTime Gelcaps 2011
Maximum Strength Tylenol Flu NightTime Liquid 2011
Maximum Strength Tylenol Flu Non-Drowsy Gelcaps 2011
Maximum Strength Tylenol Sinus NightTime Caplets 2012
Maximum Strength Tylenol Sinus Non-Drowsy Geltabs, Gelcaps, Caplets, and Tablets 2012
Vicks 44D Cough & Head Congestion Relief Liquid 724
Vicks 44M Cough, Cold & Flu Relief Liquid 725
Pediatric Vicks 44m Cough & Cold Relief 728
Vicks DayQuil LiquiCaps/Liquid Multi-Symptom Cold/Flu Relief ... 727
Children's Vicks NyQuil Cold/Cough Relief 726
Vicks NyQuil LiquiCaps/Liquid Multi-Symptom Cold/Flu Relief, Original and Cherry Flavors 727
Zephrex Tablets 3091
Zephrex LA Tablets 3092
Zyrtec-D 12 Hour Extended Relief Tablets 2758

Pseudoephedrine Sulfate (Tachycardia or arrhythmias may occur). Products include:
Chlor-Trimeton Allergy/Decongestant Tablets 736
Claritin-D 12 Hour Extended Release Tablets 3102
Claritin-D 24 Hour Extended Release Tablets 3104
Coricidin 'D' Cold, Flu & Sinus Tablets 737
Drixoral Allergy/Sinus Extended-Release Tablets 741
Drixoral Cold & Allergy Sustained-Action Tablets 740
Drixoral Cold & Flu Extended-Release Tablets 740
Drixoral Nasal Decongestant Long-Acting Non-Drowsy Tablets 740
Rynatan Tablets 3351

Quazepam (Additive sedative effects).
No products indexed under this heading.

Remifentanil Hydrochloride (Additive sedative effects).
No products indexed under this heading.

Salmeterol Xinafoate (Tachycardia or arrhythmias may occur). Products include:
Advair Diskus 100/50 1448
Advair Diskus 250/50 1448
Advair Diskus 500/50 1448
Serevent Diskus 1637
Serevent Inhalation Aerosol 1633

Secobarbital Sodium (Additive sedative effects).
No products indexed under this heading.

Selegiline Hydrochloride (Acute hypertensive crisis; concurrent use is contraindicated). Products include:
Eldepryl Capsules 3266

Sotalol Hydrochloride (Cardiostimulating effects blocked). Products include:
Betapace Tablets 950
Betapace AF Tablets 954

Sufentanil Citrate (Additive sedative effects).
No products indexed under this heading.

Temazepam (Additive sedative effects).
No products indexed under this heading.

Terazosin Hydrochloride (Decreased pressor response). Products include:
Hytrin Capsules 464

Terbutaline Sulfate (Tachycardia or arrhythmias may occur). Products include:
Brethine Ampuls 2314
Brethine Tablets 2313

Thioridazine Hydrochloride (Additive sedative effects). Products include:
Thioridazine Hydrochloride Tablets 2289

Thiothixene (Additive sedative effects). Products include:
Navane Capsules 2701
Thiothixene Capsules 2290

Timolol Hemihydrate (Cardiostimulating effects blocked). Products include:
Betimol Ophthalmic Solution .... ⊙ 324

Timolol Maleate (Cardiostimulating effects blocked). Products include:
Blocadren Tablets 2046
Cosopt Sterile Ophthalmic Solution 2065
Timolide Tablets 2187
Timolol GFS .... ⊙ 266
Timoptic in Ocudose 2192
Timoptic Sterile Ophthalmic Solution 2190
Timoptic-XE Sterile Ophthalmic Gel Forming Solution 2194

Tranylcypromine Sulfate (Acute hypertensive crisis; concurrent use is contraindicated). Products include:
Parnate Tablets 1607

Triazolam (Additive sedative effects). Products include:
Halcion Tablets 2823

Trifluoperazine Hydrochloride (Additive sedative effects). Products include:
Stelazine 1640

Trimipramine Maleate (Additive sedative effects; increased pressor response). Products include:
Surmontil Capsules 3595

Zaleplon (Additive sedative effects). Products include:
Sonata Capsules 3591

Zolpidem Tartrate (Additive sedative effects). Products include:
Ambien Tablets 3191

Food Interactions

Alcohol (Additive sedative effects).

PHENERGAN VC WITH CODEINE SYRUP

(Codeine Phosphate, Phenylephrine Hydrochloride, Promethazine Hydrochloride) 3561
May interact with alpha adrenergic blockers, beta blockers, hypnotics and sedatives, monoamine oxidase inhibitors, narcotic analgesics, sympathomimetic bronchodilators, sympathomimetics, tranquilizers, tricyclic antidepressants, and certain other agents. Compounds in these categories include:

Acebutolol Hydrochloride (Cardiostimulating effects blocked). Products include:
Sectral Capsules 3589

Albuterol (Tachycardia or arrhythmias may occur). Products include:
Proventil Inhalation Aerosol 3142
Ventolin Inhalation Aerosol and Refill 1679

Albuterol Sulfate (Tachycardia or arrhythmias may occur). Products include:
AccuNeb Inhalation Solution 1230
Combivent Inhalation Aerosol 1041
DuoNeb Inhalation Solution 1233
Proventil Inhalation Solution 0.083% 3146
Proventil Repetabs Tablets 3148
Proventil Solution for Inhalation 0.5% 3144
Proventil HFA Inhalation Aerosol 3150
Ventolin HFA Inhalation Aerosol 3618
Volmax Extended-Release Tablets .. 2276

Alfentanil Hydrochloride (Additive sedative effects).
No products indexed under this heading.

Alprazolam (Additive sedative effects). Products include:
Xanax Tablets 2865

Amitriptyline Hydrochloride (Additive sedative effects; increased pressor response). Products include:
Etrafon 3115
Limbitrol 1738

Amoxapine (Additive sedative effects; increased pressor response).
No products indexed under this heading.

Atenolol (Cardiostimulating effects blocked). Products include:
Tenoretic Tablets 690
Tenormin I.V. Injection 692

Atropine Sulfate (Enhanced pressor response; reflex bradycardia blocked). Products include:
Donnatal 2929
Donnatal Extentabs 2930
Motofen Tablets 577
Prosed/DS Tablets 3268
Urised Tablets 2876

Betaxolol Hydrochloride (Cardiostimulating effects blocked). Products include:
Betoptic S Ophthalmic Suspension 537

Bisoprolol Fumarate (Cardiostimulating effects blocked). Products include:
Zebeta Tablets 1885
Ziac Tablets 1887

Bitolterol Mesylate (Tachycardia or arrhythmias may occur).
No products indexed under this heading.

Buprenorphine Hydrochloride (Additive sedative effects). Products include:
Buprenex Injectable 2918

Buspirone Hydrochloride (Additive sedative effects).
No products indexed under this heading.

Carteolol Hydrochloride (Cardiostimulating effects blocked). Products include:
Carteolol Hydrochloride Ophthalmic Solution USP, 1% ..... ⊙ 258
Ocupress Ophthalmic Solution, 1% Sterile .... ⊙ 303

Chlordiazepoxide (Additive sedative effects). Products include:
Limbitrol 1738

Chlordiazepoxide Hydrochloride (Additive sedative effects). Products include:
Librium Capsules 1736
Librium for Injection 1737

Chlorpromazine (Additive sedative effects). Products include:
Thorazine Suppositories 1656

Chlorpromazine Hydrochloride (Additive sedative effects). Products include:
Thorazine 1656

Chlorprothixene (Additive sedative effects).
No products indexed under this heading.

Chlorprothixene Hydrochloride (Additive sedative effects).
No products indexed under this heading.

Clomipramine Hydrochloride (Additive sedative effects; increased pressor response).
No products indexed under this heading.

Clorazepate Dipotassium (Additive sedative effects). Products include:
Tranxene 511

Desipramine Hydrochloride (Additive sedative effects; increased pressor response). Products include:
Norpramin Tablets 755

Dezocine (Additive sedative effects).
No products indexed under this heading.

Diazepam (Additive sedative effects). Products include:
Valium Injectable 3026
Valium Tablets 3047

Dobutamine Hydrochloride (Tachycardia or arrhythmias may occur). Products include:
Dobutrex Solution Vials 1914

Dopamine Hydrochloride (Tachycardia or arrhythmias may occur).
No products indexed under this heading.

Doxazosin Mesylate (Pressor response decreased). Products include:
Cardura Tablets 2668

Doxepin Hydrochloride (Additive sedative effects; increased pressor response). Products include:
Sinequan 2713

Droperidol (Additive sedative effects).
No products indexed under this heading.

Ephedrine Hydrochloride (Tachycardia or arrhythmias may occur). Products include:
Primatene Tablets 780

Ephedrine Sulfate (Tachycardia or arrhythmias may occur).
No products indexed under this heading.

Ephedrine Tannate (Tachycardia or arrhythmias may occur). Products include:
Rynatuss Pediatric Suspension 3353
Rynatuss Tablets 3353

Epinephrine (Tachycardia or arrhythmias may occur). Products include:
Epifrin Sterile Ophthalmic Solution ...... ⊙235
EpiPen 1236
Primatene Mist ...... ▣779
Xylocaine with Epinephrine Injection 653

Epinephrine Bitartrate (Tachycardia or arrhythmias may occur). Products include:
Sensorcaine 643

Epinephrine Hydrochloride (Tachycardia or arrhythmias may occur).
No products indexed under this heading.

Ergotamine Tartrate (Excessive rise in blood pressure).
No products indexed under this heading.

Esmolol Hydrochloride (Cardiostimulating effects blocked). Products include:
Brevibloc Injection 858

Estazolam (Additive sedative effects). Products include:
ProSom Tablets 500

Ethchlorvynol (Additive sedative effects).
No products indexed under this heading.

Ethinamate (Additive sedative effects).
No products indexed under this heading.

Fentanyl (Additive sedative effects). Products include:
Duragesic Transdermal System 1786

Fentanyl Citrate (Additive sedative effects). Products include:
Actiq 1184

Fluphenazine Decanoate (Additive sedative effects).
No products indexed under this heading.

Fluphenazine Enanthate (Additive sedative effects).
No products indexed under this heading.

Fluphenazine Hydrochloride (Additive sedative effects).
No products indexed under this heading.

Flurazepam Hydrochloride (Additive sedative effects).
No products indexed under this heading.

Glutethimide (Additive sedative effects).
No products indexed under this heading.

Haloperidol (Additive sedative effects). Products include:
Haldol Injection, Tablets and Concentrate 2533

Haloperidol Decanoate (Additive sedative effects). Products include:
Haldol Decanoate 2535

Hydrocodone Bitartrate (Additive sedative effects). Products include:
Hycodan 1316
Hycomine Compound Tablets 1317
Hycotuss Expectorant Syrup 1318
Lortab 3319
Lortab Elixir 3317
Maxidone Tablets CIII 3399
Norco 5/325 Tablets CIII 3424
Norco 7.5/325 Tablets CIII 3425
Norco 10/325 Tablets CIII 3427
Norco 10/325 Tablets CIII 3425
Vicodin Tablets 516
Vicodin ES Tablets 517
Vicodin HP Tablets 518
Vicodin Tuss Expectorant 519
Vicoprofen Tablets 520
Zydone Tablets 1330

Hydrocodone Polistirex (Additive sedative effects). Products include:
Tussionex Pennkinetic Extended-Release Suspension 1174

Hydromorphone Hydrochloride (Additive sedative effects). Products include:
Dilaudid 441
Dilaudid Oral Liquid 445
Dilaudid Powder 441
Dilaudid Rectal Suppositories 441
Dilaudid Tablets 441
Dilaudid Tablets - 8 mg 445
Dilaudid-HP 443

Hydroxyzine Hydrochloride (Additive sedative effects). Products include:
Atarax Tablets & Syrup 2667
Vistaril Intramuscular Solution 2738

Imipramine Hydrochloride (Additive sedative effects; increased pressor response).
No products indexed under this heading.

Imipramine Pamoate (Additive sedative effects; increased pressor response).
No products indexed under this heading.

Isocarboxazid (Acute hypertensive crisis; concurrent use is contraindicated).
No products indexed under this heading.

Isoetharine (Tachycardia or arrhythmias may occur).
No products indexed under this heading.

Isoproterenol Hydrochloride (Tachycardia or arrhythmias may occur).
No products indexed under this heading.

Isoproterenol Sulfate (Tachycardia or arrhythmias may occur).
No products indexed under this heading.

Labetalol Hydrochloride (Cardiostimulating effects blocked). Products include:
Normodyne Injection 3135
Normodyne Tablets 3137

Levalbuterol Hydrochloride (Tachycardia or arrhythmias may occur). Products include:
Xopenex Inhalation Solution 3207

Levobunolol Hydrochloride (Cardiostimulating effects blocked). Products include:
Betagan ...... ⊙228

Levorphanol Tartrate (Additive sedative effects). Products include:
Levo-Dromoran 1734
Levorphanol Tartrate Tablets 3059

Lorazepam (Additive sedative effects). Products include:
Ativan Injection 3478
Ativan Tablets 3482

Loxapine Hydrochloride (Additive sedative effects).
No products indexed under this heading.

Loxapine Succinate (Additive sedative effects). Products include:
Loxitane Capsules 3398

Maprotiline Hydrochloride (Additive sedative effects; increased pressor response).
No products indexed under this heading.

Meperidine Hydrochloride (Additive sedative effects). Products include:
Demerol 3079
Mepergan Injection 3539

Meprobamate (Additive sedative effects). Products include:
Miltown Tablets 3349

Mesoridazine Besylate (Additive sedative effects). Products include:
Serentil 1057

Metaproterenol Sulfate (Tachycardia or arrhythmias may occur). Products include:
Alupent 1029

Metaraminol Bitartrate (Tachycardia or arrhythmias may occur). Products include:
Aramine Injection 2043

Methadone Hydrochloride (Additive sedative effects). Products include:
Dolophine Hydrochloride Tablets 3056

Methoxamine Hydrochloride (Tachycardia or arrhythmias may occur).
No products indexed under this heading.

Metipranolol Hydrochloride (Cardiostimulating effects blocked).
No products indexed under this heading.

Metoprolol Succinate (Cardiostimulating effects blocked). Products include:
Toprol-XL Tablets 651

Metoprolol Tartrate (Cardiostimulating effects blocked).
No products indexed under this heading.

Midazolam Hydrochloride (Additive sedative effects). Products include:
Versed Injection 3027
Versed Syrup 3033

Moclobemide (Acute hypertensive crisis; concurrent use is contraindicated).
No products indexed under this heading.

Molindone Hydrochloride (Additive sedative effects). Products include:
Moban 1320

Morphine Sulfate (Additive sedative effects). Products include:
Astramorph/PF Injection, USP (Preservative-Free) 594
Duramorph Injection 1312
Infumorph 200 and Infumorph 500 Sterile Solutions 1314
Kadian Capsules 1335
MS Contin Tablets 2896
MSIR 2898
Oramorph SR Tablets 3062
Roxanol 3066

Nadolol (Cardiostimulating effects blocked). Products include:
Corgard Tablets 2245
Corzide 40/5 Tablets 2247
Corzide 80/5 Tablets 2247
Nadolol Tablets 2288

Norepinephrine Bitartrate (Tachycardia or arrhythmias may occur).
No products indexed under this heading.

Nortriptyline Hydrochloride (Additive sedative effects; increased pressor response).
No products indexed under this heading.

Oxazepam (Additive sedative effects).
No products indexed under this heading.

Oxycodone Hydrochloride (Additive sedative effects). Products include:
OxyContin Tablets 2912
OxyFast Oral Concentrate Solution 2916
OxyIR Capsules 2916
Percocet Tablets 1326
Percodan Tablets 1327
Percolone Tablets 1327
Roxicodone 3067
Tylox Capsules 2597

Pargyline Hydrochloride (Acute hypertensive crisis; concurrent use is contraindicated).
No products indexed under this heading.

Penbutolol Sulfate (Cardiostimulating effects blocked).
No products indexed under this heading.

Perphenazine (Additive sedative effects). Products include:
Etrafon 3115
Trilafon 3160

Phenelzine Sulfate (Acute hypertensive crisis; concurrent use is contraindicated). Products include:
Nardil Tablets 2653

Phentolamine Mesylate (Decreased pressor response).
No products indexed under this heading.

Phenylephrine Bitartrate (Tachycardia or arrhythmias may occur).
No products indexed under this heading.

Phenylephrine Tannate (Tachycardia or arrhythmias may occur). Products include:
Ryna-12 S Suspension 3351
Reformulated Rynatan Pediatric Suspension 3352
Rynatuss Pediatric Suspension 3353
Rynatuss Tablets 3353

Phenylpropanolamine Hydrochloride (Tachycardia or arrhythmias may occur).
No products indexed under this heading.

Pindolol (Cardiostimulating effects blocked).
No products indexed under this heading.

Pirbuterol Acetate (Tachycardia or arrhythmias may occur). Products include:
Maxair Autohaler 1981
Maxair Inhaler 1984

Prazepam (Additive sedative effects).
No products indexed under this heading.

Prazosin Hydrochloride (Pressor response decreased). Products include:
Minipress Capsules 2699
Minizide Capsules 2700

Procarbazine Hydrochloride (Acute hypertensive crisis; concurrent use is contraindicated). Products include:
Matulane Capsules 3246

Prochlorperazine (Additive sedative effects). Products include:
Compazine 1505

Propofol (Additive sedative effects). Products include:
Diprivan Injectable Emulsion 667

Propoxyphene Hydrochloride (Additive sedative effects). Products include:
Darvon Pulvules 1909
Darvon Compound-65 Pulvules 1910

Propoxyphene Napsylate (Additive sedative effects). Products include:
Darvon-N/Darvocet-N 1907
Darvon-N Tablets 1912

Propranolol Hydrochloride (Cardiostimulating effects blocked). Products include:
Inderal 3513
Inderal LA Long-Acting Capsules 3516
Inderide Tablets 3517
Inderide LA Long-Acting Capsules 3519

Protriptyline Hydrochloride (Additive sedative effects; increased pressor response). Products include:
Vivactil Tablets 2446
Vivactil Tablets 2217

Pseudoephedrine Hydrochloride (Tachycardia or arrhythmias may occur). Products include:
Actifed Cold & Allergy Tablets ...... ▣688
Actifed Cold & Sinus Caplets and Tablets ...... ▣688
Advil Cold and Sinus Caplets ...... ▣771
Advil Cold and Sinus Tablets ...... ▣771
Advil Flu & Body Ache Caplets ...... ▣772
Aleve Cold & Sinus Caplets ...... ▣603
Alka-Seltzer Plus Liqui-Gels ...... ▣604
Alka-Seltzer Plus Cold & Flu Medicine Liqui-Gels ...... ▣604
Alka-Seltzer Plus Cold & Sinus Medicine Liqui-Gels ...... ▣604
Allegra-D Extended-Release Tablets 714
BC Cold Powder ...... ▣619
Benadryl Allergy/Cold Tablets ...... ▣691

Benadryl Allergy/Congestion Tablets ... 692
Benadryl Allergy & Sinus Liquid ... 693
Benadryl Allergy & Sinus Fastmelt Tablets ... 693
Benadryl Allergy Sinus Headache Caplets & Gelcaps ... 693
Benadryl Severe Allergy & Sinus Headache Caplets ... 694
Benadryl Children's Allergy/Cold Fastmelt Tablets ... 692
Benylin Multi-Symptom Liquid ... 697
Bromfed Capsules (Extended-Release) ... 2269
Bromfed-PD Capsules (Extended-Release) ... 2269
Children's Cēpacol Sore Throat ... 788
Comtrex Acute Head Cold & Sinus Pressure Relief Tablets ... 627
Comtrex Deep Chest Cold & Congestion Relief Softgels ... 627
Comtrex Flu Therapy & Fever Relief Daytime Caplets ... 628
Comtrex Flu Therapy & Fever Relief Nighttime Tablets ... 628
Comtrex Maximum Strength Multi-Symptom Cold & Cough Relief Tablets and Caplets ... 626
Contac Non-Drowsy 12 Hour Cold Caplets ... 745
Contac Non-Drowsy Timed Release 12 Hour Cold Caplets ... 746
Contac Severe Cold and Flu Caplets Maximum Strength ... 746
Contac Severe Cold and Flu Caplets Non-Drowsy ... 746
Dimetapp Elixir ... 777
Dimetapp Cold and Fever Suspension ... 775
Dimetapp DM Cold & Cough Elixir ... 775
Dimetapp Nighttime Flu Liquid ... 776
Dimetapp Non-Drowsy Flu Syrup ... 777
Dimetapp Infant Drops Decongestant ... 775
Dimetapp Infant Drops Decongestant Plus Cough ... 776
Guaifed ... 2272
Kronofed-A ... 1341
Children's Motrin Cold Oral Suspension ... 2007
Motrin Sinus Headache Caplets ... 2005
PediaCare Cough-Cold Liquid ... 719
PediaCare Infants' Drops Decongestant ... 719
PediaCare Infants' Drops Decongestant Plus Cough ... 719
PediaCare NightRest Cough-Cold Liquid ... 719
Robitussin Cold Caplets Cold & Congestion ... 780
Robitussin Cold Softgels Cold & Congestion ... 780
Robitussin Cold Caplets Multi-Symptom Cold & Flu ... 781
Robitussin Cold Softgels Multi-Symptom Cold & Flu ... 781
Robitussin Cold Softgels Severe Congestion ... 782
Robitussin Cough & Cold Infant Drops ... 782
Robitussin Maximum Strength Cough & Cold Liquid ... 785
Robitussin Pediatric Cough & Cold Formula Liquid ... 785
Robitussin Multi Symptom Honey Flu Liquid ... 785
Robitussin Nighttime Honey Flu Liquid ... 786
Robitussin-CF Liquid ... 783
Robitussin-DAC Syrup ... 2942
Robitussin-PE Liquid ... 782
Ryna ... 768
Semprex-D Capsules ... 1172
Singlet Caplets ... 761
Sinutab Non-Drying Liquid Caps ... 706
Sinutab Sinus Allergy Medication, Maximum Strength Formula, Tablets & Caplets ... 707
Sinutab Sinus Medication, Maximum Strength Without Drowsiness Formula, Tablets & Caplets ... 707
Sudafed 12 Hour Tablets ... 708
Sudafed 24 Hour Tablets ... 708
Children's Sudafed Cold & Cough Liquid ... 709
Children's Sudafed Nasal Decongestant Chewables ... 711
Children's Sudafed Nasal Decongestant Liquid Medication ... 711
Sudafed Cold & Allergy Tablets ... 708
Sudafed Cold & Cough Liquid Caps ... 709
Sudafed Cold & Sinus Liquid Caps ... 710
Sudafed Nasal Decongestant Tablets ... 710
Sudafed Non-Drying Sinus Liquid Caps ... 712
Sudafed Severe Cold ... 711
Sudafed Sinus Headache Caplets ... 712
Sudafed Sinus Headache Tablets ... 712
Tavist Sinus Non-Drowsy Coated Caplets ... 676
TheraFlu Regular Strength Cold & Cough Night Time Hot Liquid ... 676
TheraFlu Regular Strength Cold & Sore Throat Night Time Hot Liquid ... 676
TheraFlu Maximum Strength Flu & Congestion Non-Drowsy Hot Liquid ... 677
TheraFlu Maximum Strength Flu & Cough Night Time Hot Liquid ... 678
TheraFlu Maximum Strength Flu & Sore Throat Night Time Hot Liquid ... 677
TheraFlu Maximum Strength Severe Cold & Congestion Night Time Caplets ... 678
TheraFlu Maximum Strength Severe Cold & Congestion Night Time Hot Liquid ... 678
TheraFlu Maximum Strength Severe Cold & Congestion Non-Drowsy ... 679
Triaminic Allergy Congestion Liquid ... 680
Triaminic Chest Congestion Liquid ... 680
Triaminic Cold & Allergy Liquid ... 681
Triaminic Cold & Allergy Softchews ... 683
Triaminic Cold & Cough Liquid ... 681
Triaminic Cold & Cough Softchews ... 683
Triaminic Cold & Night Time Cough Liquid ... 681
Triaminic Cold, Cough & Fever Liquid ... 681
Triaminic Cough Liquid ... 682
Triaminic Cough & Congestion Liquid ... 682
Triaminic Cough & Sore Throat Liquid ... 682
Triaminic Cough & Sore Throat Softchews ... 684
Children's Tylenol Allergy-D Liquid ... 2014
Children's Tylenol Cold Suspension Liquid and Chewable Tablets ... 2015
Children's Tylenol Cold Plus Cough Suspension Liquid and Chewable Tablets ... 2015
Children's Tylenol Flu Suspension Liquid ... 2015
Children's Tylenol Sinus Suspension Liquid ... 2017
Infants' Tylenol Cold Decongestant and Fever Reducer Concentrated Drops ... 2015
Infants' Tylenol Cold Decongestant and Fever Reducer Concentrated Drops Plus Cough ... 2015
Tylenol Allergy Sinus ... 2010
Multi-Symptom Tylenol Cold Complete Formula Caplets ... 2010
Multi-Symptom Tylenol Cold Non-Drowsy Caplets and Gelcaps ... 2010
Multi-Symptom Tylenol Cold Severe Congestion Non-Drowsy Caplets ... 2011
Maximum Strength Tylenol Flu NightTime Gelcaps ... 2011
Maximum Strength Tylenol Flu NightTime Liquid ... 2011
Maximum Strength Tylenol Flu Non-Drowsy Gelcaps ... 2011
Maximum Strength Tylenol Sinus NightTime Caplets ... 2012
Maximum Strength Tylenol Sinus Non-Drowsy Geltabs, Gelcaps, Caplets, and Tablets ... 2012
Vicks 44D Cough & Head Congestion Relief Liquid ... 724
Vicks 44M Cough, Cold & Flu Relief Liquid ... 725
Pediatric Vicks 44m Cough & Cold Relief ... 728
Vicks DayQuil LiquiCaps/Liquid Multi-Symptom Cold/Flu Relief ... 727
Children's Vicks NyQuil Cold/Cough Relief ... 726
Vicks NyQuil LiquiCaps/Liquid Multi-Symptom Cold/Flu Relief, Original and Cherry Flavors ... 727
Zephrex Tablets ... 3091
Zephrex LA Tablets ... 3092
Zyrtec-D 12 Hour Extended Relief Tablets ... 2758

Pseudoephedrine Sulfate (Tachycardia or arrhythmias may occur). Products include:
Chlor-Trimeton Allergy/Decongestant Tablets ... 736
Claritin-D 12 Hour Extended Release Tablets ... 3102
Claritin-D 24 Hour Extended Release Tablets ... 3104
Coricidin 'D' Cold, Flu & Sinus Tablets ... 737
Drixoral Allergy/Sinus Extended-Release Tablets ... 741
Drixoral Cold & Allergy Sustained-Action Tablets ... 740
Drixoral Cold & Flu Extended-Release Tablets ... 740
Drixoral Nasal Decongestant Long-Acting Non-Drowsy Tablets ... 740
Rynatan Tablets ... 3351

Quazepam (Additive sedative effects).
No products indexed under this heading.

Remifentanil Hydrochloride (Additive sedative effects).
No products indexed under this heading.

Salmeterol Xinafoate (Tachycardia or arrhythmias may occur). Products include:
Advair Diskus 100/50 ... 1448
Advair Diskus 250/50 ... 1448
Advair Diskus 500/50 ... 1448
Serevent Diskus ... 1637
Serevent Inhalation Aerosol ... 1633

Secobarbital Sodium (Additive sedative effects).
No products indexed under this heading.

Selegiline Hydrochloride (Acute hypertensive crisis; concurrent use is contraindicated). Products include:
Eldepryl Capsules ... 3266

Sotalol Hydrochloride (Cardiostimulating effects blocked). Products include:
Betapace Tablets ... 950
Betapace AF Tablets ... 954

Sufentanil Citrate (Additive sedative effects).
No products indexed under this heading.

Temazepam (Additive sedative effects).
No products indexed under this heading.

Terazosin Hydrochloride (Pressor response decreased). Products include:
Hytrin Capsules ... 464

Terbutaline Sulfate (Tachycardia or arrhythmias may occur). Products include:
Brethine Ampuls ... 2314
Brethine Tablets ... 2313

Thioridazine Hydrochloride (Additive sedative effects). Products include:
Thioridazine Hydrochloride Tablets ... 2289

Thiothixene (Additive sedative effects). Products include:
Navane Capsules ... 2701
Thiothixene Capsules ... 2290

Timolol Hemihydrate (Cardiostimulating effects blocked). Products include:
Betimol Ophthalmic Solution ... ⊙324

Timolol Maleate (Cardiostimulating effects blocked). Products include:
Blocadren Tablets ... 2046
Cosopt Sterile Ophthalmic Solution ... 2065
Timolide Tablets ... 2187
Timolol GFS ... ⊙266
Timoptic in Ocudose ... 2192
Timoptic Sterile Ophthalmic Solution ... 2190
Timoptic-XE Sterile Ophthalmic Gel Forming Solution ... 2194

Tranylcypromine Sulfate (Acute hypertensive crisis; concurrent use is contraindicated). Products include:
Parnate Tablets ... 1607

Triazolam (Additive sedative effects). Products include:
Halcion Tablets ... 2823

Trifluoperazine Hydrochloride (Additive sedative effects). Products include:
Stelazine ... 1640

Trimipramine Maleate (Additive sedative effects; increased pressor response). Products include:
Surmontil Capsules ... 3595

Zaleplon (Additive sedative effects). Products include:
Sonata Capsules ... 3591

Zolpidem Tartrate (Additive sedative effects). Products include:
Ambien Tablets ... 3191

Food Interactions

Alcohol (Additive sedative effects).

PHILLIPS' CHEWABLE TABLETS

(Magnesium Hydroxide) ... 615
May interact with:

Prescription Drugs, unspecified (Antacids may interact with certain unspecified prescription drugs).

PHILLIPS' FIBERCAPS CAPLETS

(Calcium Polycarbophil) ... 615
May interact with tetracyclines. Compounds in these categories include:

Demeclocycline Hydrochloride (Phillips' Fibercaps contains calcium, which may impair oral absorption of tetracycline; take at least one hour before or two hours after taking tetracycline). Products include:
Declomycin Tablets ... 1855

Doxycycline Calcium (Phillips' Fibercaps contains calcium, which may impair oral absorption of tetracycline; take at least one hour before or two hours after taking tetracycline). Products include:
Vibramycin Calcium Oral Suspension Syrup ... 2735

Doxycycline Hyclate (Phillips' Fibercaps contains calcium, which may impair oral absorption of tetracycline; take at least one hour before or two hours after taking tetracycline). Products include:
Doryx Coated Pellet Filled Capsules ... 3357
Periostat Tablets ... 1208
Vibramycin Hyclate Capsules ... 2735
Vibramycin Hyclate Intravenous ... 2737
Vibra-Tabs Film Coated Tablets ... 2735

Doxycycline Monohydrate (Phillips' Fibercaps contains calcium, which may impair oral absorption of tetracycline; take at least one hour before or two hours after taking tetracycline). Products include:
Monodox Capsules ... 2442
Vibramycin Monohydrate for Oral Suspension ... 2735

Methacycline Hydrochloride (Phillips' Fibercaps contains calcium, which may impair oral absorption of tetracycline; take at least one hour before or two hours after taking tetracycline).
No products indexed under this heading.

Minocycline Hydrochloride (Phillips' Fibercaps contains calcium, which may impair oral absorption of tetracycline; take at least one hour before or two hours after taking tetracycline). Products include:
Dynacin Capsules ... 2019
Minocin Intravenous ... 1862
Minocin Oral Suspension ... 1865
Minocin Pellet-Filled Capsules ... 1863

Oxytetracycline Hydrochloride (Phillips' Fibercaps contains calcium, which may impair oral absorption of

tetracycline; take at least one hour before or two hours after taking tetracycline). Products include:

- Terra-Cortril Ophthalmic Suspension ... 2716
- Urobiotic-250 Capsules ... 2731

Tetracycline Hydrochloride (Phillips' Fibercaps contains calcium, which may impair oral absorption of tetracycline; take at least one hour before or two hours after taking tetracycline).

No products indexed under this heading.

PHILLIPS' LIQUI-GELS

(Docusate Sodium) ... ■616

May interact with:

Mineral Oil (Concurrent oral use is not recommended). Products include:

- Anusol Ointment ... ■688
- Fleet Mineral Oil Enema ... 1360
- Lubriderm Advanced Therapy Creamy Lotion ... ■703
- Lubriderm Seriously Sensitive Lotion ... ■703
- Lubriderm Skin Therapy Moisturizing Lotion ... ■703
- Moisture Eyes PM Preservative Free Eye Ointment ... ⊙253
- Preparation H Ointment ... ■778
- Refresh P.M. Lubricant Eye Ointment ... ⊙251

PHILLIPS' MILK OF MAGNESIA LIQUID (ORIGINAL, CHERRY, & MINT)

(Magnesium Hydroxide) ... ■616

May interact with:

Prescription Drugs, unspecified (Antacids may interact with certain unspecified prescription drugs).

PHOSCHOL CONCENTRATE

(Phosphatidylcholine) ... 579

None cited in PDR database.

PHOSCHOL 900 SOFTGELS

(Phosphatidylcholine) ... 579

None cited in PDR database.

PHOSLO GELCAPS

(Calcium Acetate) ... 1069

See PhosLo Tablets

PHOSLO TABLETS

(Calcium Acetate) ... 1069

May interact with calcium preparations, cardiac glycosides, tetracyclines, and certain other agents. Compounds in these categories include:

Antacids, unspecified (Concurrent use should be avoided).

Calcium Carbonate (Potential for increased risk of hypercalcemia; concurrent use with other calcium supplements is not recommended). Products include:

- Aspirin Regimen Bayer 81 mg Caplets with Calcium ... ■607
- Extra Strength Bayer Plus Caplets ... ■610
- Caltrate 600 Tablets ... ■814
- Caltrate 600 PLUS ... ■815
- Caltrate 600 + D Tablets ... ■814
- Caltrate 600 + Soy Tablets ... ■814
- D-Cal Chewable Caplets ... ■794
- Florical Capsules and Tablets ... 2223
- Quick Dissolve Maalox Max Maximum Strength Antacid/Antigas Tablets ... 2301
- Quick Dissolve Maalox Regular Strength Antacid Tablets ... 2301
- Marblen Suspension ... ■633
- Monocal Tablets ... 2223
- Mylanta Fast-Acting ... 1813
- Mylanta Calci Tabs ... ■636
- One-A-Day Bedtime & Rest Tablets ... ■805
- One-A-Day Calcium Plus Chewable Tablets ... ■805
- Os-Cal Chewable Tablets ... ■838
- Pepcid Complete Chewable Tablets ... 1815
- ReSource Wellness CalciWise Soft Chews ... ■824
- Rolaids Tablets ... ■706
- Extra Strength Rolaids Tablets ... ■706
- Slow-Mag Tablets ... ■835
- Titralac ... ■640
- 3M Titralac Plus Antacid Tablets ... ■640
- Tums ... ■763

Calcium Chloride (Potential for increased risk of hypercalcemia; concurrent use with other calcium supplements is not recommended).

No products indexed under this heading.

Calcium Citrate (Potential for increased risk of hypercalcemia; concurrent use with other calcium supplements is not recommended). Products include:

- Active Calcium Tablets ... 3335
- Citracal Liquitab Tablets ... ■823
- Citracal Tablets ... 2231
- Citracal Caplets + D ... ■823

Calcium Glubionate (Potential for increased risk of hypercalcemia; concurrent use with other calcium supplements is not recommended).

No products indexed under this heading.

Demeclocycline Hydrochloride (Bioavailability of oral tetracyclines may be decreased). Products include:

- Declomycin Tablets ... 1855

Deslanoside (Hypercalcemia may precipitate cardiac arrhythmia).

No products indexed under this heading.

Digitoxin (Hypercalcemia may precipitate cardiac arrhythmia).

No products indexed under this heading.

Digoxin (Hypercalcemia may precipitate cardiac arrhythmia). Products include:

- Digitek Tablets ... 1003
- Lanoxicaps Capsules ... 1574
- Lanoxin Injection ... 1581
- Lanoxin Tablets ... 1587
- Lanoxin Elixir Pediatric ... 1578
- Lanoxin Injection Pediatric ... 1584

Doxycycline Calcium (Bioavailability of oral tetracyclines may be decreased). Products include:

- Vibramycin Calcium Oral Suspension Syrup ... 2735

Doxycycline Hyclate (Bioavailability of oral tetracyclines may be decreased). Products include:

- Doryx Coated Pellet Filled Capsules ... 3357
- Periostat Tablets ... 1208
- Vibramycin Hyclate Capsules ... 2735
- Vibramycin Hyclate Intravenous ... 2737
- Vibra-Tabs Film Coated Tablets ... 2735

Doxycycline Monohydrate (Bioavailability of oral tetracyclines may be decreased). Products include:

- Monodox Capsules ... 2442
- Vibramycin Monohydrate for Oral Suspension ... 2735

Methacycline Hydrochloride (Bioavailability of oral tetracyclines may be decreased).

No products indexed under this heading.

Minocycline Hydrochloride (Bioavailability of oral tetracyclines may be decreased). Products include:

- Dynacin Capsules ... 2019
- Minocin Intravenous ... 1862
- Minocin Oral Suspension ... 1865
- Minocin Pellet-Filled Capsules ... 1863

Oxytetracycline Hydrochloride (Bioavailability of oral tetracyclines may be decreased). Products include:

- Terra-Cortril Ophthalmic Suspension ... 2716
- Urobiotic-250 Capsules ... 2731

Tetracycline Hydrochloride (Bioavailability of oral tetracyclines may be decreased).

No products indexed under this heading.

PHOTOFRIN FOR INJECTION

(Porfimer Sodium) ... 831

May interact with calcium channel blockers, glucocorticoids, drugs known to be photosensitizers, inhibitors of endogenous prostaglandin synthesis, and certain other agents. Compounds in these categories include:

Alatrofloxacin Mesylate (Co-administration with other photosensitizing agents could increase the photosensitivity reactions). Products include:

- Trovan I.V. ... 2722

Allopurinol (Could interfere with porfimer photodynamic therapy).

No products indexed under this heading.

Amlodipine Besylate (Could interfere with porfimer photodynamic therapy). Products include:

- Lotrel Capsules ... 2370
- Norvasc Tablets ... 2704

Aspirin (Some prostaglandin synthesis inhibitors could interfere with porfimer photodynamic therapy). Products include:

- Aggrenox Capsules ... 1026
- Alka-Seltzer ... ■603
- Alka-Seltzer Lemon Lime Antacid and Pain Reliever Effervescent Tablets ... ■603
- Alka-Seltzer Extra Strength Antacid and Pain Reliever Effervescent Tablets ... ■603
- Alka-Seltzer PM Effervescent Tablets ... ■605
- Genuine Bayer Tablets, Caplets and Gelcaps ... ■606
- Extra Strength Bayer Caplets and Gelcaps ... ■610
- Aspirin Regimen Bayer Children's Chewable Tablets (Orange or Cherry Flavored) ... ■607
- Bayer, Aspirin Regimen ... ■606
- Aspirin Regimen Bayer 81 mg Caplets with Calcium ... ■607
- Genuine Bayer Professional Labeling (Aspirin Regimen Bayer) ... ■608
- Extra Strength Bayer Arthritis Caplets ... ■610
- Extra Strength Bayer Plus Caplets ... ■610
- Extra Strength Bayer PM Caplets ... ■611
- BC Powder ... ■619
- BC Allergy Sinus Cold Powder ... ■619
- Arthritis Strength BC Powder ... ■619
- BC Sinus Cold Powder ... ■619
- Darvon Compound-65 Pulvules ... 1910
- Ecotrin Enteric Coated Aspirin Low, Regular and Maximum Strength Tablets ... 1715
- Excedrin Extra-Strength Tablets, Caplets, and Geltabs ... ■629
- Excedrin Migraine ... 1070
- Goody's Body Pain Formula Powder ... ■620
- Goody's Extra Strength Headache Powder ... ■620
- Goody's Extra Strength Pain Relief Tablets ... ■620
- Percodan Tablets ... 1327
- Robaxisal Tablets ... 2939
- Soma Compound Tablets ... 3354
- Soma Compound w/Codeine Tablets ... 3355
- Vanquish Caplets ... ■617

Bendroflumethiazide (Co-administration with other photosensitizing agents could increase the photosensitivity reactions). Products include:

- Corzide 40/5 Tablets ... 2247
- Corzide 80/5 Tablets ... 2247

Bepridil Hydrochloride (Could interfere with porfimer photodynamic therapy). Products include:

- Vascor Tablets ... 2602

Beta-Carotene (Compounds that quench active oxygen species or scavenge radicals, such as b-carotene, would be expected to decrease photodynamic therapy; no human data available to support or rebut this possibility).

No products indexed under this heading.

Betamethasone Acetate (Glucocorticoid hormone given before or concomitantly with photodynamic therapy may decrease the efficacy of the treatment). Products include:

- Celestone Soluspan Injectable Suspension ... 3097

Betamethasone Sodium Phosphate (Glucocorticoid hormone given before or concomitantly with photodynamic therapy may decrease the efficacy of the treatment). Products include:

- Celestone Soluspan Injectable Suspension ... 3097

Celecoxib (Some prostaglandin synthesis inhibitors could interfere with porfimer photodynamic therapy). Products include:

- Celebrex Capsules ... 2676
- Celebrex Capsules ... 2780

Chlorothiazide (Co-administration with other photosensitizing agents could increase the photosensitivity reactions). Products include:

- Aldoclor Tablets ... 2035
- Diuril Oral ... 2087

Chlorothiazide Sodium (Co-administration with other photosensitizing agents could increase the photosensitivity reactions). Products include:

- Diuril Sodium Intravenous ... 2086

Chlorpromazine (Co-administration with other photosensitizing agents could increase the photosensitivity reactions). Products include:

- Thorazine Suppositories ... 1656

Chlorpromazine Hydrochloride (Co-administration with other photosensitizing agents could increase the photosensitivity reactions). Products include:

- Thorazine ... 1656

Chlorpropamide (Co-administration with other photosensitizing agents could increase the photosensitivity reactions). Products include:

- Diabinese Tablets ... 2680

Ciprofloxacin (Co-administration with other photosensitizing agents could increase the photosensitivity reactions). Products include:

- Cipro I.V. ... 893
- Cipro I.V. Pharmacy Bulk Package ... 897
- Cipro Oral Suspension ... 887

Ciprofloxacin Hydrochloride (Co-administration with other photosensitizing agents could increase the photosensitivity reactions). Products include:

- Ciloxan ... 538
- Cipro HC Otic Suspension ... 540
- Cipro Tablets ... 887

Cortisone Acetate (Glucocorticoid hormone given before or concomitantly with photodynamic therapy may decrease the efficacy of the treatment). Products include:

- Cortone Acetate Injectable Suspension ... 2059
- Cortone Acetate Tablets ... 2061

Demeclocycline Hydrochloride (Co-administration with other photosensitizing agents could increase the photosensitivity reactions). Products include:

- Declomycin Tablets ... 1855

Dexamethasone (Glucocorticoid hormone given before or concomitantly with photodynamic therapy may decrease the efficacy of the treatment). Products include:

- Decadron Elixir ... 2078
- Decadron Tablets ... 2079
- TobraDex Ophthalmic Ointment ... 542
- TobraDex Ophthalmic Suspension ... 541

Dexamethasone Acetate (Glucocorticoid hormone given before or concomitantly with photodynamic

therapy may decrease the efficacy of the treatment).
No products indexed under this heading.

Dexamethasone Sodium Phosphate (Glucocorticoid hormone given before or concomitantly with photodynamic therapy may decrease the efficacy of the treatment). Products include:
- Decadron Phosphate Injection 2081
- Decadron Phosphate Sterile Ophthalmic Ointment 2083
- Decadron Phosphate Sterile Ophthalmic Solution 2084
- NeoDecadron Sterile Ophthalmic Solution 2144

Diclofenac Potassium (Some prostaglandin synthesis inhibitors could interfere with porfimer photodynamic therapy). Products include:
- Cataflam Tablets 2315

Diclofenac Sodium (Some prostaglandin synthesis inhibitors could interfere with porfimer photodynamic therapy). Products include:
- Arthrotec Tablets 3195
- Voltaren Ophthalmic Sterile Ophthalmic Solution .... ⊙ 312
- Voltaren Tablets 2315
- Voltaren-XR Tablets 2315

Diltiazem Hydrochloride (Could interfere with porfimer photodynamic therapy). Products include:
- Cardizem Injectable 1018
- Cardizem Lyo-Ject Syringe 1018
- Cardizem Monovial 1018
- Cardizem CD Capsules 1016
- Tiazac Capsules 1378

Dimethyl Sulfoxide (Compounds that quench active oxygen species or scavenge radicals, such as DMSO, would be expected to decrease photodynamic therapy; no human data available to support or rebut this possibility). Products include:
- Rimso-50 Solution 1267

Doxycycline Calcium (Co-administration with other photosensitizing agents could increase the photosensitivity reactions). Products include:
- Vibramycin Calcium Oral Suspension Syrup 2735

Doxycycline Hyclate (Co-administration with other photosensitizing agents could increase the photosensitivity reactions). Products include:
- Doryx Coated Pellet Filled Capsules 3357
- Periostat Tablets 1208
- Vibramycin Hyclate Capsules 2735
- Vibramycin Hyclate Intravenous 2737
- Vibra-Tabs Film Coated Tablets 2735

Doxycycline Monohydrate (Co-administration with other photosensitizing agents could increase the photosensitivity reactions). Products include:
- Monodox Capsules 2442
- Vibramycin Monohydrate for Oral Suspension 2735

Enoxacin (Co-administration with other photosensitizing agents could increase the photosensitivity reactions).
No products indexed under this heading.

Felodipine (Could interfere with porfimer photodynamic therapy). Products include:
- Lexxel Tablets 608
- Plendil Extended-Release Tablets ... 623

Fenoprofen Calcium (Some prostaglandin synthesis inhibitors could interfere with porfimer photodynamic therapy).
No products indexed under this heading.

Fludrocortisone Acetate (Glucocorticoid hormone given before or concomitantly with photodynamic therapy may decrease the efficacy of the treatment). Products include:
- Florinef Acetate Tablets 2250

Fluphenazine Decanoate (Co-administration with other photosensitizing agents could increase the photosensitivity reactions).
No products indexed under this heading.

Fluphenazine Enanthate (Co-administration with other photosensitizing agents could increase the photosensitivity reactions).
No products indexed under this heading.

Fluphenazine Hydrochloride (Co-administration with other photosensitizing agents could increase the photosensitivity reactions).
No products indexed under this heading.

Flurbiprofen (Some prostaglandin synthesis inhibitors could interfere with porfimer photodynamic therapy).
No products indexed under this heading.

Glipizide (Co-administration with other photosensitizing agents could increase the photosensitivity reactions). Products include:
- Glucotrol Tablets 2692
- Glucotrol XL Extended Release Tablets 2693

Glyburide (Co-administration with other photosensitizing agents could increase the photosensitivity reactions). Products include:
- DiaBeta Tablets 741
- Glucovance Tablets 1086

Grepafloxacin Hydrochloride (Co-administration with other photosensitizing agents could increase the photosensitivity reactions).
No products indexed under this heading.

Griseofulvin (Co-administration with other photosensitizing agents could increase the photosensitivity reactions). Products include:
- Grifulvin V Tablets Microsize and Oral Suspension Microsize 2518
- Gris-PEG Tablets 2661

Hydrochlorothiazide (Co-administration with other photosensitizing agents could increase the photosensitivity reactions). Products include:
- Accuretic Tablets 2614
- Aldoril Tablets 2039
- Atacand HCT Tablets 597
- Avalide Tablets 1070
- Diovan HCT Tablets 2338
- Dyazide Capsules 1515
- HydroDIURIL Tablets 2108
- Hyzaar 2109
- Inderide Tablets 3517
- Inderide LA Long-Acting Capsules .. 3519
- Lotensin HCT Tablets 2367
- Maxzide 1008
- Micardis HCT Tablets 1051
- Microzide Capsules 3414
- Moduretic Tablets 2138
- Monopril HCT 1094
- Prinzide Tablets 2168
- Timolide Tablets 2187
- Uniretic Tablets 3178
- Vaseretic Tablets 2204
- Zestoretic Tablets 695
- Ziac Tablets 1887

Hydrocortisone (Glucocorticoid hormone given before or concomitantly with photodynamic therapy may decrease the efficacy of the treatment). Products include:
- Anusol-HC Cream 2.5% 2237
- Cipro HC Otic Suspension 540
- Cortaid Intensive Therapy Cream . ⊡ 717
- Cortaid Maximum Strength Cream .... ⊡ 717
- Cortisporin Ophthalmic Suspension Sterile .... ⊙ 297
- Cortizone•5 .... ⊡ 699
- Cortizone•10 .... ⊡ 699
- Cortizone•10 Plus Creme .... ⊡ 700
- Cortizone for Kids Creme .... ⊡ 699
- Hydrocortone Tablets 2106
- Massengill Medicated Soft Cloth Towelette .... ⊡ 753
- VōSoL HC Otic Solution 3356

Hydrocortisone Acetate (Glucocorticoid hormone given before or concomitantly with photodynamic therapy may decrease the efficacy of the treatment). Products include:
- Analpram-HC 1338
- Anusol HC-1 Hydrocortisone Anti-Itch Cream .... ⊡ 689
- Anusol-HC Suppositories 2238
- Cortaid .... ⊡ 717
- Cortifoam Rectal Foam 3170
- Cortisporin-TC Otic Suspension 2246
- Hydrocortone Acetate Injectable Suspension 2103
- Pramosone 1343
- Proctocort Suppositories 2264
- ProctoFoam-HC 3177
- Terra-Cortril Ophthalmic Suspension 2716

Hydrocortisone Sodium Phosphate (Glucocorticoid hormone given before or concomitantly with photodynamic therapy may decrease the efficacy of the treatment). Products include:
- Hydrocortone Phosphate Injection, Sterile 2105

Hydrocortisone Sodium Succinate (Glucocorticoid hormone given before or concomitantly with photodynamic therapy may decrease the efficacy of the treatment).
No products indexed under this heading.

Hydroflumethiazide (Co-administration with other photosensitizing agents could increase the photosensitivity reactions). Products include:
- Diucardin Tablets 3494

Ibuprofen (Some prostaglandin synthesis inhibitors could interfere with porfimer photodynamic therapy). Products include:
- Advil .... ⊡ 771
- Children's Advil Oral Suspension ... ⊡ 773
- Children's Advil Chewable Tablets ... ⊡ 773
- Advil Cold and Sinus Caplets .... ⊡ 771
- Advil Cold and Sinus Tablets .... ⊡ 771
- Advil Flu & Body Ache Caplets .... ⊡ 772
- Infants' Advil Drops .... ⊡ 773
- Junior Strength Advil Tablets .... ⊡ 773
- Junior Strength Advil Chewable Tablets .... ⊡ 773
- Advil Migraine Liquigels .... ⊡ 772
- Children's Motrin Oral Suspension and Chewable Tablets 2006
- Children's Motrin Cold Oral Suspension 2007
- Children's Motrin Oral Suspension .... ⊡ 643
- Motrin Suspension, Oral Drops, Chewable Tablets, and Caplets 2002
- Infants' Motrin Concentrated Drops 2006
- Junior Strength Motrin Caplets and Chewable Tablets 2006
- Motrin IB Tablets, Caplets, and Gelcaps 2002
- Motrin Migraine Pain Caplets 2005
- Motrin Sinus Headache Caplets 2005
- Vicoprofen Tablets 520

Indomethacin (Some prostaglandin synthesis inhibitors could interfere with porfimer photodynamic therapy). Products include:
- Indocin 2112

Indomethacin Sodium Trihydrate (Some prostaglandin synthesis inhibitors could interfere with porfimer photodynamic therapy). Products include:
- Indocin I.V. 2115

Isradipine (Could interfere with porfimer photodynamic therapy). Products include:
- DynaCirc Capsules 2921
- DynaCirc CR Tablets 2923

Ketoprofen (Some prostaglandin synthesis inhibitors could interfere with porfimer photodynamic therapy). Products include:
- Orudis Capsules 3548
- Orudis KT Tablets .... ⊡ 778
- Oruvail Capsules 3548

Lomefloxacin Hydrochloride (Co-administration with other photosensitizing agents could increase the photosensitivity reactions).
No products indexed under this heading.

Mannitol (Compounds that quench active oxygen species or scavenge radicals, such as mannitol, would be expected to decrease photodynamic therapy; no human data available to support or rebut this possibility).
No products indexed under this heading.

Meclofenamate Sodium (Some prostaglandin synthesis inhibitors could interfere with porfimer photodynamic therapy).
No products indexed under this heading.

Mefenamic Acid (Some prostaglandin synthesis inhibitors could interfere with porfimer photodynamic therapy). Products include:
- Ponstel Capsules 1356

Mesoridazine Besylate (Co-administration with other photosensitizing agents could increase the photosensitivity reactions). Products include:
- Serentil 1057

Methacycline Hydrochloride (Co-administration with other photosensitizing agents could increase the photosensitivity reactions).
No products indexed under this heading.

Methotrimeprazine (Co-administration with other photosensitizing agents could increase the photosensitivity reactions).
No products indexed under this heading.

Methyclothiazide (Co-administration with other photosensitizing agents could increase the photosensitivity reactions).
No products indexed under this heading.

Methylprednisolone Acetate (Glucocorticoid hormone given before or concomitantly with photodynamic therapy may decrease the efficacy of the treatment). Products include:
- Depo-Medrol Injectable Suspension 2795

Methylprednisolone Sodium Succinate (Glucocorticoid hormone given before or concomitantly with photodynamic therapy may decrease the efficacy of the treatment). Products include:
- Solu-Medrol Sterile Powder 2855

Mibefradil Dihydrochloride (Could interfere with porfimer photodynamic therapy).
No products indexed under this heading.

Minocycline Hydrochloride (Co-administration with other photosensitizing agents could increase the photosensitivity reactions). Products include:
- Dynacin Capsules 2019
- Minocin Intravenous 1862
- Minocin Oral Suspension 1865
- Minocin Pellet-Filled Capsules 1863

Naproxen (Some prostaglandin synthesis inhibitors could interfere with porfimer photodynamic therapy). Products include:
- EC-Naprosyn Delayed-Release Tablets 2967
- Naprosyn Suspension 2967
- Naprosyn Tablets 2967

Naproxen Sodium (Some prostaglandin synthesis inhibitors could interfere with porfimer photodynamic therapy). Products include:
- Aleve Tablets, Caplets and Gelcaps .... ⊡ 602
- Aleve Cold & Sinus Caplets .... ⊡ 603
- Anaprox Tablets 2967
- Anaprox DS Tablets 2967
- Naprelan Tablets 1293

Nicardipine Hydrochloride (Could interfere with porfimer photodynamic therapy). Products include:

Cardene I.V. 3485

Nifedipine (Could interfere with porfimer photodynamic therapy). Products include:
Adalat CC Tablets 877
Procardia Capsules 2708
Procardia XL Extended Release Tablets 2710

Nimodipine (Could interfere with porfimer photodynamic therapy). Products include:
Nimotop Capsules 904

Nisoldipine (Could interfere with porfimer photodynamic therapy). Products include:
Sular Tablets 688

Norfloxacin (Co-administration with other photosensitizing agents could increase the photosensitivity reactions). Products include:
Chibroxin Sterile Ophthalmic Solution 2051
Noroxin Tablets 2145

Ofloxacin (Co-administration with other photosensitizing agents could increase the photosensitivity reactions). Products include:
Floxin I.V. 2526
Floxin Otic Solution 1219
Floxin Tablets 2529
Ocuflox Ophthalmic Solution 554

Oxytetracycline Hydrochloride (Co-administration with other photosensitizing agents could increase the photosensitivity reactions). Products include:
Terra-Cortril Ophthalmic Suspension 2716
Urobiotic-250 Capsules 2731

Perphenazine (Co-administration with other photosensitizing agents could increase the photosensitivity reactions). Products include:
Etrafon 3115
Trilafon 3160

Phenylbutazone (Some prostaglandin synthesis inhibitors could interfere with porfimer photodynamic therapy).
No products indexed under this heading.

Piroxicam (Some prostaglandin synthesis inhibitors could interfere with porfimer photodynamic therapy). Products include:
Feldene Capsules 2685

Polythiazide (Co-administration with other photosensitizing agents could increase the photosensitivity reactions). Products include:
Minizide Capsules 2700
Renese Tablets 2712

Prednisolone Acetate (Glucocorticoid hormone given before or concomitantly with photodynamic therapy may decrease the efficacy of the treatment). Products include:
Blephamide Ophthalmic Ointment 547
Blephamide Ophthalmic Suspension 548
Poly-Pred Liquifilm Ophthalmic Suspension .... ⊙245
Pred Forte Ophthalmic Suspension .... ⊙246
Pred Mild Sterile Ophthalmic Suspension .... ⊙249
Pred-G Ophthalmic Suspension .... ⊙247
Pred-G Sterile Ophthalmic Ointment .... ⊙248

Prednisolone Sodium Phosphate (Glucocorticoid hormone given before or concomitantly with photodynamic therapy may decrease the efficacy of the treatment). Products include:
Pediapred Oral Solution 1170

Prednisolone Tebutate (Glucocorticoid hormone given before or concomitantly with photodynamic therapy may decrease the efficacy of the treatment).
No products indexed under this heading.

Prednisone (Glucocorticoid hormone given before or concomitantly with photodynamic therapy may decrease the efficacy of the treatment). Products include:
Prednisone 3064

Prochlorperazine (Co-administration with other photosensitizing agents could increase the photosensitivity reactions). Products include:
Compazine 1505

Promethazine Hydrochloride (Co-administration with other photosensitizing agents could increase the photosensitivity reactions). Products include:
Mepergan Injection 3539
Phenergan Injection 3553
Phenergan 3556
Phenergan Syrup 3554
Phenergan with Codeine Syrup 3557
Phenergan with Dextromethorphan Syrup 3559
Phenergan VC Syrup 3560
Phenergan VC with Codeine Syrup 3561

Sulfamethizole (Co-administration with other photosensitizing agents could increase the photosensitivity reactions). Products include:
Urobiotic-250 Capsules 2731

Sulfamethoxazole (Co-administration with other photosensitizing agents could increase the photosensitivity reactions). Products include:
Bactrim 2949
Septra Suspension 2265
Septra Tablets 2265
Septra DS Tablets 2265

Sulfasalazine (Co-administration with other photosensitizing agents could increase the photosensitivity reactions). Products include:
Azulfidine EN-tabs Tablets 2775

Sulfinpyrazone (Co-administration with other photosensitizing agents could increase the photosensitivity reactions).
No products indexed under this heading.

Sulfisoxazole (Co-administration with other photosensitizing agents could increase the photosensitivity reactions).
No products indexed under this heading.

Sulfisoxazole Acetyl (Co-administration with other photosensitizing agents could increase the photosensitivity reactions). Products include:
Pediazole Suspension 3050

Sulfisoxazole Diolamine (Co-administration with other photosensitizing agents could increase the photosensitivity reactions).
No products indexed under this heading.

Sulindac (Some prostaglandin synthesis inhibitors could interfere with porfimer photodynamic therapy). Products include:
Clinoril Tablets 2053

Tetracycline Hydrochloride (Co-administration with other photosensitizing agents could increase the photosensitivity reactions).
No products indexed under this heading.

Thioridazine Hydrochloride (Co-administration with other photosensitizing agents could increase the photosensitivity reactions). Products include:
Thioridazine Hydrochloride Tablets 2289

Tolazamide (Co-administration with other photosensitizing agents could increase the photosensitivity reactions).
No products indexed under this heading.

Tolbutamide (Co-administration with other photosensitizing agents could increase the photosensitivity reactions).
No products indexed under this heading.

Tolmetin Sodium (Some prostaglandin synthesis inhibitors could interfere with porfimer photodynamic therapy). Products include:
Tolectin 2589

Triamcinolone (Glucocorticoid hormone given before or concomitantly with photodynamic therapy may decrease the efficacy of the treatment).
No products indexed under this heading.

Triamcinolone Acetonide (Glucocorticoid hormone given before or concomitantly with photodynamic therapy may decrease the efficacy of the treatment). Products include:
Azmacort Inhalation Aerosol 728
Nasacort Nasal Inhaler 750
Nasacort AQ Nasal Spray 752
Tri-Nasal Spray 2274

Triamcinolone Diacetate (Glucocorticoid hormone given before or concomitantly with photodynamic therapy may decrease the efficacy of the treatment).
No products indexed under this heading.

Triamcinolone Hexacetonide (Glucocorticoid hormone given before or concomitantly with photodynamic therapy may decrease the efficacy of the treatment).
No products indexed under this heading.

Trifluoperazine Hydrochloride (Co-administration with other photosensitizing agents could increase the photosensitivity reactions). Products include:
Stelazine 1640

Trovafloxacin Mesylate (Co-administration with other photosensitizing agents could increase the photosensitivity reactions). Products include:
Trovan Tablets 2722

Verapamil Hydrochloride (Could interfere with porfimer photodynamic therapy). Products include:
Covera-HS Tablets 3199
Isoptin SR Tablets 467
Tarka Tablets 508
Verelan Capsules 3184
Verelan PM Capsules 3186

Food Interactions

Alcohol (Compounds that quench active oxygen species or scavenge radicals, such as ethanol, would be expected to decrease photodynamic therapy; no human data available to support or rebut this possibility).

PHRENILIN FORTE CAPSULES

(Acetaminophen, Butalbital) 578

May interact with central nervous system depressants, general anesthetics, hypnotics and sedatives, monoamine oxidase inhibitors, narcotic analgesics, tranquilizers, and certain other agents. Compounds in these categories include:

Alfentanil Hydrochloride (Potential for increased CNS depression).
No products indexed under this heading.

Alprazolam (Potential for increased CNS depression). Products include:
Xanax Tablets 2865

Aprobarbital (Potential for increased CNS depression).
No products indexed under this heading.

Buprenorphine Hydrochloride (Potential for increased CNS depression). Products include:
Buprenex Injectable 2918

Buspirone Hydrochloride (Potential for increased CNS depression).
No products indexed under this heading.

Butabarbital (Potential for increased CNS depression).
No products indexed under this heading.

Chlordiazepoxide (Potential for increased CNS depression). Products include:
Limbitrol 1738

Chlordiazepoxide Hydrochloride (Potential for increased CNS depression). Products include:
Librium Capsules 1736
Librium for Injection 1737

Chlorpromazine (Potential for increased CNS depression). Products include:
Thorazine Suppositories 1656

Chlorpromazine Hydrochloride (Potential for levels of both drugs). Products include:
Thorazine 1656

Chlorprothixene (Potential for increased CNS depression).
No products indexed under this heading.

Chlorprothixene Hydrochloride (Potential for increased CNS depression).
No products indexed under this heading.

Chlorprothixene Lactate (Potential for increased CNS depression).
No products indexed under this heading.

Clorazepate Dipotassium (Potential for increased CNS depression). Products include:
Tranxene 511

Clozapine (Potential for increased CNS depression). Products include:
Clozaril Tablets 2319

Codeine Phosphate (Potential for increased CNS depression). Products include:
Phenergan with Codeine Syrup 3557
Phenergan VC with Codeine Syrup 3561
Robitussin A-C Syrup 2942
Robitussin-DAC Syrup 2942
Ryna-C Liquid .... ▣768
Soma Compound w/Codeine Tablets 3355
Tussi-Organidin NR Liquid 3350
Tussi-Organidin-S NR Liquid 3350
Tylenol with Codeine 2595

Desflurane (Potential for increased CNS depression). Products include:
Suprane Liquid for Inhalation 874

Dezocine (Potential for increased CNS depression).
No products indexed under this heading.

Diazepam (Potential for increased CNS depression). Products include:
Valium Injectable 3026
Valium Tablets 3047

Droperidol (Potential for increased CNS depression).
No products indexed under this heading.

Enflurane (Potential for increased CNS depression).
No products indexed under this heading.

Estazolam (Potential for increased CNS depression). Products include:
ProSom Tablets 500

Ethchlorvynol (Potential for increased CNS depression).
No products indexed under this heading.

Ethinamate (Potential for increased CNS depression).
No products indexed under this heading.

Fentanyl (Potential for increased CNS depression). Products include:
Duragesic Transdermal System 1786

Fentanyl Citrate (Potential for increased CNS depression). Products include:

Actiq 1184

Fluphenazine Decanoate (Potential for increased CNS depression).
No products indexed under this heading.

Fluphenazine Enanthate (Potential for increased CNS depression).
No products indexed under this heading.

Fluphenazine Hydrochloride (Potential for increased CNS depression).
No products indexed under this heading.

Flurazepam Hydrochloride (Potential for increased CNS depression).
No products indexed under this heading.

Glutethimide (Potential for increased CNS depression).
No products indexed under this heading.

Haloperidol (Potential for increased CNS depression). Products include:
Haldol Injection, Tablets and Concentrate 2533

Haloperidol Decanoate (Potential for increased CNS depression). Products include:
Haldol Decanoate 2535

Hydrocodone Bitartrate (Potential for increased CNS depression). Products include:
Hycodan 1316
Hycomine Compound Tablets 1317
Hycotuss Expectorant Syrup 1318
Lortab 3319
Lortab Elixir 3317
Maxidone Tablets CIII 3399
Norco 5/325 Tablets CIII 3424
Norco 7.5/325 Tablets CIII 3425
Norco 10/325 Tablets CIII 3427
Norco 10/325 Tablets CIII 3425
Vicodin Tablets 516
Vicodin ES Tablets 517
Vicodin HP Tablets 518
Vicodin Tuss Expectorant 519
Vicoprofen Tablets 520
Zydone Tablets 1330

Hydrocodone Polistirex (Potential for increased CNS depression). Products include:
Tussionex Pennkinetic Extended-Release Suspension 1174

Hydromorphone Hydrochloride (Potential for increased CNS depression). Products include:
Dilaudid 441
Dilaudid Oral Liquid 445
Dilaudid Powder 441
Dilaudid Rectal Suppositories 441
Dilaudid Tablets 441
Dilaudid Tablets - 8 mg 445
Dilaudid-HP 443

Hydroxyzine Hydrochloride (Potential for increased CNS depression). Products include:
Atarax Tablets & Syrup 2667
Vistaril Intramuscular Solution 2738

Isocarboxazid (Enhances the CNS effects of butalbital).
No products indexed under this heading.

Isoflurane (Potential for increased CNS depression).
No products indexed under this heading.

Ketamine Hydrochloride (Potential for increased CNS depression).
No products indexed under this heading.

Levomethadyl Acetate Hydrochloride (Potential for increased CNS depression).
No products indexed under this heading.

Levorphanol Tartrate (Potential for increased CNS depression). Products include:
Levo-Dromoran 1734
Levorphanol Tartrate Tablets 3059

Lorazepam (Potential for increased CNS depression). Products include:
Ativan Injection 3478
Ativan Tablets 3482

Loxapine Hydrochloride (Potential for increased CNS depression).
No products indexed under this heading.

Loxapine Succinate (Potential for increased CNS depression). Products include:
Loxitane Capsules 3398

Meperidine Hydrochloride (Potential for increased CNS depression). Products include:
Demerol 3079
Mepergan Injection 3539

Mephobarbital (Potential for increased CNS depression).
No products indexed under this heading.

Meprobamate (Potential for increased CNS depression). Products include:
Miltown Tablets 3349

Mesoridazine Besylate (Potential for increased CNS depression). Products include:
Serentil 1057

Methadone Hydrochloride (Potential for increased CNS depression). Products include:
Dolophine Hydrochloride Tablets 3056

Methohexital Sodium (Potential for increased CNS depression). Products include:
Brevital Sodium for Injection, USP 1815

Methotrimeprazine (Potential for increased CNS depression).
No products indexed under this heading.

Methoxyflurane (Potential for increased CNS depression).
No products indexed under this heading.

Midazolam Hydrochloride (Potential for increased CNS depression). Products include:
Versed Injection 3027
Versed Syrup 3033

Moclobemide (Enhances the CNS effects of butalbital).
No products indexed under this heading.

Molindone Hydrochloride (Potential for increased CNS depression). Products include:
Moban 1320

Morphine Sulfate (Potential for increased CNS depression). Products include:
Astramorph/PF Injection, USP (Preservative-Free) 594
Duramorph Injection 1312
Infumorph 200 and Infumorph 500 Sterile Solutions 1314
Kadian Capsules 1335
MS Contin Tablets 2896
MSIR 2898
Oramorph SR Tablets 3062
Roxanol 3066

Olanzapine (Potential for increased CNS depression). Products include:
Zyprexa Tablets 1973
Zyprexa ZYDIS Orally Disintegrating Tablets 1973

Oxazepam (Potential for increased CNS depression).
No products indexed under this heading.

Oxycodone Hydrochloride (Potential for increased CNS depression). Products include:
OxyContin Tablets 2912
OxyFast Oral Concentrate Solution 2916
OxyIR Capsules 2916
Percocet Tablets 1326
Percodan Tablets 1327
Percolone Tablets 1327
Roxicodone 3067
Tylox Capsules 2597

Pargyline Hydrochloride (Enhances the CNS effects of butalbital).
No products indexed under this heading.

Pentobarbital Sodium (Potential for increased CNS depression). Products include:
Nembutal Sodium Solution 485

Perphenazine (Potential for increased CNS depression). Products include:
Etrafon 3115
Trilafon 3160

Phenelzine Sulfate (Enhances the CNS effects of butalbital). Products include:
Nardil Tablets 2653

Phenobarbital (Potential for increased CNS depression). Products include:
Arco-Lase Plus Tablets 592
Donnatal 2929
Donnatal Extentabs 2930

Prazepam (Potential for increased CNS depression).
No products indexed under this heading.

Procarbazine Hydrochloride (Enhances the CNS effects of butalbital). Products include:
Matulane Capsules 3246

Prochlorperazine (Potential for increased CNS depression). Products include:
Compazine 1505

Promethazine Hydrochloride (Potential for increased CNS depression). Products include:
Mepergan Injection 3539
Phenergan Injection 3553
Phenergan 3556
Phenergan Syrup 3554
Phenergan with Codeine Syrup 3557
Phenergan with Dextromethorphan Syrup 3559
Phenergan VC Syrup 3560
Phenergan VC with Codeine Syrup 3561

Propofol (Potential for increased CNS depression). Products include:
Diprivan Injectable Emulsion 667

Propoxyphene Hydrochloride (Potential for increased CNS depression). Products include:
Darvon Pulvules 1909
Darvon Compound-65 Pulvules 1910

Propoxyphene Napsylate (Potential for increased CNS depression). Products include:
Darvon-N/Darvocet-N 1907
Darvon-N Tablets 1912

Quazepam (Potential for increased CNS depression).
No products indexed under this heading.

Quetiapine Fumarate (Potential for increased CNS depression). Products include:
Seroquel Tablets 684

Remifentanil Hydrochloride (Potential for increased CNS depression).
No products indexed under this heading.

Risperidone (Potential for increased CNS depression). Products include:
Risperdal 1796

Secobarbital Sodium (Potential for increased CNS depression).
No products indexed under this heading.

Selegiline Hydrochloride (Enhances the CNS effects of butalbital). Products include:
Eldepryl Capsules 3266

Sevoflurane (Potential for increased CNS depression).
No products indexed under this heading.

Sufentanil Citrate (Potential for increased CNS depression).
No products indexed under this heading.

Temazepam (Potential for increased CNS depression).
No products indexed under this heading.

Thiamylal Sodium (Potential for increased CNS depression).
No products indexed under this heading.

Thioridazine Hydrochloride (Potential for increased CNS depression). Products include:
Thioridazine Hydrochloride Tablets 2289

Thiothixene (Potential for increased CNS depression). Products include:
Navane Capsules 2701
Thiothixene Capsules 2290

Tranylcypromine Sulfate (Enhances the CNS effects of butalbital). Products include:
Parnate Tablets 1607

Triazolam (Potential for increased CNS depression). Products include:
Halcion Tablets 2823

Trifluoperazine Hydrochloride (Potential for increased CNS depression). Products include:
Stelazine 1640

Zaleplon (Potential for increased CNS depression). Products include:
Sonata Capsules 3591

Ziprasidone Hydrochloride (Potential for increased CNS depression). Products include:
Geodon Capsules 2688

Zolpidem Tartrate (Potential for increased CNS depression). Products include:
Ambien Tablets 3191

Food Interactions

Alcohol (Potential for increased CNS depression).

PHRENILIN TABLETS
(Acetaminophen, Butalbital) 578
See Phrenilin Forte Capsules

PHYTALOE CAPSULES
(Aloe vera, Herbals, Multiple) 819
None cited in PDR database.

PHYTALOE POWDER
(Aloe vera, Herbals, Multiple) 819
None cited in PDR database.

PHYTO-VITE TABLETS
(Bioflavonoids, Ginkgo biloba, Herbals with Vitamins & Minerals) 849
None cited in PDR database.

PILOPINE HS OPHTHALMIC GEL
(Pilocarpine Hydrochloride) .... ⊙217
None cited in PDR database.

PIMA SYRUP
(Potassium Iodide) 1362
None cited in PDR database.

PIN-X PINWORM TREATMENT
(Pyrantel Pamoate) 632
None cited in PDR database.

PIPRACIL
(Piperacillin Sodium) 1866
May interact with aminoglycosides, nondepolarizing neuromuscular blocking agents, and certain other agents. Compounds in these categories include:

Amikacin Sulfate (Substantial inactivation of aminoglycosides *in vitro*).
No products indexed under this heading.

Atracurium Besylate (Co-administration with vecuronium has been implicated in the prolongation of the neuromuscular blockage; due to similar mechanism of action, same interaction can be expected with other non-depolarizing muscle relaxants).
No products indexed under this heading.

IMPORTANT NOTE: Always consult each drug listing in the patient's regimen for possible interactions.

Cisatracurium Besylate (Co-administration with vecuronium has been implicated in the prolongation of the neuromuscular blockage; due to similar mechanism of action, same interaction can be expected with other non-depolarizing muscle relaxants).
No products indexed under this heading.

Gentamicin Sulfate (Substantial inactivation of aminoglycosides *in vitro*). Products include:
Genoptic Ophthalmic Ointment ...... ⊙239
Genoptic Sterile Ophthalmic Solution ...... ⊙239
Pred-G Ophthalmic Suspension ..... ⊙247
Pred-G Sterile Ophthalmic Ointment ...... ⊙248

Kanamycin Sulfate (Substantial inactivation of aminoglycosides *in vitro*).
No products indexed under this heading.

Metocurine Iodide (Co-administration with vecuronium has been implicated in the prolongation of the neuromuscular blockage; due to similar mechanism of action, same interaction can be expected with other non-depolarizing muscle relaxants).
No products indexed under this heading.

Mivacurium Chloride (Co-administration with vecuronium has been implicated in the prolongation of the neuromuscular blockage; due to similar mechanism of action, same interaction can be expected with other non-depolarizing muscle relaxants).
No products indexed under this heading.

Pancuronium Bromide (Co-administration with vecuronium has been implicated in the prolongation of the neuromuscular blockage; due to similar mechanism of action, same interaction can be expected with other non-depolarizing muscle relaxants).
No products indexed under this heading.

Probenecid (Increases peak serum level and area under the curve).
No products indexed under this heading.

Rapacuronium Bromide (Co-administration with vecuronium has been implicated in the prolongation of the neuromuscular blockage; due to similar mechanism of action, same interaction can be expected with other non-depolarizing muscle relaxants).
No products indexed under this heading.

Rocuronium Bromide (Co-administration with vecuronium has been implicated in the prolongation of the neuromuscular blockage; due to similar mechanism of action, same interaction can be expected with other non-depolarizing muscle relaxants). Products include:
Zemuron Injection 2491

Streptomycin Sulfate (Substantial inactivation of aminoglycosides *in vitro*). Products include:
Streptomycin Sulfate Injection 2714

Tobramycin (Substantial inactivation of aminoglycosides *in vitro*). Products include:
TOBI Solution for Inhalation 1206
TobraDex Ophthalmic Ointment 542
TobraDex Ophthalmic Suspension .. 541
Tobrex Ophthalmic Ointment ...... ⊙220
Tobrex Ophthalmic Solution ...... ⊙221

Tobramycin Sulfate (Substantial inactivation of aminoglycosides *in vitro*). Products include:
Nebcin Vials, Hyporets & ADD-Vantage 1955

Vecuronium Bromide (Co-administration with vecuronium has been implicated in the prolongation of the neuromuscular blockage; due to similar mechanism of action, same interaction can be expected with other non-depolarizing muscle relaxants). Products include:
Norcuron for Injection 2478

PLAQUENIL TABLETS
(Hydroxychloroquine Sulfate) 3082
May interact with:

Hepatotoxic Drugs, unspecified (Use with caution).

PLASBUMIN-5
(Albumin (human)) 939
None cited in PDR database.

PLASBUMIN-20
(Albumin (human)) 940
None cited in PDR database.

PLASBUMIN-25
(Albumin (human)) 941
None cited in PDR database.

PLASMANATE
(Plasma Protein Fraction (Human)) 942
None cited in PDR database.

PLAVIX TABLETS
(Clopidogrel Bisulfate) 1097
May interact with non-steroidal anti-inflammatory agents, phenytoin, and certain other agents. Compounds in these categories include:

Aspirin (Clopidogrel potentiates the effect of aspirin on collagen-induced platelet aggregation; co-administration did not significantly increase the prolongation of bleeding time induced by clopidogrel). Products include:
Aggrenox Capsules 1026
Alka-Seltzer ...... ■603
Alka-Seltzer Lemon Lime Antacid and Pain Reliever Effervescent Tablets ...... ■603
Alka-Seltzer Extra Strength Antacid and Pain Reliever Effervescent Tablets ...... ■603
Alka-Seltzer PM Effervescent Tablets ...... ■605
Genuine Bayer Tablets, Caplets and Gelcaps ...... ■606
Extra Strength Bayer Caplets and Gelcaps ...... ■610
Aspirin Regimen Bayer Children's Chewable Tablets (Orange or Cherry Flavored) ...... ■607
Bayer, Aspirin Regimen ...... ■606
Aspirin Regimen Bayer 81 mg Caplets with Calcium ...... ■607
Genuine Bayer Professional Labeling (Aspirin Regimen Bayer) ...... ■608
Extra Strength Bayer Arthritis Caplets ...... ■610
Extra Strength Bayer Plus Caplets ...... ■610
Extra Strength Bayer PM Caplets . ■611
BC Powder ...... ■619
BC Allergy Sinus Cold Powder ...... ■619
Arthritis Strength BC Powder ...... ■619
BC Sinus Cold Powder ...... ■619
Darvon Compound-65 Pulvules 1910
Ecotrin Enteric Coated Aspirin Low, Regular and Maximum Strength Tablets 1715
Excedrin Extra-Strength Tablets, Caplets, and Geltabs ...... ■629
Excedrin Migraine 1070
Goody's Body Pain Formula Powder ...... ■620
Goody's Extra Strength Headache Powder ...... ■620
Goody's Extra Strength Pain Relief Tablets ...... ■620
Percodan Tablets 1327
Robaxisal Tablets 2939
Soma Compound Tablets 3354
Soma Compound w/Codeine Tablets 3355
Vanquish Caplets ...... ■617

Celecoxib (Co-administration can be associated with increased occult gastrointestinal blood loss; at high concentrations in vitro, clopidogrel inhibits P450IIC9, accordingly it may interfere with the metabolism of many non-steroidal anti-inflammatory agents). Products include:
Celebrex Capsules 2676
Celebrex Capsules 2780

Diclofenac Potassium (Co-administration can be associated with increased occult gastrointestinal blood loss; at high concentrations in vitro, clopidogrel inhibits P450IIC9, accordingly it may interfere with the metabolism of many non-steroidal anti-inflammatory agents). Products include:
Cataflam Tablets 2315

Diclofenac Sodium (Co-administration can be associated with increased occult gastrointestinal blood loss; at high concentrations in vitro, clopidogrel inhibits P450IIC9, accordingly it may interfere with the metabolism of many non-steroidal anti-inflammatory agents). Products include:
Arthrotec Tablets 3195
Voltaren Ophthalmic Sterile Ophthalmic Solution ...... ⊙312
Voltaren Tablets 2315
Voltaren-XR Tablets 2315

Etodolac (Co-administration can be associated with increased occult gastrointestinal blood loss; at high concentrations in vitro, clopidogrel inhibits P450IIC9, accordingly it may interfere with the metabolism of many non-steroidal anti-inflammatory agents). Products include:
Lodine 3528
Lodine XL Extended-Release Tablets 3530

Fenoprofen Calcium (Co-administration can be associated with increased occult gastrointestinal blood loss; at high concentrations in vitro, clopidogrel inhibits P450IIC9, accordingly it may interfere with the metabolism of many non-steroidal anti-inflammatory agents).
No products indexed under this heading.

Flurbiprofen (Co-administration can be associated with increased occult gastrointestinal blood loss; at high concentrations in vitro, clopidogrel inhibits P450IIC9, accordingly it may interfere with the metabolism of many non-steroidal anti-inflammatory agents).
No products indexed under this heading.

Fluvastatin Sodium (At high concentrations in vitro, clopidogrel inhibits P450IIC9, accordingly it may interfere with the metabolism of fluvastatin). Products include:
Lescol Capsules 2361
Lescol 2925
Lescol XL Tablets 2361

Fosphenytoin Sodium (At high concentrations in vitro, clopidogrel inhibits P450IIC9, accordingly it may interfere with the metabolism of phenytoin). Products include:
Cerebyx Injection 2619

Heparin Sodium (Co-administration should be undertaken with caution; concomitant heparin has no effect on inhibition of platelet aggregation induced by clopidogrel). Products include:
Heparin Lock Flush Solution 3509
Heparin Sodium Injection 3511

Ibuprofen (Co-administration can be associated with increased occult gastrointestinal blood loss; at high concentrations in vitro, clopidogrel inhibits P450IIC9, accordingly it may interfere with the metabolism of many non-steroidal anti-inflammatory agents). Products include:
Advil ...... ■771
Children's Advil Oral Suspension ...... ■773
Children's Advil Chewable Tablets . ■773
Advil Cold and Sinus Caplets ...... ■771
Advil Cold and Sinus Tablets ...... ■771
Advil Flu & Body Ache Caplets ...... ■772
Infants' Advil Drops ...... ■773
Junior Strength Advil Tablets ...... ■773
Junior Strength Advil Chewable Tablets ...... ■773
Advil Migraine Liquigels ...... ■772
Children's Motrin Oral Suspension and Chewable Tablets 2006
Children's Motrin Cold Oral Suspension 2007
Children's Motrin Oral Suspension ...... ■643
Motrin Suspension, Oral Drops, Chewable Tablets, and Caplets 2002
Infants' Motrin Concentrated Drops 2006
Junior Strength Motrin Caplets and Chewable Tablets 2006
Motrin IB Tablets, Caplets, and Gelcaps 2002
Motrin Migraine Pain Caplets 2005
Motrin Sinus Headache Caplets 2005
Vicoprofen Tablets 520

Indomethacin (Co-administration can be associated with increased occult gastrointestinal blood loss; at high concentrations in vitro, clopidogrel inhibits P450IIC9, accordingly it may interfere with the metabolism of many non-steroidal anti-inflammatory agents). Products include:
Indocin 2112

Indomethacin Sodium Trihydrate (Co-administration can be associated with increased occult gastrointestinal blood loss; at high concentrations in vitro, clopidogrel inhibits P450IIC9, accordingly it may interfere with the metabolism of many non-steroidal anti-inflammatory agents). Products include:
Indocin I.V. 2115

Ketoprofen (Co-administration can be associated with increased occult gastrointestinal blood loss; at high concentrations in vitro, clopidogrel inhibits P450IIC9, accordingly it may interfere with the metabolism of many non-steroidal anti-inflammatory agents). Products include:
Orudis Capsules 3548
Orudis KT Tablets ...... ■778
Oruvail Capsules 3548

Ketorolac Tromethamine (Co-administration can be associated with increased occult gastrointestinal blood loss; at high concentrations in vitro, clopidogrel inhibits P450IIC9, accordingly it may interfere with the metabolism of many non-steroidal anti-inflammatory agents). Products include:
Acular Ophthalmic Solution 544
Acular PF Ophthalmic Solution 544
Toradol 3018

Meclofenamate Sodium (Co-administration can be associated with increased occult gastrointestinal blood loss; at high concentrations in vitro, clopidogrel inhibits P450IIC9, accordingly it may interfere with the metabolism of many non-steroidal anti-inflammatory agents).
No products indexed under this heading.

Mefenamic Acid (Co-administration can be associated with increased occult gastrointestinal blood loss; at high concentrations in vitro, clopidogrel inhibits P450IIC9, accordingly it may interfere with the metabolism of many non-steroidal anti-inflammatory agents). Products include:
Ponstel Capsules 1356

Meloxicam (Co-administration can be associated with increased occult gastrointestinal blood loss; at high concentrations in vitro, clopidogrel inhibits P450IIC9, accordingly it may interfere with the metabolism of many non-steroidal anti-inflammatory agents). Products include:
Mobic Tablets 1054

Nabumetone (Co-administration can be associated with increased occult gastrointestinal blood loss; at high concentrations in vitro, clopidogrel inhibits P450IIC9, accordingly it may interfere with the metabolism of many non-steroidal anti-inflammatory agents). Products include:
- Relafen Tablets 1617

Naproxen (Co-administration can be associated with increased occult gastrointestinal blood loss; at high concentrations in vitro, clopidogrel inhibits P450IIC9, accordingly it may interfere with the metabolism of many non-steroidal anti-inflammatory agents). Products include:
- EC-Naprosyn Delayed-Release Tablets 2967
- Naprosyn Suspension 2967
- Naprosyn Tablets 2967

Naproxen Sodium (Co-administration can be associated with increased occult gastrointestinal blood loss; at high concentrations in vitro, clopidogrel inhibits P450IIC9, accordingly it may interfere with the metabolism of many non-steroidal anti-inflammatory agents). Products include:
- Aleve Tablets, Caplets and Gelcaps .... ■602
- Aleve Cold & Sinus Caplets .... ■603
- Anaprox Tablets 2967
- Anaprox DS Tablets 2967
- Naprelan Tablets 1293

Oxaprozin (Co-administration can be associated with increased occult gastrointestinal blood loss; at high concentrations in vitro, clopidogrel inhibits P450IIC9, accordingly it may interfere with the metabolism of many non-steroidal anti-inflammatory agents).
- No products indexed under this heading.

Phenylbutazone (Co-administration can be associated with increased occult gastrointestinal blood loss; at high concentrations in vitro, clopidogrel inhibits P450IIC9, accordingly it may interfere with the metabolism of many non-steroidal anti-inflammatory agents).
- No products indexed under this heading.

Phenytoin (At high concentrations in vitro, clopidogrel inhibits P450IIC9, accordingly it may interfere with the metabolism of phenytoin). Products include:
- Dilantin Infatabs 2624
- Dilantin-125 Oral Suspension 2625

Phenytoin Sodium (At high concentrations in vitro, clopidogrel inhibits P450IIC9, accordingly it may interfere with the metabolism of phenytoin). Products include:
- Dilantin Kapseals 2622

Piroxicam (Co-administration can be associated with increased occult gastrointestinal blood loss; at high concentrations in vitro, clopidogrel inhibits P450IIC9, accordingly it may interfere with the metabolism of many non-steroidal anti-inflammatory agents). Products include:
- Feldene Capsules 2685

Rofecoxib (Co-administration can be associated with increased occult gastrointestinal blood loss; at high concentrations in vitro, clopidogrel inhibits P450IIC9, accordingly it may interfere with the metabolism of many non-steroidal anti-inflammatory agents). Products include:
- Vioxx 2213

Sulindac (Co-administration can be associated with increased occult gastrointestinal blood loss; at high concentrations in vitro, clopidogrel inhibits P450IIC9, accordingly it may interfere with the metabolism of many non-steroidal anti-inflammatory agents). Products include:
- Clinoril Tablets 2053

Tamoxifen Citrate (At high concentrations in vitro, clopidogrel inhibits P450IIC9, accordingly it may interfere with the metabolism of tamoxifen). Products include:
- Nolvadex Tablets 678

Tolbutamide (At high concentrations in vitro, clopidogrel inhibits P450IIC9, accordingly it may interfere with the metabolism of tolbutamide).
- No products indexed under this heading.

Tolmetin Sodium (Co-administration can be associated with increased occult gastrointestinal blood loss; at high concentrations in vitro, clopidogrel inhibits P450IIC9, accordingly it may interfere with the metabolism of many non-steroidal anti-inflammatory agents). Products include:
- Tolectin 2589

Torsemide (At high concentrations in vitro, clopidogrel inhibits P450IIC9, accordingly it may interfere with the metabolism of torsemide). Products include:
- Demadex Tablets and Injection 2965

Warfarin Sodium (Clopidogrel prolongs the bleeding time, consequently, co-administration should be undertaken with caution; at high concentrations in vitro, clopidogrel inhibits its P450IIC9, accordingly it may interfere with the metabolism of warfarin). Products include:
- Coumadin for Injection 1243
- Coumadin Tablets 1243
- Warfarin Sodium Tablets, USP 3302

PLAVIX TABLETS

(Clopidogrel Bisulfate) 3084

May interact with non-steroidal anti-inflammatory agents, phenytoin, and certain other agents. Compounds in these categories include:

Aspirin (Clopidogrel potentiates the effect of aspirin on collagen-induced platelet aggregation; co-administration did not significantly increase the prolongation of bleeding time induced by clopidogrel). Products include:
- Aggrenox Capsules 1026
- Alka-Seltzer .... ■603
- Alka-Seltzer Lemon Lime Antacid and Pain Reliever Effervescent Tablets .... ■603
- Alka-Seltzer Extra Strength Antacid and Pain Reliever Effervescent Tablets .... ■603
- Alka-Seltzer PM Effervescent Tablets .... ■605
- Genuine Bayer Tablets, Caplets and Gelcaps .... ■606
- Extra Strength Bayer Caplets and Gelcaps .... ■610
- Aspirin Regimen Bayer Children's Chewable Tablets (Orange or Cherry Flavored) .... ■607
- Bayer, Aspirin Regimen .... ■606
- Aspirin Regimen Bayer 81 mg Caplets with Calcium .... ■607
- Genuine Bayer Professional Labeling (Aspirin Regimen Bayer) .... ■608
- Extra Strength Bayer Arthritis Caplets .... ■610
- Extra Strength Bayer Plus Caplets .... ■610
- Extra Strength Bayer PM Caplets .... ■611
- BC Powder .... ■619
- BC Allergy Sinus Cold Powder .... ■619
- Arthritis Strength BC Powder .... ■619
- BC Sinus Cold Powder .... ■619
- Darvon Compound-65 Pulvules 1910
- Ecotrin Enteric Coated Aspirin Low, Regular and Maximum Strength Tablets 1715
- Excedrin Extra-Strength Tablets, Caplets, and Geltabs .... ■629
- Excedrin Migraine 1070
- Goody's Body Pain Formula Powder .... ■620
- Goody's Extra Strength Headache Powder .... ■620
- Goody's Extra Strength Pain Relief Tablets .... ■620
- Percodan Tablets 1327
- Robaxisal Tablets 2939
- Soma Compound Tablets 3354
- Soma Compound w/Codeine Tablets 3355
- Vanquish Caplets .... ■617

Celecoxib (Co-administration can be associated with increased occult gastrointestinal blood loss; at high concentrations in vitro, clopidogrel inhibits P450IIC9, accordingly it may interfere with the metabolism of many non-steroidal anti-inflammatory agents). Products include:
- Celebrex Capsules 2676
- Celebrex Capsules 2780

Diclofenac Potassium (Co-administration can be associated with increased occult gastrointestinal blood loss; at high concentrations in vitro, clopidogrel inhibits P450IIC9, accordingly it may interfere with the metabolism of many non-steroidal anti-inflammatory agents). Products include:
- Cataflam Tablets 2315

Diclofenac Sodium (Co-administration can be associated with increased occult gastrointestinal blood loss; at high concentrations in vitro, clopidogrel inhibits P450IIC9, accordingly it may interfere with the metabolism of many non-steroidal anti-inflammatory agents). Products include:
- Arthrotec Tablets 3195
- Voltaren Ophthalmic Sterile Ophthalmic Solution .... ⊙312
- Voltaren Tablets 2315
- Voltaren-XR Tablets 2315

Etodolac (Co-administration can be associated with increased occult gastrointestinal blood loss; at high concentrations in vitro, clopidogrel inhibits P450IIC9, accordingly it may interfere with the metabolism of many non-steroidal anti-inflammatory agents). Products include:
- Lodine 3528
- Lodine XL Extended-Release Tablets 3530

Fenoprofen Calcium (Co-administration can be associated with increased occult gastrointestinal blood loss; at high concentrations in vitro, clopidogrel inhibits P450IIC9, accordingly it may interfere with the metabolism of many non-steroidal anti-inflammatory agents).
- No products indexed under this heading.

Flurbiprofen (Co-administration can be associated with increased occult gastrointestinal blood loss; at high concentrations in vitro, clopidogrel inhibits P450IIC9, accordingly it may interfere with the metabolism of many non-steroidal anti-inflammatory agents).
- No products indexed under this heading.

Fluvastatin Sodium (At high concentrations in vitro, clopidogrel inhibits P450IIC9, accordingly it may interfere with the metabolism of fluvastatin). Products include:
- Lescol Capsules 2361
- Lescol 2925
- Lescol XL Tablets 2361

Fosphenytoin Sodium (At high concentrations in vitro, clopidogrel inhibits P450IIC9, accordingly it may interfere with the metabolism of phenytoin). Products include:
- Cerebyx Injection 2619

Heparin Sodium (Co-administration should be undertaken with caution; concomitant heparin has no effect on inhibition of platelet aggregation induced by clopidogrel). Products include:
- Heparin Lock Flush Solution 3509
- Heparin Sodium Injection 3511

Ibuprofen (Co-administration can be associated with increased occult gastrointestinal blood loss; at high concentrations in vitro, clopidogrel inhibits P450IIC9, accordingly it may interfere with the metabolism of many non-steroidal anti-inflammatory agents). Products include:
- Advil .... ■771
- Children's Advil Oral Suspension .... ■773
- Children's Advil Chewable Tablets .... ■773
- Advil Cold and Sinus Caplets .... ■771
- Advil Cold and Sinus Tablets .... ■771
- Advil Flu & Body Ache Caplets .... ■772
- Infants' Advil Drops .... ■773
- Junior Strength Advil Tablets .... ■773
- Junior Strength Advil Chewable Tablets .... ■773
- Advil Migraine Liquigels .... ■772
- Children's Motrin Oral Suspension and Chewable Tablets 2006
- Children's Motrin Cold Oral Suspension 2007
- Children's Motrin Oral Suspension .... ■643
- Motrin Suspension, Oral Drops, Chewable Tablets, and Caplets 2002
- Infants' Motrin Concentrated Drops 2006
- Junior Strength Motrin Caplets and Chewable Tablets 2006
- Motrin IB Tablets, Caplets, and Gelcaps 2002
- Motrin Migraine Pain Caplets 2005
- Motrin Sinus Headache Caplets 2005
- Vicoprofen Tablets 520

Indomethacin (Co-administration can be associated with increased occult gastrointestinal blood loss; at high concentrations in vitro, clopidogrel inhibits P450IIC9, accordingly it may interfere with the metabolism of many non-steroidal anti-inflammatory agents). Products include:
- Indocin 2112

Indomethacin Sodium Trihydrate (Co-administration can be associated with increased occult gastrointestinal blood loss; at high concentrations in vitro, clopidogrel inhibits P450IIC9, accordingly it may interfere with the metabolism of many non-steroidal anti-inflammatory agents). Products include:
- Indocin I.V. 2115

Ketoprofen (Co-administration can be associated with increased occult gastrointestinal blood loss; at high concentrations in vitro, clopidogrel inhibits P450IIC9, accordingly it may interfere with the metabolism of many non-steroidal anti-inflammatory agents). Products include:
- Orudis Capsules 3548
- Orudis KT Tablets .... ■778
- Oruvail Capsules 3548

Ketorolac Tromethamine (Co-administration can be associated with increased occult gastrointestinal blood loss; at high concentrations in vitro, clopidogrel inhibits P450IIC9, accordingly it may interfere with the metabolism of many non-steroidal anti-inflammatory agents). Products include:
- Acular Ophthalmic Solution 544
- Acular PF Ophthalmic Solution 544
- Toradol 3018

Meclofenamate Sodium (Co-administration can be associated with increased occult gastrointestinal blood loss; at high concentrations in vitro, clopidogrel inhibits P450IIC9, accordingly it may interfere with the metabolism of many non-steroidal anti-inflammatory agents).
- No products indexed under this heading.

Mefenamic Acid (Co-administration can be associated with increased occult gastrointestinal blood loss; at high concentrations in vitro, clopidogrel inhibits P450IIC9, accordingly it may interfere with the metabolism of many non-steroidal anti-inflammatory agents). Products include:
- Ponstel Capsules 1356

Meloxicam (Co-administration can be associated with increased occult

gastrointestinal blood loss; at high concentrations in vitro, clopidogrel inhibits P450IIC9, accordingly it may interfere with the metabolism of many non-steroidal anti-inflammatory agents). Products include:

Mobic Tablets 1054

Nabumetone (Co-administration can be associated with increased occult gastrointestinal blood loss; at high concentrations in vitro, clopidogrel inhibits P450IIC9, accordingly it may interfere with the metabolism of many non-steroidal anti-inflammatory agents). Products include:

Relafen Tablets 1617

Naproxen (Co-administration can be associated with increased occult gastrointestinal blood loss; at high concentrations in vitro, clopidogrel inhibits P450IIC9, accordingly it may interfere with the metabolism of many non-steroidal anti-inflammatory agents). Products include:

EC-Naprosyn Delayed-Release Tablets 2967
Naprosyn Suspension 2967
Naprosyn Tablets 2967

Naproxen Sodium (Co-administration can be associated with increased occult gastrointestinal blood loss; at high concentrations in vitro, clopidogrel inhibits P450IIC9, accordingly it may interfere with the metabolism of many non-steroidal anti-inflammatory agents). Products include:

Aleve Tablets, Caplets and Gelcaps .... ▣602
Aleve Cold & Sinus Caplets .... ▣603
Anaprox Tablets 2967
Anaprox DS Tablets 2967
Naprelan Tablets 1293

Oxaprozin (Co-administration can be associated with increased occult gastrointestinal blood loss; at high concentrations in vitro, clopidogrel inhibits P450IIC9, accordingly it may interfere with the metabolism of many non-steroidal anti-inflammatory agents).

No products indexed under this heading.

Phenylbutazone (Co-administration can be associated with increased occult gastrointestinal blood loss; at high concentrations in vitro, clopidogrel inhibits P450IIC9, accordingly it may interfere with the metabolism of many non-steroidal anti-inflammatory agents).

No products indexed under this heading.

Phenytoin (At high concentrations in vitro, clopidogrel inhibits P450IIC9, accordingly it may interfere with the metabolism of phenytoin). Products include:

Dilantin Infatabs 2624
Dilantin-125 Oral Suspension 2625

Phenytoin Sodium (At high concentrations in vitro, clopidogrel inhibits P450IIC9, accordingly it may interfere with the metabolism of phenytoin). Products include:

Dilantin Kapseals 2622

Piroxicam (Co-administration can be associated with increased occult gastrointestinal blood loss; at high concentrations in vitro, clopidogrel inhibits P450IIC9, accordingly it may interfere with the metabolism of many non-steroidal anti-inflammatory agents). Products include:

Feldene Capsules 2685

Rofecoxib (Co-administration can be associated with increased occult gastrointestinal blood loss; at high concentrations in vitro, clopidogrel inhibits P450IIC9, accordingly it may interfere with the metabolism of many non-steroidal anti-inflammatory agents). Products include:

Vioxx 2213

Sulindac (Co-administration can be associated with increased occult gastrointestinal blood loss; at high concentrations in vitro, clopidogrel inhibits P450IIC9, accordingly it may interfere with the metabolism of many non-steroidal anti-inflammatory agents). Products include:

Clinoril Tablets 2053

Tamoxifen Citrate (At high concentrations in vitro, clopidogrel inhibits P450IIC9, accordingly it may interfere with the metabolism of tamoxifen). Products include:

Nolvadex Tablets 678

Tolbutamide (At high concentrations in vitro, clopidogrel inhibits P450IIC9, accordingly it may interfere with the metabolism of tolbutamide).

No products indexed under this heading.

Tolmetin Sodium (Co-administration can be associated with increased occult gastrointestinal blood loss; at high concentrations in vitro, clopidogrel inhibits P450IIC9, accordingly it may interfere with the metabolism of many non-steroidal anti-inflammatory agents). Products include:

Tolectin 2589

Torsemide (At high concentrations in vitro, clopidogrel inhibits P450IIC9, accordingly it may interfere with the metabolism of torsemide). Products include:

Demadex Tablets and Injection 2965

Warfarin Sodium (Clopidogrel prolongs the bleeding time, consequently, co-administration should be undertaken with caution; at high concentrations in vitro, clopidogrel inhibits P450IIC9, accordingly it may interfere with the metabolism of warfarin). Products include:

Coumadin for Injection 1243
Coumadin Tablets 1243
Warfarin Sodium Tablets, USP 3302

PLENDIL EXTENDED-RELEASE TABLETS

(Felodipine) 623

May interact with beta blockers, anticonvulsants, erythromycin, and certain other agents. Compounds in these categories include:

Acebutolol Hydrochloride (Caution should be exercised when using Plendil in patients with heart failure or compromised ventricular function, particularly in combination with beta blocker). Products include:

Sectral Capsules 3589

Atenolol (Caution should be exercised when using Plendil in patients with heart failure or compromised ventricular function, particularly in combination with beta blocker). Products include:

Tenoretic Tablets 690
Tenormin I.V. Injection 692

Betaxolol Hydrochloride (Caution should be exercised when using Plendil in patients with heart failure or compromised ventricular function, particularly in combination with beta blocker). Products include:

Betoptic S Ophthalmic Suspension 537

Bisoprolol Fumarate (Caution should be exercised when using Plendil in patients with heart failure or compromised ventricular function, particularly in combination with beta blocker). Products include:

Zebeta Tablets 1885
Ziac Tablets 1887

Carbamazepine (Potential for low maximum plasma concentrations of felodipine in epileptic patients on long-term anticonvulsant therapy). Products include:

Carbatrol Capsules 3234
Tegretol/Tegretol-XR 2404

Carteolol Hydrochloride (Caution should be exercised when using Plendil in patients with heart failure or compromised ventricular function, particularly in combination with beta blocker). Products include:

Carteolol Hydrochloride Ophthalmic Solution USP, 1% ..... ⊙258
Ocupress Ophthalmic Solution, 1% Sterile .... ⊙303

Cimetidine (Increases AUC and Cmax by approximately 50%; low doses of Plendil should be used). Products include:

Tagamet HB 200 Suspension .... ▣762
Tagamet HB 200 Tablets .... ▣761
Tagamet Tablets 1644

Cimetidine Hydrochloride (Increases AUC and Cmax by approximately 50%; low doses of Plendil should be used). Products include:

Tagamet 1644

Digoxin (Co-administration does not significantly alter the pharmacokinetics of digoxin in patients with heart failure). Products include:

Digitek Tablets 1003
Lanoxicaps Capsules 1574
Lanoxin Injection 1581
Lanoxin Tablets 1587
Lanoxin Elixir Pediatric 1578
Lanoxin Injection Pediatric 1584

Divalproex Sodium (Potential for low maximum plasma concentrations of felodipine in epileptic patients on long-term anticonvulsant therapy). Products include:

Depakote Sprinkle Capsules 426
Depakote Tablets 430
Depakote ER Tablets 436

Erythromycin (Felodipine is metabolized by CYP3A4; co-administration of felodipine with erythromycin resulted in approximately 2.5-fold increase in the AUC and Cmax, and about 2-fold prolongation in the half-life of felodipine). Products include:

Emgel 2% Topical Gel 1285
Ery-Tab Tablets 448
Erythromycin Base Filmtab Tablets . 454
Erythromycin Delayed-Release Capsules, USP 455
PCE Dispertab Tablets 498

Erythromycin Estolate (Felodipine is metabolized by CYP3A4; co-administration of felodipine with erythromycin resulted in approximately 2.5-fold increase in the AUC and Cmax, and about 2-fold prolongation in the half-life of felodipine).

No products indexed under this heading.

Erythromycin Ethylsuccinate (Felodipine is metabolized by CYP3A4; co-administration of felodipine with erythromycin resulted in approximately 2.5-fold increase in the AUC and Cmax, and about 2-fold prolongation in the half-life of felodipine). Products include:

E.E.S. 450
EryPed 446
Pediazole Suspension 3050

Erythromycin Gluceptate (Felodipine is metabolized by CYP3A4; co-administration of felodipine with erythromycin resulted in approximately 2.5-fold increase in the AUC and Cmax, and about 2-fold prolongation in the half-life of felodipine).

No products indexed under this heading.

Erythromycin Stearate (Felodipine is metabolized by CYP3A4; co-administration of felodipine with erythromycin resulted in approximately 2.5-fold increase in the AUC and Cmax, and about 2-fold prolongation in the half-life of felodipine). Products include:

Erythrocin Stearate Filmtab Tablets 452

Esmolol Hydrochloride (Caution should be exercised when using Plendil in patients with heart failure or compromised ventricular function, particularly in combination with beta blocker). Products include:

Brevibloc Injection 858

Ethosuximide (Potential for low maximum plasma concentrations of felodipine in epileptic patients on long-term anticonvulsant therapy). Products include:

Zarontin Capsules 2659
Zarontin Syrup 2660

Ethotoin (Potential for low maximum plasma concentrations of felodipine in epileptic patients on long-term anticonvulsant therapy).

No products indexed under this heading.

Felbamate (Potential for low maximum plasma concentrations of felodipine in epileptic patients on long-term anticonvulsant therapy). Products include:

Felbatol 3343

Fosphenytoin Sodium (Potential for low maximum plasma concentrations of felodipine in epileptic patients on long-term anticonvulsant therapy). Products include:

Cerebyx Injection 2619

Itraconazole (Felodipine is metabolized by CYP3A4; co-administration of another extended release formulation of felodipine with itraconazole resulted in approximately 8-fold increase in the AUC, more than 6-fold increase in the Cmax, and 2-fold prolongation in the half-life of felodipine). Products include:

Sporanox Capsules 1800
Sporanox Injection 1804
Sporanox Injection 2509
Sporanox Oral Solution 1808
Sporanox Oral Solution 2512

Ketoconazole (Felodipine is metabolized by CYP3A4; co-administration of CYP3A4 inhibitors, such as ketoconazole, with felodipine may lead to several-fold increases in the plasma levels of felodipine, either due to an increase in bioavailability or due to a decrease in metabolism). Products include:

Nizoral 2% Cream 3620
Nizoral A-D Shampoo 2008
Nizoral 2% Shampoo 2007
Nizoral Tablets 1791

Labetalol Hydrochloride (Caution should be exercised when using Plendil in patients with heart failure or compromised ventricular function, particularly in combination with beta blocker). Products include:

Normodyne Injection 3135
Normodyne Tablets 3137

Lamotrigine (Potential for low maximum plasma concentrations of felodipine in epileptic patients on long-term anticonvulsant therapy). Products include:

Lamictal 1567

Levetiracetam (Potential for low maximum plasma concentrations of felodipine in epileptic patients on long-term anticonvulsant therapy). Products include:

Keppra Tablets 3314

Levobunolol Hydrochloride (Caution should be exercised when using Plendil in patients with heart failure or compromised ventricular function, particularly in combination with beta blocker). Products include:

Betagan .... ⊙228

Mephenytoin (Potential for low maximum plasma concentrations of felodipine in epileptic patients on long-term anticonvulsant therapy).

No products indexed under this heading.

Methsuximide (Potential for low maximum plasma concentrations of felodipine in epileptic patients on long-term anticonvulsant therapy). Products include:

Celontin Capsules 2618

Metipranolol Hydrochloride (Caution should be exercised when using Plendil in patients with heart failure or compromised ventricular function, particularly in combination with beta blocker).
No products indexed under this heading.

Metoprolol Succinate (Caution should be exercised when using Plendil in patients with heart failure or compromised ventricular function, particularly in combination with beta blocker). Products include:
Toprol-XL Tablets 651

Metoprolol Tartrate (Caution should be exercised when using Plendil in patients with heart failure or compromised ventricular function, particularly in combination with beta blocker).
No products indexed under this heading.

Nadolol (Caution should be exercised when using Plendil in patients with heart failure or compromised ventricular function, particularly in combination with beta blocker).
Products include:
Corgard Tablets 2245
Corzide 40/5 Tablets 2247
Corzide 80/5 Tablets 2247
Nadolol Tablets 2288

Oxcarbazepine (Potential for low maximum plasma concentrations of felodipine in epileptic patients on long-term anticonvulsant therapy).
Products include:
Trileptal Oral Suspension 2407
Trileptal Tablets 2407

Paramethadione (Potential for low maximum plasma concentrations of felodipine in epileptic patients on long-term anticonvulsant therapy).
No products indexed under this heading.

Penbutolol Sulfate (Caution should be exercised when using Plendil in patients with heart failure or compromised ventricular function, particularly in combination with beta blocker).
No products indexed under this heading.

Phenacemide (Potential for low maximum plasma concentrations of felodipine in epileptic patients on long-term anticonvulsant therapy).
No products indexed under this heading.

Phenobarbital (Potential for low maximum plasma concentrations of felodipine in epileptic patients on long-term anticonvulsant therapy).
Products include:
Arco-Lase Plus Tablets 592
Donnatal 2929
Donnatal Extentabs 2930

Phensuximide (Potential for low maximum plasma concentrations of felodipine in epileptic patients on long-term anticonvulsant therapy).
No products indexed under this heading.

Phenytoin (Potential for low maximum plasma concentrations of felodipine in epileptic patients on long-term anticonvulsant therapy).
Products include:
Dilantin Infatabs 2624
Dilantin-125 Oral Suspension 2625

Phenytoin Sodium (Potential for low maximum plasma concentrations of felodipine in epileptic patients on long-term anticonvulsant therapy). Products include:
Dilantin Kapseals 2622

Pindolol (Caution should be exercised when using Plendil in patients with heart failure or compromised ventricular function, particularly in combination with beta blocker).
No products indexed under this heading.

Primidone (Potential for low maximum plasma concentrations of felodipine in epileptic patients on long-term anticonvulsant therapy).
No products indexed under this heading.

Propranolol Hydrochloride (Caution should be exercised when using Plendil in patients with heart failure or compromised ventricular function, particularly in combination with beta blocker). Products include:
Inderal 3513
Inderal LA Long-Acting Capsules 3516
Inderide Tablets 3517
Inderide LA Long-Acting Capsules 3519

Sotalol Hydrochloride (Caution should be exercised when using Plendil in patients with heart failure or compromised ventricular function, particularly in combination with beta blocker). Products include:
Betapace Tablets 950
Betapace AF Tablets 954

Tiagabine Hydrochloride (Potential for low maximum plasma concentrations of felodipine in epileptic patients on long-term anticonvulsant therapy). Products include:
Gabitril Tablets 1189

Timolol Hemihydrate (Caution should be exercised when using Plendil in patients with heart failure or compromised ventricular function, particularly in combination with beta blocker). Products include:
Betimol Ophthalmic Solution .... ⊙324

Timolol Maleate (Caution should be exercised when using Plendil in patients with heart failure or compromised ventricular function, particularly in combination with beta blocker).
Products include:
Blocadren Tablets 2046
Cosopt Sterile Ophthalmic Solution 2065
Timolide Tablets 2187
Timolol GFS .... ⊙266
Timoptic in Ocudose 2192
Timoptic Sterile Ophthalmic Solution 2190
Timoptic-XE Sterile Ophthalmic Gel Forming Solution 2194

Topiramate (Potential for low maximum plasma concentrations of felodipine in epileptic patients on long-term anticonvulsant therapy).
Products include:
Topamax Sprinkle Capsules 2590
Topamax Tablets 2590

Trimethadione (Potential for low maximum plasma concentrations of felodipine in epileptic patients on long-term anticonvulsant therapy).
No products indexed under this heading.

Valproate Sodium (Potential for low maximum plasma concentrations of felodipine in epileptic patients on long-term anticonvulsant therapy). Products include:
Depacon Injection 416

Valproic Acid (Potential for low maximum plasma concentrations of felodipine in epileptic patients on long-term anticonvulsant therapy).
Products include:
Depakene 421

Zonisamide (Potential for low maximum plasma concentrations of felodipine in epileptic patients on long-term anticonvulsant therapy).
Products include:
Zonegran Capsules 1307

Food Interactions

Food, unspecified (When Plendil is administered either with high fat or carbohydrate diet, Cmax is increased by approximately 60%, AUC is unchanged; Plendil should regularly be taken either without food or with a light meal).

Grapefruit Juice (The bioavailability of felodipine is increased more than two-fold when taken with doubly concentrated grapefruit juice).

PLETAL TABLETS
(Cilostazol) 2605
May interact with erythromycin, macrolide antibiotics, and certain other agents. Compounds in these categories include:

Aspirin (Short-term co-administration has shown a 23% to 35% increase in inhibition of ADP-induced ex vivo platelet aggregation compared to aspirin alone; no clinically significant impact on bleeding time, PT, or aPTT was noted; there was no apparent greater incidence of hemorrhagic adverse effects in patients on cilostazol and aspirin compared to patients taking placebo and aspirin). Products include:
Aggrenox Capsules 1026
Alka-Seltzer .... ▣603
Alka-Seltzer Lemon Lime Antacid and Pain Reliever Effervescent Tablets .... ▣603
Alka-Seltzer Extra Strength Antacid and Pain Reliever Effervescent Tablets .... ▣603
Alka-Seltzer PM Effervescent Tablets .... ▣605
Genuine Bayer Tablets, Caplets and Gelcaps .... ▣606
Extra Strength Bayer Caplets and Gelcaps .... ▣610
Aspirin Regimen Bayer Children's Chewable Tablets (Orange or Cherry Flavored) .... ▣607
Bayer, Aspirin Regimen .... ▣606
Aspirin Regimen Bayer 81 mg Caplets with Calcium .... ▣607
Genuine Bayer Professional Labeling (Aspirin Regimen Bayer) .... ▣608
Extra Strength Bayer Arthritis Caplets .... ▣610
Extra Strength Bayer Plus Caplets .... ▣610
Extra Strength Bayer PM Caplets .... ▣611
BC Powder .... ▣619
BC Allergy Sinus Cold Powder .... ▣619
Arthritis Strength BC Powder .... ▣619
BC Sinus Cold Powder .... ▣619
Darvon Compound-65 Pulvules 1910
Ecotrin Enteric Coated Aspirin Low, Regular and Maximum Strength Tablets 1715
Excedrin Extra-Strength Tablets, Caplets, and Geltabs .... ▣629
Excedrin Migraine 1070
Goody's Body Pain Formula Powder .... ▣620
Goody's Extra Strength Headache Powder .... ▣620
Goody's Extra Strength Pain Relief Tablets .... ▣620
Percodan Tablets 1327
Robaxisal Tablets 2939
Soma Compound Tablets 3354
Soma Compound w/Codeine Tablets 3355
Vanquish Caplets .... ▣617

Azithromycin Dihydrate (Co-administration of cilostazol with inhibitors of CYP3A4, such as erythromycin, a macrolide antibiotic, has resulted in significant increases in the systemic exposure of cilostazol and/or its major metabolites; caution should be exercised if concurrently used). Products include:
Zithromax 2743
Zithromax for IV Infusion 2748
Zithromax for Oral Suspension, 300 mg, 600 mg, 900 mg, 1200 mg 2739
Zithromax Tablets, 250 mg 2739

Clarithromycin (Co-administration of cilostazol with inhibitors of CYP3A4, such as erythromycin, a macrolide antibiotic, has resulted in significant increases in the systemic exposure of cilostazol and/or its major metabolites; caution should be exercised if concurrently used).
Products include:
Biaxin/Biaxin XL 403
PREVPAC 3298

Diltiazem Hydrochloride (Co-administration with cilostazol with moderate inhibitors of CYP3A4, such as diltiazem, has been shown to increase cilostazol plasma concentrations by approximately 53%).
Products include:
Cardizem Injectable 1018
Cardizem Lyo-Ject Syringe 1018
Cardizem Monovial 1018
Cardizem CD Capsules 1016
Tiazac Capsules 1378

Diltiazem Malate (Co-administration with cilostazol with moderate inhibitors of CYP3A4, such as diltiazem, has been shown to increase cilostazol plasma concentrations by approximately 53%).
No products indexed under this heading.

Dirithromycin (Co-administration of cilostazol with inhibitors of CYP3A4, such as erythromycin, a macrolide antibiotic, has resulted in significant increases in the systemic exposure of cilostazol and/or its major metabolites; caution should be exercised if concurrently used). Products include:
Dynabac Tablets 2269

Erythromycin (Co-administration of cilostazol with inhibitors of CYP3A4, such as erythromycin, significantly increases in the systemic exposure of cilostazol and/or its major metabolites; caution should be exercised if concurrently used). Products include:
Emgel 2% Topical Gel 1285
Ery-Tab Tablets 448
Erythromycin Base Filmtab Tablets 454
Erythromycin Delayed-Release Capsules, USP 455
PCE Dispertab Tablets 498

Erythromycin Estolate (Co-administration of cilostazol with inhibitors of CYP3A4, such as erythromycin, significantly increases in the systemic exposure of cilostazol and/or its major metabolites; caution should be exercised if concurrently used).
No products indexed under this heading.

Erythromycin Ethylsuccinate (Co-administration of cilostazol with inhibitors of CYP3A4, such as erythromycin, significantly increases in the systemic exposure of cilostazol and/or its major metabolites; caution should be exercised if concurrently used). Products include:
E.E.S. 450
EryPed 446
Pediazole Suspension 3050

Erythromycin Gluceptate (Co-administration of cilostazol with inhibitors of CYP3A4, such as erythromycin, significantly increases in the systemic exposure of cilostazol and/or its major metabolites; caution should be exercised if concurrently used).
No products indexed under this heading.

Erythromycin Stearate (Co-administration of cilostazol with inhibitors of CYP3A4, such as erythromycin, significantly increases in the systemic exposure of cilostazol and/or its major metabolites; caution should be exercised if concurrently used). Products include:
Erythrocin Stearate Filmtab Tablets 452

Fluconazole (Co-administration of cilostazol with strong inhibitors of CYP3A4, such as fluconazole, would be expected to cause a greater increase in plasma levels of cilostazol and metabolites; this combination has not been studied). Products include:
Diflucan Tablets, Injection, and Oral Suspension 2681

Fluoxetine Hydrochloride (Co-administration of cilostazol with strong inhibitors of CYP3A4, such as fluoxetine, would be expected to cause a greater increase in plasma

levels of cilostazol and metabolites; this combination has not been studied). Products include:
Prozac Pulvules, Liquid, and Weekly Capsules 1238
Sarafem Pulvules 1962

Fluvoxamine Maleate (Co-administration of cilostazol with strong inhibitors of CYP3A4, such as fluvoxamine, would be expected to cause a greater increase in plasma levels of cilostazol and metabolites; this combination has not been studied). Products include:
Luvox Tablets (25, 50, 100 mg) 3256

Itraconazole (Co-administration of cilostazol with strong inhibitors of CYP3A4, such as itraconazole, would be expected to cause a greater increase in plasma levels of cilostazol and metabolites; this combination has not been studied). Products include:
Sporanox Capsules 1800
Sporanox Injection 1804
Sporanox Injection 2509
Sporanox Oral Solution 1808
Sporanox Oral Solution 2512

Ketoconazole (Co-administration of cilostazol with strong inhibitors of CYP3A4, such as ketoconazole, would be expected to cause a greater increase in plasma levels of cilostazol and metabolites; this combination has not been studied). Products include:
Nizoral 2% Cream 3620
Nizoral A-D Shampoo 2008
Nizoral 2% Shampoo 2007
Nizoral Tablets 1791

Miconazole (Co-administration of cilostazol with strong inhibitors of CYP3A4, such as miconazole, would be expected to cause a greater increase in plasma levels of cilostazol and metabolites; this combination has not been studied).
No products indexed under this heading.

Nefazodone Hydrochloride (Co-administration of cilostazol with strong inhibitors of CYP3A4, such as nefazodone, would be expected to cause a greater increase in plasma levels of cilostazol and metabolites; this combination has not been studied). Products include:
Serzone Tablets 1104

Omeprazole (Co-administration with potent inhibitor of CYP2C19, such as omeprazole, has increased the systemic exposure to 3,4 dehydro-cilostazol by 69%). Products include:
Prilosec Delayed-Release Capsules 628

Sertraline Hydrochloride (Co-administration of cilostazol with strong inhibitors of CYP3A4, such as sertraline, would be expected to cause a greater increase in plasma levels of cilostazol and metabolites; this combination has not been studied). Products include:
Zoloft 2751

Troleandomycin (Co-administration of cilostazol with inhibitors of CYP3A4, such as erythromycin, a macrolide antibiotic, has resulted in significant increases in the systemic exposure of cilostazol and/or its major metabolites; caution should be exercised if concurrently used). Products include:
Tao Capsules 2716

Food Interactions

Food, unspecified (Co-administration with high fat meal increases absorption, with an approximately 90% increase in Cmax and a 25% increase in AUC; patients should be advised to take Pletal at least one hour before or two hours after breakfast and dinner).

Grapefruit Juice (Co-administration of cilostazol with inhibitors of CYP3A4, such as grapefruit juice, may increase cilostazol plasma concentration; this interaction has not been studied, however, concurrent consumption of grapefruit juice should be avoided).

PLETAL TABLETS

(Cilostazol) 2848

May interact with erythromycin, macrolide antibiotics, and certain other agents. Compounds in these categories include:

Aspirin (Short-term co-administration has shown a 23% to 35% increase in inhibition of ADP-induced ex vivo platelet aggregation compared to aspirin alone; no clinically significant impact on bleeding time, PT, or aPTT was noted; there was no apparent greater incidence of hemorrhagic adverse effects in patients on cilostazol and aspirin compared to patients taking placebo and aspirin). Products include:
Aggrenox Capsules 1026
Alka-Seltzer .... ■603
Alka-Seltzer Lemon Lime Antacid and Pain Reliever Effervescent Tablets .... ■603
Alka-Seltzer Extra Strength Antacid and Pain Reliever Effervescent Tablets .... ■603
Alka-Seltzer PM Effervescent Tablets .... ■605
Genuine Bayer Tablets, Caplets and Gelcaps .... ■606
Extra Strength Bayer Caplets and Gelcaps .... ■610
Aspirin Regimen Bayer Children's Chewable Tablets (Orange or Cherry Flavored) .... ■607
Bayer, Aspirin Regimen .... ■606
Aspirin Regimen Bayer 81 mg Caplets with Calcium .... ■607
Genuine Bayer Professional Labeling (Aspirin Regimen Bayer) .... ■608
Extra Strength Bayer Arthritis Caplets .... ■610
Extra Strength Bayer Plus Caplets .... ■610
Extra Strength Bayer PM Caplets .... ■611
BC Powder .... ■619
BC Allergy Sinus Cold Powder .... ■619
Arthritis Strength BC Powder .... ■619
BC Sinus Cold Powder .... ■619
Darvon Compound-65 Pulvules 1910
Ecotrin Enteric Coated Aspirin Low, Regular and Maximum Strength Tablets 1715
Excedrin Extra-Strength Tablets, Caplets, and Geltabs .... ■629
Excedrin Migraine 1070
Goody's Body Pain Formula Powder .... ■620
Goody's Extra Strength Headache Powder .... ■620
Goody's Extra Strength Pain Relief Tablets .... ■620
Percodan Tablets 1327
Robaxisal Tablets 2939
Soma Compound Tablets 3354
Soma Compound w/Codeine Tablets 3355
Vanquish Caplets .... ■617

Azithromycin Dihydrate (Co-administration of cilostazol with inhibitors of CYP3A4, such as erythromycin, a macrolide antibiotic, has resulted in significant increases in the systemic exposure of cilostazol and/or its major metabolites; caution should be exercised if concurrently used). Products include:
Zithromax 2743
Zithromax for IV Infusion 2748
Zithromax for Oral Suspension, 300 mg, 600 mg, 900 mg, 1200 mg 2739
Zithromax Tablets, 250 mg 2739

Clarithromycin (Co-administration of cilostazol with inhibitors of CYP3A4, such as erythromycin, a macrolide antibiotic, has resulted in significant increases in the systemic exposure of cilostazol and/or its major metabolites; caution should be exercised if concurrently used). Products include:
Biaxin/Biaxin XL 403
PREVPAC 3298

Diltiazem Hydrochloride (Co-administration with cilostazol with moderate inhibitors of CYP3A4, such as diltiazem, has been shown to increase cilostazol plasma concentrations by approximately 53%). Products include:
Cardizem Injectable 1018
Cardizem Lyo-Ject Syringe 1018
Cardizem Monovial 1018
Cardizem CD Capsules 1016
Tiazac Capsules 1378

Diltiazem Malate (Co-administration with cilostazol with moderate inhibitors of CYP3A4, such as diltiazem, has been shown to increase cilostazol plasma concentrations by approximately 53%).
No products indexed under this heading.

Dirithromycin (Co-administration of cilostazol with inhibitors of CYP3A4, such as erythromycin, a macrolide antibiotic, has resulted in significant increases in the systemic exposure of cilostazol and/or its major metabolites; caution should be exercised if concurrently used). Products include:
Dynabac Tablets 2269

Erythromycin (Co-administration of cilostazol with inhibitors of CYP3A4, such as erythromycin, significantly increases in the systemic exposure of cilostazol and/or its major metabolites; caution should be exercised if concurrently used). Products include:
Emgel 2% Topical Gel 1285
Ery-Tab Tablets 448
Erythromycin Base Filmtab Tablets . 454
Erythromycin Delayed-Release Capsules, USP 455
PCE Dispertab Tablets 498

Erythromycin Estolate (Co-administration of cilostazol with inhibitors of CYP3A4, such as erythromycin, significantly increases in the systemic exposure of cilostazol and/or its major metabolites; caution should be exercised if concurrently used).
No products indexed under this heading.

Erythromycin Ethylsuccinate (Co-administration of cilostazol with inhibitors of CYP3A4, such as erythromycin, significantly increases in the systemic exposure of cilostazol and/or its major metabolites; caution should be exercised if concurrently used). Products include:
E.E.S. 450
EryPed 446
Pediazole Suspension 3050

Erythromycin Gluceptate (Co-administration of cilostazol with inhibitors of CYP3A4, such as erythromycin, significantly increases in the systemic exposure of cilostazol and/or its major metabolites; caution should be exercised if concurrently used).
No products indexed under this heading.

Erythromycin Stearate (Co-administration of cilostazol with inhibitors of CYP3A4, such as erythromycin, significantly increases in the systemic exposure of cilostazol and/or its major metabolites; caution should be exercised if concurrently used). Products include:
Erythrocin Stearate Filmtab Tablets 452

Fluconazole (Co-administration of cilostazol with strong inhibitors of CYP3A4, such as fluconazole, would be expected to cause a greater increase in plasma levels of cilostazol and metabolites; this combination has not been studied). Products include:
Diflucan Tablets, Injection, and Oral Suspension 2681

Fluoxetine Hydrochloride (Co-administration of cilostazol with strong inhibitors of CYP3A4, such as fluoxetine, would be expected to cause a greater increase in plasma levels of cilostazol and metabolites; this combination has not been studied). Products include:
Prozac Pulvules, Liquid, and Weekly Capsules 1238
Sarafem Pulvules 1962

Fluvoxamine Maleate (Co-administration of cilostazol with strong inhibitors of CYP3A4, such as fluvoxamine, would be expected to cause a greater increase in plasma levels of cilostazol and metabolites; this combination has not been studied). Products include:
Luvox Tablets (25, 50, 100 mg) 3256

Itraconazole (Co-administration of cilostazol with strong inhibitors of CYP3A4, such as itraconazole, would be expected to cause a greater increase in plasma levels of cilostazol and metabolites; this combination has not been studied). Products include:
Sporanox Capsules 1800
Sporanox Injection 1804
Sporanox Injection 2509
Sporanox Oral Solution 1808
Sporanox Oral Solution 2512

Ketoconazole (Co-administration of cilostazol with strong inhibitors of CYP3A4, such as ketoconazole, would be expected to cause a greater increase in plasma levels of cilostazol and metabolites; this combination has not been studied). Products include:
Nizoral 2% Cream 3620
Nizoral A-D Shampoo 2008
Nizoral 2% Shampoo 2007
Nizoral Tablets 1791

Miconazole (Co-administration of cilostazol with strong inhibitors of CYP3A4, such as miconazole, would be expected to cause a greater increase in plasma levels of cilostazol and metabolites; this combination has not been studied).
No products indexed under this heading.

Nefazodone Hydrochloride (Co-administration of cilostazol with strong inhibitors of CYP3A4, such as nefazodone, would be expected to cause a greater increase in plasma levels of cilostazol and metabolites; this combination has not been studied). Products include:
Serzone Tablets 1104

Omeprazole (Co-administration with potent inhibitor of CYP2C19, such as omeprazole, has increased the systemic exposure to 3,4 dehydro-cilostazol by 69%). Products include:
Prilosec Delayed-Release Capsules 628

Sertraline Hydrochloride (Co-administration of cilostazol with strong inhibitors of CYP3A4, such as sertraline, would be expected to cause a greater increase in plasma levels of cilostazol and metabolites; this combination has not been studied). Products include:
Zoloft 2751

Troleandomycin (Co-administration of cilostazol with inhibitors of CYP3A4, such as erythromycin, a macrolide antibiotic, has resulted in significant increases in the systemic exposure of cilostazol and/or its major metabolites; caution should be exercised if concurrently used). Products include:
Tao Capsules 2716

Food Interactions

Food, unspecified (Co-administration with high fat meal increases absorption, with an approximately 90% increase in Cmax and a 25% increase in AUC; patients should be advised to take Pletal at least one hour before or two hours after breakfast and dinner).

Grapefruit Juice (Co-administration of cilostazol with inhibitors of CYP3A4, such as grapefruit juice, may increase cilostazol plasma concentration; this interaction has not been studied, however, concurrent consumption of grapefruit juice should be avoided).

PLEXION CLEANSER
(Sodium Sulfacetamide, Sulfur) 2024
None cited in PDR database.

PLEXION TOPICAL SUSPENSION
(Sodium Sulfacetamide, Sulfur) 2024
None cited in PDR database.

PLUS CAPLETS
(Amino Acid Preparations) .... ▣820
None cited in PDR database.

PNEUMOVAX 23
(Pneumococcal Vaccine, Polyvalent) 2156
May interact with:

Azathioprine (Co-administration of vaccine in patients receiving immunosuppressive therapy may not result in expected serum antibody response; potential impairment of future immune responses to pneumoccocal antigens may occur).
No products indexed under this heading.

Cyclosporine (Co-administration of vaccine in patients receiving immunosuppressive therapy may not result in expected serum antibody response; potential impairment of future immune responses to pneumoccocal antigens may occur). Products include:
Gengraf Capsules 457
Neoral Soft Gelatin Capsules 2380
Neoral Oral Solution 2380
Sandimmune 2388

Muromonab-CD3 (Co-administration of vaccine in patients receiving immunosuppressive therapy may not result in expected serum antibody response; potential impairment of future immune responses to pneumoccocal antigens may occur). Products include:
Orthoclone OKT3 Sterile Solution ... 2498

Mycophenolate Mofetil (Co-administration of vaccine in patients receiving immunosuppressive therapy may not result in expected serum antibody response; potential impairment of future immune responses to pneumoccocal antigens may occur). Products include:
CellCept Capsules 2951
CellCept Oral Suspension 2951
CellCept Tablets 2951

Tacrolimus (Co-administration of vaccine in patients receiving immunosuppressive therapy may not result in expected serum antibody response; potential impairment of future immune responses to pneumoccocal antigens may occur). Products include:
Prograf 1393
Protopic Ointment 1397

PNU-IMUNE 23
(Pneumococcal Vaccine, Polyvalent) 1868
May interact with antineoplastics and immunosuppressive agents. Compounds in these categories include:

Altretamine (Possible impaired serum antibody response to vaccine). Products include:
Hexalen Capsules 2226

Anastrozole (Possible impaired serum antibody response to vaccine). Products include:
Arimidex Tablets 659

Asparaginase (Possible impaired serum antibody response to vaccine). Products include:
Elspar for Injection 2092

Azathioprine (Reduction of antibody levels).
No products indexed under this heading.

Basiliximab (Reduction of antibody levels). Products include:
Simulect for Injection 2399

Bicalutamide (Possible impaired serum antibody response to vaccine). Products include:
Casodex Tablets 662

Bleomycin Sulfate (Possible impaired serum antibody response to vaccine).
No products indexed under this heading.

Busulfan (Possible impaired serum antibody response to vaccine). Products include:
Myleran Tablets 1603

Carboplatin (Possible impaired serum antibody response to vaccine). Products include:
Paraplatin for Injection 1126

Carmustine (BCNU) (Possible impaired serum antibody response to vaccine). Products include:
Gliadel Wafer 1723

Chlorambucil (Possible impaired serum antibody response to vaccine). Products include:
Leukeran Tablets 1591

Cisplatin (Possible impaired serum antibody response to vaccine).
No products indexed under this heading.

Cyclophosphamide (Possible impaired serum antibody response to vaccine).
No products indexed under this heading.

Cyclosporine (Reduction of antibody levels). Products include:
Gengraf Capsules 457
Neoral Soft Gelatin Capsules 2380
Neoral Oral Solution 2380
Sandimmune 2388

Dacarbazine (Possible impaired serum antibody response to vaccine). Products include:
DTIC-Dome 902

Daunorubicin Citrate (Possible impaired serum antibody response to vaccine). Products include:
DaunoXome Injection 1442

Daunorubicin Hydrochloride (Possible impaired serum antibody response to vaccine). Products include:
Cerubidine for Injection 947

Denileukin Diftitox (Possible impaired serum antibody response to vaccine).
No products indexed under this heading.

Docetaxel (Possible impaired serum antibody response to vaccine). Products include:
Taxotere for Injection Concentrate 778

Doxorubicin Hydrochloride (Possible impaired serum antibody response to vaccine). Products include:
Adriamycin PFS/RDF Injection 2767
Doxil Injection 566

Epirubicin Hydrochloride (Possible impaired serum antibody response to vaccine). Products include:
Ellence Injection 2806

Estramustine Phosphate Sodium (Possible impaired serum antibody response to vaccine). Products include:
Emcyt Capsules 2810

Etoposide (Possible impaired serum antibody response to vaccine).
No products indexed under this heading.

Exemestane (Possible impaired serum antibody response to vaccine). Products include:
Aromasin Tablets 2769

Floxuridine (Possible impaired serum antibody response to vaccine). Products include:
Sterile FUDR 2974

Fluorouracil (Possible impaired serum antibody response to vaccine). Products include:
Carac Cream 1222
Efudex 1733
Fluoroplex 552

Flutamide (Possible impaired serum antibody response to vaccine). Products include:
Eulexin Capsules 3118

Gemcitabine Hydrochloride (Possible impaired serum antibody response to vaccine). Products include:
Gemzar for Injection 1919

Hydroxyurea (Possible impaired serum antibody response to vaccine). Products include:
Mylocel Tablets 2227

Idarubicin Hydrochloride (Possible impaired serum antibody response to vaccine). Products include:
Idamycin PFS Injection 2825

Ifosfamide (Possible impaired serum antibody response to vaccine). Products include:
Ifex for Injection 1123

Immune Globulin Intravenous (Human) (Reduction of antibody levels).
No products indexed under this heading.

Interferon alfa-2A, Recombinant (Possible impaired serum antibody response to vaccine). Products include:
Roferon-A Injection 2996

Interferon alfa-2B, Recombinant (Possible impaired serum antibody response to vaccine). Products include:
Intron A for Injection 3120
Rebetron Combination Therapy 3153

Irinotecan Hydrochloride (Possible impaired serum antibody response to vaccine).
No products indexed under this heading.

Levamisole Hydrochloride (Possible impaired serum antibody response to vaccine). Products include:
Ergamisol Tablets 1789

Lomustine (CCNU) (Possible impaired serum antibody response to vaccine).
No products indexed under this heading.

Mechlorethamine Hydrochloride (Possible impaired serum antibody response to vaccine). Products include:
Mustargen for Injection 2142

Megestrol Acetate (Possible impaired serum antibody response to vaccine). Products include:
Megace Oral Suspension 1124

Melphalan (Possible impaired serum antibody response to vaccine). Products include:
Alkeran Tablets 1466

Mercaptopurine (Possible impaired serum antibody response to vaccine). Products include:
Purinethol Tablets 1615

Methotrexate Sodium (Possible impaired serum antibody response to vaccine).
No products indexed under this heading.

Mitomycin (Mitomycin-C) (Possible impaired serum antibody response to vaccine).
No products indexed under this heading.

Mitotane (Possible impaired serum antibody response to vaccine).
No products indexed under this heading.

Mitoxantrone Hydrochloride (Possible impaired serum antibody response to vaccine). Products include:
Novantrone for Injection 1760

Muromonab-CD3 (Reduction of antibody levels). Products include:
Orthoclone OKT3 Sterile Solution ... 2498

Mycophenolate Mofetil (Reduction of antibody levels). Products include:
CellCept Capsules 2951
CellCept Oral Suspension 2951
CellCept Tablets 2951

Paclitaxel (Possible impaired serum antibody response to vaccine). Products include:
Taxol Injection 1129

Procarbazine Hydrochloride (Possible impaired serum antibody response to vaccine). Products include:
Matulane Capsules 3246

Sirolimus (Reduction of antibody levels). Products include:
Rapamune Oral Solution and Tablets 3584

Streptozocin (Possible impaired serum antibody response to vaccine).
No products indexed under this heading.

Tacrolimus (Reduction of antibody levels). Products include:
Prograf 1393
Protopic Ointment 1397

Tamoxifen Citrate (Possible impaired serum antibody response to vaccine). Products include:
Nolvadex Tablets 678

Teniposide (Possible impaired serum antibody response to vaccine).
No products indexed under this heading.

Thioguanine (Possible impaired serum antibody response to vaccine). Products include:
Tabloid Tablets 1642

Thiotepa (Possible impaired serum antibody response to vaccine). Products include:
Thioplex for Injection 1765

Topotecan Hydrochloride (Possible impaired serum antibody response to vaccine). Products include:
Hycamtin for Injection 1546

Toremifene Citrate (Possible impaired serum antibody response to vaccine). Products include:
Fareston Tablets 3237

Valrubicin (Possible impaired serum antibody response to vaccine). Products include:
Valstar Sterile Solution for Intravesical Instillation 1175

Vincristine Sulfate (Possible impaired serum antibody response to vaccine).
No products indexed under this heading.

Vinorelbine Tartrate (Possible impaired serum antibody response to vaccine). Products include:
Navelbine Injection 1604

PODOCON-25 LIQUID
(Podophyllin) 2608
None cited in PDR database.

POLOCAINE INJECTION, USP

(Mepivacaine Hydrochloride) 625

May interact with ergot-type oxytocic drugs, monoamine oxidase inhibitors, phenothiazines, and tricyclic antidepressants. Compounds in these categories include:

Amitriptyline Hydrochloride (Co-administration of local anesthetics solution containing epinephrine or norepinephrine with tricyclic antidepressants may produce severe, prolonged hypertension; concurrent use should be avoided). Products include:
- Etrafon 3115
- Limbitrol 1738

Amoxapine (Co-administration of local anesthetics solution containing epinephrine or norepinephrine with tricyclic antidepressants may produce severe, prolonged hypertension; concurrent use should be avoided).
- No products indexed under this heading.

Chlorpromazine (Co-administration of local anesthetics solution containing epinephrine and phenothiazines may reduce or reverse the pressor effect of epinephrine). Products include:
- Thorazine Suppositories 1656

Chlorpromazine Hydrochloride (Co-administration of local anesthetics solution containing epinephrine and phenothiazines may reduce or reverse the pressor effect of epinephrine). Products include:
- Thorazine 1656

Clomipramine Hydrochloride (Co-administration of local anesthetics solution containing epinephrine or norepinephrine with tricyclic antidepressants may produce severe, prolonged hypertension; concurrent use should be avoided).
- No products indexed under this heading.

Desipramine Hydrochloride (Co-administration of local anesthetics solution containing epinephrine or norepinephrine with tricyclic antidepressants may produce severe, prolonged hypertension; concurrent use should be avoided). Products include:
- Norpramin Tablets 755

Doxepin Hydrochloride (Co-administration of local anesthetics solution containing epinephrine or norepinephrine with tricyclic antidepressants may produce severe, prolonged hypertension; concurrent use should be avoided). Products include:
- Sinequan 2713

Fluphenazine Decanoate (Co-administration of local anesthetics solution containing epinephrine and phenothiazines may reduce or reverse the pressor effect of epinephrine).
- No products indexed under this heading.

Fluphenazine Enanthate (Co-administration of local anesthetics solution containing epinephrine and phenothiazines may reduce or reverse the pressor effect of epinephrine).
- No products indexed under this heading.

Fluphenazine Hydrochloride (Co-administration of local anesthetics solution containing epinephrine and phenothiazines may reduce or reverse the pressor effect of epinephrine).
- No products indexed under this heading.

Haloperidol (Co-administration of local anesthetics solution containing epinephrine and butyrophenones may reduce or reverse the pressor effect of epinephrine). Products include:
- Haldol Injection, Tablets and Concentrate 2533

Haloperidol Decanoate (Co-administration of local anesthetics solution containing epinephrine and butyrophenones may reduce or reverse the pressor effect of epinephrine). Products include:
- Haldol Decanoate 2535

Imipramine Hydrochloride (Co-administration of local anesthetics solution containing epinephrine or norepinephrine with tricyclic antidepressants may produce severe, prolonged hypertension; concurrent use should be avoided).
- No products indexed under this heading.

Imipramine Pamoate (Co-administration of local anesthetics solution containing epinephrine or norepinephrine with tricyclic antidepressants may produce severe, prolonged hypertension; concurrent use should be avoided).
- No products indexed under this heading.

Isocarboxazid (Co-administration of local anesthetics solution containing epinephrine or norepinephrine with MAO inhibitors may produce severe, prolonged hypertension; concurrent use should be avoided).
- No products indexed under this heading.

Maprotiline Hydrochloride (Co-administration of local anesthetics solution containing epinephrine or norepinephrine with tricyclic antidepressants may produce severe, prolonged hypertension; concurrent use should be avoided).
- No products indexed under this heading.

Mesoridazine Besylate (Co-administration of local anesthetics solution containing epinephrine and phenothiazines may reduce or reverse the pressor effect of epinephrine). Products include:
- Serentil 1057

Methotrimeprazine (Co-administration of local anesthetics solution containing epinephrine and phenothiazines may reduce or reverse the pressor effect of epinephrine).
- No products indexed under this heading.

Methylergonovine Maleate (Co-administration of local anesthetics solution containing vasopressors with ergot-type oxytocic drugs may cause severe, persistent hypertension or cerebrovascular accident).
- No products indexed under this heading.

Moclobemide (Co-administration of local anesthetics solution containing epinephrine or norepinephrine with MAO inhibitors may produce severe, prolonged hypertension; concurrent use should be avoided).
- No products indexed under this heading.

Nortriptyline Hydrochloride (Co-administration of local anesthetics solution containing epinephrine or norepinephrine with tricyclic antidepressants may produce severe, prolonged hypertension; concurrent use should be avoided).
- No products indexed under this heading.

Pargyline Hydrochloride (Co-administration of local anesthetics solution containing epinephrine or norepinephrine with MAO inhibitors may produce severe, prolonged hypertension; concurrent use should be avoided).
- No products indexed under this heading.

Perphenazine (Co-administration of local anesthetics solution containing epinephrine and phenothiazines may reduce or reverse the pressor effect of epinephrine). Products include:
- Etrafon 3115
- Trilafon 3160

Phenelzine Sulfate (Co-administration of local anesthetics solution containing epinephrine or norepinephrine with MAO inhibitors may produce severe, prolonged hypertension; concurrent use should be avoided). Products include:
- Nardil Tablets 2653

Procarbazine Hydrochloride (Co-administration of local anesthetics solution containing epinephrine or norepinephrine with MAO inhibitors may produce severe, prolonged hypertension; concurrent use should be avoided). Products include:
- Matulane Capsules 3246

Prochlorperazine (Co-administration of local anesthetics solution containing epinephrine and phenothiazines may reduce or reverse the pressor effect of epinephrine). Products include:
- Compazine 1505

Promethazine Hydrochloride (Co-administration of local anesthetics solution containing epinephrine and phenothiazines may reduce or reverse the pressor effect of epinephrine). Products include:
- Mepergan Injection 3539
- Phenergan Injection 3553
- Phenergan 3556
- Phenergan Syrup 3554
- Phenergan with Codeine Syrup 3557
- Phenergan with Dextromethorphan Syrup 3559
- Phenergan VC Syrup 3560
- Phenergan VC with Codeine Syrup . 3561

Protriptyline Hydrochloride (Co-administration of local anesthetics solution containing epinephrine or norepinephrine with tricyclic antidepressants may produce severe, prolonged hypertension; concurrent use should be avoided). Products include:
- Vivactil Tablets 2446
- Vivactil Tablets 2217

Selegiline Hydrochloride (Co-administration of local anesthetics solution containing epinephrine or norepinephrine with MAO inhibitors may produce severe, prolonged hypertension; concurrent use should be avoided). Products include:
- Eldepryl Capsules 3266

Thioridazine Hydrochloride (Co-administration of local anesthetics solution containing epinephrine and phenothiazines may reduce or reverse the pressor effect of epinephrine). Products include:
- Thioridazine Hydrochloride Tablets 2289

Tranylcypromine Sulfate (Co-administration of local anesthetics solution containing epinephrine or norepinephrine with MAO inhibitors may produce severe, prolonged hypertension; concurrent use should be avoided). Products include:
- Parnate Tablets 1607

Trifluoperazine Hydrochloride (Co-administration of local anesthetics solution containing epinephrine and phenothiazines may reduce or reverse the pressor effect of epinephrine). Products include:
- Stelazine 1640

Trimipramine Maleate (Co-administration of local anesthetics solution containing epinephrine or norepinephrine with tricyclic antidepressants may produce severe, prolonged hypertension; concurrent use should be avoided). Products include:
- Surmontil Capsules 3595

POLOCAINE-MPF INJECTION, USP

(Mepivacaine Hydrochloride) 625

See Polocaine Injection, USP

POLY-PRED LIQUIFILM OPHTHALMIC SUSPENSION

(Neomycin Sulfate, Polymyxin B Sulfate, Prednisolone Acetate).......... ⊙ 245

None cited in PDR database.

POLYSPORIN OINTMENT

(Bacitracin Zinc, Polymyxin B Sulfate).. ▣ 706

None cited in PDR database.

POLYSPORIN OPHTHALMIC OINTMENT STERILE

(Bacitracin Zinc, Polymyxin B Sulfate) .... ⊙ 301

None cited in PDR database.

POLYSPORIN POWDER

(Bacitracin Zinc, Polymyxin B Sulfate) .... ▣ 706

None cited in PDR database.

POLYTRIM OPHTHALMIC SOLUTION

(Polymyxin B Sulfate, Trimethoprim Sulfate) 556

None cited in PDR database.

PONSTEL CAPSULES

(Mefenamic Acid) 1356

May interact with ACE inhibitors, lithium preparations, thiazides, and certain other agents. Compounds in these categories include:

Aspirin (Co-administration is not generally recommended because of the potential of increased adverse effects). Products include:
- Aggrenox Capsules 1026
- Alka-Seltzer .... ▣ 603
- Alka-Seltzer Lemon Lime Antacid and Pain Reliever Effervescent Tablets .... ▣ 603
- Alka-Seltzer Extra Strength Antacid and Pain Reliever Effervescent Tablets .... ▣ 603
- Alka-Seltzer PM Effervescent Tablets .... ▣ 605
- Genuine Bayer Tablets, Caplets and Gelcaps .... ▣ 606
- Extra Strength Bayer Caplets and Gelcaps .... ▣ 610
- Aspirin Regimen Bayer Children's Chewable Tablets (Orange or Cherry Flavored) .... ▣ 607
- Bayer, Aspirin Regimen .... ▣ 606
- Aspirin Regimen Bayer 81 mg Caplets with Calcium .... ▣ 607
- Genuine Bayer Professional Labeling (Aspirin Regimen Bayer) .... ▣ 608
- Extra Strength Bayer Arthritis Caplets .... ▣ 610
- Extra Strength Bayer Plus Caplets .... ▣ 610
- Extra Strength Bayer PM Caplets . ▣ 611
- BC Powder .... ▣ 619
- BC Allergy Sinus Cold Powder .... ▣ 619
- Arthritis Strength BC Powder .... ▣ 619
- BC Sinus Cold Powder .... ▣ 619
- Darvon Compound-65 Pulvules 1910
- Ecotrin Enteric Coated Aspirin Low, Regular and Maximum Strength Tablets 1715
- Excedrin Extra-Strength Tablets, Caplets, and Geltabs .... ▣ 629
- Excedrin Migraine 1070
- Goody's Body Pain Formula Powder .... ▣ 620
- Goody's Extra Strength Headache Powder .... ▣ 620
- Goody's Extra Strength Pain Relief Tablets .... ▣ 620
- Percodan Tablets 1327
- Robaxisal Tablets 2939
- Soma Compound Tablets 3354

Soma Compound w/Codeine Tablets 3355
Vanquish Caplets .... ■617

Benazepril Hydrochloride (NSAIDs may diminish the antihypertensive effect of ACE inhibitors; concomitant use potentially could result in overt renal decompensation). Products include:
Lotensin Tablets 2365
Lotensin HCT Tablets 2367
Lotrel Capsules 2370

Bendroflumethiazide (NSAIDs can reduce the natriuretic effect of thiazides; concomitant use potentially could result in overt renal decompensation). Products include:
Corzide 40/5 Tablets 2247
Corzide 80/5 Tablets 2247

Captopril (NSAIDs may diminish the antihypertensive effect of ACE inhibitors; concomitant use potentially could result in overt renal decompensation). Products include:
Captopril Tablets 2281

Chlorothiazide (NSAIDs can reduce the natriuretic effect of thiazides; concomitant use potentially could result in overt renal decompensation). Products include:
Aldoclor Tablets 2035
Diuril Oral 2087

Chlorothiazide Sodium (NSAIDs can reduce the natriuretic effect of thiazides; concomitant use potentially could result in overt renal decompensation). Products include:
Diuril Sodium Intravenous 2086

Enalapril Maleate (NSAIDs may diminish the antihypertensive effect of ACE inhibitors; concomitant use potentially could result in overt renal decompensation). Products include:
Lexxel Tablets 608
Vaseretic Tablets 2204
Vasotec Tablets 2210

Enalaprilat (NSAIDs may diminish the antihypertensive effect of ACE inhibitors; concomitant use potentially could result in overt renal decompensation). Products include:
Enalaprilat Injection 863
Vasotec I.V. Injection 2207

Fosinopril Sodium (NSAIDs may diminish the antihypertensive effect of ACE inhibitors; concomitant use potentially could result in overt renal decompensation). Products include:
Monopril Tablets 1091
Monopril HCT 1094

Furosemide (NSAIDs can reduce the natriuretic effect of furosemide; concomitant use potentially could result in overt renal decompensation). Products include:
Furosemide Tablets 2284

Hydrochlorothiazide (NSAIDs can reduce the natriuretic effect of thiazides; concomitant use potentially could result in overt renal decompensation). Products include:
Accuretic Tablets 2614
Aldoril Tablets 2039
Atacand HCT Tablets 597
Avalide Tablets 1070
Diovan HCT Tablets 2338
Dyazide Capsules 1515
HydroDIURIL Tablets 2108
Hyzaar 2109
Inderide Tablets 3517
Inderide LA Long-Acting Capsules 3519
Lotensin HCT Tablets 2367
Maxzide 1008
Micardis HCT Tablets 1051
Microzide Capsules 3414
Moduretic Tablets 2138
Monopril HCT 1094
Prinzide Tablets 2168
Timolide Tablets 2187
Uniretic Tablets 3178
Vaseretic Tablets 2204
Zestoretic Tablets 695
Ziac Tablets 1887

Hydroflumethiazide (NSAIDs can reduce the natriuretic effect of thiazides; concomitant use potentially could result in overt renal decompensation). Products include:
Diucardin Tablets 3494

Lisinopril (NSAIDs may diminish the antihypertensive effect of ACE inhibitors; concomitant use potentially could result in overt renal decompensation). Products include:
Prinivil Tablets 2164
Prinzide Tablets 2168
Zestoretic Tablets 695
Zestril Tablets 698

Lithium Carbonate (NSAIDs have produced an elevation of plasma lithium levels and a redution in renal lithium clearance). Products include:
Eskalith 1527
Lithium Carbonate 3061
Lithobid Slow-Release Tablets 3255

Lithium Citrate (NSAIDs have produced an elevation of plasma lithium levels and a reduction in renal lithium clearance). Products include:
Lithium Citrate Syrup 3061

Magnesium Hydroxide (Ingestion of an antacid containing magnesium hydroxide with mefenamic acid increased the Cmax and AUC of mefenamic acid by 125% and 36% respectively). Products include:
Ex•Lax Milk of Magnesia Liquid .... ■670
Maalox Antacid/Anti-Gas Oral Suspension .... ■673
Maalox Max Maximum Strength Antacid/Anti-Gas Liquid 2300
Maalox Regular Strength Antacid/Antigas Liquid 2300
Mylanta Fast-Acting 1813
Mylanta 1813
Pepcid Complete Chewable Tablets 1815
Phillips' Chewable Tablets .... ■615
Phillips' Milk of Magnesia Liquid (Original, Cherry, & Mint) .... ■616
Rolaids Tablets .... ■706
Extra Strength Rolaids Tablets .... ■706
Vanquish Caplets .... ■617

Methotrexate Sodium (NSAIDs have been reported to competitively inhibit methotrexate accumulation in rabbit kidney slices; this may indicate that NSAIDs could enhance the toxicity of methotrexate).
No products indexed under this heading.

Methyclothiazide (NSAIDs can reduce the natriuretic effect of thiazides; concomitant use potentially could result in overt renal decompensation).
No products indexed under this heading.

Moexipril Hydrochloride (NSAIDs may diminish the antihypertensive effect of ACE inhibitors; concomitant use potentially could result in overt renal decompensation). Products include:
Uniretic Tablets 3178
Univasc Tablets 3181

Perindopril Erbumine (NSAIDs may diminish the antihypertensive effect of ACE inhibitors; concomitant use potentially could result in overt renal decompensation). Products include:
Aceon Tablets (2 mg, 4 mg, 8 mg) 3249

Polythiazide (NSAIDs can reduce the natriuretic effect of thiazides; concomitant use potentially could result in overt renal decompensation). Products include:
Minizide Capsules 2700
Renese Tablets 2712

Quinapril Hydrochloride (NSAIDs may diminish the antihypertensive effect of ACE inhibitors; concomitant use potentially could result in overt renal decompensation). Products include:
Accupril Tablets 2611
Accuretic Tablets 2614

Ramipril (NSAIDs may diminish the antihypertensive effect of ACE inhibitors; concomitant use potentially could result in overt renal decompensation). Products include:
Altace Capsules 2233

Spirapril Hydrochloride (NSAIDs may diminish the antihypertensive effect of ACE inhibitors; concomitant use potentially could result in overt renal decompensation).
No products indexed under this heading.

Trandolapril (NSAIDs may diminish the antihypertensive effect of ACE inhibitors; concomitant use potentially could result in overt renal decompensation). Products include:
Mavik Tablets 478
Tarka Tablets 508

Warfarin Sodium (Co-administration has synergistic effects on GI bleeding). Products include:
Coumadin for Injection 1243
Coumadin Tablets 1243
Warfarin Sodium Tablets, USP 3302

POTABA CAPSULES
(Aminobenzoate Potassium) 1721
May interact with:

Sulfamethoxazole (Co-administration with sulfonamides is contraindicated). Products include:
Bactrim 2949
Septra Suspension 2265
Septra Tablets 2265
Septra DS Tablets 2265

Sulfasalazine (Co-administration with sulfonamides is contraindicated). Products include:
Azulfidine EN-tabs Tablets 2775

Sulfisoxazole Acetyl (Co-administration with sulfonamides is contraindicated). Products include:
Pediazole Suspension 3050

POTABA POWDER
(Aminobenzoate Potassium) 1721
See Potaba Capsules

POTABA TABLETS
(Aminobenzoate Potassium) 1721
See Potaba Capsules

PRAMOSONE CREAM 1% AND 2.5%
(Hydrocortisone Acetate, Pramoxine Hydrochloride) 1343
None cited in PDR database.

PRAMOSONE LOTION 1% AND 2.5%
(Hydrocortisone Acetate, Pramoxine Hydrochloride) 1343
See Pramosone Cream 1% and 2.5%

PRAMOSONE OINTMENT 1% AND 2.5%
(Hydrocortisone Acetate, Pramoxine Hydrochloride) 1343
See Pramosone Cream 1% and 2.5%

PRANDIN TABLETS (0.5, 1, AND 2 MG)
(Repaglinide) 2432
May interact with barbiturates, beta blockers, calcium channel blockers, corticosteroids, oral anticoagulants, diuretics, erythromycin, estrogens, monoamine oxidase inhibitors, nonsteroidal anti-inflammatory agents, phenothiazines, phenytoin, and salicylates. Compounds in these categories include:

Acebutolol Hydrochloride (The hypoglycemic action of oral antidiabetic agents may be potentiated by beta adrenergic blocking agents; hypoglycemia may be difficult to recognize with co-administration). Products include:
Sectral Capsules 3589

Albuterol (Sympathomimetics tend to produce hyperglycemia and may lead to loss of glycemic control). Products include:
Proventil Inhalation Aerosol 3142
Ventolin Inhalation Aerosol and Refill 1679

Albuterol Sulfate (Sympathomimetics tend to produce hyperglycemia and may lead to loss of glycemic control). Products include:
AccuNeb Inhalation Solution 1230
Combivent Inhalation Aerosol 1041
DuoNeb Inhalation Solution 1233
Proventil Inhalation Solution 0.083% 3146
Proventil Repetabs Tablets 3148
Proventil Solution for Inhalation 0.5% 3144
Proventil HFA Inhalation Aerosol 3150
Ventolin HFA Inhalation Aerosol 3618
Volmax Extended-Release Tablets 2276

Amiloride Hydrochloride (Diuretics tend to produce hyperglycemia and may lead to loss of glycemic control). Products include:
Midamor Tablets 2136
Moduretic Tablets 2138

Amlodipine Besylate (Calcium channel blocking agents tend to produce hyperglycemia and may lead to loss of glycemic control). Products include:
Lotrel Capsules 2370
Norvasc Tablets 2704

Aprobarbital (Drugs that induce the CYP450 enzyme system 3A4, such as barbiturates, may increase repaglinide metabolism).
No products indexed under this heading.

Aspirin (The hypoglycemic action of oral antidiabetic agents may be potentiated by salicylates). Products include:
Aggrenox Capsules 1026
Alka-Seltzer .... ■603
Alka-Seltzer Lemon Lime Antacid and Pain Reliever Effervescent Tablets .... ■603
Alka-Seltzer Extra Strength Antacid and Pain Reliever Effervescent Tablets .... ■603
Alka-Seltzer PM Effervescent Tablets .... ■605
Genuine Bayer Tablets, Caplets and Gelcaps .... ■606
Extra Strength Bayer Caplets and Gelcaps .... ■610
Aspirin Regimen Bayer Children's Chewable Tablets (Orange or Cherry Flavored) .... ■607
Bayer, Aspirin Regimen .... ■606
Aspirin Regimen Bayer 81 mg Caplets with Calcium .... ■607
Genuine Bayer Professional Labeling (Aspirin Regimen Bayer) .... ■608
Extra Strength Bayer Arthritis Caplets .... ■610
Extra Strength Bayer Plus Caplets .... ■610
Extra Strength Bayer PM Caplets .... ■611
BC Powder .... ■619
BC Allergy Sinus Cold Powder .... ■619
Arthritis Strength BC Powder .... ■619
BC Sinus Cold Powder .... ■619
Darvon Compound-65 Pulvules 1910
Ecotrin Enteric Coated Aspirin Low, Regular and Maximum Strength Tablets 1715
Excedrin Extra-Strength Tablets, Caplets, and Geltabs .... ■629
Excedrin Migraine 1070
Goody's Body Pain Formula Powder .... ■620
Goody's Extra Strength Headache Powder .... ■620
Goody's Extra Strength Pain Relief Tablets .... ■620
Percodan Tablets 1327
Robaxisal Tablets 2939
Soma Compound Tablets 3354
Soma Compound w/Codeine Tablets 3355
Vanquish Caplets .... ■617

Atenolol (The hypoglycemic action of oral antidiabetic agents may be potentiated by beta adrenergic blocking agents; hypoglycemia may be difficult to recognize with co-administration). Products include:
Tenoretic Tablets 690
Tenormin I.V. Injection 692

IMPORTANT NOTE: Always consult each drug listing in the patient's regimen for possible interactions.

Bendroflumethiazide (Diuretics tend to produce hyperglycemia and may lead to loss of glycemic control). Products include:
- Corzide 40/5 Tablets 2247
- Corzide 80/5 Tablets 2247

Bepridil Hydrochloride (Calcium channel blocking agents tend to produce hyperglycemia and may lead to loss of glycemic control). Products include:
- Vascor Tablets 2602

Betamethasone Acetate (Corticosteroids tend to produce hyperglycemia and may lead to loss of glycemic control). Products include:
- Celestone Soluspan Injectable Suspension 3097

Betamethasone Sodium Phosphate (Corticosteroids tend to produce hyperglycemia and may lead to loss of glycemic control). Products include:
- Celestone Soluspan Injectable Suspension 3097

Betaxolol Hydrochloride (The hypoglycemic action of oral antidiabetic agents may be potentiated by beta adrenergic blocking agents; hypoglycemia may be difficult to recognize with co-administration). Products include:
- Betoptic S Ophthalmic Suspension 537

Bisoprolol Fumarate (The hypoglycemic action of oral antidiabetic agents may be potentiated by beta adrenergic blocking agents; hypoglycemia may be difficult to recognize with co-administration). Products include:
- Zebeta Tablets 1885
- Ziac Tablets 1887

Bumetanide (Diuretics tend to produce hyperglycemia and may lead to loss of glycemic control).
No products indexed under this heading.

Butabarbital (Drugs that induce the CYP450 enzyme system 3A4, such as barbiturates, may increase repaglinide metabolism).
No products indexed under this heading.

Butalbital (Drugs that induce the CYP450 enzyme system 3A4, such as barbiturates, may increase repaglinide metabolism). Products include:
- Phrenilin 578
- Sedapap Tablets 50 mg/650 mg 2225

Carbamazepine (Drugs that induce the CYP450 enzyme system 3A4, such as carbamazepine, may increase repaglinide metabolism). Products include:
- Carbatrol Capsules 3234
- Tegretol/Tegretol-XR 2404

Carteolol Hydrochloride (The hypoglycemic action of oral antidiabetic agents may be potentiated by beta adrenergic blocking agents; hypoglycemia may be difficult to recognize with co-administration). Products include:
- Carteolol Hydrochloride Ophthalmic Solution USP, 1% ..... ⊙258
- Ocupress Ophthalmic Solution, 1% Sterile .... ⊙303

Celecoxib (The hypoglycemic action of oral antidiabetic agents may be potentiated by non-steroidal anti-inflammatory agents). Products include:
- Celebrex Capsules 2676
- Celebrex Capsules 2780

Chloramphenicol Sodium Succinate (The hypoglycemic action of oral antidiabetic agents may be potentiated by chloramphenicol).
No products indexed under this heading.

Chlorothiazide (Diuretics tend to produce hyperglycemia and may lead to loss of glycemic control). Products include:
- Aldoclor Tablets 2035
- Diuril Oral 2087

Chlorothiazide Sodium (Diuretics tend to produce hyperglycemia and may lead to loss of glycemic control). Products include:
- Diuril Sodium Intravenous 2086

Chlorotrianisene (Estrogens and oral contraceptives tend to produce hyperglycemia and may lead to loss of glycemic control).
No products indexed under this heading.

Chlorpromazine (Phenothiazines tend to produce hyperglycemia and may lead to loss of glycemic control). Products include:
- Thorazine Suppositories 1656

Chlorpromazine Hydrochloride (Phenothiazines tend to produce hyperglycemia and may lead to loss of glycemic control). Products include:
- Thorazine 1656

Chlorpropamide (The hypoglycemic action of oral antidiabetic agents may be potentiated by sulfonamides). Products include:
- Diabinese Tablets 2680

Chlorthalidone (Diuretics tend to produce hyperglycemia and may lead to loss of glycemic control). Products include:
- Clorpres Tablets 1002
- Combipres Tablets 1040
- Tenoretic Tablets 690

Choline Magnesium Trisalicylate (The hypoglycemic action of oral antidiabetic agents may be potentiated by salicylates). Products include:
- Trilisate 2901

Cortisone Acetate (Corticosteroids tend to produce hyperglycemia and may lead to loss of glycemic control). Products include:
- Cortone Acetate Injectable Suspension 2059
- Cortone Acetate Tablets 2061

Dexamethasone (Corticosteroids tend to produce hyperglycemia and may lead to loss of glycemic control). Products include:
- Decadron Elixir 2078
- Decadron Tablets 2079
- TobraDex Ophthalmic Ointment 542
- TobraDex Ophthalmic Suspension .. 541

Dexamethasone Acetate (Corticosteroids tend to produce hyperglycemia and may lead to loss of glycemic control).
No products indexed under this heading.

Dexamethasone Sodium Phosphate (Corticosteroids tend to produce hyperglycemia and may lead to loss of glycemic control). Products include:
- Decadron Phosphate Injection 2081
- Decadron Phosphate Sterile Ophthalmic Ointment 2083
- Decadron Phosphate Sterile Ophthalmic Solution 2084
- NeoDecadron Sterile Ophthalmic Solution 2144

Diclofenac Potassium (The hypoglycemic action of oral antidiabetic agents may be potentiated by non-steroidal anti-inflammatory agents). Products include:
- Cataflam Tablets 2315

Diclofenac Sodium (The hypoglycemic action of oral antidiabetic agents may be potentiated by non-steroidal anti-inflammatory agents). Products include:
- Arthrotec Tablets 3195
- Voltaren Ophthalmic Sterile Ophthalmic Solution .... ⊙312
- Voltaren Tablets 2315
- Voltaren-XR Tablets 2315

Dicumarol (The hypoglycemic action of oral antidiabetic agents may be potentiated by coumarins).
No products indexed under this heading.

Dienestrol (Estrogens and oral contraceptives tend to produce hyperglycemia and may lead to loss of glycemic control). Products include:
- Ortho Dienestrol Cream 2554

Diethylstilbestrol (Estrogens and oral contraceptives tend to produce hyperglycemia and may lead to loss of glycemic control).
No products indexed under this heading.

Diflunisal (The hypoglycemic action of oral antidiabetic agents may be potentiated by salicylates). Products include:
- Dolobid Tablets 2088

Diltiazem Hydrochloride (Calcium channel blocking agents tend to produce hyperglycemia and may lead to loss of glycemic control). Products include:
- Cardizem Injectable 1018
- Cardizem Lyo-Ject Syringe 1018
- Cardizem Monovial 1018
- Cardizem CD Capsules 1016
- Tiazac Capsules 1378

Dobutamine Hydrochloride (Sympathomimetics tend to produce hyperglycemia and may lead to loss of glycemic control). Products include:
- Dobutrex Solution Vials 1914

Dopamine Hydrochloride (Sympathomimetics tend to produce hyperglycemia and may lead to loss of glycemic control).
No products indexed under this heading.

Ephedrine Hydrochloride (Sympathomimetics tend to produce hyperglycemia and may lead to loss of glycemic control). Products include:
- Primatene Tablets .... ■780

Ephedrine Sulfate (Sympathomimetics tend to produce hyperglycemia and may lead to loss of glycemic control).
No products indexed under this heading.

Ephedrine Tannate (Sympathomimetics tend to produce hyperglycemia and may lead to loss of glycemic control). Products include:
- Rynatuss Pediatric Suspension 3353
- Rynatuss Tablets 3353

Epinephrine (Sympathomimetics tend to produce hyperglycemia and may lead to loss of glycemic control). Products include:
- Epifrin Sterile Ophthalmic Solution .... ⊙235
- EpiPen 1236
- Primatene Mist .... ■779
- Xylocaine with Epinephrine Injection 653

Epinephrine Bitartrate (Sympathomimetics tend to produce hyperglycemia and may lead to loss of glycemic control). Products include:
- Sensorcaine 643

Epinephrine Hydrochloride (Sympathomimetics tend to produce hyperglycemia and may lead to loss of glycemic control).
No products indexed under this heading.

Erythromycin (In vitro data indicate that repaglinide metabolism may be inhibited by erythromycin). Products include:
- Emgel 2% Topical Gel 1285
- Ery-Tab Tablets 448
- Erythromycin Base Filmtab Tablets . 454
- Erythromycin Delayed-Release Capsules, USP 455
- PCE Dispertab Tablets 498

Erythromycin Estolate (In vitro data indicate that repaglinide metabolism may be inhibited by erythromycin).
No products indexed under this heading.

Erythromycin Ethylsuccinate (In vitro data indicate that repaglinide metabolism may be inhibited by erythromycin). Products include:
- E.E.S. 450
- EryPed 446
- Pediazole Suspension 3050

Erythromycin Gluceptate (In vitro data indicate that repaglinide metabolism may be inhibited by erythromycin).
No products indexed under this heading.

Erythromycin Stearate (In vitro data indicate that repaglinide metabolism may be inhibited by erythromycin). Products include:
- Erythrocin Stearate Filmtab Tablets 452

Esmolol Hydrochloride (The hypoglycemic action of oral antidiabetic agents may be potentiated by beta adrenergic blocking agents; hypoglycemia may be difficult to recognize with co-administration). Products include:
- Brevibloc Injection 858

Estradiol (Estrogens and oral contraceptives tend to produce hyperglycemia and may lead to loss of glycemic control). Products include:
- Activella Tablets 2764
- Alora Transdermal System 3372
- Climara Transdermal System 958
- CombiPatch Transdermal System .. 2323
- Esclim Transdermal System 3460
- Estrace Vaginal Cream 3358
- Estrace Tablets 3361
- Estring Vaginal Ring 2811
- Ortho-Prefest Tablets 2570
- Vagifem Tablets 2857
- Vivelle Transdermal System 2412
- Vivelle-Dot Transdermal System 2416

Estrogens, Conjugated (Estrogens and oral contraceptives tend to produce hyperglycemia and may lead to loss of glycemic control). Products include:
- Premarin Intravenous 3563
- Premarin Tablets 3566
- Premarin Vaginal Cream 3570
- Premphase Tablets 3572
- Prempro Tablets 3572

Estrogens, Esterified (Estrogens and oral contraceptives tend to produce hyperglycemia and may lead to loss of glycemic control). Products include:
- Estratest 3252
- Menest Tablets 2254

Estropipate (Estrogens and oral contraceptives tend to produce hyperglycemia and may lead to loss of glycemic control). Products include:
- Ogen Tablets 2846
- Ortho-Est Tablets 3464

Ethacrynic Acid (Diuretics tend to produce hyperglycemia and may lead to loss of glycemic control). Products include:
- Edecrin Tablets 2091

Ethinyl Estradiol (Estrogens and oral contraceptives tend to produce hyperglycemia and may lead to loss of glycemic control). Products include:
- Alesse-21 Tablets 3468
- Alesse-28 Tablets 3473
- Brevicon 28-Day Tablets 3380
- Cyclessa Tablets 2450
- Desogen Tablets 2458
- Estinyl Tablets 3112
- Estrostep 2627
- femhrt Tablets 2635
- Levlen 962
- Levlite 21 Tablets 962
- Levlite 28 Tablets 962
- Levora Tablets 3389
- Loestrin 21 Tablets 2642
- Loestrin Fe Tablets 2642
- Lo/Ovral Tablets 3532
- Lo/Ovral-28 Tablets 3538
- Low-Ogestrel-28 Tablets 3392
- Microgestin Fe 1.5/30 Tablets 3407
- Microgestin Fe 1/20 Tablets 3400
- Mircette Tablets 2470
- Modicon 2563

Necon ... 3415
Nordette-28 Tablets ... 2257
Norinyl 1 +35 28-Day Tablets ... 3380
Ogestrel 0.5/50-28 Tablets ... 3428
Ortho-Cept 21 Tablets ... 2546
Ortho-Cept 28 Tablets ... 2546
Ortho-Cyclen/Ortho Tri-Cyclen ... 2573
Ortho-Novum ... 2563
Ovcon ... 3364
Ovral Tablets ... 3551
Ovral-28 Tablets ... 3552
Tri-Levlen ... 962
Tri-Norinyl-28 Tablets ... 3433
Triphasil-21 Tablets ... 3600
Triphasil-28 Tablets ... 3605
Trivora Tablets ... 3439
Yasmin 28 Tablets ... 980
Zovia ... 3449

Etodolac (The hypoglycemic action of oral antidiabetic agents may be potentiated by non-steroidal anti-inflammatory agents). Products include:
Lodine ... 3528
Lodine XL Extended-Release Tablets ... 3530

Felodipine (Calcium channel blocking agents tend to produce hyperglycemia and may lead to loss of glycemic control). Products include:
Lexxel Tablets ... 608
Plendil Extended-Release Tablets ... 623

Fenoprofen Calcium (The hypoglycemic action of oral antidiabetic agents may be potentiated by non-steroidal anti-inflammatory agents).
No products indexed under this heading.

Fludrocortisone Acetate (Corticosteroids tend to produce hyperglycemia and may lead to loss of glycemic control). Products include:
Florinef Acetate Tablets ... 2250

Fluphenazine Decanoate (Phenothiazines tend to produce hyperglycemia and may lead to loss of glycemic control).
No products indexed under this heading.

Fluphenazine Enanthate (Phenothiazines tend to produce hyperglycemia and may lead to loss of glycemic control).
No products indexed under this heading.

Fluphenazine Hydrochloride (Phenothiazines tend to produce hyperglycemia and may lead to loss of glycemic control).
No products indexed under this heading.

Flurbiprofen (The hypoglycemic action of oral antidiabetic agents may be potentiated by non-steroidal anti-inflammatory agents).
No products indexed under this heading.

Fosphenytoin Sodium (Phenytoin tends to produce hyperglycemia and may lead to loss of glycemic control). Products include:
Cerebyx Injection ... 2619

Furosemide (Diuretics tend to produce hyperglycemia and may lead to loss of glycemic control). Products include:
Furosemide Tablets ... 2284

Glipizide (The hypoglycemic action of oral antidiabetic agents may be potentiated by sulfonamides). Products include:
Glucotrol Tablets ... 2692
Glucotrol XL Extended Release Tablets ... 2693

Glyburide (The hypoglycemic action of oral antidiabetic agents may be potentiated by sulfonamides). Products include:
DiaBeta Tablets ... 741
Glucovance Tablets ... 1086

Hydrochlorothiazide (Diuretics tend to produce hyperglycemia and may lead to loss of glycemic control). Products include:
Accuretic Tablets ... 2614
Aldoril Tablets ... 2039
Atacand HCT Tablets ... 597
Avalide Tablets ... 1070
Diovan HCT Tablets ... 2338
Dyazide Capsules ... 1515
HydroDIURIL Tablets ... 2108
Hyzaar ... 2109
Inderide Tablets ... 3517
Inderide LA Long-Acting Capsules ... 3519
Lotensin HCT Tablets ... 2367
Maxzide ... 1008
Micardis HCT Tablets ... 1051
Microzide Capsules ... 3414
Moduretic Tablets ... 2138
Monopril HCT ... 1094
Prinzide Tablets ... 2168
Timolide Tablets ... 2187
Uniretic Tablets ... 3178
Vaseretic Tablets ... 2204
Zestoretic Tablets ... 695
Ziac Tablets ... 1887

Hydrocortisone (Corticosteroids tend to produce hyperglycemia and may lead to loss of glycemic control). Products include:
Anusol-HC Cream 2.5% ... 2237
Cipro HC Otic Suspension ... 540
Cortaid Intensive Therapy Cream ... ▣717
Cortaid Maximum Strength Cream ... ▣717
Cortisporin Ophthalmic Suspension Sterile ... ⊙297
Cortizone•5 ... ▣699
Cortizone•10 ... ▣699
Cortizone•10 Plus Creme ... ▣700
Cortizone for Kids Creme ... ▣699
Hydrocortone Tablets ... 2106
Massengill Medicated Soft Cloth Towelette ... ▣753
VōSoL HC Otic Solution ... 3356

Hydrocortisone Acetate (Corticosteroids tend to produce hyperglycemia and may lead to loss of glycemic control). Products include:
Analpram-HC ... 1338
Anusol HC-1 Hydrocortisone Anti-Itch Cream ... ▣689
Anusol-HC Suppositories ... 2238
Cortaid ... ▣717
Cortifoam Rectal Foam ... 3170
Cortisporin-TC Otic Suspension ... 2246
Hydrocortone Acetate Injectable Suspension ... 2103
Pramosone ... 1343
Proctocort Suppositories ... 2264
ProctoFoam-HC ... 3177
Terra-Cortril Ophthalmic Suspension ... 2716

Hydrocortisone Sodium Phosphate (Corticosteroids tend to produce hyperglycemia and may lead to loss of glycemic control). Products include:
Hydrocortone Phosphate Injection, Sterile ... 2105

Hydrocortisone Sodium Succinate (Corticosteroids tend to produce hyperglycemia and may lead to loss of glycemic control).
No products indexed under this heading.

Hydroflumethiazide (Diuretics tend to produce hyperglycemia and may lead to loss of glycemic control). Products include:
Diucardin Tablets ... 3494

Ibuprofen (The hypoglycemic action of oral antidiabetic agents may be potentiated by non-steroidal anti-inflammatory agents). Products include:
Advil ... ▣771
Children's Advil Oral Suspension ... ▣773
Children's Advil Chewable Tablets ... ▣773
Advil Cold and Sinus Caplets ... ▣771
Advil Cold and Sinus Tablets ... ▣771
Advil Flu & Body Ache Caplets ... ▣772
Infants' Advil Drops ... ▣773
Junior Strength Advil Tablets ... ▣773
Junior Strength Advil Chewable Tablets ... ▣773
Advil Migraine Liquigels ... ▣772
Children's Motrin Oral Suspension and Chewable Tablets ... 2006
Children's Motrin Cold Oral Suspension ... 2007
Children's Motrin Oral Suspension ... ▣643
Motrin Suspension, Oral Drops, Chewable Tablets, and Caplets ... 2002
Infants' Motrin Concentrated Drops ... 2006
Junior Strength Motrin Caplets and Chewable Tablets ... 2006
Motrin IB Tablets, Caplets, and Gelcaps ... 2002
Motrin Migraine Pain Caplets ... 2005
Motrin Sinus Headache Caplets ... 2005
Vicoprofen Tablets ... 520

Indapamide (Diuretics tend to produce hyperglycemia and may lead to loss of glycemic control). Products include:
Indapamide Tablets ... 2286

Indomethacin (The hypoglycemic action of oral antidiabetic agents may be potentiated by non-steroidal anti-inflammatory agents). Products include:
Indocin ... 2112

Indomethacin Sodium Trihydrate (The hypoglycemic action of oral antidiabetic agents may be potentiated by non-steroidal anti-inflammatory agents). Products include:
Indocin I.V. ... 2115

Isocarboxazid (The hypoglycemic action of oral antidiabetic agents may be potentiated by MAO inhibitors).
No products indexed under this heading.

Isoniazid (INH tends to produce hyperglycemia and may lead to loss of glycemic control). Products include:
Rifamate Capsules ... 767
Rifater Tablets ... 769

Isoproterenol Hydrochloride (Sympathomimetics tend to produce hyperglycemia and may lead to loss of glycemic control).
No products indexed under this heading.

Isoproterenol Sulfate (Sympathomimetics tend to produce hyperglycemia and may lead to loss of glycemic control).
No products indexed under this heading.

Isradipine (Calcium channel blocking agents tend to produce hyperglycemia and may lead to loss of glycemic control). Products include:
DynaCirc Capsules ... 2921
DynaCirc CR Tablets ... 2923

Ketoconazole (In vitro data indicate that repaglinide metabolism may be inhibited by antifungal agent ketoconazole). Products include:
Nizoral 2% Cream ... 3620
Nizoral A-D Shampoo ... 2008
Nizoral 2% Shampoo ... 2007
Nizoral Tablets ... 1791

Ketoprofen (The hypoglycemic action of oral antidiabetic agents may be potentiated by non-steroidal anti-inflammatory agents). Products include:
Orudis Capsules ... 3548
Orudis KT Tablets ... ▣778
Oruvail Capsules ... 3548

Ketorolac Tromethamine (The hypoglycemic action of oral antidiabetic agents may be potentiated by non-steroidal anti-inflammatory agents). Products include:
Acular Ophthalmic Solution ... 544
Acular PF Ophthalmic Solution ... 544
Toradol ... 3018

Labetalol Hydrochloride (The hypoglycemic action of oral antidiabetic agents may be potentiated by beta adrenergic blocking agents; hypoglycemia may be difficult to recognize with co-administration). Products include:
Normodyne Injection ... 3135
Normodyne Tablets ... 3137

Levalbuterol Hydrochloride (Sympathomimetics tend to produce hyperglycemia and may lead to loss of glycemic control). Products include:
Xopenex Inhalation Solution ... 3207

Levobunolol Hydrochloride (The hypoglycemic action of oral antidiabetic agents may be potentiated by beta adrenergic blocking agents; hypoglycemia may be difficult to recognize with co-administration). Products include:
Betagan ... ⊙228

Levothyroxine Sodium (Thyroid products tend to produce hyperglycemia and may lead to loss of glycemic control). Products include:
Levothroid Tablets ... 1373
Levoxyl Tablets ... 1819
Synthroid ... 505
Unithroid Tablets ... 3445

Liothyronine Sodium (Thyroid products tend to produce hyperglycemia and may lead to loss of glycemic control). Products include:
Cytomel Tablets ... 1817
Triostat Injection ... 1825

Liotrix (Thyroid products tend to produce hyperglycemia and may lead to loss of glycemic control).
No products indexed under this heading.

Magnesium Salicylate (The hypoglycemic action of oral antidiabetic agents may be potentiated by salicylates). Products include:
Momentum Backache Relief Extra Strength Caplets ... ▣666

Meclofenamate Sodium (The hypoglycemic action of oral antidiabetic agents may be potentiated by non-steroidal anti-inflammatory agents).
No products indexed under this heading.

Mefenamic Acid (The hypoglycemic action of oral antidiabetic agents may be potentiated by non-steroidal anti-inflammatory agents). Products include:
Ponstel Capsules ... 1356

Meloxicam (The hypoglycemic action of oral antidiabetic agents may be potentiated by non-steroidal anti-inflammatory agents). Products include:
Mobic Tablets ... 1054

Mephobarbital (Drugs that induce the CYP450 enzyme system 3A4, such as barbiturates, may increase repaglinide metabolism).
No products indexed under this heading.

Mesoridazine Besylate (Phenothiazines tend to produce hyperglycemia and may lead to loss of glycemic control). Products include:
Serentil ... 1057

Metaproterenol Sulfate (Sympathomimetics tend to produce hyperglycemia and may lead to loss of glycemic control). Products include:
Alupent ... 1029

Metaraminol Bitartrate (Sympathomimetics tend to produce hyperglycemia and may lead to loss of glycemic control). Products include:
Aramine Injection ... 2043

Methotrimeprazine (Phenothiazines tend to produce hyperglycemia and may lead to loss of glycemic control).
No products indexed under this heading.

Methoxamine Hydrochloride (Sympathomimetics tend to produce hyperglycemia and may lead to loss of glycemic control).
No products indexed under this heading.

Methyclothiazide (Diuretics tend to produce hyperglycemia and may lead to loss of glycemic control).
No products indexed under this heading.

Methylprednisolone Acetate (Corticosteroids tend to produce

IMPORTANT NOTE: Always consult each drug listing in the patient's regimen for possible interactions.

hyperglycemia and may lead to loss of glycemic control). Products include:
Depo-Medrol Injectable Suspension ... 2795

Methylprednisolone Sodium Succinate (Corticosteroids tend to produce hyperglycemia and may lead to loss of glycemic control). Products include:
Solu-Medrol Sterile Powder ... 2855

Metipranolol Hydrochloride (The hypoglycemic action of oral antidiabetic agents may be potentiated by beta adrenergic blocking agents; hypoglycemia may be difficult to recognize with co-administration).
No products indexed under this heading.

Metolazone (Diuretics tend to produce hyperglycemia and may lead to loss of glycemic control). Products include:
Mykrox Tablets ... 1168
Zaroxolyn Tablets ... 1177

Metoprolol Succinate (The hypoglycemic action of oral antidiabetic agents may be potentiated by beta adrenergic blocking agents; hypoglycemia may be difficult to recognize with co-administration). Products include:
Toprol-XL Tablets ... 651

Metoprolol Tartrate (The hypoglycemic action of oral antidiabetic agents may be potentiated by beta adrenergic blocking agents; hypoglycemia may be difficult to recognize with co-administration).
No products indexed under this heading.

Mibefradil Dihydrochloride (Calcium channel blocking agents tend to produce hyperglycemia and may lead to loss of glycemic control).
No products indexed under this heading.

Miconazole (In vitro data indicate that repaglinide metabolism may be inhibited by antifungal agent miconazole).
No products indexed under this heading.

Moclobemide (The hypoglycemic action of oral antidiabetic agents may be potentiated by MAO inhibitors).
No products indexed under this heading.

Nabumetone (The hypoglycemic action of oral antidiabetic agents may be potentiated by non-steroidal anti-inflammatory agents). Products include:
Relafen Tablets ... 1617

Nadolol (The hypoglycemic action of oral antidiabetic agents may be potentiated by beta adrenergic blocking agents; hypoglycemia may be difficult to recognize with co-administration). Products include:
Corgard Tablets ... 2245
Corzide 40/5 Tablets ... 2247
Corzide 80/5 Tablets ... 2247
Nadolol Tablets ... 2288

Naproxen (The hypoglycemic action of oral antidiabetic agents may be potentiated by non-steroidal anti-inflammatory agents). Products include:
EC-Naprosyn Delayed-Release Tablets ... 2967
Naprosyn Suspension ... 2967
Naprosyn Tablets ... 2967

Naproxen Sodium (The hypoglycemic action of oral antidiabetic agents may be potentiated by non-steroidal anti-inflammatory agents). Products include:
Aleve Tablets, Caplets and Gelcaps ... ▣602
Aleve Cold & Sinus Caplets ... ▣603
Anaprox Tablets ... 2967
Anaprox DS Tablets ... 2967
Naprelan Tablets ... 1293

Niacin (Nicotinic acid tends to produce hyperglycemia and may lead to a loss of glycemic control). Products include:
Niaspan Extended-Release Tablets ... 1846
Nicotinex Elixir ... ▣633

Nicardipine Hydrochloride (Calcium channel blocking agents tend to produce hyperglycemia and may lead to loss of glycemic control). Products include:
Cardene I.V. ... 3485

Nifedipine (Calcium channel blocking agents tend to produce hyperglycemia and may lead to loss of glycemic control). Products include:
Adalat CC Tablets ... 877
Procardia Capsules ... 2708
Procardia XL Extended Release Tablets ... 2710

Nimodipine (Calcium channel blocking agents tend to produce hyperglycemia and may lead to loss of glycemic control). Products include:
Nimotop Capsules ... 904

Nisoldipine (Calcium channel blocking agents tend to produce hyperglycemia and may lead to loss of glycemic control). Products include:
Sular Tablets ... 688

Norepinephrine Bitartrate (Sympathomimetics tend to produce hyperglycemia and may lead to loss of glycemic control).
No products indexed under this heading.

Oxaprozin (The hypoglycemic action of oral antidiabetic agents may be potentiated by non-steroidal anti-inflammatory agents).
No products indexed under this heading.

Pargyline Hydrochloride (The hypoglycemic action of oral antidiabetic agents may be potentiated by MAO inhibitors).
No products indexed under this heading.

Penbutolol Sulfate (The hypoglycemic action of oral antidiabetic agents may be potentiated by beta adrenergic blocking agents; hypoglycemia may be difficult to recognize with co-administration).
No products indexed under this heading.

Pentobarbital Sodium (Drugs that induce the CYP450 enzyme system 3A4, such as barbiturates, may increase repaglinide metabolism). Products include:
Nembutal Sodium Solution ... 485

Perphenazine (Phenothiazines tend to produce hyperglycemia and may lead to loss of glycemic control). Products include:
Etrafon ... 3115
Trilafon ... 3160

Phenelzine Sulfate (The hypoglycemic action of oral antidiabetic agents may be potentiated by MAO inhibitors). Products include:
Nardil Tablets ... 2653

Phenobarbital (Drugs that induce the CYP450 enzyme system 3A4, such as barbiturates, may increase repaglinide metabolism). Products include:
Arco-Lase Plus Tablets ... 592
Donnatal ... 2929
Donnatal Extentabs ... 2930

Phenylbutazone (The hypoglycemic action of oral antidiabetic agents may be potentiated by non-steroidal anti-inflammatory agents).
No products indexed under this heading.

Phenylephrine Bitartrate (Sympathomimetics tend to produce hyperglycemia and may lead to loss of glycemic control).
No products indexed under this heading.

Phenylephrine Hydrochloride (Sympathomimetics tend to produce hyperglycemia and may lead to loss of glycemic control). Products include:
Afrin Nasal Decongestant Children's Pump Mist ... ▣734
Extendryl ... 1361
Hycomine Compound Tablets ... 1317
Neo-Synephrine ... ▣614
Phenergan VC Syrup ... 3560
Phenergan VC with Codeine Syrup ... 3561
Preparation H Cream ... ▣778
Preparation H Cooling Gel ... ▣778
Preparation H ... ▣778
Vicks Sinex Nasal Spray and Ultra Fine Mist ... ▣729

Phenylephrine Tannate (Sympathomimetics tend to produce hyperglycemia and may lead to loss of glycemic control). Products include:
Ryna-12 S Suspension ... 3351
Reformulated Rynatan Pediatric Suspension ... 3352
Rynatuss Pediatric Suspension ... 3353
Rynatuss Tablets ... 3353

Phenylpropanolamine Hydrochloride (Sympathomimetics tend to produce hyperglycemia and may lead to loss of glycemic control).
No products indexed under this heading.

Phenytoin (Phenytoin tends to produce hyperglycemia and may lead to loss of glycemic control). Products include:
Dilantin Infatabs ... 2624
Dilantin-125 Oral Suspension ... 2625

Phenytoin Sodium (Phenytoin tends to produce hyperglycemia and may lead to loss of glycemic control). Products include:
Dilantin Kapseals ... 2622

Pindolol (The hypoglycemic action of oral antidiabetic agents may be potentiated by beta adrenergic blocking agents; hypoglycemia may be difficult to recognize with co-administration).
No products indexed under this heading.

Pirbuterol Acetate (Sympathomimetics tend to produce hyperglycemia and may lead to loss of glycemic control). Products include:
Maxair Autohaler ... 1981
Maxair Inhaler ... 1984

Piroxicam (The hypoglycemic action of oral antidiabetic agents may be potentiated by non-steroidal anti-inflammatory agents). Products include:
Feldene Capsules ... 2685

Polyestradiol Phosphate (Estrogens and oral contraceptives tend to produce hyperglycemia and may lead to loss of glycemic control).
No products indexed under this heading.

Polythiazide (Diuretics tend to produce hyperglycemia and may lead to loss of glycemic control). Products include:
Minizide Capsules ... 2700
Renese Tablets ... 2712

Prednisolone Acetate (Corticosteroids tend to produce hyperglycemia and may lead to loss of glycemic control). Products include:
Blephamide Ophthalmic Ointment ... 547
Blephamide Ophthalmic Suspension ... 548
Poly-Pred Liquifilm Ophthalmic Suspension ... ⊙245
Pred Forte Ophthalmic Suspension ... ⊙246
Pred Mild Sterile Ophthalmic Suspension ... ⊙249
Pred-G Ophthalmic Suspension ... ⊙247
Pred-G Sterile Ophthalmic Ointment ... ⊙248

Prednisolone Sodium Phosphate (Corticosteroids tend to produce hyperglycemia and may lead to loss of glycemic control). Products include:
Pediapred Oral Solution ... 1170

Prednisolone Tebutate (Corticosteroids tend to produce hyperglycemia and may lead to loss of glycemic control).
No products indexed under this heading.

Prednisone (Corticosteroids tend to produce hyperglycemia and may lead to loss of glycemic control). Products include:
Prednisone ... 3064

Probenecid (The hypoglycemic action of oral antidiabetic agents may be potentiated by probenecid).
No products indexed under this heading.

Procarbazine Hydrochloride (The hypoglycemic action of oral antidiabetic agents may be potentiated by MAO inhibitors). Products include:
Matulane Capsules ... 3246

Prochlorperazine (Phenothiazines tend to produce hyperglycemia and may lead to loss of glycemic control). Products include:
Compazine ... 1505

Promethazine Hydrochloride (Phenothiazines tend to produce hyperglycemia and may lead to loss of glycemic control). Products include:
Mepergan Injection ... 3539
Phenergan Injection ... 3553
Phenergan ... 3556
Phenergan Syrup ... 3554
Phenergan with Codeine Syrup ... 3557
Phenergan with Dextromethorphan Syrup ... 3559
Phenergan VC Syrup ... 3560
Phenergan VC with Codeine Syrup ... 3561

Propranolol Hydrochloride (The hypoglycemic action of oral antidiabetic agents may be potentiated by beta adrenergic blocking agents; hypoglycemia may be difficult to recognize with co-administration). Products include:
Inderal ... 3513
Inderal LA Long-Acting Capsules ... 3516
Inderide Tablets ... 3517
Inderide LA Long-Acting Capsules ... 3519

Pseudoephedrine Hydrochloride (Sympathomimetics tend to produce hyperglycemia and may lead to loss of glycemic control). Products include:
Actifed Cold & Allergy Tablets ... ▣688
Actifed Cold & Sinus Caplets and Tablets ... ▣688
Advil Cold and Sinus Caplets ... ▣771
Advil Cold and Sinus Tablets ... ▣771
Advil Flu & Body Ache Caplets ... ▣772
Aleve Cold & Sinus Caplets ... ▣603
Alka-Seltzer Plus Liqui-Gels ... ▣604
Alka-Seltzer Plus Cold & Flu Medicine Liqui-Gels ... ▣604
Alka-Seltzer Plus Cold & Sinus Medicine Liqui-Gels ... ▣604
Allegra-D Extended-Release Tablets ... 714
BC Cold Powder ... ▣619
Benadryl Allergy/Cold Tablets ... ▣691
Benadryl Allergy/Congestion Tablets ... ▣692
Benadryl Allergy & Sinus Liquid ... ▣693
Benadryl Allergy & Sinus Fastmelt Tablets ... ▣693
Benadryl Allergy Sinus Headache Caplets & Gelcaps ... ▣693
Benadryl Severe Allergy & Sinus Headache Caplets ... ▣694
Benadryl Children's Allergy/Cold Fastmelt Tablets ... ▣692
Benylin Multi-Symptom Liquid ... ▣697
Bromfed Capsules (Extended-Release) ... 2269
Bromfed-PD Capsules (Extended-Release) ... 2269
Children's Cēpacol Sore Throat ... ▣788
Comtrex Acute Head Cold & Sinus Pressure Relief Tablets ... ▣627
Comtrex Deep Chest Cold & Congestion Relief Softgels ... ▣627
Comtrex Flu Therapy & Fever Relief Daytime Caplets ... ▣628
Comtrex Flu Therapy & Fever Relief Nighttime Tablets ... ▣628

Comtrex Maximum Strength Multi-Symptom Cold & Cough Relief Tablets and Caplets 626
Contac Non-Drowsy 12 Hour Cold Caplets 745
Contac Non-Drowsy Timed Release 12 Hour Cold Caplets 746
Contac Severe Cold and Flu Caplets Maximum Strength 746
Contac Severe Cold and Flu Caplets Non-Drowsy 746
Dimetapp Elixir 777
Dimetapp Cold and Fever Suspension 775
Dimetapp DM Cold & Cough Elixir . 775
Dimetapp Nighttime Flu Liquid 776
Dimetapp Non-Drowsy Flu Syrup ... 777
Dimetapp Infant Drops Decongestant 775
Dimetapp Infant Drops Decongestant Plus Cough 776
Guaifed 2272
Kronofed-A 1341
Children's Motrin Cold Oral Suspension 2007
Motrin Sinus Headache Caplets 2005
PediaCare Cough-Cold Liquid 719
PediaCare Infants' Drops Decongestant 719
PediaCare Infants' Drops Decongestant Plus Cough 719
PediaCare NightRest Cough-Cold Liquid 719
Robitussin Cold Caplets Cold & Congestion 780
Robitussin Cold Softgels Cold & Congestion 780
Robitussin Cold Caplets Multi-Symptom Cold & Flu 781
Robitussin Cold Softgels Multi-Symptom Cold & Flu 781
Robitussin Cold Softgels Severe Congestion 782
Robitussin Cough & Cold Infant Drops 782
Robitussin Maximum Strength Cough & Cold Liquid 785
Robitussin Pediatric Cough & Cold Formula Liquid 785
Robitussin Multi Symptom Honey Flu Liquid 785
Robitussin Nighttime Honey Flu Liquid 786
Robitussin-CF Liquid 783
Robitussin-DAC Syrup 2942
Robitussin-PE Liquid 782
Ryna 768
Semprex-D Capsules 1172
Singlet Caplets 761
Sinutab Non-Drying Liquid Caps 706
Sinutab Sinus Allergy Medication, Maximum Strength Formula, Tablets & Caplets 707
Sinutab Sinus Medication, Maximum Strength Without Drowsiness Formula, Tablets & Caplets 707
Sudafed 12 Hour Tablets 708
Sudafed 24 Hour Tablets 708
Children's Sudafed Cold & Cough Liquid 709
Children's Sudafed Nasal Decongestant Chewables 711
Children's Sudafed Nasal Decongestant Liquid Medication 711
Sudafed Cold & Allergy Tablets 708
Sudafed Cold & Cough Liquid Caps 709
Sudafed Cold & Sinus Liquid Caps 710
Sudafed Nasal Decongestant Tablets 710
Sudafed Non-Drying Sinus Liquid Caps 712
Sudafed Severe Cold 711
Sudafed Sinus Headache Caplets . 712
Sudafed Sinus Headache Tablets . 712
Tavist Sinus Non-Drowsy Coated Caplets 676
TheraFlu Regular Strength Cold & Cough Night Time Hot Liquid 676
TheraFlu Regular Strength Cold & Sore Throat Night Time Hot Liquid 676
TheraFlu Maximum Strength Flu & Congestion Non-Drowsy Hot Liquid 677
TheraFlu Maximum Strength Flu & Cough Night Time Hot Liquid .. 678
TheraFlu Maximum Strength Flu & Sore Throat Night Time Hot Liquid 677
TheraFlu Maximum Strength Severe Cold & Congestion Night Time Caplets 678
TheraFlu Maximum Strength Severe Cold & Congestion Night Time Hot Liquid 678
TheraFlu Maximum Strength Severe Cold & Congestion Non-Drowsy 679
Triaminic Allergy Congestion Liquid 680
Triaminic Chest Congestion Liquid 680
Triaminic Cold & Allergy Liquid 681
Triaminic Cold & Allergy Softchews 683
Triaminic Cold & Cough Liquid 681
Triaminic Cold & Cough Softchews 683
Triaminic Cold & Night Time Cough Liquid 681
Triaminic Cold, Cough & Fever Liquid 681
Triaminic Cough Liquid 682
Triaminic Cough & Congestion Liquid 682
Triaminic Cough & Sore Throat Liquid 682
Triaminic Cough & Sore Throat Softchews 684
Children's Tylenol Allergy-D Liquid ... 2014
Children's Tylenol Cold Suspension Liquid and Chewable Tablets 2015
Children's Tylenol Cold Plus Cough Suspension Liquid and Chewable Tablets 2015
Children's Tylenol Flu Suspension Liquid 2015
Children's Tylenol Sinus Suspension Liquid 2017
Infants' Tylenol Cold Decongestant and Fever Reducer Concentrated Drops 2015
Infants' Tylenol Cold Decongestant and Fever Reducer Concentrated Drops Plus Cough .. 2015
Tylenol Allergy Sinus 2010
Multi-Symptom Tylenol Cold Complete Formula Caplets 2010
Multi-Symptom Tylenol Cold Non-Drowsy Caplets and Gelcaps 2010
Multi-Symptom Tylenol Cold Severe Congestion Non-Drowsy Caplets 2011
Maximum Strength Tylenol Flu NightTime Gelcaps 2011
Maximum Strength Tylenol Flu NightTime Liquid 2011
Maximum Strength Tylenol Flu Non-Drowsy Gelcaps 2011
Maximum Strength Tylenol Sinus NightTime Caplets 2012
Maximum Strength Tylenol Sinus Non-Drowsy Geltabs, Gelcaps, Caplets, and Tablets 2012
Vicks 44D Cough & Head Congestion Relief Liquid 724
Vicks 44M Cough, Cold & Flu Relief Liquid 725
Pediatric Vicks 44m Cough & Cold Relief 728
Vicks DayQuil LiquiCaps/Liquid Multi-Symptom Cold/Flu Relief ... 727
Children's Vicks NyQuil Cold/Cough Relief 726
Vicks NyQuil LiquiCaps/Liquid Multi-Symptom Cold/Flu Relief, Original and Cherry Flavors 727
Zephrex Tablets 3091
Zephrex LA Tablets 3092
Zyrtec-D 12 Hour Extended Relief Tablets 2758

Pseudoephedrine Sulfate (Sympathomimetics tend to produce hyperglycemia and may lead to loss of glycemic control). Products include:
Chlor-Trimeton Allergy/Decongestant Tablets 736
Claritin-D 12 Hour Extended Release Tablets 3102
Claritin-D 24 Hour Extended Release Tablets 3104
Coricidin 'D' Cold, Flu & Sinus Tablets 737
Drixoral Allergy/Sinus Extended-Release Tablets 741
Drixoral Cold & Allergy Sustained-Action Tablets 740
Drixoral Cold & Flu Extended-Release Tablets 740
Drixoral Nasal Decongestant Long-Acting Non-Drowsy Tablets 740
Rynatan Tablets 3351

Quinestrol (Estrogens and oral contraceptives tend to produce hyperglycemia and may lead to loss of glycemic control).
No products indexed under this heading.

Rifampin (Drugs that induce the CYP450 enzyme system 3A4, such as rifampin, may increase repaglinide metabolism). Products include:
Rifadin 765
Rifamate Capsules 767
Rifater Tablets 769

Rofecoxib (The hypoglycemic action of oral antidiabetic agents may be potentiated by non-steroidal anti-inflammatory agents). Products include:
Vioxx 2213

Salmeterol Xinafoate (Sympathomimetics tend to produce hyperglycemia and may lead to loss of glycemic control). Products include:
Advair Diskus 100/50 1448
Advair Diskus 250/50 1448
Advair Diskus 500/50 1448
Serevent Diskus 1637
Serevent Inhalation Aerosol 1633

Salsalate (The hypoglycemic action of oral antidiabetic agents may be potentiated by salicylates).
No products indexed under this heading.

Secobarbital Sodium (Drugs that induce the CYP450 enzyme system 3A4, such as barbiturates, may increase repaglinide metabolism).
No products indexed under this heading.

Selegiline Hydrochloride (The hypoglycemic action of oral antidiabetic agents may be potentiated by MAO inhibitors). Products include:
Eldepryl Capsules 3266

Sotalol Hydrochloride (The hypoglycemic action of oral antidiabetic agents may be potentiated by beta adrenergic blocking agents; hypoglycemia may be difficult to recognize with co-administration). Products include:
Betapace Tablets 950
Betapace AF Tablets 954

Spironolactone (Diuretics tend to produce hyperglycemia and may lead to loss of glycemic control).
No products indexed under this heading.

Sulfacytine (The hypoglycemic action of oral antidiabetic agents may be potentiated by sulfonamides).

Sulfamethizole (The hypoglycemic action of oral antidiabetic agents may be potentiated by sulfonamides). Products include:
Urobiotic-250 Capsules 2731

Sulfamethoxazole (The hypoglycemic action of oral antidiabetic agents may be potentiated by sulfonamides). Products include:
Bactrim 2949
Septra Suspension 2265
Septra Tablets 2265
Septra DS Tablets 2265

Sulfasalazine (The hypoglycemic action of oral antidiabetic agents may be potentiated by sulfonamides). Products include:
Azulfidine EN-tabs Tablets 2775

Sulfinpyrazone (The hypoglycemic action of oral antidiabetic agents may be potentiated by sulfonamides).
No products indexed under this heading.

Sulfisoxazole (The hypoglycemic action of oral antidiabetic agents may be potentiated by sulfonamides).
No products indexed under this heading.

Sulfisoxazole Acetyl (The hypoglycemic action of oral antidiabetic agents may be potentiated by sulfonamides). Products include:
Pediazole Suspension 3050

Sulfisoxazole Diolamine (The hypoglycemic action of oral antidiabetic agents may be potentiated by sulfonamides).
No products indexed under this heading.

Sulindac (The hypoglycemic action of oral antidiabetic agents may be potentiated by non-steroidal anti-inflammatory agents). Products include:
Clinoril Tablets 2053

Terbutaline Sulfate (Sympathomimetics tend to produce hyperglycemia and may lead to loss of glycemic control). Products include:
Brethine Ampuls 2314
Brethine Tablets 2313

Thiamylal Sodium (Drugs that induce the CYP450 enzyme system 3A4, such as barbiturates, may increase repaglinide metabolism).
No products indexed under this heading.

Thioridazine Hydrochloride (Phenothiazines tend to produce hyperglycemia and may lead to loss of glycemic control). Products include:
Thioridazine Hydrochloride Tablets 2289

Thyroglobulin (Thyroid products tend to produce hyperglycemia and may lead to loss of glycemic control).
No products indexed under this heading.

Thyroid (Thyroid products tend to produce hyperglycemia and may lead to loss of glycemic control).
No products indexed under this heading.

Thyroxine (Thyroid products tend to produce hyperglycemia and may lead to loss of glycemic control).
No products indexed under this heading.

Thyroxine Sodium (Thyroid products tend to produce hyperglycemia and may lead to loss of glycemic control).
No products indexed under this heading.

Timolol Hemihydrate (The hypoglycemic action of oral antidiabetic agents may be potentiated by beta adrenergic blocking agents; hypoglycemia may be difficult to recognize with co-administration). Products include:
Betimol Ophthalmic Solution .... ⊙ 324

Timolol Maleate (The hypoglycemic action of oral antidiabetic agents may be potentiated by beta adrenergic blocking agents; hypoglycemia may be difficult to recognize with co-administration). Products include:
Blocadren Tablets 2046
Cosopt Sterile Ophthalmic Solution 2065
Timolide Tablets 2187
Timolol GFS .... ⊙ 266
Timoptic in Ocudose 2192
Timoptic Sterile Ophthalmic Solution 2190
Timoptic-XE Sterile Ophthalmic Gel Forming Solution 2194

Tolazamide (The hypoglycemic action of oral antidiabetic agents may be potentiated by sulfonamides).
No products indexed under this heading.

Tolbutamide (The hypoglycemic action of oral antidiabetic agents may be potentiated by sulfonamides).
No products indexed under this heading.

Tolmetin Sodium (The hypoglycemic action of oral antidiabetic agents may be potentiated by non-steroidal anti-inflammatory agents). Products include:
Tolectin 2589

Torsemide (Diuretics tend to produce hyperglycemia and may lead to loss of glycemic control). Products include:
Demadex Tablets and Injection 2965

Tranylcypromine Sulfate (The hypoglycemic action of oral antidiabetic agents may be potentiated by MAO inhibitors). Products include:
Parnate Tablets 1607

Triamcinolone (Corticosteroids tend to produce hyperglycemia and may lead to loss of glycemic control).
No products indexed under this heading.

Triamcinolone Acetonide (Corticosteroids tend to produce hyperglycemia and may lead to loss of glycemic control). Products include:
Azmacort Inhalation Aerosol 728
Nasacort Nasal Inhaler 750
Nasacort AQ Nasal Spray 752
Tri-Nasal Spray 2274

Triamcinolone Diacetate (Corticosteroids tend to produce hyperglycemia and may lead to loss of glycemic control).
No products indexed under this heading.

Triamcinolone Hexacetonide (Corticosteroids tend to produce hyperglycemia and may lead to loss of glycemic control).
No products indexed under this heading.

Triamterene (Diuretics tend to produce hyperglycemia and may lead to loss of glycemic control). Products include:
Dyazide Capsules 1515
Dyrenium Capsules 3458
Maxzide 1008

Trifluoperazine Hydrochloride (Phenothiazines tend to produce hyperglycemia and may lead to loss of glycemic control). Products include:
Stelazine 1640

Troglitazone (Drugs that induce the CYP450 enzyme system 3A4, such as troglitazone, may increase repaglinide metabolism).
No products indexed under this heading.

Verapamil Hydrochloride (Calcium channel blocking agents tend to produce hyperglycemia and may lead to loss of glycemic control). Products include:
Covera-HS Tablets 3199
Isoptin SR Tablets 467
Tarka Tablets 508
Verelan Capsules 3184
Verelan PM Capsules 3186

Warfarin Sodium (The hypoglycemic action of oral antidiabetic agents may be potentiated by coumarins). Products include:
Coumadin for Injection 1243
Coumadin Tablets 1243
Warfarin Sodium Tablets, USP 3302

Food Interactions

Food, unspecified (When repaglinide was given with food the mean Cmax and AUC were decreased 20% and 12.4% respectively; Tmax was unchanged).

PRAVACHOL TABLETS

(Pravastatin Sodium) 1099
May interact with fibrates and certain other agents. Compounds in these categories include:

Cholestyramine (Co-administration has resulted in an approximately 40% to 50% decrease in the mean AUC of pravastatin; Pravachol should be given either 1 hour or more before or at least 4 hours following the resin).
No products indexed under this heading.

Clofibrate (The use of fibrates alone may occasionally be associated with myopathy; the combined use should be avoided). Products include:
Atromid-S Capsules 3483

Colestipol Hydrochloride (Co-administration has resulted in an approximately 40% to 50% decrease in the mean AUC of pravastatin; Pravachol should be given either 1 hour or more before or at least 4 hours following the resin). Products include:
Colestid Tablets 2791

Cyclosporine (The risk of myopathy during treatment with another HMG-CoA reductase inhibitor has increased with concurrent therapy; in one single-dose study, pravastatin levels were found to be increased with concurrent therapy in cardiac transplant patients). Products include:
Gengraf Capsules 457
Neoral Soft Gelatin Capsules 2380
Neoral Oral Solution 2380
Sandimmune 2388

Digoxin (Co-administration indicates that the bioavailability parameters of digoxin are not affected, however, the AUC of pravastatin tends to increase, but the overall bioavailability of pravastatin plus its metabolites are not affected). Products include:
Digitek Tablets 1003
Lanoxicaps Capsules 1574
Lanoxin Injection 1581
Lanoxin Tablets 1587
Lanoxin Elixir Pediatric 1578
Lanoxin Injection Pediatric 1584

Fenofibrate (The use of fibrates alone may occasionally be associated with myopathy; the combined use should be avoided). Products include:
Tricor Capsules, Micronized 513

Gemfibrozil (Co-administration has resulted in a significant decrease in urinary excretion and protein binding of pravastatin; significant increase in AUC, Cmax, and Tmax for the pravastatin metabolite SQ31906; combined therapy has resulted in market CPK elevation insome patients; combination therapy is not recommended). Products include:
Lopid Tablets 2650

Itraconazole (Co-administration with itraconazole has resulted in an increase in mean AUC and Cmax for pravastatin by factors of 1.7 and 2.5 respectively compared to placebo; the mean t1/2 was not affected suggesting that the relatively small increases in Cmax and AUCwere solely due to increased bioavailability rather than a decrease in clearance). Products include:
Sporanox Capsules 1800
Sporanox Injection 1804
Sporanox Injection 2509
Sporanox Oral Solution 1808
Sporanox Oral Solution 2512

PRECARE CHEWABLE TABLETS

(Vitamins, Prenatal) 3312
None cited in PDR database.

PRECARE CONCEIVE TABLETS

(Vitamins, Prenatal) 3312
None cited in PDR database.

PRECARE PRENATAL CAPLETS

(Vitamins, Prenatal) 3313
None cited in PDR database.

PRECOSE TABLETS

(Acarbose) 906
May interact with calcium channel blockers, corticosteroids, estrogens, oral contraceptives, phenothiazines, phenytoin, sympathomimetics, thiazides, thyroid preparations, and certain other agents. Compounds in these categories include:

Albuterol (Sympathomimetics tend to produce hyperglycemia leading to loss of control; patients on concurrent therapy should be closely observed for loss of control). Products include:
Proventil Inhalation Aerosol 3142
Ventolin Inhalation Aerosol and Refill 1679

Albuterol Sulfate (Sympathomimetics tend to produce hyperglycemia leading to loss of control; patients on concurrent therapy should be closely observed for loss of control). Products include:
AccuNeb Inhalation Solution 1230
Combivent Inhalation Aerosol 1041
DuoNeb Inhalation Solution 1233
Proventil Inhalation Solution 0.083% 3146
Proventil Repetabs Tablets 3148
Proventil Solution for Inhalation 0.5% 3144
Proventil HFA Inhalation Aerosol 3150
Ventolin HFA Inhalation Aerosol 3618
Volmax Extended-Release Tablets 2276

Amlodipine Besylate (Calcium channel blockers tend to produce hyperglycemia leading to loss of control; patients on concurrent therapy should be closely observed for loss of control). Products include:
Lotrel Capsules 2370
Norvasc Tablets 2704

Amylase (Amylase, a carbohydrate splitting enzyme, may reduce the effect of acarbose and should not be taken concurrently). Products include:
Arco-Lase Tablets 592
Arco-Lase Plus Tablets 592

Bendroflumethiazide (Thiazide diuretics tend to produce hyperglycemia leading to loss of control; patients on concurrent therapy should be closely observed for loss of control). Products include:
Corzide 40/5 Tablets 2247
Corzide 80/5 Tablets 2247

Bepridil Hydrochloride (Calcium channel blockers tend to produce hyperglycemia leading to loss of control; patients on concurrent therapy should be closely observed for loss of control). Products include:
Vascor Tablets 2602

Betamethasone Acetate (Corticosteroids tend to produce hyperglycemia leading to loss of control; patients on concurrent therapy should be closely observed for loss of control). Products include:
Celestone Soluspan Injectable Suspension 3097

Betamethasone Sodium Phosphate (Corticosteroids tend to produce hyperglycemia leading to loss of control; patients on concurrent therapy should be closely observed for loss of control). Products include:
Celestone Soluspan Injectable Suspension 3097

Charcoal, Activated (Charcoal, an intestinal adsorbent, may reduce the effect of acarbose and should not be taken concurrently).
No products indexed under this heading.

Chlorothiazide (Thiazide diuretics tend to produce hyperglycemia leading to loss of control; patients on concurrent therapy should be closely observed for loss of control). Products include:
Aldoclor Tablets 2035
Diuril Oral 2087

Chlorothiazide Sodium (Thiazide diuretics tend to produce hyperglycemia leading to loss of control; patients on concurrent therapy should be closely observed for loss of control). Products include:
Diuril Sodium Intravenous 2086

Chlorotrianisene (Estrogens tend to produce hyperglycemia leading to loss of control; patients on concurrent therapy should be closely observed for loss of control).
No products indexed under this heading.

Chlorpromazine (Phenothiazines tend to produce hyperglycemia leading to loss of control; patients on concurrent therapy should be closely observed for loss of control). Products include:
Thorazine Suppositories 1656

Chlorpromazine Hydrochloride (Phenothiazines tend to produce hyperglycemia leading to loss of control; patients on concurrent therapy should be closely observed for loss of control). Products include:
Thorazine 1656

Cortisone Acetate (Corticosteroids tend to produce hyperglycemia leading to loss of control; patients on concurrent therapy should be closely observed for loss of control). Products include:
Cortone Acetate Injectable Suspension 2059
Cortone Acetate Tablets 2061

Desogestrel (Oral contraceptives tend to produce hyperglycemia leading to loss of control; patients on concurrent therapy should be closely observed for loss of control). Products include:
Cyclessa Tablets 2450
Desogen Tablets 2458
Mircette Tablets 2470
Ortho-Cept 21 Tablets 2546
Ortho-Cept 28 Tablets 2546

Dexamethasone (Corticosteroids tend to produce hyperglycemia leading to loss of control; patients on concurrent therapy should be closely observed for loss of control). Products include:
Decadron Elixir 2078
Decadron Tablets 2079
TobraDex Ophthalmic Ointment 542
TobraDex Ophthalmic Suspension 541

Dexamethasone Acetate (Corticosteroids tend to produce hyperglycemia leading to loss of control; patients on concurrent therapy should be closely observed for loss of control).
No products indexed under this heading.

Dexamethasone Sodium Phosphate (Corticosteroids tend to produce hyperglycemia leading to loss of control; patients on concurrent therapy should be closely observed for loss of control). Products include:
Decadron Phosphate Injection 2081
Decadron Phosphate Sterile Ophthalmic Ointment 2083
Decadron Phosphate Sterile Ophthalmic Solution 2084
NeoDecadron Sterile Ophthalmic Solution 2144

Dienestrol (Estrogens tend to produce hyperglycemia leading to loss of control; patients on concurrent therapy should be closely observed for loss of control). Products include:
Ortho Dienestrol Cream 2554

Diethylstilbestrol (Estrogens tend to produce hyperglycemia leading to loss of control; patients on concurrent therapy should be closely observed for loss of control).
No products indexed under this heading.

Diltiazem Hydrochloride (Calcium channel blockers tend to produce hyperglycemia leading to loss of control; patients on concurrent therapy should be closely observed for loss of control). Products include:
Cardizem Injectable 1018
Cardizem Lyo-Ject Syringe 1018
Cardizem Monovial 1018
Cardizem CD Capsules 1016
Tiazac Capsules 1378

Dobutamine Hydrochloride (Sympathomimetics tend to produce hyperglycemia leading to loss of

control; patients on concurrent therapy should be closely observed for loss of control). Products include:
Dobutrex Solution Vials 1914

Dopamine Hydrochloride (Sympathomimetics tend to produce hyperglycemia leading to loss of control; patients on concurrent therapy should be closely observed for loss of control).
No products indexed under this heading.

Ephedrine Hydrochloride (Sympathomimetics tend to produce hyperglycemia leading to loss of control; patients on concurrent therapy should be closely observed for loss of control). Products include:
Primatene Tablets .... ⊡780

Ephedrine Sulfate (Sympathomimetics tend to produce hyperglycemia leading to loss of control; patients on concurrent therapy should be closely observed for loss of control).
No products indexed under this heading.

Ephedrine Tannate (Sympathomimetics tend to produce hyperglycemia leading to loss of control; patients on concurrent therapy should be closely observed for loss of control). Products include:
Rynatuss Pediatric Suspension 3353
Rynatuss Tablets 3353

Epinephrine (Sympathomimetics tend to produce hyperglycemia leading to loss of control; patients on concurrent therapy should be closely observed for loss of control). Products include:
Epifrin Sterile Ophthalmic Solution .... ⊙235
EpiPen 1236
Primatene Mist .... ⊡779
Xylocaine with Epinephrine Injection 653

Epinephrine Bitartrate (Sympathomimetics tend to produce hyperglycemia leading to loss of control; patients on concurrent therapy should be closely observed for loss of control). Products include:
Sensorcaine 643

Epinephrine Hydrochloride (Sympathomimetics tend to produce hyperglycemia leading to loss of control; patients on concurrent therapy should be closely observed for loss of control).
No products indexed under this heading.

Estradiol (Estrogens tend to produce hyperglycemia leading to loss of control; patients on concurrent therapy should be closely observed for loss of control). Products include:
Activella Tablets 2764
Alora Transdermal System 3372
Climara Transdermal System 958
CombiPatch Transdermal System .. 2323
Esclim Transdermal System 3460
Estrace Vaginal Cream 3358
Estrace Tablets 3361
Estring Vaginal Ring 2811
Ortho-Prefest Tablets 2570
Vagifem Tablets 2857
Vivelle Transdermal System 2412
Vivelle-Dot Transdermal System 2416

Estrogens, Conjugated (Estrogens tend to produce hyperglycemia leading to loss of control; patients on concurrent therapy should be closely observed for loss of control). Products include:
Premarin Intravenous 3563
Premarin Tablets 3566
Premarin Vaginal Cream 3570
Premphase Tablets 3572
Prempro Tablets 3572

Estrogens, Esterified (Estrogens tend to produce hyperglycemia leading to loss of control; patients on concurrent therapy should be closely observed for loss of control). Products include:
Estratest 3252
Menest Tablets 2254

Estropipate (Estrogens tend to produce hyperglycemia leading to loss of control; patients on concurrent therapy should be closely observed for loss of control). Products include:
Ogen Tablets 2846
Ortho-Est Tablets 3464

Ethinyl Estradiol (Estrogens tend to produce hyperglycemia leading to loss of control; patients on concurrent therapy should be closely observed for loss of control). Products include:
Alesse-21 Tablets 3468
Alesse-28 Tablets 3473
Brevicon 28-Day Tablets 3380
Cyclessa Tablets 2450
Desogen Tablets 2458
Estinyl Tablets 3112
Estrostep 2627
femhrt Tablets 2635
Levlen 962
Levlite 21 Tablets 962
Levlite 28 Tablets 962
Levora Tablets 3389
Loestrin 21 Tablets 2642
Loestrin Fe Tablets 2642
Lo/Ovral Tablets 3532
Lo/Ovral-28 Tablets 3538
Low-Ogestrel-28 Tablets 3392
Microgestin Fe 1.5/30 Tablets 3407
Microgestin Fe 1/20 Tablets 3400
Mircette Tablets 2470
Modicon 2563
Necon 3415
Nordette-28 Tablets 2257
Norinyl 1 +35 28-Day Tablets 3380
Ogestrel 0.5/50-28 Tablets 3428
Ortho-Cept 21 Tablets 2546
Ortho-Cept 28 Tablets 2546
Ortho-Cyclen/Ortho Tri-Cyclen 2573
Ortho-Novum 2563
Ovcon 3364
Ovral Tablets 3551
Ovral-28 Tablets 3552
Tri-Levlen 962
Tri-Norinyl-28 Tablets 3433
Triphasil-21 Tablets 3600
Triphasil-28 Tablets 3605
Trivora Tablets 3439
Yasmin 28 Tablets 980
Zovia 3449

Ethynodiol Diacetate (Oral contraceptives tend to produce hyperglycemia leading to loss of control; patients on concurrent therapy should be closely observed for loss of control). Products include:
Zovia 3449

Felodipine (Calcium channel blockers tend to produce hyperglycemia leading to loss of control; patients on concurrent therapy should be closely observed for loss of control). Products include:
Lexxel Tablets 608
Plendil Extended-Release Tablets ... 623

Fludrocortisone Acetate (Corticosteroids tend to produce hyperglycemia leading to loss of control; patients on concurrent therapy should be closely observed for loss of control). Products include:
Florinef Acetate Tablets 2250

Fluphenazine Decanoate (Phenothiazines tend to produce hyperglycemia leading to loss of control; patients on concurrent therapy should be closely observed for loss of control).
No products indexed under this heading.

Fluphenazine Enanthate (Phenothiazines tend to produce hyperglycemia leading to loss of control; patients on concurrent therapy should be closely observed for loss of control).
No products indexed under this heading.

Fluphenazine Hydrochloride (Phenothiazines tend to produce hyperglycemia leading to loss of control; patients on concurrent therapy should be closely observed for loss of control).
No products indexed under this heading.

Fosphenytoin Sodium (Phenytoin tends to produce hyperglycemia leading to loss of control; patients on concurrent therapy should be closely observed for loss of control). Products include:
Cerebyx Injection 2619

Hydrochlorothiazide (Thiazide diuretics tend to produce hyperglycemia leading to loss of control; patients on concurrent therapy should be closely observed for loss of control). Products include:
Accuretic Tablets 2614
Aldoril Tablets 2039
Atacand HCT Tablets 597
Avalide Tablets 1070
Diovan HCT Tablets 2338
Dyazide Capsules 1515
HydroDIURIL Tablets 2108
Hyzaar 2109
Inderide Tablets 3517
Inderide LA Long-Acting Capsules .. 3519
Lotensin HCT Tablets 2367
Maxzide 1008
Micardis HCT Tablets 1051
Microzide Capsules 3414
Moduretic Tablets 2138
Monopril HCT 1094
Prinzide Tablets 2168
Timolide Tablets 2187
Uniretic Tablets 3178
Vaseretic Tablets 2204
Zestoretic Tablets 695
Ziac Tablets 1887

Hydrocortisone (Corticosteroids tend to produce hyperglycemia leading to loss of control; patients on concurrent therapy should be closely observed for loss of control). Products include:
Anusol-HC Cream 2.5% 2237
Cipro HC Otic Suspension 540
Cortaid Intensive Therapy Cream . ⊡717
Cortaid Maximum Strength Cream .... ⊡717
Cortisporin Ophthalmic Suspension Sterile .... ⊙297
Cortizone•5 .... ⊡699
Cortizone•10 .... ⊡699
Cortizone•10 Plus Creme .... ⊡700
Cortizone for Kids Creme .... ⊡699
Hydrocortone Tablets 2106
Massengill Medicated Soft Cloth Towelette .... ⊡753
VōSoL HC Otic Solution 3356

Hydrocortisone Acetate (Corticosteroids tend to produce hyperglycemia leading to loss of control; patients on concurrent therapy should be closely observed for loss of control). Products include:
Analpram-HC 1338
Anusol HC-1 Hydrocortisone Anti-Itch Cream .... ⊡689
Anusol-HC Suppositories 2238
Cortaid .... ⊡717
Cortifoam Rectal Foam 3170
Cortisporin-TC Otic Suspension 2246
Hydrocortone Acetate Injectable Suspension 2103
Pramosone 1343
Proctocort Suppositories 2264
ProctoFoam-HC 3177
Terra-Cortril Ophthalmic Suspension 2716

Hydrocortisone Sodium Phosphate (Corticosteroids tend to produce hyperglycemia leading to loss of control; patients on concurrent therapy should be closely observed for loss of control). Products include:
Hydrocortone Phosphate Injection, Sterile 2105

Hydrocortisone Sodium Succinate (Corticosteroids tend to produce hyperglycemia leading to loss of control; patients on concurrent therapy should be closely observed for loss of control).
No products indexed under this heading.

Hydroflumethiazide (Thiazide diuretics tend to produce hyperglycemia leading to loss of control; patients on concurrent therapy should be closely observed for loss of control). Products include:
Diucardin Tablets 3494

Isoniazid (Isoniazid tends to produce hyperglycemia leading to loss of control; patients on concurrent therapy should be closely observed for loss of control). Products include:
Rifamate Capsules 767
Rifater Tablets 769

Isoproterenol Hydrochloride (Sympathomimetics tend to produce hyperglycemia leading to loss of control; patients on concurrent therapy should be closely observed for loss of control).
No products indexed under this heading.

Isoproterenol Sulfate (Sympathomimetics tend to produce hyperglycemia leading to loss of control; patients on concurrent therapy should be closely observed for loss of control).
No products indexed under this heading.

Isradipine (Calcium channel blockers tend to produce hyperglycemia leading to loss of control; patients on concurrent therapy should be closely observed for loss of control). Products include:
DynaCirc Capsules 2921
DynaCirc CR Tablets 2923

Levalbuterol Hydrochloride (Sympathomimetics tend to produce hyperglycemia leading to loss of control; patients on concurrent therapy should be closely observed for loss of control). Products include:
Xopenex Inhalation Solution 3207

Levonorgestrel (Oral contraceptives tend to produce hyperglycemia leading to loss of control; patients on concurrent therapy should be closely observed for loss of control). Products include:
Alesse-21 Tablets 3468
Alesse-28 Tablets 3473
Levlen 962
Levlite 21 Tablets 962
Levlite 28 Tablets 962
Levora Tablets 3389
Mirena Intrauterine System 974
Nordette-28 Tablets 2257
Norplant System 3543
Tri-Levlen 962
Triphasil-21 Tablets 3600
Triphasil-28 Tablets 3605
Trivora Tablets 3439

Levothyroxine Sodium (Thyroid products tend to produce hyperglycemia leading to loss of control; patients on concurrent therapy should be closely observed for loss of control). Products include:
Levothroid Tablets 1373
Levoxyl Tablets 1819
Synthroid 505
Unithroid Tablets 3445

Liothyronine Sodium (Thyroid products tend to produce hyperglycemia leading to loss of control; patients on concurrent therapy should be closely observed for loss of control). Products include:
Cytomel Tablets 1817
Triostat Injection 1825

Liotrix (Thyroid products tend to produce hyperglycemia leading to loss of control; patients on concurrent therapy should be closely observed for loss of control).
No products indexed under this heading.

Mesoridazine Besylate (Phenothiazines tend to produce hyperglycemia leading to loss of control; patients on concurrent therapy should be closely observed for loss of control). Products include:
Serentil 1057

Mestranol (Oral contraceptives tend to produce hyperglycemia leading to loss of control; patients on

concurrent therapy should be closely observed for loss of control). Products include:

- Necon 1/50 Tablets 3415
- Norinyl 1 + 50 28-Day Tablets 3380
- Ortho-Novum 1/50▫28 Tablets 2556

Metaproterenol Sulfate (Sympathomimetics tend to produce hyperglycemia leading to loss of control; patients on concurrent therapy should be closely observed for loss of control). Products include:

- Alupent 1029

Metaraminol Bitartrate (Sympathomimetics tend to produce hyperglycemia leading to loss of control; patients on concurrent therapy should be closely observed for loss of control). Products include:

- Aramine Injection 2043

Methotrimeprazine (Phenothiazines tend to produce hyperglycemia leading to loss of control; patients on concurrent therapy should be closely observed for loss of control).

No products indexed under this heading.

Methoxamine Hydrochloride (Sympathomimetics tend to produce hyperglycemia leading to loss of control; patients on concurrent therapy should be closely observed for loss of control).

No products indexed under this heading.

Methyclothiazide (Thiazide diuretics tend to produce hyperglycemia leading to loss of control; patients on concurrent therapy should be closely observed for loss of control).

No products indexed under this heading.

Methylprednisolone Acetate (Corticosteroids tend to produce hyperglycemia leading to loss of control; patients on concurrent therapy should be closely observed for loss of control). Products include:

- Depo-Medrol Injectable Suspension 2795

Methylprednisolone Sodium Succinate (Corticosteroids tend to produce hyperglycemia leading to loss of control; patients on concurrent therapy should be closely observed for loss of control). Products include:

- Solu-Medrol Sterile Powder 2855

Mibefradil Dihydrochloride (Calcium channel blockers tend to produce hyperglycemia leading to loss of control; patients on concurrent therapy should be closely observed for loss of control).

No products indexed under this heading.

Nicardipine Hydrochloride (Calcium channel blockers tend to produce hyperglycemia leading to loss of control; patients on concurrent therapy should be closely observed for loss of control). Products include:

- Cardene I.V. 3485

Nicotinic Acid (Nicotinic acid tends to produce hyperglycemia leading to loss of control; patients on concurrent therapy should be closely observed for loss of control).

No products indexed under this heading.

Nifedipine (Calcium channel blockers tend to produce hyperglycemia leading to loss of control; patients on concurrent therapy should be closely observed for loss of control). Products include:

- Adalat CC Tablets 877
- Procardia Capsules 2708
- Procardia XL Extended Release Tablets 2710

Nimodipine (Calcium channel blockers tend to produce hyperglycemia leading to loss of control; patients on concurrent therapy should be closely observed for loss of control). Products include:

- Nimotop Capsules 904

Nisoldipine (Calcium channel blockers tend to produce hyperglycemia leading to loss of control; patients on concurrent therapy should be closely observed for loss of control). Products include:

- Sular Tablets 688

Norepinephrine Bitartrate (Sympathomimetics tend to produce hyperglycemia leading to loss of control; patients on concurrent therapy should be closely observed for loss of control).

No products indexed under this heading.

Norethindrone (Oral contraceptives tend to produce hyperglycemia leading to loss of control; patients on concurrent therapy should be closely observed for loss of control). Products include:

- Brevicon 28-Day Tablets 3380
- Micronor Tablets 2543
- Modicon 2563
- Necon 3415
- Norinyl 1 +35 28-Day Tablets 3380
- Norinyl 1 + 50 28-Day Tablets 3380
- Nor-QD Tablets 3423
- Ortho-Novum 2563
- Ortho-Novum 1/50▫28 Tablets 2556
- Ovcon 3364
- Tri-Norinyl-28 Tablets 3433

Norethynodrel (Oral contraceptives tend to produce hyperglycemia leading to loss of control; patients on concurrent therapy should be closely observed for loss of control).

No products indexed under this heading.

Norgestimate (Oral contraceptives tend to produce hyperglycemia leading to loss of control; patients on concurrent therapy should be closely observed for loss of control). Products include:

- Ortho-Cyclen/Ortho Tri-Cyclen 2573
- Ortho-Prefest Tablets 2570

Norgestrel (Oral contraceptives tend to produce hyperglycemia leading to loss of control; patients on concurrent therapy should be closely observed for loss of control). Products include:

- Lo/Ovral Tablets 3532
- Lo/Ovral-28 Tablets 3538
- Low-Ogestrel-28 Tablets 3392
- Ogestrel 0.5/50-28 Tablets 3428
- Ovral Tablets 3551
- Ovral-28 Tablets 3552
- Ovrette Tablets 3552

Pancreatin (Pancreatin, a carbohydrate splitting enzyme, may reduce the effect of acarbose and should not be taken concurrently). Products include:

- Donnazyme Tablets 2931

Perphenazine (Phenothiazines tend to produce hyperglycemia leading to loss of control; patients on concurrent therapy should be closely observed for loss of control). Products include:

- Etrafon 3115
- Trilafon 3160

Phenylephrine Bitartrate (Sympathomimetics tend to produce hyperglycemia leading to loss of control; patients on concurrent therapy should be closely observed for loss of control).

No products indexed under this heading.

Phenylephrine Hydrochloride (Sympathomimetics tend to produce hyperglycemia leading to loss of control; patients on concurrent therapy should be closely observed for loss of control). Products include:

- Afrin Nasal Decongestant Children's Pump Mist .... ▣734
- Extendryl 1361
- Hycomine Compound Tablets 1317
- Neo-Synephrine .... ▣614
- Phenergan VC Syrup 3560
- Phenergan VC with Codeine Syrup 3561
- Preparation H Cream .... ▣778
- Preparation H Cooling Gel .... ▣778
- Preparation H .... ▣778
- Vicks Sinex Nasal Spray and Ultra Fine Mist .... ▣729

Phenylephrine Tannate (Sympathomimetics tend to produce hyperglycemia leading to loss of control; patients on concurrent therapy should be closely observed for loss of control). Products include:

- Ryna-12 S Suspension 3351
- Reformulated Rynatan Pediatric Suspension 3352
- Rynatuss Pediatric Suspension 3353
- Rynatuss Tablets 3353

Phenylpropanolamine Hydrochloride (Sympathomimetics tend to produce hyperglycemia leading to loss of control; patients on concurrent therapy should be closely observed for loss of control).

No products indexed under this heading.

Phenytoin (Phenytoin tends to produce hyperglycemia leading to loss of control; patients on concurrent therapy should be closely observed for loss of control). Products include:

- Dilantin Infatabs 2624
- Dilantin-125 Oral Suspension 2625

Phenytoin Sodium (Phenytoin tends to produce hyperglycemia leading to loss of control; patients on concurrent therapy should be closely observed for loss of control). Products include:

- Dilantin Kapseals 2622

Pirbuterol Acetate (Sympathomimetics tend to produce hyperglycemia leading to loss of control; patients on concurrent therapy should be closely observed for loss of control). Products include:

- Maxair Autohaler 1981
- Maxair Inhaler 1984

Polyestradiol Phosphate (Estrogens tend to produce hyperglycemia leading to loss of control; patients on concurrent therapy should be closely observed for loss of control).

No products indexed under this heading.

Polythiazide (Thiazide diuretics tend to produce hyperglycemia leading to loss of control; patients on concurrent therapy should be closely observed for loss of control). Products include:

- Minizide Capsules 2700
- Renese Tablets 2712

Prednisolone Acetate (Corticosteroids tend to produce hyperglycemia leading to loss of control; patients on concurrent therapy should be closely observed for loss of control). Products include:

- Blephamide Ophthalmic Ointment 547
- Blephamide Ophthalmic Suspension 548
- Poly-Pred Liquifilm Ophthalmic Suspension .... ⊙245
- Pred Forte Ophthalmic Suspension .... ⊙246
- Pred Mild Sterile Ophthalmic Suspension .... ⊙249
- Pred-G Ophthalmic Suspension .... ⊙247
- Pred-G Sterile Ophthalmic Ointment .... ⊙248

Prednisolone Sodium Phosphate (Corticosteroids tend to produce hyperglycemia leading to loss of control; patients on concurrent therapy should be closely observed for loss of control). Products include:

- Pediapred Oral Solution 1170

Prednisolone Tebutate (Corticosteroids tend to produce hyperglycemia leading to loss of control; patients on concurrent therapy should be closely observed for loss of control).

No products indexed under this heading.

Prednisone (Corticosteroids tend to produce hyperglycemia leading to loss of control; patients on concurrent therapy should be closely observed for loss of control). Products include:

- Prednisone 3064

Prochlorperazine (Phenothiazines tend to produce hyperglycemia leading to loss of control; patients on concurrent therapy should be closely observed for loss of control). Products include:

- Compazine 1505

Promethazine Hydrochloride (Phenothiazines tend to produce hyperglycemia leading to loss of control; patients on concurrent therapy should be closely observed for loss of control). Products include:

- Mepergan Injection 3539
- Phenergan Injection 3553
- Phenergan 3556
- Phenergan Syrup 3554
- Phenergan with Codeine Syrup 3557
- Phenergan with Dextromethorphan Syrup 3559
- Phenergan VC Syrup 3560
- Phenergan VC with Codeine Syrup 3561

Pseudoephedrine Hydrochloride (Sympathomimetics tend to produce hyperglycemia leading to loss of control; patients on concurrent therapy should be closely observed for loss of control). Products include:

- Actifed Cold & Allergy Tablets .... ▣688
- Actifed Cold & Sinus Caplets and Tablets .... ▣688
- Advil Cold and Sinus Caplets .... ▣771
- Advil Cold and Sinus Tablets .... ▣771
- Advil Flu & Body Ache Caplets .... ▣772
- Aleve Cold & Sinus Caplets .... ▣603
- Alka-Seltzer Plus Liqui-Gels .... ▣604
- Alka-Seltzer Plus Cold & Flu Medicine Liqui-Gels .... ▣604
- Alka-Seltzer Plus Cold & Sinus Medicine Liqui-Gels .... ▣604
- Allegra-D Extended-Release Tablets 714
- BC Cold Powder .... ▣619
- Benadryl Allergy/Cold Tablets .... ▣691
- Benadryl Allergy/Congestion Tablets .... ▣692
- Benadryl Allergy & Sinus Liquid .... ▣693
- Benadryl Allergy & Sinus Fastmelt Tablets .... ▣693
- Benadryl Allergy Sinus Headache Caplets & Gelcaps .... ▣693
- Benadryl Severe Allergy & Sinus Headache Caplets .... ▣694
- Benadryl Children's Allergy/Cold Fastmelt Tablets .... ▣692
- Benylin Multi-Symptom Liquid .... ▣697
- Bromfed Capsules (Extended-Release) 2269
- Bromfed-PD Capsules (Extended-Release) 2269
- Children's Cēpacol Sore Throat .... ▣788
- Comtrex Acute Head Cold & Sinus Pressure Relief Tablets .... ▣627
- Comtrex Deep Chest Cold & Congestion Relief Softgels .... ▣627
- Comtrex Flu Therapy & Fever Relief Daytime Caplets .... ▣628
- Comtrex Flu Therapy & Fever Relief Nighttime Tablets .... ▣628
- Comtrex Maximum Strength Multi-Symptom Cold & Cough Relief Tablets and Caplets .... ▣626
- Contac Non-Drowsy 12 Hour Cold Caplets .... ▣745
- Contac Non-Drowsy Timed Release 12 Hour Cold Caplets .... ▣746
- Contac Severe Cold and Flu Caplets Maximum Strength .... ▣746
- Contac Severe Cold and Flu Caplets Non-Drowsy .... ▣746
- Dimetapp Elixir .... ▣777
- Dimetapp Cold and Fever Suspension .... ▣775
- Dimetapp DM Cold & Cough Elixir .... ▣775
- Dimetapp Nighttime Flu Liquid .... ▣776
- Dimetapp Non-Drowsy Flu Syrup .... ▣777
- Dimetapp Infant Drops Decongestant .... ▣775
- Dimetapp Infant Drops Decongestant Plus Cough .... ▣776
- Guaifed 2272
- Kronofed-A 1341
- Children's Motrin Cold Oral Suspension 2007
- Motrin Sinus Headache Caplets 2005
- PediaCare Cough-Cold Liquid .... ▣719

PediaCare Infants' Drops Decongestant.......... 719
PediaCare Infants' Drops Decongestant Plus Cough.......... 719
PediaCare NightRest Cough-Cold Liquid.......... 719
Robitussin Cold Caplets Cold & Congestion.......... 780
Robitussin Cold Softgels Cold & Congestion.......... 780
Robitussin Cold Caplets Multi-Symptom Cold & Flu.......... 781
Robitussin Cold Softgels Multi-Symptom Cold & Flu.......... 781
Robitussin Cold Softgels Severe Congestion.......... 782
Robitussin Cough & Cold Infant Drops.......... 782
Robitussin Maximum Strength Cough & Cold Liquid.......... 785
Robitussin Pediatric Cough & Cold Formula Liquid.......... 785
Robitussin Multi Symptom Honey Flu Liquid.......... 785
Robitussin Nighttime Honey Flu Liquid.......... 786
Robitussin-CF Liquid.......... 783
Robitussin-DAC Syrup.......... 2942
Robitussin-PE Liquid.......... 782
Ryna.......... 768
Semprex-D Capsules.......... 1172
Singlet Caplets.......... 761
Sinutab Non-Drying Liquid Caps.......... 706
Sinutab Sinus Allergy Medication, Maximum Strength Formula, Tablets & Caplets.......... 707
Sinutab Sinus Medication, Maximum Strength Without Drowsiness Formula, Tablets & Caplets.......... 707
Sudafed 12 Hour Tablets.......... 708
Sudafed 24 Hour Tablets.......... 708
Children's Sudafed Cold & Cough Liquid.......... 709
Children's Sudafed Nasal Decongestant Chewables.......... 711
Children's Sudafed Nasal Decongestant Liquid Medication.......... 711
Sudafed Cold & Allergy Tablets.......... 708
Sudafed Cold & Cough Liquid Caps.......... 709
Sudafed Cold & Sinus Liquid Caps.......... 710
Sudafed Nasal Decongestant Tablets.......... 710
Sudafed Non-Drying Sinus Liquid Caps.......... 712
Sudafed Severe Cold.......... 711
Sudafed Sinus Headache Caplets.......... 712
Sudafed Sinus Headache Tablets.......... 712
Tavist Sinus Non-Drowsy Coated Caplets.......... 676
TheraFlu Regular Strength Cold & Cough Night Time Hot Liquid.......... 676
TheraFlu Regular Strength Cold & Sore Throat Night Time Hot Liquid.......... 676
TheraFlu Maximum Strength Flu & Congestion Non-Drowsy Hot Liquid.......... 677
TheraFlu Maximum Strength Flu & Cough Night Time Hot Liquid.......... 678
TheraFlu Maximum Strength Flu & Sore Throat Night Time Hot Liquid.......... 677
TheraFlu Maximum Strength Severe Cold & Congestion Night Time Caplets.......... 678
TheraFlu Maximum Strength Severe Cold & Congestion Night Time Hot Liquid.......... 678
TheraFlu Maximum Strength Severe Cold & Congestion Non-Drowsy.......... 679
Triaminic Allergy Congestion Liquid.......... 680
Triaminic Chest Congestion Liquid.......... 680
Triaminic Cold & Allergy Liquid.......... 681
Triaminic Cold & Allergy Softchews.......... 683
Triaminic Cold & Cough Liquid.......... 681
Triaminic Cold & Cough Softchews.......... 683
Triaminic Cold & Night Time Cough Liquid.......... 681
Triaminic Cold, Cough & Fever Liquid.......... 681
Triaminic Cough Liquid.......... 682
Triaminic Cough & Congestion Liquid.......... 682
Triaminic Cough & Sore Throat Liquid.......... 682
Triaminic Cough & Sore Throat Softchews.......... 684
Children's Tylenol Allergy-D Liquid.......... 2014
Children's Tylenol Cold Suspension Liquid and Chewable Tablets.......... 2015
Children's Tylenol Cold Plus Cough Suspension Liquid and Chewable Tablets.......... 2015
Children's Tylenol Flu Suspension Liquid.......... 2015
Children's Tylenol Sinus Suspension Liquid.......... 2017
Infants' Tylenol Cold Decongestant and Fever Reducer Concentrated Drops.......... 2015
Infants' Tylenol Cold Decongestant and Fever Reducer Concentrated Drops Plus Cough.......... 2015
Tylenol Allergy Sinus.......... 2010
Multi-Symptom Tylenol Cold Complete Formula Caplets.......... 2010
Multi-Symptom Tylenol Cold Non-Drowsy Caplets and Gelcaps.......... 2010
Multi-Symptom Tylenol Cold Severe Congestion Non-Drowsy Caplets.......... 2011
Maximum Strength Tylenol Flu NightTime Gelcaps.......... 2011
Maximum Strength Tylenol Flu NightTime Liquid.......... 2011
Maximum Strength Tylenol Flu Non-Drowsy Gelcaps.......... 2011
Maximum Strength Tylenol Sinus NightTime Caplets.......... 2012
Maximum Strength Tylenol Sinus Non-Drowsy Geltabs, Gelcaps, Caplets, and Tablets.......... 2012
Vicks 44D Cough & Head Congestion Relief Liquid.......... 724
Vicks 44M Cough, Cold & Flu Relief Liquid.......... 725
Pediatric Vicks 44m Cough & Cold Relief.......... 728
Vicks DayQuil LiquiCaps/Liquid Multi-Symptom Cold/Flu Relief.......... 727
Children's Vicks NyQuil Cold/Cough Relief.......... 726
Vicks NyQuil LiquiCaps/Liquid Multi-Symptom Cold/Flu Relief, Original and Cherry Flavors.......... 727
Zephrex Tablets.......... 3091
Zephrex LA Tablets.......... 3092
Zyrtec-D 12 Hour Extended Relief Tablets.......... 2758

Pseudoephedrine Sulfate (Sympathomimetics tend to produce hyperglycemia leading to loss of control; patients on concurrent therapy should be closely observed for loss of control). Products include:

Chlor-Trimeton Allergy/Decongestant Tablets.......... 736
Claritin-D 12 Hour Extended Release Tablets.......... 3102
Claritin-D 24 Hour Extended Release Tablets.......... 3104
Coricidin 'D' Cold, Flu & Sinus Tablets.......... 737
Drixoral Allergy/Sinus Extended-Release Tablets.......... 741
Drixoral Cold & Allergy Sustained-Action Tablets.......... 740
Drixoral Cold & Flu Extended-Release Tablets.......... 740
Drixoral Nasal Decongestant Long-Acting Non-Drowsy Tablets.......... 740
Rynatan Tablets.......... 3351

Quinestrol (Estrogens tend to produce hyperglycemia leading to loss of control; patients on concurrent therapy should be closely observed for loss of control).

No products indexed under this heading.

Salmeterol Xinafoate (Sympathomimetics tend to produce hyperglycemia leading to loss of control; patients on concurrent therapy should be closely observed for loss of control). Products include:

Advair Diskus 100/50.......... 1448
Advair Diskus 250/50.......... 1448
Advair Diskus 500/50.......... 1448
Serevent Diskus.......... 1637
Serevent Inhalation Aerosol.......... 1633

Terbutaline Sulfate (Sympathomimetics tend to produce hyperglycemia leading to loss of control; patients on concurrent therapy should be closely observed for loss of control). Products include:

Brethine Ampuls.......... 2314
Brethine Tablets.......... 2313

Thioridazine Hydrochloride (Phenothiazines tend to produce hyperglycemia leading to loss of control; patients on concurrent therapy should be closely observed for loss of control). Products include:

Thioridazine Hydrochloride Tablets.......... 2289

Thyroglobulin (Thyroid products tend to produce hyperglycemia leading to loss of control; patients on concurrent therapy should be closely observed for loss of control).

No products indexed under this heading.

Thyroid (Thyroid products tend to produce hyperglycemia leading to loss of control; patients on concurrent therapy should be closely observed for loss of control).

No products indexed under this heading.

Thyroxine (Thyroid products tend to produce hyperglycemia leading to loss of control; patients on concurrent therapy should be closely observed for loss of control).

No products indexed under this heading.

Thyroxine Sodium (Thyroid products tend to produce hyperglycemia leading to loss of control; patients on concurrent therapy should be closely observed for loss of control).

No products indexed under this heading.

Triamcinolone (Corticosteroids tend to produce hyperglycemia leading to loss of control; patients on concurrent therapy should be closely observed for loss of control).

No products indexed under this heading.

Triamcinolone Acetonide (Corticosteroids tend to produce hyperglycemia leading to loss of control; patients on concurrent therapy should be closely observed for loss of control). Products include:

Azmacort Inhalation Aerosol.......... 728
Nasacort Nasal Inhaler.......... 750
Nasacort AQ Nasal Spray.......... 752
Tri-Nasal Spray.......... 2274

Triamcinolone Diacetate (Corticosteroids tend to produce hyperglycemia leading to loss of control; patients on concurrent therapy should be closely observed for loss of control).

No products indexed under this heading.

Triamcinolone Hexacetonide (Corticosteroids tend to produce hyperglycemia leading to loss of control; patients on concurrent therapy should be closely observed for loss of control).

No products indexed under this heading.

Trifluoperazine Hydrochloride (Phenothiazines tend to produce hyperglycemia leading to loss of control; patients on concurrent therapy should be closely observed for loss of control). Products include:

Stelazine.......... 1640

Verapamil Hydrochloride (Calcium channel blockers tend to produce hyperglycemia leading to loss of control; patients on concurrent therapy should be closely observed for loss of control). Products include:

Covera-HS Tablets.......... 3199
Isoptin SR Tablets.......... 467
Tarka Tablets.......... 508
Verelan Capsules.......... 3184
Verelan PM Capsules.......... 3186

PRED FORTE OPHTHALMIC SUSPENSION

(Prednisolone Acetate).......... ⊙246
None cited in PDR database.

PRED MILD STERILE OPHTHALMIC SUSPENSION

(Prednisolone Acetate).......... ⊙249
None cited in PDR database.

PRED-G OPHTHALMIC SUSPENSION

(Gentamicin Sulfate, Prednisolone Acetate).......... ⊙247
None cited in PDR database.

PRED-G STERILE OPHTHALMIC OINTMENT

(Gentamicin Sulfate, Prednisolone Acetate).......... ⊙248
None cited in PDR database.

PREDNISONE INTENSOL

(Prednisone).......... 3064
See Prednisone Tablets

PREDNISONE ORAL SOLUTION

(Prednisone).......... 3064
See Prednisone Tablets

PREDNISONE TABLETS

(Prednisone).......... 3064
May interact with:

Aspirin (Co-administration of corticosteroids with aspirin in hypoprothrombinemia should be undertaken with caution). Products include:

Aggrenox Capsules.......... 1026
Alka-Seltzer.......... 603
Alka-Seltzer Lemon Lime Antacid and Pain Reliever Effervescent Tablets.......... 603
Alka-Seltzer Extra Strength Antacid and Pain Reliever Effervescent Tablets.......... 603
Alka-Seltzer PM Effervescent Tablets.......... 605
Genuine Bayer Tablets, Caplets and Gelcaps.......... 606
Extra Strength Bayer Caplets and Gelcaps.......... 610
Aspirin Regimen Bayer Children's Chewable Tablets (Orange or Cherry Flavored).......... 607
Bayer, Aspirin Regimen.......... 606
Aspirin Regimen Bayer 81 mg Caplets with Calcium.......... 607
Genuine Bayer Professional Labeling (Aspirin Regimen Bayer).......... 608
Extra Strength Bayer Arthritis Caplets.......... 610
Extra Strength Bayer Plus Caplets.......... 610
Extra Strength Bayer PM Caplets.......... 611
BC Powder.......... 619
BC Allergy Sinus Cold Powder.......... 619
Arthritis Strength BC Powder.......... 619
BC Sinus Cold Powder.......... 619
Darvon Compound-65 Pulvules.......... 1910
Ecotrin Enteric Coated Aspirin Low, Regular and Maximum Strength Tablets.......... 1715
Excedrin Extra-Strength Tablets, Caplets, and Geltabs.......... 629
Excedrin Migraine.......... 1070
Goody's Body Pain Formula Powder.......... 620
Goody's Extra Strength Headache Powder.......... 620
Goody's Extra Strength Pain Relief Tablets.......... 620
Percodan Tablets.......... 1327
Robaxisal Tablets.......... 2939
Soma Compound Tablets.......... 3354
Soma Compound w/Codeine Tablets.......... 3355
Vanquish Caplets.......... 617

PREGNYL FOR INJECTION

(Chorionic Gonadotropin).......... 2482
None cited in PDR database.

PRELIEF TABLETS AND GRANULATE

(Calcium Glycerophosphate).......... 801
May interact with:

Prescription Drugs, unspecified (Calcium may interact with certain

prescription drugs; concurrent use should be undertaken with the supervision of a health professional).

PRELONE SYRUP
(Prednisolone) 2273
May interact with oral hypoglycemic agents, insulin, and certain other agents. Compounds in these categories include:

Acarbose (Potential for increased requirements of oral hypoglycemic agents). Products include:
- Precose Tablets 906

Aspirin (Aspirin should be used cautiously in conjunction with corticosteroids in hypoprothrombinemia). Products include:
- Aggrenox Capsules 1026
- Alka-Seltzer .... ▣ 603
- Alka-Seltzer Lemon Lime Antacid and Pain Reliever Effervescent Tablets .... ▣ 603
- Alka-Seltzer Extra Strength Antacid and Pain Reliever Effervescent Tablets .... ▣ 603
- Alka-Seltzer PM Effervescent Tablets .... ▣ 605
- Genuine Bayer Tablets, Caplets and Gelcaps .... ▣ 606
- Extra Strength Bayer Caplets and Gelcaps .... ▣ 610
- Aspirin Regimen Bayer Children's Chewable Tablets (Orange or Cherry Flavored) .... ▣ 607
- Bayer, Aspirin Regimen .... ▣ 606
- Aspirin Regimen Bayer 81 mg Caplets with Calcium .... ▣ 607
- Genuine Bayer Professional Labeling (Aspirin Regimen Bayer) .... ▣ 608
- Extra Strength Bayer Arthritis Caplets .... ▣ 610
- Extra Strength Bayer Plus Caplets .... ▣ 610
- Extra Strength Bayer PM Caplets .... ▣ 611
- BC Powder .... ▣ 619
- BC Allergy Sinus Cold Powder .... ▣ 619
- Arthritis Strength BC Powder .... ▣ 619
- BC Sinus Cold Powder .... ▣ 619
- Darvon Compound-65 Pulvules 1910
- Ecotrin Enteric Coated Aspirin Low, Regular and Maximum Strength Tablets 1715
- Excedrin Extra-Strength Tablets, Caplets, and Geltabs .... ▣ 629
- Excedrin Migraine 1070
- Goody's Body Pain Formula Powder .... ▣ 620
- Goody's Extra Strength Headache Powder .... ▣ 620
- Goody's Extra Strength Pain Relief Tablets .... ▣ 620
- Percodan Tablets 1327
- Robaxisal Tablets 2939
- Soma Compound Tablets 3354
- Soma Compound w/Codeine Tablets 3355
- Vanquish Caplets .... ▣ 617

Chlorpropamide (Potential for increased requirements of oral hypoglycemic agents). Products include:
- Diabinese Tablets 2680

Glimepiride (Potential for increased requirements of oral hypoglycemic agents). Products include:
- Amaryl Tablets 717

Glipizide (Potential for increased requirements of oral hypoglycemic agents). Products include:
- Glucotrol Tablets 2692
- Glucotrol XL Extended Release Tablets 2693

Glyburide (Potential for increased requirements of oral hypoglycemic agents). Products include:
- DiaBeta Tablets 741
- Glucovance Tablets 1086

Insulin, Human, Zinc Suspension (Potential for increased requirements of insulin). Products include:
- Humulin L, 100 Units 1937
- Humulin U, 100 Units 1943
- Novolin L Human Insulin 10 ml Vials 2422

Insulin, Human NPH (Potential for increased requirements of insulin). Products include:
- Humulin N, 100 Units 1939
- Humulin N NPH Pen 1940
- Novolin N Human Insulin 10 ml Vials 2422
- Novolin N PenFill 2423
- Novolin N Prefilled Syringe Disposable Insulin Delivery System 2425

Insulin, Human Regular (Potential for increased requirements of insulin). Products include:
- Humulin R Regular (U-500) 1943
- Humulin R, 100 Units 1941
- Novolin R Human Insulin 10 ml Vials 2423
- Novolin R PenFill 2423
- Novolin R Prefilled Syringe Disposable Insulin Delivery System 2425
- Velosulin BR Human Insulin 10 ml Vials 2435

Insulin, Human Regular and Human NPH Mixture (Potential for increased requirements of insulin). Products include:
- Humulin 50/50, 100 Units 1934
- Humulin 70/30, 100 Units 1935
- Humulin 70/30 Pen 1936
- Novolin 70/30 Human Insulin 10 ml Vials 2421
- Novolin 70/30 PenFill 2423
- Novolin 70/30 Prefilled Disposable Insulin Delivery System 2425

Insulin, NPH (Potential for increased requirements of insulin). Products include:
- Iletin II, NPH (Pork), 100 Units 1946

Insulin, Regular (Potential for increased requirements of insulin). Products include:
- Iletin II, Regular (Pork), 100 Units ... 1947

Insulin, Zinc Crystals (Potential for increased requirements of insulin).
No products indexed under this heading.

Insulin, Zinc Suspension (Potential for increased requirements of insulin). Products include:
- Iletin II, Lente (Pork), 100 Units 1945

Insulin Aspart, Human Regular (Potential for increased requirements of insulin).
No products indexed under this heading.

Insulin glargine (Potential for increased requirements of insulin). Products include:
- Lantus Injection 742

Insulin Lispro, Human (Potential for increased requirements of insulin). Products include:
- Humalog 1926
- Humalog Mix 75/25 Pen 1928

Insulin Lispro Protamine, Human (Potential for increased requirements of insulin). Products include:
- Humalog Mix 75/25 Pen 1928

Metformin Hydrochloride (Potential for increased requirements of oral hypoglycemic agents). Products include:
- Glucophage Tablets 1080
- Glucophage XR Tablets 1080
- Glucovance Tablets 1086

Miglitol (Potential for increased requirements of oral hypoglycemic agents). Products include:
- Glyset Tablets 2821

Pioglitazone Hydrochloride (Potential for increased requirements of oral hypoglycemic agents). Products include:
- Actos Tablets 3275

Repaglinide (Potential for increased requirements of oral hypoglycemic agents). Products include:
- Prandin Tablets (0.5, 1, and 2 mg) 2432

Rosiglitazone Maleate (Potential for increased requirements of oral hypoglycemic agents). Products include:
- Avandia Tablets 1490

Tolazamide (Potential for increased requirements of oral hypoglycemic agents).
No products indexed under this heading.

Tolbutamide (Potential for increased requirements of oral hypoglycemic agents).
No products indexed under this heading.

Troglitazone (Potential for increased requirements of oral hypoglycemic agents).
No products indexed under this heading.

PREMARIN INTRAVENOUS
(Estrogens, Conjugated) 3563
None cited in PDR database.

PREMARIN TABLETS
(Estrogens, Conjugated) 3566
May interact with:

Medroxyprogesterone Acetate (Co-administration of estrogen with progestin may include possible adverse effects on carbohydrate and lipid metabolism). Products include:
- Depo-Provera Contraceptive Injection 2798
- Lunelle Monthly Injection 2827
- Premphase Tablets 3572
- Prempro Tablets 3572
- Provera Tablets 2853

PREMARIN VAGINAL CREAM
(Estrogens, Conjugated) 3570
See Premarin Tablets

PREMESISRX TABLETS
(Vitamin B_6, Vitamins, Prenatal) 3313
None cited in PDR database.

PREMPHASE TABLETS
(Estrogens, Conjugated, Medroxyprogesterone Acetate) 3572
May interact with:

Aminoglutethimide (Aminoglutethimide administered concomitantly with medroxyprogesterone acetate (MPA) may significantly depress the bioavailability of MPA).
No products indexed under this heading.

Food Interactions

Food, unspecified (Administration with a high fat breakfast decreased total estrone Cmax and increased total equilin Cmax compared to fasting state, no other effect on rate or extent of absorption; administration with food doubles MPA Cmax and increases MPA AUC).

PREMPRO TABLETS
(Estrogens, Conjugated, Medroxyprogesterone Acetate) 3572
May interact with:

Aminoglutethimide (Aminoglutethimide administered concomitantly with medroxyprogesterone acetate (MPA) may significantly depress the bioavailability of MPA).
No products indexed under this heading.

Food Interactions

Food, unspecified (Administration with food decreased Cmax of total estrone compared to fasting state, no other effect on rate or extent of absorption; administration with food doubles MPA Cmax and increases MPA AUC).

PREPARATION H CREAM
(Glycerin, Petrolatum, Phenylephrine Hydrochloride, Shark Liver Oil) .... ▣ 778
None cited in PDR database.

PREPARATION H COOLING GEL
(Phenylephrine Hydrochloride) .... ▣ 778
None cited in PDR database.

PREPARATION H OINTMENT
(Mineral Oil, Petrolatum, Phenylephrine Hydrochloride, Shark Liver Oil) .... ▣ 778
None cited in PDR database.

PREPARATION H SUPPOSITORIES
(Cocoa Butter, Phenylephrine Hydrochloride, Shark Liver Oil) .... ▣ 778
None cited in PDR database.

PREPARATION H MEDICATED WIPES
(Witch Hazel) .... ▣ 779
None cited in PDR database.

PREPIDIL GEL
(Dinoprostone) 2851
May interact with oxytocic drugs. Compounds in these categories include:

Ergonovine Maleate (Prepidil may augment the activity of other oxytocic drugs; co-administration is not recommended).
No products indexed under this heading.

Methylergonovine Maleate (Prepidil may augment the activity of other oxytocic drugs; co-administration is not recommended).
No products indexed under this heading.

Oxytocin (Prepidil may augment the activity of other oxytocic drugs; co-administration is not recommended; allow a 6-12 hour dosing interval for sequential use of oxytocin).
No products indexed under this heading.

PREVACID DELAYED-RELEASE CAPSULES
(Lansoprazole) 3292
May interact with iron containing oral preparations, absorption of drugs where gastric ph is an important determinant in their bioavailability, theophylline, and certain other agents. Compounds in these categories include:

Aminophylline (Co-administration has resulted in a minor increase (10%) in the clearance of theophylline; this interaction is unlikely to be of clinical concern, nonetheless monitor blood levels).
No products indexed under this heading.

Bacampicillin Hydrochloride (Lansoprazole causes a profound and long-lasting inhibition of gastric acid secretion; therefore, it is theoretically possible that it may interfere with the oral absorption of drugs where gastric pH is an important determinant of bioavailability).
No products indexed under this heading.

Digoxin (Lansoprazole causes a profound and long-lasting inhibition of gastric acid secretion; therefore, it is theoretically possible that it may interfere with the oral absorption of drugs where gastric pH is an important determinant of bioavailability, such asdigoxin). Products include:
- Digitek Tablets 1003
- Lanoxicaps Capsules 1574
- Lanoxin Injection 1581
- Lanoxin Tablets 1587
- Lanoxin Elixir Pediatric 1578
- Lanoxin Injection Pediatric 1584

Dyphylline (Co-administration has resulted in a minor increase (10%) in the clearance of theophylline; this interaction is unlikely to be of clinical concern, nonetheless monitor blood levels). Products include:
- Lufyllin Tablets 3347
- Lufyllin-400 Tablets 3347

Lufyllin-GG Elixir 3348
Lufyllin-GG Tablets 3348

Ferrous Fumarate (Lansoprazole causes profound and long-lasting inhibition of gastric acid secretion; therefore it is theoretically possible that it may interfere with the absorption of drugs, such as iron salts, where gastric pH is an important determinant of bioavailability). Products include:
New Formulation Chromagen OB Capsules 3094
Loestrin Fe Tablets 2642
NataChew Tablets 3364

Ferrous Gluconate (Lansoprazole causes profound and long-lasting inhibition of gastric acid secretion; therefore it is theoretically possible that it may interfere with the absorption of drugs, such as iron salts, where gastric pH is an important determinant of bioavailability). Products include:
Fergon Iron Tablets .... ▣802

Ferrous Sulfate (Lansoprazole causes profound and long-lasting inhibition of gastric acid secretion; therefore it is theoretically possible that it may interfere with the absorption of drugs, such as iron salts, where gastric pH is an important determinant of bioavailability). Products include:
Feosol Tablets 1717
Slow Fe Tablets .... ▣827
Slow Fe with Folic Acid Tablets .... ▣828

Iron (Lansoprazole causes profound and long-lasting inhibition of gastric acid secretion; therefore it is theoretically possible that it may interfere with the absorption of drugs, such as iron salts, where gastric pH is an important determinant of bioavailability).
No products indexed under this heading.

Ketoconazole (Lansoprazole causes a profound and long-lasting inhibition of gastric acid secretion; therefore, it is theoretically possible that it may interfere with the oral absorption of drugs where gastric pH is an important determinant of bioavailability). Products include:
Nizoral 2% Cream 3620
Nizoral A-D Shampoo 2008
Nizoral 2% Shampoo 2007
Nizoral Tablets 1791

Polysaccharide-Iron Complex (Lansoprazole causes profound and long-lasting inhibition of gastric acid secretion; therefore it is theoretically possible that it may interfere with the absorption of drugs, such as iron salts, where gastric pH is an important determinant of bioavailability). Products include:
Niferex 3176
Niferex-150 Capsules 3176
Nu-Iron 150 Capsules 2224

Sucralfate (Co-administration delays absorption and reduces bioavailability of lansoprazole by about 30%, therefore lansoprazole should be taken at least 30 minutes prior to sucralfate). Products include:
Carafate Suspension 731
Carafate Tablets 730

Terfenadine (Co-administration of lansoprazole-clarithromycin combination with terfenadine in patients with pre-existing cardiac abnormalities is contraindicated).
No products indexed under this heading.

Theophylline (Co-administration has resulted in a minor increase (10%) in the clearance of theophylline; this interaction is unlikely to be of clinical concern, nonetheless monitor blood levels). Products include:
Aerolate 1361
Theo-Dur Extended-Release Tablets 1835
Uni-Dur Extended-Release Tablets 1841
Uniphyl 400 mg and 600 mg Tablets 2903

Theophylline Calcium Salicylate (Co-administration has resulted in a minor increase (10%) in the clearance of theophylline; this interaction is unlikely to be of clinical concern, nonetheless monitor blood levels).
No products indexed under this heading.

Theophylline Sodium Glycinate (Co-administration has resulted in a minor increase (10%) in the clearance of theophylline; this interaction is unlikely to be of clinical concern, nonetheless monitor blood levels).
No products indexed under this heading.

Food Interactions

Food, unspecified (Cmax and AUC are diminished by about 50% if the drug is given 30 minutes after food as opposed to the fasting condition; Prevacid should be taken before eating).

PREVNAR FOR INJECTION

(Pneumococcal vaccine, diphtheria conjugate) 1870
May interact with corticosteroids, cytotoxic drugs, and immunosuppressive agents. Compounds in these categories include:

Azathioprine (Children receiving immunosuppressive therapy may not respond optimally to active immunization).
No products indexed under this heading.

Basiliximab (Children receiving immunosuppressive therapy may not respond optimally to active immunization). Products include:
Simulect for Injection 2399

Betamethasone Acetate (Children receiving large doses of corticosteroids for immunosuppressive therapy may not respond optimally to active immunization). Products include:
Celestone Soluspan Injectable Suspension 3097

Betamethasone Sodium Phosphate (Children receiving large doses of corticosteroids for immunosuppressive therapy may not respond optimally to active immunization). Products include:
Celestone Soluspan Injectable Suspension 3097

Bleomycin Sulfate (Children receiving cytotoxic agents may not respond optimally to active immunization).
No products indexed under this heading.

Cortisone Acetate (Children receiving large doses of corticosteroids for immunosuppressive therapy may not respond optimally to active immunization). Products include:
Cortone Acetate Injectable Suspension 2059
Cortone Acetate Tablets 2061

Cyclophosphamide (Children receiving cytotoxic agents may not respond optimally to active immunization).
No products indexed under this heading.

Cyclosporine (Children receiving immunosuppressive therapy may not respond optimally to active immunization). Products include:
Gengraf Capsules 457
Neoral Soft Gelatin Capsules 2380
Neoral Oral Solution 2380
Sandimmune 2388

Daunorubicin Hydrochloride (Children receiving cytotoxic agents may not respond optimally to active immunization). Products include:
Cerubidine for Injection 947

Dexamethasone (Children receiving large doses of corticosteroids for immunosuppressive therapy may not respond optimally to active immunization). Products include:
Decadron Elixir 2078
Decadron Tablets 2079
TobraDex Ophthalmic Ointment 542
TobraDex Ophthalmic Suspension 541

Dexamethasone Acetate (Children receiving large doses of corticosteroids for immunosuppressive therapy may not respond optimally to active immunization).
No products indexed under this heading.

Dexamethasone Sodium Phosphate (Children receiving large doses of corticosteroids for immunosuppressive therapy may not respond optimally to active immunization). Products include:
Decadron Phosphate Injection 2081
Decadron Phosphate Sterile Ophthalmic Ointment 2083
Decadron Phosphate Sterile Ophthalmic Solution 2084
NeoDecadron Sterile Ophthalmic Solution 2144

Doxorubicin Hydrochloride (Children receiving cytotoxic agents may not respond optimally to active immunization). Products include:
Adriamycin PFS/RDF Injection 2767
Doxil Injection 566

Epirubicin Hydrochloride (Children receiving cytotoxic agents may not respond optimally to active immunization). Products include:
Ellence Injection 2806

Fludrocortisone Acetate (Children receiving large doses of corticosteroids for immunosuppressive therapy may not respond optimally to active immunization). Products include:
Florinef Acetate Tablets 2250

Fluorouracil (Children receiving cytotoxic agents may not respond optimally to active immunization). Products include:
Carac Cream 1222
Efudex 1733
Fluoroplex 552

Hydrocortisone (Children receiving large doses of corticosteroids for immunosuppressive therapy may not respond optimally to active immunization). Products include:
Anusol-HC Cream 2.5% 2237
Cipro HC Otic Suspension 540
Cortaid Intensive Therapy Cream .... ▣717
Cortaid Maximum Strength Cream .... ▣717
Cortisporin Ophthalmic Suspension Sterile .... ⊙297
Cortizone•5 .... ▣699
Cortizone•10 .... ▣699
Cortizone•10 Plus Creme .... ▣700
Cortizone for Kids Creme .... ▣699
Hydrocortone Tablets 2106
Massengill Medicated Soft Cloth Towelette .... ▣753
VōSoL HC Otic Solution 3356

Hydrocortisone Acetate (Children receiving large doses of corticosteroids for immunosuppressive therapy may not respond optimally to active immunization). Products include:
Analpram-HC 1338
Anusol HC-1 Hydrocortisone Anti-Itch Cream .... ▣689
Anusol-HC Suppositories 2238
Cortaid .... ▣717
Cortifoam Rectal Foam 3170
Cortisporin-TC Otic Suspension 2246
Hydrocortone Acetate Injectable Suspension 2103
Pramosone 1343
Proctocort Suppositories 2264
ProctoFoam-HC 3177
Terra-Cortril Ophthalmic Suspension 2716

Hydrocortisone Sodium Phosphate (Children receiving large doses of corticosteroids for immunosuppressive therapy may not respond optimally to active immunization). Products include:
Hydrocortone Phosphate Injection, Sterile 2105

Hydrocortisone Sodium Succinate (Children receiving large doses of corticosteroids for immunosuppressive therapy may not respond optimally to active immunization).
No products indexed under this heading.

Hydroxyurea (Children receiving cytotoxic agents may not respond optimally to active immunization). Products include:
Mylocel Tablets 2227

Methotrexate Sodium (Children receiving cytotoxic agents may not respond optimally to active immunization).
No products indexed under this heading.

Methylprednisolone Acetate (Children receiving large doses of corticosteroids for immunosuppressive therapy may not respond optimally to active immunization). Products include:
Depo-Medrol Injectable Suspension 2795

Methylprednisolone Sodium Succinate (Children receiving large doses of corticosteroids for immunosuppressive therapy may not respond optimally to active immunization). Products include:
Solu-Medrol Sterile Powder 2855

Mitotane (Children receiving cytotoxic agents may not respond optimally to active immunization).
No products indexed under this heading.

Mitoxantrone Hydrochloride (Children receiving cytotoxic agents may not respond optimally to active immunization). Products include:
Novantrone for Injection 1760

Muromonab-CD3 (Children receiving immunosuppressive therapy may not respond optimally to active immunization). Products include:
Orthoclone OKT3 Sterile Solution 2498

Mycophenolate Mofetil (Children receiving immunosuppressive therapy may not respond optimally to active immunization). Products include:
CellCept Capsules 2951
CellCept Oral Suspension 2951
CellCept Tablets 2951

Prednisolone Acetate (Children receiving large doses of corticosteroids for immunosuppressive therapy may not respond optimally to active immunization). Products include:
Blephamide Ophthalmic Ointment 547
Blephamide Ophthalmic Suspension 548
Poly-Pred Liquifilm Ophthalmic Suspension .... ⊙245
Pred Forte Ophthalmic Suspension .... ⊙246
Pred Mild Sterile Ophthalmic Suspension .... ⊙249
Pred-G Ophthalmic Suspension .... ⊙247
Pred-G Sterile Ophthalmic Ointment .... ⊙248

Prednisolone Sodium Phosphate (Children receiving large doses of corticosteroids for immunosuppressive therapy may not respond optimally to active immunization). Products include:
Pediapred Oral Solution 1170

Prednisolone Tebutate (Children receiving large doses of corticosteroids for immunosuppressive therapy may not respond optimally to active immunization).
No products indexed under this heading.

Prednisone (Children receiving large doses of corticosteroids for immunosuppressive therapy may not respond optimally to active immunization). Products include:
Prednisone 3064

Procarbazine Hydrochloride (Children receiving cytotoxic agents may not respond optimally to active immunization). Products include:
Matulane Capsules 3246

Sirolimus (Children receiving immunosuppressive therapy may not respond optimally to active immunization). Products include:
Rapamune Oral Solution and Tablets 3584

Tacrolimus (Children receiving immunosuppressive therapy may not respond optimally to active immunization). Products include:
Prograf 1393
Protopic Ointment 1397

Tamoxifen Citrate (Children receiving cytotoxic agents may not respond optimally to active immunization). Products include:
Nolvadex Tablets 678

Triamcinolone (Children receiving large doses of corticosteroids for immunosuppressive therapy may not respond optimally to active immunization).
No products indexed under this heading.

Triamcinolone Acetonide (Children receiving large doses of corticosteroids for immunosuppressive therapy may not respond optimally to active immunization). Products include:
Azmacort Inhalation Aerosol 728
Nasacort Nasal Inhaler 750
Nasacort AQ Nasal Spray 752
Tri-Nasal Spray 2274

Triamcinolone Diacetate (Children receiving large doses of corticosteroids for immunosuppressive therapy may not respond optimally to active immunization).
No products indexed under this heading.

Triamcinolone Hexacetonide (Children receiving large doses of corticosteroids for immunosuppressive therapy may not respond optimally to active immunization).
No products indexed under this heading.

Vincristine Sulfate (Children receiving cytotoxic agents may not respond optimally to active immunization).
No products indexed under this heading.

PREVPAC
(Amoxicillin, Clarithromycin, Lansoprazole) 3298
May interact with oral anticoagulants, oral hypoglycemic agents, insulin, iron containing oral preparations, absorption of drugs where gastric ph is an important determinant in their bioavailability, phenytoin, valproate, theophylline, and certain other agents. Compounds in these categories include:

Acarbose (Co-administration has resulted in rare reports of hypoglycemia, some of which occurred in patients taking oral hypoglycemia agents). Products include:
Precose Tablets 906

Alfentanil Hydrochloride (Concurrent use of erythromycin or clarithromycin in patients receiving drugs metabolized by the cytochrome P450 system may be associated with elevation in serum levels of alfentanil).
No products indexed under this heading.

Aminophylline (Co-administration of theophylline with clarithromycin in patients who are receiving high doses of theophylline may be associated with an increase in serum theophylline levels and potential theophylline toxicity).
No products indexed under this heading.

Astemizole (Concurrent use of erythromycin in patients receiving astemizole has resulted in prolonged QT interval and torsades de pointes; because clarithromycin is metabolized by P450, co-administration is not recommended).
No products indexed under this heading.

Bacampicillin Hydrochloride (Lansoprazole causes a profound and long lasting inhibition of gastric secretion; therefore, it is theoretically possible that it may interfere with oral absorption of drugs where gastric pH is an important determinant of bioavailability).
No products indexed under this heading.

Bromocriptine Mesylate (Concurrent use of erythromycin or clarithromycin in patients receiving drugs metabolized by the cytochrome P450 system may be associated with elevation in serum levels of bromocriptine).
No products indexed under this heading.

Carbamazepine (Co-administration of clarithromycin with carbamazepine has resulted in increased plasma concentrations of carbamazepine). Products include:
Carbatrol Capsules 3234
Tegretol/Tegretol-XR 2404

Chlorpropamide (Co-administration has resulted in rare reports of hypoglycemia, some of which occurred in patients taking oral hypoglycemia agents). Products include:
Diabinese Tablets 2680

Cisapride (Concurrent use of erythromycin or clarithromycin in patients receiving cisapride has been reported to result in rare cases of cardiovascular adverse events including prolonged QT interval, ventricular tachycardia, ventricular fibrillation, and torsades de pointes, and death have been reported; co-administration is contraindicated).
No products indexed under this heading.

Cyclosporine (Concurrent use of erythromycin or clarithromycin in patients receiving drugs metabolized by the cytochrome P450 system may be associated with elevation in serum levels of cyclosporine). Products include:
Gengraf Capsules 457
Neoral Soft Gelatin Capsules 2380
Neoral Oral Solution 2380
Sandimmune 2388

Dicumarol (Co-administration of clarithromycin with oral anticoagulants may result in the potentiation of oral coagulant effects).
No products indexed under this heading.

Digoxin (Co-administration of clarithromycin and digoxin has resulted in elevated digoxin serum concentrations resulting in clinical signs of digoxin toxicity including potentially fatal arrhythmias; lansoprazole causes profound and long-lasting inhibition of gastric acid secretion; therefore it is theoretically possible that it may interfere with the absorption of drugs, such as digoxin, where gastric pH is an important determinant of bioavailability). Products include:
Digitek Tablets 1003
Lanoxicaps Capsules 1574
Lanoxin Injection 1581
Lanoxin Tablets 1587
Lanoxin Elixir Pediatric 1578
Lanoxin Injection Pediatric 1584

Dihydroergotamine Mesylate (Co-administration of clarithromycin or erythromycin with dihydroergotamine has been associated in some patients with acute ergot toxicity characterized by severe peripheral vasospasm and dysesthesia). Products include:
D.H.E. 45 Injection 2334
Migranal Nasal Spray 2376

Disopyramide Phosphate (Concurrent use of erythromycin or clarithromycin in patients receiving drugs metabolized by the cytochrome P450 system may be associated with elevation in serum levels of disopyramide).
No products indexed under this heading.

Divalproex Sodium (Concurrent use of erythromycin or clarithromycin in patients receiving drugs metabolized by the cytochrome P450 system may be associated with elevation in serum levels of valproate). Products include:
Depakote Sprinkle Capsules 426
Depakote Tablets 430
Depakote ER Tablets 436

Dyphylline (Co-administration of theophylline with clarithromycin in patients who are receiving high doses of theophylline may be associated with an increase in serum theophylline levels and potential theophylline toxicity). Products include:
Lufyllin Tablets 3347
Lufyllin-400 Tablets 3347
Lufyllin-GG Elixir 3348
Lufyllin-GG Tablets 3348

Ergotamine Tartrate (Co-administration of clarithromycin or erythromycin with ergotamine has been associated in some patients with acute ergot toxicity characterized by severe peripheral vasospasm and dysesthesia).
No products indexed under this heading.

Ferrous Fumarate (Lansoprazole causes profound and long-lasting inhibition of gastric acid secretion; therefore it is theoretically possible that it may interfere with the absorption of drugs, such as iron salts, where gastric pH is an important determinant of bioavailability). Products include:
New Formulation Chromagen OB Capsules 3094
Loestrin Fe Tablets 2642
NataChew Tablets 3364

Ferrous Gluconate (Lansoprazole causes profound and long-lasting inhibition of gastric acid secretion; therefore it is theoretically possible that it may interfere with the absorption of drugs, such as iron salts, where gastric pH is an important determinant of bioavailability). Products include:
Fergon Iron Tablets .... ■ 802

Ferrous Sulfate (Lansoprazole causes profound and long-lasting inhibition of gastric acid secretion; therefore it is theoretically possible that it may interfere with the absorption of drugs, such as iron salts, where gastric pH is an important determinant of bioavailability). Products include:
Feosol Tablets 1717
Slow Fe Tablets .... ■ 827
Slow Fe with Folic Acid Tablets .... ■ 828

Fosphenytoin Sodium (Concurrent use of erythromycin or clarithromycin in patients receiving drugs metabolized by the cytochrome P450 system may be associated with elevation in serum levels of phenytoin). Products include:
Cerebyx Injection 2619

Glimepiride (Co-administration has resulted in rare reports of hypoglycemia, some of which occurred in patients taking oral hypoglycemia agents). Products include:
Amaryl Tablets 717

Glipizide (Co-administration has resulted in rare reports of hypoglycemia, some of which occurred in patients taking oral hypoglycemia agents). Products include:
Glucotrol Tablets 2692
Glucotrol XL Extended Release Tablets 2693

Glyburide (Co-administration has resulted in rare reports of hypoglycemia, some of which occurred in patients taking oral hypoglycemia agents). Products include:
DiaBeta Tablets 741
Glucovance Tablets 1086

Hexobarbital (Concurrent use of erythromycin or clarithromycin in patients receiving drugs metabolized by the cytochrome P450 system may be associated with elevation in serum levels of hexobarbital).

Insulin, Human, Zinc Suspension (Co-administration has resulted in rare reports of hypoglycemia, some of which occurred in patients taking insulin). Products include:
Humulin L, 100 Units 1937
Humulin U, 100 Units 1943
Novolin L Human Insulin 10 ml Vials 2422

Insulin, Human NPH (Co-administration has resulted in rare reports of hypoglycemia, some of which occurred in patients taking insulin). Products include:
Humulin N, 100 Units 1939
Humulin N NPH Pen 1940
Novolin N Human Insulin 10 ml Vials 2422
Novolin N PenFill 2423
Novolin N Prefilled Syringe Disposable Insulin Delivery System 2425

Insulin, Human Regular (Co-administration has resulted in rare reports of hypoglycemia, some of which occurred in patients taking insulin). Products include:
Humulin R Regular (U-500) 1943
Humulin R, 100 Units 1941
Novolin R Human Insulin 10 ml Vials 2423
Novolin R PenFill 2423
Novolin R Prefilled Syringe Disposable Insulin Delivery System 2425
Velosulin BR Human Insulin 10 ml Vials 2435

Insulin, Human Regular and Human NPH Mixture (Co-administration has resulted in rare reports of hypoglycemia, some of which occurred in patients taking insulin). Products include:
Humulin 50/50, 100 Units 1934
Humulin 70/30, 100 Units 1935
Humulin 70/30 Pen 1936
Novolin 70/30 Human Insulin 10 ml Vials 2421
Novolin 70/30 PenFill 2423
Novolin 70/30 Prefilled Disposable Insulin Delivery System 2425

Insulin, NPH (Co-administration has resulted in rare reports of hypoglycemia, some of which occurred in patients taking insulin). Products include:
Iletin II, NPH (Pork), 100 Units 1946

Insulin, Regular (Co-administration has resulted in rare reports of hypoglycemia, some of which occurred in patients taking insulin). Products include:
Iletin II, Regular (Pork), 100 Units 1947

Insulin, Zinc Crystals (Co-administration has resulted in rare reports of hypoglycemia, some of which occurred in patients taking insulin).
No products indexed under this heading.

Insulin, Zinc Suspension (Co-administration has resulted in rare

reports of hypoglycemia, some of which occurred in patients taking insulin). Products include:

Iletin II, Lente (Pork), 100 Units 1945

Insulin Aspart, Human Regular (Co-administration has resulted in rare reports of hypoglycemia, some of which occurred in patients taking insulin).

No products indexed under this heading.

Insulin glargine (Co-administration has resulted in rare reports of hypoglycemia, some of which occurred in patients taking insulin). Products include:

Lantus Injection 742

Insulin Lispro, Human (Co-administration has resulted in rare reports of hypoglycemia, some of which occurred in patients taking insulin). Products include:

Humalog 1926
Humalog Mix 75/25 Pen 1928

Insulin Lispro Protamine, Human (Co-administration has resulted in rare reports of hypoglycemia, some of which occurred in patients taking insulin). Products include:

Humalog Mix 75/25 Pen 1928

Iron (Lansoprazole causes profound and long-lasting inhibition of gastric acid secretion; therefore it is theoretically possible that it may interfere with the absorption of drugs, such as iron salts, where gastric pH is an important determinant of bioavailability).

No products indexed under this heading.

Ketoconazole (Lansoprazole causes a profound and long lasting inhibition of gastric secretion; therefore, it is theoretically possible that it may interfere with oral absorption of drugs where gastric pH is an important determinant of bioavailability). Products include:

Nizoral 2% Cream 3620
Nizoral A-D Shampoo 2008
Nizoral 2% Shampoo 2007
Nizoral Tablets 1791

Metformin Hydrochloride (Co-administration has resulted in rare reports of hypoglycemia, some of which occurred in patients taking oral hypoglycemia agents). Products include:

Glucophage Tablets 1080
Glucophage XR Tablets 1080
Glucovance Tablets 1086

Miglitol (Co-administration has resulted in rare reports of hypoglycemia, some of which occurred in patients taking oral hypoglycemia agents). Products include:

Glyset Tablets 2821

Phenytoin (Concurrent use of erythromycin or clarithromycin in patients receiving drugs metabolized by the cytochrome P450 system may be associated with elevation in serum levels of phenytoin). Products include:

Dilantin Infatabs 2624
Dilantin-125 Oral Suspension 2625

Phenytoin Sodium (Concurrent use of erythromycin or clarithromycin in patients receiving drugs metabolized by the cytochrome P450 system may be associated with elevation in serum levels of phenytoin). Products include:

Dilantin Kapseals 2622

Pimozide (Concurrent use of erythromycin or clarithromycin in patients receiving pimozide has been reported to result in rare cases of cardiovascular adverse events including prolonged QT interval, ventricular tachycardia, ventricular fibrillation, and torsades depointes, and death have been reported; co-administration is contraindicated). Products include:

Orap Tablets 1407

Pioglitazone Hydrochloride (Co-administration has resulted in rare reports of hypoglycemia, some of which occurred in patients taking oral hypoglycemia agents). Products include:

Actos Tablets 3275

Polysaccharide-Iron Complex (Lansoprazole causes profound and long-lasting inhibition of gastric acid secretion; therefore it is theoretically possible that it may interfere with the absorption of drugs, such as iron salts, where gastric pH is an important determinant of bioavailability). Products include:

Niferex 3176
Niferex-150 Capsules 3176
Nu-Iron 150 Capsules 2224

Repaglinide (Co-administration has resulted in rare reports of hypoglycemia, some of which occurred in patients taking oral hypoglycemia agents). Products include:

Prandin Tablets (0.5, 1, and 2 mg) 2432

Rosiglitazone Maleate (Co-administration has resulted in rare reports of hypoglycemia, some of which occurred in patients taking oral hypoglycemia agents). Products include:

Avandia Tablets 1490

Sucralfate (Co-administration delays absorption and reduces bioavailability by about 30%, therefore lansoprazole should be taken at least 30 minutes prior to sucralfate). Products include:

Carafate Suspension 731
Carafate Tablets 730

Tacrolimus (Concurrent use of erythromycin or clarithromycin in patients receiving drugs metabolized by the cytochrome P450 system may be associated with elevation in serum levels of tacrolimus). Products include:

Prograf 1393
Protopic Ointment 1397

Terfenadine (Co-administration has resulted in increased active acid metabolite of terfenadine by 3-fold; rare cases of cardiovascular adverse events including prolonged QT interval, ventricular tachycardia, ventricular fibrillation, and torsades de pointes, and death have been reported; co-administration of Prevpac with terfenadine is contraindicated).

No products indexed under this heading.

Theophylline (Co-administration of theophylline with clarithromycin in patients who are receiving high doses of theophylline may be associated with an increase in serum theophylline levels and potential theophylline toxicity). Products include:

Aerolate 1361
Theo-Dur Extended-Release Tablets 1835
Uni-Dur Extended-Release Tablets .. 1841
Uniphyl 400 mg and 600 mg Tablets 2903

Theophylline Calcium Salicylate (Co-administration of theophylline with clarithromycin in patients who are receiving high doses of theophylline may be associated with an increase in serum theophylline levels and potential theophylline toxicity).

No products indexed under this heading.

Theophylline Sodium Glycinate (Co-administration of theophylline with clarithromycin in patients who are receiving high doses of theophylline may be associated with an increase in serum theophylline levels and potential theophylline toxicity).

No products indexed under this heading.

Tolazamide (Co-administration has resulted in rare reports of hypoglycemia, some of which occurred in patients taking oral hypoglycemia agents).

No products indexed under this heading.

Tolbutamide (Co-administration has resulted in rare reports of hypoglycemia, some of which occurred in patients taking oral hypoglycemia agents).

No products indexed under this heading.

Triazolam (Erythromycin, another macrolide antibiotic, has been reported to decrease the clearance of triazolam and, thus, may increase the pharmacologic effect of triazolam; concomitant use has resulted in somnolence and confusion). Products include:

Halcion Tablets 2823

Troglitazone (Co-administration has resulted in rare reports of hypoglycemia, some of which occurred in patients taking oral hypoglycemia agents).

No products indexed under this heading.

Valproate Sodium (Concurrent use of erythromycin or clarithromycin in patients receiving drugs metabolized by the cytochrome P450 system may be associated with elevation in serum levels of valproate). Products include:

Depacon Injection 416

Valproic Acid (Concurrent use of erythromycin or clarithromycin in patients receiving drugs metabolized by the cytochrome P450 system may be associated with elevation in serum levels of valproate). Products include:

Depakene 421

Warfarin Sodium (Co-administration of clarithromycin with oral anticoagulants may result in the potentiation of oral coagulant effects). Products include:

Coumadin for Injection 1243
Coumadin Tablets 1243
Warfarin Sodium Tablets, USP 3302

Food Interactions

Food, unspecified (Both Cmax and AUC are diminished by about 50% if the lansoprazole is given 30 minutes after food as opposed to the fasting condition).

PRIFTIN TABLETS

(Rifapentine) 758

May interact with antacids, barbiturates, corticosteroids, doxycycline, fluoroquinolone antibiotics, cardiac glycosides, narcotic analgesics, phenytoin, protease inhibitors, quinidine, reverse transcriptase inhibitors, sulfonylureas, tricyclic antidepressants, theophylline, and certain other agents. Compounds in these categories include:

Alatrofloxacin Mesylate (Rifapentine is an inducer of cytochromes P4503A4 and P4502C8/9; therefore, rifapentine may increase the metabolism and decrease the activity of other co-administered drugs that are metabolized by these enzymes, such as fluoroquinolones). Products include:

Trovan I.V. 2722

Alfentanil Hydrochloride (Rifapentine is an inducer of cytochromes P4503A4 and P4502C8/9; therefore, rifapentine may increase the metabolism and decrease the activity of other co-administered drugs that are metabolized by these enzymes, such as narcotic analgesics).

No products indexed under this heading.

Aluminum Carbonate (Rifapentine should be taken at least 1 hour before or 2 hours after ingestion of antacids).

No products indexed under this heading.

Aluminum Hydroxide (Rifapentine should be taken at least 1 hour before or 2 hours after ingestion of antacids). Products include:

Amphojel Suspension (Mint Flavor) 789
Gaviscon Extra Strength Liquid 751
Gaviscon Extra Strength Tablets ... 751
Gaviscon Regular Strength Liquid . 751
Gaviscon Regular Strength Tablets 750
Maalox Antacid/Anti-Gas Oral Suspension 673
Maalox Max Maximum Strength Antacid/Anti-Gas Liquid 2300
Maalox Regular Strength Antacid/Antigas Liquid 2300
Mylanta 1813
Vanquish Caplets 617

Aminophylline (Rifapentine is an inducer of cytochromes P4503A4 and P4502C8/9; therefore, rifapentine may increase the metabolism and decrease the activity of other co-administered drugs that are metabolized by these enzymes, such as theophylline).

No products indexed under this heading.

Amitriptyline Hydrochloride (Rifapentine is an inducer of cytochromes P4503A4 and P4502C8/9; therefore, rifapentine may increase the metabolism and decrease the activity of other co-administered drugs that are metabolized by these enzymes, such as tricyclic antidepressants). Products include:

Etrafon 3115
Limbitrol 1738

Amoxapine (Rifapentine is an inducer of cytochromes P4503A4 and P4502C8/9; therefore, rifapentine may increase the metabolism and decrease the activity of other co-administered drugs that are metabolized by these enzymes, such as tricyclic antidepressants).

No products indexed under this heading.

Amprenavir (Rifapentine is an inducer of cytochromes P4503A4 and P4502C8/9; therefore, rifapentine may increase the metabolism and decrease the activity of other co-administered drugs that are metabolized by these enzymes, such as protease inhibitors; based on the rifapentine-indinavir interaction; rifapentine should be use with extreme caution, if at all, in patients who are also taking protease inhibitors). Products include:

Agenerase Capsules 1454
Agenerase Oral Solution 1459

Aprobarbital (Rifapentine is an inducer of cytochromes P4503A4 and P4502C8/9; therefore, rifapentine may increase the metabolism and decrease the activity of other co-administered drugs that are metabolized by these enzymes, such as barbiturates).

No products indexed under this heading.

Betamethasone Acetate (Rifapentine is an inducer of cytochromes P4503A4 and P4502C8/9; therefore, rifapentine may increase the metabolism and decrease the activity of other co-administered drugs that are metabolized by these enzymes, such as corticosteroids). Products include:

Celestone Soluspan Injectable Suspension 3097

Betamethasone Sodium Phosphate (Rifapentine is an inducer of cytochromes P4503A4 and P4502C8/9; therefore, rifapentine may increase the metabolism and

decrease the activity of other co-administered drugs that are metabolized by these enzymes, such as corticosteroids). Products include:
Celestone Soluspan Injectable Suspension 3097

Buprenorphine Hydrochloride (Rifapentine is an inducer of cytochromes P4503A4 and P4502C8/9; therefore, rifapentine may increase the metabolism and decrease the activity of other co-administered drugs that are metabolized by these enzymes, such as narcotic analgesics). Products include:
Buprenex Injectable 2918

Butabarbital (Rifapentine is an inducer of cytochromes P4503A4 and P4502C8/9; therefore, rifapentine may increase the metabolism and decrease the activity of other co-administered drugs that are metabolized by these enzymes, such as barbiturates).
No products indexed under this heading.

Butalbital (Rifapentine is an inducer of cytochromes P4503A4 and P4502C8/9; therefore, rifapentine may increase the metabolism and decrease the activity of other co-administered drugs that are metabolized by these enzymes, such as barbiturates). Products include:
Phrenilin 578
Sedapap Tablets 50 mg/650 mg 2225

Chloramphenicol Sodium Succinate (Rifapentine is an inducer of cytochromes P4503A4 and P4502C8/9; therefore, rifapentine may increase the metabolism and decrease the activity of other co-administered drugs that are metabolized by these enzymes, such as chloramphenicol).
No products indexed under this heading.

Chlorpropamide (Rifapentine is an inducer of cytochromes P4503A4 and P4502C8/9; therefore, rifapentine may increase the metabolism and decrease the activity of other co-administered drugs that are metabolized by these enzymes, such as sulfonylureas). Products include:
Diabinese Tablets 2680

Ciprofloxacin (Rifapentine is an inducer of cytochromes P4503A4 and P4502C8/9; therefore, rifapentine may increase the metabolism and decrease the activity of other co-administered drugs that are metabolized by these enzymes, such as fluoroquinolones). Products include:
Cipro I.V. 893
Cipro I.V. Pharmacy Bulk Package 897
Cipro Oral Suspension 887

Ciprofloxacin Hydrochloride (Rifapentine is an inducer of cytochromes P4503A4 and P4502C8/9; therefore, rifapentine may increase the metabolism and decrease the activity of other co-administered drugs that are metabolized by these enzymes, such as fluoroquinolones). Products include:
Ciloxan 538
Cipro HC Otic Suspension 540
Cipro Tablets 887

Clarithromycin (Rifapentine is an inducer of cytochromes P4503A4 and P4502C8/9; therefore, rifapentine may increase the metabolism and decrease the activity of other co-administered drugs that are metabolized by these enzymes, such as clarithromycin). Products include:
Biaxin/Biaxin XL 403
PREVPAC 3298

Clofibrate (Rifapentine is an inducer of cytochromes P4503A4 and P4502C8/9; therefore, rifapentine may increase the metabolism and decrease the activity of other co-administered drugs that are metabolized by these enzymes, such as clofibrate). Products include:
Atromid-S Capsules 3483

Clomipramine Hydrochloride (Rifapentine is an inducer of cytochromes P4503A4 and P4502C8/9; therefore, rifapentine may increase the metabolism and decrease the activity of other co-administered drugs that are metabolized by these enzymes, such as tricyclic antidepressants).
No products indexed under this heading.

Codeine Phosphate (Rifapentine is an inducer of cytochromes P4503A4 and P4502C8/9; therefore, rifapentine may increase the metabolism and decrease the activity of other co-administered drugs that are metabolized by these enzymes, such as narcotic analgesics). Products include:
Phenergan with Codeine Syrup 3557
Phenergan VC with Codeine Syrup 3561
Robitussin A-C Syrup 2942
Robitussin-DAC Syrup 2942
Ryna-C Liquid .... ▣ 768
Soma Compound w/Codeine Tablets 3355
Tussi-Organidin NR Liquid 3350
Tussi-Organidin-S NR Liquid 3350
Tylenol with Codeine 2595

Cortisone Acetate (Rifapentine is an inducer of cytochromes P4503A4 and P4502C8/9; therefore, rifapentine may increase the metabolism and decrease the activity of other co-administered drugs that are metabolized by these enzymes, such as corticosteroids). Products include:
Cortone Acetate Injectable Suspension 2059
Cortone Acetate Tablets 2061

Cyclosporine (Rifapentine is an inducer of cytochromes P4503A4 and P4502C8/9; therefore, rifapentine may increase the metabolism and decrease the activity of other co-administered drugs that are metabolized by these enzymes, such as cyclosporine). Products include:
Gengraf Capsules 457
Neoral Soft Gelatin Capsules 2380
Neoral Oral Solution 2380
Sandimmune 2388

Dapsone (Rifapentine is an inducer of cytochromes P4503A4 and P4502C8/9; therefore, rifapentine may increase the metabolism and decrease the activity of other co-administered drugs that are metabolized by these enzymes, such as dapsone). Products include:
Dapsone Tablets USP 1780

Desipramine Hydrochloride (Rifapentine is an inducer of cytochromes P4503A4 and P4502C8/9; therefore, rifapentine may increase the metabolism and decrease the activity of other co-administered drugs that are metabolized by these enzymes, such as tricyclic antidepressants). Products include:
Norpramin Tablets 755

Deslanoside (Rifapentine is an inducer of cytochromes P4503A4 and P4502C8/9; therefore, rifapentine may increase the metabolism and decrease the activity of other co-administered drugs that are metabolized by these enzymes, such as cardiac glycosides).
No products indexed under this heading.

Dexamethasone (Rifapentine is an inducer of cytochromes P4503A4 and P4502C8/9; therefore, rifapentine may increase the metabolism and decrease the activity of other co-administered drugs that are metabolized by these enzymes, such as corticosteroids). Products include:
Decadron Elixir 2078
Decadron Tablets 2079
TobraDex Ophthalmic Ointment 542
TobraDex Ophthalmic Suspension 541

Dexamethasone Acetate (Rifapentine is an inducer of cytochromes P4503A4 and P4502C8/9; therefore, rifapentine may increase the metabolism and decrease the activity of other co-administered drugs that are metabolized by these enzymes, such as corticosteroids).
No products indexed under this heading.

Dexamethasone Sodium Phosphate (Rifapentine is an inducer of cytochromes P4503A4 and P4502C8/9; therefore, rifapentine may increase the metabolism and decrease the activity of other co-administered drugs that are metabolized by these enzymes, such as corticosteroids). Products include:
Decadron Phosphate Injection 2081
Decadron Phosphate Sterile Ophthalmic Ointment 2083
Decadron Phosphate Sterile Ophthalmic Solution 2084
NeoDecadron Sterile Ophthalmic Solution 2144

Dezocine (Rifapentine is an inducer of cytochromes P4503A4 and P4502C8/9; therefore, rifapentine may increase the metabolism and decrease the activity of other co-administered drugs that are metabolized by these enzymes, such as narcotic analgesics).
No products indexed under this heading.

Diazepam (Rifapentine is an inducer of cytochromes P4503A4 and P4502C8/9; therefore, rifapentine may increase the metabolism and decrease the activity of other co-administered drugs that are metabolized by these enzymes, such as diazepam). Products include:
Valium Injectable 3026
Valium Tablets 3047

Didanosine (Rifapentine is an inducer of cytochromes P4503A4 and P4502C8/9; therefore, rifapentine may increase the metabolism and decrease the activity of other co-administered drugs that are metabolized by these enzymes, such as reverse transcriptase inhibitors). Products include:
Videx 1138
Videx EC Capsules 1143

Digitoxin (Rifapentine is an inducer of cytochromes P4503A4 and P4502C8/9; therefore, rifapentine may increase the metabolism and decrease the activity of other co-administered drugs that are metabolized by these enzymes, such as cardiac glycosides).
No products indexed under this heading.

Digoxin (Rifapentine is an inducer of cytochromes P4503A4 and P4502C8/9; therefore, rifapentine may increase the metabolism and decrease the activity of other co-administered drugs that are metabolized by these enzymes, such as cardiac glycosides). Products include:
Digitek Tablets 1003
Lanoxicaps Capsules 1574
Lanoxin Injection 1581
Lanoxin Tablets 1587
Lanoxin Elixir Pediatric 1578
Lanoxin Injection Pediatric 1584

Disopyramide Phosphate (Rifapentine is an inducer of cytochromes P4503A4 and P4502C8/9; therefore, rifapentine may increase the metabolism and decrease the activity of other co-administered drugs that are metabolized by these enzymes, such as disopyramide).
No products indexed under this heading.

Doxepin Hydrochloride (Rifapentine is an inducer of cytochromes P4503A4 and P4502C8/9; therefore, rifapentine may increase the metabolism and decrease the activity of other co-administered drugs that are metabolized by these enzymes, such as tricyclic antidepressants). Products include:
Sinequan 2713

Doxycycline Calcium (Rifapentine is an inducer of cytochromes P4503A4 and P4502C8/9; therefore, rifapentine may increase the metabolism and decrease the activity of other co-administered drugs that are metabolized by these enzymes, such as doxycycline). Products include:
Vibramycin Calcium Oral Suspension Syrup 2735

Doxycycline Hyclate (Rifapentine is an inducer of cytochromes P4503A4 and P4502C8/9; therefore, rifapentine may increase the metabolism and decrease the activity of other co-administered drugs that are metabolized by these enzymes, such as doxycycline). Products include:
Doryx Coated Pellet Filled Capsules 3357
Periostat Tablets 1208
Vibramycin Hyclate Capsules 2735
Vibramycin Hyclate Intravenous 2737
Vibra-Tabs Film Coated Tablets 2735

Doxycycline Monohydrate (Rifapentine is an inducer of cytochromes P4503A4 and P4502C8/9; therefore, rifapentine may increase the metabolism and decrease the activity of other co-administered drugs that are metabolized by these enzymes, such as doxycycline). Products include:
Monodox Capsules 2442
Vibramycin Monohydrate for Oral Suspension 2735

Dyphylline (Rifapentine is an inducer of cytochromes P4503A4 and P4502C8/9; therefore, rifapentine may increase the metabolism and decrease the activity of other co-administered drugs that are metabolized by these enzymes, such as theophylline). Products include:
Lufyllin Tablets 3347
Lufyllin-400 Tablets 3347
Lufyllin-GG Elixir 3348
Lufyllin-GG Tablets 3348

Enoxacin (Rifapentine is an inducer of cytochromes P4503A4 and P4502C8/9; therefore, rifapentine may increase the metabolism and decrease the activity of other co-administered drugs that are metabolized by these enzymes, such as fluoroquinolones).
No products indexed under this heading.

Ethinyl Estradiol (Rifapentine is an inducer of cytochromes P4503A4 and P4502C8/9; therefore, rifapentine may increase the metabolism and decrease the activity of other co-administered drugs that are metabolized by these enzymes, such as hormonal contraceptives; consideration should be given to using alternative contraceptive measures). Products include:
Alesse-21 Tablets 3468
Alesse-28 Tablets 3473
Brevicon 28-Day Tablets 3380
Cyclessa Tablets 2450
Desogen Tablets 2458
Estinyl Tablets 3112
Estrostep 2627
femhrt Tablets 2635
Levlen 962
Levlite 21 Tablets 962
Levlite 28 Tablets 962
Levora Tablets 3389
Loestrin 21 Tablets 2642
Loestrin Fe Tablets 2642
Lo/Ovral Tablets 3532
Lo/Ovral-28 Tablets 3538
Low-Ogestrel-28 Tablets 3392

Microgestin Fe 1.5/30 Tablets 3407
Microgestin Fe 1/20 Tablets 3400
Mircette Tablets 2470
Modicon 2563
Necon 3415
Nordette-28 Tablets 2257
Norinyl 1 +35 28-Day Tablets 3380
Ogestrel 0.5/50-28 Tablets 3428
Ortho-Cept 21 Tablets 2546
Ortho-Cept 28 Tablets 2546
Ortho-Cyclen/Ortho Tri-Cyclen 2573
Ortho-Novum 2563
Ovcon 3364
Ovral Tablets 3551
Ovral-28 Tablets 3552
Tri-Levlen 962
Tri-Norinyl-28 Tablets 3433
Triphasil-21 Tablets 3600
Triphasil-28 Tablets 3605
Trivora Tablets 3439
Yasmin 28 Tablets 980
Zovia 3449

Fentanyl (Rifapentine is an inducer of cytochromes P4503A4 and P4502C8/9; therefore, rifapentine may increase the metabolism and decrease the activity of other co-administered drugs that are metabolized by these enzymes, such as narcotic analgesics). Products include:
Duragesic Transdermal System 1786

Fentanyl Citrate (Rifapentine is an inducer of cytochromes P4503A4 and P4502C8/9; therefore, rifapentine may increase the metabolism and decrease the activity of other co-administered drugs that are metabolized by these enzymes, such as narcotic analgesics). Products include:
Actiq 1184

Fluconazole (Rifapentine is an inducer of cytochromes P4503A4 and P4502C8/9; therefore, rifapentine may increase the metabolism and decrease the activity of other co-administered drugs that are metabolized by these enzymes, such as fluconazole). Products include:
Diflucan Tablets, Injection, and Oral Suspension 2681

Fludrocortisone Acetate (Rifapentine is an inducer of cytochromes P4503A4 and P4502C8/9; therefore, rifapentine may increase the metabolism and decrease the activity of other co-administered drugs that are metabolized by these enzymes, such as corticosteroids). Products include:
Florinef Acetate Tablets 2250

Fosphenytoin Sodium (Rifapentine is an inducer of cytochromes P4503A4 and P4502C8/9; therefore, rifapentine may increase the metabolism and decrease the activity of other co-administered drugs that are metabolized by these enzymes, such as phenytoin). Products include:
Cerebyx Injection 2619

Glimepiride (Rifapentine is an inducer of cytochromes P4503A4 and P4502C8/9; therefore, rifapentine may increase the metabolism and decrease the activity of other co-administered drugs that are metabolized by these enzymes, such as sulfonylureas). Products include:
Amaryl Tablets 717

Glipizide (Rifapentine is an inducer of cytochromes P4503A4 and P4502C8/9; therefore, rifapentine may increase the metabolism and decrease the activity of other co-administered drugs that are metabolized by these enzymes, such as sulfonylureas). Products include:
Glucotrol Tablets 2692
Glucotrol XL Extended Release Tablets 2693

Glyburide (Rifapentine is an inducer of cytochromes P4503A4 and P4502C8/9; therefore, rifapentine may increase the metabolism and decrease the activity of other co-administered drugs that are metabolized by these enzymes, such as sulfonylureas). Products include:
DiaBeta Tablets 741
Glucovance Tablets 1086

Grepafloxacin Hydrochloride (Rifapentine is an inducer of cytochromes P4503A4 and P4502C8/9; therefore, rifapentine may increase the metabolism and decrease the activity of other co-administered drugs that are metabolized by these enzymes, such as fluoroquinolones).
No products indexed under this heading.

Haloperidol (Rifapentine is an inducer of cytochromes P4503A4 and P4502C8/9; therefore, rifapentine may increase the metabolism and decrease the activity of other co-administered drugs that are metabolized by these enzymes, such as haloperidol). Products include:
Haldol Injection, Tablets and Concentrate 2533

Haloperidol Decanoate (Rifapentine is an inducer of cytochromes P4503A4 and P4502C8/9; therefore, rifapentine may increase the metabolism and decrease the activity of other co-administered drugs that are metabolized by these enzymes, such as haloperidol). Products include:
Haldol Decanoate 2535

Hydrocodone Bitartrate (Rifapentine is an inducer of cytochromes P4503A4 and P4502C8/9; therefore, rifapentine may increase the metabolism and decrease the activity of other co-administered drugs that are metabolized by these enzymes, such as narcotic analgesics). Products include:
Hycodan 1316
Hycomine Compound Tablets 1317
Hycotuss Expectorant Syrup 1318
Lortab 3319
Lortab Elixir 3317
Maxidone Tablets CIII 3399
Norco 5/325 Tablets CIII 3424
Norco 7.5/325 Tablets CIII 3425
Norco 10/325 Tablets CIII 3427
Norco 10/325 Tablets CIII 3425
Vicodin Tablets 516
Vicodin ES Tablets 517
Vicodin HP Tablets 518
Vicodin Tuss Expectorant 519
Vicoprofen Tablets 520
Zydone Tablets 1330

Hydrocodone Polistirex (Rifapentine is an inducer of cytochromes P4503A4 and P4502C8/9; therefore, rifapentine may increase the metabolism and decrease the activity of other co-administered drugs that are metabolized by these enzymes, such as narcotic analgesics). Products include:
Tussionex Pennkinetic Extended-Release Suspension 1174

Hydrocortisone (Rifapentine is an inducer of cytochromes P4503A4 and P4502C8/9; therefore, rifapentine may increase the metabolism and decrease the activity of other co-administered drugs that are metabolized by these enzymes, such as corticosteroids). Products include:
Anusol-HC Cream 2.5% 2237
Cipro HC Otic Suspension 540
Cortaid Intensive Therapy Cream . ▣717
Cortaid Maximum Strength Cream .... ▣717
Cortisporin Ophthalmic Suspension Sterile .... ⊙297
Cortizone•5 .... ▣699
Cortizone•10 .... ▣699
Cortizone•10 Plus Creme .... ▣700
Cortizone for Kids Creme .... ▣699
Hydrocortone Tablets 2106
Massengill Medicated Soft Cloth Towelette .... ▣753
VōSoL HC Otic Solution 3356

Hydrocortisone Acetate (Rifapentine is an inducer of cytochromes P4503A4 and P4502C8/9; therefore, rifapentine may increase the metabolism and decrease the activity of other co-administered drugs that are metabolized by these enzymes, such as corticosteroids). Products include:
Analpram-HC 1338
Anusol HC-1 Hydrocortisone Anti-Itch Cream .... ▣689
Anusol-HC Suppositories 2238
Cortaid .... ▣717
Cortifoam Rectal Foam 3170
Cortisporin-TC Otic Suspension 2246
Hydrocortone Acetate Injectable Suspension 2103
Pramosone 1343
Proctocort Suppositories 2264
ProctoFoam-HC 3177
Terra-Cortril Ophthalmic Suspension 2716

Hydrocortisone Sodium Phosphate (Rifapentine is an inducer of cytochromes P4503A4 and P4502C8/9; therefore, rifapentine may increase the metabolism and decrease the activity of other co-administered drugs that are metabolized by these enzymes, such as corticosteroids). Products include:
Hydrocortone Phosphate Injection, Sterile 2105

Hydrocortisone Sodium Succinate (Rifapentine is an inducer of cytochromes P4503A4 and P4502C8/9; therefore, rifapentine may increase the metabolism and decrease the activity of other co-administered drugs that are metabolized by these enzymes, such as corticosteroids).
No products indexed under this heading.

Hydromorphone Hydrochloride (Rifapentine is an inducer of cytochromes P4503A4 and P4502C8/9; therefore, rifapentine may increase the metabolism and decrease the activity of other co-administered drugs that are metabolized by these enzymes, such as narcotic analgesics). Products include:
Dilaudid 441
Dilaudid Oral Liquid 445
Dilaudid Powder 441
Dilaudid Rectal Suppositories 441
Dilaudid Tablets 441
Dilaudid Tablets - 8 mg 445
Dilaudid-HP 443

Imipramine Hydrochloride (Rifapentine is an inducer of cytochromes P4503A4 and P4502C8/9; therefore, rifapentine may increase the metabolism and decrease the activity of other co-administered drugs that are metabolized by these enzymes, such as tricyclic antidepressants).
No products indexed under this heading.

Imipramine Pamoate (Rifapentine is an inducer of cytochromes P4503A4 and P4502C8/9; therefore, rifapentine may increase the metabolism and decrease the activity of other co-administered drugs that are metabolized by these enzymes, such as tricyclic antidepressants).
No products indexed under this heading.

Indinavir Sulfate (Co-administration has resulted in decreased indinavir Cmax by 55% while AUC reduced by 70% and clearance of indinavir increased by 3-fold; rifapentine should be used with extreme caution, if at all, in patients who are also taking protease inhibitors). Products include:
Crixivan Capsules 2070

Itraconazole (Rifapentine is an inducer of cytochromes P4503A4 and P4502C8/9; therefore, rifapentine may increase the metabolism and decrease the activity of other co-administered drugs that are metabolized by these enzymes, such as itraconazole). Products include:
Sporanox Capsules 1800
Sporanox Injection 1804
Sporanox Injection 2509
Sporanox Oral Solution 1808
Sporanox Oral Solution 2512

Ketoconazole (Rifapentine is an inducer of cytochromes P4503A4 and P4502C8/9; therefore, rifapentine may increase the metabolism and decrease the activity of other co-administered drugs that are metabolized by these enzymes, such as ketoconazole). Products include:
Nizoral 2% Cream 3620
Nizoral A-D Shampoo 2008
Nizoral 2% Shampoo 2007
Nizoral Tablets 1791

Lamivudine (Rifapentine is an inducer of cytochromes P4503A4 and P4502C8/9; therefore, rifapentine may increase the metabolism and decrease the activity of other co-administered drugs that are metabolized by these enzymes, such as reverse transcriptase inhibitors). Products include:
Combivir Tablets 1502
Epivir 1520
Epivir-HBV 1524
Trizivir Tablets 1669

Levonorgestrel (Rifapentine is an inducer of cytochromes P4503A4 and P4502C8/9; therefore, rifapentine may increase the metabolism and decrease the activity of other co-administered drugs that are metabolized by these enzymes, such as hormonal contraceptives; consideration should be given to using alternative contraceptive measures). Products include:
Alesse-21 Tablets 3468
Alesse-28 Tablets 3473
Levlen 962
Levlite 21 Tablets 962
Levlite 28 Tablets 962
Levora Tablets 3389
Mirena Intrauterine System 974
Nordette-28 Tablets 2257
Norplant System 3543
Tri-Levlen 962
Triphasil-21 Tablets 3600
Triphasil-28 Tablets 3605
Trivora Tablets 3439

Levorphanol Tartrate (Rifapentine is an inducer of cytochromes P4503A4 and P4502C8/9; therefore, rifapentine may increase the metabolism and decrease the activity of other co-administered drugs that are metabolized by these enzymes, such as narcotic analgesics). Products include:
Levo-Dromoran 1734
Levorphanol Tartrate Tablets 3059

Levothyroxine Sodium (Rifapentine is an inducer of cytochromes P4503A4 and P4502C8/9; therefore, rifapentine may increase the metabolism and decrease the activity of other co-administered drugs that are metabolized by these enzymes, such as levothyroxine). Products include:
Levothroid Tablets 1373
Levoxyl Tablets 1819
Synthroid 505
Unithroid Tablets 3445

Lomefloxacin Hydrochloride (Rifapentine is an inducer of cytochromes P4503A4 and P4502C8/9; therefore, rifapentine may increase the metabolism and decrease the activity of other co-administered drugs that are metabolized by these enzymes, such as fluoroquinolones).
No products indexed under this heading.

Lopinavir (Rifapentine is an inducer of cytochromes P4503A4 and P4502C8/9; therefore, rifapentine may increase the metabolism and decrease the activity of other co-administered drugs that are metabo-

lized by these enzymes, such as protease inhibitors; based on the rifapentine-indinavir interaction; rifapentine should be use with extreme caution, if at all, in patients who are also taking protease inhibitors). Products include:
- Kaletra Capsules 471
- Kaletra Oral Solution 471

Magaldrate (Rifapentine should be taken at least 1 hour before or 2 hours after ingestion of antacids).
No products indexed under this heading.

Magnesium Hydroxide (Rifapentine should be taken at least 1 hour before or 2 hours after ingestion of antacids). Products include:
- Ex•Lax Milk of Magnesia Liquid .... ■670
- Maalox Antacid/Anti-Gas Oral Suspension .... ■673
- Maalox Max Maximum Strength Antacid/Anti-Gas Liquid 2300
- Maalox Regular Strength Antacid/Antigas Liquid 2300
- Mylanta Fast-Acting 1813
- Mylanta 1813
- Pepcid Complete Chewable Tablets 1815
- Phillips' Chewable Tablets .... ■615
- Phillips' Milk of Magnesia Liquid (Original, Cherry, & Mint) .... ■616
- Rolaids Tablets .... ■706
- Extra Strength Rolaids Tablets .... ■706
- Vanquish Caplets .... ■617

Magnesium Oxide (Rifapentine should be taken at least 1 hour before or 2 hours after ingestion of antacids). Products include:
- Beelith Tablets 946
- Mag-Ox 400 Tablets 1024
- Uro-Mag Capsules 1024

Maprotiline Hydrochloride (Rifapentine is an inducer of cytochromes P4503A4 and P4502C8/9; therefore, rifapentine may increase the metabolism and decrease the activity of other co-administered drugs that are metabolized by these enzymes, such as tricyclic antidepressants).
No products indexed under this heading.

Medroxyprogesterone Acetate (Rifapentine is an inducer of cytochromes P4503A4 and P4502C8/9; therefore, rifapentine may increase the metabolism and decrease the activity of other co-administered drugs that are metabolized by these enzymes, such as progestins). Products include:
- Depo-Provera Contraceptive Injection 2798
- Lunelle Monthly Injection 2827
- Premphase Tablets 3572
- Prempro Tablets 3572
- Provera Tablets 2853

Megestrol Acetate (Rifapentine is an inducer of cytochromes P4503A4 and P4502C8/9; therefore, rifapentine may increase the metabolism and decrease the activity of other co-administered drugs that are metabolized by these enzymes, such as progestins). Products include:
- Megace Oral Suspension 1124

Meperidine Hydrochloride (Rifapentine is an inducer of cytochromes P4503A4 and P4502C8/9; therefore, rifapentine may increase the metabolism and decrease the activity of other co-administered drugs that are metabolized by these enzymes, such as narcotic analgesics). Products include:
- Demerol 3079
- Mepergan Injection 3539

Mephobarbital (Rifapentine is an inducer of cytochromes P4503A4 and P4502C8/9; therefore, rifapentine may increase the metabolism and decrease the activity of other co-administered drugs that are metabolized by these enzymes, such as barbiturates).
No products indexed under this heading.

Methadone Hydrochloride (Rifapentine is an inducer of cytochromes P4503A4 and P4502C8/9; therefore, rifapentine may increase the metabolism and decrease the activity of other co-administered drugs that are metabolized by these enzymes, such as narcotic analgesics). Products include:
- Dolophine Hydrochloride Tablets 3056

Methylprednisolone Acetate (Rifapentine is an inducer of cytochromes P4503A4 and P4502C8/9; therefore, rifapentine may increase the metabolism and decrease the activity of other co-administered drugs that are metabolized by these enzymes, such as corticosteroids). Products include:
- Depo-Medrol Injectable Suspension 2795

Methylprednisolone Sodium Succinate (Rifapentine is an inducer of cytochromes P4503A4 and P4502C8/9; therefore, rifapentine may increase the metabolism and decrease the activity of other co-administered drugs that are metabolized by these enzymes, such as corticosteroids). Products include:
- Solu-Medrol Sterile Powder 2855

Mexiletine Hydrochloride (Rifapentine is an inducer of cytochromes P4503A4 and P4502C8/9; therefore, rifapentine may increase the metabolism and decrease the activity of other co-administered drugs that are metabolized by these enzymes, such as mexiletine). Products include:
- Mexitil Capsules 1047

Morphine Sulfate (Rifapentine is an inducer of cytochromes P4503A4 and P4502C8/9; therefore, rifapentine may increase the metabolism and decrease the activity of other co-administered drugs that are metabolized by these enzymes, such as narcotic analgesics). Products include:
- Astramorph/PF Injection, USP (Preservative-Free) 594
- Duramorph Injection 1312
- Infumorph 200 and Infumorph 500 Sterile Solutions 1314
- Kadian Capsules 1335
- MS Contin Tablets 2896
- MSIR 2898
- Oramorph SR Tablets 3062
- Roxanol 3066

Moxifloxacin Hydrochloride (Rifapentine is an inducer of cytochromes P4503A4 and P4502C8/9; therefore, rifapentine may increase the metabolism and decrease the activity of other co-administered drugs that are metabolized by these enzymes, such as fluoroquinolones). Products include:
- Avelox Tablets 879

Nelfinavir Mesylate (Rifapentine is an inducer of cytochromes P4503A4 and P4502C8/9; therefore, rifapentine may increase the metabolism and decrease the activity of other co-administered drugs that are metabolized by these enzymes, such as protease inhibitors; based on the rifapentine-indinavir interaction; rifapentine should be use with extreme caution, if at all, in patients who are also taking protease inhibitors). Products include:
- Viracept 532

Norethindrone (Rifapentine is an inducer of cytochromes P4503A4 and P4502C8/9; therefore, rifapentine may increase the metabolism and decrease the activity of other co-administered drugs that are metabolized by these enzymes, such as hormonal contraceptives; consideration should be given to using alternative contraceptive measures). Products include:
- Brevicon 28-Day Tablets 3380
- Micronor Tablets 2543
- Modicon 2563
- Necon 3415
- Norinyl 1 +35 28-Day Tablets 3380
- Norinyl 1 + 50 28-Day Tablets 3380
- Nor-QD Tablets 3423
- Ortho-Novum 2563
- Ortho-Novum 1/50□28 Tablets 2556
- Ovcon 3364
- Tri-Norinyl-28 Tablets 3433

Norfloxacin (Rifapentine is an inducer of cytochromes P4503A4 and P4502C8/9; therefore, rifapentine may increase the metabolism and decrease the activity of other co-administered drugs that are metabolized by these enzymes, such as fluoroquinolones). Products include:
- Chibroxin Sterile Ophthalmic Solution 2051
- Noroxin Tablets 2145

Norgestimate (Rifapentine is an inducer of cytochromes P4503A4 and P4502C8/9; therefore, rifapentine may increase the metabolism and decrease the activity of other co-administered drugs that are metabolized by these enzymes, such as hormonal contraceptives; consideration should be given to using alternative contraceptive measures). Products include:
- Ortho-Cyclen/Ortho Tri-Cyclen 2573
- Ortho-Prefest Tablets 2570

Nortriptyline Hydrochloride (Rifapentine is an inducer of cytochromes P4503A4 and P4502C8/9; therefore, rifapentine may increase the metabolism and decrease the activity of other co-administered drugs that are metabolized by these enzymes, such as tricyclic antidepressants).
No products indexed under this heading.

Ofloxacin (Rifapentine is an inducer of cytochromes P4503A4 and P4502C8/9; therefore, rifapentine may increase the metabolism and decrease the activity of other co-administered drugs that are metabolized by these enzymes, such as fluoroquinolones). Products include:
- Floxin I.V. 2526
- Floxin Otic Solution 1219
- Floxin Tablets 2529
- Ocuflox Ophthalmic Solution 554

Oxycodone Hydrochloride (Rifapentine is an inducer of cytochromes P4503A4 and P4502C8/9; therefore, rifapentine may increase the metabolism and decrease the activity of other co-administered drugs that are metabolized by these enzymes, such as narcotic analgesics). Products include:
- OxyContin Tablets 2912
- OxyFast Oral Concentrate Solution .2916
- OxyIR Capsules 2916
- Percocet Tablets 1326
- Percodan Tablets 1327
- Percolone Tablets 1327
- Roxicodone 3067
- Tylox Capsules 2597

Pentobarbital Sodium (Rifapentine is an inducer of cytochromes P4503A4 and P4502C8/9; therefore, rifapentine may increase the metabolism and decrease the activity of other co-administered drugs that are metabolized by these enzymes, such as barbiturates). Products include:
- Nembutal Sodium Solution 485

Phenobarbital (Rifapentine is an inducer of cytochromes P4503A4 and P4502C8/9; therefore, rifapentine may increase the metabolism and decrease the activity of other co-administered drugs that are metabolized by these enzymes, such as barbiturates). Products include:
- Arco-Lase Plus Tablets 592
- Donnatal 2929
- Donnatal Extentabs 2930

Phenytoin (Rifapentine is an inducer of cytochromes P4503A4 and P4502C8/9; therefore, rifapentine may increase the metabolism and decrease the activity of other co-administered drugs that are metabolized by these enzymes, such as phenytoin). Products include:
- Dilantin Infatabs 2624
- Dilantin-125 Oral Suspension 2625

Phenytoin Sodium (Rifapentine is an inducer of cytochromes P4503A4 and P4502C8/9; therefore, rifapentine may increase the metabolism and decrease the activity of other co-administered drugs that are metabolized by these enzymes, such as phenytoin). Products include:
- Dilantin Kapseals 2622

Prednisolone Acetate (Rifapentine is an inducer of cytochromes P4503A4 and P4502C8/9; therefore, rifapentine may increase the metabolism and decrease the activity of other co-administered drugs that are metabolized by these enzymes, such as corticosteroids). Products include:
- Blephamide Ophthalmic Ointment .. 547
- Blephamide Ophthalmic Suspension 548
- Poly-Pred Liquifilm Ophthalmic Suspension .... ⊙245
- Pred Forte Ophthalmic Suspension .... ⊙246
- Pred Mild Sterile Ophthalmic Suspension .... ⊙249
- Pred-G Ophthalmic Suspension .... ⊙247
- Pred-G Sterile Ophthalmic Ointment .... ⊙248

Prednisolone Sodium Phosphate (Rifapentine is an inducer of cytochromes P4503A4 and P4502C8/9; therefore, rifapentine may increase the metabolism and decrease the activity of other co-administered drugs that are metabolized by these enzymes, such as corticosteroids). Products include:
- Pediapred Oral Solution 1170

Prednisolone Tebutate (Rifapentine is an inducer of cytochromes P4503A4 and P4502C8/9; therefore, rifapentine may increase the metabolism and decrease the activity of other co-administered drugs that are metabolized by these enzymes, such as corticosteroids).
No products indexed under this heading.

Prednisone (Rifapentine is an inducer of cytochromes P4503A4 and P4502C8/9; therefore, rifapentine may increase the metabolism and decrease the activity of other co-administered drugs that are metabolized by these enzymes, such as corticosteroids). Products include:
- Prednisone 3064

Propoxyphene Hydrochloride (Rifapentine is an inducer of cytochromes P4503A4 and P4502C8/9; therefore, rifapentine may increase the metabolism and decrease the activity of other co-administered drugs that are metabolized by these enzymes, such as narcotic analgesics). Products include:
- Darvon Pulvules 1909
- Darvon Compound-65 Pulvules 1910

Propoxyphene Napsylate (Rifapentine is an inducer of cytochromes P4503A4 and P4502C8/9; therefore, rifapentine may increase the metabolism and decrease the activity of other co-administered drugs that are metabolized by these enzymes, such as narcotic analgesics). Products include:
- Darvon-N/Darvocet-N 1907
- Darvon-N Tablets 1912

Protriptyline Hydrochloride (Rifapentine is an inducer of cytochromes P4503A4 and P4502C8/9; therefore, rifapentine may increase the metabolism and decrease the activity of other co-administered drugs

that are metabolized by these enzymes, such as tricyclic antidepressants). Products include:

Vivactil Tablets 2446
Vivactil Tablets 2217

Quinidine Gluconate (Rifapentine is an inducer of cytochromes P4503A4 and P4502C8/9; therefore, rifapentine may increase the metabolism and decrease the activity of other co-administered drugs that are metabolized by these enzymes, such as quinidine). Products include:

Quinaglute Dura-Tabs Tablets 978

Quinidine Polygalacturonate (Rifapentine is an inducer of cytochromes P4503A4 and P4502C8/9; therefore, rifapentine may increase the metabolism and decrease the activity of other co-administered drugs that are metabolized by these enzymes, such as quinidine).

No products indexed under this heading.

Quinidine Sulfate (Rifapentine is an inducer of cytochromes P4503A4 and P4502C8/9; therefore, rifapentine may increase the metabolism and decrease the activity of other co-administered drugs that are metabolized by these enzymes, such as quinidine). Products include:

Quinidex Extentabs 2933

Quinine Sulfate (Rifapentine is an inducer of cytochromes P4503A4 and P4502C8/9; therefore, rifapentine may increase the metabolism and decrease the activity of other co-administered drugs that are metabolized by these enzymes, such as quinine).

No products indexed under this heading.

Remifentanil Hydrochloride (Rifapentine is an inducer of cytochromes P4503A4 and P4502C8/9; therefore, rifapentine may increase the metabolism and decrease the activity of other co-administered drugs that are metabolized by these enzymes, such as narcotic analgesics).

No products indexed under this heading.

Ritonavir (Rifapentine is an inducer of cytochromes P4503A4 and P4502C8/9; therefore, rifapentine may increase the metabolism and decrease the activity of other co-administered drugs that are metabolized by these enzymes, such as protease inhibitors; based on the rifapentine-indinavir interaction; rifapentine should be use with extreme caution, if at all, in patients who are also taking protease inhibitors). Products include:

Kaletra Capsules 471
Kaletra Oral Solution 471
Norvir Capsules 487
Norvir Oral Solution 487

Saquinavir (Rifapentine is an inducer of cytochromes P4503A4 and P4502C8/9; therefore, rifapentine may increase the metabolism and decrease the activity of other co-administered drugs that are metabolized by these enzymes, such as protease inhibitors; based on the rifapentine-indinavir interaction; rifapentine should be use with extreme caution, if at all, in patients who are also taking protease inhibitors). Products include:

Fortovase Capsules 2970

Saquinavir Mesylate (Rifapentine is an inducer of cytochromes P4503A4 and P4502C8/9; therefore, rifapentine may increase the metabolism and decrease the activity of other co-administered drugs that are metabolized by these enzymes, such as protease inhibitors; based on the rifapentine-indinavir interaction; rifapentine should be use with extreme caution, if at all, in patients who are also taking protease inhibitors). Products include:

Invirase Capsules 2979

Secobarbital Sodium (Rifapentine is an inducer of cytochromes P4503A4 and P4502C8/9; therefore, rifapentine may increase the metabolism and decrease the activity of other co-administered drugs that are metabolized by these enzymes, such as barbiturates).

No products indexed under this heading.

Sildenafil Citrate (Rifapentine is an inducer of cytochromes P4503A4 and P4502C8/9; therefore, rifapentine may increase the metabolism and decrease the activity of other co-administered drugs that are metabolized by these enzymes, such as sildenafil). Products include:

Viagra Tablets 2732

Sodium Bicarbonate (Rifapentine should be taken at least 1 hour before or 2 hours after ingestion of antacids). Products include:

Alka-Seltzer 603
Alka-Seltzer Lemon Lime Antacid and Pain Reliever Effervescent Tablets 603
Alka-Seltzer Extra Strength Antacid and Pain Reliever Effervescent Tablets 603
Alka-Seltzer Heartburn Relief Tablets 604
Ceo-Two Evacuant Suppository 618
Colyte with Flavor Packs for Oral Solution 3170
GoLYTELY and Pineapple Flavor GoLYTELY for Oral Solution 1068
NuLYTELY, Cherry Flavor, Lemon-Lime Flavor, and Orange Flavor NuLYTELY for Oral Solution 1068

Stavudine (Rifapentine is an inducer of cytochromes P4503A4 and P4502C8/9; therefore, rifapentine may increase the metabolism and decrease the activity of other co-administered drugs that are metabolized by these enzymes, such as reverse transcriptase inhibitors). Products include:

Zerit 1147

Sufentanil Citrate (Rifapentine is an inducer of cytochromes P4503A4 and P4502C8/9; therefore, rifapentine may increase the metabolism and decrease the activity of other co-administered drugs that are metabolized by these enzymes, such as narcotic analgesics).

No products indexed under this heading.

Tacrolimus (Rifapentine is an inducer of cytochromes P4503A4 and P4502C8/9; therefore, rifapentine may increase the metabolism and decrease the activity of other co-administered drugs that are metabolized by these enzymes, such as tacrolimus). Products include:

Prograf 1393
Protopic Ointment 1397

Theophylline (Rifapentine is an inducer of cytochromes P4503A4 and P4502C8/9; therefore, rifapentine may increase the metabolism and decrease the activity of other co-administered drugs that are metabolized by these enzymes, such as theophylline). Products include:

Aerolate 1361
Theo-Dur Extended-Release Tablets 1835
Uni-Dur Extended-Release Tablets .. 1841
Uniphyl 400 mg and 600 mg Tablets 2903

Theophylline Calcium Salicylate (Rifapentine is an inducer of cytochromes P4503A4 and P4502C8/9; therefore, rifapentine may increase the metabolism and decrease the activity of other co-administered drugs that are metabolized by these enzymes, such as theophylline).

No products indexed under this heading.

Theophylline Sodium Glycinate (Rifapentine is an inducer of cytochromes P4503A4 and P4502C8/9; therefore, rifapentine may increase the metabolism and decrease the activity of other co-administered drugs that are metabolized by these enzymes, such as theophylline).

No products indexed under this heading.

Thiamylal Sodium (Rifapentine is an inducer of cytochromes P4503A4 and P4502C8/9; therefore, rifapentine may increase the metabolism and decrease the activity of other co-administered drugs that are metabolized by these enzymes, such as barbiturates).

No products indexed under this heading.

Tocainide Hydrochloride (Rifapentine is an inducer of cytochromes P4503A4 and P4502C8/9; therefore, rifapentine may increase the metabolism and decrease the activity of other co-administered drugs that are metabolized by these enzymes, such as tocainide). Products include:

Tonocard Tablets 649

Tolazamide (Rifapentine is an inducer of cytochromes P4503A4 and P4502C8/9; therefore, rifapentine may increase the metabolism and decrease the activity of other co-administered drugs that are metabolized by these enzymes, such as sulfonylureas).

No products indexed under this heading.

Tolbutamide (Rifapentine is an inducer of cytochromes P4503A4 and P4502C8/9; therefore, rifapentine may increase the metabolism and decrease the activity of other co-administered drugs that are metabolized by these enzymes, such as sulfonylureas).

No products indexed under this heading.

Triamcinolone (Rifapentine is an inducer of cytochromes P4503A4 and P4502C8/9; therefore, rifapentine may increase the metabolism and decrease the activity of other co-administered drugs that are metabolized by these enzymes, such as corticosteroids).

No products indexed under this heading.

Triamcinolone Acetonide (Rifapentine is an inducer of cytochromes P4503A4 and P4502C8/9; therefore, rifapentine may increase the metabolism and decrease the activity of other co-administered drugs that are metabolized by these enzymes, such as corticosteroids). Products include:

Azmacort Inhalation Aerosol 728
Nasacort Nasal Inhaler 750
Nasacort AQ Nasal Spray 752
Tri-Nasal Spray 2274

Triamcinolone Diacetate (Rifapentine is an inducer of cytochromes P4503A4 and P4502C8/9; therefore, rifapentine may increase the metabolism and decrease the activity of other co-administered drugs that are metabolized by these enzymes, such as corticosteroids).

No products indexed under this heading.

Triamcinolone Hexacetonide (Rifapentine is an inducer of cytochromes P4503A4 and P4502C8/9; therefore, rifapentine may increase the metabolism and decrease the activity of other co-administered drugs that are metabolized by these enzymes, such as corticosteroids).

No products indexed under this heading.

Trimipramine Maleate (Rifapentine is an inducer of cytochromes P4503A4 and P4502C8/9; therefore, rifapentine may increase the metabolism and decrease the activity of other co-administered drugs that are metabolized by these enzymes, such as tricyclic antidepressants). Products include:

Surmontil Capsules 3595

Trovafloxacin Mesylate (Rifapentine is an inducer of cytochromes P4503A4 and P4502C8/9; therefore, rifapentine may increase the metabolism and decrease the activity of other co-administered drugs that are metabolized by these enzymes, such as fluoroquinolones). Products include:

Trovan Tablets 2722

Warfarin Sodium (Rifapentine is an inducer of cytochromes P4503A4 and P4502C8/9; therefore, rifapentine may increase the metabolism and decrease the activity of other co-administered drugs that are metabolized by these enzymes, such as warfarin). Products include:

Coumadin for Injection 1243
Coumadin Tablets 1243
Warfarin Sodium Tablets, USP 3302

Zalcitabine (Rifapentine is an inducer of cytochromes P4503A4 and P4502C8/9; therefore, rifapentine may increase the metabolism and decrease the activity of other co-administered drugs that are metabolized by these enzymes, such as reverse transcriptase inhibitors). Products include:

Hivid Tablets 2975

Zidovudine (Rifapentine is an inducer of cytochromes P4503A4 and P4502C8/9; therefore, rifapentine may increase the metabolism and decrease the activity of other co-administered drugs that are metabolized by these enzymes, such as reverse transcriptase inhibitors). Products include:

Combivir Tablets 1502
Retrovir 1625
Retrovir IV Infusion 1629
Trizivir Tablets 1669

Food Interactions

Food, unspecified (Increases AUC and Cmax by 43% and 44% respectively compared to fasting conditions; administration with food may be useful to avoid gastrointestinal upset).

PRILOSEC DELAYED-RELEASE CAPSULES

(Omeprazole) 628

May interact with benzodiazepines, iron containing oral preparations, phenytoin, and certain other agents. Compounds in these categories include:

Alprazolam (Potential for metabolism interaction via cytochrome P-450 system). Products include:

Xanax Tablets 2865

Astemizole (Co-administration of omeprazole-clarithromycin combination with astemizole is not recommended because clarithromycin, like erythromycin, is also metabolized by cytochrome P450 and there have been reports of QT prolongation and torsade de pointes with concurrent use of erythromycin and astemizole).

No products indexed under this heading.

Bacampicillin Hydrochloride (Omeprazole may interfere with gastric absorption of drugs, such as ampicillin esters, where gastric pH is an important determinant of their bioavailability).

No products indexed under this heading.

Chlordiazepoxide (Potential for metabolism interaction via cytochrome P-450 system). Products include:
Limbitrol ... 1738

Chlordiazepoxide Hydrochloride (Potential for metabolism interaction via cytochrome P-450 system). Products include:
Librium Capsules ... 1736
Librium for Injection ... 1737

Cisapride (Co-administration of omeprazole-clarithromycin combination with cisapride has resulted in cardiac arrhythmias, including QT prolongation, ventricular tachycardia and fibrillation and torsade de pointes, and fatalities; concomitant use of clarithromycin and cisapride is contraindicated).
No products indexed under this heading.

Clarithromycin (Co-administration may result in increases in plasma levels of omeprazole, clarithromycin, and 14-hydroxy-clarithromycin). Products include:
Biaxin/Biaxin XL ... 403
PREVPAC ... 3298

Clonazepam (Potential for metabolism interaction via cytochrome P-450 system). Products include:
Klonopin Tablets ... 2983

Clorazepate Dipotassium (Potential for metabolism interaction via cytochrome P-450 system). Products include:
Tranxene ... 511

Cyclosporine (Potential of metabolism interaction via the cytochrome P-450 system). Products include:
Gengraf Capsules ... 457
Neoral Soft Gelatin Capsules ... 2380
Neoral Oral Solution ... 2380
Sandimmune ... 2388

Diazepam (Potential for metabolism interaction via cytochrome P-450 system; prolonged elimination of diazepam). Products include:
Valium Injectable ... 3026
Valium Tablets ... 3047

Disulfiram (Potential of metabolism interaction via the cytochrome P-450 system). Products include:
Antabuse Tablets ... 2444
Antabuse Tablets ... 3474

Estazolam (Potential for metabolism interaction via cytochrome P-450 system). Products include:
ProSom Tablets ... 500

Ferrous Fumarate (Omeprazole may interfere with gastric absorption of drugs, such as iron salts, where gastric pH is an important determinant of their bioavailability). Products include:
New Formulation Chromagen OB Capsules ... 3094
Loestrin Fe Tablets ... 2642
NataChew Tablets ... 3364

Ferrous Gluconate (Omeprazole may interfere with gastric absorption of drugs, such as iron salts, where gastric pH is an important determinant of their bioavailability). Products include:
Fergon Iron Tablets ... ▣802

Ferrous Sulfate (Omeprazole may interfere with gastric absorption of drugs, such as iron salts, where gastric pH is an important determinant of their bioavailability). Products include:
Feosol Tablets ... 1717
Slow Fe Tablets ... ▣827
Slow Fe with Folic Acid Tablets ... ▣828

Flurazepam Hydrochloride (Potential for metabolism interaction via cytochrome P-450 system).
No products indexed under this heading.

Fosphenytoin Sodium (Prolonged elimination of phenytoin). Products include:
Cerebyx Injection ... 2619

Halazepam (Potential for metabolism interaction via cytochrome P-450 system).
No products indexed under this heading.

Iron (Omeprazole may interfere with gastric absorption of drugs, such as iron salts, where gastric pH is an important determinant of their bioavailability).
No products indexed under this heading.

Ketoconazole (Omeprazole may interfere with gastric absorption of drugs, such as ketoconazole, where gastric pH is an important determinant of their bioavailability). Products include:
Nizoral 2% Cream ... 3620
Nizoral A-D Shampoo ... 2008
Nizoral 2% Shampoo ... 2007
Nizoral Tablets ... 1791

Lorazepam (Potential for metabolism interaction via cytochrome P-450 system). Products include:
Ativan Injection ... 3478
Ativan Tablets ... 3482

Midazolam Hydrochloride (Potential for metabolism interaction via cytochrome P-450 system). Products include:
Versed Injection ... 3027
Versed Syrup ... 3033

Oxazepam (Potential for metabolism interaction via cytochrome P-450 system).
No products indexed under this heading.

Phenytoin (Prolonged elimination of phenytoin). Products include:
Dilantin Infatabs ... 2624
Dilantin-125 Oral Suspension ... 2625

Phenytoin Sodium (Prolonged elimination of phenytoin). Products include:
Dilantin Kapseals ... 2622

Pimozide (Co-administration of omeprazole-clarithromycin combination with pimozide has resulted in cardiac arrhythmias, including QT prolongation, ventricular tachycardia and fibrillation and torsade de pointes, and fatalities; concomitant use of clarithromycin and pimozide is contraindicated). Products include:
Orap Tablets ... 1407

Polysaccharide-Iron Complex (Omeprazole may interfere with gastric absorption of drugs, such as iron salts, where gastric pH is an important determinant of their bioavailability). Products include:
Niferex ... 3176
Niferex-150 Capsules ... 3176
Nu-Iron 150 Capsules ... 2224

Prazepam (Potential for metabolism interaction via cytochrome P-450 system).
No products indexed under this heading.

Quazepam (Potential for metabolism interaction via cytochrome P-450 system).
No products indexed under this heading.

Temazepam (Potential for metabolism interaction via cytochrome P-450 system).
No products indexed under this heading.

Terfenadine (Co-administration of omeprazole-clarithromycin combination with terfenadine has resulted in cardiac arrhythmias, including QT prolongation, ventricular tachycardia and fibrillation and torsade de pointes, and fatalities; concomitant use of clarithromycin and terfenadine is contraindicated).
No products indexed under this heading.

Triazolam (Potential for metabolism interaction via cytochrome P-450 system). Products include:
Halcion Tablets ... 2823

Warfarin Sodium (Prolonged elimination of warfarin). Products include:
Coumadin for Injection ... 1243
Coumadin Tablets ... 1243
Warfarin Sodium Tablets, USP ... 3302

Food Interactions

Food, unspecified (Absorption of Prilosec begins only after the granules leave the stomach; it should be taken before eating).

PRIMACOR INJECTION
(Milrinone Lactate) ... 3086
May interact with:

Furosemide (Immediate chemical interaction which is evidenced by the formation of a precipitate when furosemide is injected into IV line of an infusion of Primacor). Products include:
Furosemide Tablets ... 2284

PRIMATENE MIST
(Epinephrine) ... ▣779
See Primatene Tablets

PRIMATENE TABLETS
(Ephedrine Hydrochloride, Guaifenesin) ... ▣780
May interact with monoamine oxidase inhibitors. Compounds in these categories include:

Isocarboxazid (Concurrent and/or sequential use with MAO inhibitors is not recommended).
No products indexed under this heading.

Moclobemide (Concurrent and/or sequential use with MAO inhibitors is not recommended).
No products indexed under this heading.

Pargyline Hydrochloride (Concurrent and/or sequential use with MAO inhibitors is not recommended).
No products indexed under this heading.

Phenelzine Sulfate (Concurrent and/or sequential use with MAO inhibitors is not recommended). Products include:
Nardil Tablets ... 2653

Procarbazine Hydrochloride (Concurrent and/or sequential use with MAO inhibitors is not recommended). Products include:
Matulane Capsules ... 3246

Selegiline Hydrochloride (Concurrent and/or sequential use with MAO inhibitors is not recommended). Products include:
Eldepryl Capsules ... 3266

Tranylcypromine Sulfate (Concurrent and/or sequential use with MAO inhibitors is not recommended). Products include:
Parnate Tablets ... 1607

PRIMAXIN I.M.
(Cilastatin Sodium, Imipenem) ... 2158
See Primaxin I.V.

PRIMAXIN I.V.
(Cilastatin Sodium, Imipenem) ... 2160
May interact with:

Ganciclovir Sodium (Concomitant administration may result in generalized seizures). Products include:
Cytovene-IV ... 2959

Probenecid (Concomitant administration results in only minimal increase in plasma levels of imipenem; concomitant administration not recommended).
No products indexed under this heading.

PRINIVIL TABLETS
(Lisinopril) ... 2164
May interact with diuretics, lithium preparations, non-steroidal anti-inflammatory agents, potassium preparations, potassium sparing diuretics, thiazides, and certain other agents. Compounds in these categories include:

Amiloride Hydrochloride (Potential for significant hyperkalemia; possibility of excessive reduction in blood pressure). Products include:
Midamor Tablets ... 2136
Moduretic Tablets ... 2138

Bendroflumethiazide (Thiazide-induced potassium loss attenuated; possibility of excessive reduction in blood pressure). Products include:
Corzide 40/5 Tablets ... 2247
Corzide 80/5 Tablets ... 2247

Bumetanide (Possibility of excessive reduction in blood pressure).
No products indexed under this heading.

Celecoxib (Co-administration in some patients with compromised renal function who are being treated with NSAIDs may result in a further deterioration of renal function). Products include:
Celebrex Capsules ... 2676
Celebrex Capsules ... 2780

Chlorothiazide (Thiazide-induced potassium loss attenuated; possibility of excessive reduction in blood pressure). Products include:
Aldoclor Tablets ... 2035
Diuril Oral ... 2087

Chlorothiazide Sodium (Thiazide-induced potassium loss attenuated; possibility of excessive reduction in blood pressure). Products include:
Diuril Sodium Intravenous ... 2086

Chlorthalidone (Possibility of excessive reduction in blood pressure). Products include:
Clorpres Tablets ... 1002
Combipres Tablets ... 1040
Tenoretic Tablets ... 690

Diclofenac Potassium (Co-administration in some patients with compromised renal function who are being treated with NSAIDs may result in a further deterioration of renal function). Products include:
Cataflam Tablets ... 2315

Diclofenac Sodium (Co-administration in some patients with compromised renal function who are being treated with NSAIDs may result in a further deterioration of renal function). Products include:
Arthrotec Tablets ... 3195
Voltaren Ophthalmic Sterile Ophthalmic Solution ... ⊙312
Voltaren Tablets ... 2315
Voltaren-XR Tablets ... 2315

Ethacrynic Acid (Possibility of excessive reduction in blood pressure). Products include:
Edecrin Tablets ... 2091

Etodolac (Co-administration in some patients with compromised renal function who are being treated with NSAIDs may result in a further deterioration of renal function). Products include:
Lodine ... 3528
Lodine XL Extended-Release Tablets ... 3530

Fenoprofen Calcium (Co-administration in some patients with compromised renal function who are being treated with NSAIDs may result in a further deterioration of renal function).
No products indexed under this heading.

Flurbiprofen (Co-administration in some patients with compromised renal function who are being treated with NSAIDs may result in a further

deterioration of renal function).
No products indexed under this heading.

Furosemide (Possibility of excessive reduction in blood pressure). Products include:
Furosemide Tablets ... 2284

Hydrochlorothiazide (Thiazide-induced potassium loss attenuated; possibility of excessive reduction in blood pressure). Products include:
Accuretic Tablets ... 2614
Aldoril Tablets ... 2039
Atacand HCT Tablets ... 597
Avalide Tablets ... 1070
Diovan HCT Tablets ... 2338
Dyazide Capsules ... 1515
HydroDIURIL Tablets ... 2108
Hyzaar ... 2109
Inderide Tablets ... 3517
Inderide LA Long-Acting Capsules .. 3519
Lotensin HCT Tablets ... 2367
Maxzide ... 1008
Micardis HCT Tablets ... 1051
Microzide Capsules ... 3414
Moduretic Tablets ... 2138
Monopril HCT ... 1094
Prinzide Tablets ... 2168
Timolide Tablets ... 2187
Uniretic Tablets ... 3178
Vaseretic Tablets ... 2204
Zestoretic Tablets ... 695
Ziac Tablets ... 1887

Hydroflumethiazide (Thiazide-induced potassium loss attenuated; possibility of excessive reduction in blood pressure). Products include:
Diucardin Tablets ... 3494

Ibuprofen (Co-administration in some patients with compromised renal function who are being treated with NSAIDs may result in a further deterioration of renal function). Products include:
Advil ... 771
Children's Advil Oral Suspension ... 773
Children's Advil Chewable Tablets . 773
Advil Cold and Sinus Caplets ... 771
Advil Cold and Sinus Tablets ... 771
Advil Flu & Body Ache Caplets ... 772
Infants' Advil Drops ... 773
Junior Strength Advil Tablets ... 773
Junior Strength Advil Chewable Tablets ... 773
Advil Migraine Liquigels ... 772
Children's Motrin Oral Suspension and Chewable Tablets ... 2006
Children's Motrin Cold Oral Suspension ... 2007
Children's Motrin Oral Suspension ... 643
Motrin Suspension, Oral Drops, Chewable Tablets, and Caplets ... 2002
Infants' Motrin Concentrated Drops ... 2006
Junior Strength Motrin Caplets and Chewable Tablets ... 2006
Motrin IB Tablets, Caplets, and Gelcaps ... 2002
Motrin Migraine Pain Caplets ... 2005
Motrin Sinus Headache Caplets ... 2005
Vicoprofen Tablets ... 520

Indapamide (Possibility of excessive reduction in blood pressure). Products include:
Indapamide Tablets ... 2286

Indomethacin (Co-administration in some patients with compromised renal function who are being treated with NSAIDs may result in a further deterioration of renal function). Products include:
Indocin ... 2112

Indomethacin Sodium Trihydrate (Co-administration in some patients with compromised renal function who are being treated with NSAIDs may result in a further deterioration of renal function). Products include:
Indocin I.V. ... 2115

Ketoprofen (Co-administration in some patients with compromised renal function who are being treated with NSAIDs may result in a further deterioration of renal function). Products include:
Orudis Capsules ... 3548
Orudis KT Tablets ... 778
Oruvail Capsules ... 3548

Ketorolac Tromethamine (Co-administration in some patients with compromised renal function who are being treated with NSAIDs may result in a further deterioration of renal function). Products include:
Acular Ophthalmic Solution ... 544
Acular PF Ophthalmic Solution ... 544
Toradol ... 3018

Lithium Carbonate (Potential for reversible lithium toxicity; frequent monitoring of lithium levels is recommended). Products include:
Eskalith ... 1527
Lithium Carbonate ... 3061
Lithobid Slow-Release Tablets ... 3255

Lithium Citrate (Potential for reversible lithium toxicity; frequent monitoring of lithium levels is recommended). Products include:
Lithium Citrate Syrup ... 3061

Meclofenamate Sodium (Co-administration in some patients with compromised renal function who are being treated with NSAIDs may result in a further deterioration of renal function).
No products indexed under this heading.

Mefenamic Acid (Co-administration in some patients with compromised renal function who are being treated with NSAIDs may result in a further deterioration of renal function). Products include:
Ponstel Capsules ... 1356

Meloxicam (Co-administration in some patients with compromised renal function who are being treated with NSAIDs may result in a further deterioration of renal function). Products include:
Mobic Tablets ... 1054

Methyclothiazide (Thiazide-induced potassium loss attenuated; possibility of excessive reduction in blood pressure).
No products indexed under this heading.

Metolazone (Possibility of excessive reduction in blood pressure). Products include:
Mykrox Tablets ... 1168
Zaroxolyn Tablets ... 1177

Nabumetone (Co-administration in some patients with compromised renal function who are being treated with NSAIDs may result in a further deterioration of renal function). Products include:
Relafen Tablets ... 1617

Naproxen (Co-administration in some patients with compromised renal function who are being treated with NSAIDs may result in a further deterioration of renal function). Products include:
EC-Naprosyn Delayed-Release Tablets ... 2967
Naprosyn Suspension ... 2967
Naprosyn Tablets ... 2967

Naproxen Sodium (Co-administration in some patients with compromised renal function who are being treated with NSAIDs may result in a further deterioration of renal function). Products include:
Aleve Tablets, Caplets and Gelcaps ... 602
Aleve Cold & Sinus Caplets ... 603
Anaprox Tablets ... 2967
Anaprox DS Tablets ... 2967
Naprelan Tablets ... 1293

Oxaprozin (Co-administration in some patients with compromised renal function who are being treated with NSAIDs may result in a further deterioration of renal function).
No products indexed under this heading.

Phenylbutazone (Co-administration in some patients with compromised renal function who are being treated with NSAIDs may result in a further deterioration of renal function).
No products indexed under this heading.

Piroxicam (Co-administration in some patients with compromised renal function who are being treated with NSAIDs may result in a further deterioration of renal function). Products include:
Feldene Capsules ... 2685

Polythiazide (Thiazide-induced potassium loss attenuated; possibility of excessive reduction in blood pressure). Products include:
Minizide Capsules ... 2700
Renese Tablets ... 2712

Potassium Acid Phosphate (Potential for significant hyperkalemia). Products include:
K-Phos Original (Sodium Free) Tablets ... 947

Potassium Bicarbonate (Potential for significant hyperkalemia).
No products indexed under this heading.

Potassium Chloride (Potential for significant hyperkalemia). Products include:
Chlor-3 ... 1361
Colyte with Flavor Packs for Oral Solution ... 3170
GoLYTELY and Pineapple Flavor GoLYTELY for Oral Solution ... 1068
K-Dur Microburst Release System ER Tablets ... 1832
Klor-Con M20/Klor-Con M10 Tablets ... 3329
K-Lor Powder Packets ... 469
K-Tab Filmtab Tablets ... 470
Micro-K ... 3311
NuLYTELY, Cherry Flavor, Lemon-Lime Flavor, and Orange Flavor NuLYTELY for Oral Solution ... 1068
Rum-K ... 1363

Potassium Citrate (Potential for significant hyperkalemia). Products include:
Urocit-K Tablets ... 2232

Potassium Gluconate (Potential for significant hyperkalemia).
No products indexed under this heading.

Potassium Phosphate (Potential for significant hyperkalemia). Products include:
K-Phos Neutral Tablets ... 946

Rofecoxib (Co-administration in some patients with compromised renal function who are being treated with NSAIDs may result in a further deterioration of renal function). Products include:
Vioxx ... 2213

Spironolactone (Potential for significant hyperkalemia; possibility of excessive reduction in blood pressure).
No products indexed under this heading.

Sulindac (Co-administration in some patients with compromised renal function who are being treated with NSAIDs may result in a further deterioration of renal function). Products include:
Clinoril Tablets ... 2053

Tolmetin Sodium (Co-administration in some patients with compromised renal function who are being treated with NSAIDs may result in a further deterioration of renal function). Products include:
Tolectin ... 2589

Torsemide (Possibility of excessive reduction in blood pressure). Products include:
Demadex Tablets and Injection ... 2965

Triamterene (Potential for significant hyperkalemia; possibility of excessive reduction in blood pressure). Products include:
Dyazide Capsules ... 1515
Dyrenium Capsules ... 3458
Maxzide ... 1008

PRINZIDE TABLETS

(Hydrochlorothiazide, Lisinopril) ... 2168
May interact with antihypertensives, barbiturates, corticosteroids, diuretics, cardiac glycosides, oral hypoglycemic agents, insulin, lithium preparations, narcotic analgesics, nondepolarizing neuromuscular blocking agents, non-steroidal anti-inflammatory agents, potassium preparations, potassium sparing diuretics, and certain other agents. Compounds in these categories include:

Acarbose (Hyperglycemia may occur with thiazide diuretics; dosage adjustment of oral hypoglycemic agents may be required). Products include:
Precose Tablets ... 906

Acebutolol Hydrochloride (Co-administration of thiazide and other antihypertensive agents can lead to additive effect or potentiation). Products include:
Sectral Capsules ... 3589

ACTH (Co-administration of thiazide diuretics with ACTH intensifies electrolyte depletion, particularly potassium).
No products indexed under this heading.

Alfentanil Hydrochloride (Co-administration of thiazide and narcotics may potentiate orthostatic hypotension).
No products indexed under this heading.

Amiloride Hydrochloride (Lisinopril attenuates diuretic-induced potassium loss; concomitant use can lead to hyperkalemia; frequent monitoring of serum potassium is recommended if used concurrently; co-administration can result in excessive hypotension). Products include:
Midamor Tablets ... 2136
Moduretic Tablets ... 2138

Amlodipine Besylate (Co-administration of thiazide and other antihypertensive agents can lead to additive effect or potentiation). Products include:
Lotrel Capsules ... 2370
Norvasc Tablets ... 2704

Aprobarbital (Co-administration of thiazide and barbiturates may potentiate orthostatic hypotension).
No products indexed under this heading.

Atenolol (Co-administration of thiazide and other antihypertensive agents can lead to additive effect or potentiation). Products include:
Tenoretic Tablets ... 690
Tenormin I.V. Injection ... 692

Atracurium Besylate (Co-administration with nondepolarizing skeletal muscle relaxants may result in possible increased responsiveness to the muscle relaxant).
No products indexed under this heading.

Benazepril Hydrochloride (Co-administration of thiazide and other antihypertensive agents can lead to additive effect or potentiation). Products include:
Lotensin Tablets ... 2365
Lotensin HCT Tablets ... 2367
Lotrel Capsules ... 2370

Bendroflumethiazide (Co-administration of lisinopril in patients on diuretics, especially those in whom diuretic therapy was recently instituted, may occasionally experience excessive hypotension; antihypertensive effects of lisinopril are augmented by antihypertensive agents that cause renin release). Products include:
Corzide 40/5 Tablets ... 2247
Corzide 80/5 Tablets ... 2247

Betamethasone Acetate (Co-administration of thiazide diuretics

IMPORTANT NOTE: Always consult each drug listing in the patient's regimen for possible interactions.

with corticosteroids intensifies electrolyte depletion, particularly potassium). Products include:
Celestone Soluspan Injectable Suspension ... 3097

Betamethasone Sodium Phosphate (Co-administration of thiazide diuretics with corticosteroids intensifies electrolyte depletion, particularly potassium). Products include:
Celestone Soluspan Injectable Suspension ... 3097

Betaxolol Hydrochloride (Co-administration of thiazide and other antihypertensive agents can lead to additive effect or potentiation). Products include:
Betoptic S Ophthalmic Suspension ... 537

Bisoprolol Fumarate (Co-administration of thiazide and other antihypertensive agents can lead to additive effect or potentiation). Products include:
Zebeta Tablets ... 1885
Ziac Tablets ... 1887

Bumetanide (Co-administration of lisinopril in patients on diuretics, especially those in whom diuretic therapy was recently instituted, may occasionally experience excessive hypotension; antihypertensive effects of lisinopril are augmented by antihypertensive agents that cause renin release).
No products indexed under this heading.

Buprenorphine Hydrochloride (Co-administration of thiazide and narcotics may potentiate orthostatic hypotension). Products include:
Buprenex Injectable ... 2918

Butabarbital (Co-administration of thiazide and barbiturates may potentiate orthostatic hypotension).
No products indexed under this heading.

Butalbital (Co-administration of thiazide and barbiturates may potentiate orthostatic hypotension). Products include:
Phrenilin ... 578
Sedapap Tablets 50 mg/650 mg ... 2225

Candesartan Cilexetil (Co-administration of thiazide and other antihypertensive agents can lead to additive effect or potentiation). Products include:
Atacand Tablets ... 595
Atacand HCT Tablets ... 597

Captopril (Co-administration of thiazide and other antihypertensive agents can lead to additive effect or potentiation). Products include:
Captopril Tablets ... 2281

Carteolol Hydrochloride (Co-administration of thiazide and other antihypertensive agents can lead to additive effect or potentiation). Products include:
Carteolol Hydrochloride Ophthalmic Solution USP, 1% ... ⊙258
Ocupress Ophthalmic Solution, 1% Sterile ... ⊙303

Celecoxib (Co-administration in some patients with compromised renal function who are being treated with NSAIDs may result in a further deterioration of renal function: NSAID may reduce the diuretic, natriuretic and antihypertensive effects of thiazide). Products include:
Celebrex Capsules ... 2676
Celebrex Capsules ... 2780

Chlorothiazide (Co-administration of lisinopril in patients on diuretics, especially those in whom diuretic therapy was recently instituted, may occasionally experience excessive hypotension; antihypertensive effects of lisinopril are augmented by antihypertensive agents that cause renin release). Products include:
Aldoclor Tablets ... 2035
Diuril Oral ... 2087

Chlorothiazide Sodium (Co-administration of lisinopril in patients on diuretics, especially those in whom diuretic therapy was recently instituted, may occasionally experience excessive hypotension; antihypertensive effects of lisinopril are augmented by antihypertensive agents that cause renin release). Products include:
Diuril Sodium Intravenous ... 2086

Chlorpropamide (Hyperglycemia may occur with thiazide diuretics; dosage adjustment of oral hypoglycemic agents may be required). Products include:
Diabinese Tablets ... 2680

Chlorthalidone (Co-administration of lisinopril in patients on diuretics, especially those in whom diuretic therapy was recently instituted, may occasionally experience excessive hypotension; antihypertensive effects of lisinopril are augmented by antihypertensive agents that cause renin release). Products include:
Clorpres Tablets ... 1002
Combipres Tablets ... 1040
Tenoretic Tablets ... 690

Cholestyramine (Absorption of hydrochlorothiazide is impaired in the presence of anionic exchange resins; these resins bind the hydrochlorothiazide and reduce its absorption from GI tract).
No products indexed under this heading.

Cisatracurium Besylate (Co-administration with nondepolarizing skeletal muscle relaxants may result in possible increased responsiveness to the muscle relaxant).
No products indexed under this heading.

Clonidine (Co-administration of thiazide and other antihypertensive agents can lead to additive effect or potentiation). Products include:
Catapres-TTS ... 1038

Clonidine Hydrochloride (Co-administration of thiazide and other antihypertensive agents can lead to additive effect or potentiation). Products include:
Catapres Tablets ... 1037
Clorpres Tablets ... 1002
Combipres Tablets ... 1040
Duraclon Injection ... 3057

Codeine Phosphate (Co-administration of thiazide and narcotics may potentiate orthostatic hypotension). Products include:
Phenergan with Codeine Syrup ... 3557
Phenergan VC with Codeine Syrup ... 3561
Robitussin A-C Syrup ... 2942
Robitussin-DAC Syrup ... 2942
Ryna-C Liquid ... ▣768
Soma Compound w/Codeine Tablets ... 3355
Tussi-Organidin NR Liquid ... 3350
Tussi-Organidin-S NR Liquid ... 3350
Tylenol with Codeine ... 2595

Colestipol Hydrochloride (Absorption of hydrochlorothiazide is impaired in the presence of anionic exchange resins; these resins bind the hydrochlorothiazide and reduce its absorption from GI tract). Products include:
Colestid Tablets ... 2791

Cortisone Acetate (Co-administration of thiazide diuretics with corticosteroids intensifies electrolyte depletion, particularly potassium). Products include:
Cortone Acetate Injectable Suspension ... 2059
Cortone Acetate Tablets ... 2061

Deserpidine (Co-administration of thiazide and other antihypertensive agents can lead to additive effect or potentiation).
No products indexed under this heading.

Deslanoside (Hypokalemia induced by thiazide diuretics may cause cardiac arrhythmia and may also sensitize or exaggerate the response to the heart to the toxic effects of digitalis, such as ventricular irritability).
No products indexed under this heading.

Dexamethasone (Co-administration of thiazide diuretics with corticosteroids intensifies electrolyte depletion, particularly potassium). Products include:
Decadron Elixir ... 2078
Decadron Tablets ... 2079
TobraDex Ophthalmic Ointment ... 542
TobraDex Ophthalmic Suspension ... 541

Dexamethasone Acetate (Co-administration of thiazide diuretics with corticosteroids intensifies electrolyte depletion, particularly potassium).
No products indexed under this heading.

Dexamethasone Sodium Phosphate (Co-administration of thiazide diuretics with corticosteroids intensifies electrolyte depletion, particularly potassium). Products include:
Decadron Phosphate Injection ... 2081
Decadron Phosphate Sterile Ophthalmic Ointment ... 2083
Decadron Phosphate Sterile Ophthalmic Solution ... 2084
NeoDecadron Sterile Ophthalmic Solution ... 2144

Dezocine (Co-administration of thiazide and narcotics may potentiate orthostatic hypotension).
No products indexed under this heading.

Diazoxide (Co-administration of thiazide and other antihypertensive agents can lead to additive effect or potentiation).
No products indexed under this heading.

Diclofenac Potassium (Co-administration in some patients with compromised renal function who are being treated with NSAIDs may result in a further deterioration of renal function: NSAID may reduce the diuretic, natriuretic and antihypertensive effects of thiazide). Products include:
Cataflam Tablets ... 2315

Diclofenac Sodium (Co-administration in some patients with compromised renal function who are being treated with NSAIDs may result in a further deterioration of renal function: NSAID may reduce the diuretic, natriuretic and antihypertensive effects of thiazide). Products include:
Arthrotec Tablets ... 3195
Voltaren Ophthalmic Sterile Ophthalmic Solution ... ⊙312
Voltaren Tablets ... 2315
Voltaren-XR Tablets ... 2315

Digitoxin (Hypokalemia induced by thiazide diuretics may cause cardiac arrhythmia and may also sensitize or exaggerate the response to the heart to the toxic effects of digitalis, such as ventricular irritability).
No products indexed under this heading.

Digoxin (Hypokalemia induced by thiazide diuretics may cause cardiac arrhythmia and may also sensitize or exaggerate the response to the heart to the toxic effects of digitalis, such as ventricular irritability). Products include:
Digitek Tablets ... 1003
Lanoxicaps Capsules ... 1574
Lanoxin Injection ... 1581
Lanoxin Tablets ... 1587
Lanoxin Elixir Pediatric ... 1578
Lanoxin Injection Pediatric ... 1584

Diltiazem Hydrochloride (Co-administration of thiazide and other antihypertensive agents can lead to additive effect or potentiation). Products include:
Cardizem Injectable ... 1018
Cardizem Lyo-Ject Syringe ... 1018
Cardizem Monovial ... 1018
Cardizem CD Capsules ... 1016
Tiazac Capsules ... 1378

Doxazosin Mesylate (Co-administration of thiazide and other antihypertensive agents can lead to additive effect or potentiation). Products include:
Cardura Tablets ... 2668

Enalapril Maleate (Co-administration of thiazide and other antihypertensive agents can lead to additive effect or potentiation). Products include:
Lexxel Tablets ... 608
Vaseretic Tablets ... 2204
Vasotec Tablets ... 2210

Enalaprilat (Co-administration of thiazide and other antihypertensive agents can lead to additive effect or potentiation). Products include:
Enalaprilat Injection ... 863
Vasotec I.V. Injection ... 2207

Eprosartan Mesylate (Co-administration of thiazide and other antihypertensive agents can lead to additive effect or potentiation). Products include:
Teveten Tablets ... 3327

Esmolol Hydrochloride (Co-administration of thiazide and other antihypertensive agents can lead to additive effect or potentiation). Products include:
Brevibloc Injection ... 858

Ethacrynic Acid (Co-administration of lisinopril in patients on diuretics, especially those in whom diuretic therapy was recently instituted, may occasionally experience excessive hypotension; antihypertensive effects of lisinopril are augmented by antihypertensive agents that cause renin release). Products include:
Edecrin Tablets ... 2091

Etodolac (Co-administration in some patients with compromised renal function who are being treated with NSAIDs may result in a further deterioration of renal function: NSAID may reduce the diuretic, natriuretic and antihypertensive effects of thiazide). Products include:
Lodine ... 3528
Lodine XL Extended-Release Tablets ... 3530

Felodipine (Co-administration of thiazide and other antihypertensive agents can lead to additive effect or potentiation). Products include:
Lexxel Tablets ... 608
Plendil Extended-Release Tablets ... 623

Fenoprofen Calcium (Co-administration in some patients with compromised renal function who are being treated with NSAIDs may result in a further deterioration of renal function: NSAID may reduce the diuretic, natriuretic and antihypertensive effects of thiazide).
No products indexed under this heading.

Fentanyl (Co-administration of thiazide and narcotics may potentiate orthostatic hypotension). Products include:
Duragesic Transdermal System ... 1786

Fentanyl Citrate (Co-administration of thiazide and narcotics may potentiate orthostatic hypotension). Products include:
Actiq ... 1184

Fludrocortisone Acetate (Co-administration of thiazide diuretics with corticosteroids intensifies electrolyte depletion, particularly potassium). Products include:
Florinef Acetate Tablets ... 2250

Flurbiprofen (Co-administration in some patients with compromised

renal function who are being treated with NSAIDs may result in a further deterioration of renal function: NSAID may reduce the diuretic, natriuretic and antihypertensive effects of thiazide).

No products indexed under this heading.

Fosinopril Sodium (Co-administration of thiazide and other antihypertensive agents can lead to additive effect or potentiation). Products include:

Monopril Tablets 1091
Monopril HCT 1094

Furosemide (Co-administration of lisinopril in patients on diuretics, especially those in whom diuretic therapy was recently instituted, may occasionally experience excessive hypotension; antihypertensive effects of lisinopril are augmented by antihypertensive agents that cause renin release). Products include:

Furosemide Tablets 2284

Glimepiride (Hyperglycemia may occur with thiazide diuretics; dosage adjustment of oral hypoglycemic agents may be required). Products include:

Amaryl Tablets 717

Glipizide (Hyperglycemia may occur with thiazide diuretics; dosage adjustment of oral hypoglycemic agents may be required). Products include:

Glucotrol Tablets 2692
Glucotrol XL Extended Release Tablets 2693

Glyburide (Hyperglycemia may occur with thiazide diuretics; dosage adjustment of oral hypoglycemic agents may be required). Products include:

DiaBeta Tablets 741
Glucovance Tablets 1086

Guanabenz Acetate (Co-administration of thiazide and other antihypertensive agents can lead to additive effect or potentiation).

No products indexed under this heading.

Guanethidine Monosulfate (Co-administration of thiazide and other antihypertensive agents can lead to additive effect or potentiation).

No products indexed under this heading.

Hydralazine Hydrochloride (Co-administration of thiazide and other antihypertensive agents can lead to additive effect or potentiation).

No products indexed under this heading.

Hydrocodone Bitartrate (Co-administration of thiazide and narcotics may potentiate orthostatic hypotension). Products include:

Hycodan 1316
Hycomine Compound Tablets 1317
Hycotuss Expectorant Syrup 1318
Lortab 3319
Lortab Elixir 3317
Maxidone Tablets CIII 3399
Norco 5/325 Tablets CIII 3424
Norco 7.5/325 Tablets CIII 3425
Norco 10/325 Tablets CIII 3427
Norco 10/325 Tablets CIII 3425
Vicodin Tablets 516
Vicodin ES Tablets 517
Vicodin HP Tablets 518
Vicodin Tuss Expectorant 519
Vicoprofen Tablets 520
Zydone Tablets 1330

Hydrocodone Polistirex (Co-administration of thiazide and narcotics may potentiate orthostatic hypotension). Products include:

Tussionex Pennkinetic Extended-Release Suspension 1174

Hydrocortisone (Co-administration of thiazide diuretics with corticosteroids intensifies electrolyte depletion, particularly potassium). Products include:

Anusol-HC Cream 2.5% 2237
Cipro HC Otic Suspension 540
Cortaid Intensive Therapy Cream 717
Cortaid Maximum Strength Cream 717
Cortisporin Ophthalmic Suspension Sterile 297
Cortizone•5 699
Cortizone•10 699
Cortizone•10 Plus Creme 700
Cortizone for Kids Creme 699
Hydrocortone Tablets 2106
Massengill Medicated Soft Cloth Towelette 753
VōSoL HC Otic Solution 3356

Hydrocortisone Acetate (Co-administration of thiazide diuretics with corticosteroids intensifies electrolyte depletion, particularly potassium). Products include:

Analpram-HC 1338
Anusol HC-1 Hydrocortisone Anti-Itch Cream 689
Anusol-HC Suppositories 2238
Cortaid 717
Cortifoam Rectal Foam 3170
Cortisporin-TC Otic Suspension 2246
Hydrocortone Acetate Injectable Suspension 2103
Pramosone 1343
Proctocort Suppositories 2264
ProctoFoam-HC 3177
Terra-Cortril Ophthalmic Suspension 2716

Hydrocortisone Sodium Phosphate (Co-administration of thiazide diuretics with corticosteroids intensifies electrolyte depletion, particularly potassium). Products include:

Hydrocortone Phosphate Injection, Sterile 2105

Hydrocortisone Sodium Succinate (Co-administration of thiazide diuretics with corticosteroids intensifies electrolyte depletion, particularly potassium).

No products indexed under this heading.

Hydroflumethiazide (Co-administration of lisinopril in patients on diuretics, especially those in whom diuretic therapy was recently instituted, may occasionally experience excessive hypotension; antihypertensive effects of lisinopril are augmented by antihypertensive agents that cause renin release). Products include:

Diucardin Tablets 3494

Hydromorphone Hydrochloride (Co-administration of thiazide and narcotics may potentiate orthostatic hypotension). Products include:

Dilaudid 441
Dilaudid Oral Liquid 445
Dilaudid Powder 441
Dilaudid Rectal Suppositories 441
Dilaudid Tablets 441
Dilaudid Tablets - 8 mg 445
Dilaudid-HP 443

Ibuprofen (Co-administration in some patients with compromised renal function who are being treated with NSAIDs may result in a further deterioration of renal function: NSAID may reduce the diuretic, natriuretic and antihypertensive effects of thiazide). Products include:

Advil 771
Children's Advil Oral Suspension 773
Children's Advil Chewable Tablets 773
Advil Cold and Sinus Caplets 771
Advil Cold and Sinus Tablets 771
Advil Flu & Body Ache Caplets 772
Infants' Advil Drops 773
Junior Strength Advil Tablets 773
Junior Strength Advil Chewable Tablets 773
Advil Migraine Liquigels 772
Children's Motrin Oral Suspension and Chewable Tablets 2006
Children's Motrin Cold Oral Suspension 2007
Children's Motrin Oral Suspension 643
Motrin Suspension, Oral Drops, Chewable Tablets, and Caplets 2002
Infants' Motrin Concentrated Drops 2006
Junior Strength Motrin Caplets and Chewable Tablets 2006
Motrin IB Tablets, Caplets, and Gelcaps 2002
Motrin Migraine Pain Caplets 2005
Motrin Sinus Headache Caplets 2005
Vicoprofen Tablets 520

Indapamide (Co-administration of lisinopril in patients on diuretics, especially those in whom diuretic therapy was recently instituted, may occasionally experience excessive hypotension; antihypertensive effects of lisinopril are augmented by antihypertensive agents that cause renin release). Products include:

Indapamide Tablets 2286

Indomethacin (Co-administration in some patients with compromised renal function who are being treated with NSAIDs may result in a further deterioration of renal function: NSAID may reduce the diuretic, natriuretic and antihypertensive effects of thiazide). Products include:

Indocin 2112

Indomethacin Sodium Trihydrate (Co-administration in some patients with compromised renal function who are being treated with NSAIDs may result in a further deterioration of renal function: NSAID may reduce the diuretic, natriuretic and antihypertensive effects of thiazide). Products include:

Indocin I.V. 2115

Insulin, Human, Zinc Suspension (Hyperglycemia may occur with thiazide diuretics; dosage adjustment of insulin may be required). Products include:

Humulin L, 100 Units 1937
Humulin U, 100 Units 1943
Novolin L Human Insulin 10 ml Vials 2422

Insulin, Human NPH (Hyperglycemia may occur with thiazide diuretics; dosage adjustment of insulin may be required). Products include:

Humulin N, 100 Units 1939
Humulin N NPH Pen 1940
Novolin N Human Insulin 10 ml Vials 2422
Novolin N PenFill 2423
Novolin N Prefilled Syringe Disposable Insulin Delivery System 2425

Insulin, Human Regular (Hyperglycemia may occur with thiazide diuretics; dosage adjustment of insulin may be required). Products include:

Humulin R Regular (U-500) 1943
Humulin R, 100 Units 1941
Novolin R Human Insulin 10 ml Vials 2423
Novolin R PenFill 2423
Novolin R Prefilled Syringe Disposable Insulin Delivery System 2425
Velosulin BR Human Insulin 10 ml Vials 2435

Insulin, Human Regular and Human NPH Mixture (Hyperglycemia may occur with thiazide diuretics; dosage adjustment of insulin may be required). Products include:

Humulin 50/50, 100 Units 1934
Humulin 70/30, 100 Units 1935
Humulin 70/30 Pen 1936
Novolin 70/30 Human Insulin 10 ml Vials 2421
Novolin 70/30 PenFill 2423
Novolin 70/30 Prefilled Disposable Insulin Delivery System 2425

Insulin, NPH (Hyperglycemia may occur with thiazide diuretics; dosage adjustment of insulin may be required). Products include:

Iletin II, NPH (Pork), 100 Units 1946

Insulin, Regular (Hyperglycemia may occur with thiazide diuretics; dosage adjustment of insulin may be required). Products include:

Iletin II, Regular (Pork), 100 Units 1947

Insulin, Zinc Crystals (Hyperglycemia may occur with thiazide diuretics; dosage adjustment of insulin may be required).

No products indexed under this heading.

Insulin, Zinc Suspension (Hyperglycemia may occur with thiazide diuretics; dosage adjustment of insulin may be required). Products include:

Iletin II, Lente (Pork), 100 Units 1945

Insulin Aspart, Human Regular (Hyperglycemia may occur with thiazide diuretics; dosage adjustment of insulin may be required).

No products indexed under this heading.

Insulin glargine (Hyperglycemia may occur with thiazide diuretics; dosage adjustment of insulin may be required). Products include:

Lantus Injection 742

Insulin Lispro, Human (Hyperglycemia may occur with thiazide diuretics; dosage adjustment of insulin may be required). Products include:

Humalog 1926
Humalog Mix 75/25 Pen 1928

Insulin Lispro Protamine, Human (Hyperglycemia may occur with thiazide diuretics; dosage adjustment of insulin may be required). Products include:

Humalog Mix 75/25 Pen 1928

Irbesartan (Co-administration of thiazide and other antihypertensive agents can lead to additive effect or potentiation). Products include:

Avalide Tablets 1070
Avapro Tablets 1074
Avapro Tablets 3076

Isradipine (Co-administration of thiazide and other antihypertensive agents can lead to additive effect or potentiation). Products include:

DynaCirc Capsules 2921
DynaCirc CR Tablets 2923

Ketoprofen (Co-administration in some patients with compromised renal function who are being treated with NSAIDs may result in a further deterioration of renal function: NSAID may reduce the diuretic, natriuretic and antihypertensive effects of thiazide). Products include:

Orudis Capsules 3548
Orudis KT Tablets 778
Oruvail Capsules 3548

Ketorolac Tromethamine (Co-administration in some patients with compromised renal function who are being treated with NSAIDs may result in a further deterioration of renal function: NSAID may reduce the diuretic, natriuretic and antihypertensive effects of thiazide). Products include:

Acular Ophthalmic Solution 544
Acular PF Ophthalmic Solution 544
Toradol 3018

Labetalol Hydrochloride (Co-administration of thiazide and other antihypertensive agents can lead to additive effect or potentiation). Products include:

Normodyne Injection 3135
Normodyne Tablets 3137

Levorphanol Tartrate (Co-administration of thiazide and narcotics may potentiate orthostatic hypotension). Products include:

Levo-Dromoran 1734
Levorphanol Tartrate Tablets 3059

Lithium Carbonate (Co-administration of lithium with drugs that cause elimination of sodium, including ACE inhibitors, can lead to lithium toxicity; diuretics can reduce renal clearance of lithium and add a high risk of lithium toxicity). Products include:

Eskalith 1527
Lithium Carbonate 3061
Lithobid Slow-Release Tablets 3255

Lithium Citrate (Co-administration of lithium with drugs that cause elimi-

IMPORTANT NOTE: Always consult each drug listing in the patient's regimen for possible interactions.

nation of sodium, including ACE inhibitors, can lead to lithium toxicity; diuretics can reduce renal clearance of lithium and add a high risk of lithium toxicity). Products include:

Lithium Citrate Syrup 3061

Losartan Potassium (Co-administration of thiazide and other antihypertensive agents can lead to additive effect or potentiation). Products include:

Cozaar Tablets 2067
Hyzaar 2109

Mecamylamine Hydrochloride (Co-administration of thiazide and other antihypertensive agents can lead to additive effect or potentiation). Products include:

Inversine Tablets 1850

Meclofenamate Sodium (Co-administration in some patients with compromised renal function who are being treated with NSAIDs may result in a further deterioration of renal function: NSAID may reduce the diuretic, natriuretic and antihypertensive effects of thiazide).

No products indexed under this heading.

Mefenamic Acid (Co-administration in some patients with compromised renal function who are being treated with NSAIDs may result in a further deterioration of renal function: NSAID may reduce the diuretic, natriuretic and antihypertensive effects of thiazide). Products include:

Ponstel Capsules 1356

Meloxicam (Co-administration in some patients with compromised renal function who are being treated with NSAIDs may result in a further deterioration of renal function: NSAID may reduce the diuretic, natriuretic and antihypertensive effects of thiazide). Products include:

Mobic Tablets 1054

Meperidine Hydrochloride (Co-administration of thiazide and narcotics may potentiate orthostatic hypotension). Products include:

Demerol 3079
Mepergan Injection 3539

Mephobarbital (Co-administration of thiazide and barbiturates may potentiate orthostatic hypotension).

No products indexed under this heading.

Metformin Hydrochloride (Hyperglycemia may occur with thiazide diuretics; dosage adjustment of oral hypoglycemic agents may be required). Products include:

Glucophage Tablets 1080
Glucophage XR Tablets 1080
Glucovance Tablets 1086

Methadone Hydrochloride (Co-administration of thiazide and narcotics may potentiate orthostatic hypotension). Products include:

Dolophine Hydrochloride Tablets 3056

Methyclothiazide (Co-administration of lisinopril in patients on diuretics, especially those in whom diuretic therapy was recently instituted, may occasionally experience excessive hypotension; antihypertensive effects of lisinopril are augmented by antihypertensive agents that cause renin release).

No products indexed under this heading.

Methyldopa (Co-administration of thiazide and other antihypertensive agents can lead to additive effect or potentiation). Products include:

Aldoclor Tablets 2035
Aldomet Tablets 2037
Aldoril Tablets 2039

Methyldopate Hydrochloride (Co-administration of thiazide and other antihypertensive agents can lead to additive effect or potentiation).

No products indexed under this heading.

Methylprednisolone Acetate (Co-administration of thiazide diuretics with corticosteroids intensifies electrolyte depletion, particularly potassium). Products include:

Depo-Medrol Injectable Suspension 2795

Methylprednisolone Sodium Succinate (Co-administration of thiazide diuretics with corticosteroids intensifies electrolyte depletion, particularly potassium). Products include:

Solu-Medrol Sterile Powder 2855

Metocurine Iodide (Co-administration with nondepolarizing skeletal muscle relaxants may result in possible increased responsiveness to the muscle relaxant).

No products indexed under this heading.

Metolazone (Co-administration of lisinopril in patients on diuretics, especially those in whom diuretic therapy was recently instituted, may occasionally experience excessive hypotension; antihypertensive effects of lisinopril are augmented by antihypertensive agents that cause renin release). Products include:

Mykrox Tablets 1168
Zaroxolyn Tablets 1177

Metoprolol Succinate (Co-administration of thiazide and other antihypertensive agents can lead to additive effect or potentiation). Products include:

Toprol-XL Tablets 651

Metoprolol Tartrate (Co-administration of thiazide and other antihypertensive agents can lead to additive effect or potentiation).

No products indexed under this heading.

Metyrosine (Co-administration of thiazide and other antihypertensive agents can lead to additive effect or potentiation). Products include:

Demser Capsules 2085

Mibefradil Dihydrochloride (Co-administration of thiazide and other antihypertensive agents can lead to additive effect or potentiation).

No products indexed under this heading.

Miglitol (Hyperglycemia may occur with thiazide diuretics; dosage adjustment of oral hypoglycemic agents may be required). Products include:

Glyset Tablets 2821

Minoxidil (Co-administration of thiazide and other antihypertensive agents can lead to additive effect or potentiation). Products include:

Rogaine Extra Strength for Men Topical Solution .... ■ 721
Rogaine for Women Topical Solution .... ■ 721

Mivacurium Chloride (Co-administration with nondepolarizing skeletal muscle relaxants may result in possible increased responsiveness to the muscle relaxant).

No products indexed under this heading.

Moexipril Hydrochloride (Co-administration of thiazide and other antihypertensive agents can lead to additive effect or potentiation). Products include:

Uniretic Tablets 3178
Univasc Tablets 3181

Morphine Sulfate (Co-administration of thiazide and narcotics may potentiate orthostatic hypotension). Products include:

Astramorph/PF Injection, USP (Preservative-Free) 594
Duramorph Injection 1312
Infumorph 200 and Infumorph 500 Sterile Solutions 1314
Kadian Capsules 1335
MS Contin Tablets 2896
MSIR 2898
Oramorph SR Tablets 3062
Roxanol 3066

Nabumetone (Co-administration in some patients with compromised renal function who are being treated with NSAIDs may result in a further deterioration of renal function: NSAID may reduce the diuretic, natriuretic and antihypertensive effects of thiazide). Products include:

Relafen Tablets 1617

Nadolol (Co-administration of thiazide and other antihypertensive agents can lead to additive effect or potentiation). Products include:

Corgard Tablets 2245
Corzide 40/5 Tablets 2247
Corzide 80/5 Tablets 2247
Nadolol Tablets 2288

Naproxen (Co-administration in some patients with compromised renal function who are being treated with NSAIDs may result in a further deterioration of renal function: NSAID may reduce the diuretic, natriuretic and antihypertensive effects of thiazide). Products include:

EC-Naprosyn Delayed-Release Tablets 2967
Naprosyn Suspension 2967
Naprosyn Tablets 2967

Naproxen Sodium (Co-administration in some patients with compromised renal function who are being treated with NSAIDs may result in a further deterioration of renal function: NSAID may reduce the diuretic, natriuretic and antihypertensive effects of thiazide). Products include:

Aleve Tablets, Caplets and Gelcaps .... ■ 602
Aleve Cold & Sinus Caplets .... ■ 603
Anaprox Tablets 2967
Anaprox DS Tablets 2967
Naprelan Tablets 1293

Nicardipine Hydrochloride (Co-administration of thiazide and other antihypertensive agents can lead to additive effect or potentiation). Products include:

Cardene I.V. 3485

Nifedipine (Co-administration of thiazide and other antihypertensive agents can lead to additive effect or potentiation). Products include:

Adalat CC Tablets 877
Procardia Capsules 2708
Procardia XL Extended Release Tablets 2710

Nisoldipine (Co-administration of thiazide and other antihypertensive agents can lead to additive effect or potentiation). Products include:

Sular Tablets 688

Nitroglycerin (Co-administration of thiazide and other antihypertensive agents can lead to additive effect or potentiation). Products include:

Nitro-Dur Transdermal Infusion System 3134
Nitro-Dur Transdermal Infusion System 1834
Nitrolingual Pumpspray 1355
Nitrostat Tablets 2658

Norepinephrine Bitartrate (Possible decreased response to pressor amines but not sufficient to preclude pressor amine use).

No products indexed under this heading.

Oxaprozin (Co-administration in some patients with compromised renal function who are being treated with NSAIDs may result in a further deterioration of renal function: NSAID may reduce the diuretic, natriuretic and antihypertensive effects of thiazide).

No products indexed under this heading.

Oxycodone Hydrochloride (Co-administration of thiazide and narcotics may potentiate orthostatic hypotension). Products include:

OxyContin Tablets 2912
OxyFast Oral Concentrate Solution . 2916
OxyIR Capsules 2916
Percocet Tablets 1326
Percodan Tablets 1327
Percolone Tablets 1327
Roxicodone 3067
Tylox Capsules 2597

Pancuronium Bromide (Co-administration with nondepolarizing skeletal muscle relaxants may result in possible increased responsiveness to the muscle relaxant).

No products indexed under this heading.

Penbutolol Sulfate (Co-administration of thiazide and other antihypertensive agents can lead to additive effect or potentiation).

No products indexed under this heading.

Pentobarbital Sodium (Co-administration of thiazide and barbiturates may potentiate orthostatic hypotension). Products include:

Nembutal Sodium Solution 485

Perindopril Erbumine (Co-administration of thiazide and other antihypertensive agents can lead to additive effect or potentiation). Products include:

Aceon Tablets (2 mg, 4 mg, 8 mg) 3249

Phenobarbital (Co-administration of thiazide and barbiturates may potentiate orthostatic hypotension). Products include:

Arco-Lase Plus Tablets 592
Donnatal 2929
Donnatal Extentabs 2930

Phenoxybenzamine Hydrochloride (Co-administration of thiazide and other antihypertensive agents can lead to additive effect or potentiation). Products include:

Dibenzyline Capsules 3457

Phentolamine Mesylate (Co-administration of thiazide and other antihypertensive agents can lead to additive effect or potentiation).

No products indexed under this heading.

Phenylbutazone (Co-administration in some patients with compromised renal function who are being treated with NSAIDs may result in a further deterioration of renal function: NSAID may reduce the diuretic, natriuretic and antihypertensive effects of thiazide).

No products indexed under this heading.

Pindolol (Co-administration of thiazide and other antihypertensive agents can lead to additive effect or potentiation).

No products indexed under this heading.

Pioglitazone Hydrochloride (Hyperglycemia may occur with thiazide diuretics; dosage adjustment of oral hypoglycemic agents may be required). Products include:

Actos Tablets 3275

Piroxicam (Co-administration in some patients with compromised renal function who are being treated with NSAIDs may result in a further deterioration of renal function: NSAID may reduce the diuretic, natriuretic and antihypertensive effects of thiazide). Products include:

Feldene Capsules 2685

Polythiazide (Co-administration of lisinopril in patients on diuretics, especially those in whom diuretic therapy was recently instituted, may occasionally experience excessive hypotension; antihypertensive effects of lisinopril are augmented

by antihypertensive agents that cause renin release). Products include:
Minizide Capsules 2700
Renese Tablets 2712

Potassium Acid Phosphate (Concomitant use of potassium-containing salt substitute or potassium supplements can lead to hyperkalemia; frequent monitoring of serum potassium is recommended if used concurrently). Products include:
K-Phos Original (Sodium Free) Tablets 947

Potassium Bicarbonate (Concomitant use of potassium-containing salt substitute or potassium supplements can lead to hyperkalemia; frequent monitoring of serum potassium is recommended if used concurrently).
No products indexed under this heading.

Potassium Chloride (Concomitant use of potassium-containing salt substitute or potassium supplements can lead to hyperkalemia; frequent monitoring of serum potassium is recommended if used concurrently). Products include:
Chlor-3 1361
Colyte with Flavor Packs for Oral Solution 3170
GoLYTELY and Pineapple Flavor GoLYTELY for Oral Solution 1068
K-Dur Microburst Release System ER Tablets 1832
Klor-Con M20/Klor-Con M10 Tablets 3329
K-Lor Powder Packets 469
K-Tab Filmtab Tablets 470
Micro-K 3311
NuLYTELY, Cherry Flavor, Lemon-Lime Flavor, and Orange Flavor NuLYTELY for Oral Solution 1068
Rum-K 1363

Potassium Citrate (Concomitant use of potassium-containing salt substitute or potassium supplements can lead to hyperkalemia; frequent monitoring of serum potassium is recommended if used concurrently). Products include:
Urocit-K Tablets 2232

Potassium Gluconate (Concomitant use of potassium-containing salt substitute or potassium supplements can lead to hyperkalemia; frequent monitoring of serum potassium is recommended if used concurrently).
No products indexed under this heading.

Potassium Phosphate (Concomitant use of potassium-containing salt substitute or potassium supplements can lead to hyperkalemia; frequent monitoring of serum potassium is recommended if used concurrently). Products include:
K-Phos Neutral Tablets 946

Prazosin Hydrochloride (Co-administration of thiazide and other antihypertensive agents can lead to additive effect or potentiation). Products include:
Minipress Capsules 2699
Minizide Capsules 2700

Prednisolone Acetate (Co-administration of thiazide diuretics with corticosteroids intensifies electrolyte depletion, particularly potassium). Products include:
Blephamide Ophthalmic Ointment 547
Blephamide Ophthalmic Suspension 548
Poly-Pred Liquifilm Ophthalmic Suspension .... ⊙245
Pred Forte Ophthalmic Suspension .... ⊙246
Pred Mild Sterile Ophthalmic Suspension .... ⊙249
Pred-G Ophthalmic Suspension .... ⊙247
Pred-G Sterile Ophthalmic Ointment .... ⊙248

Prednisolone Sodium Phosphate (Co-administration of thiazide diuretics with corticosteroids intensifies electrolyte depletion, particularly potassium). Products include:
Pediapred Oral Solution 1170

Prednisolone Tebutate (Co-administration of thiazide diuretics with corticosteroids intensifies electrolyte depletion, particularly potassium).
No products indexed under this heading.

Prednisone (Co-administration of thiazide diuretics with corticosteroids intensifies electrolyte depletion, particularly potassium). Products include:
Prednisone 3064

Propoxyphene Hydrochloride (Co-administration of thiazide and narcotics may potentiate orthostatic hypotension). Products include:
Darvon Pulvules 1909
Darvon Compound-65 Pulvules 1910

Propoxyphene Napsylate (Co-administration of thiazide and narcotics may potentiate orthostatic hypotension). Products include:
Darvon-N/Darvocet-N 1907
Darvon-N Tablets 1912

Propranolol Hydrochloride (Co-administration of thiazide and other antihypertensive agents can lead to additive effect or potentiation). Products include:
Inderal 3513
Inderal LA Long-Acting Capsules 3516
Inderide Tablets 3517
Inderide LA Long-Acting Capsules 3519

Quinapril Hydrochloride (Co-administration of thiazide and other antihypertensive agents can lead to additive effect or potentiation). Products include:
Accupril Tablets 2611
Accuretic Tablets 2614

Ramipril (Co-administration of thiazide and other antihypertensive agents can lead to additive effect or potentiation). Products include:
Altace Capsules 2233

Rapacuronium Bromide (Co-administration with nondepolarizing skeletal muscle relaxants may result in possible increased responsiveness to the muscle relaxant).
No products indexed under this heading.

Rauwolfia serpentina (Co-administration of thiazide and other antihypertensive agents can lead to additive effect or potentiation).
No products indexed under this heading.

Remifentanil Hydrochloride (Co-administration of thiazide and narcotics may potentiate orthostatic hypotension).
No products indexed under this heading.

Repaglinide (Hyperglycemia may occur with thiazide diuretics; dosage adjustment of oral hypoglycemic agents may be required). Products include:
Prandin Tablets (0.5, 1, and 2 mg) 2432

Rescinnamine (Co-administration of thiazide and other antihypertensive agents can lead to additive effect or potentiation).
No products indexed under this heading.

Reserpine (Co-administration of thiazide and other antihypertensive agents can lead to additive effect or potentiation).
No products indexed under this heading.

Rocuronium Bromide (Co-administration with nondepolarizing skeletal muscle relaxants may result in possible increased responsiveness to the muscle relaxant). Products include:
Zemuron Injection 2491

Rofecoxib (Co-administration in some patients with compromised renal function who are being treated with NSAIDs may result in a further deterioration of renal function: NSAID may reduce the diuretic, natriuretic and antihypertensive effects of thiazide). Products include:
Vioxx 2213

Rosiglitazone Maleate (Hyperglycemia may occur with thiazide diuretics; dosage adjustment of oral hypoglycemic agents may be required). Products include:
Avandia Tablets 1490

Secobarbital Sodium (Co-administration of thiazide and barbiturates may potentiate orthostatic hypotension).
No products indexed under this heading.

Sodium Nitroprusside (Co-administration of thiazide and other antihypertensive agents can lead to additive effect or potentiation).
No products indexed under this heading.

Sotalol Hydrochloride (Co-administration of thiazide and other antihypertensive agents can lead to additive effect or potentiation). Products include:
Betapace Tablets 950
Betapace AF Tablets 954

Spirapril Hydrochloride (Co-administration of thiazide and other antihypertensive agents can lead to additive effect or potentiation).
No products indexed under this heading.

Spironolactone (Lisinopril attenuates diuretic-induced potassium loss; concomitant use can lead to hyperkalemia; frequent monitoring of serum potassium is recommended if used concurrently; co-administration can result in excessive hypotension).
No products indexed under this heading.

Sufentanil Citrate (Co-administration of thiazide and narcotics may potentiate orthostatic hypotension).
No products indexed under this heading.

Sulindac (Co-administration in some patients with compromised renal function who are being treated with NSAIDs may result in a further deterioration of renal function: NSAID may reduce the diuretic, natriuretic and antihypertensive effects of thiazide). Products include:
Clinoril Tablets 2053

Telmisartan (Co-administration of thiazide and other antihypertensive agents can lead to additive effect or potentiation). Products include:
Micardis Tablets 1049
Micardis HCT Tablets 1051

Terazosin Hydrochloride (Co-administration of thiazide and other antihypertensive agents can lead to additive effect or potentiation). Products include:
Hytrin Capsules 464

Thiamylal Sodium (Co-administration of thiazide and barbiturates may potentiate orthostatic hypotension).
No products indexed under this heading.

Timolol Maleate (Co-administration of thiazide and other antihypertensive agents can lead to additive effect or potentiation). Products include:
Blocadren Tablets 2046
Cosopt Sterile Ophthalmic Solution 2065
Timolide Tablets 2187
Timolol GFS .... ⊙266
Timoptic in Ocudose 2192
Timoptic Sterile Ophthalmic Solution 2190
Timoptic-XE Sterile Ophthalmic Gel Forming Solution 2194

Tolazamide (Hyperglycemia may occur with thiazide diuretics; dosage adjustment of oral hypoglycemic agents may be required).
No products indexed under this heading.

Tolbutamide (Hyperglycemia may occur with thiazide diuretics; dosage adjustment of oral hypoglycemic agents may be required).
No products indexed under this heading.

Tolmetin Sodium (Co-administration in some patients with compromised renal function who are being treated with NSAIDs may result in a further deterioration of renal function: NSAID may reduce the diuretic, natriuretic and antihypertensive effects of thiazide). Products include:
Tolectin 2589

Torsemide (Co-administration of lisinopril in patients on diuretics, especially those in whom diuretic therapy was recently instituted, may occasionally experience excessive hypotension; antihypertensive effects of lisinopril are augmented by antihypertensive agents that cause renin release). Products include:
Demadex Tablets and Injection 2965

Trandolapril (Co-administration of thiazide and other antihypertensive agents can lead to additive effect or potentiation). Products include:
Mavik Tablets 478
Tarka Tablets 508

Triamcinolone (Co-administration of thiazide diuretics with corticosteroids intensifies electrolyte depletion, particularly potassium).
No products indexed under this heading.

Triamcinolone Acetonide (Co-administration of thiazide diuretics with corticosteroids intensifies electrolyte depletion, particularly potassium). Products include:
Azmacort Inhalation Aerosol 728
Nasacort Nasal Inhaler 750
Nasacort AQ Nasal Spray 752
Tri-Nasal Spray 2274

Triamcinolone Diacetate (Co-administration of thiazide diuretics with corticosteroids intensifies electrolyte depletion, particularly potassium).
No products indexed under this heading.

Triamcinolone Hexacetonide (Co-administration of thiazide diuretics with corticosteroids intensifies electrolyte depletion, particularly potassium).
No products indexed under this heading.

Triamterene (Lisinopril attenuates diuretic-induced potassium loss; concomitant use can lead to hyperkalemia; frequent monitoring of serum potassium is recommended if used concurrently; co-administration can result in excessive hypotension). Products include:
Dyazide Capsules 1515
Dyrenium Capsules 3458
Maxzide 1008

Trimethaphan Camsylate (Co-administration of thiazide and other antihypertensive agents can lead to additive effect or potentiation).
No products indexed under this heading.

Troglitazone (Hyperglycemia may occur with thiazide diuretics; dosage adjustment of oral hypoglycemic agents may be required).
No products indexed under this heading.

Valsartan (Co-administration of thiazide and other antihypertensive agents can lead to additive effect or potentiation). Products include:

Diovan Capsules 2337
Diovan HCT Tablets 2338

Vecuronium Bromide (Co-administration with nondepolarizing skeletal muscle relaxants may result in possible increased responsiveness to the muscle relaxant). Products include:

Norcuron for Injection 2478

Verapamil Hydrochloride (Co-administration of thiazide and other antihypertensive agents can lead to additive effect or potentiation). Products include:

Covera-HS Tablets 3199
Isoptin SR Tablets 467
Tarka Tablets 508
Verelan Capsules 3184
Verelan PM Capsules 3186

Food Interactions

Alcohol (Co-administration of thiazide and alcohol may potentiate orthostatic hypotension).

PROAMATINE TABLETS

(Midodrine Hydrochloride) 3241

May interact with alpha adrenergic blockers, cardiac glycosides, quinidine, and certain other agents. Compounds in these categories include:

Cimetidine (The high renal clearance of desglymidodrine is due to active tubular secretion by the base-secreting system also responsible for the secretion of cimetidine; possibility of drug interaction exists with co-administration). Products include:

Tagamet HB 200 Suspension .... ▣762
Tagamet HB 200 Tablets .... ▣761
Tagamet Tablets 1644

Deslanoside (Co-administration with cardiac glycosides may enhance or precipitate bradycardia, AV block or arrhythmia).

No products indexed under this heading.

Digitoxin (Co-administration with cardiac glycosides may enhance or precipitate bradycardia, AV block or arrhythmia).

No products indexed under this heading.

Digoxin (Co-administration with cardiac glycosides may enhance or precipitate bradycardia, AV block or arrhythmia). Products include:

Digitek Tablets 1003
Lanoxicaps Capsules 1574
Lanoxin Injection 1581
Lanoxin Tablets 1587
Lanoxin Elixir Pediatric 1578
Lanoxin Injection Pediatric 1584

Dihydroergotamine Mesylate (Co-administration with alpha-adrenergic receptor stimulants may enhance or potentiate pressor effects of midodrine). Products include:

D.H.E. 45 Injection 2334
Migranal Nasal Spray 2376

Doxazosin Mesylate (Alpha adrenergic blocking agents can antagonize the effects of midodrine). Products include:

Cardura Tablets 2668

Ephedrine Hydrochloride (Co-administration with alpha-adrenergic receptor stimulants may enhance or potentiate pressor effects of midodrine). Products include:

Primatene Tablets .... ▣780

Ephedrine Sulfate (Co-administration with alpha-adrenergic receptor stimulants may enhance or potentiate pressor effects of midodrine).

No products indexed under this heading.

Ephedrine Tannate (Co-administration with alpha-adrenergic receptor stimulants may enhance or potentiate pressor effects of midodrine). Products include:

Rynatuss Pediatric Suspension 3353
Rynatuss Tablets 3353

Flecainide Acetate (The high renal clearance of desglymidodrine is due to active tubular secretion by the base-secreting system also responsible for the secretion of flecainide; possibility of drug interaction exists with co-administration). Products include:

Tambocor Tablets 1990

Fludrocortisone Acetate (Co-administration with salt-retaining steroid therapy increases the potential for supine hypertension; this can be minimized by reducing the dose of fludrocortisone or decreasing salt intake). Products include:

Florinef Acetate Tablets 2250

Metformin (The high renal clearance of desglymidodrine is due to active tubular secretion by the base-secreting system also responsible for the secretion of metformin; possibility of drug interaction exists with co-administration).

Phenylephrine Hydrochloride (Co-administration with alpha-adrenergic receptor stimulants may enhance or potentiate pressor effects of midodrine). Products include:

Afrin Nasal Decongestant Children's Pump Mist .... ▣734
Extendryl 1361
Hycomine Compound Tablets 1317
Neo-Synephrine .... ▣614
Phenergan VC Syrup 3560
Phenergan VC with Codeine Syrup 3561
Preparation H Cream .... ▣778
Preparation H Cooling Gel .... ▣778
Preparation H .... ▣778
Vicks Sinex Nasal Spray and Ultra Fine Mist .... ▣729

Phenylephrine Tannate (Co-administration with alpha-adrenergic receptor stimulants may enhance or potentiate pressor effects of midodrine). Products include:

Ryna-12 S Suspension 3351
Reformulated Rynatan Pediatric Suspension 3352
Rynatuss Pediatric Suspension 3353
Rynatuss Tablets 3353

Prazosin Hydrochloride (Alpha adrenergic blocking agents can antagonize the effects of midodrine). Products include:

Minipress Capsules 2699
Minizide Capsules 2700

Procainamide Hydrochloride (The high renal clearance of desglymidodrine is due to active tubular secretion by the base-secreting system also responsible for the secretion of procainamide; possibility of drug interaction exists with co-administration). Products include:

Procanbid Extended-Release Tablets 2262

Pseudoephedrine Hydrochloride (Co-administration with alpha-adrenergic receptor stimulants may enhance or potentiate pressor effects of midodrine). Products include:

Actifed Cold & Allergy Tablets .... ▣688
Actifed Cold & Sinus Caplets and Tablets .... ▣688
Advil Cold and Sinus Caplets .... ▣771
Advil Cold and Sinus Tablets .... ▣771
Advil Flu & Body Ache Caplets .... ▣772
Aleve Cold & Sinus Caplets .... ▣603
Alka-Seltzer Plus Liqui-Gels .... ▣604
Alka-Seltzer Plus Cold & Flu Medicine Liqui-Gels .... ▣604
Alka-Seltzer Plus Cold & Sinus Medicine Liqui-Gels .... ▣604
Allegra-D Extended-Release Tablets 714
BC Cold Powder .... ▣619
Benadryl Allergy/Cold Tablets .... ▣691
Benadryl Allergy/Congestion Tablets .... ▣692
Benadryl Allergy & Sinus Liquid .... ▣693
Benadryl Allergy & Sinus Fastmelt Tablets .... ▣693
Benadryl Allergy Sinus Headache Caplets & Gelcaps .... ▣693
Benadryl Severe Allergy & Sinus Headache Caplets .... ▣694
Benadryl Children's Allergy/Cold Fastmelt Tablets .... ▣692
Benylin Multi-Symptom Liquid .... ▣697
Bromfed Capsules (Extended-Release) 2269
Bromfed-PD Capsules (Extended-Release) 2269
Children's Cēpacol Sore Throat .... ▣788
Comtrex Acute Head Cold & Sinus Pressure Relief Tablets .... ▣627
Comtrex Deep Chest Cold & Congestion Relief Softgels .... ▣627
Comtrex Flu Therapy & Fever Relief Daytime Caplets .... ▣628
Comtrex Flu Therapy & Fever Relief Nighttime Tablets .... ▣628
Comtrex Maximum Strength Multi-Symptom Cold & Cough Relief Tablets and Caplets .... ▣626
Contac Non-Drowsy 12 Hour Cold Caplets .... ▣745
Contac Non-Drowsy Timed Release 12 Hour Cold Caplets .... ▣746
Contac Severe Cold and Flu Caplets Maximum Strength .... ▣746
Contac Severe Cold and Flu Caplets Non-Drowsy .... ▣746
Dimetapp Elixir .... ▣777
Dimetapp Cold and Fever Suspension .... ▣775
Dimetapp DM Cold & Cough Elixir .... ▣775
Dimetapp Nighttime Flu Liquid .... ▣776
Dimetapp Non-Drowsy Flu Syrup .... ▣777
Dimetapp Infant Drops Decongestant .... ▣775
Dimetapp Infant Drops Decongestant Plus Cough .... ▣776
Guaifed 2272
Kronofed-A 1341
Children's Motrin Cold Oral Suspension 2007
Motrin Sinus Headache Caplets 2005
PediaCare Cough-Cold Liquid .... ▣719
PediaCare Infants' Drops Decongestant .... ▣719
PediaCare Infants' Drops Decongestant Plus Cough .... ▣719
PediaCare NightRest Cough-Cold Liquid .... ▣719
Robitussin Cold Caplets Cold & Congestion .... ▣780
Robitussin Cold Softgels Cold & Congestion .... ▣780
Robitussin Cold Caplets Multi-Symptom Cold & Flu .... ▣781
Robitussin Cold Softgels Multi-Symptom Cold & Flu .... ▣781
Robitussin Cold Softgels Severe Congestion .... ▣782
Robitussin Cough & Cold Infant Drops .... ▣782
Robitussin Maximum Strength Cough & Cold Liquid .... ▣785
Robitussin Pediatric Cough & Cold Formula Liquid .... ▣785
Robitussin Multi Symptom Honey Flu Liquid .... ▣785
Robitussin Nighttime Honey Flu Liquid .... ▣786
Robitussin-CF Liquid .... ▣783
Robitussin-DAC Syrup 2942
Robitussin-PE Liquid .... ▣782
Ryna .... ▣768
Semprex-D Capsules 1172
Singlet Caplets .... ▣761
Sinutab Non-Drying Liquid Caps .... ▣706
Sinutab Sinus Allergy Medication, Maximum Strength Formula, Tablets & Caplets .... ▣707
Sinutab Sinus Medication, Maximum Strength Without Drowsiness Formula, Tablets & Caplets .... ▣707
Sudafed 12 Hour Tablets .... ▣708
Sudafed 24 Hour Tablets .... ▣708
Children's Sudafed Cold & Cough Liquid .... ▣709
Children's Sudafed Nasal Decongestant Chewables .... ▣711
Children's Sudafed Nasal Decongestant Liquid Medication .... ▣711
Sudafed Cold & Allergy Tablets .... ▣708
Sudafed Cold & Cough Liquid Caps .... ▣709
Sudafed Cold & Sinus Liquid Caps .... ▣710
Sudafed Nasal Decongestant Tablets .... ▣710
Sudafed Non-Drying Sinus Liquid Caps .... ▣712
Sudafed Severe Cold .... ▣711
Sudafed Sinus Headache Caplets .... ▣712
Sudafed Sinus Headache Tablets .... ▣712
Tavist Sinus Non-Drowsy Coated Caplets .... ▣676
TheraFlu Regular Strength Cold & Cough Night Time Hot Liquid .... ▣676
TheraFlu Regular Strength Cold & Sore Throat Night Time Hot Liquid .... ▣676
TheraFlu Maximum Strength Flu & Congestion Non-Drowsy Hot Liquid .... ▣677
TheraFlu Maximum Strength Flu & Cough Night Time Hot Liquid .... ▣678
TheraFlu Maximum Strength Flu & Sore Throat Night Time Hot Liquid .... ▣677
TheraFlu Maximum Strength Severe Cold & Congestion Night Time Caplets .... ▣678
TheraFlu Maximum Strength Severe Cold & Congestion Night Time Hot Liquid .... ▣678
TheraFlu Maximum Strength Severe Cold & Congestion Non-Drowsy .... ▣679
Triaminic Allergy Congestion Liquid .... ▣680
Triaminic Chest Congestion Liquid .... ▣680
Triaminic Cold & Allergy Liquid .... ▣681
Triaminic Cold & Allergy Softchews .... ▣683
Triaminic Cold & Cough Liquid .... ▣681
Triaminic Cold & Cough Softchews .... ▣683
Triaminic Cold & Night Time Cough Liquid .... ▣681
Triaminic Cold, Cough & Fever Liquid .... ▣681
Triaminic Cough Liquid .... ▣682
Triaminic Cough & Congestion Liquid .... ▣682
Triaminic Cough & Sore Throat Liquid .... ▣682
Triaminic Cough & Sore Throat Softchews .... ▣684
Children's Tylenol Allergy-D Liquid 2014
Children's Tylenol Cold Suspension Liquid and Chewable Tablets 2015
Children's Tylenol Cold Plus Cough Suspension Liquid and Chewable Tablets 2015
Children's Tylenol Flu Suspension Liquid 2015
Children's Tylenol Sinus Suspension Liquid 2017
Infants' Tylenol Cold Decongestant and Fever Reducer Concentrated Drops 2015
Infants' Tylenol Cold Decongestant and Fever Reducer Concentrated Drops Plus Cough 2015
Tylenol Allergy Sinus 2010
Multi-Symptom Tylenol Cold Complete Formula Caplets 2010
Multi-Symptom Tylenol Cold Non-Drowsy Caplets and Gelcaps 2010
Multi-Symptom Tylenol Cold Severe Congestion Non-Drowsy Caplets 2011
Maximum Strength Tylenol Flu NightTime Gelcaps 2011
Maximum Strength Tylenol Flu NightTime Liquid 2011
Maximum Strength Tylenol Flu Non-Drowsy Gelcaps 2011
Maximum Strength Tylenol Sinus NightTime Caplets 2012
Maximum Strength Tylenol Sinus Non-Drowsy Geltabs, Gelcaps, Caplets, and Tablets 2012
Vicks 44D Cough & Head Congestion Relief Liquid .... ▣724
Vicks 44M Cough, Cold & Flu Relief Liquid .... ▣725
Pediatric Vicks 44m Cough & Cold Relief .... ▣728
Vicks DayQuil LiquiCaps/Liquid Multi-Symptom Cold/Flu Relief .... ▣727
Children's Vicks NyQuil Cold/Cough Relief .... ▣726
Vicks NyQuil LiquiCaps/Liquid Multi-Symptom Cold/Flu Relief, Original and Cherry Flavors .... ▣727
Zephrex Tablets 3091
Zephrex LA Tablets 3092
Zyrtec-D 12 Hour Extended Relief Tablets 2758

Pseudoephedrine Sulfate (Co-administration with alpha-adrenergic receptor stimulants may enhance or potentiate pressor effects of midodrine). Products include:

Chlor-Trimeton
Allergy/Decongestant Tablets .... ■736
Claritin-D 12 Hour Extended
Release Tablets 3102
Claritin-D 24 Hour Extended
Release Tablets 3104
Coricidin 'D' Cold, Flu & Sinus
Tablets .... ■737
Drixoral Allergy/Sinus
Extended-Release Tablets .... ■741
Drixoral Cold & Allergy
Sustained-Action Tablets .... ■740
Drixoral Cold & Flu
Extended-Release Tablets .... ■740
Drixoral Nasal Decongestant
Long-Acting Non-Drowsy
Tablets .... ■740
Rynatan Tablets 3351

Quinidine Gluconate (The high renal clearance of desglymidodrine is due to active tubular secretion by the base-secreting system also responsible for the secretion of quinidine; possibility of drug interaction exists with co-administration). Products include:
Quinaglute Dura-Tabs Tablets 978

Quinidine Polygalacturonate (The high renal clearance of desglymidodrine is due to active tubular secretion by the base-secreting system also responsible for the secretion of quinidine; possibility of drug interaction exists with co-administration).
No products indexed under this heading.

Quinidine Sulfate (The high renal clearance of desglymidodrine is due to active tubular secretion by the base-secreting system also responsible for the secretion of quinidine; possibility of drug interaction exists with co-administration). Products include:
Quinidex Extentabs 2933

Ranitidine Hydrochloride (The high renal clearance of desglymidodrine is due to active tubular secretion by the base-secreting system also responsible for the secretion of ranitidine; possibility of drug interaction exists with co-administration). Products include:
Zantac 1690
Zantac Injection 1688
Zantac 75 Tablets .... ■717

Terazosin Hydrochloride (Alpha adrenergic blocking agents can antagonize the effects of midodrine). Products include:
Hytrin Capsules 464

Triamterene (The high renal clearance of desglymidodrine is due to active tubular secretion by the base-secreting system also responsible for the secretion of triamterene; possibility of drug interaction exists with co-administration). Products include:
Dyazide Capsules 1515
Dyrenium Capsules 3458
Maxzide 1008

PROBIOTICA TABLETS

(Lactobacillus Reuteri) 2008
None cited in PDR database.

PROCANBID EXTENDED-RELEASE TABLETS

(Procainamide Hydrochloride) 2262
May interact with antiarrhythmics, anticholinergics, cardiac glycosides, neuromuscular blocking agents, quinidine, and certain other agents. Compounds in these categories include:

Acebutolol Hydrochloride (Co-administration with other antiarrhythmic drugs may result in additive effects on heart; dosage reduction may be necessary). Products include:
Sectral Capsules 3589

Adenosine (Co-administration with other antiarrhythmic drugs may result in additive effects on heart; dosage reduction may be necessary). Products include:
Adenocard Injection 1380
Adenoscan 1381

Amiodarone Hydrochloride (Co-administration may result in higher plasma PA concentration). Products include:
Cordarone Intravenous 3491
Cordarone Tablets 3487
Pacerone Tablets 3331

Atracurium Besylate (Co-administration may require less than usual doses of the neuromuscular blocking agent due to PA effects of reducing acetylcholine release).
No products indexed under this heading.

Atropine Sulfate (May produce additive antivagal effects on A-V nodal conduction). Products include:
Donnatal 2929
Donnatal Extentabs 2930
Motofen Tablets 577
Prosed/DS Tablets 3268
Urised Tablets 2876

Belladonna Alkaloids (May produce additive antivagal effects on A-V nodal conduction). Products include:
Hyland's Teething Tablets .... ■766
Urimax Tablets 1769

Benztropine Mesylate (May produce additive antivagal effects on A-V nodal conduction). Products include:
Cogentin 2055

Biperiden Hydrochloride (May produce additive antivagal effects on A-V nodal conduction). Products include:
Akineton 402

Bretylium Tosylate (Co-administration with other antiarrhythmic drugs may result in additive effects on heart; dosage reduction may be necessary).
No products indexed under this heading.

Cimetidine (Co-administration decreases renal clearance of procainamide, potentially leading to clinically significant increases in plasma concentrations). Products include:
Tagamet HB 200 Suspension .... ■762
Tagamet HB 200 Tablets .... ■761
Tagamet Tablets 1644

Cimetidine Hydrochloride (Co-administration decreases renal clearance of procainamide, potentially leading to clinically significant increases in plasma concentrations). Products include:
Tagamet 1644

Cisatracurium Besylate (Co-administration may require less than usual doses of the neuromuscular blocking agent due to PA effects of reducing acetylcholine release).
No products indexed under this heading.

Clidinium Bromide (May produce additive antivagal effects on A-V nodal conduction).
No products indexed under this heading.

Deslanoside (Potential for additional disturbance of conduction, ventricular asystole or fibrillation in patients with concomitant marked disturbance of A-V conduction).
No products indexed under this heading.

Dicyclomine Hydrochloride (May produce additive antivagal effects on A-V nodal conduction).
No products indexed under this heading.

Digitoxin (Potential for additional disturbance of conduction, ventricular asystole or fibrillation in patients with concomitant marked disturbance of A-V conduction).
No products indexed under this heading.

Digoxin (Potential for additional disturbance of conduction, ventricular asystole or fibrillation in patients with concomitant marked disturbance of A-V conduction). Products include:
Digitek Tablets 1003
Lanoxicaps Capsules 1574
Lanoxin Injection 1581
Lanoxin Tablets 1587
Lanoxin Elixir Pediatric 1578
Lanoxin Injection Pediatric 1584

Disopyramide Phosphate (Concurrent use may produce enhanced prolongation of conduction or depression of contractility and hypotension, especially in patients with cardiac decompensation).
No products indexed under this heading.

Dofetilide (Co-administration with other antiarrhythmic drugs may result in additive effects on heart; dosage reduction may be necessary). Products include:
Tikosyn Capsules 2717

Doxacurium Chloride (Co-administration may require less than usual doses of the neuromuscular blocking agent due to PA effects of reducing acetylcholine release).
No products indexed under this heading.

Flecainide Acetate (Co-administration with other antiarrhythmic drugs may result in additive effects on heart; dosage reduction may be necessary). Products include:
Tambocor Tablets 1990

Glycopyrrolate (May produce additive antivagal effects on A-V nodal conduction). Products include:
Robinul Forte Tablets 1358
Robinul Injectable 2940
Robinul Tablets 1358

Hyoscyamine (May produce additive antivagal effects on A-V nodal conduction). Products include:
Urised Tablets 2876

Hyoscyamine Sulfate (May produce additive antivagal effects on A-V nodal conduction). Products include:
Arco-Lase Plus Tablets 592
Donnatal 2929
Donnatal Extentabs 2930
Levsin/Levsinex/Levbid 3172
NuLev Orally Disintegrating
Tablets 3176
Prosed/DS Tablets 3268
Urimax Tablets 1769

Ipratropium Bromide (May produce additive antivagal effects on A-V nodal conduction). Products include:
Atrovent Inhalation Aerosol 1030
Atrovent Inhalation Solution 1031
Atrovent Nasal Spray 0.03% 1032
Atrovent Nasal Spray 0.06% 1033
Combivent Inhalation Aerosol 1041
DuoNeb Inhalation Solution 1233

Lidocaine Hydrochloride (Co-administration with other antiarrhythmic drugs may result in additive effects on heart; dosage reduction may be necessary). Products include:
Bactine First Aid Liquid .... ■611
Xylocaine Injections 653

Mepenzolate Bromide (May produce additive antivagal effects on A-V nodal conduction).
No products indexed under this heading.

Metocurine Iodide (Co-administration may require less than usual doses of the neuromuscular blocking agent due to PA effects of reducing acetylcholine release).
No products indexed under this heading.

Mexiletine Hydrochloride (Co-administration with other antiarrhythmic drugs may result in additive effects on heart; dosage reduction may be necessary). Products include:
Mexitil Capsules 1047

Mivacurium Chloride (Co-administration may require less than usual doses of the neuromuscular blocking agent due to PA effects of reducing acetylcholine release).
No products indexed under this heading.

Moricizine Hydrochloride (Co-administration with other antiarrhythmic drugs may result in additive effects on heart; dosage reduction may be necessary).
No products indexed under this heading.

Oxybutynin Chloride (May produce additive antivagal effects on A-V nodal conduction). Products include:
Ditropan XL Extended Release
Tablets 564

Pancuronium Bromide (Co-administration may require less than usual doses of the neuromuscular blocking agent due to PA effects of reducing acetylcholine release).
No products indexed under this heading.

Procyclidine Hydrochloride (May produce additive antivagal effects on A-V nodal conduction).
No products indexed under this heading.

Propafenone Hydrochloride (Co-administration with other antiarrhythmic drugs may result in additive effects on heart; dosage reduction may be necessary). Products include:
Rythmol Tablets – 150 mg,
225 mg, 300 mg 502

Propantheline Bromide (May produce additive antivagal effects on A-V nodal conduction).
No products indexed under this heading.

Propranolol Hydrochloride (Co-administration with other antiarrhythmic drugs may result in additive effects on heart; dosage reduction may be necessary). Products include:
Inderal 3513
Inderal LA Long-Acting Capsules 3516
Inderide Tablets 3517
Inderide LA Long-Acting Capsules 3519

Quinidine Gluconate (Concurrent use may produce enhanced prolongation of conduction or depression of contractility and hypotension, especially in patients with cardiac decompensation). Products include:
Quinaglute Dura-Tabs Tablets 978

Quinidine Polygalacturonate (Concurrent use may produce enhanced prolongation of conduction or depression of contractility and hypotension, especially in patients with cardiac decompensation).
No products indexed under this heading.

Quinidine Sulfate (Concurrent use may produce enhanced prolongation of conduction or depression of contractility and hypotension, especially in patients with cardiac decompensation). Products include:
Quinidex Extentabs 2933

Ranitidine Hydrochloride (Co-administration at large (>300 mg/day) doses of ranitidine may decrease renal clearance of procainamide). Products include:
Zantac 1690
Zantac Injection 1688
Zantac 75 Tablets .... ■717

Rapacuronium Bromide (Co-administration may require less than usual doses of the neuromuscular blocking agent due to PA effects of

reducing acetylcholine release).
No products indexed under this heading.

Rocuronium Bromide (Co-administration may require less than usual doses of the neuromuscular blocking agent due to PA effects of reducing acetylcholine release). Products include:
Zemuron Injection 2491

Scopolamine (May produce additive antivagal effects on A-V nodal conduction). Products include:
Transderm Scōp Transdermal Therapeutic System 2302

Scopolamine Hydrobromide (May produce additive antivagal effects on A-V nodal conduction). Products include:
Donnatal 2929
Donnatal Extentabs 2930

Sotalol Hydrochloride (Co-administration with other antiarrhythmic drugs may result in additive effects on heart; dosage reduction may be necessary). Products include:
Betapace Tablets 950
Betapace AF Tablets 954

Succinylcholine Chloride (Co-administration may require less than usual doses of the neuromuscular blocking agent due to PA effects of reducing acetylcholine release). Products include:
Anectine Injection 1476

Tocainide Hydrochloride (Co-administration with other antiarrhythmic drugs may result in additive effects on heart; dosage reduction may be necessary). Products include:
Tonocard Tablets 649

Tolterodine Tartrate (May produce additive antivagal effects on A-V nodal conduction). Products include:
Detrol Tablets 3623
Detrol LA Capsules 2801

Tridihexethyl Chloride (May produce additive antivagal effects on A-V nodal conduction).
No products indexed under this heading.

Trihexyphenidyl Hydrochloride (May produce additive antivagal effects on A-V nodal conduction). Products include:
Artane 1855

Trimethoprim (Co-administration may result in higher plasma PA concentration). Products include:
Bactrim 2949
Septra Suspension 2265
Septra Tablets 2265
Septra DS Tablets 2265

Vecuronium Bromide (Co-administration may require less than usual doses of the neuromuscular blocking agent due to PA effects of reducing acetylcholine release). Products include:
Norcuron for Injection 2478

Verapamil Hydrochloride (Co-administration with other antiarrhythmic drugs may result in additive effects on heart; dosage reduction may be necessary). Products include:
Covera-HS Tablets 3199
Isoptin SR Tablets 467
Tarka Tablets 508
Verelan Capsules 3184
Verelan PM Capsules 3186

Food Interactions

Alcohol (Alcohol consumption tends to decrease the half-life of procainamide in the blood through induction of its acetylation to NAPA).

PROCARDIA CAPSULES

(Nifedipine) 2708
May interact with beta blockers, oral anticoagulants, cardiac glycosides, narcotic analgesics, quinidine, and certain other agents. Compounds in these categories include:

Acebutolol Hydrochloride (Combination therapy may increase the likelihood of congestive heart failure, severe hypotension, or exacerbation of angina). Products include:
Sectral Capsules 3589

Alfentanil Hydrochloride (Severe hypotension and/or increased fluid volume requirements have been reported in patients receiving nifedipine with beta blocker who underwent coronary artery bypass surgery using high-dose fentanyl anesthesia; possibility of this interaction cannot be ruled out with other narcotic analgesics or in other surgical procedures).
No products indexed under this heading.

Atenolol (Combination therapy may increase the likelihood of congestive heart failure, severe hypotension, or exacerbation of angina). Products include:
Tenoretic Tablets 690
Tenormin I.V. Injection 692

Betaxolol Hydrochloride (Combination therapy may increase the likelihood of congestive heart failure, severe hypotension, or exacerbation of angina). Products include:
Betoptic S Ophthalmic Suspension 537

Bisoprolol Fumarate (Combination therapy may increase the likelihood of congestive heart failure, severe hypotension, or exacerbation of angina). Products include:
Zebeta Tablets 1885
Ziac Tablets 1887

Buprenorphine Hydrochloride (Severe hypotension and/or increased fluid volume requirements have been reported in patients receiving nifedipine with beta blocker who underwent coronary artery bypass surgery using high-dose fentanyl anesthesia; possibility of this interaction cannot be ruled out with other narcotic analgesics or in other surgical procedures). Products include:
Buprenex Injectable 2918

Carteolol Hydrochloride (Combination therapy may increase the likelihood of congestive heart failure, severe hypotension, or exacerbation of angina). Products include:
Carteolol Hydrochloride Ophthalmic Solution USP, 1% .... ⊙258
Ocupress Ophthalmic Solution, 1% Sterile .... ⊙303

Cimetidine (Significant increase in peak nifedipine plasma levels and AUC). Products include:
Tagamet HB 200 Suspension .... ▣762
Tagamet HB 200 Tablets .... ▣761
Tagamet Tablets 1644

Cimetidine Hydrochloride (Significant increase in peak nifedipine plasma levels and AUC). Products include:
Tagamet 1644

Codeine Phosphate (Severe hypotension and/or increased fluid volume requirements have been reported in patients receiving nifedipine with beta blocker who underwent coronary artery bypass surgery using high-dose fentanyl anesthesia; possibility of this interaction cannot be ruled out with other narcotic analgesics or in other surgical procedures). Products include:
Phenergan with Codeine Syrup 3557
Phenergan VC with Codeine Syrup . 3561
Robitussin A-C Syrup 2942
Robitussin-DAC Syrup 2942
Ryna-C Liquid .... ▣768
Soma Compound w/Codeine Tablets 3355
Tussi-Organidin NR Liquid 3350
Tussi-Organidin-S NR Liquid 3350
Tylenol with Codeine 2595

Deslanoside (Co-administration has resulted in isolated reports of increased digoxin blood levels).
No products indexed under this heading.

Dezocine (Severe hypotension and/or increased fluid volume requirements have been reported in patients receiving nifedipine with beta blocker who underwent coronary artery bypass surgery using high-dose fentanyl anesthesia; possibility of this interaction cannot be ruled out with other narcotic analgesics or in other surgical procedures).
No products indexed under this heading.

Dicumarol (Co-administration has resulted in rare reports of increased prothrombin time; relationship to nifedipine therapy is uncertain).
No products indexed under this heading.

Digitoxin (Co-administration has resulted in isolated reports of increased digoxin blood levels).
No products indexed under this heading.

Digoxin (Co-administration has resulted in isolated reports of increased digoxin blood levels). Products include:
Digitek Tablets 1003
Lanoxicaps Capsules 1574
Lanoxin Injection 1581
Lanoxin Tablets 1587
Lanoxin Elixir Pediatric 1578
Lanoxin Injection Pediatric 1584

Esmolol Hydrochloride (Combination therapy may increase the likelihood of congestive heart failure, severe hypotension, or exacerbation of angina). Products include:
Brevibloc Injection 858

Fentanyl (Severe hypotension and/or increased fluid volume requirements have been reported in patients receiving nifedipine with beta blocker who underwent coronary artery bypass surgery using high-dose fentanyl anesthesia; possibility of this interaction cannot be ruled out with low-dose fentanyl or in other surgical procedures). Products include:
Duragesic Transdermal System 1786

Fentanyl Citrate (Severe hypotension and/or increased fluid volume requirements have been reported in patients receiving nifedipine with beta blocker who underwent coronary artery bypass surgery using high-dose fentanyl anesthesia; possibility of this interaction cannot be ruled out with low-dose fentanyl or in other surgical procedures). Products include:
Actiq 1184

Hydrocodone Bitartrate (Severe hypotension and/or increased fluid volume requirements have been reported in patients receiving nifedipine with beta blocker who underwent coronary artery bypass surgery using high-dose fentanyl anesthesia; possibility of this interaction cannot be ruled out with other narcotic analgesics or in other surgical procedures). Products include:
Hycodan 1316
Hycomine Compound Tablets 1317
Hycotuss Expectorant Syrup 1318
Lortab 3319
Lortab Elixir 3317
Maxidone Tablets CIII 3399
Norco 5/325 Tablets CIII 3424
Norco 7.5/325 Tablets CIII 3425
Norco 10/325 Tablets CIII 3427
Norco 10/325 Tablets CIII 3425
Vicodin Tablets 516
Vicodin ES Tablets 517
Vicodin HP Tablets 518
Vicodin Tuss Expectorant 519
Vicoprofen Tablets 520
Zydone Tablets 1330

Hydrocodone Polistirex (Severe hypotension and/or increased fluid volume requirements have been reported in patients receiving nifedipine with beta blocker who underwent coronary artery bypass surgery using high-dose fentanyl anesthesia; possibility of this interaction cannot be ruled out with other narcotic analgesics or in other surgical procedures). Products include:
Tussionex Pennkinetic Extended-Release Suspension 1174

Hydromorphone Hydrochloride (Severe hypotension and/or increased fluid volume requirements have been reported in patients receiving nifedipine with beta blocker who underwent coronary artery bypass surgery using high-dose fentanyl anesthesia; possibility of this interaction cannot be ruled out with other narcotic analgesics or in other surgical procedures). Products include:
Dilaudid 441
Dilaudid Oral Liquid 445
Dilaudid Powder 441
Dilaudid Rectal Suppositories 441
Dilaudid Tablets 441
Dilaudid Tablets - 8 mg 445
Dilaudid-HP 443

Labetalol Hydrochloride (Combination therapy may increase the likelihood of congestive heart failure, severe hypotension, or exacerbation of angina). Products include:
Normodyne Injection 3135
Normodyne Tablets 3137

Levobunolol Hydrochloride (Combination therapy may increase the likelihood of congestive heart failure, severe hypotension, or exacerbation of angina). Products include:
Betagan .... ⊙228

Levorphanol Tartrate (Severe hypotension and/or increased fluid volume requirements have been reported in patients receiving nifedipine with beta blocker who underwent coronary artery bypass surgery using high-dose fentanyl anesthesia; possibility of this interaction cannot be ruled out with other narcotic analgesics or in other surgical procedures). Products include:
Levo-Dromoran 1734
Levorphanol Tartrate Tablets 3059

Meperidine Hydrochloride (Severe hypotension and/or increased fluid volume requirements have been reported in patients receiving nifedipine with beta blocker who underwent coronary artery bypass surgery using high-dose fentanyl anesthesia; possibility of this interaction cannot be ruled out with other narcotic analgesics or in other surgical procedures). Products include:
Demerol 3079
Mepergan Injection 3539

Methadone Hydrochloride (Severe hypotension and/or increased fluid volume requirements have been reported in patients receiving nifedipine with beta blocker who underwent coronary artery bypass surgery using high-dose fentanyl anesthesia; possibility of this interaction cannot be ruled out with other narcotic analgesics or in other surgical procedures). Products include:
Dolophine Hydrochloride Tablets 3056

Metipranolol Hydrochloride (Combination therapy may increase the likelihood of congestive heart failure, severe hypotension, or exacerbation of angina).
No products indexed under this heading.

Metoprolol Succinate (Combination therapy may increase the likeli-

hood of congestive heart failure, severe hypotension, or exacerbation of angina). Products include:

Toprol-XL Tablets 651

Metoprolol Tartrate (Combination therapy may increase the likelihood of congestive heart failure, severe hypotension, or exacerbation of angina).

No products indexed under this heading.

Morphine Sulfate (Severe hypotension and/or increased fluid volume requirements have been reported in patients receiving nifedipine with beta blocker who underwent coronary artery bypass surgery using high-dose fentanyl anesthesia; possibility of this interaction cannot be ruled out with other narcotic analgesics or in other surgical procedures). Products include:

Astramorph/PF Injection, USP (Preservative-Free) 594
Duramorph Injection 1312
Infumorph 200 and Infumorph 500 Sterile Solutions 1314
Kadian Capsules 1335
MS Contin Tablets 2896
MSIR 2898
Oramorph SR Tablets 3062
Roxanol 3066

Nadolol (Combination therapy may increase the likelihood of congestive heart failure, severe hypotension, or exacerbation of angina). Products include:

Corgard Tablets 2245
Corzide 40/5 Tablets 2247
Corzide 80/5 Tablets 2247
Nadolol Tablets 2288

Oxycodone Hydrochloride (Severe hypotension and/or increased fluid volume requirements have been reported in patients receiving nifedipine with beta blocker who underwent coronary artery bypass surgery using high-dose fentanyl anesthesia; possibility of this interaction cannot be ruled out with other narcotic analgesics or in other surgical procedures). Products include:

OxyContin Tablets 2912
OxyFast Oral Concentrate Solution 2916
OxyIR Capsules 2916
Percocet Tablets 1326
Percodan Tablets 1327
Percolone Tablets 1327
Roxicodone 3067
Tylox Capsules 2597

Penbutolol Sulfate (Combination therapy may increase the likelihood of congestive heart failure, severe hypotension, or exacerbation of angina).

No products indexed under this heading.

Pindolol (Combination therapy may increase the likelihood of congestive heart failure, severe hypotension, or exacerbation of angina).

No products indexed under this heading.

Propoxyphene Hydrochloride (Severe hypotension and/or increased fluid volume requirements have been reported in patients receiving nifedipine with beta blocker who underwent coronary artery bypass surgery using high-dose fentanyl anesthesia; possibility of this interaction cannot be ruled out with other narcotic analgesics or in other surgical procedures). Products include:

Darvon Pulvules 1909
Darvon Compound-65 Pulvules 1910

Propoxyphene Napsylate (Severe hypotension and/or increased fluid volume requirements have been reported in patients receiving nifedipine with beta blocker who underwent coronary artery bypass surgery using high-dose fentanyl anesthesia; possibility of this interaction cannot be ruled out with other narcotic analgesics or in other surgical procedures). Products include:

Darvon-N/Darvocet-N 1907
Darvon-N Tablets 1912

Propranolol Hydrochloride (Combination therapy may increase the likelihood of congestive heart failure, severe hypotension, or exacerbation of angina). Products include:

Inderal 3513
Inderal LA Long-Acting Capsules 3516
Inderide Tablets 3517
Inderide LA Long-Acting Capsules 3519

Quinidine Gluconate (Co-administration of Procardia and quinidine has resulted in rare reports of decreased plasma level of quinidine). Products include:

Quinaglute Dura-Tabs Tablets 978

Quinidine Polygalacturonate (Co-administration of Procardia and quinidine has resulted in rare reports of decreased plasma level of quinidine).

No products indexed under this heading.

Quinidine Sulfate (Co-administration of Procardia and quinidine has resulted in rare reports of decreased plasma level of quinidine). Products include:

Quinidex Extentabs 2933

Ranitidine Hydrochloride (Co-administration produces smaller non-significant increases in nifedipine level). Products include:

Zantac 1690
Zantac Injection 1688
Zantac 75 Tablets .... ▣717

Remifentanil Hydrochloride (Severe hypotension and/or increased fluid volume requirements have been reported in patients receiving nifedipine with beta blocker who underwent coronary artery bypass surgery using high-dose fentanyl anesthesia; possibility of this interaction cannot be ruled out with other narcotic analgesics or in other surgical procedures).

No products indexed under this heading.

Sotalol Hydrochloride (Combination therapy may increase the likelihood of congestive heart failure, severe hypotension, or exacerbation of angina). Products include:

Betapace Tablets 950
Betapace AF Tablets 954

Sufentanil Citrate (Severe hypotension and/or increased fluid volume requirements have been reported in patients receiving nifedipine with beta blocker who underwent coronary artery bypass surgery using high-dose fentanyl anesthesia; possibility of this interaction cannot be ruled out with other narcotic analgesics or in other surgical procedures).

No products indexed under this heading.

Timolol Hemihydrate (Combination therapy may increase the likelihood of congestive heart failure, severe hypotension, or exacerbation of angina). Products include:

Betimol Ophthalmic Solution .... ⊙324

Timolol Maleate (Combination therapy may increase the likelihood of congestive heart failure, severe hypotension, or exacerbation of angina). Products include:

Blocadren Tablets 2046
Cosopt Sterile Ophthalmic Solution 2065
Timolide Tablets 2187
Timolol GFS .... ⊙266
Timoptic in Ocudose 2192
Timoptic Sterile Ophthalmic Solution 2190
Timoptic-XE Sterile Ophthalmic Gel Forming Solution 2194

Warfarin Sodium (Co-administration has resulted in rare reports of increased prothrombin time; relationship to nifedipine therapy is uncertain). Products include:

Coumadin for Injection 1243
Coumadin Tablets 1243
Warfarin Sodium Tablets, USP 3302

Food Interactions

Grapefruit Juice (Co-administration of nifedipine with grapefruit juice has resulted in approximately a 2-fold increase in nifedipine AUC and Cmax and no change in half-life; concurrent use should be avoided).

PROCARDIA XL EXTENDED RELEASE TABLETS

(Nifedipine) 2710
See Procardia Capsules

PROCRIT FOR INJECTION

(Epoetin Alfa) 2502
None cited in PDR database.

PROCTOCORT SUPPOSITORIES

(Hydrocortisone Acetate) 2264
None cited in PDR database.

PROCTOFOAM-HC

(Hydrocortisone Acetate, Pramoxine Hydrochloride) 3177
None cited in PDR database.

PROFLAVANOL TABLETS

(Dietary Supplement) 3335
None cited in PDR database.

PROGRAF

(Tacrolimus) 1393
May interact with aminoglycosides, erythromycin, phenytoin, protease inhibitors, potassium sparing diuretics, and certain other agents. Compounds in these categories include:

Amikacin Sulfate (Potential for additive or synergistic impairment of renal function).

No products indexed under this heading.

Amiloride Hydrochloride (Mild to severe hyperkalemia has been reported with tacrolimus; concurrent use with potassium-sparing diuretics should be avoided). Products include:

Midamor Tablets 2136
Moduretic Tablets 2138

Amphotericin B (Potential for additive or synergistic impairment of renal function). Products include:

Abelcet Injection 1273
AmBisome for Injection 1383
Amphotec 1774

Amprenavir (Co-administration with drugs known to inhibit CYP3A enzyme systems, such as protease inhibitors, may increase tacrolimus blood concentrations). Products include:

Agenerase Capsules 1454
Agenerase Oral Solution 1459

Bromocriptine Mesylate (Co-administration with drugs known to inhibit CYP3A enzyme systems, such as bromocriptine, may increase tacrolimus blood concentrations).

No products indexed under this heading.

Carbamazepine (Co-administration with drugs known to induce CYP3A enzyme systems, such as carbamazepine, may result in increased metabolism of tacrolimus and decreased blood or plasma concentrations). Products include:

Carbatrol Capsules 3234
Tegretol/Tegretol-XR 2404

Cimetidine (Co-administration with drugs known to inhibit CYP3A enzyme systems, such as cimetidine, may increase tacrolimus blood concentrations). Products include:

Tagamet HB 200 Suspension .... ▣762
Tagamet HB 200 Tablets .... ▣761
Tagamet Tablets 1644

Cimetidine Hydrochloride (Co-administration with drugs known to inhibit CYP3A enzyme systems, such as cimetidine, may increase tacrolimus blood concentrations). Products include:

Tagamet 1644

Cisapride (Co-administration with drugs known to inhibit CYP3A enzyme systems, such as cisapride, may increase tacrolimus blood concentrations).

No products indexed under this heading.

Cisplatin (Potential for additive or synergistic impairment of renal function).

No products indexed under this heading.

Clarithromycin (Co-administration with drugs known to inhibit CYP3A enzyme systems, such as clarithromycin, may increase tacrolimus blood concentrations). Products include:

Biaxin/Biaxin XL 403
PREVPAC 3298

Clotrimazole (Co-administration with drugs known to inhibit CYP3A enzyme systems, such as clotrimazole, may increase tacrolimus blood concentrations). Products include:

Gyne-Lotrimin 3, 3-Day Cream .... ▣741
Lotrimin AF Cream, Lotion, Solution, and Jock Itch Cream .... ▣742
Lotrimin 3128
Lotrisone 3129
Mycelex Troche 573
Mycelex-7 Combination-Pack Vaginal Inserts & External Vulvar Cream .... ▣614
Mycelex-7 Vaginal Cream .... ▣614
Mycelex-7 Vaginal Cream with 7 Disposable Applicators .... ▣614

Cyclosporine (Increases tacrolimus blood levels resulting in additive/synergistic nephrotoxicity; Prograf should not be used simultaneously with cyclosporine; Prograf or cyclosporine should be discontinued at least 24 hours or more prior to initiating the other). Products include:

Gengraf Capsules 457
Neoral Soft Gelatin Capsules 2380
Neoral Oral Solution 2380
Sandimmune 2388

Danazol (Co-administration with drugs known to inhibit CYP3A enzyme systems, such as danazol, may increase tacrolimus blood concentrations).

No products indexed under this heading.

Diltiazem Hydrochloride (Co-administration with drugs known to inhibit CYP3A enzyme systems, such as diltiazem, may increase tacrolimus blood concentrations). Products include:

Cardizem Injectable 1018
Cardizem Lyo-Ject Syringe 1018
Cardizem Monovial 1018
Cardizem CD Capsules 1016
Tiazac Capsules 1378

Erythromycin (Co-administration with drugs known to inhibit CYP3A enzyme systems, such as erythromycin, may increase tacrolimus blood concentrations). Products include:

Emgel 2% Topical Gel 1285
Ery-Tab Tablets 448
Erythromycin Base Filmtab Tablets 454
Erythromycin Delayed-Release Capsules, USP 455
PCE Dispertab Tablets 498

Erythromycin Estolate (Co-administration with drugs known to inhibit CYP3A enzyme systems, such as erythromycin, may increase tacrolimus blood concentrations).

No products indexed under this heading.

Erythromycin Ethylsuccinate (Co-administration with drugs known to inhibit CYP3A enzyme systems, such as erythromycin, may increase tacrolimus blood concentrations). Products include:
- E.E.S. 450
- EryPed 446
- Pediazole Suspension 3050

Erythromycin Gluceptate (Co-administration with drugs known to inhibit CYP3A enzyme systems, such as erythromycin, may increase tacrolimus blood concentrations).
- No products indexed under this heading.

Erythromycin Stearate (Co-administration with drugs known to inhibit CYP3A enzyme systems, such as erythromycin, may increase tacrolimus blood concentrations). Products include:
- Erythrocin Stearate Filmtab Tablets 452

Fluconazole (Co-administration with drugs known to inhibit CYP3A enzyme systems, such as fluconazole, may increase tacrolimus blood concentrations). Products include:
- Diflucan Tablets, Injection, and Oral Suspension 2681

Fosphenytoin Sodium (Co-administration with drugs known to induce CYP3A enzyme systems, such as phenytoin, may result in increased metabolism of tacrolimus and decreased blood or plasma concentrations). Products include:
- Cerebyx Injection 2619

Ganciclovir (May increase nephrotoxicity). Products include:
- Cytovene Capsules 2959
- Vitrasert Implant .... ⊙254

Ganciclovir Sodium (May increase nephrotoxicity). Products include:
- Cytovene-IV 2959

Gentamicin Sulfate (Potential for additive or synergistic impairment of renal function). Products include:
- Genoptic Ophthalmic Ointment .... ⊙239
- Genoptic Sterile Ophthalmic Solution .... ⊙239
- Pred-G Ophthalmic Suspension .... ⊙247
- Pred-G Sterile Ophthalmic Ointment .... ⊙248

Indinavir Sulfate (Co-administration with drugs known to inhibit CYP3A enzyme systems, such as protease inhibitors, may increase tacrolimus blood concentrations). Products include:
- Crixivan Capsules 2070

Itraconazole (Co-administration with drugs known to inhibit CYP3A enzyme systems, such as itraconazole, may increase tacrolimus blood concentrations). Products include:
- Sporanox Capsules 1800
- Sporanox Injection 1804
- Sporanox Injection 2509
- Sporanox Oral Solution 1808
- Sporanox Oral Solution 2512

Kanamycin Sulfate (Potential for additive or synergistic impairment of renal function).
- No products indexed under this heading.

Ketoconazole (Co-administration with drugs known to inhibit CYP3A enzyme systems, such as ketoconazole, may increase tacrolimus blood concentrations). Products include:
- Nizoral 2% Cream 3620
- Nizoral A-D Shampoo 2008
- Nizoral 2% Shampoo 2007
- Nizoral Tablets 1791

Lopinavir (Co-administration with drugs known to inhibit CYP3A enzyme systems, such as protease inhibitors, may increase tacrolimus blood concentrations). Products include:
- Kaletra Capsules 471
- Kaletra Oral Solution 471

Measles, Mumps & Rubella Virus Vaccine, Live (During treatment with tacrolimus, vaccination may be less effective). Products include:
- M-M-R II 2118

Measles & Rubella Virus Vaccine Live (During treatment with tacrolimus, vaccination may be less effective).
- No products indexed under this heading.

Measles Virus Vaccine Live (During treatment with tacrolimus, vaccination may be less effective). Products include:
- Attenuvax 2044

Methylprednisolone (Co-administration with drugs known to inhibit CYP3A enzyme systems, such as methylprednisolone, may increase tacrolimus blood concentrations).
- No products indexed under this heading.

Metoclopramide Hydrochloride (Co-administration with drugs known to inhibit CYP3A enzyme systems, such as metoclopramide, may increase tacrolimus blood concentrations). Products include:
- Reglan 2935

Nelfinavir Mesylate (Co-administration with drugs known to inhibit CYP3A enzyme systems, such as protease inhibitors, may increase tacrolimus blood concentrations). Products include:
- Viracept 532

Nicardipine Hydrochloride (Co-administration with drugs known to inhibit CYP3A enzyme systems, such as nicardipine, may increase tacrolimus blood concentrations). Products include:
- Cardene I.V. 3485

Nifedipine (Co-administration with drugs known to inhibit CYP3A enzyme systems, such as nifedipine, may increase tacrolimus blood concentrations). Products include:
- Adalat CC Tablets 877
- Procardia Capsules 2708
- Procardia XL Extended Release Tablets 2710

Phenobarbital (Co-administration with drugs known to induce CYP3A enzyme systems, such as phenobarbital, may result in increased metabolism of tacrolimus and decreased blood or plasma concentrations). Products include:
- Arco-Lase Plus Tablets 592
- Donnatal 2929
- Donnatal Extentabs 2930

Phenytoin (Co-administration with drugs known to induce CYP3A enzyme systems, such as phenytoin, may result in increased metabolism of tacrolimus and decreased blood or plasma concentrations). Products include:
- Dilantin Infatabs 2624
- Dilantin-125 Oral Suspension 2625

Phenytoin Sodium (Co-administration with drugs known to induce CYP3A enzyme systems, such as phenytoin, may result in increased metabolism of tacrolimus and decreased blood or plasma concentrations). Products include:
- Dilantin Kapseals 2622

Poliovirus Vaccine, Live, Oral, Trivalent, Types 1,2,3 (Sabin) (During treatment with tacrolimus, vaccination may be less effective).
- No products indexed under this heading.

Poliovirus Vaccine Inactivated, Trivalent Types 1,2,3 (During treatment with tacrolimus, vaccination may be less effective). Products include:
- IPOL Vaccine 809

Rifabutin (Co-administration with drugs known to induce CYP3A enzyme systems, such as rifabutin, may result in increased metabolism of tacrolimus and decreased blood or plasma concentrations). Products include:
- Mycobutin Capsules 2838

Rifampin (Co-administration with drugs known to induce CYP3A enzyme systems, such as refampin, may result in increased metabolism of tacrolimus and decreased blood or plasma concentrations). Products include:
- Rifadin 765
- Rifamate Capsules 767
- Rifater Tablets 769

Ritonavir (Co-administration with drugs known to inhibit CYP3A enzyme systems, such as protease inhibitors, may increase tacrolimus blood concentrations). Products include:
- Kaletra Capsules 471
- Kaletra Oral Solution 471
- Norvir Capsules 487
- Norvir Oral Solution 487

Saquinavir (Co-administration with drugs known to inhibit CYP3A enzyme systems, such as protease inhibitors, may increase tacrolimus blood concentrations). Products include:
- Fortovase Capsules 2970

Saquinavir Mesylate (Co-administration with drugs known to inhibit CYP3A enzyme systems, such as protease inhibitors, may increase tacrolimus blood concentrations). Products include:
- Invirase Capsules 2979

Spironolactone (Mild to severe hyperkalemia has been reported with tacrolimus; concurrent use with potassium-sparing diuretics should be avoided).
- No products indexed under this heading.

Streptomycin Sulfate (Potential for additive or synergistic impairment of renal function). Products include:
- Streptomycin Sulfate Injection 2714

Tobramycin (Potential for additive or synergistic impairment of renal function). Products include:
- TOBI Solution for Inhalation 1206
- TobraDex Ophthalmic Ointment 542
- TobraDex Ophthalmic Suspension 541
- Tobrex Ophthalmic Ointment .... ⊙220
- Tobrex Ophthalmic Solution .... ⊙221

Tobramycin Sulfate (Potential for additive or synergistic impairment of renal function). Products include:
- Nebcin Vials, Hyporets & ADD-Vantage 1955

Triamterene (Mild to severe hyperkalemia has been reported with tacrolimus; concurrent use with potassium-sparing diuretics should be avoided). Products include:
- Dyazide Capsules 1515
- Dyrenium Capsules 3458
- Maxzide 1008

Troleandomycin (Co-administration with drugs known to inhibit CYP3A enzyme systems, such as troleandomycin, may increase tacrolimus blood concentrations). Products include:
- Tao Capsules 2716

Typhoid Vaccine Live Oral TY21a (During treatment with tacrolimus, vaccination may be less effective). Products include:
- Vivotif Berna 997

Vaccines (Live) (During treatment with tacrolimus, vaccination may be less effective).
- No products indexed under this heading.

Verapamil Hydrochloride (Co-administration with drugs known to inhibit CYP3A enzyme systems, such as verapamil, may increase tacrolimus blood concentrations). Products include:
- Covera-HS Tablets 3199
- Isoptin SR Tablets 467
- Tarka Tablets 508
- Verelan Capsules 3184
- Verelan PM Capsules 3186

Yellow Fever Vaccine (During treatment with tacrolimus, vaccination may be less effective). Products include:
- YF-VAX Vaccine 827

Food Interactions

Food, unspecified (The presence and composition of food has decreased both the rate and extent of tacrolimus absorption; this effect was most pronounced with a high-fat meal; the rate and extent of tacrolimus absorption were greatest under fasted conditions).

Grapefruit Juice (Co-administered grapefruit juice has been reported to increase tacrolimus blood trough concentrations in liver transplant patients; grapefruit juice should be avoided).

PROLASTIN

(Alpha$_1$ -Proteinase Inhibitor (Human)) 943

None cited in PDR database.

PROLEUKIN FOR INJECTION

(Aldesleukin) 1199

May interact with aminoglycosides, antihypertensives, beta blockers, cytotoxic drugs, glucocorticoids, hypnotics and sedatives, narcotic analgesics, radiographic iodinated contrast media, tranquilizers, and certain other agents. Compounds in these categories include:

Acebutolol Hydrochloride (May potentiate the hypotension seen with aldesleukin). Products include:
- Sectral Capsules 3589

Alfentanil Hydrochloride (Potential for unspecified effect on central nervous function).
- No products indexed under this heading.

Alprazolam (Potential for unspecified effect on central nervous function). Products include:
- Xanax Tablets 2865

Amikacin Sulfate (Potential for increased nephrotoxicity).
- No products indexed under this heading.

Amlodipine Besylate (May potentiate the hypotension seen with aldesleukin). Products include:
- Lotrel Capsules 2370
- Norvasc Tablets 2704

Asparaginase (Potential for increased hepatic toxicity). Products include:
- Elspar for Injection 2092

Atenolol (May potentiate the hypotension seen with aldesleukin). Products include:
- Tenoretic Tablets 690
- Tenormin I.V. Injection 692

Benazepril Hydrochloride (May potentiate the hypotension seen with aldesleukin). Products include:
- Lotensin Tablets 2365
- Lotensin HCT Tablets 2367
- Lotrel Capsules 2370

Bendroflumethiazide (May potentiate the hypotension seen with aldesleukin). Products include:
- Corzide 40/5 Tablets 2247
- Corzide 80/5 Tablets 2247

Betamethasone Acetate (May reduce the antitumor effectiveness of aldesleukin). Products include:
- Celestone Soluspan Injectable Suspension 3097

Betamethasone Sodium Phosphate (May reduce the antitumor effectiveness of aldesleukin). Products include:
- Celestone Soluspan Injectable Suspension 3097

Betaxolol Hydrochloride (May potentiate the hypotension seen with aldesleukin). Products include:

Betoptic S Ophthalmic Suspension 537

Bisoprolol Fumarate (May potentiate the hypotension seen with aldesleukin). Products include:
Zebeta Tablets 1885
Ziac Tablets 1887

Bleomycin Sulfate (Potential for increased myelotoxicity).
No products indexed under this heading.

Buprenorphine Hydrochloride (Potential for unspecified effect on central nervous function). Products include:
Buprenex Injectable 2918

Buspirone Hydrochloride (Potential for unspecified effect on central nervous function).
No products indexed under this heading.

Candesartan Cilexetil (May potentiate the hypotension seen with aldesleukin). Products include:
Atacand Tablets 595
Atacand HCT Tablets 597

Captopril (May potentiate the hypotension seen with aldesleukin). Products include:
Captopril Tablets 2281

Carteolol Hydrochloride (May potentiate the hypotension seen with aldesleukin). Products include:
Carteolol Hydrochloride Ophthalmic Solution USP, 1% .... ⊙258
Ocupress Ophthalmic Solution, 1% Sterile .... ⊙303

Chlordiazepoxide (Potential for unspecified effect on central nervous function). Products include:
Limbitrol 1738

Chlordiazepoxide Hydrochloride (Potential for unspecified effect on central nervous function). Products include:
Librium Capsules 1736
Librium for Injection 1737

Chlorothiazide (May potentiate the hypotension seen with aldesleukin). Products include:
Aldoclor Tablets 2035
Diuril Oral 2087

Chlorothiazide Sodium (May potentiate the hypotension seen with aldesleukin). Products include:
Diuril Sodium Intravenous 2086

Chlorpromazine (Potential for unspecified effect on central nervous function). Products include:
Thorazine Suppositories 1656

Chlorpromazine Hydrochloride (Potential for unspecified effect on central nervous function). Products include:
Thorazine 1656

Chlorprothixene (Potential for unspecified effect on central nervous function).
No products indexed under this heading.

Chlorprothixene Hydrochloride (Potential for unspecified effect on central nervous function).
No products indexed under this heading.

Chlorthalidone (May potentiate the hypotension seen with aldesleukin). Products include:
Clorpres Tablets 1002
Combipres Tablets 1040
Tenoretic Tablets 690

Clonidine (May potentiate the hypotension seen with aldesleukin). Products include:
Catapres-TTS 1038

Clonidine Hydrochloride (May potentiate the hypotension seen with aldesleukin). Products include:
Catapres Tablets 1037
Clorpres Tablets 1002
Combipres Tablets 1040
Duraclon Injection 3057

Clorazepate Dipotassium (Potential for unspecified effect on central nervous function). Products include:
Tranxene 511

Codeine Phosphate (Potential for unspecified effect on central nervous function). Products include:
Phenergan with Codeine Syrup 3557
Phenergan VC with Codeine Syrup 3561
Robitussin A-C Syrup 2942
Robitussin-DAC Syrup 2942
Ryna-C Liquid 768
Soma Compound w/Codeine Tablets 3355
Tussi-Organidin NR Liquid 3350
Tussi-Organidin-S NR Liquid 3350
Tylenol with Codeine 2595

Cortisone Acetate (May reduce the antitumor effectiveness of aldesleukin). Products include:
Cortone Acetate Injectable Suspension 2059
Cortone Acetate Tablets 2061

Cyclophosphamide (Potential for increased myelotoxicity).
No products indexed under this heading.

Daunorubicin Hydrochloride (Potential for increased myelotoxicity). Products include:
Cerubidine for Injection 947

Deserpidine (May potentiate the hypotension seen with aldesleukin).
No products indexed under this heading.

Dexamethasone (May reduce the antitumor effectiveness of aldesleukin). Products include:
Decadron Elixir 2078
Decadron Tablets 2079
TobraDex Ophthalmic Ointment 542
TobraDex Ophthalmic Suspension 541

Dexamethasone Acetate (May reduce the antitumor effectiveness of aldesleukin).
No products indexed under this heading.

Dexamethasone Sodium Phosphate (May reduce the antitumor effectiveness of aldesleukin). Products include:
Decadron Phosphate Injection 2081
Decadron Phosphate Sterile Ophthalmic Ointment 2083
Decadron Phosphate Sterile Ophthalmic Solution 2084
NeoDecadron Sterile Ophthalmic Solution 2144

Dezocine (Potential for unspecified effect on central nervous function).
No products indexed under this heading.

Diatrizoate Meglumine (Potential for delayed adverse reactions to iodinated contrast media including fever, chills, nausea, vomiting, pruritus, rash, diarrhea, hypotension, edema, and oliguria).
No products indexed under this heading.

Diatrizoate Sodium (Potential for delayed adverse reactions to iodinated contrast media including fever, chills, nausea, vomiting, pruritus, rash, diarrhea, hypotension, edema, and oliguria).
No products indexed under this heading.

Diazepam (Potential for unspecified effect on central nervous function). Products include:
Valium Injectable 3026
Valium Tablets 3047

Diazoxide (May potentiate the hypotension seen with aldesleukin).
No products indexed under this heading.

Diltiazem Hydrochloride (May potentiate the hypotension seen with aldesleukin). Products include:
Cardizem Injectable 1018
Cardizem Lyo-Ject Syringe 1018
Cardizem Monovial 1018
Cardizem CD Capsules 1016
Tiazac Capsules 1378

Doxazosin Mesylate (May potentiate the hypotension seen with aldesleukin). Products include:
Cardura Tablets 2668

Doxorubicin Hydrochloride (Potential for increased cardiotoxicity and myelotoxicity). Products include:
Adriamycin PFS/RDF Injection 2767
Doxil Injection 566

Droperidol (Potential for unspecified effect on central nervous function).
No products indexed under this heading.

Enalapril Maleate (May potentiate the hypotension seen with aldesleukin). Products include:
Lexxel Tablets 608
Vaseretic Tablets 2204
Vasotec Tablets 2210

Enalaprilat (May potentiate the hypotension seen with aldesleukin). Products include:
Enalaprilat Injection 863
Vasotec I.V. Injection 2207

Epirubicin Hydrochloride (Potential for increased myelotoxicity). Products include:
Ellence Injection 2806

Eprosartan Mesylate (May potentiate the hypotension seen with aldesleukin). Products include:
Teveten Tablets 3327

Esmolol Hydrochloride (May potentiate the hypotension seen with aldesleukin). Products include:
Brevibloc Injection 858

Estazolam (Potential for unspecified effect on central nervous function). Products include:
ProSom Tablets 500

Ethchlorvynol (Potential for unspecified effect on central nervous function).
No products indexed under this heading.

Ethinamate (Potential for unspecified effect on central nervous function).
No products indexed under this heading.

Ethiodized Oil (Potential for delayed adverse reactions to iodinated contrast media including fever, chills, nausea, vomiting, pruritus, rash, diarrhea, hypotension, edema, and oliguria). Products include:
Ethiodol Injection 3095

Felodipine (May potentiate the hypotension seen with aldesleukin). Products include:
Lexxel Tablets 608
Plendil Extended-Release Tablets 623

Fentanyl (Potential for unspecified effect on central nervous function). Products include:
Duragesic Transdermal System 1786

Fentanyl Citrate (Potential for unspecified effect on central nervous function). Products include:
Actiq 1184

Fludrocortisone Acetate (May reduce the antitumor effectiveness of aldesleukin). Products include:
Florinef Acetate Tablets 2250

Fluorouracil (Potential for increased myelotoxicity). Products include:
Carac Cream 1222
Efudex 1733
Fluoroplex 552

Fluphenazine Decanoate (Potential for unspecified effect on central nervous function).
No products indexed under this heading.

Fluphenazine Enanthate (Potential for unspecified effect on central nervous function).
No products indexed under this heading.

Fluphenazine Hydrochloride (Potential for unspecified effect on central nervous function).
No products indexed under this heading.

Flurazepam Hydrochloride (Potential for unspecified effect on central nervous function).
No products indexed under this heading.

Fosinopril Sodium (May potentiate the hypotension seen with aldesleukin). Products include:
Monopril Tablets 1091
Monopril HCT 1094

Furosemide (May potentiate the hypotension seen with aldesleukin). Products include:
Furosemide Tablets 2284

Gadopentetate Dimeglumine (Potential for delayed adverse reactions to iodinated contrast media including fever, chills, nausea, vomiting, pruritus, rash, diarrhea, hypotension, edema, and oliguria).
No products indexed under this heading.

Gentamicin Sulfate (Potential for increased nephrotoxicity). Products include:
Genoptic Ophthalmic Ointment .... ⊙239
Genoptic Sterile Ophthalmic Solution .... ⊙239
Pred-G Ophthalmic Suspension .... ⊙247
Pred-G Sterile Ophthalmic Ointment .... ⊙248

Glutethimide (Potential for unspecified effect on central nervous function).
No products indexed under this heading.

Guanabenz Acetate (May potentiate the hypotension seen with aldesleukin).
No products indexed under this heading.

Guanethidine Monosulfate (May potentiate the hypotension seen with aldesleukin).
No products indexed under this heading.

Haloperidol (Potential for unspecified effect on central nervous function). Products include:
Haldol Injection, Tablets and Concentrate 2533

Haloperidol Decanoate (Potential for unspecified effect on central nervous function). Products include:
Haldol Decanoate 2535

Hepatotoxic Drugs, unspecified (Potential for increased hepatic toxicity).

Hydralazine Hydrochloride (May potentiate the hypotension seen with aldesleukin).
No products indexed under this heading.

Hydrochlorothiazide (May potentiate the hypotension seen with aldesleukin). Products include:
Accuretic Tablets 2614
Aldoril Tablets 2039
Atacand HCT Tablets 597
Avalide Tablets 1070
Diovan HCT Tablets 2338
Dyazide Capsules 1515
HydroDIURIL Tablets 2108
Hyzaar 2109
Inderide Tablets 3517
Inderide LA Long-Acting Capsules 3519
Lotensin HCT Tablets 2367
Maxzide 1008
Micardis HCT Tablets 1051
Microzide Capsules 3414
Moduretic Tablets 2138
Monopril HCT 1094
Prinzide Tablets 2168
Timolide Tablets 2187
Uniretic Tablets 3178
Vaseretic Tablets 2204
Zestoretic Tablets 695
Ziac Tablets 1887

Hydrocodone Bitartrate (Potential for unspecified effect on central nervous function). Products include:
Hycodan 1316
Hycomine Compound Tablets 1317
Hycotuss Expectorant Syrup 1318
Lortab 3319
Lortab Elixir 3317

IMPORTANT NOTE: Always consult each drug listing in the patient's regimen for possible interactions.

Maxidone Tablets CIII 3399
Norco 5/325 Tablets CIII 3424
Norco 7.5/325 Tablets CIII 3425
Norco 10/325 Tablets CIII 3427
Norco 10/325 Tablets CIII 3425
Vicodin Tablets 516
Vicodin ES Tablets 517
Vicodin HP Tablets 518
Vicodin Tuss Expectorant 519
Vicoprofen Tablets 520
Zydone Tablets 1330

Hydrocodone Polistirex (Potential for unspecified effect on central nervous function). Products include:
Tussionex Pennkinetic Extended-Release Suspension 1174

Hydrocortisone (May reduce the antitumor effectiveness of aldesleukin). Products include:
Anusol-HC Cream 2.5% 2237
Cipro HC Otic Suspension 540
Cortaid Intensive Therapy Cream ..... ▣ 717
Cortaid Maximum Strength Cream ..... ▣ 717
Cortisporin Ophthalmic Suspension Sterile ..... ⊙ 297
Cortizone•5 ..... ▣ 699
Cortizone•10 ..... ▣ 699
Cortizone•10 Plus Creme ..... ▣ 700
Cortizone for Kids Creme ..... ▣ 699
Hydrocortone Tablets 2106
Massengill Medicated Soft Cloth Towelette ..... ▣ 753
VōSoL HC Otic Solution 3356

Hydrocortisone Acetate (May reduce the antitumor effectiveness of aldesleukin). Products include:
Analpram-HC 1338
Anusol HC-1 Hydrocortisone Anti-Itch Cream ..... ▣ 689
Anusol-HC Suppositories 2238
Cortaid ..... ▣ 717
Cortifoam Rectal Foam 3170
Cortisporin-TC Otic Suspension 2246
Hydrocortone Acetate Injectable Suspension 2103
Pramosone 1343
Proctocort Suppositories 2264
ProctoFoam-HC 3177
Terra-Cortril Ophthalmic Suspension 2716

Hydrocortisone Sodium Phosphate (May reduce the antitumor effectiveness of aldesleukin). Products include:
Hydrocortone Phosphate Injection, Sterile 2105

Hydrocortisone Sodium Succinate (May reduce the antitumor effectiveness of aldesleukin).
No products indexed under this heading.

Hydroflumethiazide (May potentiate the hypotension seen with aldesleukin). Products include:
Diucardin Tablets 3494

Hydromorphone Hydrochloride (Potential for unspecified effect on central nervous function). Products include:
Dilaudid 441
Dilaudid Oral Liquid 445
Dilaudid Powder 441
Dilaudid Rectal Suppositories 441
Dilaudid Tablets 441
Dilaudid Tablets - 8 mg 445
Dilaudid-HP 443

Hydroxyurea (Potential for increased myelotoxicity). Products include:
Mylocel Tablets 2227

Hydroxyzine Hydrochloride (Potential for unspecified effect on central nervous function). Products include:
Atarax Tablets & Syrup 2667
Vistaril Intramuscular Solution 2738

Indapamide (May potentiate the hypotension seen with aldesleukin). Products include:
Indapamide Tablets 2286

Indomethacin (Potential for increased nephrotoxicity). Products include:
Indocin 2112

Interferon alfa-2A, Recombinant (Co-administration of Proleukin and interferon-alfa has resulted in increased incidence of myocardial injury, including myocardial infarction, myocarditis, ventricular hypokinesia, and severe rhabdomyolysis; exacerbation or the initial presentation of a number of autoimmune and inflammatory disorders has been observed with concurrent use). Products include:
Roferon-A Injection 2996

Interferon alfa-2B, Recombinant (Co-administration of Proleukin and interferon-alfa has resulted in increased incidence of myocardial injury, including myocardial infarction, myocarditis, ventricular hypokinesia, and severe rhabdomyolysis; exacerbation or the initial presentation of a number of autoimmune and inflammatory disorders has been observed with concurrent use). Products include:
Intron A for Injection 3120
Rebetron Combination Therapy 3153

Iodamide Meglumine (Potential for delayed adverse reactions to iodinated contrast media including fever, chills, nausea, vomiting, pruritus, rash, diarrhea, hypotension, edema, and oliguria).
No products indexed under this heading.

Iohexol (Potential for delayed adverse reactions to iodinated contrast media including fever, chills, nausea, vomiting, pruritus, rash, diarrhea, hypotension, edema, and oliguria).
No products indexed under this heading.

Iopamidol (Potential for delayed adverse reactions to iodinated contrast media including fever, chills, nausea, vomiting, pruritus, rash, diarrhea, hypotension, edema, and oliguria).
No products indexed under this heading.

Iopanoic Acid (Potential for delayed adverse reactions to iodinated contrast media including fever, chills, nausea, vomiting, pruritus, rash, diarrhea, hypotension, edema, and oliguria).

Iothalamate Meglumine (Potential for delayed adverse reactions to iodinated contrast media including fever, chills, nausea, vomiting, pruritus, rash, diarrhea, hypotension, edema, and oliguria).
No products indexed under this heading.

Ioxaglate Meglumine (Potential for delayed adverse reactions to iodinated contrast media including fever, chills, nausea, vomiting, pruritus, rash, diarrhea, hypotension, edema, and oliguria).
No products indexed under this heading.

Ioxaglate Sodium (Potential for delayed adverse reactions to iodinated contrast media including fever, chills, nausea, vomiting, pruritus, rash, diarrhea, hypotension, edema, and oliguria).
No products indexed under this heading.

Irbesartan (May potentiate the hypotension seen with aldesleukin). Products include:
Avalide Tablets 1070
Avapro Tablets 1074
Avapro Tablets 3076

Isradipine (May potentiate the hypotension seen with aldesleukin). Products include:
DynaCirc Capsules 2921
DynaCirc CR Tablets 2923

Kanamycin Sulfate (Potential for increased nephrotoxicity).
No products indexed under this heading.

Labetalol Hydrochloride (May potentiate the hypotension seen with aldesleukin). Products include:
Normodyne Injection 3135
Normodyne Tablets 3137

Levobunolol Hydrochloride (May potentiate the hypotension seen with aldesleukin). Products include:
Betagan ..... ⊙ 228

Levorphanol Tartrate (Potential for unspecified effect on central nervous function). Products include:
Levo-Dromoran 1734
Levorphanol Tartrate Tablets 3059

Lisinopril (May potentiate the hypotension seen with aldesleukin). Products include:
Prinivil Tablets 2164
Prinzide Tablets 2168
Zestoretic Tablets 695
Zestril Tablets 698

Lorazepam (Potential for unspecified effect on central nervous function). Products include:
Ativan Injection 3478
Ativan Tablets 3482

Losartan Potassium (May potentiate the hypotension seen with aldesleukin). Products include:
Cozaar Tablets 2067
Hyzaar 2109

Loxapine Hydrochloride (Potential for unspecified effect on central nervous function).
No products indexed under this heading.

Loxapine Succinate (Potential for unspecified effect on central nervous function). Products include:
Loxitane Capsules 3398

Mecamylamine Hydrochloride (May potentiate the hypotension seen with aldesleukin). Products include:
Inversine Tablets 1850

Meperidine Hydrochloride (Potential for unspecified effect on central nervous function). Products include:
Demerol 3079
Mepergan Injection 3539

Meprobamate (Potential for unspecified effect on central nervous function). Products include:
Miltown Tablets 3349

Mesoridazine Besylate (Potential for unspecified effect on central nervous function). Products include:
Serentil 1057

Methadone Hydrochloride (Potential for unspecified effect on central nervous function). Products include:
Dolophine Hydrochloride Tablets 3056

Methotrexate Sodium (Potential for increased hepatic toxicity and myelotoxicity).
No products indexed under this heading.

Methyclothiazide (May potentiate the hypotension seen with aldesleukin).
No products indexed under this heading.

Methyldopa (May potentiate the hypotension seen with aldesleukin). Products include:
Aldoclor Tablets 2035
Aldomet Tablets 2037
Aldoril Tablets 2039

Methyldopate Hydrochloride (May potentiate the hypotension seen with aldesleukin).
No products indexed under this heading.

Methylprednisolone Acetate (May reduce the antitumor effectiveness of aldesleukin). Products include:
Depo-Medrol Injectable Suspension 2795

Methylprednisolone Sodium Succinate (May reduce the antitumor effectiveness of aldesleukin). Products include:
Solu-Medrol Sterile Powder 2855

Metipranolol Hydrochloride (May potentiate the hypotension seen with aldesleukin).
No products indexed under this heading.

Metolazone (May potentiate the hypotension seen with aldesleukin). Products include:
Mykrox Tablets 1168
Zaroxolyn Tablets 1177

Metoprolol Succinate (May potentiate the hypotension seen with aldesleukin). Products include:
Toprol-XL Tablets 651

Metoprolol Tartrate (May potentiate the hypotension seen with aldesleukin).
No products indexed under this heading.

Metyrosine (May potentiate the hypotension seen with aldesleukin). Products include:
Demser Capsules 2085

Mibefradil Dihydrochloride (May potentiate the hypotension seen with aldesleukin).
No products indexed under this heading.

Midazolam Hydrochloride (Potential for unspecified effect on central nervous function). Products include:
Versed Injection 3027
Versed Syrup 3033

Minoxidil (May potentiate the hypotension seen with aldesleukin). Products include:
Rogaine Extra Strength for Men Topical Solution ..... ▣ 721
Rogaine for Women Topical Solution ..... ▣ 721

Mitotane (Potential for increased myelotoxicity).
No products indexed under this heading.

Mitoxantrone Hydrochloride (Potential for increased myelotoxicity). Products include:
Novantrone for Injection 1760

Moexipril Hydrochloride (May potentiate the hypotension seen with aldesleukin). Products include:
Uniretic Tablets 3178
Univasc Tablets 3181

Molindone Hydrochloride (Potential for unspecified effect on central nervous function). Products include:
Moban 1320

Morphine Sulfate (Potential for unspecified effect on central nervous function). Products include:
Astramorph/PF Injection, USP (Preservative-Free) 594
Duramorph Injection 1312
Infumorph 200 and Infumorph 500 Sterile Solutions 1314
Kadian Capsules 1335
MS Contin Tablets 2896
MSIR 2898
Oramorph SR Tablets 3062
Roxanol 3066

Nadolol (May potentiate the hypotension seen with aldesleukin). Products include:
Corgard Tablets 2245
Corzide 40/5 Tablets 2247
Corzide 80/5 Tablets 2247
Nadolol Tablets 2288

Nephrotoxic Drugs (Potential for increased nephrotoxicity).

Nicardipine Hydrochloride (May potentiate the hypotension seen with aldesleukin). Products include:
Cardene I.V. 3485

Nifedipine (May potentiate the hypotension seen with aldesleukin). Products include:
Adalat CC Tablets 877
Procardia Capsules 2708
Procardia XL Extended Release Tablets 2710

Nisoldipine (May potentiate the hypotension seen with aldesleukin). Products include:
Sular Tablets 688

Nitroglycerin (May potentiate the hypotension seen with aldesleukin). Products include:
- Nitro-Dur Transdermal Infusion System 3134
- Nitro-Dur Transdermal Infusion System 1834
- Nitrolingual Pumpspray 1355
- Nitrostat Tablets 2658

Oxazepam (Potential for unspecified effect on central nervous function).
- No products indexed under this heading.

Oxycodone Hydrochloride (Potential for unspecified effect on central nervous function). Products include:
- OxyContin Tablets 2912
- OxyFast Oral Concentrate Solution . 2916
- OxyIR Capsules 2916
- Percocet Tablets 1326
- Percodan Tablets 1327
- Percolone Tablets 1327
- Roxicodone 3067
- Tylox Capsules 2597

Penbutolol Sulfate (May potentiate the hypotension seen with aldesleukin).
- No products indexed under this heading.

Perindopril Erbumine (May potentiate the hypotension seen with aldesleukin). Products include:
- Aceon Tablets (2 mg, 4 mg, 8 mg) 3249

Perphenazine (Potential for unspecified effect on central nervous function). Products include:
- Etrafon 3115
- Trilafon 3160

Phenoxybenzamine Hydrochloride (May potentiate the hypotension seen with aldesleukin). Products include:
- Dibenzyline Capsules 3457

Phentolamine Mesylate (May potentiate the hypotension seen with aldesleukin).
- No products indexed under this heading.

Pindolol (May potentiate the hypotension seen with aldesleukin).
- No products indexed under this heading.

Polythiazide (May potentiate the hypotension seen with aldesleukin). Products include:
- Minizide Capsules 2700
- Renese Tablets 2712

Prazepam (Potential for unspecified effect on central nervous function).
- No products indexed under this heading.

Prazosin Hydrochloride (May potentiate the hypotension seen with aldesleukin). Products include:
- Minipress Capsules 2699
- Minizide Capsules 2700

Prednisolone Acetate (May reduce the antitumor effectiveness of aldesleukin). Products include:
- Blephamide Ophthalmic Ointment .. 547
- Blephamide Ophthalmic Suspension 548
- Poly-Pred Liquifilm Ophthalmic Suspension .... ⊙245
- Pred Forte Ophthalmic Suspension .... ⊙246
- Pred Mild Sterile Ophthalmic Suspension .... ⊙249
- Pred-G Ophthalmic Suspension ..... ⊙247
- Pred-G Sterile Ophthalmic Ointment .... ⊙248

Prednisolone Sodium Phosphate (May reduce the antitumor effectiveness of aldesleukin). Products include:
- Pediapred Oral Solution 1170

Prednisolone Tebutate (May reduce the antitumor effectiveness of aldesleukin).
- No products indexed under this heading.

Prednisone (May reduce the antitumor effectiveness of aldesleukin). Products include:
- Prednisone 3064

Procarbazine Hydrochloride (Potential for increased myelotoxicity). Products include:
- Matulane Capsules 3246

Prochlorperazine (Potential for unspecified effect on central nervous function). Products include:
- Compazine 1505

Promethazine Hydrochloride (Potential for unspecified effect on central nervous function). Products include:
- Mepergan Injection 3539
- Phenergan Injection 3553
- Phenergan 3556
- Phenergan Syrup 3554
- Phenergan with Codeine Syrup 3557
- Phenergan with Dextromethorphan Syrup 3559
- Phenergan VC Syrup 3560
- Phenergan VC with Codeine Syrup .. 3561

Propofol (Potential for unspecified effect on central nervous function). Products include:
- Diprivan Injectable Emulsion 667

Propoxyphene Hydrochloride (Potential for unspecified effect on central nervous function). Products include:
- Darvon Pulvules 1909
- Darvon Compound-65 Pulvules 1910

Propoxyphene Napsylate (Potential for unspecified effect on central nervous function). Products include:
- Darvon-N/Darvocet-N 1907
- Darvon-N Tablets 1912

Propranolol Hydrochloride (May potentiate the hypotension seen with aldesleukin). Products include:
- Inderal 3513
- Inderal LA Long-Acting Capsules 3516
- Inderide Tablets 3517
- Inderide LA Long-Acting Capsules .. 3519

Quazepam (Potential for unspecified effect on central nervous function).
- No products indexed under this heading.

Quinapril Hydrochloride (May potentiate the hypotension seen with aldesleukin). Products include:
- Accupril Tablets 2611
- Accuretic Tablets 2614

Ramipril (May potentiate the hypotension seen with aldesleukin). Products include:
- Altace Capsules 2233

Rauwolfia serpentina (May potentiate the hypotension seen with aldesleukin).
- No products indexed under this heading.

Remifentanil Hydrochloride (Potential for unspecified effect on central nervous function).
- No products indexed under this heading.

Rescinnamine (May potentiate the hypotension seen with aldesleukin).
- No products indexed under this heading.

Reserpine (May potentiate the hypotension seen with aldesleukin).
- No products indexed under this heading.

Secobarbital Sodium (Potential for unspecified effect on central nervous function).
- No products indexed under this heading.

Sodium Nitroprusside (May potentiate the hypotension seen with aldesleukin).
- No products indexed under this heading.

Sotalol Hydrochloride (May potentiate the hypotension seen with aldesleukin). Products include:
- Betapace Tablets 950
- Betapace AF Tablets 954

Spirapril Hydrochloride (May potentiate the hypotension seen with aldesleukin).
- No products indexed under this heading.

Streptomycin Sulfate (Potential for increased nephrotoxicity). Products include:
- Streptomycin Sulfate Injection 2714

Sufentanil Citrate (Potential for unspecified effect on central nervous function).
- No products indexed under this heading.

Tamoxifen Citrate (Potential for increased myelotoxicity). Products include:
- Nolvadex Tablets 678

Telmisartan (May potentiate the hypotension seen with aldesleukin). Products include:
- Micardis Tablets 1049
- Micardis HCT Tablets 1051

Temazepam (Potential for unspecified effect on central nervous function).
- No products indexed under this heading.

Terazosin Hydrochloride (May potentiate the hypotension seen with aldesleukin). Products include:
- Hytrin Capsules 464

Thioridazine Hydrochloride (Potential for unspecified effect on central nervous function). Products include:
- Thioridazine Hydrochloride Tablets 2289

Thiothixene (Potential for unspecified effect on central nervous function). Products include:
- Navane Capsules 2701
- Thiothixene Capsules 2290

Timolol Hemihydrate (May potentiate the hypotension seen with aldesleukin). Products include:
- Betimol Ophthalmic Solution .... ⊙324

Timolol Maleate (May potentiate the hypotension seen with aldesleukin). Products include:
- Blocadren Tablets 2046
- Cosopt Sterile Ophthalmic Solution 2065
- Timolide Tablets 2187
- Timolol GFS .... ⊙266
- Timoptic in Ocudose 2192
- Timoptic Sterile Ophthalmic Solution 2190
- Timoptic-XE Sterile Ophthalmic Gel Forming Solution 2194

Tobramycin (Potential for increased nephrotoxicity). Products include:
- TOBI Solution for Inhalation 1206
- TobraDex Ophthalmic Ointment 542
- TobraDex Ophthalmic Suspension 541
- Tobrex Ophthalmic Ointment .... ⊙220
- Tobrex Ophthalmic Solution .... ⊙221

Tobramycin Sulfate (Potential for increased nephrotoxicity). Products include:
- Nebcin Vials, Hyporets & ADD-Vantage 1955

Torsemide (May potentiate the hypotension seen with aldesleukin). Products include:
- Demadex Tablets and Injection 2965

Trandolapril (May potentiate the hypotension seen with aldesleukin). Products include:
- Mavik Tablets 478
- Tarka Tablets 508

Triamcinolone (May reduce the antitumor effectiveness of aldesleukin).
- No products indexed under this heading.

Triamcinolone Acetonide (May reduce the antitumor effectiveness of aldesleukin). Products include:
- Azmacort Inhalation Aerosol 728
- Nasacort Nasal Inhaler 750
- Nasacort AQ Nasal Spray 752
- Tri-Nasal Spray 2274

Triamcinolone Diacetate (May reduce the antitumor effectiveness of aldesleukin).
- No products indexed under this heading.

Triamcinolone Hexacetonide (May reduce the antitumor effectiveness of aldesleukin).
- No products indexed under this heading.

Triazolam (Potential for unspecified effect on central nervous function). Products include:
- Halcion Tablets 2823

Trifluoperazine Hydrochloride (Potential for unspecified effect on central nervous function). Products include:
- Stelazine 1640

Trimethaphan Camsylate (May potentiate the hypotension seen with aldesleukin).
- No products indexed under this heading.

Tyropanoate Sodium (Potential for delayed adverse reactions to iodinated contrast media including fever, chills, nausea, vomiting, pruritus, rash, diarrhea, hypotension, edema, and oliguria).
- No products indexed under this heading.

Valsartan (May potentiate the hypotension seen with aldesleukin). Products include:
- Diovan Capsules 2337
- Diovan HCT Tablets 2338

Verapamil Hydrochloride (May potentiate the hypotension seen with aldesleukin). Products include:
- Covera-HS Tablets 3199
- Isoptin SR Tablets 467
- Tarka Tablets 508
- Verelan Capsules 3184
- Verelan PM Capsules 3186

Vincristine Sulfate (Potential for increased myelotoxicity).
- No products indexed under this heading.

Zaleplon (Potential for unspecified effect on central nervous function). Products include:
- Sonata Capsules 3591

Zolpidem Tartrate (Potential for unspecified effect on central nervous function). Products include:
- Ambien Tablets 3191

PROMETRIUM CAPSULES (100 MG, 200 MG)

(Progesterone) 3261

May interact with:

Estrogens, Conjugated (Coadministration has resulted in an increase in total estrone and equilin concentrations and decrease in circulating 17β estradiol concentrations). Products include:
- Premarin Intravenous 3563
- Premarin Tablets 3566
- Premarin Vaginal Cream 3570
- Premphase Tablets 3572
- Prempro Tablets 3572

Ketoconazole (The metabolism of progesterone by human liver microsomes is inhibited by ketoconazole, a known inhibitor of CYP4503A4; the clinical relevance of the in vitro findings is unknown). Products include:
- Nizoral 2% Cream 3620
- Nizoral A-D Shampoo 2008
- Nizoral 2% Shampoo 2007
- Nizoral Tablets 1791

Food Interactions

Food, unspecified (Concomitant food ingestion increases the bioavailability of Prometrium Capsules relative to the fasting state).

PROMOTION CAPSULES

(Glucosamine Hydrochloride) .... ■800

None cited in PDR database.

IMPORTANT NOTE: Always consult each drug listing in the patient's regimen for possible interactions.

PROPECIA TABLETS
(Finasteride) 2172
None cited in PDR database.

PROPINE OPHTHALMIC SOLUTION
(Dipivefrin Hydrochloride) .... ⊙250
None cited in PDR database.

PROPLEX T
(Factor IX Complex) 851
None cited in PDR database.

PROSCAR TABLETS
(Finasteride) 2175
None cited in PDR database.

PROSED/DS TABLETS
(Atropine Sulfate, Benzoic Acid, Hyoscyamine Sulfate, Methenamine, Methylene Blue, Phenyl Salicylate)............................. 3268
May interact with antacids, antimuscarinic drugs, monoamine oxidase inhibitors, narcotic analgesics, thiazides, and urinary alkalinizing agents. Compounds in these categories include:

Alfentanil Hydrochloride (Co-administration may result in increased risk of severe constipation).
No products indexed under this heading.

Aluminum Carbonate (Concurrent use of antacids may cause the urine to become alkaline reducing the effectiveness of methenamine by inhibiting its conversion to formaldehyde; doses of these medications should be spaced 1 hour apart from doses of atropine and hyoscyamine).
No products indexed under this heading.

Aluminum Hydroxide (Concurrent use of antacids may cause the urine to become alkaline reducing the effectiveness of methenamine by inhibiting its conversion to formaldehyde; doses of these medications should be spaced 1 hour apart from doses of atropine and hyoscyamine). Products include:
- Amphojel Suspension (Mint Flavor) .... ■789
- Gaviscon Extra Strength Liquid ..... ■751
- Gaviscon Extra Strength Tablets .... ■751
- Gaviscon Regular Strength Liquid . ■751
- Gaviscon Regular Strength Tablets .... ■750
- Maalox Antacid/Anti-Gas Oral Suspension .... ■673
- Maalox Max Maximum Strength Antacid/Anti-Gas Liquid 2300
- Maalox Regular Strength Antacid/Antigas Liquid 2300
- Mylanta 1813
- Vanquish Caplets .... ■617

Belladonna Alkaloids (Concurrent use of antimuscarinics may intensify antimuscarinic effects). Products include:
- Hyland's Teething Tablets .... ■766
- Urimax Tablets 1769

Bendroflumethiazide (Thiazide diuretics may cause the urine to become alkaline reducing the effectiveness of methenamine by inhibiting its conversion to formaldehyde). Products include:
- Corzide 40/5 Tablets 2247
- Corzide 80/5 Tablets 2247

Buprenorphine Hydrochloride (Co-administration may result in increased risk of severe constipation). Products include:
- Buprenex Injectable 2918

Chlorothiazide (Thiazide diuretics may cause the urine to become alkaline reducing the effectiveness of methenamine by inhibiting its conversion to formaldehyde). Products include:
- Aldoclor Tablets 2035
- Diuril Oral 2087

Chlorothiazide Sodium (Thiazide diuretics may cause the urine to become alkaline reducing the effectiveness of methenamine by inhibiting its conversion to formaldehyde). Products include:
- Diuril Sodium Intravenous 2086

Clidinium Bromide (Concurrent use of antimuscarinics may intensify antimuscarinic effects).
No products indexed under this heading.

Codeine Phosphate (Co-administration may result in increased risk of severe constipation). Products include:
- Phenergan with Codeine Syrup 3557
- Phenergan VC with Codeine Syrup .. 3561
- Robitussin A-C Syrup 2942
- Robitussin-DAC Syrup 2942
- Ryna-C Liquid .... ■768
- Soma Compound w/Codeine Tablets 3355
- Tussi-Organidin NR Liquid 3350
- Tussi-Organidin-S NR Liquid 3350
- Tylenol with Codeine 2595

Dezocine (Co-administration may result in increased risk of severe constipation).
No products indexed under this heading.

Dicyclomine Hydrochloride (Concurrent use of antimuscarinics may intensify antimuscarinic effects).
No products indexed under this heading.

Diphenoxylate Hydrochloride (Concurrent use with antidiarrheals may reduce the absorption of atropine and hyoscyamine resulting in decreased therapeutic effect; doses of these medications should be spaced 1 hour apart from doses of atropine and hyoscyamine).
No products indexed under this heading.

Fentanyl (Co-administration may result in increased risk of severe constipation). Products include:
- Duragesic Transdermal System 1786

Fentanyl Citrate (Co-administration may result in increased risk of severe constipation). Products include:
- Actiq 1184

Glycopyrrolate (Concurrent use of antimuscarinics may intensify antimuscarinic effects). Products include:
- Robinul Forte Tablets 1358
- Robinul Injectable 2940
- Robinul Tablets 1358

Hydrochlorothiazide (Thiazide diuretics may cause the urine to become alkaline reducing the effectiveness of methenamine by inhibiting its conversion to formaldehyde). Products include:
- Accuretic Tablets 2614
- Aldoril Tablets 2039
- Atacand HCT Tablets 597
- Avalide Tablets 1070
- Diovan HCT Tablets 2338
- Dyazide Capsules 1515
- HydroDIURIL Tablets 2108
- Hyzaar 2109
- Inderide Tablets 3517
- Inderide LA Long-Acting Capsules .. 3519
- Lotensin HCT Tablets 2367
- Maxzide 1008
- Micardis HCT Tablets 1051
- Microzide Capsules 3414
- Moduretic Tablets 2138
- Monopril HCT 1094
- Prinzide Tablets 2168
- Timolide Tablets 2187
- Uniretic Tablets 3178
- Vaseretic Tablets 2204
- Zestoretic Tablets 695
- Ziac Tablets 1887

Hydrocodone Bitartrate (Co-administration may result in increased risk of severe constipation). Products include:
- Hycodan 1316
- Hycomine Compound Tablets 1317
- Hycotuss Expectorant Syrup 1318
- Lortab 3319
- Lortab Elixir 3317
- Maxidone Tablets CIII 3399
- Norco 5/325 Tablets CIII 3424
- Norco 7.5/325 Tablets CIII 3425
- Norco 10/325 Tablets CIII 3427
- Norco 10/325 Tablets CIII 3425
- Vicodin Tablets 516
- Vicodin ES Tablets 517
- Vicodin HP Tablets 518
- Vicodin Tuss Expectorant 519
- Vicoprofen Tablets 520
- Zydone Tablets 1330

Hydrocodone Polistirex (Co-administration may result in increased risk of severe constipation). Products include:
- Tussionex Pennkinetic Extended-Release Suspension..... 1174

Hydroflumethiazide (Thiazide diuretics may cause the urine to become alkaline reducing the effectiveness of methenamine by inhibiting its conversion to formaldehyde). Products include:
- Diucardin Tablets 3494

Hydromorphone Hydrochloride (Co-administration may result in increased risk of severe constipation). Products include:
- Dilaudid 441
- Dilaudid Oral Liquid 445
- Dilaudid Powder 441
- Dilaudid Rectal Suppositories 441
- Dilaudid Tablets 441
- Dilaudid Tablets - 8 mg 445
- Dilaudid-HP 443

Hyoscyamine (Concurrent use of antimuscarinics may intensify antimuscarinic effects). Products include:
- Urised Tablets 2876

Ipratropium Bromide (Concurrent use of antimuscarinics may intensify antimuscarinic effects). Products include:
- Atrovent Inhalation Aerosol 1030
- Atrovent Inhalation Solution 1031
- Atrovent Nasal Spray 0.03% 1032
- Atrovent Nasal Spray 0.06% 1033
- Combivent Inhalation Aerosol 1041
- DuoNeb Inhalation Solution 1233

Isocarboxazid (Co-administration with MAO inhibitors may intensify antimuscarinic side effects).
No products indexed under this heading.

Ketoconazole (Atropine and hyoscyamine may cause increased gastrointestinal pH; concurrent use may result in marked reduction in the absorption of ketoconazole; patients should be advised to take this combination at least 2 hours after ketoconazole). Products include:
- Nizoral 2% Cream 3620
- Nizoral A-D Shampoo 2008
- Nizoral 2% Shampoo 2007
- Nizoral Tablets 1791

Levorphanol Tartrate (Co-administration may result in increased risk of severe constipation). Products include:
- Levo-Dromoran 1734
- Levorphanol Tartrate Tablets 3059

Loperamide Hydrochloride (Concurrent use with antidiarrheals may reduce the absorption of atropine and hyoscyamine resulting in decreased therapeutic effect; doses of these medications should be spaced 1 hour apart from doses of atropine and hyoscyamine). Products include:
- Imodium A-D Liquid and Caplets 2001
- Imodium Advanced Caplets and Chewable Tablets 2001

Magaldrate (Concurrent use of antacids may cause the urine to become alkaline reducing the effectiveness of methenamine by inhibiting its conversion to formaldehyde; doses of these medications should be spaced 1 hour apart from doses of atropine and hyoscyamine).
No products indexed under this heading.

Magnesium Hydroxide (Concurrent use of antacids may cause the urine to become alkaline reducing the effectiveness of methenamine by inhibiting its conversion to formaldehyde; doses of these medications should be spaced 1 hour apart from doses of atropine and hyoscyamine). Products include:
- Ex•Lax Milk of Magnesia Liquid .... ■670
- Maalox Antacid/Anti-Gas Oral Suspension .... ■673
- Maalox Max Maximum Strength Antacid/Anti-Gas Liquid 2300
- Maalox Regular Strength Antacid/Antigas Liquid 2300
- Mylanta Fast-Acting 1813
- Mylanta 1813
- Pepcid Complete Chewable Tablets 1815
- Phillips' Chewable Tablets .... ■615
- Phillips' Milk of Magnesia Liquid (Original, Cherry, & Mint) .... ■616
- Rolaids Tablets .... ■706
- Extra Strength Rolaids Tablets ...... ■706
- Vanquish Caplets .... ■617

Magnesium Oxide (Concurrent use of antacids may cause the urine to become alkaline reducing the effectiveness of methenamine by inhibiting its conversion to formaldehyde; doses of these medications should be spaced 1 hour apart from doses of atropine and hyoscyamine). Products include:
- Beelith Tablets 946
- Mag-Ox 400 Tablets 1024
- Uro-Mag Capsules 1024

Mepenzolate Bromide (Concurrent use of antimuscarinics may intensify antimuscarinic effects).
No products indexed under this heading.

Meperidine Hydrochloride (Co-administration may result in increased risk of severe constipation). Products include:
- Demerol 3079
- Mepergan Injection 3539

Methadone Hydrochloride (Co-administration may result in increased risk of severe constipation). Products include:
- Dolophine Hydrochloride Tablets 3056

Methyclothiazide (Thiazide diuretics may cause the urine to become alkaline reducing the effectiveness of methenamine by inhibiting its conversion to formaldehyde).
No products indexed under this heading.

Moclobemide (Co-administration with MAO inhibitors may intensify antimuscarinic side effects).
No products indexed under this heading.

Morphine Sulfate (Co-administration may result in increased risk of severe constipation). Products include:
- Astramorph/PF Injection, USP (Preservative-Free) 594
- Duramorph Injection 1312
- Infumorph 200 and Infumorph 500 Sterile Solutions 1314
- Kadian Capsules 1335
- MS Contin Tablets 2896
- MSIR 2898
- Oramorph SR Tablets 3062
- Roxanol 3066

Neostigmine Bromide (Co-administration with antimyasthenic drugs may further reduce intestinal motility). Products include:
- Prostigmin Tablets 1744

Neostigmine Methylsulfate (Co-administration with antimyasthenic drugs may further reduce intestinal motility). Products include:
- Prostigmin Injectable 1744

Oxycodone Hydrochloride (Co-administration may result in increased risk of severe constipation). Products include:
- OxyContin Tablets 2912
- OxyFast Oral Concentrate Solution . 2916
- OxyIR Capsules 2916

Percocet Tablets 1326
Percodan Tablets 1327
Percolone Tablets 1327
Roxicodone 3067
Tylox Capsules 2597

Oxyphenonium Bromide (Concurrent use of antimuscarinics may intensify antimuscarinic effects).
No products indexed under this heading.

Pargyline Hydrochloride (Co-administration with MAO inhibitors may intensify antimuscarinic side effects).
No products indexed under this heading.

Phenelzine Sulfate (Co-administration with MAO inhibitors may intensify antimuscarinic side effects). Products include:
Nardil Tablets 2653

Polythiazide (Thiazide diuretics may cause the urine to become alkaline reducing the effectiveness of methenamine by inhibiting its conversion to formaldehyde). Products include:
Minizide Capsules 2700
Renese Tablets 2712

Potassium Citrate (Urinary alkalizers may cause the urine to become alkaline reducing the effectiveness of methenamine by inhibiting its conversion to formaldehyde). Products include:
Urocit-K Tablets 2232

Procarbazine Hydrochloride (Co-administration with MAO inhibitors may intensify antimuscarinic side effects). Products include:
Matulane Capsules 3246

Propantheline Bromide (Concurrent use of antimuscarinics may intensify antimuscarinic effects).
No products indexed under this heading.

Propoxyphene Hydrochloride (Co-administration may result in increased risk of severe constipation). Products include:
Darvon Pulvules 1909
Darvon Compound-65 Pulvules 1910

Propoxyphene Napsylate (Co-administration may result in increased risk of severe constipation). Products include:
Darvon-N/Darvocet-N 1907
Darvon-N Tablets 1912

Pyridostigmine Bromide (Co-administration with antimyasthenic drugs may further reduce intestinal motility). Products include:
Mestinon 1740

Remifentanil Hydrochloride (Co-administration may result in increased risk of severe constipation).
No products indexed under this heading.

Scopolamine (Concurrent use of antimuscarinics may intensify antimuscarinic effects). Products include:
Transderm Scōp Transdermal Therapeutic System 2302

Scopolamine Hydrobromide (Concurrent use of antimuscarinics may intensify antimuscarinic effects). Products include:
Donnatal 2929
Donnatal Extentabs 2930

Selegiline Hydrochloride (Co-administration with MAO inhibitors may intensify antimuscarinic side effects). Products include:
Eldepryl Capsules 3266

Sodium Bicarbonate (Concurrent use of antacids may cause the urine to become alkaline reducing the effectiveness of methenamine by inhibiting its conversion to formaldehyde; doses of these medications should be spaced 1 hour apart from doses of atropine and hyoscyamine). Products include:
Alka-Seltzer 603
Alka-Seltzer Lemon Lime Antacid and Pain Reliever Effervescent Tablets 603
Alka-Seltzer Extra Strength Antacid and Pain Reliever Effervescent Tablets 603
Alka-Seltzer Heartburn Relief Tablets 604
Ceo-Two Evacuant Suppository 618
Colyte with Flavor Packs for Oral Solution 3170
GoLYTELY and Pineapple Flavor GoLYTELY for Oral Solution 1068
NuLYTELY, Cherry Flavor, Lemon-Lime Flavor, and Orange Flavor NuLYTELY for Oral Solution 1068

Sodium Citrate (Urinary alkalizers may cause the urine to become alkaline reducing the effectiveness of methenamine by inhibiting its conversion to formaldehyde).
No products indexed under this heading.

Sufentanil Citrate (Co-administration may result in increased risk of severe constipation).
No products indexed under this heading.

Sulfamethizole (Co-administration with sulfonamides may precipitate with formaldehyde in the urine increasing the danger of crystalluria). Products include:
Urobiotic-250 Capsules 2731

Sulfamethoxazole (Co-administration with sulfonamides may precipitate with formaldehyde in the urine increasing the danger of crystalluria). Products include:
Bactrim 2949
Septra Suspension 2265
Septra Tablets 2265
Septra DS Tablets 2265

Sulfisoxazole Acetyl (Co-administration with sulfonamides may precipitate with formaldehyde in the urine increasing the danger of crystalluria). Products include:
Pediazole Suspension 3050

Tolterodine Tartrate (Concurrent use of antimuscarinics may intensify antimuscarinic effects). Products include:
Detrol Tablets 3623
Detrol LA Capsules 2801

Tranylcypromine Sulfate (Co-administration with MAO inhibitors may intensify antimuscarinic side effects). Products include:
Parnate Tablets 1607

Tridihexethyl Chloride (Concurrent use of antimuscarinics may intensify antimuscarinic effects).
No products indexed under this heading.

PROSOM TABLES

(Estazolam) 500

May interact with antihistamines, barbiturates, central nervous system depressants, anticonvulsants, monoamine oxidase inhibitors, narcotic analgesics, phenothiazines, and certain other agents. Compounds in these categories include:

Acrivastine (Co-administration results in increased CNS depression). Products include:
Semprex-D Capsules 1172

Alfentanil Hydrochloride (Co-administration results in increased CNS depression).
No products indexed under this heading.

Alprazolam (Co-administration results in increased CNS depression). Products include:
Xanax Tablets 2865

Aprobarbital (Co-administration results in increased CNS depression).
No products indexed under this heading.

Astemizole (Co-administration results in increased CNS depression).
No products indexed under this heading.

Azatadine Maleate (Co-administration results in increased CNS depression). Products include:
Rynatan Tablets 3351

Bromodiphenhydramine Hydrochloride (Co-administration results in increased CNS depression).
No products indexed under this heading.

Brompheniramine Maleate (Co-administration results in increased CNS depression). Products include:
Bromfed Capsules (Extended-Release) 2269
Bromfed-PD Capsules (Extended-Release) 2269
Comtrex Acute Head Cold & Sinus Pressure Relief Tablets 627
Dimetapp Elixir 777
Dimetapp Cold and Fever Suspension 775
Dimetapp DM Cold & Cough Elixir 775
Dimetapp Nighttime Flu Liquid 776

Buprenorphine Hydrochloride (Co-administration results in increased CNS depression). Products include:
Buprenex Injectable 2918

Buspirone Hydrochloride (Co-administration results in increased CNS depression).
No products indexed under this heading.

Butabarbital (Co-administration results in increased CNS depression).
No products indexed under this heading.

Butalbital (Co-administration results in increased CNS depression). Products include:
Phrenilin 578
Sedapap Tablets 50 mg/650 mg 2225

Carbamazepine (Co-administration results in increased CNS depression). Products include:
Carbatrol Capsules 3234
Tegretol/Tegretol-XR 2404

Cetirizine Hydrochloride (Co-administration results in increased CNS depression). Products include:
Zyrtec 2756
Zyrtec-D 12 Hour Extended Relief Tablets 2758

Chlordiazepoxide (Co-administration results in increased CNS depression). Products include:
Limbitrol 1738

Chlordiazepoxide Hydrochloride (Co-administration results in increased CNS depression). Products include:
Librium Capsules 1736
Librium for Injection 1737

Chlorpheniramine Maleate (Co-administration results in increased CNS depression). Products include:
Actifed Cold & Sinus Caplets and Tablets 688
Alka-Seltzer Plus Liqui-Gels 604
BC Allergy Sinus Cold Powder 619
Chlor-Trimeton Allergy Tablets 735
Chlor-Trimeton Allergy/Decongestant Tablets 736
Comtrex Flu Therapy & Fever Relief Nighttime Tablets 628
Comtrex Maximum Strength Multi-Symptom Cold & Cough Relief Tablets and Caplets 626
Contac Severe Cold and Flu Caplets Maximum Strength 746
Coricidin 'D' Cold, Flu & Sinus Tablets 737
Coricidin/Coricidin D 738
Coricidin HBP Maximum Strength Flu Tablets 738
Extendryl 1361
Hycomine Compound Tablets 1317
Kronofed-A 1341
PediaCare Cough-Cold Liquid 719
PediaCare NightRest Cough-Cold Liquid 719
Robitussin Nighttime Honey Flu Liquid 786
Ryna 768
Singlet Caplets 761
Sinutab Sinus Allergy Medication, Maximum Strength Formula, Tablets & Caplets 707
Sudafed Cold & Allergy Tablets 708
TheraFlu Regular Strength Cold & Cough Night Time Hot Liquid 676
TheraFlu Regular Strength Cold & Sore Throat Night Time Hot Liquid 676
TheraFlu Maximum Strength Flu & Cough Night Time Hot Liquid 678
TheraFlu Maximum Strength Flu & Sore Throat Night Time Hot Liquid 677
TheraFlu Maximum Strength Severe Cold & Congestion Night Time Caplets 678
TheraFlu Maximum Strength Severe Cold & Congestion Night Time Hot Liquid 678
Triaminic Cold & Allergy Liquid 681
Triaminic Cold & Allergy Softchews 683
Triaminic Cold & Cough Liquid 681
Triaminic Cold & Cough Softchews 683
Triaminic Cold & Night Time Cough Liquid 681
Triaminic Cold, Cough & Fever Liquid 681
Children's Tylenol Cold Suspension Liquid and Chewable Tablets 2015
Children's Tylenol Cold Plus Cough Suspension Liquid and Chewable Tablets 2015
Children's Tylenol Flu Suspension Liquid 2015
Maximum Strength Tylenol Allergy Sinus Caplets, Gelcaps, and Geltabs 2010
Multi-Symptom Tylenol Cold Complete Formula Caplets 2010
Vicks 44M Cough, Cold & Flu Relief Liquid 725
Pediatric Vicks 44m Cough & Cold Relief 728
Children's Vicks NyQuil Cold/Cough Relief 726

Chlorpheniramine Polistirex (Co-administration results in increased CNS depression). Products include:
Tussionex Pennkinetic Extended-Release Suspension 1174

Chlorpheniramine Tannate (Co-administration results in increased CNS depression). Products include:
Reformulated Rynatan Pediatric Suspension 3352
Rynatuss Pediatric Suspension 3353
Rynatuss Tablets 3353
Tussi-12 S Suspension 3356
Tussi-12 Tablets 3356

Chlorpromazine (Co-administration results in increased CNS depression). Products include:
Thorazine Suppositories 1656

Chlorpromazine Hydrochloride (Co-administration results in increased CNS depression). Products include:
Thorazine 1656

Chlorprothixene (Co-administration results in increased CNS depression).
No products indexed under this heading.

Chlorprothixene Hydrochloride (Co-administration results in increased CNS depression).
No products indexed under this heading.

Chlorprothixene Lactate (Co-administration results in increased CNS depression).
No products indexed under this heading.

Clemastine Fumarate (Co-administration results in increased CNS depression). Products include:
Tavist 12 Hour Allergy Tablets 676

Clonazepam (Co-administration results in increased CNS depression). Products include:
Klonopin Tablets 2983

IMPORTANT NOTE: Always consult each drug listing in the patient's regimen for possible interactions.

Clorazepate Dipotassium (Co-administration results in increased CNS depression). Products include:
Tranxene 511

Clozapine (Co-administration results in increased CNS depression). Products include:
Clozaril Tablets 2319

Codeine Phosphate (Co-administration results in increased CNS depression). Products include:
Phenergan with Codeine Syrup 3557
Phenergan VC with Codeine Syrup .. 3561
Robitussin A-C Syrup 2942
Robitussin-DAC Syrup 2942
Ryna-C Liquid .... ▣768
Soma Compound w/Codeine Tablets 3355
Tussi-Organidin NR Liquid 3350
Tussi-Organidin-S NR Liquid 3350
Tylenol with Codeine 2595

Cyproheptadine Hydrochloride (Co-administration results in increased CNS depression). Products include:
Periactin Tablets 2155

Desflurane (Co-administration results in increased CNS depression). Products include:
Suprane Liquid for Inhalation 874

Dexchlorpheniramine Maleate (Co-administration results in increased CNS depression).
No products indexed under this heading.

Dezocine (Co-administration results in increased CNS depression).
No products indexed under this heading.

Diazepam (Co-administration results in increased CNS depression). Products include:
Valium Injectable 3026
Valium Tablets 3047

Diphenhydramine Citrate (Co-administration results in increased CNS depression). Products include:
Alka-Seltzer PM Effervescent Tablets .... ▣605
Benadryl Allergy & Sinus Fastmelt Tablets .... ▣693
Benadryl Children's Allergy/Cold Fastmelt Tablets .... ▣692
Excedrin PM Tablets, Caplets, and Geltabs .... ▣631
Goody's PM Powder .... ▣621

Diphenhydramine Hydrochloride (Co-administration results in increased CNS depression). Products include:
Extra Strength Bayer PM Caplets .... ▣611
Benadryl Allergy Chewables .... ▣689
Benadryl Allergy .... ▣691
Benadryl Allergy Liquid .... ▣690
Benadryl Allergy/Cold Tablets .... ▣691
Benadryl Allergy/Congestion Tablets .... ▣692
Benadryl Allergy & Sinus Liquid .... ▣693
Benadryl Allergy Sinus Headache Caplets & Gelcaps .... ▣693
Benadryl Severe Allergy & Sinus Headache Caplets .... ▣694
Benadryl Dye-Free Allergy Liquid ... ▣690
Benadryl Dye-Free Allergy Liqui-Gels Softgels .... ▣690
Benadryl Itch Relief Stick Extra Strength .... ▣695
Benadryl Cream .... ▣695
Benadryl Gel .... ▣695
Benadryl Spray .... ▣696
Benadryl Parenteral 2617
Coricidin HBP Night-Time Cold & Flu Tablets .... ▣738
Nytol QuickCaps Caplets .... ▣622
Maximum Strength Nytol QuickGels Softgels .... ▣621
Extra Strength Percogesic Aspirin-Free Coated Caplets .... ▣665
Simply Sleep Caplets 2008
Sominex Original Formula Tablets . ▣761
Children's Tylenol Allergy-D Liquid ... 2014
Maximum Strength Tylenol Allergy Sinus NightTime Caplets 2010
Tylenol Severe Allergy Caplets 2010
Maximum Strength Tylenol Flu NightTime Gelcaps 2011
Extra Strength Tylenol PM Caplets, Geltabs, and Gelcaps 2012
Unisom Maximum Strength SleepGels .... ▣713

Diphenylpyraline Hydrochloride (Co-administration results in increased CNS depression).
No products indexed under this heading.

Divalproex Sodium (Co-administration results in increased CNS depression). Products include:
Depakote Sprinkle Capsules 426
Depakote Tablets 430
Depakote ER Tablets 436

Droperidol (Co-administration results in increased CNS depression).
No products indexed under this heading.

Enflurane (Co-administration results in increased CNS depression).
No products indexed under this heading.

Ethchlorvynol (Co-administration results in increased CNS depression).
No products indexed under this heading.

Ethinamate (Co-administration results in increased CNS depression).
No products indexed under this heading.

Ethosuximide (Co-administration results in increased CNS depression). Products include:
Zarontin Capsules 2659
Zarontin Syrup 2660

Ethotoin (Co-administration results in increased CNS depression).
No products indexed under this heading.

Felbamate (Co-administration results in increased CNS depression). Products include:
Felbatol 3343

Fentanyl (Co-administration results in increased CNS depression). Products include:
Duragesic Transdermal System 1786

Fentanyl Citrate (Co-administration results in increased CNS depression). Products include:
Actiq 1184

Fexofenadine Hydrochloride (Co-administration results in increased CNS depression). Products include:
Allegra 712
Allegra-D Extended-Release Tablets 714

Fluphenazine Decanoate (Co-administration results in increased CNS depression).
No products indexed under this heading.

Fluphenazine Enanthate (Co-administration results in increased CNS depression).
No products indexed under this heading.

Fluphenazine Hydrochloride (Co-administration results in increased CNS depression).
No products indexed under this heading.

Flurazepam Hydrochloride (Co-administration results in increased CNS depression).
No products indexed under this heading.

Fosphenytoin Sodium (Co-administration results in increased CNS depression). Products include:
Cerebyx Injection 2619

Glutethimide (Co-administration results in increased CNS depression).
No products indexed under this heading.

Haloperidol (Co-administration results in increased CNS depression). Products include:
Haldol Injection, Tablets and Concentrate 2533

Haloperidol Decanoate (Co-administration results in increased CNS depression). Products include:
Haldol Decanoate 2535

Hydrocodone Bitartrate (Co-administration results in increased CNS depression). Products include:
Hycodan 1316
Hycomine Compound Tablets 1317
Hycotuss Expectorant Syrup 1318
Lortab 3319
Lortab Elixir 3317
Maxidone Tablets CIII 3399
Norco 5/325 Tablets CIII 3424
Norco 7.5/325 Tablets CIII 3425
Norco 10/325 Tablets CIII 3427
Norco 10/325 Tablets CIII 3425
Vicodin Tablets 516
Vicodin ES Tablets 517
Vicodin HP Tablets 518
Vicodin Tuss Expectorant 519
Vicoprofen Tablets 520
Zydone Tablets 1330

Hydrocodone Polistirex (Co-administration results in increased CNS depression). Products include:
Tussionex Pennkinetic Extended-Release Suspension 1174

Hydromorphone Hydrochloride (Co-administration results in increased CNS depression). Products include:
Dilaudid 441
Dilaudid Oral Liquid 445
Dilaudid Powder 441
Dilaudid Rectal Suppositories 441
Dilaudid Tablets 441
Dilaudid Tablets - 8 mg 445
Dilaudid-HP 443

Hydroxyzine Hydrochloride (Co-administration results in increased CNS depression). Products include:
Atarax Tablets & Syrup 2667
Vistaril Intramuscular Solution 2738

Isocarboxazid (Co-administration with MAO inhibitor results in increased CNS depression).
No products indexed under this heading.

Isoflurane (Co-administration results in increased CNS depression).
No products indexed under this heading.

Ketamine Hydrochloride (Co-administration results in increased CNS depression).
No products indexed under this heading.

Lamotrigine (Co-administration results in increased CNS depression). Products include:
Lamictal 1567

Levetiracetam (Co-administration results in increased CNS depression). Products include:
Keppra Tablets 3314

Levomethadyl Acetate Hydrochloride (Co-administration results in increased CNS depression).
No products indexed under this heading.

Levorphanol Tartrate (Co-administration results in increased CNS depression). Products include:
Levo-Dromoran 1734
Levorphanol Tartrate Tablets 3059

Loratadine (Co-administration results in increased CNS depression). Products include:
Claritin 3100
Claritin-D 12 Hour Extended Release Tablets 3102
Claritin-D 24 Hour Extended Release Tablets 3104

Lorazepam (Co-administration results in increased CNS depression). Products include:
Ativan Injection 3478
Ativan Tablets 3482

Loxapine Hydrochloride (Co-administration results in increased CNS depression).
No products indexed under this heading.

Loxapine Succinate (Co-administration results in increased CNS depression). Products include:
Loxitane Capsules 3398

Meperidine Hydrochloride (Co-administration results in increased CNS depression). Products include:
Demerol 3079
Mepergan Injection 3539

Mephenytoin (Co-administration results in increased CNS depression).
No products indexed under this heading.

Mephobarbital (Co-administration results in increased CNS depression).
No products indexed under this heading.

Meprobamate (Co-administration results in increased CNS depression). Products include:
Miltown Tablets 3349

Mesoridazine Besylate (Co-administration results in increased CNS depression). Products include:
Serentil 1057

Methadone Hydrochloride (Co-administration results in increased CNS depression). Products include:
Dolophine Hydrochloride Tablets 3056

Methdilazine Hydrochloride (Co-administration results in increased CNS depression).
No products indexed under this heading.

Methohexital Sodium (Co-administration results in increased CNS depression). Products include:
Brevital Sodium for Injection, USP .. 1815

Methotrimeprazine (Co-administration results in increased CNS depression).
No products indexed under this heading.

Methoxyflurane (Co-administration results in increased CNS depression).
No products indexed under this heading.

Methsuximide (Co-administration results in increased CNS depression). Products include:
Celontin Capsules 2618

Midazolam Hydrochloride (Co-administration results in increased CNS depression). Products include:
Versed Injection 3027
Versed Syrup 3033

Moclobemide (Co-administration with MAO inhibitor results in increased CNS depression).
No products indexed under this heading.

Molindone Hydrochloride (Co-administration results in increased CNS depression). Products include:
Moban 1320

Morphine Sulfate (Co-administration results in increased CNS depression). Products include:
Astramorph/PF Injection, USP (Preservative-Free) 594
Duramorph Injection 1312
Infumorph 200 and Infumorph 500 Sterile Solutions 1314
Kadian Capsules 1335
MS Contin Tablets 2896
MSIR 2898
Oramorph SR Tablets 3062
Roxanol 3066

Olanzapine (Co-administration results in increased CNS depression). Products include:
Zyprexa Tablets 1973
Zyprexa ZYDIS Orally Disintegrating Tablets 1973

Oxazepam (Co-administration results in increased CNS depression).
No products indexed under this heading.

Oxcarbazepine (Co-administration results in increased CNS depression). Products include:

Trileptal Oral Suspension 2407
Trileptal Tablets 2407

Oxycodone Hydrochloride (Co-administration results in increased CNS depression). Products include:
OxyContin Tablets 2912
OxyFast Oral Concentrate Solution . 2916
OxyIR Capsules 2916
Percocet Tablets 1326
Percodan Tablets 1327
Percolone Tablets 1327
Roxicodone 3067
Tylox Capsules 2597

Paramethadione (Co-administration results in increased CNS depression).
No products indexed under this heading.

Pargyline Hydrochloride (Co-administration with MAO inhibitor results in increased CNS depression).
No products indexed under this heading.

Pentobarbital Sodium (Co-administration results in increased CNS depression). Products include:
Nembutal Sodium Solution 485

Perphenazine (Co-administration results in increased CNS depression). Products include:
Etrafon 3115
Trilafon 3160

Phenacemide (Co-administration results in increased CNS depression).
No products indexed under this heading.

Phenelzine Sulfate (Co-administration with MAO inhibitor results in increased CNS depression). Products include:
Nardil Tablets 2653

Phenobarbital (Co-administration results in increased CNS depression). Products include:
Arco-Lase Plus Tablets 592
Donnatal 2929
Donnatal Extentabs 2930

Phensuximide (Co-administration results in increased CNS depression).
No products indexed under this heading.

Phenytoin (Co-administration results in increased CNS depression). Products include:
Dilantin Infatabs 2624
Dilantin-125 Oral Suspension 2625

Phenytoin Sodium (Co-administration results in increased CNS depression). Products include:
Dilantin Kapseals 2622

Prazepam (Co-administration results in increased CNS depression).
No products indexed under this heading.

Primidone (Co-administration results in increased CNS depression).
No products indexed under this heading.

Procarbazine Hydrochloride (Co-administration with MAO inhibitor results in increased CNS depression). Products include:
Matulane Capsules 3246

Prochlorperazine (Co-administration results in increased CNS depression). Products include:
Compazine 1505

Promethazine Hydrochloride (Co-administration results in increased CNS depression). Products include:
Mepergan Injection 3539
Phenergan Injection 3553
Phenergan 3556
Phenergan Syrup 3554
Phenergan with Codeine Syrup 3557
Phenergan with Dextromethorphan Syrup 3559
Phenergan VC Syrup 3560
Phenergan VC with Codeine Syrup .. 3561

Propofol (Co-administration results in increased CNS depression). Products include:
Diprivan Injectable Emulsion 667

Propoxyphene Hydrochloride (Co-administration results in increased CNS depression). Products include:
Darvon Pulvules 1909
Darvon Compound-65 Pulvules 1910

Propoxyphene Napsylate (Co-administration results in increased CNS depression). Products include:
Darvon-N/Darvocet-N 1907
Darvon-N Tablets 1912

Pyrilamine Maleate (Co-administration results in increased CNS depression). Products include:
Maximum Strength Midol Menstrual Caplets and Gelcaps 612
Maximum Strength Midol PMS Caplets and Gelcaps 613

Pyrilamine Tannate (Co-administration results in increased CNS depression). Products include:
Ryna-12 S Suspension 3351

Quazepam (Co-administration results in increased CNS depression).
No products indexed under this heading.

Quetiapine Fumarate (Co-administration results in increased CNS depression). Products include:
Seroquel Tablets 684

Remifentanil Hydrochloride (Co-administration results in increased CNS depression).
No products indexed under this heading.

Risperidone (Co-administration results in increased CNS depression). Products include:
Risperdal 1796

Secobarbital Sodium (Co-administration results in increased CNS depression).
No products indexed under this heading.

Selegiline Hydrochloride (Co-administration with MAO inhibitor results in increased CNS depression). Products include:
Eldepryl Capsules 3266

Sevoflurane (Co-administration results in increased CNS depression).
No products indexed under this heading.

Sufentanil Citrate (Co-administration results in increased CNS depression).
No products indexed under this heading.

Temazepam (Co-administration results in increased CNS depression).
No products indexed under this heading.

Terfenadine (Co-administration results in increased CNS depression).
No products indexed under this heading.

Thiamylal Sodium (Co-administration results in increased CNS depression).
No products indexed under this heading.

Thioridazine Hydrochloride (Co-administration results in increased CNS depression). Products include:
Thioridazine Hydrochloride Tablets 2289

Thiothixene (Co-administration results in increased CNS depression). Products include:
Navane Capsules 2701
Thiothixene Capsules 2290

Tiagabine Hydrochloride (Co-administration results in increased CNS depression). Products include:
Gabitril Tablets 1189

Topiramate (Co-administration results in increased CNS depression). Products include:
Topamax Sprinkle Capsules 2590
Topamax Tablets 2590

Tranylcypromine Sulfate (Co-administration with MAO inhibitor results in increased CNS depression). Products include:
Parnate Tablets 1607

Triazolam (Co-administration results in increased CNS depression). Products include:
Halcion Tablets 2823

Trifluoperazine Hydrochloride (Co-administration results in increased CNS depression). Products include:
Stelazine 1640

Trimeprazine Tartrate (Co-administration results in increased CNS depression).
No products indexed under this heading.

Trimethadione (Co-administration results in increased CNS depression).
No products indexed under this heading.

Tripelennamine Hydrochloride (Co-administration results in increased CNS depression).
No products indexed under this heading.

Triprolidine Hydrochloride (Co-administration results in increased CNS depression). Products include:
Actifed Cold & Allergy Tablets 688

Valproate Sodium (Co-administration results in increased CNS depression). Products include:
Depacon Injection 416

Valproic Acid (Co-administration results in increased CNS depression). Products include:
Depakene 421

Zaleplon (Co-administration results in increased CNS depression). Products include:
Sonata Capsules 3591

Ziprasidone Hydrochloride (Co-administration results in increased CNS depression). Products include:
Geodon Capsules 2688

Zolpidem Tartrate (Co-administration results in increased CNS depression). Products include:
Ambien Tablets 3191

Zonisamide (Co-administration results in increased CNS depression). Products include:
Zonegran Capsules 1307

Food Interactions

Alcohol (Co-administration results in increased CNS depression).

PROSTATONIN SOFTGEL CAPSULES

(Herbals, Multiple) 832
None cited in PDR database.

PROSTIGMIN INJECTABLE

(Neostigmine Methylsulfate) 1744
May interact with antiarrhythmics, general anesthetics, and certain other agents. Compounds in these categories include:

Acebutolol Hydrochloride (Interferes with neuromuscular transmission). Products include:
Sectral Capsules 3589

Adenosine (Interferes with neuromuscular transmission). Products include:
Adenocard Injection 1380
Adenoscan 1381

Amiodarone Hydrochloride (Interferes with neuromuscular transmission). Products include:
Cordarone Intravenous 3491
Cordarone Tablets 3487
Pacerone Tablets 3331

Bretylium Tosylate (Interferes with neuromuscular transmission).
No products indexed under this heading.

Decamethonium (Phase I block of depolarizing muscle relaxants may be prolonged).
No products indexed under this heading.

Disopyramide Phosphate (Interferes with neuromuscular transmission).
No products indexed under this heading.

Dofetilide (Interferes with neuromuscular transmission). Products include:
Tikosyn Capsules 2717

Enflurane (Caution should be exercised if used concurrently in myasthenia gravis).
No products indexed under this heading.

Flecainide Acetate (Interferes with neuromuscular transmission). Products include:
Tambocor Tablets 1990

Isoflurane (Caution should be exercised if used concurrently in myasthenia gravis).
No products indexed under this heading.

Kanamycin Sulfate (May accentuate neuromuscular block).
No products indexed under this heading.

Ketamine Hydrochloride (Caution should be exercised if used concurrently in myasthenia gravis).
No products indexed under this heading.

Lidocaine Hydrochloride (Interferes with neuromuscular transmission). Products include:
Bactine First Aid Liquid 611
Xylocaine Injections 653

Local Anesthetics (Prostigmin dosage increase may be required).
No products indexed under this heading.

Methohexital Sodium (Caution should be exercised if used concurrently in myasthenia gravis). Products include:
Brevital Sodium for Injection, USP .. 1815

Methoxyflurane (Caution should be exercised if used concurrently in myasthenia gravis).
No products indexed under this heading.

Mexiletine Hydrochloride (Interferes with neuromuscular transmission). Products include:
Mexitil Capsules 1047

Moricizine Hydrochloride (Interferes with neuromuscular transmission).
No products indexed under this heading.

Neomycin Sulfate (May accentuate neuromuscular block). Products include:
Cortisporin Ophthalmic Suspension Sterile .... ⊙297
Cortisporin-TC Otic Suspension 2246
NeoDecadron Sterile Ophthalmic Solution 2144
Neosporin G.U. Irrigant Sterile 2256
Neosporin Ophthalmic Ointment Sterile .... ⊙299
Neosporin Ophthalmic Solution Sterile .... ⊙300
Poly-Pred Liquifilm Ophthalmic Suspension .... ⊙245

Procainamide Hydrochloride (Interferes with neuromuscular transmission). Products include:
Procanbid Extended-Release Tablets 2262

Propafenone Hydrochloride (Interferes with neuromuscular transmission). Products include:
Rythmol Tablets – 150 mg, 225 mg, 300 mg 502

Propofol (Caution should be exercised if used concurrently in myasthenia gravis). Products include:
- Diprivan Injectable Emulsion 667

Propranolol Hydrochloride (Interferes with neuromuscular transmission). Products include:
- Inderal 3513
- Inderal LA Long-Acting Capsules 3516
- Inderide Tablets 3517
- Inderide LA Long-Acting Capsules .. 3519

Quinidine Gluconate (Interferes with neuromuscular transmission). Products include:
- Quinaglute Dura-Tabs Tablets 978

Quinidine Polygalacturonate (Interferes with neuromuscular transmission).
- No products indexed under this heading.

Quinidine Sulfate (Interferes with neuromuscular transmission). Products include:
- Quinidex Extentabs 2933

Sevoflurane (Caution should be exercised if used concurrently in myasthenia gravis).
- No products indexed under this heading.

Sotalol Hydrochloride (Interferes with neuromuscular transmission). Products include:
- Betapace Tablets 950
- Betapace AF Tablets 954

Streptomycin Sulfate (May accentuate neuromuscular block). Products include:
- Streptomycin Sulfate Injection 2714

Succinylcholine Chloride (Phase I block of depolarizing muscle relaxants may be prolonged). Products include:
- Anectine Injection 1476

Tocainide Hydrochloride (Interferes with neuromuscular transmission). Products include:
- Tonocard Tablets 649

Verapamil Hydrochloride (Interferes with neuromuscular transmission). Products include:
- Covera-HS Tablets 3199
- Isoptin SR Tablets 467
- Tarka Tablets 508
- Verelan Capsules 3184
- Verelan PM Capsules 3186

PROSTIGMIN TABLETS

(Neostigmine Bromide) 1744

May interact with antiarrhythmics, anticholinergics, and certain other agents. Compounds in these categories include:

Acebutolol Hydrochloride (Interferes with neuromuscular transmission). Products include:
- Sectral Capsules 3589

Adenosine (Interferes with neuromuscular transmission). Products include:
- Adenocard Injection 1380
- Adenoscan 1381

Amiodarone Hydrochloride (Interferes with neuromuscular transmission). Products include:
- Cordarone Intravenous 3491
- Cordarone Tablets 3487
- Pacerone Tablets 3331

Atropine Sulfate (Decreased intestinal motility). Products include:
- Donnatal 2929
- Donnatal Extentabs 2930
- Motofen Tablets 577
- Prosed/DS Tablets 3268
- Urised Tablets 2876

Belladonna Alkaloids (Decreased intestinal motility). Products include:
- Hyland's Teething Tablets .... ▣766
- Urimax Tablets 1769

Benztropine Mesylate (Decreased intestinal motility). Products include:
- Cogentin 2055

Biperiden Hydrochloride (Decreased intestinal motility). Products include:
- Akineton 402

Bretylium Tosylate (Interferes with neuromuscular transmission).
- No products indexed under this heading.

Clidinium Bromide (Decreased intestinal motility).
- No products indexed under this heading.

Dicyclomine Hydrochloride (Decreased intestinal motility).
- No products indexed under this heading.

Disopyramide Phosphate (Interferes with neuromuscular transmission).
- No products indexed under this heading.

Dofetilide (Interferes with neuromuscular transmission). Products include:
- Tikosyn Capsules 2717

Ethopropazine Hydrochloride (Decreased intestinal motility).
- No products indexed under this heading.

Flecainide Acetate (Interferes with neuromuscular transmission). Products include:
- Tambocor Tablets 1990

Glycopyrrolate (Decreased intestinal motility). Products include:
- Robinul Forte Tablets 1358
- Robinul Injectable 2940
- Robinul Tablets 1358

Hyoscyamine (Decreased intestinal motility). Products include:
- Urised Tablets 2876

Hyoscyamine Sulfate (Decreased intestinal motility). Products include:
- Arco-Lase Plus Tablets 592
- Donnatal 2929
- Donnatal Extentabs 2930
- Levsin/Levsinex/Levbid 3172
- NuLev Orally Disintegrating Tablets 3176
- Prosed/DS Tablets 3268
- Urimax Tablets 1769

Ipratropium Bromide (Decreased intestinal motility). Products include:
- Atrovent Inhalation Aerosol 1030
- Atrovent Inhalation Solution 1031
- Atrovent Nasal Spray 0.03% 1032
- Atrovent Nasal Spray 0.06% 1033
- Combivent Inhalation Aerosol 1041
- DuoNeb Inhalation Solution 1233

Kanamycin Sulfate (May accentuate neuromuscular block).
- No products indexed under this heading.

Lidocaine Hydrochloride (Interferes with neuromuscular transmission). Products include:
- Bactine First Aid Liquid .... ▣611
- Xylocaine Injections 653

Local Anesthetics (Prostigmin dosage increase may be required).

Mepenzolate Bromide (Decreased intestinal motility).
- No products indexed under this heading.

Mexiletine Hydrochloride (Interferes with neuromuscular transmission). Products include:
- Mexitil Capsules 1047

Moricizine Hydrochloride (Interferes with neuromuscular transmission).
- No products indexed under this heading.

Oxybutynin Chloride (Decreased intestinal motility). Products include:
- Ditropan XL Extended Release Tablets 564

Oxyphenonium Bromide (Decreased intestinal motility).
- No products indexed under this heading.

Procainamide Hydrochloride (Interferes with neuromuscular transmission). Products include:
- Procanbid Extended-Release Tablets 2262

Procyclidine Hydrochloride (Decreased intestinal motility).
- No products indexed under this heading.

Propafenone Hydrochloride (Interferes with neuromuscular transmission). Products include:
- Rythmol Tablets – 150 mg, 225 mg, 300 mg 502

Propantheline Bromide (Decreased intestinal motility).
- No products indexed under this heading.

Propranolol Hydrochloride (Interferes with neuromuscular transmission). Products include:
- Inderal 3513
- Inderal LA Long-Acting Capsules 3516
- Inderide Tablets 3517
- Inderide LA Long-Acting Capsules .. 3519

Quinidine Gluconate (Interferes with neuromuscular transmission). Products include:
- Quinaglute Dura-Tabs Tablets 978

Quinidine Polygalacturonate (Interferes with neuromuscular transmission).
- No products indexed under this heading.

Quinidine Sulfate (Interferes with neuromuscular transmission). Products include:
- Quinidex Extentabs 2933

Scopolamine (Decreased intestinal motility). Products include:
- Transderm Scōp Transdermal Therapeutic System 2302

Scopolamine Hydrobromide (Decreased intestinal motility). Products include:
- Donnatal 2929
- Donnatal Extentabs 2930

Sotalol Hydrochloride (Interferes with neuromuscular transmission). Products include:
- Betapace Tablets 950
- Betapace AF Tablets 954

Streptomycin Sulfate (May accentuate neuromuscular block). Products include:
- Streptomycin Sulfate Injection 2714

Tocainide Hydrochloride (Interferes with neuromuscular transmission). Products include:
- Tonocard Tablets 649

Tolterodine Tartrate (Decreased intestinal motility). Products include:
- Detrol Tablets 3623
- Detrol LA Capsules 2801

Tridihexethyl Chloride (Decreased intestinal motility).
- No products indexed under this heading.

Trihexyphenidyl Hydrochloride (Decreased intestinal motility). Products include:
- Artane 1855

Verapamil Hydrochloride (Interferes with neuromuscular transmission). Products include:
- Covera-HS Tablets 3199
- Isoptin SR Tablets 467
- Tarka Tablets 508
- Verelan Capsules 3184
- Verelan PM Capsules 3186

PROSTIN E2 SUPPOSITORIES

(Dinoprostone) 2852

May interact with oxytocic drugs. Compounds in these categories include:

Ergonovine Maleate (Prostin E2 may augment the activity of other oxytocic drugs; co-administration is not recommended).
- No products indexed under this heading.

Methylergonovine Maleate (Prostin E2 may augment the activity of other oxytocic drugs; co-administration is not recommended).
- No products indexed under this heading.

Oxytocin (Prostin E2 may augment the activity of other oxytocic drugs; co-administration is not recommended).
- No products indexed under this heading.

PROTONIX I.V.

(Pantoprazole Sodium) 3580

See Protonix Tablets

PROTONIX TABLETS

(Pantoprazole Sodium) 3577

May interact with iron containing oral preparations and certain other agents. Compounds in these categories include:

Bacampicillin Hydrochloride (Pantoprazole produces sustained inhibition of gastric acid secretion; pantoprazole may interfere with the absorption of certain drugs, such as ampicillin esters, where gastric pH is an important determinant of the bioavailability).
- No products indexed under this heading.

Ferrous Fumarate (Pantoprazole produces sustained inhibition of gastric acid secretion; pantoprazole may interfere with the absorption of certain drugs, such as iron salts, where gastric pH is an important determinant of the bioavailability). Products include:
- New Formulation Chromagen OB Capsules 3094
- Loestrin Fe Tablets 2642
- NataChew Tablets 3364

Ferrous Gluconate (Pantoprazole produces sustained inhibition of gastric acid secretion; pantoprazole may interfere with the absorption of certain drugs, such as iron salts, where gastric pH is an important determinant of the bioavailability). Products include:
- Fergon Iron Tablets .... ▣802

Ferrous Sulfate (Pantoprazole produces sustained inhibition of gastric acid secretion; pantoprazole may interfere with the absorption of certain drugs, such as iron salts, where gastric pH is an important determinant of the bioavailability). Products include:
- Feosol Tablets 1717
- Slow Fe Tablets .... ▣827
- Slow Fe with Folic Acid Tablets .... ▣828

Iron (Pantoprazole produces sustained inhibition of gastric acid secretion; pantoprazole may interfere with the absorption of certain drugs, such as iron salts, where gastric pH is an important determinant of the bioavailability).
- No products indexed under this heading.

Ketoconazole (Pantoprazole produces sustained inhibition of gastric acid secretion; pantoprazole may interfere with the absorption of certain drugs, such as ketoconazole, where gastric pH is an important determinant of the bioavailability). Products include:
- Nizoral 2% Cream 3620
- Nizoral A-D Shampoo 2008
- Nizoral 2% Shampoo 2007
- Nizoral Tablets 1791

Polysaccharide-Iron Complex (Pantoprazole produces sustained inhibition of gastric acid secretion; pantoprazole may interfere with the absorption of certain drugs, such as iron salts, where gastric pH is an important determinant of the bioavailability). Products include:
- Niferex 3176
- Niferex-150 Capsules 3176
- Nu-Iron 150 Capsules 2224

PROTOPAM CHLORIDE FOR INJECTION

(Pralidoxime Chloride) 3582

May interact with barbiturates, phenothiazines, theophylline, and certain other agents. Compounds in these categories include:

Aminophylline (Concurrent use should be avoided in patients with organophosphate poisoning).
- No products indexed under this heading.

Aprobarbital (Barbiturates are potentiated by the anticholinester-

ases, they should be used cautiously in the treatment of convulsions).
No products indexed under this heading.

Atropine Nitrate, Methyl (Signs of atropinization may occur earlier than expected).
No products indexed under this heading.

Atropine Sulfate (Signs of atropinization may occur earlier than expected). Products include:
Donnatal 2929
Donnatal Extentabs 2930
Motofen Tablets 577
Prosed/DS Tablets 3268
Urised Tablets 2876

Butabarbital (Barbiturates are potentiated by the anticholinesterases, they should be used cautiously in the treatment of convulsions).
No products indexed under this heading.

Butalbital (Barbiturates are potentiated by the anticholinesterases, they should be used cautiously in the treatment of convulsions). Products include:
Phrenilin 578
Sedapap Tablets 50 mg/650 mg 2225

Chlorpromazine (Concurrent use should be avoided in patients with organophosphate poisoning). Products include:
Thorazine Suppositories 1656

Chlorpromazine Hydrochloride (Concurrent use should be avoided in patients with organophosphate poisoning). Products include:
Thorazine 1656

Dyphylline (Concurrent use should be avoided in patients with organophosphate poisoning). Products include:
Lufyllin Tablets 3347
Lufyllin-400 Tablets 3347
Lufyllin-GG Elixir 3348
Lufyllin-GG Tablets 3348

Fluphenazine Decanoate (Concurrent use should be avoided in patients with organophosphate poisoning).
No products indexed under this heading.

Fluphenazine Enanthate (Concurrent use should be avoided in patients with organophosphate poisoning).
No products indexed under this heading.

Fluphenazine Hydrochloride (Concurrent use should be avoided in patients with organophosphate poisoning).
No products indexed under this heading.

Mephobarbital (Barbiturates are potentiated by the anticholinesterases, they should be used cautiously in the treatment of convulsions).
No products indexed under this heading.

Mesoridazine Besylate (Concurrent use should be avoided in patients with organophosphate poisoning). Products include:
Serentil 1057

Methotrimeprazine (Concurrent use should be avoided in patients with organophosphate poisoning).
No products indexed under this heading.

Morphine Sulfate (Concurrent use should be avoided in patients with organophosphate poisoning). Products include:
Astramorph/PF Injection, USP (Preservative-Free) 594
Duramorph Injection 1312
Infumorph 200 and Infumorph 500 Sterile Solutions 1314
Kadian Capsules 1335
MS Contin Tablets 2896
MSIR 2898
Oramorph SR Tablets 3062
Roxanol 3066

Pentobarbital Sodium (Barbiturates are potentiated by the anticholinesterases, they should be used cautiously in the treatment of convulsions). Products include:
Nembutal Sodium Solution 485

Perphenazine (Concurrent use should be avoided in patients with organophosphate poisoning). Products include:
Etrafon 3115
Trilafon 3160

Phenobarbital (Barbiturates are potentiated by the anticholinesterases, they should be used cautiously in the treatment of convulsions). Products include:
Arco-Lase Plus Tablets 592
Donnatal 2929
Donnatal Extentabs 2930

Prochlorperazine (Concurrent use should be avoided in patients with organophosphate poisoning). Products include:
Compazine 1505

Promethazine Hydrochloride (Concurrent use should be avoided in patients with organophosphate poisoning). Products include:
Mepergan Injection 3539
Phenergan Injection 3553
Phenergan 3556
Phenergan Syrup 3554
Phenergan with Codeine Syrup 3557
Phenergan with Dextromethorphan Syrup 3559
Phenergan VC Syrup 3560
Phenergan VC with Codeine Syrup 3561

Reserpine (Concurrent use should be avoided in patients with organophosphate poisoning).
No products indexed under this heading.

Secobarbital Sodium (Barbiturates are potentiated by the anticholinesterases, they should be used cautiously in the treatment of convulsions).
No products indexed under this heading.

Succinylcholine Chloride (Concurrent use should be avoided in patients with organophosphate poisoning). Products include:
Anectine Injection 1476

Theophylline (Concurrent use should be avoided in patients with organophosphate poisoning). Products include:
Aerolate 1361
Theo-Dur Extended-Release Tablets 1835
Uni-Dur Extended-Release Tablets 1841
Uniphyl 400 mg and 600 mg Tablets 2903

Theophylline Calcium Salicylate (Concurrent use should be avoided in patients with organophosphate poisoning).
No products indexed under this heading.

Theophylline Sodium Glycinate (Concurrent use should be avoided in patients with organophosphate poisoning).
No products indexed under this heading.

Thiamylal Sodium (Barbiturates are potentiated by the anticholinesterases, they should be used cautiously in the treatment of convulsions).
No products indexed under this heading.

Thioridazine Hydrochloride (Concurrent use should be avoided in patients with organophosphate poisoning). Products include:
Thioridazine Hydrochloride Tablets 2289

Trifluoperazine Hydrochloride (Concurrent use should be avoided in patients with organophosphate poisoning). Products include:
Stelazine 1640

PROTOPIC OINTMENT

(Tacrolimus) 1397

May interact with calcium channel blockers, erythromycin, and certain other agents. Compounds in these categories include:

Amlodipine Besylate (Co-administration of known CYP3A4 inhibitors, such as calcium channel blockers, in patients with widespread and/or erythrodermic disease should be done with caution; based on its minimal extent of absorption, interactions of Protopic Ointment with systemically administered drugs are unlikely to occur but cannot be ruled out). Products include:
Lotrel Capsules 2370
Norvasc Tablets 2704

Bepridil Hydrochloride (Co-administration of known CYP3A4 inhibitors, such as calcium channel blockers, in patients with widespread and/or erythrodermic disease should be done with caution; based on its minimal extent of absorption, interactions of Protopic Ointment with systemically administered drugs are unlikely to occur but cannot be ruled out). Products include:
Vascor Tablets 2602

Cimetidine (Co-administration of known CYP3A4 inhibitors, such as cimetidine, in patients with widespread and/or erythrodermic disease should be done with caution; based on its minimal extent of absorption, interactions of Protopic Ointment with systemically administered drugs are unlikely to occur but cannot be ruled out). Products include:
Tagamet HB 200 Suspension 762
Tagamet HB 200 Tablets 761
Tagamet Tablets 1644

Cimetidine Hydrochloride (Co-administration of known CYP3A4 inhibitors, such as cimetidine, in patients with widespread and/or erythrodermic disease should be done with caution; based on its minimal extent of absorption, interactions of Protopic Ointment with systemically administered drugs are unlikely to occur but cannot be ruled out). Products include:
Tagamet 1644

Diltiazem Hydrochloride (Co-administration of known CYP3A4 inhibitors, such as calcium channel blockers, in patients with widespread and/or erythrodermic disease should be done with caution; based on its minimal extent of absorption, interactions of Protopic Ointment with systemically administered drugs are unlikely to occur but cannot be ruled out). Products include:
Cardizem Injectable 1018
Cardizem Lyo-Ject Syringe 1018
Cardizem Monovial 1018
Cardizem CD Capsules 1016
Tiazac Capsules 1378

Erythromycin (Co-administration of known CYP3A4 inhibitors, such as erythromycin, in patients with widespread and/or erythrodermic disease should be done with caution; based on its minimal extent of absorption, interactions of Protopic Ointment with systemically administered drugs are unlikely to occur but cannot be ruled out). Products include:
Emgel 2% Topical Gel 1285
Ery-Tab Tablets 448
Erythromycin Base Filmtab Tablets 454
Erythromycin Delayed-Release Capsules, USP 455
PCE Dispertab Tablets 498

Erythromycin Estolate (Co-administration of known CYP3A4 inhibitors, such as erythromycin, in patients with widespread and/or erythrodermic disease should be done with caution; based on its minimal extent of absorption, interactions of Protopic Ointment with systemically administered drugs are unlikely to occur but cannot be ruled out).
No products indexed under this heading.

Erythromycin Ethylsuccinate (Co-administration of known CYP3A4 inhibitors, such as erythromycin, in patients with widespread and/or erythrodermic disease should be done with caution; based on its minimal extent of absorption, interactions of Protopic Ointment with systemically administered drugs are unlikely to occur but cannot be ruled out). Products include:
E.E.S. 450
EryPed 446
Pediazole Suspension 3050

Erythromycin Gluceptate (Co-administration of known CYP3A4 inhibitors, such as erythromycin, in patients with widespread and/or erythrodermic disease should be done with caution; based on its minimal extent of absorption, interactions of Protopic Ointment with systemically administered drugs are unlikely to occur but cannot be ruled out).
No products indexed under this heading.

Erythromycin Stearate (Co-administration of known CYP3A4 inhibitors, such as erythromycin, in patients with widespread and/or erythrodermic disease should be done with caution; based on its minimal extent of absorption, interactions of Protopic Ointment with systemically administered drugs are unlikely to occur but cannot be ruled out). Products include:
Erythrocin Stearate Filmtab Tablets 452

Felodipine (Co-administration of known CYP3A4 inhibitors, such as calcium channel blockers, in patients with widespread and/or erythrodermic disease should be done with caution; based on its minimal extent of absorption, interactions of Protopic Ointment with systemically administered drugs are unlikely to occur but cannot be ruled out). Products include:
Lexxel Tablets 608
Plendil Extended-Release Tablets 623

Fluconazole (Co-administration of known CYP3A4 inhibitors, such as fluconazole, in patients with widespread and/or erythrodermic disease should be done with caution; based on its minimal extent of absorption, interactions of Protopic Ointment with systemically administered drugs are unlikely to occur but cannot be ruled out). Products include:
Diflucan Tablets, Injection, and Oral Suspension 2681

Isradipine (Co-administration of known CYP3A4 inhibitors, such as calcium channel blockers, in patients with widespread and/or erythrodermic disease should be done with caution; based on its minimal extent of absorption, interactions of Protopic Ointment with systemically administered drugs are unlikely to occur but cannot be ruled out). Products include:
DynaCirc Capsules 2921
DynaCirc CR Tablets 2923

Itraconazole (Co-administration of known CYP3A4 inhibitors, such as itraconazole, in patients with widespread and/or erythrodermic disease should be done with caution; based on its minimal extent of absorption, interactions of Protopic Ointment with systemically adminis-

tered drugs are unlikely to occur but cannot be ruled out). Products include:

- Sporanox Capsules 1800
- Sporanox Injection 1804
- Sporanox Injection 2509
- Sporanox Oral Solution 1808
- Sporanox Oral Solution 2512

Ketoconazole (Co-administration of known CYP3A4 inhibitors, such as ketoconazole, in patients with widespread and/or erythrodermic disease should be done with caution; based on its minimal extent of absorption, interactions of Protopic Ointment with systemically administered drugs are unlikely to occur but cannot be ruled out). Products include:

- Nizoral 2% Cream 3620
- Nizoral A-D Shampoo 2008
- Nizoral 2% Shampoo 2007
- Nizoral Tablets 1791

Mibefradil Dihydrochloride (Co-administration of known CYP3A4 inhibitors, such as calcium channel blockers, in patients with widespread and/or erythrodermic disease should be done with caution; based on its minimal extent of absorption, interactions of Protopic Ointment with systemically administered drugs are unlikely to occur but cannot be ruled out).

No products indexed under this heading.

Nicardipine Hydrochloride (Co-administration of known CYP3A4 inhibitors, such as calcium channel blockers, in patients with widespread and/or erythrodermic disease should be done with caution; based on its minimal extent of absorption, interactions of Protopic Ointment with systemically administered drugs are unlikely to occur but cannot be ruled out). Products include:

- Cardene I.V. 3485

Nifedipine (Co-administration of known CYP3A4 inhibitors, such as calcium channel blockers, in patients with widespread and/or erythrodermic disease should be done with caution; based on its minimal extent of absorption, interactions of Protopic Ointment with systemically administered drugs are unlikely to occur but cannot be ruled out). Products include:

- Adalat CC Tablets 877
- Procardia Capsules 2708
- Procardia XL Extended Release Tablets 2710

Nimodipine (Co-administration of known CYP3A4 inhibitors, such as calcium channel blockers, in patients with widespread and/or erythrodermic disease should be done with caution; based on its minimal extent of absorption, interactions of Protopic Ointment with systemically administered drugs are unlikely to occur but cannot be ruled out). Products include:

- Nimotop Capsules 904

Nisoldipine (Co-administration of known CYP3A4 inhibitors, such as calcium channel blockers, in patients with widespread and/or erythrodermic disease should be done with caution; based on its minimal extent of absorption, interactions of Protopic Ointment with systemically administered drugs are unlikely to occur but cannot be ruled out). Products include:

- Sular Tablets 688

Verapamil Hydrochloride (Co-administration of known CYP3A4 inhibitors, such as calcium channel blockers, in patients with widespread and/or erythrodermic disease should be done with caution; based on its minimal extent of absorption, interactions of Protopic Ointment with systemically administered drugs are unlikely to occur but cannot be ruled out). Products include:

- Covera-HS Tablets 3199
- Isoptin SR Tablets 467
- Tarka Tablets 508
- Verelan Capsules 3184
- Verelan PM Capsules 3186

PROVENTIL INHALATION AEROSOL

(Albuterol) 3142

May interact with beta blockers, drugs that lower serum potassium (selected), monoamine oxidase inhibitors, sympathomimetics, tricyclic antidepressants, and certain other agents. Compounds in these categories include:

Acebutolol Hydrochloride (Effects of both drugs inhibited). Products include:

- Sectral Capsules 3589

Albuterol Sulfate (Concomitant use with other oral sympathomimetic agents is not recommended since such use may lead to deleterious cardiovascular effects). Products include:

- AccuNeb Inhalation Solution 1230
- Combivent Inhalation Aerosol 1041
- DuoNeb Inhalation Solution 1233
- Proventil Inhalation Solution 0.083% 3146
- Proventil Repetabs Tablets 3148
- Proventil Solution for Inhalation 0.5% 3144
- Proventil HFA Inhalation Aerosol 3150
- Ventolin HFA Inhalation Aerosol 3618
- Volmax Extended-Release Tablets 2276

Amitriptyline Hydrochloride (Potentiation of albuterol's action on vascular system). Products include:

- Etrafon 3115
- Limbitrol 1738

Amoxapine (Potentiation of albuterol's action on vascular system).

No products indexed under this heading.

Atenolol (Effects of both drugs inhibited). Products include:

- Tenoretic Tablets 690
- Tenormin I.V. Injection 692

Bendroflumethiazide (Potential for additive hypokalemic effect with concurrent use). Products include:

- Corzide 40/5 Tablets 2247
- Corzide 80/5 Tablets 2247

Betamethasone Acetate (Potential for additive hypokalemic effect with concurrent use). Products include:

- Celestone Soluspan Injectable Suspension 3097

Betamethasone Sodium Phosphate (Potential for additive hypokalemic effect with concurrent use). Products include:

- Celestone Soluspan Injectable Suspension 3097

Betaxolol Hydrochloride (Effects of both drugs inhibited). Products include:

- Betoptic S Ophthalmic Suspension 537

Bisoprolol Fumarate (Effects of both drugs inhibited). Products include:

- Zebeta Tablets 1885
- Ziac Tablets 1887

Carteolol Hydrochloride (Effects of both drugs inhibited). Products include:

- Carteolol Hydrochloride Ophthalmic Solution USP, 1% ⊙258
- Ocupress Ophthalmic Solution, 1% Sterile ⊙303

Chlorothiazide (Potential for additive hypokalemic effect with concurrent use). Products include:

- Aldoclor Tablets 2035
- Diuril Oral 2087

Chlorothiazide Sodium (Potential for additive hypokalemic effect with concurrent use). Products include:

- Diuril Sodium Intravenous 2086

Clomipramine Hydrochloride (Potentiation of albuterol's action on vascular system).

No products indexed under this heading.

Cortisone Acetate (Potential for additive hypokalemic effect with concurrent use). Products include:

- Cortone Acetate Injectable Suspension 2059
- Cortone Acetate Tablets 2061

Desipramine Hydrochloride (Potentiation of albuterol's action on vascular system). Products include:

- Norpramin Tablets 755

Dexamethasone (Potential for additive hypokalemic effect with concurrent use). Products include:

- Decadron Elixir 2078
- Decadron Tablets 2079
- TobraDex Ophthalmic Ointment 542
- TobraDex Ophthalmic Suspension 541

Dexamethasone Acetate (Potential for additive hypokalemic effect with concurrent use).

No products indexed under this heading.

Dexamethasone Sodium Phosphate (Potential for additive hypokalemic effect with concurrent use). Products include:

- Decadron Phosphate Injection 2081
- Decadron Phosphate Sterile Ophthalmic Ointment 2083
- Decadron Phosphate Sterile Ophthalmic Solution 2084
- NeoDecadron Sterile Ophthalmic Solution 2144

Digoxin (Decreased serum digoxin levels (16%-22%); the clinical significance of these findings for patients with COPD who are concurrently taking these drugs on a chronic basis is unclear). Products include:

- Digitek Tablets 1003
- Lanoxicaps Capsules 1574
- Lanoxin Injection 1581
- Lanoxin Tablets 1587
- Lanoxin Elixir Pediatric 1578
- Lanoxin Injection Pediatric 1584

Dobutamine Hydrochloride (Concomitant use with other oral sympathomimetic agents is not recommended since such use may lead to deleterious cardiovascular effects). Products include:

- Dobutrex Solution Vials 1914

Dopamine Hydrochloride (Concomitant use with other oral sympathomimetic agents is not recommended since such use may lead to deleterious cardiovascular effects).

No products indexed under this heading.

Doxepin Hydrochloride (Potentiation of albuterol's action on vascular system). Products include:

- Sinequan 2713

Ephedrine Hydrochloride (Concomitant use with other oral sympathomimetic agents is not recommended since such use may lead to deleterious cardiovascular effects). Products include:

- Primatene Tablets ▣780

Ephedrine Sulfate (Concomitant use with other oral sympathomimetic agents is not recommended since such use may lead to deleterious cardiovascular effects).

No products indexed under this heading.

Ephedrine Tannate (Concomitant use with other oral sympathomimetic agents is not recommended since such use may lead to deleterious cardiovascular effects). Products include:

- Rynatuss Pediatric Suspension 3353
- Rynatuss Tablets 3353

Epinephrine (Concomitant use with other oral sympathomimetic agents is not recommended since such use may lead to deleterious cardiovascular effects). Products include:

- Epifrin Sterile Ophthalmic Solution ⊙235
- EpiPen 1236
- Primatene Mist ▣779
- Xylocaine with Epinephrine Injection 653

Epinephrine Bitartrate (Concomitant use with other oral sympathomimetic agents is not recommended since such use may lead to deleterious cardiovascular effects). Products include:

- Sensorcaine 643

Epinephrine Hydrochloride (Concomitant use with other oral sympathomimetic agents is not recommended since such use may lead to deleterious cardiovascular effects).

No products indexed under this heading.

Esmolol Hydrochloride (Effects of both drugs inhibited). Products include:

- Brevibloc Injection 858

Hydrochlorothiazide (Potential for additive hypokalemic effect with concurrent use). Products include:

- Accuretic Tablets 2614
- Aldoril Tablets 2039
- Atacand HCT Tablets 597
- Avalide Tablets 1070
- Diovan HCT Tablets 2338
- Dyazide Capsules 1515
- HydroDIURIL Tablets 2108
- Hyzaar 2109
- Inderide Tablets 3517
- Inderide LA Long-Acting Capsules 3519
- Lotensin HCT Tablets 2367
- Maxzide 1008
- Micardis HCT Tablets 1051
- Microzide Capsules 3414
- Moduretic Tablets 2138
- Monopril HCT 1094
- Prinzide Tablets 2168
- Timolide Tablets 2187
- Uniretic Tablets 3178
- Vaseretic Tablets 2204
- Zestoretic Tablets 695
- Ziac Tablets 1887

Hydrocortisone (Potential for additive hypokalemic effect with concurrent use). Products include:

- Anusol-HC Cream 2.5% 2237
- Cipro HC Otic Suspension 540
- Cortaid Intensive Therapy Cream ▣717
- Cortaid Maximum Strength Cream ▣717
- Cortisporin Ophthalmic Suspension Sterile ⊙297
- Cortizone•5 ▣699
- Cortizone•10 ▣699
- Cortizone•10 Plus Creme ▣700
- Cortizone for Kids Creme ▣699
- Hydrocortone Tablets 2106
- Massengill Medicated Soft Cloth Towelette ▣753
- VōSoL HC Otic Solution 3356

Hydrocortisone Acetate (Potential for additive hypokalemic effect with concurrent use). Products include:

- Analpram-HC 1338
- Anusol HC-1 Hydrocortisone Anti-Itch Cream ▣689
- Anusol-HC Suppositories 2238
- Cortaid ▣717
- Cortifoam Rectal Foam 3170
- Cortisporin-TC Otic Suspension 2246
- Hydrocortone Acetate Injectable Suspension 2103
- Pramosone 1343
- Proctocort Suppositories 2264
- ProctoFoam-HC 3177
- Terra-Cortril Ophthalmic Suspension 2716

Hydrocortisone Sodium Phosphate (Potential for additive hypokalemic effect with concurrent use). Products include:

- Hydrocortone Phosphate Injection, Sterile 2105

Hydrocortisone Sodium Succinate (Potential for additive hypokalemic effect with concurrent use).

No products indexed under this heading.

Hydroflumethiazide (Potential for additive hypokalemic effect with concurrent use). Products include:

- Diucardin Tablets 3494

Imipramine Hydrochloride (Potentiation of albuterol's action on vascular system).
No products indexed under this heading.

Imipramine Pamoate (Potentiation of albuterol's action on vascular system).
No products indexed under this heading.

Isocarboxazid (Potentiation of albuterol's action on vascular system).
No products indexed under this heading.

Isoproterenol Hydrochloride (Concomitant use with other oral sympathomimetic agents is not recommended since such use may lead to deleterious cardiovascular effects).
No products indexed under this heading.

Isoproterenol Sulfate (Concomitant use with other oral sympathomimetic agents is not recommended since such use may lead to deleterious cardiovascular effects).
No products indexed under this heading.

Labetalol Hydrochloride (Effects of both drugs inhibited). Products include:
Normodyne Injection 3135
Normodyne Tablets 3137

Levalbuterol Hydrochloride (Concomitant use with other oral sympathomimetic agents is not recommended since such use may lead to deleterious cardiovascular effects). Products include:
Xopenex Inhalation Solution 3207

Levobunolol Hydrochloride (Effects of both drugs inhibited). Products include:
Betagan ..... ⊙228

Maprotiline Hydrochloride (Potentiation of albuterol's action on vascular system).
No products indexed under this heading.

Metaproterenol Sulfate (Concomitant use with other oral sympathomimetic agents is not recommended since such use may lead to deleterious cardiovascular effects). Products include:
Alupent 1029

Metaraminol Bitartrate (Concomitant use with other oral sympathomimetic agents is not recommended since such use may lead to deleterious cardiovascular effects). Products include:
Aramine Injection 2043

Methoxamine Hydrochloride (Concomitant use with other oral sympathomimetic agents is not recommended since such use may lead to deleterious cardiovascular effects).
No products indexed under this heading.

Methyclothiazide (Potential for additive hypokalemic effect with concurrent use).
No products indexed under this heading.

Methylprednisolone Acetate (Potential for additive hypokalemic effect with concurrent use). Products include:
Depo-Medrol Injectable Suspension 2795

Methylprednisolone Sodium Succinate (Potential for additive hypokalemic effect with concurrent use). Products include:
Solu-Medrol Sterile Powder 2855

Metipranolol Hydrochloride (Effects of both drugs inhibited).
No products indexed under this heading.

Metoprolol Succinate (Effects of both drugs inhibited). Products include:
Toprol-XL Tablets 651

Metoprolol Tartrate (Effects of both drugs inhibited).
No products indexed under this heading.

Moclobemide (Potentiation of albuterol's action on vascular system).
No products indexed under this heading.

Nadolol (Effects of both drugs inhibited). Products include:
Corgard Tablets 2245
Corzide 40/5 Tablets 2247
Corzide 80/5 Tablets 2247
Nadolol Tablets 2288

Norepinephrine Bitartrate (Concomitant use with other oral sympathomimetic agents is not recommended since such use may lead to deleterious cardiovascular effects).
No products indexed under this heading.

Nortriptyline Hydrochloride (Potentiation of albuterol's action on vascular system).
No products indexed under this heading.

Pargyline Hydrochloride (Potentiation of albuterol's action on vascular system).
No products indexed under this heading.

Penbutolol Sulfate (Effects of both drugs inhibited).
No products indexed under this heading.

Phenelzine Sulfate (Potentiation of albuterol's action on vascular system). Products include:
Nardil Tablets 2653

Phenylephrine Bitartrate (Concomitant use with other oral sympathomimetic agents is not recommended since such use may lead to deleterious cardiovascular effects).
No products indexed under this heading.

Phenylephrine Hydrochloride (Concomitant use with other oral sympathomimetic agents is not recommended since such use may lead to deleterious cardiovascular effects). Products include:
Afrin Nasal Decongestant Children's Pump Mist ..... ■734
Extendryl 1361
Hycomine Compound Tablets 1317
Neo-Synephrine ..... ■614
Phenergan VC Syrup 3560
Phenergan VC with Codeine Syrup 3561
Preparation H Cream ..... ■778
Preparation H Cooling Gel ..... ■778
Preparation H ..... ■778
Vicks Sinex Nasal Spray and Ultra Fine Mist ..... ■729

Phenylephrine Tannate (Concomitant use with other oral sympathomimetic agents is not recommended since such use may lead to deleterious cardiovascular effects). Products include:
Ryna-12 S Suspension 3351
Reformulated Rynatan Pediatric Suspension 3352
Rynatuss Pediatric Suspension 3353
Rynatuss Tablets 3353

Phenylpropanolamine Hydrochloride (Concomitant use with other oral sympathomimetic agents is not recommended since such use may lead to deleterious cardiovascular effects).
No products indexed under this heading.

Pindolol (Effects of both drugs inhibited).
No products indexed under this heading.

Pirbuterol Acetate (Concomitant use with other oral sympathomimetic agents is not recommended since such use may lead to deleterious cardiovascular effects). Products include:
Maxair Autohaler 1981
Maxair Inhaler 1984

Polythiazide (Potential for additive hypokalemic effect with concurrent use). Products include:
Minizide Capsules 2700
Renese Tablets 2712

Prednisolone Acetate (Potential for additive hypokalemic effect with concurrent use). Products include:
Blephamide Ophthalmic Ointment 547
Blephamide Ophthalmic Suspension 548
Poly-Pred Liquifilm Ophthalmic Suspension ..... ⊙245
Pred Forte Ophthalmic Suspension ..... ⊙246
Pred Mild Sterile Ophthalmic Suspension ..... ⊙249
Pred-G Ophthalmic Suspension ..... ⊙247
Pred-G Sterile Ophthalmic Ointment ..... ⊙248

Prednisolone Sodium Phosphate (Potential for additive hypokalemic effect with concurrent use). Products include:
Pediapred Oral Solution 1170

Prednisolone Tebutate (Potential for additive hypokalemic effect with concurrent use).
No products indexed under this heading.

Prednisone (Potential for additive hypokalemic effect with concurrent use). Products include:
Prednisone 3064

Procarbazine Hydrochloride (Potentiation of albuterol's action on vascular system). Products include:
Matulane Capsules 3246

Propranolol Hydrochloride (Effects of both drugs inhibited). Products include:
Inderal 3513
Inderal LA Long-Acting Capsules 3516
Inderide Tablets 3517
Inderide LA Long-Acting Capsules 3519

Protriptyline Hydrochloride (Potentiation of albuterol's action on vascular system). Products include:
Vivactil Tablets 2446
Vivactil Tablets 2217

Pseudoephedrine Hydrochloride (Concomitant use with other oral sympathomimetic agents is not recommended since such use may lead to deleterious cardiovascular effects). Products include:
Actifed Cold & Allergy Tablets ..... ■688
Actifed Cold & Sinus Caplets and Tablets ..... ■688
Advil Cold and Sinus Caplets ..... ■771
Advil Cold and Sinus Tablets ..... ■771
Advil Flu & Body Ache Caplets ..... ■772
Aleve Cold & Sinus Caplets ..... ■603
Alka-Seltzer Plus Liqui-Gels ..... ■604
Alka-Seltzer Plus Cold & Flu Medicine Liqui-Gels ..... ■604
Alka-Seltzer Plus Cold & Sinus Medicine Liqui-Gels ..... ■604
Allegra-D Extended-Release Tablets 714
BC Cold Powder ..... ■619
Benadryl Allergy/Cold Tablets ..... ■691
Benadryl Allergy/Congestion Tablets ..... ■692
Benadryl Allergy & Sinus Liquid ..... ■693
Benadryl Allergy & Sinus Fastmelt Tablets ..... ■693
Benadryl Allergy Sinus Headache Caplets & Gelcaps ..... ■693
Benadryl Severe Allergy & Sinus Headache Caplets ..... ■694
Benadryl Children's Allergy/Cold Fastmelt Tablets ..... ■692
Benylin Multi-Symptom Liquid ..... ■697
Bromfed Capsules (Extended-Release) 2269
Bromfed-PD Capsules (Extended-Release) 2269
Children's Cēpacol Sore Throat ..... ■788
Comtrex Acute Head Cold & Sinus Pressure Relief Tablets ..... ■627
Comtrex Deep Chest Cold & Congestion Relief Softgels ..... ■627
Comtrex Flu Therapy & Fever Relief Daytime Caplets ..... ■628
Comtrex Flu Therapy & Fever Relief Nighttime Tablets ..... ■628
Comtrex Maximum Strength Multi-Symptom Cold & Cough Relief Tablets and Caplets ..... ■626
Contac Non-Drowsy 12 Hour Cold Caplets ..... ■745
Contac Non-Drowsy Timed Release 12 Hour Cold Caplets ..... ■746
Contac Severe Cold and Flu Caplets Maximum Strength ..... ■746
Contac Severe Cold and Flu Caplets Non-Drowsy ..... ■746
Dimetapp Elixir ..... ■777
Dimetapp Cold and Fever Suspension ..... ■775
Dimetapp DM Cold & Cough Elixir ..... ■775
Dimetapp Nighttime Flu Liquid ..... ■776
Dimetapp Non-Drowsy Flu Syrup ..... ■777
Dimetapp Infant Drops Decongestant ..... ■775
Dimetapp Infant Drops Decongestant Plus Cough ..... ■776
Guaifed 2272
Kronofed-A 1341
Children's Motrin Cold Oral Suspension 2007
Motrin Sinus Headache Caplets 2005
PediaCare Cough-Cold Liquid ..... ■719
PediaCare Infants' Drops Decongestant ..... ■719
PediaCare Infants' Drops Decongestant Plus Cough ..... ■719
PediaCare NightRest Cough-Cold Liquid ..... ■719
Robitussin Cold Caplets Cold & Congestion ..... ■780
Robitussin Cold Softgels Cold & Congestion ..... ■780
Robitussin Cold Caplets Multi-Symptom Cold & Flu ..... ■781
Robitussin Cold Softgels Multi-Symptom Cold & Flu ..... ■781
Robitussin Cold Softgels Severe Congestion ..... ■782
Robitussin Cough & Cold Infant Drops ..... ■782
Robitussin Maximum Strength Cough & Cold Liquid ..... ■785
Robitussin Pediatric Cough & Cold Formula Liquid ..... ■785
Robitussin Multi Symptom Honey Flu Liquid ..... ■785
Robitussin Nighttime Honey Flu Liquid ..... ■786
Robitussin-CF Liquid ..... ■783
Robitussin-DAC Syrup 2942
Robitussin-PE Liquid ..... ■782
Ryna ..... ■768
Semprex-D Capsules 1172
Singlet Caplets ..... ■761
Sinutab Non-Drying Liquid Caps ..... ■706
Sinutab Sinus Allergy Medication, Maximum Strength Formula, Tablets & Caplets ..... ■707
Sinutab Sinus Medication, Maximum Strength Without Drowsiness Formula, Tablets & Caplets ..... ■707
Sudafed 12 Hour Tablets ..... ■708
Sudafed 24 Hour Tablets ..... ■708
Children's Sudafed Cold & Cough Liquid ..... ■709
Children's Sudafed Nasal Decongestant Chewables ..... ■711
Children's Sudafed Nasal Decongestant Liquid Medication ..... ■711
Sudafed Cold & Allergy Tablets ..... ■708
Sudafed Cold & Cough Liquid Caps ..... ■709
Sudafed Cold & Sinus Liquid Caps ..... ■710
Sudafed Nasal Decongestant Tablets ..... ■710
Sudafed Non-Drying Sinus Liquid Caps ..... ■712
Sudafed Severe Cold ..... ■711
Sudafed Sinus Headache Caplets ..... ■712
Sudafed Sinus Headache Tablets ..... ■712
Tavist Sinus Non-Drowsy Coated Caplets ..... ■676
TheraFlu Regular Strength Cold & Cough Night Time Hot Liquid ..... ■676
TheraFlu Regular Strength Cold & Sore Throat Night Time Hot Liquid ..... ■676
TheraFlu Maximum Strength Flu & Congestion Non-Drowsy Hot Liquid ..... ■677
TheraFlu Maximum Strength Flu & Cough Night Time Hot Liquid ..... ■678
TheraFlu Maximum Strength Flu & Sore Throat Night Time Hot Liquid ..... ■677

IMPORTANT NOTE: Always consult each drug listing in the patient's regimen for possible interactions.

TheraFlu Maximum Strength Severe Cold & Congestion Night Time Caplets .... ▣678
TheraFlu Maximum Strength Severe Cold & Congestion Night Time Hot Liquid .... ▣678
TheraFlu Maximum Strength Severe Cold & Congestion Non-Drowsy .... ▣679
Triaminic Allergy Congestion Liquid .... ▣680
Triaminic Chest Congestion Liquid .... ▣680
Triaminic Cold & Allergy Liquid .... ▣681
Triaminic Cold & Allergy Softchews .... ▣683
Triaminic Cold & Cough Liquid .... ▣681
Triaminic Cold & Cough Softchews .... ▣683
Triaminic Cold & Night Time Cough Liquid .... ▣681
Triaminic Cold, Cough & Fever Liquid .... ▣681
Triaminic Cough Liquid .... ▣682
Triaminic Cough & Congestion Liquid .... ▣682
Triaminic Cough & Sore Throat Liquid .... ▣682
Triaminic Cough & Sore Throat Softchews .... ▣684
Children's Tylenol Allergy-D Liquid 2014
Children's Tylenol Cold Suspension Liquid and Chewable Tablets 2015
Children's Tylenol Cold Plus Cough Suspension Liquid and Chewable Tablets 2015
Children's Tylenol Flu Suspension Liquid 2015
Children's Tylenol Sinus Suspension Liquid 2017
Infants' Tylenol Cold Decongestant and Fever Reducer Concentrated Drops 2015
Infants' Tylenol Cold Decongestant and Fever Reducer Concentrated Drops Plus Cough 2015
Tylenol Allergy Sinus 2010
Multi-Symptom Tylenol Cold Complete Formula Caplets 2010
Multi-Symptom Tylenol Cold Non-Drowsy Caplets and Gelcaps 2010
Multi-Symptom Tylenol Cold Severe Congestion Non-Drowsy Caplets 2011
Maximum Strength Tylenol Flu NightTime Gelcaps 2011
Maximum Strength Tylenol Flu NightTime Liquid 2011
Maximum Strength Tylenol Flu Non-Drowsy Gelcaps 2011
Maximum Strength Tylenol Sinus NightTime Caplets 2012
Maximum Strength Tylenol Sinus Non-Drowsy Geltabs, Gelcaps, Caplets, and Tablets 2012
Vicks 44D Cough & Head Congestion Relief Liquid .... ▣724
Vicks 44M Cough, Cold & Flu Relief Liquid .... ▣725
Pediatric Vicks 44m Cough & Cold Relief .... ▣728
Vicks DayQuil LiquiCaps/Liquid Multi-Symptom Cold/Flu Relief .... ▣727
Children's Vicks NyQuil Cold/Cough Relief .... ▣726
Vicks NyQuil LiquiCaps/Liquid Multi-Symptom Cold/Flu Relief, Original and Cherry Flavors .... ▣727
Zephrex Tablets 3091
Zephrex LA Tablets 3092
Zyrtec-D 12 Hour Extended Relief Tablets 2758

Pseudoephedrine Sulfate (Concomitant use with other oral sympathomimetic agents is not recommended since such use may lead to deleterious cardiovascular effects). Products include:
Chlor-Trimeton Allergy/Decongestant Tablets .... ▣736
Claritin-D 12 Hour Extended Release Tablets 3102
Claritin-D 24 Hour Extended Release Tablets 3104
Coricidin 'D' Cold, Flu & Sinus Tablets .... ▣737
Drixoral Allergy/Sinus Extended-Release Tablets .... ▣741
Drixoral Cold & Allergy Sustained-Action Tablets .... ▣740
Drixoral Cold & Flu Extended-Release Tablets .... ▣740
Drixoral Nasal Decongestant Long-Acting Non-Drowsy Tablets .... ▣740
Rynatan Tablets 3351

Salmeterol Xinafoate (Concomitant use with other oral sympathomimetic agents is not recommended since such use may lead to deleterious cardiovascular effects). Products include:
Advair Diskus 100/50 1448
Advair Diskus 250/50 1448
Advair Diskus 500/50 1448
Serevent Diskus 1637
Serevent Inhalation Aerosol 1633

Selegiline Hydrochloride (Potentiation of albuterol's action on vascular system). Products include:
Eldepryl Capsules 3266

Sotalol Hydrochloride (Effects of both drugs inhibited). Products include:
Betapace Tablets 950
Betapace AF Tablets 954

Terbutaline Sulfate (Concomitant use with other oral sympathomimetic agents is not recommended since such use may lead to deleterious cardiovascular effects). Products include:
Brethine Ampuls 2314
Brethine Tablets 2313

Timolol Hemihydrate (Effects of both drugs inhibited). Products include:
Betimol Ophthalmic Solution .... ⊙324

Timolol Maleate (Effects of both drugs inhibited). Products include:
Blocadren Tablets 2046
Cosopt Sterile Ophthalmic Solution 2065
Timolide Tablets 2187
Timolol GFS .... ⊙266
Timoptic in Ocudose 2192
Timoptic Sterile Ophthalmic Solution 2190
Timoptic-XE Sterile Ophthalmic Gel Forming Solution 2194

Tranylcypromine Sulfate (Potentiation of albuterol's action on vascular system). Products include:
Parnate Tablets 1607

Triamcinolone (Potential for additive hypokalemic effect with concurrent use).
No products indexed under this heading.

Triamcinolone Acetonide (Potential for additive hypokalemic effect with concurrent use). Products include:
Azmacort Inhalation Aerosol 728
Nasacort Nasal Inhaler 750
Nasacort AQ Nasal Spray 752
Tri-Nasal Spray 2274

Triamcinolone Diacetate (Potential for additive hypokalemic effect with concurrent use).
No products indexed under this heading.

Triamcinolone Hexacetonide (Potential for additive hypokalemic effect with concurrent use).
No products indexed under this heading.

Trimipramine Maleate (Potentiation of albuterol's action on vascular system). Products include:
Surmontil Capsules 3595

PROVENTIL INHALATION SOLUTION 0.083%
(Albuterol Sulfate) 3146
See Proventil Inhalation Aerosol

PROVENTIL REPETABS TABLETS
(Albuterol Sulfate) 3148
May interact with tricyclic antidepressants and certain other agents. Compounds in these categories include:

Acebutolol Hydrochloride (Co-administration with beta-blockers inhibits the effects of each other). Products include:
Sectral Capsules 3589

Albuterol (Co-administration with other sympathomimetic agents increases the risk of adverse cardiovascular effects). Products include:
Proventil Inhalation Aerosol 3142
Ventolin Inhalation Aerosol and Refill 1679

Amitriptyline Hydrochloride (Co-administration with tricyclic antidepressants can potentiate the action of albuterol on the cardiovascular system). Products include:
Etrafon 3115
Limbitrol 1738

Amoxapine (Co-administration with tricyclic antidepressants can potentiate the action of albuterol on the cardiovascular system).
No products indexed under this heading.

Atenolol (Co-administration with beta-blockers inhibits the effects of each other). Products include:
Tenoretic Tablets 690
Tenormin I.V. Injection 692

Bendroflumethiazide (Co-administration with non-potassium sparing diuretics can result in acute worsening of ECG changes and/or hypokalemia, especially when recommended dose of the beta agonist is exceeded; clinical significance of the interaction is unknown). Products include:
Corzide 40/5 Tablets 2247
Corzide 80/5 Tablets 2247

Betaxolol Hydrochloride (Co-administration with beta-blockers inhibits the effects of each other). Products include:
Betoptic S Ophthalmic Suspension 537

Bisoprolol Fumarate (Co-administration with beta-blockers inhibits the effects of each other). Products include:
Zebeta Tablets 1885
Ziac Tablets 1887

Bumetanide (Co-administration with non-potassium sparing diuretics can result in acute worsening of ECG changes and/or hypokalemia, especially when recommended dose of the beta agonist is exceeded; clinical significance of the interaction is unknown).
No products indexed under this heading.

Carteolol Hydrochloride (Co-administration with beta-blockers inhibits the effects of each other). Products include:
Carteolol Hydrochloride Ophthalmic Solution USP, 1% .... ⊙258
Ocupress Ophthalmic Solution, 1% Sterile .... ⊙303

Chlorothiazide (Co-administration with non-potassium sparing diuretics can result in acute worsening of ECG changes and/or hypokalemia, especially when recommended dose of the beta agonist is exceeded; clinical significance of the interaction is unknown). Products include:
Aldoclor Tablets 2035
Diuril Oral 2087

Chlorothiazide Sodium (Co-administration with non-potassium sparing diuretics can result in acute worsening of ECG changes and/or hypokalemia, especially when recommended dose of the beta agonist is exceeded; clinical significance of the interaction is unknown). Products include:
Diuril Sodium Intravenous 2086

Clomipramine Hydrochloride (Co-administration with tricyclic antidepressants can potentiate the action of albuterol on the cardiovascular system).
No products indexed under this heading.

Desipramine Hydrochloride (Co-administration with tricyclic antidepressants can potentiate the action of albuterol on the cardiovascular system). Products include:
Norpramin Tablets 755

Digoxin (Mean decreases of 16% to 22% in serum digoxin levels were demonstrated after single dose IV and oral albuterol, respectively; the clinical significance of this interaction is unknown). Products include:
Digitek Tablets 1003
Lanoxicaps Capsules 1574
Lanoxin Injection 1581
Lanoxin Tablets 1587
Lanoxin Elixir Pediatric 1578
Lanoxin Injection Pediatric 1584

Dobutamine Hydrochloride (Co-administration with other sympathomimetic agents increases the risk of adverse cardiovascular effects). Products include:
Dobutrex Solution Vials 1914

Dopamine Hydrochloride (Co-administration with other sympathomimetic agents increases the risk of adverse cardiovascular effects).
No products indexed under this heading.

Doxepin Hydrochloride (Co-administration with tricyclic antidepressants can potentiate the action of albuterol on the cardiovascular system). Products include:
Sinequan 2713

Ephedrine Hydrochloride (Co-administration with other sympathomimetic agents increases the risk of adverse cardiovascular effects). Products include:
Primatene Tablets .... ▣780

Ephedrine Sulfate (Co-administration with other sympathomimetic agents increases the risk of adverse cardiovascular effects).
No products indexed under this heading.

Ephedrine Tannate (Co-administration with other sympathomimetic agents increases the risk of adverse cardiovascular effects). Products include:
Rynatuss Pediatric Suspension 3353
Rynatuss Tablets 3353

Epinephrine (Co-administration with other sympathomimetic agents increases the risk of adverse cardiovascular effects). Products include:
Epifrin Sterile Ophthalmic Solution .... ⊙235
EpiPen 1236
Primatene Mist .... ▣779
Xylocaine with Epinephrine Injection 653

Epinephrine Bitartrate (Co-administration with other sympathomimetic agents increases the risk of adverse cardiovascular effects). Products include:
Sensorcaine 643

Epinephrine Hydrochloride (Co-administration with other sympathomimetic agents increases the risk of adverse cardiovascular effects).
No products indexed under this heading.

Esmolol Hydrochloride (Co-administration with beta-blockers inhibits the effects of each other). Products include:
Brevibloc Injection 858

Ethacrynic Acid (Co-administration with non-potassium sparing diuretics can result in acute worsening of ECG changes and/or hypokalemia, especially when recommended dose of the beta agonist is exceeded; clinical significance of the interaction is unknown). Products include:
Edecrin Tablets 2091

Furosemide (Co-administration with non-potassium sparing diuretics can result in acute worsening of ECG changes and/or hypokalemia, espe-

cially when recommended dose of the beta agonist is exceeded; clinical significance of the interaction is unknown). Products include:

Furosemide Tablets 2284

Hydrochlorothiazide (Co-administration with non-potassium sparing diuretics can result in acute worsening of ECG changes and/or hypokalemia, especially when recommended dose of the beta agonist is exceeded; clinical significance of the interaction is unknown). Products include:

Accuretic Tablets 2614
Aldoril Tablets 2039
Atacand HCT Tablets 597
Avalide Tablets 1070
Diovan HCT Tablets 2338
Dyazide Capsules 1515
HydroDIURIL Tablets 2108
Hyzaar 2109
Inderide Tablets 3517
Inderide LA Long-Acting Capsules .. 3519
Lotensin HCT Tablets 2367
Maxzide 1008
Micardis HCT Tablets 1051
Microzide Capsules 3414
Moduretic Tablets 2138
Monopril HCT 1094
Prinzide Tablets 2168
Timolide Tablets 2187
Uniretic Tablets 3178
Vaseretic Tablets 2204
Zestoretic Tablets 695
Ziac Tablets 1887

Hydroflumethiazide (Co-administration with non-potassium sparing diuretics can result in acute worsening of ECG changes and/or hypokalemia, especially when recommended dose of the beta agonist is exceeded; clinical significance of the interaction is unknown). Products include:

Diucardin Tablets 3494

Imipramine Hydrochloride (Co-administration with tricyclic antidepressants can potentiate the action of albuterol on the cardiovascular system).

No products indexed under this heading.

Imipramine Pamoate (Co-administration with tricyclic antidepressants can potentiate the action of albuterol on the cardiovascular system).

No products indexed under this heading.

Isocarboxazid (Co-administration with MAO inhibitors can potentiate the action of albuterol on the cardiovascular system).

No products indexed under this heading.

Isoproterenol Hydrochloride (Co-administration with other sympathomimetic agents increases the risk of adverse cardiovascular effects).

No products indexed under this heading.

Isoproterenol Sulfate (Co-administration with other sympathomimetic agents increases the risk of adverse cardiovascular effects).

No products indexed under this heading.

Labetalol Hydrochloride (Co-administration with beta-blockers inhibits the effects of each other). Products include:

Normodyne Injection 3135
Normodyne Tablets 3137

Levalbuterol Hydrochloride (Co-administration with other sympathomimetic agents increases the risk of adverse cardiovascular effects). Products include:

Xopenex Inhalation Solution 3207

Levobunolol Hydrochloride (Co-administration with beta-blockers inhibits the effects of each other). Products include:

Betagan .... ⊙228

Maprotiline Hydrochloride (Co-administration with tricyclic antidepressants can potentiate the action of albuterol on the cardiovascular system).

No products indexed under this heading.

Metaproterenol Sulfate (Co-administration with other sympathomimetic agents increases the risk of adverse cardiovascular effects). Products include:

Alupent 1029

Metaraminol Bitartrate (Co-administration with other sympathomimetic agents increases the risk of adverse cardiovascular effects). Products include:

Aramine Injection 2043

Methoxamine Hydrochloride (Co-administration with other sympathomimetic agents increases the risk of adverse cardiovascular effects).

No products indexed under this heading.

Methyclothiazide (Co-administration with non-potassium sparing diuretics can result in acute worsening of ECG changes and/or hypokalemia, especially when recommended dose of the beta agonist is exceeded; clinical significance of the interaction is unknown).

No products indexed under this heading.

Metipranolol Hydrochloride (Co-administration with beta-blockers inhibits the effects of each other).

No products indexed under this heading.

Metoprolol Succinate (Co-administration with beta-blockers inhibits the effects of each other). Products include:

Toprol-XL Tablets 651

Metoprolol Tartrate (Co-administration with beta-blockers inhibits the effects of each other).

No products indexed under this heading.

Moclobemide (Co-administration with MAO inhibitors can potentiate the action of albuterol on the cardiovascular system).

No products indexed under this heading.

Nadolol (Co-administration with beta-blockers inhibits the effects of each other). Products include:

Corgard Tablets 2245
Corzide 40/5 Tablets 2247
Corzide 80/5 Tablets 2247
Nadolol Tablets 2288

Norepinephrine Bitartrate (Co-administration with other sympathomimetic agents increases the risk of adverse cardiovascular effects).

No products indexed under this heading.

Nortriptyline Hydrochloride (Co-administration with tricyclic antidepressants can potentiate the action of albuterol on the cardiovascular system).

No products indexed under this heading.

Pargyline Hydrochloride (Co-administration with MAO inhibitors can potentiate the action of albuterol on the cardiovascular system).

No products indexed under this heading.

Penbutolol Sulfate (Co-administration with beta-blockers inhibits the effects of each other).

No products indexed under this heading.

Phenelzine Sulfate (Co-administration with MAO inhibitors can potentiate the action of albuterol on the cardiovascular system). Products include:

Nardil Tablets 2653

Phenylephrine Bitartrate (Co-administration with other sympathomimetic agents increases the risk of adverse cardiovascular effects).

No products indexed under this heading.

Phenylephrine Hydrochloride (Co-administration with other sympathomimetic agents increases the risk of adverse cardiovascular effects). Products include:

Afrin Nasal Decongestant Children's Pump Mist 734
Extendryl 1361
Hycomine Compound Tablets 1317
Neo-Synephrine 614
Phenergan VC Syrup 3560
Phenergan VC with Codeine Syrup .. 3561
Preparation H Cream 778
Preparation H Cooling Gel 778
Preparation H 778
Vicks Sinex Nasal Spray and Ultra Fine Mist 729

Phenylephrine Tannate (Co-administration with other sympathomimetic agents increases the risk of adverse cardiovascular effects). Products include:

Ryna-12 S Suspension 3351
Reformulated Rynatan Pediatric Suspension 3352
Rynatuss Pediatric Suspension 3353
Rynatuss Tablets 3353

Phenylpropanolamine Hydrochloride (Co-administration with other sympathomimetic agents increases the risk of adverse cardiovascular effects).

No products indexed under this heading.

Pindolol (Co-administration with beta-blockers inhibits the effects of each other).

No products indexed under this heading.

Pirbuterol Acetate (Co-administration with other sympathomimetic agents increases the risk of adverse cardiovascular effects). Products include:

Maxair Autohaler 1981
Maxair Inhaler 1984

Polythiazide (Co-administration with non-potassium sparing diuretics can result in acute worsening of ECG changes and/or hypokalemia, especially when recommended dose of the beta agonist is exceeded; clinical significance of the interaction is unknown). Products include:

Minizide Capsules 2700
Renese Tablets 2712

Procarbazine Hydrochloride (Co-administration with MAO inhibitors can potentiate the action of albuterol on the cardiovascular system). Products include:

Matulane Capsules 3246

Propranolol Hydrochloride (Co-administration with beta-blockers inhibits the effects of each other). Products include:

Inderal 3513
Inderal LA Long-Acting Capsules 3516
Inderide Tablets 3517
Inderide LA Long-Acting Capsules .. 3519

Protriptyline Hydrochloride (Co-administration with tricyclic antidepressants can potentiate the action of albuterol on the cardiovascular system). Products include:

Vivactil Tablets 2446
Vivactil Tablets 2217

Pseudoephedrine Hydrochloride (Co-administration with other sympathomimetic agents increases the risk of adverse cardiovascular effects). Products include:

Actifed Cold & Allergy Tablets 688
Actifed Cold & Sinus Caplets and Tablets 688
Advil Cold and Sinus Caplets 771
Advil Cold and Sinus Tablets 771
Advil Flu & Body Ache Caplets 772
Aleve Cold & Sinus Caplets 603
Alka-Seltzer Plus Liqui-Gels 604
Alka-Seltzer Plus Cold & Flu Medicine Liqui-Gels 604
Alka-Seltzer Plus Cold & Sinus Medicine Liqui-Gels 604
Allegra-D Extended-Release Tablets 714
BC Cold Powder 619
Benadryl Allergy/Cold Tablets 691
Benadryl Allergy/Congestion Tablets 692
Benadryl Allergy & Sinus Liquid 693
Benadryl Allergy & Sinus Fastmelt Tablets 693
Benadryl Allergy Sinus Headache Caplets & Gelcaps 693
Benadryl Severe Allergy & Sinus Headache Caplets 694
Benadryl Children's Allergy/Cold Fastmelt Tablets 692
Benylin Multi-Symptom Liquid 697
Bromfed Capsules (Extended-Release) 2269
Bromfed-PD Capsules (Extended-Release) 2269
Children's Cēpacol Sore Throat 788
Comtrex Acute Head Cold & Sinus Pressure Relief Tablets 627
Comtrex Deep Chest Cold & Congestion Relief Softgels 627
Comtrex Flu Therapy & Fever Relief Daytime Caplets 628
Comtrex Flu Therapy & Fever Relief Nighttime Tablets 628
Comtrex Maximum Strength Multi-Symptom Cold & Cough Relief Tablets and Caplets 626
Contac Non-Drowsy 12 Hour Cold Caplets 745
Contac Non-Drowsy Timed Release 12 Hour Cold Caplets 746
Contac Severe Cold and Flu Caplets Maximum Strength 746
Contac Severe Cold and Flu Caplets Non-Drowsy 746
Dimetapp Elixir 777
Dimetapp Cold and Fever Suspension 775
Dimetapp DM Cold & Cough Elixir 775
Dimetapp Nighttime Flu Liquid 776
Dimetapp Non-Drowsy Flu Syrup 777
Dimetapp Infant Drops Decongestant 775
Dimetapp Infant Drops Decongestant Plus Cough 776
Guaifed 2272
Kronofed-A 1341
Children's Motrin Cold Oral Suspension 2007
Motrin Sinus Headache Caplets 2005
PediaCare Cough-Cold Liquid 719
PediaCare Infants' Drops Decongestant 719
PediaCare Infants' Drops Decongestant Plus Cough 719
PediaCare NightRest Cough-Cold Liquid 719
Robitussin Cold Caplets Cold & Congestion 780
Robitussin Cold Softgels Cold & Congestion 780
Robitussin Cold Caplets Multi-Symptom Cold & Flu 781
Robitussin Cold Softgels Multi-Symptom Cold & Flu 781
Robitussin Cold Softgels Severe Congestion 782
Robitussin Cough & Cold Infant Drops 782
Robitussin Maximum Strength Cough & Cold Liquid 785
Robitussin Pediatric Cough & Cold Formula Liquid 785
Robitussin Multi Symptom Honey Flu Liquid 785
Robitussin Nighttime Honey Flu Liquid 786
Robitussin-CF Liquid 783
Robitussin-DAC Syrup 2942
Robitussin-PE Liquid 782
Ryna 768
Semprex-D Capsules 1172
Singlet Caplets 761
Sinutab Non-Drying Liquid Caps 706
Sinutab Sinus Allergy Medication, Maximum Strength Formula, Tablets & Caplets 707
Sinutab Sinus Medication, Maximum Strength Without Drowsiness Formula, Tablets & Caplets 707
Sudafed 12 Hour Tablets 708
Sudafed 24 Hour Tablets 708
Children's Sudafed Cold & Cough Liquid 709
Children's Sudafed Nasal Decongestant Chewables 711
Children's Sudafed Nasal Decongestant Liquid Medication 711
Sudafed Cold & Allergy Tablets 708

Sudafed Cold & Cough Liquid Caps ▣709
Sudafed Cold & Sinus Liquid Caps ▣710
Sudafed Nasal Decongestant Tablets ▣710
Sudafed Non-Drying Sinus Liquid Caps ▣712
Sudafed Severe Cold ▣711
Sudafed Sinus Headache Caplets ▣712
Sudafed Sinus Headache Tablets ▣712
Tavist Sinus Non-Drowsy Coated Caplets ▣676
TheraFlu Regular Strength Cold & Cough Night Time Hot Liquid ▣676
TheraFlu Regular Strength Cold & Sore Throat Night Time Hot Liquid ▣676
TheraFlu Maximum Strength Flu & Congestion Non-Drowsy Hot Liquid ▣677
TheraFlu Maximum Strength Flu & Cough Night Time Hot Liquid ▣678
TheraFlu Maximum Strength Flu & Sore Throat Night Time Hot Liquid ▣677
TheraFlu Maximum Strength Severe Cold & Congestion Night Time Caplets ▣678
TheraFlu Maximum Strength Severe Cold & Congestion Night Time Hot Liquid ▣678
TheraFlu Maximum Strength Severe Cold & Congestion Non-Drowsy ▣679
Triaminic Allergy Congestion Liquid ▣680
Triaminic Chest Congestion Liquid ▣680
Triaminic Cold & Allergy Liquid ▣681
Triaminic Cold & Allergy Softchews ▣683
Triaminic Cold & Cough Liquid ▣681
Triaminic Cold & Cough Softchews ▣683
Triaminic Cold & Night Time Cough Liquid ▣681
Triaminic Cold, Cough & Fever Liquid ▣681
Triaminic Cough Liquid ▣682
Triaminic Cough & Congestion Liquid ▣682
Triaminic Cough & Sore Throat Liquid ▣682
Triaminic Cough & Sore Throat Softchews ▣684
Children's Tylenol Allergy-D Liquid 2014
Children's Tylenol Cold Suspension Liquid and Chewable Tablets 2015
Children's Tylenol Cold Plus Cough Suspension Liquid and Chewable Tablets 2015
Children's Tylenol Flu Suspension Liquid 2015
Children's Tylenol Sinus Suspension Liquid 2017
Infants' Tylenol Cold Decongestant and Fever Reducer Concentrated Drops 2015
Infants' Tylenol Cold Decongestant and Fever Reducer Concentrated Drops Plus Cough 2015
Tylenol Allergy Sinus 2010
Multi-Symptom Tylenol Cold Complete Formula Caplets 2010
Multi-Symptom Tylenol Cold Non-Drowsy Caplets and Gelcaps 2010
Multi-Symptom Tylenol Cold Severe Congestion Non-Drowsy Caplets 2011
Maximum Strength Tylenol Flu NightTime Gelcaps 2011
Maximum Strength Tylenol Flu NightTime Liquid 2011
Maximum Strength Tylenol Flu Non-Drowsy Gelcaps 2011
Maximum Strength Tylenol Sinus NightTime Caplets 2012
Maximum Strength Tylenol Sinus Non-Drowsy Geltabs, Gelcaps, Caplets, and Tablets 2012
Vicks 44D Cough & Head Congestion Relief Liquid ▣724
Vicks 44M Cough, Cold & Flu Relief Liquid ▣725
Pediatric Vicks 44m Cough & Cold Relief ▣728
Vicks DayQuil LiquiCaps/Liquid Multi-Symptom Cold/Flu Relief ▣727
Children's Vicks NyQuil Cold/Cough Relief ▣726
Vicks NyQuil LiquiCaps/Liquid Multi-Symptom Cold/Flu Relief, Original and Cherry Flavors ▣727
Zephrex Tablets 3091
Zephrex LA Tablets 3092
Zyrtec-D 12 Hour Extended Relief Tablets 2758

Pseudoephedrine Sulfate (Co-administration with other sympathomimetic agents increases the risk of adverse cardiovascular effects). Products include:

Chlor-Trimeton Allergy/Decongestant Tablets ▣736
Claritin-D 12 Hour Extended Release Tablets 3102
Claritin-D 24 Hour Extended Release Tablets 3104
Coricidin 'D' Cold, Flu & Sinus Tablets ▣737
Drixoral Allergy/Sinus Extended-Release Tablets ▣741
Drixoral Cold & Allergy Sustained-Action Tablets ▣740
Drixoral Cold & Flu Extended-Release Tablets ▣740
Drixoral Nasal Decongestant Long-Acting Non-Drowsy Tablets ▣740
Rynatan Tablets 3351

Salmeterol Xinafoate (Co-administration with other sympathomimetic agents increases the risk of adverse cardiovascular effects). Products include:

Advair Diskus 100/50 1448
Advair Diskus 250/50 1448
Advair Diskus 500/50 1448
Serevent Diskus 1637
Serevent Inhalation Aerosol 1633

Selegiline Hydrochloride (Co-administration with MAO inhibitors can potentiate the action of albuterol on the cardiovascular system). Products include:

Eldepryl Capsules 3266

Sotalol Hydrochloride (Co-administration with beta-blockers inhibits the effects of each other). Products include:

Betapace Tablets 950
Betapace AF Tablets 954

Terbutaline Sulfate (Co-administration with other sympathomimetic agents increases the risk of adverse cardiovascular effects). Products include:

Brethine Ampuls 2314
Brethine Tablets 2313

Timolol Hemihydrate (Co-administration with beta-blockers inhibits the effects of each other). Products include:

Betimol Ophthalmic Solution ⊙324

Timolol Maleate (Co-administration with beta-blockers inhibits the effects of each other). Products include:

Blocadren Tablets 2046
Cosopt Sterile Ophthalmic Solution 2065
Timolide Tablets 2187
Timolol GFS ⊙266
Timoptic in Ocudose 2192
Timoptic Sterile Ophthalmic Solution 2190
Timoptic-XE Sterile Ophthalmic Gel Forming Solution 2194

Torsemide (Co-administration with non-potassium sparing diuretics can result in acute worsening of ECG changes and/or hypokalemia, especially when recommended dose of the beta agonist is exceeded; clinical significance of the interaction is unknown). Products include:

Demadex Tablets and Injection 2965

Tranylcypromine Sulfate (Co-administration with MAO inhibitors can potentiate the action of albuterol on the cardiovascular system). Products include:

Parnate Tablets 1607

Trimipramine Maleate (Co-administration with tricyclic antidepressants can potentiate the action of albuterol on the cardiovascular system). Products include:

Surmontil Capsules 3595

PROVENTIL SOLUTION FOR INHALATION 0.5%

(Albuterol Sulfate) 3144

See Proventil Inhalation Aerosol

PROVENTIL HFA INHALATION AEROSOL

(Albuterol Sulfate) 3150

May interact with beta blockers, loop diuretics, monoamine oxidase inhibitors, potassium-depleting diuretics, tricyclic antidepressants, and certain other agents. Compounds in these categories include:

Acebutolol Hydrochloride (Co-administration with beta adrenergic blocking agent blocks the pulmonary effect of beta agonists and may produce severe bronchospasm). Products include:

Sectral Capsules 3589

Amitriptyline Hydrochloride (Action of albuterol on the cardiovascular system may be potentiated by tricyclic antidepressants). Products include:

Etrafon 3115
Limbitrol 1738

Amoxapine (Action of albuterol on the cardiovascular system may be potentiated by tricyclic antidepressants).

No products indexed under this heading.

Atenolol (Co-administration with beta adrenergic blocking agent blocks the pulmonary effect of beta agonists and may produce severe bronchospasm). Products include:

Tenoretic Tablets 690
Tenormin I.V. Injection 692

Bendroflumethiazide (The ECG changes and hypokalemia which may result from administration of nonpotassium-sparing diuretics can be acutely worsened by beta agonists). Products include:

Corzide 40/5 Tablets 2247
Corzide 80/5 Tablets 2247

Betaxolol Hydrochloride (Co-administration with beta adrenergic blocking agent blocks the pulmonary effect of beta agonists and may produce severe bronchospasm). Products include:

Betoptic S Ophthalmic Suspension 537

Bisoprolol Fumarate (Co-administration with beta adrenergic blocking agent blocks the pulmonary effect of beta agonists and may produce severe bronchospasm). Products include:

Zebeta Tablets 1885
Ziac Tablets 1887

Bumetanide (The ECG changes and hypokalemia which may result from administration of nonpotassium-sparing diuretics can be acutely worsened by beta agonists).

No products indexed under this heading.

Carteolol Hydrochloride (Co-administration with beta adrenergic blocking agent blocks the pulmonary effect of beta agonists and may produce severe bronchospasm). Products include:

Carteolol Hydrochloride Ophthalmic Solution USP, 1% ⊙258
Ocupress Ophthalmic Solution, 1% Sterile ⊙303

Chlorothiazide (The ECG changes and hypokalemia which may result from administration of nonpotassium-sparing diuretics can be acutely worsened by beta agonists). Products include:

Aldoclor Tablets 2035
Diuril Oral 2087

Chlorothiazide Sodium (The ECG changes and hypokalemia which may result from administration of nonpotassium-sparing diuretics can be acutely worsened by beta agonists). Products include:

Diuril Sodium Intravenous 2086

Clomipramine Hydrochloride (Action of albuterol on the cardiovascular system may be potentiated by tricyclic antidepressants).

No products indexed under this heading.

Desipramine Hydrochloride (Action of albuterol on the cardiovascular system may be potentiated by tricyclic antidepressants). Products include:

Norpramin Tablets 755

Digoxin (Mean decreases in serum digoxin levels have been demonstrated with intravenous and oral albuterol). Products include:

Digitek Tablets 1003
Lanoxicaps Capsules 1574
Lanoxin Injection 1581
Lanoxin Tablets 1587
Lanoxin Elixir Pediatric 1578
Lanoxin Injection Pediatric 1584

Doxepin Hydrochloride (Action of albuterol on the cardiovascular system may be potentiated by tricyclic antidepressants). Products include:

Sinequan 2713

Esmolol Hydrochloride (Co-administration with beta adrenergic blocking agent blocks the pulmonary effect of beta agonists and may produce severe bronchospasm). Products include:

Brevibloc Injection 858

Ethacrynic Acid (The ECG changes and hypokalemia which may result from administration of nonpotassium-sparing diuretics can be acutely worsened by beta agonists). Products include:

Edecrin Tablets 2091

Furosemide (The ECG changes and hypokalemia which may result from administration of nonpotassium-sparing diuretics can be acutely worsened by beta agonists). Products include:

Furosemide Tablets 2284

Hydrochlorothiazide (The ECG changes and hypokalemia which may result from administration of nonpotassium-sparing diuretics can be acutely worsened by beta agonists). Products include:

Accuretic Tablets 2614
Aldoril Tablets 2039
Atacand HCT Tablets 597
Avalide Tablets 1070
Diovan HCT Tablets 2338
Dyazide Capsules 1515
HydroDIURIL Tablets 2108
Hyzaar 2109
Inderide Tablets 3517
Inderide LA Long-Acting Capsules 3519
Lotensin HCT Tablets 2367
Maxzide 1008
Micardis HCT Tablets 1051
Microzide Capsules 3414
Moduretic Tablets 2138
Monopril HCT 1094
Prinzide Tablets 2168
Timolide Tablets 2187
Uniretic Tablets 3178
Vaseretic Tablets 2204
Zestoretic Tablets 695
Ziac Tablets 1887

Hydroflumethiazide (The ECG changes and hypokalemia which may result from administration of nonpotassium-sparing diuretics can be acutely worsened by beta agonists). Products include:

Diucardin Tablets 3494

Imipramine Hydrochloride (Action of albuterol on the cardiovascular system may be potentiated by tricyclic antidepressants).

No products indexed under this heading.

Imipramine Pamoate (Action of albuterol on the cardiovascular system may be potentiated by tricyclic

antidepressants).
No products indexed under this heading.

Isocarboxazid (Action of albuterol on the cardiovascular system may be potentiated by MAO inhibitors).
No products indexed under this heading.

Labetalol Hydrochloride (Co-administration with beta adrenergic blocking agent blocks the pulmonary effect of beta agonists and may produce severe bronchospasm).
Products include:
Normodyne Injection 3135
Normodyne Tablets 3137

Levobunolol Hydrochloride (Co-administration with beta adrenergic blocking agent blocks the pulmonary effect of beta agonists and may produce severe bronchospasm).
Products include:
Betagan .... ⊙228

Maprotiline Hydrochloride (Action of albuterol on the cardiovascular system may be potentiated by tricyclic antidepressants).
No products indexed under this heading.

Methyclothiazide (The ECG changes and hypokalemia which may result from administration of nonpotassium-sparing diuretics can be acutely worsened by beta agonists).
No products indexed under this heading.

Metipranolol Hydrochloride (Co-administration with beta adrenergic blocking agent blocks the pulmonary effect of beta agonists and may produce severe bronchospasm).
No products indexed under this heading.

Metoprolol Succinate (Co-administration with beta adrenergic blocking agent blocks the pulmonary effect of beta agonists and may produce severe bronchospasm).
Products include:
Toprol-XL Tablets 651

Metoprolol Tartrate (Co-administration with beta adrenergic blocking agent blocks the pulmonary effect of beta agonists and may produce severe bronchospasm).
No products indexed under this heading.

Moclobemide (Action of albuterol on the cardiovascular system may be potentiated by MAO inhibitors).
No products indexed under this heading.

Nadolol (Co-administration with beta adrenergic blocking agent blocks the pulmonary effect of beta agonists and may produce severe bronchospasm). Products include:
Corgard Tablets 2245
Corzide 40/5 Tablets 2247
Corzide 80/5 Tablets 2247
Nadolol Tablets 2288

Nortriptyline Hydrochloride (Action of albuterol on the cardiovascular system may be potentiated by tricyclic antidepressants).
No products indexed under this heading.

Pargyline Hydrochloride (Action of albuterol on the cardiovascular system may be potentiated by MAO inhibitors).
No products indexed under this heading.

Penbutolol Sulfate (Co-administration with beta adrenergic blocking agent blocks the pulmonary effect of beta agonists and may produce severe bronchospasm).
No products indexed under this heading.

Phenelzine Sulfate (Action of albuterol on the cardiovascular system may be potentiated by MAO inhibitors). Products include:
Nardil Tablets 2653

Pindolol (Co-administration with beta adrenergic blocking agent blocks the pulmonary effect of beta agonists and may produce severe bronchospasm).
No products indexed under this heading.

Polythiazide (The ECG changes and hypokalemia which may result from administration of nonpotassium-sparing diuretics can be acutely worsened by beta agonists). Products include:
Minizide Capsules 2700
Renese Tablets 2712

Procarbazine Hydrochloride (Action of albuterol on the cardiovascular system may be potentiated by MAO inhibitors). Products include:
Matulane Capsules 3246

Propranolol Hydrochloride (Co-administration with beta adrenergic blocking agent blocks the pulmonary effect of beta agonists and may produce severe bronchospasm).
Products include:
Inderal 3513
Inderal LA Long-Acting Capsules 3516
Inderide Tablets 3517
Inderide LA Long-Acting Capsules .. 3519

Protriptyline Hydrochloride (Action of albuterol on the cardiovascular system may be potentiated by tricyclic antidepressants). Products include:
Vivactil Tablets 2446
Vivactil Tablets 2217

Selegiline Hydrochloride (Action of albuterol on the cardiovascular system may be potentiated by MAO inhibitors). Products include:
Eldepryl Capsules 3266

Sotalol Hydrochloride (Co-administration with beta adrenergic blocking agent blocks the pulmonary effect of beta agonists and may produce severe bronchospasm).
Products include:
Betapace Tablets 950
Betapace AF Tablets 954

Timolol Hemihydrate (Co-administration with beta adrenergic blocking agent blocks the pulmonary effect of beta agonists and may produce severe bronchospasm).
Products include:
Betimol Ophthalmic Solution .... ⊙324

Timolol Maleate (Co-administration with beta adrenergic blocking agent blocks the pulmonary effect of beta agonists and may produce severe bronchospasm). Products include:
Blocadren Tablets 2046
Cosopt Sterile Ophthalmic Solution 2065
Timolide Tablets 2187
Timolol GFS .... ⊙266
Timoptic in Ocudose 2192
Timoptic Sterile Ophthalmic Solution 2190
Timoptic-XE Sterile Ophthalmic Gel Forming Solution 2194

Torsemide (The ECG changes and hypokalemia which may result from administration of nonpotassium-sparing diuretics can be acutely worsened by beta agonists).
Products include:
Demadex Tablets and Injection 2965

Tranylcypromine Sulfate (Action of albuterol on the cardiovascular system may be potentiated by MAO inhibitors). Products include:
Parnate Tablets 1607

Trimipramine Maleate (Action of albuterol on the cardiovascular system may be potentiated by tricyclic antidepressants). Products include:
Surmontil Capsules 3595

PROVERA TABLETS

(Medroxyprogesterone Acetate) 2853
May interact with:

Aminoglutethimide (Significantly depresses the bioavailability of Provera).
No products indexed under this heading.

PROVIGIL TABLETS

(Modafinil) 1193
May interact with monoamine oxidase inhibitors, oral contraceptives, phenytoin, selective serotonin reuptake inhibitors, tricyclic antidepressants, theophylline, and certain other agents. Compounds in these categories include:

Aminophylline (Chronic administration of modafinil may cause modest induction of CYP3A4, thus reducing the levels, to a lesser degree, of co-administered substrate for that enzyme system, such as theophylline).
No products indexed under this heading.

Amitriptyline Hydrochloride (Modafinil is a reversible inhibitor of the CYP2C19; the levels of CYP2D6 substrates such as tricyclic antidepressants, which have ancillary routes of elimination through CYP2D6, may be increased by co-administration of modafinil).
Products include:
Etrafon 3115
Limbitrol 1738

Amoxapine (Modafinil is a reversible inhibitor of the CYP2C19; the levels of CYP2D6 substrates such as tricyclic antidepressants, which have ancillary routes of elimination through CYP2D6, may be increased by co-administration of modafinil).
No products indexed under this heading.

Carbamazepine (Chronic administration of modafinil may cause induction of its metabolism; co-administration of potent inducers of CYP3A4, such as carbamazepine, could alter the levels of modafinil due to the partial involvement of that enzyme in the metabolic elimination of the compound). Products include:
Carbatrol Capsules 3234
Tegretol/Tegretol-XR 2404

Citalopram Hydrobromide (Modafinil is a reversible inhibitor of the CYP2C19; the levels of CYP2D6 substrates such as selective serotonin reuptake inhibitors, which have ancillary routes of elimination through CYP2D6, may be increased by co-administration of modafinil).
Products include:
Celexa 1365

Clomipramine Hydrochloride (Co-administration has resulted in one incident of increased levels of clomipramine and its active metabolite desmethylclomipramine).
No products indexed under this heading.

Cyclosporine (Chronic administration of modafinil may cause modest induction of CYP3A4, thus reducing the levels of co-administered substrate for that enzyme system, such as cyclosporine). Products include:
Gengraf Capsules 457
Neoral Soft Gelatin Capsules 2380
Neoral Oral Solution 2380
Sandimmune 2388

Desipramine Hydrochloride (Modafinil is a reversible inhibitor of the CYP2C19; the levels of CYP2D6 substrates such as tricyclic antidepressants, which have ancillary routes of elimination through CYP2D6, may be increased by co-administration of modafinil).
Products include:
Norpramin Tablets 755

Desogestrel (Chronic administration of modafinil may cause modest induction of CYP3A4, thus reducing the levels of co-administered substrate for that enzyme system, such as steroidal contraceptives).
Products include:
Cyclessa Tablets 2450
Desogen Tablets 2458
Mircette Tablets 2470
Ortho-Cept 21 Tablets 2546
Ortho-Cept 28 Tablets 2546

Diazepam (Modafinil is a reversible inhibitor of the CYP2C19; co-administration with drugs that are largely eliminated via this pathway, such as diazepam, may increase the circulating levels of diazepam).
Products include:
Valium Injectable 3026
Valium Tablets 3047

Doxepin Hydrochloride (Modafinil is a reversible inhibitor of the CYP2C19; the levels of CYP2D6 substrates such as tricyclic antidepressants, which have ancillary routes of elimination through CYP2D6, may be increased by co-administration of modafinil). Products include:
Sinequan 2713

Dyphylline (Chronic administration of modafinil may cause modest induction of CYP3A4, thus reducing the levels, to a lesser degree, of co-administered substrate for that enzyme system, such as theophylline). Products include:
Lufyllin Tablets 3347
Lufyllin-400 Tablets 3347
Lufyllin-GG Elixir 3348
Lufyllin-GG Tablets 3348

Ethinyl Estradiol (Chronic administration of modafinil may cause modest induction of CYP3A4, thus reducing the levels of co-administered substrate for that enzyme system, such as steroidal contraceptives).
Products include:
Alesse-21 Tablets 3468
Alesse-28 Tablets 3473
Brevicon 28-Day Tablets 3380
Cyclessa Tablets 2450
Desogen Tablets 2458
Estinyl Tablets 3112
Estrostep 2627
femhrt Tablets 2635
Levlen 962
Levlite 21 Tablets 962
Levlite 28 Tablets 962
Levora Tablets 3389
Loestrin 21 Tablets 2642
Loestrin Fe Tablets 2642
Lo/Ovral Tablets 3532
Lo/Ovral-28 Tablets 3538
Low-Ogestrel-28 Tablets 3392
Microgestin Fe 1.5/30 Tablets 3407
Microgestin Fe 1/20 Tablets 3400
Mircette Tablets 2470
Modicon 2563
Necon 3415
Nordette-28 Tablets 2257
Norinyl 1 +35 28-Day Tablets 3380
Ogestrel 0.5/50-28 Tablets 3428
Ortho-Cept 21 Tablets 2546
Ortho-Cept 28 Tablets 2546
Ortho-Cyclen/Ortho Tri-Cyclen 2573
Ortho-Novum 2563
Ovcon 3364
Ovral Tablets 3551
Ovral-28 Tablets 3552
Tri-Levlen 962
Tri-Norinyl-28 Tablets 3433
Triphasil-21 Tablets 3600
Triphasil-28 Tablets 3605
Trivora Tablets 3439
Yasmin 28 Tablets 980
Zovia 3449

Ethynodiol Diacetate (Chronic administration of modafinil may cause modest induction of CYP3A4, thus reducing the levels of co-administered substrate for that enzyme system, such as steroidal contraceptives). Products include:
Zovia 3449

Fluoxetine Hydrochloride (Modafinil is a reversible inhibitor of the CYP2C19; the levels of CYP2D6 substrates such as selective serotonin reuptake inhibitors, which have ancillary routes of elimination

through CYP2D6, may be increased by co-administration of modafinil). Products include:

Prozac Pulvules, Liquid, and Weekly Capsules 1238
Sarafem Pulvules 1962

Fluvoxamine Maleate (Modafinil is a reversible inhibitor of the CYP2C19; the levels of CYP2D6 substrates such as selective serotonin reuptake inhibitors, which have ancillary routes of elimination through CYP2D6, may be increased by co-administration of modafinil). Products include:

Luvox Tablets (25, 50, 100 mg) 3256

Fosphenytoin Sodium (Modafinil is a reversible inhibitor of the CYP2C19; co-administration with drugs that are largely eliminated via this pathway, such as phenytoin, may increase the circulating levels of phenytoin). Products include:

Cerebyx Injection 2619

Imipramine Hydrochloride (Modafinil is a reversible inhibitor of the CYP2C19; the levels of CYP2D6 substrates such as tricyclic antidepressants, which have ancillary routes of elimination through CYP2D6, may be increased by co-administration of modafinil).

No products indexed under this heading.

Imipramine Pamoate (Modafinil is a reversible inhibitor of the CYP2C19; the levels of CYP2D6 substrates such as tricyclic antidepressants, which have ancillary routes of elimination through CYP2D6, may be increased by co-administration of modafinil).

No products indexed under this heading.

Isocarboxazid (Co-administration requires caution; no interaction studies have been performed).

No products indexed under this heading.

Itraconazole (Chronic administration of modafinil may cause induction of its metabolism; co-administration of potent inhibitors of CYP3A4, such as itraconazole, could alter the levels of modafinil due to the partial involvement of that enzyme in the metabolic elimination of the compound). Products include:

Sporanox Capsules 1800
Sporanox Injection 1804
Sporanox Injection 2509
Sporanox Oral Solution 1808
Sporanox Oral Solution 2512

Ketoconazole (Chronic administration of modafinil may cause induction of its metabolism; co-administration of potent inhibitors of CYP3A4, such as ketoconazole, could alter the levels of modafinil due to the partial involvement of that enzyme in the metabolic elimination of the compound). Products include:

Nizoral 2% Cream 3620
Nizoral A-D Shampoo 2008
Nizoral 2% Shampoo 2007
Nizoral Tablets 1791

Levonorgestrel (Chronic administration of modafinil may cause modest induction of CYP3A4, thus reducing the levels of co-administered substrate for that enzyme system, such as steroidal contraceptives). Products include:

Alesse-21 Tablets 3468
Alesse-28 Tablets 3473
Levlen 962
Levlite 21 Tablets 962
Levlite 28 Tablets 962
Levora Tablets 3389
Mirena Intrauterine System 974
Nordette-28 Tablets 2257
Norplant System 3543
Tri-Levlen 962
Triphasil-21 Tablets 3600
Triphasil-28 Tablets 3605
Trivora Tablets 3439

Maprotiline Hydrochloride (Modafinil is a reversible inhibitor of the CYP2C19; the levels of CYP2D6 substrates such as tricyclic antidepressants, which have ancillary routes of elimination through CYP2D6, may be increased by co-administration of modafinil).

No products indexed under this heading.

Mestranol (Chronic administration of modafinil may cause modest induction of CYP3A4, thus reducing the levels of co-administered substrate for that enzyme system, such as steroidal contraceptives). Products include:

Necon 1/50 Tablets 3415
Norinyl 1 + 50 28-Day Tablets 3380
Ortho-Novum 1/50□28 Tablets 2556

Methylphenidate Hydrochloride (May delay absorption of modafinil by approximately one hour; no significant alterations in pharmacokinetics of either drug). Products include:

Concerta Extended-Release Tablets 1998
Concerta Tablets 561
Metadate CD Capsules 1164
Metadate ER Tablets 1167
Methylin Tablets 1995
Methylin ER Tablets 1995
Ritalin 2387

Moclobemide (Co-administration requires caution; no interaction studies have been performed).

No products indexed under this heading.

Norethindrone (Chronic administration of modafinil may cause modest induction of CYP3A4, thus reducing the levels of co-administered substrate for that enzyme system, such as steroidal contraceptives). Products include:

Brevicon 28-Day Tablets 3380
Micronor Tablets 2543
Modicon 2563
Necon 3415
Norinyl 1 +35 28-Day Tablets 3380
Norinyl 1 + 50 28-Day Tablets 3380
Nor-QD Tablets 3423
Ortho-Novum 2563
Ortho-Novum 1/50□28 Tablets 2556
Ovcon 3364
Tri-Norinyl-28 Tablets 3433

Norethynodrel (Chronic administration of modafinil may cause modest induction of CYP3A4, thus reducing the levels of co-administered substrate for that enzyme system, such as steroidal contraceptives).

No products indexed under this heading.

Norgestimate (Chronic administration of modafinil may cause modest induction of CYP3A4, thus reducing the levels of co-administered substrate for that enzyme system, such as steroidal contraceptives). Products include:

Ortho-Cyclen/Ortho Tri-Cyclen 2573
Ortho-Prefest Tablets 2570

Norgestrel (Chronic administration of modafinil may cause modest induction of CYP3A4, thus reducing the levels of co-administered substrate for that enzyme system, such as steroidal contraceptives). Products include:

Lo/Ovral Tablets 3532
Lo/Ovral-28 Tablets 3538
Low-Ogestrel-28 Tablets 3392
Ogestrel 0.5/50-28 Tablets 3428
Ovral Tablets 3551
Ovral-28 Tablets 3552
Ovrette Tablets 3552

Nortriptyline Hydrochloride (Modafinil is a reversible inhibitor of the CYP2C19; the levels of CYP2D6 substrates such as tricyclic antidepressants, which have ancillary routes of elimination through CYP2D6, may be increased by co-administration of modafinil).

No products indexed under this heading.

Pargyline Hydrochloride (Co-administration requires caution; no interaction studies have been performed).

No products indexed under this heading.

Paroxetine Hydrochloride (Modafinil is a reversible inhibitor of the CYP2C19; the levels of CYP2D6 substrates such as selective serotonin reuptake inhibitors, which have ancillary routes of elimination through CYP2D6, may be increased by co-administration of modafinil). Products include:

Paxil 1609

Phenelzine Sulfate (Co-administration requires caution; no interaction studies have been performed). Products include:

Nardil Tablets 2653

Phenobarbital (Chronic administration of modafinil may cause induction of its metabolism; co-administration of potent inducers of CYP3A4, such as phenobarbital, could alter the levels of modafinil due to the partial involvement of that enzyme in the metabolic elimination of the compound). Products include:

Arco-Lase Plus Tablets 592
Donnatal 2929
Donnatal Extentabs 2930

Phenytoin (Modafinil is a reversible inhibitor of the CYP2C19; co-administration with drugs that are largely eliminated via this pathway, such as phenytoin, may increase the circulating levels of phenytoin). Products include:

Dilantin Infatabs 2624
Dilantin-125 Oral Suspension 2625

Phenytoin Sodium (Modafinil is a reversible inhibitor of the CYP2C19; co-administration with drugs that are largely eliminated via this pathway, such as phenytoin, may increase the circulating levels of phenytoin). Products include:

Dilantin Kapseals 2622

Procarbazine Hydrochloride (Co-administration requires caution; no interaction studies have been performed). Products include:

Matulane Capsules 3246

Propranolol Hydrochloride (Modafinil is a reversible inhibitor of the CYP2C19; co-administration with drugs that are largely eliminated via this pathway, such as propranolol, may increase the circulating levels of propranolol). Products include:

Inderal 3513
Inderal LA Long-Acting Capsules 3516
Inderide Tablets 3517
Inderide LA Long-Acting Capsules 3519

Protriptyline Hydrochloride (Modafinil is a reversible inhibitor of the CYP2C19; the levels of CYP2D6 substrates such as tricyclic antidepressants, which have ancillary routes of elimination through CYP2D6, may be increased by co-administration of modafinil). Products include:

Vivactil Tablets 2446
Vivactil Tablets 2217

Rifampin (Chronic administration of modafinil may cause induction of its metabolism; co-administration of potent inducers of CYP3A4, such as rifampin, could alter the levels of modafinil due to the partial involvement of that enzyme in the metabolic elimination of the compound). Products include:

Rifadin 765
Rifamate Capsules 767
Rifater Tablets 769

Selegiline Hydrochloride (Co-administration requires caution; no interaction studies have been performed). Products include:

Eldepryl Capsules 3266

Sertraline Hydrochloride (Modafinil is a reversible inhibitor of the CYP2C19; the levels of CYP2D6 substrates such as selective serotonin reuptake inhibitors, which have ancillary routes of elimination through CYP2D6, may be increased by co-administration of modafinil). Products include:

Zoloft 2751

Theophylline (Chronic administration of modafinil may cause modest induction of CYP3A4, thus reducing the levels, to a lesser degree, of co-administered substrate for that enzyme system, such as theophylline). Products include:

Aerolate 1361
Theo-Dur Extended-Release Tablets 1835
Uni-Dur Extended-Release Tablets 1841
Uniphyl 400 mg and 600 mg Tablets 2903

Theophylline Calcium Salicylate (Chronic administration of modafinil may cause modest induction of CYP3A4, thus reducing the levels, to a lesser degree, of co-administered substrate for that enzyme system, such as theophylline).

No products indexed under this heading.

Theophylline Sodium Glycinate (Chronic administration of modafinil may cause modest induction of CYP3A4, thus reducing the levels, to a lesser degree, of co-administered substrate for that enzyme system, such as theophylline).

No products indexed under this heading.

Tranylcypromine Sulfate (Co-administration requires caution; no interaction studies have been performed). Products include:

Parnate Tablets 1607

Trimipramine Maleate (Modafinil is a reversible inhibitor of the CYP2C19; the levels of CYP2D6 substrates such as tricyclic antidepressants, which have ancillary routes of elimination through CYP2D6, may be increased by co-administration of modafinil). Products include:

Surmontil Capsules 3595

Warfarin Sodium (Modafinil, in vitro, has demonstrated an apparent concentration-related suppression of CYP2C9 activity; these in vitro results suggest that there is potential for metabolic interaction between modafinil and warfarin). Products include:

Coumadin for Injection 1243
Coumadin Tablets 1243
Warfarin Sodium Tablets, USP 3302

Food Interactions

Food, unspecified (Delays the absorption (tmax) by approximately one hour; no effect on overall bioavailability).

PROXEED POWDER

(Acetyl-L-Carnitine Hydrochloride, Citric Acid, Levocarnitine Fumarate) .... ▣835
None cited in PDR database.

PRO-XTREME DRINK MIX

(Amino Acid Preparations) .... ▣845
None cited in PDR database.

PROZAC PULVULES, LIQUID, AND WEEKLY CAPSULES

(Fluoxetine Hydrochloride) 1238
May interact with oral hypoglycemic agents, insulin, lithium preparations, monoamine oxidase inhibitors, phenytoin, tricyclic antidepressants, and certain other agents. Compounds in these categories include:

Acarbose (Fluoxetine may alter glycemic control in diabetics; hypoglycemia has occurred during therapy with fluoxetine, and hyperglycemia has developed following discontinua-

tion of the drug; hypoglycemia dosage may need to be adjusted). Products include:
Precose Tablets 906

Alprazolam (Co-administration has resulted in increased alprazolam plasma concentrations and further psychomotor performance decrement due to increased alprazolam levels). Products include:
Xanax Tablets 2865

Amitriptyline Hydrochloride (Fluoxetine inhibits the activity of P450 IID6 isoenzyme making normal metabolizers resemble poor metabolizers; therapy with drugs that are predominantly metabolized by the P450 IID6, such as tricyclic antidepressants, and have relatively narrow therapeutic index should be initiated at low end of the dose range if a patient is receiving fluoxetine concurrently or has taken it in the previous 5 weeks). Products include:
Etrafon 3115
Limbitrol 1738

Amoxapine (Fluoxetine inhibits the activity of P450 IID6 isoenzyme making normal metabolizers resemble poor metabolizers; therapy with drugs that are predominantly metabolized by the P450 IID6, such as tricyclic antidepressants, and have relatively narrow therapeutic index should be initiated at low end of the dose range if a patient is receiving fluoxetine concurrently or has taken it in the previous 5 weeks).
No products indexed under this heading.

Carbamazepine (Patients stable on doses of carbamazepine have developed elevated plasma carbamazepine concentrations and clinical anticonvulsant toxicity following initiation of concomitant fluoxetine therapy). Products include:
Carbatrol Capsules 3234
Tegretol/Tegretol-XR 2404

Chlorpropamide (Fluoxetine may alter glycemic control in diabetics; hypoglycemia has occurred during therapy with fluoxetine, and hyperglycemia has developed following discontinuation of the drug; hypoglycemia dosage may need to be adjusted). Products include:
Diabinese Tablets 2680

Clomipramine Hydrochloride (Fluoxetine inhibits the activity of P450 IID6 isoenzyme making normal metabolizers resemble poor metabolizers; therapy with drugs that are predominantly metabolized by the P450 IID6, such as tricyclic antidepressants, and have relatively narrow therapeutic index should be initiated at low end of the dose range if a patient is receiving fluoxetine concurrently or has taken it in the previous 5 weeks).
No products indexed under this heading.

Clozapine (Co-administration of SSRIs, fluoxetine, and antipsychotics, such as clozapine, has resulted in elevation of blood levels of clozapine). Products include:
Clozaril Tablets 2319

Desipramine Hydrochloride (Fluoxetine inhibits the activity of P450 IID6 isoenzyme making normal metabolizers resemble poor metabolizers; therapy with drugs that are predominantly metabolized by the P450 IID6, such as tricyclic antidepressants, and have relatively narrow therapeutic index should be initiated at low end of the dose range if a patient is receiving fluoxetine concurrently or has taken it in the previous 5 weeks). Products include:
Norpramin Tablets 755

Diazepam (Co-administration results in prolonged half-life of diazepam). Products include:
Valium Injectable 3026
Valium Tablets 3047

Digitoxin (Fluoxetine is tightly bound to protein, co-administration may cause shift in plasma concentrations resulting in potential adverse effects).
No products indexed under this heading.

Doxepin Hydrochloride (Fluoxetine inhibits the activity of P450 IID6 isoenzyme making normal metabolizers resemble poor metabolizers; therapy with drugs that are predominantly metabolized by the P450 IID6, such as tricyclic antidepressants, and have relatively narrow therapeutic index should be initiated at low end of the dose range if a patient is receiving fluoxetine concurrently or has taken it in the previous 5 weeks). Products include:
Sinequan 2713

Flecainide Acetate (Fluoxetine inhibits the activity of P450 IID6 isoenzyme making normal metabolizers resemble poor metabolizers; therapy with drugs that are predominantly metabolized by the P450 IID6, such as flecainide, and have relatively narrow therapeutic index should be initiated at low end of the dose range if a patient is receiving fluoxetine concurrently or has taken it in the previous 5 weeks). Products include:
Tambocor Tablets 1990

Fosphenytoin Sodium (Patients stable on doses of phenytoin have developed elevated plasma phenytoin concentrations and clinical anticonvulsant toxicity following initiation of concomitant fluoxetine therapy). Products include:
Cerebyx Injection 2619

Glimepiride (Fluoxetine may alter glycemic control in diabetics; hypoglycemia has occurred during therapy with fluoxetine, and hyperglycemia has developed following discontinuation of the drug; hypoglycemia dosage may need to be adjusted). Products include:
Amaryl Tablets 717

Glipizide (Fluoxetine may alter glycemic control in diabetics; hypoglycemia has occurred during therapy with fluoxetine, and hyperglycemia has developed following discontinuation of the drug; hypoglycemia dosage may need to be adjusted). Products include:
Glucotrol Tablets 2692
Glucotrol XL Extended Release Tablets 2693

Glyburide (Fluoxetine may alter glycemic control in diabetics; hypoglycemia has occurred during therapy with fluoxetine, and hyperglycemia has developed following discontinuation of the drug; hypoglycemia dosage may need to be adjusted). Products include:
DiaBeta Tablets 741
Glucovance Tablets 1086

Haloperidol (Co-administration of SSRIs, fluoxetine, and antipsychotics, such as haloperidol, has resulted in elevation of blood levels of haloperidol). Products include:
Haldol Injection, Tablets and Concentrate 2533

Haloperidol Decanoate (Co-administration of SSRIs, fluoxetine, and antipsychotics, such as haloperidol, has resulted in elevation of blood levels of haloperidol). Products include:
Haldol Decanoate 2535

Imipramine Hydrochloride (Fluoxetine inhibits the activity of P450 IID6 isoenzyme making normal metabolizers resemble poor metabolizers; therapy with drugs that are predominantly metabolized by the P450 IID6, such as tricyclic antidepressants, and have relatively narrow therapeutic index should be initiated at low end of the dose range if a patient is receiving fluoxetine concurrently or has taken it in the previous 5 weeks).
No products indexed under this heading.

Imipramine Pamoate (Fluoxetine inhibits the activity of P450 IID6 isoenzyme making normal metabolizers resemble poor metabolizers; therapy with drugs that are predominantly metabolized by the P450 IID6, such as tricyclic antidepressants, and have relatively narrow therapeutic index should be initiated at low end of the dose range if a patient is receiving fluoxetine concurrently or has taken it in the previous 5 weeks).
No products indexed under this heading.

Insulin, Human, Zinc Suspension (Fluoxetine may alter glycemic control in diabetics; hypoglycemia has occurred during therapy with fluoxetine, and hyperglycemia has developed following discontinuation of the drug; insulin dosage may need to be adjusted). Products include:
Humulin L, 100 Units 1937
Humulin U, 100 Units 1943
Novolin L Human Insulin 10 ml Vials 2422

Insulin, Human NPH (Fluoxetine may alter glycemic control in diabetics; hypoglycemia has occurred during therapy with fluoxetine, and hyperglycemia has developed following discontinuation of the drug; insulin dosage may need to be adjusted). Products include:
Humulin N, 100 Units 1939
Humulin N NPH Pen 1940
Novolin N Human Insulin 10 ml Vials 2422
Novolin N PenFill 2423
Novolin N Prefilled Syringe Disposable Insulin Delivery System 2425

Insulin, Human Regular (Fluoxetine may alter glycemic control in diabetics; hypoglycemia has occurred during therapy with fluoxetine, and hyperglycemia has developed following discontinuation of the drug; insulin dosage may need to be adjusted). Products include:
Humulin R Regular (U-500) 1943
Humulin R, 100 Units 1941
Novolin R Human Insulin 10 ml Vials 2423
Novolin R PenFill 2423
Novolin R Prefilled Syringe Disposable Insulin Delivery System 2425
Velosulin BR Human Insulin 10 ml Vials 2435

Insulin, Human Regular and Human NPH Mixture (Fluoxetine may alter glycemic control in diabetics; hypoglycemia has occurred during therapy with fluoxetine, and hyperglycemia has developed following discontinuation of the drug; insulin dosage may need to be adjusted). Products include:
Humulin 50/50, 100 Units 1934
Humulin 70/30, 100 Units 1935
Humulin 70/30 Pen 1936
Novolin 70/30 Human Insulin 10 ml Vials 2421
Novolin 70/30 PenFill 2423
Novolin 70/30 Prefilled Disposable Insulin Delivery System 2425

Insulin, NPH (Fluoxetine may alter glycemic control in diabetics; hypoglycemia has occurred during therapy with fluoxetine, and hyperglycemia has developed following discontinuation of the drug; insulin dosage may need to be adjusted). Products include:
Iletin II, NPH (Pork), 100 Units 1946

Insulin, Regular (Fluoxetine may alter glycemic control in diabetics; hypoglycemia has occurred during therapy with fluoxetine, and hyperglycemia has developed following discontinuation of the drug; insulin dosage may need to be adjusted). Products include:
Iletin II, Regular (Pork), 100 Units 1947

Insulin, Zinc Crystals (Fluoxetine may alter glycemic control in diabetics; hypoglycemia has occurred during therapy with fluoxetine, and hyperglycemia has developed following discontinuation of the drug; insulin dosage may need to be adjusted).
No products indexed under this heading.

Insulin, Zinc Suspension (Fluoxetine may alter glycemic control in diabetics; hypoglycemia has occurred during therapy with fluoxetine, and hyperglycemia has developed following discontinuation of the drug; insulin dosage may need to be adjusted). Products include:
Iletin II, Lente (Pork), 100 Units 1945

Insulin Aspart, Human Regular (Fluoxetine may alter glycemic control in diabetics; hypoglycemia has occurred during therapy with fluoxetine, and hyperglycemia has developed following discontinuation of the drug; insulin dosage may need to be adjusted).
No products indexed under this heading.

Insulin glargine (Fluoxetine may alter glycemic control in diabetics; hypoglycemia has occurred during therapy with fluoxetine, and hyperglycemia has developed following discontinuation of the drug; insulin dosage may need to be adjusted). Products include:
Lantus Injection 742

Insulin Lispro, Human (Fluoxetine may alter glycemic control in diabetics; hypoglycemia has occurred during therapy with fluoxetine, and hyperglycemia has developed following discontinuation of the drug; insulin dosage may need to be adjusted). Products include:
Humalog 1926
Humalog Mix 75/25 Pen 1928

Insulin Lispro Protamine, Human (Fluoxetine may alter glycemic control in diabetics; hypoglycemia has occurred during therapy with fluoxetine, and hyperglycemia has developed following discontinuation of the drug; insulin dosage may need to be adjusted). Products include:
Humalog Mix 75/25 Pen 1928

Isocarboxazid (Co-administration with MAO inhibitors has resulted in serious, sometimes fatal, reactions including hyperthermia, rigidity, extreme agitation, delirium, coma, and features resembling neuroleptic malignant syndrome; concurrent and/or sequential use is contraindicated).
No products indexed under this heading.

Lithium Carbonate (Co-administration has resulted in reports of both increased and decreased lithium levels; cases of lithium toxicity have been reported). Products include:
Eskalith 1527
Lithium Carbonate 3061
Lithobid Slow-Release Tablets 3255

Lithium Citrate (Co-administration has resulted in reports of both increased and decreased lithium levels; cases of lithium toxicity have been reported). Products include:
Lithium Citrate Syrup 3061

Maprotiline Hydrochloride (Fluoxetine inhibits the activity of P450 IID6 isoenzyme making normal metabolizers resemble poor metabolizers; therapy with drugs that are predominantly metabolized by the P450 IID6, such as tricyclic antidepressants, and have relatively nar-

row therapeutic index should be initiated at low end of the dose range if a patient is receiving fluoxetine concurrently or has taken it in the previous 5 weeks).
No products indexed under this heading.

Metformin Hydrochloride (Fluoxetine may alter glycemic control in diabetics; hypoglycemia has occurred during therapy with fluoxetine, and hyperglycemia has developed following discontinuation of the drug; hypoglycemia dosage may need to be adjusted). Products include:
Glucophage Tablets 1080
Glucophage XR Tablets 1080
Glucovance Tablets 1086

Miglitol (Fluoxetine may alter glycemic control in diabetics; hypoglycemia has occurred during therapy with fluoxetine, and hyperglycemia has developed following discontinuation of the drug; hypoglycemia dosage may need to be adjusted). Products include:
Glyset Tablets 2821

Moclobemide (Co-administration with MAO inhibitors has resulted in serious, sometimes fatal, reactions including hyperthermia, rigidity, extreme agitation, delirium, coma, and features resembling neuroleptic malignant syndrome; concurrent and/or sequential use is contraindicated).
No products indexed under this heading.

Nortriptyline Hydrochloride (Fluoxetine inhibits the activity of P450 IID6 isoenzyme making normal metabolizers resemble poor metabolizers; therapy with drugs that are predominantly metabolized by the P450 IID6, such as tricyclic antidepressants, and have relatively narrow therapeutic index should be initiated at low end of the dose range if a patient is receiving fluoxetine concurrently or has taken it in the previous 5 weeks).
No products indexed under this heading.

Pargyline Hydrochloride (Co-administration with MAO inhibitors has resulted in serious, sometimes fatal, reactions including hyperthermia, rigidity, extreme agitation, delirium, coma, and features resembling neuroleptic malignant syndrome; concurrent and/or sequential use is contraindicated).
No products indexed under this heading.

Phenelzine Sulfate (Co-administration with MAO inhibitors has resulted in serious, sometimes fatal, reactions including hyperthermia, rigidity, extreme agitation, delirium, coma, and features resembling neuroleptic malignant syndrome; concurrent and/or sequential use is contraindicated). Products include:
Nardil Tablets 2653

Phenytoin (Patients stable on doses of phenytoin have developed elevated plasma phenytoin concentrations and clinical anticonvulsant toxicity following initiation of concomitant fluoxetine therapy). Products include:
Dilantin Infatabs 2624
Dilantin-125 Oral Suspension 2625

Phenytoin Sodium (Patients stable on doses of phenytoin have developed elevated plasma phenytoin concentrations and clinical anticonvulsant toxicity following initiation of concomitant fluoxetine therapy). Products include:
Dilantin Kapseals 2622

Pimozide (Co-administration has resulted in a single case report of possible additive effects of pimozide leading to bradycardia). Products include:
Orap Tablets 1407

Pioglitazone Hydrochloride (Fluoxetine may alter glycemic control in diabetics; hypoglycemia has occurred during therapy with fluoxetine, and hyperglycemia has developed following discontinuation of the drug; hypoglycemia dosage may need to be adjusted). Products include:
Actos Tablets 3275

Procarbazine Hydrochloride (Co-administration with MAO inhibitors has resulted in serious, sometimes fatal, reactions including hyperthermia, rigidity, extreme agitation, delirium, coma, and features resembling neuroleptic malignant syndrome; concurrent and/or sequential use is contraindicated). Products include:
Matulane Capsules 3246

Protriptyline Hydrochloride (Fluoxetine inhibits the activity of P450 IID6 isoenzyme making normal metabolizers resemble poor metabolizers; therapy with drugs that are predominantly metabolized by the P450 IID6, such as tricyclic antidepressants, and have relatively narrow therapeutic index should be initiated at low end of the dose range if a patient is receiving fluoxetine concurrently or has taken it in the previous 5 weeks). Products include:
Vivactil Tablets 2446
Vivactil Tablets 2217

Repaglinide (Fluoxetine may alter glycemic control in diabetics; hypoglycemia has occurred during therapy with fluoxetine, and hyperglycemia has developed following discontinuation of the drug; hypoglycemia dosage may need to be adjusted). Products include:
Prandin Tablets (0.5, 1, and 2 mg) 2432

Rosiglitazone Maleate (Fluoxetine may alter glycemic control in diabetics; hypoglycemia has occurred during therapy with fluoxetine, and hyperglycemia has developed following discontinuation of the drug; hypoglycemia dosage may need to be adjusted). Products include:
Avandia Tablets 1490

Selegiline Hydrochloride (Co-administration with MAO inhibitors has resulted in serious, sometimes fatal, reactions including hyperthermia, rigidity, extreme agitation, delirium, coma, and features resembling neuroleptic malignant syndrome; concurrent and/or sequential use is contraindicated). Products include:
Eldepryl Capsules 3266

Sumatriptan (Co-administration of SSRI and sumatriptan has resulted in weakness, hyperreflexia, and incoordination). Products include:
Imitrex Nasal Spray 1554

Sumatriptan Succinate (Co-administration of SSRI and sumatriptan has resulted in weakness, hyperreflexia, and incoordination). Products include:
Imitrex Injection 1549
Imitrex Tablets 1558

Thioridazine Hydrochloride (Co-administration of fluoxetine with thioridazine has produced a 2.4 fold higher Cmax and a 4.5 fold higher AUC for thioridazine; because thioridazine administration produces a dose-related prolongation of the QTc interval, which is associated with serious ventricular arrhythmias, such as torsade de pointes-type arrhythmias, and sudden death, concurrent and/or sequential use within a minimum of 5 weeks of Prozac is contraindicated). Products include:
Thioridazine Hydrochloride Tablets 2289

Tolazamide (Fluoxetine may alter glycemic control in diabetics; hypoglycemia has occurred during therapy with fluoxetine, and hyperglycemia has developed following discontinuation of the drug; hypoglycemia dosage may need to be adjusted).
No products indexed under this heading.

Tolbutamide (Fluoxetine may alter glycemic control in diabetics; hypoglycemia has occurred during therapy with fluoxetine, and hyperglycemia has developed following discontinuation of the drug; hypoglycemia dosage may need to be adjusted).
No products indexed under this heading.

Tranylcypromine Sulfate (Co-administration with MAO inhibitors has resulted in serious, sometimes fatal, reactions including hyperthermia, rigidity, extreme agitation, delirium, coma, and features resembling neuroleptic malignant syndrome; concurrent and/or sequential use is contraindicated). Products include:
Parnate Tablets 1607

Trimipramine Maleate (Fluoxetine inhibits the activity of P450 IID6 isoenzyme making normal metabolizers resemble poor metabolizers; therapy with drugs that are predominantly metabolized by the P450 IID6, such as tricyclic antidepressants, and have relatively narrow therapeutic index should be initiated at low end of the dose range if a patient is receiving fluoxetine concurrently or has taken it in the previous 5 weeks). Products include:
Surmontil Capsules 3595

Troglitazone (Fluoxetine may alter glycemic control in diabetics; hypoglycemia has occurred during therapy with fluoxetine, and hyperglycemia has developed following discontinuation of the drug; hypoglycemia dosage may need to be adjusted).
No products indexed under this heading.

L-Tryptophan (Co-administration has resulted in adverse reactions, including agitation, restlessness, and gastrointestinal distress).
No products indexed under this heading.

Vinblastine Sulfate (Fluoxetine inhibits the activity of P450 IID6 isoenzyme making normal metabolizers resemble poor metabolizers; therapy with drugs that are predominantly metabolized by the P450 IID6, such as vinblastine, and have relatively narrow therapeutic index should be initiated at low end of the dose range if a patient is receiving fluoxetine concurrently or has taken it in the previous 5 weeks).
No products indexed under this heading.

Warfarin Sodium (Fluoxetine is tightly bound to protein, co-administration may cause shift in plasma concentrations resulting in potential adverse effects). Products include:
Coumadin for Injection 1243
Coumadin Tablets 1243
Warfarin Sodium Tablets, USP 3302

Food Interactions

Alcohol (Concurrent use with CNS active agents, such as alcohol, requires caution).

Food, unspecified (May delay absorption of fluoxetine inconsequentially; Prozac may be administered with or without food).

PSORCON E CREAM
(Diflorasone Diacetate) 1227
None cited in PDR database.

PSORCON E OINTMENT
(Diflorasone Diacetate) 1228
None cited in PDR database.

PSORIATEC CREAM
(Anthralin) 3247
None cited in PDR database.

PULMICORT RESPULES
(Budesonide) 632
See Pulmicort Turbuhaler Inhalation Powder

PULMICORT TURBUHALER INHALATION POWDER
(Budesonide) 636
May interact with:

Ketoconazole (Co-administration with a potent inhibitor of cytochrome P450 3A, such as ketoconazole, may increase plasma levels of budesonide; caution is warranted). Products include:
Nizoral 2% Cream 3620
Nizoral A-D Shampoo 2008
Nizoral 2% Shampoo 2007
Nizoral Tablets 1791

PULMOZYME INHALATION SOLUTION
(Dornase Alfa) 1426
None cited in PDR database.

PURGE LIQUID
(Castor Oil) .... ▭ 633
None cited in PDR database.

PURINETHOL TABLETS
(Mercaptopurine) 1615
May interact with:

Allopurinol (Concomitant use at the regular dose results in delayed catabolism of mercaptopurine; substantial dosage reductions may be required to avoid the development of life-threatening bone marrow depression).
No products indexed under this heading.

Doxorubicin Hydrochloride (Potential for increased hepatotoxicity). Products include:
Adriamycin PFS/RDF Injection 2767
Doxil Injection 566

Hepatotoxic Drugs, unspecified (Hepatotoxicity).

Sulfamethoxazole (Enhanced bone marrow suppression has been noted in some of the patients also receiving trimethoprim-sulfamethoxazole). Products include:
Bactrim 2949
Septra Suspension 2265
Septra Tablets 2265
Septra DS Tablets 2265

Thioguanine (Complete cross-resistance). Products include:
Tabloid Tablets 1642

Trimethoprim (Enhanced bone marrow suppression has been noted in some of the patients also receiving trimethoprim-sulfamethoxazole). Products include:
Bactrim 2949
Septra Suspension 2265
Septra Tablets 2265
Septra DS Tablets 2265

PYRAZINAMIDE TABLETS
(Pyrazinamide) 1876
None cited in PDR database.

QUINAGLUTE DURA-TABS TABLETS
(Quinidine Gluconate) 978
May interact with anticholinergics, carbonic anhydrase inhibitors, cholinergic agents, negative inotropic agents, neuromuscular blocking agents, phenothiazines, phenytoin, thiazides, tricyclic antidepressants, vasopressors, vasodilators, and certain other agents. Compounds in these categories include:

Acebutolol Hydrochloride (Quinidine's negative inotropic actions may be additive to those of other similar agents). Products include:

Sectral Capsules 3589

Acetazolamide (Carbonic anhydrase inhibitors reduce renal elimination of quinidine by alkalinizing urine; following quinidine overdose, drugs that delay elimination of quinidine, such as carbonic anhydrase inhibitors, should be withdrawn unless absolutely required). Products include:
Diamox Sequels Sustained Release Capsules .... ⊙270
Diamox Tablets .... ⊙269

Amiodarone Hydrochloride (Co-administration may increase quinidine levels). Products include:
Cordarone Intravenous 3491
Cordarone Tablets 3487
Pacerone Tablets 3331

Amitriptyline Hydrochloride (Therapeutic serum levels of quinidine inhibit the action of cytochrome P450IID6 and most polycyclic antidepressants are metabolized by this enzyme; caution should be exercised). Products include:
Etrafon 3115
Limbitrol 1738

Amoxapine (Therapeutic serum levels of quinidine inhibit the action of cytochrome P450IID6 and most polycyclic antidepressants are metabolized by this enzyme; caution should be exercised).
No products indexed under this heading.

Atenolol (Quinidine's negative inotropic actions may be additive to those of other similar agents). Products include:
Tenoretic Tablets 690
Tenormin I.V. Injection 692

Atracurium Besylate (Quinidine potentiates the action of neuromuscular blocking agents).
No products indexed under this heading.

Atropine Sulfate (Quinidine's anticholinergic actions may be additive to those of other anticholinergic drugs). Products include:
Donnatal 2929
Donnatal Extentabs 2930
Motofen Tablets 577
Prosed/DS Tablets 3268
Urised Tablets 2876

Belladonna Alkaloids (Quinidine's anticholinergic actions may be additive to those of other anticholinergic drugs). Products include:
Hyland's Teething Tablets .... ▣766
Urimax Tablets 1769

Bendroflumethiazide (Thiazide diuretics reduce renal elimination of quinidine by alkalinizing urine; following quinidine overdose, drugs that delay elimination of quinidine, such as thiazide diuretics, should be withdrawn unless absolutely required). Products include:
Corzide 40/5 Tablets 2247
Corzide 80/5 Tablets 2247

Benztropine Mesylate (Quinidine's anticholinergic actions may be additive to those of other anticholinergic drugs). Products include:
Cogentin 2055

Betaxolol Hydrochloride (Quinidine's negative inotropic actions may be additive to those of other similar agents). Products include:
Betoptic S Ophthalmic Suspension 537

Bethanechol Chloride (Quinidine's anticholinergic actions may be antagonistic to those of cholinergic agents). Products include:
Urecholine 2198
Urecholine Tablets 2445

Biperiden Hydrochloride (Quinidine's anticholinergic actions may be additive to those of other anticholinergic drugs). Products include:
Akineton 402

Carteolol Hydrochloride (Quinidine's negative inotropic actions may be additive to those of other similar agents). Products include:
Carteolol Hydrochloride Ophthalmic Solution USP, 1% .... ⊙258
Ocupress Ophthalmic Solution, 1% Sterile .... ⊙303

Cevimeline Hydrochloride (Quinidine's anticholinergic actions may be antagonistic to those of cholinergic agents). Products include:
Evoxac Capsules 1217

Chlorothiazide (Thiazide diuretics reduce renal elimination of quinidine by alkalinizing urine; following quinidine overdose, drugs that delay elimination of quinidine, such as thiazide diuretics, should be withdrawn unless absolutely required). Products include:
Aldoclor Tablets 2035
Diuril Oral 2087

Chlorothiazide Sodium (Thiazide diuretics reduce renal elimination of quinidine by alkalinizing urine; following quinidine overdose, drugs that delay elimination of quinidine, such as thiazide diuretics, should be withdrawn unless absolutely required). Products include:
Diuril Sodium Intravenous 2086

Chlorpromazine (Therapeutic serum levels of quinidine inhibit the action of cytochrome P450IID6 and certain unspecified phenothiazines are metabolized by this enzyme; caution should be exercised). Products include:
Thorazine Suppositories 1656

Chlorpromazine Hydrochloride (Therapeutic serum levels of quinidine inhibit the action of cytochrome P450IID6 and certain unspecified phenothiazines are metabolized by this enzyme; caution should be exercised). Products include:
Thorazine 1656

Cimetidine (Co-administration may delay elimination thereby increase quinidine levels; following quinidine overdose, drugs that delay elimination of quinidine, such as cimetidine, should be withdrawn unless absolutely required). Products include:
Tagamet HB 200 Suspension .... ▣762
Tagamet HB 200 Tablets .... ▣761
Tagamet Tablets 1644

Cimetidine Hydrochloride (Co-administration may delay elimination thereby increase quinidine levels; following quinidine overdose, drugs that delay elimination of quinidine, such as cimetidine, should be withdrawn unless absolutely required). Products include:
Tagamet 1644

Cisatracurium Besylate (Quinidine potentiates the action of neuromuscular blocking agents).
No products indexed under this heading.

Clidinium Bromide (Quinidine's anticholinergic actions may be additive to those of other anticholinergic drugs).
No products indexed under this heading.

Clomipramine Hydrochloride (Therapeutic serum levels of quinidine inhibit the action of cytochrome P450IID6 and most polycyclic antidepressants are metabolized by this enzyme; caution should be exercised).
No products indexed under this heading.

Codeine Phosphate (Co-administration of prodrug whose actions are actually mediated by P450IID6, such as codeine and whose analgesic and antitussive effects appear to be mediated by morphine, may cause decrease in the concentrations of morphine (an active metabolite of codeine) resulting in reduced therapeutic effects of codeine). Products include:
Phenergan with Codeine Syrup 3557
Phenergan VC with Codeine Syrup 3561
Robitussin A-C Syrup 2942
Robitussin-DAC Syrup 2942
Ryna-C Liquid .... ▣768
Soma Compound w/Codeine Tablets 3355
Tussi-Organidin NR Liquid 3350
Tussi-Organidin-S NR Liquid 3350
Tylenol with Codeine 2595

Decamethonium (Quinidine potentiates the action of neuromuscular blocking agent).
No products indexed under this heading.

Desipramine Hydrochloride (Therapeutic serum levels of quinidine inhibit the action of cytochrome P450IID6 and most polycyclic antidepressants are metabolized by this enzyme; caution should be exercised). Products include:
Norpramin Tablets 755

Diazoxide (Quinidine's vasodilating actions may be additive to those of other vasodilators).
No products indexed under this heading.

Dichlorphenamide (Carbonic anhydrase inhibitors reduce renal elimination of quinidine by alkalinizing urine; following quinidine overdose, drugs that delay elimination of quinidine, such as carbonic anhydrase inhibitors, should be withdrawn unless absolutely required). Products include:
Daranide Tablets 2077

Dicyclomine Hydrochloride (Quinidine's anticholinergic actions may be additive to those of other anticholinergic drugs).
No products indexed under this heading.

Dietary salt (The rate and extent of quinidine absorption may be affected by changes in dietary salt intake; a decrease in dietary salt intake may lead to an increase in plasma quinidine concentrations).
No products indexed under this heading.

Digitoxin (Quinidine slows the elimination of digitoxin resulting in the elevation of serum levels of digitoxin when co-administered, although the effect appears to be smaller).
No products indexed under this heading.

Digoxin (Quinidine slows the elimination of digoxin and simultaneously reduces digoxin's apparent volume of distribution resulting in elevated serum digoxin levels). Products include:
Digitek Tablets 1003
Lanoxicaps Capsules 1574
Lanoxin Injection 1581
Lanoxin Tablets 1587
Lanoxin Elixir Pediatric 1578
Lanoxin Injection Pediatric 1584

Diltiazem Hydrochloride (Co-administration with diltiazem significantly decreases the clearance and increases the t1/2 of quinidine, but quinidine does not alter the kinetics of diltiazem; following quinidine overdose, drugs that delay elimination of quinidine, such as diltiazem, should be withdrawn unless absolutely required). Products include:
Cardizem Injectable 1018
Cardizem Lyo-Ject Syringe 1018
Cardizem Monovial 1018
Cardizem CD Capsules 1016
Tiazac Capsules 1378

Diltiazem Malate (Co-administration with diltiazem significantly decreases the clearance and increases the t1/2 of quinidine, but quinidine does not alter the kinetics of diltiazem; following quinidine overdose, drugs that delay elimination of quinidine, such as diltiazem, should be withdrawn unless absolutely required).
No products indexed under this heading.

Donepezil Hydrochloride (Quinidine's anticholinergic actions may be antagonistic to those of cholinergic agents). Products include:
Aricept Tablets 1270
Aricept Tablets 2665

Dopamine Hydrochloride (Quinidine's vasodilating actions may be antagonistic to those of vasopressors).
No products indexed under this heading.

Dorzolamide Hydrochloride (Carbonic anhydrase inhibitors reduce renal elimination of quinidine by alkalinizing urine; following quinidine overdose, drugs that delay elimination of quinidine, such as carbonic anhydrase inhibitors, should be withdrawn unless absolutely required). Products include:
Cosopt Sterile Ophthalmic Solution 2065
Trusopt Sterile Ophthalmic Solution 2196

Doxacurium Chloride (Quinidine potentiates the action of neuromuscular blocking agents).
No products indexed under this heading.

Doxepin Hydrochloride (Therapeutic serum levels of quinidine inhibit the action of cytochrome P450IID6 and most polycyclic antidepressants are metabolized by this enzyme; caution should be exercised). Products include:
Sinequan 2713

Edrophonium Chloride (Quinidine's anticholinergic actions may be antagonistic to those of cholinergic agents). Products include:
Tensilon Injectable 1745

Epinephrine Bitartrate (Quinidine's vasodilating actions may be antagonistic to those of vasopressors). Products include:
Sensorcaine 643

Epinephrine Hydrochloride (Quinidine's vasodilating actions may be antagonistic to those of vasopressors).
No products indexed under this heading.

Epoprostenol Sodium (Quinidine's vasodilating actions may be additive to those of other vasodilators). Products include:
Flolan for Injection 1528

Esmolol Hydrochloride (Quinidine's negative inotropic actions may be additive to those of other similar agents). Products include:
Brevibloc Injection 858

Felodipine (Potential for variable slowing of the metabolism of felodipine). Products include:
Lexxel Tablets 608
Plendil Extended-Release Tablets 623

Fluphenazine Decanoate (Therapeutic serum levels of quinidine inhibit the action of cytochrome P450IID6 and certain unspecified phenothiazines are metabolized by this enzyme; caution should be exercised).
No products indexed under this heading.

Fluphenazine Enanthate (Therapeutic serum levels of quinidine inhibit the action of cytochrome P450IID6 and certain unspecified phenothiazines are metabolized by this enzyme; caution should be exercised).
No products indexed under this heading.

Fluphenazine Hydrochloride (Therapeutic serum levels of quinidine inhibit the action of cytochrome P450IID6 and certain unspecified

phenothiazines are metabolized by this enzyme; caution should be exercised).
No products indexed under this heading.

Fosphenytoin Sodium (Co-administration with drugs that induce production of CYP450IIIA4, such as phenytoin, may accelerate hepatic elimination of quinidine). Products include:
Cerebyx Injection 2619

Galantamine Hydrobromide (Quinidine's anticholinergic actions may be antagonistic to those of cholinergic agents). Products include:
Reminyl Oral Solution 1792
Reminyl Tablets 1792

Glycopyrrolate (Quinidine's anticholinergic actions may be additive to those of other anticholinergic drugs). Products include:
Robinul Forte Tablets 1358
Robinul Injectable 2940
Robinul Tablets 1358

Haloperidol (Serum levels of haloperidol are increased when quinidine is co-administered). Products include:
Haldol Injection, Tablets and Concentrate 2533

Haloperidol Decanoate (Serum levels of haloperidol are increased when quinidine is co-administered). Products include:
Haldol Decanoate 2535

Hydralazine Hydrochloride (Quinidine's vasodilating actions may be additive to those of other vasodilators).
No products indexed under this heading.

Hydrochlorothiazide (Thiazide diuretics reduce renal elimination of quinidine by alkalinizing urine; following quinidine overdose, drugs that delay elimination of quinidine, such as thiazide diuretics, should be withdrawn unless absolutely required). Products include:
Accuretic Tablets 2614
Aldoril Tablets 2039
Atacand HCT Tablets 597
Avalide Tablets 1070
Diovan HCT Tablets 2338
Dyazide Capsules 1515
HydroDIURIL Tablets 2108
Hyzaar 2109
Inderide Tablets 3517
Inderide LA Long-Acting Capsules .. 3519
Lotensin HCT Tablets 2367
Maxzide 1008
Micardis HCT Tablets 1051
Microzide Capsules 3414
Moduretic Tablets 2138
Monopril HCT 1094
Prinzide Tablets 2168
Timolide Tablets 2187
Uniretic Tablets 3178
Vaseretic Tablets 2204
Zestoretic Tablets 695
Ziac Tablets 1887

Hydrocodone Bitartrate (Co-administration of prodrug whose actions are actually mediated by P450IID6, such as codeine and whose analgesic and antitussive effects appear to be mediated by hydromorphone, may cause decrease in the concentrations of hydromorphone (an active metabolite of hydrocodone) resulting in reduced therapeutic effects of hydrocodone). Products include:
Hycodan 1316
Hycomine Compound Tablets 1317
Hycotuss Expectorant Syrup 1318
Lortab 3319
Lortab Elixir 3317
Maxidone Tablets CIII 3399
Norco 5/325 Tablets CIII 3424
Norco 7.5/325 Tablets CIII 3425
Norco 10/325 Tablets CIII 3427
Norco 10/325 Tablets CIII 3425
Vicodin Tablets 516
Vicodin ES Tablets 517
Vicodin HP Tablets 518
Vicodin Tuss Expectorant 519
Vicoprofen Tablets 520
Zydone Tablets 1330

Hydroflumethiazide (Thiazide diuretics reduce renal elimination of quinidine by alkalinizing urine; following quinidine overdose, drugs that delay elimination of quinidine, such as thiazide diuretics, should be withdrawn unless absolutely required). Products include:
Diucardin Tablets 3494

Hyoscyamine (Quinidine's anticholinergic actions may be additive to those of other anticholinergic drugs). Products include:
Urised Tablets 2876

Hyoscyamine Sulfate (Quinidine's anticholinergic actions may be additive to those of other anticholinergic drugs). Products include:
Arco-Lase Plus Tablets 592
Donnatal 2929
Donnatal Extentabs 2930
Levsin/Levsinex/Levbid 3172
NuLev Orally Disintegrating Tablets 3176
Prosed/DS Tablets 3268
Urimax Tablets 1769

Imipramine Hydrochloride (Therapeutic serum levels of quinidine inhibit the action of cytochrome P450IID6 and most polycyclic antidepressants are metabolized by this enzyme; caution should be exercised).
No products indexed under this heading.

Imipramine Pamoate (Therapeutic serum levels of quinidine inhibit the action of cytochrome P450IID6 and most polycyclic antidepressants are metabolized by this enzyme; caution should be exercised).
No products indexed under this heading.

Ipratropium Bromide (Quinidine's anticholinergic actions may be additive to those of other anticholinergic drugs). Products include:
Atrovent Inhalation Aerosol 1030
Atrovent Inhalation Solution 1031
Atrovent Nasal Spray 0.03% 1032
Atrovent Nasal Spray 0.06% 1033
Combivent Inhalation Aerosol 1041
DuoNeb Inhalation Solution 1233

Ketoconazole (Co-administration may increase quinidine levels). Products include:
Nizoral 2% Cream 3620
Nizoral A-D Shampoo 2008
Nizoral 2% Shampoo 2007
Nizoral Tablets 1791

Labetalol Hydrochloride (Quinidine's negative inotropic actions may be additive to those of other similar agents). Products include:
Normodyne Injection 3135
Normodyne Tablets 3137

Maprotiline Hydrochloride (Therapeutic serum levels of quinidine inhibit the action of cytochrome P450IID6 and most polycyclic antidepressants are metabolized by this enzyme; caution should be exercised).
No products indexed under this heading.

Mepenzolate Bromide (Quinidine's anticholinergic actions may be additive to those of other anticholinergic drugs).
No products indexed under this heading.

Mesoridazine Besylate (Therapeutic serum levels of quinidine inhibit the action of cytochrome P450IID6 and certain unspecified phenothiazines are metabolized by this enzyme; caution should be exercised). Products include:
Serentil 1057

Metaraminol Bitartrate (Quinidine's vasodilating actions may be antagonistic to those of vasopressors). Products include:
Aramine Injection 2043

Methazolamide (Carbonic anhydrase inhibitors reduce renal elimination of quinidine by alkalinizing urine; following quinidine overdose, drugs that delay elimination of quinidine, such as carbonic anhydrase inhibitors, should be withdrawn unless absolutely required). Products include:
Neptazane Tablets .... ⊙271

Methotrimeprazine (Therapeutic serum levels of quinidine inhibit the action of cytochrome P450IID6 and certain unspecified phenothiazines are metabolized by this enzyme; caution should be exercised).
No products indexed under this heading.

Methoxamine Hydrochloride (Quinidine's vasodilating actions may be antagonistic to those of vasopressors).
No products indexed under this heading.

Methyclothiazide (Thiazide diuretics reduce renal elimination of quinidine by alkalinizing urine; following quinidine overdose, drugs that delay elimination of quinidine, such as thiazide diuretics, should be withdrawn unless absolutely required).
No products indexed under this heading.

Metocurine Iodide (Quinidine potentiates the action of neuromuscular blocking agents).
No products indexed under this heading.

Metoprolol Tartrate (Quinidine's negative inotropic actions may be additive to those of other similar agents).
No products indexed under this heading.

Mexiletine Hydrochloride (Therapeutic serum levels of quinidine inhibit the action of cytochrome P450IID6 and mexiletine is metabolized by this enzyme; caution should be exercised). Products include:
Mexitil Capsules 1047

Minoxidil (Quinidine's vasodilating actions may be additive to those of other vasodilators). Products include:
Rogaine Extra Strength for Men Topical Solution .... ■721
Rogaine for Women Topical Solution .... ■721

Mivacurium Chloride (Quinidine potentiates the action of neuromuscular blocking agents).
No products indexed under this heading.

Nadolol (Quinidine's negative inotropic actions may be additive to those of other similar agents). Products include:
Corgard Tablets 2245
Corzide 40/5 Tablets 2247
Corzide 80/5 Tablets 2247
Nadolol Tablets 2288

Neostigmine Bromide (Quinidine's anticholinergic actions may be antagonistic to those of cholinergic agents). Products include:
Prostigmin Tablets 1744

Neostigmine Methylsulfate (Quinidine's anticholinergic actions may be antagonistic to those of cholinergic agents). Products include:
Prostigmin Injectable 1744

Nicardipine Hydrochloride (Potential for variable slowing of the metabolism of nicardipine). Products include:
Cardene I.V. 3485

Nifedipine (Very rarely co-administration may decrease quinidine levels; quinidine causes variable slowing of the metabolism of nifedipine). Products include:
Adalat CC Tablets 877
Procardia Capsules 2708
Procardia XL Extended Release Tablets 2710

Nimodipine (Potential for variable slowing of the metabolism of nimodipine). Products include:
Nimotop Capsules 904

Norepinephrine Bitartrate (Quinidine's vasodilating actions may be antagonistic to those of vasopressors).
No products indexed under this heading.

Nortriptyline Hydrochloride (Therapeutic serum levels of quinidine inhibit the action of cytochrome P450IID6 and most polycyclic antidepressants are metabolized by this enzyme; caution should be exercised).
No products indexed under this heading.

Oxybutynin Chloride (Quinidine's anticholinergic actions may be additive to those of other anticholinergic drugs). Products include:
Ditropan XL Extended Release Tablets 564

Pancuronium Bromide (Quinidine potentiates the action of neuromuscular blocking agents).
No products indexed under this heading.

Penbutolol Sulfate (Quinidine's negative inotropic actions may be additive to those of other similar agents).
No products indexed under this heading.

Perphenazine (Therapeutic serum levels of quinidine inhibit the action of cytochrome P450IID6 and certain unspecified phenothiazines are metabolized by this enzyme; caution should be exercised). Products include:
Etrafon 3115
Trilafon 3160

Phenobarbital (Co-administration with drugs that induce production of CYP450IIIA4, such as phenobarbital, may accelerate hepatic elimination of quinidine). Products include:
Arco-Lase Plus Tablets 592
Donnatal 2929
Donnatal Extentabs 2930

Phenylephrine Hydrochloride (Quinidine's vasodilating actions may be antagonistic to those of vasopressors). Products include:
Afrin Nasal Decongestant Children's Pump Mist .... ■734
Extendryl 1361
Hycomine Compound Tablets 1317
Neo-Synephrine .... ■614
Phenergan VC Syrup 3560
Phenergan VC with Codeine Syrup .. 3561
Preparation H Cream .... ■778
Preparation H Cooling Gel .... ■778
Preparation H .... ■778
Vicks Sinex Nasal Spray and Ultra Fine Mist .... ■729

Phenytoin (Co-administration with drugs that induce production of CYP450IIIA4, such as phenytoin, may accelerate hepatic elimination of quinidine). Products include:
Dilantin Infatabs 2624
Dilantin-125 Oral Suspension 2625

Phenytoin Sodium (Co-administration with drugs that induce production of CYP450IIIA4, such as phenytoin, may accelerate hepatic elimination of quinidine). Products include:
Dilantin Kapseals 2622

Pindolol (Quinidine's negative inotropic actions may be additive to those of other similar agents).
No products indexed under this heading.

Polythiazide (Thiazide diuretics reduce renal elimination of quinidine by alkalinizing urine; following quinidine overdose, drugs that delay elimination of quinidine, such as thiazide

diuretics, should be withdrawn unless absolutely required). Products include:
- Minizide Capsules 2700
- Renese Tablets 2712

Procainamide Hydrochloride (Co-administration causes an increase in serum levels of procainamide). Products include:
- Procanbid Extended-Release Tablets 2262

Prochlorperazine (Therapeutic serum levels of quinidine inhibit the action of cytochrome P450IID6 and certain unspecified phenothiazines are metabolized by this enzyme; caution should be exercised). Products include:
- Compazine 1505

Procyclidine Hydrochloride (Quinidine's anticholinergic actions may be additive to those of other anticholinergic drugs).
- No products indexed under this heading.

Promethazine Hydrochloride (Therapeutic serum levels of quinidine inhibit the action of cytochrome P450IID6 and certain unspecified phenothiazines are metabolized by this enzyme; caution should be exercised). Products include:
- Mepergan Injection 3539
- Phenergan Injection 3553
- Phenergan 3556
- Phenergan Syrup 3554
- Phenergan with Codeine Syrup 3557
- Phenergan with Dextromethorphan Syrup 3559
- Phenergan VC Syrup 3560
- Phenergan VC with Codeine Syrup 3561

Propantheline Bromide (Quinidine's anticholinergic actions may be additive to those of other anticholinergic drugs).
- No products indexed under this heading.

Propranolol Hydrochloride (Co-administration in some patients may cause increase in the peak serum levels of quinidine, decrease in quinidine's volume of distribution, and decrease in total quinidine clearance). Products include:
- Inderal 3513
- Inderal LA Long-Acting Capsules 3516
- Inderide Tablets 3517
- Inderide LA Long-Acting Capsules 3519

Protriptyline Hydrochloride (Therapeutic serum levels of quinidine inhibit the action of cytochrome P450IID6 and most polycyclic antidepressants are metabolized by this enzyme; caution should be exercised). Products include:
- Vivactil Tablets 2446
- Vivactil Tablets 2217

Pyridostigmine Bromide (Quinidine's anticholinergic actions may be antagonistic to those of cholinergic agents). Products include:
- Mestinon 1740

Rapacuronium Bromide (Quinidine potentiates the action of neuromuscular blocking agents).
- No products indexed under this heading.

Rifampin (Co-administration with drugs that induce production of CYP450IIIA4, such as rifampin, may accelerate hepatic elimination of quinidine). Products include:
- Rifadin 765
- Rifamate Capsules 767
- Rifater Tablets 769

Rivastigmine Tartrate (Quinidine's anticholinergic actions may be antagonistic to those of cholinergic agents). Products include:
- Exelon Capsules 2342
- Exelon Oral Solution 2345

Rocuronium Bromide (Quinidine potentiates the action of neuromuscular blocking agents). Products include:
- Zemuron Injection 2491

Scopolamine (Quinidine's anticholinergic actions may be additive to those of other anticholinergic drugs). Products include:
- Transderm Scōp Transdermal Therapeutic System 2302

Scopolamine Hydrobromide (Quinidine's anticholinergic actions may be additive to those of other anticholinergic drugs). Products include:
- Donnatal 2929
- Donnatal Extentabs 2930

Sodium Bicarbonate (Systemic sodium bicarbonate reduces renal elimination of quinidine by alkalinizing the urine). Products include:
- Alka-Seltzer .... ⊡603
- Alka-Seltzer Lemon Lime Antacid and Pain Reliever Effervescent Tablets .... ⊡603
- Alka-Seltzer Extra Strength Antacid and Pain Reliever Effervescent Tablets .... ⊡603
- Alka-Seltzer Heartburn Relief Tablets .... ⊡604
- Ceo-Two Evacuant Suppository .... ⊡618
- Colyte with Flavor Packs for Oral Solution 3170
- GoLYTELY and Pineapple Flavor GoLYTELY for Oral Solution 1068
- NuLYTELY, Cherry Flavor, Lemon-Lime Flavor, and Orange Flavor NuLYTELY for Oral Solution 1068

Succinylcholine Chloride (Quinidine potentiates the action of neuromuscular blocking agents). Products include:
- Anectine Injection 1476

Tacrine Hydrochloride (Quinidine's anticholinergic actions may be antagonistic to those of cholinergic agents). Products include:
- Cognex Capsules 1351

Thioridazine Hydrochloride (Therapeutic serum levels of quinidine inhibit the action of cytochrome P450IID6 and certain unspecified phenothiazines are metabolized by this enzyme; caution should be exercised). Products include:
- Thioridazine Hydrochloride Tablets 2289

Timolol Maleate (Quinidine's negative inotropic actions may be additive to those of other similar agents). Products include:
- Blocadren Tablets 2046
- Cosopt Sterile Ophthalmic Solution 2065
- Timolide Tablets 2187
- Timolol GFS .... ⊙266
- Timoptic in Ocudose 2192
- Timoptic Sterile Ophthalmic Solution 2190
- Timoptic-XE Sterile Ophthalmic Gel Forming Solution 2194

Tolterodine Tartrate (Quinidine's anticholinergic actions may be additive to those of other anticholinergic drugs). Products include:
- Detrol Tablets 3623
- Detrol LA Capsules 2801

Trazodone Hydrochloride (Therapeutic serum levels of quinidine inhibit the action of cytochrome P450IID6 and most polycyclic antidepressants are metabolized by this enzyme; caution should be exercised).
- No products indexed under this heading.

Tridihexethyl Chloride (Quinidine's anticholinergic actions may be additive to those of other anticholinergic drugs).
- No products indexed under this heading.

Trifluoperazine Hydrochloride (Therapeutic serum levels of quinidine inhibit the action of cytochrome P450IID6 and certain unspecified phenothiazines are metabolized by this enzyme; caution should be exercised). Products include:
- Stelazine 1640

Trihexyphenidyl Hydrochloride (Quinidine's anticholinergic actions may be additive to those of other anticholinergic drugs). Products include:
- Artane 1855

Trimipramine Maleate (Therapeutic serum levels of quinidine inhibit the action of cytochrome P450IID6 and most polycyclic antidepressants are metabolized by this enzyme; caution should be exercised). Products include:
- Surmontil Capsules 3595

Tubocurarine Chloride (Potentiation of neuromuscular blockade).
- No products indexed under this heading..

Vecuronium Bromide (Quinidine potentiates the action of neuromuscular blocking agents). Products include:
- Norcuron for Injection 2478

Verapamil Hydrochloride (Hepatic clearance of quinidine is significantly reduced with co-administration resulting in corresponding increase in serum levels and half-life). Products include:
- Covera-HS Tablets 3199
- Isoptin SR Tablets 467
- Tarka Tablets 508
- Verelan Capsules 3184
- Verelan PM Capsules 3186

Warfarin Sodium (Quinidine may potentiate anticoagulant action of warfarin). Products include:
- Coumadin for Injection 1243
- Coumadin Tablets 1243
- Warfarin Sodium Tablets, USP 3302

Food Interactions

Food, unspecified (Increases absorption of quinidine in both rate (27%) and extent (17%)).

Grapefruit Juice (Because grapefruit juice inhibits CYPIIIA4-mediated metabolism of quinidine to 3-hydroxyquinidine, the ingestion of grapefruit juice during treatment with quinidine should be avoided; the clinical significance of this interaction is unknown).

QUINIDEX EXTENTABS

(Quinidine Sulfate) 2933

May interact with anticholinergics, carbonic anhydrase inhibitors, negative inotropic agents, neuromuscular blocking agents, phenothiazines, phenytoin, thiazides, tricyclic antidepressants, vasodilators, and certain other agents. Compounds in these categories include:

Acebutolol Hydrochloride (Negative inotropic actions of quinidine may be additive to those of other co-administered drugs with similar actions). Products include:
- Sectral Capsules 3589

Acetazolamide (Drugs that alkalinize urine, such as carbonic anhydrase inhibitors, reduce renal elimination of quinidine; following quinidine overdose, drugs that delay elimination of quinidine, such as carbonic anhydrase inhibitors, should be withdrawn). Products include:
- Diamox Sequels Sustained Release Capsules .... ⊙270
- Diamox Tablets .... ⊙269

Amiodarone Hydrochloride (Co-administration may increase quinidine levels). Products include:
- Cordarone Intravenous 3491
- Cordarone Tablets 3487
- Pacerone Tablets 3331

Amitriptyline Hydrochloride (Therapeutic serum levels of quinidine inhibit the action of CYP4502D6; this enzyme system is critical for the metabolism of polycyclic antidepressants; therefore, caution is advised). Products include:
- Etrafon 3115
- Limbitrol 1738

Amoxapine (Therapeutic serum levels of quinidine inhibit the action of CYP4502D6; this enzyme system is critical for the metabolism of polycyclic antidepressants; therefore, caution is advised).
- No products indexed under this heading.

Atenolol (Negative inotropic actions of quinidine may be additive to those of other co-administered drugs with similar actions). Products include:
- Tenoretic Tablets 690
- Tenormin I.V. Injection 692

Atracurium Besylate (Quinidine potentiates the action of neuromuscular blocking agents).
- No products indexed under this heading.

Atropine Sulfate (Anticholinergic actions of quinidine may be additive to those of other co-administered anticholinergic agents). Products include:
- Donnatal 2929
- Donnatal Extentabs 2930
- Motofen Tablets 577
- Prosed/DS Tablets 3268
- Urised Tablets 2876

Belladonna Alkaloids (Anticholinergic actions of quinidine may be additive to those of other co-administered anticholinergic agents). Products include:
- Hyland's Teething Tablets .... ⊡766
- Urimax Tablets 1769

Bendroflumethiazide (Drugs that alkalinize urine, such as thiazide diuretics, reduce renal elimination of quinidine; following quinidine overdose, drugs that delay elimination of quinidine, such as thiazide diuretics, should be withdrawn). Products include:
- Corzide 40/5 Tablets 2247
- Corzide 80/5 Tablets 2247

Benztropine Mesylate (Anticholinergic actions of quinidine may be additive to those of other co-administered anticholinergic agents). Products include:
- Cogentin 2055

Betaxolol Hydrochloride (Negative inotropic actions of quinidine may be additive to those of other co-administered drugs with similar actions). Products include:
- Betoptic S Ophthalmic Suspension 537

Biperiden Hydrochloride (Anticholinergic actions of quinidine may be additive to those of other co-administered anticholinergic agents). Products include:
- Akineton 402

Carteolol Hydrochloride (Negative inotropic actions of quinidine may be additive to those of other co-administered drugs with similar actions). Products include:
- Carteolol Hydrochloride Ophthalmic Solution USP, 1% .... ⊙258
- Ocupress Ophthalmic Solution, 1% Sterile .... ⊙303

Chlorothiazide (Drugs that alkalinize urine, such as thiazide diuretics, reduce renal elimination of quinidine; following quinidine overdose, drugs that delay elimination of quinidine, such as thiazide diuretics, should be withdrawn). Products include:
- Aldoclor Tablets 2035
- Diuril Oral 2087

Chlorothiazide Sodium (Drugs that alkalinize urine, such as thiazide diuretics, reduce renal elimination of quinidine; following quinidine overdose, drugs that delay elimination of quinidine, such as thiazide diuretics, should be withdrawn). Products include:
- Diuril Sodium Intravenous 2086

Chlorpromazine (Therapeutic serum levels of quinidine inhibit the action of CYP4502D6; this enzyme system is critical for the metabolism of phenothiazines; therefore, caution is advised). Products include:
- Thorazine Suppositories 1656

Chlorpromazine Hydrochloride (Therapeutic serum levels of quinidine inhibit the action of CYP4502D6; this enzyme system is critical for the metabolism of phenothiazines; therefore, caution is advised). Products include:
- Thorazine 1656

Cimetidine (Co-administration may increase quinidine levels; following quinidine overdose, drugs that delay elimination of quinidine, such as cimetidine, should be withdrawn). Products include:
- Tagamet HB 200 Suspension .... ▣762
- Tagamet HB 200 Tablets .... ▣761
- Tagamet Tablets 1644

Cimetidine Hydrochloride (Co-administration may increase quinidine levels; following quinidine overdose, drugs that delay elimination of quinidine, such as cimetidine, should be withdrawn). Products include:
- Tagamet 1644

Cisatracurium Besylate (Quinidine potentiates the action of neuromuscular blocking agents).
No products indexed under this heading.

Clidinium Bromide (Anticholinergic actions of quinidine may be additive to those of other co-administered anticholinergic agents).
No products indexed under this heading.

Clomipramine Hydrochloride (Therapeutic serum levels of quinidine inhibit the action of CYP4502D6; this enzyme system is critical for the metabolism of polycyclic antidepressants; therefore, caution is advised).
No products indexed under this heading.

Codeine Phosphate (Therapeutic serum levels of quinidine inhibit the action of CYP4502D6; co-administration of prodrug whose actions are actually mediated by P450IID6, such as codeine and whose analgesic and antitussive effects appear to be mediated by morphine, may cause decrease in the concentrations of morphine (an active metabolite of codeine) resulting in reduced therapeutic effects of codeine). Products include:
- Phenergan with Codeine Syrup 3557
- Phenergan VC with Codeine Syrup . 3561
- Robitussin A-C Syrup 2942
- Robitussin-DAC Syrup 2942
- Ryna-C Liquid .... ▣768
- Soma Compound w/Codeine Tablets 3355
- Tussi-Organidin NR Liquid 3350
- Tussi-Organidin-S NR Liquid 3350
- Tylenol with Codeine 2595

Desipramine Hydrochloride (Therapeutic serum levels of quinidine inhibit the action of CYP4502D6; this enzyme system is critical for the metabolism of polycyclic antidepressants; therefore, caution is advised). Products include:
- Norpramin Tablets 755

Diazoxide (Vasodilating actions of quinidine may be additive to those of other co-administered drugs with similar actions).
No products indexed under this heading.

Dichlorphenamide (Drugs that alkalinize urine, such as carbonic anhydrase inhibitors, reduce renal elimination of quinidine; following quinidine overdose, drugs that delay elimination of quinidine, such as carbonic anhydrase inhibitors, should be withdrawn). Products include:
- Daranide Tablets 2077

Dicyclomine Hydrochloride (Anticholinergic actions of quinidine may be additive to those of other co-administered anticholinergic agents).
No products indexed under this heading.

Digitoxin (Co-administration raises serum digitoxin levels).
No products indexed under this heading.

Digoxin (Quinidine slows the elimination of digoxin and simultaneously reduces digoxin's apparent volume of distribution; serum digoxin levels may be as much as doubled). Products include:
- Digitek Tablets 1003
- Lanoxicaps Capsules 1574
- Lanoxin Injection 1581
- Lanoxin Tablets 1587
- Lanoxin Elixir Pediatric 1578
- Lanoxin Injection Pediatric 1584

Diltiazem Hydrochloride (Co-administration with diltiazem significantly decreases the clearance and increases the t1/2 of quinidine; following quinidine overdose, drugs that delay elimination of quinidine, such as diltiazem, should be withdrawn). Products include:
- Cardizem Injectable 1018
- Cardizem Lyo-Ject Syringe 1018
- Cardizem Monovial 1018
- Cardizem CD Capsules 1016
- Tiazac Capsules 1378

Diltiazem Malate (Co-administration with diltiazem significantly decreases the clearance and increases the t1/2 of quinidine; following quinidine overdose, drugs that delay elimination of quinidine, such as diltiazem, should be withdrawn).
No products indexed under this heading.

Dorzolamide Hydrochloride (Drugs that alkalinize urine, such as carbonic anhydrase inhibitors, reduce renal elimination of quinidine; following quinidine overdose, drugs that delay elimination of quinidine, such as carbonic anhydrase inhibitors, should be withdrawn). Products include:
- Cosopt Sterile Ophthalmic Solution 2065
- Trusopt Sterile Ophthalmic Solution 2196

Doxacurium Chloride (Quinidine potentiates the action of neuromuscular blocking agents).
No products indexed under this heading.

Doxepin Hydrochloride (Therapeutic serum levels of quinidine inhibit the action of CYP4502D6; this enzyme system is critical for the metabolism of polycyclic antidepressants; therefore, caution is advised). Products include:
- Sinequan 2713

Epoprostenol Sodium (Vasodilating actions of quinidine may be additive to those of other co-administered drugs with similar actions). Products include:
- Flolan for Injection 1528

Esmolol Hydrochloride (Negative inotropic actions of quinidine may be additive to those of other co-administered drugs with similar actions). Products include:
- Brevibloc Injection 858

Felodipine (Dihydropyridine calcium channel blockers, such as felodipine, are dependent on P4503A4 for metabolism; potential exists for variable slowing of the metabolism of felodipine). Products include:
- Lexxel Tablets 608
- Plendil Extended-Release Tablets ... 623

Fluphenazine Decanoate (Therapeutic serum levels of quinidine inhibit the action of CYP4502D6; this enzyme system is critical for the metabolism of phenothiazines; therefore, caution is advised).
No products indexed under this heading.

Fluphenazine Enanthate (Therapeutic serum levels of quinidine inhibit the action of CYP4502D6; this enzyme system is critical for the metabolism of phenothiazines; therefore, caution is advised).
No products indexed under this heading.

Fluphenazine Hydrochloride (Therapeutic serum levels of quinidine inhibit the action of CYP4502D6; this enzyme system is critical for the metabolism of phenothiazines; therefore, caution is advised).
No products indexed under this heading.

Fosphenytoin Sodium (Co-administration with drugs that induce production of CYP4503A4, such as phenytoin, accelerates hepatic elimination of quinidine). Products include:
- Cerebyx Injection 2619

Glycopyrrolate (Anticholinergic actions of quinidine may be additive to those of other co-administered anticholinergic agents). Products include:
- Robinul Forte Tablets 1358
- Robinul Injectable 2940
- Robinul Tablets 1358

Haloperidol (Co-administration increases serum levels of haloperidol). Products include:
- Haldol Injection, Tablets and Concentrate 2533

Haloperidol Decanoate (Co-administration increases serum levels of haloperidol). Products include:
- Haldol Decanoate 2535

Hydralazine Hydrochloride (Vasodilating actions of quinidine may be additive to those of other co-administered drugs with similar actions).
No products indexed under this heading.

Hydrochlorothiazide (Drugs that alkalinize urine, such as thiazide diuretics, reduce renal elimination of quinidine; following quinidine overdose, drugs that delay elimination of quinidine, such as thiazide diuretics, should be withdrawn). Products include:
- Accuretic Tablets 2614
- Aldoril Tablets 2039
- Atacand HCT Tablets 597
- Avalide Tablets 1070
- Diovan HCT Tablets 2338
- Dyazide Capsules 1515
- HydroDIURIL Tablets 2108
- Hyzaar 2109
- Inderide Tablets 3517
- Inderide LA Long-Acting Capsules .. 3519
- Lotensin HCT Tablets 2367
- Maxzide 1008
- Micardis HCT Tablets 1051
- Microzide Capsules 3414
- Moduretic Tablets 2138
- Monopril HCT 1094
- Prinzide Tablets 2168
- Timolide Tablets 2187
- Uniretic Tablets 3178
- Vaseretic Tablets 2204
- Zestoretic Tablets 695
- Ziac Tablets 1887

Hydrocodone Bitartrate (Therapeutic serum levels of quinidine inhibit the action of CYP4502D6; co-administration of prodrug whose actions are actually mediated by P450IID6, such as codeine and whose analgesic and antitussive effects appear to be mediated by hydromorphone, may cause decrease in the concentrations of hydromorphone (an active metabolite of hydrocodone) resulting in reduced therapeutic effects of hydrocodone). Products include:
- Hycodan 1316
- Hycomine Compound Tablets 1317
- Hycotuss Expectorant Syrup 1318
- Lortab 3319
- Lortab Elixir 3317
- Maxidone Tablets CIII 3399
- Norco 5/325 Tablets CIII 3424
- Norco 7.5/325 Tablets CIII 3425
- Norco 10/325 Tablets CIII 3427
- Norco 10/325 Tablets CIII 3425
- Vicodin Tablets 516
- Vicodin ES Tablets 517
- Vicodin HP Tablets 518
- Vicodin Tuss Expectorant 519
- Vicoprofen Tablets 520
- Zydone Tablets 1330

Hydroflumethiazide (Drugs that alkalinize urine, such as thiazide diuretics, reduce renal elimination of quinidine; following quinidine overdose, drugs that delay elimination of quinidine, such as thiazide diuretics, should be withdrawn). Products include:
- Diucardin Tablets 3494

Hyoscyamine (Anticholinergic actions of quinidine may be additive to those of other co-administered anticholinergic agents). Products include:
- Urised Tablets 2876

Hyoscyamine Sulfate (Anticholinergic actions of quinidine may be additive to those of other co-administered anticholinergic agents). Products include:
- Arco-Lase Plus Tablets 592
- Donnatal 2929
- Donnatal Extentabs 2930
- Levsin/Levsinex/Levbid 3172
- NuLev Orally Disintegrating Tablets 3176
- Prosed/DS Tablets 3268
- Urimax Tablets 1769

Imipramine Hydrochloride (Therapeutic serum levels of quinidine inhibit the action of CYP4502D6; this enzyme system is critical for the metabolism of polycyclic antidepressants; therefore, caution is advised).
No products indexed under this heading.

Imipramine Pamoate (Therapeutic serum levels of quinidine inhibit the action of CYP4502D6; this enzyme system is critical for the metabolism of polycyclic antidepressants; therefore, caution is advised).
No products indexed under this heading.

Ipratropium Bromide (Anticholinergic actions of quinidine may be additive to those of other co-administered anticholinergic agents). Products include:
- Atrovent Inhalation Aerosol 1030
- Atrovent Inhalation Solution 1031
- Atrovent Nasal Spray 0.03% 1032
- Atrovent Nasal Spray 0.06% 1033
- Combivent Inhalation Aerosol 1041
- DuoNeb Inhalation Solution 1233

Ketoconazole (Co-administration may increase quinidine levels through competition for the CYP4503A4 metabolic pathway). Products include:
- Nizoral 2% Cream 3620
- Nizoral A-D Shampoo 2008
- Nizoral 2% Shampoo 2007
- Nizoral Tablets 1791

Labetalol Hydrochloride (Negative inotropic actions of quinidine may be additive to those of other co-administered drugs with similar actions). Products include:
- Normodyne Injection 3135
- Normodyne Tablets 3137

Maprotiline Hydrochloride (Therapeutic serum levels of quinidine inhibit the action of CYP4502D6; this enzyme system is critical for the metabolism of polycyclic antidepressants; therefore, caution is advised).
No products indexed under this heading.

Mepenzolate Bromide (Anticholinergic actions of quinidine may be additive to those of other co-administered anticholinergic agents).
No products indexed under this heading.

Mesoridazine Besylate (Therapeutic serum levels of quinidine inhibit the action of CYP4502D6; this

enzyme system is critical for the metabolism of phenothiazines; therefore, caution is advised). Products include:

Serentil 1057

Methazolamide (Drugs that alkalinize urine, such as carbonic anhydrase inhibitors, reduce renal elimination of quinidine; following quinidine overdose, drugs that delay elimination of quinidine, such as carbonic anhydrase inhibitors, should be withdrawn). Products include:

Neptazane Tablets .... ⊙ 271

Methotrimeprazine (Therapeutic serum levels of quinidine inhibit the action of CYP4502D6; this enzyme system is critical for the metabolism of phenothiazines; therefore, caution is advised).

No products indexed under this heading.

Methyclothiazide (Drugs that alkalinize urine, such as thiazide diuretics, reduce renal elimination of quinidine; following quinidine overdose, drugs that delay elimination of quinidine, such as thiazide diuretics, should be withdrawn).

No products indexed under this heading.

Metocurine Iodide (Quinidine potentiates the action of neuromuscular blocking agents).

No products indexed under this heading.

Metoprolol Tartrate (Negative inotropic actions of quinidine may be additive to those of other co-administered drugs with similar actions).

No products indexed under this heading.

Mexiletine Hydrochloride (Therapeutic serum levels of quinidine inhibit the action of CYP4502D6; this enzyme system is critical for the metabolism of mexiletine; therefore, caution is advised). Products include:

Mexitil Capsules 1047

Minoxidil (Vasodilating actions of quinidine may be additive to those of other co-administered drugs with similar actions). Products include:

Rogaine Extra Strength for Men Topical Solution 721

Rogaine for Women Topical Solution 721

Mivacurium Chloride (Quinidine potentiates the action of neuromuscular blocking agents).

No products indexed under this heading.

Nadolol (Negative inotropic actions of quinidine may be additive to those of other co-administered drugs with similar actions). Products include:

Corgard Tablets 2245

Corzide 40/5 Tablets 2247

Corzide 80/5 Tablets 2247

Nadolol Tablets 2288

Nicardipine Hydrochloride (Dihydropyridine calcium channel blockers, such as nicardipine, are dependent on P4503A4 for metabolism; potential exists for variable slowing of the metabolism of nicardipine). Products include:

Cardene I.V. 3485

Nifedipine (Co-administration decreases quinidine levels very rarely; quinidine causes variable slowing of the metabolism of nifedipine). Products include:

Adalat CC Tablets 877

Procardia Capsules 2708

Procardia XL Extended Release Tablets 2710

Nimodipine (Dihydropyridine calcium channel blockers, such as nimodipine, are dependent on P4503A4 for metabolism; potential exists for variable slowing of the metabolism of nimodipine). Products include:

Nimotop Capsules 904

Nortriptyline Hydrochloride (Therapeutic serum levels of quinidine inhibit the action of CYP4502D6; this enzyme system is critical for the metabolism of polycyclic antidepressants; therefore, caution is advised).

No products indexed under this heading.

Oxybutynin Chloride (Anticholinergic actions of quinidine may be additive to those of other co-administered anticholinergic agents). Products include:

Ditropan XL Extended Release Tablets 564

Pancuronium Bromide (Quinidine potentiates the action of neuromuscular blocking agents).

No products indexed under this heading.

Penbutolol Sulfate (Negative inotropic actions of quinidine may be additive to those of other co-administered drugs with similar actions).

No products indexed under this heading.

Perphenazine (Therapeutic serum levels of quinidine inhibit the action of CYP4502D6; this enzyme system is critical for the metabolism of phenothiazines; therefore, caution is advised). Products include:

Etrafon 3115

Trilafon 3160

Phenobarbital (Co-administration with drugs that induce production of CYP4503A4, such as phenobarbital, accelerates hepatic elimination of quinidine). Products include:

Arco-Lase Plus Tablets 592

Donnatal 2929

Donnatal Extentabs 2930

Phenytoin (Co-administration with drugs that induce production of CYP4503A4, such as phenytoin, accelerates hepatic elimination of quinidine). Products include:

Dilantin Infatabs 2624

Dilantin-125 Oral Suspension 2625

Phenytoin Sodium (Co-administration with drugs that induce production of CYP4503A4, such as phenytoin, accelerates hepatic elimination of quinidine). Products include:

Dilantin Kapseals 2622

Pindolol (Negative inotropic actions of quinidine may be additive to those of other co-administered drugs with similar actions).

No products indexed under this heading.

Polythiazide (Drugs that alkalinize urine, such as thiazide diuretics, reduce renal elimination of quinidine; following quinidine overdose, drugs that delay elimination of quinidine, such as thiazide diuretics, should be withdrawn). Products include:

Minizide Capsules 2700

Renese Tablets 2712

Procainamide Hydrochloride (Increased serum levels of procainamide through competition for pathways of renal clearance). Products include:

Procanbid Extended-Release Tablets 2262

Prochlorperazine (Therapeutic serum levels of quinidine inhibit the action of CYP4502D6; this enzyme system is critical for the metabolism of phenothiazines; therefore, caution is advised). Products include:

Compazine 1505

Procyclidine Hydrochloride (Anticholinergic actions of quinidine may be additive to those of other co-administered anticholinergic agents).

No products indexed under this heading.

Promethazine Hydrochloride (Therapeutic serum levels of quinidine inhibit the action of CYP4502D6; this enzyme system is critical for the metabolism of phenothiazines; therefore, caution is advised). Products include:

Mepergan Injection 3539

Phenergan Injection 3553

Phenergan 3556

Phenergan Syrup 3554

Phenergan with Codeine Syrup 3557

Phenergan with Dextromethorphan Syrup 3559

Phenergan VC Syrup 3560

Phenergan VC with Codeine Syrup 3561

Propantheline Bromide (Anticholinergic actions of quinidine may be additive to those of other co-administered anticholinergic agents).

No products indexed under this heading.

Propranolol Hydrochloride (Co-administration in some studies has resulted in increase in peak serum levels of quinidine, decreases in quinidine's volume of distribution and decrease in total quinidine clearance). Products include:

Inderal 3513

Inderal LA Long-Acting Capsules 3516

Inderide Tablets 3517

Inderide LA Long-Acting Capsules 3519

Protriptyline Hydrochloride (Therapeutic serum levels of quinidine inhibit the action of CYP4502D6; this enzyme system is critical for the metabolism of polycyclic antidepressants; therefore, caution is advised). Products include:

Vivactil Tablets 2446

Vivactil Tablets 2217

Rapacuronium Bromide (Quinidine potentiates the action of neuromuscular blocking agents).

No products indexed under this heading.

Rifampin (Co-administration with drugs that induce production of CYP4503A4, such as rifampin, accelerates hepatic elimination of quinidine). Products include:

Rifadin 765

Rifamate Capsules 767

Rifater Tablets 769

Rocuronium Bromide (Quinidine potentiates the action of neuromuscular blocking agents). Products include:

Zemuron Injection 2491

Scopolamine (Anticholinergic actions of quinidine may be additive to those of other co-administered anticholinergic agents). Products include:

Transderm Scōp Transdermal Therapeutic System 2302

Scopolamine Hydrobromide (Anticholinergic actions of quinidine may be additive to those of other co-administered anticholinergic agents). Products include:

Donnatal 2929

Donnatal Extentabs 2930

Sodium Bicarbonate (Drugs that alkalinize urine, such as systemic sodium bicarbonate, reduce renal elimination of quinidine). Products include:

Alka-Seltzer 603

Alka-Seltzer Lemon Lime Antacid and Pain Reliever Effervescent Tablets 603

Alka-Seltzer Extra Strength Antacid and Pain Reliever Effervescent Tablets 603

Alka-Seltzer Heartburn Relief Tablets 604

Ceo-Two Evacuant Suppository 618

Colyte with Flavor Packs for Oral Solution 3170

GoLYTELY and Pineapple Flavor GoLYTELY for Oral Solution 1068

NuLYTELY, Cherry Flavor, Lemon-Lime Flavor, and Orange Flavor NuLYTELY for Oral Solution 1068

Succinylcholine Chloride (Quinidine potentiates the action of neuromuscular blocking agents). Products include:

Anectine Injection 1476

Thioridazine Hydrochloride (Therapeutic serum levels of quinidine inhibit the action of CYP4502D6; this enzyme system is critical for the metabolism of phenothiazines; therefore, caution is advised). Products include:

Thioridazine Hydrochloride Tablets 2289

Timolol Maleate (Negative inotropic actions of quinidine may be additive to those of other co-administered drugs with similar actions). Products include:

Blocadren Tablets 2046

Cosopt Sterile Ophthalmic Solution 2065

Timolide Tablets 2187

Timolol GFS .... ⊙ 266

Timoptic in Ocudose 2192

Timoptic Sterile Ophthalmic Solution 2190

Timoptic-XE Sterile Ophthalmic Gel Forming Solution 2194

Tolterodine Tartrate (Anticholinergic actions of quinidine may be additive to those of other co-administered anticholinergic agents). Products include:

Detrol Tablets 3623

Detrol LA Capsules 2801

Tridihexethyl Chloride (Anticholinergic actions of quinidine may be additive to those of other co-administered anticholinergic agents).

No products indexed under this heading.

Trifluoperazine Hydrochloride (Therapeutic serum levels of quinidine inhibit the action of CYP4502D6; this enzyme system is critical for the metabolism of phenothiazines; therefore, caution is advised). Products include:

Stelazine 1640

Trihexyphenidyl Hydrochloride (Anticholinergic actions of quinidine may be additive to those of other co-administered anticholinergic agents). Products include:

Artane 1855

Trimipramine Maleate (Therapeutic serum levels of quinidine inhibit the action of CYP4502D6; this enzyme system is critical for the metabolism of polycyclic antidepressants; therefore, caution is advised). Products include:

Surmontil Capsules 3595

Vecuronium Bromide (Quinidine potentiates the action of neuromuscular blocking agents). Products include:

Norcuron for Injection 2478

Verapamil Hydrochloride (Hepatic clearance of quinidine is significantly reduced during co-administration of verapamil with corresponding increases in serum levels and half-life; hypotension attributable to additive peripheral alpha-blockade has been reported with combined therapy). Products include:

Covera-HS Tablets 3199

Isoptin SR Tablets 467

Tarka Tablets 508

Verelan Capsules 3184

Verelan PM Capsules 3186

Warfarin Sodium (Quinidine potentiates the anticoagulatory action of warfarin). Products include:

Coumadin for Injection 1243

Coumadin Tablets 1243

Warfarin Sodium Tablets, USP 3302

Food Interactions

Food, unspecified (Peak serum quinidine levels obtained from immediate-release quinidine sulfate are known to be delayed by nearly an hour without change in total absorption when these products are taken with food).

QUIXIN OPHTHALMIC SOLUTION

(Levofloxacin) 3093

May interact with theophylline and certain other agents. Compounds in these categories include:

Aminophylline (Systemic administration of some quinolones has been shown to elevate plasma concentrations of theophylline).
No products indexed under this heading.

Caffeine (Systemic administration of some quinolones has been shown to interfere with the metabolism of caffeine). Products include:
- BC Powder ..... ▣619
- Arthritis Strength BC Powder ..... ▣619
- Darvon Compound-65 Pulvules 1910
- Aspirin Free Excedrin Caplets and Geltabs ..... ▣628
- Excedrin Extra-Strength Tablets, Caplets, and Geltabs ..... ▣629
- Excedrin Migraine 1070
- Goody's Extra Strength Headache Powder ..... ▣620
- Goody's Extra Strength Pain Relief Tablets ..... ▣620
- Hycomine Compound Tablets 1317
- Maximum Strength Midol Menstrual Caplets and Gelcaps ..... ▣612
- Vanquish Caplets ..... ▣617
- Vivarin ..... ▣763

Caffeine Citrate (Systemic administration of some quinolones has been shown to interfere with the metabolism of caffeine). Products include:
- Cafcit 1035

Cyclosporine (Systemic administration of some quinolones has been associated with transient elevations of serum creatinine in patients receiving systemic cyclosporine concomitantly). Products include:
- Gengraf Capsules 457
- Neoral Soft Gelatin Capsules 2380
- Neoral Oral Solution 2380
- Sandimmune 2388

Dyphylline (Systemic administration of some quinolones has been shown to elevate plasma concentrations of theophylline). Products include:
- Lufyllin Tablets 3347
- Lufyllin-400 Tablets 3347
- Lufyllin-GG Elixir 3348
- Lufyllin-GG Tablets 3348

Theophylline (Systemic administration of some quinolones has been shown to elevate plasma concentrations of theophylline). Products include:
- Aerolate 1361
- Theo-Dur Extended-Release Tablets 1835
- Uni-Dur Extended-Release Tablets 1841
- Uniphyl 400 mg and 600 mg Tablets 2903

Theophylline Calcium Salicylate (Systemic administration of some quinolones has been shown to elevate plasma concentrations of theophylline).
No products indexed under this heading.

Theophylline Sodium Glycinate (Systemic administration of some quinolones has been shown to elevate plasma concentrations of theophylline).
No products indexed under this heading.

Warfarin Sodium (Systemic administration of some quinolones has been shown to enhance the effects of the oral anticoagulant warfarin). Products include:
- Coumadin for Injection 1243
- Coumadin Tablets 1243
- Warfarin Sodium Tablets, USP 3302

QVAR INHALATION AEROSOL

(Beclomethasone Dipropionate) 1987

None cited in PDR database.

RABIES VACCINE RABAVERT

(Rabies Vaccine) 1203

May interact with antimalarials, corticosteroids, immunosuppressive agents, and certain other agents. Compounds in these categories include:

Azathioprine (Immunosuppressive agents can interfere with the development of active immunity after vaccination, and may diminish the protective efficacy of the vaccine).
No products indexed under this heading.

Basiliximab (Immunosuppressive agents can interfere with the development of active immunity after vaccination, and may diminish the protective efficacy of the vaccine). Products include:
- Simulect for Injection 2399

Betamethasone Acetate (Corticosteroids can interfere with the development of active immunity after vaccination, and may diminish the protective efficacy of the vaccine). Products include:
- Celestone Soluspan Injectable Suspension 3097

Betamethasone Sodium Phosphate (Corticosteroids can interfere with the development of active immunity after vaccination, and may diminish the protective efficacy of the vaccine). Products include:
- Celestone Soluspan Injectable Suspension 3097

Chloroquine Hydrochloride (Antimalarials can interfere with the development of active immunity after vaccination, and may diminish the protective efficacy of the vaccine).
No products indexed under this heading.

Chloroquine Phosphate (Antimalarials can interfere with the development of active immunity after vaccination, and may diminish the protective efficacy of the vaccine). Products include:
- Aralen Tablets 3075

Cortisone Acetate (Corticosteroids can interfere with the development of active immunity after vaccination, and may diminish the protective efficacy of the vaccine). Products include:
- Cortone Acetate Injectable Suspension 2059
- Cortone Acetate Tablets 2061

Cyclosporine (Immunosuppressive agents can interfere with the development of active immunity after vaccination, and may diminish the protective efficacy of the vaccine). Products include:
- Gengraf Capsules 457
- Neoral Soft Gelatin Capsules 2380
- Neoral Oral Solution 2380
- Sandimmune 2388

Dexamethasone (Corticosteroids can interfere with the development of active immunity after vaccination, and may diminish the protective efficacy of the vaccine). Products include:
- Decadron Elixir 2078
- Decadron Tablets 2079
- TobraDex Ophthalmic Ointment 542
- TobraDex Ophthalmic Suspension 541

Dexamethasone Acetate (Corticosteroids can interfere with the development of active immunity after vaccination, and may diminish the protective efficacy of the vaccine).
No products indexed under this heading.

Dexamethasone Sodium Phosphate (Corticosteroids can interfere with the development of active immunity after vaccination, and may diminish the protective efficacy of the vaccine). Products include:
- Decadron Phosphate Injection 2081
- Decadron Phosphate Sterile Ophthalmic Ointment 2083
- Decadron Phosphate Sterile Ophthalmic Solution 2084
- NeoDecadron Sterile Ophthalmic Solution 2144

Fludrocortisone Acetate (Corticosteroids can interfere with the development of active immunity after vaccination, and may diminish the protective efficacy of the vaccine). Products include:
- Florinef Acetate Tablets 2250

Hydrocortisone (Corticosteroids can interfere with the development of active immunity after vaccination, and may diminish the protective efficacy of the vaccine). Products include:
- Anusol-HC Cream 2.5% 2237
- Cipro HC Otic Suspension 540
- Cortaid Intensive Therapy Cream ..... ▣717
- Cortaid Maximum Strength Cream ..... ▣717
- Cortisporin Ophthalmic Suspension Sterile ..... ⊙297
- Cortizone•5 ..... ▣699
- Cortizone•10 ..... ▣699
- Cortizone•10 Plus Creme ..... ▣700
- Cortizone for Kids Creme ..... ▣699
- Hydrocortone Tablets 2106
- Massengill Medicated Soft Cloth Towelette ..... ▣753
- VōSoL HC Otic Solution 3356

Hydrocortisone Acetate (Corticosteroids can interfere with the development of active immunity after vaccination, and may diminish the protective efficacy of the vaccine). Products include:
- Analpram-HC 1338
- Anusol HC-1 Hydrocortisone Anti-Itch Cream ..... ▣689
- Anusol-HC Suppositories 2238
- Cortaid ..... ▣717
- Cortifoam Rectal Foam 3170
- Cortisporin-TC Otic Suspension 2246
- Hydrocortone Acetate Injectable Suspension 2103
- Pramosone 1343
- Proctocort Suppositories 2264
- ProctoFoam-HC 3177
- Terra-Cortril Ophthalmic Suspension 2716

Hydrocortisone Sodium Phosphate (Corticosteroids can interfere with the development of active immunity after vaccination, and may diminish the protective efficacy of the vaccine). Products include:
- Hydrocortone Phosphate Injection, Sterile 2105

Hydrocortisone Sodium Succinate (Corticosteroids can interfere with the development of active immunity after vaccination, and may diminish the protective efficacy of the vaccine).
No products indexed under this heading.

Mefloquine Hydrochloride (Antimalarials can interfere with the development of active immunity after vaccination, and may diminish the protective efficacy of the vaccine). Products include:
- Lariam Tablets 2989

Methylprednisolone Acetate (Corticosteroids can interfere with the development of active immunity after vaccination, and may diminish the protective efficacy of the vaccine). Products include:
- Depo-Medrol Injectable Suspension 2795

Methylprednisolone Sodium Succinate (Corticosteroids can interfere with the development of active immunity after vaccination, and may diminish the protective efficacy of the vaccine). Products include:
- Solu-Medrol Sterile Powder 2855

Muromonab-CD3 (Immunosuppressive agents can interfere with the development of active immunity after vaccination, and may diminish the protective efficacy of the vaccine). Products include:
- Orthoclone OKT3 Sterile Solution 2498

Mycophenolate Mofetil (Immunosuppressive agents can interfere with the development of active immunity after vaccination, and may diminish the protective efficacy of the vaccine). Products include:
- CellCept Capsules 2951
- CellCept Oral Suspension 2951
- CellCept Tablets 2951

Prednisolone Acetate (Corticosteroids can interfere with the development of active immunity after vaccination, and may diminish the protective efficacy of the vaccine). Products include:
- Blephamide Ophthalmic Ointment 547
- Blephamide Ophthalmic Suspension 548
- Poly-Pred Liquifilm Ophthalmic Suspension ..... ⊙245
- Pred Forte Ophthalmic Suspension ..... ⊙246
- Pred Mild Sterile Ophthalmic Suspension ..... ⊙249
- Pred-G Ophthalmic Suspension ..... ⊙247
- Pred-G Sterile Ophthalmic Ointment ..... ⊙248

Prednisolone Sodium Phosphate (Corticosteroids can interfere with the development of active immunity after vaccination, and may diminish the protective efficacy of the vaccine). Products include:
- Pediapred Oral Solution 1170

Prednisolone Tebutate (Corticosteroids can interfere with the development of active immunity after vaccination, and may diminish the protective efficacy of the vaccine).
No products indexed under this heading.

Prednisone (Corticosteroids can interfere with the development of active immunity after vaccination, and may diminish the protective efficacy of the vaccine). Products include:
- Prednisone 3064

Pyrimethamine (Antimalarials can interfere with the development of active immunity after vaccination, and may diminish the protective efficacy of the vaccine). Products include:
- Daraprim Tablets 1511

Rabies Immune Globulin (Human) (Must not be administered at more than the recommended dose, since the response to active immunization may be impaired). Products include:
- BayRab 917
- Imogam Rabies - HT 805

Sirolimus (Immunosuppressive agents can interfere with the development of active immunity after vaccination, and may diminish the protective efficacy of the vaccine). Products include:
- Rapamune Oral Solution and Tablets 3584

Tacrolimus (Immunosuppressive agents can interfere with the development of active immunity after vaccination, and may diminish the protective efficacy of the vaccine). Products include:
- Prograf 1393
- Protopic Ointment 1397

Triamcinolone (Corticosteroids can interfere with the development of active immunity after vaccination, and may diminish the protective efficacy of the vaccine).
No products indexed under this heading.

Triamcinolone Acetonide (Corticosteroids can interfere with the development of active immunity after vaccination, and may diminish the protective efficacy of the vaccine). Products include:
- Azmacort Inhalation Aerosol 728
- Nasacort Nasal Inhaler 750
- Nasacort AQ Nasal Spray 752
- Tri-Nasal Spray 2274

Triamcinolone Diacetate (Corticosteroids can interfere with the development of active immunity after vaccination, and may diminish the protective efficacy of the vaccine).

No products indexed under this heading.

Triamcinolone Hexacetonide (Corticosteroids can interfere with the development of active immunity after vaccination, and may diminish the protective efficacy of the vaccine).

No products indexed under this heading.

RAPAMUNE ORAL SOLUTION AND TABLETS

(Sirolimus) 3584

May interact with erythromycin, HMG-CoA reductase inhibitors, phenytoin, and certain other agents. Compounds in these categories include:

Atorvastatin Calcium (Co-administration of Rapamune with cyclosporine in conjunction with an HMG-CoA reductase inhibitor should be monitored for the development of rhabdomyolysis). Products include:

Lipitor Tablets 2639
Lipitor Tablets 2696

Bromocriptine Mesylate (Sirolimus is extensively metabolized by the CYP3A4 isoenzyme; co-administration with inhibitors of CYP3A4, such as bromocriptine, may decrease the metabolism of sirolimus and increase the plasma levels of sirolimus).

No products indexed under this heading.

Carbamazepine (Sirolimus is extensively metabolized by the CYP3A4 isoenzyme; co-administration with inducers of CYP3A4, such as carbamazepine, may increase the metabolism of sirolimus and decrease the plasma levels of sirolimus). Products include:

Carbatrol Capsules 3234
Tegretol/Tegretol-XR 2404

Cerivastatin Sodium (Co-administration of Rapamune with cyclosporine in conjunction with an HMG-CoA reductase inhibitor should be monitored for the development of rhabdomyolysis). Products include:

Baycol Tablets 883

Cimetidine (Sirolimus is extensively metabolized by the CYP3A4 isoenzyme; co-administration with inhibitors of CYP3A4, such as cimetidine, may decrease the metabolism of sirolimus and increase the plasma levels of sirolimus). Products include:

Tagamet HB 200 Suspension 762
Tagamet HB 200 Tablets 761
Tagamet Tablets 1644

Cimetidine Hydrochloride (Sirolimus is extensively metabolized by the CYP3A4 isoenzyme; co-administration with inhibitors of CYP3A4, such as cimetidine, may decrease the metabolism of sirolimus and increase the plasma levels of sirolimus). Products include:

Tagamet 1644

Cisapride (Sirolimus is extensively metabolized by the CYP3A4 isoenzyme; co-administration with inhibitors of CYP3A4, such as cisapride, may decrease the metabolism of sirolimus and increase the plasma levels of sirolimus).

No products indexed under this heading.

Clarithromycin (Sirolimus is extensively metabolized by the CYP3A4 isoenzyme; co-administration with inhibitors of CYP3A4, such as clarithromycin, may decrease the metabolism of sirolimus and increase the plasma levels of sirolimus). Products include:

Biaxin/Biaxin XL 403
PREVPAC 3298

Cyclosporine (Co-administration of sirolimus simultaneously with cyclosporine capsules modified results in increased mean AUC and Cmax (116% and 230% respectively) relative to sirolimus alone; when given 4 hours apart, Cmax and AUC were increased by 37% and 80% respectively compared to sirolimus alone; because of the effect of cyclosporine capsules modified, it is recommended that sirolimus should be taken 4 hours after cyclosporine oral solution modified and/or cyclosporine capsules modified). Products include:

Gengraf Capsules 457
Neoral Soft Gelatin Capsules 2380
Neoral Oral Solution 2380
Sandimmune 2388

Danazol (Sirolimus is extensively metabolized by the CYP3A4 isoenzyme; co-administration with inhibitors of CYP3A4, such as danazol, may decrease the metabolism of sirolimus and increase the plasma levels of sirolimus).

No products indexed under this heading.

Diltiazem Hydrochloride (Co-administration in healthy individuals significantly affects the bioavailability of sirolimus; monitor sirolimus levels and dose adjustment may be necessary). Products include:

Cardizem Injectable 1018
Cardizem Lyo-Ject Syringe 1018
Cardizem Monovial 1018
Cardizem CD Capsules 1016
Tiazac Capsules 1378

Erythromycin (Sirolimus is extensively metabolized by the CYP3A4 isoenzyme; co-administration with inhibitors of CYP3A4, such as erythromycin, may decrease the metabolism of sirolimus and increase the plasma levels of sirolimus). Products include:

Emgel 2% Topical Gel 1285
Ery-Tab Tablets 448
Erythromycin Base Filmtab Tablets . 454
Erythromycin Delayed-Release Capsules, USP 455
PCE Dispertab Tablets 498

Erythromycin Estolate (Sirolimus is extensively metabolized by the CYP3A4 isoenzyme; co-administration with inhibitors of CYP3A4, such as erythromycin, may decrease the metabolism of sirolimus and increase the plasma levels of sirolimus).

No products indexed under this heading.

Erythromycin Ethylsuccinate (Sirolimus is extensively metabolized by the CYP3A4 isoenzyme; co-administration with inhibitors of CYP3A4, such as erythromycin, may decrease the metabolism of sirolimus and increase the plasma levels of sirolimus). Products include:

E.E.S. 450
EryPed 446
Pediazole Suspension 3050

Erythromycin Gluceptate (Sirolimus is extensively metabolized by the CYP3A4 isoenzyme; co-administration with inhibitors of CYP3A4, such as erythromycin, may decrease the metabolism of sirolimus and increase the plasma levels of sirolimus).

No products indexed under this heading.

Erythromycin Stearate (Sirolimus is extensively metabolized by the CYP3A4 isoenzyme; co-administration with inhibitors of CYP3A4, such as erythromycin, may decrease the metabolism of sirolimus and increase the plasma levels of sirolimus). Products include:

Erythrocin Stearate Filmtab Tablets 452

Fluconazole (Sirolimus is extensively metabolized by the CYP3A4 isoenzyme; co-administration with inhibitors of CYP3A4, such as fluconazole, may decrease the metabolism of sirolimus and increase the plasma levels of sirolimus). Products include:

Diflucan Tablets, Injection, and Oral Suspension 2681

Fluvastatin Sodium (Co-administration of Rapamune with cyclosporine in conjunction with an HMG-CoA reductase inhibitor should be monitored for the development of rhabdomyolysis). Products include:

Lescol Capsules 2361
Lescol 2925
Lescol XL Tablets 2361

Fosphenytoin Sodium (Sirolimus is extensively metabolized by the CYP3A4 isoenzyme; co-administration with inducers of CYP3A4, such as phenytoin, may increase the metabolism of sirolimus and decrease the plasma levels of sirolimus). Products include:

Cerebyx Injection 2619

Indinavir Sulfate (Sirolimus is extensively metabolized by the CYP3A4 isoenzyme; co-administration with inhibitors of CYP3A4, such as indinavir, may decrease the metabolism of sirolimus and increase the plasma levels of sirolimus). Products include:

Crixivan Capsules 2070

Itraconazole (Sirolimus is extensively metabolized by the CYP3A4 isoenzyme; co-administration with inhibitors of CYP3A4, such as itraconazole, may decrease the metabolism of sirolimus and increase the plasma levels of sirolimus). Products include:

Sporanox Capsules 1800
Sporanox Injection 1804
Sporanox Injection 2509
Sporanox Oral Solution 1808
Sporanox Oral Solution 2512

Ketoconazole (Multiple-dose ketoconazole administration significantly affected the rate and extent of absorption and sirolimus exposure; sirolimus should not be co-administered with ketoconazole). Products include:

Nizoral 2% Cream 3620
Nizoral A-D Shampoo 2008
Nizoral 2% Shampoo 2007
Nizoral Tablets 1791

Lovastatin (Co-administration of Rapamune with cyclosporine in conjunction with an HMG-CoA reductase inhibitor should be monitored for the development of rhabdomyolysis). Products include:

Mevacor Tablets 2132

Metoclopramide Hydrochloride (Sirolimus is extensively metabolized by the CYP3A4 isoenzyme; co-administration with inhibitors of CYP3A4, such as metoclopramide, may decrease the metabolism of sirolimus and increase the plasma levels of sirolimus). Products include:

Reglan 2935

Nicardipine Hydrochloride (Sirolimus is extensively metabolized by the CYP3A4 isoenzyme; co-administration with inhibitors of CYP3A4, such as nicardipine, may decrease the metabolism of sirolimus and increase the plasma levels of sirolimus). Products include:

Cardene I.V. 3485

Phenobarbital (Sirolimus is extensively metabolized by the CYP3A4 isoenzyme; co-administration with inducers of CYP3A4, such as phenobarbital, may increase the metabolism of sirolimus and decrease the plasma levels of sirolimus). Products include:

Arco-Lase Plus Tablets 592
Donnatal 2929
Donnatal Extentabs 2930

Phenytoin (Sirolimus is extensively metabolized by the CYP3A4 isoenzyme; co-administration with inducers of CYP3A4, such as phenytoin, may increase the metabolism of sirolimus and decrease the plasma levels of sirolimus). Products include:

Dilantin Infatabs 2624
Dilantin-125 Oral Suspension 2625

Phenytoin Sodium (Sirolimus is extensively metabolized by the CYP3A4 isoenzyme; co-administration with inducers of CYP3A4, such as phenytoin, may increase the metabolism of sirolimus and decrease the plasma levels of sirolimus). Products include:

Dilantin Kapseals 2622

Pravastatin Sodium (Co-administration of Rapamune with cyclosporine in conjunction with an HMG-CoA reductase inhibitor should be monitored for the development of rhabdomyolysis). Products include:

Pravachol Tablets 1099

Rifabutin (Sirolimus is extensively metabolized by the CYP3A4 isoenzyme; co-administration with inducers of CYP3A4, such as rifabutin, may increase the metabolism of sirolimus and decrease the plasma levels of sirolimus). Products include:

Mycobutin Capsules 2838

Rifampin (Pretreatment with multiple doses of rifampin greatly increased sirolimus oral dose clearance resulting in mean decrease in AUC and Cmax; alternative therapeutic agents with less enzyme induction potential than rifampin should be considered). Products include:

Rifadin 765
Rifamate Capsules 767
Rifater Tablets 769

Rifapentine (Sirolimus is extensively metabolized by the CYP3A4 isoenzyme; co-administration with inducers of CYP3A4, such as rifapentine, may increase the metabolism of sirolimus and decrease the plasma levels of sirolimus). Products include:

Priftin Tablets 758

Ritonavir (Sirolimus is extensively metabolized by the CYP3A4 isoenzyme; co-administration with inhibitors of CYP3A4, such as ritonavir, may decrease the metabolism of sirolimus and increase the plasma levels of sirolimus). Products include:

Kaletra Capsules 471
Kaletra Oral Solution 471
Norvir Capsules 487
Norvir Oral Solution 487

Simvastatin (Co-administration of Rapamune with cyclosporine in conjunction with an HMG-CoA reductase inhibitor should be monitored for the development of rhabdomyolysis). Products include:

Zocor Tablets 2219

Troleandomycin (Sirolimus is extensively metabolized by the CYP3A4 isoenzyme; co-administration with inhibitors of CYP3A4, such as troleandomycin, may decrease the metabolism of sirolimus and increase the plasma levels of sirolimus). Products include:

Tao Capsules 2716

Verapamil Hydrochloride (Sirolimus is extensively metabolized by the CYP3A4 isoenzyme; co-administration with inhibitors of CYP3A4, such as verapamil, may

decrease the metabolism of sirolimus and increase the plasma levels of sirolimus). Products include:

- Covera-HS Tablets ... 3199
- Isoptin SR Tablets ... 467
- Tarka Tablets ... 508
- Verelan Capsules ... 3184
- Verelan PM Capsules ... 3186

Food Interactions

Food, unspecified (A fat breakfast altered the bioavailability characteristics of sirolimus compared to fasting; 34% decrease in the peak blood sirolimus concentration, a 3.5 fold increase in the time-to-peak concentration and 35% increase in total exposure; to minimize variability, Rapamune should be taken consistently with or without food).

Grapefruit Juice (Induces CYP3A4-mediated metabolism of sirolimus; Rapamune must not be administered or diluted with grapefruit juice).

REBETRON COMBINATION THERAPY

(Interferon alfa-2B, Recombinant, Ribavirin) ... 3153

May interact with:

Magnesium Hydroxide (Coadministration with an antacid containing magnesium, aluminum, and simethicone resulted in a 14% decrease in ribavirin AUC; the clinical relevance of results from this single-dose study is unknown). Products include:

- Ex•Lax Milk of Magnesia Liquid ... ■670
- Maalox Antacid/Anti-Gas Oral Suspension ... ■673
- Maalox Max Maximum Strength Antacid/Anti-Gas Liquid ... 2300
- Maalox Regular Strength Antacid/Antigas Liquid ... 2300
- Mylanta Fast-Acting ... 1813
- Mylanta ... 1813
- Pepcid Complete Chewable Tablets ... 1815
- Phillips' Chewable Tablets ... ■615
- Phillips' Milk of Magnesia Liquid (Original, Cherry, & Mint) ... ■616
- Rolaids Tablets ... ■706
- Extra Strength Rolaids Tablets ... ■706
- Vanquish Caplets ... ■617

Food Interactions

Food, unspecified (Both AUC and Cmax increased by 70% when Rebetrol Capsules were administered with a high-fat meal in a single-dose pharmacokinetic study; there are insufficient data to address the clinical relevance of these results).

RECOMBINATE

(Antihemophilic Factor (Recombinant)) ... 853

None cited in PDR database.

RECOMBIVAX HB

(Hepatitis B Vaccine, Recombinant) ... 2178

None cited in PDR database.

REFACTO VIALS

(Antihemophilic Factor (Recombinant)) ... 1437

None cited in PDR database.

REFLUDAN FOR INJECTION

(Lepirudin) ... 761

May interact with oral anticoagulants, non-steroidal anti-inflammatory agents, thrombolytics, and certain other agents. Compounds in these categories include:

Alteplase, Recombinant (Concomitant therapy with thrombolytics may increase the risk of bleeding complications and considerably enhance the effect of Refludan on aPTT prolongation). Products include:

- Activase I.V. ... 1410
- Cathflo Activase ... 3611

Anistreplase (Concomitant therapy with thrombolytics may increase the risk of bleeding complications and considerably enhance the effect of Refludan on aPTT prolongation).

No products indexed under this heading.

Aspirin (Concomitant therapy with drugs that affect platelet function, such as aspirin, may increase the risk of bleeding). Products include:

- Aggrenox Capsules ... 1026
- Alka-Seltzer ... ■603
- Alka-Seltzer Lemon Lime Antacid and Pain Reliever Effervescent Tablets ... ■603
- Alka-Seltzer Extra Strength Antacid and Pain Reliever Effervescent Tablets ... ■603
- Alka-Seltzer PM Effervescent Tablets ... ■605
- Genuine Bayer Tablets, Caplets and Gelcaps ... ■606
- Extra Strength Bayer Caplets and Gelcaps ... ■610
- Aspirin Regimen Bayer Children's Chewable Tablets (Orange or Cherry Flavored) ... ■607
- Bayer, Aspirin Regimen ... ■606
- Aspirin Regimen Bayer 81 mg Caplets with Calcium ... ■607
- Genuine Bayer Professional Labeling (Aspirin Regimen Bayer) ... ■608
- Extra Strength Bayer Arthritis Caplets ... ■610
- Extra Strength Bayer Plus Caplets ... ■610
- Extra Strength Bayer PM Caplets ... ■611
- BC Powder ... ■619
- BC Allergy Sinus Cold Powder ... ■619
- Arthritis Strength BC Powder ... ■619
- BC Sinus Cold Powder ... ■619
- Darvon Compound-65 Pulvules ... 1910
- Ecotrin Enteric Coated Aspirin Low, Regular and Maximum Strength Tablets ... 1715
- Excedrin Extra-Strength Tablets, Caplets, and Geltabs ... ■629
- Excedrin Migraine ... 1070
- Goody's Body Pain Formula Powder ... ■620
- Goody's Extra Strength Headache Powder ... ■620
- Goody's Extra Strength Pain Relief Tablets ... ■620
- Percodan Tablets ... 1327
- Robaxisal Tablets ... 2939
- Soma Compound Tablets ... 3354
- Soma Compound w/Codeine Tablets ... 3355
- Vanquish Caplets ... ■617

Celecoxib (Concomitant therapy with drugs that affect platelet function, such as non-steroid anti-inflammatory agents, may increase the risk of bleeding). Products include:

- Celebrex Capsules ... 2676
- Celebrex Capsules ... 2780

Clopidogrel Bisulfate (Concomitant therapy with drugs that affect platelet function, such as clopidogrel, may increase the risk of bleeding). Products include:

- Plavix Tablets ... 1097
- Plavix Tablets ... 3084

Diclofenac Potassium (Concomitant therapy with drugs that affect platelet function, such as non-steroid anti-inflammatory agents, may increase the risk of bleeding). Products include:

- Cataflam Tablets ... 2315

Diclofenac Sodium (Concomitant therapy with drugs that affect platelet function, such as non-steroid anti-inflammatory agents, may increase the risk of bleeding). Products include:

- Arthrotec Tablets ... 3195
- Voltaren Ophthalmic Sterile Ophthalmic Solution ... ⊙312
- Voltaren Tablets ... 2315
- Voltaren-XR Tablets ... 2315

Dicumarol (Concomitant therapy with oral anticoagulants may increase the risk of bleeding).

No products indexed under this heading.

Dipyridamole (Concomitant therapy with drugs that affect platelet function, such as dipyridamole, may increase the risk of bleeding). Products include:

- Aggrenox Capsules ... 1026
- Persantine Tablets ... 1057

Etodolac (Concomitant therapy with drugs that affect platelet function, such as non-steroid anti-inflammatory agents, may increase the risk of bleeding). Products include:

- Lodine ... 3528
- Lodine XL Extended-Release Tablets ... 3530

Fenoprofen Calcium (Concomitant therapy with drugs that affect platelet function, such as non-steroid anti-inflammatory agents, may increase the risk of bleeding).

No products indexed under this heading.

Flurbiprofen (Concomitant therapy with drugs that affect platelet function, such as non-steroid anti-inflammatory agents, may increase the risk of bleeding).

No products indexed under this heading.

Ibuprofen (Concomitant therapy with drugs that affect platelet function, such as non-steroid anti-inflammatory agents, may increase the risk of bleeding). Products include:

- Advil ... ■771
- Children's Advil Oral Suspension ... ■773
- Children's Advil Chewable Tablets ... ■773
- Advil Cold and Sinus Caplets ... ■771
- Advil Cold and Sinus Tablets ... ■771
- Advil Flu & Body Ache Caplets ... ■772
- Infants' Advil Drops ... ■773
- Junior Strength Advil Tablets ... ■773
- Junior Strength Advil Chewable Tablets ... ■773
- Advil Migraine Liquigels ... ■772
- Children's Motrin Oral Suspension and Chewable Tablets ... 2006
- Children's Motrin Cold Oral Suspension ... 2007
- Children's Motrin Oral Suspension ... ■643
- Motrin Suspension, Oral Drops, Chewable Tablets, and Caplets ... 2002
- Infants' Motrin Concentrated Drops ... 2006
- Junior Strength Motrin Caplets and Chewable Tablets ... 2006
- Motrin IB Tablets, Caplets, and Gelcaps ... 2002
- Motrin Migraine Pain Caplets ... 2005
- Motrin Sinus Headache Caplets ... 2005
- Vicoprofen Tablets ... 520

Indomethacin (Concomitant therapy with drugs that affect platelet function, such as non-steroid anti-inflammatory agents, may increase the risk of bleeding). Products include:

- Indocin ... 2112

Indomethacin Sodium Trihydrate (Concomitant therapy with drugs that affect platelet function, such as non-steroid anti-inflammatory agents, may increase the risk of bleeding). Products include:

- Indocin I.V. ... 2115

Ketoprofen (Concomitant therapy with drugs that affect platelet function, such as non-steroid anti-inflammatory agents, may increase the risk of bleeding). Products include:

- Orudis Capsules ... 3548
- Orudis KT Tablets ... ■778
- Oruvail Capsules ... 3548

Ketorolac Tromethamine (Concomitant therapy with drugs that affect platelet function, such as non-steroid anti-inflammatory agents, may increase the risk of bleeding). Products include:

- Acular Ophthalmic Solution ... 544
- Acular PF Ophthalmic Solution ... 544
- Toradol ... 3018

Meclofenamate Sodium (Concomitant therapy with drugs that affect platelet function, such as non-steroid anti-inflammatory agents, may increase the risk of bleeding).

No products indexed under this heading.

Mefenamic Acid (Concomitant therapy with drugs that affect platelet function, such as non-steroid anti-inflammatory agents, may increase the risk of bleeding). Products include:

- Ponstel Capsules ... 1356

Meloxicam (Concomitant therapy with drugs that affect platelet function, such as non-steroid anti-inflammatory agents, may increase the risk of bleeding). Products include:

- Mobic Tablets ... 1054

Nabumetone (Concomitant therapy with drugs that affect platelet function, such as non-steroid anti-inflammatory agents, may increase the risk of bleeding). Products include:

- Relafen Tablets ... 1617

Naproxen (Concomitant therapy with drugs that affect platelet function, such as non-steroid anti-inflammatory agents, may increase the risk of bleeding). Products include:

- EC-Naprosyn Delayed-Release Tablets ... 2967
- Naprosyn Suspension ... 2967
- Naprosyn Tablets ... 2967

Naproxen Sodium (Concomitant therapy with drugs that affect platelet function, such as non-steroid anti-inflammatory agents, may increase the risk of bleeding). Products include:

- Aleve Tablets, Caplets and Gelcaps ... ■602
- Aleve Cold & Sinus Caplets ... ■603
- Anaprox Tablets ... 2967
- Anaprox DS Tablets ... 2967
- Naprelan Tablets ... 1293

Oxaprozin (Concomitant therapy with drugs that affect platelet function, such as non-steroid anti-inflammatory agents, may increase the risk of bleeding).

No products indexed under this heading.

Phenylbutazone (Concomitant therapy with drugs that affect platelet function, such as non-steroid anti-inflammatory agents, may increase the risk of bleeding).

No products indexed under this heading.

Piroxicam (Concomitant therapy with drugs that affect platelet function, such as non-steroid anti-inflammatory agents, may increase the risk of bleeding). Products include:

- Feldene Capsules ... 2685

Reteplase (Concomitant therapy with thrombolytics may increase the risk of bleeding complications and considerably enhance the effect of Refludan on aPTT prolongation). Products include:

- Retavase Vials ... 1182

Rofecoxib (Concomitant therapy with drugs that affect platelet function, such as non-steroid anti-inflammatory agents, may increase the risk of bleeding). Products include:

- Vioxx ... 2213

Streptokinase (Concomitant therapy with thrombolytics may increase the risk of bleeding complications and considerably enhance the effect of Refludan on aPTT prolongation). Products include:

- Streptase for Infusion ... 647

Sulindac (Concomitant therapy with drugs that affect platelet function, such as non-steroid anti-inflammatory agents, may increase the risk of bleeding). Products include:

- Clinoril Tablets ... 2053

Tolmetin Sodium (Concomitant therapy with drugs that affect platelet function, such as non-steroid anti-inflammatory agents, may increase the risk of bleeding). Products include:

- Tolectin ... 2589

Urokinase (Concomitant therapy with thrombolytics may increase the

risk of bleeding complications and considerably enhance the effect of Refludan on aPTT prolongation).
No products indexed under this heading.

Warfarin Sodium (Concomitant therapy with oral anticoagulants may increase the risk of bleeding). Products include:
Coumadin for Injection 1243
Coumadin Tablets 1243
Warfarin Sodium Tablets, USP 3302

REFRESH P.M. LUBRICANT EYE OINTMENT
(Mineral Oil, Petrolatum, White) .... ⊙251
None cited in PDR database.

REFRESH PLUS LUBRICANT EYE DROPS
(Carboxymethylcellulose Sodium) .... ⊙251
None cited in PDR database.

REFRESH TEARS LUBRICANT EYE DROPS
(Carboxymethylcellulose Sodium) .... ⊙251
None cited in PDR database.

REGLAN INJECTABLE
(Metoclopramide Hydrochloride) 2935
May interact with anticholinergics, central nervous system depressants, cardiac glycosides, hypnotics and sedatives, insulin, monoamine oxidase inhibitors, narcotic analgesics, tranquilizers, and certain other agents. Compounds in these categories include:

Acetaminophen (Increased rate and/or extent of absorption from the small bowel). Products include:
Actifed Cold & Sinus Caplets and Tablets 688
Alka-Seltzer Plus Liqui-Gels 604
Alka-Seltzer Plus Cold & Flu Medicine Liqui-Gels 604
Alka-Seltzer Plus Cold & Sinus Medicine Liqui-Gels 604
Benadryl Allergy/Cold Tablets 691
Benadryl Allergy Sinus Headache Caplets & Gelcaps 693
Benadryl Severe Allergy & Sinus Headache Caplets 694
Children's Cēpacol Sore Throat 788
Comtrex Acute Head Cold & Sinus Pressure Relief Tablets 627
Comtrex Deep Chest Cold & Congestion Relief Softgels 627
Comtrex Flu Therapy & Fever Relief Daytime Caplets 628
Comtrex Flu Therapy & Fever Relief Nighttime Tablets 628
Comtrex Maximum Strength Multi-Symptom Cold & Cough Relief Tablets and Caplets 626
Contac Severe Cold and Flu Caplets Maximum Strength 746
Contac Severe Cold and Flu Caplets Non-Drowsy 746
Coricidin 'D' Cold, Flu & Sinus Tablets 737
Coricidin HBP Cold & Flu Tablets 738
Coricidin HBP Maximum Strength Flu Tablets 738
Coricidin HBP Night-Time Cold & Flu Tablets 738
Darvon-N/Darvocet-N 1907
Dimetapp Cold and Fever Suspension 775
Dimetapp Nighttime Flu Liquid 776
Dimetapp Non-Drowsy Flu Syrup 777
Drixoral Allergy/Sinus Extended-Release Tablets 741
Drixoral Cold & Flu Extended-Release Tablets 740
Aspirin Free Excedrin Caplets and Geltabs 628
Excedrin Extra-Strength Tablets, Caplets, and Geltabs 629
Excedrin Migraine 1070
Excedrin PM Tablets, Caplets, and Geltabs 631
Goody's Body Pain Formula Powder 620
Goody's Extra Strength Headache Powder 620
Goody's Extra Strength Pain Relief Tablets 620
Goody's PM Powder 621
Hycomine Compound Tablets 1317
Lortab 3319
Lortab Elixir 3317
Maxidone Tablets CIII 3399
Maximum Strength Midol Menstrual Caplets and Gelcaps 612
Maximum Strength Midol PMS Caplets and Gelcaps 613
Maximum Strength Midol Teen Caplets 612
Midrin Capsules 3464
Norco 5/325 Tablets CIII 3424
Norco 7.5/325 Tablets CIII 3425
Norco 10/325 Tablets CIII 3427
Norco 10/325 Tablets CIII 3425
Percocet Tablets 1326
Percogesic Aspirin-Free Coated Tablets 667
Extra Strength Percogesic Aspirin-Free Coated Caplets 665
Phrenilin 578
Robitussin Cold Caplets Multi-Symptom Cold & Flu 781
Robitussin Cold Softgels Multi-Symptom Cold & Flu 781
Robitussin Multi Symptom Honey Flu Liquid 785
Robitussin Nighttime Honey Flu Liquid 786
Sedapap Tablets 50 mg/650 mg 2225
Singlet Caplets 761
Sinutab Sinus Allergy Medication, Maximum Strength Formula, Tablets & Caplets 707
Sinutab Sinus Medication, Maximum Strength Without Drowsiness Formula, Tablets & Caplets 707
Sudafed Cold & Cough Liquid Caps 709
Sudafed Cold & Sinus Liquid Caps 710
Sudafed Severe Cold 711
Sudafed Sinus Headache Caplets 712
Sudafed Sinus Headache Tablets 712
Tavist Sinus Non-Drowsy Coated Caplets 676
TheraFlu Regular Strength Cold & Cough Night Time Hot Liquid 676
TheraFlu Regular Strength Cold & Sore Throat Night Time Hot Liquid 676
TheraFlu Maximum Strength Flu & Congestion Non-Drowsy Hot Liquid 677
TheraFlu Maximum Strength Flu & Cough Night Time Hot Liquid 678
TheraFlu Maximum Strength Flu & Sore Throat Night Time Hot Liquid 677
TheraFlu Maximum Strength Severe Cold & Congestion Night Time Caplets 678
TheraFlu Maximum Strength Severe Cold & Congestion Night Time Hot Liquid 678
TheraFlu Maximum Strength Severe Cold & Congestion Non-Drowsy 679
Triaminic Cold, Cough & Fever Liquid 681
Triaminic Cough & Sore Throat Liquid 682
Triaminic Cough & Sore Throat Softchews 684
Tylenol, Children's 2014
Children's Tylenol Allergy-D Liquid 2014
Children's Tylenol Cold Suspension Liquid and Chewable Tablets 2015
Children's Tylenol Cold Plus Cough Suspension Liquid and Chewable Tablets 2015
Children's Tylenol Flu Suspension Liquid 2015
Children's Tylenol Sinus Suspension Liquid 2017
Infants' Tylenol Cold Decongestant and Fever Reducer Concentrated Drops 2015
Infants' Tylenol Cold Decongestant and Fever Reducer Concentrated Drops Plus Cough 2015
Junior Strength Tylenol Soft Chews Chewable Tablets 2014
Tylenol 2009
Tylenol Allergy Sinus 2010
Tylenol Severe Allergy Caplets 2010
Multi-Symptom Tylenol Cold Complete Formula Caplets 2010
Multi-Symptom Tylenol Cold Non-Drowsy Caplets and Gelcaps 2010
Multi-Symptom Tylenol Cold Severe Congestion Non-Drowsy Caplets 2011
Maximum Strength Tylenol Flu NightTime Gelcaps 2011
Maximum Strength Tylenol Flu NightTime Liquid 2011
Maximum Strength Tylenol Flu Non-Drowsy Gelcaps 2011
Extra Strength Tylenol PM Caplets, Geltabs, and Gelcaps 2012
Maximum Strength Tylenol Sinus NightTime Caplets 2012
Maximum Strength Tylenol Sinus Non-Drowsy Geltabs, Gelcaps, Caplets, and Tablets 2012
Maximum Strength Tylenol Sore Throat Adult Liquid 2013
Tylenol with Codeine 2595
Women's Tylenol Menstrual Relief Caplets 2013
Tylox Capsules 2597
Ultracet Tablets 2597
Vanquish Caplets 617
Vicks 44M Cough, Cold & Flu Relief Liquid 725
Vicks DayQuil LiquiCaps/Liquid Multi-Symptom Cold/Flu Relief 727
Vicks NyQuil LiquiCaps/Liquid Multi-Symptom Cold/Flu Relief, Original and Cherry Flavors 727
Vicodin Tablets 516
Vicodin ES Tablets 517
Vicodin HP Tablets 518
Zydone Tablets 1330

Alfentanil Hydrochloride (Additive sedative effects; antagonizes gastrointestinal motility effects).
No products indexed under this heading.

Alprazolam (Additive sedative effects). Products include:
Xanax Tablets 2865

Aprobarbital (Additive sedative effects).
No products indexed under this heading.

Atropine Sulfate (Antagonizes gastrointestinal motility effects). Products include:
Donnatal 2929
Donnatal Extentabs 2930
Motofen Tablets 577
Prosed/DS Tablets 3268
Urised Tablets 2876

Belladonna Alkaloids (Antagonizes gastrointestinal motility effects). Products include:
Hyland's Teething Tablets 766
Urimax Tablets 1769

Benztropine Mesylate (Antagonizes gastrointestinal motility effects). Products include:
Cogentin 2055

Biperiden Hydrochloride (Antagonizes gastrointestinal motility effects). Products include:
Akineton 402

Buprenorphine Hydrochloride (Additive sedative effects; antagonizes gastrointestinal motility effects). Products include:
Buprenex Injectable 2918

Buspirone Hydrochloride (Additive sedative effects).
No products indexed under this heading.

Butabarbital (Additive sedative effects).
No products indexed under this heading.

Butalbital (Additive sedative effects). Products include:
Phrenilin 578
Sedapap Tablets 50 mg/650 mg 2225

Chlordiazepoxide (Additive sedative effects). Products include:
Limbitrol 1738

Chlordiazepoxide Hydrochloride (Additive sedative effects). Products include:
Librium Capsules 1736
Librium for Injection 1737

Chlorpromazine (Additive sedative effects). Products include:
Thorazine Suppositories 1656

Chlorpromazine Hydrochloride (Additive sedative effects). Products include:
Thorazine 1656

Chlorprothixene (Additive sedative effects).
No products indexed under this heading.

Chlorprothixene Hydrochloride (Additive sedative effects).
No products indexed under this heading.

Chlorprothixene Lactate (Additive sedative effects).
No products indexed under this heading.

Clidinium Bromide (Antagonizes gastrointestinal motility effects).
No products indexed under this heading.

Clorazepate Dipotassium (Additive sedative effects). Products include:
Tranxene 511

Clozapine (Additive sedative effects; antagonizes gastrointestinal motility effects). Products include:
Clozaril Tablets 2319

Codeine Phosphate (Additive sedative effects; antagonizes gastrointestinal motility effects). Products include:
Phenergan with Codeine Syrup 3557
Phenergan VC with Codeine Syrup 3561
Robitussin A-C Syrup 2942
Robitussin-DAC Syrup 2942
Ryna-C Liquid 768
Soma Compound w/Codeine Tablets 3355
Tussi-Organidin NR Liquid 3350
Tussi-Organidin-S NR Liquid 3350
Tylenol with Codeine 2595

Cyclosporine (Increased rate and/or extent of absorption from the small bowel). Products include:
Gengraf Capsules 457
Neoral Soft Gelatin Capsules 2380
Neoral Oral Solution 2380
Sandimmune 2388

Desflurane (Additive sedative effects; antagonizes gastrointestinal motility effects). Products include:
Suprane Liquid for Inhalation 874

Deslanoside (Diminished absorption from the stomach).
No products indexed under this heading.

Dezocine (Additive sedative effects; antagonizes gastrointestinal motility effects).
No products indexed under this heading.

Diazepam (Additive sedative effects). Products include:
Valium Injectable 3026
Valium Tablets 3047

Dicyclomine Hydrochloride (Antagonizes gastrointestinal motility effects).
No products indexed under this heading.

Digitoxin (Diminished absorption from the stomach).
No products indexed under this heading.

Digoxin (Diminished absorption from the stomach). Products include:
Digitek Tablets 1003
Lanoxicaps Capsules 1574
Lanoxin Injection 1581
Lanoxin Tablets 1587
Lanoxin Elixir Pediatric 1578
Lanoxin Injection Pediatric 1584

Droperidol (Additive sedative effects).
No products indexed under this heading.

Enflurane (Additive sedative effects).
No products indexed under this heading.

Estazolam (Additive sedative effects; antagonizes gastrointestinal motility effects). Products include:
ProSom Tablets 500

Ethchlorvynol (Additive sedative effects).
No products indexed under this heading.

Ethinamate (Additive sedative effects).
No products indexed under this heading.

Fentanyl (Additive sedative effects; antagonizes gastrointestinal motility effects). Products include:
Duragesic Transdermal System 1786

Fentanyl Citrate (Additive sedative effects; antagonizes gastrointestinal motility effects). Products include:
Actiq 1184

Fluphenazine Decanoate (Additive sedative effects).
No products indexed under this heading.

Fluphenazine Enanthate (Additive sedative effects).
No products indexed under this heading.

Fluphenazine Hydrochloride (Additive sedative effects).
No products indexed under this heading.

Flurazepam Hydrochloride (Additive sedative effects).
No products indexed under this heading.

Glutethimide (Additive sedative effects).
No products indexed under this heading.

Glycopyrrolate (Antagonizes gastrointestinal motility effects). Products include:
Robinul Forte Tablets 1358
Robinul Injectable 2940
Robinul Tablets 1358

Haloperidol (Additive sedative effects). Products include:
Haldol Injection, Tablets and Concentrate 2533

Haloperidol Decanoate (Additive sedative effects). Products include:
Haldol Decanoate 2535

Hydrocodone Bitartrate (Additive sedative effects; antagonizes gastrointestinal motility effects). Products include:
Hycodan 1316
Hycomine Compound Tablets 1317
Hycotuss Expectorant Syrup 1318
Lortab 3319
Lortab Elixir 3317
Maxidone Tablets CIII 3399
Norco 5/325 Tablets CIII 3424
Norco 7.5/325 Tablets CIII 3425
Norco 10/325 Tablets CIII 3427
Norco 10/325 Tablets CIII 3425
Vicodin Tablets 516
Vicodin ES Tablets 517
Vicodin HP Tablets 518
Vicodin Tuss Expectorant 519
Vicoprofen Tablets 520
Zydone Tablets 1330

Hydrocodone Polistirex (Additive sedative effects; antagonizes gastrointestinal motility effects). Products include:
Tussionex Pennkinetic Extended-Release Suspension 1174

Hydromorphone Hydrochloride (Additive sedative effects; antagonizes gastrointestinal motility effects). Products include:
Dilaudid 441
Dilaudid Oral Liquid 445
Dilaudid Powder 441
Dilaudid Rectal Suppositories 441
Dilaudid Tablets 441
Dilaudid Tablets - 8 mg 445
Dilaudid-HP 443

Hydroxyzine Hydrochloride (Additive sedative effects). Products include:
Atarax Tablets & Syrup 2667
Vistaril Intramuscular Solution 2738

Hyoscyamine (Antagonizes gastrointestinal motility effects). Products include:
Urised Tablets 2876

Hyoscyamine Sulfate (Antagonizes gastrointestinal motility effects). Products include:
Arco-Lase Plus Tablets 592
Donnatal 2929
Donnatal Extentabs 2930
Levsin/Levsinex/Levbid 3172
NuLev Orally Disintegrating Tablets 3176
Prosed/DS Tablets 3268
Urimax Tablets 1769

Insulin, Human, Zinc Suspension (Exogenous insulin may begin to act before food has left the stomach and lead to hypoglycemia in diabetic patients with gastroparesis; insulin dosage or timing of dosage may require adjustment). Products include:
Humulin L, 100 Units 1937
Humulin U, 100 Units 1943
Novolin L Human Insulin 10 ml Vials 2422

Insulin, Human NPH (Exogenous insulin may begin to act before food has left the stomach and lead to hypoglycemia in diabetic patients with gastroparesis; insulin dosage or timing of dosage may require adjustment). Products include:
Humulin N, 100 Units 1939
Humulin N NPH Pen 1940
Novolin N Human Insulin 10 ml Vials 2422
Novolin N PenFill 2423
Novolin N Prefilled Syringe Disposable Insulin Delivery System 2425

Insulin, Human Regular (Exogenous insulin may begin to act before food has left the stomach and lead to hypoglycemia in diabetic patients with gastroparesis; insulin dosage or timing of dosage may require adjustment). Products include:
Humulin R Regular (U-500) 1943
Humulin R, 100 Units 1941
Novolin R Human Insulin 10 ml Vials 2423
Novolin R PenFill 2423
Novolin R Prefilled Syringe Disposable Insulin Delivery System 2425
Velosulin BR Human Insulin 10 ml Vials 2435

Insulin, Human Regular and Human NPH Mixture (Exogenous insulin may begin to act before food has left the stomach and lead to hypoglycemia in diabetic patients with gastroparesis; insulin dosage or timing of dosage may require adjustment). Products include:
Humulin 50/50, 100 Units 1934
Humulin 70/30, 100 Units 1935
Humulin 70/30 Pen 1936
Novolin 70/30 Human Insulin 10 ml Vials 2421
Novolin 70/30 PenFill 2423
Novolin 70/30 Prefilled Disposable Insulin Delivery System 2425

Insulin, NPH (Exogenous insulin may begin to act before food has left the stomach and lead to hypoglycemia in diabetic patients with gastroparesis; insulin dosage or timing of dosage may require adjustment). Products include:
Iletin II, NPH (Pork), 100 Units 1946

Insulin, Regular (Exogenous insulin may begin to act before food has left the stomach and lead to hypoglycemia in diabetic patients with gastroparesis; insulin dosage or timing of dosage may require adjustment). Products include:
Iletin II, Regular (Pork), 100 Units ... 1947

Insulin, Zinc Crystals (Exogenous insulin may begin to act before food has left the stomach and lead to hypoglycemia in diabetic patients with gastroparesis; insulin dosage or timing of dosage may require adjustment).
No products indexed under this heading.

Insulin, Zinc Suspension (Exogenous insulin may begin to act before food has left the stomach and lead to hypoglycemia in diabetic patients with gastroparesis; insulin dosage or timing of dosage may require adjustment). Products include:
Iletin II, Lente (Pork), 100 Units 1945

Insulin Aspart, Human Regular (Exogenous insulin may begin to act before food has left the stomach and lead to hypoglycemia in diabetic patients with gastroparesis; insulin dosage or timing of dosage may require adjustment).
No products indexed under this heading.

Insulin glargine (Exogenous insulin may begin to act before food has left the stomach and lead to hypoglycemia in diabetic patients with gastroparesis; insulin dosage or timing of dosage may require adjustment). Products include:
Lantus Injection 742

Insulin Lispro, Human (Exogenous insulin may begin to act before food has left the stomach and lead to hypoglycemia in diabetic patients with gastroparesis; insulin dosage or timing of dosage may require adjustment). Products include:
Humalog 1926
Humalog Mix 75/25 Pen 1928

Insulin Lispro Protamine, Human (Exogenous insulin may begin to act before food has left the stomach and lead to hypoglycemia in diabetic patients with gastroparesis; insulin dosage or timing of dosage may require adjustment). Products include:
Humalog Mix 75/25 Pen 1928

Ipratropium Bromide (Antagonizes gastrointestinal motility effects). Products include:
Atrovent Inhalation Aerosol 1030
Atrovent Inhalation Solution 1031
Atrovent Nasal Spray 0.03% 1032
Atrovent Nasal Spray 0.06% 1033
Combivent Inhalation Aerosol 1041
DuoNeb Inhalation Solution 1233

Isocarboxazid (Metoclopramide releases catecholamines in patients with essential hypertension hence it should be used cautiously in patients receiving MAO inhibitors).
No products indexed under this heading.

Isoflurane (Additive sedative effects).
No products indexed under this heading.

Ketamine Hydrochloride (Additive sedative effects; antagonizes gastrointestinal motility effects).
No products indexed under this heading.

Levodopa (Increased rate and/or extent of absorption from the small bowel). Products include:
Sinemet Tablets 1253
Sinemet CR Tablets 1255

Levomethadyl Acetate Hydrochloride (Additive sedative effects; antagonizes gastrointestinal motility effects).
No products indexed under this heading.

Levorphanol Tartrate (Additive sedative effects; antagonizes gastrointestinal motility effects). Products include:
Levo-Dromoran 1734
Levorphanol Tartrate Tablets 3059

Lorazepam (Additive sedative effects). Products include:
Ativan Injection 3478
Ativan Tablets 3482

Loxapine Hydrochloride (Additive sedative effects).
No products indexed under this heading.

Loxapine Succinate (Additive sedative effects; antagonizes gastrointestinal motility effects). Products include:
Loxitane Capsules 3398

Mepenzolate Bromide (Antagonizes gastrointestinal motility effects).
No products indexed under this heading.

Meperidine Hydrochloride (Additive sedative effects; antagonizes gastrointestinal motility effects). Products include:
Demerol 3079
Mepergan Injection 3539

Mephobarbital (Additive sedative effects).
No products indexed under this heading.

Meprobamate (Additive sedative effects). Products include:
Miltown Tablets 3349

Mesoridazine Besylate (Additive sedative effects). Products include:
Serentil 1057

Methadone Hydrochloride (Additive sedative effects; antagonizes gastrointestinal motility effects). Products include:
Dolophine Hydrochloride Tablets 3056

Methohexital Sodium (Additive sedative effects). Products include:
Brevital Sodium for Injection, USP .. 1815

Methotrimeprazine (Additive sedative effects; antagonizes gastrointestinal motility effects).
No products indexed under this heading.

Methoxyflurane (Additive sedative effects).
No products indexed under this heading.

Midazolam Hydrochloride (Additive sedative effects). Products include:
Versed Injection 3027
Versed Syrup 3033

Moclobemide (Metoclopramide releases catecholamines in patients with essential hypertension hence it should be used cautiously in patients receiving MAO inhibitors).
No products indexed under this heading.

Molindone Hydrochloride (Additive sedative effects). Products include:
Moban 1320

Morphine Sulfate (Additive sedative effects; antagonizes gastrointestinal motility effects). Products include:
Astramorph/PF Injection, USP (Preservative-Free) 594
Duramorph Injection 1312
Infumorph 200 and Infumorph 500 Sterile Solutions 1314
Kadian Capsules 1335
MS Contin Tablets 2896
MSIR 2898
Oramorph SR Tablets 3062
Roxanol 3066

Olanzapine (Additive sedative effects). Products include:
Zyprexa Tablets 1973
Zyprexa ZYDIS Orally Disintegrating Tablets 1973

Oxazepam (Additive sedative effects).
No products indexed under this heading.

Oxybutynin Chloride (Antagonizes gastrointestinal motility effects). Products include:
Ditropan XL Extended Release Tablets 564

Oxycodone Hydrochloride (Additive sedative effects; antagonizes gastrointestinal motility effects). Products include:
OxyContin Tablets 2912
OxyFast Oral Concentrate Solution . 2916
OxyIR Capsules 2916
Percocet Tablets 1326
Percodan Tablets 1327
Percolone Tablets 1327
Roxicodone 3067
Tylox Capsules 2597

Pargyline Hydrochloride (Metoclopramide releases catecholamines in patients with essential hyperten-

sion hence it should be used cautiously in patients receiving MAO inhibitors).
No products indexed under this heading.

Pentobarbital Sodium (Additive sedative effects). Products include:
Nembutal Sodium Solution 485

Perphenazine (Additive sedative effects). Products include:
Etrafon 3115
Trilafon 3160

Phenelzine Sulfate (Metoclopramide releases catecholamines in patients with essential hypertension hence it should be used cautiously in patients receiving MAO inhibitors). Products include:
Nardil Tablets 2653

Phenobarbital (Additive sedative effects). Products include:
Arco-Lase Plus Tablets 592
Donnatal 2929
Donnatal Extentabs 2930

Prazepam (Additive sedative effects).
No products indexed under this heading.

Procarbazine Hydrochloride (Metoclopramide releases catecholamines in patients with essential hypertension hence it should be used cautiously in patients receiving MAO inhibitors). Products include:
Matulane Capsules 3246

Prochlorperazine (Additive sedative effects). Products include:
Compazine 1505

Procyclidine Hydrochloride (Antagonizes gastrointestinal motility effects).
No products indexed under this heading.

Promethazine Hydrochloride (Additive sedative effects). Products include:
Mepergan Injection 3539
Phenergan Injection 3553
Phenergan 3556
Phenergan Syrup 3554
Phenergan with Codeine Syrup 3557
Phenergan with Dextromethorphan Syrup 3559
Phenergan VC Syrup 3560
Phenergan VC with Codeine Syrup 3561

Propantheline Bromide (Antagonizes gastrointestinal motility effects).
No products indexed under this heading.

Propofol (Additive sedative effects; antagonizes gastrointestinal motility effects). Products include:
Diprivan Injectable Emulsion 667

Propoxyphene Hydrochloride (Additive sedative effects; antagonizes gastrointestinal motility effects). Products include:
Darvon Pulvules 1909
Darvon Compound-65 Pulvules 1910

Propoxyphene Napsylate (Additive sedative effects; antagonizes gastrointestinal motility effects). Products include:
Darvon-N/Darvocet-N 1907
Darvon-N Tablets 1912

Quazepam (Additive sedative effects; antagonizes gastrointestinal motility effects).
No products indexed under this heading.

Quetiapine Fumarate (Additive sedative effects). Products include:
Seroquel Tablets 684

Remifentanil Hydrochloride (Additive sedative effects; antagonizes gastrointestinal motility effects).
No products indexed under this heading.

Risperidone (Additive sedative effects; antagonizes gastrointestinal motility effects). Products include:
Risperdal 1796

Scopolamine (Antagonizes gastrointestinal motility effects). Products include:
Transderm Scōp Transdermal Therapeutic System 2302

Scopolamine Hydrobromide (Antagonizes gastrointestinal motility effects). Products include:
Donnatal 2929
Donnatal Extentabs 2930

Secobarbital Sodium (Additive sedative effects; antagonizes gastrointestinal motility effects).
No products indexed under this heading.

Selegiline Hydrochloride (Metoclopramide releases catecholamines in patients with essential hypertension hence it should be used cautiously in patients receiving MAO inhibitors). Products include:
Eldepryl Capsules 3266

Sevoflurane (Additive sedative effects).
No products indexed under this heading.

Sufentanil Citrate (Additive sedative effects; antagonizes gastrointestinal motility effects).
No products indexed under this heading.

Temazepam (Additive sedative effects).
No products indexed under this heading.

Tetracycline Hydrochloride (Increased rate and/or extent of absorption from the small bowel).
No products indexed under this heading.

Thiamylal Sodium (Additive sedative effects).
No products indexed under this heading.

Thioridazine Hydrochloride (Additive sedative effects). Products include:
Thioridazine Hydrochloride Tablets 2289

Thiothixene (Additive sedative effects). Products include:
Navane Capsules 2701
Thiothixene Capsules 2290

Tolterodine Tartrate (Antagonizes gastrointestinal motility effects). Products include:
Detrol Tablets 3623
Detrol LA Capsules 2801

Tranylcypromine Sulfate (Metoclopramide releases catecholamines in patients with essential hypertension hence it should be used cautiously in patients receiving MAO inhibitors). Products include:
Parnate Tablets 1607

Triazolam (Additive sedative effects). Products include:
Halcion Tablets 2823

Tridihexethyl Chloride (Antagonizes gastrointestinal motility effects).
No products indexed under this heading.

Trifluoperazine Hydrochloride (Additive sedative effects). Products include:
Stelazine 1640

Trihexyphenidyl Hydrochloride (Antagonizes gastrointestinal motility effects). Products include:
Artane 1855

Zaleplon (Additive sedative effects). Products include:
Sonata Capsules 3591

Ziprasidone Hydrochloride (Additive sedative effects). Products include:
Geodon Capsules 2688

Zolpidem Tartrate (Additive sedative effects; antagonizes gastrointestinal motility effects). Products include:
Ambien Tablets 3191

Food Interactions

Alcohol (Increased rate and/or extent of absorption from the small bowel; additive sedative effects).

REGLAN SYRUP
(Metoclopramide Hydrochloride) 2935
See Reglan Injectable

REGLAN TABLETS
(Metoclopramide Hydrochloride) 2935
See Reglan Injectable

REGRANEX GEL
(Becaplermin) 2586
None cited in PDR database.

REHYDRALYTE ORAL ELECTROLYTE REHYDRATION SOLUTION
(Electrolyte Supplement) 3052
None cited in PDR database.

RELAFEN TABLETS
(Nabumetone) 1617
May interact with highly protein bound drugs (selected). Compounds in these categories include:

Amiodarone Hydrochloride (In vitro studies have shown that 6 MNA, an active metabolite of nabumetone, may displace other protein bound drugs from their binding site). Products include:
Cordarone Intravenous 3491
Cordarone Tablets 3487
Pacerone Tablets 3331

Amitriptyline Hydrochloride (In vitro studies have shown that 6 MNA, an active metabolite of nabumetone, may displace other protein bound drugs from their binding site). Products include:
Etrafon 3115
Limbitrol 1738

Atovaquone (In vitro studies have shown that 6 MNA, an active metabolite of nabumetone, may displace other protein bound drugs from their binding site). Products include:
Malarone 1596
Mepron Suspension 1598

Cefonicid Sodium (In vitro studies have shown that 6 MNA, an active metabolite of nabumetone, may displace other protein bound drugs from their binding site).
No products indexed under this heading.

Celecoxib (In vitro studies have shown that 6 MNA, an active metabolite of nabumetone, may displace other protein bound drugs from their binding site). Products include:
Celebrex Capsules 2676
Celebrex Capsules 2780

Chlordiazepoxide (In vitro studies have shown that 6 MNA, an active metabolite of nabumetone, may displace other protein bound drugs from their binding site). Products include:
Limbitrol 1738

Chlordiazepoxide Hydrochloride (In vitro studies have shown that 6 MNA, an active metabolite of nabumetone, may displace other protein bound drugs from their binding site). Products include:
Librium Capsules 1736
Librium for Injection 1737

Chlorpromazine (In vitro studies have shown that 6 MNA, an active metabolite of nabumetone, may displace other protein bound drugs from their binding site). Products include:
Thorazine Suppositories 1656

Chlorpromazine Hydrochloride (In vitro studies have shown that 6 MNA, an active metabolite of nabumetone, may displace other protein bound drugs from their binding site). Products include:
Thorazine 1656

Clomipramine Hydrochloride (In vitro studies have shown that 6 MNA, an active metabolite of nabumetone, may displace other protein bound drugs from their binding site).
No products indexed under this heading.

Clozapine (In vitro studies have shown that 6 MNA, an active metabolite of nabumetone, may displace other protein bound drugs from their binding site). Products include:
Clozaril Tablets 2319

Cyclosporine (In vitro studies have shown that 6 MNA, an active metabolite of nabumetone, may displace other protein bound drugs from their binding site). Products include:
Gengraf Capsules 457
Neoral Soft Gelatin Capsules 2380
Neoral Oral Solution 2380
Sandimmune 2388

Diazepam (In vitro studies have shown that 6 MNA, an active metabolite of nabumetone, may displace other protein bound drugs from their binding site). Products include:
Valium Injectable 3026
Valium Tablets 3047

Diclofenac Potassium (In vitro studies have shown that 6 MNA, an active metabolite of nabumetone, may displace other protein bound drugs from their binding site). Products include:
Cataflam Tablets 2315

Diclofenac Sodium (In vitro studies have shown that 6 MNA, an active metabolite of nabumetone, may displace other protein bound drugs from their binding site). Products include:
Arthrotec Tablets 3195
Voltaren Ophthalmic Sterile Ophthalmic Solution .... ⊙312
Voltaren Tablets 2315
Voltaren-XR Tablets 2315

Dipyridamole (In vitro studies have shown that 6 MNA, an active metabolite of nabumetone, may displace other protein bound drugs from their binding site). Products include:
Aggrenox Capsules 1026
Persantine Tablets 1057

Fenoprofen Calcium (In vitro studies have shown that 6 MNA, an active metabolite of nabumetone, may displace other protein bound drugs from their binding site).
No products indexed under this heading.

Flurazepam Hydrochloride (In vitro studies have shown that 6 MNA, an active metabolite of nabumetone, may displace other protein bound drugs from their binding site).
No products indexed under this heading.

Flurbiprofen (In vitro studies have shown that 6 MNA, an active metabolite of nabumetone, may displace other protein bound drugs from their binding site).
No products indexed under this heading.

Glipizide (In vitro studies have shown that 6 MNA, an active metabolite of nabumetone, may displace other protein bound drugs from their binding site). Products include:
Glucotrol Tablets 2692
Glucotrol XL Extended Release Tablets 2693

Ibuprofen (In vitro studies have shown that 6 MNA, an active metab-

IMPORTANT NOTE: Always consult each drug listing in the patient's regimen for possible interactions.

olite of nabumetone, may displace other protein bound drugs from their binding site). Products include:

Advil .... ▣771
Children's Advil Oral Suspension ... ▣773
Children's Advil Chewable Tablets . ▣773
Advil Cold and Sinus Caplets .... ▣771
Advil Cold and Sinus Tablets .... ▣771
Advil Flu & Body Ache Caplets ...... ▣772
Infants' Advil Drops .... ▣773
Junior Strength Advil Tablets .... ▣773
Junior Strength Advil Chewable Tablets .... ▣773
Advil Migraine Liquigels .... ▣772
Children's Motrin Oral Suspension and Chewable Tablets........ 2006
Children's Motrin Cold Oral Suspension........ 2007
Children's Motrin Oral Suspension........ ▣643
Motrin Suspension, Oral Drops, Chewable Tablets, and Caplets.... 2002
Infants' Motrin Concentrated Drops........ 2006
Junior Strength Motrin Caplets and Chewable Tablets........ 2006
Motrin IB Tablets, Caplets, and Gelcaps........ 2002
Motrin Migraine Pain Caplets 2005
Motrin Sinus Headache Caplets 2005
Vicoprofen Tablets 520

Imipramine Hydrochloride (In vitro studies have shown that 6 MNA, an active metabolite of nabumetone, may displace other protein bound drugs from their binding site).
No products indexed under this heading.

Imipramine Pamoate (In vitro studies have shown that 6 MNA, an active metabolite of nabumetone, may displace other protein bound drugs from their binding site).
No products indexed under this heading.

Indomethacin (In vitro studies have shown that 6 MNA, an active metabolite of nabumetone, may displace other protein bound drugs from their binding site). Products include:

Indocin 2112

Indomethacin Sodium Trihydrate (In vitro studies have shown that 6 MNA, an active metabolite of nabumetone, may displace other protein bound drugs from their binding site). Products include:

Indocin I.V. 2115

Ketoprofen (In vitro studies have shown that 6 MNA, an active metabolite of nabumetone, may displace other protein bound drugs from their binding site). Products include:

Orudis Capsules 3548
Orudis KT Tablets .... ▣778
Oruvail Capsules 3548

Ketorolac Tromethamine (In vitro studies have shown that 6 MNA, an active metabolite of nabumetone, may displace other protein bound drugs from their binding site). Products include:

Acular Ophthalmic Solution 544
Acular PF Ophthalmic Solution 544
Toradol 3018

Meclofenamate Sodium (In vitro studies have shown that 6 MNA, an active metabolite of nabumetone, may displace other protein bound drugs from their binding site).
No products indexed under this heading.

Mefenamic Acid (In vitro studies have shown that 6 MNA, an active metabolite of nabumetone, may displace other protein bound drugs from their binding site). Products include:

Ponstel Capsules 1356

Midazolam Hydrochloride (In vitro studies have shown that 6 MNA, an active metabolite of nabumetone, may displace other protein bound drugs from their binding site). Products include:

Versed Injection 3027
Versed Syrup 3033

Naproxen (In vitro studies have shown that 6 MNA, an active metabolite of nabumetone, may displace other protein bound drugs from their binding site). Products include:

EC-Naprosyn Delayed-Release Tablets........ 2967
Naprosyn Suspension 2967
Naprosyn Tablets 2967

Naproxen Sodium (In vitro studies have shown that 6 MNA, an active metabolite of nabumetone, may displace other protein bound drugs from their binding site). Products include:

Aleve Tablets, Caplets and Gelcaps........ ▣602
Aleve Cold & Sinus Caplets .... ▣603
Anaprox Tablets 2967
Anaprox DS Tablets 2967
Naprelan Tablets 1293

Nortriptyline Hydrochloride (In vitro studies have shown that 6 MNA, an active metabolite of nabumetone, may displace other protein bound drugs from their binding site).
No products indexed under this heading.

Oxaprozin (In vitro studies have shown that 6 MNA, an active metabolite of nabumetone, may displace other protein bound drugs from their binding site).
No products indexed under this heading.

Oxazepam (In vitro studies have shown that 6 MNA, an active metabolite of nabumetone, may displace other protein bound drugs from their binding site).
No products indexed under this heading.

Phenylbutazone (In vitro studies have shown that 6 MNA, an active metabolite of nabumetone, may displace other protein bound drugs from their binding site).
No products indexed under this heading.

Piroxicam (In vitro studies have shown that 6 MNA, an active metabolite of nabumetone, may displace other protein bound drugs from their binding site). Products include:

Feldene Capsules 2685

Propranolol Hydrochloride (In vitro studies have shown that 6 MNA, an active metabolite of nabumetone, may displace other protein bound drugs from their binding site). Products include:

Inderal 3513
Inderal LA Long-Acting Capsules 3516
Inderide Tablets 3517
Inderide LA Long-Acting Capsules .. 3519

Sulindac (In vitro studies have shown that 6 MNA, an active metabolite of nabumetone, may displace other protein bound drugs from their binding site). Products include:

Clinoril Tablets 2053

Temazepam (In vitro studies have shown that 6 MNA, an active metabolite of nabumetone, may displace other protein bound drugs from their binding site).
No products indexed under this heading.

Tolbutamide (In vitro studies have shown that 6 MNA, an active metabolite of nabumetone, may displace other protein bound drugs from their binding site).
No products indexed under this heading.

Tolmetin Sodium (In vitro studies have shown that 6 MNA, an active metabolite of nabumetone, may displace other protein bound drugs from their binding site). Products include:

Tolectin 2589

Trimipramine Maleate (In vitro studies have shown that 6 MNA, an active metabolite of nabumetone, may displace other protein bound drugs from their binding site). Products include:

Surmontil Capsules 3595

Warfarin Sodium (Effects not specified; caution should be exercised; in vitro studies have shown that 6 MNA, an active metabolite of nabumetone, may displace other protein bound drugs from their binding site). Products include:

Coumadin for Injection 1243
Coumadin Tablets 1243
Warfarin Sodium Tablets, USP 3302

Food Interactions

Dairy products (Potential for more rapid absorption, however, the total amount of GMNA in the plasma is unchanged).

Food, unspecified (Potential for more rapid absorption, however, the total amount of GMNA in the plasma is unchanged).

RELENZA ROTADISK

(Zanamivir) 1619
None cited in PDR database.

RELIEF NASAL & THROAT SPRAY

(Homeopathic Formulations) .... ▣811
None cited in PDR database.

REMERON TABLETS

(Mirtazapine) 2483
May interact with central nervous system depressants, monoamine oxidase inhibitors, and certain other agents. Compounds in these categories include:

Alfentanil Hydrochloride (Co-administration may result in an additive impairment of motor skills).
No products indexed under this heading.

Alprazolam (Co-administration may result in an additive impairment of motor skills). Products include:

Xanax Tablets 2865

Aprobarbital (Co-administration may result in an additive impairment of motor skills).
No products indexed under this heading.

Buprenorphine Hydrochloride (Co-administration may result in an additive impairment of motor skills). Products include:

Buprenex Injectable 2918

Buspirone Hydrochloride (Co-administration may result in an additive impairment of motor skills).
No products indexed under this heading.

Butabarbital (Co-administration may result in an additive impairment of motor skills).
No products indexed under this heading.

Butalbital (Co-administration may result in an additive impairment of motor skills). Products include:

Phrenilin 578
Sedapap Tablets 50 mg/650 mg ... 2225

Chlordiazepoxide (Co-administration may result in an additive impairment of motor skills). Products include:

Limbitrol 1738

Chlordiazepoxide Hydrochloride (Co-administration may result in an additive impairment of motor skills). Products include:

Librium Capsules 1736
Librium for Injection 1737

Chlorpromazine (Co-administration may result in an additive impairment of motor skills). Products include:

Thorazine Suppositories 1656

Chlorpromazine Hydrochloride (Co-administration may result in an additive impairment of motor skills). Products include:

Thorazine 1656

Chlorprothixene (Co-administration may result in an additive impairment of motor skills).
No products indexed under this heading.

Chlorprothixene Hydrochloride (Co-administration may result in an additive impairment of motor skills).
No products indexed under this heading.

Chlorprothixene Lactate (Co-administration may result in an additive impairment of motor skills).
No products indexed under this heading.

Clorazepate Dipotassium (Co-administration may result in an additive impairment of motor skills). Products include:

Tranxene 511

Clozapine (Co-administration may result in an additive impairment of motor skills). Products include:

Clozaril Tablets 2319

Codeine Phosphate (Co-administration may result in an additive impairment of motor skills). Products include:

Phenergan with Codeine Syrup 3557
Phenergan VC with Codeine Syrup .. 3561
Robitussin A-C Syrup 2942
Robitussin-DAC Syrup 2942
Ryna-C Liquid .... ▣768
Soma Compound w/Codeine Tablets........ 3355
Tussi-Organidin NR Liquid 3350
Tussi-Organidin-S NR Liquid 3350
Tylenol with Codeine 2595

Desflurane (Co-administration may result in an additive impairment of motor skills). Products include:

Suprane Liquid for Inhalation 874

Dezocine (Co-administration may result in an additive impairment of motor skills).
No products indexed under this heading.

Diazepam (Co-administration has shown to result in an additive impairment of motor skills). Products include:

Valium Injectable 3026
Valium Tablets 3047

Droperidol (Co-administration may result in an additive impairment of motor skills).
No products indexed under this heading.

Enflurane (Co-administration may result in an additive impairment of motor skills).
No products indexed under this heading.

Estazolam (Co-administration may result in an additive impairment of motor skills). Products include:

ProSom Tablets 500

Ethchlorvynol (Co-administration may result in an additive impairment of motor skills).
No products indexed under this heading.

Ethinamate (Co-administration may result in an additive impairment of motor skills).
No products indexed under this heading.

Fentanyl (Co-administration may result in an additive impairment of motor skills). Products include:

Duragesic Transdermal System 1786

Fentanyl Citrate (Co-administration may result in an additive impairment of motor skills). Products include:

Actiq 1184

Fluphenazine Decanoate (Co-administration may result in an additive impairment of motor skills).
No products indexed under this heading.

Fluphenazine Enanthate (Co-administration may result in an addi-

tive impairment of motor skills).
No products indexed under this heading.

Fluphenazine Hydrochloride (Co-administration may result in an additive impairment of motor skills).
No products indexed under this heading.

Flurazepam Hydrochloride (Co-administration may result in an additive impairment of motor skills).
No products indexed under this heading.

Glutethimide (Co-administration may result in an additive impairment of motor skills).
No products indexed under this heading.

Haloperidol (Co-administration may result in an additive impairment of motor skills). Products include:
Haldol Injection, Tablets and Concentrate 2533

Haloperidol Decanoate (Co-administration may result in an additive impairment of motor skills).
Products include:
Haldol Decanoate 2535

Hydrocodone Bitartrate (Co-administration may result in an additive impairment of motor skills).
Products include:
Hycodan 1316
Hycomine Compound Tablets 1317
Hycotuss Expectorant Syrup 1318
Lortab 3319
Lortab Elixir 3317
Maxidone Tablets CIII 3399
Norco 5/325 Tablets CIII 3424
Norco 7.5/325 Tablets CIII 3425
Norco 10/325 Tablets CIII 3427
Norco 10/325 Tablets CIII 3425
Vicodin Tablets 516
Vicodin ES Tablets 517
Vicodin HP Tablets 518
Vicodin Tuss Expectorant 519
Vicoprofen Tablets 520
Zydone Tablets 1330

Hydrocodone Polistirex (Co-administration may result in an additive impairment of motor skills).
Products include:
Tussionex Pennkinetic Extended-Release Suspension 1174

Hydromorphone Hydrochloride (Co-administration may result in an additive impairment of motor skills).
Products include:
Dilaudid 441
Dilaudid Oral Liquid 445
Dilaudid Powder 441
Dilaudid Rectal Suppositories 441
Dilaudid Tablets 441
Dilaudid Tablets - 8 mg 445
Dilaudid-HP 443

Hydroxyzine Hydrochloride (Co-administration may result in an additive impairment of motor skills).
Products include:
Atarax Tablets & Syrup 2667
Vistaril Intramuscular Solution 2738

Isocarboxazid (Co-administration of antidepressants and MAO inhibitors has resulted in serious, and sometimes fatal, reactions including hyperthermia, autonomic instability, seizures, agitation, and coma; concurrent and/or sequential use is contraindicated).
No products indexed under this heading.

Isoflurane (Co-administration may result in an additive impairment of motor skills).
No products indexed under this heading.

Ketamine Hydrochloride (Co-administration may result in an additive impairment of motor skills).
No products indexed under this heading.

Levomethadyl Acetate Hydrochloride (Co-administration may result in an additive impairment of motor skills).
No products indexed under this heading.

Levorphanol Tartrate (Co-administration may result in an additive impairment of motor skills).
Products include:
Levo-Dromoran 1734
Levorphanol Tartrate Tablets 3059

Lorazepam (Co-administration may result in an additive impairment of motor skills). Products include:
Ativan Injection 3478
Ativan Tablets 3482

Loxapine Hydrochloride (Co-administration may result in an additive impairment of motor skills).
No products indexed under this heading.

Loxapine Succinate (Co-administration may result in an additive impairment of motor skills).
Products include:
Loxitane Capsules 3398

Meperidine Hydrochloride (Co-administration may result in an additive impairment of motor skills).
Products include:
Demerol 3079
Mepergan Injection 3539

Mephobarbital (Co-administration may result in an additive impairment of motor skills).
No products indexed under this heading.

Meprobamate (Co-administration may result in an additive impairment of motor skills). Products include:
Miltown Tablets 3349

Mesoridazine Besylate (Co-administration may result in an additive impairment of motor skills).
Products include:
Serentil 1057

Methadone Hydrochloride (Co-administration may result in an additive impairment of motor skills).
Products include:
Dolophine Hydrochloride Tablets 3056

Methohexital Sodium (Co-administration may result in an additive impairment of motor skills).
Products include:
Brevital Sodium for Injection, USP .. 1815

Methotrimeprazine (Co-administration may result in an additive impairment of motor skills).
No products indexed under this heading.

Methoxyflurane (Co-administration may result in an additive impairment of motor skills).
No products indexed under this heading.

Midazolam Hydrochloride (Co-administration may result in an additive impairment of motor skills).
Products include:
Versed Injection 3027
Versed Syrup 3033

Moclobemide (Co-administration of antidepressants and MAO inhibitors has resulted in serious, and sometimes fatal, reactions including hyperthermia, autonomic instability, seizures, agitation, and coma; concurrent and/or sequential use is contraindicated).
No products indexed under this heading.

Molindone Hydrochloride (Co-administration may result in an additive impairment of motor skills).
Products include:
Moban 1320

Morphine Sulfate (Co-administration may result in an additive impairment of motor skills).
Products include:
Astramorph/PF Injection, USP (Preservative-Free) 594
Duramorph Injection 1312
Infumorph 200 and Infumorph 500 Sterile Solutions 1314
Kadian Capsules 1335
MS Contin Tablets 2896
MSIR 2898
Oramorph SR Tablets 3062
Roxanol 3066

Olanzapine (Co-administration may result in an additive impairment of motor skills). Products include:
Zyprexa Tablets 1973
Zyprexa ZYDIS Orally Disintegrating Tablets 1973

Oxazepam (Co-administration may result in an additive impairment of motor skills).
No products indexed under this heading.

Oxycodone Hydrochloride (Co-administration may result in an additive impairment of motor skills).
Products include:
OxyContin Tablets 2912
OxyFast Oral Concentrate Solution . 2916
OxyIR Capsules 2916
Percocet Tablets 1326
Percodan Tablets 1327
Percolone Tablets 1327
Roxicodone 3067
Tylox Capsules 2597

Pargyline Hydrochloride (Co-administration of antidepressants and MAO inhibitors has resulted in serious, and sometimes fatal, reactions including hyperthermia, autonomic instability, seizures, agitation, and coma; concurrent and/or sequential use is contraindicated).
No products indexed under this heading.

Pentobarbital Sodium (Co-administration may result in an additive impairment of motor skills).
Products include:
Nembutal Sodium Solution 485

Perphenazine (Co-administration may result in an additive impairment of motor skills). Products include:
Etrafon 3115
Trilafon 3160

Phenelzine Sulfate (Co-administration of antidepressants and MAO inhibitors has resulted in serious, and sometimes fatal, reactions including hyperthermia, autonomic instability, seizures, agitation, and coma; concurrent and/or sequential use is contraindicated).
Products include:
Nardil Tablets 2653

Phenobarbital (Co-administration may result in an additive impairment of motor skills). Products include:
Arco-Lase Plus Tablets 592
Donnatal 2929
Donnatal Extentabs 2930

Prazepam (Co-administration may result in an additive impairment of motor skills).
No products indexed under this heading.

Procarbazine Hydrochloride (Co-administration of antidepressants and MAO inhibitors has resulted in serious, and sometimes fatal, reactions including hyperthermia, autonomic instability, seizures, agitation, and coma; concurrent and/or sequential use is contraindicated).
Products include:
Matulane Capsules 3246

Prochlorperazine (Co-administration may result in an additive impairment of motor skills).
Products include:
Compazine 1505

Promethazine Hydrochloride (Co-administration may result in an additive impairment of motor skills).
Products include:
Mepergan Injection 3539
Phenergan Injection 3553
Phenergan 3556
Phenergan Syrup 3554
Phenergan with Codeine Syrup 3557
Phenergan with Dextromethorphan Syrup 3559
Phenergan VC Syrup 3560
Phenergan VC with Codeine Syrup .. 3561

Propofol (Co-administration may result in an additive impairment of motor skills). Products include:
Diprivan Injectable Emulsion 667

Propoxyphene Hydrochloride (Co-administration may result in an additive impairment of motor skills).
Products include:
Darvon Pulvules 1909
Darvon Compound-65 Pulvules 1910

Propoxyphene Napsylate (Co-administration may result in an additive impairment of motor skills).
Products include:
Darvon-N/Darvocet-N 1907
Darvon-N Tablets 1912

Quazepam (Co-administration may result in an additive impairment of motor skills).
No products indexed under this heading.

Quetiapine Fumarate (Co-administration may result in an additive impairment of motor skills).
Products include:
Seroquel Tablets 684

Remifentanil Hydrochloride (Co-administration may result in an additive impairment of motor skills).
No products indexed under this heading.

Risperidone (Co-administration may result in an additive impairment of motor skills). Products include:
Risperdal 1796

Secobarbital Sodium (Co-administration may result in an additive impairment of motor skills).
No products indexed under this heading.

Selegiline Hydrochloride (Co-administration of antidepressants and MAO inhibitors has resulted in serious, and sometimes fatal, reactions including hyperthermia, autonomic instability, seizures, agitation, and coma; concurrent and/or sequential use is contraindicated).
Products include:
Eldepryl Capsules 3266

Sevoflurane (Co-administration may result in an additive impairment of motor skills).
No products indexed under this heading.

Sufentanil Citrate (Co-administration may result in an additive impairment of motor skills).
No products indexed under this heading.

Temazepam (Co-administration may result in an additive impairment of motor skills).
No products indexed under this heading.

Thiamylal Sodium (Co-administration may result in an additive impairment of motor skills).
No products indexed under this heading.

Thioridazine Hydrochloride (Co-administration may result in an additive impairment of motor skills).
Products include:
Thioridazine Hydrochloride Tablets 2289

Thiothixene (Co-administration may result in an additive impairment of motor skills). Products include:
Navane Capsules 2701
Thiothixene Capsules 2290

Tranylcypromine Sulfate (Co-administration of antidepressants and MAO inhibitors has resulted in serious, and sometimes fatal, reactions including hyperthermia, autonomic instability, seizures, agitation, and coma; concurrent and/or sequential use is contraindicated).
Products include:
Parnate Tablets 1607

Triazolam (Co-administration may result in an additive impairment of motor skills). Products include:
- Halcion Tablets ... 2823

Trifluoperazine Hydrochloride (Co-administration may result in an additive impairment of motor skills). Products include:
- Stelazine ... 1640

Zaleplon (Co-administration may result in an additive impairment of motor skills). Products include:
- Sonata Capsules ... 3591

Ziprasidone Hydrochloride (Co-administration may result in an additive impairment of motor skills). Products include:
- Geodon Capsules ... 2688

Zolpidem Tartrate (Co-administration may result in an additive impairment of motor skills). Products include:
- Ambien Tablets ... 3191

Food Interactions

Alcohol (Co-administration has shown to result in an additive impairment of motor skills).

Food, unspecified (The presence of food in the stomach has a minimal effect on both the rate and extent of absorption and does not require a dosage adjustment).

REMERON SOLTAB TABLETS

(Mirtazapine) ... 2486

May interact with central nervous system depressants, monoamine oxidase inhibitors, and certain other agents. Compounds in these categories include:

Alfentanil Hydrochloride (Co-administration may result in an additive impairment of motor skills).
No products indexed under this heading.

Alprazolam (Co-administration may result in an additive impairment of motor skills). Products include:
- Xanax Tablets ... 2865

Aprobarbital (Co-administration may result in an additive impairment of motor skills).
No products indexed under this heading.

Buprenorphine Hydrochloride (Co-administration may result in an additive impairment of motor skills). Products include:
- Buprenex Injectable ... 2918

Buspirone Hydrochloride (Co-administration may result in an additive impairment of motor skills).
No products indexed under this heading.

Butabarbital (Co-administration may result in an additive impairment of motor skills).
No products indexed under this heading.

Butalbital (Co-administration may result in an additive impairment of motor skills). Products include:
- Phrenilin ... 578
- Sedapap Tablets 50 mg/650 mg ... 2225

Chlordiazepoxide (Co-administration may result in an additive impairment of motor skills). Products include:
- Limbitrol ... 1738

Chlordiazepoxide Hydrochloride (Co-administration may result in an additive impairment of motor skills). Products include:
- Librium Capsules ... 1736
- Librium for Injection ... 1737

Chlorpromazine (Co-administration may result in an additive impairment of motor skills). Products include:
- Thorazine Suppositories ... 1656

Chlorpromazine Hydrochloride (Co-administration may result in an additive impairment of motor skills). Products include:
- Thorazine ... 1656

Chlorprothixene (Co-administration may result in an additive impairment of motor skills).
No products indexed under this heading.

Chlorprothixene Hydrochloride (Co-administration may result in an additive impairment of motor skills).
No products indexed under this heading.

Chlorprothixene Lactate (Co-administration may result in an additive impairment of motor skills).
No products indexed under this heading.

Clorazepate Dipotassium (Co-administration may result in an additive impairment of motor skills). Products include:
- Tranxene ... 511

Clozapine (Co-administration may result in an additive impairment of motor skills). Products include:
- Clozaril Tablets ... 2319

Codeine Phosphate (Co-administration may result in an additive impairment of motor skills). Products include:
- Phenergan with Codeine Syrup ... 3557
- Phenergan VC with Codeine Syrup ... 3561
- Robitussin A-C Syrup ... 2942
- Robitussin-DAC Syrup ... 2942
- Ryna-C Liquid ... ▣768
- Soma Compound w/Codeine Tablets ... 3355
- Tussi-Organidin NR Liquid ... 3350
- Tussi-Organidin-S NR Liquid ... 3350
- Tylenol with Codeine ... 2595

Desflurane (Co-administration may result in an additive impairment of motor skills). Products include:
- Suprane Liquid for Inhalation ... 874

Dezocine (Co-administration may result in an additive impairment of motor skills).
No products indexed under this heading.

Diazepam (Co-administration has shown to result in an additive impairment of motor skills). Products include:
- Valium Injectable ... 3026
- Valium Tablets ... 3047

Droperidol (Co-administration may result in an additive impairment of motor skills).
No products indexed under this heading.

Enflurane (Co-administration may result in an additive impairment of motor skills).
No products indexed under this heading.

Estazolam (Co-administration may result in an additive impairment of motor skills). Products include:
- ProSom Tablets ... 500

Ethchlorvynol (Co-administration may result in an additive impairment of motor skills).
No products indexed under this heading.

Ethinamate (Co-administration may result in an additive impairment of motor skills).
No products indexed under this heading.

Fentanyl (Co-administration may result in an additive impairment of motor skills). Products include:
- Duragesic Transdermal System ... 1786

Fentanyl Citrate (Co-administration may result in an additive impairment of motor skills). Products include:
- Actiq ... 1184

Fluphenazine Decanoate (Co-administration may result in an additive impairment of motor skills).
No products indexed under this heading.

Fluphenazine Enanthate (Co-administration may result in an additive impairment of motor skills).
No products indexed under this heading.

Fluphenazine Hydrochloride (Co-administration may result in an additive impairment of motor skills).
No products indexed under this heading.

Flurazepam Hydrochloride (Co-administration may result in an additive impairment of motor skills).
No products indexed under this heading.

Glutethimide (Co-administration may result in an additive impairment of motor skills).
No products indexed under this heading.

Haloperidol (Co-administration may result in an additive impairment of motor skills). Products include:
- Haldol Injection, Tablets and Concentrate ... 2533

Haloperidol Decanoate (Co-administration may result in an additive impairment of motor skills). Products include:
- Haldol Decanoate ... 2535

Hydrocodone Bitartrate (Co-administration may result in an additive impairment of motor skills). Products include:
- Hycodan ... 1316
- Hycomine Compound Tablets ... 1317
- Hycotuss Expectorant Syrup ... 1318
- Lortab ... 3319
- Lortab Elixir ... 3317
- Maxidone Tablets CIII ... 3399
- Norco 5/325 Tablets CIII ... 3424
- Norco 7.5/325 Tablets CIII ... 3425
- Norco 10/325 Tablets CIII ... 3427
- Norco 10/325 Tablets CIII ... 3425
- Vicodin Tablets ... 516
- Vicodin ES Tablets ... 517
- Vicodin HP Tablets ... 518
- Vicodin Tuss Expectorant ... 519
- Vicoprofen Tablets ... 520
- Zydone Tablets ... 1330

Hydrocodone Polistirex (Co-administration may result in an additive impairment of motor skills). Products include:
- Tussionex Pennkinetic Extended-Release Suspension ... 1174

Hydromorphone Hydrochloride (Co-administration may result in an additive impairment of motor skills). Products include:
- Dilaudid ... 441
- Dilaudid Oral Liquid ... 445
- Dilaudid Powder ... 441
- Dilaudid Rectal Suppositories ... 441
- Dilaudid Tablets ... 441
- Dilaudid Tablets - 8 mg ... 445
- Dilaudid-HP ... 443

Hydroxyzine Hydrochloride (Co-administration may result in an additive impairment of motor skills). Products include:
- Atarax Tablets & Syrup ... 2667
- Vistaril Intramuscular Solution ... 2738

Isocarboxazid (Co-administration of antidepressants and MAO inhibitors has resulted in serious, and sometimes fatal, reactions including hyperthermia, autonomic instability, seizures, agitation, and coma; concurrent and/or sequential use is contraindicated).
No products indexed under this heading.

Isoflurane (Co-administration may result in an additive impairment of motor skills).
No products indexed under this heading.

Ketamine Hydrochloride (Co-administration may result in an additive impairment of motor skills).
No products indexed under this heading.

Levomethadyl Acetate Hydrochloride (Co-administration may result in an additive impairment of motor skills).
No products indexed under this heading.

Levorphanol Tartrate (Co-administration may result in an additive impairment of motor skills). Products include:
- Levo-Dromoran ... 1734
- Levorphanol Tartrate Tablets ... 3059

Lorazepam (Co-administration may result in an additive impairment of motor skills). Products include:
- Ativan Injection ... 3478
- Ativan Tablets ... 3482

Loxapine Hydrochloride (Co-administration may result in an additive impairment of motor skills).
No products indexed under this heading.

Loxapine Succinate (Co-administration may result in an additive impairment of motor skills). Products include:
- Loxitane Capsules ... 3398

Meperidine Hydrochloride (Co-administration may result in an additive impairment of motor skills). Products include:
- Demerol ... 3079
- Mepergan Injection ... 3539

Mephobarbital (Co-administration may result in an additive impairment of motor skills).
No products indexed under this heading.

Meprobamate (Co-administration may result in an additive impairment of motor skills). Products include:
- Miltown Tablets ... 3349

Mesoridazine Besylate (Co-administration may result in an additive impairment of motor skills). Products include:
- Serentil ... 1057

Methadone Hydrochloride (Co-administration may result in an additive impairment of motor skills). Products include:
- Dolophine Hydrochloride Tablets ... 3056

Methohexital Sodium (Co-administration may result in an additive impairment of motor skills). Products include:
- Brevital Sodium for Injection, USP ... 1815

Methotrimeprazine (Co-administration may result in an additive impairment of motor skills).
No products indexed under this heading.

Methoxyflurane (Co-administration may result in an additive impairment of motor skills).
No products indexed under this heading.

Midazolam Hydrochloride (Co-administration may result in an additive impairment of motor skills). Products include:
- Versed Injection ... 3027
- Versed Syrup ... 3033

Moclobemide (Co-administration of antidepressants and MAO inhibitors has resulted in serious, and sometimes fatal, reactions including hyperthermia, autonomic instability, seizures, agitation, and coma; concurrent and/or sequential use is contraindicated).
No products indexed under this heading.

Molindone Hydrochloride (Co-administration may result in an additive impairment of motor skills). Products include:
- Moban ... 1320

Morphine Sulfate (Co-administration may result in an additive impairment of motor skills). Products include:
- Astramorph/PF Injection, USP (Preservative-Free) ... 594

Duramorph Injection 1312
Infumorph 200 and Infumorph 500 Sterile Solutions 1314
Kadian Capsules 1335
MS Contin Tablets 2896
MSIR 2898
Oramorph SR Tablets 3062
Roxanol 3066

Olanzapine (Co-administration may result in an additive impairment of motor skills). Products include:
Zyprexa Tablets 1973
Zyprexa ZYDIS Orally Disintegrating Tablets 1973

Oxazepam (Co-administration may result in an additive impairment of motor skills).
No products indexed under this heading.

Oxycodone Hydrochloride (Co-administration may result in an additive impairment of motor skills). Products include:
OxyContin Tablets 2912
OxyFast Oral Concentrate Solution . 2916
OxyIR Capsules 2916
Percocet Tablets 1326
Percodan Tablets 1327
Percolone Tablets 1327
Roxicodone 3067
Tylox Capsules 2597

Pargyline Hydrochloride (Co-administration of antidepressants and MAO inhibitors has resulted in serious, and sometimes fatal, reactions including hyperthermia, autonomic instability, seizures, agitation, and coma; concurrent and/or sequential use is contraindicated).
No products indexed under this heading.

Pentobarbital Sodium (Co-administration may result in an additive impairment of motor skills). Products include:
Nembutal Sodium Solution 485

Perphenazine (Co-administration may result in an additive impairment of motor skills). Products include:
Etrafon 3115
Trilafon 3160

Phenelzine Sulfate (Co-administration of antidepressants and MAO inhibitors has resulted in serious, and sometimes fatal, reactions including hyperthermia, autonomic instability, seizures, agitation, and coma; concurrent and/or sequential use is contraindicated). Products include:
Nardil Tablets 2653

Phenobarbital (Co-administration may result in an additive impairment of motor skills). Products include:
Arco-Lase Plus Tablets 592
Donnatal 2929
Donnatal Extentabs 2930

Prazepam (Co-administration may result in an additive impairment of motor skills).
No products indexed under this heading.

Procarbazine Hydrochloride (Co-administration of antidepressants and MAO inhibitors has resulted in serious, and sometimes fatal, reactions including hyperthermia, autonomic instability, seizures, agitation, and coma; concurrent and/or sequential use is contraindicated). Products include:
Matulane Capsules 3246

Prochlorperazine (Co-administration may result in an additive impairment of motor skills). Products include:
Compazine 1505

Promethazine Hydrochloride (Co-administration may result in an additive impairment of motor skills). Products include:
Mepergan Injection 3539
Phenergan Injection 3553
Phenergan 3556
Phenergan Syrup 3554
Phenergan with Codeine Syrup 3557
Phenergan with Dextromethorphan Syrup 3559
Phenergan VC Syrup 3560
Phenergan VC with Codeine Syrup .. 3561

Propofol (Co-administration may result in an additive impairment of motor skills). Products include:
Diprivan Injectable Emulsion 667

Propoxyphene Hydrochloride (Co-administration may result in an additive impairment of motor skills). Products include:
Darvon Pulvules 1909
Darvon Compound-65 Pulvules 1910

Propoxyphene Napsylate (Co-administration may result in an additive impairment of motor skills). Products include:
Darvon-N/Darvocet-N 1907
Darvon-N Tablets 1912

Quazepam (Co-administration may result in an additive impairment of motor skills).
No products indexed under this heading.

Quetiapine Fumarate (Co-administration may result in an additive impairment of motor skills). Products include:
Seroquel Tablets 684

Remifentanil Hydrochloride (Co-administration may result in an additive impairment of motor skills).
No products indexed under this heading.

Risperidone (Co-administration may result in an additive impairment of motor skills). Products include:
Risperdal 1796

Secobarbital Sodium (Co-administration may result in an additive impairment of motor skills).
No products indexed under this heading.

Selegiline Hydrochloride (Co-administration of antidepressants and MAO inhibitors has resulted in serious, and sometimes fatal, reactions including hyperthermia, autonomic instability, seizures, agitation, and coma; concurrent and/or sequential use is contraindicated). Products include:
Eldepryl Capsules 3266

Sevoflurane (Co-administration may result in an additive impairment of motor skills).
No products indexed under this heading.

Sufentanil Citrate (Co-administration may result in an additive impairment of motor skills).
No products indexed under this heading.

Temazepam (Co-administration may result in an additive impairment of motor skills).
No products indexed under this heading.

Thiamylal Sodium (Co-administration may result in an additive impairment of motor skills).
No products indexed under this heading.

Thioridazine Hydrochloride (Co-administration may result in an additive impairment of motor skills). Products include:
Thioridazine Hydrochloride Tablets 2289

Thiothixene (Co-administration may result in an additive impairment of motor skills). Products include:
Navane Capsules 2701
Thiothixene Capsules 2290

Tranylcypromine Sulfate (Co-administration of antidepressants and MAO inhibitors has resulted in serious, and sometimes fatal, reactions including hyperthermia, autonomic instability, seizures, agitation, and coma; concurrent and/or sequential use is contraindicated). Products include:
Parnate Tablets 1607

Triazolam (Co-administration may result in an additive impairment of motor skills). Products include:
Halcion Tablets 2823

Trifluoperazine Hydrochloride (Co-administration may result in an additive impairment of motor skills). Products include:
Stelazine 1640

Zaleplon (Co-administration may result in an additive impairment of motor skills). Products include:
Sonata Capsules 3591

Ziprasidone Hydrochloride (Co-administration may result in an additive impairment of motor skills). Products include:
Geodon Capsules 2688

Zolpidem Tartrate (Co-administration may result in an additive impairment of motor skills). Products include:
Ambien Tablets 3191

Food Interactions

Alcohol (Co-administration has shown to result in an additive impairment of motor skills).

Food, unspecified (The presence of food in the stomach has a minimal effect on both the rate and extent of absorption and does not require a dosage adjustment).

REMICADE FOR IV INJECTION
(Infliximab) 1178
None cited in PDR database.

REMIFEMIN MENOPAUSE TABLETS
(Black Cohosh) 839
None cited in PDR database.

REMINYL ORAL SOLUTION
(Galantamine Hydrobromide) 1792
See Reminyl Tablets

REMINYL TABLETS
(Galantamine Hydrobromide) 1792
May interact with anticholinergics, cholinergic agents, erythromycin, neuromuscular blocking agents, nonsteroidal anti-inflammatory agents, and certain other agents. Compounds in these categories include:

Atracurium Besylate (Galantamine is a cholinesterase inhibitor; co-administration with neuromuscular blocking agents may exaggerate neuromuscular blockade).
No products indexed under this heading.

Atropine Sulfate (Galantamine has the potential to interfere with the activity of anticholinergic agents). Products include:
Donnatal 2929
Donnatal Extentabs 2930
Motofen Tablets 577
Prosed/DS Tablets 3268
Urised Tablets 2876

Belladonna Alkaloids (Galantamine has the potential to interfere with the activity of anticholinergic agents). Products include:
Hyland's Teething Tablets 766
Urimax Tablets 1769

Benztropine Mesylate (Galantamine has the potential to interfere with the activity of anticholinergic agents). Products include:
Cogentin 2055

Bethanechol Chloride (Co-administration with other cholinesterase inhibitors or cholinergic agonists may result in a synergistic effect). Products include:
Urecholine 2198
Urecholine Tablets 2445

Biperiden Hydrochloride (Galantamine has the potential to interfere with the activity of anticholinergic agents). Products include:
Akineton 402

Celecoxib (Cholinomimetics, such as galantamine, may be expected to increase gastric acid secretion; therefore, co-administration in patients with increased risk of developing gastric ulcers or bleeding, such as patients on NSAIDs, should be closely monitored). Products include:
Celebrex Capsules 2676
Celebrex Capsules 2780

Cevimeline Hydrochloride (Co-administration with other cholinesterase inhibitors or cholinergic agonists may result in a synergistic effect). Products include:
Evoxac Capsules 1217

Cimetidine (Co-administration with cimetidine has resulted in increased bioavailability galantamine by approximately 16%). Products include:
Tagamet HB 200 Suspension 762
Tagamet HB 200 Tablets 761
Tagamet Tablets 1644

Cimetidine Hydrochloride (Co-administration with cimetidine has resulted in increased bioavailability galantamine by approximately 16%). Products include:
Tagamet 1644

Cisatracurium Besylate (Galantamine is a cholinesterase inhibitor; co-administration with neuromuscular blocking agents may exaggerate neuromuscular blockade).
No products indexed under this heading.

Clidinium Bromide (Galantamine has the potential to interfere with the activity of anticholinergic agents).
No products indexed under this heading.

Diclofenac Potassium (Cholinomimetics, such as galantamine, may be expected to increase gastric acid secretion; therefore, co-administration in patients with increased risk of developing gastric ulcers or bleeding, such as patients on NSAIDs, should be closely monitored). Products include:
Cataflam Tablets 2315

Diclofenac Sodium (Cholinomimetics, such as galantamine, may be expected to increase gastric acid secretion; therefore, co-administration in patients with increased risk of developing gastric ulcers or bleeding, such as patients on NSAIDs, should be closely monitored). Products include:
Arthrotec Tablets 3195
Voltaren Ophthalmic Sterile Ophthalmic Solution 312
Voltaren Tablets 2315
Voltaren-XR Tablets 2315

Dicyclomine Hydrochloride (Galantamine has the potential to interfere with the activity of anticholinergic agents).
No products indexed under this heading.

Digoxin (Co-administration in a healthy subject has resulted in 2nd and 3rd degree heart block and bradycardia). Products include:
Digitek Tablets 1003
Lanoxicaps Capsules 1574
Lanoxin Injection 1581
Lanoxin Tablets 1587
Lanoxin Elixir Pediatric 1578
Lanoxin Injection Pediatric 1584

Donepezil Hydrochloride (Co-administration with other cholinesterase inhibitors or cholinergic agonists may result in a synergistic effect). Products include:
Aricept Tablets 1270
Aricept Tablets 2665

Doxacurium Chloride (Galantamine is a cholinesterase inhibitor; co-administration with neuromuscular blocking agents may exaggerate neuromuscular blockade).
No products indexed under this heading.

Edrophonium Chloride (Co-administration with other cholinesterase inhibitors or cholinergic agonists may result in a synergistic effect). Products include:

Tensilon Injectable ... 1745

Erythromycin (Co-administration with a moderate inhibitor of CYP3A4, such as erythromycin, increases the AUC of galantamine by 10%). Products include:

Emgel 2% Topical Gel ... 1285
Ery-Tab Tablets ... 448
Erythromycin Base Filmtab Tablets . 454
Erythromycin Delayed-Release Capsules, USP ... 455
PCE Dispertab Tablets ... 498

Erythromycin Estolate (Co-administration with a moderate inhibitor of CYP3A4, such as erythromycin, increases the AUC of galantamine by 10%).

No products indexed under this heading.

Erythromycin Ethylsuccinate (Co-administration with a moderate inhibitor of CYP3A4, such as erythromycin, increases the AUC of galantamine by 10%). Products include:

E.E.S. ... 450
EryPed ... 446
Pediazole Suspension ... 3050

Erythromycin Gluceptate (Co-administration with a moderate inhibitor of CYP3A4, such as erythromycin, increases the AUC of galantamine by 10%).

No products indexed under this heading.

Erythromycin Stearate (Co-administration with a moderate inhibitor of CYP3A4, such as erythromycin, increases the AUC of galantamine by 10%). Products include:

Erythrocin Stearate Filmtab Tablets ... 452

Etodolac (Cholinomimetics, such as galantamine, may be expected to increase gastric acid secretion; therefore, co-administration in patients with increased risk of developing gastric ulcers or bleeding, such as patients on NSAIDs, should be closely monitored). Products include:

Lodine ... 3528
Lodine XL Extended-Release Tablets ... 3530

Fenoprofen Calcium (Cholinomimetics, such as galantamine, may be expected to increase gastric acid secretion; therefore, co-administration in patients with increased risk of developing gastric ulcers or bleeding, such as patients on NSAIDs, should be closely monitored).

No products indexed under this heading.

Flurbiprofen (Cholinomimetics, such as galantamine, may be expected to increase gastric acid secretion; therefore, co-administration in patients with increased risk of developing gastric ulcers or bleeding, such as patients on NSAIDs, should be closely monitored).

No products indexed under this heading.

Glycopyrrolate (Galantamine has the potential to interfere with the activity of anticholinergic agents). Products include:

Robinul Forte Tablets ... 1358
Robinul Injectable ... 2940
Robinul Tablets ... 1358

Hyoscyamine (Galantamine has the potential to interfere with the activity of anticholinergic agents). Products include:

Urised Tablets ... 2876

Hyoscyamine Sulfate (Galantamine has the potential to interfere with the activity of anticholinergic agents). Products include:

Arco-Lase Plus Tablets ... 592
Donnatal ... 2929
Donnatal Extentabs ... 2930
Levsin/Levsinex/Levbid ... 3172
NuLev Orally Disintegrating Tablets ... 3176
Prosed/DS Tablets ... 3268
Urimax Tablets ... 1769

Ibuprofen (Cholinomimetics, such as galantamine, may be expected to increase gastric acid secretion; therefore, co-administration in patients with increased risk of developing gastric ulcers or bleeding, such as patients on NSAIDs, should be closely monitored). Products include:

Advil ... ■771
Children's Advil Oral Suspension ... ■773
Children's Advil Chewable Tablets ... ■773
Advil Cold and Sinus Caplets ... ■771
Advil Cold and Sinus Tablets ... ■771
Advil Flu & Body Ache Caplets ... ■772
Infants' Advil Drops ... ■773
Junior Strength Advil Tablets ... ■773
Junior Strength Advil Chewable Tablets ... ■773
Advil Migraine Liquigels ... ■772
Children's Motrin Oral Suspension and Chewable Tablets ... 2006
Children's Motrin Cold Oral Suspension ... 2007
Children's Motrin Oral Suspension ... ■643
Motrin Suspension, Oral Drops, Chewable Tablets, and Caplets ... 2002
Infants' Motrin Concentrated Drops ... 2006
Junior Strength Motrin Caplets and Chewable Tablets ... 2006
Motrin IB Tablets, Caplets, and Gelcaps ... 2002
Motrin Migraine Pain Caplets ... 2005
Motrin Sinus Headache Caplets ... 2005
Vicoprofen Tablets ... 520

Indomethacin (Cholinomimetics, such as galantamine, may be expected to increase gastric acid secretion; therefore, co-administration in patients with increased risk of developing gastric ulcers or bleeding, such as patients on NSAIDs, should be closely monitored). Products include:

Indocin ... 2112

Indomethacin Sodium Trihydrate (Cholinomimetics, such as galantamine, may be expected to increase gastric acid secretion; therefore, co-administration in patients with increased risk of developing gastric ulcers or bleeding, such as patients on NSAIDs, should be closely monitored). Products include:

Indocin I.V. ... 2115

Ipratropium Bromide (Galantamine has the potential to interfere with the activity of anticholinergic agents). Products include:

Atrovent Inhalation Aerosol ... 1030
Atrovent Inhalation Solution ... 1031
Atrovent Nasal Spray 0.03% ... 1032
Atrovent Nasal Spray 0.06% ... 1033
Combivent Inhalation Aerosol ... 1041
DuoNeb Inhalation Solution ... 1233

Ketoconazole (Co-administration with a potent inhibitor of CYP3A4, such as ketoconazole, increases the AUC of galantamine by 30%). Products include:

Nizoral 2% Cream ... 3620
Nizoral A-D Shampoo ... 2008
Nizoral 2% Shampoo ... 2007
Nizoral Tablets ... 1791

Ketoprofen (Cholinomimetics, such as galantamine, may be expected to increase gastric acid secretion; therefore, co-administration in patients with increased risk of developing gastric ulcers or bleeding, such as patients on NSAIDs, should be closely monitored). Products include:

Orudis Capsules ... 3548
Orudis KT Tablets ... ■778
Oruvail Capsules ... 3548

Ketorolac Tromethamine (Cholinomimetics, such as galantamine, may be expected to increase gastric acid secretion; therefore, co-administration in patients with increased risk of developing gastric ulcers or bleeding, such as patients on NSAIDs, should be closely monitored). Products include:

Acular Ophthalmic Solution ... 544
Acular PF Ophthalmic Solution ... 544
Toradol ... 3018

Meclofenamate Sodium (Cholinomimetics, such as galantamine, may be expected to increase gastric acid secretion; therefore, co-administration in patients with increased risk of developing gastric ulcers or bleeding, such as patients on NSAIDs, should be closely monitored).

No products indexed under this heading.

Mefenamic Acid (Cholinomimetics, such as galantamine, may be expected to increase gastric acid secretion; therefore, co-administration in patients with increased risk of developing gastric ulcers or bleeding, such as patients on NSAIDs, should be closely monitored). Products include:

Ponstel Capsules ... 1356

Meloxicam (Cholinomimetics, such as galantamine, may be expected to increase gastric acid secretion; therefore, co-administration in patients with increased risk of developing gastric ulcers or bleeding, such as patients on NSAIDs, should be closely monitored). Products include:

Mobic Tablets ... 1054

Mepenzolate Bromide (Galantamine has the potential to interfere with the activity of anticholinergic agents).

No products indexed under this heading.

Metocurine Iodide (Galantamine is a cholinesterase inhibitor; co-administration with neuromuscular blocking agents may exaggerate neuromuscular blockade).

No products indexed under this heading.

Mivacurium Chloride (Galantamine is a cholinesterase inhibitor; co-administration with neuromuscular blocking agents may exaggerate neuromuscular blockade).

No products indexed under this heading.

Nabumetone (Cholinomimetics, such as galantamine, may be expected to increase gastric acid secretion; therefore, co-administration in patients with increased risk of developing gastric ulcers or bleeding, such as patients on NSAIDs, should be closely monitored). Products include:

Relafen Tablets ... 1617

Naproxen (Cholinomimetics, such as galantamine, may be expected to increase gastric acid secretion; therefore, co-administration in patients with increased risk of developing gastric ulcers or bleeding, such as patients on NSAIDs, should be closely monitored). Products include:

EC-Naprosyn Delayed-Release Tablets ... 2967
Naprosyn Suspension ... 2967
Naprosyn Tablets ... 2967

Naproxen Sodium (Cholinomimetics, such as galantamine, may be expected to increase gastric acid secretion; therefore, co-administration in patients with increased risk of developing gastric ulcers or bleeding, such as patients on NSAIDs, should be closely monitored). Products include:

Aleve Tablets, Caplets and Gelcaps ... ■602
Aleve Cold & Sinus Caplets ... ■603
Anaprox Tablets ... 2967
Anaprox DS Tablets ... 2967
Naprelan Tablets ... 1293

Neostigmine Bromide (Co-administration with other cholinesterase inhibitors or cholinergic agonists may result in a synergistic effect). Products include:

Prostigmin Tablets ... 1744

Neostigmine Methylsulfate (Co-administration with other cholinesterase inhibitors or cholinergic agonists may result in a synergistic effect). Products include:

Prostigmin Injectable ... 1744

Oxaprozin (Cholinomimetics, such as galantamine, may be expected to increase gastric acid secretion; therefore, co-administration in patients with increased risk of developing gastric ulcers or bleeding, such as patients on NSAIDs, should be closely monitored).

No products indexed under this heading.

Oxybutynin Chloride (Galantamine has the potential to interfere with the activity of anticholinergic agents). Products include:

Ditropan XL Extended Release Tablets ... 564

Pancuronium Bromide (Galantamine is a cholinesterase inhibitor; co-administration with neuromuscular blocking agents may exaggerate neuromuscular blockade).

No products indexed under this heading.

Paroxetine Hydrochloride (Co-administration with a strong inhibitor of CYP3A4 and CYP2D6, such as ketoconazole, results in increased AUC of galantamine by 30%). Products include:

Paxil ... 1609

Phenylbutazone (Cholinomimetics, such as galantamine, may be expected to increase gastric acid secretion; therefore, co-administration in patients with increased risk of developing gastric ulcers or bleeding, such as patients on NSAIDs, should be closely monitored).

No products indexed under this heading.

Piroxicam (Cholinomimetics, such as galantamine, may be expected to increase gastric acid secretion; therefore, co-administration in patients with increased risk of developing gastric ulcers or bleeding, such as patients on NSAIDs, should be closely monitored). Products include:

Feldene Capsules ... 2685

Procyclidine Hydrochloride (Galantamine has the potential to interfere with the activity of anticholinergic agents).

No products indexed under this heading.

Propantheline Bromide (Galantamine has the potential to interfere with the activity of anticholinergic agents).

No products indexed under this heading.

Pyridostigmine Bromide (Co-administration with other cholinesterase inhibitors or cholinergic agonists may result in a synergistic effect). Products include:

Mestinon ... 1740

Rapacuronium Bromide (Galantamine is a cholinesterase inhibitor; co-administration with neuromuscular blocking agents may exaggerate

neuromuscular blockade).
No products indexed under this heading.

Rivastigmine Tartrate (Co-administration with other cholinesterase inhibitors or cholinergic agonists may result in a synergistic effect). Products include:
Exelon Capsules 2342
Exelon Oral Solution 2345

Rocuronium Bromide (Galantamine is a cholinesterase inhibitor; co-administration with neuromuscular blocking agents may exaggerate neuromuscular blockade). Products include:
Zemuron Injection 2491

Rofecoxib (Cholinomimetics, such as galantamine, may be expected to increase gastric acid secretion; therefore, co-administration in patients with increased risk of developing gastric ulcers or bleeding, such as patients on NSAIDs, should be closely monitored). Products include:
Vioxx 2213

Scopolamine (Galantamine has the potential to interfere with the activity of anticholinergic agents). Products include:
Transderm Scōp Transdermal Therapeutic System 2302

Scopolamine Hydrobromide (Galantamine has the potential to interfere with the activity of anticholinergic agents). Products include:
Donnatal 2929
Donnatal Extentabs 2930

Succinylcholine Chloride (Galantamine is a cholinesterase inhibitor; co-administration with neuromuscular blocking agents may exaggerate neuromuscular blockade). Products include:
Anectine Injection 1476

Sulindac (Cholinomimetics, such as galantamine, may be expected to increase gastric acid secretion; therefore, co-administration in patients with increased risk of developing gastric ulcers or bleeding, such as patients on NSAIDs, should be closely monitored). Products include:
Clinoril Tablets 2053

Tacrine Hydrochloride (Co-administration with other cholinesterase inhibitors or cholinergic agonists may result in a synergistic effect). Products include:
Cognex Capsules 1351

Tolmetin Sodium (Cholinomimetics, such as galantamine, may be expected to increase gastric acid secretion; therefore, co-administration in patients with increased risk of developing gastric ulcers or bleeding, such as patients on NSAIDs, should be closely monitored). Products include:
Tolectin 2589

Tolterodine Tartrate (Galantamine has the potential to interfere with the activity of anticholinergic agents). Products include:
Detrol Tablets 3623
Detrol LA Capsules 2801

Tridihexethyl Chloride (Galantamine has the potential to interfere with the activity of anticholinergic agents).
No products indexed under this heading.

Trihexyphenidyl Hydrochloride (Galantamine has the potential to interfere with the activity of anticholinergic agents). Products include:
Artane 1855

Vecuronium Bromide (Galantamine is a cholinesterase inhibitor; co-administration with neuromuscular blocking agents may exaggerate neuromuscular blockade). Products include:
Norcuron for Injection 2478

RENAGEL CAPSULES
(Sevelamer Hydrochloride) 1439
None cited in PDR database.

RENAGEL TABLETS
(Sevelamer Hydrochloride) 1439
None cited in PDR database.

RENESE TABLETS
(Polythiazide) 2712
May interact with antihypertensives, barbiturates, corticosteroids, cardiac glycosides, insulin, narcotic analgesics, and certain other agents. Compounds in these categories include:

Acebutolol Hydrochloride (Thiazides may add to or potentiate the action of other antihypertensives). Products include:
Sectral Capsules 3589

ACTH (Hypokalemia may develop with thiazides during concomitant ACTH).
No products indexed under this heading.

Alfentanil Hydrochloride (Orthostatic hypotension may be aggravated by narcotics).
No products indexed under this heading.

Amlodipine Besylate (Thiazides may add to or potentiate the action of other antihypertensives). Products include:
Lotrel Capsules 2370
Norvasc Tablets 2704

Aprobarbital (Orthostatic hypotension may be aggravated by barbiturates).
No products indexed under this heading.

Atenolol (Thiazides may add to or potentiate the action of other antihypertensives). Products include:
Tenoretic Tablets 690
Tenormin I.V. Injection 692

Benazepril Hydrochloride (Thiazides may add to or potentiate the action of other antihypertensives). Products include:
Lotensin Tablets 2365
Lotensin HCT Tablets 2367
Lotrel Capsules 2370

Bendroflumethiazide (Thiazides may add to or potentiate the action of other antihypertensives). Products include:
Corzide 40/5 Tablets 2247
Corzide 80/5 Tablets 2247

Betamethasone Acetate (Hypokalemia may develop with thiazides during concomitant corticosteroids). Products include:
Celestone Soluspan Injectable Suspension 3097

Betamethasone Sodium Phosphate (Hypokalemia may develop with thiazides during concomitant corticosteroids). Products include:
Celestone Soluspan Injectable Suspension 3097

Betaxolol Hydrochloride (Thiazides may add to or potentiate the action of other antihypertensives). Products include:
Betoptic S Ophthalmic Suspension 537

Bisoprolol Fumarate (Thiazides may add to or potentiate the action of other antihypertensives). Products include:
Zebeta Tablets 1885
Ziac Tablets 1887

Buprenorphine Hydrochloride (Orthostatic hypotension may be aggravated by narcotics). Products include:
Buprenex Injectable 2918

Butabarbital (Orthostatic hypotension may be aggravated by barbiturates).
No products indexed under this heading.

Butalbital (Orthostatic hypotension may be aggravated by barbiturates). Products include:
Phrenilin 578
Sedapap Tablets 50 mg/650 mg 2225

Candesartan Cilexetil (Thiazides may add to or potentiate the action of other antihypertensives). Products include:
Atacand Tablets 595
Atacand HCT Tablets 597

Captopril (Thiazides may add to or potentiate the action of other antihypertensives). Products include:
Captopril Tablets 2281

Carteolol Hydrochloride (Thiazides may add to or potentiate the action of other antihypertensives). Products include:
Carteolol Hydrochloride Ophthalmic Solution USP, 1% .... ⊙258
Ocupress Ophthalmic Solution, 1% Sterile .... ⊙303

Chlorothiazide (Thiazides may add to or potentiate the action of other antihypertensives). Products include:
Aldoclor Tablets 2035
Diuril Oral 2087

Chlorothiazide Sodium (Thiazides may add to or potentiate the action of other antihypertensives). Products include:
Diuril Sodium Intravenous 2086

Chlorthalidone (Thiazides may add to or potentiate the action of other antihypertensives). Products include:
Clorpres Tablets 1002
Combipres Tablets 1040
Tenoretic Tablets 690

Clonidine (Thiazides may add to or potentiate the action of other antihypertensives). Products include:
Catapres-TTS 1038

Clonidine Hydrochloride (Thiazides may add to or potentiate the action of other antihypertensives). Products include:
Catapres Tablets 1037
Clorpres Tablets 1002
Combipres Tablets 1040
Duraclon Injection 3057

Codeine Phosphate (Orthostatic hypotension may be aggravated by narcotics). Products include:
Phenergan with Codeine Syrup 3557
Phenergan VC with Codeine Syrup 3561
Robitussin A-C Syrup 2942
Robitussin-DAC Syrup 2942
Ryna-C Liquid .... ▣768
Soma Compound w/Codeine Tablets 3355
Tussi-Organidin NR Liquid 3350
Tussi-Organidin-S NR Liquid 3350
Tylenol with Codeine 2595

Cortisone Acetate (Hypokalemia may develop with thiazides during concomitant corticosteroids). Products include:
Cortone Acetate Injectable Suspension 2059
Cortone Acetate Tablets 2061

Deserpidine (Thiazides may add to or potentiate the action of other antihypertensives).
No products indexed under this heading.

Deslanoside (Digitalis therapy may exaggerate metabolic effects of hypokalemia especially with reference to myocardial activity).
No products indexed under this heading.

Dexamethasone (Hypokalemia may develop with thiazides during concomitant corticosteroids). Products include:
Decadron Elixir 2078
Decadron Tablets 2079
TobraDex Ophthalmic Ointment 542
TobraDex Ophthalmic Suspension 541

Dexamethasone Acetate (Hypokalemia may develop with thiazides during concomitant corticosteroids).
No products indexed under this heading.

Dexamethasone Sodium Phosphate (Hypokalemia may develop with thiazides during concomitant corticosteroids). Products include:
Decadron Phosphate Injection 2081
Decadron Phosphate Sterile Ophthalmic Ointment 2083
Decadron Phosphate Sterile Ophthalmic Solution 2084
NeoDecadron Sterile Ophthalmic Solution 2144

Dezocine (Orthostatic hypotension may be aggravated by narcotics).
No products indexed under this heading.

Diazoxide (Thiazides may add to or potentiate the action of other antihypertensives).
No products indexed under this heading.

Digitoxin (Digitalis therapy may exaggerate metabolic effects of hypokalemia especially with reference to myocardial activity).
No products indexed under this heading.

Digoxin (Digitalis therapy may exaggerate metabolic effects of hypokalemia especially with reference to myocardial activity). Products include:
Digitek Tablets 1003
Lanoxicaps Capsules 1574
Lanoxin Injection 1581
Lanoxin Tablets 1587
Lanoxin Elixir Pediatric 1578
Lanoxin Injection Pediatric 1584

Diltiazem Hydrochloride (Thiazides may add to or potentiate the action of other antihypertensives). Products include:
Cardizem Injectable 1018
Cardizem Lyo-Ject Syringe 1018
Cardizem Monovial 1018
Cardizem CD Capsules 1016
Tiazac Capsules 1378

Doxazosin Mesylate (Thiazides may add to or potentiate the action of other antihypertensives). Products include:
Cardura Tablets 2668

Enalapril Maleate (Thiazides may add to or potentiate the action of other antihypertensives). Products include:
Lexxel Tablets 608
Vaseretic Tablets 2204
Vasotec Tablets 2210

Enalaprilat (Thiazides may add to or potentiate the action of other antihypertensives). Products include:
Enalaprilat Injection 863
Vasotec I.V. Injection 2207

Eprosartan Mesylate (Thiazides may add to or potentiate the action of other antihypertensives). Products include:
Teveten Tablets 3327

Esmolol Hydrochloride (Thiazides may add to or potentiate the action of other antihypertensives). Products include:
Brevibloc Injection 858

Felodipine (Thiazides may add to or potentiate the action of other antihypertensives). Products include:
Lexxel Tablets 608
Plendil Extended-Release Tablets 623

Fentanyl (Orthostatic hypotension may be aggravated by narcotics). Products include:
Duragesic Transdermal System 1786

Fentanyl Citrate (Orthostatic hypotension may be aggravated by narcotics). Products include:
Actiq 1184

Fludrocortisone Acetate (Hypokalemia may develop with thiazides during concomitant corticosteroids). Products include:
Florinef Acetate Tablets 2250

IMPORTANT NOTE: Always consult each drug listing in the patient's regimen for possible interactions.

Fosinopril Sodium (Thiazides may add to or potentiate the action of other antihypertensives). Products include:
- Monopril Tablets ... 1091
- Monopril HCT ... 1094

Furosemide (Thiazides may add to or potentiate the action of other antihypertensives). Products include:
- Furosemide Tablets ... 2284

Guanabenz Acetate (Thiazides may add to or potentiate the action of other antihypertensives).
- No products indexed under this heading.

Guanethidine Monosulfate (Thiazides may add to or potentiate the action of other antihypertensives).
- No products indexed under this heading.

Hydralazine Hydrochloride (Thiazides may add to or potentiate the action of other antihypertensives).
- No products indexed under this heading.

Hydrochlorothiazide (Thiazides may add to or potentiate the action of other antihypertensives). Products include:
- Accuretic Tablets ... 2614
- Aldoril Tablets ... 2039
- Atacand HCT Tablets ... 597
- Avalide Tablets ... 1070
- Diovan HCT Tablets ... 2338
- Dyazide Capsules ... 1515
- HydroDIURIL Tablets ... 2108
- Hyzaar ... 2109
- Inderide Tablets ... 3517
- Inderide LA Long-Acting Capsules ... 3519
- Lotensin HCT Tablets ... 2367
- Maxzide ... 1008
- Micardis HCT Tablets ... 1051
- Microzide Capsules ... 3414
- Moduretic Tablets ... 2138
- Monopril HCT ... 1094
- Prinzide Tablets ... 2168
- Timolide Tablets ... 2187
- Uniretic Tablets ... 3178
- Vaseretic Tablets ... 2204
- Zestoretic Tablets ... 695
- Ziac Tablets ... 1887

Hydrocodone Bitartrate (Orthostatic hypotension may be aggravated by narcotics). Products include:
- Hycodan ... 1316
- Hycomine Compound Tablets ... 1317
- Hycotuss Expectorant Syrup ... 1318
- Lortab ... 3319
- Lortab Elixir ... 3317
- Maxidone Tablets CIII ... 3399
- Norco 5/325 Tablets CIII ... 3424
- Norco 7.5/325 Tablets CIII ... 3425
- Norco 10/325 Tablets CIII ... 3427
- Norco 10/325 Tablets CIII ... 3425
- Vicodin Tablets ... 516
- Vicodin ES Tablets ... 517
- Vicodin HP Tablets ... 518
- Vicodin Tuss Expectorant ... 519
- Vicoprofen Tablets ... 520
- Zydone Tablets ... 1330

Hydrocodone Polistirex (Orthostatic hypotension may be aggravated by narcotics). Products include:
- Tussionex Pennkinetic Extended-Release Suspension ... 1174

Hydrocortisone (Hypokalemia may develop with thiazides during concomitant corticosteroids). Products include:
- Anusol-HC Cream 2.5% ... 2237
- Cipro HC Otic Suspension ... 540
- Cortaid Intensive Therapy Cream ... ■717
- Cortaid Maximum Strength Cream ... ■717
- Cortisporin Ophthalmic Suspension Sterile ... ⊙297
- Cortizone•5 ... ■699
- Cortizone•10 ... ■699
- Cortizone•10 Plus Creme ... ■700
- Cortizone for Kids Creme ... ■699
- Hydrocortone Tablets ... 2106
- Massengill Medicated Soft Cloth Towelette ... ■753
- VōSoL HC Otic Solution ... 3356

Hydrocortisone Acetate (Hypokalemia may develop with thiazides during concomitant corticosteroids). Products include:
- Analpram-HC ... 1338
- Anusol HC-1 Hydrocortisone Anti-Itch Cream ... ■689
- Anusol-HC Suppositories ... 2238
- Cortaid ... ■717
- Cortifoam Rectal Foam ... 3170
- Cortisporin-TC Otic Suspension ... 2246
- Hydrocortone Acetate Injectable Suspension ... 2103
- Pramosone ... 1343
- Proctocort Suppositories ... 2264
- ProctoFoam-HC ... 3177
- Terra-Cortril Ophthalmic Suspension ... 2716

Hydrocortisone Sodium Phosphate (Hypokalemia may develop with thiazides during concomitant corticosteroids). Products include:
- Hydrocortone Phosphate Injection, Sterile ... 2105

Hydrocortisone Sodium Succinate (Hypokalemia may develop with thiazides during concomitant corticosteroids).
- No products indexed under this heading.

Hydroflumethiazide (Thiazides may add to or potentiate the action of other antihypertensives). Products include:
- Diucardin Tablets ... 3494

Hydromorphone Hydrochloride (Orthostatic hypotension may be aggravated by narcotics). Products include:
- Dilaudid ... 441
- Dilaudid Oral Liquid ... 445
- Dilaudid Powder ... 441
- Dilaudid Rectal Suppositories ... 441
- Dilaudid Tablets ... 441
- Dilaudid Tablets - 8 mg ... 445
- Dilaudid-HP ... 443

Indapamide (Thiazides may add to or potentiate the action of other antihypertensives). Products include:
- Indapamide Tablets ... 2286

Insulin, Human, Zinc Suspension (Thiazides can cause hyperglycemia; insulin requirements in diabetic patients may be increased, decreased or unchanged). Products include:
- Humulin L, 100 Units ... 1937
- Humulin U, 100 Units ... 1943
- Novolin L Human Insulin 10 ml Vials ... 2422

Insulin, Human NPH (Thiazides can cause hyperglycemia; insulin requirements in diabetic patients may be increased, decreased or unchanged). Products include:
- Humulin N, 100 Units ... 1939
- Humulin N NPH Pen ... 1940
- Novolin N Human Insulin 10 ml Vials ... 2422
- Novolin N PenFill ... 2423
- Novolin N Prefilled Syringe Disposable Insulin Delivery System ... 2425

Insulin, Human Regular (Thiazides can cause hyperglycemia; insulin requirements in diabetic patients may be increased, decreased or unchanged). Products include:
- Humulin R Regular (U-500) ... 1943
- Humulin R, 100 Units ... 1941
- Novolin R Human Insulin 10 ml Vials ... 2423
- Novolin R PenFill ... 2423
- Novolin R Prefilled Syringe Disposable Insulin Delivery System ... 2425
- Velosulin BR Human Insulin 10 ml Vials ... 2435

Insulin, Human Regular and Human NPH Mixture (Thiazides can cause hyperglycemia; insulin requirements in diabetic patients may be increased, decreased or unchanged). Products include:
- Humulin 50/50, 100 Units ... 1934
- Humulin 70/30, 100 Units ... 1935
- Humulin 70/30 Pen ... 1936
- Novolin 70/30 Human Insulin 10 ml Vials ... 2421
- Novolin 70/30 PenFill ... 2423
- Novolin 70/30 Prefilled Disposable Insulin Delivery System ... 2425

Insulin, NPH (Thiazides can cause hyperglycemia; insulin requirements in diabetic patients may be increased, decreased or unchanged). Products include:
- Iletin II, NPH (Pork), 100 Units ... 1946

Insulin, Regular (Thiazides can cause hyperglycemia; insulin requirements in diabetic patients may be increased, decreased or unchanged). Products include:
- Iletin II, Regular (Pork), 100 Units ... 1947

Insulin, Zinc Crystals (Thiazides can cause hyperglycemia; insulin requirements in diabetic patients may be increased, decreased or unchanged).
- No products indexed under this heading.

Insulin, Zinc Suspension (Thiazides can cause hyperglycemia; insulin requirements in diabetic patients may be increased, decreased or unchanged). Products include:
- Iletin II, Lente (Pork), 100 Units ... 1945

Insulin Aspart, Human Regular (Thiazides can cause hyperglycemia; insulin requirements in diabetic patients may be increased, decreased or unchanged).
- No products indexed under this heading.

Insulin glargine (Thiazides can cause hyperglycemia; insulin requirements in diabetic patients may be increased, decreased or unchanged). Products include:
- Lantus Injection ... 742

Insulin Lispro, Human (Thiazides can cause hyperglycemia; insulin requirements in diabetic patients may be increased, decreased or unchanged). Products include:
- Humalog ... 1926
- Humalog Mix 75/25 Pen ... 1928

Insulin Lispro Protamine, Human (Thiazides can cause hyperglycemia; insulin requirements in diabetic patients may be increased, decreased or unchanged). Products include:
- Humalog Mix 75/25 Pen ... 1928

Irbesartan (Thiazides may add to or potentiate the action of other antihypertensives). Products include:
- Avalide Tablets ... 1070
- Avapro Tablets ... 1074
- Avapro Tablets ... 3076

Isradipine (Thiazides may add to or potentiate the action of other antihypertensives). Products include:
- DynaCirc Capsules ... 2921
- DynaCirc CR Tablets ... 2923

Labetalol Hydrochloride (Thiazides may add to or potentiate the action of other antihypertensives). Products include:
- Normodyne Injection ... 3135
- Normodyne Tablets ... 3137

Levorphanol Tartrate (Orthostatic hypotension may be aggravated by narcotics). Products include:
- Levo-Dromoran ... 1734
- Levorphanol Tartrate Tablets ... 3059

Lisinopril (Thiazides may add to or potentiate the action of other antihypertensives). Products include:
- Prinivil Tablets ... 2164
- Prinzide Tablets ... 2168
- Zestoretic Tablets ... 695
- Zestril Tablets ... 698

Losartan Potassium (Thiazides may add to or potentiate the action of other antihypertensives). Products include:
- Cozaar Tablets ... 2067
- Hyzaar ... 2109

Mecamylamine Hydrochloride (Thiazides may add to or potentiate the action of other antihypertensives). Products include:
- Inversine Tablets ... 1850

Meperidine Hydrochloride (Orthostatic hypotension may be aggravated by narcotics). Products include:
- Demerol ... 3079
- Mepergan Injection ... 3539

Mephobarbital (Orthostatic hypotension may be aggravated by barbiturates).
- No products indexed under this heading.

Methadone Hydrochloride (Orthostatic hypotension may be aggravated by narcotics). Products include:
- Dolophine Hydrochloride Tablets ... 3056

Methyclothiazide (Thiazides may add to or potentiate the action of other antihypertensives).
- No products indexed under this heading.

Methyldopa (Thiazides may add to or potentiate the action of other antihypertensives). Products include:
- Aldoclor Tablets ... 2035
- Aldomet Tablets ... 2037
- Aldoril Tablets ... 2039

Methyldopate Hydrochloride (Thiazides may add to or potentiate the action of other antihypertensives).
- No products indexed under this heading.

Methylprednisolone Acetate (Hypokalemia may develop with thiazides during concomitant corticosteroids). Products include:
- Depo-Medrol Injectable Suspension ... 2795

Methylprednisolone Sodium Succinate (Hypokalemia may develop with thiazides during concomitant corticosteroids). Products include:
- Solu-Medrol Sterile Powder ... 2855

Metolazone (Thiazides may add to or potentiate the action of other antihypertensives). Products include:
- Mykrox Tablets ... 1168
- Zaroxolyn Tablets ... 1177

Metoprolol Succinate (Thiazides may add to or potentiate the action of other antihypertensives). Products include:
- Toprol-XL Tablets ... 651

Metoprolol Tartrate (Thiazides may add to or potentiate the action of other antihypertensives).
- No products indexed under this heading.

Metyrosine (Thiazides may add to or potentiate the action of other antihypertensives). Products include:
- Demser Capsules ... 2085

Mibefradil Dihydrochloride (Thiazides may add to or potentiate the action of other antihypertensives).
- No products indexed under this heading.

Minoxidil (Thiazides may add to or potentiate the action of other antihypertensives). Products include:
- Rogaine Extra Strength for Men Topical Solution ... ■721
- Rogaine for Women Topical Solution ... ■721

Moexipril Hydrochloride (Thiazides may add to or potentiate the action of other antihypertensives). Products include:
- Uniretic Tablets ... 3178
- Univasc Tablets ... 3181

Morphine Sulfate (Orthostatic hypotension may be aggravated by narcotics). Products include:
- Astramorph/PF Injection, USP (Preservative-Free) ... 594
- Duramorph Injection ... 1312
- Infumorph 200 and Infumorph 500 Sterile Solutions ... 1314
- Kadian Capsules ... 1335
- MS Contin Tablets ... 2896
- MSIR ... 2898
- Oramorph SR Tablets ... 3062
- Roxanol ... 3066

Nadolol (Thiazides may add to or potentiate the action of other antihypertensives). Products include:
- Corgard Tablets ... 2245
- Corzide 40/5 Tablets ... 2247
- Corzide 80/5 Tablets ... 2247
- Nadolol Tablets ... 2288

Nicardipine Hydrochloride (Thiazides may add to or potentiate the action of other antihypertensives). Products include:
- Cardene I.V. ... 3485

Nifedipine (Thiazides may add to or potentiate the action of other antihypertensives). Products include:
- Adalat CC Tablets ... 877
- Procardia Capsules ... 2708
- Procardia XL Extended Release Tablets ... 2710

Nisoldipine (Thiazides may add to or potentiate the action of other antihypertensives). Products include:
- Sular Tablets ... 688

Nitroglycerin (Thiazides may add to or potentiate the action of other antihypertensives). Products include:
- Nitro-Dur Transdermal Infusion System ... 3134
- Nitro-Dur Transdermal Infusion System ... 1834
- Nitrolingual Pumpspray ... 1355
- Nitrostat Tablets ... 2658

Norepinephrine Bitartrate (Thiazides may decrease arterial responsiveness to norepinephrine).
- No products indexed under this heading.

Oxycodone Hydrochloride (Orthostatic hypotension may be aggravated by narcotics). Products include:
- OxyContin Tablets ... 2912
- OxyFast Oral Concentrate Solution . 2916
- OxyIR Capsules ... 2916
- Percocet Tablets ... 1326
- Percodan Tablets ... 1327
- Percolone Tablets ... 1327
- Roxicodone ... 3067
- Tylox Capsules ... 2597

Penbutolol Sulfate (Thiazides may add to or potentiate the action of other antihypertensives).
- No products indexed under this heading.

Pentobarbital Sodium (Orthostatic hypotension may be aggravated by barbiturates). Products include:
- Nembutal Sodium Solution ... 485

Perindopril Erbumine (Thiazides may add to or potentiate the action of other antihypertensives). Products include:
- Aceon Tablets (2 mg, 4 mg, 8 mg) ... 3249

Phenobarbital (Orthostatic hypotension may be aggravated by barbiturates). Products include:
- Arco-Lase Plus Tablets ... 592
- Donnatal ... 2929
- Donnatal Extentabs ... 2930

Phenoxybenzamine Hydrochloride (Thiazides may add to or potentiate the action of other antihypertensives). Products include:
- Dibenzyline Capsules ... 3457

Phentolamine Mesylate (Thiazides may add to or potentiate the action of other antihypertensives).
- No products indexed under this heading.

Pindolol (Thiazides may add to or potentiate the action of other antihypertensives).
- No products indexed under this heading.

Prazosin Hydrochloride (Thiazides may add to or potentiate the action of other antihypertensives). Products include:
- Minipress Capsules ... 2699
- Minizide Capsules ... 2700

Prednisolone Acetate (Hypokalemia may develop with thiazides during concomitant corticosteroids). Products include:
- Blephamide Ophthalmic Ointment .. 547
- Blephamide Ophthalmic Suspension ... 548
- Poly-Pred Liquifilm Ophthalmic Suspension ... ⊙245
- Pred Forte Ophthalmic Suspension ... ⊙246
- Pred Mild Sterile Ophthalmic Suspension ... ⊙249
- Pred-G Ophthalmic Suspension ... ⊙247
- Pred-G Sterile Ophthalmic Ointment ... ⊙248

Prednisolone Sodium Phosphate (Hypokalemia may develop with thiazides during concomitant corticosteroids). Products include:
- Pediapred Oral Solution ... 1170

Prednisolone Tebutate (Hypokalemia may develop with thiazides during concomitant corticosteroids).
- No products indexed under this heading.

Prednisone (Hypokalemia may develop with thiazides during concomitant corticosteroids). Products include:
- Prednisone ... 3064

Propoxyphene Hydrochloride (Orthostatic hypotension may be aggravated by narcotics). Products include:
- Darvon Pulvules ... 1909
- Darvon Compound-65 Pulvules ... 1910

Propoxyphene Napsylate (Orthostatic hypotension may be aggravated by narcotics). Products include:
- Darvon-N/Darvocet-N ... 1907
- Darvon-N Tablets ... 1912

Propranolol Hydrochloride (Thiazides may add to or potentiate the action of other antihypertensives). Products include:
- Inderal ... 3513
- Inderal LA Long-Acting Capsules ... 3516
- Inderide Tablets ... 3517
- Inderide LA Long-Acting Capsules .. 3519

Quinapril Hydrochloride (Thiazides may add to or potentiate the action of other antihypertensives). Products include:
- Accupril Tablets ... 2611
- Accuretic Tablets ... 2614

Ramipril (Thiazides may add to or potentiate the action of other antihypertensives). Products include:
- Altace Capsules ... 2233

Rauwolfia serpentina (Thiazides may add to or potentiate the action of other antihypertensives).
- No products indexed under this heading.

Remifentanil Hydrochloride (Orthostatic hypotension may be aggravated by narcotics).
- No products indexed under this heading.

Rescinnamine (Thiazides may add to or potentiate the action of other antihypertensives).
- No products indexed under this heading.

Reserpine (Thiazides may add to or potentiate the action of other antihypertensives).
- No products indexed under this heading.

Secobarbital Sodium (Orthostatic hypotension may be aggravated by barbiturates).
- No products indexed under this heading.

Sodium Nitroprusside (Thiazides may add to or potentiate the action of other antihypertensives).
- No products indexed under this heading.

Sotalol Hydrochloride (Thiazides may add to or potentiate the action of other antihypertensives). Products include:
- Betapace Tablets ... 950
- Betapace AF Tablets ... 954

Spirapril Hydrochloride (Thiazides may add to or potentiate the action of other antihypertensives).
- No products indexed under this heading.

Sufentanil Citrate (Orthostatic hypotension may be aggravated by narcotics).
- No products indexed under this heading.

Telmisartan (Thiazides may add to or potentiate the action of other antihypertensives). Products include:
- Micardis Tablets ... 1049
- Micardis HCT Tablets ... 1051

Terazosin Hydrochloride (Thiazides may add to or potentiate the action of other antihypertensives). Products include:
- Hytrin Capsules ... 464

Thiamylal Sodium (Orthostatic hypotension may be aggravated by barbiturates).
- No products indexed under this heading.

Timolol Maleate (Thiazides may add to or potentiate the action of other antihypertensives). Products include:
- Blocadren Tablets ... 2046
- Cosopt Sterile Ophthalmic Solution ... 2065
- Timolide Tablets ... 2187
- Timolol GFS ... ⊙266
- Timoptic in Ocudose ... 2192
- Timoptic Sterile Ophthalmic Solution ... 2190
- Timoptic-XE Sterile Ophthalmic Gel Forming Solution ... 2194

Torsemide (Thiazides may add to or potentiate the action of other antihypertensives). Products include:
- Demadex Tablets and Injection ... 2965

Trandolapril (Thiazides may add to or potentiate the action of other antihypertensives). Products include:
- Mavik Tablets ... 478
- Tarka Tablets ... 508

Triamcinolone (Hypokalemia may develop with thiazides during concomitant corticosteroids).
- No products indexed under this heading.

Triamcinolone Acetonide (Hypokalemia may develop with thiazides during concomitant corticosteroids). Products include:
- Azmacort Inhalation Aerosol ... 728
- Nasacort Nasal Inhaler ... 750
- Nasacort AQ Nasal Spray ... 752
- Tri-Nasal Spray ... 2274

Triamcinolone Diacetate (Hypokalemia may develop with thiazides during concomitant corticosteroids).
- No products indexed under this heading.

Triamcinolone Hexacetonide (Hypokalemia may develop with thiazides during concomitant corticosteroids).
- No products indexed under this heading.

Trimethaphan Camsylate (Thiazides may add to or potentiate the action of other antihypertensives).
- No products indexed under this heading.

Valsartan (Thiazides may add to or potentiate the action of other antihypertensives). Products include:
- Diovan Capsules ... 2337
- Diovan HCT Tablets ... 2338

Verapamil Hydrochloride (Thiazides may add to or potentiate the action of other antihypertensives). Products include:
- Covera-HS Tablets ... 3199
- Isoptin SR Tablets ... 467
- Tarka Tablets ... 508
- Verelan Capsules ... 3184
- Verelan PM Capsules ... 3186

Food Interactions

Alcohol (Orthostatic hypotension may be aggravated by alcohol).

RENOVA 0.02% CREAM

(Tretinoin) ... 2520

See Renova 0.05% Cream

RENOVA 0.05% CREAM

(Tretinoin) ... 2519

May interact with drugs known to be photosensitizers and certain other agents. Compounds in these categories include:

Alatrofloxacin Mesylate (Co-administration with drugs known to be photosensitizers may augment phototoxicity; concurrent use with these agents is not recommended). Products include:
- Trovan I.V. ... 2722

Bendroflumethiazide (Co-administration with drugs known to be photosensitizers may augment phototoxicity; concurrent use with these agents is not recommended). Products include:
- Corzide 40/5 Tablets ... 2247
- Corzide 80/5 Tablets ... 2247

Chlorothiazide (Co-administration with drugs known to be photosensitizers may augment phototoxicity; concurrent use with these agents is not recommended). Products include:
- Aldoclor Tablets ... 2035
- Diuril Oral ... 2087

Chlorothiazide Sodium (Co-administration with drugs known to be photosensitizers may augment phototoxicity; concurrent use with these agents is not recommended). Products include:
- Diuril Sodium Intravenous ... 2086

Chlorpromazine (Co-administration with drugs known to be photosensitizers may augment phototoxicity; concurrent use with these agents is not recommended). Products include:
- Thorazine Suppositories ... 1656

Chlorpromazine Hydrochloride (Co-administration with drugs known to be photosensitizers may augment phototoxicity; concurrent use with these agents is not recommended). Products include:
- Thorazine ... 1656

Chlorpropamide (Co-administration with drugs known to be photosensitizers may augment phototoxicity; concurrent use with these agents is not recommended). Products include:
- Diabinese Tablets ... 2680

Ciprofloxacin (Co-administration with drugs known to be photosensitizers may augment phototoxicity; concurrent use with these agents is not recommended). Products include:
- Cipro I.V. ... 893
- Cipro I.V. Pharmacy Bulk Package .. 897
- Cipro Oral Suspension ... 887

Ciprofloxacin Hydrochloride (Co-administration with drugs known to be photosensitizers may augment phototoxicity; concurrent use with these agents is not recommended). Products include:
- Ciloxan ... 538
- Cipro HC Otic Suspension ... 540
- Cipro Tablets ... 887

Demeclocycline Hydrochloride (Co-administration with drugs known to be photosensitizers may augment phototoxicity; concurrent use with these agents is not recommended). Products include:
- Declomycin Tablets ... 1855

Doxycycline Calcium (Co-administration with drugs known to be photosensitizers may augment phototoxicity; concurrent use with these agents is not recommended). Products include:
- Vibramycin Calcium Oral Suspension Syrup ... 2735

IMPORTANT NOTE: Always consult each drug listing in the patient's regimen for possible interactions.

Doxycycline Hyclate (Co-administration with drugs known to be photosensitizers may augment phototoxicity; concurrent use with these agents is not recommended). Products include:

- Doryx Coated Pellet Filled Capsules 3357
- Periostat Tablets 1208
- Vibramycin Hyclate Capsules 2735
- Vibramycin Hyclate Intravenous 2737
- Vibra-Tabs Film Coated Tablets 2735

Doxycycline Monohydrate (Co-administration with drugs known to be photosensitizers may augment phototoxicity; concurrent use with these agents is not recommended). Products include:

- Monodox Capsules 2442
- Vibramycin Monohydrate for Oral Suspension 2735

Enoxacin (Co-administration with drugs known to be photosensitizers may augment phototoxicity; concurrent use with these agents is not recommended).

No products indexed under this heading.

Fluphenazine Decanoate (Co-administration with drugs known to be photosensitizers may augment phototoxicity; concurrent use with these agents is not recommended).

No products indexed under this heading.

Fluphenazine Enanthate (Co-administration with drugs known to be photosensitizers may augment phototoxicity; concurrent use with these agents is not recommended).

No products indexed under this heading.

Fluphenazine Hydrochloride (Co-administration with drugs known to be photosensitizers may augment phototoxicity; concurrent use with these agents is not recommended).

No products indexed under this heading.

Glipizide (Co-administration with drugs known to be photosensitizers may augment phototoxicity; concurrent use with these agents is not recommended). Products include:

- Glucotrol Tablets 2692
- Glucotrol XL Extended Release Tablets 2693

Glyburide (Co-administration with drugs known to be photosensitizers may augment phototoxicity; concurrent use with these agents is not recommended). Products include:

- DiaBeta Tablets 741
- Glucovance Tablets 1086

Grepafloxacin Hydrochloride (Co-administration with drugs known to be photosensitizers may augment phototoxicity; concurrent use with these agents is not recommended).

No products indexed under this heading.

Hydrochlorothiazide (Co-administration with drugs known to be photosensitizers may augment phototoxicity; concurrent use with these agents is not recommended). Products include:

- Accuretic Tablets 2614
- Aldoril Tablets 2039
- Atacand HCT Tablets 597
- Avalide Tablets 1070
- Diovan HCT Tablets 2338
- Dyazide Capsules 1515
- HydroDIURIL Tablets 2108
- Hyzaar 2109
- Inderide Tablets 3517
- Inderide LA Long-Acting Capsules 3519
- Lotensin HCT Tablets 2367
- Maxzide 1008
- Micardis HCT Tablets 1051
- Microzide Capsules 3414
- Moduretic Tablets 2138
- Monopril HCT 1094
- Prinzide Tablets 2168
- Timolide Tablets 2187
- Uniretic Tablets 3178
- Vaseretic Tablets 2204
- Zestoretic Tablets 695
- Ziac Tablets 1887

Hydroflumethiazide (Co-administration with drugs known to be photosensitizers may augment phototoxicity; concurrent use with these agents is not recommended). Products include:

- Diucardin Tablets 3494

Lomefloxacin Hydrochloride (Co-administration with drugs known to be photosensitizers may augment phototoxicity; concurrent use with these agents is not recommended).

No products indexed under this heading.

Mesoridazine Besylate (Co-administration with drugs known to be photosensitizers may augment phototoxicity; concurrent use with these agents is not recommended). Products include:

- Serentil 1057

Methacycline Hydrochloride (Co-administration with drugs known to be photosensitizers may augment phototoxicity; concurrent use with these agents is not recommended).

No products indexed under this heading.

Methotrimeprazine (Co-administration with drugs known to be photosensitizers may augment phototoxicity; concurrent use with these agents is not recommended).

No products indexed under this heading.

Methyclothiazide (Co-administration with drugs known to be photosensitizers may augment phototoxicity; concurrent use with these agents is not recommended).

No products indexed under this heading.

Minocycline Hydrochloride (Co-administration with drugs known to be photosensitizers may augment phototoxicity; concurrent use with these agents is not recommended). Products include:

- Dynacin Capsules 2019
- Minocin Intravenous 1862
- Minocin Oral Suspension 1865
- Minocin Pellet-Filled Capsules 1863

Norfloxacin (Co-administration with drugs known to be photosensitizers may augment phototoxicity; concurrent use with these agents is not recommended). Products include:

- Chibroxin Sterile Ophthalmic Solution 2051
- Noroxin Tablets 2145

Ofloxacin (Co-administration with drugs known to be photosensitizers may augment phototoxicity; concurrent use with these agents is not recommended). Products include:

- Floxin I.V. 2526
- Floxin Otic Solution 1219
- Floxin Tablets 2529
- Ocuflox Ophthalmic Solution 554

Oxytetracycline Hydrochloride (Co-administration with drugs known to be photosensitizers may augment phototoxicity; concurrent use with these agents is not recommended). Products include:

- Terra-Cortril Ophthalmic Suspension 2716
- Urobiotic-250 Capsules 2731

Perphenazine (Co-administration with drugs known to be photosensitizers may augment phototoxicity; concurrent use with these agents is not recommended). Products include:

- Etrafon 3115
- Trilafon 3160

Polythiazide (Co-administration with drugs known to be photosensitizers may augment phototoxicity; concurrent use with these agents is not recommended). Products include:

- Minizide Capsules 2700
- Renese Tablets 2712

Prochlorperazine (Co-administration with drugs known to be photosensitizers may augment phototoxicity; concurrent use with these agents is not recommended). Products include:

- Compazine 1505

Promethazine Hydrochloride (Co-administration with drugs known to be photosensitizers may augment phototoxicity; concurrent use with these agents is not recommended). Products include:

- Mepergan Injection 3539
- Phenergan Injection 3553
- Phenergan 3556
- Phenergan Syrup 3554
- Phenergan with Codeine Syrup 3557
- Phenergan with Dextromethorphan Syrup 3559
- Phenergan VC Syrup 3560
- Phenergan VC with Codeine Syrup 3561

Sulfamethizole (Co-administration with drugs known to be photosensitizers may augment phototoxicity; concurrent use with these agents is not recommended). Products include:

- Urobiotic-250 Capsules 2731

Sulfamethoxazole (Co-administration with drugs known to be photosensitizers may augment phototoxicity; concurrent use with these agents is not recommended). Products include:

- Bactrim 2949
- Septra Suspension 2265
- Septra Tablets 2265
- Septra DS Tablets 2265

Sulfasalazine (Co-administration with drugs known to be photosensitizers may augment phototoxicity; concurrent use with these agents is not recommended). Products include:

- Azulfidine EN-tabs Tablets 2775

Sulfinpyrazone (Co-administration with drugs known to be photosensitizers may augment phototoxicity; concurrent use with these agents is not recommended).

No products indexed under this heading.

Sulfisoxazole (Co-administration with drugs known to be photosensitizers may augment phototoxicity; concurrent use with these agents is not recommended).

No products indexed under this heading.

Sulfisoxazole Acetyl (Co-administration with drugs known to be photosensitizers may augment phototoxicity; concurrent use with these agents is not recommended). Products include:

- Pediazole Suspension 3050

Sulfisoxazole Diolamine (Co-administration with drugs known to be photosensitizers may augment phototoxicity; concurrent use with these agents is not recommended).

No products indexed under this heading.

Tetracycline Hydrochloride (Co-administration with drugs known to be photosensitizers may augment phototoxicity; concurrent use with these agents is not recommended).

No products indexed under this heading.

Thioridazine Hydrochloride (Co-administration with drugs known to be photosensitizers may augment phototoxicity; concurrent use with these agents is not recommended). Products include:

- Thioridazine Hydrochloride Tablets 2289

Tolazamide (Co-administration with drugs known to be photosensitizers may augment phototoxicity; concurrent use with these agents is not recommended).

No products indexed under this heading.

Tolbutamide (Co-administration with drugs known to be photosensitizers may augment phototoxicity; concurrent use with these agents is not recommended).

No products indexed under this heading.

Trifluoperazine Hydrochloride (Co-administration with drugs known to be photosensitizers may augment phototoxicity; concurrent use with these agents is not recommended). Products include:

- Stelazine 1640

Trovafloxacin Mesylate (Co-administration with drugs known to be photosensitizers may augment phototoxicity; concurrent use with these agents is not recommended). Products include:

- Trovan Tablets 2722

Food Interactions

Alcohol (Topical products with high concentration of alcohol may increase the irritation when used concurrently).

REOPRO VIALS

(Abciximab) 1958

May interact with anticoagulants, oral anticoagulants, non-steroidal anti-inflammatory agents, thrombolytics, and certain other agents. Compounds in these categories include:

Alteplase, Recombinant (Co-administration with thrombolytics may be associated with an increase in bleeding). Products include:

- Activase I.V. 1410
- Cathflo Activase 3611

Anistreplase (Co-administration with thrombolytics may be associated with an increase in bleeding).

No products indexed under this heading.

Ardeparin Sodium (Co-administration with other anticoagulant agents may be associated with an increase in bleeding).

No products indexed under this heading.

Aspirin (Co-administration with antiplatelet agents, such as aspirin, may be associated with an increase in bleeding). Products include:

- Aggrenox Capsules 1026
- Alka-Seltzer .... ▣603
- Alka-Seltzer Lemon Lime Antacid and Pain Reliever Effervescent Tablets .... ▣603
- Alka-Seltzer Extra Strength Antacid and Pain Reliever Effervescent Tablets .... ▣603
- Alka-Seltzer PM Effervescent Tablets .... ▣605
- Genuine Bayer Tablets, Caplets and Gelcaps .... ▣606
- Extra Strength Bayer Caplets and Gelcaps .... ▣610
- Aspirin Regimen Bayer Children's Chewable Tablets (Orange or Cherry Flavored) .... ▣607
- Bayer, Aspirin Regimen .... ▣606
- Aspirin Regimen Bayer 81 mg Caplets with Calcium .... ▣607
- Genuine Bayer Professional Labeling (Aspirin Regimen Bayer) .... ▣608
- Extra Strength Bayer Arthritis Caplets .... ▣610
- Extra Strength Bayer Plus Caplets .... ▣610
- Extra Strength Bayer PM Caplets .... ▣611
- BC Powder .... ▣619
- BC Allergy Sinus Cold Powder .... ▣619
- Arthritis Strength BC Powder .... ▣619
- BC Sinus Cold Powder .... ▣619
- Darvon Compound-65 Pulvules 1910
- Ecotrin Enteric Coated Aspirin Low, Regular and Maximum Strength Tablets 1715
- Excedrin Extra-Strength Tablets, Caplets, and Geltabs .... ▣629
- Excedrin Migraine 1070
- Goody's Body Pain Formula Powder .... ▣620
- Goody's Extra Strength Headache Powder .... ▣620
- Goody's Extra Strength Pain Relief Tablets .... ▣620

Percodan Tablets ... 1327
Robaxisal Tablets ... 2939
Soma Compound Tablets ... 3354
Soma Compound w/Codeine Tablets ... 3355
Vanquish Caplets ... 617

Celecoxib (Co-administration with antiplatelet agents, such as non-steroidal anti-inflammatory agents, may be associated with an increase in bleeding). Products include:
Celebrex Capsules ... 2676
Celebrex Capsules ... 2780

Clopidogrel Bisulfate (Co-administration with antiplatelet agents, such as clopidogrel, may be associated with an increase in bleeding). Products include:
Plavix Tablets ... 1097
Plavix Tablets ... 3084

Dalteparin Sodium (Co-administration with other anticoagulant agents may be associated with an increase in bleeding). Products include:
Fragmin Injection ... 2814

Danaparoid Sodium (Co-administration with other anticoagulant agents may be associated with an increase in bleeding). Products include:
Orgaran Injection ... 2480

Dextran (Co-administration with intravenous dextran before percutaneous coronary intervention, or intent to use it during an intervention is contraindicated).
No products indexed under this heading.

Diclofenac Potassium (Co-administration with antiplatelet agents, such as non-steroidal anti-inflammatory agents, may be associated with an increase in bleeding). Products include:
Cataflam Tablets ... 2315

Diclofenac Sodium (Co-administration with antiplatelet agents, such as non-steroidal anti-inflammatory agents, may be associated with an increase in bleeding). Products include:
Arthrotec Tablets ... 3195
Voltaren Ophthalmic Sterile Ophthalmic Solution ... ⊙312
Voltaren Tablets ... 2315
Voltaren-XR Tablets ... 2315

Dicumarol (Co-administration of oral anticoagulants within seven days is contraindicated unless prothrombin time is less than or equal to 1.2 times control; concurrent use with other anticoagulant agents may be associated with an increase in bleeding).
No products indexed under this heading.

Dipyridamole (Co-administration with antiplatelet agents, such as dipyridamole, may be associated with an increase in bleeding). Products include:
Aggrenox Capsules ... 1026
Persantine Tablets ... 1057

Enoxaparin (Co-administration with other anticoagulant agents may be associated with an increase in bleeding). Products include:
Lovenox Injection ... 746

Etodolac (Co-administration with antiplatelet agents, such as non-steroidal anti-inflammatory agents, may be associated with an increase in bleeding). Products include:
Lodine ... 3528
Lodine XL Extended-Release Tablets ... 3530

Fenoprofen Calcium (Co-administration with antiplatelet agents, such as non-steroidal anti-inflammatory agents, may be associated with an increase in bleeding).
No products indexed under this heading.

Flurbiprofen (Co-administration with antiplatelet agents, such as non-steroidal anti-inflammatory agents, may be associated with an increase in bleeding).
No products indexed under this heading.

Heparin Sodium (Co-administration with other anticoagulant agents may be associated with an increase in bleeding). Products include:
Heparin Lock Flush Solution ... 3509
Heparin Sodium Injection ... 3511

Ibuprofen (Co-administration with antiplatelet agents, such as non-steroidal anti-inflammatory agents, may be associated with an increase in bleeding). Products include:
Advil ... 771
Children's Advil Oral Suspension ... 773
Children's Advil Chewable Tablets ... 773
Advil Cold and Sinus Caplets ... 771
Advil Cold and Sinus Tablets ... 771
Advil Flu & Body Ache Caplets ... 772
Infants' Advil Drops ... 773
Junior Strength Advil Tablets ... 773
Junior Strength Advil Chewable Tablets ... 773
Advil Migraine Liquigels ... 772
Children's Motrin Oral Suspension and Chewable Tablets ... 2006
Children's Motrin Cold Oral Suspension ... 2007
Children's Motrin Oral Suspension ... 643
Motrin Suspension, Oral Drops, Chewable Tablets, and Caplets ... 2002
Infants' Motrin Concentrated Drops ... 2006
Junior Strength Motrin Caplets and Chewable Tablets ... 2006
Motrin IB Tablets, Caplets, and Gelcaps ... 2002
Motrin Migraine Pain Caplets ... 2005
Motrin Sinus Headache Caplets ... 2005
Vicoprofen Tablets ... 520

Indomethacin (Co-administration with antiplatelet agents, such as non-steroidal anti-inflammatory agents, may be associated with an increase in bleeding). Products include:
Indocin ... 2112

Indomethacin Sodium Trihydrate (Co-administration with antiplatelet agents, such as non-steroidal anti-inflammatory agents, may be associated with an increase in bleeding). Products include:
Indocin I.V. ... 2115

Ketoprofen (Co-administration with antiplatelet agents, such as non-steroidal anti-inflammatory agents, may be associated with an increase in bleeding). Products include:
Orudis Capsules ... 3548
Orudis KT Tablets ... 778
Oruvail Capsules ... 3548

Ketorolac Tromethamine (Co-administration with antiplatelet agents, such as non-steroidal anti-inflammatory agents, may be associated with an increase in bleeding). Products include:
Acular Ophthalmic Solution ... 544
Acular PF Ophthalmic Solution ... 544
Toradol ... 3018

Meclofenamate Sodium (Co-administration with antiplatelet agents, such as non-steroidal anti-inflammatory agents, may be associated with an increase in bleeding).
No products indexed under this heading.

Mefenamic Acid (Co-administration with antiplatelet agents, such as non-steroidal anti-inflammatory agents, may be associated with an increase in bleeding). Products include:
Ponstel Capsules ... 1356

Meloxicam (Co-administration with antiplatelet agents, such as non-steroidal anti-inflammatory agents, may be associated with an increase in bleeding). Products include:
Mobic Tablets ... 1054

Nabumetone (Co-administration with antiplatelet agents, such as non-steroidal anti-inflammatory agents, may be associated with an increase in bleeding). Products include:
Relafen Tablets ... 1617

Naproxen (Co-administration with antiplatelet agents, such as non-steroidal anti-inflammatory agents, may be associated with an increase in bleeding). Products include:
EC-Naprosyn Delayed-Release Tablets ... 2967
Naprosyn Suspension ... 2967
Naprosyn Tablets ... 2967

Naproxen Sodium (Co-administration with antiplatelet agents, such as non-steroidal anti-inflammatory agents, may be associated with an increase in bleeding). Products include:
Aleve Tablets, Caplets and Gelcaps ... 602
Aleve Cold & Sinus Caplets ... 603
Anaprox Tablets ... 2967
Anaprox DS Tablets ... 2967
Naprelan Tablets ... 1293

Oxaprozin (Co-administration with antiplatelet agents, such as non-steroidal anti-inflammatory agents, may be associated with an increase in bleeding).
No products indexed under this heading.

Phenylbutazone (Co-administration with antiplatelet agents, such as non-steroidal anti-inflammatory agents, may be associated with an increase in bleeding).
No products indexed under this heading.

Piroxicam (Co-administration with antiplatelet agents, such as non-steroidal anti-inflammatory agents, may be associated with an increase in bleeding). Products include:
Feldene Capsules ... 2685

Reteplase (Co-administration with thrombolytics may be associated with an increase in bleeding). Products include:
Retavase Vials ... 1182

Rofecoxib (Co-administration with antiplatelet agents, such as non-steroidal anti-inflammatory agents, may be associated with an increase in bleeding). Products include:
Vioxx ... 2213

Streptokinase (Co-administration with thrombolytics may be associated with an increase in bleeding). Products include:
Streptase for Infusion ... 647

Sulindac (Co-administration with antiplatelet agents, such as non-steroidal anti-inflammatory agents, may be associated with an increase in bleeding). Products include:
Clinoril Tablets ... 2053

Ticlopidine Hydrochloride (Co-administration with antiplatelet agents, such as ticlopidine, may be associated with an increase in bleeding). Products include:
Ticlid Tablets ... 3015

Tinzaparin sodium (Co-administration with other anticoagulant agents may be associated with an increase in bleeding). Products include:
Innohep Injection ... 1248

Tolmetin Sodium (Co-administration with antiplatelet agents, such as non-steroidal anti-inflammatory agents, may be associated with an increase in bleeding). Products include:
Tolectin ... 2589

Urokinase (Co-administration with thrombolytics may be associated with an increase in bleeding).
No products indexed under this heading.

Warfarin Sodium (Co-administration of oral anticoagulants within seven days is contraindicated unless prothrombin time is less than or equal to 1.2 times control; concurrent use with other anticoagulant agents may be associated with an increase in bleeding). Products include:
Coumadin for Injection ... 1243
Coumadin Tablets ... 1243
Warfarin Sodium Tablets, USP ... 3302

REPRONEX FOR INTRAMUSCULAR AND SUBCUTANEOUS INJECTION

(Menotropins) ... 1347
None cited in PDR database.

REQUIP TABLETS

(Ropinirole Hydrochloride) ... 1621
May interact with central nervous system depressants, antidepressant drugs, dopamine D2 antagonists, and certain other agents. Compounds in these categories include:

Alfentanil Hydrochloride (Possible additive sedative effects).
No products indexed under this heading.

Alprazolam (Possible additive sedative effects). Products include:
Xanax Tablets ... 2865

Amitriptyline Hydrochloride (Possible additive sedative effects). Products include:
Etrafon ... 3115
Limbitrol ... 1738

Amoxapine (Possible additive sedative effects).
No products indexed under this heading.

Aprobarbital (Possible additive sedative effects).
No products indexed under this heading.

Buprenorphine Hydrochloride (Possible additive sedative effects). Products include:
Buprenex Injectable ... 2918

Bupropion Hydrochloride (Possible additive sedative effects). Products include:
Wellbutrin Tablets ... 1680
Wellbutrin SR Sustained-Release Tablets ... 1684
Zyban Sustained-Release Tablets ... 1710

Buspirone Hydrochloride (Possible additive sedative effects).
No products indexed under this heading.

Butabarbital (Possible additive sedative effects).
No products indexed under this heading.

Butalbital (Possible additive sedative effects). Products include:
Phrenilin ... 578
Sedapap Tablets 50 mg/650 mg ... 2225

Chlordiazepoxide (Possible additive sedative effects). Products include:
Limbitrol ... 1738

Chlordiazepoxide Hydrochloride (Possible additive sedative effects). Products include:
Librium Capsules ... 1736
Librium for Injection ... 1737

Chlorpromazine (Co-administration with dopamine antagonists may diminish the effectiveness of ropinirole). Products include:
Thorazine Suppositories ... 1656

Chlorpromazine Hydrochloride (Co-administration with dopamine antagonists may diminish the effectiveness of ropinirole). Products include:
Thorazine ... 1656

Chlorprothixene (Co-administration with dopamine antagonists may diminish the effectiveness of ropinirole).
No products indexed under this heading.

Chlorprothixene Hydrochloride (Co-administration with dopamine antagonists may diminish the effectiveness of ropinirole).
No products indexed under this heading.

Chlorprothixene Lactate (Possible additive sedative effects).
No products indexed under this heading.

Ciprofloxacin (Co-administration increases ropinirole AUC by 84% on average and Cmax by 60%).
Products include:
Cipro I.V. 893
Cipro I.V. Pharmacy Bulk Package .. 897
Cipro Oral Suspension 887

Ciprofloxacin Hydrochloride (Co-administration increases ropinirole AUC by 84% on average and Cmax by 60%). Products include:
Ciloxan 538
Cipro HC Otic Suspension 540
Cipro Tablets 887

Citalopram Hydrobromide (Possible additive sedative effects).
Products include:
Celexa 1365

Clorazepate Dipotassium (Possible additive sedative effects).
Products include:
Tranxene 511

Clozapine (Possible additive sedative effects). Products include:
Clozaril Tablets 2319

Codeine Phosphate (Possible additive sedative effects). Products include:
Phenergan with Codeine Syrup 3557
Phenergan VC with Codeine Syrup .. 3561
Robitussin A-C Syrup 2942
Robitussin-DAC Syrup 2942
Ryna-C Liquid .... ▣ 768
Soma Compound w/Codeine Tablets 3355
Tussi-Organidin NR Liquid 3350
Tussi-Organidin-S NR Liquid 3350
Tylenol with Codeine 2595

Desflurane (Possible additive sedative effects). Products include:
Suprane Liquid for Inhalation 874

Desipramine Hydrochloride (Possible additive sedative effects).
Products include:
Norpramin Tablets 755

Dezocine (Possible additive sedative effects).
No products indexed under this heading.

Diazepam (Possible additive sedative effects). Products include:
Valium Injectable 3026
Valium Tablets 3047

Doxepin Hydrochloride (Possible additive sedative effects). Products include:
Sinequan 2713

Droperidol (Possible additive sedative effects).
No products indexed under this heading.

Enflurane (Possible additive sedative effects).
No products indexed under this heading.

Estazolam (Possible additive sedative effects). Products include:
ProSom Tablets 500

Ethchlorvynol (Possible additive sedative effects).
No products indexed under this heading.

Ethinamate (Possible additive sedative effects).
No products indexed under this heading.

Ethinyl Estradiol (Reduces the oral clearance of ropinirole by 36%).
Products include:
Alesse-21 Tablets 3468
Alesse-28 Tablets 3473
Brevicon 28-Day Tablets 3380
Cyclessa Tablets 2450
Desogen Tablets 2458
Estinyl Tablets 3112
Estrostep 2627
femhrt Tablets 2635
Levlen 962
Levlite 21 Tablets 962
Levlite 28 Tablets 962
Levora Tablets 3389
Loestrin 21 Tablets 2642
Loestrin Fe Tablets 2642
Lo/Ovral Tablets 3532
Lo/Ovral-28 Tablets 3538
Low-Ogestrel-28 Tablets 3392
Microgestin Fe 1.5/30 Tablets 3407
Microgestin Fe 1/20 Tablets 3400
Mircette Tablets 2470
Modicon 2563
Necon 3415
Nordette-28 Tablets 2257
Norinyl 1 +35 28-Day Tablets 3380
Ogestrel 0.5/50-28 Tablets 3428
Ortho-Cept 21 Tablets 2546
Ortho-Cept 28 Tablets 2546
Ortho-Cyclen/Ortho Tri-Cyclen 2573
Ortho-Novum 2563
Ovcon 3364
Ovral Tablets 3551
Ovral-28 Tablets 3552
Tri-Levlen 962
Tri-Norinyl-28 Tablets 3433
Triphasil-21 Tablets 3600
Triphasil-28 Tablets 3605
Trivora Tablets 3439
Yasmin 28 Tablets 980
Zovia 3449

Fentanyl (Possible additive sedative effects). Products include:
Duragesic Transdermal System 1786

Fentanyl Citrate (Possible additive sedative effects). Products include:
Actiq 1184

Fluoxetine Hydrochloride (Possible additive sedative effects).
Products include:
Prozac Pulvules, Liquid, and Weekly Capsules 1238
Sarafem Pulvules 1962

Fluphenazine Decanoate (Co-administration with dopamine antagonists may diminish the effectiveness of ropinirole).
No products indexed under this heading.

Fluphenazine Enanthate (Co-administration with dopamine antagonists may diminish the effectiveness of ropinirole).
No products indexed under this heading.

Fluphenazine Hydrochloride (Co-administration with dopamine antagonists may diminish the effectiveness of ropinirole).
No products indexed under this heading.

Flurazepam Hydrochloride (Possible additive sedative effects).
No products indexed under this heading.

Glutethimide (Possible additive sedative effects).
No products indexed under this heading.

Haloperidol (Co-administration with dopamine antagonists may diminish the effectiveness of ropinirole).
Products include:
Haldol Injection, Tablets and Concentrate 2533

Haloperidol Decanoate (Co-administration with dopamine antagonists may diminish the effectiveness of ropinirole). Products include:
Haldol Decanoate 2535

Hydrocodone Bitartrate (Possible additive sedative effects). Products include:
Hycodan 1316
Hycomine Compound Tablets 1317
Hycotuss Expectorant Syrup 1318
Lortab 3319
Lortab Elixir 3317
Maxidone Tablets CIII 3399
Norco 5/325 Tablets CIII 3424
Norco 7.5/325 Tablets CIII 3425
Norco 10/325 Tablets CIII 3427
Norco 10/325 Tablets CIII 3425
Vicodin Tablets 516
Vicodin ES Tablets 517
Vicodin HP Tablets 518
Vicodin Tuss Expectorant 519
Vicoprofen Tablets 520
Zydone Tablets 1330

Hydrocodone Polistirex (Possible additive sedative effects). Products include:
Tussionex Pennkinetic Extended-Release Suspension 1174

Hydromorphone Hydrochloride (Possible additive sedative effects).
Products include:
Dilaudid 441
Dilaudid Oral Liquid 445
Dilaudid Powder 441
Dilaudid Rectal Suppositories 441
Dilaudid Tablets 441
Dilaudid Tablets - 8 mg 445
Dilaudid-HP 443

Hydroxyzine Hydrochloride (Possible additive sedative effects).
Products include:
Atarax Tablets & Syrup 2667
Vistaril Intramuscular Solution 2738

Imipramine Hydrochloride (Possible additive sedative effects).
No products indexed under this heading.

Imipramine Pamoate (Possible additive sedative effects).
No products indexed under this heading.

Isocarboxazid (Possible additive sedative effects).
No products indexed under this heading.

Isoflurane (Possible additive sedative effects).
No products indexed under this heading.

Ketamine Hydrochloride (Possible additive sedative effects).
No products indexed under this heading.

Levodopa (Ropinirole may potentiate the dopaminergic effects of L-dopa and may cause and/or exacerbate pre-existing dyskinesia; increased mean steady state of L-dopa by 20%). Products include:
Sinemet Tablets 1253
Sinemet CR Tablets 1255

Levomethadyl Acetate Hydrochloride (Possible additive sedative effects).
No products indexed under this heading.

Levorphanol Tartrate (Possible additive sedative effects). Products include:
Levo-Dromoran 1734
Levorphanol Tartrate Tablets 3059

Lorazepam (Possible additive sedative effects). Products include:
Ativan Injection 3478
Ativan Tablets 3482

Loxapine Hydrochloride (Co-administration with dopamine antagonists may diminish the effectiveness of ropinirole).
No products indexed under this heading.

Loxapine Succinate (Co-administration with dopamine antagonists may diminish the effectiveness of ropinirole). Products include:
Loxitane Capsules 3398

Maprotiline Hydrochloride (Possible additive sedative effects).
No products indexed under this heading.

Meperidine Hydrochloride (Possible additive sedative effects).
Products include:
Demerol 3079
Mepergan Injection 3539

Mephobarbital (Possible additive sedative effects).
No products indexed under this heading.

Meprobamate (Possible additive sedative effects). Products include:
Miltown Tablets 3349

Mesoridazine Besylate (Co-administration with dopamine antagonists may diminish the effectiveness of ropinirole). Products include:
Serentil 1057

Methadone Hydrochloride (Possible additive sedative effects).
Products include:
Dolophine Hydrochloride Tablets 3056

Methohexital Sodium (Possible additive sedative effects). Products include:
Brevital Sodium for Injection, USP .. 1815

Methotrimeprazine (Co-administration with dopamine antagonists may diminish the effectiveness of ropinirole).
No products indexed under this heading.

Methoxyflurane (Possible additive sedative effects).
No products indexed under this heading.

Metoclopramide Hydrochloride (Co-administration with dopamine antagonists may diminish the effectiveness of ropinirole). Products include:
Reglan 2935

Midazolam Hydrochloride (Possible additive sedative effects).
Products include:
Versed Injection 3027
Versed Syrup 3033

Mirtazapine (Possible additive sedative effects). Products include:
Remeron Tablets 2483
Remeron SolTab Tablets 2486

Molindone Hydrochloride (Co-administration with dopamine antagonists may diminish the effectiveness of ropinirole). Products include:
Moban 1320

Morphine Sulfate (Possible additive sedative effects). Products include:
Astramorph/PF Injection, USP (Preservative-Free) 594
Duramorph Injection 1312
Infumorph 200 and Infumorph 500 Sterile Solutions 1314
Kadian Capsules 1335
MS Contin Tablets 2896
MSIR 2898
Oramorph SR Tablets 3062
Roxanol 3066

Nefazodone Hydrochloride (Possible additive sedative effects).
Products include:
Serzone Tablets 1104

Nortriptyline Hydrochloride (Possible additive sedative effects).
No products indexed under this heading.

Olanzapine (Possible additive sedative effects). Products include:
Zyprexa Tablets 1973
Zyprexa ZYDIS Orally Disintegrating Tablets 1973

Oxazepam (Possible additive sedative effects).
No products indexed under this heading.

Oxycodone Hydrochloride (Possible additive sedative effects).
Products include:
OxyContin Tablets 2912
OxyFast Oral Concentrate Solution . 2916
OxyIR Capsules 2916
Percocet Tablets 1326
Percodan Tablets 1327
Percolone Tablets 1327
Roxicodone 3067
Tylox Capsules 2597

Paroxetine Hydrochloride (Possible additive sedative effects).
Products include:
Paxil 1609

Pentobarbital Sodium (Possible additive sedative effects). Products include:
Nembutal Sodium Solution 485

Perphenazine (Co-administration with dopamine antagonists may diminish the effectiveness of ropinirole). Products include:
- Etrafon 3115
- Trilafon 3160

Phenelzine Sulfate (Possible additive sedative effects). Products include:
- Nardil Tablets 2653

Phenobarbital (Possible additive sedative effects). Products include:
- Arco-Lase Plus Tablets 592
- Donnatal 2929
- Donnatal Extentabs 2930

Prazepam (Possible additive sedative effects).
- No products indexed under this heading.

Prochlorperazine (Co-administration with dopamine antagonists may diminish the effectiveness of ropinirole). Products include:
- Compazine 1505

Promethazine Hydrochloride (Co-administration with dopamine antagonists may diminish the effectiveness of ropinirole). Products include:
- Mepergan Injection 3539
- Phenergan Injection 3553
- Phenergan 3556
- Phenergan Syrup 3554
- Phenergan with Codeine Syrup 3557
- Phenergan with Dextromethorphan Syrup 3559
- Phenergan VC Syrup 3560
- Phenergan VC with Codeine Syrup 3561

Propofol (Possible additive sedative effects). Products include:
- Diprivan Injectable Emulsion 667

Propoxyphene Hydrochloride (Possible additive sedative effects). Products include:
- Darvon Pulvules 1909
- Darvon Compound-65 Pulvules 1910

Propoxyphene Napsylate (Possible additive sedative effects). Products include:
- Darvon-N/Darvocet-N 1907
- Darvon-N Tablets 1912

Protriptyline Hydrochloride (Possible additive sedative effects). Products include:
- Vivactil Tablets 2446
- Vivactil Tablets 2217

Quazepam (Possible additive sedative effects).
- No products indexed under this heading.

Quetiapine Fumarate (Co-administration with dopamine antagonists may diminish the effectiveness of ropinirole). Products include:
- Seroquel Tablets 684

Remifentanil Hydrochloride (Possible additive sedative effects).
- No products indexed under this heading.

Risperidone (Co-administration with dopamine antagonists may diminish the effectiveness of ropinirole). Products include:
- Risperdal 1796

Secobarbital Sodium (Possible additive sedative effects).
- No products indexed under this heading.

Sertraline Hydrochloride (Possible additive sedative effects). Products include:
- Zoloft 2751

Sevoflurane (Possible additive sedative effects).
- No products indexed under this heading.

Sufentanil Citrate (Possible additive sedative effects).
- No products indexed under this heading.

Temazepam (Possible additive sedative effects).
- No products indexed under this heading.

Thiamylal Sodium (Possible additive sedative effects).
- No products indexed under this heading.

Thioridazine Hydrochloride (Co-administration with dopamine antagonists may diminish the effectiveness of ropinirole). Products include:
- Thioridazine Hydrochloride Tablets 2289

Thiothixene (Co-administration with dopamine antagonists may diminish the effectiveness of ropinirole). Products include:
- Navane Capsules 2701
- Thiothixene Capsules 2290

Tranylcypromine Sulfate (Possible additive sedative effects). Products include:
- Parnate Tablets 1607

Trazodone Hydrochloride (Possible additive sedative effects).
- No products indexed under this heading.

Triazolam (Possible additive sedative effects). Products include:
- Halcion Tablets 2823

Trifluoperazine Hydrochloride (Co-administration with dopamine antagonists may diminish the effectiveness of ropinirole). Products include:
- Stelazine 1640

Trimipramine Maleate (Possible additive sedative effects). Products include:
- Surmontil Capsules 3595

Venlafaxine Hydrochloride (Possible additive sedative effects). Products include:
- Effexor Tablets 3495
- Effexor XR Capsules 3499

Zaleplon (Possible additive sedative effects). Products include:
- Sonata Capsules 3591

Ziprasidone Hydrochloride (Possible additive sedative effects). Products include:
- Geodon Capsules 2688

Zolpidem Tartrate (Possible additive sedative effects). Products include:
- Ambien Tablets 3191

Food Interactions

Alcohol (Possible additive sedative effects).

Food, unspecified (Increases ropinirole Tmax by 2.5 hours; food does not affect the extent of absorption of ropinirole).

RESCRIPTOR TABLETS

(Delavirdine Mesylate) 526

May interact with amphetamines, antacids, dexamethasone, dihydropyridine calcium channel blockers, ergot-containing drugs, histamine H_2-receptor antagonists, phenytoin, proton pump inhibitor, quinidine, and certain other agents. Compounds in these categories include:

Alprazolam (Co-administration with drugs that are highly dependent on CYP3A for clearance and for which elevated plasma levels are associated with serious and/or life threatening events, such as prolonged or increased sedation or respiratory depression; concurrent use is contraindicated). Products include:
- Xanax Tablets 2865

Aluminum Carbonate (Co-administration with antacids results in decreased delavirdine concentrations because of reduced absorption; patients taking antacids should be advised to take them at least one hour apart).
- No products indexed under this heading.

Aluminum Hydroxide (Co-administration with antacids results in decreased delavirdine concentrations because of reduced absorption; patients taking antacids should be advised to take them at least one hour apart). Products include:
- Amphojel Suspension (Mint Flavor) ..... ▣789
- Gaviscon Extra Strength Liquid ..... ▣751
- Gaviscon Extra Strength Tablets ..... ▣751
- Gaviscon Regular Strength Liquid ..... ▣751
- Gaviscon Regular Strength Tablets ..... ▣750
- Maalox Antacid/Anti-Gas Oral Suspension ..... ▣673
- Maalox Max Maximum Strength Antacid/Anti-Gas Liquid 2300
- Maalox Regular Strength Antacid/Antigas Liquid 2300
- Mylanta 1813
- Vanquish Caplets ..... ▣617

Amiodarone Hydrochloride (Co-administration results in increased amiodarone concentrations). Products include:
- Cordarone Intravenous 3491
- Cordarone Tablets 3487
- Pacerone Tablets 3331

Amlodipine Besylate (Co-administration results in increased dihydropyridine calcium channel blockers concentrations). Products include:
- Lotrel Capsules 2370
- Norvasc Tablets 2704

Amphetamine Resins (Co-administration results in increased amphetamine concentrations).
- No products indexed under this heading.

Amphetamine Sulfate (Co-administration results in increased amphetamine concentrations). Products include:
- Adderall Tablets 3231
- Adderall XR Capsules .....

Amprenavir (Co-administration results in increased amprenavir concentrations). Products include:
- Agenerase Capsules 1454
- Agenerase Oral Solution 1459

Astemizole (Co-administration with drugs that are highly dependent on CYP3A for clearance and for which elevated plasma levels are associated with serious and/or life threatening events, such as cardiac arrhythmias; concurrent use is contraindicated).
- No products indexed under this heading.

Atorvastatin Calcium (The risk of myopathy, including rhabdomolysis, may be increased with concurrent use). Products include:
- Lipitor Tablets 2639
- Lipitor Tablets 2696

Bepridil Hydrochloride (Co-administration results in increased bepridil concentrations; increased bepridil exposure may be associated with life-threatening reactions such as cardiac arrhythmias). Products include:
- Vascor Tablets 2602

Carbamazepine (May lead to loss of virologic response and possible resistance to delavirdine or the class of non-nucleoside reverse transcriptase inhibitors). Products include:
- Carbatrol Capsules 3234
- Tegretol/Tegretol-XR 2404

Cerivastatin Sodium (The risk of myopathy, including rhabdomyolysis, may be increased with concurrent use). Products include:
- Baycol Tablets 883

Cimetidine (H2 antagonists increase gastric pH and may reduce the absorption of delavirdine; chronic use of these drugs with delavirdine is not recommended). Products include:
- Tagamet HB 200 Suspension ..... ▣762
- Tagamet HB 200 Tablets ..... ▣761
- Tagamet Tablets 1644

Cimetidine Hydrochloride (H2 antagonists increase gastric pH and may reduce the absorption of delavirdine; chronic use of these drugs with delavirdine is not recommended). Products include:
- Tagamet 1644

Cisapride (Co-administration with drugs that are highly dependent on CYP3A for clearance and for which elevated plasma levels are associated with serious and/or life threatening events, such as cardiac arrrhythmias; concurrent use is contraindicated).
- No products indexed under this heading.

Clarithromycin (Co-administrations results in increased clarithromycin concentrations). Products include:
- Biaxin/Biaxin XL 403
- PREVPAC 3298

Cyclosporine (Co-administration results in increased cyclosporine concentrations). Products include:
- Gengraf Capsules 457
- Neoral Soft Gelatin Capsules 2380
- Neoral Oral Solution 2380
- Sandimmune 2388

Dexamethasone (Co-administration results in decreased delavirdine concentrations). Products include:
- Decadron Elixir 2078
- Decadron Tablets 2079
- TobraDex Ophthalmic Ointment 542
- TobraDex Ophthalmic Suspension 541

Dexamethasone Acetate (Co-administration results in decreased delavirdine concentrations).
- No products indexed under this heading.

Dexamethasone Sodium Phosphate (Co-administration results in decreased delavirdine concentrations). Products include:
- Decadron Phosphate Injection 2081
- Decadron Phosphate Sterile Ophthalmic Ointment 2083
- Decadron Phosphate Sterile Ophthalmic Solution 2084
- NeoDecadron Sterile Ophthalmic Solution 2144

Dextroamphetamine Sulfate (Co-administration results in increased amphetamine concentrations). Products include:
- Adderall Tablets 3231
- Adderall XR Capsules .....
- Dexedrine 1512
- DextroStat Tablets 3236

Didanosine (Co-administration results in decreased didanosine and delavirdine plasma concentrations; administration of didanosine (buffered tablets) and delavirdine should be separated by at least one hour). Products include:
- Videx 1138
- Videx EC Capsules 1143

Dihydroergotamine Mesylate (Co-administration with drugs that are highly dependent on CYP3A for clearance and for which elevated plasma levels are associated with serious and/or life threatening events, such as acute ergot toxicity characterized by peripheral vasospasm and ischemiaof the extremities; concurrent use is contraindicated). Products include:
- D.H.E. 45 Injection 2334
- Migranal Nasal Spray 2376

Diltiazem Hydrochloride (Co-administration results in increased calcium channel blockers concentrations). Products include:
- Cardizem Injectable 1018
- Cardizem Lyo-Ject Syringe 1018
- Cardizem Monovial 1018
- Cardizem CD Capsules 1016

Tiazac Capsules ... 1378

Ergonovine Maleate (Co-administration with drugs that are highly dependent on CYP3A for clearance and for which elevated plasma levels are associated with serious and/or life threatening events, such as acute ergot toxicity characterized by peripheral vasospasm and ischemiaof the extremities; concurrent use is contraindicated).
No products indexed under this heading.

Ergotamine Tartrate (Co-administration with drugs that are highly dependent on CYP3A for clearance and for which elevated plasma levels are associated with serious and/or life threatening events, such as acute ergot toxicity characterized by peripheral vasospasm and ischemiaof the extremities; concurrent use is contraindicated).
No products indexed under this heading.

Esomeprazole Magnesium (Proton pump inhibitors increase gastric pH and may reduce the absorption of delavirdine; chronic use of these drugs with delavirdine is not recommended). Products include:
Nexium Delayed-Release Capsules ... 619

Ethinyl Estradiol (Co-administration results in increased ethinyl estradiol concentrations). Products include:
Alesse-21 Tablets ... 3468
Alesse-28 Tablets ... 3473
Brevicon 28-Day Tablets ... 3380
Cyclessa Tablets ... 2450
Desogen Tablets ... 2458
Estinyl Tablets ... 3112
Estrostep ... 2627
femhrt Tablets ... 2635
Levlen ... 962
Levlite 21 Tablets ... 962
Levlite 28 Tablets ... 962
Levora Tablets ... 3389
Loestrin 21 Tablets ... 2642
Loestrin Fe Tablets ... 2642
Lo/Ovral Tablets ... 3532
Lo/Ovral-28 Tablets ... 3538
Low-Ogestrel-28 Tablets ... 3392
Microgestin Fe 1.5/30 Tablets ... 3407
Microgestin Fe 1/20 Tablets ... 3400
Mircette Tablets ... 2470
Modicon ... 2563
Necon ... 3415
Nordette-28 Tablets ... 2257
Norinyl 1 +35 28-Day Tablets ... 3380
Ogestrel 0.5/50-28 Tablets ... 3428
Ortho-Cept 21 Tablets ... 2546
Ortho-Cept 28 Tablets ... 2546
Ortho-Cyclen/Ortho Tri-Cyclen ... 2573
Ortho-Novum ... 2563
Ovcon ... 3364
Ovral Tablets ... 3551
Ovral-28 Tablets ... 3552
Tri-Levlen ... 962
Tri-Norinyl-28 Tablets ... 3433
Triphasil-21 Tablets ... 3600
Triphasil-28 Tablets ... 3605
Trivora Tablets ... 3439
Yasmin 28 Tablets ... 980
Zovia ... 3449

Famotidine (H2 antagonists increase gastric pH and may reduce the absorption of delavirdine; chronic use of these drugs with delavirdine is not recommended). Products include:
Famotidine Injection ... 866
Pepcid AC ... 1814
Pepcid Complete Chewable Tablets ... 1815
Pepcid Injection ... 2153
Pepcid for Oral Suspension ... 2150
Pepcid RPD Orally Disintegrating Tablets ... 2150
Pepcid Tablets ... 2150

Felodipine (Co-administration results in increased dihydropyridine calcium channel blockers concentrations). Products include:
Lexxel Tablets ... 608
Plendil Extended-Release Tablets ... 623

Flecainide Acetate (Co-administration results in increased flecainide concentrations). Products include:
Tambocor Tablets ... 1990

Fluoxetine Hydrochloride (Co-administration has resulted in 50% change in the Cmax). Products include:
Prozac Pulvules, Liquid, and Weekly Capsules ... 1238
Sarafem Pulvules ... 1962

Fluvastatin Sodium (Co-administration results in increased fluvastatin concentrations). Products include:
Lescol Capsules ... 2361
Lescol ... 2925
Lescol XL Tablets ... 2361

Fosphenytoin Sodium (May lead to loss of virologic response and possible resistance to delavirdine or the class of non-nucleoside reverse transcriptase inhibitors). Products include:
Cerebyx Injection ... 2619

Hypericum (Co-administration with St. John's Wort or St. John's Wort-containing products and delavirdine is expected to substantially decrease delavirdine's concentrations and may result in suboptimal levels of delavirdine and lead to loss of virologic response). Products include:
Brite-Life Caplets ... ▣795
Centrum St. John's Wort Softgels ... ▣853
Metabolic Nutrition System ... ▣798
Movana Tablets ... ▣832
One-A-Day Tension & Mood Softgels ... ▣808
ReSource Wellness StayCalm Caplets ... ▣826
Satiete Tablets ... ▣846

Indinavir Sulfate (Co-administration results in increased indinavir concentrations; a dose reduction of indinavir to 600 mg t.i.d. should be considered when used concurrently). Products include:
Crixivan Capsules ... 2070

Isradipine (Co-administration results in increased dihydropyridine calcium channel blockers concentrations). Products include:
DynaCirc Capsules ... 2921
DynaCirc CR Tablets ... 2923

Lansoprazole (Proton pump inhibitors increase gastric pH and may reduce the absorption of delavirdine; chronic use of these drugs with delavirdine is not recommended). Products include:
Prevacid Delayed-Release Capsules ... 3292
PREVPAC ... 3298

Lidocaine Hydrochloride (Co-administration results in increased systemic lidocaine concentrations). Products include:
Bactine First Aid Liquid ... ▣611
Xylocaine Injections ... 653

Lopinavir (Co-administration results in increased lopinavir concentrations). Products include:
Kaletra Capsules ... 471
Kaletra Oral Solution ... 471

Lovastatin (Potential for serious reactions such as myopathy including rhabdomyolysis; concurrent use is not recommended). Products include:
Mevacor Tablets ... 2132

Magaldrate (Co-administration with antacids results in decreased delavirdine concentrations because of reduced absorption; patients taking antacids should be advised to take them at least one hour apart).
No products indexed under this heading.

Magnesium Hydroxide (Co-administration with antacids results in decreased delavirdine concentrations because of reduced absorption; patients taking antacids should be advised to take them at least one hour apart). Products include:
Ex•Lax Milk of Magnesia Liquid ... ▣670
Maalox Antacid/Anti-Gas Oral Suspension ... ▣673
Maalox Max Maximum Strength Antacid/Anti-Gas Liquid ... 2300
Maalox Regular Strength Antacid/Antigas Liquid ... 2300
Mylanta Fast-Acting ... 1813
Mylanta ... 1813
Pepcid Complete Chewable Tablets ... 1815
Phillips' Chewable Tablets ... ▣615
Phillips' Milk of Magnesia Liquid (Original, Cherry, & Mint) ... ▣616
Rolaids Tablets ... ▣706
Extra Strength Rolaids Tablets ... ▣706
Vanquish Caplets ... ▣617

Magnesium Oxide (Co-administration with antacids results in decreased delavirdine concentrations because of reduced absorption; patients taking antacids should be advised to take them at least one hour apart). Products include:
Beelith Tablets ... 946
Mag-Ox 400 Tablets ... 1024
Uro-Mag Capsules ... 1024

Methadone Hydrochloride (Co-administration results in increased methadone concentrations). Products include:
Dolophine Hydrochloride Tablets ... 3056

Methamphetamine Hydrochloride (Co-administration results in increased amphetamine concentrations). Products include:
Desoxyn Tablets ... 440

Methylergonovine Maleate (Co-administration with drugs that are highly dependent on CYP3A for clearance and for which elevated plasma levels are associated with serious and/or life threatening events, such as acute ergot toxicity characterized by peripheral vasospasm and ischemiaof the extremities; concurrent use is contraindicated).
No products indexed under this heading.

Methysergide Maleate (Co-administration with drugs that are highly dependent on CYP3A for clearance and for which elevated plasma levels are associated with serious and/or life threatening events, such as acute ergot toxicity characterized by peripheral vasospasm and ischemiaof the extremities; concurrent use is contraindicated).
No products indexed under this heading.

Midazolam Hydrochloride (Co-administration with drugs that are highly dependent on CYP3A for clearance and for which elevated plasma levels are associated with serious and/or life threatening events, such as cardiac arrhythmias; concurrent use is contraindicated). Products include:
Versed Injection ... 3027
Versed Syrup ... 3033

Nelfinavir Mesylate (Co-administration results in increased nelfinavir concentrations and decreased delavirdine concentrations). Products include:
Viracept ... 532

Nicardipine Hydrochloride (Co-administration results in increased dihydropyridine calcium channel blockers concentrations). Products include:
Cardene I.V. ... 3485

Nifedipine (Co-administration results in increased dihydropyridine calcium channel blockers concentrations). Products include:
Adalat CC Tablets ... 877
Procardia Capsules ... 2708
Procardia XL Extended Release Tablets ... 2710

Nimodipine (Co-administration results in increased dihydropyridine calcium channel blockers concentrations). Products include:
Nimotop Capsules ... 904

Nisoldipine (Co-adminstration results in increased calcium channel blockers concentrations). Products include:
Sular Tablets ... 688

Nizatidine (H2 antagonists increase gastric pH and may reduce the absorption of delavirdine; chronic use of these drugs with delavirdine is not recommended). Products include:
Axid Pulvules ... 1903
Axid Pulvules ... 2919

Omeprazole (Proton pump inhibitors increase gastric pH and may reduce the absorption of delavirdine; chronic use of these drugs with delavirdine is not recommended). Products include:
Prilosec Delayed-Release Capsules ... 628

Pantoprazole Sodium (Proton pump inhibitors increase gastric pH and may reduce the absorption of delavirdine; chronic use of these drugs with delavirdine is not recommended). Products include:
Protonix I.V. ... 3580
Protonix Tablets ... 3577

Phenobarbital (May lead to loss of virologic response and possible resistance to delavirdine or the class of non-nucleoside reverse transcriptase inhibitors). Products include:
Arco-Lase Plus Tablets ... 592
Donnatal ... 2929
Donnatal Extentabs ... 2930

Phenytoin (May lead to loss of virologic response and possible resistance to delavirdine or the class of non-nucleoside reverse transcriptase inhibitors). Products include:
Dilantin Infatabs ... 2624
Dilantin-125 Oral Suspension ... 2625

Phenytoin Sodium (May lead to loss of virologic response and possible resistance to delavirdine or the class of non-nucleoside reverse transcriptase inhibitors). Products include:
Dilantin Kapseals ... 2622

Pimozide (Co-administration with drugs that are highly dependent on CYP3A for clearance and for which elevated plasma levels are associated with serious and/or life threatening events, such as cardiac arrhythmias; concurrent use is contraindicated). Products include:
Orap Tablets ... 1407

Propafenone Hydrochloride (Co-administration results in increased propafenone concentrations). Products include:
Rythmol Tablets – 150 mg, 225 mg, 300 mg ... 502

Quinidine Gluconate (Co-administration results in increased quinidine concentrations). Products include:
Quinaglute Dura-Tabs Tablets ... 978

Quinidine Polygalacturonate (Co-administration results in increased quinidine concentrations).
No products indexed under this heading.

Quinidine Sulfate (Co-administration results in increased quinidine concentrations). Products include:
Quinidex Extentabs ... 2933

Rabeprazole Sodium (Proton pump inhibitors increase gastric pH and may reduce the absorption of delavirdine; chronic use of these drugs with delavirdine is not recommended). Products include:

Aciphex Tablets 1267
Aciphex Tablets 1783

Ranitidine Bismuth Citrate (H2 antagonists increase gastric pH and may reduce the absorption of delavirdine; chronic use of these drugs with delavirdine is not recommended).

No products indexed under this heading.

Ranitidine Hydrochloride (H2 antagonists increase gastric pH and may reduce the absorption of delavirdine; chronic use of these drugs with delavirdine is not recommended). Products include:

Zantac 1690
Zantac Injection 1688
Zantac 75 Tablets 717

Rapamycin (Co-administration results in increased rapamycin concentrations).

No products indexed under this heading.

Rifabutin (May lead to loss of virologic response and possible resistance to delavirdine or the class of non-nucleoside reverse transcriptase inhibitors or other co-administered antiviral drugs). Products include:

Mycobutin Capsules 2838

Rifampin (May lead to loss or virologic response and possible resistance to delavirdine or the class of non-nucleoside reverse transcriptase inhibitors or other co-administered antiviral drugs). Products include:

Rifadin 765
Rifamate Capsules 767
Rifater Tablets 769

Ritonavir (Co-administration results in increased ritonavir concentrations). Products include:

Kaletra Capsules 471
Kaletra Oral Solution 471
Norvir Capsules 487
Norvir Oral Solution 487

Saquinavir (Co-administration results in increased saquinavir concentrations). Products include:

Fortovase Capsules 2970

Saquinavir Mesylate (Co-administration results in increased saquinavir concentrations). Products include:

Invirase Capsules 2979

Sildenafil Citrate (Co-administration is expected to substantially increase sildenafil concentrations and may result in an increase in sildenafil-associated adverse events, including hypotension, visual changes, and priapism). Products include:

Viagra Tablets 2732

Simvastatin (Potential for serious reactions such as myopathy including rhabdomyolysis; concurrent use is not recommended). Products include:

Zocor Tablets 2219

Sodium Bicarbonate (Co-administration with antacids results in decreased delavirdine concentrations because of reduced absorption; patients taking antacids should be advised to take them at least one hour apart). Products include:

Alka-Seltzer 603
Alka-Seltzer Lemon Lime Antacid and Pain Reliever Effervescent Tablets 603
Alka-Seltzer Extra Strength Antacid and Pain Reliever Effervescent Tablets 603
Alka-Seltzer Heartburn Relief Tablets 604
Ceo-Two Evacuant Suppository 618
Colyte with Flavor Packs for Oral Solution 3170
GoLYTELY and Pineapple Flavor GoLYTELY for Oral Solution 1068
NuLYTELY, Cherry Flavor, Lemon-Lime Flavor, and Orange Flavor NuLYTELY for Oral Solution 1068

Tacrolimus (Co-administration results in increased tacrolimus concentrations). Products include:

Prograf 1393
Protopic Ointment 1397

Terfenadine (Co-administration with drugs that are highly dependent on CYP3A for clearance and for which elevated plasma levels are associated with serious and/or life threatening events, such as cardiac arrhythmias; concurrent use is contraindicated).

No products indexed under this heading.

Triazolam (Co-administration with drugs that are highly dependent on CYP3A for clearance and for which elevated plasma levels are associated with serious and/or life threatening events, such as prolonged or increased sedation or respiratory depression; concurrent use is contraindicated). Products include:

Halcion Tablets 2823

Verapamil Hydrochloride (Co-administration results in increased calcium channel blockers concentrations). Products include:

Covera-HS Tablets 3199
Isoptin SR Tablets 467
Tarka Tablets 508
Verelan Capsules 3184
Verelan PM Capsules 3186

Warfarin Sodium (Co-administration results in increased warfarin concentrations). Products include:

Coumadin for Injection 1243
Coumadin Tablets 1243
Warfarin Sodium Tablets, USP 3302

RESCULA OPHTHALMIC SOLUTION

(Unoprostone isopropyl) .... ⊙ 306
None cited in PDR database.

RESOURCE WELLNESS ALLERPRO CAPSULES

(Herbals, Multiple) 824
None cited in PDR database.

RESOURCE WELLNESS CALCIWISE SOFT CHEWS

(Calcium Carbonate, Vitamins with Minerals) 824
None cited in PDR database.

RESOURCE WELLNESS ENVIGOR CAPLETS

(Ginkgo biloba, Ginseng, Herbals with Vitamins & Minerals) 824
May interact with oral anticoagulants, monoamine oxidase inhibitors, and certain other agents. Compounds in these categories include:

Hormones, unspecified (Concurrent use with unspecified hormone drugs is not recommended).

Aspirin (Concurrent use with aspirin is not recommended). Products include:

Aggrenox Capsules 1026
Alka-Seltzer 603
Alka-Seltzer Lemon Lime Antacid and Pain Reliever Effervescent Tablets 603
Alka-Seltzer Extra Strength Antacid and Pain Reliever Effervescent Tablets 603
Alka-Seltzer PM Effervescent Tablets 605
Genuine Bayer Tablets, Caplets and Gelcaps 606
Extra Strength Bayer Caplets and Gelcaps 610
Aspirin Regimen Bayer Children's Chewable Tablets (Orange or Cherry Flavored) 607
Bayer, Aspirin Regimen 606
Aspirin Regimen Bayer 81 mg Caplets with Calcium 607
Genuine Bayer Professional Labeling (Aspirin Regimen Bayer) 608
Extra Strength Bayer Arthritis Caplets 610
Extra Strength Bayer Plus Caplets 610
Extra Strength Bayer PM Caplets 611
BC Powder 619
BC Allergy Sinus Cold Powder 619
Arthritis Strength BC Powder 619
BC Sinus Cold Powder 619
Darvon Compound-65 Pulvules 1910
Ecotrin Enteric Coated Aspirin Low, Regular and Maximum Strength Tablets 1715
Excedrin Extra-Strength Tablets, Caplets, and Geltabs 629
Excedrin Migraine 1070
Goody's Body Pain Formula Powder 620
Goody's Extra Strength Headache Powder 620
Goody's Extra Strength Pain Relief Tablets 620
Percodan Tablets 1327
Robaxisal Tablets 2939
Soma Compound Tablets 3354
Soma Compound w/Codeine Tablets 3355
Vanquish Caplets 617

Dicumarol (Concurrent use with anticoagulants is not recommended).

No products indexed under this heading.

Isocarboxazid (Concurrent use with MAO inhibitors is not recommended).

No products indexed under this heading.

Moclobemide (Concurrent use with MAO inhibitors is not recommended).

No products indexed under this heading.

Pargyline Hydrochloride (Concurrent use with MAO inhibitors is not recommended).

No products indexed under this heading.

Phenelzine Sulfate (Concurrent use with MAO inhibitors is not recommended). Products include:

Nardil Tablets 2653

Procarbazine Hydrochloride (Concurrent use with MAO inhibitors is not recommended). Products include:

Matulane Capsules 3246

Selegiline Hydrochloride (Concurrent use with MAO inhibitors is not recommended). Products include:

Eldepryl Capsules 3266

Steroids, unspecified (Concurrent use with unspecified steroids is not recommended).

No products indexed under this heading.

Tranylcypromine Sulfate (Concurrent use with MAO inhibitors is not recommended). Products include:

Parnate Tablets 1607

Warfarin Sodium (Concurrent use with anticoagulants is not recommended). Products include:

Coumadin for Injection 1243
Coumadin Tablets 1243
Warfarin Sodium Tablets, USP 3302

RESOURCE WELLNESS FLEXTEND CAPLETS

(Glucosamine Sulfate, Vitamins with Minerals) 825
None cited in PDR database.

RESOURCE WELLNESS FORSIGHT CAPLETS

(Dicalcium Phosphate, Vitamins with Minerals) 825
May interact with oral anticoagulants. Compounds in these categories include:

Dicumarol (Concurrent use with anticoagulants is not recommended).

No products indexed under this heading.

Warfarin Sodium (Concurrent use with anticoagulants is not recommended). Products include:

Coumadin for Injection 1243
Coumadin Tablets 1243
Warfarin Sodium Tablets, USP 3302

RESOURCE WELLNESS MEMORABLE SOFTGELS

(Ginkgo biloba, Herbals with Vitamins, Lecithin) 825
May interact with oral anticoagulants. Compounds in these categories include:

Dicumarol (Concurrent use with anticoagulants is not recommended).

No products indexed under this heading.

Warfarin Sodium (Concurrent use with anticoagulants is not recommended). Products include:

Coumadin for Injection 1243
Coumadin Tablets 1243
Warfarin Sodium Tablets, USP 3302

RESOURCE WELLNESS RESISTEX CAPSULES

(Echinacea, Ginseng) 826
None cited in PDR database.

RESOURCE WELLNESS 2ND WIND CAPSULES

(Ginseng) 826
May interact with oral anticoagulants. Compounds in these categories include:

Dicumarol (Concurrent use with anticoagulants is not recommended).

No products indexed under this heading.

Warfarin Sodium (Concurrent use with anticoagulants is not recommended). Products include:

Coumadin for Injection 1243
Coumadin Tablets 1243
Warfarin Sodium Tablets, USP 3302

RESOURCE WELLNESS STAYCALM CAPLETS

(Herbals with Vitamins & Minerals, Hypericum, Valeriana officinalis) 826
May interact with antidepressant drugs, hypnotics and sedatives, monoamine oxidase inhibitors, protease inhibitors, and certain other agents. Compounds in these categories include:

Amitriptyline Hydrochloride (Concurrent use with antidepressants is not recommended). Products include:

Etrafon 3115
Limbitrol 1738

Amoxapine (Concurrent use with antidepressants is not recommended).

No products indexed under this heading.

Amprenavir (Resource Wellness StayCalm contains St. John's Wort; concurrent use with protease inhibitors is not recommended). Products include:

Agenerase Capsules 1454
Agenerase Oral Solution 1459

Bupropion Hydrochloride (Concurrent use with antidepressants is not recommended). Products include:

Wellbutrin Tablets 1680
Wellbutrin SR Sustained-Release Tablets 1684
Zyban Sustained-Release Tablets 1710

Citalopram Hydrobromide (Concurrent use with antidepressants is not recommended). Products include:

Celexa 1365

Cyclosporine (Resource Wellness StayCalm contains St. John's Wort; concurrent use with cyclosporine is not recommended). Products include:

Gengraf Capsules 457
Neoral Soft Gelatin Capsules 2380
Neoral Oral Solution 2380
Sandimmune 2388

Desipramine Hydrochloride (Concurrent use with antidepressants is not recommended). Products include:
Norpramin Tablets 755

Doxepin Hydrochloride (Concurrent use with antidepressants is not recommended). Products include:
Sinequan 2713

Estazolam (Resource Wellness StayCalm contains valerian extract which causes drowsiness; concurrent use with sedatives is not recommended). Products include:
ProSom Tablets 500

Ethchlorvynol (Resource Wellness StayCalm contains valerian extract which causes drowsiness; concurrent use with sedatives is not recommended).
No products indexed under this heading.

Ethinamate (Resource Wellness StayCalm contains valerian extract which causes drowsiness; concurrent use with sedatives is not recommended).
No products indexed under this heading.

Fluoxetine Hydrochloride (Concurrent use with antidepressants is not recommended). Products include:
Prozac Pulvules, Liquid, and Weekly Capsules 1238
Sarafem Pulvules 1962

Flurazepam Hydrochloride (Resource Wellness StayCalm contains valerian extract which causes drowsiness; concurrent use with sedatives is not recommended).
No products indexed under this heading.

Glutethimide (Resource Wellness StayCalm contains valerian extract which causes drowsiness; concurrent use with sedatives is not recommended).
No products indexed under this heading.

Imipramine Hydrochloride (Concurrent use with antidepressants is not recommended).
No products indexed under this heading.

Imipramine Pamoate (Concurrent use with antidepressants is not recommended).
No products indexed under this heading.

Indinavir Sulfate (Resource Wellness StayCalm contains St. John's Wort; concurrent use with protease inhibitors is not recommended). Products include:
Crixivan Capsules 2070

Isocarboxazid (Concurrent use with MAO inhibitors is not recommended).
No products indexed under this heading.

Lopinavir (Resource Wellness StayCalm contains St. John's Wort; concurrent use with protease inhibitors is not recommended). Products include:
Kaletra Capsules 471
Kaletra Oral Solution 471

Lorazepam (Resource Wellness StayCalm contains valerian extract which causes drowsiness; concurrent use with sedatives is not recommended). Products include:
Ativan Injection 3478
Ativan Tablets 3482

Maprotiline Hydrochloride (Concurrent use with antidepressants is not recommended).
No products indexed under this heading.

Midazolam Hydrochloride (Resource Wellness StayCalm contains valerian extract which causes drowsiness; concurrent use with sedatives is not recommended). Products include:
Versed Injection 3027
Versed Syrup 3033

Mirtazapine (Concurrent use with antidepressants is not recommended). Products include:
Remeron Tablets 2483
Remeron SolTab Tablets 2486

Moclobemide (Concurrent use with MAO inhibitors is not recommended).
No products indexed under this heading.

Nefazodone Hydrochloride (Concurrent use with antidepressants is not recommended). Products include:
Serzone Tablets 1104

Nelfinavir Mesylate (Resource Wellness StayCalm contains St. John's Wort; concurrent use with protease inhibitors is not recommended). Products include:
Viracept 532

Nortriptyline Hydrochloride (Concurrent use with antidepressants is not recommended).
No products indexed under this heading.

Pargyline Hydrochloride (Concurrent use with MAO inhibitors is not recommended).
No products indexed under this heading.

Paroxetine Hydrochloride (Concurrent use with antidepressants is not recommended). Products include:
Paxil 1609

Phenelzine Sulfate (Concurrent use with MAO inhibitors is not recommended). Products include:
Nardil Tablets 2653

Procarbazine Hydrochloride (Concurrent use with MAO inhibitors is not recommended). Products include:
Matulane Capsules 3246

Propofol (Resource Wellness StayCalm contains valerian extract which causes drowsiness; concurrent use with sedatives is not recommended). Products include:
Diprivan Injectable Emulsion 667

Protriptyline Hydrochloride (Concurrent use with antidepressants is not recommended). Products include:
Vivactil Tablets 2446
Vivactil Tablets 2217

Quazepam (Resource Wellness StayCalm contains valerian extract which causes drowsiness; concurrent use with sedatives is not recommended).
No products indexed under this heading.

Ritonavir (Resource Wellness StayCalm contains St. John's Wort; concurrent use with protease inhibitors is not recommended). Products include:
Kaletra Capsules 471
Kaletra Oral Solution 471
Norvir Capsules 487
Norvir Oral Solution 487

Saquinavir (Resource Wellness StayCalm contains St. John's Wort; concurrent use with protease inhibitors is not recommended). Products include:
Fortovase Capsules 2970

Saquinavir Mesylate (Resource Wellness StayCalm contains St. John's Wort; concurrent use with protease inhibitors is not recommended). Products include:
Invirase Capsules 2979

Secobarbital Sodium (Resource Wellness StayCalm contains valerian extract which causes drowsiness; concurrent use with sedatives is not recommended).
No products indexed under this heading.

Selegiline Hydrochloride (Concurrent use with MAO inhibitors is not recommended). Products include:
Eldepryl Capsules 3266

Sertraline Hydrochloride (Concurrent use with antidepressants is not recommended). Products include:
Zoloft 2751

Temazepam (Resource Wellness StayCalm contains valerian extract which causes drowsiness; concurrent use with sedatives is not recommended).
No products indexed under this heading.

Tranylcypromine Sulfate (Concurrent use with MAO inhibitors is not recommended). Products include:
Parnate Tablets 1607

Trazodone Hydrochloride (Concurrent use with antidepressants is not recommended).
No products indexed under this heading.

Triazolam (Resource Wellness StayCalm contains valerian extract which causes drowsiness; concurrent use with sedatives is not recommended). Products include:
Halcion Tablets 2823

Trimipramine Maleate (Concurrent use with antidepressants is not recommended). Products include:
Surmontil Capsules 3595

Venlafaxine Hydrochloride (Concurrent use with antidepressants is not recommended). Products include:
Effexor Tablets 3495
Effexor XR Capsules 3499

Zaleplon (Resource Wellness StayCalm contains valerian extract which causes drowsiness; concurrent use with sedatives is not recommended). Products include:
Sonata Capsules 3591

Zolpidem Tartrate (Resource Wellness StayCalm contains valerian extract which causes drowsiness; concurrent use with sedatives is not recommended). Products include:
Ambien Tablets 3191

Food Interactions

Alcohol (Resource Wellness StayCalm contains valerian extract which causes drowsiness; concurrent use with alcohol is not recommended).

RESOURCE WELLNESS VEINTAIN CAPLETS

(Herbals with Vitamins & Minerals) ▭827
May interact with oral anticoagulants. Compounds in these categories include:

Dicumarol (Concurrent use with anticoagulants is not recommended).
No products indexed under this heading.

Warfarin Sodium (Concurrent use with anticoagulants is not recommended). Products include:
Coumadin for Injection 1243
Coumadin Tablets 1243
Warfarin Sodium Tablets, USP 3302

RESPERATE DEVICE

(Device) 1770
None cited in PDR database.

PROBIOTIC RESTORE CAPSULES

(Lactobacillus Acidophilus) ▭799
None cited in PDR database.

RETAVASE VIALS

(Reteplase) 1182
May interact with vitamin K antagonists and certain other agents. Compounds in these categories include:

Abciximab (Drugs that alter platelet function, such as abciximab, may increase the risk of bleeding if administered prior to or after reteplase therapy). Products include:
ReoPro Vials 1958

Aspirin (Drugs that alter platelet function, such as aspirin, may increase the risk of bleeding if administered prior to or after reteplase therapy). Products include:
Aggrenox Capsules 1026
Alka-Seltzer ▭603
Alka-Seltzer Lemon Lime Antacid and Pain Reliever Effervescent Tablets ▭603
Alka-Seltzer Extra Strength Antacid and Pain Reliever Effervescent Tablets ▭603
Alka-Seltzer PM Effervescent Tablets ▭605
Genuine Bayer Tablets, Caplets and Gelcaps ▭606
Extra Strength Bayer Caplets and Gelcaps ▭610
Aspirin Regimen Bayer Children's Chewable Tablets (Orange or Cherry Flavored) ▭607
Bayer, Aspirin Regimen ▭606
Aspirin Regimen Bayer 81 mg Caplets with Calcium ▭607
Genuine Bayer Professional Labeling (Aspirin Regimen Bayer) ▭608
Extra Strength Bayer Arthritis Caplets ▭610
Extra Strength Bayer Plus Caplets ▭610
Extra Strength Bayer PM Caplets ▭611
BC Powder ▭619
BC Allergy Sinus Cold Powder ▭619
Arthritis Strength BC Powder ▭619
BC Sinus Cold Powder ▭619
Darvon Compound-65 Pulvules 1910
Ecotrin Enteric Coated Aspirin Low, Regular and Maximum Strength Tablets 1715
Excedrin Extra-Strength Tablets, Caplets, and Geltabs ▭629
Excedrin Migraine 1070
Goody's Body Pain Formula Powder ▭620
Goody's Extra Strength Headache Powder ▭620
Goody's Extra Strength Pain Relief Tablets ▭620
Percodan Tablets 1327
Robaxisal Tablets 2939
Soma Compound Tablets 3354
Soma Compound w/Codeine Tablets 3355
Vanquish Caplets ▭617

Clopidogrel Bisulfate (Drugs that alter platelet function, such as clopidogrel, may increase the risk of bleeding if administered prior to or after reteplase therapy). Products include:
Plavix Tablets 1097
Plavix Tablets 3084

Dicumarol (Co-administration increases the risk of bleeding).
No products indexed under this heading.

Dipyridamole (Drugs that alter platelet function, such as dipyridamole, may increase the risk of bleeding if administered prior to or after reteplase therapy). Products include:
Aggrenox Capsules 1026
Persantine Tablets 1057

Eptifibatide (Drugs that alter platelet function, such as eptifibatide, may increase the risk of bleeding if administered prior to or after reteplase therapy). Products include:
Integrilin Injection 1213
Integrilin Injection 1828

Ticlopidine Hydrochloride (Drugs that alter platelet function, such as ticlopidine, may increase the risk of bleeding if administered prior to or after reteplase therapy). Products include:
Ticlid Tablets 3015

Tirofiban Hydrochloride (Drugs that alter platelet function, such as tirofiban, may increase the risk of bleeding if administered prior to or after reteplase therapy). Products include:
- Aggrastat 2031

Warfarin Sodium (Co-administration increases the risk of bleeding). Products include:
- Coumadin for Injection 1243
- Coumadin Tablets 1243
- Warfarin Sodium Tablets, USP 3302

RETIN-A MICRO 0.1%
(Tretinoin) 2522
May interact with:

Concomitant Topical Acne Therapy (Effect not specified).
- No products indexed under this heading.

Resorcinol (Caution should be exercised).
- No products indexed under this heading.

Salicylic Acid (Caution should be exercised). Products include:
- Clear Away Gel with Aloe Wart Remover System .... ▣736
- Clear Away Liquid Wart Remover System .... ▣736
- Clear Away One Step Wart Remover .... ▣737
- Clear Away One Step Wart Remover for Kids .... ▣737
- Clear Away One Step Plantar Wart Remover .... ▣737
- Compound W One Step Pads for Kids .... ▣664
- Compound W One Step Plantar Pads .... ▣664
- Compound W One Step Wart Remover Pads .... ▣664
- Compound W Wart Remover Gel ... ▣665
- Compound W Wart Remover Liquid .... ▣665
- Wart-Off Liquid .... ▣716

Sulfur (Caution should be exercised). Products include:
- Plexion 2024

Topical Medications (Effect not specified).
- No products indexed under this heading.

RETROVIR CAPSULES
(Zidovudine) 1625
May interact with cytotoxic drugs, Interferon alpha, phenytoin, valproate, and certain other agents. Compounds in these categories include:

Atovaquone (Co-administration results in increased AUC of zidovudine; routine dose modification of zidovudine is not warranted). Products include:
- Malarone 1596
- Mepron Suspension 1598

Bleomycin Sulfate (Co-administration with cytotoxic agents may increase the hematologic toxicity of zidovudine).
- No products indexed under this heading.

Bone Marrow Suppressants, unspecified (May increase the hematologic toxicity of zidovudine).

Cyclophosphamide (Co-administration with cytotoxic agents may increase the hematologic toxicity of zidovudine).
- No products indexed under this heading.

Daunorubicin Hydrochloride (Co-administration with cytotoxic agents may increase the hematologic toxicity of zidovudine). Products include:
- Cerubidine for Injection 947

Divalproex Sodium (Co-administration results in increased AUC of zidovudine by 80%; routine dose modification of zidovudine is not warranted unless patient is experiencing pronounced anemia or other severe zidovudine-associated events). Products include:
- Depakote Sprinkle Capsules 426
- Depakote Tablets 430
- Depakote ER Tablets 436

Doxorubicin Hydrochloride (Concomitant use should be avoided since an antagonistic relationship has been demonstrated). Products include:
- Adriamycin PFS/RDF Injection 2767
- Doxil Injection 566

Epirubicin Hydrochloride (Co-administration with cytotoxic agents may increase the hematologic toxicity of zidovudine). Products include:
- Ellence Injection 2806

Fluconazole (Co-administration results in increased AUC of zidovudine by 74%; routine dose modification of zidovudine is not warranted unless patient is experiencing pronounced anemia or other severe zidovudine-associated events). Products include:
- Diflucan Tablets, Injection, and Oral Suspension 2681

Fluorouracil (Co-administration with cytotoxic agents may increase the hematologic toxicity of zidovudine). Products include:
- Carac Cream 1222
- Efudex 1733
- Fluoroplex 552

Fosphenytoin Sodium (Co-administration has resulted in low phenytoin levels in some patients and a high level in one case; a 30% decrease in oral zidovudine clearance was observed with phenytoin). Products include:
- Cerebyx Injection 2619

Ganciclovir Sodium (May increase the hematologic toxicity of zidovudine). Products include:
- Cytovene-IV 2959

Hydroxyurea (Co-administration with cytotoxic agents may increase the hematologic toxicity of zidovudine). Products include:
- Mylocel Tablets 2227

Interferon alfa-2A, Recombinant (May increase the hematologic toxicity of zidovudine). Products include:
- Roferon-A Injection 2996

Interferon alfa-2B, Recombinant (May increase the hematologic toxicity of zidovudine). Products include:
- Intron A for Injection 3120
- Rebetron Combination Therapy 3153

Interferon alfa-N3 (Human Leukocyte Derived) (May increase the hematologic toxicity of zidovudine). Products include:
- Alferon N Injection 1770

Methadone Hydrochloride (Co-administration results in increased AUC of zidovudine; routine dose modification of zidovudine is not warranted). Products include:
- Dolophine Hydrochloride Tablets 3056

Methotrexate Sodium (Co-administration with cytotoxic agents may increase the hematologic toxicity of zidovudine).
- No products indexed under this heading.

Mitotane (Co-administration with cytotoxic agents may increase the hematologic toxicity of zidovudine).
- No products indexed under this heading.

Mitoxantrone Hydrochloride (Co-administration with cytotoxic agents may increase the hematologic toxicity of zidovudine). Products include:
- Novantrone for Injection 1760

Nelfinavir Mesylate (Co-administration results in decreased AUC of zidovudine; routine dose modification of zidovudine is not warranted). Products include:
- Viracept 532

Peginterferon Alfa-2B (May increase the hematologic toxicity of zidovudine). Products include:
- PEG-Intron Powder for Injection 3140

Phenytoin (Co-administration has resulted in low phenytoin levels in some patients and a high level in one case; a 30% decrease in oral zidovudine clearance was observed with phenytoin). Products include:
- Dilantin Infatabs 2624
- Dilantin-125 Oral Suspension 2625

Phenytoin Sodium (Co-administration has resulted in low phenytoin levels in some patients and a high level in one case; a 30% decrease in oral zidovudine clearance was observed with phenytoin). Products include:
- Dilantin Kapseals 2622

Probenecid (Co-administration results in increased AUC of zidovudine by 106%; routine dose modification of zidovudine is not warranted unless patient is experiencing pronounced anemia or other severe zidovudine-associated events).
- No products indexed under this heading.

Procarbazine Hydrochloride (Co-administration with cytotoxic agents may increase the hematologic toxicity of zidovudine). Products include:
- Matulane Capsules 3246

Ribavirin (Antagonizes the in vitro antiviral activity of zidovudine againt HIV; concomitant use should be avoided). Products include:
- Rebetron Combination Therapy 3153
- Virazole for Inhalation Solution 1747

Rifampin (Co-administration results in decreased AUC of zidovudine; routine dose modification of zidovudine is not warranted). Products include:
- Rifadin 765
- Rifamate Capsules 767
- Rifater Tablets 769

Ritonavir (Co-administration results in decreased AUC of zidovudine; routine dose modification of zidovudine is not warranted). Products include:
- Kaletra Capsules 471
- Kaletra Oral Solution 471
- Norvir Capsules 487
- Norvir Oral Solution 487

Stavudine (Concomitant use should be avoided since an antagonistic relationship has been demonstrated in vitro). Products include:
- Zerit 1147

Tamoxifen Citrate (Co-administration with cytotoxic agents may increase the hematologic toxicity of zidovudine). Products include:
- Nolvadex Tablets 678

Valproate Sodium (Co-administration results in increased AUC of zidovudine by 80%; routine dose modification of zidovudine is not warranted unless patient is experiencing pronounced anemia or other severe zidovudine-associated events). Products include:
- Depacon Injection 416

Valproic Acid (Co-administration results in increased AUC of zidovudine by 80%; routine dose modification of zidovudine is not warranted unless patient is experiencing pronounced anemia or other severe zidovudine-associated events). Products include:
- Depakene 421

Vincristine Sulfate (Co-administration with cytotoxic agents may increase the hematologic toxicity of zidovudine).
- No products indexed under this heading.

RETROVIR IV INFUSION
(Zidovudine) 1629
See Retrovir Capsules

RETROVIR SYRUP
(Zidovudine) 1625
See Retrovir Capsules

RETROVIR TABLETS
(Zidovudine) 1625
See Retrovir Capsules

RĒV-EYES STERILE OPHTHALMIC EYEDROPS 0.5%
(Dapiprazole Hydrochloride) .... ⊙265
None cited in PDR database.

RHINOCORT AQUA NASAL SPRAY
(Budesonide) 642
May interact with erythromycin and certain other agents. Compounds in these categories include:

Cimetidine (Co-administration with inhibitors of CYP4502C19, such as cimetidine, caused a slight decrease in budesonide clearance and corresponding increase in its oral bioavailability). Products include:
- Tagamet HB 200 Suspension .... ▣762
- Tagamet HB 200 Tablets .... ▣761
- Tagamet Tablets 1644

Cimetidine Hydrochloride (Co-administration with inhibitors of CYP4502C19, such as cimetidine, caused a slight decrease in budesonide clearance and corresponding increase in its oral bioavailability). Products include:
- Tagamet 1644

Clarithromycin (Co-administration with inhibitors of CYP4502C19, such as clarithromycin, may inhibit the metabolism of, and increase the systemic exposure to, budesonide). Products include:
- Biaxin/Biaxin XL 403
- PREVPAC 3298

Erythromycin (Co-administration with inhibitors of CYP4503A, such as erythromycin, may inhibit the metabolism of, and increase the systemic exposure to, budesonide). Products include:
- Emgel 2% Topical Gel 1285
- Ery-Tab Tablets 448
- Erythromycin Base Filmtab Tablets 454
- Erythromycin Delayed-Release Capsules, USP 455
- PCE Dispertab Tablets 498

Erythromycin Estolate (Co-administration with inhibitors of CYP4503A, such as erythromycin, may inhibit the metabolism of, and increase the systemic exposure to, budesonide).
- No products indexed under this heading.

Erythromycin Ethylsuccinate (Co-administration with inhibitors of CYP4503A, such as erythromycin, may inhibit the metabolism of, and increase the systemic exposure to, budesonide). Products include:
- E.E.S. 450
- EryPed 446
- Pediazole Suspension 3050

Erythromycin Gluceptate (Co-administration with inhibitors of CYP4503A, such as erythromycin, may inhibit the metabolism of, and increase the systemic exposure to, budesonide).
- No products indexed under this heading.

Erythromycin Stearate (Co-administration with inhibitors of CYP4503A, such as erythromycin, may inhibit the metabolism of, and increase the systemic exposure to, budesonide). Products include:
- Erythrocin Stearate Filmtab Tablets 452

Itraconazole (Co-administration with inhibitors of CYP4503A, such as itraconazole, may inhibit the metabolism of, and increase the systemic exposure to, budesonide). Products include:
- Sporanox Capsules 1800
- Sporanox Injection 1804
- Sporanox Injection 2509

Sporanox Oral Solution 1808
Sporanox Oral Solution 2512

Ketoconazole (The main route of metabolism of budesonide is via CYP4503A; co-administration with a potent inhibitor of CYP4503A, such as ketoconazole, has resulted in increased plasma concentration of orally administered budesonide). Products include:
Nizoral 2% Cream 3620
Nizoral A-D Shampoo 2008
Nizoral 2% Shampoo 2007
Nizoral Tablets 1791

RHINOCORT NASAL INHALER
(Budesonide) 640
None cited in PDR database.

RHOGAM INJECTION
(Rh_0 (D) Immune Globulin (Human)) 2524
None cited in PDR database.

MAXIMUM STRENGTH RID MOUSSE
(Piperonyl Butoxide, Pyrethrins) .... ▣617
None cited in PDR database.

MAXIMUM STRENGTH RID SHAMPOO
(Piperonyl Butoxide, Pyrethrum Extract) .... ▣616
None cited in PDR database.

RIFADIN CAPSULES
(Rifampin) 765
May interact with antacids, barbiturates, beta blockers, corticosteroids, oral anticoagulants, doxycycline, fluoroquinolone antibiotics, cardiac glycosides, narcotic analgesics, oral contraceptives, phenytoin, quinidine, sulfonylureas, tricyclic antidepressants, theophylline, and certain other agents. Compounds in these categories include:

Acebutolol Hydrochloride (Rifampin has been reported to accelerate the metabolism of beta blockers). Products include:
Sectral Capsules 3589

Alatrofloxacin Mesylate (Rifampin has been reported to accelerate the metabolism of fluoroquinolones). Products include:
Trovan I.V. 2722

Alfentanil Hydrochloride (Rifampin has been reported to accelerate the metabolism of narcotic analgesics).
No products indexed under this heading.

Aluminum Carbonate (Concomitant antacid administration may reduce the absorption of rifampin; daily doses of rifampin should be given at least 1 hour before the ingestion of antacids).
No products indexed under this heading.

Aluminum Hydroxide (Concomitant antacid administration may reduce the absorption of rifampin; daily doses of rifampin should be given at least 1 hour before the ingestion of antacids). Products include:
Amphojel Suspension (Mint Flavor) .... ▣789
Gaviscon Extra Strength Liquid .... ▣751
Gaviscon Extra Strength Tablets .... ▣751
Gaviscon Regular Strength Liquid .... ▣751
Gaviscon Regular Strength Tablets .... ▣750
Maalox Antacid/Anti-Gas Oral Suspension .... ▣673
Maalox Max Maximum Strength Antacid/Anti-Gas Liquid 2300
Maalox Regular Strength Antacid/Antigas Liquid 2300
Mylanta 1813
Vanquish Caplets .... ▣617

Aminophylline (Rifampin has been reported to accelerate the metabolism of theophylline).
No products indexed under this heading.

Amitriptyline Hydrochloride (Rifampin has been reported to accelerate the metabolism of tricyclic antidepressants). Products include:
Etrafon 3115
Limbitrol 1738

Amoxapine (Rifampin has been reported to accelerate the metabolism of tricyclic antidepressants).
No products indexed under this heading.

Aprobarbital (Rifampin has been reported to accelerate the metabolism of barbiturates).
No products indexed under this heading.

Atenolol (Rifampin has been reported to accelerate the metabolism of beta blockers). Products include:
Tenoretic Tablets 690
Tenormin I.V. Injection 692

Atovaquone (Co-administration results in decreased concentrations of atovaquone and increased concentrations of rifampin). Products include:
Malarone 1596
Mepron Suspension 1598

Betamethasone Acetate (Rifampin has been reported to accelerate the metabolism of corticosteroids). Products include:
Celestone Soluspan Injectable Suspension 3097

Betamethasone Sodium Phosphate (Rifampin has been reported to accelerate the metabolism of corticosteroids). Products include:
Celestone Soluspan Injectable Suspension 3097

Betaxolol Hydrochloride (Rifampin has been reported to accelerate the metabolism of beta blockers). Products include:
Betoptic S Ophthalmic Suspension 537

Bisoprolol Fumarate (Rifampin has been reported to accelerate the metabolism of beta blockers). Products include:
Zebeta Tablets 1885
Ziac Tablets 1887

Buprenorphine Hydrochloride (Rifampin has been reported to accelerate the metabolism of narcotic analgesics). Products include:
Buprenex Injectable 2918

Butabarbital (Rifampin has been reported to accelerate the metabolism of barbiturates).
No products indexed under this heading.

Butalbital (Rifampin has been reported to accelerate the metabolism of barbiturates). Products include:
Phrenilin 578
Sedapap Tablets 50 mg/650 mg 2225

Carteolol Hydrochloride (Rifampin has been reported to accelerate the metabolism of beta blockers). Products include:
Carteolol Hydrochloride Ophthalmic Solution USP, 1% .... ⊙258
Ocupress Ophthalmic Solution, 1% Sterile .... ⊙303

Chloramphenicol Sodium Succinate (Rifampin has been reported to accelerate the metabolism of chloramphenicol).
No products indexed under this heading.

Chlorpropamide (Rifampin has been reported to accelerate the metabolism of sulfonylurea hypoglycemic agents). Products include:
Diabinese Tablets 2680

Ciprofloxacin (Rifampin has been reported to accelerate the metabolism of fluoroquinolones). Products include:
Cipro I.V. 893
Cipro I.V. Pharmacy Bulk Package 897
Cipro Oral Suspension 887

Ciprofloxacin Hydrochloride (Rifampin has been reported to accelerate the metabolism of fluoroquinolones). Products include:
Ciloxan 538
Cipro HC Otic Suspension 540
Cipro Tablets 887

Clarithromycin (Rifampin has been reported to accelerate the metabolism of clarithromycin). Products include:
Biaxin/Biaxin XL 403
PREVPAC 3298

Clofibrate (Rifampin has been reported to accelerate the metabolism of clofibrate). Products include:
Atromid-S Capsules 3483

Clomipramine Hydrochloride (Rifampin has been reported to accelerate the metabolism of tricyclic antidepressants).
No products indexed under this heading.

Codeine Phosphate (Rifampin has been reported to accelerate the metabolism of narcotic analgesics). Products include:
Phenergan with Codeine Syrup 3557
Phenergan VC with Codeine Syrup 3561
Robitussin A-C Syrup 2942
Robitussin-DAC Syrup 2942
Ryna-C Liquid .... ▣768
Soma Compound w/Codeine Tablets 3355
Tussi-Organidin NR Liquid 3350
Tussi-Organidin-S NR Liquid 3350
Tylenol with Codeine 2595

Cortisone Acetate (Rifampin has been reported to accelerate the metabolism of corticosteroids). Products include:
Cortone Acetate Injectable Suspension 2059
Cortone Acetate Tablets 2061

Cyclosporine (Rifampin has been reported to accelerate the metabolism of cyclosporine). Products include:
Gengraf Capsules 457
Neoral Soft Gelatin Capsules 2380
Neoral Oral Solution 2380
Sandimmune 2388

Dapsone (Rifampin has been reported to accelerate the metabolism of dapsone). Products include:
Dapsone Tablets USP 1780

Desipramine Hydrochloride (Rifampin has been reported to accelerate the metabolism of tricyclic antidepressants). Products include:
Norpramin Tablets 755

Deslanoside (Rifampin has been reported to accelerate the metabolism of cardiac glycoside preparations)
No products indexed under this heading.

Desogestrel (Rifampin has been reported to accelerate the metabolism of oral or systemic hormone contraceptives; reliability of hormonal contraceptive may be affected and consideration should be given to using alternative contraceptive measures). Products include:
Cyclessa Tablets 2450
Desogen Tablets 2458
Mircette Tablets 2470
Ortho-Cept 21 Tablets 2546
Ortho-Cept 28 Tablets 2546

Dexamethasone (Rifampin has been reported to accelerate the metabolism of corticosteroids). Products include:
Decadron Elixir 2078
Decadron Tablets 2079
TobraDex Ophthalmic Ointment 542
TobraDex Ophthalmic Suspension 541

Dexamethasone Acetate (Rifampin has been reported to accelerate the metabolism of corticosteroids).
No products indexed under this heading.

Dexamethasone Sodium Phosphate (Rifampin has been reported to accelerate the metabolism of corticosteroids). Products include:
Decadron Phosphate Injection 2081
Decadron Phosphate Sterile Ophthalmic Ointment 2083
Decadron Phosphate Sterile Ophthalmic Solution 2084
NeoDecadron Sterile Ophthalmic Solution 2144

Dezocine (Rifampin has been reported to accelerate the metabolism of narcotic analgesics).
No products indexed under this heading.

Diazepam (Rifampin has been reported to accelerate the metabolism of diazepam). Products include:
Valium Injectable 3026
Valium Tablets 3047

Dicumarol (Rifampin has been reported to accelerate the metabolism of oral anticoagulants; rifampin increases the requirements for oral anticoagulants).
No products indexed under this heading.

Digitoxin (Rifampin has been reported to accelerate the metabolism of cardiac glycoside preparations).
No products indexed under this heading.

Digoxin (Rifampin has been reported to accelerate the metabolism of cardiac glycoside preparations). Products include:
Digitek Tablets 1003
Lanoxicaps Capsules 1574
Lanoxin Injection 1581
Lanoxin Tablets 1587
Lanoxin Elixir Pediatric 1578
Lanoxin Injection Pediatric 1584

Diltiazem Hydrochloride (Rifampin has been reported to accelerate the metabolism of calcium channel blocker, dilitiazem). Products include:
Cardizem Injectable 1018
Cardizem Lyo-Ject Syringe 1018
Cardizem Monovial 1018
Cardizem CD Capsules 1016
Tiazac Capsules 1378

Disopyramide Phosphate (Rifampin has been reported to accelerate the metabolism of disopyramide).
No products indexed under this heading.

Doxepin Hydrochloride (Rifampin has been reported to accelerate the metabolism of tricyclic antidepressants). Products include:
Sinequan 2713

Doxycycline Calcium (Rifampin has been reported to accelerate the metabolism of doxycycline). Products include:
Vibramycin Calcium Oral Suspension Syrup 2735

Doxycycline Hyclate (Rifampin has been reported to accelerate the metabolism of doxycycline). Products include:
Doryx Coated Pellet Filled Capsules 3357
Periostat Tablets 1208
Vibramycin Hyclate Capsules 2735
Vibramycin Hyclate Intravenous 2737
Vibra-Tabs Film Coated Tablets 2735

Doxycycline Monohydrate (Rifampin has been reported to accelerate the metabolism of doxycycline). Products include:
Monodox Capsules 2442
Vibramycin Monohydrate for Oral Suspension 2735

Dyphylline (Rifampin has been reported to accelerate the metabolism of theophylline). Products include:
Lufyllin Tablets 3347
Lufyllin-400 Tablets 3347

Lufyllin-GG Elixir 3348
Lufyllin-GG Tablets 3348

Enalapril Maleate (Co-administration has resulted in decreased concentrations of enalaprilat, the active metabolite of enalapril). Products include:
Lexxel Tablets 608
Vaseretic Tablets 2204
Vasotec Tablets 2210

Enoxacin (Rifampin has been reported to accelerate the metabolism of fluoroquinolones).
No products indexed under this heading.

Esmolol Hydrochloride (Rifampin has been reported to accelerate the metabolism of beta blockers). Products include:
Brevibloc Injection 858

Ethinyl Estradiol (Rifampin has been reported to accelerate the metabolism of oral or systemic hormone contraceptives; reliability of hormonal contraceptive may be affected and consideration should be given to using alternative contraceptive measures). Products include:
Alesse-21 Tablets 3468
Alesse-28 Tablets 3473
Brevicon 28-Day Tablets 3380
Cyclessa Tablets 2450
Desogen Tablets 2458
Estinyl Tablets 3112
Estrostep 2627
femhrt Tablets 2635
Levlen 962
Levlite 21 Tablets 962
Levlite 28 Tablets 962
Levora Tablets 3389
Loestrin 21 Tablets 2642
Loestrin Fe Tablets 2642
Lo/Ovral Tablets 3532
Lo/Ovral-28 Tablets 3538
Low-Ogestrel-28 Tablets 3392
Microgestin Fe 1.5/30 Tablets 3407
Microgestin Fe 1/20 Tablets 3400
Mircette Tablets 2470
Modicon 2563
Necon 3415
Nordette-28 Tablets 2257
Norinyl 1 +35 28-Day Tablets 3380
Ogestrel 0.5/50-28 Tablets 3428
Ortho-Cept 21 Tablets 2546
Ortho-Cept 28 Tablets 2546
Ortho-Cyclen/Ortho Tri-Cyclen 2573
Ortho-Novum 2563
Ovcon 3364
Ovral Tablets 3551
Ovral-28 Tablets 3552
Tri-Levlen 962
Tri-Norinyl-28 Tablets 3433
Triphasil-21 Tablets 3600
Triphasil-28 Tablets 3605
Trivora Tablets 3439
Yasmin 28 Tablets 980
Zovia 3449

Ethynodiol Diacetate (Rifampin has been reported to accelerate the metabolism of oral or systemic hormone contraceptives; reliability of hormonal contraceptive may be affected and consideration should be given to using alternative contraceptive measures). Products include:
Zovia 3449

Fentanyl (Rifampin has been reported to accelerate the metabolism of narcotic analgesics). Products include:
Duragesic Transdermal System 1786

Fentanyl Citrate (Rifampin has been reported to accelerate the metabolism of narcotic analgesics). Products include:
Actiq 1184

Fluconazole (Rifampin has been reported to accelerate the metabolism of fluconazole). Products include:
Diflucan Tablets, Injection, and Oral Suspension 2681

Fludrocortisone Acetate (Rifampin has been reported to accelerate the metabolism of corticosteroids). Products include:
Florinef Acetate Tablets 2250

Fosphenytoin Sodium (Rifampin has been reported to accelerate the metabolism of phenytoin). Products include:
Cerebyx Injection 2619

Glimepiride (Rifampin has been reported to accelerate the metabolism of sulfonylurea hypoglycemic agents). Products include:
Amaryl Tablets 717

Glipizide (Rifampin has been reported to accelerate the metabolism of sulfonylurea hypoglycemic agents). Products include:
Glucotrol Tablets 2692
Glucotrol XL Extended Release Tablets 2693

Glyburide (Rifampin has been reported to accelerate the metabolism of sulfonylurea hypoglycemic agents). Products include:
DiaBeta Tablets 741
Glucovance Tablets 1086

Grepafloxacin Hydrochloride (Rifampin has been reported to accelerate the metabolism of fluoroquinolones).
No products indexed under this heading.

Haloperidol (Rifampin has been reported to accelerate the metabolism of haloperidol). Products include:
Haldol Injection, Tablets and Concentrate 2533

Haloperidol Decanoate (Rifampin has been reported to accelerate the metabolism of haloperidol). Products include:
Haldol Decanoate 2535

Halothane (Potential for increased hepatotoxicity; concomitant use should be avoided). Products include:
Fluothane Inhalation 3508

Hydrocodone Bitartrate (Rifampin has been reported to accelerate the metabolism of narcotic analgesics). Products include:
Hycodan 1316
Hycomine Compound Tablets 1317
Hycotuss Expectorant Syrup 1318
Lortab 3319
Lortab Elixir 3317
Maxidone Tablets CIII 3399
Norco 5/325 Tablets CIII 3424
Norco 7.5/325 Tablets CIII 3425
Norco 10/325 Tablets CIII 3427
Norco 10/325 Tablets CIII 3425
Vicodin Tablets 516
Vicodin ES Tablets 517
Vicodin HP Tablets 518
Vicodin Tuss Expectorant 519
Vicoprofen Tablets 520
Zydone Tablets 1330

Hydrocodone Polistirex (Rifampin has been reported to accelerate the metabolism of narcotic analgesics). Products include:
Tussionex Pennkinetic Extended-Release Suspension 1174

Hydrocortisone (Rifampin has been reported to accelerate the metabolism of corticosteroids). Products include:
Anusol-HC Cream 2.5% 2237
Cipro HC Otic Suspension 540
Cortaid Intensive Therapy Cream .... ■717
Cortaid Maximum Strength Cream .... ■717
Cortisporin Ophthalmic Suspension Sterile .... ⊙297
Cortizone•5 .... ■699
Cortizone•10 .... ■699
Cortizone•10 Plus Creme .... ■700
Cortizone for Kids Creme .... ■699
Hydrocortone Tablets 2106
Massengill Medicated Soft Cloth Towelette .... ■753
VōSoL HC Otic Solution 3356

Hydrocortisone Acetate (Rifampin has been reported to accelerate the metabolism of corticosteroids). Products include:
Analpram-HC 1338
Anusol HC-1 Hydrocortisone Anti-Itch Cream .... ■689
Anusol-HC Suppositories 2238
Cortaid .... ■717
Cortifoam Rectal Foam 3170
Cortisporin-TC Otic Suspension 2246
Hydrocortone Acetate Injectable Suspension 2103
Pramosone 1343
Proctocort Suppositories 2264
ProctoFoam-HC 3177
Terra-Cortril Ophthalmic Suspension 2716

Hydrocortisone Sodium Phosphate (Rifampin has been reported to accelerate the metabolism of corticosteroids). Products include:
Hydrocortone Phosphate Injection, Sterile 2105

Hydrocortisone Sodium Succinate (Rifampin has been reported to accelerate the metabolism of corticosteroids).
No products indexed under this heading.

Hydromorphone Hydrochloride (Rifampin has been reported to accelerate the metabolism of narcotic analgesics). Products include:
Dilaudid 441
Dilaudid Oral Liquid 445
Dilaudid Powder 441
Dilaudid Rectal Suppositories 441
Dilaudid Tablets 441
Dilaudid Tablets - 8 mg 445
Dilaudid-HP 443

Imipramine Hydrochloride (Rifampin has been reported to accelerate the metabolism of tricyclic antidepressants).
No products indexed under this heading.

Imipramine Pamoate (Rifampin has been reported to accelerate the metabolism of tricyclic antidepressants).
No products indexed under this heading.

Isoniazid (Potential for increased hepatotoxicity). Products include:
Rifamate Capsules 767
Rifater Tablets 769

Itraconazole (Rifampin has been reported to accelerate the metabolism of itraconazole). Products include:
Sporanox Capsules 1800
Sporanox Injection 1804
Sporanox Injection 2509
Sporanox Oral Solution 1808
Sporanox Oral Solution 2512

Ketoconazole (Rifampin has been reported to accelerate the metabolism of ketoconazole; concurrent use has resulted in decreased serum concentrations of both drugs). Products include:
Nizoral 2% Cream 3620
Nizoral A-D Shampoo 2008
Nizoral 2% Shampoo 2007
Nizoral Tablets 1791

Labetalol Hydrochloride (Rifampin has been reported to accelerate the metabolism of beta blockers). Products include:
Normodyne Injection 3135
Normodyne Tablets 3137

Levobunolol Hydrochloride (Rifampin has been reported to accelerate the metabolism of beta blockers). Products include:
Betagan .... ⊙228

Levonorgestrel (Rifampin has been reported to accelerate the metabolism of oral or systemic hormone contraceptives; reliability of hormonal contraceptive may be affected and consideration should be given to using alternative contraceptive measures). Products include:
Alesse-21 Tablets 3468
Alesse-28 Tablets 3473
Levlen 962
Levlite 21 Tablets 962
Levlite 28 Tablets 962
Levora Tablets 3389
Mirena Intrauterine System 974
Nordette-28 Tablets 2257
Norplant System 3543
Tri-Levlen 962
Triphasil-21 Tablets 3600
Triphasil-28 Tablets 3605
Trivora Tablets 3439

Levorphanol Tartrate (Rifampin has been reported to accelerate the metabolism of narcotic analgesics). Products include:
Levo-Dromoran 1734
Levorphanol Tartrate Tablets 3059

Levothyroxine Sodium (Rifampin has been reported to accelerate the metabolism of levothyroxine). Products include:
Levothroid Tablets 1373
Levoxyl Tablets 1819
Synthroid 505
Unithroid Tablets 3445

Lomefloxacin Hydrochloride (Rifampin has been reported to accelerate the metabolism of fluoroquinolones).
No products indexed under this heading.

Magaldrate (Concomitant antacid administration may reduce the absorption of rifampin; daily doses of rifampin should be given at least 1 hour before the ingestion of antacids).
No products indexed under this heading.

Magnesium Hydroxide (Concomitant antacid administration may reduce the absorption of rifampin; daily doses of rifampin should be given at least 1 hour before the ingestion of antacids). Products include:
Ex•Lax Milk of Magnesia Liquid .... ■670
Maalox Antacid/Anti-Gas Oral Suspension .... ■673
Maalox Max Maximum Strength Antacid/Anti-Gas Liquid 2300
Maalox Regular Strength Antacid/Antigas Liquid 2300
Mylanta Fast-Acting 1813
Mylanta 1813
Pepcid Complete Chewable Tablets 1815
Phillips' Chewable Tablets .... ■615
Phillips' Milk of Magnesia Liquid (Original, Cherry, & Mint) .... ■616
Rolaids Tablets .... ■706
Extra Strength Rolaids Tablets .... ■706
Vanquish Caplets .... ■617

Magnesium Oxide (Concomitant antacid administration may reduce the absorption of rifampin; daily doses of rifampin should be given at least 1 hour before the ingestion of antacids). Products include:
Beelith Tablets 946
Mag-Ox 400 Tablets 1024
Uro-Mag Capsules 1024

Maprotiline Hydrochloride (Rifampin has been reported to accelerate the metabolism of tricyclic antidepressants).
No products indexed under this heading.

Medroxyprogesterone Acetate (Rifampin has been reported to accelerate the metabolism of progestins). Products include:
Depo-Provera Contraceptive Injection 2798
Lunelle Monthly Injection 2827
Premphase Tablets 3572
Prempro Tablets 3572
Provera Tablets 2853

Megestrol Acetate (Rifampin has been reported to accelerate the metabolism of progestins). Products include:
Megace Oral Suspension 1124

Meperidine Hydrochloride (Rifampin has been reported to accelerate the metabolism of narcotic analgesics). Products include:
Demerol 3079
Mepergan Injection 3539

Mephobarbital (Rifampin has been reported to accelerate the metabolism of barbiturates).
No products indexed under this heading.

Mestranol (Rifampin has been reported to accelerate the metabolism of oral or systemic hormone contraceptives; reliability of hormonal contraceptive may be affected and consideration should be given to using alternative contraceptive measures). Products include:
- Necon 1/50 Tablets 3415
- Norinyl 1 + 50 28-Day Tablets 3380
- Ortho-Novum 1/50□28 Tablets 2556

Methadone Hydrochloride (Rifampin has been reported to accelerate the metabolism of narcotic analgesics). Products include:
- Dolophine Hydrochloride Tablets 3056

Methylprednisolone Acetate (Rifampin has been reported to accelerate the metabolism of corticosteroids). Products include:
- Depo-Medrol Injectable Suspension 2795

Methylprednisolone Sodium Succinate (Rifampin has been reported to accelerate the metabolism of corticosteroids). Products include:
- Solu-Medrol Sterile Powder 2855

Metipranolol Hydrochloride (Rifampin has been reported to accelerate the metabolism of beta blockers).
- No products indexed under this heading.

Metoprolol Succinate (Rifampin has been reported to accelerate the metabolism of beta blockers). Products include:
- Toprol-XL Tablets 651

Metoprolol Tartrate (Rifampin has been reported to accelerate the metabolism of beta blockers).
- No products indexed under this heading.

Mexiletine Hydrochloride (Rifampin has been reported to accelerate the metabolism of mexiletine). Products include:
- Mexitil Capsules 1047

Morphine Sulfate (Rifampin has been reported to accelerate the metabolism of narcotic analgesics). Products include:
- Astramorph/PF Injection, USP (Preservative-Free) 594
- Duramorph Injection 1312
- Infumorph 200 and Infumorph 500 Sterile Solutions 1314
- Kadian Capsules 1335
- MS Contin Tablets 2896
- MSIR 2898
- Oramorph SR Tablets 3062
- Roxanol 3066

Moxifloxacin Hydrochloride (Rifampin has been reported to accelerate the metabolism of fluoroquinolones). Products include:
- Avelox Tablets 879

Nadolol (Rifampin has been reported to accelerate the metabolism of beta blockers). Products include:
- Corgard Tablets 2245
- Corzide 40/5 Tablets 2247
- Corzide 80/5 Tablets 2247
- Nadolol Tablets 2288

Nifedipine (Rifampin has been reported to accelerate the metabolism of calcium channel blocker, nifedipine). Products include:
- Adalat CC Tablets 877
- Procardia Capsules 2708
- Procardia XL Extended Release Tablets 2710

Norethindrone (Rifampin has been reported to accelerate the metabolism of oral or systemic hormone contraceptives; reliability of hormonal contraceptive may be affected and consideration should be given to using alternative contraceptive measures). Products include:
- Brevicon 28-Day Tablets 3380
- Micronor Tablets 2543
- Modicon 2563
- Necon 3415
- Norinyl 1 +35 28-Day Tablets 3380
- Norinyl 1 + 50 28-Day Tablets 3380
- Nor-QD Tablets 3423
- Ortho-Novum 2563
- Ortho-Novum 1/50□28 Tablets 2556
- Ovcon 3364
- Tri-Norinyl-28 Tablets 3433

Norethynodrel (Rifampin has been reported to accelerate the metabolism of oral or systemic hormone contraceptives; reliability of hormonal contraceptive may be affected and consideration should be given to using alternative contraceptive measures).
- No products indexed under this heading.

Norfloxacin (Rifampin has been reported to accelerate the metabolism of fluoroquinolones). Products include:
- Chibroxin Sterile Ophthalmic Solution 2051
- Noroxin Tablets 2145

Norgestimate (Rifampin has been reported to accelerate the metabolism of oral or systemic hormone contraceptives; reliability of hormonal contraceptive may be affected and consideration should be given to using alternative contraceptive measures). Products include:
- Ortho-Cyclen/Ortho Tri-Cyclen 2573
- Ortho-Prefest Tablets 2570

Norgestrel (Rifampin has been reported to accelerate the metabolism of oral or systemic hormone contraceptives; reliability of hormonal contraceptive may be affected and consideration should be given to using alternative contraceptive measures). Products include:
- Lo/Ovral Tablets 3532
- Lo/Ovral-28 Tablets 3538
- Low-Ogestrel-28 Tablets 3392
- Ogestrel 0.5/50-28 Tablets 3428
- Ovral Tablets 3551
- Ovral-28 Tablets 3552
- Ovrette Tablets 3552

Nortriptyline Hydrochloride (Rifampin has been reported to accelerate the metabolism of tricyclic antidepressants).
- No products indexed under this heading.

Ofloxacin (Rifampin has been reported to accelerate the metabolism of fluoroquinolones). Products include:
- Floxin I.V. 2526
- Floxin Otic Solution 1219
- Floxin Tablets 2529
- Ocuflox Ophthalmic Solution 554

Oxycodone Hydrochloride (Rifampin has been reported to accelerate the metabolism of narcotic analgesics). Products include:
- OxyContin Tablets 2912
- OxyFast Oral Concentrate Solution 2916
- OxyIR Capsules 2916
- Percocet Tablets 1326
- Percodan Tablets 1327
- Percolone Tablets 1327
- Roxicodone 3067
- Tylox Capsules 2597

Penbutolol Sulfate (Rifampin has been reported to accelerate the metabolism of beta blockers).
- No products indexed under this heading.

Pentobarbital Sodium (Rifampin has been reported to accelerate the metabolism of barbiturates). Products include:
- Nembutal Sodium Solution 485

Phenobarbital (Rifampin has been reported to accelerate the metabolism of barbiturates). Products include:
- Arco-Lase Plus Tablets 592
- Donnatal 2929
- Donnatal Extentabs 2930

Phenytoin (Rifampin has been reported to accelerate the metabolism of phenytoin). Products include:
- Dilantin Infatabs 2624
- Dilantin-125 Oral Suspension 2625

Phenytoin Sodium (Rifampin has been reported to accelerate the metabolism of phenytoin). Products include:
- Dilantin Kapseals 2622

Pindolol (Rifampin has been reported to accelerate the metabolism of beta blockers).
- No products indexed under this heading.

Prednisolone Acetate (Rifampin has been reported to accelerate the metabolism of corticosteroids). Products include:
- Blephamide Ophthalmic Ointment 547
- Blephamide Ophthalmic Suspension 548
- Poly-Pred Liquifilm Ophthalmic Suspension .... ⊙ 245
- Pred Forte Ophthalmic Suspension .... ⊙ 246
- Pred Mild Sterile Ophthalmic Suspension .... ⊙ 249
- Pred-G Ophthalmic Suspension .... ⊙ 247
- Pred-G Sterile Ophthalmic Ointment .... ⊙ 248

Prednisolone Sodium Phosphate (Rifampin has been reported to accelerate the metabolism of corticosteroids). Products include:
- Pediapred Oral Solution 1170

Prednisolone Tebutate (Rifampin has been reported to accelerate the metabolism of corticosteroids).
- No products indexed under this heading.

Prednisone (Rifampin has been reported to accelerate the metabolism of corticosteroids). Products include:
- Prednisone 3064

Probenecid (Increases the blood level rifampin).
- No products indexed under this heading.

Propoxyphene Hydrochloride (Rifampin has been reported to accelerate the metabolism of narcotic analgesics). Products include:
- Darvon Pulvules 1909
- Darvon Compound-65 Pulvules 1910

Propoxyphene Napsylate (Rifampin has been reported to accelerate the metabolism of narcotic analgesics). Products include:
- Darvon-N/Darvocet-N 1907
- Darvon-N Tablets 1912

Propranolol Hydrochloride (Rifampin has been reported to accelerate the metabolism of beta blockers). Products include:
- Inderal 3513
- Inderal LA Long-Acting Capsules 3516
- Inderide Tablets 3517
- Inderide LA Long-Acting Capsules 3519

Protriptyline Hydrochloride (Rifampin has been reported to accelerate the metabolism of tricyclic antidepressants). Products include:
- Vivactil Tablets 2446
- Vivactil Tablets 2217

Quinidine Gluconate (Rifampin has been reported to accelerate the metabolism of quinidine). Products include:
- Quinaglute Dura-Tabs Tablets 978

Quinidine Polygalacturonate (Rifampin has been reported to accelerate the metabolism of quinidine).
- No products indexed under this heading.

Quinidine Sulfate (Rifampin has been reported to accelerate the metabolism of quinidine). Products include:
- Quinidex Extentabs 2933

Quinine (Rifampin has been reported to accelerate the metabolism of quinine).
- No products indexed under this heading.

Remifentanil Hydrochloride (Rifampin has been reported to accelerate the metabolism of narcotic analgesics).
- No products indexed under this heading.

Secobarbital Sodium (Rifampin has been reported to accelerate the metabolism of barbiturates).
- No products indexed under this heading.

Sodium Bicarbonate (Concomitant antacid administration may reduce the absorption of rifampin; daily doses of rifampin should be given at least 1 hour before the ingestion of antacids). Products include:
- Alka-Seltzer .... ▣ 603
- Alka-Seltzer Lemon Lime Antacid and Pain Reliever Effervescent Tablets .... ▣ 603
- Alka-Seltzer Extra Strength Antacid and Pain Reliever Effervescent Tablets .... ▣ 603
- Alka-Seltzer Heartburn Relief Tablets .... ▣ 604
- Ceo-Two Evacuant Suppository .... ▣ 618
- Colyte with Flavor Packs for Oral Solution 3170
- GoLYTELY and Pineapple Flavor GoLYTELY for Oral Solution 1068
- NuLYTELY, Cherry Flavor, Lemon-Lime Flavor, and Orange Flavor NuLYTELY for Oral Solution 1068

Sotalol Hydrochloride (Rifampin has been reported to accelerate the metabolism of beta blockers). Products include:
- Betapace Tablets 950
- Betapace AF Tablets 954

Sufentanil Citrate (Rifampin has been reported to accelerate the metabolism of narcotic analgesics).
- No products indexed under this heading.

Sulfamethoxazole (Cotrimexazole increases the blood level rifampin). Products include:
- Bactrim 2949
- Septra Suspension 2265
- Septra Tablets 2265
- Septra DS Tablets 2265

Sulfasalazine (Plasma concentrations of sulfapyridine may be reduced following the co-administration of sulfasalazine and rifampin). Products include:
- Azulfidine EN-tabs Tablets 2775

Tacrolimus (Rifampin has been reported to accelerate the metabolism of tacrolimus). Products include:
- Prograf 1393
- Protopic Ointment 1397

Theophylline (Rifampin has been reported to accelerate the metabolism of theophylline). Products include:
- Aerolate 1361
- Theo-Dur Extended-Release Tablets 1835
- Uni-Dur Extended-Release Tablets 1841
- Uniphyl 400 mg and 600 mg Tablets 2903

Theophylline Calcium Salicylate (Rifampin has been reported to accelerate the metabolism of theophylline).
- No products indexed under this heading.

Theophylline Sodium Glycinate (Rifampin has been reported to accelerate the metabolism of theophylline).
- No products indexed under this heading.

Thiamylal Sodium (Rifampin has been reported to accelerate the metabolism of barbiturates).
- No products indexed under this heading.

Timolol Hemihydrate (Rifampin has been reported to accelerate the metabolism of beta blockers). Products include:
- Betimol Ophthalmic Solution .... ⊙ 324

Timolol Maleate (Rifampin has been reported to accelerate the metabolism of beta blockers). Products include:

Blocadren Tablets 2046
Cosopt Sterile Ophthalmic Solution 2065
Timolide Tablets 2187
Timolol GFS .... ⊙266
Timoptic in Ocudose 2192
Timoptic Sterile Ophthalmic Solution 2190
Timoptic-XE Sterile Ophthalmic Gel Forming Solution 2194

Tocainide Hydrochloride (Rifampin has been reported to accelerate the metabolism of tocainide). Products include:

Tonocard Tablets 649

Tolazamide (Rifampin has been reported to accelerate the metabolism of sulfonylurea hypoglycemic agents).

No products indexed under this heading.

Tolbutamide (Rifampin has been reported to accelerate the metabolism of sulfonylurea hypoglycemic agents).

No products indexed under this heading.

Triamcinolone (Rifampin has been reported to accelerate the metabolism of corticosteroids).

No products indexed under this heading.

Triamcinolone Acetonide (Rifampin has been reported to accelerate the metabolism of corticosteroids). Products include:

Azmacort Inhalation Aerosol 728
Nasacort Nasal Inhaler 750
Nasacort AQ Nasal Spray 752
Tri-Nasal Spray 2274

Triamcinolone Diacetate (Rifampin has been reported to accelerate the metabolism of corticosteroids).

No products indexed under this heading.

Triamcinolone Hexacetonide (Rifampin has been reported to accelerate the metabolism of corticosteroids).

No products indexed under this heading.

Trimipramine Maleate (Rifampin has been reported to accelerate the metabolism of tricyclic antidepressants). Products include:

Surmontil Capsules 3595

Trovafloxacin Mesylate (Rifampin has been reported to accelerate the metabolism of fluoroquinolones). Products include:

Trovan Tablets 2722

Verapamil Hydrochloride (Rifampin has been reported to accelerate the metabolism of calcium channel blocker, verapamil). Products include:

Covera-HS Tablets 3199
Isoptin SR Tablets 467
Tarka Tablets 508
Verelan Capsules 3184
Verelan PM Capsules 3186

Warfarin Sodium (Rifampin has been reported to accelerate the metabolism of oral anticoagulants; rifampin increases the requirements for oral anticoagulants). Products include:

Coumadin for Injection 1243
Coumadin Tablets 1243
Warfarin Sodium Tablets, USP 3302

Zidovudine (Rifampin has been reported to accelerate the metabolism of zidovudine). Products include:

Combivir Tablets 1502
Retrovir 1625
Retrovir IV Infusion 1629
Trizivir Tablets 1669

Food Interactions

Food, unspecified (Absorption of rifampin is reduced by about 30% when the drug is ingested with food; patients should be instructed to take 1 hour before or 2 hours after a meal).

RIFADIN IV

(Rifampin) 765
See Rifadin Capsules

RIFAMATE CAPSULES

(Isoniazid, Rifampin) 767

May interact with corticosteroids, oral anticoagulants, oral hypoglycemic agents, oral contraceptives, and certain other agents. Compounds in these categories include:

Acarbose (Rifampin given in combination with other antituberculosis drugs may decrease the pharmacologic activity of oral hypoglycemic agents; dosage adjustment may be required). Products include:

Precose Tablets 906

Betamethasone Acetate (Rifampin given in combination with other antituberculosis drugs may decrease the pharmacologic activity of corticosteroids; dosage adjustment may be required). Products include:

Celestone Soluspan Injectable Suspension 3097

Betamethasone Sodium Phosphate (Rifampin given in combination with other antituberculosis drugs may decrease the pharmacologic activity of corticosteroids; dosage adjustment may be required). Products include:

Celestone Soluspan Injectable Suspension 3097

Chlorpropamide (Rifampin given in combination with other antituberculosis drugs may decrease the pharmacologic activity of oral hypoglycemic agents; dosage adjustment may be required). Products include:

Diabinese Tablets 2680

Cortisone Acetate (Rifampin given in combination with other antituberculosis drugs may decrease the pharmacologic activity of corticosteroids; dosage adjustment may be required). Products include:

Cortone Acetate Injectable Suspension 2059
Cortone Acetate Tablets 2061

Dapsone (Rifampin given in combination with other antituberculosis drugs may decrease the pharmacologic activity of dapsone; dosage adjustment may be required). Products include:

Dapsone Tablets USP 1780

Desogestrel (Rifampin given in combination with other antituberculosis drugs may affect the reliability of oral contraceptives; alternative contraceptive measures may need to be considered). Products include:

Cyclessa Tablets 2450
Desogen Tablets 2458
Mircette Tablets 2470
Ortho-Cept 21 Tablets 2546
Ortho-Cept 28 Tablets 2546

Dexamethasone (Rifampin given in combination with other antituberculosis drugs may decrease the pharmacologic activity of corticosteroids; dosage adjustment may be required). Products include:

Decadron Elixir 2078
Decadron Tablets 2079
TobraDex Ophthalmic Ointment 542
TobraDex Ophthalmic Suspension 541

Dexamethasone Acetate (Rifampin given in combination with other antituberculosis drugs may decrease the pharmacologic activity of corticosteroids; dosage adjustment may be required).

No products indexed under this heading.

Dexamethasone Sodium Phosphate (Rifampin given in combination with other antituberculosis drugs may decrease the pharmacologic activity of corticosteroids; dosage adjustment may be required). Products include:

Decadron Phosphate Injection 2081
Decadron Phosphate Sterile Ophthalmic Ointment 2083
Decadron Phosphate Sterile Ophthalmic Solution 2084
NeoDecadron Sterile Ophthalmic Solution 2144

Dicumarol (Rifampin has been observed to increase the requirements of coumarin-type anticoagulant; it is recommended that prothrombin time be performed frequently and dosage adjustment may be required).

No products indexed under this heading.

Digitoxin (Rifampin given in combination with other antituberculosis drugs may decrease the pharmacologic activity of digitoxin; dosage adjustment may be required).

No products indexed under this heading.

Disopyramide Phosphate (Rifampin given in combination with other antituberculosis drugs may decrease the pharmacologic activity of disopyramide; dosage adjustment may be required).

No products indexed under this heading.

Ethinyl Estradiol (Rifampin given in combination with other antituberculosis drugs may affect the reliability of oral contraceptives; alternative contraceptive measures may need to be considered). Products include:

Alesse-21 Tablets 3468
Alesse-28 Tablets 3473
Brevicon 28-Day Tablets 3380
Cyclessa Tablets 2450
Desogen Tablets 2458
Estinyl Tablets 3112
Estrostep 2627
femhrt Tablets 2635
Levlen 962
Levlite 21 Tablets 962
Levlite 28 Tablets 962
Levora Tablets 3389
Loestrin 21 Tablets 2642
Loestrin Fe Tablets 2642
Lo/Ovral Tablets 3532
Lo/Ovral-28 Tablets 3538
Low-Ogestrel-28 Tablets 3392
Microgestin Fe 1.5/30 Tablets 3407
Microgestin Fe 1/20 Tablets 3400
Mircette Tablets 2470
Modicon 2563
Necon 3415
Nordette-28 Tablets 2257
Norinyl 1 +35 28-Day Tablets 3380
Ogestrel 0.5/50-28 Tablets 3428
Ortho-Cept 21 Tablets 2546
Ortho-Cept 28 Tablets 2546
Ortho-Cyclen/Ortho Tri-Cyclen 2573
Ortho-Novum 2563
Ovcon 3364
Ovral Tablets 3551
Ovral-28 Tablets 3552
Tri-Levlen 962
Tri-Norinyl-28 Tablets 3433
Triphasil-21 Tablets 3600
Triphasil-28 Tablets 3605
Trivora Tablets 3439
Yasmin 28 Tablets 980
Zovia 3449

Ethynodiol Diacetate (Rifampin given in combination with other antituberculosis drugs may affect the reliability of oral contraceptives; alternative contraceptive measures may need to be considered). Products include:

Zovia 3449

Fludrocortisone Acetate (Rifampin given in combination with other antituberculosis drugs may decrease the pharmacologic activity of corticosteroids; dosage adjustment may be required). Products include:

Florinef Acetate Tablets 2250

Glimepiride (Rifampin given in combination with other antituberculosis drugs may decrease the pharmacologic activity of oral hypoglycemic agents; dosage adjustment may be required). Products include:

Amaryl Tablets 717

Glipizide (Rifampin given in combination with other antituberculosis drugs may decrease the pharmacologic activity of oral hypoglycemic agents; dosage adjustment may be required). Products include:

Glucotrol Tablets 2692
Glucotrol XL Extended Release Tablets 2693

Glyburide (Rifampin given in combination with other antituberculosis drugs may decrease the pharmacologic activity of oral hypoglycemic agents; dosage adjustment may be required). Products include:

DiaBeta Tablets 741
Glucovance Tablets 1086

Hydrocortisone (Rifampin given in combination with other antituberculosis drugs may decrease the pharmacologic activity of corticosteroids; dosage adjustment may be required). Products include:

Anusol-HC Cream 2.5% 2237
Cipro HC Otic Suspension 540
Cortaid Intensive Therapy Cream .... ▣717
Cortaid Maximum Strength Cream .... ▣717
Cortisporin Ophthalmic Suspension Sterile .... ⊙297
Cortizone•5 .... ▣699
Cortizone•10 .... ▣699
Cortizone•10 Plus Creme .... ▣700
Cortizone for Kids Creme .... ▣699
Hydrocortone Tablets 2106
Massengill Medicated Soft Cloth Towelette .... ▣753
VōSoL HC Otic Solution 3356

Hydrocortisone Acetate (Rifampin given in combination with other antituberculosis drugs may decrease the pharmacologic activity of corticosteroids; dosage adjustment may be required). Products include:

Analpram-HC 1338
Anusol HC-1 Hydrocortisone Anti-Itch Cream .... ▣689
Anusol-HC Suppositories 2238
Cortaid .... ▣717
Cortifoam Rectal Foam 3170
Cortisporin-TC Otic Suspension 2246
Hydrocortone Acetate Injectable Suspension 2103
Pramosone 1343
Proctocort Suppositories 2264
ProctoFoam-HC 3177
Terra-Cortril Ophthalmic Suspension 2716

Hydrocortisone Sodium Phosphate (Rifampin given in combination with other antituberculosis drugs may decrease the pharmacologic activity of corticosteroids; dosage adjustment may be required). Products include:

Hydrocortone Phosphate Injection, Sterile 2105

Hydrocortisone Sodium Succinate (Rifampin given in combination with other antituberculosis drugs may decrease the pharmacologic activity of corticosteroids; dosage adjustment may be required).

No products indexed under this heading.

Levonorgestrel (Rifampin given in combination with other antituberculosis drugs may affect the reliability of oral contraceptives; alternative contraceptive measures may need to be considered). Products include:

Alesse-21 Tablets 3468
Alesse-28 Tablets 3473
Levlen 962
Levlite 21 Tablets 962
Levlite 28 Tablets 962
Levora Tablets 3389
Mirena Intrauterine System 974
Nordette-28 Tablets 2257
Norplant System 3543
Tri-Levlen 962
Triphasil-21 Tablets 3600

Triphasil-28 Tablets 3605
Trivora Tablets 3439

Mestranol (Rifampin given in combination with other antituberculosis drugs may affect the reliability of oral contraceptives; alternative contraceptive measures may need to be considered). Products include:
Necon 1/50 Tablets 3415
Norinyl 1 + 50 28-Day Tablets 3380
Ortho-Novum 1/50□28 Tablets 2556

Metformin Hydrochloride (Rifampin given in combination with other antituberculosis drugs may decrease the pharmacologic activity of oral hypoglycemic agents; dosage adjustment may be required). Products include:
Glucophage Tablets 1080
Glucophage XR Tablets 1080
Glucovance Tablets 1086

Methadone Hydrochloride (Rifampin given in combination with other antituberculosis drugs may decrease the pharmacologic activity of methadone; dosage adjustment may be required). Products include:
Dolophine Hydrochloride Tablets 3056

Methylprednisolone Acetate (Rifampin given in combination with other antituberculosis drugs may decrease the pharmacologic activity of corticosteroids; dosage adjustment may be required). Products include:
Depo-Medrol Injectable Suspension 2795

Methylprednisolone Sodium Succinate (Rifampin given in combination with other antituberculosis drugs may decrease the pharmacologic activity of corticosteroids; dosage adjustment may be required). Products include:
Solu-Medrol Sterile Powder 2855

Miglitol (Rifampin given in combination with other antituberculosis drugs may decrease the pharmacologic activity of oral hypoglycemic agents; dosage adjustment may be required). Products include:
Glyset Tablets 2821

Norethindrone (Rifampin given in combination with other antituberculosis drugs may affect the reliability of oral contraceptives; alternative contraceptive measures may need to be considered). Products include:
Brevicon 28-Day Tablets 3380
Micronor Tablets 2543
Modicon 2563
Necon 3415
Norinyl 1 +35 28-Day Tablets 3380
Norinyl 1 + 50 28-Day Tablets 3380
Nor-QD Tablets 3423
Ortho-Novum 2563
Ortho-Novum 1/50□28 Tablets 2556
Ovcon 3364
Tri-Norinyl-28 Tablets 3433

Norethynodrel (Rifampin given in combination with other antituberculosis drugs may affect the reliability of oral contraceptives; alternative contraceptive measures may need to be considered).
No products indexed under this heading.

Norgestimate (Rifampin given in combination with other antituberculosis drugs may affect the reliability of oral contraceptives; alternative contraceptive measures may need to be considered). Products include:
Ortho-Cyclen/Ortho Tri-Cyclen 2573
Ortho-Prefest Tablets 2570

Norgestrel (Rifampin given in combination with other antituberculosis drugs may affect the reliability of oral contraceptives; alternative contraceptive measures may need to be considered). Products include:
Lo/Ovral Tablets 3532
Lo/Ovral-28 Tablets 3538
Low-Ogestrel-28 Tablets 3392
Ogestrel 0.5/50-28 Tablets 3428
Ovral Tablets 3551
Ovral-28 Tablets 3552
Ovrette Tablets 3552

Phenytoin (Isoniazid may decrease the excretion of phenytoin or may enhance its effects; dosage adjustment may be required). Products include:
Dilantin Infatabs 2624
Dilantin-125 Oral Suspension 2625

Phenytoin Sodium (Isoniazid may decrease the excretion of phenytoin or may enhance its effects; dosage adjustment may be required). Products include:
Dilantin Kapseals 2622

Pioglitazone Hydrochloride (Rifampin given in combination with other antituberculosis drugs may decrease the pharmacologic activity of oral hypoglycemic agents; dosage adjustment may be required). Products include:
Actos Tablets 3275

Prednisolone Acetate (Rifampin given in combination with other antituberculosis drugs may decrease the pharmacologic activity of corticosteroids; dosage adjustment may be required). Products include:
Blephamide Ophthalmic Ointment .. 547
Blephamide Ophthalmic Suspension 548
Poly-Pred Liquifilm Ophthalmic Suspension .... ⊙245
Pred Forte Ophthalmic Suspension .... ⊙246
Pred Mild Sterile Ophthalmic Suspension .... ⊙249
Pred-G Ophthalmic Suspension ..... ⊙247
Pred-G Sterile Ophthalmic Ointment .... ⊙248

Prednisolone Sodium Phosphate (Rifampin given in combination with other antituberculosis drugs may decrease the pharmacologic activity of corticosteroids; dosage adjustment may be required). Products include:
Pediapred Oral Solution 1170

Prednisolone Tebutate (Rifampin given in combination with other antituberculosis drugs may decrease the pharmacologic activity of corticosteroids; dosage adjustment may be required).
No products indexed under this heading.

Prednisone (Rifampin given in combination with other antituberculosis drugs may decrease the pharmacologic activity of corticosteroids; dosage adjustment may be required). Products include:
Prednisone 3064

Quinidine Gluconate (Rifampin given in combination with other antituberculosis drugs may decrease the pharmacologic activity of quinidine; dosage adjustment may be required). Products include:
Quinaglute Dura-Tabs Tablets 978

Quinidine Polygalacturonate (Rifampin given in combination with other antituberculosis drugs may decrease the pharmacologic activity of quinidine; dosage adjustment may be required).
No products indexed under this heading.

Quinidine Sulfate (Rifampin given in combination with other antituberculosis drugs may decrease the pharmacologic activity of quinidine; dosage adjustment may be required). Products include:
Quinidex Extentabs 2933

Repaglinide (Rifampin given in combination with other antituberculosis drugs may decrease the pharmacologic activity of oral hypoglycemic agents; dosage adjustment may be required). Products include:
Prandin Tablets (0.5, 1, and 2 mg) 2432

Rosiglitazone Maleate (Rifampin given in combination with other antituberculosis drugs may decrease the pharmacologic activity of oral hypoglycemic agents; dosage adjustment may be required). Products include:
Avandia Tablets 1490

Tolazamide (Rifampin given in combination with other antituberculosis drugs may decrease the pharmacologic activity of oral hypoglycemic agents; dosage adjustment may be required).
No products indexed under this heading.

Tolbutamide (Rifampin given in combination with other antituberculosis drugs may decrease the pharmacologic activity of oral hypoglycemic agents; dosage adjustment may be required).
No products indexed under this heading.

Triamcinolone (Rifampin given in combination with other antituberculosis drugs may decrease the pharmacologic activity of corticosteroids; dosage adjustment may be required).
No products indexed under this heading.

Triamcinolone Acetonide (Rifampin given in combination with other antituberculosis drugs may decrease the pharmacologic activity of corticosteroids; dosage adjustment may be required). Products include:
Azmacort Inhalation Aerosol 728
Nasacort Nasal Inhaler 750
Nasacort AQ Nasal Spray 752
Tri-Nasal Spray 2274

Triamcinolone Diacetate (Rifampin given in combination with other antituberculosis drugs may decrease the pharmacologic activity of corticosteroids; dosage adjustment may be required).
No products indexed under this heading.

Triamcinolone Hexacetonide (Rifampin given in combination with other antituberculosis drugs may decrease the pharmacologic activity of corticosteroids; dosage adjustment may be required).
No products indexed under this heading.

Troglitazone (Rifampin given in combination with other antituberculosis drugs may decrease the pharmacologic activity of oral hypoglycemic agents; dosage adjustment may be required).
No products indexed under this heading.

Warfarin Sodium (Rifampin has been observed to increase the requirements of coumarin-type anticoagulant; it is recommended that prothrombin time be performed frequently and dosage adjustment may be required). Products include:
Coumadin for Injection 1243
Coumadin Tablets 1243
Warfarin Sodium Tablets, USP 3302

Food Interactions

Alcohol (Daily ingestion of alcohol may be associated with a higher incidence of isoniazid hepatitis).

RIFATER TABLETS

(Isoniazid, Pyrazinamide, Rifampin) 769

May interact with antacids, barbiturates, beta blockers, corticosteroids, oral anticoagulants, cardiac glycosides, narcotic analgesics, oral contraceptives, phenytoin, progestins, quinidine, sulfonylureas, valproate, theophylline, and certain other agents. Compounds in these categories include:

Acebutolol Hydrochloride (Rifampin accelerates the metabolism of beta blocker; dosage adjustment may be required when starting or stopping concomitantly administered rifampin). Products include:
Sectral Capsules 3589

Alfentanil Hydrochloride (Rifampin accelerates the metabolism of narcotic; dosage adjustment may be required when starting or stopping concomitantly administered rifampin).
No products indexed under this heading.

Aluminum Carbonate (Concomitant antacid administration may reduce the absorption of rifampin and isoniazid; daily dose of Rifater should be given at least one hour before the ingestion of antacids).
No products indexed under this heading.

Aluminum Hydroxide (Concomitant antacid administration may reduce the absorption of rifampin and isoniazid; daily dose of Rifater should be given at least one hour before the ingestion of antacids). Products include:
Amphojel Suspension (Mint Flavor) .... ■789
Gaviscon Extra Strength Liquid ..... ■751
Gaviscon Extra Strength Tablets ..... ■751
Gaviscon Regular Strength Liquid . ■751
Gaviscon Regular Strength Tablets .... ■750
Maalox Antacid/Anti-Gas Oral Suspension .... ■673
Maalox Max Maximum Strength Antacid/Anti-Gas Liquid 2300
Maalox Regular Strength Antacid/Antigas Liquid 2300
Mylanta 1813
Vanquish Caplets .... ■617

Aminophylline (Rifampin accelerates the metabolism of theophylline and isoniazid inhibits the metabolism; dosage adjustment may be required when starting or stopping concomitantly administered rifampin).
No products indexed under this heading.

Aminosalicylic Acid (Increases the plasma concentration and elimination half-life of isoniazid). Products include:
Paser Granules 1781

Aprobarbital (Rifampin accelerates the metabolism of barbiturates; dosage adjustment may be required when starting or stopping concomitantly administered rifampin).
No products indexed under this heading.

Atenolol (Rifampin accelerates the metabolism of beta blocker; dosage adjustment may be required when starting or stopping concomitantly administered rifampin). Products include:
Tenoretic Tablets 690
Tenormin I.V. Injection 692

Betamethasone Acetate (Rifampin accelerates the metabolism of corticosteroid; dosage adjustment may be required when starting or stopping concomitantly administered rifampin). Products include:
Celestone Soluspan Injectable Suspension 3097

Betamethasone Sodium Phosphate (Rifampin accelerates the metabolism of corticosteroid; dosage adjustment may be required when starting or stopping concomitantly administered rifampin). Products include:
Celestone Soluspan Injectable Suspension 3097

Betaxolol Hydrochloride (Rifampin accelerates the metabolism of beta blocker; dosage adjustment may be required when starting or stopping concomitantly administered rifampin). Products include:
Betoptic S Ophthalmic Suspension 537

Bisoprolol Fumarate (Rifampin accelerates the metabolism of beta blocker; dosage adjustment may be required when starting or stopping concomitantly administered rifampin). Products include:
- Zebeta Tablets 1885
- Ziac Tablets 1887

Buprenorphine Hydrochloride (Rifampin accelerates the metabolism of narcotic; dosage adjustment may be required when starting or stopping concomitantly administered rifampin). Products include:
- Buprenex Injectable 2918

Butabarbital (Rifampin accelerates the metabolism of barbiturates; dosage adjustment may be required when starting or stopping concomitantly administered rifampin).
- No products indexed under this heading.

Butalbital (Rifampin accelerates the metabolism of barbiturates; dosage adjustment may be required when starting or stopping concomitantly administered rifampin). Products include:
- Phrenilin 578
- Sedapap Tablets 50 mg/650 mg 2225

Carbamazepine (Isoniazid inhibits the metabolism of carbamazepine). Products include:
- Carbatrol Capsules 3234
- Tegretol/Tegretol-XR 2404

Carteolol Hydrochloride (Rifampin accelerates the metabolism of beta blocker; dosage adjustment may be required when starting or stopping concomitantly administered rifampin). Products include:
- Carteolol Hydrochloride Ophthalmic Solution USP, 1% .... ⊙258
- Ocupress Ophthalmic Solution, 1% Sterile .... ⊙303

Chloramphenicol (Rifampin accelerates the metabolism of chloramphenicol; dosage adjustment may be required when starting or stopping concomitantly administered rifampin). Products include:
- Chloromycetin Ophthalmic Ointment, 1% .... ⊙296
- Chloromycetin Ophthalmic Solution .... ⊙297
- Chloroptic Sterile Ophthalmic Ointment .... ⊙234
- Chloroptic Sterile Ophthalmic Solution .... ⊙235

Chloramphenicol Palmitate (Rifampin accelerates the metabolism of chloramphenicol; dosage adjustment may be required when starting or stopping concomitantly administered rifampin).
- No products indexed under this heading.

Chloramphenicol Sodium Succinate (Rifampin accelerates the metabolism of chloramphenicol; dosage adjustment may be required when starting or stopping concomitantly administered rifampin).
- No products indexed under this heading.

Chlorpropamide (Rifampin accelerates the metabolism of sulfonylureas; isoniazid may produce hyperglycemia and lead to loss of glucose control; dosage adjustment may be required when starting or stopping concomitantly administered rifampin). Products include:
- Diabinese Tablets 2680

Ciprofloxacin (Rifampin accelerates the metabolism of ciprofloxacin; dosage adjustment may be required when starting or stopping concomitantly administered rifampin). Products include:
- Cipro I.V. 893
- Cipro I.V. Pharmacy Bulk Package 897
- Cipro Oral Suspension 887

Ciprofloxacin Hydrochloride (Rifampin accelerates the metabolism of ciprofloxacin; dosage adjustment may be required when starting or stopping concomitantly administered rifampin). Products include:
- Ciloxan 538
- Cipro HC Otic Suspension 540
- Cipro Tablets 887

Clofibrate (Rifampin accelerates the metabolism of clofibrate; dosage adjustment may be required when starting or stopping concomitantly administered rifampin). Products include:
- Atromid-S Capsules 3483

Codeine Phosphate (Rifampin accelerates the metabolism of narcotic; dosage adjustment may be required when starting or stopping concomitantly administered rifampin). Products include:
- Phenergan with Codeine Syrup 3557
- Phenergan VC with Codeine Syrup 3561
- Robitussin A-C Syrup 2942
- Robitussin-DAC Syrup 2942
- Ryna-C Liquid .... ▣768
- Soma Compound w/Codeine Tablets 3355
- Tussi-Organidin NR Liquid 3350
- Tussi-Organidin-S NR Liquid 3350
- Tylenol with Codeine 2595

Cortisone Acetate (Rifampin accelerates the metabolism of corticosteroid; dosage adjustment may be required when starting or stopping concomitantly administered rifampin). Products include:
- Cortone Acetate Injectable Suspension 2059
- Cortone Acetate Tablets 2061

Cycloserine (Rifater exaggerates drowsiness and dizziness).
- No products indexed under this heading.

Cyclosporine (Rifampin accelerates the metabolism of cyclosporine; dosage adjustment may be required when starting or stopping concomitantly administered rifampin). Products include:
- Gengraf Capsules 457
- Neoral Soft Gelatin Capsules 2380
- Neoral Oral Solution 2380
- Sandimmune 2388

Dapsone (Rifampin accelerates the metabolism of dapsone; dosage adjustment may be required when starting or stopping concomitantly administered rifampin). Products include:
- Dapsone Tablets USP 1780

Deslanoside (Rifampin accelerates the metabolism of cardiac glycosides; dosage adjustment may be required when starting or stopping concomitantly administered rifampin).
- No products indexed under this heading.

Desogestrel (Rifampin accelerates the metabolism of oral contraceptive or progestin; dosage adjustment may be required when starting or stopping concomitantly administered rifampin). Products include:
- Cyclessa Tablets 2450
- Desogen Tablets 2458
- Mircette Tablets 2470
- Ortho-Cept 21 Tablets 2546
- Ortho-Cept 28 Tablets 2546

Dexamethasone (Rifampin accelerates the metabolism of corticosteroid; dosage adjustment may be required when starting or stopping concomitantly administered rifampin). Products include:
- Decadron Elixir 2078
- Decadron Tablets 2079
- TobraDex Ophthalmic Ointment 542
- TobraDex Ophthalmic Suspension 541

Dexamethasone Acetate (Rifampin accelerates the metabolism of corticosteroid; dosage adjustment may be required when starting or stopping concomitantly administered rifampin).
- No products indexed under this heading.

Dexamethasone Sodium Phosphate (Rifampin accelerates the metabolism of corticosteroid; dosage adjustment may be required when starting or stopping concomitantly administered rifampin). Products include:
- Decadron Phosphate Injection 2081
- Decadron Phosphate Sterile Ophthalmic Ointment 2083
- Decadron Phosphate Sterile Ophthalmic Solution 2084
- NeoDecadron Sterile Ophthalmic Solution 2144

Dezocine (Rifampin accelerates the metabolism of narcotic; dosage adjustment may be required when starting or stopping concomitantly administered rifampin).
- No products indexed under this heading.

Diazepam (Rifampin accelerates the metabolism of diazepam and isoniazid inhibits the metabolism of diazepam; dosage adjustment may be required when starting or stopping concomitantly administered rifampin). Products include:
- Valium Injectable 3026
- Valium Tablets 3047

Dicumarol (Rifampin accelerates the metabolism of anticoagulants and isoniazid inhibits the metabolism; increased requirements of coumarin type anticoagulant; dosage adjustment may be required when starting or stopping concomitantly administered rifampin).
- No products indexed under this heading.

Digitoxin (Rifampin accelerates the metabolism of cardiac glycosides; dosage adjustment may be required when starting or stopping concomitantly administered rifampin).
- No products indexed under this heading.

Digoxin (Rifampin accelerates the metabolism of cardiac glycosides; dosage adjustment may be required when starting or stopping concomitantly administered rifampin). Products include:
- Digitek Tablets 1003
- Lanoxicaps Capsules 1574
- Lanoxin Injection 1581
- Lanoxin Tablets 1587
- Lanoxin Elixir Pediatric 1578
- Lanoxin Injection Pediatric 1584

Diltiazem Hydrochloride (Rifampin accelerates the metabolism of diltiazem; dosage adjustment may be required when starting or stopping concomitantly administered rifampin). Products include:
- Cardizem Injectable 1018
- Cardizem Lyo-Ject Syringe 1018
- Cardizem Monovial 1018
- Cardizem CD Capsules 1016
- Tiazac Capsules 1378

Disopyramide Phosphate (Rifampin accelerates the metabolism of disopyramide; dosage adjustment may be required when starting or stopping concomitantly administered rifampin).
- No products indexed under this heading.

Disulfiram (Rifater exaggerates acute behavioral and coordination changes). Products include:
- Antabuse Tablets 2444
- Antabuse Tablets 3474

Divalproex Sodium (Isoniazid inhibits the metabolism of valproic acid). Products include:
- Depakote Sprinkle Capsules 426
- Depakote Tablets 430
- Depakote ER Tablets 436

Dyphylline (Rifampin accelerates the metabolism of theophylline and isoniazid inhibits the metabolism; dosage adjustment may be required when starting or stopping concomitantly administered rifampin). Products include:
- Lufyllin Tablets 3347
- Lufyllin-400 Tablets 3347
- Lufyllin-GG Elixir 3348
- Lufyllin-GG Tablets 3348

Enalapril Maleate (Concurrent use results in decreased concentrations of enalaprilat, the active metabolite). Products include:
- Lexxel Tablets 608
- Vaseretic Tablets 2204
- Vasotec Tablets 2210

Enflurane (Fast acetylation of isoniazid may produce high concentrations of hydrazine which facilitate defloration).
- No products indexed under this heading.

Esmolol Hydrochloride (Rifampin accelerates the metabolism of beta blocker; dosage adjustment may be required when starting or stopping concomitantly administered rifampin). Products include:
- Brevibloc Injection 858

Ethinyl Estradiol (Rifampin accelerates the metabolism of oral contraceptive; dosage adjustment may be required when starting or stopping concomitantly administered rifampin). Products include:
- Alesse-21 Tablets 3468
- Alesse-28 Tablets 3473
- Brevicon 28-Day Tablets 3380
- Cyclessa Tablets 2450
- Desogen Tablets 2458
- Estinyl Tablets 3112
- Estrostep 2627
- femhrt Tablets 2635
- Levlen 962
- Levlite 21 Tablets 962
- Levlite 28 Tablets 962
- Levora Tablets 3389
- Loestrin 21 Tablets 2642
- Loestrin Fe Tablets 2642
- Lo/Ovral Tablets 3532
- Lo/Ovral-28 Tablets 3538
- Low-Ogestrel-28 Tablets 3392
- Microgestin Fe 1.5/30 Tablets 3407
- Microgestin Fe 1/20 Tablets 3400
- Mircette Tablets 2470
- Modicon 2563
- Necon 3415
- Nordette-28 Tablets 2257
- Norinyl 1 +35 28-Day Tablets 3380
- Ogestrel 0.5/50-28 Tablets 3428
- Ortho-Cept 21 Tablets 2546
- Ortho-Cept 28 Tablets 2546
- Ortho-Cyclen/Ortho Tri-Cyclen 2573
- Ortho-Novum 2563
- Ovcon 3364
- Ovral Tablets 3551
- Ovral-28 Tablets 3552
- Tri-Levlen 962
- Tri-Norinyl-28 Tablets 3433
- Triphasil-21 Tablets 3600
- Triphasil-28 Tablets 3605
- Trivora Tablets 3439
- Yasmin 28 Tablets 980
- Zovia 3449

Ethynodiol Diacetate (Rifampin accelerates the metabolism of oral contraceptive; dosage adjustment may be required when starting or stopping concomitantly administered rifampin). Products include:
- Zovia 3449

Fentanyl (Rifampin accelerates the metabolism of narcotic; dosage adjustment may be required when starting or stopping concomitantly administered rifampin). Products include:
- Duragesic Transdermal System 1786

Fentanyl Citrate (Rifampin accelerates the metabolism of narcotic; dosage adjustment may be required when starting or stopping concomitantly administered rifampin). Products include:
- Actiq 1184

Fluconazole (Rifampin accelerates the metabolism of fluconazole; dosage adjustment may be required when starting or stopping concomitantly administered rifampin). Products include:
- Diflucan Tablets, Injection, and Oral Suspension 2681

Fludrocortisone Acetate (Rifampin accelerates the metabolism of corticosteroid; dosage adjustment may be required when starting or stopping concomitantly administered rifampin). Products include:
- Florinef Acetate Tablets 2250

Fosphenytoin Sodium (Rifampin accelerates the metabolism and isoniazid inhibits the metabolism of phenytoin; dosage adjustment may be required when starting or stopping concomitantly administered rifampin). Products include:
- Cerebyx Injection 2619

Glimepiride (Rifampin accelerates the metabolism of sulfonylureas; isoniazid may produce hyperglycemia and lead to loss of glucose control; dosage adjustment may be required when starting or stopping concomitantly administered rifampin). Products include:
- Amaryl Tablets 717

Glipizide (Rifampin accelerates the metabolism of sulfonylureas; isoniazid may produce hyperglycemia and lead to loss of glucose control; dosage adjustment may be required when starting or stopping concomitantly administered rifampin). Products include:
- Glucotrol Tablets 2692
- Glucotrol XL Extended Release Tablets 2693

Glyburide (Rifampin accelerates the metabolism of sulfonylureas; isoniazid may produce hyperglycemia and lead to loss of glucose control; dosage adjustment may be required when starting or stopping concomitantly administered rifampin). Products include:
- DiaBeta Tablets 741
- Glucovance Tablets 1086

Haloperidol (Rifampin accelerates the metabolism of haloperidol and isoniazid inhibits the metabolism of haloperidol; dosage adjustment may be required when starting or stopping concomitantly administered rifampin). Products include:
- Haldol Injection, Tablets and Concentrate 2533

Haloperidol Decanoate (Rifampin accelerates the metabolism of haloperidol and isoniazid inhibits the metabolism of haloperidol; dosage adjustment may be required when starting or stopping concomitantly administered rifampin). Products include:
- Haldol Decanoate 2535

Halothane (Increased potential for hepatotoxicity). Products include:
- Fluothane Inhalation 3508

Hydrocodone Bitartrate (Rifampin accelerates the metabolism of narcotic; dosage adjustment may be required when starting or stopping concomitantly administered rifampin). Products include:
- Hycodan 1316
- Hycomine Compound Tablets 1317
- Hycotuss Expectorant Syrup 1318
- Lortab 3319
- Lortab Elixir 3317
- Maxidone Tablets CIII 3399
- Norco 5/325 Tablets CIII 3424
- Norco 7.5/325 Tablets CIII 3425
- Norco 10/325 Tablets CIII 3427
- Norco 10/325 Tablets CIII 3425
- Vicodin Tablets 516
- Vicodin ES Tablets 517
- Vicodin HP Tablets 518
- Vicodin Tuss Expectorant 519
- Vicoprofen Tablets 520
- Zydone Tablets 1330

Hydrocodone Polistirex (Rifampin accelerates the metabolism of narcotic; dosage adjustment may be required when starting or stopping concomitantly administered rifampin). Products include:
- Tussionex Pennkinetic Extended-Release Suspension 1174

Hydrocortisone (Rifampin accelerates the metabolism of corticosteroid; dosage adjustment may be required when starting or stopping concomitantly administered rifampin). Products include:
- Anusol-HC Cream 2.5% 2237
- Cipro HC Otic Suspension 540
- Cortaid Intensive Therapy Cream .... ▣717
- Cortaid Maximum Strength Cream .... ▣717
- Cortisporin Ophthalmic Suspension Sterile .... ⊙297
- Cortizone•5 .... ▣699
- Cortizone•10 .... ▣699
- Cortizone•10 Plus Creme .... ▣700
- Cortizone for Kids Creme .... ▣699
- Hydrocortone Tablets 2106
- Massengill Medicated Soft Cloth Towelette .... ▣753
- VōSoL HC Otic Solution 3356

Hydrocortisone Acetate (Rifampin accelerates the metabolism of corticosteroid; dosage adjustment may be required when starting or stopping concomitantly administered rifampin). Products include:
- Analpram-HC 1338
- Anusol HC-1 Hydrocortisone Anti-Itch Cream .... ▣689
- Anusol-HC Suppositories 2238
- Cortaid .... ▣717
- Cortifoam Rectal Foam 3170
- Cortisporin-TC Otic Suspension 2246
- Hydrocortone Acetate Injectable Suspension 2103
- Pramosone 1343
- Proctocort Suppositories 2264
- ProctoFoam-HC 3177
- Terra-Cortril Ophthalmic Suspension 2716

Hydrocortisone Sodium Phosphate (Rifampin accelerates the metabolism of corticosteroid; dosage adjustment may be required when starting or stopping concomitantly administered rifampin). Products include:
- Hydrocortone Phosphate Injection, Sterile 2105

Hydrocortisone Sodium Succinate (Rifampin accelerates the metabolism of corticosteroid; dosage adjustment may be required when starting or stopping concomitantly administered rifampin).
- No products indexed under this heading.

Hydromorphone Hydrochloride (Rifampin accelerates the metabolism of narcotic; dosage adjustment may be required when starting or stopping concomitantly administered rifampin). Products include:
- Dilaudid 441
- Dilaudid Oral Liquid 445
- Dilaudid Powder 441
- Dilaudid Rectal Suppositories 441
- Dilaudid Tablets 441
- Dilaudid Tablets - 8 mg 445
- Dilaudid-HP 443

Itraconazole (Rifampin accelerates the metabolism of itraconazole; dosage adjustment may be required when starting or stopping concomitantly administered rifampin). Products include:
- Sporanox Capsules 1800
- Sporanox Injection 1804
- Sporanox Injection 2509
- Sporanox Oral Solution 1808
- Sporanox Oral Solution 2512

Ketoconazole (Rifampin accelerates the metabolism of ketoconazole; concurrent use has resulted in decreased serum concentration of both drugs; isoniazid inhibits the metabolism of ketoconazole; dosage adjustment may be required when starting or stopping concomitantly administered rifampin). Products include:
- Nizoral 2% Cream 3620
- Nizoral A-D Shampoo 2008
- Nizoral 2% Shampoo 2007
- Nizoral Tablets 1791

Labetalol Hydrochloride (Rifampin accelerates the metabolism of beta blocker; dosage adjustment may be required when starting or stopping concomitantly administered rifampin). Products include:
- Normodyne Injection 3135
- Normodyne Tablets 3137

Levobunolol Hydrochloride (Rifampin accelerates the metabolism of beta blocker; dosage adjustment may be required when starting or stopping concomitantly administered rifampin). Products include:
- Betagan .... ⊙228

Levodopa (Concurrent use may produce symptoms of excess catecholamine stimulation (agitation, flushing, palpitations) or lack of levodopa effect). Products include:
- Sinemet Tablets 1253
- Sinemet CR Tablets 1255

Levonorgestrel (Rifampin accelerates the metabolism of oral contraceptive; dosage adjustment may be required when starting or stopping concomitantly administered rifampin). Products include:
- Alesse-21 Tablets 3468
- Alesse-28 Tablets 3473
- Levlen 962
- Levlite 21 Tablets 962
- Levlite 28 Tablets 962
- Levora Tablets 3389
- Mirena Intrauterine System 974
- Nordette-28 Tablets 2257
- Norplant System 3543
- Tri-Levlen 962
- Triphasil-21 Tablets 3600
- Triphasil-28 Tablets 3605
- Trivora Tablets 3439

Levorphanol Tartrate (Rifampin accelerates the metabolism of narcotic; dosage adjustment may be required when starting or stopping concomitantly administered rifampin). Products include:
- Levo-Dromoran 1734
- Levorphanol Tartrate Tablets 3059

Magaldrate (Concomitant antacid administration may reduce the absorption of rifampin and isoniazid; daily dose of Rifater should be given at least one hour before the ingestion of antacids).
- No products indexed under this heading.

Magnesium Hydroxide (Concomitant antacid administration may reduce the absorption of rifampin and isoniazid; daily dose of Rifater should be given at least one hour before the ingestion of antacids). Products include:
- Ex•Lax Milk of Magnesia Liquid .... ▣670
- Maalox Antacid/Anti-Gas Oral Suspension .... ▣673
- Maalox Max Maximum Strength Antacid/Anti-Gas Liquid 2300
- Maalox Regular Strength Antacid/Antigas Liquid 2300
- Mylanta Fast-Acting 1813
- Mylanta 1813
- Pepcid Complete Chewable Tablets 1815
- Phillips' Chewable Tablets .... ▣615
- Phillips' Milk of Magnesia Liquid (Original, Cherry, & Mint) .... ▣616
- Rolaids Tablets .... ▣706
- Extra Strength Rolaids Tablets .... ▣706
- Vanquish Caplets .... ▣617

Magnesium Oxide (Concomitant antacid administration may reduce the absorption of rifampin and isoniazid; daily dose of Rifater should be given at least one hour before the ingestion of antacids). Products include:
- Beelith Tablets 946
- Mag-Ox 400 Tablets 1024
- Uro-Mag Capsules 1024

Medroxyprogesterone Acetate (Rifampin accelerates the metabolism of progestin; dosage adjustment may be required when starting or stopping concomitantly administered rifampin). Products include:
- Depo-Provera Contraceptive Injection 2798
- Lunelle Monthly Injection 2827
- Premphase Tablets 3572
- Prempro Tablets 3572
- Provera Tablets 2853

Megestrol Acetate (Rifampin accelerates the metabolism of progestin; dosage adjustment may be required when starting or stopping concomitantly administered rifampin). Products include:
- Megace Oral Suspension 1124

Meperidine Hydrochloride (Rifampin accelerates the metabolism of narcotic; dosage adjustment may be required when starting or stopping concomitantly administered rifampin; Rifater exaggerates drowsiness). Products include:
- Demerol 3079
- Mepergan Injection 3539

Mephobarbital (Rifampin accelerates the metabolism of barbiturates; dosage adjustment may be required when starting or stopping concomitantly administered rifampin).
- No products indexed under this heading.

Mestranol (Rifampin accelerates the metabolism of oral contraceptive; dosage adjustment may be required when starting or stopping concomitantly administered rifampin). Products include:
- Necon 1/50 Tablets 3415
- Norinyl 1 + 50 28-Day Tablets 3380
- Ortho-Novum 1/50□28 Tablets 2556

Methadone Hydrochloride (Rifampin accelerates the metabolism of narcotic; dosage adjustment may be required when starting or stopping concomitantly administered rifampin). Products include:
- Dolophine Hydrochloride Tablets 3056

Methylprednisolone Acetate (Rifampin accelerates the metabolism of corticosteroid; dosage adjustment may be required when starting or stopping concomitantly administered rifampin). Products include:
- Depo-Medrol Injectable Suspension 2795

Methylprednisolone Sodium Succinate (Rifampin accelerates the metabolism of corticosteroid; dosage adjustment may be required when starting or stopping concomitantly administered rifampin). Products include:
- Solu-Medrol Sterile Powder 2855

Metipranolol Hydrochloride (Rifampin accelerates the metabolism of beta blocker; dosage adjustment may be required when starting or stopping concomitantly administered rifampin).
- No products indexed under this heading.

Metoprolol Succinate (Rifampin accelerates the metabolism of beta blocker; dosage adjustment may be required when starting or stopping concomitantly administered rifampin). Products include:
- Toprol-XL Tablets 651

Metoprolol Tartrate (Rifampin accelerates the metabolism of beta blocker; dosage adjustment may be required when starting or stopping concomitantly administered rifampin).
- No products indexed under this heading.

Mexiletine Hydrochloride (Rifampin accelerates the metabolism of mexiletine; dosage adjustment may be required when starting or stopping concomitantly administered rifampin). Products include:
- Mexitil Capsules 1047

Morphine Sulfate (Rifampin accelerates the metabolism of narcotic; dosage adjustment may be required when starting or stopping concomitantly administered rifampin). Products include:

Astramorph/PF Injection, USP (Preservative-Free) 594
Duramorph Injection 1312
Infumorph 200 and Infumorph 500 Sterile Solutions 1314
Kadian Capsules 1335
MS Contin Tablets 2896
MSIR 2898
Oramorph SR Tablets 3062
Roxanol 3066

Nadolol (Rifampin accelerates the metabolism of beta blocker; dosage adjustment may be required when starting or stopping concomitantly administered rifampin). Products include:
Corgard Tablets 2245
Corzide 40/5 Tablets 2247
Corzide 80/5 Tablets 2247
Nadolol Tablets 2288

Nifedipine (Rifampin accelerates the metabolism of nifedipine; dosage adjustment may be required when starting or stopping concomitantly administered rifampin). Products include:
Adalat CC Tablets 877
Procardia Capsules 2708
Procardia XL Extended Release Tablets 2710

Norethindrone (Rifampin accelerates the metabolism of oral contraceptive; dosage adjustment may be required when starting or stopping concomitantly administered rifampin). Products include:
Brevicon 28-Day Tablets 3380
Micronor Tablets 2543
Modicon 2563
Necon 3415
Norinyl 1 +35 28-Day Tablets 3380
Norinyl 1 + 50 28-Day Tablets 3380
Nor-QD Tablets 3423
Ortho-Novum 2563
Ortho-Novum 1/50▫28 Tablets 2556
Ovcon 3364
Tri-Norinyl-28 Tablets 3433

Norethynodrel (Rifampin accelerates the metabolism of oral contraceptive; dosage adjustment may be required when starting or stopping concomitantly administered rifampin).
No products indexed under this heading.

Norgestimate (Rifampin accelerates the metabolism of oral contraceptive or progestin; dosage adjustment may be required when starting or stopping concomitantly administered rifampin). Products include:
Ortho-Cyclen/Ortho Tri-Cyclen 2573
Ortho-Prefest Tablets 2570

Norgestrel (Rifampin accelerates the metabolism of oral contraceptive; dosage adjustment may be required when starting or stopping concomitantly administered rifampin). Products include:
Lo/Ovral Tablets 3532
Lo/Ovral-28 Tablets 3538
Low-Ogestrel-28 Tablets 3392
Ogestrel 0.5/50-28 Tablets 3428
Ovral Tablets 3551
Ovral-28 Tablets 3552
Ovrette Tablets 3552

Nortriptyline Hydrochloride (Rifampin accelerates the metabolism of nortriptyline; dosage adjustment may be required when starting or stopping concomitantly administered rifampin).
No products indexed under this heading.

Oxycodone Hydrochloride (Rifampin accelerates the metabolism of narcotic; dosage adjustment may be required when starting or stopping concomitantly administered rifampin). Products include:
OxyContin Tablets 2912
OxyFast Oral Concentrate Solution 2916
OxyIR Capsules 2916
Percocet Tablets 1326
Percodan Tablets 1327
Percolone Tablets 1327
Roxicodone 3067
Tylox Capsules 2597

Para-Aminosalicylic Acid (Increases the plasma concentration and elimination half-life of isoniazid).
No products indexed under this heading.

Penbutolol Sulfate (Rifampin accelerates the metabolism of beta blocker; dosage adjustment may be required when starting or stopping concomitantly administered rifampin).
No products indexed under this heading.

Pentobarbital Sodium (Rifampin accelerates the metabolism of barbiturates; dosage adjustment may be required when starting or stopping concomitantly administered rifampin). Products include:
Nembutal Sodium Solution 485

Phenobarbital (Rifampin accelerates the metabolism of barbiturates; dosage adjustment may be required when starting or stopping concomitantly administered rifampin). Products include:
Arco-Lase Plus Tablets 592
Donnatal 2929
Donnatal Extentabs 2930

Phenytoin (Rifampin accelerates the metabolism and isoniazid inhibits the metabolism of phenytoin; dosage adjustment may be required when starting or stopping concomitantly administered rifampin). Products include:
Dilantin Infatabs 2624
Dilantin-125 Oral Suspension 2625

Phenytoin Sodium (Rifampin accelerates the metabolism and isoniazid inhibits the metabolism of phenytoin; dosage adjustment may be required when starting or stopping concomitantly administered rifampin). Products include:
Dilantin Kapseals 2622

Pindolol (Rifampin accelerates the metabolism of beta blocker; dosage adjustment may be required when starting or stopping concomitantly administered rifampin).
No products indexed under this heading.

Prednisolone Acetate (Rifampin accelerates the metabolism of corticosteroid; dosage adjustment may be required when starting or stopping concomitantly administered rifampin; may increase the serum concentration of isoniazid by increasing acetylation rate and/or renal clearance). Products include:
Blephamide Ophthalmic Ointment 547
Blephamide Ophthalmic Suspension 548
Poly-Pred Liquifilm Ophthalmic Suspension .... ⊙245
Pred Forte Ophthalmic Suspension .... ⊙246
Pred Mild Sterile Ophthalmic Suspension .... ⊙249
Pred-G Ophthalmic Suspension .... ⊙247
Pred-G Sterile Ophthalmic Ointment .... ⊙248

Prednisolone Sodium Phosphate (Rifampin accelerates the metabolism of corticosteroid; dosage adjustment may be required when starting or stopping concomitantly administered rifampin; may increase the serum concentration of isoniazid by increasing acetylation rate and/or renal clearance). Products include:
Pediapred Oral Solution 1170

Prednisolone Tebutate (Rifampin accelerates the metabolism of corticosteroid; dosage adjustment may be required when starting or stopping concomitantly administered rifampin; may increase the serum concentration of isoniazid by increasing acetylation rate and/or renal clearance).
No products indexed under this heading.

Prednisone (Rifampin accelerates the metabolism of corticosteroid; dosage adjustment may be required when starting or stopping concomitantly administered rifampin). Products include:
Prednisone 3064

Primidone (Isoniazid inhibits the metabolism of primidone).
No products indexed under this heading.

Probenecid (Increases blood levels of rifampin).
No products indexed under this heading.

Propoxyphene Hydrochloride (Rifampin accelerates the metabolism of narcotic; dosage adjustment may be required when starting or stopping concomitantly administered rifampin). Products include:
Darvon Pulvules 1909
Darvon Compound-65 Pulvules 1910

Propoxyphene Napsylate (Rifampin accelerates the metabolism of narcotic; dosage adjustment may be required when starting or stopping concomitantly administered rifampin). Products include:
Darvon-N/Darvocet-N 1907
Darvon-N Tablets 1912

Propranolol Hydrochloride (Rifampin accelerates the metabolism of beta blocker; dosage adjustment may be required when starting or stopping concomitantly administered rifampin). Products include:
Inderal 3513
Inderal LA Long-Acting Capsules 3516
Inderide Tablets 3517
Inderide LA Long-Acting Capsules 3519

Quinidine Gluconate (Rifampin accelerates the metabolism of quinidine; dosage adjustment may be required when starting or stopping concomitantly administered rifampin). Products include:
Quinaglute Dura-Tabs Tablets 978

Quinidine Polygalacturonate (Rifampin accelerates the metabolism of quinidine; dosage adjustment may be required when starting or stopping concomitantly administered rifampin).
No products indexed under this heading.

Quinidine Sulfate (Rifampin accelerates the metabolism of quinidine; dosage adjustment may be required when starting or stopping concomitantly administered rifampin). Products include:
Quinidex Extentabs 2933

Remifentanil Hydrochloride (Rifampin accelerates the metabolism of narcotic; dosage adjustment may be required when starting or stopping concomitantly administered rifampin).
No products indexed under this heading.

Secobarbital Sodium (Rifampin accelerates the metabolism of barbiturates; dosage adjustment may be required when starting or stopping concomitantly administered rifampin).
No products indexed under this heading.

Sodium Bicarbonate (Concomitant antacid administration may reduce the absorption of rifampin and isoniazid; daily dose of Rifater should be given at least one hour before the ingestion of antacids). Products include:
Alka-Seltzer .... ■603
Alka-Seltzer Lemon Lime Antacid and Pain Reliever Effervescent Tablets .... ■603
Alka-Seltzer Extra Strength Antacid and Pain Reliever Effervescent Tablets .... ■603
Alka-Seltzer Heartburn Relief Tablets .... ■604
Ceo-Two Evacuant Suppository .... ■618
Colyte with Flavor Packs for Oral Solution 3170
GoLYTELY and Pineapple Flavor GoLYTELY for Oral Solution 1068
NuLYTELY, Cherry Flavor, Lemon-Lime Flavor, and Orange Flavor NuLYTELY for Oral Solution 1068

Sotalol Hydrochloride (Rifampin accelerates the metabolism of beta blocker; dosage adjustment may be required when starting or stopping concomitantly administered rifampin). Products include:
Betapace Tablets 950
Betapace AF Tablets 954

Sufentanil Citrate (Rifampin accelerates the metabolism of narcotic; dosage adjustment may be required when starting or stopping concomitantly administered rifampin).
No products indexed under this heading.

Sulfamethoxazole (Cotrimoxazole has been reported to increase the blood level of rifampin). Products include:
Bactrim 2949
Septra Suspension 2265
Septra Tablets 2265
Septra DS Tablets 2265

Sulfasalazine (Reduced plasma concentration of sulfapyridine by rifampin due to alteration in colonic bacteria responsible for reduction of sulfasalazine to sulfapyridine). Products include:
Azulfidine EN-tabs Tablets 2775

Theophylline (Rifampin accelerates the metabolism of theophylline and isoniazid inhibits the metabolism; dosage adjustment may be required when starting or stopping concomitantly administered rifampin). Products include:
Aerolate 1361
Theo-Dur Extended-Release Tablets 1835
Uni-Dur Extended-Release Tablets 1841
Uniphyl 400 mg and 600 mg Tablets 2903

Theophylline Calcium Salicylate (Rifampin accelerates the metabolism of theophylline and isoniazid inhibits the metabolism; dosage adjustment may be required when starting or stopping concomitantly administered rifampin).
No products indexed under this heading.

Theophylline Sodium Glycinate (Rifampin accelerates the metabolism of theophylline and isoniazid inhibits the metabolism; dosage adjustment may be required when starting or stopping concomitantly administered rifampin).
No products indexed under this heading.

Thiamylal Sodium (Rifampin accelerates the metabolism of barbiturates; dosage adjustment may be required when starting or stopping concomitantly administered rifampin).
No products indexed under this heading.

Timolol Hemihydrate (Rifampin accelerates the metabolism of beta blocker; dosage adjustment may be required when starting or stopping concomitantly administered rifampin). Products include:
Betimol Ophthalmic Solution .... ⊙324

Timolol Maleate (Rifampin accelerates the metabolism of beta blocker; dosage adjustment may be required when starting or stopping concomitantly administered rifampin). Products include:
Blocadren Tablets 2046
Cosopt Sterile Ophthalmic Solution 2065
Timolide Tablets 2187
Timolol GFS .... ⊙266
Timoptic in Ocudose 2192
Timoptic Sterile Ophthalmic Solution 2190

IMPORTANT NOTE: Always consult each drug listing in the patient's regimen for possible interactions.

Timoptic-XE Sterile Ophthalmic Gel Forming Solution 2194

Tocainide Hydrochloride (Rifampin accelerates the metabolism of tocainide; dosage adjustment may be required when starting or stopping concomitantly administered rifampin). Products include:
- Tonocard Tablets 649

Tolazamide (Rifampin accelerates the metabolism of sulfonylureas; isoniazid may produce hyperglycemia and lead to loss of glucose control; dosage adjustment may be required when starting or stopping concomitantly administered rifampin).
- No products indexed under this heading.

Tolbutamide (Rifampin accelerates the metabolism of sulfonylureas; isoniazid may produce hyperglycemia and lead to loss of glucose control; dosage adjustment may be required when starting or stopping concomitantly administered rifampin).
- No products indexed under this heading.

Triamcinolone (Rifampin accelerates the metabolism of corticosteroid; dosage adjustment may be required when starting or stopping concomitantly administered rifampin).
- No products indexed under this heading.

Triamcinolone Acetonide (Rifampin accelerates the metabolism of corticosteroid; dosage adjustment may be required when starting or stopping concomitantly administered rifampin). Products include:
- Azmacort Inhalation Aerosol 728
- Nasacort Nasal Inhaler 750
- Nasacort AQ Nasal Spray 752
- Tri-Nasal Spray 2274

Triamcinolone Diacetate (Rifampin accelerates the metabolism of corticosteroid; dosage adjustment may be required when starting or stopping concomitantly administered rifampin).
- No products indexed under this heading.

Triamcinolone Hexacetonide (Rifampin accelerates the metabolism of corticosteroid; dosage adjustment may be required when starting or stopping concomitantly administered rifampin).
- No products indexed under this heading.

Trimethoprim (Cotrimoxazole has been reported to increase the blood level of rifampin). Products include:
- Bactrim 2949
- Septra Suspension 2265
- Septra Tablets 2265
- Septra DS Tablets 2265

Valproate Sodium (Isoniazid inhibits the metabolism of valproic acid). Products include:
- Depacon Injection 416

Valproic Acid (Isoniazid inhibits the metabolism of valproic acid). Products include:
- Depakene 421

Verapamil Hydrochloride (Rifampin accelerates the metabolism of verapamil; dosage adjustment may be required when starting or stopping concomitantly administered rifampin). Products include:
- Covera-HS Tablets 3199
- Isoptin SR Tablets 467
- Tarka Tablets 508
- Verelan Capsules 3184
- Verelan PM Capsules 3186

Warfarin Sodium (Rifampin accelerates the metabolism of anticoagulants and isoniazid inhibits the metabolism; increased requirements of coumarin type anticoagulant; dosage adjustment may be required when starting or stopping concomitantly administered rifampin). Products include:
- Coumadin for Injection 1243
- Coumadin Tablets 1243
- Warfarin Sodium Tablets, USP 3302

Food Interactions

Alcohol (Daily ingestion of alcohol may be associated with higher incidence of isoniazid hepatitis).

Cheese, unspecified (Isoniazid has some MAO inhibiting activity, an interaction with tyramine-containing food may occur).

Fish, tropical (Isoniazid may inhibit diamine oxidase, causing exaggerated response (headache, sweating, palpitations, flushing, hypotension) to food containing histamine).

Food, unspecified (Ingestion with food may reduce the absorption of isoniazid; daily dose of Rifater should be given on an empty stomach at least one hour before the ingestion of food).

Food with high concentration of tyramine (Isoniazid has some MAO inhibiting activity, an interaction with tyramine-containing food may occur).

Skipjack fish (Isoniazid may inhibit diamine oxidase, causing exaggerated response (headache, sweating, palpitations, flushing, hypotension) to food containing histamine).

Tuna Fish (Isoniazid may inhibit diamine oxidase, causing exaggerated response (headache, sweating, palpitations, flushing, hypotension) to food containing histamine).

Wine, Red (Isoniazid has some MAO inhibiting activity, an interaction with tyramine-containing food may occur).

RIGHT CHOICE A.M. MULTI FORMULA CAPLETS

(Herbals with Vitamins) .... ▣811
None cited in PDR database.

RIGHT CHOICE P.M. MULTI FORMULA CAPLETS

(Minerals, Multiple) .... ▣812
None cited in PDR database.

RILUTEK TABLETS

(Riluzole) 772
May interact with quinolones, theophylline, and certain other agents. Compounds in these categories include:

Alatrofloxacin Mesylate (Potential inhibitors of CYP1A2, such as quinolones, could decrease the rate of riluzole elimination). Products include:
- Trovan I.V. 2722

Allopurinol (Riluzole induces hepatic injury; ALS patients on concomitant hepatotoxic drugs, such as allopurinol, were excluded in the clinical trials; if such combination is used, practitioner should exercise caution).
- No products indexed under this heading.

Aminophylline (Potential inhibitors of CYP1A2, such as theophylline, could decrease the rate of riluzole elimination).
- No products indexed under this heading.

Amitriptyline Hydrochloride (Potential inhibitors of CYP1A2, such as amitriptyline, could decrease the rate of riluzole elimination). Products include:
- Etrafon 3115
- Limbitrol 1738

Caffeine (Potential inhibitors of CYP1A2, such as caffeine, could decrease the rate of riluzole elimination). Products include:
- BC Powder .... ▣619
- Arthritis Strength BC Powder .... ▣619
- Darvon Compound-65 Pulvules 1910
- Aspirin Free Excedrin Caplets and Geltabs .... ▣628
- Excedrin Extra-Strength Tablets, Caplets, and Geltabs .... ▣629
- Excedrin Migraine 1070
- Goody's Extra Strength Headache Powder .... ▣620
- Goody's Extra Strength Pain Relief Tablets .... ▣620
- Hycomine Compound Tablets 1317
- Maximum Strength Midol Menstrual Caplets and Gelcaps .... ▣612
- Vanquish Caplets .... ▣617
- Vivarin .... ▣763

Ciprofloxacin (Potential inhibitors of CYP1A2, such as quinolones, could decrease the rate of riluzole elimination). Products include:
- Cipro I.V. 893
- Cipro I.V. Pharmacy Bulk Package 897
- Cipro Oral Suspension 887

Ciprofloxacin Hydrochloride (Potential inhibitors of CYP1A2, such as quinolones, could decrease the rate of riluzole elimination). Products include:
- Ciloxan 538
- Cipro HC Otic Suspension 540
- Cipro Tablets 887

Dyphylline (Potential inhibitors of CYP1A2, such as theophylline, could decrease the rate of riluzole elimination). Products include:
- Lufyllin Tablets 3347
- Lufyllin-400 Tablets 3347
- Lufyllin-GG Elixir 3348
- Lufyllin-GG Tablets 3348

Enoxacin (Potential inhibitors of CYP1A2, such as quinolones, could decrease the rate of riluzole elimination).
- No products indexed under this heading.

Grepafloxacin Hydrochloride (Potential inhibitors of CYP1A2, such as quinolones, could decrease the rate of riluzole elimination).
- No products indexed under this heading.

Lomefloxacin Hydrochloride (Potential inhibitors of CYP1A2, such as quinolones, could decrease the rate of riluzole elimination).
- No products indexed under this heading.

Methyldopa (Riluzole induces hepatic injury; ALS patients on concomitant hepatotoxic drugs, such as methyldopa, were excluded in the clinical trials; if such combination is used, practitioner should exercise caution). Products include:
- Aldoclor Tablets 2035
- Aldomet Tablets 2037
- Aldoril Tablets 2039

Moxifloxacin Hydrochloride (Potential inhibitors of CYP1A2, such as quinolones, could decrease the rate of riluzole elimination). Products include:
- Avelox Tablets 879

Norfloxacin (Potential inhibitors of CYP1A2, such as quinolones, could decrease the rate of riluzole elimination). Products include:
- Chibroxin Sterile Ophthalmic Solution 2051
- Noroxin Tablets 2145

Ofloxacin (Potential inhibitors of CYP1A2, such as quinolones, could decrease the rate of riluzole elimination). Products include:
- Floxin I.V. 2526
- Floxin Otic Solution 1219
- Floxin Tablets 2529
- Ocuflox Ophthalmic Solution 554

Omeprazole (Potential inducers of CYP1A2, such as theophylline, could increase the rate of riluzole elimination). Products include:
- Prilosec Delayed-Release Capsules 628

Phenacetin (Potential inhibitors of CYP1A2, such as phenacetin, could decrease the rate of riluzole elimination).

Rifampin (Potential inducers of CYP1A2, such as theophylline, could increase the rate of riluzole elimination). Products include:
- Rifadin 765
- Rifamate Capsules 767
- Rifater Tablets 769

Sulfasalazine (Riluzole induces hepatic injury; ALS patients on concomitant hepatotoxic drugs, such as sulfasalazine, were excluded in the clinical trials; if such combination is used, practitioner should exercise caution). Products include:
- Azulfidine EN-tabs Tablets 2775

Tacrine Hydrochloride (CYP1A2 is the principal isoenzyme involved in the initial oxidative metabolism of riluzole; potential interaction may occur when co-administered with other agents, such as tacrine, which are also metabolized primarily by CYP1A2). Products include:
- Cognex Capsules 1351

Theophylline (Potential inhibitors of CYP1A2, such as theophylline, could decrease the rate of riluzole elimination). Products include:
- Aerolate 1361
- Theo-Dur Extended-Release Tablets 1835
- Uni-Dur Extended-Release Tablets 1841
- Uniphyl 400 mg and 600 mg Tablets 2903

Theophylline Calcium Salicylate (Potential inhibitors of CYP1A2, such as theophylline, could decrease the rate of riluzole elimination).
- No products indexed under this heading.

Theophylline Sodium Glycinate (Potential inhibitors of CYP1A2, such as theophylline, could decrease the rate of riluzole elimination).
- No products indexed under this heading.

Trovafloxacin Mesylate (Potential inhibitors of CYP1A2, such as quinolones, could decrease the rate of riluzole elimination). Products include:
- Trovan Tablets 2722

Food Interactions

Alcohol (Alcohol may increase the risk of hepatotoxicity; patients on riluzole should be discouraged from drinking excessive amounts of alcohol).

Diet, high-lipid (Co-administration with high-fat meal decreases absorption, reduces AUC by about 20% and peak blood levels by about 45%).

Food, charcoal-broiled (Potential inducers of CYP1A2, such as charcoal-broiled food, could increase the rate of riluzole elimination).

RIMSO-50 SOLUTION

(Dimethyl Sulfoxide) 1267
May interact with:

Drugs, unspecified (Some data indicate that dimethyl sulfoxide potentiates other concomitantly administered medications).

RISPERDAL ORAL SOLUTION

(Risperidone) 1796
See Risperdal Tablets

RISPERDAL TABLETS

(Risperidone) 1796
May interact with antihypertensives, central nervous system depressants, drugs that inhibit cytochrome p450iid6 and other p450 isoenzymes, dopamine agonists, and certain other agents. Compounds in these categories include:

Acebutolol Hydrochloride (Co-administration with antihypertensive

agents has resulted in clinically significant hypotension). Products include:
- Sectral Capsules 3589

Alfentanil Hydrochloride (Effects not specified; caution should be used when used concurrently).
- No products indexed under this heading.

Alprazolam (Effects not specified; caution should be used when used concurrently). Products include:
- Xanax Tablets 2865

Amitriptyline Hydrochloride (Inhibitors of cytochrome P450IID6 could interfere with the conversion of risperidone to 9-hydroxyrisperidone). Products include:
- Etrafon 3115
- Limbitrol 1738

Amlodipine Besylate (Co-administration with antihypertensive agents has resulted in clinically significant hypotension). Products include:
- Lotrel Capsules 2370
- Norvasc Tablets 2704

Aprobarbital (Effects not specified; caution should be used when used concurrently).
- No products indexed under this heading.

Atenolol (Co-administration with antihypertensive agents has resulted in clinically significant hypotension). Products include:
- Tenoretic Tablets 690
- Tenormin I.V. Injection 692

Benazepril Hydrochloride (Co-administration with antihypertensive agents has resulted in clinically significant hypotension). Products include:
- Lotensin Tablets 2365
- Lotensin HCT Tablets 2367
- Lotrel Capsules 2370

Bendroflumethiazide (Co-administration with antihypertensive agents has resulted in clinically significant hypotension). Products include:
- Corzide 40/5 Tablets 2247
- Corzide 80/5 Tablets 2247

Betaxolol Hydrochloride (Co-administration with antihypertensive agents has resulted in clinically significant hypotension). Products include:
- Betoptic S Ophthalmic Suspension 537

Bisoprolol Fumarate (Co-administration with antihypertensive agents has resulted in clinically significant hypotension). Products include:
- Zebeta Tablets 1885
- Ziac Tablets 1887

Bromocriptine Mesylate (Risperidone may antagonize the effect of dopamine agonists).
- No products indexed under this heading.

Buprenorphine Hydrochloride (Effects not specified; caution should be used when used concurrently). Products include:
- Buprenex Injectable 2918

Buspirone Hydrochloride (Effects not specified; caution should be used when used concurrently).
- No products indexed under this heading.

Butabarbital (Effects not specified; caution should be used when used concurrently).
- No products indexed under this heading.

Butalbital (Effects not specified; caution should be used when used concurrently). Products include:
- Phrenilin 578
- Sedapap Tablets 50 mg/650 mg 2225

Candesartan Cilexetil (Co-administration with antihypertensive agents has resulted in clinically significant hypotension). Products include:
- Atacand Tablets 595
- Atacand HCT Tablets 597

Captopril (Co-administration with antihypertensive agents has resulted in clinically significant hypotension). Products include:
- Captopril Tablets 2281

Carbamazepine (Chronic administration of carbamazepine may increase the clearance of risperidone). Products include:
- Carbatrol Capsules 3234
- Tegretol/Tegretol-XR 2404

Carteolol Hydrochloride (Co-administration with antihypertensive agents has resulted in clinically significant hypotension). Products include:
- Carteolol Hydrochloride Ophthalmic Solution USP, 1% .... ⊙258
- Ocupress Ophthalmic Solution, 1% Sterile .... ⊙303

Chlordiazepoxide (Effects not specified; caution should be used when used concurrently). Products include:
- Limbitrol 1738

Chlordiazepoxide Hydrochloride (Effects not specified; caution should be used when used concurrently). Products include:
- Librium Capsules 1736
- Librium for Injection 1737

Chlorothiazide (Co-administration with antihypertensive agents has resulted in clinically significant hypotension). Products include:
- Aldoclor Tablets 2035
- Diuril Oral 2087

Chlorothiazide Sodium (Co-administration with antihypertensive agents has resulted in clinically significant hypotension). Products include:
- Diuril Sodium Intravenous 2086

Chlorpromazine (Inhibitors of cytochrome P450IID6 could interfere with the conversion of risperidone to 9-hydroxyrisperidone; caution should be used when used concurrently). Products include:
- Thorazine Suppositories 1656

Chlorpromazine Hydrochloride (Inhibitors of cytochrome P450IID6 could interfere with the conversion of risperidone to 9-hydroxyrisperidone; caution should be used when used concurrently). Products include:
- Thorazine 1656

Chlorprothixene (Effects not specified; caution should be used when used concurrently).
- No products indexed under this heading.

Chlorprothixene Hydrochloride (Effects not specified; caution should be used when used concurrently).
- No products indexed under this heading.

Chlorprothixene Lactate (Effects not specified; caution should be used when used concurrently).
- No products indexed under this heading.

Chlorthalidone (Co-administration with antihypertensive agents has resulted in clinically significant hypotension). Products include:
- Clorpres Tablets 1002
- Combipres Tablets 1040
- Tenoretic Tablets 690

Clonidine (Co-administration with antihypertensive agents has resulted in clinically significant hypotension). Products include:
- Catapres-TTS 1038

Clonidine Hydrochloride (Co-administration with antihypertensive agents has resulted in clinically significant hypotension). Products include:
- Catapres Tablets 1037
- Clorpres Tablets 1002
- Combipres Tablets 1040
- Duraclon Injection 3057

Clorazepate Dipotassium (Effects not specified; caution should be used when used concurrently). Products include:
- Tranxene 511

Clozapine (Chronic administration of clozapine with risperidone may decrease the clearance of risperidone; caution should be used when used concurrently). Products include:
- Clozaril Tablets 2319

CNS-Active Drugs, unspecified (Effects not specified; caution should be used when used concurrently).

Codeine Phosphate (Effects not specified; caution should be used when used concurrently). Products include:
- Phenergan with Codeine Syrup 3557
- Phenergan VC with Codeine Syrup 3561
- Robitussin A-C Syrup 2942
- Robitussin-DAC Syrup 2942
- Ryna-C Liquid .... ▣768
- Soma Compound w/Codeine Tablets 3355
- Tussi-Organidin NR Liquid 3350
- Tussi-Organidin-S NR Liquid 3350
- Tylenol with Codeine 2595

Deserpidine (Co-administration with antihypertensive agents has resulted in clinically significant hypotension).
- No products indexed under this heading.

Desflurane (Effects not specified; caution should be used when used concurrently). Products include:
- Suprane Liquid for Inhalation 874

Dezocine (Effects not specified; caution should be used when used concurrently).
- No products indexed under this heading.

Diazepam (Effects not specified; caution should be used when used concurrently). Products include:
- Valium Injectable 3026
- Valium Tablets 3047

Diazoxide (Co-administration with antihypertensive agents has resulted in clinically significant hypotension).
- No products indexed under this heading.

Diltiazem Hydrochloride (Co-administration with antihypertensive agents has resulted in clinically significant hypotension). Products include:
- Cardizem Injectable 1018
- Cardizem Lyo-Ject Syringe 1018
- Cardizem Monovial 1018
- Cardizem CD Capsules 1016
- Tiazac Capsules 1378

Dopamine Hydrochloride (Risperidone may antagonize the effect of dopamine agonists).
- No products indexed under this heading.

Doxazosin Mesylate (Co-administration with antihypertensive agents has resulted in clinically significant hypotension). Products include:
- Cardura Tablets 2668

Droperidol (Effects not specified; caution should be used when used concurrently).
- No products indexed under this heading.

Enalapril Maleate (Co-administration with antihypertensive agents has resulted in clinically significant hypotension). Products include:
- Lexxel Tablets 608
- Vaseretic Tablets 2204
- Vasotec Tablets 2210

Enalaprilat (Co-administration with antihypertensive agents has resulted in clinically significant hypotension). Products include:
- Enalaprilat Injection 863
- Vasotec I.V. Injection 2207

Enflurane (Effects not specified; caution should be used when used concurrently).
- No products indexed under this heading.

Eprosartan Mesylate (Co-administration with antihypertensive agents has resulted in clinically significant hypotension). Products include:
- Teveten Tablets 3327

Esmolol Hydrochloride (Co-administration with antihypertensive agents has resulted in clinically significant hypotension). Products include:
- Brevibloc Injection 858

Estazolam (Effects not specified; caution should be used when used concurrently). Products include:
- ProSom Tablets 500

Ethchlorvynol (Effects not specified; caution should be used when used concurrently).
- No products indexed under this heading.

Ethinamate (Effects not specified; caution should be used when used concurrently).
- No products indexed under this heading.

Felodipine (Co-administration with antihypertensive agents has resulted in clinically significant hypotension). Products include:
- Lexxel Tablets 608
- Plendil Extended-Release Tablets 623

Fentanyl (Effects not specified; caution should be used when used concurrently). Products include:
- Duragesic Transdermal System 1786

Fentanyl Citrate (Effects not specified; caution should be used when used concurrently). Products include:
- Actiq 1184

Fluoxetine Hydrochloride (May increase the plasma concentration of the anti-psychotic fraction, risperidone plus 9-hydroxyrisperidone, by raising the concentration of resperidone, although not the active metabolite, 9-hydroxyrisperidone). Products include:
- Prozac Pulvules, Liquid, and Weekly Capsules 1238
- Sarafem Pulvules 1962

Fluphenazine Decanoate (Effects not specified; caution should be used when used concurrently).
- No products indexed under this heading.

Fluphenazine Enanthate (Effects not specified; caution should be used when used concurrently).
- No products indexed under this heading.

Fluphenazine Hydrochloride (Effects not specified; caution should be used when used concurrently).
- No products indexed under this heading.

Flurazepam Hydrochloride (Effects not specified; caution should be used when used concurrently).
- No products indexed under this heading.

Fosinopril Sodium (Co-administration with antihypertensive agents has resulted in clinically significant hypotension). Products include:
- Monopril Tablets 1091
- Monopril HCT 1094

Furosemide (Co-administration with antihypertensive agents has resulted in clinically significant hypotension). Products include:
- Furosemide Tablets 2284

Glutethimide (Effects not specified; caution should be used when used

concurrently).
No products indexed under this heading.

Guanabenz Acetate (Co-administration with antihypertensive agents has resulted in clinically significant hypotension).
No products indexed under this heading.

Guanethidine Monosulfate (Co-administration with antihypertensive agents has resulted in clinically significant hypotension).
No products indexed under this heading.

Haloperidol (Inhibitors of cytochrome P450IID6 could interfere with the conversion of risperidone to 9-hydroxyrisperidone; caution should be used when used concurrently).
Products include:
Haldol Injection, Tablets and Concentrate 2533

Haloperidol Decanoate (Inhibitors of cytochrome P450IID6 could interfere with the conversion of risperidone to 9-hydroxyrisperidone; caution should be used when used concurrently). Products include:
Haldol Decanoate 2535

Hydralazine Hydrochloride (Co-administration with antihypertensive agents has resulted in clinically significant hypotension).
No products indexed under this heading.

Hydrochlorothiazide (Co-administration with antihypertensive agents has resulted in clinically significant hypotension). Products include:
Accuretic Tablets 2614
Aldoril Tablets 2039
Atacand HCT Tablets 597
Avalide Tablets 1070
Diovan HCT Tablets 2338
Dyazide Capsules 1515
HydroDIURIL Tablets 2108
Hyzaar 2109
Inderide Tablets 3517
Inderide LA Long-Acting Capsules .. 3519
Lotensin HCT Tablets 2367
Maxzide 1008
Micardis HCT Tablets 1051
Microzide Capsules 3414
Moduretic Tablets 2138
Monopril HCT 1094
Prinzide Tablets 2168
Timolide Tablets 2187
Uniretic Tablets 3178
Vaseretic Tablets 2204
Zestoretic Tablets 695
Ziac Tablets 1887

Hydrocodone Bitartrate (Effects not specified; caution should be used when used concurrently).
Products include:
Hycodan 1316
Hycomine Compound Tablets 1317
Hycotuss Expectorant Syrup 1318
Lortab 3319
Lortab Elixir 3317
Maxidone Tablets CIII 3399
Norco 5/325 Tablets CIII 3424
Norco 7.5/325 Tablets CIII 3425
Norco 10/325 Tablets CIII 3427
Norco 10/325 Tablets CIII 3425
Vicodin Tablets 516
Vicodin ES Tablets 517
Vicodin HP Tablets 518
Vicodin Tuss Expectorant 519
Vicoprofen Tablets 520
Zydone Tablets 1330

Hydrocodone Polistirex (Effects not specified; caution should be used when used concurrently).
Products include:
Tussionex Pennkinetic Extended-Release Suspension 1174

Hydroflumethiazide (Co-administration with antihypertensive agents has resulted in clinically significant hypotension). Products include:
Diucardin Tablets 3494

Hydromorphone Hydrochloride (Effects not specified; caution should be used when used concurrently).
Products include:
Dilaudid 441
Dilaudid Oral Liquid 445
Dilaudid Powder 441
Dilaudid Rectal Suppositories 441
Dilaudid Tablets 441
Dilaudid Tablets - 8 mg 445
Dilaudid-HP 443

Hydroxyzine Hydrochloride (Effects not specified; caution should be used when used concurrently).
Products include:
Atarax Tablets & Syrup 2667
Vistaril Intramuscular Solution 2738

Imipramine Hydrochloride (Inhibitors of cytochrome P450IID6 could interfere with the conversion of risperidone to 9-hydroxyrisperidone).
No products indexed under this heading.

Indapamide (Co-administration with antihypertensive agents has resulted in clinically significant hypotension).
Products include:
Indapamide Tablets 2286

Irbesartan (Co-administration with antihypertensive agents has resulted in clinically significant hypotension).
Products include:
Avalide Tablets 1070
Avapro Tablets 1074
Avapro Tablets 3076

Isoflurane (Effects not specified; caution should be used when used concurrently).
No products indexed under this heading.

Isradipine (Co-administration with antihypertensive agents has resulted in clinically significant hypotension).
Products include:
DynaCirc Capsules 2921
DynaCirc CR Tablets 2923

Ketamine Hydrochloride (Effects not specified; caution should be used when used concurrently).
No products indexed under this heading.

Labetalol Hydrochloride (Co-administration with antihypertensive agents has resulted in clinically significant hypotension). Products include:
Normodyne Injection 3135
Normodyne Tablets 3137

Levodopa (Risperidone may antagonize the effect of levodopa).
Products include:
Sinemet Tablets 1253
Sinemet CR Tablets 1255

Levomethadyl Acetate Hydrochloride (Effects not specified; caution should be used when used concurrently).
No products indexed under this heading.

Levorphanol Tartrate (Effects not specified; caution should be used when used concurrently). Products include:
Levo-Dromoran 1734
Levorphanol Tartrate Tablets 3059

Lisinopril (Co-administration with antihypertensive agents has resulted in clinically significant hypotension).
Products include:
Prinivil Tablets 2164
Prinzide Tablets 2168
Zestoretic Tablets 695
Zestril Tablets 698

Lorazepam (Effects not specified; caution should be used when used concurrently). Products include:
Ativan Injection 3478
Ativan Tablets 3482

Losartan Potassium (Co-administration with antihypertensive agents has resulted in clinically significant hypotension). Products include:
Cozaar Tablets 2067
Hyzaar 2109

Loxapine Hydrochloride (Effects not specified; caution should be used when used concurrently).
No products indexed under this heading.

Loxapine Succinate (Effects not specified; caution should be used when used concurrently). Products include:
Loxitane Capsules 3398

Mecamylamine Hydrochloride (Co-administration with antihypertensive agents has resulted in clinically significant hypotension). Products include:
Inversine Tablets 1850

Meperidine Hydrochloride (Effects not specified; caution should be used when used concurrently).
Products include:
Demerol 3079
Mepergan Injection 3539

Mephobarbital (Effects not specified; caution should be used when used concurrently).
No products indexed under this heading.

Meprobamate (Effects not specified; caution should be used when used concurrently). Products include:
Miltown Tablets 3349

Mesoridazine Besylate (Effects not specified; caution should be used when used concurrently).
Products include:
Serentil 1057

Methadone Hydrochloride (Effects not specified; caution should be used when used concurrently).
Products include:
Dolophine Hydrochloride Tablets 3056

Methohexital Sodium (Effects not specified; caution should be used when used concurrently). Products include:
Brevital Sodium for Injection, USP .. 1815

Methotrimeprazine (Effects not specified; caution should be used when used concurrently).
No products indexed under this heading.

Methoxyflurane (Effects not specified; caution should be used when used concurrently).
No products indexed under this heading.

Methyclothiazide (Co-administration with antihypertensive agents has resulted in clinically significant hypotension).
No products indexed under this heading.

Methyldopa (Co-administration with antihypertensive agents has resulted in clinically significant hypotension).
Products include:
Aldoclor Tablets 2035
Aldomet Tablets 2037
Aldoril Tablets 2039

Methyldopate Hydrochloride (Co-administration with antihypertensive agents has resulted in clinically significant hypotension).
No products indexed under this heading.

Metolazone (Co-administration with antihypertensive agents has resulted in clinically significant hypotension).
Products include:
Mykrox Tablets 1168
Zaroxolyn Tablets 1177

Metoprolol Succinate (Co-administration with antihypertensive agents has resulted in clinically significant hypotension). Products include:
Toprol-XL Tablets 651

Metoprolol Tartrate (Co-administration with antihypertensive agents has resulted in clinically significant hypotension).
No products indexed under this heading.

Metyrosine (Co-administration with antihypertensive agents has resulted in clinically significant hypotension).
Products include:
Demser Capsules 2085

Mibefradil Dihydrochloride (Co-administration with antihypertensive agents has resulted in clinically significant hypotension).
No products indexed under this heading.

Midazolam Hydrochloride (Effects not specified; caution should be used when used concurrently).
Products include:
Versed Injection 3027
Versed Syrup 3033

Minoxidil (Co-administration with antihypertensive agents has resulted in clinically significant hypotension).
Products include:
Rogaine Extra Strength for Men Topical Solution .... ◘ 721
Rogaine for Women Topical Solution .... ◘ 721

Moexipril Hydrochloride (Co-administration with antihypertensive agents has resulted in clinically significant hypotension). Products include:
Uniretic Tablets 3178
Univasc Tablets 3181

Molindone Hydrochloride (Effects not specified; caution should be used when used concurrently).
Products include:
Moban 1320

Morphine Sulfate (Effects not specified; caution should be used when used concurrently). Products include:
Astramorph/PF Injection, USP (Preservative-Free) 594
Duramorph Injection 1312
Infumorph 200 and Infumorph 500 Sterile Solutions 1314
Kadian Capsules 1335
MS Contin Tablets 2896
MSIR 2898
Oramorph SR Tablets 3062
Roxanol 3066

Nadolol (Co-administration with antihypertensive agents has resulted in clinically significant hypotension).
Products include:
Corgard Tablets 2245
Corzide 40/5 Tablets 2247
Corzide 80/5 Tablets 2247
Nadolol Tablets 2288

Nicardipine Hydrochloride (Co-administration with antihypertensive agents has resulted in clinically significant hypotension). Products include:
Cardene I.V. 3485

Nifedipine (Co-administration with antihypertensive agents has resulted in clinically significant hypotension).
Products include:
Adalat CC Tablets 877
Procardia Capsules 2708
Procardia XL Extended Release Tablets 2710

Nisoldipine (Co-administration with antihypertensive agents has resulted in clinically significant hypotension).
Products include:
Sular Tablets 688

Nitroglycerin (Co-administration with antihypertensive agents has resulted in clinically significant hypotension). Products include:
Nitro-Dur Transdermal Infusion System 3134
Nitro-Dur Transdermal Infusion System 1834
Nitrolingual Pumpspray 1355
Nitrostat Tablets 2658

Olanzapine (Effects not specified; caution should be used when used concurrently). Products include:
Zyprexa Tablets 1973
Zyprexa ZYDIS Orally Disintegrating Tablets 1973

Oxazepam (Effects not specified; caution should be used when used

concurrently).
No products indexed under this heading.

Oxycodone Hydrochloride (Effects not specified; caution should be used when used concurrently). Products include:
- OxyContin Tablets 2912
- OxyFast Oral Concentrate Solution . 2916
- OxyIR Capsules 2916
- Percocet Tablets 1326
- Percodan Tablets 1327
- Percolone Tablets 1327
- Roxicodone 3067
- Tylox Capsules 2597

Penbutolol Sulfate (Co-administration with antihypertensive agents has resulted in clinically significant hypotension).
No products indexed under this heading.

Pentobarbital Sodium (Effects not specified; caution should be used when used concurrently). Products include:
- Nembutal Sodium Solution 485

Pergolide Mesylate (Risperidone may antagonize the effect of dopamine agonists). Products include:
- Permax Tablets 1299

Perindopril Erbumine (Co-administration with antihypertensive agents has resulted in clinically significant hypotension). Products include:
- Aceon Tablets (2 mg, 4 mg, 8 mg) 3249

Perphenazine (Effects not specified; caution should be used when used concurrently). Products include:
- Etrafon 3115
- Trilafon 3160

Phenobarbital (Effects not specified; caution should be used when used concurrently). Products include:
- Arco-Lase Plus Tablets 592
- Donnatal 2929
- Donnatal Extentabs 2930

Phenoxybenzamine Hydrochloride (Co-administration with antihypertensive agents has resulted in clinically significant hypotension). Products include:
- Dibenzyline Capsules 3457

Phentolamine Mesylate (Co-administration with antihypertensive agents has resulted in clinically significant hypotension).
No products indexed under this heading.

Pindolol (Co-administration with antihypertensive agents has resulted in clinically significant hypotension).
No products indexed under this heading.

Polythiazide (Co-administration with antihypertensive agents has resulted in clinically significant hypotension). Products include:
- Minizide Capsules 2700
- Renese Tablets 2712

Pramipexole Dihydrochloride (Risperidone may antagonize the effect of dopamine agonists). Products include:
- Mirapex Tablets 2834

Prazepam (Effects not specified; caution should be used when used concurrently).
No products indexed under this heading.

Prazosin Hydrochloride (Co-administration with antihypertensive agents has resulted in clinically significant hypotension). Products include:
- Minipress Capsules 2699
- Minizide Capsules 2700

Prochlorperazine (Effects not specified; caution should be used when used concurrently). Products include:
- Compazine 1505

Promethazine Hydrochloride (Effects not specified; caution should be used when used concurrently). Products include:
- Meperigan Injection 3539
- Phenergan Injection 3553
- Phenergan 3556
- Phenergan Syrup 3554
- Phenergan with Codeine Syrup 3557
- Phenergan with Dextromethorphan Syrup 3559
- Phenergan VC Syrup 3560
- Phenergan VC with Codeine Syrup .. 3561

Propofol (Effects not specified; caution should be used when used concurrently). Products include:
- Diprivan Injectable Emulsion 667

Propoxyphene Hydrochloride (Effects not specified; caution should be used when used concurrently). Products include:
- Darvon Pulvules 1909
- Darvon Compound-65 Pulvules 1910

Propoxyphene Napsylate (Effects not specified; caution should be used when used concurrently). Products include:
- Darvon-N/Darvocet-N 1907
- Darvon-N Tablets 1912

Propranolol Hydrochloride (Co-administration with antihypertensive agents has resulted in clinically significant hypotension). Products include:
- Inderal 3513
- Inderal LA Long-Acting Capsules 3516
- Inderide Tablets 3517
- Inderide LA Long-Acting Capsules .. 3519

Quazepam (Effects not specified; caution should be used when used concurrently).
No products indexed under this heading.

Quetiapine Fumarate (Effects not specified; caution should be used when used concurrently). Products include:
- Seroquel Tablets 684

Quinapril Hydrochloride (Co-administration with antihypertensive agents has resulted in clinically significant hypotension). Products include:
- Accupril Tablets 2611
- Accuretic Tablets 2614

Quinidine Gluconate (Inhibitors of cytochrome P450IID6 could interfere with the conversion of risperidone to 9-hydroxyrisperidone). Products include:
- Quinaglute Dura-Tabs Tablets 978

Quinidine Polygalacturonate (Inhibitors of cytochrome P450IID6 could interfere with the conversion of risperidone to 9-hydroxyrisperidone).
No products indexed under this heading.

Quinidine Sulfate (Inhibitors of cytochrome P450IID6 could interfere with the conversion of risperidone to 9-hydroxyrisperidone). Products include:
- Quinidex Extentabs 2933

Ramipril (Co-administration with antihypertensive agents has resulted in clinically significant hypotension). Products include:
- Altace Capsules 2233

Rauwolfia serpentina (Co-administration with antihypertensive agents has resulted in clinically significant hypotension).
No products indexed under this heading.

Remifentanil Hydrochloride (Effects not specified; caution should be used when used concurrently).
No products indexed under this heading.

Rescinnamine (Co-administration with antihypertensive agents has resulted in clinically significant hypotension).
No products indexed under this heading.

Reserpine (Co-administration with antihypertensive agents has resulted in clinically significant hypotension).
No products indexed under this heading.

Ropinirole Hydrochloride (Risperidone may antagonize the effect of dopamine agonists). Products include:
- Requip Tablets 1621

Secobarbital Sodium (Effects not specified; caution should be used when used concurrently).
No products indexed under this heading.

Sevoflurane (Effects not specified; caution should be used when used concurrently).
No products indexed under this heading.

Sodium Nitroprusside (Co-administration with antihypertensive agents has resulted in clinically significant hypotension).
No products indexed under this heading.

Sotalol Hydrochloride (Co-administration with antihypertensive agents has resulted in clinically significant hypotension). Products include:
- Betapace Tablets 950
- Betapace AF Tablets 954

Spirapril Hydrochloride (Co-administration with antihypertensive agents has resulted in clinically significant hypotension).
No products indexed under this heading.

Sufentanil Citrate (Effects not specified; caution should be used when used concurrently).
No products indexed under this heading.

Telmisartan (Co-administration with antihypertensive agents has resulted in clinically significant hypotension). Products include:
- Micardis Tablets 1049
- Micardis HCT Tablets 1051

Temazepam (Effects not specified; caution should be used when used concurrently).
No products indexed under this heading.

Terazosin Hydrochloride (Co-administration with antihypertensive agents has resulted in clinically significant hypotension). Products include:
- Hytrin Capsules 464

Thiamylal Sodium (Effects not specified; caution should be used when used concurrently).
No products indexed under this heading.

Thioridazine Hydrochloride (Effects not specified; caution should be used when used concurrently). Products include:
- Thioridazine Hydrochloride Tablets 2289

Thiothixene (Effects not specified; caution should be used when used concurrently). Products include:
- Navane Capsules 2701
- Thiothixene Capsules 2290

Timolol Maleate (Co-administration with antihypertensive agents has resulted in clinically significant hypotension). Products include:
- Blocadren Tablets 2046
- Cosopt Sterile Ophthalmic Solution 2065
- Timolide Tablets 2187
- Timolol GFS .... ⊙ 266
- Timoptic in Ocudose 2192
- Timoptic Sterile Ophthalmic Solution 2190
- Timoptic-XE Sterile Ophthalmic Gel Forming Solution 2194

Torsemide (Co-administration with antihypertensive agents has resulted in clinically significant hypotension). Products include:
- Demadex Tablets and Injection 2965

Trandolapril (Co-administration with antihypertensive agents has resulted in clinically significant hypotension). Products include:
- Mavik Tablets 478
- Tarka Tablets 508

Triazolam (Effects not specified; caution should be used when used concurrently). Products include:
- Halcion Tablets 2823

Trifluoperazine Hydrochloride (Effects not specified; caution should be used when used concurrently). Products include:
- Stelazine 1640

Trimethaphan Camsylate (Co-administration with antihypertensive agents has resulted in clinically significant hypotension).
No products indexed under this heading.

Valsartan (Co-administration with antihypertensive agents has resulted in clinically significant hypotension). Products include:
- Diovan Capsules 2337
- Diovan HCT Tablets 2338

Verapamil Hydrochloride (Co-administration with antihypertensive agents has resulted in clinically significant hypotension). Products include:
- Covera-HS Tablets 3199
- Isoptin SR Tablets 467
- Tarka Tablets 508
- Verelan Capsules 3184
- Verelan PM Capsules 3186

Zaleplon (Effects not specified; caution should be used when used concurrently). Products include:
- Sonata Capsules 3591

Ziprasidone Hydrochloride (Effects not specified; caution should be used when used concurrently). Products include:
- Geodon Capsules 2688

Zolpidem Tartrate (Effects not specified; caution should be used when used concurrently). Products include:
- Ambien Tablets 3191

Food Interactions

Alcohol (Effects not specified; concurrent use should be avoided).

RITALIN HYDROCHLORIDE TABLETS

(Methylphenidate Hydrochloride) 2387

May interact with oral anticoagulants, monoamine oxidase inhibitors, phenytoin, tricyclic antidepressants, vasopressors, and certain other agents. Compounds in these categories include:

Amitriptyline Hydrochloride (Methylphenidate may inhibit the metabolism of tricyclic antidepressants; downward dosage adjustments may be required if used concomitantly). Products include:
- Etrafon 3115
- Limbitrol 1738

Amoxapine (Methylphenidate may inhibit the metabolism of tricyclic antidepressants; downward dosage adjustments may be required if used concomitantly).
No products indexed under this heading.

Clomipramine Hydrochloride (Methylphenidate may inhibit the metabolism of tricyclic antidepressants; downward dosage adjustments may be required if used concomitantly).
No products indexed under this heading.

Clonidine (Co-administration has resulted in serious adverse events). Products include:
- Catapres-TTS 1038

Clonidine Hydrochloride (Co-administration has resulted in serious adverse events). Products include:
- Catapres Tablets ... 1037
- Clorpres Tablets ... 1002
- Combipres Tablets ... 1040
- Duraclon Injection ... 3057

Desipramine Hydrochloride (Methylphenidate may inhibit the metabolism of tricyclic antidepressants; downward dosage adjustments may be required if used concomitantly). Products include:
- Norpramin Tablets ... 755

Dicumarol (Methylphenidate may inhibit the metabolism of coumarin anticoagulants; downward dosage adjustments may be required if used concomitantly).
- No products indexed under this heading.

Dopamine Hydrochloride (Resultant effect of concurrent use with pressor agent is not specified; caution is advised if used concomitantly).
- No products indexed under this heading.

Doxepin Hydrochloride (Methylphenidate may inhibit the metabolism of tricyclic antidepressants; downward dosage adjustments may be required if used concomitantly). Products include:
- Sinequan ... 2713

Epinephrine Bitartrate (Resultant effect of concurrent use with pressor agent is not specified; caution is advised if used concomitantly). Products include:
- Sensorcaine ... 643

Epinephrine Hydrochloride (Resultant effect of concurrent use with pressor agent is not specified; caution is advised if used concomitantly).
- No products indexed under this heading.

Fosphenytoin Sodium (Methylphenidate may inhibit the metabolism of diphenylhydantoin; downward dosage adjustment may be required if used concomitantly). Products include:
- Cerebyx Injection ... 2619

Guanethidine Monosulfate (Methylphenidate may decrease the hypotensive effect of guanethidine).
- No products indexed under this heading.

Imipramine Hydrochloride (Methylphenidate may inhibit the metabolism of tricyclic antidepressants; downward dosage adjustments may be required if used concomitantly).
- No products indexed under this heading.

Imipramine Pamoate (Methylphenidate may inhibit the metabolism of tricyclic antidepressants; downward dosage adjustments may be required if used concomitantly).
- No products indexed under this heading.

Isocarboxazid (Concurrent and/or sequential administration with MAO inhibitors may result in hypertensive crises; concurrent use or within 14 days following discontinuation of a MAO inhibitor is contraindicated).
- No products indexed under this heading.

Maprotiline Hydrochloride (Methylphenidate may inhibit the metabolism of tricyclic antidepressants; downward dosage adjustments may be required if used concomitantly).
- No products indexed under this heading.

Metaraminol Bitartrate (Resultant effect of concurrent use with pressor agent is not specified; caution is advised if used concomitantly). Products include:
- Aramine Injection ... 2043

Methoxamine Hydrochloride (Resultant effect of concurrent use with pressor agent is not specified; caution is advised if used concomitantly).
- No products indexed under this heading.

Moclobemide (Concurrent and/or sequential administration with MAO inhibitors may result in hypertensive crises; concurrent use or within 14 days following discontinuation of a MAO inhibitor is contraindicated).
- No products indexed under this heading.

Norepinephrine Bitartrate (Resultant effect of concurrent use with pressor agent is not specified; caution is advised if used concomitantly).
- No products indexed under this heading.

Nortriptyline Hydrochloride (Methylphenidate may inhibit the metabolism of tricyclic antidepressants; downward dosage adjustments may be required if used concomitantly).
- No products indexed under this heading.

Pargyline Hydrochloride (Concurrent and/or sequential administration with MAO inhibitors may result in hypertensive crises; concurrent use or within 14 days following discontinuation of a MAO inhibitor is contraindicated).
- No products indexed under this heading.

Phenelzine Sulfate (Concurrent and/or sequential administration with MAO inhibitors may result in hypertensive crises; concurrent use or within 14 days following discontinuation of a MAO inhibitor is contraindicated). Products include:
- Nardil Tablets ... 2653

Phenobarbital (Methylphenidate may inhibit the metabolism of phenobarbitol; downward dosage adjustments may be required if used concomitantly). Products include:
- Arco-Lase Plus Tablets ... 592
- Donnatal ... 2929
- Donnatal Extentabs ... 2930

Phenylbutazone (Methylphenidate may inhibit the metabolism of phenylbutazone; downward dosage adjustments may be required if used concomitantly).
- No products indexed under this heading.

Phenylephrine Hydrochloride (Resultant effect of concurrent use with pressor agent is not specified, caution is advised if used concomitantly). Products include:
- Afrin Nasal Decongestant Children's Pump Mist ... ▣734
- Extendryl ... 1361
- Hycomine Compound Tablets ... 1317
- Neo-Synephrine ... ▣614
- Phenergan VC Syrup ... 3560
- Phenergan VC with Codeine Syrup ... 3561
- Preparation H Cream ... ▣778
- Preparation H Cooling Gel ... ▣778
- Preparation H ... ▣778
- Vicks Sinex Nasal Spray and Ultra Fine Mist ... ▣729

Phenytoin (Methylphenidate may inhibit the metabolism of diphenylhydantoin; downward dosage adjustment may be required if used concomitantly). Products include:
- Dilantin Infatabs ... 2624
- Dilantin-125 Oral Suspension ... 2625

Phenytoin Sodium (Methylphenidate may inhibit the metabolism of diphenylhydantoin; downward dosage adjustment may be required if used concomitantly). Products include:
- Dilantin Kapseals ... 2622

Primidone (Methylphenidate may inhibit the metabolism of primidone; downward dosage adjustments may be required if used concomitantly).
- No products indexed under this heading.

Procarbazine Hydrochloride (Concurrent and/or sequential administration with MAO inhibitors may result in hypertensive crises; concurrent use or within 14 days following discontinuation of a MAO inhibitor is contraindicated). Products include:
- Matulane Capsules ... 3246

Protriptyline Hydrochloride (Methylphenidate may inhibit the metabolism of tricyclic antidepressants; downward dosage adjustments may be required if used concomitantly). Products include:
- Vivactil Tablets ... 2446
- Vivactil Tablets ... 2217

Selegiline Hydrochloride (Concurrent and/or sequential administration with MAO inhibitors may result in hypertensive crises; concurrent use or within 14 days following discontinuation of a MAO inhibitor is contraindicated). Products include:
- Eldepryl Capsules ... 3266

Tranylcypromine Sulfate (Concurrent and/or sequential administration with MAO inhibitors may result in hypertensive crises; concurrent use or within 14 days following discontinuation of a MAO inhibitor is contraindicated). Products include:
- Parnate Tablets ... 1607

Trimipramine Maleate (Methylphenidate may inhibit the metabolism of tricyclic antidepressants; downward dosage adjustments may be required if used concomitantly). Products include:
- Surmontil Capsules ... 3595

Venlafaxine Hydrochloride (Co-administration of venlafaxine in a patient stabilized on methylphenidate has resulted in neuroleptic malignant syndrome; it is uncertain whether this case represents a drug-drug interaction, a response to either drug alone, or some other cause). Products include:
- Effexor Tablets ... 3495
- Effexor XR Capsules ... 3499

Warfarin Sodium (Methylphenidate may inhibit the metabolism of coumarin anticoagulants; downward dosage adjustments may be required if used concomitantly). Products include:
- Coumadin for Injection ... 1243
- Coumadin Tablets ... 1243
- Warfarin Sodium Tablets, USP ... 3302

RITALIN-SR TABLETS

(Methylphenidate Hydrochloride) ... 2387
See Ritalin Hydrochloride Tablets

RITUXAN FOR INFUSION

(Rituximab) ... 1750
None cited in PDR database.

RITUXAN I.V.

(Rituximab) ... 1428
None cited in PDR database.

ROBAXIN INJECTABLE

(Methocarbamol) ... 2938
May interact with anticholinesterase drugs, central nervous system depressants, and certain other agents. Compounds in these categories include:

Alfentanil Hydrochloride (Increased CNS depressant effect).
- No products indexed under this heading.

Alprazolam (Increased CNS depressant effect). Products include:
- Xanax Tablets ... 2865

Aprobarbital (Increased CNS depressant effect).
- No products indexed under this heading.

Buprenorphine Hydrochloride (Increased CNS depressant effect). Products include:
- Buprenex Injectable ... 2918

Buspirone Hydrochloride (Increased CNS depressant effect).
- No products indexed under this heading.

Butabarbital (Increased CNS depressant effect).
- No products indexed under this heading.

Butalbital (Increased CNS depressant effect). Products include:
- Phrenilin ... 578
- Sedapap Tablets 50 mg/650 mg ... 2225

Chlordiazepoxide (Increased CNS depressant effect). Products include:
- Limbitrol ... 1738

Chlordiazepoxide Hydrochloride (Increased CNS depressant effect). Products include:
- Librium Capsules ... 1736
- Librium for Injection ... 1737

Chlorpromazine (Increased CNS depressant effect). Products include:
- Thorazine Suppositories ... 1656

Chlorpromazine Hydrochloride (Increased CNS depressant effect). Products include:
- Thorazine ... 1656

Chlorprothixene (Increased CNS depressant effect).
- No products indexed under this heading.

Chlorprothixene Hydrochloride (Increased CNS depressant effect).
- No products indexed under this heading.

Chlorprothixene Lactate (Increased CNS depressant effect).
- No products indexed under this heading.

Clorazepate Dipotassium (Increased CNS depressant effect). Products include:
- Tranxene ... 511

Clozapine (Increased CNS depressant effect). Products include:
- Clozaril Tablets ... 2319

Codeine Phosphate (Increased CNS depressant effect). Products include:
- Phenergan with Codeine Syrup ... 3557
- Phenergan VC with Codeine Syrup ... 3561
- Robitussin A-C Syrup ... 2942
- Robitussin-DAC Syrup ... 2942
- Ryna-C Liquid ... ▣768
- Soma Compound w/Codeine Tablets ... 3355
- Tussi-Organidin NR Liquid ... 3350
- Tussi-Organidin-S NR Liquid ... 3350
- Tylenol with Codeine ... 2595

Desflurane (Increased CNS depressant effect). Products include:
- Suprane Liquid for Inhalation ... 874

Dezocine (Increased CNS depressant effect).
- No products indexed under this heading.

Diazepam (Increased CNS depressant effect). Products include:
- Valium Injectable ... 3026
- Valium Tablets ... 3047

Donepezil Hydrochloride (Methocarbamol may inhibit the effect of anticholinesterase agents, such as pyridostigmine; caution is advised in patients with myasthenia gravis receiving anticholinesterase agents). Products include:
- Aricept Tablets ... 1270
- Aricept Tablets ... 2665

Droperidol (Increased CNS depressant effect).
- No products indexed under this heading.

Enflurane (Increased CNS depressant effect).
No products indexed under this heading.

Estazolam (Increased CNS depressant effect). Products include:
ProSom Tablets 500

Ethchlorvynol (Increased CNS depressant effect).
No products indexed under this heading.

Ethinamate (Increased CNS depressant effect).
No products indexed under this heading.

Fentanyl (Increased CNS depressant effect). Products include:
Duragesic Transdermal System 1786

Fentanyl Citrate (Increased CNS depressant effect). Products include:
Actiq 1184

Fluphenazine Decanoate (Increased CNS depressant effect).
No products indexed under this heading.

Fluphenazine Enanthate (Increased CNS depressant effect).
No products indexed under this heading.

Fluphenazine Hydrochloride (Increased CNS depressant effect).
No products indexed under this heading.

Flurazepam Hydrochloride (Increased CNS depressant effect).
No products indexed under this heading.

Galantamine Hydrobromide (Methocarbamol may inhibit the effect of anticholinesterase agents, such as pyridostigmine; caution is advised in patients with myasthenia gravis receiving anticholinesterase agents). Products include:
Reminyl Oral Solution 1792
Reminyl Tablets 1792

Glutethimide (Increased CNS depressant effect).
No products indexed under this heading.

Haloperidol (Increased CNS depressant effect). Products include:
Haldol Injection, Tablets and Concentrate 2533

Haloperidol Decanoate (Increased CNS depressant effect). Products include:
Haldol Decanoate 2535

Hydrocodone Bitartrate (Increased CNS depressant effect). Products include:
Hycodan 1316
Hycomine Compound Tablets 1317
Hycotuss Expectorant Syrup 1318
Lortab 3319
Lortab Elixir 3317
Maxidone Tablets CIII 3399
Norco 5/325 Tablets CIII 3424
Norco 7.5/325 Tablets CIII 3425
Norco 10/325 Tablets CIII 3427
Norco 10/325 Tablets CIII 3425
Vicodin Tablets 516
Vicodin ES Tablets 517
Vicodin HP Tablets 518
Vicodin Tuss Expectorant 519
Vicoprofen Tablets 520
Zydone Tablets 1330

Hydrocodone Polistirex (Increased CNS depressant effect). Products include:
Tussionex Pennkinetic Extended-Release Suspension..... 1174

Hydromorphone Hydrochloride (Increased CNS depressant effect). Products include:
Dilaudid 441
Dilaudid Oral Liquid 445
Dilaudid Powder 441
Dilaudid Rectal Suppositories 441
Dilaudid Tablets 441
Dilaudid Tablets - 8 mg 445
Dilaudid-HP 443

Hydroxyzine Hydrochloride (Increased CNS depressant effect). Products include:
Atarax Tablets & Syrup 2667
Vistaril Intramuscular Solution 2738

Isoflurane (Increased CNS depressant effect).
No products indexed under this heading.

Ketamine Hydrochloride (Increased CNS depressant effect).
No products indexed under this heading.

Levomethadyl Acetate Hydrochloride (Increased CNS depressant effect).
No products indexed under this heading.

Levorphanol Tartrate (Increased CNS depressant effect). Products include:
Levo-Dromoran 1734
Levorphanol Tartrate Tablets 3059

Lorazepam (Increased CNS depressant effect). Products include:
Ativan Injection 3478
Ativan Tablets 3482

Loxapine Hydrochloride (Increased CNS depressant effect).
No products indexed under this heading.

Loxapine Succinate (Increased CNS depressant effect). Products include:
Loxitane Capsules 3398

Meperidine Hydrochloride (Increased CNS depressant effect). Products include:
Demerol 3079
Mepergan Injection 3539

Mephobarbital (Increased CNS depressant effect).
No products indexed under this heading.

Meprobamate (Increased CNS depressant effect). Products include:
Miltown Tablets 3349

Mesoridazine Besylate (Increased CNS depressant effect). Products include:
Serentil 1057

Methadone Hydrochloride (Increased CNS depressant effect). Products include:
Dolophine Hydrochloride Tablets 3056

Methohexital Sodium (Increased CNS depressant effect). Products include:
Brevital Sodium for Injection, USP .. 1815

Methotrimeprazine (Increased CNS depressant effect).
No products indexed under this heading.

Methoxyflurane (Increased CNS depressant effect).
No products indexed under this heading.

Midazolam Hydrochloride (Increased CNS depressant effect). Products include:
Versed Injection 3027
Versed Syrup 3033

Molindone Hydrochloride (Increased CNS depressant effect). Products include:
Moban 1320

Morphine Sulfate (Increased CNS depressant effect). Products include:
Astramorph/PF Injection, USP (Preservative-Free) 594
Duramorph Injection 1312
Infumorph 200 and Infumorph 500 Sterile Solutions 1314
Kadian Capsules 1335
MS Contin Tablets 2896
MSIR 2898
Oramorph SR Tablets 3062
Roxanol 3066

Neostigmine Bromide (Methocarbamol may inhibit the effect of anticholinesterase agents, such as pyridostigmine; caution is advised in patients with myasthenia gravis receiving anticholinesterase agents). Products include:
Prostigmin Tablets 1744

Neostigmine Methylsulfate (Methocarbamol may inhibit the effect of anticholinesterase agents, such as pyridostigmine; caution is advised in patients with myasthenia gravis receiving anticholinesterase agents). Products include:
Prostigmin Injectable 1744

Olanzapine (Increased CNS depressant effect). Products include:
Zyprexa Tablets 1973
Zyprexa ZYDIS Orally Disintegrating Tablets........ 1973

Oxazepam (Increased CNS depressant effect).
No products indexed under this heading.

Oxycodone Hydrochloride (Increased CNS depressant effect). Products include:
OxyContin Tablets 2912
OxyFast Oral Concentrate Solution . 2916
OxyIR Capsules 2916
Percocet Tablets 1326
Percodan Tablets 1327
Percolone Tablets 1327
Roxicodone 3067
Tylox Capsules 2597

Pentobarbital Sodium (Increased additive effect). Products include:
Nembutal Sodium Solution 485

Perphenazine (Increased CNS depressant effect). Products include:
Etrafon 3115
Trilafon 3160

Phenobarbital (Increased CNS depressant effect). Products include:
Arco-Lase Plus Tablets 592
Donnatal 2929
Donnatal Extentabs 2930

Prazepam (Increased CNS depressant effect).
No products indexed under this heading.

Prochlorperazine (Increased CNS depressant effect). Products include:
Compazine 1505

Promethazine Hydrochloride (Increased CNS depressant effect). Products include:
Mepergan Injection 3539
Phenergan Injection 3553
Phenergan 3556
Phenergan Syrup 3554
Phenergan with Codeine Syrup 3557
Phenergan with Dextromethorphan Syrup 3559
Phenergan VC Syrup 3560
Phenergan VC with Codeine Syrup .. 3561

Propofol (Increased CNS depressant effect). Products include:
Diprivan Injectable Emulsion 667

Propoxyphene Hydrochloride (Increased CNS depressant effect). Products include:
Darvon Pulvules 1909
Darvon Compound-65 Pulvules 1910

Propoxyphene Napsylate (Increased CNS depressant effect). Products include:
Darvon-N/Darvocet-N 1907
Darvon-N Tablets 1912

Pyridostigmine Bromide (Methocarbamol may inhibit the effect of anticholinesterase agents, such as pyridostigmine; caution is advised in patients with myasthenia gravis receiving anticholinesterase agents). Products include:
Mestinon 1740

Quazepam (Increased CNS depressant effect).
No products indexed under this heading.

Quetiapine Fumarate (Increased CNS depressant effect). Products include:
Seroquel Tablets 684

Remifentanil Hydrochloride (Increased CNS depressant effect).
No products indexed under this heading.

Risperidone (Increased CNS depressant effect). Products include:
Risperdal 1796

Rivastigmine Tartrate (Methocarbamol may inhibit the effect of anticholinesterase agents, such as pyridostigmine; caution is advised in patients with myasthenia gravis receiving anticholinesterase agents). Products include:
Exelon Capsules 2342
Exelon Oral Solution 2345

Secobarbital Sodium (Increased CNS depressant effect).
No products indexed under this heading.

Sevoflurane (Increased CNS depressant effect).
No products indexed under this heading.

Sufentanil Citrate (Increased CNS depressant effect).
No products indexed under this heading.

Tacrine Hydrochloride (Methocarbamol may inhibit the effect of anticholinesterase agents, such as pyridostigmine; caution is advised in patients with myasthenia gravis receiving anticholinesterase agents). Products include:
Cognex Capsules 1351

Temazepam (Increased CNS depressant effect).
No products indexed under this heading.

Thiamylal Sodium (Increased CNS depressant effect).
No products indexed under this heading.

Thioridazine Hydrochloride (Increased CNS depressant effect). Products include:
Thioridazine Hydrochloride Tablets 2289

Thiothixene (Increased CNS depressant effect). Products include:
Navane Capsules 2701
Thiothixene Capsules 2290

Triazolam (Increased CNS depressant effect). Products include:
Halcion Tablets 2823

Trifluoperazine Hydrochloride (Increased CNS depressant effect). Products include:
Stelazine 1640

Zaleplon (Increased CNS depressant effect). Products include:
Sonata Capsules 3591

Ziprasidone Hydrochloride (Increased CNS depressant effect). Products include:
Geodon Capsules 2688

Zolpidem Tartrate (Increased CNS depressant effect). Products include:
Ambien Tablets 3191

Food Interactions

Alcohol (Increased depressant effect).

ROBAXIN TABLETS

(Methocarbamol) 2939
See Robaxin Injectable

ROBAXIN-750 TABLETS

(Methocarbamol) 2939
See Robaxin Injectable

ROBAXISAL TABLETS

(Aspirin, Methocarbamol) 2939
May interact with central nervous system depressants, corticosteroids, oral anticoagulants, oral hypoglycemic agents, insulin, non-steroidal anti-inflammatory agents, and certain other agents. Compounds in these categories include:

Acarbose (Aspirin may enhance the effects of oral hypoglycemic agents causing hypoglycemia). Products include:
Precose Tablets 906

Alfentanil Hydrochloride (Increased general CNS depressant effects with concurrent use).
No products indexed under this heading.

IMPORTANT NOTE: Always consult each drug listing in the patient's regimen for possible interactions.

Alprazolam (Increased general CNS depressant effects with concurrent use). Products include:
Xanax Tablets 2865

Aprobarbital (Increased general CNS depressant effects with concurrent use).
No products indexed under this heading.

Betamethasone Acetate (Corticosteroids enhance renal clearance of salicylates; withdrawal of corticosteroids in patients on chronic aspirin therapy may result in salicylism when renal clearance returns to normal). Products include:
Celestone Soluspan Injectable Suspension 3097

Betamethasone Sodium Phosphate (Corticosteroids enhance renal clearance of salicylates; withdrawal of corticosteroids in patients on chronic aspirin therapy may result in salicylism when renal clearance returns to normal). Products include:
Celestone Soluspan Injectable Suspension 3097

Buprenorphine Hydrochloride (Increased general CNS depressant effects with concurrent use). Products include:
Buprenex Injectable 2918

Buspirone Hydrochloride (Increased general CNS depressant effects with concurrent use).
No products indexed under this heading.

Butabarbital (Increased general CNS depressant effects with concurrent use).
No products indexed under this heading.

Butalbital (Increased general CNS depressant effects with concurrent use). Products include:
Phrenilin 578
Sedapap Tablets 50 mg/650 mg 2225

Celecoxib (Co-administration increases the risk of peptic ulceration and bleeding). Products include:
Celebrex Capsules 2676
Celebrex Capsules 2780

Chlordiazepoxide (Increased general CNS depressant effects with concurrent use). Products include:
Limbitrol 1738

Chlordiazepoxide Hydrochloride (Increased general CNS depressant effects with concurrent use). Products include:
Librium Capsules 1736
Librium for Injection 1737

Chlorpromazine (Increased general CNS depressant effects with concurrent use). Products include:
Thorazine Suppositories 1656

Chlorpromazine Hydrochloride (Increased general CNS depressant effects with concurrent use). Products include:
Thorazine 1656

Chlorpropamide (Aspirin may enhance the effects of oral hypoglycemic agents causing hypoglycemia). Products include:
Diabinese Tablets 2680

Chlorprothixene (Increased general CNS depressant effects with concurrent use).
No products indexed under this heading.

Chlorprothixene Hydrochloride (Increased general CNS depressant effects with concurrent use).
No products indexed under this heading.

Chlorprothixene Lactate (Increased general CNS depressant effects with concurrent use).
No products indexed under this heading.

Clorazepate Dipotassium (Increased general CNS depressant effects with concurrent use). Products include:
Tranxene 511

Clozapine (Increased general CNS depressant effects with concurrent use). Products include:
Clozaril Tablets 2319

Codeine Phosphate (Increased general CNS depressant effects with concurrent use). Products include:
Phenergan with Codeine Syrup 3557
Phenergan VC with Codeine Syrup 3561
Robitussin A-C Syrup 2942
Robitussin-DAC Syrup 2942
Ryna-C Liquid ■768
Soma Compound w/Codeine Tablets 3355
Tussi-Organidin NR Liquid 3350
Tussi-Organidin-S NR Liquid 3350
Tylenol with Codeine 2595

Cortisone Acetate (Corticosteroids enhance renal clearance of salicylates; withdrawal of corticosteroids in patients on chronic aspirin therapy may result in salicylism when renal clearance returns to normal). Products include:
Cortone Acetate Injectable Suspension 2059
Cortone Acetate Tablets 2061

Desflurane (Increased general CNS depressant effects with concurrent use). Products include:
Suprane Liquid for Inhalation 874

Dexamethasone (Corticosteroids enhance renal clearance of salicylates; withdrawal of corticosteroids in patients on chronic aspirin therapy may result in salicylism when renal clearance returns to normal). Products include:
Decadron Elixir 2078
Decadron Tablets 2079
TobraDex Ophthalmic Ointment 542
TobraDex Ophthalmic Suspension 541

Dexamethasone Acetate (Corticosteroids enhance renal clearance of salicylates; withdrawal of corticosteroids in patients on chronic aspirin therapy may result in salicylism when renal clearance returns to normal).
No products indexed under this heading.

Dexamethasone Sodium Phosphate (Corticosteroids enhance renal clearance of salicylates; withdrawal of corticosteroids in patients on chronic aspirin therapy may result in salicylism when renal clearance returns to normal). Products include:
Decadron Phosphate Injection 2081
Decadron Phosphate Sterile Ophthalmic Ointment 2083
Decadron Phosphate Sterile Ophthalmic Solution 2084
NeoDecadron Sterile Ophthalmic Solution 2144

Dezocine (Increased general CNS depressant effects with concurrent use).
No products indexed under this heading.

Diazepam (Increased general CNS depressant effects with concurrent use). Products include:
Valium Injectable 3026
Valium Tablets 3047

Diclofenac Potassium (Co-administration increases the risk of peptic ulceration and bleeding). Products include:
Cataflam Tablets 2315

Diclofenac Sodium (Co-administration increases the risk of peptic ulceration and bleeding). Products include:
Arthrotec Tablets 3195
Voltaren Ophthalmic Sterile Ophthalmic Solution ⊙312
Voltaren Tablets 2315
Voltaren-XR Tablets 2315

Dicumarol (Aspirin may enhance the effects of oral anticoagulants resulting in bleeding).
No products indexed under this heading.

Droperidol (Increased general CNS depressant effects with concurrent use).
No products indexed under this heading.

Enflurane (Increased general CNS depressant effects with concurrent use).
No products indexed under this heading.

Estazolam (Increased general CNS depressant effects with concurrent use). Products include:
ProSom Tablets 500

Ethchlorvynol (Increased general CNS depressant effects with concurrent use).
No products indexed under this heading.

Ethinamate (Increased general CNS depressant effects with concurrent use).
No products indexed under this heading.

Etodolac (Co-administration increases the risk of peptic ulceration and bleeding). Products include:
Lodine 3528
Lodine XL Extended-Release Tablets 3530

Fenoprofen Calcium (Co-administration increases the risk of peptic ulceration and bleeding).
No products indexed under this heading.

Fentanyl (Increased general CNS depressant effects with concurrent use). Products include:
Duragesic Transdermal System 1786

Fentanyl Citrate (Increased general CNS depressant effects with concurrent use). Products include:
Actiq 1184

Fludrocortisone Acetate (Corticosteroids enhance renal clearance of salicylates; withdrawal of corticosteroids in patients on chronic aspirin therapy may result in salicylism when renal clearance returns to normal). Products include:
Florinef Acetate Tablets 2250

Fluphenazine Decanoate (Increased general CNS depressant effects with concurrent use).
No products indexed under this heading.

Fluphenazine Enanthate (Increased general CNS depressant effects with concurrent use).
No products indexed under this heading.

Fluphenazine Hydrochloride (Increased general CNS depressant effects with concurrent use).
No products indexed under this heading.

Flurazepam Hydrochloride (Increased general CNS depressant effects with concurrent use).
No products indexed under this heading.

Flurbiprofen (Co-administration increases the risk of peptic ulceration and bleeding).
No products indexed under this heading.

Glimepiride (Aspirin may enhance the effects of oral hypoglycemic agents causing hypoglycemia). Products include:
Amaryl Tablets 717

Glipizide (Aspirin may enhance the effects of oral hypoglycemic agents causing hypoglycemia). Products include:
Glucotrol Tablets 2692
Glucotrol XL Extended Release Tablets 2693

Glutethimide (Increased general CNS depressant effects with concurrent use).
No products indexed under this heading.

Glyburide (Aspirin may enhance the effects of oral hypoglycemic agents causing hypoglycemia). Products include:
DiaBeta Tablets 741
Glucovance Tablets 1086

Haloperidol (Increased general CNS depressant effects with concurrent use). Products include:
Haldol Injection, Tablets and Concentrate 2533

Haloperidol Decanoate (Increased general CNS depressant effects with concurrent use). Products include:
Haldol Decanoate 2535

Hydrocodone Bitartrate (Increased general CNS depressant effects with concurrent use). Products include:
Hycodan 1316
Hycomine Compound Tablets 1317
Hycotuss Expectorant Syrup 1318
Lortab 3319
Lortab Elixir 3317
Maxidone Tablets CIII 3399
Norco 5/325 Tablets CIII 3424
Norco 7.5/325 Tablets CIII 3425
Norco 10/325 Tablets CIII 3427
Norco 10/325 Tablets CIII 3425
Vicodin Tablets 516
Vicodin ES Tablets 517
Vicodin HP Tablets 518
Vicodin Tuss Expectorant 519
Vicoprofen Tablets 520
Zydone Tablets 1330

Hydrocodone Polistirex (Increased general CNS depressant effects with concurrent use). Products include:
Tussionex Pennkinetic Extended-Release Suspension 1174

Hydrocortisone (Corticosteroids enhance renal clearance of salicylates; withdrawal of corticosteroids in patients on chronic aspirin therapy may result in salicylism when renal clearance returns to normal). Products include:
Anusol-HC Cream 2.5% 2237
Cipro HC Otic Suspension 540
Cortaid Intensive Therapy Cream ■717
Cortaid Maximum Strength Cream ■717
Cortisporin Ophthalmic Suspension Sterile ⊙297
Cortizone•5 ■699
Cortizone•10 ■699
Cortizone•10 Plus Creme ■700
Cortizone for Kids Creme ■699
Hydrocortone Tablets 2106
Massengill Medicated Soft Cloth Towelette ■753
VōSoL HC Otic Solution 3356

Hydrocortisone Acetate (Corticosteroids enhance renal clearance of salicylates; withdrawal of corticosteroids in patients on chronic aspirin therapy may result in salicylism when renal clearance returns to normal). Products include:
Analpram-HC 1338
Anusol HC-1 Hydrocortisone Anti-Itch Cream ■689
Anusol-HC Suppositories 2238
Cortaid ■717
Cortifoam Rectal Foam 3170
Cortisporin-TC Otic Suspension 2246
Hydrocortone Acetate Injectable Suspension 2103
Pramosone 1343
Proctocort Suppositories 2264
ProctoFoam-HC 3177
Terra-Cortril Ophthalmic Suspension 2716

Hydrocortisone Sodium Phosphate (Corticosteroids enhance renal clearance of salicylates; withdrawal of corticosteroids in patients on chronic aspirin therapy may result in salicylism when renal clearance returns to normal). Products include:
Hydrocortone Phosphate Injection, Sterile 2105

Hydrocortisone Sodium Succinate (Corticosteroids enhance renal

clearance of salicylates; withdrawal of corticosteroids in patients on chronic aspirin therapy may result in salicylism when renal clearance returns to normal).
No products indexed under this heading.

Hydromorphone Hydrochloride (Increased general CNS depressant effects with concurrent use). Products include:
Dilaudid ... 441
Dilaudid Oral Liquid ... 445
Dilaudid Powder ... 441
Dilaudid Rectal Suppositories ... 441
Dilaudid Tablets ... 441
Dilaudid Tablets - 8 mg ... 445
Dilaudid-HP ... 443

Hydroxyzine Hydrochloride (Increased general CNS depressant effects with concurrent use). Products include:
Atarax Tablets & Syrup ... 2667
Vistaril Intramuscular Solution ... 2738

Ibuprofen (Co-administration increases the risk of peptic ulceration and bleeding). Products include:
Advil ... 771
Children's Advil Oral Suspension ... 773
Children's Advil Chewable Tablets ... 773
Advil Cold and Sinus Caplets ... 771
Advil Cold and Sinus Tablets ... 771
Advil Flu & Body Ache Caplets ... 772
Infants' Advil Drops ... 773
Junior Strength Advil Tablets ... 773
Junior Strength Advil Chewable Tablets ... 773
Advil Migraine Liquigels ... 772
Children's Motrin Oral Suspension and Chewable Tablets ... 2006
Children's Motrin Cold Oral Suspension ... 2007
Children's Motrin Oral Suspension ... 643
Motrin Suspension, Oral Drops, Chewable Tablets, and Caplets ... 2002
Infants' Motrin Concentrated Drops ... 2006
Junior Strength Motrin Caplets and Chewable Tablets ... 2006
Motrin IB Tablets, Caplets, and Gelcaps ... 2002
Motrin Migraine Pain Caplets ... 2005
Motrin Sinus Headache Caplets ... 2005
Vicoprofen Tablets ... 520

Indomethacin (Co-administration increases the risk of peptic ulceration and bleeding). Products include:
Indocin ... 2112

Indomethacin Sodium Trihydrate (Co-administration increases the risk of peptic ulceration and bleeding). Products include:
Indocin I.V. ... 2115

Insulin, Human, Zinc Suspension (Aspirin may enhance the effects of insulin causing hypoglycemia). Products include:
Humulin L, 100 Units ... 1937
Humulin U, 100 Units ... 1943
Novolin L Human Insulin 10 ml Vials ... 2422

Insulin, Human NPH (Aspirin may enhance the effects of insulin causing hypoglycemia). Products include:
Humulin N, 100 Units ... 1939
Humulin N NPH Pen ... 1940
Novolin N Human Insulin 10 ml Vials ... 2422
Novolin N PenFill ... 2423
Novolin N Prefilled Syringe Disposable Insulin Delivery System ... 2425

Insulin, Human Regular (Aspirin may enhance the effects of insulin causing hypoglycemia). Products include:
Humulin R Regular (U-500) ... 1943
Humulin R, 100 Units ... 1941
Novolin R Human Insulin 10 ml Vials ... 2423
Novolin R PenFill ... 2423
Novolin R Prefilled Syringe Disposable Insulin Delivery System ... 2425
Velosulin BR Human Insulin 10 ml Vials ... 2435

Insulin, Human Regular and Human NPH Mixture (Aspirin may enhance the effects of insulin causing hypoglycemia). Products include:
Humulin 50/50, 100 Units ... 1934
Humulin 70/30, 100 Units ... 1935
Humulin 70/30 Pen ... 1936
Novolin 70/30 Human Insulin 10 ml Vials ... 2421
Novolin 70/30 PenFill ... 2423
Novolin 70/30 Prefilled Disposable Insulin Delivery System ... 2425

Insulin, NPH (Aspirin may enhance the effects of insulin causing hypoglycemia). Products include:
Iletin II, NPH (Pork), 100 Units ... 1946

Insulin, Regular (Aspirin may enhance the effects of insulin causing hypoglycemia). Products include:
Iletin II, Regular (Pork), 100 Units ... 1947

Insulin, Zinc Crystals (Aspirin may enhance the effects of insulin causing hypoglycemia).
No products indexed under this heading.

Insulin, Zinc Suspension (Aspirin may enhance the effects of insulin causing hypoglycemia). Products include:
Iletin II, Lente (Pork), 100 Units ... 1945

Insulin Aspart, Human Regular (Aspirin may enhance the effects of insulin causing hypoglycemia).
No products indexed under this heading.

Insulin glargine (Aspirin may enhance the effects of insulin causing hypoglycemia). Products include:
Lantus Injection ... 742

Insulin Lispro, Human (Aspirin may enhance the effects of insulin causing hypoglycemia). Products include:
Humalog ... 1926
Humalog Mix 75/25 Pen ... 1928

Insulin Lispro Protamine, Human (Aspirin may enhance the effects of insulin causing hypoglycemia). Products include:
Humalog Mix 75/25 Pen ... 1928

Isoflurane (Increased general CNS depressant effects with concurrent use).
No products indexed under this heading.

Ketamine Hydrochloride (Increased general CNS depressant effects with concurrent use).
No products indexed under this heading.

Ketoprofen (Co-administration increases the risk of peptic ulceration and bleeding). Products include:
Orudis Capsules ... 3548
Orudis KT Tablets ... 778
Oruvail Capsules ... 3548

Ketorolac Tromethamine (Co-administration increases the risk of peptic ulceration and bleeding). Products include:
Acular Ophthalmic Solution ... 544
Acular PF Ophthalmic Solution ... 544
Toradol ... 3018

Levomethadyl Acetate Hydrochloride (Increased general CNS depressant effects with concurrent use).
No products indexed under this heading.

Levorphanol Tartrate (Increased general CNS depressant effects with concurrent use). Products include:
Levo-Dromoran ... 1734
Levorphanol Tartrate Tablets ... 3059

Lorazepam (Increased general CNS depressant effects with concurrent use). Products include:
Ativan Injection ... 3478
Ativan Tablets ... 3482

Loxapine Hydrochloride (Increased general CNS depressant effects with concurrent use).
No products indexed under this heading.

Loxapine Succinate (Increased general CNS depressant effects with concurrent use). Products include:
Loxitane Capsules ... 3398

Meclofenamate Sodium (Co-administration increases the risk of peptic ulceration and bleeding).
No products indexed under this heading.

Mefenamic Acid (Co-administration increases the risk of peptic ulceration and bleeding). Products include:
Ponstel Capsules ... 1356

Meloxicam (Co-administration increases the risk of peptic ulceration and bleeding). Products include:
Mobic Tablets ... 1054

Meperidine Hydrochloride (Increased general CNS depressant effects with concurrent use). Products include:
Demerol ... 3079
Mepergan Injection ... 3539

Mephobarbital (Increased general CNS depressant effects with concurrent use).
No products indexed under this heading.

Meprobamate (Increased general CNS depressant effects with concurrent use). Products include:
Miltown Tablets ... 3349

Mercaptopurine (Aspirin may enhance the effects of mercaptopurine resulting in bone marrow toxicity and blood dyscrasias by displacing it from binding sites). Products include:
Purinethol Tablets ... 1615

Mesoridazine Besylate (Increased general CNS depressant effects with concurrent use). Products include:
Serentil ... 1057

Metformin Hydrochloride (Aspirin may enhance the effects of oral hypoglycemic agents causing hypoglycemia). Products include:
Glucophage Tablets ... 1080
Glucophage XR Tablets ... 1080
Glucovance Tablets ... 1086

Methadone Hydrochloride (Increased general CNS depressant effects with concurrent use). Products include:
Dolophine Hydrochloride Tablets ... 3056

Methohexital Sodium (Increased general CNS depressant effects with concurrent use). Products include:
Brevital Sodium for Injection, USP ... 1815

Methotrexate Sodium (Aspirin may enhance the effects of methotrexate resulting in bone marrow toxicity and blood dyscrasias by displacing its binding sites and reducing its excretion).
No products indexed under this heading.

Methotrimeprazine (Increased general CNS depressant effects with concurrent use).
No products indexed under this heading.

Methoxyflurane (Increased general CNS depressant effects with concurrent use).
No products indexed under this heading.

Methylprednisolone Acetate (Corticosteroids enhance renal clearance of salicylates; withdrawal of corticosteroids in patients on chronic aspirin therapy may result in salicylism when renal clearance returns to normal). Products include:
Depo-Medrol Injectable Suspension ... 2795

Methylprednisolone Sodium Succinate (Corticosteroids enhance renal clearance of salicylates; withdrawal of corticosteroids in patients on chronic aspirin therapy may result in salicylism when renal clearance returns to normal). Products include:
Solu-Medrol Sterile Powder ... 2855

Midazolam Hydrochloride (Increased general CNS depressant effects with concurrent use). Products include:
Versed Injection ... 3027
Versed Syrup ... 3033

Miglitol (Aspirin may enhance the effects of oral hypoglycemic agents causing hypoglycemia). Products include:
Glyset Tablets ... 2821

Molindone Hydrochloride (Increased general CNS depressant effects with concurrent use). Products include:
Moban ... 1320

Morphine Sulfate (Increased general CNS depressant effects with concurrent use). Products include:
Astramorph/PF Injection, USP (Preservative-Free) ... 594
Duramorph Injection ... 1312
Infumorph 200 and Infumorph 500 Sterile Solutions ... 1314
Kadian Capsules ... 1335
MS Contin Tablets ... 2896
MSIR ... 2898
Oramorph SR Tablets ... 3062
Roxanol ... 3066

Nabumetone (Co-administration increases the risk of peptic ulceration and bleeding). Products include:
Relafen Tablets ... 1617

Naproxen (Co-administration increases the risk of peptic ulceration and bleeding). Products include:
EC-Naprosyn Delayed-Release Tablets ... 2967
Naprosyn Suspension ... 2967
Naprosyn Tablets ... 2967

Naproxen Sodium (Co-administration increases the risk of peptic ulceration and bleeding). Products include:
Aleve Tablets, Caplets and Gelcaps ... 602
Aleve Cold & Sinus Caplets ... 603
Anaprox Tablets ... 2967
Anaprox DS Tablets ... 2967
Naprelan Tablets ... 1293

Olanzapine (Increased general CNS depressant effects with concurrent use). Products include:
Zyprexa Tablets ... 1973
Zyprexa ZYDIS Orally Disintegrating Tablets ... 1973

Oxaprozin (Co-administration increases the risk of peptic ulceration and bleeding).
No products indexed under this heading.

Oxazepam (Increased general CNS depressant effects with concurrent use).
No products indexed under this heading.

Oxycodone Hydrochloride (Increased general CNS depressant effects with concurrent use). Products include:
OxyContin Tablets ... 2912
OxyFast Oral Concentrate Solution ... 2916
OxyIR Capsules ... 2916
Percocet Tablets ... 1326
Percodan Tablets ... 1327
Percolone Tablets ... 1327
Roxicodone ... 3067
Tylox Capsules ... 2597

Pentobarbital Sodium (Increased general CNS depressant effects with concurrent use). Products include:
Nembutal Sodium Solution ... 485

Perphenazine (Increased general CNS depressant effects with concurrent use). Products include:
Etrafon ... 3115
Trilafon ... 3160

IMPORTANT NOTE: Always consult each drug listing in the patient's regimen for possible interactions.

Phenobarbital (Increased general CNS depressant effects with concurrent use). Products include:
- Arco-Lase Plus Tablets 592
- Donnatal 2929
- Donnatal Extentabs 2930

Phenylbutazone (Co-administration increases the risk of peptic ulceration and bleeding).
No products indexed under this heading.

Pioglitazone Hydrochloride (Aspirin may enhance the effects of oral hypoglycemic agents causing hypoglycemia). Products include:
- Actos Tablets 3275

Piroxicam (Co-administration increases the risk of peptic ulceration and bleeding). Products include:
- Feldene Capsules 2685

Prazepam (Increased general CNS depressant effects with concurrent use).
No products indexed under this heading.

Prednisolone Acetate (Corticosteroids enhance renal clearance of salicylates; withdrawal of corticosteroids in patients on chronic aspirin therapy may result in salicylism when renal clearance returns to normal).
Products include:
- Blephamide Ophthalmic Ointment ... 547
- Blephamide Ophthalmic Suspension 548
- Poly-Pred Liquifilm Ophthalmic Suspension .... ⊙245
- Pred Forte Ophthalmic Suspension .... ⊙246
- Pred Mild Sterile Ophthalmic Suspension .... ⊙249
- Pred-G Ophthalmic Suspension ..... ⊙247
- Pred-G Sterile Ophthalmic Ointment .... ⊙248

Prednisolone Sodium Phosphate (Corticosteroids enhance renal clearance of salicylates; withdrawal of corticosteroids in patients on chronic aspirin therapy may result in salicylism when renal clearance returns to normal). Products include:
- Pediapred Oral Solution 1170

Prednisolone Tebutate (Corticosteroids enhance renal clearance of salicylates; withdrawal of corticosteroids in patients on chronic aspirin therapy may result in salicylism when renal clearance returns to normal).
No products indexed under this heading.

Prednisone (Corticosteroids enhance renal clearance of salicylates; withdrawal of corticosteroids in patients on chronic aspirin therapy may result in salicylism when renal clearance returns to normal).
Products include:
- Prednisone 3064

Probenecid (Aspirin may diminish the effects of uricosuric agents, such as probenecid).
No products indexed under this heading.

Prochlorperazine (Increased general CNS depressant effects with concurrent use). Products include:
- Compazine 1505

Promethazine Hydrochloride (Increased general CNS depressant effects with concurrent use).
Products include:
- Mepergan Injection 3539
- Phenergan Injection 3553
- Phenergan 3556
- Phenergan Syrup 3554
- Phenergan with Codeine Syrup 3557
- Phenergan with Dextromethorphan Syrup 3559
- Phenergan VC Syrup 3560
- Phenergan VC with Codeine Syrup .. 3561

Propofol (Increased general CNS depressant effects with concurrent use). Products include:
- Diprivan Injectable Emulsion 667

Propoxyphene Hydrochloride (Increased general CNS depressant effects with concurrent use).
Products include:
- Darvon Pulvules 1909
- Darvon Compound-65 Pulvules 1910

Propoxyphene Napsylate (Increased general CNS depressant effects with concurrent use).
Products include:
- Darvon-N/Darvocet-N 1907
- Darvon-N Tablets 1912

Quazepam (Increased general CNS depressant effects with concurrent use).
No products indexed under this heading.

Quetiapine Fumarate (Increased general CNS depressant effects with concurrent use). Products include:
- Seroquel Tablets 684

Remifentanil Hydrochloride (Increased general CNS depressant effects with concurrent use).
No products indexed under this heading.

Repaglinide (Aspirin may enhance the effects of oral hypoglycemic agents causing hypoglycemia).
Products include:
- Prandin Tablets (0.5, 1, and 2 mg) 2432

Risperidone (Increased general CNS depressant effects with concurrent use). Products include:
- Risperdal 1796

Rofecoxib (Co-administration increases the risk of peptic ulceration and bleeding). Products include:
- Vioxx 2213

Rosiglitazone Maleate (Aspirin may enhance the effects of oral hypoglycemic agents causing hypoglycemia). Products include:
- Avandia Tablets 1490

Secobarbital Sodium (Increased general CNS depressant effects with concurrent use).
No products indexed under this heading.

Sevoflurane (Increased general CNS depressant effects with concurrent use).
No products indexed under this heading.

Sufentanil Citrate (Increased general CNS depressant effects with concurrent use).
No products indexed under this heading.

Sulfinpyrazone (Aspirin may diminish the effects of uricosuric agents, such as sulfinpyrazone).
No products indexed under this heading.

Sulindac (Co-administration increases the risk of peptic ulceration and bleeding). Products include:
- Clinoril Tablets 2053

Temazepam (Increased general CNS depressant effects with concurrent use).
No products indexed under this heading.

Thiamylal Sodium (Increased general CNS depressant effects with concurrent use).
No products indexed under this heading.

Thioridazine Hydrochloride (Increased general CNS depressant effects with concurrent use).
Products include:
- Thioridazine Hydrochloride Tablets 2289

Thiothixene (Increased general CNS depressant effects with concurrent use). Products include:
- Navane Capsules 2701
- Thiothixene Capsules 2290

Tolazamide (Aspirin may enhance the effects of oral hypoglycemic agents causing hypoglycemia).
No products indexed under this heading.

Tolbutamide (Aspirin may enhance the effects of oral hypoglycemic agents causing hypoglycemia).
No products indexed under this heading.

Tolmetin Sodium (Co-administration increases the risk of peptic ulceration and bleeding).
Products include:
- Tolectin 2589

Triamcinolone (Corticosteroids enhance renal clearance of salicylates; withdrawal of corticosteroids in patients on chronic aspirin therapy may result in salicylism when renal clearance returns to normal).
No products indexed under this heading.

Triamcinolone Acetonide (Corticosteroids enhance renal clearance of salicylates; withdrawal of corticosteroids in patients on chronic aspirin therapy may result in salicylism when renal clearance returns to normal).
Products include:
- Azmacort Inhalation Aerosol 728
- Nasacort Nasal Inhaler 750
- Nasacort AQ Nasal Spray 752
- Tri-Nasal Spray 2274

Triamcinolone Diacetate (Corticosteroids enhance renal clearance of salicylates; withdrawal of corticosteroids in patients on chronic aspirin therapy may result in salicylism when renal clearance returns to normal).
No products indexed under this heading.

Triamcinolone Hexacetonide (Corticosteroids enhance renal clearance of salicylates; withdrawal of corticosteroids in patients on chronic aspirin therapy may result in salicylism when renal clearance returns to normal).
No products indexed under this heading.

Triazolam (Increased general CNS depressant effects with concurrent use). Products include:
- Halcion Tablets 2823

Trifluoperazine Hydrochloride (Increased general CNS depressant effects with concurrent use).
Products include:
- Stelazine 1640

Troglitazone (Aspirin may enhance the effects of oral hypoglycemic agents causing hypoglycemia).
No products indexed under this heading.

Warfarin Sodium (Aspirin may enhance the effects of oral anticoagulants resulting in bleeding).
Products include:
- Coumadin for Injection 1243
- Coumadin Tablets 1243
- Warfarin Sodium Tablets, USP 3302

Zaleplon (Increased general CNS depressant effects with concurrent use). Products include:
- Sonata Capsules 3591

Ziprasidone Hydrochloride (Increased general CNS depressant effects with concurrent use).
Products include:
- Geodon Capsules 2688

Zolpidem Tartrate (Increased general CNS depressant effects with concurrent use). Products include:
- Ambien Tablets 3191

Food Interactions

Alcohol (Increased general CNS depressant effects with concurrent use).

ROBINUL FORTE TABLETS
(Glycopyrrolate) 1358
None cited in PDR database.

ROBINUL INJECTABLE
(Glycopyrrolate) 2940
May interact with anticholinergics, anticholinergic-type antiparkinsonism drugs, phenothiazines, tricyclic antidepressants, and certain other agents. Compounds in these categories include:

Amitriptyline Hydrochloride (Co-administration with other drugs with anticholinergic activity may intensify the antimuscarinic effects and may result in increased anticholinergic side effects). Products include:
- Etrafon 3115
- Limbitrol 1738

Amoxapine (Co-administration with other drugs with anticholinergic activity may intensify the antimuscarinic effects and may result in increased anticholinergic side effects).
No products indexed under this heading.

Atropine Sulfate (Co-administration with other anticholinergic agents may intensify the antimuscarinic effects and may result in increased anticholinergic side effects).
Products include:
- Donnatal 2929
- Donnatal Extentabs 2930
- Motofen Tablets 577
- Prosed/DS Tablets 3268
- Urised Tablets 2876

Belladonna Alkaloids (Co-administration with other anticholinergic agents may intensify the antimuscarinic effects and may result in increased anticholinergic side effects). Products include:
- Hyland's Teething Tablets .... ▣766
- Urimax Tablets 1769

Benztropine Mesylate (Co-administration with other anticholinergic agents may intensify the antimuscarinic effects and may result in increased anticholinergic side effects). Products include:
- Cogentin 2055

Biperiden Hydrochloride (Co-administration with other anticholinergic agents may intensify the antimuscarinic effects and may result in increased anticholinergic side effects). Products include:
- Akineton 402

Chlorpromazine (Co-administration with other drugs with anticholinergic activity may intensify the antimuscarinic effects and may result in increased anticholinergic side effects). Products include:
- Thorazine Suppositories 1656

Chlorpromazine Hydrochloride (Co-administration with other drugs with anticholinergic activity may intensify the antimuscarinic effects and may result in increased anticholinergic side effects). Products include:
- Thorazine 1656

Clidinium Bromide (Co-administration with other anticholinergic agents may intensify the antimuscarinic effects and may result in increased anticholinergic side effects).
No products indexed under this heading.

Clomipramine Hydrochloride (Co-administration with other drugs with anticholinergic activity may intensify the antimuscarinic effects and may result in increased anticholinergic side effects).
No products indexed under this heading.

Desipramine Hydrochloride (Co-administration with other drugs with anticholinergic activity may intensify the antimuscarinic effects and may result in increased anticholinergic side effects). Products include:
- Norpramin Tablets 755

Dicyclomine Hydrochloride (Co-administration with other anticholinergic agents may intensify the antimuscarinic effects and may result in increased anticholinergic side effects).
No products indexed under this heading.

Doxepin Hydrochloride (Co-administration with other drugs with

anticholinergic activity may intensify the antimuscarinic effects and may result in increased anticholinergic side effects). Products include:
Sinequan 2713

Fluphenazine Decanoate (Co-administration with other drugs with anticholinergic activity may intensify the antimuscarinic effects and may result in increased anticholinergic side effects).
No products indexed under this heading.

Fluphenazine Enanthate (Co-administration with other drugs with anticholinergic activity may intensify the antimuscarinic effects and may result in increased anticholinergic side effects).
No products indexed under this heading.

Fluphenazine Hydrochloride (Co-administration with other drugs with anticholinergic activity may intensify the antimuscarinic effects and may result in increased anticholinergic side effects).
No products indexed under this heading.

Hyoscyamine (Co-administration with other anticholinergic agents may intensify the antimuscarinic effects and may result in increased anticholinergic side effects). Products include:
Urised Tablets 2876

Hyoscyamine Sulfate (Co-administration with other anticholinergic agents may intensify the antimuscarinic effects and may result in increased anticholinergic side effects). Products include:
Arco-Lase Plus Tablets 592
Donnatal 2929
Donnatal Extentabs 2930
Levsin/Levsinex/Levbid 3172
NuLev Orally Disintegrating Tablets 3176
Prosed/DS Tablets 3268
Urimax Tablets 1769

Imipramine Hydrochloride (Co-administration with other drugs with anticholinergic activity may intensify the antimuscarinic effects and may result in increased anticholinergic side effects).
No products indexed under this heading.

Imipramine Pamoate (Co-administration with other drugs with anticholinergic activity may intensify the antimuscarinic effects and may result in increased anticholinergic side effects).
No products indexed under this heading.

Ipratropium Bromide (Co-administration with other anticholinergic agents may intensify the antimuscarinic effects and may result in increased anticholinergic side effects). Products include:
Atrovent Inhalation Aerosol 1030
Atrovent Inhalation Solution 1031
Atrovent Nasal Spray 0.03% 1032
Atrovent Nasal Spray 0.06% 1033
Combivent Inhalation Aerosol 1041
DuoNeb Inhalation Solution 1233

Maprotiline Hydrochloride (Co-administration with other drugs with anticholinergic activity may intensify the antimuscarinic effects and may result in increased anticholinergic side effects).
No products indexed under this heading.

Mepenzolate Bromide (Co-administration with other anticholinergic agents may intensify the antimuscarinic effects and may result in increased anticholinergic side effects).
No products indexed under this heading.

Mesoridazine Besylate (Co-administration with other drugs with anticholinergic activity may intensify the antimuscarinic effects and may result in increased anticholinergic side effects). Products include:
Serentil 1057

Methotrimeprazine (Co-administration with other drugs with anticholinergic activity may intensify the antimuscarinic effects and may result in increased anticholinergic side effects).
No products indexed under this heading.

Nortriptyline Hydrochloride (Co-administration with other drugs with anticholinergic activity may intensify the antimuscarinic effects and may result in increased anticholinergic side effects).
No products indexed under this heading.

Oxybutynin Chloride (Co-administration with other anticholinergic agents may intensify the antimuscarinic effects and may result in increased anticholinergic side effects). Products include:
Ditropan XL Extended Release Tablets 564

Perphenazine (Co-administration with other drugs with anticholinergic activity may intensify the antimuscarinic effects and may result in increased anticholinergic side effects). Products include:
Etrafon 3115
Trilafon 3160

Potassium Chloride (Co-administration of potassium chloride in a wax matrix may increase the severity of potassium chloride-induced gastrointestinal lesions as a result of a slower gastrointestinal transit time). Products include:
Chlor-3 1361
Colyte with Flavor Packs for Oral Solution 3170
GoLYTELY and Pineapple Flavor GoLYTELY for Oral Solution 1068
K-Dur Microburst Release System ER Tablets 1832
Klor-Con M20/Klor-Con M10 Tablets 3329
K-Lor Powder Packets 469
K-Tab Filmtab Tablets 470
Micro-K 3311
NuLYTELY, Cherry Flavor, Lemon-Lime Flavor, and Orange Flavor NuLYTELY for Oral Solution 1068
Rum-K 1363

Prochlorperazine (Co-administration with other drugs with anticholinergic activity may intensify the antimuscarinic effects and may result in increased anticholinergic side effects). Products include:
Compazine 1505

Procyclidine Hydrochloride (Co-administration with other anticholinergic agents may intensify the antimuscarinic effects and may result in increased anticholinergic side effects).
No products indexed under this heading.

Promethazine Hydrochloride (Co-administration with other drugs with anticholinergic activity may intensify the antimuscarinic effects and may result in increased anticholinergic side effects). Products include:
Mepergan Injection 3539
Phenergan Injection 3553
Phenergan 3556
Phenergan Syrup 3554
Phenergan with Codeine Syrup 3557
Phenergan with Dextromethorphan Syrup 3559
Phenergan VC Syrup 3560
Phenergan VC with Codeine Syrup 3561

Propantheline Bromide (Co-administration with other anticholinergic agents may intensify the antimuscarinic effects and may result in increased anticholinergic side effects).
No products indexed under this heading.

Protriptyline Hydrochloride (Co-administration with other drugs with anticholinergic activity may intensify the antimuscarinic effects and may result in increased anticholinergic side effects). Products include:
Vivactil Tablets 2446
Vivactil Tablets 2217

Scopolamine (Co-administration with other anticholinergic agents may intensify the antimuscarinic effects and may result in increased anticholinergic side effects). Products include:
Transderm Scōp Transdermal Therapeutic System 2302

Scopolamine Hydrobromide (Co-administration with other anticholinergic agents may intensify the antimuscarinic effects and may result in increased anticholinergic side effects). Products include:
Donnatal 2929
Donnatal Extentabs 2930

Thioridazine Hydrochloride (Co-administration with other drugs with anticholinergic activity may intensify the antimuscarinic effects and may result in increased anticholinergic side effects). Products include:
Thioridazine Hydrochloride Tablets 2289

Tolterodine Tartrate (Co-administration with other anticholinergic agents may intensify the antimuscarinic effects and may result in increased anticholinergic side effects). Products include:
Detrol Tablets 3623
Detrol LA Capsules 2801

Tridihexethyl Chloride (Co-administration with other anticholinergic agents may intensify the antimuscarinic effects and may result in increased anticholinergic side effects).
No products indexed under this heading.

Trifluoperazine Hydrochloride (Co-administration with other drugs with anticholinergic activity may intensify the antimuscarinic effects and may result in increased anticholinergic side effects). Products include:
Stelazine 1640

Trihexyphenidyl Hydrochloride (Co-administration with other anticholinergic agents may intensify the antimuscarinic effects and may result in increased anticholinergic side effects). Products include:
Artane 1855

Trimipramine Maleate (Co-administration with other drugs with anticholinergic activity may intensify the antimuscarinic effects and may result in increased anticholinergic side effects). Products include:
Surmontil Capsules 3595

ROBINUL TABLETS

(Glycopyrrolate) 1358
None cited in PDR database.

ROBITUSSIN LIQUID

(Guaifenesin) .... ▣782
None cited in PDR database.

ROBITUSSIN A-C SYRUP

(Codeine Phosphate, Guaifenesin) 2942
May interact with antidepressant drugs, hypnotics and sedatives, tranquilizers, and certain other agents. Compounds in these categories include:

Alprazolam (Concurrent therapy may cause greater sedation). Products include:
Xanax Tablets 2865

Amitriptyline Hydrochloride (Concurrent therapy with antidepressants may cause greater sedation). Products include:
Etrafon 3115
Limbitrol 1738

Amoxapine (Concurrent therapy with antidepressants may cause greater sedation).
No products indexed under this heading.

Bupropion Hydrochloride (Concurrent therapy with antidepressants may cause greater sedation). Products include:
Wellbutrin Tablets 1680
Wellbutrin SR Sustained-Release Tablets 1684
Zyban Sustained-Release Tablets 1710

Buspirone Hydrochloride (Concurrent therapy may cause greater sedation).
No products indexed under this heading.

Chlordiazepoxide (Concurrent therapy may cause greater sedation). Products include:
Limbitrol 1738

Chlordiazepoxide Hydrochloride (Concurrent therapy may cause greater sedation). Products include:
Librium Capsules 1736
Librium for Injection 1737

Chlorpromazine (Concurrent therapy may cause greater sedation). Products include:
Thorazine Suppositories 1656

Chlorpromazine Hydrochloride (Concurrent therapy may cause greater sedation). Products include:
Thorazine 1656

Chlorprothixene (Concurrent therapy may cause greater sedation).
No products indexed under this heading.

Chlorprothixene Hydrochloride (Concurrent therapy may cause greater sedation).
No products indexed under this heading.

Citalopram Hydrobromide (Concurrent therapy with antidepressants may cause greater sedation). Products include:
Celexa 1365

Clorazepate Dipotassium (Concurrent therapy may cause greater sedation). Products include:
Tranxene 511

Desipramine Hydrochloride (Concurrent therapy with antidepressants may cause greater sedation). Products include:
Norpramin Tablets 755

Diazepam (Concurrent therapy may cause greater sedation). Products include:
Valium Injectable 3026
Valium Tablets 3047

Doxepin Hydrochloride (Concurrent therapy with antidepressants may cause greater sedation). Products include:
Sinequan 2713

Droperidol (Concurrent therapy may cause greater sedation).
No products indexed under this heading.

Estazolam (Concurrent therapy may cause greater sedation). Products include:
ProSom Tablets 500

Ethchlorvynol (Concurrent therapy may cause greater sedation).
No products indexed under this heading.

Ethinamate (Concurrent therapy may cause greater sedation).
No products indexed under this heading.

Fluoxetine Hydrochloride (Concurrent therapy with antidepressants may cause greater sedation). Products include:
Prozac Pulvules, Liquid, and Weekly Capsules 1238
Sarafem Pulvules 1962

Fluphenazine Decanoate (Concurrent therapy may cause greater sedation).
No products indexed under this heading.

Fluphenazine Enanthate (Concurrent therapy may cause greater sedation).
No products indexed under this heading.

Fluphenazine Hydrochloride (Concurrent therapy may cause greater sedation).
No products indexed under this heading.

Flurazepam Hydrochloride (Concurrent therapy may cause greater sedation).
No products indexed under this heading.

Glutethimide (Concurrent therapy may cause greater sedation).
No products indexed under this heading.

Haloperidol (Concurrent therapy may cause greater sedation). Products include:
Haldol Injection, Tablets and Concentrate 2533

Haloperidol Decanoate (Concurrent therapy may cause greater sedation). Products include:
Haldol Decanoate 2535

Hydroxyzine Hydrochloride (Concurrent therapy may cause greater sedation). Products include:
Atarax Tablets & Syrup 2667
Vistaril Intramuscular Solution 2738

Imipramine Hydrochloride (Concurrent therapy with antidepressants may cause greater sedation).
No products indexed under this heading.

Imipramine Pamoate (Concurrent therapy with antidepressants may cause greater sedation).
No products indexed under this heading.

Isocarboxazid (Concurrent therapy with MAO inhibitors may cause greater sedation).
No products indexed under this heading.

Lorazepam (Concurrent therapy may cause greater sedation). Products include:
Ativan Injection 3478
Ativan Tablets 3482

Loxapine Hydrochloride (Concurrent therapy may cause greater sedation).
No products indexed under this heading.

Loxapine Succinate (Concurrent therapy may cause greater sedation). Products include:
Loxitane Capsules 3398

Maprotiline Hydrochloride (Concurrent therapy with antidepressants may cause greater sedation).
No products indexed under this heading.

Meprobamate (Concurrent therapy may cause greater sedation). Products include:
Miltown Tablets 3349

Mesoridazine Besylate (Concurrent therapy may cause greater sedation). Products include:
Serentil 1057

Midazolam Hydrochloride (Concurrent therapy may cause greater sedation). Products include:
Versed Injection 3027
Versed Syrup 3033

Mirtazapine (Concurrent therapy with antidepressants may cause greater sedation). Products include:
Remeron Tablets 2483
Remeron SolTab Tablets 2486

Molindone Hydrochloride (Concurrent therapy may cause greater sedation). Products include:
Moban 1320

Nefazodone Hydrochloride (Concurrent therapy with antidepressants may cause greater sedation). Products include:
Serzone Tablets 1104

Nortriptyline Hydrochloride (Concurrent therapy with antidepressants may cause greater sedation).
No products indexed under this heading.

Oxazepam (Concurrent therapy may cause greater sedation).
No products indexed under this heading.

Paroxetine Hydrochloride (Concurrent therapy with antidepressants may cause greater sedation). Products include:
Paxil 1609

Perphenazine (Concurrent therapy may cause greater sedation). Products include:
Etrafon 3115
Trilafon 3160

Phenelzine Sulfate (Concurrent therapy with MAO inhibitors may cause greater sedation). Products include:
Nardil Tablets 2653

Prazepam (Concurrent therapy may cause greater sedation).
No products indexed under this heading.

Prochlorperazine (Concurrent therapy may cause greater sedation). Products include:
Compazine 1505

Promethazine Hydrochloride (Concurrent therapy may cause greater sedation). Products include:
Mepergan Injection 3539
Phenergan Injection 3553
Phenergan 3556
Phenergan Syrup 3554
Phenergan with Codeine Syrup 3557
Phenergan with Dextromethorphan Syrup 3559
Phenergan VC Syrup 3560
Phenergan VC with Codeine Syrup 3561

Propofol (Concurrent therapy may cause greater sedation). Products include:
Diprivan Injectable Emulsion 667

Protriptyline Hydrochloride (Concurrent therapy with antidepressants may cause greater sedation). Products include:
Vivactil Tablets 2446
Vivactil Tablets 2217

Quazepam (Concurrent therapy may cause greater sedation).
No products indexed under this heading.

Secobarbital Sodium (Concurrent therapy may cause greater sedation).
No products indexed under this heading.

Sertraline Hydrochloride (Concurrent therapy with antidepressants may cause greater sedation). Products include:
Zoloft 2751

Temazepam (Concurrent therapy may cause greater sedation).
No products indexed under this heading.

Thioridazine Hydrochloride (Concurrent therapy may cause greater sedation). Products include:
Thioridazine Hydrochloride Tablets 2289

Thiothixene (Concurrent therapy may cause greater sedation). Products include:
Navane Capsules 2701
Thiothixene Capsules 2290

Tranylcypromine Sulfate (Concurrent therapy with MAO inhibitors may cause greater sedation). Products include:
Parnate Tablets 1607

Trazodone Hydrochloride (Concurrent therapy with antidepressants may cause greater sedation).
No products indexed under this heading.

Triazolam (Concurrent therapy may cause greater sedation). Products include:
Halcion Tablets 2823

Trifluoperazine Hydrochloride (Concurrent therapy may cause greater sedation). Products include:
Stelazine 1640

Trimipramine Maleate (Concurrent therapy with antidepressants may cause greater sedation). Products include:
Surmontil Capsules 3595

Venlafaxine Hydrochloride (Concurrent therapy with antidepressants may cause greater sedation). Products include:
Effexor Tablets 3495
Effexor XR Capsules 3499

Zaleplon (Concurrent therapy may cause greater sedation). Products include:
Sonata Capsules 3591

Zolpidem Tartrate (Concurrent therapy may cause greater sedation). Products include:
Ambien Tablets 3191

ROBITUSSIN COLD CAPLETS COLD & CONGESTION

(Dextromethorphan Hydrobromide, Guaifenesin, Pseudoephedrine Hydrochloride) .... ▣780
See Robitussin-CF Liquid

ROBITUSSIN COLD SOFTGELS COLD & CONGESTION

(Dextromethorphan Hydrobromide, Guaifenesin, Pseudoephedrine Hydrochloride) .... ▣780
See Robitussin-CF Liquid

ROBITUSSIN COLD CAPLETS MULTI-SYMPTOM COLD & FLU

(Acetaminophen, Dextromethorphan Hydrobromide, Guaifenesin, Pseudoephedrine Hydrochloride) .... ▣781
See Robitussin Cold Softgels Multi-Symptom Cold & Flu

ROBITUSSIN COLD SOFTGELS MULTI-SYMPTOM COLD & FLU

(Acetaminophen, Dextromethorphan Hydrobromide, Guaifenesin, Pseudoephedrine Hydrochloride) .... ▣781
May interact with monoamine oxidase inhibitors and certain other agents. Compounds in these categories include:

Isocarboxazid (Concurrent and/or sequential use with MAO inhibitors is not recommended).
No products indexed under this heading.

Moclobemide (Concurrent and/or sequential use with MAO inhibitors is not recommended).
No products indexed under this heading.

Pargyline Hydrochloride (Concurrent and/or sequential use with MAO inhibitors is not recommended).
No products indexed under this heading.

Phenelzine Sulfate (Concurrent and/or sequential use with MAO inhibitors is not recommended). Products include:
Nardil Tablets 2653

Procarbazine Hydrochloride (Concurrent and/or sequential use with MAO inhibitors is not recommended). Products include:
Matulane Capsules 3246

Selegiline Hydrochloride (Concurrent and/or sequential use with MAO inhibitors is not recommended). Products include:
Eldepryl Capsules 3266

Tranylcypromine Sulfate (Concurrent and/or sequential use with MAO inhibitors is not recommended). Products include:
Parnate Tablets 1607

Food Interactions

Alcohol (Chronic heavy alcohol users, 3 or more drinks per day, should consult their physicians for advice on when and how they should take pain relievers/fever reducers including acetaminophen).

ROBITUSSIN COLD SOFTGELS SEVERE CONGESTION

(Guaifenesin, Pseudoephedrine Hydrochloride) .... ▣782
See Robitussin-CF Liquid

ROBITUSSIN COUGH DROPS

(Menthol) .... ▣781
None cited in PDR database.

ROBITUSSIN HONEY COUGH DROPS

(Menthol) .... ▣784
None cited in PDR database.

ROBITUSSIN COUGH & COLD INFANT DROPS

(Dextromethorphan Hydrobromide, Guaifenesin, Pseudoephedrine Hydrochloride) .... ▣782
See Robitussin-CF Liquid

ROBITUSSIN MAXIMUM STRENGTH COUGH & COLD LIQUID

(Dextromethorphan Hydrobromide, Pseudoephedrine Hydrochloride) .... ▣785
May interact with monoamine oxidase inhibitors. Compounds in these categories include:

Isocarboxazid (Concurrent and/or sequential use with MAO inhibitors is not recommended).
No products indexed under this heading.

Moclobemide (Concurrent and/or sequential use with MAO inhibitors is not recommended).
No products indexed under this heading.

Pargyline Hydrochloride (Concurrent and/or sequential use with MAO inhibitors is not recommended).
No products indexed under this heading.

Phenelzine Sulfate (Concurrent and/or sequential use with MAO inhibitors is not recommended). Products include:
Nardil Tablets 2653

Procarbazine Hydrochloride (Concurrent and/or sequential use with MAO inhibitors is not recommended). Products include:
Matulane Capsules 3246

Selegiline Hydrochloride (Concurrent and/or sequential use with MAO inhibitors is not recommended). Products include:
Eldepryl Capsules 3266

Tranylcypromine Sulfate (Concurrent and/or sequential use with MAO inhibitors is not recommended). Products include:
Parnate Tablets 1607

ROBITUSSIN PEDIATRIC COUGH & COLD FORMULA LIQUID
(Dextromethorphan Hydrobromide, Pseudoephedrine Hydrochloride)..... 785
See Robitussin Maximum Strength Cough & Cold Liquid

ROBITUSSIN MAXIMUM STRENGTH COUGH SUPPRESSANT LIQUID
(Dextromethorphan Hydrobromide)................................ 784
See Robitussin Pediatric Cough Suppressant Liquid

ROBITUSSIN PEDIATRIC COUGH SUPPRESSANT LIQUID
(Dextromethorphan Hydrobromide)................................ 784
May interact with monoamine oxidase inhibitors. Compounds in these categories include:

Isocarboxazid (Concurrent and/or sequential use with MAO inhibitors should be avoided).
No products indexed under this heading.

Moclobemide (Concurrent and/or sequential use with MAO inhibitors should be avoided).
No products indexed under this heading.

Pargyline Hydrochloride (Concurrent and/or sequential use with MAO inhibitors should be avoided).
No products indexed under this heading.

Phenelzine Sulfate (Concurrent and/or sequential use with MAO inhibitors should be avoided). Products include:
Nardil Tablets 2653

Procarbazine Hydrochloride (Concurrent and/or sequential use with MAO inhibitors should be avoided). Products include:
Matulane Capsules 3246

Selegiline Hydrochloride (Concurrent and/or sequential use with MAO inhibitors should be avoided). Products include:
Eldepryl Capsules 3266

Tranylcypromine Sulfate (Concurrent and/or sequential use with MAO inhibitors should be avoided). Products include:
Parnate Tablets 1607

ROBITUSSIN MULTI SYMPTOM HONEY FLU LIQUID
(Acetaminophen, Dextromethorphan Hydrobromide, Pseudoephedrine Hydrochloride) 785
See Robitussin Nighttime Honey Flu Liquid

ROBITUSSIN NIGHTTIME HONEY FLU LIQUID
(Acetaminophen, Chlorpheniramine Maleate, Dextromethorphan Hydrobromide, Pseudoephedrine Hydrochloride) 786
May interact with hypnotics and sedatives, monoamine oxidase inhibitors, tranquilizers, and certain other agents. Compounds in these categories include:

Alprazolam (May increase drowsiness effect). Products include:
Xanax Tablets 2865

Buspirone Hydrochloride (May increase drowsiness effect).
No products indexed under this heading.

Chlordiazepoxide (May increase drowsiness effect). Products include:
Limbitrol 1738

Chlordiazepoxide Hydrochloride (May increase drowsiness effect). Products include:
Librium Capsules 1736
Librium for Injection 1737

Chlorpromazine (May increase drowsiness effect). Products include:
Thorazine Suppositories 1656

Chlorpromazine Hydrochloride (May increase drowsiness effect). Products include:
Thorazine 1656

Chlorprothixene (May increase drowsiness effect).
No products indexed under this heading.

Chlorprothixene Hydrochloride (May increase drowsiness effect).
No products indexed under this heading.

Clorazepate Dipotassium (May increase drowsiness effect). Products include:
Tranxene 511

Diazepam (May increase drowsiness effect). Products include:
Valium Injectable 3026
Valium Tablets 3047

Droperidol (May increase drowsiness effect).
No products indexed under this heading.

Estazolam (May increase drowsiness effect). Products include:
ProSom Tablets 500

Ethchlorvynol (May increase drowsiness effect).
No products indexed under this heading.

Ethinamate (May increase drowsiness effect).
No products indexed under this heading.

Fluphenazine Decanoate (May increase drowsiness effect).
No products indexed under this heading.

Fluphenazine Enanthate (May increase drowsiness effect).
No products indexed under this heading.

Fluphenazine Hydrochloride (May increase drowsiness effect).
No products indexed under this heading.

Flurazepam Hydrochloride (May increase drowsiness effect).
No products indexed under this heading.

Glutethimide (May increase drowsiness effect).
No products indexed under this heading.

Haloperidol (May increase drowsiness effect). Products include:
Haldol Injection, Tablets and Concentrate 2533

Haloperidol Decanoate (May increase drowsiness effect). Products include:
Haldol Decanoate 2535

Hydroxyzine Hydrochloride (May increase drowsiness effect). Products include:
Atarax Tablets & Syrup 2667
Vistaril Intramuscular Solution 2738

Isocarboxazid (Concurrent and/or sequential use with MAO inhibitors is not recommended).
No products indexed under this heading.

Lorazepam (May increase drowsiness effect). Products include:
Ativan Injection 3478
Ativan Tablets 3482

Loxapine Hydrochloride (May increase drowsiness effect).
No products indexed under this heading.

Loxapine Succinate (May increase drowsiness effect). Products include:
Loxitane Capsules 3398

Meprobamate (May increase drowsiness effect). Products include:
Miltown Tablets 3349

Mesoridazine Besylate (May increase drowsiness effect). Products include:
Serentil 1057

Midazolam Hydrochloride (May increase drowsiness effect). Products include:
Versed Injection 3027
Versed Syrup 3033

Moclobemide (Concurrent and/or sequential use with MAO inhibitors is not recommended).
No products indexed under this heading.

Molindone Hydrochloride (May increase drowsiness effect). Products include:
Moban 1320

Oxazepam (May increase drowsiness effect).
No products indexed under this heading.

Pargyline Hydrochloride (Concurrent and/or sequential use with MAO inhibitors is not recommended).
No products indexed under this heading.

Perphenazine (May increase drowsiness effect). Products include:
Etrafon 3115
Trilafon 3160

Phenelzine Sulfate (Concurrent and/or sequential use with MAO inhibitors is not recommended). Products include:
Nardil Tablets 2653

Prazepam (May increase drowsiness effect).
No products indexed under this heading.

Procarbazine Hydrochloride (Concurrent and/or sequential use with MAO inhibitors is not recommended). Products include:
Matulane Capsules 3246

Prochlorperazine (May increase drowsiness effect). Products include:
Compazine 1505

Promethazine Hydrochloride (May increase drowsiness effect). Products include:
Mepergan Injection 3539
Phenergan Injection 3553
Phenergan 3556
Phenergan Syrup 3554
Phenergan with Codeine Syrup 3557
Phenergan with Dextromethorphan Syrup 3559
Phenergan VC Syrup 3560
Phenergan VC with Codeine Syrup . 3561

Propofol (May increase drowsiness effect). Products include:
Diprivan Injectable Emulsion 667

Quazepam (May increase drowsiness effect).
No products indexed under this heading.

Secobarbital Sodium (May increase drowsiness effect).
No products indexed under this heading.

Selegiline Hydrochloride (Concurrent and/or sequential use with MAO inhibitors is not recommended). Products include:
Eldepryl Capsules 3266

Temazepam (May increase drowsiness effect).
No products indexed under this heading.

Thioridazine Hydrochloride (May increase drowsiness effect). Products include:
Thioridazine Hydrochloride Tablets 2289

Thiothixene (May increase drowsiness effect). Products include:
Navane Capsules 2701
Thiothixene Capsules 2290

Tranylcypromine Sulfate (Concurrent and/or sequential use with MAO inhibitors is not recommended). Products include:
Parnate Tablets 1607

Triazolam (May increase drowsiness effect). Products include:
Halcion Tablets 2823

Trifluoperazine Hydrochloride (May increase drowsiness effect). Products include:
Stelazine 1640

Zaleplon (May increase drowsiness effect). Products include:
Sonata Capsules 3591

Zolpidem Tartrate (May increase drowsiness effect). Products include:
Ambien Tablets 3191

Food Interactions

Alcohol (Chronic heavy alcohol users, 3 or more drinks per day, should consult their physician for advice on when and how they should take pain relievers/fever reducers including acetaminophen; increases drowsiness effect; avoid alcoholic beverages).

ROBITUSSIN HONEY CALMERS THROAT DROPS
(Menthol) 783
None cited in PDR database.

ROBITUSSIN SUGAR FREE THROAT DROPS
(Menthol) 786
None cited in PDR database.

ROBITUSSIN-CF LIQUID
(Dextromethorphan Hydrobromide, Guaifenesin, Pseudoephedrine Hydrochloride) 783
May interact with monoamine oxidase inhibitors. Compounds in these categories include:

Isocarboxazid (Concurrent and/or sequential use with MAO inhibitors is not recommended).
No products indexed under this heading.

Moclobemide (Concurrent and/or sequential use with MAO inhibitors is not recommended).
No products indexed under this heading.

Pargyline Hydrochloride (Concurrent and/or sequential use with MAO inhibitors is not recommended).
No products indexed under this heading.

Phenelzine Sulfate (Concurrent and/or sequential use with MAO inhibitors is not recommended). Products include:
Nardil Tablets 2653

Procarbazine Hydrochloride (Concurrent and/or sequential use with MAO inhibitors is not recommended). Products include:
Matulane Capsules 3246

Selegiline Hydrochloride (Concurrent and/or sequential use with MAO inhibitors is not recommended). Products include:
Eldepryl Capsules 3266

Tranylcypromine Sulfate (Concurrent and/or sequential use with MAO inhibitors is not recommended). Products include:
Parnate Tablets 1607

ROBITUSSIN-DAC SYRUP
(Codeine Phosphate, Guaifenesin, Pseudoephedrine Hydrochloride) 2942
May interact with monoamine oxidase inhibitors. Compounds in these categories include:

Isocarboxazid (Concurrent use is not recommended).
No products indexed under this heading.

IMPORTANT NOTE: Always consult each drug listing in the patient's regimen for possible interactions.

Moclobemide (Concurrent use is not recommended).
No products indexed under this heading.

Pargyline Hydrochloride (Concurrent use is not recommended).
No products indexed under this heading.

Phenelzine Sulfate (Concurrent use is not recommended). Products include:
Nardil Tablets 2653

Procarbazine Hydrochloride (Concurrent use is not recommended). Products include:
Matulane Capsules 3246

Selegiline Hydrochloride (Concurrent use is not recommended). Products include:
Eldepryl Capsules 3266

Tranylcypromine Sulfate (Concurrent use is not recommended). Products include:
Parnate Tablets 1607

ROBITUSSIN DM INFANT DROPS

(Dextromethorphan Hydrobromide, Guaifenesin) .... ▣783
See Robitussin-DM Liquid

ROBITUSSIN-DM LIQUID

(Dextromethorphan Hydrobromide, Guaifenesin) .... ▣783
May interact with monoamine oxidase inhibitors. Compounds in these categories include:

Isocarboxazid (Concurrent and/or sequential use with MAO inhibitors is not recommended).
No products indexed under this heading.

Moclobemide (Concurrent and/or sequential use with MAO inhibitors is not recommended).
No products indexed under this heading.

Pargyline Hydrochloride (Concurrent and/or sequential use with MAO inhibitors is not recommended).
No products indexed under this heading.

Phenelzine Sulfate (Concurrent and/or sequential use with MAO inhibitors is not recommended). Products include:
Nardil Tablets 2653

Procarbazine Hydrochloride (Concurrent and/or sequential use with MAO inhibitors is not recommended). Products include:
Matulane Capsules 3246

Selegiline Hydrochloride (Concurrent and/or sequential use with MAO inhibitors is not recommended). Products include:
Eldepryl Capsules 3266

Tranylcypromine Sulfate (Concurrent and/or sequential use with MAO inhibitors is not recommended). Products include:
Parnate Tablets 1607

ROBITUSSIN-PE LIQUID

(Guaifenesin, Pseudoephedrine Hydrochloride) .... ▣782
See Robitussin-CF Liquid

ROCALTROL CAPSULES

(Calcitriol) 2991
May interact with cardiac glycosides, phenytoin, thiazides, and certain other agents. Compounds in these categories include:

Bendroflumethiazide (Thiazides are known to induce hypercalcemia by the reduction of calcium excretion in urine; co-administration has resulted in hypercalcemia). Products include:
Corzide 40/5 Tablets 2247
Corzide 80/5 Tablets 2247

Chlorothiazide (Thiazides are known to induce hypercalcemia by the reduction of calcium excretion in urine; co-administration has resulted in hypercalcemia). Products include:
Aldoclor Tablets 2035
Diuril Oral 2087

Chlorothiazide Sodium (Thiazides are known to induce hypercalcemia by the reduction of calcium excretion in urine; co-administration has resulted in hypercalcemia). Products include:
Diuril Sodium Intravenous 2086

Cholestyramine (Co-adminstration with cholestyramine with fat-soluble vitamins has resulted in reduced intestinal absorption of these vitamins; as such it may impair intestinal absorption of calcitriol).
No products indexed under this heading.

Deslanoside (Rocaltrol induces hypercalcemia; hypercalcemia in patients receiving digitalis may precipitate cardiac arrhythmias).
No products indexed under this heading.

Digitoxin (Rocaltrol induces hypercalcemia; hypercalcemia in patients receiving digitalis may precipitate cardiac arrhythmias).
No products indexed under this heading.

Digoxin (Rocaltrol induces hypercalcemia; hypercalcemia in patients receiving digitalis may precipitate cardiac arrhythmias). Products include:
Digitek Tablets 1003
Lanoxicaps Capsules 1574
Lanoxin Injection 1581
Lanoxin Tablets 1587
Lanoxin Elixir Pediatric 1578
Lanoxin Injection Pediatric 1584

Fosphenytoin Sodium (Co-administration may reduce endogenous plasma levels of 25(OH)D3 by inhibiting 25-hydroxylase in liver; since endogenous synthesis of calcitriol will be inhibited, higher doses of Rocaltrol may be necessary if these drugs are administered simultaneously). Products include:
Cerebyx Injection 2619

Hydrochlorothiazide (Thiazides are known to induce hypercalcemia by the reduction of calcium excretion in urine; co-administration has resulted in hypercalcemia). Products include:
Accuretic Tablets 2614
Aldoril Tablets 2039
Atacand HCT Tablets 597
Avalide Tablets 1070
Diovan HCT Tablets 2338
Dyazide Capsules 1515
HydroDIURIL Tablets 2108
Hyzaar 2109
Inderide Tablets 3517
Inderide LA Long-Acting Capsules 3519
Lotensin HCT Tablets 2367
Maxzide 1008
Micardis HCT Tablets 1051
Microzide Capsules 3414
Moduretic Tablets 2138
Monopril HCT 1094
Prinzide Tablets 2168
Timolide Tablets 2187
Uniretic Tablets 3178
Vaseretic Tablets 2204
Zestoretic Tablets 695
Ziac Tablets 1887

Hydroflumethiazide (Thiazides are known to induce hypercalcemia by the reduction of calcium excretion in urine; co-administration has resulted in hypercalcemia). Products include:
Diucardin Tablets 3494

Ketoconazole (May inhibit both synthetic and catabolic enzymes of calcitriol; reduction in serum endogenous calcitriol concentrations have been observed with co-administration). Products include:
Nizoral 2% Cream 3620
Nizoral A-D Shampoo 2008
Nizoral 2% Shampoo 2007
Nizoral Tablets 1791

Magaldrate (Co-administration with magnesium-containing antacids may lead to the development of hypermagnesemia; magnesium-containing antacids should not be used concomitantly in patients with chronic renal failure).
No products indexed under this heading.

Magnesium Hydroxide (Co-administration with magnesium-containing antacids may lead to the development of hypermagnesemia; magnesium-containing antacids should not be used concomitantly in patients with chronic renal failure). Products include:
Ex•Lax Milk of Magnesia Liquid .... ▣670
Maalox Antacid/Anti-Gas Oral Suspension .... ▣673
Maalox Max Maximum Strength Antacid/Anti-Gas Liquid 2300
Maalox Regular Strength Antacid/Antigas Liquid 2300
Mylanta Fast-Acting 1813
Mylanta 1813
Pepcid Complete Chewable Tablets 1815
Phillips' Chewable Tablets .... ▣615
Phillips' Milk of Magnesia Liquid (Original, Cherry, & Mint) .... ▣616
Rolaids Tablets .... ▣706
Extra Strength Rolaids Tablets .... ▣706
Vanquish Caplets .... ▣617

Magnesium Oxide (Co-administration with magnesium-containing antacids may lead to the development of hypermagnesemia; magnesium-containing antacids should not be used concomitantly in patients with chronic renal failure). Products include:
Beelith Tablets 946
Mag-Ox 400 Tablets 1024
Uro-Mag Capsules 1024

Methyclothiazide (Thiazides are known to induce hypercalcemia by the reduction of calcium excretion in urine; co-administration has resulted in hypercalcemia).
No products indexed under this heading.

Phenobarbital (Co-administration may reduce endogenous plasma levels of 25(OH)D3 by inhibiting 25-hydroxylase in liver; since endogenous synthesis of calcitriol will be inhibited, higher doses of Rocaltrol may be necessary if these drugs are administered simultaneously). Products include:
Arco-Lase Plus Tablets 592
Donnatal 2929
Donnatal Extentabs 2930

Phenytoin (Co-administration may reduce endogenous plasma levels of 25(OH)D3 by inhibiting 25-hydroxylase in liver; since endogenous synthesis of calcitriol will be inhibited, higher doses of Rocaltrol may be necessary if these drugs are administered simultaneously). Products include:
Dilantin Infatabs 2624
Dilantin-125 Oral Suspension 2625

Phenytoin Sodium (Co-administration may reduce endogenous plasma levels of 25(OH)D3 by inhibiting 25-hydroxylase in liver; since endogenous synthesis of calcitriol will be inhibited, higher doses of Rocaltrol may be necessary if these drugs are administered simultaneously). Products include:
Dilantin Kapseals 2622

Polythiazide (Thiazides are known to induce hypercalcemia by the reduction of calcium excretion in urine; co-administration has resulted in hypercalcemia). Products include:
Minizide Capsules 2700
Renese Tablets 2712

Vitamin D (Possible additive effect and hypercalcemia). Products include:
Active Calcium Tablets 3335
Caltrate 600 PLUS .... ▣815
Caltrate 600 + D Tablets .... ▣814
Centrum Focused Formulas Bone Health Tablets .... ▣815
Citracal Caplets + D .... ▣823
D-Cal Chewable Caplets .... ▣794
One-A-Day Calcium Plus Chewable Tablets .... ▣805
Os-Cal 250 + D Tablets .... ▣838
Os-Cal 500 + D Tablets .... ▣839

ROCALTROL ORAL SOLUTION

(Calcitriol) 2991
See Rocaltrol Capsules

ROCEPHIN INJECTABLE VIALS, ADD-VANTAGE, GALAXY, BULK

(Ceftriaxone Sodium) 2993
None cited in PDR database.

ROFERON-A INJECTION

(Interferon alfa-2A, Recombinant) 2996
May interact with theophylline and certain other agents. Compounds in these categories include:

Aldesleukin (Co-administration with interleukin-2 may potentiate risks of renal failure). Products include:
Proleukin for Injection 1199

Aminophylline (Co-administration of interferon alfa-2a with theophylline has been reported to reduce the theophylline clearance).
No products indexed under this heading.

Bone Marrow Depressants, unspecified (Caution should be exercised when administered concomitantly with myelosuppressive agents).

Dyphylline (Co-administration of interferon alfa-2a with theophylline has been reported to reduce the theophylline clearance). Products include:
Lufyllin Tablets 3347
Lufyllin-400 Tablets 3347
Lufyllin-GG Elixir 3348
Lufyllin-GG Tablets 3348

Theophylline (Co-administration of interferon alfa-2a with theophylline has been reported to reduce the theophylline clearance). Products include:
Aerolate 1361
Theo-Dur Extended-Release Tablets 1835
Uni-Dur Extended-Release Tablets 1841
Uniphyl 400 mg and 600 mg Tablets 2903

Theophylline Calcium Salicylate (Co-administration of interferon alfa-2a with theophylline has been reported to reduce the theophylline clearance).
No products indexed under this heading.

Theophylline Sodium Glycinate (Co-administration of interferon alfa-2a with theophylline has been reported to reduce the theophylline clearance).
No products indexed under this heading.

Zidovudine (Co-administration may result in synergistic toxicity, especially hematologic toxicities). Products include:
Combivir Tablets 1502
Retrovir 1625
Retrovir IV Infusion 1629
Trizivir Tablets 1669

ROGAINE EXTRA STRENGTH FOR MEN TOPICAL SOLUTION

(Minoxidil) .... ▣721
None cited in PDR database.

ROGAINE FOR WOMEN TOPICAL SOLUTION

(Minoxidil) .... ▣721
None cited in PDR database.

ROLAIDS TABLETS
(Calcium Carbonate, Magnesium Hydroxide) 706
May interact with:

Drugs, Oral, unspecified (Antacids may interact with certain unspecified prescription drugs).

EXTRA STRENGTH ROLAIDS TABLETS
(Calcium Carbonate, Magnesium Hydroxide) 706
See Rolaids Tablets

ROMAZICON INJECTION
(Flumazenil) 3000
May interact with antidepressant drugs, neuromuscular blocking agents, and certain other agents. Compounds in these categories include:

Amitriptyline Hydrochloride (Toxic effects of cyclic antidepressant may emerge with the reversal of the benzodiazepine effect). Products include:
- Etrafon 3115
- Limbitrol 1738

Amoxapine (Toxic effects of cyclic antidepressant may emerge with the reversal of the benzodiazepine effect).
No products indexed under this heading.

Atracurium Besylate (Romazicon should not be used until the effects of neuromuscular blockade have been fully reversed).
No products indexed under this heading.

Bupropion Hydrochloride (Toxic effects of cyclic antidepressant may emerge with the reversal of the benzodiazepine effect). Products include:
- Wellbutrin Tablets 1680
- Wellbutrin SR Sustained-Release Tablets 1684
- Zyban Sustained-Release Tablets ... 1710

Cisatracurium Besylate (Romazicon should not be used until the effects of neuromuscular blockade have been fully reversed).
No products indexed under this heading.

Citalopram Hydrobromide (Toxic effects of cyclic antidepressant may emerge with the reversal of the benzodiazepine effect). Products include:
- Celexa 1365

Desipramine Hydrochloride (Toxic effects of cyclic antidepressant may emerge with the reversal of the benzodiazepine effect). Products include:
- Norpramin Tablets 755

Doxacurium Chloride (Romazicon should not be used until the effects of neuromuscular blockade have been fully reversed).
No products indexed under this heading.

Doxepin Hydrochloride (Toxic effects of cyclic antidepressant may emerge with the reversal of the benzodiazepine effect). Products include:
- Sinequan 2713

Fluoxetine Hydrochloride (Toxic effects of cyclic antidepressant may emerge with the reversal of the benzodiazepine effect). Products include:
- Prozac Pulvules, Liquid, and Weekly Capsules 1238
- Sarafem Pulvules 1962

Imipramine Hydrochloride (Toxic effects of cyclic antidepressant may emerge with the reversal of the benzodiazepine effect).
No products indexed under this heading.

Imipramine Pamoate (Toxic effects of cyclic antidepressant may emerge with the reversal of the benzodiazepine effect).
No products indexed under this heading.

Isocarboxazid (Toxic effects of cyclic antidepressant may emerge with the reversal of the benzodiazepine effect).
No products indexed under this heading.

Maprotiline Hydrochloride (Toxic effects of cyclic antidepressant may emerge with the reversal of the benzodiazepine effect).
No products indexed under this heading.

Metocurine Iodide (Romazicon should not be used until the effects of neuromuscular blockade have been fully reversed).
No products indexed under this heading.

Mirtazapine (Toxic effects of cyclic antidepressant may emerge with the reversal of the benzodiazepine effect). Products include:
- Remeron Tablets 2483
- Remeron SolTab Tablets 2486

Mivacurium Chloride (Romazicon should not be used until the effects of neuromuscular blockade have been fully reversed).
No products indexed under this heading.

Nefazodone Hydrochloride (Toxic effects of cyclic antidepressant may emerge with the reversal of the benzodiazepine effect). Products include:
- Serzone Tablets 1104

Nortriptyline Hydrochloride (Toxic effects of cyclic antidepressant may emerge with the reversal of the benzodiazepine effect).
No products indexed under this heading.

Pancuronium Bromide (Romazicon should not be used until the effects of neuromuscular blockade have been fully reversed).
No products indexed under this heading.

Paroxetine Hydrochloride (Toxic effects of cyclic antidepressant may emerge with the reversal of the benzodiazepine effect). Products include:
- Paxil 1609

Phenelzine Sulfate (Toxic effects of cyclic antidepressant may emerge with the reversal of the benzodiazepine effect). Products include:
- Nardil Tablets 2653

Protriptyline Hydrochloride (Toxic effects of cyclic antidepressant may emerge with the reversal of the benzodiazepine effect). Products include:
- Vivactil Tablets 2446
- Vivactil Tablets 2217

Rapacuronium Bromide (Romazicon should not be used until the effects of neuromuscular blockade have been fully reversed).
No products indexed under this heading.

Rocuronium Bromide (Romazicon should not be used until the effects of neuromuscular blockade have been fully reversed). Products include:
- Zemuron Injection 2491

Sertraline Hydrochloride (Toxic effects of cyclic antidepressant may emerge with the reversal of the benzodiazepine effect). Products include:
- Zoloft 2751

Succinylcholine Chloride (Romazicon should not be used until the effects of neuromuscular blockade have been fully reversed). Products include:
- Anectine Injection 1476

Tranylcypromine Sulfate (Toxic effects of cyclic antidepressant may emerge with the reversal of the benzodiazepine effect). Products include:
- Parnate Tablets 1607

Trazodone Hydrochloride (Toxic effects of cyclic antidepressant may emerge with the reversal of the benzodiazepine effect).
No products indexed under this heading.

Trimipramine Maleate (Toxic effects of cyclic antidepressant may emerge with the reversal of the benzodiazepine effect). Products include:
- Surmontil Capsules 3595

Vecuronium Bromide (Romazicon should not be used until the effects of neuromuscular blockade have been fully reversed). Products include:
- Norcuron for Injection 2478

Venlafaxine Hydrochloride (Toxic effects of cyclic antidepressant may emerge with the reversal of the benzodiazepine effect). Products include:
- Effexor Tablets 3495
- Effexor XR Capsules 3499

Food Interactions

Alcohol (Concurrent use should be avoided).

ROWASA RECTAL SUSPENSION ENEMA 4.0 GRAMS/UNIT (60 ML)
(Mesalamine) 3264
May interact with:

Sulfasalazine (Patients on concurrent oral products which liberate mesalamine should be carefully monitored with urinalysis). Products include:
- Azulfidine EN-tabs Tablets 2775

ROXANOL 100 CONCENTRATED ORAL SOLUTION
(Morphine Sulfate) 3066
See Roxanol Concentrated Oral Solution

ROXANOL CONCENTRATED ORAL SOLUTION
(Morphine Sulfate) 3066
May interact with antihistamines, barbiturates, central nervous system depressants, oral anticoagulants, hypnotics and sedatives, monoamine oxidase inhibitors, narcotic analgesics, phenothiazines, tricyclic antidepressants, urinary alkalinizing agents, and certain other agents. Compounds in these categories include:

Acrivastine (May enhance the CNS depressant actions of morphine). Products include:
- Semprex-D Capsules 1172

Alfentanil Hydrochloride (May enhance the CNS depressant actions of morphine; respiratory depression, hypotension, and profound sedation or coma may result).
No products indexed under this heading.

Alprazolam (May enhance the CNS depressant actions of morphine; respiratory depression, hypotension, and profound sedation or coma may result). Products include:
- Xanax Tablets 2865

Amitriptyline Hydrochloride (May enhance the CNS depressant actions of morphine; respiratory depression, hypotension, and profound sedation or coma may result). Products include:
- Etrafon 3115
- Limbitrol 1738

Amoxapine (May enhance the CNS depressant actions of morphine; respiratory depression, hypotension, and profound sedation or coma may result).
No products indexed under this heading.

Aprobarbital (May enhance the CNS depressant actions of morphine; respiratory depression, hypotension, and profound sedation or coma may result).
No products indexed under this heading.

Astemizole (May enhance the CNS depressant actions of morphine).
No products indexed under this heading.

Azatadine Maleate (May enhance the CNS depressant actions of morphine). Products include:
- Rynatan Tablets 3351

Bromodiphenhydramine Hydrochloride (May enhance the CNS depressant actions of morphine).
No products indexed under this heading.

Brompheniramine Maleate (May enhance the CNS depressant actions of morphine). Products include:
- Bromfed Capsules (Extended-Release) 2269
- Bromfed-PD Capsules (Extended-Release) 2269
- Comtrex Acute Head Cold & Sinus Pressure Relief Tablets 627
- Dimetapp Elixir 777
- Dimetapp Cold and Fever Suspension 775
- Dimetapp DM Cold & Cough Elixir .. 775
- Dimetapp Nighttime Flu Liquid 776

Buprenorphine Hydrochloride (May enhance the CNS depressant actions of morphine; respiratory depression, hypotension, and profound sedation or coma may result). Products include:
- Buprenex Injectable 2918

Buspirone Hydrochloride (May enhance the CNS depressant actions of morphine; respiratory depression, hypotension, and profound sedation or coma may result).
No products indexed under this heading.

Butabarbital (May enhance the CNS depressant actions of morphine; respiratory depression, hypotension, and profound sedation or coma may result).
No products indexed under this heading.

Butalbital (May enhance the CNS depressant actions of morphine; respiratory depression, hypotension, and profound sedation or coma may result). Products include:
- Phrenilin 578
- Sedapap Tablets 50 mg/650 mg ... 2225

Cetirizine Hydrochloride (May enhance the CNS depressant actions of morphine). Products include:
- Zyrtec 2756
- Zyrtec-D 12 Hour Extended Relief Tablets 2758

Chloral Hydrate (May enhance the CNS depressant actions of morphine).
No products indexed under this heading.

Chlordiazepoxide (May enhance the CNS depressant actions of morphine; respiratory depression, hypotension, and profound sedation or coma may result). Products include:
- Limbitrol 1738

Chlordiazepoxide Hydrochloride (May enhance the CNS depressant actions of morphine; respiratory

depression, hypotension, and profound sedation or coma may result). Products include:
- Librium Capsules 1736
- Librium for Injection 1737

Chlorpheniramine Maleate (May enhance the CNS depressant actions of morphine). Products include:
- Actifed Cold & Sinus Caplets and Tablets .... ▣688
- Alka-Seltzer Plus Liqui-Gels .... ▣604
- BC Allergy Sinus Cold Powder .... ▣619
- Chlor-Trimeton Allergy Tablets .... ▣735
- Chlor-Trimeton Allergy/Decongestant Tablets .... ▣736
- Comtrex Flu Therapy & Fever Relief Nighttime Tablets .... ▣628
- Comtrex Maximum Strength Multi-Symptom Cold & Cough Relief Tablets and Caplets .... ▣626
- Contac Severe Cold and Flu Caplets Maximum Strength .... ▣746
- Coricidin 'D' Cold, Flu & Sinus Tablets .... ▣737
- Coricidin/Coricidin D .... ▣738
- Coricidin HBP Maximum Strength Flu Tablets .... ▣738
- Extendryl 1361
- Hycomine Compound Tablets 1317
- Kronofed-A 1341
- PediaCare Cough-Cold Liquid .... ▣719
- PediaCare NightRest Cough-Cold Liquid .... ▣719
- Robitussin Nighttime Honey Flu Liquid .... ▣786
- Ryna .... ▣768
- Singlet Caplets .... ▣761
- Sinutab Sinus Allergy Medication, Maximum Strength Formula, Tablets & Caplets .... ▣707
- Sudafed Cold & Allergy Tablets .... ▣708
- TheraFlu Regular Strength Cold & Cough Night Time Hot Liquid .... ▣676
- TheraFlu Regular Strength Cold & Sore Throat Night Time Hot Liquid .... ▣676
- TheraFlu Maximum Strength Flu & Cough Night Time Hot Liquid .... ▣678
- TheraFlu Maximum Strength Flu & Sore Throat Night Time Hot Liquid .... ▣677
- TheraFlu Maximum Strength Severe Cold & Congestion Night Time Caplets .... ▣678
- TheraFlu Maximum Strength Severe Cold & Congestion Night Time Hot Liquid .... ▣678
- Triaminic Cold & Allergy Liquid .... ▣681
- Triaminic Cold & Allergy Softchews .... ▣683
- Triaminic Cold & Cough Liquid .... ▣681
- Triaminic Cold & Cough Softchews .... ▣683
- Triaminic Cold & Night Time Cough Liquid .... ▣681
- Triaminic Cold, Cough & Fever Liquid .... ▣681
- Children's Tylenol Cold Suspension Liquid and Chewable Tablets 2015
- Children's Tylenol Cold Plus Cough Suspension Liquid and Chewable Tablets 2015
- Children's Tylenol Flu Suspension Liquid 2015
- Maximum Strength Tylenol Allergy Sinus Caplets, Gelcaps, and Geltabs 2010
- Multi-Symptom Tylenol Cold Complete Formula Caplets 2010
- Vicks 44M Cough, Cold & Flu Relief Liquid .... ▣725
- Pediatric Vicks 44m Cough & Cold Relief .... ▣728
- Children's Vicks NyQuil Cold/Cough Relief .... ▣726

Chlorpheniramine Polistirex (May enhance the CNS depressant actions of morphine). Products include:
- Tussionex Pennkinetic Extended-Release Suspension 1174

Chlorpheniramine Tannate (May enhance the CNS depressant actions of morphine). Products include:
- Reformulated Rynatan Pediatric Suspension 3352
- Rynatuss Pediatric Suspension 3353
- Rynatuss Tablets 3353
- Tussi-12 S Suspension 3356
- Tussi-12 Tablets 3356

Chlorpromazine (Potentiates analgesic effect of morphine; may enhance the CNS depressant actions of morphine; respiratory depression, hypotension, and profound sedation or coma may result). Products include:
- Thorazine Suppositories 1656

Chlorpromazine Hydrochloride (Potentiates analgesic effect of morphine; may enhance the CNS depressant actions of morphine; respiratory depression, hypotension, and profound sedation or coma may result). Products include:
- Thorazine 1656

Chlorprothixene (May enhance the CNS depressant actions of morphine; respiratory depression, hypotension, and profound sedation or coma may result).
No products indexed under this heading.

Chlorprothixene Hydrochloride (May enhance the CNS depressant actions of morphine; respiratory depression, hypotension, and profound sedation or coma may result).
No products indexed under this heading.

Chlorprothixene Lactate (May enhance the CNS depressant actions of morphine; respiratory depression, hypotension, and profound sedation or coma may result).
No products indexed under this heading.

Clemastine Fumarate (May enhance the CNS depressant actions of morphine). Products include:
- Tavist 12 Hour Allergy Tablets .... ▣676

Clomipramine Hydrochloride (May enhance the CNS depressant actions of morphine; respiratory depression, hypotension, and profound sedation or coma may result).
No products indexed under this heading.

Clorazepate Dipotassium (May enhance the CNS depressant actions of morphine; respiratory depression, hypotension, and profound sedation or coma may result). Products include:
- Tranxene 511

Clozapine (May enhance the CNS depressant actions of morphine; respiratory depression, hypotension, and profound sedation or coma may result). Products include:
- Clozaril Tablets 2319

Codeine Phosphate (May enhance the CNS depressant actions of morphine; respiratory depression, hypotension, and profound sedation or coma may result). Products include:
- Phenergan with Codeine Syrup 3557
- Phenergan VC with Codeine Syrup 3561
- Robitussin A-C Syrup 2942
- Robitussin-DAC Syrup 2942
- Ryna-C Liquid .... ▣768
- Soma Compound w/Codeine Tablets 3355
- Tussi-Organidin NR Liquid 3350
- Tussi-Organidin-S NR Liquid 3350
- Tylenol with Codeine 2595

Cyproheptadine Hydrochloride (May enhance the CNS depressant actions of morphine). Products include:
- Periactin Tablets 2155

Desflurane (May enhance the CNS depressant actions of morphine; respiratory depression, hypotension, and profound sedation or coma may result). Products include:
- Suprane Liquid for Inhalation 874

Desipramine Hydrochloride (May enhance the CNS depressant actions of morphine; respiratory depression, hypotension, and profound sedation or coma may result). Products include:
- Norpramin Tablets 755

Dexchlorpheniramine Maleate (May enhance the CNS depressant actions of morphine).
No products indexed under this heading.

Dezocine (May enhance the CNS depressant actions of morphine; respiratory depression, hypotension, and profound sedation or coma may result).
No products indexed under this heading.

Diazepam (May enhance the CNS depressant actions of morphine; respiratory depression, hypotension, and profound sedation or coma may result). Products include:
- Valium Injectable 3026
- Valium Tablets 3047

Dicumarol (Morphine may increase anticoagulant activity of coumarins and other anticoagulants).
No products indexed under this heading.

Diphenhydramine Citrate (May enhance the CNS depressant actions of morphine). Products include:
- Alka-Seltzer PM Effervescent Tablets .... ▣605
- Benadryl Allergy & Sinus Fastmelt Tablets .... ▣693
- Benadryl Children's Allergy/Cold Fastmelt Tablets .... ▣692
- Excedrin PM Tablets, Caplets, and Geltabs .... ▣631
- Goody's PM Powder .... ▣621

Diphenhydramine Hydrochloride (May enhance the CNS depressant actions of morphine). Products include:
- Extra Strength Bayer PM Caplets .... ▣611
- Benadryl Allergy Chewables .... ▣689
- Benadryl Allergy .... ▣691
- Benadryl Allergy Liquid .... ▣690
- Benadryl Allergy/Cold Tablets .... ▣691
- Benadryl Allergy/Congestion Tablets .... ▣692
- Benadryl Allergy & Sinus Liquid .... ▣693
- Benadryl Allergy Sinus Headache Caplets & Gelcaps .... ▣693
- Benadryl Severe Allergy & Sinus Headache Caplets .... ▣694
- Benadryl Dye-Free Allergy Liquid .... ▣690
- Benadryl Dye-Free Allergy Liqui-Gels Softgels .... ▣690
- Benadryl Itch Relief Stick Extra Strength .... ▣695
- Benadryl Cream .... ▣695
- Benadryl Gel .... ▣695
- Benadryl Spray .... ▣696
- Benadryl Parenteral 2617
- Coricidin HBP Night-Time Cold & Flu Tablets .... ▣738
- Nytol QuickCaps Caplets .... ▣622
- Maximum Strength Nytol QuickGels Softgels .... ▣621
- Extra Strength Percogesic Aspirin-Free Coated Caplets .... ▣665
- Simply Sleep Caplets 2008
- Sominex Original Formula Tablets .... ▣761
- Children's Tylenol Allergy-D Liquid 2014
- Maximum Strength Tylenol Allergy Sinus NightTime Caplets 2010
- Tylenol Severe Allergy Caplets 2010
- Maximum Strength Tylenol Flu NightTime Gelcaps 2011
- Extra Strength Tylenol PM Caplets, Geltabs, and Gelcaps 2012
- Unisom Maximum Strength SleepGels .... ▣713

Diphenylpyraline Hydrochloride (May enhance the CNS depressant actions of morphine).
No products indexed under this heading.

Doxepin Hydrochloride (May enhance the CNS depressant actions of morphine; respiratory depression, hypotension, and profound sedation or coma may result). Products include:
- Sinequan 2713

Droperidol (May enhance the CNS depressant actions of morphine; respiratory depression, hypotension, and profound sedation or coma may result).
No products indexed under this heading.

Enflurane (May enhance the CNS depressant actions of morphine; respiratory depression, hypotension, and profound sedation or coma may result).
No products indexed under this heading.

Estazolam (May enhance the CNS depressant actions of morphine; respiratory depression, hypotension, and profound sedation or coma may result). Products include:
- ProSom Tablets 500

Ethchlorvynol (May enhance the CNS depressant actions of morphine; respiratory depression, hypotension, and profound sedation or coma may result).
No products indexed under this heading.

Ethinamate (May enhance the CNS depressant actions of morphine; respiratory depression, hypotension, and profound sedation or coma may result).
No products indexed under this heading.

Fentanyl (May enhance the CNS depressant actions of morphine; respiratory depression, hypotension, and profound sedation or coma may result). Products include:
- Duragesic Transdermal System 1786

Fentanyl Citrate (May enhance the CNS depressant actions of morphine; respiratory depression, hypotension, and profound sedation or coma may result). Products include:
- Actiq 1184

Fexofenadine Hydrochloride (May enhance the CNS depressant actions of morphine). Products include:
- Allegra 712
- Allegra-D Extended-Release Tablets 714

Fluphenazine Decanoate (May enhance the CNS depressant actions of morphine; respiratory depression, hypotension, and profound sedation or coma may result).
No products indexed under this heading.

Fluphenazine Enanthate (May enhance the CNS depressant actions of morphine; respiratory depression, hypotension, and profound sedation or coma may result).
No products indexed under this heading.

Fluphenazine Hydrochloride (May enhance the CNS depressant actions of morphine; respiratory depression, hypotension, and profound sedation or coma may result).
No products indexed under this heading.

Flurazepam Hydrochloride (May enhance the CNS depressant actions of morphine; respiratory depression, hypotension, and profound sedation or coma may result).
No products indexed under this heading.

Furazolidone (May enhance the CNS depressant actions of morphine).
No products indexed under this heading.

Glutethimide (May enhance the CNS depressant actions of morphine; respiratory depression, hypotension, and profound sedation or coma may result).
No products indexed under this heading.

Haloperidol (May enhance the CNS depressant actions of morphine; respiratory depression, hypotension, and profound sedation or coma may result). Products include:
- Haldol Injection, Tablets and Concentrate 2533

Haloperidol Decanoate (May enhance the CNS depressant actions of morphine; respiratory depression,

hypotension, and profound sedation or coma may result). Products include:

- Haldol Decanoate 2535

Hydrocodone Bitartrate (May enhance the CNS depressant actions of morphine; respiratory depression, hypotension, and profound sedation or coma may result). Products include:

- Hycodan 1316
- Hycomine Compound Tablets 1317
- Hycotuss Expectorant Syrup 1318
- Lortab 3319
- Lortab Elixir 3317
- Maxidone Tablets CIII 3399
- Norco 5/325 Tablets CIII 3424
- Norco 7.5/325 Tablets CIII 3425
- Norco 10/325 Tablets CIII 3427
- Norco 10/325 Tablets CIII 3425
- Vicodin Tablets 516
- Vicodin ES Tablets 517
- Vicodin HP Tablets 518
- Vicodin Tuss Expectorant 519
- Vicoprofen Tablets 520
- Zydone Tablets 1330

Hydrocodone Polistirex (May enhance the CNS depressant actions of morphine; respiratory depression, hypotension, and profound sedation or coma may result). Products include:

- Tussionex Pennkinetic Extended-Release Suspension 1174

Hydromorphone Hydrochloride (May enhance the CNS depressant actions of morphine; respiratory depression, hypotension, and profound sedation or coma may result). Products include:

- Dilaudid 441
- Dilaudid Oral Liquid 445
- Dilaudid Powder 441
- Dilaudid Rectal Suppositories 441
- Dilaudid Tablets 441
- Dilaudid Tablets - 8 mg 445
- Dilaudid-HP 443

Hydroxyzine Hydrochloride (May enhance the CNS depressant actions of morphine; respiratory depression, hypotension, and profound sedation or coma may result). Products include:

- Atarax Tablets & Syrup 2667
- Vistaril Intramuscular Solution 2738

Imipramine Hydrochloride (May enhance the CNS depressant actions of morphine; respiratory depression, hypotension, and profound sedation or coma may result).

No products indexed under this heading.

Imipramine Pamoate (May enhance the CNS depressant actions of morphine; respiratory depression, hypotension, and profound sedation or coma may result).

No products indexed under this heading.

Isocarboxazid (May enhance the CNS depressant actions of morphine).

No products indexed under this heading.

Isoflurane (May enhance the CNS depressant actions of morphine; respiratory depression, hypotension, and profound sedation or coma may result).

No products indexed under this heading.

Ketamine Hydrochloride (May enhance the CNS depressant actions of morphine; respiratory depression, hypotension, and profound sedation or coma may result).

No products indexed under this heading.

Levomethadyl Acetate Hydrochloride (May enhance the CNS depressant actions of morphine; respiratory depression, hypotension, and profound sedation or coma may result).

No products indexed under this heading.

Levorphanol Tartrate (May enhance the CNS depressant actions of morphine; respiratory depression, hypotension, and profound sedation or coma may result). Products include:

- Levo-Dromoran 1734
- Levorphanol Tartrate Tablets 3059

Loratadine (May enhance the CNS depressant actions of morphine). Products include:

- Claritin 3100
- Claritin-D 12 Hour Extended Release Tablets 3102
- Claritin-D 24 Hour Extended Release Tablets 3104

Lorazepam (May enhance the CNS depressant actions of morphine; respiratory depression, hypotension, and profound sedation or coma may result). Products include:

- Ativan Injection 3478
- Ativan Tablets 3482

Loxapine Hydrochloride (May enhance the CNS depressant actions of morphine; respiratory depression, hypotension, and profound sedation or coma may result).

No products indexed under this heading.

Loxapine Succinate (May enhance the CNS depressant actions of morphine; respiratory depression, hypotension, and profound sedation or coma may result). Products include:

- Loxitane Capsules 3398

Maprotiline Hydrochloride (May enhance the CNS depressant actions of morphine; respiratory depression, hypotension, and profound sedation or coma may result).

No products indexed under this heading.

Meperidine Hydrochloride (May enhance the CNS depressant actions of morphine; respiratory depression, hypotension, and profound sedation or coma may result). Products include:

- Demerol 3079
- Mepergan Injection 3539

Mephobarbital (May enhance the CNS depressant actions of morphine; respiratory depression, hypotension, and profound sedation or coma may result).

No products indexed under this heading.

Meprobamate (May enhance the CNS depressant actions of morphine; respiratory depression, hypotension, and profound sedation or coma may result). Products include:

- Miltown Tablets 3349

Mesoridazine Besylate (May enhance the CNS depressant actions of morphine; respiratory depression, hypotension, and profound sedation or coma may result). Products include:

- Serentil 1057

Methadone Hydrochloride (May enhance the CNS depressant actions of morphine; respiratory depression, hypotension, and profound sedation or coma may result). Products include:

- Dolophine Hydrochloride Tablets 3056

Methdilazine Hydrochloride (May enhance the CNS depressant actions of morphine).

No products indexed under this heading.

Methocarbamol (Potentiates analgesic effect of morphine). Products include:

- Robaxin Injectable 2938
- Robaxin Tablets 2939
- Robaxisal Tablets 2939

Methohexital Sodium (May enhance the CNS depressant actions of morphine; respiratory depression, hypotension, and profound sedation or coma may result). Products include:

- Brevital Sodium for Injection, USP 1815

Methotrimeprazine (May enhance the CNS depressant actions of morphine; respiratory depression, hypotension, and profound sedation or coma may result).

No products indexed under this heading.

Methoxyflurane (May enhance the CNS depressant actions of morphine; respiratory depression, hypotension, and profound sedation or coma may result).

No products indexed under this heading.

Midazolam Hydrochloride (May enhance the CNS depressant actions of morphine; respiratory depression, hypotension, and profound sedation or coma may result). Products include:

- Versed Injection 3027
- Versed Syrup 3033

Moclobemide (May enhance the CNS depressant actions of morphine).

No products indexed under this heading.

Molindone Hydrochloride (May enhance the CNS depressant actions of morphine; respiratory depression, hypotension, and profound sedation or coma may result). Products include:

- Moban 1320

Nortriptyline Hydrochloride (May enhance the CNS depressant actions of morphine; respiratory depression, hypotension, and profound sedation or coma may result).

No products indexed under this heading.

Olanzapine (May enhance the CNS depressant actions of morphine; respiratory depression, hypotension, and profound sedation or coma may result). Products include:

- Zyprexa Tablets 1973
- Zyprexa ZYDIS Orally Disintegrating Tablets 1973

Oxazepam (May enhance the CNS depressant actions of morphine; respiratory depression, hypotension, and profound sedation or coma may result).

No products indexed under this heading.

Oxycodone Hydrochloride (May enhance the CNS depressant actions of morphine; respiratory depression, hypotension, and profound sedation or coma may result). Products include:

- OxyContin Tablets 2912
- OxyFast Oral Concentrate Solution 2916
- OxyIR Capsules 2916
- Percocet Tablets 1326
- Percodan Tablets 1327
- Percolone Tablets 1327
- Roxicodone 3067
- Tylox Capsules 2597

Pargyline Hydrochloride (May enhance the CNS depressant actions of morphine).

No products indexed under this heading.

Pentobarbital Sodium (May enhance the CNS depressant actions of morphine; respiratory depression, hypotension, and profound sedation or coma may result). Products include:

- Nembutal Sodium Solution 485

Perphenazine (May enhance the CNS depressant actions of morphine; respiratory depression, hypotension, and profound sedation or coma may result). Products include:

- Etrafon 3115
- Trilafon 3160

Phenelzine Sulfate (May enhance the CNS depressant actions of morphine). Products include:

- Nardil Tablets 2653

Phenobarbital (May enhance the CNS depressant actions of morphine; respiratory depression, hypotension, and profound sedation or coma may result). Products include:

- Arco-Lase Plus Tablets 592
- Donnatal 2929
- Donnatal Extentabs 2930

Potassium Acid Phosphate (Effects of morphine may be antagonized by acidifying agents). Products include:

- K-Phos Original (Sodium Free) Tablets 947

Potassium Citrate (Effects of morphine may be potentiated by alkalizing agents). Products include:

- Urocit-K Tablets 2232

Prazepam (May enhance the CNS depressant actions of morphine; respiratory depression, hypotension, and profound sedation or coma may result).

No products indexed under this heading.

Procarbazine Hydrochloride (May enhance the CNS depressant actions of morphine). Products include:

- Matulane Capsules 3246

Prochlorperazine (May enhance the CNS depressant actions of morphine; respiratory depression, hypotension, and profound sedation or coma may result). Products include:

- Compazine 1505

Promethazine Hydrochloride (May enhance the CNS depressant actions of morphine; respiratory depression, hypotension, and profound sedation or coma may result). Products include:

- Mepergan Injection 3539
- Phenergan Injection 3553
- Phenergan 3556
- Phenergan Syrup 3554
- Phenergan with Codeine Syrup 3557
- Phenergan with Dextromethorphan Syrup 3559
- Phenergan VC Syrup 3560
- Phenergan VC with Codeine Syrup 3561

Propofol (May enhance the CNS depressant actions of morphine; respiratory depression, hypotension, and profound sedation or coma may result). Products include:

- Diprivan Injectable Emulsion 667

Propoxyphene Hydrochloride (May enhance the CNS depressant actions of morphine; respiratory depression, hypotension, and profound sedation or coma may result). Products include:

- Darvon Pulvules 1909
- Darvon Compound-65 Pulvules 1910

Propoxyphene Napsylate (May enhance the CNS depressant actions of morphine; respiratory depression, hypotension, and profound sedation or coma may result). Products include:

- Darvon-N/Darvocet-N 1907
- Darvon-N Tablets 1912

Propranolol Hydrochloride (May enhance the CNS depressant actions of morphine). Products include:

- Inderal 3513
- Inderal LA Long-Acting Capsules 3516
- Inderide Tablets 3517
- Inderide LA Long-Acting Capsules 3519

Protriptyline Hydrochloride (May enhance the CNS depressant actions of morphine; respiratory depression, hypotension, and profound sedation or coma may result). Products include:

- Vivactil Tablets 2446
- Vivactil Tablets 2217

Pyrilamine Maleate (May enhance the CNS depressant actions of morphine). Products include:

- Maximum Strength Midol Menstrual Caplets and Gelcaps .... ▣612
- Maximum Strength Midol PMS Caplets and Gelcaps .... ▣613

IMPORTANT NOTE: Always consult each drug listing in the patient's regimen for possible interactions.

Pyrilamine Tannate (May enhance the CNS depressant actions of morphine). Products include:
Ryna-12 S Suspension 3351
Quazepam (May enhance the CNS depressant actions of morphine; respiratory depression, hypotension, and profound sedation or coma may result).
No products indexed under this heading.
Quetiapine Fumarate (May enhance the CNS depressant actions of morphine; respiratory depression, hypotension, and profound sedation or coma may result). Products include:
Seroquel Tablets 684
Remifentanil Hydrochloride (May enhance the CNS depressant actions of morphine; respiratory depression, hypotension, and profound sedation or coma may result).
No products indexed under this heading.
Risperidone (May enhance the CNS depressant actions of morphine; respiratory depression, hypotension, and profound sedation or coma may result). Products include:
Risperdal 1796
Secobarbital Sodium (May enhance the CNS depressant actions of morphine; respiratory depression, hypotension, and profound sedation or coma may result).
No products indexed under this heading.
Selegiline Hydrochloride (May enhance the CNS depressant actions of morphine). Products include:
Eldepryl Capsules 3266
Sevoflurane (May enhance the CNS depressant actions of morphine; respiratory depression, hypotension, and profound sedation or coma may result).
No products indexed under this heading.
Sodium Citrate (Effects of morphine may be potentiated by alkalizing agents).
No products indexed under this heading.
Sufentanil Citrate (May enhance the CNS depressant actions of morphine; respiratory depression, hypotension, and profound sedation or coma may result).
No products indexed under this heading.
Temazepam (May enhance the CNS depressant actions of morphine; respiratory depression, hypotension, and profound sedation or coma may result).
No products indexed under this heading.
Terfenadine (May enhance the CNS depressant actions of morphine).
No products indexed under this heading.
Thiamylal Sodium (May enhance the CNS depressant actions of morphine; respiratory depression, hypotension, and profound sedation or coma may result).
No products indexed under this heading.
Thioridazine Hydrochloride (May enhance the CNS depressant actions of morphine; respiratory depression, hypotension, and profound sedation or coma may result). Products include:
Thioridazine Hydrochloride Tablets 2289
Thiothixene (May enhance the CNS depressant actions of morphine; respiratory depression, hypotension, and profound sedation or coma may result). Products include:
Navane Capsules 2701
Thiothixene Capsules 2290
Tranylcypromine Sulfate (May enhance the CNS depressant actions of morphine). Products include:
Parnate Tablets 1607
Triazolam (May enhance the CNS depressant actions of morphine; respiratory depression, hypotension, and profound sedation or coma may result). Products include:
Halcion Tablets 2823
Trifluoperazine Hydrochloride (May enhance the CNS depressant actions of morphine; respiratory depression, hypotension, and profound sedation or coma may result). Products include:
Stelazine 1640
Trimeprazine Tartrate (May enhance the CNS depressant actions of morphine).
No products indexed under this heading.
Trimipramine Maleate (May enhance the CNS depressant actions of morphine; respiratory depression, hypotension, and profound sedation or coma may result). Products include:
Surmontil Capsules 3595
Tripelennamine Hydrochloride (May enhance the CNS depressant actions of morphine).
No products indexed under this heading.
Triprolidine Hydrochloride (May enhance the CNS depressant actions of morphine). Products include:
Actifed Cold & Allergy Tablets .... ▣688
Warfarin Sodium (Morphine may increase anticoagulant activity of coumarins and other anticoagulants). Products include:
Coumadin for Injection 1243
Coumadin Tablets 1243
Warfarin Sodium Tablets, USP 3302
Zaleplon (May enhance the CNS depressant actions of morphine; respiratory depression, hypotension, and profound sedation or coma may result). Products include:
Sonata Capsules 3591
Ziprasidone Hydrochloride (May enhance the CNS depressant actions of morphine; respiratory depression, hypotension, and profound sedation or coma may result). Products include:
Geodon Capsules 2688
Zolpidem Tartrate (May enhance the CNS depressant actions of morphine; respiratory depression, hypotension, and profound sedation or coma may result). Products include:
Ambien Tablets 3191

Food Interactions

Alcohol (May enhance the CNS depressant actions of morphine).

ROXANOL-T ORAL SOLUTION

(Morphine Sulfate) 3066
See Roxanol Concentrated Oral Solution

ROXICODONE INTENSOL

(Oxycodone Hydrochloride) 3067
May interact with central nervous system depressants and certain other agents. Compounds in these categories include:

Alfentanil Hydrochloride (Possible additive CNS depression).
No products indexed under this heading.
Alprazolam (Possible additive CNS depression). Products include:
Xanax Tablets 2865
Aprobarbital (Possible additive CNS depression).
No products indexed under this heading.
Buprenorphine Hydrochloride (Possible additive CNS depression). Products include:
Buprenex Injectable 2918
Buspirone Hydrochloride (Possible additive CNS depression).
No products indexed under this heading.
Butabarbital (Possible additive CNS depression).
No products indexed under this heading.
Butalbital (Possible additive CNS depression). Products include:
Phrenilin 578
Sedapap Tablets 50 mg/650 mg ... 2225
Chlordiazepoxide (Possible additive CNS depression). Products include:
Limbitrol 1738
Chlordiazepoxide Hydrochloride (Possible additive CNS depression). Products include:
Librium Capsules 1736
Librium for Injection 1737
Chlorpromazine (Possible additive CNS depression). Products include:
Thorazine Suppositories 1656
Chlorpromazine Hydrochloride (Possible additive CNS depression). Products include:
Thorazine 1656
Chlorprothixene (Possible additive CNS depression).
No products indexed under this heading.
Chlorprothixene Hydrochloride (Possible additive CNS depression).
No products indexed under this heading.
Chlorprothixene Lactate (Possible additive CNS depression).
No products indexed under this heading.
Clorazepate Dipotassium (Possible additive CNS depression). Products include:
Tranxene 511
Clozapine (Possible additive CNS depression). Products include:
Clozaril Tablets 2319
Codeine Phosphate (Possible additive CNS depression). Products include:
Phenergan with Codeine Syrup 3557
Phenergan VC with Codeine Syrup .. 3561
Robitussin A-C Syrup 2942
Robitussin-DAC Syrup 2942
Ryna-C Liquid .... ▣768
Soma Compound w/Codeine Tablets 3355
Tussi-Organidin NR Liquid 3350
Tussi-Organidin-S NR Liquid 3350
Tylenol with Codeine 2595
Desflurane (Possible additive CNS depression). Products include:
Suprane Liquid for Inhalation 874
Dezocine (Possible additive CNS depression).
No products indexed under this heading.
Diazepam (Possible additive CNS depression). Products include:
Valium Injectable 3026
Valium Tablets 3047
Droperidol (Possible additive CNS depression).
No products indexed under this heading.
Enflurane (Possible additive CNS depression).
No products indexed under this heading.
Estazolam (Possible additive CNS depression). Products include:
ProSom Tablets 500
Ethchlorvynol (Possible additive CNS depression).
No products indexed under this heading.
Ethinamate (Possible additive CNS depression).
No products indexed under this heading.
Fentanyl (Possible additive CNS depression). Products include:
Duragesic Transdermal System 1786
Fentanyl Citrate (Possible additive CNS depression). Products include:
Actiq 1184
Fluphenazine Decanoate (Possible additive CNS depression).
No products indexed under this heading.
Fluphenazine Enanthate (Possible additive CNS depression).
No products indexed under this heading.
Fluphenazine Hydrochloride (Possible additive CNS depression).
No products indexed under this heading.
Flurazepam Hydrochloride (Possible additive CNS depression).
No products indexed under this heading.
Glutethimide (Possible additive CNS depression).
No products indexed under this heading.
Haloperidol (Possible additive CNS depression). Products include:
Haldol Injection, Tablets and Concentrate 2533
Haloperidol Decanoate (Possible additive CNS depression). Products include:
Haldol Decanoate 2535
Hydrocodone Bitartrate (Possible additive CNS depression). Products include:
Hycodan 1316
Hycomine Compound Tablets 1317
Hycotuss Expectorant Syrup 1318
Lortab 3319
Lortab Elixir 3317
Maxidone Tablets CIII 3399
Norco 5/325 Tablets CIII 3424
Norco 7.5/325 Tablets CIII 3425
Norco 10/325 Tablets CIII 3427
Norco 10/325 Tablets CIII 3425
Vicodin Tablets 516
Vicodin ES Tablets 517
Vicodin HP Tablets 518
Vicodin Tuss Expectorant 519
Vicoprofen Tablets 520
Zydone Tablets 1330
Hydrocodone Polistirex (Possible additive CNS depression). Products include:
Tussionex Pennkinetic Extended-Release Suspension..... 1174
Hydromorphone Hydrochloride (Possible additive CNS depression). Products include:
Dilaudid 441
Dilaudid Oral Liquid 445
Dilaudid Powder 441
Dilaudid Rectal Suppositories 441
Dilaudid Tablets 441
Dilaudid Tablets - 8 mg 445
Dilaudid-HP 443
Hydroxyzine Hydrochloride (Possible additive CNS depression). Products include:
Atarax Tablets & Syrup 2667
Vistaril Intramuscular Solution 2738
Isoflurane (Possible additive CNS depression).
No products indexed under this heading.
Ketamine Hydrochloride (Possible additive CNS depression).
No products indexed under this heading.
Levomethadyl Acetate Hydrochloride (Possible additive CNS depression).
No products indexed under this heading.
Levorphanol Tartrate (Possible additive CNS depression). Products include:
Levo-Dromoran 1734
Levorphanol Tartrate Tablets 3059
Lorazepam (Possible additive CNS depression). Products include:
Ativan Injection 3478
Ativan Tablets 3482

Loxapine Hydrochloride (Possible additive CNS depression).
No products indexed under this heading.

Loxapine Succinate (Possible additive CNS depression). Products include:
Loxitane Capsules 3398

Meperidine Hydrochloride (Possible additive CNS depression). Products include:
Demerol 3079
Mepergan Injection 3539

Mephobarbital (Possible additive CNS depression).
No products indexed under this heading.

Meprobamate (Possible additive CNS depression). Products include:
Miltown Tablets 3349

Mesoridazine Besylate (Possible additive CNS depression). Products include:
Serentil 1057

Methadone Hydrochloride (Possible additive CNS depression). Products include:
Dolophine Hydrochloride Tablets 3056

Methohexital Sodium (Possible additive CNS depression). Products include:
Brevital Sodium for Injection, USP 1815

Methotrimeprazine (Possible additive CNS depression).
No products indexed under this heading.

Methoxyflurane (Possible additive CNS depression).
No products indexed under this heading.

Midazolam Hydrochloride (Possible additive CNS depression). Products include:
Versed Injection 3027
Versed Syrup 3033

Molindone Hydrochloride (Possible additive CNS depression). Products include:
Moban 1320

Morphine Sulfate (Possible additive CNS depression). Products include:
Astramorph/PF Injection, USP (Preservative-Free) 594
Duramorph Injection 1312
Infumorph 200 and Infumorph 500 Sterile Solutions 1314
Kadian Capsules 1335
MS Contin Tablets 2896
MSIR 2898
Oramorph SR Tablets 3062
Roxanol 3066

Olanzapine (Possible additive CNS depression). Products include:
Zyprexa Tablets 1973
Zyprexa ZYDIS Orally Disintegrating Tablets 1973

Oxazepam (Possible additive CNS depression).
No products indexed under this heading.

Pentobarbital Sodium (Possible additive CNS depression). Products include:
Nembutal Sodium Solution 485

Perphenazine (Possible additive CNS depression). Products include:
Etrafon 3115
Trilafon 3160

Phenobarbital (Possible additive CNS depression). Products include:
Arco-Lase Plus Tablets 592
Donnatal 2929
Donnatal Extentabs 2930

Prazepam (Possible additive CNS depression).
No products indexed under this heading.

Prochlorperazine (Possible additive CNS depression). Products include:
Compazine 1505

Promethazine Hydrochloride (Possible additive CNS depression). Products include:
Mepergan Injection 3539
Phenergan Injection 3553
Phenergan 3556
Phenergan Syrup 3554
Phenergan with Codeine Syrup 3557
Phenergan with Dextromethorphan Syrup 3559
Phenergan VC Syrup 3560
Phenergan VC with Codeine Syrup 3561

Propofol (Possible additive CNS depression). Products include:
Diprivan Injectable Emulsion 667

Propoxyphene Hydrochloride (Possible additive CNS depression). Products include:
Darvon Pulvules 1909
Darvon Compound-65 Pulvules 1910

Propoxyphene Napsylate (Possible additive CNS depression). Products include:
Darvon-N/Darvocet-N 1907
Darvon-N Tablets 1912

Quazepam (Possible additive CNS depression).
No products indexed under this heading.

Quetiapine Fumarate (Possible additive CNS depression). Products include:
Seroquel Tablets 684

Remifentanil Hydrochloride (Possible additive CNS depression).
No products indexed under this heading.

Risperidone (Possible additive CNS depression). Products include:
Risperdal 1796

Secobarbital Sodium (Possible additive CNS depression).
No products indexed under this heading.

Sevoflurane (Possible additive CNS depression).
No products indexed under this heading.

Sufentanil Citrate (Possible additive CNS depression).
No products indexed under this heading.

Temazepam (Possible additive CNS depression).
No products indexed under this heading.

Thiamylal Sodium (Possible additive CNS depression).
No products indexed under this heading.

Thioridazine Hydrochloride (Possible additive CNS depression). Products include:
Thioridazine Hydrochloride Tablets 2289

Thiothixene (Possible additive CNS depression). Products include:
Navane Capsules 2701
Thiothixene Capsules 2290

Triazolam (Possible additive CNS depression). Products include:
Halcion Tablets 2823

Trifluoperazine Hydrochloride (Possible additive CNS depression). Products include:
Stelazine 1640

Zaleplon (Possible additive CNS depression). Products include:
Sonata Capsules 3591

Ziprasidone Hydrochloride (Possible additive CNS depression). Products include:
Geodon Capsules 2688

Zolpidem Tartrate (Possible additive CNS depression). Products include:
Ambien Tablets 3191

Food Interactions

Alcohol (Possible additive CNS depression).

ROXICODONE ORAL SOLUTION

(Oxycodone Hydrochloride) 3067
May interact with central nervous system depressants and certain other agents. Compounds in these categories include:

Alfentanil Hydrochloride (Possible additive CNS depression).
No products indexed under this heading.

Alprazolam (Possible additive CNS depression). Products include:
Xanax Tablets 2865

Aprobarbital (Possible additive CNS depression).
No products indexed under this heading.

Buprenorphine Hydrochloride (Possible additive CNS depression). Products include:
Buprenex Injectable 2918

Buspirone Hydrochloride (Possible additive CNS depression).
No products indexed under this heading.

Butabarbital (Possible additive CNS depression).
No products indexed under this heading.

Butalbital (Possible additive CNS depression). Products include:
Phrenilin 578
Sedapap Tablets 50 mg/650 mg 2225

Chlordiazepoxide (Possible additive CNS depression). Products include:
Limbitrol 1738

Chlordiazepoxide Hydrochloride (Possible additive CNS depression). Products include:
Librium Capsules 1736
Librium for Injection 1737

Chlorpromazine (Possible additive CNS depression). Products include:
Thorazine Suppositories 1656

Chlorpromazine Hydrochloride (Possible additive CNS depression). Products include:
Thorazine 1656

Chlorprothixene (Possible additive CNS depression).
No products indexed under this heading.

Chlorprothixene Hydrochloride (Possible additive CNS depression).
No products indexed under this heading.

Chlorprothixene Lactate (Possible additive CNS depression).
No products indexed under this heading.

Clorazepate Dipotassium (Possible additive CNS depression). Products include:
Tranxene 511

Clozapine (Possible additive CNS depression). Products include:
Clozaril Tablets 2319

Codeine Phosphate (Possible additive CNS depression). Products include:
Phenergan with Codeine Syrup 3557
Phenergan VC with Codeine Syrup 3561
Robitussin A-C Syrup 2942
Robitussin-DAC Syrup 2942
Ryna-C Liquid 768
Soma Compound w/Codeine Tablets 3355
Tussi-Organidin NR Liquid 3350
Tussi-Organidin-S NR Liquid 3350
Tylenol with Codeine 2595

Desflurane (Possible additive CNS depression). Products include:
Suprane Liquid for Inhalation 874

Dezocine (Possible additive CNS depression).
No products indexed under this heading.

Diazepam (Possible additive CNS depression). Products include:
Valium Injectable 3026
Valium Tablets 3047

Droperidol (Possible additive CNS depression).
No products indexed under this heading.

Enflurane (Possible additive CNS depression).
No products indexed under this heading.

Estazolam (Possible additive CNS depression). Products include:
ProSom Tablets 500

Ethchlorvynol (Possible additive CNS depression).
No products indexed under this heading.

Ethinamate (Possible additive CNS depression).
No products indexed under this heading.

Fentanyl (Possible additive CNS depression). Products include:
Duragesic Transdermal System 1786

Fentanyl Citrate (Possible additive CNS depression). Products include:
Actiq 1184

Fluphenazine Decanoate (Possible additive CNS depression).
No products indexed under this heading.

Fluphenazine Enanthate (Possible additive CNS depression).
No products indexed under this heading.

Fluphenazine Hydrochloride (Possible additive CNS depression).
No products indexed under this heading.

Flurazepam Hydrochloride (Possible additive CNS depression).
No products indexed under this heading.

Glutethimide (Possible additive CNS depression).
No products indexed under this heading.

Haloperidol (Possible additive CNS depression). Products include:
Haldol Injection, Tablets and Concentrate 2533

Haloperidol Decanoate (Possible additive CNS depression). Products include:
Haldol Decanoate 2535

Hydrocodone Bitartrate (Possible additive CNS depression). Products include:
Hycodan 1316
Hycomine Compound Tablets 1317
Hycotuss Expectorant Syrup 1318
Lortab 3319
Lortab Elixir 3317
Maxidone Tablets CIII 3399
Norco 5/325 Tablets CIII 3424
Norco 7.5/325 Tablets CIII 3425
Norco 10/325 Tablets CIII 3427
Norco 10/325 Tablets CIII 3425
Vicodin Tablets 516
Vicodin ES Tablets 517
Vicodin HP Tablets 518
Vicodin Tuss Expectorant 519
Vicoprofen Tablets 520
Zydone Tablets 1330

Hydrocodone Polistirex (Possible additive CNS depression). Products include:
Tussionex Pennkinetic Extended-Release Suspension 1174

Hydromorphone Hydrochloride (Possible additive CNS depression). Products include:
Dilaudid 441
Dilaudid Oral Liquid 445
Dilaudid Powder 441
Dilaudid Rectal Suppositories 441
Dilaudid Tablets 441
Dilaudid Tablets - 8 mg 445
Dilaudid-HP 443

Hydroxyzine Hydrochloride (Possible additive CNS depression). Products include:
Atarax Tablets & Syrup 2667
Vistaril Intramuscular Solution 2738

Isoflurane (Possible additive CNS depression).
No products indexed under this heading.

Ketamine Hydrochloride (Possible additive CNS depression).
No products indexed under this heading.

Levomethadyl Acetate Hydrochloride (Possible additive CNS depression).
No products indexed under this heading.

Levorphanol Tartrate (Possible additive CNS depression). Products include:
Levo-Dromoran 1734
Levorphanol Tartrate Tablets 3059

Lorazepam (Possible additive CNS depression). Products include:
Ativan Injection 3478
Ativan Tablets 3482

Loxapine Hydrochloride (Possible additive CNS depression).
No products indexed under this heading.

Loxapine Succinate (Possible additive CNS depression). Products include:
Loxitane Capsules 3398

Meperidine Hydrochloride (Possible additive CNS depression). Products include:
Demerol 3079
Mepergan Injection 3539

Mephobarbital (Possible additive CNS depression).
No products indexed under this heading.

Meprobamate (Possible additive CNS depression). Products include:
Miltown Tablets 3349

Mesoridazine Besylate (Possible additive CNS depression). Products include:
Serentil 1057

Methadone Hydrochloride (Possible additive CNS depression). Products include:
Dolophine Hydrochloride Tablets 3056

Methohexital Sodium (Possible additive CNS depression). Products include:
Brevital Sodium for Injection, USP .. 1815

Methotrimeprazine (Possible additive CNS depression).
No products indexed under this heading.

Methoxyflurane (Possible additive CNS depression).
No products indexed under this heading.

Midazolam Hydrochloride (Possible additive CNS depression). Products include:
Versed Injection 3027
Versed Syrup 3033

Molindone Hydrochloride (Possible additive CNS depression). Products include:
Moban 1320

Morphine Sulfate (Possible additive CNS depression). Products include:
Astramorph/PF Injection, USP (Preservative-Free) 594
Duramorph Injection 1312
Infumorph 200 and Infumorph 500 Sterile Solutions 1314
Kadian Capsules 1335
MS Contin Tablets 2896
MSIR 2898
Oramorph SR Tablets 3062
Roxanol 3066

Olanzapine (Possible additive CNS depression). Products include:
Zyprexa Tablets 1973
Zyprexa ZYDIS Orally Disintegrating Tablets 1973

Oxazepam (Possible additive CNS depression).
No products indexed under this heading.

Pentobarbital Sodium (Possible additive CNS depression). Products include:
Nembutal Sodium Solution 485

Perphenazine (Possible additive CNS depression). Products include:
Etrafon 3115
Trilafon 3160

Phenobarbital (Possible additive CNS depression). Products include:
Arco-Lase Plus Tablets 592
Donnatal 2929
Donnatal Extentabs 2930

Prazepam (Possible additive CNS depression).
No products indexed under this heading.

Prochlorperazine (Possible additive CNS depression). Products include:
Compazine 1505

Promethazine Hydrochloride (Possible additive CNS depression). Products include:
Mepergan Injection 3539
Phenergan Injection 3553
Phenergan 3556
Phenergan Syrup 3554
Phenergan with Codeine Syrup 3557
Phenergan with Dextromethorphan Syrup 3559
Phenergan VC Syrup 3560
Phenergan VC with Codeine Syrup .. 3561

Propofol (Possible additive CNS depression). Products include:
Diprivan Injectable Emulsion 667

Propoxyphene Hydrochloride (Possible additive CNS depression). Products include:
Darvon Pulvules 1909
Darvon Compound-65 Pulvules 1910

Propoxyphene Napsylate (Possible additive CNS depression). Products include:
Darvon-N/Darvocet-N 1907
Darvon-N Tablets 1912

Quazepam (Possible additive CNS depression).
No products indexed under this heading.

Quetiapine Fumarate (Possible additive CNS depression). Products include:
Seroquel Tablets 684

Remifentanil Hydrochloride (Possible additive CNS depression).
No products indexed under this heading.

Risperidone (Possible additive CNS depression). Products include:
Risperdal 1796

Secobarbital Sodium (Possible additive CNS depression).
No products indexed under this heading.

Sevoflurane (Possible additive CNS depression).
No products indexed under this heading.

Sufentanil Citrate (Possible additive CNS depression).
No products indexed under this heading.

Temazepam (Possible additive CNS depression).
No products indexed under this heading.

Thiamylal Sodium (Possible additive CNS depression).
No products indexed under this heading.

Thioridazine Hydrochloride (Possible additive CNS depression). Products include:
Thioridazine Hydrochloride Tablets 2289

Thiothixene (Possible additive CNS depression). Products include:
Navane Capsules 2701
Thiothixene Capsules 2290

Triazolam (Possible additive CNS depression). Products include:
Halcion Tablets 2823

Trifluoperazine Hydrochloride (Possible additive CNS depression). Products include:
Stelazine 1640

Zaleplon (Possible additive CNS depression). Products include:
Sonata Capsules 3591

Ziprasidone Hydrochloride (Possible additive CNS depression). Products include:
Geodon Capsules 2688

Zolpidem Tartrate (Possible additive CNS depression). Products include:
Ambien Tablets 3191

Food Interactions

Alcohol (Possible additive CNS depression).

ROXICODONE TABLETS

(Oxycodone Hydrochloride) 3067
May interact with central nervous system depressants, monoamine oxidase inhibitors, mixed agonist/antagonist opioid analgesics, neuromuscular blocking agents, and certain other agents. Compounds in these categories include:

Alfentanil Hydrochloride (Co-administration may exhibit an additive CNS depression resulting in respiratory depression, hypotension, profound sedation or coma).
No products indexed under this heading.

Alprazolam (Co-administration may exhibit an additive CNS depression resulting in respiratory depression, hypotension, profound sedation or coma). Products include:
Xanax Tablets 2865

Aprobarbital (Co-administration may exhibit an additive CNS depression resulting in respiratory depression, hypotension, profound sedation or coma).
No products indexed under this heading.

Atracurium Besylate (Co-administration with neuromuscular agents may result in enhanced skeletal muscle relaxants and produce an increased degree of respiratory depression).
No products indexed under this heading.

Buprenorphine Hydrochloride (Mixed agonist/antagonist analgesics may reduce the analgesic effect of oxycodone and/or may precipitate withdrawal symptoms in these patients). Products include:
Buprenex Injectable 2918

Buspirone Hydrochloride (Co-administration may exhibit an additive CNS depression resulting in respiratory depression, hypotension, profound sedation or coma).
No products indexed under this heading.

Butabarbital (Co-administration may exhibit an additive CNS depression resulting in respiratory depression, hypotension, profound sedation or coma).
No products indexed under this heading.

Butalbital (Co-administration may exhibit an additive CNS depression resulting in respiratory depression, hypotension, profound sedation or coma). Products include:
Phrenilin 578
Sedapap Tablets 50 mg/650 mg ... 2225

Butorphanol Tartrate (Mixed agonist/antagonist analgesics may reduce the analgesic effect of oxycodone and/or may precipitate withdrawal symptoms in these patients). Products include:
Stadol NS Nasal Spray 1108

Chlordiazepoxide (Co-administration may exhibit an additive CNS depression resulting in respiratory depression, hypotension, profound sedation or coma). Products include:
Limbitrol 1738

Chlordiazepoxide Hydrochloride (Co-administration may exhibit an additive CNS depression resulting in respiratory depression, hypotension, profound sedation or coma). Products include:
Librium Capsules 1736
Librium for Injection 1737

Chlorpromazine (Co-administration may exhibit an additive CNS depression resulting in respiratory depression, hypotension, profound sedation or coma). Products include:
Thorazine Suppositories 1656

Chlorpromazine Hydrochloride (Co-administration may exhibit an additive CNS depression resulting in respiratory depression, hypotension, profound sedation or coma). Products include:
Thorazine 1656

Chlorprothixene (Co-administration may exhibit an additive CNS depression resulting in respiratory depression, hypotension, profound sedation or coma).
No products indexed under this heading.

Chlorprothixene Hydrochloride (Co-administration may exhibit an additive CNS depression resulting in respiratory depression, hypotension, profound sedation or coma).
No products indexed under this heading.

Chlorprothixene Lactate (Co-administration may exhibit an additive CNS depression resulting in respiratory depression, hypotension, profound sedation or coma).
No products indexed under this heading.

Cisatracurium Besylate (Co-administration with neuromuscular agents may result in enhanced skeletal muscle relaxants and produce an increased degree of respiratory depression).
No products indexed under this heading.

Clorazepate Dipotassium (Co-administration may exhibit an additive CNS depression resulting in respiratory depression, hypotension, profound sedation or coma). Products include:
Tranxene 511

Clozapine (Co-administration may exhibit an additive CNS depression resulting in respiratory depression, hypotension, profound sedation or coma). Products include:
Clozaril Tablets 2319

Codeine Phosphate (Co-administration may exhibit an additive CNS depression resulting in respiratory depression, hypotension, profound sedation or coma). Products include:
Phenergan with Codeine Syrup 3557
Phenergan VC with Codeine Syrup .. 3561
Robitussin A-C Syrup 2942
Robitussin-DAC Syrup 2942
Ryna-C Liquid .... ■768
Soma Compound w/Codeine Tablets 3355
Tussi-Organidin NR Liquid 3350
Tussi-Organidin-S NR Liquid 3350
Tylenol with Codeine 2595

Desflurane (Co-administration may exhibit an additive CNS depression resulting in respiratory depression, hypotension, profound sedation or coma). Products include:
Suprane Liquid for Inhalation 874

Dezocine (Co-administration may exhibit an additive CNS depression resulting in respiratory depression, hypotension, profound sedation or

coma).
No products indexed under this heading.

Diazepam (Co-administration may exhibit an additive CNS depression resulting in respiratory depression, hypotension, profound sedation or coma). Products include:
Valium Injectable 3026
Valium Tablets 3047

Doxacurium Chloride (Co-administration with neuromuscular agents may result in enhanced skeletal muscle relaxants and produce an increased degree of respiratory depression).
No products indexed under this heading.

Droperidol (Co-administration may exhibit an additive CNS depression resulting in respiratory depression, hypotension, profound sedation or coma).
No products indexed under this heading.

Enflurane (Co-administration may exhibit an additive CNS depression resulting in respiratory depression, hypotension, profound sedation or coma).
No products indexed under this heading.

Estazolam (Co-administration may exhibit an additive CNS depression resulting in respiratory depression, hypotension, profound sedation or coma). Products include:
ProSom Tablets 500

Ethchlorvynol (Co-administration may exhibit an additive CNS depression resulting in respiratory depression, hypotension, profound sedation or coma).
No products indexed under this heading.

Ethinamate (Co-administration may exhibit an additive CNS depression resulting in respiratory depression, hypotension, profound sedation or coma).
No products indexed under this heading.

Fentanyl (Co-administration may exhibit an additive CNS depression resulting in respiratory depression, hypotension, profound sedation or coma). Products include:
Duragesic Transdermal System 1786

Fentanyl Citrate (Co-administration may exhibit an additive CNS depression resulting in respiratory depression, hypotension, profound sedation or coma). Products include:
Actiq 1184

Fluphenazine Decanoate (Co-administration may exhibit an additive CNS depression resulting in respiratory depression, hypotension, profound sedation or coma).
No products indexed under this heading.

Fluphenazine Enanthate (Co-administration may exhibit an additive CNS depression resulting in respiratory depression, hypotension, profound sedation or coma).
No products indexed under this heading.

Fluphenazine Hydrochloride (Co-administration may exhibit an additive CNS depression resulting in respiratory depression, hypotension, profound sedation or coma).
No products indexed under this heading.

Flurazepam Hydrochloride (Co-administration may exhibit an additive CNS depression resulting in respiratory depression, hypotension, profound sedation or coma).
No products indexed under this heading.

Glutethimide (Co-administration may exhibit an additive CNS depression resulting in respiratory depression, hypotension, profound sedation or coma).
No products indexed under this heading.

Haloperidol (Co-administration may exhibit an additive CNS depression resulting in respiratory depression, hypotension, profound sedation or coma). Products include:
Haldol Injection, Tablets and Concentrate 2533

Haloperidol Decanoate (Co-administration may exhibit an additive CNS depression resulting in respiratory depression, hypotension, profound sedation or coma). Products include:
Haldol Decanoate 2535

Hydrocodone Bitartrate (Co-administration may exhibit an additive CNS depression resulting in respiratory depression, hypotension, profound sedation or coma). Products include:
Hycodan 1316
Hycomine Compound Tablets 1317
Hycotuss Expectorant Syrup 1318
Lortab 3319
Lortab Elixir 3317
Maxidone Tablets CIII 3399
Norco 5/325 Tablets CIII 3424
Norco 7.5/325 Tablets CIII 3425
Norco 10/325 Tablets CIII 3427
Norco 10/325 Tablets CIII 3425
Vicodin Tablets 516
Vicodin ES Tablets 517
Vicodin HP Tablets 518
Vicodin Tuss Expectorant 519
Vicoprofen Tablets 520
Zydone Tablets 1330

Hydrocodone Polistirex (Co-administration may exhibit an additive CNS depression resulting in respiratory depression, hypotension, profound sedation or coma). Products include:
Tussionex Pennkinetic Extended-Release Suspension 1174

Hydromorphone Hydrochloride (Co-administration may exhibit an additive CNS depression resulting in respiratory depression, hypotension, profound sedation or coma). Products include:
Dilaudid 441
Dilaudid Oral Liquid 445
Dilaudid Powder 441
Dilaudid Rectal Suppositories 441
Dilaudid Tablets 441
Dilaudid Tablets - 8 mg 445
Dilaudid-HP 443

Hydroxyzine Hydrochloride (Co-administration may exhibit an additive CNS depression resulting in respiratory depression, hypotension, profound sedation or coma). Products include:
Atarax Tablets & Syrup 2667
Vistaril Intramuscular Solution 2738

Isocarboxazid (MAO inhibitors have been reported to intensify the effects of at least one opioid drug causing anxiety, confusion, and significant respiratory depression and coma; concurrent and/or sequential use is not recommended).
No products indexed under this heading.

Isoflurane (Co-administration may exhibit an additive CNS depression resulting in respiratory depression, hypotension, profound sedation or coma).
No products indexed under this heading.

Ketamine Hydrochloride (Co-administration may exhibit an additive CNS depression resulting in respiratory depression, hypotension, profound sedation or coma).
No products indexed under this heading.

Levomethadyl Acetate Hydrochloride (Co-administration may exhibit an additive CNS depression resulting in respiratory depression, hypotension, profound sedation or coma).
No products indexed under this heading.

Levorphanol Tartrate (Co-administration may exhibit an additive CNS depression resulting in respiratory depression, hypotension, profound sedation or coma). Products include:
Levo-Dromoran 1734
Levorphanol Tartrate Tablets 3059

Lorazepam (Co-administration may exhibit an additive CNS depression resulting in respiratory depression, hypotension, profound sedation or coma). Products include:
Ativan Injection 3478
Ativan Tablets 3482

Loxapine Hydrochloride (Co-administration may exhibit an additive CNS depression resulting in respiratory depression, hypotension, profound sedation or coma).
No products indexed under this heading.

Loxapine Succinate (Co-administration may exhibit an additive CNS depression resulting in respiratory depression, hypotension, profound sedation or coma). Products include:
Loxitane Capsules 3398

Meperidine Hydrochloride (Co-administration may exhibit an additive CNS depression resulting in respiratory depression, hypotension, profound sedation or coma). Products include:
Demerol 3079
Mepergan Injection 3539

Mephobarbital (Co-administration may exhibit an additive CNS depression resulting in respiratory depression, hypotension, profound sedation or coma).
No products indexed under this heading.

Meprobamate (Co-administration may exhibit an additive CNS depression resulting in respiratory depression, hypotension, profound sedation or coma). Products include:
Miltown Tablets 3349

Mesoridazine Besylate (Co-administration may exhibit an additive CNS depression resulting in respiratory depression, hypotension, profound sedation or coma). Products include:
Serentil 1057

Methadone Hydrochloride (Co-administration may exhibit an additive CNS depression resulting in respiratory depression, hypotension, profound sedation or coma). Products include:
Dolophine Hydrochloride Tablets 3056

Methohexital Sodium (Co-administration may exhibit an additive CNS depression resulting in respiratory depression, hypotension, profound sedation or coma). Products include:
Brevital Sodium for Injection, USP .. 1815

Methotrimeprazine (Co-administration may exhibit an additive CNS depression resulting in respiratory depression, hypotension, profound sedation or coma).
No products indexed under this heading.

Methoxyflurane (Co-administration may exhibit an additive CNS depression resulting in respiratory depression, hypotension, profound sedation or coma).
No products indexed under this heading.

Metocurine Iodide (Co-administration with neuromuscular agents may result in enhanced skeletal muscle relaxants and produce an increased degree of respiratory depression).
No products indexed under this heading.

Midazolam Hydrochloride (Co-administration may exhibit an additive CNS depression resulting in respiratory depression, hypotension, profound sedation or coma). Products include:
Versed Injection 3027
Versed Syrup 3033

Mivacurium Chloride (Co-administration with neuromuscular agents may result in enhanced skeletal muscle relaxants and produce an increased degree of respiratory depression).
No products indexed under this heading.

Moclobemide (MAO inhibitors have been reported to intensify the effects of at least one opioid drug causing anxiety, confusion, and significant respiratory depression and coma; concurrent and/or sequential use is not recommended).
No products indexed under this heading.

Molindone Hydrochloride (Co-administration may exhibit an additive CNS depression resulting in respiratory depression, hypotension, profound sedation or coma). Products include:
Moban 1320

Morphine Sulfate (Co-administration may exhibit an additive CNS depression resulting in respiratory depression, hypotension, profound sedation or coma). Products include:
Astramorph/PF Injection, USP (Preservative-Free) 594
Duramorph Injection 1312
Infumorph 200 and Infumorph 500 Sterile Solutions 1314
Kadian Capsules 1335
MS Contin Tablets 2896
MSIR 2898
Oramorph SR Tablets 3062
Roxanol 3066

Nalbuphine Hydrochloride (Mixed agonist/antagonist analgesics may reduce the analgesic effect of oxycodone and/or may precipitate withdrawal symptoms in these patients). Products include:
Nubain Injection 1323

Olanzapine (Co-administration may exhibit an additive CNS depression resulting in respiratory depression, hypotension, profound sedation or coma). Products include:
Zyprexa Tablets 1973
Zyprexa ZYDIS Orally Disintegrating Tablets 1973

Oxazepam (Co-administration may exhibit an additive CNS depression resulting in respiratory depression, hypotension, profound sedation or coma).
No products indexed under this heading.

Pancuronium Bromide (Co-administration with neuromuscular agents may result in enhanced skeletal muscle relaxants and produce an increased degree of respiratory depression).
No products indexed under this heading.

Pargyline Hydrochloride (MAO inhibitors have been reported to intensify the effects of at least one opioid drug causing anxiety, confusion, and significant respiratory depression and coma; concurrent and/or sequential use is not recommended).
No products indexed under this heading.

Pentazocine Hydrochloride (Mixed agonist/antagonist analgesics may reduce the analgesic effect

of oxycodone and/or may precipitate withdrawal symptoms in these patients). Products include:
Talacen Caplets 3089
Talwin Nx Tablets 3090

Pentazocine Lactate (Mixed agonist/antagonist analgesics may reduce the analgesic effect of oxycodone and/or may precipitate withdrawal symptoms in these patients).
No products indexed under this heading.

Pentobarbital Sodium (Co-administration may exhibit an additive CNS depression resulting in respiratory depression, hypotension, profound sedation or coma). Products include:
Nembutal Sodium Solution 485

Perphenazine (Co-administration may exhibit an additive CNS depression resulting in respiratory depression, hypotension, profound sedation or coma). Products include:
Etrafon 3115
Trilafon 3160

Phenelzine Sulfate (MAO inhibitors have been reported to intensify the effects of at least one opioid drug causing anxiety, confusion, and significant respiratory depression and coma; concurrent and/or sequential use is not recommended). Products include:
Nardil Tablets 2653

Phenobarbital (Co-administration may exhibit an additive CNS depression resulting in respiratory depression, hypotension, profound sedation or coma). Products include:
Arco-Lase Plus Tablets 592
Donnatal 2929
Donnatal Extentabs 2930

Prazepam (Co-administration may exhibit an additive CNS depression resulting in respiratory depression, hypotension, profound sedation or coma).
No products indexed under this heading.

Procarbazine Hydrochloride (MAO inhibitors have been reported to intensify the effects of at least one opioid drug causing anxiety, confusion, and significant respiratory depression and coma; concurrent and/or sequential use is not recommended). Products include:
Matulane Capsules 3246

Prochlorperazine (Co-administration may exhibit an additive CNS depression resulting in respiratory depression, hypotension, profound sedation or coma). Products include:
Compazine 1505

Promethazine Hydrochloride (Co administration may exhibit an additive CNS depression resulting in respiratory depression, hypotension, profound sedation or coma). Products include:
Mepergan Injection 3539
Phenergan Injection 3553
Phenergan 3556
Phenergan Syrup 3554
Phenergan with Codeine Syrup 3557
Phenergan with Dextromethorphan Syrup 3559
Phenergan VC Syrup 3560
Phenergan VC with Codeine Syrup .. 3561

Propofol (Co-administration may exhibit an additive CNS depression resulting in respiratory depression, hypotension, profound sedation or coma). Products include:
Diprivan Injectable Emulsion 667

Propoxyphene Hydrochloride (Co-administration may exhibit an additive CNS depression resulting in respiratory depression, hypotension, profound sedation or coma). Products include:
Darvon Pulvules 1909
Darvon Compound-65 Pulvules 1910

Propoxyphene Napsylate (Co-administration may exhibit an additive CNS depression resulting in respiratory depression, hypotension, profound sedation or coma). Products include:
Darvon-N/Darvocet-N 1907
Darvon-N Tablets 1912

Quazepam (Co-administration may exhibit an additive CNS depression resulting in respiratory depression, hypotension, profound sedation or coma).
No products indexed under this heading.

Quetiapine Fumarate (Co-administration may exhibit an additive CNS depression resulting in respiratory depression, hypotension, profound sedation or coma). Products include:
Seroquel Tablets 684

Rapacuronium Bromide (Co-administration with neuromuscular agents may result in enhanced skeletal muscle relaxants and produce an increased degree of respiratory depression).
No products indexed under this heading.

Remifentanil Hydrochloride (Co-administration may exhibit an additive CNS depression resulting in respiratory depression, hypotension, profound sedation or coma).
No products indexed under this heading.

Risperidone (Co-administration may exhibit an additive CNS depression resulting in respiratory depression, hypotension, profound sedation or coma). Products include:
Risperdal 1796

Rocuronium Bromide (Co-administration with neuromuscular agents may result in enhanced skeletal muscle relaxants and produce an increased degree of respiratory depression). Products include:
Zemuron Injection 2491

Secobarbital Sodium (Co-administration may exhibit an additive CNS depression resulting in respiratory depression, hypotension, profound sedation or coma).
No products indexed under this heading.

Selegiline Hydrochloride (MAO inhibitors have been reported to intensify the effects of at least one opioid drug causing anxiety, confusion, and significant respiratory depression and coma; concurrent and/or sequential use is not recommended). Products include:
Eldepryl Capsules 3266

Sevoflurane (Co-administration may exhibit an additive CNS depression resulting in respiratory depression, hypotension, profound sedation or coma).
No products indexed under this heading.

Succinylcholine Chloride (Co-administration with neuromuscular agents may result in enhanced skeletal muscle relaxants and produce an increased degree of respiratory depression). Products include:
Anectine Injection 1476

Sufentanil Citrate (Co-administration may exhibit an additive CNS depression resulting in respiratory depression, hypotension, profound sedation or coma).
No products indexed under this heading.

Temazepam (Co-administration may exhibit an additive CNS depression resulting in respiratory depression, hypotension, profound sedation or coma).
No products indexed under this heading.

Thiamylal Sodium (Co-administration may exhibit an additive CNS depression resulting in respiratory depression, hypotension, profound sedation or coma).
No products indexed under this heading.

Thioridazine Hydrochloride (Co-administration may exhibit an additive CNS depression resulting in respiratory depression, hypotension, profound sedation or coma). Products include:
Thioridazine Hydrochloride Tablets 2289

Thiothixene (Co-administration may exhibit an additive CNS depression resulting in respiratory depression, hypotension, profound sedation or coma). Products include:
Navane Capsules 2701
Thiothixene Capsules 2290

Tranylcypromine Sulfate (MAO inhibitors have been reported to intensify the effects of at least one opioid drug causing anxiety, confusion, and significant respiratory depression and coma; concurrent and/or sequential use is not recommended). Products include:
Parnate Tablets 1607

Triazolam (Co-administration may exhibit an additive CNS depression resulting in respiratory depression, hypotension, profound sedation or coma). Products include:
Halcion Tablets 2823

Trifluoperazine Hydrochloride (Co-administration may exhibit an additive CNS depression resulting in respiratory depression, hypotension, profound sedation or coma). Products include:
Stelazine 1640

Vecuronium Bromide (Co-administration with neuromuscular agents may result in enhanced skeletal muscle relaxants and produce an increased degree of respiratory depression). Products include:
Norcuron for Injection 2478

Zaleplon (Co-administration may exhibit an additive CNS depression resulting in respiratory depression, hypotension, profound sedation or coma). Products include:
Sonata Capsules 3591

Ziprasidone Hydrochloride (Co-administration may exhibit an additive CNS depression resulting in respiratory depression, hypotension, profound sedation or coma). Products include:
Geodon Capsules 2688

Zolpidem Tartrate (Co-administration may exhibit an additive CNS depression resulting in respiratory depression, hypotension, profound sedation or coma). Products include:
Ambien Tablets 3191

Food Interactions

Alcohol (Concurrent use may exhibit an additive CNS depression).

RUM-K

(Potassium Chloride) 1363
None cited in PDR database.

RYNA LIQUID

(Chlorpheniramine Maleate, Pseudoephedrine Hydrochloride) .... ▣768
See Ryna-C Liquid

RYNA-C LIQUID

(Chlorpheniramine Maleate, Codeine Phosphate, Pseudoephedrine Hydrochloride) .... ▣768
May interact with hypnotics and sedatives, monoamine oxidase inhibitors, tranquilizers, and certain other agents. Compounds in these categories include:

Alprazolam (May increase the drowsiness effect). Products include:
Xanax Tablets 2865

Buspirone Hydrochloride (May increase the drowsiness effect).
No products indexed under this heading.

Chlordiazepoxide (May increase the drowsiness effect). Products include:
Limbitrol 1738

Chlordiazepoxide Hydrochloride (May increase the drowsiness effect). Products include:
Librium Capsules 1736
Librium for Injection 1737

Chlorpromazine (May increase the drowsiness effect). Products include:
Thorazine Suppositories 1656

Chlorpromazine Hydrochloride (May increase the drowsiness effect). Products include:
Thorazine 1656

Chlorprothixene (May increase the drowsiness effect).
No products indexed under this heading.

Chlorprothixene Hydrochloride (May increase the drowsiness effect).
No products indexed under this heading.

Clorazepate Dipotassium (May increase the drowsiness effect). Products include:
Tranxene 511

Diazepam (May increase the drowsiness effect). Products include:
Valium Injectable 3026
Valium Tablets 3047

Droperidol (May increase the drowsiness effect).
No products indexed under this heading.

Estazolam (May increase the drowsiness effect). Products include:
ProSom Tablets 500

Ethchlorvynol (May increase the drowsiness effect).
No products indexed under this heading.

Ethinamate (May increase the drowsiness effect).
No products indexed under this heading.

Fluphenazine Decanoate (May increase the drowsiness effect).
No products indexed under this heading.

Fluphenazine Enanthate (May increase the drowsiness effect).
No products indexed under this heading.

Fluphenazine Hydrochloride (May increase the drowsiness effect).
No products indexed under this heading.

Flurazepam Hydrochloride (May increase the drowsiness effect).
No products indexed under this heading.

Glutethimide (May increase the drowsiness effect).
No products indexed under this heading.

Haloperidol (May increase the drowsiness effect). Products include:
Haldol Injection, Tablets and Concentrate 2533

Haloperidol Decanoate (May increase the drowsiness effect). Products include:
Haldol Decanoate 2535

Hydroxyzine Hydrochloride (May increase the drowsiness effect). Products include:
Atarax Tablets & Syrup 2667
Vistaril Intramuscular Solution 2738

Isocarboxazid (Concurrent and/or sequential use with MAO inhibitors is not recommended).
No products indexed under this heading.

Lorazepam (May increase the drowsiness effect). Products include:
Ativan Injection 3478
Ativan Tablets 3482

Loxapine Hydrochloride (May increase the drowsiness effect).
No products indexed under this heading.

Loxapine Succinate (May increase the drowsiness effect). Products include:
Loxitane Capsules 3398

Meprobamate (May increase the drowsiness effect). Products include:
Miltown Tablets 3349

Mesoridazine Besylate (May increase the drowsiness effect). Products include:
Serentil 1057

Midazolam Hydrochloride (May increase the drowsiness effect). Products include:
Versed Injection 3027
Versed Syrup 3033

Moclobemide (Concurrent and/or sequential use with MAO inhibitors is not recommended).
No products indexed under this heading.

Molindone Hydrochloride (May increase the drowsiness effect). Products include:
Moban 1320

Oxazepam (May increase the drowsiness effect).
No products indexed under this heading.

Pargyline Hydrochloride (Concurrent and/or sequential use with MAO inhibitors is not recommended).
No products indexed under this heading.

Perphenazine (May increase the drowsiness effect). Products include:
Etrafon 3115
Trilafon 3160

Phenelzine Sulfate (Concurrent and/or sequential use with MAO inhibitors is not recommended). Products include:
Nardil Tablets 2653

Prazepam (May increase the drowsiness effect).
No products indexed under this heading.

Procarbazine Hydrochloride (Concurrent and/or sequential use with MAO inhibitors is not recommended). Products include:
Matulane Capsules 3246

Prochlorperazine (May increase the drowsiness effect). Products include:
Compazine 1505

Promethazine Hydrochloride (May increase the drowsiness effect). Products include:
Mepergan Injection 3539
Phenergan Injection 3553
Phenergan 3556
Phenergan Syrup 3554
Phenergan with Codeine Syrup 3557
Phenergan with Dextromethorphan Syrup 3559
Phenergan VC Syrup 3560
Phenergan VC with Codeine Syrup .. 3561

Propofol (May increase the drowsiness effect). Products include:
Diprivan Injectable Emulsion 667

Quazepam (May increase the drowsiness effect).
No products indexed under this heading.

Secobarbital Sodium (May increase the drowsiness effect).
No products indexed under this heading.

Selegiline Hydrochloride (Concurrent and/or sequential use with MAO inhibitors is not recommended). Products include:
Eldepryl Capsules 3266

Temazepam (May increase the drowsiness effect).
No products indexed under this heading.

Thioridazine Hydrochloride (May increase the drowsiness effect). Products include:
Thioridazine Hydrochloride Tablets 2289

Thiothixene (May increase the drowsiness effect). Products include:
Navane Capsules 2701
Thiothixene Capsules 2290

Tranylcypromine Sulfate (Concurrent and/or sequential use with MAO inhibitors is not recommended). Products include:
Parnate Tablets 1607

Triazolam (May increase the drowsiness effect). Products include:
Halcion Tablets 2823

Trifluoperazine Hydrochloride (May increase the drowsiness effect). Products include:
Stelazine 1640

Zaleplon (May increase the drowsiness effect). Products include:
Sonata Capsules 3591

Zolpidem Tartrate (May increase the drowsiness effect). Products include:
Ambien Tablets 3191

Food Interactions

Alcohol (May increase the drowsiness effect).

RYNA-12 S SUSPENSION

(Phenylephrine Tannate, Pyrilamine Tannate) 3351

May interact with central nervous system depressants, monoamine oxidase inhibitors, and certain other agents. Compounds in these categories include:

Alfentanil Hydrochloride (Ryna-12 S contains an antihistamine which may cause drowsiness and may have additive central nervous system effects with other CNS depressants).
No products indexed under this heading.

Alprazolam (Ryna-12 S contains an antihistamine which may cause drowsiness and may have additive central nervous system effects with other CNS depressants). Products include:
Xanax Tablets 2865

Aprobarbital (Ryna-12 S contains an antihistamine which may cause drowsiness and may have additive central nervous system effects with other CNS depressants).
No products indexed under this heading.

Buprenorphine Hydrochloride (Ryna-12 S contains an antihistamine which may cause drowsiness and may have additive central nervous system effects with other CNS depressants). Products include:
Buprenex Injectable 2918

Buspirone Hydrochloride (Ryna-12 S contains an antihistamine which may cause drowsiness and may have additive central nervous system effects with other CNS depressants).
No products indexed under this heading.

Butabarbital (Ryna-12 S contains an antihistamine which may cause drowsiness and may have additive central nervous system effects with other CNS depressants).
No products indexed under this heading.

Butalbital (Ryna-12 S contains an antihistamine which may cause drowsiness and may have additive central nervous system effects with other CNS depressants). Products include:
Phrenilin 578
Sedapap Tablets 50 mg/650 mg ... 2225

Chlordiazepoxide (Ryna-12 S contains an antihistamine which may cause drowsiness and may have additive central nervous system effects with other CNS depressants). Products include:
Limbitrol 1738

Chlordiazepoxide Hydrochloride (Ryna-12 S contains an antihistamine which may cause drowsiness and may have additive central nervous system effects with other CNS depressants). Products include:
Librium Capsules 1736
Librium for Injection 1737

Chlorpromazine (Ryna-12 S contains an antihistamine which may cause drowsiness and may have additive central nervous system effects with other CNS depressants). Products include:
Thorazine Suppositories 1656

Chlorpromazine Hydrochloride (Ryna-12 S contains an antihistamine which may cause drowsiness and may have additive central nervous system effects with other CNS depressants). Products include:
Thorazine 1656

Chlorprothixene (Ryna-12 S contains an antihistamine which may cause drowsiness and may have additive central nervous system effects with other CNS depressants).
No products indexed under this heading.

Chlorprothixene Hydrochloride (Ryna-12 S contains an antihistamine which may cause drowsiness and may have additive central nervous system effects with other CNS depressants).
No products indexed under this heading.

Chlorprothixene Lactate (Ryna-12 S contains an antihistamine which may cause drowsiness and may have additive central nervous system effects with other CNS depressants).
No products indexed under this heading.

Clorazepate Dipotassium (Ryna-12 S contains an antihistamine which may cause drowsiness and may have additive central nervous system effects with other CNS depressants). Products include:
Tranxene 511

Clozapine (Ryna-12 S contains an antihistamine which may cause drowsiness and may have additive central nervous system effects with other CNS depressants). Products include:
Clozaril Tablets 2319

Codeine Phosphate (Ryna-12 S contains an antihistamine which may cause drowsiness and may have additive central nervous system effects with other CNS depressants). Products include:
Phenergan with Codeine Syrup 3557
Phenergan VC with Codeine Syrup .. 3561
Robitussin A-C Syrup 2942
Robitussin-DAC Syrup 2942
Ryna-C Liquid 768
Soma Compound w/Codeine Tablets 3355
Tussi-Organidin NR Liquid 3350
Tussi-Organidin-S NR Liquid 3350
Tylenol with Codeine 2595

Desflurane (Ryna-12 S contains an antihistamine which may cause drowsiness and may have additive central nervous system effects with other CNS depressants). Products include:
Suprane Liquid for Inhalation 874

Dezocine (Ryna-12 S contains an antihistamine which may cause drowsiness and may have additive central nervous system effects with other CNS depressants).
No products indexed under this heading.

Diazepam (Ryna-12 S contains an antihistamine which may cause drowsiness and may have additive central nervous system effects with other CNS depressants). Products include:
Valium Injectable 3026
Valium Tablets 3047

Droperidol (Ryna-12 S contains an antihistamine which may cause drowsiness and may have additive central nervous system effects with other CNS depressants).
No products indexed under this heading.

Enflurane (Ryna-12 S contains an antihistamine which may cause drowsiness and may have additive central nervous system effects with other CNS depressants).
No products indexed under this heading.

Estazolam (Ryna-12 S contains an antihistamine which may cause drowsiness and may have additive central nervous system effects with other CNS depressants). Products include:
ProSom Tablets 500

Ethchlorvynol (Ryna-12 S contains an antihistamine which may cause drowsiness and may have additive central nervous system effects with other CNS depressants).
No products indexed under this heading.

Ethinamate (Ryna-12 S contains an antihistamine which may cause drowsiness and may have additive central nervous system effects with other CNS depressants).
No products indexed under this heading.

Fentanyl (Ryna-12 S contains an antihistamine which may cause drowsiness and may have additive central nervous system effects with other CNS depressants). Products include:
Duragesic Transdermal System 1786

Fentanyl Citrate (Ryna-12 S contains an antihistamine which may cause drowsiness and may have additive central nervous system effects with other CNS depressants). Products include:
Actiq 1184

Fluphenazine Decanoate (Ryna-12 S contains an antihistamine which may cause drowsiness and may have additive central nervous system effects with other CNS depressants).
No products indexed under this heading.

Fluphenazine Enanthate (Ryna-12 S contains an antihistamine which may cause drowsiness and may have additive central nervous system effects with other CNS depressants).
No products indexed under this heading.

Fluphenazine Hydrochloride (Ryna-12 S contains an antihistamine which may cause drowsiness and may have additive central nervous system effects with other CNS depressants).
No products indexed under this heading.

Flurazepam Hydrochloride (Ryna-12 S contains an antihistamine which may cause drowsiness and may have additive central nervous system effects with other CNS depressants).
No products indexed under this heading.

Glutethimide (Ryna-12 S contains an antihistamine which may cause drowsiness and may have additive central nervous system effects with other CNS depressants).
No products indexed under this heading.

Haloperidol (Ryna-12 S contains an antihistamine which may cause drowsiness and may have additive central

nervous system effects with other CNS depressants). Products include:
Haldol Injection, Tablets and Concentrate 2533

Haloperidol Decanoate (Ryna-12 S contains an antihistamine which may cause drowsiness and may have additive central nervous system effects with other CNS depressants). Products include:
Haldol Decanoate 2535

Hydrocodone Bitartrate (Ryna-12 S contains an antihistamine which may cause drowsiness and may have additive central nervous system effects with other CNS depressants). Products include:
Hycodan 1316
Hycomine Compound Tablets 1317
Hycotuss Expectorant Syrup 1318
Lortab 3319
Lortab Elixir 3317
Maxidone Tablets CIII 3399
Norco 5/325 Tablets CIII 3424
Norco 7.5/325 Tablets CIII 3425
Norco 10/325 Tablets CIII 3427
Norco 10/325 Tablets CIII 3425
Vicodin Tablets 516
Vicodin ES Tablets 517
Vicodin HP Tablets 518
Vicodin Tuss Expectorant 519
Vicoprofen Tablets 520
Zydone Tablets 1330

Hydrocodone Polistirex (Ryna-12 S contains an antihistamine which may cause drowsiness and may have additive central nervous system effects with other CNS depressants). Products include:
Tussionex Pennkinetic Extended-Release Suspension 1174

Hydromorphone Hydrochloride (Ryna-12 S contains an antihistamine which may cause drowsiness and may have additive central nervous system effects with other CNS depressants). Products include:
Dilaudid 441
Dilaudid Oral Liquid 445
Dilaudid Powder 441
Dilaudid Rectal Suppositories 441
Dilaudid Tablets 441
Dilaudid Tablets - 8 mg 445
Dilaudid-HP 443

Hydroxyzine Hydrochloride (Ryna-12 S contains an antihistamine which may cause drowsiness and may have additive central nervous system effects with other CNS depressants). Products include:
Atarax Tablets & Syrup 2667
Vistaril Intramuscular Solution 2738

Isocarboxazid (Co-administration or sequential use with MAO inhibitors may prolong and intensify the anticholinergic effects of antihistamines and the overall effects of sympathomimetic agents).
No products indexed under this heading.

Isoflurane (Ryna-12 S contains an antihistamine which may cause drowsiness and may have additive central nervous system effects with other CNS depressants).
No products indexed under this heading.

Ketamine Hydrochloride (Ryna-12 S contains an antihistamine which may cause drowsiness and may have additive central nervous system effects with other CNS depressants).
No products indexed under this heading.

Levomethadyl Acetate Hydrochloride (Ryna-12 S contains an antihistamine which may cause drowsiness and may have additive central nervous system effects with other CNS depressants).
No products indexed under this heading.

Levorphanol Tartrate (Ryna-12 S contains an antihistamine which may cause drowsiness and may have additive central nervous system effects with other CNS depressants). Products include:
Levo-Dromoran 1734
Levorphanol Tartrate Tablets 3059

Lorazepam (Ryna-12 S contains an antihistamine which may cause drowsiness and may have additive central nervous system effects with other CNS depressants). Products include:
Ativan Injection 3478
Ativan Tablets 3482

Loxapine Hydrochloride (Ryna-12 S contains an antihistamine which may cause drowsiness and may have additive central nervous system effects with other CNS depressants).
No products indexed under this heading.

Loxapine Succinate (Ryna-12 S contains an antihistamine which may cause drowsiness and may have additive central nervous system effects with other CNS depressants). Products include:
Loxitane Capsules 3398

Meperidine Hydrochloride (Ryna-12 S contains an antihistamine which may cause drowsiness and may have additive central nervous system effects with other CNS depressants). Products include:
Demerol 3079
Mepergan Injection 3539

Mephobarbital (Ryna-12 S contains an antihistamine which may cause drowsiness and may have additive central nervous system effects with other CNS depressants).
No products indexed under this heading.

Meprobamate (Ryna-12 S contains an antihistamine which may cause drowsiness and may have additive central nervous system effects with other CNS depressants). Products include:
Miltown Tablets 3349

Mesoridazine Besylate (Ryna-12 S contains an antihistamine which may cause drowsiness and may have additive central nervous system effects with other CNS depressants). Products include:
Serentil 1057

Methadone Hydrochloride (Ryna-12 S contains an antihistamine which may cause drowsiness and may have additive central nervous system effects with other CNS depressants). Products include:
Dolophine Hydrochloride Tablets 3056

Methohexital Sodium (Ryna-12 S contains an antihistamine which may cause drowsiness and may have additive central nervous system effects with other CNS depressants). Products include:
Brevital Sodium for Injection, USP 1815

Methotrimeprazine (Ryna-12 S contains an antihistamine which may cause drowsiness and may have additive central nervous system effects with other CNS depressants).
No products indexed under this heading.

Methoxyflurane (Ryna-12 S contains an antihistamine which may cause drowsiness and may have additive central nervous system effects with other CNS depressants).
No products indexed under this heading.

Midazolam Hydrochloride (Ryna-12 S contains an antihistamine which may cause drowsiness and may have additive central nervous system effects with other CNS depressants). Products include:
Versed Injection 3027
Versed Syrup 3033

Moclobemide (Co-administration or sequential use with MAO inhibitors may prolong and intensify the anticholinergic effects of antihistamines and the overall effects of sympathomimetic agents).
No products indexed under this heading.

Molindone Hydrochloride (Ryna-12 S contains an antihistamine which may cause drowsiness and may have additive central nervous system effects with other CNS depressants). Products include:
Moban 1320

Morphine Sulfate (Ryna-12 S contains an antihistamine which may cause drowsiness and may have additive central nervous system effects with other CNS depressants). Products include:
Astramorph/PF Injection, USP (Preservative-Free) 594
Duramorph Injection 1312
Infumorph 200 and Infumorph 500 Sterile Solutions 1314
Kadian Capsules 1335
MS Contin Tablets 2896
MSIR 2898
Oramorph SR Tablets 3062
Roxanol 3066

Olanzapine (Ryna-12 S contains an antihistamine which may cause drowsiness and may have additive central nervous system effects with other CNS depressants). Products include:
Zyprexa Tablets 1973
Zyprexa ZYDIS Orally Disintegrating Tablets 1973

Oxazepam (Ryna-12 S contains an antihistamine which may cause drowsiness and may have additive central nervous system effects with other CNS depressants).
No products indexed under this heading.

Oxycodone Hydrochloride (Ryna-12 S contains an antihistamine which may cause drowsiness and may have additive central nervous system effects with other CNS depressants). Products include:
OxyContin Tablets 2912
OxyFast Oral Concentrate Solution 2916
OxyIR Capsules 2916
Percocet Tablets 1326
Percodan Tablets 1327
Percolone Tablets 1327
Roxicodone 3067
Tylox Capsules 2597

Pargyline Hydrochloride (Co-administration or sequential use with MAO inhibitors may prolong and intensify the anticholinergic effects of antihistamines and the overall effects of sympathomimetic agents).
No products indexed under this heading.

Pentobarbital Sodium (Ryna-12 S contains an antihistamine which may cause drowsiness and may have additive central nervous system effects with other CNS depressants). Products include:
Nembutal Sodium Solution 485

Perphenazine (Ryna-12 S contains an antihistamine which may cause drowsiness and may have additive central nervous system effects with other CNS depressants). Products include:
Etrafon 3115
Trilafon 3160

Phenelzine Sulfate (Co-administration or sequential use with MAO inhibitors may prolong and intensify the anticholinergic effects of antihistamines and the overall effects of sympathomimetic agents). Products include:
Nardil Tablets 2653

Phenobarbital (Ryna-12 S contains an antihistamine which may cause drowsiness and may have additive central nervous system effects with other CNS depressants). Products include:
Arco-Lase Plus Tablets 592
Donnatal 2929
Donnatal Extentabs 2930

Prazepam (Ryna-12 S contains an antihistamine which may cause drowsiness and may have additive central nervous system effects with other CNS depressants).
No products indexed under this heading.

Procarbazine Hydrochloride (Co-administration or sequential use with MAO inhibitors may prolong and intensify the anticholinergic effects of antihistamines and the overall effects of sympathomimetic agents). Products include:
Matulane Capsules 3246

Prochlorperazine (Ryna-12 S contains an antihistamine which may cause drowsiness and may have additive central nervous system effects with other CNS depressants). Products include:
Compazine 1505

Promethazine Hydrochloride (Ryna-12 S contains an antihistamine which may cause drowsiness and may have additive central nervous system effects with other CNS depressants). Products include:
Mepergan Injection 3539
Phenergan Injection 3553
Phenergan 3556
Phenergan Syrup 3554
Phenergan with Codeine Syrup 3557
Phenergan with Dextromethorphan Syrup 3559
Phenergan VC Syrup 3560
Phenergan VC with Codeine Syrup 3561

Propofol (Ryna-12 S contains an antihistamine which may cause drowsiness and may have additive central nervous system effects with other CNS depressants). Products include:
Diprivan Injectable Emulsion 667

Propoxyphene Hydrochloride (Ryna-12 S contains an antihistamine which may cause drowsiness and may have additive central nervous system effects with other CNS depressants). Products include:
Darvon Pulvules 1909
Darvon Compound-65 Pulvules 1910

Propoxyphene Napsylate (Ryna-12 S contains an antihistamine which may cause drowsiness and may have additive central nervous system effects with other CNS depressants). Products include:
Darvon-N/Darvocet-N 1907
Darvon-N Tablets 1912

Quazepam (Ryna-12 S contains an antihistamine which may cause drowsiness and may have additive central nervous system effects with other CNS depressants).
No products indexed under this heading.

Quetiapine Fumarate (Ryna-12 S contains an antihistamine which may cause drowsiness and may have additive central nervous system effects with other CNS depressants). Products include:
Seroquel Tablets 684

Remifentanil Hydrochloride (Ryna-12 S contains an antihistamine which may cause drowsiness and may have additive central nervous system effects with other CNS depressants).
No products indexed under this heading.

Risperidone (Ryna-12 S contains an antihistamine which may cause drowsiness and may have additive central nervous system effects with other CNS depressants). Products include:
Risperdal 1796

Secobarbital Sodium (Ryna-12 S contains an antihistamine which may cause drowsiness and may have additive central nervous system effects with other CNS depressants).
No products indexed under this heading.

Selegiline Hydrochloride (Co-administration or sequential use with MAO inhibitors may prolong and intensify the anticholinergic effects of antihistamines and the overall effects of sympathomimetic agents). Products include:
- Eldepryl Capsules 3266

Sevoflurane (Ryna-12 S contains an antihistamine which may cause drowsiness and may have additive central nervous system effects with other CNS depressants).
- No products indexed under this heading.

Sufentanil Citrate (Ryna-12 S contains an antihistamine which may cause drowsiness and may have additive central nervous system effects with other CNS depressants).
- No products indexed under this heading.

Temazepam (Ryna-12 S contains an antihistamine which may cause drowsiness and may have additive central nervous system effects with other CNS depressants).
- No products indexed under this heading.

Thiamylal Sodium (Ryna-12 S contains an antihistamine which may cause drowsiness and may have additive central nervous system effects with other CNS depressants).
- No products indexed under this heading.

Thioridazine Hydrochloride (Ryna-12 S contains an antihistamine which may cause drowsiness and may have additive central nervous system effects with other CNS depressants). Products include:
- Thioridazine Hydrochloride Tablets 2289

Thiothixene (Ryna-12 S contains an antihistamine which may cause drowsiness and may have additive central nervous system effects with other CNS depressants). Products include:
- Navane Capsules 2701
- Thiothixene Capsules 2290

Tranylcypromine Sulfate (Co-administration or sequential use with MAO inhibitors may prolong and intensify the anticholinergic effects of antihistamines and the overall effects of sympathomimetic agents). Products include:
- Parnate Tablets 1607

Triazolam (Ryna-12 S contains an antihistamine which may cause drowsiness and may have additive central nervous system effects with other CNS depressants). Products include:
- Halcion Tablets 2823

Trifluoperazine Hydrochloride (Ryna-12 S contains an antihistamine which may cause drowsiness and may have additive central nervous system effects with other CNS depressants). Products include:
- Stelazine 1640

Zaleplon (Ryna-12 S contains an antihistamine which may cause drowsiness and may have additive central nervous system effects with other CNS depressants). Products include:
- Sonata Capsules 3591

Ziprasidone Hydrochloride (Ryna-12 S contains an antihistamine which may cause drowsiness and may have additive central nervous system effects with other CNS depressants). Products include:
- Geodon Capsules 2688

Zolpidem Tartrate (Ryna-12 S contains an antihistamine which may cause drowsiness and may have additive central nervous system effects with other CNS depressants). Products include:
- Ambien Tablets 3191

Food Interactions

Alcohol (Ryan-12 S contains an antihistamine which may cause drowsiness and may have additive central nervous system effects with alcohol).

REFORMULATED RYNATAN PEDIATRIC SUSPENSION

(Chlorpheniramine Tannate, Phenylephrine Tannate) 3352

May interact with central nervous system depressants, hypnotics and sedatives, monoamine oxidase inhibitors, tranquilizers, and certain other agents. Compounds in these categories include:

Alfentanil Hydrochloride (Antihistamines cause drowsiness and co-administration may increase drowsiness effect).
- No products indexed under this heading.

Alprazolam (Antihistamines cause drowsiness and co-administration may increase drowsiness effect). Products include:
- Xanax Tablets 2865

Aprobarbital (Antihistamines cause drowsiness and co-administration may increase drowsiness effect).
- No products indexed under this heading.

Buprenorphine Hydrochloride (Antihistamines cause drowsiness and co-administration may increase drowsiness effect). Products include:
- Buprenex Injectable 2918

Buspirone Hydrochloride (Antihistamines cause drowsiness and co-administration may increase drowsiness effect).
- No products indexed under this heading.

Butabarbital (Antihistamines cause drowsiness and co-administration may increase drowsiness effect).
- No products indexed under this heading.

Butalbital (Antihistamines cause drowsiness and co-administration may increase drowsiness effect). Products include:
- Phrenilin 578
- Sedapap Tablets 50 mg/650 mg 2225

Chlordiazepoxide (Antihistamines cause drowsiness and co-administration may increase drowsiness effect). Products include:
- Limbitrol 1738

Chlordiazepoxide Hydrochloride (Antihistamines cause drowsiness and co-administration may increase drowsiness effect). Products include:
- Librium Capsules 1736
- Librium for Injection 1737

Chlorpromazine (Antihistamines cause drowsiness and co-administration may increase drowsiness effect). Products include:
- Thorazine Suppositories 1656

Chlorpromazine Hydrochloride (Antihistamines cause drowsiness and co-administration may increase drowsiness effect). Products include:
- Thorazine 1656

Chlorprothixene (Antihistamines cause drowsiness and co-administration may increase drowsiness effect).
- No products indexed under this heading.

Chlorprothixene Hydrochloride (Antihistamines cause drowsiness and co-administration may increase drowsiness effect).
- No products indexed under this heading.

Chlorprothixene Lactate (Antihistamines cause drowsiness and co-administration may increase drowsiness effect).
- No products indexed under this heading.

Clorazepate Dipotassium (Antihistamines cause drowsiness and co-administration may increase drowsiness effect). Products include:
- Tranxene 511

Clozapine (Antihistamines cause drowsiness and co-administration may increase drowsiness effect). Products include:
- Clozaril Tablets 2319

Codeine Phosphate (Antihistamines cause drowsiness and co-administration may increase drowsiness effect). Products include:
- Phenergan with Codeine Syrup 3557
- Phenergan VC with Codeine Syrup 3561
- Robitussin A-C Syrup 2942
- Robitussin-DAC Syrup 2942
- Ryna-C Liquid 768
- Soma Compound w/Codeine Tablets 3355
- Tussi-Organidin NR Liquid 3350
- Tussi-Organidin-S NR Liquid 3350
- Tylenol with Codeine 2595

Desflurane (Antihistamines cause drowsiness and co-administration may increase drowsiness effect). Products include:
- Suprane Liquid for Inhalation 874

Dezocine (Antihistamines cause drowsiness and co-administration may increase drowsiness effect).
- No products indexed under this heading.

Diazepam (Antihistamines cause drowsiness and co-administration may increase drowsiness effect). Products include:
- Valium Injectable 3026
- Valium Tablets 3047

Droperidol (Antihistamines cause drowsiness and co-administration may increase drowsiness effect).
- No products indexed under this heading.

Enflurane (Antihistamines cause drowsiness and co-administration may increase drowsiness effect).
- No products indexed under this heading.

Estazolam (Antihistamines cause drowsiness and co-administration may increase drowsiness effect). Products include:
- ProSom Tablets 500

Ethchlorvynol (Antihistamines cause drowsiness and co-administration may increase drowsiness effect).
- No products indexed under this heading.

Ethinamate (Antihistamines cause drowsiness and co-administration may increase drowsiness effect).
- No products indexed under this heading.

Fentanyl (Antihistamines cause drowsiness and co-administration may increase drowsiness effect). Products include:
- Duragesic Transdermal System 1786

Fentanyl Citrate (Antihistamines cause drowsiness and co-administration may increase drowsiness effect). Products include:
- Actiq 1184

Fluphenazine Decanoate (Antihistamines cause drowsiness and co-administration may increase drowsiness effect).
- No products indexed under this heading.

Fluphenazine Enanthate (Antihistamines cause drowsiness and co-administration may increase drowsiness effect).
- No products indexed under this heading.

Fluphenazine Hydrochloride (Antihistamines cause drowsiness and co-administration may increase drowsiness effect).
- No products indexed under this heading.

Flurazepam Hydrochloride (Antihistamines cause drowsiness and co-administration may increase drowsiness effect).
- No products indexed under this heading.

Glutethimide (Antihistamines cause drowsiness and co-administration may increase drowsiness effect).
- No products indexed under this heading.

Haloperidol (Antihistamines cause drowsiness and co-administration may increase drowsiness effect). Products include:
- Haldol Injection, Tablets and Concentrate 2533

Haloperidol Decanoate (Antihistamines cause drowsiness and co-administration may increase drowsiness effect). Products include:
- Haldol Decanoate 2535

Hydrocodone Bitartrate (Antihistamines cause drowsiness and co-administration may increase drowsiness effect). Products include:
- Hycodan 1316
- Hycomine Compound Tablets 1317
- Hycotuss Expectorant Syrup 1318
- Lortab 3319
- Lortab Elixir 3317
- Maxidone Tablets CIII 3399
- Norco 5/325 Tablets CIII 3424
- Norco 7.5/325 Tablets CIII 3425
- Norco 10/325 Tablets CIII 3427
- Norco 10/325 Tablets CIII 3425
- Vicodin Tablets 516
- Vicodin ES Tablets 517
- Vicodin HP Tablets 518
- Vicodin Tuss Expectorant 519
- Vicoprofen Tablets 520
- Zydone Tablets 1330

Hydrocodone Polistirex (Antihistamines cause drowsiness and co-administration may increase drowsiness effect). Products include:
- Tussionex Pennkinetic Extended-Release Suspension 1174

Hydromorphone Hydrochloride (Antihistamines cause drowsiness and co-administration may increase drowsiness effect). Products include:
- Dilaudid 441
- Dilaudid Oral Liquid 445
- Dilaudid Powder 441
- Dilaudid Rectal Suppositories 441
- Dilaudid Tablets 441
- Dilaudid Tablets - 8 mg 445
- Dilaudid-HP 443

Hydroxyzine Hydrochloride (Antihistamines cause drowsiness and co-administration may increase drowsiness effect). Products include:
- Atarax Tablets & Syrup 2667
- Vistaril Intramuscular Solution 2738

Isocarboxazid (MAO inhibitors prolong and intensify the anticholinergic effects of antihistamines and the overall effects of sympathomimetics; concurrent and/or sequential use is not recommended).
- No products indexed under this heading.

Isoflurane (Antihistamines cause drowsiness and co-administration may increase drowsiness effect).
- No products indexed under this heading.

Ketamine Hydrochloride (Antihistamines cause drowsiness and co-administration may increase drowsiness effect).
- No products indexed under this heading.

Levomethadyl Acetate Hydrochloride (Antihistamines cause drowsiness and co-administration may increase drowsiness effect).
- No products indexed under this heading.

Levorphanol Tartrate (Antihistamines cause drowsiness and co-administration may increase drowsiness effect). Products include:

Levo-Dromoran 1734
Levorphanol Tartrate Tablets 3059

Lorazepam (Antihistamines cause drowsiness and co-administration may increase drowsiness effect). Products include:
Ativan Injection 3478
Ativan Tablets 3482

Loxapine Hydrochloride (Antihistamines cause drowsiness and co-administration may increase drowsiness effect).
No products indexed under this heading.

Loxapine Succinate (Antihistamines cause drowsiness and co-administration may increase drowsiness effect). Products include:
Loxitane Capsules 3398

Meperidine Hydrochloride (Antihistamines cause drowsiness and co-administration may increase drowsiness effect). Products include:
Demerol 3079
Mepergan Injection 3539

Mephobarbital (Antihistamines cause drowsiness and co-administration may increase drowsiness effect).
No products indexed under this heading.

Meprobamate (Antihistamines cause drowsiness and co-administration may increase drowsiness effect). Products include:
Miltown Tablets 3349

Mesoridazine Besylate (Antihistamines cause drowsiness and co-administration may increase drowsiness effect). Products include:
Serentil 1057

Methadone Hydrochloride (Antihistamines cause drowsiness and co-administration may increase drowsiness effect). Products include:
Dolophine Hydrochloride Tablets 3056

Methohexital Sodium (Antihistamines cause drowsiness and co-administration may increase drowsiness effect). Products include:
Brevital Sodium for Injection, USP .. 1815

Methotrimeprazine (Antihistamines cause drowsiness and co-administration may increase drowsiness effect).
No products indexed under this heading.

Methoxyflurane (Antihistamines cause drowsiness and co-administration may increase drowsiness effect).
No products indexed under this heading.

Midazolam Hydrochloride (Antihistamines cause drowsiness and co-administration may increase drowsiness effect). Products include:
Versed Injection 3027
Versed Syrup 3033

Moclobemide (MAO inhibitors prolong and intensify the anticholinergic effects of antihistamines and the overall effects of sympathomimetics; concurrent and/or sequential use is not recommended).
No products indexed under this heading.

Molindone Hydrochloride (Antihistamines cause drowsiness and co-administration may increase drowsiness effect). Products include:
Moban 1320

Morphine Sulfate (Antihistamines cause drowsiness and co-administration may increase drowsiness effect). Products include:
Astramorph/PF Injection, USP (Preservative-Free) 594
Duramorph Injection 1312
Infumorph 200 and Infumorph 500 Sterile Solutions 1314
Kadian Capsules 1335
MS Contin Tablets 2896
MSIR 2898
Oramorph SR Tablets 3062

Roxanol 3066

Olanzapine (Antihistamines cause drowsiness and co-administration may increase drowsiness effect). Products include:
Zyprexa Tablets 1973
Zyprexa ZYDIS Orally Disintegrating Tablets 1973

Oxazepam (Antihistamines cause drowsiness and co-administration may increase drowsiness effect).
No products indexed under this heading.

Oxycodone Hydrochloride (Antihistamines cause drowsiness and co-administration may increase drowsiness effect). Products include:
OxyContin Tablets 2912
OxyFast Oral Concentrate Solution . 2916
OxyIR Capsules 2916
Percocet Tablets 1326
Percodan Tablets 1327
Percolone Tablets 1327
Roxicodone 3067
Tylox Capsules 2597

Pargyline Hydrochloride (MAO inhibitors prolong and intensify the anticholinergic effects of antihistamines and the overall effects of sympathomimetics; concurrent and/or sequential use is not recommended).
No products indexed under this heading.

Pentobarbital Sodium (Antihistamines cause drowsiness and co-administration may increase drowsiness effect). Products include:
Nembutal Sodium Solution 485

Perphenazine (Antihistamines cause drowsiness and co-administration may increase drowsiness effect). Products include:
Etrafon 3115
Trilafon 3160

Phenelzine Sulfate (MAO inhibitors prolong and intensify the anticholinergic effects of antihistamines and the overall effects of sympathomimetics; concurrent and/or sequential use is not recommended). Products include:
Nardil Tablets 2653

Phenobarbital (Antihistamines cause drowsiness and co-administration may increase drowsiness effect). Products include:
Arco-Lase Plus Tablets 592
Donnatal 2929
Donnatal Extentabs 2930

Prazepam (Antihistamines cause drowsiness and co-administration may increase drowsiness effect).
No products indexed under this heading.

Procarbazine Hydrochloride (MAO inhibitors prolong and intensify the anticholinergic effects of antihistamines and the overall effects of sympathomimetics; concurrent and/or sequential use is not recommended). Products include:
Matulane Capsules 3246

Prochlorperazine (Antihistamines cause drowsiness and co-administration may increase drowsiness effect). Products include:
Compazine 1505

Promethazine Hydrochloride (Antihistamines cause drowsiness and co-administration may increase drowsiness effect). Products include:
Mepergan Injection 3539
Phenergan Injection 3553
Phenergan 3556
Phenergan Syrup 3554
Phenergan with Codeine Syrup 3557
Phenergan with Dextromethorphan Syrup 3559
Phenergan VC Syrup 3560
Phenergan VC with Codeine Syrup .. 3561

Propofol (Antihistamines cause drowsiness and co-administration may increase drowsiness effect). Products include:
Diprivan Injectable Emulsion 667

Propoxyphene Hydrochloride (Antihistamines cause drowsiness and co-administration may increase drowsiness effect). Products include:
Darvon Pulvules 1909
Darvon Compound-65 Pulvules 1910

Propoxyphene Napsylate (Antihistamines cause drowsiness and co-administration may increase drowsiness effect). Products include:
Darvon-N/Darvocet-N 1907
Darvon-N Tablets 1912

Quazepam (Antihistamines cause drowsiness and co-administration may increase drowsiness effect).
No products indexed under this heading.

Quetiapine Fumarate (Antihistamines cause drowsiness and co-administration may increase drowsiness effect). Products include:
Seroquel Tablets 684

Remifentanil Hydrochloride (Antihistamines cause drowsiness and co-administration may increase drowsiness effect).
No products indexed under this heading.

Risperidone (Antihistamines cause drowsiness and co-administration may increase drowsiness effect). Products include:
Risperdal 1796

Secobarbital Sodium (Antihistamines cause drowsiness and co-administration may increase drowsiness effect).
No products indexed under this heading.

Selegiline Hydrochloride (MAO inhibitors prolong and intensify the anticholinergic effects of antihistamines and the overall effects of sympathomimetics; concurrent and/or sequential use is not recommended). Products include:
Eldepryl Capsules 3266

Sevoflurane (Antihistamines cause drowsiness and co-administration may increase drowsiness effect).
No products indexed under this heading.

Sufentanil Citrate (Antihistamines cause drowsiness and co-administration may increase drowsiness effect).
No products indexed under this heading.

Temazepam (Antihistamines cause drowsiness and co-administration may increase drowsiness effect).
No products indexed under this heading.

Thiamylal Sodium (Antihistamines cause drowsiness and co-administration may increase drowsiness effect).
No products indexed under this heading.

Thioridazine Hydrochloride (Antihistamines cause drowsiness and co-administration may increase drowsiness effect). Products include:
Thioridazine Hydrochloride Tablets 2289

Thiothixene (Antihistamines cause drowsiness and co-administration may increase drowsiness effect). Products include:
Navane Capsules 2701
Thiothixene Capsules 2290

Tranylcypromine Sulfate (MAO inhibitors prolong and intensify the anticholinergic effects of antihistamines and the overall effects of sympathomimetics; concurrent and/or sequential use is not recommended). Products include:
Parnate Tablets 1607

Triazolam (Antihistamines cause drowsiness and co-administration may increase drowsiness effect). Products include:
Halcion Tablets 2823

Trifluoperazine Hydrochloride (Antihistamines cause drowsiness and co-administration may increase drowsiness effect). Products include:
Stelazine 1640

Zaleplon (Antihistamines cause drowsiness and co-administration may increase drowsiness effect). Products include:
Sonata Capsules 3591

Ziprasidone Hydrochloride (Antihistamines cause drowsiness and co-administration may increase drowsiness effect). Products include:
Geodon Capsules 2688

Zolpidem Tartrate (Antihistamines cause drowsiness and co-administration may increase drowsiness effect). Products include:
Ambien Tablets 3191

Food Interactions

Alcohol (Antihistamines cause drowsiness and co-administration may increase drowsiness effect).

RYNATAN TABLETS

(Azatadine Maleate, Pseudoephedrine Sulfate) 3351

May interact with antacids, barbiturates, beta blockers, central nervous system depressants, cardiac glycosides, monoamine oxidase inhibitors, tricyclic antidepressants, veratrum alkaloids, and certain other agents. Compounds in these categories include:

Acebutolol Hydrochloride (Concurrent use with beta adrenergic blocker increases the effects of sympathomimetics). Products include:
Sectral Capsules 3589

Alfentanil Hydrochloride (CNS depressants may enhance the drowsiness caused by antihistamines; potential for additive effects).
No products indexed under this heading.

Alprazolam (CNS depressants may enhance the drowsiness caused by antihistamines; potential for additive effects). Products include:
Xanax Tablets 2865

Aluminum Carbonate (Antacids increase the rate of absorption of pseudoephedrine).
No products indexed under this heading.

Aluminum Hydroxide (Antacids increase the rate of absorption of pseudoephedrine). Products include:
Amphojel Suspension (Mint Flavor) .... ■789
Gaviscon Extra Strength Liquid ..... ■751
Gaviscon Extra Strength Tablets .... ■751
Gaviscon Regular Strength Liquid . ■751
Gaviscon Regular Strength Tablets .... ■750
Maalox Antacid/Anti Gas Oral Suspension .... ■673
Maalox Max Maximum Strength Antacid/Anti-Gas Liquid 2300
Maalox Regular Strength Antacid/Antigas Liquid 2300
Mylanta 1813
Vanquish Caplets .... ■617

Amitriptyline Hydrochloride (Tricyclic antidepressants may enhance the drowsiness caused by antihistamines; potential for additive effects). Products include:
Etrafon 3115
Limbitrol 1738

Amoxapine (Tricyclic antidepressants may enhance the drowsiness caused by antihistamines; potential for additive effects).
No products indexed under this heading.

Aprobarbital (Barbiturates may enhance the drowsiness caused by antihistamines; potential for additive effects).
No products indexed under this heading.

Atenolol (Concurrent use with beta adrenergic blocker increases the effects of sympathomimetics). Products include:
Tenoretic Tablets 690
Tenormin I.V. Injection 692

Betaxolol Hydrochloride (Concurrent use with beta adrenergic blocker increases the effects of sympathomimetics). Products include:
Betoptic S Ophthalmic Suspension 537

Bisoprolol Fumarate (Concurrent use with beta adrenergic blocker increases the effects of sympathomimetics). Products include:
Zebeta Tablets 1885
Ziac Tablets 1887

Buprenorphine Hydrochloride (CNS depressants may enhance the drowsiness caused by antihistamines; potential for additive effects). Products include:
Buprenex Injectable 2918

Buspirone Hydrochloride (CNS depressants may enhance the drowsiness caused by antihistamines; potential for additive effects).
No products indexed under this heading.

Butabarbital (Barbiturates may enhance the drowsiness caused by antihistamines; potential for additive effects).
No products indexed under this heading.

Butalbital (Barbiturates may enhance the drowsiness caused by antihistamines; potential for additive effects). Products include:
Phrenilin 578
Sedapap Tablets 50 mg/650 mg 2225

Carteolol Hydrochloride (Concurrent use with beta adrenergic blocker increases the effects of sympathomimetics). Products include:
Carteolol Hydrochloride Ophthalmic Solution USP, 1% .... ⊙258
Ocupress Ophthalmic Solution, 1% Sterile .... ⊙303

Chlordiazepoxide (CNS depressants may enhance the drowsiness caused by antihistamines; potential for additive effects). Products include:
Limbitrol 1738

Chlordiazepoxide Hydrochloride (CNS depressants may enhance the drowsiness caused by antihistamines; potential for additive effects). Products include:
Librium Capsules 1736
Librium for Injection 1737

Chlorpromazine (CNS depressants may enhance the drowsiness caused by antihistamines; potential for additive effects). Products include:
Thorazine Suppositories 1656

Chlorpromazine Hydrochloride (CNS depressants may enhance the drowsiness caused by antihistamines; potential for additive effects). Products include:
Thorazine 1656

Chlorprothixene (CNS depressants may enhance the drowsiness caused by antihistamines; potential for additive effects).
No products indexed under this heading.

Chlorprothixene Hydrochloride (CNS depressants may enhance the drowsiness caused by antihistamines; potential for additive effects).
No products indexed under this heading.

Chlorprothixene Lactate (CNS depressants may enhance the drowsiness caused by antihistamines; potential for additive effects).
No products indexed under this heading.

Clomipramine Hydrochloride (Tricyclic antidepressants may enhance the drowsiness caused by antihistamines; potential for additive effects).
No products indexed under this heading.

Clorazepate Dipotassium (CNS depressants may enhance the drowsiness caused by antihistamines; potential for additive effects). Products include:
Tranxene 511

Clozapine (CNS depressants may enhance the drowsiness caused by antihistamines; potential for additive effects). Products include:
Clozaril Tablets 2319

Codeine Phosphate (CNS depressants may enhance the drowsiness caused by antihistamines; potential for additive effects). Products include:
Phenergan with Codeine Syrup 3557
Phenergan VC with Codeine Syrup 3561
Robitussin A-C Syrup 2942
Robitussin-DAC Syrup 2942
Ryna-C Liquid .... ▣768
Soma Compound w/Codeine Tablets 3355
Tussi-Organidin NR Liquid 3350
Tussi-Organidin-S NR Liquid 3350
Tylenol with Codeine 2595

Cryptenamine Preparations (Sympathomimetics may reduce the antihypertensive effects of veratrum alkaloids).
No products indexed under this heading.

Desflurane (CNS depressants may enhance the drowsiness caused by antihistamines; potential for additive effects). Products include:
Suprane Liquid for Inhalation 874

Desipramine Hydrochloride (Tricyclic antidepressants may enhance the drowsiness caused by antihistamines; potential for additive effects). Products include:
Norpramin Tablets 755

Deslanoside (Co-administration of pseudoephedrine with digitalis can result in increased ectopic pacemaker activity).
No products indexed under this heading.

Dezocine (CNS depressants may enhance the drowsiness caused by antihistamines; potential for additive effects).
No products indexed under this heading.

Diazepam (CNS depressants may enhance the drowsiness caused by antihistamines; potential for additive effects). Products include:
Valium Injectable 3026
Valium Tablets 3047

Digitoxin (Co-administration of pseudoephedrine with digitalis can result in increased ectopic pacemaker activity).
No products indexed under this heading.

Digoxin (Co-administration of pseudoephedrine with digitalis can result in increased ectopic pacemaker activity). Products include:
Digitek Tablets 1003
Lanoxicaps Capsules 1574
Lanoxin Injection 1581
Lanoxin Tablets 1587
Lanoxin Elixir Pediatric 1578
Lanoxin Injection Pediatric 1584

Doxepin Hydrochloride (Tricyclic antidepressants may enhance the drowsiness caused by antihistamines; potential for additive effects). Products include:
Sinequan 2713

Droperidol (CNS depressants may enhance the drowsiness caused by antihistamines; potential for additive effects).
No products indexed under this heading.

Enflurane (CNS depressants may enhance the drowsiness caused by antihistamines; potential for additive effects).
No products indexed under this heading.

Esmolol Hydrochloride (Concurrent use with beta adrenergic blocker increases the effects of sympathomimetics). Products include:
Brevibloc Injection 858

Estazolam (CNS depressants may enhance the drowsiness caused by antihistamines; potential for additive effects). Products include:
ProSom Tablets 500

Ethchlorvynol (CNS depressants may enhance the drowsiness caused by antihistamines; potential for additive effects).
No products indexed under this heading.

Ethinamate (CNS depressants may enhance the drowsiness caused by antihistamines; potential for additive effects).
No products indexed under this heading.

Fentanyl (CNS depressants may enhance the drowsiness caused by antihistamines; potential for additive effects). Products include:
Duragesic Transdermal System 1786

Fentanyl Citrate (CNS depressants may enhance the drowsiness caused by antihistamines; potential for additive effects). Products include:
Actiq 1184

Fluphenazine Decanoate (CNS depressants may enhance the drowsiness caused by antihistamines; potential for additive effects).
No products indexed under this heading.

Fluphenazine Enanthate (CNS depressants may enhance the drowsiness caused by antihistamines; potential for additive effects).
No products indexed under this heading.

Fluphenazine Hydrochloride (CNS depressants may enhance the drowsiness caused by antihistamines; potential for additive effects).
No products indexed under this heading.

Flurazepam Hydrochloride (CNS depressants may enhance the drowsiness caused by antihistamines; potential for additive effects).
No products indexed under this heading.

Glutethimide (CNS depressants may enhance the drowsiness caused by antihistamines; potential for additive effects).
No products indexed under this heading.

Guanethidine Monosulfate (Sympathomimetics may reduce the antihypertensive effects of guanethidine).
No products indexed under this heading.

Haloperidol (CNS depressants may enhance the drowsiness caused by antihistamines; potential for additive effects). Products include:
Haldol Injection, Tablets and Concentrate 2533

Haloperidol Decanoate (CNS depressants may enhance the drowsiness caused by antihistamines; potential for additive effects). Products include:
Haldol Decanoate 2535

Hydrocodone Bitartrate (CNS depressants may enhance the drowsiness caused by antihistamines; potential for additive effects). Products include:
Hycodan 1316
Hycomine Compound Tablets 1317
Hycotuss Expectorant Syrup 1318
Lortab 3319
Lortab Elixir 3317
Maxidone Tablets CIII 3399
Norco 5/325 Tablets CIII 3424
Norco 7.5/325 Tablets CIII 3425
Norco 10/325 Tablets CIII 3427
Norco 10/325 Tablets CIII 3425
Vicodin Tablets 516
Vicodin ES Tablets 517
Vicodin HP Tablets 518
Vicodin Tuss Expectorant 519
Vicoprofen Tablets 520
Zydone Tablets 1330

Hydrocodone Polistirex (CNS depressants may enhance the drowsiness caused by antihistamines; potential for additive effects). Products include:
Tussionex Pennkinetic Extended-Release Suspension 1174

Hydromorphone Hydrochloride (CNS depressants may enhance the drowsiness caused by antihistamines; potential for additive effects). Products include:
Dilaudid 441
Dilaudid Oral Liquid 445
Dilaudid Powder 441
Dilaudid Rectal Suppositories 441
Dilaudid Tablets 441
Dilaudid Tablets - 8 mg 445
Dilaudid-HP 443

Hydroxyzine Hydrochloride (CNS depressants may enhance the drowsiness caused by antihistamines; potential for additive effects). Products include:
Atarax Tablets & Syrup 2667
Vistaril Intramuscular Solution 2738

Imipramine Hydrochloride (Tricyclic antidepressants may enhance the drowsiness caused by antihistamines; potential for additive effects).
No products indexed under this heading.

Imipramine Pamoate (Tricyclic antidepressants may enhance the drowsiness caused by antihistamines; potential for additive effects).
No products indexed under this heading.

Isocarboxazid (Concurrent use with MAO inhibitor prolongs and intensifies the effects of antihistamines; co-administration of MAO inhibitors with sympathomimetics can result in hypertensive reactions, including hypertensive crises; co-administration and/or sequential use is contraindicated).
No products indexed under this heading.

Isoflurane (CNS depressants may enhance the drowsiness caused by antihistamines; potential for additive effects).
No products indexed under this heading.

Kaolin (Decreases the rate of absorption of pseudoephedrine).
No products indexed under this heading.

Ketamine Hydrochloride (CNS depressants may enhance the drowsiness caused by antihistamines; potential for additive effects).
No products indexed under this heading.

Labetalol Hydrochloride (Concurrent use with beta adrenergic blocker increases the effects of sympathomimetics). Products include:
Normodyne Injection 3135
Normodyne Tablets 3137

Levobunolol Hydrochloride (Concurrent use with beta adrenergic blocker increases the effects of sympathomimetics). Products include:
Betagan .... ⊙228

Levomethadyl Acetate Hydrochloride (CNS depressants may enhance the drowsiness caused by antihistamines; potential for additive effects).
No products indexed under this heading.

Levorphanol Tartrate (CNS depressants may enhance the drow-

siness caused by antihistamines; potential for additive effects). Products include:
- Levo-Dromoran 1734
- Levorphanol Tartrate Tablets 3059

Lorazepam (CNS depressants may enhance the drowsiness caused by antihistamines; potential for additive effects). Products include:
- Ativan Injection 3478
- Ativan Tablets 3482

Loxapine Hydrochloride (CNS depressants may enhance the drowsiness caused by antihistamines; potential for additive effects).
No products indexed under this heading.

Loxapine Succinate (CNS depressants may enhance the drowsiness caused by antihistamines; potential for additive effects). Products include:
- Loxitane Capsules 3398

Magaldrate (Antacids increase the rate of absorption of pseudoephedrine).
No products indexed under this heading.

Magnesium Hydroxide (Antacids increase the rate of absorption of pseudoephedrine). Products include:
- Ex•Lax Milk of Magnesia Liquid ..... ▣670
- Maalox Antacid/Anti-Gas Oral Suspension ..... ▣673
- Maalox Max Maximum Strength Antacid/Anti-Gas Liquid 2300
- Maalox Regular Strength Antacid/Antigas Liquid 2300
- Mylanta Fast-Acting 1813
- Mylanta 1813
- Pepcid Complete Chewable Tablets 1815
- Phillips' Chewable Tablets ..... ▣615
- Phillips' Milk of Magnesia Liquid (Original, Cherry, & Mint) ..... ▣616
- Rolaids Tablets ..... ▣706
- Extra Strength Rolaids Tablets ..... ▣706
- Vanquish Caplets ..... ▣617

Magnesium Oxide (Antacids increase the rate of absorption of pseudoephedrine). Products include:
- Beelith Tablets 946
- Mag-Ox 400 Tablets 1024
- Uro-Mag Capsules 1024

Maprotiline Hydrochloride (Tricyclic antidepressants may enhance the drowsiness caused by antihistamines; potential for additive effects).
No products indexed under this heading.

Meperidine Hydrochloride (CNS depressants may enhance the drowsiness caused by antihistamines; potential for additive effects). Products include:
- Demerol 3079
- Mepergan Injection 3539

Mephobarbital (Barbiturates may enhance the drowsiness caused by antihistamines; potential for additive effects).
No products indexed under this heading.

Meprobamate (CNS depressants may enhance the drowsiness caused by antihistamines; potential for additive effects). Products include:
- Miltown Tablets 3349

Mesoridazine Besylate (CNS depressants may enhance the drowsiness caused by antihistamines; potential for additive effects). Products include:
- Serentil 1057

Methadone Hydrochloride (CNS depressants may enhance the drowsiness caused by antihistamines; potential for additive effects). Products include:
- Dolophine Hydrochloride Tablets 3056

Methohexital Sodium (CNS depressants may enhance the drowsiness caused by antihistamines; potential for additive effects). Products include:
- Brevital Sodium for Injection, USP 1815

Methotrimeprazine (CNS depressants may enhance the drowsiness caused by antihistamines; potential for additive effects).
No products indexed under this heading.

Methoxyflurane (CNS depressants may enhance the drowsiness caused by antihistamines; potential for additive effects).
No products indexed under this heading.

Methyldopa (Sympathomimetics may reduce the antihypertensive effects of methyldopa). Products include:
- Aldoclor Tablets 2035
- Aldomet Tablets 2037
- Aldoril Tablets 2039

Metipranolol Hydrochloride (Concurrent use with beta adrenergic blocker increases the effects of sympathomimetics).
No products indexed under this heading.

Metoprolol Succinate (Concurrent use with beta adrenergic blocker increases the effects of sympathomimetics). Products include:
- Toprol-XL Tablets 651

Metoprolol Tartrate (Concurrent use with beta adrenergic blocker increases the effects of sympathomimetics).
No products indexed under this heading.

Midazolam Hydrochloride (CNS depressants may enhance the drowsiness caused by antihistamines; potential for additive effects). Products include:
- Versed Injection 3027
- Versed Syrup 3033

Moclobemide (Concurrent use with MAO inhibitor prolongs and intensifies the effects of antihistamines; co-administration of MAO inhibitors with sympathomimetics can result in hypertensive reactions, including hypertensive crises; co-administration and/or sequential use is contraindicated).
No products indexed under this heading.

Molindone Hydrochloride (CNS depressants may enhance the drowsiness caused by antihistamines; potential for additive effects). Products include:
- Moban 1320

Morphine Sulfate (CNS depressants may enhance the drowsiness caused by antihistamines; potential for additive effects). Products include:
- Astramorph/PF Injection, USP (Preservative-Free) 594
- Duramorph Injection 1312
- Infumorph 200 and Infumorph 500 Sterile Solutions 1314
- Kadian Capsules 1335
- MS Contin Tablets 2896
- MSIR 2898
- Oramorph SR Tablets 3062
- Roxanol 3066

Nadolol (Concurrent use with beta adrenergic blocker increases the effects of sympathomimetics). Products include:
- Corgard Tablets 2245
- Corzide 40/5 Tablets 2247
- Corzide 80/5 Tablets 2247
- Nadolol Tablets 2288

Nortriptyline Hydrochloride (Tricyclic antidepressants may enhance the drowsiness caused by antihistamines; potential for additive effects).
No products indexed under this heading.

Olanzapine (CNS depressants may enhance the drowsiness caused by antihistamines; potential for additive effects). Products include:
- Zyprexa Tablets 1973
- Zyprexa ZYDIS Orally Disintegrating Tablets 1973

Oxazepam (CNS depressants may enhance the drowsiness caused by antihistamines; potential for additive effects).
No products indexed under this heading.

Oxycodone Hydrochloride (CNS depressants may enhance the drowsiness caused by antihistamines; potential for additive effects). Products include:
- OxyContin Tablets 2912
- OxyFast Oral Concentrate Solution 2916
- OxyIR Capsules 2916
- Percocet Tablets 1326
- Percodan Tablets 1327
- Percolone Tablets 1327
- Roxicodone 3067
- Tylox Capsules 2597

Pargyline Hydrochloride (Concurrent use with MAO inhibitor prolongs and intensifies the effects of antihistamines; co-administration of MAO inhibitors with sympathomimetics can result in hypertensive reactions, including hypertensive crises; co-administration and/or sequential use is contraindicated).
No products indexed under this heading.

Penbutolol Sulfate (Concurrent use with beta adrenergic blocker increases the effects of sympathomimetics).
No products indexed under this heading.

Pentobarbital Sodium (Barbiturates may enhance the drowsiness caused by antihistamines; potential for additive effects). Products include:
- Nembutal Sodium Solution 485

Perphenazine (CNS depressants may enhance the drowsiness caused by antihistamines; potential for additive effects). Products include:
- Etrafon 3115
- Trilafon 3160

Phenelzine Sulfate (Concurrent use with MAO inhibitor prolongs and intensifies the effects of antihistamines; co-administration of MAO inhibitors with sympathomimetics can result in hypertensive reactions, including hypertensive crises; co-administration and/or sequential use is contraindicated). Products include:
- Nardil Tablets 2653

Phenobarbital (Barbiturates may enhance the drowsiness caused by antihistamines; potential for additive effects). Products include:
- Arco-Lase Plus Tablets 592
- Donnatal 2929
- Donnatal Extentabs 2930

Pindolol (Concurrent use with beta adrenergic blocker increases the effects of sympathomimetics).
No products indexed under this heading.

Prazepam (CNS depressants may enhance the drowsiness caused by antihistamines; potential for additive effects).
No products indexed under this heading.

Procarbazine Hydrochloride (Concurrent use with MAO inhibitor prolongs and intensifies the effects of antihistamines; co-administration of MAO inhibitors with sympathomimetics can result in hypertensive reactions, including hypertensive crises; co-administration and/or sequential use is contraindicated). Products include:
- Matulane Capsules 3246

Prochlorperazine (CNS depressants may enhance the drowsiness caused by antihistamines; potential for additive effects). Products include:
- Compazine 1505

Promethazine Hydrochloride (CNS depressants may enhance the drowsiness caused by antihistamines; potential for additive effects). Products include:
- Mepergan Injection 3539
- Phenergan Injection 3553
- Phenergan 3556
- Phenergan Syrup 3554
- Phenergan with Codeine Syrup 3557
- Phenergan with Dextromethorphan Syrup 3559
- Phenergan VC Syrup 3560
- Phenergan VC with Codeine Syrup 3561

Propofol (CNS depressants may enhance the drowsiness caused by antihistamines; potential for additive effects). Products include:
- Diprivan Injectable Emulsion 667

Propoxyphene Hydrochloride (CNS depressants may enhance the drowsiness caused by antihistamines; potential for additive effects). Products include:
- Darvon Pulvules 1909
- Darvon Compound-65 Pulvules 1910

Propoxyphene Napsylate (CNS depressants may enhance the drowsiness caused by antihistamines; potential for additive effects). Products include:
- Darvon-N/Darvocet-N 1907
- Darvon-N Tablets 1912

Propranolol Hydrochloride (Concurrent use with beta adrenergic blocker increases the effects of sympathomimetics). Products include:
- Inderal 3513
- Inderal LA Long-Acting Capsules 3516
- Inderide Tablets 3517
- Inderide LA Long-Acting Capsules 3519

Protriptyline Hydrochloride (Tricyclic antidepressants may enhance the drowsiness caused by antihistamines; potential for additive effects). Products include:
- Vivactil Tablets 2446
- Vivactil Tablets 2217

Quazepam (CNS depressants may enhance the drowsiness caused by antihistamines; potential for additive effects).
No products indexed under this heading.

Quetiapine Fumarate (CNS depressants may enhance the drowsiness caused by antihistamines; potential for additive effects). Products include:
- Seroquel Tablets 684

Remifentanil Hydrochloride (CNS depressants may enhance the drowsiness caused by antihistamines; potential for additive effects).
No products indexed under this heading.

Reserpine (Sympathomimetics may reduce the antihypertensive effects of reserpine).
No products indexed under this heading.

Risperidone (CNS depressants may enhance the drowsiness caused by antihistamines; potential for additive effects). Products include:
- Risperdal 1796

Secobarbital Sodium (Barbiturates may enhance the drowsiness caused by antihistamines; potential for additive effects).
No products indexed under this heading.

Selegiline Hydrochloride (Concurrent use with MAO inhibitor prolongs and intensifies the effects of antihistamines; co-administration of MAO inhibitors with sympathomimetics can result in hypertensive reactions, including hypertensive crises; co-administration and/or sequential use is contraindicated). Products include:
- Eldepryl Capsules 3266

Sevoflurane (CNS depressants may enhance the drowsiness caused

by antihistamines; potential for additive effects).
No products indexed under this heading.

Sodium Bicarbonate (Antacids increase the rate of absorption of pseudoephedrine). Products include:
- Alka-Seltzer 603
- Alka-Seltzer Lemon Lime Antacid and Pain Reliever Effervescent Tablets 603
- Alka-Seltzer Extra Strength Antacid and Pain Reliever Effervescent Tablets 603
- Alka-Seltzer Heartburn Relief Tablets 604
- Ceo-Two Evacuant Suppository 618
- Colyte with Flavor Packs for Oral Solution 3170
- GoLYTELY and Pineapple Flavor GoLYTELY for Oral Solution 1068
- NuLYTELY, Cherry Flavor, Lemon-Lime Flavor, and Orange Flavor NuLYTELY for Oral Solution 1068

Sotalol Hydrochloride (Concurrent use with beta adrenergic blocker increases the effects of sympathomimetics). Products include:
- Betapace Tablets 950
- Betapace AF Tablets 954

Sufentanil Citrate (CNS depressants may enhance the drowsiness caused by antihistamines; potential for additive effects).
No products indexed under this heading.

Temazepam (CNS depressants may enhance the drowsiness caused by antihistamines; potential for additive effects).
No products indexed under this heading.

Thiamylal Sodium (Barbiturates may enhance the drowsiness caused by antihistamines; potential for additive effects).
No products indexed under this heading.

Thioridazine Hydrochloride (CNS depressants may enhance the drowsiness caused by antihistamines; potential for additive effects). Products include:
- Thioridazine Hydrochloride Tablets 2289

Thiothixene (CNS depressants may enhance the drowsiness caused by antihistamines; potential for additive effects). Products include:
- Navane Capsules 2701
- Thiothixene Capsules 2290

Timolol Hemihydrate (Concurrent use with beta adrenergic blocker increases the effects of sympathomimetics). Products include:
- Betimol Ophthalmic Solution .... ⊙324

Timolol Maleate (Concurrent use with beta adrenergic blocker increases the effects of sympathomimetics). Products include:
- Blocadren Tablets 2046
- Cosopt Sterile Ophthalmic Solution 2065
- Timolide Tablets 2187
- Timolol GFS .... ⊙266
- Timoptic in Ocudose 2192
- Timoptic Sterile Ophthalmic Solution 2190
- Timoptic-XE Sterile Ophthalmic Gel Forming Solution 2194

Tranylcypromine Sulfate (Concurrent use with MAO inhibitor prolongs and intensifies the effects of antihistamines; co-administration of MAO inhibitors with sympathomimetics can result in hypertensive reactions, including hypertensive crises; co-administration and/or sequential use is contraindicated). Products include:
- Parnate Tablets 1607

Triazolam (CNS depressants may enhance the drowsiness caused by antihistamines; potential for additive effects). Products include:
- Halcion Tablets 2823

Trifluoperazine Hydrochloride (CNS depressants may enhance the drowsiness caused by antihistamines; potential for additive effects). Products include:
- Stelazine 1640

Trimipramine Maleate (Tricyclic antidepressants may enhance the drowsiness caused by antihistamines; potential for additive effects). Products include:
- Surmontil Capsules 3595

Zaleplon (CNS depressants may enhance the drowsiness caused by antihistamines; potential for additive effects). Products include:
- Sonata Capsules 3591

Ziprasidone Hydrochloride (CNS depressants may enhance the drowsiness caused by antihistamines; potential for additive effects). Products include:
- Geodon Capsules 2688

Zolpidem Tartrate (CNS depressants may enhance the drowsiness caused by antihistamines; potential for additive effects). Products include:
- Ambien Tablets 3191

Food Interactions

Alcohol (May enhance the drowsiness caused by antihistamines).

RYNATUSS PEDIATRIC SUSPENSION

(Carbetapentane Tannate, Chlorpheniramine Tannate, Ephedrine Tannate, Phenylephrine Tannate) 3353

May interact with central nervous system depressants, hypnotics and sedatives, monoamine oxidase inhibitors, tranquilizers, and certain other agents. Compounds in these categories include:

Alfentanil Hydrochloride (Antihistamines cause drowsiness and co-administration may increase drowsiness effect).
No products indexed under this heading.

Alprazolam (Antihistamines cause drowsiness and co-administration may increase drowsiness effect). Products include:
- Xanax Tablets 2865

Aprobarbital (Antihistamines cause drowsiness and co-administration may increase drowsiness effect).
No products indexed under this heading.

Buprenorphine Hydrochloride (Antihistamines cause drowsiness and co-administration may increase drowsiness effect). Products include:
- Buprenex Injectable 2918

Buspirone Hydrochloride (Antihistamines cause drowsiness and co-administration may increase drowsiness effect).
No products indexed under this heading.

Butabarbital (Antihistamines cause drowsiness and co-administration may increase drowsiness effect).
No products indexed under this heading.

Butalbital (Antihistamines cause drowsiness and co-administration may increase drowsiness effect). Products include:
- Phrenilin 578
- Sedapap Tablets 50 mg/650 mg 2225

Chlordiazepoxide (Antihistamines cause drowsiness and co-administration may increase drowsiness effect). Products include:
- Limbitrol 1738

Chlordiazepoxide Hydrochloride (Antihistamines cause drowsiness and co-administration may increase drowsiness effect). Products include:
- Librium Capsules 1736
- Librium for Injection 1737

Chlorpromazine (Antihistamines cause drowsiness and co-administration may increase drowsiness effect). Products include:
- Thorazine Suppositories 1656

Chlorpromazine Hydrochloride (Antihistamines cause drowsiness and co-administration may increase drowsiness effect). Products include:
- Thorazine 1656

Chlorprothixene (Antihistamines cause drowsiness and co-administration may increase drowsiness effect).
No products indexed under this heading.

Chlorprothixene Hydrochloride (Antihistamines cause drowsiness and co-administration may increase drowsiness effect).
No products indexed under this heading.

Chlorprothixene Lactate (Antihistamines cause drowsiness and co-administration may increase drowsiness effect).
No products indexed under this heading.

Clorazepate Dipotassium (Antihistamines cause drowsiness and co-administration may increase drowsiness effect). Products include:
- Tranxene 511

Clozapine (Antihistamines cause drowsiness and co-administration may increase drowsiness effect). Products include:
- Clozaril Tablets 2319

Codeine Phosphate (Antihistamines cause drowsiness and co-administration may increase drowsiness effect). Products include:
- Phenergan with Codeine Syrup 3557
- Phenergan VC with Codeine Syrup 3561
- Robitussin A-C Syrup 2942
- Robitussin-DAC Syrup 2942
- Ryna-C Liquid 768
- Soma Compound w/Codeine Tablets 3355
- Tussi-Organidin NR Liquid 3350
- Tussi-Organidin-S NR Liquid 3350
- Tylenol with Codeine 2595

Desflurane (Antihistamines cause drowsiness and co-administration may increase drowsiness effect). Products include:
- Suprane Liquid for Inhalation 874

Dezocine (Antihistamines cause drowsiness and co-administration may increase drowsiness effect).
No products indexed under this heading.

Diazepam (Antihistamines cause drowsiness and co-administration may increase drowsiness effect). Products include:
- Valium Injectable 3026
- Valium Tablets 3047

Droperidol (Antihistamines cause drowsiness and co-administration may increase drowsiness effect).
No products indexed under this heading.

Enflurane (Antihistamines cause drowsiness and co-administration may increase drowsiness effect).
No products indexed under this heading.

Estazolam (Antihistamines cause drowsiness and co-administration may increase drowsiness effect). Products include:
- ProSom Tablets 500

Ethchlorvynol (Antihistamines cause drowsiness and co-administration may increase drowsiness effect).
No products indexed under this heading.

Ethinamate (Antihistamines cause drowsiness and co-administration may increase drowsiness effect).
No products indexed under this heading.

Fentanyl (Antihistamines cause drowsiness and co-administration may increase drowsiness effect). Products include:
- Duragesic Transdermal System 1786

Fentanyl Citrate (Antihistamines cause drowsiness and co-administration may increase drowsiness effect). Products include:
- Actiq 1184

Fluphenazine Decanoate (Antihistamines cause drowsiness and co-administration may increase drowsiness effect).
No products indexed under this heading.

Fluphenazine Enanthate (Antihistamines cause drowsiness and co-administration may increase drowsiness effect).
No products indexed under this heading.

Fluphenazine Hydrochloride (Antihistamines cause drowsiness and co-administration may increase drowsiness effect).
No products indexed under this heading.

Flurazepam Hydrochloride (Antihistamines cause drowsiness and co-administration may increase drowsiness effect).
No products indexed under this heading.

Glutethimide (Antihistamines cause drowsiness and co-administration may increase drowsiness effect).
No products indexed under this heading.

Haloperidol (Antihistamines cause drowsiness and co-administration may increase drowsiness effect). Products include:
- Haldol Injection, Tablets and Concentrate 2533

Haloperidol Decanoate (Antihistamines cause drowsiness and co-administration may increase drowsiness effect). Products include:
- Haldol Decanoate 2535

Hydrocodone Bitartrate (Antihistamines cause drowsiness and co-administration may increase drowsiness effect). Products include:
- Hycodan 1316
- Hycomine Compound Tablets 1317
- Hycotuss Expectorant Syrup 1318
- Lortab 3319
- Lortab Elixir 3317
- Maxidone Tablets CIII 3399
- Norco 5/325 Tablets CIII 3424
- Norco 7.5/325 Tablets CIII 3425
- Norco 10/325 Tablets CIII 3427
- Norco 10/325 Tablets CIII 3425
- Vicodin Tablets 516
- Vicodin ES Tablets 517
- Vicodin HP Tablets 518
- Vicodin Tuss Expectorant 519
- Vicoprofen Tablets 520
- Zydone Tablets 1330

Hydrocodone Polistirex (Antihistamines cause drowsiness and co-administration may increase drowsiness effect). Products include:
- Tussionex Pennkinetic Extended-Release Suspension 1174

Hydromorphone Hydrochloride (Antihistamines cause drowsiness and co-administration may increase drowsiness effect). Products include:
- Dilaudid 441
- Dilaudid Oral Liquid 445
- Dilaudid Powder 441
- Dilaudid Rectal Suppositories 441
- Dilaudid Tablets 441
- Dilaudid Tablets - 8 mg 445
- Dilaudid-HP 443

Hydroxyzine Hydrochloride (Antihistamines cause drowsiness and co-administration may increase drowsiness effect). Products include:
- Atarax Tablets & Syrup 2667
- Vistaril Intramuscular Solution 2738

Isocarboxazid (MAO inhibitors prolong and intensify the anticholinergic effects of antihistamines and the overall effects of sympathomimetics; concurrent and/or sequential use is not recommended).
No products indexed under this heading.

Isoflurane (Antihistamines cause drowsiness and co-administration may increase drowsiness effect).
No products indexed under this heading.

Ketamine Hydrochloride (Antihistamines cause drowsiness and co-administration may increase drowsiness effect).
No products indexed under this heading.

Levomethadyl Acetate Hydrochloride (Antihistamines cause drowsiness and co-administration may increase drowsiness effect).
No products indexed under this heading.

Levorphanol Tartrate (Antihistamines cause drowsiness and co-administration may increase drowsiness effect). Products include:
- Levo-Dromoran ... 1734
- Levorphanol Tartrate Tablets ... 3059

Lorazepam (Antihistamines cause drowsiness and co-administration may increase drowsiness effect). Products include:
- Ativan Injection ... 3478
- Ativan Tablets ... 3482

Loxapine Hydrochloride (Antihistamines cause drowsiness and co-administration may increase drowsiness effect).
No products indexed under this heading.

Loxapine Succinate (Antihistamines cause drowsiness and co-administration may increase drowsiness effect). Products include:
- Loxitane Capsules ... 3398

Meperidine Hydrochloride (Antihistamines cause drowsiness and co-administration may increase drowsiness effect). Products include:
- Demerol ... 3079
- Mepergan Injection ... 3539

Mephobarbital (Antihistamines cause drowsiness and co-administration may increase drowsiness effect).
No products indexed under this heading.

Meprobamate (Antihistamines cause drowsiness and co-administration may increase drowsiness effect). Products include:
- Miltown Tablets ... 3349

Mesoridazine Besylate (Antihistamines cause drowsiness and co-administration may increase drowsiness effect). Products include:
- Serentil ... 1057

Methadone Hydrochloride (Antihistamines cause drowsiness and co-administration may increase drowsiness effect). Products include:
- Dolophine Hydrochloride Tablets ... 3056

Methohexital Sodium (Antihistamines cause drowsiness and co-administration may increase drowsiness effect). Products include:
- Brevital Sodium for Injection, USP .. 1815

Methotrimeprazine (Antihistamines cause drowsiness and co-administration may increase drowsiness effect).
No products indexed under this heading.

Methoxyflurane (Antihistamines cause drowsiness and co-administration may increase drowsiness effect).
No products indexed under this heading.

Midazolam Hydrochloride (Antihistamines cause drowsiness and co-administration may increase drowsiness effect). Products include:
- Versed Injection ... 3027
- Versed Syrup ... 3033

Moclobemide (MAO inhibitors prolong and intensify the anticholinergic effects of antihistamines and the overall effects of sympathomimetics; concurrent and/or sequential use is not recommended).
No products indexed under this heading.

Molindone Hydrochloride (Antihistamines cause drowsiness and co-administration may increase drowsiness effect). Products include:
- Moban ... 1320

Morphine Sulfate (Antihistamines cause drowsiness and co-administration may increase drowsiness effect). Products include:
- Astramorph/PF Injection, USP (Preservative-Free) ... 594
- Duramorph Injection ... 1312
- Infumorph 200 and Infumorph 500 Sterile Solutions ... 1314
- Kadian Capsules ... 1335
- MS Contin Tablets ... 2896
- MSIR ... 2898
- Oramorph SR Tablets ... 3062
- Roxanol ... 3066

Olanzapine (Antihistamines cause drowsiness and co-administration may increase drowsiness effect). Products include:
- Zyprexa Tablets ... 1973
- Zyprexa ZYDIS Orally Disintegrating Tablets ... 1973

Oxazepam (Antihistamines cause drowsiness and co-administration may increase drowsiness effect).
No products indexed under this heading.

Oxycodone Hydrochloride (Antihistamines cause drowsiness and co-administration may increase drowsiness effect). Products include:
- OxyContin Tablets ... 2912
- OxyFast Oral Concentrate Solution . 2916
- OxyIR Capsules ... 2916
- Percocet Tablets ... 1326
- Percodan Tablets ... 1327
- Percolone Tablets ... 1327
- Roxicodone ... 3067
- Tylox Capsules ... 2597

Pargyline Hydrochloride (MAO inhibitors prolong and intensify the anticholinergic effects of antihistamines and the overall effects of sympathomimetics; concurrent and/or sequential use is not recommended).
No products indexed under this heading.

Pentobarbital Sodium (Antihistamines cause drowsiness and co-administration may increase drowsiness effect). Products include:
- Nembutal Sodium Solution ... 485

Perphenazine (Antihistamines cause drowsiness and co-administration may increase drowsiness effect). Products include:
- Etrafon ... 3115
- Trilafon ... 3160

Phenelzine Sulfate (MAO inhibitors prolong and intensify the anticholinergic effects of antihistamines and the overall effects of sympathomimetics; concurrent and/or sequential use is not recommended). Products include:
- Nardil Tablets ... 2653

Phenobarbital (Antihistamines cause drowsiness and co-administration may increase drowsiness effect). Products include:
- Arco-Lase Plus Tablets ... 592
- Donnatal ... 2929
- Donnatal Extentabs ... 2930

Prazepam (Antihistamines cause drowsiness and co-administration may increase drowsiness effect).
No products indexed under this heading.

Procarbazine Hydrochloride (MAO inhibitors prolong and intensify the anticholinergic effects of antihistamines and the overall effects of sympathomimetics; concurrent and/or sequential use is not recommended). Products include:
- Matulane Capsules ... 3246

Prochlorperazine (Antihistamines cause drowsiness and co-administration may increase drowsiness effect). Products include:
- Compazine ... 1505

Promethazine Hydrochloride (Antihistamines cause drowsiness and co-administration may increase drowsiness effect). Products include:
- Mepergan Injection ... 3539
- Phenergan Injection ... 3553
- Phenergan ... 3556
- Phenergan Syrup ... 3554
- Phenergan with Codeine Syrup ... 3557
- Phenergan with Dextromethorphan Syrup ... 3559
- Phenergan VC Syrup ... 3560
- Phenergan VC with Codeine Syrup ... 3561

Propofol (Antihistamines cause drowsiness and co-administration may increase drowsiness effect). Products include:
- Diprivan Injectable Emulsion ... 667

Propoxyphene Hydrochloride (Antihistamines cause drowsiness and co-administration may increase drowsiness effect). Products include:
- Darvon Pulvules ... 1909
- Darvon Compound-65 Pulvules ... 1910

Propoxyphene Napsylate (Antihistamines cause drowsiness and co-administration may increase drowsiness effect). Products include:
- Darvon-N/Darvocet-N ... 1907
- Darvon-N Tablets ... 1912

Quazepam (Antihistamines cause drowsiness and co-administration may increase drowsiness effect).
No products indexed under this heading.

Quetiapine Fumarate (Antihistamines cause drowsiness and co-administration may increase drowsiness effect). Products include:
- Seroquel Tablets ... 684

Remifentanil Hydrochloride (Antihistamines cause drowsiness and co-administration may increase drowsiness effect).
No products indexed under this heading.

Risperidone (Antihistamines cause drowsiness and co-administration may increase drowsiness effect). Products include:
- Risperdal ... 1796

Secobarbital Sodium (Antihistamines cause drowsiness and co-administration may increase drowsiness effect).
No products indexed under this heading.

Selegiline Hydrochloride (MAO inhibitors prolong and intensify the anticholinergic effects of antihistamines and the overall effects of sympathomimetics; concurrent and/or sequential use is not recommended). Products include:
- Eldepryl Capsules ... 3266

Sevoflurane (Antihistamines cause drowsiness and co-administration may increase drowsiness effect).
No products indexed under this heading.

Sufentanil Citrate (Antihistamines cause drowsiness and co-administration may increase drowsiness effect).
No products indexed under this heading.

Temazepam (Antihistamines cause drowsiness and co-administration may increase drowsiness effect).
No products indexed under this heading.

Thiamylal Sodium (Antihistamines cause drowsiness and co-administration may increase drowsiness effect).
No products indexed under this heading.

Thioridazine Hydrochloride (Antihistamines cause drowsiness and co-administration may increase drowsiness effect). Products include:
- Thioridazine Hydrochloride Tablets ... 2289

Thiothixene (Antihistamines cause drowsiness and co-administration may increase drowsiness effect). Products include:
- Navane Capsules ... 2701
- Thiothixene Capsules ... 2290

Tranylcypromine Sulfate (MAO inhibitors prolong and intensify the anticholinergic effects of antihistamines and the overall effects of sympathomimetics; concurrent and/or sequential use is not recommended). Products include:
- Parnate Tablets ... 1607

Triazolam (Antihistamines cause drowsiness and co-administration may increase drowsiness effect). Products include:
- Halcion Tablets ... 2823

Trifluoperazine Hydrochloride (Antihistamines cause drowsiness and co-administration may increase drowsiness effect). Products include:
- Stelazine ... 1640

Zaleplon (Antihistamines cause drowsiness and co-administration may increase drowsiness effect). Products include:
- Sonata Capsules ... 3591

Ziprasidone Hydrochloride (Antihistamines cause drowsiness and co-administration may increase drowsiness effect). Products include:
- Geodon Capsules ... 2688

Zolpidem Tartrate (Antihistamines cause drowsiness and co-administration may increase drowsiness effect). Products include:
- Ambien Tablets ... 3191

Food Interactions

Alcohol (Antihistamines cause drowsiness and co-administration may increase drowsiness effect).

RYNATUSS TABLETS

(Carbetapentane Tannate, Chlorpheniramine Tannate, Ephedrine Tannate, Phenylephrine Tannate) ... 3353

See Rynatuss Pediatric Suspension

RYTHMOL TABLETS -- 150 MG, 225 MG, 300 MG

(Propafenone Hydrochloride) ... 502

May interact with cardiac glycosides, local anesthetics, quinidine, theophylline, and certain other agents. Compounds in these categories include:

Aminophylline (Combined therapy may result in an increase in theophylline concentration with the development of theophylline toxicity).
No products indexed under this heading.

Bupivacaine Hydrochloride (Concomitant use of local anesthetics may increase the risk of CNS side effects). Products include:
- Sensorcaine ... 643
- Sensorcaine-MPF Injection ... 643

Chloroprocaine Hydrochloride (Concomitant use of local anesthetics may increase the risk of CNS side effects). Products include:
- Nesacaine/Nesacaine MPF ... 617

Cimetidine (Increases steady-state plasma concentrations with no detectable changes in electrocardiographic parameters). Products include:
- Tagamet HB 200 Suspension ... ▣762
- Tagamet HB 200 Tablets ... ▣761
- Tagamet Tablets ... 1644

Cimetidine Hydrochloride (Increases steady-state plasma con-

centrations with no detectable changes in electrocardiographic parameters). Products include:

- Tagamet 1644

Cyclosporine (Propafenone therapy may increase levels of cyclosporine). Products include:

- Gengraf Capsules 457
- Neoral Soft Gelatin Capsules 2380
- Neoral Oral Solution 2380
- Sandimmune 2388

Desipramine Hydrochloride (Co-administration may result in elevated serum desipramine levels). Products include:

- Norpramin Tablets 755

Deslanoside (Potential for elevated digoxin levels; dosage reduction of digitalis may be necessary).

No products indexed under this heading.

Digitoxin (Potential for elevated digoxin levels; dosage reduction of digitalis may be necessary).

No products indexed under this heading.

Digoxin (Potential for elevated digoxin levels; dosage reduction of digitalis may be necessary).
Products include:

- Digitek Tablets 1003
- Lanoxicaps Capsules 1574
- Lanoxin Injection 1581
- Lanoxin Tablets 1587
- Lanoxin Elixir Pediatric 1578
- Lanoxin Injection Pediatric 1584

Dyphylline (Combined therapy may result in an increase in theophylline concentration with the development of theophylline toxicity). Products include:

- Lufyllin Tablets 3347
- Lufyllin-400 Tablets 3347
- Lufyllin-GG Elixir 3348
- Lufyllin-GG Tablets 3348

Etidocaine Hydrochloride (Concomitant use of local anesthetics may increase the risk of CNS side effects). Products include:

- Duranest Injections 600

Levobupivacaine Hydrochloride (Concomitant use of local anesthetics may increase the risk of CNS side effects). Products include:

- Chirocaine Injection 2909

Lidocaine Hydrochloride (Concomitant use of local anesthetics may increase the risk of CNS side effects). Products include:

- Bactine First Aid Liquid ▣611
- Xylocaine Injections 653

Mepivacaine Hydrochloride (Concomitant use of local anesthetics may increase the risk of CNS side effects). Products include:

- Polocaine Injection, USP 625
- Polocaine-MPF Injection, USP 625

Metoprolol Succinate (Co-administration can result in substantial increases in metoprolol concentration and elimination of half-life; increased plasma levels of metoprolol could overcome its cardioselectivity). Products include:

- Toprol-XL Tablets 651

Metoprolol Tartrate (Co-administration can result in substantial increases in metoprolol concentration and elimination of half-life; increased plasma levels of metoprolol could overcome its cardioselectivity).

No products indexed under this heading.

Procaine Hydrochloride (Concomitant use of local anesthetics may increase the risk of CNS side effects).

No products indexed under this heading.

Propranolol Hydrochloride (Co-administration has resulted in substantial increases in propranolol concentration and elimination of half-life). Products include:

- Inderal 3513
- Inderal LA Long-Acting Capsules 3516
- Inderide Tablets 3517
- Inderide LA Long-Acting Capsules 3519

Quinidine Gluconate (Small doses of quinidine completely inhibit the hydroxylation metabolic pathway, making all patients, in effect, slow metabolizers; there is too little information to recommend concomitant use). Products include:

- Quinaglute Dura-Tabs Tablets 978

Quinidine Polygalacturonate (Small doses of quinidine completely inhibit the hydroxylation metabolic pathway, making all patients, in effect, slow metabolizers; there is too little information to recommend concomitant use).

No products indexed under this heading.

Quinidine Sulfate (Small doses of quinidine completely inhibit the hydroxylation metabolic pathway, making all patients, in effect, slow metabolizers; there is too little information to recommend concomitant use). Products include:

- Quinidex Extentabs 2933

Rifampin (May accelerate the metabolism and decrease the plasma levels and antiarrythmic efficacy of propafenone). Products include:

- Rifadin 765
- Rifamate Capsules 767
- Rifater Tablets 769

Tetracaine Hydrochloride (Concomitant use of local anesthetics may increase the risk of CNS side effects). Products include:

- Cēpacol Viractin Cold Sore and Fever Blister Treatment, Gel ▣788
- Cetacaine Topical Anesthetic 1196

Theophylline (Combined therapy may result in an increase in theophylline concentration with the development of theophylline toxicity). Products include:

- Aerolate 1361
- Theo-Dur Extended-Release Tablets 1835
- Uni-Dur Extended-Release Tablets 1841
- Uniphyl 400 mg and 600 mg Tablets 2903

Theophylline Calcium Salicylate (Combined therapy may result in an increase in theophylline concentration with the development of theophylline toxicity).

No products indexed under this heading.

Theophylline Sodium Glycinate (Combined therapy may result in an increase in theophylline concentration with the development of theophylline toxicity).

No products indexed under this heading.

Warfarin Sodium (Increase in mean steady-state plasma levels of warfarin resulting in increased prothrombin time). Products include:

- Coumadin for Injection 1243
- Coumadin Tablets 1243
- Warfarin Sodium Tablets, USP 3302

Food Interactions

Food, unspecified (Increased peak blood level and bioavailability in a single dose study).

SAIZEN FOR INJECTION

(Somatropin) 3225
May interact with glucocorticoids. Compounds in these categories include:

Betamethasone Acetate (Concomitant glucocorticoid therapy may inhibit the growth promoting effect of somatropin). Products include:

- Celestone Soluspan Injectable Suspension 3097

Betamethasone Sodium Phosphate (Concomitant glucocorticoid therapy may inhibit the growth promoting effect of somatropin).
Products include:

- Celestone Soluspan Injectable Suspension 3097

Cortisone Acetate (Concomitant glucocorticoid therapy may inhibit the growth promoting effect of somatropin). Products include:

- Cortone Acetate Injectable Suspension 2059
- Cortone Acetate Tablets 2061

Dexamethasone (Concomitant glucocorticoid therapy may inhibit the growth promoting effect of somatropin). Products include:

- Decadron Elixir 2078
- Decadron Tablets 2079
- TobraDex Ophthalmic Ointment 542
- TobraDex Ophthalmic Suspension 541

Dexamethasone Acetate (Concomitant glucocorticoid therapy may inhibit the growth promoting effect of somatropin).

No products indexed under this heading.

Dexamethasone Sodium Phosphate (Concomitant glucocorticoid therapy may inhibit the growth promoting effect of somatropin).
Products include:

- Decadron Phosphate Injection 2081
- Decadron Phosphate Sterile Ophthalmic Ointment 2083
- Decadron Phosphate Sterile Ophthalmic Solution 2084
- NeoDecadron Sterile Ophthalmic Solution 2144

Fludrocortisone Acetate (Concomitant glucocorticoid therapy may inhibit the growth promoting effect of somatropin). Products include:

- Florinef Acetate Tablets 2250

Hydrocortisone (Concomitant glucocorticoid therapy may inhibit the growth promoting effect of somatropin). Products include:

- Anusol-HC Cream 2.5% 2237
- Cipro HC Otic Suspension 540
- Cortaid Intensive Therapy Cream ▣717
- Cortaid Maximum Strength Cream ▣717
- Cortisporin Ophthalmic Suspension Sterile ⊙297
- Cortizone•5 ▣699
- Cortizone•10 ▣699
- Cortizone•10 Plus Creme ▣700
- Cortizone for Kids Creme ▣699
- Hydrocortone Tablets 2106
- Massengill Medicated Soft Cloth Towelette ▣753
- VōSoL HC Otic Solution 3356

Hydrocortisone Acetate (Concomitant glucocorticoid therapy may inhibit the growth promoting effect of somatropin). Products include:

- Analpram-HC 1338
- Anusol HC-1 Hydrocortisone Anti-Itch Cream ▣689
- Anusol-HC Suppositories 2238
- Cortaid ▣717
- Cortifoam Rectal Foam 3170
- Cortisporin-TC Otic Suspension 2246
- Hydrocortone Acetate Injectable Suspension 2103
- Pramosone 1343
- Proctocort Suppositories 2264
- ProctoFoam-HC 3177
- Terra-Cortril Ophthalmic Suspension 2716

Hydrocortisone Sodium Phosphate (Concomitant glucocorticoid therapy may inhibit the growth promoting effect of somatropin).
Products include:

- Hydrocortone Phosphate Injection, Sterile 2105

Hydrocortisone Sodium Succinate (Concomitant glucocorticoid therapy may inhibit the growth promoting effect of somatropin).

No products indexed under this heading.

Methylprednisolone Acetate (Concomitant glucocorticoid therapy may inhibit the growth promoting effect of somatropin). Products include:

- Depo-Medrol Injectable Suspension 2795

Methylprednisolone Sodium Succinate (Concomitant glucocorticoid therapy may inhibit the growth promoting effect of somatropin).
Products include:

- Solu-Medrol Sterile Powder 2855

Prednisolone Acetate (Concomitant glucocorticoid therapy may inhibit the growth promoting effect of somatropin). Products include:

- Blephamide Ophthalmic Ointment 547
- Blephamide Ophthalmic Suspension 548
- Poly-Pred Liquifilm Ophthalmic Suspension ⊙245
- Pred Forte Ophthalmic Suspension ⊙246
- Pred Mild Sterile Ophthalmic Suspension ⊙249
- Pred-G Ophthalmic Suspension ⊙247
- Pred-G Sterile Ophthalmic Ointment ⊙248

Prednisolone Sodium Phosphate (Concomitant glucocorticoid therapy may inhibit the growth promoting effect of somatropin). Products include:

- Pediapred Oral Solution 1170

Prednisolone Tebutate (Concomitant glucocorticoid therapy may inhibit the growth promoting effect of somatropin).

No products indexed under this heading.

Prednisone (Concomitant glucocorticoid therapy may inhibit the growth promoting effect of somatropin).
Products include:

- Prednisone 3064

Triamcinolone (Concomitant glucocorticoid therapy may inhibit the growth promoting effect of somatropin).

No products indexed under this heading.

Triamcinolone Acetonide (Concomitant glucocorticoid therapy may inhibit the growth promoting effect of somatropin). Products include:

- Azmacort Inhalation Aerosol 728
- Nasacort Nasal Inhaler 750
- Nasacort AQ Nasal Spray 752
- Tri-Nasal Spray 2274

Triamcinolone Diacetate (Concomitant glucocorticoid therapy may inhibit the growth promoting effect of somatropin).

No products indexed under this heading.

Triamcinolone Hexacetonide (Concomitant glucocorticoid therapy may inhibit the growth promoting effect of somatropin).

No products indexed under this heading.

SALAGEN TABLETS

(Pilocarpine Hydrochloride) 2229
May interact with anticholinergics, beta blockers, parasympathomimetics, and certain other agents. Compounds in these categories include:

Acebutolol Hydrochloride (Co-administration of pilocarpine with beta adrenergic antagonists may result in possible conduction disturbances). Products include:

- Sectral Capsules 3589

Atenolol (Co-administration of pilocarpine with beta adrenergic antagonists may result in possible conduction disturbances). Products include:

- Tenoretic Tablets 690
- Tenormin I.V. Injection 692

Atropine Sulfate (Pilocarpine might antagonize the anticholinergic effects of drugs used concomitantly). Products include:

- Donnatal 2929
- Donnatal Extentabs 2930
- Motofen Tablets 577
- Prosed/DS Tablets 3268
- Urised Tablets 2876

IMPORTANT NOTE: Always consult each drug listing in the patient's regimen for possible interactions.

Belladonna Alkaloids (Pilocarpine might antagonize the anticholinergic effects of drugs used concomitantly). Products include:
Hyland's Teething Tablets .... ◙766
Urimax Tablets 1769

Benztropine Mesylate (Pilocarpine might antagonize the anticholinergic effects of drugs used concomitantly). Products include:
Cogentin 2055

Betaxolol Hydrochloride (Co-administration of pilocarpine with beta adrenergic antagonists may result in possible conduction disturbances). Products include:
Betoptic S Ophthalmic Suspension 537

Biperiden Hydrochloride (Pilocarpine might antagonize the anticholinergic effects of drugs used concomitantly). Products include:
Akineton 402

Bisoprolol Fumarate (Co-administration of pilocarpine with beta adrenergic antagonists may result in possible conduction disturbances). Products include:
Zebeta Tablets 1885
Ziac Tablets 1887

Carteolol Hydrochloride (Co-administration of pilocarpine with beta adrenergic antagonists may result in possible conduction disturbances). Products include:
Carteolol Hydrochloride Ophthalmic Solution USP, 1% ..... ⊙258
Ocupress Ophthalmic Solution, 1% Sterile .... ⊙303

Cevimeline Hydrochloride (Additive pharmacologic effect). Products include:
Evoxac Capsules 1217

Clidinium Bromide (Pilocarpine might antagonize the anticholinergic effects of drugs used concomitantly).
No products indexed under this heading.

Dicyclomine Hydrochloride (Pilocarpine might antagonize the anticholinergic effects of drugs used concomitantly).
No products indexed under this heading.

Edrophonium Chloride (Additive pharmacologic effect). Products include:
Tensilon Injectable 1745

Esmolol Hydrochloride (Co-administration of pilocarpine with beta adrenergic antagonists may result in possible conduction disturbances). Products include:
Brevibloc Injection 858

Glycopyrrolate (Pilocarpine might antagonize the anticholinergic effects of drugs used concomitantly). Products include:
Robinul Forte Tablets 1358
Robinul Injectable 2940
Robinul Tablets 1358

Hyoscyamine (Pilocarpine might antagonize the anticholinergic effects of drugs used concomitantly). Products include:
Urised Tablets 2876

Hyoscyamine Sulfate (Pilocarpine might antagonize the anticholinergic effects of drugs used concomitantly). Products include:
Arco-Lase Plus Tablets 592
Donnatal 2929
Donnatal Extentabs 2930
Levsin/Levsinex/Levbid 3172
NuLev Orally Disintegrating Tablets 3176
Prosed/DS Tablets 3268
Urimax Tablets 1769

Ipratropium Bromide (Pilocarpine might antagonize the anticholinergic effects of drugs used concomitantly). Products include:
Atrovent Inhalation Aerosol 1030
Atrovent Inhalation Solution 1031
Atrovent Nasal Spray 0.03% 1032
Atrovent Nasal Spray 0.06% 1033
Combivent Inhalation Aerosol 1041
DuoNeb Inhalation Solution 1233

Labetalol Hydrochloride (Co-administration of pilocarpine with beta adrenergic antagonists may result in possible conduction disturbances). Products include:
Normodyne Injection 3135
Normodyne Tablets 3137

Levobunolol Hydrochloride (Co-administration of pilocarpine with beta adrenergic antagonists may result in possible conduction disturbances). Products include:
Betagan .... ⊙228

Mepenzolate Bromide (Pilocarpine might antagonize the anticholinergic effects of drugs used concomitantly).
No products indexed under this heading.

Metipranolol Hydrochloride (Co-administration of pilocarpine with beta adrenergic antagonists may result in possible conduction disturbances).
No products indexed under this heading.

Metoprolol Succinate (Co-administration of pilocarpine with beta adrenergic antagonists may result in possible conduction disturbances). Products include:
Toprol-XL Tablets 651

Metoprolol Tartrate (Co-administration of pilocarpine with beta adrenergic antagonists may result in possible conduction disturbances).
No products indexed under this heading.

Nadolol (Co-administration of pilocarpine with beta adrenergic antagonists may result in possible conduction disturbances). Products include:
Corgard Tablets 2245
Corzide 40/5 Tablets 2247
Corzide 80/5 Tablets 2247
Nadolol Tablets 2288

Neostigmine Bromide (Additive pharmacologic effect). Products include:
Prostigmin Tablets 1744

Neostigmine Methylsulfate (Additive pharmacologic effect). Products include:
Prostigmin Injectable 1744

Oxybutynin Chloride (Pilocarpine might antagonize the anticholinergic effects of drugs used concomitantly). Products include:
Ditropan XL Extended Release Tablets 564

Penbutolol Sulfate (Co-administration of pilocarpine with beta adrenergic antagonists may result in possible conduction disturbances).
No products indexed under this heading.

Pindolol (Co-administration of pilocarpine with beta adrenergic antagonists may result in possible conduction disturbances).
No products indexed under this heading.

Procyclidine Hydrochloride (Pilocarpine might antagonize the anticholinergic effects of drugs used concomitantly).
No products indexed under this heading.

Propantheline Bromide (Pilocarpine might antagonize the anticholinergic effects of drugs used concomitantly).
No products indexed under this heading.

Propranolol Hydrochloride (Co-administration of pilocarpine with beta adrenergic antagonists may result in possible conduction disturbances). Products include:
Inderal 3513
Inderal LA Long-Acting Capsules 3516
Inderide Tablets 3517
Inderide LA Long-Acting Capsules .. 3519

Pyridostigmine Bromide (Additive pharmacologic effect). Products include:
Mestinon 1740

Scopolamine (Pilocarpine might antagonize the anticholinergic effects of drugs used concomitantly). Products include:
Transderm Scōp Transdermal Therapeutic System 2302

Scopolamine Hydrobromide (Pilocarpine might antagonize the anticholinergic effects of drugs used concomitantly). Products include:
Donnatal 2929
Donnatal Extentabs 2930

Sotalol Hydrochloride (Co-administration of pilocarpine with beta adrenergic antagonists may result in possible conduction disturbances). Products include:
Betapace Tablets 950
Betapace AF Tablets 954

Timolol Hemihydrate (Co-administration of pilocarpine with beta adrenergic antagonists may result in possible conduction disturbances). Products include:
Betimol Ophthalmic Solution .... ⊙324

Timolol Maleate (Co-administration of pilocarpine with beta adrenergic antagonists may result in possible conduction disturbances). Products include:
Blocadren Tablets 2046
Cosopt Sterile Ophthalmic Solution..................................... 2065
Timolide Tablets 2187
Timolol GFS .... ⊙266
Timoptic in Ocudose 2192
Timoptic Sterile Ophthalmic Solution..................................... 2190
Timoptic-XE Sterile Ophthalmic Gel Forming Solution 2194

Tolterodine Tartrate (Pilocarpine might antagonize the anticholinergic effects of drugs used concomitantly). Products include:
Detrol Tablets 3623
Detrol LA Capsules 2801

Tridihexethyl Chloride (Pilocarpine might antagonize the anticholinergic effects of drugs used concomitantly).
No products indexed under this heading.

Trihexyphenidyl Hydrochloride (Pilocarpine might antagonize the anticholinergic effects of drugs used concomitantly). Products include:
Artane 1855

Food Interactions

Diet, high-lipid (Decrease in the rate of absorption of pilocarpine when taken with high fat meal).

SANDIMMUNE I.V. AMPULS FOR INFUSION

(Cyclosporine) 2388
May interact with erythromycin, immunosuppressive agents, methylprednisolone, non-steroidal anti-inflammatory agents, phenytoin, prednisolone, protease inhibitors, potassium sparing diuretics, and certain other agents. Compounds in these categories include:

Allopurinol (Increases cyclosporine concentrations).
No products indexed under this heading.

Amiloride Hydrochloride (Cyclosporine may cause hyperkalemia, concurrent use should be avoided). Products include:
Midamor Tablets 2136
Moduretic Tablets 2138

Amiodarone Hydrochloride (Increases cyclosporine concentrations). Products include:
Cordarone Intravenous 3491
Cordarone Tablets 3487
Pacerone Tablets 3331

Amphotericin B (May potentiate renal dysfunction). Products include:
Abelcet Injection 1273
AmBisome for Injection 1383
Amphotec 1774

Amprenavir (The HIV protease inhibitors are known to inhibit CYP450 3A and thus could potentially increase the concentrations of cyclosporine). Products include:
Agenerase Capsules 1454
Agenerase Oral Solution 1459

Antibiotics, unspecified (Potential synergies of nephrotoxicity may occur).

Azapropazon (May potentiate renal dysfunction).
No products indexed under this heading.

Azathioprine (Increases susceptibility to infection).
No products indexed under this heading.

Basiliximab (Increases susceptibility to infection). Products include:
Simulect for Injection 2399

Bromocriptine Mesylate (Increases cyclosporine levels; dosage adjustments are essential).
No products indexed under this heading.

Carbamazepine (Decreases cyclosporine plasma concentrations; dosage adjustments are essential). Products include:
Carbatrol Capsules 3234
Tegretol/Tegretol-XR 2404

Celecoxib (Co-administration with NSAID's, particularly in the setting of dehydration, may potentiate renal dysfunction). Products include:
Celebrex Capsules 2676
Celebrex Capsules 2780

Cimetidine (May potentiate renal dysfunction). Products include:
Tagamet HB 200 Suspension .... ◙762
Tagamet HB 200 Tablets .... ◙761
Tagamet Tablets 1644

Cimetidine Hydrochloride (May potentiate renal dysfunction). Products include:
Tagamet 1644

Colchicine (Co-administration results in increased cyclosporine concentrations and potentiation of renal dysfunction).
No products indexed under this heading.

Dalfopristin (Co-administration with substrates that inhibit CYP450 3A, such as dalfopristin, could decrease metabolism and increase cyclosporine concentrations). Products include:
Synercid I.V. 775

Danazol (Increases cyclosporine plasma concentrations; dosage adjustments are essential).
No products indexed under this heading.

Diclofenac Potassium (Co-administration with NSAID's, particularly in the setting of dehydration, may potentiate renal dysfunction). Products include:
Cataflam Tablets 2315

Diclofenac Sodium (Co-administration with NSAID's, particularly in the setting of dehydration, may potentiate renal dysfunction). Products include:
Arthrotec Tablets 3195
Voltaren Ophthalmic Sterile Ophthalmic Solution .... ⊙312
Voltaren Tablets 2315
Voltaren-XR Tablets 2315

Digoxin (Reduced clearance of digoxin and potential for severe digitalis toxicity). Products include:
Digitek Tablets 1003
Lanoxicaps Capsules 1574
Lanoxin Injection 1581
Lanoxin Tablets 1587
Lanoxin Elixir Pediatric 1578
Lanoxin Injection Pediatric 1584

Diltiazem Hydrochloride (Increases cyclosporine plasma concentrations; dosage adjustments are essential). Products include:
- Cardizem Injectable ... 1018
- Cardizem Lyo-Ject Syringe ... 1018
- Cardizem Monovial ... 1018
- Cardizem CD Capsules ... 1016
- Tiazac Capsules ... 1378

Erythromycin (Co-administration with substrates that inhibit CYP450 3A, such as erythromycin, could decrease metabolism and increase cyclosporine concentrations). Products include:
- Emgel 2% Topical Gel ... 1285
- Ery-Tab Tablets ... 448
- Erythromycin Base Filmtab Tablets ... 454
- Erythromycin Delayed-Release Capsules, USP ... 455
- PCE Dispertab Tablets ... 498

Erythromycin Estolate (Co-administration with substrates that inhibit CYP450 3A, such as erythromycin, could decrease metabolism and increase cyclosporine concentrations).
No products indexed under this heading.

Erythromycin Ethylsuccinate (Co-administration with substrates that inhibit CYP450 3A, such as erythromycin, could decrease metabolism and increase cyclosporine concentrations). Products include:
- E.E.S. ... 450
- EryPed ... 446
- Pediazole Suspension ... 3050

Erythromycin Gluceptate (Co-administration with substrates that inhibit CYP450 3A, such as erythromycin, could decrease metabolism and increase cyclosporine concentrations).
No products indexed under this heading.

Erythromycin Stearate (Co-administration with substrates that inhibit CYP450 3A, such as erythromycin, could decrease metabolism and increase cyclosporine concentrations). Products include:
- Erythrocin Stearate Filmtab Tablets ... 452

Etodolac (Co-administration with NSAID's, particularly in the setting of dehydration, may potentiate renal dysfunction). Products include:
- Lodine ... 3528
- Lodine XL Extended-Release Tablets ... 3530

Fenoprofen Calcium (Co-administration with NSAID's, particularly in the setting of dehydration, may potentiate renal dysfunction).
No products indexed under this heading.

Fluconazole (Increases cyclosporine levels; dosage adjustments are essential). Products include:
- Diflucan Tablets, Injection, and Oral Suspension ... 2681

Flurbiprofen (Co-administration with NSAID's, particularly in the setting of dehydration, may potentiate renal dysfunction).
No products indexed under this heading.

Fosphenytoin Sodium (Co-administration with agents that are known to induce CYP450 system, such as phenytoin, will increase hepatic metabolism and decrease cyclosporine levels). Products include:
- Cerebyx Injection ... 2619

Gentamicin Sulfate (May potentiate renal dysfunction). Products include:
- Genoptic Ophthalmic Ointment ... ⊙239
- Genoptic Sterile Ophthalmic Solution ... ⊙239
- Pred-G Ophthalmic Suspension ... ⊙247
- Pred-G Sterile Ophthalmic Ointment ... ⊙248

Hypericum (Co-administration has been reported to produce a marked reduction in blood cyclosporine concentrations, resulting in subtherapeutic levels, rejection of transplanted organs, and graft loss). Products include:
- Brite-Life Caplets ... ⊞795
- Centrum St. John's Wort Softgels ... ⊞853
- Metabolic Nutrition System ... ⊞798
- Movana Tablets ... ⊞832
- One-A-Day Tension & Mood Softgels ... ⊞808
- ReSource Wellness StayCalm Caplets ... ⊞826
- Satiete Tablets ... ⊞846

Ibuprofen (Co-administration with NSAID's, particularly in the setting of dehydration, may potentiate renal dysfunction). Products include:
- Advil ... ⊞771
- Children's Advil Oral Suspension ... ⊞773
- Children's Advil Chewable Tablets ... ⊞773
- Advil Cold and Sinus Caplets ... ⊞771
- Advil Cold and Sinus Tablets ... ⊞771
- Advil Flu & Body Ache Caplets ... ⊞772
- Infants' Advil Drops ... ⊞773
- Junior Strength Advil Tablets ... ⊞773
- Junior Strength Advil Chewable Tablets ... ⊞773
- Advil Migraine Liquigels ... ⊞772
- Children's Motrin Oral Suspension and Chewable Tablets ... 2006
- Children's Motrin Cold Oral Suspension ... 2007
- Children's Motrin Oral Suspension ... ⊞643
- Motrin Suspension, Oral Drops, Chewable Tablets, and Caplets ... 2002
- Infants' Motrin Concentrated Drops ... 2006
- Junior Strength Motrin Caplets and Chewable Tablets ... 2006
- Motrin IB Tablets, Caplets, and Gelcaps ... 2002
- Motrin Migraine Pain Caplets ... 2005
- Motrin Sinus Headache Caplets ... 2005
- Vicoprofen Tablets ... 520

Immune Globulin Intravenous (Human) (Increases susceptibility to infection).
No products indexed under this heading.

Indinavir Sulfate (The HIV protease inhibitors are known to inhibit CYP450 3A and thus could potentially increase the concentrations of cyclosporine). Products include:
- Crixivan Capsules ... 2070

Indomethacin (Co-administration with NSAID's, particularly in the setting of dehydration, may potentiate renal dysfunction). Products include:
- Indocin ... 2112

Indomethacin Sodium Trihydrate (Co-administration with NSAID's, particularly in the setting of dehydration, may potentiate renal dysfunction). Products include:
- Indocin I.V. ... 2115

Itraconazole (Increases cyclosporine levels; dosage adjustments are essential). Products include:
- Sporanox Capsules ... 1800
- Sporanox Injection ... 1804
- Sporanox Injection ... 2509
- Sporanox Oral Solution ... 1808
- Sporanox Oral Solution ... 2512

Ketoconazole (May potentiate renal dysfunction; co-administration with substrates that inhibit CYP450 3A, such as ketoconazole, could decrease metabolism and increase cyclosporine concentrations). Products include:
- Nizoral 2% Cream ... 3620
- Nizoral A-D Shampoo ... 2008
- Nizoral 2% Shampoo ... 2007
- Nizoral Tablets ... 1791

Ketoprofen (Co-administration with NSAID's, particularly in the setting of dehydration, may potentiate renal dysfunction). Products include:
- Orudis Capsules ... 3548
- Orudis KT Tablets ... ⊞778
- Oruvail Capsules ... 3548

Ketorolac Tromethamine (Co-administration with NSAID's, particularly in the setting of dehydration, may potentiate renal dysfunction). Products include:
- Acular Ophthalmic Solution ... 544
- Acular PF Ophthalmic Solution ... 544
- Toradol ... 3018

Lopinavir (The HIV protease inhibitors are known to inhibit CYP450 3A and thus could potentially increase the concentrations of cyclosporine). Products include:
- Kaletra Capsules ... 471
- Kaletra Oral Solution ... 471

Lovastatin (Reduced clearance of lovastatin; concomitant administration associated with development of myositis). Products include:
- Mevacor Tablets ... 2132

Meclofenamate Sodium (Co-administration with NSAID's, particularly in the setting of dehydration, may potentiate renal dysfunction).
No products indexed under this heading.

Mefenamic Acid (Co-administration with NSAID's, particularly in the setting of dehydration, may potentiate renal dysfunction). Products include:
- Ponstel Capsules ... 1356

Meloxicam (Co-administration with NSAID's, particularly in the setting of dehydration, may potentiate renal dysfunction). Products include:
- Mobic Tablets ... 1054

Melphalan (May potentiate renal dysfunction). Products include:
- Alkeran Tablets ... 1466

Methotrexate Sodium (Co-administration in rheumatoid arthritis patients has resulted in increased AUC of methotrexate by approximately 30% and concentration of its metabolite decreased by approximately 80%; the clinical significance is not known).
No products indexed under this heading.

Methylprednisolone (Co-administration with agents that are known to inhibit CYP450 system, such as methylprednisolone, will decrease hepatic metabolism and increase cyclosporine levels; convulsions have been reported with concomitant high doses of methylprednisolone).
No products indexed under this heading.

Methylprednisolone Acetate (Co-administration with agents that are known to inhibit CYP450 system, such as methylprednisolone, will decrease hepatic metabolism and increase cyclosporine levels; convulsions have been reported with concomitant high doses of methylprednisolone). Products include:
- Depo-Medrol Injectable Suspension ... 2795

Methylprednisolone Sodium Succinate (Co-administration with agents that are known to inhibit CYP450 system, such as methylprednisolone, will decrease hepatic metabolism and increase cyclosporine levels; convulsions have been reported with concomitant high doses of methylprednisolone). Products include:
- Solu-Medrol Sterile Powder ... 2855

Metoclopramide Hydrochloride (Increases cyclosporine levels; dosage adjustments are essential). Products include:
- Reglan ... 2935

Muromonab-CD3 (Increased susceptibility to infection and increased risk for development of lymphomas and malignancies). Products include:
- Orthoclone OKT3 Sterile Solution ... 2498

Mycophenolate Mofetil (Increases susceptibility to infection). Products include:
- CellCept Capsules ... 2951
- CellCept Oral Suspension ... 2951
- CellCept Tablets ... 2951

Nabumetone (Co-administration with NSAID's, particularly in the setting of dehydration, may potentiate renal dysfunction). Products include:
- Relafen Tablets ... 1617

Nafcillin Sodium (Decreases cyclosporine concentrations).
No products indexed under this heading.

Naproxen (Co-administration with NSAID's, particularly in the setting of dehydration, may potentiate renal dysfunction). Products include:
- EC-Naprosyn Delayed-Release Tablets ... 2967
- Naprosyn Suspension ... 2967
- Naprosyn Tablets ... 2967

Naproxen Sodium (Co-administration with NSAID's, particularly in the setting of dehydration, may potentiate renal dysfunction). Products include:
- Aleve Tablets, Caplets and Gelcaps ... ⊞602
- Aleve Cold & Sinus Caplets ... ⊞603
- Anaprox Tablets ... 2967
- Anaprox DS Tablets ... 2967
- Naprelan Tablets ... 1293

Nelfinavir Mesylate (The HIV protease inhibitors are known to inhibit CYP450 3A and thus could potentially increase the concentrations of cyclosporine). Products include:
- Viracept ... 532

Nephrotoxic Drugs (Potential synergics of nephrotoxicity).
No products indexed under this heading.

Nicardipine Hydrochloride (Increases cyclosporine plasma concentrations; dosage adjustments are essential). Products include:
- Cardene I.V. ... 3485

Nifedipine (Potential for frequent gingival hyperplasia). Products include:
- Adalat CC Tablets ... 877
- Procardia Capsules ... 2708
- Procardia XL Extended Release Tablets ... 2710

Octreotide Acetate (Decreases cyclosporine concentrations). Products include:
- Sandostatin LAR Depot ... 2395

Orlistat (Co-administration can result in decreased absorption of cyclosporine; concomitant use should be avoided). Products include:
- Xenical Capsules ... 3043

Oxaprozin (Co-administration with NSAID's, particularly in the setting of dehydration, may potentiate renal dysfunction).
No products indexed under this heading.

Phenobarbital (Decreases cyclosporine plasma levels; dosage adjustments are essential). Products include:
- Arco-Lase Plus Tablets ... 592
- Donnatal ... 2929
- Donnatal Extentabs ... 2930

Phenylbutazone (Co-administration with NSAID's, particularly in the setting of dehydration, may potentiate renal dysfunction).
No products indexed under this heading.

Phenytoin (Co-administration with agents that are known to induce CYP450 system, such as phenytoin, will increase hepatic metabolism and decrease cyclosporine levels). Products include:
- Dilantin Infatabs ... 2624
- Dilantin-125 Oral Suspension ... 2625

Phenytoin Sodium (Co-administration with agents that are known to induce CYP450 system, such as phenytoin, will increase hepatic metabolism and decrease cyclosporine levels). Products include:
- Dilantin Kapseals ... 2622

IMPORTANT NOTE: Always consult each drug listing in the patient's regimen for possible interactions.

Piroxicam (Co-administration with NSAID's, particularly in the setting of dehydration, may potentiate renal dysfunction). Products include:
Feldene Capsules 2685

Prednisolone (Co-administration results in reduced clearance of prednisolone). Products include:
Prelone Syrup 2273

Prednisolone Acetate (Co-administration results in reduced clearance of prednisolone). Products include:
Blephamide Ophthalmic Ointment ... 547
Blephamide Ophthalmic Suspension 548
Poly-Pred Liquifilm Ophthalmic Suspension .... ⊙245
Pred Forte Ophthalmic Suspension .... ⊙246
Pred Mild Sterile Ophthalmic Suspension .... ⊙249
Pred-G Ophthalmic Suspension ..... ⊙247
Pred-G Sterile Ophthalmic Ointment .... ⊙248

Prednisolone Sodium Phosphate (Co-administration results in reduced clearance of prednisolone). Products include:
Pediapred Oral Solution 1170

Prednisolone Tebutate (Co-administration results in reduced clearance of prednisolone).
No products indexed under this heading.

Quinupristin (Co-administration with substrates that inhibit CYP450 3A, such as quinupristine, could decrease metabolism and increase cyclosporine concentrations). Products include:
Synercid I.V. 775

Ranitidine Hydrochloride (May potentiate renal dysfunction). Products include:
Zantac 1690
Zantac Injection 1688
Zantac 75 Tablets .... ▣717

Rifabutin (Rifabutin is known to increase the metabolism of other drugs metabolized by CYP450 system; the interaction between cyclosporine and rifabutin has not been studied; care should be exercised). Products include:
Mycobutin Capsules 2838

Rifampin (Decreases cyclosporine plasma levels; dosage adjustments are essential). Products include:
Rifadin 765
Rifamate Capsules 767
Rifater Tablets 769

Ritonavir (The HIV protease inhibitors are known to inhibit CYP450 3A and thus could potentially increase the concentrations of cyclosporine). Products include:
Kaletra Capsules 471
Kaletra Oral Solution 471
Norvir Capsules 487
Norvir Oral Solution 487

Rofecoxib (Co-administration with NSAID's, particularly in the setting of dehydration, may potentiate renal dysfunction). Products include:
Vioxx 2213

Saquinavir (The HIV protease inhibitors are known to inhibit CYP450 3A and thus could potentially increase the concentrations of cyclosporine). Products include:
Fortovase Capsules 2970

Saquinavir Mesylate (The HIV protease inhibitors are known to inhibit CYP450 3A and thus could potentially increase the concentrations of cyclosporine). Products include:
Invirase Capsules 2979

Sirolimus (Increases susceptibility to infection). Products include:
Rapamune Oral Solution and Tablets 3584

Spironolactone (Cyclosporine may cause hyperkalemia, concurrent use should be avoided).
No products indexed under this heading.

Sulfamethoxazole (May potentiate renal dysfunction). Products include:
Bactrim 2949
Septra Suspension 2265
Septra Tablets 2265
Septra DS Tablets 2265

Sulindac (Co-administration with NSAID's, particularly in the setting of dehydration, may potentiate renal dysfunction). Products include:
Clinoril Tablets 2053

Tacrolimus (May potentiate renal dysfunction). Products include:
Prograf 1393
Protopic Ointment 1397

Ticlopidine Hydrochloride (Decreases cyclosporine concentrations). Products include:
Ticlid Tablets 3015

Tobramycin (May potentiate renal dysfunction). Products include:
TOBI Solution for Inhalation 1206
TobraDex Ophthalmic Ointment 542
TobraDex Ophthalmic Suspension .. 541
Tobrex Ophthalmic Ointment .... ⊙220
Tobrex Ophthalmic Solution .... ⊙221

Tobramycin Sulfate (May potentiate renal dysfunction). Products include:
Nebcin Vials, Hyporets & ADD-Vantage 1955

Tolmetin Sodium (Co-administration with NSAID's, particularly in the setting of dehydration, may potentiate renal dysfunction). Products include:
Tolectin 2589

Triamterene (Cyclosporine may cause hyperkalemia, concurrent use should be avoided). Products include:
Dyazide Capsules 1515
Dyrenium Capsules 3458
Maxzide 1008

Trimethoprim (May potentiate renal dysfunction). Products include:
Bactrim 2949
Septra Suspension 2265
Septra Tablets 2265
Septra DS Tablets 2265

Vancomycin Hydrochloride (May potentiate renal dysfunction). Products include:
Vancocin HCl Capsules & Pulvules .. 1972
Vancocin HCl Oral Solution 1971
Vancocin HCl, Vials & ADD-Vantage 1970

Verapamil Hydrochloride (Increases cyclosporine levels; dosage adjustments are essential). Products include:
Covera-HS Tablets 3199
Isoptin SR Tablets 467
Tarka Tablets 508
Verelan Capsules 3184
Verelan PM Capsules 3186

Food Interactions

Grapefruit (Co-administration results in increased blood concentrations of cyclosporine; concurrent use should be avoided).

Grapefruit Juice (Co-administration results in increased blood concentrations of cyclosporine; concurrent use should be avoided).

SANDIMMUNE ORAL SOLUTION
(Cyclosporine) 2388
See Sandimmune I.V. Ampuls for Infusion

SANDIMMUNE SOFT GELATIN CAPSULES
(Cyclosporine) 2388
See Sandimmune I.V. Ampuls for Infusion

SANDOGLOBULIN I.V.
(Globulin, Immune (Human)) 2391
May interact with:

Measles, Mumps & Rubella Virus Vaccine, Live (Antibodies in Immune Globulin may interfere with the response to live viral vaccines). Products include:
M-M-R II 2118

SANDOSTATIN LAR DEPOT
(Octreotide Acetate) 2395
May interact with beta blockers, calcium channel blockers, oral hypoglycemic agents, insulin, and certain other agents. Compounds in these categories include:

Acarbose (Octreotide causes hypo- and hyperglycemia in some patients; dosage adjustments of oral hypoglycemic agents may be required). Products include:
Precose Tablets 906

Acebutolol Hydrochloride (Adjustment of the dosage of beta blockers may be required). Products include:
Sectral Capsules 3589

Amlodipine Besylate (Adjustment of the dosage of calcium channel blocker may be required). Products include:
Lotrel Capsules 2370
Norvasc Tablets 2704

Atenolol (Adjustment of the dosage of beta blockers may be required). Products include:
Tenoretic Tablets 690
Tenormin I.V. Injection 692

Bepridil Hydrochloride (Adjustment of the dosage of calcium channel blocker may be required). Products include:
Vascor Tablets 2602

Betaxolol Hydrochloride (Adjustment of the dosage of beta blockers may be required). Products include:
Betoptic S Ophthalmic Suspension 537

Bisoprolol Fumarate (Adjustment of the dosage of beta blockers may be required). Products include:
Zebeta Tablets 1885
Ziac Tablets 1887

Carteolol Hydrochloride (Adjustment of the dosage of beta blockers may be required). Products include:
Carteolol Hydrochloride Ophthalmic Solution USP, 1% ..... ⊙258
Ocupress Ophthalmic Solution, 1% Sterile .... ⊙303

Chlorpropamide (Octreotide causes hypo- and hyperglycemia in some patients; dosage adjustments of oral hypoglycemic agents may be required). Products include:
Diabinese Tablets 2680

Cyclosporine (Co-administration may decrease blood levels of cyclosporine and may result in transplant rejection). Products include:
Gengraf Capsules 457
Neoral Soft Gelatin Capsules 2380
Neoral Oral Solution 2380
Sandimmune 2388

Diazoxide (Adjustment of the dosage of diazoxide may be required).
No products indexed under this heading.

Diltiazem Hydrochloride (Adjustment of the dosage of calcium channel blocker may be required). Products include:
Cardizem Injectable 1018
Cardizem Lyo-Ject Syringe 1018
Cardizem Monovial 1018
Cardizem CD Capsules 1016
Tiazac Capsules 1378

Esmolol Hydrochloride (Adjustment of the dosage of beta blockers may be required). Products include:
Brevibloc Injection 858

Felodipine (Adjustment of the dosage of calcium channel blocker may be required). Products include:
Lexxel Tablets 608
Plendil Extended-Release Tablets ... 623

Glimepiride (Octreotide causes hypo- and hyperglycemia in some patients; dosage adjustments of oral hypoglycemic agents may be required). Products include:
Amaryl Tablets 717

Glipizide (Octreotide causes hypo- and hyperglycemia in some patients; dosage adjustments of oral hypoglycemic agents may be required). Products include:
Glucotrol Tablets 2692
Glucotrol XL Extended Release Tablets 2693

Glyburide (Octreotide causes hypo- and hyperglycemia in some patients; dosage adjustments of oral hypoglycemic agents may be required). Products include:
DiaBeta Tablets 741
Glucovance Tablets 1086

Insulin, Human, Zinc Suspension (Octreotide causes hypo- and hyperglycemia in some patients; insulin dosage adjustments may be required). Products include:
Humulin L, 100 Units 1937
Humulin U, 100 Units 1943
Novolin L Human Insulin 10 ml Vials 2422

Insulin, Human NPH (Octreotide causes hypo- and hyperglycemia in some patients; insulin dosage adjustments may be required). Products include:
Humulin N, 100 Units 1939
Humulin N NPH Pen 1940
Novolin N Human Insulin 10 ml Vials 2422
Novolin N PenFill 2423
Novolin N Prefilled Syringe Disposable Insulin Delivery System 2425

Insulin, Human Regular (Octreotide causes hypo- and hyperglycemia in some patients; insulin dosage adjustments may be required). Products include:
Humulin R Regular (U-500) 1943
Humulin R, 100 Units 1941
Novolin R Human Insulin 10 ml Vials 2423
Novolin R PenFill 2423
Novolin R Prefilled Syringe Disposable Insulin Delivery System 2425
Velosulin BR Human Insulin 10 ml Vials 2435

Insulin, Human Regular and Human NPH Mixture (Octreotide causes hypo- and hyperglycemia in some patients; insulin dosage adjustments may be required). Products include:
Humulin 50/50, 100 Units 1934
Humulin 70/30, 100 Units 1935
Humulin 70/30 Pen 1936
Novolin 70/30 Human Insulin 10 ml Vials 2421
Novolin 70/30 PenFill 2423
Novolin 70/30 Prefilled Disposable Insulin Delivery System 2425

Insulin, NPH (Octreotide causes hypo- and hyperglycemia in some patients; insulin dosage adjustments may be required). Products include:
Iletin II, NPH (Pork), 100 Units 1946

Insulin, Regular (Octreotide causes hypo- and hyperglycemia in some patients; insulin dosage adjustments may be required). Products include:
Iletin II, Regular (Pork), 100 Units ... 1947

Insulin, Zinc Crystals (Octreotide causes hypo- and hyperglycemia in some patients; insulin dosage adjustments may be required).
No products indexed under this heading.

Insulin, Zinc Suspension (Octreotide causes hypo- and hyperglycemia in some patients; insulin dosage adjustments may be required). Products include:
Iletin II, Lente (Pork), 100 Units 1945

Insulin Aspart, Human Regular (Octreotide causes hypo- and hyperglycemia in some patients; insulin dosage adjustments may be

required).
No products indexed under this heading.

Insulin glargine (Octreotide causes hypo- and hyperglycemia in some patients; insulin dosage adjustments may be required). Products include:
Lantus Injection 742

Insulin Lispro, Human (Octreotide causes hypo- and hyperglycemia in some patients; insulin dosage adjustments may be required). Products include:
Humalog 1926
Humalog Mix 75/25 Pen 1928

Insulin Lispro Protamine, Human (Octreotide causes hypo- and hyperglycemia in some patients; insulin dosage adjustments may be required). Products include:
Humalog Mix 75/25 Pen 1928

Isradipine (Adjustment of the dosage of calcium channel blocker may be required). Products include:
DynaCirc Capsules 2921
DynaCirc CR Tablets 2923

Labetalol Hydrochloride (Adjustment of the dosage of beta blockers may be required). Products include:
Normodyne Injection 3135
Normodyne Tablets 3137

Levobunolol Hydrochloride (Adjustment of the dosage of beta blockers may be required). Products include:
Betagan .... ⊙ 228

Metformin Hydrochloride (Octreotide causes hypo- and hyperglycemia in some patients; dosage adjustments of oral hypoglycemic agents may be required). Products include:
Glucophage Tablets 1080
Glucophage XR Tablets 1080
Glucovance Tablets 1086

Metipranolol Hydrochloride (Adjustment of the dosage of beta blockers may be required).
No products indexed under this heading.

Metoprolol Succinate (Adjustment of the dosage of beta blockers may be required). Products include:
Toprol-XL Tablets 651

Metoprolol Tartrate (Adjustment of the dosage of beta blockers may be required).
No products indexed under this heading.

Mibefradil Dihydrochloride (Adjustment of the dosage of calcium channel blocker may be required).
No products indexed under this heading.

Miglitol (Octreotide causes hypo- and hyperglycemia in some patients; dosage adjustments of oral hypoglycemic agents may be required). Products include:
Glyset Tablets 2821

Nadolol (Adjustment of the dosage of beta blockers may be required). Products include:
Corgard Tablets 2245
Corzide 40/5 Tablets 2247
Corzide 80/5 Tablets 2247
Nadolol Tablets 2288

Nicardipine Hydrochloride (Adjustment of the dosage of calcium channel blocker may be required). Products include:
Cardene I.V. 3485

Nifedipine (Adjustment of the dosage of calcium channel blocker may be required). Products include:
Adalat CC Tablets 877
Procardia Capsules 2708
Procardia XL Extended Release Tablets 2710

Nimodipine (Adjustment of the dosage of calcium channel blocker may be required). Products include:
Nimotop Capsules 904

Nisoldipine (Adjustment of the dosage of calcium channel blocker may be required). Products include:
Sular Tablets 688

Penbutolol Sulfate (Adjustment of the dosage of beta blockers may be required).
No products indexed under this heading.

Pindolol (Adjustment of the dosage of beta blockers may be required).
No products indexed under this heading.

Pioglitazone Hydrochloride (Octreotide causes hypo- and hyperglycemia in some patients; dosage adjustments of oral hypoglycemic agents may be required). Products include:
Actos Tablets 3275

Propranolol Hydrochloride (Adjustment of the dosage of beta blockers may be required). Products include:
Inderal 3513
Inderal LA Long-Acting Capsules 3516
Inderide Tablets 3517
Inderide LA Long-Acting Capsules 3519

Repaglinide (Octreotide causes hypo- and hyperglycemia in some patients; dosage adjustments of oral hypoglycemic agents may be required). Products include:
Prandin Tablets (0.5, 1, and 2 mg) 2432

Rosiglitazone Maleate (Octreotide causes hypo- and hyperglycemia in some patients; dosage adjustments of oral hypoglycemic agents may be required). Products include:
Avandia Tablets 1490

Sotalol Hydrochloride (Adjustment of the dosage of beta blockers may be required). Products include:
Betapace Tablets 950
Betapace AF Tablets 954

Timolol Hemihydrate (Adjustment of the dosage of beta blockers may be required). Products include:
Betimol Ophthalmic Solution .... ⊙ 324

Timolol Maleate (Adjustment of the dosage of beta blockers may be required). Products include:
Blocadren Tablets 2046
Cosopt Sterile Ophthalmic Solution 2065
Timolide Tablets 2187
Timolol GFS .... ⊙ 266
Timoptic in Ocudose 2192
Timoptic Sterile Ophthalmic Solution 2190
Timoptic-XE Sterile Ophthalmic Gel Forming Solution 2194

Tolazamide (Octreotide causes hypo- and hyperglycemia in some patients; dosage adjustments of oral hypoglycemic agents may be required).
No products indexed under this heading.

Tolbutamide (Octreotide causes hypo- and hyperglycemia in some patients; dosage adjustments of oral hypoglycemic agents may be required).
No products indexed under this heading.

Troglitazone (Octreotide causes hypo- and hyperglycemia in some patients; dosage adjustments of oral hypoglycemic agents may be required).
No products indexed under this heading.

Verapamil Hydrochloride (Adjustment of the dosage of calcium channel blocker may be required). Products include:
Covera-HS Tablets 3199
Isoptin SR Tablets 467
Tarka Tablets 508
Verelan Capsules 3184
Verelan PM Capsules 3186

SARAFEM PULVULES

(Fluoxetine Hydrochloride) 1962
May interact with oral hypoglycemic agents, insulin, lithium preparations, monoamine oxidase inhibitors, phenytoin, tricyclic antidepressants, and certain other agents. Compounds in these categories include:

Acarbose (Fluoxetine may alter glycemic control; hypoglycemia has occured during therapy with fluoxetine and hyperglycemia has developed following discontinuation of the drug; dosage of oral hypoglycemics may need to be adjusted when therapy with fluoxetine is instituted or discontinued). Products include:
Precose Tablets 906

Alprazolam (Co-administration has resulted in increased alprazolam plasma concentrations and further psychomotor performance decrement due to increased alprazolam levels). Products include:
Xanax Tablets 2865

Amitriptyline Hydrochloride (Fluoxetine inhibits the activity of CYP450IID6 making normal metabolizers resemble poor metabolizers; therapy with drugs that are predominantly metabolized by this enzyme, such as tricyclic antidepressants, and have relatively narrow therapeutic index should be initiated at low end of the dose range if a patient is receiving fluoxetine concurrently or has taken it in the previous 5 weeks). Products include:
Etrafon 3115
Limbitrol 1738

Amoxapine (Fluoxetine inhibits the activity of CYP450IID6 making normal metabolizers resemble poor metabolizers; therapy with drugs that are predominantly metabolized by this enzyme, such as tricyclic antidepressants, and have relatively narrow therapeutic index should be initiated at low end of the dose range if a patient is receiving fluoxetine concurrently or has taken it in the previous 5 weeks).
No products indexed under this heading.

Carbamazepine (Patients on stable doses of carbamazepine have developed elevated plasma carbamazepine concentrations and clinical anticonvulsant toxicity following initiation of concomitant fluoxetine treatment). Products include:
Carbatrol Capsules 3234
Tegretol/Tegretol-XR 2404

Chlorpropamide (Fluoxetine may alter glycemic control; hypoglycemia has occured during therapy with fluoxetine and hyperglycemia has developed following discontinuation of the drug; dosage of oral hypoglycemics may need to be adjusted when therapy with fluoxetine is instituted or discontinued). Products include:
Diabinese Tablets 2680

Clomipramine Hydrochloride (Fluoxetine inhibits the activity of CYP450IID6 making normal metabolizers resemble poor metabolizers; therapy with drugs that are predominantly metabolized by this enzyme, such as tricyclic antidepressants, and have relatively narrow therapeutic index should be initiated at low end of the dose range if a patient is receiving fluoxetine concurrently or has taken it in the previous 5 weeks).
No products indexed under this heading.

Clozapine (Co-administration has resulted in elevation of blood levels of clozapine). Products include:
Clozaril Tablets 2319

Desipramine Hydrochloride (Fluoxetine inhibits the activity of CYP450IID6 making normal metabolizers resemble poor metabolizers; therapy with drugs that are predominantly metabolized by this enzyme, such as tricyclic antidepressants, and have relatively narrow therapeutic index should be initiated at low end of the dose range if a patient is receiving fluoxetine concurrently or has taken it in the previous 5 weeks; previously stable plasma levels of desipramine have increased greater than 2 to 10-fold when fluoxetine was co-administered). Products include:
Norpramin Tablets 755

Diazepam (Co-administration results in prolonged half-life of diazepam). Products include:
Valium Injectable 3026
Valium Tablets 3047

Digitoxin (Fluoxetine is tightly bound to protein, co-administration may cause shift in plasma concentrations resulting in potential adverse effects).
No products indexed under this heading.

Doxepin Hydrochloride (Fluoxetine inhibits the activity of CYP450IID6 making normal metabolizers resemble poor metabolizers; therapy with drugs that are predominantly metabolized by this enzyme, such as tricyclic antidepressants, and have relatively narrow therapeutic index should be initiated at low end of the dose range if a patient is receiving fluoxetine concurrently or has taken it in the previous 5 weeks). Products include:
Sinequan 2713

Flecainide Acetate (Fluoxetine inhibits the activity of CYP450IID6 making normal metabolizers resemble poor metabolizers; therapy with drugs that are predominantly metabolized by this enzyme, such as flecainide, and have relatively narrow therapeutic index should be initiated at low end of the dose range if a patient is receiving fluoxetine concurrently or has taken it in the previous 5 weeks). Products include:
Tambocor Tablets 1990

Fosphenytoin Sodium (Patients on stable doses of phenytoin have developed elevated plasma phenytoin concentrations and clinical anticonvulsant toxicity following initiation of concomitant fluoxetine treatment). Products include:
Cerebyx Injection 2619

Glimepiride (Fluoxetine may alter glycemic control; hypoglycemia has occured during therapy with fluoxetine and hyperglycemia has developed following discontinuation of the drug; dosage of oral hypoglycemics may need to be adjusted when therapy with fluoxetine is instituted or discontinued). Products include:
Amaryl Tablets 717

Glipizide (Fluoxetine may alter glycemic control; hypoglycemia has occured during therapy with fluoxetine and hyperglycemia has developed following discontinuation of the drug; dosage of oral hypoglycemics may need to be adjusted when therapy with fluoxetine is instituted or discontinued). Products include:
Glucotrol Tablets 2692
Glucotrol XL Extended Release Tablets 2693

Glyburide (Fluoxetine may alter glycemic control; hypoglycemia has occured during therapy with fluoxetine and hyperglycemia has developed following discontinuation of the drug; dosage of oral hypoglycemics may need to be adjusted when therapy with fluoxetine is instituted or discontinued). Products include:
DiaBeta Tablets 741
Glucovance Tablets 1086

Haloperidol (Co-administration has resulted in elevation of blood levels of haloperidol). Products include:
Haldol Injection, Tablets and Concentrate ... 2533

Haloperidol Decanoate (Co-administration has resulted in elevation of blood levels of haloperidol). Products include:
Haldol Decanoate ... 2535

Imipramine Hydrochloride (Fluoxetine inhibits the activity of CYP450IID6 making normal metabolizers resemble poor metabolizers; therapy with drugs that are predominantly metabolized by this enzyme, such as tricyclic antidepressants, and have relatively narrow therapeutic index should be initiated at low end of the dose range if a patient is receiving fluoxetine concurrently or has taken it in the previous 5 weeks).
No products indexed under this heading.

Imipramine Pamoate (Fluoxetine inhibits the activity of CYP450IID6 making normal metabolizers resemble poor metabolizers; therapy with drugs that are predominantly metabolized by this enzyme, such as tricyclic antidepressants, and have relatively narrow therapeutic index should be initiated at low end of the dose range if a patient is receiving fluoxetine concurrently or has taken it in the previous 5 weeks; previously stable plasma levels of imipramine have increased 2 to 10-fold when fluoxetine was co-administered).
No products indexed under this heading.

Insulin, Human, Zinc Suspension (Fluoxetine may alter glycemic control; hypoglycemia has occurred during therapy with fluoxetine and hyperglycemia has developed following discontinuation of the drug; insulin dosage may need to be adjusted when therapy with fluoxetine is instituted or discontinued). Products include:
Humulin L, 100 Units ... 1937
Humulin U, 100 Units ... 1943
Novolin L Human Insulin 10 ml Vials ... 2422

Insulin, Human NPH (Fluoxetine may alter glycemic control; hypoglycemia has occurred during therapy with fluoxetine and hyperglycemia has developed following discontinuation of the drug; insulin dosage may need to be adjusted when therapy with fluoxetine is instituted or discontinued). Products include:
Humulin N, 100 Units ... 1939
Humulin N NPH Pen ... 1940
Novolin N Human Insulin 10 ml Vials ... 2422
Novolin N PenFill ... 2423
Novolin N Prefilled Syringe Disposable Insulin Delivery System ... 2425

Insulin, Human Regular (Fluoxetine may alter glycemic control; hypoglycemia has occurred during therapy with fluoxetine and hyperglycemia has developed following discontinuation of the drug; insulin dosage may need to be adjusted when therapy with fluoxetine is instituted or discontinued). Products include:
Humulin R Regular (U-500) ... 1943
Humulin R, 100 Units ... 1941
Novolin R Human Insulin 10 ml Vials ... 2423
Novolin R PenFill ... 2423
Novolin R Prefilled Syringe Disposable Insulin Delivery System ... 2425
Velosulin BR Human Insulin 10 ml Vials ... 2435

Insulin, Human Regular and Human NPH Mixture (Fluoxetine may alter glycemic control; hypoglycemia has occurred during therapy with fluoxetine and hyperglycemia has developed following discontinuation of the drug; insulin dosage may need to be adjusted when therapy with fluoxetine is instituted or discontinued). Products include:
Humulin 50/50, 100 Units ... 1934
Humulin 70/30, 100 Units ... 1935
Humulin 70/30 Pen ... 1936
Novolin 70/30 Human Insulin 10 ml Vials ... 2421
Novolin 70/30 PenFill ... 2423
Novolin 70/30 Prefilled Disposable Insulin Delivery System ... 2425

Insulin, NPH (Fluoxetine may alter glycemic control; hypoglycemia has occurred during therapy with fluoxetine and hyperglycemia has developed following discontinuation of the drug; insulin dosage may need to be adjusted when therapy with fluoxetine is instituted or discontinued). Products include:
Iletin II, NPH (Pork), 100 Units ... 1946

Insulin, Regular (Fluoxetine may alter glycemic control; hypoglycemia has occurred during therapy with fluoxetine and hyperglycemia has developed following discontinuation of the drug; insulin dosage may need to be adjusted when therapy with fluoxetine is instituted or discontinued). Products include:
Iletin II, Regular (Pork), 100 Units ... 1947

Insulin, Zinc Crystals (Fluoxetine may alter glycemic control; hypoglycemia has occurred during therapy with fluoxetine and hyperglycemia has developed following discontinuation of the drug; insulin dosage may need to be adjusted when therapy with fluoxetine is instituted or discontinued).
No products indexed under this heading.

Insulin, Zinc Suspension (Fluoxetine may alter glycemic control; hypoglycemia has occurred during therapy with fluoxetine and hyperglycemia has developed following discontinuation of the drug; insulin dosage may need to be adjusted when therapy with fluoxetine is instituted or discontinued). Products include:
Iletin II, Lente (Pork), 100 Units ... 1945

Insulin Aspart, Human Regular (Fluoxetine may alter glycemic control; hypoglycemia has occurred during therapy with fluoxetine and hyperglycemia has developed following discontinuation of the drug; insulin dosage may need to be adjusted when therapy with fluoxetine is instituted or discontinued).
No products indexed under this heading.

Insulin glargine (Fluoxetine may alter glycemic control; hypoglycemia has occurred during therapy with fluoxetine and hyperglycemia has developed following discontinuation of the drug; insulin dosage may need to be adjusted when therapy with fluoxetine is instituted or discontinued). Products include:
Lantus Injection ... 742

Insulin Lispro, Human (Fluoxetine may alter glycemic control; hypoglycemia has occurred during therapy with fluoxetine and hyperglycemia has developed following discontinuation of the drug; insulin dosage may need to be adjusted when therapy with fluoxetine is instituted or discontinued). Products include:
Humalog ... 1926
Humalog Mix 75/25 Pen ... 1928

Insulin Lispro Protamine, Human (Fluoxetine may alter glycemic control; hypoglycemia has occurred during therapy with fluoxetine and hyperglycemia has developed following discontinuation of the drug; insulin dosage may need to be adjusted when therapy with fluoxetine is instituted or discontinued). Products include:
Humalog Mix 75/25 Pen ... 1928

Isocarboxazid (Co-administration with MAO inhibitors has resulted in serious, sometimes fatal, reactions including hyperthermia, rigidity, myoclonus, extreme agitation progressing to delirium, coma, and features resembling neuroleptic malignant syndrome; concurrent and/or sequential use is contraindicated).
No products indexed under this heading.

Lithium Carbonate (Co-administration has resulted in both increased and decreased lithium levels; cases of toxicity and increased serotonergic effects have been reported). Products include:
Eskalith ... 1527
Lithium Carbonate ... 3061
Lithobid Slow-Release Tablets ... 3255

Lithium Citrate (Co-administration has resulted in both increased and decreased lithium levels; cases of toxicity and increased serotonergic effects have been reported). Products include:
Lithium Citrate Syrup ... 3061

Maprotiline Hydrochloride (Fluoxetine inhibits the activity of CYP450IID6 making normal metabolizers resemble poor metabolizers; therapy with drugs that are predominantly metabolized by this enzyme, such as tricyclic antidepressants, and have relatively narrow therapeutic index should be initiated at low end of the dose range if a patient is receiving fluoxetine concurrently or has taken it in the previous 5 weeks).
No products indexed under this heading.

Metformin Hydrochloride (Fluoxetine may alter glycemic control; hypoglycemia has occured during therapy with fluoxetine and hyperglycemia has developed following discontinuation of the drug; dosage of oral hypoglycemics may need to be adjusted when therapy with fluoxetine is instituted or discontinued). Products include:
Glucophage Tablets ... 1080
Glucophage XR Tablets ... 1080
Glucovance Tablets ... 1086

Miglitol (Fluoxetine may alter glycemic control; hypoglycemia has occured during therapy with fluoxetine and hyperglycemia has developed following discontinuation of the drug; dosage of oral hypoglycemics may need to be adjusted when therapy with fluoxetine is instituted or discontinued). Products include:
Glyset Tablets ... 2821

Moclobemide (Co-administration with MAO inhibitors has resulted in serious, sometimes fatal, reactions including hyperthermia, rigidity, myoclonus, extreme agitation progressing to delirium, coma, and features resembling neuroleptic malignant syndrome; concurrent and/or sequential use is contraindicated).
No products indexed under this heading.

Nortriptyline Hydrochloride (Fluoxetine inhibits the activity of CYP450IID6 making normal metabolizers resemble poor metabolizers; therapy with drugs that are predominantly metabolized by this enzyme, such as tricyclic antidepressants, and have relatively narrow therapeutic index should be initiated at low end of the dose range if a patient is receiving fluoxetine concurrently or has taken it in the previous 5 weeks).
No products indexed under this heading.

Pargyline Hydrochloride (Co-administration with MAO inhibitors has resulted in serious, sometimes fatal, reactions including hyperthermia, rigidity, myoclonus, extreme agitation progressing to delirium, coma, and features resembling neuroleptic malignant syndrome; concurrent and/or sequential use is contraindicated).
No products indexed under this heading.

Phenelzine Sulfate (Co-administration with MAO inhibitors has resulted in serious, sometimes fatal, reactions including hyperthermia, rigidity, myoclonus, extreme agitation progressing to delirium, coma, and features resembling neuroleptic malignant syndrome; concurrent and/or sequential use is contraindicated). Products include:
Nardil Tablets ... 2653

Phenytoin (Patients on stable doses of phenytoin have developed elevated plasma phenytoin concentrations and clinical anticonvulsant toxicity following initiation of concomitant fluoxetine treatment). Products include:
Dilantin Infatabs ... 2624
Dilantin-125 Oral Suspension ... 2625

Phenytoin Sodium (Patients on stable doses of phenytoin have developed elevated plasma phenytoin concentrations and clinical anticonvulsant toxicity following initiation of concomitant fluoxetine treatment). Products include:
Dilantin Kapseals ... 2622

Pimozide (Co-administration has resulted in a single case report of possible additive effects leading to bradycardia). Products include:
Orap Tablets ... 1407

Pioglitazone Hydrochloride (Fluoxetine may alter glycemic control; hypoglycemia has occured during therapy with fluoxetine and hyperglycemia has developed following discontinuation of the drug; dosage of oral hypoglycemics may need to be adjusted when therapy with fluoxetine is instituted or discontinued). Products include:
Actos Tablets ... 3275

Procarbazine Hydrochloride (Co-administration with MAO inhibitors has resulted in serious, sometimes fatal, reactions including hyperthermia, rigidity, myoclonus, extreme agitation progressing to delirium, coma, and features resembling neuroleptic malignant syndrome; concurrent and/or sequential use is contraindicated). Products include:
Matulane Capsules ... 3246

Protriptyline Hydrochloride (Fluoxetine inhibits the activity of CYP450IID6 making normal metabolizers resemble poor metabolizers; therapy with drugs that are predominantly metabolized by this enzyme, such as tricyclic antidepressants, and have relatively narrow therapeutic index should be initiated at low end of the dose range if a patient is receiving fluoxetine concurrently or has taken it in the previous 5 weeks). Products include:
Vivactil Tablets ... 2446
Vivactil Tablets ... 2217

Repaglinide (Fluoxetine may alter glycemic control; hypoglycemia has occured during therapy with fluoxetine and hyperglycemia has developed following discontinuation of the drug; dosage of oral hypoglycemics may need to be adjusted when therapy with fluoxetine is instituted or discontinued). Products include:
Prandin Tablets (0.5, 1, and 2 mg) ... 2432

Rosiglitazone Maleate (Fluoxetine may alter glycemic control; hypoglycemia has occured during therapy with fluoxetine and hyperglycemia has developed following discontinuation of the drug; dosage of oral hypoglycemics may need to be

adjusted when therapy with fluoxetine is instituted or discontinued). Products include:
Avandia Tablets 1490

Selegiline Hydrochloride (Co-administration with MAO inhibitors has resulted in serious, sometimes fatal, reactions including hyperthermia, rigidity, myoclonus, extreme agitation progressing to delirium, coma, and features resembling neuroleptic malignant syndrome; concurrent and/or sequential use is contraindicated). Products include:
Eldepryl Capsules 3266

Sumatriptan (Co-administration of SSRI and sumatriptan has resulted in rare postmarketing reports of weakness, hyperreflexia, and incoordination). Products include:
Imitrex Nasal Spray 1554

Sumatriptan Succinate (Co-administration of SSRI and sumatriptan has resulted in rare postmarketing reports of weakness, hyperreflexia, and incoordination). Products include:
Imitrex Injection 1549
Imitrex Tablets 1558

Thioridazine Hydrochloride (Co-administration of drugs which inhibit P450IID6, such as SSRIs, including fluoxetine, with thioridazine will produce elevated plasma levels of thioridazine because of inhibition of thioridazine because of thioridazine's metabolism; thioridazine administration produces a dose-related prolongation of the QTc interval, which is associated with serious ventricular arrhythmias and sudden death; concurrent and/or sequential use within a minimum of 5 weeks is contraindicated). Products include:
Thioridazine Hydrochloride Tablets 2289

Tolazamide (Fluoxetine may alter glycemic control; hypoglycemia has occured during therapy with fluoxetine and hyperglycemia has developed following discontinuation of the drug; dosage of oral hypoglycemics may need to be adjusted when therapy with fluoxetine is instituted or discontinued).
No products indexed under this heading.

Tolbutamide (Fluoxetine may alter glycemic control; hypoglycemia has occured during therapy with fluoxetine and hyperglycemia has developed following discontinuation of the drug; dosage of oral hypoglycemics may need to be adjusted when therapy with fluoxetine is instituted or discontinued).
No products indexed under this heading.

Tranylcypromine Sulfate (Co-administration with MAO inhibitors has resulted in serious, sometimes fatal, reactions including hyperthermia, rigidity, myoclonus, extreme agitation progressing to delirium, coma, and features resembling neuroleptic malignant syndrome; concurrent and/or sequential use is contraindicated). Products include:
Parnate Tablets 1607

Trimipramine Maleate (Fluoxetine inhibits the activity of CYP450IID6 making normal metabolizers resemble poor metabolizers; therapy with drugs that are predominantly metabolized by this enzyme, such as tricyclic antidepressants, and have relatively narrow therapeutic index should be initiated at low end of the dose range if a patient is receiving fluoxetine concurrently or has taken it in the previous 5 weeks). Products include:
Surmontil Capsules 3595

Troglitazone (Fluoxetine may alter glycemic control; hypoglycemia has occured during therapy with fluoxetine and hyperglycemia has developed following discontinuation of the drug; dosage of oral hypoglycemics may need to be adjusted when therapy with fluoxetine is instituted or discontinued).
No products indexed under this heading.

Vinblastine Sulfate (Fluoxetine inhibits the activity of CYP450IID6 making normal metabolizers resemble poor metabolizers; therapy with drugs that are predominantly metabolized by this enzyme, such as vinblastine, and have relatively narrow therapeutic index should be initiated at low end of the dose range if a patient is receiving fluoxetine concurrently or has taken it in the previous 5 weeks).
No products indexed under this heading.

Warfarin Sodium (Co-administration has resulted in altered anti-coagulant effects, including increased bleeding). Products include:
Coumadin for Injection 1243
Coumadin Tablets 1243
Warfarin Sodium Tablets, USP 3302

Food Interactions

Alcohol (Concurrent use with CNS active agents, such as alcohol, requires caution).

Food, unspecified (May delay fluoxetine's absorption inconsequentially, thus, fluoxetine may be administered with or without food).

SARAPIN
(Sarraceniaceae) 1727
None cited in PDR database.

SATIETE TABLETS
(Amino Acid Preparations, Ginkgo biloba, Herbals with Vitamins & Minerals, Hypericum) .... ■846
May interact with anorexiants, monoamine oxidase inhibitors, selective serotonin reuptake inhibitors, and tricyclic antidepressants. Compounds in these categories include:

Amitriptyline Hydrochloride (Concurrent use with tricyclic antidepressants is not recommended). Products include:
Etrafon 3115
Limbitrol 1738

Amoxapine (Concurrent use with tricyclic antidepressants is not recommended).
No products indexed under this heading.

Amphetamine Resins (Concurrent use with prescription diet drugs is not recommended).
No products indexed under this heading.

Benzphetamine Hydrochloride (Concurrent use with prescription diet drugs is not recommended).
No products indexed under this heading.

Citalopram Hydrobromide (Concurrent use with SSRI antidepressants is not recommended). Products include:
Celexa 1365

Clomipramine Hydrochloride (Concurrent use with tricyclic antidepressants is not recommended).
No products indexed under this heading.

Desipramine Hydrochloride (Concurrent use with tricyclic antidepressants is not recommended). Products include:
Norpramin Tablets 755

Dextroamphetamine Sulfate (Concurrent use with prescription diet drugs is not recommended). Products include:
Adderall Tablets 3231
Adderall XR Capsules ....
Dexedrine 1512
DextroStat Tablets 3236

Diethylpropion Hydrochloride (Concurrent use with prescription diet drugs is not recommended).
No products indexed under this heading.

Doxepin Hydrochloride (Concurrent use with tricyclic antidepressants is not recommended). Products include:
Sinequan 2713

Fenfluramine Hydrochloride (Concurrent use with prescription diet drugs is not recommended).
No products indexed under this heading.

Fluoxetine Hydrochloride (Concurrent use with SSRI antidepressants is not recommended). Products include:
Prozac Pulvules, Liquid, and Weekly Capsules 1238
Sarafem Pulvules 1962

Fluvoxamine Maleate (Concurrent use with SSRI antidepressants is not recommended). Products include:
Luvox Tablets (25, 50, 100 mg) 3256

Imipramine Hydrochloride (Concurrent use with tricyclic antidepressants is not recommended).
No products indexed under this heading.

Imipramine Pamoate (Concurrent use with tricyclic antidepressants is not recommended).
No products indexed under this heading.

Isocarboxazid (Concurrent use with MAO inhibitors is not recommended).
No products indexed under this heading.

Maprotiline Hydrochloride (Concurrent use with tricyclic antidepressants is not recommended).
No products indexed under this heading.

Mazindol (Concurrent use with prescription diet drugs is not recommended).
No products indexed under this heading.

Methamphetamine Hydrochloride (Concurrent use with prescription diet drugs is not recommended). Products include:
Desoxyn Tablets 440

Moclobemide (Concurrent use with MAO inhibitors is not recommended).
No products indexed under this heading.

Nortriptyline Hydrochloride (Concurrent use with tricyclic antidepressants is not recommended).
No products indexed under this heading.

Pargyline Hydrochloride (Concurrent use with MAO inhibitors is not recommended).
No products indexed under this heading.

Paroxetine Hydrochloride (Concurrent use with SSRI antidepressants is not recommended). Products include:
Paxil 1609

Phendimetrazine Tartrate (Concurrent use with prescription diet drugs is not recommended). Products include:
Bontril Slow-Release Capsules 576

Phenelzine Sulfate (Concurrent use with MAO inhibitors is not recommended). Products include:
Nardil Tablets 2653

Phenmetrazine Hydrochloride (Concurrent use with prescription diet drugs is not recommended).
No products indexed under this heading.

Procarbazine Hydrochloride (Concurrent use with MAO inhibitors is not recommended). Products include:
Matulane Capsules 3246

Protriptyline Hydrochloride (Concurrent use with tricyclic antidepressants is not recommended). Products include:
Vivactil Tablets 2446
Vivactil Tablets 2217

Selegiline Hydrochloride (Concurrent use with MAO inhibitors is not recommended). Products include:
Eldepryl Capsules 3266

Sertraline Hydrochloride (Concurrent use with SSRI antidepressants is not recommended). Products include:
Zoloft 2751

Sibutramine Hydrochloride Monohydrate (Concurrent use with prescription diet drugs is not recommended). Products include:
Meridia Capsules 481

Tranylcypromine Sulfate (Concurrent use with MAO inhibitors is not recommended). Products include:
Parnate Tablets 1607

Trimipramine Maleate (Concurrent use with tricyclic antidepressants is not recommended). Products include:
Surmontil Capsules 3595

SECTRAL CAPSULES
(Acebutolol Hydrochloride) 3589
May interact with alpha adrenergic stimulants, insulin, and non-steroidal anti-inflammatory agents. Compounds in these categories include:

Celecoxib (Blunting of the antihypertensive effect). Products include:
Celebrex Capsules 2676
Celebrex Capsules 2780

Diclofenac Potassium (Blunting of the antihypertensive effect). Products include:
Cataflam Tablets 2315

Diclofenac Sodium (Blunting of the antihypertensive effect). Products include:
Arthrotec Tablets 3195
Voltaren Ophthalmic Sterile Ophthalmic Solution .... ⊙312
Voltaren Tablets 2315
Voltaren-XR Tablets 2315

Epinephrine (Potential for unresponsiveness to epinephrine to treat allergic reactions in certain patients). Products include:
Epifrin Sterile Ophthalmic Solution .... ⊙235
EpiPen 1236
Primatene Mist .... ■779
Xylocaine with Epinephrine Injection 653

Epinephrine Hydrochloride (Potential for unresponsiveness to epinephrine to treat allergic reactions in certain patients).
No products indexed under this heading.

Etodolac (Blunting of the antihypertensive effect). Products include:
Lodine 3528
Lodine XL Extended-Release Tablets 3530

Fenoprofen Calcium (Blunting of the antihypertensive effect).
No products indexed under this heading.

Flurbiprofen (Blunting of the antihypertensive effect).
No products indexed under this heading.

Ibuprofen (Blunting of the antihypertensive effect). Products include:
Advil .... ■771
Children's Advil Oral Suspension .... ■773
Children's Advil Chewable Tablets .. ■773
Advil Cold and Sinus Caplets .... ■771
Advil Cold and Sinus Tablets .... ■771
Advil Flu & Body Ache Caplets ...... ■772
Infants' Advil Drops .... ■773

Junior Strength Advil Tablets .... ▣773
Junior Strength Advil Chewable Tablets .... ▣773
Advil Migraine Liquigels .... ▣772
Children's Motrin Oral Suspension and Chewable Tablets 2006
Children's Motrin Cold Oral Suspension 2007
Children's Motrin Oral Suspension .... ▣643
Motrin Suspension, Oral Drops, Chewable Tablets, and Caplets 2002
Infants' Motrin Concentrated Drops 2006
Junior Strength Motrin Caplets and Chewable Tablets 2006
Motrin IB Tablets, Caplets, and Gelcaps 2002
Motrin Migraine Pain Caplets 2005
Motrin Sinus Headache Caplets 2005
Vicoprofen Tablets 520

Indomethacin (Blunting of the antihypertensive effect). Products include:
Indocin 2112

Indomethacin Sodium Trihydrate (Blunting of the antihypertensive effect). Products include:
Indocin I.V. 2115

Insulin, Human, Zinc Suspension (Beta-blockers may potentiate insulin-induced hypoglycemia). Products include:
Humulin L, 100 Units 1937
Humulin U, 100 Units 1943
Novolin L Human Insulin 10 ml Vials 2422

Insulin, Human NPH (Beta-blockers may potentiate insulin-induced hypoglycemia). Products include:
Humulin N, 100 Units 1939
Humulin N NPH Pen 1940
Novolin N Human Insulin 10 ml Vials 2422
Novolin N PenFill 2423
Novolin N Prefilled Syringe Disposable Insulin Delivery System 2425

Insulin, Human Regular (Beta-blockers may potentiate insulin-induced hypoglycemia). Products include:
Humulin R Regular (U-500) 1943
Humulin R, 100 Units 1941
Novolin R Human Insulin 10 ml Vials 2423
Novolin R PenFill 2423
Novolin R Prefilled Syringe Disposable Insulin Delivery System 2425
Velosulin BR Human Insulin 10 ml Vials 2435

Insulin, Human Regular and Human NPH Mixture (Beta-blockers may potentiate insulin-induced hypoglycemia). Products include:
Humulin 50/50, 100 Units 1934
Humulin 70/30, 100 Units 1935
Humulin 70/30 Pen 1936
Novolin 70/30 Human Insulin 10 ml Vials 2421
Novolin 70/30 PenFill 2423
Novolin 70/30 Prefilled Disposable Insulin Delivery System 2425

Insulin, NPH (Beta-blockers may potentiate insulin-induced hypoglycemia). Products include:
Iletin II, NPH (Pork), 100 Units 1946

Insulin, Regular (Beta-blockers may potentiate insulin-induced hypoglycemia). Products include:
Iletin II, Regular (Pork), 100 Units 1947

Insulin, Zinc Crystals (Beta-blockers may potentiate insulin-induced hypoglycemia).
No products indexed under this heading.

Insulin, Zinc Suspension (Beta-blockers may potentiate insulin-induced hypoglycemia). Products include:
Iletin II, Lente (Pork), 100 Units 1945

Insulin Aspart, Human Regular (Beta-blockers may potentiate insulin-induced hypoglycemia).
No products indexed under this heading.

Insulin glargine (Beta-blockers may potentiate insulin-induced hypoglycemia). Products include:
Lantus Injection 742

Insulin Lispro, Human (Beta-blockers may potentiate insulin-induced hypoglycemia). Products include:
Humalog 1926
Humalog Mix 75/25 Pen 1928

Insulin Lispro Protamine, Human (Beta-blockers may potentiate insulin-induced hypoglycemia). Products include:
Humalog Mix 75/25 Pen 1928

Ketoprofen (Blunting of the antihypertensive effect). Products include:
Orudis Capsules 3548
Orudis KT Tablets .... ▣778
Oruvail Capsules 3548

Ketorolac Tromethamine (Blunting of the antihypertensive effect). Products include:
Acular Ophthalmic Solution 544
Acular PF Ophthalmic Solution 544
Toradol 3018

Meclofenamate Sodium (Blunting of the antihypertensive effect).
No products indexed under this heading.

Mefenamic Acid (Blunting of the antihypertensive effect). Products include:
Ponstel Capsules 1356

Meloxicam (Blunting of the antihypertensive effect). Products include:
Mobic Tablets 1054

Nabumetone (Blunting of the antihypertensive effect). Products include:
Relafen Tablets 1617

Naphazoline Hydrochloride (Exaggerated hypertensive responses have been reported from the combined use of beta-adrenergic antagonists and alpha-adrenergic stimulants, including those contained in cold remedies). Products include:
Albalon Ophthalmic Solution .... ⊙225
All Clear Eye Drops .... ⊙252
All Clear AR Eye Drops .... ⊙252
Clear Eyes ACR Astringent/Lubricant Eye Redness Reliever .... ⊙322
Clear Eyes Lubricant Eye Redness Reliever .... ⊙322
Naphcon-A Ophthalmic Solution 540
Opcon-A Eye Drops .... ⊙253
Vasocon-A Eye Drops .... ⊙307
Visine-A Eye Allergy Relief Eye Drops .... ⊙314
Visine-A Eye Drops .... ▣714

Naproxen (Blunting of the antihypertensive effect). Products include:
EC-Naprosyn Delayed-Release Tablets 2967
Naprosyn Suspension 2967
Naprosyn Tablets 2967

Naproxen Sodium (Blunting of the antihypertensive effect). Products include:
Aleve Tablets, Caplets and Gelcaps .... ▣602
Aleve Cold & Sinus Caplets .... ▣603
Anaprox Tablets 2967
Anaprox DS Tablets 2967
Naprelan Tablets 1293

Oxaprozin (Blunting of the antihypertensive effect).
No products indexed under this heading.

Oxymetazoline Hydrochloride (Exaggerated hypertensive responses have been reported from the combined use of beta-adrenergic antagonists and alpha-adrenergic stimulants, including those contained in cold remedies). Products include:
Afrin .... ▣733
Afrin No Drip Original Nasal Spray .... ▣735
Afrin No Drip Extra Moisturizing Nasal Spray .... ▣735
Afrin No Drip Severe Congestion Nasal Spray .... ▣735
Afrin No Drip Sinus Nasal Spray .... ▣735
Afrin Original Pump Mist .... ▣733
Neo-Synephrine 12 Hour .... ▣615
Vicks Sinex 12-Hour Nasal Spray and Ultra Fine Mist .... ▣729
Visine L.R. Long Lasting Eye Drops .... ⊙315

Phenylbutazone (Blunting of the antihypertensive effect).
No products indexed under this heading.

Phenylephrine Hydrochloride (Exaggerated hypertensive responses have been reported from the combined use of beta-adrenergic antagonists and alpha-adrenergic stimulants, including those contained in cold remedies). Products include:
Afrin Nasal Decongestant Children's Pump Mist .... ▣734
Extendryl 1361
Hycomine Compound Tablets 1317
Neo-Synephrine .... ▣614
Phenergan VC Syrup 3560
Phenergan VC with Codeine Syrup 3561
Preparation H Cream .... ▣778
Preparation H Cooling Gel .... ▣778
Preparation H .... ▣778
Vicks Sinex Nasal Spray and Ultra Fine Mist .... ▣729

Phenylpropanolamine Hydrochloride (Exaggerated hypertensive responses have been reported from the combined use of beta-adrenergic antagonists and alpha-adrenergic stimulants, including those contained in cold remedies).
No products indexed under this heading.

Piroxicam (Blunting of the antihypertensive effect). Products include:
Feldene Capsules 2685

Pseudoephedrine Hydrochloride (Exaggerated hypertensive responses have been reported from the combined use of beta-adrenergic antagonists and alpha-adrenergic stimulants, including those contained in cold remedies). Products include:
Actifed Cold & Allergy Tablets .... ▣688
Actifed Cold & Sinus Caplets and Tablets .... ▣688
Advil Cold and Sinus Caplets .... ▣771
Advil Cold and Sinus Tablets .... ▣771
Advil Flu & Body Ache Caplets .... ▣772
Aleve Cold & Sinus Caplets .... ▣603
Alka-Seltzer Plus Liqui-Gels .... ▣604
Alka-Seltzer Plus Cold & Flu Medicine Liqui-Gels .... ▣604
Alka-Seltzer Plus Cold & Sinus Medicine Liqui-Gels .... ▣604
Allegra-D Extended-Release Tablets 714
BC Cold Powder .... ▣619
Benadryl Allergy/Cold Tablets .... ▣691
Benadryl Allergy/Congestion Tablets .... ▣692
Benadryl Allergy & Sinus Liquid .... ▣693
Benadryl Allergy & Sinus Fastmelt Tablets .... ▣693
Benadryl Allergy Sinus Headache Caplets & Gelcaps .... ▣693
Benadryl Severe Allergy & Sinus Headache Caplets .... ▣694
Benadryl Children's Allergy/Cold Fastmelt Tablets .... ▣692
Benylin Multi-Symptom Liquid .... ▣697
Bromfed Capsules (Extended-Release) 2269
Bromfed-PD Capsules (Extended-Release) 2269
Children's Cēpacol Sore Throat .... ▣788
Comtrex Acute Head Cold & Sinus Pressure Relief Tablets .... ▣627
Comtrex Deep Chest Cold & Congestion Relief Softgels .... ▣627
Comtrex Flu Therapy & Fever Relief Daytime Caplets .... ▣628
Comtrex Flu Therapy & Fever Relief Nighttime Tablets .... ▣628
Comtrex Maximum Strength Multi-Symptom Cold & Cough Relief Tablets and Caplets .... ▣626
Contac Non-Drowsy 12 Hour Cold Caplets .... ▣745
Contac Non-Drowsy Timed Release 12 Hour Cold Caplets .... ▣746
Contac Severe Cold and Flu Caplets Maximum Strength .... ▣746
Contac Severe Cold and Flu Caplets Non-Drowsy .... ▣746
Dimetapp Elixir .... ▣777
Dimetapp Cold and Fever Suspension .... ▣775
Dimetapp DM Cold & Cough Elixir .... ▣775
Dimetapp Nighttime Flu Liquid .... ▣776
Dimetapp Non-Drowsy Flu Syrup .... ▣777
Dimetapp Infant Drops Decongestant .... ▣775
Dimetapp Infant Drops Decongestant Plus Cough .... ▣776
Guaifed 2272
Kronofed-A 1341
Children's Motrin Cold Oral Suspension 2007
Motrin Sinus Headache Caplets 2005
PediaCare Cough-Cold Liquid .... ▣719
PediaCare Infants' Drops Decongestant .... ▣719
PediaCare Infants' Drops Decongestant Plus Cough .... ▣719
PediaCare NightRest Cough-Cold Liquid .... ▣719
Robitussin Cold Caplets Cold & Congestion .... ▣780
Robitussin Cold Softgels Cold & Congestion .... ▣780
Robitussin Cold Caplets Multi-Symptom Cold & Flu .... ▣781
Robitussin Cold Softgels Multi-Symptom Cold & Flu .... ▣781
Robitussin Cold Softgels Severe Congestion .... ▣782
Robitussin Cough & Cold Infant Drops .... ▣782
Robitussin Maximum Strength Cough & Cold Liquid .... ▣785
Robitussin Pediatric Cough & Cold Formula Liquid .... ▣785
Robitussin Multi Symptom Honey Flu Liquid .... ▣785
Robitussin Nighttime Honey Flu Liquid .... ▣786
Robitussin-CF Liquid .... ▣783
Robitussin-DAC Syrup 2942
Robitussin-PE Liquid .... ▣782
Ryna .... ▣768
Semprex-D Capsules 1172
Singlet Caplets .... ▣761
Sinutab Non-Drying Liquid Caps .... ▣706
Sinutab Sinus Allergy Medication, Maximum Strength Formula, Tablets & Caplets .... ▣707
Sinutab Sinus Medication, Maximum Strength Without Drowsiness Formula, Tablets & Caplets .... ▣707
Sudafed 12 Hour Tablets .... ▣708
Sudafed 24 Hour Tablets .... ▣708
Children's Sudafed Cold & Cough Liquid .... ▣709
Children's Sudafed Nasal Decongestant Chewables .... ▣711
Children's Sudafed Nasal Decongestant Liquid Medication .... ▣711
Sudafed Cold & Allergy Tablets .... ▣708
Sudafed Cold & Cough Liquid Caps .... ▣709
Sudafed Cold & Sinus Liquid Caps .... ▣710
Sudafed Nasal Decongestant Tablets .... ▣710
Sudafed Non-Drying Sinus Liquid Caps .... ▣712
Sudafed Severe Cold .... ▣711
Sudafed Sinus Headache Caplets .... ▣712
Sudafed Sinus Headache Tablets .... ▣712
Tavist Sinus Non-Drowsy Coated Caplets .... ▣676
TheraFlu Regular Strength Cold & Cough Night Time Hot Liquid .... ▣676
TheraFlu Regular Strength Cold & Sore Throat Night Time Hot Liquid .... ▣676
TheraFlu Maximum Strength Flu & Congestion Non-Drowsy Hot Liquid .... ▣677
TheraFlu Maximum Strength Flu & Cough Night Time Hot Liquid .... ▣678
TheraFlu Maximum Strength Flu & Sore Throat Night Time Hot Liquid .... ▣677
TheraFlu Maximum Strength Severe Cold & Congestion Night Time Caplets .... ▣678
TheraFlu Maximum Strength Severe Cold & Congestion Night Time Hot Liquid .... ▣678
TheraFlu Maximum Strength Severe Cold & Congestion Non-Drowsy .... ▣679
Triaminic Allergy Congestion Liquid .... ▣680
Triaminic Chest Congestion Liquid .... ▣680

Triaminic Cold & Allergy Liquid ...... ■ 681
Triaminic Cold & Allergy Softchews ...... ■ 683
Triaminic Cold & Cough Liquid ...... ■ 681
Triaminic Cold & Cough Softchews ...... ■ 683
Triaminic Cold & Night Time Cough Liquid ...... ■ 681
Triaminic Cold, Cough & Fever Liquid ...... ■ 681
Triaminic Cough Liquid ...... ■ 682
Triaminic Cough & Congestion Liquid ...... ■ 682
Triaminic Cough & Sore Throat Liquid ...... ■ 682
Triaminic Cough & Sore Throat Softchews ...... ■ 684
Children's Tylenol Allergy-D Liquid ... 2014
Children's Tylenol Cold Suspension Liquid and Chewable Tablets 2015
Children's Tylenol Cold Plus Cough Suspension Liquid and Chewable Tablets 2015
Children's Tylenol Flu Suspension Liquid 2015
Children's Tylenol Sinus Suspension Liquid 2017
Infants' Tylenol Cold Decongestant and Fever Reducer Concentrated Drops 2015
Infants' Tylenol Cold Decongestant and Fever Reducer Concentrated Drops Plus Cough.. 2015
Tylenol Allergy Sinus 2010
Multi-Symptom Tylenol Cold Complete Formula Caplets 2010
Multi-Symptom Tylenol Cold Non-Drowsy Caplets and Gelcaps 2010
Multi-Symptom Tylenol Cold Severe Congestion Non-Drowsy Caplets 2011
Maximum Strength Tylenol Flu NightTime Gelcaps 2011
Maximum Strength Tylenol Flu NightTime Liquid 2011
Maximum Strength Tylenol Flu Non-Drowsy Gelcaps 2011
Maximum Strength Tylenol Sinus NightTime Caplets 2012
Maximum Strength Tylenol Sinus Non-Drowsy Geltabs, Gelcaps, Caplets, and Tablets 2012
Vicks 44D Cough & Head Congestion Relief Liquid ...... ■ 724
Vicks 44M Cough, Cold & Flu Relief Liquid ...... ■ 725
Pediatric Vicks 44m Cough & Cold Relief ...... ■ 728
Vicks DayQuil LiquiCaps/Liquid Multi-Symptom Cold/Flu Relief ... ■ 727
Children's Vicks NyQuil Cold/Cough Relief ...... ■ 726
Vicks NyQuil LiquiCaps/Liquid Multi-Symptom Cold/Flu Relief, Original and Cherry Flavors ...... ■ 727
Zephrex Tablets 3091
Zephrex LA Tablets 3092
Zyrtec-D 12 Hour Extended Relief Tablets 2758

Reserpine (Co-administration of beta blockers with catecholamine-depleting drugs, such as reserpine, may result in additive effect; patients on combined therapy should be observed for marked bradycardia or hypotension which may present as vertigo, syncope/presyncope, or orthostatic changes in blood pressure).
No products indexed under this heading.

Rofecoxib (Blunting of the antihypertensive effect). Products include:
Vioxx 2213

Sulindac (Blunting of the antihypertensive effect). Products include:
Clinoril Tablets 2053

Tetrahydrozoline Hydrochloride (Exaggerated hypertensive responses have been reported from the combined use of beta-adrenergic antagonists and alpha-adrenergic stimulants, including those contained in cold remedies). Products include:
Murine Tears Plus Lubricant Redness Reliever Eye Drops ...... ⊙ 323
Visine Original Eye Drops ...... ⊙ 315
Visine A.C. Seasonal Relief From Pollen & Dust Eye Drops ...... ⊙ 314
Advanced Relief Visine Eye Drops . ⊙ 313

Tolmetin Sodium (Blunting of the antihypertensive effect). Products include:
Tolectin 2589

Food Interactions

Food, unspecified (Slightly decreases absorption and peak concentration).

SEDAPAP TABLETS 50 MG/ 650 MG
(Acetaminophen, Butalbital) 2225
May interact with central nervous system depressants, general anesthetics, monoamine oxidase inhibitors, narcotic analgesics, psychotropics, tranquilizers, tricyclic antidepressants, and certain other agents. Compounds in these categories include:

Alfentanil Hydrochloride (Additive CNS depression).
No products indexed under this heading.

Alprazolam (Additive CNS depression). Products include:
Xanax Tablets 2865

Amitriptyline Hydrochloride (Additive CNS depression). Products include:
Etrafon 3115
Limbitrol 1738

Amoxapine (Additive CNS depression).
No products indexed under this heading.

Aprobarbital (Additive CNS depression).
No products indexed under this heading.

Buprenorphine Hydrochloride (Additive CNS depression). Products include:
Buprenex Injectable 2918

Buspirone Hydrochloride (Additive CNS depression).
No products indexed under this heading.

Butabarbital (Additive CNS depression).
No products indexed under this heading.

Chlordiazepoxide (Additive CNS depression). Products include:
Limbitrol 1738

Chlordiazepoxide Hydrochloride (Additive CNS depression). Products include:
Librium Capsules 1736
Librium for Injection 1737

Chlorpromazine (Additive CNS depression). Products include:
Thorazine Suppositories 1656

Chlorpromazine Hydrochloride (Additive CNS depression). Products include:
Thorazine 1656

Chlorprothixene (Additive CNS depression).
No products indexed under this heading.

Chlorprothixene Hydrochloride (Additive CNS depression).
No products indexed under this heading.

Chlorprothixene Lactate (Additive CNS depression).
No products indexed under this heading.

Clomipramine Hydrochloride (Additive CNS depression).
No products indexed under this heading.

Clorazepate Dipotassium (Additive CNS depression). Products include:
Tranxene 511

Clozapine (Additive CNS depression). Products include:
Clozaril Tablets 2319

Codeine Phosphate (Additive CNS depression). Products include:
Phenergan with Codeine Syrup 3557
Phenergan VC with Codeine Syrup .. 3561
Robitussin A-C Syrup 2942
Robitussin-DAC Syrup 2942
Ryna-C Liquid ...... ■ 768
Soma Compound w/Codeine Tablets 3355
Tussi-Organidin NR Liquid 3350
Tussi-Organidin-S NR Liquid 3350
Tylenol with Codeine 2595

Desflurane (Additive CNS depression). Products include:
Suprane Liquid for Inhalation 874

Desipramine Hydrochloride (Additive CNS depression). Products include:
Norpramin Tablets 755

Dezocine (Additive CNS depression).
No products indexed under this heading.

Diazepam (Additive CNS depression). Products include:
Valium Injectable 3026
Valium Tablets 3047

Doxepin Hydrochloride (Additive CNS depression). Products include:
Sinequan 2713

Droperidol (Additive CNS depression).
No products indexed under this heading.

Enflurane (Additive CNS depression).
No products indexed under this heading.

Estazolam (Additive CNS depression). Products include:
ProSom Tablets 500

Ethchlorvynol (Additive CNS depression).
No products indexed under this heading.

Ethinamate (Additive CNS depression).
No products indexed under this heading.

Fentanyl (Additive CNS depression). Products include:
Duragesic Transdermal System 1786

Fentanyl Citrate (Additive CNS depression). Products include:
Actiq 1184

Fluphenazine Decanoate (Additive CNS depression).
No products indexed under this heading.

Fluphenazine Enanthate (Additive CNS depression).
No products indexed under this heading.

Fluphenazine Hydrochloride (Additive CNS depression).
No products indexed under this heading.

Flurazepam Hydrochloride (Additive CNS depression).
No products indexed under this heading.

Glutethimide (Additive CNS depression).
No products indexed under this heading.

Haloperidol (Additive CNS depression). Products include:
Haldol Injection, Tablets and Concentrate 2533

Haloperidol Decanoate (Additive CNS depression). Products include:
Haldol Decanoate 2535

Hydrocodone Bitartrate (Additive CNS depression). Products include:
Hycodan 1316
Hycomine Compound Tablets 1317
Hycotuss Expectorant Syrup 1318
Lortab 3319
Lortab Elixir 3317
Maxidone Tablets CIII 3399
Norco 5/325 Tablets CIII 3424
Norco 7.5/325 Tablets CIII 3425
Norco 10/325 Tablets CIII 3427
Norco 10/325 Tablets CIII 3425
Vicodin Tablets 516
Vicodin ES Tablets 517
Vicodin HP Tablets 518
Vicodin Tuss Expectorant 519
Vicoprofen Tablets 520
Zydone Tablets 1330

Hydrocodone Polistirex (Additive CNS depression). Products include:
Tussionex Pennkinetic Extended-Release Suspension 1174

Hydromorphone Hydrochloride (Additive CNS depression). Products include:
Dilaudid 441
Dilaudid Oral Liquid 445
Dilaudid Powder 441
Dilaudid Rectal Suppositories 441
Dilaudid Tablets 441
Dilaudid Tablets - 8 mg 445
Dilaudid-HP 443

Hydroxyzine Hydrochloride (Additive CNS depression). Products include:
Atarax Tablets & Syrup 2667
Vistaril Intramuscular Solution 2738

Imipramine Hydrochloride (Additive CNS depression).
No products indexed under this heading.

Imipramine Pamoate (Additive CNS depression).
No products indexed under this heading.

Isocarboxazid (The effects of butalbital may be enhanced by MAO inhibitors).
No products indexed under this heading.

Isoflurane (Additive CNS depression).
No products indexed under this heading.

Ketamine Hydrochloride (Additive CNS depression).
No products indexed under this heading.

Levomethadyl Acetate Hydrochloride (Additive CNS depression).
No products indexed under this heading.

Levorphanol Tartrate (Additive CNS depression). Products include:
Levo-Dromoran 1734
Levorphanol Tartrate Tablets 3059

Lithium Carbonate (Additive CNS depression). Products include:
Eskalith 1527
Lithium Carbonate 3061
Lithobid Slow-Release Tablets 3255

Lithium Citrate (Additive CNS depression). Products include:
Lithium Citrate Syrup 3061

Lorazepam (Additive CNS depression). Products include:
Ativan Injection 3478
Ativan Tablets 3482

Loxapine Hydrochloride (Additive CNS depression).
No products indexed under this heading.

Loxapine Succinate (Additive CNS depression). Products include:
Loxitane Capsules 3398

Maprotiline Hydrochloride (Additive CNS depression).
No products indexed under this heading.

Meperidine Hydrochloride (Additive CNS depression). Products include:
Demerol 3079
Mepergan Injection 3539

Mephobarbital (Additive CNS depression).
No products indexed under this heading.

Meprobamate (Additive CNS depression). Products include:
Miltown Tablets 3349

Mesoridazine Besylate (Additive CNS depression). Products include:
Serentil 1057

Methadone Hydrochloride (Additive CNS depression). Products include:
Dolophine Hydrochloride Tablets 3056

Methohexital Sodium (Additive CNS depression). Products include:
Brevital Sodium for Injection, USP .. 1815

Methotrimeprazine (Additive CNS depression).
No products indexed under this heading.

Methoxyflurane (Additive CNS depression).
No products indexed under this heading.

Midazolam Hydrochloride (Additive CNS depression). Products include:
Versed Injection 3027
Versed Syrup 3033

Moclobemide (The effects of butalbital may be enhanced by MAO inhibitors).
No products indexed under this heading.

Molindone Hydrochloride (Additive CNS depression). Products include:
Moban 1320

Morphine Sulfate (Additive CNS depression). Products include:
Astramorph/PF Injection, USP (Preservative-Free).......... 594
Duramorph Injection 1312
Infumorph 200 and Infumorph 500 Sterile Solutions.......... 1314
Kadian Capsules 1335
MS Contin Tablets 2896
MSIR 2898
Oramorph SR Tablets 3062
Roxanol 3066

Nortriptyline Hydrochloride (Additive CNS depression).
No products indexed under this heading.

Olanzapine (Additive CNS depression). Products include:
Zyprexa Tablets 1973
Zyprexa ZYDIS Orally Disintegrating Tablets.......... 1973

Oxazepam (Additive CNS depression).
No products indexed under this heading.

Oxycodone Hydrochloride (Additive CNS depression). Products include:
OxyContin Tablets 2912
OxyFast Oral Concentrate Solution . 2916
OxyIR Capsules 2916
Percocet Tablets 1326
Percodan Tablets 1327
Percolone Tablets 1327
Roxicodone 3067
Tylox Capsules 2597

Pargyline Hydrochloride (The effects of butalbital may be enhanced by MAO inhibitors).
No products indexed under this heading.

Pentobarbital Sodium (Additive CNS depression). Products include:
Nembutal Sodium Solution 485

Perphenazine (Additive CNS depression). Products include:
Etrafon 3115
Trilafon 3160

Phenelzine Sulfate (The effects of butalbital may be enhanced by MAO inhibitors). Products include:
Nardil Tablets 2653

Phenobarbital (Additive CNS depression). Products include:
Arco-Lase Plus Tablets 592
Donnatal 2929
Donnatal Extentabs 2930

Prazepam (Additive CNS depression).
No products indexed under this heading.

Procarbazine Hydrochloride (The effects of butalbital may be enhanced by MAO inhibitors). Products include:
Matulane Capsules 3246

Prochlorperazine (Additive CNS depression). Products include:
Compazine 1505

Promethazine Hydrochloride (Additive CNS depression). Products include:
Mepergan Injection 3539
Phenergan Injection 3553
Phenergan 3556
Phenergan Syrup 3554
Phenergan with Codeine Syrup 3557
Phenergan with Dextromethorphan Syrup.......... 3559
Phenergan VC Syrup 3560
Phenergan VC with Codeine Syrup .. 3561

Propofol (Additive CNS depression). Products include:
Diprivan Injectable Emulsion 667

Propoxyphene Hydrochloride (Additive CNS depression). Products include:
Darvon Pulvules 1909
Darvon Compound-65 Pulvules 1910

Propoxyphene Napsylate (Additive CNS depression). Products include:
Darvon-N/Darvocet-N 1907
Darvon-N Tablets 1912

Protriptyline Hydrochloride (Additive CNS depression; decreased blood levels of the antidepressant). Products include:
Vivactil Tablets 2446
Vivactil Tablets 2217

Quazepam (Additive CNS depression).
No products indexed under this heading.

Quetiapine Fumarate (Additive CNS depression). Products include:
Seroquel Tablets 684

Remifentanil Hydrochloride (Additive CNS depression).
No products indexed under this heading.

Risperidone (Additive CNS depression). Products include:
Risperdal 1796

Secobarbital Sodium (Additive CNS depression).
No products indexed under this heading.

Selegiline Hydrochloride (The effects of butalbital may be enhanced by MAO inhibitors). Products include:
Eldepryl Capsules 3266

Sevoflurane (Additive CNS depression).
No products indexed under this heading.

Sufentanil Citrate (Additive CNS depression).
No products indexed under this heading.

Temazepam (Additive CNS depression).
No products indexed under this heading.

Thiamylal Sodium (Additive CNS depression).
No products indexed under this heading.

Thioridazine Hydrochloride (Additive CNS depression). Products include:
Thioridazine Hydrochloride Tablets.......... 2289

Thiothixene (Additive CNS depression). Products include:
Navane Capsules 2701
Thiothixene Capsules 2290

Tranylcypromine Sulfate (The effects of butalbital may be enhanced by MAO inhibitors). Products include:
Parnate Tablets 1607

Triazolam (Additive CNS depression). Products include:
Halcion Tablets 2823

Trifluoperazine Hydrochloride (Additive CNS depression). Products include:
Stelazine 1640

Trimipramine Maleate (Additive CNS depression). Products include:
Surmontil Capsules 3595

Zaleplon (Additive CNS depression). Products include:
Sonata Capsules 3591

Ziprasidone Hydrochloride (Additive CNS depression). Products include:
Geodon Capsules 2688

Zolpidem Tartrate (Additive CNS depression). Products include:
Ambien Tablets 3191

Food Interactions

Alcohol (Additive CNS depression).

SELSUN RX 2.5% LOTION, USP

(Selenium Sulfide) 3053
None cited in PDR database.

SEMPREX-D CAPSULES

(Acrivastine, Pseudoephedrine Hydrochloride).......... 1172
May interact with central nervous system depressants, monoamine oxidase inhibitors, sympathomimetics, veratrum alkaloids, and certain other agents. Compounds in these categories include:

Albuterol (Beta-adrenergic agonists (other sympathomimetics) increase the effects of pseudoephedrine and combined effects on cardiovascular system may be harmful). Products include:
Proventil Inhalation Aerosol 3142
Ventolin Inhalation Aerosol and Refill.......... 1679

Albuterol Sulfate (Beta-adrenergic agonists (other sympathomimetics) increase the effects of pseudoephedrine and combined effects on cardiovascular system may be harmful). Products include:
AccuNeb Inhalation Solution 1230
Combivent Inhalation Aerosol 1041
DuoNeb Inhalation Solution 1233
Proventil Inhalation Solution 0.083%.......... 3146
Proventil Repetabs Tablets 3148
Proventil Solution for Inhalation 0.5%.......... 3144
Proventil HFA Inhalation Aerosol 3150
Ventolin HFA Inhalation Aerosol 3618
Volmax Extended-Release Tablets .. 2276

Alfentanil Hydrochloride (Co-administration may result in additional reduction in alertness and impairment of CNS performance and should be avoided).
No products indexed under this heading.

Alprazolam (Co-administration may result in additional reduction in alertness and impairment of CNS performance and should be avoided). Products include:
Xanax Tablets 2865

Aprobarbital (Co-administration may result in additional reduction in alertness and impairment of CNS performance and should be avoided).
No products indexed under this heading.

Buprenorphine Hydrochloride (Co-administration may result in additional reduction in alertness and impairment of CNS performance and should be avoided). Products include:
Buprenex Injectable 2918

Buspirone Hydrochloride (Co-administration may result in additional reduction in alertness and impairment of CNS performance and should be avoided).
No products indexed under this heading.

Butabarbital (Co-administration may result in additional reduction in alertness and impairment of CNS performance and should be avoided).
No products indexed under this heading.

Butalbital (Co-administration may result in additional reduction in alertness and impairment of CNS performance and should be avoided). Products include:
Phrenilin 578
Sedapap Tablets 50 mg/650 mg ... 2225

Chlordiazepoxide (Co-administration may result in additional reduction in alertness and impairment of CNS performance and should be avoided). Products include:
Limbitrol 1738

Chlordiazepoxide Hydrochloride (Co-administration may result in additional reduction in alertness and impairment of CNS performance and should be avoided). Products include:
Librium Capsules 1736
Librium for Injection 1737

Chlorpromazine (Co-administration may result in additional reduction in alertness and impairment of CNS performance and should be avoided). Products include:
Thorazine Suppositories 1656

Chlorpromazine Hydrochloride (Co-administration may result in additional reduction in alertness and impairment of CNS performance and should be avoided). Products include:
Thorazine 1656

Chlorprothixene (Co-administration may result in additional reduction in alertness and impairment of CNS performance and should be avoided).
No products indexed under this heading.

Chlorprothixene Hydrochloride (Co-administration may result in additional reduction in alertness and impairment of CNS performance and should be avoided).
No products indexed under this heading.

Chlorprothixene Lactate (Co-administration may result in additional reduction in alertness and impairment of CNS performance and should be avoided).
No products indexed under this heading.

Clorazepate Dipotassium (Co-administration may result in additional reduction in alertness and impairment of CNS performance and should be avoided). Products include:
Tranxene 511

Clozapine (Co-administration may result in additional reduction in alertness and impairment of CNS performance and should be avoided). Products include:
Clozaril Tablets 2319

Codeine Phosphate (Co-administration may result in additional reduction in alertness and impairment of CNS performance and should be avoided). Products include:
Phenergan with Codeine Syrup 3557
Phenergan VC with Codeine Syrup .. 3561
Robitussin A-C Syrup 2942
Robitussin-DAC Syrup 2942
Ryna-C Liquid .... ▣768
Soma Compound w/Codeine Tablets.......... 3355
Tussi-Organidin NR Liquid 3350
Tussi-Organidin-S NR Liquid 3350
Tylenol with Codeine 2595

Desflurane (Co-administration may result in additional reduction in alertness and impairment of CNS performance and should be avoided). Products include:
Suprane Liquid for Inhalation 874

Dezocine (Co-administration may result in additional reduction in alertness and impairment of CNS perfor-

mance and should be avoided).
No products indexed under this heading.

Diazepam (Co-administration may result in additional reduction in alertness and impairment of CNS performance and should be avoided). Products include:
- Valium Injectable 3026
- Valium Tablets 3047

Dobutamine Hydrochloride (Beta-adrenergic agonists (other sympathomimetics) increase the effects of pseudoephedrine and combined effects on cardiovascular system may be harmful). Products include:
- Dobutrex Solution Vials 1914

Dopamine Hydrochloride (Beta-adrenergic agonists (other sympathomimetics) increase the effects of pseudoephedrine and combined effects on cardiovascular system may be harmful).
No products indexed under this heading.

Droperidol (Co-administration may result in additional reduction in alertness and impairment of CNS performance and should be avoided).
No products indexed under this heading.

Enflurane (Co-administration may result in additional reduction in alertness and impairment of CNS performance and should be avoided).
No products indexed under this heading.

Ephedrine Hydrochloride (Beta-adrenergic agonists (other sympathomimetics) increase the effects of pseudoephedrine and combined effects on cardiovascular system may be harmful). Products include:
- Primatene Tablets 780

Ephedrine Sulfate (Beta-adrenergic agonists (other sympathomimetics) increase the effects of pseudoephedrine and combined effects on cardiovascular system may be harmful).
No products indexed under this heading.

Ephedrine Tannate (Beta-adrenergic agonists (other sympathomimetics) increase the effects of pseudoephedrine and combined effects on cardiovascular system may be harmful). Products include:
- Rynatuss Pediatric Suspension 3353
- Rynatuss Tablets 3353

Epinephrine (Beta-adrenergic agonists (other sympathomimetics) increase the effects of pseudoephedrine and combined effects on cardiovascular system may be harmful). Products include:
- Epifrin Sterile Ophthalmic Solution 235
- EpiPen 1236
- Primatene Mist 779
- Xylocaine with Epinephrine Injection 653

Epinephrine Bitartrate (Beta-adrenergic agonists (other sympathomimetics) increase the effects of pseudoephedrine and combined effects on cardiovascular system may be harmful). Products include:
- Sensorcaine 643

Epinephrine Hydrochloride (Beta-adrenergic agonists (other sympathomimetics) increase the effects of pseudoephedrine and combined effects on cardiovascular system may be harmful).
No products indexed under this heading.

Estazolam (Co-administration may result in additional reduction in alertness and impairment of CNS performance and should be avoided). Products include:
- ProSom Tablets 500

Ethchlorvynol (Co-administration may result in additional reduction in alertness and impairment of CNS performance and should be avoided).
No products indexed under this heading.

Ethinamate (Co-administration may result in additional reduction in alertness and impairment of CNS performance and should be avoided).
No products indexed under this heading.

Fentanyl (Co-administration may result in additional reduction in alertness and impairment of CNS performance and should be avoided). Products include:
- Duragesic Transdermal System 1786

Fentanyl Citrate (Co-administration may result in additional reduction in alertness and impairment of CNS performance and should be avoided). Products include:
- Actiq 1184

Fluphenazine Decanoate (Co-administration may result in additional reduction in alertness and impairment of CNS performance and should be avoided).
No products indexed under this heading.

Fluphenazine Enanthate (Co-administration may result in additional reduction in alertness and impairment of CNS performance and should be avoided).
No products indexed under this heading.

Fluphenazine Hydrochloride (Co-administration may result in additional reduction in alertness and impairment of CNS performance and should be avoided).
No products indexed under this heading.

Flurazepam Hydrochloride (Co-administration may result in additional reduction in alertness and impairment of CNS performance and should be avoided).
No products indexed under this heading.

Glutethimide (Co-administration may result in additional reduction in alertness and impairment of CNS performance and should be avoided).
No products indexed under this heading.

Haloperidol (Co-administration may result in additional reduction in alertness and impairment of CNS performance and should be avoided). Products include:
- Haldol Injection, Tablets and Concentrate 2533

Haloperidol Decanoate (Co-administration may result in additional reduction in alertness and impairment of CNS performance and should be avoided). Products include:
- Haldol Decanoate 2535

Hydrocodone Bitartrate (Co-administration may result in additional reduction in alertness and impairment of CNS performance and should be avoided). Products include:
- Hycodan 1316
- Hycomine Compound Tablets 1317
- Hycotuss Expectorant Syrup 1318
- Lortab 3319
- Lortab Elixir 3317
- Maxidone Tablets CIII 3399
- Norco 5/325 Tablets CIII 3424
- Norco 7.5/325 Tablets CIII 3425
- Norco 10/325 Tablets CIII 3427
- Norco 10/325 Tablets CIII 3425
- Vicodin Tablets 516
- Vicodin ES Tablets 517
- Vicodin HP Tablets 518
- Vicodin Tuss Expectorant 519
- Vicoprofen Tablets 520
- Zydone Tablets 1330

Hydrocodone Polistirex (Co-administration may result in additional reduction in alertness and impairment of CNS performance and should be avoided). Products include:
- Tussionex Pennkinetic Extended-Release Suspension 1174

Hydromorphone Hydrochloride (Co-administration may result in additional reduction in alertness and impairment of CNS performance and should be avoided). Products include:
- Dilaudid 441
- Dilaudid Oral Liquid 445
- Dilaudid Powder 441
- Dilaudid Rectal Suppositories 441
- Dilaudid Tablets 441
- Dilaudid Tablets - 8 mg 445
- Dilaudid-HP 443

Hydroxyzine Hydrochloride (Co-administration may result in additional reduction in alertness and impairment of CNS performance and should be avoided). Products include:
- Atarax Tablets & Syrup 2667
- Vistaril Intramuscular Solution 2738

Isocarboxazid (MAO inhibitors increase the effects of sympathomimetics; potential for hypertensive crisis; concurrent and/or sequential use is contraindicated for two weeks).
No products indexed under this heading.

Isoflurane (Co-administration may result in additional reduction in alertness and impairment of CNS performance and should be avoided).
No products indexed under this heading.

Isoproterenol Hydrochloride (Beta-adrenergic agonists (other sympathomimetics) increase the effects of pseudoephedrine and combined effects on cardiovascular system may be harmful).
No products indexed under this heading.

Isoproterenol Sulfate (Beta-adrenergic agonists (other sympathomimetics) increase the effects of pseudoephedrine and combined effects on cardiovascular system may be harmful).
No products indexed under this heading.

Ketamine Hydrochloride (Co-administration may result in additional reduction in alertness and impairment of CNS performance and should be avoided).
No products indexed under this heading.

Levalbuterol Hydrochloride (Beta-adrenergic agonists (other sympathomimetics) increase the effects of pseudoephedrine and combined effects on cardiovascular system may be harmful). Products include:
- Xopenex Inhalation Solution 3207

Levomethadyl Acetate Hydrochloride (Co-administration may result in additional reduction in alertness and impairment of CNS performance and should be avoided).
No products indexed under this heading.

Levorphanol Tartrate (Co-administration may result in additional reduction in alertness and impairment of CNS performance and should be avoided). Products include:
- Levo-Dromoran 1734
- Levorphanol Tartrate Tablets 3059

Lorazepam (Co-administration may result in additional reduction in alertness and impairment of CNS performance and should be avoided). Products include:
- Ativan Injection 3478
- Ativan Tablets 3482

Loxapine Hydrochloride (Co-administration may result in additional reduction in alertness and impairment of CNS performance and should be avoided).
No products indexed under this heading.

Loxapine Succinate (Co-administration may result in additional reduction in alertness and impairment of CNS performance and should be avoided). Products include:
- Loxitane Capsules 3398

Mecamylamine Hydrochloride (Reduced antihypertensive effects of drugs that interfere with sympathetic activity). Products include:
- Inversine Tablets 1850

Meperidine Hydrochloride (Co-administration may result in additional reduction in alertness and impairment of CNS performance and should be avoided). Products include:
- Demerol 3079
- Mepergan Injection 3539

Mephobarbital (Co-administration may result in additional reduction in alertness and impairment of CNS performance and should be avoided).
No products indexed under this heading.

Meprobamate (Co-administration may result in additional reduction in alertness and impairment of CNS performance and should be avoided). Products include:
- Miltown Tablets 3349

Mesoridazine Besylate (Co-administration may result in additional reduction in alertness and impairment of CNS performance and should be avoided). Products include:
- Serentil 1057

Metaproterenol Sulfate (Beta-adrenergic agonists (other sympathomimetics) increase the effects of pseudoephedrine and combined effects on cardiovascular system may be harmful). Products include:
- Alupent 1029

Metaraminol Bitartrate (Beta-adrenergic agonists (other sympathomimetics) increase the effects of pseudoephedrine and combined effects on cardiovascular system may be harmful). Products include:
- Aramine Injection 2043

Methadone Hydrochloride (Co-administration may result in additional reduction in alertness and impairment of CNS performance and should be avoided). Products include:
- Dolophine Hydrochloride Tablets 3056

Methohexital Sodium (Co-administration may result in additional reduction in alertness and impairment of CNS performance and should be avoided). Products include:
- Brevital Sodium for Injection, USP 1815

Methotrimeprazine (Co-administration may result in additional reduction in alertness and impairment of CNS performance and should be avoided).
No products indexed under this heading.

Methoxamine Hydrochloride (Beta-adrenergic agonists (other sympathomimetics) increase the effects of pseudoephedrine and combined effects on cardiovascular system may be harmful).
No products indexed under this heading.

Methoxyflurane (Co-administration may result in additional reduction in alertness and impairment of CNS

performance and should be avoided).
No products indexed under this heading.

Methyldopa (Reduced antihypertensive effects of drugs that interfere with sympathetic activity). Products include:
Aldoclor Tablets **2035**
Aldomet Tablets **2037**
Aldoril Tablets **2039**

Methyldopate Hydrochloride (Reduced antihypertensive effects of drugs that interfere with sympathetic activity).
No products indexed under this heading.

Midazolam Hydrochloride (Co-administration may result in additional reduction in alertness and impairment of CNS performance and should be avoided). Products include:
Versed Injection **3027**
Versed Syrup **3033**

Moclobemide (MAO inhibitors increase the effects of sympathomimetics; potential for hypertensive crisis; concurrent and/or sequential use is contraindicated for two weeks).
No products indexed under this heading.

Molindone Hydrochloride (Co-administration may result in additional reduction in alertness and impairment of CNS performance and should be avoided). Products include:
Moban **1320**

Morphine Sulfate (Co-administration may result in additional reduction in alertness and impairment of CNS performance and should be avoided). Products include:
Astramorph/PF Injection, USP (Preservative-Free).......... **594**
Duramorph Injection **1312**
Infumorph 200 and Infumorph 500 Sterile Solutions.......... **1314**
Kadian Capsules **1335**
MS Contin Tablets **2896**
MSIR **2898**
Oramorph SR Tablets **3062**
Roxanol **3066**

Norepinephrine Bitartrate (Beta-adrenergic agonists (other sympathomimetics) increase the effects of pseudoephedrine and combined effects on cardiovascular system may be harmful).
No products indexed under this heading.

Olanzapine (Co-administration may result in additional reduction in alertness and impairment of CNS performance and should be avoided). Products include:
Zyprexa Tablets **1973**
Zyprexa ZYDIS Orally Disintegrating Tablets.......... **1973**

Oxazepam (Co-administration may result in additional reduction in alertness and impairment of CNS performance and should be avoided).
No products indexed under this heading.

Oxycodone Hydrochloride (Co-administration may result in additional reduction in alertness and impairment of CNS performance and should be avoided). Products include:
OxyContin Tablets **2912**
OxyFast Oral Concentrate Solution . **2916**
OxyIR Capsules **2916**
Percocet Tablets **1326**
Percodan Tablets **1327**
Percolone Tablets **1327**
Roxicodone **3067**
Tylox Capsules **2597**

Pargyline Hydrochloride (MAO inhibitors increase the effects of sympathomimetics; potential for hypertensive crisis; concurrent and/or sequential use is contraindicated for two weeks).
No products indexed under this heading.

Pentobarbital Sodium (Co-administration may result in additional reduction in alertness and impairment of CNS performance and should be avoided). Products include:
Nembutal Sodium Solution **485**

Perphenazine (Co-administration may result in additional reduction in alertness and impairment of CNS performance and should be avoided). Products include:
Etrafon **3115**
Trilafon **3160**

Phenelzine Sulfate (MAO inhibitors increase the effects of sympathomimetics; potential for hypertensive crisis; concurrent and/or sequential use is contraindicated for two weeks). Products include:
Nardil Tablets **2653**

Phenobarbital (Co-administration may result in additional reduction in alertness and impairment of CNS performance and should be avoided). Products include:
Arco-Lase Plus Tablets **592**
Donnatal **2929**
Donnatal Extentabs **2930**

Phenylephrine Bitartrate (Beta-adrenergic agonists (other sympathomimetics) increase the effects of pseudoephedrine and combined effects on cardiovascular system may be harmful).
No products indexed under this heading.

Phenylephrine Hydrochloride (Beta-adrenergic agonists (other sympathomimetics) increase the effects of pseudoephedrine and combined effects on cardiovascular system may be harmful). Products include:
Afrin Nasal Decongestant Children's Pump Mist.......... ▣ **734**
Extendryl **1361**
Hycomine Compound Tablets **1317**
Neo-Synephrine .... ▣ **614**
Phenergan VC Syrup **3560**
Phenergan VC with Codeine Syrup .. **3561**
Preparation H Cream .... ▣ **778**
Preparation H Cooling Gel .... ▣ **778**
Preparation H .... ▣ **778**
Vicks Sinex Nasal Spray and Ultra Fine Mist.......... ▣ **729**

Phenylephrine Tannate (Beta-adrenergic agonists (other sympathomimetics) increase the effects of pseudoephedrine and combined effects on cardiovascular system may be harmful). Products include:
Ryna-12 S Suspension **3351**
Reformulated Rynatan Pediatric Suspension.......... **3352**
Rynatuss Pediatric Suspension **3353**
Rynatuss Tablets **3353**

Phenylpropanolamine Hydrochloride (Beta-adrenergic agonists (other sympathomimetics) increase the effects of pseudoephedrine and combined effects on cardiovascular system may be harmful).
No products indexed under this heading.

Pirbuterol Acetate (Beta-adrenergic agonists (other sympathomimetics) increase the effects of pseudoephedrine and combined effects on cardiovascular system may be harmful). Products include:
Maxair Autohaler **1981**
Maxair Inhaler **1984**

Prazepam (Co-administration may result in additional reduction in alertness and impairment of CNS performance and should be avoided).
No products indexed under this heading.

Procarbazine Hydrochloride (MAO inhibitors increase the effects of sympathomimetics; potential for hypertensive crisis; concurrent and/or sequential use is contraindicated for two weeks). Products include:
Matulane Capsules **3246**

Prochlorperazine (Co-administration may result in additional reduction in alertness and impairment of CNS performance and should be avoided). Products include:
Compazine **1505**

Promethazine Hydrochloride (Co-administration may result in additional reduction in alertness and impairment of CNS performance and should be avoided). Products include:
Mepergan Injection **3539**
Phenergan Injection **3553**
Phenergan **3556**
Phenergan Syrup **3554**
Phenergan with Codeine Syrup **3557**
Phenergan with Dextromethorphan Syrup.......... **3559**
Phenergan VC Syrup **3560**
Phenergan VC with Codeine Syrup .. **3561**

Propofol (Co-administration may result in additional reduction in alertness and impairment of CNS performance and should be avoided). Products include:
Diprivan Injectable Emulsion **667**

Propoxyphene Hydrochloride (Co-administration may result in additional reduction in alertness and impairment of CNS performance and should be avoided). Products include:
Darvon Pulvules **1909**
Darvon Compound-65 Pulvules **1910**

Propoxyphene Napsylate (Co-administration may result in additional reduction in alertness and impairment of CNS performance and should be avoided). Products include:
Darvon-N/Darvocet-N **1907**
Darvon-N Tablets **1912**

Pseudoephedrine Sulfate (Beta-adrenergic agonists (other sympathomimetics) increase the effects of pseudoephedrine and combined effects on cardiovascular system may be harmful). Products include:
Chlor-Trimeton Allergy/Decongestant Tablets.... ▣ **736**
Claritin-D 12 Hour Extended Release Tablets.......... **3102**
Claritin-D 24 Hour Extended Release Tablets.......... **3104**
Coricidin 'D' Cold, Flu & Sinus Tablets.......... ▣ **737**
Drixoral Allergy/Sinus Extended-Release Tablets.......... ▣ **741**
Drixoral Cold & Allergy Sustained-Action Tablets.......... ▣ **740**
Drixoral Cold & Flu Extended-Release Tablets.......... ▣ **740**
Drixoral Nasal Decongestant Long-Acting Non-Drowsy Tablets.......... ▣ **740**
Rynatan Tablets **3351**

Quazepam (Co-administration may result in additional reduction in alertness and impairment of CNS performance and should be avoided).
No products indexed under this heading.

Quetiapine Fumarate (Co-administration may result in additional reduction in alertness and impairment of CNS performance and should be avoided). Products include:
Seroquel Tablets **684**

Remifentanil Hydrochloride (Co-administration may result in additional reduction in alertness and impairment of CNS performance and should be avoided).
No products indexed under this heading.

Risperidone (Co-administration may result in additional reduction in alertness and impairment of CNS performance and should be avoided). Products include:
Risperdal **1796**

Salmeterol Xinafoate (Beta-adrenergic agonists (other sympathomimetics) increase the effects of pseudoephedrine and combined effects on cardiovascular system may be harmful). Products include:
Advair Diskus 100/50 .... **1448**
Advair Diskus 250/50 .... **1448**
Advair Diskus 500/50 .... **1448**
Serevent Diskus **1637**
Serevent Inhalation Aerosol **1633**

Secobarbital Sodium (Co-administration may result in additional reduction in alertness and impairment of CNS performance and should be avoided).
No products indexed under this heading.

Selegiline Hydrochloride (MAO inhibitors increase the effects of sympathomimetics; potential for hypertensive crisis; concurrent and/or sequential use is contraindicated for two weeks). Products include:
Eldepryl Capsules **3266**

Sevoflurane (Co-administration may result in additional reduction in alertness and impairment of CNS performance and should be avoided).
No products indexed under this heading.

Sufentanil Citrate (Co-administration may result in additional reduction in alertness and impairment of CNS performance and should be avoided).
No products indexed under this heading.

Temazepam (Co-administration may result in additional reduction in alertness and impairment of CNS performance and should be avoided).
No products indexed under this heading.

Terbutaline Sulfate (Beta-adrenergic agonists (other sympathomimetics) increase the effects of pseudoephedrine and combined effects on cardiovascular system may be harmful). Products include:
Brethine Ampuls **2314**
Brethine Tablets **2313**

Thiamylal Sodium (Co-administration may result in additional reduction in alertness and impairment of CNS performance and should be avoided).
No products indexed under this heading.

Thioridazine Hydrochloride (Co-administration may result in additional reduction in alertness and impairment of CNS performance and should be avoided). Products include:
Thioridazine Hydrochloride Tablets.......... **2289**

Thiothixene (Co-administration may result in additional reduction in alertness and impairment of CNS performance and should be avoided). Products include:
Navane Capsules **2701**
Thiothixene Capsules **2290**

Tranylcypromine Sulfate (MAO inhibitors increase the effects of sympathomimetics; potential for hypertensive crisis; concurrent and/or sequential use is contraindicated for two weeks). Products include:
Parnate Tablets **1607**

Triazolam (Co-administration may result in additional reduction in alertness and impairment of CNS performance and should be avoided). Products include:
Halcion Tablets **2823**

Trifluoperazine Hydrochloride (Co-administration may result in additional reduction in alertness and

impairment of CNS performance and should be avoided). Products include:

Stelazine 1640

Zaleplon (Co-administration may result in additional reduction in alertness and impairment of CNS performance and should be avoided). Products include:

Sonata Capsules 3591

Ziprasidone Hydrochloride (Co-administration may result in additional reduction in alertness and impairment of CNS performance and should be avoided). Products include:

Geodon Capsules 2688

Zolpidem Tartrate (Co-administration may result in additional reduction in alertness and impairment of CNS performance and should be avoided). Products include:

Ambien Tablets 3191

Food Interactions

Alcohol (Co-administration may result in additional reduction in alertness and impairment of CNS performance and should be avoided).

SENOKOT GRANULES

(Senna) 2901

None cited in PDR database.

SENOKOT SYRUP

(Senna) 732

None cited in PDR database.

SENOKOT CHILDREN'S SYRUP

(Senna) 2900

None cited in PDR database.

SENOKOT TABLETS

(Senna) 2901

None cited in PDR database.

SENOKOT-S TABLETS

(Docusate Sodium, Senna) 2901

None cited in PDR database.

SENOKOTXTRA TABLETS

(Senna) 2901

None cited in PDR database.

SENSODYNE ORIGINAL FLAVOR

(Potassium Nitrate, Sodium Fluoride) 623

None cited in PDR database.

SENSODYNE COOL GEL

(Potassium Nitrate, Sodium Fluoride) 623

None cited in PDR database.

SENSODYNE EXTRA WHITENING

(Potassium Nitrate, Sodium Monofluorophosphate) 623

None cited in PDR database.

SENSODYNE FRESH MINT

(Potassium Nitrate, Sodium Fluoride) 623

None cited in PDR database.

SENSODYNE TARTAR CONTROL

(Potassium Nitrate, Sodium Fluoride) 623

None cited in PDR database.

SENSODYNE TARTAR CONTROL PLUS WHITENING

(Potassium Nitrate, Sodium Fluoride) 623

None cited in PDR database.

SENSODYNE WITH BAKING SODA

(Potassium Nitrate, Sodium Fluoride) 623

None cited in PDR database.

SENSORCAINE INJECTION

(Bupivacaine Hydrochloride) 643

See Sensorcaine with Epinephrine Injection

SENSORCAINE WITH EPINEPHRINE INJECTION

(Bupivacaine Hydrochloride, Epinephrine Bitartrate) 643

May interact with butyrophenones, ergot-type oxytocic drugs, inhalant anesthetics, monoamine oxidase inhibitors, phenothiazines, tricyclic antidepressants, and vasopressors. Compounds in these categories include:

Amitriptyline Hydrochloride (May produce severe and prolonged hypertension). Products include:

Etrafon 3115
Limbitrol 1738

Amoxapine (May produce severe and prolonged hypertension).

No products indexed under this heading.

Chlorpromazine (Reduces or reverses the pressor effect of epinephrine). Products include:

Thorazine Suppositories 1656

Chlorpromazine Hydrochloride (Reduces or reverses the pressor effect of epinephrine). Products include:

Thorazine 1656

Clomipramine Hydrochloride (May produce severe and prolonged hypertension).

No products indexed under this heading.

Desflurane (Concurrent use may produce serious dose-related cardiac arrhythmias). Products include:

Suprane Liquid for Inhalation 874

Desipramine Hydrochloride (May produce severe and prolonged hypertension). Products include:

Norpramin Tablets 755

Dopamine Hydrochloride (May produce severe and prolonged hypertension or cerebrovascular accidents).

No products indexed under this heading.

Doxepin Hydrochloride (May produce severe and prolonged hypertension). Products include:

Sinequan 2713

Enflurane (Concurrent use may produce serious dose-related cardiac arrhythmias).

No products indexed under this heading.

Epinephrine Hydrochloride (May produce severe and prolonged hypertension or cerebrovascular accidents).

No products indexed under this heading.

Fluphenazine Decanoate (Reduces or reverses the pressor effect of epinephrine).

No products indexed under this heading.

Fluphenazine Enanthate (Reduces or reverses the pressor effect of epinephrine).

No products indexed under this heading.

Fluphenazine Hydrochloride (Reduces or reverses the pressor effect of epinephrine).

No products indexed under this heading.

Haloperidol (Reduces or reverses the pressor effect of epinephrine). Products include:

Haldol Injection, Tablets and Concentrate 2533

Haloperidol Decanoate (Reduces or reverses the pressor effect of epinephrine). Products include:

Haldol Decanoate 2535

Halothane (Concurrent use may produce serious dose-related cardiac arrhythmias). Products include:

Fluothane Inhalation 3508

Imipramine Hydrochloride (May produce severe and prolonged hypertension).

No products indexed under this heading.

Imipramine Pamoate (May produce severe and prolonged hypertension).

No products indexed under this heading.

Isocarboxazid (May produce severe and prolonged hypertension).

No products indexed under this heading.

Isoflurane (Concurrent use may produce serious dose-related cardiac arrhythmias).

No products indexed under this heading.

Maprotiline Hydrochloride (May produce severe and prolonged hypertension).

No products indexed under this heading.

Mesoridazine Besylate (Reduces or reverses the pressor effect of epinephrine). Products include:

Serentil 1057

Metaraminol Bitartrate (May produce severe and prolonged hypertension or cerebrovascular accidents). Products include:

Aramine Injection 2043

Methotrimeprazine (Reduces or reverses the pressor effect of epinephrine).

No products indexed under this heading.

Methoxamine Hydrochloride (May produce severe and prolonged hypertension or cerebrovascular accidents).

No products indexed under this heading.

Methoxyflurane (Concurrent use may produce serious dose-related cardiac arrhythmias).

No products indexed under this heading.

Methylergonovine Maleate (May produce severe and prolonged hypertension or cerebrovascular accidents).

No products indexed under this heading.

Moclobemide (May produce severe and prolonged hypertension).

No products indexed under this heading.

Norepinephrine Bitartrate (May produce severe and prolonged hypertension or cerebrovascular accidents).

No products indexed under this heading.

Nortriptyline Hydrochloride (May produce severe and prolonged hypertension).

No products indexed under this heading.

Pargyline Hydrochloride (May produce severe and prolonged hypertension).

No products indexed under this heading.

Perphenazine (Reduces or reverses the pressor effect of epinephrine). Products include:

Etrafon 3115
Trilafon 3160

Phenelzine Sulfate (May produce severe and prolonged hypertension). Products include:

Nardil Tablets 2653

Phenylephrine Hydrochloride (May produce severe and prolonged hypertension or cerebrovascular accidents). Products include:

Afrin Nasal Decongestant Children's Pump Mist 734
Extendryl 1361
Hycomine Compound Tablets 1317
Neo-Synephrine 614
Phenergan VC Syrup 3560
Phenergan VC with Codeine Syrup .. 3561
Preparation H Cream 778
Preparation H Cooling Gel 778
Preparation H 778
Vicks Sinex Nasal Spray and Ultra Fine Mist 729

Procarbazine Hydrochloride (May produce severe and prolonged hypertension). Products include:

Matulane Capsules 3246

Prochlorperazine (Reduces or reverses the pressor effect of epinephrine). Products include:

Compazine 1505

Promethazine Hydrochloride (Reduces or reverses the pressor effect of epinephrine). Products include:

Mepergan Injection 3539
Phenergan Injection 3553
Phenergan 3556
Phenergan Syrup 3554
Phenergan with Codeine Syrup 3557
Phenergan with Dextromethorphan Syrup 3559
Phenergan VC Syrup 3560
Phenergan VC with Codeine Syrup .. 3561

Protriptyline Hydrochloride (May produce severe and prolonged hypertension). Products include:

Vivactil Tablets 2446
Vivactil Tablets 2217

Selegiline Hydrochloride (May produce severe and prolonged hypertension). Products include:

Eldepryl Capsules 3266

Thioridazine Hydrochloride (Reduces or reverses the pressor effect of epinephrine). Products include:

Thioridazine Hydrochloride Tablets 2289

Tranylcypromine Sulfate (May produce severe and prolonged hypertension). Products include:

Parnate Tablets 1607

Trifluoperazine Hydrochloride (Reduces or reverses the pressor effect of epinephrine). Products include:

Stelazine 1640

Trimipramine Maleate (May produce severe and prolonged hypertension). Products include:

Surmontil Capsules 3595

SENSORCAINE-MPF WITH EPINEPHRINE INJECTION

(Bupivacaine Hydrochloride, Epinephrine Bitartrate) 643

See Sensorcaine with Epinephrine Injection

SENSORCAINE-MPF INJECTION

(Bupivacaine Hydrochloride) 643

See Sensorcaine with Epinephrine Injection

SEPTRA SUSPENSION

(Sulfamethoxazole, Trimethoprim) 2265

See Septra DS Tablets

SEPTRA GRAPE SUSPENSION

(Sulfamethoxazole, Trimethoprim) 2265

See Septra DS Tablets

SEPTRA TABLETS

(Sulfamethoxazole, Trimethoprim) 2265

See Septra DS Tablets

SEPTRA DS TABLETS

(Sulfamethoxazole, Trimethoprim) 2265

May interact with phenytoin, thiazides, and certain other agents. Compounds in these categories include:

Bendroflumethiazide (Potential for thrombocytopenia with purpura in elderly). Products include:

Corzide 40/5 Tablets 2247
Corzide 80/5 Tablets 2247

Chlorothiazide (Potential for thrombocytopenia with purpura in elderly). Products include:
Aldoclor Tablets 2035
Diuril Oral 2087

Chlorothiazide Sodium (Potential for thrombocytopenia with purpura in elderly). Products include:
Diuril Sodium Intravenous 2086

Fosphenytoin Sodium (Hepatic metabolism of phenytoin may be inhibited resulting in increased phenytoin half-life and decreased metabolic clearance). Products include:
Cerebyx Injection 2619

Hydrochlorothiazide (Potential for thrombocytopenia with purpura in elderly). Products include:
Accuretic Tablets 2614
Aldoril Tablets 2039
Atacand HCT Tablets 597
Avalide Tablets 1070
Diovan HCT Tablets 2338
Dyazide Capsules 1515
HydroDIURIL Tablets 2108
Hyzaar 2109
Inderide Tablets 3517
Inderide LA Long-Acting Capsules .. 3519
Lotensin HCT Tablets 2367
Maxzide 1008
Micardis HCT Tablets 1051
Microzide Capsules 3414
Moduretic Tablets 2138
Monopril HCT 1094
Prinzide Tablets 2168
Timolide Tablets 2187
Uniretic Tablets 3178
Vaseretic Tablets 2204
Zestoretic Tablets 695
Ziac Tablets 1887

Hydroflumethiazide (Potential for thrombocytopenia with purpura in elderly). Products include:
Diucardin Tablets 3494

Leucovorin Calcium (Co-administration for the acute treatment of *Pneumocystis carinii* pneumonia in patients with HIV infection is associated with increased rates of treatment failure and morbidity).
No products indexed under this heading.

Methotrexate Sodium (Sulfonamides can displace methotrexate from plasma protein binding sites, thus increasing free methotrexate concentrations).
No products indexed under this heading.

Methyclothiazide (Potential for thrombocytopenia with purpura in elderly).
No products indexed under this heading.

Phenytoin (Hepatic metabolism of phenytoin may be inhibited resulting in increased phenytoin half-life and decreased metabolic clearance). Products include:
Dilantin Infatabs 2624
Dilantin-125 Oral Suspension 2625

Phenytoin Sodium (Hepatic metabolism of phenytoin may be inhibited resulting in increased phenytoin half-life and decreased metabolic clearance). Products include:
Dilantin Kapseals 2622

Polythiazide (Potential for thrombocytopenia with purpura in elderly). Products include:
Minizide Capsules 2700
Renese Tablets 2712

Warfarin Sodium (Co-administration results in prolonged prothrombin time). Products include:
Coumadin for Injection 1243
Coumadin Tablets 1243
Warfarin Sodium Tablets, USP 3302

SERENTIL AMPULS

(Mesoridazine Besylate) 1057
May interact with barbiturates, central nervous system depressants, general anesthetics, narcotic analgesics, drugs that prolong the QT interval, and certain other agents. Compounds in these categories include:

Alfentanil Hydrochloride (Potentiation of central nervous system depressant).
No products indexed under this heading.

Alprazolam (Potentiation of central nervous system depressant). Products include:
Xanax Tablets 2865

Amiodarone Hydrochloride (Mesoridazine has been shown to prolong the QTc interval and has been associated with torsade de pointes type arrhythmias and sudden death; co-administration with other drugs that are known to prolong the QTc interval is contraindicated). Products include:
Cordarone Intravenous 3491
Cordarone Tablets 3487
Pacerone Tablets 3331

Amitriptyline Hydrochloride (Mesoridazine has been shown to prolong the QTc interval and has been associated with torsade de pointes type arrhythmias and sudden death; co-administration with other drugs that are known to prolong the QTc interval is contraindicated). Products include:
Etrafon 3115
Limbitrol 1738

Amoxapine (Mesoridazine has been shown to prolong the QTc interval and has been associated with torsade de pointes type arrhythmias and sudden death; co-administration with other drugs that are known to prolong the QTc interval is contraindicated).
No products indexed under this heading.

Aprobarbital (Potentiation of central nervous system depressant).
No products indexed under this heading.

Astemizole (Mesoridazine has been shown to prolong the QTc interval and has been associated with torsade de pointes type arrhythmias and sudden death; co-administration with other drugs that are known to prolong the QTc interval is contraindicated).
No products indexed under this heading.

Atropine Sulfate (Potentiation of central nervous system depressant). Products include:
Donnatal 2929
Donnatal Extentabs 2930
Motofen Tablets 577
Prosed/DS Tablets 3268
Urised Tablets 2876

Bretylium Tosylate (Mesoridazine has been shown to prolong the QTc interval and has been associated with torsade de pointes type arrhythmias and sudden death; co-administration with other drugs that are known to prolong the QTc interval is contraindicated).
No products indexed under this heading.

Buprenorphine Hydrochloride (Potentiation of central nervous system depressant). Products include:
Buprenex Injectable 2918

Buspirone Hydrochloride (Potentiation of central nervous system depressant).
No products indexed under this heading.

Butabarbital (Potentiation of central nervous system depressant).
No products indexed under this heading.

Butalbital (Potentiation of central nervous system depressant). Products include:
Phrenilin 578
Sedapap Tablets 50 mg/650 mg ... 2225

Chlordiazepoxide (Potentiation of central nervous system depressant). Products include:
Limbitrol 1738

Chlordiazepoxide Hydrochloride (Potentiation of central nervous system depressant). Products include:
Librium Capsules 1736
Librium for Injection 1737

Chlorpromazine (Mesoridazine has been shown to prolong the QTc interval and has been associated with torsade de pointes type arrhythmias and sudden death; co-administration with other drugs that are known to prolong the QTc interval is contraindicated). Products include:
Thorazine Suppositories 1656

Chlorpromazine Hydrochloride (Mesoridazine has been shown to prolong the QTc interval and has been associated with torsade de pointes type arrhythmias and sudden death; co-administration with other drugs that are known to prolong the QTc interval is contraindicated). Products include:
Thorazine 1656

Chlorprothixene (Potentiation of central nervous system depressant).
No products indexed under this heading.

Chlorprothixene Hydrochloride (Potentiation of central nervous system depressant).
No products indexed under this heading.

Chlorprothixene Lactate (Potentiation of central nervous system depressant).
No products indexed under this heading.

Clomipramine Hydrochloride (Mesoridazine has been shown to prolong the QTc interval and has been associated with torsade de pointes type arrhythmias and sudden death; co-administration with other drugs that are known to prolong the QTc interval is contraindicated).
No products indexed under this heading.

Clorazepate Dipotassium (Potentiation of central nervous system depressant). Products include:
Tranxene 511

Clozapine (Potentiation of central nervous system depressant). Products include:
Clozaril Tablets 2319

Codeine Phosphate (Potentiation of central nervous system depressant). Products include:
Phenergan with Codeine Syrup 3557
Phenergan VC with Codeine Syrup .. 3561
Robitussin A-C Syrup 2942
Robitussin-DAC Syrup 2942
Ryna-C Liquid .... ▣ 768
Soma Compound w/Codeine Tablets 3355
Tussi-Organidin NR Liquid 3350
Tussi-Organidin-S NR Liquid 3350
Tylenol with Codeine 2595

Desflurane (Potentiation of central nervous system depressant). Products include:
Suprane Liquid for Inhalation 874

Desipramine Hydrochloride (Mesoridazine has been shown to prolong the QTc interval and has been associated with torsade de pointes type arrhythmias and sudden death; co-administration with other drugs that are known to prolong the QTc interval is contraindicated). Products include:
Norpramin Tablets 755

Dezocine (Potentiation of central nervous system depressant).
No products indexed under this heading.

Diazepam (Potentiation of central nervous system depressant). Products include:
Valium Injectable 3026
Valium Tablets 3047

Disopyramide Phosphate (Mesoridazine has been shown to prolong the QTc interval and has been associated with torsade de pointes type arrhythmias and sudden death; co-administration with other drugs that are known to prolong the QTc interval is contraindicated).
No products indexed under this heading.

Dofetilide (Mesoridazine has been shown to prolong the QTc interval and has been associated with torsade de pointes type arrhythmias and sudden death; co-administration with other drugs that are known to prolong the QTc interval is contraindicated). Products include:
Tikosyn Capsules 2717

Doxepin Hydrochloride (Mesoridazine has been shown to prolong the QTc interval and has been associated with torsade de pointes type arrhythmias and sudden death; co-administration with other drugs that are known to prolong the QTc interval is contraindicated). Products include:
Sinequan 2713

Droperidol (Potentiation of central nervous system depressant).
No products indexed under this heading.

Enflurane (Potentiation of central nervous system depressant).
No products indexed under this heading.

Estazolam (Potentiation of central nervous system depressant). Products include:
ProSom Tablets 500

Ethchlorvynol (Potentiation of central nervous system depressant).
No products indexed under this heading.

Ethinamate (Potentiation of central nervous system depressant).
No products indexed under this heading.

Fentanyl (Potentiation of central nervous system depressant). Products include:
Duragesic Transdermal System 1786

Fentanyl Citrate (Potentiation of central nervous system depressant). Products include:
Actiq 1184

Flecainide Acetate (Mesoridazine has been shown to prolong the QTc interval and has been associated with torsade de pointes type arrhythmias and sudden death; co-administration with other drugs that are known to prolong the QTc interval is contraindicated). Products include:
Tambocor Tablets 1990

Fluphenazine Decanoate (Mesoridazine has been shown to prolong the QTc interval and has been associated with torsade de pointes type arrhythmias and sudden death; co-administration with other drugs that are known to prolong the QTc interval is contraindicated).
No products indexed under this heading.

Fluphenazine Enanthate (Mesoridazine has been shown to prolong the QTc interval and has been associated with torsade de pointes type arrhythmias and sudden death; co-administration with other drugs that are known to prolong the

QTc interval is contraindicated).
No products indexed under this heading.

Fluphenazine Hydrochloride (Mesoridazine has been shown to prolong the QTc interval and has been associated with torsade de pointes type arrhythmias and sudden death; co-administration with other drugs that are known to prolong the QTc interval is contraindicated).
No products indexed under this heading.

Flurazepam Hydrochloride (Potentiation of central nervous system depressant).
No products indexed under this heading.

Glutethimide (Potentiation of central nervous system depressant).
No products indexed under this heading.

Haloperidol (Potentiation of central nervous system depressant).
Products include:
Haldol Injection, Tablets and Concentrate 2533

Haloperidol Decanoate (Potentiation of central nervous system depressant). Products include:
Haldol Decanoate 2535

Hydrocodone Bitartrate (Potentiation of central nervous system depressant). Products include:
Hycodan 1316
Hycomine Compound Tablets 1317
Hycotuss Expectorant Syrup 1318
Lortab 3319
Lortab Elixir 3317
Maxidone Tablets CIII 3399
Norco 5/325 Tablets CIII 3424
Norco 7.5/325 Tablets CIII 3425
Norco 10/325 Tablets CIII 3427
Norco 10/325 Tablets CIII 3425
Vicodin Tablets 516
Vicodin ES Tablets 517
Vicodin HP Tablets 518
Vicodin Tuss Expectorant 519
Vicoprofen Tablets 520
Zydone Tablets 1330

Hydrocodone Polistirex (Potentiation of central nervous system depressant). Products include:
Tussionex Pennkinetic Extended-Release Suspension 1174

Hydromorphone Hydrochloride (Potentiation of central nervous system depressant). Products include:
Dilaudid 441
Dilaudid Oral Liquid 445
Dilaudid Powder 441
Dilaudid Rectal Suppositories 441
Dilaudid Tablets 441
Dilaudid Tablets - 8 mg 445
Dilaudid-HP 443

Hydroxyzine Hydrochloride (Potentiation of central nervous system depressant). Products include:
Atarax Tablets & Syrup 2667
Vistaril Intramuscular Solution 2738

Imipramine Hydrochloride (Mesoridazine has been shown to prolong the QTc interval and has been associated with torsade de pointes type arrhythmias and sudden death; co-administration with other drugs that are known to prolong the QTc interval is contraindicated).
No products indexed under this heading.

Imipramine Pamoate (Mesoridazine has been shown to prolong the QTc interval and has been associated with torsade de pointes type arrhythmias and sudden death; co-administration with other drugs that are known to prolong the QTc interval is contraindicated).
No products indexed under this heading.

Isoflurane (Potentiation of central nervous system depressant).
No products indexed under this heading.

Ketamine Hydrochloride (Potentiation of central nervous system depressant).
No products indexed under this heading.

Levomethadyl Acetate Hydrochloride (Potentiation of central nervous system depressant).
No products indexed under this heading.

Levorphanol Tartrate (Potentiation of central nervous system depressant). Products include:
Levo-Dromoran 1734
Levorphanol Tartrate Tablets 3059

Lidocaine Hydrochloride (Mesoridazine has been shown to prolong the QTc interval and has been associated with torsade de pointes type arrhythmias and sudden death; co-administration with other drugs that are known to prolong the QTc interval is contraindicated).
Products include:
Bactine First Aid Liquid 611
Xylocaine Injections 653

Lorazepam (Potentiation of central nervous system depressant).
Products include:
Ativan Injection 3478
Ativan Tablets 3482

Loxapine Hydrochloride (Potentiation of central nervous system depressant).
No products indexed under this heading.

Loxapine Succinate (Potentiation of central nervous system depressant). Products include:
Loxitane Capsules 3398

Maprotiline Hydrochloride (Mesoridazine has been shown to prolong the QTc interval and has been associated with torsade de pointes type arrhythmias and sudden death; co-administration with other drugs that are known to prolong the QTc interval is contraindicated).
No products indexed under this heading.

Meperidine Hydrochloride (Potentiation of central nervous system depressant). Products include:
Demerol 3079
Mepergan Injection 3539

Mephobarbital (Potentiation of central nervous system depressant).
No products indexed under this heading.

Meprobamate (Potentiation of central nervous system depressant).
Products include:
Miltown Tablets 3349

Methadone Hydrochloride (Potentiation of central nervous system depressant). Products include:
Dolophine Hydrochloride Tablets 3056

Methohexital Sodium (Potentiation of central nervous system depressant). Products include:
Brevital Sodium for Injection, USP 1815

Methotrimeprazine (Potentiation of central nervous system depressant).
No products indexed under this heading.

Methoxyflurane (Potentiation of central nervous system depressant).
No products indexed under this heading.

Mexiletine Hydrochloride (Mesoridazine has been shown to prolong the QTc interval and has been associated with torsade de pointes type arrhythmias and sudden death; co-administration with other drugs that are known to prolong the QTc interval is contraindicated).
Products include:
Mexitil Capsules 1047

Midazolam Hydrochloride (Potentiation of central nervous system depressant). Products include:
Versed Injection 3027
Versed Syrup 3033

Molindone Hydrochloride (Potentiation of central nervous system depressant). Products include:
Moban 1320

Morphine Sulfate (Potentiation of central nervous system depressant).
Products include:
Astramorph/PF Injection, USP (Preservative-Free) 594
Duramorph Injection 1312
Infumorph 200 and Infumorph 500 Sterile Solutions 1314
Kadian Capsules 1335
MS Contin Tablets 2896
MSIR 2898
Oramorph SR Tablets 3062
Roxanol 3066

Nortriptyline Hydrochloride (Mesoridazine has been shown to prolong the QTc interval and has been associated with torsade de pointes type arrhythmias and sudden death; co-administration with other drugs that are known to prolong the QTc interval is contraindicated).
No products indexed under this heading.

Olanzapine (Potentiation of central nervous system depressant).
Products include:
Zyprexa Tablets 1973
Zyprexa ZYDIS Orally Disintegrating Tablets 1973

Oxazepam (Potentiation of central nervous system depressant).
No products indexed under this heading.

Oxycodone Hydrochloride (Potentiation of central nervous system depressant). Products include:
OxyContin Tablets 2912
OxyFast Oral Concentrate Solution 2916
OxyIR Capsules 2916
Percocet Tablets 1326
Percodan Tablets 1327
Percolone Tablets 1327
Roxicodone 3067
Tylox Capsules 2597

Pentobarbital Sodium (Potentiation of central nervous system depressant). Products include:
Nembutal Sodium Solution 485

Perphenazine (Mesoridazine has been shown to prolong the QTc interval and has been associated with torsade de pointes type arrhythmias and sudden death; co-administration with other drugs that are known to prolong the QTc interval is contraindicated). Products include:
Etrafon 3115
Trilafon 3160

Phenobarbital (Potentiation of central nervous system depressant).
Products include:
Arco-Lase Plus Tablets 592
Donnatal 2929
Donnatal Extentabs 2930

Prazepam (Potentiation of central nervous system depressant).
No products indexed under this heading.

Procainamide Hydrochloride (Mesoridazine has been shown to prolong the QTc interval and has been associated with torsade de pointes type arrhythmias and sudden death; co-administration with other drugs that are known to prolong the QTc interval is contraindicated).
Products include:
Procanbid Extended-Release Tablets 2262

Prochlorperazine (Mesoridazine has been shown to prolong the QTc interval and has been associated with torsade de pointes type arrhythmias and sudden death; co-administration with other drugs that are known to prolong the QTc interval is contraindicated). Products include:
Compazine 1505

Promethazine Hydrochloride (Mesoridazine has been shown to prolong the QTc interval and has been associated with torsade de pointes type arrhythmias and sudden death; co-administration with other drugs that are known to prolong the QTc interval is contraindicated).
Products include:
Mepergan Injection 3539
Phenergan Injection 3553
Phenergan 3556
Phenergan Syrup 3554
Phenergan with Codeine Syrup 3557
Phenergan with Dextromethorphan Syrup 3559
Phenergan VC Syrup 3560
Phenergan VC with Codeine Syrup 3561

Propafenone Hydrochloride (Mesoridazine has been shown to prolong the QTc interval and has been associated with torsade de pointes type arrhythmias and sudden death; co-administration with other drugs that are known to prolong the QTc interval is contraindicated).
Products include:
Rythmol Tablets – 150 mg, 225 mg, 300 mg 502

Propofol (Potentiation of central nervous system depressant).
Products include:
Diprivan Injectable Emulsion 667

Propoxyphene Hydrochloride (Potentiation of central nervous system depressant). Products include:
Darvon Pulvules 1909
Darvon Compound-65 Pulvules 1910

Propoxyphene Napsylate (Potentiation of central nervous system depressant). Products include:
Darvon-N/Darvocet-N 1907
Darvon-N Tablets 1912

Protriptyline Hydrochloride (Mesoridazine has been shown to prolong the QTc interval and has been associated with torsade de pointes type arrhythmias and sudden death; co-administration with other drugs that are known to prolong the QTc interval is contraindicated).
Products include:
Vivactil Tablets 2446
Vivactil Tablets 2217

Quazepam (Potentiation of central nervous system depressant).
No products indexed under this heading.

Quetiapine Fumarate (Potentiation of central nervous system depressant). Products include:
Seroquel Tablets 684

Quinidine Gluconate (Mesoridazine has been shown to prolong the QTc interval and has been associated with torsade de pointes type arrhythmias and sudden death; co-administration with other drugs that are known to prolong the QTc interval is contraindicated).
Products include:
Quinaglute Dura-Tabs Tablets 978

Quinidine Polygalacturonate (Mesoridazine has been shown to prolong the QTc interval and has been associated with torsade de pointes type arrhythmias and sudden death; co-administration with other drugs that are known to prolong the QTc interval is contraindicated).
No products indexed under this heading.

Quinidine Sulfate (Mesoridazine has been shown to prolong the QTc interval and has been associated with torsade de pointes type arrhythmias and sudden death; co-administration with other drugs that are known to prolong the QTc interval is contraindicated). Products include:
Quinidex Extentabs 2933

Remifentanil Hydrochloride (Potentiation of central nervous system depressant).
No products indexed under this heading.

IMPORTANT NOTE: Always consult each drug listing in the patient's regimen for possible interactions.

Risperidone (Potentiation of central nervous system depressant). Products include:
Risperdal 1796

Secobarbital Sodium (Potentiation of central nervous system depressant).
No products indexed under this heading.

Sevoflurane (Potentiation of central nervous system depressant).
No products indexed under this heading.

Sufentanil Citrate (Potentiation of central nervous system depressant).
No products indexed under this heading.

Temazepam (Potentiation of central nervous system depressant).
No products indexed under this heading.

Terfenadine (Mesoridazine has been shown to prolong the QTc interval and has been associated with torsade de pointes type arrhythmias and sudden death; co-administration with other drugs that are known to prolong the QTc interval is contraindicated).
No products indexed under this heading.

Thiamylal Sodium (Potentiation of central nervous system depressant).
No products indexed under this heading.

Thioridazine Hydrochloride (Mesoridazine has been shown to prolong the QTc interval and has been associated with torsade de pointes type arrhythmias and sudden death; co-administration with other drugs that are known to prolong the QTc interval is contraindicated). Products include:
Thioridazine Hydrochloride Tablets 2289

Thiothixene (Potentiation of central nervous system depressant). Products include:
Navane Capsules 2701
Thiothixene Capsules 2290

Tocainide Hydrochloride (Mesoridazine has been shown to prolong the QTc interval and has been associated with torsade de pointes type arrhythmias and sudden death; co-administration with other drugs that are known to prolong the QTc interval is contraindicated). Products include:
Tonocard Tablets 649

Triazolam (Potentiation of central nervous system depressant). Products include:
Halcion Tablets 2823

Trifluoperazine Hydrochloride (Mesoridazine has been shown to prolong the QTc interval and has been associated with torsade de pointes type arrhythmias and sudden death; co-administration with other drugs that are known to prolong the QTc interval is contraindicated). Products include:
Stelazine 1640

Trimipramine Maleate (Mesoridazine has been shown to prolong the QTc interval and has been associated with torsade de pointes type arrhythmias and sudden death; co-administration with other drugs that are known to prolong the QTc interval is contraindicated). Products include:
Surmontil Capsules 3595

Zaleplon (Potentiation of central nervous system depressant). Products include:
Sonata Capsules 3591

Ziprasidone Hydrochloride (Mesoridazine has been shown to prolong the QTc interval and has been associated with torsade de pointes type arrhythmias and sudden death; co-administration with other drugs that are known to prolong the QTc interval is contraindicated). Products include:
Geodon Capsules 2688

Zolpidem Tartrate (Potentiation of central nervous system depressant). Products include:
Ambien Tablets 3191

Food Interactions

Alcohol (Potentiation of central nervous system depressant).

SERENTIL CONCENTRATE
(Mesoridazine Besylate) 1057
See Serentil Ampuls

SERENTIL TABLETS
(Mesoridazine Besylate) 1057
See Serentil Ampuls

SEREVENT DISKUS
(Salmeterol Xinafoate) 1637
See Serevent Inhalation Aerosol

SEREVENT INHALATION AEROSOL
(Salmeterol Xinafoate) 1633
May interact with beta blockers, monoamine oxidase inhibitors, non-potassium-sparing diuretics, and tricyclic antidepressants. Compounds in these categories include:

Acebutolol Hydrochloride (Beta-adrenergic blockers may produce severe bronchospasm in asthmatic patients, however, beta blockers do not block the pulmonary effect of beta-agonists). Products include:
Sectral Capsules 3589

Amitriptyline Hydrochloride (The action of salmeterol on the vascular system may be potentiated by tricyclic antidepressant). Products include:
Etrafon 3115
Limbitrol 1738

Amoxapine (The action of salmeterol on the vascular system may be potentiated by tricyclic antidepressant).
No products indexed under this heading.

Atenolol (Beta-adrenergic blockers may produce severe bronchospasm in asthmatic patients, however, beta blockers do not block the pulmonary effect of beta-agonists). Products include:
Tenoretic Tablets 690
Tenormin I.V. Injection 692

Bendroflumethiazide (The ECG changes and/or hypokalemia that may result from the administration of nonpotassium-sparing diuretics can be acutely worsened by beta-agonists, especially when the recommended dose of beta-agonist is exceeded). Products include:
Corzide 40/5 Tablets 2247
Corzide 80/5 Tablets 2247

Betaxolol Hydrochloride (Beta-adrenergic blockers may produce severe bronchospasm in asthmatic patients, however, beta blockers do not block the pulmonary effect of beta-agonists). Products include:
Betoptic S Ophthalmic Suspension 537

Bisoprolol Fumarate (Beta-adrenergic blockers may produce severe bronchospasm in asthmatic patients, however, beta blockers do not block the pulmonary effect of beta-agonists). Products include:
Zebeta Tablets 1885
Ziac Tablets 1887

Bumetanide (The ECG changes and/or hypokalemia that may result from the administration of nonpotassium-sparing diuretics can be acutely worsened by beta-agonists, especially when the recommended dose of beta-agonist is exceeded).
No products indexed under this heading.

Carteolol Hydrochloride (Beta-adrenergic blockers may produce severe bronchospasm in asthmatic patients, however, beta blockers do not block the pulmonary effect of beta-agonists). Products include:
Carteolol Hydrochloride Ophthalmic Solution USP, 1% .... ⊙258
Ocupress Ophthalmic Solution, 1% Sterile .... ⊙303

Chlorothiazide (The ECG changes and/or hypokalemia that may result from the administration of nonpotassium-sparing diuretics can be acutely worsened by beta-agonists, especially when the recommended dose of beta-agonist is exceeded). Products include:
Aldoclor Tablets 2035
Diuril Oral 2087

Chlorothiazide Sodium (The ECG changes and/or hypokalemia that may result from the administration of nonpotassium-sparing diuretics can be acutely worsened by beta-agonists, especially when the recommended dose of beta-agonist is exceeded). Products include:
Diuril Sodium Intravenous 2086

Clomipramine Hydrochloride (The action of salmeterol on the vascular system may be potentiated by tricyclic antidepressant).
No products indexed under this heading.

Desipramine Hydrochloride (The action of salmeterol on the vascular system may be potentiated by tricyclic antidepressant). Products include:
Norpramin Tablets 755

Doxepin Hydrochloride (The action of salmeterol on the vascular system may be potentiated by tricyclic antidepressant). Products include:
Sinequan 2713

Esmolol Hydrochloride (Beta-adrenergic blockers may produce severe bronchospasm in asthmatic patients, however, beta blockers do not block the pulmonary effect of beta-agonists). Products include:
Brevibloc Injection 858

Ethacrynic Acid (The ECG changes and/or hypokalemia that may result from the administration of nonpotassium-sparing diuretics can be acutely worsened by beta-agonists, especially when the recommended dose of beta-agonist is exceeded). Products include:
Edecrin Tablets 2091

Furosemide (The ECG changes and/or hypokalemia that may result from the administration of nonpotassium-sparing diuretics can be acutely worsened by beta-agonists, especially when the recommended dose of beta-agonist is exceeded). Products include:
Furosemide Tablets 2284

Hydrochlorothiazide (The ECG changes and/or hypokalemia that may result from the administration of nonpotassium-sparing diuretics can be acutely worsened by beta-agonists, especially when the recommended dose of beta-agonist is exceeded). Products include:
Accuretic Tablets 2614
Aldoril Tablets 2039
Atacand HCT Tablets 597
Avalide Tablets 1070
Diovan HCT Tablets 2338
Dyazide Capsules 1515
HydroDIURIL Tablets 2108
Hyzaar 2109
Inderide Tablets 3517
Inderide LA Long-Acting Capsules 3519
Lotensin HCT Tablets 2367
Maxzide 1008
Micardis HCT Tablets 1051
Microzide Capsules 3414
Moduretic Tablets 2138
Monopril HCT 1094
Prinzide Tablets 2168
Timolide Tablets 2187
Uniretic Tablets 3178
Vaseretic Tablets 2204
Zestoretic Tablets 695
Ziac Tablets 1887

Hydroflumethiazide (The ECG changes and/or hypokalemia that may result from the administration of nonpotassium-sparing diuretics can be acutely worsened by beta-agonists, especially when the recommended dose of beta-agonist is exceeded). Products include:
Diucardin Tablets 3494

Imipramine Hydrochloride (The action of salmeterol on the vascular system may be potentiated by tricyclic antidepressant).
No products indexed under this heading.

Imipramine Pamoate (The action of salmeterol on the vascular system may be potentiated by tricyclic antidepressant).
No products indexed under this heading.

Isocarboxazid (The action of salmeterol on the vascular system may be potentiated by MAO inhibitor).
No products indexed under this heading.

Labetalol Hydrochloride (Beta-adrenergic blockers may produce severe bronchospasm in asthmatic patients, however, beta blockers do not block the pulmonary effect of beta-agonists). Products include:
Normodyne Injection 3135
Normodyne Tablets 3137

Levobunolol Hydrochloride (Beta-adrenergic blockers may produce severe bronchospasm in asthmatic patients, however, beta blockers do not block the pulmonary effect of beta-agonists). Products include:
Betagan .... ⊙228

Maprotiline Hydrochloride (The action of salmeterol on the vascular system may be potentiated by tricyclic antidepressant).
No products indexed under this heading.

Methyclothiazide (The ECG changes and/or hypokalemia that may result from the administration of nonpotassium-sparing diuretics can be acutely worsened by beta-agonists, especially when the recommended dose of beta-agonist is exceeded).
No products indexed under this heading

Metipranolol Hydrochloride (Beta-adrenergic blockers may produce severe bronchospasm in asthmatic patients, however, beta blockers do not block the pulmonary effect of beta-agonists).
No products indexed under this heading.

Metoprolol Succinate (Beta-adrenergic blockers may produce severe bronchospasm in asthmatic patients, however, beta blockers do not block the pulmonary effect of beta-agonists). Products include:
Toprol-XL Tablets 651

Metoprolol Tartrate (Beta-adrenergic blockers may produce severe bronchospasm in asthmatic patients, however, beta blockers do not block the pulmonary effect of beta-agonists).
No products indexed under this heading.

Moclobemide (The action of salmeterol on the vascular system may be

potentiated by MAO inhibitor).
No products indexed under this heading.

Nadolol (Beta-adrenergic blockers may produce severe bronchospasm in asthmatic patients, however, beta blockers do not block the pulmonary effect of beta-agonists). Products include:
Corgard Tablets 2245
Corzide 40/5 Tablets 2247
Corzide 80/5 Tablets 2247
Nadolol Tablets 2288

Nortriptyline Hydrochloride (The action of salmeterol on the vascular system may be potentiated by tricyclic antidepressant).
No products indexed under this heading.

Pargyline Hydrochloride (The action of salmeterol on the vascular system may be potentiated by MAO inhibitor).
No products indexed under this heading.

Penbutolol Sulfate (Beta-adrenergic blockers may produce severe bronchospasm in asthmatic patients, however, beta blockers do not block the pulmonary effect of beta-agonists).
No products indexed under this heading.

Phenelzine Sulfate (The action of salmeterol on the vascular system may be potentiated by MAO inhibitor). Products include:
Nardil Tablets 2653

Pindolol (Beta-adrenergic blockers may produce severe bronchospasm in asthmatic patients, however, beta blockers do not block the pulmonary effect of beta-agonists).
No products indexed under this heading.

Polythiazide (The ECG changes and/or hypokalemia that may result from the administration of nonpotassium-sparing diuretics can be acutely worsened by beta-agonists, especially when the recommended dose of beta-agonist is exceeded). Products include:
Minizide Capsules 2700
Renese Tablets 2712

Procarbazine Hydrochloride (The action of salmeterol on the vascular system may be potentiated by MAO inhibitor). Products include:
Matulane Capsules 3246

Propranolol Hydrochloride (Beta-adrenergic blockers may produce severe bronchospasm in asthmatic patients, however, beta blockers do not block the pulmonary effect of beta-agonists). Products include:
Inderal 3513
Inderal LA Long-Acting Capsules 3516
Inderide Tablets 3517
Inderide LA Long-Acting Capsules .. 3519

Protriptyline Hydrochloride (The action of salmeterol on the vascular system may be potentiated by tricyclic antidepressant). Products include:
Vivactil Tablets 2446
Vivactil Tablets 2217

Selegiline Hydrochloride (The action of salmeterol on the vascular system may be potentiated by MAO inhibitor). Products include:
Eldepryl Capsules 3266

Sotalol Hydrochloride (Beta-adrenergic blockers may produce severe bronchospasm in asthmatic patients, however, beta blockers do not block the pulmonary effect of beta-agonists). Products include:
Betapace Tablets 950
Betapace AF Tablets 954

Timolol Hemihydrate (Beta-adrenergic blockers may produce severe bronchospasm in asthmatic patients, however, beta blockers do not block the pulmonary effect of beta-agonists). Products include:
Betimol Ophthalmic Solution .... ⊙ 324

Timolol Maleate (Beta-adrenergic blockers may produce severe bronchospasm in asthmatic patients, however, beta blockers do not block the pulmonary effect of beta-agonists). Products include:
Blocadren Tablets 2046
Cosopt Sterile Ophthalmic Solution 2065
Timolide Tablets 2187
Timolol GFS .... ⊙ 266
Timoptic in Ocudose 2192
Timoptic Sterile Ophthalmic Solution 2190
Timoptic-XE Sterile Ophthalmic Gel Forming Solution 2194

Torsemide (The ECG changes and/or hypokalemia that may result from the administration of nonpotassium-sparing diuretics can be acutely worsened by beta-agonists, especially when the recommended dose of beta-agonist is exceeded). Products include:
Demadex Tablets and Injection 2965

Tranylcypromine Sulfate (The action of salmeterol on the vascular system may be potentiated by MAO inhibitor). Products include:
Parnate Tablets 1607

Trimipramine Maleate (The action of salmeterol on the vascular system may be potentiated by tricyclic antidepressant). Products include:
Surmontil Capsules 3595

SEROPHENE TABLETS

(Clomiphene Citrate) 3226
None cited in PDR database.

SEROQUEL TABLETS

(Quetiapine Fumarate) 684
May interact with antihypertensives, barbiturates, dopamine agonists, erythromycin, glucocorticoids, phenytoin, and certain other agents. Compounds in these categories include:

Acebutolol Hydrochloride (Enhanced effects of certain antihypertensive agents). Products include:
Sectral Capsules 3589

Amlodipine Besylate (Enhanced effects of certain antihypertensive agents). Products include:
Lotrel Capsules 2370
Norvasc Tablets 2704

Aprobarbital (Co-administration with hepatic enzyme inducers, such as barbiturates, may increase oral clearance).
No products indexed under this heading.

Atenolol (Enhanced effects of certain antihypertensive agents). Products include:
Tenoretic Tablets 690
Tenormin I.V. Injection 692

Benazepril Hydrochloride (Enhanced effects of certain antihypertensive agents). Products include:
Lotensin Tablets 2365
Lotensin HCT Tablets 2367
Lotrel Capsules 2370

Bendroflumethiazide (Enhanced effects of certain antihypertensive agents). Products include:
Corzide 40/5 Tablets 2247
Corzide 80/5 Tablets 2247

Betamethasone Acetate (Co-administration with hepatic enzyme inducers, such as glucocorticosteroids, may increase oral clearance). Products include:
Celestone Soluspan Injectable Suspension 3097

Betamethasone Sodium Phosphate (Co-administration with hepatic enzyme inducers, such as glucocorticosteroids, may increase oral clearance). Products include:
Celestone Soluspan Injectable Suspension 3097

Betaxolol Hydrochloride (Enhanced effects of certain antihypertensive agents). Products include:
Betoptic S Ophthalmic Suspension 537

Bisoprolol Fumarate (Enhanced effects of certain antihypertensive agents). Products include:
Zebeta Tablets 1885
Ziac Tablets 1887

Bromocriptine Mesylate (Quetiapine may antagonize the effects of dopamine agonists).
No products indexed under this heading.

Butabarbital (Co-administration with hepatic enzyme inducers, such as barbiturates, may increase oral clearance).
No products indexed under this heading.

Butalbital (Co-administration with hepatic enzyme inducers, such as barbiturates, may increase oral clearance). Products include:
Phrenilin 578
Sedapap Tablets 50 mg/650 mg ... 2225

Candesartan Cilexetil (Enhanced effects of certain antihypertensive agents). Products include:
Atacand Tablets 595
Atacand HCT Tablets 597

Captopril (Enhanced effects of certain antihypertensive agents). Products include:
Captopril Tablets 2281

Carbamazepine (Co-administration with hepatic enzyme inducers, such as carbamazepine, may increase oral clearance). Products include:
Carbatrol Capsules 3234
Tegretol/Tegretol-XR 2404

Carteolol Hydrochloride (Enhanced effects of certain antihypertensive agents). Products include:
Carteolol Hydrochloride Ophthalmic Solution USP, 1%..... ⊙ 258
Ocupress Ophthalmic Solution, 1% Sterile .... ⊙ 303

Chlorothiazide (Enhanced effects of certain antihypertensive agents). Products include:
Aldoclor Tablets 2035
Diuril Oral 2087

Chlorothiazide Sodium (Enhanced effects of certain antihypertensive agents). Products include:
Diuril Sodium Intravenous 2086

Chlorthalidone (Enhanced effects of certain antihypertensive agents). Products include:
Clorpres Tablets 1002
Combipres Tablets 1040
Tenoretic Tablets 690

Cimetidine (Co-administration has resulted in a 20% decrease in the mean oral clearance of quetiapine). Products include:
Tagamet HB 200 Suspension 762
Tagamet HB 200 Tablets 761
Tagamet Tablets 1644

Clonidine (Enhanced effects of certain antihypertensive agents). Products include:
Catapres-TTS 1038

Clonidine Hydrochloride (Enhanced effects of certain antihypertensive agents). Products include:
Catapres Tablets 1037
Clorpres Tablets 1002
Combipres Tablets 1040
Duraclon Injection 3057

Cortisone Acetate (Co-administration with hepatic enzyme inducers, such as glucocorticosteroids, may increase oral clearance). Products include:
Cortone Acetate Injectable Suspension 2059
Cortone Acetate Tablets 2061

Deserpidine (Enhanced effects of certain antihypertensive agents).
No products indexed under this heading.

Dexamethasone (Co-administration with hepatic enzyme inducers, such as glucocorticosteroids, may increase oral clearance). Products include:
Decadron Elixir 2078
Decadron Tablets 2079
TobraDex Ophthalmic Ointment 542
TobraDex Ophthalmic Suspension .. 541

Dexamethasone Acetate (Co-administration with hepatic enzyme inducers, such as glucocorticosteroids, may increase oral clearance).
No products indexed under this heading.

Dexamethasone Sodium Phosphate (Co-administration with hepatic enzyme inducers, such as glucocorticosteroids, may increase oral clearance). Products include:
Decadron Phosphate Injection 2081
Decadron Phosphate Sterile Ophthalmic Ointment 2083
Decadron Phosphate Sterile Ophthalmic Solution 2084
NeoDecadron Sterile Ophthalmic Solution 2144

Diazoxide (Enhanced effects of certain antihypertensive agents).
No products indexed under this heading.

Diltiazem Hydrochloride (Enhanced effects of certain antihypertensive agents). Products include:
Cardizem Injectable 1018
Cardizem Lyo-Ject Syringe 1018
Cardizem Monovial 1018
Cardizem CD Capsules 1016
Tiazac Capsules 1378

Dopamine Hydrochloride (Quetiapine may antagonize the effects of dopamine agonists).
No products indexed under this heading.

Doxazosin Mesylate (Enhanced effects of certain antihypertensive agents). Products include:
Cardura Tablets 2668

Enalapril Maleate (Enhanced effects of certain antihypertensive agents). Products include:
Lexxel Tablets 608
Vaseretic Tablets 2204
Vasotec Tablets 2210

Enalaprilat (Enhanced effects of certain antihypertensive agents). Products include:
Enalaprilat Injection 863
Vasotec I.V. Injection 2207

Eprosartan Mesylate (Enhanced effects of certain antihypertensive agents). Products include:
Teveten Tablets 3327

Erythromycin (Co-administration of erythromycin, an inhibitor of CYP4503A, may reduce oral clearance of quetiapine, resulting in an increase in maximum plasma concentration of quetiapine; dose adjustment of quetiapine will be necessary if it is used with erythromycin). Products include:
Emgel 2% Topical Gel 1285
Ery-Tab Tablets 448
Erythromycin Base Filmtab Tablets . 454
Erythromycin Delayed-Release Capsules, USP 455
PCE Dispertab Tablets 498

Erythromycin Estolate (Co-administration of erythromycin, an inhibitor of CYP4503A, may reduce oral clearance of quetiapine, resulting in an increase in maximum plasma concentration of quetiapine; dose adjustment of quetiapine will be necessary if it is used with erythromycin).
No products indexed under this heading.

Erythromycin Ethylsuccinate (Co-administration of erythromycin, an inhibitor of CYP4503A, may reduce oral clearance of quetiapine, resulting in an increase in maximum plasma concentration of quetiapine; dose adjustment of quetiapine will be necessary if it is used with erythromycin). Products include:

E.E.S. ... 450
EryPed ... 446
Pediazole Suspension ... 3050

Erythromycin Gluceptate (Co-administration of erythromycin, an inhibitor of CYP4503A, may reduce oral clearance of quetiapine, resulting in an increase in maximum plasma concentration of quetiapine; dose adjustment of quetiapine will be necessary if it is used with erythromycin).
No products indexed under this heading.

Erythromycin Stearate (Co-administration of erythromycin, an inhibitor of CYP4503A, may reduce oral clearance of quetiapine, resulting in an increase in maximum plasma concentration of quetiapine; dose adjustment of quetiapine will be necessary if it is used with erythromycin). Products include:
Erythrocin Stearate Filmtab Tablets ... 452

Esmolol Hydrochloride (Enhanced effects of certain antihypertensive agents). Products include:
Brevibloc Injection ... 858

Felodipine (Enhanced effects of certain antihypertensive agents). Products include:
Lexxel Tablets ... 608
Plendil Extended-Release Tablets ... 623

Fluconazole (Co-administration of fluconazole, an inhibitor of CYP4503A, may reduce oral clearance of quetiapine, resulting in an increase in maximum plasma concentration of quetiapine; dose adjustment of quetiapine will be necessary if it is used with fluconazole). Products include:
Diflucan Tablets, Injection, and Oral Suspension ... 2681

Fludrocortisone Acetate (Co-administration with hepatic enzyme inducers, such as glucocorticosteroids, may increase oral clearance). Products include:
Florinef Acetate Tablets ... 2250

Fosinopril Sodium (Enhanced effects of certain antihypertensive agents). Products include:
Monopril Tablets ... 1091
Monopril HCT ... 1094

Fosphenytoin Sodium (Co-administration has resulted in increased mean oral clearance of quetiapine by 5-fold; increased dose of quetiapine may be required). Products include:
Cerebyx Injection ... 2619

Furosemide (Enhanced effects of certain antihypertensive agents). Products include:
Furosemide Tablets ... 2284

Guanabenz Acetate (Enhanced effects of certain antihypertensive agents).
No products indexed under this heading.

Guanethidine Monosulfate (Enhanced effects of certain antihypertensive agents).
No products indexed under this heading.

Hydralazine Hydrochloride (Enhanced effects of certain antihypertensive agents).
No products indexed under this heading.

Hydrochlorothiazide (Enhanced effects of certain antihypertensive agents). Products include:
Accuretic Tablets ... 2614
Aldoril Tablets ... 2039
Atacand HCT Tablets ... 597
Avalide Tablets ... 1070
Diovan HCT Tablets ... 2338
Dyazide Capsules ... 1515
HydroDIURIL Tablets ... 2108
Hyzaar ... 2109
Inderide Tablets ... 3517
Inderide LA Long-Acting Capsules ... 3519
Lotensin HCT Tablets ... 2367
Maxzide ... 1008
Micardis HCT Tablets ... 1051
Microzide Capsules ... 3414
Moduretic Tablets ... 2138
Monopril HCT ... 1094
Prinzide Tablets ... 2168
Timolide Tablets ... 2187
Uniretic Tablets ... 3178
Vaseretic Tablets ... 2204
Zestoretic Tablets ... 695
Ziac Tablets ... 1887

Hydrocortisone (Co-administration with hepatic enzyme inducers, such as glucocorticosteroids, may increase oral clearance). Products include:
Anusol-HC Cream 2.5% ... 2237
Cipro HC Otic Suspension ... 540
Cortaid Intensive Therapy Cream ... ■717
Cortaid Maximum Strength Cream ... ■717
Cortisporin Ophthalmic Suspension Sterile ... ⊙297
Cortizone•5 ... ■699
Cortizone•10 ... ■699
Cortizone•10 Plus Creme ... ■700
Cortizone for Kids Creme ... ■699
Hydrocortone Tablets ... 2106
Massengill Medicated Soft Cloth Towelette ... ■753
VōSoL HC Otic Solution ... 3356

Hydrocortisone Acetate (Co-administration with hepatic enzyme inducers, such as glucocorticosteroids, may increase oral clearance). Products include:
Analpram-HC ... 1338
Anusol HC-1 Hydrocortisone Anti-Itch Cream ... ■689
Anusol-HC Suppositories ... 2238
Cortaid ... ■717
Cortifoam Rectal Foam ... 3170
Cortisporin-TC Otic Suspension ... 2246
Hydrocortone Acetate Injectable Suspension ... 2103
Pramosone ... 1343
Proctocort Suppositories ... 2264
ProctoFoam-HC ... 3177
Terra-Cortril Ophthalmic Suspension ... 2716

Hydrocortisone Sodium Phosphate (Co-administration with hepatic enzyme inducers, such as glucocorticosteroids, may increase oral clearance). Products include:
Hydrocortone Phosphate Injection, Sterile ... 2105

Hydrocortisone Sodium Succinate (Co-administration with hepatic enzyme inducers, such as glucocorticosteroids, may increase oral clearance).
No products indexed under this heading.

Hydroflumethiazide (Enhanced effects of certain antihypertensive agents). Products include:
Diucardin Tablets ... 3494

Indapamide (Enhanced effects of certain antihypertensive agents). Products include:
Indapamide Tablets ... 2286

Irbesartan (Enhanced effects of certain antihypertensive agents). Products include:
Avalide Tablets ... 1070
Avapro Tablets ... 1074
Avapro Tablets ... 3076

Isradipine (Enhanced effects of certain antihypertensive agents). Products include:
DynaCirc Capsules ... 2921
DynaCirc CR Tablets ... 2923

Itraconazole (Co-administration of itraconazole, an inhibitor of CYP4503A, may reduce oral clearance of quetiapine, resulting in an increase in maximum plasma concentration of quetiapine; dose adjustment of quetiapine will be necessary if it is used with itraconazole). Products include:
Sporanox Capsules ... 1800
Sporanox Injection ... 1804
Sporanox Injection ... 2509
Sporanox Oral Solution ... 1808
Sporanox Oral Solution ... 2512

Ketoconazole (Co-administration of ketoconazole, a potent inhibitor of CYP4503A, reduced oral clearance of quetiapine by 84%, resulting in a 335% increase in maximum plasma concentration of quetiapine; dose adjustment of quetiapine will be necessary if it is used with ketoconazole). Products include:
Nizoral 2% Cream ... 3620
Nizoral A-D Shampoo ... 2008
Nizoral 2% Shampoo ... 2007
Nizoral Tablets ... 1791

Labetalol Hydrochloride (Enhanced effects of certain antihypertensive agents). Products include:
Normodyne Injection ... 3135
Normodyne Tablets ... 3137

Levodopa (Quetiapine may antagonize the effects of levodopa). Products include:
Sinemet Tablets ... 1253
Sinemet CR Tablets ... 1255

Lisinopril (Enhanced effects of certain antihypertensive agents). Products include:
Prinivil Tablets ... 2164
Prinzide Tablets ... 2168
Zestoretic Tablets ... 695
Zestril Tablets ... 698

Lorazepam (Co-administration has resulted in reduced mean oral clearance of lorazepam). Products include:
Ativan Injection ... 3478
Ativan Tablets ... 3482

Losartan Potassium (Enhanced effects of certain antihypertensive agents). Products include:
Cozaar Tablets ... 2067
Hyzaar ... 2109

Mecamylamine Hydrochloride (Enhanced effects of certain antihypertensive agents). Products include:
Inversine Tablets ... 1850

Mephobarbital (Co-administration with hepatic enzyme inducers, such as barbiturates, may increase oral clearance).
No products indexed under this heading.

Methyclothiazide (Enhanced effects of certain antihypertensive agents).
No products indexed under this heading.

Methyldopa (Enhanced effects of certain antihypertensive agents). Products include:
Aldoclor Tablets ... 2035
Aldomet Tablets ... 2037
Aldoril Tablets ... 2039

Methyldopate Hydrochloride (Enhanced effects of certain antihypertensive agents).
No products indexed under this heading.

Methylprednisolone Acetate (Co-administration with hepatic enzyme inducers, such as glucocorticosteroids, may increase oral clearance). Products include:
Depo-Medrol Injectable Suspension ... 2795

Methylprednisolone Sodium Succinate (Co-administration with hepatic enzyme inducers, such as glucocorticosteroids, may increase oral clearance). Products include:
Solu-Medrol Sterile Powder ... 2855

Metolazone (Enhanced effects of certain antihypertensive agents). Products include:
Mykrox Tablets ... 1168
Zaroxolyn Tablets ... 1177

Metoprolol Succinate (Enhanced effects of certain antihypertensive agents). Products include:
Toprol-XL Tablets ... 651

Metoprolol Tartrate (Enhanced effects of certain antihypertensive agents).
No products indexed under this heading.

Metyrosine (Enhanced effects of certain antihypertensive agents). Products include:
Demser Capsules ... 2085

Mibefradil Dihydrochloride (Enhanced effects of certain antihypertensive agents).
No products indexed under this heading.

Minoxidil (Enhanced effects of certain antihypertensive agents). Products include:
Rogaine Extra Strength for Men Topical Solution ... ■721
Rogaine for Women Topical Solution ... ■721

Moexipril Hydrochloride (Enhanced effects of certain antihypertensive agents). Products include:
Uniretic Tablets ... 3178
Univasc Tablets ... 3181

Nadolol (Enhanced effects of certain antihypertensive agents). Products include:
Corgard Tablets ... 2245
Corzide 40/5 Tablets ... 2247
Corzide 80/5 Tablets ... 2247
Nadolol Tablets ... 2288

Nicardipine Hydrochloride (Enhanced effects of certain antihypertensive agents). Products include:
Cardene I.V. ... 3485

Nifedipine (Enhanced effects of certain antihypertensive agents). Products include:
Adalat CC Tablets ... 877
Procardia Capsules ... 2708
Procardia XL Extended Release Tablets ... 2710

Nisoldipine (Enhanced effects of certain antihypertensive agents). Products include:
Sular Tablets ... 688

Nitroglycerin (Enhanced effects of certain antihypertensive agents). Products include:
Nitro-Dur Transdermal Infusion System ... 3134
Nitro-Dur Transdermal Infusion System ... 1834
Nitrolingual Pumpspray ... 1355
Nitrostat Tablets ... 2658

Penbutolol Sulfate (Enhanced effects of certain antihypertensive agents).
No products indexed under this heading.

Pentobarbital Sodium (Co-administration with hepatic enzyme inducers, such as barbiturates, may increase oral clearance). Products include:
Nembutal Sodium Solution ... 485

Pergolide Mesylate (Quetiapine may antagonize the effects of dopamine agonists). Products include:
Permax Tablets ... 1299

Perindopril Erbumine (Enhanced effects of certain antihypertensive agents). Products include:
Aceon Tablets (2 mg, 4 mg, 8 mg) ... 3249

Phenobarbital (Co-administration with hepatic enzyme inducers, such as barbiturates, may increase oral clearance). Products include:
Arco-Lase Plus Tablets ... 592
Donnatal ... 2929
Donnatal Extentabs ... 2930

Phenoxybenzamine Hydrochloride (Enhanced effects of certain antihypertensive agents). Products include:
Dibenzyline Capsules ... 3457

Phentolamine Mesylate (Enhanced effects of certain antihypertensive agents).
No products indexed under this heading.

Phenytoin (Co-administration has resulted in increased mean oral

clearance of quetiapine by 5-fold; increased dose of quetiapine may be required). Products include:
- Dilantin Infatabs ... **2624**
- Dilantin-125 Oral Suspension ... **2625**

Phenytoin Sodium (Co-administration has resulted in increased mean oral clearance of quetiapine by 5-fold; increased dose of quetiapine may be required). Products include:
- Dilantin Kapseals ... **2622**

Pindolol (Enhanced effects of certain antihypertensive agents).
No products indexed under this heading.

Polythiazide (Enhanced effects of certain antihypertensive agents). Products include:
- Minizide Capsules ... **2700**
- Renese Tablets ... **2712**

Pramipexole Dihydrochloride (Quetiapine may antagonize the effects of dopamine agonists). Products include:
- Mirapex Tablets ... **2834**

Prazosin Hydrochloride (Enhanced effects of certain antihypertensive agents). Products include:
- Minipress Capsules ... **2699**
- Minizide Capsules ... **2700**

Prednisolone Acetate (Co-administration with hepatic enzyme inducers, such as glucocorticosteroids, may increase oral clearance). Products include:
- Blephamide Ophthalmic Ointment .. **547**
- Blephamide Ophthalmic Suspension ... **548**
- Poly-Pred Liquifilm Ophthalmic Suspension ... ⊙**245**
- Pred Forte Ophthalmic Suspension ... ⊙**246**
- Pred Mild Sterile Ophthalmic Suspension ... ⊙**249**
- Pred-G Ophthalmic Suspension ... ⊙**247**
- Pred-G Sterile Ophthalmic Ointment ... ⊙**248**

Prednisolone Sodium Phosphate (Co-administration with hepatic enzyme inducers, such as glucocorticosteroids, may increase oral clearance). Products include:
- Pediapred Oral Solution ... **1170**

Prednisolone Tebutate (Co-administration with hepatic enzyme inducers, such as glucocorticosteroids, may increase oral clearance).
No products indexed under this heading.

Prednisone (Co-administration with hepatic enzyme inducers, such as glucocorticosteroids, may increase oral clearance). Products include:
- Prednisone ... **3064**

Propranolol Hydrochloride (Enhanced effects of certain antihypertensive agents). Products include:
- Inderal ... **3513**
- Inderal LA Long-Acting Capsules ... **3516**
- Inderide Tablets ... **3517**
- Inderide LA Long-Acting Capsules .. **3519**

Quinapril Hydrochloride (Enhanced effects of certain antihypertensive agents). Products include:
- Accupril Tablets ... **2611**
- Accuretic Tablets ... **2614**

Ramipril (Enhanced effects of certain antihypertensive agents). Products include:
- Altace Capsules ... **2233**

Rauwolfia serpentina (Enhanced effects of certain antihypertensive agents).
No products indexed under this heading.

Rescinnamine (Enhanced effects of certain antihypertensive agents).
No products indexed under this heading.

Reserpine (Enhanced effects of certain antihypertensive agents).
No products indexed under this heading.

Rifampin (Co-administration with hepatic enzyme inducers, such as rifampin, may increase oral clearance). Products include:
- Rifadin ... **765**
- Rifamate Capsules ... **767**
- Rifater Tablets ... **769**

Ropinirole Hydrochloride (Quetiapine may antagonize the effects of dopamine agonists). Products include:
- Requip Tablets ... **1621**

Secobarbital Sodium (Co-administration with hepatic enzyme inducers, such as barbiturates, may increase oral clearance).
No products indexed under this heading.

Sodium Nitroprusside (Enhanced effects of certain antihypertensive agents).
No products indexed under this heading.

Sotalol Hydrochloride (Enhanced effects of certain antihypertensive agents). Products include:
- Betapace Tablets ... **950**
- Betapace AF Tablets ... **954**

Spirapril Hydrochloride (Enhanced effects of certain antihypertensive agents).
No products indexed under this heading.

Telmisartan (Enhanced effects of certain antihypertensive agents). Products include:
- Micardis Tablets ... **1049**
- Micardis HCT Tablets ... **1051**

Terazosin Hydrochloride (Enhanced effects of certain antihypertensive agents). Products include:
- Hytrin Capsules ... **464**

Thiamylal Sodium (Co-administration with hepatic enzyme inducers, such as barbiturates, may increase oral clearance).
No products indexed under this heading.

Thioridazine (Increases the oral clearance of quetiapine by 66%).
No products indexed under this heading.

Timolol Maleate (Enhanced effects of certain antihypertensive agents). Products include:
- Blocadren Tablets ... **2046**
- Cosopt Sterile Ophthalmic Solution ... **2065**
- Timolide Tablets ... **2187**
- Timolol GFS ... ⊙**266**
- Timoptic in Ocudose ... **2192**
- Timoptic Sterile Ophthalmic Solution ... **2190**
- Timoptic-XE Sterile Ophthalmic Gel Forming Solution ... **2194**

Torsemide (Enhanced effects of certain antihypertensive agents). Products include:
- Demadex Tablets and Injection ... **2965**

Trandolapril (Enhanced effects of certain antihypertensive agents). Products include:
- Mavik Tablets ... **478**
- Tarka Tablets ... **508**

Triamcinolone (Co-administration with hepatic enzyme inducers, such as glucocorticosteroids, may increase oral clearance).
No products indexed under this heading.

Triamcinolone Acetonide (Co-administration with hepatic enzyme inducers, such as glucocorticosteroids, may increase oral clearance). Products include:
- Azmacort Inhalation Aerosol ... **728**
- Nasacort Nasal Inhaler ... **750**
- Nasacort AQ Nasal Spray ... **752**
- Tri-Nasal Spray ... **2274**

Triamcinolone Diacetate (Co-administration with hepatic enzyme inducers, such as glucocorticosteroids, may increase oral clearance).
No products indexed under this heading.

Triamcinolone Hexacetonide (Co-administration with hepatic enzyme inducers, such as glucocorticosteroids, may increase oral clearance).
No products indexed under this heading.

Trimethaphan Camsylate (Enhanced effects of certain antihypertensive agents).
No products indexed under this heading.

Valsartan (Enhanced effects of certain antihypertensive agents). Products include:
- Diovan Capsules ... **2337**
- Diovan HCT Tablets ... **2338**

Verapamil Hydrochloride (Enhanced effects of certain antihypertensive agents). Products include:
- Covera-HS Tablets ... **3199**
- Isoptin SR Tablets ... **467**
- Tarka Tablets ... **508**
- Verelan Capsules ... **3184**
- Verelan PM Capsules ... **3186**

Food Interactions

Alcohol (The cognitive and motor effect of alcohol is potentiated; alcohol use should be avoided).

Food, unspecified (The bioavailability of quetiapine is marginally affected by administration with food, with Cmax and AUC values increased by 25% and 15% respectively).

SEROSTIM FOR INJECTION

(Somatropin) ... **3229**

May interact with oral hypoglycemic agents and insulin. Compounds in these categories include:

Acarbose (During post-marketing surveillance cases of new onset diabetes and exacerbation of pre-existing diabetes have been reported with Somatropin; adjustment of antidiabetic treatment may be required). Products include:
- Precose Tablets ... **906**

Chlorpropamide (During post-marketing surveillance cases of new onset diabetes and exacerbation of pre-existing diabetes have been reported with Somatropin; adjustment of antidiabetic treatment may be required). Products include:
- Diabinese Tablets ... **2680**

Glimepiride (During post-marketing surveillance cases of new onset diabetes and exacerbation of pre-existing diabetes have been reported with Somatropin; adjustment of antidiabetic treatment may be required). Products include:
- Amaryl Tablets ... **717**

Glipizide (During post-marketing surveillance cases of new onset diabetes and exacerbation of pre-existing diabetes have been reported with Somatropin; adjustment of antidiabetic treatment may be required). Products include:
- Glucotrol Tablets ... **2692**
- Glucotrol XL Extended Release Tablets ... **2693**

Glyburide (During post-marketing surveillance cases of new onset diabetes and exacerbation of pre-existing diabetes have been reported with Somatropin; adjustment of antidiabetic treatment may be required). Products include:
- DiaBeta Tablets ... **741**
- Glucovance Tablets ... **1086**

Insulin, Human, Zinc Suspension (During post-marketing surveillance cases of new onset diabetes and exacerbation of pre-existing diabetes have been reported with Somatropin; adjustment of antidiabetic treatment may be required). Products include:
- Humulin L, 100 Units ... **1937**
- Humulin U, 100 Units ... **1943**
- Novolin L Human Insulin 10 ml Vials ... **2422**

Insulin, Human NPH (During post-marketing surveillance cases of new onset diabetes and exacerbation of pre-existing diabetes have been reported with Somatropin; adjustment of antidiabetic treatment may be required). Products include:
- Humulin N, 100 Units ... **1939**
- Humulin N NPH Pen ... **1940**
- Novolin N Human Insulin 10 ml Vials ... **2422**
- Novolin N PenFill ... **2423**
- Novolin N Prefilled Syringe Disposable Insulin Delivery System ... **2425**

Insulin, Human Regular (During post-marketing surveillance cases of new onset diabetes and exacerbation of pre-existing diabetes have been reported with Somatropin; adjustment of antidiabetic treatment may be required). Products include:
- Humulin R Regular (U-500) ... **1943**
- Humulin R, 100 Units ... **1941**
- Novolin R Human Insulin 10 ml Vials ... **2423**
- Novolin R PenFill ... **2423**
- Novolin R Prefilled Syringe Disposable Insulin Delivery System ... **2425**
- Velosulin BR Human Insulin 10 ml Vials ... **2435**

Insulin, Human Regular and Human NPH Mixture (During post-marketing surveillance cases of new onset diabetes and exacerbation of pre-existing diabetes have been reported with Somatropin; adjustment of antidiabetic treatment may be required). Products include:
- Humulin 50/50, 100 Units ... **1934**
- Humulin 70/30, 100 Units ... **1935**
- Humulin 70/30 Pen ... **1936**
- Novolin 70/30 Human Insulin 10 ml Vials ... **2421**
- Novolin 70/30 PenFill ... **2423**
- Novolin 70/30 Prefilled Disposable Insulin Delivery System ... **2425**

Insulin, NPH (During post-marketing surveillance cases of new onset diabetes and exacerbation of pre-existing diabetes have been reported with Somatropin; adjustment of antidiabetic treatment may be required). Products include:
- Iletin II, NPH (Pork), 100 Units ... **1946**

Insulin, Regular (During post-marketing surveillance cases of new onset diabetes and exacerbation of pre-existing diabetes have been reported with Somatropin; adjustment of antidiabetic treatment may be required). Products include:
- Iletin II, Regular (Pork), 100 Units ... **1947**

Insulin, Zinc Crystals (During post-marketing surveillance cases of new onset diabetes and exacerbation of pre-existing diabetes have been reported with Somatropin; adjustment of antidiabetic treatment may be required).
No products indexed under this heading.

Insulin, Zinc Suspension (During post-marketing surveillance cases of new onset diabetes and exacerbation of pre-existing diabetes have been reported with Somatropin; adjustment of antidiabetic treatment may be required). Products include:
- Iletin II, Lente (Pork), 100 Units ... **1945**

Insulin Aspart, Human Regular (During post-marketing surveillance cases of new onset diabetes and exacerbation of pre-existing diabetes have been reported with Somatropin; adjustment of antidiabetic treat-

ment may be required).
No products indexed under this heading.

Insulin glargine (During post-marketing surveillance cases of new onset diabetes and exacerbation of pre-existing diabetes have been reported with Somatropin; adjustment of antidiabetic treatment may be required). Products include:
Lantus Injection 742

Insulin Lispro, Human (During post-marketing surveillance cases of new onset diabetes and exacerbation of pre-existing diabetes have been reported with Somatropin; adjustment of antidiabetic treatment may be required). Products include:
Humalog 1926
Humalog Mix 75/25 Pen 1928

Insulin Lispro Protamine, Human (During post-marketing surveillance cases of new onset diabetes and exacerbation of pre-existing diabetes have been reported with Somatropin; adjustment of antidiabetic treatment may be required). Products include:
Humalog Mix 75/25 Pen 1928

Metformin Hydrochloride (During post-marketing surveillance cases of new onset diabetes and exacerbation of pre-existing diabetes have been reported with Somatropin; adjustment of antidiabetic treatment may be required). Products include:
Glucophage Tablets 1080
Glucophage XR Tablets 1080
Glucovance Tablets 1086

Miglitol (During post-marketing surveillance cases of new onset diabetes and exacerbation of pre-existing diabetes have been reported with Somatropin; adjustment of antidiabetic treatment may be required). Products include:
Glyset Tablets 2821

Pioglitazone Hydrochloride (During post-marketing surveillance cases of new onset diabetes and exacerbation of pre-existing diabetes have been reported with Somatropin; adjustment of antidiabetic treatment may be required). Products include:
Actos Tablets 3275

Repaglinide (During post-marketing surveillance cases of new onset diabetes and exacerbation of pre-existing diabetes have been reported with Somatropin; adjustment of antidiabetic treatment may be required). Products include:
Prandin Tablets (0.5, 1, and 2 mg) 2432

Rosiglitazone Maleate (During post-marketing surveillance cases of new onset diabetes and exacerbation of pre-existing diabetes have been reported with Somatropin; adjustment of antidiabetic treatment may be required). Products include:
Avandia Tablets 1490

Tolazamide (During post-marketing surveillance cases of new onset diabetes and exacerbation of pre-existing diabetes have been reported with Somatropin; adjustment of antidiabetic treatment may be required).
No products indexed under this heading.

Tolbutamide (During post-marketing surveillance cases of new onset diabetes and exacerbation of pre-existing diabetes have been reported with Somatropin; adjustment of antidiabetic treatment may be required).
No products indexed under this heading.

Troglitazone (During post-marketing surveillance cases of new onset diabetes and exacerbation of pre-existing diabetes have been reported with Somatropin; adjustment of antidiabetic treatment may be required).
No products indexed under this heading.

SERZONE TABLETS

(Nefazodone Hydrochloride) 1104
May interact with monoamine oxidase inhibitors, highly protein bound drugs (selected), triazolobenzodiazepines, and certain other agents. Compounds in these categories include:

Alprazolam (Co-administration may increase steady-state peak concentrations, AUC and half-life values; potentiated effects on psychomotor performance tests; reduction in initial dosage of triazolobenzodiazepines is required). Products include:
Xanax Tablets 2865

Amiodarone Hydrochloride (Nefazodone is highly bound to the plasma protein hence co-administration with another drug that is highly protein bound may cause increased free concentrations of other drug, potentially resulting in adverse events). Products include:
Cordarone Intravenous 3491
Cordarone Tablets 3487
Pacerone Tablets 3331

Amitriptyline Hydrochloride (Nefazodone is highly bound to the plasma protein hence co-administration with another drug that is highly protein bound may cause increased free concentrations of other drug, potentially resulting in adverse events). Products include:
Etrafon 3115
Limbitrol 1738

Astemizole (Nefazodone has been shown *in vitro* to be inhibitor of cytochrome P450II4 resulting in the potential for increased plasma concentration of astemizole leading to QT prolongation and rare cases of serious cardiovascular toxicity; concurrent use is contraindicated).
No products indexed under this heading.

Atorvastatin Calcium (Co-administration has resulted in approximately 3- to 4-fold increases in plasma concentrations of atorvastatin and atorvastatin lactone to inhibition of CYP3A4 by nefazodone; there have been rare reports of rhabdomyolysis with concurrent use). Products include:
Lipitor Tablets 2639
Lipitor Tablets 2696

Atovaquone (Nefazodone is highly bound to the plasma protein hence co-administration with another drug that is highly protein bound may cause increased free concentrations of other drug, potentially resulting in adverse events). Products include:
Malarone 1596
Mepron Suspension 1598

Buspirone Hydrochloride (Co-administration has resulted in marked increases in plasma buspirone concentrations and statistically significant decreases in plasma concentrations of the buspirone metabolite).
No products indexed under this heading.

Carbamazepine (Co-administration, at steady state for both drugs, resulted in almost 95% reduction in AUCs for nefazodone and hydroxynefazodone, likely resulting in insufficient plasma nefazodone and hydroxynefazodone concentrations for achieving an antidepressant effect; concurrent use is contraindicated). Products include:
Carbatrol Capsules 3234
Tegretol/Tegretol-XR 2404

Cefonicid Sodium (Nefazodone is highly bound to the plasma protein hence co-administration with another drug that is highly protein bound may cause increased free concentrations of other drug, potentially resulting in adverse events).
No products indexed under this heading.

Celecoxib (Nefazodone is highly bound to the plasma protein hence co-administration with another drug that is highly protein bound may cause increased free concentrations of other drug, potentially resulting in adverse events). Products include:
Celebrex Capsules 2676
Celebrex Capsules 2780

Chlordiazepoxide (Nefazodone is highly bound to the plasma protein hence co-administration with another drug that is highly protein bound may cause increased free concentrations of other drug, potentially resulting in adverse events). Products include:
Limbitrol 1738

Chlordiazepoxide Hydrochloride (Nefazodone is highly bound to the plasma protein hence co-administration with another drug that is highly protein bound may cause increased free concentrations of other drug, potentially resulting in adverse events). Products include:
Librium Capsules 1736
Librium for Injection 1737

Chlorpromazine (Nefazodone is highly bound to the plasma protein hence co-administration with another drug that is highly protein bound may cause increased free concentrations of other drug, potentially resulting in adverse events). Products include:
Thorazine Suppositories 1656

Chlorpromazine Hydrochloride (Nefazodone is highly bound to the plasma protein hence co-administration with another drug that is highly protein bound may cause increased free concentrations of other drug, potentially resulting in adverse events). Products include:
Thorazine 1656

Cisapride (Nefazodone has been shown *in vitro* to be an inhibitor of cytochrome P450IIIA4 resulting in the potential for increased plasma concentration of cisapride leading to QT prolongation and rare cases of serious cardiovascular toxicity; concurrent use is contraindicated).
No products indexed under this heading.

Clomipramine Hydrochloride (Nefazodone is highly bound to the plasma protein hence co-administration with another drug that is highly protein bound may cause increased free concentrations of other drug, potentially resulting in adverse events).
No products indexed under this heading.

Clozapine (Nefazodone is highly bound to the plasma protein hence co-administration with another drug that is highly protein bound may cause increased free concentrations of other drug, potentially resulting in adverse events). Products include:
Clozaril Tablets 2319

CNS-Active Drugs, unspecified (Caution is advised if concomitant administration of nefazodone and other CNS active drugs is required).

Cyclosporine (Co-administration has resulted in rare reports of increased serum cyclosporine levels (up to seven times higher) in patients receiving combined therapy). Products include:
Gengraf Capsules 457
Neoral Soft Gelatin Capsules 2380
Neoral Oral Solution 2380
Sandimmune 2388

Diazepam (Nefazodone is highly bound to the plasma protein hence co-administration with another drug that is highly protein bound may cause increased free concentrations of other drug, potentially resulting in adverse events). Products include:
Valium Injectable 3026
Valium Tablets 3047

Diclofenac Potassium (Nefazodone is highly bound to the plasma protein hence co-administration with another drug that is highly protein bound may cause increased free concentrations of other drug, potentially resulting in adverse events). Products include:
Cataflam Tablets 2315

Diclofenac Sodium (Nefazodone is highly bound to the plasma protein hence co-administration with another drug that is highly protein bound may cause increased free concentrations of other drug, potentially resulting in adverse events). Products include:
Arthrotec Tablets 3195
Voltaren Ophthalmic Sterile Ophthalmic Solution .... ⊙ 312
Voltaren Tablets 2315
Voltaren-XR Tablets 2315

Digoxin (Potential for increased digoxin Cmax, Cmin, and AUC by 29%, 27%, and 15% respectively; caution should be exercised if used concurrently). Products include:
Digitek Tablets 1003
Lanoxicaps Capsules 1574
Lanoxin Injection 1581
Lanoxin Tablets 1587
Lanoxin Elixir Pediatric 1578
Lanoxin Injection Pediatric 1584

Dipyridamole (Nefazodone is highly bound to the plasma protein hence co-administration with another drug that is highly protein bound may cause increased free concentrations of other drug, potentially resulting in adverse events). Products include:
Aggrenox Capsules 1026
Persantine Tablets 1057

Fenoprofen Calcium (Nefazodone is highly bound to the plasma protein hence co-administration with another drug that is highly protein bound may cause increased free concentrations of other drug, potentially resulting in adverse events).
No products indexed under this heading.

Fluoxetine Hydrochloride (Co-administration of nefazodone to patients who had been receiving fluoxetine for 1 week has resulted in increased incidence of transient adverse events such as headache, lightheadedness, nausea or paresthesia, possibly due to the elevated mCPP levels; because of the long half-life of fluoxetine and its metabolites, the washout period may range from one to several weeks depending on the dose of fluoxetine and other individual patient variables). Products include:
Prozac Pulvules, Liquid, and Weekly Capsules 1238
Sarafem Pulvules 1962

Flurazepam Hydrochloride (Nefazodone is highly bound to the plasma protein hence co-administration with another drug that is highly protein bound may cause increased free concentrations of other drug, potentially resulting in adverse events).
No products indexed under this heading.

Flurbiprofen (Nefazodone is highly bound to the plasma protein hence co-administration with another drug that is highly protein bound may cause increased free concentrations of other drug, potentially resulting in adverse events).
No products indexed under this heading.

Glipizide (Nefazodone is highly bound to the plasma protein hence co-administration with another drug

that is highly protein bound may cause increased free concentrations of other drug, potentially resulting in adverse events). Products include:

Glucotrol Tablets 2692
Glucotrol XL Extended Release Tablets 2693

Haloperidol (Decreased haloperidol apparent clearance by 35% with no significant increase in peak plasma levels or time to peak; dosage adjustment may be required). Products include:

Haldol Injection, Tablets and Concentrate 2533

Haloperidol Decanoate (Decreased haloperidol apparent clearance by 35% with no significant increase in peak plasma levels or time to peak; dosage adjustment may be required). Products include:

Haldol Decanoate 2535

Ibuprofen (Nefazodone is highly bound to the plasma protein hence co-administration with another drug that is highly protein bound may cause increased free concentrations of other drug, potentially resulting in adverse events). Products include:

Advil 771
Children's Advil Oral Suspension 773
Children's Advil Chewable Tablets 773
Advil Cold and Sinus Caplets 771
Advil Cold and Sinus Tablets 771
Advil Flu & Body Ache Caplets 772
Infants' Advil Drops 773
Junior Strength Advil Tablets 773
Junior Strength Advil Chewable Tablets 773
Advil Migraine Liquigels 772
Children's Motrin Oral Suspension and Chewable Tablets 2006
Children's Motrin Cold Oral Suspension 2007
Children's Motrin Oral Suspension 643
Motrin Suspension, Oral Drops, Chewable Tablets, and Caplets 2002
Infants' Motrin Concentrated Drops 2006
Junior Strength Motrin Caplets and Chewable Tablets 2006
Motrin IB Tablets, Caplets, and Gelcaps 2002
Motrin Migraine Pain Caplets 2005
Motrin Sinus Headache Caplets 2005
Vicoprofen Tablets 520

Imipramine Hydrochloride (Nefazodone is highly bound to the plasma protein hence co-administration with another drug that is highly protein bound may cause increased free concentrations of other drug, potentially resulting in adverse events).

No products indexed under this heading.

Imipramine Pamoate (Nefazodone is highly bound to the plasma protein hence co-administration with another drug that is highly protein bound may cause increased free concentrations of other drug, potentially resulting in adverse events).

No products indexed under this heading.

Indomethacin (Nefazodone is highly bound to the plasma protein hence co-administration with another drug that is highly protein bound may cause increased free concentrations of other drug, potentially resulting in adverse events). Products include:

Indocin 2112

Indomethacin Sodium Trihydrate (Nefazodone is highly bound to the plasma protein hence co-administration with another drug that is highly protein bound may cause increased free concentrations of other drug, potentially resulting in adverse events). Products include:

Indocin I.V. 2115

Isocarboxazid (Co-administration of antidepressants with pharmacological properties similar to nefazodone and MAO inhibitors has resulted in serious, sometimes fatal, reactions including hyperthermia, rigidity, myoclonus, extreme agitation progressing to delirium and coma; effects of concurrent use have not been evaluated; therefore, nefazodone should not be used concurrently and/or sequentially with an MAO inhibitor).

No products indexed under this heading.

Ketoprofen (Nefazodone is highly bound to the plasma protein hence co-administration with another drug that is highly protein bound may cause increased free concentrations of other drug, potentially resulting in adverse events). Products include:

Orudis Capsules 3548
Orudis KT Tablets 778
Oruvail Capsules 3548

Ketorolac Tromethamine (Nefazodone is highly bound to the plasma protein hence co-administration with another drug that is highly protein bound may cause increased free concentrations of other drug, potentially resulting in adverse events). Products include:

Acular Ophthalmic Solution 544
Acular PF Ophthalmic Solution 544
Toradol 3018

Lovastatin (There have been rare reports of rhabdomyolysis in patients receiving nefazodone, a known inhibitor of the CYP450IIIA4 and HMG-CoA reductase inhibitor lovastatin, a known substrate of CYP450IIIA4). Products include:

Mevacor Tablets 2132

Meclofenamate Sodium (Nefazodone is highly bound to the plasma protein hence co-administration with another drug that is highly protein bound may cause increased free concentrations of other drug, potentially resulting in adverse events).

No products indexed under this heading.

Mefenamic Acid (Nefazodone is highly bound to the plasma protein hence co-administration with another drug that is highly protein bound may cause increased free concentrations of other drug, potentially resulting in adverse events). Products include:

Ponstel Capsules 1356

Midazolam Hydrochloride (Co-administration may increase steady-state peak concentrations, AUC and half-life values; potentiated effects on psychomotor performance tests; reduction in initial dosage of triazolobenzodiazepines is required). Products include:

Versed Injection 3027
Versed Syrup 3033

Moclobemide (Co-administration of antidepressants with pharmacological properties similar to nefazodone and MAO inhibitors has resulted in serious, sometimes fatal, reactions including hyperthermia, rigidity, myoclonus, extreme agitation progressing to delirium and coma; effects of concurrent use have not been evaluated; therefore, nefazodone should not be used concurrently and/or sequentially with an MAO inhibitor).

No products indexed under this heading.

Naproxen (Nefazodone is highly bound to the plasma protein hence co-administration with another drug that is highly protein bound may cause increased free concentrations of other drug, potentially resulting in adverse events). Products include:

EC-Naprosyn Delayed-Release Tablets 2967
Naprosyn Suspension 2967
Naprosyn Tablets 2967

Naproxen Sodium (Nefazodone is highly bound to the plasma protein hence co-administration with another drug that is highly protein bound may cause increased free concentrations of other drug, potentially resulting in adverse events). Products include:

Aleve Tablets, Caplets and Gelcaps 602
Aleve Cold & Sinus Caplets 603
Anaprox Tablets 2967
Anaprox DS Tablets 2967
Naprelan Tablets 1293

Nortriptyline Hydrochloride (Nefazodone is highly bound to the plasma protein hence co-administration with another drug that is highly protein bound may cause increased free concentrations of other drug, potentially resulting in adverse events).

No products indexed under this heading.

Oxaprozin (Nefazodone is highly bound to the plasma protein hence co-administration with another drug that is highly protein bound may cause increased free concentrations of other drug, potentially resulting in adverse events).

No products indexed under this heading.

Oxazepam (Nefazodone is highly bound to the plasma protein hence co-administration with another drug that is highly protein bound may cause increased free concentrations of other drug, potentially resulting in adverse events).

No products indexed under this heading.

Pargyline Hydrochloride (Co-administration of antidepressants with pharmacological properties similar to nefazodone and MAO inhibitors has resulted in serious, sometimes fatal, reactions including hyperthermia, rigidity, myoclonus, extreme agitation progressing to delirium and coma; effects of concurrent use have not been evaluated; therefore, nefazodone should not be used concurrently and/or sequentially with an MAO inhibitor).

No products indexed under this heading.

Phenelzine Sulfate (Co-administration of antidepressants with pharmacological properties similar to nefazodone and MAO inhibitors has resulted in serious, sometimes fatal, reactions including hyperthermia, rigidity, myoclonus, extreme agitation progressing to delirium and coma; effects of concurrent use have not been evaluated; therefore, nefazodone should not be used concurrently and/or sequentially with an MAO inhibitor). Products include:

Nardil Tablets 2653

Phenylbutazone (Nefazodone is highly bound to the plasma protein hence co-administration with another drug that is highly protein bound may cause increased free concentrations of other drug, potentially resulting in adverse events).

No products indexed under this heading.

Pimozide (Nefazodone has been shown in vitro to be an inhibitor of CYP3A4; co-administration of CYP3A4 inhibitors and drugs that are metabolized by this isoenzyme, such as pimozide, can result in increased plasma concentrations of pimozide resulting in QT prolongation and with rare cases of serious cardiovascular adverse events, including death; concurrent use is contraindicated). Products include:

Orap Tablets 1407

Piroxicam (Nefazodone is highly bound to the plasma protein hence co-administration with another drug that is highly protein bound may cause increased free concentrations of other drug, potentially resulting in adverse events). Products include:

Feldene Capsules 2685

Procarbazine Hydrochloride (Co-administration of antidepressants with pharmacological properties similar to nefazodone and MAO inhibitors has resulted in serious, sometimes fatal, reactions including hyperthermia, rigidity, myoclonus, extreme agitation progressing to delirium and coma; effects of concurrent use have not been evaluated; therefore, nefazodone should not be used concurrently and/or sequentially with an MAO inhibitor). Products include:

Matulane Capsules 3246

Propranolol Hydrochloride (Potential for reduction in Cmax and AUC of propranolol with no significant change in clinical outcome). Products include:

Inderal 3513
Inderal LA Long-Acting Capsules 3516
Inderide Tablets 3517
Inderide LA Long-Acting Capsules 3519

Selegiline Hydrochloride (Co-administration of antidepressants with pharmacological properties similar to nefazodone and MAO inhibitors has resulted in serious, sometimes fatal, reactions including hyperthermia, rigidity, myoclonus, extreme agitation progressing to delirium and coma; effects of concurrent use have not been evaluated; therefore, nefazodone should not be used concurrently and/or sequentially with an MAO inhibitor). Products include:

Eldepryl Capsules 3266

Simvastatin (Co-administration has resulted in approximately 20-fold increases in plasma concentrations of simvastatin and simvastatin acid due to inhibition of CYP3A4 by nefazodone; there have been rare reports of rhabdomyolysis with concurrent use). Products include:

Zocor Tablets 2219

Sulindac (Nefazodone is highly bound to the plasma protein hence co-administration with another drug that is highly protein bound may cause increased free concentrations of other drug, potentially resulting in adverse events). Products include:

Clinoril Tablets 2053

Tacrolimus (Co-administration has resulted in rare reports of increased blood concentrations of tacrolimus into toxic ranges). Products include:

Prograf 1393
Protopic Ointment 1397

Temazepam (Nefazodone is highly bound to the plasma protein hence co-administration with another drug that is highly protein bound may cause increased free concentrations of other drug, potentially resulting in adverse events).

No products indexed under this heading.

Terfenadine (Nefazodone has been shown *in vitro* to be an inhibitor of cytochrome P450IIIA4 resulting in the potential for increased plasma concentration of terfenadine leading to QT prolongation and rare cases of serious cardiovascular toxicity; concurrent use is contraindicated).

No products indexed under this heading.

Tolbutamide (Nefazodone is highly bound to the plasma protein hence co-administration with another drug that is highly protein bound may cause increased free concentrations of other drug, potentially resulting in adverse events).

No products indexed under this heading.

Tolmetin Sodium (Nefazodone is highly bound to the plasma protein hence co-administration with another drug that is highly protein bound may

cause increased free concentrations of other drug, potentially resulting in adverse events). Products include:

Tolectin 2589

Tranylcypromine Sulfate (Co-administration of antidepressants with pharmacological properties similar to nefazodone and MAO inhibitors has resulted in serious, sometimes fatal, reactions including hyperthermia, rigidity, myoclonus, extreme agitation progressing to delirium and coma; effects of concurrent use have not been evaluated; therefore, nefazodone should not be used concurrently and/or sequentially with an MAO inhibitor). Products include:

Parnate Tablets 1607

Triazolam (Co-administration causes a significant increase in the plasma level of triazolam, and a 75% reduction in the initial triazolam dosage is recommended if the two drugs are to be given together; because not all commercially available dosage forms of triazolam permit sufficient dosage reduction, the co-administration should be avoided). Products include:

Halcion Tablets 2823

Trimipramine Maleate (Nefazodone is highly bound to the plasma protein hence co-administration with another drug that is highly protein bound may cause increased free concentrations of other drug, potentially resulting in adverse events). Products include:

Surmontil Capsules 3595

Warfarin Sodium (Co-administration of nefazodone with warfarin decreases the exposure to S-warfarin by 12%, however, there were no effects on the prothrombin or bleeding times or upon the pharmacokinetics of R-warfarin; although these results suggest no adjustments in warfarin dosage, such patients should be monitored as required by standard medical practices). Products include:

Coumadin for Injection 1243
Coumadin Tablets 1243
Warfarin Sodium Tablets, USP 3302

Food Interactions

Alcohol (Concomitant use should be avoided).

Food, unspecified (Food delays the absorption of nefazodone and decreases the bioavailability by approximately 20%).

SILVADENE CREAM 1%

(Silver Sulfadiazine) 2267

May interact with:

Cimetidine (An increased incidence of leukopenia has been reported in patients treated concurrently with cimetidine). Products include:

Tagamet HB 200 Suspension .... ▣762
Tagamet HB 200 Tablets .... ▣761
Tagamet Tablets 1644

Cimetidine Hydrochloride (An increased incidence of leukopenia has been reported in patients treated concurrently with cimetidine). Products include:

Tagamet 1644

Protease (Concomitant use of topical proteolytic enzymes with silver sulfadiazine may result in inactivation of enzyme by silver). Products include:

Arco-Lase Tablets 592
Arco-Lase Plus Tablets 592

SIMPLY SLEEP CAPLETS

(Diphenhydramine Hydrochloride) 2008

May interact with hypnotics and sedatives, tranquilizers, and certain other agents. Compounds in these categories include:

Alprazolam (Diphenhydramine is an antihistamine with sedative properties; concurrent use should be avoided). Products include:

Xanax Tablets 2865

Buspirone Hydrochloride (Diphenhydramine is an antihistamine with sedative properties; concurrent use should be avoided).

No products indexed under this heading.

Chlordiazepoxide (Diphenhydramine is an antihistamine with sedative properties; concurrent use should be avoided). Products include:

Limbitrol 1738

Chlordiazepoxide Hydrochloride (Diphenhydramine is an antihistamine with sedative properties; concurrent use should be avoided). Products include:

Librium Capsules 1736
Librium for Injection 1737

Chlorpromazine (Diphenhydramine is an antihistamine with sedative properties; concurrent use should be avoided). Products include:

Thorazine Suppositories 1656

Chlorpromazine Hydrochloride (Diphenhydramine is an antihistamine with sedative properties; concurrent use should be avoided). Products include:

Thorazine 1656

Chlorprothixene (Diphenhydramine is an antihistamine with sedative properties; concurrent use should be avoided).

No products indexed under this heading.

Chlorprothixene Hydrochloride (Diphenhydramine is an antihistamine with sedative properties; concurrent use should be avoided).

No products indexed under this heading.

Clorazepate Dipotassium (Diphenhydramine is an antihistamine with sedative properties; concurrent use should be avoided). Products include:

Tranxene 511

Diazepam (Diphenhydramine is an antihistamine with sedative properties; concurrent use should be avoided). Products include:

Valium Injectable 3026
Valium Tablets 3047

Droperidol (Diphenhydramine is an antihistamine with sedative properties; concurrent use should be avoided).

No products indexed under this heading.

Estazolam (Diphenhydramine is an antihistamine with sedative properties; concurrent use should be avoided). Products include:

ProSom Tablets 500

Ethchlorvynol (Diphenhydramine is an antihistamine with sedative properties; concurrent use should be avoided).

No products indexed under this heading.

Ethinamate (Diphenhydramine is an antihistamine with sedative properties; concurrent use should be avoided).

No products indexed under this heading.

Fluphenazine Decanoate (Diphenhydramine is an antihistamine with sedative properties; concurrent use should be avoided).

No products indexed under this heading.

Fluphenazine Enanthate (Diphenhydramine is an antihistamine with sedative properties; concurrent use should be avoided).

No products indexed under this heading.

Fluphenazine Hydrochloride (Diphenhydramine is an antihistamine with sedative properties; concurrent use should be avoided).

No products indexed under this heading.

Flurazepam Hydrochloride (Diphenhydramine is an antihistamine with sedative properties; concurrent use should be avoided).

No products indexed under this heading.

Glutethimide (Diphenhydramine is an antihistamine with sedative properties; concurrent use should be avoided).

No products indexed under this heading.

Haloperidol (Diphenhydramine is an antihistamine with sedative properties; concurrent use should be avoided). Products include:

Haldol Injection, Tablets and Concentrate 2533

Haloperidol Decanoate (Diphenhydramine is an antihistamine with sedative properties; concurrent use should be avoided). Products include:

Haldol Decanoate 2535

Hydroxyzine Hydrochloride (Diphenhydramine is an antihistamine with sedative properties; concurrent use should be avoided). Products include:

Atarax Tablets & Syrup 2667
Vistaril Intramuscular Solution 2738

Lorazepam (Diphenhydramine is an antihistamine with sedative properties; concurrent use should be avoided). Products include:

Ativan Injection 3478
Ativan Tablets 3482

Loxapine Hydrochloride (Diphenhydramine is an antihistamine with sedative properties; concurrent use should be avoided).

No products indexed under this heading.

Loxapine Succinate (Diphenhydramine is an antihistamine with sedative properties; concurrent use should be avoided). Products include:

Loxitane Capsules 3398

Meprobamate (Diphenhydramine is an antihistamine with sedative properties; concurrent use should be avoided). Products include:

Miltown Tablets 3349

Mesoridazine Besylate (Diphenhydramine is an antihistamine with sedative properties; concurrent use should be avoided). Products include:

Serentil 1057

Midazolam Hydrochloride (Diphenhydramine is an antihistamine with sedative properties; concurrent use should be avoided). Products include:

Versed Injection 3027
Versed Syrup 3033

Molindone Hydrochloride (Diphenhydramine is an antihistamine with sedative properties; concurrent use should be avoided). Products include:

Moban 1320

Oxazepam (Diphenhydramine is an antihistamine with sedative properties; concurrent use should be avoided).

No products indexed under this heading.

Perphenazine (Diphenhydramine is an antihistamine with sedative properties; concurrent use should be avoided). Products include:

Etrafon 3115
Trilafon 3160

Prazepam (Diphenhydramine is an antihistamine with sedative properties; concurrent use should be avoided).

No products indexed under this heading.

Prochlorperazine (Diphenhydramine is an antihistamine with sedative properties; concurrent use should be avoided). Products include:

Compazine 1505

Promethazine Hydrochloride (Diphenhydramine is an antihistamine with sedative properties; concurrent use should be avoided). Products include:

Mepergan Injection 3539
Phenergan Injection 3553
Phenergan 3556
Phenergan Syrup 3554
Phenergan with Codeine Syrup 3557
Phenergan with Dextromethorphan Syrup 3559
Phenergan VC Syrup 3560
Phenergan VC with Codeine Syrup .. 3561

Propofol (Diphenhydramine is an antihistamine with sedative properties; concurrent use should be avoided). Products include:

Diprivan Injectable Emulsion 667

Quazepam (Diphenhydramine is an antihistamine with sedative properties; concurrent use should be avoided).

No products indexed under this heading.

Secobarbital Sodium (Diphenhydramine is an antihistamine with sedative properties; concurrent use should be avoided).

No products indexed under this heading.

Temazepam (Diphenhydramine is an antihistamine with sedative properties; concurrent use should be avoided).

No products indexed under this heading.

Thioridazine Hydrochloride (Diphenhydramine is an antihistamine with sedative properties; concurrent use should be avoided). Products include:

Thioridazine Hydrochloride Tablets 2289

Thiothixene (Diphenhydramine is an antihistamine with sedative properties; concurrent use should be avoided). Products include:

Navane Capsules 2701
Thiothixene Capsules 2290

Triazolam (Diphenhydramine is an antihistamine with sedative properties; concurrent use should be avoided). Products include:

Halcion Tablets 2823

Trifluoperazine Hydrochloride (Diphenhydramine is an antihistamine with sedative properties; concurrent use should be avoided). Products include:

Stelazine 1640

Zaleplon (Diphenhydramine is an antihistamine with sedative properties; concurrent use should be avoided). Products include:

Sonata Capsules 3591

Zolpidem Tartrate (Diphenhydramine is an antihistamine with sedative properties; concurrent use should be avoided). Products include:

Ambien Tablets 3191

Food Interactions

Alcohol (Diphenhydramine is an antihistamine with sedative properties; concurrent use with alcoholic beverages should be avoided).

SIMULECT FOR INJECTION

(Basiliximab) 2399

None cited in PDR database.

SINEMET TABLETS

(Carbidopa, Levodopa) 1253

See Sinemet CR Tablets

SINEMET CR TABLETS
(Carbidopa, Levodopa) 1255
May interact with antihypertensives, dopamine D2 antagonists, iron containing oral preparations, nonselective MAO inhibitors, phenytoin, tricyclic antidepressants, and certain other agents. Compounds in these categories include:

Acebutolol Hydrochloride (Co-administration with some antihypertensives has resulted in symptomatic postural hypotension). Products include:
Sectral Capsules 3589

Amitriptyline Hydrochloride (Co-administration with tricyclic antidepressants has resulted in rare reports of adverse reactions including hypertension and dyskinesia). Products include:
Etrafon 3115
Limbitrol 1738

Amlodipine Besylate (Co-administration with some antihypertensives has resulted in symptomatic postural hypotension). Products include:
Lotrel Capsules 2370
Norvasc Tablets 2704

Amoxapine (Co-administration with tricyclic antidepressants has resulted in rare reports of adverse reactions including hypertension and dyskinesia).
No products indexed under this heading.

Atenolol (Co-administration with some antihypertensives has resulted in symptomatic postural hypotension). Products include:
Tenoretic Tablets 690
Tenormin I.V. Injection 692

Benazepril Hydrochloride (Co-administration with some antihypertensives has resulted in symptomatic postural hypotension). Products include:
Lotensin Tablets 2365
Lotensin HCT Tablets 2367
Lotrel Capsules 2370

Bendroflumethiazide (Co-administration with some antihypertensives has resulted in symptomatic postural hypotension). Products include:
Corzide 40/5 Tablets 2247
Corzide 80/5 Tablets 2247

Betaxolol Hydrochloride (Co-administration with some antihypertensives has resulted in symptomatic postural hypotension). Products include:
Betoptic S Ophthalmic Suspension 537

Bisoprolol Fumarate (Co-administration with some antihypertensives has resulted in symptomatic postural hypotension). Products include:
Zebeta Tablets 1885
Ziac Tablets 1887

Candesartan Cilexetil (Co-administration with some antihypertensives has resulted in symptomatic postural hypotension). Products include:
Atacand Tablets 595
Atacand HCT Tablets 597

Captopril (Co-administration with some antihypertensives has resulted in symptomatic postural hypotension). Products include:
Captopril Tablets 2281

Carteolol Hydrochloride (Co-administration with some antihypertensives has resulted in symptomatic postural hypotension). Products include:
Carteolol Hydrochloride Ophthalmic Solution USP, 1% ..... ⊙ 258
Ocupress Ophthalmic Solution, 1% Sterile .... ⊙ 303

Chlorothiazide (Co-administration with some antihypertensives has resulted in symptomatic postural hypotension). Products include:
Aldoclor Tablets 2035
Diuril Oral 2087

Chlorothiazide Sodium (Co-administration with some antihypertensives has resulted in symptomatic postural hypotension). Products include:
Diuril Sodium Intravenous 2086

Chlorpromazine (Co-administration with dopamine D2 receptor antagonists may reduce the therapeutic effects of levodopa). Products include:
Thorazine Suppositories 1656

Chlorpromazine Hydrochloride (Co-administration with dopamine D2 receptor antagonists may reduce the therapeutic effects of levodopa). Products include:
Thorazine 1656

Chlorprothixene (Co-administration with dopamine D2 receptor antagonists may reduce the therapeutic effects of levodopa).
No products indexed under this heading.

Chlorprothixene Hydrochloride (Co-administration with dopamine D2 receptor antagonists may reduce the therapeutic effects of levodopa).
No products indexed under this heading.

Chlorthalidone (Co-administration with some antihypertensives has resulted in symptomatic postural hypotension). Products include:
Clorpres Tablets 1002
Combipres Tablets 1040
Tenoretic Tablets 690

Clomipramine Hydrochloride (Co-administration with tricyclic antidepressants has resulted in rare reports of adverse reactions including hypertension and dyskinesia).
No products indexed under this heading.

Clonidine (Co-administration with some antihypertensives has resulted in symptomatic postural hypotension). Products include:
Catapres-TTS 1038

Clonidine Hydrochloride (Co-administration with some antihypertensives has resulted in symptomatic postural hypotension). Products include:
Catapres Tablets 1037
Clorpres Tablets 1002
Combipres Tablets 1040
Duraclon Injection 3057

Deserpidine (Co-administration with some antihypertensives has resulted in symptomatic postural hypotension).
No products indexed under this heading.

Desipramine Hydrochloride (Co-administration with tricyclic antidepressants has resulted in rare reports of adverse reactions including hypertension and dyskinesia). Products include:
Norpramin Tablets 755

Diazoxide (Co-administration with some antihypertensives has resulted in symptomatic postural hypotension).
No products indexed under this heading.

Diltiazem Hydrochloride (Co-administration with some antihypertensives has resulted in symptomatic postural hypotension). Products include:
Cardizem Injectable 1018
Cardizem Lyo-Ject Syringe 1018
Cardizem Monovial 1018
Cardizem CD Capsules 1016
Tiazac Capsules 1378

Doxazosin Mesylate (Co-administration with some antihypertensives has resulted in symptomatic postural hypotension). Products include:
Cardura Tablets 2668

Doxepin Hydrochloride (Co-administration with tricyclic antidepressants has resulted in rare reports of adverse reactions including hypertension and dyskinesia). Products include:
Sinequan 2713

Enalapril Maleate (Co-administration with some antihypertensives has resulted in symptomatic postural hypotension). Products include:
Lexxel Tablets 608
Vaseretic Tablets 2204
Vasotec Tablets 2210

Enalaprilat (Co-administration with some antihypertensives has resulted in symptomatic postural hypotension). Products include:
Enalaprilat Injection 863
Vasotec I.V. Injection 2207

Eprosartan Mesylate (Co-administration with some antihypertensives has resulted in symptomatic postural hypotension). Products include:
Teveten Tablets 3327

Esmolol Hydrochloride (Co-administration with some antihypertensives has resulted in symptomatic postural hypotension). Products include:
Brevibloc Injection 858

Felodipine (Co-administration with some antihypertensives has resulted in symptomatic postural hypotension). Products include:
Lexxel Tablets 608
Plendil Extended-Release Tablets 623

Ferrous Fumarate (Iron salts may reduce the bioavailability of levodopa and carbidopa). Products include:
New Formulation Chromagen OB Capsules 3094
Loestrin Fe Tablets 2642
NataChew Tablets 3364

Ferrous Gluconate (Iron salts may reduce the bioavailability of levodopa and carbidopa). Products include:
Fergon Iron Tablets .... ▣ 802

Ferrous Sulfate (Iron salts may reduce the bioavailability of levodopa and carbidopa). Products include:
Feosol Tablets 1717
Slow Fe Tablets .... ▣ 827
Slow Fe with Folic Acid Tablets ...... ▣ 828

Fluphenazine Decanoate (Co-administration with dopamine D2 receptor antagonists may reduce the therapeutic effects of levodopa).
No products indexed under this heading.

Fluphenazine Enanthate (Co-administration with dopamine D2 receptor antagonists may reduce the therapeutic effects of levodopa).
No products indexed under this heading.

Fluphenazine Hydrochloride (Co-administration with dopamine D2 receptor antagonists may reduce the therapeutic effects of levodopa).
No products indexed under this heading.

Fosinopril Sodium (Co-administration with some antihypertensives has resulted in symptomatic postural hypotension). Products include:
Monopril Tablets 1091
Monopril HCT 1094

Fosphenytoin Sodium (The beneficial effects of levodopa in Parkinson's disease have been reported to be reversed by phenytoin). Products include:
Cerebyx Injection 2619

Furosemide (Co-administration with some antihypertensives has resulted in symptomatic postural hypotension). Products include:
Furosemide Tablets 2284

Guanabenz Acetate (Co-administration with some antihypertensives has resulted in symptomatic postural hypotension).
No products indexed under this heading.

Guanethidine Monosulfate (Co-administration with some antihypertensives has resulted in symptomatic postural hypotension).
No products indexed under this heading.

Haloperidol (Co-administration with dopamine D2 receptor antagonists may reduce the therapeutic effects of levodopa). Products include:
Haldol Injection, Tablets and Concentrate 2533

Haloperidol Decanoate (Co-administration with dopamine D2 receptor antagonists may reduce the therapeutic effects of levodopa). Products include:
Haldol Decanoate 2535

Hydralazine Hydrochloride (Co-administration with some antihypertensives has resulted in symptomatic postural hypotension).
No products indexed under this heading.

Hydrochlorothiazide (Co-administration with some antihypertensives has resulted in symptomatic postural hypotension). Products include:
Accuretic Tablets 2614
Aldoril Tablets 2039
Atacand HCT Tablets 597
Avalide Tablets 1070
Diovan HCT Tablets 2338
Dyazide Capsules 1515
HydroDIURIL Tablets 2108
Hyzaar 2109
Inderide Tablets 3517
Inderide LA Long-Acting Capsules .. 3519
Lotensin HCT Tablets 2367
Maxzide 1008
Micardis HCT Tablets 1051
Microzide Capsules 3414
Moduretic Tablets 2138
Monopril HCT 1094
Prinzide Tablets 2168
Timolide Tablets 2187
Uniretic Tablets 3178
Vaseretic Tablets 2204
Zestoretic Tablets 695
Ziac Tablets 1887

Hydroflumethiazide (Co-administration with some antihypertensives has resulted in symptomatic postural hypotension). Products include:
Diucardin Tablets 3494

Imipramine Hydrochloride (Co-administration with tricyclic antidepressants has resulted in rare reports of adverse reactions including hypertension and dyskinesia).
No products indexed under this heading.

Imipramine Pamoate (Co-administration with tricyclic antidepressants has resulted in rare reports of adverse reactions including hypertension and dyskinesia).
No products indexed under this heading.

Indapamide (Co-administration with some antihypertensives has resulted in symptomatic postural hypotension). Products include:
Indapamide Tablets 2286

Irbesartan (Co-administration with some antihypertensives has resulted in symptomatic postural hypotension). Products include:
Avalide Tablets 1070
Avapro Tablets 1074
Avapro Tablets 3076

Iron (Iron salts may reduce the bioavailability of levodopa and carbidopa).
No products indexed under this heading.

Isocarboxazid (Concurrent and/or sequential use with nonselective MAO inhibitors is contraindicated).
No products indexed under this heading.

Isoniazid (May reduce the therapeutic effects of levodopa). Products include:
Rifamate Capsules 767
Rifater Tablets 769

Isradipine (Co-administration with some antihypertensives has resulted in symptomatic postural hypotension). Products include:
DynaCirc Capsules 2921
DynaCirc CR Tablets 2923

Labetalol Hydrochloride (Co-administration with some antihypertensives has resulted in symptomatic postural hypotension). Products include:
Normodyne Injection 3135
Normodyne Tablets 3137

Lisinopril (Co-administration with some antihypertensives has resulted in symptomatic postural hypotension). Products include:
Prinivil Tablets 2164
Prinzide Tablets 2168
Zestoretic Tablets 695
Zestril Tablets 698

Losartan Potassium (Co-administration with some antihypertensives has resulted in symptomatic postural hypotension). Products include:
Cozaar Tablets 2067
Hyzaar 2109

Loxapine Hydrochloride (Co-administration with dopamine D2 receptor antagonists may reduce the therapeutic effects of levodopa).
No products indexed under this heading.

Loxapine Succinate (Co-administration with dopamine D2 receptor antagonists may reduce the therapeutic effects of levodopa). Products include:
Loxitane Capsules 3398

Maprotiline Hydrochloride (Co-administration with tricyclic antidepressants has resulted in rare reports of adverse reactions including hypertension and dyskinesia).
No products indexed under this heading.

Mecamylamine Hydrochloride (Co-administration with some antihypertensives has resulted in symptomatic postural hypotension). Products include:
Inversine Tablets 1850

Mesoridazine Besylate (Co-administration with dopamine D2 receptor antagonists may reduce the therapeutic effects of levodopa). Products include:
Serentil 1057

Methotrimeprazine (Co-administration with dopamine D2 receptor antagonists may reduce the therapeutic effects of levodopa).
No products indexed under this heading.

Methyclothiazide (Co-administration with some antihypertensives has resulted in symptomatic postural hypotension).
No products indexed under this heading.

Methyldopa (Co-administration with some antihypertensives has resulted in symptomatic postural hypotension). Products include:
Aldoclor Tablets 2035
Aldomet Tablets 2037
Aldoril Tablets 2039

Methyldopate Hydrochloride (Co-administration with some antihypertensives has resulted in symptomatic postural hypotension).
No products indexed under this heading.

Metoclopramide Hydrochloride (May increase the bioavailability of levodopa by increasing gastric emptying and also adversely affect disease control by its dopamine receptor antagonistic properties). Products include:
Reglan 2935

Metolazone (Co-administration with some antihypertensives has resulted in symptomatic postural hypotension). Products include:
Mykrox Tablets 1168
Zaroxolyn Tablets 1177

Metoprolol Succinate (Co-administration with some antihypertensives has resulted in symptomatic postural hypotension). Products include:
Toprol-XL Tablets 651

Metoprolol Tartrate (Co-administration with some antihypertensives has resulted in symptomatic postural hypotension).
No products indexed under this heading.

Metyrosine (Co-administration with some antihypertensives has resulted in symptomatic postural hypotension). Products include:
Demser Capsules 2085

Mibefradil Dihydrochloride (Co-administration with some antihypertensives has resulted in symptomatic postural hypotension).
No products indexed under this heading.

Minoxidil (Co-administration with some antihypertensives has resulted in symptomatic postural hypotension). Products include:
Rogaine Extra Strength for Men Topical Solution .... ▣ 721
Rogaine for Women Topical Solution .... ▣ 721

Moexipril Hydrochloride (Co-administration with some antihypertensives has resulted in symptomatic postural hypotension). Products include:
Uniretic Tablets 3178
Univasc Tablets 3181

Molindone Hydrochloride (Co-administration with dopamine D2 receptor antagonists may reduce the therapeutic effects of levodopa). Products include:
Moban 1320

Nadolol (Co-administration with some antihypertensives has resulted in symptomatic postural hypotension). Products include:
Corgard Tablets 2245
Corzide 40/5 Tablets 2247
Corzide 80/5 Tablets 2247
Nadolol Tablets 2288

Nicardipine Hydrochloride (Co-administration with some antihypertensives has resulted in symptomatic postural hypotension). Products include:
Cardene I.V. 3485

Nifedipine (Co-administration with some antihypertensives has resulted in symptomatic postural hypotension). Products include:
Adalat CC Tablets 877
Procardia Capsules 2708
Procardia XL Extended Release Tablets 2710

Nisoldipine (Co-administration with some antihypertensives has resulted in symptomatic postural hypotension). Products include:
Sular Tablets 688

Nitroglycerin (Co-administration with some antihypertensives has resulted in symptomatic postural hypotension). Products include:
Nitro-Dur Transdermal Infusion System 3134
Nitro-Dur Transdermal Infusion System 1834
Nitrolingual Pumpspray 1355
Nitrostat Tablets 2658

Nortriptyline Hydrochloride (Co-administration with tricyclic antidepressants has resulted in rare reports of adverse reactions including hypertension and dyskinesia).
No products indexed under this heading.

Papaverine Hydrochloride (The beneficial effects of levodopa in Parkinson's disease have been reported to be reversed by papaverine).
No products indexed under this heading.

Pargyline Hydrochloride (Concurrent and/or sequential use with nonselective MAO inhibitors is contraindicated).
No products indexed under this heading.

Penbutolol Sulfate (Co-administration with some antihypertensives has resulted in symptomatic postural hypotension).
No products indexed under this heading.

Perindopril Erbumine (Co-administration with some antihypertensives has resulted in symptomatic postural hypotension). Products include:
Aceon Tablets (2 mg, 4 mg, 8 mg) 3249

Perphenazine (Co-administration with dopamine D2 receptor antagonists may reduce the therapeutic effects of levodopa). Products include:
Etrafon 3115
Trilafon 3160

Phenelzine Sulfate (Concurrent and/or sequential use with nonselective MAO inhibitors is contraindicated). Products include:
Nardil Tablets 2653

Phenoxybenzamine Hydrochloride (Co-administration with some antihypertensives has resulted in symptomatic postural hypotension). Products include:
Dibenzyline Capsules 3457

Phentolamine Mesylate (Co-administration with some antihypertensives has resulted in symptomatic postural hypotension).
No products indexed under this heading.

Phenytoin (The beneficial effects of levodopa in Parkinson's disease have been reported to be reversed by phenytoin). Products include:
Dilantin Infatabs 2624
Dilantin-125 Oral Suspension 2625

Phenytoin Sodium (The beneficial effects of levodopa in Parkinson's disease have been reported to be reversed by phenytoin). Products include:
Dilantin Kapseals 2622

Pindolol (Co-administration with some antihypertensives has resulted in symptomatic postural hypotension).
No products indexed under this heading.

Polysaccharide-Iron Complex (Iron salts may reduce the bioavailability of levodopa and carbidopa). Products include:
Niferex 3176
Niferex-150 Capsules 3176
Nu-Iron 150 Capsules 2224

Polythiazide (Co-administration with some antihypertensives has resulted in symptomatic postural hypotension). Products include:
Minizide Capsules 2700
Renese Tablets 2712

Prazosin Hydrochloride (Co-administration with some antihypertensives has resulted in symptomatic postural hypotension). Products include:
Minipress Capsules 2699
Minizide Capsules 2700

Procarbazine Hydrochloride (Concurrent and/or sequential use with nonselective MAO inhibitors is contraindicated). Products include:
Matulane Capsules 3246

Prochlorperazine (Co-administration with dopamine D2 receptor antagonists may reduce the therapeutic effects of levodopa). Products include:
Compazine 1505

Promethazine Hydrochloride (Co-administration with dopamine D2 receptor antagonists may reduce the therapeutic effects of levodopa). Products include:
Mepergan Injection 3539
Phenergan Injection 3553
Phenergan 3556
Phenergan Syrup 3554
Phenergan with Codeine Syrup 3557
Phenergan with Dextromethorphan Syrup 3559
Phenergan VC Syrup 3560
Phenergan VC with Codeine Syrup 3561

Propranolol Hydrochloride (Co-administration with some antihypertensives has resulted in symptomatic postural hypotension). Products include:
Inderal 3513
Inderal LA Long-Acting Capsules 3516
Inderide Tablets 3517
Inderide LA Long-Acting Capsules 3519

Protriptyline Hydrochloride (Co-administration with tricyclic antidepressants has resulted in rare reports of adverse reactions including hypertension and dyskinesia). Products include:
Vivactil Tablets 2446
Vivactil Tablets 2217

Quetiapine Fumarate (Co-administration with dopamine D2 receptor antagonists may reduce the therapeutic effects of levodopa). Products include:
Seroquel Tablets 684

Quinapril Hydrochloride (Co-administration with some antihypertensives has resulted in symptomatic postural hypotension). Products include:
Accupril Tablets 2611
Accuretic Tablets 2614

Ramipril (Co-administration with some antihypertensives has resulted in symptomatic postural hypotension). Products include:
Altace Capsules 2233

Rauwolfia serpentina (Co-administration with some antihypertensives has resulted in symptomatic postural hypotension).
No products indexed under this heading.

Rescinnamine (Co-administration with some antihypertensives has resulted in symptomatic postural hypotension).
No products indexed under this heading.

Reserpine (Co-administration with some antihypertensives has resulted in symptomatic postural hypotension).
No products indexed under this heading.

Risperidone (Co-administration with dopamine D2 receptor antagonists may reduce the therapeutic effects of levodopa). Products include:
Risperdal 1796

Selegiline Hydrochloride (Concomitant therapy with selegiline and carbidopa-levodopa may be associated with severe orthostatic hypotension not attributable to carbidopa-levodopa alone). Products include:
Eldepryl Capsules 3266

Sodium Nitroprusside (Co-administration with some antihypertensives has resulted in symptomatic

postural hypotension).
No products indexed under this heading.

Sotalol Hydrochloride (Co-administration with some antihypertensives has resulted in symptomatic postural hypotension). Products include:
Betapace Tablets 950
Betapace AF Tablets 954

Spirapril Hydrochloride (Co-administration with some antihypertensives has resulted in symptomatic postural hypotension).
No products indexed under this heading.

Telmisartan (Co-administration with some antihypertensives has resulted in symptomatic postural hypotension). Products include:
Micardis Tablets 1049
Micardis HCT Tablets 1051

Terazosin Hydrochloride (Co-administration with some antihypertensives has resulted in symptomatic postural hypotension). Products include:
Hytrin Capsules 464

Thioridazine Hydrochloride (Co-administration with dopamine D2 receptor antagonists may reduce the therapeutic effects of levodopa). Products include:
Thioridazine Hydrochloride Tablets 2289

Thiothixene (Co-administration with dopamine D2 receptor antagonists may reduce the therapeutic effects of levodopa). Products include:
Navane Capsules 2701
Thiothixene Capsules 2290

Timolol Maleate (Co-administration with some antihypertensives has resulted in symptomatic postural hypotension). Products include:
Blocadren Tablets 2046
Cosopt Sterile Ophthalmic Solution 2065
Timolide Tablets 2187
Timolol GFS .... ⊙266
Timoptic in Ocudose 2192
Timoptic Sterile Ophthalmic Solution 2190
Timoptic-XE Sterile Ophthalmic Gel Forming Solution 2194

Torsemide (Co-administration with some antihypertensives has resulted in symptomatic postural hypotension). Products include:
Demadex Tablets and Injection 2965

Trandolapril (Co-administration with some antihypertensives has resulted in symptomatic postural hypotension). Products include:
Mavik Tablets 478
Tarka Tablets 508

Tranylcypromine Sulfate (Concurrent and/or sequential use with non-selective MAO inhibitors is contraindicated). Products include:
Parnate Tablets 1607

Trifluoperazine Hydrochloride (Co-administration with dopamine D2 receptor antagonists may reduce the therapeutic effects of levodopa). Products include:
Stelazine 1640

Trimethaphan Camsylate (Co-administration with some antihypertensives has resulted in symptomatic postural hypotension).
No products indexed under this heading.

Trimipramine Maleate (Co-administration with tricyclic antidepressants has resulted in rare reports of adverse reactions including hypertension and dyskinesia). Products include:
Surmontil Capsules 3595

Valsartan (Co-administration with some antihypertensives has resulted in symptomatic postural hypotension). Products include:
Diovan Capsules 2337
Diovan HCT Tablets 2338

Verapamil Hydrochloride (Co-administration with some antihypertensives has resulted in symptomatic postural hypotension). Products include:
Covera-HS Tablets 3199
Isoptin SR Tablets 467
Tarka Tablets 508
Verelan Capsules 3184
Verelan PM Capsules 3186

Food Interactions

Food, unspecified (The extent of availability and peak concentrations of levodopa after a single dose of Sinemet CR increased by about 50% and 25% respectively when administered with food; foods that are high in protein may delay the absorption of levodopa and may reduce the amount taken up in the circulation).

SINEQUAN CAPSULES

(Doxepin Hydrochloride) 2713
May interact with anticholinergics, drugs that inhibit cytochrome p450iid6, antidepressant drugs, monoamine oxidase inhibitors, phenothiazines, selective serotonin reuptake inhibitors, and certain other agents. Compounds in these categories include:

Amitriptyline Hydrochloride (Concurrent use with drugs that are substrate for cytochrome P450IID6 may make normal metabolizer resemble poor metabolizer leading to higher than expected plasma concentrations of TCA with resultant toxicity). Products include:
Etrafon 3115
Limbitrol 1738

Amoxapine (Concurrent use with drugs that are substrate for cytochrome P450IID6 may make normal metabolizer resemble poor metabolizer leading to higher than expected plasma concentrations of TCA with resultant toxicity).
No products indexed under this heading.

Atropine Sulfate (Caution is advised when co-administered due to doxepin-induced anticholinergic effects). Products include:
Donnatal 2929
Donnatal Extentabs 2930
Motofen Tablets 577
Prosed/DS Tablets 3268
Urised Tablets 2876

Belladonna Alkaloids (Caution is advised when co-administered due to doxepin-induced anticholinergic effects). Products include:
Hyland's Teething Tablets .... ▣766
Urimax Tablets 1769

Benztropine Mesylate (Caution is advised when co-administered due to doxepin-induced anticholinergic effects). Products include:
Cogentin 2055

Biperiden Hydrochloride (Caution is advised when co-administered due to doxepin-induced anticholinergic effects). Products include:
Akineton 402

Bupropion Hydrochloride (Concurrent use with drugs that are substrate for cytochrome P450IID6 may make normal metabolizer resemble poor metabolizer leading to higher than expected plasma concentrations of TCA with resultant toxicity). Products include:
Wellbutrin Tablets 1680
Wellbutrin SR Sustained-Release Tablets 1684
Zyban Sustained-Release Tablets ... 1710

Chlorpromazine (Concurrent use with drugs that are substrate for cytochrome P450IID6 may make normal metabolizer resemble poor metabolizer leading to higher than expected plasma concentrations of TCA with resultant toxicity). Products include:
Thorazine Suppositories 1656

Chlorpromazine Hydrochloride (Concurrent use with drugs that are substrate for cytochrome P450IID6 may make normal metabolizer resemble poor metabolizer leading to higher than expected plasma concentrations of TCA with resultant toxicity). Products include:
Thorazine 1656

Cimetidine (Produces clinically significant fluctuations in steady-state serum concentrations of various tricyclic antidepressants resulting in frequency and severity of side effects, particularly anticholinergic). Products include:
Tagamet HB 200 Suspension .... ▣762
Tagamet HB 200 Tablets .... ▣761
Tagamet Tablets 1644

Cimetidine Hydrochloride (Produces clinically significant fluctuations in steady-state serum concentrations of various tricyclic antidepressants resulting in frequency and severity of side effects, particularly anticholinergic). Products include:
Tagamet 1644

Citalopram Hydrobromide (Concurrent use with drugs that are substrate for cytochrome P450IID6 may make normal metabolizer resemble poor metabolizer leading to higher than expected plasma concentrations of TCA with resultant toxicity; due to variation in the extent of inhibition of P450IID6 caution is indicated if co-administered). Products include:
Celexa 1365

Clidinium Bromide (Caution is advised when co-administered due to doxepin-induced anticholinergic effects).
No products indexed under this heading.

Desipramine Hydrochloride (Concurrent use with drugs that are substrate for cytochrome P450IID6 may make normal metabolizer resemble poor metabolizer leading to higher than expected plasma concentrations of TCA with resultant toxicity). Products include:
Norpramin Tablets 755

Dicyclomine Hydrochloride (Caution is advised when co-administered due to doxepin-induced anticholinergic effects).
No products indexed under this heading.

Flecainide Acetate (Concurrent use with drugs that are substrate for cytochrome P450IID6 may make normal metabolizer resemble poor metabolizer leading to higher than expected plasma concentrations of TCA with resultant toxicity). Products include:
Tambocor Tablets 1990

Fluoxetine Hydrochloride (Concurrent use with drugs that are substrate for cytochrome P450IID6 may make normal metabolizer resemble poor metabolizer leading to higher than expected plasma concentrations of TCA with resultant toxicity; due to variation in the extent of inhibition of P450IID6 caution is indicated if co-administered). Products include:
Prozac Pulvules, Liquid, and Weekly Capsules 1238
Sarafem Pulvules 1962

Fluphenazine Decanoate (Concurrent use with drugs that are substrate for cytochrome P450IID6 may make normal metabolizer resemble poor metabolizer leading to higher than expected plasma concentrations of TCA with resultant toxicity).
No products indexed under this heading.

Fluphenazine Enanthate (Concurrent use with drugs that are substrate for cytochrome P450IID6 may make normal metabolizer resemble poor metabolizer leading to higher than expected plasma concentrations of TCA with resultant toxicity).
No products indexed under this heading.

Fluphenazine Hydrochloride (Concurrent use with drugs that are substrate for cytochrome P450IID6 may make normal metabolizer resemble poor metabolizer leading to higher than expected plasma concentrations of TCA with resultant toxicity).
No products indexed under this heading.

Fluvoxamine Maleate (Concurrent use with drugs that are substrate for cytochrome P450IID6 may make normal metabolizer resemble poor metabolizer leading to higher than expected plasma concentrations of TCA with resultant toxicity; due to variation in the extent of inhibition of P450IID6 caution is indicated if co-administered). Products include:
Luvox Tablets (25, 50, 100 mg) 3256

Glycopyrrolate (Caution is advised when co-administered due to doxepin-induced anticholinergic effects). Products include:
Robinul Forte Tablets 1358
Robinul Injectable 2940
Robinul Tablets 1358

Hyoscyamine (Caution is advised when co-administered due to doxepin-induced anticholinergic effects). Products include:
Urised Tablets 2876

Hyoscyamine Sulfate (Caution is advised when co-administered due to doxepin-induced anticholinergic effects). Products include:
Arco-Lase Plus Tablets 592
Donnatal 2929
Donnatal Extentabs 2930
Levsin/Levsinex/Levbid 3172
NuLev Orally Disintegrating Tablets 3176
Prosed/DS Tablets 3268
Urimax Tablets 1769

Imipramine Hydrochloride (Concurrent use with drugs that are substrate for cytochrome P450IID6 may make normal metabolizer resemble poor metabolizer leading to higher than expected plasma concentrations of TCA with resultant toxicity).
No products indexed under this heading.

Imipramine Pamoate (Concurrent use with drugs that are substrate for cytochrome P450IID6 may make normal metabolizer resemble poor metabolizer leading to higher than expected plasma concentrations of TCA with resultant toxicity).
No products indexed under this heading.

Ipratropium Bromide (Caution is advised when co-administered due to doxepin-induced anticholinergic effects). Products include:
Atrovent Inhalation Aerosol 1030
Atrovent Inhalation Solution 1031
Atrovent Nasal Spray 0.03% 1032
Atrovent Nasal Spray 0.06% 1033
Combivent Inhalation Aerosol 1041
DuoNeb Inhalation Solution 1233

Isocarboxazid (Concurrent use is not recommended; potential for serious adverse effects).
No products indexed under this heading.

Maprotiline Hydrochloride (Concurrent use with drugs that are substrate for cytochrome P450IID6 may make normal metabolizer resemble poor metabolizer leading to higher than expected plasma concentrations of TCA with resultant toxicity).
No products indexed under this heading.

Mepenzolate Bromide (Caution is advised when co-administered due to doxepin-induced anticholinergic effects).
No products indexed under this heading.

Mesoridazine Besylate (Concurrent use with drugs that are substrate for cytochrome P450IID6 may make normal metabolizer resemble poor metabolizer leading to higher than expected plasma concentrations of TCA with resultant toxicity). Products include:
Serentil 1057

Methotrimeprazine (Concurrent use with drugs that are substrate for cytochrome P450IID6 may make normal metabolizer resemble poor metabolizer leading to higher than expected plasma concentrations of TCA with resultant toxicity).
No products indexed under this heading.

Mirtazapine (Concurrent use with drugs that are substrate for cytochrome P450IID6 may make normal metabolizer resemble poor metabolizer leading to higher than expected plasma concentrations of TCA with resultant toxicity). Products include:
Remeron Tablets 2483
Remeron SolTab Tablets 2486

Moclobemide (Concurrent use is not recommended; potential for serious adverse effects).
No products indexed under this heading.

Nefazodone Hydrochloride (Concurrent use with drugs that are substrate for cytochrome P450IID6 may make normal metabolizer resemble poor metabolizer leading to higher than expected plasma concentrations of TCA with resultant toxicity). Products include:
Serzone Tablets 1104

Nortriptyline Hydrochloride (Concurrent use with drugs that are substrate for cytochrome P450IID6 may make normal metabolizer resemble poor metabolizer leading to higher than expected plasma concentrations of TCA with resultant toxicity).
No products indexed under this heading.

Oxybutynin Chloride (Caution is advised when co-administered due to doxepin-induced anticholinergic effects). Products include:
Ditropan XL Extended Release Tablets 564

Pargyline Hydrochloride (Concurrent use is not recommended; potential for serious adverse effects).
No products indexed under this heading.

Paroxetine Hydrochloride (Concurrent use with drugs that are substrate for cytochrome P450IID6 may make normal metabolizer resemble poor metabolizer leading to higher than expected plasma concentrations of TCA with resultant toxicity; due to variation in the extent of inhibition of P450IID6 caution is indicated if co-administered). Products include:
Paxil 1609

Perphenazine (Concurrent use with drugs that are substrate for cytochrome P450IID6 may make normal metabolizer resemble poor metabolizer leading to higher than expected plasma concentrations of TCA with resultant toxicity). Products include:
Etrafon 3115
Trilafon 3160

Phenelzine Sulfate (Concurrent use is not recommended; potential for serious adverse effects). Products include:
Nardil Tablets 2653

Procarbazine Hydrochloride (Concurrent use is not recommended; potential for serious adverse effects). Products include:
Matulane Capsules 3246

Prochlorperazine (Concurrent use with drugs that are substrate for cytochrome P450IID6 may make normal metabolizer resemble poor metabolizer leading to higher than expected plasma concentrations of TCA with resultant toxicity). Products include:
Compazine 1505

Procyclidine Hydrochloride (Caution is advised when co-administered due to doxepin-induced anticholinergic effects).
No products indexed under this heading.

Promethazine Hydrochloride (Concurrent use with drugs that are substrate for cytochrome P450IID6 may make normal metabolizer resemble poor metabolizer leading to higher than expected plasma concentrations of TCA with resultant toxicity). Products include:
Mepergan Injection 3539
Phenergan Injection 3553
Phenergan 3556
Phenergan Syrup 3554
Phenergan with Codeine Syrup 3557
Phenergan with Dextromethorphan Syrup 3559
Phenergan VC Syrup 3560
Phenergan VC with Codeine Syrup 3561

Propafenone Hydrochloride (Concurrent use with drugs that are substrate for cytochrome P450IID6 may make normal metabolizer resemble poor metabolizer leading to higher than expected plasma concentrations of TCA with resultant toxicity). Products include:
Rythmol Tablets – 150 mg, 225 mg, 300 mg 502

Propantheline Bromide (Caution is advised when co-administered due to doxepin-induced anticholinergic effects).
No products indexed under this heading.

Protriptyline Hydrochloride (Concurrent use with drugs that are substrate for cytochrome P450IID6 may make normal metabolizer resemble poor metabolizer leading to higher than expected plasma concentrations of TCA with resultant toxicity). Products include:
Vivactil Tablets 2446
Vivactil Tablets 2217

Quinidine Gluconate (Concurrent use with drugs that inhibit cytochrome P450IID6 may make normal metabolizer resemble poor metabolizer leading to higher than expected plasma concentrations of TCA with resultant toxicity). Products include:
Quinaglute Dura-Tabs Tablets 978

Quinidine Polygalacturonate (Concurrent use with drugs that inhibit cytochrome P450IID6 may make normal metabolizer resemble poor metabolizer leading to higher than expected plasma concentrations of TCA with resultant toxicity).
No products indexed under this heading.

Quinidine Sulfate (Concurrent use with drugs that inhibit cytochrome P450IID6 may make normal metabolizer resemble poor metabolizer leading to higher than expected plasma concentrations of TCA with resultant toxicity). Products include:
Quinidex Extentabs 2933

Scopolamine (Caution is advised when co-administered due to doxepin-induced anticholinergic effects). Products include:
Transderm Scōp Transdermal Therapeutic System 2302

Scopolamine Hydrobromide (Caution is advised when co-administered due to doxepin-induced anticholinergic effects). Products include:
Donnatal 2929
Donnatal Extentabs 2930

Selegiline Hydrochloride (Concurrent use is not recommended; potential for serious adverse effects). Products include:
Eldepryl Capsules 3266

Sertraline Hydrochloride (Concurrent use with drugs that are substrate for cytochrome P450IID6 may make normal metabolizer resemble poor metabolizer leading to higher than expected plasma concentrations of TCA with resultant toxicity; due to variation in the extent of inhibition of P450IID6 caution is indicated if co-administered). Products include:
Zoloft 2751

Thioridazine Hydrochloride (Concurrent use with drugs that are substrate for cytochrome P450IID6 may make normal metabolizer resemble poor metabolizer leading to higher than expected plasma concentrations of TCA with resultant toxicity). Products include:
Thioridazine Hydrochloride Tablets 2289

Tolazamide (A case of severe hypoglycemia has been reported in a type II diabetic patient maintained on tolazamide (1 gm/day) 11 days after the addition of doxepin (75 mg/day)).
No products indexed under this heading.

Tolterodine Tartrate (Caution is advised when co-administered due to doxepin-induced anticholinergic effects). Products include:
Detrol Tablets 3623
Detrol LA Capsules 2801

Tranylcypromine Sulfate (Concurrent use is not recommended; potential for serious adverse effects). Products include:
Parnate Tablets 1607

Trazodone Hydrochloride (Concurrent use with drugs that are substrate for cytochrome P450IID6 may make normal metabolizer resemble poor metabolizer leading to higher than expected plasma concentrations of TCA with resultant toxicity).
No products indexed under this heading.

Tridihexethyl Chloride (Caution is advised when co-administered due to doxepin-induced anticholinergic effects).
No products indexed under this heading.

Trifluoperazine Hydrochloride (Concurrent use with drugs that are substrate for cytochrome P450IID6 may make normal metabolizer resemble poor metabolizer leading to higher than expected plasma concentrations of TCA with resultant toxicity). Products include:
Stelazine 1640

Trihexyphenidyl Hydrochloride (Caution is advised when co-administered due to doxepin-induced anticholinergic effects). Products include:
Artane 1855

Trimipramine Maleate (Concurrent use with drugs that are substrate for cytochrome P450IID6 may make normal metabolizer resemble poor metabolizer leading to higher than expected plasma concentrations of TCA with resultant toxicity). Products include:
Surmontil Capsules 3595

Venlafaxine Hydrochloride (Concurrent use with drugs that are substrate for cytochrome P450IID6 may make normal metabolizer resemble poor metabolizer leading to higher than expected plasma concentrations of TCA with resultant toxicity). Products include:
Effexor Tablets 3495
Effexor XR Capsules 3499

Food Interactions

Alcohol (Doxepin may enhance the response to alcohol).

SINEQUAN ORAL CONCENTRATE

(Doxepin Hydrochloride) 2713
See Sinequan Capsules

SINGLET CAPLETS

(Acetaminophen, Chlorpheniramine Maleate, Pseudoephedrine Hydrochloride) .... ▣761
May interact with hypnotics and sedatives, monoamine oxidase inhibitors, tranquilizers, and certain other agents. Compounds in these categories include:

Alprazolam (May increase drowsiness effect). Products include:
Xanax Tablets 2865

Buspirone Hydrochloride (May increase drowsiness effect).
No products indexed under this heading.

Chlordiazepoxide (May increase drowsiness effect). Products include:
Limbitrol 1738

Chlordiazepoxide Hydrochloride (May increase drowsiness effect). Products include:
Librium Capsules 1736
Librium for Injection 1737

Chlorpromazine (May increase drowsiness effect). Products include:
Thorazine Suppositories 1656

Chlorpromazine Hydrochloride (May increase drowsiness effect). Products include:
Thorazine 1656

Chlorprothixene (May increase drowsiness effect).
No products indexed under this heading.

Chlorprothixene Hydrochloride (May increase drowsiness effect).
No products indexed under this heading.

Clorazepate Dipotassium (May increase drowsiness effect). Products include:
Tranxene 511

Diazepam (May increase drowsiness effect). Products include:
Valium Injectable 3026
Valium Tablets 3047

Droperidol (May increase drowsiness effect).
No products indexed under this heading.

Estazolam (May increase drowsiness effect). Products include:
ProSom Tablets 500

Ethchlorvynol (May increase drowsiness effect).
No products indexed under this heading.

Ethinamate (May increase drowsiness effect).
No products indexed under this heading.

Fluphenazine Decanoate (May increase drowsiness effect).
No products indexed under this heading.

Fluphenazine Enanthate (May increase drowsiness effect).
No products indexed under this heading.

Fluphenazine Hydrochloride (May increase drowsiness effect).
No products indexed under this heading.

Flurazepam Hydrochloride (May increase drowsiness effect).
No products indexed under this heading.

Glutethimide (May increase drowsiness effect).
No products indexed under this heading.

Haloperidol (May increase drowsiness effect). Products include:
Haldol Injection, Tablets and Concentrate 2533

Haloperidol Decanoate (May increase drowsiness effect). Products include:
Haldol Decanoate 2535

Hydroxyzine Hydrochloride (May increase drowsiness effect). Products include:
Atarax Tablets & Syrup 2667
Vistaril Intramuscular Solution 2738

Isocarboxazid (Concurrent and/or sequential use with MAO inhibitors is not recommended).
No products indexed under this heading.

Lorazepam (May increase drowsiness effect). Products include:
Ativan Injection 3478
Ativan Tablets 3482

Loxapine Hydrochloride (May increase drowsiness effect).
No products indexed under this heading.

Loxapine Succinate (May increase drowsiness effect). Products include:
Loxitane Capsules 3398

Meprobamate (May increase drowsiness effect). Products include:
Miltown Tablets 3349

Mesoridazine Besylate (May increase drowsiness effect). Products include:
Serentil 1057

Midazolam Hydrochloride (May increase drowsiness effect). Products include:
Versed Injection 3027
Versed Syrup 3033

Moclobemide (Concurrent and/or sequential use with MAO inhibitors is not recommended).
No products indexed under this heading.

Molindone Hydrochloride (May increase drowsiness effect). Products include:
Moban 1320

Oxazepam (May increase drowsiness effect).
No products indexed under this heading.

Pargyline Hydrochloride (Concurrent and/or sequential use with MAO inhibitors is not recommended).
No products indexed under this heading.

Perphenazine (May increase drowsiness effect). Products include:
Etrafon 3115
Trilafon 3160

Phenelzine Sulfate (Concurrent and/or sequential use with MAO inhibitors is not recommended). Products include:
Nardil Tablets 2653

Prazepam (May increase drowsiness effect).
No products indexed under this heading.

Procarbazine Hydrochloride (Concurrent and/or sequential use with MAO inhibitors is not recommended). Products include:
Matulane Capsules 3246

Prochlorperazine (May increase drowsiness effect). Products include:
Compazine 1505

Promethazine Hydrochloride (May increase drowsiness effect). Products include:
Mepergan Injection 3539
Phenergan Injection 3553
Phenergan 3556
Phenergan Syrup 3554
Phenergan with Codeine Syrup 3557
Phenergan with Dextromethorphan Syrup 3559
Phenergan VC Syrup 3560
Phenergan VC with Codeine Syrup 3561

Propofol (May increase drowsiness effect). Products include:
Diprivan Injectable Emulsion 667

Quazepam (May increase drowsiness effect).
No products indexed under this heading.

Secobarbital Sodium (May increase drowsiness effect).
No products indexed under this heading.

Selegiline Hydrochloride (Concurrent and/or sequential use with MAO inhibitors is not recommended). Products include:
Eldepryl Capsules 3266

Temazepam (May increase drowsiness effect).
No products indexed under this heading.

Thioridazine Hydrochloride (May increase drowsiness effect). Products include:
Thioridazine Hydrochloride Tablets 2289

Thiothixene (May increase drowsiness effect). Products include:
Navane Capsules 2701
Thiothixene Capsules 2290

Tranylcypromine Sulfate (Concurrent and/or sequential use with MAO inhibitors is not recommended). Products include:
Parnate Tablets 1607

Triazolam (May increase drowsiness effect). Products include:
Halcion Tablets 2823

Trifluoperazine Hydrochloride (May increase drowsiness effect). Products include:
Stelazine 1640

Zaleplon (May increase drowsiness effect). Products include:
Sonata Capsules 3591

Zolpidem Tartrate (May increase drowsiness effect). Products include:
Ambien Tablets 3191

Food Interactions

Alcohol (Chronic heavy alcohol users, 3 or more drinks per day, should consult their physicians for advice on when and how they should take pain relievers/fever reducers including acetaminophen; increases drowsiness effect).

SINGULAIR TABLETS

(Montelukast Sodium) 2181
May interact with:

Phenobarbital (Induces hepatic metabolism and decreases the AUC of montelukast approximately 40%; no dosage adjustment for Singulair is recommended). Products include:
Arco-Lase Plus Tablets 592
Donnatal 2929
Donnatal Extentabs 2930

Rifampin (Co-administration with CYP450 enzyme inducers, such as rifampin, may alter metabolism of montelukast; it is reasonable to employ appropriate clinical monitoring). Products include:
Rifadin 765
Rifamate Capsules 767
Rifater Tablets 769

SINGULAIR CHEWABLE TABLETS

(Montelukast Sodium) 2181
See Singulair Tablets

SINUTAB NON-DRYING LIQUID CAPS

(Guaifenesin, Pseudoephedrine Hydrochloride) 706
May interact with monoamine oxidase inhibitors. Compounds in these categories include:

Isocarboxazid (Concurrent and/or sequential use not recommended).
No products indexed under this heading.

Moclobemide (Concurrent and/or sequential use not recommended).
No products indexed under this heading.

Pargyline Hydrochloride (Concurrent and/or sequential use not recommended).
No products indexed under this heading.

Phenelzine Sulfate (Concurrent and/or sequential use not recommended). Products include:
Nardil Tablets 2653

Procarbazine Hydrochloride (Concurrent and/or sequential use not recommended). Products include:
Matulane Capsules 3246

Selegiline Hydrochloride (Concurrent and/or sequential use not recommended). Products include:
Eldepryl Capsules 3266

Tranylcypromine Sulfate (Concurrent and/or sequential use not recommended). Products include:
Parnate Tablets 1607

SINUTAB SINUS ALLERGY MEDICATION, MAXIMUM STRENGTH FORMULA, TABLETS & CAPLETS

(Acetaminophen, Chlorpheniramine Maleate, Pseudoephedrine Hydrochloride) 707
May interact with hypnotics and sedatives, monoamine oxidase inhibitors, tranquilizers, and certain other agents. Compounds in these categories include:

Alprazolam (May increase drowsiness effect). Products include:
Xanax Tablets 2865

Buspirone Hydrochloride (May increase drowsiness effect).
No products indexed under this heading.

Chlordiazepoxide (May increase drowsiness effect). Products include:
Limbitrol 1738

Chlordiazepoxide Hydrochloride (May increase drowsiness effect). Products include:
Librium Capsules 1736
Librium for Injection 1737

Chlorpromazine (May increase drowsiness effect). Products include:
Thorazine Suppositories 1656

Chlorpromazine Hydrochloride (May increase drowsiness effect). Products include:
Thorazine 1656

Chlorprothixene (May increase drowsiness effect).
No products indexed under this heading.

Chlorprothixene Hydrochloride (May increase drowsiness effect).
No products indexed under this heading.

Clorazepate Dipotassium (May increase drowsiness effect). Products include:
Tranxene 511

Diazepam (May increase drowsiness effect). Products include:
Valium Injectable 3026
Valium Tablets 3047

Droperidol (May increase drowsiness effect).
No products indexed under this heading.

Estazolam (May increase drowsiness effect). Products include:
ProSom Tablets 500

Ethchlorvynol (May increase drowsiness effect).
No products indexed under this heading.

Ethinamate (May increase drowsiness effect).
No products indexed under this heading.

Fluphenazine Decanoate (May increase drowsiness effect).
No products indexed under this heading.

Fluphenazine Enanthate (May increase drowsiness effect).
No products indexed under this heading.

Fluphenazine Hydrochloride (May increase drowsiness effect).
No products indexed under this heading.

Flurazepam Hydrochloride (May increase drowsiness effect).
No products indexed under this heading.

Glutethimide (May increase drowsiness effect).
No products indexed under this heading.

Haloperidol (May increase drowsiness effect). Products include:
Haldol Injection, Tablets and Concentrate 2533

Haloperidol Decanoate (May increase drowsiness effect). Products include:
Haldol Decanoate 2535

Hydroxyzine Hydrochloride (May increase drowsiness effect). Products include:
Atarax Tablets & Syrup 2667
Vistaril Intramuscular Solution 2738

Isocarboxazid (Concurrent and/or sequential use is not recommended).
No products indexed under this heading.

Lorazepam (May increase drowsiness effect). Products include:
Ativan Injection 3478
Ativan Tablets 3482

Loxapine Hydrochloride (May increase drowsiness effect).
No products indexed under this heading.

Loxapine Succinate (May increase drowsiness effect). Products include:
Loxitane Capsules 3398

Meprobamate (May increase drowsiness effect). Products include:
Miltown Tablets 3349

Mesoridazine Besylate (May increase drowsiness effect). Products include:
Serentil 1057

Midazolam Hydrochloride (May increase drowsiness effect). Products include:
Versed Injection 3027
Versed Syrup 3033

Moclobemide (Concurrent and/or sequential use is not recommended).
No products indexed under this heading.

Molindone Hydrochloride (May increase drowsiness effect). Products include:
Moban 1320

Oxazepam (May increase drowsiness effect).
No products indexed under this heading.

Pargyline Hydrochloride (Concurrent and/or sequential use is not recommended).
No products indexed under this heading.

Perphenazine (May increase drowsiness effect). Products include:
Etrafon 3115
Trilafon 3160

Phenelzine Sulfate (Concurrent and/or sequential use is not recommended). Products include:
- Nardil Tablets 2653

Prazepam (May increase drowsiness effect).
- No products indexed under this heading.

Procarbazine Hydrochloride (Concurrent and/or sequential use is not recommended). Products include:
- Matulane Capsules 3246

Prochlorperazine (May increase drowsiness effect). Products include:
- Compazine 1505

Promethazine Hydrochloride (May increase drowsiness effect). Products include:
- Mepergan Injection 3539
- Phenergan Injection 3553
- Phenergan 3556
- Phenergan Syrup 3554
- Phenergan with Codeine Syrup 3557
- Phenergan with Dextromethorphan Syrup 3559
- Phenergan VC Syrup 3560
- Phenergan VC with Codeine Syrup 3561

Propofol (May increase drowsiness effect). Products include:
- Diprivan Injectable Emulsion 667

Quazepam (May increase drowsiness effect).
- No products indexed under this heading.

Secobarbital Sodium (May increase drowsiness effect).
- No products indexed under this heading.

Selegiline Hydrochloride (Concurrent and/or sequential use is not recommended). Products include:
- Eldepryl Capsules 3266

Temazepam (May increase drowsiness effect).
- No products indexed under this heading.

Thioridazine Hydrochloride (May increase drowsiness effect). Products include:
- Thioridazine Hydrochloride Tablets 2289

Thiothixene (May increase drowsiness effect). Products include:
- Navane Capsules 2701
- Thiothixene Capsules 2290

Tranylcypromine Sulfate (Concurrent and/or sequential use is not recommended). Products include:
- Parnate Tablets 1607

Triazolam (May increase drowsiness effect). Products include:
- Halcion Tablets 2823

Trifluoperazine Hydrochloride (May increase drowsiness effect). Products include:
- Stelazine 1640

Zaleplon (May increase drowsiness effect). Products include:
- Sonata Capsules 3591

Zolpidem Tartrate (May increase drowsiness effect). Products include:
- Ambien Tablets 3191

Food Interactions

Alcohol (May increase drowsiness effect; patients consuming 3 or more alcoholic beverages a day should consult a physician for advice on when and how they should take this medication).

SINUTAB SINUS MEDICATION, MAXIMUM STRENGTH WITHOUT DROWSINESS FORMULA, TABLETS & CAPLETS

(Acetaminophen, Pseudoephedrine Hydrochloride) .... ▣707

May interact with monoamine oxidase inhibitors. Compounds in these categories include:

Isocarboxazid (Concurrent and/or sequential use is not recommended).
- No products indexed under this heading.

Moclobemide (Concurrent and/or sequential use is not recommended).
- No products indexed under this heading.

Pargyline Hydrochloride (Concurrent and/or sequential use is not recommended).
- No products indexed under this heading.

Phenelzine Sulfate (Concurrent and/or sequential use is not recommended). Products include:
- Nardil Tablets 2653

Procarbazine Hydrochloride (Concurrent and/or sequential use is not recommended). Products include:
- Matulane Capsules 3246

Selegiline Hydrochloride (Concurrent and/or sequential use is not recommended). Products include:
- Eldepryl Capsules 3266

Tranylcypromine Sulfate (Concurrent and/or sequential use is not recommended). Products include:
- Parnate Tablets 1607

Food Interactions

Alcohol (Patients consuming 3 or more alcohol-containing drinks per day should consult physician for advice on when and how they should take this product).

SKELAXIN TABLETS

(Metaxalone) 1301

None cited in PDR database.

SKELID TABLETS

(Tiludronate Disodium) 3088

May interact with antacids containing aluminum, calcium and magnesium, calcium preparations, and certain other agents. Compounds in these categories include:

Aluminum Carbonate (Some aluminum- or magnesium-containing antacids decrease bioavailability by 60% when administered 1 hour before Skelid; these antacids should be taken, if needed, at least 2 hours after taking Skelid).
- No products indexed under this heading.

Aluminum Hydroxide (Some aluminum- or magnesium-containing antacids decrease bioavailability by 60% when administered 1 hour before Skelid; these antacids should be taken, if needed, at least 2 hours after taking Skelid). Products include:
- Amphojel Suspension (Mint Flavor) .... ▣789
- Gaviscon Extra Strength Liquid .... ▣751
- Gaviscon Extra Strength Tablets .... ▣751
- Gaviscon Regular Strength Liquid .... ▣751
- Gaviscon Regular Strength Tablets .... ▣750
- Maalox Antacid/Anti-Gas Oral Suspension .... ▣673
- Maalox Max Maximum Strength Antacid/Anti-Gas Liquid 2300
- Maalox Regular Strength Antacid/Antigas Liquid 2300
- Mylanta 1813
- Vanquish Caplets .... ▣617

Aspirin (May decrease bioavailability by up to 50% when taken 2 hours after Skelid; aspirin should not be taken within 2 hours before or 2 hours after Skelid). Products include:
- Aggrenox Capsules 1026
- Alka-Seltzer .... ▣603
- Alka-Seltzer Lemon Lime Antacid and Pain Reliever Effervescent Tablets .... ▣603
- Alka-Seltzer Extra Strength Antacid and Pain Reliever Effervescent Tablets .... ▣603
- Alka-Seltzer PM Effervescent Tablets .... ▣605
- Genuine Bayer Tablets, Caplets and Gelcaps .... ▣606
- Extra Strength Bayer Caplets and Gelcaps .... ▣610
- Aspirin Regimen Bayer Children's Chewable Tablets (Orange or Cherry Flavored) .... ▣607
- Bayer, Aspirin Regimen .... ▣606
- Aspirin Regimen Bayer 81 mg Caplets with Calcium .... ▣607
- Genuine Bayer Professional Labeling (Aspirin Regimen Bayer) .... ▣608
- Extra Strength Bayer Arthritis Caplets .... ▣610
- Extra Strength Bayer Plus Caplets .... ▣610
- Extra Strength Bayer PM Caplets .... ▣611
- BC Powder .... ▣619
- BC Allergy Sinus Cold Powder .... ▣619
- Arthritis Strength BC Powder .... ▣619
- BC Sinus Cold Powder .... ▣619
- Darvon Compound-65 Pulvules 1910
- Ecotrin Enteric Coated Aspirin Low, Regular and Maximum Strength Tablets 1715
- Excedrin Extra-Strength Tablets, Caplets, and Geltabs .... ▣629
- Excedrin Migraine 1070
- Goody's Body Pain Formula Powder .... ▣620
- Goody's Extra Strength Headache Powder .... ▣620
- Goody's Extra Strength Pain Relief Tablets .... ▣620
- Percodan Tablets 1327
- Robaxisal Tablets 2939
- Soma Compound Tablets 3354
- Soma Compound w/Codeine Tablets 3355
- Vanquish Caplets .... ▣617

Calcium Carbonate (Decreases bioavailability by 80% when Skelid and calcium are administered at the same time; calcium supplements should not be taken within 2 hours before or 2 hours after Skelid, however, adequate calcium and vitamin D intake should be maintained). Products include:
- Aspirin Regimen Bayer 81 mg Caplets with Calcium .... ▣607
- Extra Strength Bayer Plus Caplets .... ▣610
- Caltrate 600 Tablets .... ▣814
- Caltrate 600 PLUS .... ▣815
- Caltrate 600 + D Tablets .... ▣814
- Caltrate 600 + Soy Tablets .... ▣814
- D-Cal Chewable Caplets .... ▣794
- Florical Capsules and Tablets 2223
- Quick Dissolve Maalox Max Maximum Strength Antacid/Antigas Tablets 2301
- Quick Dissolve Maalox Regular Strength Antacid Tablets 2301
- Marblen Suspension .... ▣633
- Monocal Tablets 2223
- Mylanta Fast-Acting 1813
- Mylanta Calci Tabs .... ▣636
- One-A-Day Bedtime & Rest Tablets .... ▣805
- One-A-Day Calcium Plus Chewable Tablets .... ▣805
- Os-Cal Chewable Tablets .... ▣838
- Pepcid Complete Chewable Tablets 1815
- ReSource Wellness CalciWise Soft Chews .... ▣824
- Rolaids Tablets .... ▣706
- Extra Strength Rolaids Tablets .... ▣706
- Slow-Mag Tablets .... ▣835
- Titralac .... ▣640
- 3M Titralac Plus Antacid Tablets .... ▣640
- Tums .... ▣763

Calcium Chloride (Decreases bioavailability by 80% when Skelid and calcium are administered at the same time; calcium supplements should not be taken within 2 hours before or 2 hours after Skelid, however, adequate calcium and vitamin D intake should be maintained).
- No products indexed under this heading.

Calcium Citrate (Decreases bioavailability by 80% when Skelid and calcium are administered at the same time; calcium supplements should not be taken within 2 hours before or 2 hours after Skelid, however, adequate calcium and vitamin D intake should be maintained). Products include:
- Active Calcium Tablets 3335
- Citracal Liquitab Tablets .... ▣823
- Citracal Tablets 2231
- Citracal Caplets + D .... ▣823

Calcium Glubionate (Decreases bioavailability by 80% when Skelid and calcium are administered at the same time; calcium supplements should not be taken within 2 hours before or 2 hours after Skelid, however, adequate calcium and vitamin D intake should be maintained).
- No products indexed under this heading.

Indomethacin (Increases bioavailability by 2-4 fold; indomethacin should not be taken within 2 hours before or 2 hours after Skelid). Products include:
- Indocin 2112

Magaldrate (Some aluminum- or magnesium-containing antacids decrease bioavailability by 60% when administered 1 hour before Skelid; these antacids should be taken, if needed, at least 2 hours after taking Skelid).
- No products indexed under this heading.

Magnesium Hydroxide (Some aluminum- or magnesium-containing antacids decrease bioavailability by 60% when administered 1 hour before Skelid; these antacids should be taken, if needed, at least 2 hours after taking Skelid). Products include:
- Ex•Lax Milk of Magnesia Liquid .... ▣670
- Maalox Antacid/Anti-Gas Oral Suspension .... ▣673
- Maalox Max Maximum Strength Antacid/Anti-Gas Liquid 2300
- Maalox Regular Strength Antacid/Antigas Liquid 2300
- Mylanta Fast-Acting 1813
- Mylanta 1813
- Pepcid Complete Chewable Tablets 1815
- Phillips' Chewable Tablets .... ▣615
- Phillips' Milk of Magnesia Liquid (Original, Cherry, & Mint) .... ▣616
- Rolaids Tablets .... ▣706
- Extra Strength Rolaids Tablets .... ▣706
- Vanquish Caplets .... ▣617

Magnesium Oxide (Some aluminum- or magnesium-containing antacids decrease bioavailability by 60% when administered 1 hour before Skelid; these antacids should be taken, if needed, at least 2 hours after taking Skelid). Products include:
- Beelith Tablets 946
- Mag-Ox 400 Tablets 1024
- Uro-Mag Capsules 1024

Food Interactions

Food, unspecified (Reduces bioavailability by 90% when an oral dose equivalent to 400 mg tiludronic acid was administered with, or 2 hours after, a standard breakfast compared to the same dose administered after an overnight fast and 4 hours before a standard breakfast; Skelid should not be taken within 2 hours of food).

SLEEP-TITE CAPLETS

(Herbals, Multiple) .... ▣850

May interact with antidepressant drugs, hypnotics and sedatives, monoamine oxidase inhibitors, and certain other agents. Compounds in these categories include:

Amitriptyline Hydrochloride (Concurrent use with antidepressants is not recommended unless directed by physician). Products include:
- Etrafon 3115
- Limbitrol 1738

Amoxapine (Concurrent use with antidepressants is not recommended unless directed by physician).
- No products indexed under this heading.

Bupropion Hydrochloride (Concurrent use with antidepressants is not recommended unless directed by physician). Products include:
- Wellbutrin Tablets 1680
- Wellbutrin SR Sustained-Release Tablets 1684

Zyban Sustained-Release Tablets ... 1710

Citalopram Hydrobromide (Concurrent use with antidepressants is not recommended unless directed by physician). Products include:

Celexa ... 1365

Desipramine Hydrochloride (Concurrent use with antidepressants is not recommended unless directed by physician). Products include:

Norpramin Tablets ... 755

Doxepin Hydrochloride (Concurrent use with antidepressants is not recommended unless directed by physician). Products include:

Sinequan ... 2713

Estazolam (Concurrent use with hypnotic or sedative is not recommended unless directed by physician). Products include:

ProSom Tablets ... 500

Ethchlorvynol (Concurrent use with hypnotic or sedative is not recommended unless directed by physician).

No products indexed under this heading.

Ethinamate (Concurrent use with hypnotic or sedative is not recommended unless directed by physician).

No products indexed under this heading.

Fluoxetine Hydrochloride (Concurrent use with antidepressants is not recommended unless directed by physician). Products include:

Prozac Pulvules, Liquid, and Weekly Capsules ... 1238
Sarafem Pulvules ... 1962

Flurazepam Hydrochloride (Concurrent use with hypnotic or sedative is not recommended unless directed by physician).

No products indexed under this heading.

Glutethimide (Concurrent use with hypnotic or sedative is not recommended unless directed by physician).

No products indexed under this heading.

Imipramine Hydrochloride (Concurrent use with antidepressants is not recommended unless directed by physician).

No products indexed under this heading.

Imipramine Pamoate (Concurrent use with antidepressants is not recommended unless directed by physician).

No products indexed under this heading.

Isocarboxazid (Concurrent use with monoamine oxidase inhibitors is not recommended).

No products indexed under this heading.

Lorazepam (Concurrent use with hypnotic or sedative is not recommended unless directed by physician). Products include:

Ativan Injection ... 3478
Ativan Tablets ... 3482

Maprotiline Hydrochloride (Concurrent use with antidepressants is not recommended unless directed by physician).

No products indexed under this heading.

Midazolam Hydrochloride (Concurrent use with hypnotic or sedative is not recommended unless directed by physician). Products include:

Versed Injection ... 3027
Versed Syrup ... 3033

Mirtazapine (Concurrent use with antidepressants is not recommended unless directed by physician). Products include:

Remeron Tablets ... 2483
Remeron SolTab Tablets ... 2486

Moclobemide (Concurrent use with monoamine oxidase inhibitors is not recommended).

No products indexed under this heading.

Nefazodone Hydrochloride (Concurrent use with antidepressants is not recommended unless directed by physician). Products include:

Serzone Tablets ... 1104

Nortriptyline Hydrochloride (Concurrent use with antidepressants is not recommended unless directed by physician).

No products indexed under this heading.

Pargyline Hydrochloride (Concurrent use with monoamine oxidase inhibitors is not recommended).

No products indexed under this heading.

Paroxetine Hydrochloride (Concurrent use with antidepressants is not recommended unless directed by physician). Products include:

Paxil ... 1609

Phenelzine Sulfate (Concurrent use with monoamine oxidase inhibitors is not recommended). Products include:

Nardil Tablets ... 2653

Procarbazine Hydrochloride (Concurrent use with monoamine oxidase inhibitors is not recommended). Products include:

Matulane Capsules ... 3246

Propofol (Concurrent use with hypnotic or sedative is not recommended unless directed by physician). Products include:

Diprivan Injectable Emulsion ... 667

Protriptyline Hydrochloride (Concurrent use with antidepressants is not recommended unless directed by physician). Products include:

Vivactil Tablets ... 2446
Vivactil Tablets ... 2217

Quazepam (Concurrent use with hypnotic or sedative is not recommended unless directed by physician).

No products indexed under this heading.

Secobarbital Sodium (Concurrent use with hypnotic or sedative is not recommended unless directed by physician).

No products indexed under this heading.

Selegiline Hydrochloride (Concurrent use with monoamine oxidase inhibitors is not recommended). Products include:

Eldepryl Capsules ... 3266

Sertraline Hydrochloride (Concurrent use with antidepressants is not recommended unless directed by physician). Products include:

Zoloft ... 2751

Temazepam (Concurrent use with hypnotic or sedative is not recommended unless directed by physician).

No products indexed under this heading.

Tranylcypromine Sulfate (Concurrent use with monoamine oxidase inhibitors is not recommended). Products include:

Parnate Tablets ... 1607

Trazodone Hydrochloride (Concurrent use with antidepressants is not recommended unless directed by physician).

No products indexed under this heading.

Triazolam (Concurrent use with hypnotic or sedative is not recommended unless directed by physician). Products include:

Halcion Tablets ... 2823

Trimipramine Maleate (Concurrent use with antidepressants is not recommended unless directed by physician). Products include:

Surmontil Capsules ... 3595

Venlafaxine Hydrochloride (Concurrent use with antidepressants is not recommended unless directed by physician). Products include:

Effexor Tablets ... 3495
Effexor XR Capsules ... 3499

Zaleplon (Concurrent use with hypnotic or sedative is not recommended unless directed by physician). Products include:

Sonata Capsules ... 3591

Zolpidem Tartrate (Concurrent use with hypnotic or sedative is not recommended unless directed by physician). Products include:

Ambien Tablets ... 3191

Food Interactions

Alcohol (Concurrent use is not recommended).

SLOW FE TABLETS

(Ferrous Sulfate) ... 827

May interact with tetracyclines. Compounds in these categories include:

Demeclocycline Hydrochloride (Absorption of oral tetracycline impaired). Products include:

Declomycin Tablets ... 1855

Doxycycline Calcium (Absorption of oral tetracycline impaired). Products include:

Vibramycin Calcium Oral Suspension Syrup ... 2735

Doxycycline Hyclate (Absorption of oral tetracycline impaired). Products include:

Doryx Coated Pellet Filled Capsules ... 3357
Periostat Tablets ... 1208
Vibramycin Hyclate Capsules ... 2735
Vibramycin Hyclate Intravenous ... 2737
Vibra-Tabs Film Coated Tablets ... 2735

Doxycycline Monohydrate (Absorption of oral tetracycline impaired). Products include:

Monodox Capsules ... 2442
Vibramycin Monohydrate for Oral Suspension ... 2735

Methacycline Hydrochloride (Absorption of oral tetracycline impaired).

No products indexed under this heading.

Minocycline Hydrochloride (Absorption of oral tetracycline impaired). Products include:

Dynacin Capsules ... 2019
Minocin Intravenous ... 1862
Minocin Oral Suspension ... 1865
Minocin Pellet-Filled Capsules ... 1863

Oxytetracycline (Absorption of oral tetracycline impaired).

No products indexed under this heading.

Oxytetracycline Hydrochloride (Absorption of oral tetracycline impaired). Products include:

Terra-Cortril Ophthalmic Suspension ... 2716
Urobiotic-250 Capsules ... 2731

Tetracycline Hydrochloride (Absorption of oral tetracycline impaired).

No products indexed under this heading.

SLOW FE WITH FOLIC ACID TABLETS

(Ferrous Sulfate, Folic Acid) ... 828

May interact with tetracyclines. Compounds in these categories include:

Demeclocycline Hydrochloride (Oral iron products interfere with oral absorption of tetracycline; do not take within two hours of each other). Products include:

Declomycin Tablets ... 1855

Doxycycline Calcium (Oral iron products interfere with oral absorption of tetracycline; do not take within two hours of each other). Products include:

Vibramycin Calcium Oral Suspension Syrup ... 2735

Doxycycline Hyclate (Oral iron products interfere with oral absorption of tetracycline; do not take within two hours of each other). Products include:

Doryx Coated Pellet Filled Capsules ... 3357
Periostat Tablets ... 1208
Vibramycin Hyclate Capsules ... 2735
Vibramycin Hyclate Intravenous ... 2737
Vibra-Tabs Film Coated Tablets ... 2735

Doxycycline Monohydrate (Oral iron products interfere with oral absorption of tetracycline; do not take within two hours of each other). Products include:

Monodox Capsules ... 2442
Vibramycin Monohydrate for Oral Suspension ... 2735

Methacycline Hydrochloride (Oral iron products interfere with oral absorption of tetracycline; do not take within two hours of each other).

No products indexed under this heading.

Minocycline Hydrochloride (Oral iron products interfere with oral absorption of tetracycline; do not take within two hours of each other). Products include:

Dynacin Capsules ... 2019
Minocin Intravenous ... 1862
Minocin Oral Suspension ... 1865
Minocin Pellet-Filled Capsules ... 1863

Oxytetracycline Hydrochloride (Oral iron products interfere with oral absorption of tetracycline; do not take within two hours of each other). Products include:

Terra-Cortril Ophthalmic Suspension ... 2716
Urobiotic-250 Capsules ... 2731

Tetracycline Hydrochloride (Oral iron products interfere with oral absorption of tetracycline; do not take within two hours of each other).

No products indexed under this heading.

SLOW-MAG TABLETS

(Calcium Carbonate, Magnesium Chloride) ... 835

None cited in PDR database.

SMILE'S PRID SALVE

(Homeopathic Formulations) ... 766

None cited in PDR database.

SOLAQUIN FORTE 4% CREAM

(Dioxybenzone, Hydroquinone, Oxybenzone, Padimate O (Octyl Dimethyl Paba)) ... 1734

None cited in PDR database.

SOLAQUIN FORTE 4% GEL

(Dioxybenzone, Hydroquinone, Padimate O (Octyl Dimethyl Paba)) ... 1734

None cited in PDR database.

SOLU-MEDROL STERILE POWDER

(Methylprednisolone Sodium Succinate) ... 2855

May interact with oral anticoagulants, phenytoin, and certain other agents. Compounds in these categories include:

Aspirin (Methylprednisolone may increase the clearance of chronic high dose aspirin; potential for decreased salicylate serum levels of increased risk of salicylate toxicity when methylprednisolone is withdrawn; aspirin should be used cau-

tiously in conjunction with corticosteroids in patients with hypoprothrombinemia). Products include:

- Aggrenox Capsules 1026
- Alka-Seltzer .... ▣603
- Alka-Seltzer Lemon Lime Antacid and Pain Reliever Effervescent Tablets .... ▣603
- Alka-Seltzer Extra Strength Antacid and Pain Reliever Effervescent Tablets .... ▣603
- Alka-Seltzer PM Effervescent Tablets .... ▣605
- Genuine Bayer Tablets, Caplets and Gelcaps .... ▣606
- Extra Strength Bayer Caplets and Gelcaps .... ▣610
- Aspirin Regimen Bayer Children's Chewable Tablets (Orange or Cherry Flavored) .... ▣607
- Bayer, Aspirin Regimen .... ▣606
- Aspirin Regimen Bayer 81 mg Caplets with Calcium .... ▣607
- Genuine Bayer Professional Labeling (Aspirin Regimen Bayer) .... ▣608
- Extra Strength Bayer Arthritis Caplets .... ▣610
- Extra Strength Bayer Plus Caplets .... ▣610
- Extra Strength Bayer PM Caplets .. ▣611
- BC Powder .... ▣619
- BC Allergy Sinus Cold Powder .... ▣619
- Arthritis Strength BC Powder .... ▣619
- BC Sinus Cold Powder .... ▣619
- Darvon Compound-65 Pulvules 1910
- Ecotrin Enteric Coated Aspirin Low, Regular and Maximum Strength Tablets 1715
- Excedrin Extra-Strength Tablets, Caplets, and Geltabs .... ▣629
- Excedrin Migraine 1070
- Goody's Body Pain Formula Powder .... ▣620
- Goody's Extra Strength Headache Powder .... ▣620
- Goody's Extra Strength Pain Relief Tablets .... ▣620
- Percodan Tablets 1327
- Robaxisal Tablets 2939
- Soma Compound Tablets 3354
- Soma Compound w/Codeine Tablets 3355
- Vanquish Caplets .... ▣617

Cyclosporine (Mutual inhibition of metabolism occurs with concurrent use of cyclosporine and methylprednisolone; convulsions have been reported with co-administration). Products include:

- Gengraf Capsules 457
- Neoral Soft Gelatin Capsules 2380
- Neoral Oral Solution 2380
- Sandimmune 2388

Dicumarol (The effect of methylprednisolone on oral anticoagulants is variable; there are reports of enhanced as well as diminished effects of anticoagulants when given concurrently with corticosteroids).

No products indexed under this heading.

Fosphenytoin Sodium (Drugs that induce hepatic enzymes, such as phenytoin, may increase the clearance of methylprednisolone and may require increases in methylprednisolone dose to achieve the desired response). Products include:

- Cerebyx Injection 2619

Ketoconazole (May inhibit the metabolism of methylprednisolone and thus decrease its clearance; therefore, the dose of methylprednisolone should be titrated to avoid steroid toxicity). Products include:

- Nizoral 2% Cream 3620
- Nizoral A-D Shampoo 2008
- Nizoral 2% Shampoo 2007
- Nizoral Tablets 1791

Phenobarbital (Drugs that induce hepatic enzymes, such as phenobarbital, may increase the clearance of methylprednisolone and may require increases in methylprednisolone dose to achieve the desired response). Products include:

- Arco-Lase Plus Tablets 592
- Donnatal 2929
- Donnatal Extentabs 2930

Phenytoin (Drugs that induce hepatic enzymes, such as phenytoin, may increase the clearance of methylprednisolone and may require increases in methylprednisolone dose to achieve the desired response). Products include:

- Dilantin Infatabs 2624
- Dilantin-125 Oral Suspension 2625

Phenytoin Sodium (Drugs that induce hepatic enzymes, such as phenytoin, may increase the clearance of methylprednisolone and may require increases in methylprednisolone dose to achieve the desired response). Products include:

- Dilantin Kapseals 2622

Rifampin (Drugs that induce hepatic enzymes, such as rifampin, may increase the clearance of methylprednisolone and may require increases in methylprednisolone dose to achieve the desired response). Products include:

- Rifadin 765
- Rifamate Capsules 767
- Rifater Tablets 769

Troleandomycin (May inhibit the metabolism of methylprednisolone and thus decrease its clearance; therefore, the dose of methylprednisolone should be titrated to avoid steroid toxicity). Products include:

- Tao Capsules 2716

Warfarin Sodium (The effect of methylprednisolone on oral anticoagulants is variable; there are reports of enhanced as well as diminished effects of anticoagulants when given concurrently with corticosteroids). Products include:

- Coumadin for Injection 1243
- Coumadin Tablets 1243
- Warfarin Sodium Tablets, USP 3302

SOMA TABLETS

(Carisoprodol) 3353

May interact with central nervous system depressants and certain other agents. Compounds in these categories include:

Alfentanil Hydrochloride (Carisoprodol causes drowsiness and co-administration may increase drowsiness effect).

No products indexed under this heading.

Alprazolam (Carisoprodol causes drowsiness and co-administration may increase drowsiness effect). Products include:

- Xanax Tablets 2865

Aprobarbital (Carisoprodol causes drowsiness and co-administration may increase drowsiness effect).

No products indexed under this heading.

Buprenorphine Hydrochloride (Carisoprodol causes drowsiness and co-administration may increase drowsiness effect). Products include:

- Buprenex Injectable 2918

Buspirone Hydrochloride (Carisoprodol causes drowsiness and co-administration may increase drowsiness effect).

No products indexed under this heading.

Butabarbital (Carisoprodol causes drowsiness and co-administration may increase drowsiness effect).

No products indexed under this heading.

Butalbital (Carisoprodol causes drowsiness and co-administration may increase drowsiness effect). Products include:

- Phrenilin 578
- Sedapap Tablets 50 mg/650 mg 2225

Chlordiazepoxide (Carisoprodol causes drowsiness and co-administration may increase drowsiness effect). Products include:

- Limbitrol 1738

Chlordiazepoxide Hydrochloride (Carisoprodol causes drowsiness and co-administration may increase drowsiness effect). Products include:

- Librium Capsules 1736
- Librium for Injection 1737

Chlorpromazine (Carisoprodol causes drowsiness and co-administration may increase drowsiness effect). Products include:

- Thorazine Suppositories 1656

Chlorpromazine Hydrochloride (Carisoprodol causes drowsiness and co-administration may increase drowsiness effect). Products include:

- Thorazine 1656

Chlorprothixene (Carisoprodol causes drowsiness and co-administration may increase drowsiness effect).

No products indexed under this heading.

Chlorprothixene Hydrochloride (Carisoprodol causes drowsiness and co-administration may increase drowsiness effect).

No products indexed under this heading.

Chlorprothixene Lactate (Carisoprodol causes drowsiness and co-administration may increase drowsiness effect).

No products indexed under this heading.

Clorazepate Dipotassium (Carisoprodol causes drowsiness and co-administration may increase drowsiness effect). Products include:

- Tranxene 511

Clozapine (Carisoprodol causes drowsiness and co-administration may increase drowsiness effect). Products include:

- Clozaril Tablets 2319

Codeine Phosphate (Carisoprodol causes drowsiness and co-administration may increase drowsiness effect). Products include:

- Phenergan with Codeine Syrup 3557
- Phenergan VC with Codeine Syrup .. 3561
- Robitussin A-C Syrup 2942
- Robitussin-DAC Syrup 2942
- Ryna-C Liquid .... ▣768
- Soma Compound w/Codeine Tablets 3355
- Tussi-Organidin NR Liquid 3350
- Tussi-Organidin-S NR Liquid 3350
- Tylenol with Codeine 2595

Desflurane (Carisoprodol causes drowsiness and co-administration may increase drowsiness effect). Products include:

- Suprane Liquid for Inhalation 874

Dezocine (Carisoprodol causes drowsiness and co-administration may increase drowsiness effect).

No products indexed under this heading.

Diazepam (Carisoprodol causes drowsiness and co-administration may increase drowsiness effect). Products include:

- Valium Injectable 3026
- Valium Tablets 3047

Droperidol (Carisoprodol causes drowsiness and co-administration may increase drowsiness effect).

No products indexed under this heading.

Enflurane (Carisoprodol causes drowsiness and co-administration may increase drowsiness effect).

No products indexed under this heading.

Estazolam (Carisoprodol causes drowsiness and co-administration may increase drowsiness effect). Products include:

- ProSom Tablets 500

Ethchlorvynol (Carisoprodol causes drowsiness and co-administration may increase drowsiness effect).

No products indexed under this heading.

Ethinamate (Carisoprodol causes drowsiness and co-administration may increase drowsiness effect).

No products indexed under this heading.

Fentanyl (Carisoprodol causes drowsiness and co-administration may increase drowsiness effect). Products include:

- Duragesic Transdermal System 1786

Fentanyl Citrate (Carisoprodol causes drowsiness and co-administration may increase drowsiness effect). Products include:

- Actiq 1184

Fluphenazine Decanoate (Carisoprodol causes drowsiness and co-administration may increase drowsiness effect).

No products indexed under this heading.

Fluphenazine Enanthate (Carisoprodol causes drowsiness and co-administration may increase drowsiness effect).

No products indexed under this heading.

Fluphenazine Hydrochloride (Carisoprodol causes drowsiness and co-administration may increase drowsiness effect).

No products indexed under this heading.

Flurazepam Hydrochloride (Carisoprodol causes drowsiness and co-administration may increase drowsiness effect).

No products indexed under this heading.

Glutethimide (Carisoprodol causes drowsiness and co-administration may increase drowsiness effect).

No products indexed under this heading.

Haloperidol (Carisoprodol causes drowsiness and co-administration may increase drowsiness effect). Products include:

- Haldol Injection, Tablets and Concentrate 2533

Haloperidol Decanoate (Carisoprodol causes drowsiness and co-administration may increase drowsiness effect). Products include:

- Haldol Decanoate 2535

Hydrocodone Bitartrate (Carisoprodol causes drowsiness and co-administration may increase drowsiness effect). Products include:

- Hycodan 1316
- Hycomine Compound Tablets 1317
- Hycotuss Expectorant Syrup 1318
- Lortab 3319
- Lortab Elixir 3317
- Maxidone Tablets CIII 3399
- Norco 5/325 Tablets CIII 3424
- Norco 7.5/325 Tablets CIII 3425
- Norco 10/325 Tablets CIII 3427
- Norco 10/325 Tablets CIII 3425
- Vicodin Tablets 516
- Vicodin ES Tablets 517
- Vicodin HP Tablets 518
- Vicodin Tuss Expectorant 519
- Vicoprofen Tablets 520
- Zydone Tablets 1330

Hydrocodone Polistirex (Carisoprodol causes drowsiness and co-administration may increase drowsiness effect). Products include:

- Tussionex Pennkinetic Extended-Release Suspension 1174

Hydromorphone Hydrochloride (Carisoprodol causes drowsiness and co-administration may increase drowsiness effect). Products include:

- Dilaudid 441
- Dilaudid Oral Liquid 445
- Dilaudid Powder 441
- Dilaudid Rectal Suppositories 441
- Dilaudid Tablets 441
- Dilaudid Tablets - 8 mg 445
- Dilaudid-HP 443

Hydroxyzine Hydrochloride (Carisoprodol causes drowsiness and co-administration may increase drowsiness effect). Products include:

Atarax Tablets & Syrup 2667
Vistaril Intramuscular Solution 2738

Isoflurane (Carisoprodol causes drowsiness and co-administration may increase drowsiness effect).
No products indexed under this heading.

Ketamine Hydrochloride (Carisoprodol causes drowsiness and co-administration may increase drowsiness effect).
No products indexed under this heading.

Levomethadyl Acetate Hydrochloride (Carisoprodol causes drowsiness and co-administration may increase drowsiness effect).
No products indexed under this heading.

Levorphanol Tartrate (Carisoprodol causes drowsiness and co-administration may increase drowsiness effect). Products include:
Levo-Dromoran 1734
Levorphanol Tartrate Tablets 3059

Lorazepam (Carisoprodol causes drowsiness and co-administration may increase drowsiness effect). Products include:
Ativan Injection 3478
Ativan Tablets 3482

Loxapine Hydrochloride (Carisoprodol causes drowsiness and co-administration may increase drowsiness effect).
No products indexed under this heading.

Loxapine Succinate (Carisoprodol causes drowsiness and co-administration may increase drowsiness effect). Products include:
Loxitane Capsules 3398

Meperidine Hydrochloride (Carisoprodol causes drowsiness and co-administration may increase drowsiness effect). Products include:
Demerol 3079
Mepergan Injection 3539

Mephobarbital (Carisoprodol causes drowsiness and co-administration may increase drowsiness effect).
No products indexed under this heading.

Meprobamate (Carisoprodol causes drowsiness and co-administration may increase drowsiness effect). Products include:
Miltown Tablets 3349

Mesoridazine Besylate (Carisoprodol causes drowsiness and co-administration may increase drowsiness effect). Products include:
Serentil 1057

Methadone Hydrochloride (Carisoprodol causes drowsiness and co-administration may increase drowsiness effect). Products include:
Dolophine Hydrochloride Tablets 3056

Methohexital Sodium (Carisoprodol causes drowsiness and co-administration may increase drowsiness effect). Products include:
Brevital Sodium for Injection, USP .. 1815

Methotrimeprazine (Carisoprodol causes drowsiness and co-administration may increase drowsiness effect).
No products indexed under this heading.

Methoxyflurane (Carisoprodol causes drowsiness and co-administration may increase drowsiness effect).
No products indexed under this heading.

Midazolam Hydrochloride (Carisoprodol causes drowsiness and co-administration may increase drowsiness effect). Products include:
Versed Injection 3027
Versed Syrup 3033

Molindone Hydrochloride (Carisoprodol causes drowsiness and co-administration may increase drowsiness effect). Products include:
Moban 1320

Morphine Sulfate (Carisoprodol causes drowsiness and co-administration may increase drowsiness effect). Products include:
Astramorph/PF Injection, USP (Preservative-Free)................. 594
Duramorph Injection 1312
Infumorph 200 and Infumorph 500 Sterile Solutions 1314
Kadian Capsules 1335
MS Contin Tablets 2896
MSIR 2898
Oramorph SR Tablets 3062
Roxanol 3066

Olanzapine (Carisoprodol causes drowsiness and co-administration may increase drowsiness effect). Products include:
Zyprexa Tablets 1973
Zyprexa ZYDIS Orally Disintegrating Tablets................. 1973

Oxazepam (Carisoprodol causes drowsiness and co-administration may increase drowsiness effect).
No products indexed under this heading.

Oxycodone Hydrochloride (Carisoprodol causes drowsiness and co-administration may increase drowsiness effect). Products include:
OxyContin Tablets 2912
OxyFast Oral Concentrate Solution . 2916
OxyIR Capsules 2916
Percocet Tablets 1326
Percodan Tablets 1327
Percolone Tablets 1327
Roxicodone 3067
Tylox Capsules 2597

Pentobarbital Sodium (Carisoprodol causes drowsiness and co-administration may increase drowsiness effect). Products include:
Nembutal Sodium Solution 485

Perphenazine (Carisoprodol causes drowsiness and co-administration may increase drowsiness effect). Products include:
Etrafon 3115
Trilafon 3160

Phenobarbital (Carisoprodol causes drowsiness and co-administration may increase drowsiness effect). Products include:
Arco-Lase Plus Tablets 592
Donnatal 2929
Donnatal Extentabs 2930

Prazepam (Carisoprodol causes drowsiness and co-administration may increase drowsiness effect).
No products indexed under this heading.

Prochlorperazine (Carisoprodol causes drowsiness and co-administration may increase drowsiness effect). Products include:
Compazine 1505

Promethazine Hydrochloride (Carisoprodol causes drowsiness and co-administration may increase drowsiness effect). Products include:
Mepergan Injection 3539
Phenergan Injection 3553
Phenergan 3556
Phenergan Syrup 3554
Phenergan with Codeine Syrup 3557
Phenergan with Dextromethorphan Syrup 3559
Phenergan VC Syrup 3560
Phenergan VC with Codeine Syrup .. 3561

Propofol (Carisoprodol causes drowsiness and co-administration may increase drowsiness effect). Products include:
Diprivan Injectable Emulsion 667

Propoxyphene Hydrochloride (Carisoprodol causes drowsiness and co-administration may increase drowsiness effect). Products include:
Darvon Pulvules 1909
Darvon Compound-65 Pulvules 1910

Propoxyphene Napsylate (Carisoprodol causes drowsiness and co-administration may increase drowsiness effect). Products include:
Darvon-N/Darvocet-N 1907
Darvon-N Tablets 1912

Quazepam (Carisoprodol causes drowsiness and co-administration may increase drowsiness effect).
No products indexed under this heading.

Quetiapine Fumarate (Carisoprodol causes drowsiness and co-administration may increase drowsiness effect). Products include:
Seroquel Tablets 684

Remifentanil Hydrochloride (Carisoprodol causes drowsiness and co-administration may increase drowsiness effect).
No products indexed under this heading.

Risperidone (Carisoprodol causes drowsiness and co-administration may increase drowsiness effect). Products include:
Risperdal 1796

Secobarbital Sodium (Carisoprodol causes drowsiness and co-administration may increase drowsiness effect).
No products indexed under this heading.

Sevoflurane (Carisoprodol causes drowsiness and co-administration may increase drowsiness effect).
No products indexed under this heading.

Sufentanil Citrate (Carisoprodol causes drowsiness and co-administration may increase drowsiness effect).
No products indexed under this heading.

Temazepam (Carisoprodol causes drowsiness and co-administration may increase drowsiness effect).
No products indexed under this heading.

Thiamylal Sodium (Carisoprodol causes drowsiness and co-administration may increase drowsiness effect).
No products indexed under this heading.

Thioridazine Hydrochloride (Carisoprodol causes drowsiness and co-administration may increase drowsiness effect). Products include:
Thioridazine Hydrochloride Tablets 2289

Thiothixene (Carisoprodol causes drowsiness and co-administration may increase drowsiness effect). Products include:
Navane Capsules 2701
Thiothixene Capsules 2290

Triazolam (Carisoprodol causes drowsiness and co-administration may increase drowsiness effect). Products include:
Halcion Tablets 2823

Trifluoperazine Hydrochloride (Carisoprodol causes drowsiness and co-administration may increase drowsiness effect). Products include:
Stelazine 1640

Zaleplon (Carisoprodol causes drowsiness and co-administration may increase drowsiness effect). Products include:
Sonata Capsules 3591

Ziprasidone Hydrochloride (Carisoprodol causes drowsiness and co-administration may increase drowsiness effect). Products include:
Geodon Capsules 2688

Zolpidem Tartrate (Carisoprodol causes drowsiness and co-administration may increase drowsiness effect). Products include:
Ambien Tablets 3191

Food Interactions

Alcohol (Carisoprodol causes drowsiness and co-administration may increase drowsiness effect).

SOMA COMPOUND TABLETS

(Aspirin, Carisoprodol) 3354
May interact with antacids, central nervous system depressants, corticosteroids, oral anticoagulants, oral hypoglycemic agents, psychotropics, and certain other agents. Compounds in these categories include:

Acarbose (Possible enhancement of hypoglycemia). Products include:
Precose Tablets 906

Alfentanil Hydrochloride (Additive effects).
No products indexed under this heading.

Alprazolam (Additive effects). Products include:
Xanax Tablets 2865

Aluminum Carbonate (May substantially decrease plasma salicylate concentration).
No products indexed under this heading.

Aluminum Hydroxide (May substantially decrease plasma salicylate concentration). Products include:
Amphojel Suspension (Mint Flavor).. 789
Gaviscon Extra Strength Liquid 751
Gaviscon Extra Strength Tablets 751
Gaviscon Regular Strength Liquid . 751
Gaviscon Regular Strength Tablets 750
Maalox Antacid/Anti-Gas Oral Suspension................................ 673
Maalox Max Maximum Strength Antacid/Anti-Gas Liquid 2300
Maalox Regular Strength Antacid/Antigas Liquid 2300
Mylanta 1813
Vanquish Caplets 617

Amitriptyline Hydrochloride (Additive effects). Products include:
Etrafon 3115
Limbitrol 1738

Ammonium Chloride (Elevated plasma salicylate concentrations).
No products indexed under this heading.

Amoxapine (Additive effects).
No products indexed under this heading.

Aprobarbital (Additive effects).
No products indexed under this heading.

Betamethasone Acetate (May decrease salicylate plasma levels). Products include:
Celestone Soluspan Injectable Suspension 3097

Betamethasone Sodium Phosphate (May decrease salicylate plasma levels). Products include:
Celestone Soluspan Injectable Suspension 3097

Buprenorphine Hydrochloride (Additive effects). Products include:
Buprenex Injectable 2918

Buspirone Hydrochloride (Additive effects).
No products indexed under this heading.

Butabarbital (Additive effects).
No products indexed under this heading.

Butalbital (Additive effects). Products include:
Phrenilin 578
Sedapap Tablets 50 mg/650 mg ... 2225

Chlordiazepoxide (Additive effects). Products include:
Limbitrol 1738

Chlordiazepoxide Hydrochloride (Additive effects). Products include:
Librium Capsules 1736
Librium for Injection 1737

Chlorpromazine (Additive effects). Products include:

Thorazine Suppositories 1656

Chlorpromazine Hydrochloride (Additive effects). Products include:
Thorazine 1656

Chlorpropamide (Possible enhancement of hypoglycemia). Products include:
Diabinese Tablets 2680

Chlorprothixene (Additive effects).
No products indexed under this heading.

Chlorprothixene Hydrochloride (Additive effects).
No products indexed under this heading.

Chlorprothixene Lactate (Additive effects).
No products indexed under this heading.

Clorazepate Dipotassium (Additive effects). Products include:
Tranxene 511

Clozapine (Additive effects). Products include:
Clozaril Tablets 2319

Codeine Phosphate (Additive effects). Products include:
Phenergan with Codeine Syrup 3557
Phenergan VC with Codeine Syrup 3561
Robitussin A-C Syrup 2942
Robitussin-DAC Syrup 2942
Ryna-C Liquid .... ▣768
Soma Compound w/Codeine Tablets 3355
Tussi-Organidin NR Liquid 3350
Tussi-Organidin-S NR Liquid 3350
Tylenol with Codeine 2595

Cortisone Acetate (May decrease salicylate plasma levels). Products include:
Cortone Acetate Injectable Suspension 2059
Cortone Acetate Tablets 2061

Desflurane (Additive effects). Products include:
Suprane Liquid for Inhalation 874

Desipramine Hydrochloride (Additive effects). Products include:
Norpramin Tablets 755

Dexamethasone (May decrease salicylate plasma levels). Products include:
Decadron Elixir 2078
Decadron Tablets 2079
TobraDex Ophthalmic Ointment 542
TobraDex Ophthalmic Suspension 541

Dexamethasone Acetate (May decrease salicylate plasma levels).
No products indexed under this heading.

Dexamethasone Sodium Phosphate (May decrease salicylate plasma levels). Products include:
Decadron Phosphate Injection 2081
Decadron Phosphate Sterile Ophthalmic Ointment 2083
Decadron Phosphate Sterile Ophthalmic Solution 2084
NeoDecadron Sterile Ophthalmic Solution 2144

Dezocine (Additive effects).
No products indexed under this heading.

Diazepam (Additive effects). Products include:
Valium Injectable 3026
Valium Tablets 3047

Dicumarol (Enhanced potential for bleeding).
No products indexed under this heading.

Doxepin Hydrochloride (Additive effects). Products include:
Sinequan 2713

Droperidol (Additive effects).
No products indexed under this heading.

Enflurane (Additive effects).
No products indexed under this heading.

Estazolam (Additive effects). Products include:
ProSom Tablets 500

Ethchlorvynol (Additive effects).
No products indexed under this heading.

Ethinamate (Additive effects).
No products indexed under this heading.

Fentanyl (Additive effects). Products include:
Duragesic Transdermal System 1786

Fentanyl Citrate (Additive effects). Products include:
Actiq 1184

Fludrocortisone Acetate (May decrease salicylate plasma levels). Products include:
Florinef Acetate Tablets 2250

Fluphenazine Decanoate (Additive effects).
No products indexed under this heading.

Fluphenazine Enanthate (Additive effects).
No products indexed under this heading.

Fluphenazine Hydrochloride (Additive effects).
No products indexed under this heading.

Flurazepam Hydrochloride (Additive effects).
No products indexed under this heading.

Glimepiride (Possible enhancement of hypoglycemia). Products include:
Amaryl Tablets 717

Glipizide (Possible enhancement of hypoglycemia). Products include:
Glucotrol Tablets 2692
Glucotrol XL Extended Release Tablets 2693

Glutethimide (Additive effects).
No products indexed under this heading.

Glyburide (Possible enhancement of hypoglycemia). Products include:
DiaBeta Tablets 741
Glucovance Tablets 1086

Haloperidol (Additive effects). Products include:
Haldol Injection, Tablets and Concentrate 2533

Haloperidol Decanoate (Additive effects). Products include:
Haldol Decanoate 2535

Hydrocodone Bitartrate (Additive effects). Products include:
Hycodan 1316
Hycomine Compound Tablets 1317
Hycotuss Expectorant Syrup 1318
Lortab 3319
Lortab Elixir 3317
Maxidone Tablets CIII 3399
Norco 5/325 Tablets CIII 3424
Norco 7.5/325 Tablets CIII 3425
Norco 10/325 Tablets CIII 3427
Norco 10/325 Tablets CIII 3425
Vicodin Tablets 516
Vicodin ES Tablets 517
Vicodin HP Tablets 518
Vicodin Tuss Expectorant 519
Vicoprofen Tablets 520
Zydone Tablets 1330

Hydrocodone Polistirex (Additive effects). Products include:
Tussionex Pennkinetic Extended-Release Suspension 1174

Hydrocortisone (May decrease salicylate plasma levels). Products include:
Anusol-HC Cream 2.5% 2237
Cipro HC Otic Suspension 540
Cortaid Intensive Therapy Cream .... ▣717
Cortaid Maximum Strength Cream .... ▣717
Cortisporin Ophthalmic Suspension Sterile .... ⊙297
Cortizone•5 .... ▣699
Cortizone•10 .... ▣699
Cortizone•10 Plus Creme .... ▣700
Cortizone for Kids Creme .... ▣699
Hydrocortone Tablets 2106
Massengill Medicated Soft Cloth Towelette .... ▣753
VōSoL HC Otic Solution 3356

Hydrocortisone Acetate (May decrease salicylate plasma levels). Products include:
Analpram-HC 1338
Anusol HC-1 Hydrocortisone Anti-Itch Cream .... ▣689
Anusol-HC Suppositories 2238
Cortaid .... ▣717
Cortifoam Rectal Foam 3170
Cortisporin-TC Otic Suspension 2246
Hydrocortone Acetate Injectable Suspension 2103
Pramosone 1343
Proctocort Suppositories 2264
ProctoFoam-HC 3177
Terra-Cortril Ophthalmic Suspension 2716

Hydrocortisone Sodium Phosphate (May decrease salicylate plasma levels). Products include:
Hydrocortone Phosphate Injection, Sterile 2105

Hydrocortisone Sodium Succinate (May decrease salicylate plasma levels).
No products indexed under this heading.

Hydromorphone Hydrochloride (Additive effects). Products include:
Dilaudid 441
Dilaudid Oral Liquid 445
Dilaudid Powder 441
Dilaudid Rectal Suppositories 441
Dilaudid Tablets 441
Dilaudid Tablets - 8 mg 445
Dilaudid-HP 443

Hydroxyzine Hydrochloride (Additive effects). Products include:
Atarax Tablets & Syrup 2667
Vistaril Intramuscular Solution 2738

Imipramine Hydrochloride (Additive effects).
No products indexed under this heading.

Imipramine Pamoate (Additive effects).
No products indexed under this heading.

Isocarboxazid (Additive effects).
No products indexed under this heading.

Isoflurane (Additive effects).
No products indexed under this heading.

Ketamine Hydrochloride (Additive effects).
No products indexed under this heading.

Levomethadyl Acetate Hydrochloride (Additive effects).
No products indexed under this heading.

Levorphanol Tartrate (Additive effects). Products include:
Levo-Dromoran 1734
Levorphanol Tartrate Tablets 3059

Lithium Carbonate (Additive effects). Products include:
Eskalith 1527
Lithium Carbonate 3061
Lithobid Slow-Release Tablets 3255

Lithium Citrate (Additive effects). Products include:
Lithium Citrate Syrup 3061

Lorazepam (Additive effects). Products include:
Ativan Injection 3478
Ativan Tablets 3482

Loxapine Hydrochloride (Additive effects).
No products indexed under this heading.

Loxapine Succinate (Additive effects). Products include:
Loxitane Capsules 3398

Magaldrate (May substantially decrease plasma salicylate concentration).
No products indexed under this heading.

Magnesium Hydroxide (May substantially decrease plasma salicylate concentration). Products include:
Ex•Lax Milk of Magnesia Liquid .... ▣670
Maalox Antacid/Anti-Gas Oral Suspension .... ▣673
Maalox Max Maximum Strength Antacid/Anti-Gas Liquid 2300
Maalox Regular Strength Antacid/Antigas Liquid 2300
Mylanta Fast-Acting 1813
Mylanta 1813
Pepcid Complete Chewable Tablets 1815
Phillips' Chewable Tablets .... ▣615
Phillips' Milk of Magnesia Liquid (Original, Cherry, & Mint) .... ▣616
Rolaids Tablets .... ▣706
Extra Strength Rolaids Tablets .... ▣706
Vanquish Caplets .... ▣617

Magnesium Oxide (May substantially decrease plasma salicylate concentration). Products include:
Beelith Tablets 946
Mag-Ox 400 Tablets 1024
Uro-Mag Capsules 1024

Maprotiline Hydrochloride (Additive effects).
No products indexed under this heading.

Meperidine Hydrochloride (Additive effects). Products include:
Demerol 3079
Mepergan Injection 3539

Mephobarbital (Additive effects).
No products indexed under this heading.

Meprobamate (Additive effects). Products include:
Miltown Tablets 3349

Mesoridazine Besylate (Additive effects). Products include:
Serentil 1057

Metformin Hydrochloride (Possible enhancement of hypoglycemia). Products include:
Glucophage Tablets 1080
Glucophage XR Tablets 1080
Glucovance Tablets 1086

Methadone Hydrochloride (Additive effects). Products include:
Dolophine Hydrochloride Tablets 3056

Methohexital Sodium (Additive effects). Products include:
Brevital Sodium for Injection, USP 1815

Methotrexate Sodium (Toxic effects of metotrexate enhanced).
No products indexed under this heading.

Methotrimeprazine (Additive effects).
No products indexed under this heading.

Methoxyflurane (Additive effects).
No products indexed under this heading.

Methylprednisolone Acetate (May decrease salicylate plasma levels). Products include:
Depo-Medrol Injectable Suspension 2795

Methylprednisolone Sodium Succinate (May decrease salicylate plasma levels). Products include:
Solu-Medrol Sterile Powder 2855

Midazolam Hydrochloride (Additive effects). Products include:
Versed Injection 3027
Versed Syrup 3033

Miglitol (Possible enhancement of hypoglycemia). Products include:
Glyset Tablets 2821

Molindone Hydrochloride (Additive effects). Products include:
Moban 1320

Morphine Sulfate (Additive effects). Products include:
Astramorph/PF Injection, USP (Preservative-Free) 594
Duramorph Injection 1312
Infumorph 200 and Infumorph 500 Sterile Solutions 1314
Kadian Capsules 1335
MS Contin Tablets 2896
MSIR 2898
Oramorph SR Tablets 3062
Roxanol 3066

Nortriptyline Hydrochloride (Additive effects).
No products indexed under this heading.

Olanzapine (Additive effects). Products include:
Zyprexa Tablets 1973
Zyprexa ZYDIS Orally Disintegrating Tablets 1973

Oxazepam (Additive effects).
No products indexed under this heading.

Oxycodone Hydrochloride (Additive effects). Products include:
OxyContin Tablets 2912
OxyFast Oral Concentrate Solution 2916
OxyIR Capsules 2916
Percocet Tablets 1326
Percodan Tablets 1327
Percolone Tablets 1327
Roxicodone 3067
Tylox Capsules 2597

Pentobarbital Sodium (Additive effects). Products include:
Nembutal Sodium Solution 485

Perphenazine (Additive effects). Products include:
Etrafon 3115
Trilafon 3160

Phenelzine Sulfate (Additive effects). Products include:
Nardil Tablets 2653

Phenobarbital (Additive effects). Products include:
Arco-Lase Plus Tablets 592
Donnatal 2929
Donnatal Extentabs 2930

Pioglitazone Hydrochloride (Possible enhancement of hypoglycemia). Products include:
Actos Tablets 3275

Potassium Acid Phosphate (Elevated plasma salicylate concentrations). Products include:
K-Phos Original (Sodium Free) Tablets 947

Prazepam (Additive effects).
No products indexed under this heading.

Prednisolone Acetate (May decrease salicylate plasma levels). Products include:
Blephamide Ophthalmic Ointment 547
Blephamide Ophthalmic Suspension 548
Poly-Pred Liquifilm Ophthalmic Suspension .... ⊙245
Pred Forte Ophthalmic Suspension .... ⊙246
Pred Mild Sterile Ophthalmic Suspension .... ⊙249
Pred-G Ophthalmic Suspension .... ⊙247
Pred-G Sterile Ophthalmic Ointment .... ⊙248

Prednisolone Sodium Phosphate (May decrease salicylate plasma levels). Products include:
Pediapred Oral Solution 1170

Prednisolone Tebutate (May decrease salicylate plasma levels).
No products indexed under this heading.

Prednisone (May decrease salicylate plasma levels). Products include:
Prednisone 3064

Probenecid (Reduced uricosuric effect of both drugs; possible reduced renal excretion of salicylate).
No products indexed under this heading.

Prochlorperazine (Additive effects). Products include:
Compazine 1505

Promethazine Hydrochloride (Additive effects). Products include:
Mepergan Injection 3539
Phenergan Injection 3553
Phenergan 3556
Phenergan Syrup 3554
Phenergan with Codeine Syrup 3557
Phenergan with Dextromethorphan Syrup 3559
Phenergan VC Syrup 3560
Phenergan VC with Codeine Syrup 3561

Propofol (Additive effects). Products include:
Diprivan Injectable Emulsion 667

Propoxyphene Hydrochloride (Additive effects). Products include:
Darvon Pulvules 1909
Darvon Compound-65 Pulvules 1910

Propoxyphene Napsylate (Additive effects). Products include:
Darvon-N/Darvocet-N 1907
Darvon-N Tablets 1912

Protriptyline Hydrochloride (Additive effects). Products include:
Vivactil Tablets 2446
Vivactil Tablets 2217

Quazepam (Additive effects).
No products indexed under this heading.

Quetiapine Fumarate (Additive effects). Products include:
Seroquel Tablets 684

Remifentanil Hydrochloride (Additive effects).
No products indexed under this heading.

Repaglinide (Possible enhancement of hypoglycemia). Products include:
Prandin Tablets (0.5, 1, and 2 mg) 2432

Risperidone (Additive effects). Products include:
Risperdal 1796

Rosiglitazone Maleate (Possible enhancement of hypoglycemia). Products include:
Avandia Tablets 1490

Secobarbital Sodium (Additive effects).
No products indexed under this heading.

Sevoflurane (Additive effects).
No products indexed under this heading.

Sodium Acid Phosphate (Elevated plasma salicylate concentrations). Products include:
Uroqid-Acid No. 2 Tablets 947

Sodium Bicarbonate (May substantially decrease plasma salicylate concentration). Products include:
Alka-Seltzer .... ▣603
Alka-Seltzer Lemon Lime Antacid and Pain Reliever Effervescent Tablets .... ▣603
Alka-Seltzer Extra Strength Antacid and Pain Reliever Effervescent Tablets .... ▣603
Alka-Seltzer Heartburn Relief Tablets .... ▣604
Ceo-Two Evacuant Suppository .... ▣618
Colyte with Flavor Packs for Oral Solution 3170
GoLYTELY and Pineapple Flavor GoLYTELY for Oral Solution 1068
NuLYTELY, Cherry Flavor, Lemon-Lime Flavor, and Orange Flavor NuLYTELY for Oral Solution 1068

Sufentanil Citrate (Additive effects).
No products indexed under this heading.

Sulfinpyrazone (Reduced uricosuric effect of both drugs; possible reduced renal excretion of salicylate).
No products indexed under this heading.

Temazepam (Additive effects).
No products indexed under this heading.

Thiamylal Sodium (Additive effects).
No products indexed under this heading.

Thioridazine Hydrochloride (Additive effects). Products include:
Thioridazine Hydrochloride Tablets 2289

Thiothixene (Additive effects). Products include:
Navane Capsules 2701
Thiothixene Capsules 2290

Tolazamide (Possible enhancement of hypoglycemia).
No products indexed under this heading.

Tolbutamide (Possible enhancement of hypoglycemia).
No products indexed under this heading.

Tranylcypromine Sulfate (Additive effects). Products include:
Parnate Tablets 1607

Triamcinolone (May decrease salicylate plasma levels).
No products indexed under this heading.

Triamcinolone Acetonide (May decrease salicylate plasma levels). Products include:
Azmacort Inhalation Aerosol 728
Nasacort Nasal Inhaler 750
Nasacort AQ Nasal Spray 752
Tri-Nasal Spray 2274

Triamcinolone Diacetate (May decrease salicylate plasma levels).
No products indexed under this heading.

Triamcinolone Hexacetonide (May decrease salicylate plasma levels).
No products indexed under this heading.

Triazolam (Additive effects). Products include:
Halcion Tablets 2823

Trifluoperazine Hydrochloride (Additive effects). Products include:
Stelazine 1640

Trimipramine Maleate (Additive effects). Products include:
Surmontil Capsules 3595

Troglitazone (Possible enhancement of hypoglycemia).
No products indexed under this heading.

Warfarin Sodium (Enhanced potential for bleeding). Products include:
Coumadin for Injection 1243
Coumadin Tablets 1243
Warfarin Sodium Tablets, USP 3302

Zaleplon (Additive effects). Products include:
Sonata Capsules 3591

Ziprasidone Hydrochloride (Additive effects). Products include:
Geodon Capsules 2688

Zolpidem Tartrate (Additive effects). Products include:
Ambien Tablets 3191

Food Interactions

Alcohol (Additive effects including enhanced aspirin-induced fecal blood loss).

SOMA COMPOUND W/ CODEINE TABLETS

(Aspirin, Carisoprodol, Codeine Phosphate) 3355

May interact with antacids, central nervous system depressants, corticosteroids, oral anticoagulants, oral hypoglycemic agents, psychotropics, and certain other agents. Compounds in these categories include:

Acarbose (Possible enhancement of hypoglycemia). Products include:
Precose Tablets 906

Alfentanil Hydrochloride (Additive effects).
No products indexed under this heading.

Alprazolam (Additive effects). Products include:
Xanax Tablets 2865

Aluminum Carbonate (May substantially decrease plasma salicylate concentration).
No products indexed under this heading.

Aluminum Hydroxide (May substantially decrease plasma salicylate concentration). Products include:
Amphojel Suspension (Mint Flavor) .... ▣789
Gaviscon Extra Strength Liquid .... ▣751
Gaviscon Extra Strength Tablets .... ▣751
Gaviscon Regular Strength Liquid .... ▣751
Gaviscon Regular Strength Tablets .... ▣750
Maalox Antacid/Anti-Gas Oral Suspension .... ▣673
Maalox Max Maximum Strength Antacid/Anti-Gas Liquid 2300
Maalox Regular Strength Antacid/Antigas Liquid 2300
Mylanta 1813
Vanquish Caplets .... ▣617

Amitriptyline Hydrochloride (Additive effects). Products include:
Etrafon 3115
Limbitrol 1738

Ammonium Chloride (Elevated plasma salicylate concentrations).
No products indexed under this heading.

Amoxapine (Additive effects).
No products indexed under this heading.

Aprobarbital (Additive effects).
No products indexed under this heading.

Betamethasone Acetate (May decrease salicylate plasma levels). Products include:
Celestone Soluspan Injectable Suspension 3097

Betamethasone Sodium Phosphate (May decrease salicylate plasma levels). Products include:
Celestone Soluspan Injectable Suspension 3097

Buprenorphine Hydrochloride (Additive effects). Products include:
Buprenex Injectable 2918

Buspirone Hydrochloride (Additive effects).
No products indexed under this heading.

Butabarbital (Additive effects).
No products indexed under this heading.

Butalbital (Additive effects). Products include:
Phrenilin 578
Sedapap Tablets 50 mg/650 mg 2225

Chlordiazepoxide (Additive effects). Products include:
Limbitrol 1738

Chlordiazepoxide Hydrochloride (Additive effects). Products include:
Librium Capsules 1736
Librium for Injection 1737

Chlorpromazine (Additive effects). Products include:
Thorazine Suppositories 1656

Chlorpromazine Hydrochloride (Additive effects). Products include:
Thorazine 1656

Chlorpropamide (Possible enhancement of hypoglycemia). Products include:
Diabinese Tablets 2680

Chlorprothixene (Additive effects).
No products indexed under this heading.

Chlorprothixene Hydrochloride (Additive effects).
No products indexed under this heading.

Chlorprothixene Lactate (Additive effects).
No products indexed under this heading.

Clorazepate Dipotassium (Additive effects). Products include:
Tranxene 511

Clozapine (Additive effects). Products include:
Clozaril Tablets 2319

Cortisone Acetate (May decrease salicylate plasma levels). Products include:
Cortone Acetate Injectable Suspension 2059
Cortone Acetate Tablets 2061

Desflurane (Additive effects). Products include:

Suprane Liquid for Inhalation 874

Desipramine Hydrochloride (Additive effects). Products include:
Norpramin Tablets 755

Dexamethasone (May decrease salicylate plasma levels). Products include:
Decadron Elixir 2078
Decadron Tablets 2079
TobraDex Ophthalmic Ointment 542
TobraDex Ophthalmic Suspension .. 541

Dexamethasone Acetate (May decrease salicylate plasma levels).
No products indexed under this heading.

Dexamethasone Sodium Phosphate (May decrease salicylate plasma levels). Products include:
Decadron Phosphate Injection 2081
Decadron Phosphate Sterile Ophthalmic Ointment 2083
Decadron Phosphate Sterile Ophthalmic Solution 2084
NeoDecadron Sterile Ophthalmic Solution..................................... 2144

Dezocine (Additive effects).
No products indexed under this heading.

Diazepam (Additive effects). Products include:
Valium Injectable 3026
Valium Tablets 3047

Dicumarol (Enhanced potential for bleeding).
No products indexed under this heading.

Doxepin Hydrochloride (Additive effects). Products include:
Sinequan 2713

Droperidol (Additive effects).
No products indexed under this heading.

Enflurane (Additive effects).
No products indexed under this heading.

Estazolam (Additive effects). Products include:
ProSom Tablets 500

Ethchlorvynol (Additive effects).
No products indexed under this heading.

Ethinamate (Additive effects).
No products indexed under this heading.

Fentanyl (Additive effects). Products include:
Duragesic Transdermal System 1786

Fentanyl Citrate (Additive effects). Products include:
Actiq 1184

Fludrocortisone Acetate (May decrease salicylate plasma levels). Products include:
Florinef Acetate Tablets 2250

Fluphenazine Decanoate (Additive effects).
No products indexed under this heading.

Fluphenazine Enanthate (Additive effects).
No products indexed under this heading.

Fluphenazine Hydrochloride (Additive effects).
No products indexed under this heading.

Flurazepam Hydrochloride (Additive effects).
No products indexed under this heading.

Glimepiride (Possible enhancement of hypoglycemia). Products include:
Amaryl Tablets 717

Glipizide (Possible enhancement of hypoglycemia). Products include:
Glucotrol Tablets 2692
Glucotrol XL Extended Release Tablets.. 2693

Glutethimide (Additive effects).
No products indexed under this heading.

Glyburide (Possible enhancement of hypoglycemia). Products include:
DiaBeta Tablets 741
Glucovance Tablets 1086

Haloperidol (Additive effects). Products include:
Haldol Injection, Tablets and Concentrate 2533

Haloperidol Decanoate (Additive effects). Products include:
Haldol Decanoate 2535

Hydrocodone Bitartrate (Additive effects). Products include:
Hycodan 1316
Hycomine Compound Tablets 1317
Hycotuss Expectorant Syrup 1318
Lortab 3319
Lortab Elixir 3317
Maxidone Tablets CIII 3399
Norco 5/325 Tablets CIII 3424
Norco 7.5/325 Tablets CIII 3425
Norco 10/325 Tablets CIII 3427
Norco 10/325 Tablets CIII 3425
Vicodin Tablets 516
Vicodin ES Tablets 517
Vicodin HP Tablets 518
Vicodin Tuss Expectorant 519
Vicoprofen Tablets 520
Zydone Tablets 1330

Hydrocodone Polistirex (Additive effects). Products include:
Tussionex Pennkinetic Extended-Release Suspension..... 1174

Hydrocortisone (May decrease salicylate plasma levels). Products include:
Anusol-HC Cream 2.5% 2237
Cipro HC Otic Suspension 540
Cortaid Intensive Therapy Cream .. ▣717
Cortaid Maximum Strength Cream.. ▣717
Cortisporin Ophthalmic Suspension Sterile .... ⊙297
Cortizone•5 .... ▣699
Cortizone•10 .... ▣699
Cortizone•10 Plus Creme .... ▣700
Cortizone for Kids Creme .... ▣699
Hydrocortone Tablets 2106
Massengill Medicated Soft Cloth Towelette... ▣753
VōSoL HC Otic Solution 3356

Hydrocortisone Acetate (May decrease salicylate plasma levels). Products include:
Analpram-HC 1338
Anusol HC-1 Hydrocortisone Anti-Itch Cream .... ▣689
Anusol-HC Suppositories 2238
Cortaid .... ▣717
Cortifoam Rectal Foam 3170
Cortisporin-TC Otic Suspension 2246
Hydrocortone Acetate Injectable Suspension 2103
Pramosone 1343
Proctocort Suppositories 2264
ProctoFoam-HC 3177
Terra-Cortril Ophthalmic Suspension 2716

Hydrocortisone Sodium Phosphate (May decrease salicylate plasma levels). Products include:
Hydrocortone Phosphate Injection, Sterile 2105

Hydrocortisone Sodium Succinate (May decrease salicylate plasma levels).
No products indexed under this heading.

Hydromorphone Hydrochloride (Additive effects). Products include:
Dilaudid 441
Dilaudid Oral Liquid 445
Dilaudid Powder 441
Dilaudid Rectal Suppositories 441
Dilaudid Tablets 441
Dilaudid Tablets - 8 mg 445
Dilaudid-HP 443

Hydroxyzine Hydrochloride (Additive effects). Products include:
Atarax Tablets & Syrup 2667
Vistaril Intramuscular Solution 2738

Imipramine Hydrochloride (Additive effects).
No products indexed under this heading.

Imipramine Pamoate (Additive effects).
No products indexed under this heading.

Isocarboxazid (Additive effects).
No products indexed under this heading.

Isoflurane (Additive effects).
No products indexed under this heading.

Ketamine Hydrochloride (Additive effects).
No products indexed under this heading.

Levomethadyl Acetate Hydrochloride (Additive effects).
No products indexed under this heading.

Levorphanol Tartrate (Additive effects). Products include:
Levo-Dromoran 1734
Levorphanol Tartrate Tablets 3059

Lithium Carbonate (Additive effects). Products include:
Eskalith 1527
Lithium Carbonate 3061
Lithobid Slow-Release Tablets 3255

Lithium Citrate (Additive effects). Products include:
Lithium Citrate Syrup 3061

Lorazepam (Additive effects). Products include:
Ativan Injection 3478
Ativan Tablets 3482

Loxapine Hydrochloride (Additive effects).
No products indexed under this heading.

Loxapine Succinate (Additive effects). Products include:
Loxitane Capsules 3398

Magaldrate (May substantially decrease plasma salicylate concentration).
No products indexed under this heading.

Magnesium Hydroxide (May substantially decrease plasma salicylate concentration). Products include:
Ex•Lax Milk of Magnesia Liquid .... ▣670
Maalox Antacid/Anti-Gas Oral Suspension.. ▣673
Maalox Max Maximum Strength Antacid/Anti-Gas Liquid 2300
Maalox Regular Strength Antacid/Antigas Liquid 2300
Mylanta Fast-Acting 1813
Mylanta 1813
Pepcid Complete Chewable Tablets 1815
Phillips' Chewable Tablets .... ▣615
Phillips' Milk of Magnesia Liquid (Original, Cherry, & Mint)............. ▣616
Rolaids Tablets .... ▣706
Extra Strength Rolaids Tablets .... ▣706
Vanquish Caplets .... ▣617

Magnesium Oxide (May substantially decrease plasma salicylate concentration). Products include:
Beelith Tablets 946
Mag-Ox 400 Tablets 1024
Uro-Mag Capsules 1024

Maprotiline Hydrochloride (Additive effects).
No products indexed under this heading.

Meperidine Hydrochloride (Additive effects). Products include:
Demerol 3079
Mepergan Injection 3539

Mephobarbital (Additive effects).
No products indexed under this heading.

Meprobamate (Additive effects). Products include:
Miltown Tablets 3349

Mesoridazine Besylate (Additive effects). Products include:
Serentil 1057

Metformin Hydrochloride (Possible enhancement of hypoglycemia). Products include:
Glucophage Tablets 1080
Glucophage XR Tablets 1080
Glucovance Tablets 1086

Methadone Hydrochloride (Additive effects). Products include:
Dolophine Hydrochloride Tablets 3056

Methohexital Sodium (Additive effects). Products include:
Brevital Sodium for Injection, USP .. 1815

Methotrexate Sodium (Toxic effects of methotrexate enhanced).
No products indexed under this heading.

Methotrimeprazine (Additive effects).
No products indexed under this heading.

Methoxyflurane (Additive effects).
No products indexed under this heading.

Methylprednisolone Acetate (May decrease salicylate plasma levels). Products include:
Depo-Medrol Injectable Suspension 2795

Methylprednisolone Sodium Succinate (May decrease salicylate plasma levels). Products include:
Solu-Medrol Sterile Powder 2855

Midazolam Hydrochloride (Additive effects). Products include:
Versed Injection 3027
Versed Syrup 3033

Miglitol (Possible enhancement of hypoglycemia). Products include:
Glyset Tablets 2821

Molindone Hydrochloride (Additive effects). Products include:
Moban 1320

Morphine Sulfate (Additive effects). Products include:
Astramorph/PF Injection, USP (Preservative-Free)...................... 594
Duramorph Injection 1312
Infumorph 200 and Infumorph 500 Sterile Solutions 1314
Kadian Capsules 1335
MS Contin Tablets 2896
MSIR 2898
Oramorph SR Tablets 3062
Roxanol 3066

Nortriptyline Hydrochloride (Additive effects).
No products indexed under this heading.

Olanzapine (Additive effects). Products include:
Zyprexa Tablets 1973
Zyprexa ZYDIS Orally Disintegrating Tablets.................... 1973

Oxazepam (Additive effects).
No products indexed under this heading.

Oxycodone Hydrochloride (Additive effects). Products include:
OxyContin Tablets 2912
OxyFast Oral Concentrate Solution . 2916
OxyIR Capsules 2916
Percocet Tablets 1326
Percodan Tablets 1327
Percolone Tablets 1327
Roxicodone 3067
Tylox Capsules 2597

Pentobarbital Sodium (Additive effects). Products include:
Nembutal Sodium Solution 485

Perphenazine (Additive effects). Products include:
Etrafon 3115
Trilafon 3160

Phenelzine Sulfate (Additive effects). Products include:
Nardil Tablets 2653

Phenobarbital (Additive effects). Products include:
Arco-Lase Plus Tablets 592
Donnatal 2929
Donnatal Extentabs 2930

Pioglitazone Hydrochloride (Possible enhancement of hypoglycemia). Products include:
Actos Tablets 3275

Potassium Acid Phosphate (Elevated plasma salicylate concentrations). Products include:
K-Phos Original (Sodium Free) Tablets.. 947

Prazepam (Additive effects).
No products indexed under this heading.

Prednisolone Acetate (May decrease salicylate plasma levels). Products include:
- Blephamide Ophthalmic Ointment 547
- Blephamide Ophthalmic Suspension 548
- Poly-Pred Liquifilm Ophthalmic Suspension .... ⊙ 245
- Pred Forte Ophthalmic Suspension .... ⊙ 246
- Pred Mild Sterile Ophthalmic Suspension .... ⊙ 249
- Pred-G Ophthalmic Suspension .... ⊙ 247
- Pred-G Sterile Ophthalmic Ointment .... ⊙ 248

Prednisolone Sodium Phosphate (May decrease salicylate plasma levels). Products include:
- Pediapred Oral Solution 1170

Prednisolone Tebutate (May decrease salicylate plasma levels).
No products indexed under this heading.

Prednisone (May decrease salicylate plasma levels). Products include:
- Prednisone 3064

Probenecid (Possible reduced renal excretion of salicylate).
No products indexed under this heading.

Prochlorperazine (Additive effects). Products include:
- Compazine 1505

Promethazine Hydrochloride (Additive effects). Products include:
- Mepergan Injection 3539
- Phenergan Injection 3553
- Phenergan 3556
- Phenergan Syrup 3554
- Phenergan with Codeine Syrup 3557
- Phenergan with Dextromethorphan Syrup 3559
- Phenergan VC Syrup 3560
- Phenergan VC with Codeine Syrup .. 3561

Propofol (Additive effects). Products include:
- Diprivan Injectable Emulsion 667

Propoxyphene Hydrochloride (Additive effects). Products include:
- Darvon Pulvules 1909
- Darvon Compound-65 Pulvules 1910

Propoxyphene Napsylate (Additive effects). Products include:
- Darvon-N/Darvocet-N 1907
- Darvon-N Tablets 1912

Protriptyline Hydrochloride (Additive effects). Products include:
- Vivactil Tablets 2446
- Vivactil Tablets 2217

Quazepam (Additive effects).
No products indexed under this heading.

Quetiapine Fumarate (Additive effects). Products include:
- Seroquel Tablets 684

Remifentanil Hydrochloride (Additive effects).
No products indexed under this heading.

Repaglinide (Possible enhancement of hypoglycemia). Products include:
- Prandin Tablets (0.5, 1, and 2 mg) 2432

Risperidone (Additive effects). Products include:
- Risperdal 1796

Rosiglitazone Maleate (Possible enhancement of hypoglycemia). Products include:
- Avandia Tablets 1490

Secobarbital Sodium (Additive effects).
No products indexed under this heading.

Sevoflurane (Additive effects).
No products indexed under this heading.

Sodium Acid Phosphate (Elevated plasma salicylate concentrations). Products include:
- Uroqid-Acid No. 2 Tablets 947

Sodium Bicarbonate (May substantially decrease plasma salicylate concentration). Products include:
- Alka-Seltzer 603
- Alka-Seltzer Lemon Lime Antacid and Pain Reliever Effervescent Tablets 603
- Alka-Seltzer Extra Strength Antacid and Pain Reliever Effervescent Tablets 603
- Alka-Seltzer Heartburn Relief Tablets 604
- Ceo-Two Evacuant Suppository 618
- Colyte with Flavor Packs for Oral Solution 3170
- GoLYTELY and Pineapple Flavor GoLYTELY for Oral Solution 1068
- NuLYTELY, Cherry Flavor, Lemon-Lime Flavor, and Orange Flavor NuLYTELY for Oral Solution 1068

Sufentanil Citrate (Additive effects).
No products indexed under this heading.

Sulfinpyrazone (Reduced uricosuric effect of both drugs; possible reduced renal excretion of salicylate).
No products indexed under this heading.

Temazepam (Additive effects).
No products indexed under this heading.

Thiamylal Sodium (Additive effects).
No products indexed under this heading.

Thioridazine Hydrochloride (Additive effects). Products include:
- Thioridazine Hydrochloride Tablets 2289

Thiothixene (Additive effects). Products include:
- Navane Capsules 2701
- Thiothixene Capsules 2290

Tolazamide (Possible enhancement of hypoglycemia).
No products indexed under this heading.

Tolbutamide (Possible enhancement of hypoglycemia).
No products indexed under this heading.

Tranylcypromine Sulfate (Additive effects). Products include:
- Parnate Tablets 1607

Triamcinolone (May decrease salicylate plasma levels).
No products indexed under this heading.

Triamcinolone Acetonide (May decrease salicylate plasma levels). Products include:
- Azmacort Inhalation Aerosol 728
- Nasacort Nasal Inhaler 750
- Nasacort AQ Nasal Spray 752
- Tri-Nasal Spray 2274

Triamcinolone Diacetate (May decrease salicylate plasma levels).
No products indexed under this heading.

Triamcinolone Hexacetonide (May decrease salicylate plasma levels).
No products indexed under this heading.

Triazolam (Additive effects). Products include:
- Halcion Tablets 2823

Trifluoperazine Hydrochloride (Additive effects). Products include:
- Stelazine 1640

Trimipramine Maleate (Additive effects). Products include:
- Surmontil Capsules 3595

Troglitazone (Possible enhancement of hypoglycemia).
No products indexed under this heading.

Warfarin Sodium (Enhanced potential for bleeding). Products include:
- Coumadin for Injection 1243
- Coumadin Tablets 1243
- Warfarin Sodium Tablets, USP 3302

Zaleplon (Additive effects). Products include:
- Sonata Capsules 3591

Ziprasidone Hydrochloride (Additive effects). Products include:
- Geodon Capsules 2688

Zolpidem Tartrate (Additive effects). Products include:
- Ambien Tablets 3191

Food Interactions

Alcohol (Additive effects including gastrointestinal bleeding).

SOMINEX ORIGINAL FORMULA TABLETS

(Diphenhydramine Hydrochloride) 761

May interact with hypnotics and sedatives, tranquilizers, and certain other agents. Compounds in these categories include:

Alprazolam (Concurrent use with tranquilizers is not recommended unless directed by a physician). Products include:
- Xanax Tablets 2865

Buspirone Hydrochloride (Concurrent use with tranquilizers is not recommended unless directed by a physician).
No products indexed under this heading.

Chlordiazepoxide (Concurrent use with tranquilizers is not recommended unless directed by a physician). Products include:
- Limbitrol 1738

Chlordiazepoxide Hydrochloride (Concurrent use with tranquilizers is not recommended unless directed by a physician). Products include:
- Librium Capsules 1736
- Librium for Injection 1737

Chlorpromazine (Concurrent use with tranquilizers is not recommended unless directed by a physician). Products include:
- Thorazine Suppositories 1656

Chlorpromazine Hydrochloride (Concurrent use with tranquilizers is not recommended unless directed by a physician). Products include:
- Thorazine 1656

Chlorprothixene (Concurrent use with tranquilizers is not recommended unless directed by a physician).
No products indexed under this heading.

Chlorprothixene Hydrochloride (Concurrent use with tranquilizers is not recommended unless directed by a physician).
No products indexed under this heading.

Clorazepate Dipotassium (Concurrent use with tranquilizers is not recommended unless directed by a physician). Products include:
- Tranxene 511

Diazepam (Concurrent use with tranquilizers is not recommended unless directed by a physician). Products include:
- Valium Injectable 3026
- Valium Tablets 3047

Droperidol (Concurrent use with tranquilizers is not recommended unless directed by a physician).
No products indexed under this heading.

Estazolam (Concurrent use with sedatives is not recommended unless directed by a physician). Products include:
- ProSom Tablets 500

Ethchlorvynol (Concurrent use with sedatives is not recommended unless directed by a physician).
No products indexed under this heading.

Ethinamate (Concurrent use with sedatives is not recommended unless directed by a physician).
No products indexed under this heading.

Fluphenazine Decanoate (Concurrent use with tranquilizers is not recommended unless directed by a physician).
No products indexed under this heading.

Fluphenazine Enanthate (Concurrent use with tranquilizers is not recommended unless directed by a physician).
No products indexed under this heading.

Fluphenazine Hydrochloride (Concurrent use with tranquilizers is not recommended unless directed by a physician).
No products indexed under this heading.

Flurazepam Hydrochloride (Concurrent use with sedatives is not recommended unless directed by a physician).
No products indexed under this heading.

Glutethimide (Concurrent use with sedatives is not recommended unless directed by a physician).
No products indexed under this heading.

Haloperidol (Concurrent use with tranquilizers is not recommended unless directed by a physician). Products include:
- Haldol Injection, Tablets and Concentrate 2533

Haloperidol Decanoate (Concurrent use with tranquilizers is not recommended unless directed by a physician). Products include:
- Haldol Decanoate 2535

Hydroxyzine Hydrochloride (Concurrent use with tranquilizers is not recommended unless directed by a physician). Products include:
- Atarax Tablets & Syrup 2667
- Vistaril Intramuscular Solution 2738

Lorazepam (Concurrent use with tranquilizers is not recommended unless directed by a physician). Products include:
- Ativan Injection 3478
- Ativan Tablets 3482

Loxapine Hydrochloride (Concurrent use with tranquilizers is not recommended unless directed by a physician).
No products indexed under this heading.

Loxapine Succinate (Concurrent use with tranquilizers is not recommended unless directed by a physician). Products include:
- Loxitane Capsules 3398

Meprobamate (Concurrent use with tranquilizers is not recommended unless directed by a physician). Products include:
- Miltown Tablets 3349

Mesoridazine Besylate (Concurrent use with tranquilizers is not recommended unless directed by a physician). Products include:
- Serentil 1057

Midazolam Hydrochloride (Concurrent use with sedatives is not recommended unless directed by a physician). Products include:
- Versed Injection 3027
- Versed Syrup 3033

Molindone Hydrochloride (Concurrent use with tranquilizers is not recommended unless directed by a physician). Products include:
- Moban 1320

Oxazepam (Concurrent use with tranquilizers is not recommended unless directed by a physician).
No products indexed under this heading.

Perphenazine (Concurrent use with tranquilizers is not recommended unless directed by a physician). Products include:
- Etrafon 3115
- Trilafon 3160

Prazepam (Concurrent use with tranquilizers is not recommended unless directed by a physician).
No products indexed under this heading.

Prochlorperazine (Concurrent use with tranquilizers is not recommended unless directed by a physician). Products include:

Compazine ... 1505

Promethazine Hydrochloride (Concurrent use with tranquilizers is not recommended unless directed by a physician). Products include:
- Mepergan Injection ... 3539
- Phenergan Injection ... 3553
- Phenergan ... 3556
- Phenergan Syrup ... 3554
- Phenergan with Codeine Syrup ... 3557
- Phenergan with Dextromethorphan Syrup ... 3559
- Phenergan VC Syrup ... 3560
- Phenergan VC with Codeine Syrup .. 3561

Propofol (Concurrent use with sedatives is not recommended unless directed by a physician). Products include:
- Diprivan Injectable Emulsion ... 667

Quazepam (Concurrent use with sedatives is not recommended unless directed by a physician).
- No products indexed under this heading.

Secobarbital Sodium (Concurrent use with sedatives is not recommended unless directed by a physician).
- No products indexed under this heading.

Temazepam (Concurrent use with sedatives is not recommended unless directed by a physician).
- No products indexed under this heading.

Thioridazine Hydrochloride (Concurrent use with tranquilizers is not recommended unless directed by a physician). Products include:
- Thioridazine Hydrochloride Tablets ... 2289

Thiothixene (Concurrent use with tranquilizers is not recommended unless directed by a physician). Products include:
- Navane Capsules ... 2701
- Thiothixene Capsules ... 2290

Triazolam (Concurrent use with sedatives is not recommended unless directed by a physician). Products include:
- Halcion Tablets ... 2823

Trifluoperazine Hydrochloride (Concurrent use with tranquilizers is not recommended unless directed by a physician). Products include:
- Stelazine ... 1640

Zaleplon (Concurrent use with sedatives is not recommended unless directed by a physician). Products include:
- Sonata Capsules ... 3591

Zolpidem Tartrate (Concurrent use with sedatives is not recommended unless directed by a physician). Products include:
- Ambien Tablets ... 3191

Food Interactions

Alcohol (Concurrent use of alcoholic beverages is not recommended).

SONATA CAPSULES

(Zaleplon) ... 3591

May interact with antihistamines, central nervous system depressants, anticonvulsants, phenytoin, psychotropics, and certain other agents. Compounds in these categories include:

Acrivastine (Concurrent use may produce additive CNS depressant effects). Products include:
- Semprex-D Capsules ... 1172

Alfentanil Hydrochloride (Concurrent use may produce additive CNS depressant effects).
- No products indexed under this heading.

Alprazolam (Concurrent use may produce additive CNS depressant effects). Products include:
- Xanax Tablets ... 2865

Amitriptyline Hydrochloride (Concurrent use may produce additive CNS depressant effects). Products include:
- Etrafon ... 3115
- Limbitrol ... 1738

Amoxapine (Concurrent use may produce additive CNS depressant effects).
- No products indexed under this heading.

Aprobarbital (Concurrent use may produce additive CNS depressant effects).
- No products indexed under this heading.

Astemizole (Concurrent use may produce additive CNS depressant effects).
- No products indexed under this heading.

Azatadine Maleate (Concurrent use may produce additive CNS depressant effects). Products include:
- Rynatan Tablets ... 3351

Bromodiphenhydramine Hydrochloride (Concurrent use may produce additive CNS depressant effects).
- No products indexed under this heading.

Brompheniramine Maleate (Concurrent use may produce additive CNS depressant effects). Products include:
- Bromfed Capsules (Extended-Release) ... 2269
- Bromfed-PD Capsules (Extended-Release) ... 2269
- Comtrex Acute Head Cold & Sinus Pressure Relief Tablets ... ▣627
- Dimetapp Elixir ... ▣777
- Dimetapp Cold and Fever Suspension ... ▣775
- Dimetapp DM Cold & Cough Elixir . ▣775
- Dimetapp Nighttime Flu Liquid ... ▣776

Buprenorphine Hydrochloride (Concurrent use may produce additive CNS depressant effects). Products include:
- Buprenex Injectable ... 2918

Buspirone Hydrochloride (Concurrent use may produce additive CNS depressant effects).
- No products indexed under this heading.

Butabarbital (Concurrent use may produce additive CNS depressant effects).
- No products indexed under this heading.

Butalbital (Concurrent use may produce additive CNS depressant effects). Products include:
- Phrenilin ... 578
- Sedapap Tablets 50 mg/650 mg ... 2225

Carbamazepine (CYP3A4 is ordinarily a minor metabolizing enzyme of zaleplon, the co-administration of a potent inducer, such as carbamazepine, although not posing a safety concern, could lead to ineffectiveness of zaleplon; concurrent use with anticonvulsants may produce additive CNS depressant effects). Products include:
- Carbatrol Capsules ... 3234
- Tegretol/Tegretol-XR ... 2404

Cetirizine Hydrochloride (Concurrent use may produce additive CNS depressant effects). Products include:
- Zyrtec ... 2756
- Zyrtec-D 12 Hour Extended Relief Tablets ... 2758

Chlordiazepoxide (Concurrent use may produce additive CNS depressant effects). Products include:
- Limbitrol ... 1738

Chlordiazepoxide Hydrochloride (Concurrent use may produce additive CNS depressant effects). Products include:
- Librium Capsules ... 1736
- Librium for Injection ... 1737

Chlorpheniramine Maleate (Concurrent use may produce additive CNS depressant effects). Products include:
- Actifed Cold & Sinus Caplets and Tablets ... ▣688
- Alka-Seltzer Plus Liqui-Gels ... ▣604
- BC Allergy Sinus Cold Powder ... ▣619
- Chlor-Trimeton Allergy Tablets ... ▣735
- Chlor-Trimeton Allergy/Decongestant Tablets ... ▣736
- Comtrex Flu Therapy & Fever Relief Nighttime Tablets ... ▣628
- Comtrex Maximum Strength Multi-Symptom Cold & Cough Relief Tablets and Caplets ... ▣626
- Contac Severe Cold and Flu Caplets Maximum Strength ... ▣746
- Coricidin 'D' Cold, Flu & Sinus Tablets ... ▣737
- Coricidin/Coricidin D ... ▣738
- Coricidin HBP Maximum Strength Flu Tablets ... ▣738
- Extendryl ... 1361
- Hycomine Compound Tablets ... 1317
- Kronofed-A ... 1341
- PediaCare Cough-Cold Liquid ... ▣719
- PediaCare NightRest Cough-Cold Liquid ... ▣719
- Robitussin Nighttime Honey Flu Liquid ... ▣786
- Ryna ... ▣768
- Singlet Caplets ... ▣761
- Sinutab Sinus Allergy Medication, Maximum Strength Formula, Tablets & Caplets ... ▣707
- Sudafed Cold & Allergy Tablets ... ▣708
- TheraFlu Regular Strength Cold & Cough Night Time Hot Liquid ... ▣676
- TheraFlu Regular Strength Cold & Sore Throat Night Time Hot Liquid ... ▣676
- TheraFlu Maximum Strength Flu & Cough Night Time Hot Liquid .. ▣678
- TheraFlu Maximum Strength Flu & Sore Throat Night Time Hot Liquid ... ▣677
- TheraFlu Maximum Strength Severe Cold & Congestion Night Time Caplets ... ▣678
- TheraFlu Maximum Strength Severe Cold & Congestion Night Time Hot Liquid ... ▣678
- Triaminic Cold & Allergy Liquid ... ▣681
- Triaminic Cold & Allergy Softchews ... ▣683
- Triaminic Cold & Cough Liquid ... ▣681
- Triaminic Cold & Cough Softchews ... ▣683
- Triaminic Cold & Night Time Cough Liquid ... ▣681
- Triaminic Cold, Cough & Fever Liquid ... ▣681
- Children's Tylenol Cold Suspension Liquid and Chewable Tablets ... 2015
- Children's Tylenol Cold Plus Cough Suspension Liquid and Chewable Tablets ... 2015
- Children's Tylenol Flu Suspension Liquid ... 2015
- Maximum Strength Tylenol Allergy Sinus Caplets, Gelcaps, and Geltabs ... 2010
- Multi-Symptom Tylenol Cold Complete Formula Caplets ... 2010
- Vicks 44M Cough, Cold & Flu Relief Liquid ... ▣725
- Pediatric Vicks 44m Cough & Cold Relief ... ▣728
- Children's Vicks NyQuil Cold/Cough Relief ... ▣726

Chlorpheniramine Polistirex (Concurrent use may produce additive CNS depressant effects). Products include:
- Tussionex Pennkinetic Extended-Release Suspension ... 1174

Chlorpheniramine Tannate (Concurrent use may produce additive CNS depressant effects). Products include:
- Reformulated Rynatan Pediatric Suspension ... 3352
- Rynatuss Pediatric Suspension ... 3353
- Rynatuss Tablets ... 3353
- Tussi-12 S Suspension ... 3356
- Tussi-12 Tablets ... 3356

Chlorpromazine (Concurrent use may produce additive CNS depressant effects). Products include:
- Thorazine Suppositories ... 1656

Chlorpromazine Hydrochloride (Concurrent use may produce additive CNS depressant effects). Products include:
- Thorazine ... 1656

Chlorprothixene (Concurrent use may produce additive CNS depressant effects).
- No products indexed under this heading.

Chlorprothixene Hydrochloride (Concurrent use may produce additive CNS depressant effects).
- No products indexed under this heading.

Chlorprothixene Lactate (Concurrent use may produce additive CNS depressant effects).
- No products indexed under this heading.

Cimetidine (Co-administration has produced an 85% increase in the mean Cmax and AUC of zaleplon; an initial dose of 5 mg should be given to patients who are concomitantly being treated with cimetidine). Products include:
- Tagamet HB 200 Suspension ... ▣762
- Tagamet HB 200 Tablets ... ▣761
- Tagamet Tablets ... 1644

Cimetidine Hydrochloride (Co-administration has produced an 85% increase in the mean Cmax and AUC of zaleplon; an initial dose of 5 mg should be given to patients who are concomitantly being treated with cimetidine). Products include:
- Tagamet ... 1644

Clemastine Fumarate (Concurrent use may produce additive CNS depressant effects). Products include:
- Tavist 12 Hour Allergy Tablets ... ▣676

Clorazepate Dipotassium (Concurrent use may produce additive CNS depressant effects). Products include:
- Tranxene ... 511

Clozapine (Concurrent use may produce additive CNS depressant effects). Products include:
- Clozaril Tablets ... 2319

Codeine Phosphate (Concurrent use may produce additive CNS depressant effects). Products include:
- Phenergan with Codeine Syrup ... 3557
- Phenergan VC with Codeine Syrup .. 3561
- Robitussin A-C Syrup ... 2942
- Robitussin-DAC Syrup ... 2942
- Ryna-C Liquid ... ▣768
- Soma Compound w/Codeine Tablets ... 3355
- Tussi-Organidin NR Liquid ... 3350
- Tussi-Organidin-S NR Liquid ... 3350
- Tylenol with Codeine ... 2595

Cyproheptadine Hydrochloride (Concurrent use may produce additive CNS depressant effects). Products include:
- Periactin Tablets ... 2155

Desflurane (Concurrent use may produce additive CNS depressant effects). Products include:
- Suprane Liquid for Inhalation ... 874

Desipramine Hydrochloride (Concurrent use may produce additive CNS depressant effects). Products include:
- Norpramin Tablets ... 755

Dexchlorpheniramine Maleate (Concurrent use may produce additive CNS depressant effects).
- No products indexed under this heading.

Dezocine (Concurrent use may produce additive CNS depressant effects).
- No products indexed under this heading.

Diazepam (Concurrent use may produce additive CNS depressant effects). Products include:
- Valium Injectable ... 3026
- Valium Tablets ... 3047

Diphenhydramine Citrate (Concurrent use may produce additive CNS depressant effects). Products include:
- Alka-Seltzer PM Effervescent Tablets ... 605
- Benadryl Allergy & Sinus Fastmelt Tablets ... 693
- Benadryl Children's Allergy/Cold Fastmelt Tablets ... 692
- Excedrin PM Tablets, Caplets, and Geltabs ... 631
- Goody's PM Powder ... 621

Diphenhydramine Hydrochloride (Concurrent use may produce additive CNS depressant effects). Products include:
- Extra Strength Bayer PM Caplets ... 611
- Benadryl Allergy Chewables ... 689
- Benadryl Allergy ... 691
- Benadryl Allergy Liquid ... 690
- Benadryl Allergy/Cold Tablets ... 691
- Benadryl Allergy/Congestion Tablets ... 692
- Benadryl Allergy & Sinus Liquid ... 693
- Benadryl Allergy Sinus Headache Caplets & Gelcaps ... 693
- Benadryl Severe Allergy & Sinus Headache Caplets ... 694
- Benadryl Dye-Free Allergy Liquid ... 690
- Benadryl Dye-Free Allergy Liqui-Gels Softgels ... 690
- Benadryl Itch Relief Stick Extra Strength ... 695
- Benadryl Cream ... 695
- Benadryl Gel ... 695
- Benadryl Spray ... 696
- Benadryl Parenteral ... 2617
- Coricidin HBP Night-Time Cold & Flu Tablets ... 738
- Nytol QuickCaps Caplets ... 622
- Maximum Strength Nytol QuickGels Softgels ... 621
- Extra Strength Percogesic Aspirin-Free Coated Caplets ... 665
- Simply Sleep Caplets ... 2008
- Sominex Original Formula Tablets ... 761
- Children's Tylenol Allergy-D Liquid ... 2014
- Maximum Strength Tylenol Allergy Sinus NightTime Caplets ... 2010
- Tylenol Severe Allergy Caplets ... 2010
- Maximum Strength Tylenol Flu NightTime Gelcaps ... 2011
- Extra Strength Tylenol PM Caplets, Geltabs, and Gelcaps ... 2012
- Unisom Maximum Strength SleepGels ... 713

Diphenylpyraline Hydrochloride (Concurrent use may produce additive CNS depressant effects).
No products indexed under this heading.

Divalproex Sodium (Concurrent use with anticonvulsants may produce additive CNS depressant effects). Products include:
- Depakote Sprinkle Capsules ... 426
- Depakote Tablets ... 430
- Depakote ER Tablets ... 436

Doxepin Hydrochloride (Concurrent use may produce additive CNS depressant effects). Products include:
- Sinequan ... 2713

Droperidol (Concurrent use may produce additive CNS depressant effects).
No products indexed under this heading.

Enflurane (Concurrent use may produce additive CNS depressant effects).
No products indexed under this heading.

Estazolam (Concurrent use may produce additive CNS depressant effects). Products include:
- ProSom Tablets ... 500

Ethchlorvynol (Concurrent use may produce additive CNS depressant effects).
No products indexed under this heading.

Ethinamate (Concurrent use may produce additive CNS depressant effects).
No products indexed under this heading.

Ethosuximide (Concurrent use with anticonvulsants may produce additive CNS depressant effects). Products include:
- Zarontin Capsules ... 2659
- Zarontin Syrup ... 2660

Ethotoin (Concurrent use with anticonvulsants may produce additive CNS depressant effects).
No products indexed under this heading.

Felbamate (Concurrent use with anticonvulsants may produce additive CNS depressant effects). Products include:
- Felbatol ... 3343

Fentanyl (Concurrent use may produce additive CNS depressant effects). Products include:
- Duragesic Transdermal System ... 1786

Fentanyl Citrate (Concurrent use may produce additive CNS depressant effects). Products include:
- Actiq ... 1184

Fexofenadine Hydrochloride (Concurrent use may produce additive CNS depressant effects). Products include:
- Allegra ... 712
- Allegra-D Extended-Release Tablets ... 714

Fluphenazine Decanoate (Concurrent use may produce additive CNS depressant effects).
No products indexed under this heading.

Fluphenazine Enanthate (Concurrent use may produce additive CNS depressant effects).
No products indexed under this heading.

Fluphenazine Hydrochloride (Concurrent use may produce additive CNS depressant effects).
No products indexed under this heading.

Flurazepam Hydrochloride (Concurrent use may produce additive CNS depressant effects).
No products indexed under this heading.

Fosphenytoin Sodium (CYP3A4 is ordinarily a minor metabolizing enzyme of zaleplon, the co-administration of a potent inducer, such as phenytoin, although not posing a safety concern, could lead to ineffectiveness of zaleplon; concurrent use with anticonvulsants may produce additive CNS depressant effects). Products include:
- Cerebyx Injection ... 2619

Glutethimide (Concurrent use may produce additive CNS depressant effects).
No products indexed under this heading.

Haloperidol (Concurrent use may produce additive CNS depressant effects). Products include:
- Haldol Injection, Tablets and Concentrate ... 2533

Haloperidol Decanoate (Concurrent use may produce additive CNS depressant effects). Products include:
- Haldol Decanoate ... 2535

Hydrocodone Bitartrate (Concurrent use may produce additive CNS depressant effects). Products include:
- Hycodan ... 1316
- Hycomine Compound Tablets ... 1317
- Hycotuss Expectorant Syrup ... 1318
- Lortab ... 3319
- Lortab Elixir ... 3317
- Maxidone Tablets CIII ... 3399
- Norco 5/325 Tablets CIII ... 3424
- Norco 7.5/325 Tablets CIII ... 3425
- Norco 10/325 Tablets CIII ... 3427
- Norco 10/325 Tablets CIII ... 3425
- Vicodin Tablets ... 516
- Vicodin ES Tablets ... 517
- Vicodin HP Tablets ... 518
- Vicodin Tuss Expectorant ... 519
- Vicoprofen Tablets ... 520
- Zydone Tablets ... 1330

Hydrocodone Polistirex (Concurrent use may produce additive CNS depressant effects). Products include:
- Tussionex Pennkinetic Extended-Release Suspension ... 1174

Hydromorphone Hydrochloride (Concurrent use may produce additive CNS depressant effects). Products include:
- Dilaudid ... 441
- Dilaudid Oral Liquid ... 445
- Dilaudid Powder ... 441
- Dilaudid Rectal Suppositories ... 441
- Dilaudid Tablets ... 441
- Dilaudid Tablets - 8 mg ... 445
- Dilaudid-HP ... 443

Hydroxyzine Hydrochloride (Concurrent use may produce additive CNS depressant effects). Products include:
- Atarax Tablets & Syrup ... 2667
- Vistaril Intramuscular Solution ... 2738

Imipramine Hydrochloride (Concurrent use may produce additive CNS depressant effects).
No products indexed under this heading.

Imipramine Pamoate (Concurrent use may produce additive CNS depressant effects).
No products indexed under this heading.

Isocarboxazid (Concurrent use may produce additive CNS depressant effects).
No products indexed under this heading.

Isoflurane (Concurrent use may produce additive CNS depressant effects).
No products indexed under this heading.

Ketamine Hydrochloride (Concurrent use may produce additive CNS depressant effects).
No products indexed under this heading.

Lamotrigine (Concurrent use with anticonvulsants may produce additive CNS depressant effects). Products include:
- Lamictal ... 1567

Levetiracetam (Concurrent use with anticonvulsants may produce additive CNS depressant effects). Products include:
- Keppra Tablets ... 3314

Levomethadyl Acetate Hydrochloride (Concurrent use may produce additive CNS depressant effects).
No products indexed under this heading.

Levorphanol Tartrate (Concurrent use may produce additive CNS depressant effects). Products include:
- Levo-Dromoran ... 1734
- Levorphanol Tartrate Tablets ... 3059

Lithium Carbonate (Concurrent use may produce additive CNS depressant effects). Products include:
- Eskalith ... 1527
- Lithium Carbonate ... 3061
- Lithobid Slow-Release Tablets ... 3255

Lithium Citrate (Concurrent use may produce additive CNS depressant effects). Products include:
- Lithium Citrate Syrup ... 3061

Loratadine (Concurrent use may produce additive CNS depressant effects). Products include:
- Claritin ... 3100
- Claritin-D 12 Hour Extended Release Tablets ... 3102
- Claritin-D 24 Hour Extended Release Tablets ... 3104

Lorazepam (Concurrent use may produce additive CNS depressant effects). Products include:
- Ativan Injection ... 3478
- Ativan Tablets ... 3482

Loxapine Hydrochloride (Concurrent use may produce additive CNS depressant effects).
No products indexed under this heading.

Loxapine Succinate (Concurrent use may produce additive CNS depressant effects). Products include:
- Loxitane Capsules ... 3398

Maprotiline Hydrochloride (Concurrent use may produce additive CNS depressant effects).
No products indexed under this heading.

Meperidine Hydrochloride (Concurrent use may produce additive CNS depressant effects). Products include:
- Demerol ... 3079
- Mepergan Injection ... 3539

Mephenytoin (Concurrent use with anticonvulsants may produce additive CNS depressant effects).
No products indexed under this heading.

Mephobarbital (Concurrent use may produce additive CNS depressant effects).
No products indexed under this heading.

Meprobamate (Concurrent use may produce additive CNS depressant effects). Products include:
- Miltown Tablets ... 3349

Mesoridazine Besylate (Concurrent use may produce additive CNS depressant effects). Products include:
- Serentil ... 1057

Methadone Hydrochloride (Concurrent use may produce additive CNS depressant effects). Products include:
- Dolophine Hydrochloride Tablets ... 3056

Methdilazine Hydrochloride (Concurrent use may produce additive CNS depressant effects).
No products indexed under this heading.

Methohexital Sodium (Concurrent use may produce additive CNS depressant effects). Products include:
- Brevital Sodium for Injection, USP ... 1815

Methotrimeprazine (Concurrent use may produce additive CNS depressant effects).
No products indexed under this heading.

Methoxyflurane (Concurrent use may produce additive CNS depressant effects).
No products indexed under this heading.

Methsuximide (Concurrent use with anticonvulsants may produce additive CNS depressant effects). Products include:
- Celontin Capsules ... 2618

Midazolam Hydrochloride (Concurrent use may produce additive CNS depressant effects). Products include:
- Versed Injection ... 3027
- Versed Syrup ... 3033

Molindone Hydrochloride (Concurrent use may produce additive CNS depressant effects). Products include:
- Moban ... 1320

Morphine Sulfate (Concurrent use may produce additive CNS depressant effects). Products include:
- Astramorph/PF Injection, USP (Preservative-Free) ... 594
- Duramorph Injection ... 1312
- Infumorph 200 and Infumorph 500 Sterile Solutions ... 1314
- Kadian Capsules ... 1335
- MS Contin Tablets ... 2896
- MSIR ... 2898
- Oramorph SR Tablets ... 3062

IMPORTANT NOTE: Always consult each drug listing in the patient's regimen for possible interactions.

Roxanol 3066

Nortriptyline Hydrochloride (Concurrent use may produce additive CNS depressant effects).
No products indexed under this heading.

Olanzapine (Concurrent use may produce additive CNS depressant effects). Products include:
Zyprexa Tablets 1973
Zyprexa ZYDIS Orally Disintegrating Tablets 1973

Oxazepam (Concurrent use may produce additive CNS depressant effects).
No products indexed under this heading.

Oxcarbazepine (Concurrent use with anticonvulsants may produce additive CNS depressant effects). Products include:
Trileptal Oral Suspension 2407
Trileptal Tablets 2407

Oxycodone Hydrochloride (Concurrent use may produce additive CNS depressant effects). Products include:
OxyContin Tablets 2912
OxyFast Oral Concentrate Solution . 2916
OxyIR Capsules 2916
Percocet Tablets 1326
Percodan Tablets 1327
Percolone Tablets 1327
Roxicodone 3067
Tylox Capsules 2597

Paramethadione (Concurrent use with anticonvulsants may produce additive CNS depressant effects).
No products indexed under this heading.

Pentobarbital Sodium (Concurrent use may produce additive CNS depressant effects). Products include:
Nembutal Sodium Solution 485

Perphenazine (Concurrent use may produce additive CNS depressant effects). Products include:
Etrafon 3115
Trilafon 3160

Phenacemide (Concurrent use with anticonvulsants may produce additive CNS depressant effects).
No products indexed under this heading.

Phenelzine Sulfate (Concurrent use may produce additive CNS depressant effects). Products include:
Nardil Tablets 2653

Phenobarbital (CYP3A4 is ordinarily a minor metabolizing enzyme of zaleplon, the co-administration of a potent inducer, such as phenobarbital, although not posing a safety concern, could lead to ineffectiveness of zaleplon; concurrent use may produce additive CNS depressant effects). Products include:
Arco-Lase Plus Tablets 592
Donnatal 2929
Donnatal Extentabs 2930

Phensuximide (Concurrent use with anticonvulsants may produce additive CNS depressant effects).
No products indexed under this heading.

Phenytoin (CYP3A4 is ordinarily a minor metabolizing enzyme of zaleplon, the co-administration of a potent inducer, such as phenytoin, although not posing a safety concern, could lead to ineffectiveness of zaleplon; concurrent use with anticonvulsants may produce additive CNS depressant effects). Products include:
Dilantin Infatabs 2624
Dilantin-125 Oral Suspension 2625

Phenytoin Sodium (CYP3A4 is ordinarily a minor metabolizing enzyme of zaleplon, the co-administration of a potent inducer, such as phenytoin, although not posing a safety concern, could lead to ineffectiveness of zaleplon; concurrent use with anticonvulsants may produce additive CNS depressant effects). Products include:
Dilantin Kapseals 2622

Prazepam (Concurrent use may produce additive CNS depressant effects).
No products indexed under this heading.

Primidone (Concurrent use with anticonvulsants may produce additive CNS depressant effects).
No products indexed under this heading.

Prochlorperazine (Concurrent use may produce additive CNS depressant effects). Products include:
Compazine 1505

Promethazine Hydrochloride (Concurrent use may produce additive CNS depressant effects). Products include:
Mepergan Injection 3539
Phenergan Injection 3553
Phenergan 3556
Phenergan Syrup 3554
Phenergan with Codeine Syrup 3557
Phenergan with Dextromethorphan Syrup 3559
Phenergan VC Syrup 3560
Phenergan VC with Codeine Syrup .. 3561

Propofol (Concurrent use may produce additive CNS depressant effects). Products include:
Diprivan Injectable Emulsion 667

Propoxyphene Hydrochloride (Concurrent use may produce additive CNS depressant effects). Products include:
Darvon Pulvules 1909
Darvon Compound-65 Pulvules 1910

Propoxyphene Napsylate (Concurrent use may produce additive CNS depressant effects). Products include:
Darvon-N/Darvocet-N 1907
Darvon-N Tablets 1912

Protriptyline Hydrochloride (Concurrent use may produce additive CNS depressant effects). Products include:
Vivactil Tablets 2446
Vivactil Tablets 2217

Pyrilamine Maleate (Concurrent use may produce additive CNS depressant effects). Products include:
Maximum Strength Midol Menstrual Caplets and Gelcaps .... ■612
Maximum Strength Midol PMS Caplets and Gelcaps .... ■613

Pyrilamine Tannate (Concurrent use may produce additive CNS depressant effects). Products include:
Ryna-12 S Suspension 3351

Quazepam (Concurrent use may produce additive CNS depressant effects).
No products indexed under this heading.

Quetiapine Fumarate (Concurrent use may produce additive CNS depressant effects). Products include:
Seroquel Tablets 684

Remifentanil Hydrochloride (Concurrent use may produce additive CNS depressant effects).
No products indexed under this heading.

Rifampin (Co-administration with multiple-dose of rifampin, a CYP3A4 inducer, has reduced zaleplon Cmax and AUC by approximately 80%). Products include:
Rifadin 765
Rifamate Capsules 767
Rifater Tablets 769

Risperidone (Concurrent use may produce additive CNS depressant effects). Products include:
Risperdal 1796

Secobarbital Sodium (Concurrent use may produce additive CNS depressant effects).
No products indexed under this heading.

Sevoflurane (Concurrent use may produce additive CNS depressant effects).
No products indexed under this heading.

Sufentanil Citrate (Concurrent use may produce additive CNS depressant effects).
No products indexed under this heading.

Temazepam (Concurrent use may produce additive CNS depressant effects).
No products indexed under this heading.

Terfenadine (Concurrent use may produce additive CNS depressant effects).
No products indexed under this heading.

Thiamylal Sodium (Concurrent use may produce additive CNS depressant effects).
No products indexed under this heading.

Thioridazine Hydrochloride (Co-administration has produced additive effects of decreased alertness and impaired psychomotor performance for 2 to 4 hours). Products include:
Thioridazine Hydrochloride Tablets 2289

Thiothixene (Concurrent use may produce additive CNS depressant effects). Products include:
Navane Capsules 2701
Thiothixene Capsules 2290

Tiagabine Hydrochloride (Concurrent use with anticonvulsants may produce additive CNS depressant effects). Products include:
Gabitril Tablets 1189

Topiramate (Concurrent use with anticonvulsants may produce additive CNS depressant effects). Products include:
Topamax Sprinkle Capsules 2590
Topamax Tablets 2590

Tranylcypromine Sulfate (Concurrent use may produce additive CNS depressant effects). Products include:
Parnate Tablets 1607

Triazolam (Concurrent use may produce additive CNS depressant effects). Products include:
Halcion Tablets 2823

Trifluoperazine Hydrochloride (Concurrent use may produce additive CNS depressant effects). Products include:
Stelazine 1640

Trimeprazine Tartrate (Concurrent use may produce additive CNS depressant effects).
No products indexed under this heading.

Trimethadione (Concurrent use with anticonvulsants may produce additive CNS depressant effects).
No products indexed under this heading.

Trimipramine Maleate (Concurrent use may produce additive CNS depressant effects). Products include:
Surmontil Capsules 3595

Tripelennamine Hydrochloride (Concurrent use may produce additive CNS depressant effects).
No products indexed under this heading.

Triprolidine Hydrochloride (Concurrent use may produce additive CNS depressant effects). Products include:
Actifed Cold & Allergy Tablets .... ■688

Valproate Sodium (Concurrent use with anticonvulsants may produce additive CNS depressant effects). Products include:
Depacon Injection 416

Valproic Acid (Concurrent use with anticonvulsants may produce additive CNS depressant effects). Products include:
Depakene 421

Ziprasidone Hydrochloride (Concurrent use may produce additive CNS depressant effects). Products include:
Geodon Capsules 2688

Zolpidem Tartrate (Concurrent use may produce additive CNS depressant effects). Products include:
Ambien Tablets 3191

Zonisamide (Concurrent use with anticonvulsants may produce additive CNS depressant effects). Products include:
Zonegran Capsules 1307

Food Interactions

Alcohol (Concurrent use may produce additive CNS depressant effects).

Food, unspecified (A high-fat/heavy meal prolongs the absorption of zaleplon compared to fasting state, delays tmax by approximately 2 hours and reduces Cmax approximately 35%; the effect of Sonata on sleep onset may be reduced if it is taken with or immediately after a high-fat/heavy meal).

SORIATANE CAPSULES

(Acitretin) 3003
May interact with:

Glibenclamide (Co-administration has resulted in enhanced clearance of blood glucose).
No products indexed under this heading.

Methotrexate Sodium (Possibility of an increased risk of hepatotoxicity in patients treated with etretinate and methotrexate concomitantly; consequently concomitant use of acitretin and methotrexate should be avoided).
No products indexed under this heading.

Norethindrone (Acitretin interferes with the contraceptive effect of microdosed progestin minipill preparations). Products include:
Brevicon 28-Day Tablets 3380
Micronor Tablets 2543
Modicon 2563
Necon 3415
Norinyl 1 +35 28-Day Tablets 3380
Norinyl 1 + 50 28-Day Tablets 3380
Nor-QD Tablets 3423
Ortho-Novum 2563
Ortho-Novum 1/50□28 Tablets 2556
Ovcon 3364
Tri-Norinyl-28 Tablets 3433

Vitamin A (Because of the relationship of acitretin to vitamin A, patients should be advised against taking vitamin A supplements in excess of minimum recommended daily allowances). Products include:
Aquasol A Parenteral 593
Beta-C Tablets .... ■811
Centrum Focused Formulas Prostate Softgels .... ■816

Food Interactions

Alcohol (Concurrent ingestion has been associated with the formation of etretinate, which has a longer elimination half-life than acitretin; longer elimination half-life increases the duration of teratogenic potential for female patients; alcohol must not be ingested during or for 2 months after the cessation of therapy).

SPARK! BEVERAGE MIX

(Amino Acid Preparations, Vitamins with Minerals) .... ■800
None cited in PDR database.

SPORANOX CAPSULES
(Itraconazole) 1800
May interact with antacids, dihydropyridine calcium channel blockers, erythromycin, histamine H_2-receptor antagonists, oral hypoglycemic agents, methylprednisolone, phenytoin, proton pump inhibitor, quinidine, vinca alkaloids, and certain other agents. Compounds in these categories include:

Esomeprazole Magnesium (Decreases plasma concentrations of itraconazole). Products include:
Nexium Delayed-Release Capsules 619

Acarbose (Severe hypoglycemia has been reported in patients concomitantly receiving azole antifungal agents and oral hypoglycemic agents). Products include:
Precose Tablets 906

Alfentanil Hydrochloride (Co-administration may result in increased plasma concentrations of alfentanil).
No products indexed under this heading.

Alprazolam (Co-administration with alprazolam could lead to increased plasma concentrations of alprazolam; increased plasma concentrations could potentiate and prolong hypnotic and sedative effects). Products include:
Xanax Tablets 2865

Aluminum Carbonate (Absorption of itraconazole is impaired when gastric acidity is decreased; antacid should not be administered for at least two hours after itraconazole administration).
No products indexed under this heading.

Aluminum Hydroxide (Absorption of itraconazole is impaired when gastric acidity is decreased; antacid should not be administered for at least two hours after itraconazole administration). Products include:
Amphojel Suspension (Mint Flavor) 789
Gaviscon Extra Strength Liquid 751
Gaviscon Extra Strength Tablets 751
Gaviscon Regular Strength Liquid 751
Gaviscon Regular Strength Tablets 750
Maalox Antacid/Anti-Gas Oral Suspension 673
Maalox Max Maximum Strength Antacid/Anti-Gas Liquid 2300
Maalox Regular Strength Antacid/Antigas Liquid 2300
Mylanta 1813
Vanquish Caplets 617

Amlodipine Besylate (Co-administration has resulted in edema; calcium channel blockers can have negative inotropic effect which may be additive to those of itraconazole; itraconazole can inhibit metabolism of calcium channel blockers such as dihydropyridines). Products include:
Lotrel Capsules 2370
Norvasc Tablets 2704

Amphotericin B (Prior treatment with itraconazole may reduce or inhibit the activity of polyenes such as amphotericin B). Products include:
Abelcet Injection 1273
AmBisome for Injection 1383
Amphotec 1774

Astemizole (Itraconazole is a potent inhibitor of the CYP4503A4 system and may raise plasma concentrations of drugs metabolized by this pathway, such as astemizole; serious cardiovascular events, including ventricular tachycardia, QT prolongation, torsade de pointes, cardiac arrest, and/or death have occurred in patients using astemizole with itraconazole and/or other CYP3A4 inhibitors; concurrent use is contraindicated).
No products indexed under this heading.

Atorvastatin Calcium (Co-administration results in inhibition of the metabolism of atorvastatin leading to increased plasma concentrations of atorvastatin; increased risk of skeletal muscle toxicity, including rhabdomyolysis). Products include:
Lipitor Tablets 2639
Lipitor Tablets 2696

Buspirone Hydrochloride (Co-administration results in significant increases in plasma concentrations of buspirone).
No products indexed under this heading.

Busulfan (Itraconazole may inhibit the metabolism of busulfan). Products include:
Myleran Tablets 1603

Carbamazepine (Co-administration would be expected to result in decreased plasma concentrations of itraconazole; concurrent use may result in inhibition of the metabolism of carbamazepine resulting in increased plasma concentrations of carbamazepine). Products include:
Carbatrol Capsules 3234
Tegretol/Tegretol-XR 2404

Cerivastatin Sodium (Co-administration results in inhibition of the metabolism of cerivastatin leading to increased plasma concentrations of cerivastatin; increased risk of skeletal muscle toxicity, including rhabdomyolysis). Products include:
Baycol Tablets 883

Chlorpropamide (Severe hypoglycemia has been reported in patients concomitantly receiving azole antifungal agents and oral hypoglycemic agents). Products include:
Diabinese Tablets 2680

Cimetidine (Decreases plasma concentrations of itraconazole). Products include:
Tagamet HB 200 Suspension 762
Tagamet HB 200 Tablets 761
Tagamet Tablets 1644

Cimetidine Hydrochloride (Decreases plasma concentrations of itraconazole). Products include:
Tagamet 1644

Cisapride (Itraconazole is a potent inhibitor of the CYP4503A4 system and may raise plasma concentrations of drugs metabolized by this pathway, such as cisapride; serious cardiovascular events, including ventricular tachycardia, QT prolongation, torsade de pointes, cardiac arrest, and/or death have occurred in patients using cisapride with itraconazole and/or other CYP3A4 inhibitors; concurrent use is contraindicated).
No products indexed under this heading.

Clarithromycin (Increases plasma concentrations of itraconazole). Products include:
Biaxin/Biaxin XL 403
PREVPAC 3298

Cyclosporine (Co-administration has led to increased plasma concentrations of cyclosporine). Products include:
Gengraf Capsules 457
Neoral Soft Gelatin Capsules 2380
Neoral Oral Solution 2380
Sandimmune 2388

Diazepam (Co-administration with diazepam could lead to increased plasma concentrations of diazepam; increased plasma concentrations could potentiate and prolong hypnotic and sedative effects). Products include:
Valium Injectable 3026
Valium Tablets 3047

Digoxin (Co-administration results in increased plasma concentrations of digoxin). Products include:
Digitek Tablets 1003
Lanoxicaps Capsules 1574
Lanoxin Injection 1581
Lanoxin Tablets 1587
Lanoxin Elixir Pediatric 1578
Lanoxin Injection Pediatric 1584

Docetaxel (Itraconazole may inhibit the metabolism of docetaxel). Products include:
Taxotere for Injection Concentrate 778

Dofetilide (Itraconazole is a potent inhibitor of CYP4503A4 system and may raise plasma concentrations of drugs metabolized by this pathway, such as dofetilide, serious cardiovascular events, including ventricular tachycardia, QT prolongation, torsade de pointes, cardiac arrest, and/or death have occurred in patients concurrently on CYP4503A4 inhibitors; co-administration is contraindicated). Products include:
Tikosyn Capsules 2717

Erythromycin (Increases the plasma concentration of itraconazole). Products include:
Emgel 2% Topical Gel 1285
Ery-Tab Tablets 448
Erythromycin Base Filmtab Tablets 454
Erythromycin Delayed-Release Capsules, USP 455
PCE Dispertab Tablets 498

Erythromycin Estolate (Increases the plasma concentration of itraconazole).
No products indexed under this heading.

Erythromycin Ethylsuccinate (Increases the plasma concentration of itraconazole). Products include:
E.E.S. 450
EryPed 446
Pediazole Suspension 3050

Erythromycin Gluceptate (Increases the plasma concentration of itraconazole).
No products indexed under this heading.

Erythromycin Stearate (Increases the plasma concentration of itraconazole). Products include:
Erythrocin Stearate Filmtab Tablets 452

Famotidine (Decreases plasma concentrations of itraconazole). Products include:
Famotidine Injection 866
Pepcid AC 1814
Pepcid Complete Chewable Tablets 1815
Pepcid Injection 2153
Pepcid for Oral Suspension 2150
Pepcid RPD Orally Disintegrating Tablets 2150
Pepcid Tablets 2150

Felodipine (Co-administration has resulted in edema; calcium channel blockers can have negative inotropic effect which may be additive to those of itraconazole; itraconazole can inhibit metabolism of calcium channel blockers such as dihydropyridines). Products include:
Lexxel Tablets 608
Plendil Extended-Release Tablets 623

Fosphenytoin Sodium (Co-administration with inducers of CYP3A4, such as phenytoin, results in reduced plasma concentrations of itraconazole). Products include:
Cerebyx Injection 2619

Glimepiride (Severe hypoglycemia has been reported in patients concomitantly receiving azole antifungal agents and oral hypoglycemic agents). Products include:
Amaryl Tablets 717

Glipizide (Severe hypoglycemia has been reported in patients concomitantly receiving azole antifungal agents and oral hypoglycemic agents). Products include:
Glucotrol Tablets 2692
Glucotrol XL Extended Release Tablets 2693

Glyburide (Severe hypoglycemia has been reported in patients concomitantly receiving azole antifungal agents and oral hypoglycemic agents). Products include:
DiaBeta Tablets 741
Glucovance Tablets 1086

Indinavir Sulfate (Co-administration with protease inhibitors metabolized by CYP3A4, such as indinavir, may increase plasma concentrations of indinavir; indinavir administration also increases the plasma concentrations of itraconazole). Products include:
Crixivan Capsules 2070

Isoniazid (Co-administration may result in reduced plasma levels of itraconazole; efficacy of itraconazole could be substantially reduced if used concurrently; co-administration is not recommended). Products include:
Rifamate Capsules 767
Rifater Tablets 769

Isradipine (Co-administration has resulted in edema; calcium channel blockers can have negative inotropic effect which may be additive to those of itraconazole; itraconazole can inhibit metabolism of calcium channel blockers such as dihydropyridines). Products include:
DynaCirc Capsules 2921
DynaCirc CR Tablets 2923

Lansoprazole (Decreases plasma concentrations of itraconazole). Products include:
Prevacid Delayed-Release Capsules 3292
PREVPAC 3298

Lovastatin (Co-administration results in inhibition of the metabolism of lovastatin leading to increased plasma concentrations of lovastatin; increased risk of skeletal muscle toxicity, including rhabdomyolysis; concurrent use is contraindicated). Products include:
Mevacor Tablets 2132

Magaldrate (Absorption of itraconazole is impaired when gastric acidity is decreased; antacid should not be administered for at least two hours after itraconazole administration).
No products indexed under this heading.

Magnesium Hydroxide (Absorption of itraconazole is impaired when gastric acidity is decreased; antacid should not be administered for at least two hours after itraconazole administration). Products include:
Ex•Lax Milk of Magnesia Liquid 670
Maalox Antacid/Anti-Gas Oral Suspension 673
Maalox Max Maximum Strength Antacid/Anti-Gas Liquid 2300
Maalox Regular Strength Antacid/Antigas Liquid 2300
Mylanta Fast-Acting 1813
Mylanta 1813
Pepcid Complete Chewable Tablets 1815
Phillips' Chewable Tablets 615
Phillips' Milk of Magnesia Liquid (Original, Cherry, & Mint) 616
Rolaids Tablets 706
Extra Strength Rolaids Tablets 706
Vanquish Caplets 617

Magnesium Oxide (Absorption of itraconazole is impaired when gastric acidity is decreased; antacid should not be administered for at least two hours after itraconazole administration). Products include:
Beelith Tablets 946
Mag-Ox 400 Tablets 1024
Uro-Mag Capsules 1024

Metformin Hydrochloride (Severe hypoglycemia has been reported in patients concomitantly receiving

IMPORTANT NOTE: Always consult each drug listing in the patient's regimen for possible interactions.

azole antifungal agents and oral hypoglycemic agents). Products include:

- Glucophage Tablets 1080
- Glucophage XR Tablets 1080
- Glucovance Tablets 1086

Methylprednisolone (Itraconazole may inhibit the metabolism of methylprednisolone).

No products indexed under this heading.

Methylprednisolone Acetate (Itraconazole may inhibit the metabolism of methylprednisolone). Products include:

- Depo-Medrol Injectable Suspension 2795

Methylprednisolone Sodium Succinate (Itraconazole may inhibit the metabolism of methylprednisolone). Products include:

- Solu-Medrol Sterile Powder 2855

Midazolam Hydrochloride (Co-administration with oral midazolam could lead to increased plasma concentrations of midazolam; increased plasma concentrations could potentiate and prolong hypnotic and sedative effects; concurrent use of oral midazolam is contraindicated). Products include:

- Versed Injection 3027
- Versed Syrup 3033

Miglitol (Severe hypoglycemia has been reported in patients concomitantly receiving azole antifungal agents and oral hypoglycemic agents). Products include:

- Glyset Tablets 2821

Nevirapine (In vivo studies have shown that nevirapine induces the metabolism of ketoconazole, significantly reducing the bioavailability of ketoconazole; because of the similarities between ketoconazole and itraconazole, co-administration is not recommended). Products include:

- Viramune Oral Suspension 1060
- Viramune Tablets 1060

Nicardipine Hydrochloride (Co-administration has resulted in edema; calcium channel blockers can have negative inotropic effect which may be additive to those of itraconazole; itraconazole can inhibit metabolism of calcium channel blockers such as dihydropyridines). Products include:

- Cardene I.V. 3485

Nifedipine (Co-administration has resulted in edema; calcium channel blockers can have negative inotropic effect which may be additive to those of itraconazole; itraconazole can inhibit metabolism of calcium channel blockers such as dihydropyridines). Products include:

- Adalat CC Tablets 877
- Procardia Capsules 2708
- Procardia XL Extended Release Tablets 2710

Nimodipine (Co-administration has resulted in edema; calcium channel blockers can have negative inotropic effect which may be additive to those of itraconazole; itraconazole can inhibit metabolism of calcium channel blockers such as dihydropyridines). Products include:

- Nimotop Capsules 904

Nizatidine (Decreases plasma concentrations of itraconazole). Products include:

- Axid Pulvules 1903
- Axid Pulvules 2919

Omeprazole (Decreases plasma concentrations of itraconazole). Products include:

- Prilosec Delayed-Release Capsules 628

Pantoprazole Sodium (Decreases plasma concentrations of itraconazole). Products include:

- Protonix I.V. 3580
- Protonix Tablets 3577

Phenobarbital (Co-administration would be expected to result in decreased plasma concentrations of itraconazole). Products include:

- Arco-Lase Plus Tablets 592
- Donnatal 2929
- Donnatal Extentabs 2930

Phenytoin (Co-administration with inducers of CYP3A4, such as phenytoin, results in reduced plasma concentrations of itraconazole). Products include:

- Dilantin Infatabs 2624
- Dilantin-125 Oral Suspension 2625

Phenytoin Sodium (Co-administration with inducers of CYP3A4, such as phenytoin, results in reduced plasma concentrations of itraconazole). Products include:

- Dilantin Kapseals 2622

Pimozide (Itraconazole is a potent inhibitor of the CYP4503A4 system and may raise plasma concentrations of drugs metabolized by this pathway, such as pimozide; serious cardiovascular events, including ventricular tachycardia, QT prolongation, torsade de pointes, cardiac arrest, and/or death have occurred in patients using pimozide with itraconazole and/or other CYP3A4 inhibitors; concurrent use is contraindicated). Products include:

- Orap Tablets 1407

Pioglitazone Hydrochloride (Severe hypoglycemia has been reported in patients concomitantly receiving azole antifungal agents and oral hypoglycemic agents). Products include:

- Actos Tablets 3275

Quinidine Gluconate (Itraconazole is a potent inhibitor of the CYP4503A4 system and may raise plasma concentrations of drugs metabolized by this pathway, such as quinidine; serious cardiovascular events, including ventricular tachycardia, QT prolongation, torsade de pointes, cardiac arrest, and/or death have occurred in patients using quinidine with itraconazole and/or other CYP3A4 inhibitors; concurrent use is contraindicated). Products include:

- Quinaglute Dura-Tabs Tablets 978

Quinidine Polygalacturonate (Itraconazole is a potent inhibitor of the CYP4503A4 system and may raise plasma concentrations of drugs metabolized by this pathway, such as quinidine; serious cardiovascular events, including ventricular tachycardia, QT prolongation, torsade de pointes, cardiac arrest, and/or death have occurred in patients using quinidine with itraconazole and/or other CYP3A4 inhibitors; concurrent use is contraindicated).

No products indexed under this heading.

Quinidine Sulfate (Itraconazole is a potent inhibitor of the CYP4503A4 system and may raise plasma concentrations of drugs metabolized by this pathway, such as quinidine; serious cardiovascular events, including ventricular tachycardia, QT prolongation, torsade de pointes, cardiac arrest, and/or death have occurred in patients using quinidine with itraconazole and/or other CYP3A4 inhibitors; concurrent use is contraindicated). Products include:

- Quinidex Extentabs 2933

Rabeprazole Sodium (Decreases plasma concentrations of itraconazole). Products include:

- Aciphex Tablets 1267
- Aciphex Tablets 1783

Ranitidine Bismuth Citrate (Decreases plasma concentrations of itraconazole).

No products indexed under this heading.

Ranitidine Hydrochloride (Decreases plasma concentrations of itraconazole). Products include:

- Zantac 1690
- Zantac Injection 1688
- Zantac 75 Tablets .... ▣717

Repaglinide (Severe hypoglycemia has been reported in patients concomitantly receiving azole antifungal agents and oral hypoglycemic agents). Products include:

- Prandin Tablets (0.5, 1, and 2 mg) 2432

Rifabutin (Co-administration has resulted in significantly reduced plasma levels of itraconazole and its metabolite, hydroxyitraconazole; efficacy of itraconazole could be substantially reduced if used concurrently; co-administration is not recommended; itraconazole may inhibit the metabolism of rifabutin). Products include:

- Mycobutin Capsules 2838

Rifampin (Co-administration has resulted in significantly reduced plasma levels of itraconazole and its metabolite, hydroxyitraconazole; efficacy of itraconazole could be substantially reduced if used concurrently; co-administration is not recommended). Products include:

- Rifadin 765
- Rifamate Capsules 767
- Rifater Tablets 769

Ritonavir (Co-administration with protease inhibitors metabolized by CYP3A4, such as ritonavir, may increase plasma concentrations of ritonavir; ritonavir administration also increases the plasma concentrations of itraconazole). Products include:

- Kaletra Capsules 471
- Kaletra Oral Solution 471
- Norvir Capsules 487
- Norvir Oral Solution 487

Rosiglitazone Maleate (Severe hypoglycemia has been reported in patients concomitantly receiving azole antifungal agents and oral hypoglycemic agents). Products include:

- Avandia Tablets 1490

Saquinavir (Co-administration with protease inhibitors metabolized by CYP3A4, such as saquinavir, may increase plasma concentrations of saquinavir). Products include:

- Fortovase Capsules 2970

Saquinavir Mesylate (Co-administration with protease inhibitors metabolized by CYP3A4, such as saquinavir, may increase plasma concentrations of saquinavir). Products include:

- Invirase Capsules 2979

Simvastatin (Co-administration results in inhibition of the metabolism of simvastatin leading to increased plasma concentrations of simvastatin; increased risk of skeletal muscle toxicity, including rhabdomyolysis; concurrent use is contraindicated). Products include:

- Zocor Tablets 2219

Sirolimus (Co-administration could increase plasma concentrations of sirolimus). Products include:

- Rapamune Oral Solution and Tablets 3584

Sodium Bicarbonate (Absorption of itraconazole is impaired when gastric acidity is decreased; antacid should not be administered for at least two hours after itraconazole administration). Products include:

- Alka-Seltzer .... ▣603
- Alka-Seltzer Lemon Lime Antacid and Pain Reliever Effervescent Tablets .... ▣603
- Alka-Seltzer Extra Strength Antacid and Pain Reliever Effervescent Tablets .... ▣603
- Alka-Seltzer Heartburn Relief Tablets .... ▣604
- Ceo-Two Evacuant Suppository .... ▣618
- Colyte with Flavor Packs for Oral Solution 3170
- GoLYTELY and Pineapple Flavor GoLYTELY for Oral Solution 1068
- NuLYTELY, Cherry Flavor, Lemon-Lime Flavor, and Orange Flavor NuLYTELY for Oral Solution 1068

Tacrolimus (Co-administration has led to increased plasma concentrations of tacrolimus). Products include:

- Prograf 1393
- Protopic Ointment 1397

Terfenadine (Itraconazole is a potent inhibitor of the cytochrome P450 3A system and may raise plasma concentrations of drugs metabolized by this pathway, such as terfenadine; co-administration has resulted in serious cardiovascular events, including death, ventricular tachycardia, and torsade de pointes; concurrent use is contraindicated).

No products indexed under this heading.

Tolazamide (Severe hypoglycemia has been reported in patients concomitantly receiving azole antifungal agents and oral hypoglycemic agents).

No products indexed under this heading.

Tolbutamide (Severe hypoglycemia has been reported in patients concomitantly receiving azole antifungal agents and oral hypoglycemic agents).

No products indexed under this heading.

Triazolam (Co-administration with triazolam could lead to increased plasma concentrations of triazolam; increased plasma concentrations could potentiate and prolong hypnotic and sedative effects; concurrent use of triazolam is contraindicated). Products include:

- Halcion Tablets 2823

Trimetrexate Glucuronate (Because of the similarities between ketoconazole and itraconazole, co-administration may inhibit the metabolism of trimetrexate).

No products indexed under this heading.

Troglitazone (Severe hypoglycemia has been reported in patients concomitantly receiving azole antifungal agents and oral hypoglycemic agents).

No products indexed under this heading.

Verapamil Hydrochloride (Co-administration has resulted in edema; calcium channel blockers can have negative inotropic effect which may be additive to those of itraconazole; itraconazole can inhibit metabolism of calcium channel blockers such as verapamil). Products include:

- Covera-HS Tablets 3199
- Isoptin SR Tablets 467
- Tarka Tablets 508
- Verelan Capsules 3184
- Verelan PM Capsules 3186

Vinblastine Sulfate (Itraconazole may inhibit the metabolism of vinca alkaloids).

No products indexed under this heading.

Vincristine Sulfate (Itraconazole may inhibit the metabolism of vinca alkaloids).

No products indexed under this heading.

Vinorelbine Tartrate (Itraconazole may inhibit the metabolism of vinca alkaloids). Products include:

- Navelbine Injection 1604

Warfarin Sodium (Itraconazole enhances the anticoagulant effect of warfarin). Products include:

- Coumadin for Injection 1243
- Coumadin Tablets 1243

Warfarin Sodium Tablets, USP 3302

Food Interactions

Cola (Absorption of oral itraconazole is enhanced when administered with a cola beverage in patients with achlorhydria, such as AIDS or patients taking acid suppressors, e.g., H_2 inhibitors and proton pump inhibitors).

Food, unspecified (Presence of food increases systemic bioavailability; when taken on an empty stomach the systemic bioavailability is reduced; Sporanox Capsules should be taken with a full meal to ensure maximal absorption).

SPORANOX INJECTION

(Itraconazole) 2509

See Sporanox Capsules

SPORANOX INJECTION

(Itraconazole) 1804

See Sporanox Capsules

SPORANOX ORAL SOLUTION

(Itraconazole) 1808

See Sporanox Capsules

SPORANOX ORAL SOLUTION

(Itraconazole) 2512

See Sporanox Capsules

STADOL NS NASAL SPRAY

(Butorphanol Tartrate) 1108

May interact with antihistamines, barbiturates, central nervous system depressants, erythromycin, tranquilizers, theophylline, and certain other agents. Compounds in these categories include:

Acrivastine (Co-administration may result in increased CNS depressant effects, such as drowsiness, dizziness, and impaired mental function). Products include:

Semprex-D Capsules 1172

Alfentanil Hydrochloride (Co-administration may result in increased CNS depressant effects, such as drowsiness, dizziness, and impaired mental function).

No products indexed under this heading.

Alprazolam (Co-administration may result in increased CNS depressant effects, such as drowsiness, dizziness, and impaired mental function). Products include:

Xanax Tablets 2865

Aminophylline (It is not known if the effects of butorphanol are altered by co-administration of drugs that affect hepatic metabolism, such as theophylline, but physician should be alert to the possibility that a smaller initial dose and longer intervals between doses may be needed).

No products indexed under this heading.

Aprobarbital (Co-administration may result in increased CNS depressant effects, such as drowsiness, dizziness, and impaired mental function).

No products indexed under this heading.

Astemizole (Co-administration may result in increased CNS depressant effects, such as drowsiness, dizziness, and impaired mental function).

No products indexed under this heading.

Azatadine Maleate (Co-administration may result in increased CNS depressant effects, such as drowsiness, dizziness, and impaired mental function). Products include:

Rynatan Tablets 3351

Bromodiphenhydramine Hydrochloride (Co-administration may result in increased CNS depressant effects, such as drowsiness, dizziness, and impaired mental function).

No products indexed under this heading.

Brompheniramine Maleate (Co-administration may result in increased CNS depressant effects, such as drowsiness, dizziness, and impaired mental function). Products include:

Bromfed Capsules (Extended-Release).................... 2269

Bromfed-PD Capsules (Extended-Release).................... 2269

Comtrex Acute Head Cold & Sinus Pressure Relief Tablets..... 627

Dimetapp Elixir 777

Dimetapp Cold and Fever Suspension.................................. 775

Dimetapp DM Cold & Cough Elixir . 775

Dimetapp Nighttime Flu Liquid 776

Buprenorphine Hydrochloride (Co-administration may result in increased CNS depressant effects, such as drowsiness, dizziness, and impaired mental function). Products include:

Buprenex Injectable 2918

Buspirone Hydrochloride (Co-administration may result in increased CNS depressant effects, such as drowsiness, dizziness, and impaired mental function).

No products indexed under this heading.

Butabarbital (Co-administration may result in increased CNS depressant effects, such as drowsiness, dizziness, and impaired mental function).

No products indexed under this heading.

Butalbital (Co-administration may result in increased CNS depressant effects, such as drowsiness, dizziness, and impaired mental function). Products include:

Phrenilin 578

Sedapap Tablets 50 mg/650 mg ... 2225

Cetirizine Hydrochloride (Co-administration may result in increased CNS depressant effects, such as drowsiness, dizziness, and impaired mental function). Products include:

Zyrtec 2756

Zyrtec-D 12 Hour Extended Relief Tablets.. 2758

Chlordiazepoxide (Co-administration may result in increased CNS depressant effects, such as drowsiness, dizziness, and impaired mental function). Products include:

Limbitrol 1738

Chlordiazepoxide Hydrochloride (Co-administration may result in increased CNS depressant effects, such as drowsiness, dizziness, and impaired mental function). Products include:

Librium Capsules 1736

Librium for Injection 1737

Chlorpheniramine Maleate (Co-administration may result in increased CNS depressant effects, such as drowsiness, dizziness, and impaired mental function). Products include:

Actifed Cold & Sinus Caplets and Tablets.................................. 688

Alka-Seltzer Plus Liqui-Gels 604

BC Allergy Sinus Cold Powder 619

Chlor-Trimeton Allergy Tablets 735

Chlor-Trimeton Allergy/Decongestant Tablets.... 736

Comtrex Flu Therapy & Fever Relief Nighttime Tablets.............. 628

Comtrex Maximum Strength Multi-Symptom Cold & Cough Relief Tablets and Caplets........... 626

Contac Severe Cold and Flu Caplets Maximum Strength........ 746

Coricidin 'D' Cold, Flu & Sinus Tablets 737

Coricidin/Coricidin D 738

Coricidin HBP Maximum Strength Flu Tablets 738

Extendryl 1361

Hycomine Compound Tablets 1317

Kronofed-A 1341

PediaCare Cough-Cold Liquid 719

PediaCare NightRest Cough-Cold Liquid 719

Robitussin Nighttime Honey Flu Liquid 786

Ryna 768

Singlet Caplets 761

Sinutab Sinus Allergy Medication, Maximum Strength Formula, Tablets & Caplets......................... 707

Sudafed Cold & Allergy Tablets 708

TheraFlu Regular Strength Cold & Cough Night Time Hot Liquid....... 676

TheraFlu Regular Strength Cold & Sore Throat Night Time Hot Liquid 676

TheraFlu Maximum Strength Flu & Cough Night Time Hot Liquid.. 678

TheraFlu Maximum Strength Flu & Sore Throat Night Time Hot Liquid 677

TheraFlu Maximum Strength Severe Cold & Congestion Night Time Caplets................... 678

TheraFlu Maximum Strength Severe Cold & Congestion Night Time Hot Liquid 678

Triaminic Cold & Allergy Liquid 681

Triaminic Cold & Allergy Softchews..................................... 683

Triaminic Cold & Cough Liquid 681

Triaminic Cold & Cough Softchews..................................... 683

Triaminic Cold & Night Time Cough Liquid 681

Triaminic Cold, Cough & Fever Liquid 681

Children's Tylenol Cold Suspension Liquid and Chewable Tablets 2015

Children's Tylenol Cold Plus Cough Suspension Liquid and Chewable Tablets....................... 2015

Children's Tylenol Flu Suspension Liquid.. 2015

Maximum Strength Tylenol Allergy Sinus Caplets, Gelcaps, and Geltabs 2010

Multi-Symptom Tylenol Cold Complete Formula Caplets 2010

Vicks 44M Cough, Cold & Flu Relief Liquid.............................. 725

Pediatric Vicks 44m Cough & Cold Relief.................................. 728

Children's Vicks NyQuil Cold/Cough Relief 726

Chlorpheniramine Polistirex (Co-administration may result in increased CNS depressant effects, such as drowsiness, dizziness, and impaired mental function). Products include:

Tussionex Pennkinetic Extended-Release Suspension........ 1174

Chlorpheniramine Tannate (Co-administration may result in increased CNS depressant effects, such as drowsiness, dizziness, and impaired mental function). Products include:

Reformulated Rynatan Pediatric Suspension 3352

Rynatuss Pediatric Suspension 3353

Rynatuss Tablets 3353

Tussi-12 S Suspension 3356

Tussi-12 Tablets 3356

Chlorpromazine (Co-administration may result in increased CNS depressant effects, such as drowsiness, dizziness, and impaired mental function). Products include:

Thorazine Suppositories 1656

Chlorpromazine Hydrochloride (Co-administration may result in increased CNS depressant effects, such as drowsiness, dizziness, and impaired mental function). Products include:

Thorazine 1656

Chlorprothixene (Co-administration may result in increased CNS depressant effects, such as drowsiness, dizziness, and impaired mental function).

No products indexed under this heading.

Chlorprothixene Hydrochloride (Co-administration may result in increased CNS depressant effects, such as drowsiness, dizziness, and impaired mental function).

No products indexed under this heading.

Chlorprothixene Lactate (Co-administration may result in increased CNS depressant effects, such as drowsiness, dizziness, and impaired mental function).

No products indexed under this heading.

Cimetidine (It is not known if the effects of butorphanol are altered by co-administration of drugs that affect hepatic metabolism, such as cimetidine, but physician should be alert to the possibility that a smaller initial dose and longer intervals between doses may be needed). Products include:

Tagamet HB 200 Suspension 762

Tagamet HB 200 Tablets 761

Tagamet Tablets 1644

Clemastine Fumarate (Co-administration may result in increased CNS depressant effects, such as drowsiness, dizziness, and impaired mental function). Products include:

Tavist 12 Hour Allergy Tablets 676

Clorazepate Dipotassium (Co-administration may result in increased CNS depressant effects, such as drowsiness, dizziness, and impaired mental function). Products include:

Tranxene 511

Clozapine (Co-administration may result in increased CNS depressant effects, such as drowsiness, dizziness, and impaired mental function). Products include:

Clozaril Tablets 2319

Codeine Phosphate (Co-administration may result in increased CNS depressant effects, such as drowsiness, dizziness, and impaired mental function). Products include:

Phenergan with Codeine Syrup 3557

Phenergan VC with Codeine Syrup .. 3561

Robitussin A-C Syrup 2942

Robitussin-DAC Syrup 2942

Ryna-C Liquid 768

Soma Compound w/Codeine Tablets.. 3355

Tussi-Organidin NR Liquid 3350

Tussi-Organidin-S NR Liquid 3350

Tylenol with Codeine 2595

Cyproheptadine Hydrochloride (Co-administration may result in increased CNS depressant effects, such as drowsiness, dizziness, and impaired mental function). Products include:

Periactin Tablets 2155

Desflurane (Co-administration may result in increased CNS depressant effects, such as drowsiness, dizziness, and impaired mental function). Products include:

Suprane Liquid for Inhalation 874

Dexchlorpheniramine Maleate (Co-administration may result in increased CNS depressant effects, such as drowsiness, dizziness, and impaired mental function).

No products indexed under this heading.

Dezocine (Co-administration may result in increased CNS depressant effects, such as drowsiness, dizziness, and impaired mental function).

No products indexed under this heading.

Diazepam (Co-administration may result in increased CNS depressant effects, such as drowsiness, dizziness, and impaired mental function). Products include:

Valium Injectable 3026

Valium Tablets 3047

Diphenhydramine Citrate (Co-administration may result in

increased CNS depressant effects, such as drowsiness, dizziness, and impaired mental function). Products include:

Alka-Seltzer PM Effervescent Tablets ■605
Benadryl Allergy & Sinus Fastmelt Tablets ■693
Benadryl Children's Allergy/Cold Fastmelt Tablets ■692
Excedrin PM Tablets, Caplets, and Geltabs ■631
Goody's PM Powder ■621

Diphenhydramine Hydrochloride (Co-administration may result in increased CNS depressant effects, such as drowsiness, dizziness, and impaired mental function). Products include:

Extra Strength Bayer PM Caplets ■611
Benadryl Allergy Chewables ■689
Benadryl Allergy ■691
Benadryl Allergy Liquid ■690
Benadryl Allergy/Cold Tablets ■691
Benadryl Allergy/Congestion Tablets ■692
Benadryl Allergy & Sinus Liquid ■693
Benadryl Allergy Sinus Headache Caplets & Gelcaps ■693
Benadryl Severe Allergy & Sinus Headache Caplets ■694
Benadryl Dye-Free Allergy Liquid ■690
Benadryl Dye-Free Allergy Liqui-Gels Softgels ■690
Benadryl Itch Relief Stick Extra Strength ■695
Benadryl Cream ■695
Benadryl Gel ■695
Benadryl Spray ■696
Benadryl Parenteral 2617
Coricidin HBP Night-Time Cold & Flu Tablets ■738
Nytol QuickCaps Caplets ■622
Maximum Strength Nytol QuickGels Softgels ■621
Extra Strength Percogesic Aspirin-Free Coated Caplets ■665
Simply Sleep Caplets 2008
Sominex Original Formula Tablets ■761
Children's Tylenol Allergy-D Liquid 2014
Maximum Strength Tylenol Allergy Sinus NightTime Caplets 2010
Tylenol Severe Allergy Caplets 2010
Maximum Strength Tylenol Flu NightTime Gelcaps 2011
Extra Strength Tylenol PM Caplets, Geltabs, and Gelcaps 2012
Unisom Maximum Strength SleepGels ■713

Diphenylpyraline Hydrochloride (Co-administration may result in increased CNS depressant effects, such as drowsiness, dizziness, and impaired mental function).

No products indexed under this heading.

Droperidol (Co-administration may result in increased CNS depressant effects, such as drowsiness, dizziness, and impaired mental function).

No products indexed under this heading.

Dyphylline (It is not known if the effects of butorphanol are altered by co-administration of drugs that affect hepatic metabolism, such as theophylline, but physician should be alert to the possibility that a smaller initial dose and longer intervals between doses may be needed). Products include:

Lufyllin Tablets 3347
Lufyllin-400 Tablets 3347
Lufyllin-GG Elixir 3348
Lufyllin-GG Tablets 3348

Enflurane (Co-administration may result in increased CNS depressant effects, such as drowsiness, dizziness, and impaired mental function).

No products indexed under this heading.

Erythromycin (It is not known if the effects of butorphanol are altered by co-administration of drugs that affect hepatic metabolism, such as erythromycin, but physician should be alert to the possibility that a smaller initial dose and longer intervals between doses may be needed). Products include:

Emgel 2% Topical Gel 1285
Ery-Tab Tablets 448
Erythromycin Base Filmtab Tablets 454
Erythromycin Delayed-Release Capsules, USP 455
PCE Dispertab Tablets 498

Erythromycin Estolate (It is not known if the effects of butorphanol are altered by co-administration of drugs that affect hepatic metabolism, such as erythromycin, but physician should be alert to the possibility that a smaller initial dose and longer intervals between doses may be needed).

No products indexed under this heading.

Erythromycin Ethylsuccinate (It is not known if the effects of butorphanol are altered by co-administration of drugs that affect hepatic metabolism, such as erythromycin, but physician should be alert to the possibility that a smaller initial dose and longer intervals between doses may be needed). Products include:

E.E.S. 450
EryPed 446
Pediazole Suspension 3050

Erythromycin Gluceptate (It is not known if the effects of butorphanol are altered by co-administration of drugs that affect hepatic metabolism, such as erythromycin, but physician should be alert to the possibility that a smaller initial dose and longer intervals between doses may be needed).

No products indexed under this heading.

Erythromycin Stearate (It is not known if the effects of butorphanol are altered by co-administration of drugs that affect hepatic metabolism, such as erythromycin, but physician should be alert to the possibility that a smaller initial dose and longer intervals between doses may be needed). Products include:

Erythrocin Stearate Filmtab Tablets 452

Estazolam (Co-administration may result in increased CNS depressant effects, such as drowsiness, dizziness, and impaired mental function). Products include:

ProSom Tablets 500

Ethchlorvynol (Co-administration may result in increased CNS depressant effects, such as drowsiness, dizziness, and impaired mental function).

No products indexed under this heading.

Ethinamate (Co-administration may result in increased CNS depressant effects, such as drowsiness, dizziness, and impaired mental function).

No products indexed under this heading.

Fentanyl (Co-administration may result in increased CNS depressant effects, such as drowsiness, dizziness, and impaired mental function). Products include:

Duragesic Transdermal System 1786

Fentanyl Citrate (Co-administration may result in increased CNS depressant effects, such as drowsiness, dizziness, and impaired mental function). Products include:

Actiq 1184

Fexofenadine Hydrochloride (Co-administration may result in increased CNS depressant effects, such as drowsiness, dizziness, and impaired mental function). Products include:

Allegra 712
Allegra-D Extended-Release Tablets 714

Fluphenazine Decanoate (Co-administration may result in increased CNS depressant effects, such as drowsiness, dizziness, and impaired mental function).

No products indexed under this heading.

Fluphenazine Enanthate (Co-administration may result in increased CNS depressant effects, such as drowsiness, dizziness, and impaired mental function).

No products indexed under this heading.

Fluphenazine Hydrochloride (Co-administration may result in increased CNS depressant effects, such as drowsiness, dizziness, and impaired mental function).

No products indexed under this heading.

Flurazepam Hydrochloride (Co-administration may result in increased CNS depressant effects, such as drowsiness, dizziness, and impaired mental function).

No products indexed under this heading.

Glutethimide (Co-administration may result in increased CNS depressant effects, such as drowsiness, dizziness, and impaired mental function).

No products indexed under this heading.

Haloperidol (Co-administration may result in increased CNS depressant effects, such as drowsiness, dizziness, and impaired mental function). Products include:

Haldol Injection, Tablets and Concentrate 2533

Haloperidol Decanoate (Co-administration may result in increased CNS depressant effects, such as drowsiness, dizziness, and impaired mental function). Products include:

Haldol Decanoate 2535

Hydrocodone Bitartrate (Co-administration may result in increased CNS depressant effects, such as drowsiness, dizziness, and impaired mental function). Products include:

Hycodan 1316
Hycomine Compound Tablets 1317
Hycotuss Expectorant Syrup 1318
Lortab 3319
Lortab Elixir 3317
Maxidone Tablets CIII 3399
Norco 5/325 Tablets CIII 3424
Norco 7.5/325 Tablets CIII 3425
Norco 10/325 Tablets CIII 3427
Norco 10/325 Tablets CIII 3425
Vicodin Tablets 516
Vicodin ES Tablets 517
Vicodin HP Tablets 518
Vicodin Tuss Expectorant 519
Vicoprofen Tablets 520
Zydone Tablets 1330

Hydrocodone Polistirex (Co-administration may result in increased CNS depressant effects, such as drowsiness, dizziness, and impaired mental function). Products include:

Tussionex Pennkinetic Extended-Release Suspension 1174

Hydromorphone Hydrochloride (Co-administration may result in increased CNS depressant effects, such as drowsiness, dizziness, and impaired mental function). Products include:

Dilaudid 441
Dilaudid Oral Liquid 445
Dilaudid Powder 441
Dilaudid Rectal Suppositories 441
Dilaudid Tablets 441
Dilaudid Tablets - 8 mg 445
Dilaudid-HP 443

Hydroxyzine Hydrochloride (Co-administration may result in increased CNS depressant effects, such as drowsiness, dizziness, and impaired mental function). Products include:

Atarax Tablets & Syrup 2667
Vistaril Intramuscular Solution 2738

Isoflurane (Co-administration may result in increased CNS depressant effects, such as drowsiness, dizziness, and impaired mental function).

No products indexed under this heading.

Ketamine Hydrochloride (Co-administration may result in increased CNS depressant effects, such as drowsiness, dizziness, and impaired mental function).

No products indexed under this heading.

Levomethadyl Acetate Hydrochloride (Co-administration may result in increased CNS depressant effects, such as drowsiness, dizziness, and impaired mental function).

No products indexed under this heading.

Levorphanol Tartrate (Co-administration may result in increased CNS depressant effects, such as drowsiness, dizziness, and impaired mental function). Products include:

Levo-Dromoran 1734
Levorphanol Tartrate Tablets 3059

Loratadine (Co-administration may result in increased CNS depressant effects, such as drowsiness, dizziness, and impaired mental function). Products include:

Claritin 3100
Claritin-D 12 Hour Extended Release Tablets 3102
Claritin-D 24 Hour Extended Release Tablets 3104

Lorazepam (Co-administration may result in increased CNS depressant effects, such as drowsiness, dizziness, and impaired mental function). Products include:

Ativan Injection 3478
Ativan Tablets 3482

Loxapine Hydrochloride (Co-administration may result in increased CNS depressant effects, such as drowsiness, dizziness, and impaired mental function).

No products indexed under this heading.

Loxapine Succinate (Co-administration may result in increased CNS depressant effects, such as drowsiness, dizziness, and impaired mental function). Products include:

Loxitane Capsules 3398

Meperidine Hydrochloride (Co-administration may result in increased CNS depressant effects, such as drowsiness, dizziness, and impaired mental function). Products include:

Demerol 3079
Mepergan Injection 3539

Mephobarbital (Co-administration may result in increased CNS depressant effects, such as drowsiness, dizziness, and impaired mental function).

No products indexed under this heading.

Meprobamate (Co-administration may result in increased CNS depressant effects, such as drowsiness, dizziness, and impaired mental function). Products include:

Miltown Tablets 3349

Mesoridazine Besylate (Co-administration may result in increased CNS depressant effects, such as drowsiness, dizziness, and impaired mental function). Products include:

Serentil 1057

Methadone Hydrochloride (Co-administration may result in increased CNS depressant effects,

such as drowsiness, dizziness, and impaired mental function). Products include:

Dolophine Hydrochloride Tablets 3056

Methdilazine Hydrochloride (Co-administration may result in increased CNS depressant effects, such as drowsiness, dizziness, and impaired mental function).

No products indexed under this heading.

Methohexital Sodium (Co-administration may result in increased CNS depressant effects, such as drowsiness, dizziness, and impaired mental function). Products include:

Brevital Sodium for Injection, USP .. 1815

Methotrimeprazine (Co-administration may result in increased CNS depressant effects, such as drowsiness, dizziness, and impaired mental function).

No products indexed under this heading.

Methoxyflurane (Co-administration may result in increased CNS depressant effects, such as drowsiness, dizziness, and impaired mental function).

No products indexed under this heading.

Midazolam Hydrochloride (Co-administration may result in increased CNS depressant effects, such as drowsiness, dizziness, and impaired mental function). Products include:

Versed Injection 3027
Versed Syrup 3033

Molindone Hydrochloride (Co-administration may result in increased CNS depressant effects, such as drowsiness, dizziness, and impaired mental function). Products include:

Moban 1320

Morphine Sulfate (Co-administration may result in increased CNS depressant effects, such as drowsiness, dizziness, and impaired mental function). Products include:

Astramorph/PF Injection, USP (Preservative-Free) 594
Duramorph Injection 1312
Infumorph 200 and Infumorph 500 Sterile Solutions 1314
Kadian Capsules 1335
MS Contin Tablets 2896
MSIR 2898
Oramorph SR Tablets 3062
Roxanol 3066

Olanzapine (Co-administration may result in increased CNS depressant effects, such as drowsiness, dizziness, and impaired mental function). Products include:

Zyprexa Tablets 1973
Zyprexa ZYDIS Orally Disintegrating Tablets 1973

Oxazepam (Co-administration may result in increased CNS depressant effects, such as drowsiness, dizziness, and impaired mental function).

No products indexed under this heading.

Oxycodone Hydrochloride (Co-administration may result in increased CNS depressant effects, such as drowsiness, dizziness, and impaired mental function). Products include:

OxyContin Tablets 2912
OxyFast Oral Concentrate Solution 2916
OxyIR Capsules 2916
Percocet Tablets 1326
Percodan Tablets 1327
Percolone Tablets 1327
Roxicodone 3067
Tylox Capsules 2597

Oxymetazoline Hydrochloride (Co-administration with nasal vasoconstrictors, such as oxymetazoline, with Stadol NS may decrease the rate of absorption resulting in slower onset of action). Products include:

Afrin 733
Afrin No Drip Original Nasal Spray 735
Afrin No Drip Extra Moisturizing Nasal Spray 735
Afrin No Drip Severe Congestion Nasal Spray 735
Afrin No Drip Sinus Nasal Spray 735
Afrin Original Pump Mist 733
Neo-Synephrine 12 Hour 615
Vicks Sinex 12-Hour Nasal Spray and Ultra Fine Mist 729
Visine L.R. Long Lasting Eye Drops .... ⊙ 315

Pentobarbital Sodium (Co-administration may result in increased CNS depressant effects, such as drowsiness, dizziness, and impaired mental function). Products include:

Nembutal Sodium Solution 485

Perphenazine (Co-administration may result in increased CNS depressant effects, such as drowsiness, dizziness, and impaired mental function). Products include:

Etrafon 3115
Trilafon 3160

Phenobarbital (Co-administration may result in increased CNS depressant effects, such as drowsiness, dizziness, and impaired mental function). Products include:

Arco-Lase Plus Tablets 592
Donnatal 2929
Donnatal Extentabs 2930

Prazepam (Co-administration may result in increased CNS depressant effects, such as drowsiness, dizziness, and impaired mental function).

No products indexed under this heading.

Prochlorperazine (Co-administration may result in increased CNS depressant effects, such as drowsiness, dizziness, and impaired mental function). Products include:

Compazine 1505

Promethazine Hydrochloride (Co-administration may result in increased CNS depressant effects, such as drowsiness, dizziness, and impaired mental function). Products include:

Mepergan Injection 3539
Phenergan Injection 3553
Phenergan 3556
Phenergan Syrup 3554
Phenergan with Codeine Syrup 3557
Phenergan with Dextromethorphan Syrup 3559
Phenergan VC Syrup 3560
Phenergan VC with Codeine Syrup .. 3561

Propofol (Co-administration may result in increased CNS depressant effects, such as drowsiness, dizziness, and impaired mental function). Products include:

Diprivan Injectable Emulsion 667

Propoxyphene Hydrochloride (Co-administration may result in increased CNS depressant effects, such as drowsiness, dizziness, and impaired mental function). Products include:

Darvon Pulvules 1909
Darvon Compound-65 Pulvules 1910

Propoxyphene Napsylate (Co-administration may result in increased CNS depressant effects, such as drowsiness, dizziness, and impaired mental function). Products include:

Darvon-N/Darvocet-N 1907
Darvon-N Tablets 1912

Pyrilamine Maleate (Co-administration may result in increased CNS depressant effects, such as drowsiness, dizziness, and impaired mental function). Products include:

Maximum Strength Midol Menstrual Caplets and Gelcaps 612
Maximum Strength Midol PMS Caplets and Gelcaps 613

Pyrilamine Tannate (Co-administration may result in increased CNS depressant effects, such as drowsiness, dizziness, and impaired mental function). Products include:

Ryna-12 S Suspension 3351

Quazepam (Co-administration may result in increased CNS depressant effects, such as drowsiness, dizziness, and impaired mental function).

No products indexed under this heading.

Quetiapine Fumarate (Co-administration may result in increased CNS depressant effects, such as drowsiness, dizziness, and impaired mental function). Products include:

Seroquel Tablets 684

Remifentanil Hydrochloride (Co-administration may result in increased CNS depressant effects, such as drowsiness, dizziness, and impaired mental function).

No products indexed under this heading.

Risperidone (Co-administration may result in increased CNS depressant effects, such as drowsiness, dizziness, and impaired mental function). Products include:

Risperdal 1796

Secobarbital Sodium (Co-administration may result in increased CNS depressant effects, such as drowsiness, dizziness, and impaired mental function).

No products indexed under this heading.

Sevoflurane (Co-administration may result in increased CNS depressant effects, such as drowsiness, dizziness, and impaired mental function).

No products indexed under this heading.

Sufentanil Citrate (Co-administration may result in increased CNS depressant effects, such as drowsiness, dizziness, and impaired mental function).

No products indexed under this heading.

Temazepam (Co-administration may result in increased CNS depressant effects, such as drowsiness, dizziness, and impaired mental function).

No products indexed under this heading.

Terfenadine (Co-administration may result in increased CNS depressant effects, such as drowsiness, dizziness, and impaired mental function).

No products indexed under this heading.

Theophylline (It is not known if the effects of butorphanol are altered by co-administration of drugs that affect hepatic metabolism, such as theophylline, but physician should be alert to the possibility that a smaller initial dose and longer intervals between doses may be needed). Products include:

Aerolate 1361
Theo-Dur Extended-Release Tablets 1835
Uni-Dur Extended-Release Tablets .. 1841
Uniphyl 400 mg and 600 mg Tablets 2903

Theophylline Calcium Salicylate (It is not known if the effects of butorphanol are altered by co-administration of drugs that affect hepatic metabolism, such as theophylline, but physician should be alert to the possibility that a smaller initial dose and longer intervals between doses may be needed).

No products indexed under this heading.

Theophylline Sodium Glycinate (It is not known if the effects of butorphanol are altered by co-administration of drugs that affect hepatic metabolism, such as theophylline, but physician should be alert to the possibility that a smaller initial dose and longer intervals between doses may be needed).

No products indexed under this heading.

Thiamylal Sodium (Co-administration may result in increased CNS depressant effects, such as drowsiness, dizziness, and impaired mental function).

No products indexed under this heading.

Thioridazine Hydrochloride (Co-administration may result in increased CNS depressant effects, such as drowsiness, dizziness, and impaired mental function). Products include:

Thioridazine Hydrochloride Tablets 2289

Thiothixene (Co-administration may result in increased CNS depressant effects, such as drowsiness, dizziness, and impaired mental function). Products include:

Navane Capsules 2701
Thiothixene Capsules 2290

Triazolam (Co-administration may result in increased CNS depressant effects, such as drowsiness, dizziness, and impaired mental function). Products include:

Halcion Tablets 2823

Trifluoperazine Hydrochloride (Co-administration may result in increased CNS depressant effects, such as drowsiness, dizziness, and impaired mental function). Products include:

Stelazine 1640

Trimeprazine Tartrate (Co-administration may result in increased CNS depressant effects, such as drowsiness, dizziness, and impaired mental function).

No products indexed under this heading.

Tripelennamine Hydrochloride (Co-administration may result in increased CNS depressant effects, such as drowsiness, dizziness, and impaired mental function).

No products indexed under this heading.

Triprolidine Hydrochloride (Co-administration may result in increased CNS depressant effects, such as drowsiness, dizziness, and impaired mental function). Products include:

Actifed Cold & Allergy Tablets 688

Zaleplon (Co-administration may result in increased CNS depressant effects, such as drowsiness, dizziness, and impaired mental function). Products include:

Sonata Capsules 3591

Ziprasidone Hydrochloride (Co-administration may result in increased CNS depressant effects, such as drowsiness, dizziness, and impaired mental function). Products include:

Geodon Capsules 2688

Zolpidem Tartrate (Co-administration may result in increased CNS depressant effects, such as drowsiness, dizziness, and impaired mental function). Products include:

Ambien Tablets 3191

Food Interactions

Alcohol (Concurrent use may result in increased CNS depressant effects, such as drowsiness, dizziness, and impaired mental function).

STARLIX TABLETS

(Nateglinide) 2401
May interact with beta blockers, corticosteroids, monoamine oxidase inhibitors, non-steroidal anti-inflammatory agents, salicylates, sympathomimetics, thiazides, thyroid preparations, and certain other agents. Compounds in these categories include:

Acebutolol Hydrochloride (The hypoglycemic action of nateglinide may be potentiated by non-selective beta-adrenergic-blocking agents). Products include:
- Sectral Capsules 3589

Albuterol (Co-administration with certain drugs, such as sympathomimetics, may reduce the hypoglycemic action of nateglinide and other oral antidiabetic drugs; when these drugs are administered to or withdrawn from patients receiving nateglinide, the patient should be observed closely for changes in glycemic control). Products include:
- Proventil Inhalation Aerosol 3142
- Ventolin Inhalation Aerosol and Refill 1679

Albuterol Sulfate (Co-administration with certain drugs, such as sympathomimetics, may reduce the hypoglycemic action of nateglinide and other oral antidiabetic drugs; when these drugs are administered to or withdrawn from patients receiving nateglinide, the patient should be observed closely for changes in glycemic control). Products include:
- AccuNeb Inhalation Solution 1230
- Combivent Inhalation Aerosol 1041
- DuoNeb Inhalation Solution 1233
- Proventil Inhalation Solution 0.083% 3146
- Proventil Repetabs Tablets 3148
- Proventil Solution for Inhalation 0.5% 3144
- Proventil HFA Inhalation Aerosol 3150
- Ventolin HFA Inhalation Aerosol 3618
- Volmax Extended-Release Tablets 2276

Aspirin (The hypoglycemic action of nateglinide may be potentiated by salicylates). Products include:
- Aggrenox Capsules 1026
- Alka-Seltzer ...... ▣603
- Alka-Seltzer Lemon Lime Antacid and Pain Reliever Effervescent Tablets ...... ▣603
- Alka-Seltzer Extra Strength Antacid and Pain Reliever Effervescent Tablets ...... ▣603
- Alka-Seltzer PM Effervescent Tablets ...... ▣605
- Genuine Bayer Tablets, Caplets and Gelcaps ...... ▣606
- Extra Strength Bayer Caplets and Gelcaps ...... ▣610
- Aspirin Regimen Bayer Children's Chewable Tablets (Orange or Cherry Flavored) ...... ▣607
- Bayer, Aspirin Regimen ...... ▣606
- Aspirin Regimen Bayer 81 mg Caplets with Calcium ...... ▣607
- Genuine Bayer Professional Labeling (Aspirin Regimen Bayer) ...... ▣608
- Extra Strength Bayer Arthritis Caplets ...... ▣610
- Extra Strength Bayer Plus Caplets ...... ▣610
- Extra Strength Bayer PM Caplets ...... ▣611
- BC Powder ...... ▣619
- BC Allergy Sinus Cold Powder ...... ▣619
- Arthritis Strength BC Powder ...... ▣619
- BC Sinus Cold Powder ...... ▣619
- Darvon Compound-65 Pulvules 1910
- Ecotrin Enteric Coated Aspirin Low, Regular and Maximum Strength Tablets 1715
- Excedrin Extra-Strength Tablets, Caplets, and Geltabs ...... ▣629
- Excedrin Migraine 1070
- Goody's Body Pain Formula Powder ...... ▣620
- Goody's Extra Strength Headache Powder ...... ▣620
- Goody's Extra Strength Pain Relief Tablets ...... ▣620
- Percodan Tablets 1327
- Robaxisal Tablets 2939
- Soma Compound Tablets 3354
- Soma Compound w/Codeine Tablets 3355
- Vanquish Caplets ...... ▣617

Atenolol (The hypoglycemic action of nateglinide may be potentiated by non-selective beta-adrenergic-blocking agents). Products include:
- Tenoretic Tablets 690
- Tenormin I.V. Injection 692

Bendroflumethiazide (Co-administration with certain drugs, such as thiazides, may reduce the hypoglycemic action of nateglinide and other oral antidiabetic drugs; when these drugs are administered to or withdrawn from patients receiving nateglinide, the patient should be observed closely for changes in glycemic control). Products include:
- Corzide 40/5 Tablets 2247
- Corzide 80/5 Tablets 2247

Betamethasone Acetate (Co-administration with certain drugs, such as corticosteroids, may reduce the hypoglycemic action of nateglinide and other oral antidiabetic drugs; when these drugs are administered to or withdrawn from patients receiving nateglinide, the patient should be observed closely for changes in glycemic control). Products include:
- Celestone Soluspan Injectable Suspension 3097

Betamethasone Sodium Phosphate (Co-administration with certain drugs, such as corticosteroids, may reduce the hypoglycemic action of nateglinide and other oral antidiabetic drugs; when these drugs are administered to or withdrawn from patients receiving nateglinide, the patient should be observed closely for changes in glycemic control). Products include:
- Celestone Soluspan Injectable Suspension 3097

Betaxolol Hydrochloride (The hypoglycemic action of nateglinide may be potentiated by non-selective beta-adrenergic-blocking agents). Products include:
- Betoptic S Ophthalmic Suspension 537

Bisoprolol Fumarate (The hypoglycemic action of nateglinide may be potentiated by non-selective beta-adrenergic-blocking agents). Products include:
- Zebeta Tablets 1885
- Ziac Tablets 1887

Carteolol Hydrochloride (The hypoglycemic action of nateglinide may be potentiated by non-selective beta-adrenergic-blocking agents). Products include:
- Carteolol Hydrochloride Ophthalmic Solution USP, 1% ...... ⊙258
- Ocupress Ophthalmic Solution, 1% Sterile ...... ⊙303

Celecoxib (The hypoglycemic action of nateglinide may be potentiated by non-steroidal anti-inflammatory agents). Products include:
- Celebrex Capsules 2676
- Celebrex Capsules 2780

Chlorothiazide (Co-administration with certain drugs, such as thiazides, may reduce the hypoglycemic action of nateglinide and other oral antidiabetic drugs; when these drugs are administered to or withdrawn from patients receiving nateglinide, the patient should be observed closely for changes in glycemic control). Products include:
- Aldoclor Tablets 2035
- Diuril Oral 2087

Chlorothiazide Sodium (Co-administration with certain drugs, such as thiazides, may reduce the hypoglycemic action of nateglinide and other oral antidiabetic drugs; when these drugs are administered to or withdrawn from patients receiving nateglinide, the patient should be observed closely for changes in glycemic control). Products include:
- Diuril Sodium Intravenous 2086

Choline Magnesium Trisalicylate (The hypoglycemic action of nateglinide may be potentiated by salicylates). Products include:
- Trilisate 2901

Cortisone Acetate (Co-administration with certain drugs, such as corticosteroids, may reduce the hypoglycemic action of nateglinide and other oral antidiabetic drugs; when these drugs are administered to or withdrawn from patients receiving nateglinide, the patient should be observed closely for changes in glycemic control). Products include:
- Cortone Acetate Injectable Suspension 2059
- Cortone Acetate Tablets 2061

Dexamethasone (Co-administration with certain drugs, such as corticosteroids, may reduce the hypoglycemic action of nateglinide and other oral antidiabetic drugs; when these drugs are administered to or withdrawn from patients receiving nateglinide, the patient should be observed closely for changes in glycemic control). Products include:
- Decadron Elixir 2078
- Decadron Tablets 2079
- TobraDex Ophthalmic Ointment 542
- TobraDex Ophthalmic Suspension 541

Dexamethasone Acetate (Co-administration with certain drugs, such as corticosteroids, may reduce the hypoglycemic action of nateglinide and other oral antidiabetic drugs; when these drugs are administered to or withdrawn from patients receiving nateglinide, the patient should be observed closely for changes in glycemic control).

No products indexed under this heading.

Dexamethasone Sodium Phosphate (Co-administration with certain drugs, such as corticosteroids, may reduce the hypoglycemic action of nateglinide and other oral antidiabetic drugs; when these drugs are administered to or withdrawn from patients receiving nateglinide, the patient should be observed closely for changes in glycemic control). Products include:
- Decadron Phosphate Injection 2081
- Decadron Phosphate Sterile Ophthalmic Ointment 2083
- Decadron Phosphate Sterile Ophthalmic Solution 2084
- NeoDecadron Sterile Ophthalmic Solution 2144

Diclofenac Potassium (The hypoglycemic action of nateglinide may be potentiated by non-steroidal anti-inflammatory agents). Products include:
- Cataflam Tablets 2315

Diclofenac Sodium (The hypoglycemic action of nateglinide may be potentiated by non-steroidal anti-inflammatory agents). Products include:
- Arthrotec Tablets 3195
- Voltaren Ophthalmic Sterile Ophthalmic Solution ...... ⊙312
- Voltaren Tablets 2315
- Voltaren-XR Tablets 2315

Diflunisal (The hypoglycemic action of nateglinide may be potentiated by salicylates). Products include:
- Dolobid Tablets 2088

Dobutamine Hydrochloride (Co-administration with certain drugs, such as sympathomimetics, may reduce the hypoglycemic action of nateglinide and other oral antidiabetic drugs; when these drugs are administered to or withdrawn from patients receiving nateglinide, the patient should be observed closely for changes in glycemic control). Products include:
- Dobutrex Solution Vials 1914

Dopamine Hydrochloride (Co-administration with certain drugs, such as sympathomimetics, may reduce the hypoglycemic action of nateglinide and other oral antidiabetic drugs; when these drugs are administered to or withdrawn from patients receiving nateglinide, the patient should be observed closely for changes in glycemic control).

No products indexed under this heading.

Ephedrine Hydrochloride (Co-administration with certain drugs, such as sympathomimetics, may reduce the hypoglycemic action of nateglinide and other oral antidiabetic drugs; when these drugs are administered to or withdrawn from patients receiving nateglinide, the patient should be observed closely for changes in glycemic control). Products include:
- Primatene Tablets ...... ▣780

Ephedrine Sulfate (Co-administration with certain drugs, such as sympathomimetics, may reduce the hypoglycemic action of nateglinide and other oral antidiabetic drugs; when these drugs are administered to or withdrawn from patients receiving nateglinide, the patient should be observed closely for changes in glycemic control).

No products indexed under this heading.

Ephedrine Tannate (Co-administration with certain drugs, such as sympathomimetics, may reduce the hypoglycemic action of nateglinide and other oral antidiabetic drugs; when these drugs are administered to or withdrawn from patients receiving nateglinide, the patient should be observed closely for changes in glycemic control). Products include:
- Rynatuss Pediatric Suspension 3353
- Rynatuss Tablets 3353

Epinephrine (Co-administration with certain drugs, such as sympathomimetics, may reduce the hypoglycemic action of nateglinide and other oral antidiabetic drugs; when these drugs are administered to or withdrawn from patients receiving nateglinide, the patient should be observed closely for changes in glycemic control). Products include:
- Epifrin Sterile Ophthalmic Solution ...... ⊙235
- EpiPen 1236
- Primatene Mist ...... ▣779
- Xylocaine with Epinephrine Injection 653

Epinephrine Bitartrate (Co-administration with certain drugs, such as sympathomimetics, may reduce the hypoglycemic action of nateglinide and other oral antidiabetic drugs; when these drugs are administered to or withdrawn from patients receiving nateglinide, the patient should be observed closely for changes in glycemic control). Products include:
- Sensorcaine 643

Epinephrine Hydrochloride (Co-administration with certain drugs, such as sympathomimetics, may reduce the hypoglycemic action of nateglinide and other oral antidiabetic drugs; when these drugs are administered to or withdrawn from patients receiving nateglinide, the patient should be observed closely for changes in glycemic control).

No products indexed under this heading.

Esmolol Hydrochloride (The hypoglycemic action of nateglinide may be potentiated by non-selective beta-adrenergic-blocking agents). Products include:
- Brevibloc Injection 858

Etodolac (The hypoglycemic action of nateglinide may be potentiated by non-steroidal anti-inflammatory agents). Products include:
- Lodine 3528
- Lodine XL Extended-Release Tablets 3530

Fenoprofen Calcium (The hypoglycemic action of nateglinide may be potentiated by non-steroidal anti-inflammatory agents).
- No products indexed under this heading.

Fludrocortisone Acetate (Co-administration with certain drugs, such as corticosteroids, may reduce the hypoglycemic action of nateglinide and other oral antidiabetic drugs; when these drugs are administered to or withdrawn from patients receiving nateglinide, the patient should be observed closely for changes in glycemic control). Products include:
- Florinef Acetate Tablets 2250

Flurbiprofen (The hypoglycemic action of nateglinide may be potentiated by non-steroidal anti-inflammatory agents).
- No products indexed under this heading.

Hydrochlorothiazide (Co-administration with certain drugs, such as thiazides, may reduce the hypoglycemic action of nateglinide and other oral antidiabetic drugs; when these drugs are administered to or withdrawn from patients receiving nateglinide, the patient should be observed closely for changes in glycemic control). Products include:
- Accuretic Tablets 2614
- Aldoril Tablets 2039
- Atacand HCT Tablets 597
- Avalide Tablets 1070
- Diovan HCT Tablets 2338
- Dyazide Capsules 1515
- HydroDIURIL Tablets 2108
- Hyzaar 2109
- Inderide Tablets 3517
- Inderide LA Long-Acting Capsules 3519
- Lotensin HCT Tablets 2367
- Maxzide 1008
- Micardis HCT Tablets 1051
- Microzide Capsules 3414
- Moduretic Tablets 2138
- Monopril HCT 1094
- Prinzide Tablets 2168
- Timolide Tablets 2187
- Uniretic Tablets 3178
- Vaseretic Tablets 2204
- Zestoretic Tablets 695
- Ziac Tablets 1887

Hydrocortisone (Co-administration with certain drugs, such as corticosteroids, may reduce the hypoglycemic action of nateglinide and other oral antidiabetic drugs; when these drugs are administered to or withdrawn from patients receiving nateglinide, the patient should be observed closely for changes in glycemic control). Products include:
- Anusol-HC Cream 2.5% 2237
- Cipro HC Otic Suspension 540
- Cortaid Intensive Therapy Cream .... ◘717
- Cortaid Maximum Strength Cream .... ◘717
- Cortisporin Ophthalmic Suspension Sterile .... ⊙297
- Cortizone•5 .... ◘699
- Cortizone•10 .... ◘699
- Cortizone•10 Plus Creme .... ◘700
- Cortizone for Kids Creme .... ◘699
- Hydrocortone Tablets 2106
- Massengill Medicated Soft Cloth Towelette .... ◘753
- VōSoL HC Otic Solution 3356

Hydrocortisone Acetate (Co-administration with certain drugs, such as corticosteroids, may reduce the hypoglycemic action of nateglinide and other oral antidiabetic drugs; when these drugs are administered to or withdrawn from patients receiving nateglinide, the patient should be observed closely for changes in glycemic control). Products include:
- Analpram-HC 1338
- Anusol HC-1 Hydrocortisone Anti-Itch Cream .... ◘689
- Anusol-HC Suppositories 2238
- Cortaid .... ◘717
- Cortifoam Rectal Foam 3170
- Cortisporin-TC Otic Suspension 2246
- Hydrocortone Acetate Injectable Suspension 2103
- Pramosone 1343
- Proctocort Suppositories 2264
- ProctoFoam-HC 3177
- Terra-Cortril Ophthalmic Suspension 2716

Hydrocortisone Sodium Phosphate (Co-administration with certain drugs, such as corticosteroids, may reduce the hypoglycemic action of nateglinide and other oral antidiabetic drugs; when these drugs are administered to or withdrawn from patients receiving nateglinide, the patient should be observed closely for changes in glycemic control). Products include:
- Hydrocortone Phosphate Injection, Sterile 2105

Hydrocortisone Sodium Succinate (Co-administration with certain drugs, such as corticosteroids, may reduce the hypoglycemic action of nateglinide and other oral antidiabetic drugs; when these drugs are administered to or withdrawn from patients receiving nateglinide, the patient should be observed closely for changes in glycemic control).
- No products indexed under this heading.

Hydroflumethiazide (Co-administration with certain drugs, such as thiazides, may reduce the hypoglycemic action of nateglinide and other oral antidiabetic drugs; when these drugs are administered to or withdrawn from patients receiving nateglinide, the patient should be observed closely for changes in glycemic control). Products include:
- Diucardin Tablets 3494

Ibuprofen (The hypoglycemic action of nateglinide may be potentiated by non-steroidal anti-inflammatory agents). Products include:
- Advil .... ◘771
- Children's Advil Oral Suspension .... ◘773
- Children's Advil Chewable Tablets .... ◘773
- Advil Cold and Sinus Caplets .... ◘771
- Advil Cold and Sinus Tablets .... ◘771
- Advil Flu & Body Ache Caplets .... ◘772
- Infants' Advil Drops .... ◘773
- Junior Strength Advil Tablets .... ◘773
- Junior Strength Advil Chewable Tablets .... ◘773
- Advil Migraine Liquigels .... ◘772
- Children's Motrin Oral Suspension and Chewable Tablets 2006
- Children's Motrin Cold Oral Suspension 2007
- Children's Motrin Oral Suspension .... ◘643
- Motrin Suspension, Oral Drops, Chewable Tablets, and Caplets 2002
- Infants' Motrin Concentrated Drops 2006
- Junior Strength Motrin Caplets and Chewable Tablets 2006
- Motrin IB Tablets, Caplets, and Gelcaps 2002
- Motrin Migraine Pain Caplets 2005
- Motrin Sinus Headache Caplets 2005
- Vicoprofen Tablets 520

Indomethacin (The hypoglycemic action of nateglinide may be potentiated by non-steroidal anti-inflammatory agents). Products include:
- Indocin 2112

Indomethacin Sodium Trihydrate (The hypoglycemic action of nateglinide may be potentiated by non-steroidal anti-inflammatory agents). Products include:
- Indocin I.V. 2115

Isocarboxazid (The hypoglycemic action of nateglinide may be potentiated by MAO inhibitors).
- No products indexed under this heading.

Isoproterenol Hydrochloride (Co-administration with certain drugs, such as sympathomimetics, may reduce the hypoglycemic action of nateglinide and other oral antidiabetic drugs; when these drugs are administered to or withdrawn from patients receiving nateglinide, the patient should be observed closely for changes in glycemic control).
- No products indexed under this heading.

Isoproterenol Sulfate (Co-administration with certain drugs, such as sympathomimetics, may reduce the hypoglycemic action of nateglinide and other oral antidiabetic drugs; when these drugs are administered to or withdrawn from patients receiving nateglinide, the patient should be observed closely for changes in glycemic control).
- No products indexed under this heading.

Ketoprofen (The hypoglycemic action of nateglinide may be potentiated by non-steroidal anti-inflammatory agents). Products include:
- Orudis Capsules 3548
- Orudis KT Tablets .... ◘778
- Oruvail Capsules 3548

Ketorolac Tromethamine (The hypoglycemic action of nateglinide may be potentiated by non-steroidal anti-inflammatory agents). Products include:
- Acular Ophthalmic Solution 544
- Acular PF Ophthalmic Solution 544
- Toradol 3018

Labetalol Hydrochloride (The hypoglycemic action of nateglinide may be potentiated by non-selective beta-adrenergic-blocking agents). Products include:
- Normodyne Injection 3135
- Normodyne Tablets 3137

Levalbuterol Hydrochloride (Co-administration with certain drugs, such as sympathomimetics, may reduce the hypoglycemic action of nateglinide and other oral antidiabetic drugs; when these drugs are administered to or withdrawn from patients receiving nateglinide, the patient should be observed closely for changes in glycemic control). Products include:
- Xopenex Inhalation Solution 3207

Levobunolol Hydrochloride (The hypoglycemic action of nateglinide may be potentiated by non-selective beta-adrenergic-blocking agents). Products include:
- Betagan .... ⊙228

Levothyroxine Sodium (Co-administration with certain drugs, such as thyroid products, may reduce the hypoglycemic action of nateglinide and other oral antidiabetic drugs; when these drugs are administered to or withdrawn from patients receiving nateglinide, the patient should be observed closely for changes in glycemic control). Products include:
- Levothroid Tablets 1373
- Levoxyl Tablets 1819
- Synthroid 505
- Unithroid Tablets 3445

Liothyronine Sodium (Co-administration with certain drugs, such as thyroid products, may reduce the hypoglycemic action of nateglinide and other oral antidiabetic drugs; when these drugs are administered to or withdrawn from patients receiving nateglinide, the patient should be observed closely for changes in glycemic control). Products include:
- Cytomel Tablets 1817
- Triostat Injection 1825

Liotrix (Co-administration with certain drugs, such as thyroid products, may reduce the hypoglycemic action of nateglinide and other oral antidiabetic drugs; when these drugs are administered to or withdrawn from patients receiving nateglinide, the patient should be observed closely for changes in glycemic control).
- No products indexed under this heading.

Magnesium Salicylate (The hypoglycemic action of nateglinide may be potentiated by salicylates). Products include:
- Momentum Backache Relief Extra Strength Caplets .... ◘666

Meclofenamate Sodium (The hypoglycemic action of nateglinide may be potentiated by non-steroidal anti-inflammatory agents).
- No products indexed under this heading.

Mefenamic Acid (The hypoglycemic action of nateglinide may be potentiated by non-steroidal anti-inflammatory agents). Products include:
- Ponstel Capsules 1356

Meloxicam (The hypoglycemic action of nateglinide may be potentiated by non-steroidal anti-inflammatory agents). Products include:
- Mobic Tablets 1054

Metaproterenol Sulfate (Co-administration with certain drugs, such as sympathomimetics, may reduce the hypoglycemic action of nateglinide and other oral antidiabetic drugs; when these drugs are administered to or withdrawn from patients receiving nateglinide, the patient should be observed closely for changes in glycemic control). Products include:
- Alupent 1029

Metaraminol Bitartrate (Co-administration with certain drugs, such as sympathomimetics, may reduce the hypoglycemic action of nateglinide and other oral antidiabetic drugs; when these drugs are administered to or withdrawn from patients receiving nateglinide, the patient should be observed closely for changes in glycemic control). Products include:
- Aramine Injection 2043

Methoxamine Hydrochloride (Co-administration with certain drugs, such as sympathomimetics, may reduce the hypoglycemic action of nateglinide and other oral antidiabetic drugs; when these drugs are administered to or withdrawn from patients receiving nateglinide, the patient should be observed closely for changes in glycemic control).
- No products indexed under this heading.

Methyclothiazide (Co-administration with certain drugs, such as thiazides, may reduce the hypoglycemic action of nateglinide and other oral antidiabetic drugs; when these drugs are administered to or withdrawn from patients receiving nateglinide, the patient should be observed closely for changes in glycemic control).
- No products indexed under this heading.

Methylprednisolone Acetate (Co-administration with certain drugs, such as corticosteroids, may reduce the hypoglycemic action of nateglinide and other oral antidiabetic drugs; when these drugs are administered to or withdrawn from patients receiving nateglinide, the patient should be observed closely for changes in glycemic control). Products include:
- Depo-Medrol Injectable Suspension 2795

Methylprednisolone Sodium Succinate (Co-administration with certain drugs, such as corticosteroids, may reduce the hypoglycemic action of nateglinide and other oral antidiabetic drugs; when these drugs are administered to or withdrawn

from patients receiving nateglinide, the patient should be observed closely for changes in glycemic control). Products include:

Solu-Medrol Sterile Powder 2855

Metipranolol Hydrochloride (The hypoglycemic action of nateglinide may be potentiated by non-selective beta-adrenergic-blocking agents).

No products indexed under this heading.

Metoprolol Succinate (The hypoglycemic action of nateglinide may be potentiated by non-selective beta-adrenergic-blocking agents). Products include:

Toprol-XL Tablets 651

Metoprolol Tartrate (The hypoglycemic action of nateglinide may be potentiated by non-selective beta-adrenergic-blocking agents).

No products indexed under this heading.

Moclobemide (The hypoglycemic action of nateglinide may be potentiated by MAO inhibitors).

No products indexed under this heading.

Nabumetone (The hypoglycemic action of nateglinide may be potentiated by non-steroidal anti-inflammatory agents). Products include:

Relafen Tablets 1617

Nadolol (The hypoglycemic action of nateglinide may be potentiated by non-selective beta-adrenergic-blocking agents). Products include:

Corgard Tablets 2245
Corzide 40/5 Tablets 2247
Corzide 80/5 Tablets 2247
Nadolol Tablets 2288

Naproxen (The hypoglycemic action of nateglinide may be potentiated by non-steroidal anti-inflammatory agents). Products include:

EC-Naprosyn Delayed-Release Tablets 2967
Naprosyn Suspension 2967
Naprosyn Tablets 2967

Naproxen Sodium (The hypoglycemic action of nateglinide may be potentiated by non-steroidal anti-inflammatory agents). Products include:

Aleve Tablets, Caplets and Gelcaps .... ▣602
Aleve Cold & Sinus Caplets .... ▣603
Anaprox Tablets 2967
Anaprox DS Tablets 2967
Naprelan Tablets 1293

Norepinephrine Bitartrate (Co-administration with certain drugs, such as sympathomimetics, may reduce the hypoglycemic action of nateglinide and other oral antidiabetic drugs; when these drugs are administered to or withdrawn from patients receiving nateglinide, the patient should be observed closely for changes in glycemic control).

No products indexed under this heading.

Oxaprozin (The hypoglycemic action of nateglinide may be potentiated by non-steroidal anti-inflammatory agents).

No products indexed under this heading.

Pargyline Hydrochloride (The hypoglycemic action of nateglinide may be potentiated by MAO inhibitors).

No products indexed under this heading.

Penbutolol Sulfate (The hypoglycemic action of nateglinide may be potentiated by non-selective beta-adrenergic-blocking agents).

No products indexed under this heading.

Phenelzine Sulfate (The hypoglycemic action of nateglinide may be potentiated by MAO inhibitors). Products include:

Nardil Tablets 2653

Phenylbutazone (The hypoglycemic action of nateglinide may be potentiated by non-steroidal anti-inflammatory agents).

No products indexed under this heading.

Phenylephrine Bitartrate (Co-administration with certain drugs, such as sympathomimetics, may reduce the hypoglycemic action of nateglinide and other oral antidiabetic drugs; when these drugs are administered to or withdrawn from patients receiving nateglinide, the patient should be observed closely for changes in glycemic control).

No products indexed under this heading.

Phenylephrine Hydrochloride (Co-administration with certain drugs, such as sympathomimetics, may reduce the hypoglycemic action of nateglinide and other oral antidiabetic drugs; when these drugs are administered to or withdrawn from patients receiving nateglinide, the patient should be observed closely for changes in glycemic control). Products include:

Afrin Nasal Decongestant Children's Pump Mist .... ▣734
Extendryl 1361
Hycomine Compound Tablets 1317
Neo-Synephrine .... ▣614
Phenergan VC Syrup 3560
Phenergan VC with Codeine Syrup . 3561
Preparation H Cream .... ▣778
Preparation H Cooling Gel .... ▣778
Preparation H .... ▣778
Vicks Sinex Nasal Spray and Ultra Fine Mist .... ▣729

Phenylephrine Tannate (Co-administration with certain drugs, such as sympathomimetics, may reduce the hypoglycemic action of nateglinide and other oral antidiabetic drugs; when these drugs are administered to or withdrawn from patients receiving nateglinide, the patient should be observed closely for changes in glycemic control). Products include:

Ryna-12 S Suspension 3351
Reformulated Rynatan Pediatric Suspension 3352
Rynatuss Pediatric Suspension 3353
Rynatuss Tablets 3353

Phenylpropanolamine Hydrochloride (Co-administration with certain drugs, such as sympathomimetics, may reduce the hypoglycemic action of nateglinide and other oral antidiabetic drugs; when these drugs are administered to or withdrawn from patients receiving nateglinide, the patient should be observed closely for changes in glycemic control).

No products indexed under this heading.

Pindolol (The hypoglycemic action of nateglinide may be potentiated by non-selective beta-adrenergic-blocking agents).

No products indexed under this heading.

Pirbuterol Acetate (Co-administration with certain drugs, such as sympathomimetics, may reduce the hypoglycemic action of nateglinide and other oral antidiabetic drugs; when these drugs are administered to or withdrawn from patients receiving nateglinide, the patient should be observed closely for changes in glycemic control). Products include:

Maxair Autohaler 1981
Maxair Inhaler 1984

Piroxicam (The hypoglycemic action of nateglinide may be potentiated by non-steroidal anti-inflammatory agents). Products include:

Feldene Capsules 2685

Polythiazide (Co-administration with certain drugs, such as thiazides, may reduce the hypoglycemic action of nateglinide and other oral antidiabetic drugs; when these drugs are administered to or withdrawn from patients receiving nateglinide, the patient should be observed closely for changes in glycemic control). Products include:

Minizide Capsules 2700
Renese Tablets 2712

Prednisolone Acetate (Co-administration with certain drugs, such as corticosteroids, may reduce the hypoglycemic action of nateglinide and other oral antidiabetic drugs; when these drugs are administered to or withdrawn from patients receiving nateglinide, the patient should be observed closely for changes in glycemic control). Products include:

Blephamide Ophthalmic Ointment ... 547
Blephamide Ophthalmic Suspension 548
Poly-Pred Liquifilm Ophthalmic Suspension .... ⊙245
Pred Forte Ophthalmic Suspension .... ⊙246
Pred Mild Sterile Ophthalmic Suspension .... ⊙249
Pred-G Ophthalmic Suspension .... ⊙247
Pred-G Sterile Ophthalmic Ointment .... ⊙248

Prednisolone Sodium Phosphate (Co-administration with certain drugs, such as corticosteroids, may reduce the hypoglycemic action of nateglinide and other oral antidiabetic drugs; when these drugs are administered to or withdrawn from patients receiving nateglinide, the patient should be observed closely for changes in glycemic control). Products include:

Pediapred Oral Solution 1170

Prednisolone Tebutate (Co-administration with certain drugs, such as corticosteroids, may reduce the hypoglycemic action of nateglinide and other oral antidiabetic drugs; when these drugs are administered to or withdrawn from patients receiving nateglinide, the patient should be observed closely for changes in glycemic control).

No products indexed under this heading.

Prednisone (Co-administration with certain drugs, such as corticosteroids, may reduce the hypoglycemic action of nateglinide and other oral antidiabetic drugs; when these drugs are administered to or withdrawn from patients receiving nateglinide, the patient should be observed closely for changes in glycemic control). Products include:

Prednisone 3064

Procarbazine Hydrochloride (The hypoglycemic action of nateglinide may be potentiated by MAO inhibitors). Products include:

Matulane Capsules 3246

Propranolol Hydrochloride (The hypoglycemic action of nateglinide may be potentiated by non-selective beta-adrenergic-blocking agents). Products include:

Inderal 3513
Inderal LA Long-Acting Capsules 3516
Inderide Tablets 3517
Inderide LA Long-Acting Capsules .. 3519

Pseudoephedrine Hydrochloride (Co-administration with certain drugs, such as sympathomimetics, may reduce the hypoglycemic action of nateglinide and other oral antidiabetic drugs; when these drugs are administered to or withdrawn from patients receiving nateglinide, the patient should be observed closely for changes in glycemic control). Products include:

Actifed Cold & Allergy Tablets .... ▣688
Actifed Cold & Sinus Caplets and Tablets .... ▣688
Advil Cold and Sinus Caplets .... ▣771
Advil Cold and Sinus Tablets .... ▣771
Advil Flu & Body Ache Caplets .... ▣772
Aleve Cold & Sinus Caplets .... ▣603
Alka-Seltzer Plus Liqui-Gels .... ▣604
Alka-Seltzer Plus Cold & Flu Medicine Liqui-Gels .... ▣604
Alka-Seltzer Plus Cold & Sinus Medicine Liqui-Gels .... ▣604
Allegra-D Extended-Release Tablets 714
BC Cold Powder .... ▣619
Benadryl Allergy/Cold Tablets .... ▣691
Benadryl Allergy/Congestion Tablets .... ▣692
Benadryl Allergy & Sinus Liquid .... ▣693
Benadryl Allergy & Sinus Fastmelt Tablets .... ▣693
Benadryl Allergy Sinus Headache Caplets & Gelcaps .... ▣693
Benadryl Severe Allergy & Sinus Headache Caplets .... ▣694
Benadryl Children's Allergy/Cold Fastmelt Tablets .... ▣692
Benylin Multi-Symptom Liquid .... ▣697
Bromfed Capsules (Extended-Release) 2269
Bromfed-PD Capsules (Extended-Release) 2269
Children's Cēpacol Sore Throat .... ▣788
Comtrex Acute Head Cold & Sinus Pressure Relief Tablets .... ▣627
Comtrex Deep Chest Cold & Congestion Relief Softgels .... ▣627
Comtrex Flu Therapy & Fever Relief Daytime Caplets .... ▣628
Comtrex Flu Therapy & Fever Relief Nighttime Tablets .... ▣628
Comtrex Maximum Strength Multi-Symptom Cold & Cough Relief Tablets and Caplets .... ▣626
Contac Non-Drowsy 12 Hour Cold Caplets .... ▣745
Contac Non-Drowsy Timed Release 12 Hour Cold Caplets ... ▣746
Contac Severe Cold and Flu Caplets Maximum Strength .... ▣746
Contac Severe Cold and Flu Caplets Non-Drowsy .... ▣746
Dimetapp Elixir .... ▣777
Dimetapp Cold and Fever Suspension .... ▣775
Dimetapp DM Cold & Cough Elixir .. ▣775
Dimetapp Nighttime Flu Liquid .... ▣776
Dimetapp Non-Drowsy Flu Syrup ... ▣777
Dimetapp Infant Drops Decongestant .... ▣775
Dimetapp Infant Drops Decongestant Plus Cough .... ▣776
Guaifed 2272
Kronofed-A 1341
Children's Motrin Cold Oral Suspension 2007
Motrin Sinus Headache Caplets 2005
PediaCare Cough-Cold Liquid .... ▣719
PediaCare Infants' Drops Decongestant .... ▣719
PediaCare Infants' Drops Decongestant Plus Cough .... ▣719
PediaCare NightRest Cough-Cold Liquid .... ▣719
Robitussin Cold Caplets Cold & Congestion .... ▣780
Robitussin Cold Softgels Cold & Congestion .... ▣780
Robitussin Cold Caplets Multi-Symptom Cold & Flu .... ▣781
Robitussin Cold Softgels Multi-Symptom Cold & Flu .... ▣781
Robitussin Cold Softgels Severe Congestion .... ▣782
Robitussin Cough & Cold Infant Drops .... ▣782
Robitussin Maximum Strength Cough & Cold Liquid .... ▣785
Robitussin Pediatric Cough & Cold Formula Liquid .... ▣785
Robitussin Multi Symptom Honey Flu Liquid .... ▣785
Robitussin Nighttime Honey Flu Liquid .... ▣786
Robitussin-CF Liquid .... ▣783
Robitussin-DAC Syrup 2942
Robitussin-PE Liquid .... ▣782
Ryna .... ▣768
Semprex-D Capsules 1172
Singlet Caplets .... ▣761
Sinutab Non-Drying Liquid Caps .... ▣706
Sinutab Sinus Allergy Medication, Maximum Strength Formula, Tablets & Caplets .... ▣707
Sinutab Sinus Medication, Maximum Strength Without Drowsiness Formula, Tablets & Caplets .... ▣707
Sudafed 12 Hour Tablets .... ▣708
Sudafed 24 Hour Tablets .... ▣708

Children's Sudafed Cold & Cough Liquid 709
Children's Sudafed Nasal Decongestant Chewables 711
Children's Sudafed Nasal Decongestant Liquid Medication 711
Sudafed Cold & Allergy Tablets 708
Sudafed Cold & Cough Liquid Caps 709
Sudafed Cold & Sinus Liquid Caps 710
Sudafed Nasal Decongestant Tablets 710
Sudafed Non-Drying Sinus Liquid Caps 712
Sudafed Severe Cold 711
Sudafed Sinus Headache Caplets 712
Sudafed Sinus Headache Tablets 712
Tavist Sinus Non-Drowsy Coated Caplets 676
TheraFlu Regular Strength Cold & Cough Night Time Hot Liquid 676
TheraFlu Regular Strength Cold & Sore Throat Night Time Hot Liquid 676
TheraFlu Maximum Strength Flu & Congestion Non-Drowsy Hot Liquid 677
TheraFlu Maximum Strength Flu & Cough Night Time Hot Liquid 678
TheraFlu Maximum Strength Flu & Sore Throat Night Time Hot Liquid 677
TheraFlu Maximum Strength Severe Cold & Congestion Night Time Caplets 678
TheraFlu Maximum Strength Severe Cold & Congestion Night Time Hot Liquid 678
TheraFlu Maximum Strength Severe Cold & Congestion Non-Drowsy 679
Triaminic Allergy Congestion Liquid 680
Triaminic Chest Congestion Liquid 680
Triaminic Cold & Allergy Liquid 681
Triaminic Cold & Allergy Softchews 683
Triaminic Cold & Cough Liquid 681
Triaminic Cold & Cough Softchews 683
Triaminic Cold & Night Time Cough Liquid 681
Triaminic Cold, Cough & Fever Liquid 681
Triaminic Cough Liquid 682
Triaminic Cough & Congestion Liquid 682
Triaminic Cough & Sore Throat Liquid 682
Triaminic Cough & Sore Throat Softchews 684
Children's Tylenol Allergy-D Liquid 2014
Children's Tylenol Cold Suspension Liquid and Chewable Tablets 2015
Children's Tylenol Cold Plus Cough Suspension Liquid and Chewable Tablets 2015
Children's Tylenol Flu Suspension Liquid 2015
Children's Tylenol Sinus Suspension Liquid 2017
Infants' Tylenol Cold Decongestant and Fever Reducer Concentrated Drops 2015
Infants' Tylenol Cold Decongestant and Fever Reducer Concentrated Drops Plus Cough 2015
Tylenol Allergy Sinus 2010
Multi-Symptom Tylenol Cold Complete Formula Caplets 2010
Multi-Symptom Tylenol Cold Non-Drowsy Caplets and Gelcaps 2010
Multi-Symptom Tylenol Cold Severe Congestion Non-Drowsy Caplets 2011
Maximum Strength Tylenol Flu NightTime Gelcaps 2011
Maximum Strength Tylenol Flu NightTime Liquid 2011
Maximum Strength Tylenol Flu Non-Drowsy Gelcaps 2011
Maximum Strength Tylenol Sinus NightTime Caplets 2012
Maximum Strength Tylenol Sinus Non-Drowsy Geltabs, Gelcaps, Caplets, and Tablets 2012
Vicks 44D Cough & Head Congestion Relief Liquid 724
Vicks 44M Cough, Cold & Flu Relief Liquid 725
Pediatric Vicks 44m Cough & Cold Relief 728
Vicks DayQuil LiquiCaps/Liquid Multi-Symptom Cold/Flu Relief 727
Children's Vicks NyQuil Cold/Cough Relief 726
Vicks NyQuil LiquiCaps/Liquid Multi-Symptom Cold/Flu Relief, Original and Cherry Flavors 727
Zephrex Tablets 3091
Zephrex LA Tablets 3092
Zyrtec-D 12 Hour Extended Relief Tablets 2758

Pseudoephedrine Sulfate (Co-administration with certain drugs, such as sympathomimetics, may reduce the hypoglycemic action of nateglinide and other oral antidiabetic drugs; when these drugs are administered to or withdrawn from patients receiving nateglinide, the patient should be observed closely for changes in glycemic control). Products include:
Chlor-Trimeton Allergy/Decongestant Tablets 736
Claritin-D 12 Hour Extended Release Tablets 3102
Claritin-D 24 Hour Extended Release Tablets 3104
Coricidin 'D' Cold, Flu & Sinus Tablets 737
Drixoral Allergy/Sinus Extended-Release Tablets 741
Drixoral Cold & Allergy Sustained-Action Tablets 740
Drixoral Cold & Flu Extended-Release Tablets 740
Drixoral Nasal Decongestant Long-Acting Non-Drowsy Tablets 740
Rynatan Tablets 3351

Rofecoxib (The hypoglycemic action of nateglinide may be potentiated by non-steroidal anti-inflammatory agents). Products include:
Vioxx 2213

Salmeterol Xinafoate (Co-administration with certain drugs, such as sympathomimetics, may reduce the hypoglycemic action of nateglinide and other oral antidiabetic drugs; when these drugs are administered to or withdrawn from patients receiving nateglinide, the patient should be observed closely for changes in glycemic control). Products include:
Advair Diskus 100/50 1448
Advair Diskus 250/50 1448
Advair Diskus 500/50 1448
Serevent Diskus 1637
Serevent Inhalation Aerosol 1633

Salsalate (The hypoglycemic action of nateglinide may be potentiated by salicylates).
No products indexed under this heading.

Selegiline Hydrochloride (The hypoglycemic action of nateglinide may be potentiated by MAO inhibitors). Products include:
Eldepryl Capsules 3266

Sotalol Hydrochloride (The hypoglycemic action of nateglinide may be potentiated by non-selective beta-adrenergic-blocking agents). Products include:
Betapace Tablets 950
Betapace AF Tablets 954

Sulindac (The hypoglycemic action of nateglinide may be potentiated by non-steroidal anti-inflammatory agents). Products include:
Clinoril Tablets 2053

Terbutaline Sulfate (Co-administration with certain drugs, such as sympathomimetics, may reduce the hypoglycemic action of nateglinide and other oral antidiabetic drugs; when these drugs are administered to or withdrawn from patients receiving nateglinide, the patient should be observed closely for changes in glycemic control). Products include:
Brethine Ampuls 2314
Brethine Tablets 2313

Thyroglobulin (Co-administration with certain drugs, such as thyroid products, may reduce the hypoglycemic action of nateglinide and other oral antidiabetic drugs; when these drugs are administered to or withdrawn from patients receiving nateglinide, the patient should be observed closely for changes in glycemic control).
No products indexed under this heading.

Thyroid (Co-administration with certain drugs, such as thyroid products, may reduce the hypoglycemic action of nateglinide and other oral antidiabetic drugs; when these drugs are administered to or withdrawn from patients receiving nateglinide, the patient should be observed closely for changes in glycemic control).
No products indexed under this heading.

Thyroxine (Co-administration with certain drugs, such as thyroid products, may reduce the hypoglycemic action of nateglinide and other oral antidiabetic drugs; when these drugs are administered to or withdrawn from patients receiving nateglinide, the patient should be observed closely for changes in glycemic control).
No products indexed under this heading.

Thyroxine Sodium (Co-administration with certain drugs, such as thyroid products, may reduce the hypoglycemic action of nateglinide and other oral antidiabetic drugs; when these drugs are administered to or withdrawn from patients receiving nateglinide, the patient should be observed closely for changes in glycemic control).
No products indexed under this heading.

Timolol Hemihydrate (The hypoglycemic action of nateglinide may be potentiated by non-selective beta-adrenergic-blocking agents). Products include:
Betimol Ophthalmic Solution .... ⊙ 324

Timolol Maleate (The hypoglycemic action of nateglinide may be potentiated by non-selective beta-adrenergic-blocking agents). Products include:
Blocadren Tablets 2046
Cosopt Sterile Ophthalmic Solution 2065
Timolide Tablets 2187
Timolol GFS .... ⊙ 266
Timoptic in Ocudose 2192
Timoptic Sterile Ophthalmic Solution 2190
Timoptic-XE Sterile Ophthalmic Gel Forming Solution 2194

Tolmetin Sodium (The hypoglycemic action of nateglinide may be potentiated by non-steroidal anti-inflammatory agents). Products include:
Tolectin 2589

Tranylcypromine Sulfate (The hypoglycemic action of nateglinide may be potentiated by MAO inhibitors). Products include:
Parnate Tablets 1607

Triamcinolone (Co-administration with certain drugs, such as corticosteroids, may reduce the hypoglycemic action of nateglinide and other oral antidiabetic drugs; when these drugs are administered to or withdrawn from patients receiving nateglinide, the patient should be observed closely for changes in glycemic control).
No products indexed under this heading.

Triamcinolone Acetonide (Co-administration with certain drugs, such as corticosteroids, may reduce the hypoglycemic action of nateglinide and other oral antidiabetic drugs; when these drugs are administered to or withdrawn from patients receiving nateglinide, the patient should be observed closely for changes in glycemic control). Products include:
Azmacort Inhalation Aerosol 728
Nasacort Nasal Inhaler 750
Nasacort AQ Nasal Spray 752
Tri-Nasal Spray 2274

Triamcinolone Diacetate (Co-administration with certain drugs, such as corticosteroids, may reduce the hypoglycemic action of nateglinide and other oral antidiabetic drugs; when these drugs are administered to or withdrawn from patients receiving nateglinide, the patient should be observed closely for changes in glycemic control).
No products indexed under this heading.

Triamcinolone Hexacetonide (Co-administration with certain drugs, such as corticosteroids, may reduce the hypoglycemic action of nateglinide and other oral antidiabetic drugs; when these drugs are administered to or withdrawn from patients receiving nateglinide, the patient should be observed closely for changes in glycemic control).
No products indexed under this heading.

Food Interactions

Food, unspecified (Administration of nateglinide with liquid meal significantly reduces peak plasma levels).

STELAZINE INJECTION

(Trifluoperazine Hydrochloride) 1640
May interact with central nervous system depressants, oral anticoagulants, anticonvulsants, thiazides, vasopressors, and certain other agents. Compounds in these categories include:

Alfentanil Hydrochloride (Additive depressant effects).
No products indexed under this heading.

Alprazolam (Additive depressant effects). Products include:
Xanax Tablets 2865

Aprobarbital (Additive depressant effects).
No products indexed under this heading.

Bendroflumethiazide (Orthostatic hypotension that occurs with phenothiazines may be accentuated). Products include:
Corzide 40/5 Tablets 2247
Corzide 80/5 Tablets 2247

Buprenorphine Hydrochloride (Additive depressant effects). Products include:
Buprenex Injectable 2918

Buspirone Hydrochloride (Additive depressant effects).
No products indexed under this heading.

Butabarbital (Additive depressant effects).
No products indexed under this heading.

Butalbital (Additive depressant effects). Products include:
Phrenilin 578
Sedapap Tablets 50 mg/650 mg 2225

Carbamazepine (Stelazine may lower convulsive thresholds; dosage adjustments of anticonvulsants may be necessary). Products include:
Carbatrol Capsules 3234
Tegretol/Tegretol-XR 2404

Chlordiazepoxide (Additive depressant effects). Products include:
Limbitrol 1738

Chlordiazepoxide Hydrochloride (Additive depressant effects). Products include:
Librium Capsules 1736
Librium for Injection 1737

Chlorothiazide (Orthostatic hypotension that occurs with phenothiazines may be accentuated). Products include:
Aldoclor Tablets ... 2035
Diuril Oral ... 2087

Chlorothiazide Sodium (Orthostatic hypotension that occurs with phenothiazines may be accentuated). Products include:
Diuril Sodium Intravenous ... 2086

Chlorpromazine (Additive depressant effects). Products include:
Thorazine Suppositories ... 1656

Chlorpromazine Hydrochloride (Additive depressant effects). Products include:
Thorazine ... 1656

Chlorprothixene (Additive depressant effects).
No products indexed under this heading.

Chlorprothixene Hydrochloride (Additive depressant effects).
No products indexed under this heading.

Chlorprothixene Lactate (Additive depressant effects).
No products indexed under this heading.

Clorazepate Dipotassium (Additive depressant effects). Products include:
Tranxene ... 511

Clozapine (Additive depressant effects). Products include:
Clozaril Tablets ... 2319

Codeine Phosphate (Additive depressant effects). Products include:
Phenergan with Codeine Syrup ... 3557
Phenergan VC with Codeine Syrup .. 3561
Robitussin A-C Syrup ... 2942
Robitussin-DAC Syrup ... 2942
Ryna-C Liquid ... ▣ 768
Soma Compound w/Codeine Tablets ... 3355
Tussi-Organidin NR Liquid ... 3350
Tussi-Organidin-S NR Liquid ... 3350
Tylenol with Codeine ... 2595

Desflurane (Additive depressant effects). Products include:
Suprane Liquid for Inhalation ... 874

Dezocine (Additive depressant effects).
No products indexed under this heading.

Diazepam (Additive depressant effects). Products include:
Valium Injectable ... 3026
Valium Tablets ... 3047

Dicumarol (Effect may be diminished).
No products indexed under this heading.

Divalproex Sodium (Stelazine may lower convulsive thresholds; dosage adjustments of anticonvulsants may be necessary). Products include:
Depakote Sprinkle Capsules ... 426
Depakote Tablets ... 430
Depakote ER Tablets ... 436

Dopamine Hydrochloride (May cause a paradoxical further lowering of blood pressure).
No products indexed under this heading.

Droperidol (Additive depressant effects).
No products indexed under this heading.

Enflurane (Additive depressant effects).
No products indexed under this heading.

Epinephrine Bitartrate (Reversed epinephrine effect; may cause a paradoxical further lowering of blood pressure). Products include:
Sensorcaine ... 643

Epinephrine Hydrochloride (Reversed epinephrine effect; may cause a paradoxical further lowering of blood pressure).
No products indexed under this heading.

Estazolam (Additive depressant effects). Products include:
ProSom Tablets ... 500

Ethchlorvynol (Additive depressant effects).
No products indexed under this heading.

Ethinamate (Additive depressant effects).
No products indexed under this heading.

Ethosuximide (Stelazine may lower convulsive thresholds; dosage adjustments of anticonvulsants may be necessary). Products include:
Zarontin Capsules ... 2659
Zarontin Syrup ... 2660

Ethotoin (Stelazine may lower convulsive thresholds; dosage adjustments of anticonvulsants may be necessary).
No products indexed under this heading.

Felbamate (Stelazine may lower convulsive thresholds; dosage adjustments of anticonvulsants may be necessary). Products include:
Felbatol ... 3343

Fentanyl (Additive depressant effects). Products include:
Duragesic Transdermal System ... 1786

Fentanyl Citrate (Additive depressant effects). Products include:
Actiq ... 1184

Fluphenazine Decanoate (Additive depressant effects).
No products indexed under this heading.

Fluphenazine Enanthate (Additive depressant effects).
No products indexed under this heading.

Fluphenazine Hydrochloride (Additive depressant effects).
No products indexed under this heading.

Flurazepam Hydrochloride (Additive depressant effects).
No products indexed under this heading.

Fosphenytoin Sodium (Stelazine may lower convulsive thresholds; dosage adjustments of anticonvulsants may be necessary). Products include:
Cerebyx Injection ... 2619

Glutethimide (Additive depressant effects).
No products indexed under this heading.

Guanethidine Monosulfate (Antihypertensive effects of guanethidine and related compounds may be counteracted when used concurrently).
No products indexed under this heading.

Haloperidol (Additive depressant effects). Products include:
Haldol Injection, Tablets and Concentrate ... 2533

Haloperidol Decanoate (Additive depressant effects). Products include:
Haldol Decanoate ... 2535

Hydrochlorothiazide (Orthostatic hypotension that occurs with Stelazine may be accentuated). Products include:
Accuretic Tablets ... 2614
Aldoril Tablets ... 2039
Atacand HCT Tablets ... 597
Avalide Tablets ... 1070
Diovan HCT Tablets ... 2338
Dyazide Capsules ... 1515
HydroDIURIL Tablets ... 2108
Hyzaar ... 2109
Inderide Tablets ... 3517
Inderide LA Long-Acting Capsules .. 3519
Lotensin HCT Tablets ... 2367
Maxzide ... 1008
Micardis HCT Tablets ... 1051
Microzide Capsules ... 3414
Moduretic Tablets ... 2138
Monopril HCT ... 1094
Prinzide Tablets ... 2168
Timolide Tablets ... 2187
Uniretic Tablets ... 3178
Vaseretic Tablets ... 2204
Zestoretic Tablets ... 695
Ziac Tablets ... 1887

Hydrocodone Bitartrate (Additive depressant effects). Products include:
Hycodan ... 1316
Hycomine Compound Tablets ... 1317
Hycotuss Expectorant Syrup ... 1318
Lortab ... 3319
Lortab Elixir ... 3317
Maxidone Tablets CIII ... 3399
Norco 5/325 Tablets CIII ... 3424
Norco 7.5/325 Tablets CIII ... 3425
Norco 10/325 Tablets CIII ... 3427
Norco 10/325 Tablets CIII ... 3425
Vicodin Tablets ... 516
Vicodin ES Tablets ... 517
Vicodin HP Tablets ... 518
Vicodin Tuss Expectorant ... 519
Vicoprofen Tablets ... 520
Zydone Tablets ... 1330

Hydrocodone Polistirex (Additive depressant effects). Products include:
Tussionex Pennkinetic Extended-Release Suspension ... 1174

Hydroflumethiazide (Orthostatic hypotension that occurs with Stelazine may be accentuated). Products include:
Diucardin Tablets ... 3494

Hydromorphone Hydrochloride (Additive depressant effects). Products include:
Dilaudid ... 441
Dilaudid Oral Liquid ... 445
Dilaudid Powder ... 441
Dilaudid Rectal Suppositories ... 441
Dilaudid Tablets ... 441
Dilaudid Tablets - 8 mg ... 445
Dilaudid-HP ... 443

Hydroxyzine Hydrochloride (Additive depressant effects). Products include:
Atarax Tablets & Syrup ... 2667
Vistaril Intramuscular Solution ... 2738

Isoflurane (Additive depressant effects).
No products indexed under this heading.

Ketamine Hydrochloride (Additive depressant effects).
No products indexed under this heading.

Lamotrigine (Stelazine may lower convulsive thresholds; dosage adjustments of anticonvulsants may be necessary). Products include:
Lamictal ... 1567

Levetiracetam (Stelazine may lower convulsive thresholds; dosage adjustments of anticonvulsants may be necessary). Products include:
Keppra Tablets ... 3314

Levomethadyl Acetate Hydrochloride (Additive depressant effects).
No products indexed under this heading.

Levorphanol Tartrate (Additive depressant effects). Products include:
Levo-Dromoran ... 1734
Levorphanol Tartrate Tablets ... 3059

Lorazepam (Additive depressant effects). Products include:
Ativan Injection ... 3478
Ativan Tablets ... 3482

Loxapine Hydrochloride (Additive depressant effects).
No products indexed under this heading.

Loxapine Succinate (Additive depressant effects). Products include:
Loxitane Capsules ... 3398

Meperidine Hydrochloride (Additive depressant effects). Products include:
Demerol ... 3079
Mepergan Injection ... 3539

Mephenytoin (Stelazine may lower convulsive thresholds; dosage adjustments of anticonvulsants may be necessary).
No products indexed under this heading.

Mephobarbital (Additive depressant effects).
No products indexed under this heading.

Meprobamate (Additive depressant effects). Products include:
Miltown Tablets ... 3349

Mesoridazine Besylate (Additive depressant effects). Products include:
Serentil ... 1057

Metaraminol Bitartrate (May cause a paradoxical further lowering of blood pressure). Products include:
Aramine Injection ... 2043

Methadone Hydrochloride (Additive depressant effects). Products include:
Dolophine Hydrochloride Tablets ... 3056

Methohexital Sodium (Additive depressant effects). Products include:
Brevital Sodium for Injection, USP .. 1815

Methotrimeprazine (Additive depressant effects).
No products indexed under this heading.

Methoxamine Hydrochloride (May cause a paradoxical further lowering of blood pressure).
No products indexed under this heading.

Methoxyflurane (Additive depressant effects).
No products indexed under this heading.

Methsuximide (Stelazine may lower convulsive thresholds; dosage adjustments of anticonvulsants may be necessary). Products include:
Celontin Capsules ... 2618

Methyclothiazide (Orthostatic hypotension that occurs with Stelazine may be accentuated).
No products indexed under this heading.

Metrizamide (Stelazine may lower the seizure threshold; do not use concurrently).
No products indexed under this heading.

Midazolam Hydrochloride (Additive depressant effects). Products include:
Versed Injection ... 3027
Versed Syrup ... 3033

Molindone Hydrochloride (Additive depressant effects). Products include:
Moban ... 1320

Morphine Sulfate (Additive depressant effects). Products include:
Astramorph/PF Injection, USP (Preservative-Free) ... 594
Duramorph Injection ... 1312
Infumorph 200 and Infumorph 500 Sterile Solutions ... 1314
Kadian Capsules ... 1335
MS Contin Tablets ... 2896
MSIR ... 2898
Oramorph SR Tablets ... 3062
Roxanol ... 3066

Norepinephrine Bitartrate (May cause a paradoxical further lowering of blood pressure).
No products indexed under this heading.

Olanzapine (Additive depressant effects). Products include:
Zyprexa Tablets ... 1973
Zyprexa ZYDIS Orally Disintegrating Tablets ... 1973

Oxazepam (Additive depressant effects).
No products indexed under this heading.

Oxcarbazepine (Stelazine may lower convulsive thresholds; dosage adjustments of anticonvulsants may be necessary). Products include:
Trileptal Oral Suspension 2407
Trileptal Tablets 2407

Oxycodone Hydrochloride (Additive depressant effects). Products include:
OxyContin Tablets 2912
OxyFast Oral Concentrate Solution . 2916
OxyIR Capsules 2916
Percocet Tablets 1326
Percodan Tablets 1327
Percolone Tablets 1327
Roxicodone 3067
Tylox Capsules 2597

Paramethadione (Stelazine may lower convulsive thresholds; dosage adjustments of anticonvulsants may be necessary).
No products indexed under this heading.

Pentobarbital Sodium (Additive depressant effects). Products include:
Nembutal Sodium Solution 485

Perphenazine (Additive depressant effects). Products include:
Etrafon 3115
Trilafon 3160

Phenacemide (Stelazine may lower convulsive thresholds; dosage adjustments of anticonvulsants may be necessary).
No products indexed under this heading.

Phenobarbital (Additive depressant effects). Products include:
Arco-Lase Plus Tablets 592
Donnatal 2929
Donnatal Extentabs 2930

Phensuximide (Phenothiazines may lower convulsive thresholds; dosage adjustments of anticonvulsants may be necessary).
No products indexed under this heading.

Phenylephrine Hydrochloride (May cause a paradoxical further lowering of blood pressure). Products include:
Afrin Nasal Decongestant Children's Pump Mist 734
Extendryl 1361
Hycomine Compound Tablets 1317
Neo-Synephrine 614
Phenergan VC Syrup 3560
Phenergan VC with Codeine Syrup .. 3561
Preparation H Cream 778
Preparation H Cooling Gel 778
Preparation H 778
Vicks Sinex Nasal Spray and Ultra Fine Mist 729

Phenytoin (Phenytoin toxicity may be precipitated; Stelazine may lower convulsive thresholds; dosage adjustments of anticonvulsants may be necessary). Products include:
Dilantin Infatabs 2624
Dilantin-125 Oral Suspension 2625

Phenytoin Sodium (Phenytoin toxicity may be precipitated; Stelazine may lower convulsive thresholds; dosage adjustments of anticonvulsants may be necessary). Products include:
Dilantin Kapseals 2622

Polythiazide (Orthostatic hypotension that occurs with Stelazine may be accentuated). Products include:
Minizide Capsules 2700
Renese Tablets 2712

Prazepam (Additive depressant effects).
No products indexed under this heading.

Primidone (Stelazine may lower convulsive thresholds; dosage adjustments of anticonvulsants may be necessary).
No products indexed under this heading.

Prochlorperazine (Additive depressant effects). Products include:
Compazine 1505

Promethazine Hydrochloride (Additive depressant effects). Products include:
Mepergan Injection 3539
Phenergan Injection 3553
Phenergan 3556
Phenergan Syrup 3554
Phenergan with Codeine Syrup 3557
Phenergan with Dextromethorphan Syrup 3559
Phenergan VC Syrup 3560
Phenergan VC with Codeine Syrup .. 3561

Propofol (Additive depressant effects). Products include:
Diprivan Injectable Emulsion 667

Propoxyphene Hydrochloride (Additive depressant effects). Products include:
Darvon Pulvules 1909
Darvon Compound-65 Pulvules 1910

Propoxyphene Napsylate (Additive depressant effects). Products include:
Darvon-N/Darvocet-N 1907
Darvon-N Tablets 1912

Propranolol Hydrochloride (Concomitant administration results in increased plasma levels of both drugs). Products include:
Inderal 3513
Inderal LA Long-Acting Capsules 3516
Inderide Tablets 3517
Inderide LA Long-Acting Capsules .. 3519

Quazepam (Additive depressant effects).
No products indexed under this heading.

Quetiapine Fumarate (Additive depressant effects). Products include:
Seroquel Tablets 684

Remifentanil Hydrochloride (Additive depressant effects).
No products indexed under this heading.

Risperidone (Additive depressant effects). Products include:
Risperdal 1796

Secobarbital Sodium (Additive depressant effects).
No products indexed under this heading.

Sevoflurane (Additive depressant effects).
No products indexed under this heading.

Sufentanil Citrate (Additive depressant effects).
No products indexed under this heading.

Temazepam (Additive depressant effects).
No products indexed under this heading.

Thiamylal Sodium (Additive depressant effects).
No products indexed under this heading.

Thioridazine Hydrochloride (Additive depressant effects). Products include:
Thioridazine Hydrochloride Tablets 2289

Thiothixene (Additive depressant effects). Products include:
Navane Capsules 2701
Thiothixene Capsules 2290

Tiagabine Hydrochloride (Stelazine may lower convulsive thresholds; dosage adjustments of anticonvulsants may be necessary). Products include:
Gabitril Tablets 1189

Topiramate (Stelazine may lower convulsive thresholds; dosage adjustments of anticonvulsants may be necessary). Products include:
Topamax Sprinkle Capsules 2590
Topamax Tablets 2590

Triazolam (Additive depressant effects). Products include:
Halcion Tablets 2823

Trimethadione (Stelazine may lower convulsive thresholds; dosage adjustments of anticonvulsants may be necessary).
No products indexed under this heading.

Valproate Sodium (Stelazine may lower convulsive thresholds; dosage adjustments of anticonvulsants may be necessary). Products include:
Depacon Injection 416

Valproic Acid (Stelazine may lower convulsive thresholds; dosage adjustments of anticonvulsants may be necessary). Products include:
Depakene 421

Warfarin Sodium (Effect may be diminished). Products include:
Coumadin for Injection 1243
Coumadin Tablets 1243
Warfarin Sodium Tablets, USP 3302

Zaleplon (Additive depressant effects). Products include:
Sonata Capsules 3591

Ziprasidone Hydrochloride (Additive depressant effects). Products include:
Geodon Capsules 2688

Zolpidem Tartrate (Additive depressant effects). Products include:
Ambien Tablets 3191

Zonisamide (Stelazine may lower convulsive thresholds; dosage adjustments of anticonvulsants may be necessary). Products include:
Zonegran Capsules 1307

Food Interactions

Alcohol (Additive depressant effects).

STELAZINE TABLETS
(Trifluoperazine Hydrochloride) 1640
See Stelazine Injection

STEPHAN BIO-NUTRITIONAL DAYTIME HYDRATING CREME
(Vitamin E) 770
None cited in PDR database.

STEPHAN BIO-NUTRITIONAL EYE-FIRMING CONCENTRATE
(Moisturizing Formula) 770
None cited in PDR database.

STEPHAN BIO-NUTRITIONAL NIGHTIME MOISTURE CREME
(Moisturizing Formula) 770
None cited in PDR database.

STEPHAN BIO-NUTRITIONAL REFRESHING MOISTURE GEL
(Moisturizing Formula) 770
None cited in PDR database.

STEPHAN BIO-NUTRITIONAL ULTRA HYDRATING FLUID
(Moisturizing Formula) 770
None cited in PDR database.

STEPHAN CLARITY CAPSULES
(Amino Acid Preparations, Ginkgo biloba, Herbals with Vitamins) 844
None cited in PDR database.

STEPHAN ELASTICITY CAPSULES
(Amino Acid Preparations, Herbals with Vitamins & Minerals) 847
None cited in PDR database.

STEPHAN ELIXIR CAPSULES
(Amino Acid Preparations, Ginkgo biloba, Herbals with Vitamins & Minerals) 848
None cited in PDR database.

STEPHAN ESSENTIAL CAPSULES
(Amino Acid Preparations, Vitamins with Minerals) 848
None cited in PDR database.

STEPHAN FEMININE CAPSULES
(Amino Acid Preparations, Vitamin E) 848
None cited in PDR database.

STEPHAN FLEXIBILITY CAPSULES
(Amino Acid Preparations, Vitamins with Minerals) 848
None cited in PDR database.

STEPHAN LOVPIL CAPSULES
(Amino Acid Preparations, Herbals with Vitamins & Minerals) 849
None cited in PDR database.

STEPHAN MASCULINE CAPSULES
(Amino Acid Preparations, Herbals with Minerals) 849
None cited in PDR database.

STEPHAN PROTECTOR CAPSULES
(Amino Acid Preparations, Astragalus) 850
None cited in PDR database.

STEPHAN RELIEF CAPSULES
(Amino Acid Preparations, Herbals with Vitamins, Psyllium Preparations) 850
None cited in PDR database.

STEPHAN TRANQUILITY CAPSULES
(Amino Acid Preparations, Herbals with Vitamins & Minerals, Valeriana officinalis) 851
None cited in PDR database.

STIMATE NASAL SPRAY
(Desmopressin Acetate) 796
May interact with vasopressors. Compounds in these categories include:

Dopamine Hydrochloride (Although the pressor activity of desmopressin is very low, its use with other pressor agents should be done with careful monitoring).
No products indexed under this heading.

Epinephrine Bitartrate (Although the pressor activity of desmopressin is very low, its use with other pressor agents should be done with careful monitoring). Products include:
Sensorcaine 643

Epinephrine Hydrochloride (Although the pressor activity of desmopressin is very low, its use with other pressor agents should be done with careful monitoring).
No products indexed under this heading.

Metaraminol Bitartrate (Although the pressor activity of desmopressin is very low, its use with other pressor agents should be done with careful monitoring). Products include:
Aramine Injection 2043

Methoxamine Hydrochloride (Although the pressor activity of des-

mopressin is very low, its use with other pressor agents should be done with careful monitoring).
No products indexed under this heading.

Norepinephrine Bitartrate (Although the pressor activity of desmopressin is very low, its use with other pressor agents should be done with careful monitoring).
No products indexed under this heading.

Phenylephrine Hydrochloride (Although the pressor activity of desmopressin is very low, its use with other pressor agents should be done with careful monitoring). Products include:
- Afrin Nasal Decongestant Children's Pump Mist .... ■734
- Extendryl 1361
- Hycomine Compound Tablets 1317
- Neo-Synephrine .... ■614
- Phenergan VC Syrup 3560
- Phenergan VC with Codeine Syrup .. 3561
- Preparation H Cream .... ■778
- Preparation H Cooling Gel .... ■778
- Preparation H .... ■778
- Vicks Sinex Nasal Spray and Ultra Fine Mist .... ■729

STREPTASE FOR INFUSION

(Streptokinase) 647

May interact with anticoagulants and platelet inhibitors. Compounds in these categories include:

Ardeparin Sodium (Streptokinase, alone or in combination with antiplatelet and anticoagulants, may cause bleeding complications).
No products indexed under this heading.

Aspirin (Streptokinase, alone or in combination with antiplatelet and anticoagulants, may cause bleeding complications). Products include:
- Aggrenox Capsules 1026
- Alka-Seltzer .... ■603
- Alka-Seltzer Lemon Lime Antacid and Pain Reliever Effervescent Tablets .... ■603
- Alka-Seltzer Extra Strength Antacid and Pain Reliever Effervescent Tablets .... ■603
- Alka-Seltzer PM Effervescent Tablets .... ■605
- Genuine Bayer Tablets, Caplets and Gelcaps .... ■606
- Extra Strength Bayer Caplets and Gelcaps .... ■610
- Aspirin Regimen Bayer Children's Chewable Tablets (Orange or Cherry Flavored) .... ■607
- Bayer, Aspirin Regimen .... ■606
- Aspirin Regimen Bayer 81 mg Caplets with Calcium .... ■607
- Genuine Bayer Professional Labeling (Aspirin Regimen Bayer) .... ■608
- Extra Strength Bayer Arthritis Caplets .... ■610
- Extra Strength Bayer Plus Caplets .... ■610
- Extra Strength Bayer PM Caplets .. ■611
- BC Powder .... ■619
- BC Allergy Sinus Cold Powder .... ■619
- Arthritis Strength BC Powder .... ■619
- BC Sinus Cold Powder .... ■619
- Darvon Compound-65 Pulvules 1910
- Ecotrin Enteric Coated Aspirin Low, Regular and Maximum Strength Tablets 1715
- Excedrin Extra-Strength Tablets, Caplets, and Geltabs .... ■629
- Excedrin Migraine 1070
- Goody's Body Pain Formula Powder .... ■620
- Goody's Extra Strength Headache Powder .... ■620
- Goody's Extra Strength Pain Relief Tablets .... ■620
- Percodan Tablets 1327
- Robaxisal Tablets 2939
- Soma Compound Tablets 3354
- Soma Compound w/Codeine Tablets 3355
- Vanquish Caplets .... ■617

Azlocillin Sodium (Streptokinase, alone or in combination with antiplatelet and anticoagulants, may cause bleeding complications).
No products indexed under this heading.

Carbenicillin Indanyl Sodium (Streptokinase, alone or in combination with antiplatelet and anticoagulants, may cause bleeding complications). Products include:
- Geocillin Tablets 2687

Choline Magnesium Trisalicylate (Streptokinase, alone or in combination with antiplatelet and anticoagulants, may cause bleeding complications). Products include:
- Trilisate 2901

Clopidogrel Bisulfate (Streptokinase, alone or in combination with antiplatelet and anticoagulants, may cause bleeding complications). Products include:
- Plavix Tablets 1097
- Plavix Tablets 3084

Dalteparin Sodium (Streptokinase, alone or in combination with antiplatelet and anticoagulants, may cause bleeding complications). Products include:
- Fragmin Injection 2814

Danaparoid Sodium (Streptokinase, alone or in combination with antiplatelet and anticoagulants, may cause bleeding complications). Products include:
- Orgaran Injection 2480

Diclofenac Potassium (Streptokinase, alone or in combination with antiplatelet and anticoagulants, may cause bleeding complications). Products include:
- Cataflam Tablets 2315

Diclofenac Sodium (Streptokinase, alone or in combination with antiplatelet and anticoagulants, may cause bleeding complications). Products include:
- Arthrotec Tablets 3195
- Voltaren Ophthalmic Sterile Ophthalmic Solution .... ⊙312
- Voltaren Tablets 2315
- Voltaren-XR Tablets 2315

Dicumarol (Streptokinase, alone or in combination with antiplatelet and anticoagulants, may cause bleeding complications).
No products indexed under this heading.

Diflunisal (Streptokinase, alone or in combination with antiplatelet and anticoagulants, may cause bleeding complications). Products include:
- Dolobid Tablets 2088

Dipyridamole (Streptokinase, alone or in combination with antiplatelet and anticoagulants, may cause bleeding complications). Products include:
- Aggrenox Capsules 1026
- Persantine Tablets 1057

Enoxaparin (Streptokinase, alone or in combination with antiplatelet and anticoagulants, may cause bleeding complications). Products include:
- Lovenox Injection 746

Fenoprofen Calcium (Streptokinase, alone or in combination with antiplatelet and anticoagulants, may cause bleeding complications).
No products indexed under this heading.

Flurbiprofen (Streptokinase, alone or in combination with antiplatelet and anticoagulants, may cause bleeding complications).
No products indexed under this heading.

Heparin Sodium (Streptokinase, alone or in combination with antiplatelet and anticoagulants, may cause bleeding complications). Products include:
- Heparin Lock Flush Solution 3509
- Heparin Sodium Injection 3511

Ibuprofen (Streptokinase, alone or in combination with antiplatelet and anticoagulants, may cause bleeding complications). Products include:
- Advil .... ■771
- Children's Advil Oral Suspension .... ■773
- Children's Advil Chewable Tablets . ■773
- Advil Cold and Sinus Caplets .... ■771
- Advil Cold and Sinus Tablets .... ■771
- Advil Flu & Body Ache Caplets .... ■772
- Infants' Advil Drops .... ■773
- Junior Strength Advil Tablets .... ■773
- Junior Strength Advil Chewable Tablets .... ■773
- Advil Migraine Liquigels .... ■772
- Children's Motrin Oral Suspension and Chewable Tablets 2006
- Children's Motrin Cold Oral Suspension 2007
- Children's Motrin Oral Suspension .... ■643
- Motrin Suspension, Oral Drops, Chewable Tablets, and Caplets 2002
- Infants' Motrin Concentrated Drops 2006
- Junior Strength Motrin Caplets and Chewable Tablets 2006
- Motrin IB Tablets, Caplets, and Gelcaps 2002
- Motrin Migraine Pain Caplets 2005
- Motrin Sinus Headache Caplets 2005
- Vicoprofen Tablets 520

Indomethacin (Streptokinase, alone or in combination with antiplatelet and anticoagulants, may cause bleeding complications). Products include:
- Indocin 2112

Indomethacin Sodium Trihydrate (Streptokinase, alone or in combination with antiplatelet and anticoagulants, may cause bleeding complications). Products include:
- Indocin I.V. 2115

Ketoprofen (Streptokinase, alone or in combination with antiplatelet and anticoagulants, may cause bleeding complications). Products include:
- Orudis Capsules 3548
- Orudis KT Tablets .... ■778
- Oruvail Capsules 3548

Magnesium Salicylate (Streptokinase, alone or in combination with antiplatelet and anticoagulants, may cause bleeding complications). Products include:
- Momentum Backache Relief Extra Strength Caplets .... ■666

Meclofenamate Sodium (Streptokinase, alone or in combination with antiplatelet and anticoagulants, may cause bleeding complications).
No products indexed under this heading.

Mefenamic Acid (Streptokinase, alone or in combination with antiplatelet and anticoagulants, may cause bleeding complications). Products include:
- Ponstel Capsules 1356

Mezlocillin Sodium (Streptokinase, alone or in combination with antiplatelet and anticoagulants, may cause bleeding complications).
No products indexed under this heading.

Nafcillin Sodium (Streptokinase, alone or in combination with antiplatelet and anticoagulants, may cause bleeding complications).
No products indexed under this heading.

Naproxen (Streptokinase, alone or in combination with antiplatelet and anticoagulants, may cause bleeding complications). Products include:
- EC-Naprosyn Delayed-Release Tablets 2967
- Naprosyn Suspension 2967
- Naprosyn Tablets 2967

Naproxen Sodium (Streptokinase, alone or in combination with antiplatelet and anticoagulants, may cause bleeding complications). Products include:
- Aleve Tablets, Caplets and Gelcaps .... ■602
- Aleve Cold & Sinus Caplets .... ■603
- Anaprox Tablets 2967
- Anaprox DS Tablets 2967
- Naprelan Tablets 1293

Penicillin G Benzathine (Streptokinase, alone or in combination with antiplatelet and anticoagulants, may cause bleeding complications). Products include:
- Bicillin C-R 900/300 Injection 2240
- Bicillin C-R Injection 2238
- Bicillin L-A Injection 2242
- Permapen Isoject 2706

Penicillin G Procaine (Streptokinase, alone or in combination with antiplatelet and anticoagulants, may cause bleeding complications). Products include:
- Bicillin C-R 900/300 Injection 2240
- Bicillin C-R Injection 2238

Phenylbutazone (Streptokinase, alone or in combination with antiplatelet and anticoagulants, may cause bleeding complications).
No products indexed under this heading.

Piroxicam (Streptokinase, alone or in combination with antiplatelet and anticoagulants, may cause bleeding complications). Products include:
- Feldene Capsules 2685

Salsalate (Streptokinase, alone or in combination with antiplatelet and anticoagulants, may cause bleeding complications).
No products indexed under this heading.

Sulindac (Streptokinase, alone or in combination with antiplatelet and anticoagulants, may cause bleeding complications). Products include:
- Clinoril Tablets 2053

Ticarcillin Disodium (Streptokinase, alone or in combination with antiplatelet and anticoagulants, may cause bleeding complications). Products include:
- Timentin Injection- ADD-Vantage Vial 1661
- Timentin Injection-Galaxy Container 1664
- Timentin Injection-Pharmacy Bulk Package 1666
- Timentin for Intravenous Administration 1658

Ticlopidine Hydrochloride (Streptokinase, alone or in combination with antiplatelet and anticoagulants, may cause bleeding complications). Products include:
- Ticlid Tablets 3015

Tinzaparin sodium (Streptokinase, alone or in combination with antiplatelet and anticoagulants, may cause bleeding complications). Products include:
- Innohep Injection 1248

Tolmetin Sodium (Streptokinase, alone or in combination with antiplatelet and anticoagulants, may cause bleeding complications). Products include:
- Tolectin 2589

Warfarin Sodium (Streptokinase, alone or in combination with antiplatelet and anticoagulants, may cause bleeding complications). Products include:
- Coumadin for Injection 1243
- Coumadin Tablets 1243
- Warfarin Sodium Tablets, USP 3302

STREPTOMYCIN SULFATE INJECTION

(Streptomycin Sulfate) 2714

May interact with anesthetics, diuretics, muscle relaxants, and certain other agents. Compounds in these categories include:

Alfentanil Hydrochloride (Potential for respiratory paralysis from neuromuscular blockage due to neurotoxicity, especially when given soon after the use of anesthesia).
No products indexed under this heading.

Amiloride Hydrochloride (Interaction with furosemide is extrapolated to other diuretics where co-administration may possibly result in the potentiation of ototoxic effects). Products include:
- Midamor Tablets 2136
- Moduretic Tablets 2138

Atracurium Besylate (Potential for respiratory paralysis from neuromuscular blockage due to neurotoxicity, especially when given soon after the use of muscle relaxants).
No products indexed under this heading.

Baclofen (Potential for respiratory paralysis from neuromuscular blockage due to neurotoxicity, especially when given soon after the use of muscle relaxants).
No products indexed under this heading.

Bendroflumethiazide (Interaction with furosemide is extrapolated to other diuretics where co-administration may possibly result in the potentiation of ototoxic effects). Products include:
- Corzide 40/5 Tablets 2247
- Corzide 80/5 Tablets 2247

Bumetanide (Interaction with furosemide is extrapolated to other diuretics where co-administration may possibly result in the potentiation of ototoxic effects).
No products indexed under this heading.

Carisoprodol (Potential for respiratory paralysis from neuromuscular blockage due to neurotoxicity, especially when given soon after the use of muscle relaxants). Products include:
- Soma Tablets 3353
- Soma Compound Tablets 3354
- Soma Compound w/Codeine Tablets 3355

Cephaloridine (Concurrent and/or sequential use may increase the potential for increased toxicity; co-administration should be avoided).
No products indexed under this heading.

Chlorothiazide (Interaction with furosemide is extrapolated to other diuretics where co-administration may possibly result in the potentiation of ototoxic effects). Products include:
- Aldoclor Tablets 2035
- Diuril Oral 2087

Chlorothiazide Sodium (Interaction with furosemide is extrapolated to other diuretics where co-administration may possibly result in the potentiation of ototoxic effects). Products include:
- Diuril Sodium Intravenous 2086

Chlorthalidone (Interaction with furosemide is extrapolated to other diuretics where co-administration may possibly result in the potentiation of ototoxic effects). Products include:
- Clorpres Tablets 1002
- Combipres Tablets 1040
- Tenoretic Tablets 690

Chlorzoxazone (Potential for respiratory paralysis from neuromuscular blockage due to neurotoxicity, especially when given soon after the use of muscle relaxants). Products include:
- Parafon Forte DSC Caplets 2582

Cisatracurium Besylate (Potential for respiratory paralysis from neuromuscular blockage due to neurotoxicity, especially when given soon after the use of muscle relaxants).
No products indexed under this heading.

Colistin Sulfate (Concurrent and/or sequential use may increase the potential for increased toxicity; co-administration should be avoided). Products include:
- Cortisporin-TC Otic Suspension 2246

Cyclobenzaprine Hydrochloride (Potential for respiratory paralysis from neuromuscular blockage due to neurotoxicity, especially when given soon after the use of muscle relaxants). Products include:
- Flexeril Tablets 572
- Flexeril Tablets 2094

Cyclosporine (Concurrent and/or sequential use may increase the potential for increased toxicity; co-administration should be avoided). Products include:
- Gengraf Capsules 457
- Neoral Soft Gelatin Capsules 2380
- Neoral Oral Solution 2380
- Sandimmune 2388

Dantrolene Sodium (Potential for respiratory paralysis from neuromuscular blockage due to neurotoxicity, especially when given soon after the use of muscle relaxants). Products include:
- Dantrium Capsules 2885
- Dantrium Intravenous 2886

Doxacurium Chloride (Potential for respiratory paralysis from neuromuscular blockage due to neurotoxicity, especially when given soon after the use of muscle relaxants).
No products indexed under this heading.

Enflurane (Potential for respiratory paralysis from neuromuscular blockage due to neurotoxicity, especially when given soon after the use of anesthesia).
No products indexed under this heading.

Ethacrynic Acid (Interaction with furosemide is extrapolated to other diuretics where co-administration may possibly result in the potentiation of ototoxic effects). Products include:
- Edecrin Tablets 2091

Fentanyl Citrate (Potential for respiratory paralysis from neuromuscular blockage due to neurotoxicity, especially when given soon after the use of anesthesia). Products include:
- Actiq 1184

Furosemide (Interaction with furosemide is extrapolated to other diuretics where co-administration may possibly result in the potentiation of ototoxic effects). Products include:
- Furosemide Tablets 2284

Gentamicin Sulfate (Concurrent and/or sequential use may increase the potential for increased toxicity; co-administration should be avoided). Products include:
- Genoptic Ophthalmic Ointment .... ⊙239
- Genoptic Sterile Ophthalmic Solution .... ⊙239
- Pred-G Ophthalmic Suspension .... ⊙247
- Pred-G Sterile Ophthalmic Ointment .... ⊙248

Halothane (Potential for respiratory paralysis from neuromuscular blockage due to neurotoxicity, especially when given soon after the use of anesthesia). Products include:
- Fluothane Inhalation 3508

Hydrochlorothiazide (Interaction with furosemide is extrapolated to other diuretics where co-administration may possibly result in the potentiation of ototoxic effects). Products include:
- Accuretic Tablets 2614
- Aldoril Tablets 2039
- Atacand HCT Tablets 597
- Avalide Tablets 1070
- Diovan HCT Tablets 2338
- Dyazide Capsules 1515
- HydroDIURIL Tablets 2108
- Hyzaar 2109
- Inderide Tablets 3517
- Inderide LA Long-Acting Capsules 3519
- Lotensin HCT Tablets 2367
- Maxzide 1008
- Micardis HCT Tablets 1051
- Microzide Capsules 3414
- Moduretic Tablets 2138
- Monopril HCT 1094
- Prinzide Tablets 2168
- Timolide Tablets 2187
- Uniretic Tablets 3178
- Vaseretic Tablets 2204
- Zestoretic Tablets 695
- Ziac Tablets 1887

Hydroflumethiazide (Interaction with furosemide is extrapolated to other diuretics where co-administration may possibly result in the potentiation of ototoxic effects). Products include:
- Diucardin Tablets 3494

Indapamide (Interaction with furosemide is extrapolated to other diuretics where co-administration may possibly result in the potentiation of ototoxic effects). Products include:
- Indapamide Tablets 2286

Isoflurane (Potential for respiratory paralysis from neuromuscular blockage due to neurotoxicity, especially when given soon after the use of anesthesia).
No products indexed under this heading.

Kanamycin Sulfate (Concurrent and/or sequential use may increase the potential for increased toxicity; co-administration should be avoided).
No products indexed under this heading.

Ketamine Hydrochloride (Potential for respiratory paralysis from neuromuscular blockage due to neurotoxicity, especially when given soon after the use of anesthesia).
No products indexed under this heading.

Mannitol (Co-administration results in the potentiation of ototoxic effects).
No products indexed under this heading.

Metaxalone (Potential for respiratory paralysis from neuromuscular blockage due to neurotoxicity, especially when given soon after the use of muscle relaxants). Products include:
- Skelaxin Tablets 1301

Methocarbamol (Potential for respiratory paralysis from neuromuscular blockage due to neurotoxicity, especially when given soon after the use of muscle relaxants). Products include:
- Robaxin Injectable 2938
- Robaxin Tablets 2939
- Robaxisal Tablets 2939

Methohexital Sodium (Potential for respiratory paralysis from neuromuscular blockage due to neurotoxicity, especially when given soon after the use of anesthesia). Products include:
- Brevital Sodium for Injection, USP .. 1815

Methyclothiazide (Interaction with furosemide is extrapolated to other diuretics where co-administration may possibly result in the potentiation of ototoxic effects).
No products indexed under this heading.

Metocurine Iodide (Potential for respiratory paralysis from neuromuscular blockage due to neurotoxicity, especially when given soon after the use of muscle relaxants).
No products indexed under this heading.

Metolazone (Interaction with furosemide is extrapolated to other diuretics where co-administration may possibly result in the potentiation of ototoxic effects). Products include:
- Mykrox Tablets 1168
- Zaroxolyn Tablets 1177

Midazolam Hydrochloride (Potential for respiratory paralysis from neuromuscular blockage due to neurotoxicity, especially when given soon after the use of anesthesia). Products include:
- Versed Injection 3027
- Versed Syrup 3033

Mivacurium Chloride (Potential for respiratory paralysis from neuromuscular blockage due to neurotoxicity, especially when given soon after the use of muscle relaxants).
No products indexed under this heading.

Neomycin, oral (Concurrent and/or sequential use may increase the potential for increased toxicity; co-administration should be avoided).
No products indexed under this heading.

Neomycin Sulfate (Concurrent and/or sequential use may increase the potential for increased toxicity; co-administration should be avoided). Products include:
- Cortisporin Ophthalmic Suspension Sterile .... ⊙297
- Cortisporin-TC Otic Suspension 2246
- NeoDecadron Sterile Ophthalmic Solution 2144
- Neosporin G.U. Irrigant Sterile 2256
- Neosporin Ophthalmic Ointment Sterile .... ⊙299
- Neosporin Ophthalmic Solution Sterile .... ⊙300
- Poly-Pred Liquifilm Ophthalmic Suspension .... ⊙245

Orphenadrine Citrate (Potential for respiratory paralysis from neuromuscular blockage due to neurotoxicity, especially when given soon after the use of muscle relaxants). Products include:
- Norflex 1987

Pancuronium Bromide (Potential for respiratory paralysis from neuromuscular blockage due to neurotoxicity, especially when given soon after the use of muscle relaxants).
No products indexed under this heading.

Paromomycin Sulfate (Concurrent and/or sequential use may increase the potential for increased toxicity; co-administration should be avoided).
No products indexed under this heading.

Polymyxin B Sulfate (Concurrent and/or sequential use may increase the potential for increased toxicity; co-administration should be avoided). Products include:
- Betadine Brand First Aid Antibiotics & Moisturizer Ointment 2894
- Betadine Brand Plus First Aid Antibiotics & Pain Reliever Ointment 2894
- Cortisporin Ophthalmic Suspension Sterile .... ⊙297
- Neosporin G.U. Irrigant Sterile 2256
- Neosporin Ointment .... ▣704
- Neosporin Ophthalmic Ointment Sterile .... ⊙299
- Neosporin Ophthalmic Solution Sterile .... ⊙300
- Neosporin + Pain Relief Maximum Strength Cream .... ▣704
- Neosporin + Pain Relief Maximum Strength Ointment .... ▣704
- Poly-Pred Liquifilm Ophthalmic Suspension .... ⊙245
- Polysporin Ointment .... ▣706
- Polysporin Ophthalmic Ointment Sterile .... ⊙301
- Polysporin Powder .... ▣706
- Polytrim Ophthalmic Solution 556

Polythiazide (Interaction with furosemide is extrapolated to other diuretics where co-administration may possibly result in the potentiation of ototoxic effects). Products include:
- Minizide Capsules 2700
- Renese Tablets 2712

Propofol (Potential for respiratory paralysis from neuromuscular blockage due to neurotoxicity, especially when given soon after the use of anesthesia). Products include:
- Diprivan Injectable Emulsion 667

IMPORTANT NOTE: Always consult each drug listing in the patient's regimen for possible interactions.

Rapacuronium Bromide (Potential for respiratory paralysis from neuromuscular blockage due to neurotoxicity, especially when given soon after the use of muscle relaxants).
No products indexed under this heading.

Remifentanil Hydrochloride (Potential for respiratory paralysis from neuromuscular blockage due to neurotoxicity, especially when given soon after the use of anesthesia).
No products indexed under this heading.

Rocuronium Bromide (Potential for respiratory paralysis from neuromuscular blockage due to neurotoxicity, especially when given soon after the use of muscle relaxants). Products include:
Zemuron Injection 2491

Spironolactone (Interaction with furosemide is extrapolated to other diuretics where co-administration may possibly result in the potentiation of ototoxic effects).
No products indexed under this heading.

Succinylcholine Chloride (Potential for respiratory paralysis from neuromuscular blockage due to neurotoxicity, especially when given soon after the use of muscle relaxants). Products include:
Anectine Injection 1476

Sufentanil Citrate (Potential for respiratory paralysis from neuromuscular blockage due to neurotoxicity, especially when given soon after the use of anesthesia).
No products indexed under this heading.

Thiamylal Sodium (Potential for respiratory paralysis from neuromuscular blockage due to neurotoxicity, especially when given soon after the use of anesthesia).
No products indexed under this heading.

Tobramycin (Concurrent and/or sequential use may increase the potential for increased toxicity; co-administration should be avoided). Products include:
TOBI Solution for Inhalation 1206
TobraDex Ophthalmic Ointment 542
TobraDex Ophthalmic Suspension .. 541
Tobrex Ophthalmic Ointment .... ⊙220
Tobrex Ophthalmic Solution .... ⊙221

Tobramycin Sulfate (Concurrent and/or sequential use may increase the potential for increased toxicity; co-administration should be avoided). Products include:
Nebcin Vials, Hyporets & ADD-Vantage 1955

Torsemide (Interaction with furosemide is extrapolated to other diuretics where co-administration may possibly result in the potentiation of ototoxic effects). Products include:
Demadex Tablets and Injection 2965

Triamterene (Interaction with furosemide is extrapolated to other diuretics where co-administration may possibly result in the potentiation of ototoxic effects). Products include:
Dyazide Capsules 1515
Dyrenium Capsules 3458
Maxzide 1008

Vecuronium Bromide (Potential for respiratory paralysis from neuromuscular blockage due to neurotoxicity, especially when given soon after the use of muscle relaxants). Products include:
Norcuron for Injection 2478

Viomycin (Concurrent and/or sequential use may increase the potential for increased toxicity; co-administration should be avoided).

STROMECTOL TABLETS
(Ivermectin) 2185
None cited in PDR database.

STRONGSTART CAPLETS
(Vitamins, Prenatal, Vitamins with Minerals) 3096
None cited in PDR database.

STRONGSTART CHEWABLE
(Vitamins, Prenatal, Vitamins with Minerals) 3097
None cited in PDR database.

STUARTNATAL PLUS 3 TABLETS
(Vitamins, Prenatal) 1769
None cited in PDR database.

SUDAFED 12 HOUR TABLETS
(Pseudoephedrine Hydrochloride) .... ▣708
May interact with monoamine oxidase inhibitors. Compounds in these categories include:

Isocarboxazid (Concurrent and/or sequential use with MAO inhibitors is not recommended).
No products indexed under this heading.

Moclobemide (Concurrent and/or sequential use with MAO inhibitors is not recommended).
No products indexed under this heading.

Pargyline Hydrochloride (Concurrent and/or sequential use with MAO inhibitors is not recommended).
No products indexed under this heading.

Phenelzine Sulfate (Concurrent and/or sequential use with MAO inhibitors is not recommended). Products include:
Nardil Tablets 2653

Procarbazine Hydrochloride (Concurrent and/or sequential use with MAO inhibitors is not recommended). Products include:
Matulane Capsules 3246

Selegiline Hydrochloride (Concurrent and/or sequential use with MAO inhibitors is not recommended). Products include:
Eldepryl Capsules 3266

Tranylcypromine Sulfate (Concurrent and/or sequential use with MAO inhibitors is not recommended). Products include:
Parnate Tablets 1607

SUDAFED 24 HOUR TABLETS
(Pseudoephedrine Hydrochloride) .... ▣708
See Sudafed 12 Hour Tablets

CHILDREN'S SUDAFED COLD & COUGH LIQUID
(Dextromethorphan Hydrobromide, Pseudoephedrine Hydrochloride) ..... ▣709
May interact with monoamine oxidase inhibitors. Compounds in these categories include:

Isocarboxazid (Concurrent and/or sequential use with MAO inhibitors is not recommended).
No products indexed under this heading.

Moclobemide (Concurrent and/or sequential use with MAO inhibitors is not recommended).
No products indexed under this heading.

Pargyline Hydrochloride (Concurrent and/or sequential use with MAO inhibitors is not recommended).
No products indexed under this heading.

Phenelzine Sulfate (Concurrent and/or sequential use with MAO inhibitors is not recommended). Products include:
Nardil Tablets 2653

Procarbazine Hydrochloride (Concurrent and/or sequential use with MAO inhibitors is not recommended). Products include:
Matulane Capsules 3246

Selegiline Hydrochloride (Concurrent and/or sequential use with MAO inhibitors is not recommended). Products include:
Eldepryl Capsules 3266

Tranylcypromine Sulfate (Concurrent and/or sequential use with MAO inhibitors is not recommended). Products include:
Parnate Tablets 1607

CHILDREN'S SUDAFED NASAL DECONGESTANT CHEWABLES
(Pseudoephedrine Hydrochloride) .... ▣711
See Sudafed 12 Hour Tablets

CHILDREN'S SUDAFED NASAL DECONGESTANT LIQUID MEDICATION
(Pseudoephedrine Hydrochloride) .... ▣711
May interact with monoamine oxidase inhibitors. Compounds in these categories include:

Isocarboxazid (Concurrent and/or sequential use is not recommended).
No products indexed under this heading.

Moclobemide (Concurrent and/or sequential use is not recommended).
No products indexed under this heading.

Pargyline Hydrochloride (Concurrent and/or sequential use is not recommended).
No products indexed under this heading.

Phenelzine Sulfate (Concurrent and/or sequential use is not recommended). Products include:
Nardil Tablets 2653

Procarbazine Hydrochloride (Concurrent and/or sequential use is not recommended). Products include:
Matulane Capsules 3246

Selegiline Hydrochloride (Concurrent and/or sequential use is not recommended). Products include:
Eldepryl Capsules 3266

Tranylcypromine Sulfate (Concurrent and/or sequential use is not recommended). Products include:
Parnate Tablets 1607

SUDAFED COLD & ALLERGY TABLETS
(Chlorpheniramine Maleate, Pseudoephedrine Hydrochloride) ..... ▣708
May interact with hypnotics and sedatives, monoamine oxidase inhibitors, tranquilizers, and certain other agents. Compounds in these categories include:

Alprazolam (May increase drowsiness effect). Products include:
Xanax Tablets 2865

Buspirone Hydrochloride (May increase drowsiness effect).
No products indexed under this heading.

Chlordiazepoxide (May increase drowsiness effect). Products include:
Limbitrol 1738

Chlordiazepoxide Hydrochloride (May increase drowsiness effect). Products include:
Librium Capsules 1736
Librium for Injection 1737

Chlorpromazine (May increase drowsiness effect). Products include:
Thorazine Suppositories 1656

Chlorpromazine Hydrochloride (May increase drowsiness effect). Products include:
Thorazine 1656

Chlorprothixene (May increase drowsiness effect).
No products indexed under this heading.

Chlorprothixene Hydrochloride (May increase drowsiness effect).
No products indexed under this heading.

Clorazepate Dipotassium (May increase drowsiness effect). Products include:
Tranxene 511

Diazepam (May increase drowsiness effect). Products include:
Valium Injectable 3026
Valium Tablets 3047

Droperidol (May increase drowsiness effect).
No products indexed under this heading.

Estazolam (May increase drowsiness effect). Products include:
ProSom Tablets 500

Ethchlorvynol (May increase drowsiness effect).
No products indexed under this heading.

Ethinamate (May increase drowsiness effect).
No products indexed under this heading.

Fluphenazine Decanoate (May increase drowsiness effect).
No products indexed under this heading.

Fluphenazine Enanthate (May increase drowsiness effect).
No products indexed under this heading.

Fluphenazine Hydrochloride (May increase drowsiness effect).
No products indexed under this heading.

Flurazepam Hydrochloride (May increase drowsiness effect).
No products indexed under this heading.

Glutethimide (May increase drowsiness effect).
No products indexed under this heading.

Haloperidol (May increase drowsiness effect). Products include:
Haldol Injection, Tablets and Concentrate 2533

Haloperidol Decanoate (May increase drowsiness effect). Products include:
Haldol Decanoate 2535

Hydroxyzine Hydrochloride (May increase drowsiness effect). Products include:
Atarax Tablets & Syrup 2667
Vistaril Intramuscular Solution 2738

Isocarboxazid (Concurrent and/or sequential use is not recommended).
No products indexed under this heading.

Lorazepam (May increase drowsiness effect). Products include:
Ativan Injection 3478
Ativan Tablets 3482

Loxapine Hydrochloride (May increase drowsiness effect).
No products indexed under this heading.

Loxapine Succinate (May increase drowsiness effect). Products include:
Loxitane Capsules 3398

Meprobamate (May increase drowsiness effect). Products include:
Miltown Tablets 3349

Mesoridazine Besylate (May increase drowsiness effect). Products include:
Serentil 1057

Midazolam Hydrochloride (May increase drowsiness effect). Products include:
- Versed Injection 3027
- Versed Syrup 3033

Moclobemide (Concurrent and/or sequential use is not recommended).
No products indexed under this heading.

Molindone Hydrochloride (May increase drowsiness effect). Products include:
- Moban 1320

Oxazepam (May increase drowsiness effect).
No products indexed under this heading.

Pargyline Hydrochloride (Concurrent and/or sequential use is not recommended).
No products indexed under this heading.

Perphenazine (May increase drowsiness effect). Products include:
- Etrafon 3115
- Trilafon 3160

Phenelzine Sulfate (Concurrent and/or sequential use is not recommended). Products include:
- Nardil Tablets 2653

Prazepam (May increase drowsiness effect).
No products indexed under this heading.

Procarbazine Hydrochloride (Concurrent and/or sequential use is not recommended). Products include:
- Matulane Capsules 3246

Prochlorperazine (May increase drowsiness effect). Products include:
- Compazine 1505

Promethazine Hydrochloride (May increase drowsiness effect). Products include:
- Mepergan Injection 3539
- Phenergan Injection 3553
- Phenergan 3556
- Phenergan Syrup 3554
- Phenergan with Codeine Syrup 3557
- Phenergan with Dextromethorphan Syrup 3559
- Phenergan VC Syrup 3560
- Phenergan VC with Codeine Syrup 3561

Propofol (May increase drowsiness effect). Products include:
- Diprivan Injectable Emulsion 667

Quazepam (May increase drowsiness effect).
No products indexed under this heading.

Secobarbital Sodium (May increase drowsiness effect).
No products indexed under this heading.

Selegiline Hydrochloride (Concurrent and/or sequential use is not recommended). Products include:
- Eldepryl Capsules 3266

Temazepam (May increase drowsiness effect).
No products indexed under this heading.

Thioridazine Hydrochloride (May increase drowsiness effect). Products include:
- Thioridazine Hydrochloride Tablets 2289

Thiothixene (May increase drowsiness effect). Products include:
- Navane Capsules 2701
- Thiothixene Capsules 2290

Tranylcypromine Sulfate (Concurrent and/or sequential use is not recommended). Products include:
- Parnate Tablets 1607

Triazolam (May increase drowsiness effect). Products include:
- Halcion Tablets 2823

Trifluoperazine Hydrochloride (May increase drowsiness effect). Products include:
- Stelazine 1640

Zaleplon (May increase drowsiness effect). Products include:
- Sonata Capsules 3591

Zolpidem Tartrate (May increase drowsiness effect). Products include:
- Ambien Tablets 3191

Food Interactions

Alcohol (May increase drowsiness effect).

SUDAFED COLD & COUGH LIQUID CAPS

(Acetaminophen, Dextromethorphan Hydrobromide, Guaifenesin, Pseudoephedrine Hydrochloride) .... ■ 709
May interact with monoamine oxidase inhibitors. Compounds in these categories include:

Isocarboxazid (Concurrent and/or sequential use is not recommended).
No products indexed under this heading.

Moclobemide (Concurrent and/or sequential use is not recommended).
No products indexed under this heading.

Pargyline Hydrochloride (Concurrent and/or sequential use is not recommended).
No products indexed under this heading.

Phenelzine Sulfate (Concurrent and/or sequential use is not recommended). Products include:
- Nardil Tablets 2653

Procarbazine Hydrochloride (Concurrent and/or sequential use is not recommended). Products include:
- Matulane Capsules 3246

Selegiline Hydrochloride (Concurrent and/or sequential use is not recommended). Products include:
- Eldepryl Capsules 3266

Tranylcypromine Sulfate (Concurrent and/or sequential use is not recommended). Products include:
- Parnate Tablets 1607

Food Interactions

Alcohol (Patients consuming 3 or more alcohol-containing drinks per day should consult physician for advice on when and how they should take this product).

SUDAFED COLD & SINUS LIQUID CAPS

(Acetaminophen, Pseudoephedrine Hydrochloride) .... ■ 710
May interact with monoamine oxidase inhibitors and certain other agents. Compounds in these categories include:

Isocarboxazid (Concurrent and/or sequential use with MAO inhibitors is not recommended).
No products indexed under this heading.

Moclobemide (Concurrent and/or sequential use with MAO inhibitors is not recommended).
No products indexed under this heading.

Pargyline Hydrochloride (Concurrent and/or sequential use with MAO inhibitors is not recommended).
No products indexed under this heading.

Phenelzine Sulfate (Concurrent and/or sequential use with MAO inhibitors is not recommended). Products include:
- Nardil Tablets 2653

Procarbazine Hydrochloride (Concurrent and/or sequential use with MAO inhibitors is not recommended). Products include:
- Matulane Capsules 3246

Selegiline Hydrochloride (Concurrent and/or sequential use with MAO inhibitors is not recommended). Products include:
- Eldepryl Capsules 3266

Tranylcypromine Sulfate (Concurrent and/or sequential use with MAO inhibitors is not recommended). Products include:
- Parnate Tablets 1607

Food Interactions

Alcohol (Patients consuming 3 or more alcohol-containing drinks per day should consult physician for advice on when and how they should take this product).

SUDAFED NASAL DECONGESTANT TABLETS

(Pseudoephedrine Hydrochloride) .... ■ 710
May interact with monoamine oxidase inhibitors. Compounds in these categories include:

Isocarboxazid (Concurrent and/or sequential use is not recommended).
No products indexed under this heading.

Moclobemide (Concurrent and/or sequential use is not recommended).
No products indexed under this heading.

Pargyline Hydrochloride (Concurrent and/or sequential use is not recommended).
No products indexed under this heading.

Phenelzine Sulfate (Concurrent and/or sequential use is not recommended). Products include:
- Nardil Tablets 2653

Procarbazine Hydrochloride (Concurrent and/or sequential use is not recommended). Products include:
- Matulane Capsules 3246

Selegiline Hydrochloride (Concurrent and/or sequential use is not recommended). Products include:
- Eldepryl Capsules 3266

Tranylcypromine Sulfate (Concurrent and/or sequential use is not recommended). Products include:
- Parnate Tablets 1607

SUDAFED NON-DRYING SINUS LIQUID CAPS

(Guaifenesin, Pseudoephedrine Hydrochloride) .... ■ 712
May interact with monoamine oxidase inhibitors. Compounds in these categories include:

Isocarboxazid (Concurrent and/or sequential use is not recommended).
No products indexed under this heading.

Moclobemide (Concurrent and/or sequential use is not recommended).
No products indexed under this heading.

Pargyline Hydrochloride (Concurrent and/or sequential use is not recommended).
No products indexed under this heading.

Phenelzine Sulfate (Concurrent and/or sequential use is not recommended). Products include:
- Nardil Tablets 2653

Procarbazine Hydrochloride (Concurrent and/or sequential use is not recommended). Products include:
- Matulane Capsules 3246

Selegiline Hydrochloride (Concurrent and/or sequential use is not recommended). Products include:
- Eldepryl Capsules 3266

Tranylcypromine Sulfate (Concurrent and/or sequential use is not recommended). Products include:
- Parnate Tablets 1607

- Eldepryl Capsules 3266

Tranylcypromine Sulfate (Concurrent and/or sequential use with MAO inhibitors is not recommended). Products include:
- Parnate Tablets 1607

Food Interactions

Alcohol (Patients consuming 3 or more alcohol-containing drinks per day should consult physician for advice on when and how they should take this product).

SUDAFED SEVERE COLD FORMULA CAPLETS

(Acetaminophen, Dextromethorphan Hydrobromide, Pseudoephedrine Hydrochloride) .... ■ 711
May interact with monoamine oxidase inhibitors. Compounds in these categories include:

Isocarboxazid (Concurrent and/or sequential use is not recommended).
No products indexed under this heading.

Moclobemide (Concurrent and/or sequential use is not recommended).
No products indexed under this heading.

Pargyline Hydrochloride (Concurrent and/or sequential use is not recommended).
No products indexed under this heading.

Phenelzine Sulfate (Concurrent and/or sequential use is not recommended). Products include:
- Nardil Tablets 2653

Procarbazine Hydrochloride (Concurrent and/or sequential use is not recommended). Products include:
- Matulane Capsules 3246

Selegiline Hydrochloride (Concurrent and/or sequential use is not recommended). Products include:
- Eldepryl Capsules 3266

Tranylcypromine Sulfate (Concurrent and/or sequential use is not recommended). Products include:
- Parnate Tablets 1607

SUDAFED SEVERE COLD FORMULA TABLETS

(Acetaminophen, Dextromethorphan Hydrobromide, Pseudoephedrine Hydrochloride) .... ■ 711
See Sudafed Severe Cold Formula Caplets

SUDAFED SINUS HEADACHE CAPLETS

(Acetaminophen, Pseudoephedrine Hydrochloride) .... ■ 712
May interact with monoamine oxidase inhibitors. Compounds in these categories include:

Isocarboxazid (Concurrent and/or sequential use is not recommended).
No products indexed under this heading.

Moclobemide (Concurrent and/or sequential use is not recommended).
No products indexed under this heading.

Pargyline Hydrochloride (Concurrent and/or sequential use is not recommended).
No products indexed under this heading.

Phenelzine Sulfate (Concurrent and/or sequential use is not recommended). Products include:
- Nardil Tablets 2653

Procarbazine Hydrochloride (Concurrent and/or sequential use is not recommended). Products include:
- Matulane Capsules 3246

Selegiline Hydrochloride (Concurrent and/or sequential use is not recommended). Products include:
- Eldepryl Capsules 3266

Tranylcypromine Sulfate (Concurrent and/or sequential use is not recommended). Products include:
- Parnate Tablets 1607

Food Interactions

Alcohol (Patients consuming 3 or more alcohol-containing drinks per day should consult physician for advice on when and how they should take this product).

SUDAFED SINUS HEADACHE TABLETS
(Acetaminophen, Pseudoephedrine Hydrochloride)..... ■712
May interact with monoamine oxidase inhibitors. Compounds in these categories include:

Isocarboxazid (Concurrent and/or sequential use is not recommended).
No products indexed under this heading.

Moclobemide (Concurrent and/or sequential use is not recommended).
No products indexed under this heading.

Pargyline Hydrochloride (Concurrent and/or sequential use is not recommended).
No products indexed under this heading.

Phenelzine Sulfate (Concurrent and/or sequential use is not recommended). Products include:
Nardil Tablets 2653

Procarbazine Hydrochloride (Concurrent and/or sequential use is not recommended). Products include:
Matulane Capsules 3246

Selegiline Hydrochloride (Concurrent and/or sequential use is not recommended). Products include:
Eldepryl Capsules 3266

Tranylcypromine Sulfate (Concurrent and/or sequential use is not recommended). Products include:
Parnate Tablets 1607

SUI-SHEN-AN LIQUID
(Herbals, Multiple) 1725
None cited in PDR database.

SULAR TABLETS
(Nisoldipine) 688
May interact with dexamethasone, phenytoin, quinidine, and certain other agents. Compounds in these categories include:

Atenolol (Greater blood pressure effect of Sular with concomitant use). Products include:
Tenoretic Tablets 690
Tenormin I.V. Injection 692

Carbamazepine (Co-administration of nisoldipine with known CYP3A4 inducer, such as carbamazepine, should be avoided because of possible reduced nisoldipine plasma concentrations). Products include:
Carbatrol Capsules 3234
Tegretol/Tegretol-XR 2404

Cimetidine (Concomitant use increases nisoldipine AUC and Cmax by 30% to 45%). Products include:
Tagamet HB 200 Suspension .... ■762
Tagamet HB 200 Tablets .... ■761
Tagamet Tablets 1644

Cimetidine Hydrochloride (Concomitant use increases nisoldipine AUC and Cmax by 30% to 45%). Products include:
Tagamet 1644

Dexamethasone (Co-administration of nisoldipine with known CYP3A4 inducer, such as dexamethasone, should be avoided because of possible reduced nisoldipine plasma concentrations). Products include:
Decadron Elixir 2078
Decadron Tablets 2079
TobraDex Ophthalmic Ointment 542
TobraDex Ophthalmic Suspension .. 541

Dexamethasone Acetate (Co-administration of nisoldipine with known CYP3A4 inducer, such as dexamethasone, should be avoided because of possible reduced nisoldipine plasma concentrations).
No products indexed under this heading.

Dexamethasone Sodium Phosphate (Co-administration of nisoldipine with known CYP3A4 inducer, such as dexamethasone, should be avoided because of possible reduced nisoldipine plasma concentrations). Products include:
Decadron Phosphate Injection 2081
Decadron Phosphate Sterile Ophthalmic Ointment................. 2083
Decadron Phosphate Sterile Ophthalmic Solution.................. 2084
NeoDecadron Sterile Ophthalmic Solution...................................... 2144

Fosphenytoin Sodium (Co-administration in epileptic patients has resulted in reduced nisoldipine plasma concentrations to undetectable levels). Products include:
Cerebyx Injection 2619

Phenobarbital (Co-administration of nisoldipine with known CYP3A4 inducer, such as phenobarbital, should be avoided because of possible reduced nisoldipine plasma concentrations). Products include:
Arco-Lase Plus Tablets 592
Donnatal 2929
Donnatal Extentabs 2930

Phenytoin (Co-administration in epileptic patients has resulted in reduced nisoldipine plasma concentrations to undetectable levels). Products include:
Dilantin Infatabs 2624
Dilantin-125 Oral Suspension 2625

Phenytoin Sodium (Co-administration in epileptic patients has resulted in reduced nisoldipine plasma concentrations to undetectable levels). Products include:
Dilantin Kapseals 2622

Propranolol Hydrochloride (Propanolol attenuates the heart rate increase following the administration of immediate-release nisoldipine). Products include:
Inderal 3513
Inderal LA Long-Acting Capsules 3516
Inderide Tablets 3517
Inderide LA Long-Acting Capsules .. 3519

Quinidine Gluconate (May decrease the bioavailability (AUC) of nisoldipine by 26%, but not the peak concentration; clinical significance is not known). Products include:
Quinaglute Dura-Tabs Tablets 978

Quinidine Polygalacturonate (May decrease the bioavailability (AUC) of nisoldipine by 26%, but not the peak concentration; clinical significance is not known).
No products indexed under this heading.

Quinidine Sulfate (May decrease the bioavailability (AUC) of nisoldipine by 26%, but not the peak concentration; clinical significance is not known). Products include:
Quinidex Extentabs 2933

Ranitidine Hydrochloride (Concomitant use decreases AUC by 15% to 20%). Products include:
Zantac 1690
Zantac Injection 1688
Zantac 75 Tablets .... ■717

Rifampin (Co-administration of nisoldipine with known CYP3A4 inducer, such as rifampin, should be avoided because of possible reduced nisoldipine plasma concentrations). Products include:
Rifadin 765
Rifamate Capsules 767
Rifater Tablets 769

Food Interactions

Diet, high-lipid (Food with a high fat content has a pronounced effect on the release of nisoldipine resulting in a significant increase in peak concentration (Cmax) by up to 300%; concomitant intake of high-fat meal should be avoided).

SULFAMYLON CREAM
(Mafenide Acetate).............................1011
None cited in PDR database.

SULFAMYLON TOPICAL SOLUTION
(Mafenide Acetate) 1011
None cited in PDR database.

SULTRIN TRIPLE SULFA CREAM
(Sulfabenzamide, Sulfacetamide, Sulfathiazole)................................... 2587
None cited in PDR database.

SUPER ANTI-OXIDANT CELL PROTECTOR CAPSULES
(Herbals, Multiple) .... ■854
None cited in PDR database.

SUPER FOOD SOY SHAKE
(Amino Acid Preparations, Herbals with Vitamins & Minerals, Lactobacillus Acidophilus)...................................... ■854
None cited in PDR database.

SUPEREPA 2000 SOFTGELS
(Docosahexaenoic Acid (DHA), EPA (Eicosapentaenoic Acid)) 526
None cited in PDR database.

SUPRANE LIQUID FOR INHALATION
(Desflurane) 874
May interact with:

Atracurium Besylate (Anesthetic concentrations of desflurane reduce the ED_{95} of atracurium by approximately 50%).
No products indexed under this heading.

Fentanyl (Decreases the minimum alveolar concentration (MAC) of desflurane by 50%). Products include:
Duragesic Transdermal System 1786

Fentanyl Citrate (Decreases the minimum alveolar concentration (MAC) of desflurane by 50%). Products include:
Actiq 1184

Midazolam Hydrochloride (Decreases the minimum alveolar concentration (MAC) of desflurane by 16%). Products include:
Versed Injection 3027
Versed Syrup 3033

Pancuronium Bromide (Anesthetic concentrations of desflurane reduce the ED_{95} of pancuronium by approximately 50%).
No products indexed under this heading.

Succinylcholine Chloride (Anesthetic concentrations of desflurane reduce the ED_{95} of succinylcholine by approximately 30%). Products include:
Anectine Injection 1476

SUPRAX FOR ORAL SUSPENSION
(Cefixime) 1877
See Suprax Tablets

SUPRAX TABLETS
(Cefixime) 1877
May interact with oral anticoagulants and certain other agents. Compounds in these categories include:

Carbamazepine (Co-administration has resulted in elevated carbamazepine levels). Products include:
Carbatrol Capsules 3234
Tegretol/Tegretol-XR 2404

Dicumarol (Co-administration has resulted in increased prothrombin time, with or without clinical bleeding).
No products indexed under this heading.

Warfarin Sodium (Co-administration has resulted in increased prothrombin time, with or without clinical bleeding). Products include:
Coumadin for Injection 1243
Coumadin Tablets 1243
Warfarin Sodium Tablets, USP 3302

Food Interactions

Food, unspecified (Increases time to maximal absorption approximately 0.8 hour).

SURE2ENDURE TABLETS
(Glucosamine Hydrochloride, Herbals with Vitamins & Minerals).. ■851
None cited in PDR database.

SURFAK LIQUI-GELS
(Docusate Calcium) .... ■721
May interact with:

Mineral Oil (Concurrent use with oral mineral oil is not recommended unless directed by a doctor). Products include:
Anusol Ointment .... ■688
Fleet Mineral Oil Enema 1360
Lubriderm Advanced Therapy Creamy Lotion .... ■703
Lubriderm Seriously Sensitive Lotion .... ■703
Lubriderm Skin Therapy Moisturizing Lotion .... ■703
Moisture Eyes PM Preservative Free Eye Ointment .... ⊙253
Preparation H Ointment .... ■778
Refresh P.M. Lubricant Eye Ointment .... ⊙251

SURMONTIL CAPSULES
(Trimipramine Maleate) 3595
May interact with anticholinergics, drugs that inhibit cytochrome p450iid6, antidepressant drugs, monoamine oxidase inhibitors, phenothiazines, selective serotonin reuptake inhibitors, sympathomimetics, thyroid preparations, and certain other agents. Compounds in these categories include:

Albuterol (Potentiated effects of catecholamines; careful adjustment of dosage and close supervision are required). Products include:
Proventil Inhalation Aerosol 3142
Ventolin Inhalation Aerosol and Refill 1679

Albuterol Sulfate (Potentiated effects of catecholamines; careful adjustment of dosage and close supervision are required). Products include:
AccuNeb Inhalation Solution 1230
Combivent Inhalation Aerosol 1041
DuoNeb Inhalation Solution 1233
Proventil Inhalation Solution 0.083% 3146
Proventil Repetabs Tablets 3148
Proventil Solution for Inhalation 0.5% 3144
Proventil HFA Inhalation Aerosol 3150
Ventolin HFA Inhalation Aerosol 3618
Volmax Extended-Release Tablets .. 2276

Amitriptyline Hydrochloride (Concurrent use with drugs that are substrate for cytochrome P450IID6 may make normal metabolizer resemble poor metabolizer leading to higher than expected plasma concentrations of TCA with resultant toxicity). Products include:
Etrafon 3115
Limbitrol 1738

Amoxapine (Concurrent use with drugs that are substrate for cytochrome P450IID6 may make normal metabolizer resemble poor metabolizer leading to higher than expected plasma concentrations of TCA with resultant toxicity).
No products indexed under this heading.

Atropine Sulfate (Concurrent use may result in pronounced atropine-like effects). Products include:
Donnatal 2929
Donnatal Extentabs 2930

Motofen Tablets ... 577
Prosed/DS Tablets ... 3268
Urised Tablets ... 2876

Belladonna Alkaloids (Concurrent use may result in pronounced atropinelike effects). Products include:
Hyland's Teething Tablets ... 766
Urimax Tablets ... 1769

Benztropine Mesylate (Concurrent use may result in pronounced atropinelike effects). Products include:
Cogentin ... 2055

Biperiden Hydrochloride (Concurrent use may result in pronounced atropinelike effects). Products include:
Akineton ... 402

Bupropion Hydrochloride (Concurrent use with drugs that are substrate for cytochrome P450IID6 may make normal metabolizer resemble poor metabolizer leading to higher than expected plasma concentrations of TCA with resultant toxicity). Products include:
Wellbutrin Tablets ... 1680
Wellbutrin SR Sustained-Release Tablets ... 1684
Zyban Sustained-Release Tablets ... 1710

Chlorpromazine (Concurrent use with drugs that are substrate for cytochrome P450IID6 may make normal metabolizer resemble poor metabolizer leading to higher than expected plasma concentrations of TCA with resultant toxicity). Products include:
Thorazine Suppositories ... 1656

Chlorpromazine Hydrochloride (Concurrent use with drugs that are substrate for cytochrome P450IID6 may make normal metabolizer resemble poor metabolizer leading to higher than expected plasma concentrations of TCA with resultant toxicity). Products include:
Thorazine ... 1656

Cimetidine (Inhibits the elimination of tricyclic antidepressants; downward adjustment of Surmontil dosage may be required if cimetidine therapy is initiated; upward adjustment if cimetidine therapy is discontinued). Products include:
Tagamet HB 200 Suspension ... 762
Tagamet HB 200 Tablets ... 761
Tagamet Tablets ... 1644

Cimetidine Hydrochloride (Inhibits the elimination of tricyclic antidepressants; downward adjustment of Surmontil dosage may be required if cimetidine therapy is initiated; upward adjustment if cimetidine therapy is discontinued). Products include:
Tagamet ... 1644

Citalopram Hydrobromide (Concurrent use with drugs that are substrate for cytochrome P450IID6 may make normal metabolizer resemble poor metabolizer leading to higher than expected plasma concentrations of TCA with resultant toxicity; due to variation in the extent of inhibition of P450IID6 caution is indicated; if co-administered sufficient time must elapse). Products include:
Celexa ... 1365

Clidinium Bromide (Concurrent use may result in pronounced atropinelike effects).
No products indexed under this heading.

Desipramine Hydrochloride (Concurrent use with drugs that are substrate for cytochrome P450IID6 may make normal metabolizer resemble poor metabolizer leading to higher than expected plasma concentrations of TCA with resultant toxicity). Products include:
Norpramin Tablets ... 755

Dicyclomine Hydrochloride (Concurrent use may result in pronounced atropinelike effects).
No products indexed under this heading.

Dobutamine Hydrochloride (Potentiated effects of catecholamines; careful adjustment of dosage and close supervision are required). Products include:
Dobutrex Solution Vials ... 1914

Dopamine Hydrochloride (Potentiated effects of catecholamines; careful adjustment of dosage and close supervision are required).
No products indexed under this heading.

Doxepin Hydrochloride (Concurrent use with drugs that are substrate for cytochrome P450IID6 may make normal metabolizer resemble poor metabolizer leading to higher than expected plasma concentrations of TCA with resultant toxicity). Products include:
Sinequan ... 2713

Ephedrine Hydrochloride (Potentiated effects of catecholamines; careful adjustment of dosage and close supervision are required). Products include:
Primatene Tablets ... 780

Ephedrine Sulfate (Potentiated effects of catecholamines; careful adjustment of dosage and close supervision are required).
No products indexed under this heading.

Ephedrine Tannate (Potentiated effects of catecholamines; careful adjustment of dosage and close supervision are required). Products include:
Rynatuss Pediatric Suspension ... 3353
Rynatuss Tablets ... 3353

Epinephrine (Potentiated effects of catecholamines; careful adjustment of dosage and close supervision are required). Products include:
Epifrin Sterile Ophthalmic Solution ... ⊙235
EpiPen ... 1236
Primatene Mist ... 779
Xylocaine with Epinephrine Injection ... 653

Epinephrine Bitartrate (Potentiated effects of catecholamines; careful adjustment of dosage and close supervision are required). Products include:
Sensorcaine ... 643

Epinephrine Hydrochloride (Potentiated effects of catecholamines; careful adjustment of dosage and close supervision are required).
No products indexed under this heading.

Flecainide Acetate (Concurrent use with drugs that are substrate for cytochrome P450IID6 may make normal metabolizer resemble poor metabolizer leading to higher than expected plasma concentrations of TCA with resultant toxicity). Products include:
Tambocor Tablets ... 1990

Fluoxetine Hydrochloride (Concurrent use with drugs that are substrate for cytochrome P450IID6 may make normal metabolizer resemble poor metabolizer leading to higher than expected plasma concentrations of TCA with resultant toxicity; due to variation in the extent of inhibition of P450IID6 and long half-life of the parent (fluoxetine) and active metabolite sufficient time must elapse, at least 5 weeks before switching to TCA). Products include:
Prozac Pulvules, Liquid, and Weekly Capsules ... 1238
Sarafem Pulvules ... 1962

Fluphenazine Decanoate (Concurrent use with drugs that are substrate for cytochrome P450IID6 may make normal metabolizer resemble poor metabolizer leading to higher than expected plasma concentrations of TCA with resultant toxicity).
No products indexed under this heading.

Fluphenazine Enanthate (Concurrent use with drugs that are substrate for cytochrome P450IID6 may make normal metabolizer resemble poor metabolizer leading to higher than expected plasma concentrations of TCA with resultant toxicity).
No products indexed under this heading.

Fluphenazine Hydrochloride (Concurrent use with drugs that are substrate for cytochrome P450IID6 may make normal metabolizer resemble poor metabolizer leading to higher than expected plasma concentrations of TCA with resultant toxicity).
No products indexed under this heading.

Fluvoxamine Maleate (Concurrent use with drugs that are substrate for cytochrome P450IID6 may make normal metabolizer resemble poor metabolizer leading to higher than expected plasma concentrations of TCA with resultant toxicity; due to variation in the extent of inhibition of P450IID6 caution is indicated; if co-administered sufficient time must elapse). Products include:
Luvox Tablets (25, 50, 100 mg) ... 3256

Glycopyrrolate (Concurrent use may result in pronounced atropinelike effects). Products include:
Robinul Forte Tablets ... 1358
Robinul Injectable ... 2940
Robinul Tablets ... 1358

Guanadrel Sulfate (Trimipramine may block the antihypertensive effect).
No products indexed under this heading.

Guanethidine Monosulfate (Trimipramine may block the antihypertensive effect of guanethidine or similarly acting compounds).
No products indexed under this heading.

Hyoscyamine (Concurrent use may result in pronounced atropinelike effects). Products include:
Urised Tablets ... 2876

Hyoscyamine Sulfate (Concurrent use may result in pronounced atropinelike effects). Products include:
Arco-Lase Plus Tablets ... 592
Donnatal ... 2929
Donnatal Extentabs ... 2930
Levsin/Levsinex/Levbid ... 3172
NuLev Orally Disintegrating Tablets ... 3176
Prosed/DS Tablets ... 3268
Urimax Tablets ... 1769

Imipramine Hydrochloride (Concurrent use with drugs that are substrate for cytochrome P450IID6 may make normal metabolizer resemble poor metabolizer leading to higher than expected plasma concentrations of TCA with resultant toxicity).
No products indexed under this heading.

Imipramine Pamoate (Concurrent use with drugs that are substrate for cytochrome P450IID6 may make normal metabolizer resemble poor metabolizer leading to higher than expected plasma concentrations of TCA with resultant toxicity).
No products indexed under this heading.

Ipratropium Bromide (Concurrent use may result in pronounced atropinelike effects). Products include:
Atrovent Inhalation Aerosol ... 1030
Atrovent Inhalation Solution ... 1031
Atrovent Nasal Spray 0.03% ... 1032
Atrovent Nasal Spray 0.06% ... 1033
Combivent Inhalation Aerosol ... 1041
DuoNeb Inhalation Solution ... 1233

Isocarboxazid (Potential for hyperpyretic crises, severe convulsions, and death; concurrent and/or sequential use is contraindicated).
No products indexed under this heading.

Isoproterenol Hydrochloride (Potentiated effects of catecholamines; careful adjustment of dosage and close supervision are required).
No products indexed under this heading.

Isoproterenol Sulfate (Potentiated effects of catecholamines; careful adjustment of dosage and close supervision are required).
No products indexed under this heading.

Levalbuterol Hydrochloride (Potentiated effects of catecholamines; careful adjustment of dosage and close supervision are required). Products include:
Xopenex Inhalation Solution ... 3207

Levothyroxine Sodium (Potential for cardiovascular toxicity). Products include:
Levothroid Tablets ... 1373
Levoxyl Tablets ... 1819
Synthroid ... 505
Unithroid Tablets ... 3445

Liothyronine Sodium (Potential for cardiovascular toxicity). Products include:
Cytomel Tablets ... 1817
Triostat Injection ... 1825

Liotrix (Potential for cardiovascular toxicity).
No products indexed under this heading.

Maprotiline Hydrochloride (Concurrent use with drugs that are substrate for cytochrome P450IID6 may make normal metabolizer resemble poor metabolizer leading to higher than expected plasma concentrations of TCA with resultant toxicity).
No products indexed under this heading.

Mepenzolate Bromide (Concurrent use may result in pronounced atropinelike effects).
No products indexed under this heading.

Mesoridazine Besylate (Concurrent use with drugs that are substrate for cytochrome P450IID6 may make normal metabolizer resemble poor metabolizer leading to higher than expected plasma concentrations of TCA with resultant toxicity). Products include:
Serentil ... 1057

Metaproterenol Sulfate (Potentiated effects of catecholamines; careful adjustment of dosage and close supervision are required). Products include:
Alupent ... 1029

Metaraminol Bitartrate (Potentiated effects of catecholamines; careful adjustment of dosage and close supervision are required). Products include:
Aramine Injection ... 2043

Methotrimeprazine (Concurrent use with drugs that are substrate for cytochrome P450IID6 may make normal metabolizer resemble poor metabolizer leading to higher than expected plasma concentrations of TCA with resultant toxicity).
No products indexed under this heading.

Methoxamine Hydrochloride (Potentiated effects of catecholamines; careful adjustment of dosage and close supervision are required).
No products indexed under this heading.

Mirtazapine (Concurrent use with drugs that are substrate for cytochrome P450IID6 may make normal metabolizer resemble poor metabo-

lizer leading to higher than expected plasma concentrations of TCA with resultant toxicity). Products include:
- Remeron Tablets 2483
- Remeron SolTab Tablets 2486

Moclobemide (Potential for hyperpyretic crises, severe convulsions, and death; concurrent and/or sequential use is contraindicated).
No products indexed under this heading.

Nefazodone Hydrochloride (Concurrent use with drugs that are substrate for cytochrome P450IID6 may make normal metabolizer resemble poor metabolizer leading to higher than expected plasma concentrations of TCA with resultant toxicity). Products include:
- Serzone Tablets 1104

Norepinephrine Bitartrate (Potentiated effects of catecholamines; careful adjustment of dosage and close supervision are required).
No products indexed under this heading.

Nortriptyline Hydrochloride (Concurrent use with drugs that are substrate for cytochrome P450IID6 may make normal metabolizer resemble poor metabolizer leading to higher than expected plasma concentrations of TCA with resultant toxicity).
No products indexed under this heading.

Oxybutynin Chloride (Concurrent use may result in pronounced atropinelike effects). Products include:
- Ditropan XL Extended Release Tablets 564

Pargyline Hydrochloride (Potential for hyperpyretic crises, severe convulsions, and death; concurrent and/or sequential use is contraindicated).
No products indexed under this heading.

Paroxetine Hydrochloride (Concurrent use with drugs that are substrate for cytochrome P450IID6 may make normal metabolizer resemble poor metabolizer leading to higher than expected plasma concentrations of TCA with resultant toxicity; due to variation in the extent of inhibition of P450IID6 caution is indicated; if co-administered sufficient time must elapse). Products include:
- Paxil 1609

Perphenazine (Concurrent use with drugs that are substrate for cytochrome P450IID6 may make normal metabolizer resemble poor metabolizer leading to higher than expected plasma concentrations of TCA with resultant toxicity). Products include:
- Etrafon 3115
- Trilafon 3160

Phenelzine Sulfate (Potential for hyperpyretic crises, severe convulsions, and death; concurrent and/or sequential use is contraindicated). Products include:
- Nardil Tablets 2653

Phenylephrine Bitartrate (Potentiated effects of catecholamines; careful adjustment of dosage and close supervision are required).
No products indexed under this heading.

Phenylephrine Hydrochloride (Potentiated effects of catecholamines; careful adjustment of dosage and close supervision are required). Products include:
- Afrin Nasal Decongestant Children's Pump Mist ..... ▣734
- Extendryl 1361
- Hycomine Compound Tablets 1317
- Neo-Synephrine ..... ▣614
- Phenergan VC Syrup 3560
- Phenergan VC with Codeine Syrup 3561
- Preparation H Cream ..... ▣778
- Preparation H Cooling Gel ..... ▣778
- Preparation H ..... ▣778
- Vicks Sinex Nasal Spray and Ultra Fine Mist ..... ▣729

Phenylephrine Tannate (Potentiated effects of catecholamines; careful adjustment of dosage and close supervision are required). Products include:
- Ryna-12 S Suspension 3351
- Reformulated Rynatan Pediatric Suspension 3352
- Rynatuss Pediatric Suspension 3353
- Rynatuss Tablets 3353

Phenylpropanolamine Hydrochloride (Potentiated effects of catecholamines; careful adjustment of dosage and close supervision are required).
No products indexed under this heading.

Pirbuterol Acetate (Potentiated effects of catecholamines; careful adjustment of dosage and close supervision are required). Products include:
- Maxair Autohaler 1981
- Maxair Inhaler 1984

Procarbazine Hydrochloride (Potential for hyperpyretic crises, severe convulsions, and death; concurrent and/or sequential use is contraindicated). Products include:
- Matulane Capsules 3246

Prochlorperazine (Concurrent use with drugs that are substrate for cytochrome P450IID6 may make normal metabolizer resemble poor metabolizer leading to higher than expected plasma concentrations of TCA with resultant toxicity). Products include:
- Compazine 1505

Procyclidine Hydrochloride (Concurrent use may result in pronounced atropinelike effects).
No products indexed under this heading.

Promethazine Hydrochloride (Concurrent use with drugs that are substrate for cytochrome P450IID6 may make normal metabolizer resemble poor metabolizer leading to higher than expected plasma concentrations of TCA with resultant toxicity). Products include:
- Mepergan Injection 3539
- Phenergan Injection 3553
- Phenergan 3556
- Phenergan Syrup 3554
- Phenergan with Codeine Syrup 3557
- Phenergan with Dextromethorphan Syrup 3559
- Phenergan VC Syrup 3560
- Phenergan VC with Codeine Syrup 3561

Propafenone Hydrochloride (Concurrent use with drugs that are substrate for cytochrome P450IID6 may make normal metabolizer resemble poor metabolizer leading to higher than expected plasma concentrations of TCA with resultant toxicity). Products include:
- Rythmol Tablets – 150 mg, 225 mg, 300 mg 502

Propantheline Bromide (Concurrent use may result in pronounced atropinelike effects).
No products indexed under this heading.

Protriptyline Hydrochloride (Concurrent use with drugs that are substrate for cytochrome P450IID6 may make normal metabolizer resemble poor metabolizer leading to higher than expected plasma concentrations of TCA with resultant toxicity). Products include:
- Vivactil Tablets 2446
- Vivactil Tablets 2217

Pseudoephedrine Hydrochloride (Potentiated effects of catecholamines; careful adjustment of dosage and close supervision are required). Products include:
- Actifed Cold & Allergy Tablets ..... ▣688
- Actifed Cold & Sinus Caplets and Tablets ..... ▣688
- Advil Cold and Sinus Caplets ..... ▣771
- Advil Cold and Sinus Tablets ..... ▣771
- Advil Flu & Body Ache Caplets ..... ▣772
- Aleve Cold & Sinus Caplets ..... ▣603
- Alka-Seltzer Plus Liqui-Gels ..... ▣604
- Alka-Seltzer Plus Cold & Flu Medicine Liqui-Gels ..... ▣604
- Alka-Seltzer Plus Cold & Sinus Medicine Liqui-Gels ..... ▣604
- Allegra-D Extended-Release Tablets 714
- BC Cold Powder ..... ▣619
- Benadryl Allergy/Cold Tablets ..... ▣691
- Benadryl Allergy/Congestion Tablets ..... ▣692
- Benadryl Allergy & Sinus Liquid ..... ▣693
- Benadryl Allergy & Sinus Fastmelt Tablets ..... ▣693
- Benadryl Allergy Sinus Headache Caplets & Gelcaps ..... ▣693
- Benadryl Severe Allergy & Sinus Headache Caplets ..... ▣694
- Benadryl Children's Allergy/Cold Fastmelt Tablets ..... ▣692
- Benylin Multi-Symptom Liquid ..... ▣697
- Bromfed Capsules (Extended-Release) 2269
- Bromfed-PD Capsules (Extended-Release) 2269
- Children's Cēpacol Sore Throat ..... ▣788
- Comtrex Acute Head Cold & Sinus Pressure Relief Tablets ..... ▣627
- Comtrex Deep Chest Cold & Congestion Relief Softgels ..... ▣627
- Comtrex Flu Therapy & Fever Relief Daytime Caplets ..... ▣628
- Comtrex Flu Therapy & Fever Relief Nighttime Tablets ..... ▣628
- Comtrex Maximum Strength Multi-Symptom Cold & Cough Relief Tablets and Caplets ..... ▣626
- Contac Non-Drowsy 12 Hour Cold Caplets ..... ▣745
- Contac Non-Drowsy Timed Release 12 Hour Cold Caplets ..... ▣746
- Contac Severe Cold and Flu Caplets Maximum Strength ..... ▣746
- Contac Severe Cold and Flu Caplets Non-Drowsy ..... ▣746
- Dimetapp Elixir ..... ▣777
- Dimetapp Cold and Fever Suspension ..... ▣775
- Dimetapp DM Cold & Cough Elixir ..... ▣775
- Dimetapp Nighttime Flu Liquid ..... ▣776
- Dimetapp Non-Drowsy Flu Syrup ..... ▣777
- Dimetapp Infant Drops Decongestant ..... ▣775
- Dimetapp Infant Drops Decongestant Plus Cough ..... ▣776
- Guaifed 2272
- Kronofed-A 1341
- Children's Motrin Cold Oral Suspension 2007
- Motrin Sinus Headache Caplets 2005
- PediaCare Cough-Cold Liquid ..... ▣719
- PediaCare Infants' Drops Decongestant ..... ▣719
- PediaCare Infants' Drops Decongestant Plus Cough ..... ▣719
- PediaCare NightRest Cough-Cold Liquid ..... ▣719
- Robitussin Cold Caplets Cold & Congestion ..... ▣780
- Robitussin Cold Softgels Cold & Congestion ..... ▣780
- Robitussin Cold Caplets Multi-Symptom Cold & Flu ..... ▣781
- Robitussin Cold Softgels Multi-Symptom Cold & Flu ..... ▣781
- Robitussin Cold Softgels Severe Congestion ..... ▣782
- Robitussin Cough & Cold Infant Drops ..... ▣782
- Robitussin Maximum Strength Cough & Cold Liquid ..... ▣785
- Robitussin Pediatric Cough & Cold Formula Liquid ..... ▣785
- Robitussin Multi Symptom Honey Flu Liquid ..... ▣785
- Robitussin Nighttime Honey Flu Liquid ..... ▣786
- Robitussin-CF Liquid ..... ▣783
- Robitussin-DAC Syrup 2942
- Robitussin-PE Liquid ..... ▣782
- Ryna ..... ▣768
- Semprex-D Capsules 1172
- Singlet Caplets ..... ▣761
- Sinutab Non-Drying Liquid Caps ..... ▣706
- Sinutab Sinus Allergy Medication, Maximum Strength Formula, Tablets & Caplets ..... ▣707
- Sinutab Sinus Medication, Maximum Strength Without Drowsiness Formula, Tablets & Caplets ..... ▣707
- Sudafed 12 Hour Tablets ..... ▣708
- Sudafed 24 Hour Tablets ..... ▣708
- Children's Sudafed Cold & Cough Liquid ..... ▣709
- Children's Sudafed Nasal Decongestant Chewables ..... ▣711
- Children's Sudafed Nasal Decongestant Liquid Medication ..... ▣711
- Sudafed Cold & Allergy Tablets ..... ▣708
- Sudafed Cold & Cough Liquid Caps ..... ▣709
- Sudafed Cold & Sinus Liquid Caps ..... ▣710
- Sudafed Nasal Decongestant Tablets ..... ▣710
- Sudafed Non-Drying Sinus Liquid Caps ..... ▣712
- Sudafed Severe Cold ..... ▣711
- Sudafed Sinus Headache Caplets ..... ▣712
- Sudafed Sinus Headache Tablets ..... ▣712
- Tavist Sinus Non-Drowsy Coated Caplets ..... ▣676
- TheraFlu Regular Strength Cold & Cough Night Time Hot Liquid ..... ▣676
- TheraFlu Regular Strength Cold & Sore Throat Night Time Hot Liquid ..... ▣676
- TheraFlu Maximum Strength Flu & Congestion Non-Drowsy Hot Liquid ..... ▣677
- TheraFlu Maximum Strength Flu & Cough Night Time Hot Liquid ..... ▣678
- TheraFlu Maximum Strength Flu & Sore Throat Night Time Hot Liquid ..... ▣677
- TheraFlu Maximum Strength Severe Cold & Congestion Night Time Caplets ..... ▣678
- TheraFlu Maximum Strength Severe Cold & Congestion Night Time Hot Liquid ..... ▣678
- TheraFlu Maximum Strength Severe Cold & Congestion Non-Drowsy ..... ▣679
- Triaminic Allergy Congestion Liquid ..... ▣680
- Triaminic Chest Congestion Liquid ..... ▣680
- Triaminic Cold & Allergy Liquid ..... ▣681
- Triaminic Cold & Allergy Softchews ..... ▣683
- Triaminic Cold & Cough Liquid ..... ▣681
- Triaminic Cold & Cough Softchews ..... ▣683
- Triaminic Cold & Night Time Cough Liquid ..... ▣681
- Triaminic Cold, Cough & Fever Liquid ..... ▣681
- Triaminic Cough Liquid ..... ▣682
- Triaminic Cough & Congestion Liquid ..... ▣682
- Triaminic Cough & Sore Throat Liquid ..... ▣682
- Triaminic Cough & Sore Throat Softchews ..... ▣684
- Children's Tylenol Allergy-D Liquid 2014
- Children's Tylenol Cold Suspension Liquid and Chewable Tablets 2015
- Children's Tylenol Cold Plus Cough Suspension Liquid and Chewable Tablets 2015
- Children's Tylenol Flu Suspension Liquid 2015
- Children's Tylenol Sinus Suspension Liquid 2017
- Infants' Tylenol Cold Decongestant and Fever Reducer Concentrated Drops 2015
- Infants' Tylenol Cold Decongestant and Fever Reducer Concentrated Drops Plus Cough 2015
- Tylenol Allergy Sinus 2010
- Multi-Symptom Tylenol Cold Complete Formula Caplets 2010
- Multi-Symptom Tylenol Cold Non-Drowsy Caplets and Gelcaps 2010
- Multi-Symptom Tylenol Cold Severe Congestion Non-Drowsy Caplets 2011
- Maximum Strength Tylenol Flu NightTime Gelcaps 2011
- Maximum Strength Tylenol Flu NightTime Liquid 2011
- Maximum Strength Tylenol Flu Non-Drowsy Gelcaps 2011
- Maximum Strength Tylenol Sinus NightTime Caplets 2012
- Maximum Strength Tylenol Sinus Non-Drowsy Geltabs, Gelcaps, Caplets, and Tablets 2012
- Vicks 44D Cough & Head Congestion Relief Liquid ..... ▣724
- Vicks 44M Cough, Cold & Flu Relief Liquid ..... ▣725

Pediatric Vicks 44m Cough & Cold Relief 728
Vicks DayQuil LiquiCaps/Liquid Multi-Symptom Cold/Flu Relief ... 727
Children's Vicks NyQuil Cold/Cough Relief 726
Vicks NyQuil LiquiCaps/Liquid Multi-Symptom Cold/Flu Relief, Original and Cherry Flavors 727
Zephrex Tablets 3091
Zephrex LA Tablets 3092
Zyrtec-D 12 Hour Extended Relief Tablets 2758

Pseudoephedrine Sulfate (Potentiated effects of catecholamines; careful adjustment of dosage and close supervision are required). Products include:
Chlor-Trimeton Allergy/Decongestant Tablets 736
Claritin-D 12 Hour Extended Release Tablets 3102
Claritin-D 24 Hour Extended Release Tablets 3104
Coricidin 'D' Cold, Flu & Sinus Tablets 737
Drixoral Allergy/Sinus Extended-Release Tablets 741
Drixoral Cold & Allergy Sustained-Action Tablets 740
Drixoral Cold & Flu Extended-Release Tablets 740
Drixoral Nasal Decongestant Long-Acting Non-Drowsy Tablets 740
Rynatan Tablets 3351

Quinidine Gluconate (Concurrent use with drugs that inhibit cytochrome P450IID6 may make normal metabolizer resemble poor metabolizer leading to higher than expected plasma concentrations of TCA with resultant toxicity). Products include:
Quinaglute Dura-Tabs Tablets 978

Quinidine Polygalacturonate (Concurrent use with drugs that inhibit cytochrome P450IID6 may make normal metabolizer resemble poor metabolizer leading to higher than expected plasma concentrations of TCA with resultant toxicity).
No products indexed under this heading.

Quinidine Sulfate (Concurrent use with drugs that inhibit cytochrome P450IID6 may make normal metabolizer resemble poor metabolizer leading to higher than expected plasma concentrations of TCA with resultant toxicity). Products include:
Quinidex Extentabs 2933

Salmeterol Xinafoate (Potentiated effects of catecholamines; careful adjustment of dosage and close supervision are required). Products include:
Advair Diskus 100/50 1448
Advair Diskus 250/50 1448
Advair Diskus 500/50 1448
Serevent Diskus 1637
Serevent Inhalation Aerosol 1633

Scopolamine (Concurrent use may result in pronounced atropinelike effects). Products include:
Transderm Scōp Transdermal Therapeutic System 2302

Scopolamine Hydrobromide (Concurrent use may result in pronounced atropinelike effects). Products include:
Donnatal 2929
Donnatal Extentabs 2930

Selegiline Hydrochloride (Potential for hyperpyretic crises, severe convulsions, and death; concurrent and/or sequential use is contraindicated). Products include:
Eldepryl Capsules 3266

Sertraline Hydrochloride (Concurrent use with drugs that are substrate for cytochrome P450IID6 may make normal metabolizer resemble poor metabolizer leading to higher than expected plasma concentrations of TCA with resultant toxicity; due to variation in the extent of inhibition of P450IID6 caution is indicated; if co-administered sufficient time must elapse). Products include:
Zoloft 2751

Terbutaline Sulfate (Potentiated effects of catecholamines; careful adjustment of dosage and close supervision are required). Products include:
Brethine Ampuls 2314
Brethine Tablets 2313

Thioridazine Hydrochloride (Concurrent use with drugs that are substrate for cytochrome P450IID6 may make normal metabolizer resemble poor metabolizer leading to higher than expected plasma concentrations of TCA with resultant toxicity). Products include:
Thioridazine Hydrochloride Tablets 2289

Thyroglobulin (Potential for cardiovascular toxicity).
No products indexed under this heading.

Thyroid (Potential for cardiovascular toxicity).
No products indexed under this heading.

Thyroxine (Potential for cardiovascular toxicity).
No products indexed under this heading.

Thyroxine Sodium (Potential for cardiovascular toxicity).
No products indexed under this heading.

Tolterodine Tartrate (Concurrent use may result in pronounced atropinelike effects). Products include:
Detrol Tablets 3623
Detrol LA Capsules 2801

Tranylcypromine Sulfate (Potential for hyperpyretic crises, severe convulsions, and death; concurrent and/or sequential use is contraindicated). Products include:
Parnate Tablets 1607

Trazodone Hydrochloride (Concurrent use with drugs that are substrate for cytochrome P450IID6 may make normal metabolizer resemble poor metabolizer leading to higher than expected plasma concentrations of TCA with resultant toxicity).
No products indexed under this heading.

Tridihexethyl Chloride (Concurrent use may result in pronounced atropinelike effects).
No products indexed under this heading.

Trifluoperazine Hydrochloride (Concurrent use with drugs that are substrate for cytochrome P450IID6 may make normal metabolizer resemble poor metabolizer leading to higher than expected plasma concentrations of TCA with resultant toxicity). Products include:
Stelazine 1640

Trihexyphenidyl Hydrochloride (Concurrent use may result in pronounced atropinelike effects). Products include:
Artane 1855

Food Interactions

Alcohol (Concomitant use of alcoholic beverages and trimipramine may be associated with exaggerated effects).

SURVANTA INTRATRACHEAL SUSPENSION

(Beractant) 3053
None cited in PDR database.

SUSTIVA CAPSULES

(Efavirenz) 1258
May interact with central nervous system depressants, ergot-containing drugs, and certain other agents. Compounds in these categories include:

Alfentanil Hydrochloride (Potential for additive central nervous system effects when Sustiva is used concomitantly with other CNS depressants).
No products indexed under this heading.

Alprazolam (Potential for additive central nervous system effects when Sustiva is used concomitantly with other CNS depressants). Products include:
Xanax Tablets 2865

Amprenavir (Efavirenz has the potential to decrease serum concentrations of amprenavir). Products include:
Agenerase Capsules 1454
Agenerase Oral Solution 1459

Aprobarbital (Potential for additive central nervous system effects when Sustiva is used concomitantly with other CNS depressants).
No products indexed under this heading.

Astemizole (Efavirenz has been shown *in vivo* to induce CYP3A4, other compounds that are substrates of CYP3A4, such as astemizole, may have decreased plasma concentrations when co-administered; *in vitro* efavirenz inhibits 3A4, co-administration with the drugs primarily metabolized by this isoenzyme, such as astemizole, may result in altered plasma concentrations of astemizole; concurrent use should be avoided).
No products indexed under this heading.

Azithromycin Dihydrate (Co-administration has resulted in increases in azithromycin Cmax (22%) with no change in AUC; no dosage adjustment is necessary). Products include:
Zithromax 2743
Zithromax for IV Infusion 2748
Zithromax for Oral Suspension, 300 mg, 600 mg, 900 mg, 1200 mg 2739
Zithromax Tablets, 250 mg 2739

Buprenorphine Hydrochloride (Potential for additive central nervous system effects when Sustiva is used concomitantly with other CNS depressants). Products include:
Buprenex Injectable 2918

Buspirone Hydrochloride (Potential for additive central nervous system effects when Sustiva is used concomitantly with other CNS depressants).
No products indexed under this heading.

Butabarbital (Potential for additive central nervous system effects when Sustiva is used concomitantly with other CNS depressants).
No products indexed under this heading.

Butalbital (Potential for additive central nervous system effects when Sustiva is used concomitantly with other CNS depressants). Products include:
Phrenilin 578
Sedapap Tablets 50 mg/650 mg ... 2225

Chlordiazepoxide (Potential for additive central nervous system effects when Sustiva is used concomitantly with other CNS depressants). Products include:
Limbitrol 1738

Chlordiazepoxide Hydrochloride (Potential for additive central nervous system effects when Sustiva is used concomitantly with other CNS depressants). Products include:
Librium Capsules 1736
Librium for Injection 1737

Chlorpromazine (Potential for additive central nervous system effects when Sustiva is used concomitantly with other CNS depressants). Products include:
Thorazine Suppositories 1656

Chlorpromazine Hydrochloride (Potential for additive central nervous system effects when Sustiva is used concomitantly with other CNS depressants). Products include:
Thorazine 1656

Chlorprothixene (Potential for additive central nervous system effects when Sustiva is used concomitantly with other CNS depressants).
No products indexed under this heading.

Chlorprothixene Hydrochloride (Potential for additive central nervous system effects when Sustiva is used concomitantly with other CNS depressants).
No products indexed under this heading.

Chlorprothixene Lactate (Potential for additive central nervous system effects when Sustiva is used concomitantly with other CNS depressants).
No products indexed under this heading.

Cisapride (Efavirenz has been shown *in vivo* to induce CYP3A4, other compounds that are substrates of CYP3A4, such as cisapride, may have decreased plasma concentrations when co-administered; *in vitro* efavirenz inhibits 3A4, co-administration with the drugs primarily metabolized by this isoenzyme, such as cisapride, may result in altered plasma concentrations of cisapride; concurrent use should be avoided).
No products indexed under this heading.

Clarithromycin (Co-administration has resulted in decreased AUC (39%) and Cmax (26%) of clarithromycin; AUC and Cmax of the clarithromycin hydroxymetabolite were increased 34% and 49% respectively; the clinical significance is unknown). Products include:
Biaxin/Biaxin XL 403
PREVPAC 3298

Clorazepate Dipotassium (Potential for additive central nervous system effects when Sustiva is used concomitantly with other CNS depressants). Products include:
Tranxene 511

Clozapine (Potential for additive central nervous system effects when Sustiva is used concomitantly with other CNS depressants). Products include:
Clozaril Tablets 2319

Codeine Phosphate (Potential for additive central nervous system effects when Sustiva is used concomitantly with other CNS depressants). Products include:
Phenergan with Codeine Syrup 3557
Phenergan VC with Codeine Syrup .. 3561
Robitussin A-C Syrup 2942
Robitussin-DAC Syrup 2942
Ryna-C Liquid 768
Soma Compound w/Codeine Tablets 3355
Tussi-Organidin NR Liquid 3350
Tussi-Organidin-S NR Liquid 3350
Tylenol with Codeine 2595

Desflurane (Potential for additive central nervous system effects when Sustiva is used concomitantly with other CNS depressants). Products include:
Suprane Liquid for Inhalation 874

Dezocine (Potential for additive central nervous system effects when Sustiva is used concomitantly with other CNS depressants).
No products indexed under this heading.

Diazepam (Potential for additive central nervous system effects when Sustiva is used concomitantly with other CNS depressants). Products include:

Valium Injectable 3026
Valium Tablets 3047

Dihydroergotamine Mesylate (Efavirenz has been shown *in vivo* to induce CYP3A4, other compounds that are substrates of CYP3A4, such as ergot derivatives, may have decreased plasma concentrations when co-administered; *in vitro* efavirenz inhibits 3A4, co-administration with the drugs primarily metabolized by this isoenzyme, such as ergot derivatives, may result in altered plasma concentrations of ergot derivatives; concurrent use should be avoided). Products include:
D.H.E. 45 Injection 2334
Migranal Nasal Spray 2376

Droperidol (Potential for additive central nervous system effects when Sustiva is used concomitantly with other CNS depressants).
No products indexed under this heading.

Enflurane (Potential for additive central nervous system effects when Sustiva is used concomitantly with other CNS depressants).
No products indexed under this heading.

Ergonovine Maleate (Efavirenz has been shown in vivo to induce CYP3A4, other compounds that are substrates of CYP3A4, such as ergot derivatives, may have decreased plasma concentrations when co-administered; in vitro efavirenz inhibits 3A4, co-administration with the drugs primarily metabolized by this isoenzyme, such as ergot derivatives, may result in altered plasma concentrations of ergot derivatives; concurrent use should be avoided).
No products indexed under this heading.

Ergotamine Tartrate (Efavirenz has been shown *in vivo* to induce CYP3A4, other compounds that are substrates of CYP3A4, such as ergot derivatives, may have decreased plasma concentrations when co-administered; *in vitro* efavirenz inhibits 3A4, co-administration with the drugs primarily metabolized by this isoenzyme, such as ergot derivatives, may result in altered plasma concentrations of ergot derivatives; concurrent use should be avoided).
No products indexed under this heading.

Estazolam (Potential for additive central nervous system effects when Sustiva is used concomitantly with other CNS depressants). Products include:
ProSom Tablets 500

Ethchlorvynol (Potential for additive central nervous system effects when Sustiva is used concomitantly with other CNS depressants).
No products indexed under this heading.

Ethinamate (Potential for additive central nervous system effects when Sustiva is used concomitantly with other CNS depressants).
No products indexed under this heading.

Ethinyl Estradiol (Co-administration has resulted in increased AUC for ethinyl estradiol; there was no effect on efavirenz AUC or Cmax; clinical significance is unknown). Products include:
Alesse-21 Tablets 3468
Alesse-28 Tablets 3473
Brevicon 28-Day Tablets 3380
Cyclessa Tablets 2450
Desogen Tablets 2458
Estinyl Tablets 3112
Estrostep 2627
femhrt Tablets 2635
Levlen 962
Levlite 21 Tablets 962
Levlite 28 Tablets 962
Levora Tablets 3389
Loestrin 21 Tablets 2642
Loestrin Fe Tablets 2642
Lo/Ovral Tablets 3532
Lo/Ovral-28 Tablets 3538
Low-Ogestrel-28 Tablets 3392
Microgestin Fe 1.5/30 Tablets 3407
Microgestin Fe 1/20 Tablets 3400
Mircette Tablets 2470
Modicon 2563
Necon 3415
Nordette-28 Tablets 2257
Norinyl 1 +35 28-Day Tablets 3380
Ogestrel 0.5/50-28 Tablets 3428
Ortho-Cept 21 Tablets 2546
Ortho-Cept 28 Tablets 2546
Ortho-Cyclen/Ortho Tri-Cyclen 2573
Ortho-Novum 2563
Ovcon 3364
Ovral Tablets 3551
Ovral-28 Tablets 3552
Tri-Levlen 962
Tri-Norinyl-28 Tablets 3433
Triphasil-21 Tablets 3600
Triphasil-28 Tablets 3605
Trivora Tablets 3439
Yasmin 28 Tablets 980
Zovia 3449

Fentanyl (Potential for additive central nervous system effects when Sustiva is used concomitantly with other CNS depressants). Products include:
Duragesic Transdermal System 1786

Fentanyl Citrate (Potential for additive central nervous system effects when Sustiva is used concomitantly with other CNS depressants). Products include:
Actiq 1184

Fluconazole (Co-administration has resulted in increase in 16% AUC for efavirenz; there was no change in fluconazole Cmax or AUC). Products include:
Diflucan Tablets, Injection, and Oral Suspension 2681

Fluphenazine Decanoate (Potential for additive central nervous system effects when Sustiva is used concomitantly with other CNS depressants).
No products indexed under this heading.

Fluphenazine Enanthate (Potential for additive central nervous system effects when Sustiva is used concomitantly with other CNS depressants).
No products indexed under this heading.

Fluphenazine Hydrochloride (Potential for additive central nervous system effects when Sustiva is used concomitantly with other CNS depressants).
No products indexed under this heading.

Flurazepam Hydrochloride (Potential for additive central nervous system effects when Sustiva is used concomitantly with other CNS depressants).
No products indexed under this heading.

Glutethimide (Potential for additive central nervous system effects when Sustiva is used concomitantly with other CNS depressants).
No products indexed under this heading.

Haloperidol (Potential for additive central nervous system effects when Sustiva is used concomitantly with other CNS depressants). Products include:
Haldol Injection, Tablets and Concentrate 2533

Haloperidol Decanoate (Potential for additive central nervous system effects when Sustiva is used concomitantly with other CNS depressants). Products include:
Haldol Decanoate 2535

Hydrocodone Bitartrate (Potential for additive central nervous system effects when Sustiva is used concomitantly with other CNS depressants). Products include:
Hycodan 1316
Hycomine Compound Tablets 1317
Hycotuss Expectorant Syrup 1318
Lortab 3319
Lortab Elixir 3317
Maxidone Tablets CIII 3399
Norco 5/325 Tablets CIII 3424
Norco 7.5/325 Tablets CIII 3425
Norco 10/325 Tablets CIII 3427
Norco 10/325 Tablets CIII 3425
Vicodin Tablets 516
Vicodin ES Tablets 517
Vicodin HP Tablets 518
Vicodin Tuss Expectorant 519
Vicoprofen Tablets 520
Zydone Tablets 1330

Hydrocodone Polistirex (Potential for additive central nervous system effects when Sustiva is used concomitantly with other CNS depressants). Products include:
Tussionex Pennkinetic Extended-Release Suspension 1174

Hydromorphone Hydrochloride (Potential for additive central nervous system effects when Sustiva is used concomitantly with other CNS depressants). Products include:
Dilaudid 441
Dilaudid Oral Liquid 445
Dilaudid Powder 441
Dilaudid Rectal Suppositories 441
Dilaudid Tablets 441
Dilaudid Tablets - 8 mg 445
Dilaudid-HP 443

Hydroxyzine Hydrochloride (Potential for additive central nervous system effects when Sustiva is used concomitantly with other CNS depressants). Products include:
Atarax Tablets & Syrup 2667
Vistaril Intramuscular Solution 2738

Indinavir Sulfate (Co-administration has resulted in decreases in AUC (31%) and Cmax (16%) for indinavir; indinavir dose of indinavir should be increased from 800 mg to 1000 mg every 8 hours). Products include:
Crixivan Capsules 2070

Isoflurane (Potential for additive central nervous system effects when Sustiva is used concomitantly with other CNS depressants).
No products indexed under this heading.

Ketamine Hydrochloride (Potential for additive central nervous system effects when Sustiva is used concomitantly with other CNS depressants).
No products indexed under this heading.

Levomethadyl Acetate Hydrochloride (Potential for additive central nervous system effects when Sustiva is used concomitantly with other CNS depressants).
No products indexed under this heading.

Levorphanol Tartrate (Potential for additive central nervous system effects when Sustiva is used concomitantly with other CNS depressants). Products include:
Levo-Dromoran 1734
Levorphanol Tartrate Tablets 3059

Lorazepam (Potential for additive central nervous system effects when Sustiva is used concomitantly with other CNS depressants). Products include:
Ativan Injection 3478
Ativan Tablets 3482

Loxapine Hydrochloride (Potential for additive central nervous system effects when Sustiva is used concomitantly with other CNS depressants).
No products indexed under this heading.

Loxapine Succinate (Potential for additive central nervous system effects when Sustiva is used concomitantly with other CNS depressants). Products include:
Loxitane Capsules 3398

Meperidine Hydrochloride (Potential for additive central nervous system effects when Sustiva is used concomitantly with other CNS depressants). Products include:
Demerol 3079
Mepergan Injection 3539

Mephobarbital (Potential for additive central nervous system effects when Sustiva is used concomitantly with other CNS depressants).
No products indexed under this heading.

Meprobamate (Potential for additive central nervous system effects when Sustiva is used concomitantly with other CNS depressants). Products include:
Miltown Tablets 3349

Mesoridazine Besylate (Potential for additive central nervous system effects when Sustiva is used concomitantly with other CNS depressants). Products include:
Serentil 1057

Methadone Hydrochloride (Potential for additive central nervous system effects when Sustiva is used concomitantly with other CNS depressants). Products include:
Dolophine Hydrochloride Tablets 3056

Methohexital Sodium (Potential for additive central nervous system effects when Sustiva is used concomitantly with other CNS depressants). Products include:
Brevital Sodium for Injection, USP .. 1815

Methotrimeprazine (Potential for additive central nervous system effects when Sustiva is used concomitantly with other CNS depressants).
No products indexed under this heading.

Methoxyflurane (Potential for additive central nervous system effects when Sustiva is used concomitantly with other CNS depressants).
No products indexed under this heading.

Methylergonovine Maleate (Efavirenz has been shown *in vivo* to induce CYP3A4, other compounds that are substrates of CYP3A4, such as ergot derivatives, may have decreased plasma concentrations when co-administered; *in vitro* efavirenz inhibits 3A4, co-administration with the drugs primarily metabolized by this isoenzyme, such as ergot derivatives, may result in altered plasma concentrations of ergot derivatives; concurrent use should be avoided).
No products indexed under this heading.

Methysergide Maleate (Efavirenz has been shown *in vivo* to induce CYP3A4, other compounds that are substrates of CYP3A4, such as ergot derivatives, may have decreased plasma concentrations when co-administered; *in vitro* efavirenz inhibits 3A4, co-administration with the drugs primarily metabolized by this isoenzyme, such as ergot derivatives, may result in altered plasma concentrations of ergot derivatives; concurrent use should be avoided).
No products indexed under this heading.

Midazolam Hydrochloride (Efavirenz has been shown *in vivo* to induce CYP3A4, other compounds that are substrates of CYP3A4, such as midazolam, may have decreased plasma concentrations when co-administered; *in vitro* efavirenz inhib-

its 3A4, co-administration with the drugs primarily metabolized by this isoenzyme, such as midazolam, may result in altered plasma concentrations of midazolam; concurrent use should be avoided). Products include:

- Versed Injection 3027
- Versed Syrup 3033

Molindone Hydrochloride (Potential for additive central nervous system effects when Sustiva is used concomitantly with other CNS depressants). Products include:

- Moban 1320

Morphine Sulfate (Potential for additive central nervous system effects when Sustiva is used concomitantly with other CNS depressants). Products include:

- Astramorph/PF Injection, USP (Preservative-Free) 594
- Duramorph Injection 1312
- Infumorph 200 and Infumorph 500 Sterile Solutions 1314
- Kadian Capsules 1335
- MS Contin Tablets 2896
- MSIR 2898
- Oramorph SR Tablets 3062
- Roxanol 3066

Nelfinavir Mesylate (Co-administration in uninfected individuals has resulted in increases in AUC (20%) and Cmax (21%) for nelfinavir; no dose adjustment is necessary). Products include:

- Viracept 532

Olanzapine (Potential for additive central nervous system effects when Sustiva is used concomitantly with other CNS depressants). Products include:

- Zyprexa Tablets 1973
- Zyprexa ZYDIS Orally Disintegrating Tablets 1973

Oxazepam (Potential for additive central nervous system effects when Sustiva is used concomitantly with other CNS depressants).

No products indexed under this heading.

Oxycodone Hydrochloride (Potential for additive central nervous system effects when Sustiva is used concomitantly with other CNS depressants). Products include:

- OxyContin Tablets 2912
- OxyFast Oral Concentrate Solution 2916
- OxyIR Capsules 2916
- Percocet Tablets 1326
- Percodan Tablets 1327
- Percolone Tablets 1327
- Roxicodone 3067
- Tylox Capsules 2597

Pentobarbital Sodium (Potential for additive central nervous system effects when Sustiva is used concomitantly with other CNS depressants). Products include:

- Nembutal Sodium Solution 485

Perphenazine (Potential for additive central nervous system effects when Sustiva is used concomitantly with other CNS depressants). Products include:

- Etrafon 3115
- Trilafon 3160

Phenobarbital (Co-administration with CYP3A4 inducers, such as phenobarbital, would be expected to increase the clearance of efavirenz resulting in lowered plasma concentrations; potential for additive central nervous system effects when Sustiva is used with concomitantly with other CNS depressants). Products include:

- Arco-Lase Plus Tablets 592
- Donnatal 2929
- Donnatal Extentabs 2930

Prazepam (Potential for additive central nervous system effects when Sustiva is used concomitantly with other CNS depressants).

No products indexed under this heading.

Prochlorperazine (Potential for additive central nervous system effects when Sustiva is used concomitantly with other CNS depressants). Products include:

- Compazine 1505

Promethazine Hydrochloride (Potential for additive central nervous system effects when Sustiva is used concomitantly with other CNS depressants). Products include:

- Mepergan Injection 3539
- Phenergan Injection 3553
- Phenergan 3556
- Phenergan Syrup 3554
- Phenergan with Codeine Syrup 3557
- Phenergan with Dextromethorphan Syrup 3559
- Phenergan VC Syrup 3560
- Phenergan VC with Codeine Syrup 3561

Propofol (Potential for additive central nervous system effects when Sustiva is used concomitantly with other CNS depressants). Products include:

- Diprivan Injectable Emulsion 667

Propoxyphene Hydrochloride (Potential for additive central nervous system effects when Sustiva is used concomitantly with other CNS depressants). Products include:

- Darvon Pulvules 1909
- Darvon Compound-65 Pulvules 1910

Propoxyphene Napsylate (Potential for additive central nervous system effects when Sustiva is used concomitantly with other CNS depressants). Products include:

- Darvon-N/Darvocet-N 1907
- Darvon-N Tablets 1912

Quazepam (Potential for additive central nervous system effects when Sustiva is used concomitantly with other CNS depressants).

No products indexed under this heading.

Quetiapine Fumarate (Potential for additive central nervous system effects when Sustiva is used concomitantly with other CNS depressants). Products include:

- Seroquel Tablets 684

Remifentanil Hydrochloride (Potential for additive central nervous system effects when Sustiva is used concomitantly with other CNS depressants).

No products indexed under this heading.

Rifabutin (Co-administration with CYP3A4 inducers, such as rifabutin, would be expected to increase the clearance of efavirenz resulting in lowered plasma concentrations; rifabutin has not been studied in combination with Sustiva). Products include:

- Mycobutin Capsules 2838

Rifampin (Co-administration has resulted in decreased efavirenz plasma concentrations; clinical significance is unknown). Products include:

- Rifadin 765
- Rifamate Capsules 767
- Rifater Tablets 769

Risperidone (Potential for additive central nervous system effects when Sustiva is used concomitantly with other CNS depressants). Products include:

- Risperdal 1796

Ritonavir (Co-administration has resulted in increases in AUC for each drug by 20%; the combination was associated with a higher frequency of adverse clinical experiences including dizziness, nausea, paresthesia, and laboratory abnormalities (elevated liver enzymes)). Products include:

- Kaletra Capsules 471
- Kaletra Oral Solution 471
- Norvir Capsules 487
- Norvir Oral Solution 487

Saquinavir (Co-administration with saquinavir soft gelatin capsule has resulted in decreases in AUC (62%) and Cmax (50%) for saquinavir; saquinavir should not be used as sole protease inhibitor in combination with Sustiva). Products include:

- Fortovase Capsules 2970

Saquinavir Mesylate (Co-administration with saquinavir soft gelatin capsule has resulted in decreases in AUC (62%) and Cmax (50%) for saquinavir; saquinavir should not be used as sole protease inhibitor in combination with Sustiva). Products include:

- Invirase Capsules 2979

Secobarbital Sodium (Potential for additive central nervous system effects when Sustiva is used concomitantly with other CNS depressants).

No products indexed under this heading.

Sevoflurane (Potential for additive central nervous system effects when Sustiva is used concomitantly with other CNS depressants).

No products indexed under this heading.

Sufentanil Citrate (Potential for additive central nervous system effects when Sustiva is used concomitantly with other CNS depressants).

No products indexed under this heading.

Temazepam (Potential for additive central nervous system effects when Sustiva is used concomitantly with other CNS depressants).

No products indexed under this heading.

Thiamylal Sodium (Potential for additive central nervous system effects when Sustiva is used concomitantly with other CNS depressants).

No products indexed under this heading.

Thioridazine Hydrochloride (Potential for additive central nervous system effects when Sustiva is used concomitantly with other CNS depressants). Products include:

- Thioridazine Hydrochloride Tablets 2289

Thiothixene (Potential for additive central nervous system effects when Sustiva is used concomitantly with other CNS depressants). Products include:

- Navane Capsules 2701
- Thiothixene Capsules 2290

Triazolam (Efavirenz has been shown *in vivo* to induce CYP3A4, other compounds that are substrates of CYP3A4, such as triazolam, may have decreased plasma concentrations when co-administered; *in vitro* efavirenz inhibits its 3A4, co-administration with the drugs primarily metabolized by this isoenzyme, such as triazolam, may result in altered plasma concentrations of triazolam; concurrent use should be avoided). Products include:

- Halcion Tablets 2823

Trifluoperazine Hydrochloride (Potential for additive central nervous system effects when Sustiva is used concomitantly with other CNS depressants). Products include:

- Stelazine 1640

Warfarin Sodium (Co-administration may result in increased or decreased plasma concentrations and effects of warfarin). Products include:

- Coumadin for Injection 1243
- Coumadin Tablets 1243
- Warfarin Sodium Tablets, USP 3302

Zaleplon (Potential for additive central nervous system effects when Sustiva is used concomitantly with other CNS depressants). Products include:

- Sonata Capsules 3591

Ziprasidone Hydrochloride (Potential for additive central nervous system effects when Sustiva is used concomitantly with other CNS depressants). Products include:

- Geodon Capsules 2688

Zolpidem Tartrate (Potential for additive central nervous system effects when Sustiva is used concomitantly with other CNS depressants). Products include:

- Ambien Tablets 3191

Food Interactions

Alcohol (Potential for additive central nervous system effects when Sustiva is used concomitantly with alcohol).

Food, unspecified (High fat meal may increase the absorption of Sustiva and should be avoided; it can be taken with or without meals of normal composition).

SYMMETREL SYRUP

(Amantadine Hydrochloride) 1328

See Symmetrel Tablets

SYMMETREL TABLETS

(Amantadine Hydrochloride) 1328

May interact with anticholinergics, central nervous system stimulants, quinidine, and certain other agents. Compounds in these categories include:

Amphetamine Resins (Co-administration with central nervous system stimulants requires careful observation).

No products indexed under this heading.

Atropine Sulfate (Agents with anticholinergic properties may potentiate the anticholinergic-like side effects of amantadine). Products include:

- Donnatal 2929
- Donnatal Extentabs 2930
- Motofen Tablets 577
- Prosed/DS Tablets 3268
- Urised Tablets 2876

Belladonna Alkaloids (Agents with anticholinergic properties may potentiate the anticholinergic-like side effects of amantadine). Products include:

- Hyland's Teething Tablets 766
- Urimax Tablets 1769

Benztropine Mesylate (Agents with anticholinergic properties may potentiate the anticholinergic-like side effects of amantadine). Products include:

- Cogentin 2055

Biperiden Hydrochloride (Agents with anticholinergic properties may potentiate the anticholinergic-like side effects of amantadine). Products include:

- Akineton 402

Clidinium Bromide (Agents with anticholinergic properties may potentiate the anticholinergic-like side effects of amantadine).

No products indexed under this heading.

Dextroamphetamine Sulfate (Co-administration with central nervous system stimulants requires careful observation). Products include:

- Adderall Tablets 3231
- Adderall XR Capsules
- Dexedrine 1512
- DextroStat Tablets 3236

Dicyclomine Hydrochloride (Agents with anticholinergic properties may potentiate the anticholinergic-like side effects of amantadine).

No products indexed under this heading.

Glycopyrrolate (Agents with anticholinergic properties may potenti-

ate the anticholinergic-like side effects of amantadine). Products include:

- Robinul Forte Tablets ... 1358
- Robinul Injectable ... 2940
- Robinul Tablets ... 1358

Hydrochlorothiazide (Co-administration with triamterene-hydrochlorothiazide capsules has resulted in a higher plasma amantadine concentration in a patient with Parkinsonism; it is not known which components of triamterene-hydrochlorothiazide capsules contributed to this interaction). Products include:

- Accuretic Tablets ... 2614
- Aldoril Tablets ... 2039
- Atacand HCT Tablets ... 597
- Avalide Tablets ... 1070
- Diovan HCT Tablets ... 2338
- Dyazide Capsules ... 1515
- HydroDIURIL Tablets ... 2108
- Hyzaar ... 2109
- Inderide Tablets ... 3517
- Inderide LA Long-Acting Capsules ... 3519
- Lotensin HCT Tablets ... 2367
- Maxzide ... 1008
- Micardis HCT Tablets ... 1051
- Microzide Capsules ... 3414
- Moduretic Tablets ... 2138
- Monopril HCT ... 1094
- Prinzide Tablets ... 2168
- Timolide Tablets ... 2187
- Uniretic Tablets ... 3178
- Vaseretic Tablets ... 2204
- Zestoretic Tablets ... 695
- Ziac Tablets ... 1887

Hyoscyamine (Agents with anticholinergic properties may potentiate the anticholinergic-like side effects of amantadine). Products include:

- Urised Tablets ... 2876

Hyoscyamine Sulfate (Agents with anticholinergic properties may potentiate the anticholinergic-like side effects of amantadine). Products include:

- Arco-Lase Plus Tablets ... 592
- Donnatal ... 2929
- Donnatal Extentabs ... 2930
- Levsin/Levsinex/Levbid ... 3172
- NuLev Orally Disintegrating Tablets ... 3176
- Prosed/DS Tablets ... 3268
- Urimax Tablets ... 1769

Ipratropium Bromide (Agents with anticholinergic properties may potentiate the anticholinergic-like side effects of amantadine). Products include:

- Atrovent Inhalation Aerosol ... 1030
- Atrovent Inhalation Solution ... 1031
- Atrovent Nasal Spray 0.03% ... 1032
- Atrovent Nasal Spray 0.06% ... 1033
- Combivent Inhalation Aerosol ... 1041
- DuoNeb Inhalation Solution ... 1233

Mepenzolate Bromide (Agents with anticholinergic properties may potentiate the anticholinergic-like side effects of amantadine).

No products indexed under this heading.

Methamphetamine Hydrochloride (Co-administration with central nervous system stimulants requires careful observation). Products include:

- Desoxyn Tablets ... 440

Methylphenidate Hydrochloride (Co-administration with central nervous system stimulants requires careful observation). Products include:

- Concerta Extended-Release Tablets ... 1998
- Concerta Tablets ... 561
- Metadate CD Capsules ... 1164
- Metadate ER Tablets ... 1167
- Methylin Tablets ... 1995
- Methylin ER Tablets ... 1995
- Ritalin ... 2387

Oxybutynin Chloride (Agents with anticholinergic properties may potentiate the anticholinergic-like side effects of amantadine). Products include:

- Ditropan XL Extended Release Tablets ... 564

Pemoline (Co-administration with central nervous system stimulants requires careful observation). Products include:

- Cylert Tablets ... 415

Procyclidine Hydrochloride (Agents with anticholinergic properties may potentiate the anticholinergic-like side effects of amantadine).

No products indexed under this heading.

Propantheline Bromide (Agents with anticholinergic properties may potentiate the anticholinergic-like side effects of amantadine).

No products indexed under this heading.

Quinidine Gluconate (Co-administration of quinidine with amantadine has been shown to reduce the renal clearance of amantadine). Products include:

- Quinaglute Dura-Tabs Tablets ... 978

Quinidine Polygalacturonate (Co-administration of quinidine with amantadine has been shown to reduce the renal clearance of amantadine).

No products indexed under this heading.

Quinidine Sulfate (Co-administration of quinidine with amantadine has been shown to reduce the renal clearance of amantadine). Products include:

- Quinidex Extentabs ... 2933

Quinine (Co-administration of quinine with amantadine has been shown to reduce the renal clearance of amantadine).

No products indexed under this heading.

Scopolamine (Agents with anticholinergic properties may potentiate the anticholinergic-like side effects of amantadine). Products include:

- Transderm Scōp Transdermal Therapeutic System ... 2302

Scopolamine Hydrobromide (Agents with anticholinergic properties may potentiate the anticholinergic-like side effects of amantadine). Products include:

- Donnatal ... 2929
- Donnatal Extentabs ... 2930

Sulfamethoxazole (Co-administration of trimethoprim-sulfamethoxazole may impair renal clearance of amantadine). Products include:

- Bactrim ... 2949
- Septra Suspension ... 2265
- Septra Tablets ... 2265
- Septra DS Tablets ... 2265

Thioridazine Hydrochloride (Co-administration has been reported to worsen the tremor in elderly patients with Parkinson's disease). Products include:

- Thioridazine Hydrochloride Tablets ... 2289

Tolterodine Tartrate (Agents with anticholinergic properties may potentiate the anticholinergic-like side effects of amantadine). Products include:

- Detrol Tablets ... 3623
- Detrol LA Capsules ... 2801

Triamterene (Co-administration with triamterene-hydrochlorothiazide capsules has resulted in a higher plasma amantadine concentration in a patient with Parkinsonism; it is not known which components of triamterene-hydrochlorothiazide capsules contributed to this interaction). Products include:

- Dyazide Capsules ... 1515
- Dyrenium Capsules ... 3458
- Maxzide ... 1008

Tridihexethyl Chloride (Agents with anticholinergic properties may potentiate the anticholinergic-like side effects of amantadine).

No products indexed under this heading.

Trihexyphenidyl Hydrochloride (Agents with anticholinergic properties may potentiate the anticholinergic-like side effects of amantadine). Products include:

- Artane ... 1855

Trimethoprim (Co-administration of trimethoprim-sulfamethoxazole may impair renal clearance of amantadine). Products include:

- Bactrim ... 2949
- Septra Suspension ... 2265
- Septra Tablets ... 2265
- Septra DS Tablets ... 2265

Food Interactions

Alcohol (May increase the potential for CNS effects such as dizziness, confusion, light-headedness and orthostatic hypotension; avoid excessive alcohol usage).

SYNAGIS INTRAMUSCULAR

(Palivizumab) ... 2028

None cited in PDR database.

SYNALAR CREAM

(Fluocinolone Acetonide) ... 2020

None cited in PDR database.

SYNALAR OINTMENT

(Fluocinolone Acetonide) ... 2020

None cited in PDR database.

SYNALAR TOPICAL SOLUTION

(Fluocinolone Acetonide) ... 2020

None cited in PDR database.

SYNAREL NASAL SOLUTION FOR CENTRAL PRECOCIOUS PUBERTY

(Nafarelin Acetate) ... 3204

None cited in PDR database.

SYNAREL NASAL SOLUTION FOR ENDOMETRIOSIS

(Nafarelin Acetate) ... 3205

None cited in PDR database.

SYNERCID I.V.

(Dalfopristin, Quinupristin) ... 775

May interact with HMG-CoA reductase inhibitors, methylprednisolone, quinidine, vinca alkaloids, and certain other agents. Compounds in these categories include:

Astemizole (Quinupristin/dalfopristin inhibits CYP4503A4, therefore, it is reasonable to expect that the co-administration with other drugs primarily metabolized by this enzyme system, such as astemizole, is likely to result in increased plasma concentrations of astemizole that could increase or prolong its therapeutic effects and /or increased adverse reactions).

No products indexed under this heading.

Atorvastatin Calcium (Quinupristin/dalfopristin inhibits CYP4503A4, therefore, it is reasonable to expect that the co-administration with other drugs primarily metabolized by this enzyme system, such as HMG-CoA reductase inhibitors, is likely to result in increased plasma concentrations of HMG-CoA reductase inhibitors that could increase or prolong its therapeutic effects and/or increased adverse reactions). Products include:

- Lipitor Tablets ... 2639
- Lipitor Tablets ... 2696

Carbamazepine (Quinupristin/dalfopristin inhibits CYP4503A4, therefore, it is reasonable to expect that the co-administration with other drugs primarily metabolized by this enzyme system, such as carbamazepine, is likely to result in increased plasma concentrations of carbamazepine that could increase and/or increased adverse reactions). Products include:

- Carbatrol Capsules ... 3234
- Tegretol/Tegretol-XR ... 2404

Cerivastatin Sodium (Quinupristin/dalfopristin inhibits CYP4503A4, therefore, it is reasonable to expect that the co-administration with other drugs primarily metabolized by this enzyme system, such as HMG-CoA reductase inhibitors, is likely to result in increased plasma concentrations of HMG-CoA reductase inhibitors that could increase or prolong its therapeutic effects and/or increased adverse reactions). Products include:

- Baycol Tablets ... 883

Cisapride (Quinupristin/dalfopristin inhibits CYP4503A4, therefore, it is reasonable to expect that the co-administration with other drugs primarily metabolized by this enzyme system, such as cisapride, is likely to result in increased plasma concentrations of cisapride that could increase or prolong its therapeutic effects and/or increased adverse reactions).

No products indexed under this heading.

Cyclosporine (Quinupristin/dalfopristin significantly inhibits CYP4503A4 metabolism of cyclosporine; co-administration has resulted in an increase of 63% in the AUC, 30% in the Cmax, and a 77% increase in t1/2 of cyclosporine and a decrease of 34% in the clearance of cyclosporine). Products include:

- Gengraf Capsules ... 457
- Neoral Soft Gelatin Capsules ... 2380
- Neoral Oral Solution ... 2380
- Sandimmune ... 2388

Delavirdine Mesylate (Quinupristin/dalfopristin inhibits CYP4503A4, therefore, it is reasonable to expect that the co-administration with other drugs primarily metabolized by this enzyme system, such as delavirdine, is likely to result in increased plasma concentrations of delavirdine that could increase or prolong its therapeutic effects and/or increased adverse reactions). Products include:

- Rescriptor Tablets ... 526

Diazepam (Quinupristin/dalfopristin inhibits CYP4503A4, therefore, it is reasonable to expect that the co-administration with other drugs primarily metabolized by this enzyme system, such as diazepam, is likely to result in increased plasma concentrations of diazepam that could increase or prolong its therapeutic effects and/or increased adverse reactions). Products include:

- Valium Injectable ... 3026
- Valium Tablets ... 3047

Digoxin (Quinupristin/dalfopristin has shown in vitro activity against Eubacterium lentum, digoxin is metabolized in part by bacteria in the gut and as such, a drug interaction based on Quinupristin/dalfopristin's inhibition of digoxin's gut metabolism (by Eubacterium lentum) may be possible). Products include:

- Digitek Tablets ... 1003
- Lanoxicaps Capsules ... 1574
- Lanoxin Injection ... 1581
- Lanoxin Tablets ... 1587
- Lanoxin Elixir Pediatric ... 1578
- Lanoxin Injection Pediatric ... 1584

Diltiazem Hydrochloride (Quinupristin/dalfopristin inhibits

CYP4503A4, therefore, it is reasonable to expect that the co-administration with other drugs primarily metabolized by this enzyme system, such as diltiazem, is likely to result in increased plasma concentrations of diltiazem that could increase or prolong its therapeutic effects and/or increased adverse reactions). Products include:

Cardizem Injectable 1018
Cardizem Lyo-Ject Syringe 1018
Cardizem Monovial 1018
Cardizem CD Capsules 1016
Tiazac Capsules 1378

Disopyramide Phosphate (Quinupristin/dalfopristin inhibits CYP4503A4, therefore, it is reasonable to expect that the co-administration with other drugs metabolized by this enzyme system, such as disopyramide, is likely to result in increased plasma concentrations of disopyramide that could increase or prolong its therapeutic effects and/or increased adverse reactions).

No products indexed under this heading.

Docetaxel (Quinupristin/dalfopristin inhibits CYP4503A4, therefore, it is reasonable to expect that the co-administration with other drugs primarily metabolized by this enzyme system, such as docetaxel, is likely to result in increased plasma concentrations of docetaxel that could increase or prolong its therapeutic effects and/or increased adverse reactions). Products include:

Taxotere for Injection Concentrate 778

Fluvastatin Sodium (Quinupristin/dalfopristin inhibits CYP4503A4, therefore, it is reasonable to expect that the co-administration with other drugs primarily metabolized by this enzyme system, such as HMG-CoA reductase inhibitors, is likely to result in increased plasma concentrations of HMG-CoA reductase inhibitors that could increase or prolong its therapeutic effects and/or increased adverse reactions). Products include:

Lescol Capsules 2361
Lescol 2925
Lescol XL Tablets 2361

Indinavir Sulfate (Quinupristin/dalfopristin inhibits CYP4503A4, therefore, it is reasonable to expect that the co-administration with other drugs primarily metabolized by this enzyme system, such as indinavir, is likely to result in increased plasma concentrations of indinavir that could increase or prolong its therapeutic effects and/or increased adverse reactions). Products include:

Crixivan Capsules 2070

Lidocaine Hydrochloride (Quinupristin/dalfopristin inhibits CYP4503A4, therefore, it is reasonable to expect that the co-administration with other drugs primarily metabolized by this enzyme system, such as lidocaine, is likely to result in increased plasma concentrations of lidocaine that could increase or prolong its therapeutic effects and/or increased adverse reactions). Products include:

Bactine First Aid Liquid 611
Xylocaine Injections 653

Lovastatin (Quinupristin/dalfopristin inhibits CYP4503A4, therefore, it is reasonable to expect that the co-administration with other drugs primarily metabolized by this enzyme system, such as HMG-CoA reductase inhibitors, is likely to result in increased plasma concentrations of HMG-CoA reductase inhibitors that could increase or prolong its therapeutic effects and/or increased adverse reactions). Products include:

Mevacor Tablets 2132

Methylprednisolone (Quinupristin/dalfopristin inhibits CYP4503A4, therefore it is reasonable to expect that the co-administration with other drugs primarily metabolized by this enzyme system, such as methylprednisolone, is likely to result in increased plasma concentrationsof methylprednisolone that could increase or prolong its therapeutic affects and/or increased adverse reactions).

No products indexed under this heading.

Methylprednisolone Acetate (Quinupristin/dalfopristin inhibits CYP4503A4, therefore it is reasonable to expect that the co-administration with other drugs primarily metabolized by this enzyme system, such as methylprednisolone, is likely to result in increased plasma concentrationsof methylprednisolone that could increase or prolong its therapeutic affects and/or increased adverse reactions). Products include:

Depo-Medrol Injectable Suspension 2795

Methylprednisolone Sodium Succinate (Quinupristin/dalfopristin inhibits CYP4503A4, therefore it is reasonable to expect that the co-administration with other drugs primarily metabolized by this enzyme system, such as methylprednisolone, is likely to result in increased plasma concentrationsof methylprednisolone that could increase or prolong its therapeutic affects and/or increased adverse reactions). Products include:

Solu-Medrol Sterile Powder 2855

Midazolam Hydrochloride (Quinupristin/dalfopristin significantly inhibits CYP4503A4 metabolism of midazolam; co-administration of midazolam (intravenous bolus dose) in healthy volunteers resulted in elevated plasma concentrations of midazolam). Products include:

Versed Injection 3027
Versed Syrup 3033

Nevirapine (Quinupristin/dalfopristin inhibits CYP4503A4, therefore, it is reasonable to expect that the co-administration with other drugs primarily metabolized by this enzyme system, such as nevirapine, is likely to result in increased plasma concentrations of nevirapine that could increase or prolong its therapeutic effects and/or increased adverse reactions). Products include:

Viramune Oral Suspension 1060
Viramune Tablets 1060

Nifedipine (Quinupristin/dalfopristin significantly inhibits CYP4503A4 metabolism of nifedipine; co-administration of nifedipine (repeated oral doses) in healthy volunteers resulted in elevated plasma concentrations of nifedipine). Products include:

Adalat CC Tablets 877
Procardia Capsules 2708
Procardia XL Extended Release Tablets 2710

Paclitaxel (Quinupristin/dalfopristin inhibits CYP4503A4, therefore, it is reasonable to expect that the co-administration with other drugs primarily metabolized by this enzyme system, such as paclitaxel, is likely to result in increased plasma concentrations of paclitaxel that could increase or prolong its therapeutic effects and/or increased adverse reactions). Products include:

Taxol Injection 1129

Pravastatin Sodium (Quinupristin/dalfopristin inhibits CYP4503A4, therefore, it is reasonable to expect that the co-administration with other drugs primarily metabolized by this enzyme system, such as HMG-CoA reductase inhibitors, is likely to result in increased plasma concentrations of HMG-CoA reductase inhibitors that could increase or prolong its therapeutic effects and/or increased adverse reactions). Products include:

Pravachol Tablets 1099

Quinidine Gluconate (Quinupristin/dalfopristin inhibits CTP4503A4, therefore, it is reasonable to expect that the co-administration with other drugs primarily metabolized by this enzyme system, such as quinidine, is likely to result in increased plasma concentrations of quinidine that could increase or prolong its therapeutic effects and/or increased adverse reactions). Products include:

Quinaglute Dura-Tabs Tablets 978

Quinidine Polygalacturonate (Quinupristin/dalfopristin inhibits CTP4503A4, therefore, it is reasonable to expect that the co-administration with other drugs primarily metabolized by this enzyme system, such as quinidine, is likely to result in increased plasma concentrations of quinidine that could increase or prolong its therapeutic effects and/or increased adverse reactions).

No products indexed under this heading.

Quinidine Sulfate (Quinupristin/dalfopristin inhibits CTP4503A4, therefore, it is reasonable to expect that the co-administration with other drugs primarily metabolized by this enzyme system, such as quinidine, is likely to result in increased plasma concentrations of quinidine that could increase or prolong its therapeutic effects and/or increased adverse reactions). Products include:

Quinidex Extentabs 2933

Ritonavir (Quinupristin/dalfopristin inhibits CYP4503A4, therefore, it is reasonable to expect that the co-administration with other drugs primarily metabolized by this enzyme system, such as ritonavir, is likely to result in increased plasma concentrations of ritonavir that could increase or prolong its therapeutic effects and/or increased adverse reactions). Products include:

Kaletra Capsules 471
Kaletra Oral Solution 471
Norvir Capsules 487
Norvir Oral Solution 487

Simvastatin (Quinupristin/dalfopristin inhibits CYP4503A4, therefore, it is reasonable to expect that the co-administration with other drugs primarily metabolized by this enzyme system, such as HMG-CoA reductase inhibitors, is likely to result in increased plasma concentrations of HMG-CoA reductase inhibitors that could increase or prolong its therapeutic effects and/or increased adverse reactions). Products include:

Zocor Tablets 2219

Tacrolimus (Quinupristin/dalfopristin significantly inhibits CYP4503A4, therefore, it is reasonable to expect that the co-administration with other drugs primarily metabolized by this enzyme system, such as tacrolimus, is likely to result in increased plasma concentrations of tacrolimus that could increase or prolong its therapeutic effects and/or adverse reactions). Products include:

Prograf 1393
Protopic Ointment 1397

Terfenadine (Quinupristin/dalfopristin significantly inhibits CYP4503A4 metabolism of terfenadine; co-administration is likely to result in increased plasma concentrations of terfenadine that could increase or prolong its therapeutic effects and/or increased adverse reactions).

No products indexed under this heading.

Verapamil Hydrochloride (Quinupristin/dalfopristin inhibits CYP4503A4, therefore, it is reasonable to expect that the co-administration with other drugs primarily metabolized by this enzyme system, such as verapamil, is likely to result in increased plasma concentrations of verapamil that could increase or prolong its therapeutic effects and/or adverse reactions). Products include:

Covera-HS Tablets 3199
Isoptin SR Tablets 467
Tarka Tablets 508
Verelan Capsules 3184
Verelan PM Capsules 3186

Vinblastine Sulfate (Quinupristin/dalfopristin inhibits CYP4503A4, therefore, it is reasonable to expect that the co-administration with other drugs primarily metabolized by this enzyme system, such as vinca alkaloids that could increase or prolong its therapeutic effects and/or increased adverse reactions).

No products indexed under this heading.

Vincristine Sulfate (Quinupristin/dalfopristin inhibits CYP4503A4, therefore, it is reasonable to expect that the co-administration with other drugs primarily metabolized by this enzyme system, such as vinca alkaloids that could increase or prolong its therapeutic effects and/or increased adverse reactions).

No products indexed under this heading.

Vinorelbine Tartrate (Quinupristin/dalfopristin inhibits CYP4503A4, therefore, it is reasonable to expect that the co-administration with other drugs primarily metabolized by this enzyme system, such as vinca alkaloids that could increase or prolong its therapeutic effects and/or increased adverse reactions). Products include:

Navelbine Injection 1604

SYNTHROID INJECTION

(Levothyroxine Sodium) 505

See Synthroid Tablets

SYNTHROID TABLETS

(Levothyroxine Sodium) 505

May interact with androgens, antithyroid agents, beta blockers, oral anticoagulants, cytokines, dopamine agonists, estrogens, glucocorticoids, cardiac glycosides, hepatic microsomal enzyme inducers, oral hypoglycemic agents, insulin, lithium preparations, phenytoin, radiographic iodinated contrast media, salicylates, sulfonamides, sulfonylureas, sympathomimetics, thiazides, tricyclic antidepressants, theophylline, and certain other agents. Compounds in these categories include:

Acarbose (Requirements of oral antidiabetic agents may be reduced in hypothyroid patients with diabetes and may be subsequently increased with initiation of thyroid hormone therapy). Products include:

Precose Tablets 906

Acebutolol Hydrochloride (Alters thyroid hormone or TSH levels; actions of some beta blockers may be impaired when hypothyroid patients become euthyroid). Products include:

Sectral Capsules 3589

Albuterol (Possible increased risk of coronary insufficiency in patients with coronary artery disease). Products include:

Proventil Inhalation Aerosol 3142
Ventolin Inhalation Aerosol and Refill.. 1679

Albuterol Sulfate (Possible increased risk of coronary insufficiency in patients with coronary artery disease). Products include:
AccuNeb Inhalation Solution 1230
Combivent Inhalation Aerosol 1041
DuoNeb Inhalation Solution 1233
Proventil Inhalation Solution 0.083%.. 3146
Proventil Repetabs Tablets 3148
Proventil Solution for Inhalation 0.5%.. 3144
Proventil HFA Inhalation Aerosol 3150
Ventolin HFA Inhalation Aerosol 3618
Volmax Extended-Release Tablets .. 2276

Aldesleukin (Cytokines have been reported to induce both hyperthyroidism or hypothyroidism; dosage adjustment may be necessary). Products include:
Proleukin for Injection 1199

Aluminum Hydroxide (Binds and decreases absorption of levothyroxine sodium from the gastrointestinal tract). Products include:
Amphojel Suspension (Mint Flavor).. ▣789
Gaviscon Extra Strength Liquid ..... ▣751
Gaviscon Extra Strength Tablets ... ▣751
Gaviscon Regular Strength Liquid . ▣751
Gaviscon Regular Strength Tablets... ▣750
Maalox Antacid/Anti-Gas Oral Suspension.................................. ▣673
Maalox Max Maximum Strength Antacid/Anti-Gas Liquid 2300
Maalox Regular Strength Antacid/Antigas Liquid 2300
Mylanta 1813
Vanquish Caplets .... ▣617

Aminoglutethimide (Alters thyroid hormone or TSH levels).
No products indexed under this heading.

Aminophylline (Theophylline clearance may be decreased in hypothyroid patients and return toward normal when euthyroid state is achieved).
No products indexed under this heading.

p-Aminosalicylic Acid (Alters thyroid hormone or TSH levels).
No products indexed under this heading.

Amiodarone Hydrochloride (Amiodarone therapy alone can cause hypothyroidism or hyperthyroidism). Products include:
Cordarone Intravenous 3491
Cordarone Tablets 3487
Pacerone Tablets 3331

Amitriptyline Hydrochloride (Concurrent use may increase the therapeutic and toxic effects of both drugs; onset of action of tricyclics may be accelerated). Products include:
Etrafon 3115
Limbitrol 1738

Amoxapine (Concurrent use may increase the therapeutic and toxic effects of both drugs; onset of action of tricyclics may be accelerated).
No products indexed under this heading.

Asparaginase (May inhibit levothyroxine sodium binding to serum proteins or alter the concentrations of serum proteins). Products include:
Elspar for Injection 2092

Aspirin (May inhibit levothyroxine sodium binding to serum proteins or alter the concentrations of serum proteins). Products include:
Aggrenox Capsules 1026
Alka-Seltzer .... ▣603
Alka-Seltzer Lemon Lime Antacid and Pain Reliever Effervescent Tablets .... ▣603
Alka-Seltzer Extra Strength Antacid and Pain Reliever Effervescent Tablets................ ▣603
Alka-Seltzer PM Effervescent Tablets .... ▣605
Genuine Bayer Tablets, Caplets and Gelcaps .... ▣606
Extra Strength Bayer Caplets and Gelcaps.. ▣610
Aspirin Regimen Bayer Children's Chewable Tablets (Orange or Cherry Flavored)....................... ▣607
Bayer, Aspirin Regimen .... ▣606
Aspirin Regimen Bayer 81 mg Caplets with Calcium .... ▣607
Genuine Bayer Professional Labeling (Aspirin Regimen Bayer).. ▣608
Extra Strength Bayer Arthritis Caplets.. ▣610
Extra Strength Bayer Plus Caplets.. ▣610
Extra Strength Bayer PM Caplets .. ▣611
BC Powder .... ▣619
BC Allergy Sinus Cold Powder ...... ▣619
Arthritis Strength BC Powder .... ▣619
BC Sinus Cold Powder .... ▣619
Darvon Compound-65 Pulvules 1910
Ecotrin Enteric Coated Aspirin Low, Regular and Maximum Strength Tablets.......................... 1715
Excedrin Extra-Strength Tablets, Caplets, and Geltabs .... ▣629
Excedrin Migraine 1070
Goody's Body Pain Formula Powder.. ▣620
Goody's Extra Strength Headache Powder .... ▣620
Goody's Extra Strength Pain Relief Tablets .... ▣620
Percodan Tablets 1327
Robaxisal Tablets 2939
Soma Compound Tablets 3354
Soma Compound w/Codeine Tablets.. 3355
Vanquish Caplets .... ▣617

Atenolol (Alters thyroid hormone or TSH levels; actions of some beta blockers may be impaired when hypothyroid patients become euthyroid). Products include:
Tenoretic Tablets 690
Tenormin I.V. Injection 692

Bendroflumethiazide (Alters thyroid hormone or TSH levels). Products include:
Corzide 40/5 Tablets 2247
Corzide 80/5 Tablets 2247

Betamethasone Acetate (May inhibit levothyroxine sodium binding to serum proteins or alter the concentrations of serum proteins). Products include:
Celestone Soluspan Injectable Suspension................................ 3097

Betamethasone Sodium Phosphate (May inhibit levothyroxine sodium binding to serum proteins or alter the concentrations of serum proteins). Products include:
Celestone Soluspan Injectable Suspension................................ 3097

Betaxolol Hydrochloride (Alters thyroid hormone or TSH levels; actions of some beta blockers may be impaired when hypothyroid patients become euthyroid). Products include:
Betoptic S Ophthalmic Suspension................................ 537

Bisoprolol Fumarate (Alters thyroid hormone or TSH levels; actions of some beta blockers may be impaired when hypothyroid patients become euthyroid). Products include:
Zebeta Tablets 1885
Ziac Tablets 1887

Bromocriptine Mesylate (Alters thyroid hormone or TSH levels).
No products indexed under this heading.

Carbamazepine (Alters thyroid hormone or TSH levels). Products include:
Carbatrol Capsules 3234
Tegretol/Tegretol-XR 2404

Carteolol Hydrochloride (Alters thyroid hormone or TSH levels; actions of some beta blockers may be impaired when hypothyroid patients become euthyroid). Products include:
Carteolol Hydrochloride Ophthalmic Solution USP, 1%..... ⊙258
Ocupress Ophthalmic Solution, 1% Sterile .... ⊙303

Chloral Hydrate (Alters thyroid hormone or TSH levels).
No products indexed under this heading.

Chlorothiazide (Alters thyroid hormone or TSH levels). Products include:
Aldoclor Tablets 2035
Diuril Oral 2087

Chlorothiazide Sodium (Alters thyroid hormone or TSH levels). Products include:
Diuril Sodium Intravenous 2086

Chlorotrianisene (Estrogens or estrogen-containing compounds may inhibit levothyroxine sodium binding to serum proteins or alter the concentrations of serum proteins).
No products indexed under this heading.

Chlorpropamide (Alters thyroid hormone or TSH levels; requirements of oral antidiabetic agents may be reduced in hypothyroid patients with diabetes and may be subsequently increased with initiation of thyroid hormone therapy). Products include:
Diabinese Tablets 2680

Cholestyramine (Binds and decreases absorption of levothyroxine sodium from the gastrointestinal tract).
No products indexed under this heading.

Choline Magnesium Trisalicylate (May inhibit levothyroxine sodium binding to serum proteins or alter the concentrations of serum proteins). Products include:
Trilisate 2901

Clofibrate (May inhibit levothyroxine sodium binding to serum proteins or alter the concentrations of serum proteins). Products include:
Atromid-S Capsules 3483

Clomipramine Hydrochloride (Concurrent use may increase the therapeutic and toxic effects of both drugs; onset of action of tricyclics may be accelerated).
No products indexed under this heading.

Colestipol Hydrochloride (Binds and decreases absorption of levothyroxine sodium from the gastrointestinal tract). Products include:
Colestid Tablets 2791

Cortisone Acetate (May inhibit levothyroxine sodium binding to serum proteins or alter the concentrations of serum proteins). Products include:
Cortone Acetate Injectable Suspension................................ 2059
Cortone Acetate Tablets 2061

Desipramine Hydrochloride (Concurrent use may increase the therapeutic and toxic effects of both drugs; onset of action of tricyclics may be accelerated). Products include:
Norpramin Tablets 755

Deslanoside (Therapeutic effects of digitalis glycosides may be reduced; serum digitalis levels may be decreased in hyperthyroidism or when a hypothyroid patient becomes euthyroid).
No products indexed under this heading.

Dexamethasone (May inhibit levothyroxine sodium binding to serum proteins or alter the concentrations of serum proteins). Products include:
Decadron Elixir 2078
Decadron Tablets 2079
TobraDex Ophthalmic Ointment 542
TobraDex Ophthalmic Suspension .. 541

Dexamethasone Acetate (May inhibit levothyroxine sodium binding to serum proteins or alter the concentrations of serum proteins).
No products indexed under this heading.

Dexamethasone Sodium Phosphate (May inhibit levothyroxine sodium binding to serum proteins or alter the concentrations of serum proteins). Products include:
Decadron Phosphate Injection 2081
Decadron Phosphate Sterile Ophthalmic Ointment.................. 2083
Decadron Phosphate Sterile Ophthalmic Solution.................. 2084
NeoDecadron Sterile Ophthalmic Solution.. 2144

Diatrizoate Meglumine (Alters thyroid hormone or TSH levels).
No products indexed under this heading.

Diatrizoate Sodium (Alters thyroid hormone or TSH levels).
No products indexed under this heading.

Diazepam (Alters thyroid hormone or TSH levels). Products include:
Valium Injectable 3026
Valium Tablets 3047

Dicumarol (The hypoprothrombinemic effect of anticoagulants may be potentiated).
No products indexed under this heading.

Dienestrol (Estrogens or estrogen-containing compounds may inhibit levothyroxine sodium binding to serum proteins or alter the concentrations of serum proteins). Products include:
Ortho Dienestrol Cream 2554

Diethylstilbestrol (Estrogens or estrogen-containing compounds may inhibit levothyroxine sodium binding to serum proteins or alter the concentrations of serum proteins).
No products indexed under this heading.

Diflunisal (May inhibit levothyroxine sodium binding to serum proteins or alter the concentrations of serum proteins). Products include:
Dolobid Tablets 2088

Digitoxin (Therapeutic effects of digitalis glycosides may be reduced; serum digitalis levels may be decreased in hyperthyroidism or when a hypothyroid patient becomes euthyroid).
No products indexed under this heading.

Digoxin (Therapeutic effects of digitalis glycosides may be reduced; serum digitalis levels may be decreased in hyperthyroidism or when a hypothyroid patient becomes euthyroid). Products include:
Digitek Tablets 1003
Lanoxicaps Capsules 1574
Lanoxin Injection 1581
Lanoxin Tablets 1587
Lanoxin Elixir Pediatric 1578
Lanoxin Injection Pediatric 1584

Dobutamine Hydrochloride (Possible increased risk of coronary insufficiency in patients with coronary artery disease). Products include:
Dobutrex Solution Vials 1914

Dopamine Hydrochloride (Alters thyroid hormone or TSH levels).
No products indexed under this heading.

Doxepin Hydrochloride (Concurrent use may increase the therapeutic and toxic effects of both drugs; onset of action of tricyclics may be accelerated). Products include:
Sinequan 2713

Dyphylline (Theophylline clearance may be decreased in hypothyroid patients and return toward normal when euthyroid state is achieved). Products include:
Lufyllin Tablets 3347
Lufyllin-400 Tablets 3347
Lufyllin-GG Elixir 3348
Lufyllin-GG Tablets 3348

Ephedrine Hydrochloride (Possible increased risk of coronary insufficiency in patients with coronary artery disease). Products include:

Primatene Tablets ⊡780

Ephedrine Sulfate (Possible increased risk of coronary insufficiency in patients with coronary artery disease).

No products indexed under this heading.

Ephedrine Tannate (Possible increased risk of coronary insufficiency in patients with coronary artery disease). Products include:

Rynatuss Pediatric Suspension 3353
Rynatuss Tablets 3353

Epinephrine (Possible increased risk of coronary insufficiency in patients with coronary artery disease). Products include:

Epifrin Sterile Ophthalmic Solution ⊙235
EpiPen 1236
Primatene Mist ⊡779
Xylocaine with Epinephrine Injection 653

Epinephrine Bitartrate (Possible increased risk of coronary insufficiency in patients with coronary artery disease). Products include:

Sensorcaine 643

Epinephrine Hydrochloride (Possible increased risk of coronary insufficiency in patients with coronary artery disease).

No products indexed under this heading.

Esmolol Hydrochloride (Alters thyroid hormone or TSH levels; actions of some beta blockers may be impaired when hypothyroid patients become euthyroid). Products include:

Brevibloc Injection 858

Estradiol (Estrogens or estrogen-containing compounds may inhibit levothyroxine sodium binding to serum proteins or alter the concentrations of serum proteins). Products include:

Activella Tablets 2764
Alora Transdermal System 3372
Climara Transdermal System 958
CombiPatch Transdermal System 2323
Esclim Transdermal System 3460
Estrace Vaginal Cream 3358
Estrace Tablets 3361
Estring Vaginal Ring 2811
Ortho-Prefest Tablets 2570
Vagifem Tablets 2857
Vivelle Transdermal System 2412
Vivelle-Dot Transdermal System 2416

Estrogens, Conjugated (Estrogens or estrogen-containing compounds may inhibit levothyroxine sodium binding to serum proteins or alter the concentrations of serum proteins). Products include:

Premarin Intravenous 3563
Premarin Tablets 3566
Premarin Vaginal Cream 3570
Premphase Tablets 3572
Prempro Tablets 3572

Estrogens, Esterified (Estrogens or estrogen-containing compounds may inhibit levothyroxine sodium binding to serum proteins or alter the concentrations of serum proteins). Products include:

Estratest 3252
Menest Tablets 2254

Estropipate (Estrogens or estrogen-containing compounds may inhibit levothyroxine sodium binding to serum proteins or alter the concentrations of serum proteins). Products include:

Ogen Tablets 2846
Ortho-Est Tablets 3464

Ethinyl Estradiol (Estrogens or estrogen-containing compounds may inhibit levothyroxine sodium binding to serum proteins or alter the concentrations of serum proteins). Products include:

Alesse-21 Tablets 3468
Alesse-28 Tablets 3473
Brevicon 28-Day Tablets 3380
Cyclessa Tablets 2450
Desogen Tablets 2458
Estinyl Tablets 3112
Estrostep 2627
femhrt Tablets 2635
Levlen 962
Levlite 21 Tablets 962
Levlite 28 Tablets 962
Levora Tablets 3389
Loestrin 21 Tablets 2642
Loestrin Fe Tablets 2642
Lo/Ovral Tablets 3532
Lo/Ovral-28 Tablets 3538
Low-Ogestrel-28 Tablets 3392
Microgestin Fe 1.5/30 Tablets 3407
Microgestin Fe 1/20 Tablets 3400
Mircette Tablets 2470
Modicon 2563
Necon 3415
Nordette-28 Tablets 2257
Norinyl 1 +35 28-Day Tablets 3380
Ogestrel 0.5/50-28 Tablets 3428
Ortho-Cept 21 Tablets 2546
Ortho-Cept 28 Tablets 2546
Ortho-Cyclen/Ortho Tri-Cyclen 2573
Ortho-Novum 2563
Ovcon 3364
Ovral Tablets 3551
Ovral-28 Tablets 3552
Tri-Levlen 962
Tri-Norinyl-28 Tablets 3433
Triphasil-21 Tablets 3600
Triphasil-28 Tablets 3605
Trivora Tablets 3439
Yasmin 28 Tablets 980
Zovia 3449

Ethiodized Oil (Alters thyroid hormone or TSH levels). Products include:

Ethiodol Injection 3095

Ethionamide (Alters thyroid hormone or TSH levels). Products include:

Trecator-SC Tablets 3598

Ferrous Sulfate (Binds and decreases absorption of levothyroxine sodium from the gastrointestinal tract). Products include:

Feosol Tablets 1717
Slow Fe Tablets ⊡827
Slow Fe with Folic Acid Tablets ⊡828

Fludrocortisone Acetate (May inhibit levothyroxine sodium binding to serum proteins or alter the concentrations of serum proteins). Products include:

Florinef Acetate Tablets 2250

Fluorouracil (May inhibit levothyroxine sodium binding to serum proteins or alter the concentrations of serum proteins). Products include:

Carac Cream 1222
Efudex 1733
Fluoroplex 552

Fluoxymesterone (May inhibit levothyroxine sodium binding to serum proteins or alter the concentrations of serum proteins; alters TSH or thyroid hormone levels).

No products indexed under this heading.

Fosphenytoin Sodium (Alters thyroid hormone or TSH levels). Products include:

Cerebyx Injection 2619

Furosemide (May inhibit levothyroxine sodium binding to serum proteins or alter the concentrations of serum proteins). Products include:

Furosemide Tablets 2284

Gadopentetate Dimeglumine (Alters thyroid hormone or TSH levels).

No products indexed under this heading.

Glimepiride (Alters thyroid hormone or TSH levels; requirements of oral antidiabetic agents may be reduced in hypothyroid patients with diabetes and may be subsequently increased with initiation of thyroid hormone therapy). Products include:

Amaryl Tablets 717

Glipizide (Alters thyroid hormone or TSH levels; requirements of oral antidiabetic agents may be reduced in hypothyroid patients with diabetes and may be subsequently increased with initiation of thyroid hormone therapy). Products include:

Glucotrol Tablets 2692
Glucotrol XL Extended Release Tablets 2693

Glyburide (Alters thyroid hormone or TSH levels; requirements of oral antidiabetic agents may be reduced in hypothyroid patients with diabetes and may be subsequently increased with initiation of thyroid hormone therapy). Products include:

DiaBeta Tablets 741
Glucovance Tablets 1086

Heparin Sodium (Alters thyroid hormone or TSH levels). Products include:

Heparin Lock Flush Solution 3509
Heparin Sodium Injection 3511

Hydrochlorothiazide (Alters thyroid hormone or TSH levels). Products include:

Accuretic Tablets 2614
Aldoril Tablets 2039
Atacand HCT Tablets 597
Avalide Tablets 1070
Diovan HCT Tablets 2338
Dyazide Capsules 1515
HydroDIURIL Tablets 2108
Hyzaar 2109
Inderide Tablets 3517
Inderide LA Long-Acting Capsules 3519
Lotensin HCT Tablets 2367
Maxzide 1008
Micardis HCT Tablets 1051
Microzide Capsules 3414
Moduretic Tablets 2138
Monopril HCT 1094
Prinzide Tablets 2168
Timolide Tablets 2187
Uniretic Tablets 3178
Vaseretic Tablets 2204
Zestoretic Tablets 695
Ziac Tablets 1887

Hydrocortisone (May inhibit levothyroxine sodium binding to serum proteins or alter the concentrations of serum proteins). Products include:

Anusol-HC Cream 2.5% 2237
Cipro HC Otic Suspension 540
Cortaid Intensive Therapy Cream ⊡717
Cortaid Maximum Strength Cream ⊡717
Cortisporin Ophthalmic Suspension Sterile ⊙297
Cortizone•5 ⊡699
Cortizone•10 ⊡699
Cortizone•10 Plus Creme ⊡700
Cortizone for Kids Creme ⊡699
Hydrocortone Tablets 2106
Massengill Medicated Soft Cloth Towelette ⊡753
VōSoL HC Otic Solution 3356

Hydrocortisone Acetate (May inhibit levothyroxine sodium binding to serum proteins or alter the concentrations of serum proteins). Products include:

Analpram-HC 1338
Anusol HC-1 Hydrocortisone Anti-Itch Cream ⊡689
Anusol-HC Suppositories 2238
Cortaid ⊡717
Cortifoam Rectal Foam 3170
Cortisporin-TC Otic Suspension 2246
Hydrocortone Acetate Injectable Suspension 2103
Pramosone 1343
Proctocort Suppositories 2264
ProctoFoam-HC 3177
Terra-Cortril Ophthalmic Suspension 2716

Hydrocortisone Sodium Phosphate (May inhibit levothyroxine sodium binding to serum proteins or alter the concentrations of serum proteins). Products include:

Hydrocortone Phosphate Injection, Sterile 2105

Hydrocortisone Sodium Succinate (May inhibit levothyroxine sodium binding to serum proteins or alter the concentrations of serum proteins).

No products indexed under this heading.

Hydroflumethiazide (Alters thyroid hormone or TSH levels). Products include:

Diucardin Tablets 3494

Imipramine Hydrochloride (Concurrent use may increase the therapeutic and toxic effects of both drugs; onset of action of tricyclics may be accelerated).

No products indexed under this heading.

Imipramine Pamoate (Concurrent use may increase the therapeutic and toxic effects of both drugs; onset of action of tricyclics may be accelerated).

No products indexed under this heading.

Insulin, Human, Zinc Suspension (Requirements of insulin may be reduced in hypothyroid patients with diabetes and may be subsequently increased with initiation of thyroid hormone therapy). Products include:

Humulin L, 100 Units 1937
Humulin U, 100 Units 1943
Novolin L Human Insulin 10 ml Vials 2422

Insulin, Human NPH (Requirements of insulin may be reduced in hypothyroid patients with diabetes and may be subsequently increased with initiation of thyroid hormone therapy). Products include:

Humulin N, 100 Units 1939
Humulin N NPH Pen 1940
Novolin N Human Insulin 10 ml Vials 2422
Novolin N PenFill 2423
Novolin N Prefilled Syringe Disposable Insulin Delivery System 2425

Insulin, Human Regular (Requirements of insulin may be reduced in hypothyroid patients with diabetes and may be subsequently increased with initiation of thyroid hormone therapy). Products include:

Humulin R Regular (U-500) 1943
Humulin R, 100 Units 1941
Novolin R Human Insulin 10 ml Vials 2423
Novolin R PenFill 2423
Novolin R Prefilled Syringe Disposable Insulin Delivery System 2425
Velosulin BR Human Insulin 10 ml Vials 2435

Insulin, Human Regular and Human NPH Mixture (Requirements of insulin may be reduced in hypothyroid patients with diabetes and may be subsequently increased with initiation of thyroid hormone therapy). Products include:

Humulin 50/50, 100 Units 1934
Humulin 70/30, 100 Units 1935
Humulin 70/30 Pen 1936
Novolin 70/30 Human Insulin 10 ml Vials 2421
Novolin 70/30 PenFill 2423
Novolin 70/30 Prefilled Disposable Insulin Delivery System 2425

Insulin, NPH (Requirements of insulin may be reduced in hypothyroid patients with diabetes and may be subsequently increased with initiation of thyroid hormone therapy). Products include:

Iletin II, NPH (Pork), 100 Units 1946

Insulin, Regular (Requirements of insulin may be reduced in hypothyroid patients with diabetes and may be subsequently increased with initiation of thyroid hormone therapy). Products include:

Iletin II, Regular (Pork), 100 Units 1947

Insulin, Zinc Crystals (Requirements of insulin may be reduced in hypothyroid patients with diabetes and may be subsequently increased with initiation of thyroid hormone therapy).

No products indexed under this heading.

Insulin, Zinc Suspension (Requirements of insulin may be reduced in

hypothyroid patients with diabetes and may be subsequently increased with initiation of thyroid hormone therapy). Products include:
Iletin II, Lente (Pork), 100 Units 1945

Insulin Aspart, Human Regular (Requirements of insulin may be reduced in hypothyroid patients with diabetes and may be subsequently increased with initiation of thyroid hormone therapy).
No products indexed under this heading.

Insulin glargine (Requirements of insulin may be reduced in hypothyroid patients with diabetes and may be subsequently increased with initiation of thyroid hormone therapy). Products include:
Lantus Injection 742

Insulin Lispro, Human (Requirements of insulin may be reduced in hypothyroid patients with diabetes and may be subsequently increased with initiation of thyroid hormone therapy). Products include:
Humalog 1926
Humalog Mix 75/25 Pen 1928

Insulin Lispro Protamine, Human (Requirements of insulin may be reduced in hypothyroid patients with diabetes and may be subsequently increased with initiation of thyroid hormone therapy). Products include:
Humalog Mix 75/25 Pen 1928

Interferon alfa-2A, Recombinant (Cytokines have been reported to induce both hyperthyroidism or hypothyroidism; dosage adjustment may be necessary). Products include:
Roferon-A Injection 2996

Interferon alfa-2B, Recombinant (Cytokines have been reported to induce both hyperthyroidism or hypothyroidism; dosage adjustment may be necessary). Products include:
Intron A for Injection 3120
Rebetron Combination Therapy 3153

Interferon alfa-N3 (Human Leukocyte Derived) (Cytokines have been reported to induce both hyperthyroidism or hypothyroidism; dosage adjustment may be necessary). Products include:
Alferon N Injection 1770

Interferon Beta-1b (Cytokines have been reported to induce both hyperthyroidism or hypothyroidism; dosage adjustment may be necessary). Products include:
Betaseron for SC Injection 988

Interferon Gamma-1B (Cytokines have been reported to induce both hyperthyroidism or hypothyroidism; dosage adjustment may be necessary). Products include:
Actimmune 1772

Iodamide Meglumine (Alters thyroid hormone or TSH levels).
No products indexed under this heading.

Iodinated Glycerol (Alters thyroid hormone or TSH levels).
No products indexed under this heading.

Iodine, radiolabeled (Uptake of radiolabeled ions may be decreased).

Iohexol (Alters thyroid hormone or TSH levels).
No products indexed under this heading.

Iopamidol (Alters thyroid hormone or TSH levels).
No products indexed under this heading.

Iopanoic Acid (Alters thyroid hormone or TSH levels).
No products indexed under this heading.

Iothalamate Meglumine (Alters thyroid hormone or TSH levels).
No products indexed under this heading.

Ioxaglate Meglumine (Alters thyroid hormone or TSH levels).
No products indexed under this heading.

Ioxaglate Sodium (Alters thyroid hormone or TSH levels).
No products indexed under this heading.

Isoproterenol Hydrochloride (Possible increased risk of coronary insufficiency in patients with coronary artery disease).
No products indexed under this heading.

Isoproterenol Sulfate (Possible increased risk of coronary insufficiency in patients with coronary artery disease).
No products indexed under this heading.

Ketamine Hydrochloride (Coadministration produces marked hypertension and tachycardia).
No products indexed under this heading.

Labetalol Hydrochloride (Alters thyroid hormone or TSH levels; actions of some beta blockers may be impaired when hypothyroid patients become euthyroid). Products include:
Normodyne Injection 3135
Normodyne Tablets 3137

Levalbuterol Hydrochloride (Possible increased risk of coronary insufficiency in patients with coronary artery disease). Products include:
Xopenex Inhalation Solution 3207

Levobunolol Hydrochloride (Alters thyroid hormone or TSH levels; actions of some beta blockers may be impaired when hypothyroid patients become euthyroid). Products include:
Betagan .... ⊙228

Levodopa (Alters thyroid hormone or TSH levels). Products include:
Sinemet Tablets 1253
Sinemet CR Tablets 1255

Lithium Carbonate (Blocks the TSH-mediated release of T4 and T3; thyroid function should therefore be carefully monitored during lithium initiation, stablization, and maintenence; if hypothyroidism occurs during lithium treatment, a higher than usual Synthroid dose may be required). Products include:
Eskalith 1527
Lithium Carbonate 3061
Lithobid Slow-Release Tablets 3255

Lithium Citrate (Blocks the TSH-mediated release of T4 and T3; thyroid function should therefore be carefully monitored during lithium initiation, stablization, and maintenence; if hypothyroidism occurs during lithium treatment, a higher than usual Synthroid dose may be required). Products include:
Lithium Citrate Syrup 3061

Lovastatin (Alters thyroid hormone or TSH levels). Products include:
Mevacor Tablets 2132

Magnesium Salicylate (May inhibit levothyroxine sodium binding to serum proteins or alter the concentrations of serum proteins). Products include:
Momentum Backache Relief Extra Strength Caplets .... ■666

Maprotiline Hydrochloride (Risk of cardiac arrhythmias may increase).
No products indexed under this heading.

Meclofenamate Sodium (Meclofenamic acid may inhibit levothyroxine sodium binding to serum proteins or alter the concentrations of serum proteins).
No products indexed under this heading.

Mefenamic Acid (May inhibit levothyroxine sodium binding to serum proteins or alter the concentrations of serum proteins). Products include:
Ponstel Capsules 1356

Mercaptopurine (Alters thyroid hormone or TSH levels). Products include:
Purinethol Tablets 1615

Metaproterenol Sulfate (Possible increased risk of coronary insufficiency in patients with coronary artery disease). Products include:
Alupent 1029

Metaraminol Bitartrate (Possible increased risk of coronary insufficiency in patients with coronary artery disease). Products include:
Aramine Injection 2043

Metformin Hydrochloride (Requirements of oral antidiabetic agents may be reduced in hypothyroid patients with diabetes and may be subsequently increased with initiation of thyroid hormone therapy). Products include:
Glucophage Tablets 1080
Glucophage XR Tablets 1080
Glucovance Tablets 1086

Methadone Hydrochloride (May inhibit levothyroxine sodium binding to serum proteins or alter the concentrations of serum proteins). Products include:
Dolophine Hydrochloride Tablets 3056

Methimazole (Alters thyroid hormone or TSH levels).
No products indexed under this heading.

Methoxamine Hydrochloride (Possible increased risk of coronary insufficiency in patients with coronary artery disease).
No products indexed under this heading.

Methyclothiazide (Alters thyroid hormone or TSH levels).
No products indexed under this heading.

Methylprednisolone Acetate (May inhibit levothyroxine sodium binding to serum proteins or alter the concentrations of serum proteins). Products include:
Depo-Medrol Injectable Suspension 2795

Methylprednisolone Sodium Succinate (May inhibit levothyroxine sodium binding to serum proteins or alter the concentrations of serum proteins). Products include:
Solu-Medrol Sterile Powder 2855

Methyltestosterone (May inhibit levothyroxine sodium binding to serum proteins or alter the concentrations of serum proteins; alters TSH or thyroid hormone levels). Products include:
Android Capsules, 10 mg 1731
Estratest 3252
Testred Capsules, 10 mg 1746

Metipranolol Hydrochloride (Alters thyroid hormone or TSH levels; actions of some beta blockers may be impaired when hypothyroid patients become euthyroid).
No products indexed under this heading.

Metoclopramide Hydrochloride (Alters thyroid hormone or TSH levels). Products include:
Reglan 2935

Metoprolol Succinate (Alters thyroid hormone or TSH levels; actions of some beta blockers may be impaired when hypothyroid patients become euthyroid). Products include:
Toprol-XL Tablets 651

Metoprolol Tartrate (Alters thyroid hormone or TSH levels; actions of some beta blockers may be impaired when hypothyroid patients become euthyroid).
No products indexed under this heading.

Miglitol (Requirements of oral antidiabetic agents may be reduced in hypothyroid patients with diabetes and may be subsequently increased with initiation of thyroid hormone therapy). Products include:
Glyset Tablets 2821

Mitotane (Alters thyroid hormone or TSH levels).
No products indexed under this heading.

Nadolol (Alters thyroid hormone or TSH levels; actions of some beta blockers may be impaired when hypothyroid patients become euthyroid). Products include:
Corgard Tablets 2245
Corzide 40/5 Tablets 2247
Corzide 80/5 Tablets 2247
Nadolol Tablets 2288

Norepinephrine Bitartrate (Possible increased risk of coronary insufficiency in patients with coronary artery disease).
No products indexed under this heading.

Nortriptyline Hydrochloride (Concurrent use may increase the therapeutic and toxic effects of both drugs; onset of action of tricyclics may be accelerated).
No products indexed under this heading.

Octreotide Acetate (Alters thyroid hormone or TSH levels). Products include:
Sandostatin LAR Depot 2395

Oxandrolone (May inhibit levothyroxine sodium binding to serum proteins or alter the concentrations of serum proteins; alters TSH or thyroid hormone levels). Products include:
Oxandrin Tablets 1153

Oxymetholone (May inhibit levothyroxine sodium binding to serum proteins or alter the concentrations of serum proteins; alters TSH or thyroid hormone levels). Products include:
Anadrol-50 Tablets 3321

Penbutolol Sulfate (Alters thyroid hormone or TSH levels; actions of some beta blockers may be impaired when hypothyroid patients become euthyroid).
No products indexed under this heading.

Pergolide Mesylate (Alters thyroid hormone or TSH levels). Products include:
Permax Tablets 1299

Perphenazine (May inhibit levothyroxine sodium binding to serum proteins or alter the concentrations of serum proteins). Products include:
Etrafon 3115
Trilafon 3160

Phenobarbital (Alters thyroid hormone or TSH levels). Products include:
Arco-Lase Plus Tablets 592
Donnatal 2929
Donnatal Extentabs 2930

Phenylbutazone (May inhibit levothyroxine sodium binding to serum proteins or alter the concentrations of serum proteins; alters thyroid hormone or TSH levels).
No products indexed under this heading.

Phenylephrine Bitartrate (Possible increased risk of coronary insufficiency in patients with coronary artery disease).
No products indexed under this heading.

Phenylephrine Hydrochloride (Possible increased risk of coronary

insufficiency in patients with coronary artery disease). Products include:
- Afrin Nasal Decongestant Children's Pump Mist 734
- Extendryl 1361
- Hycomine Compound Tablets 1317
- Neo-Synephrine 614
- Phenergan VC Syrup 3560
- Phenergan VC with Codeine Syrup .. 3561
- Preparation H Cream 778
- Preparation H Cooling Gel 778
- Preparation H 778
- Vicks Sinex Nasal Spray and Ultra Fine Mist 729

Phenylephrine Tannate (Possible increased risk of coronary insufficiency in patients with coronary artery disease). Products include:
- Ryna-12 S Suspension 3351
- Reformulated Rynatan Pediatric Suspension 3352
- Rynatuss Pediatric Suspension 3353
- Rynatuss Tablets 3353

Phenylpropanolamine Hydrochloride (Possible increased risk of coronary insufficiency in patients with coronary artery disease).
- No products indexed under this heading.

Phenytoin (May inhibit levothyroxine sodium binding to serum proteins or alter the concentrations of serum proteins; alters thyroid hormone or TSH levels). Products include:
- Dilantin Infatabs 2624
- Dilantin-125 Oral Suspension 2625

Phenytoin Sodium (May inhibit levothyroxine sodium binding to serum proteins or alter the concentrations of serum proteins; alters thyroid hormone or TSH levels). Products include:
- Dilantin Kapseals 2622

Pindolol (Alters thyroid hormone or TSH levels; actions of some beta blockers may be impaired when hypothyroid patients become euthyroid).
- No products indexed under this heading.

Pioglitazone Hydrochloride (Requirements of oral antidiabetic agents may be reduced in hypothyroid patients with diabetes and may be subsequently increased with initiation of thyroid hormone therapy). Products include:
- Actos Tablets 3275

Pirbuterol Acetate (Possible increased risk of coronary insufficiency in patients with coronary artery disease). Products include:
- Maxair Autohaler 1981
- Maxair Inhaler 1984

Polyestradiol Phosphate (Estrogens or estrogen-containing compounds may inhibit levothyroxine sodium binding to serum proteins or alter the concentrations of serum proteins).
- No products indexed under this heading.

Polythiazide (Alters thyroid hormone or TSH levels). Products include:
- Minizide Capsules 2700
- Renese Tablets 2712

Pramipexole Dihydrochloride (Alters thyroid hormone or TSH levels). Products include:
- Mirapex Tablets 2834

Prednisolone Acetate (May inhibit levothyroxine sodium binding to serum proteins or alter the concentrations of serum proteins). Products include:
- Blephamide Ophthalmic Ointment .. 547
- Blephamide Ophthalmic Suspension 548
- Poly-Pred Liquifilm Ophthalmic Suspension .... ⊙ 245
- Pred Forte Ophthalmic Suspension .... ⊙ 246
- Pred Mild Sterile Ophthalmic Suspension .... ⊙ 249
- Pred-G Ophthalmic Suspension .... ⊙ 247
- Pred-G Sterile Ophthalmic Ointment .... ⊙ 248

Prednisolone Sodium Phosphate (May inhibit levothyroxine sodium binding to serum proteins or alter the concentrations of serum proteins). Products include:
- Pediapred Oral Solution 1170

Prednisolone Tebutate (May inhibit levothyroxine sodium binding to serum proteins or alter the concentrations of serum proteins).
- No products indexed under this heading.

Prednisone (May inhibit levothyroxine sodium binding to serum proteins or alter the concentrations of serum proteins). Products include:
- Prednisone 3064

Propranolol Hydrochloride (Alters thyroid hormone or TSH levels; actions of some beta blockers may be impaired when hypothyroid patients become euthyroid). Products include:
- Inderal 3513
- Inderal LA Long-Acting Capsules 3516
- Inderide Tablets 3517
- Inderide LA Long-Acting Capsules .. 3519

Protriptyline Hydrochloride (Concurrent use may increase the therapeutic and toxic effects of both drugs; onset of action of tricyclics may be accelerated). Products include:
- Vivactil Tablets 2446
- Vivactil Tablets 2217

Pseudoephedrine Hydrochloride (Possible increased risk of coronary insufficiency in patients with coronary artery disease). Products include:
- Actifed Cold & Allergy Tablets 688
- Actifed Cold & Sinus Caplets and Tablets 688
- Advil Cold and Sinus Caplets 771
- Advil Cold and Sinus Tablets 771
- Advil Flu & Body Ache Caplets 772
- Aleve Cold & Sinus Caplets 603
- Alka-Seltzer Plus Liqui-Gels 604
- Alka-Seltzer Plus Cold & Flu Medicine Liqui-Gels 604
- Alka-Seltzer Plus Cold & Sinus Medicine Liqui-Gels 604
- Allegra-D Extended-Release Tablets 714
- BC Cold Powder 619
- Benadryl Allergy/Cold Tablets 691
- Benadryl Allergy/Congestion Tablets 692
- Benadryl Allergy & Sinus Liquid 693
- Benadryl Allergy & Sinus Fastmelt Tablets 693
- Benadryl Allergy Sinus Headache Caplets & Gelcaps 693
- Benadryl Severe Allergy & Sinus Headache Caplets 694
- Benadryl Children's Allergy/Cold Fastmelt Tablets 692
- Benylin Multi-Symptom Liquid 697
- Bromfed Capsules (Extended-Release) 2269
- Bromfed-PD Capsules (Extended-Release) 2269
- Children's Cēpacol Sore Throat 788
- Comtrex Acute Head Cold & Sinus Pressure Relief Tablets 627
- Comtrex Deep Chest Cold & Congestion Relief Softgels 627
- Comtrex Flu Therapy & Fever Relief Daytime Caplets 628
- Comtrex Flu Therapy & Fever Relief Nighttime Tablets 628
- Comtrex Maximum Strength Multi-Symptom Cold & Cough Relief Tablets and Caplets 626
- Contac Non-Drowsy 12 Hour Cold Caplets 745
- Contac Non-Drowsy Timed Release 12 Hour Cold Caplets ... 746
- Contac Severe Cold and Flu Caplets Maximum Strength 746
- Contac Severe Cold and Flu Caplets Non-Drowsy 746
- Dimetapp Elixir 777
- Dimetapp Cold and Fever Suspension 775
- Dimetapp DM Cold & Cough Elixir ... 775
- Dimetapp Nighttime Flu Liquid 776
- Dimetapp Non-Drowsy Flu Syrup 777
- Dimetapp Infant Drops Decongestant 775
- Dimetapp Infant Drops Decongestant Plus Cough 776
- Guaifed 2272
- Kronofed-A 1341
- Children's Motrin Cold Oral Suspension 2007
- Motrin Sinus Headache Caplets 2005
- PediaCare Cough-Cold Liquid 719
- PediaCare Infants' Drops Decongestant 719
- PediaCare Infants' Drops Decongestant Plus Cough 719
- PediaCare NightRest Cough-Cold Liquid 719
- Robitussin Cold Caplets Cold & Congestion 780
- Robitussin Cold Softgels Cold & Congestion 780
- Robitussin Cold Caplets Multi-Symptom Cold & Flu 781
- Robitussin Cold Softgels Multi-Symptom Cold & Flu 781
- Robitussin Cold Softgels Severe Congestion 782
- Robitussin Cough & Cold Infant Drops 782
- Robitussin Maximum Strength Cough & Cold Liquid 785
- Robitussin Pediatric Cough & Cold Formula Liquid 785
- Robitussin Multi Symptom Honey Flu Liquid 785
- Robitussin Nighttime Honey Flu Liquid 786
- Robitussin-CF Liquid 783
- Robitussin-DAC Syrup 2942
- Robitussin-PE Liquid 782
- Ryna 768
- Semprex-D Capsules 1172
- Singlet Caplets 761
- Sinutab Non-Drying Liquid Caps 706
- Sinutab Sinus Allergy Medication, Maximum Strength Formula, Tablets & Caplets 707
- Sinutab Sinus Medication, Maximum Strength Without Drowsiness Formula, Tablets & Caplets 707
- Sudafed 12 Hour Tablets 708
- Sudafed 24 Hour Tablets 708
- Children's Sudafed Cold & Cough Liquid 709
- Children's Sudafed Nasal Decongestant Chewables 711
- Children's Sudafed Nasal Decongestant Liquid Medication 711
- Sudafed Cold & Allergy Tablets 708
- Sudafed Cold & Cough Liquid Caps 709
- Sudafed Cold & Sinus Liquid Caps 710
- Sudafed Nasal Decongestant Tablets 710
- Sudafed Non-Drying Sinus Liquid Caps 712
- Sudafed Severe Cold 711
- Sudafed Sinus Headache Caplets 712
- Sudafed Sinus Headache Tablets 712
- Tavist Sinus Non-Drowsy Coated Caplets 676
- TheraFlu Regular Strength Cold & Cough Night Time Hot Liquid 676
- TheraFlu Regular Strength Cold & Sore Throat Night Time Hot Liquid 676
- TheraFlu Maximum Strength Flu & Congestion Non-Drowsy Hot Liquid 677
- TheraFlu Maximum Strength Flu & Cough Night Time Hot Liquid 678
- TheraFlu Maximum Strength Flu & Sore Throat Night Time Hot Liquid 677
- TheraFlu Maximum Strength Severe Cold & Congestion Night Time Caplets 678
- TheraFlu Maximum Strength Severe Cold & Congestion Night Time Hot Liquid 678
- TheraFlu Maximum Strength Severe Cold & Congestion Non-Drowsy 679
- Triaminic Allergy Congestion Liquid 680
- Triaminic Chest Congestion Liquid 680
- Triaminic Cold & Allergy Liquid 681
- Triaminic Cold & Allergy Softchews 683
- Triaminic Cold & Cough Liquid 681
- Triaminic Cold & Cough Softchews 683
- Triaminic Cold & Night Time Cough Liquid 681
- Triaminic Cold, Cough & Fever Liquid 681
- Triaminic Cough Liquid 682
- Triaminic Cough & Congestion Liquid 682
- Triaminic Cough & Sore Throat Liquid 682
- Triaminic Cough & Sore Throat Softchews 684
- Children's Tylenol Allergy-D Liquid ... 2014
- Children's Tylenol Cold Suspension Liquid and Chewable Tablets 2015
- Children's Tylenol Cold Plus Cough Suspension Liquid and Chewable Tablets 2015
- Children's Tylenol Flu Suspension Liquid 2015
- Children's Tylenol Sinus Suspension Liquid 2017
- Infants' Tylenol Cold Decongestant and Fever Reducer Concentrated Drops 2015
- Infants' Tylenol Cold Decongestant and Fever Reducer Concentrated Drops Plus Cough .. 2015
- Tylenol Allergy Sinus 2010
- Multi-Symptom Tylenol Cold Complete Formula Caplets 2010
- Multi-Symptom Tylenol Cold Non-Drowsy Caplets and Gelcaps 2010
- Multi-Symptom Tylenol Cold Severe Congestion Non-Drowsy Caplets 2011
- Maximum Strength Tylenol Flu NightTime Gelcaps 2011
- Maximum Strength Tylenol Flu NightTime Liquid 2011
- Maximum Strength Tylenol Flu Non-Drowsy Gelcaps 2011
- Maximum Strength Tylenol Sinus NightTime Caplets 2012
- Maximum Strength Tylenol Sinus Non-Drowsy Geltabs, Gelcaps, Caplets, and Tablets 2012
- Vicks 44D Cough & Head Congestion Relief Liquid 724
- Vicks 44M Cough, Cold & Flu Relief Liquid 725
- Pediatric Vicks 44m Cough & Cold Relief 728
- Vicks DayQuil LiquiCaps/Liquid Multi-Symptom Cold/Flu Relief ... 727
- Children's Vicks NyQuil Cold/Cough Relief 726
- Vicks NyQuil LiquiCaps/Liquid Multi-Symptom Cold/Flu Relief, Original and Cherry Flavors 727
- Zephrex Tablets 3091
- Zephrex LA Tablets 3092
- Zyrtec-D 12 Hour Extended Relief Tablets 2758

Pseudoephedrine Sulfate (Possible increased risk of coronary insufficiency in patients with coronary artery disease). Products include:
- Chlor-Trimeton Allergy/Decongestant Tablets 736
- Claritin-D 12 Hour Extended Release Tablets 3102
- Claritin-D 24 Hour Extended Release Tablets 3104
- Coricidin 'D' Cold, Flu & Sinus Tablets 737
- Drixoral Allergy/Sinus Extended-Release Tablets 741
- Drixoral Cold & Allergy Sustained-Action Tablets 740
- Drixoral Cold & Flu Extended-Release Tablets 740
- Drixoral Nasal Decongestant Long-Acting Non-Drowsy Tablets 740
- Rynatan Tablets 3351

Quinestrol (Estrogens or estrogen-containing compounds may inhibit levothyroxine sodium binding to serum proteins or alter the concentrations of serum proteins).
- No products indexed under this heading.

Repaglinide (Requirements of oral antidiabetic agents may be reduced in hypothyroid patients with diabetes and may be subsequently increased with initiation of thyroid hormone therapy). Products include:
- Prandin Tablets (0.5, 1, and 2 mg) 2432

Resorcinol (Alters thyroid hormone or TSH levels).
- No products indexed under this heading.

IMPORTANT NOTE: Always consult each drug listing in the patient's regimen for possible interactions.

Rifampin (Alters thyroid hormone or TSH levels). Products include:
Rifadin ... 765
Rifamate Capsules ... 767
Rifater Tablets ... 769
Rifapentine (Alters thyroid hormone or TSH levels). Products include:
Priftin Tablets ... 758
Ropinirole Hydrochloride (Alters thyroid hormone or TSH levels). Products include:
Requip Tablets ... 1621
Rosiglitazone Maleate (Requirements of oral antidiabetic agents may be reduced in hypothyroid patients with diabetes and may be subsequently increased with initiation of thyroid hormone therapy). Products include:
Avandia Tablets ... 1490
Salmeterol Xinafoate (Possible increased risk of coronary insufficiency in patients with coronary artery disease). Products include:
Advair Diskus 100/50 ... 1448
Advair Diskus 250/50 ... 1448
Advair Diskus 500/50 ... 1448
Serevent Diskus ... 1637
Serevent Inhalation Aerosol ... 1633
Salsalate (May inhibit levothyroxine sodium binding to serum proteins or alter the concentrations of serum proteins).
No products indexed under this heading.
Sodium Iodide I 123 (Uptake of radiolabeled ions may be decreased).
No products indexed under this heading.
Sodium Iodide I 131 (Uptake of radiolabeled ions may be decreased).
No products indexed under this heading.
Sodium Nitroprusside (Alters thyroid hormone or TSH levels).
No products indexed under this heading.
Sodium Pertechnetate (Alters thyroid hormone or TSH levels).
No products indexed under this heading.
Sodium Polystyrene Sulfonate (Binds and decreases absorption of levothyroxine sodium from the gastrointestinal tract).
No products indexed under this heading.
Somatrem (Excessive concurrent use of thyroid hormone may accelerate epiphyseal closure; untreated hypothyroidism may interfere with the growth response to somatrem).
No products indexed under this heading.
Somatropin (Excessive concurrent use of thyroid hormone may accelerate epiphyseal closure; untreated hypothyroidism may interfere with the growth response to somatrem). Products include:
Genotropin Lyophilized Powder ... 2818
Humatrope Vials and Cartridges ... 1930
Norditropin Cartridges ... 2420
Norditropin for Injection ... 2419
Nutropin AQ Injection ... 1420
Nutropin Depot for Injectable Suspension ... 1423
Nutropin for Injection ... 1417
Saizen for Injection ... 3225
Serostim for Injection ... 3229
Sotalol Hydrochloride (Alters thyroid hormone or TSH levels; actions of some beta blockers may be impaired when hypothyroid patients become euthyroid). Products include:
Betapace Tablets ... 950
Betapace AF Tablets ... 954
Stanozolol (May inhibit levothyroxine sodium binding to serum proteins or alter the concentrations of serum proteins; alters TSH or thyroid hormone levels).
No products indexed under this heading.
Sucralfate (Binds and decreases absorption of levothyroxine sodium from the gastrointestinal tract). Products include:
Carafate Suspension ... 731
Carafate Tablets ... 730
Sulfacytine (Alters thyroid hormone or TSH levels).
Sulfamethizole (Alters thyroid hormone or TSH levels). Products include:
Urobiotic-250 Capsules ... 2731
Sulfamethoxazole (Alters thyroid hormone or TSH levels). Products include:
Bactrim ... 2949
Septra Suspension ... 2265
Septra Tablets ... 2265
Septra DS Tablets ... 2265
Sulfasalazine (Alters thyroid hormone or TSH levels). Products include:
Azulfidine EN-tabs Tablets ... 2775
Sulfinpyrazone (Alters thyroid hormone or TSH levels).
No products indexed under this heading.
Sulfisoxazole (Alters thyroid hormone or TSH levels).
No products indexed under this heading.
Sulfisoxazole Acetyl (Alters thyroid hormone or TSH levels). Products include:
Pediazole Suspension ... 3050
Sulfisoxazole Diolamine (Alters thyroid hormone or TSH levels).
No products indexed under this heading.
Tamoxifen Citrate (May inhibit levothyroxine sodium binding to serum proteins or alter the concentrations of serum proteins). Products include:
Nolvadex Tablets ... 678
Terbutaline Sulfate (Possible increased risk of coronary insufficiency in patients with coronary artery disease). Products include:
Brethine Ampuls ... 2314
Brethine Tablets ... 2313
Theophylline (Theophylline clearance may be decreased in hypothyroid patients and return toward normal when euthyroid state is achieved). Products include:
Aerolate ... 1361
Theo-Dur Extended-Release Tablets ... 1835
Uni-Dur Extended-Release Tablets ... 1841
Uniphyl 400 mg and 600 mg Tablets ... 2903
Theophylline Calcium Salicylate (Theophylline clearance may be decreased in hypothyroid patients and return toward normal when euthyroid state is achieved).
No products indexed under this heading.
Theophylline Sodium Glycinate (Theophylline clearance may be decreased in hypothyroid patients and return toward normal when euthyroid state is achieved).
No products indexed under this heading.
Timolol Hemihydrate (Alters thyroid hormone or TSH levels; actions of some beta blockers may be impaired when hypothyroid patients become euthyroid). Products include:
Betimol Ophthalmic Solution ... ⊙324
Timolol Maleate (Alters thyroid hormone or TSH levels; actions of some beta blockers may be impaired when hypothyroid patients become euthyroid). Products include:
Blocadren Tablets ... 2046
Cosopt Sterile Ophthalmic Solution ... 2065
Timolide Tablets ... 2187
Timolol GFS ... ⊙266
Timoptic in Ocudose ... 2192
Timoptic Sterile Ophthalmic Solution ... 2190
Timoptic-XE Sterile Ophthalmic Gel Forming Solution ... 2194
Tolazamide (Alters thyroid hormone or TSH levels; requirements of oral antidiabetic agents may be reduced in hypothyroid patients with diabetes and may be subsequently increased with initiation of thyroid hormone therapy).
No products indexed under this heading.
Tolbutamide (Alters thyroid hormone or TSH levels; requirements of oral antidiabetic agents may be reduced in hypothyroid patients with diabetes and may be subsequently increased with initiation of thyroid hormone therapy).
No products indexed under this heading.
Triamcinolone (May inhibit levothyroxine sodium binding to serum proteins or alter the concentrations of serum proteins).
No products indexed under this heading.
Triamcinolone Acetonide (May inhibit levothyroxine sodium binding to serum proteins or alter the concentrations of serum proteins). Products include:
Azmacort Inhalation Aerosol ... 728
Nasacort Nasal Inhaler ... 750
Nasacort AQ Nasal Spray ... 752
Tri-Nasal Spray ... 2274
Triamcinolone Diacetate (May inhibit levothyroxine sodium binding to serum proteins or alter the concentrations of serum proteins).
No products indexed under this heading.
Triamcinolone Hexacetonide (May inhibit levothyroxine sodium binding to serum proteins or alter the concentrations of serum proteins).
No products indexed under this heading.
Trimipramine Maleate (Concurrent use may increase the therapeutic and toxic effects of both drugs; onset of action of tricyclics may be accelerated). Products include:
Surmontil Capsules ... 3595
Troglitazone (Requirements of oral antidiabetic agents may be reduced in hypothyroid patients with diabetes and may be subsequently increased with initiation of thyroid hormone therapy).
No products indexed under this heading.
Tyropanoate Sodium (Alters thyroid hormone or TSH levels).
No products indexed under this heading.
Warfarin Sodium (The hypoprothrombinemic effect of anticoagulants may be potentiated). Products include:
Coumadin for Injection ... 1243
Coumadin Tablets ... 1243
Warfarin Sodium Tablets, USP ... 3302

Food Interactions

Soybean Formula, Children's (Binds and decreases absorption of levothyroxine sodium from the gastrointestinal tract).

SYNVISC

(Hylan G-F 20) ... 3596
May interact with:

Quaternary Aluminum Salts (Hyaluronan can precipitate in the presence of disinfectants containing quaternary aluminum salts; concurrent use should be avoided).
No products indexed under this heading.

SYPRINE CAPSULES

(Trientine Hydrochloride) ... 2186
None cited in PDR database.

SYSTEM 3-4-3 CAPSULES

(Allium sativum, Echinacea, Herbals, Multiple, Herbals with Vitamins & Minerals, Lactobacillus Acidophilus, Psyllium Preparations, Senna) ... ■800
None cited in PDR database.

TABLOID TABLETS

(Thioguanine) ... 1642
May interact with cytotoxic drugs and certain other agents. Compounds in these categories include:

Bleomycin Sulfate (Combination therapy may produce hepatic disease).
No products indexed under this heading.
Busulfan (Potential for esophageal varices associated with abnormal liver function tests). Products include:
Myleran Tablets ... 1603
Cyclophosphamide (Combination therapy may produce hepatic disease).
No products indexed under this heading.
Daunorubicin Hydrochloride (Combination therapy may produce hepatic disease). Products include:
Cerubidine for Injection ... 947
Doxorubicin Hydrochloride (Combination therapy may produce hepatic disease). Products include:
Adriamycin PFS/RDF Injection ... 2767
Doxil Injection ... 566
Epirubicin Hydrochloride (Combination therapy may produce hepatic disease). Products include:
Ellence Injection ... 2806
Fluorouracil (Combination therapy may produce hepatic disease). Products include:
Carac Cream ... 1222
Efudex ... 1733
Fluoroplex ... 552
Hydroxyurea (Combination therapy may produce hepatic disease). Products include:
Mylocel Tablets ... 2227
Mercaptopurine (Complete cross-resistance). Products include:
Purinethol Tablets ... 1615
Methotrexate Sodium (Combination therapy may produce hepatic disease).
No products indexed under this heading.
Mitotane (Combination therapy may produce hepatic disease).
No products indexed under this heading.
Mitoxantrone Hydrochloride (Combination therapy may produce hepatic disease). Products include:
Novantrone for Injection ... 1760
Procarbazine Hydrochloride (Combination therapy may produce hepatic disease). Products include:
Matulane Capsules ... 3246
Tamoxifen Citrate (Combination therapy may produce hepatic disease). Products include:
Nolvadex Tablets ... 678
Vincristine Sulfate (Combination therapy may produce hepatic disease).
No products indexed under this heading.

TAGAMET HB 200 SUSPENSION

(Cimetidine) ... ■762
See Tagamet HB 200 Tablets

TAGAMET HB 200 TABLETS

(Cimetidine) 761

May interact with dihydropyridine calcium channel blockers, theophylline, and certain other agents. Compounds in these categories include:

Aminophylline (Increased AUC of theophylline by 14% and peak levels by 15% when used concurrently at the maximum recommended OTC dose level; clinically significant pharmacokinetic interactions have been reported at prescription doses).
- No products indexed under this heading.

Amlodipine Besylate (Clinically significant pharmacokinetic interactions have been reported with concurrent use at prescription doses of cimetidine; patients are advised to consult their physician). Products include:
- Lotrel Capsules 2370
- Norvasc Tablets 2704

Dyphylline (Increased AUC of theophylline by 14% and peak levels by 15% when used concurrently at the maximum recommended OTC dose level; clinically significant pharmacokinetic interactions have been reported at prescription doses). Products include:
- Lufyllin Tablets 3347
- Lufyllin-400 Tablets 3347
- Lufyllin-GG Elixir 3348
- Lufyllin-GG Tablets 3348

Felodipine (Clinically significant pharmacokinetic interactions have been reported with concurrent use at prescription doses of cimetidine; patients are advised to consult their physician). Products include:
- Lexxel Tablets 608
- Plendil Extended-Release Tablets 623

Isradipine (Clinically significant pharmacokinetic interactions have been reported with concurrent use at prescription doses of cimetidine; patients are advised to consult their physician). Products include:
- DynaCirc Capsules 2921
- DynaCirc CR Tablets 2923

Nicardipine Hydrochloride (Clinically significant pharmacokinetic interactions have been reported with concurrent use at prescription doses of cimetidine; patients are advised to consult their physician). Products include:
- Cardene I.V. 3485

Nifedipine (Clinically significant pharmacokinetic interactions have been reported with concurrent use at prescription doses of cimetidine; patients are advised to consult their physician). Products include:
- Adalat CC Tablets 877
- Procardia Capsules 2708
- Procardia XL Extended Release Tablets 2710

Nimodipine (Clinically significant pharmacokinetic interactions have been reported with concurrent use at prescription doses of cimetidine; patients are advised to consult their physician). Products include:
- Nimotop Capsules 904

Phenytoin (Clinically significant pharmacokinetic interactions have been reported with concurrent use at prescription doses of cimetidine; patients are advised to consult their physician). Products include:
- Dilantin Infatabs 2624
- Dilantin-125 Oral Suspension 2625

Phenytoin Sodium (Clinically significant pharmacokinetic interactions have been reported with concurrent use at prescription doses of cimetidine; patients are advised to consult their physician). Products include:
- Dilantin Kapseals 2622

Theophylline (Increased AUC of theophylline by 14% and peak levels by 15% when used concurrently at the maximum recommended OTC dose level; clinically significant pharmacokinetic interactions have been reported at prescription doses). Products include:
- Aerolate 1361
- Theo-Dur Extended-Release Tablets 1835
- Uni-Dur Extended-Release Tablets .. 1841
- Uniphyl 400 mg and 600 mg Tablets 2903

Theophylline Calcium Salicylate (Increased AUC of theophylline by 14% and peak levels by 15% when used concurrently at the maximum recommended OTC dose level; clinically significant pharmacokinetic interactions have been reported at prescription doses).
- No products indexed under this heading.

Theophylline Sodium Glycinate (Increased AUC of theophylline by 14% and peak levels by 15% when used concurrently at the maximum recommended OTC dose level; clinically significant pharmacokinetic interactions have been reported at prescription doses).
- No products indexed under this heading.

Triazolam (Potential for increased AUC of triazolam by 26-28% and increased peak levels by 11-23%). Products include:
- Halcion Tablets 2823

Warfarin Sodium (Clinically significant pharmacokinetic interactions have been reported with concurrent use at prescription doses of cimetidine; patients are advised to consult their physician). Products include:
- Coumadin for Injection 1243
- Coumadin Tablets 1243
- Warfarin Sodium Tablets, USP 3302

TAGAMET INJECTION

(Cimetidine Hydrochloride) 1644

See Tagamet Tablets

TAGAMET LIQUID

(Cimetidine Hydrochloride) 1644

See Tagamet Tablets

TAGAMET TABLETS

(Cimetidine) 1644

May interact with antacids, oral anticoagulants, tricyclic antidepressants, theophylline, and certain other agents. Compounds in these categories include:

Aluminum Carbonate (Simultaneous administration is not recommended since antacids may interfere with the absorption of cimetidine).
- No products indexed under this heading.

Aluminum Hydroxide (Simultaneous administration is not recommended since antacids may interfere with the absorption of cimetidine). Products include:
- Amphojel Suspension (Mint Flavor) 789
- Gaviscon Extra Strength Liquid 751
- Gaviscon Extra Strength Tablets 751
- Gaviscon Regular Strength Liquid .. 751
- Gaviscon Regular Strength Tablets 750
- Maalox Antacid/Anti-Gas Oral Suspension 673
- Maalox Max Maximum Strength Antacid/Anti-Gas Liquid 2300
- Maalox Regular Strength Antacid/Antigas Liquid 2300
- Mylanta 1813
- Vanquish Caplets 617

Aminophylline (Reduces hepatic metabolism of theophylline resulting in delayed elimination and increased blood levels of theophylline).
- No products indexed under this heading.

Amitriptyline Hydrochloride (Reduces hepatic metabolism of certain unspecified tricyclic antidepressants resulting in delayed elimination and increased blood levels of these drugs). Products include:
- Etrafon 3115
- Limbitrol 1738

Amoxapine (Reduces hepatic metabolism of certain unspecified tricyclic antidepressants resulting in delayed elimination and increased blood levels of these drugs).
- No products indexed under this heading.

Chlordiazepoxide (Reduces hepatic metabolism of chlordiazepoxide resulting in delayed elimination and increased blood levels of chlordiazepoxide). Products include:
- Limbitrol 1738

Chlordiazepoxide Hydrochloride (Reduces hepatic metabolism of chlordiazepoxide resulting in delayed elimination and increased blood levels of chlordiazepoxide). Products include:
- Librium Capsules 1736
- Librium for Injection 1737

Clomipramine Hydrochloride (Reduces hepatic metabolism of certain unspecified tricyclic antidepressants resulting in delayed elimination and increased blood levels of these drugs).
- No products indexed under this heading.

Desipramine Hydrochloride (Reduces hepatic metabolism of certain unspecified tricyclic antidepressants resulting in delayed elimination and increased blood levels of these drugs). Products include:
- Norpramin Tablets 755

Diazepam (Reduces hepatic metabolism of diazepam resulting in delayed elimination and increased blood levels of diazepam). Products include:
- Valium Injectable 3026
- Valium Tablets 3047

Dicumarol (Reduces hepatic metabolism of warfarin-type anticoagulants resulting in clinically significant effects; close monitoring of prothrombin time of these recommended).
- No products indexed under this heading.

Doxepin Hydrochloride (Reduces hepatic metabolism of certain unspecified tricyclic antidepressants resulting in delayed elimination and increased blood levels of these drugs). Products include:
- Sinequan 2713

Dyphylline (Reduces hepatic metabolism of theophylline resulting in delayed elimination and increased blood levels of theophylline). Products include:
- Lufyllin Tablets 3347
- Lufyllin-400 Tablets 3347
- Lufyllin-GG Elixir 3348
- Lufyllin-GG Tablets 3348

Imipramine Hydrochloride (Reduces hepatic metabolism of certain unspecified tricyclic antidepressants resulting in delayed elimination and increased blood levels of these drugs).
- No products indexed under this heading.

Imipramine Pamoate (Reduces hepatic metabolism of certain unspecified tricyclic antidepressants resulting in delayed elimination and increased blood levels of these drugs).
- No products indexed under this heading.

Ketoconazole (Alteration of pH may affect absorption of ketoconazole; administer oral ketoconazole at least 2 hours before cimetidine). Products include:
- Nizoral 2% Cream 3620
- Nizoral A-D Shampoo 2008
- Nizoral 2% Shampoo 2007
- Nizoral Tablets 1791

Lidocaine Hydrochloride (Reduces hepatic metabolism of lidocaine resulting in delayed elimination and increased blood levels of lidocaine). Products include:
- Bactine First Aid Liquid 611
- Xylocaine Injections 653

Magaldrate (Simultaneous administration is not recommended since antacids may interfere with the absorption of cimetidine).
- No products indexed under this heading.

Magnesium Hydroxide (Simultaneous administration is not recommended since antacids may interfere with the absorption of cimetidine). Products include:
- Ex•Lax Milk of Magnesia Liquid 670
- Maalox Antacid/Anti-Gas Oral Suspension 673
- Maalox Max Maximum Strength Antacid/Anti-Gas Liquid 2300
- Maalox Regular Strength Antacid/Antigas Liquid 2300
- Mylanta Fast-Acting 1813
- Mylanta 1813
- Pepcid Complete Chewable Tablets 1815
- Phillips' Chewable Tablets 615
- Phillips' Milk of Magnesia Liquid (Original, Cherry, & Mint) 616
- Rolaids Tablets 706
- Extra Strength Rolaids Tablets 706
- Vanquish Caplets 617

Magnesium Oxide (Simultaneous administration is not recommended since antacids may interfere with the absorption of cimetidine). Products include:
- Beelith Tablets 946
- Mag-Ox 400 Tablets 1024
- Uro-Mag Capsules 1024

Maprotiline Hydrochloride (Reduces hepatic metabolism of certain unspecified tricyclic antidepressants resulting in delayed elimination and increased blood levels of these drugs).
- No products indexed under this heading.

Metronidazole (Reduces hepatic metabolism of metronidazole resulting in delayed elimination and increased blood levels of metronidazole). Products include:
- MetroCream 1404
- MetroGel 1405
- MetroGel-Vaginal Gel 1986
- MetroLotion 1405
- Noritate Cream 1224

Metronidazole Hydrochloride (Reduces hepatic metabolism of metronidazole resulting in delayed elimination and increased blood levels of metronidazole).
- No products indexed under this heading.

Nifedipine (Reduces hepatic metabolism of nifedipine resulting in delayed elimination and increased blood levels of nifedipine). Products include:
- Adalat CC Tablets 877
- Procardia Capsules 2708
- Procardia XL Extended Release Tablets 2710

Nortriptyline Hydrochloride (Reduces hepatic metabolism of certain unspecified tricyclic antidepressants resulting in delayed elimination and increased blood levels of these drugs).
- No products indexed under this heading.

Phenytoin (Reduces hepatic metabolism of phenytoin resulting in delayed elimination and increased blood levels of phenytoin). Products include:
- Dilantin Infatabs 2624
- Dilantin-125 Oral Suspension 2625

Phenytoin Sodium (Reduces hepatic metabolism of phenytoin

IMPORTANT NOTE: Always consult each drug listing in the patient's regimen for possible interactions.

resulting in delayed elimination and increased blood levels of phenytoin). Products include:
- Dilantin Kapseals 2622

Propranolol Hydrochloride (Reduces hepatic metabolism of propranolol resulting in delayed elimination and increased blood levels of propranolol). Products include:
- Inderal 3513
- Inderal LA Long-Acting Capsules 3516
- Inderide Tablets 3517
- Inderide LA Long-Acting Capsules .. 3519

Protriptyline Hydrochloride (Reduces hepatic metabolism of certain unspecified tricyclic antidepressants resulting in delayed elimination and increased blood levels of these drugs). Products include:
- Vivactil Tablets 2446
- Vivactil Tablets 2217

Sodium Bicarbonate (Simultaneous administration is not recommended since antacids may interfere with the absorption of cimetidine). Products include:
- Alka-Seltzer .... ▣603
- Alka-Seltzer Lemon Lime Antacid and Pain Reliever Effervescent Tablets .... ▣603
- Alka-Seltzer Extra Strength Antacid and Pain Reliever Effervescent Tablets .... ▣603
- Alka-Seltzer Heartburn Relief Tablets .... ▣604
- Ceo-Two Evacuant Suppository .... ▣618
- Colyte with Flavor Packs for Oral Solution 3170
- GoLYTELY and Pineapple Flavor GoLYTELY for Oral Solution 1068
- NuLYTELY, Cherry Flavor, Lemon-Lime Flavor, and Orange Flavor NuLYTELY for Oral Solution 1068

Theophylline (Reduces hepatic metabolism of theophylline resulting in delayed elimination and increased blood levels of theophylline). Products include:
- Aerolate 1361
- Theo-Dur Extended-Release Tablets 1835
- Uni-Dur Extended-Release Tablets .. 1841
- Uniphyl 400 mg and 600 mg Tablets 2903

Theophylline Calcium Salicylate (Reduces hepatic metabolism of theophylline resulting in delayed elimination and increased blood levels of theophylline).
- No products indexed under this heading.

Theophylline Sodium Glycinate (Reduces hepatic metabolism of theophylline resulting in delayed elimination and increased blood levels of theophylline).
- No products indexed under this heading.

Trimipramine Maleate (Reduces hepatic metabolism of certain unspecified tricyclic antidepressants resulting in delayed elimination and increased blood levels of these drugs). Products include:
- Surmontil Capsules 3595

Warfarin Sodium (Reduces hepatic metabolism of warfarin-type anticoagulants resulting in clinically significant effects; close monitoring of prothrombin time of these recommended). Products include:
- Coumadin for Injection 1243
- Coumadin Tablets 1243
- Warfarin Sodium Tablets, USP 3302

TALACEN CAPLETS

(Pentazocine Hydrochloride) 3089

May interact with central nervous system depressants, narcotic analgesics, and certain other agents. Compounds in these categories include:

Alfentanil Hydrochloride (Potential for withdrawal symptoms; additive CNS depressant effects).
- No products indexed under this heading.

Alprazolam (Additive CNS depressant effects). Products include:
- Xanax Tablets 2865

Aprobarbital (Additive CNS depressant effects).
- No products indexed under this heading.

Buprenorphine Hydrochloride (Potential for withdrawal symptoms; additive CNS depressant effects). Products include:
- Buprenex Injectable 2918

Buspirone Hydrochloride (Additive CNS depressant effects).
- No products indexed under this heading.

Butabarbital (Additive CNS depressant effects).
- No products indexed under this heading.

Butalbital (Additive CNS depressant effects). Products include:
- Phrenilin 578
- Sedapap Tablets 50 mg/650 mg ... 2225

Chlordiazepoxide (Additive CNS depressant effects). Products include:
- Limbitrol 1738

Chlordiazepoxide Hydrochloride (Additive CNS depressant effects). Products include:
- Librium Capsules 1736
- Librium for Injection 1737

Chlorpromazine (Additive CNS depressant effects). Products include:
- Thorazine Suppositories 1656

Chlorpromazine Hydrochloride (Additive CNS depressant effects). Products include:
- Thorazine 1656

Chlorprothixene (Additive CNS depressant effects).
- No products indexed under this heading.

Chlorprothixene Hydrochloride (Additive CNS depressant effects).
- No products indexed under this heading.

Chlorprothixene Lactate (Additive CNS depressant effects).
- No products indexed under this heading.

Clorazepate Dipotassium (Additive CNS depressant effects). Products include:
- Tranxene 511

Clozapine (Potential for withdrawal symptoms; additive CNS depressant effects). Products include:
- Clozaril Tablets 2319

Codeine Phosphate (Potential for withdrawal symptoms; additive CNS depressant effects). Products include:
- Phenergan with Codeine Syrup 3557
- Phenergan VC with Codeine Syrup .. 3561
- Robitussin A-C Syrup 2942
- Robitussin-DAC Syrup 2942
- Ryna-C Liquid .... ▣768
- Soma Compound w/Codeine Tablets 3355
- Tussi-Organidin NR Liquid 3350
- Tussi-Organidin-S NR Liquid 3350
- Tylenol with Codeine 2595

Desflurane (Potential for withdrawal symptoms; additive CNS depressant effects). Products include:
- Suprane Liquid for Inhalation 874

Dezocine (Potential for withdrawal symptoms).
- No products indexed under this heading.

Diazepam (Additive CNS depressant effects). Products include:
- Valium Injectable 3026
- Valium Tablets 3047

Diphenoxylate Hydrochloride (Potential for withdrawal symptoms).
- No products indexed under this heading.

Droperidol (Additive CNS depressant effects).
- No products indexed under this heading.

Enflurane (Additive CNS depressant effects).
- No products indexed under this heading.

Estazolam (Potential for withdrawal symptoms; additive CNS depressant effects). Products include:
- ProSom Tablets 500

Ethchlorvynol (Additive CNS depressant effects).
- No products indexed under this heading.

Ethinamate (Additive CNS depressant effects).
- No products indexed under this heading.

Fentanyl (Potential for withdrawal symptoms). Products include:
- Duragesic Transdermal System 1786

Fentanyl Citrate (Potential for withdrawal symptoms; additive CNS depressant effects). Products include:
- Actiq 1184

Fluphenazine Decanoate (Additive CNS depressant effects).
- No products indexed under this heading.

Fluphenazine Enanthate (Additive CNS depressant effects).
- No products indexed under this heading.

Fluphenazine Hydrochloride (Additive CNS depressant effects).
- No products indexed under this heading.

Flurazepam Hydrochloride (Additive CNS depressant effects).
- No products indexed under this heading.

Glutethimide (Additive CNS depressant effects).
- No products indexed under this heading.

Haloperidol (Additive CNS depressant effects). Products include:
- Haldol Injection, Tablets and Concentrate 2533

Haloperidol Decanoate (Additive CNS depressant effects). Products include:
- Haldol Decanoate 2535

Hydrocodone Bitartrate (Potential for withdrawal symptoms; additive CNS depressant effects). Products include:
- Hycodan 1316
- Hycomine Compound Tablets 1317
- Hycotuss Expectorant Syrup 1318
- Lortab 3319
- Lortab Elixir 3317
- Maxidone Tablets CIII 3399
- Norco 5/325 Tablets CIII 3424
- Norco 7.5/325 Tablets CIII 3425
- Norco 10/325 Tablets CIII 3427
- Norco 10/325 Tablets CIII 3425
- Vicodin Tablets 516
- Vicodin ES Tablets 517
- Vicodin HP Tablets 518
- Vicodin Tuss Expectorant 519
- Vicoprofen Tablets 520
- Zydone Tablets 1330

Hydrocodone Polistirex (Potential for withdrawal symptoms; additive CNS depressant effects). Products include:
- Tussionex Pennkinetic Extended-Release Suspension..... 1174

Hydromorphone Hydrochloride (Potential for withdrawal symptoms; additive CNS depressant effects). Products include:
- Dilaudid 441
- Dilaudid Oral Liquid 445
- Dilaudid Powder 441
- Dilaudid Rectal Suppositories 441
- Dilaudid Tablets 441
- Dilaudid Tablets - 8 mg 445
- Dilaudid-HP 443

Hydroxyzine Hydrochloride (Additive CNS depressant effects). Products include:
- Atarax Tablets & Syrup 2667
- Vistaril Intramuscular Solution 2738

Isoflurane (Additive CNS depressant effects).
- No products indexed under this heading.

Ketamine Hydrochloride (Additive CNS depressant effects).
- No products indexed under this heading.

Levomethadyl Acetate Hydrochloride (Potential for withdrawal symptoms; additive CNS depressant effects).
- No products indexed under this heading.

Levorphanol Tartrate (Potential for withdrawal symptoms; additive CNS depressant effects). Products include:
- Levo-Dromoran 1734
- Levorphanol Tartrate Tablets 3059

Lorazepam (Additive CNS depressant effects). Products include:
- Ativan Injection 3478
- Ativan Tablets 3482

Loxapine Hydrochloride (Additive CNS depressant effects).
- No products indexed under this heading.

Loxapine Succinate (Additive CNS depressant effects). Products include:
- Loxitane Capsules 3398

Meperidine Hydrochloride (Potential for withdrawal symptoms; additive CNS depressant effects). Products include:
- Demerol 3079
- Mepergan Injection 3539

Mephobarbital (Additive CNS depressant effects).
- No products indexed under this heading.

Meprobamate (Additive CNS depressant effects). Products include:
- Miltown Tablets 3349

Mesoridazine Besylate (Additive CNS depressant effects). Products include:
- Serentil 1057

Methadone Hydrochloride (Potential for withdrawal symptoms; additive CNS depressant effects). Products include:
- Dolophine Hydrochloride Tablets 3056

Methohexital Sodium (Additive CNS depressant effects). Products include:
- Brevital Sodium for Injection, USP .. 1815

Methotrimeprazine (Potential for withdrawal symptoms; additive CNS depressant effects).
- No products indexed under this heading.

Methoxyflurane (Additive CNS depressant effects).
- No products indexed under this heading.

Midazolam Hydrochloride (Additive CNS depressant effects). Products include:
- Versed Injection 3027
- Versed Syrup 3033

Molindone Hydrochloride (Additive CNS depressant effects). Products include:
- Moban 1320

Morphine Sulfate (Potential for withdrawal symptoms; additive CNS depressant effects). Products include:
- Astramorph/PF Injection, USP (Preservative-Free) 594
- Duramorph Injection 1312
- Infumorph 200 and Infumorph 500 Sterile Solutions 1314
- Kadian Capsules 1335
- MS Contin Tablets 2896
- MSIR 2898

Oramorph SR Tablets ... 3062
Roxanol ... 3066

Olanzapine (Additive CNS depressant effects). Products include:
Zyprexa Tablets ... 1973
Zyprexa ZYDIS Orally Disintegrating Tablets ... 1973

Oxazepam (Additive CNS depressant effects).
No products indexed under this heading.

Oxycodone Hydrochloride (Potential for withdrawal symptoms; additive CNS depressant effects). Products include:
OxyContin Tablets ... 2912
OxyFast Oral Concentrate Solution ... 2916
OxyIR Capsules ... 2916
Percocet Tablets ... 1326
Percodan Tablets ... 1327
Percolone Tablets ... 1327
Roxicodone ... 3067
Tylox Capsules ... 2597

Paregoric (Potential for withdrawal symptoms).
No products indexed under this heading.

Pentobarbital Sodium (Additive CNS depressant effects). Products include:
Nembutal Sodium Solution ... 485

Perphenazine (Additive CNS depressant effects). Products include:
Etrafon ... 3115
Trilafon ... 3160

Phenobarbital (Additive CNS depressant effects). Products include:
Arco-Lase Plus Tablets ... 592
Donnatal ... 2929
Donnatal Extentabs ... 2930

Prazepam (Additive CNS depressant effects).
No products indexed under this heading.

Prochlorperazine (Additive CNS depressant effects). Products include:
Compazine ... 1505

Promethazine Hydrochloride (Potential for withdrawal symptoms; additive CNS depressant effects). Products include:
Mepergan Injection ... 3539
Phenergan Injection ... 3553
Phenergan ... 3556
Phenergan Syrup ... 3554
Phenergan with Codeine Syrup ... 3557
Phenergan with Dextromethorphan Syrup ... 3559
Phenergan VC Syrup ... 3560
Phenergan VC with Codeine Syrup ... 3561

Propofol (Additive CNS depressant effects). Products include:
Diprivan Injectable Emulsion ... 667

Propoxyphene Hydrochloride (Potential for withdrawal symptoms; additive CNS depressant effects). Products include:
Darvon Pulvules ... 1909
Darvon Compound-65 Pulvules ... 1910

Propoxyphene Napsylate (Potential for withdrawal symptoms; additive CNS depressant effects). Products include:
Darvon-N/Darvocet-N ... 1907
Darvon-N Tablets ... 1912

Quazepam (Additive CNS depressant effects).
No products indexed under this heading.

Quetiapine Fumarate (Additive CNS depressant effects). Products include:
Seroquel Tablets ... 684

Remifentanil Hydrochloride (Potential for withdrawal symptoms; additive CNS depressant effects).
No products indexed under this heading.

Risperidone (Potential for withdrawal symptoms; additive CNS depressant effects). Products include:
Risperdal ... 1796

Secobarbital Sodium (Potential for withdrawal symptoms; additive CNS depressant effects).
No products indexed under this heading.

Sevoflurane (Additive CNS depressant effects).
No products indexed under this heading.

Sufentanil Citrate (Potential for withdrawal symptoms; additive CNS depressant effects).
No products indexed under this heading.

Temazepam (Potential for withdrawal symptoms; additive CNS depressant effects).
No products indexed under this heading.

Thiamylal Sodium (Potential for withdrawal symptoms; additive CNS depressant effects).
No products indexed under this heading.

Thioridazine Hydrochloride (Potential for withdrawal symptoms; additive CNS depressant effects). Products include:
Thioridazine Hydrochloride Tablets ... 2289

Thiothixene (Potential for withdrawal symptoms; additive CNS depressant effects). Products include:
Navane Capsules ... 2701
Thiothixene Capsules ... 2290

Triazolam (Potential for withdrawal symptoms; additive CNS depressant effects). Products include:
Halcion Tablets ... 2823

Trifluoperazine Hydrochloride (Potential for withdrawal symptoms; additive CNS depressant effects). Products include:
Stelazine ... 1640

Zaleplon (Additive CNS depressant effects). Products include:
Sonata Capsules ... 3591

Ziprasidone Hydrochloride (Additive CNS depressant effects). Products include:
Geodon Capsules ... 2688

Zolpidem Tartrate (Potential for withdrawal symptoms; additive CNS depressant effects). Products include:
Ambien Tablets ... 3191

Food Interactions

Alcohol (Potential for increased CNS depressant effects).

TALWIN NX TABLETS

(Naloxone Hydrochloride, Pentazocine Hydrochloride) ... 3090

May interact with central nervous system depressants, narcotic analgesics, and certain other agents. Compounds in these categories include:

Alfentanil Hydrochloride (Pentazocine is a mild narcotic antagonist and concurrent use may lead to withdrawal symptoms; potential for additive CNS depressant properties).
No products indexed under this heading.

Alprazolam (Potential for additive CNS depressant properties). Products include:
Xanax Tablets ... 2865

Aprobarbital (Potential for additive CNS depressant properties).
No products indexed under this heading.

Buprenorphine Hydrochloride (Pentazocine is a mild narcotic antagonist and concurrent use may lead to withdrawal symptoms; potential for additive CNS depressant properties). Products include:
Buprenex Injectable ... 2918

Buspirone Hydrochloride (Potential for additive CNS depressant properties).
No products indexed under this heading.

Butabarbital (Potential for additive CNS depressant properties).
No products indexed under this heading.

Butalbital (Potential for additive CNS depressant properties). Products include:
Phrenilin ... 578
Sedapap Tablets 50 mg/650 mg ... 2225

Chlordiazepoxide (Potential for additive CNS depressant properties). Products include:
Limbitrol ... 1738

Chlordiazepoxide Hydrochloride (Potential for additive CNS depressant properties). Products include:
Librium Capsules ... 1736
Librium for Injection ... 1737

Chlorpromazine (Potential for additive CNS depressant properties). Products include:
Thorazine Suppositories ... 1656

Chlorpromazine Hydrochloride (Potential for additive CNS depressant properties). Products include:
Thorazine ... 1656

Chlorprothixene (Potential for additive CNS depressant properties).
No products indexed under this heading.

Chlorprothixene Hydrochloride (Potential for additive CNS depressant properties).
No products indexed under this heading.

Chlorprothixene Lactate (Potential for additive CNS depressant properties).
No products indexed under this heading.

Clorazepate Dipotassium (Potential for additive CNS depressant properties). Products include:
Tranxene ... 511

Clozapine (Potential for additive CNS depressant properties). Products include:
Clozaril Tablets ... 2319

Codeine Phosphate (Pentazocine is a mild narcotic antagonist and concurrent use may lead to withdrawal symptoms; potential for additive CNS depressant properties). Products include:
Phenergan with Codeine Syrup ... 3557
Phenergan VC with Codeine Syrup ... 3561
Robitussin A-C Syrup ... 2942
Robitussin-DAC Syrup ... 2942
Ryna-C Liquid ... 768
Soma Compound w/Codeine Tablets ... 3355
Tussi-Organidin NR Liquid ... 3350
Tussi-Organidin-S NR Liquid ... 3350
Tylenol with Codeine ... 2595

Desflurane (Potential for additive CNS depressant properties). Products include:
Suprane Liquid for Inhalation ... 874

Dezocine (Pentazocine is a mild narcotic antagonist and concurrent use may lead to withdrawal symptoms; potential for additive CNS depressant properties).
No products indexed under this heading.

Diazepam (Potential for additive CNS depressant properties). Products include:
Valium Injectable ... 3026
Valium Tablets ... 3047

Droperidol (Potential for additive CNS depressant properties).
No products indexed under this heading.

Enflurane (Potential for additive CNS depressant properties).
No products indexed under this heading.

Estazolam (Potential for additive CNS depressant properties). Products include:
ProSom Tablets ... 500

Ethchlorvynol (Potential for additive CNS depressant properties).
No products indexed under this heading.

Ethinamate (Potential for additive CNS depressant properties).
No products indexed under this heading.

Fentanyl (Pentazocine is a mild narcotic antagonist and concurrent use may lead to withdrawal symptoms; potential for additive CNS depressant properties). Products include:
Duragesic Transdermal System ... 1786

Fentanyl Citrate (Pentazocine is a mild narcotic antagonist and concurrent use may lead to withdrawal symptoms; potential for additive CNS depressant properties). Products include:
Actiq ... 1184

Fluphenazine Decanoate (Potential for additive CNS depressant properties).
No products indexed under this heading.

Fluphenazine Enanthate (Potential for additive CNS depressant properties).
No products indexed under this heading.

Fluphenazine Hydrochloride (Potential for additive CNS depressant properties).
No products indexed under this heading.

Flurazepam Hydrochloride (Potential for additive CNS depressant properties).
No products indexed under this heading.

Glutethimide (Potential for additive CNS depressant properties).
No products indexed under this heading.

Haloperidol (Potential for additive CNS depressant properties). Products include:
Haldol Injection, Tablets and Concentrate ... 2533

Haloperidol Decanoate (Potential for additive CNS depressant properties). Products include:
Haldol Decanoate ... 2535

Hydrocodone Bitartrate (Pentazocine is a mild narcotic antagonist and concurrent use may lead to withdrawal symptoms; potential for additive CNS depressant properties). Products include:
Hycodan ... 1316
Hycomine Compound Tablets ... 1317
Hycotuss Expectorant Syrup ... 1318
Lortab ... 3319
Lortab Elixir ... 3317
Maxidone Tablets CIII ... 3399
Norco 5/325 Tablets CIII ... 3424
Norco 7.5/325 Tablets CIII ... 3425
Norco 10/325 Tablets CIII ... 3427
Norco 10/325 Tablets CIII ... 3425
Vicodin Tablets ... 516
Vicodin ES Tablets ... 517
Vicodin HP Tablets ... 518
Vicodin Tuss Expectorant ... 519
Vicoprofen Tablets ... 520
Zydone Tablets ... 1330

Hydrocodone Polistirex (Pentazocine is a mild narcotic antagonist and concurrent use may lead to withdrawal symptoms; potential for additive CNS depressant properties). Products include:
Tussionex Pennkinetic Extended-Release Suspension ... 1174

Hydromorphone Hydrochloride (Pentazocine is a mild narcotic antagonist and concurrent use may lead to withdrawal symptoms). Products include:
Dilaudid ... 441
Dilaudid Oral Liquid ... 445
Dilaudid Powder ... 441
Dilaudid Rectal Suppositories ... 441
Dilaudid Tablets ... 441
Dilaudid Tablets - 8 mg ... 445

Dilaudid-HP ... 443

Hydroxyzine Hydrochloride (Potential for additive CNS depressant properties). Products include:
- Atarax Tablets & Syrup ... 2667
- Vistaril Intramuscular Solution ... 2738

Isoflurane (Potential for additive CNS depressant properties).
No products indexed under this heading.

Ketamine Hydrochloride (Potential for additive CNS depressant properties).
No products indexed under this heading.

Levomethadyl Acetate Hydrochloride (Potential for additive CNS depressant properties).
No products indexed under this heading.

Levorphanol Tartrate (Pentazocine is a mild narcotic antagonist and concurrent use may lead to withdrawal symptoms; potential for additive CNS depressant properties). Products include:
- Levo-Dromoran ... 1734
- Levorphanol Tartrate Tablets ... 3059

Lorazepam (Potential for additive CNS depressant properties). Products include:
- Ativan Injection ... 3478
- Ativan Tablets ... 3482

Loxapine Hydrochloride (Potential for additive CNS depressant properties).
No products indexed under this heading.

Loxapine Succinate (Potential for additive CNS depressant properties). Products include:
- Loxitane Capsules ... 3398

Meperidine Hydrochloride (Pentazocine is a mild narcotic antagonist and concurrent use may lead to withdrawal symptoms; potential for additive CNS depressant properties). Products include:
- Demerol ... 3079
- Mepergan Injection ... 3539

Mephobarbital (Potential for additive CNS depressant properties).
No products indexed under this heading.

Meprobamate (Potential for additive CNS depressant properties). Products include:
- Miltown Tablets ... 3349

Mesoridazine Besylate (Potential for additive CNS depressant properties). Products include:
- Serentil ... 1057

Methadone Hydrochloride (Pentazocine is a mild narcotic antagonist and concurrent use may lead to withdrawal symptoms; potential for additive CNS depressant properties). Products include:
- Dolophine Hydrochloride Tablets ... 3056

Methohexital Sodium (Potential for additive CNS depressant properties). Products include:
- Brevital Sodium for Injection, USP .. 1815

Methotrimeprazine (Potential for additive CNS depressant properties).
No products indexed under this heading.

Methoxyflurane (Potential for additive CNS depressant properties).
No products indexed under this heading.

Midazolam Hydrochloride (Potential for additive CNS depressant properties). Products include:
- Versed Injection ... 3027
- Versed Syrup ... 3033

Molindone Hydrochloride (Potential for additive CNS depressant properties). Products include:
- Moban ... 1320

Morphine Sulfate (Pentazocine is a mild narcotic antagonist and concurrent use may lead to withdrawal symptoms; potential for additive CNS depressant properties). Products include:
- Astramorph/PF Injection, USP (Preservative-Free) ... 594
- Duramorph Injection ... 1312
- Infumorph 200 and Infumorph 500 Sterile Solutions ... 1314
- Kadian Capsules ... 1335
- MS Contin Tablets ... 2896
- MSIR ... 2898
- Oramorph SR Tablets ... 3062
- Roxanol ... 3066

Olanzapine (Potential for additive CNS depressant properties). Products include:
- Zyprexa Tablets ... 1973
- Zyprexa ZYDIS Orally Disintegrating Tablets ... 1973

Oxazepam (Potential for additive CNS depressant properties).
No products indexed under this heading.

Oxycodone Hydrochloride (Pentazocine is a mild narcotic antagonist and concurrent use may lead to withdrawal symptoms; potential for additive CNS depressant properties). Products include:
- OxyContin Tablets ... 2912
- OxyFast Oral Concentrate Solution . 2916
- OxyIR Capsules ... 2916
- Percocet Tablets ... 1326
- Percodan Tablets ... 1327
- Percolone Tablets ... 1327
- Roxicodone ... 3067
- Tylox Capsules ... 2597

Pentobarbital Sodium (Potential for additive CNS depressant properties). Products include:
- Nembutal Sodium Solution ... 485

Perphenazine (Potential for additive CNS depressant properties). Products include:
- Etrafon ... 3115
- Trilafon ... 3160

Phenobarbital (Potential for additive CNS depressant properties). Products include:
- Arco-Lase Plus Tablets ... 592
- Donnatal ... 2929
- Donnatal Extentabs ... 2930

Prazepam (Potential for additive CNS depressant properties).
No products indexed under this heading.

Prochlorperazine (Potential for additive CNS depressant properties). Products include:
- Compazine ... 1505

Promethazine Hydrochloride (Potential for additive CNS depressant properties). Products include:
- Mepergan Injection ... 3539
- Phenergan Injection ... 3553
- Phenergan ... 3556
- Phenergan Syrup ... 3554
- Phenergan with Codeine Syrup ... 3557
- Phenergan with Dextromethorphan Syrup ... 3559
- Phenergan VC Syrup ... 3560
- Phenergan VC with Codeine Syrup .. 3561

Propofol (Potential for additive CNS depressant properties). Products include:
- Diprivan Injectable Emulsion ... 667

Propoxyphene Hydrochloride (Pentazocine is a mild narcotic antagonist and concurrent use may lead to withdrawal symptoms; potential for additive CNS depressant properties). Products include:
- Darvon Pulvules ... 1909
- Darvon Compound-65 Pulvules ... 1910

Propoxyphene Napsylate (Pentazocine is a mild narcotic antagonist and concurrent use may lead to withdrawal symptoms; potential for additive CNS depressant properties). Products include:
- Darvon-N/Darvocet-N ... 1907
- Darvon-N Tablets ... 1912

Quazepam (Potential for additive CNS depressant properties).
No products indexed under this heading.

Quetiapine Fumarate (Potential for additive CNS depressant properties). Products include:
- Seroquel Tablets ... 684

Remifentanil Hydrochloride (Pentazocine is a mild narcotic antagonist and concurrent use may lead to withdrawal symptoms).
No products indexed under this heading.

Risperidone (Potential for additive CNS depressant properties). Products include:
- Risperdal ... 1796

Secobarbital Sodium (Potential for additive CNS depressant properties).
No products indexed under this heading.

Sevoflurane (Potential for additive CNS depressant properties).
No products indexed under this heading.

Sufentanil Citrate (Pentazocine is a mild narcotic antagonist and concurrent use may lead to withdrawal symptoms; potential for additive CNS depressant properties).
No products indexed under this heading.

Temazepam (Potential for additive CNS depressant properties).
No products indexed under this heading.

Thiamylal Sodium (Potential for additive CNS depressant properties).
No products indexed under this heading.

Thioridazine Hydrochloride (Potential for additive CNS depressant properties). Products include:
- Thioridazine Hydrochloride Tablets ... 2289

Thiothixene (Potential for additive CNS depressant properties). Products include:
- Navane Capsules ... 2701
- Thiothixene Capsules ... 2290

Triazolam (Potential for additive CNS depressant properties). Products include:
- Halcion Tablets ... 2823

Trifluoperazine Hydrochloride (Potential for additive CNS depressant properties). Products include:
- Stelazine ... 1640

Zaleplon (Potential for additive CNS depressant properties). Products include:
- Sonata Capsules ... 3591

Ziprasidone Hydrochloride (Potential for additive CNS depressant properties). Products include:
- Geodon Capsules ... 2688

Zolpidem Tartrate (Potential for additive CNS depressant properties). Products include:
- Ambien Tablets ... 3191

Food Interactions

Alcohol (May increase CNS depression).

TAMBOCOR TABLETS

(Flecainide Acetate) ... 1990

May interact with beta blockers, phenytoin, quinidine, and certain other agents. Compounds in these categories include:

Acebutolol Hydrochloride (Co-administration of flecainide with beta adrenergic blocking agents may result in possible additive negative inotropic effects; combined therapy has not resulted in adverse effects). Products include:
- Sectral Capsules ... 3589

Amiodarone Hydrochloride (When amiodarone is added to flecainide therapy, plasma flecainide levels may increase two-fold or more in some patients, if flecainide dosage is not reduced). Products include:
- Cordarone Intravenous ... 3491
- Cordarone Tablets ... 3487
- Pacerone Tablets ... 3331

Atenolol (Co-administration of flecainide with beta adrenergic blocking agents may result in possible additive negative inotropic effects; combined therapy has not resulted in adverse effects). Products include:
- Tenoretic Tablets ... 690
- Tenormin I.V. Injection ... 692

Betaxolol Hydrochloride (Co-administration of flecainide with beta adrenergic blocking agents may result in possible additive negative inotropic effects; combined therapy has not resulted in adverse effects). Products include:
- Betoptic S Ophthalmic Suspension ... 537

Bisoprolol Fumarate (Co-administration of flecainide with beta adrenergic blocking agents may result in possible additive negative inotropic effects; combined therapy has not resulted in adverse effects). Products include:
- Zebeta Tablets ... 1885
- Ziac Tablets ... 1887

Carbamazepine (Limited data in patients receiving known enzyme inducers, such as carbamazepine, indicate only a 30% increase in the rate of flecainide elimination). Products include:
- Carbatrol Capsules ... 3234
- Tegretol/Tegretol-XR ... 2404

Carteolol Hydrochloride (Co-administration of flecainide with beta adrenergic blocking agents may result in possible additive negative inotropic effects; combined therapy has not resulted in adverse effects). Products include:
- Carteolol Hydrochloride Ophthalmic Solution USP, 1% ... ⊙258
- Ocupress Ophthalmic Solution, 1% Sterile ... ⊙303

Cimetidine (Increases plasma levels by about 30% and half-life by about 10%). Products include:
- Tagamet HB 200 Suspension ... ▣762
- Tagamet HB 200 Tablets ... ▣761
- Tagamet Tablets ... 1644

Cimetidine Hydrochloride (Increases plasma levels by about 30% and half-life by about 10%). Products include:
- Tagamet ... 1644

Digoxin (Co-administration in individuals stabilized on a maintenance dose of digoxin has resulted in increased plasma digoxin levels by 13% to 19% at six hours postdose). Products include:
- Digitek Tablets ... 1003
- Lanoxicaps Capsules ... 1574
- Lanoxin Injection ... 1581
- Lanoxin Tablets ... 1587
- Lanoxin Elixir Pediatric ... 1578
- Lanoxin Injection Pediatric ... 1584

Disopyramide Phosphate (Co-administration is not recommended because both drugs have negative inotropic properties).
No products indexed under this heading.

Esmolol Hydrochloride (Co-administration of flecainide with beta adrenergic blocking agents may result in possible additive negative inotropic effects; combined therapy has not resulted in adverse effects). Products include:
- Brevibloc Injection ... 858

Fosphenytoin Sodium (Limited data in patients receiving known enzyme inducers, such as phenytoin, indicate only a 30% increase in the rate of flecainide elimination). Products include:

Cerebyx Injection 2619

Labetalol Hydrochloride (Co-administration of flecainide with beta adrenergic blocking agents may result in possible additive negative inotropic effects; combined therapy has not resulted in adverse effects). Products include:

Normodyne Injection 3135
Normodyne Tablets 3137

Levobunolol Hydrochloride (Co-administration of flecainide with beta adrenergic blocking agents may result in possible additive negative inotropic effects; combined therapy has not resulted in adverse effects). Products include:

Betagan .... ⊙ 228

Metipranolol Hydrochloride (Co-administration of flecainide with beta adrenergic blocking agents may result in possible additive negative inotropic effects; combined therapy has not resulted in adverse effects).

No products indexed under this heading.

Metoprolol Succinate (Co-administration of flecainide with beta adrenergic blocking agents may result in possible additive negative inotropic effects; combined therapy has not resulted in adverse effects). Products include:

Toprol-XL Tablets 651

Metoprolol Tartrate (Co-administration of flecainide with beta adrenergic blocking agents may result in possible additive negative inotropic effects; combined therapy has not resulted in adverse effects).

No products indexed under this heading.

Nadolol (Co-administration of flecainide with beta adrenergic blocking agents may result in possible additive negative inotropic effects; combined therapy has not resulted in adverse effects). Products include:

Corgard Tablets 2245
Corzide 40/5 Tablets 2247
Corzide 80/5 Tablets 2247
Nadolol Tablets 2288

Penbutolol Sulfate (Co-administration of flecainide with beta adrenergic blocking agents may result in possible additive negative inotropic effects; combined therapy has not resulted in adverse effects).

No products indexed under this heading.

Phenobarbital (Limited data in patients receiving known enzyme inducers, such as phenobarbital, indicate only a 30% increase in the rate of flecainide elimination). Products include:

Arco-Lase Plus Tablets 592
Donnatal 2929
Donnatal Extentabs 2930

Phenytoin (Limited data in patients receiving known enzyme inducers, such as phenytoin, indicate only a 30% increase in the rate of flecainide elimination). Products include:

Dilantin Infatabs 2624
Dilantin-125 Oral Suspension 2625

Phenytoin Sodium (Limited data in patients receiving known enzyme inducers, such as phenytoin, indicate only a 30% increase in the rate of flecainide elimination). Products include:

Dilantin Kapseals 2622

Pindolol (Co-administration of flecainide with beta adrenergic blocking agents may result in possible additive negative inotropic effects; combined therapy has not resulted in adverse effects).

No products indexed under this heading.

Propranolol Hydrochloride (Co-administration has resulted in increased flecainide and propranolol levels by about 20% and 30% respectively; concurrent use in this study has resulted in additive negative inotropic effects). Products include:

Inderal 3513
Inderal LA Long-Acting Capsules 3516
Inderide Tablets 3517
Inderide LA Long-Acting Capsules .. 3519

Quinidine Gluconate (Drugs that inhibit cytochrome P4502D6, such as quinidine, might increase the plasma-concentrations of flecainide in patients who are on chronic flecainide therapy). Products include:

Quinaglute Dura-Tabs Tablets 978

Quinidine Polygalacturonate (Drugs that inhibit cytochrome P4502D6, such as quinidine, might increase the plasma-concentrations of flecainide in patients who are on chronic flecainide therapy).

No products indexed under this heading.

Quinidine Sulfate (Drugs that inhibit cytochrome P4502D6, such as quinidine, might increase the plasma-concentrations of flecainide in patients who are on chronic flecainide therapy). Products include:

Quinidex Extentabs 2933

Sotalol Hydrochloride (Co-administration of flecainide with beta adrenergic blocking agents may result in possible additive negative inotropic effects; combined therapy has not resulted in adverse effects). Products include:

Betapace Tablets 950
Betapace AF Tablets 954

Timolol Hemihydrate (Co-administration of flecainide with beta adrenergic blocking agents may result in possible additive negative inotropic effects; combined therapy has not resulted in adverse effects). Products include:

Betimol Ophthalmic Solution .... ⊙ 324

Timolol Maleate (Co-administration of flecainide with beta adrenergic blocking agents may result in possible additive negative inotropic effects; combined therapy has not resulted in adverse effects). Products include:

Blocadren Tablets 2046
Cosopt Sterile Ophthalmic Solution 2065
Timolide Tablets 2187
Timolol GFS .... ⊙ 266
Timoptic in Ocudose 2192
Timoptic Sterile Ophthalmic Solution 2190
Timoptic-XE Sterile Ophthalmic Gel Forming Solution 2194

Verapamil Hydrochloride (Co-administration is not recommended because both drugs have negative inotropic properties). Products include:

Covera-HS Tablets 3199
Isoptin SR Tablets 467
Tarka Tablets 508
Verelan Capsules 3184
Verelan PM Capsules 3186

Food Interactions

Dairy products (Milk may inhibit absorption in infants; a reduction in Tambocor dosage should be considered when milk is removed from the diet of infants).

TAMIFLU CAPSULES

(Oseltamivir Phosphate) 3008
May interact with:

Probenecid (Co-administration with probenecid results in an approximate twofold increase in exposure to oseltamivir carboxylate due to a decrease in active anionic tubular secretion in the kidneys; no dose adjustments are required due to the safety margin of oseltamivir carboxylate).

No products indexed under this heading.

TAMIFLU ORAL SUSPENSION

(Oseltamivir Phosphate) 3008
See Tamiflu Capsules

TAO CAPSULES

(Troleandomycin) 2716
May interact with ergot-containing drugs, theophylline, and certain other agents. Compounds in these categories include:

Aminophylline (Elevated serum concentrations of theophylline).

No products indexed under this heading.

Dihydroergotamine Mesylate (Co-administration with ergot-containing drugs and troleandomycin may result in ischemic reactions; concurrent use should be avoided). Products include:

D.H.E. 45 Injection 2334
Migranal Nasal Spray 2376

Dyphylline (Elevated serum concentrations of theophylline). Products include:

Lufyllin Tablets 3347
Lufyllin-400 Tablets 3347
Lufyllin-GG Elixir 3348
Lufyllin-GG Tablets 3348

Ergonovine Maleate (Co-administration with ergot-containing drugs and troleandomycin may result in ischemic reactions; concurrent use should be avoided).

No products indexed under this heading.

Ergotamine Tartrate (Co-administration with ergot-containing drugs and troleandomycin may result in ischemic reactions; concurrent use should be avoided).

No products indexed under this heading.

Ethinyl Estradiol (Troleandomycin should be administered with caution to patients concurrently receiving estrogen containing oral contraceptives). Products include:

Alesse-21 Tablets 3468
Alesse-28 Tablets 3473
Brevicon 28-Day Tablets 3380
Cyclessa Tablets 2450
Desogen Tablets 2458
Estinyl Tablets 3112
Estrostep 2627
femhrt Tablets 2635
Levlen 962
Levlite 21 Tablets 962
Levlite 28 Tablets 962
Levora Tablets 3389
Loestrin 21 Tablets 2642
Loestrin Fe Tablets 2642
Lo/Ovral Tablets 3532
Lo/Ovral-28 Tablets 3538
Low-Ogestrel-28 Tablets 3392
Microgestin Fe 1.5/30 Tablets 3407
Microgestin Fe 1/20 Tablets 3400
Mircette Tablets 2470
Modicon 2563
Necon 3415
Nordette-28 Tablets 2257
Norinyl 1 +35 28-Day Tablets 3380
Ogestrel 0.5/50-28 Tablets 3428
Ortho-Cept 21 Tablets 2546
Ortho-Cept 28 Tablets 2546
Ortho-Cyclen/Ortho Tri-Cyclen 2573
Ortho-Novum 2563
Ovcon 3364
Ovral Tablets 3551
Ovral-28 Tablets 3552
Tri-Levlen 962
Tri-Norinyl-28 Tablets 3433
Triphasil-21 Tablets 3600
Triphasil-28 Tablets 3605
Trivora Tablets 3439
Yasmin 28 Tablets 980
Zovia 3449

Mestranol (Troleandomycin should be administered with caution to patients concurrently receiving estrogen containing oral contraceptives). Products include:

Necon 1/50 Tablets 3415
Norinyl 1 + 50 28-Day Tablets 3380
Ortho-Novum 1/50□28 Tablets 2556

Methylergonovine Maleate (Co-administration with ergot-containing drugs and troleandomycin may result in ischemic reactions; concurrent use should be avoided).

No products indexed under this heading.

Methysergide Maleate (Co-administration with ergot-containing drugs and troleandomycin may result in ischemic reactions; concurrent use should be avoided).

No products indexed under this heading.

Metoclopramide Hydrochloride (May induce ischemic reactions). Products include:

Reglan 2935

Theophylline (Elevated serum concentrations of theophylline). Products include:

Aerolate 1361
Theo-Dur Extended-Release Tablets 1835
Uni-Dur Extended-Release Tablets .. 1841
Uniphyl 400 mg and 600 mg Tablets 2903

Theophylline Calcium Salicylate (Elevated serum concentrations of theophylline).

No products indexed under this heading.

Theophylline Sodium Glycinate (Elevated serum concentrations of theophylline).

No products indexed under this heading.

TARKA TABLETS

(Trandolapril, Verapamil Hydrochloride) 508
May interact with beta blockers, diuretics, cardiac glycosides, inhalant anesthetics, lithium preparations, neuromuscular blocking agents, potassium preparations, potassium sparing diuretics, quinidine, and theophylline. Compounds in these categories include:

Acebutolol Hydrochloride (Co-administration of beta blockers and verapamil may result in additive effects on heart rate, atrioventricular conduction, and/or cardiac contractility). Products include:

Sectral Capsules 3589

Amiloride Hydrochloride (Increased risk of hyperkalemia; patients on diuretics, especially those on recently instituted diuretic therapy, may occasionally experience an excessive reduction of blood pressure after initiation of therapy with Tarka). Products include:

Midamor Tablets 2136
Moduretic Tablets 2138

Aminophylline (Verapamil may inhibit the clearance and increase the plasma levels of theophylline).

No products indexed under this heading.

Atenolol (Co-administration of beta blockers and verapamil may result in additive effects on heart rate, atrioventricular conduction, and/or cardiac contractility). Products include:

Tenoretic Tablets 690
Tenormin I.V. Injection 692

Atracurium Besylate (Verapamil may potentiate the activity of neuromuscular blocking agents).

No products indexed under this heading.

Bendroflumethiazide (Patients on diuretics, especially those on recently instituted diuretic therapy, may occasionally experience an excessive reduction of blood pressure after initiation of therapy with Tarka). Products include:

Corzide 40/5 Tablets 2247
Corzide 80/5 Tablets 2247

Betaxolol Hydrochloride (Co-administration of beta blockers and verapamil may result in additive

effects on heart rate, atrioventricular conduction, and/or cardiac contractility). Products include:
- Betoptic S Ophthalmic Suspension 537

Bisoprolol Fumarate (Co-administration of beta blockers and verapamil may result in additive effects on heart rate, atrioventricular conduction, and/or cardiac contractility). Products include:
- Zebeta Tablets 1885
- Ziac Tablets 1887

Bumetanide (Patients on diuretics, especially those on recently instituted diuretic therapy, may occasionally experience an excessive reduction of blood pressure after initiation of therapy with Tarka).
- No products indexed under this heading.

Carbamazepine (Combined therapy of verapamil and carbamazepine may increase carbamazepine concentrations resulting in side effects such as diplopia, ataxia, and headache). Products include:
- Carbatrol Capsules 3234
- Tegretol/Tegretol-XR 2404

Carteolol Hydrochloride (Co-administration of beta blockers and verapamil may result in additive effects on heart rate, atrioventricular conduction, and/or cardiac contractility). Products include:
- Carteolol Hydrochloride Ophthalmic Solution USP, 1% .... ⊙258
- Ocupress Ophthalmic Solution, 1% Sterile .... ⊙303

Chlorothiazide (Patients on diuretics, especially those on recently instituted diuretic therapy, may occasionally experience an excessive reduction of blood pressure after initiation of therapy with Tarka). Products include:
- Aldoclor Tablets 2035
- Diuril Oral 2087

Chlorothiazide Sodium (Patients on diuretics, especially those on recently instituted diuretic therapy, may occasionally experience an excessive reduction of blood pressure after initiation of therapy with Tarka). Products include:
- Diuril Sodium Intravenous 2086

Chlorthalidone (Patients on diuretics, especially those on recently instituted diuretic therapy, may occasionally experience an excessive reduction of blood pressure after initiation of therapy with Tarka). Products include:
- Clorpres Tablets 1002
- Combipres Tablets 1040
- Tenoretic Tablets 690

Cimetidine (Variable results on clearance have been obtained in acute studies during concomitant therapy; clearance of verapamil may be reduced or unchanged). Products include:
- Tagamet HB 200 Suspension .... ▣762
- Tagamet HB 200 Tablets .... ▣761
- Tagamet Tablets 1644

Cimetidine Hydrochloride (Variable results on clearance have been obtained in acute studies during concomitant therapy; clearance of verapamil may be reduced or unchanged). Products include:
- Tagamet 1644

Cisatracurium Besylate (Verapamil may potentiate the activity of neuromuscular blocking agents).
- No products indexed under this heading.

Cyclosporine (Increased serum levels of cyclosporine). Products include:
- Gengraf Capsules 457
- Neoral Soft Gelatin Capsules 2380
- Neoral Oral Solution 2380
- Sandimmune 2388

Desflurane (Potential for excessive cardiovascular depression). Products include:
- Suprane Liquid for Inhalation 874

Deslanoside (Chronic verapamil therapy can increase serum digoxin levels by 50% to 75% during the first week, and this can result in digoxin toxicity; patient should be carefully monitored to avoid over- or under-digitalization).
- No products indexed under this heading.

Digitoxin (Chronic verapamil therapy can increase serum digoxin levels by 50% to 75% during the first week, and this can result in digoxin toxicity; patient should be carefully monitored to avoid over- or under-digitalization).
- No products indexed under this heading.

Digoxin (Chronic verapamil therapy can increase serum digoxin levels by 50% to 75% during the first week, and this can result in digoxin toxicity; patient should be carefully monitored to avoid over- or under-digitalization). Products include:
- Digitek Tablets 1003
- Lanoxicaps Capsules 1574
- Lanoxin Injection 1581
- Lanoxin Tablets 1587
- Lanoxin Elixir Pediatric 1578
- Lanoxin Injection Pediatric 1584

Doxacurium Chloride (Verapamil may potentiate the activity of neuromuscular blocking agents).
- No products indexed under this heading.

Dyphylline (Verapamil may inhibit the clearance and increase the plasma levels of theophylline). Products include:
- Lufyllin Tablets 3347
- Lufyllin-400 Tablets 3347
- Lufyllin-GG Elixir 3348
- Lufyllin-GG Tablets 3348

Enflurane (Potential for excessive cardiovascular depression).
- No products indexed under this heading.

Esmolol Hydrochloride (Co-administration of beta blockers and verapamil may result in additive effects on heart rate, atrioventricular conduction, and/or cardiac contractility). Products include:
- Brevibloc Injection 858

Ethacrynic Acid (Patients on diuretics, especially those on recently instituted diuretic therapy, may occasionally experience an excessive reduction of blood pressure after initiation of therapy with Tarka). Products include:
- Edecrin Tablets 2091

Flecainide Acetate (Concomitant use may result in additive effects on myocardial contractility, AV conduction and repolarization; concurrent use of flecainide and verapamil may result in additive inotropic effect and prolongation of atrioventricular conduction). Products include:
- Tambocor Tablets 1990

Furosemide (Patients on diuretics, especially those on recently instituted diuretic therapy, may occasionally experience an excessive reduction of blood pressure after initiation of therapy with Tarka). Products include:
- Furosemide Tablets 2284

Halothane (Potential for excessive cardiovascular depression). Products include:
- Fluothane Inhalation 3508

Hydrochlorothiazide (Patients on diuretics, especially those on recently instituted diuretic therapy, may occasionally experience an excessive reduction of blood pressure after initiation of therapy with Tarka). Products include:
- Accuretic Tablets 2614
- Aldoril Tablets 2039
- Atacand HCT Tablets 597
- Avalide Tablets 1070
- Diovan HCT Tablets 2338
- Dyazide Capsules 1515
- HydroDIURIL Tablets 2108
- Hyzaar 2109
- Inderide Tablets 3517
- Inderide LA Long-Acting Capsules .. 3519
- Lotensin HCT Tablets 2367
- Maxzide 1008
- Micardis HCT Tablets 1051
- Microzide Capsules 3414
- Moduretic Tablets 2138
- Monopril HCT 1094
- Prinzide Tablets 2168
- Timolide Tablets 2187
- Uniretic Tablets 3178
- Vaseretic Tablets 2204
- Zestoretic Tablets 695
- Ziac Tablets 1887

Hydroflumethiazide (Patients on diuretics, especially those on recently instituted diuretic therapy, may occasionally experience an excessive reduction of blood pressure after initiation of therapy with Tarka). Products include:
- Diucardin Tablets 3494

Indapamide (Patients on diuretics, especially those on recently instituted diuretic therapy, may occasionally experience an excessive reduction of blood pressure after initiation of therapy with Tarka). Products include:
- Indapamide Tablets 2286

Isoflurane (Potential for excessive cardiovascular depression).
- No products indexed under this heading.

Labetalol Hydrochloride (Co-administration of beta blockers and verapamil may result in additive effects on heart rate, atrioventricular conduction, and/or cardiac contractility). Products include:
- Normodyne Injection 3135
- Normodyne Tablets 3137

Levobunolol Hydrochloride (Co-administration of beta blockers and verapamil may result in additive effects on heart rate, atrioventricular conduction, and/or cardiac contractility). Products include:
- Betagan .... ⊙228

Lithium Carbonate (Co-administration results in increased sensitivity to the effects of lithium (neurotoxicity) with either no change or increase in serum lithium levels; increased lithium levels have been reported in patients receiving lithium and ACE inhibitor). Products include:
- Eskalith 1527
- Lithium Carbonate 3061
- Lithobid Slow-Release Tablets 3255

Lithium Citrate (Co-administration results in increased sensitivity to the effects of lithium (neurotoxicity) with either no change or increase in serum lithium levels; increased lithium levels have been reported in patients receiving lithium and ACE inhibitor). Products include:
- Lithium Citrate Syrup 3061

Methoxyflurane (Potential for excessive cardiovascular depression).
- No products indexed under this heading.

Methyclothiazide (Patients on diuretics, especially those on recently instituted diuretic therapy, may occasionally experience an excessive reduction of blood pressure after initiation of therapy with Tarka).
- No products indexed under this heading.

Metipranolol Hydrochloride (Co-administration of beta blockers and verapamil may result in additive effects on heart rate, atrioventricular conduction, and/or cardiac contractility).
- No products indexed under this heading.

Metocurine Iodide (Verapamil may potentiate the activity of neuromuscular blocking agents).
- No products indexed under this heading.

Metolazone (Patients on diuretics, especially those on recently instituted diuretic therapy, may occasionally experience an excessive reduction of blood pressure after initiation of therapy with Tarka). Products include:
- Mykrox Tablets 1168
- Zaroxolyn Tablets 1177

Metoprolol Succinate (Co-administration of beta blockers and verapamil may result in additive effects on heart rate, atrioventricular conduction, and/or cardiac contractility). Products include:
- Toprol-XL Tablets 651

Metoprolol Tartrate (Co-administration of beta blockers and verapamil may result in additive effects on heart rate, atrioventricular conduction, and/or cardiac contractility).
- No products indexed under this heading.

Mivacurium Chloride (Verapamil may potentiate the activity of neuromuscular blocking agents).
- No products indexed under this heading.

Nadolol (Co-administration of beta blockers and verapamil may result in additive effects on heart rate, atrioventricular conduction, and/or cardiac contractility). Products include:
- Corgard Tablets 2245
- Corzide 40/5 Tablets 2247
- Corzide 80/5 Tablets 2247
- Nadolol Tablets 2288

Pancuronium Bromide (Verapamil may potentiate the activity of neuromuscular blocking agents).
- No products indexed under this heading.

Penbutolol Sulfate (Co-administration of beta blockers and verapamil may result in additive effects on heart rate, atrioventricular conduction, and/or cardiac contractility).
- No products indexed under this heading.

Phenobarbital (May increase verapamil clearance). Products include:
- Arco-Lase Plus Tablets 592
- Donnatal 2929
- Donnatal Extentabs 2930

Pindolol (Co-administration of beta blockers and verapamil may result in additive effects on heart rate, atrioventricular conduction, and/or cardiac contractility).
- No products indexed under this heading.

Polythiazide (Patients on diuretics, especially those on recently instituted diuretic therapy, may occasionally experience an excessive reduction of blood pressure after initiation of therapy with Tarka). Products include:
- Minizide Capsules 2700
- Renese Tablets 2712

Potassium Acid Phosphate (Increased risk of hyperkalemia). Products include:
- K-Phos Original (Sodium Free) Tablets 947

Potassium Bicarbonate (Increased risk of hyperkalemia).
- No products indexed under this heading.

Potassium Chloride (Increased risk of hyperkalemia). Products include:
- Chlor-3 1361
- Colyte with Flavor Packs for Oral Solution 3170
- GoLYTELY and Pineapple Flavor GoLYTELY for Oral Solution 1068

K-Dur Microburst Release System ER Tablets ... 1832
Klor-Con M20/Klor-Con M10 Tablets ... 3329
K-Lor Powder Packets ... 469
K-Tab Filmtab Tablets ... 470
Micro-K ... 3311
NuLYTELY, Cherry Flavor, Lemon-Lime Flavor, and Orange Flavor NuLYTELY for Oral Solution ... 1068
Rum-K ... 1363

Potassium Citrate (Increased risk of hyperkalemia). Products include:
Urocit-K Tablets ... 2232

Potassium Gluconate (Increased risk of hyperkalemia).
No products indexed under this heading.

Potassium Phosphate (Increased risk of hyperkalemia). Products include:
K-Phos Neutral Tablets ... 946

Propranolol Hydrochloride (Co-administration of beta blockers and verapamil may result in additive effects on heart rate, atrioventricular conduction, and/or cardiac contractility). Products include:
Inderal ... 3513
Inderal LA Long-Acting Capsules ... 3516
Inderide Tablets ... 3517
Inderide LA Long-Acting Capsules ... 3519

Quinidine Gluconate (Concomitant use of verapamil and quinidine has resulted in significant hypotension and/or increased quinidine levels during verapamil therapy). Products include:
Quinaglute Dura-Tabs Tablets ... 978

Quinidine Polygalacturonate (Concomitant use of verapamil and quinidine has resulted in significant hypotension and/or increased quinidine levels during verapamil therapy).
No products indexed under this heading.

Quinidine Sulfate (Concomitant use of verapamil and quinidine has resulted in significant hypotension and/or increased quinidine levels during verapamil therapy). Products include:
Quinidex Extentabs ... 2933

Rapacuronium Bromide (Verapamil may potentiate the activity of neuromuscular blocking agents).
No products indexed under this heading.

Rifampin (May markedly reduce oral verapamil bioavailability). Products include:
Rifadin ... 765
Rifamate Capsules ... 767
Rifater Tablets ... 769

Rocuronium Bromide (Verapamil may potentiate the activity of neuromuscular blocking agents). Products include:
Zemuron Injection ... 2491

Sotalol Hydrochloride (Co-administration of beta blockers and verapamil may result in additive effects on heart rate, atrioventricular conduction, and/or cardiac contractility). Products include:
Betapace Tablets ... 950
Betapace AF Tablets ... 954

Spironolactone (Increased risk of hyperkalemia; patients on diuretics, especially those on recently instituted diuretic therapy, may occasionally experience an excessive reduction of blood pressure after initiation of therapy with Tarka).
No products indexed under this heading.

Succinylcholine Chloride (Verapamil may potentiate the activity of neuromuscular blocking agents). Products include:
Anectine Injection ... 1476

Theophylline (Verapamil may inhibit the clearance and increase the plasma levels of theophylline). Products include:
Aerolate ... 1361
Theo-Dur Extended-Release Tablets ... 1835
Uni-Dur Extended-Release Tablets ... 1841
Uniphyl 400 mg and 600 mg Tablets ... 2903

Theophylline Calcium Salicylate (Verapamil may inhibit the clearance and increase the plasma levels of theophylline).
No products indexed under this heading.

Theophylline Sodium Glycinate (Verapamil may inhibit the clearance and increase the plasma levels of theophylline).
No products indexed under this heading.

Timolol Hemihydrate (Concomitant use of timolol eye drops and verapamil has resulted in asymptomatic bradycardia with wandering atrial pacemaker). Products include:
Betimol Ophthalmic Solution ... ⊙324

Timolol Maleate (Concomitant use of timolol eye drops and verapamil has resulted in asymptomatic bradycardia with wandering atrial pacemaker). Products include:
Blocadren Tablets ... 2046
Cosopt Sterile Ophthalmic Solution ... 2065
Timolide Tablets ... 2187
Timolol GFS ... ⊙266
Timoptic in Ocudose ... 2192
Timoptic Sterile Ophthalmic Solution ... 2190
Timoptic-XE Sterile Ophthalmic Gel Forming Solution ... 2194

Torsemide (Patients on diuretics, especially those on recently instituted diuretic therapy, may occasionally experience an excessive reduction of blood pressure after initiation of therapy with Tarka). Products include:
Demadex Tablets and Injection ... 2965

Triamterene (Increased risk of hyperkalemia; patients on diuretics, especially those on recently instituted diuretic therapy, may occasionally experience an excessive reduction of blood pressure after initiation of therapy with Tarka). Products include:
Dyazide Capsules ... 1515
Dyrenium Capsules ... 3458
Maxzide ... 1008

Vecuronium Bromide (Verapamil may potentiate the activity of neuromuscular blocking agents). Products include:
Norcuron for Injection ... 2478

Food Interactions

Food, unspecified (Co-administration with food decreases verapamil bioavailability and the time to peak plasma concentration is delayed; bioavailability of trandolapril is not altered; Tarka should be administered with food).

TASMAR TABLETS

(Tolcapone) ... 3010
May interact with central nervous system depressants, nonselective MAO inhibitors, and certain other agents. Compounds in these categories include:

Alfentanil Hydrochloride (Possible additive sedative effects when used in combination with CNS depressants).
No products indexed under this heading.

Alprazolam (Possible additive sedative effects when used in combination with CNS depressants). Products include:
Xanax Tablets ... 2865

Apomorphine (Tolcapone may influence the pharmacokinetics of drugs metabolized by COMT; dosage adjustments should be considered when co-administered).

Aprobarbital (Possible additive sedative effects when used in combination with CNS depressants).
No products indexed under this heading.

Buprenorphine Hydrochloride (Possible additive sedative effects when used in combination with CNS depressants). Products include:
Buprenex Injectable ... 2918

Buspirone Hydrochloride (Possible additive sedative effects when used in combination with CNS depressants).
No products indexed under this heading.

Butabarbital (Possible additive sedative effects when used in combination with CNS depressants).
No products indexed under this heading.

Butalbital (Possible additive sedative effects when used in combination with CNS depressants). Products include:
Phrenilin ... 578
Sedapap Tablets 50 mg/650 mg ... 2225

Chlordiazepoxide (Possible additive sedative effects when used in combination with CNS depressants). Products include:
Limbitrol ... 1738

Chlordiazepoxide Hydrochloride (Possible additive sedative effects when used in combination with CNS depressants). Products include:
Librium Capsules ... 1736
Librium for Injection ... 1737

Chlorpromazine (Possible additive sedative effects when used in combination with CNS depressants). Products include:
Thorazine Suppositories ... 1656

Chlorpromazine Hydrochloride (Possible additive sedative effects when used in combination with CNS depressants). Products include:
Thorazine ... 1656

Chlorprothixene (Possible additive sedative effects when used in combination with CNS depressants).
No products indexed under this heading.

Chlorprothixene Hydrochloride (Possible additive sedative effects when used in combination with CNS depressants).
No products indexed under this heading.

Chlorprothixene Lactate (Possible additive sedative effects when used in combination with CNS depressants).
No products indexed under this heading.

Clorazepate Dipotassium (Possible additive sedative effects when used in combination with CNS depressants). Products include:
Tranxene ... 511

Clozapine (Possible additive sedative effects when used in combination with CNS depressants). Products include:
Clozaril Tablets ... 2319

Codeine Phosphate (Possible additive sedative effects when used in combination with CNS depressants). Products include:
Phenergan with Codeine Syrup ... 3557
Phenergan VC with Codeine Syrup ... 3561
Robitussin A-C Syrup ... 2942
Robitussin-DAC Syrup ... 2942
Ryna-C Liquid ... ▣768
Soma Compound w/Codeine Tablets ... 3355
Tussi-Organidin NR Liquid ... 3350
Tussi-Organidin-S NR Liquid ... 3350
Tylenol with Codeine ... 2595

Desflurane (Possible additive sedative effects when used in combination with CNS depressants). Products include:
Suprane Liquid for Inhalation ... 874

Desipramine Hydrochloride (Co-administration of tolcapone with levodopa/carbidopa and desipramine has resulted in slight increase in frequency of adverse events; caution should be exercised when co-administered). Products include:
Norpramin Tablets ... 755

Dezocine (Possible additive sedative effects when used in combination with CNS depressants).
No products indexed under this heading.

Diazepam (Possible additive sedative effects when used in combination with CNS depressants). Products include:
Valium Injectable ... 3026
Valium Tablets ... 3047

Dobutamine Hydrochloride (Tolcapone may influence the pharmacokinetics of drugs metabolized by COMT; dosage adjustments should be considered when co-administered). Products include:
Dobutrex Solution Vials ... 1914

Droperidol (Possible additive sedative effects when used in combination with CNS depressants).
No products indexed under this heading.

Enflurane (Possible additive sedative effects when used in combination with CNS depressants).
No products indexed under this heading.

Estazolam (Possible additive sedative effects when used in combination with CNS depressants). Products include:
ProSom Tablets ... 500

Ethchlorvynol (Possible additive sedative effects when used in combination with CNS depressants).
No products indexed under this heading.

Ethinamate (Possible additive sedative effects when used in combination with CNS depressants).
No products indexed under this heading.

Fentanyl (Possible additive sedative effects when used in combination with CNS depressants). Products include:
Duragesic Transdermal System ... 1786

Fentanyl Citrate (Possible additive sedative effects when used in combination with CNS depressants). Products include:
Actiq ... 1184

Fluphenazine Decanoate (Possible additive sedative effects when used in combination with CNS depressants).
No products indexed under this heading.

Fluphenazine Enanthate (Possible additive sedative effects when used in combination with CNS depressants).
No products indexed under this heading.

Fluphenazine Hydrochloride (Possible additive sedative effects when used in combination with CNS depressants).
No products indexed under this heading.

Flurazepam Hydrochloride (Possible additive sedative effects when used in combination with CNS depressants).
No products indexed under this heading.

Glutethimide (Possible additive sedative effects when used in combi-

nation with CNS depressants).
No products indexed under this heading.

Haloperidol (Possible additive sedative effects when used in combination with CNS depressants). Products include:
Haldol Injection, Tablets and Concentrate 2533

Haloperidol Decanoate (Possible additive sedative effects when used in combination with CNS depressants). Haldol Decanoate 2535

Hydrocodone Bitartrate (Possible additive sedative effects when used in combination with CNS depressants). Products include:
Hycodan 1316
Hycomine Compound Tablets 1317
Hycotuss Expectorant Syrup 1318
Lortab 3319
Lortab Elixir 3317
Maxidone Tablets CIII 3399
Norco 5/325 Tablets CIII 3424
Norco 7.5/325 Tablets CIII 3425
Norco 10/325 Tablets CIII 3427
Norco 10/325 Tablets CIII 3425
Vicodin Tablets 516
Vicodin ES Tablets 517
Vicodin HP Tablets 518
Vicodin Tuss Expectorant 519
Vicoprofen Tablets 520
Zydone Tablets 1330

Hydrocodone Polistirex (Possible additive sedative effects when used in combination with CNS depressants). Products include:
Tussionex Pennkinetic Extended-Release Suspension 1174

Hydromorphone Hydrochloride (Possible additive sedative effects when used in combination with CNS depressants). Products include:
Dilaudid 441
Dilaudid Oral Liquid 445
Dilaudid Powder 441
Dilaudid Rectal Suppositories 441
Dilaudid Tablets 441
Dilaudid Tablets - 8 mg 445
Dilaudid-HP 443

Hydroxyzine Hydrochloride (Possible additive sedative effects when used in combination with CNS depressants). Products include:
Atarax Tablets & Syrup 2667
Vistaril Intramuscular Solution 2738

Isocarboxazid (The combination, in theory, of tolcapone and non-selective MAO inhibitor may result in inhibition of the majority of the pathways responsible for normal catecholamine metabolism; patients should ordinarily not be treated concomitantly).
No products indexed under this heading.

Isoflurane (Possible additive sedative effects when used in combination with CNS depressants).
No products indexed under this heading.

Isoproterenol Hydrochloride (Tolcapone may influence the pharmacokinetics of drugs metabolized by COMT; dosage adjustments should be considered when co-administered).
No products indexed under this heading.

Ketamine Hydrochloride (Possible additive sedative effects when used in combination with CNS depressants).
No products indexed under this heading.

Levodopa (Tolcapone enhances levodopa bioavailability and, therefore, may increase the occurence of orthostatic hypotension; tolcapone may potentiate the dopaminergic side effects of levodopa and may cause and/or exacerbate preexisting dyskinesia). Products include:
Sinemet Tablets 1253
Sinemet CR Tablets 1255

Levomethadyl Acetate Hydrochloride (Possible additive sedative effects when used in combination with CNS depressants).
No products indexed under this heading.

Levorphanol Tartrate (Possible additive sedative effects when used in combination with CNS depressants). Products include:
Levo-Dromoran 1734
Levorphanol Tartrate Tablets 3059

Lorazepam (Possible additive sedative effects when used in combination with CNS depressants). Products include:
Ativan Injection 3478
Ativan Tablets 3482

Loxapine Hydrochloride (Possible additive sedative effects when used in combination with CNS depressants).
No products indexed under this heading.

Loxapine Succinate (Possible additive sedative effects when used in combination with CNS depressants). Products include:
Loxitane Capsules 3398

Meperidine Hydrochloride (Possible additive sedative effects when used in combination with CNS depressants). Products include:
Demerol 3079
Mepergan Injection 3539

Mephobarbital (Possible additive sedative effects when used in combination with CNS depressants).
No products indexed under this heading.

Meprobamate (Possible additive sedative effects when used in combination with CNS depressants). Products include:
Miltown Tablets 3349

Mesoridazine Besylate (Possible additive sedative effects when used in combination with CNS depressants). Products include:
Serentil 1057

Methadone Hydrochloride (Possible additive sedative effects when used in combination with CNS depressants). Products include:
Dolophine Hydrochloride Tablets 3056

Methohexital Sodium (Possible additive sedative effects when used in combination with CNS depressants). Products include:
Brevital Sodium for Injection, USP 1815

Methotrimeprazine (Possible additive sedative effects when used in combination with CNS depressants).
No products indexed under this heading.

Methoxyflurane (Possible additive sedative effects when used in combination with CNS depressants).
No products indexed under this heading.

Methyldopa (Tolcapone may influence the pharmacokinetics of drugs metabolized by COMT; dosage adjustments should be considered when co-administered). Products include:
Aldoclor Tablets 2035
Aldomet Tablets 2037
Aldoril Tablets 2039

Midazolam Hydrochloride (Possible additive sedative effects when used in combination with CNS depressants). Products include:
Versed Injection 3027
Versed Syrup 3033

Molindone Hydrochloride (Possible additive sedative effects when used in combination with CNS depressants). Products include:
Moban 1320

Morphine Sulfate (Possible additive sedative effects when used in combination with CNS depressants). Products include:
Astramorph/PF Injection, USP (Preservative-Free) 594
Duramorph Injection 1312
Infumorph 200 and Infumorph 500 Sterile Solutions 1314
Kadian Capsules 1335
MS Contin Tablets 2896
MSIR 2898
Oramorph SR Tablets 3062
Roxanol 3066

Olanzapine (Possible additive sedative effects when used in combination with CNS depressants). Products include:
Zyprexa Tablets 1973
Zyprexa ZYDIS Orally Disintegrating Tablets 1973

Oxazepam (Possible additive sedative effects when used in combination with CNS depressants).
No products indexed under this heading.

Oxycodone Hydrochloride (Possible additive sedative effects when used in combination with CNS depressants). Products include:
OxyContin Tablets 2912
OxyFast Oral Concentrate Solution 2916
OxyIR Capsules 2916
Percocet Tablets 1326
Percodan Tablets 1327
Percolone Tablets 1327
Roxicodone 3067
Tylox Capsules 2597

Pargyline Hydrochloride (The combination, in theory, of tolcapone and non-selective MAO inhibitor may result in inhibition of the majority of the pathways responsible for normal catecholamine metabolism; patients should ordinarily not be treated concomitantly).
No products indexed under this heading.

Pentobarbital Sodium (Possible additive sedative effects when used in combination with CNS depressants). Products include:
Nembutal Sodium Solution 485

Perphenazine (Possible additive sedative effects when used in combination with CNS depressants). Products include:
Etrafon 3115
Trilafon 3160

Phenelzine Sulfate (The combination, in theory, of tolcapone and non-selective MAO inhibitor may result in inhibition of the majority of the pathways responsible for normal catecholamine metabolism; patients should ordinarily not be treated concomitantly). Products include:
Nardil Tablets 2653

Phenobarbital (Possible additive sedative effects when used in combination with CNS depressants). Products include:
Arco-Lase Plus Tablets 592
Donnatal 2929
Donnatal Extentabs 2930

Prazepam (Possible additive sedative effects when used in combination with CNS depressants).
No products indexed under this heading.

Procarbazine Hydrochloride (The combination, in theory, of tolcapone and non-selective MAO inhibitor may result in inhibition of the majority of the pathways responsible for normal catecholamine metabolism; patients should ordinarily not be treated concomitantly). Products include:
Matulane Capsules 3246

Prochlorperazine (Possible additive sedative effects when used in combination with CNS depressants). Products include:
Compazine 1505

Promethazine Hydrochloride (Possible additive sedative effects when used in combination with CNS depressants). Products include:
Mepergan Injection 3539
Phenergan Injection 3553
Phenergan 3556
Phenergan Syrup 3554
Phenergan with Codeine Syrup 3557
Phenergan with Dextromethorphan Syrup 3559
Phenergan VC Syrup 3560
Phenergan VC with Codeine Syrup 3561

Propofol (Possible additive sedative effects when used in combination with CNS depressants). Products include:
Diprivan Injectable Emulsion 667

Propoxyphene Hydrochloride (Possible additive sedative effects when used in combination with CNS depressants). Products include:
Darvon Pulvules 1909
Darvon Compound-65 Pulvules 1910

Propoxyphene Napsylate (Possible additive sedative effects when used in combination with CNS depressants). Products include:
Darvon-N/Darvocet-N 1907
Darvon-N Tablets 1912

Quazepam (Possible additive sedative effects when used in combination with CNS depressants).
No products indexed under this heading.

Quetiapine Fumarate (Possible additive sedative effects when used in combination with CNS depressants). Products include:
Seroquel Tablets 684

Remifentanil Hydrochloride (Possible additive sedative effects when used in combination with CNS depressants).
No products indexed under this heading.

Risperidone (Possible additive sedative effects when used in combination with CNS depressants). Products include:
Risperdal 1796

Secobarbital Sodium (Possible additive sedative effects when used in combination with CNS depressants).
No products indexed under this heading.

Sevoflurane (Possible additive sedative effects when used in combination with CNS depressants).
No products indexed under this heading.

Sufentanil Citrate (Possible additive sedative effects when used in combination with CNS depressants).
No products indexed under this heading.

Temazepam (Possible additive sedative effects when used in combination with CNS depressants).
No products indexed under this heading.

Thiamylal Sodium (Possible additive sedative effects when used in combination with CNS depressants).
No products indexed under this heading.

Thioridazine Hydrochloride (Possible additive sedative effects when used in combination with CNS depressants). Products include:
Thioridazine Hydrochloride Tablets 2289

Thiothixene (Possible additive sedative effects when used in combination with CNS depressants). Products include:
Navane Capsules 2701
Thiothixene Capsules 2290

Tranylcypromine Sulfate (The combination, in theory, of tolcapone and non-selective MAO inhibitor may result in inhibition of the majority of the pathways responsible for normal catecholamine metabolism; patients should ordinarily not be treated concomitantly). Products include:
Parnate Tablets 1607

Triazolam (Possible additive sedative effects when used in combination with CNS depressants). Products include:
Halcion Tablets 2823

Trifluoperazine Hydrochloride (Possible additive sedative effects when used in combination with CNS depressants). Products include:
Stelazine 1640

Zaleplon (Possible additive sedative effects when used in combination with CNS depressants). Products include:
Sonata Capsules 3591

Ziprasidone Hydrochloride (Possible additive sedative effects when used in combination with CNS depressants). Products include:
Geodon Capsules 2688

Zolpidem Tartrate (Possible additive sedative effects when used in combination with CNS depressants). Products include:
Ambien Tablets 3191

Food Interactions

Alcohol (Possible additive sedative effects when used in combination with CNS depressants, such as alcohol).

Food, unspecified (Food given within 1 hour before and 2 hours after dosing of tolcapone decreases the relative bioavailability by 10% to 20%; Tasmar may be taken with or without food).

TAVIST 12 HOUR ALLERGY TABLETS

(Clemastine Fumarate) 676
May interact with hypnotics and sedatives, tranquilizers, and certain other agents. Compounds in these categories include:

Alprazolam (May increase drowsiness effect). Products include:
Xanax Tablets 2865

Buspirone Hydrochloride (May increase drowsiness effect).
No products indexed under this heading.

Chlordiazepoxide (May increase drowsiness effect). Products include:
Limbitrol 1738

Chlordiazepoxide Hydrochloride (May increase drowsiness effect). Products include:
Librium Capsules 1736
Librium for Injection 1737

Chlorpromazine (May increase drowsiness effect). Products include:
Thorazine Suppositories 1656

Chlorpromazine Hydrochloride (May increase drowsiness effect). Products include:
Thorazine 1656

Chlorprothixene (May increase drowsiness effect).
No products indexed under this heading.

Chlorprothixene Hydrochloride (May increase drowsiness effect).
No products indexed under this heading.

Clorazepate Dipotassium (May increase drowsiness effect). Products include:
Tranxene 511

Diazepam (May increase drowsiness effect). Products include:
Valium Injectable 3026
Valium Tablets 3047

Droperidol (May increase drowsiness effect).
No products indexed under this heading.

Estazolam (May increase drowsiness effect). Products include:
ProSom Tablets 500

Ethchlorvynol (May increase drowsiness effect).
No products indexed under this heading.

Ethinamate (May increase drowsiness effect).
No products indexed under this heading.

Fluphenazine Decanoate (May increase drowsiness effect).
No products indexed under this heading.

Fluphenazine Enanthate (May increase drowsiness effect).
No products indexed under this heading.

Fluphenazine Hydrochloride (May increase drowsiness effect).
No products indexed under this heading.

Flurazepam Hydrochloride (May increase drowsiness effect).
No products indexed under this heading.

Glutethimide (May increase drowsiness effect).
No products indexed under this heading.

Haloperidol (May increase drowsiness effect). Products include:
Haldol Injection, Tablets and Concentrate 2533

Haloperidol Decanoate (May increase drowsiness effect). Products include:
Haldol Decanoate 2535

Hydroxyzine Hydrochloride (May increase drowsiness effect). Products include:
Atarax Tablets & Syrup 2667
Vistaril Intramuscular Solution 2738

Lorazepam (May increase drowsiness effect). Products include:
Ativan Injection 3478
Ativan Tablets 3482

Loxapine Hydrochloride (May increase drowsiness effect).
No products indexed under this heading.

Loxapine Succinate (May increase drowsiness effect). Products include:
Loxitane Capsules 3398

Meprobamate (May increase drowsiness effect). Products include:
Miltown Tablets 3349

Mesoridazine Besylate (May increase drowsiness effect). Products include:
Serentil 1057

Midazolam Hydrochloride (May increase drowsiness effect). Products include:
Versed Injection 3027
Versed Syrup 3033

Molindone Hydrochloride (May increase drowsiness effect). Products include:
Moban 1320

Oxazepam (May increase drowsiness effect).
No products indexed under this heading.

Perphenazine (May increase drowsiness effect). Products include:
Etrafon 3115
Trilafon 3160

Prazepam (May increase drowsiness effect).
No products indexed under this heading.

Prochlorperazine (May increase drowsiness effect). Products include:
Compazine 1505

Promethazine Hydrochloride (May increase drowsiness effect). Products include:
Mepergan Injection 3539
Phenergan Injection 3553
Phenergan 3556
Phenergan Syrup 3554
Phenergan with Codeine Syrup 3557
Phenergan with Dextromethorphan Syrup 3559
Phenergan VC Syrup 3560
Phenergan VC with Codeine Syrup 3561

Propofol (May increase drowsiness effect). Products include:
Diprivan Injectable Emulsion 667

Quazepam (May increase drowsiness effect).
No products indexed under this heading.

Secobarbital Sodium (May increase drowsiness effect).
No products indexed under this heading.

Temazepam (May increase drowsiness effect).
No products indexed under this heading.

Thioridazine Hydrochloride (May increase drowsiness effect). Products include:
Thioridazine Hydrochloride Tablets 2289

Thiothixene (May increase drowsiness effect). Products include:
Navane Capsules 2701
Thiothixene Capsules 2290

Triazolam (May increase drowsiness effect). Products include:
Halcion Tablets 2823

Trifluoperazine Hydrochloride (May increase drowsiness effect). Products include:
Stelazine 1640

Zaleplon (May increase drowsiness effect). Products include:
Sonata Capsules 3591

Zolpidem Tartrate (May increase drowsiness effect). Products include:
Ambien Tablets 3191

Food Interactions

Alcohol (May increase drowsiness effect).

TAVIST SINUS NON-DROWSY COATED CAPLETS

(Acetaminophen, Pseudoephedrine Hydrochloride) 676
May interact with monoamine oxidase inhibitors. Compounds in these categories include:

Isocarboxazid (Concurrent and/or sequential use with MAO inhibitors is not recommended).
No products indexed under this heading.

Moclobemide (Concurrent and/or sequential use with MAO inhibitors is not recommended).
No products indexed under this heading.

Pargyline Hydrochloride (Concurrent and/or sequential use with MAO inhibitors is not recommended).
No products indexed under this heading.

Phenelzine Sulfate (Concurrent and/or sequential use with MAO inhibitors is not recommended). Products include:
Nardil Tablets 2653

Procarbazine Hydrochloride (Concurrent and/or sequential use with MAO inhibitors is not recommended). Products include:
Matulane Capsules 3246

Selegiline Hydrochloride (Concurrent and/or sequential use with MAO inhibitors is not recommended). Products include:
Eldepryl Capsules 3266

Tranylcypromine Sulfate (Concurrent and/or sequential use with MAO inhibitors is not recommended). Products include:
Parnate Tablets 1607

Food Interactions

Alcohol (Chronic heavy alcohol users, 3 or more drinks per day, should consult their physicians for advice on when and how they should take pain relievers/fever reducers including acetaminophen).

TAXOL INJECTION

(Paclitaxel) 1129
May interact with erythromycin, quinidine, and certain other agents. Compounds in these categories include:

Cisplatin (Decreases paclitaxel clearance approximately 33% when Taxol is administered following cisplatin; concurrent administration given as sequential infusion results in profound myelosuppression when Taxol is given after cisplatin).
No products indexed under this heading.

Cyclosporine (The metabolism of paclitaxel is catalyzed by cytochrome P450 isoenzymes; based on *in vitro* studies, cyclosporine inhibits the metabolism of paclitaxel to 6-alpha-hydroxypaclitaxel, but the concentrations used exceeded those found *in vivo* following normaltherapeutic doses). Products include:
Gengraf Capsules 457
Neoral Soft Gelatin Capsules 2380
Neoral Oral Solution 2380
Sandimmune 2388

Dexamethasone (The metabolism of paclitaxel is catalyzed by cytochrome P450 isoenzymes; based on *in vitro* studies, dexamethasone inhibits the metabolism of paclitaxel to 6-alpha-hydroxypaclitaxel, but the concentrations used exceeded those found *in vivo* following normal therapeutic doses). Products include:
Decadron Elixir 2078
Decadron Tablets 2079
TobraDex Ophthalmic Ointment 542
TobraDex Ophthalmic Suspension 541

Dexamethasone Acetate (The metabolism of paclitaxel is catalyzed by cytochrome P450 isoenzymes; based on *in vitro* studies, dexamethasone inhibits the metabolism of paclitaxel to 6-alpha-hydroxypaclitaxel, but the concentrations used exceeded those found *in vivo* following normal therapeutic doses).
No products indexed under this heading.

Dexamethasone Sodium Phosphate (The metabolism of paclitaxel is catalyzed by cytochrome P450 isoenzymes; based on *in vitro* studies, dexamethasone inhibits the metabolism of paclitaxel to 6-alpha-hydroxypaclitaxel, but the concentrations used exceeded those found *in vivo* following normal therapeutic doses). Products include:
Decadron Phosphate Injection 2081
Decadron Phosphate Sterile Ophthalmic Ointment 2083
Decadron Phosphate Sterile Ophthalmic Solution 2084
NeoDecadron Sterile Ophthalmic Solution 2144

Diazepam (The metabolism of paclitaxel is catalyzed by cytochrome P450 isoenzymes; based on *in vitro* studies, diazepam inhibits the metabolism of paclitaxel to 6-alpha-hydroxypaclitaxel, but the concentrations used exceeded those found *in vivo* following normal therapeutic doses). Products include:
Valium Injectable 3026
Valium Tablets 3047

Doxorubicin Hydrochloride (Coadministration may result in increased plasma levels of doxorubicin and its active metabolite doxorubicinol). Products include:
Adriamycin PFS/RDF Injection 2767
Doxil Injection 566

Erythromycin (The metabolism of paclitaxel is catalyzed by cytochrome P450 isoenzymes; based on *in vitro* studies, erythromycin inhibits the metabolism of paclitaxel to 6-alpha-hydroxypaclitaxel). Products include:
Emgel 2% Topical Gel 1285
Ery-Tab Tablets 448
Erythromycin Base Filmtab Tablets 454
Erythromycin Delayed-Release Capsules, USP 455
PCE Dispertab Tablets 498

Erythromycin Estolate (The metabolism of paclitaxel is catalyzed by cytochrome P450 isoenzymes; based on *in vitro* studies, erythromy-

cin inhibits the metabolism of paclitaxel to 6-alpha-hydroxypaclitaxel).
No products indexed under this heading.

Erythromycin Ethylsuccinate (The metabolism of paclitaxel is catalyzed by cytochrome P450 isoenzymes; based on *in vitro* studies, erythromycin inhibits the metabolism of paclitaxel to 6-alpha-hydroxypaclitaxel). Products include:
E.E.S. **450**
EryPed **446**
Pediazole Suspension **3050**

Erythromycin Gluceptate (The metabolism of paclitaxel is catalyzed by cytochrome P450 isoenzymes; based on *in vitro* studies, erythromycin inhibits the metabolism of paclitaxel to 6-alpha-hydroxypaclitaxel).
No products indexed under this heading.

Erythromycin Stearate (The metabolism of paclitaxel is catalyzed by cytochrome P450 isoenzymes; based on *in vitro* studies, erythromycin inhibits the metabolism of paclitaxel to 6-alpha-hydroxypaclitaxel). Products include:
Erythrocin Stearate Filmtab Tablets **452**

Ethinyl Estradiol (The metabolism of paclitaxel is catalyzed by cytochrome P450 isoenzymes; based on *in vitro* studies, 17-alpha ethinyl estradiol inhibits the metabolism of paclitaxel to 6-alpha-hydroxypaclitaxel). Products include:
Alesse-21 Tablets **3468**
Alesse-28 Tablets **3473**
Brevicon 28-Day Tablets **3380**
Cyclessa Tablets **2450**
Desogen Tablets **2458**
Estinyl Tablets **3112**
Estrostep **2627**
femhrt Tablets **2635**
Levlen **962**
Levlite 21 Tablets **962**
Levlite 28 Tablets **962**
Levora Tablets **3389**
Loestrin 21 Tablets **2642**
Loestrin Fe Tablets **2642**
Lo/Ovral Tablets **3532**
Lo/Ovral-28 Tablets **3538**
Low-Ogestrel-28 Tablets **3392**
Microgestin Fe 1.5/30 Tablets **3407**
Microgestin Fe 1/20 Tablets **3400**
Mircette Tablets **2470**
Modicon **2563**
Necon **3415**
Nordette-28 Tablets **2257**
Norinyl 1 +35 28-Day Tablets **3380**
Ogestrel 0.5/50-28 Tablets **3428**
Ortho-Cept 21 Tablets **2546**
Ortho-Cept 28 Tablets **2546**
Ortho-Cyclen/Ortho Tri-Cyclen **2573**
Ortho-Novum **2563**
Ovcon **3364**
Ovral Tablets **3551**
Ovral-28 Tablets **3552**
Tri-Levlen **962**
Tri-Norinyl-28 Tablets **3433**
Triphasil-21 Tablets **3600**
Triphasil-28 Tablets **3605**
Trivora Tablets **3439**
Yasmin 28 Tablets **980**
Zovia **3449**

Etoposide (The metabolism of paclitaxel is catalyzed by cytochrome P450 isoenzymes; based on *in vitro* studies, etoposide inhibits the metabolism of paclitaxel to 6-alpha-hydroxypaclitaxel, but the concentrations used exceeded those found *in vivo* following normal therapeutic doses).
No products indexed under this heading.

Etoposide Phosphate (The metabolism of paclitaxel is catalyzed by cytochrome P450 isoenzymes; based on *in vitro* studies, etoposide inhibits the metabolism of paclitaxel to 6-alpha-hydroxypaclitaxel, but the concentrations used exceeded those found *in vivo* following normal therapeutic doses).
No products indexed under this heading.

Etretinate (The metabolism of paclitaxel is catalyzed by cytochrome P450 isoenzymes; based on *in vitro* studies, retinoic acid inhibits the metabolism of paclitaxel to 6-alpha-hydroxypaclitaxel).
No products indexed under this heading.

Isotretinoin (The metabolism of paclitaxel is catalyzed by cytochrome P450 isoenzymes; based on *in vitro* studies, retinoic acid inhibits the metabolism of paclitaxel to 6-alpha-hydroxypaclitaxel). Products include:
Accutane Capsules **2944**

Ketoconazole (The metabolism of paclitaxel is catalyzed by cytochrome P450 isoenzymes; based on *in vitro* studies, ketoconazole inhibits the metabolism of paclitaxel to 6-alpha-hydroxypaclitaxel, but the concentrations used exceeded those found *in vivo* following normal therapeutic doses). Products include:
Nizoral 2% Cream **3620**
Nizoral A-D Shampoo **2008**
Nizoral 2% Shampoo **2007**
Nizoral Tablets **1791**

Quercetin (The metabolism of paclitaxel is catalyzed by cytochrome P450 isoenzymes; based on *in vitro* studies, quercetin, a, specific inhibitor of CYP2C8, inhibits the metabolism of paclitaxel to 6-alpha-hydroxypaclitaxel).
No products indexed under this heading.

Quinidine Gluconate (The metabolism of paclitaxel is catalyzed by cytochrome P450 isoenzymes; based on *in vitro* studies, quinidine inhibits the metabolism of paclitaxel to 6-alpha-hydroxypaclitaxel, but the concentrations used exceeded those found in vivo following normal therapeutic doses). Products include:
Quinaglute Dura-Tabs Tablets **978**

Quinidine Polygalacturonate (The metabolism of paclitaxel is catalyzed by cytochrome P450 isoenzymes; based on *in vitro* studies, quinidine inhibits the metabolism of paclitaxel to 6-alpha-hydroxypaclitaxel, but the concentrations used exceeded those found in vivo following normal therapeutic doses).
No products indexed under this heading.

Quinidine Sulfate (The metabolism of paclitaxel is catalyzed by cytochrome P450 isoenzymes; based on *in vitro* studies, quinidine inhibits the metabolism of paclitaxel to 6-alpha-hydroxypaclitaxel, but the concentrations used exceeded those found in vivo following normal therapeutic doses). Products include:
Quinidex Extentabs **2933**

Teniposide (The metabolism of paclitaxel is catalyzed by cytochrome P450 isoenzymes; based on *in vitro* studies, teniposide inhibits the metabolism of paclitaxel to 6-alpha-hydroxypaclitaxel, but the concentrations used exceeded those found *in vivo* following normal therapeutic doses).
No products indexed under this heading.

Testosterone (The metabolism of paciltaxel is catalyzed by cytochrome P450 isoenzymes; based on *in vitro* studies, testosterone inhibits the metabolism of paclitaxel to 6-alpha-hydroxpaclitaxel). Products include:
Androderm Transdermal System CIII **3377**
AndroGel **3322**
Testoderm Transdermal Systems **574**
Testopel Pellets **3610**

Tretinoin (The metabolism of paclitaxel is catalyzed by cytochrome P450 isoenzymes; based on *in vitro* studies, retinoic acid inhibits the metabolism of paclitaxel to 6-alpha-hydroxypaclitaxel). Products include:
Avita Cream **999**
Avita Gel **1000**
Renova 0.02% Cream **2520**
Renova 0.05% Cream **2519**
Retin-A Micro 0.1% **2522**
Vesanoid Capsules **3037**

Verapamil Hydrochloride (The metabolism of paclitaxel is catalyzed by cytochrome P450 isoenzymes; based on *in vitro* studies, verapamil inhibits the metabolism of paclitaxel to 6-alpha-hydroxypaclitaxel, but the concentrations used exceeded those found *in vivo* following normal therapeutic doses). Products include:
Covera-HS Tablets **3199**
Isoptin SR Tablets **467**
Tarka Tablets **508**
Verelan Capsules **3184**
Verelan PM Capsules **3186**

Vincristine Sulfate (The metabolism of paclitaxel is catalyzed by cytochrome P450 isoenzymes; based on *in vitro* studies, vincristine inhibits the metabolism of paclitaxel to 6-alpha-hydroxypaclitaxel, but the concentrations used exceeded those found *in vivo* following normal therapeutic doses).
No products indexed under this heading.

TAXOTERE FOR INJECTION CONCENTRATE

(Docetaxel) **778**
May interact with erythromycin and certain other agents. Compounds in these categories include:

Cyclosporine (*in vitro* studies have shown that the metabolism of docetaxel may be modified by co-administration of compounds that induce, inhibit, or are metabolized by cytochrome P450 3A4, such as cyclosporine). Products include:
Gengraf Capsules **457**
Neoral Soft Gelatin Capsules **2380**
Neoral Oral Solution **2380**
Sandimmune **2388**

Erythromycin (*in vitro* studies have shown that the metabolism of docetaxel may be modified by co-administration of compounds that induce, inhibit, or are metabolized by cytochrome P450 3A4, such as erythromycin). Products include:
Emgel 2% Topical Gel **1285**
Ery-Tab Tablets **448**
Erythromycin Base Filmtab Tablets **454**
Erythromycin Delayed-Release Capsules, USP **455**
PCE Dispertab Tablets **498**

Erythromycin Estolate (*in vitro* studies have shown that the metabolism of docetaxel may be modified by co-administration of compounds that induce, inhibit, or are metabolized by cytochrome P450 3A4, such as erythromycin).
No products indexed under this heading.

Erythromycin Ethylsuccinate (*in vitro* studies have shown that the metabolism of docetaxel may be modified by co-administration of compounds that induce, inhibit, or are metabolized by cytochrome P450 3A4, such as erythromycin). Products include:
E.E.S. **450**
EryPed **446**
Pediazole Suspension **3050**

Erythromycin Gluceptate (*in vitro* studies have shown that the metabolism of docetaxel may be modified by co-administration of compounds that induce, inhibit, or are metabolized by cytochrome P450 3A4, such as erythromycin).
No products indexed under this heading.

Erythromycin Stearate (*in vitro* studies have shown that the metabolism of docetaxel may be modified by co-administration of compounds that induce, inhibit, or are metabolized by cytochrome P450 3A4, such as erythromycin). Products include:
Erythrocin Stearate Filmtab Tablets **452**

Ketoconazole (*in vitro* studies have shown that the metabolism of docetaxel may be modified by co-administration of compounds that induce, inhibit, or are metabolized by cytochrome P450 3A4, such as ketoconazole). Products include:
Nizoral 2% Cream **3620**
Nizoral A-D Shampoo **2008**
Nizoral 2% Shampoo **2007**
Nizoral Tablets **1791**

Terfenadine (*in vitro* studies have shown that the metabolism of docetaxel may be modified by co-administration of compounds that induce, inhibit, or are metabolized by cytochrome P450 3A4, such as terfenadine).
No products indexed under this heading.

Troleandomycin (*in vitro* studies have shown that the metabolism of docetaxel may be modified by co-administration of compounds that induce, inhibit, or are metabolized by cytochrome P450 3A4, such as troleandomycin). Products include:
Tao Capsules **2716**

TAZICEF FOR INJECTION

(Ceftazidime) **1647**
May interact with aminoglycosides, chloramphenicol, and certain other agents. Compounds in these categories include:

Amikacin Sulfate (Concomitant administration may result in nephrotoxicity).
No products indexed under this heading.

Chloramphenicol (Co-administration should be avoided due to the fact that chloramphenicol is shown to be antagonistic to beta-lactam antibiotics based on in vitro studies and time to kill curves with enteric gram-negative bacilli). Products include:
Chloromycetin Ophthalmic Ointment, 1% .... ⊙ **296**
Chloromycetin Ophthalmic Solution .... ⊙ **297**
Chloroptic Sterile Ophthalmic Ointment .... ⊙ **234**
Chloroptic Sterile Ophthalmic Solution .... ⊙ **235**

Chloramphenicol Palmitate (Co-administration should be avoided due to the fact that chloramphenicol is shown to be antagonistic to beta-lactam antibiotics based on in vitro studies and time to kill curves with enteric gram-negative bacilli).
No products indexed under this heading.

Chloramphenicol Sodium Succinate (Co-administration should be avoided due to the fact that chloramphenicol is shown to be antagonistic to beta-lactam antibiotics based on in vitro studies and time to kill curves with enteric gram-negative bacilli).
No products indexed under this heading.

Furosemide (Concomitant administration may result in nephrotoxicity). Products include:
Furosemide Tablets **2284**

Gentamicin Sulfate (Concomitant administration may result in nephrotoxicity). Products include:
Genoptic Ophthalmic Ointment .... ⊙ **239**
Genoptic Sterile Ophthalmic Solution .... ⊙ **239**
Pred-G Ophthalmic Suspension .... ⊙ **247**

Pred-G Sterile Ophthalmic Ointment .... ⊙248

Kanamycin Sulfate (Concomitant administration may result in nephrotoxicity).
No products indexed under this heading.

Streptomycin Sulfate (Concomitant administration may result in nephrotoxicity). Products include:
Streptomycin Sulfate Injection 2714

Tobramycin (Concomitant administration may result in nephrotoxicity). Products include:
TOBI Solution for Inhalation 1206
TobraDex Ophthalmic Ointment 542
TobraDex Ophthalmic Suspension 541
Tobrex Ophthalmic Ointment .... ⊙220
Tobrex Ophthalmic Solution .... ⊙221

Tobramycin Sulfate (Concomitant administration may result in nephrotoxicity). Products include:
Nebcin Vials, Hyporets & ADD-Vantage 1955

TAZICEF GALAXY CONTAINER
(Ceftazidime Sodium) 1650
See Tazicef for Injection

TAZICEF PHARMACY BULK PACKAGE
(Ceftazidime) 1653
See Tazicef for Injection

TAZIDIME VIALS, FASPAK & ADD-VANTAGE
(Ceftazidime) 1966
May interact with aminoglycosides and certain other agents. Compounds in these categories include:

Amikacin Sulfate (Potential for nephrotoxicity and ototoxicity; monitor renal function).
No products indexed under this heading.

Chloramphenicol Sodium Succinate (Chloramphenicol has been shown to be antagonistic to cephalosporins, including ceftazidime, based on in vitro studies; this combination therapy should be avoided).
No products indexed under this heading.

Furosemide (Potential for nephrotoxicity with potent diuretics, such as furosemide). Products include:
Furosemide Tablets 2284

Gentamicin Sulfate (Potential for nephrotoxicity and ototoxicity; monitor renal function). Products include:
Genoptic Ophthalmic Ointment .... ⊙239
Genoptic Sterile Ophthalmic Solution .... ⊙239
Pred-G Ophthalmic Suspension .... ⊙247
Pred-G Sterile Ophthalmic Ointment .... ⊙248

Kanamycin Sulfate (Potential for nephrotoxicity and ototoxicity; monitor renal function).
No products indexed under this heading.

Streptomycin Sulfate (Potential for nephrotoxicity and ototoxicity; monitor renal function). Products include:
Streptomycin Sulfate Injection 2714

Tobramycin (Potential for nephrotoxicity and ototoxicity; monitor renal function). Products include:
TOBI Solution for Inhalation 1206
TobraDex Ophthalmic Ointment 542
TobraDex Ophthalmic Suspension 541
Tobrex Ophthalmic Ointment .... ⊙220
Tobrex Ophthalmic Solution .... ⊙221

Tobramycin Sulfate (Potential for nephrotoxicity and ototoxicity; monitor renal function). Products include:
Nebcin Vials, Hyporets & ADD-Vantage 1955

TAZORAC GEL
(Tazarotene) 556
May interact with drugs known to be photosensitizers. Compounds in these categories include:

Alatrofloxacin Mesylate (Co-administration with drugs known to be photosensitizers may increase the possibility of augmented photosensitivity). Products include:
Trovan I.V. 2722

Bendroflumethiazide (Co-administration with drugs known to be photosensitizers may increase the possibility of augmented photosensitivity). Products include:
Corzide 40/5 Tablets 2247
Corzide 80/5 Tablets 2247

Chlorothiazide (Co-administration with drugs known to be photosensitizers may increase the possibility of augmented photosensitivity). Products include:
Aldoclor Tablets 2035
Diuril Oral 2087

Chlorothiazide Sodium (Co-administration with drugs known to be photosensitizers may increase the possibility of augmented photosensitivity). Products include:
Diuril Sodium Intravenous 2086

Chlorpromazine (Co-administration with drugs known to be photosensitizers may increase the possibility of augmented photosensitivity). Products include:
Thorazine Suppositories 1656

Chlorpromazine Hydrochloride (Co-administration with drugs known to be photosensitizers may increase the possibility of augmented photosensitivity). Products include:
Thorazine 1656

Chlorpropamide (Co-administration with drugs known to be photosensitizers may increase the possibility of augmented photosensitivity). Products include:
Diabinese Tablets 2680

Ciprofloxacin (Co-administration with drugs known to be photosensitizers may increase the possibility of augmented photosensitivity). Products include:
Cipro I.V. 893
Cipro I.V. Pharmacy Bulk Package 897
Cipro Oral Suspension 887

Ciprofloxacin Hydrochloride (Co-administration with drugs known to be photosensitizers may increase the possibility of augmented photosensitivity). Products include:
Ciloxan 538
Cipro HC Otic Suspension 540
Cipro Tablets 887

Demeclocycline Hydrochloride (Co-administration with drugs known to be photosensitizers may increase the possibility of augmented photosensitivity). Products include:
Declomycin Tablets 1855

Doxycycline Calcium (Co-administration with drugs known to be photosensitizers may increase the possibility of augmented photosensitivity). Products include:
Vibramycin Calcium Oral Suspension Syrup 2735

Doxycycline Hyclate (Co-administration with drugs known to be photosensitizers may increase the possibility of augmented photosensitivity). Products include:
Doryx Coated Pellet Filled Capsules 3357
Periostat Tablets 1208
Vibramycin Hyclate Capsules 2735
Vibramycin Hyclate Intravenous 2737
Vibra-Tabs Film Coated Tablets 2735

Doxycycline Monohydrate (Co-administration with drugs known to be photosensitizers may increase the possibility of augmented photosensitivity). Products include:
Monodox Capsules 2442
Vibramycin Monohydrate for Oral Suspension 2735

Enoxacin (Co-administration with drugs known to be photosensitizers may increase the possibility of augmented photosensitivity).
No products indexed under this heading.

Fluphenazine Decanoate (Co-administration with drugs known to be photosensitizers may increase the possibility of augmented photosensitivity).
No products indexed under this heading.

Fluphenazine Enanthate (Co-administration with drugs known to be photosensitizers may increase the possibility of augmented photosensitivity).
No products indexed under this heading.

Fluphenazine Hydrochloride (Co-administration with drugs known to be photosensitizers may increase the possibility of augmented photosensitivity).
No products indexed under this heading.

Glipizide (Co-administration with drugs known to be photosensitizers may increase the possibility of augmented photosensitivity). Products include:
Glucotrol Tablets 2692
Glucotrol XL Extended Release Tablets 2693

Glyburide (Co-administration with drugs known to be photosensitizers may increase the possibility of augmented photosensitivity). Products include:
DiaBeta Tablets 741
Glucovance Tablets 1086

Grepafloxacin Hydrochloride (Co-administration with drugs known to be photosensitizers may increase the possibility of augmented photosensitivity).
No products indexed under this heading.

Hydrochlorothiazide (Co-administration with drugs known to be photosensitizers may increase the possibility of augmented photosensitivity). Products include:
Accuretic Tablets 2614
Aldoril Tablets 2039
Atacand HCT Tablets 597
Avalide Tablets 1070
Diovan HCT Tablets 2338
Dyazide Capsules 1515
HydroDIURIL Tablets 2108
Hyzaar 2109
Inderide Tablets 3517
Inderide LA Long-Acting Capsules 3519
Lotensin HCT Tablets 2367
Maxzide 1008
Micardis HCT Tablets 1051
Microzide Capsules 3414
Moduretic Tablets 2138
Monopril HCT 1094
Prinzide Tablets 2168
Timolide Tablets 2187
Uniretic Tablets 3178
Vaseretic Tablets 2204
Zestoretic Tablets 695
Ziac Tablets 1887

Hydroflumethiazide (Co-administration with drugs known to be photosensitizers may increase the possibility of augmented photosensitivity). Products include:
Diucardin Tablets 3494

Lomefloxacin Hydrochloride (Co-administration with drugs known to be photosensitizers may increase the possibility of augmented photosensitivity).
No products indexed under this heading.

Mesoridazine Besylate (Co-administration with drugs known to be photosensitizers may increase the possibility of augmented photosensitivity). Products include:
Serentil 1057

Methacycline Hydrochloride (Co-administration with drugs known to be photosensitizers may increase the possibility of augmented photosensitivity).
No products indexed under this heading.

Methotrimeprazine (Co-administration with drugs known to be photosensitizers may increase the possibility of augmented photosensitivity).
No products indexed under this heading.

Methyclothiazide (Co-administration with drugs known to be photosensitizers may increase the possibility of augmented photosensitivity).
No products indexed under this heading.

Minocycline Hydrochloride (Co-administration with drugs known to be photosensitizers may increase the possibility of augmented photosensitivity). Products include:
Dynacin Capsules 2019
Minocin Intravenous 1862
Minocin Oral Suspension 1865
Minocin Pellet-Filled Capsules 1863

Norfloxacin (Co-administration with drugs known to be photosensitizers may increase the possibility of augmented photosensitivity). Products include:
Chibroxin Sterile Ophthalmic Solution 2051
Noroxin Tablets 2145

Ofloxacin (Co-administration with drugs known to be photosensitizers may increase the possibility of augmented photosensitivity). Products include:
Floxin I.V. 2526
Floxin Otic Solution 1219
Floxin Tablets 2529
Ocuflox Ophthalmic Solution 554

Oxytetracycline Hydrochloride (Co-administration with drugs known to be photosensitizers may increase the possibility of augmented photosensitivity). Products include:
Terra-Cortril Ophthalmic Suspension 2716
Urobiotic-250 Capsules 2731

Perphenazine (Co-administration with drugs known to be photosensitizers may increase the possibility of augmented photosensitivity). Products include:
Etrafon 3115
Trilafon 3160

Polythiazide (Co-administration with drugs known to be photosensitizers may increase the possibility of augmented photosensitivity). Products include:
Minizide Capsules 2700
Renese Tablets 2712

Prochlorperazine (Co-administration with drugs known to be photosensitizers may increase the possibility of augmented photosensitivity). Products include:
Compazine 1505

Promethazine Hydrochloride (Co-administration with drugs known to be photosensitizers may increase the possibility of augmented photosensitivity). Products include:
Mepergan Injection 3539
Phenergan Injection 3553
Phenergan 3556
Phenergan Syrup 3554
Phenergan with Codeine Syrup 3557
Phenergan with Dextromethorphan Syrup 3559
Phenergan VC Syrup 3560
Phenergan VC with Codeine Syrup 3561

Sulfamethizole (Co-administration with drugs known to be photosensitizers may increase the possibility of augmented photosensitivity). Products include:
Urobiotic-250 Capsules 2731

Sulfamethoxazole (Co-administration with drugs known to be photosensitizers may increase the possibility of augmented photosensitivity). Products include:
- Bactrim 2949
- Septra Suspension 2265
- Septra Tablets 2265
- Septra DS Tablets 2265

Sulfasalazine (Co-administration with drugs known to be photosensitizers may increase the possibility of augmented photosensitivity). Products include:
- Azulfidine EN-tabs Tablets 2775

Sulfinpyrazone (Co-administration with drugs known to be photosensitizers may increase the possibility of augmented photosensitivity).
No products indexed under this heading.

Sulfisoxazole (Co-administration with drugs known to be photosensitizers may increase the possibility of augmented photosensitivity).
No products indexed under this heading.

Sulfisoxazole Acetyl (Co-administration with drugs known to be photosensitizers may increase the possibility of augmented photosensitivity). Products include:
- Pediazole Suspension 3050

Sulfisoxazole Diolamine (Co-administration with drugs known to be photosensitizers may increase the possibility of augmented photosensitivity).
No products indexed under this heading.

Tetracycline Hydrochloride (Co-administration with drugs known to be photosensitizers may increase the possibility of augmented photosensitivity).
No products indexed under this heading.

Thioridazine Hydrochloride (Co-administration with drugs known to be photosensitizers may increase the possibility of augmented photosensitivity). Products include:
- Thioridazine Hydrochloride Tablets 2289

Tolazamide (Co-administration with drugs known to be photosensitizers may increase the possibility of augmented photosensitivity).
No products indexed under this heading.

Tolbutamide (Co-administration with drugs known to be photosensitizers may increase the possibility of augmented photosensitivity).
No products indexed under this heading.

Trifluoperazine Hydrochloride (Co-administration with drugs known to be photosensitizers may increase the possibility of augmented photosensitivity). Products include:
- Stelazine 1640

Trovafloxacin Mesylate (Co-administration with drugs known to be photosensitizers may increase the possibility of augmented photosensitivity). Products include:
- Trovan Tablets 2722

TEARS NATURALE FORTE LUBRICANT EYE DROPS
(Dextran 70, Hydroxypropyl Methylcellulose) 541
None cited in PDR database.

TEARS NATURALE FREE LUBRICANT EYE DROPS
(Dextran 70, Hydroxypropyl Methylcellulose) 541
None cited in PDR database.

TECHNI-CARE SURGICAL SCRUB, PREP AND WOUND DECONTAMINANT
(Chloroxylenol, Cocamidopropyl PG-Dimonium Chloride Phosphate) .... ▣632
None cited in PDR database.

TEGRETOL CHEWABLE TABLETS
(Carbamazepine) 2404
See Tegretol-XR Tablets

TEGRETOL SUSPENSION
(Carbamazepine) 2404
See Tegretol-XR Tablets

TEGRETOL TABLETS
(Carbamazepine) 2404
See Tegretol-XR Tablets

TEGRETOL-XR TABLETS
(Carbamazepine) 2404
May interact with doxycycline, anticonvulsants, erythromycin, lithium preparations, macrolide antibiotics, monoamine oxidase inhibitors, oral contraceptives, phenytoin, valproate, theophylline, and certain other agents. Compounds in these categories include:

Acetaminophen (Carbamazepine induces hepatic CYP activity; carbamazepine causes, or would be expected to cause, decreased levels of acetaminophen). Products include:
- Actifed Cold & Sinus Caplets and Tablets .... ▣688
- Alka-Seltzer Plus Liqui-Gels .... ▣604
- Alka-Seltzer Plus Cold & Flu Medicine Liqui-Gels .... ▣604
- Alka-Seltzer Plus Cold & Sinus Medicine Liqui-Gels .... ▣604
- Benadryl Allergy/Cold Tablets .... ▣691
- Benadryl Allergy Sinus Headache Caplets & Gelcaps .... ▣693
- Benadryl Severe Allergy & Sinus Headache Caplets .... ▣694
- Children's Cepacol Sore Throat .... ▣788
- Comtrex Acute Head Cold & Sinus Pressure Relief Tablets .... ▣627
- Comtrex Deep Chest Cold & Congestion Relief Softgels .... ▣627
- Comtrex Flu Therapy & Fever Relief Daytime Caplets .... ▣628
- Comtrex Flu Therapy & Fever Relief Nighttime Tablets .... ▣628
- Comtrex Maximum Strength Multi-Symptom Cold & Cough Relief Tablets and Caplets .... ▣626
- Contac Severe Cold and Flu Caplets Maximum Strength .... ▣746
- Contac Severe Cold and Flu Caplets Non-Drowsy .... ▣718
- Coricidin 'D' Cold, Flu & Sinus Tablets .... ▣737
- Coricidin HBP Cold & Flu Tablets .... ▣738
- Coricidin HBP Maximum Strength Flu Tablets .... ▣738
- Coricidin HBP Night-Time Cold & Flu Tablets .... ▣738
- Darvon-N/Darvocet-N 1907
- Dimetapp Cold and Fever Suspension .... ▣775
- Dimetapp Nighttime Flu Liquid .... ▣776
- Dimetapp Non-Drowsy Flu Syrup .... ▣777
- Drixoral Allergy/Sinus Extended-Release Tablets .... ▣741
- Drixoral Cold & Flu Extended-Release Tablets .... ▣740
- Aspirin Free Excedrin Caplets and Geltabs .... ▣628
- Excedrin Extra-Strength Tablets, Caplets, and Geltabs .... ▣629
- Excedrin Migraine 1070
- Excedrin PM Tablets, Caplets, and Geltabs .... ▣631
- Goody's Body Pain Formula Powder .... ▣620
- Goody's Extra Strength Headache Powder .... ▣620
- Goody's Extra Strength Pain Relief Tablets .... ▣620
- Goody's PM Powder .... ▣621
- Hycomine Compound Tablets 1317
- Lortab 3319
- Lortab Elixir 3317
- Maxidone Tablets CIII 3399
- Maximum Strength Midol Menstrual Caplets and Gelcaps .... ▣612
- Maximum Strength Midol PMS Caplets and Gelcaps .... ▣613
- Maximum Strength Midol Teen Caplets .... ▣612
- Midrin Capsules 3464
- Norco 5/325 Tablets CIII 3424
- Norco 7.5/325 Tablets CIII 3425
- Norco 10/325 Tablets CIII 3427
- Norco 10/325 Tablets CIII 3425
- Percocet Tablets 1326
- Percogesic Aspirin-Free Coated Tablets .... ▣667
- Extra Strength Percogesic Aspirin-Free Coated Caplets .... ▣665
- Phrenilin 578
- Robitussin Cold Caplets Multi-Symptom Cold & Flu .... ▣781
- Robitussin Cold Softgels Multi-Symptom Cold & Flu .... ▣781
- Robitussin Multi Symptom Honey Flu Liquid .... ▣785
- Robitussin Nighttime Honey Flu Liquid .... ▣786
- Sedapap Tablets 50 mg/650 mg 2225
- Singlet Caplets .... ▣761
- Sinutab Sinus Allergy Medication, Maximum Strength Formula, Tablets & Caplets .... ▣707
- Sinutab Sinus Medication, Maximum Strength Without Drowsiness Formula, Tablets & Caplets .... ▣707
- Sudafed Cold & Cough Liquid Caps .... ▣709
- Sudafed Cold & Sinus Liquid Caps .... ▣710
- Sudafed Severe Cold .... ▣711
- Sudafed Sinus Headache Caplets .... ▣712
- Sudafed Sinus Headache Tablets .... ▣712
- Tavist Sinus Non-Drowsy Coated Caplets .... ▣676
- TheraFlu Regular Strength Cold & Cough Night Time Hot Liquid .... ▣676
- TheraFlu Regular Strength Cold & Sore Throat Night Time Hot Liquid .... ▣676
- TheraFlu Maximum Strength Flu & Congestion Non-Drowsy Hot Liquid .... ▣677
- TheraFlu Maximum Strength Flu & Cough Night Time Hot Liquid .... ▣678
- TheraFlu Maximum Strength Flu & Sore Throat Night Time Hot Liquid .... ▣677
- TheraFlu Maximum Strength Severe Cold & Congestion Night Time Caplets .... ▣678
- TheraFlu Maximum Strength Severe Cold & Congestion Night Time Hot Liquid .... ▣678
- TheraFlu Maximum Strength Severe Cold & Congestion Non-Drowsy .... ▣679
- Triaminic Cold, Cough & Fever Liquid .... ▣681
- Triaminic Cough & Sore Throat Liquid .... ▣682
- Triaminic Cough & Sore Throat Softchews .... ▣684
- Tylenol, Children's 2014
- Children's Tylenol Allergy-D Liquid 2014
- Children's Tylenol Cold Suspension Liquid and Chewable Tablets 2015
- Children's Tylenol Cold Plus Cough Suspension Liquid and Chewable Tablets 2015
- Children's Tylenol Flu Suspension Liquid 2015
- Children's Tylenol Sinus Suspension Liquid 2017
- Infants' Tylenol Cold Decongestant and Fever Reducer Concentrated Drops 2015
- Infants' Tylenol Cold Decongestant and Fever Reducer Concentrated Drops Plus Cough 2015
- Junior Strength Tylenol Soft Chews Chewable Tablets 2014
- Tylenol 2009
- Tylenol Allergy Sinus 2010
- Tylenol Severe Allergy Caplets 2010
- Multi-Symptom Tylenol Cold Complete Formula Caplets 2010
- Multi-Symptom Tylenol Cold Non-Drowsy Caplets and Gelcaps 2010
- Multi-Symptom Tylenol Cold Severe Congestion Non-Drowsy Caplets 2011
- Maximum Strength Tylenol Flu NightTime Gelcaps 2011
- Maximum Strength Tylenol Flu NightTime Liquid 2011
- Maximum Strength Tylenol Flu Non-Drowsy Gelcaps 2011
- Extra Strength Tylenol PM Caplets, Geltabs, and Gelcaps 2012
- Maximum Strength Tylenol Sinus NightTime Caplets 2012
- Maximum Strength Tylenol Sinus Non-Drowsy Geltabs, Gelcaps, Caplets, and Tablets 2012
- Maximum Strength Tylenol Sore Throat Adult Liquid 2013
- Tylenol with Codeine 2595
- Women's Tylenol Menstrual Relief Caplets 2013
- Tylox Capsules 2597
- Ultracet Tablets 2597
- Vanquish Caplets .... ▣617
- Vicks 44M Cough, Cold & Flu Relief Liquid .... ▣725
- Vicks DayQuil LiquiCaps/Liquid Multi-Symptom Cold/Flu Relief .... ▣727
- Vicks NyQuil LiquiCaps/Liquid Multi-Symptom Cold/Flu Relief, Original and Cherry Flavors .... ▣727
- Vicodin Tablets 516
- Vicodin ES Tablets 517
- Vicodin HP Tablets 518
- Zydone Tablets 1330

Alprazolam (Carbamazepine induces hepatic CYP activity; carbamazepine causes, or would be expected to cause, decreased levels of alprazolam). Products include:
- Xanax Tablets 2865

Aminophylline (Co-administration with CYP3A4 inducers, such as theophylline, has been shown, or that would be expected, to decrease carbamazepine plasma levels; carbamazepine induces hepatic CYP activity; carbamazepine causes, or would be expected to cause decreased levels of theophylline).
No products indexed under this heading.

Azithromycin Dihydrate (Co-administration with CYP3A4 inhibitors, such as macrolides, inhibits carbamazepine metabolism and has been shown, or would be expected to increase carbamazepine plasma levels). Products include:
- Zithromax 2743
- Zithromax for IV Infusion 2748
- Zithromax for Oral Suspension, 300 mg, 600 mg, 900 mg, 1200 mg 2739
- Zithromax Tablets, 250 mg 2739

Chlorpromazine Hydrochloride (Concurrent use of Thorazine solution and Tegretol Suspension has resulted in an orange rubbery precipitate in stool; Tegretol Suspension should not be administered simultaneously with other liquid medications). Products include:
- Thorazine 1656

Cimetidine (Co-administration with CYP3A4 inhibitors, such as cimetidine, inhibits carbamazepine metabolism and has been shown, or would be expected to increase carbamazepine plasma levels). Products include:
- Tagamet HB 200 Suspension .... ▣762
- Tagamet HB 200 Tablets .... ▣761
- Tagamet Tablets 1644

Cimetidine Hydrochloride (Co-administration with CYP3A4 inhibitors, such as cimetidine inhibits carbamazepine metabolism and has been shown, or would be expected to increase carbamazepine plasma levels). Products include:
- Tagamet 1644

Cisplatin (Co-administration with CYP3A4 inducers, such as cisplatin, has been shown, or that would be expected, to decrease carbamazepine plasma levels).
No products indexed under this heading.

Clarithromycin (Co-administration with CYP3A4 inhibitors, such as macrolides, inhibits carbamazepine metabolism and has been shown, or would be expected to increase carbamazepine plasma levels). Products include:

Biaxin/Biaxin XL 403
PREVPAC 3298

Clomipramine Hydrochloride (Carbamazepine increases clomipramine plasma levels).
No products indexed under this heading.

Clonazepam (Carbamazepine induces hepatic CYP activity; carbamazepine causes, or would be expected to cause, decreased levels of clonazepam; combination therapy with other anticonvulsant drugs has resulted in alterations in thyroid function). Products include:
Klonopin Tablets 2983

Clozapine (Carbamazepine induces hepatic CYP activity: carbamazepine causes, or would be expected to cause decreased levels of clozapine). Products include:
Clozaril Tablets 2319

Danazol (Co-administration with CYP3A4 inhibitors, such as danazol, inhibits carbamazepine metabolism and has been shown, or would be expected to increase carbamazepine plasma levels).
No products indexed under this heading.

Desogestrel (Carbamazepine induces hepatic CYP activity; carbamazepine causes, or would be expected to cause, decreased levels of oral contraceptives; breakthrough bleeding has been reported among patients receiving concomitant oral and subdermal contraceptives and their reliability may be adversely affected). Products include:
Cyclessa Tablets 2450
Desogen Tablets 2458
Mircette Tablets 2470
Ortho-Cept 21 Tablets 2546
Ortho-Cept 28 Tablets 2546

Dicumarol (Carbamazepine induces hepatic CYP activity; carbamazepine causes, or would be expected to cause, decreased levels of dicumarol).
No products indexed under this heading.

Diltiazem Hydrochloride (Co-administration with CYP3A4 inhibitors, such as diltiazem, inhibits carbamazepine metabolism and has been shown, or would be expected to increase carbamazepine plasma levels). Products include:
Cardizem Injectable 1018
Cardizem Lyo-Ject Syringe 1018
Cardizem Monovial 1018
Cardizem CD Capsules 1016
Tiazac Capsules 1378

Dirithromycin (Co-administration with CYP3A4 inhibitors, such as macrolides, inhibits carbamazepine metabolism and has been shown, or would be expected to increase carbamazepine plasma levels).
Products include:
Dynabac Tablets 2269

Divalproex Sodium (Co-administration with CYP3A4 inhibitors, such as valproate, inhibits carbamazepine metabolism and has been shown, or would be expected to increase carbamazepine (active 10, 11-epoxide) plasma levels; carbamazepine causes, or would be expected to cause, decreased levels of valproate; combination therapy with other anticonvulsant drugs has resulted in alterations in thyroid function). Products include:
Depakote Sprinkle Capsules 426
Depakote Tablets 430
Depakote ER Tablets 436

Doxorubicin Hydrochloride (Co-administration with CYP3A4 inducers, such as doxorubicin, has been shown, or that would be expected, to decrease carbamazepine plasma levels). Products include:
Adriamycin PFS/RDF Injection 2767
Doxil Injection 566

Doxycycline Calcium (Carbamazepine induces hepatic CYP activity; carbamazepine causes, or would be expected to cause, decreased levels of doxycycline). Products include:
Vibramycin Calcium Oral Suspension Syrup 2735

Doxycycline Hyclate (Carbamazepine induces hepatic CYP activity; carbamazepine causes, or would be expected to cause, decreased levels of doxycycline). Products include:
Doryx Coated Pellet Filled Capsules 3357
Periostat Tablets 1208
Vibramycin Hyclate Capsules 2735
Vibramycin Hyclate Intravenous 2737
Vibra-Tabs Film Coated Tablets 2735

Doxycycline Monohydrate (Carbamazepine induces hepatic CYP activity; carbamazepine causes, or would be expected to cause, decreased levels of doxycycline). Products include:
Monodox Capsules 2442
Vibramycin Monohydrate for Oral Suspension 2735

Dyphylline (Co-administration with CYP3A4 inducers, such as theophylline, has been shown, or that would be expected, to decrease carbamazepine plasma levels; carbamazepine induces hepatic CYP activity; carbamazepine causes, or would be expected to cause decreased levels of theophylline). Products include:
Lufyllin Tablets 3347
Lufyllin-400 Tablets 3347
Lufyllin-GG Elixir 3348
Lufyllin-GG Tablets 3348

Erythromycin (Co-administration with CYP3A4 inhibitors, such as erythromycin, inhibits carbamazepine metabolism and has been shown, or would be expected to increase carbamazepine plasma levels). Products include:
Emgel 2% Topical Gel 1285
Ery-Tab Tablets 448
Erythromycin Base Filmtab Tablets 454
Erythromycin Delayed-Release Capsules, USP 455
PCE Dispertab Tablets 498

Erythromycin Estolate (Co-administration with CYP3A4 inhibitors, such as erythromycin, inhibits carbamazepine metabolism and has been shown, or would be expected to increase carbamazepine plasma levels).
No products indexed under this heading.

Erythromycin Ethylsuccinate (Co-administration with CYP3A4 inhibitors, such as erythromycin, inhibits carbamazepine metabolism and has been shown, or would be expected to increase carbamazepine plasma levels). Products include:
E.E.S. 450
EryPed 446
Pediazole Suspension 3050

Erythromycin Gluceptate (Co-administration with CYP3A4 inhibitors, such as erythromycin, inhibits carbamazepine metabolism and has been shown, or would be expected to increase carbamazepine plasma levels).
No products indexed under this heading.

Erythromycin Stearate (Co-administration with CYP3A4 inhibitors, such as erythromycin, inhibits carbamazepine metabolism and has been shown, or would be expected to increase carbamazepine plasma levels). Products include:
Erythrocin Stearate Filmtab Tablets 452

Ethinyl Estradiol (Carbamazepine induces hepatic CYP activity; carbamazepine causes, or would be expected to cause, decreased levels of oral contraceptives; breakthrough bleeding has been reported among patients receiving concomitant oral and subdermal contraceptives and their reliability may be adversely affected). Products include:
Alesse-21 Tablets 3468
Alesse-28 Tablets 3473
Brevicon 28-Day Tablets 3380
Cyclessa Tablets 2450
Desogen Tablets 2458
Estinyl Tablets 3112
Estrostep 2627
femhrt Tablets 2635
Levlen 962
Levlite 21 Tablets 962
Levlite 28 Tablets 962
Levora Tablets 3389
Loestrin 21 Tablets 2642
Loestrin Fe Tablets 2642
Lo/Ovral Tablets 3532
Lo/Ovral-28 Tablets 3538
Low-Ogestrel-28 Tablets 3392
Microgestin Fe 1.5/30 Tablets 3407
Microgestin Fe 1/20 Tablets 3400
Mircette Tablets 2470
Modicon 2563
Necon 3415
Nordette-28 Tablets 2257
Norinyl 1 +35 28-Day Tablets 3380
Ogestrel 0.5/50-28 Tablets 3428
Ortho-Cept 21 Tablets 2546
Ortho-Cept 28 Tablets 2546
Ortho-Cyclen/Ortho Tri-Cyclen 2573
Ortho-Novum 2563
Ovcon 3364
Ovral Tablets 3551
Ovral-28 Tablets 3552
Tri-Levlen 962
Tri-Norinyl-28 Tablets 3433
Triphasil-21 Tablets 3600
Triphasil-28 Tablets 3605
Trivora Tablets 3439
Yasmin 28 Tablets 980
Zovia 3449

Ethosuximide (Carbamazepine induces hepatic CYP activity; carbamazepine causes, or would be expected to cause, decreased levels of ethosuximide; combination therapy with other anticonvulsant drugs has resulted in alterations in thyroid function). Products include:
Zarontin Capsules 2659
Zarontin Syrup 2660

Ethotoin (Combination therapy with other anticonvulsant drugs has resulted in alterations in thyroid function).
No products indexed under this heading.

Ethynodiol Diacetate (Carbamazepine induces hepatic CYP activity; carbamazepine causes, or would be expected to cause, decreased levels of oral contraceptives; breakthrough bleeding has been reported among patients receiving concomitant oral and subdermal contraceptives and their reliability may be adversely affected). Products include:
Zovia 3449

Felbamate (Co-administration with CYP3A4 inducers, such as felbamate, has been shown, or that would be expected, to decrease carbamazepine and increased levels of the 10, 11-epoxide plasma levels; combination therapy with other anticonvulsant drugs has resulted in alterations in thyroid function). Products include:
Felbatol 3343

Fluoxetine Hydrochloride (Co-administration with CYP3A4 inhibitors, such as fluoxetine, inhibits carbamazepine metabolism and has been shown, or would be expected to increase carbamazepine plasma levels). Products include:
Prozac Pulvules, Liquid, and Weekly Capsules 1238
Sarafem Pulvules 1962

Fosphenytoin Sodium (Co-administration with CYP3A4 inducers, such as phenytoin, has been shown, or that would be expected, to decrease carbamazepine plasma levels; carbamazepine increases phenytoin plasma levels; carbamazepine induces hepatic CYP activity; carbamazepine causes, or would be expected to cause, decreased levels of phenytoin; combination therapy with other anticonvulsant drugs has resulted in alterations in thyroid function). Products include:
Cerebyx Injection 2619

Haloperidol (Carbamazepine induces hepatic CYP activity; carbamazepine causes, or would be expected to cause, decreased levels of haloperidol). Products include:
Haldol Injection, Tablets and Concentrate 2533

Haloperidol Decanoate (Carbamazepine induces hepatic CYP activity; carbamazepine causes, or would be expected to cause, decreased levels of haloperidol). Products include:
Haldol Decanoate 2535

Isocarboxazid (Because of the relationship of carbamazepine to other tricyclic compounds, on theoretical grounds, co-administration with MAO inhibitors is contraindicated).
No products indexed under this heading.

Isoniazid (Co-administration with CYP3A4 inhibitors, such as isoniazid, inhibits carbamazepine metabolism and has been shown, or would be expected to increase carbamazepine plasma levels). Products include:
Rifamate Capsules 767
Rifater Tablets 769

Itraconazole (Co-administration with CYP3A4 inhibitors, such as itraconazole, inhibits carbamazepine metabolism and has been shown, or would be expected to increase carbamazepine plasma levels).
Products include:
Sporanox Capsules 1800
Sporanox Injection 1804
Sporanox Injection 2509
Sporanox Oral Solution 1808
Sporanox Oral Solution 2512

Ketoconazole (Co-administration with CYP3A4 inhibitors, such as ketoconazole, inhibits carbamazepine metabolism and has been sown, or would be expected to increase carbamazepine plasma levels).
Products include:
Nizoral 2% Cream 3620
Nizoral A-D Shampoo 2008
Nizoral 2% Shampoo 2007
Nizoral Tablets 1791

Lamotrigine (Carbamazepine induces hepatic CYP activity; carbamazepine causes, or would be expected to cause, decreased levels of lamotrigine; combination therapy with other anticonvulsant drugs has resulted in alterations in thyroid function). Products include:
Lamictal 1567

Levetiracetam (Combination therapy with other anticonvulsant drugs has resulted in alterations in thyroid function). Products include:
Keppra Tablets 3314

Levonorgestrel (Carbamazepine induces hepatic CYP activity; carbamazepine causes, or would be expected to cause, decreased levels of oral contraceptives; breakthrough bleeding has been reported among patients receiving concomitant oral and subdermal contraceptives and their reliability may be adversely affected). Products include:
Alesse-21 Tablets 3468
Alesse-28 Tablets 3473
Levlen 962
Levlite 21 Tablets 962
Levlite 28 Tablets 962
Levora Tablets 3389
Mirena Intrauterine System 974
Nordette-28 Tablets 2257
Norplant System 3543
Tri-Levlen 962
Triphasil-21 Tablets 3600
Triphasil-28 Tablets 3605
Trivora Tablets 3439

Lithium Carbonate (Co-administration may increase the risk of nuerotoxic side effects). Products include:
- Eskalith 1527
- Lithium Carbonate 3061
- Lithobid Slow-Release Tablets 3255

Lithium Citrate (Co-administration may increase the risk of nuerotoxic side effects). Products include:
- Lithium Citrate Syrup 3061

Loratadine (Co-administration with CYP3A4 inhibitors, such as loratadine, inhibits carbamazepine metabolism and has been shown, or would be expected to increase carbamazepine plasma levels). Products include:
- Claritin 3100
- Claritin-D 12 Hour Extended Release Tablets 3102
- Claritin-D 24 Hour Extended Release Tablets 3104

Mephenytoin (Combination therapy with other anticonvulsant drugs has resulted in alterations in thyroid function).
- No products indexed under this heading.

Mestranol (Carbamazepine induces hepatic CYP activity; carbamazepine causes, or would be expected to cause, decreased levels of oral contraceptives; breakthrough bleeding has been reported among patients receiving concomitant oral and subdermal contraceptives and their reliability may be adversely affected). Products include:
- Necon 1/50 Tablets 3415
- Norinyl 1 + 50 28-Day Tablets 3380
- Ortho-Novum 1/50□28 Tablets 2556

Methsuximide (Carbamazepine induces hepatic CYP activity; carbamazepine causes, or would be expected to cause, decreased levels of methsuximide; combination therapy with other anticonvulsant drugs has resulted in alterations in thyroid function). Products include:
- Celontin Capsules 2618

Moclobemide (Because of the relationship of carbamazepine to other tricyclic compounds, on theoretical grounds, co-administration with MAO inhibitors is contraindicated).
- No products indexed under this heading.

Niacinamide (Co-administration with CYP3A4 inhibitors, such as niacinamide, inhibits carbamazepine metabolism and has been shown, or would be expected to increase carbamazepine plasma levels).
- No products indexed under this heading.

Nicotinamide (Co-administration with CYP3A4 inhibitors, such as nicotinamide, inhibits carbamazepine metabolism and has been shown, or would be expected to increase carbamazepine plasma levels). Products include:
- Nicomide Tablets 3247

Norethindrone (Carbamazepine induces hepatic CYP activity; carbamazepine causes, or would be expected to cause, decreased levels of oral contraceptives; breakthrough bleeding has been reported among patients receiving concomitant oral and subdermal contraceptives and their reliability may be adversely affected). Products include:
- Brevicon 28-Day Tablets 3380
- Micronor Tablets 2543
- Modicon 2563
- Necon 3415
- Norinyl 1 +35 28-Day Tablets 3380
- Norinyl 1 + 50 28-Day Tablets 3380
- Nor-QD Tablets 3423
- Ortho-Novum 2563
- Ortho-Novum 1/50□28 Tablets 2556
- Ovcon 3364
- Tri-Norinyl-28 Tablets 3433

Norethynodrel (Carbamazepine induces hepatic CYP activity; carbamazepine causes, or would be expected to cause, decreased levels of oral contraceptives; breakthrough bleeding has been reported among patients receiving concomitant oral and subdermal contraceptives and their reliability may be adversely affected).
- No products indexed under this heading.

Norgestimate (Carbamazepine induces hepatic CYP activity; carbamazepine causes, or would be expected to cause, decreased levels of oral contraceptives; breakthrough bleeding has been reported among patients receiving concomitant oral and subdermal contraceptives and their reliability may be adversely affected). Products include:
- Ortho-Cyclen/Ortho Tri-Cyclen 2573
- Ortho-Prefest Tablets 2570

Norgestrel (Carbamazepine induces hepatic CYP activity; carbamazepine causes, or would be expected to cause, decreased levels of oral contraceptives; breakthrough bleeding has been reported among patients receiving concomitant oral and subdermal contraceptives and their reliability may be adversely affected). Products include:
- Lo/Ovral Tablets 3532
- Lo/Ovral-28 Tablets 3538
- Low-Ogestrel-28 Tablets 3392
- Ogestrel 0.5/50-28 Tablets 3428
- Ovral Tablets 3551
- Ovral-28 Tablets 3552
- Ovrette Tablets 3552

Oxcarbazepine (Combination therapy with other anticonvulsant drugs has resulted in alterations in thyroid function). Products include:
- Trileptal Oral Suspension 2407
- Trileptal Tablets 2407

Paramethadione (Combination therapy with other anticonvulsant drugs has resulted in alterations in thyroid function).
- No products indexed under this heading.

Pargyline Hydrochloride (Because of the relationship of carbamazepine to other tricyclic compounds, on theoretical grounds, co-administration with MAO inhibitors is contraindicated).
- No products indexed under this heading.

Phenacemide (Combination therapy with other anticonvulsant drugs has resulted in alterations in thyroid function).
- No products indexed under this heading.

Phenelzine Sulfate (Because of the relationship of carbamazepine to other tricyclic compounds, on theoretical grounds, co-administration with MAO inhibitors is contraindicated). Products include:
- Nardil Tablets 2653

Phenobarbital (Co-administration with CYP3A4 inducers, such as phenobarbital, has been shown, or that would be expected, to decrease carbamazepine plasma levels; carbamezepine increases phenobarbital plasma levels; combination therapy with other anticonvulsant drugs has resulted in alterations of thyroid function). Products include:
- Arco-Lase Plus Tablets 592
- Donnatal 2929
- Donnatal Extentabs 2930

Phensuximide (Carbamazepine induces hepatic CYP activity; carbamazepine causes, or would be expected to cause, decreased levels of phensuximide; combination therapy with other anticonvulsant drugs has resulted in alterations in thyroid function).
- No products indexed under this heading.

Phenytoin (Co-administration with CYP3A4 inducers, such as phenytoin, has been shown, or that would be expected, to decrease carbamazepine plasma levels; carbamazepine increases phenytoin plasma levels; carbamazepine induces hepatic CYP activity; carbamazepine causes, or would be expected to cause, decreased levels of phenytoin; combination therapy with other anticonvulsant drugs has resulted in alterations in thyroid function). Products include:
- Dilantin Infatabs 2624
- Dilantin-125 Oral Suspension 2625

Phenytoin Sodium (Co-administration with CYP3A4 inducers, such as phenytoin, has been shown, or that would be expected, to decrease carbamazepine plasma levels; carbamazepine increases phenytoin plasma levels; carbamazepine induces hepatic CYP activity; carbamazepine causes, or would be expected to cause, decreased levels of phenytoin; combination therapy with other anticonvulsant drugs has resulted in alterations in thyroid function). Products include:
- Dilantin Kapseals 2622

Primidone (Co-administration with CYP3A4 inducers, such as primidone, has been shown, or that would be expected, to decrease carbamazepine plasma levels; carbamazepine increases primidone plasma levels; combination therapy with other anticonvulsant drugs has resulted in alterations in thyroid function).
- No products indexed under this heading.

Procarbazine Hydrochloride (Because of the relationship of carbamazepine to other tricyclic compounds, on theoretical grounds, co-administration with MAO inhibitors is contraindicated). Products include:
- Matulane Capsules 3246

Propoxyphene Hydrochloride (Co-administration with CYP3A4 inhibitors, such as propoxyphene, inhibits carbamazepine metabolism and has been shown, or would be expected to increase carbamazepine plasma levels). Products include:
- Darvon Pulvules 1909
- Darvon Compound-65 Pulvules 1910

Propoxyphene Napsylate (Co-administration with CYP3A4 inhibitors, such as propoxyphene, inhibits carbamazepine metabolism and has been shown, or would be expected to increase carbamazepine plasma levels). Products include:
- Darvon-N/Darvocet-N 1907
- Darvon-N Tablets 1912

Rifampin (Co-administration with CYP3A4 inducers, such as rifampin, has been shown, or that would be expected, to decrease carbamazepine plasma levels). Products include:
- Rifadin 765
- Rifamate Capsules 767
- Rifater Tablets 769

Selegiline Hydrochloride (Because of the relationship of carbamazepine to other tricyclic compounds, on theoretical grounds, co-administration with MAO inhibitors is contraindicated). Products include:
- Eldepryl Capsules 3266

Terfenadine (Co-administration with CYP3A4 inhibitors, such as terfenadine, inhibits carbamazepine metabolism and has been shown, or would be expected to increase carbamazepine plasma levels).
- No products indexed under this heading.

Theophylline (Co-administration with CYP3A4 inducers, such as theophylline, has been shown, or that would be expected, to decrease carbamazepine plasma levels; carbamazepine induces hepatic CYP activity; carbamazepine causes, or would be expected to cause decreased levels of theophylline). Products include:
- Aerolate 1361
- Theo-Dur Extended-Release Tablets 1835
- Uni-Dur Extended-Release Tablets .. 1841
- Uniphyl 400 mg and 600 mg Tablets 2903

Theophylline Calcium Salicylate (Co-administration with CYP3A4 inducers, such as theophylline, has been shown, or that would be expected, to decrease carbamazepine plasma levels; carbamazepine induces hepatic CYP activity; carbamazepine causes, or would be expected to cause decreased levels of theophylline).
- No products indexed under this heading.

Theophylline Sodium Glycinate (Co-administration with CYP3A4 inducers, such as theophylline, has been shown, or that would be expected, to decrease carbamazepine plasma levels; carbamazepine induces hepatic CYP activity; carbamazepine causes, or would be expected to cause decreased levels of theophylline).
- No products indexed under this heading.

Thioridazine Hydrochloride (Concurrent use of Mellaril Solution and Tegretol Suspension has resulted in an orange rubbery precipitate in stool; Tegretol Suspension should not be administered simultaneously with other liquid medications). Products include:
- Thioridazine Hydrochloride Tablets 2289

Tiagabine Hydrochloride (Carbamazepine induces hepatic CYP activity; carbamazepine causes, or would be expected to cause, decreased levels of tiagabine; combination therapy with other anticonvulsant drugs has resulted in alterations in thyroid function). Products include:
- Gabitril Tablets 1189

Topiramate (Carbamazepine induces hepatic CYP activity; carbamazepine causes, or would be expected to cause, decreased levels of topiramate; combination therapy with other anticonvulsant drugs has resulted in alterations in thyroid function). Products include:
- Topamax Sprinkle Capsules 2590
- Topamax Tablets 2590

Tranylcypromine Sulfate (Because of the relationship of carbamazepine to other tricyclic compounds, on theoretical grounds, co-administration with MAO inhibitors is contraindicated). Products include:
- Parnate Tablets 1607

Trimethadione (Combination therapy with other anticonvulsant drugs has resulted in alterations in thyroid function).
- No products indexed under this heading.

Troleandomycin (Co-administration with CYP3A4 inhibitors, such as macrolides, inhibits carbamazepine metabolism and has been shown, or would be expected to increase carbamazepine plasma levels). Products include:
- Tao Capsules 2716

Valproate Sodium (Co-administration with CYP3A4 inhibitors, such as valproate, inhibits carbamazepine metabolism and has been shown, or would be expected to increase carbamazepine (active 10, 11-epoxide) plasma levels; car-

bamazepine causes, or would be expected to cause, decreased levels of valproate; combination therapy with other anticonvulsant drugs has resulted in alterations in thyroid function). Products include:

Depacon Injection ... 416

Valproic Acid (Co-administration with CYP3A4 inhibitors, such as valproate, inhibits carbamazepine metabolism and has been shown, or would be expected to increase carbamazepine (active 10, 11-epoxide) plasma levels; carbamazepine causes, or would be expected to cause, decreased levels of valproate; combination therapy with other anticonvulsant drugs has resulted in alterations in thyroid function). Products include:

Depakene ... 421

Verapamil Hydrochloride (Co-administration with CYP3A4 inhibitors, such as verapamil, inhibits carbamazepine metabolism and has been shown, or would be expected to increase carbamazepine plasma levels). Products include:

Covera-HS Tablets ... 3199
Isoptin SR Tablets ... 467
Tarka Tablets ... 508
Verelan Capsules ... 3184
Verelan PM Capsules ... 3186

Warfarin Sodium (Carbamazepine induces hepatic CYP activity; carbamazepine causes, or would be expected to cause, decreased levels of warfarin). Products include:

Coumadin for Injection ... 1243
Coumadin Tablets ... 1243
Warfarin Sodium Tablets, USP ... 3302

Zonisamide (Combination therapy with other anticonvulsant drugs has resulted in alterations in thyroid function). Products include:

Zonegran Capsules ... 1307

TEGRIN DANDRUFF SHAMPOO - EXTRA CONDITIONING

(Coal Tar) ... 623
None cited in PDR database.

TEGRIN DANDRUFF SHAMPOO - FRESH HERBAL

(Coal Tar) ... 624
None cited in PDR database.

TEGRIN SKIN CREAM

(Coal Tar) ... 624
None cited in PDR database.

TEMODAR CAPSULES

(Temozolomide) ... 3157
May interact with valproate and certain other agents. Compounds in these categories include:

Divalproex Sodium (Co-administration with valproic acid decreases oral clearance of temozolomide by about 5%; the clinical implication of this effect is not known). Products include:

Depakote Sprinkle Capsules ... 426
Depakote Tablets ... 430
Depakote ER Tablets ... 436

Valproate Sodium (Co-administration with valproic acid decreases oral clearance of temozolomide by about 5%; the clinical implication of this effect is not known). Products include:

Depacon Injection ... 416

Valproic Acid (Co-administration with valproic acid decreases oral clearance of temozolomide by about 5%; the clinical implication of this effect is not known). Products include:

Depakene ... 421

Food Interactions

Food, unspecified (Co-administration with a modified high-fat breakfast has resulted in decrease in mean plasma concentration and AUC by 32% and 9% respectively, and 2-fold increase in Tmax).

TEMOVATE CREAM

(Clobetasol Propionate) ... 1301
None cited in PDR database.

TEMOVATE GEL

(Clobetasol Propionate) ... 1303
None cited in PDR database.

TEMOVATE OINTMENT

(Clobetasol Propionate) ... 1301
None cited in PDR database.

TEMOVATE SCALP APPLICATION

(Clobetasol Propionate) ... 1304
None cited in PDR database.

TEMOVATE E EMOLLIENT

(Clobetasol Propionate) ... 1302
None cited in PDR database.

TENEX TABLETS

(Guanfacine Hydrochloride) ... 2942
May interact with central nervous system depressants and certain other agents. Compounds in these categories include:

Alfentanil Hydrochloride (Potential for increased sedation).
No products indexed under this heading.

Alprazolam (Potential for increased sedation). Products include:

Xanax Tablets ... 2865

Aprobarbital (Potential for increased sedation).
No products indexed under this heading.

Buprenorphine Hydrochloride (Potential for increased sedation). Products include:

Buprenex Injectable ... 2918

Buspirone Hydrochloride (Potential for increased sedation).
No products indexed under this heading.

Butabarbital (Potential for increased sedation).
No products indexed under this heading.

Butalbital (Potential for increased sedation). Products include:

Phrenilin ... 578
Sedapap Tablets 50 mg/650 mg ... 2225

Chlordiazepoxide (Potential for increased sedation). Products include:

Limbitrol ... 1738

Chlordiazepoxide Hydrochloride (Potential for increased sedation). Products include:

Librium Capsules ... 1736
Librium for Injection ... 1737

Chlorpromazine (Potential for increased sedation). Products include:

Thorazine Suppositories ... 1656

Chlorpromazine Hydrochloride (Potential for increased sedation). Products include:

Thorazine ... 1656

Chlorprothixene (Potential for increased sedation).
No products indexed under this heading.

Chlorprothixene Hydrochloride (Potential for increased sedation).
No products indexed under this heading.

Chlorprothixene Lactate (Potential for increased sedation).
No products indexed under this heading.

Clorazepate Dipotassium (Potential for increased sedation). Products include:

Tranxene ... 511

Clozapine (Potential for increased sedation). Products include:

Clozaril Tablets ... 2319

Codeine Phosphate (Potential for increased sedation). Products include:

Phenergan with Codeine Syrup ... 3557
Phenergan VC with Codeine Syrup ... 3561
Robitussin A-C Syrup ... 2942
Robitussin-DAC Syrup ... 2942
Ryna-C Liquid ... 768
Soma Compound w/Codeine Tablets ... 3355
Tussi-Organidin NR Liquid ... 3350
Tussi-Organidin-S NR Liquid ... 3350
Tylenol with Codeine ... 2595

Desflurane (Potential for increased sedation). Products include:

Suprane Liquid for Inhalation ... 874

Dezocine (Potential for increased sedation).
No products indexed under this heading.

Diazepam (Potential for increased sedation). Products include:

Valium Injectable ... 3026
Valium Tablets ... 3047

Droperidol (Potential for increased sedation).
No products indexed under this heading.

Enflurane (Potential for increased sedation).
No products indexed under this heading.

Estazolam (Potential for increased sedation). Products include:

ProSom Tablets ... 500

Ethchlorvynol (Potential for increased sedation).
No products indexed under this heading.

Ethinamate (Potential for increased sedation).
No products indexed under this heading.

Fentanyl (Potential for increased sedation). Products include:

Duragesic Transdermal System ... 1786

Fentanyl Citrate (Potential for increased sedation). Products include:

Actiq ... 1184

Fluphenazine Decanoate (Potential for increased sedation).
No products indexed under this heading.

Fluphenazine Enanthate (Potential for increased sedation).
No products indexed under this heading.

Fluphenazine Hydrochloride (Potential for increased sedation).
No products indexed under this heading.

Flurazepam Hydrochloride (Potential for increased sedation).
No products indexed under this heading.

Glutethimide (Potential for increased sedation).
No products indexed under this heading.

Haloperidol (Potential for increased sedation). Products include:

Haldol Injection, Tablets and Concentrate ... 2533

Haloperidol Decanoate (Potential for increased sedation). Products include:

Haldol Decanoate ... 2535

Hydrocodone Bitartrate (Potential for increased sedation). Products include:

Hycodan ... 1316
Hycomine Compound Tablets ... 1317
Hycotuss Expectorant Syrup ... 1318
Lortab ... 3319
Lortab Elixir ... 3317
Maxidone Tablets CIII ... 3399
Norco 5/325 Tablets CIII ... 3424
Norco 7.5/325 Tablets CIII ... 3425
Norco 10/325 Tablets CIII ... 3427
Norco 10/325 Tablets CIII ... 3425
Vicodin Tablets ... 516
Vicodin ES Tablets ... 517
Vicodin HP Tablets ... 518
Vicodin Tuss Expectorant ... 519
Vicoprofen Tablets ... 520
Zydone Tablets ... 1330

Hydrocodone Polistirex (Potential for increased sedation). Products include:

Tussionex Pennkinetic Extended-Release Suspension ... 1174

Hydromorphone Hydrochloride (Potential for increased sedation). Products include:

Dilaudid ... 441
Dilaudid Oral Liquid ... 445
Dilaudid Powder ... 441
Dilaudid Rectal Suppositories ... 441
Dilaudid Tablets ... 441
Dilaudid Tablets - 8 mg ... 445
Dilaudid-HP ... 443

Hydroxyzine Hydrochloride (Potential for increased sedation). Products include:

Atarax Tablets & Syrup ... 2667
Vistaril Intramuscular Solution ... 2738

Isoflurane (Potential for increased sedation).
No products indexed under this heading.

Ketamine Hydrochloride (Potential for increased sedation).
No products indexed under this heading.

Levomethadyl Acetate Hydrochloride (Potential for increased sedation).
No products indexed under this heading.

Levorphanol Tartrate (Potential for increased sedation). Products include:

Levo-Dromoran ... 1734
Levorphanol Tartrate Tablets ... 3059

Lorazepam (Potential for increased sedation). Products include:

Ativan Injection ... 3478
Ativan Tablets ... 3482

Loxapine Hydrochloride (Potential for increased sedation).
No products indexed under this heading.

Loxapine Succinate (Potential for increased sedation). Products include:

Loxitane Capsules ... 3398

Meperidine Hydrochloride (Potential for increased sedation). Products include:

Demerol ... 3079
Mepergan Injection ... 3539

Mephobarbital (Potential for increased sedation).
No products indexed under this heading.

Meprobamate (Potential for increased sedation). Products include:

Miltown Tablets ... 3349

Mesoridazine Besylate (Potential for increased sedation). Products include:

Serentil ... 1057

Methadone Hydrochloride (Potential for increased sedation). Products include:

Dolophine Hydrochloride Tablets ... 3056

Methohexital Sodium (Potential for increased sedation). Products include:

Brevital Sodium for Injection, USP ... 1815

Methotrimeprazine (Potential for increased sedation).
No products indexed under this heading.

Methoxyflurane (Potential for increased sedation).
No products indexed under this heading.

Midazolam Hydrochloride (Potential for increased sedation). Products include:

Versed Injection ... 3027
Versed Syrup ... 3033

Molindone Hydrochloride (Potential for increased sedation). Products include:

Moban 1320

Morphine Sulfate (Potential for increased sedation). Products include:
- Astramorph/PF Injection, USP (Preservative-Free) 594
- Duramorph Injection 1312
- Infumorph 200 and Infumorph 500 Sterile Solutions 1314
- Kadian Capsules 1335
- MS Contin Tablets 2896
- MSIR 2898
- Oramorph SR Tablets 3062
- Roxanol 3066

Olanzapine (Potential for increased sedation). Products include:
- Zyprexa Tablets 1973
- Zyprexa ZYDIS Orally Disintegrating Tablets 1973

Oxazepam (Potential for increased sedation).
No products indexed under this heading.

Oxycodone Hydrochloride (Potential for increased sedation). Products include:
- OxyContin Tablets 2912
- OxyFast Oral Concentrate Solution 2916
- OxyIR Capsules 2916
- Percocet Tablets 1326
- Percodan Tablets 1327
- Percolone Tablets 1327
- Roxicodone 3067
- Tylox Capsules 2597

Pentobarbital Sodium (Potential for increased sedation). Products include:
- Nembutal Sodium Solution 485

Perphenazine (Potential for increased sedation). Products include:
- Etrafon 3115
- Trilafon 3160

Phenobarbital (Potential for increased sedation; concurrent administration may result in significant reductions in elimination half-life and plasma concentration). Products include:
- Arco-Lase Plus Tablets 592
- Donnatal 2929
- Donnatal Extentabs 2930

Phenytoin (Concurrent administration may result in significant reductions in elimination half-life and plasma concentration). Products include:
- Dilantin Infatabs 2624
- Dilantin-125 Oral Suspension 2625

Phenytoin Sodium (Concurrent administration may result in significant reductions in elimination half-life and plasma concentration). Products include:
- Dilantin Kapseals 2622

Prazepam (Potential for increased sedation).
No products indexed under this heading.

Prochlorperazine (Potential for increased sedation). Products include:
- Compazine 1505

Promethazine Hydrochloride (Potential for increased sedation). Products include:
- Mepergan Injection 3539
- Phenergan Injection 3553
- Phenergan 3556
- Phenergan Syrup 3554
- Phenergan with Codeine Syrup 3557
- Phenergan with Dextromethorphan Syrup 3559
- Phenergan VC Syrup 3560
- Phenergan VC with Codeine Syrup 3561

Propofol (Potential for increased sedation). Products include:
- Diprivan Injectable Emulsion 667

Propoxyphene Hydrochloride (Potential for increased sedation). Products include:
- Darvon Pulvules 1909
- Darvon Compound-65 Pulvules 1910

Propoxyphene Napsylate (Potential for increased sedation). Products include:
- Darvon-N/Darvocet-N 1907
- Darvon-N Tablets 1912

Quazepam (Potential for increased sedation).
No products indexed under this heading.

Quetiapine Fumarate (Potential for increased sedation). Products include:
- Seroquel Tablets 684

Remifentanil Hydrochloride (Potential for increased sedation).
No products indexed under this heading.

Risperidone (Potential for increased sedation). Products include:
- Risperdal 1796

Secobarbital Sodium (Potential for increased sedation).
No products indexed under this heading.

Sevoflurane (Potential for increased sedation).
No products indexed under this heading.

Sufentanil Citrate (Potential for increased sedation).
No products indexed under this heading.

Temazepam (Potential for increased sedation).
No products indexed under this heading.

Thiamylal Sodium (Potential for increased sedation).
No products indexed under this heading.

Thioridazine Hydrochloride (Potential for increased sedation). Products include:
- Thioridazine Hydrochloride Tablets 2289

Thiothixene (Potential for increased sedation). Products include:
- Navane Capsules 2701
- Thiothixene Capsules 2290

Triazolam (Potential for increased sedation). Products include:
- Halcion Tablets 2823

Trifluoperazine Hydrochloride (Potential for increased sedation). Products include:
- Stelazine 1640

Zaleplon (Potential for increased sedation). Products include:
- Sonata Capsules 3591

Ziprasidone Hydrochloride (Potential for increased sedation). Products include:
- Geodon Capsules 2688

Zolpidem Tartrate (Potential for increased sedation). Products include:
- Ambien Tablets 3191

TENORETIC TABLETS

(Atenolol, Chlorthalidone) 690
May interact with antihypertensives, calcium channel blockers, corticosteroids, cardiac glycosides, insulin, lithium preparations, and certain other agents. Compounds in these categories include:

Acebutolol Hydrochloride (Tenoretic may potentiate the action of other antihypertensive agents). Products include:
- Sectral Capsules 3589

ACTH (Co-administration with ACTH may result in increased risk of hypokalemia).
No products indexed under this heading.

Amlodipine Besylate (Calcium channel blocker may also have an additive effect when given with Tenoretic). Products include:
- Lotrel Capsules 2370
- Norvasc Tablets 2704

Benazepril Hydrochloride (Tenoretic may potentiate the action of other antihypertensive agents). Products include:
- Lotensin Tablets 2365
- Lotensin HCT Tablets 2367
- Lotrel Capsules 2370

Bendroflumethiazide (Tenoretic may potentiate the action of other antihypertensive agents). Products include:
- Corzide 40/5 Tablets 2247
- Corzide 80/5 Tablets 2247

Bepridil Hydrochloride (Calcium channel blocker may also have an additive effect when given with Tenoretic). Products include:
- Vascor Tablets 2602

Betamethasone Acetate (Co-administration with corticosteroids may result in increased risk of hypokalemia). Products include:
- Celestone Soluspan Injectable Suspension 3097

Betamethasone Sodium Phosphate (Co-administration with corticosteroids may result in increased risk of hypokalemia). Products include:
- Celestone Soluspan Injectable Suspension 3097

Betaxolol Hydrochloride (Tenoretic may potentiate the action of other antihypertensive agents). Products include:
- Betoptic S Ophthalmic Suspension 537

Bisoprolol Fumarate (Tenoretic may potentiate the action of other antihypertensive agents). Products include:
- Zebeta Tablets 1885
- Ziac Tablets 1887

Candesartan Cilexetil (Tenoretic may potentiate the action of other antihypertensive agents). Products include:
- Atacand Tablets 595
- Atacand HCT Tablets 597

Captopril (Tenoretic may potentiate the action of other antihypertensive agents). Products include:
- Captopril Tablets 2281

Carteolol Hydrochloride (Tenoretic may potentiate the action of other antihypertensive agents). Products include:
- Carteolol Hydrochloride Ophthalmic Solution USP, 1% ⊙258
- Ocupress Ophthalmic Solution, 1% Sterile ⊙303

Chlorothiazide (Tenoretic may potentiate the action of other antihypertensive agents). Products include:
- Aldoclor Tablets 2035
- Diuril Oral 2087

Chlorothiazide Sodium (Tenoretic may potentiate the action of other antihypertensive agents). Products include:
- Diuril Sodium Intravenous 2086

Clonidine (Beta-blockers may exacerbate the rebound hypertension which can follow the withdrawal of clonidine). Products include:
- Catapres-TTS 1038

Clonidine Hydrochloride (Beta-blockers may exacerbate the rebound hypertension which can follow the withdrawal of clonidine). Products include:
- Catapres Tablets 1037
- Clorpres Tablets 1002
- Combipres Tablets 1040
- Duraclon Injection 3057

Cortisone Acetate (Co-administration with corticosteroids may result in increased risk of hypokalemia). Products include:
- Cortone Acetate Injectable Suspension 2059
- Cortone Acetate Tablets 2061

Deserpidine (Tenoretic may potentiate the action of other antihypertensive agents).
No products indexed under this heading.

Deslanoside (Hypokalemia induced by digitalis can sensitize or exaggerate the response of the heart to the toxic effects of digitalis, such as ventricular irritability).
No products indexed under this heading.

Dexamethasone (Co-administration with corticosteroids may result in increased risk of hypokalemia). Products include:
- Decadron Elixir 2078
- Decadron Tablets 2079
- TobraDex Ophthalmic Ointment 542
- TobraDex Ophthalmic Suspension 541

Dexamethasone Acetate (Co-administration with corticosteroids may result in increased risk of hypokalemia).
No products indexed under this heading.

Dexamethasone Sodium Phosphate (Co-administration with corticosteroids may result in increased risk of hypokalemia). Products include:
- Decadron Phosphate Injection 2081
- Decadron Phosphate Sterile Ophthalmic Ointment 2083
- Decadron Phosphate Sterile Ophthalmic Solution 2084
- NeoDecadron Sterile Ophthalmic Solution 2144

Diazoxide (Tenoretic may potentiate the action of other antihypertensive agents).
No products indexed under this heading.

Digitoxin (Hypokalemia induced by digitalis can sensitize or exaggerate the response of the heart to the toxic effects of digitalis, such as ventricular irritability).
No products indexed under this heading.

Digoxin (Hypokalemia induced by digitalis can sensitize or exaggerate the response of the heart to the toxic effects of digitalis, such as ventricular irritability). Products include:
- Digitek Tablets 1003
- Lanoxicaps Capsules 1574
- Lanoxin Injection 1581
- Lanoxin Tablets 1587
- Lanoxin Elixir Pediatric 1578
- Lanoxin Injection Pediatric 1584

Diltiazem Hydrochloride (Co-administration of beta-blocker with diltiazem may result in bradycardia and heart block and the left ventricular and end diastolic pressure can rise). Products include:
- Cardizem Injectable 1018
- Cardizem Lyo-Ject Syringe 1018
- Cardizem Monovial 1018
- Cardizem CD Capsules 1016
- Tiazac Capsules 1378

Doxazosin Mesylate (Tenoretic may potentiate the action of other antihypertensive agents). Products include:
- Cardura Tablets 2668

Enalapril Maleate (Tenoretic may potentiate the action of other antihypertensive agents). Products include:
- Lexxel Tablets 608
- Vaseretic Tablets 2204
- Vasotec Tablets 2210

Enalaprilat (Tenoretic may potentiate the action of other antihypertensive agents). Products include:
- Enalaprilat Injection 863
- Vasotec I.V. Injection 2207

Epinephrine (While taking beta-blocker, patients with a history of anaphylactic reaction may be unresponsive to the usual dose of epinephrine). Products include:
- Epifrin Sterile Ophthalmic Solution ⊙235
- EpiPen 1236
- Primatene Mist ▣779

(▣ Described in PDR For Nonprescription Drugs) (⊙ Described in PDR For Ophthalmic Medicines™)

Xylocaine with Epinephrine Injection 653

Epinephrine Hydrochloride (While taking beta-blocker, patients with a history of anaphylactic reaction may be unresponsive to the usual dose of epinephrine).
No products indexed under this heading.

Eprosartan Mesylate (Tenoretic may potentiate the action of other antihypertensive agents). Products include:
Teveten Tablets 3327

Esmolol Hydrochloride (Tenoretic may potentiate the action of other antihypertensive agents). Products include:
Brevibloc Injection 858

Felodipine (Calcium channel blocker may also have an additive effect when given with Tenoretic). Products include:
Lexxel Tablets 608
Plendil Extended-Release Tablets 623

Fludrocortisone Acetate (Co-administration with corticosteroids may result in increased risk of hypokalemia). Products include:
Florinef Acetate Tablets 2250

Fosinopril Sodium (Tenoretic may potentiate the action of other antihypertensive agents). Products include:
Monopril Tablets 1091
Monopril HCT 1094

Furosemide (Tenoretic may potentiate the action of other antihypertensive agents). Products include:
Furosemide Tablets 2284

Guanabenz Acetate (Tenoretic may potentiate the action of other antihypertensive agents).
No products indexed under this heading.

Guanethidine Monosulfate (Tenoretic may potentiate the action of other antihypertensive agents).
No products indexed under this heading.

Hydralazine Hydrochloride (Tenoretic may potentiate the action of other antihypertensive agents).
No products indexed under this heading.

Hydrochlorothiazide (Tenoretic may potentiate the action of other antihypertensive agents). Products include:
Accuretic Tablets 2614
Aldoril Tablets 2039
Atacand HCT Tablets 597
Avalide Tablets 1070
Diovan HCT Tablets 2338
Dyazide Capsules 1515
HydroDIURIL Tablets 2108
Hyzaar 2109
Inderide Tablets 3517
Inderide LA Long-Acting Capsules 3519
Lotensin HCT Tablets 2367
Maxzide 1008
Micardis HCT Tablets 1051
Microzide Capsules 3414
Moduretic Tablets 2138
Monopril HCT 1094
Prinzide Tablets 2168
Timolide Tablets 2187
Uniretic Tablets 3178
Vaseretic Tablets 2204
Zestoretic Tablets 695
Ziac Tablets 1887

Hydrocortisone (Co-administration with corticosteroids may result in increased risk of hypokalemia). Products include:
Anusol-HC Cream 2.5% 2237
Cipro HC Otic Suspension 540
Cortaid Intensive Therapy Cream .... ▣717
Cortaid Maximum Strength Cream .... ▣717
Cortisporin Ophthalmic Suspension Sterile .... ⊙297
Cortizone•5 .... ▣699
Cortizone•10 .... ▣699
Cortizone•10 Plus Creme .... ▣700
Cortizone for Kids Creme .... ▣699
Hydrocortone Tablets 2106
Massengill Medicated Soft Cloth Towelette .... ▣753
VōSoL HC Otic Solution 3356

Hydrocortisone Acetate (Co-administration with corticosteroids may result in increased risk of hypokalemia). Products include:
Analpram-HC 1338
Anusol HC-1 Hydrocortisone Anti-Itch Cream .... ▣689
Anusol-HC Suppositories 2238
Cortaid .... ▣717
Cortifoam Rectal Foam 3170
Cortisporin-TC Otic Suspension 2246
Hydrocortone Acetate Injectable Suspension 2103
Pramosone 1343
Proctocort Suppositories 2264
ProctoFoam-HC 3177
Terra-Cortril Ophthalmic Suspension 2716

Hydrocortisone Sodium Phosphate (Co-administration with corticosteroids may result in increased risk of hypokalemia). Products include:
Hydrocortone Phosphate Injection, Sterile 2105

Hydrocortisone Sodium Succinate (Co-administration with corticosteroids may result in increased risk of hypokalemia).
No products indexed under this heading.

Hydroflumethiazide (Tenoretic may potentiate the action of other antihypertensive agents). Products include:
Diucardin Tablets 3494

Indapamide (Tenoretic may potentiate the action of other antihypertensive agents). Products include:
Indapamide Tablets 2286

Indomethacin (Co-administration of prostaglandin synthase inhibiting drugs, such as indomethacin, may decrease the hypotensive effects of beta-blockers). Products include:
Indocin 2112

Insulin, Human, Zinc Suspension (Chlorthalidone causes hyperglycemia; insulin requirements in diabetic patients may be altered; at recommended doses atenolol does not potentiate insulin-induced hypoglycemia). Products include:
Humulin L, 100 Units 1937
Humulin U, 100 Units 1943
Novolin L Human Insulin 10 ml Vials 2422

Insulin, Human NPH (Chlorthalidone causes hyperglycemia; insulin requirements in diabetic patients may be altered; at recommended doses atenolol does not potentiate insulin-induced hypoglycemia). Products include:
Humulin N, 100 Units 1939
Humulin N NPH Pen 1940
Novolin N Human Insulin 10 ml Vials 2422
Novolin N PenFill 2423
Novolin N Prefilled Syringe Disposable Insulin Delivery System 2425

Insulin, Human Regular (Chlorthalidone causes hyperglycemia; insulin requirements in diabetic patients may be altered; at recommended doses atenolol does not potentiate insulin-induced hypoglycemia). Products include:
Humulin R Regular (U-500) 1943
Humulin R, 100 Units 1941
Novolin R Human Insulin 10 ml Vials 2423
Novolin R PenFill 2423
Novolin R Prefilled Syringe Disposable Insulin Delivery System 2425
Velosulin BR Human Insulin 10 ml Vials 2435

Insulin, Human Regular and Human NPH Mixture (Chlorthalidone causes hyperglycemia; insulin requirements in diabetic patients may be altered; at recommended doses atenolol does not potentiate insulin-induced hypoglycemia). Products include:
Humulin 50/50, 100 Units 1934
Humulin 70/30, 100 Units 1935
Humulin 70/30 Pen 1936
Novolin 70/30 Human Insulin 10 ml Vials 2421
Novolin 70/30 PenFill 2423
Novolin 70/30 Prefilled Disposable Insulin Delivery System 2425

Insulin, NPH (Chlorthalidone causes hyperglycemia; insulin requirements in diabetic patients may be altered; at recommended doses atenolol does not potentiate insulin-induced hypoglycemia). Products include:
Iletin II, NPH (Pork), 100 Units 1946

Insulin, Regular (Chlorthalidone causes hyperglycemia; insulin requirements in diabetic patients may be altered; at recommended doses atenolol does not potentiate insulin-induced hypoglycemia). Products include:
Iletin II, Regular (Pork), 100 Units 1947

Insulin, Zinc Crystals (Chlorthalidone causes hyperglycemia; insulin requirements in diabetic patients may be altered; at recommended doses atenolol does not potentiate insulin-induced hypoglycemia).
No products indexed under this heading.

Insulin, Zinc Suspension (Chlorthalidone causes hyperglycemia; insulin requirements in diabetic patients may be altered; at recommended doses atenolol does not potentiate insulin-induced hypoglycemia). Products include:
Iletin II, Lente (Pork), 100 Units 1945

Insulin Aspart, Human Regular (Chlorthalidone causes hyperglycemia; insulin requirements in diabetic patients may be altered; at recommended doses atenolol does not potentiate insulin-induced hypoglycemia).
No products indexed under this heading.

Insulin glargine (Chlorthalidone causes hyperglycemia; insulin requirements in diabetic patients may be altered; at recommended doses atenolol does not potentiate insulin-induced hypoglycemia). Products include:
Lantus Injection 742

Insulin Lispro, Human (Chlorthalidone causes hyperglycemia; insulin requirements in diabetic patients may be altered; at recommended doses atenolol does not potentiate insulin-induced hypoglycemia). Products include:
Humalog 1926
Humalog Mix 75/25 Pen 1928

Insulin Lispro Protamine, Human (Chlorthalidone causes hyperglycemia; insulin requirements in diabetic patients may be altered; at recommended doses atenolol does not potentiate insulin-induced hypoglycemia). Products include:
Humalog Mix 75/25 Pen 1928

Irbesartan (Tenoretic may potentiate the action of other antihypertensive agents). Products include:
Avalide Tablets 1070
Avapro Tablets 1074
Avapro Tablets 3076

Isradipine (Calcium channel blocker may also have an additive effect when given with Tenoretic). Products include:
DynaCirc Capsules 2921
DynaCirc CR Tablets 2923

Labetalol Hydrochloride (Tenoretic may potentiate the action of other antihypertensive agents). Products include:
Normodyne Injection 3135
Normodyne Tablets 3137

Lisinopril (Tenoretic may potentiate the action of other antihypertensive agents). Products include:
Prinivil Tablets 2164
Prinzide Tablets 2168
Zestoretic Tablets 695
Zestril Tablets 698

Lithium Carbonate (Co-administration of diuretics with lithium may reduce the renal clearance of lithium and add a high risk of lithium toxicity). Products include:
Eskalith 1527
Lithium Carbonate 3061
Lithobid Slow-Release Tablets 3255

Lithium Citrate (Co-administration of diuretics with lithium may reduce the renal clearance of lithium and add a high risk of lithium toxicity). Products include:
Lithium Citrate Syrup 3061

Losartan Potassium (Tenoretic may potentiate the action of other antihypertensive agents). Products include:
Cozaar Tablets 2067
Hyzaar 2109

Mecamylamine Hydrochloride (Tenoretic may potentiate the action of other antihypertensive agents). Products include:
Inversine Tablets 1850

Methyclothiazide (Tenoretic may potentiate the action of other antihypertensive agents).
No products indexed under this heading.

Methyldopa (Tenoretic may potentiate the action of other antihypertensive agents). Products include:
Aldoclor Tablets 2035
Aldomet Tablets 2037
Aldoril Tablets 2039

Methyldopate Hydrochloride (Tenoretic may potentiate the action of other antihypertensive agents).
No products indexed under this heading.

Methylprednisolone Acetate (Co-administration with corticosteroids may result in increased risk of hypokalemia). Products include:
Depo-Medrol Injectable Suspension 2795

Methylprednisolone Sodium Succinate (Co-administration with corticosteroids may result in increased risk of hypokalemia). Products include:
Solu-Medrol Sterile Powder 2855

Metolazone (Tenoretic may potentiate the action of other antihypertensive agents). Products include:
Mykrox Tablets 1168
Zaroxolyn Tablets 1177

Metoprolol Succinate (Tenoretic may potentiate the action of other antihypertensive agents). Products include:
Toprol-XL Tablets 651

Metoprolol Tartrate (Tenoretic may potentiate the action of other antihypertensive agents).
No products indexed under this heading.

Metyrosine (Tenoretic may potentiate the action of other antihypertensive agents). Products include:
Demser Capsules 2085

Mibefradil Dihydrochloride (Calcium channel blocker may also have an additive effect when given with Tenoretic).
No products indexed under this heading.

Minoxidil (Tenoretic may potentiate the action of other antihypertensive agents). Products include:
Rogaine Extra Strength for Men Topical Solution .... ▣721
Rogaine for Women Topical Solution .... ▣721

Moexipril Hydrochloride (Tenoretic may potentiate the action of other antihypertensive agents). Products include:
- Uniretic Tablets 3178
- Univasc Tablets 3181

Nadolol (Tenoretic may potentiate the action of other antihypertensive agents). Products include:
- Corgard Tablets 2245
- Corzide 40/5 Tablets 2247
- Corzide 80/5 Tablets 2247
- Nadolol Tablets 2288

Nicardipine Hydrochloride (Calcium channel blocker may also have an additive effect when given with Tenoretic). Products include:
- Cardene I.V. 3485

Nifedipine (Calcium channel blocker may also have an additive effect when given with Tenoretic). Products include:
- Adalat CC Tablets 877
- Procardia Capsules 2708
- Procardia XL Extended Release Tablets 2710

Nimodipine (Calcium channel blocker may also have an additive effect when given with Tenoretic). Products include:
- Nimotop Capsules 904

Nisoldipine (Calcium channel blocker may also have an additive effect when given with Tenoretic). Products include:
- Sular Tablets 688

Nitroglycerin (Tenoretic may potentiate the action of other antihypertensive agents). Products include:
- Nitro-Dur Transdermal Infusion System 3134
- Nitro-Dur Transdermal Infusion System 1834
- Nitrolingual Pumpspray 1355
- Nitrostat Tablets 2658

Norepinephrine Bitartrate (Thiazides may decrease arterial responsiveness to norepinephrine).
No products indexed under this heading.

Penbutolol Sulfate (Tenoretic may potentiate the action of other antihypertensive agents).
No products indexed under this heading.

Perindopril Erbumine (Tenoretic may potentiate the action of other antihypertensive agents). Products include:
- Aceon Tablets (2 mg, 4 mg, 8 mg) 3249

Phenoxybenzamine Hydrochloride (Tenoretic may potentiate the action of other antihypertensive agents). Products include:
- Dibenzyline Capsules 3457

Phentolamine Mesylate (Tenoretic may potentiate the action of other antihypertensive agents).
No products indexed under this heading.

Pindolol (Tenoretic may potentiate the action of other antihypertensive agents).
No products indexed under this heading.

Polythiazide (Tenoretic may potentiate the action of other antihypertensive agents). Products include:
- Minizide Capsules 2700
- Renese Tablets 2712

Prazosin Hydrochloride (Tenoretic may potentiate the action of other antihypertensive agents). Products include:
- Minipress Capsules 2699
- Minizide Capsules 2700

Prednisolone Acetate (Co-administration with corticosteroids may result in increased risk of hypokalemia). Products include:
- Blephamide Ophthalmic Ointment .. 547
- Blephamide Ophthalmic Suspension 548
- Poly-Pred Liquifilm Ophthalmic Suspension .... ⊙245
- Pred Forte Ophthalmic Suspension .... ⊙246
- Pred Mild Sterile Ophthalmic Suspension .... ⊙249
- Pred-G Ophthalmic Suspension ..... ⊙247
- Pred-G Sterile Ophthalmic Ointment .... ⊙248

Prednisolone Sodium Phosphate (Co-administration with corticosteroids may result in increased risk of hypokalemia). Products include:
- Pediapred Oral Solution 1170

Prednisolone Tebutate (Co-administration with corticosteroids may result in increased risk of hypokalemia).
No products indexed under this heading.

Prednisone (Co-administration with corticosteroids may result in increased risk of hypokalemia). Products include:
- Prednisone 3064

Propranolol Hydrochloride (Tenoretic may potentiate the action of other antihypertensive agents). Products include:
- Inderal 3513
- Inderal LA Long-Acting Capsules 3516
- Inderide Tablets 3517
- Inderide LA Long-Acting Capsules .. 3519

Quinapril Hydrochloride (Tenoretic may potentiate the action of other antihypertensive agents). Products include:
- Accupril Tablets 2611
- Accuretic Tablets 2614

Ramipril (Tenoretic may potentiate the action of other antihypertensive agents). Products include:
- Altace Capsules 2233

Rauwolfia serpentina (Tenoretic may potentiate the action of other antihypertensive agents).
No products indexed under this heading.

Rescinnamine (Tenoretic may potentiate the action of other antihypertensive agents).
No products indexed under this heading.

Reserpine (Co-administration of catecholamine depletor, such as reserpine, may result in hypotension and/or marked tachycardia which may produce vertigo, syncope or postural hypotension).
No products indexed under this heading.

Sodium Nitroprusside (Tenoretic may potentiate the action of other antihypertensive agents).
No products indexed under this heading.

Sotalol Hydrochloride (Tenoretic may potentiate the action of other antihypertensive agents). Products include:
- Betapace Tablets 950
- Betapace AF Tablets 954

Spirapril Hydrochloride (Tenoretic may potentiate the action of other antihypertensive agents).
No products indexed under this heading.

Telmisartan (Tenoretic may potentiate the action of other antihypertensive agents). Products include:
- Micardis Tablets 1049
- Micardis HCT Tablets 1051

Terazosin Hydrochloride (Tenoretic may potentiate the action of other antihypertensive agents). Products include:
- Hytrin Capsules 464

Timolol Maleate (Tenoretic may potentiate the action of other antihypertensive agents). Products include:
- Blocadren Tablets 2046
- Cosopt Sterile Ophthalmic Solution 2065
- Timolide Tablets 2187
- Timolol GFS .... ⊙266
- Timoptic in Ocudose 2192
- Timoptic Sterile Ophthalmic Solution 2190
- Timoptic-XE Sterile Ophthalmic Gel Forming Solution 2194

Torsemide (Tenoretic may potentiate the action of other antihypertensive agents). Products include:
- Demadex Tablets and Injection 2965

Trandolapril (Tenoretic may potentiate the action of other antihypertensive agents). Products include:
- Mavik Tablets 478
- Tarka Tablets 508

Triamcinolone (Co-administration with corticosteroids may result in increased risk of hypokalemia).
No products indexed under this heading.

Triamcinolone Acetonide (Co-administration with corticosteroids may result in increased risk of hypokalemia). Products include:
- Azmacort Inhalation Aerosol 728
- Nasacort Nasal Inhaler 750
- Nasacort AQ Nasal Spray 752
- Tri-Nasal Spray 2274

Triamcinolone Diacetate (Co-administration with corticosteroids may result in increased risk of hypokalemia).
No products indexed under this heading.

Triamcinolone Hexacetonide (Co-administration with corticosteroids may result in increased risk of hypokalemia).
No products indexed under this heading.

Trimethaphan Camsylate (Tenoretic may potentiate the action of other antihypertensive agents).
No products indexed under this heading.

Tubocurarine Chloride (Thiazides may increase the responsiveness to tubocurarine).
No products indexed under this heading.

Valsartan (Tenoretic may potentiate the action of other antihypertensive agents). Products include:
- Diovan Capsules 2337
- Diovan HCT Tablets 2338

Verapamil Hydrochloride (Co-administration of beta-blocker with verapamil may result in bradycardia and heart block and the left ventricular and end diastolic pressure can rise). Products include:
- Covera-HS Tablets 3199
- Isoptin SR Tablets 467
- Tarka Tablets 508
- Verelan Capsules 3184
- Verelan PM Capsules 3186

TENORMIN I.V. INJECTION

(Atenolol) 692

May interact with calcium channel blockers and certain other agents. Compounds in these categories include:

Amlodipine Besylate (Calcium channel blocker may also have an additive effect when given with Tenormin). Products include:
- Lotrel Capsules 2370
- Norvasc Tablets 2704

Bepridil Hydrochloride (Calcium channel blocker may also have an additive effect when given with Tenormin). Products include:
- Vascor Tablets 2602

Clonidine (Beta-blockers may exacerbate the rebound hypertension which can follow the withdrawal of clonidine). Products include:
- Catapres-TTS 1038

Clonidine Hydrochloride (Beta-blockers may exacerbate the rebound hypertension which can follow the withdrawal of clonidine). Products include:
- Catapres Tablets 1037
- Clorpres Tablets 1002
- Combipres Tablets 1040
- Duraclon Injection 3057

Diltiazem Hydrochloride (Co-administration of beta-blocker with diltiazem may result in bradycardia and heart block and the left ventricular and end diastolic pressure can rise). Products include:
- Cardizem Injectable 1018
- Cardizem Lyo-Ject Syringe 1018
- Cardizem Monovial 1018
- Cardizem CD Capsules 1016
- Tiazac Capsules 1378

Epinephrine (While taking beta-blocker, patients with a history of anaphylactic reaction may be unresponsive to the usual dose of epinephrine). Products include:
- Epifrin Sterile Ophthalmic Solution .... ⊙235
- EpiPen 1236
- Primatene Mist .... ▣779
- Xylocaine with Epinephrine Injection 653

Epinephrine Hydrochloride (While taking beta-blocker, patients with a history of anaphylactic reaction may be unresponsive to the usual dose of epinephrine).
No products indexed under this heading.

Felodipine (Calcium channel blocker may also have an additive effect when given with Tenormin). Products include:
- Lexxel Tablets 608
- Plendil Extended-Release Tablets ... 623

Indomethacin (Co-administration of prostaglandin synthase inhibiting drugs, such as indomethacin, may decrease the hypotensive effects of beta-blockers). Products include:
- Indocin 2112

Isradipine (Calcium channel blocker may also have an additive effect when given with Tenormin). Products include:
- DynaCirc Capsules 2921
- DynaCirc CR Tablets 2923

Mibefradil Dihydrochloride (Calcium channel blocker may also have an additive effect when given with Tenormin).
No products indexed under this heading.

Nicardipine Hydrochloride (Calcium channel blocker may also have an additive effect when given with Tenormin). Products include:
- Cardene I.V. 3485

Nifedipine (Calcium channel blocker may also have an additive effect when given with Tenormin). Products include:
- Adalat CC Tablets 877
- Procardia Capsules 2708
- Procardia XL Extended Release Tablets 2710

Nimodipine (Calcium channel blocker may also have an additive effect when given with Tenormin). Products include:
- Nimotop Capsules 904

Nisoldipine (Calcium channel blocker may also have an additive effect when given with Tenormin). Products include:
- Sular Tablets 688

Reserpine (Co-administration of catecholamine depletor, such as reserpine, may result in hypotension and/or marked tachycardia which may produce vertigo, syncope or postural hypotension).
No products indexed under this heading.

Verapamil Hydrochloride (Co-administration of beta-blocker with verapamil may result in bradycardia and heart block and the left ventricular and end diastolic pressure can rise; caution should be exercised with Tenormin I.V. Injection when given in close proximity with drugs that may also have a depressant effect on myocardial contractility).
Products include:

Covera-HS Tablets 3199
Isoptin SR Tablets 467
Tarka Tablets 508
Verelan Capsules 3184
Verelan PM Capsules 3186

TENSILON INJECTABLE

(Edrophonium Chloride) 1745
None cited in PDR database.

TEQUIN INJECTION

(Gatifloxacin) 1110
See Tequin Tablets

TEQUIN TABLETS

(Gatifloxacin) 1110
May interact with oral hypoglycemic agents, insulin, iron containing oral preparations, non-steroidal anti-inflammatory agents, and certain other agents. Compounds in these categories include:

Acarbose (As with other quinolones, disturbances of blood glucose, including symptomatic hyper- and hypoglycemia have been reported, usually in diabetic patients receiving oral hypoglycemic agents). Products include:
Precose Tablets 906

Aluminum Hydroxide (Systemic exposure to Tequin Tablets is reduced by co-administration of Tequin Tablets with antacids containing aluminum salts; Tequin Tablets can be administered 4 hours before the administration of antacids). Products include:
Amphojel Suspension (Mint Flavor) .... ▣789
Gaviscon Extra Strength Liquid .... ▣751
Gaviscon Extra Strength Tablets .... ▣751
Gaviscon Regular Strength Liquid .... ▣751
Gaviscon Regular Strength Tablets .... ▣750
Maalox Antacid/Anti-Gas Oral Suspension .... ▣673
Maalox Max Maximum Strength Antacid/Anti-Gas Liquid 2300
Maalox Regular Strength Antacid/Antigas Liquid 2300
Mylanta 1813
Vanquish Caplets .... ▣617

Celecoxib (Co-administration of non-steroidal anti-inflammatory agents with quinolones may increase the risks of CNS stimulation and convulsions; these events have not been observed with gatifloxacin in pre-clinical and clinical trials). Products include:
Celebrex Capsules 2676
Celebrex Capsules 2780

Chlorpropamide (As with other quinolones, disturbances of blood glucose, including symptomatic hyper- and hypoglycemia have been reported, usually in diabetic patients receiving oral hypoglycemic agents). Products include:
Diabinese Tablets 2680

Diclofenac Potassium (Co-administration of non-steroidal anti-inflammatory agents with quinolones may increase the risks of CNS stimulation and convulsions; these events have not been observed with gatifloxacin in pre-clinical and clinical trials). Products include:
Cataflam Tablets 2315

Diclofenac Sodium (Co-administration of non-steroidal anti-inflammatory agents with quinolones may increase the risks of CNS stimulation and convulsions; these events have not been observed with gatifloxacin in pre-clinical and clinical trials). Products include:
Arthrotec Tablets 3195
Voltaren Ophthalmic Sterile Ophthalmic Solution .... ⊙312
Voltaren Tablets 2315
Voltaren-XR Tablets 2315

Digoxin (Co-administration has resulted in modest increases in Cmax and AUC of digoxin; although dose adjustments for digoxin are not warranted with initiation of gatifloxacin treatment, patients taking digoxin should be monitored for signs and symptoms of toxicity). Products include:
Digitek Tablets 1003
Lanoxicaps Capsules 1574
Lanoxin Injection 1581
Lanoxin Tablets 1587
Lanoxin Elixir Pediatric 1578
Lanoxin Injection Pediatric 1584

Etodolac (Co-administration of non-steroidal anti-inflammatory agents with quinolones may increase the risks of CNS stimulation and convulsions; these events have not been observed with gatifloxacin in pre-clinical and clinical trials). Products include:
Lodine 3528
Lodine XL Extended-Release Tablets 3530

Fenoprofen Calcium (Co-administration of non-steroidal anti-inflammatory agents with quinolones may increase the risks of CNS stimulation and convulsions; these events have not been observed with gatifloxacin in pre-clinical and clinical trials).
No products indexed under this heading.

Ferrous Fumarate (Systemic exposure to Tequin Tablets is reduced by co-administration of Tequin Tablets with iron-containing products; Tequin Tablets can be administered 4 hours before the administration of iron containing products). Products include:
New Formulation Chromagen OB Capsules 3094
Loestrin Fe Tablets 2642
NataChew Tablets 3364

Ferrous Gluconate (Systemic exposure to Tequin Tablets is reduced by co-administration of Tequin Tablets with iron-containing products; Tequin Tablets can be administered 4 hours before the administration of iron containing products). Products include:
Fergon Iron Tablets .... ▣802

Ferrous Sulfate (Systemic exposure to Tequin Tablets is reduced by co-administration of Tequin Tablets with ferrous sulfate; Tequin Tablets can be administered 4 hours before the administration of iron containing products). Products include:
Feosol Tablets 1717
Slow Fe Tablets .... ▣827
Slow Fe with Folic Acid Tablets .... ▣828

Flurbiprofen (Co-administration of non-steroidal anti-inflammatory agents with quinolones may increase the risks of CNS stimulation and convulsions; these events have not been observed with gatifloxacin in pre-clinical and clinical trials).
No products indexed under this heading.

Glimepiride (As with other quinolones, disturbances of blood glucose, including symptomatic hyper- and hypoglycemia have been reported, usually in diabetic patients receiving oral hypoglycemic agents). Products include:
Amaryl Tablets 717

Glipizide (As with other quinolones, disturbances of blood glucose, including symptomatic hyper- and hypoglycemia have been reported, usually in diabetic patients receiving oral hypoglycemic agents). Products include:
Glucotrol Tablets 2692
Glucotrol XL Extended Release Tablets 2693

Glyburide (As with other quinolones, disturbances of blood glucose, including symptomatic hyper- and hypoglycemia have been reported, usually in diabetic patients receiving oral hypoglycemic agents). Products include:
DiaBeta Tablets 741
Glucovance Tablets 1086

Ibuprofen (Co-administration of non-steroidal anti-inflammatory agents with quinolones may increase the risks of CNS stimulation and convulsions; these events have not been observed with gatifloxacin in pre-clinical and clinical trials). Products include:
Advil .... ▣771
Children's Advil Oral Suspension .... ▣773
Children's Advil Chewable Tablets .... ▣773
Advil Cold and Sinus Caplets .... ▣771
Advil Cold and Sinus Tablets .... ▣771
Advil Flu & Body Ache Caplets .... ▣772
Infants' Advil Drops .... ▣773
Junior Strength Advil Tablets .... ▣773
Junior Strength Advil Chewable Tablets .... ▣773
Advil Migraine Liquigels .... ▣772
Children's Motrin Oral Suspension and Chewable Tablets 2006
Children's Motrin Cold Oral Suspension 2007
Children's Motrin Oral Suspension .... ▣643
Motrin Suspension, Oral Drops, Chewable Tablets, and Caplets 2002
Infants' Motrin Concentrated Drops 2006
Junior Strength Motrin Caplets and Chewable Tablets 2006
Motrin IB Tablets, Caplets, and Gelcaps 2002
Motrin Migraine Pain Caplets 2005
Motrin Sinus Headache Caplets 2005
Vicoprofen Tablets 520

Indomethacin (Co-administration of non-steroidal anti-inflammatory agents with quinolones may increase the risks of CNS stimulation and convulsions; these events have not been observed with gatifloxacin in pre-clinical and clinical trials). Products include:
Indocin 2112

Indomethacin Sodium Trihydrate (Co-administration of non-steroidal anti-inflammatory agents with quinolones may increase the risks of CNS stimulation and convulsions; these events have not been observed with gatifloxacin in pre-clinical and clinical trials). Products include:
Indocin I.V. 2115

Insulin, Human, Zinc Suspension (As with other quinolones, disturbances of blood glucose, including symptomatic hyper- and hypoglycemia have been reported, usually in diabetic patients receiving insulin). Products include:
Humulin L, 100 Units 1937
Humulin U, 100 Units 1943
Novolin L Human Insulin 10 ml Vials 2422

Insulin, Human NPH (As with other quinolones, disturbances of blood glucose, including symptomatic hyper- and hypoglycemia have been reported, usually in diabetic patients receiving insulin). Products include:
Humulin N, 100 Units 1939
Humulin N NPH Pen 1940
Novolin N Human Insulin 10 ml Vials 2422
Novolin N PenFill 2423
Novolin N Prefilled Syringe Disposable Insulin Delivery System 2425

Insulin, Human Regular (As with other quinolones, disturbances of blood glucose, including symptomatic hyper- and hypoglycemia have been reported, usually in diabetic patients receiving insulin). Products include:
Humulin R Regular (U-500) 1943
Humulin R, 100 Units 1941
Novolin R Human Insulin 10 ml Vials 2423
Novolin R PenFill 2423
Novolin R Prefilled Syringe Disposable Insulin Delivery System 2425
Velosulin BR Human Insulin 10 ml Vials 2435

Insulin, Human Regular and Human NPH Mixture (As with other quinolones, disturbances of blood glucose, including symptomatic hyper- and hypoglycemia have been reported, usually in diabetic patients receiving insulin). Products include:
Humulin 50/50, 100 Units 1934
Humulin 70/30, 100 Units 1935
Humulin 70/30 Pen 1936
Novolin 70/30 Human Insulin 10 ml Vials 2421
Novolin 70/30 PenFill 2423
Novolin 70/30 Prefilled Disposable Insulin Delivery System 2425

Insulin, NPH (As with other quinolones, disturbances of blood glucose, including symptomatic hyper- and hypoglycemia have been reported, usually in diabetic patients receiving insulin). Products include:
Iletin II, NPH (Pork), 100 Units 1946

Insulin, Regular (As with other quinolones, disturbances of blood glucose, including symptomatic hyper- and hypoglycemia have been reported, usually in diabetic patients receiving insulin). Products include:
Iletin II, Regular (Pork), 100 Units 1947

Insulin, Zinc Crystals (As with other quinolones, disturbances of blood glucose, including symptomatic hyper- and hypoglycemia have been reported, usually in diabetic patients receiving insulin).
No products indexed under this heading.

Insulin, Zinc Suspension (As with other quinolones, disturbances of blood glucose, including symptomatic hyper- and hypoglycemia have been reported, usually in diabetic patients receiving insulin). Products include:
Iletin II, Lente (Pork), 100 Units 1945

Insulin Aspart, Human Regular (As with other quinolones, disturbances of blood glucose, including symptomatic hyper- and hypoglycemia have been reported, usually in diabetic patients receiving insulin).
No products indexed under this heading.

Insulin glargine (As with other quinolones, disturbances of blood glucose, including symptomatic hyper- and hypoglycemia have been reported, usually in diabetic patients receiving insulin). Products include:
Lantus Injection 742

Insulin Lispro, Human (As with other quinolones, disturbances of blood glucose, including symptomatic hyper- and hypoglycemia have been reported, usually in diabetic patients receiving insulin). Products include:
Humalog 1926
Humalog Mix 75/25 Pen 1928

Insulin Lispro Protamine, Human (As with other quinolones, disturbances of blood glucose, including symptomatic hyper- and hypoglycemia have been reported, usually in diabetic patients receiving insulin). Products include:
Humalog Mix 75/25 Pen 1928

Iron (Systemic exposure to Tequin Tablets is reduced by co-administration of Tequin Tablets with iron-containing products; Tequin Tablets can be administered 4 hours before the administration of iron containing products).
No products indexed under this heading.

Ketoprofen (Co-administration of non-steroidal anti-inflammatory agents with quinolones may increase the risks of CNS stimulation and convulsions; these events have not been observed with gatifloxacin in pre-clinical and clinical trials). Products include:
Orudis Capsules 3548

Orudis KT Tablets .... ▣778
Oruvail Capsules 3548

Ketorolac Tromethamine (Co-administration of non-steroidal anti-inflammatory agents with quinolones may increase the risks of CNS stimulation and convulsions; these events have not been observed with gatifloxacin in pre-clinical and clinical trials). Products include:
Acular Ophthalmic Solution 544
Acular PF Ophthalmic Solution 544
Toradol 3018

Magaldrate (Systemic exposure to Tequin Tablets is reduced by co-administration of Tequin Tablets with antacids containing magnesium salts; Tequin Tablets can be administered 4 hours before the administration of antacids).
No products indexed under this heading.

Magnesium Hydroxide (Systemic exposure to Tequin Tablets is reduced by co-administration of Tequin Tablets with antacids containing magnesium salts; Tequin Tablets can be administered 4 hours before the administration of antacids). Products include:
Ex•Lax Milk of Magnesia Liquid .... ▣670
Maalox Antacid/Anti-Gas Oral Suspension .... ▣673
Maalox Max Maximum Strength Antacid/Anti-Gas Liquid 2300
Maalox Regular Strength Antacid/Antigas Liquid 2300
Mylanta Fast-Acting 1813
Mylanta 1813
Pepcid Complete Chewable Tablets 1815
Phillips' Chewable Tablets .... ▣615
Phillips' Milk of Magnesia Liquid (Original, Cherry, & Mint) .... ▣616
Rolaids Tablets .... ▣706
Extra Strength Rolaids Tablets ...... ▣706
Vanquish Caplets .... ▣617

Magnesium Oxide (Systemic exposure to Tequin Tablets is reduced by co-administration of Tequin Tablets with antacids containing magnesium salts; Tequin Tablets can be administered 4 hours before the administration of antacids). Products include:
Beelith Tablets 946
Mag-Ox 400 Tablets 1024
Uro-Mag Capsules 1024

Meclofenamate Sodium (Co-administration of non-steroidal anti-inflammatory agents with quinolones may increase the risks of CNS stimulation and convulsions; these events have not been observed with gatifloxacin in pre-clinical and clinical trials).
No products indexed under this heading.

Mefenamic Acid (Co-administration of non-steroidal anti-inflammatory agents with quinolones may increase the risks of CNS stimulation and convulsions; these events have not been observed with gatifloxacin in pre-clinical and clinical trials). Products include:
Ponstel Capsules 1356

Meloxicam (Co-administration of non-steroidal anti-inflammatory agents with quinolones may increase the risks of CNS stimulation and convulsions; these events have not been observed with gatifloxacin in pre-clinical and clinical trials). Products include:
Mobic Tablets 1054

Metformin Hydrochloride (As with other quinolones, disturbances of blood glucose, including symptomatic hyper- and hypoglycemia have been reported, usually in diabetic patients receiving oral hypoglycemic agents). Products include:
Glucophage Tablets 1080
Glucophage XR Tablets 1080
Glucovance Tablets 1086

Miglitol (As with other quinolones, disturbances of blood glucose, including symptomatic hyper- and hypoglycemia have been reported, usually in diabetic patients receiving oral hypoglycemic agents). Products include:
Glyset Tablets 2821

Nabumetone (Co-administration of non-steroidal anti-inflammatory agents with quinolones may increase the risks of CNS stimulation and convulsions; these events have not been observed with gatifloxacin in pre-clinical and clinical trials). Products include:
Relafen Tablets 1617

Naproxen (Co-administration of non-steroidal anti-inflammatory agents with quinolones may increase the risks of CNS stimulation and convulsions; these events have not been observed with gatifloxacin in pre-clinical and clinical trials). Products include:
EC-Naprosyn Delayed-Release Tablets 2967
Naprosyn Suspension 2967
Naprosyn Tablets 2967

Naproxen Sodium (Co-administration of non-steroidal anti-inflammatory agents with quinolones may increase the risks of CNS stimulation and convulsions; these events have not been observed with gatifloxacin in pre-clinical and clinical trials). Products include:
Aleve Tablets, Caplets and Gelcaps .... ▣602
Aleve Cold & Sinus Caplets .... ▣603
Anaprox Tablets 2967
Anaprox DS Tablets 2967
Naprelan Tablets 1293

Oxaprozin (Co-administration of non-steroidal anti-inflammatory agents with quinolones may increase the risks of CNS stimulation and convulsions; these events have not been observed with gatifloxacin in pre-clinical and clinical trials).
No products indexed under this heading.

Phenylbutazone (Co-administration of non-steroidal anti-inflammatory agents with quinolones may increase the risks of CNS stimulation and convulsions; these events have not been observed with gatifloxacin in pre-clinical and clinical trials).
No products indexed under this heading.

Pioglitazone Hydrochloride (As with other quinolones, disturbances of blood glucose, including symptomatic hyper- and hypoglycemia have been reported, usually in diabetic patients receiving oral hypoglycemic agents). Products include:
Actos Tablets 3275

Piroxicam (Co-administration of non-steroidal anti-inflammatory agents with quinolones may increase the risks of CNS stimulation and convulsions; these events have not been observed with gatifloxacin in pre-clinical and clinical trials). Products include:
Feldene Capsules 2685

Polysaccharide-Iron Complex (Systemic exposure to Tequin Tablets is reduced by co-administration of Tequin Tablets with iron-containing products; Tequin Tablets can be administered 4 hours before the administration of iron containing products). Products include:
Niferex 3176
Niferex-150 Capsules 3176
Nu-Iron 150 Capsules 2224

Probenecid (Systemic exposure to Tequin is increased following co-administration of Tequin with probenecid resulting in a 42% increase in AUC and a 44% longer half-life of gatifloxacin).
No products indexed under this heading.

Repaglinide (As with other quinolones, disturbances of blood glucose, including symptomatic hyper- and hypoglycemia have been reported, usually in diabetic patients receiving oral hypoglycemic agents). Products include:
Prandin Tablets (0.5, 1, and 2 mg) 2432

Rofecoxib (Co-administration of non-steroidal anti-inflammatory agents with quinolones may increase the risks of CNS stimulation and convulsions; these events have not been observed with gatifloxacin in pre-clinical and clinical trials). Products include:
Vioxx 2213

Rosiglitazone Maleate (As with other quinolones, disturbances of blood glucose, including symptomatic hyper- and hypoglycemia have been reported, usually in diabetic patients receiving oral hypoglycemic agents). Products include:
Avandia Tablets 1490

Sulindac (Co-administration of non-steroidal anti-inflammatory agents with quinolones may increase the risks of CNS stimulation and convulsions; these events have not been observed with gatifloxacin in pre-clinical and clinical trials). Products include:
Clinoril Tablets 2053

Tolazamide (As with other quinolones, disturbances of blood glucose, including symptomatic hyper- and hypoglycemia have been reported, usually in diabetic patients receiving oral hypoglycemic agents).
No products indexed under this heading.

Tolbutamide (As with other quinolones, disturbances of blood glucose, including symptomatic hyper- and hypoglycemia have been reported, usually in diabetic patients receiving oral hypoglycemic agents).
No products indexed under this heading.

Tolmetin Sodium (Co-administration of non-steroidal anti-inflammatory agents with quinolones may increase the risks of CNS stimulation and convulsions; these events have not been observed with gatifloxacin in pre-clinical and clinical trials). Products include:
Tolectin 2589

Troglitazone (As with other quinolones, disturbances of blood glucose, including symptomatic hyper- and hypoglycemia have been reported, usually in diabetic patients receiving oral hypoglycemic agents).
No products indexed under this heading.

Zinc Sulfate (Tequin Tablets can be administered 4 hours before the administration of zinc-containing supplements). Products include:
Clear Eyes ACR Astringent/Lubricant Eye Redness Reliever .... ⊙322
Visine A.C. Seasonal Relief From Pollen & Dust Eye Drops .... ⊙314

TERAZOL 3 VAGINAL CREAM
(Terconazole) 2587
None cited in PDR database.

TERAZOL 3 VAGINAL SUPPOSITORIES
(Terconazole) 2587
None cited in PDR database.

TERAZOL 7 VAGINAL CREAM
(Terconazole) 2587
None cited in PDR database.

TERRA-CORTRIL OPHTHALMIC SUSPENSION
(Hydrocortisone Acetate, Oxytetracycline Hydrochloride) 2716
None cited in PDR database.

TESSALON CAPSULES
(Benzonatate) 1377
None cited in PDR database.

TESTODERM TRANSDERMAL SYSTEMS
(Testosterone) 574
May interact with corticosteroids, oral anticoagulants, insulin, and certain other agents. Compounds in these categories include:

ACTH (Co-administration of ACTH may enhance edema formation).
No products indexed under this heading.

Betamethasone Acetate (Co-administration of corticosteroids may enhance edema formation). Products include:
Celestone Soluspan Injectable Suspension 3097

Betamethasone Sodium Phosphate (Co-administration of corticosteroids may enhance edema formation). Products include:
Celestone Soluspan Injectable Suspension 3097

Cortisone Acetate (Co-administration of corticosteroids may enhance edema formation). Products include:
Cortone Acetate Injectable Suspension 2059
Cortone Acetate Tablets 2061

Dexamethasone (Co-administration of corticosteroids may enhance edema formation). Products include:
Decadron Elixir 2078
Decadron Tablets 2079
TobraDex Ophthalmic Ointment 542
TobraDex Ophthalmic Suspension .. 541

Dexamethasone Acetate (Co-administration of corticosteroids may enhance edema formation).
No products indexed under this heading.

Dexamethasone Sodium Phosphate (Co-administration of corticosteroids may enhance edema formation). Products include:
Decadron Phosphate Injection 2081
Decadron Phosphate Sterile Ophthalmic Ointment 2083
Decadron Phosphate Sterile Ophthalmic Solution 2084
NeoDecadron Sterile Ophthalmic Solution 2144

Dicumarol (Potential for decreased requirements of oral anticoagulants).
No products indexed under this heading.

Fludrocortisone Acetate (Co-administration of corticosteroids may enhance edema formation). Products include:
Florinef Acetate Tablets 2250

Hydrocortisone (Co-administration of corticosteroids may enhance edema formation). Products include:
Anusol-HC Cream 2.5% 2237
Cipro HC Otic Suspension 540
Cortaid Intensive Therapy Cream . ▣717
Cortaid Maximum Strength Cream .... ▣717
Cortisporin Ophthalmic Suspension Sterile .... ⊙297
Cortizone•5 .... ▣699
Cortizone•10 .... ▣699
Cortizone•10 Plus Creme .... ▣700
Cortizone for Kids Creme .... ▣699
Hydrocortone Tablets 2106
Massengill Medicated Soft Cloth Towelette .... ▣753
VōSoL HC Otic Solution 3356

Hydrocortisone Acetate (Co-administration of corticosteroids may enhance edema formation). Products include:

Analpram-HC 1338
Anusol HC-1 Hydrocortisone Anti-Itch Cream .... ⊡689
Anusol-HC Suppositories 2238
Cortaid .... ⊡717
Cortifoam Rectal Foam 3170
Cortisporin-TC Otic Suspension 2246
Hydrocortone Acetate Injectable Suspension 2103
Pramosone 1343
Proctocort Suppositories 2264
ProctoFoam-HC 3177
Terra-Cortril Ophthalmic Suspension 2716

Hydrocortisone Sodium Phosphate (Co-administration of corticosteroids may enhance edema formation). Products include:
Hydrocortone Phosphate Injection, Sterile 2105

Hydrocortisone Sodium Succinate (Co-administration of corticosteroids may enhance edema formation).
No products indexed under this heading.

Insulin, Human, Zinc Suspension (Possible decrease in insulin requirements). Products include:
Humulin L, 100 Units 1937
Humulin U, 100 Units 1943
Novolin L Human Insulin 10 ml Vials 2422

Insulin, Human NPH (Possible decrease in insulin requirements). Products include:
Humulin N, 100 Units 1939
Humulin N NPH Pen 1940
Novolin N Human Insulin 10 ml Vials 2422
Novolin N PenFill 2423
Novolin N Prefilled Syringe Disposable Insulin Delivery System 2425

Insulin, Human Regular (Possible decrease in insulin requirements). Products include:
Humulin R Regular (U-500) 1943
Humulin R, 100 Units 1941
Novolin R Human Insulin 10 ml Vials 2423
Novolin R PenFill 2423
Novolin R Prefilled Syringe Disposable Insulin Delivery System 2425
Velosulin BR Human Insulin 10 ml Vials 2435

Insulin, Human Regular and Human NPH Mixture (Possible decrease in insulin requirements). Products include:
Humulin 50/50, 100 Units 1934
Humulin 70/30, 100 Units 1935
Humulin 70/30 Pen 1936
Novolin 70/30 Human Insulin 10 ml Vials 2421
Novolin 70/30 PenFill 2423
Novolin 70/30 Prefilled Disposable Insulin Delivery System 2425

Insulin, NPH (Possible decrease in insulin requirements). Products include:
Iletin II, NPH (Pork), 100 Units 1946

Insulin, Regular (Possible decrease in insulin requirements). Products include:
Iletin II, Regular (Pork), 100 Units ... 1947

Insulin, Zinc Crystals (Possible decrease in insulin requirements).
No products indexed under this heading.

Insulin, Zinc Suspension (Possible decrease in insulin requirements). Products include:
Iletin II, Lente (Pork), 100 Units 1945

Insulin Aspart, Human Regular (Possible decrease in insulin requirements).
No products indexed under this heading.

Insulin glargine (Possible decrease in insulin requirements). Products include:
Lantus Injection 742

Insulin Lispro, Human (Possible decrease in insulin requirements). Products include:
Humalog 1926
Humalog Mix 75/25 Pen 1928

Insulin Lispro Protamine, Human (Possible decrease in insulin requirements). Products include:
Humalog Mix 75/25 Pen 1928

Methylprednisolone Acetate (Co-administration of corticosteroids may enhance edema formation). Products include:
Depo-Medrol Injectable Suspension 2795

Methylprednisolone Sodium Succinate (Co-administration of corticosteroids may enhance edema formation). Products include:
Solu-Medrol Sterile Powder 2855

Oxyphenbutazone (Concurrent administration may result in elevated serum levels of oxyphenbutazone).
No products indexed under this heading.

Prednisolone Acetate (Co-administration of corticosteroids may enhance edema formation). Products include:
Blephamide Ophthalmic Ointment .. 547
Blephamide Ophthalmic Suspension 548
Poly-Pred Liquifilm Ophthalmic Suspension .... ⊙245
Pred Forte Ophthalmic Suspension .... ⊙246
Pred Mild Sterile Ophthalmic Suspension .... ⊙249
Pred-G Ophthalmic Suspension .... ⊙247
Pred-G Sterile Ophthalmic Ointment .... ⊙248

Prednisolone Sodium Phosphate (Co-administration of corticosteroids may enhance edema formation). Products include:
Pediapred Oral Solution 1170

Prednisolone Tebutate (Co-administration of corticosteroids may enhance edema formation).
No products indexed under this heading.

Prednisone (Co-administration of corticosteroids may enhance edema formation). Products include:
Prednisone 3064

Propranolol Hydrochloride (In a published pharmacokinetic study of an injectable testosterone product, administration of testosterone cypionte led to an increased clearance of propranolol in majority of men tested). Products include:
Inderal 3513
Inderal LA Long-Acting Capsules 3516
Inderide Tablets 3517
Inderide LA Long-Acting Capsules .. 3519

Triamcinolone (Co-administration of corticosteroids may enhance edema formation).
No products indexed under this heading.

Triamcinolone Acetonide (Co-administration of corticosteroids may enhance edema formation). Products include:
Azmacort Inhalation Aerosol 728
Nasacort Nasal Inhaler 750
Nasacort AQ Nasal Spray 752
Tri-Nasal Spray 2274

Triamcinolone Diacetate (Co-administration of corticosteroids may enhance edema formation).
No products indexed under this heading.

Triamcinolone Hexacetonide (Co-administration of corticosteroids may enhance edema formation).
No products indexed under this heading.

Warfarin Sodium (Potential for decreased requirements of oral anticoagulants). Products include:
Coumadin for Injection 1243
Coumadin Tablets 1243
Warfarin Sodium Tablets, USP 3302

TESTOPEL PELLETS

(Testosterone) 3610
May interact with oral anticoagulants, insulin, and certain other agents. Compounds in these categories include:

Dicumarol (Anabolic steroids have been reported to decrease the anticoagulant requirements of patients receiving oral anticoagulants; bleeding has been reported with concurrent use).
No products indexed under this heading.

Insulin, Human, Zinc Suspension (Metabolic effects of androgens may decrease blood glucose and insulin requirements). Products include:
Humulin L, 100 Units 1937
Humulin U, 100 Units 1943
Novolin L Human Insulin 10 ml Vials 2422

Insulin, Human NPH (Metabolic effects of androgens may decrease blood glucose and insulin requirements). Products include:
Humulin N, 100 Units 1939
Humulin N NPH Pen 1940
Novolin N Human Insulin 10 ml Vials 2422
Novolin N PenFill 2423
Novolin N Prefilled Syringe Disposable Insulin Delivery System 2425

Insulin, Human Regular (Metabolic effects of androgens may decrease blood glucose and insulin requirements). Products include:
Humulin R Regular (U-500) 1943
Humulin R, 100 Units 1941
Novolin R Human Insulin 10 ml Vials 2423
Novolin R PenFill 2423
Novolin R Prefilled Syringe Disposable Insulin Delivery System 2425
Velosulin BR Human Insulin 10 ml Vials 2435

Insulin, Human Regular and Human NPH Mixture (Metabolic effects of androgens may decrease blood glucose and insulin requirements). Products include:
Humulin 50/50, 100 Units 1934
Humulin 70/30, 100 Units 1935
Humulin 70/30 Pen 1936
Novolin 70/30 Human Insulin 10 ml Vials 2421
Novolin 70/30 PenFill 2423
Novolin 70/30 Prefilled Disposable Insulin Delivery System 2425

Insulin, NPH (Metabolic effects of androgens may decrease blood glucose and insulin requirements). Products include:
Iletin II, NPH (Pork), 100 Units 1946

Insulin, Regular (Metabolic effects of androgens may decrease blood glucose and insulin requirements). Products include:
Iletin II, Regular (Pork), 100 Units ... 1947

Insulin, Zinc Crystals (Metabolic effects of androgens may decrease blood glucose and insulin requirements).
No products indexed under this heading.

Insulin, Zinc Suspension (Metabolic effects of androgens may decrease blood glucose and insulin requirements). Products include:
Iletin II, Lente (Pork), 100 Units 1945

Insulin Aspart, Human Regular (Metabolic effects of androgens may decrease blood glucose and insulin requirements).
No products indexed under this heading.

Insulin glargine (Metabolic effects of androgens may decrease blood glucose and insulin requirements). Products include:
Lantus Injection 742

Insulin Lispro, Human (Metabolic effects of androgens may decrease blood glucose and insulin requirements). Products include:
Humalog 1926
Humalog Mix 75/25 Pen 1928

Insulin Lispro Protamine, Human (Metabolic effects of androgens may decrease blood glucose and insulin requirements). Products include:
Humalog Mix 75/25 Pen 1928

Oxyphenbutazone (May result in elevated serum levels of oxyphenbutazone).
No products indexed under this heading.

Warfarin Sodium (Anabolic steroids have been reported to decrease the anticoagulant requirements of patients receiving oral anticoagulants; bleeding has been reported with concurrent use). Products include:
Coumadin for Injection 1243
Coumadin Tablets 1243
Warfarin Sodium Tablets, USP 3302

TESTRED CAPSULES, 10 MG

(Methyltestosterone) 1746
May interact with oral anticoagulants, insulin, and certain other agents. Compounds in these categories include:

Dicumarol (Decreased need for anticoagulants).
No products indexed under this heading.

Insulin, Human, Zinc Suspension (Possibly decreased insulin requirements). Products include:
Humulin L, 100 Units 1937
Humulin U, 100 Units 1943
Novolin L Human Insulin 10 ml Vials 2422

Insulin, Human NPH (Possibly decreased insulin requirements). Products include:
Humulin N, 100 Units 1939
Humulin N NPH Pen 1940
Novolin N Human Insulin 10 ml Vials 2422
Novolin N PenFill 2423
Novolin N Prefilled Syringe Disposable Insulin Delivery System 2425

Insulin, Human Regular (Possibly decreased insulin requirements). Products include:
Humulin R Regular (U-500) 1943
Humulin R, 100 Units 1941
Novolin R Human Insulin 10 ml Vials 2423
Novolin R PenFill 2423
Novolin R Prefilled Syringe Disposable Insulin Delivery System 2425
Velosulin BR Human Insulin 10 ml Vials 2435

Insulin, Human Regular and Human NPH Mixture (Possibly decreased insulin requirements). Products include:
Humulin 50/50, 100 Units 1934
Humulin 70/30, 100 Units 1935
Humulin 70/30 Pen 1936
Novolin 70/30 Human Insulin 10 ml Vials 2421
Novolin 70/30 PenFill 2423
Novolin 70/30 Prefilled Disposable Insulin Delivery System 2425

Insulin, NPH (Possibly decreased insulin requirements). Products include:
Iletin II, NPH (Pork), 100 Units 1946

Insulin, Regular (Possibly decreased insulin requirements). Products include:
Iletin II, Regular (Pork), 100 Units ... 1947

Insulin, Zinc Crystals (Possibly decreased insulin requirements).
No products indexed under this heading.

Insulin, Zinc Suspension (Possibly decreased insulin requirements). Products include:

Iletin II, Lente (Pork), 100 Units 1945

Insulin Aspart, Human Regular (Possibly decreased insulin requirements).
No products indexed under this heading.

Insulin glargine (Possibly decreased insulin requirements). Products include:
Lantus Injection ... 742

Insulin Lispro, Human (Possibly decreased insulin requirements). Products include:
Humalog ... 1926
Humalog Mix 75/25 Pen ... 1928

Insulin Lispro Protamine, Human (Possibly decreased insulin requirements). Products include:
Humalog Mix 75/25 Pen ... 1928

Oxyphenbutazone (Elevated serum levels of oxyphenbutazone).
No products indexed under this heading.

Warfarin Sodium (Decreased need for anticoagulants). Products include:
Coumadin for Injection ... 1243
Coumadin Tablets ... 1243
Warfarin Sodium Tablets, USP ... 3302

TETANUS & DIPHTHERIA TOXOIDS ADSORBED FOR ADULT USE

(Tetanus & Diphtheria Toxoids Adsorbed) ... 1880

May interact with alkylating agents, anticoagulants, corticosteroids, and cytotoxic drugs. Compounds in these categories include:

Ardeparin Sodium (As with other intramuscular injections, tetanus and diphtheria toxoids should be given with caution to patients on anticoagulant therapy).
No products indexed under this heading.

Betamethasone Acetate (Immunosuppressive therapy with corticosteroids may reduce the immune response to vaccine). Products include:
Celestone Soluspan Injectable Suspension ... 3097

Betamethasone Sodium Phosphate (Immunosuppressive therapy with corticosteroids may reduce the immune response to vaccine). Products include:
Celestone Soluspan Injectable Suspension ... 3097

Bleomycin Sulfate (Immunosuppressive therapy may reduce the immune response to vaccine).
No products indexed under this heading.

Busulfan (Immunosuppressive therapy may reduce the immune response to vaccine). Products include:
Myleran Tablets ... 1603

Carmustine (BCNU) (Immunosuppressive therapy may reduce the immune response to vaccine). Products include:
Gliadel Wafer ... 1723

Chlorambucil (Immunosuppressive therapy may reduce the immune response to vaccine). Products include:
Leukeran Tablets ... 1591

Cortisone Acetate (Immunosuppressive therapy with corticosteroids may reduce the immune response to vaccine). Products include:
Cortone Acetate Injectable Suspension ... 2059
Cortone Acetate Tablets ... 2061

Cyclophosphamide (Immunosuppressive therapy may reduce the immune response to vaccine).
No products indexed under this heading.

Dacarbazine (Immunosuppressive therapy may reduce the immune response to vaccine). Products include:
DTIC-Dome ... 902

Dalteparin Sodium (As with other intramuscular injections, tetanus and diphtheria toxoids should be given with caution to patients on anticoagulant therapy). Products include:
Fragmin Injection ... 2814

Danaparoid Sodium (As with other intramuscular injections, tetanus and diphtheria toxoids should be given with caution to patients on anticoagulant therapy). Products include:
Orgaran Injection ... 2480

Daunorubicin Hydrochloride (Immunosuppressive therapy may reduce the immune response to vaccine). Products include:
Cerubidine for Injection ... 947

Dexamethasone (Immunosuppressive therapy with corticosteroids may reduce the immune response to vaccine). Products include:
Decadron Elixir ... 2078
Decadron Tablets ... 2079
TobraDex Ophthalmic Ointment ... 542
TobraDex Ophthalmic Suspension ... 541

Dexamethasone Acetate (Immunosuppressive therapy with corticosteroids may reduce the immune response to vaccine).
No products indexed under this heading.

Dexamethasone Sodium Phosphate (Immunosuppressive therapy with corticosteroids may reduce the immune response to vaccine). Products include:
Decadron Phosphate Injection ... 2081
Decadron Phosphate Sterile Ophthalmic Ointment ... 2083
Decadron Phosphate Sterile Ophthalmic Solution ... 2084
NeoDecadron Sterile Ophthalmic Solution ... 2144

Dicumarol (As with other intramuscular injections, tetanus and diphtheria toxoids should be given with caution to patients on anticoagulant therapy).
No products indexed under this heading.

Doxorubicin Hydrochloride (Immunosuppressive therapy may reduce the immune response to vaccine). Products include:
Adriamycin PFS/RDF Injection ... 2767
Doxil Injection ... 566

Enoxaparin (As with other intramuscular injections, tetanus and diphtheria toxoids should be given with caution to patients on anticoagulant therapy). Products include:
Lovenox Injection ... 746

Epirubicin Hydrochloride (Immunosuppressive therapy may reduce the immune response to vaccine). Products include:
Ellence Injection ... 2806

Fludrocortisone Acetate (Immunosuppressive therapy with corticosteroids may reduce the immune response to vaccine). Products include:
Florinef Acetate Tablets ... 2250

Fluorouracil (Immunosuppressive therapy may reduce the immune response to vaccine). Products include:
Carac Cream ... 1222
Efudex ... 1733
Fluoroplex ... 552

Heparin Sodium (As with other intramuscular injections, tetanus and diphtheria toxoids should be given with caution to patients on anticoagulant therapy). Products include:
Heparin Lock Flush Solution ... 3509
Heparin Sodium Injection ... 3511

Hydrocortisone (Immunosuppressive therapy with corticosteroids may reduce the immune response to vaccine). Products include:
Anusol-HC Cream 2.5% ... 2237
Cipro HC Otic Suspension ... 540
Cortaid Intensive Therapy Cream ... ▣717
Cortaid Maximum Strength Cream ... ▣717
Cortisporin Ophthalmic Suspension Sterile ... ⊙297
Cortizone•5 ... ▣699
Cortizone•10 ... ▣699
Cortizone•10 Plus Creme ... ▣700
Cortizone for Kids Creme ... ▣699
Hydrocortone Tablets ... 2106
Massengill Medicated Soft Cloth Towelette ... ▣753
VōSoL HC Otic Solution ... 3356

Hydrocortisone Acetate (Immunosuppressive therapy with corticosteroids may reduce the immune response to vaccine). Products include:
Analpram-HC ... 1338
Anusol HC-1 Hydrocortisone Anti-Itch Cream ... ▣689
Anusol-HC Suppositories ... 2238
Cortaid ... ▣717
Cortifoam Rectal Foam ... 3170
Cortisporin-TC Otic Suspension ... 2246
Hydrocortone Acetate Injectable Suspension ... 2103
Pramosone ... 1343
Proctocort Suppositories ... 2264
ProctoFoam-HC ... 3177
Terra-Cortril Ophthalmic Suspension ... 2716

Hydrocortisone Sodium Phosphate (Immunosuppressive therapy with corticosteroids may reduce the immune response to vaccine). Products include:
Hydrocortone Phosphate Injection, Sterile ... 2105

Hydrocortisone Sodium Succinate (Immunosuppressive therapy with corticosteroids may reduce the immune response to vaccine).
No products indexed under this heading.

Hydroxyurea (Immunosuppressive therapy may reduce the immune response to vaccine). Products include:
Mylocel Tablets ... 2227

Lomustine (CCNU) (Immunosuppressive therapy may reduce the immune response to vaccine).
No products indexed under this heading.

Mechlorethamine Hydrochloride (Immunosuppressive therapy may reduce the immune response to vaccine). Products include:
Mustargen for Injection ... 2142

Melphalan (Immunosuppressive therapy may reduce the immune response to vaccine). Products include:
Alkeran Tablets ... 1466

Methotrexate Sodium (Immunosuppressive therapy may reduce the immune response to vaccine).
No products indexed under this heading.

Methylprednisolone Acetate (Immunosuppressive therapy with corticosteroids may reduce the immune response to vaccine). Products include:
Depo-Medrol Injectable Suspension ... 2795

Methylprednisolone Sodium Succinate (Immunosuppressive therapy with corticosteroids may reduce the immune response to vaccine). Products include:
Solu-Medrol Sterile Powder ... 2855

Mitotane (Immunosuppressive therapy may reduce the immune response to vaccine).
No products indexed under this heading.

Mitoxantrone Hydrochloride (Immunosuppressive therapy may reduce the immune response to vaccine). Products include:
Novantrone for Injection ... 1760

Prednisolone Acetate (Immunosuppressive therapy with corticosteroids may reduce the immune response to vaccine). Products include:
Blephamide Ophthalmic Ointment ... 547
Blephamide Ophthalmic Suspension ... 548
Poly-Pred Liquifilm Ophthalmic Suspension ... ⊙245
Pred Forte Ophthalmic Suspension ... ⊙246
Pred Mild Sterile Ophthalmic Suspension ... ⊙249
Pred-G Ophthalmic Suspension ... ⊙247
Pred-G Sterile Ophthalmic Ointment ... ⊙248

Prednisolone Sodium Phosphate (Immunosuppressive therapy with corticosteroids may reduce the immune response to vaccine). Products include:
Pediapred Oral Solution ... 1170

Prednisolone Tebutate (Immunosuppressive therapy with corticosteroids may reduce the immune response to vaccine).
No products indexed under this heading.

Prednisone (Immunosuppressive therapy with corticosteroids may reduce the immune response to vaccine). Products include:
Prednisone ... 3064

Procarbazine Hydrochloride (Immunosuppressive therapy may reduce the immune response to vaccine). Products include:
Matulane Capsules ... 3246

Tamoxifen Citrate (Immunosuppressive therapy may reduce the immune response to vaccine). Products include:
Nolvadex Tablets ... 678

Thiotepa (Immunosuppressive therapy may reduce the immune response to vaccine). Products include:
Thioplex for Injection ... 1765

Tinzaparin sodium (As with other intramuscular injections, tetanus and diphtheria toxoids should be given with caution to patients on anticoagulant therapy). Products include:
Innohep Injection ... 1248

Triamcinolone (Immunosuppressive therapy with corticosteroids may reduce the immune response to vaccine).
No products indexed under this heading.

Triamcinolone Acetonide (Immunosuppressive therapy with corticosteroids may reduce the immune response to vaccine). Products include:
Azmacort Inhalation Aerosol ... 728
Nasacort Nasal Inhaler ... 750
Nasacort AQ Nasal Spray ... 752
Tri-Nasal Spray ... 2274

Triamcinolone Diacetate (Immunosuppressive therapy with corticosteroids may reduce the immune response to vaccine).
No products indexed under this heading.

Triamcinolone Hexacetonide (Immunosuppressive therapy with corticosteroids may reduce the immune response to vaccine).
No products indexed under this heading.

Vincristine Sulfate (Immunosuppressive therapy may reduce the immune response to vaccine).
No products indexed under this heading.

Warfarin Sodium (As with other intramuscular injections, tetanus and diphtheria toxoids should be given with caution to patients on anticoagulant therapy). Products include:
Coumadin for Injection ... 1243
Coumadin Tablets ... 1243
Warfarin Sodium Tablets, USP ... 3302

TETANUS AND DIPHTHERIA TOXOIDS ADSORBED FOR ADULT USE

(Tetanus & Diphtheria Toxoids Adsorbed).. 815
May interact with alkylating agents, anticoagulants, corticosteroids, and cytotoxic drugs. Compounds in these categories include:

Ardeparin Sodium (As with other intramuscular injections, tetanus and diphtheria toxoids should be given with caution to patients on anticoagulant therapy).
No products indexed under this heading.

Betamethasone Acetate (Immunosuppressive therapy with corticosteroids may reduce the immune response to vaccine). Products include:
Celestone Soluspan Injectable Suspension.................................. 3097

Betamethasone Sodium Phosphate (Immunosuppressive therapy with corticosteroids may reduce the immune response to vaccine). Products include:
Celestone Soluspan Injectable Suspension.................................. 3097

Bleomycin Sulfate (Immunosuppressive therapy may reduce the immune response to vaccine).
No products indexed under this heading.

Busulfan (Immunosuppressive therapy may reduce the immune response to vaccine). Products include:
Myleran Tablets.................................. 1603

Carmustine (BCNU) (Immunosuppressive therapy may reduce the immune response to vaccine). Products include:
Gliadel Wafer.................................. 1723

Chlorambucil (Immunosuppressive therapy may reduce the immune response to vaccine). Products include:
Leukeran Tablets.................................. 1591

Cortisone Acetate (Immunosuppressive therapy with corticosteroids may reduce the immune response to vaccine). Products include:
Cortone Acetate Injectable Suspension.................................. 2059
Cortone Acetate Tablets.................................. 2061

Cyclophosphamide (Immunosuppressive therapy may reduce the immune response to vaccine).
No products indexed under this heading.

Dacarbazine (Immunosuppressive therapy may reduce the immune response to vaccine). Products include:
DTIC-Dome.................................. 902

Dalteparin Sodium (As with other intramuscular injections, tetanus and diphtheria toxoids should be given with caution to patients on anticoagulant therapy). Products include:
Fragmin Injection.................................. 2814

Danaparoid Sodium (As with other intramuscular injections, tetanus and diphtheria toxoids should be given with caution to patients on anticoagulant therapy). Products include:
Orgaran Injection.................................. 2480

Daunorubicin Hydrochloride (Immunosuppressive therapy may reduce the immune response to vaccine). Products include:
Cerubidine for Injection.................................. 947

Dexamethasone (Immunosuppressive therapy with corticosteroids may reduce the immune response to vaccine). Products include:
Decadron Elixir.................................. 2078
Decadron Tablets.................................. 2079
TobraDex Ophthalmic Ointment.................................. 542
TobraDex Ophthalmic Suspension.................................. 541

Dexamethasone Acetate (Immunosuppressive therapy with corticosteroids may reduce the immune response to vaccine).
No products indexed under this heading.

Dexamethasone Sodium Phosphate (Immunosuppressive therapy with corticosteroids may reduce the immune response to vaccine). Products include:
Decadron Phosphate Injection.................................. 2081
Decadron Phosphate Sterile Ophthalmic Ointment.................................. 2083
Decadron Phosphate Sterile Ophthalmic Solution.................................. 2084
NeoDecadron Sterile Ophthalmic Solution.................................. 2144

Dicumarol (As with other intramuscular injections, tetanus and diphtheria toxoids should be given with caution to patients on anticoagulant therapy).
No products indexed under this heading.

Doxorubicin Hydrochloride (Immunosuppressive therapy may reduce the immune response to vaccine). Products include:
Adriamycin PFS/RDF Injection.................................. 2767
Doxil Injection.................................. 566

Enoxaparin (As with other intramuscular injections, tetanus and diphtheria toxoids should be given with caution to patients on anticoagulant therapy). Products include:
Lovenox Injection.................................. 746

Epirubicin Hydrochloride (Immunosuppressive therapy may reduce the immune response to vaccine). Products include:
Ellence Injection.................................. 2806

Fludrocortisone Acetate (Immunosuppressive therapy with corticosteroids may reduce the immune response to vaccine). Products include:
Florinef Acetate Tablets.................................. 2250

Fluorouracil (Immunosuppressive therapy may reduce the immune response to vaccine). Products include:
Carac Cream.................................. 1222
Efudex.................................. 1733
Fluoroplex.................................. 552

Heparin Sodium (As with other intramuscular injections, tetanus and diphtheria toxoids should be given with caution to patients on anticoagulant therapy). Products include:
Heparin Lock Flush Solution.................................. 3509
Heparin Sodium Injection.................................. 3511

Hydrocortisone (Immunosuppressive therapy with corticosteroids may reduce the immune response to vaccine). Products include:
Anusol-HC Cream 2.5%.................................. 2237
Cipro HC Otic Suspension.................................. 540
Cortaid Intensive Therapy Cream.................................. ▣717
Cortaid Maximum Strength Cream.................................. ▣717
Cortisporin Ophthalmic Suspension Sterile.................................. ⊙297
Cortizone•5.................................. ▣699
Cortizone•10.................................. ▣699
Cortizone•10 Plus Creme.................................. ▣700
Cortizone for Kids Creme.................................. ▣699
Hydrocortone Tablets.................................. 2106
Massengill Medicated Soft Cloth Towelette.................................. ▣753
VōSoL HC Otic Solution.................................. 3356

Hydrocortisone Acetate (Immunosuppressive therapy with corticosteroids may reduce the immune response to vaccine). Products include:
Analpram-HC.................................. 1338
Anusol HC-1 Hydrocortisone Anti-Itch Cream.................................. ▣689
Anusol-HC Suppositories.................................. 2238
Cortaid.................................. ▣717
Cortifoam Rectal Foam.................................. 3170
Cortisporin-TC Otic Suspension.................................. 2246
Hydrocortone Acetate Injectable Suspension.................................. 2103
Pramosone.................................. 1343
Proctocort Suppositories.................................. 2264
ProctoFoam-HC.................................. 3177
Terra-Cortril Ophthalmic Suspension.................................. 2716

Hydrocortisone Sodium Phosphate (Immunosuppressive therapy with corticosteroids may reduce the immune response to vaccine). Products include:
Hydrocortone Phosphate Injection, Sterile.................................. 2105

Hydrocortisone Sodium Succinate (Immunosuppressive therapy with corticosteroids may reduce the immune response to vaccine).
No products indexed under this heading.

Hydroxyurea (Immunosuppressive therapy may reduce the immune response to vaccine). Products include:
Mylocel Tablets.................................. 2227

Lomustine (CCNU) (Immunosuppressive therapy may reduce the immune response to vaccine).
No products indexed under this heading.

Mechlorethamine Hydrochloride (Immunosuppressive therapy may reduce the immune response to vaccine). Products include:
Mustargen for Injection.................................. 2142

Melphalan (Immunosuppressive therapy may reduce the immune response to vaccine). Products include:
Alkeran Tablets.................................. 1466

Methotrexate Sodium (Immunosuppressive therapy may reduce the immune response to vaccine).
No products indexed under this heading.

Methylprednisolone Acetate (Immunosuppressive therapy with corticosteroids may reduce the immune response to vaccine). Products include:
Depo-Medrol Injectable Suspension.................................. 2795

Methylprednisolone Sodium Succinate (Immunosuppressive therapy with corticosteroids may reduce the immune response to vaccine). Products include:
Solu-Medrol Sterile Powder.................................. 2855

Mitotane (Immunosuppressive therapy may reduce the immune response to vaccine).
No products indexed under this heading.

Mitoxantrone Hydrochloride (Immunosuppressive therapy may reduce the immune response to vaccine). Products include:
Novantrone for Injection.................................. 1760

Prednisolone Acetate (Immunosuppressive therapy with corticosteroids may reduce the immune response to vaccine). Products include:
Blephamide Ophthalmic Ointment.................................. 547
Blephamide Ophthalmic Suspension.................................. 548
Poly-Pred Liquifilm Ophthalmic Suspension.................................. ⊙245
Pred Forte Ophthalmic Suspension.................................. ⊙246
Pred Mild Sterile Ophthalmic Suspension.................................. ⊙249
Pred-G Ophthalmic Suspension.................................. ⊙247
Pred-G Sterile Ophthalmic Ointment.................................. ⊙248

Prednisolone Sodium Phosphate (Immunosuppressive therapy with corticosteroids may reduce the immune response to vaccine). Products include:
Pediapred Oral Solution.................................. 1170

Prednisolone Tebutate (Immunosuppressive therapy with corticosteroids may reduce the immune response to vaccine).
No products indexed under this heading.

Prednisone (Immunosuppressive therapy with corticosteroids may reduce the immune response to vaccine). Products include:
Prednisone.................................. 3064

Procarbazine Hydrochloride (Immunosuppressive therapy may reduce the immune response to vaccine). Products include:
Matulane Capsules.................................. 3246

Tamoxifen Citrate (Immunosuppressive therapy may reduce the immune response to vaccine). Products include:
Nolvadex Tablets.................................. 678

Thiotepa (Immunosuppressive therapy may reduce the immune response to vaccine). Products include:
Thioplex for Injection.................................. 1765

Tinzaparin sodium (As with other intramuscular injections, tetanus and diphtheria toxoids should be given with caution to patients on anticoagulant therapy). Products include:
Innohep Injection.................................. 1248

Triamcinolone (Immunosuppressive therapy with corticosteroids may reduce the immune response to vaccine).
No products indexed under this heading.

Triamcinolone Acetonide (Immunosuppressive therapy with corticosteroids may reduce the immune response to vaccine). Products include:
Azmacort Inhalation Aerosol.................................. 728
Nasacort Nasal Inhaler.................................. 750
Nasacort AQ Nasal Spray.................................. 752
Tri-Nasal Spray.................................. 2274

Triamcinolone Diacetate (Immunosuppressive therapy with corticosteroids may reduce the immune response to vaccine).
No products indexed under this heading.

Triamcinolone Hexacetonide (Immunosuppressive therapy with corticosteroids may reduce the immune response to vaccine).
No products indexed under this heading.

Vincristine Sulfate (Immunosuppressive therapy may reduce the immune response to vaccine).
No products indexed under this heading.

Warfarin Sodium (As with other intramuscular injections, tetanus and diphtheria toxoids should be given with caution to patients on anticoagulant therapy). Products include:
Coumadin for Injection.................................. 1243
Coumadin Tablets.................................. 1243
Warfarin Sodium Tablets, USP.................................. 3302

TETANUS TOXOID ADSORBED PUROGENATED

(Tetanus Toxoid, Adsorbed).................................. 1882
May interact with immunosuppressive agents and certain other agents. Compounds in these categories include:

Azathioprine (Concurrent use should be avoided).
No products indexed under this heading.

Basiliximab (Concurrent use should be avoided). Products include:
Simulect for Injection.................................. 2399

Cyclosporine (Concurrent use should be avoided). Products include:
Gengraf Capsules.................................. 457
Neoral Soft Gelatin Capsules.................................. 2380
Neoral Oral Solution.................................. 2380
Sandimmune.................................. 2388

Immune Globulin Intravenous (Human) (Concurrent use should be avoided).
No products indexed under this heading.

Muromonab-CD3 (Concurrent use should be avoided). Products include:
Orthoclone OKT3 Sterile Solution.................................. 2498

IMPORTANT NOTE: Always consult each drug listing in the patient's regimen for possible interactions.

Mycophenolate Mofetil (Concurrent use should be avoided).
Products include:
CellCept Capsules 2951
CellCept Oral Suspension 2951
CellCept Tablets 2951

Sirolimus (Concurrent use should be avoided). Products include:
Rapamune Oral Solution and Tablets 3584

Tacrolimus (Concurrent use should be avoided). Products include:
Prograf 1393
Protopic Ointment 1397

TEVETEN TABLETS

(Eprosartan Mesylate) 3327

Food Interactions

Food, unspecified (Co-administration with food delays absorption, and causes variable changes in Cmax and AUC values which do not appear clinically important).

THALOMID CAPSULES

(Thalidomide) 1154

May interact with barbiturates, drugs that may exacerbate peripheral neuropathy (selected), phenytoin, protease inhibitors, and certain other agents. Compounds in these categories include:

Amprenavir (Concomitant use of HIV-protease inhibitors with hormonal contraceptives may reduce the effectiveness of contraception; women requiring treatment with HIV-protease inhibitors must use two other highly effective methods of contraception or abstain from heterosexual sexual intercourse during treatment with thalidomide).
Products include:
Agenerase Capsules 1454
Agenerase Oral Solution 1459

Aprobarbital (Thalidomide has been reported to enhance the sedative activity of barbiturates).
No products indexed under this heading.

Butabarbital (Thalidomide has been reported to enhance the sedative activity of barbiturates).
No products indexed under this heading.

Butalbital (Thalidomide has been reported to enhance the sedative activity of barbiturates). Products include:
Phrenilin 578
Sedapap Tablets 50 mg/650 mg ... 2225

Carbamazepine (Concomitant use of carbamazepine with hormonal contraceptives may reduce the effectiveness of contraception; women requiring treatment with carbamazepine must use two other highly effective methods of contraception or abstain from heterosexual sexual intercourse during treatment with thalidomide). Products include:
Carbatrol Capsules 3234
Tegretol/Tegretol-XR 2404

Carboplatin (Peripheral neuropathy is a common, potentially severe, side effect of treatment with thalidomide; therefore, concomitant use of drugs known to be associated with peripheral neuropathy should be undertaken with caution). Products include:
Paraplatin for Injection 1126

Chlorpromazine (Thalidomide has been reported to enhance the sedative activity of chlorpromazine).
Products include:
Thorazine Suppositories 1656

Chlorpromazine Hydrochloride (Thalidomide has been reported to enhance the sedative activity of chlorpromazine). Products include:
Thorazine 1656

Didanosine (Peripheral neuropathy is a common, potentially severe, side effect of treatment with thalidomide; therefore, concomitant use of drugs known to be associated with peripheral neuropathy should be undertaken with caution). Products include:
Videx 1138
Videx EC Capsules 1143

Fosphenytoin Sodium (Concomitant use of phenytoin with hormonal contraceptives may reduce the effectiveness of contraception; women requiring treatment with phenytoin must use two other highly effective methods of contraception or abstain from heterosexual sexual intercourse during treatment with thalidomide). Products include:
Cerebyx Injection 2619

Griseofulvin (Concomitant use of griseofulvin with hormonal contraceptives may reduce the effectiveness of contraception; women requiring treatment with griseofulvin must use two other highly effective methods of contraception or abstain from heterosexual sexual intercourse during treatment with thalidomide).
Products include:
Grifulvin V Tablets Microsize and Oral Suspension Microsize 2518
Gris-PEG Tablets 2661

Indinavir Sulfate (Concomitant use of HIV-protease inhibitors with hormonal contraceptives may reduce the effectiveness of contraception; women requiring treatment with HIV-protease inhibitors must use two other highly effective methods of contraception or abstain from heterosexual sexual intercourse during treatment with thalidomide).
Products include:
Crixivan Capsules 2070

Isoniazid (Peripheral neuropathy is a common, potentially severe, side effect of treatment with thalidomide; therefore, concomitant use of drugs known to be associated with peripheral neuropathy should be undertaken with caution). Products include:
Rifamate Capsules 767
Rifater Tablets 769

Lopinavir (Concomitant use of HIV-protease inhibitors with hormonal contraceptives may reduce the effectiveness of contraception; women requiring treatment with HIV-protease inhibitors must use two other highly effective methods of contraception or abstain from heterosexual sexual intercourse during treatment with thalidomide).
Products include:
Kaletra Capsules 471
Kaletra Oral Solution 471

Mephobarbital (Thalidomide has been reported to enhance the sedative activity of barbiturates).
No products indexed under this heading.

Nelfinavir Mesylate (Concomitant use of HIV-protease inhibitors with hormonal contraceptives may reduce the effectiveness of contraception; women requiring treatment with HIV-protease inhibitors must use two other highly effective methods of contraception or abstain from heterosexual sexual intercourse during treatment with thalidomide).
Products include:
Viracept 532

Paclitaxel (Peripheral neuropathy is a common, potentially severe, side effect of treatment with thalidomide; therefore, concomitant use of drugs known to be associated with peripheral neuropathy should be undertaken with caution). Products include:
Taxol Injection 1129

Pentobarbital Sodium (Thalidomide has been reported to enhance the sedative activity of barbiturates).
Products include:
Nembutal Sodium Solution 485

Phenobarbital (Thalidomide has been reported to enhance the sedative activity of barbiturates).
Products include:
Arco-Lase Plus Tablets 592
Donnatal 2929
Donnatal Extentabs 2930

Phenytoin (Concomitant use of phenytoin with hormonal contraceptives may reduce the effectiveness of contraception; women requiring treatment with phenytoin must use two other highly effective methods of contraception or abstain from heterosexual sexual intercourse during treatment with thalidomide).
Products include:
Dilantin Infatabs 2624
Dilantin-125 Oral Suspension 2625

Phenytoin Sodium (Concomitant use of phenytoin with hormonal contraceptives may reduce the effectiveness of contraception; women requiring treatment with phenytoin must use two other highly effective methods of contraception or abstain from heterosexual sexual intercourse during treatment with thalidomide).
Products include:
Dilantin Kapseals 2622

Reserpine (Thalidomide has been reported to enhance the sedative activity of reserpine).
No products indexed under this heading.

Rifabutin (Concomitant use of rifabutin with hormonal contraceptives may reduce the effectiveness of contraception; women requiring treatment with rifabutin must use two other highly effective methods of contraception or abstain from heterosexual sexual intercourse during treatment with thalidomide).
Products include:
Mycobutin Capsules 2838

Rifampin (Concomitant use of rifampin with hormonal contraceptives may reduce the effectiveness of contraception; women requiring treatment with rifampin must use two other highly effective methods of contraception or abstain from heterosexual sexual intercourse during treatment with thalidomide).
Products include:
Rifadin 765
Rifamate Capsules 767
Rifater Tablets 769

Ritonavir (Concomitant use of HIV-protease inhibitors with hormonal contraceptives may reduce the effectiveness of contraception; women requiring treatment with HIV-protease inhibitors must use two other highly effective methods of contraception or abstain from heterosexual sexual intercourse during treatment with thalidomide).
Products include:
Kaletra Capsules 471
Kaletra Oral Solution 471
Norvir Capsules 487
Norvir Oral Solution 487

Saquinavir (Concomitant use of HIV-protease inhibitors with hormonal contraceptives may reduce the effectiveness of contraception; women requiring treatment with HIV-protease inhibitors must use two other highly effective methods of contraception or abstain from heterosexual sexual intercourse during treatment with thalidomide).
Products include:
Fortovase Capsules 2970

Saquinavir Mesylate (Concomitant use of HIV-protease inhibitors with hormonal contraceptives may reduce the effectiveness of contraception; women requiring treatment with HIV-protease inhibitors must use two other highly effective methods of contraception or abstain from heterosexual sexual intercourse during treatment with thalidomide).
Products include:
Invirase Capsules 2979

Secobarbital Sodium (Thalidomide has been reported to enhance the sedative activity of barbiturates).
No products indexed under this heading.

Stavudine (Peripheral neuropathy is a common, potentially severe, side effect of treatment with thalidomide; therefore, concomitant use of drugs known to be associated with peripheral neuropathy should be undertaken with caution). Products include:
Zerit 1147

Thiamylal Sodium (Thalidomide has been reported to enhance the sedative activity of barbiturates).
No products indexed under this heading.

Zalcitabine (Peripheral neuropathy is a common, potentially severe, side effect of treatment with thalidomide; therefore, concomitant use of drugs known to be associated with peripheral neuropathy should be undertaken with caution). Products include:
Hivid Tablets 2975

Food Interactions

Alcohol (Thalidomide has been reported to enhance the sedative activity of alcohol).

Food, unspecified (Co-administration of Thalomid with a high fat meal causes minor changes in the observed AUC and Cmax values; however, it causes an increase in Tmax to approximately 6 hours).

THEO-DUR EXTENDED-RELEASE TABLETS

(Theophylline) 1835

May interact with erythromycin, lithium preparations, phenytoin, and certain other agents. Compounds in these categories include:

Adenosine (Theophylline blocks adenosine receptors; higher doses of adenosine may be required to achieve desired effect). Products include:
Adenocard Injection 1380
Adenoscan 1381

Allopurinol (Decreases theophylline clearance at allopurinol doses greater than or equal to 600 mg/day).
No products indexed under this heading.

Aminoglutethimide (Increases theophylline clearance by induction of microsomal enzyme).
No products indexed under this heading.

Carbamazepine (Increases theophylline clearance by induction of microsomal enzyme). Products include:
Carbatrol Capsules 3234
Tegretol/Tegretol-XR 2404

Cimetidine (Decreases theophylline clearance by inhibiting cytochrome P450 1A2). Products include:
Tagamet HB 200 Suspension .... ▣762
Tagamet HB 200 Tablets .... ▣761
Tagamet Tablets 1644

Cimetidine Hydrochloride (Decreases theophylline clearance by inhibiting cytochrome P450 1A2).
Products include:
Tagamet 1644

Ciprofloxacin (Decreases theophylline clearance by inhibiting cytochrome P450 1A2). Products include:
Cipro I.V. 893
Cipro I.V. Pharmacy Bulk Package .. 897
Cipro Oral Suspension 887

Ciprofloxacin Hydrochloride (Decreases theophylline clearance by inhibiting cytochrome P450 1A2). Products include:
Ciloxan 538
Cipro HC Otic Suspension 540
Cipro Tablets 887

Clarithromycin (Decreases theophylline clearance by inhibiting cytochrome P450 3A3). Products include:
Biaxin/Biaxin XL 403
PREVPAC 3298

Diazepam (Benzodiazepines increase CNS concentrations of adenosine, a potent CNS depressant, while theophylline blocks adenosine receptors; larger diazepam doses may be required to produce desired level of sedation; discontinuation of theophylline without reduction of diazepam dose may result in respiratory depression). Products include:
Valium Injectable 3026
Valium Tablets 3047

Disulfiram (Decreases theophylline clearance by inhibiting hydroxylation and demethylation). Products include:
Antabuse Tablets 2444
Antabuse Tablets 3474

Enoxacin (Decreases theophylline clearance by inhibiting cytochrome P450 1A2).
No products indexed under this heading.

Ephedrine Hydrochloride (Co-administration results in synergistic CNS effects resulting in increased frequency of nausea, nervousness, and insomnia). Products include:
Primatene Tablets 780

Ephedrine Sulfate (Co-administration results in synergistic CNS effects resulting in increased frequency of nausea, nervousness, and insomnia).
No products indexed under this heading.

Ephedrine Tannate (Co-administration results in synergistic CNS effects resulting in increased frequency of nausea, nervousness, and insomnia). Products include:
Rynatuss Pediatric Suspension 3353
Rynatuss Tablets 3353

Erythromycin (Erythromycin metabolite decreases theophylline clearance by inhibiting cytochrome P450 3A3; decreased erythromycin steady-state serum concentrations). Products include:
Emgel 2% Topical Gel 1285
Ery-Tab Tablets 448
Erythromycin Base Filmtab Tablets 454
Erythromycin Delayed-Release Capsules, USP 455
PCE Dispertab Tablets 498

Erythromycin Estolate (Erythromycin metabolite decreases theophylline clearance by inhibiting cytochrome P450 3A3; decreased erythromycin steady-state serum concentrations).
No products indexed under this heading.

Erythromycin Ethylsuccinate (Erythromycin metabolite decreases theophylline clearance by inhibiting cytochrome P450 3A3; decreased erythromycin steady-state serum concentrations). Products include:
E.E.S. 450
EryPed 446
Pediazole Suspension 3050

Erythromycin Gluceptate (Erythromycin metabolite decreases theophylline clearance by inhibiting cytochrome P450 3A3; decreased erythromycin steady-state serum concentrations).
No products indexed under this heading.

Erythromycin Stearate (Erythromycin metabolite decreases theophylline clearance by inhibiting cytochrome P450 3A3; decreased erythromycin steady-state serum concentrations). Products include:
Erythrocin Stearate Filmtab Tablets 452

Ethinyl Estradiol (Estrogen-containing oral contraceptives decrease theophylline clearance in dose dependent fashion). Products include:
Alesse-21 Tablets 3468
Alesse-28 Tablets 3473
Brevicon 28-Day Tablets 3380
Cyclessa Tablets 2450
Desogen Tablets 2458
Estinyl Tablets 3112
Estrostep 2627
femhrt Tablets 2635
Levlen 962
Levlite 21 Tablets 962
Levlite 28 Tablets 962
Levora Tablets 3389
Loestrin 21 Tablets 2642
Loestrin Fe Tablets 2642
Lo/Ovral Tablets 3532
Lo/Ovral-28 Tablets 3538
Low-Ogestrel-28 Tablets 3392
Microgestin Fe 1.5/30 Tablets 3407
Microgestin Fe 1/20 Tablets 3400
Mircette Tablets 2470
Modicon 2563
Necon 3415
Nordette-28 Tablets 2257
Norinyl 1 +35 28-Day Tablets 3380
Ogestrel 0.5/50-28 Tablets 3428
Ortho-Cept 21 Tablets 2546
Ortho-Cept 28 Tablets 2546
Ortho-Cyclen/Ortho Tri-Cyclen 2573
Ortho-Novum 2563
Ovcon 3364
Ovral Tablets 3551
Ovral-28 Tablets 3552
Tri-Levlen 962
Tri-Norinyl-28 Tablets 3433
Triphasil-21 Tablets 3600
Triphasil-28 Tablets 3605
Trivora Tablets 3439
Yasmin 28 Tablets 980
Zovia 3449

Flurazepam Hydrochloride (Benzodiazepines increase CNS concentrations of adenosine, a potent CNS depressant, while theophylline blocks adenosine receptors; larger flurazepam doses may be required to produce desired level of sedation; discontinuation of theophylline without reduction of flurazepam dose may result in respiratory depression).
No products indexed under this heading.

Fluvoxamine Maleate (Decreases theophylline clearance by inhibiting cytochrome P450 1A2). Products include:
Luvox Tablets (25, 50, 100 mg) 3256

Fosphenytoin Sodium (Increases theophylline clearance by increasing microsomal enzyme activity; theophylline decreases phenytoin absorption; these interactions result in decreased serum theophylline and phenytoin concentrations by about 40%). Products include:
Cerebyx Injection 2619

Halothane (Halothane sensitizes the myocardium to catecholamines; theophylline increases release of endogenous catecholamines resulting in increased risk of ventricular arrhythmias). Products include:
Fluothane Inhalation 3508

Interferon alfa-2A, Recombinant (Decreases theophylline clearance). Products include:
Roferon-A Injection 2996

Isoproterenol Hydrochloride (Co-administration with intravenous isoproterenol decreases theophylline clearance).
No products indexed under this heading.

Ketamine Hydrochloride (May lower theophylline seizure threshold).
No products indexed under this heading.

Lithium Carbonate (Theophylline increases renal lithium clearance; increase in lithium dose may be required to achieve a therapeutic serum concentration). Products include:
Eskalith 1527
Lithium Carbonate 3061
Lithobid Slow-Release Tablets 3255

Lithium Citrate (Theophylline increases renal lithium clearance; increase in lithium dose may be required to achieve a therapeutic serum concentration). Products include:
Lithium Citrate Syrup 3061

Lomefloxacin Hydrochloride (Co-administration with some quinolones has increased the plasma levels of theophylline by affecting the rate of theophylline clearance).
No products indexed under this heading.

Lorazepam (Benzodiazepines increase CNS concentrations of adenosine, a potent CNS depressant, while theophylline blocks adenosine receptors; larger lorazepam doses may be required to produce desired level of sedation; discontinuation of theophylline without reduction of lorazepam dose may result in respiratory depression). Products include:
Ativan Injection 3478
Ativan Tablets 3482

Mestranol (Estrogen-containing oral contraceptives decrease theophylline clearance in dose dependent fashion). Products include:
Necon 1/50 Tablets 3415
Norinyl 1 + 50 28-Day Tablets 3380
Ortho-Novum 1/50□28 Tablets 2556

Methotrexate Sodium (Decreases theophylline clearance).
No products indexed under this heading.

Mexiletine Hydrochloride (Decreases theophylline clearance by inhibiting hydroxylation and demethylation). Products include:
Mexitil Capsules 1047

Midazolam Hydrochloride (Benzodiazepines increase CNS concentrations of adenosine, a potent CNS depressant, while theophylline blocks adenosine receptors; larger midazolam doses may be required to produce desired level of sedation; discontinuation of theophylline without reduction of midazolam dose may result in respiratory depression). Products include:
Versed Injection 3027
Versed Syrup 3033

Moricizine Hydrochloride (Increases theophylline clearance).
No products indexed under this heading.

Norfloxacin (Co-administration with some quinolones has increased the plasma levels of theophylline by affecting the rate of theophylline clearance). Products include:
Chibroxin Sterile Ophthalmic Solution 2051
Noroxin Tablets 2145

Ofloxacin (Co-administration with some quinolones has increased the plasma levels of theophylline by affecting the rate of theophylline clearance). Products include:
Floxin I.V. 2526
Floxin Otic Solution 1219
Floxin Tablets 2529
Ocuflox Ophthalmic Solution 554

Pancuronium Bromide (Theophylline may antagonize non-depolarizing neuromuscular blocking effects; possibly due to phosphodiesterase inhibition; larger pancuronium doses may be required to achieve neuromuscular blockade).
No products indexed under this heading.

Pentoxifylline (Decreases theophylline clearance). Products include:
Trental Tablets 784

Phenobarbital (Increases theophylline clearance by induction of microsomal enzyme). Products include:
Arco-Lase Plus Tablets 592
Donnatal 2929
Donnatal Extentabs 2930

Phenytoin (Increases theophylline clearance by increasing microsomal enzyme activity; theophylline decreases phenytoin absorption; these interactions result in decreased serum theophylline and phenytoin concentrations by about 40%). Products include:
Dilantin Infatabs 2624
Dilantin-125 Oral Suspension 2625

Phenytoin Sodium (Increases theophylline clearance by increasing microsomal enzyme activity; theophylline decreases phenytoin absorption; these interactions result in decreased serum theophylline and phenytoin concentrations by about 40%). Products include:
Dilantin Kapseals 2622

Propafenone Hydrochloride (Decreases theophylline clearance). Products include:
Rythmol Tablets – 150 mg, 225 mg, 300 mg 502

Propranolol Hydrochloride (Decreases theophylline clearance by inhibiting cytochrome P450 1A2). Products include:
Inderal 3513
Inderal LA Long-Acting Capsules 3516
Inderide Tablets 3517
Inderide LA Long-Acting Capsules 3519

Rifampin (Increases theophylline clearance by increasing cytochrome P450 1A2 and 3A3 activity). Products include:
Rifadin 765
Rifamate Capsules 767
Rifater Tablets 769

Ritonavir (Increases theophylline clearance resulting in 43% decrease in AUC). Products include:
Kaletra Capsules 471
Kaletra Oral Solution 471
Norvir Capsules 487
Norvir Oral Solution 487

Sucralfate (Reduces absorption of theophylline). Products include:
Carafate Suspension 731
Carafate Tablets 730

Sulfinpyrazone (Increases theophylline clearance by increasing demethylation and hydoxylation; decreases renal clearance of theophylline).
No products indexed under this heading.

Tacrine Hydrochloride (Decreases theophylline clearance by inhibiting cytochrome P450 1A2 and also increases renal clearance of theophylline). Products include:
Cognex Capsules 1351

Thiabendazole (Decreases theophylline clearance). Products include:
Mintezol 2137

Ticlopidine Hydrochloride (Decreases theophylline clearance). Products include:
Ticlid Tablets 3015

Troleandomycin (Decreases theophylline clearance by inhibiting cytochrome P450 3A3). Products include:
Tao Capsules 2716

Verapamil Hydrochloride (Decreases theophylline clearance by inhibiting hydroxylation and demethylation). Products include:
Covera-HS Tablets 3199
Isoptin SR Tablets 467
Tarka Tablets 508
Verelan Capsules 3184
Verelan PM Capsules 3186

IMPORTANT NOTE: Always consult each drug listing in the patient's regimen for possible interactions.

Food Interactions

Alcohol (Concurrent use with a single dose of alcohol (3mL/kg of whiskey) decreases theophylline clearance for up to 24 hours).

Food, unspecified (Available data suggests that co-administration with food may influence the absorption characteristics of controlled-release theophylline formulations).

THERACYS INJECTION

(BCG, Live (Intravesical)) 823

May interact with immunosuppressive agents and certain other agents. Compounds in these categories include:

Azathioprine (May impair the response to TheraCys or increase the risk of osteomyelitis or disseminated BCG infection).
No products indexed under this heading.

Basiliximab (May impair the response to TheraCys or increase the risk of osteomyelitis or disseminated BCG infection). Products include:
Simulect for Injection 2399

Cyclosporine (May impair the response to TheraCys or increase the risk of osteomyelitis or disseminated BCG infection). Products include:
Gengraf Capsules 457
Neoral Soft Gelatin Capsules 2380
Neoral Oral Solution 2380
Sandimmune 2388

Muromonab-CD3 (May impair the response to TheraCys or increase the risk of osteomyelitis or disseminated BCG infection). Products include:
Orthoclone OKT3 Sterile Solution ... 2498

Mycophenolate Mofetil (May impair the response to TheraCys or increase the risk of osteomyelitis or disseminated BCG infection). Products include:
CellCept Capsules 2951
CellCept Oral Suspension 2951
CellCept Tablets 2951

Sirolimus (May impair the response to TheraCys or increase the risk of osteomyelitis or disseminated BCG infection). Products include:
Rapamune Oral Solution and Tablets 3584

Tacrolimus (May impair the response to TheraCys or increase the risk of osteomyelitis or disseminated BCG infection). Products include:
Prograf 1393
Protopic Ointment 1397

THERAFLU REGULAR STRENGTH COLD & COUGH NIGHT TIME HOT LIQUID

(Acetaminophen, Chlorpheniramine Maleate, Dextromethorphan Hydrobromide, Pseudoephedrine Hydrochloride)..... ▣676

May interact with hypnotics and sedatives, monoamine oxidase inhibitors, tranquilizers, and certain other agents. Compounds in these categories include:

Alprazolam (May increase the drowsiness effect). Products include:
Xanax Tablets 2865

Buspirone Hydrochloride (May increase the drowsiness effect).
No products indexed under this heading.

Chlordiazepoxide (May increase the drowsiness effect). Products include:
Limbitrol 1738

Chlordiazepoxide Hydrochloride (May increase the drowsiness effect). Products include:
Librium Capsules 1736
Librium for Injection 1737

Chlorpromazine (May increase the drowsiness effect). Products include:
Thorazine Suppositories 1656

Chlorpromazine Hydrochloride (May increase the drowsiness effect). Products include:
Thorazine 1656

Chlorprothixene (May increase the drowsiness effect).
No products indexed under this heading.

Chlorprothixene Hydrochloride (May increase the drowsiness effect).
No products indexed under this heading.

Clorazepate Dipotassium (May increase the drowsiness effect). Products include:
Tranxene 511

Diazepam (May increase the drowsiness effect). Products include:
Valium Injectable 3026
Valium Tablets 3047

Droperidol (May increase the drowsiness effect).
No products indexed under this heading.

Estazolam (May increase the drowsiness effect). Products include:
ProSom Tablets 500

Ethchlorvynol (May increase the drowsiness effect).
No products indexed under this heading.

Ethinamate (May increase the drowsiness effect).
No products indexed under this heading.

Fluphenazine Decanoate (May increase the drowsiness effect).
No products indexed under this heading.

Fluphenazine Enanthate (May increase the drowsiness effect).
No products indexed under this heading.

Fluphenazine Hydrochloride (May increase the drowsiness effect).
No products indexed under this heading.

Flurazepam Hydrochloride (May increase the drowsiness effect).
No products indexed under this heading.

Glutethimide (May increase the drowsiness effect).
No products indexed under this heading.

Haloperidol (May increase the drowsiness effect). Products include:
Haldol Injection, Tablets and Concentrate 2533

Haloperidol Decanoate (May increase the drowsiness effect). Products include:
Haldol Decanoate 2535

Hydroxyzine Hydrochloride (May increase the drowsiness effect). Products include:
Atarax Tablets & Syrup 2667
Vistaril Intramuscular Solution 2738

Isocarboxazid (Concurrent and/or sequential use with MAO inhibitors is not recommended).
No products indexed under this heading.

Lorazepam (May increase the drowsiness effect). Products include:
Ativan Injection 3478
Ativan Tablets 3482

Loxapine Hydrochloride (May increase the drowsiness effect).
No products indexed under this heading.

Loxapine Succinate (May increase the drowsiness effect). Products include:
Loxitane Capsules 3398

Meprobamate (May increase the drowsiness effect). Products include:
Miltown Tablets 3349

Mesoridazine Besylate (May increase the drowsiness effect). Products include:
Serentil 1057

Midazolam Hydrochloride (May increase the drowsiness effect). Products include:
Versed Injection 3027
Versed Syrup 3033

Moclobemide (Concurrent and/or sequential use with MAO inhibitors is not recommended).
No products indexed under this heading.

Molindone Hydrochloride (May increase the drowsiness effect). Products include:
Moban 1320

Oxazepam (May increase the drowsiness effect).
No products indexed under this heading.

Pargyline Hydrochloride (Concurrent and/or sequential use with MAO inhibitors is not recommended).
No products indexed under this heading.

Perphenazine (May increase the drowsiness effect). Products include:
Etrafon 3115
Trilafon 3160

Phenelzine Sulfate (Concurrent and/or sequential use with MAO inhibitors is not recommended). Products include:
Nardil Tablets 2653

Prazepam (May increase the drowsiness effect).
No products indexed under this heading.

Procarbazine Hydrochloride (Concurrent and/or sequential use with MAO inhibitors is not recommended). Products include:
Matulane Capsules 3246

Prochlorperazine (May increase the drowsiness effect). Products include:
Compazine 1505

Promethazine Hydrochloride (May increase the drowsiness effect). Products include:
Mepergan Injection 3539
Phenergan Injection 3553
Phenergan 3556
Phenergan Syrup 3554
Phenergan with Codeine Syrup 3557
Phenergan with Dextromethorphan Syrup 3559
Phenergan VC Syrup 3560
Phenergan VC with Codeine Syrup .. 3561

Propofol (May increase the drowsiness effect). Products include:
Diprivan Injectable Emulsion 667

Quazepam (May increase the drowsiness effect).
No products indexed under this heading.

Secobarbital Sodium (May increase the drowsiness effect).
No products indexed under this heading.

Selegiline Hydrochloride (Concurrent and/or sequential use with MAO inhibitors is not recommended). Products include:
Eldepryl Capsules 3266

Temazepam (May increase the drowsiness effect).
No products indexed under this heading.

Thioridazine Hydrochloride (May increase the drowsiness effect). Products include:
Thioridazine Hydrochloride Tablets 2289

Thiothixene (May increase the drowsiness effect). Products include:
Navane Capsules 2701
Thiothixene Capsules 2290

Tranylcypromine Sulfate (Concurrent and/or sequential use with MAO inhibitors is not recommended). Products include:
Parnate Tablets 1607

Triazolam (May increase the drowsiness effect). Products include:
Halcion Tablets 2823

Trifluoperazine Hydrochloride (May increase the drowsiness effect). Products include:
Stelazine 1640

Zaleplon (May increase the drowsiness effect). Products include:
Sonata Capsules 3591

Zolpidem Tartrate (May increase the drowsiness effect). Products include:
Ambien Tablets 3191

Food Interactions

Alcohol (Chronic heavy alcohol users, 3 or more drinks per day, should consult their physicians for advice on when and how they should take pain relievers/fever reducers including acetaminophen; may increase the drowsiness effect).

THERAFLU REGULAR STRENGTH COLD & SORE THROAT NIGHT TIME HOT LIQUID

(Acetaminophen, Chlorpheniramine Maleate, Pseudoephedrine Hydrochloride)..... ▣676

See TheraFlu Regular Strength Cold & Cough Night Time Hot Liquid

THERAFLU MAXIMUM STRENGTH FLU & CONGESTION NON-DROWSY HOT LIQUID

(Acetaminophen, Dextromethorphan Hydrobromide, Guaifenesin, Pseudoephedrine Hydrochloride)..... ▣677

May interact with monoamine oxidase inhibitors and certain other agents. Compounds in these categories include:

Isocarboxazid (Concurrent and/or sequential use with MAO inhibitors is not recommended).
No products indexed under this heading.

Moclobemide (Concurrent and/or sequential use with MAO inhibitors is not recommended).
No products indexed under this heading.

Pargyline Hydrochloride (Concurrent and/or sequential use with MAO inhibitors is not recommended).
No products indexed under this heading.

Phenelzine Sulfate (Concurrent and/or sequential use with MAO inhibitors is not recommended). Products include:
Nardil Tablets 2653

Procarbazine Hydrochloride (Concurrent and/or sequential use with MAO inhibitors is not recommended). Products include:
Matulane Capsules 3246

Selegiline Hydrochloride (Concurrent and/or sequential use with MAO inhibitors is not recommended). Products include:
Eldepryl Capsules 3266

Tranylcypromine Sulfate (Concurrent and/or sequential use with MAO inhibitors is not recommended). Products include:
Parnate Tablets 1607

Food Interactions

Alcohol (Chronic heavy alcohol users, 3 or more drinks per day, should consult their physicians for advice on when and how they should take pain relievers/

fever reducers including acetaminophen).

THERAFLU MAXIMUM STRENGTH FLU & COUGH NIGHT TIME HOT LIQUID
(Acetaminophen, Chlorpheniramine Maleate, Dextromethorphan Hydrobromide, Pseudoephedrine Hydrochloride)..... 678
See TheraFlu Maximum Strength Flu & Sore Throat Night Time Hot Liquid

THERAFLU MAXIMUM STRENGTH FLU & SORE THROAT NIGHT TIME HOT LIQUID
(Acetaminophen, Chlorpheniramine Maleate, Pseudoephedrine Hydrochloride)..... 677
May interact with hypnotics and sedatives, monoamine oxidase inhibitors, tranquilizers, and certain other agents. Compounds in these categories include:

Alprazolam (May increase drowsiness effect). Products include:
Xanax Tablets 2865

Buspirone Hydrochloride (May increase drowsiness effect).
No products indexed under this heading.

Chlordiazepoxide (May increase drowsiness effect). Products include:
Limbitrol 1738

Chlordiazepoxide Hydrochloride (May increase drowsiness effect). Products include:
Librium Capsules 1736
Librium for Injection 1737

Chlorpromazine (May increase drowsiness effect). Products include:
Thorazine Suppositories 1656

Chlorpromazine Hydrochloride (May increase drowsiness effect). Products include:
Thorazine 1656

Chlorprothixene (May increase drowsiness effect).
No products indexed under this heading.

Chlorprothixene Hydrochloride (May increase drowsiness effect).
No products indexed under this heading.

Clorazepate Dipotassium (May increase drowsiness effect). Products include:
Tranxene 511

Diazepam (May increase drowsiness effect). Products include:
Valium Injectable 3026
Valium Tablets 3047

Droperidol (May increase drowsiness effect).
No products indexed under this heading.

Estazolam (May increase drowsiness effect). Products include:
ProSom Tablets 500

Ethchlorvynol (May increase drowsiness effect).
No products indexed under this heading.

Ethinamate (May increase drowsiness effect).
No products indexed under this heading.

Fluphenazine Decanoate (May increase drowsiness effect).
No products indexed under this heading.

Fluphenazine Enanthate (May increase drowsiness effect).
No products indexed under this heading.

Fluphenazine Hydrochloride (May increase drowsiness effect).
No products indexed under this heading.

Flurazepam Hydrochloride (May increase drowsiness effect).
No products indexed under this heading.

Glutethimide (May increase drowsiness effect).
No products indexed under this heading.

Haloperidol (May increase drowsiness effect). Products include:
Haldol Injection, Tablets and Concentrate 2533

Haloperidol Decanoate (May increase drowsiness effect). Products include:
Haldol Decanoate 2535

Hydroxyzine Hydrochloride (May increase drowsiness effect). Products include:
Atarax Tablets & Syrup 2667
Vistaril Intramuscular Solution 2738

Isocarboxazid (Concurrent and/or sequential use with MAO inhibitors is not recommended).
No products indexed under this heading.

Lorazepam (May increase drowsiness effect). Products include:
Ativan Injection 3478
Ativan Tablets 3482

Loxapine Hydrochloride (May increase drowsiness effect).
No products indexed under this heading.

Loxapine Succinate (May increase drowsiness effect). Products include:
Loxitane Capsules 3398

Meprobamate (May increase drowsiness effect). Products include:
Miltown Tablets 3349

Mesoridazine Besylate (May increase drowsiness effect). Products include:
Serentil 1057

Midazolam Hydrochloride (May increase drowsiness effect). Products include:
Versed Injection 3027
Versed Syrup 3033

Moclobemide (Concurrent and/or sequential use with MAO inhibitors is not recommended).
No products indexed under this heading.

Molindone Hydrochloride (May increase drowsiness effect). Products include:
Moban 1320

Oxazepam (May increase drowsiness effect).
No products indexed under this heading.

Pargyline Hydrochloride (Concurrent and/or sequential use with MAO inhibitors is not recommended).
No products indexed under this heading.

Perphenazine (May increase drowsiness effect). Products include:
Etrafon 3115
Trilafon 3160

Phenelzine Sulfate (Concurrent and/or sequential use with MAO inhibitors is not recommended). Products include:
Nardil Tablets 2653

Prazepam (May increase drowsiness effect).
No products indexed under this heading.

Procarbazine Hydrochloride (Concurrent and/or sequential use with MAO inhibitors is not recommended). Products include:
Matulane Capsules 3246

Prochlorperazine (May increase drowsiness effect). Products include:
Compazine 1505

Promethazine Hydrochloride (May increase drowsiness effect). Products include:
Mepergan Injection 3539
Phenergan Injection 3553
Phenergan 3556
Phenergan Syrup 3554
Phenergan with Codeine Syrup 3557
Phenergan with Dextromethorphan Syrup 3559
Phenergan VC Syrup 3560
Phenergan VC with Codeine Syrup .. 3561

Propofol (May increase drowsiness effect). Products include:
Diprivan Injectable Emulsion 667

Quazepam (May increase drowsiness effect).
No products indexed under this heading.

Secobarbital Sodium (May increase drowsiness effect).
No products indexed under this heading.

Selegiline Hydrochloride (Concurrent and/or sequential use with MAO inhibitors is not recommended). Products include:
Eldepryl Capsules 3266

Temazepam (May increase drowsiness effect).
No products indexed under this heading.

Thioridazine Hydrochloride (May increase drowsiness effect). Products include:
Thioridazine Hydrochloride Tablets 2289

Thiothixene (May increase drowsiness effect). Products include:
Navane Capsules 2701
Thiothixene Capsules 2290

Tranylcypromine Sulfate (Concurrent and/or sequential use with MAO inhibitors is not recommended). Products include:
Parnate Tablets 1607

Triazolam (May increase drowsiness effect). Products include:
Halcion Tablets 2823

Trifluoperazine Hydrochloride (May increase drowsiness effect). Products include:
Stelazine 1640

Zaleplon (May increase drowsiness effect). Products include:
Sonata Capsules 3591

Zolpidem Tartrate (May increase drowsiness effect). Products include:
Ambien Tablets 3191

Food Interactions

Alcohol (Chronic heavy alcohol users, 3 or more drinks per day, should consult their physicians for advice on when and how they should take pain relievers/fever reducers including acetaminophen; increases drowsiness effect).

THERAFLU MAXIMUM STRENGTH SEVERE COLD & CONGESTION NIGHT TIME CAPLETS
(Acetaminophen, Chlorpheniramine Maleate, Dextromethorphan Hydrobromide, Pseudoephedrine Hydrochloride)..... 678
See TheraFlu Maximum Strength Severe Cold & Congestion Night Time Hot Liquid

THERAFLU MAXIMUM STRENGTH SEVERE COLD & CONGESTION NIGHT TIME HOT LIQUID
(Acetaminophen, Chlorpheniramine Maleate, Dextromethorphan Hydrobromide, Pseudoephedrine Hydrochloride)..... 678
May interact with hypnotics and sedatives, monoamine oxidase inhibitors, tranquilizers, and certain other agents. Compounds in these categories include:

Alprazolam (May increase drowsiness effect). Products include:
Xanax Tablets 2865

Buspirone Hydrochloride (May increase drowsiness effect).
No products indexed under this heading.

Chlordiazepoxide (May increase drowsiness effect). Products include:
Limbitrol 1738

Chlordiazepoxide Hydrochloride (May increase drowsiness effect). Products include:
Librium Capsules 1736
Librium for Injection 1737

Chlorpromazine (May increase drowsiness effect). Products include:
Thorazine Suppositories 1656

Chlorpromazine Hydrochloride (May increase drowsiness effect). Products include:
Thorazine 1656

Chlorprothixene (May increase drowsiness effect).
No products indexed under this heading.

Chlorprothixene Hydrochloride (May increase drowsiness effect).
No products indexed under this heading.

Clorazepate Dipotassium (May increase drowsiness effect). Products include:
Tranxene 511

Diazepam (May increase drowsiness effect). Products include:
Valium Injectable 3026
Valium Tablets 3047

Droperidol (May increase drowsiness effect).
No products indexed under this heading.

Estazolam (May increase drowsiness effect). Products include:
ProSom Tablets 500

Ethchlorvynol (May increase drowsiness effect).
No products indexed under this heading.

Ethinamate (May increase drowsiness effect).
No products indexed under this heading.

Fluphenazine Decanoate (May increase drowsiness effect).
No products indexed under this heading.

Fluphenazine Enanthate (May increase drowsiness effect).
No products indexed under this heading.

Fluphenazine Hydrochloride (May increase drowsiness effect).
No products indexed under this heading.

Flurazepam Hydrochloride (May increase drowsiness effect).
No products indexed under this heading.

Glutethimide (May increase drowsiness effect).
No products indexed under this heading.

Haloperidol (May increase drowsiness effect). Products include:
Haldol Injection, Tablets and Concentrate 2533

Haloperidol Decanoate (May increase drowsiness effect). Products include:
Haldol Decanoate 2535

Hydroxyzine Hydrochloride (May increase drowsiness effect). Products include:
Atarax Tablets & Syrup 2667
Vistaril Intramuscular Solution 2738

Isocarboxazid (Concurrent and/or sequential use with MAO inhibitors is not recommended).
No products indexed under this heading.

Lorazepam (May increase drowsiness effect). Products include:
Ativan Injection 3478
Ativan Tablets 3482

Loxapine Hydrochloride (May increase drowsiness effect).
No products indexed under this heading.

Loxapine Succinate (May increase drowsiness effect). Products include:
Loxitane Capsules 3398

Meprobamate (May increase drowsiness effect). Products include:
Miltown Tablets 3349

Mesoridazine Besylate (May increase drowsiness effect). Products include:
Serentil 1057

Midazolam Hydrochloride (May increase drowsiness effect). Products include:
Versed Injection 3027
Versed Syrup 3033

Moclobemide (Concurrent and/or sequential use with MAO inhibitors is not recommended).
No products indexed under this heading.

Molindone Hydrochloride (May increase drowsiness effect). Products include:
Moban 1320

Oxazepam (May increase drowsiness effect).
No products indexed under this heading.

Pargyline Hydrochloride (Concurrent and/or sequential use with MAO inhibitors is not recommended).
No products indexed under this heading.

Perphenazine (May increase drowsiness effect). Products include:
Etrafon 3115
Trilafon 3160

Phenelzine Sulfate (Concurrent and/or sequential use with MAO inhibitors is not recommended). Products include:
Nardil Tablets 2653

Prazepam (May increase drowsiness effect).
No products indexed under this heading.

Procarbazine Hydrochloride (Concurrent and/or sequential use with MAO inhibitors is not recommended). Products include:
Matulane Capsules 3246

Prochlorperazine (May increase drowsiness effect). Products include:
Compazine 1505

Promethazine Hydrochloride (May increase drowsiness effect). Products include:
Mepergan Injection 3539
Phenergan Injection 3553
Phenergan 3556
Phenergan Syrup 3554
Phenergan with Codeine Syrup 3557
Phenergan with Dextromethorphan Syrup 3559
Phenergan VC Syrup 3560
Phenergan VC with Codeine Syrup .. 3561

Propofol (May increase drowsiness effect). Products include:
Diprivan Injectable Emulsion 667

Quazepam (May increase drowsiness effect).
No products indexed under this heading.

Secobarbital Sodium (May increase drowsiness effect).
No products indexed under this heading.

Selegiline Hydrochloride (Concurrent and/or sequential use with MAO inhibitors is not recommended). Products include:
Eldepryl Capsules 3266

Temazepam (May increase drowsiness effect).
No products indexed under this heading.

Thioridazine Hydrochloride (May increase drowsiness effect). Products include:
Thioridazine Hydrochloride Tablets 2289

Thiothixene (May increase drowsiness effect). Products include:
Navane Capsules 2701
Thiothixene Capsules 2290

Tranylcypromine Sulfate (Concurrent and/or sequential use with MAO inhibitors is not recommended). Products include:
Parnate Tablets 1607

Triazolam (May increase drowsiness effect). Products include:
Halcion Tablets 2823

Trifluoperazine Hydrochloride (May increase drowsiness effect). Products include:
Stelazine 1640

Zaleplon (May increase drowsiness effect). Products include:
Sonata Capsules 3591

Zolpidem Tartrate (May increase drowsiness effect). Products include:
Ambien Tablets 3191

Food Interactions

Alcohol (Chronic heavy alcohol users, 3 or more drinks per day, should consult their physicians for advice on when and how they should take pain relievers/fever reducers including acetaminophen; increases drowsiness effect).

THERAFLU MAXIMUM STRENGTH SEVERE COLD & CONGESTION NON-DROWSY CAPLETS

(Acetaminophen, Dextromethorphan Hydrobromide, Pseudoephedrine Hydrochloride)..... ▣679
See TheraFlu Maximum Strength Severe Cold & Congestion Non-Drowsy Hot Liquid

THERAFLU MAXIMUM STRENGTH SEVERE COLD & CONGESTION NON-DROWSY HOT LIQUID

(Acetaminophen, Dextromethorphan Hydrobromide, Pseudoephedrine Hydrochloride)..... ▣679
May interact with monoamine oxidase inhibitors. Compounds in these categories include:

Isocarboxazid (Concurrent and/or sequential use with MAO inhibitors is not recommended).
No products indexed under this heading.

Moclobemide (Concurrent and/or sequential use with MAO inhibitors is not recommended).
No products indexed under this heading

Pargyline Hydrochloride (Concurrent and/or sequential use with MAO inhibitors is not recommended).
No products indexed under this heading.

Phenelzine Sulfate (Concurrent and/or sequential use with MAO inhibitors is not recommended). Products include:
Nardil Tablets 2653

Procarbazine Hydrochloride (Concurrent and/or sequential use with MAO inhibitors is not recommended). Products include:
Matulane Capsules 3246

Selegiline Hydrochloride (Concurrent and/or sequential use with MAO inhibitors is not recommended). Products include:
Eldepryl Capsules 3266

Tranylcypromine Sulfate (Concurrent and/or sequential use with MAO inhibitors is not recommended). Products include:
Parnate Tablets 1607

Food Interactions

Alcohol (Chronic heavy alcohol users, 3 or more drinks per day, should consult their physicians for advice on when and how they should take pain relievers/fever reducers including acetaminophen).

THERA-GESIC CREME

(Menthol, Methyl Salicylate) 2233
None cited in PDR database.

THERMO-E CAPLETS

(Ephedra, Herbals with Vitamins & Minerals) .... ▣801
May interact with anorexiants, monoamine oxidase inhibitors, and certain other agents. Compounds in these categories include:

Amphetamine Resins (Concurrent use with prescription anoretics is not recommended).
No products indexed under this heading.

Benzphetamine Hydrochloride (Concurrent use with prescription anoretics is not recommended).
No products indexed under this heading.

Dextroamphetamine Sulfate (Concurrent use with prescription anoretics is not recommended). Products include:
Adderall Tablets 3231
Adderall XR Capsules ....
Dexedrine 1512
DextroStat Tablets 3236

Diethylpropion Hydrochloride (Concurrent use with prescription anoretics is not recommended).
No products indexed under this heading.

Fenfluramine Hydrochloride (Concurrent use with prescription anoretics is not recommended).
No products indexed under this heading.

Isocarboxazid (Thermo-E contains ephedra extract; concurrent and/or sequential use with MAO inhibitors is not recommended).
No products indexed under this heading.

Mazindol (Concurrent use with prescription anoretics is not recommended).
No products indexed under this heading.

Methamphetamine Hydrochloride (Concurrent use with prescription anoretics is not recommended). Products include:
Desoxyn Tablets 440

Moclobemide (Thermo-E contains ephedra extract; concurrent and/or sequential use with MAO inhibitors is not recommended).
No products indexed under this heading.

Pargyline Hydrochloride (Thermo-E contains ephedra extract; concurrent and/or sequential use with MAO inhibitors is not recommended).
No products indexed under this heading.

Phendimetrazine Tartrate (Concurrent use with prescription anoretics is not recommended). Products include:
Bontril Slow-Release Capsules 576

Phenelzine Sulfate (Thermo-E contains ephedra extract; concurrent and/or sequential use with MAO inhibitors is not recommended). Products include:
Nardil Tablets 2653

Phenmetrazine Hydrochloride (Concurrent use with prescription anoretics is not recommended).
No products indexed under this heading.

Phenylpropanolamine Hydrochloride (Thermo-E contains ephedra extract; concurrent use with phenylpropanolamine containing products is not recommended).
No products indexed under this heading.

Procarbazine Hydrochloride (Thermo-E contains ephedra extract; concurrent and/or sequential use with MAO inhibitors is not recommended). Products include:
Matulane Capsules 3246

Selegiline Hydrochloride (Thermo-E contains ephedra extract; concurrent and/or sequential use with MAO inhibitors is not recommended). Products include:
Eldepryl Capsules 3266

Sibutramine Hydrochloride Monohydrate (Concurrent use with prescription anoretics is not recommended). Products include:
Meridia Capsules 481

Tranylcypromine Sulfate (Thermo-E contains ephedra extract; concurrent and/or sequential use with MAO inhibitors is not recommended). Products include:
Parnate Tablets 1607

THIOPLEX FOR INJECTION

(Thiotepa) 1765
May interact with nitrogen-mustard-type alkylating agents and certain other agents. Compounds in these categories include:

Bone Marrow Depressants, unspecified (Avoid concurrent use).

Chlorambucil (Intensified toxicity). Products include:
Leukeran Tablets 1591

Cyclophosphamide (Intensified toxicity).
No products indexed under this heading.

Estramustine Phosphate Sodium (Intensified toxicity). Products include:
Emcyt Capsules 2810

Mechlorethamine Hydrochloride (Intensified toxicity). Products include:
Mustargen for Injection 2142

Melphalan (Intensified toxicity). Products include:
Alkeran Tablets 1466

Succinylcholine Chloride (Prolonged apnea after succinylcholine administration to patients receiving thiotepa and other cancer drugs). Products include:
Anectine Injection 1476

THIORIDAZINE HYDROCHLORIDE TABLETS

(Thioridazine Hydrochloride) 2289
May interact with:

Epinephrine (Thioridazine causes orthostatic hypotension, especially in female patients; use of epinephrine should be avoided in view of the fact that phenothiazines may induce a reversed epinephrine effect). Products include:
Epifrin Sterile Ophthalmic Solution .... ⊙235
EpiPen 1236
Primatene Mist .... ▣779
Xylocaine with Epinephrine Injection 653

Epinephrine Hydrochloride (Thioridazine causes orthostatic hypotension, especially in female patients; use of epinephrine should be avoided in view of the fact that phenothiazines may induce a reversed epinephrine effect).
No products indexed under this heading.

Propranolol Hydrochloride (Coadministration has resulted in increase in plasma levels of thiorida-

zine (approximately 50% to 400%) and its metabolites (approximately 80% to 300%)). Products include:

- Inderal 3513
- Inderal LA Long-Acting Capsules 3516
- Inderide Tablets 3517
- Inderide LA Long-Acting Capsules 3519

THIOTHIXENE CAPSULES

(Thiothixene) 2290

May interact with belladona products, central nervous system depressants, and certain other agents. Compounds in these categories include:

Alfentanil Hydrochloride (Possible additive effects which may include hypotension).
No products indexed under this heading.

Alprazolam (Possible additive effects which may include hypotension). Products include:
- Xanax Tablets 2865

Aprobarbital (Possible additive effects which may include hypotension).
No products indexed under this heading.

Atropine Sulfate (Thiothixene exhibits weak anticholinergic properties; concurrent use with atropine or related drugs requires caution). Products include:
- Donnatal 2929
- Donnatal Extentabs 2930
- Motofen Tablets 577
- Prosed/DS Tablets 3268
- Urised Tablets 2876

Belladonna Alkaloids (Thiothixene exhibits weak anticholinergic properties; concurrent use with atropine or related drugs requires caution). Products include:
- Hyland's Teething Tablets 766
- Urimax Tablets 1769

Buprenorphine Hydrochloride (Possible additive effects which may include hypotension). Products include:
- Buprenex Injectable 2918

Buspirone Hydrochloride (Possible additive effects which may include hypotension).
No products indexed under this heading.

Butabarbital (Possible additive effects which may include hypotension).
No products indexed under this heading.

Butalbital (Possible additive effects which may include hypotension). Products include:
- Phrenilin 578
- Sedapap Tablets 50 mg/650 mg 2225

Chlordiazepoxide (Possible additive effects which may include hypotension). Products include:
- Limbitrol 1738

Chlordiazepoxide Hydrochloride (Possible additive effects which may include hypotension). Products include:
- Librium Capsules 1736
- Librium for Injection 1737

Chlorpromazine (Possible additive effects which may include hypotension). Products include:
- Thorazine Suppositories 1656

Chlorpromazine Hydrochloride (Possible additive effects which may include hypotension). Products include:
- Thorazine 1656

Chlorprothixene (Possible additive effects which may include hypotension).
No products indexed under this heading.

Chlorprothixene Hydrochloride (Possible additive effects which may include hypotension).
No products indexed under this heading.

Chlorprothixene Lactate (Possible additive effects which may include hypotension).
No products indexed under this heading.

Clorazepate Dipotassium (Possible additive effects which may include hypotension). Products include:
- Tranxene 511

Clozapine (Possible additive effects which may include hypotension). Products include:
- Clozaril Tablets 2319

Codeine Phosphate (Possible additive effects which may include hypotension). Products include:
- Phenergan with Codeine Syrup 3557
- Phenergan VC with Codeine Syrup 3561
- Robitussin A-C Syrup 2942
- Robitussin-DAC Syrup 2942
- Ryna-C Liquid 768
- Soma Compound w/Codeine Tablets 3355
- Tussi-Organidin NR Liquid 3350
- Tussi-Organidin-S NR Liquid 3350
- Tylenol with Codeine 2595

Desflurane (Possible additive effects which may include hypotension). Products include:
- Suprane Liquid for Inhalation 874

Dezocine (Possible additive effects which may include hypotension).
No products indexed under this heading.

Diazepam (Possible additive effects which may include hypotension). Products include:
- Valium Injectable 3026
- Valium Tablets 3047

Droperidol (Possible additive effects which may include hypotension).
No products indexed under this heading.

Enflurane (Possible additive effects which may include hypotension).
No products indexed under this heading.

Estazolam (Possible additive effects which may include hypotension). Products include:
- ProSom Tablets 500

Ethchlorvynol (Possible additive effects which may include hypotension).
No products indexed under this heading.

Ethinamate (Possible additive effects which may include hypotension).
No products indexed under this heading.

Fentanyl (Possible additive effects which may include hypotension). Products include:
- Duragesic Transdermal System 1786

Fentanyl Citrate (Possible additive effects which may include hypotension). Products include:
- Actiq 1184

Fluphenazine Decanoate (Possible additive effects which may include hypotension).
No products indexed under this heading.

Fluphenazine Enanthate (Possible additive effects which may include hypotension).
No products indexed under this heading.

Fluphenazine Hydrochloride (Possible additive effects which may include hypotension).
No products indexed under this heading.

Flurazepam Hydrochloride (Possible additive effects which may include hypotension).
No products indexed under this heading.

Glutethimide (Possible additive effects which may include hypotension).
No products indexed under this heading.

Haloperidol (Possible additive effects which may include hypotension). Products include:
- Haldol Injection, Tablets and Concentrate 2533

Haloperidol Decanoate (Possible additive effects which may include hypotension). Products include:
- Haldol Decanoate 2535

Hydrocodone Bitartrate (Possible additive effects which may include hypotension). Products include:
- Hycodan 1316
- Hycomine Compound Tablets 1317
- Hycotuss Expectorant Syrup 1318
- Lortab 3319
- Lortab Elixir 3317
- Maxidone Tablets CIII 3399
- Norco 5/325 Tablets CIII 3424
- Norco 7.5/325 Tablets CIII 3425
- Norco 10/325 Tablets CIII 3427
- Norco 10/325 Tablets CIII 3425
- Vicodin Tablets 516
- Vicodin ES Tablets 517
- Vicodin HP Tablets 518
- Vicodin Tuss Expectorant 519
- Vicoprofen Tablets 520
- Zydone Tablets 1330

Hydrocodone Polistirex (Possible additive effects which may include hypotension). Products include:
- Tussionex Pennkinetic Extended-Release Suspension 1174

Hydromorphone Hydrochloride (Possible additive effects which may include hypotension). Products include:
- Dilaudid 441
- Dilaudid Oral Liquid 445
- Dilaudid Powder 441
- Dilaudid Rectal Suppositories 441
- Dilaudid Tablets 441
- Dilaudid Tablets - 8 mg 445
- Dilaudid-HP 443

Hydroxyzine Hydrochloride (Possible additive effects which may include hypotension). Products include:
- Atarax Tablets & Syrup 2667
- Vistaril Intramuscular Solution 2738

Hyoscyamine (Thiothixene exhibits weak anticholinergic properties; concurrent use with atropine or related drugs requires caution). Products include:
- Urised Tablets 2876

Hyoscyamine Sulfate (Thiothixene exhibits weak anticholinergic properties; concurrent use with atropine or related drugs requires caution). Products include:
- Arco-Lase Plus Tablets 592
- Donnatal 2929
- Donnatal Extentabs 2930
- Levsin/Levsinex/Levbid 3172
- NuLev Orally Disintegrating Tablets 3176
- Prosed/DS Tablets 3268
- Urimax Tablets 1769

Isoflurane (Possible additive effects which may include hypotension).
No products indexed under this heading.

Ketamine Hydrochloride (Possible additive effects which may include hypotension).
No products indexed under this heading.

Levomethadyl Acetate Hydrochloride (Possible additive effects which may include hypotension).
No products indexed under this heading.

Levorphanol Tartrate (Possible additive effects which may include hypotension). Products include:
- Levo-Dromoran 1734
- Levorphanol Tartrate Tablets 3059

Lorazepam (Possible additive effects which may include hypotension). Products include:
- Ativan Injection 3478
- Ativan Tablets 3482

Loxapine Hydrochloride (Possible additive effects which may include hypotension).
No products indexed under this heading.

Loxapine Succinate (Possible additive effects which may include hypotension). Products include:
- Loxitane Capsules 3398

Meperidine Hydrochloride (Possible additive effects which may include hypotension). Products include:
- Demerol 3079
- Mepergan Injection 3539

Mephobarbital (Possible additive effects which may include hypotension).
No products indexed under this heading.

Meprobamate (Possible additive effects which may include hypotension). Products include:
- Miltown Tablets 3349

Mesoridazine Besylate (Possible additive effects which may include hypotension). Products include:
- Serentil 1057

Methadone Hydrochloride (Possible additive effects which may include hypotension). Products include:
- Dolophine Hydrochloride Tablets 3056

Methohexital Sodium (Possible additive effects which may include hypotension). Products include:
- Brevital Sodium for Injection, USP 1815

Methotrimeprazine (Possible additive effects which may include hypotension).
No products indexed under this heading.

Methoxyflurane (Possible additive effects which may include hypotension).
No products indexed under this heading.

Midazolam Hydrochloride (Possible additive effects which may include hypotension). Products include:
- Versed Injection 3027
- Versed Syrup 3033

Molindone Hydrochloride (Possible additive effects which may include hypotension). Products include:
- Moban 1320

Morphine Sulfate (Possible additive effects which may include hypotension). Products include:
- Astramorph/PF Injection, USP (Preservative-Free) 594
- Duramorph Injection 1312
- Infumorph 200 and Infumorph 500 Sterile Solutions 1314
- Kadian Capsules 1335
- MS Contin Tablets 2896
- MSIR 2898
- Oramorph SR Tablets 3062
- Roxanol 3066

Olanzapine (Possible additive effects which may include hypotension). Products include:
- Zyprexa Tablets 1973
- Zyprexa ZYDIS Orally Disintegrating Tablets 1973

Oxazepam (Possible additive effects which may include hypotension).
No products indexed under this heading.

Oxycodone Hydrochloride (Possible additive effects which may include hypotension). Products include:
- OxyContin Tablets 2912
- OxyFast Oral Concentrate Solution 2916
- OxyIR Capsules 2916
- Percocet Tablets 1326
- Percodan Tablets 1327
- Percolone Tablets 1327
- Roxicodone 3067
- Tylox Capsules 2597

Pentobarbital Sodium (Possible additive effects which may include hypotension). Products include:
Nembutal Sodium Solution 485

Perphenazine (Possible additive effects which may include hypotension). Products include:
Etrafon 3115
Trilafon 3160

Phenobarbital (Possible additive effects which may include hypotension). Products include:
Arco-Lase Plus Tablets 592
Donnatal 2929
Donnatal Extentabs 2930

Prazepam (Possible additive effects which may include hypotension).
No products indexed under this heading.

Prochlorperazine (Possible additive effects which may include hypotension). Products include:
Compazine 1505

Promethazine Hydrochloride (Possible additive effects which may include hypotension). Products include:
Mepergan Injection 3539
Phenergan Injection 3553
Phenergan 3556
Phenergan Syrup 3554
Phenergan with Codeine Syrup 3557
Phenergan with Dextromethorphan Syrup 3559
Phenergan VC Syrup 3560
Phenergan VC with Codeine Syrup 3561

Propofol (Possible additive effects which may include hypotension). Products include:
Diprivan Injectable Emulsion 667

Propoxyphene Hydrochloride (Possible additive effects which may include hypotension). Products include:
Darvon Pulvules 1909
Darvon Compound-65 Pulvules 1910

Propoxyphene Napsylate (Possible additive effects which may include hypotension). Products include:
Darvon-N/Darvocet-N 1907
Darvon-N Tablets 1912

Quazepam (Possible additive effects which may include hypotension).
No products indexed under this heading.

Quetiapine Fumarate (Possible additive effects which may include hypotension). Products include:
Seroquel Tablets 684

Remifentanil Hydrochloride (Possible additive effects which may include hypotension).
No products indexed under this heading.

Risperidone (Possible additive effects which may include hypotension). Products include:
Risperdal 1796

Scopolamine (Thiothixene exhibits weak anticholinergic properties; concurrent use with atropine or related drugs requires caution). Products include:
Transderm Scōp Transdermal Therapeutic System 2302

Scopolamine Hydrobromide (Thiothixene exhibits weak anticholinergic properties; concurrent use with atropine or related drugs requires caution). Products include:
Donnatal 2929
Donnatal Extentabs 2930

Secobarbital Sodium (Possible additive effects which may include hypotension).
No products indexed under this heading.

Sevoflurane (Possible additive effects which may include hypotension).
No products indexed under this heading.

Sufentanil Citrate (Possible additive effects which may include hypotension).
No products indexed under this heading.

Temazepam (Possible additive effects which may include hypotension).
No products indexed under this heading.

Thiamylal Sodium (Possible additive effects which may include hypotension).
No products indexed under this heading.

Thioridazine Hydrochloride (Possible additive effects which may include hypotension). Products include:
Thioridazine Hydrochloride Tablets 2289

Triazolam (Possible additive effects which may include hypotension). Products include:
Halcion Tablets 2823

Trifluoperazine Hydrochloride (Possible additive effects which may include hypotension). Products include:
Stelazine 1640

Zaleplon (Possible additive effects which may include hypotension). Products include:
Sonata Capsules 3591

Ziprasidone Hydrochloride (Possible additive effects which may include hypotension). Products include:
Geodon Capsules 2688

Zolpidem Tartrate (Possible additive effects which may include hypotension). Products include:
Ambien Tablets 3191

Food Interactions

Alcohol (Possible additive effects which may include hypotension).

THORAZINE AMPULS
(Chlorpromazine Hydrochloride) 1656
See Thorazine Tablets

THORAZINE MULTI-DOSE VIALS
(Chlorpromazine Hydrochloride) 1656
See Thorazine Tablets

THORAZINE SPANSULE CAPSULES
(Chlorpromazine Hydrochloride) 1656
See Thorazine Tablets

THORAZINE SUPPOSITORIES
(Chlorpromazine) 1656
See Thorazine Tablets

THORAZINE SYRUP
(Chlorpromazine Hydrochloride) 1656
See Thorazine Tablets

THORAZINE TABLETS
(Chlorpromazine Hydrochloride) 1656
May interact with:

Alfentanil Hydrochloride (Prolonged and intensified action of CNS depressants).
No products indexed under this heading.

Alprazolam (Prolonged and intensified action of CNS depressants). Products include:
Xanax Tablets 2865

Aprobarbital (Prolonged and intensified action of CNS depressants).
No products indexed under this heading.

Atropine Sulfate (Use with caution). Products include:
Donnatal 2929
Donnatal Extentabs 2930
Motofen Tablets 577
Prosed/DS Tablets 3268
Urised Tablets 2876

Bendroflumethiazide (Orthostatic hypotension that may occur with chlorpromazine may be accentuated). Products include:
Corzide 40/5 Tablets 2247
Corzide 80/5 Tablets 2247

Buprenorphine Hydrochloride (Prolonged and intensified action of CNS depressants). Products include:
Buprenex Injectable 2918

Buspirone Hydrochloride (Prolonged and intensified action of CNS depressants).
No products indexed under this heading.

Butabarbital (Prolonged and intensified action of CNS depressants).
No products indexed under this heading.

Butalbital (Prolonged and intensified action of CNS depressants). Products include:
Phrenilin 578
Sedapap Tablets 50 mg/650 mg 2225

Carbamazepine (Chlorpromazine may lower convulsive threshold; dosage adjustments of anticonvulsants may be necessary). Products include:
Carbatrol Capsules 3234
Tegretol/Tegretol-XR 2404

Carmustine (BCNU) (Antiemetic action of chlorpromazine may obscure vomiting as a sign of toxicity). Products include:
Gliadel Wafer 1723

Chlordiazepoxide (Prolonged and intensified action of CNS depressants). Products include:
Limbitrol 1738

Chlordiazepoxide Hydrochloride (Prolonged and intensified action of CNS depressants). Products include:
Librium Capsules 1736
Librium for Injection 1737

Chlorothiazide (Orthostatic hypotension that may occur with chlorpromazine may be accentuated). Products include:
Aldoclor Tablets 2035
Diuril Oral 2087

Chlorothiazide Sodium (Orthostatic hypotension that may occur with chlorpromazine may be accentuated). Products include:
Diuril Sodium Intravenous 2086

Chlorprothixene (Prolonged and intensified action of CNS depressants).
No products indexed under this heading.

Chlorprothixene Hydrochloride (Prolonged and intensified action of CNS depressants).
No products indexed under this heading.

Chlorprothixene Lactate (Prolonged and intensified action of CNS depressants).
No products indexed under this heading.

Clorazepate Dipotassium (Prolonged and intensified action of CNS depressants). Products include:
Tranxene 511

Clozapine (Prolonged and intensified action of CNS depressants). Products include:
Clozaril Tablets 2319

Codeine Phosphate (Prolonged and intensified action of CNS depressants). Products include:
Phenergan with Codeine Syrup 3557
Phenergan VC with Codeine Syrup 3561
Robitussin A-C Syrup 2942
Robitussin-DAC Syrup 2942
Ryna-C Liquid .... ■ 768
Soma Compound w/Codeine Tablets 3355
Tussi-Organidin NR Liquid 3350
Tussi-Organidin-S NR Liquid 3350
Tylenol with Codeine 2595

Desflurane (Prolonged and intensified action of CNS depressants). Products include:
Suprane Liquid for Inhalation 874

Dezocine (Prolonged and intensified action of CNS depressants).
No products indexed under this heading.

Diazepam (Prolonged and intensified action of CNS depressants). Products include:
Valium Injectable 3026
Valium Tablets 3047

Dicumarol (Chlorpromazine diminishes the effects of oral anticoagulants).
No products indexed under this heading.

Divalproex Sodium (Chlorpromazine may lower convulsive threshold; dosage adjustments of anticonvulsants may be necessary). Products include:
Depakote Sprinkle Capsules 426
Depakote Tablets 430
Depakote ER Tablets 436

Droperidol (Prolonged and intensified action of CNS depressants).
No products indexed under this heading.

Enflurane (Prolonged and intensified action of CNS depressants).
No products indexed under this heading.

Estazolam (Prolonged and intensified action of CNS depressants). Products include:
ProSom Tablets 500

Estramustine Phosphate Sodium (Antiemetic action of chlorpromazine may obscure vomiting as a sign of toxicity). Products include:
Emcyt Capsules 2810

Ethchlorvynol (Prolonged and intensified action of CNS depressants).
No products indexed under this heading.

Ethinamate (Prolonged and intensified action of CNS depressants).
No products indexed under this heading.

Ethosuximide (Chlorpromazine may lower convulsive threshold; dosage adjustments of anticonvulsants may be necessary). Products include:
Zarontin Capsules 2659
Zarontin Syrup 2660

Ethotoin (Chlorpromazine may lower convulsive threshold; dosage adjustments of anticonvulsants may be necessary).
No products indexed under this heading.

Felbamate (Chlorpromazine may lower convulsive threshold; dosage adjustments of anticonvulsants may be necessary). Products include:
Felbatol 3343

Fentanyl (Prolonged and intensified action of CNS depressants). Products include:
Duragesic Transdermal System 1786

Fentanyl Citrate (Prolonged and intensified action of CNS depressants). Products include:
Actiq 1184

Fluphenazine Decanoate (Prolonged and intensified action of CNS depressants).
No products indexed under this heading.

Fluphenazine Enanthate (Prolonged and intensified action of CNS depressants).
No products indexed under this heading.

Fluphenazine Hydrochloride (Prolonged and intensified action of

CNS depressants).
No products indexed under this heading.

Flurazepam Hydrochloride (Prolonged and intensified action of CNS depressants).
No products indexed under this heading.

Fosphenytoin Sodium (Chlorpromazine may lower convulsive threshold; dosage adjustments of anticonvulsants may be necessary). Products include:
Cerebyx Injection 2619

Glutethimide (Prolonged and intensified action of CNS depressants).
No products indexed under this heading.

Guanethidine Monosulfate (Antihypertensive effect of guanethidine and related compounds may be counteracted).
No products indexed under this heading.

Haloperidol (Prolonged and intensified action of CNS depressants). Products include:
Haldol Injection, Tablets and Concentrate 2533

Haloperidol Decanoate (Prolonged and intensified action of CNS depressants). Products include:
Haldol Decanoate 2535

Hydrochlorothiazide (Orthostatic hypotension that may occur with chlorpromazine may be accentuated). Products include:
Accuretic Tablets 2614
Aldoril Tablets 2039
Atacand HCT Tablets 597
Avalide Tablets 1070
Diovan HCT Tablets 2338
Dyazide Capsules 1515
HydroDIURIL Tablets 2108
Hyzaar 2109
Inderide Tablets 3517
Inderide LA Long-Acting Capsules .. 3519
Lotensin HCT Tablets 2367
Maxzide 1008
Micardis HCT Tablets 1051
Microzide Capsules 3414
Moduretic Tablets 2138
Monopril HCT 1094
Prinzide Tablets 2168
Timolide Tablets 2187
Uniretic Tablets 3178
Vaseretic Tablets 2204
Zestoretic Tablets 695
Ziac Tablets 1887

Hydrocodone Bitartrate (Prolonged and intensified action of CNS depressants). Products include:
Hycodan 1316
Hycomine Compound Tablets 1317
Hycotuss Expectorant Syrup 1318
Lortab 3319
Lortab Elixir 3317
Maxidone Tablets CIII 3399
Norco 5/325 Tablets CIII 3424
Norco 7.5/325 Tablets CIII 3425
Norco 10/325 Tablets CIII 3427
Norco 10/325 Tablets CIII 3425
Vicodin Tablets 516
Vicodin ES Tablets 517
Vicodin HP Tablets 518
Vicodin Tuss Expectorant 519
Vicoprofen Tablets 520
Zydone Tablets 1330

Hydrocodone Polistirex (Prolonged and intensified action of CNS depressants). Products include:
Tussionex Pennkinetic Extended-Release Suspension 1174

Hydroflumethiazide (Orthostatic hypotension that may occur with chlorpromazine may be accentuated). Products include:
Diucardin Tablets 3494

Hydromorphone Hydrochloride (Prolonged and intensified action of CNS depressants). Products include:
Dilaudid 441
Dilaudid Oral Liquid 445
Dilaudid Powder 441
Dilaudid Rectal Suppositories 441
Dilaudid Tablets 441
Dilaudid Tablets - 8 mg 445
Dilaudid-HP 443

Hydroxyurea (Antiemetic action of chlorpromazine may obscure vomiting as a sign of toxicity). Products include:
Mylocel Tablets 2227

Hydroxyzine Hydrochloride (Prolonged and intensified action of CNS depressants). Products include:
Atarax Tablets & Syrup 2667
Vistaril Intramuscular Solution 2738

Isoflurane (Prolonged and intensified action of CNS depressants).
No products indexed under this heading.

Ketamine Hydrochloride (Prolonged and intensified action of CNS depressants).
No products indexed under this heading.

Lamotrigine (Chlorpromazine may lower convulsive threshold; dosage adjustments of anticonvulsants may be necessary). Products include:
Lamictal 1567

Levetiracetam (Chlorpromazine may lower convulsive threshold; dosage adjustments of anticonvulsants may be necessary). Products include:
Keppra Tablets 3314

Levomethadyl Acetate Hydrochloride (Prolonged and intensified action of CNS depressants).
No products indexed under this heading.

Levorphanol Tartrate (Prolonged and intensified action of CNS depressants). Products include:
Levo-Dromoran 1734
Levorphanol Tartrate Tablets 3059

Lorazepam (Prolonged and intensified action of CNS depressants). Products include:
Ativan Injection 3478
Ativan Tablets 3482

Loxapine Hydrochloride (Prolonged and intensified action of CNS depressants).
No products indexed under this heading.

Loxapine Succinate (Prolonged and intensified action of CNS depressants). Products include:
Loxitane Capsules 3398

Mechlorethamine Hydrochloride (Antiemetic action of chlorpromazine may obscure vomiting as a sign of toxicity). Products include:
Mustargen for Injection 2142

Melphalan (Antiemetic action of chlorpromazine may obscure vomiting as a sign of toxicity). Products include:
Alkeran Tablets 1466

Meperidine Hydrochloride (Prolonged and intensified action of CNS depressants). Products include:
Demerol 3079
Mepergan Injection 3539

Mephenytoin (Chlorpromazine may lower convulsive threshold; dosage adjustments of anticonvulsants may be necessary).
No products indexed under this heading.

Mephobarbital (Prolonged and intensified action of CNS depressants).
No products indexed under this heading.

Meprobamate (Prolonged and intensified action of CNS depressants). Products include:
Miltown Tablets 3349

Mesoridazine Besylate (Prolonged and intensified action of CNS depressants). Products include:
Serentil 1057

Methadone Hydrochloride (Prolonged and intensified action of CNS depressants). Products include:
Dolophine Hydrochloride Tablets 3056

Methohexital Sodium (Prolonged and intensified action of CNS depressants). Products include:
Brevital Sodium for Injection, USP .. 1815

Methotrimeprazine (Prolonged and intensified action of CNS depressants).
No products indexed under this heading.

Methoxyflurane (Prolonged and intensified action of CNS depressants).
No products indexed under this heading.

Methsuximide (Chlorpromazine may lower convulsive threshold; dosage adjustments of anticonvulsants may be necessary). Products include:
Celontin Capsules 2618

Methyclothiazide (Orthostatic hypotension that may occur with chlorpromazine may be accentuated).
No products indexed under this heading.

Metrizamide (Chlorpromazine may lower convulsive threshold; avoid concurrent use).
No products indexed under this heading.

Midazolam Hydrochloride (Prolonged and intensified action of CNS depressants). Products include:
Versed Injection 3027
Versed Syrup 3033

Molindone Hydrochloride (Prolonged and intensified action of CNS depressants). Products include:
Moban 1320

Morphine Sulfate (Prolonged and intensified action of CNS depressants). Products include:
Astramorph/PF Injection, USP (Preservative-Free) 594
Duramorph Injection 1312
Infumorph 200 and Infumorph 500 Sterile Solutions 1314
Kadian Capsules 1335
MS Contin Tablets 2896
MSIR 2898
Oramorph SR Tablets 3062
Roxanol 3066

Olanzapine (Prolonged and intensified action of CNS depressants). Products include:
Zyprexa Tablets 1973
Zyprexa ZYDIS Orally Disintegrating Tablets 1973

Oxazepam (Prolonged and intensified action of CNS depressants).
No products indexed under this heading.

Oxcarbazepine (Chlorpromazine may lower convulsive threshold; dosage adjustments of anticonvulsants may be necessary). Products include:
Trileptal Oral Suspension 2407
Trileptal Tablets 2407

Oxycodone Hydrochloride (Prolonged and intensified action of CNS depressants). Products include:
OxyContin Tablets 2912
OxyFast Oral Concentrate Solution . 2916
OxyIR Capsules 2916
Percocet Tablets 1326
Percodan Tablets 1327
Percolone Tablets 1327
Roxicodone 3067
Tylox Capsules 2597

Paramethadione (Chlorpromazine may lower convulsive threshold; dosage adjustments of anticonvulsants may be necessary).
No products indexed under this heading.

Pentobarbital Sodium (Prolonged and intensified action of CNS depressants). Products include:
Nembutal Sodium Solution 485

Perphenazine (Prolonged and intensified action of CNS depressants). Products include:
Etrafon 3115
Trilafon 3160

Phenacemide (Chlorpromazine may lower convulsive threshold; dosage adjustments of anticonvulsants may be necessary).
No products indexed under this heading.

Phenobarbital (Chlorpromazine may lower convulsive threshold and does not potentiate anti-convulsant action of barbiturates). Products include:
Arco-Lase Plus Tablets 592
Donnatal 2929
Donnatal Extentabs 2930

Phensuximide (Chlorpromazine may lower convulsive threshold; dosage adjustments of anticonvulsants may be necessary).
No products indexed under this heading.

Phenytoin (Chlorpromazine may interfere with the metabolism of phenytoin and thus precipitate phenytoin toxicity). Products include:
Dilantin Infatabs 2624
Dilantin-125 Oral Suspension 2625

Phenytoin Sodium (Chlorpromazine may interfere with the metabolism of phenytoin and thus precipitate phenytoin toxicity). Products include:
Dilantin Kapseals 2622

Polythiazide (Orthostatic hypotension that may occur with chlorpromazine may be accentuated). Products include:
Minizide Capsules 2700
Renese Tablets 2712

Prazepam (Prolonged and intensified action of CNS depressants).
No products indexed under this heading.

Primidone (Chlorpromazine may lower convulsive threshold; dosage adjustments of anticonvulsants may be necessary).
No products indexed under this heading.

Prochlorperazine (Prolonged and intensified action of CNS depressants). Products include:
Compazine 1505

Promethazine Hydrochloride (Prolonged and intensified action of CNS depressants). Products include:
Mepergan Injection 3539
Phenergan Injection 3553
Phenergan 3556
Phenergan Syrup 3554
Phenergan with Codeine Syrup 3557
Phenergan with Dextromethorphan Syrup 3559
Phenergan VC Syrup 3560
Phenergan VC with Codeine Syrup . 3561

Propofol (Prolonged and intensified action of CNS depressants). Products include:
Diprivan Injectable Emulsion 667

Propoxyphene Hydrochloride (Prolonged and intensified action of CNS depressants). Products include:
Darvon Pulvules 1909
Darvon Compound-65 Pulvules 1910

Propoxyphene Napsylate (Prolonged and intensified action of CNS depressants). Products include:
Darvon-N/Darvocet-N 1907
Darvon-N Tablets 1912

Propranolol Hydrochloride (Concomitant administration results in increased plasma levels of both drugs). Products include:
Inderal 3513
Inderal LA Long-Acting Capsules 3516
Inderide Tablets 3517
Inderide LA Long-Acting Capsules .. 3519

Quazepam (Prolonged and intensified action of CNS depressants).
No products indexed under this heading.

Quetiapine Fumarate (Prolonged and intensified action of CNS depressants). Products include:
Seroquel Tablets 684

Remifentanil Hydrochloride (Prolonged and intensified action of CNS depressants).
No products indexed under this heading.

Risperidone (Prolonged and intensified action of CNS depressants). Products include:
Risperdal **1796**

Secobarbital Sodium (Prolonged and intensified action of CNS depressants).
No products indexed under this heading.

Sevoflurane (Prolonged and intensified action of CNS depressants).
No products indexed under this heading.

Sufentanil Citrate (Prolonged and intensified action of CNS depressants).
No products indexed under this heading.

Temazepam (Prolonged and intensified action of CNS depressants).
No products indexed under this heading.

Thiamylal Sodium (Prolonged and intensified action of CNS depressants).
No products indexed under this heading.

Thioridazine Hydrochloride (Prolonged and intensified action of CNS depressants). Products include:
Thioridazine Hydrochloride Tablets **2289**

Thiothixene (Prolonged and intensified action of CNS depressants). Products include:
Navane Capsules **2701**
Thiothixene Capsules **2290**

Tiagabine Hydrochloride (Chlorpromazine may lower convulsive threshold; dosage adjustments of anticonvulsants may be necessary). Products include:
Gabitril Tablets **1189**

Topiramate (Chlorpromazine may lower convulsive threshold; dosage adjustments of anticonvulsants may be necessary). Products include:
Topamax Sprinkle Capsules **2590**
Topamax Tablets **2590**

Triazolam (Prolonged and intensified action of CNS depressants). Products include:
Halcion Tablets **2823**

Trifluoperazine Hydrochloride (Prolonged and intensified action of CNS depressants). Products include:
Stelazine **1640**

Trimethadione (Chlorpromazine may lower convulsive threshold; dosage adjustments of anticonvulsants may be necessary).
No products indexed under this heading.

Valproate Sodium (Chlorpromazine may lower convulsive threshold; dosage adjustments of anticonvulsants may be necessary). Products include:
Depacon Injection **416**

Valproic Acid (Chlorpromazine may lower convulsive threshold; dosage adjustments of anticonvulsants may be necessary). Products include:
Depakene **421**

Warfarin Sodium (Chlorpromazine diminishes the effects of oral anticoagulants). Products include:
Coumadin for Injection **1243**
Coumadin Tablets **1243**
Warfarin Sodium Tablets, USP **3302**

Zaleplon (Prolonged and intensified action of CNS depressants). Products include:
Sonata Capsules **3591**

Zolpidem Tartrate (Prolonged and intensified action of CNS depressants). Products include:
Ambien Tablets **3191**

THROMBATE III
(Antithrombin III) **944**
May interact with:

Heparin Sodium (The anticoagulant effect of heparin is enhanced by concurrent treatment with antithrombin III; reduced dosage of heparin may be required). Products include:
Heparin Lock Flush Solution **3509**
Heparin Sodium Injection **3511**

THROMBIN-JMI
(Thrombin) **1824**
None cited in PDR database.

THYMOGLOBULIN FOR INJECTION
(Anti-thymocyte Globulin) **3071**
May interact with immunosuppressive agents and certain other agents. Compounds in these categories include:

Azathioprine (Co-administration with standard immunosuppressive regimen may predispose patients to over-immunosuppression; decrease in maintenance immunosuppression therapy during the period of antibody therapy may be needed).
No products indexed under this heading.

Basiliximab (Co-administration with standard immunosuppressive regimen may predispose patients to over-immunosuppression; decrease in maintenance immunosuppression therapy during the period of antibody therapy may be needed). Products include:
Simulect for Injection **2399**

Cyclosporine (Co-administration with standard immunosuppressive regimen may predispose patients to over-immunosuppression; decrease in maintenance immunosuppression therapy during the period of antibody therapy may be needed). Products include:
Gengraf Capsules **457**
Neoral Soft Gelatin Capsules **2380**
Neoral Oral Solution **2380**
Sandimmune **2388**

Globulin, immune (rabbit) (Thymoglobulin can stimulate the production of antibodies which cross-react with rabbit immune globulin).
No products indexed under this heading.

Muromonab-CD3 (Co-administration with standard immunosuppressive regimen may predispose patients to over-immunosuppression; decrease in maintenance immunosuppression therapy during the period of antibody therapy may be needed). Products include:
Orthoclone OKT3 Sterile Solution **2498**

Mycophenolate Mofetil (Co-administration with standard immunosuppressive regimen may predispose patients to over-immunosuppression; decrease in maintenance immunosuppression therapy during the period of antibody therapy may be needed). Products include:
CellCept Capsules **2951**
CellCept Oral Suspension **2951**
CellCept Tablets **2951**

Sirolimus (Co-administration with standard immunosuppressive regimen may predispose patients to over-immunosuppression; decrease in maintenance immunosuppression therapy during the period of antibody therapy may be needed). Products include:
Rapamune Oral Solution and Tablets **3584**

Tacrolimus (Co-administration with standard immunosuppressive regimen may predispose patients to over-immunosuppression; decrease in maintenance immunosuppression therapy during the period of antibody therapy may be needed). Products include:
Prograf **1393**
Protopic Ointment **1397**

THYREL TRH FOR INJECTION
(Protirelin) **3630**
May interact with glucocorticoids, thyroid preparations, and certain other agents. Compounds in these categories include:

Aspirin (Inhibits the TSH response to protirelin when aspirin is given at 2 to 3 g/day). Products include:
Aggrenox Capsules **1026**
Alka-Seltzer .... ■**603**
Alka-Seltzer Lemon Lime Antacid and Pain Reliever Effervescent Tablets .... ■**603**
Alka-Seltzer Extra Strength Antacid and Pain Reliever Effervescent Tablets .... ■**603**
Alka-Seltzer PM Effervescent Tablets .... ■**605**
Genuine Bayer Tablets, Caplets and Gelcaps .... ■**606**
Extra Strength Bayer Caplets and Gelcaps .... ■**610**
Aspirin Regimen Bayer Children's Chewable Tablets (Orange or Cherry Flavored) .... ■**607**
Bayer, Aspirin Regimen .... ■**606**
Aspirin Regimen Bayer 81 mg Caplets with Calcium .... ■**607**
Genuine Bayer Professional Labeling (Aspirin Regimen Bayer) .... ■**608**
Extra Strength Bayer Arthritis Caplets .... ■**610**
Extra Strength Bayer Plus Caplets .... ■**610**
Extra Strength Bayer PM Caplets .... ■**611**
BC Powder .... ■**619**
BC Allergy Sinus Cold Powder .... ■**619**
Arthritis Strength BC Powder .... ■**619**
BC Sinus Cold Powder .... ■**619**
Darvon Compound-65 Pulvules **1910**
Ecotrin Enteric Coated Aspirin Low, Regular and Maximum Strength Tablets **1715**
Excedrin Extra-Strength Tablets, Caplets, and Geltabs .... ■**629**
Excedrin Migraine **1070**
Goody's Body Pain Formula Powder .... ■**620**
Goody's Extra Strength Headache Powder .... ■**620**
Goody's Extra Strength Pain Relief Tablets .... ■**620**
Percodan Tablets **1327**
Robaxisal Tablets **2939**
Soma Compound Tablets **3354**
Soma Compound w/Codeine Tablets **3355**
Vanquish Caplets .... ■**617**

Betamethasone Acetate (Pharmacologic doses of steroids reduce the TSH response). Products include:
Celestone Soluspan Injectable Suspension **3097**

Betamethasone Sodium Phosphate (Pharmacologic doses of steroids reduce the TSH response). Products include:
Celestone Soluspan Injectable Suspension **3097**

Cortisone Acetate (Pharmacologic doses of steroids reduce the TSH response). Products include:
Cortone Acetate Injectable Suspension **2059**
Cortone Acetate Tablets **2061**

Dexamethasone (Pharmacologic doses of steroids reduce the TSH response). Products include:
Decadron Elixir **2078**
Decadron Tablets **2079**
TobraDex Ophthalmic Ointment **542**
TobraDex Ophthalmic Suspension **541**

Dexamethasone Acetate (Pharmacologic doses of steroids reduce the TSH response).
No products indexed under this heading.

Dexamethasone Sodium Phosphate (Pharmacologic doses of steroids reduce the TSH response). Products include:
Decadron Phosphate Injection **2081**
Decadron Phosphate Sterile Ophthalmic Ointment **2083**
Decadron Phosphate Sterile Ophthalmic Solution **2084**
NeoDecadron Sterile Ophthalmic Solution **2144**

Fludrocortisone Acetate (Pharmacologic doses of steroids reduce the TSH response). Products include:
Florinef Acetate Tablets **2250**

Hydrocortisone (Pharmacologic doses of steroids reduce the TSH response). Products include:
Anusol-HC Cream 2.5% **2237**
Cipro HC Otic Suspension **540**
Cortaid Intensive Therapy Cream .... ■**717**
Cortaid Maximum Strength Cream .... ■**717**
Cortisporin Ophthalmic Suspension Sterile .... ⊙**297**
Cortizone•5 .... ■**699**
Cortizone•10 .... ■**699**
Cortizone•10 Plus Creme .... ■**700**
Cortizone for Kids Creme .... ■**699**
Hydrocortone Tablets **2106**
Massengill Medicated Soft Cloth Towelette .... ■**753**
VōSoL HC Otic Solution **3356**

Hydrocortisone Acetate (Pharmacologic doses of steroids reduce the TSH response). Products include:
Analpram-HC **1338**
Anusol HC-1 Hydrocortisone Anti-Itch Cream .... ■**689**
Anusol-HC Suppositories **2238**
Cortaid .... ■**717**
Cortifoam Rectal Foam **3170**
Cortisporin-TC Otic Suspension **2246**
Hydrocortone Acetate Injectable Suspension **2103**
Pramosone **1343**
Proctocort Suppositories **2264**
ProctoFoam-HC **3177**
Terra-Cortril Ophthalmic Suspension **2716**

Hydrocortisone Sodium Phosphate (Pharmacologic doses of steroids reduce the TSH response). Products include:
Hydrocortone Phosphate Injection, Sterile **2105**

Hydrocortisone Sodium Succinate (Pharmacologic doses of steroids reduce the TSH response).
No products indexed under this heading.

Levodopa (Chronic administration of levodopa inhibits the TSH response). Products include:
Sinemet Tablets **1253**
Sinemet CR Tablets **1255**

Levothyroxine Sodium (Thyroid hormones reduce the TSH response). Products include:
Levothroid Tablets **1373**
Levoxyl Tablets **1819**
Synthroid **505**
Unithroid Tablets **3445**

Liothyronine Sodium (Thyroid hormones reduce the TSH response). Products include:
Cytomel Tablets **1817**
Triostat Injection **1825**

Liotrix (Thyroid hormones reduce the TSH response).
No products indexed under this heading.

Methylprednisolone Acetate (Pharmacologic doses of steroids reduce the TSH response). Products include:
Depo-Medrol Injectable Suspension **2795**

Methylprednisolone Sodium Succinate (Pharmacologic doses of steroids reduce the TSH response). Products include:
Solu-Medrol Sterile Powder **2855**

Prednisolone Acetate (Pharmacologic doses of steroids reduce the TSH response). Products include:
Blephamide Ophthalmic Ointment **547**
Blephamide Ophthalmic Suspension **548**
Poly-Pred Liquifilm Ophthalmic Suspension .... ⊙**245**
Pred Forte Ophthalmic Suspension .... ⊙**246**

Pred Mild Sterile Ophthalmic Suspension .... ⊙249
Pred-G Ophthalmic Suspension ..... ⊙247
Pred-G Sterile Ophthalmic Ointment .... ⊙248

Prednisolone Sodium Phosphate (Pharmacologic doses of steroids reduce the TSH response). Products include:
Pediapred Oral Solution 1170

Prednisolone Tebutate (Pharmacologic doses of steroids reduce the TSH response).
No products indexed under this heading.

Prednisone (Pharmacologic doses of steroids reduce the TSH response). Products include:
Prednisone 3064

Thyroglobulin (Thyroid hormones reduce the TSH response).
No products indexed under this heading.

Thyroid (Thyroid hormones reduce the TSH response).
No products indexed under this heading.

Thyroxine (Thyroid hormones reduce the TSH response).
No products indexed under this heading.

Thyroxine Sodium (Thyroid hormones reduce the TSH response).
No products indexed under this heading.

Triamcinolone (Pharmacologic doses of steroids reduce the TSH response).
No products indexed under this heading.

Triamcinolone Acetonide (Pharmacologic doses of steroids reduce the TSH response). Products include:
Azmacort Inhalation Aerosol 728
Nasacort Nasal Inhaler 750
Nasacort AQ Nasal Spray 752
Tri-Nasal Spray 2274

Triamcinolone Diacetate (Pharmacologic doses of steroids reduce the TSH response).
No products indexed under this heading.

Triamcinolone Hexacetonide (Pharmacologic doses of steroids reduce the TSH response).
No products indexed under this heading.

THYROGEN FOR INJECTION

(Thyrotropin alfa) 1441
None cited in PDR database.

TIAZAC CAPSULES

(Diltiazem Hydrochloride) 1378
May interact with anesthetics, beta blockers, erythromycin, cardiac glycosides, phenytoin, and certain other agents. Compounds in these categories include:

Acebutolol Hydrochloride (Concomitant use of diltiazem with beta blockers may result in additive effects on cardiac conduction). Products include:
Sectral Capsules 3589

Alfentanil Hydrochloride (Calcium channel blockers potentiate the depression of cardiac contractility, conductivity, and automaticity as well as vascular dilation associated with anesthetics).
No products indexed under this heading.

Amiodarone Hydrochloride (Agents known to affect cardiac contractility, such as amiodarone, may produce additive inhibition of cardiac conduction leading to increased risk of AV block). Products include:
Cordarone Intravenous 3491
Cordarone Tablets 3487
Pacerone Tablets 3331

Atenolol (Concomitant use of diltiazem with beta blockers may result in additive effects on cardiac conduction). Products include:
Tenoretic Tablets 690
Tenormin I.V. Injection 692

Betaxolol Hydrochloride (Concomitant use of diltiazem with beta blockers may result in additive effects on cardiac conduction). Products include:
Betoptic S Ophthalmic Suspension 537

Bisoprolol Fumarate (Concomitant use of diltiazem with beta blockers may result in additive effects on cardiac conduction). Products include:
Zebeta Tablets 1885
Ziac Tablets 1887

Carbamazepine (Co-administration has resulted in increased serum levels of carbamazepine resulting in toxicity in some patients). Products include:
Carbatrol Capsules 3234
Tegretol/Tegretol-XR 2404

Carteolol Hydrochloride (Concomitant use of diltiazem with beta blockers may result in additive effects on cardiac conduction). Products include:
Carteolol Hydrochloride Ophthalmic Solution USP, 1% ..... ⊙258
Ocupress Ophthalmic Solution, 1% Sterile .... ⊙303

Cimetidine (Co-administration has resulted in inhibition of hepatic cytochrome P450 by cimetidine producing significant increase in peak diltiazem plasma levels and AUC; am adjustment in diltiazem dosage may be warranted). Products include:
Tagamet HB 200 Suspension .... ▣762
Tagamet HB 200 Tablets .... ▣761
Tagamet Tablets 1644

Cimetidine Hydrochloride (Co-administration has resulted in inhibition of hepatic cytochrome P450 by cimetidine producing significant increase in peak diltiazem plasma levels and AUC; am adjustment in diltiazem dosage may be warranted). Products include:
Tagamet 1644

Cyclosporine (Diltiazem inhibits cytochrome P450 3A enzyme and co-administration may result in increased cyclosporine concentrations; a reduction in cyclosporine dose may be required, especially in renal and cardiac transplant recipients). Products include:
Gengraf Capsules 457
Neoral Soft Gelatin Capsules 2380
Neoral Oral Solution 2380
Sandimmune 2388

Deslanoside (Concomitant use of diltiazem with digitalis may result in additive effects on cardiac conduction).
No products indexed under this heading.

Digitoxin (Concomitant use of diltiazem with digitalis may result in additive effects on cardiac conduction).
No products indexed under this heading.

Digoxin (Co-administration has resulted in increased plasma digoxin concentrations in some patients; concomitant use of diltiazem with digitalis may result in additive effects on cardiac conduction). Products include:
Digitek Tablets 1003
Lanoxicaps Capsules 1574
Lanoxin Injection 1581
Lanoxin Tablets 1587
Lanoxin Elixir Pediatric 1578
Lanoxin Injection Pediatric 1584

Enflurane (Calcium channel blockers potentiate the depression of cardiac contractility, conductivity, and automaticity as well as vascular dilation associated with anesthetics).
No products indexed under this heading.

Erythromycin (Diltiazem is both a substrate and inhibitor of the CYP4503A4; co-administration with inhibitors of this enzyme system, such as erythromycin, may have significant impact on the side effect profile of diltiazem). Products include:
Emgel 2% Topical Gel 1285
Ery-Tab Tablets 448
Erythromycin Base Filmtab Tablets . 454
Erythromycin Delayed-Release Capsules, USP 455
PCE Dispertab Tablets 498

Erythromycin Estolate (Diltiazem is both a substrate and inhibitor of the CYP4503A4; co-administration with inhibitors of this enzyme system, such as erythromycin, may have significant impact on the side effect profile of diltiazem).
No products indexed under this heading.

Erythromycin Ethylsuccinate (Diltiazem is both a substrate and inhibitor of the CYP4503A4; co-administration with inhibitors of this enzyme system, such as erythromycin, may have significant impact on the side effect profile of diltiazem). Products include:
E.E.S. 450
EryPed 446
Pediazole Suspension 3050

Erythromycin Gluceptate (Diltiazem is both a substrate and inhibitor of the CYP4503A4; co-administration with inhibitors of this enzyme system, such as erythromycin, may have significant impact on the side effect profile of diltiazem).
No products indexed under this heading.

Erythromycin Stearate (Diltiazem is both a substrate and inhibitor of the CYP4503A4; co-administration with inhibitors of this enzyme system, such as erythromycin, may have significant impact on the side effect profile of diltiazem). Products include:
Erythrocin Stearate Filmtab Tablets 452

Esmolol Hydrochloride (Concomitant use of diltiazem with beta blockers may result in additive effects on cardiac conduction). Products include:
Brevibloc Injection 858

Fentanyl Citrate (Calcium channel blockers potentiate the depression of cardiac contractility, conductivity, and automaticity as well as vascular dilation associated with anesthetics). Products include:
Actiq 1184

Fluoxetine Hydrochloride (Diltiazem undergoes biotransformation by cytochrome P450 mixed funciton oxidase; co-administration with other agents which follow the same route of biotransformation may result in competitve inhibition of metabolism). Products include:
Prozac Pulvules, Liquid, and Weekly Capsules 1238
Sarafem Pulvules 1962

Fluvoxamine Maleate (Diltiazem undergoes biotransformation by cytochrome P450 mixed funciton oxidase; co-administration with other agents which follow the same route of biotransformation may result in competitive inhibition of metabolism). Products include:
Luvox Tablets (25, 50, 100 mg) 3256

Fosphenytoin Sodium (Diltiazem is both a substrate and inhibitor of the CYP4503A4; co-administration with inducers of this enzyme system, such as phenytoin, may have significant impact on the efficacy of diltiazem). Products include:
Cerebyx Injection 2619

Halothane (Calcium channel blockers potentiate the depression of cardiac contractility, conductivity, and automaticity as well as vascular dilation associated with anesthetics). Products include:
Fluothane Inhalation 3508

Isoflurane (Calcium channel blockers potentiate the depression of cardiac contractility, conductivity, and automaticity as well as vascular dilation associated with anesthetics).
No products indexed under this heading.

Ketamine Hydrochloride (Calcium channel blockers potentiate the depression of cardiac contractility, conductivity, and automaticity as well as vascular dilation associated with anesthetics).
No products indexed under this heading.

Ketoconazole (Diltiazem is both a substrate and inhibitor of the CYP4503A4; co-administration with inhibitors of this enzyme system, such as ketoconazole, may have significant impact on the side effect profile of diltiazem). Products include:
Nizoral 2% Cream 3620
Nizoral A-D Shampoo 2008
Nizoral 2% Shampoo 2007
Nizoral Tablets 1791

Labetalol Hydrochloride (Concomitant use of diltiazem with beta blockers may result in additive effects on cardiac conduction). Products include:
Normodyne Injection 3135
Normodyne Tablets 3137

Levobunolol Hydrochloride (Concomitant use of diltiazem with beta blockers may result in additive effects on cardiac conduction). Products include:
Betagan .... ⊙228

Lovastatin (Co-administration has resulted in a 3-4 times increase in mean lovastatin AUC and Cmax). Products include:
Mevacor Tablets 2132

Methohexital Sodium (Calcium channel blockers potentiate the depression of cardiac contractility, conductivity, and automaticity as well as vascular dilation associated with anesthetics). Products include:
Brevital Sodium for Injection, USP .. 1815

Metipranolol Hydrochloride (Concomitant use of diltiazem with beta blockers may result in additive effects on cardiac conduction).
No products indexed under this heading.

Metoprolol Succinate (Concomitant use of diltiazem with beta blockers may result in additive effects on cardiac conduction). Products include:
Toprol-XL Tablets 651

Metoprolol Tartrate (Concomitant use of diltiazem with beta blockers may result in additive effects on cardiac conduction).
No products indexed under this heading.

Midazolam Hydrochloride (Co-administration has resulted in increased AUC of midazolam by 3-4 fold and the Cmax by 2-fold; the elimination half-life of midazolam also increased during co-administration). Products include:
Versed Injection 3027
Versed Syrup 3033

Nadolol (Concomitant use of diltiazem with beta blockers may result in additive effects on cardiac conduction). Products include:
Corgard Tablets 2245
Corzide 40/5 Tablets 2247
Corzide 80/5 Tablets 2247
Nadolol Tablets 2288

Penbutolol Sulfate (Concomitant use of diltiazem with beta blockers may result in additive effects on cardiac conduction).
No products indexed under this heading.

Phenobarbital (Diltiazem is both a substrate and inhibitor of the CYP4503A4; co-administration with inducers of this enzyme system, such as phenobarbital, may have significant impact on the efficacy of diltiazem). Products include:
Arco-Lase Plus Tablets ... 592
Donnatal ... 2929
Donnatal Extentabs ... 2930

Phenytoin (Diltiazem is both a substrate and inhibitor of the CYP4503A4; co-administration with inducers of this enzyme system, such as phenytoin, may have significant impact on the efficacy of diltiazem). Products include:
Dilantin Infatabs ... 2624
Dilantin-125 Oral Suspension ... 2625

Phenytoin Sodium (Diltiazem is both a substrate and inhibitor of the CYP4503A4; co-administration with inducers of this enzyme system, such as phenytoin, may have significant impact on the efficacy of diltiazem). Products include:
Dilantin Kapseals ... 2622

Pindolol (Concomitant use of diltiazem with beta blockers may result in additive effects on cardiac conduction).
No products indexed under this heading.

Propofol (Calcium channel blockers potentiate the depression of cardiac contractility, conductivity, and automaticity as well as vascular dilation associated with anesthetics). Products include:
Diprivan Injectable Emulsion ... 667

Propranolol Hydrochloride (Concomitant use of diltiazem with propranolol resulted in increased propranolol levels and bioavailability of propranolol was increased by approximately 50%; Concurrent therapy of diltiazem with beta blockers may result in additive effects on cardiac conduction). Products include:
Inderal ... 3513
Inderal LA Long-Acting Capsules ... 3516
Inderide Tablets ... 3517
Inderide LA Long-Acting Capsules ... 3519

Ranitidine Hydrochloride (Co-administration produces smaller, nonsignificant increase in diltiazem plasma levels). Products include:
Zantac ... 1690
Zantac Injection ... 1688
Zantac 75 Tablets ... ▣717

Remifentanil Hydrochloride (Calcium channel blockers potentiate the depression of cardiac contractility, conductivity, and automaticity as well as vascular dilation associated with anesthetics).
No products indexed under this heading.

Rifampin (Co-administration has resulted in lowered diltiazem plasma concentrations to undetectable levels; co-administration should be avoided). Products include:
Rifadin ... 765
Rifamate Capsules ... 767
Rifater Tablets ... 769

Ritonavir (Diltiazem is both a substrate and inhibitor of the CYP4503A4; co-administration with inhibitors of this enzyme system, such as ritonavir, may have significant impact on the side effect profile of diltiazem). Products include:
Kaletra Capsules ... 471
Kaletra Oral Solution ... 471
Norvir Capsules ... 487
Norvir Oral Solution ... 487

Sotalol Hydrochloride (Concomitant use of diltiazem with beta blockers may result in additive effects on cardiac conduction). Products include:
Betapace Tablets ... 950
Betapace AF Tablets ... 954

Sufentanil Citrate (Calcium channel blockers potentiate the depression of cardiac contractility, conductivity, and automaticity as well as vascular dilation associated with anesthetics).
No products indexed under this heading.

Thiamylal Sodium (Calcium channel blockers potentiate the depression of cardiac contractility, conductivity, and automaticity as well as vascular dilation associated with anesthetics).
No products indexed under this heading.

Timolol Hemihydrate (Concomitant use of diltiazem with beta blockers may result in additive effects on cardiac conduction). Products include:
Betimol Ophthalmic Solution ... ⊙324

Timolol Maleate (Concomitant use of diltiazem with beta blockers may result in additive effects on cardiac conduction). Products include:
Blocadren Tablets ... 2046
Cosopt Sterile Ophthalmic Solution ... 2065
Timolide Tablets ... 2187
Timolol GFS ... ⊙266
Timoptic in Ocudose ... 2192
Timoptic Sterile Ophthalmic Solution ... 2190
Timoptic-XE Sterile Ophthalmic Gel Forming Solution ... 2194

Triazolam (Co-administration has resulted in increased AUC of triazolam by 3-4 fold and the Cmax by 2-fold; the elimination half-life of triazolam also increased during co-administration). Products include:
Halcion Tablets ... 2823

TICE BCG, BCG LIVE

(BCG Vaccine) ... 2489
May interact with immunosuppressive agents and certain other agents. Compounds in these categories include:

Antimicrobial therapy, unspecified (May interfere with the effectiveness of TICE BCG therapy).

Azathioprine (May interfere with development of immune response).
No products indexed under this heading.

Basiliximab (May interfere with development of immune response). Products include:
Simulect for Injection ... 2399

Cyclosporine (May interfere with development of immune response). Products include:
Gengraf Capsules ... 457
Neoral Soft Gelatin Capsules ... 2380
Neoral Oral Solution ... 2380
Sandimmune ... 2388

Isoniazid (Should not be used to prevent or treat the local, irritative toxicities of TICE BCG). Products include:
Rifamate Capsules ... 767
Rifater Tablets ... 769

Muromonab-CD3 (May interfere with development of immune response). Products include:
Orthoclone OKT3 Sterile Solution ... 2498

Mycophenolate Mofetil (May interfere with development of immune response). Products include:
CellCept Capsules ... 2951
CellCept Oral Suspension ... 2951
CellCept Tablets ... 2951

Sirolimus (May interfere with development of immune response). Products include:
Rapamune Oral Solution and Tablets ... 3584

Tacrolimus (May interfere with development of immune response). Products include:
Prograf ... 1393
Protopic Ointment ... 1397

TICLID TABLETS

(Ticlopidine Hydrochloride) ... 3015
May interact with antacids, anticoagulants, non-steroidal anti-inflammatory agents, phenytoin, theophylline, and certain other agents. Compounds in these categories include:

Aluminum Carbonate (18% decrease in plasma levels of ticlopidine when administered after antacids).
No products indexed under this heading.

Aluminum Hydroxide (18% decrease in plasma levels of ticlopidine when administered after antacids). Products include:
Amphojel Suspension (Mint Flavor) ... ▣789
Gaviscon Extra Strength Liquid ... ▣751
Gaviscon Extra Strength Tablets ... ▣751
Gaviscon Regular Strength Liquid ... ▣751
Gaviscon Regular Strength Tablets ... ▣750
Maalox Antacid/Anti-Gas Oral Suspension ... ▣673
Maalox Max Maximum Strength Antacid/Anti-Gas Liquid ... 2300
Maalox Regular Strength Antacid/Antigas Liquid ... 2300
Mylanta ... 1813
Vanquish Caplets ... ▣617

Aminophylline (Co-administration may result in significant increase in the theophylline elimination half-life and a comparable reduction in total plasma clearance of theophylline).
No products indexed under this heading.

Ardeparin Sodium (The tolerance and safety of co-administration has not been established; anticoagulant should be discontinued prior to Ticlid administration).
No products indexed under this heading.

Aspirin (Ticlopidine potentiates the effect of aspirin on collagen-induced platelet aggregation; concurrent use is not recommended). Products include:
Aggrenox Capsules ... 1026
Alka-Seltzer ... ▣603
Alka-Seltzer Lemon Lime Antacid and Pain Reliever Effervescent Tablets ... ▣603
Alka-Seltzer Extra Strength Antacid and Pain Reliever Effervescent Tablets ... ▣603
Alka-Seltzer PM Effervescent Tablets ... ▣605
Genuine Bayer Tablets, Caplets and Gelcaps ... ▣606
Extra Strength Bayer Caplets and Gelcaps ... ▣610
Aspirin Regimen Bayer Children's Chewable Tablets (Orange or Cherry Flavored) ... ▣607
Bayer, Aspirin Regimen ... ▣606
Aspirin Regimen Bayer 81 mg Caplets with Calcium ... ▣607
Genuine Bayer Professional Labeling (Aspirin Regimen Bayer) ... ▣608
Extra Strength Bayer Arthritis Caplets ... ▣610
Extra Strength Bayer Plus Caplets ... ▣610
Extra Strength Bayer PM Caplets ... ▣611
BC Powder ... ▣619
BC Allergy Sinus Cold Powder ... ▣619
Arthritis Strength BC Powder ... ▣619
BC Sinus Cold Powder ... ▣619
Darvon Compound-65 Pulvules ... 1910
Ecotrin Enteric Coated Aspirin Low, Regular and Maximum Strength Tablets ... 1715
Excedrin Extra-Strength Tablets, Caplets, and Geltabs ... ▣629
Excedrin Migraine ... 1070
Goody's Body Pain Formula Powder ... ▣620
Goody's Extra Strength Headache Powder ... ▣620
Goody's Extra Strength Pain Relief Tablets ... ▣620
Percodan Tablets ... 1327
Robaxisal Tablets ... 2939
Soma Compound Tablets ... 3354
Soma Compound w/Codeine Tablets ... 3355
Vanquish Caplets ... ▣617

Celecoxib (Ticlopidine potentiates the effect of NSAIDS on platelet aggregation). Products include:
Celebrex Capsules ... 2676
Celebrex Capsules ... 2780

Cimetidine (Chronic administration of cimetidine reduces the clearance of a single dose of ticlopidine by 50%). Products include:
Tagamet HB 200 Suspension ... ▣762
Tagamet HB 200 Tablets ... ▣761
Tagamet Tablets ... 1644

Cimetidine Hydrochloride (Chronic administration of cimetidine reduces the clearance of a single dose of ticlopidine by 50%). Products include:
Tagamet ... 1644

Dalteparin Sodium (The tolerance and safety of co-administration has not been established; anticoagulant should be discontinued prior to Ticlid administration). Products include:
Fragmin Injection ... 2814

Danaparoid Sodium (The tolerance and safety of co-administration has not been established; anticoagulant should be discontinued prior to Ticlid administration). Products include:
Orgaran Injection ... 2480

Diclofenac Potassium (Ticlopidine potentiates the effect of NSAIDS on platelet aggregation). Products include:
Cataflam Tablets ... 2315

Diclofenac Sodium (Ticlopidine potentiates the effect of NSAIDS on platelet aggregation). Products include:
Arthrotec Tablets ... 3195
Voltaren Ophthalmic Sterile Ophthalmic Solution ... ⊙312
Voltaren Tablets ... 2315
Voltaren-XR Tablets ... 2315

Dicumarol (The tolerance and safety of co-administration has not been established; anticoagulant should be discontinued prior to Ticlid administration).
No products indexed under this heading.

Digoxin (Co-administration resulted in slight decrease in digoxin plasma levels; little or no change in efficacy of digoxin). Products include:
Digitek Tablets ... 1003
Lanoxicaps Capsules ... 1574
Lanoxin Injection ... 1581
Lanoxin Tablets ... 1587
Lanoxin Elixir Pediatric ... 1578
Lanoxin Injection Pediatric ... 1584

Dyphylline (Co-administration may result in significant increase in the theophylline elimination half-life and a comparable reduction in total plasma clearance of theophylline). Products include:
Lufyllin Tablets ... 3347
Lufyllin-400 Tablets ... 3347
Lufyllin-GG Elixir ... 3348
Lufyllin-GG Tablets ... 3348

Enoxaparin (The tolerance and safety of co-administration has not been established; anticoagulant should be discontinued prior to Ticlid administration). Products include:
Lovenox Injection ... 746

Etodolac (Ticlopidine potentiates the effect of NSAIDS on platelet aggregation). Products include:
Lodine ... 3528
Lodine XL Extended-Release Tablets ... 3530

Fenoprofen Calcium (Ticlopidine potentiates the effect of NSAIDS on platelet aggregation).
No products indexed under this heading.

Flurbiprofen (Ticlopidine potentiates the effect of NSAIDS on platelet aggregation).
No products indexed under this heading.

Fosphenytoin Sodium (Co-administration has resulted in several cases of elevated phenytoin plasma levels with associated somnolence and lethargy; caution is advised). Products include:
Cerebyx Injection 2619

Heparin Sodium (The tolerance and safety of co-administration has not been established; anticoagulant should be discontinued prior to Ticlid administration). Products include:
Heparin Lock Flush Solution 3509
Heparin Sodium Injection 3511

Ibuprofen (Ticlopidine potentiates the effect of NSAIDS on platelet aggregation). Products include:
Advil 771
Children's Advil Oral Suspension 773
Children's Advil Chewable Tablets 773
Advil Cold and Sinus Caplets 771
Advil Cold and Sinus Tablets 771
Advil Flu & Body Ache Caplets 772
Infants' Advil Drops 773
Junior Strength Advil Tablets 773
Junior Strength Advil Chewable Tablets 773
Advil Migraine Liquigels 772
Children's Motrin Oral Suspension and Chewable Tablets 2006
Children's Motrin Cold Oral Suspension 2007
Children's Motrin Oral Suspension 643
Motrin Suspension, Oral Drops, Chewable Tablets, and Caplets 2002
Infants' Motrin Concentrated Drops 2006
Junior Strength Motrin Caplets and Chewable Tablets 2006
Motrin IB Tablets, Caplets, and Gelcaps 2002
Motrin Migraine Pain Caplets 2005
Motrin Sinus Headache Caplets 2005
Vicoprofen Tablets 520

Indomethacin (Ticlopidine potentiates the effect of NSAIDS on platelet aggregation). Products include:
Indocin 2112

Indomethacin Sodium Trihydrate (Ticlopidine potentiates the effect of NSAIDS on platelet aggregation). Products include:
Indocin I.V. 2115

Ketoprofen (Ticlopidine potentiates the effect of NSAIDS on platelet aggregation). Products include:
Orudis Capsules 3548
Orudis KT Tablets 778
Oruvail Capsules 3548

Ketorolac Tromethamine (Ticlopidine potentiates the effect of NSAIDS on platelet aggregation). Products include:
Acular Ophthalmic Solution 544
Acular PF Ophthalmic Solution 544
Toradol 3018

Magaldrate (18% decrease in plasma levels of ticlopidine when administered after antacids).
No products indexed under this heading.

Magnesium Hydroxide (18% decrease in plasma levels of ticlopidine when administered after antacids). Products include:
Ex•Lax Milk of Magnesia Liquid 670
Maalox Antacid/Anti-Gas Oral Suspension 673
Maalox Max Maximum Strength Antacid/Anti-Gas Liquid 2300
Maalox Regular Strength Antacid/Antigas Liquid 2300
Mylanta Fast-Acting 1813
Mylanta 1813
Pepcid Complete Chewable Tablets 1815
Phillips' Chewable Tablets 615
Phillips' Milk of Magnesia Liquid (Original, Cherry, & Mint) 616
Rolaids Tablets 706
Extra Strength Rolaids Tablets 706
Vanquish Caplets 617

Magnesium Oxide (18% decrease in plasma levels of ticlopidine when administered after antacids). Products include:
Beelith Tablets 946
Mag-Ox 400 Tablets 1024
Uro-Mag Capsules 1024

Meclofenamate Sodium (Ticlopidine potentiates the effect of NSAIDS on platelet aggregation).
No products indexed under this heading.

Mefenamic Acid (Ticlopidine potentiates the effect of NSAIDS on platelet aggregation). Products include:
Ponstel Capsules 1356

Meloxicam (Ticlopidine potentiates the effect of NSAIDS on platelet aggregation). Products include:
Mobic Tablets 1054

Nabumetone (Ticlopidine potentiates the effect of NSAIDS on platelet aggregation). Products include:
Relafen Tablets 1617

Naproxen (Ticlopidine potentiates the effect of NSAIDS on platelet aggregation). Products include:
EC-Naprosyn Delayed-Release Tablets 2967
Naprosyn Suspension 2967
Naprosyn Tablets 2967

Naproxen Sodium (Ticlopidine potentiates the effect of NSAIDS on platelet aggregation). Products include:
Aleve Tablets, Caplets and Gelcaps 602
Aleve Cold & Sinus Caplets 603
Anaprox Tablets 2967
Anaprox DS Tablets 2967
Naprelan Tablets 1293

Oxaprozin (Ticlopidine potentiates the effect of NSAIDS on platelet aggregation).
No products indexed under this heading.

Phenylbutazone (Ticlopidine potentiates the effect of NSAIDS on platelet aggregation).
No products indexed under this heading.

Phenytoin (Co-administration has resulted in several cases of elevated phenytoin plasma levels with associated somnolence and lethargy; caution is advised). Products include:
Dilantin Infatabs 2624
Dilantin-125 Oral Suspension 2625

Phenytoin Sodium (Co-administration has resulted in several cases of elevated phenytoin plasma levels with associated somnolence and lethargy; caution is advised). Products include:
Dilantin Kapseals 2622

Piroxicam (Ticlopidine potentiates the effect of NSAIDS on platelet aggregation). Products include:
Feldene Capsules 2685

Propranolol Hydrochloride (Exercise caution if co-administered; *in vitro* studies indicate no alteration of plasma protein binding of propranolol). Products include:
Inderal 3513
Inderal LA Long-Acting Capsules 3516
Inderide Tablets 3517
Inderide LA Long-Acting Capsules 3519

Rofecoxib (Ticlopidine potentiates the effect of NSAIDS on platelet aggregation). Products include:
Vioxx 2213

Sodium Bicarbonate (18% decrease in plasma levels of ticlopidine when administered after antacids). Products include:
Alka-Seltzer 603
Alka-Seltzer Lemon Lime Antacid and Pain Reliever Effervescent Tablets 603
Alka-Seltzer Extra Strength Antacid and Pain Reliever Effervescent Tablets 603
Alka-Seltzer Heartburn Relief Tablets 604
Ceo-Two Evacuant Suppository 618
Colyte with Flavor Packs for Oral Solution 3170
GoLYTELY and Pineapple Flavor GoLYTELY for Oral Solution 1068
NuLYTELY, Cherry Flavor, Lemon-Lime Flavor, and Orange Flavor NuLYTELY for Oral Solution 1068

Sulindac (Ticlopidine potentiates the effect of NSAIDS on platelet aggregation). Products include:
Clinoril Tablets 2053

Theophylline (Co-administration may result in significant increase in the theophylline elimination half-life and a comparable reduction in total plasma clearance of theophylline). Products include:
Aerolate 1361
Theo-Dur Extended-Release Tablets 1835
Uni-Dur Extended-Release Tablets 1841
Uniphyl 400 mg and 600 mg Tablets 2903

Theophylline Calcium Salicylate (Co-administration may result in significant increase in the theophylline elimination half-life and a comparable reduction in total plasma clearance of theophylline).
No products indexed under this heading.

Theophylline Sodium Glycinate (Co-administration may result in significant increase in the theophylline elimination half-life and a comparable reduction in total plasma clearance of theophylline).
No products indexed under this heading.

Tinzaparin sodium (The tolerance and safety of co-administration has not been established; anticoagulant should be discontinued prior to Ticlid administration). Products include:
Innohep Injection 1248

Tolmetin Sodium (Ticlopidine potentiates the effect of NSAIDS on platelet aggregation). Products include:
Tolectin 2589

Warfarin Sodium (The tolerance and safety of co-administration has not been established; anticoagulant should be discontinued prior to Ticlid administration). Products include:
Coumadin for Injection 1243
Coumadin Tablets 1243
Warfarin Sodium Tablets, USP 3302

Food Interactions

Meal, unspecified (Administration after meals results in a 20% increase in the AUC of ticlopidine).

TIKOSYN CAPSULES

(Dofetilide) 2717

May interact with azole antifungals, macrolide antibiotics, phenothiazines, potassium-depleting diuretics, protease inhibitors, selective serotonin reuptake inhibitors, thiazides, tricyclic antidepressants, type 1 antiarrhythmic drugs, and certain other agents. Compounds in these categories include:

Amiloride Hydrochloride (Dofetilide is eliminated in the kidney by cationic secretion; co-administration with drugs that are actively secreted via this route, such as amiloride, should be undertaken with care as they might increase dofetilide levels). Products include:
Midamor Tablets 2136
Moduretic Tablets 2138

Amiodarone Hydrochloride (Dofetilide is metabolized to a small extent by the CYP4503A4 system; co-administration with inhibitors of this isoenzyme, such as amiodarone, could increase systemic dofetilide exposure; in clinical trials dofetilide was administered to patients previously treated with oral amiodarone only if serum amiodarone levels were below 0.3 mg/L or amiodarone had been withdrawn for at least three months). Products include:
Cordarone Intravenous 3491
Cordarone Tablets 3487
Pacerone Tablets 3331

Amitriptyline Hydrochloride (Dofetilide can cause serious ventricular arrhythmias associated with QT interval prolongation; concomitant use with other drugs that prolong the QT interval, such as tricyclic antidepressants, has not been studied and is not recommended). Products include:
Etrafon 3115
Limbitrol 1738

Amoxapine (Dofetilide can cause serious ventricular arrhythmias associated with QT interval prolongation; concomitant use with other drugs that prolong the QT interval, such as tricyclic antidepressants, has not been studied and is not recommended).
No products indexed under this heading.

Amprenavir (Dofetilide is metabolized to a small extent by the CYP4503A4 system; co-administration with inhibitors of this isoenzyme, such as protease inhibitors, could increase systemic dofetilide exposure). Products include:
Agenerase Capsules 1454
Agenerase Oral Solution 1459

Azithromycin Dihydrate (Dofetilide can cause serious ventricular arrhythmias associated with QT interval prolongation; concomitant use with other drugs that prolong the QT interval, such as certain oral macrolides, has not been studied and is not recommended; Dofetilide is metabolized to a small extent by the CYP4503A4 system; co-administration with inhibitors of this isoenzyme, such as macrolide antibiotics, could increase systemic dofetilide exposure). Products include:
Zithromax 2743
Zithromax for IV Infusion 2748
Zithromax for Oral Suspension, 300 mg, 600 mg, 900 mg, 1200 mg 2739
Zithromax Tablets, 250 mg 2739

Bendroflumethiazide (Hypokalemia and hypomagnesemia may occur with potassium-depleting diuretics, increasing the potential for torsade de pointes). Products include:
Corzide 40/5 Tablets 2247
Corzide 80/5 Tablets 2247

Bepridil Hydrochloride (Dofetilide can cause serious ventricular arrhythmias associated with QT interval prolongation; concomitant use with other drugs that prolong the QT interval, such as bepridil, has not been studied and is not recommended). Products include:
Vascor Tablets 2602

Bumetanide (Hypokalemia and hypomagnesemia may occur with potassium-depleting diuretics, increasing the potential for torsade de pointes).
No products indexed under this heading.

Chlorothiazide (Hypokalemia and hypomagnesemia may occur with potassium-depleting diuretics, increasing the potential for torsade de pointes). Products include:
Aldoclor Tablets 2035
Diuril Oral 2087

Chlorothiazide Sodium (Hypokalemia and hypomagnesemia may occur with potassium-depleting diuretics, increasing the potential for torsade de pointes). Products include:
Diuril Sodium Intravenous 2086

Chlorpromazine (Dofetilide can cause serious ventricular arrhythmias associated with QT interval prolongation; concomitant use with other drugs that prolong the QT interval, such as phenothiazines, has not been studied and is not recommended). Products include:
- Thorazine Suppositories 1656

Chlorpromazine Hydrochloride (Dofetilide can cause serious ventricular arrhythmias associated with QT interval prolongation; concomitant use with other drugs that prolong the QT interval, such as phenothiazines, has not been studied and is not recommended). Products include:
- Thorazine 1656

Cimetidine (Co-administration with cation transport inhibitor, cimetidine, has been shown to increase dofetilide plasma levels by 13% to 58%; concomitant use is contraindicated). Products include:
- Tagamet HB 200 Suspension ....■ 762
- Tagamet HB 200 Tablets ....■ 761
- Tagamet Tablets 1644

Cimetidine Hydrochloride (Co-administration with cation transport inhibitor, cimetidine, has been shown to increase dofetilide plasma levels by 13% to 58%; concomitant use is contraindicated). Products include:
- Tagamet 1644

Cisapride (Dofetilide can sause serious ventricular arrhythmias associated with QT interval prolongation; concomitant use with other drugs that prolong the QT interval, such as cisapride, has not been studied and is not recommended).
- No products indexed under this heading.

Citalopram Hydrobromide (Dofetilide is metabolized to a small extent by the CYP4503A4 system; co-administration with inhibitors of this isoenzyme, such as serotonin reuptake inhibitors, could increase systemic dofetilide exposure). Products include:
- Celexa 1365

Clarithromycin (Dofetilide can cause serious ventricular arrhythmias associated with QT interval prolongation; concomitant use with other drugs that prolong the QT interval, such as certain oral macrolides, has not been studied and is not recommended; Dofetilide is metabolized to a small extent by the CYP4503A4 system; co-administration with inhibitors of this isoenzyme, such as macrolide antibiotics, could increase systemic dofetilide exposure). Products include:
- Biaxin/Biaxin XL 403
- PREVPAC 3298

Clomipramine Hydrochloride (Dofetilide can cause serious ventricular arrhythmias associated with QT interval prolongation; concomitant use with other drugs that prolong the QT interval, such as tricyclic antidepressants, has not been studied and is not recommended).
- No products indexed under this heading.

Clotrimazole (Dofetilide is metabolized to a small extent by the CYP4503A4 system; co-administration with inhibitors of this isoenzyme, such as azole antifungal agents, could increase systemic dofetilide exposure). Products include:
- Gyne-Lotrimin 3, 3-Day Cream ....■ 741
- Lotrimin AF Cream, Lotion, Solution, and Jock Itch Cream ....■ 742
- Lotrimin 3128
- Lotrisone 3129
- Mycelex Troche 573
- Mycelex-7 Combination-Pack Vaginal Inserts & External Vulvar Cream ....■ 614
- Mycelex-7 Vaginal Cream ....■ 614
- Mycelex-7 Vaginal Cream with 7 Disposable Applicators ....■ 614

Desipramine Hydrochloride (Dofetilide can cause serious ventricular arrhythmias associated with QT interval prolongation; concomitant use with other drugs that prolong the QT interval, such as tricyclic antidepressants, has not been studied and is not recommended). Products include:
- Norpramin Tablets 755

Digoxin (Co-administration of digoxin with dofetilide was associated with a higher occurrence of torsade de pointes; it is not clear whether this represents an interaction with dofetilide or the presence of more severe structural heart disease in patients on digoxin). Products include:
- Digitek Tablets 1003
- Lanoxicaps Capsules 1574
- Lanoxin Injection 1581
- Lanoxin Tablets 1587
- Lanoxin Elixir Pediatric 1578
- Lanoxin Injection Pediatric 1584

Diltiazem Hydrochloride (Dofetilide is metabolized to a small extent by the CYP4503A4 system; co-administration with inhibitors of this isoenzyme, such as diltiazem, could increase systemic dofetilide exposure). Products include:
- Cardizem Injectable 1018
- Cardizem Lyo-Ject Syringe 1018
- Cardizem Monovial 1018
- Cardizem CD Capsules 1016
- Tiazac Capsules 1378

Dirithromycin (Dofetilide can cause serious ventricular arrhythmias associated with QT interval prolongation; concomitant use with other drugs that prolong the QT interval, such as certain oral macrolides, has not been studied and is not recommended; Dofetilide is metabolized to a small extent by the CYP4503A4 system; co-administration with inhibitors of this isoenzyme, such as macrolide antibiotics, could increase systemic dofetilide exposure). Products include:
- Dynabac Tablets 2269

Disopyramide Phosphate (Class I antiarrhythmic agents should be withheld for at least three half-lives prior to dosing with dofetilide).
- No products indexed under this heading.

Doxepin Hydrochloride (Dofetilide can cause serious ventricular arrhythmias associated with QT interval prolongation; concomitant use with other drugs that prolong the QT interval, such as tricyclic antidepressants, has not been studied and is not recommended). Products include:
- Sinequan 2713

Dronabinol (Dofetilide is metabolized to a small extent by the CYP4503A4 system; co-administration with inhibitors of this isoenzyme, such as dronabinol (cannabinoids), could increase systemic dofetilide exposure). Products include:
- Marinol Capsules 3325

Erythromycin (Dofetilide can cause serious ventricular arrhythmias associated with QT interval prolongation; concomitant use with other drugs that prolong the QT interval, such as certain oral macrolides, has not been studied and is not recommended; Dofetilide is metabolized to a small extent by the CYP4503A4 system; co-administration with inhibitors of this isoenzyme, such as macrolide antibiotics, could increase systemic dofetilide exposure). Products include:
- Emgel 2% Topical Gel 1285
- Ery-Tab Tablets 448
- Erythromycin Base Filmtab Tablets . 454
- Erythromycin Delayed-Release Capsules, USP 455
- PCE Dispertab Tablets 498

Erythromycin Estolate (Dofetilide can cause serious ventricular arrhythmias associated with QT interval prolongation; concomitant use with other drugs that prolong the QT interval, such as certain oral macrolides, has not been studied and is not recommended; Dofetilide is metabolized to a small extent by the CYP4503A4 system; co-administration with inhibitors of this isoenzyme, such as macrolide antibiotics, could increase systemic dofetilide exposure).
- No products indexed under this heading.

Erythromycin Ethylsuccinate (Dofetilide can cause serious ventricular arrhythmias associated with QT interval prolongation; concomitant use with other drugs that prolong the QT interval, such as certain oral macrolides, has not been studied and is not recommended; Dofetilide is metabolized to a small extent by the CYP4503A4 system; co-administration with inhibitors of this isoenzyme, such as macrolide antibiotics, could increase systemic dofetilide exposure). Products include:
- E.E.S. 450
- EryPed 446
- Pediazole Suspension 3050

Erythromycin Gluceptate (Dofetilide can cause serious ventricular arrhythmias associated with QT interval prolongation; concomitant use with other drugs that prolong the QT interval, such as certain oral macrolides, has not been studied and is not recommended; Dofetilide is metabolized to a small extent by the CYP4503A4 system; co-administration with inhibitors of this isoenzyme, such as macrolide antibiotics, could increase systemic dofetilide exposure).
- No products indexed under this heading.

Erythromycin Stearate (Dofetilide can cause serious ventricular arrhythmias associated with QT interval prolongation; concomitant use with other drugs that prolong the QT interval, such as certain oral macrolides, has not been studied and is not recommended; Dofetilide is metabolized to a small extent by the CYP4503A4 system; co-administration with inhibitors of this isoenzyme, such as macrolide antibiotics, could increase systemic dofetilide exposure). Products include:
- Erythrocin Stearate Filmtab Tablets 452

Ethacrynic Acid (Hypokalemia and hypomagnesemia may occur with potassium-depleting diuretics, increasing the potential for torsade de pointes). Products include:
- Edecrin Tablets 2091

Fluconazole (Dofetilide is metabolized to a small extent by the CYP4503A4 system; co-administration with inhibitors of this isoenzyme, such as azole antifungal agents, could increase systemic dofetilide exposure). Products include:
- Diflucan Tablets, Injection, and Oral Suspension 2681

Fluoxetine Hydrochloride (Dofetilide is metabolized to a small extent by the CYP4503A4 system; co-administration with inhibitors of this isoenzyme, such as serotonin reuptake inhibitors, could increase systemic dofetilide exposure). Products include:
- Prozac Pulvules, Liquid, and Weekly Capsules 1238
- Sarafem Pulvules 1962

Fluphenazine Decanoate (Dofetilide can cause serious ventricular arrhythmias associated with QT interval prolongation; concomitant use with other drugs that prolong the QT interval, such as phenothiazines, has not been studied and is not recommended).
- No products indexed under this heading.

Fluphenazine Enanthate (Dofetilide can cause serious ventricular arrhythmias associated with QT interval prolongation; concomitant use with other drugs that prolong the QT interval, such as phenothiazines, has not been studied and is not recommended).
- No products indexed under this heading.

Fluphenazine Hydrochloride (Dofetilide can cause serious ventricular arrhythmias associated with QT interval prolongation; concomitant use with other drugs that prolong the QT interval, such as phenothiazines, has not been studied and is not recommended).
- No products indexed under this heading.

Fluvoxamine Maleate (Dofetilide is metabolized to a small extent by the CYP4503A4 system; co-administration with inhibitors of this isoenzyme, such as serotonin reuptake inhibitors, could increase systemic dofetilide exposure). Products include:
- Luvox Tablets (25, 50, 100 mg) 3256

Furosemide (Hypokalemia and hypomagnesemia may occur with potassium-depleting diuretics, increasing the potential for torsade de pointes). Products include:
- Furosemide Tablets 2284

Hydrochlorothiazide (Hypokalemia and hypomagnesemia may occur with potassium-depleting diuretics, increasing the potential for torsade de pointes). Products include:
- Accuretic Tablets 2614
- Aldoril Tablets 2039
- Atacand HCT Tablets 597
- Avalide Tablets 1070
- Diovan HCT Tablets 2338
- Dyazide Capsules 1515
- HydroDIURIL Tablets 2108
- Hyzaar 2109
- Inderide Tablets 3517
- Inderide LA Long-Acting Capsules .. 3519
- Lotensin HCT Tablets 2367
- Maxzide 1008
- Micardis HCT Tablets 1051
- Microzide Capsules 3414
- Moduretic Tablets 2138
- Monopril HCT 1094
- Prinzide Tablets 2168
- Timolide Tablets 2187
- Uniretic Tablets 3178
- Vaseretic Tablets 2204
- Zestoretic Tablets 695
- Ziac Tablets 1887

Hydroflumethiazide (Hypokalemia and hypomagnesemia may occur with potassium-depleting diuretics, increasing the potential for torsade de pointes). Products include:
- Diucardin Tablets 3494

Imipramine Hydrochloride (Dofetilide can cause serious ventricular arrhythmias associated with QT interval prolongation; concomitant use with other drugs that prolong the QT interval, such as tricyclic antidepressants, has not been studied and is not recommended).
- No products indexed under this heading.

Imipramine Pamoate (Dofetilide can cause serious ventricular arrhythmias associated with QT interval prolongation; concomitant use with other drugs that prolong the QT interval, such as tricyclic antidepressants, has not been studied and

is not recommended).
No products indexed under this heading.

Indinavir Sulfate (Dofetilide is metabolized to a small extent by the CYP4503A4 system; co-administration with inhibitors of this isoenzyme, such as protease inhibitors, could increase systemic dofetilide exposure). Products include:
Crixivan Capsules 2070

Itraconazole (Dofetilide is metabolized to a small extent by the CYP4503A4 system; co-administration with inhibitors of this isoenzyme, such as azole antifungal agents, could increase systemic dofetilide exposure). Products include:
Sporanox Capsules 1800
Sporanox Injection 1804
Sporanox Injection 2509
Sporanox Oral Solution 1808
Sporanox Oral Solution 2512

Ketoconazole (Co-administration with ketoconazole has been shown to increase dofetilide Cmax by 53% in males and 97% in females, and AUC by 41% in males and 69% in females; concomitant use is contraindicated). Products include:
Nizoral 2% Cream 3620
Nizoral A-D Shampoo 2008
Nizoral 2% Shampoo 2007
Nizoral Tablets 1791

Lopinavir (Dofetilide is metabolized to a small extent by the CYP4503A4 system; co-administration with inhibitors of this isoenzyme, such as protease inhibitors, could increase systemic dofetilide exposure). Products include:
Kaletra Capsules 471
Kaletra Oral Solution 471

Maprotiline Hydrochloride (Dofetilide can cause serious ventricular arrhythmias associated with QT interval prolongation; concomitant use with other drugs that prolong the QT interval, such as tricyclic antidepressants, has not been studied and is not recommended).
No products indexed under this heading.

Megestrol Acetate (Dofetilide is eliminated in the kidney by cationic secretion; co-administration with inhibitors of renal cationic transport system, such as megestrol, may increase plasma levels; concurrent use is not recommended). Products include:
Megace Oral Suspension 1124

Mesoridazine Besylate (Dofetilide can cause serious ventricular arrhythmias associated with QT interval prolongation; concomitant use with other drugs that prolong the QT interval, such as phenothiazines, has not been studied and is not recommended). Products include:
Serentil 1057

Metformin Hydrochloride (Dofetilide is eliminated in the kidney by cationic secretion; co-administration with drugs that are actively secreted via this route, such as metformin, should be undertaken with care as they might increase dofetilide levels). Products include:
Glucophage Tablets 1080
Glucophage XR Tablets 1080
Glucovance Tablets 1086

Methotrimeprazine (Dofetilide can cause serious ventricular arrhythmias associated with QT interval prolongation; concomitant use with other drugs that prolong the QT interval, such as phenothiazines, has not been studied and is not recommended).
No products indexed under this heading.

Methyclothiazide (Hypokalemia and hypomagnesemia may occur with potassium-depleting diuretics, increasing the potential for torsade de pointes).
No products indexed under this heading.

Miconazole (Dofetilide is metabolized to a small extent by the CYP4503A4 system; co-administration with inhibitors of this isoenzyme, such as azole antifungal agents, could increase systemic dofetilide exposure).
No products indexed under this heading.

Moricizine Hydrochloride (Class I antiarrhythmic agents should be withheld for at least three half-lives prior to dosing with dofetilide).
No products indexed under this heading.

Nefazodone Hydrochloride (Dofetilide is metabolized to a small extent by the CYP4503A4 system; co-administration with inhibitors of this isoenzyme, such as nefazodone, could increase systemic dofetilide exposure). Products include:
Serzone Tablets 1104

Nelfinavir Mesylate (Dofetilide is metabolized to a small extent by the CYP4503A4 system; co-administration with inhibitors of this isoenzyme, such as protease inhibitors, could increase systemic dofetilide exposure). Products include:
Viracept 532

Norfloxacin (Dofetilide is metabolized to a small extent by the CYP4503A4 system; co-administration with inhibitors of this isoenzyme, such as norfloxacin, could increase systemic dofetilide exposure). Products include:
Chibroxin Sterile Ophthalmic Solution 2051
Noroxin Tablets 2145

Nortriptyline Hydrochloride (Dofetilide can cause serious ventricular arrhythmias associated with QT interval prolongation; concomitant use with other drugs that prolong the QT interval, such as tricyclic antidepressants, has not been studied and is not recommended).
No products indexed under this heading.

Oxiconazole Nitrate (Dofetilide is metabolized to a small extent by the CYP4503A4 system; co-administration with inhibitors of this isoenzyme, such as azole antifungal agents, could increase systemic dofetilide exposure). Products include:
Oxistat 1298

Paroxetine Hydrochloride (Dofetilide is metabolized to a small extent by the CYP4503A4 system; co-administration with inhibitors of this isoenzyme, such as serotonin reuptake inhibitors, could increase systemic dofetilide exposure). Products include:
Paxil 1609

Perphenazine (Dofetilide can cause serious ventricular arrhythmias associated with QT interval prolongation; concomitant use with other drugs that prolong the QT interval, such as phenothiazines, has not been studied and is not recommended). Products include:
Etrafon 3115
Trilafon 3160

Polythiazide (Hypokalemia and hypomagnesemia may occur with potassium-depleting diuretics, increasing the potential for torsade de pointes). Products include:
Minizide Capsules 2700
Renese Tablets 2712

Procainamide Hydrochloride (Class I antiarrhythmic agents should be withheld for at least three half-lives prior to dosing with dofetilide). Products include:
Procanbid Extended-Release Tablets 2262

Prochlorperazine (Dofetilide is eliminated in the kidney by cationic secretion; co-administration with inhibtors of renal cationic transport system, such as prochlorperazine, may increase plasma levels; concurrent use is not recommended). Products include:
Compazine 1505

Promethazine Hydrochloride (Dofetilide can cause serious ventricular arrhythmias associated with QT interval prolongation; concomitant use with other drugs that prolong the QT interval, such as phenothiazines, has not been studied and is not recommended). Products include:
Mepergan Injection 3539
Phenergan Injection 3553
Phenergan 3556
Phenergan Syrup 3554
Phenergan with Codeine Syrup 3557
Phenergan with Dextromethorphan Syrup 3559
Phenergan VC Syrup 3560
Phenergan VC with Codeine Syrup 3561

Propafenone Hydrochloride (Class I antiarrhythmic agents should be withheld for at least three half-lives prior to dosing with dofetilide). Products include:
Rythmol Tablets – 150 mg, 225 mg, 300 mg 502

Protriptyline Hydrochloride (Dofetilide can cause serious ventricular arrhythmias associated with QT interval prolongation; concomitant use with other drugs that prolong the QT interval, such as tricyclic antidepressants, has not been studied and is not recommended). Products include:
Vivactil Tablets 2446
Vivactil Tablets 2217

Quinidine Gluconate (Class I antiarrhythmic agents should be withheld for at least three half-lives prior to dosing with dofetilide). Products include:
Quinaglute Dura-Tabs Tablets 978

Quinidine Polygalacturonate (Class I antiarrhythmic agents should be withheld for at least three half-lives prior to dosing with dofetilide).
No products indexed under this heading.

Quinidine Sulfate (Class I antiarrhythmic agents should be withheld for at least three half-lives prior to dosing with dofetilide). Products include:
Quinidex Extentabs 2933

Quinine (Dofetilide is metabolized to a small extent by the CYP4503A4 system; co-administration with inhibitors of this isoenzyme, such as quinine, could increase systemic dofetilide exposure).
No products indexed under this heading.

Ritonavir (Dofetilide is metabolized to a small extent by the CYP4503A4 system; co-administration with inhibitors of this isoenzyme, such as protease inhibitors, could increase systemic dofetilide exposure). Products include:
Kaletra Capsules 471
Kaletra Oral Solution 471
Norvir Capsules 487
Norvir Oral Solution 487

Saquinavir (Dofetilide is metabolized to a small extent by the CYP4503A4 system; co-administration with inhibitors of this isoenzyme, such as protease inhibitors, could increase systemic dofetilide exposure). Products include:
Fortovase Capsules 2970

Saquinavir Mesylate (Dofetilide is metabolized to a small extent by the CYP4503A4 system; co-administration with inhibitors of this isoenzyme, such as protease inhibitors, could increase systemic dofetilide exposure). Products include:
Invirase Capsules 2979

Sertraline Hydrochloride (Dofetilide is metabolized to a small extent by the CYP4503A4 system; co-administration with inhibitors of this isoenzyme, such as serotonin reuptake inhibitors, could increase systemic dofetilide exposure). Products include:
Zoloft 2751

Sotalol Hydrochloride (Class III antiarrhythmic agents, such as sotalol, should be withheld for at least three half-lives prior to dosing with dofetilide). Products include:
Betapace Tablets 950
Betapace AF Tablets 954

Terconazole (Dofetilide is metabolized to a small extent by the CYP4503A4 system; co-administration with inhibitors of this isoenzyme, such as azole antifungal agents, could increase systemic dofetilide exposure). Products include:
Terazol 3 Vaginal Cream 2587
Terazol 3 Vaginal Suppositories 2587
Terazol 7 Vaginal Cream 2587

Thioridazine Hydrochloride (Dofetilide can cause serious ventricular arrhythmias associated with QT interval prolongation; concomitant use with other drugs that prolong the QT interval, such as phenothiazines, has not been studied and is not recommended). Products include:
Thioridazine Hydrochloride Tablets 2289

Torsemide (Hypokalemia and hypomagnesemia may occur with potassium-depleting diuretics, increasing the potential for torsade de pointes). Products include:
Demadex Tablets and Injection 2965

Triamterene (Dofetilide is eliminated in the kidney by cationic secretion; co-administration with drugs that are actively secreted via this route, such as triamterene, should be undertaken with care as they might increase dofetilide levels). Products include:
Dyazide Capsules 1515
Dyrenium Capsules 3458
Maxzide 1008

Trifluoperazine Hydrochloride (Dofetilide can cause serious ventricular arrhythmias associated with QT interval prolongation; concomitant use with other drugs that prolong the QT interval, such as phenothiazines, has not been studied and is not recommended). Products include:
Stelazine 1640

Trimethoprim (Co-administration with trimethoprim alone or in combination with sulfamethoxazole has been shown to increase dofetilide AUC by 103% and Cmax by 93%; concomitant use is contraindicated). Products include:
Bactrim 2949
Septra Suspension 2265
Septra Tablets 2265
Septra DS Tablets 2265

Trimipramine Maleate (Dofetilide can cause serious ventricular arrhythmias associated with QT interval prolongation; concomitant use with other drugs that prolong the QT interval, such as tricyclic antidepressants, has not been studied and is not recommended). Products include:
Surmontil Capsules 3595

Troleandomycin (Dofetilide can cause serious ventricular arrhythmias associated with QT interval prolongation; concomitant use with other drugs that prolong the QT interval, such as certain oral macrolides, has not been studied and is not recommended; Dofetilide is

metabolized to a small extent by the CYP4503A4 system; co-administration with inhibitors of this isoenzyme, such as macrolide antibiotics, could increase systemic dofetilide exposure). Products include:
Tao Capsules 2716

Verapamil Hydrochloride (Co-administration has resulted in increases in dofetilide peak plasma levels of 42%, although overall exposure to dofetilide was not significantly increased; concomitant use is contraindicated). Products include:
Covera-HS Tablets 3199
Isoptin SR Tablets 467
Tarka Tablets 508
Verelan Capsules 3184
Verelan PM Capsules 3186

Zafirlukast (Dofetilide is metabolized to a small extent by the CYP4503A4 system; co-administration with inhibitors of this isoenzyme, such as zafirlukast, could increase systemic dofetilide exposure). Products include:
Accolate Tablets 657

Food Interactions

Grapefruit Juice (Dofetilide is metabolized to a small extent by the CYP4503A4 system; co-administration with inhibitors of this isoenzyme, such as grapefruit juice, could increase systemic dofetilide exposure).

TIMENTIN INJECTION-ADD-VANTAGE VIAL
(Clavulanate Potassium, Ticarcillin Disodium) 1661
See Timentin for Intravenous Administration

TIMENTIN INJECTION-GALAXY CONTAINER
(Clavulanate Potassium, Ticarcillin Disodium) 1664
See Timentin for Intravenous Administration

TIMENTIN INJECTION-PHARMACY BULK PACKAGE
(Clavulanate Potassium, Ticarcillin Disodium) 1666
See Timentin for Intravenous Administration

TIMENTIN FOR INTRAVENOUS ADMINISTRATION
(Clavulanate Potassium, Ticarcillin Disodium) 1658
May interact with:

Probenecid (Interferes with the renal tubular secretion of ticarcillin, thereby increasing serum concentrations and prolonged serum half-life of the antibiotic).
No products indexed under this heading.

TIMOLIDE TABLETS
(Hydrochlorothiazide, Timolol Maleate) 2187
May interact with antihypertensives, catecholamine depleting drugs, corticosteroids, cardiac glycosides, insulin, lithium preparations, non-steroidal anti-inflammatory agents, quinidine, and certain other agents. Compounds in these categories include:

Acebutolol Hydrochloride (Potentiated). Products include:
Sectral Capsules 3589

ACTH (Hypokalemia).
No products indexed under this heading.

Amlodipine Besylate (Potentiated). Products include:
Lotrel Capsules 2370
Norvasc Tablets 2704

Atenolol (Potentiated). Products include:
Tenoretic Tablets 690
Tenormin I.V. Injection 692

Benazepril Hydrochloride (Potentiated). Products include:
Lotensin Tablets 2365
Lotensin HCT Tablets 2367
Lotrel Capsules 2370

Bendroflumethiazide (Potentiated). Products include:
Corzide 40/5 Tablets 2247
Corzide 80/5 Tablets 2247

Betamethasone Acetate (Hypokalemia). Products include:
Celestone Soluspan Injectable Suspension 3097

Betamethasone Sodium Phosphate (Hypokalemia). Products include:
Celestone Soluspan Injectable Suspension 3097

Betaxolol Hydrochloride (Potentiated). Products include:
Betoptic S Ophthalmic Suspension 537

Bisoprolol Fumarate (Potentiated). Products include:
Zebeta Tablets 1885
Ziac Tablets 1887

Candesartan Cilexetil (Potentiated). Products include:
Atacand Tablets 595
Atacand HCT Tablets 597

Captopril (Potentiated). Products include:
Captopril Tablets 2281

Carteolol Hydrochloride (Potentiated). Products include:
Carteolol Hydrochloride Ophthalmic Solution USP, 1% .... ⊙258
Ocupress Ophthalmic Solution, 1% Sterile .... ⊙303

Celecoxib (Reduced diuretic, natriuretic, and antihypertensive effects of Timolide). Products include:
Celebrex Capsules 2676
Celebrex Capsules 2780

Chlorothiazide (Potentiated). Products include:
Aldoclor Tablets 2035
Diuril Oral 2087

Chlorothiazide Sodium (Potentiated). Products include:
Diuril Sodium Intravenous 2086

Chlorthalidone (Potentiated). Products include:
Clorpres Tablets 1002
Combipres Tablets 1040
Tenoretic Tablets 690

Cholestyramine (Cholestyramine resin has potential of binding hydrochlorothiazide and reducing its absorption from the GI tract by up to 85%).
No products indexed under this heading.

Clonidine (Beta adrenergic blocking agents may exacerbate the rebound hypertension which can follow the withdrawal of clonidine). Products include:
Catapres-TTS 1038

Clonidine Hydrochloride (Beta adrenergic blocking agents may exacerbate the rebound hypertension which can follow the withdrawal of clonidine). Products include:
Catapres Tablets 1037
Clorpres Tablets 1002
Combipres Tablets 1040
Duraclon Injection 3057

Colestipol Hydrochloride (Colestipol resin has potential of binding hydrochlorothiazide and reducing its absorption from the GI tract by up to 43%). Products include:
Colestid Tablets 2791

Cortisone Acetate (Hypokalemia). Products include:
Cortone Acetate Injectable Suspension 2059
Cortone Acetate Tablets 2061

Deserpidine (Potentiated; hypotension; marked bradycardia).
No products indexed under this heading.

Deslanoside (Hypokalemia can lead to increased cardiac toxicity of digitalis).
No products indexed under this heading.

Dexamethasone (Hypokalemia). Products include:
Decadron Elixir 2078
Decadron Tablets 2079
TobraDex Ophthalmic Ointment 542
TobraDex Ophthalmic Suspension 541

Dexamethasone Acetate (Hypokalemia).
No products indexed under this heading.

Dexamethasone Sodium Phosphate (Hypokalemia). Products include:
Decadron Phosphate Injection 2081
Decadron Phosphate Sterile Ophthalmic Ointment 2083
Decadron Phosphate Sterile Ophthalmic Solution 2084
NeoDecadron Sterile Ophthalmic Solution 2144

Diazoxide (Potentiated).
No products indexed under this heading.

Diclofenac Potassium (Reduced diuretic, natriuretic, and antihypertensive effects of Timolide). Products include:
Cataflam Tablets 2315

Diclofenac Sodium (Reduced diuretic, natriuretic, and antihypertensive effects of Timolide). Products include:
Arthrotec Tablets 3195
Voltaren Ophthalmic Sterile Ophthalmic Solution .... ⊙312
Voltaren Tablets 2315
Voltaren-XR Tablets 2315

Digitoxin (Hypokalemia can lead to increased cardiac toxicity of digitalis).
No products indexed under this heading.

Digoxin (Hypokalemia can lead to increased cardiac toxicity of digitalis). Products include:
Digitek Tablets 1003
Lanoxicaps Capsules 1574
Lanoxin Injection 1581
Lanoxin Tablets 1587
Lanoxin Elixir Pediatric 1578
Lanoxin Injection Pediatric 1584

Diltiazem Hydrochloride (Left ventricular failure and AV conduction disturbances). Products include:
Cardizem Injectable 1018
Cardizem Lyo-Ject Syringe 1018
Cardizem Monovial 1018
Cardizem CD Capsules 1016
Tiazac Capsules 1378

Doxazosin Mesylate (Potentiated). Products include:
Cardura Tablets 2668

Enalapril Maleate (Potentiated). Products include:
Lexxel Tablets 608
Vaseretic Tablets 2204
Vasotec Tablets 2210

Enalaprilat (Potentiated). Products include:
Enalaprilat Injection 863
Vasotec I.V. Injection 2207

Eprosartan Mesylate (Potentiated). Products include:
Teveten Tablets 3327

Esmolol Hydrochloride (Potentiated). Products include:
Brevibloc Injection 858

Etodolac (Reduced diuretic, natriuretic, and antihypertensive effects of Timolide). Products include:
Lodine 3528
Lodine XL Extended-Release Tablets 3530

Felodipine (Potentiated). Products include:
Lexxel Tablets 608
Plendil Extended-Release Tablets 623

Fenoprofen Calcium (Reduced diuretic, natriuretic, and antihypertensive effects of Timolide).
No products indexed under this heading.

Fludrocortisone Acetate (Hypokalemia). Products include:
Florinef Acetate Tablets 2250

Flurbiprofen (Reduced diuretic, natriuretic, and antihypertensive effects of Timolide).
No products indexed under this heading.

Fosinopril Sodium (Potentiated). Products include:
Monopril Tablets 1091
Monopril HCT 1094

Furosemide (Potentiated). Products include:
Furosemide Tablets 2284

Guanabenz Acetate (Potentiated).
No products indexed under this heading.

Guanethidine Monosulfate (Potentiated).
No products indexed under this heading.

Hydralazine Hydrochloride (Potentiated).
No products indexed under this heading.

Hydrocortisone (Hypokalemia). Products include:
Anusol-HC Cream 2.5% 2237
Cipro HC Otic Suspension 540
Cortaid Intensive Therapy Cream .... ▣717
Cortaid Maximum Strength Cream .... ▣717
Cortisporin Ophthalmic Suspension Sterile .... ⊙297
Cortizone•5 .... ▣699
Cortizone•10 .... ▣699
Cortizone•10 Plus Creme .... ▣700
Cortizone for Kids Creme .... ▣699
Hydrocortone Tablets 2106
Massengill Medicated Soft Cloth Towelette .... ▣753
VōSoL HC Otic Solution 3356

Hydrocortisone Acetate (Hypokalemia). Products include:
Analpram-HC 1338
Anusol HC-1 Hydrocortisone Anti-Itch Cream .... ▣689
Anusol-HC Suppositories 2238
Cortaid .... ▣717
Cortifoam Rectal Foam 3170
Cortisporin-TC Otic Suspension 2246
Hydrocortone Acetate Injectable Suspension 2103
Pramosone 1343
Proctocort Suppositories 2264
ProctoFoam-HC 3177
Terra-Cortril Ophthalmic Suspension 2716

Hydrocortisone Sodium Phosphate (Hypokalemia). Products include:
Hydrocortone Phosphate Injection, Sterile 2105

Hydrocortisone Sodium Succinate (Hypokalemia).
No products indexed under this heading.

Hydroflumethiazide (Potentiated). Products include:
Diucardin Tablets 3494

Ibuprofen (Reduced diuretic, natriuretic, and antihypertensive effects of Timolide). Products include:
Advil .... ▣771
Children's Advil Oral Suspension .... ▣773
Children's Advil Chewable Tablets .... ▣773
Advil Cold and Sinus Caplets .... ▣771
Advil Cold and Sinus Tablets .... ▣771
Advil Flu & Body Ache Caplets .... ▣772
Infants' Advil Drops .... ▣773
Junior Strength Advil Tablets .... ▣773
Junior Strength Advil Chewable Tablets .... ▣773
Advil Migraine Liquigels .... ▣772
Children's Motrin Oral Suspension and Chewable Tablets 2006
Children's Motrin Cold Oral Suspension 2007
Children's Motrin Oral Suspension .... ▣643
Motrin Suspension, Oral Drops, Chewable Tablets, and Caplets 2002

Infants' Motrin Concentrated Drops 2006
Junior Strength Motrin Caplets and Chewable Tablets 2006
Motrin IB Tablets, Caplets, and Gelcaps 2002
Motrin Migraine Pain Caplets 2005
Motrin Sinus Headache Caplets 2005
Vicoprofen Tablets 520

Indapamide (Potentiated). Products include:
Indapamide Tablets 2286

Indomethacin (Reduced diuretic, natriuretic, and antihypertensive effects of Timolide). Products include:
Indocin 2112

Indomethacin Sodium Trihydrate (Reduced diuretic, natriuretic, and antihypertensive effects of Timolide). Products include:
Indocin I.V. 2115

Insulin, Human, Zinc Suspension (Insulin requirements may be altered). Products include:
Humulin L, 100 Units 1937
Humulin U, 100 Units 1943
Novolin L Human Insulin 10 ml Vials 2422

Insulin, Human NPH (Insulin requirements may be altered). Products include:
Humulin N, 100 Units 1939
Humulin N NPH Pen 1940
Novolin N Human Insulin 10 ml Vials 2422
Novolin N PenFill 2423
Novolin N Prefilled Syringe Disposable Insulin Delivery System 2425

Insulin, Human Regular (Insulin requirements may be altered). Products include:
Humulin R Regular (U-500) 1943
Humulin R, 100 Units 1941
Novolin R Human Insulin 10 ml Vials 2423
Novolin R PenFill 2423
Novolin R Prefilled Syringe Disposable Insulin Delivery System 2425
Velosulin BR Human Insulin 10 ml Vials 2435

Insulin, Human Regular and Human NPH Mixture (Insulin requirements may be altered). Products include:
Humulin 50/50, 100 Units 1934
Humulin 70/30, 100 Units 1935
Humulin 70/30 Pen 1936
Novolin 70/30 Human Insulin 10 ml Vials 2421
Novolin 70/30 PenFill 2423
Novolin 70/30 Prefilled Disposable Insulin Delivery System 2425

Insulin, NPH (Insulin requirements may be altered). Products include:
Iletin II, NPH (Pork), 100 Units 1946

Insulin, Regular (Insulin requirements may be altered). Products include:
Iletin II, Regular (Pork), 100 Units 1947

Insulin, Zinc Crystals (Insulin requirements may be altered).
No products indexed under this heading.

Insulin, Zinc Suspension (Insulin requirements may be altered). Products include:
Iletin II, Lente (Pork), 100 Units 1945

Insulin Aspart, Human Regular (Insulin requirements may be altered).
No products indexed under this heading.

Insulin glargine (Insulin requirements may be altered). Products include:
Lantus Injection 742

Insulin Lispro, Human (Insulin requirements may be altered). Products include:
Humalog 1926
Humalog Mix 75/25 Pen 1928

Insulin Lispro Protamine, Human (Insulin requirements may be altered). Products include:
Humalog Mix 75/25 Pen 1928

Irbesartan (Potentiated). Products include:
Avalide Tablets 1070
Avapro Tablets 1074
Avapro Tablets 3076

Isradipine (Potentiated). Products include:
DynaCirc Capsules 2921
DynaCirc CR Tablets 2923

Ketoprofen (Reduced diuretic, natriuretic, and antihypertensive effects of Timolide). Products include:
Orudis Capsules 3548
Orudis KT Tablets .... ⊡778
Oruvail Capsules 3548

Ketorolac Tromethamine (Reduced diuretic, natriuretic, and antihypertensive effects of Timolide). Products include:
Acular Ophthalmic Solution 544
Acular PF Ophthalmic Solution 544
Toradol 3018

Labetalol Hydrochloride (Potentiated). Products include:
Normodyne Injection 3135
Normodyne Tablets 3137

Lisinopril (Potentiated). Products include:
Prinivil Tablets 2164
Prinzide Tablets 2168
Zestoretic Tablets 695
Zestril Tablets 698

Lithium Carbonate (High risk of lithium toxicity). Products include:
Eskalith 1527
Lithium Carbonate 3061
Lithobid Slow-Release Tablets 3255

Lithium Citrate (High risk of lithium toxicity). Products include:
Lithium Citrate Syrup 3061

Losartan Potassium (Potentiated). Products include:
Cozaar Tablets 2067
Hyzaar 2109

Mecamylamine Hydrochloride (Potentiated). Products include:
Inversine Tablets 1850

Meclofenamate Sodium (Reduced diuretic, natriuretic, and antihypertensive effects of Timolide).
No products indexed under this heading.

Mefenamic Acid (Reduced diuretic, natriuretic, and antihypertensive effects of Timolide). Products include:
Ponstel Capsules 1356

Meloxicam (Reduced diuretic, natriuretic, and antihypertensive effects of Timolide). Products include:
Mobic Tablets 1054

Methyclothiazide (Potentiated).
No products indexed under this heading.

Methyldopa (Potentiated). Products include:
Aldoclor Tablets 2035
Aldomet Tablets 2037
Aldoril Tablets 2039

Methyldopate Hydrochloride (Potentiated).
No products indexed under this heading.

Methylprednisolone (Hypokalemia).
No products indexed under this heading.

Methylprednisolone Acetate (Hypokalemia). Products include:
Depo-Medrol Injectable Suspension 2795

Methylprednisolone Sodium Succinate (Hypokalemia). Products include:
Solu-Medrol Sterile Powder 2855

Metolazone (Potentiated). Products include:
Mykrox Tablets 1168
Zaroxolyn Tablets 1177

Metoprolol Succinate (Potentiated). Products include:
Toprol-XL Tablets 651

Metoprolol Tartrate (Potentiated).
No products indexed under this heading.

Metyrosine (Potentiated). Products include:
Demser Capsules 2085

Mibefradil Dihydrochloride (Potentiated).
No products indexed under this heading.

Minoxidil (Potentiated). Products include:
Rogaine Extra Strength for Men Topical Solution .... ⊡721
Rogaine for Women Topical Solution .... ⊡721

Moexipril Hydrochloride (Potentiated). Products include:
Uniretic Tablets 3178
Univasc Tablets 3181

Nabumetone (Reduced diuretic, natriuretic, and antihypertensive effects of Timolide). Products include:
Relafen Tablets 1617

Nadolol (Potentiated). Products include:
Corgard Tablets 2245
Corzide 40/5 Tablets 2247
Corzide 80/5 Tablets 2247
Nadolol Tablets 2288

Naproxen (Reduced diuretic, natriuretic, and antihypertensive effects of Timolide). Products include:
EC-Naprosyn Delayed-Release Tablets 2967
Naprosyn Suspension 2967
Naprosyn Tablets 2967

Naproxen Sodium (Reduced diuretic, natriuretic, and antihypertensive effects of Timolide). Products include:
Aleve Tablets, Caplets and Gelcaps .... ⊡602
Aleve Cold & Sinus Caplets .... ⊡603
Anaprox Tablets 2967
Anaprox DS Tablets 2967
Naprelan Tablets 1293

Nicardipine Hydrochloride (Potentiated). Products include:
Cardene I.V. 3485

Nifedipine (Potentiated). Products include:
Adalat CC Tablets 877
Procardia Capsules 2708
Procardia XL Extended Release Tablets 2710

Nisoldipine (Potentiated). Products include:
Sular Tablets 688

Nitroglycerin (Potentiated). Products include:
Nitro-Dur Transdermal Infusion System 3134
Nitro-Dur Transdermal Infusion System 1834
Nitrolingual Pumpspray 1355
Nitrostat Tablets 2658

Norepinephrine Bitartrate (Decreased arterial responsiveness to norepinephrine).
No products indexed under this heading.

Oxaprozin (Reduced diuretic, natriuretic, and antihypertensive effects of Timolide).
No products indexed under this heading.

Penbutolol Sulfate (Potentiated).
No products indexed under this heading.

Perindopril Erbumine (Potentiated). Products include:
Aceon Tablets (2 mg, 4 mg, 8 mg) 3249

Phenoxybenzamine Hydrochloride (Potentiated). Products include:
Dibenzyline Capsules 3457

Phentolamine Mesylate (Potentiated).
No products indexed under this heading.

Phenylbutazone (Reduced diuretic, natriuretic, and antihypertensive effects of Timolide).
No products indexed under this heading.

Pindolol (Potentiated).
No products indexed under this heading.

Piroxicam (Reduced diuretic, natriuretic, and antihypertensive effects of Timolide). Products include:
Feldene Capsules 2685

Polythiazide (Potentiated). Products include:
Minizide Capsules 2700
Renese Tablets 2712

Prazosin Hydrochloride (Potentiated). Products include:
Minipress Capsules 2699
Minizide Capsules 2700

Prednisolone Acetate (Hypokalemia). Products include:
Blephamide Ophthalmic Ointment 547
Blephamide Ophthalmic Suspension 548
Poly-Pred Liquifilm Ophthalmic Suspension .... ⊙245
Pred Forte Ophthalmic Suspension .... ⊙246
Pred Mild Sterile Ophthalmic Suspension .... ⊙249
Pred-G Ophthalmic Suspension .... ⊙247
Pred-G Sterile Ophthalmic Ointment .... ⊙248

Prednisolone Sodium Phosphate (Hypokalemia). Products include:
Pediapred Oral Solution 1170

Prednisolone Tebutate (Hypokalemia).
No products indexed under this heading.

Prednisone (Hypokalemia). Products include:
Prednisone 3064

Propranolol Hydrochloride (Potentiated). Products include:
Inderal 3513
Inderal LA Long-Acting Capsules 3516
Inderide Tablets 3517
Inderide LA Long-Acting Capsules 3519

Quinapril Hydrochloride (Potentiated). Products include:
Accupril Tablets 2611
Accuretic Tablets 2614

Quinidine Gluconate (Co-administration has resulted in potentiated systemic beta-blockade, e.g., decreased heart rate). Products include:
Quinaglute Dura-Tabs Tablets 978

Quinidine Polygalacturonate (Co-administration has resulted in potentiated systemic beta-blockade, e.g., decreased heart rate).
No products indexed under this heading.

Quinidine Sulfate (Co-administration has resulted in potentiated systemic beta-blockade, e.g., decreased heart rate). Products include:
Quinidex Extentabs 2933

Ramipril (Potentiated). Products include:
Altace Capsules 2233

Rauwolfia serpentina (Potentiated; hypotension; marked bradycardia).
No products indexed under this heading.

Rescinnamine (Potentiated; hypotension; marked bradycardia).
No products indexed under this heading.

Reserpine (Potentiated; hypotension; marked bradycardia).
No products indexed under this heading.

Rofecoxib (Reduced diuretic, natriuretic, and antihypertensive effects of Timolide). Products include:
Vioxx 2213

Sodium Nitroprusside (Potentiated).
No products indexed under this heading.

Sotalol Hydrochloride (Potentiated). Products include:
Betapace Tablets ... 950
Betapace AF Tablets ... 954

Spirapril Hydrochloride (Potentiated).
No products indexed under this heading.

Sulindac (Reduced diuretic, natriuretic, and antihypertensive effects of Timolide). Products include:
Clinoril Tablets ... 2053

Telmisartan (Potentiated). Products include:
Micardis Tablets ... 1049
Micardis HCT Tablets ... 1051

Terazosin Hydrochloride (Potentiation of other antihypertensives). Products include:
Hytrin Capsules ... 464

Tolmetin Sodium (Reduced diuretic, natriuretic, and antihypertensive effects of Timolide). Products include:
Tolectin ... 2589

Torsemide (Potentiated). Products include:
Demadex Tablets and Injection ... 2965

Trandolapril (Potentiated). Products include:
Mavik Tablets ... 478
Tarka Tablets ... 508

Triamcinolone (Hypokalemia).
No products indexed under this heading.

Triamcinolone Acetonide (Hypokalemia). Products include:
Azmacort Inhalation Aerosol ... 728
Nasacort Nasal Inhaler ... 750
Nasacort AQ Nasal Spray ... 752
Tri-Nasal Spray ... 2274

Triamcinolone Diacetate (Hypokalemia).
No products indexed under this heading.

Triamcinolone Hexacetonide (Hypokalemia).
No products indexed under this heading.

Trimethaphan Camsylate (Potentiated).
No products indexed under this heading.

Tubocurarine Chloride (Increased responsiveness to tubocurarine).
No products indexed under this heading.

Valsartan (Potentiated). Products include:
Diovan Capsules ... 2337
Diovan HCT Tablets ... 2338

Vorapamil Hydrochloride (Left ventricular failure and AV conduction disturbances). Products include:
Covera-HS Tablets ... 3199
Isoptin SR Tablets ... 467
Tarka Tablets ... 508
Verelan Capsules ... 3184
Verelan PM Capsules ... 3186

TIMOLOL GFS

(Timolol Maleate) ... ⊙266
May interact with beta blockers, catecholamine depleting drugs, calcium channel blockers, cardiac glycosides, oral hypoglycemic agents, insulin, quinidine, and certain other agents. Compounds in these categories include:

Acarbose (Beta blocking agents, usually systemic, may mask the signs and symptoms of acute hypoglycemia). Products include:
Precose Tablets ... 906

Acebutolol Hydrochloride (Co-administration with systemic beta blockers may result in additive effects of beta blockade, both systemic and intraocular). Products include:
Sectral Capsules ... 3589

Amlodipine Besylate (Possible atrioventricular conduction disturbances, left ventricular failure, or hypotension when used concurrently). Products include:
Lotrel Capsules ... 2370
Norvasc Tablets ... 2704

Atenolol (Co-administration with systemic beta blockers may result in additive effects of beta blockade, both systemic and intraocular). Products include:
Tenoretic Tablets ... 690
Tenormin I.V. Injection ... 692

Bepridil Hydrochloride (Possible atrioventricular conduction disturbances, left ventricular failure, or hypotension when used concurrently). Products include:
Vascor Tablets ... 2602

Betaxolol Hydrochloride (Co-administration with systemic beta blockers may result in additive effects of beta blockade, both systemic and intraocular). Products include:
Betoptic S Ophthalmic Suspension ... 537

Bisoprolol Fumarate (Co-administration with systemic beta blockers may result in additive effects of beta blockade, both systemic and intraocular). Products include:
Zebeta Tablets ... 1885
Ziac Tablets ... 1887

Carteolol Hydrochloride (Co-administration with systemic beta blockers may result in additive effects of beta blockade, both systemic and intraocular). Products include:
Carteolol Hydrochloride Ophthalmic Solution USP, 1% ... ⊙258
Ocupress Ophthalmic Solution, 1% Sterile ... ⊙303

Chlorpropamide (Beta blocking agents, usually systemic, may mask the signs and symptoms of acute hypoglycemia). Products include:
Diabinese Tablets ... 2680

Deserpidine (Possible additive effects and the production of hypotension and/or bradycardia).
No products indexed under this heading.

Deslanoside (Co-administration with digitalis and calcium antagonists may have additive effects in prolonging atrioventricular conduction time).
No products indexed under this heading.

Digitoxin (Co-administration with digitalis and calcium antagonists may have additive effects in prolonging atrioventricular conduction time).
No products indexed under this heading.

Digoxin (Co-administration with digitalis and calcium antagonists may have additive effects in prolonging atrioventricular conduction time). Products include:
Digitek Tablets ... 1003
Lanoxicaps Capsules ... 1574
Lanoxin Injection ... 1581
Lanoxin Tablets ... 1587
Lanoxin Elixir Pediatric ... 1578
Lanoxin Injection Pediatric ... 1584

Diltiazem Hydrochloride (Possible atrioventricular conduction disturbances, left ventricular failure, or hypotension when used concurrently). Products include:
Cardizem Injectable ... 1018
Cardizem Lyo-Ject Syringe ... 1018
Cardizem Monovial ... 1018
Cardizem CD Capsules ... 1016
Tiazac Capsules ... 1378

Epinephrine (Patients with a history of atopy or anaphylactic reactions to a variety of allergens may be unresponsive to the usual dose of injectable epinephrine used to treat allergic reactions). Products include:
Epifrin Sterile Ophthalmic Solution ... ⊙235
EpiPen ... 1236
Primatene Mist ... ▣779
Xylocaine with Epinephrine Injection ... 653

Epinephrine Hydrochloride (Patients with a history of atopy or anaphylactic reactions to a variety of allergens may be unresponsive to the usual dose of injectable epinephrine used to treat allergic reactions).
No products indexed under this heading.

Esmolol Hydrochloride (Co-administration with systemic beta blockers may result in additive effects of beta blockade, both systemic and intraocular). Products include:
Brevibloc Injection ... 858

Felodipine (Possible atrioventricular conduction disturbances, left ventricular failure, or hypotension when used concurrently). Products include:
Lexxel Tablets ... 608
Plendil Extended-Release Tablets ... 623

Glimepiride (Beta blocking agents, usually systemic, may mask the signs and symptoms of acute hypoglycemia). Products include:
Amaryl Tablets ... 717

Glipizide (Beta blocking agents, usually systemic, may mask the signs and symptoms of acute hypoglycemia). Products include:
Glucotrol Tablets ... 2692
Glucotrol XL Extended Release Tablets ... 2693

Glyburide (Beta blocking agents, usually systemic, may mask the signs and symptoms of acute hypoglycemia). Products include:
DiaBeta Tablets ... 741
Glucovance Tablets ... 1086

Guanethidine Monosulfate (Possible additive effects and the production of hypotension and/or bradycardia).
No products indexed under this heading.

Insulin, Human, Zinc Suspension (Beta blocking agents, usually systemic, may mask the signs and symptoms of acute hypoglycemia). Products include:
Humulin L, 100 Units ... 1937
Humulin U, 100 Units ... 1943
Novolin L Human Insulin 10 ml Vials ... 2422

Insulin, Human NPH (Beta blocking agents, usually systemic, may mask the signs and symptoms of acute hypoglycemia). Products include:
Humulin N, 100 Units ... 1939
Humulin N NPH Pen ... 1940
Novolin N Human Insulin 10 ml Vials ... 2422
Novolin N PenFill ... 2423
Novolin N Prefilled Syringe Disposable Insulin Delivery System ... 2425

Insulin, Human Regular (Beta blocking agents, usually systemic, may mask the signs and symptoms of acute hypoglycemia). Products include:
Humulin R Regular (U-500) ... 1943
Humulin R, 100 Units ... 1941
Novolin R Human Insulin 10 ml Vials ... 2423
Novolin R PenFill ... 2423
Novolin R Prefilled Syringe Disposable Insulin Delivery System ... 2425
Velosulin BR Human Insulin 10 ml Vials ... 2435

Insulin, Human Regular and Human NPH Mixture (Beta blocking agents, usually systemic, may mask the signs and symptoms of acute hypoglycemia). Products include:
Humulin 50/50, 100 Units ... 1934
Humulin 70/30, 100 Units ... 1935
Humulin 70/30 Pen ... 1936
Novolin 70/30 Human Insulin 10 ml Vials ... 2421
Novolin 70/30 PenFill ... 2423
Novolin 70/30 Prefilled Disposable Insulin Delivery System ... 2425

Insulin, NPH (Beta blocking agents, usually systemic, may mask the signs and symptoms of acute hypoglycemia). Products include:
Iletin II, NPH (Pork), 100 Units ... 1946

Insulin, Regular (Beta blocking agents, usually systemic, may mask the signs and symptoms of acute hypoglycemia). Products include:
Iletin II, Regular (Pork), 100 Units ... 1947

Insulin, Zinc Crystals (Beta blocking agents, usually systemic, may mask the signs and symptoms of acute hypoglycemia).
No products indexed under this heading.

Insulin, Zinc Suspension (Beta blocking agents, usually systemic, may mask the signs and symptoms of acute hypoglycemia). Products include:
Iletin II, Lente (Pork), 100 Units ... 1945

Insulin Aspart, Human Regular (Beta blocking agents, usually systemic, may mask the signs and symptoms of acute hypoglycemia).
No products indexed under this heading.

Insulin glargine (Beta blocking agents, usually systemic, may mask the signs and symptoms of acute hypoglycemia). Products include:
Lantus Injection ... 742

Insulin Lispro, Human (Beta blocking agents, usually systemic, may mask the signs and symptoms of acute hypoglycemia). Products include:
Humalog ... 1926
Humalog Mix 75/25 Pen ... 1928

Insulin Lispro Protamine, Human (Beta blocking agents, usually systemic, may mask the signs and symptoms of acute hypoglycemia). Products include:
Humalog Mix 75/25 Pen ... 1928

Isradipine (Possible atrioventricular conduction disturbances, left ventricular failure, or hypotension when used concurrently). Products include:
DynaCirc Capsules ... 2921
DynaCirc CR Tablets ... 2923

Labetalol Hydrochloride (Co-administration with systemic beta blockers may result in additive effects of beta blockade, both systemic and intraocular). Products include:
Normodyne Injection ... 3135
Normodyne Tablets ... 3137

Levobunolol Hydrochloride (Co-administration with systemic beta blockers may result in additive effects of beta blockade, both systemic and intraocular). Products include:
Betagan ... ⊙228

Metformin Hydrochloride (Beta blocking agents, usually systemic, may mask the signs and symptoms of acute hypoglycemia). Products include:
Glucophage Tablets ... 1080
Glucophage XR Tablets ... 1080
Glucovance Tablets ... 1086

Metipranolol Hydrochloride (Co-administration with systemic beta blockers may result in additive effects of beta blockade, both systemic and intraocular).
No products indexed under this heading.

Metoprolol Succinate (Co-administration with systemic beta blockers may result in additive effects of beta blockade, both systemic and intraocular). Products include:
Toprol-XL Tablets ... 651

Metoprolol Tartrate (Co-administration with systemic beta blockers may result in additive effects of beta blockade, both systemic and intraocular).
No products indexed under this heading.

Mibefradil Dihydrochloride (Possible atrioventricular conduction disturbances, left ventricular failure, or hypotension when used concurrently).
No products indexed under this heading.

Miglitol (Beta blocking agents, usually systemic, may mask the signs and symptoms of acute hypoglycemia). Products include:
Glyset Tablets 2821

Nadolol (Co-administration with systemic beta blockers may result in additive effects of beta blockade, both systemic and intraocular). Products include:
Corgard Tablets 2245
Corzide 40/5 Tablets 2247
Corzide 80/5 Tablets 2247
Nadolol Tablets 2288

Nicardipine Hydrochloride (Possible atrioventricular conduction disturbances, left ventricular failure, or hypotension when used concurrently). Products include:
Cardene I.V. 3485

Nifedipine (Possible atrioventricular conduction disturbances, left ventricular failure, or hypotension when used concurrently). Products include:
Adalat CC Tablets 877
Procardia Capsules 2708
Procardia XL Extended Release Tablets 2710

Nimodipine (Possible atrioventricular conduction disturbances, left ventricular failure, or hypotension when used concurrently). Products include:
Nimotop Capsules 904

Nisoldipine (Possible atrioventricular conduction disturbances, left ventricular failure, or hypotension when used concurrently). Products include:
Sular Tablets 688

Penbutolol Sulfate (Co-administration with systemic beta blockers may result in additive effects of beta blockade, both systemic and intraocular).
No products indexed under this heading.

Pindolol (Co-administration with systemic beta blockers may result in additive effects of beta blockade, both systemic and intraocular).
No products indexed under this heading.

Pioglitazone Hydrochloride (Beta blocking agents, usually systemic, may mask the signs and symptoms of acute hypoglycemia). Products include:
Actos Tablets 3275

Propranolol Hydrochloride (Co-administration with systemic beta blockers may result in additive effects of beta blockade, both systemic and intraocular). Products include:
Inderal 3513
Inderal LA Long-Acting Capsules 3516
Inderide Tablets 3517
Inderide LA Long-Acting Capsules 3519

Quinidine Gluconate (Co-administration has resulted in potentiated systemic beta blockade, e.g., decreased heart rate). Products include:
Quinaglute Dura-Tabs Tablets 978

Quinidine Polygalacturonate (Co-administration has resulted in potentiated systemic beta blockade, e.g., decreased heart rate).
No products indexed under this heading.

Quinidine Sulfate (Co-administration has resulted in potentiated systemic beta blockade, e.g., decreased heart rate). Products include:
Quinidex Extentabs 2933

Rauwolfia serpentina (Possible additive effects and the production of hypotension and/or bradycardia).
No products indexed under this heading.

Repaglinide (Beta blocking agents, usually systemic, may mask the signs and symptoms of acute hypoglycemia). Products include:
Prandin Tablets (0.5, 1, and 2 mg) 2432

Rescinnamine (Possible additive effects and the production of hypotension and/or bradycardia).
No products indexed under this heading.

Reserpine (Possible additive effects and the production of hypotension and/or bradycardia).
No products indexed under this heading.

Rosiglitazone Maleate (Beta blocking agents, usually systemic, may mask the signs and symptoms of acute hypoglycemia). Products include:
Avandia Tablets 1490

Sotalol Hydrochloride (Co-administration with systemic beta blockers may result in additive effects of beta blockade, both systemic and intraocular). Products include:
Betapace Tablets 950
Betapace AF Tablets 954

Timolol Hemihydrate (Co-administration with systemic beta blockers may result in additive effects of beta blockade, both systemic and intraocular). Products include:
Betimol Ophthalmic Solution .... ⊙324

Tolazamide (Beta blocking agents, usually systemic, may mask the signs and symptoms of acute hypoglycemia).
No products indexed under this heading.

Tolbutamide (Beta blocking agents, usually systemic, may mask the signs and symptoms of acute hypoglycemia).
No products indexed under this heading.

Troglitazone (Beta blocking agents, usually systemic, may mask the signs and symptoms of acute hypoglycemia).
No products indexed under this heading.

Verapamil Hydrochloride (Possible atrioventricular conduction disturbances, left ventricular failure, or hypotension when used concurrently). Products include:
Covera-HS Tablets 3199
Isoptin SR Tablets 467
Tarka Tablets 508
Verelan Capsules 3184
Verelan PM Capsules 3186

TIMOPTIC IN OCUDOSE

(Timolol Maleate) 2192
May interact with beta blockers, catecholamine depleting drugs, calcium channel blockers, cardiac glycosides, oral hypoglycemic agents, insulin, quinidine, and certain other agents. Compounds in these categories include:

Acarbose (Beta blocking agents, usually systemic, may mask the sign and symptoms of acute hypoglycemia). Products include:
Precose Tablets 906

Acebutolol Hydrochloride (Concurrent use with systemic beta blocker may have additive effects of beta blockade, both systemic and on intraocular pressure). Products include:
Sectral Capsules 3589

Amlodipine Besylate (Possible atrioventricular conduction disturbances, left ventricular failure, or hypotension when used concurrently). Products include:
Lotrel Capsules 2370
Norvasc Tablets 2704

Atenolol (Concurrent use with systemic beta blocker may have additive effects of beta blockade, both systemic and on intraocular pressure). Products include:
Tenoretic Tablets 690
Tenormin I.V. Injection 692

Bepridil Hydrochloride (Possible atrioventricular conduction disturbances, left ventricular failure, or hypotension when used concurrently). Products include:
Vascor Tablets 2602

Betaxolol Hydrochloride (Concurrent use with systemic beta blocker may have additive effects of beta blockade, both systemic and on intraocular pressure; concurrent use of two topical beta blockers is not recommended). Products include:
Betoptic S Ophthalmic Suspension 537

Bisoprolol Fumarate (Concurrent use with systemic beta blocker may have additive effects of beta blockade, both systemic and on intraocular pressure). Products include:
Zebeta Tablets 1885
Ziac Tablets 1887

Carteolol Hydrochloride (Concurrent use with systemic beta blocker may have additive effects of beta blockade, both systemic and on intraocular pressure; concurrent use of two topical beta blockers is not recommended). Products include:
Carteolol Hydrochloride Ophthalmic Solution USP, 1% .... ⊙258
Ocupress Ophthalmic Solution, 1% Sterile .... ⊙303

Chlorpropamide (Beta blocking agents, usually systemic, may mask the sign and symptoms of acute hypoglycemia). Products include:
Diabinese Tablets 2680

Clonidine (Oral beta-adrenergic blocking agents may exacerbate the rebound hypertension which can follow the withdrawal of clonidine; there have been no reports of exacerbation of rebound hypertension with ophthalmic timolol). Products include:
Catapres-TTS 1038

Clonidine Hydrochloride (Oral beta-adrenergic blocking agents may exacerbate the rebound hypertension which can follow the withdrawal of clonidine; there have been no reports of exacerbation of rebound hypertension with ophthalmic timolol). Products include:
Catapres Tablets 1037
Clorpres Tablets 1002
Combipres Tablets 1040
Duraclon Injection 3057

Deserpidine (Possible additive effects and the production of hypotension and/or bradycardia).
No products indexed under this heading.

Deslanoside (Co-administration with digitalis and calcium antagonists may have additive effects in prolonging atrioventricular conduction time).
No products indexed under this heading.

Digitoxin (Co-administration with digitalis and calcium antagonists may have additive effects in prolonging atrioventricular conduction time).
No products indexed under this heading.

Digoxin (Co-administration with digitalis and calcium antagonists may have additive effects in prolonging atrioventricular conduction time). Products include:
Digitek Tablets 1003
Lanoxicaps Capsules 1574
Lanoxin Injection 1581
Lanoxin Tablets 1587
Lanoxin Elixir Pediatric 1578
Lanoxin Injection Pediatric 1584

Diltiazem Hydrochloride (Possible atrioventricular conduction disturbances, left ventricular failure, or hypotension when used concurrently). Products include:
Cardizem Injectable 1018
Cardizem Lyo-Ject Syringe 1018
Cardizem Monovial 1018
Cardizem CD Capsules 1016
Tiazac Capsules 1378

Epinephrine (Patients with a history of atopy or anaphylactic reactions to a variety of allergens may be unresponsive to the usual dose of injectable epinephrine used to treat allergic reactions). Products include:
Epifrin Sterile Ophthalmic Solution .... ⊙235
EpiPen 1236
Primatene Mist .... ◼779
Xylocaine with Epinephrine Injection 653

Epinephrine Bitartrate (Patients with a history of atopy or anaphylactic reactions to a variety of allergens may be unresponsive to the usual dose of injectable epinephrine used to treat allergic reactions). Products include:
Sensorcaine 643

Esmolol Hydrochloride (Concurrent use with systemic beta blocker may have additive effects of beta blockade, both systemic and on intraocular pressure). Products include:
Brevibloc Injection 858

Felodipine (Possible atrioventricular conduction disturbances, left ventricular failure, or hypotension when used concurrently). Products include:
Lexxel Tablets 608
Plendil Extended-Release Tablets 623

Glimepiride (Beta blocking agents, usually systemic, may mask the sign and symptoms of acute hypoglycemia). Products include:
Amaryl Tablets 717

Glipizide (Beta blocking agents, usually systemic, may mask the sign and symptoms of acute hypoglycemia). Products include:
Glucotrol Tablets 2692
Glucotrol XL Extended Release Tablets 2693

Glyburide (Beta blocking agents, usually systemic, may mask the sign and symptoms of acute hypoglycemia). Products include:
DiaBeta Tablets 741
Glucovance Tablets 1086

Guanethidine Monosulfate (Possible additive effects and the production of hypotension and/or bradycardia).
No products indexed under this heading.

Insulin, Human, Zinc Suspension (Beta blocking agents, usually systemic, may mask the sign and symptoms of acute hypoglycemia). Products include:
Humulin L, 100 Units 1937
Humulin U, 100 Units 1943
Novolin L Human Insulin 10 ml Vials 2422

Insulin, Human NPH (Beta blocking agents, usually systemic, may mask the sign and symptoms of acute hypoglycemia). Products include:
Humulin N, 100 Units 1939
Humulin N NPH Pen 1940
Novolin N Human Insulin 10 ml Vials 2422

IMPORTANT NOTE: Always consult each drug listing in the patient's regimen for possible interactions.

Novolin N PenFill 2423
Novolin N Prefilled Syringe Disposable Insulin Delivery System 2425

Insulin, Human Regular (Beta blocking agents, usually systemic, may mask the sign and symptoms of acute hypoglycemia). Products include:
Humulin R Regular (U-500) 1943
Humulin R, 100 Units 1941
Novolin R Human Insulin 10 ml Vials 2423
Novolin R PenFill 2423
Novolin R Prefilled Syringe Disposable Insulin Delivery System 2425
Velosulin BR Human Insulin 10 ml Vials 2435

Insulin, Human Regular and Human NPH Mixture (Beta blocking agents, usually systemic, may mask the sign and symptoms of acute hypoglycemia). Products include:
Humulin 50/50, 100 Units 1934
Humulin 70/30, 100 Units 1935
Humulin 70/30 Pen 1936
Novolin 70/30 Human Insulin 10 ml Vials 2421
Novolin 70/30 PenFill 2423
Novolin 70/30 Prefilled Disposable Insulin Delivery System 2425

Insulin, NPH (Beta blocking agents, usually systemic, may mask the sign and symptoms of acute hypoglycemia). Products include:
Iletin II, NPH (Pork), 100 Units 1946

Insulin, Regular (Beta blocking agents, usually systemic, may mask the sign and symptoms of acute hypoglycemia). Products include:
Iletin II, Regular (Pork), 100 Units 1947

Insulin, Zinc Crystals (Beta blocking agents, usually systemic, may mask the sign and symptoms of acute hypoglycemia).
No products indexed under this heading.

Insulin, Zinc Suspension (Beta blocking agents, usually systemic, may mask the sign and symptoms of acute hypoglycemia). Products include:
Iletin II, Lente (Pork), 100 Units 1945

Insulin Aspart, Human Regular (Beta blocking agents, usually systemic, may mask the sign and symptoms of acute hypoglycemia).
No products indexed under this heading.

Insulin glargine (Beta blocking agents, usually systemic, may mask the sign and symptoms of acute hypoglycemia). Products include:
Lantus Injection 742

Insulin Lispro, Human (Beta blocking agents, usually systemic, may mask the sign and symptoms of acute hypoglycemia). Products include:
Humalog 1926
Humalog Mix 75/25 Pen 1928

Insulin Lispro Protamine, Human (Beta blocking agents, usually systemic, may mask the sign and symptoms of acute hypoglycemia). Products include:
Humalog Mix 75/25 Pen 1928

Isradipine (Possible atrioventricular conduction disturbances, left ventricular failure, or hypotension when used concurrently). Products include:
DynaCirc Capsules 2921
DynaCirc CR Tablets 2923

Labetalol Hydrochloride (Concurrent use with systemic beta blocker may have additive effects of beta blockade, both systemic and on intraocular pressure). Products include:
Normodyne Injection 3135
Normodyne Tablets 3137

Levobunolol Hydrochloride (Concurrent use of two topical beta blockers is not recommended). Products include:
Betagan .... ⊙ 228

Metformin Hydrochloride (Beta blocking agents, usually systemic, may mask the sign and symptoms of acute hypoglycemia). Products include:
Glucophage Tablets 1080
Glucophage XR Tablets 1080
Glucovance Tablets 1086

Metipranolol Hydrochloride (Concurrent use of two topical beta blockers is not recommended).
No products indexed under this heading.

Metoprolol Succinate (Concurrent use with systemic beta blocker may have additive effects of beta blockade, both systemic and on intraocular pressure). Products include:
Toprol-XL Tablets 651

Metoprolol Tartrate (Concurrent use with systemic beta blocker may have additive effects of beta blockade, both systemic and on intraocular pressure).
No products indexed under this heading.

Mibefradil Dihydrochloride (Possible atrioventricular conduction disturbances, left ventricular failure, or hypotension when used concurrently).
No products indexed under this heading.

Miglitol (Beta blocking agents, usually systemic, may mask the sign and symptoms of acute hypoglycemia). Products include:
Glyset Tablets 2821

Nadolol (Concurrent use with systemic beta blocker may have additive effects of beta blockade, both systemic and on intraocular pressure). Products include:
Corgard Tablets 2245
Corzide 40/5 Tablets 2247
Corzide 80/5 Tablets 2247
Nadolol Tablets 2288

Nicardipine Hydrochloride (Possible atrioventricular conduction disturbances, left ventricular failure, or hypotension when used concurrently). Products include:
Cardene I.V. 3485

Nifedipine (Possible atrioventricular conduction disturbances, left ventricular failure, or hypotension when used concurrently). Products include:
Adalat CC Tablets 877
Procardia Capsules 2708
Procardia XL Extended Release Tablets 2710

Nimodipine (Possible atrioventricular conduction disturbances, left ventricular failure, or hypotension when used concurrently). Products include:
Nimotop Capsules 904

Nisoldipine (Possible atrioventricular conduction disturbances, left ventricular failure, or hypotension when used concurrently). Products include:
Sular Tablets 688

Penbutolol Sulfate (Concurrent use with systemic beta blocker may have additive effects of beta blockade, both systemic and on intraocular pressure).
No products indexed under this heading.

Pindolol (Concurrent use with systemic beta blocker may have additive effects of beta blockade, both systemic and on intraocular pressure).
No products indexed under this heading.

Pioglitazone Hydrochloride (Beta blocking agents, usually systemic, may mask the sign and symptoms of acute hypoglycemia). Products include:
Actos Tablets 3275

Propranolol Hydrochloride (Concurrent use with systemic beta blocker may have additive effects of beta blockade, both systemic and on intraocular pressure). Products include:
Inderal 3513
Inderal LA Long-Acting Capsules 3516
Inderide Tablets 3517
Inderide LA Long-Acting Capsules 3519

Quinidine Gluconate (Co-administration has resulted in potentiated systemic beta-blockade, e.g., decreased heart rate). Products include:
Quinaglute Dura-Tabs Tablets 978

Quinidine Polygalacturonate (Co-administration has resulted in potentiated systemic beta-blockade, e.g., decreased heart rate).
No products indexed under this heading.

Quinidine Sulfate (Co-administration has resulted in potentiated systemic beta-blockade, e.g., decreased heart rate). Products include:
Quinidex Extentabs 2933

Rauwolfia serpentina (Possible additive effects and the production of hypotension and/or bradycardia).
No products indexed under this heading.

Repaglinide (Beta blocking agents, usually systemic, may mask the sign and symptoms of acute hypoglycemia). Products include:
Prandin Tablets (0.5, 1, and 2 mg) 2432

Rescinnamine (Possible additive effects and the production of hypotension and/or bradycardia).
No products indexed under this heading.

Reserpine (Possible additive effects and the production of hypotension and/or bradycardia).
No products indexed under this heading.

Rosiglitazone Maleate (Beta blocking agents, usually systemic, may mask the sign and symptoms of acute hypoglycemia). Products include:
Avandia Tablets 1490

Sotalol Hydrochloride (Concurrent use with systemic beta blocker may have additive effects of beta blockade, both systemic and on intraocular pressure). Products include:
Betapace Tablets 950
Betapace AF Tablets 954

Timolol Hemihydrate (Concurrent use of two topical beta blockers is not recommended). Products include:
Betimol Ophthalmic Solution .... ⊙ 324

Tolazamide (Beta blocking agents, usually systemic, may mask the sign and symptoms of acute hypoglycemia).
No products indexed under this heading.

Tolbutamide (Beta blocking agents, usually systemic, may mask the sign and symptoms of acute hypoglycemia).
No products indexed under this heading.

Troglitazone (Beta blocking agents, usually systemic, may mask the sign and symptoms of acute hypoglycemia).
No products indexed under this heading.

Verapamil Hydrochloride (Possible atrioventricular conduction disturbances, left ventricular failure, or hypotension when used concurrently). Products include:
Covera-HS Tablets 3199
Isoptin SR Tablets 467
Tarka Tablets 508
Verelan Capsules 3184
Verelan PM Capsules 3186

TIMOPTIC STERILE OPHTHALMIC SOLUTION
(Timolol Maleate) 2190
See Timoptic in Ocudose

TIMOPTIC-XE STERILE OPHTHALMIC GEL FORMING SOLUTION
(Timolol Maleate) 2194
See Timoptic in Ocudose

TINE TEST, TUBERCULIN, OLD
(Tuberculin, Old) 3631
May interact with corticosteroids, immunosuppressive agents, and certain other agents. Compounds in these categories include:

Azathioprine (Reactivity to the test may be suppressed).
No products indexed under this heading.

Basiliximab (Reactivity to the test may be suppressed). Products include:
Simulect for Injection 2399

Betamethasone Acetate (Reactivity to the test may be suppressed). Products include:
Celestone Soluspan Injectable Suspension 3097

Betamethasone Sodium Phosphate (Reactivity to the test may be suppressed). Products include:
Celestone Soluspan Injectable Suspension 3097

Cortisone Acetate (Reactivity to the test may be suppressed). Products include:
Cortone Acetate Injectable Suspension 2059
Cortone Acetate Tablets 2061

Cyclosporine (Reactivity to the test may be suppressed). Products include:
Gengraf Capsules 457
Neoral Soft Gelatin Capsules 2380
Neoral Oral Solution 2380
Sandimmune 2388

Desoximetasone (Reactivity to the test may be suppressed). Products include:
Topicort 2025

Dexamethasone (Reactivity to the test may be suppressed). Products include:
Decadron Elixir 2078
Decadron Tablets 2079
TobraDex Ophthalmic Ointment 542
TobraDex Ophthalmic Suspension 541

Dexamethasone Acetate (Reactivity to the test may be suppressed).
No products indexed under this heading.

Dexamethasone Sodium Phosphate (Reactivity to the test may be suppressed). Products include:
Decadron Phosphate Injection 2081
Decadron Phosphate Sterile Ophthalmic Ointment 2083
Decadron Phosphate Sterile Ophthalmic Solution 2084
NeoDecadron Sterile Ophthalmic Solution 2144

Fludrocortisone Acetate (Reactivity to the test may be suppressed). Products include:
Florinef Acetate Tablets 2250

Hydrocortisone (Reactivity to the test may be suppressed). Products include:
Anusol-HC Cream 2.5% 2237
Cipro HC Otic Suspension 540
Cortaid Intensive Therapy Cream .... ▣ 717
Cortaid Maximum Strength Cream .... ▣ 717
Cortisporin Ophthalmic Suspension Sterile .... ⊙ 297
Cortizone•5 .... ▣ 699

Cortizone•10 .... ■ 699
Cortizone•10 Plus Creme .... ■ 700
Cortizone for Kids Creme .... ■ 699
Hydrocortone Tablets 2106
Massengill Medicated Soft Cloth Towelette.................................. ■ 753
VōSoL HC Otic Solution 3356

Hydrocortisone Acetate (Reactivity to the test may be suppressed). Products include:
Analpram-HC 1338
Anusol HC-1 Hydrocortisone Anti-Itch Cream.............................. ■ 689
Anusol-HC Suppositories 2238
Cortaid .... ■ 717
Cortifoam Rectal Foam 3170
Cortisporin-TC Otic Suspension 2246
Hydrocortone Acetate Injectable Suspension 2103
Pramosone 1343
Proctocort Suppositories 2264
ProctoFoam-HC 3177
Terra-Cortril Ophthalmic Suspension 2716

Hydrocortisone Sodium Phosphate (Reactivity to the test may be suppressed). Products include:
Hydrocortone Phosphate Injection, Sterile 2105

Hydrocortisone Sodium Succinate (Reactivity to the test may be suppressed).
No products indexed under this heading.

Immune Globulin Intravenous (Human) (Reactivity to the test may be suppressed).
No products indexed under this heading.

Methylprednisolone Acetate (Reactivity to the test may be suppressed). Products include:
Depo-Medrol Injectable Suspension 2795

Methylprednisolone Sodium Succinate (Reactivity to the test may be suppressed). Products include:
Solu-Medrol Sterile Powder 2855

Muromonab-CD3 (Reactivity to the test may be suppressed). Products include:
Orthoclone OKT3 Sterile Solution ... 2498

Mycophenolate Mofetil (Reactivity to the test may be suppressed). Products include:
CellCept Capsules 2951
CellCept Oral Suspension 2951
CellCept Tablets 2951

Prednisolone Acetate (Reactivity to the test may be suppressed). Products include:
Blephamide Ophthalmic Ointment .. 547
Blephamide Ophthalmic Suspension 548
Poly-Pred Liquifilm Ophthalmic Suspension .... ⊙ 245
Pred Forte Ophthalmic Suspension .... ⊙ 246
Pred Mild Sterile Ophthalmic Suspension .... ⊙ 249
Pred-G Ophthalmic Suspension ...... ⊙ 247
Pred-G Sterile Ophthalmic Ointment .... ⊙ 248

Prednisolone Sodium Phosphate (Reactivity to the test may be suppressed). Products include:
Pediapred Oral Solution 1170

Prednisolone Tebutate (Reactivity to the test may be suppressed).
No products indexed under this heading.

Prednisone (Reactivity to the test may be suppressed). Products include:
Prednisone 3064

Sirolimus (Reactivity to the test may be suppressed). Products include:
Rapamune Oral Solution and Tablets 3584

Tacrolimus (Reactivity to the test may be suppressed). Products include:
Prograf 1393
Protopic Ointment 1397

Triamcinolone (Reactivity to the test may be suppressed).
No products indexed under this heading.

Triamcinolone Acetonide (Reactivity to the test may be suppressed). Products include:
Azmacort Inhalation Aerosol 728
Nasacort Inhalation Aerosol 728
Nasacort Nasal Inhaler 750
Nasacort AQ Nasal Spray 752
Tri-Nasal Spray 2274

Triamcinolone Diacetate (Reactivity to the test may be suppressed).
No products indexed under this heading.

Triamcinolone Hexacetonide (Reactivity to the test may be suppressed).
No products indexed under this heading.

TISSEEL VH

(Fibrin Sealant) 854
None cited in PDR database.

3M TITRALAC ANTACID TABLETS

(Calcium Carbonate) .... ■ 640
May interact with:

Prescription Drugs, unspecified (Antacids may interact with certain unspecified prescription drugs; consult your physician).

3M TITRALAC EXTRA STRENGTH ANTACID TABLETS

(Calcium Carbonate) .... ■ 640
See 3M Titralac Antacid Tablets

3M TITRALAC PLUS ANTACID TABLETS

(Calcium Carbonate, Simethicone) .... ■ 640
May interact with:

Prescription Drugs, unspecified (Antacids may interact with certain unspecified prescription drugs; consult your physician).

TNKASE I.V.

(Tenecteplase) 1430
May interact with vitamin K antagonists and certain other agents. Compounds in these categories include:

Abciximab (Drugs that alter platelet function, such as abciximab, may increase the risk of bleeding if administered prior to or after tenecteplase therapy). Products include:
ReoPro Vials 1958

Aspirin (Drugs that alter platelet function, such as aspirin, may increase the risk of bleeding if administered prior to or after tenecteplase therapy). Products include:
Aggrenox Capsules 1026
Alka-Seltzer .... ■ 603
Alka-Seltzer Lemon Lime Antacid and Pain Reliever Effervescent Tablets .... ■ 603
Alka-Seltzer Extra Strength Antacid and Pain Reliever Effervescent Tablets .... ■ 603
Alka-Seltzer PM Effervescent Tablets .... ■ 605
Genuine Bayer Tablets, Caplets and Gelcaps .... ■ 606
Extra Strength Bayer Caplets and Gelcaps .... ■ 610
Aspirin Regimen Bayer Children's Chewable Tablets (Orange or Cherry Flavored) .... ■ 607
Bayer, Aspirin Regimen .... ■ 606
Aspirin Regimen Bayer 81 mg Caplets with Calcium .... ■ 607
Genuine Bayer Professional Labeling (Aspirin Regimen Bayer) .... ■ 608
Extra Strength Bayer Arthritis Caplets .... ■ 610
Extra Strength Bayer Plus Caplets .... ■ 610
Extra Strength Bayer PM Caplets .... ■ 611
BC Powder .... ■ 619
BC Allergy Sinus Cold Powder ...... ■ 619
Arthritis Strength BC Powder .... ■ 619
BC Sinus Cold Powder .... ■ 619
Darvon Compound-65 Pulvules 1910
Ecotrin Enteric Coated Aspirin Low, Regular and Maximum Strength Tablets 1715
Excedrin Extra-Strength Tablets, Caplets, and Geltabs .... ■ 629
Excedrin Migraine 1070
Goody's Body Pain Formula Powder .... ■ 620
Goody's Extra Strength Headache Powder .... ■ 620
Goody's Extra Strength Pain Relief Tablets .... ■ 620
Percodan Tablets 1327
Robaxisal Tablets 2939
Soma Compound Tablets 3354
Soma Compound w/Codeine Tablets 3355
Vanquish Caplets .... ■ 617

Clopidogrel Bisulfate (Drugs that alter platelet function, such as clopidogrel, may increase the risk of bleeding if administered prior to or after tenecteplase therapy). Products include:
Plavix Tablets 1097
Plavix Tablets 3084

Dicumarol (Co-administration increases the risk of bleeding).
No products indexed under this heading.

Dipyridamole (Drugs that alter platelet function, such as dipyridamole, may increase the risk of bleeding if administered prior to or after tenecteplase therapy). Products include:
Aggrenox Capsules 1026
Persantine Tablets 1057

Epitifibatide (Drugs that alter platelet function, such as epitifibatide, may increase the risk of bleeding if administered prior to or after tenecteplase therapy).
No products indexed under this heading.

Ticlopidine Hydrochloride (Drugs that alter platelet function, such as ticlopidine, may increase the risk of bleeding if administered prior to or after tenecteplase therapy). Products include:
Ticlid Tablets 3015

Tirofiban Hydrochloride (Drugs that alter platelet function, such as tirofiban, may increase the risk of bleeding if administered prior to or after tenecteplase therapy). Products include:
Aggrastat 2031

Warfarin Sodium (Co-administration increases the risk of bleeding). Products include:
Coumadin for Injection 1243
Coumadin Tablets 1243
Warfarin Sodium Tablets, USP 3302

TOBI SOLUTION FOR INHALATION

(Tobramycin) 1206
May interact with aminoglycosides and certain other agents. Compounds in these categories include:

Amikacin Sulfate (Co-administration in some patients receiving TOBI and extensive previous or concomitant parenteral aminoglycosides has resulted in hearing loss; potential for increased risk of neurotoxicity and/or ototoxicity).
No products indexed under this heading.

Ethacrynic Acid (Some diuretics, such as ethacrynic acid, can enhance aminoglycoside toxicity by altering antibiotic concentrations in serum and tissue; TOBI should not be administered with ethacrynic acid). Products include:
Edecrin Tablets 2091

Furosemide (Some diuretics, such as furosemide, can enhance aminoglycoside toxicity by altering antibiotic concentrations in serum and tissue; TOBI should not be administered with furosemide). Products include:
Furosemide Tablets 2284

Gentamicin Sulfate (Co-administration in some patients receiving TOBI and extensive previous or concomitant parenteral aminoglycosides has resulted in hearing loss; potential for increased risk of neurotoxicity and/or ototoxicity). Products include:
Genoptic Ophthalmic Ointment ...... ⊙ 239
Genoptic Sterile Ophthalmic Solution .... ⊙ 239
Pred-G Ophthalmic Suspension ...... ⊙ 247
Pred-G Sterile Ophthalmic Ointment .... ⊙ 248

Kanamycin Sulfate (Co-administration in some patients receiving TOBI and extensive previous or concomitant parenteral aminoglycosides has resulted in hearing loss; potential for increased risk of neurotoxicity and/or ototoxicity).
No products indexed under this heading.

Mannitol (Some diuretics, such as mannitol, can enhance aminoglycoside toxicity by altering antibiotic concentrations in serum and tissue; TOBI should not be administered with mannitol).
No products indexed under this heading.

Streptomycin Sulfate (Co-administration in some patients receiving TOBI and extensive previous or concomitant parenteral aminoglycosides has resulted in hearing loss; potential for increased risk of neurotoxicity and/or ototoxicity). Products include:
Streptomycin Sulfate Injection 2714

Tobramycin Sulfate (Co-administration in some patients receiving TOBI and extensive previous or concomitant parenteral aminoglycosides has resulted in hearing loss; potential for increased risk of neurotoxicity and/or ototoxicity). Products include:
Nebcin Vials, Hyporets & ADD-Vantage 1955

Urea (Some diuretics, such as systemic urea, can enhance aminoglycoside toxicity by altering antibiotic concentrations in serum and tissue; TOBI should not be administered with urea). Products include:
Accuzyme Debriding Ointment 1725
Amino-Cerv Creme 2231
Panafil Ointment 1726

TOBRADEX OPHTHALMIC OINTMENT

(Dexamethasone, Tobramycin) 542
See TobraDex Ophthalmic Suspension

TOBRADEX OPHTHALMIC SUSPENSION

(Dexamethasone, Tobramycin) 541
May interact with aminoglycosides. Compounds in these categories include:

Amikacin Sulfate (Monitor the total serum concentration if administered with systemic aminoglycoside).
No products indexed under this heading.

Gentamicin Sulfate (Monitor the total serum concentration if administered with systemic aminoglycoside). Products include:
Genoptic Ophthalmic Ointment ...... ⊙ 239
Genoptic Sterile Ophthalmic Solution .... ⊙ 239
Pred-G Ophthalmic Suspension ...... ⊙ 247
Pred-G Sterile Ophthalmic Ointment .... ⊙ 248

Kanamycin Sulfate (Monitor the total serum concentration if administered with systemic aminoglycoside).
No products indexed under this heading.

Streptomycin Sulfate (Monitor the total serum concentration if administered with systemic aminoglycoside). Products include:
- Streptomycin Sulfate Injection 2714

Tobramycin Sulfate (Monitor the total serum concentration if administered with systemic aminoglycoside). Products include:
- Nebcin Vials, Hyporets & ADD-Vantage 1955

TOBREX OPHTHALMIC OINTMENT
(Tobramycin) .... ⊙220
May interact with aminoglycosides. Compounds in these categories include:

Amikacin Sulfate (If topical ocular tobramycin is administered concomitantly with systemic aminoglycosides, care should be taken to monitor the total serum concentration).
No products indexed under this heading.

Gentamicin Sulfate (If topical ocular tobramycin is administered concomitantly with systemic aminoglycosides, care should be taken to monitor the total serum concentration). Products include:
- Genoptic Ophthalmic Ointment .... ⊙239
- Genoptic Sterile Ophthalmic Solution .... ⊙239
- Pred-G Ophthalmic Suspension .... ⊙247
- Pred-G Sterile Ophthalmic Ointment .... ⊙248

Kanamycin Sulfate (If topical ocular tobramycin is administered concomitantly with systemic aminoglycosides, care should be taken to monitor the total serum concentration).
No products indexed under this heading.

Streptomycin Sulfate (If topical ocular tobramycin is administered concomitantly with systemic aminoglycosides, care should be taken to monitor the total serum concentration). Products include:
- Streptomycin Sulfate Injection 2714

Tobramycin Sulfate (If topical ocular tobramycin is administered concomitantly with systemic aminoglycosides, care should be taken to monitor the total serum concentration). Products include:
- Nebcin Vials, Hyporets & ADD-Vantage 1955

TOBREX OPHTHALMIC SOLUTION
(Tobramycin) .... ⊙221
See Tobrex Ophthalmic Ointment

TOLECTIN 200 TABLETS
(Tolmetin Sodium) 2589
May interact with oral anticoagulants and certain other agents. Compounds in these categories include:

Dicumarol (Increased prothrombin time and bleeding).
No products indexed under this heading.

Methotrexate Sodium (Reduced tubular secretion of methotrexate in an animal model).
No products indexed under this heading.

Warfarin Sodium (Increased prothrombin time and bleeding). Products include:
- Coumadin for Injection 1243
- Coumadin Tablets 1243
- Warfarin Sodium Tablets, USP 3302

Food Interactions

Dairy products (Decreases total tolmetin bioavailability by 16%).

Meal, unspecified (Decreases total tolmetin bioavailability by 16%; reduces peak plasma concentrations by 50%).

TOLECTIN 600 TABLETS
(Tolmetin Sodium) 2589
See Tolectin 200 Tablets

TOLECTIN DS CAPSULES
(Tolmetin Sodium) 2589
See Tolectin 200 Tablets

TONOCARD TABLETS
(Tocainide Hydrochloride) 649
May interact with:

Lidocaine Hydrochloride (Co-administration of these pharmacodynamically similar agents may cause an increased incidence of adverse reactions, including CNS adverse reactions such as seizures). Products include:
- Bactine First Aid Liquid .... ▣611
- Xylocaine Injections 653

Metoprolol Succinate (Co-administration has produced additive effects on wedge pressure and cardiac index). Products include:
- Toprol-XL Tablets 651

Metoprolol Tartrate (Co-administration has produced additive effects on wedge pressure and cardiac index).
No products indexed under this heading.

TOPAMAX SPRINKLE CAPSULES
(Topiramate) 2590
See Topamax Tablets

TOPAMAX TABLETS
(Topiramate) 2590
May interact with carbonic anhydrase inhibitors, central nervous system depressants, phenytoin, valproate, and certain other agents. Compounds in these categories include:

Acetazolamide (Co-administration of topiramate with carbonic anhydrase inhibitors may create a physiological environment that increases the risk of kidney stone formation; concurrent use should be avoided). Products include:
- Diamox Sequels Sustained Release Capsules .... ⊙270
- Diamox Tablets .... ⊙269

Alfentanil Hydrochloride (Potential for increased CNS depression).
No products indexed under this heading.

Alprazolam (Potential for increased CNS depression). Products include:
- Xanax Tablets 2865

Aprobarbital (Potential for increased CNS depression).
No products indexed under this heading.

Buprenorphine Hydrochloride (Potential for increased CNS depression). Products include:
- Buprenex Injectable 2918

Buspirone Hydrochloride (Potential for increased CNS depression).
No products indexed under this heading.

Butabarbital (Potential for increased CNS depression).
No products indexed under this heading.

Butalbital (Potential for increased CNS depression). Products include:
- Phrenilin 578
- Sedapap Tablets 50 mg/650 mg 2225

Carbamazepine (Co-administration has resulted in 40% decrease in topiramate concentration and no change in carbamazepine concentration). Products include:
- Carbatrol Capsules 3234
- Tegretol/Tegretol-XR 2404

Chlordiazepoxide (Potential for increased CNS depression). Products include:
- Limbitrol 1738

Chlordiazepoxide Hydrochloride (Potential for increased CNS depression). Products include:
- Librium Capsules 1736
- Librium for Injection 1737

Chlorpromazine (Potential for increased CNS depression). Products include:
- Thorazine Suppositories 1656

Chlorpromazine Hydrochloride (Potential for increased CNS depression). Products include:
- Thorazine 1656

Chlorprothixene (Potential for increased CNS depression).
No products indexed under this heading.

Chlorprothixene Hydrochloride (Potential for increased CNS depression).
No products indexed under this heading.

Chlorprothixene Lactate (Potential for increased CNS depression).
No products indexed under this heading.

Clorazepate Dipotassium (Potential for increased CNS depression). Products include:
- Tranxene 511

Clozapine (Potential for increased CNS depression). Products include:
- Clozaril Tablets 2319

Codeine Phosphate (Potential for increased CNS depression). Products include:
- Phenergan with Codeine Syrup 3557
- Phenergan VC with Codeine Syrup 3561
- Robitussin A-C Syrup 2942
- Robitussin-DAC Syrup 2942
- Ryna-C Liquid .... ▣768
- Soma Compound w/Codeine Tablets 3355
- Tussi-Organidin NR Liquid 3350
- Tussi-Organidin-S NR Liquid 3350
- Tylenol with Codeine 2595

Desflurane (Potential for increased CNS depression). Products include:
- Suprane Liquid for Inhalation 874

Dezocine (Potential for increased CNS depression).
No products indexed under this heading.

Diazepam (Potential for increased CNS depression). Products include:
- Valium Injectable 3026
- Valium Tablets 3047

Dichlorphenamide (Co-administration of topiramate with carbonic anhydrase inhibitors may create a physiological environment that increases the risk of kidney stone formation; concurrent use should be avoided). Products include:
- Daranide Tablets 2077

Digoxin (Co-administration has resulted in decreased serum digoxin AUC by 12%; clinical significance of this interaction is unknown). Products include:
- Digitek Tablets 1003
- Lanoxicaps Capsules 1574
- Lanoxin Injection 1581
- Lanoxin Tablets 1587
- Lanoxin Elixir Pediatric 1578
- Lanoxin Injection Pediatric 1584

Divalproex Sodium (Co-administration has resulted in 11% decrease in valproic acid concentration and 14% decrease in topiramate concentration). Products include:
- Depakote Sprinkle Capsules 426
- Depakote Tablets 430
- Depakote ER Tablets 436

Dorzolamide Hydrochloride (Co-administration of topiramate with carbonic anhydrase inhibitors may create a physiological environment that increases the risk of kidney stone formation; concurrent use should be avoided). Products include:
- Cosopt Sterile Ophthalmic Solution 2065
- Trusopt Sterile Ophthalmic Solution 2196

Droperidol (Potential for increased CNS depression).
No products indexed under this heading.

Enflurane (Potential for increased CNS depression).
No products indexed under this heading.

Estazolam (Potential for increased CNS depression). Products include:
- ProSom Tablets 500

Ethchlorvynol (Potential for increased CNS depression).
No products indexed under this heading.

Ethinamate (Potential for increased CNS depression).
No products indexed under this heading.

Ethinyl Estradiol (Co-administration of topiramate with oral contraceptive containing ethinyl estradiol/norethindrone has resulted in decreased total exposure in the estrogenic component; efficacy of oral contraceptive may be compromised). Products include:
- Alesse-21 Tablets 3468
- Alesse-28 Tablets 3473
- Brevicon 28-Day Tablets 3380
- Cyclessa Tablets 2450
- Desogen Tablets 2458
- Estinyl Tablets 3112
- Estrostep 2627
- femhrt Tablets 2635
- Levlen 962
- Levlite 21 Tablets 962
- Levlite 28 Tablets 962
- Levora Tablets 3389
- Loestrin 21 Tablets 2642
- Loestrin Fe Tablets 2642
- Lo/Ovral Tablets 3532
- Lo/Ovral-28 Tablets 3538
- Low-Ogestrel-28 Tablets 3392
- Microgestin Fe 1.5/30 Tablets 3407
- Microgestin Fe 1/20 Tablets 3400
- Mircette Tablets 2470
- Modicon 2563
- Necon 3415
- Nordette-28 Tablets 2257
- Norinyl 1 +35 28-Day Tablets 3380
- Ogestrel 0.5/50-28 Tablets 3428
- Ortho-Cept 21 Tablets 2546
- Ortho-Cept 28 Tablets 2546
- Ortho-Cyclen/Ortho Tri-Cyclen 2573
- Ortho-Novum 2563
- Ovcon 3364
- Ovral Tablets 3551
- Ovral-28 Tablets 3552
- Tri-Levlen 962
- Tri-Norinyl-28 Tablets 3433
- Triphasil-21 Tablets 3600
- Triphasil-28 Tablets 3605
- Trivora Tablets 3439
- Yasmin 28 Tablets 980
- Zovia 3449

Fentanyl (Potential for increased CNS depression). Products include:
- Duragesic Transdermal System 1786

Fentanyl Citrate (Potential for increased CNS depression). Products include:
- Actiq 1184

Fluphenazine Decanoate (Potential for increased CNS depression).
No products indexed under this heading.

Fluphenazine Enanthate (Potential for increased CNS depression).
No products indexed under this heading.

Fluphenazine Hydrochloride (Potential for increased CNS depression).
No products indexed under this heading.

Flurazepam Hydrochloride (Potential for increased CNS depression).
No products indexed under this heading.

Fosphenytoin Sodium (Co-administration has resulted in 48% decrease in topiramate concentra-

tion and no change or 25% increase in phenytoin concentration). Products include:
Cerebyx Injection 2619

Glutethimide (Potential for increased CNS depression).
No products indexed under this heading.

Haloperidol (Potential for increased CNS depression). Products include:
Haldol Injection, Tablets and Concentrate 2533

Haloperidol Decanoate (Potential for increased CNS depression). Products include:
Haldol Decanoate 2535

Hydrocodone Bitartrate (Potential for increased CNS depression). Products include:
Hycodan 1316
Hycomine Compound Tablets 1317
Hycotuss Expectorant Syrup 1318
Lortab 3319
Lortab Elixir 3317
Maxidone Tablets CIII 3399
Norco 5/325 Tablets CIII 3424
Norco 7.5/325 Tablets CIII 3425
Norco 10/325 Tablets CIII 3427
Norco 10/325 Tablets CIII 3425
Vicodin Tablets 516
Vicodin ES Tablets 517
Vicodin HP Tablets 518
Vicodin Tuss Expectorant 519
Vicoprofen Tablets 520
Zydone Tablets 1330

Hydrocodone Polistirex (Potential for increased CNS depression). Products include:
Tussionex Pennkinetic Extended-Release Suspension 1174

Hydromorphone Hydrochloride (Potential for increased CNS depression). Products include:
Dilaudid 441
Dilaudid Oral Liquid 445
Dilaudid Powder 441
Dilaudid Rectal Suppositories 441
Dilaudid Tablets 441
Dilaudid Tablets - 8 mg 445
Dilaudid-HP 443

Hydroxyzine Hydrochloride (Potential for increased CNS depression). Products include:
Atarax Tablets & Syrup 2667
Vistaril Intramuscular Solution 2738

Isoflurane (Potential for increased CNS depression).
No products indexed under this heading.

Ketamine Hydrochloride (Potential for increased CNS depression).
No products indexed under this heading.

Levomethadyl Acetate Hydrochloride (Potential for increased CNS depression).
No products indexed under this heading.

Levorphanol Tartrate (Potential for increased CNS depression). Products include:
Levo-Dromoran 1734
Levorphanol Tartrate Tablets 3059

Lorazepam (Potential for increased CNS depression). Products include:
Ativan Injection 3478
Ativan Tablets 3482

Loxapine Hydrochloride (Potential for increased CNS depression).
No products indexed under this heading.

Loxapine Succinate (Potential for increased CNS depression). Products include:
Loxitane Capsules 3398

Meperidine Hydrochloride (Potential for increased CNS depression). Products include:
Demerol 3079
Mepergan Injection 3539

Mephobarbital (Potential for increased CNS depression).
No products indexed under this heading.

Meprobamate (Potential for increased CNS depression). Products include:
Miltown Tablets 3349

Mesoridazine Besylate (Potential for increased CNS depression). Products include:
Serentil 1057

Methadone Hydrochloride (Potential for increased CNS depression). Products include:
Dolophine Hydrochloride Tablets 3056

Methazolamide (Co-administration of topiramate with carbonic anhydrase inhibitors may create a physiological environment that increases the risk of kidney stone formation; concurrent use should be avoided). Products include:
Neptazane Tablets ⊙271

Methohexital Sodium (Potential for increased CNS depression). Products include:
Brevital Sodium for Injection, USP 1815

Methotrimeprazine (Potential for increased CNS depression).
No products indexed under this heading.

Methoxyflurane (Potential for increased CNS depression).
No products indexed under this heading.

Midazolam Hydrochloride (Potential for increased CNS depression). Products include:
Versed Injection 3027
Versed Syrup 3033

Molindone Hydrochloride (Potential for increased CNS depression). Products include:
Moban 1320

Morphine Sulfate (Potential for increased CNS depression). Products include:
Astramorph/PF Injection, USP (Preservative-Free) 594
Duramorph Injection 1312
Infumorph 200 and Infumorph 500 Sterile Solutions 1314
Kadian Capsules 1335
MS Contin Tablets 2896
MSIR 2898
Oramorph SR Tablets 3062
Roxanol 3066

Olanzapine (Potential for increased CNS depression). Products include:
Zyprexa Tablets 1973
Zyprexa ZYDIS Orally Disintegrating Tablets 1973

Oxazepam (Potential for increased CNS depression).
No products indexed under this heading.

Oxycodone Hydrochloride (Potential for increased CNS depression). Products include:
OxyContin Tablets 2912
OxyFast Oral Concentrate Solution 2916
OxyIR Capsules 2916
Percocet Tablets 1326
Percodan Tablets 1327
Percolone Tablets 1327
Roxicodone 3067
Tylox Capsules 2597

Pentobarbital Sodium (Potential for increased CNS depression). Products include:
Nembutal Sodium Solution 485

Perphenazine (Potential for increased CNS depression). Products include:
Etrafon 3115
Trilafon 3160

Phenobarbital (Potential for increased CNS depression). Products include:
Arco-Lase Plus Tablets 592
Donnatal 2929
Donnatal Extentabs 2930

Phenytoin (Co-administration has resulted in 48% decrease in topiramate concentration and no change or 25% increase in phenytoin concentration). Products include:
Dilantin Infatabs 2624
Dilantin-125 Oral Suspension 2625

Phenytoin Sodium (Co-administration has resulted in 48% decrease in topiramate concentration and no change or 25% increase in phenytoin concentration). Products include:
Dilantin Kapseals 2622

Prazepam (Potential for increased CNS depression).
No products indexed under this heading.

Prochlorperazine (Potential for increased CNS depression). Products include:
Compazine 1505

Promethazine Hydrochloride (Potential for increased CNS depression). Products include:
Mepergan Injection 3539
Phenergan Injection 3553
Phenergan 3556
Phenergan Syrup 3554
Phenergan with Codeine Syrup 3557
Phenergan with Dextromethorphan Syrup 3559
Phenergan VC Syrup 3560
Phenergan VC with Codeine Syrup 3561

Propofol (Potential for increased CNS depression). Products include:
Diprivan Injectable Emulsion 667

Propoxyphene Hydrochloride (Potential for increased CNS depression). Products include:
Darvon Pulvules 1909
Darvon Compound-65 Pulvules 1910

Propoxyphene Napsylate (Potential for increased CNS depression). Products include:
Darvon-N/Darvocet-N 1907
Darvon-N Tablets 1912

Quazepam (Potential for increased CNS depression).
No products indexed under this heading.

Quetiapine Fumarate (Potential for increased CNS depression). Products include:
Seroquel Tablets 684

Remifentanil Hydrochloride (Potential for increased CNS depression).
No products indexed under this heading.

Risperidone (Potential for increased CNS depression). Products include:
Risperdal 1796

Secobarbital Sodium (Potential for increased CNS depression).
No products indexed under this heading.

Sevoflurane (Potential for increased CNS depression).
No products indexed under this heading.

Sufentanil Citrate (Potential for increased CNS depression).
No products indexed under this heading.

Temazepam (Potential for increased CNS depression).
No products indexed under this heading.

Thiamylal Sodium (Potential for increased CNS depression).
No products indexed under this heading.

Thioridazine Hydrochloride (Potential for increased CNS depression). Products include:
Thioridazine Hydrochloride Tablets 2289

Thiothixene (Potential for increased CNS depression). Products include:
Navane Capsules 2701
Thiothixene Capsules 2290

Triazolam (Potential for increased CNS depression). Products include:
Halcion Tablets 2823

Trifluoperazine Hydrochloride (Potential for increased CNS depression). Products include:
Stelazine 1640

Valproate Sodium (Co-administration has resulted in 11% decrease in valproic acid concentration and 14% decrease in topiramate concentration). Products include:
Depacon Injection 416

Valproic Acid (Co-administration has resulted in 11% decrease in valproic acid concentration and 14% decrease in topiramate concentration). Products include:
Depakene 421

Zaleplon (Potential for increased CNS depression). Products include:
Sonata Capsules 3591

Ziprasidone Hydrochloride (Potential for increased CNS depression). Products include:
Geodon Capsules 2688

Zolpidem Tartrate (Potential for increased CNS depression). Products include:
Ambien Tablets 3191

Food Interactions

Alcohol (Potential for increased CNS depression).

TOPICORT CREAM
(Desoximetasone) 2025
None cited in PDR database.

TOPICORT GEL
(Desoximetasone) 2025
None cited in PDR database.

TOPICORT OINTMENT
(Desoximetasone) 2025
None cited in PDR database.

TOPICORT LP CREAM
(Desoximetasone) 2025
None cited in PDR database.

TOPROL-XL TABLETS
(Metoprolol Succinate) 651
May interact with catecholamine depleting drugs, cardiac glycosides, quinidine, and certain other agents. Compounds in these categories include:

Deserpidine (Potential for additive effect; hypotension or marked bradycardia).
No products indexed under this heading.

Deslanoside (Metoprolol should be used cautiously in patients with hypertension and angina who have congestive heart failure and are on digitalis and diuretics since both digitalis and metoprolol slow AV conduction).
No products indexed under this heading.

Digitoxin (Metoprolol should be used cautiously in patients with hypertension and angina who have congestive heart failure and are on digitalis and diuretics since both digitalis and metoprolol slow AV conduction).
No products indexed under this heading.

Digoxin (Metoprolol should be used cautiously in patients with hypertension and angina who have congestive heart failure and are on digitalis and diuretics since both digitalis and metoprolol slow AV conduction). Products include:
Digitek Tablets 1003
Lanoxicaps Capsules 1574
Lanoxin Injection 1581
Lanoxin Tablets 1587
Lanoxin Elixir Pediatric 1578
Lanoxin Injection Pediatric 1584

Epinephrine Hydrochloride (Potential unresponsiveness to the usual dose of epinephrine to treat allergic reactions in certain patients).
No products indexed under this heading.

Fluoxetine Hydrochloride (Co-administration with drugs that inhibit

CYP2D6, such as fluoxetine, are likely to increase metoprolol concentrations; these increases in plasma concentration would decrease the cardioselectivity of metoprolol). Products include:
- Prozac Pulvules, Liquid, and Weekly Capsules 1238
- Sarafem Pulvules 1962

Guanethidine Monosulfate (Potential for additive effect; hypotension or marked bradycardia).
- No products indexed under this heading.

Paroxetine Hydrochloride (Co-administration with drugs that inhibit CYP2D6, such as paroxetine, are likely to increase metoprolol concentrations; these increases in plasma concentration would decrease the cardioselectivity of metoprolol). Products include:
- Paxil 1609

Propafenone Hydrochloride (Co-administration with drugs that inhibit CYP2D6, such as propafenone, are likely to increase metoprolol concentrations; these increases in plasma concentration would decrease the cardioselectivity of metoprolol). Products include:
- Rythmol Tablets – 150 mg, 225 mg, 300 mg 502

Quinidine Gluconate (Co-administration with drugs that inhibit CYP2D6, such as quinidine, are likely to increase metoprolol concentrations; these increases in plasma concentration would decrease the cardioselectivity of metoprolol). Products include:
- Quinaglute Dura-Tabs Tablets 978

Quinidine Polygalacturonate (Co-administration with drugs that inhibit CYP2D6, such as quinidine, are likely to increase metoprolol concentrations; these increases in plasma concentration would decrease the cardioselectivity of metoprolol).
- No products indexed under this heading.

Quinidine Sulfate (Co-administration with drugs that inhibit CYP2D6, such as quinidine, are likely to increase metoprolol concentrations; these increases in plasma concentration would decrease the cardioselectivity of metoprolol). Products include:
- Quinidex Extentabs 2933

Rauwolfia serpentina (Potential for additive effect; hypotension or marked bradycardia).
- No products indexed under this heading.

Rescinnamine (Potential for additive effect; hypotension or marked bradycardia).
- No products indexed under this heading.

Reserpine (Potential for additive effect; hypotension or marked bradycardia).
- No products indexed under this heading.

TORADOL IM INJECTION, IV INJECTION

(Ketorolac Tromethamine) 3018
See Toradol Tablets

TORADOL TABLETS

(Ketorolac Tromethamine) 3018
May interact with ACE inhibitors, lithium preparations, nondepolarizing neuromuscular blocking agents, nonsteroidal anti-inflammatory agents, salicylates, and certain other agents. Compounds in these categories include:

Alprazolam (Concurrent use may produce hallucinations). Products include:
- Xanax Tablets 2865

Aspirin (Concurrent use is contraindicated because of the cumulative risk of inducing serious NSAID-related side effects). Products include:
- Aggrenox Capsules 1026
- Alka-Seltzer .... ▣603
- Alka-Seltzer Lemon Lime Antacid and Pain Reliever Effervescent Tablets .... ▣603
- Alka-Seltzer Extra Strength Antacid and Pain Reliever Effervescent Tablets .... ▣603
- Alka-Seltzer PM Effervescent Tablets .... ▣605
- Genuine Bayer Tablets, Caplets and Gelcaps .... ▣606
- Extra Strength Bayer Caplets and Gelcaps .... ▣610
- Aspirin Regimen Bayer Children's Chewable Tablets (Orange or Cherry Flavored) .... ▣607
- Bayer, Aspirin Regimen .... ▣606
- Aspirin Regimen Bayer 81 mg Caplets with Calcium .... ▣607
- Genuine Bayer Professional Labeling (Aspirin Regimen Bayer) .... ▣608
- Extra Strength Bayer Arthritis Caplets .... ▣610
- Extra Strength Bayer Plus Caplets .... ▣610
- Extra Strength Bayer PM Caplets .... ▣611
- BC Powder .... ▣619
- BC Allergy Sinus Cold Powder .... ▣619
- Arthritis Strength BC Powder .... ▣619
- BC Sinus Cold Powder .... ▣619
- Darvon Compound-65 Pulvules 1910
- Ecotrin Enteric Coated Aspirin Low, Regular and Maximum Strength Tablets 1715
- Excedrin Extra-Strength Tablets, Caplets, and Geltabs .... ▣629
- Excedrin Migraine 1070
- Goody's Body Pain Formula Powder .... ▣620
- Goody's Extra Strength Headache Powder .... ▣620
- Goody's Extra Strength Pain Relief Tablets .... ▣620
- Percodan Tablets 1327
- Robaxisal Tablets 2939
- Soma Compound Tablets 3354
- Soma Compound w/Codeine Tablets 3355
- Vanquish Caplets .... ▣617

Atracurium Besylate (Concurrent use with parenteral form of Toradol has resulted in apnea).
- No products indexed under this heading.

Benazepril Hydrochloride (Concomitant use may increase the risk of renal impairment, particularly in volume-depleted patients). Products include:
- Lotensin Tablets 2365
- Lotensin HCT Tablets 2367
- Lotrel Capsules 2370

Captopril (Concomitant use may increase the risk of renal impairment, particularly in volume-depleted patients). Products include:
- Captopril Tablets 2281

Carbamazepine (Concomitant use has resulted in sporadic cases of seizures). Products include:
- Carbatrol Capsules 3234
- Tegretol/Tegretol-XR 2404

Celecoxib (Concurrent use is contraindicated because of the cumulative risk of inducing serious NSAID-related side effects). Products include:
- Celebrex Capsules 2676
- Celebrex Capsules 2780

Choline Magnesium Trisalicylate (*in vitro* studies indicate that, at therapeutic concentrations of salicylates, the binding of ketorolac was reduced from approximately 99.2% to 97.5%, representing a potential two-fold increase in unbound ketorolac plasma levels). Products include:
- Trilisate 2901

Cisatracurium Besylate (Concurrent use with parenteral form of Toradol has resulted in apnea).
- No products indexed under this heading.

Diclofenac Potassium (Concurrent use is contraindicated because of the cumulative risk of inducing serious NSAID-related side effects). Products include:
- Cataflam Tablets 2315

Diclofenac Sodium (Concurrent use is contraindicated because of the cumulative risk of inducing serious NSAID-related side effects). Products include:
- Arthrotec Tablets 3195
- Voltaren Ophthalmic Sterile Ophthalmic Solution .... ⊙312
- Voltaren Tablets 2315
- Voltaren-XR Tablets 2315

Diflunisal (*in vitro* studies indicate that, at therapeutic concentrations of salicylates, the binding of ketorolac was reduced from approximately 99.2% to 97.5%, representing a potential two-fold increase in unbound ketorolac plasma levels). Products include:
- Dolobid Tablets 2088

Enalapril Maleate (Concomitant use may increase the risk of renal impairment, particularly in volume-depleted patients). Products include:
- Lexxel Tablets 608
- Vaseretic Tablets 2204
- Vasotec Tablets 2210

Enalaprilat (Concomitant use may increase the risk of renal impairment, particularly in volume-depleted patients). Products include:
- Enalaprilat Injection 863
- Vasotec I.V. Injection 2207

Etodolac (Concurrent use is contraindicated because of the cumulative risk of inducing serious NSAID-related side effects). Products include:
- Lodine 3528
- Lodine XL Extended-Release Tablets 3530

Fenoprofen Calcium (Concurrent use is contraindicated because of the cumulative risk of inducing serious NSAID-related side effects).
- No products indexed under this heading.

Fluoxetine Hydrochloride (Concurrent use may produce hallucinations). Products include:
- Prozac Pulvules, Liquid, and Weekly Capsules 1238
- Sarafem Pulvules 1962

Flurbiprofen (Concurrent use is contraindicated because of the cumulative risk of inducing serious NSAID-related side effects).
- No products indexed under this heading.

Fosinopril Sodium (Concomitant use may increase the risk of renal impairment, particularly in volume-depleted patients). Products include:
- Monopril Tablets 1091
- Monopril HCT 1094

Furosemide (Potential for reduced diuretic response in normovolemic healthy subjects by 20%). Products include:
- Furosemide Tablets 2284

Heparin Sodium (Co-administration results in mean template bleeding time of 6.4 minutes compared to 6.0 minutes, however extreme caution and close monitoring is recommended). Products include:
- Heparin Lock Flush Solution 3509
- Heparin Sodium Injection 3511

Ibuprofen (Concurrent use is contraindicated because of the cumulative risk of inducing serious NSAID-related side effects). Products include:
- Advil .... ▣771
- Children's Advil Oral Suspension .... ▣773
- Children's Advil Chewable Tablets .... ▣773
- Advil Cold and Sinus Caplets .... ▣771
- Advil Cold and Sinus Tablets .... ▣771
- Advil Flu & Body Ache Caplets .... ▣772
- Infants' Advil Drops .... ▣773
- Junior Strength Advil Tablets .... ▣773
- Junior Strength Advil Chewable Tablets .... ▣773
- Advil Migraine Liquigels .... ▣772
- Children's Motrin Oral Suspension and Chewable Tablets 2006
- Children's Motrin Cold Oral Suspension 2007
- Children's Motrin Oral Suspension .... ▣643
- Motrin Suspension, Oral Drops, Chewable Tablets, and Caplets 2002
- Infants' Motrin Concentrated Drops 2006
- Junior Strength Motrin Caplets and Chewable Tablets 2006
- Motrin IB Tablets, Caplets, and Gelcaps 2002
- Motrin Migraine Pain Caplets 2005
- Motrin Sinus Headache Caplets 2005
- Vicoprofen Tablets 520

Indomethacin (Concurrent use is contraindicated because of the cumulative risk of inducing serious NSAID-related side effects). Products include:
- Indocin 2112

Indomethacin Sodium Trihydrate (Concurrent use is contraindicated because of the cumulative risk of inducing serious NSAID-related side effects). Products include:
- Indocin I.V. 2115

Ketoprofen (Concurrent use is contraindicated because of the cumulative risk of inducing serious NSAID-related side effects). Products include:
- Orudis Capsules 3548
- Orudis KT Tablets .... ▣778
- Oruvail Capsules 3548

Lisinopril (Concomitant use may increase the risk of renal impairment, particularly in volume-depleted patients). Products include:
- Prinivil Tablets 2164
- Prinzide Tablets 2168
- Zestoretic Tablets 695
- Zestril Tablets 698

Lithium Carbonate (Co-administration can result in inhibition of renal lithium clearance leading to an increase in plasma lithium concentrations). Products include:
- Eskalith 1527
- Lithium Carbonate 3061
- Lithobid Slow-Release Tablets 3255

Lithium Citrate (Co-administration can result in inhibition of renal lithium clearance leading to an increase in plasma lithium concentrations). Products include:
- Lithium Citrate Syrup 3061

Magnesium Salicylate (*in vitro* studies indicate that, at therapeutic concentrations of salicylates, the binding of ketorolac was reduced from approximately 99.2% to 97.5%, representing a potential two-fold increase in unbound ketorolac plasma levels). Products include:
- Momentum Backache Relief Extra Strength Caplets .... ▣666

Meclofenamate Sodium (Concurrent use is contraindicated because of the cumulative risk of inducing serious NSAID-related side effects).
- No products indexed under this heading.

Mefenamic Acid (Concurrent use is contraindicated because of the cumulative risk of inducing serious NSAID-related side effects). Products include:
- Ponstel Capsules 1356

Meloxicam (Concurrent use is contraindicated because of the cumulative risk of inducing serious NSAID-related side effects). Products include:
- Mobic Tablets 1054

Methotrexate Sodium (Co-administration may result in reduced clearance of methotrexate thereby enhancing the toxicity).
- No products indexed under this heading.

Metocurine Iodide (Concurrent use with parenteral form of Toradol

has resulted in apnea).
No products indexed under this heading.

Mivacurium Chloride (Concurrent use with parenteral form of Toradol has resulted in apnea).
No products indexed under this heading.

Moexipril Hydrochloride (Concomitant use may increase the risk of renal impairment, particularly in volume-depleted patients). Products include:
Uniretic Tablets 3178
Univasc Tablets 3181

Nabumetone (Concurrent use is contraindicated because of the cumulative risk of inducing serious NSAID-related side effects). Products include:
Relafen Tablets 1617

Naproxen (Concurrent use is contraindicated because of the cumulative risk of inducing serious NSAID-related side effects). Products include:
EC-Naprosyn Delayed-Release Tablets 2967
Naprosyn Suspension 2967
Naprosyn Tablets 2967

Naproxen Sodium (Concurrent use is contraindicated because of the cumulative risk of inducing serious NSAID-related side effects). Products include:
Aleve Tablets, Caplets and Gelcaps .... ▣602
Aleve Cold & Sinus Caplets .... ▣603
Anaprox Tablets 2967
Anaprox DS Tablets 2967
Naprelan Tablets 1293

Oxaprozin (Concurrent use is contraindicated because of the cumulative risk of inducing serious NSAID-related side effects).
No products indexed under this heading.

Pancuronium Bromide (Concurrent use with parenteral form of Toradol has resulted in apnea).
No products indexed under this heading.

Perindopril Erbumine (Concomitant use may increase the risk of renal impairment, particularly in volume-depleted patients). Products include:
Aceon Tablets (2 mg, 4 mg, 8 mg) 3249

Phenylbutazone (Concurrent use is contraindicated because of the cumulative risk of inducing serious NSAID-related side effects).
No products indexed under this heading.

Phenytoin (Concomitant use has resulted in sporadic cases of seizures). Products include:
Dilantin Infatabs 2624
Dilantin-125 Oral Suspension 2625

Phenytoin Sodium (Concomitant use has resulted in sporadic cases of seizures). Products include:
Dilantin Kapseals 2622

Piroxicam (Concurrent use is contraindicated because of the cumulative risk of inducing serious NSAID-related side effects). Products include:
Feldene Capsules 2685

Probenecid (Co-administration of oral ketorolac and probenecid has resulted in decreased clearance of ketorolac and a significant increase in plasma levels, AUC increased by three-fold, and terminal half-life increased by two-fold; concomitant use is contraindicated).
No products indexed under this heading.

Quinapril Hydrochloride (Concomitant use may increase the risk of renal impairment, particularly in volume-depleted patients). Products include:
Accupril Tablets 2611
Accuretic Tablets 2614

Ramipril (Concomitant use may increase the risk of renal impairment, particularly in volume-depleted patients). Products include:
Altace Capsules 2233

Rapacuronium Bromide (Concurrent use with parenteral form of Toradol has resulted in apnea).
No products indexed under this heading.

Rocuronium Bromide (Concurrent use with parenteral form of Toradol has resulted in apnea). Products include:
Zemuron Injection 2491

Rofecoxib (Concurrent use is contraindicated because of the cumulative risk of inducing serious NSAID-related side effects). Products include:
Vioxx 2213

Salsalate (*in vitro* studies indicate that, at therapeutic concentrations of salicylates, the binding of ketorolac was reduced from approximately 99.2% to 97.5%, representing a potential two-fold increase in unbound ketorolac plasma levels).
No products indexed under this heading.

Spirapril Hydrochloride (Concomitant use may increase the risk of renal impairment, particularly in volume-depleted patients).
No products indexed under this heading.

Sulindac (Concurrent use is contraindicated because of the cumulative risk of inducing serious NSAID-related side effects). Products include:
Clinoril Tablets 2053

Thiothixene (Concurrent use may produce hallucinations). Products include:
Navane Capsules 2701
Thiothixene Capsules 2290

Thiothixene Hydrochloride (Concurrent use may produce hallucinations). Products include:
Navane Concentrate 2701
Navane Intramuscular 2703

Tolmetin Sodium (Concurrent use is contraindicated because of the cumulative risk of inducing serious NSAID-related side effects). Products include:
Tolectin 2589

Trandolapril (Concomitant use may increase the risk of renal impairment, particularly in volume-depleted patients). Products include:
Mavik Tablets 478
Tarka Tablets 508

Vecuronium Bromide (Concurrent use with parenteral form of Toradol has resulted in apnea). Products include:
Norcuron for Injection 2478

Warfarin Sodium (*in vitro* binding of warfarin to plasma proteins is slightly reduced by ketorolac; extreme caution and close monitoring is recommended). Products include:
Coumadin for Injection 1243
Coumadin Tablets 1243
Warfarin Sodium Tablets, USP 3302

Food Interactions

Diet, high-lipid (Oral administration of Toradol after a high-fat meal resulted in decreased peak and delayed time-to-peak concentrations of Toradol by about 1 hour).

TRANSDERM SCOP TRANSDERMAL THERAPEUTIC SYSTEM

(Scopolamine) 2302

May interact with anticholinergics, antihistamines, central nervous system depressants, tricyclic antidepressants, and certain other agents. Compounds in these categories include:

Acrivastine (Antihistamines have anticholinergic properties and co-administration may result in additive effects). Products include:
Semprex-D Capsules 1172

Alfentanil Hydrochloride (Scopolamine is an anticholinergic agent and causes certain CNS effects, such as drowsiness and dizziness, and hence it should be used with care in patients on concomitant therapy).
No products indexed under this heading.

Alprazolam (Scopolamine is an anticholinergic agent and causes certain CNS effects, such as drowsiness and dizziness, and hence it should be used with care in patients on concomitant therapy). Products include:
Xanax Tablets 2865

Amitriptyline Hydrochloride (Tricyclic antidepressants have anticholinergic properties and co-administration may result in additive effects). Products include:
Etrafon 3115
Limbitrol 1738

Amoxapine (Tricyclic antidepressants have anticholinergic properties and co-administration may result in additive effects).
No products indexed under this heading.

Aprobarbital (Scopolamine is an anticholinergic agent and causes certain CNS effects, such as drowsiness and dizziness, and hence it should be used with care in patients on concomitant therapy).
No products indexed under this heading.

Astemizole (Antihistamines have anticholinergic properties and co-administration may result in additive effects).
No products indexed under this heading.

Atropine Sulfate (Co-administration may result in additive anticholinergic effects). Products include:
Donnatal 2929
Donnatal Extentabs 2930
Motofen Tablets 577
Prosed/DS Tablets 3268
Urised Tablets 2876

Azatadine Maleate (Antihistamines have anticholinergic properties and co-administration may result in additive effects). Products include:
Rynatan Tablets 3351

Belladonna Alkaloids (Co-administration may result in additive anticholinergic effects). Products include:
Hyland's Teething Tablets .... ▣766
Urimax Tablets 1769

Benztropine Mesylate (Co-administration may result in additive anticholinergic effects). Products include:
Cogentin 2055

Biperiden Hydrochloride (Co-administration may result in additive anticholinergic effects). Products include:
Akineton 402

Bromodiphenhydramine Hydrochloride (Antihistamines have anticholinergic properties and co-administration may result in additive effects).
No products indexed under this heading.

Brompheniramine Maleate (Antihistamines have anticholinergic properties and co-administration may result in additive effects). Products include:
Bromfed Capsules (Extended-Release) 2269
Bromfed-PD Capsules (Extended-Release) 2269
Comtrex Acute Head Cold & Sinus Pressure Relief Tablets .... ▣627
Dimetapp Elixir .... ▣777
Dimetapp Cold and Fever Suspension .... ▣775
Dimetapp DM Cold & Cough Elixir .... ▣775
Dimetapp Nighttime Flu Liquid .... ▣776

Buprenorphine Hydrochloride (Scopolamine is an anticholinergic agent and causes certain CNS effects, such as drowsiness and dizziness, and hence it should be used with care in patients on concomitant therapy). Products include:
Buprenex Injectable 2918

Buspirone Hydrochloride (Scopolamine is an anticholinergic agent and causes certain CNS effects, such as drowsiness and dizziness, and hence it should be used with care in patients on concomitant therapy).
No products indexed under this heading.

Butabarbital (Scopolamine is an anticholinergic agent and causes certain CNS effects, such as drowsiness and dizziness, and hence it should be used with care in patients on concomitant therapy).
No products indexed under this heading.

Butalbital (Scopolamine is an anticholinergic agent and causes certain CNS effects, such as drowsiness and dizziness, and hence it should be used with care in patients on concomitant therapy). Products include:
Phrenilin 578
Sedapap Tablets 50 mg/650 mg 2225

Cetirizine Hydrochloride (Antihistamines have anticholinergic properties and co-administration may result in additive effects). Products include:
Zyrtec 2756
Zyrtec-D 12 Hour Extended Relief Tablets 2758

Chlordiazepoxide (Scopolamine is an anticholinergic agent and causes certain CNS effects, such as drowsiness and dizziness, and hence it should be used with care in patients on concomitant therapy). Products include:
Limbitrol 1738

Chlordiazepoxide Hydrochloride (Scopolamine is an anticholinergic agent and causes certain CNS effects, such as drowsiness and dizziness, and hence it should be used with care in patients on concomitant therapy). Products include:
Librium Capsules 1736
Librium for Injection 1737

Chlorpheniramine Maleate (Antihistamines have anticholinergic properties and co-administration may result in additive effects). Products include:
Actifed Cold & Sinus Caplets and Tablets .... ▣688
Alka-Seltzer Plus Liqui-Gels .... ▣604
BC Allergy Sinus Cold Powder .... ▣619
Chlor-Trimeton Allergy Tablets .... ▣735
Chlor-Trimeton Allergy/Decongestant Tablets .... ▣736
Comtrex Flu Therapy & Fever Relief Nighttime Tablets .... ▣628
Comtrex Maximum Strength Multi-Symptom Cold & Cough Relief Tablets and Caplets .... ▣626
Contac Severe Cold and Flu Caplets Maximum Strength .... ▣746
Coricidin 'D' Cold, Flu & Sinus Tablets .... ▣737
Coricidin/Coricidin D .... ▣738
Coricidin HBP Maximum Strength Flu Tablets .... ▣738
Extendryl 1361
Hycomine Compound Tablets 1317
Kronofed-A 1341
PediaCare Cough-Cold Liquid .... ▣719
PediaCare NightRest Cough-Cold Liquid .... ▣719
Robitussin Nighttime Honey Flu Liquid .... ▣786
Ryna .... ▣768
Singlet Caplets .... ▣761
Sinutab Sinus Allergy Medication, Maximum Strength Formula, Tablets & Caplets .... ▣707
Sudafed Cold & Allergy Tablets .... ▣708
TheraFlu Regular Strength Cold & Cough Night Time Hot Liquid .... ▣676
TheraFlu Regular Strength Cold & Sore Throat Night Time Hot Liquid .... ▣676

TheraFlu Maximum Strength Flu & Cough Night Time Hot Liquid.. ▣678
TheraFlu Maximum Strength Flu & Sore Throat Night Time Hot Liquid ▣677
TheraFlu Maximum Strength Severe Cold & Congestion Night Time Caplets ▣678
TheraFlu Maximum Strength Severe Cold & Congestion Night Time Hot Liquid ▣678
Triaminic Cold & Allergy Liquid ▣681
Triaminic Cold & Allergy Softchews ▣683
Triaminic Cold & Cough Liquid ▣681
Triaminic Cold & Cough Softchews ▣683
Triaminic Cold & Night Time Cough Liquid ▣681
Triaminic Cold, Cough & Fever Liquid ▣681
Children's Tylenol Cold Suspension Liquid and Chewable Tablets 2015
Children's Tylenol Cold Plus Cough Suspension Liquid and Chewable Tablets 2015
Children's Tylenol Flu Suspension Liquid 2015
Maximum Strength Tylenol Allergy Sinus Caplets, Gelcaps, and Geltabs 2010
Multi-Symptom Tylenol Cold Complete Formula Caplets 2010
Vicks 44M Cough, Cold & Flu Relief Liquid ▣725
Pediatric Vicks 44m Cough & Cold Relief ▣728
Children's Vicks NyQuil Cold/Cough Relief ▣726

Chlorpheniramine Polistirex (Antihistamines have anticholinergic properties and co-administration may result in additive effects). Products include:
Tussionex Pennkinetic Extended-Release Suspension 1174

Chlorpheniramine Tannate (Antihistamines have anticholinergic properties and co-administration may result in additive effects). Products include:
Reformulated Rynatan Pediatric Suspension 3352
Rynatuss Pediatric Suspension 3353
Rynatuss Tablets 3353
Tussi-12 S Suspension 3356
Tussi-12 Tablets 3356

Chlorpromazine (Scopolamine is an anticholinergic agent and causes certain CNS effects, such as drowsiness and dizziness, and hence it should be used with care in patients on concomitant therapy). Products include:
Thorazine Suppositories 1656

Chlorpromazine Hydrochloride (Scopolamine is an anticholinergic agent and causes certain CNS effects, such as drowsiness and dizziness, and hence it should be used with care in patients on concomitant therapy) Products include:
Thorazine 1656

Chlorprothixene (Scopolamine is an anticholinergic agent and causes certain CNS effects, such as drowsiness and dizziness, and hence it should be used with care in patients on concomitant therapy).
No products indexed under this heading.

Chlorprothixene Hydrochloride (Scopolamine is an anticholinergic agent and causes certain CNS effects, such as drowsiness and dizziness, and hence it should be used with care in patients on concomitant therapy).
No products indexed under this heading.

Chlorprothixene Lactate (Scopolamine is an anticholinergic agent and causes certain CNS effects, such as drowsiness and dizziness, and hence it should be used with care in patients on concomitant therapy).
No products indexed under this heading.

Clemastine Fumarate (Antihistamines have anticholinergic properties and co-administration may result in additive effects). Products include:
Tavist 12 Hour Allergy Tablets ▣676

Clidinium Bromide (Co-administration may result in additive anticholinergic effects).
No products indexed under this heading.

Clomipramine Hydrochloride (Tricyclic antidepressants have anticholinergic properties and co-administration may result in additive effects).
No products indexed under this heading.

Clorazepate Dipotassium (Scopolamine is an anticholinergic agent and causes certain CNS effects, such as drowsiness and dizziness, and hence it should be used with care in patients on concomitant therapy). Products include:
Tranxene 511

Clozapine (Scopolamine is an anticholinergic agent and causes certain CNS effects, such as drowsiness and dizziness, and hence it should be used with care in patients on concomitant therapy). Products include:
Clozaril Tablets 2319

Codeine Phosphate (Scopolamine is an anticholinergic agent and causes certain CNS effects, such as drowsiness and dizziness, and hence it should be used with care in patients on concomitant therapy). Products include:
Phenergan with Codeine Syrup 3557
Phenergan VC with Codeine Syrup .. 3561
Robitussin A-C Syrup 2942
Robitussin-DAC Syrup 2942
Ryna-C Liquid ▣768
Soma Compound w/Codeine Tablets 3355
Tussi-Organidin NR Liquid 3350
Tussi-Organidin-S NR Liquid 3350
Tylenol with Codeine 2595

Cyproheptadine Hydrochloride (Antihistamines have anticholinergic properties and co-administration may result in additive effects). Products include:
Periactin Tablets 2155

Desflurane (Scopolamine is an anticholinergic agent and causes certain CNS effects, such as drowsiness and dizziness, and hence it should be used with care in patients on concomitant therapy). Products include:
Suprane Liquid for Inhalation 874

Desipramine Hydrochloride (Tricyclic antidepressants have anticholinergic properties and co-administration may result in additive effects). Products include:
Norpramin Tablets 755

Dexchlorpheniramine Maleate (Antihistamines have anticholinergic properties and co-administration may result in additive effects).
No products indexed under this heading.

Dezocine (Scopolamine is an anticholinergic agent and causes certain CNS effects, such as drowsiness and dizziness, and hence it should be used with care in patients on concomitant therapy).
No products indexed under this heading.

Diazepam (Scopolamine is an anticholinergic agent and causes certain CNS effects, such as drowsiness and dizziness, and hence it should be used with care in patients on concomitant therapy). Products include:
Valium Injectable 3026
Valium Tablets 3047

Dicyclomine Hydrochloride (Co-administration may result in additive anticholinergic effects).
No products indexed under this heading.

Diphenhydramine Citrate (Antihistamines have anticholinergic properties and co-administration may result in additive effects). Products include:
Alka-Seltzer PM Effervescent Tablets ▣605
Benadryl Allergy & Sinus Fastmelt Tablets ▣693
Benadryl Children's Allergy/Cold Fastmelt Tablets ▣692
Excedrin PM Tablets, Caplets, and Geltabs ▣631
Goody's PM Powder ▣621

Diphenhydramine Hydrochloride (Antihistamines have anticholinergic properties and co-administration may result in additive effects). Products include:
Extra Strength Bayer PM Caplets ▣611
Benadryl Allergy Chewables ▣689
Benadryl Allergy ▣691
Benadryl Allergy Liquid ▣690
Benadryl Allergy/Cold Tablets ▣691
Benadryl Allergy/Congestion Tablets ▣692
Benadryl Allergy & Sinus Liquid ▣693
Benadryl Allergy Sinus Headache Caplets & Gelcaps ▣693
Benadryl Severe Allergy & Sinus Headache Caplets ▣694
Benadryl Dye-Free Allergy Liquid ▣690
Benadryl Dye-Free Allergy Liqui-Gels Softgels ▣690
Benadryl Itch Relief Stick Extra Strength ▣695
Benadryl Cream ▣695
Benadryl Gel ▣695
Benadryl Spray ▣696
Benadryl Parenteral 2617
Coricidin HBP Night-Time Cold & Flu Tablets ▣738
Nytol QuickCaps Caplets ▣622
Maximum Strength Nytol QuickGels Softgels ▣621
Extra Strength Percogesic Aspirin-Free Coated Caplets ▣665
Simply Sleep Caplets 2008
Sominex Original Formula Tablets . ▣761
Children's Tylenol Allergy-D Liquid ... 2014
Maximum Strength Tylenol Allergy Sinus NightTime Caplets 2010
Tylenol Severe Allergy Caplets 2010
Maximum Strength Tylenol Flu NightTime Gelcaps 2011
Extra Strength Tylenol PM Caplets, Geltabs, and Gelcaps 2012
Unisom Maximum Strength SleepGels ▣713

Diphenylpyraline Hydrochloride (Antihistamines have anticholinergic properties and co-administration may result in additive effects).
No products indexed under this heading.

Doxepin Hydrochloride (Tricyclic antidepressants have anticholinergic properties and co-administration may result in additive effects). Products include:
Sinequan 2713

Droperidol (Scopolamine is an anticholinergic agent and causes certain CNS effects, such as drowsiness and dizziness, and hence it should be used with care in patients on concomitant therapy).
No products indexed under this heading.

Enflurane (Scopolamine is an anticholinergic agent and causes certain CNS effects, such as drowsiness and dizziness, and hence it should be used with care in patients on concomitant therapy).
No products indexed under this heading.

Estazolam (Scopolamine is an anticholinergic agent and causes certain CNS effects, such as drowsiness and dizziness, and hence it should be used with care in patients on concomitant therapy). Products include:
ProSom Tablets 500

Ethchlorvynol (Scopolamine is an anticholinergic agent and causes certain CNS effects, such as drowsiness and dizziness, and hence it should be used with care in patients on concomitant therapy).
No products indexed under this heading.

Ethinamate (Scopolamine is an anticholinergic agent and causes certain CNS effects, such as drowsiness and dizziness, and hence it should be used with care in patients on concomitant therapy).
No products indexed under this heading.

Fentanyl (Scopolamine is an anticholinergic agent and causes certain CNS effects, such as drowsiness and dizziness, and hence it should be used with care in patients on concomitant therapy). Products include:
Duragesic Transdermal System 1786

Fentanyl Citrate (Scopolamine is an anticholinergic agent and causes certain CNS effects, such as drowsiness and dizziness, and hence it should be used with care in patients on concomitant therapy). Products include:
Actiq 1184

Fexofenadine Hydrochloride (Antihistamines have anticholinergic properties and co-administration may result in additive effects). Products include:
Allegra 712
Allegra-D Extended-Release Tablets 714

Fluphenazine Decanoate (Scopolamine is an anticholinergic agent and causes certain CNS effects, such as drowsiness and dizziness, and hence it should be used with care in patients on concomitant therapy).
No products indexed under this heading.

Fluphenazine Enanthate (Scopolamine is an anticholinergic agent and causes certain CNS effects, such as drowsiness and dizziness, and hence it should be used with care in patients on concomitant therapy).
No products indexed under this heading.

Fluphenazine Hydrochloride (Scopolamine is an anticholinergic agent and causes certain CNS effects, such as drowsiness and dizziness, and hence it should be used with care in patients on concomitant therapy).
No products indexed under this heading.

Flurazepam Hydrochloride (Scopolamine is an anticholinergic agent and causes certain CNS effects, such as drowsiness and dizziness, and hence it should be used with care in patients on concomitant therapy).
No products indexed under this heading.

Glutethimide (Scopolamine is an anticholinergic agent and causes certain CNS effects, such as drowsiness and dizziness, and hence it should be used with care in patients on concomitant therapy).
No products indexed under this heading.

Glycopyrrolate (Co-administration may result in additive anticholinergic effects). Products include:
Robinul Forte Tablets 1358
Robinul Injectable 2940
Robinul Tablets 1358

Haloperidol (Scopolamine is an anticholinergic agent and causes certain CNS effects, such as drowsiness and dizziness, and hence it should be used with care in patients on concomitant therapy). Products include:
Haldol Injection, Tablets and Concentrate 2533

Haloperidol Decanoate (Scopolamine is an anticholinergic agent and causes certain CNS effects, such as drowsiness and dizziness, and

hence it should be used with care in patients on concomitant therapy). Products include:

Haldol Decanoate **2535**

Hydrocodone Bitartrate (Scopolamine is an anticholinergic agent and causes certain CNS effects, such as drowsiness and dizziness, and hence it should be used with care in patients on concomitant therapy). Products include:

Hycodan **1316**
Hycomine Compound Tablets **1317**
Hycotuss Expectorant Syrup **1318**
Lortab **3319**
Lortab Elixir **3317**
Maxidone Tablets CIII **3399**
Norco 5/325 Tablets CIII **3424**
Norco 7.5/325 Tablets CIII **3425**
Norco 10/325 Tablets CIII **3427**
Norco 10/325 Tablets CIII **3425**
Vicodin Tablets **516**
Vicodin ES Tablets **517**
Vicodin HP Tablets **518**
Vicodin Tuss Expectorant **519**
Vicoprofen Tablets **520**
Zydone Tablets **1330**

Hydrocodone Polistirex (Scopolamine is an anticholinergic agent and causes certain CNS effects, such as drowsiness and dizziness, and hence it should be used with care in patients on concomitant therapy). Products include:

Tussionex Pennkinetic Extended-Release Suspension **1174**

Hydromorphone Hydrochloride (Scopolamine is an anticholinergic agent and causes certain CNS effects, such as drowsiness and dizziness, and hence it should be used with care in patients on concomitant therapy). Products include:

Dilaudid **441**
Dilaudid Oral Liquid **445**
Dilaudid Powder **441**
Dilaudid Rectal Suppositories **441**
Dilaudid Tablets **441**
Dilaudid Tablets - 8 mg **445**
Dilaudid-HP **443**

Hydroxyzine Hydrochloride (Scopolamine is an anticholinergic agent and causes certain CNS effects, such as drowsiness and dizziness, and hence it should be used with care in patients on concomitant therapy). Products include:

Atarax Tablets & Syrup **2667**
Vistaril Intramuscular Solution **2738**

Hyoscyamine (Co-administration may result in additive anticholinergic effects). Products include:

Urised Tablets **2876**

Hyoscyamine Sulfate (Co-administration may result in additive anticholinergic effects). Products include:

Arco-Lase Plus Tablets **592**
Donnatal **2929**
Donnatal Extentabs **2930**
Levsin/Levsinex/Levbid **3172**
NuLev Orally Disintegrating Tablets **3176**
Prosed/DS Tablets **3268**
Urimax Tablets **1769**

Imipramine Hydrochloride (Tricyclic antidepressants have anticholinergic properties and co-administration may result in additive effects).

No products indexed under this heading.

Imipramine Pamoate (Tricyclic antidepressants have anticholinergic properties and co-administration may result in additive effects).

No products indexed under this heading.

Ipratropium Bromide (Co-administration may result in additive anticholinergic effects). Products include:

Atrovent Inhalation Aerosol **1030**
Atrovent Inhalation Solution **1031**
Atrovent Nasal Spray 0.03% **1032**
Atrovent Nasal Spray 0.06% **1033**
Combivent Inhalation Aerosol **1041**
DuoNeb Inhalation Solution **1233**

Isoflurane (Scopolamine is an anticholinergic agent and causes certain CNS effects, such as drowsiness and dizziness, and hence it should be used with care in patients on concomitant therapy).

No products indexed under this heading.

Ketamine Hydrochloride (Scopolamine is an anticholinergic agent and causes certain CNS effects, such as drowsiness and dizziness, and hence it should be used with care in patients on concomitant therapy).

No products indexed under this heading.

Levomethadyl Acetate Hydrochloride (Scopolamine is an anticholinergic agent and causes certain CNS effects, such as drowsiness and dizziness, and hence it should be used with care in patients on concomitant therapy).

No products indexed under this heading.

Levorphanol Tartrate (Scopolamine is an anticholinergic agent and causes certain CNS effects, such as drowsiness and dizziness, and hence it should be used with care in patients on concomitant therapy). Products include:

Levo-Dromoran **1734**
Levorphanol Tartrate Tablets **3059**

Loratadine (Antihistamines have anticholinergic properties and co-administration may result in additive effects). Products include:

Claritin **3100**
Claritin-D 12 Hour Extended Release Tablets **3102**
Claritin-D 24 Hour Extended Release Tablets **3104**

Lorazepam (Scopolamine is an anticholinergic agent and causes certain CNS effects, such as drowsiness and dizziness, and hence it should be used with care in patients on concomitant therapy). Products include:

Ativan Injection **3478**
Ativan Tablets **3482**

Loxapine Hydrochloride (Scopolamine is an anticholinergic agent and causes certain CNS effects, such as drowsiness and dizziness, and hence it should be used with care in patients on concomitant therapy).

No products indexed under this heading.

Loxapine Succinate (Scopolamine is an anticholinergic agent and causes certain CNS effects, such as drowsiness and dizziness, and hence it should be used with care in patients on concomitant therapy). Products include:

Loxitane Capsules **3398**

Maprotiline Hydrochloride (Tricyclic antidepressants have anticholinergic properties and co-administration may result in additive effects).

No products indexed under this heading.

Meclizine Hydrochloride (Antihistamines have anticholinergic properties and co-administration may result in additive effects). Products include:

Antivert, Antivert/25, & Antivert/50 Tablets **2664**
Dramamine Less Drowsy Tablets **718**

Mepenzolate Bromide (Co-administration may result in additive anticholinergic effects).

No products indexed under this heading.

Meperidine Hydrochloride (Scopolamine is an anticholinergic agent and causes certain CNS effects, such as drowsiness and dizziness, and hence it should be used with care in patients on concomitant therapy). Products include:

Demerol **3079**
Mepergan Injection **3539**

Mephobarbital (Scopolamine is an anticholinergic agent and causes certain CNS effects, such as drowsiness and dizziness, and hence it should be used with care in patients on concomitant therapy).

No products indexed under this heading.

Meprobamate (Scopolamine is an anticholinergic agent and causes certain CNS effects, such as drowsiness and dizziness, and hence it should be used with care in patients on concomitant therapy). Products include:

Miltown Tablets **3349**

Mesoridazine Besylate (Scopolamine is an anticholinergic agent and causes certain CNS effects, such as drowsiness and dizziness, and hence it should be used with care in patients on concomitant therapy). Products include:

Serentil **1057**

Methadone Hydrochloride (Scopolamine is an anticholinergic agent and causes certain CNS effects, such as drowsiness and dizziness, and hence it should be used with care in patients on concomitant therapy). Products include:

Dolophine Hydrochloride Tablets **3056**

Methdilazine Hydrochloride (Antihistamines have anticholinergic properties and co-administration may result in additive effects).

No products indexed under this heading.

Methohexital Sodium (Scopolamine is an anticholinergic agent and causes certain CNS effects, such as drowsiness and dizziness, and hence it should be used with care in patients on concomitant therapy). Products include:

Brevital Sodium for Injection, USP **1815**

Methotrimeprazine (Scopolamine is an anticholinergic agent and causes certain CNS effects, such as drowsiness and dizziness, and hence it should be used with care in patients on concomitant therapy).

No products indexed under this heading.

Methoxyflurane (Scopolamine is an anticholinergic agent and causes certain CNS effects, such as drowsiness and dizziness, and hence it should be used with care in patients on concomitant therapy).

No products indexed under this heading.

Midazolam Hydrochloride (Scopolamine is an anticholinergic agent and causes certain CNS effects, such as drowsiness and dizziness, and hence it should be used with care in patients on concomitant therapy). Products include:

Versed Injection **3027**
Versed Syrup **3033**

Molindone Hydrochloride (Scopolamine is an anticholinergic agent and causes certain CNS effects, such as drowsiness and dizziness, and hence it should be used with care in patients on concomitant therapy). Products include:

Moban **1320**

Morphine Sulfate (Scopolamine is an anticholinergic agent and causes certain CNS effects, such as drowsiness and dizziness, and hence it should be used with care in patients on concomitant therapy). Products include:

Astramorph/PF Injection, USP (Preservative-Free) **594**
Duramorph Injection **1312**
Infumorph 200 and Infumorph 500 Sterile Solutions **1314**
Kadian Capsules **1335**
MS Contin Tablets **2896**
MSIR **2898**
Oramorph SR Tablets **3062**
Roxanol **3066**

Nortriptyline Hydrochloride (Tricyclic antidepressants have anticholinergic properties and co-administration may result in additive effects).

No products indexed under this heading.

Olanzapine (Scopolamine is an anticholinergic agent and causes certain CNS effects, such as drowsiness and dizziness, and hence it should be used with care in patients on concomitant therapy). Products include:

Zyprexa Tablets **1973**
Zyprexa ZYDIS Orally Disintegrating Tablets **1973**

Oxazepam (Scopolamine is an anticholinergic agent and causes certain CNS effects, such as drowsiness and dizziness, and hence it should be used with care in patients on concomitant therapy).

No products indexed under this heading.

Oxybutynin Chloride (Co-administration may result in additive anticholinergic effects). Products include:

Ditropan XL Extended Release Tablets **564**

Oxycodone Hydrochloride (Scopolamine is an anticholinergic agent and causes certain CNS effects, such as drowsiness and dizziness, and hence it should be used with care in patients on concomitant therapy). Products include:

OxyContin Tablets **2912**
OxyFast Oral Concentrate Solution **2916**
OxyIR Capsules **2916**
Percocet Tablets **1326**
Percodan Tablets **1327**
Percolone Tablets **1327**
Roxicodone **3067**
Tylox Capsules **2597**

Pentobarbital Sodium (Scopolamine is an anticholinergic agent and causes certain CNS effects, such as drowsiness and dizziness, and hence it should be used with care in patients on concomitant therapy). Products include:

Nembutal Sodium Solution **485**

Perphenazine (Scopolamine is an anticholinergic agent and causes certain CNS effects, such as drowsiness and dizziness, and hence it should be used with care in patients on concomitant therapy). Products include:

Etrafon **3115**
Trilafon **3160**

Phenobarbital (Scopolamine is an anticholinergic agent and causes certain CNS effects, such as drowsiness and dizziness, and hence it should be used with care in patients on concomitant therapy). Products include:

Arco-Lase Plus Tablets **592**
Donnatal **2929**
Donnatal Extentabs **2930**

Prazepam (Scopolamine is an anticholinergic agent and causes certain CNS effects, such as drowsiness and dizziness, and hence it should be used with care in patients on concomitant therapy).

No products indexed under this heading.

Prochlorperazine (Scopolamine is an anticholinergic agent and causes certain CNS effects, such as drowsiness and dizziness, and hence it should be used with care in patients on concomitant therapy). Products include:

Compazine **1505**

Procyclidine Hydrochloride (Co-administration may result in additive anticholinergic effects).

No products indexed under this heading.

Promethazine Hydrochloride (Antihistamines have anticholinergic properties and co-administration may result in additive effects). Products include:
- Mepergan Injection 3539
- Phenergan Injection 3553
- Phenergan 3556
- Phenergan Syrup 3554
- Phenergan with Codeine Syrup 3557
- Phenergan with Dextromethorphan Syrup 3559
- Phenergan VC Syrup 3560
- Phenergan VC with Codeine Syrup .. 3561

Propantheline Bromide (Co-administration may result in additive anticholinergic effects).
No products indexed under this heading.

Propofol (Scopolamine is an anticholinergic agent and causes certain CNS effects, such as drowsiness and dizziness, and hence it should be used with care in patients on concomitant therapy). Products include:
- Diprivan Injectable Emulsion 667

Propoxyphene Hydrochloride (Scopolamine is an anticholinergic agent and causes certain CNS effects, such as drowsiness and dizziness, and hence it should be used with care in patients on concomitant therapy). Products include:
- Darvon Pulvules 1909
- Darvon Compound-65 Pulvules 1910

Propoxyphene Napsylate (Scopolamine is an anticholinergic agent and causes certain CNS effects, such as drowsiness and dizziness, and hence it should be used with care in patients on concomitant therapy). Products include:
- Darvon-N/Darvocet-N 1907
- Darvon-N Tablets 1912

Protriptyline Hydrochloride (Tricyclic antidepressants have anticholinergic properties and co-administration may result in additive effects). Products include:
- Vivactil Tablets 2446
- Vivactil Tablets 2217

Pyrilamine Maleate (Antihistamines have anticholinergic properties and co-administration may result in additive effects). Products include:
- Maximum Strength Midol Menstrual Caplets and Gelcaps .... ▣612
- Maximum Strength Midol PMS Caplets and Gelcaps .... ▣613

Pyrilamine Tannate (Antihistamines have anticholinergic properties and co-administration may result in additive effects). Products include:
- Ryna-12 S Suspension 3351

Quazepam (Scopolamine is an anticholinergic agent and causes certain CNS effects, such as drowsiness and dizziness, and hence it should be used with care in patients on concomitant therapy).
No products indexed under this heading.

Quetiapine Fumarate (Scopolamine is an anticholinergic agent and causes certain CNS effects, such as drowsiness and dizziness, and hence it should be used with care in patients on concomitant therapy). Products include:
- Seroquel Tablets 684

Remifentanil Hydrochloride (Scopolamine is an anticholinergic agent and causes certain CNS effects, such as drowsiness and dizziness, and hence it should be used with care in patients on concomitant therapy).
No products indexed under this heading.

Risperidone (Scopolamine is an anticholinergic agent and causes certain CNS effects, such as drowsiness and dizziness, and hence it should be used with care in patients on concomitant therapy). Products include:
- Risperdal 1796

Scopolamine Hydrobromide (Co-administration may result in additive anticholinergic effects). Products include:
- Donnatal 2929
- Donnatal Extentabs 2930

Secobarbital Sodium (Scopolamine is an anticholinergic agent and causes certain CNS effects, such as drowsiness and dizziness, and hence it should be used with care in patients on concomitant therapy).
No products indexed under this heading.

Sevoflurane (Scopolamine is an anticholinergic agent and causes certain CNS effects, such as drowsiness and dizziness, and hence it should be used with care in patients on concomitant therapy).
No products indexed under this heading.

Sufentanil Citrate (Scopolamine is an anticholinergic agent and causes certain CNS effects, such as drowsiness and dizziness, and hence it should be used with care in patients on concomitant therapy).
No products indexed under this heading.

Temazepam (Scopolamine is an anticholinergic agent and causes certain CNS effects, such as drowsiness and dizziness, and hence it should be used with care in patients on concomitant therapy).
No products indexed under this heading.

Terfenadine (Antihistamines have anticholinergic properties and co-administration may result in additive effects).
No products indexed under this heading.

Thiamylal Sodium (Scopolamine is an anticholinergic agent and causes certain CNS effects, such as drowsiness and dizziness, and hence it should be used with care in patients on concomitant therapy).
No products indexed under this heading.

Thioridazine Hydrochloride (Scopolamine is an anticholinergic agent and causes certain CNS effects, such as drowsiness and dizziness, and hence it should be used with care in patients on concomitant therapy). Products include:
- Thioridazine Hydrochloride Tablets 2289

Thiothixene (Scopolamine is an anticholinergic agent and causes certain CNS effects, such as drowsiness and dizziness, and hence it should be used with care in patients on concomitant therapy). Products include:
- Navane Capsules 2701
- Thiothixene Capsules 2290

Tolterodine Tartrate (Co-administration may result in additive anticholinergic effects). Products include:
- Detrol Tablets 3623
- Detrol LA Capsules 2801

Triazolam (Scopolamine is an anticholinergic agent and causes certain CNS effects, such as drowsiness and dizziness, and hence it should be used with care in patients on concomitant therapy). Products include:
- Halcion Tablets 2823

Tridihexethyl Chloride (Co-administration may result in additive anticholinergic effects).
No products indexed under this heading.

Trifluoperazine Hydrochloride (Scopolamine is an anticholinergic agent and causes certain CNS effects, such as drowsiness and dizziness, and hence it should be used with care in patients on concomitant therapy). Products include:
- Stelazine 1640

Trihexyphenidyl Hydrochloride (Co-administration may result in additive anticholinergic effects). Products include:
- Artane 1855

Trimeprazine Tartrate (Antihistamines have anticholinergic properties and co-administration may result in additive effects).
No products indexed under this heading.

Trimipramine Maleate (Tricyclic antidepressants have anticholinergic properties and co-administration may result in additive effects). Products include:
- Surmontil Capsules 3595

Tripelennamine Hydrochloride (Antihistamines have anticholinergic properties and co-administration may result in additive effects).
No products indexed under this heading.

Triprolidine Hydrochloride (Antihistamines have anticholinergic properties and co-administration may result in additive effects). Products include:
- Actifed Cold & Allergy Tablets .... ▣688

Zaleplon (Scopolamine is an anticholinergic agent and causes certain CNS effects, such as drowsiness and dizziness, and hence it should be used with care in patients on concomitant therapy). Products include:
- Sonata Capsules 3591

Ziprasidone Hydrochloride (Scopolamine is an anticholinergic agent and causes certain CNS effects, such as drowsiness and dizziness, and hence it should be used with care in patients on concomitant therapy). Products include:
- Geodon Capsules 2688

Zolpidem Tartrate (Scopolamine is an anticholinergic agent and causes certain CNS effects, such as drowsiness and dizziness, and hence it should be used with care in patients on concomitant therapy). Products include:
- Ambien Tablets 3191

Food Interactions

Alcohol (Scopolamine is an anticholinergic agent and causes certain CNS effects, such as drowsiness and dizziness, and hence it should be used with care in patients on concomitant therapy).

TRANSFER FACTOR CAPSULES

(Colostrum) .... ▣814
None cited in PDR database.

TRANXENE T-TAB TABLETS

(Clorazepate Dipotassium) 511
May interact with barbiturates, central nervous system depressants, antidepressant drugs, hypnotics and sedatives, monoamine oxidase inhibitors, narcotic analgesics, phenothiazines, and certain other agents. Compounds in these categories include:

Alfentanil Hydrochloride (Actions of benzodiazepines may be potentiated).
No products indexed under this heading.

Alprazolam (Actions of benzodiazepines may be potentiated). Products include:
- Xanax Tablets 2865

Amitriptyline Hydrochloride (Actions of benzodiazepines may be potentiated). Products include:
- Etrafon 3115
- Limbitrol 1738

Amoxapine (Actions of benzodiazepines may be potentiated).
No products indexed under this heading.

Aprobarbital (Actions of benzodiazepines may be potentiated).
No products indexed under this heading.

Buprenorphine Hydrochloride (Actions of benzodiazepines may be potentiated). Products include:
- Buprenex Injectable 2918

Bupropion Hydrochloride (Actions of benzodiazepines may be potentiated). Products include:
- Wellbutrin Tablets 1680
- Wellbutrin SR Sustained-Release Tablets 1684
- Zyban Sustained-Release Tablets ... 1710

Buspirone Hydrochloride (Actions of benzodiazepines may be potentiated).
No products indexed under this heading.

Butabarbital (Actions of benzodiazepines may be potentiated).
No products indexed under this heading.

Butalbital (Actions of benzodiazepines may be potentiated). Products include:
- Phrenilin 578
- Sedapap Tablets 50 mg/650 mg ... 2225

Chlordiazepoxide (Actions of benzodiazepines may be potentiated). Products include:
- Limbitrol 1738

Chlordiazepoxide Hydrochloride (Actions of benzodiazepines may be potentiated). Products include:
- Librium Capsules 1736
- Librium for Injection 1737

Chlorpromazine (Actions of benzodiazepines may be potentiated). Products include:
- Thorazine Suppositories 1656

Chlorpromazine Hydrochloride (Actions of benzodiazepines may be potentiated). Products include:
- Thorazine 1656

Chlorprothixene (Actions of benzodiazepines may be potentiated).
No products indexed under this heading.

Chlorprothixene Hydrochloride (Actions of benzodiazepines may be potentiated).
No products indexed under this heading.

Chlorprothixene Lactate (Actions of benzodiazepines may be potentiated).
No products indexed under this heading.

Citalopram Hydrobromide (Actions of benzodiazepines may be potentiated). Products include:
- Celexa 1365

Clozapine (Actions of benzodiazepines may be potentiated). Products include:
- Clozaril Tablets 2319

Codeine Phosphate (Actions of benzodiazepines may be potentiated). Products include:
- Phenergan with Codeine Syrup 3557
- Phenergan VC with Codeine Syrup .. 3561
- Robitussin A-C Syrup 2942
- Robitussin-DAC Syrup 2942
- Ryna-C Liquid .... ▣768
- Soma Compound w/Codeine Tablets 3355
- Tussi-Organidin NR Liquid 3350
- Tussi-Organidin-S NR Liquid 3350
- Tylenol with Codeine 2595

Desflurane (Actions of benzodiazepines may be potentiated). Products include:
- Suprane Liquid for Inhalation 874

Desipramine Hydrochloride (Actions of benzodiazepines may be potentiated). Products include:

Norpramin Tablets 755

Dezocine (Actions of benzodiazepines may be potentiated).
No products indexed under this heading.

Diazepam (Actions of benzodiazepines may be potentiated). Products include:
Valium Injectable 3026
Valium Tablets 3047

Doxepin Hydrochloride (Actions of benzodiazepines may be potentiated). Products include:
Sinequan 2713

Droperidol (Actions of benzodiazepines may be potentiated).
No products indexed under this heading.

Enflurane (Actions of benzodiazepines may be potentiated).
No products indexed under this heading.

Estazolam (Actions of benzodiazepines may be potentiated; increased sedation with concurrent use). Products include:
ProSom Tablets 500

Ethchlorvynol (Actions of benzodiazepines may be potentiated; increased sedation with concurrent use).
No products indexed under this heading.

Ethinamate (Actions of benzodiazepines may be potentiated; increased sedation with concurrent use).
No products indexed under this heading.

Fentanyl (Actions of benzodiazepines may be potentiated). Products include:
Duragesic Transdermal System 1786

Fentanyl Citrate (Actions of benzodiazepines may be potentiated). Products include:
Actiq 1184

Fluoxetine Hydrochloride (Actions of benzodiazepines may be potentiated). Products include:
Prozac Pulvules, Liquid, and Weekly Capsules 1238
Sarafem Pulvules 1962

Fluphenazine Decanoate (Actions of benzodiazepines may be potentiated).
No products indexed under this heading.

Fluphenazine Enanthate (Actions of benzodiazepines may be potentiated).
No products indexed under this heading.

Fluphenazine Hydrochloride (Actions of benzodiazepines may be potentiated).
No products indexed under this heading.

Flurazepam Hydrochloride (Actions of benzodiazepines may be potentiated; increased sedation with concurrent use).
No products indexed under this heading.

Glutethimide (Actions of benzodiazepines may be potentiated; increased sedation with concurrent use).
No products indexed under this heading.

Haloperidol (Actions of benzodiazepines may be potentiated). Products include:
Haldol Injection, Tablets and Concentrate 2533

Haloperidol Decanoate (Actions of benzodiazepines may be potentiated). Products include:
Haldol Decanoate 2535

Hydrocodone Bitartrate (Actions of benzodiazepines may be potentiated). Products include:
Hycodan 1316
Hycomine Compound Tablets 1317
Hycotuss Expectorant Syrup 1318
Lortab 3319
Lortab Elixir 3317
Maxidone Tablets CIII 3399
Norco 5/325 Tablets CIII 3424
Norco 7.5/325 Tablets CIII 3425
Norco 10/325 Tablets CIII 3427
Norco 10/325 Tablets CIII 3425
Vicodin Tablets 516
Vicodin ES Tablets 517
Vicodin HP Tablets 518
Vicodin Tuss Expectorant 519
Vicoprofen Tablets 520
Zydone Tablets 1330

Hydrocodone Polistirex (Actions of benzodiazepines may be potentiated). Products include:
Tussionex Pennkinetic Extended-Release Suspension 1174

Hydromorphone Hydrochloride (Actions of benzodiazepines may be potentiated). Products include:
Dilaudid 441
Dilaudid Oral Liquid 445
Dilaudid Powder 441
Dilaudid Rectal Suppositories 441
Dilaudid Tablets 441
Dilaudid Tablets - 8 mg 445
Dilaudid-HP 443

Hydroxyzine Hydrochloride (Actions of benzodiazepines may be potentiated). Products include:
Atarax Tablets & Syrup 2667
Vistaril Intramuscular Solution 2738

Imipramine Hydrochloride (Actions of benzodiazepines may be potentiated).
No products indexed under this heading.

Imipramine Pamoate (Actions of benzodiazepines may be potentiated).
No products indexed under this heading.

Isocarboxazid (Actions of benzodiazepines may be potentiated).
No products indexed under this heading.

Isoflurane (Actions of benzodiazepines may be potentiated).
No products indexed under this heading.

Ketamine Hydrochloride (Actions of benzodiazepines may be potentiated).
No products indexed under this heading.

Levomethadyl Acetate Hydrochloride (Actions of benzodiazepines may be potentiated).
No products indexed under this heading.

Levorphanol Tartrate (Actions of benzodiazepines may be potentiated). Products include:
Levo-Dromoran 1734
Levorphanol Tartrate Tablets 3059

Lorazepam (Actions of benzodiazepines may be potentiated; increased sedation with concurrent use). Products include:
Ativan Injection 3478
Ativan Tablets 3482

Loxapine Hydrochloride (Actions of benzodiazepines may be potentiated).
No products indexed under this heading.

Loxapine Succinate (Actions of benzodiazepines may be potentiated). Products include:
Loxitane Capsules 3398

Maprotiline Hydrochloride (Actions of benzodiazepines may be potentiated).
No products indexed under this heading.

Meperidine Hydrochloride (Actions of benzodiazepines may be potentiated). Products include:
Demerol 3079
Mepergan Injection 3539

Mephobarbital (Actions of benzodiazepines may be potentiated).
No products indexed under this heading.

Meprobamate (Actions of benzodiazepines may be potentiated). Products include:
Miltown Tablets 3349

Mesoridazine Besylate (Actions of benzodiazepines may be potentiated). Products include:
Serentil 1057

Methadone Hydrochloride (Actions of benzodiazepines may be potentiated). Products include:
Dolophine Hydrochloride Tablets 3056

Methohexital Sodium (Actions of benzodiazepines may be potentiated). Products include:
Brevital Sodium for Injection, USP 1815

Methotrimeprazine (Actions of benzodiazepines may be potentiated).
No products indexed under this heading.

Methoxyflurane (Actions of benzodiazepines may be potentiated).
No products indexed under this heading.

Midazolam Hydrochloride (Actions of benzodiazepines may be potentiated; increased sedation with concurrent use). Products include:
Versed Injection 3027
Versed Syrup 3033

Mirtazapine (Actions of benzodiazepines may be potentiated). Products include:
Remeron Tablets 2483
Remeron SolTab Tablets 2486

Moclobemide (Actions of benzodiazepines may be potentiated).
No products indexed under this heading.

Molindone Hydrochloride (Actions of benzodiazepines may be potentiated). Products include:
Moban 1320

Morphine Sulfate (Actions of benzodiazepines may be potentiated). Products include:
Astramorph/PF Injection, USP (Preservative-Free) 594
Duramorph Injection 1312
Infumorph 200 and Infumorph 500 Sterile Solutions 1314
Kadian Capsules 1335
MS Contin Tablets 2896
MSIR 2898
Oramorph SR Tablets 3062
Roxanol 3066

Nefazodone Hydrochloride (Actions of benzodiazepines may be potentiated). Products include:
Serzone Tablets 1104

Nortriptyline Hydrochloride (Actions of benzodiazepines may be potentiated).
No products indexed under this heading.

Olanzapine (Actions of benzodiazepines may be potentiated). Products include:
Zyprexa Tablets 1973
Zyprexa ZYDIS Orally Disintegrating Tablets 1973

Oxazepam (Actions of benzodiazepines may be potentiated).
No products indexed under this heading.

Oxycodone Hydrochloride (Actions of benzodiazepines may be potentiated). Products include:
OxyContin Tablets 2912
OxyFast Oral Concentrate Solution 2916
OxyIR Capsules 2916
Percocet Tablets 1326
Percodan Tablets 1327
Percolone Tablets 1327
Roxicodone 3067
Tylox Capsules 2597

Pargyline Hydrochloride (Actions of benzodiazepines may be potentiated).
No products indexed under this heading.

Paroxetine Hydrochloride (Actions of benzodiazepines may be potentiated). Products include:
Paxil 1609

Pentobarbital Sodium (Actions of benzodiazepines may be potentiated). Products include:
Nembutal Sodium Solution 485

Perphenazine (Actions of benzodiazepines may be potentiated). Products include:
Etrafon 3115
Trilafon 3160

Phenelzine Sulfate (Actions of benzodiazepines may be potentiated). Products include:
Nardil Tablets 2653

Phenobarbital (Actions of benzodiazepines may be potentiated). Products include:
Arco-Lase Plus Tablets 592
Donnatal 2929
Donnatal Extentabs 2930

Prazepam (Actions of benzodiazepines may be potentiated).
No products indexed under this heading.

Procarbazine Hydrochloride (Actions of benzodiazepines may be potentiated). Products include:
Matulane Capsules 3246

Prochlorperazine (Actions of benzodiazepines may be potentiated). Products include:
Compazine 1505

Promethazine Hydrochloride (Actions of benzodiazepines may be potentiated). Products include:
Mepergan Injection 3539
Phenergan Injection 3553
Phenergan 3556
Phenergan Syrup 3554
Phenergan with Codeine Syrup 3557
Phenergan with Dextromethorphan Syrup 3559
Phenergan VC Syrup 3560
Phenergan VC with Codeine Syrup 3561

Propofol (Actions of benzodiazepines may be potentiated; increased sedation with concurrent use). Products include:
Diprivan Injectable Emulsion 667

Propoxyphene Hydrochloride (Actions of benzodiazepines may be potentiated). Products include:
Darvon Pulvules 1909
Darvon Compound-65 Pulvules 1910

Propoxyphene Napsylate (Actions of benzodiazepines may be potentiated). Products include:
Darvon-N/Darvocet-N 1907
Darvon-N Tablets 1912

Protriptyline Hydrochloride (Actions of benzodiazepines may be potentiated). Products include:
Vivactil Tablets 2446
Vivactil Tablets 2217

Quazepam (Actions of benzodiazepines may be potentiated; increased sedation with concurrent use).
No products indexed under this heading.

Quetiapine Fumarate (Actions of benzodiazepines may be potentiated). Products include:
Seroquel Tablets 684

Remifentanil Hydrochloride (Actions of benzodiazepines may be potentiated).
No products indexed under this heading.

Risperidone (Actions of benzodiazepines may be potentiated). Products include:
Risperdal 1796

Secobarbital Sodium (Actions of benzodiazepines may be potentiated).
No products indexed under this heading.

IMPORTANT NOTE: Always consult each drug listing in the patient's regimen for possible interactions.

Selegiline Hydrochloride (Actions of benzodiazepines may be potentiated). Products include:
Eldepryl Capsules 3266

Sertraline Hydrochloride (Actions of benzodiazepines may be potentiated). Products include:
Zoloft 2751

Sevoflurane (Actions of benzodiazepines may be potentiated).
No products indexed under this heading.

Sufentanil Citrate (Actions of benzodiazepines may be potentiated).
No products indexed under this heading.

Temazepam (Actions of benzodiazepines may be potentiated; increased sedation with concurrent use).
No products indexed under this heading.

Thiamylal Sodium (Actions of benzodiazepines may be potentiated).
No products indexed under this heading.

Thioridazine Hydrochloride (Actions of benzodiazepines may be potentiated). Products include:
Thioridazine Hydrochloride Tablets 2289

Thiothixene (Actions of benzodiazepines may be potentiated). Products include:
Navane Capsules 2701
Thiothixene Capsules 2290

Tranylcypromine Sulfate (Actions of benzodiazepines may be potentiated). Products include:
Parnate Tablets 1607

Trazodone Hydrochloride (Actions of benzodiazepines may be potentiated).
No products indexed under this heading.

Triazolam (Actions of benzodiazepines may be potentiated; increased sedation with concurrent use). Products include:
Halcion Tablets 2823

Trifluoperazine Hydrochloride (Actions of benzodiazepines may be potentiated). Products include:
Stelazine 1640

Trimipramine Maleate (Actions of benzodiazepines may be potentiated). Products include:
Surmontil Capsules 3595

Venlafaxine Hydrochloride (Actions of benzodiazepines may be potentiated). Products include:
Effexor Tablets 3495
Effexor XR Capsules 3499

Zaleplon (Actions of benzodiazepines may be potentiated). Products include:
Sonata Capsules 3591

Ziprasidone Hydrochloride (Actions of benzodiazepines may be potentiated). Products include:
Geodon Capsules 2688

Zolpidem Tartrate (Actions of benzodiazepines may be potentiated; increased sedation with concurrent use). Products include:
Ambien Tablets 3191

Food Interactions

Alcohol (Actions of benzodiazepines may be potentiated; prolonged sleeping time).

TRANXENE-SD TABLETS
(Clorazepate Dipotassium) 511
See Tranxene T-TAB Tablets

TRANXENE-SD HALF STRENGTH TABLETS
(Clorazepate Dipotassium) 511
See Tranxene T-TAB Tablets

TRASYLOL INJECTION
(Aprotinin) 909
May interact with fibrinolytic agents and certain other agents. Compounds in these categories include:

Alteplase, Recombinant (Aprotinin may inhibit the effects of fibrinolytic agents). Products include:
Activase I.V. 1410
Cathflo Activase 3611

Anistreplase (Aprotinin may inhibit the effects of fibrinolytic agents).
No products indexed under this heading.

Captopril (Aprotinin may block the acute hypotensive effects of captopril). Products include:
Captopril Tablets 2281

Heparin Sodium (Aprotinin, in the presence of heparin, has been found to prolong the activated clotting time (ACT) as measured by surface activation methods). Products include:
Heparin Lock Flush Solution 3509
Heparin Sodium Injection 3511

Streptokinase (Aprotinin may inhibit the effects of fibrinolytic agents). Products include:
Streptase for Infusion 647

Urokinase (Aprotinin may inhibit the effects of fibrinolytic agents).
No products indexed under this heading.

TRAUMEEL INJECTION SOLUTION
(Homeopathic Formulations) 1726
None cited in PDR database.

TRAVATAN OPHTHALMIC SOLUTION
(Travoprost) 543
None cited in PDR database.

TRECATOR-SC TABLETS
(Ethionamide) 3598
May interact with antituberculosis drugs and certain other agents. Compounds in these categories include:

Aminosalicylic Acid (Ethionamide may potentiate the adverse effects of other antituberculosis drugs administered concomitantly). Products include:
Paser Granules 1781

p-Aminosalicylic Acid (Ethionamide may potentiate the adverse effects of other antituberculosis drugs administered concomitantly).
No products indexed under this heading.

Cycloserine (Co-administration has resulted in convulsions).
No products indexed under this heading.

Ethambutol Hydrochloride (Ethionamide may potentiate the adverse effects of other antituberculosis drugs administered concomitantly). Products include:
Myambutol Tablets 1290

Isoniazid (Ethionamide has been found to temporarily raise serum concentrations of isoniazid). Products include:
Rifamate Capsules 767
Rifater Tablets 769

Pyrazinamide (Ethionamide may potentiate the adverse effects of other antituberculosis drugs administered concomitantly). Products include:
Pyrazinamide Tablets 1876
Rifater Tablets 769

Rifampin (Ethionamide may potentiate the adverse effects of other antituberculosis drugs administered concomitantly). Products include:
Rifadin 765
Rifamate Capsules 767
Rifater Tablets 769

Rifapentine (Ethionamide may potentiate the adverse effects of other antituberculosis drugs administered concomitantly). Products include:
Priftin Tablets 758

Food Interactions

Alcohol (Excessive ingestion of alcohol should be avoided because a psychotic reaction has been reported).

TRENTAL TABLETS
(Pentoxifylline) 784
May interact with antihypertensives, anticoagulants, non-steroidal anti-inflammatory agents, theophylline, and certain other agents. Compounds in these categories include:

Acebutolol Hydrochloride (Pentoxifylline causes a small decrease in blood pressure in some patients; periodic monitoring of blood pressure is recommended in patients receiving concomitant antihypertensive therapy). Products include:
Sectral Capsules 3589

Aminophylline (Co-administration with theophylline-containing products leads to increased theophylline levels and theophylline toxicity).
No products indexed under this heading.

Amlodipine Besylate (Pentoxifylline causes a small decrease in blood pressure in some patients; periodic monitoring of blood pressure is recommended in patients receiving concomitant antihypertensive therapy). Products include:
Lotrel Capsules 2370
Norvasc Tablets 2704

Ardeparin Sodium (Co-administration has resulted in reports of bleeding and/or prolonged prothrombin time in patients treated with anticoagulants).
No products indexed under this heading.

Aspirin (Co-administration has resulted in reports of bleeding and/or prolonged prothrombin time in patients treated with platelet aggregation inhibitors). Products include:
Aggrenox Capsules 1026
Alka-Seltzer .... ■603
Alka-Seltzer Lemon Lime Antacid and Pain Reliever Effervescent Tablets .... ■603
Alka-Seltzer Extra Strength Antacid and Pain Reliever Effervescent Tablets .... ■603
Alka-Seltzer PM Effervescent Tablets .... ■605
Genuine Bayer Tablets, Caplets and Gelcaps .... ■000
Extra Strength Bayer Caplets and Gelcaps .... ■610
Aspirin Regimen Bayer Children's Chewable Tablets (Orange or Cherry Flavored) .... ■607
Bayer, Aspirin Regimen .... ■606
Aspirin Regimen Bayer 81 mg Caplets with Calcium .... ■607
Genuine Bayer Professional Labeling (Aspirin Regimen Bayer) .... ■608
Extra Strength Bayer Arthritis Caplets .... ■610
Extra Strength Bayer Plus Caplets .... ■610
Extra Strength Bayer PM Caplets .. ■611
BC Powder .... ■619
BC Allergy Sinus Cold Powder ...... ■619
Arthritis Strength BC Powder .... ■619
BC Sinus Cold Powder .... ■619
Darvon Compound-65 Pulvules 1910
Ecotrin Enteric Coated Aspirin Low, Regular and Maximum Strength Tablets 1715
Excedrin Extra-Strength Tablets, Caplets, and Geltabs .... ■629
Excedrin Migraine 1070
Goody's Body Pain Formula Powder .... ■620
Goody's Extra Strength Headache Powder .... ■620
Goody's Extra Strength Pain Relief Tablets .... ■620
Percodan Tablets 1327
Robaxisal Tablets 2939
Soma Compound Tablets 3354
Soma Compound w/Codeine Tablets 3355
Vanquish Caplets .... ■617

Atenolol (Pentoxifylline causes a small decrease in blood pressure in some patients; periodic monitoring of blood pressure is recommended in patients receiving concomitant antihypertensive therapy). Products include:
Tenoretic Tablets 690
Tenormin I.V. Injection 692

Benazepril Hydrochloride (Pentoxifylline causes a small decrease in blood pressure in some patients; periodic monitoring of blood pressure is recommended in patients receiving concomitant antihypertensive therapy). Products include:
Lotensin Tablets 2365
Lotensin HCT Tablets 2367
Lotrel Capsules 2370

Bendroflumethiazide (Pentoxifylline causes a small decrease in blood pressure in some patients; periodic monitoring of blood pressure is recommended in patients receiving concomitant antihypertensive therapy). Products include:
Corzide 40/5 Tablets 2247
Corzide 80/5 Tablets 2247

Betaxolol Hydrochloride (Pentoxifylline causes a small decrease in blood pressure in some patients; periodic monitoring of blood pressure is recommended in patients receiving concomitant antihypertensive therapy). Products include:
Betoptic S Ophthalmic Suspension 537

Bisoprolol Fumarate (Pentoxifylline causes a small decrease in blood pressure in some patients; periodic monitoring of blood pressure is recommended in patients receiving concomitant antihypertensive therapy). Products include:
Zebeta Tablets 1885
Ziac Tablets 1887

Candesartan Cilexetil (Pentoxifylline causes a small decrease in blood pressure in some patients; periodic monitoring of blood pressure is recommended in patients receiving concomitant antihypertensive therapy). Products include:
Atacand Tablets 595
Atacand HCT Tablets 597

Captopril (Pentoxifylline causes a small decrease in blood pressure in some patients; periodic monitoring of blood pressure is recommended in patients receiving concomitant antihypertensive therapy). Products include:
Captopril Tablets 2281

Carteolol Hydrochloride (Pentoxifylline causes a small decrease in blood pressure in some patients; periodic monitoring of blood pressure is recommended in patients receiving concomitant antihypertensive therapy). Products include:
Carteolol Hydrochloride Ophthalmic Solution USP, 1% ..... ⊙258
Ocupress Ophthalmic Solution, 1% Sterile .... ⊙303

Celecoxib (Co-administration has resulted in reports of bleeding and/or prolonged prothrombin time in patients treated with platelet aggregation inhibitors). Products include:
Celebrex Capsules 2676
Celebrex Capsules 2780

Chlorothiazide (Pentoxifylline causes a small decrease in blood pressure in some patients; periodic monitoring of blood pressure is recommended in patients receiving concomitant antihypertensive therapy). Products include:
Aldoclor Tablets 2035
Diuril Oral 2087

Chlorothiazide Sodium (Pentoxifylline causes a small decrease in

blood pressure in some patients; periodic monitoring of blood pressure is recommended in patients receiving concomitant antihypertensive therapy). Products include:

Diuril Sodium Intravenous 2086

Chlorthalidone (Pentoxifylline causes a small decrease in blood pressure in some patients; periodic monitoring of blood pressure is recommended in patients receiving concomitant antihypertensive therapy). Products include:

Clorpres Tablets 1002
Combipres Tablets 1040
Tenoretic Tablets 690

Clonidine (Pentoxifylline causes a small decrease in blood pressure in some patients; periodic monitoring of blood pressure is recommended in patients receiving concomitant antihypertensive therapy). Products include:

Catapres-TTS 1038

Clonidine Hydrochloride (Pentoxifylline causes a small decrease in blood pressure in some patients; periodic monitoring of blood pressure is recommended in patients receiving concomitant antihypertensive therapy). Products include:

Catapres Tablets 1037
Clorpres Tablets 1002
Combipres Tablets 1040
Duraclon Injection 3057

Clopidogrel Bisulfate (Co-administration has resulted in reports of bleeding and/or prolonged prothrombin time in patients treated with platelet aggregation inhibitors). Products include:

Plavix Tablets 1097
Plavix Tablets 3084

Dalteparin Sodium (Co-administration has resulted in reports of bleeding and/or prolonged prothrombin time in patients treated with anticoagulants). Products include:

Fragmin Injection 2814

Danaparoid Sodium (Co-administration has resulted in reports of bleeding and/or prolonged prothrombin time in patients treated with anticoagulants). Products include:

Orgaran Injection 2480

Deserpidine (Pentoxifylline causes a small decrease in blood pressure in some patients; periodic monitoring of blood pressure is recommended in patients receiving concomitant antihypertensive therapy).

No products indexed under this heading.

Diazoxide (Pentoxifylline causes a small decrease in blood pressure in some patients; periodic monitoring of blood pressure is recommended in patients receiving concomitant antihypertensive therapy).

No products indexed under this heading.

Diclofenac Potassium (Co-administration has resulted in reports of bleeding and/or prolonged prothrombin time in patients treated with platelet aggregation inhibitors). Products include:

Cataflam Tablets 2315

Diclofenac Sodium (Co-administration has resulted in reports of bleeding and/or prolonged prothrombin time in patients treated with platelet aggregation inhibitors). Products include:

Arthrotec Tablets 3195
Voltaren Ophthalmic Sterile Ophthalmic Solution .... ⊙ 312
Voltaren Tablets 2315
Voltaren-XR Tablets 2315

Dicumarol (Co-administration has resulted in reports of bleeding and/or prolonged prothrombin time in patients treated with anticoagulants).

No products indexed under this heading.

Diltiazem Hydrochloride (Pentoxifylline causes a small decrease in blood pressure in some patients; periodic monitoring of blood pressure is recommended in patients receiving concomitant antihypertensive therapy). Products include:

Cardizem Injectable 1018
Cardizem Lyo-Ject Syringe 1018
Cardizem Monovial 1018
Cardizem CD Capsules 1016
Tiazac Capsules 1378

Dipyridamole (Co-administration has resulted in reports of bleeding and/or prolonged prothrombin time in patients treated with platelet aggregation inhibitors). Products include:

Aggrenox Capsules 1026
Persantine Tablets 1057

Doxazosin Mesylate (Pentoxifylline causes a small decrease in blood pressure in some patients; periodic monitoring of blood pressure is recommended in patients receiving concomitant antihypertensive therapy). Products include:

Cardura Tablets 2668

Dyphylline (Co-administration with theophylline-containing products leads to increased theophylline levels and theophylline toxicity). Products include:

Lufyllin Tablets 3347
Lufyllin-400 Tablets 3347
Lufyllin-GG Elixir 3348
Lufyllin-GG Tablets 3348

Enalapril Maleate (Pentoxifylline causes a small decrease in blood pressure in some patients; periodic monitoring of blood pressure is recommended in patients receiving concomitant antihypertensive therapy). Products include:

Lexxel Tablets 608
Vaseretic Tablets 2204
Vasotec Tablets 2210

Enalaprilat (Pentoxifylline causes a small decrease in blood pressure in some patients; periodic monitoring of blood pressure is recommended in patients receiving concomitant antihypertensive therapy). Products include:

Enalaprilat Injection 863
Vasotec I.V. Injection 2207

Enoxaparin (Co-administration has resulted in reports of bleeding and/or prolonged prothrombin time in patients treated with anticoagulants). Products include:

Lovenox Injection 746

Eprosartan Mesylate (Pentoxifylline causes a small decrease in blood pressure in some patients; periodic monitoring of blood pressure is recommended in patients receiving concomitant antihypertensive therapy). Products include:

Teveten Tablets 3327

Eptifibatide (Co-administration has resulted in reports of bleeding and/or prolonged prothrombin time in patients treated with platelet aggregation inhibitors). Products include:

Integrilin Injection 1213
Integrilin Injection 1828

Esmolol Hydrochloride (Pentoxifylline causes a small decrease in blood pressure in some patients; periodic monitoring of blood pressure is recommended in patients receiving concomitant antihypertensive therapy). Products include:

Brevibloc Injection 858

Etodolac (Co-administration has resulted in reports of bleeding and/or prolonged prothrombin time in patients treated with platelet aggregation inhibitors). Products include:

Lodine 3528
Lodine XL Extended-Release Tablets 3530

Felodipine (Pentoxifylline causes a small decrease in blood pressure in some patients; periodic monitoring of blood pressure is recommended in patients receiving concomitant antihypertensive therapy). Products include:

Lexxel Tablets 608
Plendil Extended-Release Tablets ... 623

Fenoprofen Calcium (Co-administration has resulted in reports of bleeding and/or prolonged prothrombin time in patients treated with platelet aggregation inhibitors).

No products indexed under this heading.

Flurbiprofen (Co-administration has resulted in reports of bleeding and/or prolonged prothrombin time in patients treated with platelet aggregation inhibitors).

No products indexed under this heading.

Fosinopril Sodium (Pentoxifylline causes a small decrease in blood pressure in some patients; periodic monitoring of blood pressure is recommended in patients receiving concomitant antihypertensive therapy). Products include:

Monopril Tablets 1091
Monopril HCT 1094

Furosemide (Pentoxifylline causes a small decrease in blood pressure in some patients; periodic monitoring of blood pressure is recommended in patients receiving concomitant antihypertensive therapy). Products include:

Furosemide Tablets 2284

Guanabenz Acetate (Pentoxifylline causes a small decrease in blood pressure in some patients; periodic monitoring of blood pressure is recommended in patients receiving concomitant antihypertensive therapy).

No products indexed under this heading.

Guanethidine Monosulfate (Pentoxifylline causes a small decrease in blood pressure in some patients; periodic monitoring of blood pressure is recommended in patients receiving concomitant antihypertensive therapy).

No products indexed under this heading.

Heparin Sodium (Co-administration has resulted in reports of bleeding and/or prolonged prothrombin time in patients treated with anticoagulants). Products include:

Heparin Lock Flush Solution 3509
Heparin Sodium Injection 3511

Hydralazine Hydrochloride (Pentoxifylline causes a small decrease in blood pressure in some patients; periodic monitoring of blood pressure is recommended in patients receiving concomitant antihypertensive therapy).

No products indexed under this heading.

Hydrochlorothiazide (Pentoxifylline causes a small decrease in blood pressure in some patients; periodic monitoring of blood pressure is recommended in patients receiving concomitant antihypertensive therapy). Products include:

Accuretic Tablets 2614
Aldoril Tablets 2039
Atacand HCT Tablets 597
Avalide Tablets 1070
Diovan HCT Tablets 2338
Dyazide Capsules 1515
HydroDIURIL Tablets 2108
Hyzaar 2109
Inderide Tablets 3517
Inderide LA Long-Acting Capsules .. 3519
Lotensin HCT Tablets 2367
Maxzide 1008
Micardis HCT Tablets 1051
Microzide Capsules 3414
Moduretic Tablets 2138
Monopril HCT 1094
Prinzide Tablets 2168
Timolide Tablets 2187
Uniretic Tablets 3178
Vaseretic Tablets 2204
Zestoretic Tablets 695
Ziac Tablets 1887

Hydroflumethiazide (Pentoxifylline causes a small decrease in blood pressure in some patients; periodic monitoring of blood pressure is recommended in patients receiving concomitant antihypertensive therapy). Products include:

Diucardin Tablets 3494

Ibuprofen (Co-administration has resulted in reports of bleeding and/or prolonged prothrombin time in patients treated with platelet aggregation inhibitors). Products include:

Advil .... ▣771
Children's Advil Oral Suspension ... ▣773
Children's Advil Chewable Tablets ... ▣773
Advil Cold and Sinus Caplets .... ▣771
Advil Cold and Sinus Tablets .... ▣771
Advil Flu & Body Ache Caplets ...... ▣772
Infants' Advil Drops .... ▣773
Junior Strength Advil Tablets .... ▣773
Junior Strength Advil Chewable Tablets .... ▣773
Advil Migraine Liquigels .... ▣772
Children's Motrin Oral Suspension and Chewable Tablets 2006
Children's Motrin Cold Oral Suspension 2007
Children's Motrin Oral Suspension .... ▣643
Motrin Suspension, Oral Drops, Chewable Tablets, and Caplets 2002
Infants' Motrin Concentrated Drops 2006
Junior Strength Motrin Caplets and Chewable Tablets 2006
Motrin IB Tablets, Caplets, and Gelcaps 2002
Motrin Migraine Pain Caplets 2005
Motrin Sinus Headache Caplets 2005
Vicoprofen Tablets 520

Indapamide (Pentoxifylline causes a small decrease in blood pressure in some patients; periodic monitoring of blood pressure is recommended in patients receiving concomitant antihypertensive therapy). Products include:

Indapamide Tablets 2286

Indomethacin (Co-administration has resulted in reports of bleeding and/or prolonged prothrombin time in patients treated with platelet aggregation inhibitors). Products include:

Indocin 2112

Indomethacin Sodium Trihydrate (Co-administration has resulted in reports of bleeding and/or prolonged prothrombin time in patients treated with platelet aggregation inhibitors). Products include:

Indocin I.V. 2115

Irbesartan (Pentoxifylline causes a small decrease in blood pressure in some patients; periodic monitoring of blood pressure is recommended in patients receiving concomitant antihypertensive therapy). Products include:

Avalide Tablets 1070
Avapro Tablets 1074
Avapro Tablets 3076

Isradipine (Pentoxifylline causes a small decrease in blood pressure in some patients; periodic monitoring of blood pressure is recommended in patients receiving concomitant antihypertensive therapy). Products include:

DynaCirc Capsules 2921
DynaCirc CR Tablets 2923

Ketoprofen (Co-administration has resulted in reports of bleeding and/or prolonged prothrombin time in patients treated with platelet aggregation inhibitors). Products include:

Orudis Capsules 3548
Orudis KT Tablets .... ▣778
Oruvail Capsules 3548

Ketorolac Tromethamine (Co-administration has resulted in reports of bleeding and/or prolonged prothrombin time in patients treated with platelet aggregation inhibitors). Products include:

Acular Ophthalmic Solution 544
Acular PF Ophthalmic Solution 544
Toradol 3018

Labetalol Hydrochloride (Pentoxifylline causes a small decrease in blood pressure in some patients; periodic monitoring of blood pressure is recommended in patients receiving concomitant antihypertensive therapy). Products include:

Normodyne Injection 3135
Normodyne Tablets 3137

Lisinopril (Pentoxifylline causes a small decrease in blood pressure in some patients; periodic monitoring of blood pressure is recommended in patients receiving concomitant antihypertensive therapy). Products include:

Prinivil Tablets 2164
Prinzide Tablets 2168
Zestoretic Tablets 695
Zestril Tablets 698

Losartan Potassium (Pentoxifylline causes a small decrease in blood pressure in some patients; periodic monitoring of blood pressure is recommended in patients receiving concomitant antihypertensive therapy). Products include:

Cozaar Tablets 2067
Hyzaar 2109

Mecamylamine Hydrochloride (Pentoxifylline causes a small decrease in blood pressure in some patients; periodic monitoring of blood pressure is recommended in patients receiving concomitant antihypertensive therapy). Products include:

Inversine Tablets 1850

Meclofenamate Sodium (Co-administration has resulted in reports of bleeding and/or prolonged prothrombin time in patients treated with platelet aggregation inhibitors).

No products indexed under this heading.

Mefenamic Acid (Co-administration has resulted in reports of bleeding and/or prolonged prothrombin time in patients treated with platelet aggregation inhibitors). Products include:

Ponstel Capsules 1356

Meloxicam (Co-administration has resulted in reports of bleeding and/or prolonged prothrombin time in patients treated with platelet aggregation inhibitors). Products include:

Mobic Tablets 1054

Methyclothiazide (Pentoxifylline causes a small decrease in blood pressure in some patients; periodic monitoring of blood pressure is recommended in patients receiving concomitant antihypertensive therapy).

No products indexed under this heading.

Methyldopa (Pentoxifylline causes a small decrease in blood pressure in some patients; periodic monitoring of blood pressure is recommended in patients receiving concomitant antihypertensive therapy). Products include:

Aldoclor Tablets 2035
Aldomet Tablets 2037
Aldoril Tablets 2039

Methyldopate Hydrochloride (Pentoxifylline causes a small decrease in blood pressure in some patients; periodic monitoring of blood pressure is recommended in patients receiving concomitant antihypertensive therapy).

No products indexed under this heading.

Metolazone (Pentoxifylline causes a small decrease in blood pressure in some patients; periodic monitoring of blood pressure is recommended in patients receiving concomitant antihypertensive therapy). Products include:

Mykrox Tablets 1168
Zaroxolyn Tablets 1177

Metoprolol Succinate (Pentoxifylline causes a small decrease in blood pressure in some patients; periodic monitoring of blood pressure is recommended in patients receiving concomitant antihypertensive therapy). Products include:

Toprol-XL Tablets 651

Metoprolol Tartrate (Pentoxifylline causes a small decrease in blood pressure in some patients; periodic monitoring of blood pressure is recommended in patients receiving concomitant antihypertensive therapy).

No products indexed under this heading.

Metyrosine (Pentoxifylline causes a small decrease in blood pressure in some patients; periodic monitoring of blood pressure is recommended in patients receiving concomitant antihypertensive therapy). Products include:

Demser Capsules 2085

Mibefradil Dihydrochloride (Pentoxifylline causes a small decrease in blood pressure in some patients; periodic monitoring of blood pressure is recommended in patients receiving concomitant antihypertensive therapy).

No products indexed under this heading.

Minoxidil (Pentoxifylline causes a small decrease in blood pressure in some patients; periodic monitoring of blood pressure is recommended in patients receiving concomitant antihypertensive therapy). Products include:

Rogaine Extra Strength for Men Topical Solution .... ■ 721
Rogaine for Women Topical Solution .... ■ 721

Moexipril Hydrochloride (Pentoxifylline causes a small decrease in blood pressure in some patients; periodic monitoring of blood pressure is recommended in patients receiving concomitant antihypertensive therapy). Products include:

Uniretic Tablets 3178
Univasc Tablets 3181

Nabumetone (Co-administration has resulted in reports of bleeding and/or prolonged prothrombin time in patients treated with platelet aggregation inhibitors). Products include:

Relafen Tablets 1617

Nadolol (Pentoxifylline causes a small decrease in blood pressure in some patients; periodic monitoring of blood pressure is recommended in patients receiving concomitant antihypertensive therapy). Products include:

Corgard Tablets 2245
Corzide 40/5 Tablets 2247
Corzide 80/5 Tablets 2247
Nadolol Tablets 2288

Naproxen (Co-administration has resulted in reports of bleeding and/or prolonged prothrombin time in patients treated with platelet aggregation inhibitors). Products include:

EC-Naprosyn Delayed-Release Tablets 2967
Naprosyn Suspension 2967
Naprosyn Tablets 2967

Naproxen Sodium (Co-administration has resulted in reports of bleeding and/or prolonged prothrombin time in patients treated with platelet aggregation inhibitors). Products include:

Aleve Tablets, Caplets and Gelcaps .... ■ 602
Aleve Cold & Sinus Caplets .... ■ 603
Anaprox Tablets 2967
Anaprox DS Tablets 2967
Naprelan Tablets 1293

Nicardipine Hydrochloride (Pentoxifylline causes a small decrease in blood pressure in some patients; periodic monitoring of blood pressure is recommended in patients receiving concomitant antihypertensive therapy). Products include:

Cardene I.V. 3485

Nifedipine (Pentoxifylline causes a small decrease in blood pressure in some patients; periodic monitoring of blood pressure is recommended in patients receiving concomitant antihypertensive therapy). Products include:

Adalat CC Tablets 877
Procardia Capsules 2708
Procardia XL Extended Release Tablets 2710

Nisoldipine (Pentoxifylline causes a small decrease in blood pressure in some patients; periodic monitoring of blood pressure is recommended in patients receiving concomitant antihypertensive therapy). Products include:

Sular Tablets 688

Nitroglycerin (Pentoxifylline causes a small decrease in blood pressure in some patients; periodic monitoring of blood pressure is recommended in patients receiving concomitant antihypertensive therapy). Products include:

Nitro-Dur Transdermal Infusion System 3134
Nitro-Dur Transdermal Infusion System 1834
Nitrolingual Pumpspray 1355
Nitrostat Tablets 2658

Oxaprozin (Co-administration has resulted in reports of bleeding and/or prolonged prothrombin time in patients treated with platelet aggregation inhibitors).

No products indexed under this heading.

Penbutolol Sulfate (Pentoxifylline causes a small decrease in blood pressure in some patients; periodic monitoring of blood pressure is recommended in patients receiving concomitant antihypertensive therapy).

No products indexed under this heading.

Perindopril Erbumine (Pentoxifylline causes a small decrease in blood pressure in some patients; periodic monitoring of blood pressure is recommended in patients receiving concomitant antihypertensive therapy). Products include:

Aceon Tablets (2 mg, 4 mg, 8 mg) 3249

Phenoxybenzamine Hydrochloride (Pentoxifylline causes a small decrease in blood pressure in some patients; periodic monitoring of blood pressure is recommended in patients receiving concomitant antihypertensive therapy). Products include:

Dibenzyline Capsules 3457

Phentolamine Mesylate (Pentoxifylline causes a small decrease in blood pressure in some patients; periodic monitoring of blood pressure is recommended in patients receiving concomitant antihypertensive therapy).

No products indexed under this heading.

Phenylbutazone (Co-administration has resulted in reports of bleeding and/or prolonged prothrombin time in patients treated with platelet aggregation inhibitors).

No products indexed under this heading.

Pindolol (Pentoxifylline causes a small decrease in blood pressure in some patients; periodic monitoring of blood pressure is recommended in patients receiving concomitant antihypertensive therapy).

No products indexed under this heading.

Piroxicam (Co-administration has resulted in reports of bleeding and/or prolonged prothrombin time in patients treated with platelet aggregation inhibitors). Products include:

Feldene Capsules 2685

Polythiazide (Pentoxifylline causes a small decrease in blood pressure in some patients; periodic monitoring of blood pressure is recommended in patients receiving concomitant antihypertensive therapy). Products include:

Minizide Capsules 2700
Renese Tablets 2712

Prazosin Hydrochloride (Pentoxifylline causes a small decrease in blood pressure in some patients; periodic monitoring of blood pressure is recommended in patients receiving concomitant antihypertensive therapy). Products include:

Minipress Capsules 2699
Minizide Capsules 2700

Propranolol Hydrochloride (Pentoxifylline causes a small decrease in blood pressure in some patients; periodic monitoring of blood pressure is recommended in patients receiving concomitant antihypertensive therapy). Products include:

Inderal 3513
Inderal LA Long-Acting Capsules 3516
Inderide Tablets 3517
Inderide LA Long-Acting Capsules 3519

Quinapril Hydrochloride (Pentoxifylline causes a small decrease in blood pressure in some patients; periodic monitoring of blood pressure is recommended in patients receiving concomitant antihypertensive therapy). Products include:

Accupril Tablets 2611
Accuretic Tablets 2614

Ramipril (Pentoxifylline causes a small decrease in blood pressure in some patients; periodic monitoring of blood pressure is recommended in patients receiving concomitant antihypertensive therapy). Products include:

Altace Capsules 2233

Rauwolfia serpentina (Pentoxifylline causes a small decrease in blood pressure in some patients; periodic monitoring of blood pressure is recommended in patients receiving concomitant antihypertensive therapy).

No products indexed under this heading.

Rescinnamine (Pentoxifylline causes a small decrease in blood pressure in some patients; periodic monitoring of blood pressure is recommended in patients receiving concomitant antihypertensive therapy).

No products indexed under this heading.

Reserpine (Pentoxifylline causes a small decrease in blood pressure in some patients; periodic monitoring of blood pressure is recommended in patients receiving concomitant antihypertensive therapy).

No products indexed under this heading.

Rofecoxib (Co-administration has resulted in reports of bleeding and/or prolonged prothrombin time in patients treated with platelet aggregation inhibitors). Products include:

Vioxx 2213

Sodium Nitroprusside (Pentoxifylline causes a small decrease in blood pressure in some patients;

periodic monitoring of blood pressure is recommended in patients receiving concomitant antihypertensive therapy).
No products indexed under this heading.

Sotalol Hydrochloride (Pentoxifylline causes a small decrease in blood pressure in some patients; periodic monitoring of blood pressure is recommended in patients receiving concomitant antihypertensive therapy). Products include:
Betapace Tablets 950
Betapace AF Tablets 954

Spirapril Hydrochloride (Pentoxifylline causes a small decrease in blood pressure in some patients; periodic monitoring of blood pressure is recommended in patients receiving concomitant antihypertensive therapy).
No products indexed under this heading.

Sulindac (Co-administration has resulted in reports of bleeding and/or prolonged prothrombin time in patients treated with platelet aggregation inhibitors). Products include:
Clinoril Tablets 2053

Telmisartan (Pentoxifylline causes a small decrease in blood pressure in some patients; periodic monitoring of blood pressure is recommended in patients receiving concomitant antihypertensive therapy). Products include:
Micardis Tablets 1049
Micardis HCT Tablets 1051

Terazosin Hydrochloride (Pentoxifylline causes a small decrease in blood pressure in some patients; periodic monitoring of blood pressure is recommended in patients receiving concomitant antihypertensive therapy). Products include:
Hytrin Capsules 464

Theophylline (Co-administration with theophylline-containing products leads to increased theophylline levels and theophylline toxicity). Products include:
Aerolate 1361
Theo-Dur Extended-Release Tablets 1835
Uni-Dur Extended-Release Tablets .. 1841
Uniphyl 400 mg and 600 mg Tablets 2903

Theophylline Calcium Salicylate (Co-administration with theophylline-containing products leads to increased theophylline levels and theophylline toxicity).
No products indexed under this heading.

Theophylline Sodium Glycinate (Co-administration with theophylline-containing products leads to increased theophylline levels and theophylline toxicity).
No products indexed under this heading.

Ticlopidine Hydrochloride (Co-administration has resulted in reports of bleeding and/or prolonged prothrombin time in patients treated with platelet aggregation inhibitors). Products include:
Ticlid Tablets 3015

Timolol Maleate (Pentoxifylline causes a small decrease in blood pressure in some patients; periodic monitoring of blood pressure is recommended in patients receiving concomitant antihypertensive therapy). Products include:
Blocadren Tablets 2046
Cosopt Sterile Ophthalmic Solution 2065
Timolide Tablets 2187
Timolol GFS .... ⊙266
Timoptic in Ocudose 2192
Timoptic Sterile Ophthalmic Solution 2190
Timoptic-XE Sterile Ophthalmic Gel Forming Solution 2194

Tinzaparin sodium (Co-administration has resulted in reports of bleeding and/or prolonged prothrombin time in patients treated with anticoagulants). Products include:
Innohep Injection 1248

Tirofiban Hydrochloride (Co-administration has resulted in reports of bleeding and/or prolonged prothrombin time in patients treated with platelet aggregation inhibitors). Products include:
Aggrastat 2031

Tolmetin Sodium (Co-administration has resulted in reports of bleeding and/or prolonged prothrombin time in patients treated with platelet aggregation inhibitors). Products include:
Tolectin 2589

Torsemide (Pentoxifylline causes a small decrease in blood pressure in some patients; periodic monitoring of blood pressure is recommended in patients receiving concomitant antihypertensive therapy). Products include:
Demadex Tablets and Injection 2965

Trandolapril (Pentoxifylline causes a small decrease in blood pressure in some patients; periodic monitoring of blood pressure is recommended in patients receiving concomitant antihypertensive therapy). Products include:
Mavik Tablets 478
Tarka Tablets 508

Trimethaphan Camsylate (Pentoxifylline causes a small decrease in blood pressure in some patients; periodic monitoring of blood pressure is recommended in patients receiving concomitant antihypertensive therapy).
No products indexed under this heading.

Valsartan (Pentoxifylline causes a small decrease in blood pressure in some patients; periodic monitoring of blood pressure is recommended in patients receiving concomitant antihypertensive therapy). Products include:
Diovan Capsules 2337
Diovan HCT Tablets 2338

Verapamil Hydrochloride (Pentoxifylline causes a small decrease in blood pressure in some patients; periodic monitoring of blood pressure is recommended in patients receiving concomitant antihypertensive therapy). Products include:
Covera-HS Tablets 3199
Isoptin SR Tablets 467
Tarka Tablets 508
Verelan Capsules 3184
Verelan PM Capsules 3186

Warfarin Sodium (Co-administration has resulted in reports of bleeding and/or prolonged prothrombin time in patients treated with anticoagulants; frequent monitoring of prothrombin time is recommended). Products include:
Coumadin for Injection 1243
Coumadin Tablets 1243
Warfarin Sodium Tablets, USP 3302

Food Interactions

Food, unspecified (Co-administration of Trental tablets with meals resulted in an increase in mean Cmax and AUC by about 28% and 13% for pentoxifylline, respectively; Cmax for Metabolite 1 also increased by about 20%).

TRIAMINIC ALLERGY CONGESTION LIQUID

(Pseudoephedrine Hydrochloride) .... ▣680
May interact with monoamine oxidase inhibitors. Compounds in these categories include:

Isocarboxazid (Concurrent and/or sequential use with MAO inhibitors is not recommended).
No products indexed under this heading.

Moclobemide (Concurrent and/or sequential use with MAO inhibitors is not recommended).
No products indexed under this heading.

Pargyline Hydrochloride (Concurrent and/or sequential use with MAO inhibitors is not recommended).
No products indexed under this heading.

Phenelzine Sulfate (Concurrent and/or sequential use with MAO inhibitors is not recommended). Products include:
Nardil Tablets 2653

Procarbazine Hydrochloride (Concurrent and/or sequential use with MAO inhibitors is not recommended). Products include:
Matulane Capsules 3246

Selegiline Hydrochloride (Concurrent and/or sequential use with MAO inhibitors is not recommended). Products include:
Eldepryl Capsules 3266

Tranylcypromine Sulfate (Concurrent and/or sequential use with MAO inhibitors is not recommended). Products include:
Parnate Tablets 1607

TRIAMINIC CHEST CONGESTION LIQUID

(Guaifenesin, Pseudoephedrine Hydrochloride) .... ▣680
May interact with monoamine oxidase inhibitors. Compounds in these categories include:

Isocarboxazid (Concurrent and/or sequential use with MAO inhibitors is not recommended).
No products indexed under this heading.

Moclobemide (Concurrent and/or sequential use with MAO inhibitors is not recommended).
No products indexed under this heading.

Pargyline Hydrochloride (Concurrent and/or sequential use with MAO inhibitors is not recommended).
No products indexed under this heading.

Phenelzine Sulfate (Concurrent and/or sequential use with MAO inhibitors is not recommended). Products include:
Nardil Tablets 2653

Procarbazine Hydrochloride (Concurrent and/or sequential use with MAO inhibitors is not recommended). Products include:
Matulane Capsules 3246

Selegiline Hydrochloride (Concurrent and/or sequential use with MAO inhibitors is not recommended). Products include:
Eldepryl Capsules 3266

Tranylcypromine Sulfate (Concurrent and/or sequential use with MAO inhibitors is not recommended). Products include:
Parnate Tablets 1607

TRIAMINIC COLD & ALLERGY LIQUID

(Chlorpheniramine Maleate, Pseudoephedrine Hydrochloride) .... ▣681
See Triaminic Cold & Night Time Cough Liquid

TRIAMINIC COLD & ALLERGY SOFTCHEWS

(Chlorpheniramine Maleate, Pseudoephedrine Hydrochloride) .... ▣683
See Triaminic Cold & Cough Softchews

TRIAMINIC COLD & COUGH LIQUID

(Chlorpheniramine Maleate, Dextromethorphan Hydrobromide, Pseudoephedrine Hydrochloride) .... ▣681
See Triaminic Cold & Night Time Cough Liquid

TRIAMINIC COLD & COUGH SOFTCHEWS

(Chlorpheniramine Maleate, Dextromethorphan Hydrobromide, Pseudoephedrine Hydrochloride) .... ▣683
May interact with hypnotics and sedatives, monoamine oxidase inhibitors, tranquilizers, and certain other agents. Compounds in these categories include:

Alprazolam (May increase drowsiness effect). Products include:
Xanax Tablets 2865

Buspirone Hydrochloride (May increase drowsiness effect).
No products indexed under this heading.

Chlordiazepoxide (May increase drowsiness effect). Products include:
Limbitrol 1738

Chlordiazepoxide Hydrochloride (May increase drowsiness effect). Products include:
Librium Capsules 1736
Librium for Injection 1737

Chlorpromazine (May increase drowsiness effect). Products include:
Thorazine Suppositories 1656

Chlorpromazine Hydrochloride (May increase drowsiness effect). Products include:
Thorazine 1656

Chlorprothixene (May increase drowsiness effect).
No products indexed under this heading.

Chlorprothixene Hydrochloride (May increase drowsiness effect).
No products indexed under this heading.

Clorazepate Dipotassium (May increase drowsiness effect). Products include:
Tranxene 511

Diazepam (May increase drowsiness effect). Products include:
Valium Injectable 3026
Valium Tablets 3047

Droperidol (May increase drowsiness effect).
No products indexed under this heading.

Estazolam (May increase drowsiness effect). Products include:
ProSom Tablets 500

Ethchlorvynol (May increase drowsiness effect).
No products indexed under this heading.

Ethinamate (May increase drowsiness effect).
No products indexed under this heading.

Fluphenazine Decanoate (May increase drowsiness effect).
No products indexed under this heading.

Fluphenazine Enanthate (May increase drowsiness effect).
No products indexed under this heading.

Fluphenazine Hydrochloride (May increase drowsiness effect).
No products indexed under this heading.

Flurazepam Hydrochloride (May increase drowsiness effect).
No products indexed under this heading.

IMPORTANT NOTE: Always consult each drug listing in the patient's regimen for possible interactions.

Glutethimide (May increase drowsiness effect).
No products indexed under this heading.

Haloperidol (May increase drowsiness effect). Products include:
Haldol Injection, Tablets and Concentrate 2533

Haloperidol Decanoate (May increase drowsiness effect). Products include:
Haldol Decanoate 2535

Hydroxyzine Hydrochloride (May increase drowsiness effect). Products include:
Atarax Tablets & Syrup 2667
Vistaril Intramuscular Solution 2738

Isocarboxazid (Concurrent and/or sequential use with MAO inhibitors is not recommended).
No products indexed under this heading.

Lorazepam (May increase drowsiness effect). Products include:
Ativan Injection 3478
Ativan Tablets 3482

Loxapine Hydrochloride (May increase drowsiness effect).
No products indexed under this heading.

Loxapine Succinate (May increase drowsiness effect). Products include:
Loxitane Capsules 3398

Meprobamate (May increase drowsiness effect). Products include:
Miltown Tablets 3349

Mesoridazine Besylate (May increase drowsiness effect). Products include:
Serentil 1057

Midazolam Hydrochloride (May increase drowsiness effect). Products include:
Versed Injection 3027
Versed Syrup 3033

Moclobemide (Concurrent and/or sequential use with MAO inhibitors is not recommended).
No products indexed under this heading.

Molindone Hydrochloride (May increase drowsiness effect). Products include:
Moban 1320

Oxazepam (May increase drowsiness effect).
No products indexed under this heading.

Pargyline Hydrochloride (Concurrent and/or sequential use with MAO inhibitors is not recommended).
No products indexed under this heading.

Perphenazine (May increase drowsiness effect). Products include:
Etrafon 3115
Trilafon 3160

Phenelzine Sulfate (Concurrent and/or sequential use with MAO inhibitors is not recommended). Products include:
Nardil Tablets 2653

Prazepam (May increase drowsiness effect).
No products indexed under this heading.

Procarbazine Hydrochloride (Concurrent and/or sequential use with MAO inhibitors is not recommended). Products include:
Matulane Capsules 3246

Prochlorperazine (May increase drowsiness effect). Products include:
Compazine 1505

Promethazine Hydrochloride (May increase drowsiness effect). Products include:
Mepergan Injection 3539
Phenergan Injection 3553
Phenergan 3556
Phenergan Syrup 3554
Phenergan with Codeine Syrup 3557
Phenergan with Dextromethorphan Syrup 3559
Phenergan VC Syrup 3560
Phenergan VC with Codeine Syrup .. 3561

Propofol (May increase drowsiness effect). Products include:
Diprivan Injectable Emulsion 667

Quazepam (May increase drowsiness effect).
No products indexed under this heading.

Secobarbital Sodium (May increase drowsiness effect).
No products indexed under this heading.

Selegiline Hydrochloride (Concurrent and/or sequential use with MAO inhibitors is not recommended). Products include:
Eldepryl Capsules 3266

Temazepam (May increase drowsiness effect).
No products indexed under this heading.

Thioridazine Hydrochloride (May increase drowsiness effect). Products include:
Thioridazine Hydrochloride Tablets 2289

Thiothixene (May increase drowsiness effect). Products include:
Navane Capsules 2701
Thiothixene Capsules 2290

Tranylcypromine Sulfate (Concurrent and/or sequential use with MAO inhibitors is not recommended). Products include:
Parnate Tablets 1607

Triazolam (May increase drowsiness effect). Products include:
Halcion Tablets 2823

Trifluoperazine Hydrochloride (May increase drowsiness effect). Products include:
Stelazine 1640

Zaleplon (May increase drowsiness effect). Products include:
Sonata Capsules 3591

Zolpidem Tartrate (May increase drowsiness effect). Products include:
Ambien Tablets 3191

Food Interactions

Alcohol (May increase drowsiness effect).

TRIAMINIC COLD & NIGHT TIME COUGH LIQUID

(Chlorpheniramine Maleate, Dextromethorphan Hydrobromide, Pseudoephedrine Hydrochloride) .... ▣681
May interact with hypnotics and sedatives, monoamine oxidase inhibitors, and tranquilizers. Compounds in these categories include:

Alprazolam (May increase drowsiness). Products include:
Xanax Tablets 2865

Buspirone Hydrochloride (May increase drowsiness).
No products indexed under this heading.

Chlordiazepoxide (May increase drowsiness). Products include:
Limbitrol 1738

Chlordiazepoxide Hydrochloride (May increase drowsiness). Products include:
Librium Capsules 1736
Librium for Injection 1737

Chlorpromazine (May increase drowsiness). Products include:
Thorazine Suppositories 1656

Chlorpromazine Hydrochloride (May increase drowsiness). Products include:
Thorazine 1656

Chlorprothixene (May increase drowsiness).
No products indexed under this heading.

Chlorprothixene Hydrochloride (May increase drowsiness).
No products indexed under this heading.

Clorazepate Dipotassium (May increase drowsiness). Products include:
Tranxene 511

Diazepam (May increase drowsiness). Products include:
Valium Injectable 3026
Valium Tablets 3047

Droperidol (May increase drowsiness).
No products indexed under this heading.

Estazolam (May increase drowsiness). Products include:
ProSom Tablets 500

Ethchlorvynol (May increase drowsiness).
No products indexed under this heading.

Ethinamate (May increase drowsiness).
No products indexed under this heading.

Fluphenazine Decanoate (May increase drowsiness).
No products indexed under this heading.

Fluphenazine Enanthate (May increase drowsiness).
No products indexed under this heading.

Fluphenazine Hydrochloride (May increase drowsiness).
No products indexed under this heading.

Flurazepam Hydrochloride (May increase drowsiness).
No products indexed under this heading.

Glutethimide (May increase drowsiness).
No products indexed under this heading.

Haloperidol (May increase drowsiness). Products include:
Haldol Injection, Tablets and Concentrate 2533

Haloperidol Decanoate (May increase drowsiness). Products include:
Haldol Decanoate 2535

Hydroxyzine Hydrochloride (May increase drowsiness). Products include:
Atarax Tablets & Syrup 2667
Vistaril Intramuscular Solution 2738

Isocarboxazid (Concurrent and/or sequential use with MAO inhibitors is not recommended).
No products indexed under this heading.

Lorazepam (May increase drowsiness). Products include:
Ativan Injection 3478
Ativan Tablets 3482

Loxapine Hydrochloride (May increase drowsiness).
No products indexed under this heading.

Loxapine Succinate (May increase drowsiness). Products include:
Loxitane Capsules 3398

Meprobamate (May increase drowsiness). Products include:
Miltown Tablets 3349

Mesoridazine Besylate (May increase drowsiness). Products include:
Serentil 1057

Midazolam Hydrochloride (May increase drowsiness). Products include:
Versed Injection 3027
Versed Syrup 3033

Moclobemide (Concurrent and/or sequential use with MAO inhibitors is not recommended).
No products indexed under this heading.

Molindone Hydrochloride (May increase drowsiness). Products include:
Moban 1320

Oxazepam (May increase drowsiness).
No products indexed under this heading.

Pargyline Hydrochloride (Concurrent and/or sequential use with MAO inhibitors is not recommended).
No products indexed under this heading.

Perphenazine (May increase drowsiness). Products include:
Etrafon 3115
Trilafon 3160

Phenelzine Sulfate (Concurrent and/or sequential use with MAO inhibitors is not recommended). Products include:
Nardil Tablets 2653

Prazepam (May increase drowsiness).
No products indexed under this heading.

Procarbazine Hydrochloride (Concurrent and/or sequential use with MAO inhibitors is not recommended). Products include:
Matulane Capsules 3246

Prochlorperazine (May increase drowsiness). Products include:
Compazine 1505

Promethazine Hydrochloride (May increase drowsiness). Products include:
Mepergan Injection 3539
Phenergan Injection 3553
Phenergan 3556
Phenergan Syrup 3554
Phenergan with Codeine Syrup 3557
Phenergan with Dextromethorphan Syrup 3559
Phenergan VC Syrup 3560
Phenergan VC with Codeine Syrup .. 3561

Propofol (May increase drowsiness). Products include:
Diprivan Injectable Emulsion 667

Quazepam (May increase drowsiness).
No products indexed under this heading.

Secobarbital Sodium (May increase drowsiness).
No products indexed under this heading.

Selegiline Hydrochloride (Concurrent and/or sequential use with MAO inhibitors is not recommended). Products include:
Eldepryl Capsules 3266

Temazepam (May increase drowsiness).
No products indexed under this heading.

Thioridazine Hydrochloride (May increase drowsiness). Products include:
Thioridazine Hydrochloride Tablets 2289

Thiothixene (May increase drowsiness). Products include:
Navane Capsules 2701
Thiothixene Capsules 2290

Tranylcypromine Sulfate (Concurrent and/or sequential use with MAO inhibitors is not recommended). Products include:
Parnate Tablets 1607

Triazolam (May increase drowsiness). Products include:
Halcion Tablets 2823

Trifluoperazine Hydrochloride (May increase drowsiness). Products include:
Stelazine 1640

Zaleplon (May increase drowsiness). Products include:
Sonata Capsules 3591

Zolpidem Tartrate (May increase drowsiness). Products include:
Ambien Tablets 3191

TRIAMINIC COLD, COUGH & FEVER LIQUID
(Acetaminophen, Chlorpheniramine Maleate, Dextromethorphan Hydrobromide, Pseudoephedrine Hydrochloride) 681
See Triaminic Cold & Night Time Cough Liquid

TRIAMINIC COUGH LIQUID
(Dextromethorphan Hydrobromide, Pseudoephedrine Hydrochloride) 682
See Triaminic Cough & Sore Throat Liquid

TRIAMINIC COUGH SOFTCHEWS
(Dextromethorphan Hydrobromide) 684
See Triaminic Cough & Sore Throat Softchews

TRIAMINIC COUGH & CONGESTION LIQUID
(Dextromethorphan Hydrobromide, Pseudoephedrine Hydrochloride) 682
See Triaminic Cough & Sore Throat Liquid

TRIAMINIC COUGH & SORE THROAT LIQUID
(Acetaminophen, Dextromethorphan Hydrobromide, Pseudoephedrine Hydrochloride) 682
May interact with monoamine oxidase inhibitors. Compounds in these categories include:

Isocarboxazid (Concurrent and/or sequential use with MAO inhibitors is not recommened).
No products indexed under this heading.

Moclobemide (Concurrent and/or sequential use with MAO inhibitors is not recommened).
No products indexed under this heading.

Pargyline Hydrochloride (Concurrent and/or sequential use with MAO inhibitors is not recommened).
No products indexed under this heading.

Phenelzine Sulfate (Concurrent and/or sequential use with MAO inhibitors is not recommened). Products include:
Nardil Tablets 2653

Procarbazine Hydrochloride (Concurrent and/or sequential use with MAO inhibitors is not recommened). Products include:
Matulane Capsules 3246

Selegiline Hydrochloride (Concurrent and/or sequential use with MAO inhibitors is not recommened). Products include:
Eldepryl Capsules 3266

Tranylcypromine Sulfate (Concurrent and/or sequential use with MAO inhibitors is not recommened). Products include:
Parnate Tablets 1607

TRIAMINIC COUGH & SORE THROAT SOFTCHEWS
(Acetaminophen, Dextromethorphan Hydrobromide, Pseudoephedrine Hydrochloride) 684
May interact with monoamine oxidase inhibitors. Compounds in these categories include:

Isocarboxazid (Concurrent and/or sequential use with MAO inhibitors is not recommened).
No products indexed under this heading.

Moclobemide (Concurrent and/or sequential use with MAO inhibitors is not recommended).
No products indexed under this heading.

Pargyline Hydrochloride (Concurrent and/or sequential use with MAO inhibitors is not recommended).
No products indexed under this heading.

Phenelzine Sulfate (Concurrent and/or sequential use with MAO inhibitors is not recommended). Products include:
Nardil Tablets 2653

Procarbazine Hydrochloride (Concurrent and/or sequential use with MAO inhibitors is not recommended). Products include:
Matulane Capsules 3246

Selegiline Hydrochloride (Concurrent and/or sequential use with MAO inhibitors is not recommended). Products include:
Eldepryl Capsules 3266

Tranylcypromine Sulfate (Concurrent and/or sequential use with MAO inhibitors is not recommended). Products include:
Parnate Tablets 1607

TRIAMINIC VAPOR PATCH-CHERRY SCENT
(Camphor, Menthol) 684
None cited in PDR database.

TRIAMINIC VAPOR PATCH-MENTHOL SCENT
(Camphor, Menthol) 684
None cited in PDR database.

TRIAZ CLEANSER
(Benzoyl Peroxide) 2026
None cited in PDR database.

TRIAZ GEL
(Benzoyl Peroxide) 2026
None cited in PDR database.

TRICOR CAPSULES, MICRONIZED
(Fenofibrate) 513
May interact with bile acid sequestering agents, oral anticoagulants, HMG-CoA reductase inhibitors, and certain other agents. Compounds in these categories include:

Atorvastatin Calcium (Co-administration of fibric acid derivatives and HMG-CoA reductase inhibitors has been associated, in numerous case reports, with rhabdomyolysis, markedly elevated creatine kinase (CK) levels and myoglobulinuria, leading in a high proportion of cases to acute renal failure; the combined use should be avoided unless the benefit of further alterations in lipid levels is likely to outweigh the increased risk of this combination). Products include:
Lipitor Tablets 2639
Lipitor Tablets 2696

Cerivastatin Sodium (Co-administration of fibric acid derivatives and HMG-CoA reductase inhibitors has been associated, in numerous case reports, with rhabdomyolysis, markedly elevated creatine kinase (CK) levels and myoglobulinuria, leading in a high proportion of cases to acute renal failure; the combined use should be avoided unless the benefit of further alterations in lipid levels is likely to outweigh the increased risk of this combination). Products include:
Baycol Tablets 883

Cholestyramine (Bile acid sequestrants may bind fenofibrate; Tricor should be taken at least 1 hour before or 4-6 hours after a bile acid binding resin to avoid impeding its absorption).
No products indexed under this heading.

Colestipol Hydrochloride (Bile acid sequestrants may bind fenofibrate; Tricor should be taken at least 1 hour before or 4-6 hours after a bile acid binding resin to avoid impeding its absorption). Products include:
Colestid Tablets 2791

Cyclosporine (Renal excretion is the primary elimination route for fibrates and because cyclosporine can produce nephrotoxicity with decrease in creatinine clearance and rise in serum creatinine, there is a risk that an interaction will lead to deterioration). Products include:
Gengraf Capsules 457
Neoral Soft Gelatin Capsules 2380
Neoral Oral Solution 2380
Sandimmune 2388

Dicumarol (Co-administration with coumarin-type anticoagulants has resulted in potentiation of oral anticoagulants resulting in prolonged prothrombin time; the dosage of the anticoagulant should be reduced to maintain the PT at the desired level).
No products indexed under this heading.

Fluvastatin Sodium (Co-administration of fibric acid derivatives and HMG-CoA reductase inhibitors has been associated, in numerous case reports, with rhabdomyolysis, markedly elevated creatine kinase (CK) levels and myoglobulinuria, leading in a high proportion of cases to acute renal failure; the combined use should be avoided unless the benefit of further alterations in lipid levels is likely to outweigh the increased risk of this combination). Products include:
Lescol Capsules 2361
Lescol 2925
Lescol XL Tablets 2361

Lovastatin (Co-administration of fibric acid derivatives and HMG-CoA reductase inhibitors has been associated, in numerous case reports, with rhabdomyolysis, markedly elevated creatine kinase (CK) levels and myoglobulinuria, leading in a high proportion of cases to acute renal failure; the combined use should be avoided unless the benefit of further alterations in lipid levels is likely to outweigh the increased risk of this combination). Products include:
Mevacor Tablets 2132

Pravastatin Sodium (Co-administration of fibric acid derivatives and HMG-CoA reductase inhibitors has been associated, in numerous case reports, with rhabdomyolysis, markedly elevated creatine kinase (CK) levels and myoglobulinuria, leading in a high proportion of cases to acute renal failure; the combined use should be avoided unless the benefit of further alterations in lipid levels is likely to outweigh the increased risk of this combination). Products include:
Pravachol Tablets 1099

Simvastatin (Co-administration of fibric acid derivatives and HMG-CoA reductase inhibitors has been associated, in numerous case reports, with rhabdomyolysis, markedly elevated creatine kinase (CK) levels and myoglobulinuria, leading in a high proportion of cases to acute renal failure; the combined use should be avoided unless the benefit of further alterations in lipid levels is likely to outweigh the increased risk of this combination). Products include:
Zocor Tablets 2219

Warfarin Sodium (Co-administration with coumarin-type anticoagulants has resulted in potentiation of oral anticoagulants resulting in prolonged prothrombin time; the dosage of the anticoagulant should be reduced to maintain the PT at the desired level). Products include:
Coumadin for Injection 1243
Coumadin Tablets 1243
Warfarin Sodium Tablets, USP 3302

Food Interactions

Food, unspecified (The absorption of fenofibrate is increased when administered with food; Tricor should be given with meals).

TRIDENT ADVANTAGE MINTS
(Breath Freshener) 687
None cited in PDR database.

TRIDENT ADVANTAGE SUGARLESS GUM
(Breath Freshener) 687
None cited in PDR database.

TRILAFON INJECTION
(Perphenazine) 3160
See Trilafon Tablets

TRILAFON TABLETS
(Perphenazine) 3160
May interact with anticholinergics, antihistamines, central nervous system depressants, anticonvulsants, and certain other agents. Compounds in these categories include:

Acrivastine (Co-administration can potentiate each other resulting in additive effects; concurrent use of perphenazine in patients receiving large doses of antihistimines is contraindicated). Products include:
Semprex-D Capsules 1172

Alfentanil Hydrochloride (Co-administration can potentiate each other resulting in additive effects; concurrent use of perphenazine in patients receiving large doses of CNS depressants is contraindicated).
No products indexed under this heading.

Alprazolam (Co-administration can potentiate each other resulting in additive effects; concurrent use of perphenazine in patients receiving large doses of CNS depressants is contraindicated). Products include:
Xanax Tablets 2865

Aprobarbital (Co-administration can potentiate each other resulting in additive effects; concurrent use of perphenazine in patients receiving large doses of CNS depressants is contraindicated).
No products indexed under this heading.

Astemizole (Co-administration can potentiate each other resulting in additive effects; concurrent use of perphenazine in patients receiving large doses of antihistimines is contraindicated).
No products indexed under this heading.

Atropine Sulfate (Co-administration with atropine or other anticholinergic agents may result in additive anticholinergic effects). Products include:
Donnatal 2929
Donnatal Extentabs 2930
Motofen Tablets 577
Prosed/DS Tablets 3268
Urised Tablets 2876

Azatadine Maleate (Co-administration can potentiate each other resulting in additive effects; concurrent use of perphenazine in patients receiving large doses of antihistimines is contraindicated). Products include:
Rynatan Tablets 3351

Belladonna Alkaloids (Co-administration with atropine or other anticholinergic agents may result in additive anticholinergic effects). Products include:

Hyland's Teething Tablets .... ▣766
Urimax Tablets 1769

Benztropine Mesylate (Co-administration with atropine or other anticholinergic agents may result in additive anticholinergic effects). Products include:
Cogentin 2055

Biperiden Hydrochloride (Co-administration with atropine or other anticholinergic agents may result in additive anticholinergic effects). Products include:
Akineton 402

Bromodiphenhydramine Hydrochloride (Co-administration can potentiate each other resulting in additive effects; concurrent use of perphenazine in patients receiving large doses of antihistimines is contraindicated).
No products indexed under this heading.

Brompheniramine Maleate (Co-administration can potentiate each other resulting in additive effects; concurrent use of perphenazine in patients receiving large doses of antihistimines is contraindicated). Products include:
Bromfed Capsules (Extended-Release).................... 2269
Bromfed-PD Capsules (Extended-Release).................... 2269
Comtrex Acute Head Cold & Sinus Pressure Relief Tablets.... ▣627
Dimetapp Elixir .... ▣777
Dimetapp Cold and Fever Suspension .... ▣775
Dimetapp DM Cold & Cough Elixir . ▣775
Dimetapp Nighttime Flu Liquid ..... ▣776

Buprenorphine Hydrochloride (Co-administration can potentiate each other resulting in additive effects; concurrent use of perphenazine in patients receiving large doses of CNS depressants is contraindicated). Products include:
Buprenex Injectable 2918

Buspirone Hydrochloride (Co-administration can potentiate each other resulting in additive effects; concurrent use of perphenazine in patients receiving large doses of CNS depressants is contraindicated).
No products indexed under this heading.

Butabarbital (Co-administration can potentiate each other resulting in additive effects; concurrent use of perphenazine in patients receiving large doses of CNS depressants is contraindicated).
No products indexed under this heading.

Butalbital (Co-administration can potentiate each other resulting in additive effects; concurrent use of perphenazine in patients receiving large doses of CNS depressants is contraindicated). Products include:
Phrenilin 578
Sedapap Tablets 50 mg/650 mg ... 2225

Carbamazepine (Perphenazine can lower the convulsive threshold in susceptible individuals; increase in dosage of anticonvulsant agent may be required if patient is being treated with anticonvulsant). Products include:
Carbatrol Capsules 3234
Tegretol/Tegretol-XR 2404

Cetirizine Hydrochloride (Co-administration can potentiate each other resulting in additive effects; concurrent use of perphenazine in patients receiving large doses of antihistimines is contraindicated). Products include:
Zyrtec 2756
Zyrtec-D 12 Hour Extended Relief Tablets 2758

Chlordiazepoxide (Co-administration can potentiate each other resulting in additive effects; concurrent use of perphenazine in patients receiving large doses of CNS depressants is contraindicated). Products include:
Limbitrol 1738

Chlordiazepoxide Hydrochloride (Co-administration can potentiate each other resulting in additive effects; concurrent use of perphenazine in patients receiving large doses of CNS depressants is contraindicated). Products include:
Librium Capsules 1736
Librium for Injection 1737

Chlorpheniramine Maleate (Co-administration can potentiate each other resulting in additive effects; concurrent use of perphenazine in patients receiving large doses of antihistimines is contraindicated). Products include:
Actifed Cold & Sinus Caplets and Tablets .... ▣688
Alka-Seltzer Plus Liqui-Gels .... ▣604
BC Allergy Sinus Cold Powder ...... ▣619
Chlor-Trimeton Allergy Tablets ...... ▣735
Chlor-Trimeton Allergy/Decongestant Tablets.... ▣736
Comtrex Flu Therapy & Fever Relief Nighttime Tablets .... ▣628
Comtrex Maximum Strength Multi-Symptom Cold & Cough Relief Tablets and Caplets .... ▣626
Contac Severe Cold and Flu Caplets Maximum Strength........ ▣746
Coricidin 'D' Cold, Flu & Sinus Tablets .... ▣737
Coricidin/Coricidin D .... ▣738
Coricidin HBP Maximum Strength Flu Tablets .... ▣738
Extendryl 1361
Hycomine Compound Tablets 1317
Kronofed-A 1341
PediaCare Cough-Cold Liquid .... ▣719
PediaCare NightRest Cough-Cold Liquid .... ▣719
Robitussin Nighttime Honey Flu Liquid .... ▣786
Ryna .... ▣768
Singlet Caplets .... ▣761
Sinutab Sinus Allergy Medication, Maximum Strength Formula, Tablets & Caplets...................... ▣707
Sudafed Cold & Allergy Tablets ..... ▣708
TheraFlu Regular Strength Cold & Cough Night Time Hot Liquid...... ▣676
TheraFlu Regular Strength Cold & Sore Throat Night Time Hot Liquid .... ▣676
TheraFlu Maximum Strength Flu & Cough Night Time Hot Liquid.. ▣678
TheraFlu Maximum Strength Flu & Sore Throat Night Time Hot Liquid .... ▣677
TheraFlu Maximum Strength Severe Cold & Congestion Night Time Caplets.................... ▣678
TheraFlu Maximum Strength Severe Cold & Congestion Night Time Hot Liquid .... ▣678
Triaminic Cold & Allergy Liquid ...... ▣681
Triaminic Cold & Allergy Softchews .... ▣683
Triaminic Cold & Cough Liquid ...... ▣681
Triaminic Cold & Cough Softchews .... ▣683
Triaminic Cold & Night Time Cough Liquid .... ▣681
Triaminic Cold, Cough & Fever Liquid .... ▣681
Children's Tylenol Cold Suspension Liquid and Chewable Tablets 2015
Children's Tylenol Cold Plus Cough Suspension Liquid and Chewable Tablets 2015
Children's Tylenol Flu Suspension Liquid 2015
Maximum Strength Tylenol Allergy Sinus Caplets, Gelcaps, and Geltabs 2010
Multi-Symptom Tylenol Cold Complete Formula Caplets.......... 2010
Vicks 44M Cough, Cold & Flu Relief Liquid .... ▣725
Pediatric Vicks 44m Cough & Cold Relief .... ▣728
Children's Vicks NyQuil Cold/Cough Relief .... ▣726

Chlorpheniramine Polistirex (Co-administration can potentiate each other resulting in additive effects; concurrent use of perphenazine in patients receiving large doses of antihistimines is contraindicated). Products include:
Tussionex Pennkinetic Extended-Release Suspension..... 1174

Chlorpheniramine Tannate (Co-administration can potentiate each other resulting in additive effects; concurrent use of perphenazine in patients receiving large doses of antihistimines is contraindicated). Products include:
Reformulated Rynatan Pediatric Suspension 3352
Rynatuss Pediatric Suspension 3353
Rynatuss Tablets 3353
Tussi-12 S Suspension 3356
Tussi-12 Tablets 3356

Chlorpromazine (Co-administration can potentiate each other resulting in additive effects; concurrent use of perphenazine in patients receiving large doses of CNS depressants is contraindicated). Products include:
Thorazine Suppositories 1656

Chlorpromazine Hydrochloride (Co-administration can potentiate each other resulting in additive effects; concurrent use of perphenazine in patients receiving large doses of CNS depressants is contraindicated). Products include:
Thorazine 1656

Chlorprothixene (Co-administration can potentiate each other resulting in additive effects; concurrent use of perphenazine in patients receiving large doses of CNS depressants is contraindicated).
No products indexed under this heading.

Chlorprothixene Hydrochloride (Co-administration can potentiate each other resulting in additive effects; concurrent use of perphenazine in patients receiving large doses of CNS depressants is contraindicated).
No products indexed under this heading.

Chlorprothixene Lactate (Co-administration can potentiate each other resulting in additive effects; concurrent use of perphenazine in patients receiving large doses of CNS depressants is contraindicated).
No products indexed under this heading.

Clemastine Fumarate (Co-administration can potentiate each other resulting in additive effects; concurrent use of perphenazine in patients receiving large doses of antihistimines is contraindicated). Products include:
Tavist 12 Hour Allergy Tablets .... ▣676

Clidinium Bromide (Co-administration with atropine or other anticholinergic agents may result in additive anticholinergic effects).
No products indexed under this heading.

Clorazepate Dipotassium (Co-administration can potentiate each other resulting in additive effects; concurrent use of perphenazine in patients receiving large doses of CNS depressants is contraindicated). Products include:
Tranxene 511

Clozapine (Co-administration can potentiate each other resulting in additive effects; concurrent use of perphenazine in patients receiving large doses of CNS depressants is contraindicated). Products include:
Clozaril Tablets 2319

Codeine Phosphate (Co-administration can potentiate each other resulting in additive effects; concurrent use of perphenazine in patients receiving large doses of CNS depressants is contraindicated). Products include:
Phenergan with Codeine Syrup 3557
Phenergan VC with Codeine Syrup .. 3561
Robitussin A-C Syrup 2942
Robitussin-DAC Syrup 2942
Ryna-C Liquid .... ▣768
Soma Compound w/Codeine Tablets 3355
Tussi-Organidin NR Liquid 3350
Tussi-Organidin-S NR Liquid 3350
Tylenol with Codeine 2595

Cyproheptadine Hydrochloride (Co-administration can potentiate each other resulting in additive effects; concurrent use of perphenazine in patients receiving large doses of antihistimines is contraindicated). Products include:
Periactin Tablets 2155

Desflurane (Co-administration can potentiate each other resulting in additive effects; concurrent use of perphenazine in patients receiving large doses of CNS depressants is contraindicated). Products include:
Suprane Liquid for Inhalation 874

Dexchlorpheniramine Maleate (Co-administration can potentiate each other resulting in additive effects; concurrent use of perphenazine in patients receiving large doses of antihistimines is contraindicated).
No products indexed under this heading.

Dezocine (Co-administration can potentiate each other resulting in additive effects; concurrent use of perphenazine in patients receiving large doses of CNS depressants is contraindicated).
No products indexed under this heading.

Diazepam (Co-administration can potentiate each other resulting in additive effects; concurrent use of perphenazine in patients receiving large doses of CNS depressants is contraindicated). Products include:
Valium Injectable 3026
Valium Tablets 3047

Dicyclomine Hydrochloride (Co-administration with atropine or other anticholinergic agents may result in additive anticholinergic effects).
No products indexed under this heading.

Diphenhydramine Citrate (Co-administration can potentiate each other resulting in additive effects; concurrent use of perphenazine in patients receiving large doses of antihistimines is contraindicated). Products include:
Alka-Seltzer PM Effervescent Tablets .... ▣605
Benadryl Allergy & Sinus Fastmelt Tablets .... ▣693
Benadryl Children's Allergy/Cold Fastmelt Tablets .... ▣692
Excedrin PM Tablets, Caplets, and Geltabs .... ▣631
Goody's PM Powder .... ▣621

Diphenhydramine Hydrochloride (Co-administration can potentiate each other resulting in additive effects; concurrent use of perphenazine in patients receiving large doses of antihistimines is contraindicated). Products include:
Extra Strength Bayer PM Caplets.. ▣611
Benadryl Allergy Chewables .... ▣689
Benadryl Allergy .... ▣691
Benadryl Allergy Liquid .... ▣690
Benadryl Allergy/Cold Tablets .... ▣691
Benadryl Allergy/Congestion Tablets .... ▣692
Benadryl Allergy & Sinus Liquid ..... ▣693
Benadryl Allergy Sinus Headache Caplets & Gelcaps .... ▣693
Benadryl Severe Allergy & Sinus Headache Caplets .... ▣694
Benadryl Dye-Free Allergy Liquid ... ▣690
Benadryl Dye-Free Allergy Liqui-Gels Softgels .... ▣690
Benadryl Itch Relief Stick Extra Strength .... ▣695
Benadryl Cream .... ▣695
Benadryl Gel .... ▣695
Benadryl Spray .... ▣696

Benadryl Parenteral 2617
Coricidin HBP Night-Time Cold & Flu Tablets 738
Nytol QuickCaps Caplets 622
Maximum Strength Nytol QuickGels Softgels 621
Extra Strength Percogesic Aspirin-Free Coated Caplets 665
Simply Sleep Caplets 2008
Sominex Original Formula Tablets 761
Children's Tylenol Allergy-D Liquid 2014
Maximum Strength Tylenol Allergy Sinus NightTime Caplets 2010
Tylenol Severe Allergy Caplets 2010
Maximum Strength Tylenol Flu NightTime Gelcaps 2011
Extra Strength Tylenol PM Caplets, Geltabs, and Gelcaps 2012
Unisom Maximum Strength SleepGels 713

Diphenylpyraline Hydrochloride (Co-administration can potentiate each other resulting in additive effects; concurrent use of perphenazine in patients receiving large doses of antihistimines is contraindicated).
No products indexed under this heading.

Divalproex Sodium (Perphenazine can lower the convulsive threshold in susceptible individuals; increase in dosage of anticonvulsant agent may be required if patient is being treated with anticonvulsant). Products include:
Depakote Sprinkle Capsules 426
Depakote Tablets 430
Depakote ER Tablets 436

Droperidol (Co-administration can potentiate each other resulting in additive effects; concurrent use of perphenazine in patients receiving large doses of CNS depressants is contraindicated).
No products indexed under this heading.

Enflurane (Co-administration can potentiate each other resulting in additive effects; concurrent use of perphenazine in patients receiving large doses of CNS depressants is contraindicated).
No products indexed under this heading.

Estazolam (Co-administration can potentiate each other resulting in additive effects; concurrent use of perphenazine in patients receiving large doses of CNS depressants is contraindicated). Products include:
ProSom Tablets 500

Ethchlorvynol (Co-administration can potentiate each other resulting in additive effects; concurrent use of perphenazine in patients receiving large doses of CNS depressants is contraindicated).
No products indexed under this heading.

Ethinamate (Co-administration can potentiate each other resulting in additive effects; concurrent use of perphenazine in patients receiving large doses of CNS depressants is contraindicated).
No products indexed under this heading.

Ethosuximide (Perphenazine can lower the convulsive threshold in susceptible individuals; increase in dosage of anticonvulsant agent may be required if patient is being treated with anticonvulsant). Products include:
Zarontin Capsules 2659
Zarontin Syrup 2660

Ethotoin (Perphenazine can lower the convulsive threshold in susceptible individuals; increase in dosage of anticonvulsant agent may be required if patient is being treated with anticonvulsant).
No products indexed under this heading.

Felbamate (Perphenazine can lower the convulsive threshold in susceptible individuals; increase in dosage of anticonvulsant agent may be required if patient is being treated with anticonvulsant). Products include:
Felbatol 3343

Fentanyl (Co-administration can potentiate each other resulting in additive effects; concurrent use of perphenazine in patients receiving large doses of CNS depressants is contraindicated). Products include:
Duragesic Transdermal System 1786

Fentanyl Citrate (Co-administration can potentiate each other resulting in additive effects; concurrent use of perphenazine in patients receiving large doses of CNS depressants is contraindicated). Products include:
Actiq 1184

Fexofenadine Hydrochloride (Co-administration can potentiate each other resulting in additive effects; concurrent use of perphenazine in patients receiving large doses of antihistimines is contraindicated). Products include:
Allegra 712
Allegra-D Extended-Release Tablets 714

Fluphenazine Decanoate (Co-administration can potentiate each other resulting in additive effects; concurrent use of perphenazine in patients receiving large doses of CNS depressants is contraindicated).
No products indexed under this heading.

Fluphenazine Enanthate (Co-administration can potentiate each other resulting in additive effects; concurrent use of perphenazine in patients receiving large doses of CNS depressants is contraindicated).
No products indexed under this heading.

Fluphenazine Hydrochloride (Co-administration can potentiate each other resulting in additive effects; concurrent use of perphenazine in patients receiving large doses of CNS depressants is contraindicated).
No products indexed under this heading.

Flurazepam Hydrochloride (Co-administration can potentiate each other resulting in additive effects; concurrent use of perphenazine in patients receiving large doses of CNS depressants is contraindicated).
No products indexed under this heading.

Fosphenytoin Sodium (Perphenazine can lower the convulsive threshold in susceptible individuals; increase in dosage of anticonvulsant agent may be required if patient is being treated with anticonvulsant). Products include:
Cerebyx Injection 2619

Glutethimide (Co-administration can potentiate each other resulting in additive effects; concurrent use of perphenazine in patients receiving large doses of CNS depressants is contraindicated).
No products indexed under this heading.

Glycopyrrolate (Co-administration with atropine or other anticholinergic agents may result in additive anticholinergic effects). Products include:
Robinul Forte Tablets 1358
Robinul Injectable 2940
Robinul Tablets 1358

Haloperidol (Co-administration can potentiate each other resulting in additive effects; concurrent use of perphenazine in patients receiving large doses of CNS depressants is contraindicated). Products include:
Haldol Injection, Tablets and Concentrate 2533

Haloperidol Decanoate (Co-administration can potentiate each other resulting in additive effects; concurrent use of perphenazine in patients receiving large doses of CNS depressants is contraindicated). Products include:
Haldol Decanoate 2535

Hydrocodone Bitartrate (Co-administration can potentiate each other resulting in additive effects; concurrent use of perphenazine in patients receiving large doses of CNS depressants is contraindicated). Products include:
Hycodan 1316
Hycomine Compound Tablets 1317
Hycotuss Expectorant Syrup 1318
Lortab 3319
Lortab Elixir 3317
Maxidone Tablets CIII 3399
Norco 5/325 Tablets CIII 3424
Norco 7.5/325 Tablets CIII 3425
Norco 10/325 Tablets CIII 3427
Norco 10/325 Tablets CIII 3425
Vicodin Tablets 516
Vicodin ES Tablets 517
Vicodin HP Tablets 518
Vicodin Tuss Expectorant 519
Vicoprofen Tablets 520
Zydone Tablets 1330

Hydrocodone Polistirex (Co-administration can potentiate each other resulting in additive effects; concurrent use of perphenazine in patients receiving large doses of CNS depressants is contraindicated). Products include:
Tussionex Pennkinetic Extended-Release Suspension 1174

Hydromorphone Hydrochloride (Co-administration can potentiate each other resulting in additive effects; concurrent use of perphenazine in patients receiving large doses of CNS depressants is contraindicated). Products include:
Dilaudid 441
Dilaudid Oral Liquid 445
Dilaudid Powder 441
Dilaudid Rectal Suppositories 441
Dilaudid Tablets 441
Dilaudid Tablets - 8 mg 445
Dilaudid-HP 443

Hydroxyzine Hydrochloride (Co-administration can potentiate each other resulting in additive effects; concurrent use of perphenazine in patients receiving large doses of CNS depressants is contraindicated). Products include:
Atarax Tablets & Syrup 2667
Vistaril Intramuscular Solution 2738

Hyoscyamine (Co-administration with atropine or other anticholinergic agents may result in additive anticholinergic effects). Products include:
Urised Tablets 2876

Hyoscyamine Sulfate (Co-administration with atropine or other anticholinergic agents may result in additive anticholinergic effects). Products include:
Arco-Lase Plus Tablets 592
Donnatal 2929
Donnatal Extentabs 2930
Levsin/Levsinex/Levbid 3172
NuLev Orally Disintegrating Tablets 3176
Prosed/DS Tablets 3268
Urimax Tablets 1769

Ipratropium Bromide (Co-administration with atropine or other anticholinergic agents may result in additive anticholinergic effects). Products include:
Atrovent Inhalation Aerosol 1030
Atrovent Inhalation Solution 1031
Atrovent Nasal Spray 0.03% 1032
Atrovent Nasal Spray 0.06% 1033
Combivent Inhalation Aerosol 1041
DuoNeb Inhalation Solution 1233

Isoflurane (Co-administration can potentiate each other resulting in additive effects; concurrent use of perphenazine in patients receiving large doses of CNS depressants is contraindicated).
No products indexed under this heading.

Ketamine Hydrochloride (Co-administration can potentiate each other resulting in additive effects; concurrent use of perphenazine in patients receiving large doses of CNS depressants is contraindicated).
No products indexed under this heading.

Lamotrigine (Perphenazine can lower the convulsive threshold in susceptible individuals; increase in dosage of anticonvulsant agent may be required if patient is being treated with anticonvulsant). Products include:
Lamictal 1567

Levetiracetam (Perphenazine can lower the convulsive threshold in susceptible individuals; increase in dosage of anticonvulsant agent may be required if patient is being treated with anticonvulsant). Products include:
Keppra Tablets 3314

Levomethadyl Acetate Hydrochloride (Co-administration can potentiate each other resulting in additive effects; concurrent use of perphenazine in patients receiving large doses of CNS depressants is contraindicated).
No products indexed under this heading.

Levorphanol Tartrate (Co-administration can potentiate each other resulting in additive effects; concurrent use of perphenazine in patients receiving large doses of CNS depressants is contraindicated). Products include:
Levo-Dromoran 1734
Levorphanol Tartrate Tablets 3059

Loratadine (Co-administration can potentiate each other resulting in additive effects; concurrent use of perphenazine in patients receiving large doses of antihistimines is contraindicated). Products include:
Claritin 3100
Claritin-D 12 Hour Extended Release Tablets 3102
Claritin-D 24 Hour Extended Release Tablets 3104

Lorazepam (Co-administration can potentiate each other resulting in additive effects; concurrent use of perphenazine in patients receiving large doses of CNS depressants is contraindicated). Products include:
Ativan Injection 3478
Ativan Tablets 3482

Loxapine Hydrochloride (Co-administration can potentiate each other resulting in additive effects; concurrent use of perphenazine in patients receiving large doses of CNS depressants is contraindicated).
No products indexed under this heading.

Loxapine Succinate (Co-administration can potentiate each other resulting in additive effects; concurrent use of perphenazine in patients receiving large doses of CNS depressants is contraindicated). Products include:
Loxitane Capsules 3398

Mepenzolate Bromide (Co-administration with atropine or other anticholinergic agents may result in additive anticholinergic effects).
No products indexed under this heading.

Meperidine Hydrochloride (Co-administration can potentiate each other resulting in additive effects; concurrent use of perphenazine in patients receiving large doses of CNS depressants is contraindicated). Products include:

Demerol 3079
Mepergan Injection 3539

Mephenytoin (Perphenazine can lower the convulsive threshold in susceptible individuals; increase in dosage of anticonvulsant agent may be required if patient is being treated with anticonvulsant).
No products indexed under this heading.

Mephobarbital (Co-administration can potentiate each other resulting in additive effects; concurrent use of perphenazine in patients receiving large doses of CNS depressants is contraindicated).
No products indexed under this heading.

Meprobamate (Co-administration can potentiate each other resulting in additive effects; concurrent use of perphenazine in patients receiving large doses of CNS depressants is contraindicated). Products include:
Miltown Tablets 3349

Mesoridazine Besylate (Co-administration can potentiate each other resulting in additive effects; concurrent use of perphenazine in patients receiving large doses of CNS depressants is contraindicated). Products include:
Serentil 1057

Methadone Hydrochloride (Co-administration can potentiate each other resulting in additive effects; concurrent use of perphenazine in patients receiving large doses of CNS depressants is contraindicated). Products include:
Dolophine Hydrochloride Tablets 3056

Methdilazine Hydrochloride (Co-administration can potentiate each other resulting in additive effects; concurrent use of perphenazine in patients receiving large doses of antihistimines is contraindicated).
No products indexed under this heading.

Methohexital Sodium (Co-administration can potentiate each other resulting in additive effects; concurrent use of perphenazine in patients receiving large doses of CNS depressants is contraindicated). Products include:
Brevital Sodium for Injection, USP .. 1815

Methotrimeprazine (Co-administration can potentiate each other resulting in additive effects; concurrent use of perphenazine in patients receiving large doses of CNS depressants is contraindicated).
No products indexed under this heading.

Methoxyflurane (Co-administration can potentiate each other resulting in additive effects; concurrent use of perphenazine in patients receiving large doses of CNS depressants is contraindicated).
No products indexed under this heading.

Methsuximide (Perphenazine can lower the convulsive threshold in susceptible individuals; increase in dosage of anticonvulsant agent may be required if patient is being treated with anticonvulsant). Products include:
Celontin Capsules 2618

Midazolam Hydrochloride (Co-administration can potentiate each other resulting in additive effects; concurrent use of perphenazine in patients receiving large doses of CNS depressants is contraindicated). Products include:
Versed Injection 3027
Versed Syrup 3033

Molindone Hydrochloride (Co-administration can potentiate each other resulting in additive effects; concurrent use of perphenazine in patients receiving large doses of CNS depressants is contraindicated). Products include:
Moban 1320

Morphine Sulfate (Co-administration can potentiate each other resulting in additive effects; concurrent use of perphenazine in patients receiving large doses of CNS depressants is contraindicated). Products include:
Astramorph/PF Injection, USP (Preservative-Free)...................... 594
Duramorph Injection 1312
Infumorph 200 and Infumorph 500 Sterile Solutions 1314
Kadian Capsules 1335
MS Contin Tablets 2896
MSIR 2898
Oramorph SR Tablets 3062
Roxanol 3066

Olanzapine (Co-administration can potentiate each other resulting in additive effects; concurrent use of perphenazine in patients receiving large doses of CNS depressants is contraindicated). Products include:
Zyprexa Tablets 1973
Zyprexa ZYDIS Orally Disintegrating Tablets................. 1973

Oxazepam (Co-administration can potentiate each other resulting in additive effects; concurrent use of perphenazine in patients receiving large doses of CNS depressants is contraindicated).
No products indexed under this heading.

Oxcarbazepine (Perphenazine can lower the convulsive threshold in susceptible individuals; increase in dosage of anticonvulsant agent may be required if patient is being treated with anticonvulsant). Products include:
Trileptal Oral Suspension 2407
Trileptal Tablets 2407

Oxybutynin Chloride (Co-administration with atropine or other anticholinergic agents may result in additive anticholinergic effects). Products include:
Ditropan XL Extended Release Tablets 564

Oxycodone Hydrochloride (Co-administration can potentiate each other resulting in additive effects; concurrent use of perphenazine in patients receiving large doses of CNS depressants is contraindicated). Products include:
OxyContin Tablets 2912
OxyFast Oral Concentrate Solution . 2916
OxyIR Capsules 2916
Percocet Tablets 1326
Percodan Tablets 1327
Percolone Tablets 1327
Roxicodone 3067
Tylox Capsules 2597

Paramethadione (Perphenazine can lower the convulsive threshold in susceptible individuals; increase in dosage of anticonvulsant agent may be required if patient is being treated with anticonvulsant).
No products indexed under this heading.

Pentobarbital Sodium (Co-administration can potentiate each other resulting in additive effects; concurrent use of perphenazine in patients receiving large doses of CNS depressants is contraindicated). Products include:
Nembutal Sodium Solution 485

Phenacemide (Perphenazine can lower the convulsive threshold in susceptible individuals; increase in dosage of anticonvulsant agent may be required if patient is being treated with anticonvulsant).
No products indexed under this heading.

Phenobarbital (Perphenazine can lower the convulsive threshold in susceptible individuals; increase in dosage of anticonvulsant agent may be required if patient is being treated with anticonvulsant; co-administration can potentiate each other resulting in additive effects; concurrent use of perphenazine in patients receiving large doses of CNS depressants is contraindicated). Products include:
Arco-Lase Plus Tablets 592
Donnatal 2929
Donnatal Extentabs 2930

Phensuximide (Perphenazine can lower the convulsive threshold in susceptible individuals; increase in dosage of anticonvulsant agent may be required if patient is being treated with anticonvulsant).
No products indexed under this heading.

Phenytoin (Perphenazine can lower the convulsive threshold in susceptible individuals; increase in dosage of anticonvulsant agent may be required if patient is being treated with anticonvulsant). Products include:
Dilantin Infatabs 2624
Dilantin-125 Oral Suspension 2625

Phenytoin Sodium (Perphenazine can lower the convulsive threshold in susceptible individuals; increase in dosage of anticonvulsant agent may be required if patient is being treated with anticonvulsant). Products include:
Dilantin Kapseals 2622

Prazepam (Co-administration can potentiate each other resulting in additive effects; concurrent use of perphenazine in patients receiving large doses of CNS depressants is contraindicated).
No products indexed under this heading.

Primidone (Perphenazine can lower the convulsive threshold in susceptible individuals; increase in dosage of anticonvulsant agent may be required if patient is being treated with anticonvulsant).
No products indexed under this heading.

Prochlorperazine (Co-administration can potentiate each other resulting in additive effects; concurrent use of perphenazine in patients receiving large doses of CNS depressants is contraindicated). Products include:
Compazine 1505

Procyclidine Hydrochloride (Co-administration with atropine or other anticholinergic agents may result in additive anticholinergic effects).
No products indexed under this heading.

Promethazine Hydrochloride (Co-administration can potentiate each other resulting in additive effects; concurrent use of perphenazine in patients receiving large doses of CNS depressants is contraindicated). Products include:
Mepergan Injection 3539
Phenergan Injection 3553
Phenergan 3556
Phenergan Syrup 3554
Phenergan with Codeine Syrup 3557
Phenergan with Dextromethorphan Syrup 3559
Phenergan VC Syrup 3560
Phenergan VC with Codeine Syrup .. 3561

Propantheline Bromide (Co-administration with atropine or other anticholinergic agents may result in additive anticholinergic effects).
No products indexed under this heading.

Propofol (Co-administration can potentiate each other resulting in additive effects; concurrent use of perphenazine in patients receiving large doses of CNS depressants is contraindicated). Products include:
Diprivan Injectable Emulsion 667

Propoxyphene Hydrochloride (Co-administration can potentiate each other resulting in additive effects; concurrent use of perphenazine in patients receiving large doses of CNS depressants is contraindicated). Products include:
Darvon Pulvules 1909
Darvon Compound-65 Pulvules 1910

Propoxyphene Napsylate (Co-administration can potentiate each other resulting in additive effects; concurrent use of perphenazine in patients receiving large doses of CNS depressants is contraindicated). Products include:
Darvon-N/Darvocet-N 1907
Darvon-N Tablets 1912

Pyrilamine Maleate (Co-administration can potentiate each other resulting in additive effects; concurrent use of perphenazine in patients receiving large doses of antihistimines is contraindicated). Products include:
Maximum Strength Midol Menstrual Caplets and Gelcaps.......................................■■612
Maximum Strength Midol PMS Caplets and Gelcaps....................■■613

Pyrilamine Tannate (Co-administration can potentiate each other resulting in additive effects; concurrent use of perphenazine in patients receiving large doses of antihistimines is contraindicated). Products include:
Ryna-12 S Suspension 3351

Quazepam (Co-administration can potentiate each other resulting in additive effects; concurrent use of perphenazine in patients receiving large doses of CNS depressants is contraindicated).
No products indexed under this heading.

Quetiapine Fumarate (Co-administration can potentiate each other resulting in additive effects; concurrent use of perphenazine in patients receiving large doses of CNS depressants is contraindicated). Products include:
Seroquel Tablets 684

Remifentanil Hydrochloride (Co-administration can potentiate each other resulting in additive effects; concurrent use of perphenazine in patients receiving large doses of CNS depressants is contraindicated).
No products indexed under this heading.

Risperidone (Co-administration can potentiate each other resulting in additive effects; concurrent use of perphenazine in patients receiving large doses of CNS depressants is contraindicated). Products include:
Risperdal 1796

Scopolamine (Co-administration with atropine or other anticholinergic agents may result in additive anticholinergic effects). Products include:
Transderm Scōp Transdermal Therapeutic System 2302

Scopolamine Hydrobromide (Co-administration with atropine or other anticholinergic agents may result in additive anticholinergic effects). Products include:
Donnatal 2929
Donnatal Extentabs 2930

Secobarbital Sodium (Co-administration can potentiate each other resulting in additive effects; concurrent use of perphenazine in patients receiving large doses of CNS depressants is contraindicated).
No products indexed under this heading.

Sevoflurane (Co-administration can potentiate each other resulting in additive effects; concurrent use of

perphenazine in patients receiving large doses of CNS depressants is contraindicated).
No products indexed under this heading.

Sufentanil Citrate (Co-administration can potentiate each other resulting in additive effects; concurrent use of perphenazine in patients receiving large doses of CNS depressants is contraindicated).
No products indexed under this heading.

Temazepam (Co-administration can potentiate each other resulting in additive effects; concurrent use of perphenazine in patients receiving large doses of CNS depressants is contraindicated).
No products indexed under this heading.

Terfenadine (Co-administration can potentiate each other resulting in additive effects; concurrent use of perphenazine in patients receiving large doses of antihistimines is contraindicated).
No products indexed under this heading.

Thiamylal Sodium (Co-administration can potentiate each other resulting in additive effects; concurrent use of perphenazine in patients receiving large doses of CNS depressants is contraindicated).
No products indexed under this heading.

Thioridazine Hydrochloride (Co-administration can potentiate each other resulting in additive effects; concurrent use of perphenazine in patients receiving large doses of CNS depressants is contraindicated). Products include:
Thioridazine Hydrochloride Tablets 2289

Thiothixene (Co-administration can potentiate each other resulting in additive effects; concurrent use of perphenazine in patients receiving large doses of CNS depressants is contraindicated). Products include:
Navane Capsules 2701
Thiothixene Capsules 2290

Tiagabine Hydrochloride (Perphenazine can lower the convulsive threshold in susceptible individuals; increase in dosage of anticonvulsant agent may be required if patient is being treated with anticonvulsant). Products include:
Gabitril Tablets 1189

Tolterodine Tartrate (Co-administration with atropine or other anticholinergic agents may result in additive anticholinergic effects). Products include:
Detrol Tablets 3623
Detrol LA Capsules 2801

Topiramate (Perphenazine can lower the convulsive threshold in susceptible individuals; increase in dosage of anticonvulsant agent may be required if patient is being treated with anticonvulsant). Products include:
Topamax Sprinkle Capsules 2590
Topamax Tablets 2590

Triazolam (Co-administration can potentiate each other resulting in additive effects; concurrent use of perphenazine in patients receiving large doses of CNS depressants is contraindicated). Products include:
Halcion Tablets 2823

Tridihexethyl Chloride (Co-administration with atropine or other anticholinergic agents may result in additive anticholinergic effects).
No products indexed under this heading.

Trifluoperazine Hydrochloride (Co-administration can potentiate each other resulting in additive effects; concurrent use of perphenazine in patients receiving large doses of CNS depressants is contraindicated). Products include:
Stelazine 1640

Trihexyphenidyl Hydrochloride (Co-administration with atropine or other anticholinergic agents may result in additive anticholinergic effects). Products include:
Artane 1855

Trimeprazine Tartrate (Co-administration can potentiate each other resulting in additive effects; concurrent use of perphenazine in patients receiving large doses of antihistimines is contraindicated).
No products indexed under this heading.

Trimethadione (Perphenazine can lower the convulsive threshold in susceptible individuals; increase in dosage of anticonvulsant agent may be required if patient is being treated with anticonvulsant).
No products indexed under this heading.

Tripelennamine Hydrochloride (Co-administration can potentiate each other resulting in additive effects; concurrent use of perphenazine in patients receiving large doses of antihistimines is contraindicated).
No products indexed under this heading.

Triprolidine Hydrochloride (Co-administration can potentiate each other resulting in additive effects; concurrent use of perphenazine in patients receiving large doses of antihistimines is contraindicated). Products include:
Actifed Cold & Allergy Tablets 688

Valproate Sodium (Perphenazine can lower the convulsive threshold in susceptible individuals; increase in dosage of anticonvulsant agent may be required if patient is being treated with anticonvulsant). Products include:
Depacon Injection 416

Valproic Acid (Perphenazine can lower the convulsive threshold in susceptible individuals; increase in dosage of anticonvulsant agent may be required if patient is being treated with anticonvulsant). Products include:
Depakene 421

Zaleplon (Co-administration can potentiate each other resulting in additive effects; concurrent use of perphenazine in patients receiving large doses of CNS depressants is contraindicated). Products include:
Sonata Capsules 3591

Ziprasidone Hydrochloride (Co-administration can potentiate each other resulting in additive effects; concurrent use of perphenazine in patients receiving large doses of CNS depressants is contraindicated). Products include:
Geodon Capsules 2688

Zolpidem Tartrate (Co-administration can potentiate each other resulting in additive effects; concurrent use of perphenazine in patients receiving large doses of CNS depressants is contraindicated). Products include:
Ambien Tablets 3191

Zonisamide (Perphenazine can lower the convulsive threshold in susceptible individuals; increase in dosage of anticonvulsant agent may be required if patient is being treated with anticonvulsant). Products include:
Zonegran Capsules 1307

Food Interactions

Alcohol (Concurrent use may result in additive effects and hypotension; the use of alcohol should be avoided).

TRILEPTAL ORAL SUSPENSION
(Oxcarbazepine) 2407
See Trileptal Tablets

TRILEPTAL TABLETS
(Oxcarbazepine) 2407
May interact with dihydropyridine calcium channel blockers, phenytoin, valproate, and certain other agents. Compounds in these categories include:

Amlodipine Besylate (Oxcarbazepine and MHD induce a subgroup of the CYP4503A family responsible for the metabolism of dihydropyridine calcium channel antagonists, resulting in a lower plasma concentration of these drugs). Products include:
Lotrel Capsules 2370
Norvasc Tablets 2704

Carbamazepine (Co-administration with carbamazepine decreases the plasma levels of MHD (29% to 40%)). Products include:
Carbatrol Capsules 3234
Tegretol/Tegretol-XR 2404

Divalproex Sodium (Co-administration decreases MHD concentration by 18%). Products include:
Depakote Sprinkle Capsules 426
Depakote Tablets 430
Depakote ER Tablets 436

Ethinyl Estradiol (Co-administration with an oral contraceptive containing ethinyl estradiol and levonorgestrel results in the decreased mean AUC value of EE by 48% to 52%, therefore, concurrent use of Trileptal with hormonal contraceptives may render these contraceptives less effective; studies with other oral or implant contraceptives have not been studied). Products include:
Alesse-21 Tablets 3468
Alesse-28 Tablets 3473
Brevicon 28-Day Tablets 3380
Cyclessa Tablets 2450
Desogen Tablets 2458
Estinyl Tablets 3112
Estrostep 2627
femhrt Tablets 2635
Levlen 962
Levlite 21 Tablets 962
Levlite 28 Tablets 962
Levora Tablets 3389
Loestrin 21 Tablets 2642
Loestrin Fe Tablets 2642
Lo/Ovral Tablets 3532
Lo/Ovral-28 Tablets 3538
Low-Ogestrel-28 Tablets 3392
Microgestin Fe 1.5/30 Tablets 3407
Microgestin Fe 1/20 Tablets 3400
Mircette Tablets 2470
Modicon 2563
Necon 3415
Nordette-28 Tablets 2257
Norinyl 1 +35 28-Day Tablets 3380
Ogestrel 0.5/50-28 Tablets 3428
Ortho-Cept 21 Tablets 2546
Ortho-Cept 28 Tablets 2546
Ortho-Cyclen/Ortho Tri-Cyclen 2573
Ortho-Novum 2563
Ovcon 3364
Ovral Tablets 3551
Ovral-28 Tablets 3552
Tri-Levlen 962
Tri-Norinyl-28 Tablets 3433
Triphasil-21 Tablets 3600
Triphasil-28 Tablets 3605
Trivora Tablets 3439
Yasmin 28 Tablets 980
Zovia 3449

Felodipine (Repeated co-administration of Trileptal lowers felodipine AUC by 28%). Products include:
Lexxel Tablets 608
Plendil Extended-Release Tablets 623

Fosphenytoin Sodium (Co-administration increases the plasma phenytoin levels by up to 40%; phenytoin decreases the plasma levels of its active metabolite monohydroxy metabolite (MHD); a decrease in the dose of phenytoin may be required). Products include:
Cerebyx Injection 2619

Isradipine (Oxcarbazepine and MHD induce a subgroup of the CYP4503A family responsible for the metabolism of dihydropyridine calcium channel antagonists, resulting in a lower plasma concentration of these drugs). Products include:
DynaCirc Capsules 2921
DynaCirc CR Tablets 2923

Levonorgestrel (Co-administration with an oral contraceptive containing ethinyl estradiol and levonorgestrel results in the decreased mean AUC value of EE by 48% to 52%, therefore, concurrent use of Trileptal with hormonal contraceptives may render these contraceptives less effective; studies with other oral or implant contraceptives have not been studied). Products include:
Alesse-21 Tablets 3468
Alesse-28 Tablets 3473
Levlen 962
Levlite 21 Tablets 962
Levlite 28 Tablets 962
Levora Tablets 3389
Mirena Intrauterine System 974
Nordette-28 Tablets 2257
Norplant System 3543
Tri-Levlen 962
Triphasil-21 Tablets 3600
Triphasil-28 Tablets 3605
Trivora Tablets 3439

Nicardipine Hydrochloride (Oxcarbazepine and MHD induce a subgroup of the CYP4503A family responsible for the metabolism of dihydropyridine calcium channel antagonists, resulting in a lower plasma concentration of these drugs). Products include:
Cardene I.V. 3485

Nifedipine (Oxcarbazepine and MHD induce a subgroup of the CYP4503A family responsible for the metabolism of dihydropyridine calcium channel antagonists, resulting in a lower plasma concentration of these drugs). Products include:
Adalat CC Tablets 877
Procardia Capsules 2708
Procardia XL Extended Release Tablets 2710

Nimodipine (Oxcarbazepine and MHD induce a subgroup of the CYP4503A family responsible for the metabolism of dihydropyridine calcium channel antagonists, resulting in a lower plasma concentration of these drugs). Products include:
Nimotop Capsules 904

Phenobarbital (Co-administration with phenobarbital decreases the plasma levels of MHD (29% to 40%); concurrent use increases the phenobarbital level by approximately 15%). Products include:
Arco-Lase Plus Tablets 592
Donnatal 2929
Donnatal Extentabs 2930

Phenytoin (Co-administration increases the plasma phenytoin levels by up to 40%; phenytoin decreases the plasma levels of its active metabolite monohydroxy metabolite (MHD); a decrease in the dose of phenytoin may be required). Products include:
Dilantin Infatabs 2624
Dilantin-125 Oral Suspension 2625

Phenytoin Sodium (Co-administration increases the plasma phenytoin levels by up to 40%; phenytoin decreases the plasma levels of its active metabolite monohydroxy metabolite (MHD); a decrease in the dose of phenytoin may be required). Products include:

Dilantin Kapseals **2622**

Valproate Sodium (Co-administration decreases MHD concentration by 18%). Products include:

Depacon Injection **416**

Valproic Acid (Co-administration decreases MHD concentration by 18%). Products include:

Depakene **421**

Verapamil Hydrochloride (Produces a decrease of 20% of the plasma levels of MHD). Products include:

Covera-HS Tablets **3199**
Isoptin SR Tablets **467**
Tarka Tablets **508**
Verelan Capsules **3184**
Verelan PM Capsules **3186**

Food Interactions

Alcohol (Oxcarbazepine causes dizziness and somnolence, concurrent use with alcohol could result in possible additive sedative effect).

TRI-LEVLEN 21 TABLETS

(Ethinyl Estradiol, Levonorgestrel) **962**
See Levlite 21 Tablets

TRI-LEVLEN 28 TABLETS

(Ethinyl Estradiol, Levonorgestrel) **962**
See Levlite 21 Tablets

TRILISATE LIQUID

(Choline Magnesium Trisalicylate) **2901**
May interact with antacids, carbonic anhydrase inhibitors, corticosteroids, insulin, phenytoin, salicylates, sulfonylureas, thiazides, urinary alkalinizing agents, valproate, and certain other agents. Compounds in these categories include:

Acetazolamide (Raising urine pH, as with carbonic anhydrase inhibitors, can enhance renal salicylate clearance and diminish plasma salicylate concentration; salicylates compete for protein binding sites and plasma concentration or free fraction of carbonic anhydrase inhibitors may be altered). Products include:

Diamox Sequels Sustained Release Capsules .... ⊙**270**
Diamox Tablets .... ⊙**269**

Aluminum Carbonate (Raising urine pH, as with chronic antacids use, can enhance renal salicylate clearance and diminish plasma salicylate concentration).

No products indexed under this heading.

Aluminum Hydroxide (Raising urine pH, as with chronic antacids use, can enhance renal salicylate clearance and diminish plasma salicylate concentration). Products include:

Amphojel Suspension (Mint Flavor) .... ▣**789**
Gaviscon Extra Strength Liquid ..... ▣**751**
Gaviscon Extra Strength Tablets ..... ▣**751**
Gaviscon Regular Strength Liquid .. ▣**751**
Gaviscon Regular Strength Tablets .... ▣**750**
Maalox Antacid/Anti-Gas Oral Suspension .... ▣**673**
Maalox Max Maximum Strength Antacid/Anti-Gas Liquid **2300**
Maalox Regular Strength Antacid/Antigas Liquid **2300**
Mylanta **1813**
Vanquish Caplets .... ▣**617**

Aspirin (Concurrent use of other salicylate-containing products and choline magnesium trisalicylate can lead to an increase in plasma salicylate concentration and may result in potentially toxic salicylate levels). Products include:

Aggrenox Capsules **1026**
Alka-Seltzer .... ▣**603**
Alka-Seltzer Lemon Lime Antacid and Pain Reliever Effervescent Tablets .... ▣**603**
Alka-Seltzer Extra Strength Antacid and Pain Reliever Effervescent Tablets .... ▣**603**
Alka-Seltzer PM Effervescent Tablets .... ▣**605**
Genuine Bayer Tablets, Caplets and Gelcaps .... ▣**606**
Extra Strength Bayer Caplets and Gelcaps .... ▣**610**
Aspirin Regimen Bayer Children's Chewable Tablets (Orange or Cherry Flavored) .... ▣**607**
Bayer, Aspirin Regimen .... ▣**606**
Aspirin Regimen Bayer 81 mg Caplets with Calcium .... ▣**607**
Genuine Bayer Professional Labeling (Aspirin Regimen Bayer) .... ▣**608**
Extra Strength Bayer Arthritis Caplets .... ▣**610**
Extra Strength Bayer Plus Caplets .... ▣**610**
Extra Strength Bayer PM Caplets .. ▣**611**
BC Powder .... ▣**619**
BC Allergy Sinus Cold Powder ...... ▣**619**
Arthritis Strength BC Powder .... ▣**619**
BC Sinus Cold Powder .... ▣**619**
Darvon Compound-65 Pulvules **1910**
Ecotrin Enteric Coated Aspirin Low, Regular and Maximum Strength Tablets **1715**
Excedrin Extra-Strength Tablets, Caplets, and Geltabs .... ▣**629**
Excedrin Migraine **1070**
Goody's Body Pain Formula Powder .... ▣**620**
Goody's Extra Strength Headache Powder .... ▣**620**
Goody's Extra Strength Pain Relief Tablets .... ▣**620**
Percodan Tablets **1327**
Robaxisal Tablets **2939**
Soma Compound Tablets **3354**
Soma Compound w/Codeine Tablets **3355**
Vanquish Caplets .... ▣**617**

Bendroflumethiazide (Raising urine pH, as with thiazide diuretics, can enhance renal salicylate clearance and diminish plasma salicylate concentration). Products include:

Corzide 40/5 Tablets **2247**
Corzide 80/5 Tablets **2247**

Betamethasone Acetate (Corticosteroids can reduce plasma salicylate levels by increasing renal elimination and perhaps by also stimulating hepatic metabolism of salicylates). Products include:

Celestone Soluspan Injectable Suspension **3097**

Betamethasone Sodium Phosphate (Corticosteroids can reduce plasma salicylate levels by increasing renal elimination and perhaps by also stimulating hepatic metabolism of salicylates). Products include:

Celestone Soluspan Injectable Suspension **3097**

Chlorothiazide (Raising urine pH, as with thiazide diuretics, can enhance renal salicylate clearance and diminish plasma salicylate concentration). Products include:

Aldoclor Tablets **2035**
Diuril Oral **2087**

Chlorothiazide Sodium (Raising urine pH, as with thiazide diuretics, can enhance renal salicylate clearance and diminish plasma salicylate concentration). Products include:

Diuril Sodium Intravenous **2086**

Chlorpropamide (When sulonylurea oral hypoglycemic agents are co-administered with salicylates, the hypoglycemic effects may be enhanced via increased insulin secretion or by displacement of sulfonylurea agents from binding sites). Products include:

Diabinese Tablets **2680**

Cortisone Acetate (Corticosteroids can reduce plasma salicylate levels by increasing renal elimination and perhaps by also stimulating hepatic metabolism of salicylates). Products include:

Cortone Acetate Injectable Suspension **2059**
Cortone Acetate Tablets **2061**

Dexamethasone (Corticosteroids can reduce plasma salicylate levels by increasing renal elimination and perhaps by also stimulating hepatic metabolism of salicylates). Products include:

Decadron Elixir **2078**
Decadron Tablets **2079**
TobraDex Ophthalmic Ointment **542**
TobraDex Ophthalmic Suspension .. **541**

Dexamethasone Acetate (Corticosteroids can reduce plasma salicylate levels by increasing renal elimination and perhaps by also stimulating hepatic metabolism of salicylates).

No products indexed under this heading.

Dexamethasone Sodium Phosphate (Corticosteroids can reduce plasma salicylate levels by increasing renal elimination and perhaps by also stimulating hepatic metabolism of salicylates). Products include:

Decadron Phosphate Injection **2081**
Decadron Phosphate Sterile Ophthalmic Ointment **2083**
Decadron Phosphate Sterile Ophthalmic Solution **2084**
NeoDecadron Sterile Ophthalmic Solution **2144**

Dichlorphenamide (Raising urine pH, as with carbonic anhydrase inhibitors, can enhance renal salicylate clearance and diminish plasma salicylate concentration; salicylates compete for protein binding sites and plasma concentration or free fraction of carbonic anhydrase inhibitors may be altered). Products include:

Daranide Tablets **2077**

Diflunisal (Concurrent use of other salicylate-containing products and choline magnesium trisalicylate can lead to an increase in plasma salicylate concentration and may result in potentially toxic salicylate levels). Products include:

Dolobid Tablets **2088**

Divalproex Sodium (Salicylates compete for protein binding sites and plasma concentration or free fraction of valproic acid inhibitors may be altered). Products include:

Depakote Sprinkle Capsules **426**
Depakote Tablets **430**
Depakote ER Tablets **436**

Dorzolamide Hydrochloride (Raising urine pH, as with carbonic anhydrase inhibitors, can enhance renal salicylate clearance and diminish plasma salicylate concentration; salicylates compete for protein binding sites and plasma concentration or free fraction of carbonic anhydrase inhibitors may be altered). Products include:

Cosopt Sterile Ophthalmic Solution **2065**
Trusopt Sterile Ophthalmic Solution **2196**

Fludrocortisone Acetate (Corticosteroids can reduce plasma salicylate levels by increasing renal elimination and perhaps by also stimulating hepatic metabolism of salicylates). Products include:

Florinef Acetate Tablets **2250**

Fosphenytoin Sodium (Salicylates compete for protein binding sites and plasma concentration or free fraction of phenytoin may be altered). Products include:

Cerebyx Injection **2619**

Glimepiride (When sulonylurea oral hypoglycemic agents are co-administered with salicylates, the hypoglycemic effects may be enhanced via increased insulin secretion or by displacement of sulfonylurea agents from binding sites). Products include:

Amaryl Tablets **717**

Glipizide (When sulonylurea oral hypoglycemic agents are co-administered with salicylates, the hypoglycemic effects may be enhanced via increased insulin secretion or by displacement of sulfonylurea agents from binding sites). Products include:

Glucotrol Tablets **2692**
Glucotrol XL Extended Release Tablets **2693**

Glyburide (When sulonylurea oral hypoglycemic agents are co-administered with salicylates, the hypoglycemic effects may be enhanced via increased insulin secretion or by displacement of sulfonylurea agents from binding sites). Products include:

DiaBeta Tablets **741**
Glucovance Tablets **1086**

Hydrochlorothiazide (Raising urine pH, as with thiazide diuretics, can enhance renal salicylate clearance and diminish plasma salicylate concentration). Products include:

Accuretic Tablets **2614**
Aldoril Tablets **2039**
Atacand HCT Tablets **597**
Avalide Tablets **1070**
Diovan HCT Tablets **2338**
Dyazide Capsules **1515**
HydroDIURIL Tablets **2108**
Hyzaar **2109**
Inderide Tablets **3517**
Inderide LA Long-Acting Capsules .. **3519**
Lotensin HCT Tablets **2367**
Maxzide **1008**
Micardis HCT Tablets **1051**
Microzide Capsules **3414**
Moduretic Tablets **2138**
Monopril HCT **1094**
Prinzide Tablets **2168**
Timolide Tablets **2187**
Uniretic Tablets **3178**
Vaseretic Tablets **2204**
Zestoretic Tablets **695**
Ziac Tablets **1887**

Hydrocortisone (Corticosteroids can reduce plasma salicylate levels by increasing renal elimination and perhaps by also stimulating hepatic metabolism of salicylates). Products include:

Anusol-HC Cream 2.5% **2237**
Cipro HC Otic Suspension **540**
Cortaid Intensive Therapy Cream . ▣**717**
Cortaid Maximum Strength Cream .... ▣**717**
Cortisporin Ophthalmic Suspension Sterile .... ⊙**297**
Cortizone•5 .... ▣**699**
Cortizone•10 .... ▣**699**
Cortizone•10 Plus Creme .... ▣**700**
Cortizone for Kids Creme .... ▣**699**
Hydrocortone Tablets **2106**
Massengill Medicated Soft Cloth Towelette .... ▣**753**
VōSoL HC Otic Solution **3356**

Hydrocortisone Acetate (Corticosteroids can reduce plasma salicylate levels by increasing renal elimination and perhaps by also stimulating hepatic metabolism of salicylates). Products include:

Analpram-HC **1338**
Anusol HC-1 Hydrocortisone Anti-Itch Cream .... ▣**689**
Anusol-HC Suppositories **2238**
Cortaid .... ▣**717**
Cortifoam Rectal Foam **3170**
Cortisporin-TC Otic Suspension **2246**
Hydrocortone Acetate Injectable Suspension **2103**
Pramosone **1343**
Proctocort Suppositories **2264**
ProctoFoam-HC **3177**
Terra-Cortril Ophthalmic Suspension **2716**

Hydrocortisone Sodium Phosphate (Corticosteroids can reduce plasma salicylate levels by increasing renal elimination and perhaps by also stimulating hepatic metabolism of salicylates). Products include:

Hydrocortone Phosphate Injection, Sterile **2105**

Hydrocortisone Sodium Succinate (Corticosteroids can reduce plasma salicylate levels by increasing renal elimination and perhaps by also stimulating hepatic metabolism

of salicylates).
No products indexed under this heading.

Hydroflumethiazide (Raising urine pH, as with thiazide diuretics, can enhance renal salicylate clearance and diminish plasma salicylate concentration). Products include:
Diucardin Tablets 3494

Insulin, Human, Zinc Suspension (Co-administration of insulin and high doses of salicylates may enhance hypoglycemic effects). Products include:
Humulin L, 100 Units 1937
Humulin U, 100 Units 1943
Novolin L Human Insulin 10 ml Vials 2422

Insulin, Human NPH (Co-administration of insulin and high doses of salicylates may enhance hypoglycemic effects). Products include:
Humulin N, 100 Units 1939
Humulin N NPH Pen 1940
Novolin N Human Insulin 10 ml Vials 2422
Novolin N PenFill 2423
Novolin N Prefilled Syringe Disposable Insulin Delivery System 2425

Insulin, Human Regular (Co-administration of insulin and high doses of salicylates may enhance hypoglycemic effects). Products include:
Humulin R Regular (U-500) 1943
Humulin R, 100 Units 1941
Novolin R Human Insulin 10 ml Vials 2423
Novolin R PenFill 2423
Novolin R Prefilled Syringe Disposable Insulin Delivery System 2425
Velosulin BR Human Insulin 10 ml Vials 2435

Insulin, Human Regular and Human NPH Mixture (Co-administration of insulin and high doses of salicylates may enhance hypoglycemic effects). Products include:
Humulin 50/50, 100 Units 1934
Humulin 70/30, 100 Units 1935
Humulin 70/30 Pen 1936
Novolin 70/30 Human Insulin 10 ml Vials 2421
Novolin 70/30 PenFill 2423
Novolin 70/30 Prefilled Disposable Insulin Delivery System 2425

Insulin, NPH (Co-administration of insulin and high doses of salicylates may enhance hypoglycemic effects). Products include:
Iletin II, NPH (Pork), 100 Units 1946

Insulin, Regular (Co-administration of insulin and high doses of salicylates may enhance hypoglycemic effects). Products include:
Iletin II, Regular (Pork), 100 Units ... 1947

Insulin, Zinc Crystals (Co-administration of insulin and high doses of salicylates may enhance hypoglycemic effects).
No products indexed under this heading.

Insulin, Zinc Suspension (Co-administration of insulin and high doses of salicylates may enhance hypoglycemic effects). Products include:
Iletin II, Lente (Pork), 100 Units 1945

Insulin Aspart, Human Regular (Co-administration of insulin and high doses of salicylates may enhance hypoglycemic effects).
No products indexed under this heading.

Insulin glargine (Co-administration of insulin and high doses of salicylates may enhance hypoglycemic effects). Products include:
Lantus Injection 742

Insulin Lispro, Human (Co-administration of insulin and high doses of salicylates may enhance hypoglycemic effects). Products include:
Humalog 1926
Humalog Mix 75/25 Pen 1928

Insulin Lispro Protamine, Human (Co-administration of insulin and high doses of salicylates may enhance hypoglycemic effects). Products include:
Humalog Mix 75/25 Pen 1928

Magaldrate (Raising urine pH, as with chronic antacids use, can enhance renal salicylate clearance and diminish plasma salicylate concentration).
No products indexed under this heading.

Magnesium Hydroxide (Raising urine pH, as with chronic antacids use, can enhance renal salicylate clearance and diminish plasma salicylate concentration). Products include:
Ex•Lax Milk of Magnesia Liquid ..... ⊞670
Maalox Antacid/Anti-Gas Oral Suspension .... ⊞673
Maalox Max Maximum Strength Antacid/Anti-Gas Liquid 2300
Maalox Regular Strength Antacid/Antigas Liquid 2300
Mylanta Fast-Acting 1813
Mylanta 1813
Pepcid Complete Chewable Tablets 1815
Phillips' Chewable Tablets .... ⊞615
Phillips' Milk of Magnesia Liquid (Original, Cherry, & Mint) .... ⊞616
Rolaids Tablets .... ⊞706
Extra Strength Rolaids Tablets ...... ⊞706
Vanquish Caplets .... ⊞617

Magnesium Oxide (Raising urine pH, as with chronic antacids use, can enhance renal salicylate clearance and diminish plasma salicylate concentration). Products include:
Beelith Tablets 946
Mag-Ox 400 Tablets 1024
Uro-Mag Capsules 1024

Magnesium Salicylate (Concurrent use of other salicylate-containing products and choline magnesium trisalicylate can lead to an increase in plasma salicylate concentration and may result in potentially toxic salicylate levels). Products include:
Momentum Backache Relief Extra Strength Caplets .... ⊞666

Methazolamide (Raising urine pH, as with carbonic anhydrase inhibitors, can enhance renal salicylate clearance and diminish plasma salicylate concentration; salicylates compete for protein binding sites and plasma concentration or free fraction of carbonic anhydrase inhibitors may be altered). Products include:
Neptazane Tablets .... ⊙271

Methotrexate Sodium (Salicylates may increase the therapeutic as well as toxic effects of methotrexate, particularly when administered in chemotherapeutic doses, by inhibition of renal methotrexate excretion and displacement of plasma protein bound methotrexate).
No products indexed under this heading.

Methyclothiazide (Raising urine pH, as with thiazide diuretics, can enhance renal salicylate clearance and diminish plasma salicylate concentration).
No products indexed under this heading.

Methylprednisolone Acetate (Corticosteroids can reduce plasma salicylate levels by increasing renal elimination and perhaps by also stimulating hepatic metabolism of salicylates). Products include:
Depo-Medrol Injectable Suspension 2795

Methylprednisolone Sodium Succinate (Corticosteroids can reduce plasma salicylate levels by increasing renal elimination and perhaps by also stimulating hepatic metabolism of salicylates). Products include:
Solu-Medrol Sterile Powder 2855

Phenytoin (Salicylates compete for protein binding sites and plasma concentration or free fraction of phenytoin may be altered). Products include:
Dilantin Infatabs 2624
Dilantin-125 Oral Suspension 2625

Phenytoin Sodium (Salicylates compete for protein binding sites and plasma concentration or free fraction of phenytoin may be altered). Products include:
Dilantin Kapseals 2622

Polythiazide (Raising urine pH, as with thiazide diuretics, can enhance renal salicylate clearance and diminish plasma salicylate concentration). Products include:
Minizide Capsules 2700
Renese Tablets 2712

Potassium Acid Phosphate (Acidification of the urine can significantly diminish the renal clearance of salicylate and increase plasma salicylate concentrations). Products include:
K-Phos Original (Sodium Free) Tablets 947

Potassium Citrate (Raising urine pH, as with urinary alkalinizers, can enhance renal salicylate clearance and diminish plasma salicylate concentration). Products include:
Urocit-K Tablets 2232

Prednisolone Acetate (Corticosteroids can reduce plasma salicylate levels by increasing renal elimination and perhaps by also stimulating hepatic metabolism of salicylates). Products include:
Blephamide Ophthalmic Ointment .. 547
Blephamide Ophthalmic Suspension 548
Poly-Pred Liquifilm Ophthalmic Suspension .... ⊙245
Pred Forte Ophthalmic Suspension .... ⊙246
Pred Mild Sterile Ophthalmic Suspension .... ⊙249
Pred-G Ophthalmic Suspension .... ⊙247
Pred-G Sterile Ophthalmic Ointment .... ⊙248

Prednisolone Sodium Phosphate (Corticosteroids can reduce plasma salicylate levels by increasing renal elimination and perhaps by also stimulating hepatic metabolism of salicylates). Products include:
Pediapred Oral Solution 1170

Prednisolone Tebutate (Corticosteroids can reduce plasma salicylate levels by increasing renal elimination and perhaps by also stimulating hepatic metabolism of salicylates).
No products indexed under this heading.

Prednisone (Corticosteroids can reduce plasma salicylate levels by increasing renal elimination and perhaps by also stimulating hepatic metabolism of salicylates). Products include:
Prednisone 3064

Probenecid (The efficacy of uricosuric agents may be decreased when administered with salicylates).
No products indexed under this heading.

Salsalate (Concurrent use of other salicylate-containing products and choline magnesium trisalicylate can lead to an increase in plasma salicylate concentration and may result in potentially toxic salicylate levels).
No products indexed under this heading.

Sodium Bicarbonate (Raising urine pH, as with chronic antacids use, can enhance renal salicylate clearance and diminish plasma salicylate concentration). Products include:
Alka-Seltzer .... ⊞603
Alka-Seltzer Lemon Lime Antacid and Pain Reliever Effervescent Tablets .... ⊞603
Alka-Seltzer Extra Strength Antacid and Pain Reliever Effervescent Tablets .... ⊞603
Alka-Seltzer Heartburn Relief Tablets .... ⊞604
Ceo-Two Evacuant Suppository .... ⊞618
Colyte with Flavor Packs for Oral Solution 3170
GoLYTELY and Pineapple Flavor GoLYTELY for Oral Solution 1068
NuLYTELY, Cherry Flavor, Lemon-Lime Flavor, and Orange Flavor NuLYTELY for Oral Solution 1068

Sodium Citrate (Raising urine pH, as with urinary alkalinizers, can enhance renal salicylate clearance and diminish plasma salicylate concentration).
No products indexed under this heading.

Sulfinpyrazone (The efficacy of uricosuric agents may be decreased when administered with salicylates).
No products indexed under this heading.

Tolazamide (When sulonylurea oral hypoglycemic agents are co-administered with salicylates, the hypoglycemic effects may be enhanced via increased insulin secretion or by displacement of sulfonylurea agents from binding sites).
No products indexed under this heading.

Tolbutamide (When sulonylurea oral hypoglycemic agents are co-administered with salicylates, the hypoglycemic effects may be enhanced via increased insulin secretion or by displacement of sulfonylurea agents from binding sites).
No products indexed under this heading.

Triamcinolone (Corticosteroids can reduce plasma salicylate levels by increasing renal elimination and perhaps by also stimulating hepatic metabolism of salicylates).
No products indexed under this heading.

Triamcinolone Acetonide (Corticosteroids can reduce plasma salicylate levels by increasing renal elimination and perhaps by also stimulating hepatic metabolism of salicylates). Products include:
Azmacort Inhalation Aerosol 728
Nasacort Nasal Inhaler 750
Nasacort AQ Nasal Spray 752
Tri-Nasal Spray 2274

Triamcinolone Diacetate (Corticosteroids can reduce plasma salicylate levels by increasing renal elimination and perhaps by also stimulating hepatic metabolism of salicylates).
No products indexed under this heading.

Triamcinolone Hexacetonide (Corticosteroids can reduce plasma salicylate levels by increasing renal elimination and perhaps by also stimulating hepatic metabolism of salicylates).
No products indexed under this heading.

Valproate Sodium (Salicylates compete for protein binding sites and plasma concentration or free fraction of valproic acid inhibitors may be altered). Products include:
Depacon Injection 416

Valproic Acid (Salicylates compete for protein binding sites and plasma concentration or free fraction of valproic acid inhibitors may be altered). Products include:
Depakene 421

Warfarin Sodium (Potential exists for increased levels of unbound warfarin with concurrent use). Products include:
- Coumadin for Injection 1243
- Coumadin Tablets 1243
- Warfarin Sodium Tablets, USP 3302

Food Interactions

Alcohol (Chronic heavy alcohol users, 3 or more drinks per day, in combination with analgesic/antipyretic drug products containing NSAID ingredients, including choline and magnesium salicylates increases the risk of adverse GI events, including stomach bleeding).

Food that lowers urinary pH (Decreases urinary salicylate excretion and increases plasma levels).

Food that raises urinary pH (Enhances renal salicylate clearance and diminishes plasma salicylate concentration).

TRILISATE TABLETS

(Choline Magnesium Trisalicylate) 2901
See Trilisate Liquid

TRI-NASAL SPRAY

(Triamcinolone Acetonide) 2274
None cited in PDR database.

TRI-NORINYL-28 TABLETS

(Ethinyl Estradiol, Norethindrone) 3433
May interact with barbiturates, tetracyclines, and certain other agents. Compounds in these categories include:

Ampicillin (Potential for reduced efficacy and increased incidence of breakthrough bleeding and menstrual irregularities with concomitant use).
No products indexed under this heading.

Ampicillin Sodium (Potential for reduced efficacy and increased incidence of breakthrough bleeding and menstrual irregularities with concomitant use). Products include:
- Unasyn for Injection 2728

Aprobarbital (Potential for reduced efficacy and increased incidence of breakthrough bleeding and menstrual irregularities with concomitant use).
No products indexed under this heading.

Butabarbital (Potential for reduced efficacy and increased incidence of breakthrough bleeding and menstrual irregularities with concomitant use).
No products indexed under this heading.

Butalbital (Potential for reduced efficacy and increased incidence of breakthrough bleeding and menstrual irregularities with concomitant use). Products include:
- Phrenilin 578
- Sedapap Tablets 50 mg/650 mg ... 2225

Demeclocycline Hydrochloride (Potential for reduced efficacy and increased incidence of breakthrough bleeding and menstrual irregularities with concomitant use). Products include:
- Declomycin Tablets 1855

Doxycycline Calcium (Potential for reduced efficacy and increased incidence of breakthrough bleeding and menstrual irregularities with concomitant use). Products include:
- Vibramycin Calcium Oral Suspension Syrup 2735

Doxycycline Hyclate (Potential for reduced efficacy and increased incidence of breakthrough bleeding and menstrual irregularities with concomitant use). Products include:
- Doryx Coated Pellet Filled Capsules 3357
- Periostat Tablets 1208
- Vibramycin Hyclate Capsules 2735
- Vibramycin Hyclate Intravenous 2737
- Vibra-Tabs Film Coated Tablets 2735

Doxycycline Monohydrate (Potential for reduced efficacy and increased incidence of breakthrough bleeding and menstrual irregularities with concomitant use). Products include:
- Monodox Capsules 2442
- Vibramycin Monohydrate for Oral Suspension 2735

Fosphenytoin Sodium (Potential for reduced efficacy and increased incidence of breakthrough bleeding and menstrual irregularities with concomitant use). Products include:
- Cerebyx Injection 2619

Griseofulvin (Potential for reduced efficacy and increased incidence of breakthrough bleeding and menstrual irregularities with concomitant use). Products include:
- Grifulvin V Tablets Microsize and Oral Suspension Microsize 2518
- Gris-PEG Tablets 2661

Mephobarbital (Potential for reduced efficacy and increased incidence of breakthrough bleeding and menstrual irregularities with concomitant use).
No products indexed under this heading.

Methacycline Hydrochloride (Potential for reduced efficacy and increased incidence of breakthrough bleeding and menstrual irregularities with concomitant use).
No products indexed under this heading.

Minocycline Hydrochloride (Potential for reduced efficacy and increased incidence of breakthrough bleeding and menstrual irregularities with concomitant use). Products include:
- Dynacin Capsules 2019
- Minocin Intravenous 1862
- Minocin Oral Suspension 1865
- Minocin Pellet-Filled Capsules 1863

Oxytetracycline Hydrochloride (Potential for reduced efficacy and increased incidence of breakthrough bleeding and menstrual irregularities with concomitant use). Products include:
- Terra-Cortril Ophthalmic Suspension 2716
- Urobiotic-250 Capsules 2731

Pentobarbital Sodium (Potential for reduced efficacy and increased incidence of breakthrough bleeding and menstrual irregularities with concomitant use). Products include:
- Nembutal Sodium Solution 485

Phenobarbital (Potential for reduced efficacy and increased incidence of breakthrough bleeding and menstrual irregularities with concomitant use). Products include:
- Arco-Lase Plus Tablets 592
- Donnatal 2929
- Donnatal Extentabs 2930

Phenylbutazone (Potential for reduced efficacy and increased incidence of breakthrough bleeding and menstrual irregularities with concomitant use).
No products indexed under this heading.

Phenytoin (Potential for reduced efficacy and increased incidence of breakthrough bleeding and menstrual irregularities with concomitant use). Products include:
- Dilantin Infatabs 2624
- Dilantin-125 Oral Suspension 2625

Phenytoin Sodium (Potential for reduced efficacy and increased incidence of breakthrough bleeding and menstrual irregularities with concomitant use). Products include:
- Dilantin Kapseals 2622

Rifampin (Co-administration has been associated with reduced efficacy and increased incidence of breakthrough bleeding and menstrual irregularities). Products include:
- Rifadin 765
- Rifamate Capsules 767
- Rifater Tablets 769

Secobarbital Sodium (Potential for reduced efficacy and increased incidence of breakthrough bleeding and menstrual irregularities with concomitant use).
No products indexed under this heading.

Tetracycline Hydrochloride (Potential for reduced efficacy and increased incidence of breakthrough bleeding and menstrual irregularities with concomitant use).
No products indexed under this heading.

Thiamylal Sodium (Potential for reduced efficacy and increased incidence of breakthrough bleeding and menstrual irregularities with concomitant use).
No products indexed under this heading.

TRIOSTAT INJECTION

(Liothyronine Sodium) 1825
May interact with oral anticoagulants, estrogens, cardiac glycosides, oral hypoglycemic agents, insulin, tricyclic antidepressants, vasopressors, and certain other agents. Compounds in these categories include:

Acarbose (Initiating thyroid replacement therapy may cause increase in oral hypoglycemic requirements). Products include:
- Precose Tablets 906

Amitriptyline Hydrochloride (Co-administration may increase receptor sensitivity and enhance antidepressant activity; transient cardiac arrhythmias have been reported; thyroid hormone activity may be enhanced). Products include:
- Etrafon 3115
- Limbitrol 1738

Amoxapine (Co-administration may increase receptor sensitivity and enhance antidepressant activity; transient cardiac arrhythmias have been reported; thyroid hormone activity may be enhanced).
No products indexed under this heading.

Chlorotrianisene (Estrogens tend to increase serum thyroid-binding globulin in patients with nonfunctioning thyroid gland who are given thyroid replacement therapy).
No products indexed under this heading.

Chlorpropamide (Initiating thyroid replacement therapy may cause increase in oral hypoglycemic requirements). Products include:
- Diabinese Tablets 2680

Clomipramine Hydrochloride (Co-administration may increase receptor sensitivity and enhance antidepressant activity; transient cardiac arrhythmias have been reported; thyroid hormone activity may be enhanced).
No products indexed under this heading.

Desipramine Hydrochloride (Co-administration may increase receptor sensitivity and enhance antidepressant activity; transient cardiac arrhythmias have been reported; thyroid hormone activity may be enhanced). Products include:
- Norpramin Tablets 755

Deslanoside (Thyroid preparations may potentiate the toxic effects of digitalis).
No products indexed under this heading.

Dicumarol (Thyroid hormones appear to increase catabolism of vitamin K dependent clotting factors; if oral anticoagulants are also given, compensatory increase in clotting factor synthesis are impaired).
No products indexed under this heading.

Dienestrol (Estrogens tend to increase serum thyroid-binding globulin in patients with nonfunctioning thyroid gland who are given thyroid replacement therapy). Products include:
- Ortho Dienestrol Cream 2554

Diethylstilbestrol (Estrogens tend to increase serum thyroid-binding globulin in patients with nonfunctioning thyroid gland who are given thyroid replacement therapy).
No products indexed under this heading.

Digitoxin (Thyroid preparations may potentiate the toxic effects of digitalis).
No products indexed under this heading.

Digoxin (Thyroid preparations may potentiate the toxic effects of digitalis). Products include:
- Digitek Tablets 1003
- Lanoxicaps Capsules 1574
- Lanoxin Injection 1581
- Lanoxin Tablets 1587
- Lanoxin Elixir Pediatric 1578
- Lanoxin Injection Pediatric 1584

Dopamine Hydrochloride (Increased adrenergic effect).
No products indexed under this heading.

Doxepin Hydrochloride (Co-administration may increase receptor sensitivity and enhance antidepressant activity; transient cardiac arrhythmias have been reported; thyroid hormone activity may be enhanced). Products include:
- Sinequan 2713

Epinephrine Bitartrate (Increased adrenergic effect). Products include:
- Sensorcaine 643

Epinephrine Hydrochloride (Increased adrenergic effect).
No products indexed under this heading.

Estradiol (Estrogens tend to increase serum thyroid-binding globulin in patients with nonfunctioning thyroid gland who are given thyroid replacement therapy). Products include:
- Activella Tablets 2764
- Alora Transdermal System 3372
- Climara Transdermal System 958
- CombiPatch Transdermal System .. 2323
- Esclim Transdermal System 3460
- Estrace Vaginal Cream 3358
- Estrace Tablets 3361
- Estring Vaginal Ring 2811
- Ortho-Prefest Tablets 2570
- Vagifem Tablets 2857
- Vivelle Transdermal System 2412
- Vivelle-Dot Transdermal System 2416

Estrogens, Conjugated (Estrogens tend to increase serum thyroid-binding globulin in patients with nonfunctioning thyroid gland who are given thyroid replacement therapy). Products include:
- Premarin Intravenous 3563
- Premarin Tablets 3566
- Premarin Vaginal Cream 3570
- Premphase Tablets 3572
- Prempro Tablets 3572

Estrogens, Esterified (Estrogens tend to increase serum thyroid-binding globulin in patients with nonfunctioning thyroid gland who are given thyroid replacement therapy). Products include:
- Estratest 3252
- Menest Tablets 2254

Estropipate (Estrogens tend to increase serum thyroid-binding globulin in patients with nonfunctioning

thyroid gland who are given thyroid replacement therapy). Products include:
- Ogen Tablets **2846**
- Ortho-Est Tablets **3464**

Ethinyl Estradiol (Estrogens tend to increase serum thyroid-binding globulin in patients with nonfunctioning thyroid gland who are given thyroid replacement therapy). Products include:
- Alesse-21 Tablets **3468**
- Alesse-28 Tablets **3473**
- Brevicon 28-Day Tablets **3380**
- Cyclessa Tablets **2450**
- Desogen Tablets **2458**
- Estinyl Tablets **3112**
- Estrostep **2627**
- femhrt Tablets **2635**
- Levlen **962**
- Levlite 21 Tablets **962**
- Levlite 28 Tablets **962**
- Levora Tablets **3389**
- Loestrin 21 Tablets **2642**
- Loestrin Fe Tablets **2642**
- Lo/Ovral Tablets **3532**
- Lo/Ovral-28 Tablets **3538**
- Low-Ogestrel-28 Tablets **3392**
- Microgestin Fe 1.5/30 Tablets **3407**
- Microgestin Fe 1/20 Tablets **3400**
- Mircette Tablets **2470**
- Modicon **2563**
- Necon **3415**
- Nordette-28 Tablets **2257**
- Norinyl 1 +35 28-Day Tablets **3380**
- Ogestrel 0.5/50-28 Tablets **3428**
- Ortho-Cept 21 Tablets **2546**
- Ortho-Cept 28 Tablets **2546**
- Ortho-Cyclen/Ortho Tri-Cyclen **2573**
- Ortho-Novum **2563**
- Ovcon **3364**
- Ovral Tablets **3551**
- Ovral-28 Tablets **3552**
- Tri-Levlen **962**
- Tri-Norinyl-28 Tablets **3433**
- Triphasil-21 Tablets **3600**
- Triphasil-28 Tablets **3605**
- Trivora Tablets **3439**
- Yasmin 28 Tablets **980**
- Zovia **3449**

Glimepiride (Initiating thyroid replacement therapy may cause increase in oral hypoglycemic requirements). Products include:
- Amaryl Tablets **717**

Glipizide (Initiating thyroid replacement therapy may cause increase in oral hypoglycemic requirements). Products include:
- Glucotrol Tablets **2692**
- Glucotrol XL Extended Release Tablets **2693**

Glyburide (Initiating thyroid replacement therapy may cause increase in oral hypoglycemic requirements). Products include:
- DiaBeta Tablets **741**
- Glucovance Tablets **1086**

Imipramine Hydrochloride (Co-administration may increase receptor sensitivity and enhance antidepressant activity; transient cardiac arrhythmias have been reported; thyroid hormone activity may be enhanced).
No products indexed under this heading.

Imipramine Pamoate (Co-administration may increase receptor sensitivity and enhance antidepressant activity; transient cardiac arrhythmias have been reported; thyroid hormone activity may be enhanced).
No products indexed under this heading.

Insulin, Human, Zinc Suspension (Initiating thyroid replacement therapy may cause increase in insulin requirements). Products include:
- Humulin L, 100 Units **1937**
- Humulin U, 100 Units **1943**
- Novolin L Human Insulin 10 ml Vials **2422**

Insulin, Human NPH (Initiating thyroid replacement therapy may cause increase in insulin requirements). Products include:
- Humulin N, 100 Units **1939**
- Humulin N NPH Pen **1940**
- Novolin N Human Insulin 10 ml Vials **2422**
- Novolin N PenFill **2423**
- Novolin N Prefilled Syringe Disposable Insulin Delivery System **2425**

Insulin, Human Regular (Initiating thyroid replacement therapy may cause increase in insulin requirements). Products include:
- Humulin R Regular (U-500) **1943**
- Humulin R, 100 Units **1941**
- Novolin R Human Insulin 10 ml Vials **2423**
- Novolin R PenFill **2423**
- Novolin R Prefilled Syringe Disposable Insulin Delivery System **2425**
- Velosulin BR Human Insulin 10 ml Vials **2435**

Insulin, Human Regular and Human NPH Mixture (Initiating thyroid replacement therapy may cause increase in insulin requirements). Products include:
- Humulin 50/50, 100 Units **1934**
- Humulin 70/30, 100 Units **1935**
- Humulin 70/30 Pen **1936**
- Novolin 70/30 Human Insulin 10 ml Vials **2421**
- Novolin 70/30 PenFill **2423**
- Novolin 70/30 Prefilled Disposable Insulin Delivery System **2425**

Insulin, NPH (Initiating thyroid replacement therapy may cause increase in insulin requirements). Products include:
- Iletin II, NPH (Pork), 100 Units **1946**

Insulin, Regular (Initiating thyroid replacement therapy may cause increase in insulin requirements). Products include:
- Iletin II, Regular (Pork), 100 Units **1947**

Insulin, Zinc Crystals (Initiating thyroid replacement therapy may cause increase in insulin requirements).
No products indexed under this heading.

Insulin, Zinc Suspension (Initiating thyroid replacement therapy may cause increase in insulin requirements). Products include:
- Iletin II, Lente (Pork), 100 Units **1945**

Insulin Aspart, Human Regular (Initiating thyroid replacement therapy may cause increase in insulin requirements).
No products indexed under this heading.

Insulin glargine (Initiating thyroid replacement therapy may cause increase in insulin requirements). Products include:
- Lantus Injection **742**

Insulin Lispro, Human (Initiating thyroid replacement therapy may cause increase in insulin requirements). Products include:
- Humalog **1926**
- Humalog Mix 75/25 Pen **1928**

Insulin Lispro Protamine, Human (Initiating thyroid replacement therapy may cause increase in insulin requirements). Products include:
- Humalog Mix 75/25 Pen **1928**

Ketamine Hydrochloride (Potential for hypertension and tachycardia).
No products indexed under this heading.

Maprotiline Hydrochloride (Co-administration may increase receptor sensitivity and enhance antidepressant activity; transient cardiac arrhythmias have been reported; thyroid hormone activity may be enhanced).
No products indexed under this heading.

Metaraminol Bitartrate (Increased adrenergic effect). Products include:
- Aramine Injection **2043**

Metformin Hydrochloride (Initiating thyroid replacement therapy may cause increase in oral hypoglycemic requirements). Products include:
- Glucophage Tablets **1080**
- Glucophage XR Tablets **1080**
- Glucovance Tablets **1086**

Methoxamine Hydrochloride (Increased adrenergic effect).
No products indexed under this heading.

Miglitol (Initiating thyroid replacement therapy may cause increase in oral hypoglycemic requirements). Products include:
- Glyset Tablets **2821**

Norepinephrine Bitartrate (Increased adrenergic effect).
No products indexed under this heading.

Nortriptyline Hydrochloride (Co-administration may increase receptor sensitivity and enhance antidepressant activity; transient cardiac arrhythmias have been reported; thyroid hormone activity may be enhanced).
No products indexed under this heading.

Phenylephrine Hydrochloride (Increased adrenergic effect). Products include:
- Afrin Nasal Decongestant Children's Pump Mist **734**
- Extendryl **1361**
- Hycomine Compound Tablets **1317**
- Neo-Synephrine **614**
- Phenergan VC Syrup **3560**
- Phenergan VC with Codeine Syrup **3561**
- Preparation H Cream **778**
- Preparation H Cooling Gel **778**
- Preparation H **778**
- Vicks Sinex Nasal Spray and Ultra Fine Mist **729**

Pioglitazone Hydrochloride (Initiating thyroid replacement therapy may cause increase in oral hypoglycemic requirements). Products include:
- Actos Tablets **3275**

Polyestradiol Phosphate (Estrogens tend to increase serum thyroid-binding globulin in patients with nonfunctioning thyroid gland who are given thyroid replacement therapy).
No products indexed under this heading.

Protriptyline Hydrochloride (Co-administration may increase receptor sensitivity and enhance antidepressant activity; transient cardiac arrhythmias have been reported; thyroid hormone activity may be enhanced). Products include:
- Vivactil Tablets **2446**
- Vivactil Tablets **2217**

Quinestrol (Estrogens tend to increase serum thyroid-binding globulin in patients with nonfunctioning thyroid gland who are given thyroid replacement therapy).
No products indexed under this heading.

Repaglinide (Initiating thyroid replacement therapy may cause increase in oral hypoglycemic requirements). Products include:
- Prandin Tablets (0.5, 1, and 2 mg) **2432**

Rosiglitazone Maleate (Initiating thyroid replacement therapy may cause increase in oral hypoglycemic requirements). Products include:
- Avandia Tablets **1490**

Tolazamide (Initiating thyroid replacement therapy may cause increase in oral hypoglycemic requirements).
No products indexed under this heading.

Tolbutamide (Initiating thyroid replacement therapy may cause increase in oral hypoglycemic requirements).
No products indexed under this heading.

Trimipramine Maleate (Co-administration may increase receptor sensitivity and enhance antidepressant activity; transient cardiac arrhythmias have been reported; thyroid hormone activity may be enhanced). Products include:
- Surmontil Capsules **3595**

Troglitazone (Initiating thyroid replacement therapy may cause increase in oral hypoglycemic requirements).
No products indexed under this heading.

Warfarin Sodium (Thyroid hormones appear to increase catabolism of vitamin K dependent clotting factors; if oral anticoagulants are also given, compensatory increase in clotting factor synthesis are impaired). Products include:
- Coumadin for Injection **1243**
- Coumadin Tablets **1243**
- Warfarin Sodium Tablets, USP **3302**

TRIPEDIA VACCINE

(Diphtheria & Tetanus Toxoids and Acellular Pertussis Vaccine Adsorbed) **817**

May interact with alkylating agents, anticoagulants, corticosteroids, cytotoxic drugs, immunosuppressive agents, and certain other agents. Compounds in these categories include:

Ardeparin Sodium (Concurrent use requires caution).
No products indexed under this heading.

Azathioprine (An adequate immunologic response may not be obtained if used concurrently).
No products indexed under this heading.

Basiliximab (An adequate immunologic response may not be obtained if used concurrently). Products include:
- Simulect for Injection **2399**

Betamethasone Acetate (Corticosteroids, used in greater than physiologic doses, may reduce the immune response to vaccine). Products include:
- Celestone Soluspan Injectable Suspension **3097**

Betamethasone Sodium Phosphate (Corticosteroids, used in greater than physiologic doses, may reduce the immune response to vaccine). Products include:
- Celestone Soluspan Injectable Suspension **3097**

Bleomycin Sulfate (May reduce the immune response to vaccine).
No products indexed under this heading.

Busulfan (May reduce the immune response to vaccine). Products include:
- Myleran Tablets **1603**

Carmustine (BCNU) (May reduce the immune response to vaccine). Products include:
- Gliadel Wafer **1723**

Chlorambucil (May reduce the immune response to vaccine). Products include:
- Leukeran Tablets **1591**

Cortisone Acetate (Corticosteroids, used in greater than physiologic doses, may reduce the immune response to vaccine). Products include:
- Cortone Acetate Injectable Suspension **2059**
- Cortone Acetate Tablets **2061**

Cyclophosphamide (May reduce the immune response to vaccine).
No products indexed under this heading.

Cyclosporine (An adequate immunologic response may not be obtained if used concurrently). Products include:
- Gengraf Capsules ... 457
- Neoral Soft Gelatin Capsules ... 2380
- Neoral Oral Solution ... 2380
- Sandimmune ... 2388

Cytarabine Liposome (May reduce the immune response to vaccine). Products include:
- DepoCyt Injection ... 1197

Dacarbazine (May reduce the immune response to vaccine). Products include:
- DTIC-Dome ... 902

Dalteparin Sodium (Concurrent use requires caution). Products include:
- Fragmin Injection ... 2814

Danaparoid Sodium (Concurrent use requires caution). Products include:
- Orgaran Injection ... 2480

Daunorubicin Hydrochloride (May reduce the immune response to vaccine). Products include:
- Cerubidine for Injection ... 947

Dexamethasone (Corticosteroids, used in greater than physiologic doses, may reduce the immune response to vaccine). Products include:
- Decadron Elixir ... 2078
- Decadron Tablets ... 2079
- TobraDex Ophthalmic Ointment ... 542
- TobraDex Ophthalmic Suspension ... 541

Dexamethasone Acetate (Corticosteroids, used in greater than physiologic doses, may reduce the immune response to vaccine).
- No products indexed under this heading.

Dexamethasone Sodium Phosphate (Corticosteroids, used in greater than physiologic doses, may reduce the immune response to vaccine). Products include:
- Decadron Phosphate Injection ... 2081
- Decadron Phosphate Sterile Ophthalmic Ointment ... 2083
- Decadron Phosphate Sterile Ophthalmic Solution ... 2084
- NeoDecadron Sterile Ophthalmic Solution ... 2144

Dicumarol (Concurrent use requires caution).
- No products indexed under this heading.

Doxorubicin Hydrochloride (May reduce the immune response to vaccine). Products include:
- Adriamycin PFS/RDF Injection ... 2767
- Doxil Injection ... 566

Enoxaparin (Concurrent use requires caution). Products include:
- Lovenox Injection ... 746

Epirubicin Hydrochloride (May reduce the immune response to vaccine). Products include:
- Ellence Injection ... 2806

Floxuridine (May reduce the immune response to vaccine). Products include:
- Sterile FUDR ... 2974

Fludarabine Phosphate (May reduce the immune response to vaccine). Products include:
- Fludara for Injection ... 995

Fludrocortisone Acetate (Corticosteroids, used in greater than physiologic doses, may reduce the immune response to vaccine). Products include:
- Florinef Acetate Tablets ... 2250

Fluorouracil (May reduce the immune response to vaccine). Products include:
- Carac Cream ... 1222
- Efudex ... 1733
- Fluoroplex ... 552

Heparin Sodium (Concurrent use requires caution). Products include:
- Heparin Lock Flush Solution ... 3509
- Heparin Sodium Injection ... 3511

Hydrocortisone (Corticosteroids, used in greater than physiologic doses, may reduce the immune response to vaccine). Products include:
- Anusol-HC Cream 2.5% ... 2237
- Cipro HC Otic Suspension ... 540
- Cortaid Intensive Therapy Cream ... ▣717
- Cortaid Maximum Strength Cream ... ▣717
- Cortisporin Ophthalmic Suspension Sterile ... ⊙297
- Cortizone•5 ... ▣699
- Cortizone•10 ... ▣699
- Cortizone•10 Plus Creme ... ▣700
- Cortizone for Kids Creme ... ▣699
- Hydrocortone Tablets ... 2106
- Massengill Medicated Soft Cloth Towelette ... ▣753
- VōSoL HC Otic Solution ... 3356

Hydrocortisone Acetate (Corticosteroids, used in greater than physiologic doses, may reduce the immune response to vaccine). Products include:
- Analpram-HC ... 1338
- Anusol HC-1 Hydrocortisone Anti-Itch Cream ... ▣689
- Anusol-HC Suppositories ... 2238
- Cortaid ... ▣717
- Cortifoam Rectal Foam ... 3170
- Cortisporin-TC Otic Suspension ... 2246
- Hydrocortone Acetate Injectable Suspension ... 2103
- Pramosone ... 1343
- Proctocort Suppositories ... 2264
- ProctoFoam-HC ... 3177
- Terra-Cortril Ophthalmic Suspension ... 2716

Hydrocortisone Sodium Phosphate (Corticosteroids, used in greater than physiologic doses, may reduce the immune response to vaccine). Products include:
- Hydrocortone Phosphate Injection, Sterile ... 2105

Hydrocortisone Sodium Succinate (Corticosteroids, used in greater than physiologic doses, may reduce the immune response to vaccine).
- No products indexed under this heading.

Hydroxyurea (May reduce the immune response to vaccine). Products include:
- Mylocel Tablets ... 2227

Immune Globulin Intravenous (Human) (An adequate immunologic response may not be obtained if used concurrently).
- No products indexed under this heading.

Influenza Virus Vaccine (Influenza Virus Vaccine should not be given within three days of the administration of Tripedia). Products include:
- FluShield Influenza Vaccine ... 3521
- Fluzone Vaccine ... 802

Lomustine (CCNU) (May reduce the immune response to vaccine).
- No products indexed under this heading.

Mechlorethamine Hydrochloride (May reduce the immune response to vaccine). Products include:
- Mustargen for Injection ... 2142

Melphalan (May reduce the immune response to vaccine). Products include:
- Alkeran Tablets ... 1466

Methotrexate Sodium (May reduce the immune response to vaccine).
- No products indexed under this heading.

Methylprednisolone Acetate (Corticosteroids, used in greater than physiologic doses, may reduce the immune response to vaccine). Products include:
- Depo-Medrol Injectable Suspension ... 2795

Methylprednisolone Sodium Succinate (Corticosteroids, used in greater than physiologic doses, may reduce the immune response to vaccine). Products include:
- Solu-Medrol Sterile Powder ... 2855

Mitotane (May reduce the immune response to vaccine).
- No products indexed under this heading.

Mitoxantrone Hydrochloride (May reduce the immune response to vaccine). Products include:
- Novantrone for Injection ... 1760

Muromonab-CD3 (An adequate immunologic response may not be obtained if used concurrently). Products include:
- Orthoclone OKT3 Sterile Solution ... 2498

Mycophenolate Mofetil (An adequate immunologic response may not be obtained if used concurrently). Products include:
- CellCept Capsules ... 2951
- CellCept Oral Suspension ... 2951
- CellCept Tablets ... 2951

Prednisolone Acetate (Corticosteroids, used in greater than physiologic doses, may reduce the immune response to vaccine). Products include:
- Blephamide Ophthalmic Ointment ... 547
- Blephamide Ophthalmic Suspension ... 548
- Poly-Pred Liquifilm Ophthalmic Suspension ... ⊙245
- Pred Forte Ophthalmic Suspension ... ⊙246
- Pred Mild Sterile Ophthalmic Suspension ... ⊙249
- Pred-G Ophthalmic Suspension ... ⊙247
- Pred-G Sterile Ophthalmic Ointment ... ⊙248

Prednisolone Sodium Phosphate (Corticosteroids, used in greater than physiologic doses, may reduce the immune response to vaccine). Products include:
- Pediapred Oral Solution ... 1170

Prednisolone Tebutate (Corticosteroids, used in greater than physiologic doses, may reduce the immune response to vaccine).
- No products indexed under this heading.

Prednisone (Corticosteroids, used in greater than physiologic doses, may reduce the immune response to vaccine). Products include:
- Prednisone ... 3064

Procarbazine Hydrochloride (May reduce the immune response to vaccine). Products include:
- Matulane Capsules ... 3246

Sirolimus (An adequate immunologic response may not be obtained if used concurrently). Products include:
- Rapamune Oral Solution and Tablets ... 3584

Tacrolimus (An adequate immunologic response may not be obtained if used concurrently). Products include:
- Prograf ... 1393
- Protopic Ointment ... 1397

Tamoxifen Citrate (May reduce the immune response to vaccine). Products include:
- Nolvadex Tablets ... 678

Thioguanine (May reduce the immune response to vaccine). Products include:
- Tabloid Tablets ... 1642

Thiotepa (May reduce the immune response to vaccine). Products include:
- Thioplex for Injection ... 1765

Tinzaparin sodium (Concurrent use requires caution). Products include:
- Innohep Injection ... 1248

Triamcinolone (Corticosteroids, used in greater than physiologic doses, may reduce the immune response to vaccine).
- No products indexed under this heading.

Triamcinolone Acetonide (Corticosteroids, used in greater than physiologic doses, may reduce the immune response to vaccine). Products include:
- Azmacort Inhalation Aerosol ... 728
- Nasacort Nasal Inhaler ... 750
- Nasacort AQ Nasal Spray ... 752
- Tri-Nasal Spray ... 2274

Triamcinolone Diacetate (Corticosteroids, used in greater than physiologic doses, may reduce the immune response to vaccine).
- No products indexed under this heading.

Triamcinolone Hexacetonide (Corticosteroids, used in greater than physiologic doses, may reduce the immune response to vaccine).
- No products indexed under this heading.

Vincristine Sulfate (May reduce the immune response to vaccine).
- No products indexed under this heading.

Warfarin Sodium (Concurrent use requires caution). Products include:
- Coumadin for Injection ... 1243
- Coumadin Tablets ... 1243
- Warfarin Sodium Tablets, USP ... 3302

TRIPHASIL-21 TABLETS

(Ethinyl Estradiol, Levonorgestrel) ... 3600

May interact with barbiturates, phenytoin, tetracyclines, and certain other agents. Compounds in these categories include:

Ampicillin (Potential for reduced efficacy and increased incidence of breakthrough bleeding and menstrual irregularities with concomitant use).
- No products indexed under this heading.

Ampicillin Sodium (Potential for reduced efficacy and increased incidence of breakthrough bleeding and menstrual irregularities with concomitant use). Products include:
- Unasyn for Injection ... 2728

Aprobarbital (Potential for reduced efficacy and increased incidence of breakthrough bleeding and menstrual irregularities with concomitant use).
- No products indexed under this heading.

Butabarbital (Potential for reduced efficacy and increased incidence of breakthrough bleeding and menstrual irregularities with concomitant use).
- No products indexed under this heading.

Butalbital (Potential for reduced efficacy and increased incidence of breakthrough bleeding and menstrual irregularities with concomitant use). Products include:
- Phrenilin ... 578
- Sedapap Tablets 50 mg/650 mg ... 2225

Demeclocycline Hydrochloride (Potential for reduced efficacy and increased incidence of breakthrough bleeding and menstrual irregularities with concomitant use). Products include:
- Declomycin Tablets ... 1855

Doxycycline Calcium (Potential for reduced efficacy and increased incidence of breakthrough bleeding and menstrual irregularities with concomitant use). Products include:
- Vibramycin Calcium Oral Suspension Syrup ... 2735

Doxycycline Hyclate (Potential for reduced efficacy and increased incidence of breakthrough bleeding and menstrual irregularities with concomitant use). Products include:
- Doryx Coated Pellet Filled Capsules ... 3357
- Periostat Tablets ... 1208
- Vibramycin Hyclate Capsules ... 2735
- Vibramycin Hyclate Intravenous ... 2737
- Vibra-Tabs Film Coated Tablets ... 2735

Doxycycline Monohydrate (Potential for reduced efficacy and increased incidence of breakthrough bleeding and menstrual irregularities with concomitant use). Products include:

Monodox Capsules 2442
Vibramycin Monohydrate for Oral Suspension 2735

Fosphenytoin Sodium (Potential for reduced efficacy and increased incidence of breakthrough bleeding and menstrual irregularities with concomitant use). Products include:

Cerebyx Injection 2619

Griseofulvin (Potential for reduced efficacy and increased incidence of breakthrough bleeding and menstrual irregularities with concomitant use). Products include:

Grifulvin V Tablets Microsize and Oral Suspension Microsize 2518
Gris-PEG Tablets 2661

Mephobarbital (Potential for reduced efficacy and increased incidence of breakthrough bleeding and menstrual irregularities with concomitant use).

No products indexed under this heading.

Methacycline Hydrochloride (Potential for reduced efficacy and increased incidence of breakthrough bleeding and menstrual irregularities with concomitant use).

No products indexed under this heading.

Minocycline Hydrochloride (Potential for reduced efficacy and increased incidence of breakthrough bleeding and menstrual irregularities with concomitant use). Products include:

Dynacin Capsules 2019
Minocin Intravenous 1862
Minocin Oral Suspension 1865
Minocin Pellet-Filled Capsules 1863

Oxytetracycline Hydrochloride (Potential for reduced efficacy and increased incidence of breakthrough bleeding and menstrual irregularities with concomitant use). Products include:

Terra-Cortril Ophthalmic Suspension 2716
Urobiotic-250 Capsules 2731

Pentobarbital Sodium (Potential for reduced efficacy and increased incidence of breakthrough bleeding and menstrual irregularities with concomitant use). Products include:

Nembutal Sodium Solution 485

Phenobarbital (Potential for reduced efficacy and increased incidence of breakthrough bleeding and menstrual irregularities with concomitant use). Products include:

Arco-Lase Plus Tablets 592
Donnatal 2929
Donnatal Extentabs 2930

Phenylbutazone (Potential for reduced efficacy and increased incidence of breakthrough bleeding and menstrual irregularities with concomitant use).

No products indexed under this heading.

Phenytoin (Potential for reduced efficacy and increased incidence of breakthrough bleeding and menstrual irregularities with concomitant use). Products include:

Dilantin Infatabs 2624
Dilantin-125 Oral Suspension 2625

Phenytoin Sodium (Potential for reduced efficacy and increased incidence of breakthrough bleeding and menstrual irregularities with concomitant use). Products include:

Dilantin Kapseals 2622

Rifampin (Co-administration has been associated with reduced efficacy and increased incidence of breakthrough bleeding and menstrual irregularities). Products include:

Rifadin 765
Rifamate Capsules 767
Rifater Tablets 769

Secobarbital Sodium (Potential for reduced efficacy and increased incidence of breakthrough bleeding and menstrual irregularities with concomitant use).

No products indexed under this heading.

Tetracycline Hydrochloride (Potential for reduced efficacy and increased incidence of breakthrough bleeding and menstrual irregularities with concomitant use).

No products indexed under this heading.

Thiamylal Sodium (Potential for reduced efficacy and increased incidence of breakthrough bleeding and menstrual irregularities with concomitant use).

No products indexed under this heading.

Troleandomycin (Co-administration may increase the risk of intrahepatic cholestasis). Products include:

Tao Capsules 2716

TRIPHASIL-28 TABLETS

(Ethinyl Estradiol, Levonorgestrel) 3605
See Triphasil-21 Tablets

TRISENOX INJECTION

(Arsenic Trioxide) 1158

May interact with potassium-depleting diuretics, quinidine, and certain other agents. Compounds in these categories include:

Amiodarone Hydrochloride (Arsenic trioxide can cause QT interval prolongation and complete AV block; QT prolongation can lead to torsade de pointes-type ventricular arrhythmias, which can be fatal; co-administration with other drugs that can prolong the QT interval, such as certain anti-arrhythmics, increases the risk and extent of QT prolongation). Products include:

Cordarone Intravenous 3491
Cordarone Tablets 3487
Pacerone Tablets 3331

Amphotericin B (Arsenic trioxide can cause QT interval prolongation and complete AV block; QT prolongation can lead to torsade de pointes-type ventricular arrhythmias, which can be fatal; co-administration with other drugs that can prolong the QT interval, such as amphotericin B, increases the risk and extent of QT prolongation). Products include:

Abelcet Injection 1273
AmBisome for Injection 1383
Amphotec 1774

Bendroflumethiazide (Arsenic trioxide can cause QT interval prolongation and complete AV block; QT prolongation can lead to torsade de pointes-type ventricular arrhythmias, which can be fatal; co-administration with other drugs that cause hypokalemia or hypomagnesemia resulting in prolongation of the QT interval, such as potassium-wasting diuretics, increases the risk and extent of QT prolongation). Products include:

Corzide 40/5 Tablets 2247
Corzide 80/5 Tablets 2247

Bumetanide (Arsenic trioxide can cause QT interval prolongation and complete AV block; QT prolongation can lead to torsade de pointes-type ventricular arrhythmias, which can be fatal; co-administration with other drugs that cause hypokalemia or hypomagnesemia resulting in prolongation of the QT interval, such as potassium-wasting diuretics, increases the risk and extent of QT prolongation).

No products indexed under this heading.

Chlorothiazide (Arsenic trioxide can cause QT interval prolongation and complete AV block; QT prolongation can lead to torsade de pointes-type ventricular arrhythmias, which can be fatal; co-administration with other drugs that cause hypokalemia or hypomagnesemia resulting in prolongation of the QT interval, such as potassium-wasting diuretics, increases the risk and extent of QT prolongation). Products include:

Aldoclor Tablets 2035
Diuril Oral 2087

Chlorothiazide Sodium (Arsenic trioxide can cause QT interval prolongation and complete AV block; QT prolongation can lead to torsade de pointes-type ventricular arrhythmias, which can be fatal; co-administration with other drugs that cause hypokalemia or hypomagnesemia resulting in prolongation of the QT interval, such as potassium-wasting diuretics, increases the risk and extent of QT prolongation). Products include:

Diuril Sodium Intravenous 2086

Ethacrynic Acid (Arsenic trioxide can cause QT interval prolongation and complete AV block; QT prolongation can lead to torsade de pointes-type ventricular arrhythmias, which can be fatal; co-administration with other drugs that cause hypokalemia or hypomagnesemia resulting in prolongation of the QT interval, such as potassium-wasting diuretics, increases the risk and extent of QT prolongation). Products include:

Edecrin Tablets 2091

Furosemide (Arsenic trioxide can cause QT interval prolongation and complete AV block; QT prolongation can lead to torsade de pointes-type ventricular arrhythmias, which can be fatal; co-administration with other drugs that cause hypokalemia or hypomagnesemia resulting in prolongation of the QT interval, such as potassium-wasting diuretics, increases the risk and extent of QT prolongation). Products include:

Furosemide Tablets 2284

Hydrochlorothiazide (Arsenic trioxide can cause QT interval prolongation and complete AV block; QT prolongation can lead to torsade de pointes-type ventricular arrhythmias, which can be fatal; co-administration with other drugs that cause hypokalemia or hypomagnesemia resulting in prolongation of the QT interval, such as potassium-wasting diuretics, increases the risk and extent of QT prolongation). Products include:

Accuretic Tablets 2614
Aldoril Tablets 2039
Atacand HCT Tablets 597
Avalide Tablets 1070
Diovan HCT Tablets 2338
Dyazide Capsules 1515
HydroDIURIL Tablets 2108
Hyzaar 2109
Inderide Tablets 3517
Inderide LA Long-Acting Capsules .. 3519
Lotensin HCT Tablets 2367
Maxzide 1008
Micardis HCT Tablets 1051
Microzide Capsules 3414
Moduretic Tablets 2138
Monopril HCT 1094
Prinzide Tablets 2168
Timolide Tablets 2187
Uniretic Tablets 3178
Vaseretic Tablets 2204
Zestoretic Tablets 695
Ziac Tablets 1887

Hydroflumethiazide (Arsenic trioxide can cause QT interval prolongation and complete AV block; QT prolongation can lead to torsade de pointes-type ventricular arrhythmias, which can be fatal; co-administration with other drugs that cause hypokalemia or hypomagnesemia resulting in prolongation of the QT interval, such as potassium-wasting diuretics, increases the risk and extent of QT prolongation). Products include:

Diucardin Tablets 3494

Methyclothiazide (Arsenic trioxide can cause QT interval prolongation and complete AV block; QT prolongation can lead to torsade de pointes-type ventricular arrhythmias, which can be fatal; co-administration with other drugs that cause hypokalemia or hypomagnesemia resulting in prolongation of the QT interval, such as potassium-wasting diuretics, increases the risk and extent of QT prolongation).

No products indexed under this heading.

Polythiazide (Arsenic trioxide can cause QT interval prolongation and complete AV block; QT prolongation can lead to torsade de pointes-type ventricular arrhythmias, which can be fatal; co-administration with other drugs that cause hypokalemia or hypomagnesemia resulting in prolongation of the QT interval, such as potassium-wasting diuretics, increases the risk and extent of QT prolongation). Products include:

Minizide Capsules 2700
Renese Tablets 2712

Procainamide Hydrochloride (Arsenic trioxide can cause QT interval prolongation and complete AV block; QT prolongation can lead to torsade de pointes-type ventricular arrhythmias, which can be fatal; co-administration with other drugs that can prolong the QT interval, such as certain antiarrhythmics, increases the risk and extent of QT prolongation). Products include:

Procanbid Extended-Release Tablets 2262

Quinidine Gluconate (Arsenic trioxide can cause QT interval prolongation and complete AV block; QT prolongation can lead to torsade de pointes-type ventricular arrhythmias, which can be fatal; co-administration with other drugs that can prolong the QT interval, such as certain anti-arrhythmic quinidine, increases the risk and extent of QT prolongation). Products include:

Quinaglute Dura-Tabs Tablets 978

Quinidine Polygalacturonate (Arsenic trioxide can cause QT interval prolongation and complete AV block; QT prolongation can lead to torsade de pointes-type ventricular arrhythmias, which can be fatal; co-administration with other drugs that can prolong the QT interval, such as certain anti-arrhythmic quinidine, increases the risk and extent of QT prolongation).

No products indexed under this heading.

Quinidine Sulfate (Arsenic trioxide can cause QT interval prolongation and complete AV block; QT prolongation can lead to torsade de pointes-type ventricular arrhythmias, which can be fatal; co-administration with other drugs that can prolong the QT interval, such as certain anti-arrhythmic quinidine, increases the risk and extent of QT prolongation). Products include:

Quinidex Extentabs 2933

Sotalol Hydrochloride (Arsenic trioxide can cause QT interval prolongation and complete AV block; QT prolongation can lead to torsade de pointes-type ventricular arrhythmias, which can be fatal; co-administration with other drugs that can prolong the QT interval, such as certain anti-arrhythmics, increases the risk and extent of QT prolongation). Products include:

Betapace Tablets 950
Betapace AF Tablets 954

Thioridazine Hydrochloride (Arsenic trioxide can cause QT interval prolongation and complete AV block; QT prolongation can lead to torsade de pointes-type ventricular

arrhythmias, which can be fatal; co-administration with other drugs that can prolong the QT interval, such as thioridazine, increases the risk and extent of QT prolongation). Products include:
- Thioridazine Hydrochloride Tablets 2289

Torsemide (Arsenic trioxide can cause QT interval prolongation and complete AV block; QT prolongation can lead to torsade de pointes-type ventricular arrhythmias, which can be fatal; co-administration with other drugs that cause hypokalemia or hypomagnesemia resulting in prolongation of the QT interval, such as potassium-wasting diuretics, increases the risk and extent of QT prolongation). Products include:
- Demadex Tablets and Injection 2965

TRIVORA TABLETS

(Ethinyl Estradiol, Levonorgestrel) 3439

May interact with barbiturates, phenytoin, tetracyclines, and certain other agents. Compounds in these categories include:

Ampicillin (Potential for reduced efficacy and increased incidence of breakthrough bleeding and menstrual irregularities with concomitant use).
- No products indexed under this heading.

Ampicillin Sodium (Potential for reduced efficacy and increased incidence of breakthrough bleeding and menstrual irregularities with concomitant use). Products include:
- Unasyn for Injection 2728

Aprobarbital (Potential for reduced efficacy and increased incidence of breakthrough bleeding and menstrual irregularities with concomitant use).
- No products indexed under this heading.

Butabarbital (Potential for reduced efficacy and increased incidence of breakthrough bleeding and menstrual irregularities with concomitant use).
- No products indexed under this heading.

Butalbital (Potential for reduced efficacy and increased incidence of breakthrough bleeding and menstrual irregularities with concomitant use). Products include:
- Phrenilin 578
- Sedapap Tablets 50 mg/650 mg ... 2225

Demeclocycline Hydrochloride (Potential for reduced efficacy and increased incidence of breakthrough bleeding and menstrual irregularities with concomitant use). Products include:
- Declomycin Tablets 1855

Doxycycline Calcium (Potential for reduced efficacy and increased incidence of breakthrough bleeding and menstrual irregularities with concomitant use). Products include:
- Vibramycin Calcium Oral Suspension Syrup 2735

Doxycycline Hyclate (Potential for reduced efficacy and increased incidence of breakthrough bleeding and menstrual irregularities with concomitant use). Products include:
- Doryx Coated Pellet Filled Capsules 3357
- Periostat Tablets 1208
- Vibramycin Hyclate Capsules 2735
- Vibramycin Hyclate Intravenous 2737
- Vibra-Tabs Film Coated Tablets 2735

Doxycycline Monohydrate (Potential for reduced efficacy and increased incidence of breakthrough bleeding and menstrual irregularities with concomitant use). Products include:
- Monodox Capsules 2442
- Vibramycin Monohydrate for Oral Suspension 2735

Fosphenytoin Sodium (Potential for reduced efficacy and increased incidence of breakthrough bleeding and menstrual irregularities with concomitant use). Products include:
- Cerebyx Injection 2619

Griseofulvin (Potential for reduced efficacy and increased incidence of breakthrough bleeding and menstrual irregularities with concomitant use). Products include:
- Grifulvin V Tablets Microsize and Oral Suspension Microsize 2518
- Gris-PEG Tablets 2661

Mephobarbital (Potential for reduced efficacy and increased incidence of breakthrough bleeding and menstrual irregularities with concomitant use).
- No products indexed under this heading.

Methacycline Hydrochloride (Potential for reduced efficacy and increased incidence of breakthrough bleeding and menstrual irregularities with concomitant use).
- No products indexed under this heading.

Minocycline Hydrochloride (Potential for reduced efficacy and increased incidence of breakthrough bleeding and menstrual irregularities with concomitant use). Products include:
- Dynacin Capsules 2019
- Minocin Intravenous 1862
- Minocin Oral Suspension 1865
- Minocin Pellet-Filled Capsules 1863

Oxytetracycline Hydrochloride (Potential for reduced efficacy and increased incidence of breakthrough bleeding and menstrual irregularities with concomitant use). Products include:
- Terra-Cortril Ophthalmic Suspension 2716
- Urobiotic-250 Capsules 2731

Pentobarbital Sodium (Potential for reduced efficacy and increased incidence of breakthrough bleeding and menstrual irregularities with concomitant use). Products include:
- Nembutal Sodium Solution 485

Phenobarbital (Potential for reduced efficacy and increased incidence of breakthrough bleeding and menstrual irregularities with concomitant use). Products include:
- Arco-Lase Plus Tablets 592
- Donnatal 2929
- Donnatal Extentabs 2930

Phenylbutazone (Potential for reduced efficacy and increased incidence of breakthrough bleeding and menstrual irregularities with concomitant use).
- No products indexed under this heading.

Phenytoin (Potential for reduced efficacy and increased incidence of breakthrough bleeding and menstrual irregularities with concomitant use). Products include:
- Dilantin Infatabs 2624
- Dilantin-125 Oral Suspension 2625

Phenytoin Sodium (Potential for reduced efficacy and increased incidence of breakthrough bleeding and menstrual irregularities with concomitant use). Products include:
- Dilantin Kapseals 2622

Rifampin (Co-administration has been associated with reduced efficacy and increased incidence of breakthrough bleeding and menstrual irregularities). Products include:
- Rifadin 765
- Rifamate Capsules 767
- Rifater Tablets 769

Secobarbital Sodium (Potential for reduced efficacy and increased incidence of breakthrough bleeding and menstrual irregularities with concomitant use).
- No products indexed under this heading.

Tetracycline Hydrochloride (Potential for reduced efficacy and increased incidence of breakthrough bleeding and menstrual irregularities with concomitant use).
- No products indexed under this heading.

Thiamylal Sodium (Potential for reduced efficacy and increased incidence of breakthrough bleeding and menstrual irregularities with concomitant use).
- No products indexed under this heading.

TRIZIVIR TABLETS

(Abacavir Sulfate, Lamivudine, Zidovudine) 1669

May interact with cytotoxic drugs, valproate, and certain other agents. Compounds in these categories include:

Atovaquone (Co-administration may alter zidovudine blood concentrations; routine dose modification is not warranted). Products include:
- Malarone 1596
- Mepron Suspension 1598

Bleomycin Sulfate (Co-administration with cytotoxic agents may increase the hematologic toxicity of zidovudine).
- No products indexed under this heading.

Cyclophosphamide (Co-administration with cytotoxic agents may increase the hematologic toxicity of zidovudine).
- No products indexed under this heading.

Daunorubicin Hydrochloride (Co-administration with cytotoxic agents may increase the hematologic toxicity of zidovudine). Products include:
- Cerubidine for Injection 947

Divalproex Sodium (Co-administration may alter zidovudine blood concentrations; routine dose modification is not warranted). Products include:
- Depakote Sprinkle Capsules 426
- Depakote Tablets 430
- Depakote ER Tablets 436

Doxorubicin Hydrochloride (Co-administration with cytotoxic agents may increase the hematologic toxicity of zidovudine). Products include:
- Adriamycin PFS/RDF Injection 2767
- Doxil Injection 566

Epirubicin Hydrochloride (Co-administration with cytotoxic agents may increase the hematologic toxicity of zidovudine). Products include:
- Ellence Injection 2806

Fluconazole (Co-administration may alter zidovudine blood concentrations; routine dose modification is not warranted). Products include:
- Diflucan Tablets, Injection, and Oral Suspension 2681

Fluorouracil (Co-administration with cytotoxic agents may increase the hematologic toxicity of zidovudine). Products include:
- Carac Cream 1222
- Efudex 1733
- Fluoroplex 552

Ganciclovir (Co-administration may increase the hematologic toxicity of zidovudine). Products include:
- Cytovene Capsules 2959
- Vitrasert Implant .... ⊙254

Ganciclovir Sodium (Co-administration may increase the hematologic toxicity of zidovudine). Products include:
- Cytovene-IV 2959

Hydroxyurea (Co-administration with cytotoxic agents may increase the hematologic toxicity of zidovudine). Products include:
- Mylocel Tablets 2227

Interferon alfa-2A, Recombinant (Co-administration may increase the hematologic toxicity of zidovudine). Products include:
- Roferon-A Injection 2996

Interferon alfa-2B, Recombinant (Co-administration may increase the hematologic toxicity of zidovudine). Products include:
- Intron A for Injection 3120
- Rebetron Combination Therapy 3153

Methadone Hydrochloride (Co-administration may alter zidovudine blood concentrations; routine dose modification is not warranted). Products include:
- Dolophine Hydrochloride Tablets 3056

Methotrexate Sodium (Co-administration with cytotoxic agents may increase the hematologic toxicity of zidovudine).
- No products indexed under this heading.

Mitotane (Co-administration with cytotoxic agents may increase the hematologic toxicity of zidovudine).
- No products indexed under this heading.

Mitoxantrone Hydrochloride (Co-administration with cytotoxic agents may increase the hematologic toxicity of zidovudine). Products include:
- Novantrone for Injection 1760

Nelfinavir Mesylate (Co-administration may alter lamivudine and zidovudine blood concentrations; routine dose modification is not warranted). Products include:
- Viracept 532

Probenecid (Co-administration may alter zidovudine blood concentrations; routine dose modification is not warranted).
- No products indexed under this heading.

Procarbazine Hydrochloride (Co-administration with cytotoxic agents may increase the hematologic toxicity of zidovudine). Products include:
- Matulane Capsules 3246

Ribavirin (Co-administration of zidovudine with ribavirin should be avoided since an antagonistic relationship has been demonstrated in vitro). Products include:
- Rebetron Combination Therapy 3153
- Virazole for Inhalation Solution 1747

Ritonavir (Co-administration may alter zidovudine blood concentrations; routine dose modification is not warranted). Products include:
- Kaletra Capsules 471
- Kaletra Oral Solution 471
- Norvir Capsules 487
- Norvir Oral Solution 487

Stavudine (Co-administration of zidovudine with stavudine should be avoided since an antagonistic relationship has been demonstrated in vitro). Products include:
- Zerit 1147

Sulfamethoxazole (Co-administration with trimethoprim/sulfamethoxazole may alter lamivudine blood concentrations; routine dose modification is not warranted). Products include:
- Bactrim 2949
- Septra Suspension 2265
- Septra Tablets 2265
- Septra DS Tablets 2265

Tamoxifen Citrate (Co-administration with cytotoxic agents may increase the hematologic toxicity of zidovudine). Products include:
- Nolvadex Tablets 678

Trimethoprim (Co-administration with trimethoprim/sulfamethoxazole may alter lamivudine blood concentrations; routine dose modification is not warranted). Products include:
- Bactrim 2949
- Septra Suspension 2265
- Septra Tablets 2265

Septra DS Tablets 2265

Valproate Sodium (Co-administration may alter zidovudine blood concentrations; routine dose modification is not warranted). Products include:
- Depacon Injection 416

Valproic Acid (Co-administration may alter zidovudine blood concentrations; routine dose modification is not warranted). Products include:
- Depakene 421

Vincristine Sulfate (Co-administration with cytotoxic agents may increase the hematologic toxicity of zidovudine).
- No products indexed under this heading.

Food Interactions

Alcohol (Concurrent use decreases the elimination of abacavir causing an increase in overall exposure).

TROVAN I.V.

(Alatrofloxacin Mesylate) 2722
See Trovan Tablets

TROVAN TABLETS

(Trovafloxacin Mesylate) 2722
May interact with antacids containing aluminum, calcium and magnesium, iron containing oral preparations, and certain other agents. Compounds in these categories include:

Aluminum Carbonate (The absorption of oral trovafloxacin is significantly reduced by the concomitant administration of some antacids containing aluminum or magnesium; antacids should be taken at least 2 hours before or 2 hours after oral trovafloxacin).
- No products indexed under this heading.

Aluminum Hydroxide (Administration of oral trovafloxacin 30 minutes after administration of aluminum hydroxide and magnesium hydroxide antacid has resulted in reductions in trovafloxacin AUC by 66% and Cmax by 60%; antacids should be taken at least 2 hours before or 2 hours after oral trovafloxacin). Products include:
- Amphojel Suspension (Mint Flavor) .... ■789
- Gaviscon Extra Strength Liquid .... ■751
- Gaviscon Extra Strength Tablets .... ■751
- Gaviscon Regular Strength Liquid .... ■751
- Gaviscon Regular Strength Tablets .... ■750
- Maalox Antacid/Anti-Gas Oral Suspension .... ■673
- Maalox Max Maximum Strength Antacid/Anti-Gas Liquid 2300
- Maalox Regular Strength Antacid/Antigas Liquid 2300
- Mylanta 1813
- Vanquish Caplets .... ■617

Caffeine (Co-administration of caffeine with oral trovafloxacin has resulted in a 17% increase in caffeine AUC and a 15% increase in caffeine Cmax; these changes in caffeine exposure are not considered clinically significant). Products include:
- BC Powder .... ■619
- Arthritis Strength BC Powder .... ■619
- Darvon Compound-65 Pulvules 1910
- Aspirin Free Excedrin Caplets and Geltabs .... ■628
- Excedrin Extra-Strength Tablets, Caplets, and Geltabs .... ■629
- Excedrin Migraine 1070
- Goody's Extra Strength Headache Powder .... ■620
- Goody's Extra Strength Pain Relief Tablets .... ■620
- Hycomine Compound Tablets 1317
- Maximum Strength Midol Menstrual Caplets and Gelcaps .... ■612
- Vanquish Caplets .... ■617
- Vivarin .... ■763

Calcium Carbonate (Co-administration of calcium carbonate with oral trovafloxacin has resulted in a 20% reduction in trovafloxacin AUC and a 17% reduction in peak serum trovafloxacin concentration; these changes in pharmacokinetics are not considered clinically significant). Products include:
- Aspirin Regimen Bayer 81 mg Caplets with Calcium .... ■607
- Extra Strength Bayer Plus Caplets .... ■610
- Caltrate 600 Tablets .... ■814
- Caltrate 600 PLUS .... ■815
- Caltrate 600 + D Tablets .... ■814
- Caltrate 600 + Soy Tablets .... ■814
- D-Cal Chewable Caplets .... ■794
- Florical Capsules and Tablets 2223
- Quick Dissolve Maalox Max Maximum Strength Antacid/Antigas Tablets 2301
- Quick Dissolve Maalox Regular Strength Antacid Tablets 2301
- Marblen Suspension .... ■633
- Monocal Tablets 2223
- Mylanta Fast-Acting 1813
- Mylanta Calci Tabs .... ■636
- One-A-Day Bedtime & Rest Tablets .... ■805
- One-A-Day Calcium Plus Chewable Tablets .... ■805
- Os-Cal Chewable Tablets .... ■838
- Pepcid Complete Chewable Tablets 1815
- ReSource Wellness CalciWise Soft Chews .... ■824
- Rolaids Tablets .... ■706
- Extra Strength Rolaids Tablets .... ■706
- Slow-Mag Tablets .... ■835
- Titralac .... ■640
- 3M Titralac Plus Antacid Tablets .... ■640
- Tums .... ■763

Ferrous Fumarate (The absorption of oral trovafloxacin is significantly reduced by the concomitant administration of oral iron-containing products; these products should be taken at least 2 hours before or 2 hours after oral trovafloxacin). Products include:
- New Formulation Chromagen OB Capsules 3094
- Loestrin Fe Tablets 2642
- NataChew Tablets 3364

Ferrous Gluconate (The absorption of oral trovafloxacin is significantly reduced by the concomitant administration of oral iron-containing products; these products should be taken at least 2 hours before or 2 hours after oral trovafloxacin). Products include:
- Fergon Iron Tablets .... ■802

Ferrous Sulfate (Co-administration of ferrous sulfate with oral trovafloxacin has resulted in a 40% decrease in trovafloxacin AUC and a 48% decrease in Cmax; ferrous sulfate-containing preparations should be taken at least 2 hours before or 2 hours after oral trovafloxacin). Products include:
- Feosol Tablets 1717
- Slow Fe Tablets .... ■827
- Slow Fe with Folic Acid Tablets .... ■828

Iron (The absorption of oral trovafloxacin is significantly reduced by the concomitant administration of oral iron-containing products; these products should be taken at least 2 hours before or 2 hours after oral trovafloxacin).
- No products indexed under this heading.

Magaldrate (The absorption of oral trovafloxacin is significantly reduced by the concomitant administration of some antacids containing aluminum or magnesium; antacids should be taken at least 2 hours before or 2 hours after oral trovafloxacin).
- No products indexed under this heading.

Magnesium Hydroxide (Administration of oral trovafloxacin 30 minutes after administration of aluminum hydroxide and magnesium hydroxide antacid has resulted in reductions in trovafloxacin AUC by 66% and Cmax by 60%; antacids should be taken at least 2 hours before or 2 hours after oral trovafloxacin). Products include:
- Ex•Lax Milk of Magnesia Liquid .... ■670
- Maalox Antacid/Anti-Gas Oral Suspension .... ■673
- Maalox Max Maximum Strength Antacid/Anti-Gas Liquid 2300
- Maalox Regular Strength Antacid/Antigas Liquid 2300
- Mylanta Fast-Acting 1813
- Mylanta 1813
- Pepcid Complete Chewable Tablets 1815
- Phillips' Chewable Tablets .... ■615
- Phillips' Milk of Magnesia Liquid (Original, Cherry, & Mint) .... ■616
- Rolaids Tablets .... ■706
- Extra Strength Rolaids Tablets .... ■706
- Vanquish Caplets .... ■617

Magnesium Oxide (The absorption of oral trovafloxacin is significantly reduced by the concomitant administration of some antacids containing aluminum or magnesium; antacids should be taken at least 2 hours before or 2 hours after oral trovafloxacin). Products include:
- Beelith Tablets 946
- Mag-Ox 400 Tablets 1024
- Uro-Mag Capsules 1024

Morphine Sulfate (Co-administration of intravenous morphine with oral trovafloxacin has resulted in a 36% reduction in trovafloxacin AUC and a 46% decrease in Cmax; intravenous morphine should be administered at least 2 hours after oral Trovan dosing in the fasted state and at least 4 hours after oral Trovan is taken with food). Products include:
- Astramorph/PF Injection, USP (Preservative-Free) 594
- Duramorph Injection 1312
- Infumorph 200 and Infumorph 500 Sterile Solutions 1314
- Kadian Capsules 1335
- MS Contin Tablets 2896
- MSIR 2898
- Oramorph SR Tablets 3062
- Roxanol 3066

Omeprazole (Co-administration of omeprazole given two hours prior to oral trovafloxacin has resulted in a 17% reduction in trovafloxacin AUC and a 17% reduction in peak serum trovafloxacin concentration; these changes in pharmacokinetics are not considered clinically significant). Products include:
- Prilosec Delayed-Release Capsules 628

Polysaccharide-Iron Complex (The absorption of oral trovafloxacin is significantly reduced by the concomitant administration of oral iron-containing products; these products should be taken at least 2 hours before or 2 hours after oral trovafloxacin). Products include:
- Niferex 3176
- Niferex-150 Capsules 3176
- Nu-Iron 150 Capsules 2224

Sodium Citrate (The absorption of oral trovafloxacin is significantly reduced by the concomitant administration of antacids containing citric acid/sodium citrate; these products should be taken at least 2 hours before or 2 hours after oral trovafloxacin).
- No products indexed under this heading.

Sucralfate (Co-administration of sucralfate with oral trovafloxacin has resulted in a 70% decrease in trovafloxacin AUC and a 77% decrease in Cmax; sucralfate should be taken at least 2 hours before or 2 hours after oral trovafloxacin). Products include:
- Carafate Suspension 731
- Carafate Tablets 730

Warfarin Sodium (Trovafloxacin/alatrofloxacin enhance the effects of warfarin if co-administered). Products include:
- Coumadin for Injection 1243
- Coumadin Tablets 1243
- Warfarin Sodium Tablets, USP 3302

TRUSOPT STERILE OPHTHALMIC SOLUTION

(Dorzolamide Hydrochloride) 2196
May interact with carbonic anhydrase inhibitors and certain other agents. Compounds in these categories include:

Acetazolamide (Potential for an additive effect on the known systemic effects of carbonic anhydrase inhibition in patients receiving a systemic carbonic anhydrase inhibitor and Trusopt). Products include:
- Diamox Sequels Sustained Release Capsules .... ⊙270
- Diamox Tablets .... ⊙269

Acetazolamide Sodium (Potential for an additive effect on the known systemic effects of carbonic anhydrase inhibition in patients receiving a systemic carbonic anhydrase inhibitor and Trusopt). Products include:
- Diamox Intravenous .... ⊙269

Aspirin (Potential for acid-base and electrolyte disturbances with concomitant use; these disturbances have been reported with oral agent and have not been reported during clinical trials with Trusopt). Products include:
- Aggrenox Capsules 1026
- Alka-Seltzer .... ■603
- Alka-Seltzer Lemon Lime Antacid and Pain Reliever Effervescent Tablets .... ■603
- Alka-Seltzer Extra Strength Antacid and Pain Reliever Effervescent Tablets .... ■603
- Alka-Seltzer PM Effervescent Tablets .... ■605
- Genuine Bayer Tablets, Caplets and Gelcaps .... ■606
- Extra Strength Bayer Caplets and Gelcaps .... ■610
- Aspirin Regimen Bayer Children's Chewable Tablets (Orange or Cherry Flavored) .... ■607
- Bayer, Aspirin Regimen .... ■606
- Aspirin Regimen Bayer 81 mg Caplets with Calcium .... ■607
- Genuine Bayer Professional Labeling (Aspirin Regimen Bayer) .... ■608
- Extra Strength Bayer Arthritis Caplets .... ■610
- Extra Strength Bayer Plus Caplets .... ■610
- Extra Strength Bayer PM Caplets .... ■611
- BC Powder .... ■619
- BC Allergy Sinus Cold Powder .... ■619
- Arthritis Strength BC Powder .... ■619
- BC Sinus Cold Powder .... ■619
- Darvon Compound-65 Pulvules 1910
- Ecotrin Enteric Coated Aspirin Low, Regular and Maximum Strength Tablets 1715
- Excedrin Extra-Strength Tablets, Caplets, and Geltabs .... ■629
- Excedrin Migraine 1070
- Goody's Body Pain Formula Powder .... ■620
- Goody's Extra Strength Headache Powder .... ■620
- Goody's Extra Strength Pain Relief Tablets .... ■620
- Percodan Tablets 1327
- Robaxisal Tablets 2939
- Soma Compound Tablets 3354
- Soma Compound w/Codeine Tablets 3355
- Vanquish Caplets .... ■617

Dichlorphenamide (Potential for an additive effect on the known systemic effects of carbonic anhydrase inhibition in patients receiving a systemic carbonic anhydrase inhibitor and Trusopt). Products include:
- Daranide Tablets 2077

Methazolamide (Potential for an additive effect on the known systemic effects of carbonic anhydrase inhibition in patients receiving a systemic carbonic anhydrase inhibitor and Trusopt). Products include:
- Neptazane Tablets .... ⊙271

TUBERSOL DIAGNOSTIC ANTIGEN
(Tuberculin, Purified Protein Derivative For Mantoux Test)........ 3628
May interact with corticosteroids, immunosuppressive agents, and certain other agents. Compounds in these categories include:

Azathioprine (Reactivity to the test may be depressed or suppressed in individuals who are receiving immunosuppressive agents).
No products indexed under this heading.

Basiliximab (Reactivity to the test may be depressed or suppressed in individuals who are receiving immunosuppressive agents). Products include:
Simulect for Injection 2399

Betamethasone Acetate (Reactivity to the test may be depressed or suppressed in individuals who are receiving corticosteroids). Products include:
Celestone Soluspan Injectable Suspension........ 3097

Betamethasone Sodium Phosphate (Reactivity to the test may be depressed or suppressed in individuals who are receiving corticosteroids). Products include:
Celestone Soluspan Injectable Suspension........ 3097

Cortisone Acetate (Reactivity to the test may be depressed or suppressed in individuals who are receiving corticosteroids). Products include:
Cortone Acetate Injectable Suspension........ 2059
Cortone Acetate Tablets 2061

Cyclosporine (Reactivity to the test may be depressed or suppressed in individuals who are receiving immunosuppressive agents). Products include:
Gengraf Capsules 457
Neoral Soft Gelatin Capsules........ 2380
Neoral Oral Solution 2380
Sandimmune 2388

Dexamethasone (Reactivity to the test may be depressed or suppressed in individuals who are receiving corticosteroids). Products include:
Decadron Elixir 2078
Decadron Tablets 2079
TobraDex Ophthalmic Ointment 542
TobraDex Ophthalmic Suspension 541

Dexamethasone Acetate (Reactivity to the test may be depressed or suppressed in individuals who are receiving corticosteroids).
No products indexed under this heading.

Dexamethasone Sodium Phosphate (Reactivity to the test may be depressed or suppressed in individuals who are receiving corticosteroids). Products include:
Decadron Phosphate Injection 2081
Decadron Phosphate Sterile Ophthalmic Ointment........ 2083
Decadron Phosphate Sterile Ophthalmic Solution........ 2084
NeoDecadron Sterile Ophthalmic Solution........ 2144

Fludrocortisone Acetate (Reactivity to the test may be depressed or suppressed in individuals who are receiving corticosteroids). Products include:
Florinef Acetate Tablets........ 2250

Hydrocortisone (Reactivity to the test may be depressed or suppressed in individuals who are receiving corticosteroids). Products include:
Anusol-HC Cream 2.5% 2237
Cipro HC Otic Suspension 540
Cortaid Intensive Therapy Cream .... ▣717
Cortaid Maximum Strength Cream........ ▣717
Cortisporin Ophthalmic Suspension Sterile........ ⊙297
Cortizone•5 .... ▣699
Cortizone•10 .... ▣699
Cortizone•10 Plus Creme .... ▣700
Cortizone for Kids Creme .... ▣699
Hydrocortone Tablets 2106
Massengill Medicated Soft Cloth Towelette........ ▣753
VōSoL HC Otic Solution 3356

Hydrocortisone Acetate (Reactivity to the test may be depressed or suppressed in individuals who are receiving corticosteroids). Products include:
Analpram-HC 1338
Anusol HC-1 Hydrocortisone Anti-Itch Cream........ ▣689
Anusol-HC Suppositories 2238
Cortaid .... ▣717
Cortifoam Rectal Foam 3170
Cortisporin-TC Otic Suspension........ 2246
Hydrocortone Acetate Injectable Suspension........ 2103
Pramosone 1343
Proctocort Suppositories 2264
ProctoFoam-HC 3177
Terra-Cortril Ophthalmic Suspension........ 2716

Hydrocortisone Sodium Phosphate (Reactivity to the test may be depressed or suppressed in individuals who are receiving corticosteroids). Products include:
Hydrocortone Phosphate Injection, Sterile........ 2105

Hydrocortisone Sodium Succinate (Reactivity to the test may be depressed or suppressed in individuals who are receiving corticosteroids).
No products indexed under this heading.

Measles, Mumps & Rubella Virus Vaccine, Live (Reactivity to the test may be temporarily depressed). Products include:
M-M-R II 2118

Methylprednisolone Acetate (Reactivity to the test may be depressed or suppressed in individuals who are receiving corticosteroids). Products include:
Depo-Medrol Injectable Suspension........ 2795

Methylprednisolone Sodium Succinate (Reactivity to the test may be depressed or suppressed in individuals who are receiving corticosteroids). Products include:
Solu-Medrol Sterile Powder 2855

Muromonab-CD3 (Reactivity to the test may be depressed or suppressed in individuals who are receiving immunosuppressive agents). Products include:
Orthoclone OKT3 Sterile Solution 2498

Mycophenolate Mofetil (Reactivity to the test may be depressed or suppressed in individuals who are receiving immunosuppressive agents). Products include:
CellCept Capsules 2951
CellCept Oral Suspension 2951
CellCept Tablets 2951

Prednisolone Acetate (Reactivity to the test may be depressed or suppressed in individuals who are receiving corticosteroids). Products include:
Blephamide Ophthalmic Ointment........ 547
Blephamide Ophthalmic Suspension........ 548
Poly-Pred Liquifilm Ophthalmic Suspension........ ⊙245
Pred Forte Ophthalmic Suspension........ ⊙246
Pred Mild Sterile Ophthalmic Suspension........ ⊙249
Pred-G Ophthalmic Suspension .... ⊙247
Pred-G Sterile Ophthalmic Ointment........ ⊙248

Prednisolone Sodium Phosphate (Reactivity to the test may be depressed or suppressed in individuals who are receiving corticosteroids). Products include:
Pediapred Oral Solution 1170

Prednisolone Tebutate (Reactivity to the test may be depressed or suppressed in individuals who are receiving corticosteroids).
No products indexed under this heading.

Prednisone (Reactivity to the test may be depressed or suppressed in individuals who are receiving corticosteroids). Products include:
Prednisone 3064

Sirolimus (Reactivity to the test may be depressed or suppressed in individuals who are receiving immunosuppressive agents). Products include:
Rapamune Oral Solution and Tablets........ 3584

Tacrolimus (Reactivity to the test may be depressed or suppressed in individuals who are receiving immunosuppressive agents). Products include:
Prograf 1393
Protopic Ointment 1397

Triamcinolone (Reactivity to the test may be depressed or suppressed in individuals who are receiving corticosteroids).
No products indexed under this heading.

Triamcinolone Acetonide (Reactivity to the test may be depressed or suppressed in individuals who are receiving corticosteroids). Products include:
Azmacort Inhalation Aerosol 728
Nasacort Nasal Inhaler 750
Nasacort AQ Nasal Spray 752
Tri-Nasal Spray 2274

Triamcinolone Diacetate (Reactivity to the test may be depressed or suppressed in individuals who are receiving corticosteroids).
No products indexed under this heading.

Triamcinolone Hexacetonide (Reactivity to the test may be depressed or suppressed in individuals who are receiving corticosteroids).
No products indexed under this heading.

TUCKS PRE-MOISTENED PADS
(Witch Hazel) .... ▣713
None cited in PDR database.

TUMS E-X ANTACID/ CALCIUM TABLETS
(Calcium Carbonate) .... ▣763
See Tums Regular Antacid/Calcium Tablets

TUMS E-X SUGAR FREE ANTACID/CALCIUM TABLETS
(Calcium Carbonate) .... ▣763
See Tums Regular Antacid/Calcium Tablets

TUMS REGULAR ANTACID/ CALCIUM TABLETS
(Calcium Carbonate) .... ▣763
May interact with:

Prescription Drugs, unspecified (Antacids may interact with certain unspecified prescription drugs).

TUMS ULTRA ANTACID/ CALCIUM TABLETS
(Calcium Carbonate) .... ▣763
See Tums Regular Antacid/Calcium Tablets

TUSSI-12 S SUSPENSION
(Carbetapentane Tannate, Chlorpheniramine Tannate)........ 3356
May interact with central nervous system depressants, monoamine oxidase inhibitors, and certain other agents. Compounds in these categories include:

Alfentanil Hydrochloride (Tussi-12 contains antihistamine which may cause drowsiness and co-administration may result in additive CNS effects).
No products indexed under this heading.

Alprazolam (Tussi-12 contains antihistamine which may cause drowsiness and co-administration may result in additive CNS effects). Products include:
Xanax Tablets 2865

Aprobarbital (Tussi-12 contains antihistamine which may cause drowsiness and co-administration may result in additive CNS effects).
No products indexed under this heading.

Buprenorphine Hydrochloride (Tussi-12 contains antihistamine which may cause drowsiness and co-administration may result in additive CNS effects). Products include:
Buprenex Injectable 2918

Buspirone Hydrochloride (Tussi-12 contains antihistamine which may cause drowsiness and co-administration may result in additive CNS effects).
No products indexed under this heading.

Butabarbital (Tussi-12 contains antihistamine which may cause drowsiness and co-administration may result in additive CNS effects).
No products indexed under this heading.

Butalbital (Tussi-12 contains antihistamine which may cause drowsiness and co-administration may result in additive CNS effects). Products include:
Phrenilin 578
Sedapap Tablets 50 mg/650 mg ... 2225

Chlordiazepoxide (Tussi-12 contains antihistamine which may cause drowsiness and co-administration may result in additive CNS effects). Products include:
Limbitrol 1738

Chlordiazepoxide Hydrochloride (Tussi-12 contains antihistamine which may cause drowsiness and co-administration may result in additive CNS effects). Products include:
Librium Capsules 1736
Librium for Injection 1737

Chlorpromazine (Tussi-12 contains antihistamine which may cause drowsiness and co-administration may result in additive CNS effects). Products include:
Thorazine Suppositories 1656

Chlorpromazine Hydrochloride (Tussi-12 contains antihistamine which may cause drowsiness and co-administration may result in additive CNS effects). Products include:
Thorazine 1656

Chlorprothixene (Tussi-12 contains antihistamine which may cause drowsiness and co-administration may result in additive CNS effects).
No products indexed under this heading.

Chlorprothixene Hydrochloride (Tussi-12 contains antihistamine which may cause drowsiness and co-administration may result in additive CNS effects).
No products indexed under this heading.

Chlorprothixene Lactate (Tussi-12 contains antihistamine which may cause drowsiness and co-administration may result in additive CNS effects).
No products indexed under this heading.

Clorazepate Dipotassium (Tussi-12 contains antihistamine which may cause drowsiness and co-administration may result in additive CNS effects). Products include:
Tranxene 511

Clozapine (Tussi-12 contains antihistamine which may cause drowsiness and co-administration may result in additive CNS effects). Products include:
Clozaril Tablets ... 2319

Codeine Phosphate (Tussi-12 contains antihistamine which may cause drowsiness and co-administration may result in additive CNS effects). Products include:
Phenergan with Codeine Syrup ... 3557
Phenergan VC with Codeine Syrup .. 3561
Robitussin A-C Syrup ... 2942
Robitussin-DAC Syrup ... 2942
Ryna-C Liquid ... 768
Soma Compound w/Codeine Tablets ... 3355
Tussi-Organidin NR Liquid ... 3350
Tussi-Organidin-S NR Liquid ... 3350
Tylenol with Codeine ... 2595

Desflurane (Tussi-12 contains antihistamine which may cause drowsiness and co-administration may result in additive CNS effects). Products include:
Suprane Liquid for Inhalation ... 874

Dezocine (Tussi-12 contains antihistamine which may cause drowsiness and co-administration may result in additive CNS effects).
No products indexed under this heading.

Diazepam (Tussi-12 contains antihistamine which may cause drowsiness and co-administration may result in additive CNS effects). Products include:
Valium Injectable ... 3026
Valium Tablets ... 3047

Droperidol (Tussi-12 contains antihistamine which may cause drowsiness and co-administration may result in additive CNS effects).
No products indexed under this heading.

Enflurane (Tussi-12 contains antihistamine which may cause drowsiness and co-administration may result in additive CNS effects).
No products indexed under this heading.

Estazolam (Tussi-12 contains antihistamine which may cause drowsiness and co-administration may result in additive CNS effects). Products include:
ProSom Tablets ... 500

Ethchlorvynol (Tussi-12 contains antihistamine which may cause drowsiness and co-administration may result in additive CNS effects).
No products indexed under this heading.

Ethinamate (Tussi-12 contains antihistamine which may cause drowsiness and co-administration may result in additive CNS effects).
No products indexed under this heading.

Fentanyl (Tussi-12 contains antihistamine which may cause drowsiness and co-administration may result in additive CNS effects). Products include:
Duragesic Transdermal System ... 1786

Fentanyl Citrate (Tussi-12 contains antihistamine which may cause drowsiness and co-administration may result in additive CNS effects). Products include:
Actiq ... 1184

Fluphenazine Decanoate (Tussi-12 contains antihistamine which may cause drowsiness and co-administration may result in additive CNS effects).
No products indexed under this heading.

Fluphenazine Enanthate (Tussi-12 contains antihistamine which may cause drowsiness and co-administration may result in additive CNS effects).
No products indexed under this heading.

Fluphenazine Hydrochloride (Tussi-12 contains antihistamine which may cause drowsiness and co-administration may result in additive CNS effects).
No products indexed under this heading.

Flurazepam Hydrochloride (Tussi-12 contains antihistamine which may cause drowsiness and co-administration may result in additive CNS effects).
No products indexed under this heading.

Glutethimide (Tussi-12 contains antihistamine which may cause drowsiness and co-administration may result in additive CNS effects).
No products indexed under this heading.

Haloperidol (Tussi-12 contains antihistamine which may cause drowsiness and co-administration may result in additive CNS effects). Products include:
Haldol Injection, Tablets and Concentrate ... 2533

Haloperidol Decanoate (Tussi-12 contains antihistamine which may cause drowsiness and co-administration may result in additive CNS effects). Products include:
Haldol Decanoate ... 2535

Hydrocodone Bitartrate (Tussi-12 contains antihistamine which may cause drowsiness and co-administration may result in additive CNS effects). Products include:
Hycodan ... 1316
Hycomine Compound Tablets ... 1317
Hycotuss Expectorant Syrup ... 1318
Lortab ... 3319
Lortab Elixir ... 3317
Maxidone Tablets CIII ... 3399
Norco 5/325 Tablets CIII ... 3424
Norco 7.5/325 Tablets CIII ... 3425
Norco 10/325 Tablets CIII ... 3427
Norco 10/325 Tablets CIII ... 3425
Vicodin Tablets ... 516
Vicodin ES Tablets ... 517
Vicodin HP Tablets ... 518
Vicodin Tuss Expectorant ... 519
Vicoprofen Tablets ... 520
Zydone Tablets ... 1330

Hydrocodone Polistirex (Tussi-12 contains antihistamine which may cause drowsiness and co-administration may result in additive CNS effects). Products include:
Tussionex Pennkinetic Extended-Release Suspension ... 1174

Hydromorphone Hydrochloride (Tussi-12 contains antihistamine which may cause drowsiness and co-administration may result in additive CNS effects). Products include:
Dilaudid ... 441
Dilaudid Oral Liquid ... 445
Dilaudid Powder ... 441
Dilaudid Rectal Suppositories ... 441
Dilaudid Tablets ... 441
Dilaudid Tablets - 8 mg ... 445
Dilaudid-HP ... 443

Hydroxyzine Hydrochloride (Tussi-12 contains antihistamine which may cause drowsiness and co-administration may result in additive CNS effects). Products include:
Atarax Tablets & Syrup ... 2667
Vistaril Intramuscular Solution ... 2738

Isocarboxazid (Co-administration with MAO inhibitors may prolong and intensify the anticholinergic effects of antihistamines; concurrent and/or sequential use should be avoided).
No products indexed under this heading.

Isoflurane (Tussi-12 contains antihistamine which may cause drowsiness and co-administration may result in additive CNS effects).
No products indexed under this heading.

Ketamine Hydrochloride (Tussi-12 contains antihistamine which may cause drowsiness and co-administration may result in additive CNS effects).
No products indexed under this heading.

Levomethadyl Acetate Hydrochloride (Tussi-12 contains antihistamine which may cause drowsiness and co-administration may result in additive CNS effects).
No products indexed under this heading.

Levorphanol Tartrate (Tussi-12 contains antihistamine which may cause drowsiness and co-administration may result in additive CNS effects). Products include:
Levo-Dromoran ... 1734
Levorphanol Tartrate Tablets ... 3059

Lorazepam (Tussi-12 contains antihistamine which may cause drowsiness and co-administration may result in additive CNS effects). Products include:
Ativan Injection ... 3478
Ativan Tablets ... 3482

Loxapine Hydrochloride (Tussi-12 contains antihistamine which may cause drowsiness and co-administration may result in additive CNS effects).
No products indexed under this heading.

Loxapine Succinate (Tussi-12 contains antihistamine which may cause drowsiness and co-administration may result in additive CNS effects). Products include:
Loxitane Capsules ... 3398

Meperidine Hydrochloride (Tussi-12 contains antihistamine which may cause drowsiness and co-administration may result in additive CNS effects). Products include:
Demerol ... 3079
Mepergan Injection ... 3539

Mephobarbital (Tussi-12 contains antihistamine which may cause drowsiness and co-administration may result in additive CNS effects).
No products indexed under this heading.

Meprobamate (Tussi-12 contains antihistamine which may cause drowsiness and co-administration may result in additive CNS effects). Products include:
Miltown Tablets ... 3349

Mesoridazine Besylate (Tussi-12 contains antihistamine which may cause drowsiness and co-administration may result in additive CNS effects). Products include:
Serentil ... 1057

Methadone Hydrochloride (Tussi-12 contains antihistamine which may cause drowsiness and co-administration may result in additive CNS effects). Products include:
Dolophine Hydrochloride Tablets ... 3056

Methohexital Sodium (Tussi-12 contains antihistamine which may cause drowsiness and co-administration may result in additive CNS effects). Products include:
Brevital Sodium for Injection, USP .. 1815

Methotrimeprazine (Tussi-12 contains antihistamine which may cause drowsiness and co-administration may result in additive CNS effects).
No products indexed under this heading.

Methoxyflurane (Tussi-12 contains antihistamine which may cause drowsiness and co-administration may result in additive CNS effects).
No products indexed under this heading.

Midazolam Hydrochloride (Tussi-12 contains antihistamine which may cause drowsiness and co-administration may result in additive CNS effects). Products include:
Versed Injection ... 3027
Versed Syrup ... 3033

Moclobemide (Co-administration with MAO inhibitors may prolong and intensify the anticholinergic effects of antihistamines; concurrent and/or sequential use should be avoided).
No products indexed under this heading.

Molindone Hydrochloride (Tussi-12 contains antihistamine which may cause drowsiness and co-administration may result in additive CNS effects). Products include:
Moban ... 1320

Morphine Sulfate (Tussi-12 contains antihistamine which may cause drowsiness and co-administration may result in additive CNS effects). Products include:
Astramorph/PF Injection, USP (Preservative-Free) ... 594
Duramorph Injection ... 1312
Infumorph 200 and Infumorph 500 Sterile Solutions ... 1314
Kadian Capsules ... 1335
MS Contin Tablets ... 2896
MSIR ... 2898
Oramorph SR Tablets ... 3062
Roxanol ... 3066

Olanzapine (Tussi-12 contains antihistamine which may cause drowsiness and co-administration may result in additive CNS effects). Products include:
Zyprexa Tablets ... 1973
Zyprexa ZYDIS Orally Disintegrating Tablets ... 1973

Oxazepam (Tussi-12 contains antihistamine which may cause drowsiness and co-administration may result in additive CNS effects).
No products indexed under this heading.

Oxycodone Hydrochloride (Tussi-12 contains antihistamine which may cause drowsiness and co-administration may result in additive CNS effects). Products include:
OxyContin Tablets ... 2912
OxyFast Oral Concentrate Solution . 2916
OxyIR Capsules ... 2916
Percocet Tablets ... 1326
Percodan Tablets ... 1327
Percolone Tablets ... 1327
Roxicodone ... 3067
Tylox Capsules ... 2597

Pargyline Hydrochloride (Co-administration with MAO inhibitors may prolong and intensify the anticholinergic effects of antihistamines; concurrent and/or sequential use should be avoided).
No products indexed under this heading.

Pentobarbital Sodium (Tussi-12 contains antihistamine which may cause drowsiness and co-administration may result in additive CNS effects). Products include:
Nembutal Sodium Solution ... 485

Perphenazine (Tussi-12 contains antihistamine which may cause drowsiness and co-administration may result in additive CNS effects). Products include:
Etrafon ... 3115
Trilafon ... 3160

Phenelzine Sulfate (Co-administration with MAO inhibitors may prolong and intensify the anticholinergic effects of antihistamines; concurrent and/or sequential use should be avoided). Products include:
Nardil Tablets ... 2653

Phenobarbital (Tussi-12 contains antihistamine which may cause drowsiness and co-administration may result in additive CNS effects). Products include:
Arco-Lase Plus Tablets ... 592
Donnatal ... 2929
Donnatal Extentabs ... 2930

IMPORTANT NOTE: Always consult each drug listing in the patient's regimen for possible interactions.

Prazepam (Tussi-12 contains antihistamine which may cause drowsiness and co-administration may result in additive CNS effects).
No products indexed under this heading.

Procarbazine Hydrochloride (Co-administration with MAO inhibitors may prolong and intensify the anticholinergic effects of antihistamines; concurrent and/or sequential use should be avoided). Products include:
Matulane Capsules 3246

Prochlorperazine (Tussi-12 contains antihistamine which may cause drowsiness and co-administration may result in additive CNS effects). Products include:
Compazine 1505

Promethazine Hydrochloride (Tussi-12 contains antihistamine which may cause drowsiness and co-administration may result in additive CNS effects). Products include:
Mepergan Injection 3539
Phenergan Injection 3553
Phenergan 3556
Phenergan Syrup 3554
Phenergan with Codeine Syrup 3557
Phenergan with Dextromethorphan Syrup 3559
Phenergan VC Syrup 3560
Phenergan VC with Codeine Syrup .. 3561

Propofol (Tussi-12 contains antihistamine which may cause drowsiness and co-administration may result in additive CNS effects). Products include:
Diprivan Injectable Emulsion 667

Propoxyphene Hydrochloride (Tussi-12 contains antihistamine which may cause drowsiness and co-administration may result in additive CNS effects). Products include:
Darvon Pulvules 1909
Darvon Compound-65 Pulvules 1910

Propoxyphene Napsylate (Tussi-12 contains antihistamine which may cause drowsiness and co-administration may result in additive CNS effects). Products include:
Darvon-N/Darvocet-N 1907
Darvon-N Tablets 1912

Quazepam (Tussi-12 contains antihistamine which may cause drowsiness and co-administration may result in additive CNS effects).
No products indexed under this heading.

Quetiapine Fumarate (Tussi-12 contains antihistamine which may cause drowsiness and co-administration may result in additive CNS effects). Products include:
Seroquel Tablets 684

Remifentanil Hydrochloride (Tussi-12 contains antihistamine which may cause drowsiness and co-administration may result in additive CNS effects).
No products indexed under this heading.

Risperidone (Tussi-12 contains antihistamine which may cause drowsiness and co-administration may result in additive CNS effects). Products include:
Risperdal 1796

Secobarbital Sodium (Tussi-12 contains antihistamine which may cause drowsiness and co-administration may result in additive CNS effects).
No products indexed under this heading.

Selegiline Hydrochloride (Co-administration with MAO inhibitors may prolong and intensify the anticholinergic effects of antihistamines; concurrent and/or sequential use should be avoided). Products include:
Eldepryl Capsules 3266

Sevoflurane (Tussi-12 contains antihistamine which may cause drowsiness and co-administration may result in additive CNS effects).
No products indexed under this heading.

Sufentanil Citrate (Tussi-12 contains antihistamine which may cause drowsiness and co-administration may result in additive CNS effects).
No products indexed under this heading.

Temazepam (Tussi-12 contains antihistamine which may cause drowsiness and co-administration may result in additive CNS effects).
No products indexed under this heading.

Thiamylal Sodium (Tussi-12 contains antihistamine which may cause drowsiness and co-administration may result in additive CNS effects).
No products indexed under this heading.

Thioridazine Hydrochloride (Tussi-12 contains antihistamine which may cause drowsiness and co-administration may result in additive CNS effects). Products include:
Thioridazine Hydrochloride Tablets 2289

Thiothixene (Tussi-12 contains antihistamine which may cause drowsiness and co-administration may result in additive CNS effects). Products include:
Navane Capsules 2701
Thiothixene Capsules 2290

Tranylcypromine Sulfate (Co-administration with MAO inhibitors may prolong and intensify the anticholinergic effects of antihistamines; concurrent and/or sequential use should be avoided). Products include:
Parnate Tablets 1607

Triazolam (Tussi-12 contains antihistamine which may cause drowsiness and co-administration may result in additive CNS effects). Products include:
Halcion Tablets 2823

Trifluoperazine Hydrochloride (Tussi-12 contains antihistamine which may cause drowsiness and co-administration may result in additive CNS effects). Products include:
Stelazine 1640

Zaleplon (Tussi-12 contains antihistamine which may cause drowsiness and co-administration may result in additive CNS effects). Products include:
Sonata Capsules 3591

Ziprasidone Hydrochloride (Tussi-12 contains antihistamine which may cause drowsiness and co-administration may result in additive CNS effects). Products include:
Geodon Capsules 2688

Zolpidem Tartrate (Tussi-12 contains antihistamine which may cause drowsiness and co-administration may result in additive CNS effects). Products include:
Ambien Tablets 3191

Food Interactions

Alcohol (Tussi-12 contains antihistamine which may cause drowsiness and co-administration may result in additive CNS effects).

TUSSI-12 TABLETS
(Carbetapentane Tannate, Chlorpheniramine Tannate) 3356
See Tussi-12 S Suspension

TUSSIONEX PENNKINETIC EXTENDED-RELEASE SUSPENSION
(Chlorpheniramine Polistirex, Hydrocodone Polistirex) 1174
May interact with anticholinergics, antihistamines, central nervous system depressants, monoamine oxidase inhibitors, tricyclic antidepressants, and certain other agents. Compounds in these categories include:

Acrivastine (Combined therapy may result in additive CNS depression). Products include:
Semprex-D Capsules 1172

Alfentanil Hydrochloride (Combined therapy may result in additive CNS depression).
No products indexed under this heading.

Alprazolam (Combined therapy may result in additive CNS depression). Products include:
Xanax Tablets 2865

Amitriptyline Hydrochloride (Co-administration of hydrocodone with MAO inhibitors may increase the effect of tricyclic antidepressant or hydrocodone). Products include:
Etrafon 3115
Limbitrol 1738

Amoxapine (Co-administration of hydrocodone with MAO inhibitors may increase the effect of tricyclic antidepressant or hydrocodone).
No products indexed under this heading.

Aprobarbital (Combined therapy may result in additive CNS depression).
No products indexed under this heading.

Astemizole (Combined therapy may result in additive CNS depression).
No products indexed under this heading.

Atropine Sulfate (Concurrent use of other anticholinergic agents with hydrocodone may produce paralytic ileus). Products include:
Donnatal 2929
Donnatal Extentabs 2930
Motofen Tablets 577
Prosed/DS Tablets 3268
Urised Tablets 2876

Azatadine Maleate (Combined therapy may result in additive CNS depression). Products include:
Rynatan Tablets 3351

Belladonna Alkaloids (Concurrent use of other anticholinergic agents with hydrocodone may produce paralytic ileus). Products include:
Hyland's Teething Tablets .... ⊡766
Urimax Tablets 1769

Benztropine Mesylate (Concurrent use of other anticholinergic agents with hydrocodone may produce paralytic ileus). Products include:
Cogentin 2055

Biperiden Hydrochloride (Concurrent use of other anticholinergic agents with hydrocodone may produce paralytic ileus). Products include:
Akineton 402

Bromodiphenhydramine Hydrochloride (Combined therapy may result in additive CNS depression).
No products indexed under this heading.

Brompheniramine Maleate (Combined therapy may result in additive CNS depression). Products include:
Bromfed Capsules (Extended-Release) 2269
Bromfed-PD Capsules (Extended-Release) 2269
Comtrex Acute Head Cold & Sinus Pressure Relief Tablets .... ⊡627
Dimetapp Elixir .... ⊡777
Dimetapp Cold and Fever Suspension .... ⊡775
Dimetapp DM Cold & Cough Elixir . ⊡775
Dimetapp Nighttime Flu Liquid .... ⊡776

Buprenorphine Hydrochloride (Combined therapy may result in additive CNS depression). Products include:
Buprenex Injectable 2918

Buspirone Hydrochloride (Combined therapy may result in additive CNS depression).
No products indexed under this heading.

Butabarbital (Combined therapy may result in additive CNS depression).
No products indexed under this heading.

Butalbital (Combined therapy may result in additive CNS depression). Products include:
Phrenilin 578
Sedapap Tablets 50 mg/650 mg ... 2225

Cetirizine Hydrochloride (Combined therapy may result in additive CNS depression). Products include:
Zyrtec 2756
Zyrtec-D 12 Hour Extended Relief Tablets 2758

Chlordiazepoxide (Combined therapy may result in additive CNS depression). Products include:
Limbitrol 1738

Chlordiazepoxide Hydrochloride (Combined therapy may result in additive CNS depression). Products include:
Librium Capsules 1736
Librium for Injection 1737

Chlorpheniramine Maleate (Combined therapy may result in additive CNS depression). Products include:
Actifed Cold & Sinus Caplets and Tablets .... ⊡688
Alka-Seltzer Plus Liqui-Gels .... ⊡604
BC Allergy Sinus Cold Powder .... ⊡619
Chlor-Trimeton Allergy Tablets .... ⊡735
Chlor-Trimeton Allergy/Decongestant Tablets .... ⊡736
Comtrex Flu Therapy & Fever Relief Nighttime Tablets .... ⊡628
Comtrex Maximum Strength Multi-Symptom Cold & Cough Relief Tablets and Caplets .... ⊡626
Contac Severe Cold and Flu Caplets Maximum Strength .... ⊡746
Coricidin 'D' Cold, Flu & Sinus Tablets .... ⊡737
Coricidin/Coricidin D .... ⊡738
Coricidin HBP Maximum Strength Flu Tablets .... ⊡738
Extendryl 1361
Hycomine Compound Tablets 1317
Kronofed-A 1341
PediaCare Cough-Cold Liquid .... ⊡719
PediaCare NightRest Cough-Cold Liquid .... ⊡719
Robitussin Nighttime Honey Flu Liquid .... ⊡786
Ryna .... ⊡768
Singlet Caplets .... ⊡761
Sinutab Sinus Allergy Medication, Maximum Strength Formula, Tablets & Caplets .... ⊡707
Sudafed Cold & Allergy Tablets .... ⊡708
TheraFlu Regular Strength Cold & Cough Night Time Hot Liquid .... ⊡676
TheraFlu Regular Strength Cold & Sore Throat Night Time Hot Liquid .... ⊡676
TheraFlu Maximum Strength Flu & Cough Night Time Hot Liquid .. ⊡678
TheraFlu Maximum Strength Flu & Sore Throat Night Time Hot Liquid .... ⊡677
TheraFlu Maximum Strength Severe Cold & Congestion Night Time Caplets .... ⊡678
TheraFlu Maximum Strength Severe Cold & Congestion Night Time Hot Liquid .... ⊡678
Triaminic Cold & Allergy Liquid .... ⊡681
Triaminic Cold & Allergy Softchews .... ⊡683
Triaminic Cold & Cough Liquid .... ⊡681
Triaminic Cold & Cough Softchews .... ⊡683
Triaminic Cold & Night Time Cough Liquid .... ⊡681
Triaminic Cold, Cough & Fever Liquid .... ⊡681
Children's Tylenol Cold Suspension Liquid and Chewable Tablets 2015
Children's Tylenol Cold Plus Cough Suspension Liquid and Chewable Tablets 2015
Children's Tylenol Flu Suspension Liquid 2015
Maximum Strength Tylenol Allergy Sinus Caplets, Gelcaps, and Geltabs 2010
Multi-Symptom Tylenol Cold Complete Formula Caplets 2010
Vicks 44M Cough, Cold & Flu Relief Liquid .... ⊡725
Pediatric Vicks 44m Cough & Cold Relief .... ⊡728

Children's Vicks NyQuil Cold/Cough Relief 726

Chlorpheniramine Tannate (Combined therapy may result in additive CNS depression). Products include:
- Reformulated Rynatan Pediatric Suspension 3352
- Rynatuss Pediatric Suspension 3353
- Rynatuss Tablets 3353
- Tussi-12 S Suspension 3356
- Tussi-12 Tablets 3356

Chlorpromazine (Combined therapy may result in additive CNS depression). Products include:
- Thorazine Suppositories 1656

Chlorpromazine Hydrochloride (Combined therapy may result in additive CNS depression). Products include:
- Thorazine 1656

Chlorprothixene (Combined therapy may result in additive CNS depression).
No products indexed under this heading.

Chlorprothixene Hydrochloride (Combined therapy may result in additive CNS depression).
No products indexed under this heading.

Chlorprothixene Lactate (Combined therapy may result in additive CNS depression).
No products indexed under this heading.

Clemastine Fumarate (Combined therapy may result in additive CNS depression). Products include:
- Tavist 12 Hour Allergy Tablets 676

Clidinium Bromide (Concurrent use of other anticholinergic agents with hydrocodone may produce paralytic ileus).
No products indexed under this heading.

Clomipramine Hydrochloride (Co-administration of hydrocodone with MAO inhibitors may increase the effect of tricyclic antidepressant or hydrocodone).
No products indexed under this heading.

Clorazepate Dipotassium (Combined therapy may result in additive CNS depression). Products include:
- Tranxene 511

Clozapine (Combined therapy may result in additive CNS depression). Products include:
- Clozaril Tablets 2319

Codeine Phosphate (Combined therapy may result in additive CNS depression). Products include:
- Phenergan with Codeine Syrup 3557
- Phenergan VC with Codeine Syrup 3561
- Robitussin A-C Syrup 2942
- Robitussin-DAC Syrup 2942
- Ryna-C Liquid 768
- Soma Compound w/Codeine Tablets 3355
- Tussi-Organidin NR Liquid 3350
- Tussi-Organidin-S NR Liquid 3350
- Tylenol with Codeine 2595

Cyproheptadine Hydrochloride (Combined therapy may result in additive CNS depression). Products include:
- Periactin Tablets 2155

Desflurane (Combined therapy may result in additive CNS depression). Products include:
- Suprane Liquid for Inhalation 874

Desipramine Hydrochloride (Co-administration of hydrocodone with MAO inhibitors may increase the effect of tricyclic antidepressant or hydrocodone). Products include:
- Norpramin Tablets 755

Dexchlorpheniramine Maleate (Combined therapy may result in additive CNS depression).
No products indexed under this heading.

Dezocine (Combined therapy may result in additive CNS depression).
No products indexed under this heading.

Diazepam (Combined therapy may result in additive CNS depression). Products include:
- Valium Injectable 3026
- Valium Tablets 3047

Dicyclomine Hydrochloride (Concurrent use of other anticholinergic agents with hydrocodone may produce paralytic ileus).
No products indexed under this heading.

Diphenhydramine Citrate (Combined therapy may result in additive CNS depression). Products include:
- Alka-Seltzer PM Effervescent Tablets 605
- Benadryl Allergy & Sinus Fastmelt Tablets 693
- Benadryl Children's Allergy/Cold Fastmelt Tablets 692
- Excedrin PM Tablets, Caplets, and Geltabs 631
- Goody's PM Powder 621

Diphenhydramine Hydrochloride (Combined therapy may result in additive CNS depression). Products include:
- Extra Strength Bayer PM Caplets 611
- Benadryl Allergy Chewables 689
- Benadryl Allergy 691
- Benadryl Allergy Liquid 690
- Benadryl Allergy/Cold Tablets 691
- Benadryl Allergy/Congestion Tablets 692
- Benadryl Allergy & Sinus Liquid 693
- Benadryl Allergy Sinus Headache Caplets & Gelcaps 693
- Benadryl Severe Allergy & Sinus Headache Caplets 694
- Benadryl Dye-Free Allergy Liquid 690
- Benadryl Dye-Free Allergy Liqui-Gels Softgels 690
- Benadryl Itch Relief Stick Extra Strength 695
- Benadryl Cream 695
- Benadryl Gel 695
- Benadryl Spray 696
- Benadryl Parenteral 2617
- Coricidin HBP Night-Time Cold & Flu Tablets 738
- Nytol QuickCaps Caplets 622
- Maximum Strength Nytol QuickGels Softgels 621
- Extra Strength Percogesic Aspirin-Free Coated Caplets 665
- Simply Sleep Caplets 2008
- Sominex Original Formula Tablets 761
- Children's Tylenol Allergy-D Liquid 2014
- Maximum Strength Tylenol Allergy Sinus NightTime Caplets 2010
- Tylenol Severe Allergy Caplets 2010
- Maximum Strength Tylenol Flu NightTime Gelcaps 2011
- Extra Strength Tylenol PM Caplets, Geltabs, and Gelcaps 2012
- Unisom Maximum Strength SleepGels 713

Diphenylpyraline Hydrochloride (Combined therapy may result in additive CNS depression).
No products indexed under this heading.

Doxepin Hydrochloride (Co-administration of hydrocodone with MAO inhibitors may increase the effect of tricyclic antidepressant or hydrocodone). Products include:
- Sinequan 2713

Droperidol (Combined therapy may result in additive CNS depression).
No products indexed under this heading.

Enflurane (Combined therapy may result in additive CNS depression).
No products indexed under this heading.

Estazolam (Combined therapy may result in additive CNS depression). Products include:
- ProSom Tablets 500

Ethchlorvynol (Combined therapy may result in additive CNS depression).
No products indexed under this heading.

Ethinamate (Combined therapy may result in additive CNS depression).
No products indexed under this heading.

Fentanyl (Combined therapy may result in additive CNS depression). Products include:
- Duragesic Transdermal System 1786

Fentanyl Citrate (Combined therapy may result in additive CNS depression). Products include:
- Actiq 1184

Fexofenadine Hydrochloride (Combined therapy may result in additive CNS depression). Products include:
- Allegra 712
- Allegra-D Extended-Release Tablets 714

Fluphenazine Decanoate (Combined therapy may result in additive CNS depression).
No products indexed under this heading.

Fluphenazine Enanthate (Combined therapy may result in additive CNS depression).
No products indexed under this heading.

Fluphenazine Hydrochloride (Combined therapy may result in additive CNS depression).
No products indexed under this heading.

Flurazepam Hydrochloride (Combined therapy may result in additive CNS depression).
No products indexed under this heading.

Glutethimide (Combined therapy may result in additive CNS depression).
No products indexed under this heading.

Glycopyrrolate (Concurrent use of other anticholinergic agents with hydrocodone may produce paralytic ileus). Products include:
- Robinul Forte Tablets 1358
- Robinul Injectable 2940
- Robinul Tablets 1358

Haloperidol (Combined therapy may result in additive CNS depression). Products include:
- Haldol Injection, Tablets and Concentrate 2533

Haloperidol Decanoate (Combined therapy may result in additive CNS depression). Products include:
- Haldol Decanoate 2535

Hydrocodone Bitartrate (Combined therapy may result in additive CNS depression). Products include:
- Hycodan 1316
- Hycomine Compound Tablets 1317
- Hycotuss Expectorant Syrup 1318
- Lortab 3319
- Lortab Elixir 3317
- Maxidone Tablets CIII 3399
- Norco 5/325 Tablets CIII 3424
- Norco 7.5/325 Tablets CIII 3425
- Norco 10/325 Tablets CIII 3427
- Norco 10/325 Tablets CIII 3425
- Vicodin Tablets 516
- Vicodin ES Tablets 517
- Vicodin HP Tablets 518
- Vicodin Tuss Expectorant 519
- Vicoprofen Tablets 520
- Zydone Tablets 1330

Hydromorphone Hydrochloride (Combined therapy may result in additive CNS depression). Products include:
- Dilaudid 441
- Dilaudid Oral Liquid 445
- Dilaudid Powder 441
- Dilaudid Rectal Suppositories 441
- Dilaudid Tablets 441
- Dilaudid Tablets - 8 mg 445
- Dilaudid-HP 443

Hydroxyzine Hydrochloride (Combined therapy may result in additive CNS depression). Products include:
- Atarax Tablets & Syrup 2667
- Vistaril Intramuscular Solution 2738

Hyoscyamine (Concurrent use of other anticholinergic agents with hydrocodone may produce paralytic ileus). Products include:
- Urised Tablets 2876

Hyoscyamine Sulfate (Concurrent use of other anticholinergic agents with hydrocodone may produce paralytic ileus). Products include:
- Arco-Lase Plus Tablets 592
- Donnatal 2929
- Donnatal Extentabs 2930
- Levsin/Levsinex/Levbid 3172
- NuLev Orally Disintegrating Tablets 3176
- Prosed/DS Tablets 3268
- Urimax Tablets 1769

Imipramine Hydrochloride (Co-administration of hydrocodone with MAO inhibitors may increase the effect of tricyclic antidepressant or hydrocodone).
No products indexed under this heading.

Imipramine Pamoate (Co-administration of hydrocodone with MAO inhibitors may increase the effect of tricyclic antidepressant or hydrocodone).
No products indexed under this heading.

Ipratropium Bromide (Concurrent use of other anticholinergic agents with hydrocodone may produce paralytic ileus). Products include:
- Atrovent Inhalation Aerosol 1030
- Atrovent Inhalation Solution 1031
- Atrovent Nasal Spray 0.03% 1032
- Atrovent Nasal Spray 0.06% 1033
- Combivent Inhalation Aerosol 1041
- DuoNeb Inhalation Solution 1233

Isocarboxazid (Co-administration of hydrocodone with MAO inhibitors may increase the effect of MAOI or hydrocodone).
No products indexed under this heading.

Isoflurane (Combined therapy may result in additive CNS depression).
No products indexed under this heading.

Ketamine Hydrochloride (Combined therapy may result in additive CNS depression).
No products indexed under this heading.

Levomethadyl Acetate Hydrochloride (Combined therapy may result in additive CNS depression).
No products indexed under this heading.

Levorphanol Tartrate (Combined therapy may result in additive CNS depression). Products include:
- Levo-Dromoran 1734
- Levorphanol Tartrate Tablets 3059

Loratadine (Combined therapy may result in additive CNS depression). Products include:
- Claritin 3100
- Claritin-D 12 Hour Extended Release Tablets 3102
- Claritin-D 24 Hour Extended Release Tablets 3104

Lorazepam (Combined therapy may result in additive CNS depression). Products include:
- Ativan Injection 3478
- Ativan Tablets 3482

Loxapine Hydrochloride (Combined therapy may result in additive CNS depression).
No products indexed under this heading.

Loxapine Succinate (Combined therapy may result in additive CNS depression). Products include:
- Loxitane Capsules 3398

Maprotiline Hydrochloride (Co-administration of hydrocodone with MAO inhibitors may increase the effect of tricyclic antidepressant or hydrocodone).
No products indexed under this heading.

Mepenzolate Bromide (Concurrent use of other anticholinergic agents with hydrocodone may produce paralytic ileus).
No products indexed under this heading.

Meperidine Hydrochloride (Combined therapy may result in additive CNS depression). Products include:
Demerol 3079
Mepergan Injection 3539

Mephobarbital (Combined therapy may result in additive CNS depression).
No products indexed under this heading.

Meprobamate (Combined therapy may result in additive CNS depression). Products include:
Miltown Tablets 3349

Mesoridazine Besylate (Combined therapy may result in additive CNS depression). Products include:
Serentil 1057

Methadone Hydrochloride (Combined therapy may result in additive CNS depression). Products include:
Dolophine Hydrochloride Tablets 3056

Methdilazine Hydrochloride (Combined therapy may result in additive CNS depression).
No products indexed under this heading.

Methohexital Sodium (Combined therapy may result in additive CNS depression). Products include:
Brevital Sodium for Injection, USP .. 1815

Methotrimeprazine (Combined therapy may result in additive CNS depression).
No products indexed under this heading.

Methoxyflurane (Combined therapy may result in additive CNS depression).
No products indexed under this heading.

Midazolam Hydrochloride (Combined therapy may result in additive CNS depression). Products include:
Versed Injection 3027
Versed Syrup 3033

Moclobemide (Co-administration of hydrocodone with MAO inhibitors may increase the effect of MAOI or hydrocodone).
No products indexed under this heading.

Molindone Hydrochloride (Combined therapy may result in additive CNS depression). Products include:
Moban 1320

Morphine Sulfate (Combined therapy may result in additive CNS depression). Products include:
Astramorph/PF Injection, USP (Preservative-Free) 594
Duramorph Injection 1312
Infumorph 200 and Infumorph 500 Sterile Solutions 1314
Kadian Capsules 1335
MS Contin Tablets 2896
MSIR 2898
Oramorph SR Tablets 3062
Roxanol 3066

Nortriptyline Hydrochloride (Co-administration of hydrocodone with MAO inhibitors may increase the effect of tricyclic antidepressant or hydrocodone).
No products indexed under this heading.

Olanzapine (Combined therapy may result in additive CNS depression). Products include:
Zyprexa Tablets 1973
Zyprexa ZYDIS Orally Disintegrating Tablets 1973

Oxazepam (Combined therapy may result in additive CNS depression).
No products indexed under this heading.

Oxybutynin Chloride (Concurrent use of other anticholinergic agents with hydrocodone may produce paralytic ileus). Products include:
Ditropan XL Extended Release Tablets 564

Oxycodone Hydrochloride (Combined therapy may result in additive CNS depression). Products include:
OxyContin Tablets 2912
OxyFast Oral Concentrate Solution . 2916
OxyIR Capsules 2916
Percocet Tablets 1326
Percodan Tablets 1327
Percolone Tablets 1327
Roxicodone 3067
Tylox Capsules 2597

Pargyline Hydrochloride (Co-administration of hydrocodone with MAO inhibitors may increase the effect of MAOI or hydrocodone).
No products indexed under this heading.

Pentobarbital Sodium (Combined therapy may result in additive CNS depression). Products include:
Nembutal Sodium Solution 485

Perphenazine (Combined therapy may result in additive CNS depression). Products include:
Etrafon 3115
Trilafon 3160

Phenelzine Sulfate (Co-administration of hydrocodone with MAO inhibitors may increase the effect of MAOI or hydrocodone). Products include:
Nardil Tablets 2653

Phenobarbital (Combined therapy may result in additive CNS depression). Products include:
Arco-Lase Plus Tablets 592
Donnatal 2929
Donnatal Extentabs 2930

Prazepam (Combined therapy may result in additive CNS depression).
No products indexed under this heading.

Procarbazine Hydrochloride (Co-administration of hydrocodone with MAO inhibitors may increase the effect of MAOI or hydrocodone). Products include:
Matulane Capsules 3246

Prochlorperazine (Combined therapy may result in additive CNS depression). Products include:
Compazine 1505

Procyclidine Hydrochloride (Concurrent use of other anticholinergic agents with hydrocodone may produce paralytic ileus).
No products indexed under this heading.

Promethazine Hydrochloride (Combined therapy may result in additive CNS depression). Products include:
Mepergan Injection 3539
Phenergan Injection 3553
Phenergan 3556
Phenergan Syrup 3554
Phenergan with Codeine Syrup 3557
Phenergan with Dextromethorphan Syrup 3559
Phenergan VC Syrup 3560
Phenergan VC with Codeine Syrup .. 3561

Propantheline Bromide (Concurrent use of other anticholinergic agents with hydrocodone may produce paralytic ileus).
No products indexed under this heading.

Propofol (Combined therapy may result in additive CNS depression). Products include:
Diprivan Injectable Emulsion 667

Propoxyphene Hydrochloride (Combined therapy may result in additive CNS depression). Products include:
Darvon Pulvules 1909
Darvon Compound-65 Pulvules 1910

Propoxyphene Napsylate (Combined therapy may result in additive CNS depression). Products include:
Darvon-N/Darvocet-N 1907
Darvon-N Tablets 1912

Protriptyline Hydrochloride (Co-administration of hydrocodone with MAO inhibitors may increase the effect of tricyclic antidepressant or hydrocodone). Products include:
Vivactil Tablets 2446
Vivactil Tablets 2217

Pyrilamine Maleate (Combined therapy may result in additive CNS depression). Products include:
Maximum Strength Midol Menstrual Caplets and Gelcaps .... ▣612
Maximum Strength Midol PMS Caplets and Gelcaps .... ▣613

Pyrilamine Tannate (Combined therapy may result in additive CNS depression). Products include:
Ryna-12 S Suspension 3351

Quazepam (Combined therapy may result in additive CNS depression).
No products indexed under this heading.

Quetiapine Fumarate (Combined therapy may result in additive CNS depression). Products include:
Seroquel Tablets 684

Remifentanil Hydrochloride (Combined therapy may result in additive CNS depression).
No products indexed under this heading.

Risperidone (Combined therapy may result in additive CNS depression). Products include:
Risperdal 1796

Scopolamine (Concurrent use of other anticholinergic agents with hydrocodone may produce paralytic ileus). Products include:
Transderm Scōp Transdermal Therapeutic System 2302

Scopolamine Hydrobromide (Concurrent use of other anticholinergic agents with hydrocodone may produce paralytic ileus). Products include:
Donnatal 2929
Donnatal Extentabs 2930

Secobarbital Sodium (Combined therapy may result in additive CNS depression).
No products indexed under this heading.

Selegiline Hydrochloride (Co-administration of hydrocodone with MAO inhibitors may increase the effect of MAOI or hydrocodone). Products include:
Eldepryl Capsules 3266

Sevoflurane (Combined therapy may result in additive CNS depression).
No products indexed under this heading.

Sufentanil Citrate (Combined therapy may result in additive CNS depression).
No products indexed under this heading.

Temazepam (Combined therapy may result in additive CNS depression).
No products indexed under this heading.

Terfenadine (Combined therapy may result in additive CNS depression).
No products indexed under this heading.

Thiamylal Sodium (Combined therapy may result in additive CNS depression).
No products indexed under this heading.

Thioridazine Hydrochloride (Combined therapy may result in additive CNS depression). Products include:
Thioridazine Hydrochloride Tablets 2289

Thiothixene (Combined therapy may result in additive CNS depression). Products include:
Navane Capsules 2701
Thiothixene Capsules 2290

Tolterodine Tartrate (Concurrent use of other anticholinergic agents with hydrocodone may produce paralytic ileus). Products include:
Detrol Tablets 3623
Detrol LA Capsules 2801

Tranylcypromine Sulfate (Co-administration of hydrocodone with MAO inhibitors may increase the effect of MAOI or hydrocodone). Products include:
Parnate Tablets 1607

Triazolam (Combined therapy may result in additive CNS depression). Products include:
Halcion Tablets 2823

Tridihexethyl Chloride (Concurrent use of other anticholinergic agents with hydrocodone may produce paralytic ileus).
No products indexed under this heading.

Trifluoperazine Hydrochloride (Combined therapy may result in additive CNS depression). Products include:
Stelazine 1640

Trihexyphenidyl Hydrochloride (Concurrent use of other anticholinergic agents with hydrocodone may produce paralytic ileus). Products include:
Artane 1855

Trimeprazine Tartrate (Combined therapy may result in additive CNS depression).
No products indexed under this heading.

Trimipramine Maleate (Co-administration of hydrocodone with MAO inhibitors may increase the effect of tricyclic antidepressant or hydrocodone). Products include:
Surmontil Capsules 3595

Tripelennamine Hydrochloride (Combined therapy may result in additive CNS depression).
No products indexed under this heading.

Triprolidine Hydrochloride (Combined therapy may result in additive CNS depression). Products include:
Actifed Cold & Allergy Tablets .... ▣688

Zaleplon (Combined therapy may result in additive CNS depression). Products include:
Sonata Capsules 3591

Ziprasidone Hydrochloride (Combined therapy may result in additive CNS depression). Products include:
Geodon Capsules 2688

Zolpidem Tartrate (Combined therapy may result in additive CNS depression). Products include:
Ambien Tablets 3191

Food Interactions

Alcohol (Combined use may result in additive CNS depression).

TUSSI-ORGANIDIN NR LIQUID

(Codeine Phosphate, Guaifenesin) 3350
See Tussi-Organidin DM NR Liquid

TUSSI-ORGANIDIN DM NR LIQUID

(Dextromethorphan Hydrobromide, Guaifenesin) 3350
May interact with antihistamines, central nervous system depressants, monoamine oxidase inhibitors, psychotropics, and certain other agents. Compounds in these categories include:

Acrivastine (Potential for additive CNS depressant effects). Products include:

Semprex-D Capsules 1172

Alfentanil Hydrochloride (Potential for additive CNS depressant effects).
No products indexed under this heading.

Alprazolam (Potential for additive CNS depressant effects). Products include:
Xanax Tablets 2865

Amitriptyline Hydrochloride (Potential for additive CNS depressant effects). Products include:
Etrafon 3115
Limbitrol 1738

Amoxapine (Potential for additive CNS depressant effects).
No products indexed under this heading.

Aprobarbital (Potential for additive CNS depressant effects).
No products indexed under this heading.

Astemizole (Potential for additive CNS depressant effects).
No products indexed under this heading.

Azatadine Maleate (Potential for additive CNS depressant effects). Products include:
Rynatan Tablets 3351

Bromodiphenhydramine Hydrochloride (Potential for additive CNS depressant effects).
No products indexed under this heading.

Brompheniramine Maleate (Potential for additive CNS depressant effects). Products include:
Bromfed Capsules (Extended-Release) 2269
Bromfed-PD Capsules (Extended-Release) 2269
Comtrex Acute Head Cold & Sinus Pressure Relief Tablets 627
Dimetapp Elixir 777
Dimetapp Cold and Fever Suspension 775
Dimetapp DM Cold & Cough Elixir 775
Dimetapp Nighttime Flu Liquid 776

Buprenorphine Hydrochloride (Potential for additive CNS depressant effects). Products include:
Buprenex Injectable 2918

Buspirone Hydrochloride (Potential for additive CNS depressant effects).
No products indexed under this heading.

Butabarbital (Potential for additive CNS depressant effects).
No products indexed under this heading.

Butalbital (Potential for additive CNS depressant effects). Products include:
Phrenilin 578
Sedapap Tablets 50 mg/650 mg 2225

Cetirizine Hydrochloride (Potential for additive CNS depressant effects). Products include:
Zyrtec 2756
Zyrtec-D 12 Hour Extended Relief Tablets 2758

Chlordiazepoxide (Potential for additive CNS depressant effects). Products include:
Limbitrol 1738

Chlordiazepoxide Hydrochloride (Potential for additive CNS depressant effects). Products include:
Librium Capsules 1736
Librium for Injection 1737

Chlorpheniramine Maleate (Potential for additive CNS depressant effects). Products include:
Actifed Cold & Sinus Caplets and Tablets 688
Alka-Seltzer Plus Liqui-Gels 604
BC Allergy Sinus Cold Powder 619
Chlor-Trimeton Allergy Tablets 735
Chlor-Trimeton Allergy/Decongestant Tablets 736
Comtrex Flu Therapy & Fever Relief Nighttime Tablets 628
Comtrex Maximum Strength Multi-Symptom Cold & Cough Relief Tablets and Caplets 626
Contac Severe Cold and Flu Caplets Maximum Strength 746
Coricidin 'D' Cold, Flu & Sinus Tablets 737
Coricidin/Coricidin D 738
Coricidin HBP Maximum Strength Flu Tablets 738
Extendryl 1361
Hycomine Compound Tablets 1317
Kronofed-A 1341
PediaCare Cough-Cold Liquid 719
PediaCare NightRest Cough-Cold Liquid 719
Robitussin Nighttime Honey Flu Liquid 786
Ryna 768
Singlet Caplets 761
Sinutab Sinus Allergy Medication, Maximum Strength Formula, Tablets & Caplets 707
Sudafed Cold & Allergy Tablets 708
TheraFlu Regular Strength Cold & Cough Night Time Hot Liquid 676
TheraFlu Regular Strength Cold & Sore Throat Night Time Hot Liquid 676
TheraFlu Maximum Strength Flu & Cough Night Time Hot Liquid 678
TheraFlu Maximum Strength Flu & Sore Throat Night Time Hot Liquid 677
TheraFlu Maximum Strength Severe Cold & Congestion Night Time Caplets 678
TheraFlu Maximum Strength Severe Cold & Congestion Night Time Hot Liquid 678
Triaminic Cold & Allergy Liquid 681
Triaminic Cold & Allergy Softchews 683
Triaminic Cold & Cough Liquid 681
Triaminic Cold & Cough Softchews 683
Triaminic Cold & Night Time Cough Liquid 681
Triaminic Cold, Cough & Fever Liquid 681
Children's Tylenol Cold Suspension Liquid and Chewable Tablets 2015
Children's Tylenol Cold Plus Cough Suspension Liquid and Chewable Tablets 2015
Children's Tylenol Flu Suspension Liquid 2015
Maximum Strength Tylenol Allergy Sinus Caplets, Gelcaps, and Geltabs 2010
Multi-Symptom Tylenol Cold Complete Formula Caplets 2010
Vicks 44M Cough, Cold & Flu Relief Liquid 725
Pediatric Vicks 44m Cough & Cold Relief 728
Children's Vicks NyQuil Cold/Cough Relief 726

Chlorpheniramine Polistirex (Potential for additive CNS depressant effects). Products include:
Tussionex Pennkinetic Extended-Release Suspension 1174

Chlorpheniramine Tannate (Potential for additive CNS depressant effects). Products include:
Reformulated Rynatan Pediatric Suspension 3352
Rynatuss Pediatric Suspension 3353
Rynatuss Tablets 3353
Tussi-12 S Suspension 3356
Tussi-12 Tablets 3356

Chlorpromazine (Potential for additive CNS depressant effects). Products include:
Thorazine Suppositories 1656

Chlorpromazine Hydrochloride (Potential for additive CNS depressant effects). Products include:
Thorazine 1656

Chlorprothixene (Potential for additive CNS depressant effects).
No products indexed under this heading.

Chlorprothixene Hydrochloride (Potential for additive CNS depressant effects).
No products indexed under this heading.

Chlorprothixene Lactate (Potential for additive CNS depressant effects).
No products indexed under this heading.

Clemastine Fumarate (Potential for additive CNS depressant effects). Products include:
Tavist 12 Hour Allergy Tablets 676

Clorazepate Dipotassium (Potential for additive CNS depressant effects). Products include:
Tranxene 511

Clozapine (Potential for additive CNS depressant effects). Products include:
Clozaril Tablets 2319

Codeine Phosphate (Potential for additive CNS depressant effects). Products include:
Phenergan with Codeine Syrup 3557
Phenergan VC with Codeine Syrup 3561
Robitussin A-C Syrup 2942
Robitussin-DAC Syrup 2942
Ryna-C Liquid 768
Soma Compound w/Codeine Tablets 3355
Tussi-Organidin NR Liquid 3350
Tussi-Organidin-S NR Liquid 3350
Tylenol with Codeine 2595

Cyproheptadine Hydrochloride (Potential for additive CNS depressant effects). Products include:
Periactin Tablets 2155

Desflurane (Potential for additive CNS depressant effects). Products include:
Suprane Liquid for Inhalation 874

Desipramine Hydrochloride (Potential for additive CNS depressant effects). Products include:
Norpramin Tablets 755

Dexchlorpheniramine Maleate (Potential for additive CNS depressant effects).
No products indexed under this heading.

Dezocine (Potential for additive CNS depressant effects).
No products indexed under this heading.

Diazepam (Potential for additive CNS depressant effects). Products include:
Valium Injectable 3026
Valium Tablets 3047

Diphenhydramine Citrate (Potential for additive CNS depressant effects). Products include:
Alka-Seltzer PM Effervescent Tablets 605
Benadryl Allergy & Sinus Fastmelt Tablets 693
Benadryl Children's Allergy/Cold Fastmelt Tablets 692
Excedrin PM Tablets, Caplets, and Geltabs 631
Goody's PM Powder 621

Diphenhydramine Hydrochloride (Potential for additive CNS depressant effects). Products include:
Extra Strength Bayer PM Caplets 611
Benadryl Allergy Chewables 689
Benadryl Allergy 691
Benadryl Allergy Liquid 690
Benadryl Allergy/Cold Tablets 691
Benadryl Allergy/Congestion Tablets 692
Benadryl Allergy & Sinus Liquid 693
Benadryl Allergy Sinus Headache Caplets & Gelcaps 693
Benadryl Severe Allergy & Sinus Headache Caplets 694
Benadryl Dye-Free Allergy Liquid 690
Benadryl Dye-Free Allergy Liqui-Gels Softgels 690
Benadryl Itch Relief Stick Extra Strength 695
Benadryl Cream 695
Benadryl Gel 695
Benadryl Spray 696
Benadryl Parenteral 2617
Coricidin HBP Night-Time Cold & Flu Tablets 738
Nytol QuickCaps Caplets 622
Maximum Strength Nytol QuickGels Softgels 621
Extra Strength Percogesic Aspirin-Free Coated Caplets 665
Simply Sleep Caplets 2008
Sominex Original Formula Tablets 761
Children's Tylenol Allergy-D Liquid 2014
Maximum Strength Tylenol Allergy Sinus NightTime Caplets 2010
Tylenol Severe Allergy Caplets 2010
Maximum Strength Tylenol Flu NightTime Gelcaps 2011
Extra Strength Tylenol PM Caplets, Geltabs, and Gelcaps 2012
Unisom Maximum Strength SleepGels 713

Diphenylpyraline Hydrochloride (Potential for additive CNS depressant effects).
No products indexed under this heading.

Doxepin Hydrochloride (Potential for additive CNS depressant effects). Products include:
Sinequan 2713

Droperidol (Potential for additive CNS depressant effects).
No products indexed under this heading.

Enflurane (Potential for additive CNS depressant effects).
No products indexed under this heading.

Estazolam (Potential for additive CNS depressant effects). Products include:
ProSom Tablets 500

Ethchlorvynol (Potential for additive CNS depressant effects).
No products indexed under this heading.

Ethinamate (Potential for additive CNS depressant effects).
No products indexed under this heading.

Fentanyl (Potential for additive CNS depressant effects). Products include:
Duragesic Transdermal System 1786

Fentanyl Citrate (Potential for additive CNS depressant effects). Products include:
Actiq 1184

Fexofenadine Hydrochloride (Potential for additive CNS depressant effects). Products include:
Allegra 712
Allegra-D Extended-Release Tablets 714

Fluphenazine Decanoate (Potential for additive CNS depressant effects).
No products indexed under this heading.

Fluphenazine Enanthate (Potential for additive CNS depressant effects).
No products indexed under this heading.

Fluphenazine Hydrochloride (Potential for additive CNS depressant effects).
No products indexed under this heading.

Flurazepam Hydrochloride (Potential for additive CNS depressant effects).
No products indexed under this heading.

Glutethimide (Potential for additive CNS depressant effects).
No products indexed under this heading.

Haloperidol (Potential for additive CNS depressant effects). Products include:
Haldol Injection, Tablets and Concentrate 2533

Haloperidol Decanoate (Potential for additive CNS depressant effects). Products include:
Haldol Decanoate 2535

Hydrocodone Bitartrate (Potential for additive CNS depressant effects). Products include:
Hycodan 1316
Hycomine Compound Tablets 1317
Hycotuss Expectorant Syrup 1318
Lortab 3319

IMPORTANT NOTE: Always consult each drug listing in the patient's regimen for possible interactions.

Lortab Elixir ... 3317
Maxidone Tablets CIII ... 3399
Norco 5/325 Tablets CIII ... 3424
Norco 7.5/325 Tablets CIII ... 3425
Norco 10/325 Tablets CIII ... 3427
Norco 10/325 Tablets CIII ... 3425
Vicodin Tablets ... 516
Vicodin ES Tablets ... 517
Vicodin HP Tablets ... 518
Vicodin Tuss Expectorant ... 519
Vicoprofen Tablets ... 520
Zydone Tablets ... 1330

Hydrocodone Polistirex (Potential for additive CNS depressant effects). Products include:
Tussionex Pennkinetic Extended-Release Suspension ... 1174

Hydromorphone Hydrochloride (Potential for additive CNS depressant effects). Products include:
Dilaudid ... 441
Dilaudid Oral Liquid ... 445
Dilaudid Powder ... 441
Dilaudid Rectal Suppositories ... 441
Dilaudid Tablets ... 441
Dilaudid Tablets - 8 mg ... 445
Dilaudid-HP ... 443

Hydroxyzine Hydrochloride (Potential for additive CNS depressant effects). Products include:
Atarax Tablets & Syrup ... 2667
Vistaril Intramuscular Solution ... 2738

Imipramine Hydrochloride (Potential for additive CNS depressant effects).
No products indexed under this heading.

Imipramine Pamoate (Potential for additive CNS depressant effects).
No products indexed under this heading.

Isocarboxazid (Co-administration with MAO inhibitors may result in serious toxicity; concurrent use is contraindicated).
No products indexed under this heading.

Isoflurane (Potential for additive CNS depressant effects).
No products indexed under this heading.

Ketamine Hydrochloride (Potential for additive CNS depressant effects).
No products indexed under this heading.

Levomethadyl Acetate Hydrochloride (Potential for additive CNS depressant effects).
No products indexed under this heading.

Levorphanol Tartrate (Potential for additive CNS depressant effects). Products include:
Levo-Dromoran ... 1734
Levorphanol Tartrate Tablets ... 3059

Lithium Carbonate (Potential for additive CNS depressant effects). Products include:
Eskalith ... 1527
Lithium Carbonate ... 3061
Lithobid Slow-Release Tablets ... 3255

Lithium Citrate (Potential for additive CNS depressant effects). Products include:
Lithium Citrate Syrup ... 3061

Loratadine (Potential for additive CNS depressant effects). Products include:
Claritin ... 3100
Claritin-D 12 Hour Extended Release Tablets ... 3102
Claritin-D 24 Hour Extended Release Tablets ... 3104

Lorazepam (Potential for additive CNS depressant effects). Products include:
Ativan Injection ... 3478
Ativan Tablets ... 3482

Loxapine Hydrochloride (Potential for additive CNS depressant effects).
No products indexed under this heading.

Loxapine Succinate (Potential for additive CNS depressant effects). Products include:
Loxitane Capsules ... 3398

Maprotiline Hydrochloride (Potential for additive CNS depressant effects).
No products indexed under this heading.

Meperidine Hydrochloride (Potential for additive CNS depressant effects). Products include:
Demerol ... 3079
Mepergan Injection ... 3539

Mephobarbital (Potential for additive CNS depressant effects).
No products indexed under this heading.

Meprobamate (Potential for additive CNS depressant effects). Products include:
Miltown Tablets ... 3349

Mesoridazine Besylate (Potential for additive CNS depressant effects). Products include:
Serentil ... 1057

Methadone Hydrochloride (Potential for additive CNS depressant effects). Products include:
Dolophine Hydrochloride Tablets ... 3056

Methdilazine Hydrochloride (Potential for additive CNS depressant effects).
No products indexed under this heading.

Methohexital Sodium (Potential for additive CNS depressant effects). Products include:
Brevital Sodium for Injection, USP .. 1815

Methotrimeprazine (Potential for additive CNS depressant effects).
No products indexed under this heading.

Methoxyflurane (Potential for additive CNS depressant effects).
No products indexed under this heading.

Midazolam Hydrochloride (Potential for additive CNS depressant effects). Products include:
Versed Injection ... 3027
Versed Syrup ... 3033

Mirtazapine (Potential for additive CNS depressant effects). Products include:
Remeron Tablets ... 2483
Remeron SolTab Tablets ... 2486

Moclobemide (Co-administration with MAO inhibitors may result in serious toxicity; concurrent use is contraindicated).
No products indexed under this heading.

Molindone Hydrochloride (Potential for additive CNS depressant effects). Products include:
Moban ... 1320

Morphine Sulfate (Potential for additive CNS depressant effects). Products include:
Astramorph/PF Injection, USP (Preservative-Free) ... 594
Duramorph Injection ... 1312
Infumorph 200 and Infumorph 500 Sterile Solutions ... 1314
Kadian Capsules ... 1335
MS Contin Tablets ... 2896
MSIR ... 2898
Oramorph SR Tablets ... 3062
Roxanol ... 3066

Nortriptyline Hydrochloride (Potential for additive CNS depressant effects).
No products indexed under this heading.

Olanzapine (Potential for additive CNS depressant effects). Products include:
Zyprexa Tablets ... 1973
Zyprexa ZYDIS Orally Disintegrating Tablets ... 1973

Oxazepam (Potential for additive CNS depressant effects).
No products indexed under this heading.

Oxycodone Hydrochloride (Potential for additive CNS depressant effects). Products include:
OxyContin Tablets ... 2912
OxyFast Oral Concentrate Solution . 2916
OxyIR Capsules ... 2916
Percocet Tablets ... 1326
Percodan Tablets ... 1327
Percolone Tablets ... 1327
Roxicodone ... 3067
Tylox Capsules ... 2597

Pargyline Hydrochloride (Co-administration with MAO inhibitors may result in serious toxicity; concurrent use is contraindicated).
No products indexed under this heading.

Pentobarbital Sodium (Potential for additive CNS depressant effects). Products include:
Nembutal Sodium Solution ... 485

Perphenazine (Potential for additive CNS depressant effects). Products include:
Etrafon ... 3115
Trilafon ... 3160

Phenelzine Sulfate (Co-administration with MAO inhibitors may result in serious toxicity; concurrent use is contraindicated). Products include:
Nardil Tablets ... 2653

Phenobarbital (Potential for additive CNS depressant effects). Products include:
Arco-Lase Plus Tablets ... 592
Donnatal ... 2929
Donnatal Extentabs ... 2930

Prazepam (Potential for additive CNS depressant effects).
No products indexed under this heading.

Procarbazine Hydrochloride (Co-administration with MAO inhibitors may result in serious toxicity; concurrent use is contraindicated). Products include:
Matulane Capsules ... 3246

Prochlorperazine (Potential for additive CNS depressant effects). Products include:
Compazine ... 1505

Promethazine Hydrochloride (Potential for additive CNS depressant effects). Products include:
Mepergan Injection ... 3539
Phenergan Injection ... 3553
Phenergan ... 3556
Phenergan Syrup ... 3554
Phenergan with Codeine Syrup ... 3557
Phenergan with Dextromethorphan Syrup ... 3559
Phenergan VC Syrup ... 3560
Phenergan VC with Codeine Syrup .. 3561

Propofol (Potential for additive CNS depressant effects). Products include:
Diprivan Injectable Emulsion ... 667

Propoxyphene Hydrochloride (Potential for additive CNS depressant effects). Products include:
Darvon Pulvules ... 1909
Darvon Compound-65 Pulvules ... 1910

Propoxyphene Napsylate (Potential for additive CNS depressant effects). Products include:
Darvon-N/Darvocet-N ... 1907
Darvon-N Tablets ... 1912

Protriptyline Hydrochloride (Potential for additive CNS depressant effects). Products include:
Vivactil Tablets ... 2446
Vivactil Tablets ... 2217

Pyrilamine Maleate (Potential for additive CNS depressant effects). Products include:
Maximum Strength Midol Menstrual Caplets and Gelcaps ... ■612
Maximum Strength Midol PMS Caplets and Gelcaps ... ■613

Pyrilamine Tannate (Potential for additive CNS depressant effects). Products include:
Ryna-12 S Suspension ... 3351

Quazepam (Potential for additive CNS depressant effects).
No products indexed under this heading.

Quetiapine Fumarate (Potential for additive CNS depressant effects). Products include:
Seroquel Tablets ... 684

Remifentanil Hydrochloride (Potential for additive CNS depressant effects).
No products indexed under this heading.

Risperidone (Potential for additive CNS depressant effects). Products include:
Risperdal ... 1796

Secobarbital Sodium (Potential for additive CNS depressant effects).
No products indexed under this heading.

Selegiline Hydrochloride (Co-administration with MAO inhibitors may result in serious toxicity; concurrent use is contraindicated). Products include:
Eldepryl Capsules ... 3266

Sevoflurane (Potential for additive CNS depressant effects).
No products indexed under this heading.

Sufentanil Citrate (Potential for additive CNS depressant effects).
No products indexed under this heading.

Temazepam (Potential for additive CNS depressant effects).
No products indexed under this heading.

Terfenadine (Potential for additive CNS depressant effects).
No products indexed under this heading.

Thiamylal Sodium (Potential for additive CNS depressant effects).
No products indexed under this heading.

Thioridazine Hydrochloride (Potential for additive CNS depressant effects). Products include:
Thioridazine Hydrochloride Tablets ... 2289

Thiothixene (Potential for additive CNS depressant effects). Products include:
Navane Capsules ... 2701
Thiothixene Capsules ... 2290

Tranylcypromine Sulfate (Co-administration with MAO inhibitors may result in serious toxicity; concurrent use is contraindicated). Products include:
Parnate Tablets ... 1607

Triazolam (Potential for additive CNS depressant effects). Products include:
Halcion Tablets ... 2823

Trifluoperazine Hydrochloride (Potential for additive CNS depressant effects). Products include:
Stelazine ... 1640

Trimeprazine Tartrate (Potential for additive CNS depressant effects).
No products indexed under this heading.

Trimipramine Maleate (Potential for additive CNS depressant effects). Products include:
Surmontil Capsules ... 3595

Tripelennamine Hydrochloride (Potential for additive CNS depressant effects).
No products indexed under this heading.

Triprolidine Hydrochloride (Potential for additive CNS depressant effects). Products include:
Actifed Cold & Allergy Tablets ... ■688

Zaleplon (Potential for additive CNS depressant effects). Products include:

Sonata Capsules 3591

Ziprasidone Hydrochloride (Potential for additive CNS depressant effects). Products include:

Geodon Capsules 2688

Zolpidem Tartrate (Potential for additive CNS depressant effects). Products include:

Ambien Tablets 3191

Food Interactions

Alcohol (Potential for additive CNS depressant effects).

TUSSI-ORGANIDIN DM-S NR LIQUID

(Dextromethorphan Hydrobromide, Guaifenesin) 3350

See Tussi-Organidin DM NR Liquid

TUSSI-ORGANIDIN-S NR LIQUID

(Codeine Phosphate, Guaifenesin) 3350

See Tussi-Organidin DM NR Liquid

TWINRIX VACCINE

(Hepatitis A Vaccine, Inactivated, Hepatitis B Vaccine, Recombinant) 1674

None cited in PDR database.

CHILDREN'S TYLENOL SUSPENSION LIQUID AND SOFT CHEWS CHEWABLE TABLETS

(Acetaminophen) 2014

None cited in PDR database.

CHILDREN'S TYLENOL ALLERGY-D LIQUID

(Acetaminophen, Diphenhydramine Hydrochloride, Pseudoephedrine Hydrochloride) 2014

See Children's Tylenol Flu Suspension Liquid

CHILDREN'S TYLENOL COLD SUSPENSION LIQUID AND CHEWABLE TABLETS

(Acetaminophen, Chlorpheniramine Maleate, Pseudoephedrine Hydrochloride) 2015

See Children's Tylenol Flu Suspension Liquid

CHILDREN'S TYLENOL COLD PLUS COUGH SUSPENSION LIQUID AND CHEWABLE TABLETS

(Acetaminophen, Chlorpheniramine Maleate, Dextromethorphan Hydrobromide, Pseudoephedrine Hydrochloride) 2015

See Children's Tylenol Flu Suspension Liquid

CHILDREN'S TYLENOL FLU SUSPENSION LIQUID

(Acetaminophen, Chlorpheniramine Maleate, Dextromethorphan Hydrobromide, Pseudoephedrine Hydrochloride) 2015

May interact with hypnotics and sedatives, monoamine oxidase inhibitors, and tranquilizers. Compounds in these categories include:

Alprazolam (May increase the drowsiness effect). Products include:

Xanax Tablets 2865

Buspirone Hydrochloride (May increase the drowsiness effect).

No products indexed under this heading.

Chlordiazepoxide (May increase the drowsiness effect). Products include:

Limbitrol 1738

Chlordiazepoxide Hydrochloride (May increase the drowsiness effect). Products include:

Librium Capsules 1736
Librium for Injection 1737

Chlorpromazine (May increase the drowsiness effect). Products include:

Thorazine Suppositories 1656

Chlorpromazine Hydrochloride (May increase the drowsiness effect). Products include:

Thorazine 1656

Chlorprothixene (May increase the drowsiness effect).

No products indexed under this heading.

Chlorprothixene Hydrochloride (May increase the drowsiness effect).

No products indexed under this heading.

Clorazepate Dipotassium (May increase the drowsiness effect). Products include:

Tranxene 511

Diazepam (May increase the drowsiness effect). Products include:

Valium Injectable 3026
Valium Tablets 3047

Droperidol (May increase the drowsiness effect).

No products indexed under this heading.

Estazolam (May increase the drowsiness effect). Products include:

ProSom Tablets 500

Ethchlorvynol (May increase the drowsiness effect).

No products indexed under this heading.

Ethinamate (May increase the drowsiness effect).

No products indexed under this heading.

Fluphenazine Decanoate (May increase the drowsiness effect).

No products indexed under this heading.

Fluphenazine Enanthate (May increase the drowsiness effect).

No products indexed under this heading.

Fluphenazine Hydrochloride (May increase the drowsiness effect).

No products indexed under this heading.

Flurazepam Hydrochloride (May increase the drowsiness effect).

No products indexed under this heading.

Glutethimide (May increase the drowsiness effect).

No products indexed under this heading.

Haloperidol (May increase the drowsiness effect). Products include:

Haldol Injection, Tablets and Concentrate 2533

Haloperidol Decanoate (May increase the drowsiness effect). Products include:

Haldol Decanoate 2535

Hydroxyzine Hydrochloride (May increase the drowsiness effect). Products include:

Atarax Tablets & Syrup 2667
Vistaril Intramuscular Solution 2738

Isocarboxazid (Concurrent and/or sequential use with MAO inhibitor is not recommended).

No products indexed under this heading.

Lorazepam (May increase the drowsiness effect). Products include:

Ativan Injection 3478
Ativan Tablets 3482

Loxapine Hydrochloride (May increase the drowsiness effect).

No products indexed under this heading.

Loxapine Succinate (May increase the drowsiness effect). Products include:

Loxitane Capsules 3398

Meprobamate (May increase the drowsiness effect). Products include:

Miltown Tablets 3349

Mesoridazine Besylate (May increase the drowsiness effect). Products include:

Serentil 1057

Midazolam Hydrochloride (May increase the drowsiness effect). Products include:

Versed Injection 3027
Versed Syrup 3033

Moclobemide (Concurrent and/or sequential use with MAO inhibitor is not recommended).

No products indexed under this heading.

Molindone Hydrochloride (May increase the drowsiness effect). Products include:

Moban 1320

Oxazepam (May increase the drowsiness effect).

No products indexed under this heading.

Pargyline Hydrochloride (Concurrent and/or sequential use with MAO inhibitor is not recommended).

No products indexed under this heading.

Perphenazine (May increase the drowsiness effect). Products include:

Etrafon 3115
Trilafon 3160

Phenelzine Sulfate (Concurrent and/or sequential use with MAO inhibitor is not recommended). Products include:

Nardil Tablets 2653

Prazepam (May increase the drowsiness effect).

No products indexed under this heading.

Procarbazine Hydrochloride (Concurrent and/or sequential use with MAO inhibitor is not recommended). Products include:

Matulane Capsules 3246

Prochlorperazine (May increase the drowsiness effect). Products include:

Compazine 1505

Promethazine Hydrochloride (May increase the drowsiness effect). Products include:

Mepergan Injection 3539
Phenergan Injection 3553
Phenergan 3556
Phenergan Syrup 3554
Phenergan with Codeine Syrup 3557
Phenergan with Dextromethorphan Syrup 3559
Phenergan VC Syrup 3560
Phenergan VC with Codeine Syrup .. 3561

Propofol (May increase the drowsiness effect). Products include:

Diprivan Injectable Emulsion 667

Quazepam (May increase the drowsiness effect).

No products indexed under this heading.

Secobarbital Sodium (May increase the drowsiness effect).

No products indexed under this heading.

Selegiline Hydrochloride (Concurrent and/or sequential use with MAO inhibitor is not recommended). Products include:

Eldepryl Capsules 3266

Temazepam (May increase the drowsiness effect).

No products indexed under this heading.

Thioridazine Hydrochloride (May increase the drowsiness effect). Products include:

Thioridazine Hydrochloride Tablets 2289

Thiothixene (May increase the drowsiness effect). Products include:

Navane Capsules 2701
Thiothixene Capsules 2290

Tranylcypromine Sulfate (Concurrent and/or sequential use with MAO inhibitor is not recommended). Products include:

Parnate Tablets 1607

Triazolam (May increase the drowsiness effect). Products include:

Halcion Tablets 2823

Trifluoperazine Hydrochloride (May increase the drowsiness effect). Products include:

Stelazine 1640

Zaleplon (May increase the drowsiness effect). Products include:

Sonata Capsules 3591

Zolpidem Tartrate (May increase the drowsiness effect). Products include:

Ambien Tablets 3191

CHILDREN'S TYLENOL SINUS SUSPENSION LIQUID

(Acetaminophen, Pseudoephedrine Hydrochloride)....... 2017

See Infants' Tylenol Cold Decongestant and Fever Reducer Concentrated Drops Plus Cough

INFANTS' TYLENOL COLD DECONGESTANT AND FEVER REDUCER CONCENTRATED DROPS

(Acetaminophen, Pseudoephedrine Hydrochloride)....... 2015

See Infants' Tylenol Cold Decongestant and Fever Reducer Concentrated Drops Plus Cough

INFANTS' TYLENOL COLD DECONGESTANT AND FEVER REDUCER CONCENTRATED DROPS PLUS COUGH

(Acetaminophen, Dextromethorphan Hydrobromide, Pseudoephedrine Hydrochloride) 2015

May interact with monoamine oxidase inhibitors. Compounds in these categories include:

Isocarboxazid (Concurrent and/or sequential use with MAO inhibitors is contraindicated).

No products indexed under this heading.

Moclobemide (Concurrent and/or sequential use with MAO inhibitors is contraindicated).

No products indexed under this heading.

Pargyline Hydrochloride (Concurrent and/or sequential use with MAO inhibitors is contraindicated).

No products indexed under this heading.

Phenelzine Sulfate (Concurrent and/or sequential use with MAO inhibitors is contraindicated). Products include:

Nardil Tablets 2653

Procarbazine Hydrochloride (Concurrent and/or sequential use with MAO inhibitors is contraindicated). Products include:

Matulane Capsules 3246

Selegiline Hydrochloride (Concurrent and/or sequential use with MAO inhibitors is contraindicated). Products include:

Eldepryl Capsules 3266

Tranylcypromine Sulfate (Concurrent and/or sequential use with MAO inhibitors is contraindicated). Products include:

Parnate Tablets 1607

INFANTS' TYLENOL CONCENTRATED DROPS

(Acetaminophen) 2014

None cited in PDR database.

JUNIOR STRENGTH TYLENOL SOFT CHEWS CHEWABLE TABLETS
(Acetaminophen) 2014
None cited in PDR database.

EXTRA STRENGTH TYLENOL ADULT LIQUID PAIN RELIEVER
(Acetaminophen) 2009
See Regular Strength Tylenol Tablets

EXTRA STRENGTH TYLENOL GELCAPS, GELTABS, CAPLETS, AND TABLETS
(Acetaminophen) 2009
See Regular Strength Tylenol Tablets

REGULAR STRENGTH TYLENOL TABLETS
(Acetaminophen) 2009

Food Interactions

Alcohol (Chronic heavy alcohol users, 3 or more drinks per day, should consult their physicians for advice on when and how they should take pain relievers including acetaminophen).

MAXIMUM STRENGTH TYLENOL ALLERGY SINUS CAPLETS, GELCAPS, AND GELTABS
(Acetaminophen, Chlorpheniramine Maleate, Pseudoephedrine Hydrochloride) 2010
See Maximum Strength Tylenol Allergy Sinus NightTime Caplets

MAXIMUM STRENGTH TYLENOL ALLERGY SINUS NIGHTTIME CAPLETS
(Acetaminophen, Diphenhydramine Hydrochloride, Pseudoephedrine Hydrochloride) 2010
May interact with hypnotics and sedatives, monoamine oxidase inhibitors, tranquilizers, and certain other agents. Compounds in these categories include:

Alprazolam (Concurrent use may increase drowsiness effect). Products include:
Xanax Tablets 2865

Buspirone Hydrochloride (Concurrent use may increase drowsiness effect).
No products indexed under this heading.

Chlordiazepoxide (Concurrent use may increase drowsiness effect). Products include:
Limbitrol 1738

Chlordiazepoxide Hydrochloride (Concurrent use may increase drowsiness effect). Products include:
Librium Capsules 1736
Librium for Injection 1737

Chlorpromazine (Concurrent use may increase drowsiness effect). Products include:
Thorazine Suppositories 1656

Chlorpromazine Hydrochloride (Concurrent use may increase drowsiness effect). Products include:
Thorazine 1656

Chlorprothixene (Concurrent use may increase drowsiness effect).
No products indexed under this heading.

Chlorprothixene Hydrochloride (Concurrent use may increase drowsiness effect).
No products indexed under this heading.

Clorazepate Dipotassium (Concurrent use may increase drowsiness effect). Products include:
Tranxene 511

Diazepam (Concurrent use may increase drowsiness effect). Products include:
Valium Injectable 3026
Valium Tablets 3047

Droperidol (Concurrent use may increase drowsiness effect).
No products indexed under this heading.

Estazolam (Concurrent use may increase drowsiness effect). Products include:
ProSom Tablets 500

Ethchlorvynol (Concurrent use may increase drowsiness effect).
No products indexed under this heading.

Ethinamate (Concurrent use may increase drowsiness effect).
No products indexed under this heading.

Fluphenazine Decanoate (Concurrent use may increase drowsiness effect).
No products indexed under this heading.

Fluphenazine Enanthate (Concurrent use may increase drowsiness effect).
No products indexed under this heading.

Fluphenazine Hydrochloride (Concurrent use may increase drowsiness effect).
No products indexed under this heading.

Flurazepam Hydrochloride (Concurrent use may increase drowsiness effect).
No products indexed under this heading.

Glutethimide (Concurrent use may increase drowsiness effect).
No products indexed under this heading.

Haloperidol (Concurrent use may increase drowsiness effect). Products include:
Haldol Injection, Tablets and Concentrate 2533

Haloperidol Decanoate (Concurrent use may increase drowsiness effect). Products include:
Haldol Decanoate 2535

Hydroxyzine Hydrochloride (Concurrent use may increase drowsiness effect). Products include:
Atarax Tablets & Syrup 2667
Vistaril Intramuscular Solution 2738

Isocarboxazid (Concurrent and/or sequential use with MAO inhibitors is not recommended).
No products indexed under this heading.

Lorazepam (Concurrent use may increase drowsiness effect). Products include:
Ativan Injection 3478
Ativan Tablets 3482

Loxapine Hydrochloride (Concurrent use may increase drowsiness effect).
No products indexed under this heading.

Loxapine Succinate (Concurrent use may increase drowsiness effect). Products include:
Loxitane Capsules 3398

Meprobamate (Concurrent use may increase drowsiness effect). Products include:
Miltown Tablets 3349

Mesoridazine Besylate (Concurrent use may increase drowsiness effect). Products include:
Serentil 1057

Midazolam Hydrochloride (Concurrent use may increase drowsiness effect). Products include:
Versed Injection 3027
Versed Syrup 3033

Moclobemide (Concurrent and/or sequential use with MAO inhibitors is not recommended).
No products indexed under this heading.

Molindone Hydrochloride (Concurrent use may increase drowsiness effect). Products include:
Moban 1320

Oxazepam (Concurrent use may increase drowsiness effect).
No products indexed under this heading.

Pargyline Hydrochloride (Concurrent and/or sequential use with MAO inhibitors is not recommended).
No products indexed under this heading.

Perphenazine (Concurrent use may increase drowsiness effect). Products include:
Etrafon 3115
Trilafon 3160

Phenelzine Sulfate (Concurrent and/or sequential use with MAO inhibitors is not recommended). Products include:
Nardil Tablets 2653

Prazepam (Concurrent use may increase drowsiness effect).
No products indexed under this heading.

Procarbazine Hydrochloride (Concurrent and/or sequential use with MAO inhibitors is not recommended). Products include:
Matulane Capsules 3246

Prochlorperazine (Concurrent use may increase drowsiness effect). Products include:
Compazine 1505

Promethazine Hydrochloride (Concurrent use may increase drowsiness effect). Products include:
Mepergan Injection 3539
Phenergan Injection 3553
Phenergan 3556
Phenergan Syrup 3554
Phenergan with Codeine Syrup 3557
Phenergan with Dextromethorphan Syrup 3559
Phenergan VC Syrup 3560
Phenergan VC with Codeine Syrup . 3561

Propofol (Concurrent use may increase drowsiness effect). Products include:
Diprivan Injectable Emulsion 667

Quazepam (Concurrent use may increase drowsiness effect).
No products indexed under this heading.

Secobarbital Sodium (Concurrent use may increase drowsiness effect).
No products indexed under this heading.

Selegiline Hydrochloride (Concurrent and/or sequential use with MAO inhibitors is not recommended). Products include:
Eldepryl Capsules 3266

Temazepam (Concurrent use may increase drowsiness effect).
No products indexed under this heading.

Thioridazine Hydrochloride (Concurrent use may increase drowsiness effect). Products include:
Thioridazine Hydrochloride Tablets 2289

Thiothixene (Concurrent use may increase drowsiness effect). Products include:
Navane Capsules 2701
Thiothixene Capsules 2290

Tranylcypromine Sulfate (Concurrent and/or sequential use with MAO inhibitors is not recommended). Products include:
Parnate Tablets 1607

Triazolam (Concurrent use may increase drowsiness effect). Products include:
Halcion Tablets 2823

Trifluoperazine Hydrochloride (Concurrent use may increase drowsiness effect). Products include:
Stelazine 1640

Zaleplon (Concurrent use may increase drowsiness effect). Products include:
Sonata Capsules 3591

Zolpidem Tartrate (Concurrent use may increase drowsiness effect). Products include:
Ambien Tablets 3191

Food Interactions

Alcohol (Concurrent use may increase drowsiness effect; chronic heavy alcohol abusers, 3 or more drinks per day, may be at increased risk of liver toxicity from excessive acetaminophen use).

TYLENOL SEVERE ALLERGY CAPLETS
(Acetaminophen, Diphenhydramine Hydrochloride)....... 2010
See Maximum Strength Tylenol Allergy Sinus NightTime Caplets

TYLENOL ARTHRITIS PAIN EXTENDED RELIEF CAPLETS
(Acetaminophen) 2009
See Regular Strength Tylenol Tablets

MULTI-SYMPTOM TYLENOL COLD COMPLETE FORMULA CAPLETS
(Acetaminophen, Chlorpheniramine Maleate, Dextromethorphan Hydrobromide, Pseudoephedrine Hydrochloride) 2010
See Maximum Strength Tylenol Allergy Sinus NightTime Caplets

MULTI-SYMPTOM TYLENOL COLD NON-DROWSY CAPLETS AND GELCAPS
(Acetaminophen, Dextromethorphan Hydrobromide, Pseudoephedrine Hydrochloride) 2010
See Maximum Strength Tylenol Allergy Sinus NightTime Caplets

MULTI-SYMPTOM TYLENOL COLD SEVERE CONGESTION NON-DROWSY CAPLETS
(Acetaminophen, Dextromethorphan Hydrobromide, Guaifenesin, Pseudoephedrine Hydrochloride) 2011
May interact with monoamine oxidase inhibitors and certain other agents. Compounds in these categories include:

Isocarboxazid (Concurrent and/or sequential use with MAO inhibitors is not recommended).
No products indexed under this heading.

Moclobemide (Concurrent and/or sequential use with MAO inhibitors is not recommended).
No products indexed under this heading.

Pargyline Hydrochloride (Concurrent and/or sequential use with MAO inhibitors is not recommended).
No products indexed under this heading.

Phenelzine Sulfate (Concurrent and/or sequential use with MAO inhibitors is not recommended). Products include:
Nardil Tablets 2653

Procarbazine Hydrochloride (Concurrent and/or sequential use with MAO inhibitors is not recommended). Products include:
Matulane Capsules 3246

Selegiline Hydrochloride (Concurrent and/or sequential use with MAO inhibitors is not recommended). Products include:

Eldepryl Capsules 3266

Tranylcypromine Sulfate (Concurrent and/or sequential use with MAO inhibitors is not recommended). Products include:

Parnate Tablets 1607

Food Interactions

Alcohol (Chronic heavy alcohol abusers, 3 or more drinks per day, may be at increased risk of liver toxicity from acetaminophen use).

MAXIMUM STRENGTH TYLENOL FLU NIGHTTIME GELCAPS

(Acetaminophen, Diphenhydramine Hydrochloride, Pseudoephedrine Hydrochloride) 2011

May interact with hypnotics and sedatives, monoamine oxidase inhibitors, tranquilizers, and certain other agents. Compounds in these categories include:

Alprazolam (Concurrent use may increase drowsiness effect). Products include:

Xanax Tablets 2865

Buspirone Hydrochloride (Concurrent use may increase drowsiness effect).

No products indexed under this heading.

Chlordiazepoxide (Concurrent use may increase drowsiness effect). Products include:

Limbitrol 1738

Chlordiazepoxide Hydrochloride (Concurrent use may increase drowsiness effect). Products include:

Librium Capsules 1736
Librium for Injection 1737

Chlorpromazine (Concurrent use may increase drowsiness effect). Products include:

Thorazine Suppositories 1656

Chlorpromazine Hydrochloride (Concurrent use may increase drowsiness effect). Products include:

Thorazine 1656

Chlorprothixene (Concurrent use may increase drowsiness effect).

No products indexed under this heading.

Chlorprothixene Hydrochloride (Concurrent use may increase drowsiness effect).

No products indexed under this heading.

Clorazepate Dipotassium (Concurrent use may increase drowsiness effect). Products include:

Tranxene 511

Diazepam (Concurrent use may increase drowsiness effect). Products include:

Valium Injectable 3026
Valium Tablets 3047

Droperidol (Concurrent use may increase drowsiness effect).

No products indexed under this heading.

Estazolam (Concurrent use may increase drowsiness effect). Products include:

ProSom Tablets 500

Ethchlorvynol (Concurrent use may increase drowsiness effect).

No products indexed under this heading.

Ethinamate (Concurrent use may increase drowsiness effect).

No products indexed under this heading.

Fluphenazine Decanoate (Concurrent use may increase drowsiness effect).

No products indexed under this heading.

Fluphenazine Enanthate (Concurrent use may increase drowsiness effect).

No products indexed under this heading.

Fluphenazine Hydrochloride (Concurrent use may increase drowsiness effect).

No products indexed under this heading.

Flurazepam Hydrochloride (Concurrent use may increase drowsiness effect).

No products indexed under this heading.

Glutethimide (Concurrent use may increase drowsiness effect).

No products indexed under this heading.

Haloperidol (Concurrent use may increase drowsiness effect). Products include:

Haldol Injection, Tablets and Concentrate 2533

Haloperidol Decanoate (Concurrent use may increase drowsiness effect). Products include:

Haldol Decanoate 2535

Hydroxyzine Hydrochloride (Concurrent use may increase drowsiness effect). Products include:

Atarax Tablets & Syrup 2667
Vistaril Intramuscular Solution 2738

Isocarboxazid (Concurrent and/or sequential use with MAO inhibitors is not recommended).

No products indexed under this heading.

Lorazepam (Concurrent use may increase drowsiness effect). Products include:

Ativan Injection 3478
Ativan Tablets 3482

Loxapine Hydrochloride (Concurrent use may increase drowsiness effect).

No products indexed under this heading.

Loxapine Succinate (Concurrent use may increase drowsiness effect). Products include:

Loxitane Capsules 3398

Meprobamate (Concurrent use may increase drowsiness effect). Products include:

Miltown Tablets 3349

Mesoridazine Besylate (Concurrent use may increase drowsiness effect). Products include:

Serentil 1057

Midazolam Hydrochloride (Concurrent use may increase drowsiness effect). Products include:

Versed Injection 3027
Versed Syrup 3033

Moclobemide (Concurrent and/or sequential use with MAO inhibitors is not recommended).

No products indexed under this heading.

Molindone Hydrochloride (Concurrent use may increase drowsiness effect). Products include:

Moban 1320

Oxazepam (Concurrent use may increase drowsiness effect).

No products indexed under this heading.

Pargyline Hydrochloride (Concurrent and/or sequential use with MAO inhibitors is not recommended).

No products indexed under this heading.

Perphenazine (Concurrent use may increase drowsiness effect). Products include:

Etrafon 3115
Trilafon 3160

Phenelzine Sulfate (Concurrent and/or sequential use with MAO inhibitors is not recommended). Products include:

Nardil Tablets 2653

Prazepam (Concurrent use may increase drowsiness effect).

No products indexed under this heading.

Procarbazine Hydrochloride (Concurrent and/or sequential use with MAO inhibitors is not recommended). Products include:

Matulane Capsules 3246

Prochlorperazine (Concurrent use may increase drowsiness effect). Products include:

Compazine 1505

Promethazine Hydrochloride (Concurrent use may increase drowsiness effect). Products include:

Mepergan Injection 3539
Phenergan Injection 3553
Phenergan 3556
Phenergan Syrup 3554
Phenergan with Codeine Syrup 3557
Phenergan with Dextromethorphan Syrup 3559
Phenergan VC Syrup 3560
Phenergan VC with Codeine Syrup 3561

Propofol (Concurrent use may increase drowsiness effect). Products include:

Diprivan Injectable Emulsion 667

Quazepam (Concurrent use may increase drowsiness effect).

No products indexed under this heading.

Secobarbital Sodium (Concurrent use may increase drowsiness effect).

No products indexed under this heading.

Selegiline Hydrochloride (Concurrent and/or sequential use with MAO inhibitors is not recommended). Products include:

Eldepryl Capsules 3266

Temazepam (Concurrent use may increase drowsiness effect).

No products indexed under this heading.

Thioridazine Hydrochloride (Concurrent use may increase drowsiness effect). Products include:

Thioridazine Hydrochloride Tablets 2289

Thiothixene (Concurrent use may increase drowsiness effect). Products include:

Navane Capsules 2701
Thiothixene Capsules 2290

Tranylcypromine Sulfate (Concurrent and/or sequential use with MAO inhibitors is not recommended). Products include:

Parnate Tablets 1607

Triazolam (Concurrent use may increase drowsiness effect). Products include:

Halcion Tablets 2823

Trifluoperazine Hydrochloride (Concurrent use may increase drowsiness effect). Products include:

Stelazine 1640

Zaleplon (Concurrent use may increase drowsiness effect). Products include:

Sonata Capsules 3591

Zolpidem Tartrate (Concurrent use may increase drowsiness effect). Products include:

Ambien Tablets 3191

Food Interactions

Alcohol (Concurrent use may increase drowsiness effect; chronic heavy alcohol abusers, 3 or more drinks per day, may be at increased risk of liver toxicity from excessive acetaminophen use).

MAXIMUM STRENGTH TYLENOL FLU NIGHTTIME LIQUID

(Acetaminophen, Dextromethorphan Hydrobromide, Doxylamine Succinate, Pseudoephedrine Hydrochloride) 2011

See Maximum Strength Tylenol Flu Night-Time Gelcaps

MAXIMUM STRENGTH TYLENOL FLU NON-DROWSY GELCAPS

(Acetaminophen, Dextromethorphan Hydrobromide, Pseudoephedrine Hydrochloride) 2011

See Maximum Strength Tylenol Flu Night-Time Gelcaps

EXTRA STRENGTH TYLENOL PM CAPLETS, GELTABS, AND GELCAPS

(Acetaminophen, Diphenhydramine Hydrochloride) 2012

May interact with hypnotics and sedatives, tranquilizers, and certain other agents. Compounds in these categories include:

Alprazolam (Tylenol PM causes drowsiness; concurrent use may increase the drowsiness effect). Products include:

Xanax Tablets 2865

Buspirone Hydrochloride (Tylenol PM causes drowsiness; concurrent use may increase the drowsiness effect).

No products indexed under this heading.

Chlordiazepoxide (Tylenol PM causes drowsiness; concurrent use may increase the drowsiness effect). Products include:

Limbitrol 1738

Chlordiazepoxide Hydrochloride (Tylenol PM causes drowsiness; concurrent use may increase the drowsiness effect). Products include:

Librium Capsules 1736
Librium for Injection 1737

Chlorpromazine (Tylenol PM causes drowsiness; concurrent use may increase the drowsiness effect). Products include:

Thorazine Suppositories 1656

Chlorpromazine Hydrochloride (Tylenol PM causes drowsiness; concurrent use may increase the drowsiness effect). Products include:

Thorazine 1656

Chlorprothixene (Tylenol PM causes drowsiness; concurrent use may increase the drowsiness effect).

No products indexed under this heading.

Chlorprothixene Hydrochloride (Tylenol PM causes drowsiness; concurrent use may increase the drowsiness effect).

No products indexed under this heading.

Clorazepate Dipotassium (Tylenol PM causes drowsiness; concurrent use may increase the drowsiness effect). Products include:

Tranxene 511

Diazepam (Tylenol PM causes drowsiness; concurrent use may increase the drowsiness effect). Products include:

Valium Injectable 3026
Valium Tablets 3047

Droperidol (Tylenol PM causes drowsiness; concurrent use may increase the drowsiness effect).

No products indexed under this heading.

Estazolam (Tylenol PM causes drowsiness; concurrent use may increase the drowsiness effect). Products include:

ProSom Tablets 500

Ethchlorvynol (Tylenol PM causes drowsiness; concurrent use may increase the drowsiness effect).
No products indexed under this heading.

Ethinamate (Tylenol PM causes drowsiness; concurrent use may increase the drowsiness effect).
No products indexed under this heading.

Fluphenazine Decanoate (Tylenol PM causes drowsiness; concurrent use may increase the drowsiness effect).
No products indexed under this heading.

Fluphenazine Enanthate (Tylenol PM causes drowsiness; concurrent use may increase the drowsiness effect).
No products indexed under this heading.

Fluphenazine Hydrochloride (Tylenol PM causes drowsiness; concurrent use may increase the drowsiness effect).
No products indexed under this heading.

Flurazepam Hydrochloride (Tylenol PM causes drowsiness; concurrent use may increase the drowsiness effect).
No products indexed under this heading.

Glutethimide (Tylenol PM causes drowsiness; concurrent use may increase the drowsiness effect).
No products indexed under this heading.

Haloperidol (Tylenol PM causes drowsiness; concurrent use may increase the drowsiness effect). Products include:
Haldol Injection, Tablets and Concentrate 2533

Haloperidol Decanoate (Tylenol PM causes drowsiness; concurrent use may increase the drowsiness effect). Products include:
Haldol Decanoate 2535

Hydroxyzine Hydrochloride (Tylenol PM causes drowsiness; concurrent use may increase the drowsiness effect). Products include:
Atarax Tablets & Syrup 2667
Vistaril Intramuscular Solution 2738

Lorazepam (Tylenol PM causes drowsiness; concurrent use may increase the drowsiness effect). Products include:
Ativan Injection 3478
Ativan Tablets 3482

Loxapine Hydrochloride (Tylenol PM causes drowsiness; concurrent use may increase the drowsiness effect).
No products indexed under this heading.

Loxapine Succinate (Tylenol PM causes drowsiness; concurrent use may increase the drowsiness effect). Products include:
Loxitane Capsules 3398

Meprobamate (Tylenol PM causes drowsiness; concurrent use may increase the drowsiness effect). Products include:
Miltown Tablets 3349

Mesoridazine Besylate (Tylenol PM causes drowsiness; concurrent use may increase the drowsiness effect). Products include:
Serentil 1057

Midazolam Hydrochloride (Tylenol PM causes drowsiness; concurrent use may increase the drowsiness effect). Products include:
Versed Injection 3027
Versed Syrup 3033

Molindone Hydrochloride (Tylenol PM causes drowsiness; concurrent use may increase the drowsiness effect). Products include:
Moban 1320

Oxazepam (Tylenol PM causes drowsiness; concurrent use may increase the drowsiness effect).
No products indexed under this heading.

Perphenazine (Tylenol PM causes drowsiness; concurrent use may increase the drowsiness effect). Products include:
Etrafon 3115
Trilafon 3160

Prazepam (Tylenol PM causes drowsiness; concurrent use may increase the drowsiness effect).
No products indexed under this heading.

Prochlorperazine (Tylenol PM causes drowsiness; concurrent use may increase the drowsiness effect). Products include:
Compazine 1505

Promethazine Hydrochloride (Tylenol PM causes drowsiness; concurrent use may increase the drowsiness effect). Products include:
Mepergan Injection 3539
Phenergan Injection 3553
Phenergan 3556
Phenergan Syrup 3554
Phenergan with Codeine Syrup 3557
Phenergan with Dextromethorphan Syrup 3559
Phenergan VC Syrup 3560
Phenergan VC with Codeine Syrup 3561

Propofol (Tylenol PM causes drowsiness; concurrent use may increase the drowsiness effect). Products include:
Diprivan Injectable Emulsion 667

Quazepam (Tylenol PM causes drowsiness; concurrent use may increase the drowsiness effect).
No products indexed under this heading.

Secobarbital Sodium (Tylenol PM causes drowsiness; concurrent use may increase the drowsiness effect).
No products indexed under this heading.

Temazepam (Tylenol PM causes drowsiness; concurrent use may increase the drowsiness effect).
No products indexed under this heading.

Thioridazine Hydrochloride (Tylenol PM causes drowsiness; concurrent use may increase the drowsiness effect). Products include:
Thioridazine Hydrochloride Tablets 2289

Thiothixene (Tylenol PM causes drowsiness; concurrent use may increase the drowsiness effect). Products include:
Navane Capsules 2701
Thiothixene Capsules 2290

Triazolam (Tylenol PM causes drowsiness; concurrent use may increase the drowsiness effect). Products include:
Halcion Tablets 2823

Trifluoperazine Hydrochloride (Tylenol PM causes drowsiness; concurrent use may increase the drowsiness effect). Products include:
Stelazine 1640

Zaleplon (Tylenol PM causes drowsiness; concurrent use may increase the drowsiness effect). Products include:
Sonata Capsules 3591

Zolpidem Tartrate (Tylenol PM causes drowsiness; concurrent use may increase the drowsiness effect). Products include:
Ambien Tablets 3191

Food Interactions

Alcohol (Avoid concurrent use; chronic heavy alcohol abusers, 3 or more drinks per day, may be at increased risk of liver toxicity from acetaminophen use).

MAXIMUM STRENGTH TYLENOL SINUS NIGHTTIME CAPLETS

(Acetaminophen, Doxylamine Succinate, Pseudoephedrine Hydrochloride) 2012
May interact with hypnotics and sedatives, monoamine oxidase inhibitors, tranquilizers, and certain other agents. Compounds in these categories include:

Alprazolam (May increase drowsiness effect). Products include:
Xanax Tablets 2865

Buspirone Hydrochloride (May increase drowsiness effect).
No products indexed under this heading.

Chlordiazepoxide (May increase drowsiness effect). Products include:
Limbitrol 1738

Chlordiazepoxide Hydrochloride (May increase drowsiness effect). Products include:
Librium Capsules 1736
Librium for Injection 1737

Chlorpromazine (May increase drowsiness effect). Products include:
Thorazine Suppositories 1656

Chlorpromazine Hydrochloride (May increase drowsiness effect). Products include:
Thorazine 1656

Chlorprothixene (May increase drowsiness effect).
No products indexed under this heading.

Chlorprothixene Hydrochloride (May increase drowsiness effect).
No products indexed under this heading.

Clorazepate Dipotassium (May increase drowsiness effect). Products include:
Tranxene 511

Diazepam (May increase drowsiness effect). Products include:
Valium Injectable 3026
Valium Tablets 3047

Droperidol (May increase drowsiness effect).
No products indexed under this heading.

Estazolam (May increase drowsiness effect). Products include:
ProSom Tablets 500

Ethchlorvynol (May increase drowsiness effect).
No products indexed under this heading.

Ethinamate (May increase drowsiness effect).
No products indexed under this heading.

Fluphenazine Decanoate (May increase drowsiness effect).
No products indexed under this heading.

Fluphenazine Enanthate (May increase drowsiness effect).
No products indexed under this heading.

Fluphenazine Hydrochloride (May increase drowsiness effect).
No products indexed under this heading.

Flurazepam Hydrochloride (May increase drowsiness effect).
No products indexed under this heading.

Glutethimide (May increase drowsiness effect).
No products indexed under this heading.

Haloperidol (May increase drowsiness effect). Products include:
Haldol Injection, Tablets and Concentrate 2533

Haloperidol Decanoate (May increase drowsiness effect). Products include:
Haldol Decanoate 2535

Hydroxyzine Hydrochloride (May increase drowsiness effect). Products include:
Atarax Tablets & Syrup 2667
Vistaril Intramuscular Solution 2738

Isocarboxazid (Concurrent and/or sequential use with MAO inhibitors is not recommended).
No products indexed under this heading.

Lorazepam (May increase drowsiness effect). Products include:
Ativan Injection 3478
Ativan Tablets 3482

Loxapine Hydrochloride (May increase drowsiness effect).
No products indexed under this heading.

Loxapine Succinate (May increase drowsiness effect). Products include:
Loxitane Capsules 3398

Meprobamate (May increase drowsiness effect). Products include:
Miltown Tablets 3349

Mesoridazine Besylate (May increase drowsiness effect). Products include:
Serentil 1057

Midazolam Hydrochloride (May increase drowsiness effect). Products include:
Versed Injection 3027
Versed Syrup 3033

Moclobemide (Concurrent and/or sequential use with MAO inhibitors is not recommended).
No products indexed under this heading.

Molindone Hydrochloride (May increase drowsiness effect). Products include:
Moban 1320

Oxazepam (May increase drowsiness effect).
No products indexed under this heading.

Pargyline Hydrochloride (Concurrent and/or sequential use with MAO inhibitors is not recommended).
No products indexed under this heading.

Perphenazine (May increase drowsiness effect). Products include:
Etrafon 3115
Trilafon 3160

Phenelzine Sulfate (Concurrent and/or sequential use with MAO inhibitors is not recommended). Products include:
Nardil Tablets 2653

Prazepam (May increase drowsiness effect).
No products indexed under this heading.

Procarbazine Hydrochloride (Concurrent and/or sequential use with MAO inhibitors is not recommended). Products include:
Matulane Capsules 3246

Prochlorperazine (May increase drowsiness effect). Products include:
Compazine 1505

Promethazine Hydrochloride (May increase drowsiness effect). Products include:
Mepergan Injection 3539
Phenergan Injection 3553
Phenergan 3556
Phenergan Syrup 3554
Phenergan with Codeine Syrup 3557
Phenergan with Dextromethorphan Syrup 3559
Phenergan VC Syrup 3560
Phenergan VC with Codeine Syrup 3561

Propofol (May increase drowsiness effect). Products include:
Diprivan Injectable Emulsion 667

Quazepam (May increase drowsiness effect).
No products indexed under this heading.

Secobarbital Sodium (May increase drowsiness effect).
No products indexed under this heading.

Selegiline Hydrochloride (Concurrent and/or sequential use with MAO inhibitors is not recommended). Products include:
Eldepryl Capsules 3266

Temazepam (May increase drowsiness effect).
No products indexed under this heading.

Thioridazine Hydrochloride (May increase drowsiness effect). Products include:
Thioridazine Hydrochloride Tablets 2289

Thiothixene (May increase drowsiness effect). Products include:
Navane Capsules 2701
Thiothixene Capsules 2290

Tranylcypromine Sulfate (Concurrent and/or sequential use with MAO inhibitors is not recommended). Products include:
Parnate Tablets 1607

Triazolam (May increase drowsiness effect). Products include:
Halcion Tablets 2823

Trifluoperazine Hydrochloride (May increase drowsiness effect). Products include:
Stelazine 1640

Zaleplon (May increase drowsiness effect). Products include:
Sonata Capsules 3591

Zolpidem Tartrate (May increase drowsiness effect). Products include:
Ambien Tablets 3191

Food Interactions

Alcohol (Chronic heavy alcohol users, 3 or more drinks per day, are at increased risk of liver toxicity from excessive acetaminophen use; alcohol increases drowsiness effect and concurrent use of alcoholic beverages should be avoided).

MAXIMUM STRENGTH TYLENOL SINUS NON-DROWSY GELTABS, GELCAPS, CAPLETS, AND TABLETS

(Acetaminophen, Pseudoephedrine Hydrochloride) 2012
See Maximum Strength Tylenol Sinus Night-Time Caplets

MAXIMUM STRENGTH TYLENOL SORE THROAT ADULT LIQUID

(Acetaminophen) 2013
See Regular Strength Tylenol Tablets

TYLENOL WITH CODEINE ELIXIR

(Acetaminophen, Codeine Phosphate) 2595
May interact with anticholinergics and central nervous system depressants. Compounds in these categories include:

Alfentanil Hydrochloride (Co-administration with other CNS depressants may exhibit an additive CNS depression).
No products indexed under this heading.

Alprazolam (Co-administration with other CNS depressants may exhibit an additive CNS depression). Products include:
Xanax Tablets 2865

Aprobarbital (Co-administration with other CNS depressants may exhibit an additive CNS depression).
No products indexed under this heading.

Atropine Sulfate (Co-administration of codeine with anticholinergics may produce paralytic ileus). Products include:
Donnatal 2929
Donnatal Extentabs 2930
Motofen Tablets 577
Prosed/DS Tablets 3268
Urised Tablets 2876

Belladonna Alkaloids (Co-administration of codeine with anticholinergics may produce paralytic ileus). Products include:
Hyland's Teething Tablets 766
Urimax Tablets 1769

Benztropine Mesylate (Co-administration of codeine with anticholinergics may produce paralytic ileus). Products include:
Cogentin 2055

Biperiden Hydrochloride (Co-administration of codeine with anticholinergics may produce paralytic ileus). Products include:
Akineton 402

Buprenorphine Hydrochloride (Co-administration with other CNS depressants may exhibit an additive CNS depression). Products include:
Buprenex Injectable 2918

Buspirone Hydrochloride (Co-administration with other CNS depressants may exhibit an additive CNS depression).
No products indexed under this heading.

Butabarbital (Co-administration with other CNS depressants may exhibit an additive CNS depression).
No products indexed under this heading.

Butalbital (Co-administration with other CNS depressants may exhibit an additive CNS depression). Products include:
Phrenilin 578
Sedapap Tablets 50 mg/650 mg 2225

Chlordiazepoxide (Co-administration with other CNS depressants may exhibit an additive CNS depression). Products include:
Limbitrol 1738

Chlordiazepoxide Hydrochloride (Co-administration with other CNS depressants may exhibit an additive CNS depression). Products include:
Librium Capsules 1736
Librium for Injection 1737

Chlorpromazine (Co-administration with other CNS depressants may exhibit an additive CNS depression). Products include:
Thorazine Suppositories 1656

Chlorpromazine Hydrochloride (Co-administration with other CNS depressants may exhibit an additive CNS depression). Products include:
Thorazine 1656

Chlorprothixene (Co-administration with other CNS depressants may exhibit an additive CNS depression).
No products indexed under this heading.

Chlorprothixene Hydrochloride (Co-administration with other CNS depressants may exhibit an additive CNS depression).
No products indexed under this heading.

Chlorprothixene Lactate (Co-administration with other CNS depressants may exhibit an additive CNS depression).
No products indexed under this heading.

Clidinium Bromide (Co-administration of codeine with anticholinergics may produce paralytic ileus).
No products indexed under this heading.

Clorazepate Dipotassium (Co-administration with other CNS depressants may exhibit an additive CNS depression). Products include:
Tranxene 511

Clozapine (Co-administration with other CNS depressants may exhibit an additive CNS depression). Products include:
Clozaril Tablets 2319

Desflurane (Co-administration with other CNS depressants may exhibit an additive CNS depression). Products include:
Suprane Liquid for Inhalation 874

Dezocine (Co-administration with other CNS depressants may exhibit an additive CNS depression).
No products indexed under this heading.

Diazepam (Co-administration with other CNS depressants may exhibit an additive CNS depression). Products include:
Valium Injectable 3026
Valium Tablets 3047

Dicyclomine Hydrochloride (Co-administration of codeine with anticholinergics may produce paralytic ileus).
No products indexed under this heading.

Droperidol (Co-administration with other CNS depressants may exhibit an additive CNS depression).
No products indexed under this heading.

Enflurane (Co-administration with other CNS depressants may exhibit an additive CNS depression).
No products indexed under this heading.

Estazolam (Co-administration with other CNS depressants may exhibit an additive CNS depression). Products include:
ProSom Tablets 500

Ethchlorvynol (Co-administration with other CNS depressants may exhibit an additive CNS depression).
No products indexed under this heading.

Ethinamate (Co-administration with other CNS depressants may exhibit an additive CNS depression).
No products indexed under this heading.

Fentanyl (Co-administration with other CNS depressants may exhibit an additive CNS depression). Products include:
Duragesic Transdermal System 1786

Fentanyl Citrate (Co-administration with other CNS depressants may exhibit an additive CNS depression). Products include:
Actiq 1184

Fluphenazine Decanoate (Co-administration with other CNS depressants may exhibit an additive CNS depression).
No products indexed under this heading.

Fluphenazine Enanthate (Co-administration with other CNS depressants may exhibit an additive CNS depression).
No products indexed under this heading.

Fluphenazine Hydrochloride (Co-administration with other CNS depressants may exhibit an additive CNS depression).
No products indexed under this heading.

Flurazepam Hydrochloride (Co-administration with other CNS depressants may exhibit an additive CNS depression).
No products indexed under this heading.

Glutethimide (Co-administration with other CNS depressants may exhibit an additive CNS depression).
No products indexed under this heading.

Glycopyrrolate (Co-administration of codeine with anticholinergics may produce paralytic ileus). Products include:
Robinul Forte Tablets 1358
Robinul Injectable 2940
Robinul Tablets 1358

Haloperidol (Co-administration with other CNS depressants may exhibit an additive CNS depression). Products include:
Haldol Injection, Tablets and Concentrate 2533

Haloperidol Decanoate (Co-administration with other CNS depressants may exhibit an additive CNS depression). Products include:
Haldol Decanoate 2535

Hydrocodone Bitartrate (Co-administration with other CNS depressants may exhibit an additive CNS depression). Products include:
Hycodan 1316
Hycomine Compound Tablets 1317
Hycotuss Expectorant Syrup 1318
Lortab 3319
Lortab Elixir 3317
Maxidone Tablets CIII 3399
Norco 5/325 Tablets CIII 3424
Norco 7.5/325 Tablets CIII 3425
Norco 10/325 Tablets CIII 3427
Norco 10/325 Tablets CIII 3425
Vicodin Tablets 516
Vicodin ES Tablets 517
Vicodin HP Tablets 518
Vicodin Tuss Expectorant 519
Vicoprofen Tablets 520
Zydone Tablets 1330

Hydrocodone Polistirex (Co-administration with other CNS depressants may exhibit an additive CNS depression). Products include:
Tussionex Pennkinetic Extended-Release Suspension 1174

Hydromorphone Hydrochloride (Co-administration with other CNS depressants may exhibit an additive CNS depression). Products include:
Dilaudid 441
Dilaudid Oral Liquid 445
Dilaudid Powder 441
Dilaudid Rectal Suppositories 441
Dilaudid Tablets 441
Dilaudid Tablets - 8 mg 445
Dilaudid-HP 443

Hydroxyzine Hydrochloride (Co-administration with other CNS depressants may exhibit an additive CNS depression). Products include:
Atarax Tablets & Syrup 2667
Vistaril Intramuscular Solution 2738

Hyoscyamine (Co-administration of codeine with anticholinergics may produce paralytic ileus). Products include:
Urised Tablets 2876

Hyoscyamine Sulfate (Co-administration of codeine with anticholinergics may produce paralytic ileus). Products include:
Arco-Lase Plus Tablets 592
Donnatal 2929
Donnatal Extentabs 2930
Levsin/Levsinex/Levbid 3172
NuLev Orally Disintegrating Tablets 3176
Prosed/DS Tablets 3268
Urimax Tablets 1769

Ipratropium Bromide (Co-administration of codeine with anticholinergics may produce paralytic ileus). Products include:
Atrovent Inhalation Aerosol 1030
Atrovent Inhalation Solution 1031
Atrovent Nasal Spray 0.03% 1032
Atrovent Nasal Spray 0.06% 1033
Combivent Inhalation Aerosol 1041
DuoNeb Inhalation Solution 1233

Isoflurane (Co-administration with other CNS depressants may exhibit an additive CNS depression).
No products indexed under this heading.

Ketamine Hydrochloride (Co-administration with other CNS depressants may exhibit an additive

CNS depression).
No products indexed under this heading.

Levomethadyl Acetate Hydrochloride (Co-administration with other CNS depressants may exhibit an additive CNS depression).
No products indexed under this heading.

Levorphanol Tartrate (Co-administration with other CNS depressants may exhibit an additive CNS depression). Products include:
Levo-Dromoran 1734
Levorphanol Tartrate Tablets 3059

Lorazepam (Co-administration with other CNS depressants may exhibit an additive CNS depression). Products include:
Ativan Injection 3478
Ativan Tablets 3482

Loxapine Hydrochloride (Co-administration with other CNS depressants may exhibit an additive CNS depression).
No products indexed under this heading.

Loxapine Succinate (Co-administration with other CNS depressants may exhibit an additive CNS depression). Products include:
Loxitane Capsules 3398

Mepenzolate Bromide (Co-administration of codeine with anticholinergics may produce paralytic ileus).
No products indexed under this heading.

Meperidine Hydrochloride (Co-administration with other CNS depressants may exhibit an additive CNS depression). Products include:
Demerol 3079
Mepergan Injection 3539

Mephobarbital (Co-administration with other CNS depressants may exhibit an additive CNS depression).
No products indexed under this heading.

Meprobamate (Co-administration with other CNS depressants may exhibit an additive CNS depression). Products include:
Miltown Tablets 3349

Mesoridazine Besylate (Co-administration with other CNS depressants may exhibit an additive CNS depression). Products include:
Serentil 1057

Methadone Hydrochloride (Co-administration with other CNS depressants may exhibit an additive CNS depression). Products include:
Dolophine Hydrochloride Tablets 3056

Methohexital Sodium (Co-administration with other CNS depressants may exhibit an additive CNS depression). Products include:
Brevital Sodium for Injection, USP .. 1815

Methotrimeprazine (Co-administration with other CNS depressants may exhibit an additive CNS depression).
No products indexed under this heading.

Methoxyflurane (Co-administration with other CNS depressants may exhibit an additive CNS depression).
No products indexed under this heading.

Midazolam Hydrochloride (Co-administration with other CNS depressants may exhibit an additive CNS depression). Products include:
Versed Injection 3027
Versed Syrup 3033

Molindone Hydrochloride (Co-administration with other CNS depressants may exhibit an additive CNS depression). Products include:
Moban 1320

Morphine Sulfate (Co-administration with other CNS depressants may exhibit an additive CNS depression). Products include:
Astramorph/PF Injection, USP (Preservative-Free) 594
Duramorph Injection 1312
Infumorph 200 and Infumorph 500 Sterile Solutions 1314
Kadian Capsules 1335
MS Contin Tablets 2896
MSIR 2898
Oramorph SR Tablets 3062
Roxanol 3066

Olanzapine (Co-administration with other CNS depressants may exhibit an additive CNS depression). Products include:
Zyprexa Tablets 1973
Zyprexa ZYDIS Orally Disintegrating Tablets 1973

Oxazepam (Co-administration with other CNS depressants may exhibit an additive CNS depression).
No products indexed under this heading.

Oxybutynin Chloride (Co-administration of codeine with anticholinergics may produce paralytic ileus). Products include:
Ditropan XL Extended Release Tablets 564

Oxycodone Hydrochloride (Co-administration with other CNS depressants may exhibit an additive CNS depression). Products include:
OxyContin Tablets 2912
OxyFast Oral Concentrate Solution . 2916
OxyIR Capsules 2916
Percocet Tablets 1326
Percodan Tablets 1327
Percolone Tablets 1327
Roxicodone 3067
Tylox Capsules 2597

Pentobarbital Sodium (Co-administration with other CNS depressants may exhibit an additive CNS depression). Products include:
Nembutal Sodium Solution 485

Perphenazine (Co-administration with other CNS depressants may exhibit an additive CNS depression). Products include:
Etrafon 3115
Trilafon 3160

Phenobarbital (Co-administration with other CNS depressants may exhibit an additive CNS depression). Products include:
Arco-Lase Plus Tablets 592
Donnatal 2929
Donnatal Extentabs 2930

Prazepam (Co-administration with other CNS depressants may exhibit an additive CNS depression).
No products indexed under this heading.

Prochlorperazine (Co-administration with other CNS depressants may exhibit an additive CNS depression). Products include:
Compazine 1505

Procyclidine Hydrochloride (Co-administration of codeine with anticholinergics may produce paralytic ileus).
No products indexed under this heading.

Promethazine Hydrochloride (Co-administration with other CNS depressants may exhibit an additive CNS depression). Products include:
Mepergan Injection 3539
Phenergan Injection 3553
Phenergan 3556
Phenergan Syrup 3554
Phenergan with Codeine Syrup 3557
Phenergan with Dextromethorphan Syrup 3559
Phenergan VC Syrup 3560
Phenergan VC with Codeine Syrup .. 3561

Propantheline Bromide (Co-administration of codeine with anticholinergics may produce paralytic ileus).
No products indexed under this heading.

Propofol (Co-administration with other CNS depressants may exhibit an additive CNS depression). Products include:
Diprivan Injectable Emulsion 667

Propoxyphene Hydrochloride (Co-administration with other CNS depressants may exhibit an additive CNS depression). Products include:
Darvon Pulvules 1909
Darvon Compound-65 Pulvules 1910

Propoxyphene Napsylate (Co-administration with other CNS depressants may exhibit an additive CNS depression). Products include:
Darvon-N/Darvocet-N 1907
Darvon-N Tablets 1912

Quazepam (Co-administration with other CNS depressants may exhibit an additive CNS depression).
No products indexed under this heading.

Quetiapine Fumarate (Co-administration with other CNS depressants may exhibit an additive CNS depression). Products include:
Seroquel Tablets 684

Remifentanil Hydrochloride (Co-administration with other CNS depressants may exhibit an additive CNS depression).
No products indexed under this heading.

Risperidone (Co-administration with other CNS depressants may exhibit an additive CNS depression). Products include:
Risperdal 1796

Scopolamine (Co-administration of codeine with anticholinergics may produce paralytic ileus). Products include:
Transderm Scōp Transdermal Therapeutic System 2302

Scopolamine Hydrobromide (Co-administration of codeine with anticholinergics may produce paralytic ileus). Products include:
Donnatal 2929
Donnatal Extentabs 2930

Secobarbital Sodium (Co-administration with other CNS depressants may exhibit an additive CNS depression).
No products indexed under this heading.

Sevoflurane (Co-administration with other CNS depressants may exhibit an additive CNS depression).
No products indexed under this heading.

Sufentanil Citrate (Co-administration with other CNS depressants may exhibit an additive CNS depression).
No products indexed under this heading.

Temazepam (Co-administration with other CNS depressants may exhibit an additive CNS depression).
No products indexed under this heading.

Thiamylal Sodium (Co-administration with other CNS depressants may exhibit an additive CNS depression).
No products indexed under this heading.

Thioridazine Hydrochloride (Co-administration with other CNS depressants may exhibit an additive CNS depression). Products include:
Thioridazine Hydrochloride Tablets 2289

Thiothixene (Co-administration with other CNS depressants may exhibit an additive CNS depression). Products include:
Navane Capsules 2701
Thiothixene Capsules 2290

Tolterodine Tartrate (Co-administration of codeine with anticholinergics may produce paralytic ileus). Products include:
Detrol Tablets 3623
Detrol LA Capsules 2801

Triazolam (Co-administration with other CNS depressants may exhibit an additive CNS depression). Products include:
Halcion Tablets 2823

Tridihexethyl Chloride (Co-administration of codeine with anticholinergics may produce paralytic ileus).
No products indexed under this heading.

Trifluoperazine Hydrochloride (Co-administration with other CNS depressants may exhibit an additive CNS depression). Products include:
Stelazine 1640

Trihexyphenidyl Hydrochloride (Co-administration of codeine with anticholinergics may produce paralytic ileus). Products include:
Artane 1855

Zaleplon (Co-administration with other CNS depressants may exhibit an additive CNS depression). Products include:
Sonata Capsules 3591

Ziprasidone Hydrochloride (Co-administration with other CNS depressants may exhibit an additive CNS depression). Products include:
Geodon Capsules 2688

Zolpidem Tartrate (Co-administration with other CNS depressants may exhibit an additive CNS depression). Products include:
Ambien Tablets 3191

Food Interactions

Alcohol (Concurrent use with other CNS depressants may exhibit an additive CNS depression).

TYLENOL WITH CODEINE TABLETS
(Acetaminophen, Codeine Phosphate) 2595
See Tylenol with Codeine Elixir

WOMEN'S TYLENOL MENSTRUAL RELIEF CAPLETS
(Acetaminophen, Pamabrom) 2013
May interact with:

Food Interactions

Alcohol (Chronic heavy alcohol users, 3 or more drinks per day, should consult their physicians for advice on when and how they should take pain relievers, including acetaminophen).

MAXIMUM STRENGTH TYLENOL SINUS NIGHTTIME CAPLETS
(Acetaminophen, Doxylamine Succinate, Pseudoephedrine Hydrochloride) .... ▣655

TYLOX CAPSULES
(Acetaminophen, Oxycodone Hydrochloride) 2597
May interact with anticholinergics, central nervous system depressants, general anesthetics, hypnotics and sedatives, narcotic analgesics, antipsychotic agents, phenothiazines, tranquilizers, and certain other agents. Compounds in these categories include:

Alfentanil Hydrochloride (Additive CNS depression).
No products indexed under this heading.

Alprazolam (Additive CNS depression). Products include:
Xanax Tablets 2865

Aprobarbital (Additive CNS depression).
No products indexed under this heading.

Atropine Sulfate (May produce paralytic ileus). Products include:
Donnatal 2929
Donnatal Extentabs 2930
Motofen Tablets 577
Prosed/DS Tablets 3268
Urised Tablets 2876

Belladonna Alkaloids (May produce paralytic ileus). Products include:
Hyland's Teething Tablets 766
Urimax Tablets 1769

Benztropine Mesylate (May produce paralytic ileus). Products include:
Cogentin 2055

Biperiden Hydrochloride (May produce paralytic ileus). Products include:
Akineton 402

Buprenorphine Hydrochloride (Additive CNS depression). Products include:
Buprenex Injectable 2918

Buspirone Hydrochloride (Additive CNS depression).
No products indexed under this heading.

Butabarbital (Additive CNS depression).
No products indexed under this heading.

Butalbital (Additive CNS depression). Products include:
Phrenilin 578
Sedapap Tablets 50 mg/650 mg 2225

Chlordiazepoxide (Additive CNS depression). Products include:
Limbitrol 1738

Chlordiazepoxide Hydrochloride (Additive CNS depression). Products include:
Librium Capsules 1736
Librium for Injection 1737

Chlorpromazine (Additive CNS depression). Products include:
Thorazine Suppositories 1656

Chlorpromazine Hydrochloride (Additive CNS depression). Products include:
Thorazine 1656

Chlorprothixene (Additive CNS depression).
No products indexed under this heading.

Chlorprothixene Hydrochloride (Additive CNS depression).
No products indexed under this heading.

Chlorprothixene Lactate (Additive CNS depression).
No products indexed under this heading.

Clidinium Bromide (May produce paralytic ileus).
No products indexed under this heading.

Clorazepate Dipotassium (Additive CNS depression). Products include:
Tranxene 511

Clozapine (Additive CNS depression). Products include:
Clozaril Tablets 2319

Codeine Phosphate (Additive CNS depression). Products include:
Phenergan with Codeine Syrup 3557
Phenergan VC with Codeine Syrup 3561
Robitussin A-C Syrup 2942
Robitussin-DAC Syrup 2942
Ryna-C Liquid 768
Soma Compound w/Codeine Tablets 3355
Tussi-Organidin NR Liquid 3350
Tussi-Organidin-S NR Liquid 3350
Tylenol with Codeine 2595

Desflurane (Additive CNS depression). Products include:
Suprane Liquid for Inhalation 874

Dezocine (Additive CNS depression).
No products indexed under this heading.

Diazepam (Additive CNS depression). Products include:
Valium Injectable 3026
Valium Tablets 3047

Dicyclomine Hydrochloride (May produce paralytic ileus).
No products indexed under this heading.

Droperidol (Additive CNS depression).
No products indexed under this heading.

Enflurane (Additive CNS depression).
No products indexed under this heading.

Estazolam (Additive CNS depression). Products include:
ProSom Tablets 500

Ethchlorvynol (Additive CNS depression).
No products indexed under this heading.

Ethinamate (Additive CNS depression).
No products indexed under this heading.

Fentanyl (Additive CNS depression). Products include:
Duragesic Transdermal System 1786

Fentanyl Citrate (Additive CNS depression). Products include:
Actiq 1184

Fluphenazine Decanoate (Additive CNS depression).
No products indexed under this heading.

Fluphenazine Enanthate (Additive CNS depression).
No products indexed under this heading.

Fluphenazine Hydrochloride (Additive CNS depression).
No products indexed under this heading.

Flurazepam Hydrochloride (Additive CNS depression).
No products indexed under this heading.

Glutethimide (Additive CNS depression).
No products indexed under this heading.

Glycopyrrolate (May produce paralytic ileus). Products include:
Robinul Forte Tablets 1358
Robinul Injectable 2940
Robinul Tablets 1358

Haloperidol (Additive CNS depression). Products include:
Haldol Injection, Tablets and Concentrate 2533

Haloperidol Decanoate (Additive CNS depression). Products include:
Haldol Decanoate 2535

Hydrocodone Bitartrate (Additive CNS depression). Products include:
Hycodan 1316
Hycomine Compound Tablets 1317
Hycotuss Expectorant Syrup 1318
Lortab 3319
Lortab Elixir 3317
Maxidone Tablets CIII 3399
Norco 5/325 Tablets CIII 3424
Norco 7.5/325 Tablets CIII 3425
Norco 10/325 Tablets CIII 3427
Norco 10/325 Tablets CIII 3425
Vicodin Tablets 516
Vicodin ES Tablets 517
Vicodin HP Tablets 518
Vicodin Tuss Expectorant 519
Vicoprofen Tablets 520
Zydone Tablets 1330

Hydrocodone Polistirex (Additive CNS depression). Products include:
Tussionex Pennkinetic Extended-Release Suspension 1174

Hydromorphone Hydrochloride (Additive CNS depression). Products include:
Dilaudid 441
Dilaudid Oral Liquid 445
Dilaudid Powder 441
Dilaudid Rectal Suppositories 441
Dilaudid Tablets 441
Dilaudid Tablets - 8 mg 445
Dilaudid-HP 443

Hydroxyzine Hydrochloride (Additive CNS depression). Products include:
Atarax Tablets & Syrup 2667
Vistaril Intramuscular Solution 2738

Hyoscyamine (May produce paralytic ileus). Products include:
Urised Tablets 2876

Hyoscyamine Sulfate (May produce paralytic ileus). Products include:
Arco-Lase Plus Tablets 592
Donnatal 2929
Donnatal Extentabs 2930
Levsin/Levsinex/Levbid 3172
NuLev Orally Disintegrating Tablets 3176
Prosed/DS Tablets 3268
Urimax Tablets 1769

Ipratropium Bromide (May produce paralytic ileus). Products include:
Atrovent Inhalation Aerosol 1030
Atrovent Inhalation Solution 1031
Atrovent Nasal Spray 0.03% 1032
Atrovent Nasal Spray 0.06% 1033
Combivent Inhalation Aerosol 1041
DuoNeb Inhalation Solution 1233

Isoflurane (Additive CNS depression).
No products indexed under this heading.

Ketamine Hydrochloride (Additive CNS depression).
No products indexed under this heading.

Levomethadyl Acetate Hydrochloride (Additive CNS depression).
No products indexed under this heading.

Levorphanol Tartrate (Additive CNS depression). Products include:
Levo-Dromoran 1734
Levorphanol Tartrate Tablets 3059

Lithium Carbonate (Additive CNS depression). Products include:
Eskalith 1527
Lithium Carbonate 3061
Lithobid Slow-Release Tablets 3255

Lithium Citrate (Additive CNS depression). Products include:
Lithium Citrate Syrup 3061

Lorazepam (Additive CNS depression). Products include:
Ativan Injection 3478
Ativan Tablets 3482

Loxapine Hydrochloride (Additive CNS depression).
No products indexed under this heading.

Loxapine Succinate (Additive CNS depression). Products include:
Loxitane Capsules 3398

Mepenzolate Bromide (May produce paralytic ileus).
No products indexed under this heading.

Meperidine Hydrochloride (Additive CNS depression). Products include:
Demerol 3079
Mepergan Injection 3539

Mephobarbital (Additive CNS depression).
No products indexed under this heading.

Meprobamate (Additive CNS depression). Products include:
Miltown Tablets 3349

Mesoridazine Besylate (Additive CNS depression). Products include:
Serentil 1057

Methadone Hydrochloride (Additive CNS depression). Products include:
Dolophine Hydrochloride Tablets 3056

Methohexital Sodium (Additive CNS depression). Products include:
Brevital Sodium for Injection, USP 1815

Methotrimeprazine (Additive CNS depression).
No products indexed under this heading.

Methoxyflurane (Additive CNS depression).
No products indexed under this heading.

Midazolam Hydrochloride (Additive CNS depression). Products include:
Versed Injection 3027
Versed Syrup 3033

Molindone Hydrochloride (Additive CNS depression). Products include:
Moban 1320

Morphine Sulfate (Additive CNS depression). Products include:
Astramorph/PF Injection, USP (Preservative-Free) 594
Duramorph Injection 1312
Infumorph 200 and Infumorph 500 Sterile Solutions 1314
Kadian Capsules 1335
MS Contin Tablets 2896
MSIR 2898
Oramorph SR Tablets 3062
Roxanol 3066

Olanzapine (Additive CNS depression). Products include:
Zyprexa Tablets 1973
Zyprexa ZYDIS Orally Disintegrating Tablets 1973

Oxazepam (Additive CNS depression).
No products indexed under this heading.

Oxybutynin Chloride (May produce paralytic ileus). Products include:
Ditropan XL Extended Release Tablets 564

Pentobarbital Sodium (Additive CNS depression). Products include:
Nembutal Sodium Solution 485

Perphenazine (Additive CNS depression). Products include:
Etrafon 3115
Trilafon 3160

Phenobarbital (Additive CNS depression). Products include:
Arco-Lase Plus Tablets 592
Donnatal 2929
Donnatal Extentabs 2930

Pimozide (Additive CNS depression). Products include:
Orap Tablets 1407

Prazepam (Additive CNS depression).
No products indexed under this heading.

Prochlorperazine (Additive CNS depression). Products include:
Compazine 1505

Procyclidine Hydrochloride (May produce paralytic ileus).
No products indexed under this heading.

Promethazine Hydrochloride (Additive CNS depression). Products include:
Mepergan Injection 3539
Phenergan Injection 3553
Phenergan 3556
Phenergan Syrup 3554
Phenergan with Codeine Syrup 3557
Phenergan with Dextromethorphan Syrup 3559
Phenergan VC Syrup 3560
Phenergan VC with Codeine Syrup 3561

Propantheline Bromide (May produce paralytic ileus).
No products indexed under this heading.

Propofol (Additive CNS depression). Products include:
Diprivan Injectable Emulsion 667

Propoxyphene Hydrochloride (Additive CNS depression). Products include:
Darvon Pulvules 1909
Darvon Compound-65 Pulvules 1910

IMPORTANT NOTE: Always consult each drug listing in the patient's regimen for possible interactions.

Propoxyphene Napsylate (Additive CNS depression). Products include:
- Darvon-N/Darvocet-N 1907
- Darvon-N Tablets 1912

Quazepam (Additive CNS depression).
No products indexed under this heading.

Quetiapine Fumarate (Additive CNS depression). Products include:
- Seroquel Tablets 684

Remifentanil Hydrochloride (Additive CNS depression).
No products indexed under this heading.

Risperidone (Additive CNS depression). Products include:
- Risperdal 1796

Scopolamine (May produce paralytic ileus). Products include:
- Transderm Scōp Transdermal Therapeutic System 2302

Scopolamine Hydrobromide (May produce paralytic ileus). Products include:
- Donnatal 2929
- Donnatal Extentabs 2930

Secobarbital Sodium (Additive CNS depression).
No products indexed under this heading.

Sevoflurane (Additive CNS depression).
No products indexed under this heading.

Sufentanil Citrate (Additive CNS depression).
No products indexed under this heading.

Temazepam (Additive CNS depression).
No products indexed under this heading.

Thiamylal Sodium (Additive CNS depression).
No products indexed under this heading.

Thioridazine Hydrochloride (Additive CNS depression). Products include:
- Thioridazine Hydrochloride Tablets 2289

Thiothixene (Additive CNS depression). Products include:
- Navane Capsules 2701
- Thiothixene Capsules 2290

Tolterodine Tartrate (May produce paralytic ileus). Products include:
- Detrol Tablets 3623
- Detrol LA Capsules 2801

Triazolam (Additive CNS depression). Products include:
- Halcion Tablets 2823

Tridihexethyl Chloride (May produce paralytic ileus).
No products indexed under this heading.

Trifluoperazine Hydrochloride (Additive CNS depression). Products include:
- Stelazine 1640

Trihexyphenidyl Hydrochloride (May produce paralytic ileus). Products include:
- Artane 1855

Zaleplon (Additive CNS depression). Products include:
- Sonata Capsules 3591

Ziprasidone Hydrochloride (Additive CNS depression). Products include:
- Geodon Capsules 2688

Zolpidem Tartrate (Additive CNS depression). Products include:
- Ambien Tablets 3191

Food Interactions

Alcohol (Additive CNS depression).

TYPHIM VI VACCINE

(Typhoid Vi Polysaccharide Vaccine) 825

May interact with alkylating agents, anticoagulants, corticosteroids, and immunosuppressive agents. Compounds in these categories include:

Ardeparin Sodium (Typhim VI should be given with caution to individuals on anticoagulant therapy).
No products indexed under this heading.

Azathioprine (The expected immune response may not be obtained in individuals whose immune system has been compromised by treatment with corticosteroids).
No products indexed under this heading.

Basiliximab (The expected immune response may not be obtained in individuals whose immune system has been compromised by treatment with corticosteroids). Products include:
- Simulect for Injection 2399

Betamethasone Acetate (The expected immune response may not be obtained in individuals whose immune system has been compromised by treatment with corticosteroids). Products include:
- Celestone Soluspan Injectable Suspension 3097

Betamethasone Sodium Phosphate (The expected immune response may not be obtained in individuals whose immune system has been compromised by treatment with corticosteroids). Products include:
- Celestone Soluspan Injectable Suspension 3097

Busulfan (The expected immune response may not be obtained in individuals whose immune system has been compromised by treatment with alkylating drugs). Products include:
- Myleran Tablets 1603

Carmustine (BCNU) (The expected immune response may not be obtained in individuals whose immune system has been compromised by treatment with alkylating drugs). Products include:
- Gliadel Wafer 1723

Chlorambucil (The expected immune response may not be obtained in individuals whose immune system has been compromised by treatment with alkylating drugs). Products include:
- Leukeran Tablets 1591

Cortisone Acetate (The expected immune response may not be obtained in individuals whose immune system has been compromised by treatment with corticosteroids). Products include:
- Cortone Acetate Injectable Suspension 2059
- Cortone Acetate Tablets 2061

Cyclophosphamide (The expected immune response may not be obtained in individuals whose immune system has been compromised by treatment with alkylating drugs).
No products indexed under this heading.

Cyclosporine (The expected immune response may not be obtained in individuals whose immune system has been compromised by treatment with corticosteroids). Products include:
- Gengraf Capsules 457
- Neoral Soft Gelatin Capsules 2380
- Neoral Oral Solution 2380
- Sandimmune 2388

Dacarbazine (The expected immune response may not be obtained in individuals whose immune system has been compromised by treatment with alkylating drugs). Products include:
- DTIC-Dome 902

Dalteparin Sodium (Typhim VI should be given with caution to individuals on anticoagulant therapy). Products include:
- Fragmin Injection 2814

Danaparoid Sodium (Typhim VI should be given with caution to individuals on anticoagulant therapy). Products include:
- Orgaran Injection 2480

Dexamethasone (The expected immune response may not be obtained in individuals whose immune system has been compromised by treatment with corticosteroids). Products include:
- Decadron Elixir 2078
- Decadron Tablets 2079
- TobraDex Ophthalmic Ointment 542
- TobraDex Ophthalmic Suspension 541

Dexamethasone Acetate (The expected immune response may not be obtained in individuals whose immune system has been compromised by treatment with corticosteroids).
No products indexed under this heading.

Dexamethasone Sodium Phosphate (The expected immune response may not be obtained in individuals whose immune system has been compromised by treatment with corticosteroids). Products include:
- Decadron Phosphate Injection 2081
- Decadron Phosphate Sterile Ophthalmic Ointment 2083
- Decadron Phosphate Sterile Ophthalmic Solution 2084
- NeoDecadron Sterile Ophthalmic Solution 2144

Dicumarol (Typhim VI should be given with caution to individuals on anticoagulant therapy).
No products indexed under this heading.

Enoxaparin (Typhim VI should be given with caution to individuals on anticoagulant therapy). Products include:
- Lovenox Injection 746

Fludrocortisone Acetate (The expected immune response may not be obtained in individuals whose immune system has been compromised by treatment with corticosteroids). Products include:
- Florinef Acetate Tablets 2250

Heparin Sodium (Typhim VI should be given with caution to individuals on anticoagulant therapy). Products include:
- Heparin Lock Flush Solution 3509
- Heparin Sodium Injection 3511

Hydrocortisone (The expected immune response may not be obtained in individuals whose immune system has been compromised by treatment with corticosteroids). Products include:
- Anusol-HC Cream 2.5% 2237
- Cipro HC Otic Suspension 540
- Cortaid Intensive Therapy Cream .... ■717
- Cortaid Maximum Strength Cream .... ■717
- Cortisporin Ophthalmic Suspension Sterile .... ⊙297
- Cortizone•5 .... ■699
- Cortizone•10 .... ■699
- Cortizone•10 Plus Creme .... ■700
- Cortizone for Kids Creme .... ■699
- Hydrocortone Tablets 2106
- Massengill Medicated Soft Cloth Towelette .... ■753
- VōSoL HC Otic Solution 3356

Hydrocortisone Acetate (The expected immune response may not be obtained in individuals whose immune system has been compromised by treatment with corticosteroids). Products include:
- Analpram-HC 1338
- Anusol HC-1 Hydrocortisone Anti-Itch Cream .... ■689
- Anusol-HC Suppositories 2238
- Cortaid .... ■717
- Cortifoam Rectal Foam 3170
- Cortisporin-TC Otic Suspension 2246
- Hydrocortone Acetate Injectable Suspension 2103
- Pramosone 1343
- Proctocort Suppositories 2264
- ProctoFoam-HC 3177
- Terra-Cortril Ophthalmic Suspension 2716

Hydrocortisone Sodium Phosphate (The expected immune response may not be obtained in individuals whose immune system has been compromised by treatment with corticosteroids). Products include:
- Hydrocortone Phosphate Injection, Sterile 2105

Hydrocortisone Sodium Succinate (The expected immune response may not be obtained in individuals whose immune system has been compromised by treatment with corticosteroids).
No products indexed under this heading.

Lomustine (CCNU) (The expected immune response may not be obtained in individuals whose immune system has been compromised by treatment with alkylating drugs).
No products indexed under this heading.

Mechlorethamine Hydrochloride (The expected immune response may not be obtained in individuals whose immune system has been compromised by treatment with alkylating drugs). Products include:
- Mustargen for Injection 2142

Melphalan (The expected immune response may not be obtained in individuals whose immune system has been compromised by treatment with alkylating drugs). Products include:
- Alkeran Tablets 1466

Methylprednisolone Acetate (The expected immune response may not be obtained in individuals whose immune system has been compromised by treatment with corticosteroids). Products include:
- Depo-Medrol Injectable Suspension 2795

Methylprednisolone Sodium Succinate (The expected immune response may not be obtained in individuals whose immune system has been compromised by treatment with corticosteroids). Products include:
- Solu-Medrol Sterile Powder 2855

Muromonab-CD3 (The expected immune response may not be obtained in individuals whose immune system has been compromised by treatment with corticosteroids). Products include:
- Orthoclone OKT3 Sterile Solution 2498

Mycophenolate Mofetil (The expected immune response may not be obtained in individuals whose immune system has been compromised by treatment with corticosteroids). Products include:
- CellCept Capsules 2951
- CellCept Oral Suspension 2951
- CellCept Tablets 2951

Prednisolone Acetate (The expected immune response may not be obtained in individuals whose immune system has been compromised by treatment with corticosteroids). Products include:
- Blephamide Ophthalmic Ointment 547
- Blephamide Ophthalmic Suspension 548
- Poly-Pred Liquifilm Ophthalmic Suspension .... ⊙245
- Pred Forte Ophthalmic Suspension .... ⊙246

Pred Mild Sterile Ophthalmic Suspension ... ⊙249
Pred-G Ophthalmic Suspension ... ⊙247
Pred-G Sterile Ophthalmic Ointment ... ⊙248

Prednisolone Sodium Phosphate (The expected immune response may not be obtained in individuals whose immune system has been compromised by treatment with corticosteroids). Products include:
Pediapred Oral Solution ... 1170

Prednisolone Tebutate (The expected immune response may not be obtained in individuals whose immune system has been compromised by treatment with corticosteroids).
No products indexed under this heading.

Prednisone (The expected immune response may not be obtained in individuals whose immune system has been compromised by treatment with corticosteroids). Products include:
Prednisone ... 3064

Sirolimus (The expected immune response may not be obtained in individuals whose immune system has been compromised by treatment with corticosteroids). Products include:
Rapamune Oral Solution and Tablets ... 3584

Tacrolimus (The expected immune response may not be obtained in individuals whose immune system has been compromised by treatment with corticosteroids). Products include:
Prograf ... 1393
Protopic Ointment ... 1397

Thiotepa (The expected immune response may not be obtained in individuals whose immune system has been compromised by treatment with alkylating drugs). Products include:
Thioplex for Injection ... 1765

Tinzaparin sodium (Typhim Vi should be given with caution to individuals on anticoagulant therapy). Products include:
Innohep Injection ... 1248

Triamcinolone (The expected immune response may not be obtained in individuals whose immune system has been compromised by treatment with corticosteroids).
No products indexed under this heading.

Triamcinolone Acetonide (The expected immune response may not be obtained in individuals whose immune system has been compromised by treatment with corticosteroids). Products include:
Azmacort Inhalation Aerosol ... 728
Nasacort Nasal Inhaler ... 750
Nasacort AQ Nasal Spray ... 752
Tri-Nasal Spray ... 2274

Triamcinolone Diacetate (The expected immune response may not be obtained in individuals whose immune system has been compromised by treatment with corticosteroids).
No products indexed under this heading.

Triamcinolone Hexacetonide (The expected immune response may not be obtained in individuals whose immune system has been compromised by treatment with corticosteroids).
No products indexed under this heading.

Warfarin Sodium (Typhim Vi should be given with caution to individuals on anticoagulant therapy). Products include:
Coumadin for Injection ... 1243
Coumadin Tablets ... 1243
Warfarin Sodium Tablets, USP ... 3302

ULTRA ZN TABLETS

(Herbals, Multiple) ... 526
None cited in PDR database.

ULTRACET TABLETS

(Acetaminophen, Tramadol Hydrochloride) ... 2597
May interact with central nervous system depressants, monoamine oxidase inhibitors, narcotic analgesics, antipsychotic agents, phenothiazines, quinidine, drugs which lower seizure threshold, selective serotonin reuptake inhibitors, and tricyclic antidepressants. Compounds in these categories include:

Acetaminophen-containing products (Due to the potential for acetaminophen hepatotoxicity at doses higher than the recommended dose, Ultracet should not be used concomitantly with other acetaminophen-containing products).
No products indexed under this heading.

Alfentanil Hydrochloride (Co-administration increases the risk of CNS and respiratory depression).
No products indexed under this heading.

Alprazolam (Co-administration enhances the risk of seizures). Products include:
Xanax Tablets ... 2865

Amitriptyline Hydrochloride (Co-administration with tricyclic antidepressants may enhance the risk of seizures; inhibitors of CYP2D6, such as amitriptyline could inhibit metabolism of tramadol). Products include:
Etrafon ... 3115
Limbitrol ... 1738

Amoxapine (Co-administration with tricyclic antidepressants may enhance the risk of seizures).
No products indexed under this heading.

Aprobarbital (Co-administration increases the risk of CNS and respiratory depression).
No products indexed under this heading.

Buprenorphine Hydrochloride (Co-administration increases the risk of CNS and respiratory depression). Products include:
Buprenex Injectable ... 2918

Buspirone Hydrochloride (Co-administration increases the risk of CNS and respiratory depression).
No products indexed under this heading.

Butabarbital (Co-administration increases the risk of CNS and respiratory depression).
No products indexed under this heading.

Butalbital (Co-administration increases the risk of CNS and respiratory depression). Products include:
Phrenilin ... 578
Sedapap Tablets 50 mg/650 mg ... 2225

Carbamazepine (Co-administration may result in a significant reduction in analgesic effect of tramadol due to increased tramadol metabolism; concurrent use is not recommended). Products include:
Carbatrol Capsules ... 3234
Tegretol/Tegretol-XR ... 2404

Chlordiazepoxide (Co-administration enhances the risk of seizures). Products include:
Limbitrol ... 1738

Chlordiazepoxide Hydrochloride (Co-administration enhances the risk of seizures). Products include:
Librium Capsules ... 1736
Librium for Injection ... 1737

Chlorpromazine (Co-administration enhances the risk of seizures; increased risk of CNS and respiratory depression). Products include:
Thorazine Suppositories ... 1656

Chlorpromazine Hydrochloride (Co-administration enhances the risk of seizures; increased risk of CNS and respiratory depression). Products include:
Thorazine ... 1656

Chlorprothixene (Co-administration enhances the risk of seizures; increased risk of CNS and respiratory depression).
No products indexed under this heading.

Chlorprothixene Hydrochloride (Co-administration enhances the risk of seizures; increased risk of CNS and respiratory depression).
No products indexed under this heading.

Chlorprothixene Lactate (Co-administration increases the risk of CNS and respiratory depression).
No products indexed under this heading.

Citalopram Hydrobromide (Co-administration with SSRI may enhance the risk of seizures). Products include:
Celexa ... 1365

Clomipramine Hydrochloride (Co-administration with tricyclic antidepressants may enhance the risk of seizures).
No products indexed under this heading.

Clorazepate Dipotassium (Co-administration increases the risk of CNS and respiratory depression). Products include:
Tranxene ... 511

Clozapine (Co-administration enhances the risk of seizures; increased risk of CNS and respiratory depression). Products include:
Clozaril Tablets ... 2319

Codeine Phosphate (Co-administration increases the risk of CNS and respiratory depression). Products include:
Phenergan with Codeine Syrup ... 3557
Phenergan VC with Codeine Syrup ... 3561
Robitussin A-C Syrup ... 2942
Robitussin-DAC Syrup ... 2942
Ryna-C Liquid ... ▣768
Soma Compound w/Codeine Tablets ... 3355
Tussi-Organidin NR Liquid ... 3350
Tussi-Organidin-S NR Liquid ... 3350
Tylenol with Codeine ... 2595

Desflurane (Co-administration increases the risk of CNS and respiratory depression). Products include:
Suprane Liquid for Inhalation ... 874

Desipramine Hydrochloride (Co-administration with tricyclic antidepressants may enhance the risk of seizures). Products include:
Norpramin Tablets ... 755

Dezocine (Co-administration increases the risk of CNS and respiratory depression).
No products indexed under this heading.

Diazepam (Co-administration enhances the risk of seizures). Products include:
Valium Injectable ... 3026
Valium Tablets ... 3047

Digoxin (Post-marketing surveillance of tramadol has revealed rare reports of digoxin toxicity). Products include:
Digitek Tablets ... 1003
Lanoxicaps Capsules ... 1574
Lanoxin Injection ... 1581
Lanoxin Tablets ... 1587
Lanoxin Elixir Pediatric ... 1578
Lanoxin Injection Pediatric ... 1584

Doxepin Hydrochloride (Co-administration with tricyclic antidepressants may enhance the risk of seizures). Products include:
Sinequan ... 2713

Droperidol (Co-administration increases the risk of CNS and respiratory depression).
No products indexed under this heading.

Enflurane (Co-administration increases the risk of CNS and respiratory depression).
No products indexed under this heading.

Estazolam (Co-administration increases the risk of CNS and respiratory depression). Products include:
ProSom Tablets ... 500

Ethchlorvynol (Co-administration increases the risk of CNS and respiratory depression).
No products indexed under this heading.

Ethinamate (Co-administration increases the risk of CNS and respiratory depression).
No products indexed under this heading.

Fentanyl (Co-administration increases the risk of CNS and respiratory depression). Products include:
Duragesic Transdermal System ... 1786

Fentanyl Citrate (Co-administration increases the risk of CNS and respiratory depression). Products include:
Actiq ... 1184

Fluoxetine Hydrochloride (Co-administration with SSRI may enhance the risk of seizures; inhibitors of CYP2D6, such as fluoxetine, could inhibit metabolism of tramadol). Products include:
Prozac Pulvules, Liquid, and Weekly Capsules ... 1238
Sarafem Pulvules ... 1962

Fluphenazine Decanoate (Co-administration enhances the risk of seizures; increased risk of CNS and respiratory depression).
No products indexed under this heading.

Fluphenazine Enanthate (Co-administration enhances the risk of seizures; increased risk of CNS and respiratory depression).
No products indexed under this heading.

Fluphenazine Hydrochloride (Co-administration enhances the risk of seizures; increased risk of CNS and respiratory depression).
No products indexed under this heading.

Flurazepam Hydrochloride (Co-administration increases the risk of CNS and respiratory depression).
No products indexed under this heading.

Fluvoxamine Maleate (Co-administration with SSRI may enhance the risk of seizures). Products include:
Luvox Tablets (25, 50, 100 mg) ... 3256

Glutethimide (Co-administration increases the risk of CNS and respiratory depression).
No products indexed under this heading.

Haloperidol (Co-administration enhances the risk of seizures). Products include:
Haldol Injection, Tablets and Concentrate ... 2533

Haloperidol Decanoate (Co-administration enhances the risk of seizures). Products include:
Haldol Decanoate ... 2535

Hydrocodone Bitartrate (Co-administration increases the risk of CNS and respiratory depression). Products include:
Hycodan ... 1316
Hycomine Compound Tablets ... 1317
Hycotuss Expectorant Syrup ... 1318
Lortab ... 3319
Lortab Elixir ... 3317
Maxidone Tablets CIII ... 3399
Norco 5/325 Tablets CIII ... 3424
Norco 7.5/325 Tablets CIII ... 3425
Norco 10/325 Tablets CIII ... 3427
Norco 10/325 Tablets CIII ... 3425
Vicodin Tablets ... 516
Vicodin ES Tablets ... 517
Vicodin HP Tablets ... 518

IMPORTANT NOTE: Always consult each drug listing in the patient's regimen for possible interactions.

Vicodin Tuss Expectorant 519
Vicoprofen Tablets 520
Zydone Tablets 1330

Hydrocodone Polistirex (Co-administration increases the risk of CNS and respiratory depression). Products include:
Tussionex Pennkinetic Extended-Release Suspension 1174

Hydromorphone Hydrochloride (Co-administration increases the risk of CNS and respiratory depression). Products include:
Dilaudid 441
Dilaudid Oral Liquid 445
Dilaudid Powder 441
Dilaudid Rectal Suppositories 441
Dilaudid Tablets 441
Dilaudid Tablets - 8 mg 445
Dilaudid-HP 443

Hydroxyzine Hydrochloride (Co-administration increases the risk of CNS and respiratory depression). Products include:
Atarax Tablets & Syrup 2667
Vistaril Intramuscular Solution 2738

Imipramine Hydrochloride (Co-administration with tricyclic antidepressants may enhance the risk of seizures).
No products indexed under this heading.

Imipramine Pamoate (Co-administration with tricyclic antidepressants may enhance the risk of seizures).
No products indexed under this heading.

Isocarboxazid (Co-administration with MAO inhibitors may enhance the risk of seizures; animal studies have shown increased deaths with combined use; interference with detoxification mechanism has been reported with combined use of MAO inhibitors and centrally acting drugs).
No products indexed under this heading.

Isoflurane (Co-administration increases the risk of CNS and respiratory depression).
No products indexed under this heading.

Ketamine Hydrochloride (Co-administration increases the risk of CNS and respiratory depression).
No products indexed under this heading.

Levomethadyl Acetate Hydrochloride (Co-administration increases the risk of CNS and respiratory depression).
No products indexed under this heading.

Levorphanol Tartrate (Co-administration increases the risk of CNS and respiratory depression). Products include:
Levo-Dromoran 1734
Levorphanol Tartrate Tablets 3059

Lithium Carbonate (Co-administration enhances the risk of seizures; increased risk of CNS and respiratory depression). Products include:
Eskalith 1527
Lithium Carbonate 3061
Lithobid Slow-Release Tablets 3255

Lithium Citrate (Co-administration enhances the risk of seizures; increased risk of CNS and respiratory depression). Products include:
Lithium Citrate Syrup 3061

Lorazepam (Co-administration enhances the risk of seizures). Products include:
Ativan Injection 3478
Ativan Tablets 3482

Loxapine Hydrochloride (Co-administration enhances the risk of seizures; increased risk of CNS and respiratory depression).
No products indexed under this heading.

Loxapine Succinate (Co-administration enhances the risk of seizures; increased risk of CNS and respiratory depression). Products include:
Loxitane Capsules 3398

Maprotiline Hydrochloride (Co-administration with tricyclic antidepressants may enhance the risk of seizures).
No products indexed under this heading.

Meperidine Hydrochloride (Co-administration increases the risk of CNS and respiratory depression). Products include:
Demerol 3079
Mepergan Injection 3539

Mephobarbital (Co-administration increases the risk of CNS and respiratory depression).
No products indexed under this heading.

Meprobamate (Co-administration increases the risk of CNS and respiratory depression). Products include:
Miltown Tablets 3349

Mesoridazine Besylate (Co-administration enhances the risk of seizures; increased risk of CNS and respiratory depression). Products include:
Serentil 1057

Methadone Hydrochloride (Co-administration increases the risk of CNS and respiratory depression). Products include:
Dolophine Hydrochloride Tablets 3056

Methohexital Sodium (Co-administration increases the risk of CNS and respiratory depression). Products include:
Brevital Sodium for Injection, USP 1815

Methotrimeprazine (Co-administration enhances the risk of seizures; increased risk of CNS and respiratory depression).
No products indexed under this heading.

Methoxyflurane (Co-administration increases the risk of CNS and respiratory depression).
No products indexed under this heading.

Midazolam Hydrochloride (Co-administration increases the risk of CNS and respiratory depression). Products include:
Versed Injection 3027
Versed Syrup 3033

Moclobemide (Co-administration with MAO inhibitors may enhance the risk of seizures; animal studies have shown increased deaths with combined use; interference with detoxification mechanism has been reported with combined use of MAO inhibitors and centrally acting drugs).
No products indexed under this heading.

Molindone Hydrochloride (Co-administration enhances the risk of seizures; increased risk of CNS and respiratory depression). Products include:
Moban 1320

Morphine Sulfate (Co-administration increases the risk of CNS and respiratory depression). Products include:
Astramorph/PF Injection, USP (Preservative-Free) 594
Duramorph Injection 1312
Infumorph 200 and Infumorph 500 Sterile Solutions 1314
Kadian Capsules 1335
MS Contin Tablets 2896
MSIR 2898
Oramorph SR Tablets 3062
Roxanol 3066

Nortriptyline Hydrochloride (Co-administration with tricyclic antidepressants may enhance the risk of seizures).
No products indexed under this heading.

Olanzapine (Co-administration enhances the risk of seizures; increased risk of CNS and respiratory depression). Products include:
Zyprexa Tablets 1973
Zyprexa ZYDIS Orally Disintegrating Tablets 1973

Oxazepam (Co-administration enhances the risk of seizures).
No products indexed under this heading.

Oxycodone Hydrochloride (Co-administration increases the risk of CNS and respiratory depression). Products include:
OxyContin Tablets 2912
OxyFast Oral Concentrate Solution 2916
OxyIR Capsules 2916
Percocet Tablets 1326
Percodan Tablets 1327
Percolone Tablets 1327
Roxicodone 3067
Tylox Capsules 2597

Pargyline Hydrochloride (Co-administration with MAO inhibitors may enhance the risk of seizures; animal studies have shown increased deaths with combined use; interference with detoxification mechanism has been reported with combined use of MAO inhibitors and centrally acting drugs).
No products indexed under this heading.

Paroxetine Hydrochloride (Co-administration with SSRI may enhance the risk of seizures; inhibitors of CYP2D6, such as paroxetine, could inhibit metabolism of tramadol). Products include:
Paxil 1609

Pentobarbital Sodium (Co-administration increases the risk of CNS and respiratory depression). Products include:
Nembutal Sodium Solution 485

Perphenazine (Co-administration enhances the risk of seizures; increased risk of CNS and respiratory depression). Products include:
Etrafon 3115
Trilafon 3160

Phenelzine Sulfate (Co-administration with MAO inhibitors may enhance the risk of seizures; animal studies have shown increased deaths with combined use; interference with detoxification mechanism has been reported with combined use of MAO inhibitors and centrally acting drugs). Products include:
Nardil Tablets 2653

Phenobarbital (Co-administration increases the risk of CNS and respiratory depression). Products include:
Arco-Lase Plus Tablets 592
Donnatal 2929
Donnatal Extentabs 2930

Pimozide (Co-administration enhances the risk of seizures; increased risk of CNS and respiratory depression). Products include:
Orap Tablets 1407

Prazepam (Co-administration enhances the risk of seizures).
No products indexed under this heading.

Procarbazine Hydrochloride (Co-administration with MAO inhibitors may enhance the risk of seizures; animal studies have shown increased deaths with combined use; interference with detoxification mechanism has been reported with combined use of MAO inhibitors and centrally acting drugs). Products include:
Matulane Capsules 3246

Prochlorperazine (Co-administration enhances the risk of seizures; increased risk of CNS and respiratory depression). Products include:
Compazine 1505

Promethazine Hydrochloride (Co-administration enhances the risk of seizures; increased risk of CNS and respiratory depression). Products include:
Mepergan Injection 3539
Phenergan Injection 3553
Phenergan 3556
Phenergan Syrup 3554
Phenergan with Codeine Syrup 3557
Phenergan with Dextromethorphan Syrup 3559
Phenergan VC Syrup 3560
Phenergan VC with Codeine Syrup 3561

Propofol (Co-administration increases the risk of CNS and respiratory depression). Products include:
Diprivan Injectable Emulsion 667

Propoxyphene Hydrochloride (Co-administration increases the risk of CNS and respiratory depression). Products include:
Darvon Pulvules 1909
Darvon Compound-65 Pulvules 1910

Propoxyphene Napsylate (Co-administration increases the risk of CNS and respiratory depression). Products include:
Darvon-N/Darvocet-N 1907
Darvon-N Tablets 1912

Protriptyline Hydrochloride (Co-administration with tricyclic antidepressants may enhance the risk of seizures). Products include:
Vivactil Tablets 2446
Vivactil Tablets 2217

Quazepam (Co-administration increases the risk of CNS and respiratory depression).
No products indexed under this heading.

Quetiapine Fumarate (Co-administration enhances the risk of seizures; increased risk of CNS and respiratory depression). Products include:
Seroquel Tablets 684

Quinidine Gluconate (Co-administration results in increased concentrations of tramadol and reduced concentrations of its metabolite, M1). Products include:
Quinaglute Dura-Tabs Tablets 978

Quinidine Polygalacturonate (Co-administration results in increased concentrations of tramadol and reduced concentrations of its metabolite, M1).
No products indexed under this heading.

Quinidine Sulfate (Co-administration results in increased concentrations of tramadol and reduced concentrations of its metabolite, M1). Products include:
Quinidex Extentabs 2933

Remifentanil Hydrochloride (Co-administration increases the risk of CNS and respiratory depression).
No products indexed under this heading.

Risperidone (Co-administration enhances the risk of seizures; increased risk of CNS and respiratory depression). Products include:
Risperdal 1796

Secobarbital Sodium (Co-administration increases the risk of CNS and respiratory depression).
No products indexed under this heading.

Selegiline Hydrochloride (Co-administration with MAO inhibitors may enhance the risk of seizures; animal studies have shown increased deaths with combined use; interference with detoxification mechanism has been reported with combined use of MAO inhibitors and centrally acting drugs). Products include:
Eldepryl Capsules 3266

Sertraline Hydrochloride (Co-administration with SSRI may enhance the risk of seizures).
Products include:
Zoloft 2751

Sevoflurane (Co-administration increases the risk of CNS and respiratory depression).
No products indexed under this heading.

Sufentanil Citrate (Co-administration increases the risk of CNS and respiratory depression).
No products indexed under this heading.

Temazepam (Co-administration increases the risk of CNS and respiratory depression).
No products indexed under this heading.

Thiamylal Sodium (Co-administration increases the risk of CNS and respiratory depression).
No products indexed under this heading.

Thioridazine Hydrochloride (Co-administration enhances the risk of seizures; increased risk of CNS and respiratory depression). Products include:
Thioridazine Hydrochloride Tablets 2289

Thiothixene (Co-administration enhances the risk of seizures; increased risk of CNS and respiratory depression). Products include:
Navane Capsules 2701
Thiothixene Capsules 2290

Tranylcypromine Sulfate (Co-administration with MAO inhibitors may enhance the risk of seizures; animal studies have shown increased deaths with combined use; interference with detoxification mechanism has been reported with combined use of MAO inhibitors and centrally acting drugs). Products include:
Parnate Tablets 1607

Trazodone Hydrochloride (Co-administration enhances the risk of seizures).
No products indexed under this heading.

Triazolam (Co-administration increases the risk of CNS and respiratory depression). Products include:
Halcion Tablets 2823

Trifluoperazine Hydrochloride (Co-administration enhances the risk of seizures; increased risk of CNS and respiratory depression).
Products include:
Stelazine 1640

Trimipramine Maleate (Co-administration with tricyclic antidepressants may enhance the risk of seizures). Products include:
Surmontil Capsules 3595

Warfarin Sodium (Post-marketing surveillance of both tramadol and acetaminophen individual products has revealed rare alterations of warfarin effect, including elevation of prothrombin time). Products include:
Coumadin for Injection 1243
Coumadin Tablets 1243
Warfarin Sodium Tablets, USP 3302

Zaleplon (Co-administration increases the risk of CNS and respiratory depression). Products include:
Sonata Capsules 3591

Ziprasidone Hydrochloride (Co-administration enhances the risk of seizures; increased risk of CNS and respiratory depression). Products include:
Geodon Capsules 2688

Zolpidem Tartrate (Co-administration increases the risk of CNS and respiratory depression).
Products include:
Ambien Tablets 3191

Food Interactions

Alcohol (Tramadol increases the risk of CNS and respiratory depression with concurrent use; alcohol consumption with Ultracet is not recommended).

ULTRAM TABLETS

(Tramadol Hydrochloride) 2600
May interact with central nervous system depressants, monoamine oxidase inhibitors, narcotic analgesics, quinidine, drugs which lower seizure threshold, selective serotonin reuptake inhibitors, tricyclic antidepressants, and certain other agents. Compounds in these categories include:

Alfentanil Hydrochloride (Co-administration of tramadol with opioids increases the seizure risk; tramadol causes CNS effects, such as dizziness and somnolence, and may impair mental and physical abilities; Ultram should be used with caution and in reduced dosages when administered with CNS depressants).
No products indexed under this heading.

Alprazolam (Co-administration with tramadol may enhance the seizure risk). Products include:
Xanax Tablets 2865

Amitriptyline Hydrochloride (Co-administration with CYP2D6, such as amitriptyline, could result in some inhibition of the metabolism of tramadol; concurrent use may enhance the seizure risk). Products include:
Etrafon 3115
Limbitrol 1738

Amoxapine (Co-administration with tramadol may enhance the seizure risk).
No products indexed under this heading.

Aprobarbital (Tramadol causes CNS effects, such as dizziness and somnolence, and may impair mental and physical abilities; Ultram should be used with caution and in reduced dosages when administered with CNS depressants).
No products indexed under this heading.

Buprenorphine Hydrochloride (Co-administration of tramadol with opioids increases the seizure risk; tramadol causes CNS effects, such as dizziness and somnolence, and may impair mental and physical abilities; Ultram should be used with caution and in reduced dosages when administered with CNS depressants).
Products include:
Buprenex Injectable 2918

Buspirone Hydrochloride (Tramadol causes CNS effects, such as dizziness and somnolence, and may impair mental and physical abilities; Ultram should be used with caution and in reduced dosages when administered with CNS depressants).
No products indexed under this heading.

Butabarbital (Tramadol causes CNS effects, such as dizziness and somnolence, and may impair mental and physical abilities; Ultram should be used with caution and in reduced dosages when administered with CNS depressants).
No products indexed under this heading.

Butalbital (Tramadol causes CNS effects, such as dizziness and somnolence, and may impair mental and physical abilities; Ultram should be used with caution and in reduced dosages when administered with CNS depressants). Products include:
Phrenilin 578
Sedapap Tablets 50 mg/650 mg 2225

Carbamazepine (Co-administration causes a significant increase in tramadol metabolism, presumably through metabolic induction by carbamazepine; patients receiving chronic carbamazepine doses may require higher, up to twice the recommended, doses of tramadol).
Products include:
Carbatrol Capsules 3234
Tegretol/Tegretol-XR 2404

Chlordiazepoxide (Co-administration with tramadol may enhance the seizure risk). Products include:
Limbitrol 1738

Chlordiazepoxide Hydrochloride (Co-administration with tramadol may enhance the seizure risk).
Products include:
Librium Capsules 1736
Librium for Injection 1737

Chlorpromazine (Co-administration with tramadol may enhance the seizure risk). Products include:
Thorazine Suppositories 1656

Chlorpromazine Hydrochloride (Co-administration with tramadol may enhance the seizure risk).
Products include:
Thorazine 1656

Chlorprothixene (Tramadol causes CNS effects, such as dizziness and somnolence, and may impair mental and physical abilities; Ultram should be used with caution and in reduced dosages when administered with CNS depressants).
No products indexed under this heading.

Chlorprothixene Hydrochloride (Tramadol causes CNS effects, such as dizziness and somnolence, and may impair mental and physical abilities; Ultram should be used with caution and in reduced dosages when administered with CNS depressants).
No products indexed under this heading.

Chlorprothixene Lactate (Tramadol causes CNS effects, such as dizziness and somnolence, and may impair mental and physical abilities; Ultram should be used with caution and in reduced dosages when administered with CNS depressants).
No products indexed under this heading.

Citalopram Hydrobromide (Co-administration with SSRI has resulted in serotonin syndrome, fever, excitation, shivering and agitation; potential for increased risk of seizure).
Products include:
Celexa 1365

Clomipramine Hydrochloride (Co-administration with tramadol may enhance the seizure risk).
No products indexed under this heading.

Clorazepate Dipotassium (Tramadol causes CNS effects, such as dizziness and somnolence, and may impair mental and physical abilities; Ultram should be used with caution and in reduced dosages when administered with CNS depressants).
Products include:
Tranxene 511

Clozapine (Tramadol causes CNS effects, such as dizziness and somnolence, and may impair mental and physical abilities; Ultram should be used with caution and in reduced dosages when administered with CNS depressants). Products include:
Clozaril Tablets 2319

Codeine Phosphate (Co-administration of tramadol with opioids increases the seizure risk; tramadol causes CNS effects, such as dizziness and somnolence, and may impair mental and physical abilities; Ultram should be used with caution and in reduced dosages when administered with CNS depressants).
Products include:
Phenergan with Codeine Syrup 3557
Phenergan VC with Codeine Syrup 3561
Robitussin A-C Syrup 2942
Robitussin-DAC Syrup 2942
Ryna-C Liquid 768
Soma Compound w/Codeine Tablets 3355
Tussi-Organidin NR Liquid 3350
Tussi-Organidin-S NR Liquid 3350
Tylenol with Codeine 2595

Cyclobenzaprine Hydrochloride (Co-administration with tramadol may enhance the seizure risk).
Products include:
Flexeril Tablets 572
Flexeril Tablets 2094

Desflurane (Tramadol causes CNS effects, such as dizziness and somnolence, and may impair mental and physical abilities; Ultram should be used with caution and in reduced dosages when administered with CNS depressants). Products include:
Suprane Liquid for Inhalation 874

Desipramine Hydrochloride (Co-administration with tramadol may enhance the seizure risk). Products include:
Norpramin Tablets 755

Dezocine (Co-administration of tramadol with opioids increases the seizure risk; tramadol causes CNS effects, such as dizziness and somnolence, and may impair mental and physical abilities; Ultram should be used with caution and in reduced dosages when administered with CNS depressants).
No products indexed under this heading.

Diazepam (Co-administration with tramadol may enhance the seizure risk). Products include:
Valium Injectable 3026
Valium Tablets 3047

Digoxin (Rare reports of digoxin toxicity). Products include:
Digitek Tablets 1003
Lanoxicaps Capsules 1574
Lanoxin Injection 1581
Lanoxin Tablets 1587
Lanoxin Elixir Pediatric 1578
Lanoxin Injection Pediatric 1584

Doxepin Hydrochloride (Co-administration with tramadol may enhance the seizure risk). Products include:
Sinequan 2713

Droperidol (Tramadol causes CNS effects, such as dizziness and somnolence, and may impair mental and physical abilities; Ultram should be used with caution and in reduced dosages when administered with CNS depressants).
No products indexed under this heading.

Enflurane (Tramadol causes CNS effects, such as dizziness and somnolence, and may impair mental and physical abilities; Ultram should be used with caution and in reduced dosages when administered with CNS depressants).
No products indexed under this heading.

Estazolam (Tramadol causes CNS effects, such as dizziness and somnolence, and may impair mental and physical abilities; Ultram should be used with caution and in reduced dosages when administered with CNS depressants). Products include:
ProSom Tablets 500

Ethchlorvynol (Tramadol causes CNS effects, such as dizziness and somnolence, and may impair mental and physical abilities; Ultram should be used with caution and in reduced dosages when administered with CNS depressants).
No products indexed under this heading.

Ethinamate (Tramadol causes CNS effects, such as dizziness and somnolence, and may impair mental and physical abilities; Ultram should be

used with caution and in reduced dosages when administered with CNS depressants).
No products indexed under this heading.

Fentanyl (Co-administration of tramadol with opioids increases the seizure risk; tramadol causes CNS effects, such as dizziness and somnolence, and may impair mental and physical abilities; Ultram should be used with caution and in reduced dosages when administered with CNS depressants). Products include:
Duragesic Transdermal System **1786**

Fentanyl Citrate (Co-administration of tramadol with opioids increases the seizure risk; tramadol causes CNS effects, such as dizziness and somnolence, and may impair mental and physical abilities; Ultram should be used with caution and in reduced dosages when administered with CNS depressants). Products include:
Actiq **1184**

Fluoxetine Hydrochloride (Co-administration with CYP2D6, such as fluoxetine, could result in some inhibition of the metabolism of tramadol; concurrent use may enhance the seizure risk). Products include:
Prozac Pulvules, Liquid, and Weekly Capsules **1238**
Sarafem Pulvules **1962**

Fluphenazine Decanoate (Co-administration with tramadol may enhance the seizure risk).
No products indexed under this heading.

Fluphenazine Enanthate (Co-administration with tramadol may enhance the seizure risk).
No products indexed under this heading.

Fluphenazine Hydrochloride (Co-administration with tramadol may enhance the seizure risk).
No products indexed under this heading.

Flurazepam Hydrochloride (Tramadol causes CNS effects, such as dizziness and somnolence, and may impair mental and physical abilities; Ultram should be used with caution and in reduced dosages when administered with CNS depressants).
No products indexed under this heading.

Fluvoxamine Maleate (Co-administration with SSRI has resulted in serotonin syndrome, fever, excitation, shivering and agitation; potential for increased risk of seizure). Products include:
Luvox Tablets (25, 50, 100 mg) **3256**

Glutethimide (Tramadol causes CNS effects, such as dizziness and somnolence, and may impair mental and physical abilities; Ultram should be used with caution and in reduced dosages when administered with CNS depressants).
No products indexed under this heading.

Haloperidol (Co-administration with tramadol may enhance the seizure risk). Products include:
Haldol Injection, Tablets and Concentrate **2533**

Haloperidol Decanoate (Co-administration with tramadol may enhance the seizure risk). Products include:
Haldol Decanoate **2535**

Hydrocodone Bitartrate (Co-administration of tramadol with opioids increases the seizure risk; tramadol causes CNS effects, such as dizziness and somnolence, and may impair mental and physical abilities; Ultram should be used with caution and in reduced dosages when administered with CNS depressants). Products include:
Hycodan **1316**
Hycomine Compound Tablets **1317**
Hycotuss Expectorant Syrup **1318**
Lortab **3319**
Lortab Elixir **3317**
Maxidone Tablets CIII **3399**
Norco 5/325 Tablets CIII **3424**
Norco 7.5/325 Tablets CIII **3425**
Norco 10/325 Tablets CIII **3427**
Norco 10/325 Tablets CIII **3425**
Vicodin Tablets **516**
Vicodin ES Tablets **517**
Vicodin HP Tablets **518**
Vicodin Tuss Expectorant **519**
Vicoprofen Tablets **520**
Zydone Tablets **1330**

Hydrocodone Polistirex (Co-administration of tramadol with opioids increases the seizure risk; tramadol causes CNS effects, such as dizziness and somnolence, and may impair mental and physical abilities; Ultram should be used with caution and in reduced dosages when administered with CNS depressants). Products include:
Tussionex Pennkinetic Extended-Release Suspension **1174**

Hydromorphone Hydrochloride (Co-administration of tramadol with opioids increases the seizure risk; tramadol causes CNS effects, such as dizziness and somnolence, and may impair mental and physical abilities; Ultram should be used with caution and in reduced dosages when administered with CNS depressants). Products include:
Dilaudid **441**
Dilaudid Oral Liquid **445**
Dilaudid Powder **441**
Dilaudid Rectal Suppositories **441**
Dilaudid Tablets **441**
Dilaudid Tablets - 8 mg **445**
Dilaudid-HP **443**

Hydroxyzine Hydrochloride (Tramadol causes CNS effects, such as dizziness and somnolence, and may impair mental and physical abilities; Ultram should be used with caution and in reduced dosages when administered with CNS depressants). Products include:
Atarax Tablets & Syrup **2667**
Vistaril Intramuscular Solution **2738**

Imipramine Hydrochloride (Co-administration with tramadol may enhance the seizure risk).
No products indexed under this heading.

Imipramine Pamoate (Co-administration with tramadol may enhance the seizure risk).
No products indexed under this heading.

Isocarboxazid (Co-administration with MAO inhibitors has resulted in serotonin syndrome, fever, excitation, shivering and agitation; potential for increased risk of seizure).
No products indexed under this heading.

Isoflurane (Tramadol causes CNS effects, such as dizziness and somnolence, and may impair mental and physical abilities; Ultram should be used with caution and in reduced dosages when administered with CNS depressants).
No products indexed under this heading.

Ketamine Hydrochloride (Tramadol causes CNS effects, such as dizziness and somnolence, and may impair mental and physical abilities; Ultram should be used with caution and in reduced dosages when administered with CNS depressants).
No products indexed under this heading.

Levomethadyl Acetate Hydrochloride (Tramadol causes CNS effects, such as dizziness and somnolence, and may impair mental and physical abilities; Ultram should be used with caution and in reduced dosages when administered with CNS depressants).
No products indexed under this heading.

Levorphanol Tartrate (Co-administration of tramadol with opioids increases the seizure risk; tramadol causes CNS effects, such as dizziness and somnolence, and may impair mental and physical abilities; Ultram should be used with caution and in reduced dosages when administered with CNS depressants). Products include:
Levo-Dromoran **1734**
Levorphanol Tartrate Tablets **3059**

Lorazepam (Co-administration with tramadol may enhance the seizure risk). Products include:
Ativan Injection **3478**
Ativan Tablets **3482**

Loxapine Hydrochloride (Tramadol causes CNS effects, such as dizziness and somnolence, and may impair mental and physical abilities; Ultram should be used with caution and in reduced dosages when administered with CNS depressants).
No products indexed under this heading.

Loxapine Succinate (Tramadol causes CNS effects, such as dizziness and somnolence, and may impair mental and physical abilities; Ultram should be used with caution and in reduced dosages when administered with CNS depressants). Products include:
Loxitane Capsules **3398**

Maprotiline Hydrochloride (Co-administration with tramadol may enhance the seizure risk).
No products indexed under this heading.

Meperidine Hydrochloride (Co-administration of tramadol with opioids increases the seizure risk; tramadol causes CNS effects, such as dizziness and somnolence, and may impair mental and physical abilities; Ultram should be used with caution and in reduced dosages when administered with CNS depressants). Products include:
Demerol **3079**
Mepergan Injection **3539**

Mephobarbital (Tramadol causes CNS effects, such as dizziness and somnolence, and may impair mental and physical abilities; Ultram should be used with caution and in reduced dosages when administered with CNS depressants).
No products indexed under this heading.

Meprobamate (Tramadol causes CNS effects, such as dizziness and somnolence, and may impair mental and physical abilities; Ultram should be used with caution and in reduced dosages when administered with CNS depressants). Products include:
Miltown Tablets **3349**

Mesoridazine Besylate (Co-administration with tramadol may enhance the seizure risk). Products include:
Serentil **1057**

Methadone Hydrochloride (Co-administration of tramadol with opioids increases the seizure risk; tramadol causes CNS effects, such as dizziness and somnolence, and may impair mental and physical abilities; Ultram should be used with caution and in reduced dosages when administered with CNS depressants). Products include:
Dolophine Hydrochloride Tablets **3056**

Methohexital Sodium (Tramadol causes CNS effects, such as dizziness and somnolence, and may impair mental and physical abilities; Ultram should be used with caution and in reduced dosages when administered with CNS depressants). Products include:
Brevital Sodium for Injection, USP **1815**

Methotrimeprazine (Tramadol causes CNS effects, such as dizziness and somnolence, and may impair mental and physical abilities; Ultram should be used with caution and in reduced dosages when administered with CNS depressants).
No products indexed under this heading.

Methoxyflurane (Tramadol causes CNS effects, such as dizziness and somnolence, and may impair mental and physical abilities; Ultram should be used with caution and in reduced dosages when administered with CNS depressants).
No products indexed under this heading.

Midazolam Hydrochloride (Tramadol causes CNS effects, such as dizziness and somnolence, and may impair mental and physical abilities; Ultram should be used with caution and in reduced dosages when administered with CNS depressants). Products include:
Versed Injection **3027**
Versed Syrup **3033**

Moclobemide (Co-administration with MAO inhibitors has resulted in serotonin syndrome, fever, excitation, shivering and agitation; potential for increased risk of seizure).
No products indexed under this heading.

Molindone Hydrochloride (Tramadol causes CNS effects, such as dizziness and somnolence, and may impair mental and physical abilities; Ultram should be used with caution and in reduced dosages when administered with CNS depressants). Products include:
Moban **1320**

Morphine Sulfate (Co-administration of tramadol with opioids increases the seizure risk; tramadol causes CNS effects, such as dizziness and somnolence, and may impair mental and physical abilities; Ultram should be used with caution and in reduced dosages when administered with CNS depressants). Products include:
Astramorph/PF Injection, USP (Preservative-Free) **594**
Duramorph Injection **1312**
Infumorph 200 and Infumorph 500 Sterile Solutions **1314**
Kadian Capsules **1335**
MS Contin Tablets **2896**
MSIR **2898**
Oramorph SR Tablets **3062**
Roxanol **3066**

Nortriptyline Hydrochloride (Co-administration with tramadol may enhance the seizure risk).
No products indexed under this heading.

Olanzapine (Tramadol causes CNS effects, such as dizziness and somnolence, and may impair mental and physical abilities; Ultram should be used with caution and in reduced dosages when administered with CNS depressants). Products include:
Zyprexa Tablets **1973**
Zyprexa ZYDIS Orally Disintegrating Tablets **1973**

Oxazepam (Co-administration with tramadol may enhance the seizure risk).
No products indexed under this heading.

Oxycodone Hydrochloride (Co-administration of tramadol with opioids increases the seizure risk; tramadol causes CNS effects, such as dizziness and somnolence, and may impair mental and physical abilities; Ultram should be used with caution

and in reduced dosages when administered with CNS depressants). Products include:

- OxyContin Tablets ... 2912
- OxyFast Oral Concentrate Solution . 2916
- OxyIR Capsules ... 2916
- Percocet Tablets ... 1326
- Percodan Tablets ... 1327
- Percolone Tablets ... 1327
- Roxicodone ... 3067
- Tylox Capsules ... 2597

Pargyline Hydrochloride (Co-administration with MAO inhibitors has resulted in serotonin syndrome, fever, excitation, shivering and agitation; potential for increased risk of seizure).

No products indexed under this heading.

Paroxetine Hydrochloride (Co-administration with CYP2D6, such as paroxetine, could result in some inhibition of the metabolism of tramadol; concurrent use may enhance the seizure risk). Products include:

- Paxil ... 1609

Pentobarbital Sodium (Tramadol causes CNS effects, such as dizziness and somnolence, and may impair mental and physical abilities; Ultram should be used with caution and in reduced dosages when administered with CNS depressants). Products include:

- Nembutal Sodium Solution ... 485

Perphenazine (Co-administration with tramadol may enhance the seizure risk). Products include:

- Etrafon ... 3115
- Trilafon ... 3160

Phenelzine Sulfate (Co-administration with MAO inhibitors has resulted in serotonin syndrome, fever, excitation, shivering and agitation; potential for increased risk of seizure). Products include:

- Nardil Tablets ... 2653

Phenobarbital (Tramadol causes CNS effects, such as dizziness and somnolence, and may impair mental and physical abilities; Ultram should be used with caution and in reduced dosages when administered with CNS depressants). Products include:

- Arco-Lase Plus Tablets ... 592
- Donnatal ... 2929
- Donnatal Extentabs ... 2930

Prazepam (Co-administration with tramadol may enhance the seizure risk).

No products indexed under this heading.

Procarbazine Hydrochloride (Co-administration with MAO inhibitors has resulted in serotonin syndrome, fever, excitation, shivering and agitation; potential for increased risk of seizure). Products include:

- Matulane Capsules ... 3246

Prochlorperazine (Co-administration with tramadol may enhance the seizure risk). Products include:

- Compazine ... 1505

Promethazine Hydrochloride (Co-administration increases the seizure risk in patients taking promethazine; tramadol causes CNS effects, such as dizziness and somnolence, and may impair mental and physical abilities; Ultram should be used with caution and in reduced dosages when administered with CNS depressants). Products include:

- Mepergan Injection ... 3539
- Phenergan Injection ... 3553
- Phenergan ... 3556
- Phenergan Syrup ... 3554
- Phenergan with Codeine Syrup ... 3557
- Phenergan with Dextromethorphan Syrup ... 3559
- Phenergan VC Syrup ... 3560
- Phenergan VC with Codeine Syrup .. 3561

Propofol (Tramadol causes CNS effects, such as dizziness and somnolence, and may impair mental and physical abilities; Ultram should be used with caution and in reduced dosages when administered with CNS depressants). Products include:

- Diprivan Injectable Emulsion ... 667

Propoxyphene Hydrochloride (Co-administration of tramadol with opioids increases the seizure risk; tramadol causes CNS effects, such as dizziness and somnolence, and may impair mental and physical abilities; Ultram should be used with caution and in reduced dosages when administered with CNS depressants). Products include:

- Darvon Pulvules ... 1909
- Darvon Compound-65 Pulvules ... 1910

Propoxyphene Napsylate (Co-administration of tramadol with opioids increases the seizure risk; tramadol causes CNS effects, such as dizziness and somnolence, and may impair mental and physical abilities; Ultram should be used with caution and in reduced dosages when administered with CNS depressants). Products include:

- Darvon-N/Darvocet-N ... 1907
- Darvon-N Tablets ... 1912

Protriptyline Hydrochloride (Co-administration with tramadol may enhance the seizure risk). Products include:

- Vivactil Tablets ... 2446
- Vivactil Tablets ... 2217

Quazepam (Tramadol causes CNS effects, such as dizziness and somnolence, and may impair mental and physical abilities; Ultram should be used with caution and in reduced dosages when administered with CNS depressants).

No products indexed under this heading.

Quetiapine Fumarate (Tramadol causes CNS effects, such as dizziness and somnolence, and may impair mental and physical abilities; Ultram should be used with caution and in reduced dosages when administered with CNS depressants). Products include:

- Seroquel Tablets ... 684

Quinidine Gluconate (Co-administration results in increased concentrations of tramadol and reduced concentrations of M1 (o-desmethyltramadol); clinical consequences of these are unknown). Products include:

- Quinaglute Dura-Tabs Tablets ... 978

Quinidine Polygalacturonate (Co-administration results in increased concentrations of tramadol and reduced concentrations of M1 (o-desmethyltramadol); clinical consequences of these are unknown).

No products indexed under this heading.

Quinidine Sulfate (Co-administration results in increased concentrations of tramadol and reduced concentrations of M1 (o-desmethyltramadol); clinical consequences of these are unknown). Products include:

- Quinidex Extentabs ... 2933

Remifentanil Hydrochloride (Co-administration of tramadol with opioids increases the seizure risk; tramadol causes CNS effects, such as dizziness and somnolence, and may impair mental and physical abilities; Ultram should be used with caution and in reduced dosages when administered with CNS depressants).

No products indexed under this heading.

Risperidone (Tramadol causes CNS effects, such as dizziness and somnolence, and may impair mental and physical abilities; Ultram should be used with caution and in reduced dosages when administered with CNS depressants). Products include:

- Risperdal ... 1796

Secobarbital Sodium (Tramadol causes CNS effects, such as dizziness and somnolence, and may impair mental and physical abilities; Ultram should be used with caution and in reduced dosages when administered with CNS depressants).

No products indexed under this heading.

Selegiline Hydrochloride (Co-administration with MAO inhibitors has resulted in serotonin syndrome, fever, excitation, shivering and agitation; potential for increased risk of seizure). Products include:

- Eldepryl Capsules ... 3266

Sertraline Hydrochloride (Co-administration with SSRI has resulted in serotonin syndrome, fever, excitation, shivering and agitation; potential for increased risk of seizure). Products include:

- Zoloft ... 2751

Sevoflurane (Tramadol causes CNS effects, such as dizziness and somnolence, and may impair mental and physical abilities; Ultram should be used with caution and in reduced dosages when administered with CNS depressants).

No products indexed under this heading.

Sufentanil Citrate (Co-administration of tramadol with opioids increases the seizure risk; tramadol causes CNS effects, such as dizziness and somnolence, and may impair mental and physical abilities; Ultram should be used with caution and in reduced dosages when administered with CNS depressants).

No products indexed under this heading.

Temazepam (Tramadol causes CNS effects, such as dizziness and somnolence, and may impair mental and physical abilities; Ultram should be used with caution and in reduced dosages when administered with CNS depressants).

No products indexed under this heading.

Thiamylal Sodium (Tramadol causes CNS effects, such as dizziness and somnolence, and may impair mental and physical abilities; Ultram should be used with caution and in reduced dosages when administered with CNS depressants).

No products indexed under this heading.

Thioridazine Hydrochloride (Co-administration with tramadol may enhance the seizure risk). Products include:

- Thioridazine Hydrochloride Tablets ... 2289

Thiothixene (Tramadol causes CNS effects, such as dizziness and somnolence, and may impair mental and physical abilities; Ultram should be used with caution and in reduced dosages when administered with CNS depressants). Products include:

- Navane Capsules ... 2701
- Thiothixene Capsules ... 2290

Tranylcypromine Sulfate (Co-administration with MAO inhibitors has resulted in serotonin syndrome, fever, excitation, shivering and agitation; potential for increased risk of seizure). Products include:

- Parnate Tablets ... 1607

Trazodone Hydrochloride (Co-administration with tramadol may enhance the seizure risk).

No products indexed under this heading.

Triazolam (Tramadol causes CNS effects, such as dizziness and somnolence, and may impair mental and physical abilities; Ultram should be used with caution and in reduced dosages when administered with CNS depressants). Products include:

- Halcion Tablets ... 2823

Trifluoperazine Hydrochloride (Co-administration with tramadol may enhance the seizure risk). Products include:

- Stelazine ... 1640

Trimipramine Maleate (Co-administration with tramadol may enhance the seizure risk). Products include:

- Surmontil Capsules ... 3595

Warfarin Sodium (Rare reports of alteration of warfarin effect, including elevation of prothrombin times). Products include:

- Coumadin for Injection ... 1243
- Coumadin Tablets ... 1243
- Warfarin Sodium Tablets, USP ... 3302

Zaleplon (Tramadol causes CNS effects, such as dizziness and somnolence, and may impair mental and physical abilities; Ultram should be used with caution and in reduced dosages when administered with CNS depressants). Products include:

- Sonata Capsules ... 3591

Ziprasidone Hydrochloride (Tramadol causes CNS effects, such as dizziness and somnolence, and may impair mental and physical abilities; Ultram should be used with caution and in reduced dosages when administered with CNS depressants). Products include:

- Geodon Capsules ... 2688

Zolpidem Tartrate (Tramadol causes CNS effects, such as dizziness and somnolence, and may impair mental and physical abilities; Ultram should be used with caution and in reduced dosages when administered with CNS depressants). Products include:

- Ambien Tablets ... 3191

Food Interactions

Alcohol (Concurrent use should be avoided; contraindicated in cases of acute alcohol intoxication).

ULTRASE CAPSULES

(Pancrelipase) ... 835

May interact with:

Food Interactions

Food having a pH greater than 5.5 (Can dissolve the protective coating resulting in early release of enzymes, irritation of oral mucosa, and/or loss of enzyme activity).

ULTRASE MT CAPSULES

(Pancrelipase) ... 835

May interact with:

Food Interactions

Food having a pH greater than 5.5 (Can dissolve the protective enteric shell).

UNASYN FOR INJECTION

(Ampicillin Sodium, Sulbactam Sodium) ... 2728

May interact with aminoglycosides and certain other agents. Compounds in these categories include:

Allopurinol (Co-administration of allopurinol and ampicillin increases substantially the incidence of rashes).

No products indexed under this heading.

Amikacin Sulfate (In vitro inactivation of aminoglycosides when reconstituted with Unasyn).

No products indexed under this heading.

Gentamicin Sulfate (In vitro inactivation of aminoglycosides when reconstituted with Unasyn). Products include:

- Genoptic Ophthalmic Ointment ... ⊙239

Genoptic Sterile Ophthalmic Solution ⊙239
Pred-G Ophthalmic Suspension ⊙247
Pred-G Sterile Ophthalmic Ointment ⊙248

Kanamycin Sulfate (In vitro inactivation of aminoglycosides when reconstituted with Unasyn).
No products indexed under this heading.

Probenecid (Decreases the renal tubular secretion of ampicillin and sulbactam; co-administration of probenecid with Unasyn may result in increased and prolonged blood levels of ampicillin and sulbactam).
No products indexed under this heading.

Streptomycin Sulfate (In vitro inactivation of aminoglycosides when reconstituted with Unasyn). Products include:
Streptomycin Sulfate Injection 2714

Tobramycin (In vitro inactivation of aminoglycosides when reconstituted with Unasyn). Products include:
TOBI Solution for Inhalation 1206
TobraDex Ophthalmic Ointment 542
TobraDex Ophthalmic Suspension 541
Tobrex Ophthalmic Ointment ⊙220
Tobrex Ophthalmic Solution ⊙221

Tobramycin Sulfate (In vitro inactivation of aminoglycosides when reconstituted with Unasyn). Products include:
Nebcin Vials, Hyporets & ADD-Vantage 1955

UNI-DUR EXTENDED-RELEASE TABLETS

(Theophylline) 1841
May interact with erythromycin, lithium preparations, phenytoin, and certain other agents. Compounds in these categories include:

Adenosine (Theophylline blocks adenosine receptors; higher doses of adenosine may be required to achieve desired effect). Products include:
Adenocard Injection 1380
Adenoscan 1381

Allopurinol (Decreases theophylline clearance at allopurinol doses greater than or equal to 600 mg/day).
No products indexed under this heading.

Aminoglutethimide (Increases theophylline clearance by induction of microsomal enzyme).
No products indexed under this heading.

Carbamazepine (Increases theophylline clearance by induction of microsomal enzyme). Products include:
Carbatrol Capsules 3234
Tegretol/Tegretol-XR 2404

Cimetidine (Decreases theophylline clearance by inhibiting cytochrome P450 1A2). Products include:
Tagamet HB 200 Suspension ▣762
Tagamet HB 200 Tablets ▣761
Tagamet Tablets 1644

Cimetidine Hydrochloride (Decreases theophylline clearance by inhibiting cytochrome P450 1A2). Products include:
Tagamet 1644

Ciprofloxacin (Decreases theophylline clearance by inhibiting cytochrome P450 1A2). Products include:
Cipro I.V. 893
Cipro I.V. Pharmacy Bulk Package 897
Cipro Oral Suspension 887

Ciprofloxacin Hydrochloride (Decreases theophylline clearance by inhibiting cytochrome P450 1A2). Products include:
Ciloxan 538
Cipro HC Otic Suspension 540
Cipro Tablets 887

Clarithromycin (Decreases theophylline clearance by inhibiting cytochrome P450 3A3). Products include:
Biaxin/Biaxin XL 403
PREVPAC 3298

Diazepam (Benzodiazepines increase CNS concentrations of adenosine, a potent CNS depressant, while theophylline blocks adenosine receptors; larger diazepam doses may be required to produce desired level of sedation; discontinuation of theophylline without reduction of diazepam dose may result in respiratory depression). Products include:
Valium Injectable 3026
Valium Tablets 3047

Disulfiram (Decreases theophylline clearance by inhibiting hydroxylation and demethylation). Products include:
Antabuse Tablets 2444
Antabuse Tablets 3474

Enoxacin (Decreases theophylline clearance by inhibiting cytochrome P450 1A2).
No products indexed under this heading.

Ephedrine Hydrochloride (Co-administration results in synergistic CNS effects resulting in increased frequency of nausea, nervousness, and insomnia). Products include:
Primatene Tablets ▣780

Ephedrine Sulfate (Co-administration results in synergistic CNS effects resulting in increased frequency of nausea, nervousness, and insomnia).
No products indexed under this heading.

Ephedrine Tannate (Co-administration results in synergistic CNS effects resulting in increased frequency of nausea, nervousness, and insomnia). Products include:
Rynatuss Pediatric Suspension 3353
Rynatuss Tablets 3353

Erythromycin (Erythromycin metabolite decreases theophylline clearance by inhibiting cytochrome P450 3A3; decreased erythromycin steady-state serum concentrations). Products include:
Emgel 2% Topical Gel 1285
Ery-Tab Tablets 448
Erythromycin Base Filmtab Tablets 454
Erythromycin Delayed-Release Capsules, USP 455
PCE Dispertab Tablets 498

Erythromycin Estolate (Erythromycin metabolite decreases theophylline clearance by inhibiting cytochrome P450 3A3; decreased erythromycin steady-state serum concentrations).
No products indexed under this heading.

Erythromycin Ethylsuccinate (Erythromycin metabolite decreases theophylline clearance by inhibiting cytochrome P450 3A3; decreased erythromycin steady-state serum concentrations). Products include:
E.E.S. 450
EryPed 446
Pediazole Suspension 3050

Erythromycin Gluceptate (Erythromycin metabolite decreases theophylline clearance by inhibiting cytochrome P450 3A3; decreased erythromycin steady-state serum concentrations).
No products indexed under this heading.

Erythromycin Stearate (Erythromycin metabolite decreases theophylline clearance by inhibiting cytochrome P450 3A3; decreased erythromycin steady-state serum concentrations). Products include:
Erythrocin Stearate Filmtab Tablets 452

Ethinyl Estradiol (Estrogen-containing oral contraceptives decrease theophylline clearance in dose dependent fashion). Products include:
Alesse-21 Tablets 3468
Alesse-28 Tablets 3473
Brevicon 28-Day Tablets 3380
Cyclessa Tablets 2450
Desogen Tablets 2458
Estinyl Tablets 3112
Estrostep 2627
femhrt Tablets 2635
Levlen 962
Levlite 21 Tablets 962
Levlite 28 Tablets 962
Levora Tablets 3389
Loestrin 21 Tablets 2642
Loestrin Fe Tablets 2642
Lo/Ovral Tablets 3532
Lo/Ovral-28 Tablets 3538
Low-Ogestrel-28 Tablets 3392
Microgestin Fe 1.5/30 Tablets 3407
Microgestin Fe 1/20 Tablets 3400
Mircette Tablets 2470
Modicon 2563
Necon 3415
Nordette-28 Tablets 2257
Norinyl 1 +35 28-Day Tablets 3380
Ogestrel 0.5/50-28 Tablets 3428
Ortho-Cept 21 Tablets 2546
Ortho-Cept 28 Tablets 2546
Ortho-Cyclen/Ortho Tri-Cyclen 2573
Ortho-Novum 2563
Ovcon 3364
Ovral Tablets 3551
Ovral-28 Tablets 3552
Tri-Levlen 962
Tri-Norinyl-28 Tablets 3433
Triphasil-21 Tablets 3600
Triphasil-28 Tablets 3605
Trivora Tablets 3439
Yasmin 28 Tablets 980
Zovia 3449

Flurazepam Hydrochloride (Benzodiazepines increase CNS concentrations of adenosine, a potent CNS depressant, while theophylline blocks adenosine receptors; larger flurazepam doses may be required to produce desired level of sedation; discontinuation of theophylline without reduction of flurazepam dose may result in respiratory depression).
No products indexed under this heading.

Fluvoxamine Maleate (Decreases theophylline clearance by inhibiting cytochrome P450 1A2). Products include:
Luvox Tablets (25, 50, 100 mg) 3256

Fosphenytoin Sodium (Increases theophylline clearance by increasing microsomal enzyme activity; theophylline decreases phenytoin absorption; these interactions result in decreased serum theophylline and phenytoin concentrations by about 40%). Products include:
Cerebyx Injection 2619

Halothane (Halothane sensitizes the myocardium to catecholamines; theophylline increases release of endogenous catecholamines resulting in increased risk of ventricular arrhythmias). Products include:
Fluothane Inhalation 3508

Interferon alfa-2A, Recombinant (Decreases theophylline clearance). Products include:
Roferon-A Injection 2996

Isoproterenol Hydrochloride (Co-administration with intravenous isoproterenol decreases theophylline clearance).
No products indexed under this heading.

Ketamine Hydrochloride (May lower theophylline seizure threshold).
No products indexed under this heading.

Lithium Carbonate (Theophylline increases renal lithium clearance; increase in lithium dose may be required to achieve a therapeutic serum concentration). Products include:
Eskalith 1527
Lithium Carbonate 3061
Lithobid Slow-Release Tablets 3255

Lithium Citrate (Theophylline increases renal lithium clearance; increase in lithium dose may be required to achieve a therapeutic serum concentration). Products include:
Lithium Citrate Syrup 3061

Lomefloxacin Hydrochloride (Co-administration with some quinolones has increased the plasma levels of theophylline by affecting the rate of theophylline clearance).
No products indexed under this heading.

Lorazepam (Benzodiazepines increase CNS concentrations of adenosine, a potent CNS depressant, while theophylline blocks adenosine receptors; larger lorazepam doses may be required to produce desired level of sedation; discontinuation of theophylline without reduction of lorazepam dose may result in respiratory depression). Products include:
Ativan Injection 3478
Ativan Tablets 3482

Mestranol (Estrogen-containing oral contraceptives decrease theophylline clearance in dose dependent fashion). Products include:
Necon 1/50 Tablets 3415
Norinyl 1 + 50 28-Day Tablets 3380
Ortho-Novum 1/50▫28 Tablets 2556

Methotrexate Sodium (Decreases theophylline clearance).
No products indexed under this heading.

Mexiletine Hydrochloride (Decreases theophylline clearance by inhibiting hydroxylation and demethylation). Products include:
Mexitil Capsules 1047

Moricizine Hydrochloride (Increases theophylline clearance).
No products indexed under this heading.

Norfloxacin (Co-administration with some quinolones has increased the plasma levels of theophylline by affecting the rate of theophylline clearance). Products include:
Chibroxin Sterile Ophthalmic Solution 2051
Noroxin Tablets 2145

Ofloxacin (Co-administration with some quinolones has increased the plasma levels of theophylline by affecting the rate of theophylline clearance). Products include:
Floxin I.V. 2526
Floxin Otic Solution 1219
Floxin Tablets 2529
Ocuflox Ophthalmic Solution 554

Pentoxifylline (Decreases theophylline clearance). Products include:
Trental Tablets 784

Phenytoin (Increases theophylline clearance by increasing microsomal enzyme activity; theophylline decreases phenytoin absorption; these interactions result in decreased serum theophylline and phenytoin concentrations by about 40%). Products include:
Dilantin Infatabs 2624
Dilantin-125 Oral Suspension 2625

Phenytoin Sodium (Increases theophylline clearance by increasing microsomal enzyme activity; theophylline decreases phenytoin absorption; these interactions result in decreased serum theophylline and phenytoin concentrations by about 40%). Products include:
Dilantin Kapseals 2622

Ritonavir (Increases theophylline clearance resulting in 43% decrease in AUC). Products include:
Kaletra Capsules 471
Kaletra Oral Solution 471
Norvir Capsules 487

Norvir Oral Solution 487

Sucralfate (Reduces absorption of theophylline). Products include:
Carafate Suspension 731
Carafate Tablets 730

Sulfinpyrazone (Increases theophylline clearance by increasing demethylation and hydroxylation; decreases renal clearance of theophylline).
No products indexed under this heading.

Tacrine Hydrochloride (Decreases theophylline clearance by inhibiting cytochrome P450 1A2 and also increases renal clearance of theophylline). Products include:
Cognex Capsules 1351

Thiabendazole (Decreases theophylline clearance). Products include:
Mintezol 2137

Ticlopidine Hydrochloride (Decreases theophylline clearance). Products include:
Ticlid Tablets 3015

Troleandomycin (Decreases theophylline clearance by inhibiting cytochrome P450 3A3). Products include:
Tao Capsules 2716

Verapamil Hydrochloride (Decreases theophylline clearance by inhibiting hydroxylation and demethylation). Products include:
Covera-HS Tablets 3199
Isoptin SR Tablets 467
Tarka Tablets 508
Verelan Capsules 3184
Verelan PM Capsules 3186

Food Interactions

Alcohol (Concurrent use with a single dose of alcohol (3 mL/kg of whiskey) decreases theophylline clearance for up to 24 hours).

Diet, high-lipid (Co-administration with a high-fat breakfast delays the time to peak concentration, however, the extent of theophylline absorption is similar when administered fasting or immediately after a high-fat breakfast).

UNIPHYL 400 MG AND 600 MG TABLETS

(Theophylline) 2903
May interact with erythromycin, lithium preparations, and certain other agents. Compounds in these categories include:

Adenosine (Theophylline blocks adenosine receptors; higher doses of adenosine may be required to achieve desired effect). Products include:
Adenocard Injection 1380
Adenoscan 1381

Allopurinol (Decreases theophylline clearance at allopurinol doses greater than or equal to 600 mg/day).
No products indexed under this heading.

Aminoglutethimide (Increases theophylline clearance by induction of microsomal enzyme).
No products indexed under this heading.

Carbamazepine (Increases theophylline clearance by induction of microsomal enzyme). Products include:
Carbatrol Capsules 3234
Tegretol/Tegretol-XR 2404

Cimetidine (Decreases theophylline clearance by inhibiting cytochrome P450 1A2). Products include:
Tagamet HB 200 Suspension 762
Tagamet HB 200 Tablets 761
Tagamet Tablets 1644

Cimetidine Hydrochloride (Decreases theophylline clearance by inhibiting cytochrome P450 1A2). Products include:
Tagamet 1644

Ciprofloxacin (Decreases theophylline clearance by inhibiting cytochrome P450 1A2). Products include:
Cipro I.V. 893
Cipro I.V. Pharmacy Bulk Package 897
Cipro Oral Suspension 887

Ciprofloxacin Hydrochloride (Decreases theophylline clearance by inhibiting cytochrome P450 1A2). Products include:
Ciloxan 538
Cipro HC Otic Suspension 540
Cipro Tablets 887

Clarithromycin (Decreases theophylline clearance by inhibiting cytochrome P450 3A3). Products include:
Biaxin/Biaxin XL 403
PREVPAC 3298

Diazepam (Benzodiazepines increase CNS concentrations of adenosine, a potent CNS depressant, while theophylline blocks adenosine receptors; larger diazepam doses may be required to produce desired level of sedation; discontinuation of theophylline without reduction of diazepam dose may result in respiratory depression). Products include:
Valium Injectable 3026
Valium Tablets 3047

Disulfiram (Decreases theophylline clearance by inhibiting hydroxylation and demethylation). Products include:
Antabuse Tablets 2444
Antabuse Tablets 3474

Enoxacin (Decreases theophylline clearance by inhibiting cytochrome P450 1A2).
No products indexed under this heading.

Ephedrine Hydrochloride (Co-administration results in synergistic CNS effects resulting in increased frequency of nausea, nervousness, and insomnia). Products include:
Primatene Tablets 780

Ephedrine Sulfate (Co-administration results in synergistic CNS effects resulting in increased frequency of nausea, nervousness, and insomnia).
No products indexed under this heading.

Ephedrine Tannate (Co-administration results in synergistic CNS effects resulting in increased frequency of nausea, nervousness, and insomnia). Products include:
Rynatuss Pediatric Suspension 3353
Rynatuss Tablets 3353

Erythromycin (Erythromycin metabolite decreases theophylline clearance by inhibiting cytochrome P450 3A3; decreased erythromycin steady-state serum concentrations). Products include:
Emgel 2% Topical Gel 1285
Ery-Tab Tablets 448
Erythromycin Base Filmtab Tablets 454
Erythromycin Delayed-Release Capsules, USP 455
PCE Dispertab Tablets 498

Erythromycin Estolate (Erythromycin metabolite decreases theophylline clearance by inhibiting cytochrome P450 3A3; decreased erythromycin steady-state serum concentrations).
No products indexed under this heading.

Erythromycin Ethylsuccinate (Erythromycin metabolite decreases theophylline clearance by inhibiting cytochrome P450 3A3; decreased erythromycin steady-state serum concentrations). Products include:
E.E.S. 450
EryPed 446
Pediazole Suspension 3050

Erythromycin Gluceptate (Erythromycin metabolite decreases theophylline clearance by inhibiting cytochrome P450 3A3; decreased erythromycin steady-state serum concentrations).
No products indexed under this heading.

Erythromycin Stearate (Erythromycin metabolite decreases theophylline clearance by inhibiting cytochrome P450 3A3; decreased erythromycin steady-state serum concentrations). Products include:
Erythrocin Stearate Filmtab Tablets 452

Ethinyl Estradiol (Estrogen containing oral contraceptives decreases theophylline clearance in dose dependent fashion). Products include:
Alesse-21 Tablets 3468
Alesse-28 Tablets 3473
Brevicon 28-Day Tablets 3380
Cyclessa Tablets 2450
Desogen Tablets 2458
Estinyl Tablets 3112
Estrostep 2627
femhrt Tablets 2635
Levlen 962
Levlite 21 Tablets 962
Levlite 28 Tablets 962
Levora Tablets 3389
Loestrin 21 Tablets 2642
Loestrin Fe Tablets 2642
Lo/Ovral Tablets 3532
Lo/Ovral-28 Tablets 3538
Low-Ogestrel-28 Tablets 3392
Microgestin Fe 1.5/30 Tablets 3407
Microgestin Fe 1/20 Tablets 3400
Mircette Tablets 2470
Modicon 2563
Necon 3415
Nordette-28 Tablets 2257
Norinyl 1 +35 28-Day Tablets 3380
Ogestrel 0.5/50-28 Tablets 3428
Ortho-Cept 21 Tablets 2546
Ortho-Cept 28 Tablets 2546
Ortho-Cyclen/Ortho Tri-Cyclen 2573
Ortho-Novum 2563
Ovcon 3364
Ovral Tablets 3551
Ovral-28 Tablets 3552
Tri-Levlen 962
Tri-Norinyl-28 Tablets 3433
Triphasil-21 Tablets 3600
Triphasil-28 Tablets 3605
Trivora Tablets 3439
Yasmin 28 Tablets 980
Zovia 3449

Flurazepam Hydrochloride (Benzodiazepines increase CNS concentrations of adenosine, a potent CNS depressant, while theophylline blocks adenosine receptors; larger flurazepam doses may be required to produce desired level of sedation; discontinuation of theophylline without reduction of flurazepam dose may result in respiratory depression).
No products indexed under this heading.

Fluvoxamine Maleate (Decreases theophylline clearance by inhibiting cytochrome P450 1A2). Products include:
Luvox Tablets (25, 50, 100 mg) 3256

Halothane (Halothane sensitizes the myocardium to catecholamines; theophylline increases release of endogenous catecholamines resulting in increased risk of ventricular arrhythmias). Products include:
Fluothane Inhalation 3508

Interferon alfa-2A, Recombinant (Decreases theophylline clearance). Products include:
Roferon-A Injection 2996

Isoproterenol Hydrochloride (Co-administration with intravenous isoproterenol decreases theophylline clearance).
No products indexed under this heading.

Ketamine Hydrochloride (May lower theophylline seizure threshold).
No products indexed under this heading.

Lithium Carbonate (Theophylline increases renal lithium clearance; increase in lithium dose may be required to achieve a therapeutic serum concentration). Products include:
Eskalith 1527
Lithium Carbonate 3061
Lithobid Slow-Release Tablets 3255

Lithium Citrate (Theophylline increases renal lithium clearance; increase in lithium dose may be required to achieve a therapeutic serum concentration). Products include:
Lithium Citrate Syrup 3061

Lorazepam (Benzodiazepines increase CNS concentrations of adenosine, a potent CNS depressant, while theophylline blocks adenosine receptors; larger lorazepam doses may be required to produce desired level of sedation; discontinuation of theophylline without reduction of lorazepam dose may result in respiratory depression). Products include:
Ativan Injection 3478
Ativan Tablets 3482

Mestranol (Estrogen containing oral contraceptives decreases theophylline clearance in dose dependent fashion). Products include:
Necon 1/50 Tablets 3415
Norinyl 1 + 50 28-Day Tablets 3380
Ortho-Novum 1/50□28 Tablets 2556

Methotrexate Sodium (Decreases theophylline clearance).
No products indexed under this heading.

Mexiletine Hydrochloride (Decreases theophylline clearance by inhibiting hydroxylation and demethylation). Products include:
Mexitil Capsules 1047

Midazolam Hydrochloride (Benzodiazepines increase CNS concentrations of adenosine, a potent CNS depressant, while theophylline blocks adenosine receptors; larger midazolam doses may be required to produce desired level of sedation; discontinuation of theophylline without reduction of midazolam dose may result in respiratory depression). Products include:
Versed Injection 3027
Versed Syrup 3033

Moricizine Hydrochloride (Increases theophylline clearance).
No products indexed under this heading.

Pancuronium Bromide (Theophylline may antagonize non-depolarizing neuromuscular blocking effects; possibly due to phosphodiesterase inhibition; larger pancuronium doses may be required to achieve neuromuscular blockade).
No products indexed under this heading.

Pentoxifylline (Decreases theophylline clearance). Products include:
Trental Tablets 784

Phenobarbital (Increases theophylline clearance by induction of microsomal enzyme). Products include:
Arco-Lase Plus Tablets 592
Donnatal 2929
Donnatal Extentabs 2930

Phenytoin (Phenytoin increases theophylline clearance by increasing microsomal enzyme activity; theophylline decreases phenytoin absorption). Products include:
Dilantin Infatabs 2624
Dilantin-125 Oral Suspension 2625

Phenytoin Sodium (Phenytoin increases theophylline clearance by increasing microsomal enzyme activity; theophylline decreases phenytoin absorption). Products include:
Dilantin Kapseals 2622

Propafenone Hydrochloride (Decreases theophylline clearance). Products include:

Rythmol Tablets – 150 mg, 225 mg, 300 mg 502

Propranolol Hydrochloride (Decreases theophylline clearance by inhibiting cytochrome P450 1A2). Products include:

Inderal 3513
Inderal LA Long-Acting Capsules 3516
Inderide Tablets 3517
Inderide LA Long-Acting Capsules .. 3519

Rifampin (Increases theophylline clearance by increasing cytochrome P450 1A2 and 3A3 activity). Products include:

Rifadin 765
Rifamate Capsules 767
Rifater Tablets 769

Sulfinpyrazone (Increases theophylline clearance by increasing demethylation and hydroxylation; decreases renal clearance of theophylline).

No products indexed under this heading.

Tacrine Hydrochloride (Decreases theophylline clearance by inhibiting cytochrome P450 1A2 and also increases renal clearance of theophylline). Products include:

Cognex Capsules 1351

Thiabendazole (Decreases theophylline clearance). Products include:

Mintezol 2137

Ticlopidine Hydrochloride (Decreases theophylline clearance). Products include:

Ticlid Tablets 3015

Troleandomycin (Decreases theophylline clearance by inhibiting cytochrome P450 3A3). Products include:

Tao Capsules 2716

Verapamil Hydrochloride (Decreases theophylline clearance by inhibiting hydroxylation and demethylation). Products include:

Covera-HS Tablets 3199
Isoptin SR Tablets 467
Tarka Tablets 508
Verelan Capsules 3184
Verelan PM Capsules 3186

Food Interactions

Alcohol (Concurrent use with a single dose of alcohol (3mL/kg of whiskey) decreases theophylline clearance for up to 24 hours).

Diet, high-lipid (Co-administration with a standardized high-fat meal results in increased peak plasma concentration and bioavailability; however, a precipitous increase in the rate and extent of absorption was not evident; the dosing should be ideally administered consistently either with or without food).

UNIQUE E VITAMIN E CAPSULES

(Vitamin E) 1723

None cited in PDR database.

UNIRETIC TABLETS

(Hydrochlorothiazide, Moexipril Hydrochloride) 3178

May interact with barbiturates, beta blockers, corticosteroids, oral hypoglycemic agents, insulin, lithium preparations, narcotic analgesics, non-steroidal anti-inflammatory agents, potassium preparations, potassium sparing diuretics, and certain other agents. Compounds in these categories include:

Acarbose (Thiazide diuretic may reduce glucose tolerance; concomitant use may require dosage adjustment of oral hypoglycemic agents). Products include:

Precose Tablets 906

Acebutolol Hydrochloride (ACE inhibitors have less than additive effects with beta-adrenergic blockers, presumably because both work by inhibiting the renin-angiotensin system). Products include:

Sectral Capsules 3589

ACTH (Concomitant use of thiazides with ACTH may intensify electrolyte depletion, particularly hypokalemia).

No products indexed under this heading.

Alfentanil Hydrochloride (Co-administration of narcotics with thiazide diuretics may result in potentiation of orthostatic hypotension).

No products indexed under this heading.

Amiloride Hydrochloride (Potassium-sparing diuretics can increase the risk of hyperkalemia). Products include:

Midamor Tablets 2136
Moduretic Tablets 2138

Aprobarbital (Co-administration of barbiturate with thiazide diuretics may result in potentiation of orthostatic hypotension).

No products indexed under this heading.

Atenolol (ACE inhibitors have less than additive effects with beta-adrenergic blockers, presumably because both work by inhibiting the renin-angiotensin system). Products include:

Tenoretic Tablets 690
Tenormin I.V. Injection 692

Betamethasone Acetate (Concomitant use of thiazides with corticosteroids may intensify electrolyte depletion, particularly hypokalemia). Products include:

Celestone Soluspan Injectable Suspension 3097

Betamethasone Sodium Phosphate (Concomitant use of thiazides with corticosteroids may intensify electrolyte depletion, particularly hypokalemia). Products include:

Celestone Soluspan Injectable Suspension 3097

Betaxolol Hydrochloride (ACE inhibitors have less than additive effects with beta-adrenergic blockers, presumably because both work by inhibiting the renin-angiotensin system). Products include:

Betoptic S Ophthalmic Suspension 537

Bisoprolol Fumarate (ACE inhibitors have less than additive effects with beta-adrenergic blockers, presumably because both work by inhibiting the renin-angiotensin system). Products include:

Zebeta Tablets 1885
Ziac Tablets 1887

Buprenorphine Hydrochloride (Co-administration of narcotics with thiazide diuretics may result in potentiation of orthostatic hypotension). Products include:

Buprenex Injectable 2918

Butabarbital (Co-administration of barbiturate with thiazide diuretics may result in potentiation of orthostatic hypotension).

No products indexed under this heading.

Butalbital (Co-administration of barbiturate with thiazide diuretics may result in potentiation of orthostatic hypotension). Products include:

Phrenilin 578
Sedapap Tablets 50 mg/650 mg 2225

Carteolol Hydrochloride (ACE inhibitors have less than additive effects with beta-adrenergic blockers, presumably because both work by inhibiting the renin-angiotensin system). Products include:

Carteolol Hydrochloride Ophthalmic Solution USP, 1% ..... ⊙258
Ocupress Ophthalmic Solution, 1% Sterile .... ⊙303

Celecoxib (NSAIDs can reduce the diuretic, natriuretic, and antihypertensive effects of thiazides). Products include:

Celebrex Capsules 2676
Celebrex Capsules 2780

Chlorpropamide (Thiazide diuretic may reduce glucose tolerance; concomitant use may require dosage adjustment of oral hypoglycemic agents). Products include:

Diabinese Tablets 2680

Cholestyramine (Absorption of hydrochlorothiazide is impaired in the presence of anionic exchange resins; binds the hydrochlorothiazide and reduces its absorption from GI tract by up to 85%).

No products indexed under this heading.

Codeine Phosphate (Co-administration of narcotics with thiazide diuretics may result in potentiation of orthostatic hypotension). Products include:

Phenergan with Codeine Syrup 3557
Phenergan VC with Codeine Syrup . 3561
Robitussin A-C Syrup 2942
Robitussin-DAC Syrup 2942
Ryna-C Liquid .... ⊡768
Soma Compound w/Codeine Tablets 3355
Tussi-Organidin NR Liquid 3350
Tussi-Organidin-S NR Liquid 3350
Tylenol with Codeine 2595

Colestipol Hydrochloride (Absorption of hydrochlorothiazide is impaired in the presence of anionic exchange resins; binds the hydrochlorothiazide and reduces its absorption from GI tract by up to 43%). Products include:

Colestid Tablets 2791

Cortisone Acetate (Concomitant use of thiazides with corticosteroids may intensify electrolyte depletion, particularly hypokalemia). Products include:

Cortone Acetate Injectable Suspension 2059
Cortone Acetate Tablets 2061

Dexamethasone (Concomitant use of thiazides with corticosteroids may intensify electrolyte depletion, particularly hypokalemia). Products include:

Decadron Elixir 2078
Decadron Tablets 2079
TobraDex Ophthalmic Ointment 542
TobraDex Ophthalmic Suspension .. 541

Dexamethasone Acetate (Concomitant use of thiazides with corticosteroids may intensify electrolyte depletion, particularly hypokalemia).

No products indexed under this heading.

Dexamethasone Sodium Phosphate (Concomitant use of thiazides with corticosteroids may intensify electrolyte depletion, particularly hypokalemia). Products include:

Decadron Phosphate Injection 2081
Decadron Phosphate Sterile Ophthalmic Ointment 2083
Decadron Phosphate Sterile Ophthalmic Solution 2084
NeoDecadron Sterile Ophthalmic Solution 2144

Dezocine (Co-administration of narcotics with thiazide diuretics may result in potentiation of orthostatic hypotension).

No products indexed under this heading.

Diclofenac Potassium (NSAIDs can reduce the diuretic, natriuretic, and antihypertensive effects of thiazides). Products include:

Cataflam Tablets 2315

Diclofenac Sodium (NSAIDs can reduce the diuretic, natriuretic, and antihypertensive effects of thiazides). Products include:

Arthrotec Tablets 3195
Voltaren Ophthalmic Sterile Ophthalmic Solution .... ⊙312
Voltaren Tablets 2315
Voltaren-XR Tablets 2315

Esmolol Hydrochloride (ACE inhibitors have less than additive effects with beta-adrenergic blockers, presumably because both work by inhibiting the renin-angiotensin system). Products include:

Brevibloc Injection 858

Etodolac (NSAIDs can reduce the diuretic, natriuretic, and antihypertensive effects of thiazides). Products include:

Lodine 3528
Lodine XL Extended-Release Tablets 3530

Fenoprofen Calcium (NSAIDs can reduce the diuretic, natriuretic, and antihypertensive effects of thiazides).

No products indexed under this heading.

Fentanyl (Co-administration of narcotics with thiazide diuretics may result in potentiation of orthostatic hypotension). Products include:

Duragesic Transdermal System 1786

Fentanyl Citrate (Co-administration of narcotics with thiazide diuretics may result in potentiation of orthostatic hypotension). Products include:

Actiq 1184

Fludrocortisone Acetate (Concomitant use of thiazides with corticosteroids may intensify electrolyte depletion, particularly hypokalemia). Products include:

Florinef Acetate Tablets 2250

Flurbiprofen (NSAIDs can reduce the diuretic, natriuretic, and antihypertensive effects of thiazides).

No products indexed under this heading.

Glimepiride (Thiazide diuretic may reduce glucose tolerance; concomitant use may require dosage adjustment of oral hypoglycemic agents). Products include:

Amaryl Tablets 717

Glipizide (Thiazide diuretic may reduce glucose tolerance; concomitant use may require dosage adjustment of oral hypoglycemic agents). Products include:

Glucotrol Tablets 2692
Glucotrol XL Extended Release Tablets 2693

Glyburide (Thiazide diuretic may reduce glucose tolerance; concomitant use may require dosage adjustment of oral hypoglycemic agents). Products include:

DiaBeta Tablets 741
Glucovance Tablets 1000

Guanabenz Acetate (Co-administration increases the absorption of hydrochlorothiazide).

No products indexed under this heading.

Hydrocodone Bitartrate (Co-administration of narcotics with thiazide diuretics may result in potentiation of orthostatic hypotension). Products include:

Hycodan 1316
Hycomine Compound Tablets 1317
Hycotuss Expectorant Syrup 1318
Lortab 3319
Lortab Elixir 3317
Maxidone Tablets CIII 3399
Norco 5/325 Tablets CIII 3424
Norco 7.5/325 Tablets CIII 3425
Norco 10/325 Tablets CIII 3427
Norco 10/325 Tablets CIII 3425
Vicodin Tablets 516
Vicodin ES Tablets 517
Vicodin HP Tablets 518
Vicodin Tuss Expectorant 519
Vicoprofen Tablets 520
Zydone Tablets 1330

Hydrocodone Polistirex (Co-administration of narcotics with thiazide diuretics may result in potentiation of orthostatic hypotension). Products include:

Tussionex Pennkinetic Extended-Release Suspension 1174

Hydrocortisone (Concomitant use of thiazides with corticosteroids may intensify electrolyte depletion, particularly hypokalemia). Products include:
- Anusol-HC Cream 2.5% 2237
- Cipro HC Otic Suspension 540
- Cortaid Intensive Therapy Cream 717
- Cortaid Maximum Strength Cream 717
- Cortisporin Ophthalmic Suspension Sterile ..... ⊙297
- Cortizone•5 699
- Cortizone•10 699
- Cortizone•10 Plus Creme 700
- Cortizone for Kids Creme 699
- Hydrocortone Tablets 2106
- Massengill Medicated Soft Cloth Towelette 753
- VōSoL HC Otic Solution 3356

Hydrocortisone Acetate (Concomitant use of thiazides with corticosteroids may intensify electrolyte depletion, particularly hypokalemia). Products include:
- Analpram-HC 1338
- Anusol HC-1 Hydrocortisone Anti-Itch Cream 689
- Anusol-HC Suppositories 2238
- Cortaid 717
- Cortifoam Rectal Foam 3170
- Cortisporin-TC Otic Suspension 2246
- Hydrocortone Acetate Injectable Suspension 2103
- Pramosone 1343
- Proctocort Suppositories 2264
- ProctoFoam-HC 3177
- Terra-Cortril Ophthalmic Suspension 2716

Hydrocortisone Sodium Phosphate (Concomitant use of thiazides with corticosteroids may intensify electrolyte depletion, particularly hypokalemia). Products include:
- Hydrocortone Phosphate Injection, Sterile 2105

Hydrocortisone Sodium Succinate (Concomitant use of thiazides with corticosteroids may intensify electrolyte depletion, particularly hypokalemia).
No products indexed under this heading.

Hydromorphone Hydrochloride (Co-administration of narcotics with thiazide diuretics may result in potentiation of orthostatic hypotension). Products include:
- Dilaudid 441
- Dilaudid Oral Liquid 445
- Dilaudid Powder 441
- Dilaudid Rectal Suppositories 441
- Dilaudid Tablets 441
- Dilaudid Tablets - 8 mg 445
- Dilaudid-HP 443

Ibuprofen (NSAIDs can reduce the diuretic, natriuretic, and antihypertensive effects of thiazides). Products include:
- Advil 771
- Children's Advil Oral Suspension 773
- Children's Advil Chewable Tablets 773
- Advil Cold and Sinus Caplets 771
- Advil Cold and Sinus Tablets 771
- Advil Flu & Body Ache Caplets 772
- Infants' Advil Drops 773
- Junior Strength Advil Tablets 773
- Junior Strength Advil Chewable Tablets 773
- Advil Migraine Liquigels 772
- Children's Motrin Oral Suspension and Chewable Tablets 2006
- Children's Motrin Cold Oral Suspension 2007
- Children's Motrin Oral Suspension 643
- Motrin Suspension, Oral Drops, Chewable Tablets, and Caplets 2002
- Infants' Motrin Concentrated Drops 2006
- Junior Strength Motrin Caplets and Chewable Tablets 2006
- Motrin IB Tablets, Caplets, and Gelcaps 2002
- Motrin Migraine Pain Caplets 2005
- Motrin Sinus Headache Caplets 2005
- Vicoprofen Tablets 520

Indomethacin (NSAIDs can reduce the diuretic, natriuretic, and antihypertensive effects of thiazides). Products include:
- Indocin 2112

Indomethacin Sodium Trihydrate (NSAIDs can reduce the diuretic, natriuretic, and antihypertensive effects of thiazides). Products include:
- Indocin I.V. 2115

Insulin, Human, Zinc Suspension (Thiazide diuretic may reduce glucose tolerance; concomitant use may require dosage adjustment of insulin). Products include:
- Humulin L, 100 Units 1937
- Humulin U, 100 Units 1943
- Novolin L Human Insulin 10 ml Vials 2422

Insulin, Human NPH (Thiazide diuretic may reduce glucose tolerance; concomitant use may require dosage adjustment of insulin). Products include:
- Humulin N, 100 Units 1939
- Humulin N NPH Pen 1940
- Novolin N Human Insulin 10 ml Vials 2422
- Novolin N PenFill 2423
- Novolin N Prefilled Syringe Disposable Insulin Delivery System 2425

Insulin, Human Regular (Thiazide diuretic may reduce glucose tolerance; concomitant use may require dosage adjustment of insulin). Products include:
- Humulin R Regular (U-500) 1943
- Humulin R, 100 Units 1941
- Novolin R Human Insulin 10 ml Vials 2423
- Novolin R PenFill 2423
- Novolin R Prefilled Syringe Disposable Insulin Delivery System 2425
- Velosulin BR Human Insulin 10 ml Vials 2435

Insulin, Human Regular and Human NPH Mixture (Thiazide diuretic may reduce glucose tolerance; concomitant use may require dosage adjustment of insulin). Products include:
- Humulin 50/50, 100 Units 1934
- Humulin 70/30, 100 Units 1935
- Humulin 70/30 Pen 1936
- Novolin 70/30 Human Insulin 10 ml Vials 2421
- Novolin 70/30 PenFill 2423
- Novolin 70/30 Prefilled Disposable Insulin Delivery System 2425

Insulin, NPH (Thiazide diuretic may reduce glucose tolerance; concomitant use may require dosage adjustment of insulin). Products include:
- Iletin II, NPH (Pork), 100 Units 1946

Insulin, Regular (Thiazide diuretic may reduce glucose tolerance; concomitant use may require dosage adjustment of insulin). Products include:
- Iletin II, Regular (Pork), 100 Units 1947

Insulin, Zinc Crystals (Thiazide diuretic may reduce glucose tolerance; concomitant use may require dosage adjustment of insulin).
No products indexed under this heading.

Insulin, Zinc Suspension (Thiazide diuretic may reduce glucose tolerance; concomitant use may require dosage adjustment of insulin). Products include:
- Iletin II, Lente (Pork), 100 Units 1945

Insulin Aspart, Human Regular (Thiazide diuretic may reduce glucose tolerance; concomitant use may require dosage adjustment of insulin).
No products indexed under this heading.

Insulin glargine (Thiazide diuretic may reduce glucose tolerance; concomitant use may require dosage adjustment of insulin). Products include:
- Lantus Injection 742

Insulin Lispro, Human (Thiazide diuretic may reduce glucose tolerance; concomitant use may require dosage adjustment of insulin). Products include:
- Humalog 1926
- Humalog Mix 75/25 Pen 1928

Insulin Lispro Protamine, Human (Thiazide diuretic may reduce glucose tolerance; concomitant use may require dosage adjustment of insulin). Products include:
- Humalog Mix 75/25 Pen 1928

Ketoprofen (NSAIDs can reduce the diuretic, natriuretic, and antihypertensive effects of thiazides). Products include:
- Orudis Capsules 3548
- Orudis KT Tablets 778
- Oruvail Capsules 3548

Ketorolac Tromethamine (NSAIDs can reduce the diuretic, natriuretic, and antihypertensive effects of thiazides). Products include:
- Acular Ophthalmic Solution 544
- Acular PF Ophthalmic Solution 544
- Toradol 3018

Labetalol Hydrochloride (ACE inhibitors have less than additive effects with beta-adrenergic blockers, presumably because both work by inhibiting the renin-angiotension system). Products include:
- Normodyne Injection 3135
- Normodyne Tablets 3137

Levobunolol Hydrochloride (ACE inhibitors have less than additive effects with beta-adrenergic blockers, presumably because both work by inhibiting the renin-angiotension system). Products include:
- Betagan ..... ⊙228

Levorphanol Tartrate (Co-administration of narcotics with thiazide diuretics may result in potentiation of orthostatic hypotension). Products include:
- Levo-Dromoran 1734
- Levorphanol Tartrate Tablets 3059

Lithium Carbonate (Co-administration of ACE inhibitors and lithium has resulted in increased serum lithium levels and symptoms of lithium toxicity). Products include:
- Eskalith 1527
- Lithium Carbonate 3061
- Lithobid Slow-Release Tablets 3255

Lithium Citrate (Co-administration of ACE inhibitors and lithium has resulted in increased serum lithium levels and symptoms of lithium toxicity). Products include:
- Lithium Citrate Syrup 3061

Meclofenamate Sodium (NSAIDs can reduce the diuretic, natriuretic, and antihypertensive effects of thiazides).
No products indexed under this heading.

Mefenamic Acid (NSAIDs can reduce the diuretic, natriuretic, and antihypertensive effects of thiazides). Products include:
- Ponstel Capsules 1356

Meloxicam (NSAIDs can reduce the diuretic, natriuretic, and antihypertensive effects of thiazides). Products include:
- Mobic Tablets 1054

Meperidine Hydrochloride (Co-administration of narcotics with thiazide diuretics may result in potentiation of orthostatic hypotension). Products include:
- Demerol 3079
- Mepergan Injection 3539

Mephobarbital (Co-administration of barbiturate with thiazide diuretics may result in potentiation of orthostatic hypotension).
No products indexed under this heading.

Metformin Hydrochloride (Thiazide diuretic may reduce glucose tolerance; concomitant use may require dosage adjustment of oral hypoglycemic agents). Products include:
- Glucophage Tablets 1080
- Glucophage XR Tablets 1080
- Glucovance Tablets 1086

Methadone Hydrochloride (Co-administration of narcotics with thiazide diuretics may result in potentiation of orthostatic hypotension). Products include:
- Dolophine Hydrochloride Tablets 3056

Methylprednisolone Acetate (Concomitant use of thiazides with corticosteroids may intensify electrolyte depletion, particularly hypokalemia). Products include:
- Depo-Medrol Injectable Suspension 2795

Methylprednisolone Sodium Succinate (Concomitant use of thiazides with corticosteroids may intensify electrolyte depletion, particularly hypokalemia). Products include:
- Solu-Medrol Sterile Powder 2855

Metipranolol Hydrochloride (ACE inhibitors have less than additive effects with beta-adrenergic blockers, presumably because both work by inhibiting the renin-angiotension system).
No products indexed under this heading.

Metoprolol Succinate (ACE inhibitors have less than additive effects with beta-adrenergic blockers, presumably because both work by inhibiting the renin-angiotension system). Products include:
- Toprol-XL Tablets 651

Metoprolol Tartrate (ACE inhibitors have less than additive effects with beta-adrenergic blockers, presumably because both work by inhibiting the renin-angiotension system).
No products indexed under this heading.

Miglitol (Thiazide diuretic may reduce glucose tolerance; concomitant use may require dosage adjustment of oral hypoglycemic agents). Products include:
- Glyset Tablets 2821

Morphine Sulfate (Co-administration of narcotics with thiazide diuretics may result in potentiation of orthostatic hypotension). Products include:
- Astramorph/PF Injection, USP (Preservative-Free) 594
- Duramorph Injection 1312
- Infumorph 200 and Infumorph 500 Sterile Solutions 1314
- Kadian Capsules 1335
- MS Contin Tablets 2896
- MSIR 2898
- Oramorph SR Tablets 3062
- Roxanol 3066

Nabumetone (NSAIDs can reduce the diuretic, natriuretic, and antihypertensive effects of thiazides). Products include:
- Relafen Tablets 1617

Nadolol (ACE inhibitors have less than additive effects with beta-adrenergic blockers, presumably because both work by inhibiting the renin-angiotension system). Products include:
- Corgard Tablets 2245
- Corzide 40/5 Tablets 2247
- Corzide 80/5 Tablets 2247
- Nadolol Tablets 2288

Naproxen (NSAIDs can reduce the diuretic, natriuretic, and antihypertensive effects of thiazides). Products include:
- EC-Naprosyn Delayed-Release Tablets 2967
- Naprosyn Suspension 2967
- Naprosyn Tablets 2967

Naproxen Sodium (NSAIDs can reduce the diuretic, natriuretic, and antihypertensive effects of thiazides). Products include:
- Aleve Tablets, Caplets and Gelcaps .... ▣ 602
- Aleve Cold & Sinus Caplets .... ▣ 603
- Anaprox Tablets 2967
- Anaprox DS Tablets 2967
- Naprelan Tablets 1293

Norepinephrine Bitartrate (Thiazide diuretics may decrease arterial responsiveness to pressor amines).
No products indexed under this heading.

Oxaprozin (NSAIDs can reduce the diuretic, natriuretic, and antihypertensive effects of thiazides).
No products indexed under this heading.

Oxycodone Hydrochloride (Co-administration of narcotics with thiazide diuretics may result in potentiation of orthostatic hypotension).
Products include:
- OxyContin Tablets 2912
- OxyFast Oral Concentrate Solution 2916
- OxyIR Capsules 2916
- Percocet Tablets 1326
- Percodan Tablets 1327
- Percolone Tablets 1327
- Roxicodone 3067
- Tylox Capsules 2597

Penbutolol Sulfate (ACE inhibitors have less than additive effects with beta-adrenergic blockers, presumably because both work by inhibiting the renin-angiotension system).
No products indexed under this heading.

Pentobarbital Sodium (Co-administration of barbiturate with thiazide diuretics may result in potentiation of orthostatic hypotension).
Products include:
- Nembutal Sodium Solution 485

Phenobarbital (Co-administration of barbiturate with thiazide diuretics may result in potentiation of orthostatic hypotension). Products include:
- Arco-Lase Plus Tablets 592
- Donnatal 2929
- Donnatal Extentabs 2930

Phenylbutazone (NSAIDs can reduce the diuretic, natriuretic, and antihypertensive effects of thiazides).
No products indexed under this heading.

Pindolol (ACE inhibitors have less than additive effects with beta-adrenergic blockers, presumably because both work by inhibiting the renin-angiotension system).
No products indexed under this heading.

Pioglitazone Hydrochloride (Thiazide diuretic may reduce glucose tolerance; concomitant use may require dosage adjustment of oral hypoglycemic agents). Products include:
- Actos Tablets 3275

Piroxicam (NSAIDs can reduce the diuretic, natriuretic, and antihypertensive effects of thiazides).
Products include:
- Feldene Capsules 2685

Potassium Acid Phosphate (Potassium supplements can increase the risk of hyperkalemia).
Products include:
- K-Phos Original (Sodium Free) Tablets 947

Potassium Bicarbonate (Potassium supplements can increase the risk of hyperkalemia).
No products indexed under this heading.

Potassium Chloride (Potassium supplements can increase the risk of hyperkalemia). Products include:
- Chlor-3 1361
- Colyte with Flavor Packs for Oral Solution 3170
- GoLYTELY and Pineapple Flavor GoLYTELY for Oral Solution 1068
- K-Dur Microburst Release System ER Tablets 1832
- Klor-Con M20/Klor-Con M10 Tablets 3329
- K-Lor Powder Packets 469
- K-Tab Filmtab Tablets 470
- Micro-K 3311
- NuLYTELY, Cherry Flavor, Lemon-Lime Flavor, and Orange Flavor NuLYTELY for Oral Solution 1068
- Rum-K 1363

Potassium Citrate (Potassium supplements can increase the risk of hyperkalemia). Products include:
- Urocit-K Tablets 2232

Potassium Gluconate (Potassium supplements can increase the risk of hyperkalemia).
No products indexed under this heading.

Potassium Phosphate (Potassium supplements can increase the risk of hyperkalemia). Products include:
- K-Phos Neutral Tablets 946

Prednisolone Acetate (Concomitant use of thiazides with corticosteroids may intensify electrolyte depletion, particularly hypokalemia).
Products include:
- Blephamide Ophthalmic Ointment 547
- Blephamide Ophthalmic Suspension 548
- Poly-Pred Liquifilm Ophthalmic Suspension .... ⊙ 245
- Pred Forte Ophthalmic Suspension .... ⊙ 246
- Pred Mild Sterile Ophthalmic Suspension .... ⊙ 249
- Pred-G Ophthalmic Suspension .... ⊙ 247
- Pred-G Sterile Ophthalmic Ointment .... ⊙ 248

Prednisolone Sodium Phosphate (Concomitant use of thiazides with corticosteroids may intensify electrolyte depletion, particularly hypokalemia). Products include:
- Pediapred Oral Solution 1170

Prednisolone Tebutate (Concomitant use of thiazides with corticosteroids may intensify electrolyte depletion, particularly hypokalemia).
No products indexed under this heading.

Prednisone (Concomitant use of thiazides with corticosteroids may intensify electrolyte depletion, particularly hypokalemia). Products include:
- Prednisone 3064

Propantheline Bromide (Co-administration increases the absorption of hydrochlorothiazide).
No products indexed under this heading.

Propoxyphene Hydrochloride (Co-administration of narcotics with thiazide diuretics may result in potentiation of orthostatic hypotension).
Products include:
- Darvon Pulvules 1909
- Darvon Compound-65 Pulvules 1910

Propoxyphene Napsylate (Co-administration of narcotics with thiazide diuretics may result in potentiation of orthostatic hypotension).
Products include:
- Darvon-N/Darvocet-N 1907
- Darvon-N Tablets 1912

Propranolol Hydrochloride (ACE inhibitors have less than additive effects with beta-adrenergic blockers, presumably because both work by inhibiting the renin-angiotension system). Products include:
- Inderal 3513
- Inderal LA Long-Acting Capsules 3516
- Inderide Tablets 3517
- Inderide LA Long-Acting Capsules 3519

Remifentanil Hydrochloride (Co-administration of narcotics with thiazide diuretics may result in potentiation of orthostatic hypotension).
No products indexed under this heading.

Repaglinide (Thiazide diuretic may reduce glucose tolerance; concomitant use may require dosage adjustment of oral hypoglycemic agents).
Products include:
- Prandin Tablets (0.5, 1, and 2 mg) 2432

Rofecoxib (NSAIDs can reduce the diuretic, natriuretic, and antihypertensive effects of thiazides).
Products include:
- Vioxx 2213

Rosiglitazone Maleate (Thiazide diuretic may reduce glucose tolerance; concomitant use may require dosage adjustment of oral hypoglycemic agents). Products include:
- Avandia Tablets 1490

Secobarbital Sodium (Co-administration of barbiturate with thiazide diuretics may result in potentiation of orthostatic hypotension).
No products indexed under this heading.

Sotalol Hydrochloride (ACE inhibitors have less than additive effects with beta-adrenergic blockers, presumably because both work by inhibiting the renin-angiotension system).
Products include:
- Betapace Tablets 950
- Betapace AF Tablets 954

Spironolactone (Potassium-sparing diuretics can increase the risk of hyperkalemia).
No products indexed under this heading.

Sufentanil Citrate (Co-administration of narcotics with thiazide diuretics may result in potentiation of orthostatic hypotension).
No products indexed under this heading.

Sulindac (NSAIDs can reduce the diuretic, natriuretic, and antihypertensive effects of thiazides).
Products include:
- Clinoril Tablets 2053

Thiamylal Sodium (Co-administration of barbiturate with thiazide diuretics may result in potentiation of orthostatic hypotension).
No products indexed under this heading.

Timolol Hemihydrate (ACE inhibitors have less than additive effects with beta-adrenergic blockers, presumably because both work by inhibiting the renin-angiotension system).
Products include:
- Betimol Ophthalmic Solution .... ⊙ 324

Timolol Maleate (ACE inhibitors have less than additive effects with beta-adrenergic blockers, presumably because both work by inhibiting the renin-angiotension system).
Products include:
- Blocadren Tablets 2046
- Cosopt Sterile Ophthalmic Solution 2065
- Timolide Tablets 2187
- Timolol GFS .... ⊙ 266
- Timoptic in Ocudose 2192
- Timoptic Sterile Ophthalmic Solution 2190
- Timoptic-XE Sterile Ophthalmic Gel Forming Solution 2194

Tolazamide (Thiazide diuretic may reduce glucose tolerance; concomitant use may require dosage adjustment of oral hypoglycemic agents).
No products indexed under this heading.

Tolbutamide (Thiazide diuretic may reduce glucose tolerance; concomitant use may require dosage adjustment of oral hypoglycemic agents).
No products indexed under this heading.

Tolmetin Sodium (NSAIDs can reduce the diuretic, natriuretic, and antihypertensive effects of thiazides). Products include:
- Tolectin 2589

Triamcinolone (Concomitant use of thiazides with corticosteroids may intensify electrolyte depletion, particularly hypokalemia).
No products indexed under this heading.

Triamcinolone Acetonide (Concomitant use of thiazides with corticosteroids may intensify electrolyte depletion, particularly hypokalemia).
Products include:
- Azmacort Inhalation Aerosol 728
- Nasacort Nasal Inhaler 750
- Nasacort AQ Nasal Spray 752
- Tri-Nasal Spray 2274

Triamcinolone Diacetate (Concomitant use of thiazides with corticosteroids may intensify electrolyte depletion, particularly hypokalemia).
No products indexed under this heading.

Triamcinolone Hexacetonide (Concomitant use of thiazides with corticosteroids may intensify electrolyte depletion, particularly hypokalemia).
No products indexed under this heading.

Triamterene (Potassium-sparing diuretics can increase the risk of hyperkalemia). Products include:
- Dyazide Capsules 1515
- Dyrenium Capsules 3458
- Maxzide 1008

Troglitazone (Thiazide diuretic may reduce glucose tolerance; concomitant use may require dosage adjustment of oral hypoglycemic agents).
No products indexed under this heading.

Tubocurarine Chloride (Thiazide diuretics may increase the responsiveness to tubocurarine).
No products indexed under this heading.

Food Interactions

Alcohol (Co-administration of alcohol with thiazide diuretics may result in potentiation of orthostatic hypotension).

Food, unspecified (Bioavailability varies with formulation and food intake which reduces Cmax and AUC of moexipril at by about 70% and 40% respectively after ingestion of low-fat breakfast or by 80% and 50% respectively after the ingestion of a high-fat breakfast; patients should be advised to take Uniretic one hour before a meal).

UNISOM SLEEPTABS

(Doxylamine Succinate) .... ▣ 713
May interact with:

Food Interactions

Alcohol (Use Unisom cautiously).

UNISOM MAXIMUM STRENGTH SLEEPGELS

(Diphenhydramine Hydrochloride) .... ▣ 713
May interact with hypnotics and sedatives, tranquilizers, and certain other agents. Compounds in these categories include:

Alprazolam (Concurrent use with tranquilizers should be avoided).
Products include:
- Xanax Tablets 2865

Buspirone Hydrochloride (Concurrent use with tranquilizers should be avoided).
No products indexed under this heading.

Chlordiazepoxide (Concurrent use with tranquilizers should be avoided).
Products include:
- Limbitrol 1738

Chlordiazepoxide Hydrochloride (Concurrent use with tranquilizers should be avoided). Products include:
- Librium Capsules 1736
- Librium for Injection 1737

Chlorpromazine (Concurrent use with tranquilizers should be avoided). Products include:
- Thorazine Suppositories 1656

Chlorpromazine Hydrochloride (Concurrent use with tranquilizers should be avoided). Products include:
- Thorazine 1656

Chlorprothixene (Concurrent use with tranquilizers should be avoided).
- No products indexed under this heading.

Chlorprothixene Hydrochloride (Concurrent use with tranquilizers should be avoided).
- No products indexed under this heading.

Clorazepate Dipotassium (Concurrent use with tranquilizers should be avoided). Products include:
- Tranxene 511

Diazepam (Concurrent use with tranquilizers should be avoided). Products include:
- Valium Injectable 3026
- Valium Tablets 3047

Droperidol (Concurrent use with tranquilizers should be avoided).
- No products indexed under this heading.

Estazolam (Concurrent use with sedatives should be avoided). Products include:
- ProSom Tablets 500

Ethchlorvynol (Concurrent use with sedatives should be avoided).
- No products indexed under this heading.

Ethinamate (Concurrent use with sedatives should be avoided).
- No products indexed under this heading.

Fluphenazine Decanoate (Concurrent use with tranquilizers should be avoided).
- No products indexed under this heading.

Fluphenazine Enanthate (Concurrent use with tranquilizers should be avoided).
- No products indexed under this heading.

Fluphenazine Hydrochloride (Concurrent use with tranquilizers should be avoided).
- No products indexed under this heading.

Flurazepam Hydrochloride (Concurrent use with sedatives should be avoided).
- No products indexed under this heading.

Glutethimide (Concurrent use with sedatives should be avoided).
- No products indexed under this heading.

Haloperidol (Concurrent use with tranquilizers should be avoided). Products include:
- Haldol Injection, Tablets and Concentrate 2533

Haloperidol Decanoate (Concurrent use with tranquilizers should be avoided). Products include:
- Haldol Decanoate 2535

Hydroxyzine Hydrochloride (Concurrent use with tranquilizers should be avoided). Products include:
- Atarax Tablets & Syrup 2667
- Vistaril Intramuscular Solution 2738

Lorazepam (Concurrent use with sedatives should be avoided). Products include:
- Ativan Injection 3478
- Ativan Tablets 3482

Loxapine Hydrochloride (Concurrent use with tranquilizers should be avoided).
- No products indexed under this heading.

Loxapine Succinate (Concurrent use with tranquilizers should be avoided). Products include:
- Loxitane Capsules 3398

Meprobamate (Concurrent use with tranquilizers should be avoided). Products include:
- Miltown Tablets 3349

Mesoridazine Besylate (Concurrent use with tranquilizers should be avoided). Products include:
- Serentil 1057

Midazolam Hydrochloride (Concurrent use with sedatives should be avoided). Products include:
- Versed Injection 3027
- Versed Syrup 3033

Molindone Hydrochloride (Concurrent use with tranquilizers should be avoided). Products include:
- Moban 1320

Oxazepam (Concurrent use with tranquilizers should be avoided).
- No products indexed under this heading.

Perphenazine (Concurrent use with tranquilizers should be avoided). Products include:
- Etrafon 3115
- Trilafon 3160

Prazepam (Concurrent use with tranquilizers should be avoided).
- No products indexed under this heading.

Prochlorperazine (Concurrent use with tranquilizers should be avoided). Products include:
- Compazine 1505

Promethazine Hydrochloride (Concurrent use with tranquilizers should be avoided). Products include:
- Mepergan Injection 3539
- Phenergan Injection 3553
- Phenergan 3556
- Phenergan Syrup 3554
- Phenergan with Codeine Syrup 3557
- Phenergan with Dextromethorphan Syrup 3559
- Phenergan VC Syrup 3560
- Phenergan VC with Codeine Syrup 3561

Propofol (Concurrent use with sedatives should be avoided). Products include:
- Diprivan Injectable Emulsion 667

Quazepam (Concurrent use with sedatives should be avoided).
- No products indexed under this heading.

Secobarbital Sodium (Concurrent use with sedatives should be avoided).
- No products indexed under this heading.

Temazepam (Concurrent use with sedatives should be avoided).
- No products indexed under this heading.

Thioridazine Hydrochloride (Concurrent use with tranquilizers should be avoided). Products include:
- Thioridazine Hydrochloride Tablets 2289

Thiothixene (Concurrent use with tranquilizers should be avoided). Products include:
- Navane Capsules 2701
- Thiothixene Capsules 2290

Triazolam (Concurrent use with sedatives should be avoided). Products include:
- Halcion Tablets 2823

Trifluoperazine Hydrochloride (Concurrent use with tranquilizers should be avoided). Products include:
- Stelazine 1640

Zaleplon (Concurrent use with sedatives should be avoided). Products include:
- Sonata Capsules 3591

Zolpidem Tartrate (Concurrent use with sedatives should be avoided). Products include:
- Ambien Tablets 3191

Food Interactions

Alcohol (Concurrent use of alcoholic beverages should be avoided).

UNITHROID TABLETS

(Levothyroxine Sodium) 3445

May interact with androgens, antacids containing aluminum, calcium and magnesium, beta blockers, oral anticoagulants, dopamine agonists, estrogens, glucocorticoids, cardiac glycosides, hydantoin anticonvulsants, oral hypoglycemic agents, insulin, lithium preparations, phenytoin, radiographic iodinated contrast media, salicylates, sympathomimetics, thiazides, tricyclic antidepressants, theophylline, and certain other agents. Compounds in these categories include:

Cotton seed meal (Concurrent use of cotton seed meal may bind and decrease the absorption of levothyroxine sodium from GI tract).
- No products indexed under this heading.

Heroin (Co-administration may result in increased serum TBG concentrations).
- No products indexed under this heading.

Walnuts (Concurrent use of walnuts may bind and decrease the absorption of levothyroxine sodium from GI tract).
- No products indexed under this heading.

Acarbose (Addition of levothyroxine to antidiabetic therapy may result in increased antidiabetic agent requirements). Products include:
- Precose Tablets 906

Acebutolol Hydrochloride (Co-administration with beta-blockers may decrease T_4 5′-deiodinase activity; action of beta-blocker may be impaired when the hypothyroid patient is converted to euthyroid). Products include:
- Sectral Capsules 3589

Albuterol (Co-administration of sympathomimetic agents may increase the effects of sympathomimetics or thyroid hormone; thyroid hormones may increase risk of coronary insufficiency when sympathomimetic agents are administered to patients with coronary disease). Products include:
- Proventil Inhalation Aerosol 3142
- Ventolin Inhalation Aerosol and Refill 1679

Albuterol Sulfate (Co-administration of sympathomimetic agents may increase the effects of sympathomimetics or thyroid hormone; thyroid hormones may increase risk of coronary insufficiency when sympathomimetic agents are administered to patients with coronary disease). Products include:
- AccuNeb Inhalation Solution 1230
- Combivent Inhalation Aerosol 1041
- DuoNeb Inhalation Solution 1233
- Proventil Inhalation Solution 0.083% 3146
- Proventil Repetabs Tablets 3148
- Proventil Solution for Inhalation 0.5% 3144
- Proventil HFA Inhalation Aerosol 3150
- Ventolin HFA Inhalation Aerosol 3618
- Volmax Extended-Release Tablets 2276

Aldesleukin (Co-administration has been associated with transient painless thyroiditis in 20% of patients). Products include:
- Proleukin for Injection 1199

Aluminum Carbonate (Co-administration with antacids may reduce the efficacy of levothyroxine by binding and delaying or preventing absorption, potentially resulting in hypothyroidism; administer levothyroxine at least 4 hours apart from these agents).
- No products indexed under this heading.

Aluminum Hydroxide (Co-administration with antacids may reduce the efficacy of levothyroxine by binding and delaying or preventing absorption, potentially resulting in hypothyroidism; administer levothyroxine at least 4 hours apart from these agents). Products include:
- Amphojel Suspension (Mint Flavor) 789
- Gaviscon Extra Strength Liquid 751
- Gaviscon Extra Strength Tablets 751
- Gaviscon Regular Strength Liquid 751
- Gaviscon Regular Strength Tablets 750
- Maalox Antacid/Anti-Gas Oral Suspension 673
- Maalox Max Maximum Strength Antacid/Anti-Gas Liquid 2300
- Maalox Regular Strength Antacid/Antigas Liquid 2300
- Mylanta 1813
- Vanquish Caplets 617

Aminoglutethimide (May decrease thyroid hormone secretion, which may result in hypothyroidism).
- No products indexed under this heading.

Aminophylline (Decreased theophylline clearance may occur in hypothyroid patients; clearance returns to normal when euthyroid state is achieved).
- No products indexed under this heading.

p-Aminosalicylic Acid (Co-administration has been associated with thyroid hormone and/or TSH level alterations by various mechanisms).
- No products indexed under this heading.

Amiodarone Hydrochloride (May decrease thyroid hormone secretion, which may result in hypothyroidism; amiodarone is slowly excreted, producing more prolonged hypothyroidism; amiodarone may induce hyperthyroidism by causing thyroiditis). Products include:
- Cordarone Intravenous 3491
- Cordarone Tablets 3487
- Pacerone Tablets 3331

Amitriptyline Hydrochloride (Co-administration may increase the therapeutic and toxic effects of both drugs possibly due to increased receptor sensitivity to catecholamines; toxic effects may include increased risk of arrhythmias and CNS stimulation; onset of tricyclics may be accelerated). Products include:
- Etrafon 3115
- Limbitrol 1738

Amoxapine (Co-administration may increase the therapeutic and toxic effects of both drugs possibly due to increased receptor sensitivity to catecholamines; toxic effects may include increased risk of arrhythmias and CNS stimulation; onset of tricyclics may be accelerated).
- No products indexed under this heading.

Asparaginase (Co-administration may result in decreased serum TBG concentrations). Products include:
- Elspar for Injection 2092

Aspirin (Co-administration with salicylates at greater than 2 gm inhibit binding of T4 and T3 to TBG and transthyrelin; an initial increase in serum FT4 is followed by return of FT4 to normal levels with sustained therapeutic salicylate concentrations, although total T4 levels may decrease by as much as 30%). Products include:
- Aggrenox Capsules 1026
- Alka-Seltzer 603
- Alka-Seltzer Lemon Lime Antacid and Pain Reliever Effervescent Tablets 603

Alka-Seltzer Extra Strength Antacid and Pain Reliever Effervescent Tablets ▣603
Alka-Seltzer PM Effervescent Tablets ▣605
Genuine Bayer Tablets, Caplets and Gelcaps ▣606
Extra Strength Bayer Caplets and Gelcaps ▣610
Aspirin Regimen Bayer Children's Chewable Tablets (Orange or Cherry Flavored) ▣607
Bayer, Aspirin Regimen ▣606
Aspirin Regimen Bayer 81 mg Caplets with Calcium ▣607
Genuine Bayer Professional Labeling (Aspirin Regimen Bayer) ▣608
Extra Strength Bayer Arthritis Caplets ▣610
Extra Strength Bayer Plus Caplets ▣610
Extra Strength Bayer PM Caplets ▣611
BC Powder ▣619
BC Allergy Sinus Cold Powder ▣619
Arthritis Strength BC Powder ▣619
BC Sinus Cold Powder ▣619
Darvon Compound-65 Pulvules 1910
Ecotrin Enteric Coated Aspirin Low, Regular and Maximum Strength Tablets 1715
Excedrin Extra-Strength Tablets, Caplets, and Geltabs ▣629
Excedrin Migraine 1070
Goody's Body Pain Formula Powder ▣620
Goody's Extra Strength Headache Powder ▣620
Goody's Extra Strength Pain Relief Tablets ▣620
Percodan Tablets 1327
Robaxisal Tablets 2939
Soma Compound Tablets 3354
Soma Compound w/Codeine Tablets 3355
Vanquish Caplets ▣617

Atenolol (Co-administration with beta-blockers may decrease T_4 5'-deiodinase activity; action of beta-blocker may be impaired when the hypothyroid patient is converted to euthyroid). Products include:
Tenoretic Tablets 690
Tenormin I.V. Injection 692

Bendroflumethiazide (Co-administration has been associated with thyroid hormone and/or TSH level alterations by various mechanisms). Products include:
Corzide 40/5 Tablets 2247
Corzide 80/5 Tablets 2247

Betamethasone Acetate (Co-administration with glucocorticoids may result in a transient reduction in TSH secretion; the reduction is not sustained, therefore, hypothyroidism does not occur; glucocorticoids may decrease serum TBG concentrations). Products include:
Celestone Soluspan Injectable Suspension 3097

Betamethasone Sodium Phosphate (Co-administration with glucocorticoids may result in a transient reduction in TSH secretion; the reduction is not sustained, therefore, hypothyroidism does not occur; glucocorticoids may decrease serum TBG concentrations). Products include:
Celestone Soluspan Injectable Suspension 3097

Betaxolol Hydrochloride (Co-administration with beta-blockers may decrease T_4 5'-deiodinase activity; action of beta-blocker may be impaired when the hypothyroid patient is converted to euthyroid). Products include:
Betoptic S Ophthalmic Suspension 537

Bisoprolol Fumarate (Co-administration with beta-blockers may decrease T4 5'-deiodinase activity; action of beta-blocker may be impaired when the hypothyroid patient is converted to euthyroid). Products include:
Zebeta Tablets 1885
Ziac Tablets 1887

Bromocriptine Mesylate (Co-administration with dopamine agonists may result in a transient reduction in TSH secretion; the reduction is not sustained, therefore, hypothyroidism does not occur).
No products indexed under this heading.

Calcium Carbonate (Co-administration with calcium carbonate may form insoluble chelate with levothyroxine, which may result in hypothyroidism; administer levothyroxine at least 4 hours apart from these agents). Products include:
Aspirin Regimen Bayer 81 mg Caplets with Calcium ▣607
Extra Strength Bayer Plus Caplets ▣610
Caltrate 600 Tablets ▣814
Caltrate 600 PLUS ▣815
Caltrate 600 + D Tablets ▣814
Caltrate 600 + Soy Tablets ▣814
D-Cal Chewable Caplets ▣794
Florical Capsules and Tablets 2223
Quick Dissolve Maalox Max Maximum Strength Antacid/Antigas Tablets 2301
Quick Dissolve Maalox Regular Strength Antacid Tablets 2301
Marblen Suspension ▣633
Monocal Tablets 2223
Mylanta Fast-Acting 1813
Mylanta Calci Tabs ▣636
One-A-Day Bedtime & Rest Tablets ▣805
One-A-Day Calcium Plus Chewable Tablets ▣805
Os-Cal Chewable Tablets ▣838
Pepcid Complete Chewable Tablets 1815
ReSource Wellness CalciWise Soft Chews ▣824
Rolaids Tablets ▣706
Extra Strength Rolaids Tablets ▣706
Slow-Mag Tablets ▣835
Titralac ▣640
3M Titralac Plus Antacid Tablets ▣640
Tums ▣763

Carbamazepine (Co-administration may increase hepatic metabolism, which may result in hypothyroidism, resulting in increased levothyroxine requirements; carbamazepine reduces serum protein binding of levothyroxine, and total-and free-T_4 may be reduced by 20% to 40%, but most patients have normal serum TSH levels and are clinically euthyroid). Products include:
Carbatrol Capsules 3234
Tegretol/Tegretol-XR 2404

Carteolol Hydrochloride (Co-administration with beta-blockers may decrease T_4 5'-deiodinase activity; action of beta-blocker may be impaired when the hypothyroid patient is converted to euthyroid). Products include:
Carteolol Hydrochloride Ophthalmic Solution USP, 1% ⊙258
Ocupress Ophthalmic Solution, 1% Sterile ⊙303

Chloral Hydrate (Co-administration has been associated with thyroid hormone and/or TSH level alterations by various mechanisms).
No products indexed under this heading.

Chlorothiazide (Co-administration has been associated with thyroid hormone and/or TSH level alterations by various mechanisms). Products include:
Aldoclor Tablets 2035
Diuril Oral 2087

Chlorothiazide Sodium (Co-administration has been associated with thyroid hormone and/or TSH level alterations by various mechanisms). Products include:
Diuril Sodium Intravenous 2086

Chlorotrianisene (Co-administration with oral estrogens may result in increased serum TBG concentrations).
No products indexed under this heading.

Chlorpropamide (Addition of levothyroxine to antidiabetic therapy may result in increased antidiabetic agent requirements). Products include:
Diabinese Tablets 2680

Cholestyramine (Co-administration may result in decreased T_4 absorption, which may result in hypothyroidism; administer levothyroxine at least 4 hours apart from these agents).
No products indexed under this heading.

Choline Magnesium Trisalicylate (Co-administration with salicylates at greater than 2 gm inhibit binding of T4 and T3 to TBG and transthyrelin; an initial increase in serum FT4 is followed by return of FT4 to normal levels with sustained therapeutic salicylate concentrations, although total T4 levels may decrease by as much as 30%). Products include:
Trilisate 2901

Clofibrate (Co-administration may result in increased serum TBG concentrations). Products include:
Atromid-S Capsules 3483

Clomipramine Hydrochloride (Co-administration may increase the therapeutic and toxic effects of both drugs possibly due to increased receptor sensitivity to catecholamines; toxic effects may include increased risk of arrhythmias and CNS stimulation; onset of tricyclics may be accelerated).
No products indexed under this heading.

Colestipol Hydrochloride (Co-administration may result in decreased T_4 absorption, which may result in hypothyroidism; administer levothyroxine at least 4 hours apart from these agents). Products include:
Colestid Tablets 2791

Cortisone Acetate (Co-administration with glucocorticoids may result in a transient reduction in TSH secretion; the reduction is not sustained, therefore, hypothyroidism does not occur; glucocorticoids may decrease serum TBG concentrations). Products include:
Cortone Acetate Injectable Suspension 2059
Cortone Acetate Tablets 2061

Desipramine Hydrochloride (Co-administration may increase the therapeutic and toxic effects of both drugs possibly due to increased receptor sensitivity to catecholamines; toxic effects may include increased risk of arrhythmias and CNS stimulation; onset of tricyclics may be accelerated). Products include:
Norpramin Tablets 755

Deslanoside (Co-administration may result in reduced serum digitalis glycosides in hyperthyroidism or when the hypothyroid patient is converted to the euthyroid state; therapeutic effect of digitalis glycoside may be reduced).
No products indexed under this heading.

Dexamethasone (Co-administration with glucocorticoids may result in a transient reduction in TSH secretion; the reduction is not sustained, therefore, hypothyroidism does not occur; glucocorticoids may decrease serum TBG concentrations). Products include:
Decadron Elixir 2078
Decadron Tablets 2079
TobraDex Ophthalmic Ointment 542
TobraDex Ophthalmic Suspension 541

Dexamethasone Acetate (Co-administration with glucocorticoids may result in a transient reduction in TSH secretion; the reduction is not sustained, therefore, hypothyroidism does not occur; glucocorticoids may decrease serum TBG concentrations).
No products indexed under this heading.

Dexamethasone Sodium Phosphate (Co-administration with glucocorticoids may result in a transient reduction in TSH secretion; the reduction is not sustained, therefore, hypothyroidism does not occur; glucocorticoids may decrease serum TBG concentrations). Products include:
Decadron Phosphate Injection 2081
Decadron Phosphate Sterile Ophthalmic Ointment 2083
Decadron Phosphate Sterile Ophthalmic Solution 2084
NeoDecadron Sterile Ophthalmic Solution 2144

Diatrizoate Meglumine (May decrease thyroid hormone secretion, which may result in hypothyroidism; the fetus, elderly, and euthyroid patients with underlying thyroid disease are among those individuals who are susceptible to iodine-induced hypothyroidism; oral cholecytographicagents slowly excreted, producing more prolonged hypothyroidism; iodide drugs that contain pharmacologic amounts of iodide may cause hypothyroidism in euthyroid patients with Grave's disease previously treated with thyroid autonomy; hyperthyroidism may develop over several weeks and may persist for several months after therapy discontinuation).
No products indexed under this heading.

Diatrizoate Sodium (May decrease thyroid hormone secretion, which may result in hypothyroidism; the fetus, elderly, and euthyroid patients with underlying thyroid disease are among those individuals who are susceptible to iodine-induced hypothyroidism; oral cholecytographicagents slowly excreted, producing more prolonged hypothyroidism; iodide drugs that contain pharmacologic amounts of iodide may cause hypothyroidism in euthyroid patients with Grave's disease previously treated with thyroid autonomy; hyperthyroidism may develop over several weeks and may persist for several months after therapy discontinuation).
No products indexed under this heading.

Diazepam (Co-administration has been associated with thyroid hormone and/or TSH level alterations by various mechanisms). Products include:
Valium Injectable 3020
Valium Tablets 3047

Dicumarol (Thyroid hormones appear to increase the catabolism of vitamin-K dependent clotting factors, thereby increasing the anticoagulant activity of oral anticoagulants).
No products indexed under this heading.

Dienestrol (Co-administration with oral estrogens may result in increased serum TBG concentrations). Products include:
Ortho Dienestrol Cream 2554

Diethylstilbestrol (Co-administration with oral estrogens may result in increased serum TBG concentrations).
No products indexed under this heading.

Diflunisal (Co-administration with salicylates at greater than 2 gm inhibit binding of T4 and T3 to TBG and transthyrelin; an initial increase in serum FT4 is followed by return of FT4 to normal levels with sustained therapeutic salicylate concentrations, although total T4 levels may decrease by as much as 30%). Products include:
Dolobid Tablets 2088

Digitoxin (Co-administration may result in reduced serum digitalis glycosides in hyperthyroidism or when the hypothyroid patient is converted to the euthyroid state; therapeutic effect of digitalis glycoside may be reduced).
No products indexed under this heading.

Digoxin (Co-administration may result in reduced serum digitalis glycosides in hyperthyroidism or when the hypothyroid patient is converted to the euthyroid state; therapeutic effect of digitalis glycoside may be reduced). Products include:
Digitek Tablets 1003
Lanoxicaps Capsules 1574
Lanoxin Injection 1581
Lanoxin Tablets 1587
Lanoxin Elixir Pediatric 1578
Lanoxin Injection Pediatric 1584

Dobutamine Hydrochloride (Co-administration of sympathomimetic agents may increase the effects of sympathomimetics or thyroid hormone; thyroid hormones may increase risk of coronary insufficiency when sympathomimetic agents are administered to patients with coronary disease). Products include:
Dobutrex Solution Vials 1914

Dopamine Hydrochloride (Co-administration with dopamine may result in a transient reduction in TSH secretion; the reduction is not sustained, therefore, hypothyroidism does not occur).
No products indexed under this heading.

Doxepin Hydrochloride (Co-administration may increase the therapeutic and toxic effects of both drugs possibly due to increased receptor sensitivity to catecholamines; toxic effects may include increased risk of arrhythmias and CNS stimulation; onset of tricyclics may be accelerated). Products include:
Sinequan 2713

Dyphylline (Decreased theophylline clearance may occur in hypothyroid patients; clearance returns to normal when euthyroid state is achieved). Products include:
Lufyllin Tablets 3347
Lufyllin-400 Tablets 3347
Lufyllin-GG Elixir 3348
Lufyllin-GG Tablets 3348

Ephedrine Hydrochloride (Co-administration of sympathomimetic agents may increase the effects of sympathomimetics or thyroid hormone; thyroid hormones may increase risk of coronary insufficiency when sympathomimetic agents are administered to patients with coronary disease). Products include:
Primatene Tablets 780

Ephedrine Sulfate (Co-administration of sympathomimetic agents may increase the effects of sympathomimetics or thyroid hormone; thyroid hormones may increase risk of coronary insufficiency when sympathomimetic agents are administered to patients with coronary disease).
No products indexed under this heading.

Ephedrine Tannate (Co-administration of sympathomimetic agents may increase the effects of sympathomimetics or thyroid hormone; thyroid hormones may increase risk of coronary insufficiency when sympathomimetic agents are administered to patients with coronary disease). Products include:
Rynatuss Pediatric Suspension 3353
Rynatuss Tablets 3353

Epinephrine (Co-administration of sympathomimetic agents may increase the effects of sympathomimetics or thyroid hormone; thyroid hormones may increase risk of coronary insufficiency when sympathomimetic agents are administered to patients with coronary disease). Products include:
Epifrin Sterile Ophthalmic Solution .... ⊙ 235
EpiPen 1236
Primatene Mist 779
Xylocaine with Epinephrine Injection 653

Epinephrine Bitartrate (Co-administration of sympathomimetic agents may increase the effects of sympathomimetics or thyroid hormone; thyroid hormones may increase risk of coronary insufficiency when sympathomimetic agents are administered to patients with coronary disease). Products include:
Sensorcaine 643

Epinephrine Hydrochloride (Co-administration of sympathomimetic agents may increase the effects of sympathomimetics or thyroid hormone; thyroid hormones may increase risk of coronary insufficiency when sympathomimetic agents are administered to patients with coronary disease).
No products indexed under this heading.

Esmolol Hydrochloride (Co-administration with beta-blockers may decrease T_4 5'-deiodinase activity; action of beta-blocker may be impaired when the hypothyroid patient is converted to euthyroid). Products include:
Brevibloc Injection 858

Estradiol (Co-administration with oral estrogens may result in increased serum TBG concentrations). Products include:
Activella Tablets 2764
Alora Transdermal System 3372
Climara Transdermal System 958
CombiPatch Transdermal System 2323
Esclim Transdermal System 3460
Estrace Vaginal Cream 3358
Estrace Tablets 3361
Estring Vaginal Ring 2811
Ortho-Prefest Tablets 2570
Vagifem Tablets 2857
Vivelle Transdermal System 2412
Vivelle-Dot Transdermal System 2416

Estrogens, Conjugated (Co-administration with oral estrogens may result in increased serum TBG concentrations). Products include:
Premarin Intravenous 3563
Premarin Tablets 3566
Premarin Vaginal Cream 3570
Premphase Tablets 3572
Prempro Tablets 3572

Estrogens, Esterified (Co-administration with oral estrogens may result in increased serum TBG concentrations). Products include:
Estratest 3252
Menest Tablets 2254

Estropipate (Co-administration with oral estrogens may result in increased serum TBG concentrations). Products include:
Ogen Tablets 2846
Ortho-Est Tablets 3464

Ethinyl Estradiol (Co-administration with estrogen containing oral contraceptives may result in increased serum TBG concentrations). Products include:
Alesse-21 Tablets 3468
Alesse-28 Tablets 3473
Brevicon 28-Day Tablets 3380
Cyclessa Tablets 2450
Desogen Tablets 2458
Estinyl Tablets 3112
Estrostep 2627
femhrt Tablets 2635
Levlen 962
Levlite 21 Tablets 962
Levlite 28 Tablets 962
Levora Tablets 3389
Loestrin 21 Tablets 2642
Loestrin Fe Tablets 2642
Lo/Ovral Tablets 3532
Lo/Ovral-28 Tablets 3538
Low-Ogestrel-28 Tablets 3392
Microgestin Fe 1.5/30 Tablets 3407
Microgestin Fe 1/20 Tablets 3400
Mircette Tablets 2470
Modicon 2563
Necon 3415
Nordette-28 Tablets 2257
Norinyl 1 +35 28-Day Tablets 3380
Ogestrel 0.5/50-28 Tablets 3428
Ortho-Cept 21 Tablets 2546
Ortho-Cept 28 Tablets 2546
Ortho-Cyclen/Ortho Tri-Cyclen 2573
Ortho-Novum 2563
Ovcon 3364
Ovral Tablets 3551
Ovral-28 Tablets 3552
Tri-Levlen 962
Tri-Norinyl-28 Tablets 3433
Triphasil-21 Tablets 3600
Triphasil-28 Tablets 3605
Trivora Tablets 3439
Yasmin 28 Tablets 980
Zovia 3449

Ethiodized Oil (May decrease thyroid hormone secretion, which may result in hypothyroidism; the fetus, elderly, and euthyroid patients with underlying thyroid disease are among those individuals who are susceptible to iodine-induced hypothyroidism; oral cholecytographicagents slowly excreted, producing more prolonged hypothyroidism; iodide drugs that contain pharmacologic amounts of iodide may cause hypothyroidism in euthyroid patients with Grave's disease previously treated with thyroid autonomy; hyperthyroidism may develop over several weeks and may persist for several months after therapy discontinuation). Products include:
Ethiodol Injection 3095

Ethionamide (Co-administration has been associated with thyroid hormone and/or TSH level alterations by various mechanisms). Products include:
Trecator-SC Tablets 3598

Ethotoin (Hydantoins may cause protein-binding site displacement; co-administration results in an initial transient increase in FT_4; continued administration results in a decrease in serum T_4 and normal FT_4 and TSH concentrations and, therefore, patients are clinically euthyroid).
No products indexed under this heading.

Ferrous Sulfate (Co-administration may result in decreased T_4 absorption, which may result in hypothyroidism; ferrous sulfate may form a ferric-thyroxine complex; administer levothyroxine at least 4 hours apart from these agents). Products include:
Feosol Tablets 1717
Slow Fe Tablets 827
Slow Fe with Folic Acid Tablets 828

Fiber Supplement (Concurrent use of dietary fiber may bind and decrease the absorption of levothyroxine sodium from GI tract).
No products indexed under this heading.

Fludrocortisone Acetate (Co-administration with glucocorticoids may result in a transient reduction in TSH secretion; the reduction is not sustained, therefore, hypothyroidism does not occur; glucocorticoids may decrease serum TBG concentrations). Products include:
Florinef Acetate Tablets 2250

Fluorouracil (Co-administration with 5-FU may result in increased serum TBG concentrations). Products include:
Carac Cream 1222
Efudex 1733
Fluoroplex 552

Fluoxymesterone (Co-administration with androgens/anabolic steroids may result in decreased serum TBG concentrations).
No products indexed under this heading.

Fosphenytoin Sodium (Hydantoins may cause protein-binding site displacement; co-administration results in an initial transient increase in FT_4; co-administration may increase hepatic metabolism, which may result in hypothyroidism, resulting in increased levothyroxine requirements; phenytoin reduces serum protein binding of levothyroxine, and total- and free-T_4 may be reduced by 20% to 40%, but most patients have normal serum TSH levels and are clinically euthyroid). Products include:
Cerebyx Injection 2619

Furosemide (May cause protein-binding site displacement at greater than 80 mg IV; co-administration results in an initial transient increase in FT_4; continued administration results in a decrease in serum T_4 and normal FT_4 and TSH concentrations and, therefore, patients are clinically euthyroid). Products include:
Furosemide Tablets 2284

Gadopentetate Dimeglumine (May decrease thyroid hormone secretion, which may result in hypothyroidism; the fetus, elderly, and euthyroid patients with underlying thyroid disease are among those individuals who are susceptible to iodine-induced hypothyroidism; oral cholecytographicagents slowly excreted, producing more prolonged hypothyroidism; iodide drugs that contain pharmacologic amounts of iodide may cause hypothyroidism in euthyroid patients with Grave's disease previously treated with thyroid autonomy; hyperthyroidism may develop over several weeks and may persist for several months after therapy discontinuation).
No products indexed under this heading.

Glimepiride (Addition of levothyroxine to antidiabetic therapy may result in increased antidiabetic agent requirements). Products include:
Amaryl Tablets 717

Glipizide (Addition of levothyroxine to antidiabetic therapy may result in increased antidiabetic agent requirements). Products include:
Glucotrol Tablets 2692
Glucotrol XL Extended Release Tablets 2693

Glyburide (Addition of levothyroxine to antidiabetic therapy may result in increased antidiabetic agent requirements). Products include:
DiaBeta Tablets 741
Glucovance Tablets 1086

Heparin Sodium (May cause protein-binding site displacement; co-administration results in an initial transient increase in FT_4; continued administration results in a decrease in serum T_4 and normal FT_4 and TSH concentrations and, therefore, patients are clinically euthyroid). Products include:
Heparin Lock Flush Solution 3509
Heparin Sodium Injection 3511

Hydrochlorothiazide (Co-administration has been associated with thyroid hormone and/or TSH level alterations by various mechanisms). Products include:
Accuretic Tablets 2614
Aldoril Tablets 2039
Atacand HCT Tablets 597
Avalide Tablets 1070
Diovan HCT Tablets 2338
Dyazide Capsules 1515
HydroDIURIL Tablets 2108

Hyzaar 2109
Inderide Tablets 3517
Inderide LA Long-Acting Capsules .. 3519
Lotensin HCT Tablets 2367
Maxzide 1008
Micardis HCT Tablets 1051
Microzide Capsules 3414
Moduretic Tablets 2138
Monopril HCT 1094
Prinzide Tablets 2168
Timolide Tablets 2187
Uniretic Tablets 3178
Vaseretic Tablets 2204
Zestoretic Tablets 695
Ziac Tablets 1887

Hydrocortisone (Co-administration with glucocorticoids may result in a transient reduction in TSH secretion; the reduction is not sustained, therefore, hypothyroidism does not occur; glucocorticoids may decrease serum TBG concentrations). Products include:

Anusol-HC Cream 2.5% 2237
Cipro HC Otic Suspension 540
Cortaid Intensive Therapy Cream . ■717
Cortaid Maximum Strength Cream .... ■717
Cortisporin Ophthalmic Suspension Sterile .... ⊙297
Cortizone•5 .... ■699
Cortizone•10 .... ■699
Cortizone•10 Plus Creme .... ■700
Cortizone for Kids Creme .... ■699
Hydrocortone Tablets 2106
Massengill Medicated Soft Cloth Towelette .... ■753
VōSoL HC Otic Solution 3356

Hydrocortisone Acetate (Co-administration with glucocorticoids may result in a transient reduction in TSH secretion; the reduction is not sustained, therefore, hypothyroidism does not occur; glucocorticoids may decrease serum TBG concentrations). Products include:

Analpram-HC 1338
Anusol HC-1 Hydrocortisone Anti-Itch Cream .... ■689
Anusol-HC Suppositories 2238
Cortaid .... ■717
Cortifoam Rectal Foam 3170
Cortisporin-TC Otic Suspension 2246
Hydrocortone Acetate Injectable Suspension 2103
Pramosone 1343
Proctocort Suppositories 2264
ProctoFoam-HC 3177
Terra-Cortril Ophthalmic Suspension 2716

Hydrocortisone Sodium Phosphate (Co-administration with glucocorticoids may result in a transient reduction in TSH secretion; the reduction is not sustained, therefore, hypothyroidism does not occur; glucocorticoids may decrease serum TBG concentrations). Products include:

Hydrocortone Phosphate Injection, Sterile 2105

Hydrocortisone Sodium Succinate (Co-administration with glucocorticoids may result in a transient reduction in TSH secretion; the reduction is not sustained, therefore, hypothyroidism does not occur; glucocorticoids may decrease serum TBG concentrations).

No products indexed under this heading.

Hydroflumethiazide (Co-administration has been associated with thyroid hormone and/or TSH level alterations by various mechanisms). Products include:

Diucardin Tablets 3494

Imipramine Hydrochloride (Co-administration may increase the therapeutic and toxic effects of both drugs possibly due to increased receptor sensitivity to catecholamines; toxic effects may include increased risk of arrhythmias and CNS stimulation; onset of tricyclics may be accelerated).

No products indexed under this heading.

Imipramine Pamoate (Co-administration may increase the therapeutic and toxic effects of both drugs possibly due to increased receptor sensitivity to catecholamines; toxic effects may include increased risk of arrhythmias and CNS stimulation; onset of tricyclics may be accelerated).

No products indexed under this heading.

Infant Formula (Concurrent use of soybean flour may bind and decrease the absorption of levothyroxine sodium from GI tract).

Insulin, Human, Zinc Suspension (Addition of levothyroxine to insulin therapy may result in increased insulin requirements). Products include:

Humulin L, 100 Units 1937
Humulin U, 100 Units 1943
Novolin L Human Insulin 10 ml Vials 2422

Insulin, Human NPH (Addition of levothyroxine to insulin therapy may result in increased insulin requirements). Products include:

Humulin N, 100 Units 1939
Humulin N NPH Pen 1940
Novolin N Human Insulin 10 ml Vials 2422
Novolin N PenFill 2423
Novolin N Prefilled Syringe Disposable Insulin Delivery System 2425

Insulin, Human Regular (Addition of levothyroxine to insulin therapy may result in increased insulin requirements). Products include:

Humulin R Regular (U-500) 1943
Humulin R, 100 Units 1941
Novolin R Human Insulin 10 ml Vials 2423
Novolin R PenFill 2423
Novolin R Prefilled Syringe Disposable Insulin Delivery System 2425
Velosulin BR Human Insulin 10 ml Vials 2435

Insulin, Human Regular and Human NPH Mixture (Addition of levothyroxine to insulin therapy may result in increased insulin requirements). Products include:

Humulin 50/50, 100 Units 1934
Humulin 70/30, 100 Units 1935
Humulin 70/30 Pen 1936
Novolin 70/30 Human Insulin 10 ml Vials 2421
Novolin 70/30 PenFill 2423
Novolin 70/30 Prefilled Disposable Insulin Delivery System 2425

Insulin, NPH (Addition of levothyroxine to insulin therapy may result in increased insulin requirements). Products include:

Iletin II, NPH (Pork), 100 Units 1946

Insulin, Regular (Addition of levothyroxine to insulin therapy may result in increased insulin requirements). Products include:

Iletin II, Regular (Pork), 100 Units ... 1947

Insulin, Zinc Crystals (Addition of levothyroxine to insulin therapy may result in increased insulin requirements).

No products indexed under this heading.

Insulin, Zinc Suspension (Addition of levothyroxine to insulin therapy may result in increased insulin requirements). Products include:

Iletin II, Lente (Pork), 100 Units 1945

Insulin Aspart, Human Regular (Addition of levothyroxine to insulin therapy may result in increased insulin requirements).

No products indexed under this heading.

Insulin glargine (Addition of levothyroxine to insulin therapy may result in increased insulin requirements). Products include:

Lantus Injection 742

Insulin Lispro, Human (Addition of levothyroxine to insulin therapy may result in increased insulin requirements). Products include:

Humalog 1926
Humalog Mix 75/25 Pen 1928

Insulin Lispro Protamine, Human (Addition of levothyroxine to insulin therapy may result in increased insulin requirements). Products include:

Humalog Mix 75/25 Pen 1928

Interferon alfa-2A, Recombinant (Co-administration with interferon alpha has been associated with the development of antithyroid microsomal antibodies in 20% of patients and some have transient hypothyroidism, hyperthyroidism, or both; patients who have antithyroid antibodies before treatment are at higher risk for thyroid dysfunction). Products include:

Roferon-A Injection 2996

Interferon alfa-2B, Recombinant (Co-administration with interferon alpha has been associated with the development of antithyroid microsomal antibodies in 20% of patients and some have transient hypothyroidism, hyperthyroidism, or both; patients who have antithyroid antibodies before treatment are at higher risk for thyroid dysfunction). Products include:

Intron A for Injection 3120
Rebetron Combination Therapy 3153

Interferon alfa-N3 (Human Leukocyte Derived) (Co-administration with interferon alpha has been associated with the development of antithyroid microsomal antibodies in 20% of patients and some have transient hypothyroidism, hyperthyroidism, or both; patients who have antithyroid antibodies before treatment are at higher risk for thyroid dysfunction). Products include:

Alferon N Injection 1770

Iodamide Meglumine (May decrease thyroid hormone secretion, which may result in hypothyroidism; the fetus, elderly, and euthyroid patients with underlying thyroid disease are among those individuals who are susceptible to iodine-induced hypothyroidism; oral cholecytographicagents slowly excreted, producing more prolonged hypothyroidism; iodide drugs that contain pharmacologic amounts of iodide may cause hypothyroidism in euthyroid patients with Grave's disease previously treated with thyroid autonomy; hyperthyroidism may develop over several weeks and may persist for several months after therapy discontinuation).

No products indexed under this heading.

Iohexol (May decrease thyroid hormone secretion, which may result in hypothyroidism; the fetus, elderly, and euthyroid patients with underlying thyroid disease are among those individuals who are susceptible to iodine-induced hypothyroidism; oral cholecytographicagents slowly excreted, producing more prolonged hypothyroidism; iodide drugs that contain pharmacologic amounts of iodide may cause hypothyroidism in euthyroid patients with Grave's disease previously treated with thyroid autonomy; hyperthyroidism may develop over several weeks and may persist for several months after therapy discontinuation).

No products indexed under this heading.

Iopamidol (May decrease thyroid hormone secretion, which may result in hypothyroidism; the fetus, elderly, and euthyroid patients with underlying thyroid disease are among those individuals who are susceptible to iodine-induced hypothyroidism; oral cholecytographicagents slowly excreted, producing more prolonged hypothyroidism; iodide drugs that contain pharmacologic amounts of iodide may cause hypothyroidism in euthyroid patients with Grave's disease previously treated with thyroid autonomy; hyperthyroidism may develop over several weeks and may persist for several months after therapy discontinuation).

No products indexed under this heading.

Iopanoic Acid (May decrease thyroid hormone secretion, which may result in hypothyroidism; the fetus, elderly, and euthyroid patients with underlying thyroid disease are among those individuals who are susceptible to iodine-induced hypothyroidism; oral cholecytographicagents slowly excreted, producing more prolonged hypothyroidism; iodide drugs that contain pharmacologic amounts of iodide may cause hypothyroidism in euthyroid patients with Grave's disease previously treated with thyroid autonomy; hyperthyroidism may develop over several weeks and may persist for several months after therapy discontinuation).

Iothalamate Meglumine (May decrease thyroid hormone secretion, which may result in hypothyroidism; the fetus, elderly, and euthyroid patients with underlying thyroid disease are among those individuals who are susceptible to iodine-induced hypothyroidism; oral cholecytographicagents slowly excreted, producing more prolonged hypothyroidism; iodide drugs that contain pharmacologic amounts of iodide may cause hypothyroidism in euthyroid patients with Grave's disease previously treated with thyroid autonomy; hyperthyroidism may develop over several weeks and may persist for several months after therapy discontinuation).

No products indexed under this heading.

Ioxaglate Meglumine (May decrease thyroid hormone secretion, which may result in hypothyroidism; the fetus, elderly, and euthyroid patients with underlying thyroid disease are among those individuals who are susceptible to iodine-induced hypothyroidism; oral cholecytographicagents slowly excreted, producing more prolonged hypothyroidism; iodide drugs that contain pharmacologic amounts of iodide may cause hypothyroidism in euthyroid patients with Grave's disease previously treated with thyroid autonomy; hyperthyroidism may develop over several weeks and may persist for several months after therapy discontinuation).

No products indexed under this heading.

Ioxaglate Sodium (May decrease thyroid hormone secretion, which may result in hypothyroidism; the fetus, elderly, and euthyroid patients with underlying thyroid disease are among those individuals who are susceptible to iodine-induced hypothyroidism; oral cholecytographicagents slowly excreted, producing more prolonged hypothyroidism; iodide drugs that contain pharmacologic amounts of iodide may cause hypothyroidism in euthyroid patients with Grave's disease previously treated with thyroid autonomy; hyperthyroidism may develop over several weeks and may persist for several months after therapy discontinuation).

No products indexed under this heading.

Isoproterenol Hydrochloride (Co-administration of sympathomimetic agents may increase the effects of sympathomimetics or thyroid hormone; thyroid hormones may increase risk of coronary insufficiency when sympathomimetic agents are administered to patients with coronary disease).
No products indexed under this heading.

Isoproterenol Sulfate (Co-administration of sympathomimetic agents may increase the effects of sympathomimetics or thyroid hormone; thyroid hormones may increase risk of coronary insufficiency when sympathomimetic agents are administered to patients with coronary disease).
No products indexed under this heading.

Ketamine Hydrochloride (Co-administration may produce marked hypertension and tachycardia).
No products indexed under this heading.

Labetalol Hydrochloride (Co-administration with beta-blockers may decrease T_4 5'-deiodinase activity; action of beta-blocker may be impaired when the hypothyroid patient is converted to euthyroid). Products include:
Normodyne Injection 3135
Normodyne Tablets 3137

Levalbuterol Hydrochloride (Co-administration of sympathomimetic agents may increase the effects of sympathomimetics or thyroid hormone; thyroid hormones may increase risk of coronary insufficiency when sympathomimetic agents are administered to patients with coronary disease). Products include:
Xopenex Inhalation Solution 3207

Levobunolol Hydrochloride (Co-administration with beta-blockers may decrease T_4 5'-deiodinase activity; action of beta-blocker may be impaired when the hypothyroid patient is converted to euthyroid). Products include:
Betagan .... ⊙228

Lithium Carbonate (May decrease thyroid hormone secretion, which may result in hypothyroidism; long-term lithium therapy can result in goiter in up to 50% of patients, and either subclinical or overt hypothyroidism, each in up to 20% of patients). Products include:
Eskalith 1527
Lithium Carbonate 3061
Lithobid Slow-Release Tablets 3255

Lithium Citrate (May decrease thyroid hormone secretion, which may result in hypothyroidism; long-term lithium therapy can result in goiter in up to 50% of patients, and either subclinical or overt hypothyroidism, each in up to 20% of patients). Products include:
Lithium Citrate Syrup 3061

Lovastatin (Co-administration has been associated with thyroid hormone and/or TSH level alterations by various mechanisms). Products include:
Mevacor Tablets 2132

Magaldrate (Co-administration with antacids may reduce the efficacy of levothyroxine by binding and delaying or preventing absorption, potentially resulting in hypothyroidism; administer levothyroxine at least 4 hours apart from these agents).
No products indexed under this heading.

Magnesium Hydroxide (Co-administration with antacids may reduce the efficacy of levothyroxine by binding and delaying or preventing absorption, potentially resulting in hypothyroidism; administer levothyroxine at least 4 hours apart from these agents). Products include:
Ex•Lax Milk of Magnesia Liquid 670
Maalox Antacid/Anti-Gas Oral Suspension 673
Maalox Max Maximum Strength Antacid/Anti-Gas Liquid 2300
Maalox Regular Strength Antacid/Antigas Liquid 2300
Mylanta Fast-Acting 1813
Mylanta 1813
Pepcid Complete Chewable Tablets 1815
Phillips' Chewable Tablets 615
Phillips' Milk of Magnesia Liquid (Original, Cherry, & Mint) 616
Rolaids Tablets 706
Extra Strength Rolaids Tablets 706
Vanquish Caplets 617

Magnesium Oxide (Co-administration with antacids may reduce the efficacy of levothyroxine by binding and delaying or preventing absorption, potentially resulting in hypothyroidism; administer levothyroxine at least 4 hours apart from these agents). Products include:
Beelith Tablets 946
Mag-Ox 400 Tablets 1024
Uro-Mag Capsules 1024

Magnesium Salicylate (Co-administration with salicylates at greater than 2 gm inhibit binding of T4 and T3 to TBG and transthyrelin; an initial increase in serum FT4 is followed by return of FT4 to normal levels with sustained therapeutic salicylate concentrations, although total T4 levels may decrease by as much as 30%). Products include:
Momentum Backache Relief Extra Strength Caplets 666

Maprotiline Hydrochloride (Co-administration may increase the therapeutic and toxic effects of both drugs possibly due to increased receptor sensitivity to catecholamines; toxic effects may include increased risk of arrhythmias and CNS stimulation; onset of tricyclics may be accelerated).
No products indexed under this heading.

Meclofenamate Sodium (Co-administration with fenamate NSAID may result in decreased serum TBG concentrations).
No products indexed under this heading.

Mefenamic Acid (Co-administration with fenamate NSAID may result in decreased serum TBG concentrations). Products include:
Ponstel Capsules 1356

Mephenytoin (Hydantoins may cause protein-binding site displacement; co-administration results in an initial transient increase in FT_4; continued administration results in a decrease in serum T_4 and normal FT_4 and TSH concentrations and, therefore, patients are clinically euthyroid).
No products indexed under this heading.

Mercaptopurine (Co-administration has been associated with thyroid hormone and/or TSH level alterations by various mechanisms). Products include:
Purinethol Tablets 1615

Mestranol (Co-administration with estrogen containing oral contraceptives may result in increased serum TBG concentrations). Products include:
Necon 1/50 Tablets 3415
Norinyl 1 + 50 28-Day Tablets 3380
Ortho-Novum 1/50▫28 Tablets 2556

Metaproterenol Sulfate (Co-administration of sympathomimetic agents may increase the effects of sympathomimetics or thyroid hormone; thyroid hormones may increase risk of coronary insufficiency when sympathomimetic agents are administered to patients with coronary disease). Products include:
Alupent 1029

Metaraminol Bitartrate (Co-administration of sympathomimetic agents may increase the effects of sympathomimetics or thyroid hormone; thyroid hormones may increase risk of coronary insufficiency when sympathomimetic agents are administered to patients with coronary disease). Products include:
Aramine Injection 2043

Metformin Hydrochloride (Addition of levothyroxine to antidiabetic therapy may result in increased antidiabetic agent requirements). Products include:
Glucophage Tablets 1080
Glucophage XR Tablets 1080
Glucovance Tablets 1086

Methadone Hydrochloride (Co-administration may result in increased serum TBG concentrations). Products include:
Dolophine Hydrochloride Tablets 3056

Methimazole (May decrease thyroid hormone secretion, which may result in hypothyroidism).
No products indexed under this heading.

Methoxamine Hydrochloride (Co-administration of sympathomimetic agents may increase the effects of sympathomimetics or thyroid hormone; thyroid hormones may increase risk of coronary insufficiency when sympathomimetic agents are administered to patients with coronary disease).
No products indexed under this heading.

Methyclothiazide (Co-administration has been associated with thyroid hormone and/or TSH level alterations by various mechanisms).
No products indexed under this heading.

Methylprednisolone Acetate (Co-administration with glucocorticoids may result in a transient reduction in TSH secretion; the reduction is not sustained, therefore, hypothyroidism does not occur; glucocorticoids may decrease serum TBG concentrations). Products include:
Depo-Medrol Injectable Suspension 2795

Methylprednisolone Sodium Succinate (Co-administration with glucocorticoids may result in a transient reduction in TSH secretion; the reduction is not sustained, therefore, hypothyroidism does not occur; glucocorticoids may decrease serum TBG concentrations). Products include:
Solu-Medrol Sterile Powder 2855

Methyltestosterone (Co-administration with androgens/anabolic steroids may result in decreased serum TBG concentrations). Products include:
Android Capsules, 10 mg 1731
Estratest 3252
Testred Capsules, 10 mg 1746

Metipranolol Hydrochloride (Co-administration with beta-blockers may decrease T_4 5'-deiodinase activity; action of beta-blocker may be impaired when the hypothyroid patient is converted to euthyroid).
No products indexed under this heading.

Metoclopramide Hydrochloride (Co-administration has been associated with thyroid hormone and/or TSH level alterations by various mechanisms). Products include:
Reglan 2935

Metoprolol Succinate (Co-administration with beta-blockers may decrease T_4 5'-deiodinase activity; action of beta-blocker may be impaired when the hypothyroid patient is converted to euthyroid). Products include:
Toprol-XL Tablets 651

Metoprolol Tartrate (Co-administration with beta-blockers may decrease T_4 5'-deiodinase activity; action of beta-blocker may be impaired when the hypothyroid patient is converted to euthyroid).
No products indexed under this heading.

Miglitol (Addition of levothyroxine to antidiabetic therapy may result in increased antidiabetic agent requirements). Products include:
Glyset Tablets 2821

Mitotane (Co-administration may result in increased serum TBG concentrations).
No products indexed under this heading.

Nadolol (Co-administration with beta-blockers may decrease T_4 5'-deiodinase activity; action of beta-blocker may be impaired when the hypothyroid patient is converted to euthyroid). Products include:
Corgard Tablets 2245
Corzide 40/5 Tablets 2247
Corzide 80/5 Tablets 2247
Nadolol Tablets 2288

Niacin (Co-administration with slow-release nicotinic acid may result in decreased serum TBG concentrations). Products include:
Niaspan Extended-Release Tablets 1846
Nicotinex Elixir 633

Norepinephrine Bitartrate (Co-administration of sympathomimetic agents may increase the effects of sympathomimetics or thyroid hormone; thyroid hormones may increase risk of coronary insufficiency when sympathomimetic agents are administered to patients with coronary disease).
No products indexed under this heading.

Nortriptyline Hydrochloride (Co-administration may increase the therapeutic and toxic effects of both drugs possibly due to increased receptor sensitivity to catecholamines; toxic effects may include increased risk of arrhythmias and CNS stimulation; onset of tricyclics may be accelerated).
No products indexed under this heading.

Octreotide Acetate (Co-administration with octreotide may result in a transient reduction in TSH secretion; the reduction is not sustained, therefore, hypothyroidism does not occur). Products include:
Sandostatin LAR Depot 2395

Oxandrolone (Co-administration with androgens/anabolic steroids may result in decreased serum TBG concentrations). Products include:
Oxandrin Tablets 1153

Oxymetholone (Co-administration with androgens/anabolic steroids may result in decreased serum TBG concentrations). Products include:
Anadrol-50 Tablets 3321

Penbutolol Sulfate (Co-administration with beta-blockers may decrease T_4 5'-deiodinase activity; action of beta-blocker may be impaired when the hypothyroid patient is converted to euthyroid).
No products indexed under this heading.

Pergolide Mesylate (Co-administration with dopamine agonists may result in a transient reduction in TSH secretion; the reduction is not sustained, therefore, hypothyroidism does not occur). Products include:

Permax Tablets 1299

Perphenazine (Co-administration has been associated with thyroid hormone and/or TSH level alterations by various mechanisms). Products include:

Etrafon 3115
Trilafon 3160

Phenobarbital (Co-administration may increase hepatic metabolism, which may result in hypothyroidism, resulting in increased levothyroxine requirements). Products include:

Arco-Lase Plus Tablets 592
Donnatal 2929
Donnatal Extentabs 2930

Phenylephrine Bitartrate (Co-administration of sympathomimetic agents may increase the effects of sympathomimetics or thyroid hormone; thyroid hormones may increase risk of coronary insufficiency when sympathomimetic agents are administered to patients with coronary disease).

No products indexed under this heading.

Phenylephrine Hydrochloride (Co-administration of sympathomimetic agents may increase the effects of sympathomimetics or thyroid hormone; thyroid hormones may increase risk of coronary insufficiency when sympathomimetic agents are administered to patients with coronary disease). Products include:

Afrin Nasal Decongestant Children's Pump Mist ▣734
Extendryl 1361
Hycomine Compound Tablets 1317
Neo-Synephrine ▣614
Phenergan VC Syrup 3560
Phenergan VC with Codeine Syrup 3561
Preparation H Cream ▣778
Preparation H Cooling Gel ▣778
Preparation H ▣778
Vicks Sinex Nasal Spray and Ultra Fine Mist ▣729

Phenylephrine Tannate (Co-administration of sympathomimetic agents may increase the effects of sympathomimetics or thyroid hormone; thyroid hormones may increase risk of coronary insufficiency when sympathomimetic agents are administered to patients with coronary disease). Products include:

Ryna-12 S Suspension 3351
Reformulated Rynatan Pediatric Suspension 3352
Rynatuss Pediatric Suspension 3353
Rynatuss Tablets 3353

Phenylpropanolamine Hydrochloride (Co-administration of sympathomimetic agents may increase the effects of sympathomimetics or thyroid hormone; thyroid hormones may increase risk of coronary insufficiency when sympathomimetic agents are administered to patients with coronary disease).

No products indexed under this heading.

Phenytoin (Hydantoins may cause protein-binding site displacement; co-administration results in an initial transient increase in FT_4; co-administration may increase hepatic metabolism, which may result in hypothyroidism, resulting in increased levothyroxine requirements; phenytoin reduces serum protein binding of levothyroxine, and total- and free-T_4 may be reduced by 20% to 40%, but most patients have normal serum TSH levels and are clinically euthyroid). Products include:

Dilantin Infatabs 2624
Dilantin-125 Oral Suspension 2625

Phenytoin Sodium (Hydantoins may cause protein-binding site displacement; co-administration results in an initial transient increase in FT_4; co-administration may increase hepatic metabolism, which may result in hypothyroidism, resulting in increased levothyroxine requirements; phenytoin reduces serum protein binding of levothyroxine, and total- and free-T_4 may be reduced by 20% to 40%, but most patients have normal serum TSH levels and are clinically euthyroid). Products include:

Dilantin Kapseals 2622

Pindolol (Co-administration with beta-blockers may decrease T_4 5'-deiodinase activity; action of beta-blocker may be impaired when the hypothyroid patient is converted to euthyroid).

No products indexed under this heading.

Pioglitazone Hydrochloride (Addition of levothyroxine to antidiabetic therapy may result in increased antidiabetic agent requirements). Products include:

Actos Tablets 3275

Pirbuterol Acetate (Co-administration of sympathomimetic agents may increase the effects of sympathomimetics or thyroid hormone; thyroid hormones may increase risk of coronary insufficiency when sympathomimetic agents are administered to patients with coronary disease). Products include:

Maxair Autohaler 1981
Maxair Inhaler 1984

Polyestradiol Phosphate (Co-administration with oral estrogens may result in increased serum TBG concentrations).

No products indexed under this heading.

Polythiazide (Co-administration has been associated with thyroid hormone and/or TSH level alterations by various mechanisms). Products include:

Minizide Capsules 2700
Renese Tablets 2712

Potassium Iodide (May decrease thyroid hormone secretion, which may result in hypothyroidism; iodide drugs that contain pharmacologic amounts of iodide may cause hypothyroidism in euthyroid patients with Grave's disease previously treated with thyroid autonomy; hyperthyroidism may develop over several weeks and may persist for several months after therapy discontinuation). Products include:

Pima Syrup 1362

Pramipexole Dihydrochloride (Co-administration with dopamine agonists may result in a transient reduction in TSH secretion; the reduction is not sustained, therefore, hypothyroidism does not occur). Products include:

Mirapex Tablets 2834

Prednisolone Acetate (Co-administration with glucocorticoids may result in a transient reduction in TSH secretion; the reduction is not sustained, therefore, hypothyroidism does not occur; glucocorticoids may decrease serum TBG concentrations). Products include:

Blephamide Ophthalmic Ointment 547
Blephamide Ophthalmic Suspension 548
Poly-Pred Liquifilm Ophthalmic Suspension ⊙245
Pred Forte Ophthalmic Suspension ⊙246
Pred Mild Sterile Ophthalmic Suspension ⊙249
Pred-G Ophthalmic Suspension ⊙247
Pred-G Sterile Ophthalmic Ointment ⊙248

Prednisolone Sodium Phosphate (Co-administration with glucocorticoids may result in a transient reduction in TSH secretion; the reduction is not sustained, therefore, hypothyroidism does not occur; glucocorticoids may decrease serum TBG concentrations). Products include:

Pediapred Oral Solution 1170

Prednisolone Tebutate (Co-administration with glucocorticoids may result in a transient reduction in TSH secretion; the reduction is not sustained, therefore, hypothyroidism does not occur; glucocorticoids may decrease serum TBG concentrations).

No products indexed under this heading.

Prednisone (Co-administration with glucocorticoids may result in a transient reduction in TSH secretion; the reduction is not sustained, therefore, hypothyroidism does not occur; glucocorticoids may decrease serum TBG concentrations). Products include:

Prednisone 3064

Propranolol Hydrochloride (Co-administration with beta-blockers may decrease T_4 5'-deiodinase activity; in patients treated with large doses of propranolol, greater than 160 mg/day, T_3 and T_4 levels change slightly, TSH levels remain normal, and patients are clinically euthyroid; action of beta-blocker may be impaired when the hypothyroid patient is converted to euthyroid). Products include:

Inderal 3513
Inderal LA Long-Acting Capsules 3516
Inderide Tablets 3517
Inderide LA Long-Acting Capsules 3519

Propylthiouracil (May decrease thyroid hormone secretion, which may result in hypothyroidism).

No products indexed under this heading.

Protriptyline Hydrochloride (Co-administration may increase the therapeutic and toxic effects of both drugs possibly due to increased receptor sensitivity to catecholamines; toxic effects may include increased risk of arrhythmias and CNS stimulation; onset of tricyclics may be accelerated). Products include:

Vivactil Tablets 2446
Vivactil Tablets 2217

Pseudoephedrine Hydrochloride (Co-administration of sympathomimetic agents may increase the effects of sympathomimetics or thyroid hormone; thyroid hormones may increase risk of coronary insufficiency when sympathomimetic agents are administered to patients with coronary disease). Products include:

Actifed Cold & Allergy Tablets ▣688
Actifed Cold & Sinus Caplets and Tablets ▣688
Advil Cold and Sinus Caplets ▣771
Advil Cold and Sinus Tablets ▣771
Advil Flu & Body Ache Caplets ▣772
Aleve Cold & Sinus Caplets ▣603
Alka-Seltzer Plus Liqui-Gels ▣604
Alka-Seltzer Plus Cold & Flu Medicine Liqui-Gels ▣604
Alka-Seltzer Plus Cold & Sinus Medicine Liqui-Gels ▣604
Allegra-D Extended-Release Tablets 714
BC Cold Powder ▣619
Benadryl Allergy/Cold Tablets ▣691
Benadryl Allergy/Congestion Tablets ▣692
Benadryl Allergy & Sinus Liquid ▣693
Benadryl Allergy & Sinus Fastmelt Tablets ▣693
Benadryl Allergy Sinus Headache Caplets & Gelcaps ▣693
Benadryl Severe Allergy & Sinus Headache Caplets ▣694
Benadryl Children's Allergy/Cold Fastmelt Tablets ▣692
Benylin Multi-Symptom Liquid ▣697
Bromfed Capsules (Extended-Release) 2269
Bromfed-PD Capsules (Extended-Release) 2269
Children's Cēpacol Sore Throat ▣788
Comtrex Acute Head Cold & Sinus Pressure Relief Tablets ▣627
Comtrex Deep Chest Cold & Congestion Relief Softgels ▣627
Comtrex Flu Therapy & Fever Relief Daytime Caplets ▣628
Comtrex Flu Therapy & Fever Relief Nighttime Tablets ▣628
Comtrex Maximum Strength Multi-Symptom Cold & Cough Relief Tablets and Caplets ▣626
Contac Non-Drowsy 12 Hour Cold Caplets ▣745
Contac Non-Drowsy Timed Release 12 Hour Cold Caplets ▣746
Contac Severe Cold and Flu Caplets Maximum Strength ▣746
Contac Severe Cold and Flu Caplets Non-Drowsy ▣746
Dimetapp Elixir ▣777
Dimetapp Cold and Fever Suspension ▣775
Dimetapp DM Cold & Cough Elixir ▣775
Dimetapp Nighttime Flu Liquid ▣776
Dimetapp Non-Drowsy Flu Syrup ▣777
Dimetapp Infant Drops Decongestant ▣775
Dimetapp Infant Drops Decongestant Plus Cough ▣776
Guaifed 2272
Kronofed-A 1341
Children's Motrin Cold Oral Suspension 2007
Motrin Sinus Headache Caplets 2005
PediaCare Cough-Cold Liquid ▣719
PediaCare Infants' Drops Decongestant ▣719
PediaCare Infants' Drops Decongestant Plus Cough ▣719
PediaCare NightRest Cough-Cold Liquid ▣719
Robitussin Cold Caplets Cold & Congestion ▣780
Robitussin Cold Softgels Cold & Congestion ▣780
Robitussin Cold Caplets Multi-Symptom Cold & Flu ▣781
Robitussin Cold Softgels Multi-Symptom Cold & Flu ▣781
Robitussin Cold Softgels Severe Congestion ▣782
Robitussin Cough & Cold Infant Drops ▣782
Robitussin Maximum Strength Cough & Cold Liquid ▣785
Robitussin Pediatric Cough & Cold Formula Liquid ▣785
Robitussin Multi Symptom Honey Flu Liquid ▣785
Robitussin Nighttime Honey Flu Liquid ▣786
Robitussin-CF Liquid ▣783
Robitussin-DAC Syrup 2942
Robitussin-PE Liquid ▣782
Ryna ▣768
Semprex-D Capsules 1172
Singlet Caplets ▣761
Sinutab Non-Drying Liquid Caps ▣706
Sinutab Sinus Allergy Medication, Maximum Strength Formula, Tablets & Caplets ▣707
Sinutab Sinus Medication, Maximum Strength Without Drowsiness Formula, Tablets & Caplets ▣707
Sudafed 12 Hour Tablets ▣708
Sudafed 24 Hour Tablets ▣708
Children's Sudafed Cold & Cough Liquid ▣709
Children's Sudafed Nasal Decongestant Chewables ▣711
Children's Sudafed Nasal Decongestant Liquid Medication ▣711
Sudafed Cold & Allergy Tablets ▣708
Sudafed Cold & Cough Liquid Caps ▣709
Sudafed Cold & Sinus Liquid Caps ▣710
Sudafed Nasal Decongestant Tablets ▣710
Sudafed Non-Drying Sinus Liquid Caps ▣712
Sudafed Severe Cold ▣711
Sudafed Sinus Headache Caplets ▣712
Sudafed Sinus Headache Tablets ▣712
Tavist Sinus Non-Drowsy Coated Caplets ▣676
TheraFlu Regular Strength Cold & Cough Night Time Hot Liquid ▣676
TheraFlu Regular Strength Cold & Sore Throat Night Time Hot Liquid ▣676
TheraFlu Maximum Strength Flu & Congestion Non-Drowsy Hot Liquid ▣677

TheraFlu Maximum Strength Flu & Cough Night Time Hot Liquid .. 678
TheraFlu Maximum Strength Flu & Sore Throat Night Time Hot Liquid 677
TheraFlu Maximum Strength Severe Cold & Congestion Night Time Caplets 678
TheraFlu Maximum Strength Severe Cold & Congestion Night Time Hot Liquid 678
TheraFlu Maximum Strength Severe Cold & Congestion Non-Drowsy 679
Triaminic Allergy Congestion Liquid 680
Triaminic Chest Congestion Liquid 680
Triaminic Cold & Allergy Liquid 681
Triaminic Cold & Allergy Softchews 683
Triaminic Cold & Cough Liquid 681
Triaminic Cold & Cough Softchews 683
Triaminic Cold & Night Time Cough Liquid 681
Triaminic Cold, Cough & Fever Liquid 681
Triaminic Cough Liquid 682
Triaminic Cough & Congestion Liquid 682
Triaminic Cough & Sore Throat Liquid 682
Triaminic Cough & Sore Throat Softchews 684
Children's Tylenol Allergy-D Liquid ... 2014
Children's Tylenol Cold Suspension Liquid and Chewable Tablets 2015
Children's Tylenol Cold Plus Cough Suspension Liquid and Chewable Tablets 2015
Children's Tylenol Flu Suspension Liquid 2015
Children's Tylenol Sinus Suspension Liquid 2017
Infants' Tylenol Cold Decongestant and Fever Reducer Concentrated Drops 2015
Infants' Tylenol Cold Decongestant and Fever Reducer Concentrated Drops Plus Cough .. 2015
Tylenol Allergy Sinus 2010
Multi-Symptom Tylenol Cold Complete Formula Caplets 2010
Multi-Symptom Tylenol Cold Non-Drowsy Caplets and Gelcaps 2010
Multi-Symptom Tylenol Cold Severe Congestion Non-Drowsy Caplets 2011
Maximum Strength Tylenol Flu NightTime Gelcaps 2011
Maximum Strength Tylenol Flu NightTime Liquid 2011
Maximum Strength Tylenol Flu Non-Drowsy Gelcaps 2011
Maximum Strength Tylenol Sinus NightTime Caplets 2012
Maximum Strength Tylenol Sinus Non-Drowsy Geltabs, Gelcaps, Caplets, and Tablets 2012
Vicks 44D Cough & Head Congestion Relief Liquid 724
Vicks 44M Cough, Cold & Flu Relief Liquid 725
Pediatric Vicks 44m Cough & Cold Relief 728
Vicks DayQuil LiquiCaps/Liquid Multi-Symptom Cold/Flu Relief 727
Children's Vicks NyQuil Cold/Cough Relief 726
Vicks NyQuil LiquiCaps/Liquid Multi-Symptom Cold/Flu Relief, Original and Cherry Flavors 727
Zephrex Tablets 3091
Zephrex LA Tablets 3092
Zyrtec-D 12 Hour Extended Relief Tablets 2758

Pseudoephedrine Sulfate (Co-administration of sympathomimetic agents may increase the effects of sympathomimetics or thyroid hormone; thyroid hormones may increase risk of coronary insufficiency when sympathomimetic agents are administered to patients with coronary disease). Products include:
Chlor-Trimeton Allergy/Decongestant Tablets 736
Claritin-D 12 Hour Extended Release Tablets 3102
Claritin-D 24 Hour Extended Release Tablets 3104
Coricidin 'D' Cold, Flu & Sinus Tablets 737
Drixoral Allergy/Sinus Extended-Release Tablets 741
Drixoral Cold & Allergy Sustained-Action Tablets 740
Drixoral Cold & Flu Extended-Release Tablets 740
Drixoral Nasal Decongestant Long-Acting Non-Drowsy Tablets 740
Rynatan Tablets 3351

Quinestrol (Co-administration with oral estrogens may result in increased serum TBG concentrations).
No products indexed under this heading.

Repaglinide (Addition of levothyroxine to antidiabetic therapy may result in increased antidiabetic agent requirements). Products include:
Prandin Tablets (0.5, 1, and 2 mg) 2432

Resorcinol (Co-administration of excessive topical use of resorcinol has been associated with thyroid hormone and/or TSH level alterations by various mechanisms).
No products indexed under this heading.

Rifampin (Co-administration may increase hepatic metabolism, which may result in hypothyroidism, resulting in increased levothyroxine requirements). Products include:
Rifadin 765
Rifamate Capsules 767
Rifater Tablets 769

Ropinirole Hydrochloride (Co-administration with dopamine agonists may result in a transient reduction in TSH secretion; the reduction is not sustained, therefore, hypothyroidism does not occur). Products include:
Requip Tablets 1621

Rosiglitazone Maleate (Addition of levothyroxine to antidiabetic therapy may result in increased antidiabetic agent requirements). Products include:
Avandia Tablets 1490

Salmeterol Xinafoate (Co-administration of sympathomimetic agents may increase the effects of sympathomimetics or thyroid hormone; thyroid hormones may increase risk of coronary insufficiency when sympathomimetic agents are administered to patients with coronary disease). Products include:
Advair Diskus 100/50 1448
Advair Diskus 250/50 1448
Advair Diskus 500/50 1448
Serevent Diskus 1637
Serevent Inhalation Aerosol 1633

Salsalate (Co-administration with salicylates at greater than 2 gm inhibit binding of T4 and T3 to TBG and transthyretin; an initial increase in serum FT4 is followed by return of FT4 to normal levels with sustained therapeutic salicylate concentrations, although total T4 levels may decrease by as much as 30%).
No products indexed under this heading.

Sertraline Hydrochloride (Co-administration of sertraline in patients stabilized on levothyroxine may result in increased levothyroxine requirements). Products include:
Zoloft 2751

Sodium Nitroprusside (Co-administration has been associated with thyroid hormone and/or TSH level alterations by various mechanisms).
No products indexed under this heading.

Sodium Polystyrene Sulfonate (Co-administration may result in decreased T_4 absorption, which may result in hypothyroidism; administer levothyroxine at least 4 hours apart from these agents).
No products indexed under this heading.

Somatrem (Excessive use of thyroid hormone with growth hormones may accelerate epiphyseal closure; however, untreated hypothyroidism may interfere with growth response to growth hormone).
No products indexed under this heading.

Somatropin (Excessive use of thyroid hormone with growth hormones may accelerate epiphyseal closure; however, untreated hypothyroidism may interfere with growth response to growth hormone). Products include:
Genotropin Lyophilized Powder 2818
Humatrope Vials and Cartridges 1930
Norditropin Cartridges 2420
Norditropin for Injection 2419
Nutropin AQ Injection 1420
Nutropin Depot for Injectable Suspension 1423
Nutropin for Injection 1417
Saizen for Injection 3225
Serostim for Injection 3229

Sotalol Hydrochloride (Co-administration with beta-blockers may decrease T_4 5'-deiodinase activity; action of beta-blocker may be impaired when the hypothyroid patient is converted to euthyroid). Products include:
Betapace Tablets 950
Betapace AF Tablets 954

Soybean Preparations (Concurrent use of soybean flour may bind and decrease the absorption of levothyroxine sodium from GI tract).
No products indexed under this heading.

Stanozolol (Co-administration with androgens/anabolic steroids may result in decreased serum TBG concentrations).
No products indexed under this heading.

Sucralfate (Co-administration may result in decreased T_4 absorption, which may result in hypothyroidism; administer levothyroxine at least 4 hours apart from these agents). Products include:
Carafate Suspension 731
Carafate Tablets 730

Sulfamethoxazole (May decrease thyroid hormone secretion, which may result in hypothyroidism). Products include:
Bactrim 2949
Septra Suspension 2265
Septra Tablets 2265
Septra DS Tablets 2265

Sulfisoxazole Acetyl (May decrease thyroid hormone secretion, which may result in hypothyroidism). Products include:
Pediazole Suspension 3050

Tamoxifen Citrate (Co-administration may result in increased serum TBG concentrations). Products include:
Nolvadex Tablets 678

Terbutaline Sulfate (Co-administration of sympathomimetic agents may increase the effects of sympathomimetics or thyroid hormone; thyroid hormones may increase risk of coronary insufficiency when sympathomimetic agents are administered to patients with coronary disease). Products include:
Brethine Ampuls 2314
Brethine Tablets 2313

Theophylline (Decreased theophylline clearance may occur in hypothyroid patients; clearance returns to normal when euthyroid state is achieved). Products include:
Aerolate 1361
Theo-Dur Extended-Release Tablets 1835
Uni-Dur Extended-Release Tablets .. 1841
Uniphyl 400 mg and 600 mg Tablets 2903

Theophylline Calcium Salicylate (Decreased theophylline clearance may occur in hypothyroid patients; clearance returns to normal when euthyroid state is achieved).
No products indexed under this heading.

Theophylline Sodium Glycinate (Decreased theophylline clearance may occur in hypothyroid patients; clearance returns to normal when euthyroid state is achieved).
No products indexed under this heading.

Timolol Hemihydrate (Co-administration with beta-blockers may decrease T_4 5'-deiodinase activity; action of beta-blocker may be impaired when the hypothyroid patient is converted to euthyroid). Products include:
Betimol Ophthalmic Solution .... ⊙324

Timolol Maleate (Co-administration with beta-blockers may decrease T_4 5'-deiodinase activity; action of beta-blocker may be impaired when the hypothyroid patient is converted to euthyroid). Products include:
Blocadren Tablets 2046
Cosopt Sterile Ophthalmic Solution 2065
Timolide Tablets 2187
Timolol GFS .... ⊙266
Timoptic in Ocudose 2192
Timoptic Sterile Ophthalmic Solution 2190
Timoptic-XE Sterile Ophthalmic Gel Forming Solution 2194

Tolazamide (Addition of levothyroxine to antidiabetic therapy may result in increased antidiabetic agent requirements).
No products indexed under this heading.

Tolbutamide (May decrease thyroid hormone secretion, which may result in hypothyroidism).
No products indexed under this heading.

Triamcinolone (Co-administration with glucocorticoids may result in a transient reduction in TSH secretion; the reduction is not sustained, therefore, hypothyroidism does not occur; glucocorticoids may decrease serum TBG concentrations).
No products indexed under this heading.

Triamcinolone Acetonide (Co-administration with glucocorticoids may result in a transient reduction in TSH secretion; the reduction is not sustained, therefore, hypothyroidism does not occur; glucocorticoids may decrease serum TBG concentrations). Products include:
Azmacort Inhalation Aerosol 728
Nasacort Nasal Inhaler 750
Nasacort AQ Nasal Spray 752
Tri-Nasal Spray 2274

Triamcinolone Diacetate (Co-administration with glucocorticoids may result in a transient reduction in TSH secretion; the reduction is not sustained, therefore, hypothyroidism does not occur; glucocorticoids may decrease serum TBG concentrations).
No products indexed under this heading.

Triamcinolone Hexacetonide (Co-administration with glucocorticoids may result in a transient reduction in TSH secretion; the reduction is not sustained, therefore, hypothyroidism does not occur; glucocorticoids may decrease serum TBG concentrations).
No products indexed under this heading.

Trimipramine Maleate (Co-administration may increase the therapeutic and toxic effects of both

IMPORTANT NOTE: Always consult each drug listing in the patient's regimen for possible interactions.

drugs possibly due to increased receptor sensitivity to catecholamines; toxic effects may include increased risk of arrhythmias and CNS stimulation; onset of tricyclics may be accelerated). Products include:

Surmontil Capsules 3595

Troglitazone (Addition of levothyroxine to antidiabetic therapy may result in increased antidiabetic agent requirements).

No products indexed under this heading.

Tyropanoate Sodium (May decrease thyroid hormone secretion, which may result in hypothyroidism; the fetus, elderly, and euthyroid patients with underlying thyroid disease are among those individuals who are susceptible to iodine-induced hypothyroidism; oral cholecytographicagents slowly excreted, producing more prolonged hypothyroidism; iodide drugs that contain pharmacologic amounts of iodide may cause hypothyroidism in euthyroid patients with Grave's disease previously treated with thyroid autonomy; hyperthyroidism may develop over several weeks and may persist for several months after therapy discontinuation).

No products indexed under this heading.

Warfarin Sodium (Thyroid hormones appear to increase the catabolism of vitamin-K dependent clotting factors, thereby increasing the anticoagulant activity of oral anticoagulants). Products include:

Coumadin for Injection 1243
Coumadin Tablets 1243
Warfarin Sodium Tablets, USP 3302

Food Interactions

Dietary Fiber (Concurrent use of dietary fiber may bind and decrease the absorption of levothyroxine sodium from GI tract).

Soybean Formula, Children's (Concurrent use of soybean flour may bind and decrease the absorption of levothyroxine sodium from GI tract).

UNIVASC TABLETS

(Moexipril Hydrochloride) 3181

May interact with diuretics, lithium preparations, potassium preparations, potassium sparing diuretics, and certain other agents. Compounds in these categories include:

Amiloride Hydrochloride (ACE inhibitors can increase the risk of hyperkalemia with concomitant use). Products include:

Midamor Tablets 2136
Moduretic Tablets 2138

Bendroflumethiazide (Excessive reduction in blood pressure may occur in patients on diuretic therapy when ACE inhibitors are started). Products include:

Corzide 40/5 Tablets 2247
Corzide 80/5 Tablets 2247

Bumetanide (Excessive reduction in blood pressure may occur in patients on diuretic therapy when ACE inhibitors are started).

No products indexed under this heading.

Chlorothiazide (Excessive reduction in blood pressure may occur in patients on diuretic therapy when ACE inhibitors are started). Products include:

Aldoclor Tablets 2035
Diuril Oral 2087

Chlorothiazide Sodium (Excessive reduction in blood pressure may occur in patients on diuretic therapy when ACE inhibitors are started). Products include:

Diuril Sodium Intravenous 2086

Chlorthalidone (Excessive reduction in blood pressure may occur in patients on diuretic therapy when ACE inhibitors are started). Products include:

Clorpres Tablets 1002
Combipres Tablets 1040
Tenoretic Tablets 690

Ethacrynic Acid (Excessive reduction in blood pressure may occur in patients on diuretic therapy when ACE inhibitors are started). Products include:

Edecrin Tablets 2091

Furosemide (Excessive reduction in blood pressure may occur in patients on diuretic therapy when ACE inhibitors are started). Products include:

Furosemide Tablets 2284

Hydrochlorothiazide (Excessive reduction in blood pressure may occur in patients on diuretic therapy when ACE inhibitors are started). Products include:

Accuretic Tablets 2614
Aldoril Tablets 2039
Atacand HCT Tablets 597
Avalide Tablets 1070
Diovan HCT Tablets 2338
Dyazide Capsules 1515
HydroDIURIL Tablets 2108
Hyzaar 2109
Inderide Tablets 3517
Inderide LA Long-Acting Capsules .. 3519
Lotensin HCT Tablets 2367
Maxzide 1008
Micardis HCT Tablets 1051
Microzide Capsules 3414
Moduretic Tablets 2138
Monopril HCT 1094
Prinzide Tablets 2168
Timolide Tablets 2187
Uniretic Tablets 3178
Vaseretic Tablets 2204
Zestoretic Tablets 695
Ziac Tablets 1887

Hydroflumethiazide (Excessive reduction in blood pressure may occur in patients on diuretic therapy when ACE inhibitors are started). Products include:

Diucardin Tablets 3494

Indapamide (Excessive reduction in blood pressure may occur in patients on diuretic therapy when ACE inhibitors are started). Products include:

Indapamide Tablets 2286

Lithium Carbonate (Potential for increased serum lithium levels and risk of lithium toxicity). Products include:

Eskalith 1527
Lithium Carbonate 3061
Lithobid Slow-Release Tablets 3255

Lithium Citrate (Potential for increased serum lithium levels and risk of lithium toxicity). Products include:

Lithium Citrate Syrup 3061

Methyclothiazide (Excessive reduction in blood pressure may occur in patients on diuretic therapy when ACE inhibitors are started).

No products indexed under this heading.

Metolazone (Excessive reduction in blood pressure may occur in patients on diuretic therapy when ACE inhibitors are started). Products include:

Mykrox Tablets 1168
Zaroxolyn Tablets 1177

Polythiazide (Excessive reduction in blood pressure may occur in patients on diuretic therapy when ACE inhibitors are started). Products include:

Minizide Capsules 2700
Renese Tablets 2712

Potassium Acid Phosphate (ACE inhibitors can increase the risk of hyperkalemia with concomitant use). Products include:

K-Phos Original (Sodium Free) Tablets 947

Potassium Bicarbonate (ACE inhibitors can increase the risk of hyperkalemia with concomitant use).

No products indexed under this heading.

Potassium Chloride (ACE inhibitors can increase the risk of hyperkalemia with concomitant use). Products include:

Chlor-3 1361
Colyte with Flavor Packs for Oral Solution 3170
GoLYTELY and Pineapple Flavor GoLYTELY for Oral Solution 1068
K-Dur Microburst Release System ER Tablets 1832
Klor-Con M20/Klor-Con M10 Tablets 3329
K-Lor Powder Packets 469
K-Tab Filmtab Tablets 470
Micro-K 3311
NuLYTELY, Cherry Flavor, Lemon-Lime Flavor, and Orange Flavor NuLYTELY for Oral Solution 1068
Rum-K 1363

Potassium Citrate (ACE inhibitors can increase the risk of hyperkalemia with concomitant use). Products include:

Urocit-K Tablets 2232

Potassium Gluconate (ACE inhibitors can increase the risk of hyperkalemia with concomitant use).

No products indexed under this heading.

Potassium Phosphate (ACE inhibitors can increase the risk of hyperkalemia with concomitant use). Products include:

K-Phos Neutral Tablets 946

Spironolactone (ACE inhibitors can increase the risk of hyperkalemia with concomitant use).

No products indexed under this heading.

Torsemide (Excessive reduction in blood pressure may occur in patients on diuretic therapy when ACE inhibitors are started). Products include:

Demadex Tablets and Injection 2965

Triamterene (ACE inhibitors can increase the risk of hyperkalemia with concomitant use). Products include:

Dyazide Capsules 1515
Dyrenium Capsules 3458
Maxzide 1008

Food Interactions

Food, unspecified (Food reduces Cmax and AUC by about 70% and 40% respectively after ingestion of a low-fat breakfast or by 80% and 50% respectively after the ingestion of high-fat breakfast).

URECHOLINE INJECTION

(Bethanechol Chloride) 2198

See Urecholine Tablets

URECHOLINE TABLETS

(Bethanechol Chloride) 2445

May interact with ganglionic blocking agents. Compounds in these categories include:

Mecamylamine Hydrochloride (Co-administration with ganglion blocking compounds may result in a critical fall in blood pressure). Products include:

Inversine Tablets 1850

Trimethaphan Camsylate (Co-administration with ganglion blocking compounds may result in a critical fall in blood pressure).

No products indexed under this heading.

URECHOLINE TABLETS

(Bethanechol Chloride) 2198

May interact with ganglionic blocking agents. Compounds in these categories include:

Mecamylamine Hydrochloride (Critical fall in blood pressure). Products include:

Inversine Tablets 1850

Trimethaphan Camsylate (Critical fall in blood pressure).

No products indexed under this heading.

URIMAX TABLETS

(Belladonna Alkaloids, Hyoscyamine Sulfate, Methenamine, Methylene Blue, Phenyl Salicylate, Sodium Biphosphate) 1769

May interact with antacids, antimuscarinic drugs, antimyasthenics, monoamine oxidase inhibitors, narcotic analgesics, thiazides, urinary alkalinizing agents, and certain other agents. Compounds in these categories include:

Alfentanil Hydrochloride (Co-administration with narcotic analgesics may result in increased risk of severe constipation).

No products indexed under this heading.

Aluminum Carbonate (Co-administration with antacids may cause urine to become alkaline reducing effectiveness of methenamine by inhibiting its conversion to formaldehyde).

No products indexed under this heading.

Aluminum Hydroxide (Co-administration with antacids may cause urine to become alkaline reducing effectiveness of methenamine by inhibiting its conversion to formaldehyde). Products include:

Amphojel Suspension (Mint Flavor) .... ■789
Gaviscon Extra Strength Liquid ...... ■751
Gaviscon Extra Strength Tablets .... ■751
Gaviscon Regular Strength Liquid .. ■751
Gaviscon Regular Strength Tablets .... ■750
Maalox Antacid/Anti-Gas Oral Suspension .... ■673
Maalox Max Maximum Strength Antacid/Anti-Gas Liquid 2300
Maalox Regular Strength Antacid/Antigas Liquid 2300
Mylanta 1813
Vanquish Caplets .... ■617

Atropine Sulfate (Concurrent use with antimuscarinics may intensify effects of hyoscyamine). Products include:

Donnatal 2929
Donnatal Extentabs 2930
Motofen Tablets 577
Prosed/DS Tablets 3268
Urised Tablets 2876

Bendroflumethiazide (Co-administration may result in decreased absorption of thiazides; thiazide diuretics may cause the urine to become alkaline reducing the effectiveness of methenamine by inhibiting its conversion to formaldehyde). Products include:

Corzide 40/5 Tablets 2247
Corzide 80/5 Tablets 2247

Buprenorphine Hydrochloride (Co-administration with narcotic analgesics may result in increased risk of severe constipation). Products include:

Buprenex Injectable 2918

Chlorothiazide (Co-administration may result in decreased absorption of thiazides; thiazide diuretics may cause the urine to become alkaline reducing the effectiveness of methenamine by inhibiting its conversion to formaldehyde). Products include:

Aldoclor Tablets 2035
Diuril Oral 2087

Chlorothiazide Sodium (Co-administration may result in decreased absorption of thiazides; thiazide diuretics may cause the urine to become alkaline reducing the effectiveness of methenamine by inhibiting its conversion to formaldehyde). Products include:

Diuril Sodium Intravenous 2086

Clidinium Bromide (Concurrent use with antimuscarinics may intensify effects of hyoscyamine).
No products indexed under this heading.

Codeine Phosphate (Co-administration with narcotic analgesics may result in increased risk of severe constipation). Products include:
Phenergan with Codeine Syrup 3557
Phenergan VC with Codeine Syrup .. 3561
Robitussin A-C Syrup 2942
Robitussin-DAC Syrup 2942
Ryna-C Liquid 768
Soma Compound w/Codeine Tablets 3355
Tussi-Organidin NR Liquid 3350
Tussi-Organidin-S NR Liquid 3350
Tylenol with Codeine 2595

Dezocine (Co-administration with narcotic analgesics may result in increased risk of severe constipation).
No products indexed under this heading.

Dicyclomine Hydrochloride (Concurrent use with antimuscarinics may intensify effects of hyoscyamine).
No products indexed under this heading.

Diphenoxylate Hydrochloride (Co-administration with antidiarrheals may reduce the absorption of hyoscyamine).
No products indexed under this heading.

Edrophonium Chloride (Co-administration of hyoscyamine with antimyasthenics may further reduce intestinal motility). Products include:
Tensilon Injectable 1745

Fentanyl (Co-administration with narcotic analgesics may result in increased risk of severe constipation). Products include:
Duragesic Transdermal System 1786

Fentanyl Citrate (Co-administration with narcotic analgesics may result in increased risk of severe constipation). Products include:
Actiq 1184

Glycopyrrolate (Concurrent use with antimuscarinics may intensify effects of hyoscyamine). Products include:
Robinul Forte Tablets 1358
Robinul Injectable 2940
Robinul Tablets 1358

Hydrochlorothiazide (Co-administration may result in decreased absorption of thiazides; thiazide diuretics may cause the urine to become alkaline reducing the effectiveness of methenamine by inhibiting its conversion to formaldehyde). Products include:
Accuretic Tablets 2614
Aldoril Tablets 2039
Atacand HCT Tablets 597
Avalide Tablets 1070
Diovan HCT Tablets 2338
Dyazide Capsules 1515
HydroDIURIL Tablets 2108
Hyzaar 2109
Inderide Tablets 3517
Inderide LA Long-Acting Capsules .. 3519
Lotensin HCT Tablets 2367
Maxzide 1008
Micardis HCT Tablets 1051
Microzide Capsules 3414
Moduretic Tablets 2138
Monopril HCT 1094
Prinzide Tablets 2168
Timolide Tablets 2187
Uniretic Tablets 3178
Vaseretic Tablets 2204
Zestoretic Tablets 695
Ziac Tablets 1887

Hydrocodone Bitartrate (Co-administration with narcotic analgesics may result in increased risk of severe constipation). Products include:
Hycodan 1316
Hycomine Compound Tablets 1317
Hycotuss Expectorant Syrup 1318
Lortab 3319
Lortab Elixir 3317
Maxidone Tablets CIII 3399
Norco 5/325 Tablets CIII 3424
Norco 7.5/325 Tablets CIII 3425
Norco 10/325 Tablets CIII 3427
Norco 10/325 Tablets CIII 3425
Vicodin Tablets 516
Vicodin ES Tablets 517
Vicodin HP Tablets 518
Vicodin Tuss Expectorant 519
Vicoprofen Tablets 520
Zydone Tablets 1330

Hydrocodone Polistirex (Co-administration with narcotic analgesics may result in increased risk of severe constipation). Products include:
Tussionex Pennkinetic Extended-Release Suspension 1174

Hydroflumethiazide (Co-administration may result in decreased absorption of thiazides; thiazide diuretics may cause the urine to become alkaline reducing the effectiveness of methenamine by inhibiting its conversion to formaldehyde). Products include:
Diucardin Tablets 3494

Hydromorphone Hydrochloride (Co-administration with narcotic analgesics may result in increased risk of severe constipation). Products include:
Dilaudid 441
Dilaudid Oral Liquid 445
Dilaudid Powder 441
Dilaudid Rectal Suppositories 441
Dilaudid Tablets 441
Dilaudid Tablets - 8 mg 445
Dilaudid-HP 443

Hyoscyamine (Concurrent use with antimuscarinics may intensify effects of hyoscyamine). Products include:
Urised Tablets 2876

Ipratropium Bromide (Concurrent use with antimuscarinics may intensify effects of hyoscyamine). Products include:
Atrovent Inhalation Aerosol 1030
Atrovent Inhalation Solution 1031
Atrovent Nasal Spray 0.03% 1032
Atrovent Nasal Spray 0.06% 1033
Combivent Inhalation Aerosol 1041
DuoNeb Inhalation Solution 1233

Isocarboxazid (Co-administration with MAO inhibitors may intensify antimuscarinic side effects).
No products indexed under this heading.

Ketoconazole (Simultaneous administration should be avoided; patients should be advised to take this combination at least 2 hours after ketoconazole). Products include:
Nizoral 2% Cream 3620
Nizoral A-D Shampoo 2008
Nizoral 2% Shampoo 2007
Nizoral Tablets 1791

Levorphanol Tartrate (Co-administration with narcotic analgesics may result in increased risk of severe constipation). Products include:
Levo-Dromoran 1734
Levorphanol Tartrate Tablets 3059

Magaldrate (Co-administration with antacids may cause urine to become alkaline reducing effectiveness of methenamine by inhibiting its conversion to formaldehyde).
No products indexed under this heading.

Magnesium Hydroxide (Co-administration with antacids may cause urine to become alkaline reducing effectiveness of methenamine by inhibiting its conversion to formaldehyde). Products include:
Ex•Lax Milk of Magnesia Liquid 670
Maalox Antacid/Anti-Gas Oral Suspension 673
Maalox Max Maximum Strength Antacid/Anti-Gas Liquid 2300
Maalox Regular Strength Antacid/Antigas Liquid 2300
Mylanta Fast-Acting 1813
Mylanta 1813
Pepcid Complete Chewable Tablets 1815
Phillips' Chewable Tablets 615
Phillips' Milk of Magnesia Liquid (Original, Cherry, & Mint) 616
Rolaids Tablets 706
Extra Strength Rolaids Tablets 706
Vanquish Caplets 617

Magnesium Oxide (Co-administration with antacids may cause urine to become alkaline reducing effectiveness of methenamine by inhibiting its conversion to formaldehyde). Products include:
Beelith Tablets 946
Mag-Ox 400 Tablets 1024
Uro-Mag Capsules 1024

Mepenzolate Bromide (Concurrent use with antimuscarinics may intensify effects of hyoscyamine).
No products indexed under this heading.

Meperidine Hydrochloride (Co-administration with narcotic analgesics may result in increased risk of severe constipation). Products include:
Demerol 3079
Mepergan Injection 3539

Methadone Hydrochloride (Co-administration with narcotic analgesics may result in increased risk of severe constipation). Products include:
Dolophine Hydrochloride Tablets 3056

Methyclothiazide (Co-administration may result in decreased absorption of thiazides; thiazide diuretics may cause the urine to become alkaline reducing the effectiveness of methenamine by inhibiting its conversion to formaldehyde).
No products indexed under this heading.

Moclobemide (Co-administration with MAO inhibitors may intensify antimuscarinic side effects).
No products indexed under this heading.

Morphine Sulfate (Co-administration with narcotic analgesics may result in increased risk of severe constipation). Products include:
Astramorph/PF Injection, USP (Preservative-Free)........................... 594
Duramorph Injection 1312
Infumorph 200 and Infumorph 500 Sterile Solutions 1314
Kadian Capsules 1335
MS Contin Tablets 2896
MSIR 2898
Oramorph SR Tablets 3062
Roxanol 3066

Neostigmine Bromide (Co-administration of hyoscyamine with antimyasthenics may further reduce intestinal motility). Products include:
Prostigmin Tablets 1744

Oxycodone Hydrochloride (Co-administration with narcotic analgesics may result in increased risk of severe constipation). Products include:
OxyContin Tablets 2912
OxyFast Oral Concentrate Solution . 2916
OxyIR Capsules 2916
Percocet Tablets 1326
Percodan Tablets 1327
Percolone Tablets 1327
Roxicodone 3067
Tylox Capsules 2597

Oxyphenonium Bromide (Concurrent use with antimuscarinics may intensify effects of hyoscyamine).
No products indexed under this heading.

Pargyline Hydrochloride (Co-administration with MAO inhibitors may intensify antimuscarinic side effects).
No products indexed under this heading.

Phenelzine Sulfate (Co-administration with MAO inhibitors may intensify antimuscarinic side effects). Products include:
Nardil Tablets 2653

Polythiazide (Co-administration may result in decreased absorption of thiazides; thiazide diuretics may cause the urine to become alkaline reducing the effectiveness of methenamine by inhibiting its conversion to formaldehyde). Products include:
Minizide Capsules 2700
Renese Tablets 2712

Potassium Citrate (Urinary alkalizers cause urine to become alkaline reducing the effectiveness of methenamine by inhibiting its conversion to formaldehyde). Products include:
Urocit-K Tablets 2232

Procarbazine Hydrochloride (Co-administration with MAO inhibitors may intensify antimuscarinic side effects). Products include:
Matulane Capsules 3246

Propantheline Bromide (Concurrent use with antimuscarinics may intensify effects of hyoscyamine).
No products indexed under this heading.

Propoxyphene Hydrochloride (Co-administration with narcotic analgesics may result in increased risk of severe constipation). Products include:
Darvon Pulvules 1909
Darvon Compound-65 Pulvules 1910

Propoxyphene Napsylate (Co-administration with narcotic analgesics may result in increased risk of severe constipation). Products include:
Darvon-N/Darvocet-N 1907
Darvon-N Tablets 1912

Pyridostigmine Bromide (Co-administration of hyoscyamine with antimyasthenics may further reduce intestinal motility). Products include:
Mestinon 1740

Remifentanil Hydrochloride (Co-administration with narcotic analgesics may result in increased risk of severe constipation).
No products indexed under this heading.

Scopolamine (Concurrent use with antimuscarinics may intensify effects of hyoscyamine). Products include:
Transderm Scōp Transdermal Therapeutic System 2302

Scopolamine Hydrobromide (Concurrent use with antimuscarinics may intensify effects of hyoscyamine). Products include:
Donnatal 2929
Donnatal Extentabs 2930

Selegiline Hydrochloride (Co-administration with MAO inhibitors may intensify antimuscarinic side effects). Products include:
Eldepryl Capsules 3266

Sodium Bicarbonate (Co-administration with antacids may cause urine to become alkaline reducing effectiveness of methenamine by inhibiting its conversion to formaldehyde). Products include:
Alka-Seltzer 603
Alka-Seltzer Lemon Lime Antacid and Pain Reliever Effervescent Tablets 603
Alka-Seltzer Extra Strength Antacid and Pain Reliever Effervescent Tablets 603
Alka-Seltzer Heartburn Relief Tablets 604
Ceo-Two Evacuant Suppository 618
Colyte with Flavor Packs for Oral Solution 3170
GoLYTELY and Pineapple Flavor GoLYTELY for Oral Solution 1068
NuLYTELY, Cherry Flavor, Lemon-Lime Flavor, and Orange Flavor NuLYTELY for Oral Solution 1068

Sodium Citrate (Urinary alkalizers cause urine to become alkaline

reducing the effectiveness of methenamine by inhibiting its conversion to formaldehyde).
No products indexed under this heading.

Sufentanil Citrate (Co-administration with narcotic analgesics may result in increased risk of severe constipation).
No products indexed under this heading.

Sulfamethizole (Co-administration with sulfonamides may precipitate with formaldehyde in the urine, increasing the danger of crystaluria). Products include:
Urobiotic-250 Capsules 2731

Sulfamethoxazole (Co-administration with sulfonamides may precipitate with formaldehyde in the urine, increasing the danger of crystaluria). Products include:
Bactrim 2949
Septra Suspension 2265
Septra Tablets 2265
Septra DS Tablets 2265

Tolterodine Tartrate (Concurrent use with antimuscarinics may intensify effects of hyoscyamine). Products include:
Detrol Tablets 3623
Detrol LA Capsules 2801

Tranylcypromine Sulfate (Co-administration with MAO inhibitors may intensify antimuscarinic side effects). Products include:
Parnate Tablets 1607

Tridihexethyl Chloride (Concurrent use with antimuscarinics may intensify effects of hyoscyamine).
No products indexed under this heading.

URISED TABLETS
(Atropine Sulfate, Benzoic Acid, Hyoscyamine, Methenamine, Methylene Blue, Phenyl Salicylate)..... 2876
May interact with urinary alkalinizing agents and certain other agents. Compounds in these categories include:

Potassium Citrate (Methenamine has therapeutic activity in acidic urine; concurrent use with drugs which produce an alkaline urine should be restricted). Products include:
Urocit-K Tablets 2232

Sodium Citrate (Methenamine has therapeutic activity in acidic urine; concurrent use with drugs which produce an alkaline urine should be restricted).
No products indexed under this heading.

Sulfamethizole (In acid urine methenamine breaks down into formaldehyde that may form an insoluble precipitate with certain sulfonamides and may also increase the dangers of crystaluria; concurrent use is not recommended). Products include:
Urobiotic-250 Capsules 2731

Sulfamethoxazole (In acid urine methenamine breaks down into formaldehyde that may form an insoluble precipitate with certain sulfonamides and may also increase the dangers of crystaluria; concurrent use is not recommended). Products include:
Bactrim 2949
Septra Suspension 2265
Septra Tablets 2265
Septra DS Tablets 2265

Sulfisoxazole (In acid urine methenamine breaks down into formaldehyde that may form an insoluble precipitate with certain sulfonamides and may also increase the dangers of crystaluria; concurrent use is not recommended).
No products indexed under this heading.

Sulfisoxazole Acetyl (In acid urine methenamine breaks down into formaldehyde that may form an insoluble precipitate with certain sulfonamides and may also increase the dangers of crystaluria; concurrent use is not recommended). Products include:
Pediazole Suspension 3050

Food Interactions

Food that raises urinary pH (Methenamine has therapeutic activity in acidic urine; concurrent use with foods which produce an alkaline urine should be restricted).

UROBIOTIC-250 CAPSULES
(Oxytetracycline Hydrochloride, Phenazopyridine Hydrochloride, Sulfamethizole)........................... 2731
May interact with:

Aluminum Hydroxide (Decreases absorption of Urobiotic). Products include:
Amphojel Suspension (Mint Flavor) .... ■789
Gaviscon Extra Strength Liquid ....■751
Gaviscon Extra Strength Tablets ...■751
Gaviscon Regular Strength Liquid .■751
Gaviscon Regular Strength Tablets .... ■750
Maalox Antacid/Anti-Gas Oral Suspension .... ■673
Maalox Max Maximum Strength Antacid/Anti-Gas Liquid 2300
Maalox Regular Strength Antacid/Antigas Liquid 2300
Mylanta 1813
Vanquish Caplets .... ■617

UROCIT-K TABLETS
(Potassium Citrate) 2232
May interact with anticholinergics and potassium sparing diuretics. Compounds in these categories include:

Amiloride Hydrochloride (Co-administration can produce severe hyperkalemia; concurrent use should be avoided). Products include:
Midamor Tablets 2136
Moduretic Tablets 2138

Atropine Sulfate (Co-administration with drugs that slow gastrointestinal transit time, such as anticholinergics, can be expected to increase the gastrointestinal irritation produced by potassium salts; concurrent use is contraindicated). Products include:
Donnatal 2929
Donnatal Extentabs 2930
Motofen Tablets 577
Prosed/DS Tablets 3268
Urised Tablets 2876

Belladonna Alkaloids (Co-administration with drugs that slow gastrointestinal transit time, such as anticholinergics, can be expected to increase the gastrointestinal irritation produced by potassium salts; concurrent use is contraindicated). Products include:
Hyland's Teething Tablets ....■766
Urimax Tablets 1769

Benztropine Mesylate (Co-administration with drugs that slow gastrointestinal transit time, such as anticholinergics, can be expected to increase the gastrointestinal irritation produced by potassium salts; concurrent use is contraindicated). Products include:
Cogentin 2055

Biperiden Hydrochloride (Co-administration with drugs that slow gastrointestinal transit time, such as anticholinergics, can be expected to increase the gastrointestinal irritation produced by potassium salts; concurrent use is contraindicated). Products include:
Akineton 402

Clidinium Bromide (Co-administration with drugs that slow gastrointestinal transit time, such as anticholinergics, can be expected to increase the gastrointestinal irritation produced by potassium salts; concurrent use is contraindicated).
No products indexed under this heading.

Dicyclomine Hydrochloride (Co-administration with drugs that slow gastrointestinal transit time, such as anticholinergics, can be expected to increase the gastrointestinal irritation produced by potassium salts; concurrent use is contraindicated).
No products indexed under this heading.

Glycopyrrolate (Co-administration with drugs that slow gastrointestinal transit time, such as anticholinergics, can be expected to increase the gastrointestinal irritation produced by potassium salts; concurrent use is contraindicated). Products include:
Robinul Forte Tablets 1358
Robinul Injectable 2940
Robinul Tablets 1358

Hyoscyamine (Co-administration with drugs that slow gastrointestinal transit time, such as anticholinergics, can be expected to increase the gastrointestinal irritation produced by potassium salts; concurrent use is contraindicated). Products include:
Urised Tablets 2876

Hyoscyamine Sulfate (Co-administration with drugs that slow gastrointestinal transit time, such as anticholinergics, can be expected to increase the gastrointestinal irritation produced by potassium salts; concurrent use is contraindicated). Products include:
Arco-Lase Plus Tablets 592
Donnatal 2929
Donnatal Extentabs 2930
Levsin/Levsinex/Levbid 3172
NuLev Orally Disintegrating Tablets 3176
Prosed/DS Tablets 3268
Urimax Tablets 1769

Ipratropium Bromide (Co-administration with drugs that slow gastrointestinal transit time, such as anticholinergics, can be expected to increase the gastrointestinal irritation produced by potassium salts; concurrent use is contraindicated). Products include:
Atrovent Inhalation Aerosol 1030
Atrovent Inhalation Solution 1031
Atrovent Nasal Spray 0.03% 1032
Atrovent Nasal Spray 0.06% 1033
Combivent Inhalation Aerosol 1041
DuoNeb Inhalation Solution 1233

Mepenzolate Bromide (Co-administration with drugs that slow gastrointestinal transit time, such as anticholinergics, can be expected to increase the gastrointestinal irritation produced by potassium salts; concurrent use is contraindicated).
No products indexed under this heading.

Oxybutynin Chloride (Co-administration with drugs that slow gastrointestinal transit time, such as anticholinergics, can be expected to increase the gastrointestinal irritation produced by potassium salts; concurrent use is contraindicated). Products include:
Ditropan XL Extended Release Tablets 564

Procyclidine Hydrochloride (Co-administration with drugs that slow gastrointestinal transit time, such as anticholinergics, can be expected to increase the gastrointestinal irritation produced by potassium salts; concurrent use is contraindicated).
No products indexed under this heading.

Propantheline Bromide (Co-administration with drugs that slow gastrointestinal transit time, such as anticholinergics, can be expected to increase the gastrointestinal irritation produced by potassium salts; concurrent use is contraindicated).
No products indexed under this heading.

Scopolamine (Co-administration with drugs that slow gastrointestinal transit time, such as anticholinergics, can be expected to increase the gastrointestinal irritation produced by potassium salts; concurrent use is contraindicated). Products include:
Transderm Scōp Transdermal Therapeutic System 2302

Scopolamine Hydrobromide (Co-administration with drugs that slow gastrointestinal transit time, such as anticholinergics, can be expected to increase the gastrointestinal irritation produced by potassium salts; concurrent use is contraindicated). Products include:
Donnatal 2929
Donnatal Extentabs 2930

Spironolactone (Co-administration can produce severe hyperkalemia; concurrent use should be avoided).
No products indexed under this heading.

Tolterodine Tartrate (Co-administration with drugs that slow gastrointestinal transit time, such as anticholinergics, can be expected to increase the gastrointestinal irritation produced by potassium salts; concurrent use is contraindicated). Products include:
Detrol Tablets 3623
Detrol LA Capsules 2801

Triamterene (Co-administration can produce severe hyperkalemia; concurrent use should be avoided). Products include:
Dyazide Capsules 1515
Dyrenium Capsules 3458
Maxzide 1008

Tridihexethyl Chloride (Co-administration with drugs that slow gastrointestinal transit time, such as anticholinergics, can be expected to increase the gastrointestinal irritation produced by potassium salts; concurrent use is contraindicated).
No products indexed under this heading.

Trihexyphenidyl Hydrochloride (Co-administration with drugs that slow gastrointestinal transit time, such as anticholinergics, can be expected to increase the gastrointestinal irritation produced by potassium salts; concurrent use is contraindicated). Products include:
Artane 1855

URO-MAG CAPSULES
(Magnesium Oxide) 1024
None cited in PDR database.

UROQID-ACID NO. 2 TABLETS
(Methenamine Mandelate, Sodium Acid Phosphate)............................... 947
May interact with:

Acetazolamide (Reduces the effectiveness of methenamine by causing urine to become alkaline). Products include:
Diamox Sequels Sustained Release Capsules .... ⊙270
Diamox Tablets .... ⊙269

ACTH (Concurrent use with sodium phosphate may result in hypernatremia).
No products indexed under this heading.

Aluminum Carbonate (Reduces the effectiveness of methenamine by causing urine to become alkaline).
No products indexed under this heading.

Aluminum Hydroxide (Reduces the effectiveness of methenamine by causing urine to become alkaline). Products include:
- Amphojel Suspension (Mint Flavor) ▣789
- Gaviscon Extra Strength Liquid ▣751
- Gaviscon Extra Strength Tablets ▣751
- Gaviscon Regular Strength Liquid ▣751
- Gaviscon Regular Strength Tablets ▣750
- Maalox Antacid/Anti-Gas Oral Suspension ▣673
- Maalox Max Maximum Strength Antacid/Anti-Gas Liquid 2300
- Maalox Regular Strength Antacid/Antigas Liquid 2300
- Mylanta 1813
- Vanquish Caplets ▣617

Aspirin (Concurrent use may lead to increased serum salicylate levels since excretion of salicylates is reduced in acidic urine). Products include:
- Aggrenox Capsules 1026
- Alka-Seltzer ▣603
- Alka-Seltzer Lemon Lime Antacid and Pain Reliever Effervescent Tablets ▣603
- Alka-Seltzer Extra Strength Antacid and Pain Reliever Effervescent Tablets ▣603
- Alka-Seltzer PM Effervescent Tablets ▣605
- Genuine Bayer Tablets, Caplets and Gelcaps ▣606
- Extra Strength Bayer Caplets and Gelcaps ▣610
- Aspirin Regimen Bayer Children's Chewable Tablets (Orange or Cherry Flavored) ▣607
- Bayer, Aspirin Regimen ▣606
- Aspirin Regimen Bayer 81 mg Caplets with Calcium ▣607
- Genuine Bayer Professional Labeling (Aspirin Regimen Bayer) ▣608
- Extra Strength Bayer Arthritis Caplets ▣610
- Extra Strength Bayer Plus Caplets ▣610
- Extra Strength Bayer PM Caplets ▣611
- BC Powder ▣619
- BC Allergy Sinus Cold Powder ▣619
- Arthritis Strength BC Powder ▣619
- BC Sinus Cold Powder ▣619
- Darvon Compound-65 Pulvules 1910
- Ecotrin Enteric Coated Aspirin Low, Regular and Maximum Strength Tablets 1715
- Excedrin Extra-Strength Tablets, Caplets, and Geltabs ▣629
- Excedrin Migraine 1070
- Goody's Body Pain Formula Powder ▣620
- Goody's Extra Strength Headache Powder ▣620
- Goody's Extra Strength Pain Relief Tablets ▣620
- Percodan Tablets 1327
- Robaxisal Tablets 2939
- Soma Compound Tablets 3354
- Soma Compound w/Codeine Tablets 3355
- Vanquish Caplets ▣617

Bendroflumethiazide (Reduces the effectiveness of methenamine by causing urine to become alkaline). Products include:
- Corzide 40/5 Tablets 2247
- Corzide 80/5 Tablets 2247

Betamethasone Acetate (Concurrent use with sodium phosphate may result in hypernatremia). Products include:
- Celestone Soluspan Injectable Suspension 3097

Betamethasone Sodium Phosphate (Concurrent use with sodium phosphate may result in hypernatremia). Products include:
- Celestone Soluspan Injectable Suspension 3097

Chlorothiazide (Reduces the effectiveness of methenamine by causing urine to become alkaline). Products include:
- Aldoclor Tablets 2035
- Diuril Oral 2087

Chlorothiazide Sodium (Reduces the effectiveness of methenamine by causing urine to become alkaline). Products include:
- Diuril Sodium Intravenous 2086

Choline Magnesium Trisalicylate (Concurrent use may lead to increased serum salicylate levels since excretion of salicylates is reduced in acidic urine). Products include:
- Trilisate 2901

Cortisone Acetate (Concurrent use with sodium phosphate may result in hypernatremia). Products include:
- Cortone Acetate Injectable Suspension 2059
- Cortone Acetate Tablets 2061

Deserpidine (Concurrent use with sodium phosphate may result in hypernatremia).
No products indexed under this heading.

Desoxycorticosterone Acetate (Concurrent use with sodium phosphate may result in hypernatremia).
No products indexed under this heading.

Desoxycorticosterone Pivalate (Concurrent use with sodium phosphate may result in hypernatremia).
No products indexed under this heading.

Dexamethasone (Concurrent use with sodium phosphate may result in hypernatremia). Products include:
- Decadron Elixir 2078
- Decadron Tablets 2079
- TobraDex Ophthalmic Ointment 542
- TobraDex Ophthalmic Suspension 541

Dexamethasone Acetate (Concurrent use with sodium phosphate may result in hypernatremia).
No products indexed under this heading.

Dexamethasone Sodium Phosphate (Concurrent use with sodium phosphate may result in hypernatremia). Products include:
- Decadron Phosphate Injection 2081
- Decadron Phosphate Sterile Ophthalmic Ointment 2083
- Decadron Phosphate Sterile Ophthalmic Solution 2084
- NeoDecadron Sterile Ophthalmic Solution 2144

Diazoxide (Concurrant use with sodium phosphate may result in hypernatremia).
No products indexed under this heading.

Dichlorphenamide (Reduces the effectiveness of methenamine by causing urine to become alkaline). Products include:
- Daranide Tablets 2077

Diflunisal (Concurrent use may lead to increased serum salicylate levels since excretion of salicylates is reduced in acidic urine). Products include:
- Dolobid Tablets 2088

Fludrocortisone Acetate (Concurrent use with sodium phosphate may result in hypernatremia). Products include:
- Florinef Acetate Tablets 2250

Guanethidine Monosulfate (Concurrent use with sodium phosphate may result in hypernatremia).
No products indexed under this heading.

Hydralazine Hydrochloride (Concurrent use with sodium phosphate may result in hypernatremia).
No products indexed under this heading.

Hydrochlorothiazide (Reduces the effectiveness of methenamine by causing urine to become alkaline). Products include:
- Accuretic Tablets 2614
- Aldoril Tablets 2039
- Atacand HCT Tablets 597
- Avalide Tablets 1070
- Diovan HCT Tablets 2338
- Dyazide Capsules 1515
- HydroDIURIL Tablets 2108
- Hyzaar 2109
- Inderide Tablets 3517
- Inderide LA Long-Acting Capsules 3519
- Lotensin HCT Tablets 2367
- Maxzide 1008
- Micardis HCT Tablets 1051
- Microzide Capsules 3414
- Moduretic Tablets 2138
- Monopril HCT 1094
- Prinzide Tablets 2168
- Timolide Tablets 2187
- Uniretic Tablets 3178
- Vaseretic Tablets 2204
- Zestoretic Tablets 695
- Ziac Tablets 1887

Hydrocortisone (Concurrent use with sodium phosphate may result in hypernatremia). Products include:
- Anusol-HC Cream 2.5% 2237
- Cipro HC Otic Suspension 540
- Cortaid Intensive Therapy Cream ▣717
- Cortaid Maximum Strength Cream ▣717
- Cortisporin Ophthalmic Suspension Sterile ⊙297
- Cortizone•5 ▣699
- Cortizone•10 ▣699
- Cortizone•10 Plus Creme ▣700
- Cortizone for Kids Creme ▣699
- Hydrocortone Tablets 2106
- Massengill Medicated Soft Cloth Towelette ▣753
- VōSoL HC Otic Solution 3356

Hydrocortisone Acetate (Concurrent use with sodium phosphate may result in hypernatremia). Products include:
- Analpram-HC 1338
- Anusol HC-1 Hydrocortisone Anti-Itch Cream ▣689
- Anusol-HC Suppositories 2238
- Cortaid ▣717
- Cortifoam Rectal Foam 3170
- Cortisporin-TC Otic Suspension 2246
- Hydrocortone Acetate Injectable Suspension 2103
- Pramosone 1343
- Proctocort Suppositories 2264
- ProctoFoam-HC 3177
- Terra-Cortril Ophthalmic Suspension 2716

Hydrocortisone Sodium Phosphate (Concurrent use with sodium phosphate may result in hypernatremia). Products include:
- Hydrocortone Phosphate Injection, Sterile 2105

Hydrocortisone Sodium Succinate (Concurrent use with sodium phosphate may result in hypernatremia).
No products indexed under this heading.

Hydroflumethiazide (Reduces the effectiveness of methenamine by causing urine to become alkaline). Products include:
- Diucardin Tablets 3494

Magaldrate (Reduces the effectiveness of methenamine by causing urine to become alkaline).
No products indexed under this heading.

Magnesium Hydroxide (Reduces the effectiveness of methenamine by causing urine to become alkaline). Products include:
- Ex•Lax Milk of Magnesia Liquid ▣670
- Maalox Antacid/Anti-Gas Oral Suspension ▣673
- Maalox Max Maximum Strength Antacid/Anti-Gas Liquid 2300
- Maalox Regular Strength Antacid/Antigas Liquid 2300
- Mylanta Fast-Acting 1813
- Mylanta 1813
- Pepcid Complete Chewable Tablets 1815
- Phillips' Chewable Tablets ▣615
- Phillips' Milk of Magnesia Liquid (Original, Cherry, & Mint) ▣616
- Rolaids Tablets ▣706
- Extra Strength Rolaids Tablets ▣706
- Vanquish Caplets ▣617

Magnesium Oxide (Reduces the effectiveness of methenamine by causing urine to become alkaline). Products include:
- Beelith Tablets 946
- Mag-Ox 400 Tablets 1024
- Uro-Mag Capsules 1024

Magnesium Salicylate (Concurrent use may lead to increased serum salicylate levels since excretion of salicylates is reduced in acidic urine). Products include:
- Momentum Backache Relief Extra Strength Caplets ▣666

Methazolamide (Reduces the effectiveness of methenamine by causing urine to become alkaline). Products include:
- Neptazane Tablets ⊙271

Methyclothiazide (Reduces the effectiveness of methenamine by causing urine to become alkaline).
No products indexed under this heading.

Methyldopa (Concurrent use with sodium phosphate may result in hypernatremia). Products include:
- Aldoclor Tablets 2035
- Aldomet Tablets 2037
- Aldoril Tablets 2039

Methylprednisolone Acetate (Concurrent use with sodium phosphate may result in hypernatremia). Products include:
- Depo-Medrol Injectable Suspension 2795

Methylprednisolone Sodium Succinate (Concurrent use with sodium phosphate may result in hypernatremia). Products include:
- Solu-Medrol Sterile Powder 2855

Polythiazide (Reduces the effectiveness of methenamine by causing urine to become alkaline). Products include:
- Minizide Capsules 2700
- Renese Tablets 2712

Potassium Citrate (Reduces the effectiveness of methenamine by causing urine to become alkaline). Products include:
- Urocit-K Tablets 2232

Prednisolone Acetate (Concurrent use with sodium phosphate may result in hypernatremia). Products include:
- Blephamide Ophthalmic Ointment 547
- Blephamide Ophthalmic Suspension 548
- Poly-Pred Liquifilm Ophthalmic Suspension ⊙245
- Pred Forte Ophthalmic Suspension ⊙246
- Pred Mild Sterile Ophthalmic Suspension ⊙249
- Pred-G Ophthalmic Suspension ⊙247
- Pred-G Sterile Ophthalmic Ointment ⊙248

Prednisolone Sodium Phosphate (Concurrent use with sodium phosphate may result in hypernatremia). Products include:
- Pediapred Oral Solution 1170

Prednisolone Tebutate (Concurrent use with sodium phosphate may result in hypernatremia).
No products indexed under this heading.

Prednisone (Concurrent use with sodium phosphate may result in hypernatremia). Products include:
- Prednisone 3064

Rauwolfia serpentina (Concurrent use with sodium phosphate may result in hypernatremia).
No products indexed under this heading.

Rescinnamine (Concurrent use with sodium phosphate may result in hypernatremia).
No products indexed under this heading.

Reserpine (Concurrent use with sodium phosphate may result in hypernatremia).
No products indexed under this heading.

Salsalate (Concurrent use may lead to increased serum salicylate levels since excretion of salicylates is

reduced in acidic urine).
No products indexed under this heading.

Sodium Bicarbonate (Reduces the effectiveness of methenamine by causing urine to become alkaline). Products include:
- Alka-Seltzer ▣603
- Alka-Seltzer Lemon Lime Antacid and Pain Reliever Effervescent Tablets ▣603
- Alka-Seltzer Extra Strength Antacid and Pain Reliever Effervescent Tablets ▣603
- Alka-Seltzer Heartburn Relief Tablets ▣604
- Ceo-Two Evacuant Suppository ▣618
- Colyte with Flavor Packs for Oral Solution 3170
- GoLYTELY and Pineapple Flavor GoLYTELY for Oral Solution 1068
- NuLYTELY, Cherry Flavor, Lemon-Lime Flavor, and Orange Flavor NuLYTELY for Oral Solution 1068

Sodium Citrate (Reduces the effectiveness of methenamine by causing urine to become alkaline).
No products indexed under this heading.

Sulfamethizole (Concurrent use with sulfamethizole and formaldehyde forms an insoluble precipitate in acid urine and increases the risk of crystaluria). Products include:
- Urobiotic-250 Capsules 2731

Triamcinolone (Concurrent use with sodium phosphate may result in hypernatremia).
No products indexed under this heading.

Triamcinolone Acetonide (Concurrent use with sodium phosphate may result in hypernatremia). Products include:
- Azmacort Inhalation Aerosol 728
- Nasacort Nasal Inhaler 750
- Nasacort AQ Nasal Spray 752
- Tri-Nasal Spray 2274

Triamcinolone Diacetate (Concurrent use with sodium phosphate may result in hypernatremia).
No products indexed under this heading.

Triamcinolone Hexacetonide (Concurrent use with sodium phosphate may result in hypernatremia).
No products indexed under this heading.

URSO TABLETS

(Ursodiol) 836

May interact with bile acid sequestering agents, estrogens, lipid-lowering drugs, oral contraceptives, and certain other agents. Compounds in these categories include:

Aluminum Hydroxide (Aluminum-based antacids have been shown to adsorb bile acid in vitro and may be expected to interfere with ursodiol in the same manner as the bile acid sequestering agents). Products include:
- Amphojel Suspension (Mint Flavor) ▣789
- Gaviscon Extra Strength Liquid ▣751
- Gaviscon Extra Strength Tablets ▣751
- Gaviscon Regular Strength Liquid ▣751
- Gaviscon Regular Strength Tablets ▣750
- Maalox Antacid/Anti-Gas Oral Suspension ▣673
- Maalox Max Maximum Strength Antacid/Anti-Gas Liquid 2300
- Maalox Regular Strength Antacid/Antigas Liquid 2300
- Mylanta 1813
- Vanquish Caplets ▣617

Atorvastatin Calcium (Lipid-lowering drugs increase hepatic cholesterol secretion and encourage cholesterol gallstone formation and hence may counteract the effectiveness of ursodiol). Products include:
- Lipitor Tablets 2639
- Lipitor Tablets 2696

Cerivastatin Sodium (Lipid-lowering drugs increase hepatic cholesterol secretion and encourage cholesterol gallstone formation and hence may counteract the effectiveness of ursodiol). Products include:
- Baycol Tablets 883

Chlorotrianisene (Estrogens and oral contraceptives increase hepatic cholesterol excretion and encourage cholesterol gallstone formation and hence may counteract the effectiveness of ursodiol).
No products indexed under this heading.

Cholestyramine (Lipid-lowering drugs increase hepatic cholesterol secretion and encourage cholesterol gallstone formation and hence may counteract the effectiveness of ursodiol).
No products indexed under this heading.

Clofibrate (Lipid-lowering drugs increase hepatic cholesterol secretion and encourage cholesterol gallstone formation and hence may counteract the effectiveness of ursodiol). Products include:
- Atromid-S Capsules 3483

Colestipol Hydrochloride (Lipid-lowering drugs increase hepatic cholesterol secretion and encourage cholesterol gallstone formation and hence may counteract the effectiveness of ursodiol). Products include:
- Colestid Tablets 2791

Desogestrel (Estrogens and oral contraceptives increase hepatic cholesterol excretion and encourage cholesterol gallstone formation and hence may counteract the effectiveness of ursodiol). Products include:
- Cyclessa Tablets 2450
- Desogen Tablets 2458
- Mircette Tablets 2470
- Ortho-Cept 21 Tablets 2546
- Ortho-Cept 28 Tablets 2546

Dienestrol (Estrogens and oral contraceptives increase hepatic cholesterol excretion and encourage cholesterol gallstone formation and hence may counteract the effectiveness of ursodiol). Products include:
- Ortho Dienestrol Cream 2554

Diethylstilbestrol (Estrogens and oral contraceptives increase hepatic cholesterol excretion and encourage cholesterol gallstone formation and hence may counteract the effectiveness of ursodiol).
No products indexed under this heading.

Estradiol (Estrogens and oral contraceptives increase hepatic cholesterol excretion and encourage cholesterol gallstone formation and hence may counteract the effectiveness of ursodiol). Products include:
- Activella Tablets 2764
- Alora Transdermal System 3372
- Climara Transdermal System 958
- CombiPatch Transdermal System 2323
- Esclim Transdermal System 3460
- Estrace Vaginal Cream 3358
- Estrace Tablets 3361
- Estring Vaginal Ring 2811
- Ortho-Prefest Tablets 2570
- Vagifem Tablets 2857
- Vivelle Transdermal System 2412
- Vivelle-Dot Transdermal System 2416

Estrogens, Conjugated (Estrogens and oral contraceptives increase hepatic cholesterol excretion and encourage cholesterol gallstone formation and hence may counteract the effectiveness of ursodiol). Products include:
- Premarin Intravenous 3563
- Premarin Tablets 3566
- Premarin Vaginal Cream 3570
- Premphase Tablets 3572
- Prempro Tablets 3572

Estrogens, Esterified (Estrogens and oral contraceptives increase hepatic cholesterol excretion and encourage cholesterol gallstone formation and hence may counteract the effectiveness of ursodiol). Products include:
- Estratest 3252
- Menest Tablets 2254

Estropipate (Estrogens and oral contraceptives increase hepatic cholesterol excretion and encourage cholesterol gallstone formation and hence may counteract the effectiveness of ursodiol). Products include:
- Ogen Tablets 2846
- Ortho-Est Tablets 3464

Ethinyl Estradiol (Estrogens and oral contraceptives increase hepatic cholesterol secretion and encourage cholesterol gallstone formation and hence may counteract the effectiveness of ursodiol). Products include:
- Alesse-21 Tablets 3468
- Alesse-28 Tablets 3473
- Brevicon 28-Day Tablets 3380
- Cyclessa Tablets 2450
- Desogen Tablets 2458
- Estinyl Tablets 3112
- Estrostep 2627
- femhrt Tablets 2635
- Levlen 962
- Levlite 21 Tablets 962
- Levlite 28 Tablets 962
- Levora Tablets 3389
- Loestrin 21 Tablets 2642
- Loestrin Fe Tablets 2642
- Lo/Ovral Tablets 3532
- Lo/Ovral-28 Tablets 3538
- Low-Ogestrel-28 Tablets 3392
- Microgestin Fe 1.5/30 Tablets 3407
- Microgestin Fe 1/20 Tablets 3400
- Mircette Tablets 2470
- Modicon 2563
- Necon 3415
- Nordette-28 Tablets 2257
- Norinyl 1 +35 28-Day Tablets 3380
- Ogestrel 0.5/50-28 Tablets 3428
- Ortho-Cept 21 Tablets 2546
- Ortho-Cept 28 Tablets 2546
- Ortho-Cyclen/Ortho Tri-Cyclen 2573
- Ortho-Novum 2563
- Ovcon 3364
- Ovral Tablets 3551
- Ovral-28 Tablets 3552
- Tri-Levlen 962
- Tri-Norinyl-28 Tablets 3433
- Triphasil-21 Tablets 3600
- Triphasil-28 Tablets 3605
- Trivora Tablets 3439
- Yasmin 28 Tablets 980
- Zovia 3449

Ethynodiol Diacetate (Estrogens and oral contraceptives increase hepatic cholesterol secretion and encourage cholesterol gallstone formation and hence may counteract the effectiveness of ursodiol). Products include:
- Zovia 3449

Fenofibrate (Lipid-lowering drugs increase hepatic cholesterol secretion and encourage cholesterol gallstone formation and hence may counteract the effectiveness of ursodiol). Products include:
- Tricor Capsules, Micronized 513

Fluvastatin Sodium (Lipid-lowering drugs increase hepatic cholesterol secretion and encourage cholesterol gallstone formation and hence may counteract the effectiveness of ursodiol). Products include:
- Lescol Capsules 2361
- Lescol 2925
- Lescol XL Tablets 2361

Gemfibrozil (Lipid-lowering drugs increase hepatic cholesterol secretion and encourage cholesterol gallstone formation and hence may counteract the effectiveness of ursodiol). Products include:
- Lopid Tablets 2650

Levonorgestrel (Estrogens and oral contraceptives increase hepatic cholesterol secretion and encourage cholesterol gallstone formation and hence may counteract the effectiveness of ursodiol). Products include:
- Alesse-21 Tablets 3468
- Alesse-28 Tablets 3473
- Levlen 962
- Levlite 21 Tablets 962
- Levlite 28 Tablets 962
- Levora Tablets 3389
- Mirena Intrauterine System 974
- Nordette-28 Tablets 2257
- Norplant System 3543
- Tri-Levlen 962
- Triphasil-21 Tablets 3600
- Triphasil-28 Tablets 3605
- Trivora Tablets 3439

Lovastatin (Lipid-lowering drugs increase hepatic cholesterol secretion and encourage cholesterol gallstone formation and hence may counteract the effectiveness of ursodiol). Products include:
- Mevacor Tablets 2132

Mestranol (Estrogens and oral contraceptives increase hepatic cholesterol excretion and encourage cholesterol gallstone formation and hence may counteract the effectiveness of ursodiol). Products include:
- Necon 1/50 Tablets 3415
- Norinyl 1 + 50 28-Day Tablets 3380
- Ortho-Novum 1/50□28 Tablets 2556

Norethindrone (Estrogens and oral contraceptives increase hepatic cholesterol secretion and encourage cholesterol gallstone formation and hence may counteract the effectiveness of ursodiol). Products include:
- Brevicon 28-Day Tablets 3380
- Micronor Tablets 2543
- Modicon 2563
- Necon 3415
- Norinyl 1 +35 28-Day Tablets 3380
- Norinyl 1 + 50 28-Day Tablets 3380
- Nor-QD Tablets 3423
- Ortho-Novum 2563
- Ortho-Novum 1/50□28 Tablets 2556
- Ovcon 3364
- Tri-Norinyl-28 Tablets 3433

Norethynodrel (Estrogens and oral contraceptives increase hepatic cholesterol secretion and encourage cholesterol gallstone formation and hence may counteract the effectiveness of ursodiol).
No products indexed under this heading.

Norgestimate (Estrogens and oral contraceptives increase hepatic cholesterol secretion and encourage cholesterol gallstone formation and hence may counteract the effectiveness of ursodiol). Products include:
- Ortho-Cyclen/Ortho Tri-Cyclen 2573
- Ortho-Prefest Tablets 2570

Norgestrel (Estrogens and oral contraceptives increase hepatic cholesterol secretion and encourage cholesterol gallstone formation and hence may counteract the effectiveness of ursodiol). Products include:
- Lo/Ovral Tablets 3532
- Lo/Ovral-28 Tablets 3538
- Low-Ogestrel-28 Tablets 3392
- Ogestrel 0.5/50-28 Tablets 3428
- Ovral Tablets 3551
- Ovral-28 Tablets 3552
- Ovrette Tablets 3552

Polyestradiol Phosphate (Estrogens and oral contraceptives increase hepatic cholesterol excretion and encourage cholesterol gallstone formation and hence may counteract the effectiveness of ursodiol).
No products indexed under this heading.

Pravastatin Sodium (Lipid-lowering drugs increase hepatic cholesterol secretion and encourage cholesterol gallstone formation and hence may counteract the effectiveness of ursodiol). Products include:
- Pravachol Tablets 1099

Probucol (Lipid-lowering drugs increase hepatic cholesterol secretion and encourage cholesterol gallstone formation and hence may counteract the effectiveness of ursodiol).
No products indexed under this heading.

Quinestrol (Estrogens and oral contraceptives increase hepatic cholesterol excretion and encourage cholesterol gallstone formation and hence may counteract the effectiveness of ursodiol).
No products indexed under this heading.

Simvastatin (Lipid-lowering drugs increase hepatic cholesterol secretion and encourage cholesterol gallstone formation and hence may counteract the effectiveness of ursodiol). Products include:
Zocor Tablets 2219

VAGIFEM TABLETS
(Estradiol) 2857
None cited in PDR database.

VALCYTE TABLETS
(Valganciclovir Hydrochloride) 3022
May interact with:

Didanosine (Valganciclovir is extensively converted to ganciclovir; co-administration of ganciclovir with didanosine has resulted in decreased AUC of ganciclovir and increased AUC of didanosine; patients should be monitored for didanosine toxicity). Products include:
Videx 1138
Videx EC Capsules 1143

Mycophenolate Mofetil (Valganciclovir is extensively converted to ganciclovir; co-administration of ganciclovir with mycophenolate in patients with normal renal function has not resulted in any effect on PK parameters, however, patients with renal impairment should be monitored carefully as levels of metabolites or both drugs may increase). Products include:
CellCept Capsules 2951
CellCept Oral Suspension 2951
CellCept Tablets 2951

Probenecid (Valganciclovir is extensively converted to ganciclovir; co-administration of ganciclovir with probenecid results in increase in AUC of ganciclovir and decrease in ganciclovir renal cleareance; patients on concomitant therapy should be monitored for evidence of ganciclovir toxicity).
No products indexed under this heading.

Trimethoprim (Valganciclovir is extensively converted to ganciclovir; co-administration of ganciclovir with trimethoprim has resulted in decreased renal clearance and increased half-life of ganciclovir and an increase in Cmax of trimethoprim; effects of this interaction are not likely to be clinically significant). Products include:
Bactrim 2949
Septra Suspension 2265
Septra Tablets 2265
Septra DS Tablets 2265

Zalcitabine (Valganciclovir is extensively converted to ganciclovir; co-administration of ganciclovir with zalcitabine has resulted in increased AUC of ganciclovir; effects of this interaction are not likely to be clinically significant). Products include:
Hivid Tablets 2975

Zidovudine (Valganciclovir is extensively converted to ganciclovir; co-administration of ganciclovir with zidovudine has resulted in decreased AUC of ganciclovir and increased AUC of zidovudine; zidovudine and valganciclovir each have the potential to cause neutropenia and anemia; some patients may not tolerate concomitant therapy at full dosage). Products include:
Combivir Tablets 1502
Retrovir 1625
Retrovir IV Infusion 1629
Trizivir Tablets 1669

Food Interactions

Food, unspecified (Co-administration with high fat meals has resulted in increased steady-state ganciclovir AUC and Cmax without any prolongation in time to peak plasma concentrations; Valcyte should be administered with food).

VALIUM INJECTABLE
(Diazepam) 3026
May interact with barbiturates, central nervous system depressants, antidepressant drugs, monoamine oxidase inhibitors, narcotic analgesics, phenothiazines, and certain other agents. Compounds in these categories include:

Alfentanil Hydrochloride (Concomitant use increases central nervous system depression with increased risk of apnea; dosage of narcotic analgesics should be reduced by at least one-third).
No products indexed under this heading.

Alprazolam (Concomitant use increases central nervous system depression with increased risk of apnea). Products include:
Xanax Tablets 2865

Amitriptyline Hydrochloride (May potentiate the actions of diazepam). Products include:
Etrafon 3115
Limbitrol 1738

Amoxapine (May potentiate the actions of diazepam).
No products indexed under this heading.

Aprobarbital (Concomitant use increases central nervous system depression with increased risk of apnea).
No products indexed under this heading.

Buprenorphine Hydrochloride (Concomitant use increases central nervous system depression with increased risk of apnea; dosage of narcotic analgesics should be reduced by at least one-third). Products include:
Buprenex Injectable 2918

Bupropion Hydrochloride (May potentiate the actions of diazepam). Products include:
Wellbutrin Tablets 1680
Wellbutrin SR Sustained-Release Tablets 1684
Zyban Sustained-Release Tablets 1710

Buspirone Hydrochloride (Concomitant use increases central nervous system depression with increased risk of apnea).
No products indexed under this heading.

Butabarbital (Concomitant use increases central nervous system depression with increased risk of apnea).
No products indexed under this heading.

Butalbital (Concomitant use increases central nervous system depression with increased risk of apnea). Products include:
Phrenilin 578
Sedapap Tablets 50 mg/650 mg 2225

Chlordiazepoxide (Concomitant use increases central nervous system depression with increased risk of apnea). Products include:
Limbitrol 1738

Chlordiazepoxide Hydrochloride (Concomitant use increases central nervous system depression with increased risk of apnea). Products include:
Librium Capsules 1736
Librium for Injection 1737

Chlorpromazine (May potentiate the actions of diazepam). Products include:
Thorazine Suppositories 1656

Chlorpromazine Hydrochloride (May potentiate the actions of diazepam). Products include:
Thorazine 1656

Chlorprothixene (Concomitant use increases central nervous system depression with increased risk of apnea).
No products indexed under this heading.

Chlorprothixene Hydrochloride (Concomitant use increases central nervous system depression with increased risk of apnea).
No products indexed under this heading.

Chlorprothixene Lactate (Concomitant use increases central nervous system depression with increased risk of apnea).
No products indexed under this heading.

Cimetidine (Co-administration delays diazepam clearance; clinical significance of this interaction is unclear). Products include:
Tagamet HB 200 Suspension 762
Tagamet HB 200 Tablets 761
Tagamet Tablets 1644

Cimetidine Hydrochloride (Co-administration delays diazepam clearance; clinical significance of this interaction is unclear). Products include:
Tagamet 1644

Citalopram Hydrobromide (May potentiate the actions of diazepam). Products include:
Celexa 1365

Clonazepam (May potentiate the CNS depression caused by diazepam). Products include:
Klonopin Tablets 2983

Clorazepate Dipotassium (Concomitant use increases central nervous system depression with increased risk of apnea). Products include:
Tranxene 511

Clozapine (Concomitant use increases central nervous system depression with increased risk of apnea). Products include:
Clozaril Tablets 2319

Codeine Phosphate (Concomitant use increases central nervous system depression with increased risk of apnea; dosage of narcotic analgesics should be reduced by at least one-third). Products include:
Phenergan with Codeine Syrup 3557
Phenergan VC with Codeine Syrup 3561
Robitussin A-C Syrup 2942
Robitussin-DAC Syrup 2942
Ryna-C Liquid 768
Soma Compound w/Codeine Tablets 3355
Tussi-Organidin NR Liquid 3350
Tussi-Organidin-S NR Liquid 3350
Tylenol with Codeine 2595

Desflurane (Concomitant use increases central nervous system depression with increased risk of apnea). Products include:
Suprane Liquid for Inhalation 874

Desipramine Hydrochloride (May potentiate the actions of diazepam). Products include:
Norpramin Tablets 755

Dezocine (Concomitant use increases central nervous system depression with increased risk of apnea; dosage of narcotic analgesics should be reduced by at least one-third).
No products indexed under this heading.

Doxepin Hydrochloride (May potentiate the actions of diazepam). Products include:
Sinequan 2713

Droperidol (Concomitant use increases central nervous system depression with increased risk of apnea).
No products indexed under this heading.

Enflurane (Concomitant use increases central nervous system depression with increased risk of apnea).
No products indexed under this heading.

Estazolam (Concomitant use increases central nervous system depression with increased risk of apnea). Products include:
ProSom Tablets 500

Ethchlorvynol (Concomitant use increases central nervous system depression with increased risk of apnea).
No products indexed under this heading.

Ethinamate (Concomitant use increases central nervous system depression with increased risk of apnea).
No products indexed under this heading.

Fentanyl (Concomitant use increases central nervous system depression with increased risk of apnea; dosage of narcotic analgesics should be reduced by at least one-third). Products include:
Duragesic Transdermal System 1786

Fentanyl Citrate (Concomitant use increases central nervous system depression with increased risk of apnea; dosage of narcotic analgesics should be reduced by at least one-third). Products include:
Actiq 1184

Fluoxetine Hydrochloride (May potentiate the actions of diazepam). Products include:
Prozac Pulvules, Liquid, and Weekly Capsules 1238
Sarafem Pulvules 1962

Fluphenazine Decanoate (May potentiate the actions of diazepam).
No products indexed under this heading.

Fluphenazine Enanthate (May potentiate the actions of diazepam).
No products indexed under this heading.

Fluphenazine Hydrochloride (May potentiate the actions of diazepam).
No products indexed under this heading.

Flurazepam Hydrochloride (Concomitant use increases central nervous system depression with increased risk of apnea).
No products indexed under this heading.

Glutethimide (Concomitant use increases central nervous system depression with increased risk of apnea).
No products indexed under this heading.

Haloperidol (Concomitant use increases central nervous system depression with increased risk of apnea). Products include:
Haldol Injection, Tablets and Concentrate 2533

Haloperidol Decanoate (Concomitant use increases central nervous system depression with increased risk of apnea). Products include:
Haldol Decanoate 2535

Hydrocodone Bitartrate (Concomitant use increases central nervous system depression with increased risk of apnea; dosage of narcotic analgesics should be reduced by at least one-third). Products include:
Hycodan 1316
Hycomine Compound Tablets 1317
Hycotuss Expectorant Syrup 1318

IMPORTANT NOTE: Always consult each drug listing in the patient's regimen for possible interactions.

Lortab 3319
Lortab Elixir 3317
Maxidone Tablets CIII 3399
Norco 5/325 Tablets CIII 3424
Norco 7.5/325 Tablets CIII 3425
Norco 10/325 Tablets CIII 3427
Norco 10/325 Tablets CIII 3425
Vicodin Tablets 516
Vicodin ES Tablets 517
Vicodin HP Tablets 518
Vicodin Tuss Expectorant 519
Vicoprofen Tablets 520
Zydone Tablets 1330

Hydrocodone Polistirex (Concomitant use increases central nervous system depression with increased risk of apnea; dosage of narcotic analgesics should be reduced by at least one-third). Products include:
Tussionex Pennkinetic Extended-Release Suspension 1174

Hydromorphone Hydrochloride (Concomitant use increases central nervous system depression with increased risk of apnea; dosage of narcotic analgesics should be reduced by at least one-third). Products include:
Dilaudid 441
Dilaudid Oral Liquid 445
Dilaudid Powder 441
Dilaudid Rectal Suppositories 441
Dilaudid Tablets 441
Dilaudid Tablets - 8 mg 445
Dilaudid-HP 443

Hydroxyzine Hydrochloride (Concomitant use increases central nervous system depression with increased risk of apnea). Products include:
Atarax Tablets & Syrup 2667
Vistaril Intramuscular Solution 2738

Imipramine Hydrochloride (May potentiate the actions of diazepam).
No products indexed under this heading.

Imipramine Pamoate (May potentiate the actions of diazepam).
No products indexed under this heading.

Isocarboxazid (May potentiate the actions of diazepam).
No products indexed under this heading.

Isoflurane (Concomitant use increases central nervous system depression with increased risk of apnea).
No products indexed under this heading.

Ketamine Hydrochloride (Concomitant use increases central nervous system depression with increased risk of apnea).
No products indexed under this heading.

Levomethadyl Acetate Hydrochloride (Concomitant use increases central nervous system depression with increased risk of apnea).
No products indexed under this heading.

Levorphanol Tartrate (Concomitant use increases central nervous system depression with increased risk of apnea; dosage of narcotic analgesics should be reduced by at least one-third). Products include:
Levo-Dromoran 1734
Levorphanol Tartrate Tablets 3059

Lorazepam (Concomitant use increases central nervous system depression with increased risk of apnea). Products include:
Ativan Injection 3478
Ativan Tablets 3482

Loxapine Hydrochloride (Concomitant use increases central nervous system depression with increased risk of apnea).
No products indexed under this heading.

Loxapine Succinate (Concomitant use increases central nervous system depression with increased risk of apnea). Products include:
Loxitane Capsules 3398

Maprotiline Hydrochloride (May potentiate the actions of diazepam).
No products indexed under this heading.

Meperidine Hydrochloride (Concomitant use increases central nervous system depression with increased risk of apnea; dosage of narcotic analgesics should be reduced by at least one-third). Products include:
Demerol 3079
Mepergan Injection 3539

Mephobarbital (Concomitant use increases central nervous system depression with increased risk of apnea).
No products indexed under this heading.

Meprobamate (Concomitant use increases central nervous system depression with increased risk of apnea). Products include:
Miltown Tablets 3349

Mesoridazine Besylate (May potentiate the actions of diazepam). Products include:
Serentil 1057

Methadone Hydrochloride (Concomitant use increases central nervous system depression with increased risk of apnea; dosage of narcotic analgesics should be reduced by at least one-third). Products include:
Dolophine Hydrochloride Tablets 3056

Methohexital Sodium (Concomitant use increases central nervous system depression with increased risk of apnea). Products include:
Brevital Sodium for Injection, USP 1815

Methotrimeprazine (May potentiate the actions of diazepam).
No products indexed under this heading.

Methoxyflurane (Concomitant use increases central nervous system depression with increased risk of apnea).
No products indexed under this heading.

Midazolam Hydrochloride (Concomitant use increases central nervous system depression with increased risk of apnea). Products include:
Versed Injection 3027
Versed Syrup 3033

Mirtazapine (May potentiate the actions of diazepam). Products include:
Remeron Tablets 2483
Remeron SolTab Tablets 2486

Moclobemide (May potentiate the actions of diazepam).
No products indexed under this heading.

Molindone Hydrochloride (Concomitant use increases central nervous system depression with increased risk of apnea). Products include:
Moban 1320

Morphine Sulfate (Concomitant use increases central nervous system depression with increased risk of apnea; dosage of narcotic analgesics should be reduced by at least one-third). Products include:
Astramorph/PF Injection, USP (Preservative-Free) 594
Duramorph Injection 1312
Infumorph 200 and Infumorph 500 Sterile Solutions 1314
Kadian Capsules 1335
MS Contin Tablets 2896
MSIR 2898
Oramorph SR Tablets 3062
Roxanol 3066

Nefazodone Hydrochloride (May potentiate the actions of diazepam). Products include:
Serzone Tablets 1104

Nortriptyline Hydrochloride (May potentiate the actions of diazepam).
No products indexed under this heading.

Olanzapine (Concomitant use increases central nervous system depression with increased risk of apnea). Products include:
Zyprexa Tablets 1973
Zyprexa ZYDIS Orally Disintegrating Tablets 1973

Oxazepam (Concomitant use increases central nervous system depression with increased risk of apnea).
No products indexed under this heading.

Oxycodone Hydrochloride (Concomitant use increases central nervous system depression with increased risk of apnea; dosage of narcotic analgesics should be reduced by at least one-third). Products include:
OxyContin Tablets 2912
OxyFast Oral Concentrate Solution 2916
OxyIR Capsules 2916
Percocet Tablets 1326
Percodan Tablets 1327
Percolone Tablets 1327
Roxicodone 3067
Tylox Capsules 2597

Pargyline Hydrochloride (May potentiate the actions of diazepam).
No products indexed under this heading.

Paroxetine Hydrochloride (May potentiate the actions of diazepam). Products include:
Paxil 1609

Pentobarbital Sodium (Concomitant use increases central nervous system depression with increased risk of apnea). Products include:
Nembutal Sodium Solution 485

Perphenazine (May potentiate the actions of diazepam). Products include:
Etrafon 3115
Trilafon 3160

Phenelzine Sulfate (May potentiate the actions of diazepam). Products include:
Nardil Tablets 2653

Phenobarbital (Concomitant use increases central nervous system depression with increased risk of apnea). Products include:
Arco-Lase Plus Tablets 592
Donnatal 2929
Donnatal Extentabs 2930

Prazepam (Concomitant use increases central nervous system depression with increased risk of apnea).
No products indexed under this heading.

Procarbazine Hydrochloride (May potentiate the actions of diazepam). Products include:
Matulane Capsules 3246

Prochlorperazine (May potentiate the actions of diazepam). Products include:
Compazine 1505

Promethazine Hydrochloride (May potentiate the actions of diazepam). Products include:
Mepergan Injection 3539
Phenergan Injection 3553
Phenergan 3556
Phenergan Syrup 3554
Phenergan with Codeine Syrup 3557
Phenergan with Dextromethorphan Syrup 3559
Phenergan VC Syrup 3560
Phenergan VC with Codeine Syrup 3561

Propofol (Concomitant use increases central nervous system depression with increased risk of apnea). Products include:
Diprivan Injectable Emulsion 667

Propoxyphene Hydrochloride (Concomitant use increases central nervous system depression with increased risk of apnea; dosage of narcotic analgesics should be reduced by at least one-third). Products include:
Darvon Pulvules 1909
Darvon Compound-65 Pulvules 1910

Propoxyphene Napsylate (Concomitant use increases central nervous system depression with increased risk of apnea; dosage of narcotic analgesics should be reduced by at least one-third). Products include:
Darvon-N/Darvocet-N 1907
Darvon-N Tablets 1912

Protriptyline Hydrochloride (May potentiate the actions of diazepam). Products include:
Vivactil Tablets 2446
Vivactil Tablets 2217

Quazepam (Concomitant use increases central nervous system depression with increased risk of apnea).
No products indexed under this heading.

Quetiapine Fumarate (Concomitant use increases central nervous system depression with increased risk of apnea). Products include:
Seroquel Tablets 684

Remifentanil Hydrochloride (Concomitant use increases central nervous system depression with increased risk of apnea; dosage of narcotic analgesics should be reduced by at least one-third).
No products indexed under this heading.

Risperidone (Concomitant use increases central nervous system depression with increased risk of apnea). Products include:
Risperdal 1796

Secobarbital Sodium (Concomitant use increases central nervous system depression with increased risk of apnea).
No products indexed under this heading.

Selegiline Hydrochloride (May potentiate the actions of diazepam). Products include:
Eldepryl Capsules 3266

Sertraline Hydrochloride (May potentiate the actions of diazepam). Products include:
Zoloft 2751

Sevoflurane (Concomitant use increases central nervous system depression with increased risk of apnea).
No products indexed under this heading.

Sufentanil Citrate (Concomitant use increases central nervous system depression with increased risk of apnea; dosage of narcotic analgesics should be reduced by at least one-third).
No products indexed under this heading.

Temazepam (Concomitant use increases central nervous system depression with increased risk of apnea).
No products indexed under this heading.

Thiamylal Sodium (Concomitant use increases central nervous system depression with increased risk of apnea).
No products indexed under this heading.

Thioridazine Hydrochloride (May potentiate the actions of diazepam). Products include:
Thioridazine Hydrochloride Tablets 2289

Thiothixene (Concomitant use increases central nervous system depression with increased risk of apnea). Products include:
Navane Capsules 2701
Thiothixene Capsules 2290

Tranylcypromine Sulfate (May potentiate the actions of diazepam). Products include:
Parnate Tablets 1607

Trazodone Hydrochloride (May potentiate the actions of diazepam).
No products indexed under this heading.

Triazolam (Concomitant use increases central nervous system depression with increased risk of apnea). Products include:
Halcion Tablets 2823

Trifluoperazine Hydrochloride (May potentiate the actions of diazepam). Products include:
Stelazine 1640

Trimipramine Maleate (May potentiate the actions of diazepam). Products include:
Surmontil Capsules 3595

Venlafaxine Hydrochloride (May potentiate the actions of diazepam). Products include:
Effexor Tablets 3495
Effexor XR Capsules 3499

Zaleplon (Concomitant use increases central nervous system depression with increased risk of apnea). Products include:
Sonata Capsules 3591

Ziprasidone Hydrochloride (Concomitant use increases central nervous system depression with increased risk of apnea). Products include:
Geodon Capsules 2688

Zolpidem Tartrate (Concomitant use increases central nervous system depression with increased risk of apnea). Products include:
Ambien Tablets 3191

Food Interactions

Alcohol (Concomitant use increases central nervous system depression with increased risk of apnea; injectable diazepam should not be administered in acute alcoholic intoxication).

VALIUM TABLETS

(Diazepam) 3047
May interact with barbiturates, central nervous system depressants, antidepressant drugs, anticonvulsants, monoamine oxidase inhibitors, narcotic analgesics, phenothiazines, and certain other agents. Compounds in these categories include:

Alfentanil Hydrochloride (May potentiate the actions of diazepam).
No products indexed under this heading.

Alprazolam (May potentiate the actions of diazepam). Products include:
Xanax Tablets 2865

Amitriptyline Hydrochloride (May potentiate the actions of diazepam). Products include:
Etrafon 3115
Limbitrol 1738

Amoxapine (May potentiate the actions of diazepam).
No products indexed under this heading.

Aprobarbital (May potentiate the actions of diazepam).
No products indexed under this heading.

Buprenorphine Hydrochloride (May potentiate the actions of diazepam). Products include:
Buprenex Injectable 2918

Bupropion Hydrochloride (May potentiate the actions of diazepam). Products include:
Wellbutrin Tablets 1680
Wellbutrin SR Sustained-Release Tablets 1684
Zyban Sustained-Release Tablets 1710

Buspirone Hydrochloride (May potentiate the actions of diazepam).
No products indexed under this heading.

Butabarbital (May potentiate the actions of diazepam).
No products indexed under this heading.

Butalbital (May potentiate the actions of diazepam). Products include:
Phrenilin 578
Sedapap Tablets 50 mg/650 mg 2225

Carbamazepine (Co-administration of diazepam as an adjunct in treating convulsive disorders results in possibility of an increase in the frequency and/or severity of grand mal seizures which may require an increase in the dosage of standard anticonvulsant agent). Products include:
Carbatrol Capsules 3234
Tegretol/Tegretol-XR 2404

Chlordiazepoxide (May potentiate the actions of diazepam). Products include:
Limbitrol 1738

Chlordiazepoxide Hydrochloride (May potentiate the actions of diazepam). Products include:
Librium Capsules 1736
Librium for Injection 1737

Chlorpromazine (May potentiate the actions of diazepam). Products include:
Thorazine Suppositories 1656

Chlorpromazine Hydrochloride (May potentiate the actions of diazepam). Products include:
Thorazine 1656

Chlorprothixene (May potentiate the actions of diazepam).
No products indexed under this heading.

Chlorprothixene Hydrochloride (May potentiate the actions of diazepam).
No products indexed under this heading.

Chlorprothixene Lactate (May potentiate the actions of diazepam).
No products indexed under this heading.

Cimetidine (Co-administration delays diazepam clearance; clinical significance of this interaction is unclear). Products include:
Tagamet HB 200 Suspension .... ▣762
Tagamet HB 200 Tablets .... ▣761
Tagamet Tablets 1644

Cimetidine Hydrochloride (Co-administration delays diazepam clearance; clinical significance of this interaction is unclear). Products include:
Tagamet 1644

Citalopram Hydrobromide (May potentiate the actions of diazepam). Products include:
Celexa 1365

Clonazepam (Co-administration of diazepam as an adjunct in treating convulsive disorders results in possibility of an increase in the frequency and/or severity of grand mal seizures which may require an increase in the dosage of standard anticonvulsant agent; may potentiate the CNS depression caused by diazepam). Products include:
Klonopin Tablets 2983

Clorazepate Dipotassium (May potentiate the actions of diazepam). Products include:
Tranxene 511

Clozapine (May potentiate the actions of diazepam). Products include:
Clozaril Tablets 2319

Codeine Phosphate (May potentiate the actions of diazepam). Products include:
Phenergan with Codeine Syrup 3557
Phenergan VC with Codeine Syrup 3561
Robitussin A-C Syrup 2942
Robitussin-DAC Syrup 2942
Ryna-C Liquid .... ▣768
Soma Compound w/Codeine Tablets 3355
Tussi-Organidin NR Liquid 3350
Tussi-Organidin-S NR Liquid 3350
Tylenol with Codeine 2595

Desflurane (May potentiate the actions of diazepam). Products include:
Suprane Liquid for Inhalation 874

Desipramine Hydrochloride (May potentiate the actions of diazepam). Products include:
Norpramin Tablets 755

Dezocine (May potentiate the actions of diazepam).
No products indexed under this heading.

Divalproex Sodium (Co-administration of diazepam as an adjunct in treating convulsive disorders results in possibility of an increase in the frequency and/or severity of grand mal seizures which may require an increase in the dosage of standard anticonvulsant agent). Products include:
Depakote Sprinkle Capsules 426
Depakote Tablets 430
Depakote ER Tablets 436

Doxepin Hydrochloride (May potentiate the actions of diazepam). Products include:
Sinequan 2713

Droperidol (May potentiate the actions of diazepam).
No products indexed under this heading.

Enflurane (May potentiate the actions of diazepam).
No products indexed under this heading.

Estazolam (May potentiate the actions of diazepam). Products include:
ProSom Tablets 500

Ethchlorvynol (May potentiate the actions of diazepam).
No products indexed under this heading.

Ethinamate (May potentiate the actions of diazepam).
No products indexed under this heading.

Ethosuximide (Co-administration of diazepam as an adjunct in treating convulsive disorders results in possibility of an increase in the frequency and/or severity of grand mal seizures which may require an increase in the dosage of standard anticonvulsant agent). Products include:
Zarontin Capsules 2659
Zarontin Syrup 2660

Ethotoin (Co-administration of diazepam as an adjunct in treating convulsive disorders results in possibility of an increase in the frequency and/or severity of grand mal seizures which may require an increase in the dosage of standard anticonvulsant agent).
No products indexed under this heading.

Felbamate (Co-administration of diazepam as an adjunct in treating convulsive disorders results in possibility of an increase in the frequency and/or severity of grand mal seizures which may require an increase in the dosage of standard anticonvulsant agent). Products include:
Felbatol 3343

Fentanyl (May potentiate the actions of diazepam). Products include:
Duragesic Transdermal System 1786

Fentanyl Citrate (May potentiate the actions of diazepam). Products include:
Actiq 1184

Fluoxetine Hydrochloride (May potentiate the actions of diazepam). Products include:
Prozac Pulvules, Liquid, and Weekly Capsules 1238
Sarafem Pulvules 1962

Fluphenazine Decanoate (May potentiate the actions of diazepam).
No products indexed under this heading.

Fluphenazine Enanthate (May potentiate the actions of diazepam).
No products indexed under this heading.

Fluphenazine Hydrochloride (May potentiate the actions of diazepam).
No products indexed under this heading.

Flurazepam Hydrochloride (May potentiate the actions of diazepam).
No products indexed under this heading.

Fosphenytoin Sodium (Co-administration of diazepam as an adjunct in treating convulsive disorders results in possibility of an increase in the frequency and/or severity of grand mal seizures which may require an increase in the dosage of standard anticonvulsant agent). Products include:
Cerebyx Injection 2619

Glutethimide (May potentiate the actions of diazepam).
No products indexed under this heading.

Haloperidol (May potentiate the actions of diazepam). Products include:
Haldol Injection, Tablets and Concentrate 2533

Haloperidol Decanoate (May potentiate the actions of diazepam). Products include:
Haldol Decanoate 2535

Hydrocodone Bitartrate (May potentiate the actions of diazepam). Products include:
Hycodan 1316
Hycomine Compound Tablets 1317
Hycotuss Expectorant Syrup 1318
Lortab 3319
Lortab Elixir 3317
Maxidone Tablets CIII 3399
Norco 5/325 Tablets CIII 3424
Norco 7.5/325 Tablets CIII 3425
Norco 10/325 Tablets CIII 3427
Norco 10/325 Tablets CIII 3425
Vicodin Tablets 516
Vicodin ES Tablets 517
Vicodin HP Tablets 518
Vicodin Tuss Expectorant 519
Vicoprofen Tablets 520
Zydone Tablets 1330

Hydrocodone Polistirex (May potentiate the actions of diazepam). Products include:
Tussionex Pennkinetic Extended-Release Suspension 1174

Hydromorphone Hydrochloride (May potentiate the actions of diazepam). Products include:
Dilaudid 441
Dilaudid Oral Liquid 445
Dilaudid Powder 441
Dilaudid Rectal Suppositories 441
Dilaudid Tablets 441
Dilaudid Tablets - 8 mg 445
Dilaudid-HP 443

Hydroxyzine Hydrochloride (May potentiate the actions of diazepam). Products include:
Atarax Tablets & Syrup 2667
Vistaril Intramuscular Solution 2738

Imipramine Hydrochloride (May potentiate the actions of diazepam).
No products indexed under this heading.

Imipramine Pamoate (May potentiate the actions of diazepam).
No products indexed under this heading.

Isocarboxazid (May potentiate the actions of diazepam).
No products indexed under this heading.

Isoflurane (May potentiate the actions of diazepam).
No products indexed under this heading.

Ketamine Hydrochloride (May potentiate the actions of diazepam).
No products indexed under this heading.

Lamotrigine (Co-administration of diazepam as an adjunct in treating convulsive disorders results in possibility of an increase in the frequency and/or severity of grand mal seizures which may require an increase in the dosage of standard anticonvulsant agent). Products include:
Lamictal 1567

Levetiracetam (Co-administration of diazepam as an adjunct in treating convulsive disorders results in possibility of an increase in the frequency and/or severity of grand mal seizures which may require an increase in the dosage of standard anticonvulsant agent). Products include:
Keppra Tablets 3314

Levomethadyl Acetate Hydrochloride (May potentiate the actions of diazepam).
No products indexed under this heading.

Levorphanol Tartrate (May potentiate the actions of diazepam). Products include:
Levo-Dromoran 1734
Levorphanol Tartrate Tablets 3059

Lorazepam (May potentiate the actions of diazepam). Products include:
Ativan Injection 3478
Ativan Tablets 3482

Loxapine Hydrochloride (May potentiate the actions of diazepam).
No products indexed under this heading.

Loxapine Succinate (May potentiate the actions of diazepam). Products include:
Loxitane Capsules 3398

Maprotiline Hydrochloride (May potentiate the actions of diazepam).
No products indexed under this heading.

Meperidine Hydrochloride (May potentiate the actions of diazepam). Products include:
Demerol 3079
Mepergan Injection 3539

Mephenytoin (Co-administration of diazepam as an adjunct in treating convulsive disorders results in possibility of an increase in the frequency and/or severity of grand mal seizures which may require an increase in the dosage of standard anticonvulsant agent).
No products indexed under this heading.

Mephobarbital (May potentiate the actions of diazepam).
No products indexed under this heading.

Meprobamate (May potentiate the actions of diazepam). Products include:
Miltown Tablets 3349

Mesoridazine Besylate (May potentiate the actions of diazepam). Products include:
Serentil 1057

Methadone Hydrochloride (May potentiate the actions of diazepam). Products include:
Dolophine Hydrochloride Tablets 3056

Methohexital Sodium (May potentiate the actions of diazepam). Products include:
Brevital Sodium for Injection, USP .. 1815

Methotrimeprazine (May potentiate the actions of diazepam).
No products indexed under this heading.

Methoxyflurane (May potentiate the actions of diazepam).
No products indexed under this heading.

Methsuximide (Co-administration of diazepam as an adjunct in treating convulsive disorders results in possibility of an increase in the frequency and/or severity of grand mal seizures which may require an increase in the dosage of standard anticonvulsant agent). Products include:
Celontin Capsules 2618

Midazolam Hydrochloride (May potentiate the actions of diazepam). Products include:
Versed Injection 3027
Versed Syrup 3033

Mirtazapine (May potentiate the actions of diazepam). Products include:
Remeron Tablets 2483
Remeron SolTab Tablets 2486

Moclobemide (May potentiate the actions of diazepam).
No products indexed under this heading.

Molindone Hydrochloride (May potentiate the actions of diazepam). Products include:
Moban 1320

Morphine Sulfate (May potentiate the actions of diazepam). Products include:
Astramorph/PF Injection, USP (Preservative-Free) 594
Duramorph Injection 1312
Infumorph 200 and Infumorph 500 Sterile Solutions 1314
Kadian Capsules 1335
MS Contin Tablets 2896
MSIR 2898
Oramorph SR Tablets 3062
Roxanol 3066

Nefazodone Hydrochloride (May potentiate the actions of diazepam). Products include:
Serzone Tablets 1104

Nortriptyline Hydrochloride (May potentiate the actions of diazepam).
No products indexed under this heading.

Olanzapine (May potentiate the actions of diazepam). Products include:
Zyprexa Tablets 1973
Zyprexa ZYDIS Orally Disintegrating Tablets 1973

Oxazepam (May potentiate the actions of diazepam).
No products indexed under this heading.

Oxcarbazepine (Co-administration of diazepam as an adjunct in treating convulsive disorders results in possibility of an increase in the frequency and/or severity of grand mal seizures which may require an increase in the dosage of standard anticonvulsant agent). Products include:
Trileptal Oral Suspension 2407
Trileptal Tablets 2407

Oxycodone Hydrochloride (May potentiate the actions of diazepam). Products include:
OxyContin Tablets 2912
OxyFast Oral Concentrate Solution . 2916
OxyIR Capsules 2916
Percocet Tablets 1326
Percodan Tablets 1327
Percolone Tablets 1327
Roxicodone 3067
Tylox Capsules 2597

Paramethadione (Co-administration of diazepam as an adjunct in treating convulsive disorders results in possibility of an increase in the frequency and/or severity of grand mal seizures which may require an increase in the dosage of standard anticonvulsant agent).
No products indexed under this heading.

Pargyline Hydrochloride (May potentiate the actions of diazepam).
No products indexed under this heading.

Paroxetine Hydrochloride (May potentiate the actions of diazepam). Products include:
Paxil 1609

Pentobarbital Sodium (May potentiate the actions of diazepam). Products include:
Nembutal Sodium Solution 485

Perphenazine (May potentiate the actions of diazepam). Products include:
Etrafon 3115
Trilafon 3160

Phenacemide (Co-administration of diazepam as an adjunct in treating convulsive disorders results in possibility of an increase in the frequency and/or severity of grand mal seizures which may require an increase in the dosage of standard anticonvulsant agent).
No products indexed under this heading.

Phenelzine Sulfate (May potentiate the actions of diazepam). Products include:
Nardil Tablets 2653

Phenobarbital (Co-administration of diazepam as an adjunct in treating convulsive disorders results in possibility of an increase in the frequency and/or severity of grand mal seizures which may require an increase in the dosage of standard anticonvulsant agent; may potentiate the CNS depression caused by diazepam). Products include:
Arco-Lase Plus Tablets 592
Donnatal 2929
Donnatal Extentabs 2930

Phensuximide (Co-administration of diazepam as an adjunct in treating convulsive disorders results in possibility of an increase in the frequency and/or severity of grand mal seizures which may require an increase in the dosage of standard anticonvulsant agent).
No products indexed under this heading.

Phenytoin (Co-administration of diazepam as an adjunct in treating convulsive disorders results in possibility of an increase in the frequency and/or severity of grand mal seizures which may require an increase in the dosage of standard anticonvulsant agent). Products Include:
Dilantin Infatabs 2624
Dilantin-125 Oral Suspension 2625

Phenytoin Sodium (Co-administration of diazepam as an adjunct in treating convulsive disorders results in possibility of an increase in the frequency and/or severity of grand mal seizures which may require an increase in the dosage of standard anticonvulsant agent). Products include:
Dilantin Kapseals 2622

Prazepam (May potentiate the actions of diazepam).
No products indexed under this heading.

Primidone (Co-administration of diazepam as an adjunct in treating convulsive disorders results in possibility of an increase in the frequency and/or severity of grand mal seizures which may require an increase in the dosage of standard anticonvulsant agent).
No products indexed under this heading.

Procarbazine Hydrochloride (May potentiate the actions of diazepam). Products include:
Matulane Capsules 3246

Prochlorperazine (May potentiate the actions of diazepam). Products include:
Compazine 1505

Promethazine Hydrochloride (May potentiate the actions of diazepam). Products include:
Mepergan Injection 3539
Phenergan Injection 3553
Phenergan 3556
Phenergan Syrup 3554
Phenergan with Codeine Syrup 3557
Phenergan with Dextromethorphan Syrup 3559
Phenergan VC Syrup 3560
Phenergan VC with Codeine Syrup .. 3561

Propofol (May potentiate the actions of diazepam). Products include:
Diprivan Injectable Emulsion 667

Propoxyphene Hydrochloride (May potentiate the actions of diazepam). Products include:
Darvon Pulvules 1909
Darvon Compound-65 Pulvules 1910

Propoxyphene Napsylate (May potentiate the actions of diazepam). Products include:
Darvon-N/Darvocet-N 1907
Darvon-N Tablets 1912

Protriptyline Hydrochloride (May potentiate the actions of diazepam). Products include:
Vivactil Tablets 2446
Vivactil Tablets 2217

Quazepam (May potentiate the actions of diazepam).
No products indexed under this heading.

Quetiapine Fumarate (May potentiate the actions of diazepam). Products include:
Seroquel Tablets 684

Remifentanil Hydrochloride (May potentiate the actions of diazepam).
No products indexed under this heading.

Risperidone (May potentiate the actions of diazepam). Products include:
Risperdal 1796

Secobarbital Sodium (May potentiate the actions of diazepam).
No products indexed under this heading.

Selegiline Hydrochloride (May potentiate the actions of diazepam). Products include:
Eldepryl Capsules 3266

Sertraline Hydrochloride (May potentiate the actions of diazepam). Products include:
Zoloft 2751

Sevoflurane (May potentiate the actions of diazepam).
No products indexed under this heading.

Sufentanil Citrate (May potentiate the actions of diazepam).
No products indexed under this heading.

Temazepam (May potentiate the actions of diazepam).
No products indexed under this heading.

Thiamylal Sodium (May potentiate the actions of diazepam).
No products indexed under this heading.

Thioridazine Hydrochloride (May potentiate the actions of diazepam). Products include:
Thioridazine Hydrochloride Tablets 2289

Thiothixene (May potentiate the actions of diazepam). Products include:
Navane Capsules 2701
Thiothixene Capsules 2290

Tiagabine Hydrochloride (Co-administration of diazepam as an adjunct in treating convulsive disorders results in possibility of an increase in the frequency and/or severity of grand mal seizures which may require an increase in the dosage of standard anticonvulsant agent). Products include:
Gabitril Tablets 1189

Topiramate (Co-administration of diazepam as an adjunct in treating convulsive disorders results in possibility of an increase in the frequency and/or severity of grand mal seizures which may require an increase in the dosage of standard anticonvulsant agent). Products include:
Topamax Sprinkle Capsules 2590
Topamax Tablets 2590

Tranylcypromine Sulfate (May potentiate the actions of diazepam). Products include:
Parnate Tablets 1607

Trazodone Hydrochloride (May potentiate the actions of diazepam).
No products indexed under this heading.

Triazolam (May potentiate the actions of diazepam). Products include:
Halcion Tablets 2823

Trifluoperazine Hydrochloride (May potentiate the actions of diazepam). Products include:
Stelazine 1640

Trimethadione (Co-administration of diazepam as an adjunct in treating convulsive disorders results in possibility of an increase in the frequency and/or severity of grand mal seizures which may require an increase in the dosage of standard anticonvulsant agent).
No products indexed under this heading.

Trimipramine Maleate (May potentiate the actions of diazepam). Products include:
Surmontil Capsules 3595

Valproate Sodium (Co-administration of diazepam as an adjunct in treating convulsive disorders results in possibility of an increase in the frequency and/or severity of grand mal seizures which may require an increase in the dosage of standard anticonvulsant agent). Products include:
Depacon Injection 416

Valproic Acid (Co-administration of diazepam as an adjunct in treating convulsive disorders results in possibility of an increase in the frequency and/or severity of grand mal seizures which may require an increase in the dosage of standard anticonvulsant agent). Products include:
Depakene 421

Venlafaxine Hydrochloride (May potentiate the actions of diazepam). Products include:
Effexor Tablets 3495
Effexor XR Capsules 3499

Zaleplon (May potentiate the actions of diazepam). Products include:
Sonata Capsules 3591

Ziprasidone Hydrochloride (May potentiate the actions of diazepam). Products include:
Geodon Capsules 2688

Zolpidem Tartrate (May potentiate the actions of diazepam). Products include:
Ambien Tablets 3191

Zonisamide (Co-administration of diazepam as an adjunct in treating convulsive disorders results in possibility of an increase in the frequency and/or severity of grand mal seizures which may require an increase in the dosage of standard anticonvulsant agent). Products include:
Zonegran Capsules 1307

Food Interactions

Alcohol (May potentiate the actions of diazepam).

VALSTAR STERILE SOLUTION FOR INTRAVESICAL INSTILLATION

(Valrubicin) 1175
None cited in PDR database.

VALTREX CAPLETS

(Valacyclovir Hydrochloride) 1676
May interact with:

Cimetidine (Co-administration reduces the rate but not the extent of conversion of valacyclovir to acyclovir; additive increase in acyclovir AUC and Cmax). Products include:
Tagamet HB 200 Suspension .... ▣762
Tagamet HB 200 Tablets .... ▣761
Tagamet Tablets 1644

Cimetidine Hydrochloride (Co-administration reduces the rate but not the extent of conversion of valacyclovir to acyclovir; additive increase in acyclovir AUC and Cmax). Products include:
Tagamet 1644

Probenecid (Co-administration reduces the rate but not the extent of conversion of valacyclovir to acyclovir; additive increase in acyclovir AUC and Cmax).
No products indexed under this heading.

VANCENASE POCKETHALER NASAL INHALER

(Beclomethasone Dipropionate) 3162
May interact with:

Prednisone (Combined administration of alternate day prednisone systemic treatment and orally inhaled beclomethasone increases the likelihood of HPA suppression to a therapeutic dose of either one alone). Products include:
Prednisone 3064

VANCENASE AQ NASAL SPRAY 0.084%

(Beclomethasone Dipropionate) 3163
None cited in PDR database.

VANCERIL INHALATION AEROSOL

(Beclomethasone Dipropionate) 3165
None cited in PDR database.

VANCERIL DOUBLE STRENGTH INHALATION AEROSOL

(Beclomethasone Dipropionate) 3167
None cited in PDR database.

VANCOCIN HCL CAPSULES & PULVULES

(Vancomycin Hydrochloride) 1972
See Vancocin HCl, Vials & ADD-Vantage

VANCOCIN HCL ORAL SOLUTION

(Vancomycin Hydrochloride) 1971
May interact with aminoglycosides and ototoxic drugs. Compounds in these categories include:

Amikacin Sulfate (Concurrent use may result in increased ototoxicity and/or nephrotoxicity).
No products indexed under this heading.

Cisplatin (Concurrent use may result in increased ototoxicity and/or nephrotoxicity).
No products indexed under this heading.

Gentamicin Sulfate (Concurrent use may result in increased ototoxicity and/or nephrotoxicity). Products include:
Genoptic Ophthalmic Ointment .... ⊙239
Genoptic Sterile Ophthalmic Solution .... ⊙239
Pred-G Ophthalmic Suspension .... ⊙247
Pred-G Sterile Ophthalmic Ointment .... ⊙248

Kanamycin Sulfate (Concurrent use may result in increased ototoxicity and/or nephrotoxicity).
No products indexed under this heading.

Streptomycin Sulfate (Concurrent use may result in increased ototoxicity and/or nephrotoxicity). Products include:
Streptomycin Sulfate Injection 2714

Tobramycin (Concurrent use may result in increased ototoxicity and/or nephrotoxicity). Products include:
TOBI Solution for Inhalation 1206
TobraDex Ophthalmic Ointment 542
TobraDex Ophthalmic Suspension 541
Tobrex Ophthalmic Ointment .... ⊙220
Tobrex Ophthalmic Solution .... ⊙221

Tobramycin Sulfate (Concurrent use may result in increased ototoxicity and/or nephrotoxicity). Products include:
Nebcin Vials, Hyporets & ADD-Vantage 1955

VANCOCIN HCL, VIALS & ADD-VANTAGE

(Vancomycin Hydrochloride) 1970
May interact with aminoglycosides, anesthetics, and certain other agents. Compounds in these categories include:

Alfentanil Hydrochloride (Co-administration with anesthetic agents has been associated with erythema and histamine-like flushing in children).
No products indexed under this heading.

Amikacin Sulfate (Concurrent and/or sequential use may result in increased potential for neurotoxicity and/or nephrotoxicity).
No products indexed under this heading.

Amphotericin B (Concurrent and/or sequential use may result in increased potential for neurotoxicity and/or nephrotoxicity). Products include:
Abelcet Injection 1273
AmBisome for Injection 1383
Amphotec 1774

Bacitracin Zinc (Concurrent and/or sequential use may result in increased potential for neurotoxicity and/or nephrotoxicity). Products include:
Betadine Brand First Aid Antibiotics & Moisturizer Ointment 2894
Betadine Brand Plus First Aid Antibiotics & Pain Reliever Ointment 2894
Neosporin Ointment .... ▣704
Neosporin Ophthalmic Ointment Sterile .... ⊙299
Neosporin + Pain Relief Maximum Strength Ointment .... ▣704
Polysporin Ointment .... ▣706
Polysporin Ophthalmic Ointment Sterile .... ⊙301
Polysporin Powder .... ▣706

Cisplatin (Concurrent and/or sequential use may result in increased potential for neurotoxicity and/or nephrotoxicity).
No products indexed under this heading.

Colistin Sulfate (Concurrent and/or sequential use may result in increased potential for neurotoxicity and/or nephrotoxicity). Products include:
Cortisporin-TC Otic Suspension 2246

Enflurane (Co-administration with anesthetic agents has been associated with erythema and histamine-like flushing in children).
No products indexed under this heading.

Fentanyl Citrate (Co-administration with anesthetic agents has been associated with erythema and histamine-like flushing in children). Products include:
Actiq 1184

Gentamicin Sulfate (Concurrent and/or sequential use may result in increased potential for neurotoxicity and/or nephrotoxicity). Products include:
Genoptic Ophthalmic Ointment .... ⊙239
Genoptic Sterile Ophthalmic Solution .... ⊙239
Pred-G Ophthalmic Suspension .... ⊙247
Pred-G Sterile Ophthalmic Ointment .... ⊙248

Halothane (Co-administration with anesthetic agents has been associated with erythema and histamine-like flushing in children). Products include:
Fluothane Inhalation 3508

Isoflurane (Co-administration with anesthetic agents has been associated with erythema and histamine-like flushing in children).
No products indexed under this heading.

Kanamycin Sulfate (Concurrent and/or sequential use may result in increased potential for neurotoxicity and/or nephrotoxicity).
No products indexed under this heading.

Ketamine Hydrochloride (Co-administration with anesthetic agents has been associated with erythema and histamine-like flushing in children).
No products indexed under this heading.

Methohexital Sodium (Co-administration with anesthetic agents has been associated with erythema and histamine-like flushing in children). Products include:
Brevital Sodium for Injection, USP 1815

Midazolam Hydrochloride (Co-administration with anesthetic agents has been associated with erythema and histamine-like flushing in children). Products include:
Versed Injection 3027
Versed Syrup 3033

Polymyxin B Sulfate (Concurrent and/or sequential use may result in increased potential for neurotoxicity and/or nephrotoxicity). Products include:
Betadine Brand First Aid Antibiotics & Moisturizer Ointment 2894
Betadine Brand Plus First Aid Antibiotics & Pain Reliever Ointment 2894
Cortisporin Ophthalmic Suspension Sterile .... ⊙297
Neosporin G.U. Irrigant Sterile 2256
Neosporin Ointment .... ▣704
Neosporin Ophthalmic Ointment Sterile .... ⊙299
Neosporin Ophthalmic Solution Sterile .... ⊙300
Neosporin + Pain Relief Maximum Strength Cream .... ▣704
Neosporin + Pain Relief Maximum Strength Ointment .... ▣704
Poly-Pred Liquifilm Ophthalmic Suspension .... ⊙245
Polysporin Ointment .... ▣706
Polysporin Ophthalmic Ointment Sterile .... ⊙301
Polysporin Powder .... ▣706
Polytrim Ophthalmic Solution 556

Propofol (Co-administration with anesthetic agents has been associated with erythema and histamine-like flushing in children). Products include:
Diprivan Injectable Emulsion 667

Remifentanil Hydrochloride (Co-administration with anesthetic

agents has been associated with erythema and histamine-like flushing in children).
No products indexed under this heading.

Streptomycin Sulfate (Concurrent and/or sequential use may result in increased potential for neurotoxicity and/or nephrotoxicity). Products include:
Streptomycin Sulfate Injection ... 2714

Sufentanil Citrate (Co-administration with anesthetic agents has been associated with erythema and histamine-like flushing in children).
No products indexed under this heading.

Thiamylal Sodium (Co-administration with anesthetic agents has been associated with erythema and histamine-like flushing in children).
No products indexed under this heading.

Tobramycin (Concurrent and/or sequential use may result in increased potential for neurotoxicity and/or nephrotoxicity). Products include:
TOBI Solution for Inhalation ... 1206
TobraDex Ophthalmic Ointment ... 542
TobraDex Ophthalmic Suspension .. 541
Tobrex Ophthalmic Ointment ... ⊙220
Tobrex Ophthalmic Solution ... ⊙221

Tobramycin Sulfate (Concurrent and/or sequential use may result in increased potential for neurotoxicity and/or nephrotoxicity). Products include:
Nebcin Vials, Hyporets & ADD-Vantage ... 1955

Viomycin (Concurrent and/or sequential use may result in increased potential for neurotoxicity and/or nephrotoxicity).
No products indexed under this heading.

VANIQA CREAM

(Eflornithine Hydrochloride) ... 1121
None cited in PDR database.

VANQUISH CAPLETS

(Acetaminophen, Aluminum Hydroxide, Aspirin, Caffeine, Magnesium Hydroxide) ... ■617
May interact with oral anticoagulants, oral hypoglycemic agents, and certain other agents. Compounds in these categories include:

Acarbose (Concurrent use with diabetes drugs should be avoided unless directed by a doctor). Products include:
Precose Tablets ... 906

Antiarthritic Drugs, unspecified (Concurrent use with arthritis medications should be avoided unless directed by a doctor).

Chlorpropamide (Concurrent use with diabetes drugs should be avoided unless directed by a doctor). Products include:
Diabinese Tablets ... 2680

Dicumarol (Concurrent use with anticoagulants should be avoided unless directed by a doctor).
No products indexed under this heading.

Glimepiride (Concurrent use with diabetes drugs should be avoided unless directed by a doctor). Products include:
Amaryl Tablets ... 717

Glipizide (Concurrent use with diabetes drugs should be avoided unless directed by a doctor). Products include:
Glucotrol Tablets ... 2692
Glucotrol XL Extended Release Tablets ... 2693

Glyburide (Concurrent use with diabetes drugs should be avoided unless directed by a doctor). Products include:
DiaBeta Tablets ... 741
Glucovance Tablets ... 1086

Metformin Hydrochloride (Concurrent use with diabetes drugs should be avoided unless directed by a doctor). Products include:
Glucophage Tablets ... 1080
Glucophage XR Tablets ... 1080
Glucovance Tablets ... 1086

Miglitol (Concurrent use with diabetes drugs should be avoided unless directed by a doctor). Products include:
Glyset Tablets ... 2821

Pioglitazone Hydrochloride (Concurrent use with diabetes drugs should be avoided unless directed by a doctor). Products include:
Actos Tablets ... 3275

Probenecid (Concurrent use with gout medications should be avoided unless directed by a doctor).
No products indexed under this heading.

Repaglinide (Concurrent use with diabetes drugs should be avoided unless directed by a doctor). Products include:
Prandin Tablets (0.5, 1, and 2 mg) ... 2432

Rosiglitazone Maleate (Concurrent use with diabetes drugs should be avoided unless directed by a doctor). Products include:
Avandia Tablets ... 1490

Sulfinpyrazone (Concurrent use with gout medications should be avoided unless directed by a doctor).
No products indexed under this heading.

Tolazamide (Concurrent use with diabetes drugs should be avoided unless directed by a doctor).
No products indexed under this heading.

Tolbutamide (Concurrent use with diabetes drugs should be avoided unless directed by a doctor).
No products indexed under this heading.

Troglitazone (Concurrent use with diabetes drugs should be avoided unless directed by a doctor).
No products indexed under this heading.

Warfarin Sodium (Concurrent use with anticoagulants should be avoided unless directed by a doctor). Products include:
Coumadin for Injection ... 1243
Coumadin Tablets ... 1243
Warfarin Sodium Tablets, USP ... 3302

Food Interactions

Alcohol (Chronic heavy alcohol users, 3 or more drinks per day, should consult their physicians for advice on when and how they should take pain relievers/fever reducers including acetaminophen and aspirin).

VANTIN TABLETS AND ORAL SUSPENSION

(Cefpodoxime Proxetil) ... 2860
May interact with aminoglycosides, antacids, anticholinergics, histamine H_2-receptor antagonists, and certain other agents. Compounds in these categories include:

Aluminum Carbonate (High doses of antacids reduces peak plasma levels by 24% and the extent of absorption by 27%; the rate of absorption is not altered).
No products indexed under this heading.

Aluminum Hydroxide (High doses of antacids reduces peak plasma levels by 24% and the extent of absorption by 27%; the rate of absorption is not altered). Products include:
Amphojel Suspension (Mint Flavor) ... ■789
Gaviscon Extra Strength Liquid ... ■751
Gaviscon Extra Strength Tablets ... ■751
Gaviscon Regular Strength Liquid . ■751
Gaviscon Regular Strength Tablets ... ■750
Maalox Antacid/Anti-Gas Oral Suspension ... ■673
Maalox Max Maximum Strength Antacid/Anti-Gas Liquid ... 2300
Maalox Regular Strength Antacid/Antigas Liquid ... 2300
Mylanta ... 1813
Vanquish Caplets ... ■617

Amikacin Sulfate (Close monitoring of renal function is required when co-administered with compounds of known nephrotoxicity potential, such as aminoglycosides).
No products indexed under this heading.

Atropine Sulfate (Oral anticholinergics delay peak plasma levels but do not affect the extent of absorption). Products include:
Donnatal ... 2929
Donnatal Extentabs ... 2930
Motofen Tablets ... 577
Prosed/DS Tablets ... 3268
Urised Tablets ... 2876

Belladonna Alkaloids (Oral anticholinergics delay peak plasma levels but do not affect the extent of absorption). Products include:
Hyland's Teething Tablets ... ■766
Urimax Tablets ... 1769

Benztropine Mesylate (Oral anticholinergics delay peak plasma levels but do not affect the extent of absorption). Products include:
Cogentin ... 2055

Biperiden Hydrochloride (Oral anti-cholinergics delay peak plasma levels but do not affect the extent of absorption). Products include:
Akineton ... 402

Cimetidine (High doses of H_2 blockers reduces peak plasma levels by 42% and the extent of absorption by 32%; the rate of absorption is not altered). Products include:
Tagamet HB 200 Suspension ... ■762
Tagamet HB 200 Tablets ... ■761
Tagamet Tablets ... 1644

Cimetidine Hydrochloride (High doses of H_2 blockers reduces peak plasma levels by 42% and the extent of absorption by 32%; the rate of absorption is not altered). Products include:
Tagamet ... 1644

Clidinium Bromide (Oral anticholinergics delay peak plasma levels but do not affect the extent of absorption).
No products indexed under this heading.

Dicyclomine Hydrochloride (Oral anti-cholinergics delay peak plasma levels but do not affect the extent of absorption).
No products indexed under this heading.

Famotidine (High doses of H_2 blockers reduces peak plasma levels by 42% and the extent of absorption by 32%; the rate of absorption is not altered). Products include:
Famotidine Injection ... 866
Pepcid AC ... 1814
Pepcid Complete Chewable Tablets ... 1815
Pepcid Injection ... 2153
Pepcid for Oral Suspension ... 2150
Pepcid RPD Orally Disintegrating Tablets ... 2150
Pepcid Tablets ... 2150

Gentamicin Sulfate (Close monitoring of renal function is required when co-administered with compounds of known nephrotoxicity potential, such as aminoglycosides). Products include:
Genoptic Ophthalmic Ointment ... ⊙239
Genoptic Sterile Ophthalmic Solution ... ⊙239
Pred-G Ophthalmic Suspension ... ⊙247
Pred-G Sterile Ophthalmic Ointment ... ⊙248

Glycopyrrolate (Oral anticholinergics delay peak plasma levels but do not affect the extent of absorption). Products include:
Robinul Forte Tablets ... 1358
Robinul Injectable ... 2940
Robinul Tablets ... 1358

Hyoscyamine (Oral anticholinergics delay peak plasma levels but do not affect the extent of absorption). Products include:
Urised Tablets ... 2876

Hyoscyamine Sulfate (Oral anticholinergics delay peak plasma levels but do not affect the extent of absorption). Products include:
Arco-Lase Plus Tablets ... 592
Donnatal ... 2929
Donnatal Extentabs ... 2930
Levsin/Levsinex/Levbid ... 3172
NuLev Orally Disintegrating Tablets ... 3176
Prosed/DS Tablets ... 3268
Urimax Tablets ... 1769

Ipratropium Bromide (Oral anticholinergics delay peak plasma levels but do not affect the extent of absorption). Products include:
Atrovent Inhalation Aerosol ... 1030
Atrovent Inhalation Solution ... 1031
Atrovent Nasal Spray 0.03% ... 1032
Atrovent Nasal Spray 0.06% ... 1033
Combivent Inhalation Aerosol ... 1041
DuoNeb Inhalation Solution ... 1233

Kanamycin Sulfate (Close monitoring of renal function is required when co-administered with compounds of known nephrotoxicity potential, such as aminoglycosides).
No products indexed under this heading.

Magaldrate (High doses of antacids reduces peak plasma levels by 24% and the extent of absorption by 27%; the rate of absorption is not altered).
No products indexed under this heading.

Magnesium Hydroxide (High doses of antacids reduces peak plasma levels by 24% and the extent of absorption by 27%; the rate of absorption is not altered). Products include:
Ex•Lax Milk of Magnesia Liquid ... ■670
Maalox Antacid/Anti-Gas Oral Suspension ... ■673
Maalox Max Maximum Strength Antacid/Anti-Gas Liquid ... 2300
Maalox Regular Strength Antacid/Antigas Liquid ... 2300
Mylanta Fast-Acting ... 1813
Mylanta ... 1813
Pepcid Complete Chewable Tablets ... 1815
Phillips' Chewable Tablets ... ■615
Phillips' Milk of Magnesia Liquid (Original, Cherry, & Mint) ... ■616
Rolaids Tablets ... ■706
Extra Strength Rolaids Tablets ... ■706
Vanquish Caplets ... ■617

Magnesium Oxide (High doses of antacids reduces peak plasma levels by 24% and the extent of absorption by 27%; the rate of absorption is not altered). Products include:
Beelith Tablets ... 946
Mag-Ox 400 Tablets ... 1024
Uro-Mag Capsules ... 1024

Mepenzolate Bromide (Oral anticholinergics delay peak plasma levels but do not affect the extent of absorption).
No products indexed under this heading.

Nephrotoxic Drugs (Close monitoring of renal function is required when co-administered with compounds of known nephrotoxicity potential).

Nizatidine (High doses of H_2 blockers reduces peak plasma levels by 42% and the extent of absorption by 32%; the rate of absorption is not altered). Products include:

Axid Pulvules 1903
Axid Pulvules 2919

Oxybutynin Chloride (Oral anti-cholinergics delay peak plasma levels but do not affect the extent of absorption). Products include:
Ditropan XL Extended Release Tablets 564

Probenecid (Renal excretion of cefpodoxime is inhibited by probenecid and resulting in an approximately 31% increase in AUC and 20% increase in peak plasma levels).
No products indexed under this heading.

Procyclidine Hydrochloride (Oral anti-cholinergics delay peak plasma levels but do not affect the extent of absorption).
No products indexed under this heading.

Propantheline Bromide (Oral anti-cholinergics delay peak plasma levels but do not affect the extent of absorption).
No products indexed under this heading.

Ranitidine Bismuth Citrate (High doses of H_2 blockers reduces peak plasma levels by 42% and the extent of absorption by 32%; the rate of absorption is not altered).
No products indexed under this heading.

Ranitidine Hydrochloride (High doses of H_2 blockers reduces peak plasma levels by 42% and the extent of absorption by 32%; the rate of absorption is not altered). Products include:
Zantac 1690
Zantac Injection 1688
Zantac 75 Tablets .... ▣717

Scopolamine (Oral anti-cholinergics delay peak plasma levels but do not affect the extent of absorption). Products include:
Transderm Scōp Transdermal Therapeutic System 2302

Scopolamine Hydrobromide (Oral anti-cholinergics delay peak plasma levels but do not affect the extent of absorption). Products include:
Donnatal 2929
Donnatal Extentabs 2930

Sodium Bicarbonate (High doses of antacids reduces peak plasma levels by 24% and the extent of absorption by 27%; the rate of absorption is not altered). Products include:
Alka-Seltzer .... ▣603
Alka-Seltzer Lemon Lime Antacid and Pain Reliever Effervescent Tablets .... ▣603
Alka-Seltzer Extra Strength Antacid and Pain Reliever Effervescent Tablets .... ▣603
Alka-Seltzer Heartburn Relief Tablets .... ▣604
Ceo-Two Evacuant Suppository .... ▣618
Colyte with Flavor Packs for Oral Solution 3170
GoLYTELY and Pineapple Flavor GoLYTELY for Oral Solution 1068
NuLYTELY, Cherry Flavor, Lemon-Lime Flavor, and Orange Flavor NuLYTELY for Oral Solution 1068

Streptomycin Sulfate (Close monitoring of renal function is required when co-administered with compounds of known nephrotoxicity potential, such as aminoglycosides). Products include:
Streptomycin Sulfate Injection 2714

Tobramycin (Close monitoring of renal function is required when co-administered with compounds of known nephrotoxicity potential, such as aminoglycosides). Products include:
TOBI Solution for Inhalation 1206
TobraDex Ophthalmic Ointment 542
TobraDex Ophthalmic Suspension 541
Tobrex Ophthalmic Ointment .... ⊙220
Tobrex Ophthalmic Solution .... ⊙221

Tobramycin Sulfate (Close monitoring of renal function is required when co-administered with compounds of known nephrotoxicity potential, such as aminoglycosides). Products include:
Nebcin Vials, Hyporets & ADD-Vantage 1955

Tolterodine Tartrate (Oral anti-cholinergics delay peak plasma levels but do not affect the extent of absorption). Products include:
Detrol Tablets 3623
Detrol LA Capsules 2801

Tridihexethyl Chloride (Oral anti-cholinergics delay peak plasma levels but do not affect the extent of absorption).
No products indexed under this heading.

Trihexyphenidyl Hydrochloride (Oral anti-cholinergics delay peak plasma levels but do not affect the extent of absorption). Products include:
Artane 1855

Food Interactions

Food, unspecified (The extent of absorption and the mean peak plasma concentration increased when film-coated tablets were administered with food).

VAQTA

(Hepatitis A Vaccine, Inactivated) 2199
May interact with typhoid vaccine and certain other agents. Compounds in these categories include:

Typhoid Vaccine (Co-administration of Vaqta, typhoid and yellow fever vaccines has resulted in reduced GMTs for hepatitis A compared to Vaqta alone; however, following the receipt of the booster dose of Vaqta the GMTs for hepatits A in these two groups were observed to be comparable).
No products indexed under this heading.

Typhoid Vaccine Live Oral TY21a (Co-administration of Vaqta, typhoid and yellow fever vaccines has resulted in reduced GMTs for hepatitis A compared to Vaqta alone; however, following the receipt of the booster dose of Vaqta the GMTs for hepatits A in these two groups were observed to be comparable). Products include:
Vivotif Berna 997

Typhoid Vi Polysaccharide Vaccine (Co-administration of Vaqta, typhoid and yellow fever vaccines has resulted in reduced GMTs for hepatitis A compared to Vaqta alone; however, following the receipt of the booster dose of Vaqta the GMTs for hepatits A in these two groups were observed to be comparable). Products include:
TYPHIM Vi Vaccine 825

Yellow Fever Vaccine (Co-administration of Vaqta, typhoid and yellow fever vaccines has resulted in reduced GMTs for hepatitis A compared to Vaqta alone; however, following the receipt of the booster dose of Vaqta the GMTs for hepatits A in these two groups were observed to be comparable). Products include:
YF-VAX Vaccine 827

VARIVAX

(Varicella Virus Vaccine Live) 2202
May interact with corticosteroids, salicylates, and certain other agents. Compounds in these categories include:

Aspirin (Vaccine recipients should avoid use of salicylates for 6 weeks after vaccination with Varivax because of the potential for Reye's syndrome). Products include:
Aggrenox Capsules 1026
Alka-Seltzer .... ▣603
Alka-Seltzer Lemon Lime Antacid and Pain Reliever Effervescent Tablets .... ▣603
Alka-Seltzer Extra Strength Antacid and Pain Reliever Effervescent Tablets .... ▣603
Alka-Seltzer PM Effervescent Tablets .... ▣605
Genuine Bayer Tablets, Caplets and Gelcaps .... ▣606
Extra Strength Bayer Caplets and Gelcaps .... ▣610
Aspirin Regimen Bayer Children's Chewable Tablets (Orange or Cherry Flavored) .... ▣607
Bayer, Aspirin Regimen .... ▣606
Aspirin Regimen Bayer 81 mg Caplets with Calcium .... ▣607
Genuine Bayer Professional Labeling (Aspirin Regimen Bayer) .... ▣608
Extra Strength Bayer Arthritis Caplets .... ▣610
Extra Strength Bayer Plus Caplets .... ▣610
Extra Strength Bayer PM Caplets .... ▣611
BC Powder .... ▣619
BC Allergy Sinus Cold Powder .... ▣619
Arthritis Strength BC Powder .... ▣619
BC Sinus Cold Powder .... ▣619
Darvon Compound-65 Pulvules 1910
Ecotrin Enteric Coated Aspirin Low, Regular and Maximum Strength Tablets 1715
Excedrin Extra-Strength Tablets, Caplets, and Geltabs .... ▣629
Excedrin Migraine 1070
Goody's Body Pain Formula Powder .... ▣620
Goody's Extra Strength Headache Powder .... ▣620
Goody's Extra Strength Pain Relief Tablets .... ▣620
Percodan Tablets 1327
Robaxisal Tablets 2939
Soma Compound Tablets 3354
Soma Compound w/Codeine Tablets 3355
Vanquish Caplets .... ▣617

Azathioprine (Concurrent use in individuals who are on immunosuppressant drugs are more susceptible to infections; co-administration is contraindicated).
No products indexed under this heading.

Betamethasone Acetate (Co-administration in individuals on immunosuppressant doses of corticosteroids can result in more extensive vaccine-associated rash or disseminated disease). Products include:
Celestone Soluspan Injectable Suspension 3097

Betamethasone Sodium Phosphate (Co-administration in individuals on immunosuppressant doses of corticosteroids can result in more extensive vaccine-associated rash or disseminated disease). Products include:
Celestone Soluspan Injectable Suspension 3097

Choline Magnesium Trisalicylate (Vaccine recipients should avoid use of salicylates for 6 weeks after vaccination with Varivax because of the potential for Reye's syndrome). Products include:
Trilisate 2901

Cortisone Acetate (Co-administration in individuals on immunosuppressant doses of corticosteroids can result in more extensive vaccine-associated rash or disseminated disease). Products include:
Cortone Acetate Injectable Suspension 2059
Cortone Acetate Tablets 2061

Cyclosporine (Concurrent use in individuals who are on immunosuppressant drugs are more susceptible to infections; co-administration is contraindicated). Products include:
Gengraf Capsules 457
Neoral Soft Gelatin Capsules 2380
Neoral Oral Solution 2380
Sandimmune 2388

Dexamethasone (Co-administration in individuals on immunosuppressant doses of corticosteroids can result in more extensive vaccine-associated rash or disseminated disease). Products include:
Decadron Elixir 2078
Decadron Tablets 2079
TobraDex Ophthalmic Ointment 542
TobraDex Ophthalmic Suspension 541

Dexamethasone Acetate (Co-administration in individuals on immunosuppressant doses of corticosteroids can result in more extensive vaccine-associated rash or disseminated disease).
No products indexed under this heading.

Dexamethasone Sodium Phosphate (Co-administration in individuals on immunosuppressant doses of corticosteroids can result in more extensive vaccine-associated rash or disseminated disease). Products include:
Decadron Phosphate Injection 2081
Decadron Phosphate Sterile Ophthalmic Ointment 2083
Decadron Phosphate Sterile Ophthalmic Solution 2084
NeoDecadron Sterile Ophthalmic Solution 2144

Diflunisal (Vaccine recipients should avoid use of salicylates for 6 weeks after vaccination with Varivax because of the potential for Reye's syndrome). Products include:
Dolobid Tablets 2088

Fludrocortisone Acetate (Co-administration in individuals on immunosuppressant doses of corticosteroids can result in more extensive vaccine-associated rash or disseminated disease). Products include:
Florinef Acetate Tablets 2250

Globulin, Immune (Human) (Vaccination should be deferred for at least 5 months following immune globulin administration; following administration of Varivax, immune globulin should not be given for 2 months). Products include:
BayGam 914
Gamimune N, 5% Solvent/Detergent Treated 925
Gamimune N, 10% Solvent/Detergent Treated 928
Gammagard S/D 845
Iveegam EN 849
Sandoglobulin I.V. 2391

Hydrocortisone (Co-administration in individuals on immunosuppressant doses of corticosteroids can result in more extensive vaccine-associated rash or disseminated disease). Products include:
Anusol-HC Cream 2.5% 2237
Cipro HC Otic Suspension 540
Cortaid Intensive Therapy Cream .... ▣717
Cortaid Maximum Strength Cream .... ▣717
Cortisporin Ophthalmic Suspension Sterile .... ⊙297
Cortizone•5 .... ▣699
Cortizone•10 .... ▣699
Cortizone•10 Plus Creme .... ▣700
Cortizone for Kids Creme .... ▣699
Hydrocortone Tablets 2106
Massengill Medicated Soft Cloth Towelette .... ▣753
VōSoL HC Otic Solution 3356

Hydrocortisone Acetate (Co-administration in individuals on immunosuppressant doses of corticosteroids can result in more extensive vaccine-associated rash or disseminated disease). Products include:
Analpram-HC 1338
Anusol HC-1 Hydrocortisone Anti-Itch Cream .... ▣689
Anusol-HC Suppositories 2238

Cortaid .... ▣ 717
Cortifoam Rectal Foam 3170
Cortisporin-TC Otic Suspension 2246
Hydrocortone Acetate Injectable
Suspension 2103
Pramosone 1343
Proctocort Suppositories 2264
ProctoFoam-HC 3177
Terra-Cortril Ophthalmic
Suspension 2716

Hydrocortisone Sodium Phosphate (Co-administration in individuals on immunosuppressant doses of corticosteroids can result in more extensive vaccine-associated rash or disseminated disease). Products include:
Hydrocortone Phosphate
Injection, Sterile 2105

Hydrocortisone Sodium Succinate (Co-administration in individuals on immunosuppressant doses of corticosteroids can result in more extensive vaccine-associated rash or disseminated disease).
No products indexed under this heading.

Magnesium Salicylate (Vaccine recipients should avoid use of salicylates for 6 weeks after vaccination with Varivax because of the potential for Reye's syndrome). Products include:
Momentum Backache Relief
Extra Strength Caplets .... ▣ 666

Methylprednisolone Acetate (Co-administration in individuals on immunosuppressant doses of corticosteroids can result in more extensive vaccine-associated rash or disseminated disease). Products include:
Depo-Medrol Injectable
Suspension 2795

Methylprednisolone Sodium Succinate (Co-administration in individuals on immunosuppressant doses of corticosteroids can result in more extensive vaccine-associated rash or disseminated disease). Products include:
Solu-Medrol Sterile Powder 2855

Muromonab-CD3 (Concurrent use in individuals who are on immunosuppressant drugs are more susceptible to infections; co-administration is contraindicated). Products include:
Orthoclone OKT3 Sterile Solution ... 2498

Mycophenolate Mofetil (Concurrent use in individuals who are on immunosuppressant drugs are more susceptible to infections; co-administration is contraindicated). Products include:
CellCept Capsules 2951
CellCept Oral Suspension 2951
CellCept Tablets 2951

Prednisolone Acetate (Co-administration in individuals on immunosuppressant doses of corticosteroids can result in more extensive vaccine-associated rash or disseminated disease). Products include:
Blephamide Ophthalmic Ointment .. 547
Blephamide Ophthalmic
Suspension 548
Poly-Pred Liquifilm Ophthalmic
Suspension .... ⊙ 245
Pred Forte Ophthalmic
Suspension .... ⊙ 246
Pred Mild Sterile Ophthalmic
Suspension .... ⊙ 249
Pred-G Ophthalmic Suspension ..... ⊙ 247
Pred-G Sterile Ophthalmic
Ointment .... ⊙ 248

Prednisolone Sodium Phosphate (Co-administration in individuals on immunosuppressant doses of corticosteroids can result in more extensive vaccine-associated rash or disseminated disease). Products include:
Pediapred Oral Solution 1170

Prednisolone Tebutate (Co-administration in individuals on immunosuppressant doses of corticosteroids can result in more extensive vaccine-associated rash or disseminated disease).
No products indexed under this heading.

Prednisone (Co-administration in individuals on immunosuppressant doses of corticosteroids can result in more extensive vaccine-associated rash or disseminated disease). Products include:
Prednisone 3064

Salsalate (Vaccine recipients should avoid use of salicylates for 6 weeks after vaccination with Varivax because of the potential for Reye's syndrome).
No products indexed under this heading.

Tacrolimus (Concurrent use in individuals who are on immunosuppressant drugs are more susceptible to infections; co-administration is contraindicated). Products include:
Prograf 1393
Protopic Ointment 1397

Triamcinolone (Co-administration in individuals on immunosuppressant doses of corticosteroids can result in more extensive vaccine-associated rash or disseminated disease).
No products indexed under this heading.

Triamcinolone Acetonide (Co-administration in individuals on immunosuppressant doses of corticosteroids can result in more extensive vaccine-associated rash or disseminated disease). Products include:
Azmacort Inhalation Aerosol 728
Nasacort Nasal Inhaler 750
Nasacort AQ Nasal Spray 752
Tri-Nasal Spray 2274

Triamcinolone Diacetate (Co-administration in individuals on immunosuppressant doses of corticosteroids can result in more extensive vaccine-associated rash or disseminated disease).
No products indexed under this heading.

Triamcinolone Hexacetonide (Co-administration in individuals on immunosuppressant doses of corticosteroids can result in more extensive vaccine-associated rash or disseminated disease).
No products indexed under this heading.

VASCOR TABLETS
(Bepridil Hydrochloride) 2602
May interact with beta blockers, cardiac glycosides, tricyclic antidepressants, type 1 antiarrhythmic drugs, and certain other agents. Compounds in these categories include:

Acebutolol Hydrochloride (Available data are not sufficient to predict the effects of concomitant medication on patients with impaired ventricular function or cardiac conduction abnormalities). Products include:
Sectral Capsules 3589

Amitriptyline Hydrochloride (Potential for exaggeration of the QT interval prolongation). Products include:
Etrafon 3115
Limbitrol 1738

Amoxapine (Potential for exaggeration of the QT interval prolongation).
No products indexed under this heading.

Atenolol (Available data are not sufficient to predict the effects of concomitant medication on patients with impaired ventricular function or cardiac conduction abnormalities). Products include:
Tenoretic Tablets 690
Tenormin I.V. Injection 692

Betaxolol Hydrochloride (Available data are not sufficient to predict the effects of concomitant medication on patients with impaired ventricular function or cardiac conduction abnormalities). Products include:
Betoptic S Ophthalmic
Suspension 537

Bisoprolol Fumarate (Available data are not sufficient to predict the effects of concomitant medication on patients with impaired ventricular function or cardiac conduction abnormalities). Products include:
Zebeta Tablets 1885
Ziac Tablets 1887

Carteolol Hydrochloride (Available data are not sufficient to predict the effects of concomitant medication on patients with impaired ventricular function or cardiac conduction abnormalities). Products include:
Carteolol Hydrochloride
Ophthalmic Solution USP, 1% ..... ⊙ 258
Ocupress Ophthalmic Solution,
1% Sterile .... ⊙ 303

Clomipramine Hydrochloride (Potential for exaggeration of the QT interval prolongation).
No products indexed under this heading.

Desipramine Hydrochloride (Potential for exaggeration of the QT interval prolongation). Products include:
Norpramin Tablets 755

Deslanoside (Cardiac glycosides could exaggerate the depression of AV nodal conduction).
No products indexed under this heading.

Digitoxin (Cardiac glycosides could exaggerate the depression of AV nodal conduction).
No products indexed under this heading.

Digoxin (May be associated with modest increases in steady-state serum digoxin concentrations; cardiac glycosides could exaggerate the depression of AV nodal conduction). Products include:
Digitek Tablets 1003
Lanoxicaps Capsules 1574
Lanoxin Injection 1581
Lanoxin Tablets 1587
Lanoxin Elixir Pediatric 1578
Lanoxin Injection Pediatric 1584

Disopyramide Phosphate (Potential for exaggeration of the QT interval prolongation).
No products indexed under this heading.

Doxepin Hydrochloride (Potential for exaggeration of the QT interval prolongation). Products include:
Sinequan 2713

Esmolol Hydrochloride (Available data are not sufficient to predict the effects of concomitant medication on patients with impaired ventricular function or cardiac conduction abnormalities). Products include:
Brevibloc Injection 858

Imipramine Hydrochloride (Potential for exaggeration of the QT interval prolongation).
No products indexed under this heading.

Imipramine Pamoate (Potential for exaggeration of the QT interval prolongation).
No products indexed under this heading.

Labetalol Hydrochloride (Available data are not sufficient to predict the effects of concomitant medication on patients with impaired ventricular function or cardiac conduction abnormalities). Products include:
Normodyne Injection 3135
Normodyne Tablets 3137

Levobunolol Hydrochloride (Available data are not sufficient to predict the effects of concomitant medication on patients with impaired ventricular function or cardiac conduction abnormalities). Products include:
Betagan .... ⊙ 228

Maprotiline Hydrochloride (Potential for exaggeration of the QT interval prolongation).
No products indexed under this heading.

Metipranolol Hydrochloride (Available data are not sufficient to predict the effects of concomitant medication on patients with impaired ventricular function or cardiac conduction abnormalities).
No products indexed under this heading.

Metoprolol Succinate (Available data are not sufficient to predict the effects of concomitant medication on patients with impaired ventricular function or cardiac conduction abnormalities). Products include:
Toprol-XL Tablets 651

Metoprolol Tartrate (Available data are not sufficient to predict the effects of concomitant medication on patients with impaired ventricular function or cardiac conduction abnormalities).
No products indexed under this heading.

Moricizine Hydrochloride (Potential for exaggeration of the QT interval prolongation).
No products indexed under this heading.

Nadolol (Available data are not sufficient to predict the effects of concomitant medication on patients with impaired ventricular function or cardiac conduction abnormalities). Products include:
Corgard Tablets 2245
Corzide 40/5 Tablets 2247
Corzide 80/5 Tablets 2247
Nadolol Tablets 2288

Nortriptyline Hydrochloride (Potential for exaggeration of the QT interval prolongation).
No products indexed under this heading.

Penbutolol Sulfate (Available data are not sufficient to predict the effects of concomitant medication on patients with impaired ventricular function or cardiac conduction abnormalities).
No products indexed under this heading.

Pindolol (Available data are not sufficient to predict the effects of concomitant medication on patients with impaired ventricular function or cardiac conduction abnormalities).
No products indexed under this heading.

Procainamide Hydrochloride (Potential for exaggeration of the QT interval prolongation). Products include:
Procanbid Extended-Release
Tablets 2262

Propafenone Hydrochloride (Potential for exaggeration of the QT interval prolongation). Products include:
Rythmol Tablets – 150 mg,
225 mg, 300 mg 502

Propranolol Hydrochloride (Available data are not sufficient to predict the effects of concomitant medication on patients with impaired ventricular function or cardiac conduction abnormalities). Products include:
Inderal 3513
Inderal LA Long-Acting Capsules 3516
Inderide Tablets 3517
Inderide LA Long-Acting Capsules .. 3519

Protriptyline Hydrochloride (Potential for exaggeration of the QT interval prolongation). Products include:
Vivactil Tablets 2446
Vivactil Tablets 2217

Quinidine Gluconate (Potential for exaggeration of the QT interval prolongation). Products include:
Quinaglute Dura-Tabs Tablets 978

Quinidine Polygalacturonate (Potential for exaggeration of the QT interval prolongation).
No products indexed under this heading.

Quinidine Sulfate (Potential for exaggeration of the QT interval prolongation). Products include:
Quinidex Extentabs 2933

Sotalol Hydrochloride (Available data are not sufficient to predict the effects of concomitant medication on patients with impaired ventricular function or cardiac conduction abnormalities). Products include:
Betapace Tablets 950
Betapace AF Tablets 954

Timolol Hemihydrate (Available data are not sufficient to predict the effects of concomitant medication on patients with impaired ventricular function or cardiac conduction abnormalities). Products include:
Betimol Ophthalmic Solution .... ⊙324

Timolol Maleate (Available data are not sufficient to predict the effects of concomitant medication on patients with impaired ventricular function or cardiac conduction abnormalities). Products include:
Blocadren Tablets 2046
Cosopt Sterile Ophthalmic Solution 2065
Timolide Tablets 2187
Timolol GFS .... ⊙266
Timoptic in Ocudose 2192
Timoptic Sterile Ophthalmic Solution 2190
Timoptic-XE Sterile Ophthalmic Gel Forming Solution 2194

Trimipramine Maleate (Potential for exaggeration of the QT interval prolongation). Products include:
Surmontil Capsules 3595

Food Interactions

Meal, unspecified (May result in a clinically insignificant delay in time to peak concentration, but neither peak plasma levels nor the extent of absorption was changed).

VASERETIC TABLETS

(Enalapril Maleate, Hydrochlorothiazide) 2204
May interact with antihypertensives, barbiturates, corticosteroids, diuretics, cardiac glycosides, oral hypoglycemic agents, insulin, lithium preparations, narcotic analgesics, nondepolarizing neuromuscular blocking agents, non-steroidal anti-inflammatory agents, potassium preparations, potassium sparing diuretics, and certain other agents. Compounds in these categories include:

Acarbose (Hyperglycemia may occur with thiazide diuretics; dosage adjustment of oral hypoglycemic agents may be required). Products include:
Precose Tablets 906

Acebutolol Hydrochloride (Co-administration of thiazide and other antihypertensive agents can lead to additive effect or potentiation). Products include:
Sectral Capsules 3589

ACTH (Co-administration of thiazide diuretics with ACTH intensifies electrolyte depletion, particularly potassium).
No products indexed under this heading.

Alfentanil Hydrochloride (Co-administration of thiazide and narcotics may potentiate orthostatic hypotension).
No products indexed under this heading.

Amiloride Hydrochloride (Enalapril attenuates diuretic-induced potassium loss; concomitant use can lead to hyperkalemia; frequent monitoring of serum potassium is recommended if used concurrently; co-administration can result in excessive hypotension). Products include:
Midamor Tablets 2136
Moduretic Tablets 2138

Amlodipine Besylate (Co-administration of thiazide and other antihypertensive agents can lead to additive effect or potentiation). Products include:
Lotrel Capsules 2370
Norvasc Tablets 2704

Aprobarbital (Co-administration of thiazide and barbiturates may potentiate orthostatic hypotension).
No products indexed under this heading.

Atenolol (Co-administration of thiazide and other antihypertensive agents can lead to additive effect or potentiation). Products include:
Tenoretic Tablets 690
Tenormin I.V. Injection 692

Atracurium Besylate (Co-administration with nondepolarizing skeletal muscle relaxants may result in possible increased responsiveness to the muscle relaxant).
No products indexed under this heading.

Benazepril Hydrochloride (Co-administration of thiazide and other antihypertensive agents can lead to additive effect or potentiation). Products include:
Lotensin Tablets 2365
Lotensin HCT Tablets 2367
Lotrel Capsules 2370

Bendroflumethiazide (Co-administration of enalapril in patients on diuretics, especially those in whom diuretic therapy was recently instituted, may occasionally experience excessive hypotension; antihypertensive effects of enalapril are augmented by antihypertensive agents that cause renin release). Products include:
Corzide 40/5 Tablets 2247
Corzide 80/5 Tablets 2247

Betamethasone Acetate (Co-administration of thiazide diuretics with corticosteroids intensifies electrolyte depletion, particularly potassium). Products include:
Celestone Soluspan Injectable Suspension 3097

Betamethasone Sodium Phosphate (Co-administration of thiazide diuretics with corticosteroids intensifies electrolyte depletion, particularly potassium). Products include:
Celestone Soluspan Injectable Suspension 3097

Betaxolol Hydrochloride (Co-administration of thiazide and other antihypertensive agents can lead to additive effect or potentiation). Products include:
Betoptic S Ophthalmic Suspension 537

Bisoprolol Fumarate (Co-administration of thiazide and other antihypertensive agents can lead to additive effect or potentiation). Products include:
Zebeta Tablets 1885
Ziac Tablets 1887

Bumetanide (Co-administration of enalapril in patients on diuretics, especially those in whom diuretic therapy was recently instituted, may occasionally experience excessive hypotension; antihypertensive effects of enalapril are augmented by antihypertensive agents that cause renin release).
No products indexed under this heading.

Buprenorphine Hydrochloride (Co-administration of thiazide and narcotics may potentiate orthostatic hypotension). Products include:
Buprenex Injectable 2918

Butabarbital (Co-administration of thiazide and barbiturates may potentiate orthostatic hypotension).
No products indexed under this heading.

Butalbital (Co-administration of thiazide and barbiturates may potentiate orthostatic hypotension). Products include:
Phrenilin 578
Sedapap Tablets 50 mg/650 mg 2225

Candesartan Cilexetil (Co-administration of thiazide and other antihypertensive agents can lead to additive effect or potentiation). Products include:
Atacand Tablets 595
Atacand HCT Tablets 597

Captopril (Co-administration of thiazide and other antihypertensive agents can lead to additive effect or potentiation). Products include:
Captopril Tablets 2281

Carteolol Hydrochloride (Co-administration of thiazide and other antihypertensive agents can lead to additive effect or potentiation). Products include:
Carteolol Hydrochloride Ophthalmic Solution USP, 1% .... ⊙258
Ocupress Ophthalmic Solution, 1% Sterile .... ⊙303

Celecoxib (Co-administration in some patients with compromised renal function who are being treated with NSAIDS may result in a further deterioration of renal function; NSAID may reduce the diuretic, natriuretic and antihypertensive effects of thiazide). Products include:
Celebrex Capsules 2676
Celebrex Capsules 2780

Chlorothiazide (Co-administration of enalapril in patients on diuretics, especially those in whom diuretic therapy was recently instituted, may occasionally experience excessive hypotension; antihypertensive effects of enalapril are augmented by antihypertensive agents that cause renin release). Products include:
Aldoclor Tablets 2035
Diuril Oral 2087

Chlorothiazide Sodium (Co-administration of enalapril in patients on diuretics, especially those in whom diuretic therapy was recently instituted, may occasionally experience excessive hypotension; antihypertensive effects of enalapril are augmented by antihypertensive agents that cause renin release). Products include:
Diuril Sodium Intravenous 2086

Chlorpropamide (Hyperglycemia may occur with thiazide diuretics; dosage adjustment of oral hypoglycemic agents may be required). Products include:
Diabinese Tablets 2680

Chlorthalidone (Co-administration of enalapril in patients on diuretics, especially those in whom diuretic therapy was recently instituted, may occasionally experience excessive hypotension; antihypertensive effects of enalapril are augmented by antihypertensive agents that cause renin release). Products include:
Clorpres Tablets 1002
Combipres Tablets 1040
Tenoretic Tablets 690

Cholestyramine (Absorption of hydrochlorothiazide is impaired in the presence of anionic exchange resins; these resins bind the hydrochlorothiazide and reduce its absorption from GI tract).
No products indexed under this heading.

Cisatracurium Besylate (Co-administration with nondepolarizing skeletal muscle relaxants may result in possible increased responsiveness to the muscle relaxant).
No products indexed under this heading.

Clonidine (Co-administration of thiazide and other antihypertensive agents can lead to additive effect or potentiation). Products include:
Catapres-TTS 1038

Clonidine Hydrochloride (Co-administration of thiazide and other antihypertensive agents can lead to additive effect or potentiation). Products include:
Catapres Tablets 1037
Clorpres Tablets 1002
Combipres Tablets 1040
Duraclon Injection 3057

Codeine Phosphate (Co-administration of thiazide and narcotics may potentiate orthostatic hypotension). Products include:
Phenergan with Codeine Syrup 3557
Phenergan VC with Codeine Syrup 3561
Robitussin A-C Syrup 2942
Robitussin-DAC Syrup 2942
Ryna-C Liquid .... ▣768
Soma Compound w/Codeine Tablets 3355
Tussi-Organidin NR Liquid 3350
Tussi-Organidin-S NR Liquid 3350
Tylenol with Codeine 2595

Colestipol Hydrochloride (Absorption of hydrochlorothiazide is impaired in the presence of anionic exchange resins; these resins bind the hydrochlorothiazide and reduce its absorption from GI tract). Products include:
Colestid Tablets 2791

Cortisone Acetate (Co-administration of thiazide diuretics with corticosteroids intensifies electrolyte depletion, particularly potassium). Products include:
Cortone Acetate Injectable Suspension 2059
Cortone Acetate Tablets 2061

Deserpidine (Co-administration of thiazide and other antihypertensive agents can lead to additive effect or potentiation).
No products indexed under this heading.

Deslanoside (Hypokalemia induced by thiazide diuretics may cause cardiac arrhythmia and may also sensitize or exaggerate the response to the heart to the toxic effects of digitalis, such as ventricular irritability).
No products indexed under this heading.

Dexamethasone (Co-administration of thiazide diuretics with corticosteroids intensifies electrolyte depletion, particularly potassium). Products include:
Decadron Elixir 2078
Decadron Tablets 2079
TobraDex Ophthalmic Ointment 542
TobraDex Ophthalmic Suspension 541

Dexamethasone Acetate (Co-administration of thiazide diuretics with corticosteroids intensifies electrolyte depletion, particularly potassium).
No products indexed under this heading.

Dexamethasone Sodium Phosphate (Co-administration of thiazide diuretics with corticosteroids intensifies electrolyte depletion, particularly potassium). Products include:
Decadron Phosphate Injection 2081
Decadron Phosphate Sterile Ophthalmic Ointment 2083

Decadron Phosphate Sterile Ophthalmic Solution 2084
NeoDecadron Sterile Ophthalmic Solution 2144

Dezocine (Co-administration of thiazide and narcotics may potentiate orthostatic hypotension).
No products indexed under this heading.

Diazoxide (Co-administration of thiazide and other antihypertensive agents can lead to additive effect or potentiation).
No products indexed under this heading.

Diclofenac Potassium (Co-administration in some patients with compromised renal function who are being treated with NSAIDS may result in a further deterioration of renal function; NSAID may reduce the diuretic, natriuretic and antihypertensive effects of thiazide). Products include:
Cataflam Tablets 2315

Diclofenac Sodium (Co-administration in some patients with compromised renal function who are being treated with NSAIDS may result in a further deterioration of renal function; NSAID may reduce the diuretic, natriuretic and antihypertensive effects of thiazide). Products include:
Arthrotec Tablets 3195
Voltaren Ophthalmic Sterile Ophthalmic Solution .... ⊙ 312
Voltaren Tablets 2315
Voltaren-XR Tablets 2315

Digitoxin (Hypokalemia induced by thiazide diuretics may cause cardiac arrhythmia and may also sensitize or exaggerate the response to the heart to the toxic effects of digitalis, such as ventricular irritability).
No products indexed under this heading.

Digoxin (Hypokalemia induced by thiazide diuretics may cause cardiac arrhythmia and may also sensitize or exaggerate the response to the heart to the toxic effects of digitalis, such as ventricular irritability). Products include:
Digitek Tablets 1003
Lanoxicaps Capsules 1574
Lanoxin Injection 1581
Lanoxin Tablets 1587
Lanoxin Elixir Pediatric 1578
Lanoxin Injection Pediatric 1584

Diltiazem Hydrochloride (Co-administration of thiazide and other antihypertensive agents can lead to additive effect or potentiation). Products include:
Cardizem Injectable 1018
Cardizem Lyo-Ject Syringe 1018
Cardizem Monovial 1018
Cardizem CD Capsules 1016
Tiazac Capsules 1378

Doxazosin Mesylate (Co-administration of thiazide and other antihypertensive agents can lead to additive effect or potentiation). Products include:
Cardura Tablets 2668

Enalaprilat (Co-administration of thiazide and other antihypertensive agents can lead to additive effect or potentiation). Products include:
Enalaprilat Injection 863
Vasotec I.V. Injection 2207

Eprosartan Mesylate (Co-administration of thiazide and other antihypertensive agents can lead to additive effect or potentiation). Products include:
Teveten Tablets 3327

Esmolol Hydrochloride (Co-administration of thiazide and other antihypertensive agents can lead to additive effect or potentiation). Products include:
Brevibloc Injection 858

Ethacrynic Acid (Co-administration of enalapril in patients on diuretics, especially those in whom diuretic therapy was recently instituted, may occasionally experience excessive hypotension; antihypertensive effects of enalapril are augmented by antihypertensive agents that cause renin release). Products include:
Edecrin Tablets 2091

Etodolac (Co-administration in some patients with compromised renal function who are being treated with NSAIDS may result in a further deterioration of renal function; NSAID may reduce the diuretic, natriuretic and antihypertensive effects of thiazide). Products include:
Lodine 3528
Lodine XL Extended-Release Tablets 3530

Felodipine (Co-administration of thiazide and other antihypertensive agents can lead to additive effect or potentiation). Products include:
Lexxel Tablets 608
Plendil Extended-Release Tablets 623

Fenoprofen Calcium (Co-administration in some patients with compromised renal function who are being treated with NSAIDS may result in a further deterioration of renal function; NSAID may reduce the diuretic, natriuretic and antihypertensive effects of thiazide).
No products indexed under this heading.

Fentanyl (Co-administration of thiazide and narcotics may potentiate orthostatic hypotension). Products include:
Duragesic Transdermal System 1786

Fentanyl Citrate (Co-administration of thiazide and narcotics may potentiate orthostatic hypotension). Products include:
Actiq 1184

Fludrocortisone Acetate (Co-administration of thiazide diuretics with corticosteroids intensifies electrolyte depletion, particularly potassium). Products include:
Florinef Acetate Tablets 2250

Flurbiprofen (Co-administration in some patients with compromised renal function who are being treated with NSAIDS may result in a further deterioration of renal function; NSAID may reduce the diuretic, natriuretic and antihypertensive effects of thiazide).
No products indexed under this heading.

Fosinopril Sodium (Co-administration of thiazide and other antihypertensive agents can lead to additive effect or potentiation). Products include:
Monopril Tablets 1091
Monopril HCT 1094

Furosemide (Co-administration of enalapril in patients on diuretics, especially those in whom diuretic therapy was recently instituted, may occasionally experience excessive hypotension; antihypertensive effects of enalapril are augmented by antihypertensive agents that cause renin release). Products include:
Furosemide Tablets 2284

Glimepiride (Hyperglycemia may occur with thiazide diuretics; dosage adjustment of oral hypoglycemic agents may be required). Products include:
Amaryl Tablets 717

Glipizide (Hyperglycemia may occur with thiazide diuretics; dosage adjustment of oral hypoglycemic agents may be required). Products include:
Glucotrol Tablets 2692
Glucotrol XL Extended Release Tablets 2693

Glyburide (Hyperglycemia may occur with thiazide diuretics; dosage adjustment of oral hypoglycemic agents may be required). Products include:
DiaBeta Tablets 741
Glucovance Tablets 1086

Guanabenz Acetate (Co-administration of thiazide and other antihypertensive agents can lead to additive effect or potentiation).
No products indexed under this heading.

Guanethidine Monosulfate (Co-administration of thiazide and other antihypertensive agents can lead to additive effect or potentiation).
No products indexed under this heading.

Hydralazine Hydrochloride (Co-administration of thiazide and other antihypertensive agents can lead to additive effect or potentiation).
No products indexed under this heading.

Hydrocodone Bitartrate (Co-administration of thiazide and narcotics may potentiate orthostatic hypotension). Products include:
Hycodan 1316
Hycomine Compound Tablets 1317
Hycotuss Expectorant Syrup 1318
Lortab 3319
Lortab Elixir 3317
Maxidone Tablets CIII 3399
Norco 5/325 Tablets CIII 3424
Norco 7.5/325 Tablets CIII 3425
Norco 10/325 Tablets CIII 3427
Norco 10/325 Tablets CIII 3425
Vicodin Tablets 516
Vicodin ES Tablets 517
Vicodin HP Tablets 518
Vicodin Tuss Expectorant 519
Vicoprofen Tablets 520
Zydone Tablets 1330

Hydrocodone Polistirex (Co-administration of thiazide and narcotics may potentiate orthostatic hypotension). Products include:
Tussionex Pennkinetic Extended-Release Suspension 1174

Hydrocortisone (Co-administration of thiazide diuretics with corticosteroids intensifies electrolyte depletion, particularly potassium). Products include:
Anusol-HC Cream 2.5% 2237
Cipro HC Otic Suspension 540
Cortaid Intensive Therapy Cream .... ▣ 717
Cortaid Maximum Strength Cream .... ▣ 717
Cortisporin Ophthalmic Suspension Sterile .... ⊙ 297
Cortizone•5 .... ▣ 699
Cortizone•10 .... ▣ 699
Cortizone•10 Plus Creme .... ▣ 700
Cortizone for Kids Creme .... ▣ 699
Hydrocortone Tablets 2106
Massengill Medicated Soft Cloth Towelette .... ▣ 753
VōSoL HC Otic Solution 3356

Hydrocortisone Acetate (Co-administration of thiazide diuretics with corticosteroids intensifies electrolyte depletion, particularly potassium). Products include:
Analpram-HC 1338
Anusol HC-1 Hydrocortisone Anti-Itch Cream .... ▣ 689
Anusol-HC Suppositories 2238
Cortaid .... ▣ 717
Cortifoam Rectal Foam 3170
Cortisporin-TC Otic Suspension 2246
Hydrocortone Acetate Injectable Suspension 2103
Pramosone 1343
Proctocort Suppositories 2264
ProctoFoam-HC 3177
Terra-Cortril Ophthalmic Suspension 2716

Hydrocortisone Sodium Phosphate (Co-administration of thiazide diuretics with corticosteroids intensifies electrolyte depletion, particularly potassium). Products include:
Hydrocortone Phosphate Injection, Sterile 2105

Hydrocortisone Sodium Succinate (Co-administration of thiazide diuretics with corticosteroids intensifies electrolyte depletion, particularly potassium).
No products indexed under this heading.

Hydroflumethiazide (Co-administration of enalapril in patients on diuretics, especially those in whom diuretic therapy was recently instituted, may occasionally experience excessive hypotension; antihypertensive effects of enalapril are augmented by antihypertensive agents that cause renin release). Products include:
Diucardin Tablets 3494

Hydromorphone Hydrochloride (Co-administration of thiazide and narcotics may potentiate orthostatic hypotension). Products include:
Dilaudid 441
Dilaudid Oral Liquid 445
Dilaudid Powder 441
Dilaudid Rectal Suppositories 441
Dilaudid Tablets 441
Dilaudid Tablets - 8 mg 445
Dilaudid-HP 443

Ibuprofen (Co-administration in some patients with compromised renal function who are being treated with NSAIDS may result in a further deterioration of renal function; NSAID may reduce the diuretic, natriuretic and antihypertensive effects of thiazide). Products include:
Advil .... ▣ 771
Children's Advil Oral Suspension .... ▣ 773
Children's Advil Chewable Tablets .... ▣ 773
Advil Cold and Sinus Caplets .... ▣ 771
Advil Cold and Sinus Tablets .... ▣ 771
Advil Flu & Body Ache Caplets .... ▣ 772
Infants' Advil Drops .... ▣ 773
Junior Strength Advil Tablets .... ▣ 773
Junior Strength Advil Chewable Tablets .... ▣ 773
Advil Migraine Liquigels .... ▣ 772
Children's Motrin Oral Suspension and Chewable Tablets 2006
Children's Motrin Cold Oral Suspension 2007
Children's Motrin Oral Suspension .... ▣ 643
Motrin Suspension, Oral Drops, Chewable Tablets, and Caplets 2002
Infants' Motrin Concentrated Drops 2006
Junior Strength Motrin Caplets and Chewable Tablets 2006
Motrin IB Tablets, Caplets, and Gelcaps 2002
Motrin Migraine Pain Caplets 2005
Motrin Sinus Headache Caplets 2005
Vicoprofen Tablets 520

Indapamide (Co-administration of enalapril in patients on diuretics, especially those in whom diuretic therapy was recently instituted, may occasionally experience excessive hypotension; antihypertensive effects of enalapril are augmented by antihypertensive agents that cause renin release). Products include:
Indapamide Tablets 2286

Indomethacin (Co-administration in some patients with compromised renal function who are being treated with NSAIDS may result in a further deterioration of renal function; NSAID may reduce the diuretic, natriuretic and antihypertensive effects of thiazide). Products include:
Indocin 2112

Indomethacin Sodium Trihydrate (Co-administration in some patients with compromised renal function who are being treated with NSAIDS may result in a further deterioration of renal function; NSAID may reduce the diuretic, natriuretic and antihypertensive effects of thiazide). Products include:
Indocin I.V. 2115

Insulin, Human, Zinc Suspension (Hyperglycemia may occur with thiazide diuretics; dosage adjustment of insulin may be required). Products include:

Humulin L, 100 Units 1937
Humulin U, 100 Units 1943
Novolin L Human Insulin 10 ml Vials 2422

Insulin, Human NPH (Hyperglycemia may occur with thiazide diuretics; dosage adjustment of insulin may be required). Products include:
Humulin N, 100 Units 1939
Humulin N NPH Pen 1940
Novolin N Human Insulin 10 ml Vials 2422
Novolin N PenFill 2423
Novolin N Prefilled Syringe Disposable Insulin Delivery System 2425

Insulin, Human Regular (Hyperglycemia may occur with thiazide diuretics; dosage adjustment of insulin may be required). Products include:
Humulin R Regular (U-500) 1943
Humulin R, 100 Units 1941
Novolin R Human Insulin 10 ml Vials 2423
Novolin R PenFill 2423
Novolin R Prefilled Syringe Disposable Insulin Delivery System 2425
Velosulin BR Human Insulin 10 ml Vials 2435

Insulin, Human Regular and Human NPH Mixture (Hyperglycemia may occur with thiazide diuretics; dosage adjustment of insulin may be required). Products include:
Humulin 50/50, 100 Units 1934
Humulin 70/30, 100 Units 1935
Humulin 70/30 Pen 1936
Novolin 70/30 Human Insulin 10 ml Vials 2421
Novolin 70/30 PenFill 2423
Novolin 70/30 Prefilled Disposable Insulin Delivery System 2425

Insulin, NPH (Hyperglycemia may occur with thiazide diuretics; dosage adjustment of insulin may be required). Products include:
Iletin II, NPH (Pork), 100 Units 1946

Insulin, Regular (Hyperglycemia may occur with thiazide diuretics; dosage adjustment of insulin may be required). Products include:
Iletin II, Regular (Pork), 100 Units 1947

Insulin, Zinc Crystals (Hyperglycemia may occur with thiazide diuretics; dosage adjustment of insulin may be required).
No products indexed under this heading.

Insulin, Zinc Suspension (Hyperglycemia may occur with thiazide diuretics; dosage adjustment of insulin may be required). Products include:
Iletin II, Lente (Pork), 100 Units 1945

Insulin Aspart, Human Regular (Hyperglycemia may occur with thiazide diuretics; dosage adjustment of insulin may be required).
No products indexed under this heading.

Insulin glargine (Hyperglycemia may occur with thiazide diuretics; dosage adjustment of insulin may be required). Products include:
Lantus Injection 742

Insulin Lispro, Human (Hyperglycemia may occur with thiazide diuretics; dosage adjustment of insulin may be required). Products include:
Humalog 1926
Humalog Mix 75/25 Pen 1928

Insulin Lispro Protamine, Human (Hyperglycemia may occur with thiazide diuretics; dosage adjustment of insulin may be required). Products include:
Humalog Mix 75/25 Pen 1928

Irbesartan (Co-administration of thiazide and other antihypertensive agents can lead to additive effect or potentiation). Products include:
Avalide Tablets 1070
Avapro Tablets 1074
Avapro Tablets 3076

Isradipine (Co-administration of thiazide and other antihypertensive agents can lead to additive effect or potentiation). Products include:
DynaCirc Capsules 2921
DynaCirc CR Tablets 2923

Ketoprofen (Co-administration in some patients with compromised renal function who are being treated with NSAIDS may result in a further deterioration of renal function; NSAID may reduce the diuretic, natriuretic and antihypertensive effects of thiazide). Products include:
Orudis Capsules 3548
Orudis KT Tablets 778
Oruvail Capsules 3548

Ketorolac Tromethamine (Co-administration in some patients with compromised renal function who are being treated with NSAIDS may result in a further deterioration of renal function; NSAID may reduce the diuretic, natriuretic and antihypertensive effects of thiazide). Products include:
Acular Ophthalmic Solution 544
Acular PF Ophthalmic Solution 544
Toradol 3018

Labetalol Hydrochloride (Co-administration of thiazide and other antihypertensive agents can lead to additive effect or potentiation). Products include:
Normodyne Injection 3135
Normodyne Tablets 3137

Levorphanol Tartrate (Co-administration of thiazide and narcotics may potentiate orthostatic hypotension). Products include:
Levo-Dromoran 1734
Levorphanol Tartrate Tablets 3059

Lisinopril (Co-administration of thiazide and other antihypertensive agents can lead to additive effect or potentiation). Products include:
Prinivil Tablets 2164
Prinzide Tablets 2168
Zestoretic Tablets 695
Zestril Tablets 698

Lithium Carbonate (Co-administration of lithium with drugs that cause elimination of sodium, including ACE inhibitors, can lead to lithium toxicity; diuretics can reduce renal clearance of lithium and add a high risk of lithium toxicity). Products include:
Eskalith 1527
Lithium Carbonate 3061
Lithobid Slow-Release Tablets 3255

Lithium Citrate (Co-administration of lithium with drugs that cause elimination of sodium, including ACE inhibitors, can lead to lithium toxicity; diuretics can reduce renal clearance of lithium and add a high risk of lithium toxicity). Products include:
Lithium Citrate Syrup 3061

Losartan Potassium (Co-administration of thiazide and other antihypertensive agents can lead to additive effect or potentiation). Products include:
Cozaar Tablets 2067
Hyzaar 2109

Mecamylamine Hydrochloride (Co-administration of thiazide and other antihypertensive agents can lead to additive effect or potentiation). Products include:
Inversine Tablets 1850

Meclofenamate Sodium (Co-administration in some patients with compromised renal function who are being treated with NSAIDS may result in a further deterioration of renal function; NSAID may reduce the diuretic, natriuretic and antihypertensive effects of thiazide).
No products indexed under this heading.

Mefenamic Acid (Co-administration in some patients with compromised renal function who are being treated with NSAIDS may result in a further deterioration of renal function; NSAID may reduce the diuretic, natriuretic and antihypertensive effects of thiazide). Products include:
Ponstel Capsules 1356

Meloxicam (Co-administration in some patients with compromised renal function who are being treated with NSAIDS may result in a further deterioration of renal function; NSAID may reduce the diuretic, natriuretic and antihypertensive effects of thiazide). Products include:
Mobic Tablets 1054

Meperidine Hydrochloride (Co-administration of thiazide and narcotics may potentiate orthostatic hypotension). Products include:
Demerol 3079
Mepergan Injection 3539

Mephobarbital (Co-administration of thiazide and barbiturates may potentiate orthostatic hypotension).
No products indexed under this heading.

Metformin Hydrochloride (Hyperglycemia may occur with thiazide diuretics; dosage adjustment of oral hypoglycemic agents may be required). Products include:
Glucophage Tablets 1080
Glucophage XR Tablets 1080
Glucovance Tablets 1086

Methadone Hydrochloride (Co-administration of thiazide and narcotics may potentiate orthostatic hypotension). Products include:
Dolophine Hydrochloride Tablets 3056

Methyclothiazide (Co-administration of enalapril in patients on diuretics, especially those in whom diuretic therapy was recently instituted, may occasionally experience excessive hypotension; antihypertensive effects of enalapril are augmented by antihypertensive agents that cause renin release).
No products indexed under this heading.

Methyldopa (Co-administration of thiazide and other antihypertensive agents can lead to additive effect or potentiation). Products include:
Aldoclor Tablets 2035
Aldomet Tablets 2037
Aldoril Tablets 2039

Methyldopate Hydrochloride (Co-administration of thiazide and other antihypertensive agents can lead to additive effect or potentiation).
No products indexed under this heading.

Methylprednisolone Acetate (Co-administration of thiazide diuretics with corticosteroids intensifies electrolyte depletion, particularly potassium). Products include:
Depo-Medrol Injectable Suspension 2795

Methylprednisolone Sodium Succinate (Co-administration of thiazide diuretics with corticosteroids intensifies electrolyte depletion, particularly potassium). Products include:
Solu-Medrol Sterile Powder 2855

Metocurine Iodide (Co-administration with nondepolarizing skeletal muscle relaxants may result in possible increased responsiveness to the muscle relaxant).
No products indexed under this heading.

Metolazone (Co-administration of enalapril in patients on diuretics, especially those in whom diuretic therapy was recently instituted, may occasionally experience excessive hypotension; antihypertensive effects of enalapril are augmented by antihypertensive agents that cause renin release). Products include:
Mykrox Tablets 1168
Zaroxolyn Tablets 1177

Metoprolol Succinate (Co-administration of thiazide and other antihypertensive agents can lead to additive effect or potentiation). Products include:
Toprol-XL Tablets 651

Metoprolol Tartrate (Co-administration of thiazide and other antihypertensive agents can lead to additive effect or potentiation).
No products indexed under this heading.

Metyrosine (Co-administration of thiazide and other antihypertensive agents can lead to additive effect or potentiation). Products include:
Demser Capsules 2085

Mibefradil Dihydrochloride (Co-administration of thiazide and other antihypertensive agents can lead to additive effect or potentiation).
No products indexed under this heading.

Miglitol (Hyperglycemia may occur with thiazide diuretics; dosage adjustment of oral hypoglycemic agents may be required). Products include:
Glyset Tablets 2821

Minoxidil (Co-administration of thiazide and other antihypertensive agents can lead to additive effect or potentiation). Products include:
Rogaine Extra Strength for Men Topical Solution 721
Rogaine for Women Topical Solution 721

Mivacurium Chloride (Co-administration with nondepolarizing skeletal muscle relaxants may result in possible increased responsiveness to the muscle relaxant).
No products indexed under this heading.

Moexipril Hydrochloride (Co-administration of thiazide and other antihypertensive agents can lead to additive effect or potentiation). Products include:
Uniretic Tablets 3178
Univasc Tablets 3181

Morphine Sulfate (Co-administration of thiazide and narcotics may potentiate orthostatic hypotension). Products include:
Astramorph/PF Injection, USP (Preservative-Free) 594
Duramorph Injection 1312
Infumorph 200 and Infumorph 500 Sterile Solutions 1314
Kadian Capsules 1335
MS Contin Tablets 2896
MSIR 2898
Oramorph SR Tablets 3062
Roxanol 3066

Nabumetone (Co-administration in some patients with compromised renal function who are being treated with NSAIDS may result in a further deterioration of renal function; NSAID may reduce the diuretic, natriuretic and antihypertensive effects of thiazide). Products include:
Relafen Tablets 1617

Nadolol (Co-administration of thiazide and other antihypertensive agents can lead to additive effect or potentiation). Products include:
Corgard Tablets 2245
Corzide 40/5 Tablets 2247
Corzide 80/5 Tablets 2247
Nadolol Tablets 2288

Naproxen (Co-administration in some patients with compromised renal function who are being treated with NSAIDS may result in a further deterioration of renal function; NSAID may reduce the diuretic, natriuretic and antihypertensive effects of thiazide). Products include:
EC-Naprosyn Delayed-Release Tablets 2967
Naprosyn Suspension 2967
Naprosyn Tablets 2967

Naproxen Sodium (Co-administration in some patients with compromised renal function who are being treated with NSAIDS may result in a further deterioration of renal function; NSAID may reduce the diuretic, natriuretic and antihypertensive effects of thiazide). Products include:

Aleve Tablets, Caplets and Gelcaps ▣ 602
Aleve Cold & Sinus Caplets ▣ 603
Anaprox Tablets 2967
Anaprox DS Tablets 2967
Naprelan Tablets 1293

Nicardipine Hydrochloride (Co-administration of thiazide and other antihypertensive agents can lead to additive effect or potentiation). Products include:

Cardene I.V. 3485

Nifedipine (Co-administration of thiazide and other antihypertensive agents can lead to additive effect or potentiation). Products include:

Adalat CC Tablets 877
Procardia Capsules 2708
Procardia XL Extended Release Tablets 2710

Nisoldipine (Co-administration of thiazide and other antihypertensive agents can lead to additive effect or potentiation). Products include:

Sular Tablets 688

Nitroglycerin (Co-administration of thiazide and other antihypertensive agents can lead to additive effect or potentiation). Products include:

Nitro-Dur Transdermal Infusion System 3134
Nitro-Dur Transdermal Infusion System 1834
Nitrolingual Pumpspray 1355
Nitrostat Tablets 2658

Norepinephrine Bitartrate (Possible decreased response to pressor amines but not sufficient to preclude pressor amine use).

No products indexed under this heading.

Oxaprozin (Co-administration in some patients with compromised renal function who are being treated with NSAIDS may result in a further deterioration of renal function; NSAID may reduce the diuretic, natriuretic and antihypertensive effects of thiazide).

No products indexed under this heading.

Oxycodone Hydrochloride (Co-administration of thiazide and narcotics may potentiate orthostatic hypotension). Products include:

OxyContin Tablets 2912
OxyFast Oral Concentrate Solution 2916
OxyIR Capsules 2916
Percocet Tablets 1326
Percodan Tablets 1327
Percolone Tablets 1327
Roxicodone 3067
Tylox Capsules 2597

Pancuronium Bromide (Co-administration with nondepolarizing skeletal muscle relaxants may result in possible increased responsiveness to the muscle relaxant).

No products indexed under this heading.

Penbutolol Sulfate (Co-administration of thiazide and other antihypertensive agents can lead to additive effect or potentiation).

No products indexed under this heading.

Pentobarbital Sodium (Co-administration of thiazide and barbiturates may potentiate orthostatic hypotension). Products include:

Nembutal Sodium Solution 485

Perindopril Erbumine (Co-administration of thiazide and other antihypertensive agents can lead to additive effect or potentiation). Products include:

Aceon Tablets (2 mg, 4 mg, 8 mg) 3249

Phenobarbital (Co-administration of thiazide and barbiturates may potentiate orthostatic hypotension). Products include:

Arco-Lase Plus Tablets 592
Donnatal 2929
Donnatal Extentabs 2930

Phenoxybenzamine Hydrochloride (Co-administration of thiazide and other antihypertensive agents can lead to additive effect or potentiation). Products include:

Dibenzyline Capsules 3457

Phentolamine Mesylate (Co-administration of thiazide and other antihypertensive agents can lead to additive effect or potentiation).

No products indexed under this heading.

Phenylbutazone (Co-administration in some patients with compromised renal function who are being treated with NSAIDS may result in a further deterioration of renal function; NSAID may reduce the diuretic, natriuretic and antihypertensive effects of thiazide).

No products indexed under this heading.

Pindolol (Co-administration of thiazide and other antihypertensive agents can lead to additive effect or potentiation).

No products indexed under this heading.

Pioglitazone Hydrochloride (Hyperglycemia may occur with thiazide diuretics; dosage adjustment of oral hypoglycemic agents may be required). Products include:

Actos Tablets 3275

Piroxicam (Co-administration in some patients with compromised renal function who are being treated with NSAIDS may result in a further deterioration of renal function; NSAID may reduce the diuretic, natriuretic and antihypertensive effects of thiazide). Products include:

Feldene Capsules 2685

Polythiazide (Co-administration of enalapril in patients on diuretics, especially those in whom diuretic therapy was recently instituted, may occasionally experience excessive hypotension; antihypertensive effects of enalapril are augmented by antihypertensive agents that cause renin release). Products include:

Minizide Capsules 2700
Renese Tablets 2712

Potassium Acid Phosphate (Concomitant use of potassium-containing salt substitute or potassium supplements can lead to hyperkalemia; frequent monitoring of serum potassium is recommended if used concurrently). Products include:

K-Phos Original (Sodium Free) Tablets 947

Potassium Bicarbonate (Concomitant use of potassium-containing salt substitute or potassium supplements can lead to hyperkalemia; frequent monitoring of serum potassium is recommended if used concurrently).

No products indexed under this heading.

Potassium Chloride (Concomitant use of potassium-containing salt substitute or potassium supplements can lead to hyperkalemia; frequent monitoring of serum potassium is recommended if used concurrently). Products include:

Chlor-3 1361
Colyte with Flavor Packs for Oral Solution 3170
GoLYTELY and Pineapple Flavor GoLYTELY for Oral Solution 1068
K-Dur Microburst Release System ER Tablets 1832
Klor-Con M20/Klor-Con M10 Tablets 3329
K-Lor Powder Packets 469
K-Tab Filmtab Tablets 470
Micro-K 3311
NuLYTELY, Cherry Flavor, Lemon-Lime Flavor, and Orange Flavor NuLYTELY for Oral Solution 1068
Rum-K 1363

Potassium Citrate (Concomitant use of potassium-containing salt substitute or potassium supplements can lead to hyperkalemia; frequent monitoring of serum potassium is recommended if used concurrently). Products include:

Urocit-K Tablets 2232

Potassium Gluconate (Concomitant use of potassium-containing salt substitute or potassium supplements can lead to hyperkalemia; frequent monitoring of serum potassium is recommended if used concurrently).

No products indexed under this heading.

Potassium Phosphate (Concomitant use of potassium-containing salt substitute or potassium supplements can lead to hyperkalemia; frequent monitoring of serum potassium is recommended if used concurrently). Products include:

K-Phos Neutral Tablets 946

Prazosin Hydrochloride (Co-administration of thiazide and other antihypertensive agents can lead to additive effect or potentiation). Products include:

Minipress Capsules 2699
Minizide Capsules 2700

Prednisolone Acetate (Co-administration of thiazide diuretics with corticosteroids intensifies electrolyte depletion, particularly potassium). Products include:

Blephamide Ophthalmic Ointment 547
Blephamide Ophthalmic Suspension 548
Poly-Pred Liquifilm Ophthalmic Suspension ⊙ 245
Pred Forte Ophthalmic Suspension ⊙ 246
Pred Mild Sterile Ophthalmic Suspension ⊙ 249
Pred-G Ophthalmic Suspension ⊙ 247
Pred-G Sterile Ophthalmic Ointment ⊙ 248

Prednisolone Sodium Phosphate (Co-administration of thiazide diuretics with corticosteroids intensifies electrolyte depletion, particularly potassium). Products include:

Pediapred Oral Solution 1170

Prednisolone Tebutate (Co-administration of thiazide diuretics with corticosteroids intensifies electrolyte depletion, particularly potassium).

No products indexed under this heading.

Prednisone (Co-administration of thiazide diuretics with corticosteroids intensifies electrolyte depletion, particularly potassium). Products include:

Prednisone 3064

Propoxyphene Hydrochloride (Co-administration of thiazide and narcotics may potentiate orthostatic hypotension). Products include:

Darvon Pulvules 1909
Darvon Compound-65 Pulvules 1910

Propoxyphene Napsylate (Co-administration of thiazide and narcotics may potentiate orthostatic hypotension). Products include:

Darvon-N/Darvocet-N 1907
Darvon-N Tablets 1912

Propranolol Hydrochloride (Co-administration of thiazide and other antihypertensive agents can lead to additive effect or potentiation). Products include:

Inderal 3513
Inderal LA Long-Acting Capsules 3516
Inderide Tablets 3517
Inderide LA Long-Acting Capsules 3519

Quinapril Hydrochloride (Co-administration of thiazide and other antihypertensive agents can lead to additive effect or potentiation). Products include:

Accupril Tablets 2611
Accuretic Tablets 2614

Ramipril (Co-administration of thiazide and other antihypertensive agents can lead to additive effect or potentiation). Products include:

Altace Capsules 2233

Rapacuronium Bromide (Co-administration with nondepolarizing skeletal muscle relaxants may result in possible increased responsiveness to the muscle relaxant).

No products indexed under this heading.

Rauwolfia serpentina (Co-administration of thiazide and other antihypertensive agents can lead to additive effect or potentiation).

No products indexed under this heading.

Remifentanil Hydrochloride (Co-administration of thiazide and narcotics may potentiate orthostatic hypotension).

No products indexed under this heading.

Repaglinide (Hyperglycemia may occur with thiazide diuretics; dosage adjustment of oral hypoglycemic agents may be required). Products include:

Prandin Tablets (0.5, 1, and 2 mg) 2432

Rescinnamine (Co-administration of thiazide and other antihypertensive agents can lead to additive effect or potentiation).

No products indexed under this heading.

Reserpine (Co-administration of thiazide and other antihypertensive agents can lead to additive effect or potentiation).

No products indexed under this heading.

Rocuronium Bromide (Co-administration with nondepolarizing skeletal muscle relaxants may result in possible increased responsiveness to the muscle relaxant). Products include:

Zemuron Injection 2491

Rofecoxib (Co-administration in some patients with compromised renal function who are being treated with NSAIDS may result in a further deterioration of renal function; NSAID may reduce the diuretic, natriuretic and antihypertensive effects of thiazide). Products include:

Vioxx 2213

Rosiglitazone Maleate (Hyperglycemia may occur with thiazide diuretics; dosage adjustment of oral hypoglycemic agents may be required). Products include:

Avandia Tablets 1490

Secobarbital Sodium (Co-administration of thiazide and barbiturates may potentiate orthostatic hypotension).

No products indexed under this heading.

Sodium Nitroprusside (Co-administration of thiazide and other antihypertensive agents can lead to additive effect or potentiation).

No products indexed under this heading.

Sotalol Hydrochloride (Co-administration of thiazide and other antihypertensive agents can lead to additive effect or potentiation). Products include:

Betapace Tablets 950
Betapace AF Tablets 954

Spirapril Hydrochloride (Co-administration of thiazide and other antihypertensive agents can lead to additive effect or potentiation).
No products indexed under this heading.

Spironolactone (Enalapril attenuates diuretic-induced potassium loss; concomitant use can lead to hyperkalemia; frequent monitoring of serum potassium is recommended if used concurrently; co-administration can result in excessive hypotension).
No products indexed under this heading.

Sufentanil Citrate (Co-administration of thiazide and narcotics may potentiate orthostatic hypotension).
No products indexed under this heading.

Sulindac (Co-administration in some patients with compromised renal function who are being treated with NSAIDS may result in a further deterioration of renal function; NSAID may reduce the diuretic, natriuretic and antihypertensive effects of thiazide). Products include:
Clinoril Tablets 2053

Telmisartan (Co-administration of thiazide and other antihypertensive agents can lead to additive effect or potentiation). Products include:
Micardis Tablets 1049
Micardis HCT Tablets 1051

Terazosin Hydrochloride (Co-administration of thiazide and other antihypertensive agents can lead to additive effect or potentiation). Products include:
Hytrin Capsules 464

Thiamylal Sodium (Co-administration of thiazide and barbiturates may potentiate orthostatic hypotension).
No products indexed under this heading.

Timolol Maleate (Co-administration of thiazide and other antihypertensive agents can lead to additive effect or potentiation). Products include:
Blocadren Tablets 2046
Cosopt Sterile Ophthalmic Solution 2065
Timolide Tablets 2187
Timolol GFS .... ⊙266
Timoptic in Ocudose 2192
Timoptic Sterile Ophthalmic Solution 2190
Timoptic-XE Sterile Ophthalmic Gel Forming Solution 2194

Tolazamide (Hyperglycemia may occur with thiazide diuretics; dosage adjustment of oral hypoglycemic agents may be required).
No products indexed under this heading.

Tolbutamide (Hyperglycemia may occur with thiazide diuretics; dosage adjustment of oral hypoglycemic agents may be required).
No products indexed under this heading.

Tolmetin Sodium (Co-administration in some patients with compromised renal function who are being treated with NSAIDS may result in a further deterioration of renal function; NSAID may reduce the diuretic, natriuretic and antihypertensive effects of thiazide). Products include:
Tolectin 2589

Torsemide (Co-administration of enalapril in patients on diuretics, especially those in whom diuretic therapy was recently instituted, may occasionally experience excessive hypotension; antihypertensive effects of enalapril are augmented by antihypertensive agents that cause renin release). Products include:
Demadex Tablets and Injection 2965

Trandolapril (Co-administration of thiazide and other antihypertensive agents can lead to additive effect or potentiation). Products include:
Mavik Tablets 478
Tarka Tablets 508

Triamcinolone (Co-administration of thiazide diuretics with corticosteroids intensifies electrolyte depletion, particularly potassium).
No products indexed under this heading.

Triamcinolone Acetonide (Co-administration of thiazide diuretics with corticosteroids intensifies electrolyte depletion, particularly potassium). Products include:
Azmacort Inhalation Aerosol 728
Nasacort Nasal Inhaler 750
Nasacort AQ Nasal Spray 752
Tri-Nasal Spray 2274

Triamcinolone Diacetate (Co-administration of thiazide diuretics with corticosteroids intensifies electrolyte depletion, particularly potassium).
No products indexed under this heading.

Triamcinolone Hexacetonide (Co-administration of thiazide diuretics with corticosteroids intensifies electrolyte depletion, particularly potassium).
No products indexed under this heading.

Triamterene (Enalapril attenuates diuretic-induced potassium loss; concomitant use can lead to hyperkalemia; frequent monitoring of serum potassium is recommended if used concurrently; co-administration can result in excessive hypotension). Products include:
Dyazide Capsules 1515
Dyrenium Capsules 3458
Maxzide 1008

Trimethaphan Camsylate (Co-administration of thiazide and other antihypertensive agents can lead to additive effect or potentiation).
No products indexed under this heading.

Troglitazone (Hyperglycemia may occur with thiazide diuretics; dosage adjustment of oral hypoglycemic agents may be required).
No products indexed under this heading.

Valsartan (Co-administration of thiazide and other antihypertensive agents can lead to additive effect or potentiation). Products include:
Diovan Capsules 2337
Diovan HCT Tablets 2338

Vecuronium Bromide (Co-administration with nondepolarizing skeletal muscle relaxants may result in possible increased responsiveness to the muscle relaxant). Products include:
Norcuron for Injection 2478

Verapamil Hydrochloride (Co-administration of thiazide and other antihypertensive agents can lead to additive effect or potentiation). Products include:
Covera-HS Tablets 3199
Isoptin SR Tablets 467
Tarka Tablets 508
Verelan Capsules 3184
Verelan PM Capsules 3186

Food Interactions

Alcohol (Co-administration of thiazide and alcohol may potentiate orthostatic hypotension).

VASOCON-A EYE DROPS

(Antazoline Phosphate, Naphazoline Hydrochloride) .... ⊙307
None cited in PDR database.

VASOTEC I.V. INJECTION

(Enalaprilat) 2207
See Vasotec Tablets

VASOTEC TABLETS

(Enalapril Maleate) 2210
May interact with diuretics, lithium preparations, non-steroidal anti-inflammatory agents, potassium preparations, and potassium sparing diuretics. Compounds in these categories include:

Amiloride Hydrochloride (Enalapril attenuates diuretic-induced potassium loss; concomitant use can lead to hyperkalemia; frequent monitoring of serum potassium is recommended if used concurrently; co-administration can result in excessive hypotension). Products include:
Midamor Tablets 2136
Moduretic Tablets 2138

Bendroflumethiazide (Co-administration of enalapril in patients on diuretics, especially those in whom diuretic therapy was recently instituted, may occasionally experience excessive hypotension; antihypertensive effects of enalapril are augmented by antihypertensive agents that cause renin release). Products include:
Corzide 40/5 Tablets 2247
Corzide 80/5 Tablets 2247

Bumetanide (Co-administration of enalapril in patients on diuretics, especially those in whom diuretic therapy was recently instituted, may occasionally experience excessive hypotension; antihypertensive effects of enalapril are augmented by antihypertensive agents that cause renin release).
No products indexed under this heading.

Celecoxib (Co-administration in some patients with compromised renal function who are being treated with NSAIDs may result in a further deterioration of renal function). Products include:
Celebrex Capsules 2676
Celebrex Capsules 2780

Chlorothiazide (Co-administration of enalapril in patients on diuretics, especially those in whom diuretic therapy was recently instituted, may occasionally experience excessive hypotension; antihypertensive effects of enalapril are augmented by antihypertensive agents that cause renin release). Products include:
Aldoclor Tablets 2035
Diuril Oral 2087

Chlorothiazide Sodium (Co-administration of enalapril in patients on diuretics, especially those in whom diuretic therapy was recently instituted, may occasionally experience excessive hypotension; antihypertensive effects of enalapril are augmented by antihypertensive agents that cause renin release). Products include:
Diuril Sodium Intravenous 2086

Chlorthalidone (Co-administration of enalapril in patients on diuretics, especially those in whom diuretic therapy was recently instituted, may occasionally experience excessive hypotension; antihypertensive effects of enalapril are augmented by antihypertensive agents that cause renin release). Products include:
Clorpres Tablets 1002
Combipres Tablets 1040
Tenoretic Tablets 690

Diclofenac Potassium (Co-administration in some patients with compromised renal function who are being treated with NSAIDs may result in a further deterioration of renal function). Products include:
Cataflam Tablets 2315

Diclofenac Sodium (Co-administration in some patients with compromised renal function who are being treated with NSAIDs may result in a further deterioration of renal function). Products include:
Arthrotec Tablets 3195
Voltaren Ophthalmic Sterile Ophthalmic Solution .... ⊙312
Voltaren Tablets 2315
Voltaren-XR Tablets 2315

Ethacrynic Acid (Co-administration of enalapril in patients on diuretics, especially those in whom diuretic therapy was recently instituted, may occasionally experience excessive hypotension; antihypertensive effects of enalapril are augmented by antihypertensive agents that cause renin release). Products include:
Edecrin Tablets 2091

Etodolac (Co-administration in some patients with compromised renal function who are being treated with NSAIDs may result in a further deterioration of renal function). Products include:
Lodine 3528
Lodine XL Extended-Release Tablets 3530

Fenoprofen Calcium (Co-administration in some patients with compromised renal function who are being treated with NSAIDs may result in a further deterioration of renal function).
No products indexed under this heading.

Flurbiprofen (Co-administration in some patients with compromised renal function who are being treated with NSAIDs may result in a further deterioration of renal function).
No products indexed under this heading.

Furosemide (Co-administration of enalapril in patients on diuretics, especially those in whom diuretic therapy was recently instituted, may occasionally experience excessive hypotension; antihypertensive effects of enalapril are augmented by antihypertensive agents that cause renin release). Products include:
Furosemide Tablets 2284

Hydrochlorothiazide (Co-administration of enalapril in patients on diuretics, especially those in whom diuretic therapy was recently instituted, may occasionally experience excessive hypotension; antihypertensive effects of enalapril are augmented by antihypertensive agents that cause renin release). Products include:
Accuretic Tablets 2614
Aldoril Tablets 2039
Atacand HCT Tablets 597
Avalide Tablets 1070
Diovan HCT Tablets 2338
Dyazide Capsules 1515
HydroDIURIL Tablets 2108
Hyzaar 2109
Inderide Tablets 3517
Inderide LA Long-Acting Capsules 3519
Lotensin HCT Tablets 2367
Maxzide 1008
Micardis HCT Tablets 1051
Microzide Capsules 3414
Moduretic Tablets 2138
Monopril HCT 1094
Prinzide Tablets 2168
Timolide Tablets 2187
Uniretic Tablets 3178
Vaseretic Tablets 2204
Zestoretic Tablets 695
Ziac Tablets 1887

Hydroflumethiazide (Co-administration of enalapril in patients on diuretics, especially those in whom diuretic therapy was recently instituted, may occasionally experience excessive hypotension; antihypertensive effects of enalapril are augmented by antihypertensive agents that cause renin release). Products include:
Diucardin Tablets 3494

Ibuprofen (Co-administration in some patients with compromised renal function who are being treated with NSAIDs may result in a further deterioration of renal function). Products include:
- Advil ■771
- Children's Advil Oral Suspension ■773
- Children's Advil Chewable Tablets ■773
- Advil Cold and Sinus Caplets ■771
- Advil Cold and Sinus Tablets ■771
- Advil Flu & Body Ache Caplets ■772
- Infants' Advil Drops ■773
- Junior Strength Advil Tablets ■773
- Junior Strength Advil Chewable Tablets ■773
- Advil Migraine Liquigels ■772
- Children's Motrin Oral Suspension and Chewable Tablets 2006
- Children's Motrin Cold Oral Suspension 2007
- Children's Motrin Oral Suspension ■643
- Motrin Suspension, Oral Drops, Chewable Tablets, and Caplets 2002
- Infants' Motrin Concentrated Drops 2006
- Junior Strength Motrin Caplets and Chewable Tablets 2006
- Motrin IB Tablets, Caplets, and Gelcaps 2002
- Motrin Migraine Pain Caplets 2005
- Motrin Sinus Headache Caplets 2005
- Vicoprofen Tablets 520

Indapamide (Co-administration of enalapril in patients on diuretics, especially those in whom diuretic therapy was recently instituted, may occasionally experience excessive hypotension; antihypertensive effects of enalapril are augmented by antihypertensive agents that cause renin release). Products include:
- Indapamide Tablets 2286

Indomethacin (Co-administration in some patients with compromised renal function who are being treated with NSAIDs may result in a further deterioration of renal function). Products include:
- Indocin 2112

Indomethacin Sodium Trihydrate (Co-administration in some patients with compromised renal function who are being treated with NSAIDs may result in a further deterioration of renal function). Products include:
- Indocin I.V. 2115

Ketoprofen (Co-administration in some patients with compromised renal function who are being treated with NSAIDs may result in a further deterioration of renal function). Products include:
- Orudis Capsules 3548
- Orudis KT Tablets ■778
- Oruvail Capsules 3548

Ketorolac Tromethamine (Co-administration in some patients with compromised renal function who are being treated with NSAIDs may result in a further deterioration of renal function). Products include:
- Acular Ophthalmic Solution 544
- Acular PF Ophthalmic Solution 544
- Toradol 3018

Lithium Carbonate (Co-administration of lithium with drugs that cause elimination of sodium, including ACE inhibitors, can lead to lithium toxicity). Products include:
- Eskalith 1527
- Lithium Carbonate 3061
- Lithobid Slow-Release Tablets 3255

Lithium Citrate (Co-administration of lithium with drugs that cause elimination of sodium, including ACE inhibitors, can lead to lithium toxicity). Products include:
- Lithium Citrate Syrup 3061

Meclofenamate Sodium (Co-administration in some patients with compromised renal function who are being treated with NSAIDs may result in a further deterioration of renal function).

No products indexed under this heading.

Mefenamic Acid (Co-administration in some patients with compromised renal function who are being treated with NSAIDs may result in a further deterioration of renal function). Products include:
- Ponstel Capsules 1356

Meloxicam (Co-administration in some patients with compromised renal function who are being treated with NSAIDs may result in a further deterioration of renal function). Products include:
- Mobic Tablets 1054

Methyclothiazide (Co-administration of enalapril in patients on diuretics, especially those in whom diuretic therapy was recently instituted, may occasionally experience excessive hypotension; antihypertensive effects of enalapril are augmented by antihypertensive agents that cause renin release).

No products indexed under this heading.

Metolazone (Co-administration of enalapril in patients on diuretics, especially those in whom diuretic therapy was recently instituted, may occasionally experience excessive hypotension; antihypertensive effects of enalapril are augmented by antihypertensive agents that cause renin release). Products include:
- Mykrox Tablets 1168
- Zaroxolyn Tablets 1177

Nabumetone (Co-administration in some patients with compromised renal function who are being treated with NSAIDs may result in a further deterioration of renal function). Products include:
- Relafen Tablets 1617

Naproxen (Co-administration in some patients with compromised renal function who are being treated with NSAIDs may result in a further deterioration of renal function). Products include:
- EC-Naprosyn Delayed-Release Tablets 2967
- Naprosyn Suspension 2967
- Naprosyn Tablets 2967

Naproxen Sodium (Co-administration in some patients with compromised renal function who are being treated with NSAIDs may result in a further deterioration of renal function). Products include:
- Aleve Tablets, Caplets and Gelcaps ■602
- Aleve Cold & Sinus Caplets ■603
- Anaprox Tablets 2967
- Anaprox DS Tablets 2967
- Naprelan Tablets 1293

Oxaprozin (Co-administration in some patients with compromised renal function who are being treated with NSAIDs may result in a further deterioration of renal function).

No products indexed under this heading.

Phenylbutazone (Co-administration in some patients with compromised renal function who are being treated with NSAIDs may result in a further deterioration of renal function).

No products indexed under this heading.

Piroxicam (Co-administration in some patients with compromised renal function who are being treated with NSAIDs may result in a further deterioration of renal function). Products include:
- Feldene Capsules 2685

Polythiazide (Co-administration of enalapril in patients on diuretics, especially those in whom diuretic therapy was recently instituted, may occasionally experience excessive hypotension; antihypertensive effects of enalapril are augmented by antihypertensive agents that cause renin release). Products include:
- Minizide Capsules 2700
- Renese Tablets 2712

Potassium Acid Phosphate (Concomitant use of potassium-containing salt substitute or potassium supplements can lead to hyperkalemia; frequent monitoring of serum potassium is recommended if used concurrently). Products include:
- K-Phos Original (Sodium Free) Tablets 947

Potassium Bicarbonate (Concomitant use of potassium-containing salt substitute or potassium supplements can lead to hyperkalemia; frequent monitoring of serum potassium is recommended if used concurrently).

No products indexed under this heading.

Potassium Chloride (Concomitant use of potassium-containing salt substitute or potassium supplements can lead to hyperkalemia; frequent monitoring of serum potassium is recommended if used concurrently). Products include:
- Chlor-3 1361
- Colyte with Flavor Packs for Oral Solution 3170
- GoLYTELY and Pineapple Flavor GoLYTELY for Oral Solution 1068
- K-Dur Microburst Release System ER Tablets 1832
- Klor-Con M20/Klor-Con M10 Tablets 3329
- K-Lor Powder Packets 469
- K-Tab Filmtab Tablets 470
- Micro-K 3311
- NuLYTELY, Cherry Flavor, Lemon-Lime Flavor, and Orange Flavor NuLYTELY for Oral Solution 1068
- Rum-K 1363

Potassium Citrate (Concomitant use of potassium-containing salt substitute or potassium supplements can lead to hyperkalemia; frequent monitoring of serum potassium is recommended if used concurrently). Products include:
- Urocit-K Tablets 2232

Potassium Gluconate (Concomitant use of potassium-containing salt substitute or potassium supplements can lead to hyperkalemia; frequent monitoring of serum potassium is recommended if used concurrently).

No products indexed under this heading.

Potassium Phosphate (Concomitant use of potassium-containing salt substitute or potassium supplements can lead to hyperkalemia; frequent monitoring of serum potassium is recommended if used concurrently). Products include:
- K-Phos Neutral Tablets 946

Rofecoxib (Co-administration in some patients with compromised renal function who are being treated with NSAIDs may result in a further deterioration of renal function). Products include:
- Vioxx 2213

Spironolactone (Enalapril attenuates diuretic-induced potassium loss; concomitant use can lead to hyperkalemia; frequent monitoring of serum potassium is recommended if used concurrently; co-administration can result in excessive hypotension).

No products indexed under this heading.

Sulindac (Co-administration in some patients with compromised renal function who are being treated with NSAIDs may result in a further deterioration of renal function). Products include:
- Clinoril Tablets 2053

Tolmetin Sodium (Co-administration in some patients with compromised renal function who are being treated with NSAIDs may result in a further deterioration of renal function). Products include:
- Tolectin 2589

Torsemide (Co-administration of enalapril in patients on diuretics, especially those in whom diuretic therapy was recently instituted, may occasionally experience excessive hypotension; antihypertensive effects of enalapril are augmented by antihypertensive agents that cause renin release). Products include:
- Demadex Tablets and Injection 2965

Triamterene (Enalapril attenuates diuretic-induced potassium loss; concomitant use can lead to hyperkalemia; frequent monitoring of serum potassium is recommended if used concurrently; co-administration can result in excessive hypotension). Products include:
- Dyazide Capsules 1515
- Dyrenium Capsules 3458
- Maxzide 1008

VELOSULIN BR HUMAN INSULIN 10 ML VIALS

(Insulin, Human Regular) 2435

None cited in PDR database.

VENASTAT SUPPLI-CAP CAPSULES

(Horse Chestnut Seed Extract) ■833

None cited in PDR database.

VENOFER INJECTION

(Iron Sucrose) 580

May interact with iron containing oral preparations. Compounds in these categories include:

Ferrous Fumarate (Co-administration with oral iron preparations should be avoided because the absorption of oral iron is reduced). Products include:
- New Formulation Chromagen OB Capsules 3094
- Loestrin Fe Tablets 2642
- NataChew Tablets 3364

Ferrous Gluconate (Co-administration with oral iron preparations should be avoided because the absorption of oral iron is reduced). Products include:
- Fergon Iron Tablets ■802

Ferrous Sulfate (Co-administration with oral iron preparations should be avoided because the absorption of oral iron is reduced). Products include:
- Feosol Tablets 1717
- Slow Fe Tablets ■827
- Slow Fe with Folic Acid Tablets ■828

Iron (Co-administration with oral iron preparations should be avoided because the absorption of oral iron is reduced).

No products indexed under this heading.

Polysaccharide-Iron Complex (Co-administration with oral iron preparations should be avoided because the absorption of oral iron is reduced). Products include:
- Niferex 3176
- Niferex-150 Capsules 3176
- Nu-Iron 150 Capsules 2224

VENTOLIN INHALATION AEROSOL AND REFILL

(Albuterol) 1679

May interact with monoamine oxidase inhibitors, nonpotassium-sparing diuretics, sympathomimetic bronchodilators, sympathomimetics, tricyclic antidepressants, and certain other agents. Compounds in these categories include:

Albuterol (Co-administration with other short-acting sympathomimetic

aerosol bronchodilators should not be used concomitantly with albuterol). Products include:
- Proventil Inhalation Aerosol 3142
- Ventolin Inhalation Aerosol and Refill.. 1679

Amitriptyline Hydrochloride (Co-administration with tricyclic antidepressants may potentiate action of albuterol on the vascular system). Products include:
- Etrafon 3115
- Limbitrol 1738

Amoxapine (Co-administration with tricyclic antidepressants may potentiate action of albuterol on the vascular system).
- No products indexed under this heading.

Bendroflumethiazide (The ECG changes and/or hypokalemia that may result from the adminstration of nonpotassium-sparing diuretics can be acutely worsened by beta-agonists, especially when the recommended dose of beta-agonist is exceeded). Products include:
- Corzide 40/5 Tablets 2247
- Corzide 80/5 Tablets 2247

Bitolterol Mesylate (Co-administration with other short-acting sympathomimetic aerosol bronchodilators should not be used concomitantly with albuterol).
- No products indexed under this heading.

Bumetanide (The ECG changes and/or hypokalemia that may result from the adminstration of nonpotassium-sparing diuretics can be acutely worsened by beta-agonists, especially when the recommended dose of beta-agonist is exceeded).
- No products indexed under this heading.

Chlorothiazide (The ECG changes and/or hypokalemia that may result from the adminstration of nonpotassium-sparing diuretics can be acutely worsened by beta-agonists, especially when the recommended dose of beta-agonist is exceeded). Products include:
- Aldoclor Tablets 2035
- Diuril Oral 2087

Chlorothiazide Sodium (The ECG changes and/or hypokalemia that may result from the adminstration of nonpotassium-sparing diuretics can be acutely worsened by beta-agonists, especially when the recommended dose of beta-agonist is exceeded). Products include:
- Diuril Sodium Intravenous 2086

Clomipramine Hydrochloride (Co-administration with tricyclic antidepressants may potentiate action of albuterol on the vascular system).
- No products indexed under this heading.

Desipramine Hydrochloride (Co-administration with tricyclic antidepressants may potentiate action of albuterol on the vascular system). Products include:
- Norpramin Tablets 755

Digoxin (Co-administration of intravenous and oral administration of albuterol to volunteers who had received digoxin for 10 days has resulted in mean decrease in digoxin levels; the clinical significance of this finding is unknown). Products include:
- Digitek Tablets 1003
- Lanoxicaps Capsules 1574
- Lanoxin Injection 1581
- Lanoxin Tablets 1587
- Lanoxin Elixir Pediatric 1578
- Lanoxin Injection Pediatric 1584

Dobutamine Hydrochloride (Co-administration with other adrenergic agents may result in deleterious cardiovascular events). Products include:
- Dobutrex Solution Vials 1914

Dopamine Hydrochloride (Co-administration with other adrenergic agents may result in deleterious cardiovascular events).
- No products indexed under this heading.

Doxepin Hydrochloride (Co-administration with tricyclic antidepressants may potentiate action of albuterol on the vascular system). Products include:
- Sinequan 2713

Ephedrine Hydrochloride (Co-administration with other short-acting sympathomimetic aerosol bronchodilators should not be used concomitantly with albuterol). Products include:
- Primatene Tablets .... ▣780

Ephedrine Sulfate (Co-administration with other short-acting sympathomimetic aerosol bronchodilators should not be used concomitantly with albuterol).
- No products indexed under this heading.

Ephedrine Tannate (Co-administration with other short-acting sympathomimetic aerosol bronchodilators should not be used concomitantly with albuterol). Products include:
- Rynatuss Pediatric Suspension 3353
- Rynatuss Tablets 3353

Epinephrine (Co-administration with other short-acting sympathomimetic aerosol bronchodilators should not be used concomitantly with albuterol). Products include:
- Epifrin Sterile Ophthalmic Solution .... ⊙235
- EpiPen 1236
- Primatene Mist ....▣779
- Xylocaine with Epinephrine Injection 653

Epinephrine Bitartrate (Co-administration with other adrenergic agents may result in deleterious cardiovascular events). Products include:
- Sensorcaine 643

Epinephrine Hydrochloride (Co-administration with other short-acting sympathomimetic aerosol bronchodilators should not be used concomitantly with albuterol).
- No products indexed under this heading.

Ethacrynic Acid (The ECG changes and/or hypokalemia that may result from the adminstration of nonpotassium-sparing diuretics can be acutely worsened by beta-agonists, especially when the recommended dose of beta-agonist is exceeded). Products include:
- Edecrin Tablets 2091

Furosemide (The ECG changes and/or hypokalemia that may result from the adminstration of nonpotassium-sparing diuretics can be acutely worsened by beta-agonists, especially when the recommended dose of beta-agonist is exceeded). Products include:
- Furosemide Tablets 2284

Hydrochlorothiazide (The ECG changes and/or hypokalemia that may result from the adminstration of nonpotassium-sparing diuretics can be acutely worsened by beta-agonists, especially when the recommended dose of beta-agonist is exceeded). Products include:
- Accuretic Tablets 2614
- Aldoril Tablets 2039
- Atacand HCT Tablets 597
- Avalide Tablets 1070
- Diovan HCT Tablets 2338
- Dyazide Capsules 1515
- HydroDIURIL Tablets 2108
- Hyzaar 2109
- Inderide Tablets 3517
- Inderide LA Long-Acting Capsules .. 3519
- Lotensin HCT Tablets 2367
- Maxzide 1008
- Micardis HCT Tablets 1051
- Microzide Capsules 3414
- Moduretic Tablets 2138
- Monopril HCT 1094
- Prinzide Tablets 2168
- Timolide Tablets 2187
- Uniretic Tablets 3178
- Vaseretic Tablets 2204
- Zestoretic Tablets 695
- Ziac Tablets 1887

Hydroflumethiazide (The ECG changes and/or hypokalemia that may result from the adminstration of nonpotassium-sparing diuretics can be acutely worsened by beta-agonists, especially when the recommended dose of beta-agonist is exceeded). Products include:
- Diucardin Tablets 3494

Imipramine Hydrochloride (Co-administration with tricyclic antidepressants may potentiate action of albuterol on the vascular system).
- No products indexed under this heading.

Imipramine Pamoate (Co-administration with tricyclic antidepressants may potentiate action of albuterol on the vascular system).
- No products indexed under this heading.

Isocarboxazid (Co-administration with MAO inhibitors may potentiate action of albuterol on the vascular system).
- No products indexed under this heading.

Isoetharine (Co-administration with other short-acting sympathomimetic aerosol bronchodilators should not be used concomitantly with albuterol).
- No products indexed under this heading.

Isoproterenol Hydrochloride (Co-administration with other short-acting sympathomimetic aerosol bronchodilators should not be used concomitantly with albuterol).
- No products indexed under this heading.

Isoproterenol Sulfate (Co-administration with other short-acting sympathomimetic aerosol bronchodilators should not be used concomitantly with albuterol).
- No products indexed under this heading.

Levalbuterol Hydrochloride (Co-administration with other short-acting sympathomimetic aerosol bronchodilators should not be used concomitantly with albuterol). Products include:
- Xopenex Inhalation Solution 3207

Maprotiline Hydrochloride (Co-administration with tricyclic antidepressants may potentiate action of albuterol on the vascular system).
- No products indexed under this heading.

Metaproterenol Sulfate (Co-administration with other short-acting sympathomimetic aerosol bronchodilators should not be used concomitantly with albuterol). Products include:
- Alupent 1029

Metaraminol Bitartrate (Co-administration with other adrenergic agents may result in deleterious cardiovascular events). Products include:
- Aramine Injection 2043

Methoxamine Hydrochloride (Co-administration with other adrenergic agents may result in deleterious cardiovascular events).
- No products indexed under this heading.

Methyclothiazide (The ECG changes and/or hypokalemia that may result from the adminstration of nonpotassium-sparing diuretics can be acutely worsened by beta-agonists, especially when the recommended dose of beta-agonist is exceeded).
- No products indexed under this heading.

Moclobemide (Co-administration with MAO inhibitors may potentiate action of albuterol on the vascular system).
- No products indexed under this heading.

Norepinephrine Bitartrate (Co-administration with other adrenergic agents may result in deleterious cardiovascular events).
- No products indexed under this heading.

Nortriptyline Hydrochloride (Co-administration with tricyclic antidepressants may potentiate action of albuterol on the vascular system).
- No products indexed under this heading.

Pargyline Hydrochloride (Co-administration with MAO inhibitors may potentiate action of albuterol on the vascular system).
- No products indexed under this heading.

Phenelzine Sulfate (Co-administration with MAO inhibitors may potentiate action of albuterol on the vascular system). Products include:
- Nardil Tablets 2653

Phenylephrine Bitartrate (Co-administration with other adrenergic agents may result in deleterious cardiovascular events).
- No products indexed under this heading.

Phenylephrine Hydrochloride (Co-administration with other adrenergic agents may result in deleterious cardiovascular events). Products include:
- Afrin Nasal Decongestant Children's Pump Mist .... ▣734
- Extendryl 1361
- Hycomine Compound Tablets 1317
- Neo-Synephrine ....▣614
- Phenergan VC Syrup 3560
- Phenergan VC with Codeine Syrup . 3561
- Preparation H Cream ....▣778
- Preparation H Cooling Gel ....▣778
- Preparation H ....▣778
- Vicks Sinex Nasal Spray and Ultra Fine Mist ....▣729

Phenylephrine Tannate (Co-administration with other adrenergic agents may result in deleterious cardiovascular events). Products include:
- Ryna-12 S Suspension 3351
- Reformulated Rynatan Pediatric Suspension 3352
- Rynatuss Pediatric Suspension 3353
- Rynatuss Tablets 3353

Phenylpropanolamine Hydrochloride (Co-administration with other adrenergic agents may result in deleterious cardiovascular events).
- No products indexed under this heading.

Pirbuterol Acetate (Co-administration with other short-acting sympathomimetic aerosol bronchodilators should not be used concomitantly with albuterol). Products include:
- Maxair Autohaler 1981
- Maxair Inhaler 1984

Polythiazide (The ECG changes and/or hypokalemia that may result from the adminstration of nonpotassium-sparing diuretics can be acutely worsened by beta-agonists, especially when the recommended dose of beta-agonist is exceeded). Products include:
- Minizide Capsules 2700
- Renese Tablets 2712

Procarbazine Hydrochloride (Co-administration with MAO inhibitors

may potentiate action of albuterol on the vascular system). Products include:
- Matulane Capsules **3246**

Protriptyline Hydrochloride (Co-administration with tricyclic antidepressants may potentiate action of albuterol on the vascular system). Products include:
- Vivactil Tablets **2446**
- Vivactil Tablets **2217**

Pseudoephedrine Hydrochloride (Co-administration with other adrenergic agents may result in deleterious cardiovascular events). Products include:
- Actifed Cold & Allergy Tablets ...... ▣**688**
- Actifed Cold & Sinus Caplets and Tablets .... ▣**688**
- Advil Cold and Sinus Caplets .... ▣**771**
- Advil Cold and Sinus Tablets .... ▣**771**
- Advil Flu & Body Ache Caplets ...... ▣**772**
- Aleve Cold & Sinus Caplets .... ▣**603**
- Alka-Seltzer Plus Liqui-Gels .... ▣**604**
- Alka-Seltzer Plus Cold & Flu Medicine Liqui-Gels .... ▣**604**
- Alka-Seltzer Plus Cold & Sinus Medicine Liqui-Gels .... ▣**604**
- Allegra-D Extended-Release Tablets **714**
- BC Cold Powder .... ▣**619**
- Benadryl Allergy/Cold Tablets .... ▣**691**
- Benadryl Allergy/Congestion Tablets .... ▣**692**
- Benadryl Allergy & Sinus Liquid ..... ▣**693**
- Benadryl Allergy & Sinus Fastmelt Tablets .... ▣**693**
- Benadryl Allergy Sinus Headache Caplets & Gelcaps .... ▣**693**
- Benadryl Severe Allergy & Sinus Headache Caplets .... ▣**694**
- Benadryl Children's Allergy/Cold Fastmelt Tablets .... ▣**692**
- Benylin Multi-Symptom Liquid .... ▣**697**
- Bromfed Capsules (Extended-Release) **2269**
- Bromfed-PD Capsules (Extended-Release) **2269**
- Children's Cēpacol Sore Throat ..... ▣**788**
- Comtrex Acute Head Cold & Sinus Pressure Relief Tablets ..... ▣**627**
- Comtrex Deep Chest Cold & Congestion Relief Softgels .... ▣**627**
- Comtrex Flu Therapy & Fever Relief Daytime Caplets .... ▣**628**
- Comtrex Flu Therapy & Fever Relief Nighttime Tablets .... ▣**628**
- Comtrex Maximum Strength Multi-Symptom Cold & Cough Relief Tablets and Caplets .... ▣**626**
- Contac Non-Drowsy 12 Hour Cold Caplets .... ▣**745**
- Contac Non-Drowsy Timed Release 12 Hour Cold Caplets ... ▣**746**
- Contac Severe Cold and Flu Caplets Maximum Strength .... ▣**746**
- Contac Severe Cold and Flu Caplets Non-Drowsy .... ▣**746**
- Dimetapp Elixir .... ▣**777**
- Dimetapp Cold and Fever Suspension .... ▣**775**
- Dimetapp DM Cold & Cough Elixir . ▣**775**
- Dimetapp Nighttime Flu Liquid ...... ▣**776**
- Dimetapp Non-Drowsy Flu Syrup .. ▣**777**
- Dimetapp Infant Drops Decongestant .... ▣**775**
- Dimetapp Infant Drops Decongestant Plus Cough .... ▣**776**
- Guaifed **2272**
- Kronofed-A **1341**
- Children's Motrin Cold Oral Suspension **2007**
- Motrin Sinus Headache Caplets **2005**
- PediaCare Cough-Cold Liquid .... ▣**719**
- PediaCare Infants' Drops Decongestant .... ▣**719**
- PediaCare Infants' Drops Decongestant Plus Cough .... ▣**719**
- PediaCare NightRest Cough-Cold Liquid .... ▣**719**
- Robitussin Cold Caplets Cold & Congestion .... ▣**780**
- Robitussin Cold Softgels Cold & Congestion .... ▣**780**
- Robitussin Cold Caplets Multi-Symptom Cold & Flu .... ▣**781**
- Robitussin Cold Softgels Multi-Symptom Cold & Flu .... ▣**781**
- Robitussin Cold Softgels Severe Congestion .... ▣**782**
- Robitussin Cough & Cold Infant Drops .... ▣**782**
- Robitussin Maximum Strength Cough & Cold Liquid .... ▣**785**
- Robitussin Pediatric Cough & Cold Formula Liquid .... ▣**785**
- Robitussin Multi Symptom Honey Flu Liquid .... ▣**785**
- Robitussin Nighttime Honey Flu Liquid .... ▣**786**
- Robitussin-CF Liquid .... ▣**783**
- Robitussin-DAC Syrup **2942**
- Robitussin-PE Liquid .... ▣**782**
- Ryna .... ▣**768**
- Semprex-D Capsules **1172**
- Singlet Caplets .... ▣**761**
- Sinutab Non-Drying Liquid Caps .... ▣**706**
- Sinutab Sinus Allergy Medication, Maximum Strength Formula, Tablets & Caplets .... ▣**707**
- Sinutab Sinus Medication, Maximum Strength Without Drowsiness Formula, Tablets & Caplets .... ▣**707**
- Sudafed 12 Hour Tablets .... ▣**708**
- Sudafed 24 Hour Tablets .... ▣**708**
- Children's Sudafed Cold & Cough Liquid .... ▣**709**
- Children's Sudafed Nasal Decongestant Chewables .... ▣**711**
- Children's Sudafed Nasal Decongestant Liquid Medication .... ▣**711**
- Sudafed Cold & Allergy Tablets ..... ▣**708**
- Sudafed Cold & Cough Liquid Caps .... ▣**709**
- Sudafed Cold & Sinus Liquid Caps .... ▣**710**
- Sudafed Nasal Decongestant Tablets .... ▣**710**
- Sudafed Non-Drying Sinus Liquid Caps .... ▣**712**
- Sudafed Severe Cold .... ▣**711**
- Sudafed Sinus Headache Caplets . ▣**712**
- Sudafed Sinus Headache Tablets ... ▣**712**
- Tavist Sinus Non-Drowsy Coated Caplets .... ▣**676**
- TheraFlu Regular Strength Cold & Cough Night Time Hot Liquid ..... ▣**676**
- TheraFlu Regular Strength Cold & Sore Throat Night Time Hot Liquid .... ▣**676**
- TheraFlu Maximum Strength Flu & Congestion Non-Drowsy Hot Liquid .... ▣**677**
- TheraFlu Maximum Strength Flu & Cough Night Time Hot Liquid ▣**678**
- TheraFlu Maximum Strength Flu & Sore Throat Night Time Hot Liquid .... ▣**677**
- TheraFlu Maximum Strength Severe Cold & Congestion Night Time Caplets .... ▣**678**
- TheraFlu Maximum Strength Severe Cold & Congestion Night Time Hot Liquid .... ▣**678**
- TheraFlu Maximum Strength Severe Cold & Congestion Non-Drowsy .... ▣**679**
- Triaminic Allergy Congestion Liquid .... ▣**680**
- Triaminic Chest Congestion Liquid .... ▣**680**
- Triaminic Cold & Allergy Liquid ...... ▣**681**
- Triaminic Cold & Allergy Softchews .... ▣**683**
- Triaminic Cold & Cough Liquid ...... ▣**681**
- Triaminic Cold & Cough Softchews .... ▣**683**
- Triaminic Cold & Night Time Cough Liquid .... ▣**681**
- Triaminic Cold, Cough & Fever Liquid .... ▣**681**
- Triaminic Cough Liquid .... ▣**682**
- Triaminic Cough & Congestion Liquid .... ▣**682**
- Triaminic Cough & Sore Throat Liquid .... ▣**682**
- Triaminic Cough & Sore Throat Softchews .... ▣**684**
- Children's Tylenol Allergy-D Liquid ... **2014**
- Children's Tylenol Cold Suspension Liquid and Chewable Tablets **2015**
- Children's Tylenol Cold Plus Cough Suspension Liquid and Chewable Tablets **2015**
- Children's Tylenol Flu Suspension Liquid **2015**
- Children's Tylenol Sinus Suspension Liquid **2017**
- Infants' Tylenol Cold Decongestant and Fever Reducer Concentrated Drops **2015**
- Infants' Tylenol Cold Decongestant and Fever Reducer Concentrated Drops Plus Cough .. **2015**
- Tylenol Allergy Sinus **2010**
- Multi-Symptom Tylenol Cold Complete Formula Caplets **2010**
- Multi-Symptom Tylenol Cold Non-Drowsy Caplets and Gelcaps **2010**
- Multi-Symptom Tylenol Cold Severe Congestion Non-Drowsy Caplets **2011**
- Maximum Strength Tylenol Flu NightTime Gelcaps **2011**
- Maximum Strength Tylenol Flu NightTime Liquid **2011**
- Maximum Strength Tylenol Flu Non-Drowsy Gelcaps **2011**
- Maximum Strength Tylenol Sinus NightTime Caplets **2012**
- Maximum Strength Tylenol Sinus Non-Drowsy Geltabs, Gelcaps, Caplets, and Tablets **2012**
- Vicks 44D Cough & Head Congestion Relief Liquid .... ▣**724**
- Vicks 44M Cough, Cold & Flu Relief Liquid .... ▣**725**
- Pediatric Vicks 44m Cough & Cold Relief .... ▣**728**
- Vicks DayQuil LiquiCaps/Liquid Multi-Symptom Cold/Flu Relief ... ▣**727**
- Children's Vicks NyQuil Cold/Cough Relief .... ▣**726**
- Vicks NyQuil LiquiCaps/Liquid Multi-Symptom Cold/Flu Relief, Original and Cherry Flavors .... ▣**727**
- Zephrex Tablets **3091**
- Zephrex LA Tablets **3092**
- Zyrtec-D 12 Hour Extended Relief Tablets **2758**

Pseudoephedrine Sulfate (Co-administration with other adrenergic agents may result in deleterious cardiovascular events). Products include:
- Chlor-Trimeton Allergy/Decongestant Tablets .... ▣**736**
- Claritin-D 12 Hour Extended Release Tablets **3102**
- Claritin-D 24 Hour Extended Release Tablets **3104**
- Coricidin 'D' Cold, Flu & Sinus Tablets .... ▣**737**
- Drixoral Allergy/Sinus Extended-Release Tablets .... ▣**741**
- Drixoral Cold & Allergy Sustained-Action Tablets .... ▣**740**
- Drixoral Cold & Flu Extended-Release Tablets .... ▣**740**
- Drixoral Nasal Decongestant Long-Acting Non-Drowsy Tablets .... ▣**740**
- Rynatan Tablets **3351**

Salmeterol Xinafoate (Co-administration with other short-acting sympathomimetic aerosol bronchodilators should not be used concomitantly with albuterol). Products include:
- Advair Diskus 100/50 .... **1448**
- Advair Diskus 250/50 .... **1448**
- Advair Diskus 500/50 .... **1448**
- Serevent Diskus **1637**
- Serevent Inhalation Aerosol **1633**

Selegiline Hydrochloride (Co-administration with MAO inhibitors may potentiate action of albuterol on the vascular system). Products include:
- Eldepryl Capsules **3266**

Terbutaline Sulfate (Co-administration with other short-acting sympathomimetic aerosol bronchodilators should not be used concomitantly with albuterol). Products include:
- Brethine Ampuls **2314**
- Brethine Tablets **2313**

Torsemide (The ECG changes and/or hypokalemia that may result from the adminstration of nonpotassium-sparing diuretics can be acutely worsened by beta-agonists, especially when the recommended dose of beta-agonist is exceeded). Products include:
- Demadex Tablets and Injection **2965**

Tranylcypromine Sulfate (Co-administration with MAO inhibitors may potentiate action of albuterol on the vascular system). Products include:
- Parnate Tablets **1607**

Trimipramine Maleate (Co-administration with tricyclic antidepressants may potentiate action of albuterol on the vascular system). Products include:
- Surmontil Capsules **3595**

VENTOLIN HFA INHALATION AEROSOL

(Albuterol Sulfate) **3618**

See Ventolin Inhalation Aerosol and Refill

VERELAN CAPSULES

(Verapamil Hydrochloride) **3184**

May interact with ACE inhibitors, antihypertensives, beta blockers, cardiac glycosides, inhalant anesthetics, lithium preparations, neuromuscular blocking agents, quinidine, and certain other agents. Compounds in these categories include:

Acebutolol Hydrochloride (Concomitant therapy may result in additive negative effects on heart rate, AV conduction, and/or cardiac contractility; excessive bradycardia and AV block has been reported with concurrent use in hypertensive patients; possible additive effect on blood pressure). Products include:
- Sectral Capsules **3589**

Amlodipine Besylate (Co-administration with oral antihypertensive agents will usually have an additive effect on lowering blood pressure). Products include:
- Lotrel Capsules **2370**
- Norvasc Tablets **2704**

Aspirin (Co-administration, in a few reported cases, has led to increased bleeding times greater than those observed with aspirin alone). Products include:
- Aggrenox Capsules **1026**
- Alka-Seltzer .... ▣**603**
- Alka-Seltzer Lemon Lime Antacid and Pain Reliever Effervescent Tablets .... ▣**603**
- Alka-Seltzer Extra Strength Antacid and Pain Reliever Effervescent Tablets .... ▣**603**
- Alka-Seltzer PM Effervescent Tablets .... ▣**605**
- Genuine Bayer Tablets, Caplets and Gelcaps .... ▣**606**
- Extra Strength Bayer Caplets and Gelcaps .... ▣**610**
- Aspirin Regimen Bayer Children's Chewable Tablets (Orange or Cherry Flavored) .... ▣**607**
- Bayer, Aspirin Regimen .... ▣**606**
- Aspirin Regimen Bayer 81 mg Caplets with Calcium .... ▣**607**
- Genuine Bayer Professional Labeling (Aspirin Regimen Bayer) .... ▣**608**
- Extra Strength Bayer Arthritis Caplets .... ▣**610**
- Extra Strength Bayer Plus Caplets .... ▣**610**
- Extra Strength Bayer PM Caplets ... ▣**611**
- BC Powder .... ▣**619**
- BC Allergy Sinus Cold Powder ...... ▣**619**
- Arthritis Strength BC Powder .... ▣**619**
- BC Sinus Cold Powder .... ▣**619**
- Darvon Compound-65 Pulvules **1910**
- Ecotrin Enteric Coated Aspirin Low, Regular and Maximum Strength Tablets **1715**
- Excedrin Extra-Strength Tablets, Caplets, and Geltabs .... ▣**629**
- Excedrin Migraine **1070**
- Goody's Body Pain Formula Powder .... ▣**620**
- Goody's Extra Strength Headache Powder .... ▣**620**
- Goody's Extra Strength Pain Relief Tablets .... ▣**620**
- Percodan Tablets **1327**
- Robaxisal Tablets **2939**
- Soma Compound Tablets **3354**
- Soma Compound w/Codeine Tablets **3355**
- Vanquish Caplets .... ▣**617**

Atenolol (Concomitant therapy may result in additive negative effects on heart rate, AV conduction, and/or cardiac contractility; excessive bradycardia and AV block has been reported with concurrent use in

hypertensive patients; possible additive effect on blood pressure). Products include:

Tenoretic Tablets 690
Tenormin I.V. Injection 692

Atracurium Besylate (Verapamil may potentiate the activity of neuromuscular blocking drugs).

No products indexed under this heading.

Benazepril Hydrochloride (Co-administration with oral antihypertensive agents will usually have an additive effect on lowering blood pressure). Products include:

Lotensin Tablets 2365
Lotensin HCT Tablets 2367
Lotrel Capsules 2370

Bendroflumethiazide (Co-administration with oral antihypertensive agents will usually have an additive effect on lowering blood pressure). Products include:

Corzide 40/5 Tablets 2247
Corzide 80/5 Tablets 2247

Betaxolol Hydrochloride (Concomitant therapy may result in additive negative effects on heart rate, AV conduction, and/or cardiac contractility; excessive bradycardia and AV block has been reported with concurrent use in hypertensive patients; possible additive effect on blood pressure). Products include:

Betoptic S Ophthalmic Suspension 537

Bisoprolol Fumarate (Concomitant therapy may result in additive negative effects on heart rate, AV conduction, and/or cardiac contractility; excessive bradycardia and AV block has been reported with concurrent use in hypertensive patients; possible additive effect on blood pressure). Products include:

Zebeta Tablets 1885
Ziac Tablets 1887

Candesartan Cilexetil (Co-administration with oral antihypertensive agents will usually have an additive effect on lowering blood pressure). Products include:

Atacand Tablets 595
Atacand HCT Tablets 597

Captopril (Co-administration with oral antihypertensive agents will usually have an additive effect on lowering blood pressure). Products include:

Captopril Tablets 2281

Carbamazepine (Verapamil therapy may increase carbamazepine concentrations during combined therapy resulting in side effects such as diplopia, headache, ataxia, or dizziness). Products include:

Carbatrol Capsules 3234
Tegretol/Tegretol-XR 2404

Carteolol Hydrochloride (Concomitant therapy may result in additive negative effects on heart rate, AV conduction, and/or cardiac contractility; excessive bradycardia and AV block has been reported with concurrent use in hypertensive patients; possible additive effect on blood pressure). Products include:

Carteolol Hydrochloride Ophthalmic Solution USP, 1% ⊙258
Ocupress Ophthalmic Solution, 1% Sterile ⊙303

Chlorothiazide (Co-administration with oral antihypertensive agents will usually have an additive effect on lowering blood pressure). Products include:

Aldoclor Tablets 2035
Diuril Oral 2087

Chlorothiazide Sodium (Co-administration with oral antihypertensive agents will usually have an additive effect on lowering blood pressure). Products include:

Diuril Sodium Intravenous 2086

Chlorthalidone (Co-administration with oral antihypertensive agents will usually have an additive effect on lowering blood pressure). Products include:

Clorpres Tablets 1002
Combipres Tablets 1040
Tenoretic Tablets 690

Cimetidine (Variable results on verapamil clearance acute studies, either reduced or unchanged). Products include:

Tagamet HB 200 Suspension ⊞762
Tagamet HB 200 Tablets ⊞761
Tagamet Tablets 1644

Cimetidine Hydrochloride (Variable results on verapamil clearance acute studies, either reduced or unchanged). Products include:

Tagamet 1644

Cisatracurium Besylate (Verapamil may potentiate the activity of neuromuscular blocking drugs).

No products indexed under this heading.

Clonidine (Co-administration with oral antihypertensive agents will usually have an additive effect on lowering blood pressure). Products include:

Catapres-TTS 1038

Clonidine Hydrochloride (Co-administration with oral antihypertensive agents will usually have an additive effect on lowering blood pressure). Products include:

Catapres Tablets 1037
Clorpres Tablets 1002
Combipres Tablets 1040
Duraclon Injection 3057

Cyclosporine (Verapamil therapy may increase serum levels of cyclosporine). Products include:

Gengraf Capsules 457
Neoral Soft Gelatin Capsules 2380
Neoral Oral Solution 2380
Sandimmune 2388

Deserpidine (Co-administration with oral antihypertensive agents will usually have an additive effect on lowering blood pressure).

No products indexed under this heading.

Desflurane (Potential for excessive cardiovascular depression based on animal studies). Products include:

Suprane Liquid for Inhalation 874

Deslanoside (Chronic verapamil treatment can increase serum digoxin levels by 50% to 70% resulting in digitalis toxicity; influence on digoxin kinetics is magnified in hepatic cirrhosis patients).

No products indexed under this heading.

Diazoxide (Co-administration with oral antihypertensive agents will usually have an additive effect on lowering blood pressure).

No products indexed under this heading.

Digitoxin (Chronic verapamil treatment can increase serum digoxin levels by 50% to 70% resulting in digitalis toxicity; influence on digoxin kinetics is magnified in hepatic cirrhosis patients).

No products indexed under this heading.

Digoxin (Chronic verapamil treatment can increase serum digoxin levels by 50% to 70% resulting in digitalis toxicity; influence on digoxin kinetics is magnified in hepatic cirrhosis patients). Products include:

Digitek Tablets 1003
Lanoxicaps Capsules 1574
Lanoxin Injection 1581
Lanoxin Tablets 1587
Lanoxin Elixir Pediatric 1578
Lanoxin Injection Pediatric 1584

Diltiazem Hydrochloride (Co-administration with oral antihypertensive agents will usually have an additive effect on lowering blood pressure). Products include:

Cardizem Injectable 1018
Cardizem Lyo-Ject Syringe 1018
Cardizem Monovial 1018
Cardizem CD Capsules 1016
Tiazac Capsules 1378

Disopyramide Phosphate (Disopyramide should not be administered within 48 hours before or 24 hours after verapamil administration).

No products indexed under this heading.

Doxacurium Chloride (Verapamil may potentiate the activity of neuromuscular blocking drugs).

No products indexed under this heading.

Doxazosin Mesylate (Concomitant use of agents that attenuate alpha-adrenergic function, such as doxazosin, may result in excessive reduction in blood pressure). Products include:

Cardura Tablets 2668

Enalapril Maleate (Co-administration with oral antihypertensive agents will usually have an additive effect on lowering blood pressure). Products include:

Lexxel Tablets 608
Vaseretic Tablets 2204
Vasotec Tablets 2210

Enalaprilat (Co-administration with oral antihypertensive agents will usually have an additive effect on lowering blood pressure). Products include:

Enalaprilat Injection 863
Vasotec I.V. Injection 2207

Enflurane (Potential for excessive cardiovascular depression based on animal studies).

No products indexed under this heading.

Eprosartan Mesylate (Co-administration with oral antihypertensive agents will usually have an additive effect on lowering blood pressure). Products include:

Teveten Tablets 3327

Esmolol Hydrochloride (Concomitant therapy may result in additive negative effects on heart rate, AV conduction, and/or cardiac contractility; excessive bradycardia and AV block has been reported with concurrent use in hypertensive patients; possible additive effect on blood pressure). Products include:

Brevibloc Injection 858

Felodipine (Co-administration with oral antihypertensive agents will usually have an additive effect on lowering blood pressure). Products include:

Lexxel Tablets 608
Plendil Extended-Release Tablets 623

Flecainide Acetate (Co-administration may have additive effects on myocardial contractility, AV conduction, and repolarization). Products include:

Tambocor Tablets 1990

Fosinopril Sodium (Co-administration with oral antihypertensive agents will usually have an additive effect on lowering blood pressure). Products include:

Monopril Tablets 1091
Monopril HCT 1094

Furosemide (Co-administration with oral antihypertensive agents will usually have an additive effect on lowering blood pressure). Products include:

Furosemide Tablets 2284

Guanabenz Acetate (Co-administration with oral antihypertensive agents will usually have an additive effect on lowering blood pressure).

No products indexed under this heading.

Guanethidine Monosulfate (Co-administration with oral antihypertensive agents will usually have an additive effect on lowering blood pressure).

No products indexed under this heading.

Halothane (Potential for excessive cardiovascular depression based on animal studies). Products include:

Fluothane Inhalation 3508

Hydralazine Hydrochloride (Co-administration with oral antihypertensive agents will usually have an additive effect on lowering blood pressure).

No products indexed under this heading.

Hydrochlorothiazide (Co-administration with oral antihypertensive agents will usually have an additive effect on lowering blood pressure). Products include:

Accuretic Tablets 2614
Aldoril Tablets 2039
Atacand HCT Tablets 597
Avalide Tablets 1070
Diovan HCT Tablets 2338
Dyazide Capsules 1515
HydroDIURIL Tablets 2108
Hyzaar 2109
Inderide Tablets 3517
Inderide LA Long-Acting Capsules 3519
Lotensin HCT Tablets 2367
Maxzide 1008
Micardis HCT Tablets 1051
Microzide Capsules 3414
Moduretic Tablets 2138
Monopril HCT 1094
Prinzide Tablets 2168
Timolide Tablets 2187
Uniretic Tablets 3178
Vaseretic Tablets 2204
Zestoretic Tablets 695
Ziac Tablets 1887

Hydroflumethiazide (Co-administration with oral antihypertensive agents will usually have an additive effect on lowering blood pressure). Products include:

Diucardin Tablets 3494

Indapamide (Co-administration with oral antihypertensive agents will usually have an additive effect on lowering blood pressure). Products include:

Indapamide Tablets 2286

Irbesartan (Co-administration with oral antihypertensive agents will usually have an additive effect on lowering blood pressure). Products include:

Avalide Tablets 1070
Avapro Tablets 1074
Avapro Tablets 3076

Isoflurane (Potential for excessive cardiovascular depression based on animal studies).

No products indexed under this heading.

Isradipine (Co-administration with oral antihypertensive agents will usually have an additive effect on lowering blood pressure). Products include:

DynaCirc Capsules 2921
DynaCirc CR Tablets 2923

Labetalol Hydrochloride (Concomitant therapy may result in additive negative effects on heart rate, AV conduction, and/or cardiac contractility; excessive bradycardia and AV block has been reported with concurrent use in hypertensive patients; possible additive effect on blood pressure). Products include:

Normodyne Injection 3135
Normodyne Tablets 3137

Levobunolol Hydrochloride (Concomitant therapy may result in additive negative effects on heart rate, AV conduction, and/or cardiac contractility; excessive bradycardia and AV block has been reported with concurrent use in hypertensive patients; possible additive effect on blood pressure). Products include:

Betagan ⊙228

Lisinopril (Co-administration with oral antihypertensive agents will usu-

ally have an additive effect on lowering blood pressure). Products include:
- Prinivil Tablets ... 2164
- Prinzide Tablets ... 2168
- Zestoretic Tablets ... 695
- Zestril Tablets ... 698

Lithium Carbonate (Combined therapy of oral verapamil and lithium may result in a lowering of serum lithium levels in patients receiving chronic stable oral lithium; potential for increased sensitivity to the effect of lithium). Products include:
- Eskalith ... 1527
- Lithium Carbonate ... 3061
- Lithobid Slow-Release Tablets ... 3255

Lithium Citrate (Combined therapy of oral verapamil and lithium may result in a lowering of serum lithium levels in patients receiving chronic stable oral lithium; potential for increased sensitivity to the effect of lithium). Products include:
- Lithium Citrate Syrup ... 3061

Losartan Potassium (Co-administration with oral antihypertensive agents will usually have an additive effect on lowering blood pressure). Products include:
- Cozaar Tablets ... 2067
- Hyzaar ... 2109

Mecamylamine Hydrochloride (Co-administration with oral antihypertensive agents will usually have an additive effect on lowering blood pressure). Products include:
- Inversine Tablets ... 1850

Methoxyflurane (Potential for excessive cardiovascular depression based on animal studies).
No products indexed under this heading.

Methyclothiazide (Co-administration with oral antihypertensive agents will usually have an additive effect on lowering blood pressure).
No products indexed under this heading.

Methyldopa (Co-administration with oral antihypertensive agents will usually have an additive effect on lowering blood pressure). Products include:
- Aldoclor Tablets ... 2035
- Aldomet Tablets ... 2037
- Aldoril Tablets ... 2039

Methyldopate Hydrochloride (Co-administration with oral antihypertensive agents will usually have an additive effect on lowering blood pressure).
No products indexed under this heading.

Metipranolol Hydrochloride (Concomitant therapy may result in additive negative effects on heart rate, AV conduction, and/or cardiac contractility; excessive bradycardia and AV block has been reported with concurrent use in hypertensive patients; possible additive effect on blood pressure).
No products indexed under this heading.

Metocurine Iodide (Verapamil may potentiate the activity of neuromuscular blocking drugs).
No products indexed under this heading.

Metolazone (Co-administration with oral antihypertensive agents will usually have an additive effect on lowering blood pressure). Products include:
- Mykrox Tablets ... 1168
- Zaroxolyn Tablets ... 1177

Metoprolol Succinate (Co-administration has resulted in a decrease in metoprolol clearance; concomitant therapy may result in additive negative effects on heart rate, AV conduction, and/or cardiac contractility; excessive bradycardia and AV block has been reported with concurrent use in hypertensive patients). Products include:
- Toprol-XL Tablets ... 651

Metoprolol Tartrate (Co-administration has resulted in a decrease in metoprolol clearance; concomitant therapy may result in additive negative effects on heart rate, AV conduction, and/or cardiac contractility; excessive bradycardia and AV block has been reported with concurrent use in hypertensive patients).
No products indexed under this heading.

Metyrosine (Co-administration with oral antihypertensive agents will usually have an additive effect on lowering blood pressure). Products include:
- Demser Capsules ... 2085

Mibefradil Dihydrochloride (Co-administration with oral antihypertensive agents will usually have an additive effect on lowering blood pressure).
No products indexed under this heading.

Minoxidil (Co-administration with oral antihypertensive agents will usually have an additive effect on lowering blood pressure). Products include:
- Rogaine Extra Strength for Men Topical Solution ... ▣721
- Rogaine for Women Topical Solution ... ▣721

Mivacurium Chloride (Verapamil may potentiate the activity of neuromuscular blocking drugs).
No products indexed under this heading.

Moexipril Hydrochloride (Co-administration with oral antihypertensive agents will usually have an additive effect on lowering blood pressure). Products include:
- Uniretic Tablets ... 3178
- Univasc Tablets ... 3181

Nadolol (Concomitant therapy may result in additive negative effects on heart rate, AV conduction, and/or cardiac contractility; excessive bradycardia and AV block has been reported with concurrent use in hypertensive patients; possible additive effect on blood pressure). Products include:
- Corgard Tablets ... 2245
- Corzide 40/5 Tablets ... 2247
- Corzide 80/5 Tablets ... 2247
- Nadolol Tablets ... 2288

Nicardipine Hydrochloride (Co-administration with oral antihypertensive agents will usually have an additive effect on lowering blood pressure). Products include:
- Cardene I.V. ... 3485

Nifedipine (Co-administration with oral antihypertensive agents will usually have an additive effect on lowering blood pressure). Products include:
- Adalat CC Tablets ... 877
- Procardia Capsules ... 2708
- Procardia XL Extended Release Tablets ... 2710

Nisoldipine (Co-administration with oral antihypertensive agents will usually have an additive effect on lowering blood pressure). Products include:
- Sular Tablets ... 688

Nitroglycerin (Co-administration with oral antihypertensive agents will usually have an additive effect on lowering blood pressure). Products include:
- Nitro-Dur Transdermal Infusion System ... 3134
- Nitro-Dur Transdermal Infusion System ... 1834
- Nitrolingual Pumpspray ... 1355
- Nitrostat Tablets ... 2658

Pancuronium Bromide (Verapamil may potentiate the activity of neuromuscular blocking drugs).
No products indexed under this heading.

Penbutolol Sulfate (Concomitant therapy may result in additive negative effects on heart rate, AV conduction, and/or cardiac contractility; excessive bradycardia and AV block has been reported with concurrent use in hypertensive patients; possible additive effect on blood pressure).
No products indexed under this heading.

Perindopril Erbumine (Co-administration with oral antihypertensive agents will usually have an additive effect on lowering blood pressure). Products include:
- Aceon Tablets (2 mg, 4 mg, 8 mg) ... 3249

Phenobarbital (Combined therapy with phenobarbital may increase verapamil clearance). Products include:
- Arco-Lase Plus Tablets ... 592
- Donnatal ... 2929
- Donnatal Extentabs ... 2930

Phenoxybenzamine Hydrochloride (Co-administration with oral antihypertensive agents will usually have an additive effect on lowering blood pressure). Products include:
- Dibenzyline Capsules ... 3457

Phentolamine Mesylate (Co-administration with oral antihypertensive agents will usually have an additive effect on lowering blood pressure).
No products indexed under this heading.

Pindolol (Concomitant therapy may result in additive negative effects on heart rate, AV conduction, and/or cardiac contractility; excessive bradycardia and AV block has been reported with concurrent use in hypertensive patients; possible additive effect on blood pressure).
No products indexed under this heading.

Polythiazide (Co-administration with oral antihypertensive agents will usually have an additive effect on lowering blood pressure). Products include:
- Minizide Capsules ... 2700
- Renese Tablets ... 2712

Prazosin Hydrochloride (Concomitant use of agents that attenuate alpha-adrenergic function, such as prazosin, may result in excessive reduction in blood pressure). Products include:
- Minipress Capsules ... 2699
- Minizide Capsules ... 2700

Propranolol Hydrochloride (Concomitant therapy may result in additive negative effects on heart rate, AV conduction, and/or cardiac contractility; excessive bradycardia and AV block has been reported with concurrent use in hypertensive patients; possible additive effect on blood pressure). Products include:
- Inderal ... 3513
- Inderal LA Long-Acting Capsules ... 3516
- Inderide Tablets ... 3517
- Inderide LA Long-Acting Capsules .. 3519

Quinapril Hydrochloride (Co-administration with oral antihypertensive agents will usually have an additive effect on lowering blood pressure). Products include:
- Accupril Tablets ... 2611
- Accuretic Tablets ... 2614

Quinidine Gluconate (In a small number of patients with hypertrophic cardiomyopathy, co-administration has resulted in significant hypotension; combined use in these patients should probably be avoided). Products include:
- Quinaglute Dura-Tabs Tablets ... 978

Quinidine Polygalacturonate (In a small number of patients with hypertrophic cardiomyopathy, co-administration has resulted in significant hypotension; combined use in these patients should probably be avoided).
No products indexed under this heading.

Quinidine Sulfate (In a small number of patients with hypertrophic cardiomyopathy, co-administration has resulted in significant hypotension; combined use in these patients should probably be avoided). Products include:
- Quinidex Extentabs ... 2933

Ramipril (Co-administration with oral antihypertensive agents will usually have an additive effect on lowering blood pressure). Products include:
- Altace Capsules ... 2233

Rapacuronium Bromide (Verapamil may potentiate the activity of neuromuscular blocking drugs).
No products indexed under this heading.

Rauwolfia serpentina (Co-administration with oral antihypertensive agents will usually have an additive effect on lowering blood pressure).
No products indexed under this heading.

Rescinnamine (Co-administration with oral antihypertensive agents will usually have an additive effect on lowering blood pressure).
No products indexed under this heading.

Reserpine (Co-administration with oral antihypertensive agents will usually have an additive effect on lowering blood pressure).
No products indexed under this heading.

Rifampin (Combined therapy with rifampin may markedly reduce oral verapamil bioavailability). Products include:
- Rifadin ... 765
- Rifamate Capsules ... 767
- Rifater Tablets ... 769

Rocuronium Bromide (Verapamil may potentiate the activity of neuromuscular blocking drugs). Products include:
- Zemuron Injection ... 2491

Sodium Nitroprusside (Co-administration with oral antihypertensive agents will usually have an additive effect on lowering blood pressure).
No products indexed under this heading.

Sotalol Hydrochloride (Concomitant therapy may result in additive negative effects on heart rate, AV conduction, and/or cardiac contractility; excessive bradycardia and AV block has been reported with concurrent use in hypertensive patients; possible additive effect on blood pressure). Products include:
- Betapace Tablets ... 950
- Betapace AF Tablets ... 954

Spirapril Hydrochloride (Co-administration with oral antihypertensive agents will usually have an additive effect on lowering blood pressure).
No products indexed under this heading.

Succinylcholine Chloride (Verapamil may potentiate the activity of neuromuscular blocking drugs). Products include:
- Anectine Injection ... 1476

Telmisartan (Co-administration with oral antihypertensive agents will usu-

ally have an additive effect on lowering blood pressure). Products include:
- Micardis Tablets 1049
- Micardis HCT Tablets 1051

Terazosin Hydrochloride (Concomitant use of agents that attenuate alpha-adrenergic function, such as terazosin, may result in excessive reduction in blood pressure). Products include:
- Hytrin Capsules 464

Timolol Hemihydrate (Co-administration of oral verapamil and timolol eye drops has resulted in asymptomatic bradycardia with a wandering atrial pacemaker). Products include:
- Betimol Ophthalmic Solution .... ⊙324

Timolol Maleate (Co-administration of oral verapamil and timolol eye drops has resulted in asymptomatic bradycardia with a wandering atrial pacemaker; concomitant therapy may result in additive negative effects on heart rate, AV conduction, and/or cardiac contractility; excessive bradycardia and AV block has been reported with concurrent use in hypertensive patients). Products include:
- Blocadren Tablets 2046
- Cosopt Sterile Ophthalmic Solution 2065
- Timolide Tablets 2187
- Timolol GFS .... ⊙266
- Timoptic in Ocudose 2192
- Timoptic Sterile Ophthalmic Solution 2190
- Timoptic-XE Sterile Ophthalmic Gel Forming Solution 2194

Torsemide (Co-administration with oral antihypertensive agents will usually have an additive effect on lowering blood pressure). Products include:
- Demadex Tablets and Injection 2965

Trandolapril (Co-administration with oral antihypertensive agents will usually have an additive effect on lowering blood pressure). Products include:
- Mavik Tablets 478
- Tarka Tablets 508

Trimethaphan Camsylate (Co-administration with oral antihypertensive agents will usually have an additive effect on lowering blood pressure).
- No products indexed under this heading.

Tubocurarine Chloride (Verapamil may potentiate the activity of neuromuscular blocking drugs).
- No products indexed under this heading.

Valsartan (Co-administration with oral antihypertensive agents will usually have an additive effect on lowering blood pressure). Products include:
- Diovan Capsules 2337
- Diovan HCT Tablets 2338

Vecuronium Bromide (Verapamil may potentiate the activity of neuromuscular blocking drugs). Products include:
- Norcuron for Injection 2478

Food Interactions

Alcohol (Verapamil has been found to significantly inhibit ethanol elimination resulting in elevated blood ethanol concentration that may prolong the intoxicating effects of alcohol).

VERELAN PM CAPSULES

(Verapamil Hydrochloride) 3186
See Verelan Capsules

VERMOX CHEWABLE TABLETS

(Mebendazole) 2017
May interact with:

Cimetidine (Inhibits mebendazole metabolism and may result in an increase in plasma concentrations of mebendazole). Products include:
- Tagamet HB 200 Suspension .... ⊞762
- Tagamet HB 200 Tablets .... ⊞761
- Tagamet Tablets 1644

Cimetidine Hydrochloride (Inhibits mebendazole metabolism and may result in an increase in plasma concentrations of mebendazole). Products include:
- Tagamet 1644

VERSED INJECTION

(Midazolam Hydrochloride) 3027
See Versed Syrup

VERSED SYRUP

(Midazolam Hydrochloride) 3033
May interact with barbiturates, calcium channel blockers, central nervous system depressants, dexamethasone, erythromycin, macrolide antibiotics, phenytoin, protease inhibitors, and certain other agents. Compounds in these categories include:

Alfentanil Hydrochloride (Co-administration increases the risk of hypoventilation, airway obstruction, desaturation or apnea, and may contribute to profound and/or prolonged effect).
- No products indexed under this heading.

Alprazolam (Co-administration increases the risk of hypoventilation, airway obstruction, desaturation or apnea, and may contribute to profound and/or prolonged effect). Products include:
- Xanax Tablets 2865

Amlodipine Besylate (Co-administration with drugs known to inhibit CYP3A4, such as calcium channel blockers, may increase oral midazolam Cmax and AUC; this interaction may result in increased and prolonged sedation due to a decrease in plasma clearance of midazolam). Products include:
- Lotrel Capsules 2370
- Norvasc Tablets 2704

Amprenavir (Co-administration with drugs known to inhibit CYP3A4, such as protease inhibitors, may increase oral midazolam Cmax and AUC; this interaction may result in increased and prolonged sedation due to a decrease in plasma clearance of midazolam). Products include:
- Agenerase Capsules 1454
- Agenerase Oral Solution 1459

Aprobarbital (Co-administration increases the risk of hypoventilation, airway obstruction, desaturation or apnea, and may contribute to profound and/or prolonged effect).
- No products indexed under this heading.

Azithromycin Dihydrate (Co-administration with drugs known to inhibit CYP3A4, such as macrolide antibiotics, may increase oral midazolam Cmax and AUC; this interaction may result in increased and prolonged sedation due to a decrease in plasma clearance of midazolam; in clinicalstudies, azithromycin did not affect pharmacokinetics of midazolam). Products include:
- Zithromax 2743
- Zithromax for IV Infusion 2748
- Zithromax for Oral Suspension, 300 mg, 600 mg, 900 mg, 1200 mg 2739
- Zithromax Tablets, 250 mg 2739

Bepridil Hydrochloride (Co-administration with drugs known to inhibit CYP3A4, such as calcium channel blockers, may increase oral midazolam Cmax and AUC; this interaction may result in increased and prolonged sedation due to a decrease in plasma clearance of midazolam). Products include:
- Vascor Tablets 2602

Buprenorphine Hydrochloride (Co-administration increases the risk of hypoventilation, airway obstruction, desaturation or apnea, and may contribute to profound and/or prolonged effect). Products include:
- Buprenex Injectable 2918

Buspirone Hydrochloride (Co-administration increases the risk of hypoventilation, airway obstruction, desaturation or apnea, and may contribute to profound and/or prolonged effect).
- No products indexed under this heading.

Butabarbital (Co-administration increases the risk of hypoventilation, airway obstruction, desaturation or apnea, and may contribute to profound and/or prolonged effect).
- No products indexed under this heading.

Butalbital (Co-administration increases the risk of hypoventilation, airway obstruction, desaturation or apnea, and may contribute to profound and/or prolonged effect). Products include:
- Phrenilin 578
- Sedapap Tablets 50 mg/650 mg 2225

Carbamazepine (Co-administration with drugs known to induce CYP3A4, such as carbamazepine, decreases oral midazolam Cmax by 93% and AUC by 94%). Products include:
- Carbatrol Capsules 3234
- Tegretol/Tegretol-XR 2404

Chlordiazepoxide (Co-administration increases the risk of hypoventilation, airway obstruction, desaturation or apnea, and may contribute to profound and/or prolonged effect). Products include:
- Limbitrol 1738

Chlordiazepoxide Hydrochloride (Co-administration increases the risk of hypoventilation, airway obstruction, desaturation or apnea, and may contribute to profound and/or prolonged effect). Products include:
- Librium Capsules 1736
- Librium for Injection 1737

Chlorpromazine (Co-administration increases the risk of hypoventilation, airway obstruction, desaturation or apnea, and may contribute to profound and/or prolonged effect). Products include:
- Thorazine Suppositories 1656

Chlorpromazine Hydrochloride (Co-administration increases the risk of hypoventilation, airway obstruction, desaturation or apnea, and may contribute to profound and/or prolonged effect). Products include:
- Thorazine 1656

Chlorprothixene (Co-administration increases the risk of hypoventilation, airway obstruction, desaturation or apnea, and may contribute to profound and/or prolonged effect).
- No products indexed under this heading.

Chlorprothixene Hydrochloride (Co-administration increases the risk of hypoventilation, airway obstruction, desaturation or apnea, and may contribute to profound and/or prolonged effect).
- No products indexed under this heading.

Chlorprothixene Lactate (Co-administration increases the risk of hypoventilation, airway obstruction, desaturation or apnea, and may contribute to profound and/or prolonged effect).
- No products indexed under this heading.

Cimetidine (Co-administration with drugs known to inhibit CYP3A4, such as cimetidine, increases oral midazolam Cmax by 6% to 138% and AUC by 10% to 102%). Products include:
- Tagamet HB 200 Suspension .... ⊞762
- Tagamet HB 200 Tablets .... ⊞761
- Tagamet Tablets 1644

Cimetidine Hydrochloride (Co-administration with drugs known to inhibit CYP3A4, such as cimetidine, increases oral midazolam Cmax by 6% to 138% and AUC by 10% to 102%). Products include:
- Tagamet 1644

Clarithromycin (Co-administration with drugs known to inhibit CYP3A4, such as macrolide antibiotics, may increase oral midazolam Cmax and AUC; this interaction may result in increased and prolonged sedation due to a decrease in plasma clearance of midazolam). Products include:
- Biaxin/Biaxin XL 403
- PREVPAC 3298

Clorazepate Dipotassium (Co-administration increases the risk of hypoventilation, airway obstruction, desaturation or apnea, and may contribute to profound and/or prolonged effect). Products include:
- Tranxene 511

Clozapine (Co-administration increases the risk of hypoventilation, airway obstruction, desaturation or apnea, and may contribute to profound and/or prolonged effect). Products include:
- Clozaril Tablets 2319

Codeine Phosphate (Co-administration increases the risk of hypoventilation, airway obstruction, desaturation or apnea, and may contribute to profound and/or prolonged effect). Products include:
- Phenergan with Codeine Syrup 3557
- Phenergan VC with Codeine Syrup 3561
- Robitussin A-C Syrup 2942
- Robitussin-DAC Syrup 2942
- Ryna-C Liquid .... ⊞768
- Soma Compound w/Codeine Tablets 3355
- Tussi-Organidin NR Liquid 3350
- Tussi-Organidin-S NR Liquid 3350
- Tylenol with Codeine 2595

Desflurane (Co-administration increases the risk of hypoventilation, airway obstruction, desaturation or apnea, and may contribute to profound and/or prolonged effect). Products include:
- Suprane Liquid for Inhalation 874

Dexamethasone (Co-administration with drugs known to induce CYP3A4, such as dexamethasone, would be expected to decrease Cmax and AUC of oral midazolam; this interaction has not been tested). Products include:
- Decadron Elixir 2078
- Decadron Tablets 2079
- TobraDex Ophthalmic Ointment 542
- TobraDex Ophthalmic Suspension 541

Dexamethasone Acetate (Co-administration with drugs known to induce CYP3A4, such as dexamethasone, would be expected to decrease Cmax and AUC of oral midazolam; this interaction has not been tested).
- No products indexed under this heading.

Dexamethasone Sodium Phosphate (Co-administration with drugs known to induce CYP3A4, such as dexamethasone, would be expected to decrease Cmax and AUC of oral midazolam; this interaction has not been tested). Products include:
- Decadron Phosphate Injection 2081
- Decadron Phosphate Sterile Ophthalmic Ointment 2083
- Decadron Phosphate Sterile Ophthalmic Solution 2084
- NeoDecadron Sterile Ophthalmic Solution 2144

Dezocine (Co-administration increases the risk of hypoventilation, airway obstruction, desaturation or apnea, and may contribute to pro-

found and/or prolonged effect).
No products indexed under this heading.

Diazepam (Co-administration increases the risk of hypoventilation, airway obstruction, desaturation or apnea, and may contribute to profound and/or prolonged effect). Products include:
Valium Injectable ... 3026
Valium Tablets ... 3047

Diltiazem Hydrochloride (Co-administration with drugs known to inhibit CYP3A4, such as diltiazem, increases oral midazolam Cmax by 150% and AUC by 275%; this interaction may result in increased and prolonged sedation due to a decrease in plasma clearance of midazolam). Products include:
Cardizem Injectable ... 1018
Cardizem Lyo-Ject Syringe ... 1018
Cardizem Monovial ... 1018
Cardizem CD Capsules ... 1016
Tiazac Capsules ... 1378

Diltiazem Malate (Co-administration with drugs known to inhibit CYP3A4, such as diltiazem, increases oral midazolam Cmax by 150% and AUC by 275%; this interaction may result in increased and prolonged sedation due to a decrease in plasma clearance of midazolam).
No products indexed under this heading.

Dirithromycin (Co-administration with drugs known to inhibit CYP3A4, such as macrolide antibiotics, may increase oral midazolam Cmax and AUC; this interaction may result in increased and prolonged sedation due to a decrease in plasma clearance of midazolam). Products include:
Dynabac Tablets ... 2269

Droperidol (Co-administration increases the risk of hypoventilation, airway obstruction, desaturation or apnea, and may contribute to profound and/or prolonged effect).
No products indexed under this heading.

Enflurane (Co-administration increases the risk of hypoventilation, airway obstruction, desaturation or apnea, and may contribute to profound and/or prolonged effect).
No products indexed under this heading.

Erythromycin (Co-administration with drugs known to inhibit CYP3A4, such as erythromycin, increases oral midazolam Cmax by 170% to 171% and AUC by 281% to 341%; this interaction may result in increased and prolonged sedation due to a decrease in plasma clearance of midazolam). Products include:
Emgel 2% Topical Gel ... 1285
Ery-Tab Tablets ... 448
Erythromycin Base Filmtab Tablets . 454
Erythromycin Delayed-Release Capsules, USP ... 455
PCE Dispertab Tablets ... 498

Erythromycin Estolate (Co-administration with drugs known to inhibit CYP3A4, such as erythromycin, increases oral midazolam Cmax by 170% to 171% and AUC by 281% to 341%; this interaction may result in increased and prolonged sedation due to a decrease in plasma clearance of midazolam).
No products indexed under this heading.

Erythromycin Ethylsuccinate (Co-administration with drugs known to inhibit CYP3A4, such as erythromycin, increases oral midazolam Cmax by 170% to 171% and AUC by 281% to 341%; this interaction may result in increased and prolonged sedation due to a decrease in plasma clearance of midazolam). Products include:
E.E.S. ... 450
EryPed ... 446
Pediazole Suspension ... 3050

Erythromycin Gluceptate (Co-administration with drugs known to inhibit CYP3A4, such as erythromycin, increases oral midazolam Cmax by 170% to 171% and AUC by 281% to 341%; this interaction may result in increased and prolonged sedation due to a decrease in plasma clearance of midazolam).
No products indexed under this heading.

Erythromycin Stearate (Co-administration with drugs known to inhibit CYP3A4, such as erythromycin, increases oral midazolam Cmax by 170% to 171% and AUC by 281% to 341%; this interaction may result in increased and prolonged sedation due to a decrease in plasma clearance of midazolam). Products include:
Erythrocin Stearate Filmtab Tablets ... 452

Estazolam (Co-administration increases the risk of hypoventilation, airway obstruction, desaturation or apnea, and may contribute to profound and/or prolonged effect). Products include:
ProSom Tablets ... 500

Ethchlorvynol (Co-administration increases the risk of hypoventilation, airway obstruction, desaturation or apnea, and may contribute to profound and/or prolonged effect).
No products indexed under this heading.

Ethinamate (Co-administration increases the risk of hypoventilation, airway obstruction, desaturation or apnea, and may contribute to profound and/or prolonged effect).
No products indexed under this heading.

Felodipine (Co-administration with drugs known to inhibit CYP3A4, such as calcium channel blockers, may increase oral midazolam Cmax and AUC; this interaction may result in increased and prolonged sedation due to a decrease in plasma clearance of midazolam). Products include:
Lexxel Tablets ... 608
Plendil Extended-Release Tablets ... 623

Fentanyl (Co-administration increases the risk of hypoventilation, airway obstruction, desaturation or apnea, and may contribute to profound and/or prolonged effect). Products include:
Duragesic Transdermal System ... 1786

Fentanyl Citrate (Co-administration increases the risk of hypoventilation, airway obstruction, desaturation or apnea, and may contribute to profound and/or prolonged effect). Products include:
Actiq ... 1184

Fluconazole (Co-administration with drugs known to inhibit CYP3A4, such as fluconazole, increases oral midazolam Cmax by 150% and AUC by 250%; this interaction may result in increased and prolonged sedation due to a decrease in plasma clearance of midazolam). Products include:
Diflucan Tablets, Injection, and Oral Suspension ... 2681

Fluphenazine Decanoate (Co-administration increases the risk of hypoventilation, airway obstruction, desaturation or apnea, and may contribute to profound and/or prolonged effect).
No products indexed under this heading.

Fluphenazine Enanthate (Co-administration increases the risk of hypoventilation, airway obstruction, desaturation or apnea, and may contribute to profound and/or prolonged effect).
No products indexed under this heading.

Fluphenazine Hydrochloride (Co-administration increases the risk of hypoventilation, airway obstruction, desaturation or apnea, and may contribute to profound and/or prolonged effect).
No products indexed under this heading.

Flurazepam Hydrochloride (Co-administration increases the risk of hypoventilation, airway obstruction, desaturation or apnea, and may contribute to profound and/or prolonged effect).
No products indexed under this heading.

Fosphenytoin Sodium (Co-administration with drugs known to induce CYP3A4, such as phenytoin, decreases oral midazolam Cmax by 93% and AUC by 94%). Products include:
Cerebyx Injection ... 2619

Glutethimide (Co-administration increases the risk of hypoventilation, airway obstruction, desaturation or apnea, and may contribute to profound and/or prolonged effect).
No products indexed under this heading.

Haloperidol (Co-administration increases the risk of hypoventilation, airway obstruction, desaturation or apnea, and may contribute to profound and/or prolonged effect). Products include:
Haldol Injection, Tablets and Concentrate ... 2533

Haloperidol Decanoate (Co-administration increases the risk of hypoventilation, airway obstruction, desaturation or apnea, and may contribute to profound and/or prolonged effect). Products include:
Haldol Decanoate ... 2535

Hydrocodone Bitartrate (Co-administration increases the risk of hypoventilation, airway obstruction, desaturation or apnea, and may contribute to profound and/or prolonged effect). Products include:
Hycodan ... 1316
Hycomine Compound Tablets ... 1317
Hycotuss Expectorant Syrup ... 1318
Lortab ... 3319
Lortab Elixir ... 3317
Maxidone Tablets CIII ... 3399
Norco 5/325 Tablets CIII ... 3424
Norco 7.5/325 Tablets CIII ... 3425
Norco 10/325 Tablets CIII ... 3427
Norco 10/325 Tablets CIII ... 3425
Vicodin Tablets ... 516
Vicodin ES Tablets ... 517
Vicodin HP Tablets ... 518
Vicodin Tuss Expectorant ... 519
Vicoprofen Tablets ... 520
Zydone Tablets ... 1330

Hydrocodone Polistirex (Co-administration increases the risk of hypoventilation, airway obstruction, desaturation or apnea, and may contribute to profound and/or prolonged effect). Products include:
Tussionex Pennkinetic Extended-Release Suspension ... 1174

Hydromorphone Hydrochloride (Co-administration increases the risk of hypoventilation, airway obstruction, desaturation or apnea, and may contribute to profound and/or prolonged effect). Products include:
Dilaudid ... 441
Dilaudid Oral Liquid ... 445
Dilaudid Powder ... 441
Dilaudid Rectal Suppositories ... 441
Dilaudid Tablets ... 441
Dilaudid Tablets - 8 mg ... 445
Dilaudid-HP ... 443

Hydroxyzine Hydrochloride (Co-administration increases the risk of hypoventilation, airway obstruction, desaturation or apnea, and may contribute to profound and/or prolonged effect). Products include:
Atarax Tablets & Syrup ... 2667
Vistaril Intramuscular Solution ... 2738

Indinavir Sulfate (Co-administration with drugs known to inhibit CYP3A4, such as protease inhibitors, may increase oral midazolam Cmax and AUC; this interaction may result in increased and prolonged sedation due to a decrease in plasma clearance of midazolam). Products include:
Crixivan Capsules ... 2070

Isoflurane (Co-administration increases the risk of hypoventilation, airway obstruction, desaturation or apnea, and may contribute to profound and/or prolonged effect).
No products indexed under this heading.

Isradipine (Co-administration with drugs known to inhibit CYP3A4, such as calcium channel blockers, may increase oral midazolam Cmax and AUC; this interaction may result in increased and prolonged sedation due to a decrease in plasma clearance of midazolam). Products include:
DynaCirc Capsules ... 2921
DynaCirc CR Tablets ... 2923

Itraconazole (Co-administration with drugs known to inhibit CYP3A4, such as itraconazole, increases oral midazolam Cmax by 80% to 240% and AUC by 240% to 980%; this interaction may result in increased and prolonged sedation due to a decrease in plasma clearance of midazolam). Products include:
Sporanox Capsules ... 1800
Sporanox Injection ... 1804
Sporanox Injection ... 2509
Sporanox Oral Solution ... 1808
Sporanox Oral Solution ... 2512

Ketamine Hydrochloride (Co-administration increases the risk of hypoventilation, airway obstruction, desaturation or apnea, and may contribute to profound and/or prolonged effect).
No products indexed under this heading.

Ketoconazole (Co-administration with drugs known to inhibit CYP3A4, such as ketoconazole, increases oral midazolam Cmax by 309% and AUC by 1490%; this interaction may result in increased and prolonged sedation due to a decrease in plasma clearance of midazolam). Products include:
Nizoral 2% Cream ... 3620
Nizoral A-D Shampoo ... 2008
Nizoral 2% Shampoo ... 2007
Nizoral Tablets ... 1791

Levomethadyl Acetate Hydrochloride (Co-administration increases the risk of hypoventilation, airway obstruction, desaturation or apnea, and may contribute to profound and/or prolonged effect).
No products indexed under this heading.

Levorphanol Tartrate (Co-administration increases the risk of hypoventilation, airway obstruction, desaturation or apnea, and may contribute to profound and/or prolonged effect). Products include:
Levo-Dromoran ... 1734
Levorphanol Tartrate Tablets ... 3059

Lopinavir (Co-administration with drugs known to inhibit CYP3A4, such as protease inhibitors, may increase oral midazolam Cmax and AUC; this interaction may result in increased and prolonged sedation due to a decrease in plasma clearance of midazolam). Products include:
Kaletra Capsules ... 471
Kaletra Oral Solution ... 471

Lorazepam (Co-administration increases the risk of hypoventilation,

airway obstruction, desaturation or apnea, and may contribute to profound and/or prolonged effect). Products include:

Ativan Injection 3478
Ativan Tablets 3482

Loxapine Hydrochloride (Co-administration increases the risk of hypoventilation, airway obstruction, desaturation or apnea, and may contribute to profound and/or prolonged effect).

No products indexed under this heading.

Loxapine Succinate (Co-administration increases the risk of hypoventilation, airway obstruction, desaturation or apnea, and may contribute to profound and/or prolonged effect). Products include:

Loxitane Capsules 3398

Meperidine Hydrochloride (Co-administration increases the risk of hypoventilation, airway obstruction, desaturation or apnea, and may contribute to profound and/or prolonged effect). Products include:

Demerol 3079
Mepergan Injection 3539

Mephobarbital (Co-administration increases the risk of hypoventilation, airway obstruction, desaturation or apnea, and may contribute to profound and/or prolonged effect).

No products indexed under this heading.

Meprobamate (Co-administration increases the risk of hypoventilation, airway obstruction, desaturation or apnea, and may contribute to profound and/or prolonged effect). Products include:

Miltown Tablets 3349

Mesoridazine Besylate (Co-administration increases the risk of hypoventilation, airway obstruction, desaturation or apnea, and may contribute to profound and/or prolonged effect). Products include:

Serentil 1057

Methadone Hydrochloride (Co-administration increases the risk of hypoventilation, airway obstruction, desaturation or apnea, and may contribute to profound and/or prolonged effect). Products include:

Dolophine Hydrochloride Tablets 3056

Methohexital Sodium (Co-administration increases the risk of hypoventilation, airway obstruction, desaturation or apnea, and may contribute to profound and/or prolonged effect). Products include:

Brevital Sodium for Injection, USP .. 1815

Methotrimeprazine (Co-administration increases the risk of hypoventilation, airway obstruction, desaturation or apnea, and may contribute to profound and/or prolonged effect).

No products indexed under this heading.

Methoxyflurane (Co-administration increases the risk of hypoventilation, airway obstruction, desaturation or apnea, and may contribute to profound and/or prolonged effect).

No products indexed under this heading.

Methylphenidate Hydrochloride (Co-administration in a child with Williams syndrome on chronic methylphenidate therapy has resulted in inadequate sedation with chloral hydrate and later with midazolam; possible decreased absorption of the sedatives due to both the gastrointestinal effects and stimulant effect of methylphenidate). Products include:

Concerta Extended-Release Tablets 1998
Concerta Tablets 561
Metadate CD Capsules 1164
Metadate ER Tablets 1167
Methylin Tablets 1995
Methylin ER Tablets 1995
Ritalin 2387

Mibefradil Dihydrochloride (Co-administration with drugs known to inhibit CYP3A4, such as calcium channel blockers, may increase oral midazolam Cmax and AUC; this interaction may result in increased and prolonged sedation due to a decrease in plasma clearance of midazolam).

No products indexed under this heading.

Molindone Hydrochloride (Co-administration increases the risk of hypoventilation, airway obstruction, desaturation or apnea, and may contribute to profound and/or prolonged effect). Products include:

Moban 1320

Morphine Sulfate (Co-administration increases the risk of hypoventilation, airway obstruction, desaturation or apnea, and may contribute to profound and/or prolonged effect). Products include:

Astramorph/PF Injection, USP (Preservative-Free) 594
Duramorph Injection 1312
Infumorph 200 and Infumorph 500 Sterile Solutions 1314
Kadian Capsules 1335
MS Contin Tablets 2896
MSIR 2898
Oramorph SR Tablets 3062
Roxanol 3066

Nelfinavir Mesylate (Co-administration with drugs known to be potent inhibitors of CYP3A4, such as nelfinavir, may cause intense and prolonged sedation due to a decrease in plasma clearance of midazolam; this interaction has not been studied). Products include:

Viracept 532

Nicardipine Hydrochloride (Co-administration with drugs known to inhibit CYP3A4, such as calcium channel blockers, may increase oral midazolam Cmax and AUC; this interaction may result in increased and prolonged sedation due to a decrease in plasma clearance of midazolam). Products include:

Cardene I.V. 3485

Nifedipine (Co-administration with drugs known to inhibit CYP3A4, such as calcium channel blockers, may increase oral midazolam Cmax and AUC; this interaction may result in increased and prolonged sedation due to a decrease in plasma clearance of midazolam). Products include:

Adalat CC Tablets 877
Procardia Capsules 2708
Procardia XL Extended Release Tablets 2710

Nimodipine (Co-administration with drugs known to inhibit CYP3A4, such as calcium channel blockers, may increase oral midazolam Cmax and AUC; this interaction may result in increased and prolonged sedation due to a decrease in plasma clearance of midazolam). Products include:

Nimotop Capsules 904

Nisoldipine (Co-administration with drugs known to inhibit CYP3A4, such as calcium channel blockers, may increase oral midazolam Cmax and AUC; this interaction may result in increased and prolonged sedation due to a decrease in plasma clearance of midazolam). Products include:

Sular Tablets 688

Olanzapine (Co-administration increases the risk of hypoventilation, airway obstruction, desaturation or apnea, and may contribute to profound and/or prolonged effect). Products include:

Zyprexa Tablets 1973
Zyprexa ZYDIS Orally Disintegrating Tablets 1973

Oxazepam (Co-administration increases the risk of hypoventilation, airway obstruction, desaturation or apnea, and may contribute to profound and/or prolonged effect).

No products indexed under this heading.

Oxycodone Hydrochloride (Co-administration increases the risk of hypoventilation, airway obstruction, desaturation or apnea, and may contribute to profound and/or prolonged effect). Products include:

OxyContin Tablets 2912
OxyFast Oral Concentrate Solution . 2916
OxyIR Capsules 2916
Percocet Tablets 1326
Percodan Tablets 1327
Percolone Tablets 1327
Roxicodone 3067
Tylox Capsules 2597

Pentobarbital Sodium (Co-administration increases the risk of hypoventilation, airway obstruction, desaturation or apnea, and may contribute to profound and/or prolonged effect). Products include:

Nembutal Sodium Solution 485

Perphenazine (Co-administration increases the risk of hypoventilation, airway obstruction, desaturation or apnea, and may contribute to profound and/or prolonged effect). Products include:

Etrafon 3115
Trilafon 3160

Phenobarbital (Co-administration with drugs known to induce CYP3A4, such as phenobarbital, would be expected to decrease Cmax and AUC of oral midazolam; this interaction has not been tested; concurrent use increases the risk of hypoventilation, airway obstruction, desaturation or apnea, and may contribute to profound and/or prolonged effect). Products include:

Arco-Lase Plus Tablets 592
Donnatal 2929
Donnatal Extentabs 2930

Phenytoin (Co-administration with drugs known to induce CYP3A4, such as phenytoin, decreases oral midazolam Cmax by 93% and AUC by 94%). Products include:

Dilantin Infatabs 2624
Dilantin-125 Oral Suspension 2625

Phenytoin Sodium (Co-administration with drugs known to induce CYP3A4, such as phenytoin, decreases oral midazolam Cmax by 93% and AUC by 94%). Products include:

Dilantin Kapseals 2622

Prazepam (Co-administration increases the risk of hypoventilation, airway obstruction, desaturation or apnea, and may contribute to profound and/or prolonged effect).

No products indexed under this heading.

Prochlorperazine (Co-administration increases the risk of hypoventilation, airway obstruction, desaturation or apnea, and may contribute to profound and/or prolonged effect). Products include:

Compazine 1505

Promethazine Hydrochloride (Co-administration increases the risk of hypoventilation, airway obstruction, desaturation or apnea, and may contribute to profound and/or prolonged effect). Products include:

Mepergan Injection 3539
Phenergan Injection 3553
Phenergan 3556
Phenergan Syrup 3554
Phenergan with Codeine Syrup 3557
Phenergan with Dextromethorphan Syrup 3559
Phenergan VC Syrup 3560
Phenergan VC with Codeine Syrup .. 3561

Propofol (Co-administration increases the risk of hypoventilation, airway obstruction, desaturation or apnea, and may contribute to profound and/or prolonged effect). Products include:

Diprivan Injectable Emulsion 667

Propoxyphene Hydrochloride (Co-administration increases the risk of hypoventilation, airway obstruction, desaturation or apnea, and may contribute to profound and/or prolonged effect). Products include:

Darvon Pulvules 1909
Darvon Compound-65 Pulvules 1910

Propoxyphene Napsylate (Co-administration increases the risk of hypoventilation, airway obstruction, desaturation or apnea, and may contribute to profound and/or prolonged effect). Products include:

Darvon-N/Darvocet-N 1907
Darvon-N Tablets 1912

Quazepam (Co-administration increases the risk of hypoventilation, airway obstruction, desaturation or apnea, and may contribute to profound and/or prolonged effect).

No products indexed under this heading.

Quetiapine Fumarate (Co-administration increases the risk of hypoventilation, airway obstruction, desaturation or apnea, and may contribute to profound and/or prolonged effect). Products include:

Seroquel Tablets 684

Ranitidine Hydrochloride (Co-administration with drugs known to inhibit CYP3A4, such as ranitidine, increases oral midazolam Cmax by 15% to 67% and AUC by 9% to 66%). Products include:

Zantac 1690
Zantac Injection 1688
Zantac 75 Tablets 717

Remifentanil Hydrochloride (Co-administration increases the risk of hypoventilation, airway obstruction, desaturation or apnea, and may contribute to profound and/or prolonged effect).

No products indexed under this heading.

Rifabutin (Co-administration with drugs known to induce CYP3A4, such as rifabutin, would be expected to decrease Cmax and AUC of oral midazolam; this interaction has not been tested). Products include:

Mycobutin Capsules 2838

Rifampin (Co-administration with drugs known to induce CYP3A4, such as rifampin, decreases oral midazolam Cmax by 94% and AUC by 96%). Products include:

Rifadin 765
Rifamate Capsules 767
Rifater Tablets 769

Risperidone (Co-administration increases the risk of hypoventilation, airway obstruction, desaturation or apnea, and may contribute to profound and/or prolonged effect). Products include:

Risperdal 1796

Ritonavir (Co-administration with drugs known to be potent inhibitors of CYP3A4, such as ritonavir, may cause intense and prolonged sedation due to a decrease in plasma clearance of midazolam; this interaction has not been studied). Products include:

Kaletra Capsules 471
Kaletra Oral Solution 471
Norvir Capsules 487
Norvir Oral Solution 487

Roxithromycin (Co-administration with drugs known to inhibit CYP3A4, such as roxithromycin, increases oral midazolam Cmax by 37% and AUC by 47%).

No products indexed under this heading.

Saquinavir (Co-administration with drugs known to inhibit CYP3A4, such as protease inhibitors, may increase oral midazolam Cmax and AUC; this interaction may result in increased and prolonged sedation due to a decrease in plasma clearance of midazolam). Products include:
Fortovase Capsules 2970

Saquinavir Mesylate (Co-administration with drugs known to inhibit CYP3A4, such as protease inhibitors, may increase oral midazolam Cmax and AUC; this interaction may result in increased and prolonged sedation due to a decrease in plasma clearance of midazolam). Products include:
Invirase Capsules 2979

Secobarbital Sodium (Co-administration increases the risk of hypoventilation, airway obstruction, desaturation or apnea, and may contribute to profound and/or prolonged effect).
No products indexed under this heading.

Sevoflurane (Co-administration increases the risk of hypoventilation, airway obstruction, desaturation or apnea, and may contribute to profound and/or prolonged effect).
No products indexed under this heading.

Sufentanil Citrate (Co-administration increases the risk of hypoventilation, airway obstruction, desaturation or apnea, and may contribute to profound and/or prolonged effect).
No products indexed under this heading.

Temazepam (Co-administration increases the risk of hypoventilation, airway obstruction, desaturation or apnea, and may contribute to profound and/or prolonged effect).
No products indexed under this heading.

Thiamylal Sodium (Co-administration increases the risk of hypoventilation, airway obstruction, desaturation or apnea, and may contribute to profound and/or prolonged effect).
No products indexed under this heading.

Thioridazine Hydrochloride (Co-administration increases the risk of hypoventilation, airway obstruction, desaturation or apnea, and may contribute to profound and/or prolonged effect). Products include:
Thioridazine Hydrochloride Tablets 2289

Thiothixene (Co-administration increases the risk of hypoventilation, airway obstruction, desaturation or apnea, and may contribute to profound and/or prolonged effect). Products include:
Navane Capsules 2701
Thiothixene Capsules 2290

Triazolam (Co-administration increases the risk of hypoventilation, airway obstruction, desaturation or apnea, and may contribute to profound and/or prolonged effect). Products include:
Halcion Tablets 2823

Trifluoperazine Hydrochloride (Co-administration increases the risk of hypoventilation, airway obstruction, desaturation or apnea, and may contribute to profound and/or prolonged effect). Products include:
Stelazine 1640

Troglitazone (Co-administration with drugs known to induce CYP3A4, such as troglitazone, would be expected to decrease Cmax and AUC of oral midazolam; this interaction has not been tested).
No products indexed under this heading.

Troleandomycin (Co-administration with drugs known to inhibit CYP3A4, such as macrolide antibiotics, may increase oral midazolam Cmax and AUC; this interaction may result in increased and prolonged sedation due to a decrease in plasma clearance of midazolam). Products include:
Tao Capsules 2716

Verapamil Hydrochloride (Co-administration with drugs known to inhibit CYP3A4, such as verapamil, increases oral midazolam Cmax by 97% and AUC by 192%; this interaction may result in increased and prolonged sedation due to a decrease in plasma clearance of midazolam). Products include:
Covera-HS Tablets 3199
Isoptin SR Tablets 467
Tarka Tablets 508
Verelan Capsules 3184
Verelan PM Capsules 3186

Zaleplon (Co-administration increases the risk of hypoventilation, airway obstruction, desaturation or apnea, and may contribute to profound and/or prolonged effect). Products include:
Sonata Capsules 3591

Ziprasidone Hydrochloride (Co-administration increases the risk of hypoventilation, airway obstruction, desaturation or apnea, and may contribute to profound and/or prolonged effect). Products include:
Geodon Capsules 2688

Zolpidem Tartrate (Co-administration increases the risk of hypoventilation, airway obstruction, desaturation or apnea, and may contribute to profound and/or prolonged effect). Products include:
Ambien Tablets 3191

Food Interactions

Alcohol (Concurrent use with alcohol increases effects of alcohol).

Grapefruit Juice (Co-administration with agents known to inhibit CYP3A4, such as grapefruit juice, increases oral midazolam Cmax by 56% and AUC by 52%; Versed Syrup should not be taken with grapefruit juice).

VESANOID CAPSULES

(Tretinoin) 3037
May interact with erythromycin and glucocorticoids. Compounds in these categories include:

Betamethasone Acetate (Potential for alteration of pharmacokinetic parameters in patients on concomitant drugs that are inducers of hepatic CYP enzymes). Products include:
Celestone Soluspan Injectable Suspension 3097

Betamethasone Sodium Phosphate (Potential for alteration of pharmacokinetic parameters in patients on concomitant drugs that are inducers of hepatic CYP enzymes). Products include:
Celestone Soluspan Injectable Suspension 3097

Cimetidine (Potential for alteration of pharmacokinetic parameters in patients on concomitant drugs that inhibit hepatic CYP enzymes). Products include:
Tagamet HB 200 Suspension .... ▣762
Tagamet HB 200 Tablets .... ▣761
Tagamet Tablets 1644

Cimetidine Hydrochloride (Potential for alteration of pharmacokinetic parameters in patients on concomitant drugs that inhibit hepatic CYP enzymes). Products include:
Tagamet 1644

Cortisone Acetate (Potential for alteration of pharmacokinetic parameters in patients on concomitant drugs that are inducers of hepatic CYP enzymes). Products include:
Cortone Acetate Injectable Suspension 2059
Cortone Acetate Tablets 2061

Cyclosporine (Potential for alteration of pharmacokinetic parameters in patients on concomitant drugs that inhibit hepatic CYP enzymes). Products include:
Gengraf Capsules 457
Neoral Soft Gelatin Capsules 2380
Neoral Oral Solution 2380
Sandimmune 2388

Dexamethasone (Potential for alteration of pharmacokinetic parameters in patients on concomitant drugs that are inducers of hepatic CYP enzymes). Products include:
Decadron Elixir 2078
Decadron Tablets 2079
TobraDex Ophthalmic Ointment 542
TobraDex Ophthalmic Suspension .. 541

Dexamethasone Acetate (Potential for alteration of pharmacokinetic parameters in patients on concomitant drugs that are inducers of hepatic CYP enzymes).
No products indexed under this heading.

Dexamethasone Sodium Phosphate (Potential for alteration of pharmacokinetic parameters in patients on concomitant drugs that are inducers of hepatic CYP enzymes). Products include:
Decadron Phosphate Injection 2081
Decadron Phosphate Sterile Ophthalmic Ointment 2083
Decadron Phosphate Sterile Ophthalmic Solution 2084
NeoDecadron Sterile Ophthalmic Solution 2144

Diltiazem Hydrochloride (Potential for alteration of pharmacokinetic parameters in patients on concomitant drugs that inhibit hepatic CYP enzymes). Products include:
Cardizem Injectable 1018
Cardizem Lyo-Ject Syringe 1018
Cardizem Monovial 1018
Cardizem CD Capsules 1016
Tiazac Capsules 1378

Erythromycin (Potential for alteration of pharmacokinetic parameters in patients on concomitant drugs that inhibit hepatic CYP enzymes). Products include:
Emgel 2% Topical Gel 1285
Ery-Tab Tablets 448
Erythromycin Base Filmtab Tablets . 454
Erythromycin Delayed-Release Capsules, USP 455
PCE Dispertab Tablets 498

Erythromycin Estolate (Potential for alteration of pharmacokinetic parameters in patients on concomitant drugs that inhibit hepatic CYP enzymes).
No products indexed under this heading.

Erythromycin Ethylsuccinate (Potential for alteration of pharmacokinetic parameters in patients on concomitant drugs that inhibit hepatic CYP enzymes). Products include:
E.E.S. 450
EryPed 446
Pediazole Suspension 3050

Erythromycin Gluceptate (Potential for alteration of pharmacokinetic parameters in patients on concomitant drugs that inhibit hepatic CYP enzymes).
No products indexed under this heading.

Erythromycin Stearate (Potential for alteration of pharmacokinetic parameters in patients on concomitant drugs that inhibit hepatic CYP enzymes). Products include:
Erythrocin Stearate Filmtab Tablets 452

Fludrocortisone Acetate (Potential for alteration of pharmacokinetic parameters in patients on concomitant drugs that are inducers of hepatic CYP enzymes). Products include:
Florinef Acetate Tablets 2250

Hydrocortisone (Potential for alteration of pharmacokinetic parameters in patients on concomitant drugs that are inducers of hepatic CYP enzymes). Products include:
Anusol-HC Cream 2.5% 2237
Cipro HC Otic Suspension 540
Cortaid Intensive Therapy Cream .. ▣717
Cortaid Maximum Strength Cream .... ▣717
Cortisporin Ophthalmic Suspension Sterile .... ⊙297
Cortizone•5 .... ▣699
Cortizone•10 .... ▣699
Cortizone•10 Plus Creme .... ▣700
Cortizone for Kids Creme .... ▣699
Hydrocortone Tablets 2106
Massengill Medicated Soft Cloth Towelette .... ▣753
VōSoL HC Otic Solution 3356

Hydrocortisone Acetate (Potential for alteration of pharmacokinetic parameters in patients on concomitant drugs that are inducers of hepatic CYP enzymes). Products include:
Analpram-HC 1338
Anusol HC-1 Hydrocortisone Anti-Itch Cream .... ▣689
Anusol-HC Suppositories 2238
Cortaid .... ▣717
Cortifoam Rectal Foam 3170
Cortisporin-TC Otic Suspension 2246
Hydrocortone Acetate Injectable Suspension 2103
Pramosone 1343
Proctocort Suppositories 2264
ProctoFoam-HC 3177
Terra-Cortril Ophthalmic Suspension 2716

Hydrocortisone Sodium Phosphate (Potential for alteration of pharmacokinetic parameters in patients on concomitant drugs that are inducers of hepatic CYP enzymes). Products include:
Hydrocortone Phosphate Injection, Sterile 2105

Hydrocortisone Sodium Succinate (Potential for alteration of pharmacokinetic parameters in patients on concomitant drugs that are inducers of hepatic CYP enzymes).
No products indexed under this heading.

Ketoconazole (Potential for alteration of pharmacokinetic parameters in patients on concomitant drugs that inhibit hepatic CYP enzymes). Products include:
Nizoral 2% Cream 3620
Nizoral A-D Shampoo 2008
Nizoral 2% Shampoo 2007
Nizoral Tablets 1791

Methylprednisolone Acetate (Potential for alteration of pharmacokinetic parameters in patients on concomitant drugs that are inducers of hepatic CYP enzymes). Products include:
Depo-Medrol Injectable Suspension 2795

Methylprednisolone Sodium Succinate (Potential for alteration of pharmacokinetic parameters in patients on concomitant drugs that are inducers of hepatic CYP enzymes). Products include:
Solu-Medrol Sterile Powder 2855

Pentobarbital Sodium (Potential for alteration of pharmacokinetic parameters in patients on concomitant drugs that are inducers of hepatic CYP enzymes). Products include:
Nembutal Sodium Solution 485

Phenobarbital (Potential for alteration of pharmacokinetic parameters in patients on concomitant drugs that are inducers of hepatic CYP enzymes). Products include:
Arco-Lase Plus Tablets 592
Donnatal 2929
Donnatal Extentabs 2930

Prednisolone Acetate (Potential for alteration of pharmacokinetic parameters in patients on concomitant drugs that are inducers of hepatic CYP enzymes). Products include:
- Blephamide Ophthalmic Ointment ... 547
- Blephamide Ophthalmic Suspension ... 548
- Poly-Pred Liquifilm Ophthalmic Suspension ... ⊙ 245
- Pred Forte Ophthalmic Suspension ... ⊙ 246
- Pred Mild Sterile Ophthalmic Suspension ... ⊙ 249
- Pred-G Ophthalmic Suspension ... ⊙ 247
- Pred-G Sterile Ophthalmic Ointment ... ⊙ 248

Prednisolone Sodium Phosphate (Potential for alteration of pharmacokinetic parameters in patients on concomitant drugs that are inducers of hepatic CYP enzymes). Products include:
- Pediapred Oral Solution ... 1170

Prednisolone Tebutate (Potential for alteration of pharmacokinetic parameters in patients on concomitant drugs that are inducers of hepatic CYP enzymes).
No products indexed under this heading.

Prednisone (Potential for alteration of pharmacokinetic parameters in patients on concomitant drugs that are inducers of hepatic CYP enzymes). Products include:
- Prednisone ... 3064

Rifampin (Potential for alteration of pharmacokinetic parameters in patients on concomitant drugs that are inducers of hepatic CYP enzymes). Products include:
- Rifadin ... 765
- Rifamate Capsules ... 767
- Rifater Tablets ... 769

Triamcinolone (Potential for alteration of pharmacokinetic parameters in patients on concomitant drugs that are inducers of hepatic CYP enzymes).
No products indexed under this heading.

Triamcinolone Acetonide (Potential for alteration of pharmacokinetic parameters in patients on concomitant drugs that are inducers of hepatic CYP enzymes). Products include:
- Azmacort Inhalation Aerosol ... 728
- Nasacort Nasal Inhaler ... 750
- Nasacort AQ Nasal Spray ... 752
- Tri-Nasal Spray ... 2274

Triamcinolone Diacetate (Potential for alteration of pharmacokinetic parameters in patients on concomitant drugs that are inducers of hepatic CYP enzymes).
No products indexed under this heading.

Triamcinolone Hexacetonide (Potential for alteration of pharmacokinetic parameters in patients on concomitant drugs that are inducers of hepatic CYP enzymes).
No products indexed under this heading.

Verapamil Hydrochloride (Potential for alteration of pharmacokinetic parameters in patients on concomitant drugs that inhibit hepatic CYP enzymes). Products include:
- Covera-HS Tablets ... 3199
- Isoptin SR Tablets ... 467
- Tarka Tablets ... 508
- Verelan Capsules ... 3184
- Verelan PM Capsules ... 3186

Food Interactions

Food, unspecified (The absorption of retinoids as a class has been shown to be enhanced when taken with food).

VEXOL 1% OPHTHALMIC SUSPENSION

(Rimexolone) ... ⊙ 222
None cited in PDR database.

VIADUR IMPLANT

(Leuprolide Acetate) ... 912
None cited in PDR database.

VIAGRA TABLETS

(Sildenafil Citrate) ... 2732
May interact with nonspecific beta-blockers, erythromycin, loop diuretics, protease inhibitors, potassium sparing diuretics, and certain other agents. Compounds in these categories include:

Alprostadil (The safety and efficacy of combinations of Viagra with other treatments for erectile dysfunction have not been studied, therefore, the use of such combinations is not recommended). Products include:
- Caverject Sterile Powder ... 2777
- MUSE Urethral Suppository ... 3335

Amiloride Hydrochloride (The AUC of the active metabolite, N-desmethyl sildenafil, was increased 62% by potassium-sparing diuretics; these effects on the metabolite are not expected to be of clinical consequence). Products include:
- Midamor Tablets ... 2136
- Moduretic Tablets ... 2138

Amlodipine Besylate (Co-administration in hypertensive patients has resulted in mean additional reduction on supine blood pressure by 8 mmHg systolic and 7 mmHg diastolic). Products include:
- Lotrel Capsules ... 2370
- Norvasc Tablets ... 2704

Amprenavir (Although the interaction between other protease inhibitors and sildenafil has not been studied, their concomitant use is expected to increase sildenafil levels). Products include:
- Agenerase Capsules ... 1454
- Agenerase Oral Solution ... 1459

Amyl Nitrite (Viagra has been shown to potentiate the hypotensive effects of nitrates, and its administration to patients who are using organic nitrates, either regularly and/or intermittently, in any form is therefore contraindicated).
No products indexed under this heading.

Bumetanide (The AUC of the active metabolite, N-desmethyl sildenafil, was increased 62% by loop diuretics; these effects on the metabolite are not expected to be of clinical consequence).
No products indexed under this heading.

Cimetidine (Co-administration of sildenafil with non-specific CYP inhibitors, such as cimetidine, has caused a 56% increase in plasma sildenafil concentrations; potential for reduction in sildenafil clearance). Products include:
- Tagamet HB 200 Suspension ... 762
- Tagamet HB 200 Tablets ... 761
- Tagamet Tablets ... 1644

Cimetidine Hydrochloride (Co-administration of sildenafil with nonspecific CYP inhibitors, such as cimetidine, has caused a 56% increase in plasma sildenafil concentrations; potential for reduction in sildenafil clearance). Products include:
- Tagamet ... 1644

Erythromycin (Co-administration of sildenafil with a specific CYP3A4 inhibitor, such as erythromycin, at steady state has resulted in a 182% increase in sildenafil systemic exposure; potential for reduction in sildenafil clearance). Products include:
- Emgel 2% Topical Gel ... 1285
- Ery-Tab Tablets ... 448
- Erythromycin Base Filmtab Tablets ... 454
- Erythromycin Delayed-Release Capsules, USP ... 455
- PCE Dispertab Tablets ... 498

Erythromycin Estolate (Co-administration of sildenafil with a specific CYP3A4 inhibitor, such as erythromycin, at steady state has resulted in a 182% increase in sildenafil systemic exposure; potential for reduction in sildenafil clearance).
No products indexed under this heading.

Erythromycin Ethylsuccinate (Co-administration of sildenafil with a specific CYP3A4 inhibitor, such as erythromycin, at steady state has resulted in a 182% increase in sildenafil systemic exposure; potential for reduction in sildenafil clearance). Products include:
- E.E.S. ... 450
- EryPed ... 446
- Pediazole Suspension ... 3050

Erythromycin Gluceptate (Co-administration of sildenafil with a specific CYP3A4 inhibitor, such as erythromycin, at steady state has resulted in a 182% increase in sildenafil systemic exposure; potential for reduction in sildenafil clearance).
No products indexed under this heading.

Erythromycin Stearate (Co-administration of sildenafil with a specific CYP3A4 inhibitor, such as erythromycin, at steady state has resulted in a 182% increase in sildenafil systemic exposure; potential for reduction in sildenafil clearance). Products include:
- Erythrocin Stearate Filmtab Tablets ... 452

Ethacrynic Acid (The AUC of the active metabolite, N-desmethyl sildenafil, was increased 62% by loop diuretics; these effects on the metabolite are not expected to be of clinical consequence). Products include:
- Edecrin Tablets ... 2091

Furosemide (The AUC of the active metabolite, N-desmethyl sildenafil, was increased 62% by loop diuretics; these effects on the metabolite are not expected to be of clinical consequence). Products include:
- Furosemide Tablets ... 2284

Indinavir Sulfate (Although the interaction between other protease inhibitors and sildenafil has not been studied, their concomitant use is expected to increase sildenafil levels). Products include:
- Crixivan Capsules ... 2070

Isosorbide Dinitrate (Viagra has been shown to potentiate the hypotensive effects of nitrates, and its administration to patients who are using organic nitrates, either regularly and/or intermittently, in any form is therefore contraindicated). Products include:
- Isordil Sublingual Tablets ... 3525
- Isordil Titradose Tablets ... 3526

Isosorbide Mononitrate (Viagra has been shown to potentiate the hypotensive effects of nitrates, and its administration to patients who are using organic nitrates, either regularly and/or intermittently, in any form is therefore contraindicated). Products include:
- Imdur Tablets ... 1826
- Ismo Tablets ... 3524

Itraconazole (Co-administration of sildenafil with a stronger CYP3A4 inhibitor, such as itraconazole, would be expected to have a greater effect on the increase in sildenafil systemic exposure and a reduction in sildenafil clearance). Products include:
- Sporanox Capsules ... 1800
- Sporanox Injection ... 1804
- Sporanox Injection ... 2509
- Sporanox Oral Solution ... 1808
- Sporanox Oral Solution ... 2512

Ketoconazole (Co-administration of sildenafil with a stronger CYP3A4 inhibitor, such as ketoconazole, would be expected to have a greater effect on the increase in sildenafil systemic exposure and a reduction in sildenafil clearance). Products include:
- Nizoral 2% Cream ... 3620
- Nizoral A-D Shampoo ... 2008
- Nizoral 2% Shampoo ... 2007
- Nizoral Tablets ... 1791

Labetalol Hydrochloride (Co-administration with nonspecific beta-blockers has resulted in the AUC of the active metabolite, N-desmethyl sildenafil by 102%; these effects on the metabolite are not expected to be of clinical consequences). Products include:
- Normodyne Injection ... 3135
- Normodyne Tablets ... 3137

Lopinavir (Although the interaction between other protease inhibitors and sildenafil has not been studied, their concomitant use is expected to increase sildenafil levels). Products include:
- Kaletra Capsules ... 471
- Kaletra Oral Solution ... 471

Nadolol (Co-administration with nonspecific beta-blockers has resulted in the AUC of the active metabolite, N-desmethyl sildenafil by 102%; these effects on the metabolite are not expected to be of clinical consequences). Products include:
- Corgard Tablets ... 2245
- Corzide 40/5 Tablets ... 2247
- Corzide 80/5 Tablets ... 2247
- Nadolol Tablets ... 2288

Nelfinavir Mesylate (Although the interaction between other protease inhibitors and sildenafil has not been studied, their concomitant use is expected to increase sildenafil levels). Products include:
- Viracept ... 532

Nitroglycerin (Viagra has been shown to potentiate the hypotensive effects of nitrates, and its administration to patients who are using organic nitrates, either regularly and/or intermittently, in any form is therefore contraindicated). Products include:
- Nitro-Dur Transdermal Infusion System ... 3134
- Nitro-Dur Transdermal Infusion System ... 1834
- Nitrolingual Pumpspray ... 1355
- Nitrostat Tablets ... 2658

Pindolol (Co-administration with nonspecific beta-blockers has resulted in the AUC of the active metabolite, N-desmethyl sildenafil by 102%; these effects on the metabolite are not expected to be of clinical consequences).
No products indexed under this heading.

Propranolol Hydrochloride (Co-administration with nonspecific beta-blockers has resulted in the AUC of the active metabolite, N-desmethyl sildenafil by 102%; these effects on the metabolite are not expected to be of clinical consequences). Products include:
- Inderal ... 3513
- Inderal LA Long-Acting Capsules ... 3516
- Inderide Tablets ... 3517
- Inderide LA Long-Acting Capsules ... 3519

Rifampin (Co-administration of sildenafil with CYP3A4 inducers, such as rifampin, would be expected to result in decreased plasma levels of sildenafil). Products include:
- Rifadin ... 765
- Rifamate Capsules ... 767
- Rifater Tablets ... 769

Ritonavir (Co-administration of ritonavir substantially increases serum concentrations of sildenafil, 11-fold increase in AUC; visual disturbances have occurred more com-

monly at higher systemic levels of sildenafil; decreased blood pressure, syncope, and prolonged erection have been reported in some healthy subjects exposed to high doses of sildenafil; a decrease in sildenafil dosage is recommended). Products include:
Kaletra Capsules 471
Kaletra Oral Solution 471
Norvir Capsules 487
Norvir Oral Solution 487

Saquinavir (Co-administration of HIV protease inhibitor saquinavir, CYP3A4 inhibitor, at steady-state has resulted in a 140% increase in sildenafil Cmax and a 210% increase in sildenafil plasma AUC). Products include:
Fortovase Capsules 2970

Saquinavir Mesylate (Although the interaction between other protease inhibitors and sildenafil has not been studied, their concomitant use is expected to increase sildenafil levels). Products include:
Invirase Capsules 2979

Spironolactone (The AUC of the active metabolite, N-desmethyl sildenafil, was increased 62% by potassium-sparing diuretics; these effects on the metabolite are not expected to be of clinical consequence).
No products indexed under this heading.

Timolol Maleate (Co-administration with nonspecific beta-blockers has resulted in the AUC of the active metabolite, N-desmethyl sildenafil by 102%; these effects on the metabolite are not expected to be of clinical consequences). Products include:
Blocadren Tablets 2046
Cosopt Sterile Ophthalmic Solution 2065
Timolide Tablets 2187
Timolol GFS .... ⊙266
Timoptic in Ocudose 2192
Timoptic Sterile Ophthalmic Solution 2190
Timoptic-XE Sterile Ophthalmic Gel Forming Solution 2194

Torsemide (The AUC of the active metabolite, N-desmethyl sildenafil, was increased 62% by loop diuretics; these effects on the metabolite are not expected to be of clinical consequence). Products include:
Demadex Tablets and Injection 2965

Triamterene (The AUC of the active metabolite, N-desmethyl sildenafil, was increased 62% by potassium-sparing diuretics; these effects on the metabolite are not expected to be of clinical consequence). Products include:
Dyazide Capsules 1515
Dyrenium Capsules 3458
Maxzide 1008

Food Interactions

Food, unspecified (When Viagra is taken with a high fat meal, the rate of absorption is reduced with a mean delay in Tmax of 60 minutes and a mean reduction in Cmax of 29%).

VIBRAMYCIN CALCIUM ORAL SUSPENSION SYRUP

(Doxycycline Calcium) 2735
See Vibramycin Hyclate Capsules

VIBRAMYCIN HYCLATE CAPSULES

(Doxycycline Hyclate) 2735
May interact with antacids containing aluminum, calcium and magnesium, barbiturates, oral anticoagulants, iron containing oral preparations, oral contraceptives, penicillins, and certain other agents. Compounds in these categories include:

Aluminum Carbonate (Co-administration with antacids containing aluminum, magnesium, and calcium may impair oral absorption of tetracyclines).
No products indexed under this heading.

Aluminum Hydroxide (Co-administration with antacids containing aluminum, magnesium, and calcium may impair oral absorption of tetracyclines). Products include:
Amphojel Suspension (Mint Flavor) .... ▣789
Gaviscon Extra Strength Liquid ..... ▣751
Gaviscon Extra Strength Tablets ... ▣751
Gaviscon Regular Strength Liquid . ▣751
Gaviscon Regular Strength Tablets .... ▣750
Maalox Antacid/Anti-Gas Oral Suspension .... ▣673
Maalox Max Maximum Strength Antacid/Anti-Gas Liquid 2300
Maalox Regular Strength Antacid/Antigas Liquid 2300
Mylanta 1813
Vanquish Caplets .... ▣617

Amoxicillin Trihydrate (Bacteriostatic drugs may interfere with bactericidal action of penicillin).

Ampicillin (Bacteriostatic drugs may interfere with bactericidal action of penicillin).
No products indexed under this heading.

Ampicillin Sodium (Bacteriostatic drugs may interfere with bactericidal action of penicillin). Products include:
Unasyn for Injection 2728

Ampicillin Trihydrate (Bacteriostatic drugs may interfere with bactericidal action of penicillin).
No products indexed under this heading.

Aprobarbital (Co-administration with barbiturates decreases the half-life of doxycycline).
No products indexed under this heading.

Azlocillin Sodium (Bacteriostatic drugs may interfere with bactericidal action of penicillin).
No products indexed under this heading.

Bacampicillin Hydrochloride (Bacteriostatic drugs may interfere with bactericidal action of penicillin).
No products indexed under this heading.

Bismuth Subsalicylate (Absorption of tetracyclines is impaired by bismuth subsalicylate). Products include:
Pepto-Bismol Maximum Strength Liquid 2878
Pepto-Bismol Original Liquid, Original and Cherry Tablets and Easy-To-Swallow Caplets 2878

Butabarbital (Co-administration with barbiturates decreases the half-life of doxycycline).
No products indexed under this heading.

Butalbital (Co-administration with barbiturates decreases the half-life of doxycycline). Products include:
Phrenilin 578
Sedapap Tablets 50 mg/650 mg ... 2225

Calcium Carbonate (Co-administration with antacids containing aluminum, magnesium, and calcium may impair oral absorption of tetracyclines). Products include:
Aspirin Regimen Bayer 81 mg Caplets with Calcium .... ▣607
Extra Strength Bayer Plus Caplets .... ▣610
Caltrate 600 Tablets .... ▣814
Caltrate 600 PLUS .... ▣815
Caltrate 600 + D Tablets .... ▣814
Caltrate 600 + Soy Tablets .... ▣814
D-Cal Chewable Caplets .... ▣794
Florical Capsules and Tablets 2223
Quick Dissolve Maalox Max Maximum Strength Antacid/Antigas Tablets 2301
Quick Dissolve Maalox Regular Strength Antacid Tablets 2301
Marblen Suspension .... ▣633
Monocal Tablets 2223
Mylanta Fast-Acting 1813
Mylanta Calci Tabs .... ▣636
One-A-Day Bedtime & Rest Tablets .... ▣805
One-A-Day Calcium Plus Chewable Tablets .... ▣805
Os-Cal Chewable Tablets .... ▣838
Pepcid Complete Chewable Tablets 1815
ReSource Wellness CalciWise Soft Chews .... ▣824
Rolaids Tablets .... ▣706
Extra Strength Rolaids Tablets ...... ▣706
Slow-Mag Tablets .... ▣835
Titralac .... ▣640
3M Titralac Plus Antacid Tablets ... ▣640
Tums .... ▣763

Carbamazepine (Decreases the half-life of doxycycline). Products include:
Carbatrol Capsules 3234
Tegretol/Tegretol-XR 2404

Carbenicillin Disodium (Bacteriostatic drugs may interfere with bactericidal action of penicillin).
No products indexed under this heading.

Carbenicillin Indanyl Sodium (Bacteriostatic drugs may interfere with bactericidal action of penicillin). Products include:
Geocillin Tablets 2687

Desogestrel (Concurrent use may render oral contraceptive less effective). Products include:
Cyclessa Tablets 2450
Desogen Tablets 2458
Mircette Tablets 2470
Ortho-Cept 21 Tablets 2546
Ortho-Cept 28 Tablets 2546

Dicloxacillin Sodium (Bacteriostatic drugs may interfere with bactericidal action of penicillin).
No products indexed under this heading.

Dicumarol (Depressed plasma prothrombin activity; may require downward adjustment of the anticoagulant dosage).
No products indexed under this heading.

Ethinyl Estradiol (Concurrent use may render oral contraceptive less effective). Products include:
Alesse-21 Tablets 3468
Alesse-28 Tablets 3473
Brevicon 28-Day Tablets 3380
Cyclessa Tablets 2450
Desogen Tablets 2458
Estinyl Tablets 3112
Estrostep 2627
femhrt Tablets 2635
Levlen 962
Levlite 21 Tablets 962
Levlite 28 Tablets 962
Levora Tablets 3389
Loestrin 21 Tablets 2642
Loestrin Fe Tablets 2642
Lo/Ovral Tablets 3532
Lo/Ovral-28 Tablets 3538
Low-Ogestrel-28 Tablets 3392
Microgestin Fe 1.5/30 Tablets 3407
Microgestin Fe 1/20 Tablets 3400
Mircette Tablets 2470
Modicon 2563
Necon 3415
Nordette-28 Tablets 2257
Norinyl 1 +35 28-Day Tablets 3380
Ogestrel 0.5/50-28 Tablets 3428
Ortho-Cept 21 Tablets 2546
Ortho-Cept 28 Tablets 2546
Ortho-Cyclen/Ortho Tri-Cyclen 2573
Ortho-Novum 2563
Ovcon 3364
Ovral Tablets 3551
Ovral-28 Tablets 3552
Tri-Levlen 962
Tri-Norinyl-28 Tablets 3433
Triphasil-21 Tablets 3600
Triphasil-28 Tablets 3605
Trivora Tablets 3439
Yasmin 28 Tablets 980
Zovia 3449

Ethynodiol Diacetate (Concurrent use may render oral contraceptive less effective). Products include:
Zovia 3449

Ferrous Fumarate (Co-administration with iron-containing preparations may impair oral absorption of tetracyclines). Products include:
New Formulation Chromagen OB Capsules 3094
Loestrin Fe Tablets 2642
NataChew Tablets 3364

Ferrous Gluconate (Co-administration with iron-containing preparations may impair oral absorption of tetracyclines). Products include:
Fergon Iron Tablets .... ▣802

Ferrous Sulfate (Co-administration with iron-containing preparations may impair oral absorption of tetracyclines). Products include:
Feosol Tablets 1717
Slow Fe Tablets .... ▣827
Slow Fe with Folic Acid Tablets ..... ▣828

Iron (Co-administration with iron-containing preparations may impair oral absorption of tetracyclines).
No products indexed under this heading.

Levonorgestrel (Concurrent use may render oral contraceptive less effective). Products include:
Alesse-21 Tablets 3468
Alesse-28 Tablets 3473
Levlen 962
Levlite 21 Tablets 962
Levlite 28 Tablets 962
Levora Tablets 3389
Mirena Intrauterine System 974
Nordette-28 Tablets 2257
Norplant System 3543
Tri-Levlen 962
Triphasil-21 Tablets 3600
Triphasil-28 Tablets 3605
Trivora Tablets 3439

Magaldrate (Co-administration with antacids containing aluminum, magnesium, and calcium may impair oral absorption of tetracyclines).
No products indexed under this heading.

Magnesium Hydroxide (Co-administration with antacids containing aluminum, magnesium, and calcium may impair oral absorption of tetracyclines). Products include:
Ex•Lax Milk of Magnesia Liquid .... ▣670
Maalox Antacid/Anti-Gas Oral Suspension .... ▣673
Maalox Max Maximum Strength Antacid/Anti-Gas Liquid 2300
Maalox Regular Strength Antacid/Antigas Liquid 2300
Mylanta Fast-Acting 1813
Mylanta 1813
Pepcid Complete Chewable Tablets 1815
Phillips' Chewable Tablets .... ▣615
Phillips' Milk of Magnesia Liquid (Original, Cherry, & Mint) .... ▣616
Rolaids Tablets .... ▣706
Extra Strength Rolaids Tablets ...... ▣706
Vanquish Caplets .... ▣617

Magnesium Oxide (Co-administration with antacids containing aluminum, magnesium, and calcium may impair oral absorption of tetracyclines). Products include:
Beelith Tablets 946
Mag-Ox 400 Tablets 1024
Uro-Mag Capsules 1024

Mephobarbital (Co-administration with barbiturates decreases the half-life of doxycycline).
No products indexed under this heading.

Mestranol (Concurrent use may render oral contraceptive less effective). Products include:
Necon 1/50 Tablets 3415
Norinyl 1 + 50 28-Day Tablets 3380
Ortho-Novum 1/50▫28 Tablets 2556

Methoxyflurane (Potential for fatal renal toxicity).
No products indexed under this heading.

Mezlocillin Sodium (Bacteriostatic drugs may interfere with bactericidal

action of penicillin).
No products indexed under this heading.

Nafcillin Sodium (Bacteriostatic drugs may interfere with bactericidal action of penicillin).
No products indexed under this heading.

Norethindrone (Concurrent use may render oral contraceptive less effective). Products include:
Brevicon 28-Day Tablets 3380
Micronor Tablets 2543
Modicon 2563
Necon 3415
Norinyl 1 +35 28-Day Tablets 3380
Norinyl 1 + 50 28-Day Tablets 3380
Nor-QD Tablets 3423
Ortho-Novum 2563
Ortho-Novum 1/50□28 Tablets 2556
Ovcon 3364
Tri-Norinyl-28 Tablets 3433

Norethynodrel (Concurrent use may render oral contraceptive less effective).
No products indexed under this heading.

Norgestimate (Concurrent use may render oral contraceptive less effective). Products include:
Ortho-Cyclen/Ortho Tri-Cyclen 2573
Ortho-Prefest Tablets 2570

Norgestrel (Concurrent use may render oral contraceptive less effective). Products include:
Lo/Ovral Tablets 3532
Lo/Ovral-28 Tablets 3538
Low-Ogestrel-28 Tablets 3392
Ogestrel 0.5/50-28 Tablets 3428
Ovral Tablets 3551
Ovral-28 Tablets 3552
Ovrette Tablets 3552

Penicillin G Benzathine (Bacteriostatic drugs may interfere with bactericidal action of penicillin). Products include:
Bicillin C-R 900/300 Injection 2240
Bicillin C-R Injection 2238
Bicillin L-A Injection 2242
Permapen Isoject 2706

Penicillin G Potassium (Bacteriostatic drugs may interfere with bactericidal action of penicillin). Products include:
Pfizerpen for Injection 2707

Penicillin G Procaine (Bacteriostatic drugs may interfere with bactericidal action of penicillin). Products include:
Bicillin C-R 900/300 Injection 2240
Bicillin C-R Injection 2238

Penicillin G Sodium (Bacteriostatic drugs may interfere with bactericidal action of penicillin).
No products indexed under this heading.

Penicillin V Potassium (Bacteriostatic drugs may interfere with bactericidal action of penicillin).
No products indexed under this heading.

Pentobarbital Sodium (Co-administration with barbiturates decreases the half-life of doxycycline). Products include:
Nembutal Sodium Solution 485

Phenobarbital (Co-administration with barbiturates decreases the half-life of doxycycline). Products include:
Arco-Lase Plus Tablets 592
Donnatal 2929
Donnatal Extentabs 2930

Phenytoin (Decreases the half-life of doxycycline). Products include:
Dilantin Infatabs 2624
Dilantin-125 Oral Suspension 2625

Phenytoin Sodium (Decreases the half-life of doxycycline). Products include:
Dilantin Kapseals 2622

Polysaccharide-Iron Complex (Co-administration with iron-containing preparations may impair oral absorption of tetracyclines). Products include:
Niferex 3176
Niferex-150 Capsules 3176
Nu-Iron 150 Capsules 2224

Secobarbital Sodium (Co-administration with barbiturates decreases the half-life of doxycycline).
No products indexed under this heading.

Thiamylal Sodium (Co-administration with barbiturates decreases the half-life of doxycycline).
No products indexed under this heading.

Ticarcillin Disodium (Bacteriostatic drugs may interfere with bactericidal action of penicillin). Products include:
Timentin Injection- ADD-Vantage Vial 1661
Timentin Injection-Galaxy Container 1664
Timentin Injection-Pharmacy Bulk Package 1666
Timentin for Intravenous Administration 1658

Warfarin Sodium (Depressed plasma prothrombin activity; may require downward adjustment of the anticoagulant dosage). Products include:
Coumadin for Injection 1243
Coumadin Tablets 1243
Warfarin Sodium Tablets, USP 3302

Food Interactions

Dairy products (Absorption of doxycycline is not markedly influenced by simultaneous ingestion of milk).

Food, unspecified (Absorption of doxycycline is not markedly influenced by simultaneous ingestion of food).

VIBRAMYCIN HYCLATE INTRAVENOUS
(Doxycycline Hyclate) 2737
May interact with anticoagulants and penicillins. Compounds in these categories include:

Amoxicillin Trihydrate (Interference with bactericidal action of penicillin).

Ampicillin (Interference with bactericidal action of penicillin).
No products indexed under this heading.

Ampicillin Sodium (Interference with bactericidal action of penicillin). Products include:
Unasyn for Injection 2728

Ampicillin Trihydrate (Interference with bactericidal action of penicillin).
No products indexed under this heading.

Ardeparin Sodium (Depressed plasma prothrombin activity; downward adjustment of anticoagulant dosage may be necessary).
No products indexed under this heading.

Azlocillin Sodium (Interference with bactericidal action of penicillin).
No products indexed under this heading.

Bacampicillin Hydrochloride (Interference with bactericidal action of penicillin).
No products indexed under this heading.

Carbenicillin Disodium (Interference with bactericidal action of penicillin).
No products indexed under this heading.

Carbenicillin Indanyl Sodium (Interference with bactericidal action of penicillin). Products include:
Geocillin Tablets 2687

Dalteparin Sodium (Depressed plasma prothrombin activity; downward adjustment of anticoagulant dosage may be necessary). Products include:
Fragmin Injection 2814

Danaparoid Sodium (Depressed plasma prothrombin activity; downward adjustment of anticoagulant dosage may be necessary). Products include:
Orgaran Injection 2480

Dicloxacillin Sodium (Interference with bactericidal action of penicillin).
No products indexed under this heading.

Dicumarol (Depressed plasma prothrombin activity; downward adjustment of anticoagulant dosage may be necessary).
No products indexed under this heading.

Enoxaparin (Depressed plasma prothrombin activity; downward adjustment of anticoagulant dosage may be necessary). Products include:
Lovenox Injection 746

Heparin Sodium (Depressed plasma prothrombin activity; downward adjustment of anticoagulant dosage may be necessary). Products include:
Heparin Lock Flush Solution 3509
Heparin Sodium Injection 3511

Mezlocillin Sodium (Interference with bactericidal action of penicillin).
No products indexed under this heading.

Nafcillin Sodium (Interference with bactericidal action of penicillin).
No products indexed under this heading.

Penicillin G Benzathine (Interference with bactericidal action of penicillin). Products include:
Bicillin C-R 900/300 Injection 2240
Bicillin C-R Injection 2238
Bicillin L-A Injection 2242
Permapen Isoject 2706

Penicillin G Potassium (Interference with bactericidal action of penicillin). Products include:
Pfizerpen for Injection 2707

Penicillin G Procaine (Interference with bactericidal action of penicillin). Products include:
Bicillin C-R 900/300 Injection 2240
Bicillin C-R Injection 2238

Penicillin G Sodium (Interference with bactericidal action of penicillin).
No products indexed under this heading.

Penicillin V Potassium (Interference with bactericidal action of penicillin).
No products indexed under this heading.

Ticarcillin Disodium (Interference with bactericidal action of penicillin). Products include:
Timentin Injection- ADD-Vantage Vial 1661
Timentin Injection-Galaxy Container 1664
Timentin Injection-Pharmacy Bulk Package 1666
Timentin for Intravenous Administration 1658

Tinzaparin sodium (Depressed plasma prothrombin activity; downward adjustment of anticoagulant dosage may be necessary). Products include:
Innohep Injection 1248

Warfarin Sodium (Depressed plasma prothrombin activity; downward adjustment of anticoagulant dosage may be necessary). Products include:
Coumadin for Injection 1243
Coumadin Tablets 1243
Warfarin Sodium Tablets, USP 3302

VIBRAMYCIN MONOHYDRATE FOR ORAL SUSPENSION
(Doxycycline Monohydrate) 2735
See Vibramycin Hyclate Capsules

VIBRA-TABS FILM COATED TABLETS
(Doxycycline Hyclate) 2735
See Vibramycin Hyclate Capsules

VICKS 44 COUGH RELIEF LIQUID
(Dextromethorphan Hydrobromide) .... □724
May interact with monoamine oxidase inhibitors. Compounds in these categories include:

Isocarboxazid (Concurrent or sequential use not recommended).
No products indexed under this heading.

Moclobemide (Concurrent or sequential use not recommended).
No products indexed under this heading.

Pargyline Hydrochloride (Concurrent or sequential use not recommended).
No products indexed under this heading.

Phenelzine Sulfate (Concurrent or sequential use not recommended). Products include:
Nardil Tablets 2653

Procarbazine Hydrochloride (Concurrent or sequential use not recommended). Products include:
Matulane Capsules 3246

Selegiline Hydrochloride (Concurrent or sequential use not recommended). Products include:
Eldepryl Capsules 3266

Tranylcypromine Sulfate (Concurrent or sequential use not recommended). Products include:
Parnate Tablets 1607

VICKS 44D COUGH & HEAD CONGESTION RELIEF LIQUID
(Dextromethorphan Hydrobromide, Pseudoephedrine Hydrochloride) .... □724
May interact with monoamine oxidase inhibitors. Compounds in these categories include:

Isocarboxazid (Concurrent and/or sequential use is not recommended).
No products indexed under this heading.

Moclobemide (Concurrent and/or sequential use is not recommended).
No products indexed under this heading.

Pargyline Hydrochloride (Concurrent and/or sequential use is not recommended).
No products indexed under this heading.

Phenelzine Sulfate (Concurrent and/or sequential use is not recommended). Products include:
Nardil Tablets 2653

Procarbazine Hydrochloride (Concurrent and/or sequential use is not recommended). Products include:
Matulane Capsules 3246

Selegiline Hydrochloride (Concurrent and/or sequential use is not recommended). Products include:
Eldepryl Capsules 3266

Tranylcypromine Sulfate (Concurrent and/or sequential use is not recommended). Products include:
Parnate Tablets 1607

VICKS 44E COUGH & CHEST CONGESTION RELIEF LIQUID
(Dextromethorphan Hydrobromide, Guaifenesin) .... □725
May interact with monoamine oxidase inhibitors. Compounds in these categories include:

Isocarboxazid (Concurrent and/or sequential use is not recommended).
No products indexed under this heading.

IMPORTANT NOTE: Always consult each drug listing in the patient's regimen for possible interactions.

Moclobemide (Concurrent and/or sequential use is not recommended).
No products indexed under this heading.

Pargyline Hydrochloride (Concurrent and/or sequential use is not recommended).
No products indexed under this heading.

Phenelzine Sulfate (Concurrent and/or sequential use is not recommended). Products include:
Nardil Tablets 2653

Procarbazine Hydrochloride (Concurrent and/or sequential use is not recommended). Products include:
Matulane Capsules 3246

Selegiline Hydrochloride (Concurrent and/or sequential use is not recommended). Products include:
Eldepryl Capsules 3266

Tranylcypromine Sulfate (Concurrent and/or sequential use is not recommended). Products include:
Parnate Tablets 1607

PEDIATRIC VICKS 44E COUGH & CHEST CONGESTION RELIEF LIQUID

(Dextromethorphan Hydrobromide, Guaifenesin) ....▣728
May interact with monoamine oxidase inhibitors. Compounds in these categories include:

Isocarboxazid (Concurrent and/or sequential use is not recommended).
No products indexed under this heading.

Moclobemide (Concurrent and/or sequential use is not recommended).
No products indexed under this heading.

Pargyline Hydrochloride (Concurrent and/or sequential use is not recommended).
No products indexed under this heading.

Phenelzine Sulfate (Concurrent and/or sequential use is not recommended). Products include:
Nardil Tablets 2653

Procarbazine Hydrochloride (Concurrent and/or sequential use is not recommended). Products include:
Matulane Capsules 3246

Selegiline Hydrochloride (Concurrent and/or sequential use is not recommended). Products include:
Eldepryl Capsules 3266

Tranylcypromine Sulfate (Concurrent and/or sequential use is not recommended). Products include:
Parnate Tablets 1607

VICKS 44M COUGH, COLD & FLU RELIEF LIQUID

(Acetaminophen, Chlorpheniramine Maleate, Dextromethorphan Hydrobromide, Pseudoephedrine Hydrochloride) .....▣725
May interact with hypnotics and sedatives, monoamine oxidase inhibitors, tranquilizers, and certain other agents. Compounds in these categories include:

Alprazolam (May increase drowsiness effect). Products include:
Xanax Tablets 2865

Buspirone Hydrochloride (May increase drowsiness effect).
No products indexed under this heading.

Chlordiazepoxide (May increase drowsiness effect). Products include:
Limbitrol 1738

Chlordiazepoxide Hydrochloride (May increase drowsiness effect). Products include:
Librium Capsules 1736
Librium for Injection 1737

Chlorpromazine (May increase drowsiness effect). Products include:
Thorazine Suppositories 1656

Chlorpromazine Hydrochloride (May increase drowsiness effect). Products include:
Thorazine 1656

Chlorprothixene (May increase drowsiness effect).
No products indexed under this heading.

Chlorprothixene Hydrochloride (May increase drowsiness effect).
No products indexed under this heading.

Clorazepate Dipotassium (May increase drowsiness effect). Products include:
Tranxene 511

Diazepam (May increase drowsiness effect). Products include:
Valium Injectable 3026
Valium Tablets 3047

Droperidol (May increase drowsiness effect).
No products indexed under this heading.

Estazolam (May increase drowsiness effect). Products include:
ProSom Tablets 500

Ethchlorvynol (May increase drowsiness effect).
No products indexed under this heading.

Ethinamate (May increase drowsiness effect).
No products indexed under this heading.

Fluphenazine Decanoate (May increase drowsiness effect).
No products indexed under this heading.

Fluphenazine Enanthate (May increase drowsiness effect).
No products indexed under this heading.

Fluphenazine Hydrochloride (May increase drowsiness effect).
No products indexed under this heading.

Flurazepam Hydrochloride (May increase drowsiness effect).
No products indexed under this heading.

Glutethimide (May increase drowsiness effect).
No products indexed under this heading.

Haloperidol (May increase drowsiness effect). Products include:
Haldol Injection, Tablets and Concentrate 2533

Haloperidol Decanoate (May increase drowsiness effect). Products include:
Haldol Decanoate 2535

Hydroxyzine Hydrochloride (May increase drowsiness effect). Products include:
Atarax Tablets & Syrup 2667
Vistaril Intramuscular Solution 2738

Isocarboxazid (Concurrent and/or sequential use with MAO inhibitors is not recommended).
No products indexed under this heading.

Lorazepam (May increase drowsiness effect). Products include:
Ativan Injection 3478
Ativan Tablets 3482

Loxapine Hydrochloride (May increase drowsiness effect).
No products indexed under this heading.

Loxapine Succinate (May increase drowsiness effect). Products include:
Loxitane Capsules 3398

Meprobamate (May increase drowsiness effect). Products include:
Miltown Tablets 3349

Mesoridazine Besylate (May increase drowsiness effect). Products include:
Serentil 1057

Midazolam Hydrochloride (May increase drowsiness effect). Products include:
Versed Injection 3027
Versed Syrup 3033

Moclobemide (Concurrent and/or sequential use with MAO inhibitors is not recommended).
No products indexed under this heading.

Molindone Hydrochloride (May increase drowsiness effect). Products include:
Moban 1320

Oxazepam (May increase drowsiness effect).
No products indexed under this heading.

Pargyline Hydrochloride (Concurrent and/or sequential use with MAO inhibitors is not recommended).
No products indexed under this heading.

Perphenazine (May increase drowsiness effect). Products include:
Etrafon 3115
Trilafon 3160

Phenelzine Sulfate (Concurrent and/or sequential use with MAO inhibitors is not recommended). Products include:
Nardil Tablets 2653

Prazepam (May increase drowsiness effect).
No products indexed under this heading.

Procarbazine Hydrochloride (Concurrent and/or sequential use with MAO inhibitors is not recommended). Products include:
Matulane Capsules 3246

Prochlorperazine (May increase drowsiness effect). Products include:
Compazine 1505

Promethazine Hydrochloride (May increase drowsiness effect). Products include:
Mepergan Injection 3539
Phenergan Injection 3553
Phenergan 3556
Phenergan Syrup 3554
Phenergan with Codeine Syrup 3557
Phenergan with Dextromethorphan Syrup 3559
Phenergan VC Syrup 3560
Phenergan VC with Codeine Syrup . 3561

Propofol (May increase drowsiness effect). Products include:
Diprivan Injectable Emulsion 667

Quazepam (May increase drowsiness effect).
No products indexed under this heading.

Secobarbital Sodium (May increase drowsiness effect).
No products indexed under this heading.

Selegiline Hydrochloride (Concurrent and/or sequential use with MAO inhibitors is not recommended). Products include:
Eldepryl Capsules 3266

Temazepam (May increase drowsiness effect).
No products indexed under this heading.

Thioridazine Hydrochloride (May increase drowsiness effect). Products include:
Thioridazine Hydrochloride Tablets 2289

Thiothixene (May increase drowsiness effect). Products include:
Navane Capsules 2701
Thiothixene Capsules 2290

Tranylcypromine Sulfate (Concurrent and/or sequential use with MAO inhibitors is not recommended). Products include:
Parnate Tablets 1607

Triazolam (May increase drowsiness effect). Products include:
Halcion Tablets 2823

Trifluoperazine Hydrochloride (May increase drowsiness effect). Products include:
Stelazine 1640

Zaleplon (May increase drowsiness effect). Products include:
Sonata Capsules 3591

Zolpidem Tartrate (May increase drowsiness effect). Products include:
Ambien Tablets 3191

Food Interactions

Alcohol (May increase drowsiness effect; patients consuming 3 or more alcoholic drinks per day should consult their physician for advice on when and how they should take this medication).

PEDIATRIC VICKS 44M COUGH & COLD RELIEF

(Chlorpheniramine Maleate, Dextromethorphan Hydrobromide, Pseudoephedrine Hydrochloride) .....▣728
May interact with hypnotics and sedatives, monoamine oxidase inhibitors, tranquilizers, and certain other agents. Compounds in these categories include:

Alprazolam (May increase drowsiness effect). Products include:
Xanax Tablets 2865

Buspirone Hydrochloride (May increase drowsiness effect).
No products indexed under this heading.

Chlordiazepoxide (May increase drowsiness effect). Products include:
Limbitrol 1738

Chlordiazepoxide Hydrochloride (May increase drowsiness effect). Products include:
Librium Capsules 1736
Librium for Injection 1737

Chlorpromazine (May increase drowsiness effect). Products include:
Thorazine Suppositories 1656

Chlorpromazine Hydrochloride (May increase drowsiness effect). Products include:
Thorazine 1656

Chlorprothixene (May increase drowsiness effect).
No products indexed under this heading.

Chlorprothixene Hydrochloride (May increase drowsiness effect).
No products indexed under this heading.

Clorazepate Dipotassium (May increase drowsiness effect). Products include:
Tranxene 511

Diazepam (May increase drowsiness effect). Products include:
Valium Injectable 3026
Valium Tablets 3047

Droperidol (May increase drowsiness effect).
No products indexed under this heading.

Estazolam (May increase drowsiness effect). Products include:
ProSom Tablets 500

Ethchlorvynol (May increase drowsiness effect).
No products indexed under this heading.

Ethinamate (May increase drowsiness effect).
No products indexed under this heading.

Fluphenazine Decanoate (May increase drowsiness effect).
No products indexed under this heading.

Fluphenazine Enanthate (May increase drowsiness effect).
No products indexed under this heading.

Fluphenazine Hydrochloride (May increase drowsiness effect).
No products indexed under this heading.

Flurazepam Hydrochloride (May increase drowsiness effect).
No products indexed under this heading.

Glutethimide (May increase drowsiness effect).
No products indexed under this heading.

Haloperidol (May increase drowsiness effect). Products include:
Haldol Injection, Tablets and Concentrate 2533

Haloperidol Decanoate (May increase drowsiness effect). Products include:
Haldol Decanoate 2535

Hydroxyzine Hydrochloride (May increase drowsiness effect). Products include:
Atarax Tablets & Syrup 2667
Vistaril Intramuscular Solution 2738

Isocarboxazid (Concurrent and/or sequential use is not recommended).
No products indexed under this heading.

Lorazepam (May increase drowsiness effect). Products include:
Ativan Injection 3478
Ativan Tablets 3482

Loxapine Hydrochloride (May increase drowsiness effect).
No products indexed under this heading.

Loxapine Succinate (May increase drowsiness effect). Products include:
Loxitane Capsules 3398

Meprobamate (May increase drowsiness effect). Products include:
Miltown Tablets 3349

Mesoridazine Besylate (May increase drowsiness effect). Products include:
Serentil 1057

Midazolam Hydrochloride (May increase drowsiness effect). Products include:
Versed Injection 3027
Versed Syrup 3033

Moclobemide (Concurrent and/or sequential use is not recommended).
No products indexed under this heading.

Molindone Hydrochloride (May increase drowsiness effect). Products include:
Moban 1320

Oxazepam (May increase drowsiness effect).
No products indexed under this heading.

Pargyline Hydrochloride (Concurrent and/or sequential use is not recommended).
No products indexed under this heading.

Perphenazine (May increase drowsiness effect). Products include:
Etrafon 3115
Trilafon 3160

Phenelzine Sulfate (Concurrent and/or sequential use is not recommended). Products include:
Nardil Tablets 2653

Prazepam (May increase drowsiness effect).
No products indexed under this heading.

Procarbazine Hydrochloride (Concurrent and/or sequential use is not recommended). Products include:
Matulane Capsules 3246

Prochlorperazine (May increase drowsiness effect). Products include:
Compazine 1505

Promethazine Hydrochloride (May increase drowsiness effect). Products include:
Mepergan Injection 3539
Phenergan Injection 3553
Phenergan 3556
Phenergan Syrup 3554
Phenergan with Codeine Syrup 3557
Phenergan with Dextromethorphan Syrup 3559
Phenergan VC Syrup 3560
Phenergan VC with Codeine Syrup 3561

Propofol (May increase drowsiness effect). Products include:
Diprivan Injectable Emulsion 667

Quazepam (May increase drowsiness effect).
No products indexed under this heading.

Secobarbital Sodium (May increase drowsiness effect).
No products indexed under this heading.

Selegiline Hydrochloride (Concurrent and/or sequential use is not recommended). Products include:
Eldepryl Capsules 3266

Temazepam (May increase drowsiness effect).
No products indexed under this heading.

Thioridazine Hydrochloride (May increase drowsiness effect). Products include:
Thioridazine Hydrochloride Tablets 2289

Thiothixene (May increase drowsiness effect). Products include:
Navane Capsules 2701
Thiothixene Capsules 2290

Tranylcypromine Sulfate (Concurrent and/or sequential use is not recommended). Products include:
Parnate Tablets 1607

Triazolam (May increase drowsiness effect). Products include:
Halcion Tablets 2823

Trifluoperazine Hydrochloride (May increase drowsiness effect). Products include:
Stelazine 1640

Zaleplon (May increase drowsiness effect). Products include:
Sonata Capsules 3591

Zolpidem Tartrate (May increase drowsiness effect). Products include:
Ambien Tablets 3191

Food Interactions

Alcohol (May increase drowsiness effect).

VICKS COUGH DROPS, MENTHOL AND CHERRY FLAVORS

(Menthol) .... ▣726
None cited in PDR database.

VICKS DAYQUIL LIQUICAPS/LIQUID MULTI-SYMPTOM COLD/FLU RELIEF

(Acetaminophen, Dextromethorphan Hydrobromide, Pseudoephedrine Hydrochloride) .... ▣727
May interact with monoamine oxidase inhibitors and certain other agents. Compounds in these categories include:

Isocarboxazid (Concurrent and/or sequential use with MAO inhibitors is not recommended).
No products indexed under this heading.

Moclobemide (Concurrent and/or sequential use with MAO inhibitors is not recommended).
No products indexed under this heading.

Pargyline Hydrochloride (Concurrent and/or sequential use with MAO inhibitors is not recommended).
No products indexed under this heading.

Phenelzine Sulfate (Concurrent and/or sequential use with MAO inhibitors is not recommended). Products include:
Nardil Tablets 2653

Procarbazine Hydrochloride (Concurrent and/or sequential use with MAO inhibitors is not recommended). Products include:
Matulane Capsules 3246

Selegiline Hydrochloride (Concurrent and/or sequential use with MAO inhibitors is not recommended). Products include:
Eldepryl Capsules 3266

Tranylcypromine Sulfate (Concurrent and/or sequential use with MAO inhibitors is not recommended). Products include:
Parnate Tablets 1607

Food Interactions

Alcohol (Patients consuming 3 or more alcoholic drinks per day should consult their physician for advice on when and how they should take this medication).

CHILDREN'S VICKS NYQUIL COLD/COUGH RELIEF

(Chlorpheniramine Maleate, Dextromethorphan Hydrobromide, Pseudoephedrine Hydrochloride) .... ▣726
May interact with hypnotics and sedatives, monoamine oxidase inhibitors, tranquilizers, and certain other agents. Compounds in these categories include:

Alprazolam (May increase drowsiness effect). Products include:
Xanax Tablets 2865

Buspirone Hydrochloride (May increase drowsiness effect).
No products indexed under this heading.

Chlordiazepoxide (May increase drowsiness effect). Products include:
Limbitrol 1738

Chlordiazepoxide Hydrochloride (May increase drowsiness effect). Products include:
Librium Capsules 1736
Librium for Injection 1737

Chlorpromazine (May increase drowsiness effect). Products include:
Thorazine Suppositories 1656

Chlorpromazine Hydrochloride (May increase drowsiness effect). Products include:
Thorazine 1656

Chlorprothixene (May increase drowsiness effect).
No products indexed under this heading.

Chlorprothixene Hydrochloride (May increase drowsiness effect).
No products indexed under this heading.

Clorazepate Dipotassium (May increase drowsiness effect). Products include:
Tranxene 511

Diazepam (May increase drowsiness effect). Products include:
Valium Injectable 3026
Valium Tablets 3047

Droperidol (May increase drowsiness effect).
No products indexed under this heading.

Estazolam (May increase drowsiness effect). Products include:
ProSom Tablets 500

Ethchlorvynol (May increase drowsiness effect).
No products indexed under this heading.

Ethinamate (May increase drowsiness effect).
No products indexed under this heading.

Fluphenazine Decanoate (May increase drowsiness effect).
No products indexed under this heading.

Fluphenazine Enanthate (May increase drowsiness effect).
No products indexed under this heading.

Fluphenazine Hydrochloride (May increase drowsiness effect).
No products indexed under this heading.

Flurazepam Hydrochloride (May increase drowsiness effect).
No products indexed under this heading.

Glutethimide (May increase drowsiness effect).
No products indexed under this heading.

Haloperidol (May increase drowsiness effect). Products include:
Haldol Injection, Tablets and Concentrate 2533

Haloperidol Decanoate (May increase drowsiness effect). Products include:
Haldol Decanoate 2535

Hydroxyzine Hydrochloride (May increase drowsiness effect). Products include:
Atarax Tablets & Syrup 2667
Vistaril Intramuscular Solution 2738

Isocarboxazid (Concurrent and/or sequential use with MAO inhibitors is not recommended).
No products indexed under this heading.

Lorazepam (May increase drowsiness effect). Products include:
Ativan Injection 3478
Ativan Tablets 3482

Loxapine Hydrochloride (May increase drowsiness effect).
No products indexed under this heading.

Loxapine Succinate (May increase drowsiness effect). Products include:
Loxitane Capsules 3398

Meprobamate (May increase drowsiness effect). Products include:
Miltown Tablets 3349

Mesoridazine Besylate (May increase drowsiness effect). Products include:
Serentil 1057

Midazolam Hydrochloride (May increase drowsiness effect). Products include:
Versed Injection 3027
Versed Syrup 3033

Moclobemide (Concurrent and/or sequential use with MAO inhibitors is not recommended).
No products indexed under this heading.

Molindone Hydrochloride (May increase drowsiness effect). Products include:
Moban 1320

Oxazepam (May increase drowsiness effect).
No products indexed under this heading.

Pargyline Hydrochloride (Concurrent and/or sequential use with MAO inhibitors is not recommended).
No products indexed under this heading.

Perphenazine (May increase drowsiness effect). Products include:
Etrafon 3115
Trilafon 3160

Phenelzine Sulfate (Concurrent and/or sequential use with MAO inhibitors is not recommended). Products include:
Nardil Tablets 2653

IMPORTANT NOTE: Always consult each drug listing in the patient's regimen for possible interactions.

Prazepam (May increase drowsiness effect).
No products indexed under this heading.

Procarbazine Hydrochloride (Concurrent and/or sequential use with MAO inhibitors is not recommended). Products include:
Matulane Capsules 3246

Prochlorperazine (May increase drowsiness effect). Products include:
Compazine 1505

Promethazine Hydrochloride (May increase drowsiness effect). Products include:
Mepergan Injection 3539
Phenergan Injection 3553
Phenergan 3556
Phenergan Syrup 3554
Phenergan with Codeine Syrup 3557
Phenergan with Dextromethorphan Syrup 3559
Phenergan VC Syrup 3560
Phenergan VC with Codeine Syrup .. 3561

Propofol (May increase drowsiness effect). Products include:
Diprivan Injectable Emulsion 667

Quazepam (May increase drowsiness effect).
No products indexed under this heading.

Secobarbital Sodium (May increase drowsiness effect).
No products indexed under this heading.

Selegiline Hydrochloride (Concurrent and/or sequential use with MAO inhibitors is not recommended). Products include:
Eldepryl Capsules 3266

Temazepam (May increase drowsiness effect).
No products indexed under this heading.

Thioridazine Hydrochloride (May increase drowsiness effect). Products include:
Thioridazine Hydrochloride Tablets 2289

Thiothixene (May increase drowsiness effect). Products include:
Navane Capsules 2701
Thiothixene Capsules 2290

Tranylcypromine Sulfate (Concurrent and/or sequential use with MAO inhibitors is not recommended). Products include:
Parnate Tablets 1607

Triazolam (May increase drowsiness effect). Products include:
Halcion Tablets 2823

Trifluoperazine Hydrochloride (May increase drowsiness effect). Products include:
Stelazine 1640

Zaleplon (May increase drowsiness effect). Products include:
Sonata Capsules 3591

Zolpidem Tartrate (May increase drowsiness effect). Products include:
Ambien Tablets 3191

Food Interactions

Alcohol (May increase drowsiness effect).

VICKS NYQUIL LIQUICAPS/LIQUID MULTI-SYMPTOM COLD/FLU RELIEF, ORIGINAL AND CHERRY FLAVORS

(Acetaminophen, Dextromethorphan Hydrobromide, Doxylamine Succinate, Pseudoephedrine Hydrochloride) .... ▣727
May interact with hypnotics and sedatives, monoamine oxidase inhibitors, tranquilizers, and certain other agents. Compounds in these categories include:

Alprazolam (May increase drowsiness effect). Products include:
Xanax Tablets 2865

Buspirone Hydrochloride (May increase drowsiness effect).
No products indexed under this heading.

Chlordiazepoxide (May increase drowsiness effect). Products include:
Limbitrol 1738

Chlordiazepoxide Hydrochloride (May increase drowsiness effect). Products include:
Librium Capsules 1736
Librium for Injection 1737

Chlorpromazine (May increase drowsiness effect). Products include:
Thorazine Suppositories 1656

Chlorpromazine Hydrochloride (May increase drowsiness effect). Products include:
Thorazine 1656

Chlorprothixene (May increase drowsiness effect).
No products indexed under this heading.

Chlorprothixene Hydrochloride (May increase drowsiness effect).
No products indexed under this heading.

Clorazepate Dipotassium (May increase drowsiness effect). Products include:
Tranxene 511

Diazepam (May increase drowsiness effect). Products include:
Valium Injectable 3026
Valium Tablets 3047

Droperidol (May increase drowsiness effect).
No products indexed under this heading.

Estazolam (May increase drowsiness effect). Products include:
ProSom Tablets 500

Ethchlorvynol (May increase drowsiness effect).
No products indexed under this heading.

Ethinamate (May increase drowsiness effect).
No products indexed under this heading.

Fluphenazine Decanoate (May increase drowsiness effect).
No products indexed under this heading.

Fluphenazine Enanthate (May increase drowsiness effect).
No products indexed under this heading.

Fluphenazine Hydrochloride (May increase drowsiness effect).
No products indexed under this heading.

Flurazepam Hydrochloride (May increase drowsiness effect).
No products indexed under this heading.

Glutethimide (May increase drowsiness effect).
No products indexed under this heading.

Haloperidol (May increase drowsiness effect). Products include:
Haldol Injection, Tablets and Concentrate 2533

Haloperidol Decanoate (May increase drowsiness effect). Products include:
Haldol Decanoate 2535

Hydroxyzine Hydrochloride (May increase drowsiness effect). Products include:
Atarax Tablets & Syrup 2667
Vistaril Intramuscular Solution 2738

Isocarboxazid (Concurrent and/or sequential use with MAO inhibitors is not recommended).
No products indexed under this heading.

Lorazepam (May increase drowsiness effect). Products include:
Ativan Injection 3478
Ativan Tablets 3482

Loxapine Hydrochloride (May increase drowsiness effect).
No products indexed under this heading.

Loxapine Succinate (May increase drowsiness effect). Products include:
Loxitane Capsules 3398

Meprobamate (May increase drowsiness effect). Products include:
Miltown Tablets 3349

Mesoridazine Besylate (May increase drowsiness effect). Products include:
Serentil 1057

Midazolam Hydrochloride (May increase drowsiness effect). Products include:
Versed Injection 3027
Versed Syrup 3033

Moclobemide (Concurrent and/or sequential use with MAO inhibitors is not recommended).
No products indexed under this heading.

Molindone Hydrochloride (May increase drowsiness effect). Products include:
Moban 1320

Oxazepam (May increase drowsiness effect).
No products indexed under this heading.

Pargyline Hydrochloride (Concurrent and/or sequential use with MAO inhibitors is not recommended).
No products indexed under this heading.

Perphenazine (May increase drowsiness effect). Products include:
Etrafon 3115
Trilafon 3160

Phenelzine Sulfate (Concurrent and/or sequential use with MAO inhibitors is not recommended). Products include:
Nardil Tablets 2653

Prazepam (May increase drowsiness effect).
No products indexed under this heading.

Procarbazine Hydrochloride (Concurrent and/or sequential use with MAO inhibitors is not recommended). Products include:
Matulane Capsules 3246

Prochlorperazine (May increase drowsiness effect). Products include:
Compazine 1505

Promethazine Hydrochloride (May increase drowsiness effect). Products include:
Mepergan Injection 3539
Phenergan Injection 3553
Phenergan 3556
Phenergan Syrup 3554
Phenergan with Codeine Syrup 3557
Phenergan with Dextromethorphan Syrup 3559
Phenergan VC Syrup 3560
Phenergan VC with Codeine Syrup .. 3561

Propofol (May increase drowsiness effect). Products include:
Diprivan Injectable Emulsion 667

Quazepam (May increase drowsiness effect).
No products indexed under this heading.

Secobarbital Sodium (May increase drowsiness effect).
No products indexed under this heading.

Selegiline Hydrochloride (Concurrent and/or sequential use with MAO inhibitors is not recommended). Products include:
Eldepryl Capsules 3266

Temazepam (May increase drowsiness effect).
No products indexed under this heading.

Thioridazine Hydrochloride (May increase drowsiness effect). Products include:
Thioridazine Hydrochloride Tablets 2289

Thiothixene (May increase drowsiness effect). Products include:
Navane Capsules 2701
Thiothixene Capsules 2290

Tranylcypromine Sulfate (Concurrent and/or sequential use with MAO inhibitors is not recommended). Products include:
Parnate Tablets 1607

Triazolam (May increase drowsiness effect). Products include:
Halcion Tablets 2823

Trifluoperazine Hydrochloride (May increase drowsiness effect). Products include:
Stelazine 1640

Zaleplon (May increase drowsiness effect). Products include:
Sonata Capsules 3591

Zolpidem Tartrate (May increase drowsiness effect). Products include:
Ambien Tablets 3191

Food Interactions

Alcohol (May increase drowsiness effect; patients consuming 3 or more alcoholic drinks per day should consult their physician for advice on when and how they should take this medication).

VICKS SINEX NASAL SPRAY AND ULTRA FINE MIST

(Phenylephrine Hydrochloride) .... ▣729
None cited in PDR database.

VICKS SINEX 12-HOUR NASAL SPRAY AND ULTRA FINE MIST

(Oxymetazoline Hydrochloride) .... ▣729
None cited in PDR database.

VICKS VAPOR INHALER

(Levmetamfetamine) .... ▣730
None cited in PDR database.

VICKS VAPORUB CREAM

(Camphor, Menthol) .... ▣730
None cited in PDR database.

VICKS VAPORUB OINTMENT

(Camphor, Eucalyptus, Oil of, Menthol) .... ▣730
None cited in PDR database.

VICKS VAPOSTEAM

(Camphor) .... ▣730
None cited in PDR database.

VICODIN TABLETS

(Acetaminophen, Hydrocodone Bitartrate) 516
May interact with antihistamines, central nervous system depressants, monoamine oxidase inhibitors, narcotic analgesics, tricyclic antidepressants, and certain other agents. Compounds in these categories include:

Acrivastine (May exhibit an additive CNS depression). Products include:
Semprex-D Capsules 1172

Alfentanil Hydrochloride (May exhibit an additive CNS depression).
No products indexed under this heading.

Alprazolam (May exhibit an additive CNS depression). Products include:
Xanax Tablets 2865

Amitriptyline Hydrochloride (Co-administration may increase the effect of either antidepressant or hydrocodone). Products include:
Etrafon 3115
Limbitrol 1738

Amoxapine (Co-administration may increase the effect of either antide-

pressant or hydrocodone).
No products indexed under this heading.

Aprobarbital (May exhibit an additive CNS depression).
No products indexed under this heading.

Astemizole (May exhibit an additive CNS depression).
No products indexed under this heading.

Azatadine Maleate (May exhibit an additive CNS depression). Products include:
Rynatan Tablets 3351

Bromodiphenhydramine Hydrochloride (May exhibit an additive CNS depression).
No products indexed under this heading.

Brompheniramine Maleate (May exhibit an additive CNS depression). Products include:
Bromfed Capsules (Extended-Release)........ 2269
Bromfed-PD Capsules (Extended-Release)........ 2269
Comtrex Acute Head Cold & Sinus Pressure Relief Tablets........ 627
Dimetapp Elixir........ 777
Dimetapp Cold and Fever Suspension........ 775
Dimetapp DM Cold & Cough Elixir........ 775
Dimetapp Nighttime Flu Liquid........ 776

Buprenorphine Hydrochloride (May exhibit an additive CNS depression). Products include:
Buprenex Injectable 2918

Buspirone Hydrochloride (May exhibit an additive CNS depression).
No products indexed under this heading.

Butabarbital (May exhibit an additive CNS depression).
No products indexed under this heading.

Butalbital (May exhibit an additive CNS depression). Products include:
Phrenilin 578
Sedapap Tablets 50 mg/650 mg 2225

Cetirizine Hydrochloride (May exhibit an additive CNS depression). Products include:
Zyrtec 2756
Zyrtec-D 12 Hour Extended Relief Tablets........ 2758

Chlordiazepoxide (May exhibit an additive CNS depression). Products include:
Limbitrol 1738

Chlordiazepoxide Hydrochloride (May exhibit an additive CNS depression). Products include:
Librium Capsules 1736
Librium for Injection 1737

Chlorpheniramine Maleate (May exhibit an additive CNS depression). Products include:
Actifed Cold & Sinus Caplets and Tablets........ 688
Alka-Seltzer Plus Liqui-Gels 604
BC Allergy Sinus Cold Powder 619
Chlor-Trimeton Allergy Tablets 735
Chlor-Trimeton Allergy/Decongestant Tablets........ 736
Comtrex Flu Therapy & Fever Relief Nighttime Tablets........ 628
Comtrex Maximum Strength Multi-Symptom Cold & Cough Relief Tablets and Caplets........ 626
Contac Severe Cold and Flu Caplets Maximum Strength........ 746
Coricidin 'D' Cold, Flu & Sinus Tablets........ 737
Coricidin/Coricidin D 738
Coricidin HBP Maximum Strength Flu Tablets........ 738
Extendryl 1361
Hycomine Compound Tablets 1317
Kronofed-A 1341
PediaCare Cough-Cold Liquid 719
PediaCare NightRest Cough-Cold Liquid........ 719
Robitussin Nighttime Honey Flu Liquid........ 786
Ryna 768
Singlet Caplets 761
Sinutab Sinus Allergy Medication, Maximum Strength Formula, Tablets & Caplets........ 707
Sudafed Cold & Allergy Tablets 708
TheraFlu Regular Strength Cold & Cough Night Time Hot Liquid........ 676
TheraFlu Regular Strength Cold & Sore Throat Night Time Hot Liquid........ 676
TheraFlu Maximum Strength Flu & Cough Night Time Hot Liquid........ 678
TheraFlu Maximum Strength Flu & Sore Throat Night Time Hot Liquid........ 677
TheraFlu Maximum Strength Severe Cold & Congestion Night Time Caplets........ 678
TheraFlu Maximum Strength Severe Cold & Congestion Night Time Hot Liquid........ 678
Triaminic Cold & Allergy Liquid 681
Triaminic Cold & Allergy Softchews........ 683
Triaminic Cold & Cough Liquid 681
Triaminic Cold & Cough Softchews........ 683
Triaminic Cold & Night Time Cough Liquid........ 681
Triaminic Cold, Cough & Fever Liquid........ 681
Children's Tylenol Cold Suspension Liquid and Chewable Tablets........ 2015
Children's Tylenol Cold Plus Cough Suspension Liquid and Chewable Tablets........ 2015
Children's Tylenol Flu Suspension Liquid........ 2015
Maximum Strength Tylenol Allergy Sinus Caplets, Gelcaps, and Geltabs........ 2010
Multi-Symptom Tylenol Cold Complete Formula Caplets........ 2010
Vicks 44M Cough, Cold & Flu Relief Liquid........ 725
Pediatric Vicks 44m Cough & Cold Relief........ 728
Children's Vicks NyQuil Cold/Cough Relief........ 726

Chlorpheniramine Polistirex (May exhibit an additive CNS depression). Products include:
Tussionex Pennkinetic Extended-Release Suspension........ 1174

Chlorpheniramine Tannate (May exhibit an additive CNS depression). Products include:
Reformulated Rynatan Pediatric Suspension........ 3352
Rynatuss Pediatric Suspension 3353
Rynatuss Tablets 3353
Tussi-12 S Suspension 3356
Tussi-12 Tablets 3356

Chlorpromazine (May exhibit an additive CNS depression). Products include:
Thorazine Suppositories 1656

Chlorpromazine Hydrochloride (May exhibit an additive CNS depression). Products include:
Thorazine 1656

Chlorprothixene (May exhibit an additive CNS depression).
No products indexed under this heading.

Chlorprothixene Hydrochloride (May exhibit an additive CNS depression).
No products indexed under this heading.

Chlorprothixene Lactate (May exhibit an additive CNS depression).
No products indexed under this heading.

Clemastine Fumarate (May exhibit an additive CNS depression). Products include:
Tavist 12 Hour Allergy Tablets........ 676

Clomipramine Hydrochloride (Co-administration may increase the effect of either antidepressant or hydrocodone).
No products indexed under this heading.

Clorazepate Dipotassium (May exhibit an additive CNS depression). Products include:
Tranxene 511

Clozapine (May exhibit an additive CNS depression). Products include:
Clozaril Tablets 2319

Codeine Phosphate (May exhibit an additive CNS depression). Products include:
Phenergan with Codeine Syrup 3557
Phenergan VC with Codeine Syrup 3561
Robitussin A-C Syrup 2942
Robitussin-DAC Syrup 2942
Ryna-C Liquid 768
Soma Compound w/Codeine Tablets........ 3355
Tussi-Organidin NR Liquid 3350
Tussi-Organidin-S NR Liquid 3350
Tylenol with Codeine 2595

Cyproheptadine Hydrochloride (May exhibit an additive CNS depression). Products include:
Periactin Tablets 2155

Desflurane (May exhibit an additive CNS depression). Products include:
Suprane Liquid for Inhalation 874

Desipramine Hydrochloride (Co-administration may increase the effect of either antidepressant or hydrocodone). Products include:
Norpramin Tablets 755

Dexchlorpheniramine Maleate (May exhibit an additive CNS depression).
No products indexed under this heading.

Dezocine (May exhibit an additive CNS depression).
No products indexed under this heading.

Diazepam (May exhibit an additive CNS depression). Products include:
Valium Injectable 3026
Valium Tablets 3047

Diphenhydramine Citrate (May exhibit an additive CNS depression). Products include:
Alka-Seltzer PM Effervescent Tablets........ 605
Benadryl Allergy & Sinus Fastmelt Tablets........ 693
Benadryl Children's Allergy/Cold Fastmelt Tablets........ 692
Excedrin PM Tablets, Caplets, and Geltabs........ 631
Goody's PM Powder 621

Diphenhydramine Hydrochloride (May exhibit an additive CNS depression). Products include:
Extra Strength Bayer PM Caplets........ 611
Benadryl Allergy Chewables 689
Benadryl Allergy 691
Benadryl Allergy Liquid 690
Benadryl Allergy/Cold Tablets 691
Benadryl Allergy/Congestion Tablets........ 692
Benadryl Allergy & Sinus Liquid 693
Benadryl Allergy Sinus Headache Caplets & Gelcaps........ 693
Benadryl Severe Allergy & Sinus Headache Caplets........ 694
Benadryl Dye-Free Allergy Liquid 690
Benadryl Dye-Free Allergy Liqui-Gels Softgels........ 690
Benadryl Itch Relief Stick Extra Strength........ 695
Benadryl Cream 695
Benadryl Gel 695
Benadryl Spray 696
Benadryl Parenteral 2617
Coricidin HBP Night-Time Cold & Flu Tablets........ 738
Nytol QuickCaps Caplets 622
Maximum Strength Nytol QuickGels Softgels........ 621
Extra Strength Percogesic Aspirin-Free Coated Caplets........ 665
Simply Sleep Caplets 2008
Sominex Original Formula Tablets 761
Children's Tylenol Allergy-D Liquid 2014
Maximum Strength Tylenol Allergy Sinus NightTime Caplets........ 2010
Tylenol Severe Allergy Caplets 2010
Maximum Strength Tylenol Flu NightTime Gelcaps........ 2011
Extra Strength Tylenol PM Caplets, Geltabs, and Gelcaps........ 2012
Unisom Maximum Strength SleepGels........ 713

Diphenylpyraline Hydrochloride (May exhibit an additive CNS depression).
No products indexed under this heading.

Doxepin Hydrochloride (Co-administration may increase the effect of either antidepressant or hydrocodone). Products include:
Sinequan 2713

Droperidol (May exhibit an additive CNS depression).
No products indexed under this heading.

Enflurane (May exhibit an additive CNS depression).
No products indexed under this heading.

Estazolam (May exhibit an additive CNS depression). Products include:
ProSom Tablets 500

Ethchlorvynol (May exhibit an additive CNS depression).
No products indexed under this heading.

Ethinamate (May exhibit an additive CNS depression).
No products indexed under this heading.

Fentanyl (May exhibit an additive CNS depression). Products include:
Duragesic Transdermal System 1786

Fentanyl Citrate (May exhibit an additive CNS depression). Products include:
Actiq 1184

Fexofenadine Hydrochloride (May exhibit an additive CNS depression). Products include:
Allegra 712
Allegra-D Extended-Release Tablets........ 714

Fluphenazine Decanoate (May exhibit an additive CNS depression).
No products indexed under this heading.

Fluphenazine Enanthate (May exhibit an additive CNS depression).
No products indexed under this heading.

Fluphenazine Hydrochloride (May exhibit an additive CNS depression).
No products indexed under this heading.

Flurazepam Hydrochloride (May exhibit an additive CNS depression).
No products indexed under this heading.

Glutethimide (May exhibit an additive CNS depression).
No products indexed under this heading.

Haloperidol (May exhibit an additive CNS depression). Products include:
Haldol Injection, Tablets and Concentrate........ 2533

Haloperidol Decanoate (May exhibit an additive CNS depression). Products include:
Haldol Decanoate 2535

Hydrocodone Polistirex (May exhibit an additive CNS depression). Products include:
Tussionex Pennkinetic Extended-Release Suspension........ 1174

Hydromorphone Hydrochloride (May exhibit an additive CNS depression). Products include:
Dilaudid 441
Dilaudid Oral Liquid 445
Dilaudid Powder 441
Dilaudid Rectal Suppositories 441
Dilaudid Tablets 441
Dilaudid Tablets - 8 mg 445
Dilaudid-HP 443

Hydroxyzine Hydrochloride (May exhibit an additive CNS depression). Products include:
Atarax Tablets & Syrup 2667
Vistaril Intramuscular Solution 2738

Imipramine Hydrochloride (Co-administration may increase the effect of either antidepressant or hydrocodone).
No products indexed under this heading.

Imipramine Pamoate (Co-administration may increase the effect of either antidepressant or hydrocodone).
No products indexed under this heading.

Isocarboxazid (Co-administration may increase the effect of either the MAO inhibitor or hydrocodone).
No products indexed under this heading.

Isoflurane (May exhibit an additive CNS depression).
No products indexed under this heading.

Ketamine Hydrochloride (May exhibit an additive CNS depression).
No products indexed under this heading.

Levomethadyl Acetate Hydrochloride (May exhibit an additive CNS depression).
No products indexed under this heading.

Levorphanol Tartrate (May exhibit an additive CNS depression). Products include:
Levo-Dromoran 1734
Levorphanol Tartrate Tablets 3059

Loratadine (May exhibit an additive CNS depression). Products include:
Claritin 3100
Claritin-D 12 Hour Extended Release Tablets 3102
Claritin-D 24 Hour Extended Release Tablets 3104

Lorazepam (May exhibit an additive CNS depression). Products include:
Ativan Injection 3478
Ativan Tablets 3482

Loxapine Hydrochloride (May exhibit an additive CNS depression).
No products indexed under this heading.

Loxapine Succinate (May exhibit an additive CNS depression). Products include:
Loxitane Capsules 3398

Maprotiline Hydrochloride (Co-administration may increase the effect of either antidepressant or hydrocodone).
No products indexed under this heading.

Meperidine Hydrochloride (May exhibit an additive CNS depression). Products include:
Demerol 3079
Mepergan Injection 3539

Mephobarbital (May exhibit an additive CNS depression).
No products indexed under this heading.

Meprobamate (May exhibit an additive CNS depression). Products include:
Miltown Tablets 3349

Mesoridazine Besylate (May exhibit an additive CNS depression). Products include:
Serentil 1057

Methadone Hydrochloride (May exhibit an additive CNS depression). Products include:
Dolophine Hydrochloride Tablets 3056

Methdilazine Hydrochloride (May exhibit an additive CNS depression).
No products indexed under this heading.

Methohexital Sodium (May exhibit an additive CNS depression). Products include:
Brevital Sodium for Injection, USP .. 1815

Methotrimeprazine (May exhibit an additive CNS depression).
No products indexed under this heading.

Methoxyflurane (May exhibit an additive CNS depression).
No products indexed under this heading.

Midazolam Hydrochloride (May exhibit an additive CNS depression). Products include:
Versed Injection 3027
Versed Syrup 3033

Moclobemide (Co-administration may increase the effect of either the MAO inhibitor or hydrocodone).
No products indexed under this heading.

Molindone Hydrochloride (May exhibit an additive CNS depression). Products include:
Moban 1320

Morphine Sulfate (May exhibit an additive CNS depression). Products include:
Astramorph/PF Injection, USP (Preservative-Free) 594
Duramorph Injection 1312
Infumorph 200 and Infumorph 500 Sterile Solutions 1314
Kadian Capsules 1335
MS Contin Tablets 2896
MSIR 2898
Oramorph SR Tablets 3062
Roxanol 3066

Nortriptyline Hydrochloride (Co-administration may increase the effect of either antidepressant or hydrocodone).
No products indexed under this heading.

Olanzapine (May exhibit an additive CNS depression). Products include:
Zyprexa Tablets 1973
Zyprexa ZYDIS Orally Disintegrating Tablets 1973

Oxazepam (May exhibit an additive CNS depression).
No products indexed under this heading.

Oxycodone Hydrochloride (May exhibit an additive CNS depression). Products include:
OxyContin Tablets 2912
OxyFast Oral Concentrate Solution . 2916
OxyIR Capsules 2916
Percocet Tablets 1326
Percodan Tablets 1327
Percolone Tablets 1327
Roxicodone 3067
Tylox Capsules 2597

Pargyline Hydrochloride (Co-administration may increase the effect of either the MAO inhibitor or hydrocodone).
No products indexed under this heading.

Pentobarbital Sodium (May exhibit an additive CNS depression). Products include:
Nembutal Sodium Solution 485

Perphenazine (May exhibit an additive CNS depression). Products include:
Etrafon 3115
Trilafon 3160

Phenelzine Sulfate (Co-administration may increase the effect of either the MAO inhibitor or hydrocodone). Products include:
Nardil Tablets 2653

Phenobarbital (May exhibit an additive CNS depression). Products include:
Arco-Lase Plus Tablets 592
Donnatal 2929
Donnatal Extentabs 2930

Prazepam (May exhibit an additive CNS depression).
No products indexed under this heading.

Procarbazine Hydrochloride (Co-administration may increase the effect of either the MAO inhibitor or hydrocodone). Products include:
Matulane Capsules 3246

Prochlorperazine (May exhibit an additive CNS depression). Products include:
Compazine 1505

Promethazine Hydrochloride (May exhibit an additive CNS depression). Products include:
Mepergan Injection 3539
Phenergan Injection 3553
Phenergan 3556
Phenergan Syrup 3554
Phenergan with Codeine Syrup 3557
Phenergan with Dextromethorphan Syrup 3559
Phenergan VC Syrup 3560
Phenergan VC with Codeine Syrup .. 3561

Propofol (May exhibit an additive CNS depression). Products include:
Diprivan Injectable Emulsion 667

Propoxyphene Hydrochloride (May exhibit an additive CNS depression). Products include:
Darvon Pulvules 1909
Darvon Compound-65 Pulvules 1910

Propoxyphene Napsylate (May exhibit an additive CNS depression). Products include:
Darvon-N/Darvocet-N 1907
Darvon-N Tablets 1912

Protriptyline Hydrochloride (Co-administration may increase the effect of either antidepressant or hydrocodone). Products include:
Vivactil Tablets 2446
Vivactil Tablets 2217

Pyrilamine Maleate (May exhibit an additive CNS depression). Products include:
Maximum Strength Midol Menstrual Caplets and Gelcaps .... ▣612
Maximum Strength Midol PMS Caplets and Gelcaps .... ▣613

Pyrilamine Tannate (May exhibit an additive CNS depression). Products include:
Ryna-12 S Suspension 3351

Quazepam (May exhibit an additive CNS depression).
No products indexed under this heading.

Quetiapine Fumarate (May exhibit an additive CNS depression). Products include:
Seroquel Tablets 684

Remifentanil Hydrochloride (May exhibit an additive CNS depression).
No products indexed under this heading.

Risperidone (May exhibit an additive CNS depression). Products include:
Risperdal 1796

Secobarbital Sodium (May exhibit an additive CNS depression).
No products indexed under this heading.

Selegiline Hydrochloride (Co-administration may increase the effect of either the MAO inhibitor or hydrocodone). Products include:
Eldepryl Capsules 3266

Sevoflurane (May exhibit an additive CNS depression).
No products indexed under this heading.

Sufentanil Citrate (May exhibit an additive CNS depression).
No products indexed under this heading.

Temazepam (May exhibit an additive CNS depression).
No products indexed under this heading.

Terfenadine (May exhibit an additive CNS depression).
No products indexed under this heading.

Thiamylal Sodium (May exhibit an additive CNS depression).
No products indexed under this heading.

Thioridazine Hydrochloride (May exhibit an additive CNS depression). Products include:
Thioridazine Hydrochloride Tablets 2289

Thiothixene (May exhibit an additive CNS depression). Products include:
Navane Capsules 2701
Thiothixene Capsules 2290

Tranylcypromine Sulfate (Co-administration may increase the effect of either the MAO inhibitor or hydrocodone). Products include:
Parnate Tablets 1607

Triazolam (May exhibit an additive CNS depression). Products include:
Halcion Tablets 2823

Trifluoperazine Hydrochloride (May exhibit an additive CNS depression). Products include:
Stelazine 1640

Trimeprazine Tartrate (May exhibit an additive CNS depression).
No products indexed under this heading.

Trimipramine Maleate (Co-administration may increase the effect of either antidepressant or hydrocodone). Products include:
Surmontil Capsules 3595

Tripelennamine Hydrochloride (May exhibit an additive CNS depression).
No products indexed under this heading.

Triprolidine Hydrochloride (May exhibit an additive CNS depression). Products include:
Actifed Cold & Allergy Tablets .... ▣688

Zaleplon (May exhibit an additive CNS depression). Products include:
Sonata Capsules 3591

Ziprasidone Hydrochloride (May exhibit an additive CNS depression). Products include:
Geodon Capsules 2688

Zolpidem Tartrate (May exhibit an additive CNS depression). Products include:
Ambien Tablets 3191

Food Interactions

Alcohol (May exhibit an additive CNS depression).

VICODIN ES TABLETS

(Acetaminophen, Hydrocodone Bitartrate) 517

May interact with anticholinergics, central nervous system depressants, narcotic analgesics, psychotropics, tranquilizers, tricyclic antidepressants, and certain other agents. Compounds in these categories include:

Alfentanil Hydrochloride (Additive CNS depression; the dose of one or both agents should be reduced).
No products indexed under this heading.

Alprazolam (Additive CNS depression; the dose of one or both agents should be reduced). Products include:
Xanax Tablets 2865

Amitriptyline Hydrochloride (Concurrent use of tricyclic antidepressants and hydrocodone preparations may increase the effect of either the antidepressant or hydrocodone). Products include:
Etrafon 3115
Limbitrol 1738

Amoxapine (Concurrent use of tricyclic antidepressants and hydrocodone preparations may increase the effect of either the antidepressant or hydrocodone).
No products indexed under this heading.

Aprobarbital (Additive CNS depression; the dose of one or both agents should be reduced).
No products indexed under this heading.

Atropine Sulfate (May produce paralytic ileus). Products include:
Donnatal 2929
Donnatal Extentabs 2930
Motofen Tablets 577
Prosed/DS Tablets 3268
Urised Tablets 2876

Belladonna Alkaloids (May produce paralytic ileus). Products include:
Hyland's Teething Tablets 766
Urimax Tablets 1769

Benztropine Mesylate (May produce paralytic ileus). Products include:
Cogentin 2055

Biperiden Hydrochloride (May produce paralytic ileus). Products include:
Akineton 402

Buprenorphine Hydrochloride (Additive CNS depression; the dose of one or both agents should be reduced). Products include:
Buprenex Injectable 2918

Buspirone Hydrochloride (Additive CNS depression; the dose of one or both agents should be reduced).
No products indexed under this heading.

Butabarbital (Additive CNS depression; the dose of one or both agents should be reduced).
No products indexed under this heading.

Butalbital (Additive CNS depression; the dose of one or both agents should be reduced). Products include:
Phrenilin 578
Sedapap Tablets 50 mg/650 mg ... 2225

Chlordiazepoxide (Additive CNS depression; the dose of one or both agents should be reduced). Products include:
Limbitrol 1738

Chlordiazepoxide Hydrochloride (Additive CNS depression; the dose of one or both agents should be reduced). Products include:
Librium Capsules 1736
Librium for Injection 1737

Chlorpromazine (Additive CNS depression; the dose of one or both agents should be reduced). Products include:
Thorazine Suppositories 1656

Chlorpromazine Hydrochloride (Additive CNS depression; the dose of one or both agents should be reduced). Products include:
Thorazine 1656

Chlorprothixene (Additive CNS depression; the dose of one or both agents should be reduced).
No products indexed under this heading.

Chlorprothixene Hydrochloride (Additive CNS depression; the dose of one or both agents should be reduced).
No products indexed under this heading.

Chlorprothixene Lactate (Additive CNS depression; the dose of one or both agents should be reduced).
No products indexed under this heading.

Clidinium Bromide (May produce paralytic ileus).
No products indexed under this heading.

Clomipramine Hydrochloride (Concurrent use of tricyclic antidepressants and hydrocodone preparations may increase the effect of either the antidepressant or hydrocodone).
No products indexed under this heading.

Clorazepate Dipotassium (Additive CNS depression; the dose of one or both agents should be reduced). Products include:
Tranxene 511

Clozapine (Additive CNS depression; the dose of one or both agents should be reduced). Products include:
Clozaril Tablets 2319

Codeine Phosphate (Additive CNS depression; the dose of one or both agents should be reduced). Products include:
Phenergan with Codeine Syrup 3557
Phenergan VC with Codeine Syrup .. 3561
Robitussin A-C Syrup 2942
Robitussin-DAC Syrup 2942
Ryna-C Liquid 768
Soma Compound w/Codeine Tablets 3355
Tussi-Organidin NR Liquid 3350
Tussi-Organidin-S NR Liquid 3350
Tylenol with Codeine 2595

Desflurane (Additive CNS depression; the dose of one or both agents should be reduced). Products include:
Suprane Liquid for Inhalation 874

Desipramine Hydrochloride (Concurrent use of tricyclic antidepressants and hydrocodone preparations may increase the effect of either the antidepressant or hydrocodone). Products include:
Norpramin Tablets 755

Dezocine (Additive CNS depression; the dose of one or both agents should be reduced).
No products indexed under this heading.

Diazepam (Additive CNS depression; the dose of one or both agents should be reduced). Products include:
Valium Injectable 3026
Valium Tablets 3047

Dicyclomine Hydrochloride (May produce paralytic ileus).
No products indexed under this heading.

Doxepin Hydrochloride (Concurrent use of tricyclic antidepressants and hydrocodone preparations may increase the effect of either the antidepressant or hydrocodone). Products include:
Sinequan 2713

Droperidol (Additive CNS depression; the dose of one or both agents should be reduced).
No products indexed under this heading.

Enflurane (Additive CNS depression; the dose of one or both agents should be reduced).
No products indexed under this heading.

Estazolam (Additive CNS depression; the dose of one or both agents should be reduced). Products include:
ProSom Tablets 500

Ethchlorvynol (Additive CNS depression; the dose of one or both agents should be reduced).
No products indexed under this heading.

Ethinamate (Additive CNS depression; the dose of one or both agents should be reduced).
No products indexed under this heading.

Fentanyl (Additive CNS depression; the dose of one or both agents should be reduced). Products include:
Duragesic Transdermal System 1786

Fentanyl Citrate (Additive CNS depression; the dose of one or both agents should be reduced). Products include:
Actiq 1184

Fluphenazine Decanoate (Additive CNS depression; the dose of one or both agents should be reduced).
No products indexed under this heading.

Fluphenazine Enanthate (Additive CNS depression; the dose of one or both agents should be reduced).
No products indexed under this heading.

Fluphenazine Hydrochloride (Additive CNS depression; the dose of one or both agents should be reduced).
No products indexed under this heading.

Flurazepam Hydrochloride (Additive CNS depression; the dose of one or both agents should be reduced).
No products indexed under this heading.

Glutethimide (Additive CNS depression; the dose of one or both agents should be reduced).
No products indexed under this heading.

Glycopyrrolate (May produce paralytic ileus). Products include:
Robinul Forte Tablets 1358
Robinul Injectable 2940
Robinul Tablets 1358

Haloperidol (Additive CNS depression; the dose of one or both agents should be reduced). Products include:
Haldol Injection, Tablets and Concentrate 2533

Haloperidol Decanoate (Additive CNS depression; the dose of one or both agents should be reduced). Products include:
Haldol Decanoate 2535

Hydrocodone Polistirex (Additive CNS depression; the dose of one or both agents should be reduced). Products include:
Tussionex Pennkinetic Extended-Release Suspension 1174

Hydromorphone Hydrochloride (Additive CNS depression; the dose of one or both agents should be reduced). Products include:
Dilaudid 441
Dilaudid Oral Liquid 445
Dilaudid Powder 441
Dilaudid Rectal Suppositories 441
Dilaudid Tablets 441
Dilaudid Tablets - 8 mg 445
Dilaudid-HP 443

Hydroxyzine Hydrochloride (Additive CNS depression; the dose of one or both agents should be reduced). Products include:
Atarax Tablets & Syrup 2667
Vistaril Intramuscular Solution 2738

Hyoscyamine (May produce paralytic ileus). Products include:
Urised Tablets 2876

Hyoscyamine Sulfate (May produce paralytic ileus). Products include:
Arco-Lase Plus Tablets 592
Donnatal 2929
Donnatal Extentabs 2930
Levsin/Levsinex/Levbid 3172
NuLev Orally Disintegrating Tablets 3176
Prosed/DS Tablets 3268
Urimax Tablets 1769

Imipramine Hydrochloride (Concurrent use of tricyclic antidepressants and hydrocodone preparations may increase the effect of either the antidepressant or hydrocodone).
No products indexed under this heading.

Imipramine Pamoate (Concurrent use of tricyclic antidepressants and hydrocodone preparations may increase the effect of either the antidepressant or hydrocodone).
No products indexed under this heading.

Ipratropium Bromide (May produce paralytic ileus). Products include:
Atrovent Inhalation Aerosol 1030
Atrovent Inhalation Solution 1031
Atrovent Nasal Spray 0.03% 1032
Atrovent Nasal Spray 0.06% 1033
Combivent Inhalation Aerosol 1041
DuoNeb Inhalation Solution 1233

Isocarboxazid (Concurrent use of MAO inhibitor and hydrocodone preparations may increase the effect of either the MAO inhibitor or hydrocodone).
No products indexed under this heading.

Isoflurane (Additive CNS depression; the dose of one or both agents should be reduced).
No products indexed under this heading.

Ketamine Hydrochloride (Additive CNS depression; the dose of one or both agents should be reduced).
No products indexed under this heading.

Levomethadyl Acetate Hydrochloride (Additive CNS depression; the dose of one or both agents should be reduced).
No products indexed under this heading.

Levorphanol Tartrate (Additive CNS depression; the dose of one or both agents should be reduced). Products include:
Levo-Dromoran 1734
Levorphanol Tartrate Tablets 3059

Lithium Carbonate (Additive CNS depression; the dose of one or both agents should be reduced). Products include:
Eskalith 1527
Lithium Carbonate 3061
Lithobid Slow-Release Tablets 3255

Lithium Citrate (Additive CNS depression; the dose of one or both agents should be reduced). Products include:
Lithium Citrate Syrup 3061

Lorazepam (Additive CNS depression; the dose of one or both agents should be reduced). Products include:
Ativan Injection 3478
Ativan Tablets 3482

Loxapine Hydrochloride (Additive CNS depression; the dose of one or both agents should be reduced).
No products indexed under this heading.

Loxapine Succinate (Additive CNS depression; the dose of one or both agents should be reduced). Products include:
Loxitane Capsules 3398

Maprotiline Hydrochloride (Concurrent use of tricyclic antidepressants and hydrocodone preparations may increase the effect of either the antidepressant or hydrocodone).
No products indexed under this heading.

Mepenzolate Bromide (May produce paralytic ileus).
No products indexed under this heading.

Meperidine Hydrochloride (Additive CNS depression; the dose of one or both agents should be reduced). Products include:
Demerol 3079
Mepergan Injection 3539

Mephobarbital (Additive CNS depression; the dose of one or both agents should be reduced).
No products indexed under this heading.

Meprobamate (Additive CNS depression; the dose of one or both agents should be reduced). Products include:
Miltown Tablets 3349

Mesoridazine Besylate (Additive CNS depression; the dose of one or both agents should be reduced). Products include:
Serentil 1057

Methadone Hydrochloride (Additive CNS depression; the dose of one or both agents should be reduced). Products include:
Dolophine Hydrochloride Tablets 3056

Methohexital Sodium (Additive CNS depression; the dose of one or both agents should be reduced). Products include:
Brevital Sodium for Injection, USP .. 1815

Methotrimeprazine (Additive CNS depression; the dose of one or both agents should be reduced).
No products indexed under this heading.

Methoxyflurane (Additive CNS depression; the dose of one or both agents should be reduced).
No products indexed under this heading.

Midazolam Hydrochloride (Additive CNS depression; the dose of one or both agents should be reduced). Products include:
Versed Injection 3027
Versed Syrup 3033

Molindone Hydrochloride (Additive CNS depression; the dose of one or both agents should be reduced). Products include:
Moban 1320

Morphine Sulfate (Additive CNS depression; the dose of one or both agents should be reduced). Products include:
Astramorph/PF Injection, USP (Preservative-Free)........................ 594
Duramorph Injection 1312
Infumorph 200 and Infumorph 500 Sterile Solutions........................ 1314
Kadian Capsules 1335
MS Contin Tablets 2896
MSIR 2898
Oramorph SR Tablets 3062
Roxanol 3066

Nortriptyline Hydrochloride (Concurrent use of tricyclic antidepressants and hydrocodone preparations may increase the effect of either the antidepressant or hydrocodone).
No products indexed under this heading.

Olanzapine (Additive CNS depression; the dose of one or both agents should be reduced). Products include:
Zyprexa Tablets 1973
Zyprexa ZYDIS Orally Disintegrating Tablets...................... 1973

Oxazepam (Additive CNS depression; the dose of one or both agents should be reduced).
No products indexed under this heading.

Oxybutynin Chloride (May produce paralytic ileus). Products include:
Ditropan XL Extended Release Tablets... 564

Oxycodone Hydrochloride (Additive CNS depression; the dose of one or both agents should be reduced). Products include:
OxyContin Tablets 2912
OxyFast Oral Concentrate Solution . 2916
OxyIR Capsules 2916
Percocet Tablets 1326
Percodan Tablets 1327
Percolone Tablets 1327
Roxicodone 3067
Tylox Capsules 2597

Pentobarbital Sodium (Additive CNS depression; the dose of one or both agents should be reduced). Products include:
Nembutal Sodium Solution 485

Perphenazine (Additive CNS depression; the dose of one or both agents should be reduced). Products include:
Etrafon 3115
Trilafon 3160

Phenelzine Sulfate (Concurrent use of MAO inhibitor and hydrocodone preparations may increase the effect of either the MAO inhibitor or hydrocodone). Products include:
Nardil Tablets 2653

Phenobarbital (Additive CNS depression; the dose of one or both agents should be reduced). Products include:
Arco-Lase Plus Tablets 592
Donnatal 2929
Donnatal Extentabs 2930

Prazepam (Additive CNS depression; the dose of one or both agents should be reduced).
No products indexed under this heading.

Prochlorperazine (Additive CNS depression; the dose of one or both agents should be reduced). Products include:
Compazine 1505

Procyclidine Hydrochloride (May produce paralytic ileus).
No products indexed under this heading.

Promethazine Hydrochloride (Additive CNS depression; the dose of one or both agents should be reduced). Products include:
Mepergan Injection 3539
Phenergan Injection 3553
Phenergan 3556
Phenergan Syrup 3554
Phenergan with Codeine Syrup 3557
Phenergan with Dextromethorphan Syrup... 3559
Phenergan VC Syrup 3560
Phenergan VC with Codeine Syrup .. 3561

Propantheline Bromide (May produce paralytic ileus).
No products indexed under this heading.

Propofol (Additive CNS depression; the dose of one or both agents should be reduced). Products include:
Diprivan Injectable Emulsion 667

Propoxyphene Hydrochloride (Additive CNS depression; the dose of one or both agents should be reduced). Products include:
Darvon Pulvules 1909
Darvon Compound-65 Pulvules 1910

Propoxyphene Napsylate (Additive CNS depression; the dose of one or both agents should be reduced). Products include:
Darvon-N/Darvocet-N 1907
Darvon-N Tablets 1912

Protriptyline Hydrochloride (Concurrent use of tricyclic antidepressants and hydrocodone preparations may increase the effect of either the antidepressant or hydrocodone). Products include:
Vivactil Tablets 2446
Vivactil Tablets 2217

Quazepam (Additive CNS depression; the dose of one or both agents should be reduced).
No products indexed under this heading.

Quetiapine Fumarate (Additive CNS depression; the dose of one or both agents should be reduced). Products include:
Seroquel Tablets 684

Remifentanil Hydrochloride (Additive CNS depression; the dose of one or both agents should be reduced).
No products indexed under this heading.

Risperidone (Additive CNS depression; the dose of one or both agents should be reduced). Products include:
Risperdal 1796

Scopolamine (May produce paralytic ileus). Products include:
Transderm Scōp Transdermal Therapeutic System.................. 2302

Scopolamine Hydrobromide (May produce paralytic ileus). Products include:
Donnatal 2929
Donnatal Extentabs 2930

Secobarbital Sodium (Additive CNS depression; the dose of one or both agents should be reduced).
No products indexed under this heading.

Selegiline Hydrochloride (Concurrent use of MAO inhibitor and hydrocodone preparations may increase the effect of either the MAO inhibitor or hydrocodone). Products include:
Eldepryl Capsules 3266

Sevoflurane (Additive CNS depression; the dose of one or both agents should be reduced).
No products indexed under this heading.

Sufentanil Citrate (Additive CNS depression; the dose of one or both agents should be reduced).
No products indexed under this heading.

Temazepam (Additive CNS depression; the dose of one or both agents should be reduced).
No products indexed under this heading.

Thiamylal Sodium (Additive CNS depression; the dose of one or both agents should be reduced).
No products indexed under this heading.

Thioridazine Hydrochloride (Additive CNS depression; the dose of one or both agents should be reduced). Products include:
Thioridazine Hydrochloride Tablets... 2289

Thiothixene (Additive CNS depression; the dose of one or both agents should be reduced). Products include:
Navane Capsules 2701
Thiothixene Capsules 2290

Tolterodine Tartrate (May produce paralytic ileus). Products include:
Detrol Tablets 3623
Detrol LA Capsules 2801

Tranylcypromine Sulfate (Concurrent use of MAO inhibitor and hydrocodone preparations may increase the effect of either the MAO inhibitor or hydrocodone). Products include:
Parnate Tablets 1607

Triazolam (Additive CNS depression; the dose of one or both agents should be reduced). Products include:
Halcion Tablets 2823

Tridihexethyl Chloride (May produce paralytic ileus).
No products indexed under this heading.

Trifluoperazine Hydrochloride (Additive CNS depression; the dose of one or both agents should be reduced). Products include:
Stelazine 1640

Trihexyphenidyl Hydrochloride (May produce paralytic ileus). Products include:
Artane 1855

Trimipramine Maleate (Concurrent use of tricyclic antidepressants and hydrocodone preparations may increase the effect of either the antidepressant or hydrocodone). Products include:
Surmontil Capsules 3595

Zaleplon (Additive CNS depression; the dose of one or both agents should be reduced). Products include:
Sonata Capsules 3591

Ziprasidone Hydrochloride (Additive CNS depression; the dose of one or both agents should be reduced). Products include:
Geodon Capsules 2688

Zolpidem Tartrate (Additive CNS depression; the dose of one or both agents should be reduced). Products include:
Ambien Tablets 3191

Food Interactions

Alcohol (Additive CNS depression).

VICODIN HP TABLETS

(Acetaminophen, Hydrocodone Bitartrate)... 518

May interact with antihistamines, central nervous system depressants, monoamine oxidase inhibitors, narcotic analgesics, tranquilizers, tricyclic antidepressants, and certain other agents. Compounds in these categories include:

Acrivastine (Co-administration may result in an additive CNS depression). Products include:
Semprex-D Capsules 1172

Alfentanil Hydrochloride (Co-administration may result in an additive CNS depression).
No products indexed under this heading.

Alprazolam (Co-administration may result in an additive CNS depression). Products include:
Xanax Tablets 2865

Amitriptyline Hydrochloride (Co-administration with tricyclic antidepressants may increase the effect of either hydrocodone or the tricyclic antidepressant). Products include:
Etrafon 3115
Limbitrol 1738

Amoxapine (Co-administration with tricyclic antidepressants may increase the effect of either hydrocodone or the tricyclic antidepressant).
No products indexed under this heading.

Aprobarbital (Co-administration may result in an additive CNS depression).
No products indexed under this heading.

Astemizole (Co-administration may result in an additive CNS depression).
No products indexed under this heading.

Azatadine Maleate (Co-administration may result in an additive CNS depression). Products include:
Rynatan Tablets 3351

Bromodiphenhydramine Hydrochloride (Co-administration may result in an additive CNS depression).
No products indexed under this heading.

Brompheniramine Maleate (Co-administration may result in an additive CNS depression). Products include:
Bromfed Capsules (Extended-Release)...................... 2269
Bromfed-PD Capsules (Extended-Release)...................... 2269
Comtrex Acute Head Cold & Sinus Pressure Relief Tablets..... ▣627
Dimetapp Elixir .... ▣777
Dimetapp Cold and Fever Suspension................................... ▣775
Dimetapp DM Cold & Cough Elixir . ▣775
Dimetapp Nighttime Flu Liquid ...... ▣776

Buprenorphine Hydrochloride (Co-administration may result in an additive CNS depression). Products include:
Buprenex Injectable 2918

Buspirone Hydrochloride (Co-administration may result in an additive CNS depression).
No products indexed under this heading.

Butabarbital (Co-administration may result in an additive CNS depression).
No products indexed under this heading.

Butalbital (Co-administration may result in an additive CNS depression). Products include:
Phrenilin 578
Sedapap Tablets 50 mg/650 mg ... 2225

Cetirizine Hydrochloride (Co-administration may result in an additive CNS depression). Products include:
- Zyrtec ... 2756
- Zyrtec-D 12 Hour Extended Relief Tablets ... 2758

Chlordiazepoxide (Co-administration may result in an additive CNS depression). Products include:
- Limbitrol ... 1738

Chlordiazepoxide Hydrochloride (Co-administration may result in an additive CNS depression). Products include:
- Librium Capsules ... 1736
- Librium for Injection ... 1737

Chlorpheniramine Maleate (Co-administration may result in an additive CNS depression). Products include:
- Actifed Cold & Sinus Caplets and Tablets ... 688
- Alka-Seltzer Plus Liqui-Gels ... 604
- BC Allergy Sinus Cold Powder ... 619
- Chlor-Trimeton Allergy Tablets ... 735
- Chlor-Trimeton Allergy/Decongestant Tablets ... 736
- Comtrex Flu Therapy & Fever Relief Nighttime Tablets ... 628
- Comtrex Maximum Strength Multi-Symptom Cold & Cough Relief Tablets and Caplets ... 626
- Contac Severe Cold and Flu Caplets Maximum Strength ... 746
- Coricidin 'D' Cold, Flu & Sinus Tablets ... 737
- Coricidin/Coricidin D ... 738
- Coricidin HBP Maximum Strength Flu Tablets ... 738
- Extendryl ... 1361
- Hycomine Compound Tablets ... 1317
- Kronofed-A ... 1341
- PediaCare Cough-Cold Liquid ... 719
- PediaCare NightRest Cough-Cold Liquid ... 719
- Robitussin Nighttime Honey Flu Liquid ... 786
- Ryna ... 768
- Singlet Caplets ... 761
- Sinutab Sinus Allergy Medication, Maximum Strength Formula, Tablets & Caplets ... 707
- Sudafed Cold & Allergy Tablets ... 708
- TheraFlu Regular Strength Cold & Cough Night Time Hot Liquid ... 676
- TheraFlu Regular Strength Cold & Sore Throat Night Time Hot Liquid ... 676
- TheraFlu Maximum Strength Flu & Cough Night Time Hot Liquid ... 678
- TheraFlu Maximum Strength Flu & Sore Throat Night Time Hot Liquid ... 677
- TheraFlu Maximum Strength Severe Cold & Congestion Night Time Caplets ... 678
- TheraFlu Maximum Strength Severe Cold & Congestion Night Time Hot Liquid ... 678
- Triaminic Cold & Allergy Liquid ... 681
- Triaminic Cold & Allergy Softchews ... 683
- Triaminic Cold & Cough Liquid ... 681
- Triaminic Cold & Cough Softchews ... 683
- Triaminic Cold & Night Time Cough Liquid ... 681
- Triaminic Cold, Cough & Fever Liquid ... 681
- Children's Tylenol Cold Suspension Liquid and Chewable Tablets ... 2015
- Children's Tylenol Cold Plus Cough Suspension Liquid and Chewable Tablets ... 2015
- Children's Tylenol Flu Suspension Liquid ... 2015
- Maximum Strength Tylenol Allergy Sinus Caplets, Gelcaps, and Geltabs ... 2010
- Multi-Symptom Tylenol Cold Complete Formula Caplets ... 2010
- Vicks 44M Cough, Cold & Flu Relief Liquid ... 725
- Pediatric Vicks 44m Cough & Cold Relief ... 728
- Children's Vicks NyQuil Cold/Cough Relief ... 726

Chlorpheniramine Polistirex (Co-administration may result in an additive CNS depression). Products include:
- Tussionex Pennkinetic Extended-Release Suspension ... 1174

Chlorpheniramine Tannate (Co-administration may result in an additive CNS depression). Products include:
- Reformulated Rynatan Pediatric Suspension ... 3352
- Rynatuss Pediatric Suspension ... 3353
- Rynatuss Tablets ... 3353
- Tussi-12 S Suspension ... 3356
- Tussi-12 Tablets ... 3356

Chlorpromazine (Co-administration may result in an additive CNS depression). Products include:
- Thorazine Suppositories ... 1656

Chlorpromazine Hydrochloride (Co-administration may result in an additive CNS depression). Products include:
- Thorazine ... 1656

Chlorprothixene (Co-administration may result in an additive CNS depression).
No products indexed under this heading.

Chlorprothixene Hydrochloride (Co-administration may result in an additive CNS depression).
No products indexed under this heading.

Chlorprothixene Lactate (Co-administration may result in an additive CNS depression).
No products indexed under this heading.

Clemastine Fumarate (Co-administration may result in an additive CNS depression). Products include:
- Tavist 12 Hour Allergy Tablets ... 676

Clomipramine Hydrochloride (Co-administration with tricyclic antidepressants may increase the effect of either hydrocodone or the tricyclic antidepressant).
No products indexed under this heading.

Clorazepate Dipotassium (Co-administration may result in an additive CNS depression). Products include:
- Tranxene ... 511

Clozapine (Co-administration may result in an additive CNS depression). Products include:
- Clozaril Tablets ... 2319

Codeine Phosphate (Co-administration may result in an additive CNS depression). Products include:
- Phenergan with Codeine Syrup ... 3557
- Phenergan VC with Codeine Syrup ... 3561
- Robitussin A-C Syrup ... 2942
- Robitussin-DAC Syrup ... 2942
- Ryna-C Liquid ... 768
- Soma Compound w/Codeine Tablets ... 3355
- Tussi-Organidin NR Liquid ... 3350
- Tussi-Organidin-S NR Liquid ... 3350
- Tylenol with Codeine ... 2595

Cyproheptadine Hydrochloride (Co-administration may result in an additive CNS depression). Products include:
- Periactin Tablets ... 2155

Desflurane (Co-administration may result in an additive CNS depression). Products include:
- Suprane Liquid for Inhalation ... 874

Desipramine Hydrochloride (Co-administration with tricyclic antidepressants may increase the effect of either hydrocodone or the tricyclic antidepressant). Products include:
- Norpramin Tablets ... 755

Dexchlorpheniramine Maleate (Co-administration may result in an additive CNS depression).
No products indexed under this heading.

Dezocine (Co-administration may result in an additive CNS depression).
No products indexed under this heading.

Diazepam (Co-administration may result in an additive CNS depression). Products include:
- Valium Injectable ... 3026
- Valium Tablets ... 3047

Diphenhydramine Citrate (Co-administration may result in an additive CNS depression). Products include:
- Alka-Seltzer PM Effervescent Tablets ... 605
- Benadryl Allergy & Sinus Fastmelt Tablets ... 693
- Benadryl Children's Allergy/Cold Fastmelt Tablets ... 692
- Excedrin PM Tablets, Caplets, and Geltabs ... 631
- Goody's PM Powder ... 621

Diphenhydramine Hydrochloride (Co-administration may result in an additive CNS depression). Products include:
- Extra Strength Bayer PM Caplets ... 611
- Benadryl Allergy Chewables ... 689
- Benadryl Allergy ... 691
- Benadryl Allergy Liquid ... 690
- Benadryl Allergy/Cold Tablets ... 691
- Benadryl Allergy/Congestion Tablets ... 692
- Benadryl Allergy & Sinus Liquid ... 693
- Benadryl Allergy Sinus Headache Caplets & Gelcaps ... 693
- Benadryl Severe Allergy & Sinus Headache Caplets ... 694
- Benadryl Dye-Free Allergy Liquid ... 690
- Benadryl Dye-Free Allergy Liqui-Gels Softgels ... 690
- Benadryl Itch Relief Stick Extra Strength ... 695
- Benadryl Cream ... 695
- Benadryl Gel ... 695
- Benadryl Spray ... 696
- Benadryl Parenteral ... 2617
- Coricidin HBP Night-Time Cold & Flu Tablets ... 738
- Nytol QuickCaps Caplets ... 622
- Maximum Strength Nytol QuickGels Softgels ... 621
- Extra Strength Percogesic Aspirin-Free Coated Caplets ... 665
- Simply Sleep Caplets ... 2008
- Sominex Original Formula Tablets ... 761
- Children's Tylenol Allergy-D Liquid ... 2014
- Maximum Strength Tylenol Allergy Sinus NightTime Caplets ... 2010
- Tylenol Severe Allergy Caplets ... 2010
- Maximum Strength Tylenol Flu NightTime Gelcaps ... 2011
- Extra Strength Tylenol PM Caplets, Geltabs, and Gelcaps ... 2012
- Unisom Maximum Strength SleepGels ... 713

Diphenylpyraline Hydrochloride (Co-administration may result in an additive CNS depression).
No products indexed under this heading.

Doxepin Hydrochloride (Co-administration with tricyclic antidepressants may increase the effect of either hydrocodone or the tricyclic antidepressant). Products include:
- Sinequan ... 2713

Droperidol (Co-administration may result in an additive CNS depression).
No products indexed under this heading.

Enflurane (Co-administration may result in an additive CNS depression).
No products indexed under this heading.

Estazolam (Co-administration may result in an additive CNS depression). Products include:
- ProSom Tablets ... 500

Ethchlorvynol (Co-administration may result in an additive CNS depression).
No products indexed under this heading.

Ethinamate (Co-administration may result in an additive CNS depression).
No products indexed under this heading.

Fentanyl (Co-administration may result in an additive CNS depression). Products include:
- Duragesic Transdermal System ... 1786

Fentanyl Citrate (Co-administration may result in an additive CNS depression). Products include:
- Actiq ... 1184

Fexofenadine Hydrochloride (Co-administration may result in an additive CNS depression). Products include:
- Allegra ... 712
- Allegra-D Extended-Release Tablets ... 714

Fluphenazine Decanoate (Co-administration may result in an additive CNS depression).
No products indexed under this heading.

Fluphenazine Enanthate (Co-administration may result in an additive CNS depression).
No products indexed under this heading.

Fluphenazine Hydrochloride (Co-administration may result in an additive CNS depression).
No products indexed under this heading.

Flurazepam Hydrochloride (Co-administration may result in an additive CNS depression).
No products indexed under this heading.

Glutethimide (Co-administration may result in an additive CNS depression).
No products indexed under this heading.

Haloperidol (Co-administration may result in an additive CNS depression). Products include:
- Haldol Injection, Tablets and Concentrate ... 2533

Haloperidol Decanoate (Co-administration may result in an additive CNS depression). Products include:
- Haldol Decanoate ... 2535

Hydrocodone Polistirex (Co-administration may result in an additive CNS depression). Products include:
- Tussionex Pennkinetic Extended-Release Suspension ... 1174

Hydromorphone Hydrochloride (Co-administration may result in an additive CNS depression). Products include:
- Dilaudid ... 441
- Dilaudid Oral Liquid ... 445
- Dilaudid Powder ... 441
- Dilaudid Rectal Suppositories ... 441
- Dilaudid Tablets ... 441
- Dilaudid Tablets - 8 mg ... 445
- Dilaudid-HP ... 443

Hydroxyzine Hydrochloride (Co-administration may result in an additive CNS depression). Products include:
- Atarax Tablets & Syrup ... 2667
- Vistaril Intramuscular Solution ... 2738

Imipramine Hydrochloride (Co-administration with tricyclic antidepressants may increase the effect of either hydrocodone or the tricyclic antidepressant).
No products indexed under this heading.

Imipramine Pamoate (Co-administration with tricyclic antidepressants may increase the effect of either hydrocodone or the tricyclic antidepressant).
No products indexed under this heading.

Isocarboxazid (Co-administration with an MAO inhibitor may increase the effect of either hydrocodone or

the MAO inhibitor).
No products indexed under this heading.

Isoflurane (Co-administration may result in an additive CNS depression).
No products indexed under this heading.

Ketamine Hydrochloride (Co-administration may result in an additive CNS depression).
No products indexed under this heading.

Levomethadyl Acetate Hydrochloride (Co-administration may result in an additive CNS depression).
No products indexed under this heading.

Levorphanol Tartrate (Co-administration may result in an additive CNS depression). Products include:
Levo-Dromoran 1734
Levorphanol Tartrate Tablets 3059

Loratadine (Co-administration may result in an additive CNS depression). Products include:
Claritin 3100
Claritin-D 12 Hour Extended Release Tablets 3102
Claritin-D 24 Hour Extended Release Tablets 3104

Lorazepam (Co-administration may result in an additive CNS depression). Products include:
Ativan Injection 3478
Ativan Tablets 3482

Loxapine Hydrochloride (Co-administration may result in an additive CNS depression).
No products indexed under this heading.

Loxapine Succinate (Co-administration may result in an additive CNS depression). Products include:
Loxitane Capsules 3398

Maprotiline Hydrochloride (Co-administration with tricyclic antidepressants may increase the effect of either hydrocodone or the tricyclic antidepressant).
No products indexed under this heading.

Meperidine Hydrochloride (Co-administration may result in an additive CNS depression). Products include:
Demerol 3079
Mepergan Injection 3539

Mephobarbital (Co-administration may result in an additive CNS depression).
No products indexed under this heading.

Meprobamate (Co-administration may result in an additive CNS depression). Products include:
Miltown Tablets 3349

Mesoridazine Besylate (Co-administration may result in an additive CNS depression). Products include:
Serentil 1057

Methadone Hydrochloride (Co-administration may result in an additive CNS depression). Products include:
Dolophine Hydrochloride Tablets 3056

Methdilazine Hydrochloride (Co-administration may result in an additive CNS depression).
No products indexed under this heading.

Methohexital Sodium (Co-administration may result in an additive CNS depression). Products include:
Brevital Sodium for Injection, USP .. 1815

Methotrimeprazine (Co-administration may result in an additive CNS depression).
No products indexed under this heading.

Methoxyflurane (Co-administration may result in an additive CNS depression).
No products indexed under this heading.

Midazolam Hydrochloride (Co-administration may result in an additive CNS depression). Products include:
Versed Injection 3027
Versed Syrup 3033

Moclobemide (Co-administration with an MAO inhibitor may increase the effect of either hydrocodone or the MAO inhibitor).
No products indexed under this heading.

Molindone Hydrochloride (Co-administration may result in an additive CNS depression). Products include:
Moban 1320

Morphine Sulfate (Co-administration may result in an additive CNS depression). Products include:
Astramorph/PF Injection, USP (Preservative-Free) 594
Duramorph Injection 1312
Infumorph 200 and Infumorph 500 Sterile Solutions 1314
Kadian Capsules 1335
MS Contin Tablets 2896
MSIR 2898
Oramorph SR Tablets 3062
Roxanol 3066

Nortriptyline Hydrochloride (Co-administration with tricyclic antidepressants may increase the effect of either hydrocodone or the tricyclic antidepressant).
No products indexed under this heading.

Olanzapine (Co-administration may result in an additive CNS depression). Products include:
Zyprexa Tablets 1973
Zyprexa ZYDIS Orally Disintegrating Tablets 1973

Oxazepam (Co-administration may result in an additive CNS depression).
No products indexed under this heading.

Oxycodone Hydrochloride (Co-administration may result in an additive CNS depression). Products include:
OxyContin Tablets 2912
OxyFast Oral Concentrate Solution . 2916
OxyIR Capsules 2916
Percocet Tablets 1326
Percodan Tablets 1327
Percolone Tablets 1327
Roxicodone 3067
Tylox Capsules 2597

Pargyline Hydrochloride (Co-administration with an MAO inhibitor may increase the effect of either hydrocodone or the MAO inhibitor).
No products indexed under this heading.

Pentobarbital Sodium (Co-administration may result in an additive CNS depression). Products include:
Nembutal Sodium Solution 485

Perphenazine (Co-administration may result in an additive CNS depression). Products include:
Etrafon 3115
Trilafon 3160

Phenelzine Sulfate (Co-administration with an MAO inhibitor may increase the effect of either hydrocodone or the MAO inhibitor). Products include:
Nardil Tablets 2653

Phenobarbital (Co-administration may result in an additive CNS depression). Products include:
Arco-Lase Plus Tablets 592
Donnatal 2929
Donnatal Extentabs 2930

Prazepam (Co-administration may result in an additive CNS depression).
No products indexed under this heading.

Procarbazine Hydrochloride (Co-administration with an MAO inhibitor may increase the effect of either hydrocodone or the MAO inhibitor). Products include:
Matulane Capsules 3246

Prochlorperazine (Co-administration may result in an additive CNS depression). Products include:
Compazine 1505

Promethazine Hydrochloride (Co-administration may result in an additive CNS depression). Products include:
Mepergan Injection 3539
Phenergan Injection 3553
Phenergan 3556
Phenergan Syrup 3554
Phenergan with Codeine Syrup 3557
Phenergan with Dextromethorphan Syrup 3559
Phenergan VC Syrup 3560
Phenergan VC with Codeine Syrup .. 3561

Propofol (Co-administration may result in an additive CNS depression). Products include:
Diprivan Injectable Emulsion 667

Propoxyphene Hydrochloride (Co-administration may result in an additive CNS depression). Products include:
Darvon Pulvules 1909
Darvon Compound-65 Pulvules 1910

Propoxyphene Napsylate (Co-administration may result in an additive CNS depression). Products include:
Darvon-N/Darvocet-N 1907
Darvon-N Tablets 1912

Protriptyline Hydrochloride (Co-administration with tricyclic antidepressants may increase the effect of either hydrocodone or the tricyclic antidepressant). Products include:
Vivactil Tablets 2446
Vivactil Tablets 2217

Pyrilamine Maleate (Co-administration may result in an additive CNS depression). Products include:
Maximum Strength Midol Menstrual Caplets and Gelcaps .... ▣612
Maximum Strength Midol PMS Caplets and Gelcaps .... ▣613

Pyrilamine Tannate (Co-administration may result in an additive CNS depression). Products include:
Ryna-12 S Suspension 3351

Quazepam (Co-administration may result in an additive CNS depression).
No products indexed under this heading.

Quetiapine Fumarate (Co-administration may result in an additive CNS depression). Products include:
Seroquel Tablets 684

Remifentanil Hydrochloride (Co-administration may result in an additive CNS depression).
No products indexed under this heading.

Risperidone (Co-administration may result in an additive CNS depression). Products include:
Risperdal 1796

Secobarbital Sodium (Co-administration may result in an additive CNS depression).
No products indexed under this heading.

Selegiline Hydrochloride (Co-administration with an MAO inhibitor may increase the effect of either hydrocodone or the MAO inhibitor). Products include:
Eldepryl Capsules 3266

Sevoflurane (Co-administration may result in an additive CNS depression).
No products indexed under this heading.

Sufentanil Citrate (Co-administration may result in an additive CNS depression).
No products indexed under this heading.

Temazepam (Co-administration may result in an additive CNS depression).
No products indexed under this heading.

Terfenadine (Co-administration may result in an additive CNS depression).
No products indexed under this heading.

Thiamylal Sodium (Co-administration may result in an additive CNS depression).
No products indexed under this heading.

Thioridazine Hydrochloride (Co-administration may result in an additive CNS depression). Products include:
Thioridazine Hydrochloride Tablets 2289

Thiothixene (Co-administration may result in an additive CNS depression). Products include:
Navane Capsules 2701
Thiothixene Capsules 2290

Tranylcypromine Sulfate (Co-administration with an MAO inhibitor may increase the effect of either hydrocodone or the MAO inhibitor). Products include:
Parnate Tablets 1607

Triazolam (Co-administration may result in an additive CNS depression). Products include:
Halcion Tablets 2823

Trifluoperazine Hydrochloride (Co-administration may result in an additive CNS depression). Products include:
Stelazine 1640

Trimeprazine Tartrate (Co-administration may result in an additive CNS depression).
No products indexed under this heading.

Trimipramine Maleate (Co-administration with tricyclic antidepressants may increase the effect of either hydrocodone or the tricyclic antidepressant). Products include:
Surmontil Capsules 3595

Tripelennamine Hydrochloride (Co-administration may result in an additive CNS depression).
No products indexed under this heading.

Triprolidine Hydrochloride (Co-administration may result in an additive CNS depression). Products include:
Actifed Cold & Allergy Tablets .... ▣688

Zaleplon (Co-administration may result in an additive CNS depression). Products include:
Sonata Capsules 3591

Ziprasidone Hydrochloride (Co-administration may result in an additive CNS depression). Products include:
Geodon Capsules 2688

Zolpidem Tartrate (Co-administration may result in an additive CNS depression). Products include:
Ambien Tablets 3191

Food Interactions

Alcohol (Concurrent use results in an additive CNS depression).

VICODIN TUSS EXPECTORANT
(Guaifenesin, Hydrocodone Bitartrate).......... 519
May interact with central nervous system depressants, general anesthetics, hypnotics and sedatives, narcotic analgesics, phenothiazines, tranquilizers, and certain other agents. Compounds in these categories include:

Alfentanil Hydrochloride (Co-administration may exhibit an additive CNS depression; the dose of one or both agents should be reduced).
No products indexed under this heading.

Alprazolam (Co-administration may exhibit an additive CNS depression; the dose of one or both agents should be reduced). Products include:
Xanax Tablets 2865

Aprobarbital (Co-administration may exhibit an additive CNS depression; the dose of one or both agents should be reduced).
No products indexed under this heading.

Buprenorphine Hydrochloride (Co-administration may exhibit an additive CNS depression; the dose of one or both agents should be reduced). Products include:
Buprenex Injectable 2918

Buspirone Hydrochloride (Co-administration may exhibit an additive CNS depression; the dose of one or both agents should be reduced).
No products indexed under this heading.

Butabarbital (Co-administration may exhibit an additive CNS depression; the dose of one or both agents should be reduced).
No products indexed under this heading.

Butalbital (Co-administration may exhibit an additive CNS depression; the dose of one or both agents should be reduced). Products include:
Phrenilin 578
Sedapap Tablets 50 mg/650 mg 2225

Chlordiazepoxide (Co-administration may exhibit an additive CNS depression; the dose of one or both agents should be reduced). Products include:
Limbitrol 1738

Chlordiazepoxide Hydrochloride (Co-administration may exhibit an additive CNS depression; the dose of one or both agents should be reduced). Products include:
Librium Capsules 1736
Librium for Injection 1737

Chlorpromazine (Co-administration may exhibit an additive CNS depression; the dose of one or both agents should be reduced). Products include:
Thorazine Suppositories 1656

Chlorpromazine Hydrochloride (Co-administration may exhibit an additive CNS depression; the dose of one or both agents should be reduced). Products include:
Thorazine 1656

Chlorprothixene (Co-administration may exhibit an additive CNS depression; the dose of one or both agents should be reduced).
No products indexed under this heading.

Chlorprothixene Hydrochloride (Co-administration may exhibit an additive CNS depression; the dose of one or both agents should be reduced).
No products indexed under this heading.

Chlorprothixene Lactate (Co-administration may exhibit an additive CNS depression; the dose of one or both agents should be reduced).
No products indexed under this heading.

Clorazepate Dipotassium (Co-administration may exhibit an additive CNS depression; the dose of one or both agents should be reduced). Products include:
Tranxene 511

Clozapine (Co-administration may exhibit an additive CNS depression; the dose of one or both agents should be reduced). Products include:
Clozaril Tablets 2319

Codeine Phosphate (Co-administration may exhibit an additive CNS depression; the dose of one or both agents should be reduced). Products include:
Phenergan with Codeine Syrup 3557
Phenergan VC with Codeine Syrup 3561
Robitussin A-C Syrup 2942
Robitussin-DAC Syrup 2942
Ryna-C Liquid 768
Soma Compound w/Codeine Tablets 3355
Tussi-Organidin NR Liquid 3350
Tussi-Organidin-S NR Liquid 3350
Tylenol with Codeine 2595

Desflurane (Co-administration may exhibit an additive CNS depression; the dose of one or both agents should be reduced). Products include:
Suprane Liquid for Inhalation 874

Dezocine (Co-administration may exhibit an additive CNS depression; the dose of one or both agents should be reduced).
No products indexed under this heading.

Diazepam (Co-administration may exhibit an additive CNS depression; the dose of one or both agents should be reduced). Products include:
Valium Injectable 3026
Valium Tablets 3047

Droperidol (Co-administration may exhibit an additive CNS depression; the dose of one or both agents should be reduced).
No products indexed under this heading.

Enflurane (Co-administration may exhibit an additive CNS depression; the dose of one or both agents should be reduced).
No products indexed under this heading.

Estazolam (Co-administration may exhibit an additive CNS depression; the dose of one or both agents should be reduced). Products include:
ProSom Tablets 500

Ethchlorvynol (Co-administration may exhibit an additive CNS depression; the dose of one or both agents should be reduced).
No products indexed under this heading.

Ethinamate (Co-administration may exhibit an additive CNS depression; the dose of one or both agents should be reduced).
No products indexed under this heading.

Fentanyl (Co-administration may exhibit an additive CNS depression; the dose of one or both agents should be reduced). Products include:
Duragesic Transdermal System 1786

Fentanyl Citrate (Co-administration may exhibit an additive CNS depression; the dose of one or both agents should be reduced). Products include:
Actiq 1184

Fluphenazine Decanoate (Co-administration may exhibit an additive CNS depression; the dose of one or both agents should be reduced).
No products indexed under this heading.

Fluphenazine Enanthate (Co-administration may exhibit an additive CNS depression; the dose of one or both agents should be reduced).
No products indexed under this heading.

Fluphenazine Hydrochloride (Co-administration may exhibit an additive CNS depression; the dose of one or both agents should be reduced).
No products indexed under this heading.

Flurazepam Hydrochloride (Co-administration may exhibit an additive CNS depression; the dose of one or both agents should be reduced).
No products indexed under this heading.

Glutethimide (Co-administration may exhibit an additive CNS depression; the dose of one or both agents should be reduced).
No products indexed under this heading.

Haloperidol (Co-administration may exhibit an additive CNS depression; the dose of one or both agents should be reduced). Products include:
Haldol Injection, Tablets and Concentrate 2533

Haloperidol Decanoate (Co-administration may exhibit an additive CNS depression; the dose of one or both agents should be reduced). Products include:
Haldol Decanoate 2535

Hydrocodone Polistirex (Co-administration may exhibit an additive CNS depression; the dose of one or both agents should be reduced). Products include:
Tussionex Pennkinetic Extended-Release Suspension 1174

Hydromorphone Hydrochloride (Co-administration may exhibit an additive CNS depression; the dose of one or both agents should be reduced). Products include:
Dilaudid 441
Dilaudid Oral Liquid 445
Dilaudid Powder 441
Dilaudid Rectal Suppositories 441
Dilaudid Tablets 441
Dilaudid Tablets - 8 mg 445
Dilaudid-HP 443

Hydroxyzine Hydrochloride (Co-administration may exhibit an additive CNS depression; the dose of one or both agents should be reduced). Products include:
Atarax Tablets & Syrup 2667
Vistaril Intramuscular Solution 2738

Isoflurane (Co-administration may exhibit an additive CNS depression; the dose of one or both agents should be reduced).
No products indexed under this heading.

Ketamine Hydrochloride (Co-administration may exhibit an additive CNS depression; the dose of one or both agents should be reduced).
No products indexed under this heading.

Levomethadyl Acetate Hydrochloride (Co-administration may exhibit an additive CNS depression; the dose of one or both agents should be reduced).
No products indexed under this heading.

Levorphanol Tartrate (Co-administration may exhibit an additive CNS depression; the dose of one or both agents should be reduced). Products include:
Levo-Dromoran 1734
Levorphanol Tartrate Tablets 3059

Lorazepam (Co-administration may exhibit an additive CNS depression; the dose of one or both agents should be reduced). Products include:
Ativan Injection 3478
Ativan Tablets 3482

Loxapine Hydrochloride (Co-administration may exhibit an additive CNS depression; the dose of one or both agents should be reduced).
No products indexed under this heading.

Loxapine Succinate (Co-administration may exhibit an additive CNS depression; the dose of one or both agents should be reduced). Products include:
Loxitane Capsules 3398

Meperidine Hydrochloride (Co-administration may exhibit an additive CNS depression; the dose of one or both agents should be reduced). Products include:
Demerol 3079
Mepergan Injection 3539

Mephobarbital (Co-administration may exhibit an additive CNS depression; the dose of one or both agents should be reduced).
No products indexed under this heading.

Meprobamate (Co-administration may exhibit an additive CNS depression; the dose of one or both agents should be reduced). Products include:
Miltown Tablets 3349

Mesoridazine Besylate (Co-administration may exhibit an additive CNS depression; the dose of one or both agents should be reduced). Products include:
Serentil 1057

Methadone Hydrochloride (Co-administration may exhibit an additive CNS depression; the dose of one or both agents should be reduced). Products include:
Dolophine Hydrochloride Tablets 3056

Methohexital Sodium (Co-administration may exhibit an additive CNS depression; the dose of one or both agents should be reduced). Products include:
Brevital Sodium for Injection, USP 1815

Methotrimeprazine (Co-administration may exhibit an additive CNS depression; the dose of one or both agents should be reduced).
No products indexed under this heading.

Methoxyflurane (Co-administration may exhibit an additive CNS depression; the dose of one or both agents should be reduced).
No products indexed under this heading.

Midazolam Hydrochloride (Co-administration may exhibit an additive CNS depression; the dose of one or both agents should be reduced). Products include:
Versed Injection 3027
Versed Syrup 3033

Molindone Hydrochloride (Co-administration may exhibit an additive CNS depression; the dose of one or both agents should be reduced). Products include:
Moban 1320

Morphine Sulfate (Co-administration may exhibit an addi-

tive CNS depression; the dose of one or both agents should be reduced). Products include:
Astramorph/PF Injection, USP (Preservative-Free) ... 594
Duramorph Injection ... 1312
Infumorph 200 and Infumorph 500 Sterile Solutions ... 1314
Kadian Capsules ... 1335
MS Contin Tablets ... 2896
MSIR ... 2898
Oramorph SR Tablets ... 3062
Roxanol ... 3066

Olanzapine (Co-administration may exhibit an additive CNS depression; the dose of one or both agents should be reduced). Products include:
Zyprexa Tablets ... 1973
Zyprexa ZYDIS Orally Disintegrating Tablets ... 1973

Oxazepam (Co-administration may exhibit an additive CNS depression; the dose of one or both agents should be reduced).
No products indexed under this heading.

Oxycodone Hydrochloride (Co-administration may exhibit an additive CNS depression; the dose of one or both agents should be reduced). Products include:
OxyContin Tablets ... 2912
OxyFast Oral Concentrate Solution ... 2916
OxyIR Capsules ... 2916
Percocet Tablets ... 1326
Percodan Tablets ... 1327
Percolone Tablets ... 1327
Roxicodone ... 3067
Tylox Capsules ... 2597

Pentobarbital Sodium (Co-administration may exhibit an additive CNS depression; the dose of one or both agents should be reduced). Products include:
Nembutal Sodium Solution ... 485

Perphenazine (Co-administration may exhibit an additive CNS depression; the dose of one or both agents should be reduced). Products include:
Etrafon ... 3115
Trilafon ... 3160

Phenobarbital (Co-administration may exhibit an additive CNS depression; the dose of one or both agents should be reduced). Products include:
Arco-Lase Plus Tablets ... 592
Donnatal ... 2929
Donnatal Extentabs ... 2930

Prazepam (Co-administration may exhibit an additive CNS depression; the dose of one or both agents should be reduced).
No products indexed under this heading.

Prochlorperazine (Co-administration may exhibit an additive CNS depression; the dose of one or both agents should be reduced). Products include:
Compazine ... 1505

Promethazine Hydrochloride (Co-administration may exhibit an additive CNS depression; the dose of one or both agents should be reduced). Products include:
Mepergan Injection ... 3539
Phenergan Injection ... 3553
Phenergan ... 3556
Phenergan Syrup ... 3554
Phenergan with Codeine Syrup ... 3557
Phenergan with Dextromethorphan Syrup ... 3559
Phenergan VC Syrup ... 3560
Phenergan VC with Codeine Syrup ... 3561

Propofol (Co-administration may exhibit an additive CNS depression; the dose of one or both agents should be reduced). Products include:
Diprivan Injectable Emulsion ... 667

Propoxyphene Hydrochloride (Co-administration may exhibit an additive CNS depression; the dose of one or both agents should be reduced). Products include:
Darvon Pulvules ... 1909
Darvon Compound-65 Pulvules ... 1910

Propoxyphene Napsylate (Co-administration may exhibit an additive CNS depression; the dose of one or both agents should be reduced). Products include:
Darvon-N/Darvocet-N ... 1907
Darvon-N Tablets ... 1912

Quazepam (Co-administration may exhibit an additive CNS depression; the dose of one or both agents should be reduced).
No products indexed under this heading.

Quetiapine Fumarate (Co-administration may exhibit an additive CNS depression; the dose of one or both agents should be reduced). Products include:
Seroquel Tablets ... 684

Remifentanil Hydrochloride (Co-administration may exhibit an additive CNS depression; the dose of one or both agents should be reduced).
No products indexed under this heading.

Risperidone (Co-administration may exhibit an additive CNS depression; the dose of one or both agents should be reduced). Products include:
Risperdal ... 1796

Secobarbital Sodium (Co-administration may exhibit an additive CNS depression; the dose of one or both agents should be reduced).
No products indexed under this heading.

Sevoflurane (Co-administration may exhibit an additive CNS depression; the dose of one or both agents should be reduced).
No products indexed under this heading.

Sufentanil Citrate (Co-administration may exhibit an additive CNS depression; the dose of one or both agents should be reduced).
No products indexed under this heading.

Temazepam (Co-administration may exhibit an additive CNS depression; the dose of one or both agents should be reduced).
No products indexed under this heading.

Thiamylal Sodium (Co-administration may exhibit an additive CNS depression; the dose of one or both agents should be reduced).
No products indexed under this heading.

Thioridazine Hydrochloride (Co-administration may exhibit an additive CNS depression; the dose of one or both agents should be reduced). Products include:
Thioridazine Hydrochloride Tablets ... 2289

Thiothixene (Co-administration may exhibit an additive CNS depression; the dose of one or both agents should be reduced). Products include:
Navane Capsules ... 2701
Thiothixene Capsules ... 2290

Triazolam (Co-administration may exhibit an additive CNS depression; the dose of one or both agents should be reduced). Products include:
Halcion Tablets ... 2823

Trifluoperazine Hydrochloride (Co-administration may exhibit an additive CNS depression; the dose of one or both agents should be reduced). Products include:
Stelazine ... 1640

Zaleplon (Co-administration may exhibit an additive CNS depression; the dose of one or both agents should be reduced). Products include:
Sonata Capsules ... 3591

Ziprasidone Hydrochloride (Co-administration may exhibit an additive CNS depression; the dose of one or both agents should be reduced). Products include:
Geodon Capsules ... 2688

Zolpidem Tartrate (Co-administration may exhibit an additive CNS depression; the dose of one or both agents should be reduced). Products include:
Ambien Tablets ... 3191

Food Interactions

Alcohol (Co-administration may exhibit an additive CNS depression).

VICOPROFEN TABLETS

(Hydrocodone Bitartrate, Ibuprofen) ... 520

May interact with ACE inhibitors, anticholinergics, central nervous system depressants, lithium preparations, monoamine oxidase inhibitors, thiazides, tricyclic antidepressants, and certain other agents. Compounds in these categories include:

Alfentanil Hydrochloride (May exhibit additive CNS depression).
No products indexed under this heading.

Alprazolam (May exhibit additive CNS depression). Products include:
Xanax Tablets ... 2865

Amitriptyline Hydrochloride (Co-administration of tricyclic antidepressants with hydrocodone preparations may increase the effect of either the antidepressant or hydrocodone). Products include:
Etrafon ... 3115
Limbitrol ... 1738

Amoxapine (Co-administration of tricyclic antidepressants with hydrocodone preparations may increase the effect of either the antidepressant or hydrocodone).
No products indexed under this heading.

Aprobarbital (May exhibit additive CNS depression).
No products indexed under this heading.

Aspirin (Co-administration of Vicoprofen and aspirin may increase the risk of adverse effects; concurrent use should be avoided). Products include:
Aggrenox Capsules ... 1026
Alka-Seltzer ... ▣603
Alka-Seltzer Lemon Lime Antacid and Pain Reliever Effervescent Tablets ... ▣603
Alka-Seltzer Extra Strength Antacid and Pain Reliever Effervescent Tablets ... ▣603
Alka-Seltzer PM Effervescent Tablets ... ▣605
Genuine Bayer Tablets, Caplets and Gelcaps ... ▣606
Extra Strength Bayer Caplets and Gelcaps ... ▣610
Aspirin Regimen Bayer Children's Chewable Tablets (Orange or Cherry Flavored) ... ▣607
Bayer, Aspirin Regimen ... ▣606
Aspirin Regimen Bayer 81 mg Caplets with Calcium ... ▣607
Genuine Bayer Professional Labeling (Aspirin Regimen Bayer) ... ▣608
Extra Strength Bayer Arthritis Caplets ... ▣610
Extra Strength Bayer Plus Caplets ... ▣610
Extra Strength Bayer PM Caplets ... ▣611
BC Powder ... ▣619
BC Allergy Sinus Cold Powder ... ▣619
Arthritis Strength BC Powder ... ▣619
BC Sinus Cold Powder ... ▣619
Darvon Compound-65 Pulvules ... 1910
Ecotrin Enteric Coated Aspirin Low, Regular and Maximum Strength Tablets ... 1715
Excedrin Extra-Strength Tablets, Caplets, and Geltabs ... ▣629
Excedrin Migraine ... 1070
Goody's Body Pain Formula Powder ... ▣620
Goody's Extra Strength Headache Powder ... ▣620
Goody's Extra Strength Pain Relief Tablets ... ▣620
Percodan Tablets ... 1327
Robaxisal Tablets ... 2939
Soma Compound Tablets ... 3354
Soma Compound w/Codeine Tablets ... 3355
Vanquish Caplets ... ▣617

Atropine Sulfate (Concurrent use of anticholinergics with hydrocodone preparations may produce paralytic ileus). Products include:
Donnatal ... 2929
Donnatal Extentabs ... 2930
Motofen Tablets ... 577
Prosed/DS Tablets ... 3268
Urised Tablets ... 2876

Belladonna Alkaloids (Concurrent use of anticholinergics with hydrocodone preparations may produce paralytic ileus). Products include:
Hyland's Teething Tablets ... ▣766
Urimax Tablets ... 1769

Benazepril Hydrochloride (NSAIDs may diminish the antihypertensive effect of ACE inhibitors). Products include:
Lotensin Tablets ... 2365
Lotensin HCT Tablets ... 2367
Lotrel Capsules ... 2370

Bendroflumethiazide (Ibuprofen has been shown to reduce the natriuretic effect of thiazides in some patients). Products include:
Corzide 40/5 Tablets ... 2247
Corzide 80/5 Tablets ... 2247

Benztropine Mesylate (Concurrent use of anticholinergics with hydrocodone preparations may produce paralytic ileus). Products include:
Cogentin ... 2055

Biperiden Hydrochloride (Concurrent use of anticholinergics with hydrocodone preparations may produce paralytic ileus). Products include:
Akineton ... 402

Buprenorphine Hydrochloride (May exhibit additive CNS depression). Products include:
Buprenex Injectable ... 2918

Buspirone Hydrochloride (May exhibit additive CNS depression).
No products indexed under this heading.

Butabarbital (May exhibit additive CNS depression).
No products indexed under this heading.

Butalbital (May exhibit additive CNS depression). Products include:
Phrenilin ... 578
Sedapap Tablets 50 mg/650 mg ... 2225

Captopril (NSAIDs may diminish the antihypertensive effect of ACE inhibitors). Products include:
Captopril Tablets ... 2281

Chlordiazepoxide (May exhibit additive CNS depression). Products include:
Limbitrol ... 1738

Chlordiazepoxide Hydrochloride (May exhibit additive CNS depression). Products include:
Librium Capsules ... 1736
Librium for Injection ... 1737

Chlorothiazide (Ibuprofen has been shown to reduce the natriuretic effect of thiazides in some patients). Products include:
Aldoclor Tablets ... 2035
Diuril Oral ... 2087

Chlorothiazide Sodium (Ibuprofen has been shown to reduce the natriuretic effect of thiazides in some patients). Products include:
Diuril Sodium Intravenous 2086

Chlorpromazine (May exhibit additive CNS depression). Products include:
Thorazine Suppositories 1656

Chlorpromazine Hydrochloride (May exhibit additive CNS depression). Products include:
Thorazine 1656

Chlorprothixene (May exhibit additive CNS depression).
No products indexed under this heading.

Chlorprothixene Hydrochloride (May exhibit additive CNS depression).
No products indexed under this heading.

Chlorprothixene Lactate (May exhibit additive CNS depression).
No products indexed under this heading.

Clidinium Bromide (Concurrent use of anticholinergics with hydrocodone preparations may produce paralytic ileus).
No products indexed under this heading.

Clomipramine Hydrochloride (Co-administration of tricyclic antidepressants with hydrocodone preparations may increase the effect of either the antidepressant or hydrocodone).
No products indexed under this heading.

Clorazepate Dipotassium (May exhibit additive CNS depression). Products include:
Tranxene 511

Clozapine (May exhibit additive CNS depression). Products include:
Clozaril Tablets 2319

Codeine Phosphate (May exhibit additive CNS depression). Products include:
Phenergan with Codeine Syrup 3557
Phenergan VC with Codeine Syrup .. 3561
Robitussin A-C Syrup 2942
Robitussin-DAC Syrup 2942
Ryna-C Liquid 768
Soma Compound w/Codeine Tablets 3355
Tussi-Organidin NR Liquid 3350
Tussi-Organidin-S NR Liquid 3350
Tylenol with Codeine 2595

Desflurane (May exhibit additive CNS depression). Products include:
Suprane Liquid for Inhalation 874

Desipramine Hydrochloride (Co-administration of tricyclic antidepressants with hydrocodone preparations may increase the effect of either the antidepressant or hydrocodone). Products include:
Norpramin Tablets 755

Dezocine (May exhibit additive CNS depression).
No products indexed under this heading.

Diazepam (May exhibit additive CNS depression). Products include:
Valium Injectable 3026
Valium Tablets 3047

Dicyclomine Hydrochloride (Concurrent use of anticholinergics with hydrocodone preparations may produce paralytic ileus).
No products indexed under this heading.

Doxepin Hydrochloride (Co-administration of tricyclic antidepressants with hydrocodone preparations may increase the effect of either the antidepressant or hydrocodone). Products include:
Sinequan 2713

Droperidol (May exhibit additive CNS depression).
No products indexed under this heading.

Enalapril Maleate (NSAIDs may diminish the antihypertensive effect of ACE inhibitors). Products include:
Lexxel Tablets 608
Vaseretic Tablets 2204
Vasotec Tablets 2210

Enalaprilat (NSAIDs may diminish the antihypertensive effect of ACE inhibitors). Products include:
Enalaprilat Injection 863
Vasotec I.V. Injection 2207

Enflurane (May exhibit additive CNS depression).
No products indexed under this heading.

Estazolam (May exhibit additive CNS depression). Products include:
ProSom Tablets 500

Ethchlorvynol (May exhibit additive CNS depression).
No products indexed under this heading.

Ethinamate (May exhibit additive CNS depression).
No products indexed under this heading.

Fentanyl (May exhibit additive CNS depression). Products include:
Duragesic Transdermal System 1786

Fentanyl Citrate (May exhibit additive CNS depression). Products include:
Actiq 1184

Fluphenazine Decanoate (May exhibit additive CNS depression).
No products indexed under this heading.

Fluphenazine Enanthate (May exhibit additive CNS depression).
No products indexed under this heading.

Fluphenazine Hydrochloride (May exhibit additive CNS depression).
No products indexed under this heading.

Flurazepam Hydrochloride (May exhibit additive CNS depression).
No products indexed under this heading.

Fosinopril Sodium (NSAIDs may diminish the antihypertensive effect of ACE inhibitors). Products include:
Monopril Tablets 1091
Monopril HCT 1094

Furosemide (Ibuprofen has been shown to reduce the natriuretic effect of furosemide). Products include:
Furosemide Tablets 2284

Glutethimide (May exhibit additive CNS depression).
No products indexed under this heading.

Glycopyrrolate (Concurrent use of anticholinergics with hydrocodone preparations may produce paralytic ileus). Products include:
Robinul Forte Tablets 1358
Robinul Injectable 2940
Robinul Tablets 1358

Haloperidol (May exhibit additive CNS depression). Products include:
Haldol Injection, Tablets and Concentrate 2533

Haloperidol Decanoate (May exhibit additive CNS depression). Products include:
Haldol Decanoate 2535

Hydrochlorothiazide (Ibuprofen has been shown to reduce the natriuretic effect of thiazides in some patients). Products include:
Accuretic Tablets 2614
Aldoril Tablets 2039
Atacand HCT Tablets 597
Avalide Tablets 1070
Diovan HCT Tablets 2338
Dyazide Capsules 1515
HydroDIURIL Tablets 2108
Hyzaar 2109
Inderide Tablets 3517
Inderide LA Long-Acting Capsules .. 3519
Lotensin HCT Tablets 2367
Maxzide 1008
Micardis HCT Tablets 1051
Microzide Capsules 3414
Moduretic Tablets 2138
Monopril HCT 1094
Prinzide Tablets 2168
Timolide Tablets 2187
Uniretic Tablets 3178
Vaseretic Tablets 2204
Zestoretic Tablets 695
Ziac Tablets 1887

Hydrocodone Polistirex (May exhibit additive CNS depression). Products include:
Tussionex Pennkinetic Extended-Release Suspension 1174

Hydroflumethiazide (Ibuprofen has been shown to reduce the natriuretic effect of thiazides in some patients). Products include:
Diucardin Tablets 3494

Hydromorphone Hydrochloride (May exhibit additive CNS depression). Products include:
Dilaudid 441
Dilaudid Oral Liquid 445
Dilaudid Powder 441
Dilaudid Rectal Suppositories 441
Dilaudid Tablets 441
Dilaudid Tablets - 8 mg 445
Dilaudid-HP 443

Hydroxyzine Hydrochloride (May exhibit additive CNS depression). Products include:
Atarax Tablets & Syrup 2667
Vistaril Intramuscular Solution 2738

Hyoscyamine (Concurrent use of anticholinergics with hydrocodone preparations may produce paralytic ileus). Products include:
Urised Tablets 2876

Hyoscyamine Sulfate (Concurrent use of anticholinergics with hydrocodone preparations may produce paralytic ileus). Products include:
Arco-Lase Plus Tablets 592
Donnatal 2929
Donnatal Extentabs 2930
Levsin/Levsinex/Levbid 3172
NuLev Orally Disintegrating Tablets 3176
Prosed/DS Tablets 3268
Urimax Tablets 1769

Imipramine Hydrochloride (Co-administration of tricyclic antidepressants with hydrocodone preparations may increase the effect of either the antidepressant or hydrocodone).
No products indexed under this heading.

Imipramine Pamoate (Co-administration of tricyclic antidepressants with hydrocodone preparations may increase the effect of either the antidepressant or hydrocodone).
No products indexed under this heading.

Ipratropium Bromide (Concurrent use of anticholinergics with hydrocodone preparations may produce paralytic ileus). Products include:
Atrovent Inhalation Aerosol 1030
Atrovent Inhalation Solution 1031
Atrovent Nasal Spray 0.03% 1032
Atrovent Nasal Spray 0.06% 1033
Combivent Inhalation Aerosol 1041
DuoNeb Inhalation Solution 1233

Isocarboxazid (Co-administration of MAO inhibitors with hydrocodone preparations may increase the effect of either the MAO inhibitors or hydrocodone).
No products indexed under this heading.

Isoflurane (May exhibit additive CNS depression).
No products indexed under this heading.

Ketamine Hydrochloride (May exhibit additive CNS depression).
No products indexed under this heading.

Levomethadyl Acetate Hydrochloride (May exhibit additive CNS depression).
No products indexed under this heading.

Levorphanol Tartrate (May exhibit additive CNS depression). Products include:
Levo-Dromoran 1734
Levorphanol Tartrate Tablets 3059

Lisinopril (NSAIDs may diminish the antihypertensive effect of ACE inhibitors). Products include:
Prinivil Tablets 2164
Prinzide Tablets 2168
Zestoretic Tablets 695
Zestril Tablets 698

Lithium Carbonate (Ibuprofen has been shown to elevate plasma lithium concentration and reduce renal clearance). Products include:
Eskalith 1527
Lithium Carbonate 3061
Lithobid Slow-Release Tablets 3255

Lithium Citrate (Ibuprofen has been shown to elevate plasma lithium concentration and reduce renal clearance). Products include:
Lithium Citrate Syrup 3061

Lorazepam (May exhibit additive CNS depression). Products include:
Ativan Injection 3478
Ativan Tablets 3482

Loxapine Hydrochloride (May exhibit additive CNS depression).
No products indexed under this heading.

Loxapine Succinate (May exhibit additive CNS depression). Products include:
Loxitane Capsules 3398

Maprotiline Hydrochloride (Co-administration of tricyclic antidepressants with hydrocodone preparations may increase the effect of either the antidepressant or hydrocodone).
No products indexed under this heading.

Mepenzolate Bromide (Concurrent use of anticholinergics with hydrocodone preparations may produce paralytic ileus).
No products indexed under this heading.

Meperidine Hydrochloride (May exhibit additive CNS depression). Products include:
Demerol 3079
Mepergan Injection 3539

Mephobarbital (May exhibit additive CNS depression).
No products indexed under this heading.

Meprobamate (May exhibit additive CNS depression). Products include:
Miltown Tablets 3349

Mesoridazine Besylate (May exhibit additive CNS depression). Products include:
Serentil 1057

Methadone Hydrochloride (May exhibit additive CNS depression). Products include:
Dolophine Hydrochloride Tablets 3056

Methohexital Sodium (May exhibit additive CNS depression). Products include:
Brevital Sodium for Injection, USP .. 1815

Methotrexate Sodium (Ibuprofen, in animal studies, has been reported to competitively inhibit methotrexate accumulation; this could lead to enhanced toxicity of methotrexate).
No products indexed under this heading.

Methotrimeprazine (May exhibit additive CNS depression).
No products indexed under this heading.

Methoxyflurane (May exhibit additive CNS depression).
No products indexed under this heading.

Methyclothiazide (Ibuprofen has been shown to reduce the natriuretic

effect of thiazides in some patients).
No products indexed under this heading.

Midazolam Hydrochloride (May exhibit additive CNS depression). Products include:
Versed Injection **3027**
Versed Syrup **3033**

Moclobemide (Co-administration of MAO inhibitors with hydrocodone preparations may increase the effect of either the MAO inhibitors or hydrocodone).
No products indexed under this heading.

Moexipril Hydrochloride (NSAIDs may diminish the antihypertensive effect of ACE inhibitors). Products include:
Uniretic Tablets **3178**
Univasc Tablets **3181**

Molindone Hydrochloride (May exhibit additive CNS depression). Products include:
Moban **1320**

Morphine Sulfate (May exhibit additive CNS depression). Products include:
Astramorph/PF Injection, USP (Preservative-Free) **594**
Duramorph Injection **1312**
Infumorph 200 and Infumorph 500 Sterile Solutions **1314**
Kadian Capsules **1335**
MS Contin Tablets **2896**
MSIR **2898**
Oramorph SR Tablets **3062**
Roxanol **3066**

Nortriptyline Hydrochloride (Co-administration of tricyclic antidepressants with hydrocodone preparations may increase the effect of either the antidepressant or hydrocodone).
No products indexed under this heading.

Olanzapine (May exhibit additive CNS depression). Products include:
Zyprexa Tablets **1973**
Zyprexa ZYDIS Orally Disintegrating Tablets **1973**

Oxazepam (May exhibit additive CNS depression).
No products indexed under this heading.

Oxybutynin Chloride (Concurrent use of anticholinergics with hydrocodone preparations may produce paralytic ileus). Products include:
Ditropan XL Extended Release Tablets **564**

Oxycodone Hydrochloride (May exhibit additive CNS depression). Products include:
OxyContin Tablets **2912**
OxyFast Oral Concentrate Solution . **2916**
OxyIR Capsules **2916**
Percocet Tablets **1326**
Percodan Tablets **1327**
Percolone Tablets **1327**
Roxicodone **3067**
Tylox Capsules **2597**

Pargyline Hydrochloride (Co-administration of MAO inhibitors with hydrocodone preparations may increase the effect of either the MAO inhibitors or hydrocodone).
No products indexed under this heading.

Pentobarbital Sodium (May exhibit additive CNS depression). Products include:
Nembutal Sodium Solution **485**

Perindopril Erbumine (NSAIDs may diminish the antihypertensive effect of ACE inhibitors). Products include:
Aceon Tablets (2 mg, 4 mg, 8 mg) **3249**

Perphenazine (May exhibit additive CNS depression). Products include:
Etrafon **3115**
Trilafon **3160**

Phenelzine Sulfate (Co-administration of MAO inhibitors with hydrocodone preparations may increase the effect of either the MAO inhibitors or hydrocodone). Products include:
Nardil Tablets **2653**

Phenobarbital (May exhibit additive CNS depression). Products include:
Arco-Lase Plus Tablets **592**
Donnatal **2929**
Donnatal Extentabs **2930**

Polythiazide (Ibuprofen has been shown to reduce the natriuretic effect of thiazides in some patients). Products include:
Minizide Capsules **2700**
Renese Tablets **2712**

Prazepam (May exhibit additive CNS depression).
No products indexed under this heading.

Procarbazine Hydrochloride (Co-administration of MAO inhibitors with hydrocodone preparations may increase the effect of either the MAO inhibitors or hydrocodone). Products include:
Matulane Capsules **3246**

Prochlorperazine (May exhibit additive CNS depression). Products include:
Compazine **1505**

Procyclidine Hydrochloride (Concurrent use of anticholinergics with hydrocodone preparations may produce paralytic ileus).
No products indexed under this heading.

Promethazine Hydrochloride (May exhibit additive CNS depression). Products include:
Mepergan Injection **3539**
Phenergan Injection **3553**
Phenergan **3556**
Phenergan Syrup **3554**
Phenergan with Codeine Syrup **3557**
Phenergan with Dextromethorphan Syrup **3559**
Phenergan VC Syrup **3560**
Phenergan VC with Codeine Syrup .. **3561**

Propantheline Bromide (Concurrent use of anticholinergics with hydrocodone preparations may produce paralytic ileus).
No products indexed under this heading.

Propofol (May exhibit additive CNS depression). Products include:
Diprivan Injectable Emulsion **667**

Propoxyphene Hydrochloride (May exhibit additive CNS depression). Products include:
Darvon Pulvules **1909**
Darvon Compound-65 Pulvules **1910**

Propoxyphene Napsylate (May exhibit additive CNS depression). Products include:
Darvon-N/Darvocet-N **1907**
Darvon-N Tablets **1912**

Protriptyline Hydrochloride (Co-administration of tricyclic antidepressants with hydrocodone preparations may increase the effect of either the antidepressant or hydrocodone). Products include:
Vivactil Tablets **2446**
Vivactil Tablets **2217**

Quazepam (May exhibit additive CNS depression).
No products indexed under this heading.

Quetiapine Fumarate (May exhibit additive CNS depression). Products include:
Seroquel Tablets **684**

Quinapril Hydrochloride (NSAIDs may diminish the antihypertensive effect of ACE inhibitors). Products include:
Accupril Tablets **2611**
Accuretic Tablets **2614**

Ramipril (NSAIDs may diminish the antihypertensive effect of ACE inhibitors). Products include:
Altace Capsules **2233**

Remifentanil Hydrochloride (May exhibit additive CNS depression).
No products indexed under this heading.

Risperidone (May exhibit additive CNS depression). Products include:
Risperdal **1796**

Scopolamine (Concurrent use of anticholinergics with hydrocodone preparations may produce paralytic ileus). Products include:
Transderm Scōp Transdermal Therapeutic System **2302**

Scopolamine Hydrobromide (Concurrent use of anticholinergics with hydrocodone preparations may produce paralytic ileus). Products include:
Donnatal **2929**
Donnatal Extentabs **2930**

Secobarbital Sodium (May exhibit additive CNS depression).
No products indexed under this heading.

Selegiline Hydrochloride (Co-administration of MAO inhibitors with hydrocodone preparations may increase the effect of either the MAO inhibitors or hydrocodone). Products include:
Eldepryl Capsules **3266**

Sevoflurane (May exhibit additive CNS depression).
No products indexed under this heading.

Spirapril Hydrochloride (NSAIDs may diminish the antihypertensive effect of ACE inhibitors).
No products indexed under this heading.

Sufentanil Citrate (May exhibit additive CNS depression).
No products indexed under this heading.

Temazepam (May exhibit additive CNS depression).
No products indexed under this heading.

Thiamylal Sodium (May exhibit additive CNS depression).
No products indexed under this heading.

Thioridazine Hydrochloride (May exhibit additive CNS depression). Products include:
Thioridazine Hydrochloride Tablets **2289**

Thiothixene (May exhibit additive CNS depression). Products include:
Navane Capsules **2701**
Thiothixene Capsules **2290**

Tolterodine Tartrate (Concurrent use of anticholinergics with hydrocodone preparations may produce paralytic ileus). Products include:
Detrol Tablets **3623**
Detrol LA Capsules **2801**

Trandolapril (NSAIDs may diminish the antihypertensive effect of ACE inhibitors). Products include:
Mavik Tablets **478**
Tarka Tablets **508**

Tranylcypromine Sulfate (Co-administration of MAO inhibitors with hydrocodone preparations may increase the effect of either the MAO inhibitors or hydrocodone). Products include:
Parnate Tablets **1607**

Triazolam (May exhibit additive CNS depression). Products include:
Halcion Tablets **2823**

Tridihexethyl Chloride (Concurrent use of anticholinergics with hydrocodone preparations may produce paralytic ileus).
No products indexed under this heading.

Trifluoperazine Hydrochloride (May exhibit additive CNS depression). Products include:
Stelazine **1640**

Trihexyphenidyl Hydrochloride (Concurrent use of anticholinergics with hydrocodone preparations may produce paralytic ileus). Products include:
Artane **1855**

Trimipramine Maleate (Co-administration of tricyclic antidepressants with hydrocodone preparations may increase the effect of either the antidepressant or hydrocodone). Products include:
Surmontil Capsules **3595**

Warfarin Sodium (The effects of warfarin and NSAIDs on GI bleeding are synergistic). Products include:
Coumadin for Injection **1243**
Coumadin Tablets **1243**
Warfarin Sodium Tablets, USP **3302**

Zaleplon (May exhibit additive CNS depression). Products include:
Sonata Capsules **3591**

Ziprasidone Hydrochloride (May exhibit additive CNS depression). Products include:
Geodon Capsules **2688**

Zolpidem Tartrate (May exhibit additive CNS depression). Products include:
Ambien Tablets **3191**

Food Interactions

Alcohol (May exhibit additive CNS depression).

VIDEX POWDER FOR ORAL SOLUTION

(Didanosine) **1138**
See Videx EC Capsules

VIDEX PEDIATRIC POWDER FOR ORAL SOLUTION

(Didanosine) **1138**
See Videx EC Capsules

VIDEX CHEWABLE TABLETS

(Didanosine) **1138**
See Videx EC Capsules

VIDEX EC CAPSULES

(Didanosine) **1143**
May interact with antacids containing aluminum, calcium and magnesium, drugs that are known to cause peripheral neuropathy and pancreatitis (selected), tetracyclines, and certain other agents. Compounds in these categories include:

Allopurinol (Co-administration results in increased didanosine concentration; concurrent use is not recommended).
No products indexed under this heading.

Altretamine (Co-administration with drugs that are known to cause pancreatitis and peripheral neuropathy may increase the risk of these toxicities). Products include:
Hexalen Capsules **2226**

Aluminum Carbonate (Co-administration of these antacids with Videx chewable/dispersible buffered tablets or pediatric powder for oral solution may potentiate adverse effects associated with the antacid component).
No products indexed under this heading.

Aluminum Hydroxide (Co-administration of these antacids with Videx chewable/dispersible buffered tablets or pediatric powder for oral solution may potentiate adverse effects associated with the antacid component). Products include:
Amphojel Suspension (Mint Flavor) .... ▣**789**
Gaviscon Extra Strength Liquid .... ▣**751**
Gaviscon Extra Strength Tablets .... ▣**751**
Gaviscon Regular Strength Liquid . ▣**751**
Gaviscon Regular Strength Tablets .... ▣**750**
Maalox Antacid/Anti-Gas Oral Suspension .... ▣**673**
Maalox Max Maximum Strength Antacid/Anti-Gas Liquid **2300**
Maalox Regular Strength Antacid/Antigas Liquid **2300**

Mylanta 1813
Vanquish Caplets .... ⊡617

Auranofin (Co-administration with drugs that are known to cause pancreatitis and peripheral neuropathy may increase the risk of these toxicities).
No products indexed under this heading.

Carboplatin (Co-administration with drugs that are known to cause pancreatitis and peripheral neuropathy may increase the risk of these toxicities). Products include:
Paraplatin for Injection 1126

Chloramphenicol (Co-administration with drugs that are known to cause pancreatitis and peripheral neuropathy may increase the risk of these toxicities). Products include:
Chloromycetin Ophthalmic Ointment, 1% .... ⊙296
Chloromycetin Ophthalmic Solution .... ⊙297
Chloroptic Sterile Ophthalmic Ointment .... ⊙234
Chloroptic Sterile Ophthalmic Solution .... ⊙235

Chloramphenicol Palmitate (Co-administration with drugs that are known to cause pancreatitis and peripheral neuropathy may increase the risk of these toxicities).
No products indexed under this heading.

Chloramphenicol Sodium Succinate (Co-administration with drugs that are known to cause pancreatitis and peripheral neuropathy may increase the risk of these toxicities).
No products indexed under this heading.

Cisplatin (Co-administration with drugs that are known to cause pancreatitis and peripheral neuropathy may increase the risk of these toxicities).
No products indexed under this heading.

Dapsone (Co-administration with drugs that are known to cause pancreatitis and peripheral neuropathy may increase the risk of these toxicities). Products include:
Dapsone Tablets USP 1780

Demeclocycline Hydrochloride (Due to the magnesium and aluminum component of antacids present in Videx, concurrent use with any oral form of tetracycline should be avoided). Products include:
Declomycin Tablets 1855

Disulfiram (Co-administration with drugs that are known to cause pancreatitis and peripheral neuropathy may increase the risk of these toxicities). Products include:
Antabuse Tablets 2444
Antabuse Tablets 3474

Doxycycline Calcium (Due to the magnesium and aluminum component of antacids present in Videx, concurrent use with any oral form of tetracycline should be avoided). Products include:
Vibramycin Calcium Oral Suspension Syrup 2735

Doxycycline Hyclate (Due to the magnesium and aluminum component of antacids present in Videx, concurrent use with any oral form of tetracycline should be avoided). Products include:
Doryx Coated Pellet Filled Capsules 3357
Periostat Tablets 1208
Vibramycin Hyclate Capsules 2735
Vibramycin Hyclate Intravenous 2737
Vibra-Tabs Film Coated Tablets 2735

Doxycycline Monohydrate (Due to the magnesium and aluminum component of antacids present in Videx, concurrent use with any oral form of tetracycline should be avoided). Products include:
Monodox Capsules 2442
Vibramycin Monohydrate for Oral Suspension 2735

Ethionamide (Co-administration with drugs that are known to cause pancreatitis and peripheral neuropathy may increase the risk of these toxicities). Products include:
Trecator-SC Tablets 3598

Ganciclovir (Co-administration results in increased didanosine concentration; appropriate doses for this combination with respect to efficacy and safety have not been established). Products include:
Cytovene Capsules 2959
Vitrasert Implant .... ⊙254

Glutethimide (Co-administration with drugs that are known to cause pancreatitis and peripheral neuropathy may increase the risk of these toxicities).
No products indexed under this heading.

Gold Sodium Thiomalate (Co-administration with drugs that are known to cause pancreatitis and peripheral neuropathy may increase the risk of these toxicities).
No products indexed under this heading.

Hydralazine Hydrochloride (Co-administration with drugs that are known to cause pancreatitis and peripheral neuropathy may increase the risk of these toxicities).
No products indexed under this heading.

Iodoquinol (Co-administration with drugs that are known to cause pancreatitis and peripheral neuropathy may increase the risk of these toxicities). Products include:
Yodoxin Tablets 1722

Isoniazid (Co-administration with drugs that are known to cause pancreatitis and peripheral neuropathy may increase the risk of these toxicities). Products include:
Rifamate Capsules 767
Rifater Tablets 769

Leuprolide Acetate (Co-administration with drugs that are known to cause pancreatitis and peripheral neuropathy may increase the risk of these toxicities). Products include:
Lupron Depot 3.75 mg 3281
Lupron Depot 7.5 mg 3284
Lupron Depot–3 Month 11.25 mg 3285
Lupron Depot–3 Month 22.5 mg 3288
Lupron Depot–4 Month 30 mg 3289
Lupron Depot-PED 7.5 mg, 11.25 mg and 15 mg 3291
Lupron Injection 3279
Lupron Injection Pediatric 3280
Viadur Implant 912

Magaldrate (Co-administration of these antacids with Videx chewable/dispersible buffered tablets or pediatric powder for oral solution may potentiate adverse effects associated with the antacid component).
No products indexed under this heading.

Magnesium Hydroxide (Co-administration of these antacids with Videx chewable/dispersible buffered tablets or pediatric powder for oral solution may potentiate adverse effects associated with the antacid component). Products include:
Ex•Lax Milk of Magnesia Liquid .... ⊡670
Maalox Antacid/Anti-Gas Oral Suspension .... ⊡673
Maalox Max Maximum Strength Antacid/Anti-Gas Liquid 2300
Maalox Regular Strength Antacid/Antigas Liquid 2300
Mylanta Fast-Acting 1813
Mylanta 1813
Pepcid Complete Chewable Tablets 1815
Phillips' Chewable Tablets .... ⊡615
Phillips' Milk of Magnesia Liquid (Original, Cherry, & Mint) .... ⊡616
Rolaids Tablets .... ⊡706
Extra Strength Rolaids Tablets ...... ⊡706
Vanquish Caplets .... ⊡617

Magnesium Oxide (Co-administration of these antacids with Videx chewable/dispersible buffered tablets or pediatric powder for oral solution may potentiate adverse effects associated with the antacid component). Products include:
Beelith Tablets 946
Mag-Ox 400 Tablets 1024
Uro-Mag Capsules 1024

Methacycline Hydrochloride (Due to the magnesium and aluminum component of antacids present in Videx, concurrent use with any oral form of tetracycline should be avoided).
No products indexed under this heading.

Methadone Hydrochloride (Co-administration results in decreased didanosine concentration; appropriate doses for this combination with respect to efficacy and safety have not been established). Products include:
Dolophine Hydrochloride Tablets 3056

Metronidazole (Co-administration with drugs that are known to cause pancreatitis and peripheral neuropathy may increase the risk of these toxicities). Products include:
MetroCream 1404
MetroGel 1405
MetroGel-Vaginal Gel 1986
MetroLotion 1405
Noritate Cream 1224

Minocycline Hydrochloride (Due to the magnesium and aluminum component of antacids present in Videx, concurrent use with any oral form of tetracycline should be avoided). Products include:
Dynacin Capsules 2019
Minocin Intravenous 1862
Minocin Oral Suspension 1865
Minocin Pellet-Filled Capsules 1863

Nitrofurantoin (Co-administration with drugs that are known to cause pancreatitis and peripheral neuropathy may increase the risk of these toxicities). Products include:
Macrodantin Capsules 2891

Oxytetracycline Hydrochloride (Due to the magnesium and aluminum component of antacids present in Videx, concurrent use with any oral form of tetracycline should be avoided). Products include:
Terra-Cortril Ophthalmic Suspension 2716
Urobiotic-250 Capsules 2731

Pentamidine Isethionate (Co-administration with drugs that are known to cause pancreatitis and peripheral neuropathy may increase the risk of these toxicities).
No products indexed under this heading.

Phenytoin (Co-administration with drugs that are known to cause pancreatitis and peripheral neuropathy may increase the risk of these toxicities). Products include:
Dilantin Infatabs 2624
Dilantin-125 Oral Suspension 2625

Phenytoin Sodium (Co-administration with drugs that are known to cause pancreatitis and peripheral neuropathy may increase the risk of these toxicities). Products include:
Dilantin Kapseals 2622

Ribavirin (Co-administration with drugs that are known to cause pancreatitis and peripheral neuropathy may increase the risk of these toxicities). Products include:
Rebetron Combination Therapy 3153
Virazole for Inhalation Solution 1747

Sulfamethoxazole (Co-administration with drugs that are known to cause pancreatitis and peripheral neuropathy may increase the risk of these toxicities). Products include:
Bactrim 2949
Septra Suspension 2265
Septra Tablets 2265
Septra DS Tablets 2265

Tetracycline Hydrochloride (Due to the magnesium and aluminum component of antacids present in Videx, concurrent use with any oral form of tetracycline should be avoided).
No products indexed under this heading.

Vincristine Sulfate (Co-administration with drugs that are known to cause pancreatitis and peripheral neuropathy may increase the risk of these toxicities).
No products indexed under this heading.

Food Interactions

Food, unspecified (In the presence of food, the Cmax and AUC for Videx EC were reduced by approximately 46% and 19%, respectively; Videx EC should be taken on an empty stomach).

VIOKASE POWDER
(Pancrelipase) 837
None cited in PDR database.

VIOKASE TABLETS
(Pancrelipase) 837
None cited in PDR database.

VIOXX ORAL SUSPENSION
(Rofecoxib) 2213
See Vioxx Tablets

VIOXX TABLETS
(Rofecoxib) 2213
May interact with ACE inhibitors, lithium preparations, thiazides, and certain other agents. Compounds in these categories include:

Aspirin (Co-administration with low-dose aspirin may result in an increased rate of GI ulceration or other complications; at steady-state Vioxx had no effect on the anti-platelet activity of low-dose aspirin). Products include:
Aggrenox Capsules 1026
Alka-Seltzer .... ⊡603
Alka-Seltzer Lemon Lime Antacid and Pain Reliever Effervescent Tablets .... ⊡603
Alka-Seltzer Extra Strength Antacid and Pain Reliever Effervescent Tablets .... ⊡603
Alka-Seltzer PM Effervescent Tablets .... ⊡605
Genuine Bayer Tablets, Caplets and Gelcaps .... ⊡606
Extra Strength Bayer Caplets and Gelcaps .... ⊡610
Aspirin Regimen Bayer Children's Chewable Tablets (Orange or Cherry Flavored) .... ⊡607
Bayer, Aspirin Regimen .... ⊡606
Aspirin Regimen Bayer 81 mg Caplets with Calcium .... ⊡607
Genuine Bayer Professional Labeling (Aspirin Regimen Bayer) .... ⊡608
Extra Strength Bayer Arthritis Caplets .... ⊡610
Extra Strength Bayer Plus Caplets .... ⊡610
Extra Strength Bayer PM Caplets ... ⊡611
BC Powder .... ⊡619
BC Allergy Sinus Cold Powder ...... ⊡619
Arthritis Strength BC Powder .... ⊡619
BC Sinus Cold Powder .... ⊡619
Darvon Compound-65 Pulvules 1910
Ecotrin Enteric Coated Aspirin Low, Regular and Maximum Strength Tablets 1715
Excedrin Extra-Strength Tablets, Caplets, and Geltabs .... ⊡629
Excedrin Migraine 1070
Goody's Body Pain Formula Powder .... ⊡620
Goody's Extra Strength Headache Powder .... ⊡620
Goody's Extra Strength Pain Relief Tablets .... ⊡620

Percodan Tablets 1327
Robaxisal Tablets 2939
Soma Compound Tablets 3354
Soma Compound w/Codeine Tablets 3355
Vanquish Caplets .... ⊡617

Benazepril Hydrochloride (Co-administration was associated with an average increase in mean arterial pressure of about 3 mm Hg compared to ACE inhibitor alone). Products include:
Lotensin Tablets 2365
Lotensin HCT Tablets 2367
Lotrel Capsules 2370

Bendroflumethiazide (NSAIDs can reduce the natriuretic effect of thiazide in some patients). Products include:
Corzide 40/5 Tablets 2247
Corzide 80/5 Tablets 2247

Captopril (NSAIDs may diminish the antihypertensive effect of ACE inhibitors). Products include:
Captopril Tablets 2281

Chlorothiazide (NSAIDs can reduce the natriuretic effect of thiazide in some patients). Products include:
Aldoclor Tablets 2035
Diuril Oral 2087

Chlorothiazide Sodium (NSAIDs can reduce the natriuretic effect of thiazide in some patients). Products include:
Diuril Sodium Intravenous 2086

Cimetidine (Co-administration with high-dose cimetidine increases the Cmax of rofecoxib by 21%, the AUC by 23% and t1/2 by 15%). Products include:
Tagamet HB 200 Suspension .... ⊡762
Tagamet HB 200 Tablets .... ⊡761
Tagamet Tablets 1644

Cimetidine Hydrochloride (Co-administration with high-dose cimetidine increases the Cmax of rofecoxib by 21%, the AUC by 23% and t1/2 by 15%). Products include:
Tagamet 1644

Enalapril Maleate (NSAIDs may diminish the antihypertensive effect of ACE inhibitors). Products include:
Lexxel Tablets 608
Vaseretic Tablets 2204
Vasotec Tablets 2210

Enalaprilat (NSAIDs may diminish the antihypertensive effect of ACE inhibitors). Products include:
Enalaprilat Injection 863
Vasotec I.V. Injection 2207

Fosinopril Sodium (NSAIDs may diminish the antihypertensive effect of ACE inhibitors). Products include:
Monopril Tablets 1091
Monopril HCT 1094

Furosemide (NSAIDs can reduce the natriuretic effect of furosemide in some patients). Products include:
Furosemide Tablets 2284

Hydrochlorothiazide (NSAIDs can reduce the natriuretic effect of thiazide in some patients). Products include:
Accuretic Tablets 2614
Aldoril Tablets 2039
Atacand HCT Tablets 597
Avalide Tablets 1070
Diovan HCT Tablets 2338
Dyazide Capsules 1515
HydroDIURIL Tablets 2108
Hyzaar 2109
Inderide Tablets 3517
Inderide LA Long-Acting Capsules 3519
Lotensin HCT Tablets 2367
Maxzide 1008
Micardis HCT Tablets 1051
Microzide Capsules 3414
Moduretic Tablets 2138
Monopril HCT 1094
Prinzide Tablets 2168
Timolide Tablets 2187
Uniretic Tablets 3178
Vaseretic Tablets 2204
Zestoretic Tablets 695
Ziac Tablets 1887

Hydroflumethiazide (NSAIDs can reduce the natriuretic effect of thiazide in some patients). Products include:
Diucardin Tablets 3494

Lisinopril (NSAIDs may diminish the antihypertensive effect of ACE inhibitors). Products include:
Prinivil Tablets 2164
Prinzide Tablets 2168
Zestoretic Tablets 695
Zestril Tablets 698

Lithium Carbonate (Co-administration has resulted in post marketing reports of increased plasma lithium levels; concurrent use of NSAIDs and lithium has produced reduction in renal lithium clearance). Products include:
Eskalith 1527
Lithium Carbonate 3061
Lithobid Slow-Release Tablets 3255

Lithium Citrate (Co-administration has resulted in post marketing reports of increased plasma lithium levels; concurrent use of NSAIDs and lithium has produced reduction in renal lithium clearance). Products include:
Lithium Citrate Syrup 3061

Methotrexate Sodium (Potential for increased methotrexate plasma concentrations and reduction in methotrexate renal clearance).
No products indexed under this heading.

Methyclothiazide (NSAIDs can reduce the natriuretic effect of thiazide in some patients).
No products indexed under this heading.

Midazolam Hydrochloride (A 30% reduction of the AUC of midazolam was observed with rofecoxib when co-administered). Products include:
Versed Injection 3027
Versed Syrup 3033

Moexipril Hydrochloride (NSAIDs may diminish the antihypertensive effect of ACE inhibitors). Products include:
Uniretic Tablets 3178
Univasc Tablets 3181

Perindopril Erbumine (NSAIDs may diminish the antihypertensive effect of ACE inhibitors). Products include:
Aceon Tablets (2 mg, 4 mg, 8 mg) 3249

Polythiazide (NSAIDs can reduce the natriuretic effect of thiazide in some patients). Products include:
Minizide Capsules 2700
Renese Tablets 2712

Quinapril Hydrochloride (NSAIDs may diminish the antihypertensive effect of ACE inhibitors). Products include:
Accupril Tablets 2611
Accuretic Tablets 2614

Ramipril (NSAIDs may diminish the antihypertensive effect of ACE inhibitors). Products include:
Altace Capsules 2233

Rifampin (Co-administration with rifampin, a potent inducer of hepatic metabolism, produced an approximate 50% decrease in rofecoxib plasma concentrations). Products include:
Rifadin 765
Rifamate Capsules 767
Rifater Tablets 769

Spirapril Hydrochloride (NSAIDs may diminish the antihypertensive effect of ACE inhibitors).
No products indexed under this heading.

Trandolapril (NSAIDs may diminish the antihypertensive effect of ACE inhibitors). Products include:
Mavik Tablets 478
Tarka Tablets 508

Warfarin Sodium (Co-administration in healthy subjects has resulted in increased prothrombin time (measured as INR) by 8% to 11%; bleeding events have been reported, predominantly in elderly, in post-marketing experience). Products include:
Coumadin for Injection 1243
Coumadin Tablets 1243
Warfarin Sodium Tablets, USP 3302

Food Interactions

Food, unspecified (The time to peak plasma concentration (Tmax) was delayed by 1 to 2 hours when administered with high fat meal; Vioxx tablets can be administered without regard to timing of meals).

VIRACEPT ORAL POWDER

(Nelfinavir Mesylate) 532
See Viracept Tablets

VIRACEPT TABLETS

(Nelfinavir Mesylate) 532
May interact with dihydrofolate reductase inhibitors, ergot-containing drugs, phenytoin, quinidine, and certain other agents. Compounds in these categories include:

Amiodarone Hydrochloride (Nelfinavir is an inhibitor of CYP3A and co-administration with drugs primarily metabolized by CYP3A, such as amiodarone, could result in competition for CYP3A by nelfinavir; inhibition of the metabolism of amiodarone could create a potential for serious cardiac arrhythmias or prolong adverse events; concurrent use should be avoided). Products include:
Cordarone Intravenous 3491
Cordarone Tablets 3487
Pacerone Tablets 3331

Atorvastatin Calcium (Nelfinavir is an inhibitor of CYP3A and co-administration with drugs primarily metabolized by CYP3A, such as atorvastatin, could increase the risk of moypathy including rhabdomyolysis). Products include:
Lipitor Tablets 2639
Lipitor Tablets 2696

Carbamazepine (May decrease nelfinavir plasma concentrations; Viracept may not be effective due to decreased nelfinavir plasma concentrations in patients taking carbamazepine). Products include:
Carbatrol Capsules 3234
Tegretol/Tegretol-XR 2404

Cerivastatin Sodium (Nelfinavir is an inhibitor of CYP3A and co-administration with drugs primarily metabolized by CYP3A, such as cerivastatin, could increase the risk of myopathy including rhabdomyolysis). Products include:
Baycol Tablets 883

Cisapride (Nelfinavir is an inhibitor of CYP3A and co-administration with drugs primarily metabolized by CYP3A, such as cisapride, could affect hepatic metabolism of cisapride and create the potential for serious and/or life threatening adverse events; concurrent use is contraindicated).
No products indexed under this heading.

Cyclosporine (Nelfinavir is an inhibitor of CYP3A and co-administration with drugs primarily metabolized by CYP3A, such as cyclosporine, may result in increased plasma concentrations of cyclosporine that could increase or prolong both its therapeutic and adverse effects). Products include:
Gengraf Capsules 457
Neoral Soft Gelatin Capsules 2380
Neoral Oral Solution 2380
Sandimmune 2388

Didanosine (Co-administration with didanosine indicates no change in AUC or Cmax of nelfinavir; however, it is recommended that didanosine be administered on an empty stomach; therefore, nelfinavir should be administered with food one hour after or more than 2 hours before didanosine). Products include:
Videx 1138
Videx EC Capsules 1143

Dihydroergotamine Mesylate (Nelfinavir is an inhibitor of CYP3A and co-administration with drugs primarily metabolized by CYP3A, such as ergot derivatives, could result in competition for CYP3A by nelfinavir; inhibition of the metabolism of ergot derivatives could create a potential for serious cardiac arrhythmias or prolong adverse events; concurrent use should be avoided). Products include:
D.H.E. 45 Injection 2334
Migranal Nasal Spray 2376

Ergonovine Maleate (Nelfinavir is an inhibitor of CYP3A and co-administration with drugs primarily metabolized by CYP3A, such as ergot derivatives, could result in competition for CYP3A by nelfinavir; inhibition of the metabolism of ergot derivatives could create a potential for serious cardiac arrhythmias or prolong adverse events; concurrent use should be avoided).
No products indexed under this heading.

Ergotamine Tartrate (Nelfinavir is an inhibitor of CYP3A and co-administration with drugs primarily metabolized by CYP3A, such as ergot derivatives, could result in competition for CYP3A by nelfinavir; inhibition of the metabolism of ergot derivatives could create a potential for serious cardiac arrhythmias or prolong adverse events; concurrent use should be avoided).
No products indexed under this heading.

Ethinyl Estradiol (Co-administration with oral contraceptives containing ethinyl estradiol results in decreased ethinyl estradiol plasma concentrations; alternative or additional contraceptive measures should be used when oral contraceptives and Viracept are co-administered). Products include:
Alesse-21 Tablets 3468
Alesse-28 Tablets 3473
Brevicon 28-Day Tablets 3380
Cyclessa Tablets 2450
Desogen Tablets 2458
Estinyl Tablets 3112
Estrostep 2627
femhrt Tablets 2635
Levlen 962
Levlite 21 Tablets 962
Levlite 28 Tablets 962
Levora Tablets 3389
Loestrin 21 Tablets 2642
Loestrin Fe Tablets 2642
Lo/Ovral Tablets 3532
Lo/Ovral-28 Tablets 3538
Low-Ogestrel-28 Tablets 3392
Microgestin Fe 1.5/30 Tablets 3407
Microgestin Fe 1/20 Tablets 3400
Mircette Tablets 2470
Modicon 2563
Necon 3415
Nordette-28 Tablets 2257
Norinyl 1 +35 28-Day Tablets 3380
Ogestrel 0.5/50-28 Tablets 3428
Ortho-Cept 21 Tablets 2546
Ortho-Cept 28 Tablets 2546
Ortho-Cyclen/Ortho Tri-Cyclen 2573
Ortho-Novum 2563
Ovcon 3364
Ovral Tablets 3551
Ovral-28 Tablets 3552
Tri-Levlen 962
Tri-Norinyl-28 Tablets 3433
Triphasil-21 Tablets 3600
Triphasil-28 Tablets 3605
Trivora Tablets 3439
Yasmin 28 Tablets 980
Zovia 3449

Fosphenytoin Sodium (May decrease nelfinavir plasma concentrations; Viracept may not be effec-

tive due to decreased nelfinavir plasma concentrations in patients taking phenytoin). Products include:

Cerebyx Injection 2619

Hypericum (Concomitant use of St. John's wort or products containing St. John's wort and nelfinavir is expected to substantially decrease protease inhibitor concentrations and may result in sub-optimal levels of nelfinavir and lead to loss of virologic response andpossible resistance to nelfinavir). Products include:

Brite-Life Caplets .... ▣795
Centrum St. John's Wort Softgels . ▣853
Metabolic Nutrition System .... ▣798
Movana Tablets .... ▣832
One-A-Day Tension & Mood Softgels .... ▣808
ReSource Wellness StayCalm Caplets .... ▣826
Satiete Tablets .... ▣846

Indinavir Sulfate (Co-administration results in increases in both nelfinavir and indinavir plasma concentrations; appropriate doses for this combination, with respect to safety and efficacy, have not been established). Products include:

Crixivan Capsules 2070

Lovastatin (Nelfinavir is an inhibitor of CYP3A and co-administration with drugs primarily metabolized by CYP3A, such as lovastatin, could increase the risk of myopathy including rhabdomyolysis; concurrent use is not recommended). Products include:

Mevacor Tablets 2132

Methotrexate Sodium (Nelfinavir is an inhibitor of CYP3A and co-administration with drugs primarily metabolized by CYP3A, such as dihydropyridine calcium channel blockers, may result in increased plasma concentrations of dihydropyridine calcium channel blockers that could increase or prolong both its therapeutic and adverse effects).

No products indexed under this heading.

Methylergonovine Maleate (Nelfinavir is an inhibitor of CYP3A and co-administration with drugs primarily metabolized by CYP3A, such as ergot derivatives, could result in competition for CYP3A by nelfinavir; inhibition of the metabolism of ergot derivatives could create a potential for serious cardiac arrhythmias or prolong adverse events; concurrent use should be avoided).

No products indexed under this heading.

Methysergide Maleate (Nelfinavir is an inhibitor of CYP3A and co-administration with drugs primarily metabolized by CYP3A, such as ergot derivatives, could result in competition for CYP3A by nelfinavir; inhibition of the metabolism of ergot derivatives could create a potential for serious cardiac arrhythmias or prolong adverse events; concurrent use should be avoided).

No products indexed under this heading.

Midazolam Hydrochloride (Nelfinavir is an inhibitor of CYP3A and co-administration with drugs primarily metabolized by CYP3A, such as midazolam, could affect hepatic metabolism of midazolam and create the potential for serious and/or life threatening adverse events; concurrent use is contraindicated). Products include:

Versed Injection 3027
Versed Syrup 3033

Norethindrone (Co-administration with oral contraceptives containing norethindrone results in decreased norethindrone AUC by approximately 18%; alternative or additional contraceptive measures should be used when oral contraceptives and Viracept are co-administered). Products include:

Brevicon 28-Day Tablets 3380
Micronor Tablets 2543
Modicon 2563
Necon 3415
Norinyl 1 +35 28-Day Tablets 3380
Norinyl 1 + 50 28-Day Tablets 3380
Nor-QD Tablets 3423
Ortho-Novum 2563
Ortho-Novum 1/50□28 Tablets 2556
Ovcon 3364
Tri-Norinyl-28 Tablets 3433

Norethindrone Acetate (Co-administration with oral contraceptives containing norethindrone results in decreased norethindrone AUC by approximately 18%; alternative or additional contraceptive measures should be used when oral contraceptives and Viracept are co-administered). Products include:

Activella Tablets 2764
Aygestin Tablets 1333
CombiPatch Transdermal System .. 2323
Estrostep 2627
femhrt Tablets 2635
Loestrin 21 Tablets 2642
Loestrin Fe Tablets 2642
Microgestin Fe 1.5/30 Tablets 3407
Microgestin Fe 1/20 Tablets 3400

Phenobarbital (May decrease nelfinavir plasma concentrations; Viracept may not be effective due to decreased nelfinavir plasma concentrations in patients taking phenobarbital). Products include:

Arco-Lase Plus Tablets 592
Donnatal 2929
Donnatal Extentabs 2930

Phenytoin (May decrease nelfinavir plasma concentrations; Viracept may not be effective due to decreased nelfinavir plasma concentrations in patients taking phenytoin). Products include:

Dilantin Infatabs 2624
Dilantin-125 Oral Suspension 2625

Phenytoin Sodium (May decrease nelfinavir plasma concentrations; Viracept may not be effective due to decreased nelfinavir plasma concentrations in patients taking phenytoin). Products include:

Dilantin Kapseals 2622

Quinidine Gluconate (Nelfinavir is an inhibitor of CYP3A and co-administration with drugs primarily metabolized by CYP3A, such as quinidine, could result in competition for CYP3A by nelfinavir; inhibition of the metabolism of quinidine could create a potential for serious cardiac arrhythmias or prolong adverse events; concurrent use should be avoided). Products include:

Quinaglute Dura-Tabs Tablets 978

Quinidine Polygalacturonate (Nelfinavir is an inhibitor of CYP3A and co-administration with drugs primarily metabolized by CYP3A, such as quinidine, could result in competition for CYP3A by nelfinavir; inhibition of the metabolism of quinidine could create a potential for serious cardiac arrhythmias or prolong adverse events; concurrent use should be avoided).

No products indexed under this heading.

Quinidine Sulfate (Nelfinavir is an inhibitor of CYP3A and co-administration with drugs primarily metabolized by CYP3A, such as quinidine, could result in competition for CYP3A by nelfinavir; inhibition of the metabolism of quinidine could create a potential for serious cardiac arrhythmias or prolong adverse events; concurrent use should be avoided). Products include:

Quinidex Extentabs 2933

Rifabutin (Co-administration results in increased rifabutin plasma AUC and Cmax and decrease in nelfinavir plasma AUC; it is recommended that the dose of rifabutin be reduced in one-half the usual dose when administered with nelfinavir). Products include:

Mycobutin Capsules 2838

Rifampin (Co-administration with rifampin results in decreased nelfinavir AUC and Cmax; concurrent use is not recommended). Products include:

Rifadin 765
Rifamate Capsules 767
Rifater Tablets 769

Ritonavir (Co-administration results in increased nelfinavir plasma concentrations; appropriate doses for this combination, with respect to safety and efficacy, have not been established). Products include:

Kaletra Capsules 471
Kaletra Oral Solution 471
Norvir Capsules 487
Norvir Oral Solution 487

Saquinavir (Co-administration results in increase in saquinavir plasma concentrations; appropriate doses for this combination, with respect to safety and efficacy, have not been established). Products include:

Fortovase Capsules 2970

Saquinavir Mesylate (Co-administration results in increase in saquinavir plasma concentrations; appropriate doses for this combination, with respect to safety and efficacy, have not been established). Products include:

Invirase Capsules 2979

Sildenafil Citrate (Co-administration of a protease inhibitor with sildenafil is expected to substantially increase sildenafil concentrations and may result in an increase in sildenafil associated adverse events, including hypotension, visual changes, and priapism; sildenafil should not exceed a maximum single dose of 25 mg in a 48 hour period when administered in patients receiving protease inhibitors). Products include:

Viagra Tablets 2732

Simvastatin (Nelfinavir is an inhibitor of CYP3A and co-administration with drugs primarily metabolized by CYP3A, such as simvastatin, could increase the risk of myopathy including rhabdomyolysis; concurrent use is not recommended). Products include:

Zocor Tablets 2219

Tacrolimus (Nelfinavir is an inhibitor of CYP3A and co-administration with drugs primarily metabolized by CYP3A, such as tacrolimus, may result in increased plasma concentrations of cyclosporine that could increase or prolong both its therapeutic and adverse effects). Products include:

Prograf 1393
Protopic Ointment 1397

Triazolam (Nelfinavir is an inhibitor of CYP3A and co-administration with drugs primarily metabolized by CYP3A, such as triazolam, could affect hepatic metabolism of triazolam and create the potential for serious and/or life threatening adverse events; concurrent use is contraindicated). Products include:

Halcion Tablets 2823

Trimethoprim (Nelfinavir is an inhibitor of CYP3A and co-administration with drugs primarily metabolized by CYP3A, such as dihydropyridine calcium channel blockers, may result in increased plasma concentrations of dihydropyridine calcium channel blockers that could increase or prolong both its therapeutic and adverse effects). Products include:

Bactrim 2949
Septra Suspension 2265
Septra Tablets 2265
Septra DS Tablets 2265

Trimetrexate Glucuronate (Nelfinavir is an inhibitor of CYP3A and co-administration with drugs primarily metabolized by CYP3A, such as dihydropyridine calcium channel blockers, may result in increased plasma concentrations of dihydropyridine calcium channel blockers that could increase or prolong both its therapeutic and adverse effects).

No products indexed under this heading.

Food Interactions

Food, unspecified (Maximum plasma concentrations and AUC were 2- to 3-fold higher under fed conditions compared to fasting; Viracept should be taken with a meal or light snack).

VIRAMUNE ORAL SUSPENSION

(Nevirapine) 1060

See Viramune Tablets

VIRAMUNE TABLETS

(Nevirapine) 1060

May interact with macrolide antibiotics, oral contraceptives, and certain other agents. Compounds in these categories include:

Azithromycin Dihydrate (Co-administration with macrolides has resulted in elevated steady-state nevirapine trough plasma concentrations). Products include:

Zithromax 2743
Zithromax for IV Infusion 2748
Zithromax for Oral Suspension, 300 mg, 600 mg, 900 mg, 1200 mg 2739
Zithromax Tablets, 250 mg 2739

Cimetidine (Co-administration has resulted in elevated steady-state nevirapine trough plasma concentrations). Products include:

Tagamet HB 200 Suspension .... ▣762
Tagamet HB 200 Tablets .... ▣761
Tagamet Tablets 1644

Cimetidine Hydrochloride (Co-administration has resulted in elevated steady-state nevirapine trough plasma concentrations). Products include:

Tagamet 1644

Clarithromycin (Co-administration with macrolides has resulted in elevated steady-state nevirapine trough plasma concentrations). Products include:

Biaxin/Biaxin XL 403
PREVPAC 3298

Desogestrel (Nevirapine may decrease plasma concentrations of oral contraceptives and other hormonal contraceptives; concurrent use is not recommended). Products include:

Cyclessa Tablets 2450
Desogen Tablets 2458
Mircette Tablets 2470
Ortho-Cept 21 Tablets 2546
Ortho-Cept 28 Tablets 2546

Dirithromycin (Co-administration with macrolides has resulted in elevated steady-state nevirapine trough plasma concentrations). Products include:

Dynabac Tablets 2269

Erythromycin (Co-administration with macrolides has resulted in elevated steady-state nevirapine trough plasma concentrations). Products include:

Emgel 2% Topical Gel 1285
Ery-Tab Tablets 448
Erythromycin Base Filmtab Tablets . 454
Erythromycin Delayed-Release Capsules, USP 455
PCE Dispertab Tablets 498

Erythromycin Estolate (Co-administration with macrolides has resulted in elevated steady-state nevirapine trough plasma

concentrations).
No products indexed under this heading.

Erythromycin Ethylsuccinate (Co-administration with macrolides has resulted in elevated steady-state nevirapine trough plasma concentrations). Products include:

E.E.S. 450
EryPed 446
Pediazole Suspension 3050

Erythromycin Gluceptate (Co-administration with macrolides has resulted in elevated steady-state nevirapine trough plasma concentrations).
No products indexed under this heading.

Erythromycin Stearate (Co-administration with macrolides has resulted in elevated steady-state nevirapine trough plasma concentrations). Products include:

Erythrocin Stearate Filmtab Tablets 452

Ethinyl Estradiol (Nevirapine may decrease plasma concentrations of oral contraceptives and other hormonal contraceptives; concurrent use is not recommended). Products include:

Alesse-21 Tablets 3468
Alesse-28 Tablets 3473
Brevicon 28-Day Tablets 3380
Cyclessa Tablets 2450
Desogen Tablets 2458
Estinyl Tablets 3112
Estrostep 2627
femhrt Tablets 2635
Levlen 962
Levlite 21 Tablets 962
Levlite 28 Tablets 962
Levora Tablets 3389
Loestrin 21 Tablets 2642
Loestrin Fe Tablets 2642
Lo/Ovral Tablets 3532
Lo/Ovral-28 Tablets 3538
Low-Ogestrel-28 Tablets 3392
Microgestin Fe 1.5/30 Tablets 3407
Microgestin Fe 1/20 Tablets 3400
Mircette Tablets 2470
Modicon 2563
Necon 3415
Nordette-28 Tablets 2257
Norinyl 1 +35 28-Day Tablets 3380
Ogestrel 0.5/50-28 Tablets 3428
Ortho-Cept 21 Tablets 2546
Ortho-Cept 28 Tablets 2546
Ortho-Cyclen/Ortho Tri-Cyclen 2573
Ortho-Novum 2563
Ovcon 3364
Ovral Tablets 3551
Ovral-28 Tablets 3552
Tri-Levlen 962
Tri-Norinyl-28 Tablets 3433
Triphasil-21 Tablets 3600
Triphasil-28 Tablets 3605
Trivora Tablets 3439
Yasmin 28 Tablets 980
Zovia 3449

Ethynodiol Diacetate (Nevirapine may decrease plasma concentrations of oral contraceptives and other hormonal contraceptives; concurrent use is not recommended). Products include:

Zovia 3449

Indinavir Sulfate (Co-administration has resulted in a 28% mean decrease in indinavir AUC and an 11% mean decrease in indinavir Cmax; the clinical significance of this interaction is unknown). Products include:

Crixivan Capsules 2070

Ketoconazole (Co-administration has resulted in a significant reduction in ketoconazole plasma concentration; ketoconazole significantly inhibited the formation of nevirapine hydroxylated metabolites; concurrent use is not recommended). Products include:

Nizoral 2% Cream 3620
Nizoral A-D Shampoo 2008
Nizoral 2% Shampoo 2007
Nizoral Tablets 1791

Levonorgestrel (Nevirapine may decrease plasma concentrations of oral contraceptives and other hormonal contraceptives; concurrent use is not recommended). Products include:

Alesse-21 Tablets 3468
Alesse-28 Tablets 3473
Levlen 962
Levlite 21 Tablets 962
Levlite 28 Tablets 962
Levora Tablets 3389
Mirena Intrauterine System 974
Nordette-28 Tablets 2257
Norplant System 3543
Tri-Levlen 962
Triphasil-21 Tablets 3600
Triphasil-28 Tablets 3605
Trivora Tablets 3439

Mestranol (Nevirapine may decrease plasma concentrations of oral contraceptives and other hormonal contraceptives; concurrent use is not recommended). Products include:

Necon 1/50 Tablets 3415
Norinyl 1 + 50 28-Day Tablets 3380
Ortho-Novum 1/50▫28 Tablets 2556

Methadone Hydrochloride (Nevirapine may decrease plasma concentrations of methadone by increasing its hepatic metabolism; narcotic withdrawal syndrome has been reported in patients treated with Viramune and methadone concomitantly). Products include:

Dolophine Hydrochloride Tablets 3056

Norethindrone (Nevirapine may decrease plasma concentrations of oral contraceptives and other hormonal contraceptives; concurrent use is not recommended). Products include:

Brevicon 28-Day Tablets 3380
Micronor Tablets 2543
Modicon 2563
Necon 3415
Norinyl 1 +35 28-Day Tablets 3380
Norinyl 1 + 50 28-Day Tablets 3380
Nor-QD Tablets 3423
Ortho-Novum 2563
Ortho-Novum 1/50▫28 Tablets 2556
Ovcon 3364
Tri-Norinyl-28 Tablets 3433

Norethynodrel (Nevirapine may decrease plasma concentrations of oral contraceptives and other hormonal contraceptives; concurrent use is not recommended).
No products indexed under this heading.

Norgestimate (Nevirapine may decrease plasma concentrations of oral contraceptives and other hormonal contraceptives; concurrent use is not recommended). Products include:

Ortho-Cyclen/Ortho Tri-Cyclen 2573
Ortho-Prefest Tablets 2570

Norgestrel (Nevirapine may decrease plasma concentrations of oral contraceptives and other hormonal contraceptives; concurrent use is not recommended). Products include:

Lo/Ovral Tablets 3532
Lo/Ovral-28 Tablets 3538
Low-Ogestrel-28 Tablets 3392
Ogestrel 0.5/50-28 Tablets 3428
Ovral Tablets 3551
Ovral-28 Tablets 3552
Ovrette Tablets 3552

Rifabutin (Steady-state nevirapine trough concentrations were reduced in patients who received rifabutin, known inducer of CYP3A; these drugs should only be used in combination if clearly indicated and with careful monitoring). Products include:

Mycobutin Capsules 2838

Rifampin (Steady-state nevirapine trough concentrations were reduced in patients who received rifampin, known inducer of CYP3A; these drugs should only be used in combination if clearly indicated and with careful monitoring). Products include:

Rifadin 765
Rifamate Capsules 767
Rifater Tablets 769

Saquinavir Mesylate (Co-administration of saquinavir hard gelatin capsules, 600 mg tid with nevirapine has resulted in a 24% mean decrease in saquinavir AUC and a 28% mean decrease in indinavir Cmax; the clinical significance of this interaction is unknown). Products include:

Invirase Capsules 2979

Troleandomycin (Co-administration with macrolides has resulted in elevated steady-state nevirapine trough plasma concentrations). Products include:

Tao Capsules 2716

VIRAZOLE FOR INHALATION SOLUTION

(Ribavirin) 1747
None cited in PDR database.

VIROPTIC OPHTHALMIC SOLUTION STERILE

(Trifluridine) .... ⊙301
None cited in PDR database.

VISICOL TABLETS

(Sodium Phosphate) 1767
May interact with drugs that prolong the QT interval and certain other agents. Compounds in these categories include:

Amiodarone Hydrochloride (Prolongation of QT interval has been observed in patients who were dosed with Visicol due to electrolyte imbalances, such as hypokalemia and hypocalcemia; co-administration with drugs that prolong QT interval may result in serious complication). Products include:

Cordarone Intravenous 3491
Cordarone Tablets 3487
Pacerone Tablets 3331

Amitriptyline Hydrochloride (Prolongation of QT interval has been observed in patients who were dosed with Visicol due to electrolyte imbalances, such as hypokalemia and hypocalcemia; co-administration with drugs that prolong QT interval may result in serious complication). Products include:

Etrafon 3115
Limbitrol 1738

Amoxapine (Prolongation of QT interval has been observed in patients who were dosed with Visicol due to electrolyte imbalances, such as hypokalemia and hypocalcemia; co-administration with drugs that prolong QT interval may result in serious complication).
No products indexed under this heading.

Astemizole (Prolongation of QT interval has been observed in patients who were dosed with Visicol due to electrolyte imbalances, such as hypokalemia and hypocalcemia; co-administration with drugs that prolong QT interval may result in serious complication).
No products indexed under this heading.

Bretylium Tosylate (Prolongation of QT interval has been observed in patients who were dosed with Visicol due to electrolyte imbalances, such as hypokalemia and hypocalcemia; co-administration with drugs that prolong QT interval may result in serious complication).
No products indexed under this heading.

Chlorpromazine (Prolongation of QT interval has been observed in patients who were dosed with Visicol due to electrolyte imbalances, such as hypokalemia and hypocalcemia; co-administration with drugs that prolong QT interval may result in serious complication). Products include:

Thorazine Suppositories 1656

Chlorpromazine Hydrochloride (Prolongation of QT interval has been observed in patients who were dosed with Visicol due to electrolyte imbalances, such as hypokalemia and hypocalcemia; co-administration with drugs that prolong QT interval may result in serious complication). Products include:

Thorazine 1656

Clomipramine Hydrochloride (Prolongation of QT interval has been observed in patients who were dosed with Visicol due to electrolyte imbalances, such as hypokalemia and hypocalcemia; co-administration with drugs that prolong QT interval may result in serious complication).
No products indexed under this heading.

Desipramine Hydrochloride (Prolongation of QT interval has been observed in patients who were dosed with Visicol due to electrolyte imbalances, such as hypokalemia and hypocalcemia; co-administration with drugs that prolong QT interval may result in serious complication). Products include:

Norpramin Tablets 755

Disopyramide Phosphate (Prolongation of QT interval has been observed in patients who were dosed with Visicol due to electrolyte imbalances, such as hypokalemia and hypocalcemia; co-administration with drugs that prolong QT interval may result in serious complication).
No products indexed under this heading.

Dofetilide (Prolongation of QT interval has been observed in patients who were dosed with Visicol due to electrolyte imbalances, such as hypokalemia and hypocalcemia; co-administration with drugs that prolong QT interval may result in serious complication). Products include:

Tikosyn Capsules 2717

Doxepin Hydrochloride (Prolongation of QT interval has been observed in patients who were dosed with Visicol due to electrolyte imbalances, such as hypokalemia and hypocalcemia; co-administration with drugs that prolong QT interval may result in serious complication). Products include:

Sinequan 2713

Flecainide Acetate (Prolongation of QT interval has been observed in patients who were dosed with Visicol due to electrolyte imbalances, such as hypokalemia and hypocalcemia; co-administration with drugs that prolong QT interval may result in serious complication). Products include:

Tambocor Tablets 1990

Fluphenazine Decanoate (Prolongation of QT interval has been observed in patients who were dosed with Visicol due to electrolyte imbalances, such as hypokalemia and hypocalcemia; co-administration with drugs that prolong QT interval may result in serious complication).
No products indexed under this heading.

Fluphenazine Enanthate (Prolongation of QT interval has been observed in patients who were dosed with Visicol due to electrolyte imbalances, such as hypokalemia and hypocalcemia; co-administration with drugs that prolong QT interval

may result in serious complication).
No products indexed under this heading.

Fluphenazine Hydrochloride (Prolongation of QT interval has been observed in patients who were dosed with Visicol due to electrolyte imbalances, such as hypokalemia and hypocalcemia; co-administration with drugs that prolong QT interval may result in serious complication).
No products indexed under this heading.

Imipramine Hydrochloride (Prolongation of QT interval has been observed in patients who were dosed with Visicol due to electrolyte imbalances, such as hypokalemia and hypocalcemia; co-administration with drugs that prolong QT interval may result in serious complication).
No products indexed under this heading.

Imipramine Pamoate (Prolongation of QT interval has been observed in patients who were dosed with Visicol due to electrolyte imbalances, such as hypokalemia and hypocalcemia; co-administration with drugs that prolong QT interval may result in serious complication).
No products indexed under this heading.

Lidocaine Hydrochloride (Prolongation of QT interval has been observed in patients who were dosed with Visicol due to electrolyte imbalances, such as hypokalemia and hypocalcemia; co-administration with drugs that prolong QT interval may result in serious complication). Products include:
Bactine First Aid Liquid 611
Xylocaine Injections 653

Maprotiline Hydrochloride (Prolongation of QT interval has been observed in patients who were dosed with Visicol due to electrolyte imbalances, such as hypokalemia and hypocalcemia; co-administration with drugs that prolong QT interval may result in serious complication).
No products indexed under this heading.

Mesoridazine Besylate (Prolongation of QT interval has been observed in patients who were dosed with Visicol due to electrolyte imbalances, such as hypokalemia and hypocalcemia; co-administration with drugs that prolong QT interval may result in serious complication). Products include:
Serentil 1057

Mexiletine Hydrochloride (Prolongation of QT interval has been observed in patients who were dosed with Visicol due to electrolyte imbalances, such as hypokalemia and hypocalcemia; co-administration with drugs that prolong QT interval may result in serious complication). Products include:
Mexitil Capsules 1047

Nortriptyline Hydrochloride (Prolongation of QT interval has been observed in patients who were dosed with Visicol due to electrolyte imbalances, such as hypokalemia and hypocalcemia; co-administration with drugs that prolong QT interval may result in serious complication).
No products indexed under this heading.

Oral Medications, unspecified (Medications administered in close-proximity to Visicol may not be absorbed from the GI tract due to rapid intestinal peristalsis and watery diarrhea induced by purgative agent).

Perphenazine (Prolongation of QT interval has been observed in patients who were dosed with Visicol due to electrolyte imbalances, such as hypokalemia and hypocalcemia; co-administration with drugs that prolong QT interval may result in serious complication). Products include:
Etrafon 3115
Trilafon 3160

Procainamide Hydrochloride (Prolongation of QT interval has been observed in patients who were dosed with Visicol due to electrolyte imbalances, such as hypokalemia and hypocalcemia; co-administration with drugs that prolong QT interval may result in serious complication). Products include:
Procanbid Extended-Release Tablets 2262

Prochlorperazine (Prolongation of QT interval has been observed in patients who were dosed with Visicol due to electrolyte imbalances, such as hypokalemia and hypocalcemia; co-administration with drugs that prolong QT interval may result in serious complication). Products include:
Compazine 1505

Promethazine Hydrochloride (Prolongation of QT interval has been observed in patients who were dosed with Visicol due to electrolyte imbalances, such as hypokalemia and hypocalcemia; co-administration with drugs that prolong QT interval may result in serious complication). Products include:
Mepergan Injection 3539
Phenergan Injection 3553
Phenergan 3556
Phenergan Syrup 3554
Phenergan with Codeine Syrup 3557
Phenergan with Dextromethorphan Syrup 3559
Phenergan VC Syrup 3560
Phenergan VC with Codeine Syrup 3561

Propafenone Hydrochloride (Prolongation of QT interval has been observed in patients who were dosed with Visicol due to electrolyte imbalances, such as hypokalemia and hypocalcemia; co-administration with drugs that prolong QT interval may result in serious complication). Products include:
Rythmol Tablets – 150 mg, 225 mg, 300 mg 502

Protriptyline Hydrochloride (Prolongation of QT interval has been observed in patients who were dosed with Visicol due to electrolyte imbalances, such as hypokalemia and hypocalcemia; co-administration with drugs that prolong QT interval may result in serious complication). Products include:
Vivactil Tablets 2446
Vivactil Tablets 2217

Quinidine Gluconate (Prolongation of QT interval has been observed in patients who were dosed with Visicol due to electrolyte imbalances, such as hypokalemia and hypocalcemia; co-administration with drugs that prolong QT interval may result in serious complication). Products include:
Quinaglute Dura-Tabs Tablets 978

Quinidine Polygalacturonate (Prolongation of QT interval has been observed in patients who were dosed with Visicol due to electrolyte imbalances, such as hypokalemia and hypocalcemia; co-administration with drugs that prolong QT interval may result in serious complication).
No products indexed under this heading.

Quinidine Sulfate (Prolongation of QT interval has been observed in patients who were dosed with Visicol due to electrolyte imbalances, such as hypokalemia and hypocalcemia; co-administration with drugs that prolong QT interval may result in serious complication). Products include:
Quinidex Extentabs 2933

Terfenadine (Prolongation of QT interval has been observed in patients who were dosed with Visicol due to electrolyte imbalances, such as hypokalemia and hypocalcemia; co-administration with drugs that prolong QT interval may result in serious complication).
No products indexed under this heading.

Thioridazine Hydrochloride (Prolongation of QT interval has been observed in patients who were dosed with Visicol due to electrolyte imbalances, such as hypokalemia and hypocalcemia; co-administration with drugs that prolong QT interval may result in serious complication). Products include:
Thioridazine Hydrochloride Tablets 2289

Tocainide Hydrochloride (Prolongation of QT interval has been observed in patients who were dosed with Visicol due to electrolyte imbalances, such as hypokalemia and hypocalcemia; co-administration with drugs that prolong QT interval may result in serious complication). Products include:
Tonocard Tablets 649

Trifluoperazine Hydrochloride (Prolongation of QT interval has been observed in patients who were dosed with Visicol due to electrolyte imbalances, such as hypokalemia and hypocalcemia; co-administration with drugs that prolong QT interval may result in serious complication). Products include:
Stelazine 1640

Trimipramine Maleate (Prolongation of QT interval has been observed in patients who were dosed with Visicol due to electrolyte imbalances, such as hypokalemia and hypocalcemia; co-administration with drugs that prolong QT interval may result in serious complication). Products include:
Surmontil Capsules 3595

Ziprasidone Hydrochloride (Prolongation of QT interval has been observed in patients who were dosed with Visicol due to electrolyte imbalances, such as hypokalemia and hypocalcemia; co-administration with drugs that prolong QT interval may result in serious complication). Products include:
Geodon Capsules 2688

VISINE ORIGINAL EYE DROPS
(Tetrahydrozoline Hydrochloride) .... ⊙315
None cited in PDR database.

VISINE A.C. SEASONAL RELIEF FROM POLLEN & DUST EYE DROPS
(Tetrahydrozoline Hydrochloride, Zinc Sulfate) .... ⊙314
None cited in PDR database.

ADVANCED RELIEF VISINE EYE DROPS
(Dextran 70, Polyethylene Glycol, Povidone, Tetrahydrozoline Hydrochloride) .... ⊙313
None cited in PDR database.

VISINE FOR CONTACTS REWETTING DROPS
(Glycerin, Hydroxypropyl Methylcellulose) .... ⊙314
None cited in PDR database.

VISINE L.R. LONG LASTING EYE DROPS
(Oxymetazoline Hydrochloride) .... ⊙315
None cited in PDR database.

VISINE TEARS EYE DROPS
(Glycerin, Hydroxypropyl Methylcellulose, Polyethylene Glycol) .... ⊙315
None cited in PDR database.

VISINE TEARS PRESERVATIVE FREE EYE DROPS
(Glycerin, Hydroxypropyl Methylcellulose, Polyethylene Glycol) .... ⊙315
None cited in PDR database.

VISINE-A EYE ALLERGY RELIEF EYE DROPS
(Naphazoline Hydrochloride, Pheniramine Maleate) .... ⊙314
None cited in PDR database.

VISINE-A EYE DROPS
(Naphazoline Hydrochloride, Pheniramine Maleate) 714
None cited in PDR database.

VISTARIL CAPSULES
(Hydroxyzine Pamoate) 2738
May interact with barbiturates, central nervous system depressants, narcotic analgesics, and certain other agents. Compounds in these categories include:

Alfentanil Hydrochloride (Potential for increased CNS depression when used concurrently).
No products indexed under this heading.

Alprazolam (Potential for increased CNS depression when used concurrently). Products include:
Xanax Tablets 2865

Aprobarbital (Potential for increased CNS depression when used concurrently).
No products indexed under this heading.

Buprenorphine Hydrochloride (Potential for increased CNS depression when used concurrently). Products include:
Buprenex Injectable 2918

Buspirone Hydrochloride (Potential for increased CNS depression when used concurrently).
No products indexed under this heading.

Butabarbital (Potential for increased CNS depression when used concurrently).
No products indexed under this heading.

Butalbital (Potential for increased CNS depression when used concurrently). Products include:
Phrenilin 578
Sedapap Tablets 50 mg/650 mg 2225

Chlordiazepoxide (Potential for increased CNS depression when used concurrently). Products include:
Limbitrol 1738

Chlordiazepoxide Hydrochloride (Potential for increased CNS depression when used concurrently). Products include:
Librium Capsules 1736
Librium for Injection 1737

Chlorpromazine (Potential for increased CNS depression when used concurrently). Products include:
Thorazine Suppositories 1656

Chlorpromazine Hydrochloride (Potential for increased CNS depression when used concurrently). Products include:
Thorazine 1656

Chlorprothixene (Potential for increased CNS depression when used concurrently).
No products indexed under this heading.

Chlorprothixene Hydrochloride (Potential for increased CNS depression when used concurrently).
No products indexed under this heading.

Chlorprothixene Lactate (Potential for increased CNS depression when used concurrently).
No products indexed under this heading.

Clorazepate Dipotassium (Potential for increased CNS depression when used concurrently). Products include:
Tranxene 511

Clozapine (Potential for increased CNS depression when used concurrently). Products include:
Clozaril Tablets 2319

Codeine Phosphate (Potential for increased CNS depression when used concurrently). Products include:
Phenergan with Codeine Syrup 3557
Phenergan VC with Codeine Syrup 3561
Robitussin A-C Syrup 2942
Robitussin-DAC Syrup 2942
Ryna-C Liquid .... ▣768
Soma Compound w/Codeine Tablets 3355
Tussi-Organidin NR Liquid 3350
Tussi-Organidin-S NR Liquid 3350
Tylenol with Codeine 2595

Desflurane (Potential for increased CNS depression when used concurrently). Products include:
Suprane Liquid for Inhalation 874

Dezocine (Potential for increased CNS depression when used concurrently).
No products indexed under this heading.

Diazepam (Potential for increased CNS depression when used concurrently). Products include:
Valium Injectable 3026
Valium Tablets 3047

Droperidol (Potential for increased CNS depression when used concurrently).
No products indexed under this heading.

Enflurane (Potential for increased CNS depression when used concurrently).
No products indexed under this heading.

Estazolam (Potential for increased CNS depression when used concurrently). Products include:
ProSom Tablets 500

Ethchlorvynol (Potential for increased CNS depression when used concurrently).
No products indexed under this heading.

Ethinamate (Potential for increased CNS depression when used concurrently).
No products indexed under this heading.

Fentanyl (Potential for increased CNS depression when used concurrently). Products include:
Duragesic Transdermal System 1786

Fentanyl Citrate (Potential for increased CNS depression when used concurrently). Products include:
Actiq 1184

Fluphenazine Decanoate (Potential for increased CNS depression when used concurrently).
No products indexed under this heading.

Fluphenazine Enanthate (Potential for increased CNS depression when used concurrently).
No products indexed under this heading.

Fluphenazine Hydrochloride (Potential for increased CNS depression when used concurrently).
No products indexed under this heading.

Flurazepam Hydrochloride (Potential for increased CNS depression when used concurrently).
No products indexed under this heading.

Glutethimide (Potential for increased CNS depression when used concurrently).
No products indexed under this heading.

Haloperidol (Potential for increased CNS depression when used concurrently). Products include:
Haldol Injection, Tablets and Concentrate 2533

Haloperidol Decanoate (Potential for increased CNS depression when used concurrently). Products include:
Haldol Decanoate 2535

Hydrocodone Bitartrate (Potential for increased CNS depression when used concurrently). Products include:
Hycodan 1316
Hycomine Compound Tablets 1317
Hycotuss Expectorant Syrup 1318
Lortab 3319
Lortab Elixir 3317
Maxidone Tablets CIII 3399
Norco 5/325 Tablets CIII 3424
Norco 7.5/325 Tablets CIII 3425
Norco 10/325 Tablets CIII 3427
Norco 10/325 Tablets CIII 3425
Vicodin Tablets 516
Vicodin ES Tablets 517
Vicodin HP Tablets 518
Vicodin Tuss Expectorant 519
Vicoprofen Tablets 520
Zydone Tablets 1330

Hydrocodone Polistirex (Potential for increased CNS depression when used concurrently). Products include:
Tussionex Pennkinetic Extended-Release Suspension 1174

Hydromorphone Hydrochloride (Potential for increased CNS depression when used concurrently). Products include:
Dilaudid 441
Dilaudid Oral Liquid 445
Dilaudid Powder 441
Dilaudid Rectal Suppositories 441
Dilaudid Tablets 441
Dilaudid Tablets - 8 mg 445
Dilaudid-HP 443

Hydroxyzine Hydrochloride (Potential for increased CNS depression when used concurrently). Products include:
Atarax Tablets & Syrup 2667
Vistaril Intramuscular Solution 2738

Isoflurane (Potential for increased CNS depression when used concurrently).
No products indexed under this heading.

Ketamine Hydrochloride (Potential for increased CNS depression when used concurrently).
No products indexed under this heading.

Levomethadyl Acetate Hydrochloride (Potential for increased CNS depression when used concurrently).
No products indexed under this heading.

Levorphanol Tartrate (Potential for increased CNS depression when used concurrently). Products include:
Levo-Dromoran 1734
Levorphanol Tartrate Tablets 3059

Lorazepam (Potential for increased CNS depression when used concurrently). Products include:
Ativan Injection 3478
Ativan Tablets 3482

Loxapine Hydrochloride (Potential for increased CNS depression when used concurrently).
No products indexed under this heading.

Loxapine Succinate (Potential for increased CNS depression when used concurrently). Products include:
Loxitane Capsules 3398

Meperidine Hydrochloride (Potential for increased CNS depression when used concurrently). Products include:
Demerol 3079
Mepergan Injection 3539

Mephobarbital (Potential for increased CNS depression when used concurrently).
No products indexed under this heading.

Meprobamate (Potential for increased CNS depression when used concurrently). Products include:
Miltown Tablets 3349

Mesoridazine Besylate (Potential for increased CNS depression when used concurrently). Products include:
Serentil 1057

Methadone Hydrochloride (Potential for increased CNS depression when used concurrently). Products include:
Dolophine Hydrochloride Tablets 3056

Methohexital Sodium (Potential for increased CNS depression when used concurrently). Products include:
Brevital Sodium for Injection, USP 1815

Methotrimeprazine (Potential for increased CNS depression when used concurrently).
No products indexed under this heading.

Methoxyflurane (Potential for increased CNS depression when used concurrently).
No products indexed under this heading.

Midazolam Hydrochloride (Potential for increased CNS depression when used concurrently). Products include:
Versed Injection 3027
Versed Syrup 3033

Molindone Hydrochloride (Potential for increased CNS depression when used concurrently). Products include:
Moban 1320

Morphine Sulfate (Potential for increased CNS depression when used concurrently). Products include:
Astramorph/PF Injection, USP (Preservative-Free) 594
Duramorph Injection 1312
Infumorph 200 and Infumorph 500 Sterile Solutions 1314
Kadian Capsules 1335
MS Contin Tablets 2896
MSIR 2898
Oramorph SR Tablets 3062
Roxanol 3066

Olanzapine (Potential for increased CNS depression when used concurrently). Products include:
Zyprexa Tablets 1973
Zyprexa ZYDIS Orally Disintegrating Tablets 1973

Oxazepam (Potential for increased CNS depression when used concurrently).
No products indexed under this heading.

Oxycodone Hydrochloride (Potential for increased CNS depression when used concurrently). Products include:
OxyContin Tablets 2912
OxyFast Oral Concentrate Solution 2916
OxyIR Capsules 2916
Percocet Tablets 1326
Percodan Tablets 1327
Percolone Tablets 1327
Roxicodone 3067
Tylox Capsules 2597

Pentobarbital Sodium (Potential for increased CNS depression when used concurrently). Products include:
Nembutal Sodium Solution 485

Perphenazine (Potential for increased CNS depression when used concurrently). Products include:
Etrafon 3115
Trilafon 3160

Phenobarbital (Potential for increased CNS depression when used concurrently). Products include:
Arco-Lase Plus Tablets 592
Donnatal 2929
Donnatal Extentabs 2930

Prazepam (Potential for increased CNS depression when used concurrently).
No products indexed under this heading.

Prochlorperazine (Potential for increased CNS depression when used concurrently). Products include:
Compazine 1505

Promethazine Hydrochloride (Potential for increased CNS depression when used concurrently). Products include:
Mepergan Injection 3539
Phenergan Injection 3553
Phenergan 3556
Phenergan Syrup 3554
Phenergan with Codeine Syrup 3557
Phenergan with Dextromethorphan Syrup 3559
Phenergan VC Syrup 3560
Phenergan VC with Codeine Syrup 3561

Propofol (Potential for increased CNS depression when used concurrently). Products include:
Diprivan Injectable Emulsion 667

Propoxyphene Hydrochloride (Potential for increased CNS depression when used concurrently). Products include:
Darvon Pulvules 1909
Darvon Compound-65 Pulvules 1910

Propoxyphene Napsylate (Potential for increased CNS depression when used concurrently). Products include:
Darvon-N/Darvocet-N 1907
Darvon-N Tablets 1912

Quazepam (Potential for increased CNS depression when used concurrently).
No products indexed under this heading.

Quetiapine Fumarate (Potential for increased CNS depression when used concurrently). Products include:
Seroquel Tablets 684

Remifentanil Hydrochloride (Potential for increased CNS depression when used concurrently).
No products indexed under this heading.

Risperidone (Potential for increased CNS depression when used concurrently). Products include:
Risperdal 1796

Secobarbital Sodium (Potential for increased CNS depression when used concurrently).
No products indexed under this heading.

Sevoflurane (Potential for increased CNS depression when used concurrently).
No products indexed under this heading.

Sufentanil Citrate (Potential for increased CNS depression when used concurrently).
No products indexed under this heading.

Temazepam (Potential for increased CNS depression when used concurrently).
No products indexed under this heading.

Thiamylal Sodium (Potential for increased CNS depression when used concurrently).
No products indexed under this heading.

Thioridazine Hydrochloride (Potential for increased CNS depression when used concurrently). Products include:
Thioridazine Hydrochloride Tablets 2289

Thiothixene (Potential for increased CNS depression when used concurrently). Products include:
Navane Capsules 2701
Thiothixene Capsules 2290

Triazolam (Potential for increased CNS depression when used concurrently). Products include:
Halcion Tablets 2823

Trifluoperazine Hydrochloride (Potential for increased CNS depression when used concurrently). Products include:
Stelazine 1640

Zaleplon (Potential for increased CNS depression when used concurrently). Products include:
Sonata Capsules 3591

Ziprasidone Hydrochloride (Potential for increased CNS depression when used concurrently). Products include:
Geodon Capsules 2688

Zolpidem Tartrate (Potential for increased CNS depression when used concurrently). Products include:
Ambien Tablets 3191

Food Interactions

Alcohol (Increased effect of alcohol).

VISTARIL INTRAMUSCULAR SOLUTION

(Hydroxyzine Hydrochloride) 2738

May interact with barbiturates, central nervous system depressants, narcotic analgesics, and certain other agents. Compounds in these categories include:

Alfentanil Hydrochloride (May be potentiated; dosage should be decreased by up to 50%; rare potential for cardiac arrest and death).
No products indexed under this heading.

Alprazolam (May be potentiated; dosage should be decreased by up to 50%; rare potential for cardiac arrest and death). Products include:
Xanax Tablets 2865

Aprobarbital (May be potentiated; dosage should be decreased by up to 50%; rare potential for cardiac arrest and death).
No products indexed under this heading.

Buprenorphine Hydrochloride (May be potentiated; dosage should be decreased by up to 50%; rare potential for cardiac arrest and death). Products include:
Buprenex Injectable 2918

Buspirone Hydrochloride (May be potentiated; dosage should be decreased by up to 50%; rare potential for cardiac arrest and death).
No products indexed under this heading.

Butabarbital (May be potentiated; dosage should be decreased by up to 50%; rare potential for cardiac arrest and death).
No products indexed under this heading.

Butalbital (May be potentiated; dosage should be decreased by up to 50%; rare potential for cardiac arrest and death). Products include:
Phrenilin 578
Sedapap Tablets 50 mg/650 mg 2225

Chlordiazepoxide (May be potentiated; dosage should be decreased by up to 50%; rare potential for cardiac arrest and death). Products include:
Limbitrol 1738

Chlordiazepoxide Hydrochloride (May be potentiated; dosage should be decreased by up to 50%; rare potential for cardiac arrest and death). Products include:
Librium Capsules 1736
Librium for Injection 1737

Chlorpromazine (May be potentiated; dosage should be decreased by up to 50%; rare potential for cardiac arrest and death). Products include:
Thorazine Suppositories 1656

Chlorpromazine Hydrochloride (May be potentiated; dosage should be decreased by up to 50%; rare potential for cardiac arrest and death). Products include:
Thorazine 1656

Chlorprothixene (May be potentiated; dosage should be decreased by up to 50%; rare potential for cardiac arrest and death).
No products indexed under this heading.

Chlorprothixene Hydrochloride (May be potentiated; dosage should be decreased by up to 50%; rare potential for cardiac arrest and death).
No products indexed under this heading.

Chlorprothixene Lactate (May be potentiated; dosage should be decreased by up to 50%; rare potential for cardiac arrest and death).
No products indexed under this heading.

Clorazepate Dipotassium (May be potentiated; dosage should be decreased by up to 50%; rare potential for cardiac arrest and death). Products include:
Tranxene 511

Clozapine (May be potentiated; dosage should be decreased by up to 50%; rare potential for cardiac arrest and death). Products include:
Clozaril Tablets 2319

Codeine Phosphate (May be potentiated; dosage should be decreased by up to 50%; rare potential for cardiac arrest and death). Products include:
Phenergan with Codeine Syrup 3557
Phenergan VC with Codeine Syrup 3561
Robitussin A-C Syrup 2942
Robitussin-DAC Syrup 2942
Ryna-C Liquid 768
Soma Compound w/Codeine Tablets 3355
Tussi-Organidin NR Liquid 3350
Tussi-Organidin-S NR Liquid 3350
Tylenol with Codeine 2595

Desflurane (May be potentiated; dosage should be decreased by up to 50%; rare potential for cardiac arrest and death). Products include:
Suprane Liquid for Inhalation 874

Dezocine (May be potentiated; dosage should be decreased by up to 50%; rare potential for cardiac arrest and death).
No products indexed under this heading.

Diazepam (May be potentiated; dosage should be decreased by up to 50%; rare potential for cardiac arrest and death). Products include:
Valium Injectable 3026
Valium Tablets 3047

Droperidol (May be potentiated; dosage should be decreased by up to 50%; rare potential for cardiac arrest and death).
No products indexed under this heading.

Enflurane (May be potentiated; dosage should be decreased by up to 50%; rare potential for cardiac arrest and death).
No products indexed under this heading.

Estazolam (May be potentiated; dosage should be decreased by up to 50%; rare potential for cardiac arrest and death). Products include:
ProSom Tablets 500

Ethchlorvynol (May be potentiated; dosage should be decreased by up to 50%; rare potential for cardiac arrest and death).
No products indexed under this heading.

Ethinamate (May be potentiated; dosage should be decreased by up to 50%; rare potential for cardiac arrest and death).
No products indexed under this heading.

Fentanyl (May be potentiated; dosage should be decreased by up to 50%; rare potential for cardiac arrest and death). Products include:
Duragesic Transdermal System 1786

Fentanyl Citrate (May be potentiated; dosage should be decreased by up to 50%; rare potential for cardiac arrest and death). Products include:
Actiq 1184

Fluphenazine Decanoate (May be potentiated; dosage should be decreased by up to 50%; rare potential for cardiac arrest and death).
No products indexed under this heading.

Fluphenazine Enanthate (May be potentiated; dosage should be decreased by up to 50%; rare potential for cardiac arrest and death).
No products indexed under this heading.

Fluphenazine Hydrochloride (May be potentiated; dosage should be decreased by up to 50%; rare potential for cardiac arrest and death).
No products indexed under this heading.

Flurazepam Hydrochloride (May be potentiated; dosage should be decreased by up to 50%; rare potential for cardiac arrest and death).
No products indexed under this heading.

Glutethimide (May be potentiated; dosage should be decreased by up to 50%; rare potential for cardiac arrest and death).
No products indexed under this heading.

Haloperidol (May be potentiated; dosage should be decreased by up to 50%; rare potential for cardiac arrest and death). Products include:
Haldol Injection, Tablets and Concentrate 2533

Haloperidol Decanoate (May be potentiated; dosage should be decreased by up to 50%; rare potential for cardiac arrest and death). Products include:
Haldol Decanoate 2535

Hydrocodone Bitartrate (May be potentiated; dosage should be decreased by up to 50%; rare potential for cardiac arrest and death). Products include:
Hycodan 1316
Hycomine Compound Tablets 1317
Hycotuss Expectorant Syrup 1318
Lortab 3319
Lortab Elixir 3317
Maxidone Tablets CIII 3399
Norco 5/325 Tablets CIII 3424
Norco 7.5/325 Tablets CIII 3425
Norco 10/325 Tablets CIII 3427
Norco 10/325 Tablets CIII 3425
Vicodin Tablets 516
Vicodin ES Tablets 517
Vicodin HP Tablets 518
Vicodin Tuss Expectorant 519
Vicoprofen Tablets 520
Zydone Tablets 1330

Hydrocodone Polistirex (May be potentiated; dosage should be decreased by up to 50%; rare potential for cardiac arrest and death). Products include:
Tussionex Pennkinetic Extended-Release Suspension 1174

Hydromorphone Hydrochloride (May be potentiated; dosage should be decreased by up to 50%; rare potential for cardiac arrest and death). Products include:
Dilaudid 441
Dilaudid Oral Liquid 445
Dilaudid Powder 441
Dilaudid Rectal Suppositories 441
Dilaudid Tablets 441
Dilaudid Tablets - 8 mg 445
Dilaudid-HP 443

Isoflurane (May be potentiated; dosage should be decreased by up to 50%; rare potential for cardiac arrest and death).
No products indexed under this heading.

Ketamine Hydrochloride (May be potentiated; dosage should be decreased by up to 50%; rare potential for cardiac arrest and death).
No products indexed under this heading.

Levomethadyl Acetate Hydrochloride (May be potentiated; dosage should be decreased by up to 50%; rare potential for cardiac arrest and death).
No products indexed under this heading.

Levorphanol Tartrate (May be potentiated; dosage should be decreased by up to 50%; rare potential for cardiac arrest and death). Products include:
Levo-Dromoran 1734
Levorphanol Tartrate Tablets 3059

Lorazepam (May be potentiated; dosage should be decreased by up to 50%; rare potential for cardiac arrest and death). Products include:
Ativan Injection 3478
Ativan Tablets 3482

Loxapine Hydrochloride (May be potentiated; dosage should be decreased by up to 50%; rare potential for cardiac arrest and death).
No products indexed under this heading.

Loxapine Succinate (May be potentiated; dosage should be decreased by up to 50%; rare potential for cardiac arrest and death). Products include:
Loxitane Capsules 3398

Meperidine Hydrochloride (May be potentiated; dosage should be decreased by up to 50%; rare potential for cardiac arrest and death). Products include:
Demerol 3079
Mepergan Injection 3539

Mephobarbital (May be potentiated; dosage should be decreased by up to 50%; rare potential for cardiac arrest and death).
No products indexed under this heading.

Meprobamate (May be potentiated; dosage should be decreased by up to 50%; rare potential for cardiac arrest and death). Products include:
Miltown Tablets 3349

Mesoridazine Besylate (May be potentiated; dosage should be decreased by up to 50%; rare potential for cardiac arrest and death). Products include:
Serentil 1057

Methadone Hydrochloride (May be potentiated; dosage should be

decreased by up to 50%; rare potential for cardiac arrest and death). Products include:
Dolophine Hydrochloride Tablets 3056

Methohexital Sodium (May be potentiated; dosage should be decreased by up to 50%; rare potential for cardiac arrest and death). Products include:
Brevital Sodium for Injection, USP .. 1815

Methotrimeprazine (May be potentiated; dosage should be decreased by up to 50%; rare potential for cardiac arrest and death).
No products indexed under this heading.

Methoxyflurane (May be potentiated; dosage should be decreased by up to 50%; rare potential for cardiac arrest and death).
No products indexed under this heading.

Midazolam Hydrochloride (May be potentiated; dosage should be decreased by up to 50%; rare potential for cardiac arrest and death). Products include:
Versed Injection 3027
Versed Syrup 3033

Molindone Hydrochloride (May be potentiated; dosage should be decreased by up to 50%; rare potential for cardiac arrest and death). Products include:
Moban 1320

Morphine Sulfate (May be potentiated; dosage should be decreased by up to 50%; rare potential for cardiac arrest and death). Products include:
Astramorph/PF Injection, USP (Preservative-Free) 594
Duramorph Injection 1312
Infumorph 200 and Infumorph 500 Sterile Solutions 1314
Kadian Capsules 1335
MS Contin Tablets 2896
MSIR 2898
Oramorph SR Tablets 3062
Roxanol 3066

Olanzapine (May be potentiated; dosage should be decreased by up to 50%; rare potential for cardiac arrest and death). Products include:
Zyprexa Tablets 1973
Zyprexa ZYDIS Orally Disintegrating Tablets 1973

Oxazepam (May be potentiated; dosage should be decreased by up to 50%; rare potential for cardiac arrest and death).
No products indexed under this heading.

Oxycodone Hydrochloride (May be potentiated; dosage should be decreased by up to 50%; rare potential for cardiac arrest and death). Products include:
OxyContin Tablets 2912
OxyFast Oral Concentrate Solution . 2916
OxyIR Capsules 2916
Percocet Tablets 1326
Percodan Tablets 1327
Percolone Tablets 1327
Roxicodone 3067
Tylox Capsules 2597

Pentobarbital Sodium (May be potentiated; dosage should be decreased by up to 50%; rare potential for cardiac arrest and death). Products include:
Nembutal Sodium Solution 485

Perphenazine (May be potentiated; dosage should be decreased by up to 50%; rare potential for cardiac arrest and death). Products include:
Etrafon 3115
Trilafon 3160

Phenobarbital (May be potentiated; dosage should be decreased by up to 50%; rare potential for cardiac arrest and death). Products include:
Arco-Lase Plus Tablets 592
Donnatal 2929
Donnatal Extentabs 2930

Prazepam (May be potentiated; dosage should be decreased by up to 50%; rare potential for cardiac arrest and death).
No products indexed under this heading.

Prochlorperazine (May be potentiated; dosage should be decreased by up to 50%; rare potential for cardiac arrest and death). Products include:
Compazine 1505

Promethazine Hydrochloride (May be potentiated; dosage should be decreased by up to 50%; rare potential for cardiac arrest and death). Products include:
Mepergan Injection 3539
Phenergan Injection 3553
Phenergan 3556
Phenergan Syrup 3554
Phenergan with Codeine Syrup 3557
Phenergan with Dextromethorphan Syrup 3559
Phenergan VC Syrup 3560
Phenergan VC with Codeine Syrup .. 3561

Propofol (May be potentiated; dosage should be decreased by up to 50%; rare potential for cardiac arrest and death). Products include:
Diprivan Injectable Emulsion 667

Propoxyphene Hydrochloride (May be potentiated; dosage should be decreased by up to 50%; rare potential for cardiac arrest and death). Products include:
Darvon Pulvules 1909
Darvon Compound-65 Pulvules 1910

Propoxyphene Napsylate (May be potentiated; dosage should be decreased by up to 50%; rare potential for cardiac arrest and death). Products include:
Darvon-N/Darvocet-N 1907
Darvon-N Tablets 1912

Quazepam (May be potentiated; dosage should be decreased by up to 50%; rare potential for cardiac arrest and death).
No products indexed under this heading.

Quetiapine Fumarate (May be potentiated; dosage should be decreased by up to 50%; rare potential for cardiac arrest and death). Products include:
Seroquel Tablets 684

Remifentanil Hydrochloride (May be potentiated; dosage should be decreased by up to 50%; rare potential for cardiac arrest and death).
No products indexed under this heading.

Risperidone (May be potentiated; dosage should be decreased by up to 50%; rare potential for cardiac arrest and death). Products include:
Risperdal 1796

Secobarbital Sodium (May be potentiated; dosage should be decreased by up to 50%; rare potential for cardiac arrest and death).
No products indexed under this heading.

Sevoflurane (May be potentiated; dosage should be decreased by up to 50%; rare potential for cardiac arrest and death).
No products indexed under this heading.

Sufentanil Citrate (May be potentiated; dosage should be decreased by up to 50%; rare potential for cardiac arrest and death).
No products indexed under this heading.

Temazepam (May be potentiated; dosage should be decreased by up to 50%; rare potential for cardiac arrest and death).
No products indexed under this heading.

Thiamylal Sodium (May be potentiated; dosage should be decreased by up to 50%; rare potential for cardiac arrest and death).
No products indexed under this heading.

Thioridazine Hydrochloride (May be potentiated; dosage should be decreased by up to 50%; rare potential for cardiac arrest and death). Products include:
Thioridazine Hydrochloride Tablets 2289

Thiothixene (May be potentiated; dosage should be decreased by up to 50%; rare potential for cardiac arrest and death). Products include:
Navane Capsules 2701
Thiothixene Capsules 2290

Triazolam (May be potentiated; dosage should be decreased by up to 50%; rare potential for cardiac arrest and death). Products include:
Halcion Tablets 2823

Trifluoperazine Hydrochloride (May be potentiated; dosage should be decreased by up to 50%; rare potential for cardiac arrest and death). Products include:
Stelazine 1640

Zaleplon (May be potentiated; dosage should be decreased by up to 50%; rare potential for cardiac arrest and death). Products include:
Sonata Capsules 3591

Ziprasidone Hydrochloride (May be potentiated; dosage should be decreased by up to 50%; rare potential for cardiac arrest and death). Products include:
Geodon Capsules 2688

Zolpidem Tartrate (May be potentiated; dosage should be decreased by up to 50%; rare potential for cardiac arrest and death). Products include:
Ambien Tablets 3191

Food Interactions

Alcohol (May be potentiated).

VISTARIL ORAL SUSPENSION

(Hydroxyzine Pamoate) 2738
See Vistaril Capsules

VISTIDE INJECTION

(Cidofovir) 1445
May interact with ACE inhibitors, aminoglycosides, barbiturates, benzodiazepines, non-steroidal anti-inflammatory agents, theophylline, and certain other agents. Compounds in these categories include:

Acetaminophen (Probenecid must be used with each cidofovir infusion; probenecid is known to interact with the metabolism or renal tubular excretion of acetaminophen; concomitant use should be carefully assessed). Products include:
Actifed Cold & Sinus Caplets and Tablets .... ▣688
Alka-Seltzer Plus Liqui-Gels .... ▣604
Alka-Seltzer Plus Cold & Flu Medicine Liqui-Gels .... ▣604
Alka-Seltzer Plus Cold & Sinus Medicine Liqui-Gels .... ▣604
Benadryl Allergy/Cold Tablets .... ▣691
Benadryl Allergy Sinus Headache Caplets & Gelcaps .... ▣693
Benadryl Severe Allergy & Sinus Headache Caplets .... ▣694
Children's Cēpacol Sore Throat .... ▣788
Comtrex Acute Head Cold & Sinus Pressure Relief Tablets .... ▣627
Comtrex Deep Chest Cold & Congestion Relief Softgels .... ▣627
Comtrex Flu Therapy & Fever Relief Daytime Caplets .... ▣628
Comtrex Flu Therapy & Fever Relief Nighttime Tablets .... ▣628
Comtrex Maximum Strength Multi-Symptom Cold & Cough Relief Tablets and Caplets .... ▣626
Contac Severe Cold and Flu Caplets Maximum Strength .... ▣746
Contac Severe Cold and Flu Caplets Non-Drowsy .... ▣746
Coricidin 'D' Cold, Flu & Sinus Tablets .... ▣737
Coricidin HBP Cold & Flu Tablets .... ▣738
Coricidin HBP Maximum Strength Flu Tablets .... ▣738
Coricidin HBP Night-Time Cold & Flu Tablets .... ▣738
Darvon-N/Darvocet-N 1907
Dimetapp Cold and Fever Suspension .... ▣775
Dimetapp Nighttime Flu Liquid .... ▣776
Dimetapp Non-Drowsy Flu Syrup .... ▣777
Drixoral Allergy/Sinus Extended-Release Tablets .... ▣741
Drixoral Cold & Flu Extended-Release Tablets .... ▣740
Aspirin Free Excedrin Caplets and Geltabs .... ▣628
Excedrin Extra-Strength Tablets, Caplets, and Geltabs .... ▣629
Excedrin Migraine 1070
Excedrin PM Tablets, Caplets, and Geltabs .... ▣631
Goody's Body Pain Formula Powder .... ▣620
Goody's Extra Strength Headache Powder .... ▣620
Goody's Extra Strength Pain Relief Tablets .... ▣620
Goody's PM Powder .... ▣621
Hycomine Compound Tablets 1317
Lortab 3319
Lortab Elixir 3317
Maxidone Tablets CIII 3399
Maximum Strength Midol Menstrual Caplets and Gelcaps .. ▣612
Maximum Strength Midol PMS Caplets and Gelcaps .... ▣613
Maximum Strength Midol Teen Caplets .... ▣612
Midrin Capsules 3464
Norco 5/325 Tablets CIII 3424
Norco 7.5/325 Tablets CIII 3425
Norco 10/325 Tablets CIII 3427
Norco 10/325 Tablets CIII 3425
Percocet Tablets 1326
Percogesic Aspirin-Free Coated Tablets .... ▣667
Extra Strength Percogesic Aspirin-Free Coated Caplets .... ▣665
Phrenilin 578
Robitussin Cold Caplets Multi-Symptom Cold & Flu .... ▣781
Robitussin Cold Softgels Multi-Symptom Cold & Flu .... ▣781
Robitussin Multi Symptom Honey Flu Liquid .... ▣785
Robitussin Nighttime Honey Flu Liquid .... ▣786
Sedapap Tablets 50 mg/650 mg 2225
Singlet Caplets .... ▣761
Sinutab Sinus Allergy Medication, Maximum Strength Formula, Tablets & Caplets .... ▣707
Sinutab Sinus Medication, Maximum Strength Without Drowsiness Formula, Tablets & Caplets .... ▣707
Sudafed Cold & Cough Liquid Caps .... ▣709
Sudafed Cold & Sinus Liquid Caps .... ▣710
Sudafed Severe Cold .... ▣711
Sudafed Sinus Headache Caplets .... ▣712
Sudafed Sinus Headache Tablets .... ▣712
Tavist Sinus Non-Drowsy Coated Caplets .... ▣676
TheraFlu Regular Strength Cold & Cough Night Time Hot Liquid .... ▣676
TheraFlu Regular Strength Cold & Sore Throat Night Time Hot Liquid .... ▣676
TheraFlu Maximum Strength Flu & Congestion Non-Drowsy Hot Liquid .... ▣677
TheraFlu Maximum Strength Flu & Cough Night Time Hot Liquid .. ▣678
TheraFlu Maximum Strength Flu & Sore Throat Night Time Hot Liquid .... ▣677
TheraFlu Maximum Strength Severe Cold & Congestion Night Time Caplets .... ▣678
TheraFlu Maximum Strength Severe Cold & Congestion Night Time Hot Liquid .... ▣678
TheraFlu Maximum Strength Severe Cold & Congestion Non-Drowsy .... ▣679
Triaminic Cold, Cough & Fever Liquid .... ▣681
Triaminic Cough & Sore Throat Liquid .... ▣682
Triaminic Cough & Sore Throat Softchews .... ▣684
Tylenol, Children's 2014
Children's Tylenol Allergy-D Liquid 2014
Children's Tylenol Cold Suspension Liquid and Chewable Tablets 2015

Children's Tylenol Cold Plus Cough Suspension Liquid and Chewable Tablets 2015
Children's Tylenol Flu Suspension Liquid 2015
Children's Tylenol Sinus Suspension Liquid 2017
Infants' Tylenol Cold Decongestant and Fever Reducer Concentrated Drops 2015
Infants' Tylenol Cold Decongestant and Fever Reducer Concentrated Drops Plus Cough.. 2015
Junior Strength Tylenol Soft Chews Chewable Tablets 2014
Tylenol 2009
Tylenol Allergy Sinus 2010
Tylenol Severe Allergy Caplets 2010
Multi-Symptom Tylenol Cold Complete Formula Caplets 2010
Multi-Symptom Tylenol Cold Non-Drowsy Caplets and Gelcaps 2010
Multi-Symptom Tylenol Cold Severe Congestion Non-Drowsy Caplets 2011
Maximum Strength Tylenol Flu NightTime Gelcaps 2011
Maximum Strength Tylenol Flu NightTime Liquid 2011
Maximum Strength Tylenol Flu Non-Drowsy Gelcaps 2011
Extra Strength Tylenol PM Caplets, Geltabs, and Gelcaps 2012
Maximum Strength Tylenol Sinus NightTime Caplets 2012
Maximum Strength Tylenol Sinus Non-Drowsy Geltabs, Gelcaps, Caplets, and Tablets 2012
Maximum Strength Tylenol Sore Throat Adult Liquid 2013
Tylenol with Codeine 2595
Women's Tylenol Menstrual Relief Caplets 2013
Tylox Capsules 2597
Ultracet Tablets 2597
Vanquish Caplets .... ⊡617
Vicks 44M Cough, Cold & Flu Relief Liquid .... ⊡725
Vicks DayQuil LiquiCaps/Liquid Multi-Symptom Cold/Flu Relief .... ⊡727
Vicks NyQuil LiquiCaps/Liquid Multi-Symptom Cold/Flu Relief, Original and Cherry Flavors .... ⊡727
Vicodin Tablets 516
Vicodin ES Tablets 517
Vicodin HP Tablets 518
Zydone Tablets 1330

Acyclovir (Probenecid must be used with each cidofovir infusion; probenecid is known to interact with the metabolism or renal tubular excretion of acyclovir; concomitant use should be carefully assessed). Products include:
Zovirax 1706
Zovirax Ointment 1707

Acyclovir Sodium (Probenecid must be used with each cidofovir infusion; probenecid is known to interact with the metabolism or renal tubular excretion of acyclovir; concomitant use should be carefully assessed). Products include:
Zovirax for Injection 1708

Alprazolam (Probenecid must be used with each cidofovir infusion; probenecid is known to interact with the metabolism or renal tubular excretion of benzodiazepines; concomitant use should be carefully assessed). Products include:
Xanax Tablets 2865

Amikacin Sulfate (Renal impairment is the major toxicity of cidofovir; co-administration with potential nephrotoxic agents should be avoided).
No products indexed under this heading.

Aminophylline (Probenecid must be used with each cidofovir infusion; probenecid is known to interact with the metabolism or renal tubular excretion of theophylline; concomitant use should be carefully assessed).
No products indexed under this heading.

Amphotericin B (Renal impairment is the major toxicity of cidofovir; co-administration with potential nephrotoxic agents should be avoided). Products include:
Abelcet Injection 1273
AmBisome for Injection 1383
Amphotec 1774

Aprobarbital (Probenecid must be used with each cidofovir infusion; probenecid is known to interact with the metabolism or renal tubular excretion of barbiturates; concomitant use should be carefully assessed).
No products indexed under this heading.

Benazepril Hydrochloride (Probenecid must be used with each cidofovir infusion; probenecid is known to interact with the metabolism or renal tubular excretion of ACE inhibitors; concomitant use should be carefully assessed). Products include:
Lotensin Tablets 2365
Lotensin HCT Tablets 2367
Lotrel Capsules 2370

Bumetanide (Probenecid must be used with each cidofovir infusion; probenecid is known to interact with the metabolism or renal tubular excretion of bumetanide; concomitant use should be carefully assessed).
No products indexed under this heading.

Butabarbital (Probenecid must be used with each cidofovir infusion; probenecid is known to interact with the metabolism or renal tubular excretion of barbiturates; concomitant use should be carefully assessed).
No products indexed under this heading.

Butalbital (Probenecid must be used with each cidofovir infusion; probenecid is known to interact with the metabolism or renal tubular excretion of barbiturates; concomitant use should be carefully assessed). Products include:
Phrenilin 578
Sedapap Tablets 50 mg/650 mg 2225

Captopril (Probenecid must be used with each cidofovir infusion; probenecid is known to interact with the metabolism or renal tubular excretion of ACE inhibitors; concomitant use should be carefully assessed). Products include:
Captopril Tablets 2281

Celecoxib (Probenecid must be used with each cidofovir infusion; probenecid is known to interact with the metabolism or renal tubular excretion of non-steroidal anti-inflammatory agents; concomitant use should be carefully assessed). Products include:
Celebrex Capsules 2676
Celebrex Capsules 2780

Chlordiazepoxide (Probenecid must be used with each cidofovir infusion; probenecid is known to interact with the metabolism or renal tubular excretion of benzodiazepines; concomitant use should be carefully assessed). Products include:
Limbitrol 1738

Chlordiazepoxide Hydrochloride (Probenecid must be used with each cidofovir infusion; probenecid is known to interact with the metabolism or renal tubular excretion of benzodiazepines; concomitant use should be carefully assessed). Products include:
Librium Capsules 1736
Librium for Injection 1737

Clofibrate (Probenecid must be used with each cidofovir infusion; probenecid is known to interact with the metabolism or renal tubular excretion of clofibrate; concomitant use should be carefully assessed). Products include:
Atromid-S Capsules 3483

Clonazepam (Probenecid must be used with each cidofovir infusion; probenecid is known to interact with the metabolism or renal tubular excretion of benzodiazepines; concomitant use should be carefully assessed). Products include:
Klonopin Tablets 2983

Clorazepate Dipotassium (Probenecid must be used with each cidofovir infusion; probenecid is known to interact with the metabolism or renal tubular excretion of benzodiazepines; concomitant use should be carefully assessed). Products include:
Tranxene 511

Diazepam (Probenecid must be used with each cidofovir infusion; probenecid is known to interact with the metabolism or renal tubular excretion of benzodiazepines; concomitant use should be carefully assessed). Products include:
Valium Injectable 3026
Valium Tablets 3047

Diclofenac Potassium (Probenecid must be used with each cidofovir infusion; probenecid is known to interact with the metabolism or renal tubular excretion of non-steroidal anti-inflammatory agents; concomitant use should be carefully assessed). Products include:
Cataflam Tablets 2315

Diclofenac Sodium (Probenecid must be used with each cidofovir infusion; probenecid is known to interact with the metabolism or renal tubular excretion of non-steroidal anti-inflammatory agents; concomitant use should be carefully assessed). Products include:
Arthrotec Tablets 3195
Voltaren Ophthalmic Sterile Ophthalmic Solution .... ⊙312
Voltaren Tablets 2315
Voltaren-XR Tablets 2315

Dyphylline (Probenecid must be used with each cidofovir infusion; probenecid is known to interact with the metabolism or renal tubular excretion of theophylline; concomitant use should be carefully assessed). Products include:
Lufyllin Tablets 3347
Lufyllin-400 Tablets 3347
Lufyllin-GG Elixir 3348
Lufyllin-GG Tablets 3348

Enalapril Maleate (Probenecid must be used with each cidofovir infusion; probenecid is known to interact with the metabolism or renal tubular excretion of ACE inhibitors; concomitant use should be carefully assessed). Products include:
Lexxel Tablets 608
Vaseretic Tablets 2204
Vasotec Tablets 2210

Enalaprilat (Probenecid must be used with each cidofovir infusion; probenecid is known to interact with the metabolism or renal tubular excretion of ACE inhibitors; concomitant use should be carefully assessed). Products include:
Enalaprilat Injection 863
Vasotec I.V. Injection 2207

Estazolam (Probenecid must be used with each cidofovir infusion; probenecid is known to interact with the metabolism or renal tubular excretion of benzodiazepines; concomitant use should be carefully assessed). Products include:
ProSom Tablets 500

Etodolac (Probenecid must be used with each cidofovir infusion; probenecid is known to interact with the metabolism or renal tubular excretion of non-steroidal anti-inflammatory agents; concomitant use should be carefully assessed). Products include:
Lodine 3528
Lodine XL Extended-Release Tablets 3530

Famotidine (Probenecid must be used with each cidofovir infusion; probenecid is known to interact with the metabolism or renal tubular excretion of famotidine; concomitant use should be carefully assessed). Products include:
Famotidine Injection 866
Pepcid AC 1814
Pepcid Complete Chewable Tablets 1815
Pepcid Injection 2153
Pepcid for Oral Suspension 2150
Pepcid RPD Orally Disintegrating Tablets 2150
Pepcid Tablets 2150

Fenoprofen Calcium (Probenecid must be used with each cidofovir infusion; probenecid is known to interact with the metabolism or renal tubular excretion of non-steroidal anti-inflammatory agents; concomitant use should be carefully assessed).
No products indexed under this heading.

Flurazepam Hydrochloride (Probenecid must be used with each cidofovir infusion; probenecid is known to interact with the metabolism or renal tubular excretion of benzodiazepines; concomitant use should be carefully assessed).
No products indexed under this heading.

Flurbiprofen (Probenecid must be used with each cidofovir infusion; probenecid is known to interact with the metabolism or renal tubular excretion of non-steroidal anti-inflammatory agents; concomitant use should be carefully assessed).
No products indexed under this heading.

Foscarnet Sodium (Renal impairment is the major toxicity of cidofovir; co-administration with potential nephrotoxic agents should be avoided). Products include:
Foscavir Injection 605

Fosinopril Sodium (Probenecid must be used with each cidofovir infusion; probenecid is known to interact with the metabolism or renal tubular excretion of ACE inhibitors; concomitant use should be carefully assessed). Products include:
Monopril Tablets 1091
Monopril HCT 1094

Furosemide (Probenecid must be used with each cidofovir infusion; probenecid is known to interact with the metabolism or renal tubular excretion of furosemide; concomitant use should be carefully assessed). Products include:
Furosemide Tablets 2284

Gentamicin Sulfate (Renal impairment is the major toxicity of cidofovir; co-administration with potential nephrotoxic agents should be avoided). Products include:
Genoptic Ophthalmic Ointment .... ⊙239
Genoptic Sterile Ophthalmic Solution .... ⊙239
Pred-G Ophthalmic Suspension .... ⊙247
Pred-G Sterile Ophthalmic Ointment .... ⊙248

Halazepam (Probenecid must be used with each cidofovir infusion; probenecid is known to interact with the metabolism or renal tubular excretion of benzodiazepines; concomitant use should be carefully assessed).
No products indexed under this heading.

Ibuprofen (Probenecid must be used with each cidofovir infusion; probenecid is known to interact with

the metabolism or renal tubular excretion of non-steroidal anti-inflammatory agents; concomitant use should be carefully assessed). Products include:

- Advil ▣771
- Children's Advil Oral Suspension ▣773
- Children's Advil Chewable Tablets ▣773
- Advil Cold and Sinus Caplets ▣771
- Advil Cold and Sinus Tablets ▣771
- Advil Flu & Body Ache Caplets ▣772
- Infants' Advil Drops ▣773
- Junior Strength Advil Tablets ▣773
- Junior Strength Advil Chewable Tablets ▣773
- Advil Migraine Liquigels ▣772
- Children's Motrin Oral Suspension and Chewable Tablets 2006
- Children's Motrin Cold Oral Suspension 2007
- Children's Motrin Oral Suspension ▣643
- Motrin Suspension, Oral Drops, Chewable Tablets, and Caplets 2002
- Infants' Motrin Concentrated Drops 2006
- Junior Strength Motrin Caplets and Chewable Tablets 2006
- Motrin IB Tablets, Caplets, and Gelcaps 2002
- Motrin Migraine Pain Caplets 2005
- Motrin Sinus Headache Caplets 2005
- Vicoprofen Tablets 520

Indomethacin (Probenecid must be used with each cidofovir infusion; probenecid is known to interact with the metabolism or renal tubular excretion of non-steroidal anti-inflammatory agents; concomitant use should be carefully assessed). Products include:

- Indocin 2112

Indomethacin Sodium Trihydrate (Probenecid must be used with each cidofovir infusion; probenecid is known to interact with the metabolism or renal tubular excretion of non-steroidal anti-inflammatory agents; concomitant use should be carefully assessed). Products include:

- Indocin I.V. 2115

Kanamycin Sulfate (Renal impairment is the major toxicity of cidofovir; co-administration with potential nephrotoxic agents should be avoided).

No products indexed under this heading.

Ketoprofen (Probenecid must be used with each cidofovir infusion; probenecid is known to interact with the metabolism or renal tubular excretion of non-steroidal anti-inflammatory agents; concomitant use should be carefully assessed). Products include:

- Orudis Capsules 3548
- Orudis KT Tablets ▣778
- Oruvail Capsules 3548

Ketorolac Tromethamine (Probenecid must be used with each cidofovir infusion; probenecid is known to interact with the metabolism or renal tubular excretion of non-steroidal anti-inflammatory agents; concomitant use should be carefully assessed). Products include:

- Acular Ophthalmic Solution 544
- Acular PF Ophthalmic Solution 544
- Toradol 3018

Lisinopril (Probenecid must be used with each cidofovir infusion; probenecid is known to interact with the metabolism or renal tubular excretion of ACE inhibitors; concomitant use should be carefully assessed). Products include:

- Prinivil Tablets 2164
- Prinzide Tablets 2168
- Zestoretic Tablets 695
- Zestril Tablets 698

Lorazepam (Probenecid must be used with each cidofovir infusion; probenecid is known to interact with the metabolism or renal tubular excretion of benzodiazepines; concomitant use should be carefully assessed). Products include:

- Ativan Injection 3478
- Ativan Tablets 3482

Meclofenamate Sodium (Probenecid must be used with each cidofovir infusion; probenecid is known to interact with the metabolism or renal tubular excretion of non-steroidal anti-inflammatory agents; concomitant use should be carefully assessed).

No products indexed under this heading.

Mefenamic Acid (Probenecid must be used with each cidofovir infusion; probenecid is known to interact with the metabolism or renal tubular excretion of non-steroidal anti-inflammatory agents; concomitant use should be carefully assessed). Products include:

- Ponstel Capsules 1356

Meloxicam (Probenecid must be used with each cidofovir infusion; probenecid is known to interact with the metabolism or renal tubular excretion of non-steroidal anti-inflammatory agents; concomitant use should be carefully assessed). Products include:

- Mobic Tablets 1054

Mephobarbital (Probenecid must be used with each cidofovir infusion; probenecid is known to interact with the metabolism or renal tubular excretion of barbiturates; concomitant use should be carefully assessed).

No products indexed under this heading.

Methotrexate Sodium (Probenecid must be used with each cidofovir infusion; probenecid is known to interact with the metabolism and renal tubular excretion of methotrexate; concomitant use should be carefully assessed).

No products indexed under this heading.

Midazolam Hydrochloride (Probenecid must be used with each cidofovir infusion; probenecid is known to interact with the metabolism or renal tubular excretion of benzodiazepines; concomitant use should be carefully assessed). Products include:

- Versed Injection 3027
- Versed Syrup 3033

Moexipril Hydrochloride (Probenecid must be used with each cidofovir infusion; probenecid is known to interact with the metabolism or renal tubular excretion of ACE inhibitors; concomitant use should be carefully assessed). Products include:

- Uniretic Tablets 3178
- Univasc Tablets 3181

Nabumetone (Probenecid must be used with each cidofovir infusion; probenecid is known to interact with the metabolism or renal tubular excretion of non-steroidal anti-inflammatory agents; concomitant use should be carefully assessed). Products include:

- Relafen Tablets 1617

Naproxen (Probenecid must be used with each cidofovir infusion; probenecid is known to interact with the metabolism or renal tubular excretion of non-steroidal anti-inflammatory agents; concomitant use should be carefully assessed). Products include:

- EC-Naprosyn Delayed-Release Tablets 2967
- Naprosyn Suspension 2967
- Naprosyn Tablets 2967

Naproxen Sodium (Probenecid must be used with each cidofovir infusion; probenecid is known to interact with the metabolism or renal tubular excretion of non-steroidal anti-inflammatory agents; concomitant use should be carefully assessed). Products include:

- Aleve Tablets, Caplets and Gelcaps ▣602
- Aleve Cold & Sinus Caplets ▣603
- Anaprox Tablets 2967
- Anaprox DS Tablets 2967
- Naprelan Tablets 1293

Oxaprozin (Probenecid must be used with each cidofovir infusion; probenecid is known to interact with the metabolism or renal tubular excretion of non-steroidal anti-inflammatory agents; concomitant use should be carefully assessed).

No products indexed under this heading.

Oxazepam (Probenecid must be used with each cidofovir infusion; probenecid is known to interact with the metabolism or renal tubular excretion of benzodiazepines; concomitant use should be carefully assessed).

No products indexed under this heading.

Pentamidine Isethionate (Renal impairment is the major toxicity of cidofovir; co-administration with potential nephrotoxic agents, such as intravenous pentamidine, should be avoided).

No products indexed under this heading.

Pentobarbital Sodium (Probenecid must be used with each cidofovir infusion; probenecid is known to interact with the metabolism or renal tubular excretion of barbiturates; concomitant use should be carefully assessed). Products include:

- Nembutal Sodium Solution 485

Perindopril Erbumine (Probenecid must be used with each cidofovir infusion; probenecid is known to interact with the metabolism or renal tubular excretion of ACE inhibitors; concomitant use should be carefully assessed). Products include:

- Aceon Tablets (2 mg, 4 mg, 8 mg) 3249

Phenobarbital (Probenecid must be used with each cidofovir infusion; probenecid is known to interact with the metabolism or renal tubular excretion of barbiturates; concomitant use should be carefully assessed). Products include:

- Arco-Lase Plus Tablets 592
- Donnatal 2929
- Donnatal Extentabs 2930

Phenylbutazone (Probenecid must be used with each cidofovir infusion; probenecid is known to interact with the metabolism or renal tubular excretion of non-steroidal anti-inflammatory agents; concomitant use should be carefully assessed).

No products indexed under this heading.

Piroxicam (Probenecid must be used with each cidofovir infusion; probenecid is known to interact with the metabolism or renal tubular excretion of non-steroidal anti-inflammatory agents; concomitant use should be carefully assessed). Products include:

- Feldene Capsules 2685

Prazepam (Probenecid must be used with each cidofovir infusion; probenecid is known to interact with the metabolism or renal tubular excretion of benzodiazepines; concomitant use should be carefully assessed).

No products indexed under this heading.

Quazepam (Probenecid must be used with each cidofovir infusion; probenecid is known to interact with the metabolism or renal tubular excretion of benzodiazepines; concomitant use should be carefully assessed).

No products indexed under this heading.

Quinapril Hydrochloride (Probenecid must be used with each cidofovir infusion; probenecid is known to interact with the metabolism or renal tubular excretion of ACE inhibitors; concomitant use should be carefully assessed). Products include:

- Accupril Tablets 2611
- Accuretic Tablets 2614

Ramipril (Probenecid must be used with each cidofovir infusion; probenecid is known to interact with the metabolism or renal tubular excretion of ACE inhibitors; concomitant use should be carefully assessed). Products include:

- Altace Capsules 2233

Rofecoxib (Probenecid must be used with each cidofovir infusion; probenecid is known to interact with the metabolism or renal tubular excretion of non-steroidal anti-inflammatory agents; concomitant use should be carefully assessed). Products include:

- Vioxx 2213

Secobarbital Sodium (Probenecid must be used with each cidofovir infusion; probenecid is known to interact with the metabolism or renal tubular excretion of barbiturates; concomitant use should be carefully assessed).

No products indexed under this heading.

Spirapril Hydrochloride (Probenecid must be used with each cidofovir infusion; probenecid is known to interact with the metabolism or renal tubular excretion of ACE inhibitors; concomitant use should be carefully assessed).

No products indexed under this heading.

Streptomycin Sulfate (Renal impairment is the major toxicity of cidofovir; co-administration with potential nephrotoxic agents should be avoided). Products include:

- Streptomycin Sulfate Injection 2714

Sulindac (Probenecid must be used with each cidofovir infusion; probenecid is known to interact with the metabolism or renal tubular excretion of non-steroidal anti-inflammatory agents; concomitant use should be carefully assessed). Products include:

- Clinoril Tablets 2053

Temazepam (Probenecid must be used with each cidofovir infusion; probenecid is known to interact with the metabolism or renal tubular excretion of benzodiazepines; concomitant use should be carefully assessed).

No products indexed under this heading.

Theophylline (Probenecid must be used with each cidofovir infusion; probenecid is known to interact with the metabolism or renal tubular excretion of theophylline; concomitant use should be carefully assessed). Products include:

- Aerolate 1361
- Theo-Dur Extended-Release Tablets 1835
- Uni-Dur Extended-Release Tablets 1841
- Uniphyl 400 mg and 600 mg Tablets 2903

Theophylline Calcium Salicylate (Probenecid must be used with each cidofovir infusion; probenecid is known to interact with the metabolism or renal tubular excretion of theophylline; concomitant use should be carefully assessed).

No products indexed under this heading.

Theophylline Sodium Glycinate (Probenecid must be used with each cidofovir infusion; probenecid is known to interact with the metabolism or renal tubular excretion of theophylline; concomitant use should be carefully assessed).
No products indexed under this heading.

Thiamylal Sodium (Probenecid must be used with each cidofovir infusion; probenecid is known to interact with the metabolism or renal tubular excretion of barbiturates; concomitant use should be carefully assessed).
No products indexed under this heading.

Tobramycin (Renal impairment is the major toxicity of cidofovir; co-administration with potential nephrotoxic agents should be avoided). Products include:
TOBI Solution for Inhalation ... 1206
TobraDex Ophthalmic Ointment ... 542
TobraDex Ophthalmic Suspension ... 541
Tobrex Ophthalmic Ointment ... ⊙ 220
Tobrex Ophthalmic Solution ... ⊙ 221

Tobramycin Sulfate (Renal impairment is the major toxicity of cidofovir; co-administration with potential nephrotoxic agents should be avoided). Products include:
Nebcin Vials, Hyporets & ADD-Vantage ... 1955

Tolmetin Sodium (Probenecid must be used with each cidofovir infusion; probenecid is known to interact with the metabolism or renal tubular excretion of non-steroidal anti-inflammatory agents; concomitant use should be carefully assessed). Products include:
Tolectin ... 2589

Trandolapril (Probenecid must be used with each cidofovir infusion; probenecid is known to interact with the metabolism or renal tubular excretion of ACE inhibitors; concomitant use should be carefully assessed). Products include:
Mavik Tablets ... 478
Tarka Tablets ... 508

Triazolam (Probenecid must be used with each cidofovir infusion; probenecid is known to interact with the metabolism or renal tubular excretion of benzodiazepines; concomitant use should be carefully assessed). Products include:
Halcion Tablets ... 2823

Zidovudine (Probenecid must be used with each cidofovir infusion; probenecid is known to interact with the metabolism or renal tubular excretion of zidovudine; therefore, zidovudine should either be temporarily discontinued or decreased by 50% when co-administered with probenecid on the day of Vistide infusion). Products include:
Combivir Tablets ... 1502
Retrovir ... 1625
Retrovir IV Infusion ... 1629
Trizivir Tablets ... 1669

VISUDYNE FOR INJECTION

(Verteporfin) ... ⊙ 308
May interact with calcium channel blockers, anticoagulants, phenothiazines, sulfonamides, sulfonylureas, tetracyclines, thiazides, and certain other agents. Compounds in these categories include:

Amlodipine Besylate (Co-administration with calcium channel blockers could enhance the rate of verteporfin's uptake by the vascular endothelium). Products include:
Lotrel Capsules ... 2370
Norvasc Tablets ... 2704

Ardeparin Sodium (Co-administration with drugs that decrease clotting would be expected to decrease verteporfin activity).
No products indexed under this heading.

Aspirin (Co-administration with drugs that decrease platelet aggregation would be expected to decrease verteporfin activity). Products include:
Aggrenox Capsules ... 1026
Alka-Seltzer ... 603
Alka-Seltzer Lemon Lime Antacid and Pain Reliever Effervescent Tablets ... 603
Alka-Seltzer Extra Strength Antacid and Pain Reliever Effervescent Tablets ... 603
Alka-Seltzer PM Effervescent Tablets ... 605
Genuine Bayer Tablets, Caplets and Gelcaps ... 606
Extra Strength Bayer Caplets and Gelcaps ... 610
Aspirin Regimen Bayer Children's Chewable Tablets (Orange or Cherry Flavored) ... 607
Bayer, Aspirin Regimen ... 606
Aspirin Regimen Bayer 81 mg Caplets with Calcium ... 607
Genuine Bayer Professional Labeling (Aspirin Regimen Bayer) ... 608
Extra Strength Bayer Arthritis Caplets ... 610
Extra Strength Bayer Plus Caplets ... 610
Extra Strength Bayer PM Caplets ... 611
BC Powder ... 619
BC Allergy Sinus Cold Powder ... 619
Arthritis Strength BC Powder ... 619
BC Sinus Cold Powder ... 619
Darvon Compound-65 Pulvules ... 1910
Ecotrin Enteric Coated Aspirin Low, Regular and Maximum Strength Tablets ... 1715
Excedrin Extra-Strength Tablets, Caplets, and Geltabs ... 629
Excedrin Migraine ... 1070
Goody's Body Pain Formula Powder ... 620
Goody's Extra Strength Headache Powder ... 620
Goody's Extra Strength Pain Relief Tablets ... 620
Percodan Tablets ... 1327
Robaxisal Tablets ... 2939
Soma Compound Tablets ... 3354
Soma Compound w/Codeine Tablets ... 3355
Vanquish Caplets ... 617

Bendroflumethiazide (Co-administration with other photosensitizing agents, such as thiazide diuretics, could increase the potential for skin photosensitivity reactions). Products include:
Corzide 40/5 Tablets ... 2247
Corzide 80/5 Tablets ... 2247

Bepridil Hydrochloride (Co-administration with calcium channel blockers could enhance the rate of verteporfin's uptake by the vascular endothelium). Products include:
Vascor Tablets ... 2602

Chlorothiazide (Co-administration with other photosensitizing agents, such as thiazide diuretics, could increase the potential for skin photosensitivity reactions). Products include:
Aldoclor Tablets ... 2035
Diuril Oral ... 2087

Chlorothiazide Sodium (Co-administration with other photosensitizing agents, such as thiazide diuretics, could increase the potential for skin photosensitivity reactions). Products include:
Diuril Sodium Intravenous ... 2086

Chlorpromazine (Co-administration with other photosensitizing agents, such as phenothiazines, could increase the potential for skin photosensitivity reactions). Products include:
Thorazine Suppositories ... 1656

Chlorpromazine Hydrochloride (Co-administration with other photosensitizing agents, such as phenothiazines, could increase the potential for skin photosensitivity reactions). Products include:
Thorazine ... 1656

Chlorpropamide (Co-administration with other photosensitizing agents, such as sulfonylurea hypoglycemic agents, could increase the potential for skin photosensitivity reactions). Products include:
Diabinese Tablets ... 2680

Clopidogrel Bisulfate (Co-administration with drugs that decrease platelet aggregation would be expected to decrease verteporfin activity). Products include:
Plavix Tablets ... 1097
Plavix Tablets ... 3084

Dalteparin Sodium (Co-administration with drugs that decrease clotting would be expected to decrease verteporfin activity). Products include:
Fragmin Injection ... 2814

Danaparoid Sodium (Co-administration with drugs that decrease clotting would be expected to decrease verteporfin activity). Products include:
Orgaran Injection ... 2480

Demeclocycline Hydrochloride (Co-administration with other photosensitizing agents, such as tetracyclines, could increase the potential for skin photosensitivity reactions). Products include:
Declomycin Tablets ... 1855

Dicumarol (Co-administration with drugs that decrease clotting would be expected to decrease verteporfin activity).
No products indexed under this heading.

Diltiazem Hydrochloride (Co-administration with calcium channel blockers could enhance the rate of verteporfin's uptake by the vascular endothelium). Products include:
Cardizem Injectable ... 1018
Cardizem Lyo-Ject Syringe ... 1018
Cardizem Monovial ... 1018
Cardizem CD Capsules ... 1016
Tiazac Capsules ... 1378

Dimethyl Sulfoxide (Co-administration with compounds that quench active oxygen species or scavenge radicals, such as dimethyl sulfoxide, would be expected to decrease verteporfin activity). Products include:
Rimso-50 Solution ... 1267

Dipyridamole (Co-administration with drugs that decrease platelet aggregation would be expected to decrease verteporfin activity). Products include:
Aggrenox Capsules ... 1026
Persantine Tablets ... 1057

Doxycycline Calcium (Co-administration with other photosensitizing agents, such as tetracyclines, could increase the potential for skin photosensitivity reactions). Products include:
Vibramycin Calcium Oral Suspension Syrup ... 2735

Doxycycline Hyclate (Co-administration with other photosensitizing agents, such as tetracyclines, could increase the potential for skin photosensitivity reactions). Products include:
Doryx Coated Pellet Filled Capsules ... 3357
Periostat Tablets ... 1208
Vibramycin Hyclate Capsules ... 2735
Vibramycin Hyclate Intravenous ... 2737
Vibra-Tabs Film Coated Tablets ... 2735

Doxycycline Monohydrate (Co-administration with other photosensitizing agents, such as tetracyclines, could increase the potential for skin photosensitivity reactions). Products include:
Monodox Capsules ... 2442
Vibramycin Monohydrate for Oral Suspension ... 2735

Enoxaparin (Co-administration with drugs that decrease clotting would be expected to decrease verteporfin activity). Products include:
Lovenox Injection ... 746

Felodipine (Co-administration with calcium channel blockers could enhance the rate of verteporfin's uptake by the vascular endothelium). Products include:
Lexxel Tablets ... 608
Plendil Extended-Release Tablets ... 623

Fluphenazine Decanoate (Co-administration with other photosensitizing agents, such as phenothiazines, could increase the potential for skin photosensitivity reactions).
No products indexed under this heading.

Fluphenazine Enanthate (Co-administration with other photosensitizing agents, such as phenothiazines, could increase the potential for skin photosensitivity reactions).
No products indexed under this heading.

Fluphenazine Hydrochloride (Co-administration with other photosensitizing agents, such as phenothiazines, could increase the potential for skin photosensitivity reactions).
No products indexed under this heading.

Glimepiride (Co-administration with other photosensitizing agents, such as sulfonylurea hypoglycemic agents, could increase the potential for skin photosensitivity reactions). Products include:
Amaryl Tablets ... 717

Glipizide (Co-administration with other photosensitizing agents, such as sulfonylurea hypoglycemic agents, could increase the potential for skin photosensitivity reactions). Products include:
Glucotrol Tablets ... 2692
Glucotrol XL Extended Release Tablets ... 2693

Glyburide (Co-administration with other photosensitizing agents, such as sulfonylurea hypoglycemic agents, could increase the potential for skin photosensitivity reactions). Products include:
DiaBeta Tablets ... 741
Glucovance Tablets ... 1086

Griseofulvin (Co-administration with other photosensitizing agents, such as griseofulvin, could increase the potential for skin photosensitivity reactions). Products include:
Grifulvin V Tablets Microsize and Oral Suspension Microsize ... 2518
Gris-PEG Tablets ... 2661

Heparin Sodium (Co-administration with drugs that decrease clotting would be expected to decrease verteporfin activity). Products include:
Heparin Lock Flush Solution ... 3509
Heparin Sodium Injection ... 3511

Hydrochlorothiazide (Co-administration with other photosensitizing agents, such as thiazide diuretics, could increase the potential for skin photosensitivity reactions). Products include:
Accuretic Tablets ... 2614
Aldoril Tablets ... 2039
Atacand HCT Tablets ... 597
Avalide Tablets ... 1070
Diovan HCT Tablets ... 2338
Dyazide Capsules ... 1515
HydroDIURIL Tablets ... 2108
Hyzaar ... 2109
Inderide Tablets ... 3517
Inderide LA Long-Acting Capsules ... 3519
Lotensin HCT Tablets ... 2367
Maxzide ... 1008
Micardis HCT Tablets ... 1051
Microzide Capsules ... 3414
Moduretic Tablets ... 2138
Monopril HCT ... 1094
Prinzide Tablets ... 2168
Timolide Tablets ... 2187
Uniretic Tablets ... 3178

Vaseretic Tablets 2204
Zestoretic Tablets 695
Ziac Tablets 1887

Hydroflumethiazide (Co-administration with other photosensitizing agents, such as thiazide diuretics, could increase the potential for skin photosensitivity reactions). Products include:
Diucardin Tablets 3494

Isradipine (Co-administration with calcium channel blockers could enhance the rate of verteporfin's uptake by the vascular endothelium). Products include:
DynaCirc Capsules 2921
DynaCirc CR Tablets 2923

Mannitol (Co-administration with compounds that quench active oxygen species or scavenge radicals, such as mannitol, would be expected to decrease verteporfin activity).
No products indexed under this heading.

Mesoridazine Besylate (Co-administration with other photosensitizing agents, such as phenothiazines, could increase the potential for skin photosensitivity reactions). Products include:
Serentil 1057

Methacycline Hydrochloride (Co-administration with other photosensitizing agents, such as tetracyclines, could increase the potential for skin photosensitivity reactions).
No products indexed under this heading.

Methotrimeprazine (Co-administration with other photosensitizing agents, such as phenothiazines, could increase the potential for skin photosensitivity reactions).
No products indexed under this heading.

Methyclothiazide (Co-administration with other photosensitizing agents, such as thiazide diuretics, could increase the potential for skin photosensitivity reactions).
No products indexed under this heading.

Mibefradil Dihydrochloride (Co-administration with calcium channel blockers could enhance the rate of verteporfin's uptake by the vascular endothelium).
No products indexed under this heading.

Minocycline Hydrochloride (Co-administration with other photosensitizing agents, such as tetracyclines, could increase the potential for skin photosensitivity reactions). Products include:
Dynacin Capsules 2019
Minocin Intravenous 1862
Minocin Oral Suspension 1865
Minocin Pellet-Filled Capsules 1863

Nicardipine Hydrochloride (Co-administration with calcium channel blockers could enhance the rate of verteporfin's uptake by the vascular endothelium). Products include:
Cardene I.V. 3485

Nifedipine (Co-administration with calcium channel blockers could enhance the rate of verteporfin's uptake by the vascular endothelium). Products include:
Adalat CC Tablets 877
Procardia Capsules 2708
Procardia XL Extended Release Tablets 2710

Nimodipine (Co-administration with calcium channel blockers could enhance the rate of verteporfin's uptake by the vascular endothelium). Products include:
Nimotop Capsules 904

Nisoldipine (Co-administration with calcium channel blockers could enhance the rate of verteporfin's uptake by the vascular endothelium). Products include:
Sular Tablets 688

Oxytetracycline Hydrochloride (Co-administration with other photosensitizing agents, such as tetracyclines, could increase the potential for skin photosensitivity reactions). Products include:
Terra-Cortril Ophthalmic Suspension 2716
Urobiotic-250 Capsules 2731

Perphenazine (Co-administration with other photosensitizing agents, such as phenothiazines, could increase the potential for skin photosensitivity reactions). Products include:
Etrafon 3115
Trilafon 3160

Polymyxin B Sulfate (Co-administration with polymyxin B could enhance the rate of verteporfin's uptake by the vascular endothelium). Products include:
Betadine Brand First Aid Antibiotics & Moisturizer Ointment 2894
Betadine Brand Plus First Aid Antibiotics & Pain Reliever Ointment 2894
Cortisporin Ophthalmic Suspension Sterile .... ⊙297
Neosporin G.U. Irrigant Sterile 2256
Neosporin Ointment .... ▣704
Neosporin Ophthalmic Ointment Sterile .... ⊙299
Neosporin Ophthalmic Solution Sterile .... ⊙300
Neosporin + Pain Relief Maximum Strength Cream .... ▣704
Neosporin + Pain Relief Maximum Strength Ointment .... ▣704
Poly-Pred Liquifilm Ophthalmic Suspension .... ⊙245
Polysporin Ointment .... ▣706
Polysporin Ophthalmic Ointment Sterile .... ⊙301
Polysporin Powder .... ▣706
Polytrim Ophthalmic Solution 556

Polythiazide (Co-administration with other photosensitizing agents, such as thiazide diuretics, could increase the potential for skin photosensitivity reactions). Products include:
Minizide Capsules 2700
Renese Tablets 2712

Prochlorperazine (Co-administration with other photosensitizing agents, such as phenothiazines, could increase the potential for skin photosensitivity reactions). Products include:
Compazine 1505

Promethazine Hydrochloride (Co-administration with other photosensitizing agents, such as phenothiazines, could increase the potential for skin photosensitivity reactions). Products include:
Mepergan Injection 3539
Phenergan Injection 3553
Phenergan 3556
Phenergan Syrup 3554
Phenergan with Codeine Syrup 3557
Phenergan with Dextromethorphan Syrup 3559
Phenergan VC Syrup 3560
Phenergan VC with Codeine Syrup 3561

Sulfacytine (Co-administration with other photosensitizing agents, such as sulfonamides, could increase the potential for skin photosensitivity reactions).
No products indexed under this heading.

Sulfamethizole (Co-administration with other photosensitizing agents, such as sulfonamides, could increase the potential for skin photosensitivity reactions). Products include:
Urobiotic-250 Capsules 2731

Sulfamethoxazole (Co-administration with other photosensitizing agents, such as sulfonamides, could increase the potential for skin photosensitivity reactions). Products include:
Bactrim 2949
Septra Suspension 2265
Septra Tablets 2265
Septra DS Tablets 2265

Sulfasalazine (Co-administration with other photosensitizing agents, such as sulfonamides, could increase the potential for skin photosensitivity reactions). Products include:
Azulfidine EN-tabs Tablets 2775

Sulfinpyrazone (Co-administration with other photosensitizing agents, such as sulfonamides, could increase the potential for skin photosensitivity reactions).
No products indexed under this heading.

Sulfisoxazole (Co-administration with other photosensitizing agents, such as sulfonamides, could increase the potential for skin photosensitivity reactions).
No products indexed under this heading.

Sulfisoxazole Acetyl (Co-administration with other photosensitizing agents, such as sulfonamides, could increase the potential for skin photosensitivity reactions). Products include:
Pediazole Suspension 3050

Sulfisoxazole Diolamine (Co-administration with other photosensitizing agents, such as sulfonamides, could increase the potential for skin photosensitivity reactions).
No products indexed under this heading.

Tetracycline Hydrochloride (Co-administration with other photosensitizing agents, such as tetracyclines, could increase the potential for skin photosensitivity reactions).
No products indexed under this heading.

Thioridazine Hydrochloride (Co-administration with other photosensitizing agents, such as phenothiazines, could increase the potential for skin photosensitivity reactions). Products include:
Thioridazine Hydrochloride Tablets 2289

Tinzaparin sodium (Co-administration with drugs that decrease clotting would be expected to decrease verteporfin activity). Products include:
Innohep Injection 1248

Tolazamide (Co-administration with other photosensitizing agents, such as sulfonylurea hypoglycemic agents, could increase the potential for skin photosensitivity reactions).
No products indexed under this heading.

Tolbutamide (Co-administration with other photosensitizing agents, such as sulfonylurea hypoglycemic agents, could increase the potential for skin photosensitivity reactions).
No products indexed under this heading.

Trifluoperazine Hydrochloride (Co-administration with other photosensitizing agents, such as phenothiazines, could increase the potential for skin photosensitivity reactions). Products include:
Stelazine 1640

Verapamil Hydrochloride (Co-administration with calcium channel blockers could enhance the rate of verteporfin's uptake by the vascular endothelium). Products include:
Covera-HS Tablets 3199
Isoptin SR Tablets 467
Tarka Tablets 508
Verelan Capsules 3184
Verelan PM Capsules 3186

Warfarin Sodium (Co-administration with drugs that decrease clotting would be expected to decrease verteporfin activity). Products include:
Coumadin for Injection 1243
Coumadin Tablets 1243
Warfarin Sodium Tablets, USP 3302

Food Interactions

Alcohol (Co-administration with compounds that quench active oxygen species or scavenge radicals, such as ethanol, would be expected to decrease verteporfin activity).

VITAMIST INTRA-ORAL SPRAY

(Vitamins with Minerals) .... ▣821
None cited in PDR database.

VITARA CREAM

(Dehydroepiandrosterone (DHEA), N-Methylnicotinate) .... ▣731
None cited in PDR database.

VITASANA GELCAPS

(Ginseng, Herbals with Vitamins & Minerals) .... ▣834
None cited in PDR database.

VITRASERT IMPLANT

(Ganciclovir) .... ⊙254
None cited in PDR database.

VITRAVENE FOR INJECTION

(Fomivirsen Sodium) .... ⊙310
None cited in PDR database.

VIVACTIL TABLETS

(Protriptyline Hydrochloride) 2446
May interact with anticholinergics, barbiturates, central nervous system depressants, antidepressant drugs, monoamine oxidase inhibitors, phenothiazines, quinidine, selective serotonin reuptake inhibitors, sympathomimetics, thyroid preparations, and certain other agents. Compounds in these categories include:

Albuterol (Effects of concurrent use not specified; careful adjustment of dosage and close supervision are required). Products include:
Proventil Inhalation Aerosol 3142
Ventolin Inhalation Aerosol and Refill 1679

Albuterol Sulfate (Effects of concurrent use not specified; careful adjustment of dosage and close supervision are required). Products include:
AccuNeb Inhalation Solution 1230
Combivent Inhalation Aerosol 1041
DuoNeb Inhalation Solution 1233
Proventil Inhalation Solution 0.083% 3146
Proventil Repetabs Tablets 3148
Proventil Solution for Inhalation 0.5% 3144
Proventil HFA Inhalation Aerosol 3150
Ventolin HFA Inhalation Aerosol 3618
Volmax Extended-Release Tablets 2276

Alfentanil Hydrochloride (Co-administration results in enhanced response to CNS depressants).
No products indexed under this heading.

Alprazolam (Co-administration results in enhanced response to CNS depressants). Products include:
Xanax Tablets 2865

Amitriptyline Hydrochloride (Co-administration with cytochrome P4502D6 inhibitors, such as antidepressants, may make normal metabolizer resemble poor metabolizer leading to higher than expected plasma concentration of TCA with resultant toxicity; lower than usual doses of either drug may be required). Products include:
Etrafon 3115
Limbitrol 1738

Amoxapine (Co-administration with cytochrome P4502D6 inhibitors, such as antidepressants, may make normal metabolizer resemble poor metabolizer leading to higher than expected plasma concentration of TCA with resultant toxicity; lower

than usual doses of either drug may be required).
No products indexed under this heading.

Aprobarbital (Co-administration results in enhanced response to CNS depressants).
No products indexed under this heading.

Atropine Sulfate (Co-administration may result in hyperpyrexia, particularly during hot weather). Products include:
Donnatal 2929
Donnatal Extentabs 2930
Motofen Tablets 577
Prosed/DS Tablets 3268
Urised Tablets 2876

Belladonna Alkaloids (Co-administration may result in hyperpyrexia, particularly during hot weather). Products include:
Hyland's Teething Tablets .... ■766
Urimax Tablets 1769

Benztropine Mesylate (Co-administration may result in hyperpyrexia, particularly during hot weather). Products include:
Cogentin 2055

Biperiden Hydrochloride (Co-administration may result in hyperpyrexia, particularly during hot weather). Products include:
Akineton 402

Buprenorphine Hydrochloride (Co-administration results in enhanced response to CNS depressants). Products include:
Buprenex Injectable 2918

Bupropion Hydrochloride (Co-administration with cytochrome P4502D6 inhibitors, such as antidepressants, may make normal metabolizer resemble poor metabolizer leading to higher than expected plasma concentration of TCA with resultant toxicity; lower than usual doses of either drug may be required). Products include:
Wellbutrin Tablets 1680
Wellbutrin SR Sustained-Release Tablets 1684
Zyban Sustained-Release Tablets ... 1710

Buspirone Hydrochloride (Co-administration results in enhanced response to CNS depressants).
No products indexed under this heading.

Butabarbital (Co-administration results in enhanced response to CNS depressants).
No products indexed under this heading.

Butalbital (Co-administration results in enhanced response to CNS depressants). Products include:
Phrenilin 578
Sedapap Tablets 50 mg/650 mg ... 2225

Chlordiazepoxide (Co-administration results in enhanced response to CNS depressants). Products include:
Limbitrol 1738

Chlordiazepoxide Hydrochloride (Co-administration results in enhanced response to CNS depressants). Products include:
Librium Capsules 1736
Librium for Injection 1737

Chlorpromazine (Co-administration with cytochrome P4502D6 inhibitors, such as phenothiazines, may make normal metabolizer resemble poor metabolizer leading to higher than expected plasma concentration of TCA with resultant toxicity; lower than usual doses of either drug may be required; co-administration results in enhanced response to CNS depressants). Products include:
Thorazine Suppositories 1656

Chlorpromazine Hydrochloride (Co-administration with cytochrome P4502D6 inhibitors, such as phenothiazines, may make normal metabolizer resemble poor metabolizer leading to higher than expected plasma concentration of TCA with resultant toxicity; lower than usual doses of either drug may be required; co-administration results in enhanced response to CNS depressants). Products include:
Thorazine 1656

Chlorprothixene (Co-administration results in enhanced response to CNS depressants).
No products indexed under this heading.

Chlorprothixene Hydrochloride (Co-administration results in enhanced response to CNS depressants).
No products indexed under this heading.

Chlorprothixene Lactate (Co-administration results in enhanced response to CNS depressants).
No products indexed under this heading.

Cimetidine (Co-administration has been reported to reduce hepatic metabolism of certain tricyclic antidepressants, thereby delaying elimination and increasing steady-state concentrations of TCA resulting in the frequency and severity of side effects, particularly anticholinergic). Products include:
Tagamet HB 200 Suspension .... ■762
Tagamet HB 200 Tablets .... ■761
Tagamet Tablets 1644

Cimetidine Hydrochloride (Co-administration has been reported to reduce hepatic metabolism of certain tricyclic antidepressants, thereby delaying elimination and increasing steady-state concentrations of TCA resulting in the frequency and severity of side effects, particularly anticholinergic). Products include:
Tagamet 1644

Cisapride (Co-administration can result in possible adverse cardiac interactions including prolongation of the QT interval, cardiac arrhythmias and conduction system disturbances; concurrent use in contraindicated).
No products indexed under this heading.

Citalopram Hydrobromide (Co-administration with cytochrome P4502D6 inhibitors, such as antidepressants, may make normal metabolizer resemble poor metabolizer leading to higher than expected plasma concentration of TCA with resultant toxicity; lower than usual doses of either drug may be required). Products include:
Celexa 1365

Clidinium Bromide (Co-administration may result in hyperpyrexia, particularly during hot weather).
No products indexed under this heading.

Clorazepate Dipotassium (Co-administration results in enhanced response to CNS depressants). Products include:
Tranxene 511

Clozapine (Co-administration results in enhanced response to CNS depressants). Products include:
Clozaril Tablets 2319

Codeine Phosphate (Co-administration results in enhanced response to CNS depressants). Products include:
Phenergan with Codeine Syrup 3557
Phenergan VC with Codeine Syrup .. 3561
Robitussin A-C Syrup 2942
Robitussin-DAC Syrup 2942
Ryna-C Liquid .... ■768
Soma Compound w/Codeine Tablets 3355
Tussi-Organidin NR Liquid 3350
Tussi-Organidin-S NR Liquid 3350
Tylenol with Codeine 2595

Desflurane (Co-administration results in enhanced response to CNS depressants). Products include:
Suprane Liquid for Inhalation 874

Desipramine Hydrochloride (Co-administration with cytochrome P4502D6 inhibitors, such as antidepressants, may make normal metabolizer resemble poor metabolizer leading to higher than expected plasma concentration of TCA with resultant toxicity; lower than usual doses of either drug may be required). Products include:
Norpramin Tablets 755

Dezocine (Co-administration results in enhanced response to CNS depressants).
No products indexed under this heading.

Diazepam (Co-administration results in enhanced response to CNS depressants). Products include:
Valium Injectable 3026
Valium Tablets 3047

Dicyclomine Hydrochloride (Co-administration may result in hyperpyrexia, particularly during hot weather).
No products indexed under this heading.

Dobutamine Hydrochloride (Effects of concurrent use not specified; careful adjustment of dosage and close supervision are required). Products include:
Dobutrex Solution Vials 1914

Dopamine Hydrochloride (Effects of concurrent use not specified; careful adjustment of dosage and close supervision are required).
No products indexed under this heading.

Doxepin Hydrochloride (Co-administration with cytochrome P4502D6 inhibitors, such as antidepressants, may make normal metabolizer resemble poor metabolizer leading to higher than expected plasma concentration of TCA with resultant toxicity; lower than usual doses of either drug may be required). Products include:
Sinequan 2713

Droperidol (Co-administration results in enhanced response to CNS depressants).
No products indexed under this heading.

Enflurane (Co-administration results in enhanced response to CNS depressants).
No products indexed under this heading.

Ephedrine Hydrochloride (Effects of concurrent use not specified; careful adjustment of dosage and close supervision are required). Products include:
Primatene Tablets .... ■780

Ephedrine Sulfate (Effects of concurrent use not specified; careful adjustment of dosage and close supervision are required).
No products indexed under this heading.

Ephedrine Tannate (Effects of concurrent use not specified; careful adjustment of dosage and close supervision are required). Products include:
Rynatuss Pediatric Suspension 3353
Rynatuss Tablets 3353

Epinephrine (Effects of concurrent use not specified; careful adjustment of dosage and close supervision are required). Products include:
Epifrin Sterile Ophthalmic Solution .... ⊙235
EpiPen 1236
Primatene Mist .... ■779
Xylocaine with Epinephrine Injection 653

Epinephrine Bitartrate (Effects of concurrent use not specified; careful adjustment of dosage and close supervision are required). Products include:
Sensorcaine 643

Epinephrine Hydrochloride (Effects of concurrent use not specified; careful adjustment of dosage and close supervision are required).
No products indexed under this heading.

Estazolam (Co-administration results in enhanced response to CNS depressants). Products include:
ProSom Tablets 500

Ethchlorvynol (Co-administration results in enhanced response to CNS depressants).
No products indexed under this heading.

Ethinamate (Co-administration results in enhanced response to CNS depressants).
No products indexed under this heading.

Fentanyl (Co-administration results in enhanced response to CNS depressants). Products include:
Duragesic Transdermal System 1786

Fentanyl Citrate (Co-administration results in enhanced response to CNS depressants). Products include:
Actiq 1184

Flecainide Acetate (Co-administration with cytochrome P4502D6 inhibitors, such as flecainide, may make normal metabolizer resemble poor metabolizer leading to higher than expected plasma concentration of TCA with resultant toxicity; lower than usual doses of either drug may be required). Products include:
Tambocor Tablets 1990

Fluoxetine Hydrochloride (Co-administration with cytochrome P4502D6 inhibitors, such as antidepressants, may make normal metabolizer resemble poor metabolizer leading to higher than expected plasma concentration of TCA with resultant toxicity; due to variation in the extent of inhibition of P4502D6 and long half-life of fluoxetine, sufficient time, at least 5 weeks, should elapse in switching to TCA). Products include:
Prozac Pulvules, Liquid, and Weekly Capsules 1238
Sarafem Pulvules 1962

Fluphenazine Decanoate (Co-administration with cytochrome P4502D6 inhibitors, such as phenothiazines, may make normal metabolizer resemble poor metabolizer leading to higher than expected plasma concentration of TCA with resultant toxicity; lower than usual doses of either drug may be required; co-administration results in enhanced response to CNS depressants).
No products indexed under this heading.

Fluphenazine Enanthate (Co-administration with cytochrome P4502D6 inhibitors, such as phenothiazines, may make normal metabolizer resemble poor metabolizer leading to higher than expected plasma concentration of TCA with resultant toxicity; lower than usual doses of either drug may be required; co-administration results in enhanced response to CNS depressants).
No products indexed under this heading.

Fluphenazine Hydrochloride (Co-administration with cytochrome P4502D6 inhibitors, such as phenothiazines, may make normal metabolizer resemble poor metabolizer leading to higher than expected plasma concentration of TCA with resultant toxicity; lower than usual doses

of either drug may be required; co-administration results in enhanced response to CNS depressants).
No products indexed under this heading.

Flurazepam Hydrochloride (Co-administration results in enhanced response to CNS depressants).
No products indexed under this heading.

Fluvoxamine Maleate (Co-administration with cytochrome P4502D6 inhibitors, such as antidepressants, may make normal metabolizer resemble poor metabolizer leading to higher than expected plasma concentration of TCA with resultant toxicity; due to variation in the extent of inhibition of P4502D6, sufficient time should elapse in switching from one class to the other). Products include:
Luvox Tablets (25, 50, 100 mg) **3256**

Glutethimide (Co-administration results in enhanced response to CNS depressants).
No products indexed under this heading.

Glycopyrrolate (Co-administration may result in hyperpyrexia, particularly during hot weather). Products include:
Robinul Forte Tablets **1358**
Robinul Injectable **2940**
Robinul Tablets **1358**

Guanadrel Sulfate (Protriptyline may block the antihypertensive action of guanadrel).
No products indexed under this heading.

Guanethidine Monosulfate (Protriptyline may block the antihypertensive action of guanethidine).
No products indexed under this heading.

Haloperidol (Co-administration results in enhanced response to CNS depressants). Products include:
Haldol Injection, Tablets and Concentrate **2533**

Haloperidol Decanoate (Co-administration results in enhanced response to CNS depressants).
Products include:
Haldol Decanoate **2535**

Hydrocodone Bitartrate (Co-administration results in enhanced response to CNS depressants).
Products include:
Hycodan **1316**
Hycomine Compound Tablets **1317**
Hycotuss Expectorant Syrup **1318**
Lortab **3319**
Lortab Elixir **3317**
Maxidone Tablets CIII **3399**
Norco 5/325 Tablets CIII **3424**
Norco 7.5/325 Tablets CIII **3425**
Norco 10/325 Tablets CIII **3427**
Norco 10/325 Tablets CIII **3425**
Vicodin Tablets **516**
Vicodin ES Tablets **517**
Vicodin HP Tablets **518**
Vicodin Tuss Expectorant **519**
Vicoprofen Tablets **520**
Zydone Tablets **1330**

Hydrocodone Polistirex (Co-administration results in enhanced response to CNS depressants).
Products include:
Tussionex Pennkinetic Extended-Release Suspension **1174**

Hydromorphone Hydrochloride (Co-administration results in enhanced response to CNS depressants). Products include:
Dilaudid **441**
Dilaudid Oral Liquid **445**
Dilaudid Powder **441**
Dilaudid Rectal Suppositories **441**
Dilaudid Tablets **441**
Dilaudid Tablets - 8 mg **445**
Dilaudid-HP **443**

Hydroxyzine Hydrochloride (Co-administration results in enhanced response to CNS depressants).
Products include:
Atarax Tablets & Syrup **2667**
Vistaril Intramuscular Solution **2738**

Hyoscyamine (Co-administration may result in hyperpyrexia, particularly during hot weather). Products include:
Urised Tablets **2876**

Hyoscyamine Sulfate (Co-administration may result in hyperpyrexia, particularly during hot weather). Products include:
Arco-Lase Plus Tablets **592**
Donnatal **2929**
Donnatal Extentabs **2930**
Levsin/Levsinex/Levbid **3172**
NuLev Orally Disintegrating Tablets **3176**
Prosed/DS Tablets **3268**
Urimax Tablets **1769**

Imipramine Hydrochloride (Co-administration with cytochrome P4502D6 inhibitors, such as antidepressants, may make normal metabolizer resemble poor metabolizer leading to higher than expected plasma concentration of TCA with resultant toxicity; lower than usual doses of either drug may be required).
No products indexed under this heading.

Imipramine Pamoate (Co-administration with cytochrome P4502D6 inhibitors, such as antidepressants, may make normal metabolizer resemble poor metabolizer leading to higher than expected plasma concentration of TCA with resultant toxicity; lower than usual doses of either drug may be required).
No products indexed under this heading.

Ipratropium Bromide (Co-administration may result in hyperpyrexia, particularly during hot weather). Products include:
Atrovent Inhalation Aerosol **1030**
Atrovent Inhalation Solution **1031**
Atrovent Nasal Spray 0.03% **1032**
Atrovent Nasal Spray 0.06% **1033**
Combivent Inhalation Aerosol **1041**
DuoNeb Inhalation Solution **1233**

Isocarboxazid (Co-administration of tricyclic antidepressants and MAO inhibitors has resulted in hyperpyretic crises, severe convulsions, and deaths; concurrent and/or sequential use is contraindicated).
No products indexed under this heading.

Isoflurane (Co-administration results in enhanced response to CNS depressants).
No products indexed under this heading.

Isoproterenol Hydrochloride (Effects of concurrent use not specified; careful adjustment of dosage and close supervision are required).
No products indexed under this heading.

Isoproterenol Sulfate (Effects of concurrent use not specified; careful adjustment of dosage and close supervision are required).
No products indexed under this heading.

Ketamine Hydrochloride (Co-administration results in enhanced response to CNS depressants).
No products indexed under this heading.

Levalbuterol Hydrochloride (Effects of concurrent use not specified; careful adjustment of dosage and close supervision are required).
Products include:
Xopenex Inhalation Solution **3207**

Levomethadyl Acetate Hydrochloride (Co-administration results in enhanced response to CNS depressants).
No products indexed under this heading.

Levorphanol Tartrate (Co-administration results in enhanced response to CNS depressants).
Products include:
Levo-Dromoran **1734**
Levorphanol Tartrate Tablets **3059**

Levothyroxine Sodium (On rare occasions, concurrent use may result in arrhythmias). Products include:
Levothroid Tablets **1373**
Levoxyl Tablets **1819**
Synthroid **505**
Unithroid Tablets **3445**

Liothyronine Sodium (On rare occasions, concurrent use may result in arrhythmias). Products include:
Cytomel Tablets **1817**
Triostat Injection **1825**

Liotrix (On rare occasions, concurrent use may result in arrhythmias).
No products indexed under this heading.

Lorazepam (Co-administration results in enhanced response to CNS depressants). Products include:
Ativan Injection **3478**
Ativan Tablets **3482**

Loxapine Hydrochloride (Co-administration results in enhanced response to CNS depressants).
No products indexed under this heading.

Loxapine Succinate (Co-administration results in enhanced response to CNS depressants).
Products include:
Loxitane Capsules **3398**

Maprotiline Hydrochloride (Co-administration with cytochrome P4502D6 inhibitors, such as antidepressants, may make normal metabolizer resemble poor metabolizer leading to higher than expected plasma concentration of TCA with resultant toxicity; lower than usual doses of either drug may be required).
No products indexed under this heading.

Mepenzolate Bromide (Co-administration may result in hyperpyrexia, particularly during hot weather).
No products indexed under this heading.

Meperidine Hydrochloride (Co-administration results in enhanced response to CNS depressants).
Products include:
Demerol **3079**
[illegible] Injection **3539**

Mephobarbital (Co-administration results in enhanced response to CNS depressants).
No products indexed under this heading.

Meprobamate (Co-administration results in enhanced response to CNS depressants). Products include:
Miltown Tablets **3349**

Mesoridazine Besylate (Co-administration with cytochrome P4502D6 inhibitors, such as phenothiazines, may make normal metabolizer resemble poor metabolizer leading to higher than expected plasma concentration of TCA with resultant toxicity; lower than usual doses of either drug may be required; co-administration results in enhanced response to CNS depressants).
Products include:
Serentil **1057**

Metaproterenol Sulfate (Effects of concurrent use not specified; careful adjustment of dosage and close supervision are required).
Products include:
Alupent **1029**

Metaraminol Bitartrate (Effects of concurrent use not specified; careful adjustment of dosage and close supervision are required).
Products include:
Aramine Injection **2043**

Methadone Hydrochloride (Co-administration results in enhanced response to CNS depressants).
Products include:
Dolophine Hydrochloride Tablets **3056**

Methohexital Sodium (Co-administration results in enhanced response to CNS depressants).
Products include:
Brevital Sodium for Injection, USP .. **1815**

Methotrimeprazine (Co-administration with cytochrome P4502D6 inhibitors, such as phenothiazines, may make normal metabolizer resemble poor metabolizer leading to higher than expected plasma concentration of TCA with resultant toxicity; lower than usual doses of either drug may be required; co-administration results in enhanced response to CNS depressants).
No products indexed under this heading.

Methoxamine Hydrochloride (Effects of concurrent use not specified; careful adjustment of dosage and close supervision are required).
No products indexed under this heading.

Methoxyflurane (Co-administration results in enhanced response to CNS depressants).
No products indexed under this heading.

Midazolam Hydrochloride (Co-administration results in enhanced response to CNS depressants).
Products include:
Versed Injection **3027**
Versed Syrup **3033**

Mirtazapine (Co-administration with cytochrome P4502D6 inhibitors, such as antidepressants, may make normal metabolizer resemble poor metabolizer leading to higher than expected plasma concentration of TCA with resultant toxicity; lower than usual doses of either drug may be required). Products include:
Remeron Tablets **2483**
Remeron SolTab Tablets **2486**

Moclobemide (Co-administration of tricyclic antidepressants and MAO inhibitors has resulted in hyperpyretic crises, severe convulsions, and deaths; concurrent and/or sequential use is contraindicated).
No products indexed under this heading.

Molindone Hydrochloride (Co-administration results in enhanced response to CNS depressants).
Products include:
Moban **1320**

Morphine Sulfate (Co-administration results in enhanced response to CNS depressants).
Products include:
Astramorph/PF Injection, USP (Preservative-Free) **594**
Duramorph Injection **1312**
Infumorph 200 and Infumorph 500 Sterile Solutions **1314**
Kadian Capsules **1335**
MS Contin Tablets **2896**
MSIR **2898**
Oramorph SR Tablets **3062**
Roxanol **3066**

Nefazodone Hydrochloride (Co-administration with cytochrome P4502D6 inhibitors, such as antidepressants, may make normal metabolizer resemble poor metabolizer leading to higher than expected plasma concentration of TCA with resultant toxicity; lower than usual doses of either drug may be required). Products include:
Serzone Tablets **1104**

Norepinephrine Bitartrate (Effects of concurrent use not speci-

fied; careful adjustment of dosage and close supervision are required).
No products indexed under this heading.

Nortriptyline Hydrochloride (Co-administration with cytochrome P4502D6 inhibitors, such as antidepressants, may make normal metabolizer resemble poor metabolizer leading to higher than expected plasma concentration of TCA with resultant toxicity; lower than usual doses of either drug may be required).
No products indexed under this heading.

Olanzapine (Co-administration results in enhanced response to CNS depressants). Products include:
Zyprexa Tablets 1973
Zyprexa ZYDIS Orally Disintegrating Tablets........ 1973

Oxazepam (Co-administration results in enhanced response to CNS depressants).
No products indexed under this heading.

Oxybutynin Chloride (Co-administration may result in hyperpyrexia, particularly during hot weather). Products include:
Ditropan XL Extended Release Tablets........ 564

Oxycodone Hydrochloride (Co-administration results in enhanced response to CNS depressants). Products include:
OxyContin Tablets 2912
OxyFast Oral Concentrate Solution . 2916
OxyIR Capsules 2916
Percocet Tablets 1326
Percodan Tablets 1327
Percolone Tablets 1327
Roxicodone 3067
Tylox Capsules 2597

Pargyline Hydrochloride (Co-administration of tricyclic antidepressants and MAO inhibitors has resulted in hyperpyretic crises, severe convulsions, and deaths; concurrent and/or sequential use is contraindicated).
No products indexed under this heading.

Paroxetine Hydrochloride (Co-administration with cytochrome P4502D6 inhibitors, such as antidepressants, may make normal metabolizer resemble poor metabolizer leading to higher than expected plasma concentration of TCA with resultant toxicity; lower than usual doses of either drug may be required). Products include:
Paxil 1609

Pentobarbital Sodium (Co-administration results in enhanced response to CNS depressants). Products include:
Nembutal Sodium Solution 485

Perphenazine (Co-administration with cytochrome P4502D6 inhibitors, such as phenothiazines, may make normal metabolizer resemble poor metabolizer leading to higher than expected plasma concentration of TCA with resultant toxicity; lower than usual doses of either drug may be required; co-administration results in enhanced response to CNS depressants). Products include:
Etrafon 3115
Trilafon 3160

Phenelzine Sulfate (Co-administration of tricyclic antidepressants and MAO inhibitors has resulted in hyperpyretic crises, severe convulsions, and deaths; concurrent and/or sequential use is contraindicated). Products include:
Nardil Tablets 2653

Phenobarbital (Co-administration results in enhanced response to CNS depressants). Products include:
Arco-Lase Plus Tablets 592
Donnatal 2929
Donnatal Extentabs 2930

Phenylephrine Bitartrate (Effects of concurrent use not specified; careful adjustment of dosage and close supervision are required).
No products indexed under this heading.

Phenylephrine Hydrochloride (Effects of concurrent use not specified; careful adjustment of dosage and close supervision are required). Products include:
Afrin Nasal Decongestant Children's Pump Mist........ ▣734
Extendryl 1361
Hycomine Compound Tablets 1317
Neo-Synephrine .... ▣614
Phenergan VC Syrup 3560
Phenergan VC with Codeine Syrup .. 3561
Preparation H Cream .... ▣778
Preparation H Cooling Gel .... ▣778
Preparation H .... ▣778
Vicks Sinex Nasal Spray and Ultra Fine Mist........ ▣729

Phenylephrine Tannate (Effects of concurrent use not specified; careful adjustment of dosage and close supervision are required). Products include:
Ryna-12 S Suspension 3351
Reformulated Rynatan Pediatric Suspension 3352
Rynatuss Pediatric Suspension 3353
Rynatuss Tablets 3353

Phenylpropanolamine Hydrochloride (Effects of concurrent use not specified; careful adjustment of dosage and close supervision are required).
No products indexed under this heading.

Pirbuterol Acetate (Effects of concurrent use not specified; careful adjustment of dosage and close supervision are required). Products include:
Maxair Autohaler 1981
Maxair Inhaler 1984

Prazepam (Co-administration results in enhanced response to CNS depressants).
No products indexed under this heading.

Procarbazine Hydrochloride (Co-administration of tricyclic antidepressants and MAO inhibitors has resulted in hyperpyretic crises, severe convulsions, and deaths; concurrent and/or sequential use is contraindicated). Products include:
Matulane Capsules 3246

Prochlorperazine (Co-administration with cytochrome P4502D6 inhibitors, such as phenothiazines, may make normal metabolizer resemble poor metabolizer leading to higher than expected plasma concentration of TCA with resultant toxicity; lower than usual doses of either drug may be required; co-administration results in enhanced response to CNS depressants). Products include:
Compazine 1505

Procyclidine Hydrochloride (Co-administration may result in hyperpyrexia, particularly during hot weather).
No products indexed under this heading.

Promethazine Hydrochloride (Co-administration with cytochrome P4502D6 inhibitors, such as phenothiazines, may make normal metabolizer resemble poor metabolizer leading to higher than expected plasma concentration of TCA with resultant toxicity; lower than usual doses of either drug may be required; co-administration results in enhanced response to CNS depressants). Products include:
Mepergan Injection 3539
Phenergan Injection 3553
Phenergan 3556
Phenergan Syrup 3554
Phenergan with Codeine Syrup 3557
Phenergan with Dextromethorphan Syrup 3559
Phenergan VC Syrup 3560
Phenergan VC with Codeine Syrup .. 3561

Propafenone Hydrochloride (Co-administration with cytochrome P4502D6 inhibitors, such as propafenone, may make normal metabolizer resemble poor metabolizer leading to higher than expected plasma concentration of TCA with resultant toxicity; lower than usual doses of either drug may be required). Products include:
Rythmol Tablets – 150 mg, 225 mg, 300 mg 502

Propantheline Bromide (Co-administration may result in hyperpyrexia, particularly during hot weather).
No products indexed under this heading.

Propofol (Co-administration results in enhanced response to CNS depressants). Products include:
Diprivan Injectable Emulsion 667

Propoxyphene Hydrochloride (Co-administration results in enhanced response to CNS depressants). Products include:
Darvon Pulvules 1909
Darvon Compound-65 Pulvules 1910

Propoxyphene Napsylate (Co-administration results in enhanced response to CNS depressants). Products include:
Darvon-N/Darvocet-N 1907
Darvon-N Tablets 1912

Pseudoephedrine Hydrochloride (Effects of concurrent use not specified; careful adjustment of dosage and close supervision are required). Products include:
Actifed Cold & Allergy Tablets .... ▣688
Actifed Cold & Sinus Caplets and Tablets .... ▣688
Advil Cold and Sinus Caplets .... ▣771
Advil Cold and Sinus Tablets .... ▣771
Advil Flu & Body Ache Caplets .... ▣772
Aleve Cold & Sinus Caplets .... ▣603
Alka-Seltzer Plus Liqui-Gels .... ▣604
Alka-Seltzer Plus Cold & Flu Medicine Liqui-Gels........ ▣604
Alka-Seltzer Plus Cold & Sinus Medicine Liqui-Gels........ ▣604
Allegra-D Extended-Release Tablets 714
BC Cold Powder .... ▣619
Benadryl Allergy/Cold Tablets .... ▣691
Benadryl Allergy/Congestion Tablets .... ▣692
Benadryl Allergy & Sinus Liquid .... ▣693
Benadryl Allergy & Sinus Fastmelt Tablets .... ▣693
Benadryl Allergy Sinus Headache Caplets & Gelcaps........ ▣693
Benadryl Severe Allergy & Sinus Headache Caplets .... ▣694
Benadryl Children's Allergy/Cold Fastmelt Tablets........ ▣692
Benylin Multi-Symptom Liquid .... ▣697
Bromfed Capsules (Extended-Release)........ 2269
Bromfed-PD Capsules (Extended-Release)........ 2269
Children's Cēpacol Sore Throat .... ▣788
Comtrex Acute Head Cold & Sinus Pressure Relief Tablets........ ▣627
Comtrex Deep Chest Cold & Congestion Relief Softgels........ ▣627
Comtrex Flu Therapy & Fever Relief Daytime Caplets........ ▣628
Comtrex Flu Therapy & Fever Relief Nighttime Tablets .... ▣628
Comtrex Maximum Strength Multi-Symptom Cold & Cough Relief Tablets and Caplets........ ▣626
Contac Non-Drowsy 12 Hour Cold Caplets........ ▣745
Contac Non-Drowsy Timed Release 12 Hour Cold Caplets........ ▣746
Contac Severe Cold and Flu Caplets Maximum Strength........ ▣746
Contac Severe Cold and Flu Caplets Non-Drowsy........ ▣746
Dimetapp Elixir .... ▣777
Dimetapp Cold and Fever Suspension........ ▣775
Dimetapp DM Cold & Cough Elixir . ▣775
Dimetapp Nighttime Flu Liquid .... ▣776
Dimetapp Non-Drowsy Flu Syrup ... ▣777
Dimetapp Infant Drops Decongestant........ ▣775
Dimetapp Infant Drops Decongestant Plus Cough........ ▣776
Guaifed 2272
Kronofed-A 1341
Children's Motrin Cold Oral Suspension 2007
Motrin Sinus Headache Caplets 2005
PediaCare Cough-Cold Liquid .... ▣719
PediaCare Infants' Drops Decongestant........ ▣719
PediaCare Infants' Drops Decongestant Plus Cough........ ▣719
PediaCare NightRest Cough-Cold Liquid .... ▣719
Robitussin Cold Caplets Cold & Congestion........ ▣780
Robitussin Cold Softgels Cold & Congestion........ ▣780
Robitussin Cold Caplets Multi-Symptom Cold & Flu........ ▣781
Robitussin Cold Softgels Multi-Symptom Cold & Flu........ ▣781
Robitussin Cold Softgels Severe Congestion........ ▣782
Robitussin Cough & Cold Infant Drops .... ▣782
Robitussin Maximum Strength Cough & Cold Liquid .... ▣785
Robitussin Pediatric Cough & Cold Formula Liquid........ ▣785
Robitussin Multi Symptom Honey Flu Liquid .... ▣785
Robitussin Nighttime Honey Flu Liquid .... ▣786
Robitussin-CF Liquid .... ▣783
Robitussin-DAC Syrup 2942
Robitussin-PE Liquid .... ▣782
Ryna .... ▣768
Semprex-D Capsules 1172
Singlet Caplets .... ▣761
Sinutab Non-Drying Liquid Caps .... ▣706
Sinutab Sinus Allergy Medication, Maximum Strength Formula, Tablets & Caplets........ ▣707
Sinutab Sinus Medication, Maximum Strength Without Drowsiness Formula, Tablets & Caplets........ ▣707
Sudafed 12 Hour Tablets .... ▣708
Sudafed 24 Hour Tablets .... ▣708
Children's Sudafed Cold & Cough Liquid .... ▣709
Children's Sudafed Nasal Decongestant Chewables........ ▣711
Children's Sudafed Nasal Decongestant Liquid Medication........ ▣711
Sudafed Cold & Allergy Tablets .... ▣708
Sudafed Cold & Cough Liquid Caps .... ▣709
Sudafed Cold & Sinus Liquid Caps .... ▣710
Sudafed Nasal Decongestant Tablets .... ▣710
Sudafed Non-Drying Sinus Liquid Caps .... ▣712
Sudafed Severe Cold .... ▣711
Sudafed Sinus Headache Caplets . ▣712
Sudafed Sinus Headache Tablets .. ▣712
Tavist Sinus Non-Drowsy Coated Caplets........ ▣676
TheraFlu Regular Strength Cold & Cough Night Time Hot Liquid........ ▣676
TheraFlu Regular Strength Cold & Sore Throat Night Time Hot Liquid .... ▣676
TheraFlu Maximum Strength Flu & Congestion Non-Drowsy Hot Liquid .... ▣677
TheraFlu Maximum Strength Flu & Cough Night Time Hot Liquid.. ▣678
TheraFlu Maximum Strength Flu & Sore Throat Night Time Hot Liquid .... ▣677
TheraFlu Maximum Strength Severe Cold & Congestion Night Time Caplets .... ▣678
TheraFlu Maximum Strength Severe Cold & Congestion Night Time Hot Liquid .... ▣678
TheraFlu Maximum Strength Severe Cold & Congestion Non-Drowsy .... ▣679
Triaminic Allergy Congestion Liquid .... ▣680
Triaminic Chest Congestion Liquid .... ▣680
Triaminic Cold & Allergy Liquid .... ▣681
Triaminic Cold & Allergy Softchews .... ▣683
Triaminic Cold & Cough Liquid .... ▣681
Triaminic Cold & Cough Softchews .... ▣683

IMPORTANT NOTE: Always consult each drug listing in the patient's regimen for possible interactions.

Triaminic Cold & Night Time Cough Liquid .... ▣681
Triaminic Cold, Cough & Fever Liquid .... ▣681
Triaminic Cough Liquid .... ▣682
Triaminic Cough & Congestion Liquid .... ▣682
Triaminic Cough & Sore Throat Liquid .... ▣682
Triaminic Cough & Sore Throat Softchews .... ▣684
Children's Tylenol Allergy-D Liquid ... 2014
Children's Tylenol Cold Suspension Liquid and Chewable Tablets 2015
Children's Tylenol Cold Plus Cough Suspension Liquid and Chewable Tablets 2015
Children's Tylenol Flu Suspension Liquid 2015
Children's Tylenol Sinus Suspension Liquid 2017
Infants' Tylenol Cold Decongestant and Fever Reducer Concentrated Drops 2015
Infants' Tylenol Cold Decongestant and Fever Reducer Concentrated Drops Plus Cough.. 2015
Tylenol Allergy Sinus 2010
Multi-Symptom Tylenol Cold Complete Formula Caplets 2010
Multi-Symptom Tylenol Cold Non-Drowsy Caplets and Gelcaps 2010
Multi-Symptom Tylenol Cold Severe Congestion Non-Drowsy Caplets 2011
Maximum Strength Tylenol Flu NightTime Gelcaps 2011
Maximum Strength Tylenol Flu NightTime Liquid 2011
Maximum Strength Tylenol Flu Non-Drowsy Gelcaps 2011
Maximum Strength Tylenol Sinus NightTime Caplets 2012
Maximum Strength Tylenol Sinus Non-Drowsy Geltabs, Gelcaps, Caplets, and Tablets 2012
Vicks 44D Cough & Head Congestion Relief Liquid .... ▣724
Vicks 44M Cough, Cold & Flu Relief Liquid .... ▣725
Pediatric Vicks 44m Cough & Cold Relief .... ▣728
Vicks DayQuil LiquiCaps/Liquid Multi-Symptom Cold/Flu Relief ... ▣727
Children's Vicks NyQuil Cold/Cough Relief .... ▣726
Vicks NyQuil LiquiCaps/Liquid Multi-Symptom Cold/Flu Relief, Original and Cherry Flavors .... ▣727
Zephrex Tablets 3091
Zephrex LA Tablets 3092
Zyrtec-D 12 Hour Extended Relief Tablets 2758

Pseudoephedrine Sulfate (Effects of concurrent use not specified; careful adjustment of dosage and close supervision are required). Products include:
Chlor-Trimeton Allergy/Decongestant Tablets .... ▣736
Claritin-D 12 Hour Extended Release Tablets 3102
Claritin-D 24 Hour Extended Release Tablets 3104
Coricidin 'D' Cold, Flu & Sinus Tablets .... ▣737
Drixoral Allergy/Sinus Extended-Release Tablets .... ▣741
Drixoral Cold & Allergy Sustained-Action Tablets .... ▣740
Drixoral Cold & Flu Extended-Release Tablets .... ▣740
Drixoral Nasal Decongestant Long-Acting Non-Drowsy Tablets .... ▣740
Rynatan Tablets 3351

Quazepam (Co-administration results in enhanced response to CNS depressants).
No products indexed under this heading.

Quetiapine Fumarate (Co-administration results in enhanced response to CNS depressants). Products include:
Seroquel Tablets 684

Quinidine Gluconate (Co-administration with cytochrome P4502D6 inhibitors, such as quinidine, may make normal metabolizer resemble poor metabolizer leading to higher than expected plasma concentration of TCA with resultant toxicity; lower than usual doses of either drug may be required). Products include:
Quinaglute Dura-Tabs Tablets 978

Quinidine Polygalacturonate (Co-administration with cytochrome P4502D6 inhibitors, such as quinidine, may make normal metabolizer resemble poor metabolizer leading to higher than expected plasma concentration of TCA with resultant toxicity; lower than usual doses of either drug may be required).
No products indexed under this heading.

Quinidine Sulfate (Co-administration with cytochrome P4502D6 inhibitors, such as quinidine, may make normal metabolizer resemble poor metabolizer leading to higher than expected plasma concentration of TCA with resultant toxicity; lower than usual doses of either drug may be required). Products include:
Quinidex Extentabs 2933

Remifentanil Hydrochloride (Co-administration results in enhanced response to CNS depressants).
No products indexed under this heading.

Risperidone (Co-administration results in enhanced response to CNS depressants). Products include:
Risperdal 1796

Salmeterol Xinafoate (Effects of concurrent use not specified; careful adjustment of dosage and close supervision are required). Products include:
Advair Diskus 100/50 1448
Advair Diskus 250/50 1448
Advair Diskus 500/50 1448
Serevent Diskus 1637
Serevent Inhalation Aerosol 1633

Scopolamine (Co-administration may result in hyperpyrexia, particularly during hot weather). Products include:
Transderm Scōp Transdermal Therapeutic System 2302

Scopolamine Hydrobromide (Co-administration may result in hyperpyrexia, particularly during hot weather). Products include:
Donnatal 2929
Donnatal Extentabs 2930

Secobarbital Sodium (Co-administration results in enhanced response to CNS depressants).
No products indexed under this heading.

Selegiline Hydrochloride (Co-administration of tricyclic antidepressants and MAO inhibitors has resulted in hyperpyretic crises, severe convulsions, and deaths; concurrent and/or sequential use is contraindicated). Products include:
Eldepryl Capsules 3266

Sertraline Hydrochloride (Co-administration with cytochrome P4502D6 inhibitors, such as antidepressants, may make normal metabolizer resemble poor metabolizer leading to higher than expected plasma concentration of TCA with resultant toxicity; lower than usual doses of either drug may be required). Products include:
Zoloft 2751

Sevoflurane (Co-administration results in enhanced response to CNS depressants).
No products indexed under this heading.

Sufentanil Citrate (Co-administration results in enhanced response to CNS depressants).
No products indexed under this heading.

Temazepam (Co-administration results in enhanced response to CNS depressants).
No products indexed under this heading.

Terbutaline Sulfate (Effects of concurrent use not specified; careful adjustment of dosage and close supervision are required). Products include:
Brethine Ampuls 2314
Brethine Tablets 2313

Thiamylal Sodium (Co-administration results in enhanced response to CNS depressants).
No products indexed under this heading.

Thioridazine Hydrochloride (Co-administration with cytochrome P4502D6 inhibitors, such as phenothiazines, may make normal metabolizer resemble poor metabolizer leading to higher than expected plasma concentration of TCA with resultant toxicity; lower than usual doses of either drug may be required; co-administration results in enhanced response to CNS depressants). Products include:
Thioridazine Hydrochloride Tablets 2289

Thiothixene (Co-administration results in enhanced response to CNS depressants). Products include:
Navane Capsules 2701
Thiothixene Capsules 2290

Thyroglobulin (On rare occasions, concurrent use may result in arrhythmias).
No products indexed under this heading.

Thyroid (On rare occasions, concurrent use may result in arrhythmias).
No products indexed under this heading.

Thyroxine (On rare occasions, concurrent use may result in arrhythmias).
No products indexed under this heading.

Thyroxine Sodium (On rare occasions, concurrent use may result in arrhythmias).
No products indexed under this heading.

Tolterodine Tartrate (Co-administration may result in hyperpyrexia, particularly during hot weather). Products include:
Detrol Tablets 3623
Detrol LA Capsules 2801

Tramadol Hydrochloride (Tricyclic antidepressants may enhance the seizure risk in patients taking tramadol). Products include:
Ultracet Tablets 2597
Ultram Tablets 2600

Tranylcypromine Sulfate (Co-administration of tricyclic antidepressants and MAO inhibitors has resulted in hyperpyretic crises, severe convulsions, and deaths; concurrent and/or sequential use is contraindicated). Products include:
Parnate Tablets 1607

Trazodone Hydrochloride (Co-administration with cytochrome P4502D6 inhibitors, such as antidepressants, may make normal metabolizer resemble poor metabolizer leading to higher than expected plasma concentration of TCA with resultant toxicity; lower than usual doses of either drug may be required).
No products indexed under this heading.

Triazolam (Co-administration results in enhanced response to CNS depressants). Products include:
Halcion Tablets 2823

Tridihexethyl Chloride (Co-administration may result in hyperpyrexia, particularly during hot weather).
No products indexed under this heading.

Trifluoperazine Hydrochloride (Co-administration with cytochrome P4502D6 inhibitors, such as phenothiazines, may make normal metabolizer resemble poor metabolizer leading to higher than expected plasma concentration of TCA with resultant toxicity; lower than usual doses of either drug may be required; co-administration results in enhanced response to CNS depressants). Products include:
Stelazine 1640

Trihexyphenidyl Hydrochloride (Co-administration may result in hyperpyrexia, particularly during hot weather). Products include:
Artane 1855

Trimipramine Maleate (Co-administration with cytochrome P4502D6 inhibitors, such as antidepressants, may make normal metabolizer resemble poor metabolizer leading to higher than expected plasma concentration of TCA with resultant toxicity; lower than usual doses of either drug may be required). Products include:
Surmontil Capsules 3595

Venlafaxine Hydrochloride (Co-administration with cytochrome P4502D6 inhibitors, such as antidepressants, may make normal metabolizer resemble poor metabolizer leading to higher than expected plasma concentration of TCA with resultant toxicity; lower than usual doses of either drug may be required). Products include:
Effexor Tablets 3495
Effexor XR Capsules 3499

Zaleplon (Co-administration results in enhanced response to CNS depressants). Products include:
Sonata Capsules 3591

Ziprasidone Hydrochloride (Co-administration results in enhanced response to CNS depressants). Products include:
Geodon Capsules 2688

Zolpidem Tartrate (Co-administration results in enhanced response to CNS depressants). Products include:
Ambien Tablets 3191

Food Interactions

Alcohol (Co-administration results in enhanced response to alcohol).

VIVACTIL TABLETS

(Protriptyline Hydrochloride) 2217
May interact with anticholinergics, barbiturates, central nervous system depressants, antidepressant drugs, monoamine oxidase inhibitors, phenothiazines, quinidine, selective serotonin reuptake inhibitors, sympathomimetics, thyroid preparations, and certain other agents. Compounds in these categories include:

Albuterol (Effects of concurrent use not specified; careful adjustment of dosage and close supervision are required). Products include:
Proventil Inhalation Aerosol 3142
Ventolin Inhalation Aerosol and Refill 1679

Albuterol Sulfate (Effects of concurrent use not specified; careful adjustment of dosage and close supervision are required). Products include:
AccuNeb Inhalation Solution 1230
Combivent Inhalation Aerosol 1041
DuoNeb Inhalation Solution 1233
Proventil Inhalation Solution 0.083% 3146
Proventil Repetabs Tablets 3148
Proventil Solution for Inhalation 0.5% 3144
Proventil HFA Inhalation Aerosol 3150
Ventolin HFA Inhalation Aerosol 3618

Volmax Extended-Release Tablets .. 2276

Alfentanil Hydrochloride (Co-administration results in enhanced response to CNS depressants).
No products indexed under this heading.

Alprazolam (Co-administration results in enhanced response to CNS depressants). Products include:
Xanax Tablets 2865

Amitriptyline Hydrochloride (Co-administration with cytochrome P4502D6 inhibitors, such as antidepressants, may make normal metabolizer resemble poor metabolizer leading to higher than expected plasma concentration of TCA with resultant toxicity; lower than usual doses of either drug may be required). Products include:
Etrafon 3115
Limbitrol 1738

Amoxapine (Co-administration with cytochrome P4502D6 inhibitors, such as antidepressants, may make normal metabolizer resemble poor metabolizer leading to higher than expected plasma concentration of TCA with resultant toxicity; lower than usual doses of either drug may be required).
No products indexed under this heading.

Aprobarbital (Co-administration results in enhanced response to CNS depressants).
No products indexed under this heading.

Atropine Sulfate (Co-administration may result in hyperpyrexia, particularly during hot weather). Products include:
Donnatal 2929
Donnatal Extentabs 2930
Motofen Tablets 577
Prosed/DS Tablets 3268
Urised Tablets 2876

Belladonna Alkaloids (Co-administration may result in hyperpyrexia, particularly during hot weather). Products include:
Hyland's Teething Tablets 766
Urimax Tablets 1769

Benztropine Mesylate (Co-administration may result in hyperpyrexia, particularly during hot weather). Products include:
Cogentin 2055

Biperiden Hydrochloride (Co-administration may result in hyperpyrexia, particularly during hot weather). Products include:
Akineton 402

Buprenorphine Hydrochloride (Co-administration results in enhanced response to CNS depressants). Products include:
Buprenex Injectable 2918

Bupropion Hydrochloride (Co-administration with cytochrome P4502D6 inhibitors, such as antidepressants, may make normal metabolizer resemble poor metabolizer leading to higher than expected plasma concentration of TCA with resultant toxicity; lower than usual doses of either drug may be required). Products include:
Wellbutrin Tablets 1680
Wellbutrin SR Sustained-Release Tablets 1684
Zyban Sustained-Release Tablets 1710

Buspirone Hydrochloride (Co-administration results in enhanced response to CNS depressants).
No products indexed under this heading.

Butabarbital (Co-administration results in enhanced response to CNS depressants).
No products indexed under this heading.

Butalbital (Co-administration results in enhanced response to CNS depressants). Products include:
Phrenilin 578
Sedapap Tablets 50 mg/650 mg 2225

Chlordiazepoxide (Co-administration results in enhanced response to CNS depressants). Products include:
Limbitrol 1738

Chlordiazepoxide Hydrochloride (Co-administration results in enhanced response to CNS depressants). Products include:
Librium Capsules 1736
Librium for Injection 1737

Chlorpromazine (Co-administration with cytochrome P4502D6 inhibitors, such as phenothiazines, may make normal metabolizer resemble poor metabolizer leading to higher than expected plasma concentration of TCA with resultant toxicity; lower than usual doses of either drug may be required; co-administration results in enhanced response to CNS depressants). Products include:
Thorazine Suppositories 1656

Chlorpromazine Hydrochloride (Co-administration with cytochrome P4502D6 inhibitors, such as phenothiazines, may make normal metabolizer resemble poor metabolizer leading to higher than expected plasma concentration of TCA with resultant toxicity; lower than usual doses of either drug may be required; co-administration results in enhanced response to CNS depressants). Products include:
Thorazine 1656

Chlorprothixene (Co-administration results in enhanced response to CNS depressants).
No products indexed under this heading.

Chlorprothixene Hydrochloride (Co-administration results in enhanced response to CNS depressants).
No products indexed under this heading.

Chlorprothixene Lactate (Co-administration results in enhanced response to CNS depressants).
No products indexed under this heading.

Cimetidine (Co-administration has been reported to reduce hepatic metabolism of certain tricyclic antidepressants, thereby delaying elimination and increasing steady-state concentrations of TCA resulting in the frequency and severity of side effects, particularly anticholinergic). Products include:
Tagamet HB 200 Suspension 762
Tagamet HB 200 Tablets 761
Tagamet Tablets 1644

Cimetidine Hydrochloride (Co-administration has been reported to reduce hepatic metabolism of certain tricyclic antidepressants, thereby delaying elimination and increasing steady-state concentrations of TCA resulting in the frequency and severity of side effects, particularly anticholinergic). Products include:
Tagamet 1644

Cisapride (Co-administration can result in possible adverse cardiac interactions including prolongation of the QT interval, cardiac arrhythmias and conduction system disturbances; concurrent use in contraindicated).
No products indexed under this heading.

Citalopram Hydrobromide (Co-administration with cytochrome P4502D6 inhibitors, such as antidepressants, may make normal metabolizer resemble poor metabolizer leading to higher than expected plasma concentration of TCA with resultant toxicity; lower than usual doses of either drug may be required). Products include:
Celexa 1365

Clidinium Bromide (Co-administration may result in hyperpyrexia, particularly during hot weather).
No products indexed under this heading.

Clorazepate Dipotassium (Co-administration results in enhanced response to CNS depressants). Products include:
Tranxene 511

Clozapine (Co-administration results in enhanced response to CNS depressants). Products include:
Clozaril Tablets 2319

Codeine Phosphate (Co-administration results in enhanced response to CNS depressants). Products include:
Phenergan with Codeine Syrup 3557
Phenergan VC with Codeine Syrup .. 3561
Robitussin A-C Syrup 2942
Robitussin-DAC Syrup 2942
Ryna-C Liquid 768
Soma Compound w/Codeine Tablets 3355
Tussi-Organidin NR Liquid 3350
Tussi-Organidin-S NR Liquid 3350
Tylenol with Codeine 2595

Desflurane (Co-administration results in enhanced response to CNS depressants). Products include:
Suprane Liquid for Inhalation 874

Desipramine Hydrochloride (Co-administration with cytochrome P4502D6 inhibitors, such as antidepressants, may make normal metabolizer resemble poor metabolizer leading to higher than expected plasma concentration of TCA with resultant toxicity; lower than usual doses of either drug may be required). Products include:
Norpramin Tablets 755

Dezocine (Co-administration results in enhanced response to CNS depressants).
No products indexed under this heading.

Diazepam (Co-administration results in enhanced response to CNS depressants). Products include:
Valium Injectable 3026
Valium Tablets 3047

Dicyclomine Hydrochloride (Co-administration may result in hyperpyrexia, particularly during hot weather).
No products indexed under this heading.

Dobutamine Hydrochloride (Effects of concurrent use not specified; careful adjustment of dosage and close supervision are required). Products include:
Dobutrex Solution Vials 1914

Dopamine Hydrochloride (Effects of concurrent use not specified; careful adjustment of dosage and close supervision are required).
No products indexed under this heading.

Doxepin Hydrochloride (Co-administration with cytochrome P4502D6 inhibitors, such as antidepressants, may make normal metabolizer resemble poor metabolizer leading to higher than expected plasma concentration of TCA with resultant toxicity; lower than usual doses of either drug may be required). Products include:
Sinequan 2713

Droperidol (Co-administration results in enhanced response to CNS depressants).
No products indexed under this heading.

Enflurane (Co-administration results in enhanced response to CNS depressants).
No products indexed under this heading.

Ephedrine Hydrochloride (Effects of concurrent use not specified; careful adjustment of dosage and close supervision are required). Products include:
Primatene Tablets 780

Ephedrine Sulfate (Effects of concurrent use not specified; careful adjustment of dosage and close supervision are required).
No products indexed under this heading.

Ephedrine Tannate (Effects of concurrent use not specified; careful adjustment of dosage and close supervision are required). Products include:
Rynatuss Pediatric Suspension 3353
Rynatuss Tablets 3353

Epinephrine (Effects of concurrent use not specified; careful adjustment of dosage and close supervision are required). Products include:
Epifrin Sterile Ophthalmic Solution .... ⊙235
EpiPen 1236
Primatene Mist 779
Xylocaine with Epinephrine Injection 653

Epinephrine Bitartrate (Effects of concurrent use not specified; careful adjustment of dosage and close supervision are required). Products include:
Sensorcaine 643

Epinephrine Hydrochloride (Effects of concurrent use not specified; careful adjustment of dosage and close supervision are required).
No products indexed under this heading.

Estazolam (Co-administration results in enhanced response to CNS depressants). Products include:
ProSom Tablets 500

Ethchlorvynol (Co-administration results in enhanced response to CNS depressants).
No products indexed under this heading.

Ethinamate (Co-administration results in enhanced response to CNS depressants).
No products indexed under this heading.

Fentanyl (Co-administration results in enhanced response to CNS depressants). Products include:
Duragesic Transdermal System 1786

Fentanyl Citrate (Co-administration results in enhanced response to CNS depressants). Products include:
Actiq 1184

Flecainide Acetate (Co-administration with cytochrome P4502D6 inhibitors, such as flecainide, may make normal metabolizer resemble poor metabolizer leading to higher than expected plasma concentration of TCA with resultant toxicity; lower than usual doses of either drug may be required). Products include:
Tambocor Tablets 1990

Fluoxetine Hydrochloride (Co-administration with cytochrome P4502D6 inhibitors, such as antidepressants, may make normal metabolizer resemble poor metabolizer leading to higher than expected plasma concentration of TCA with resultant toxicity; due to variation in the extent of inhibition of P4502D6 and long half-life of fluoxetine, sufficient time, at least 5 weeks, should elapse in switching to TCA). Products include:
Prozac Pulvules, Liquid, and Weekly Capsules 1238
Sarafem Pulvules 1962

Fluphenazine Decanoate (Co-administration with cytochrome P4502D6 inhibitors, such as phenothiazines, may make normal metabolizer resemble poor metabolizer

leading to higher than expected plasma concentration of TCA with resultant toxicity; lower than usual doses of either drug may be required; co-administration results in enhanced response to CNS depressants).
No products indexed under this heading.

Fluphenazine Enanthate (Co-administration with cytochrome P4502D6 inhibitors, such as phenothiazines, may make normal metabolizer resemble poor metabolizer leading to higher than expected plasma concentration of TCA with resultant toxicity; lower than usual doses of either drug may be required; co-administration results in enhanced response to CNS depressants).
No products indexed under this heading.

Fluphenazine Hydrochloride (Co-administration with cytochrome P4502D6 inhibitors, such as phenothiazines, may make normal metabolizer resemble poor metabolizer leading to higher than expected plasma concentration of TCA with resultant toxicity; lower than usual doses of either drug may be required; co-administration results in enhanced response to CNS depressants).
No products indexed under this heading.

Flurazepam Hydrochloride (Co-administration results in enhanced response to CNS depressants).
No products indexed under this heading.

Fluvoxamine Maleate (Co-administration with cytochrome P4502D6 inhibitors, such as antidepressants, may make normal metabolizer resemble poor metabolizer leading to higher than expected plasma concentration of TCA with resultant toxicity; due to variation in the extent of inhibition of P4502D6, sufficient time should elapse in switching from one class to the other). Products include:
Luvox Tablets (25, 50, 100 mg) 3256

Glutethimide (Co-administration results in enhanced response to CNS depressants).
No products indexed under this heading.

Glycopyrrolate (Co-administration may result in hyperpyrexia, particularly during hot weather). Products include:
Robinul Forte Tablets 1358
Robinul Injectable 2940
Robinul Tablets 1358

Guanadrel Sulfate (Protriptyline may block the antihypertensive action).
No products indexed under this heading.

Guanethidine Monosulfate (Protriptyline may block the antihypertensive action of guanethidine).
No products indexed under this heading.

Haloperidol (Co-administration results in enhanced response to CNS depressants). Products include:
Haldol Injection, Tablets and Concentrate 2533

Haloperidol Decanoate (Co-administration results in enhanced response to CNS depressants). Products include:
Haldol Decanoate 2535

Hydrocodone Bitartrate (Co-administration results in enhanced response to CNS depressants). Products include:
Hycodan 1316
Hycomine Compound Tablets 1317
Hycotuss Expectorant Syrup 1318
Lortab 3319
Lortab Elixir 3317
Maxidone Tablets CIII 3399
Norco 5/325 Tablets CIII 3424
Norco 7.5/325 Tablets CIII 3425
Norco 10/325 Tablets CIII 3427
Norco 10/325 Tablets CIII 3425
Vicodin Tablets 516
Vicodin ES Tablets 517
Vicodin HP Tablets 518
Vicodin Tuss Expectorant 519
Vicoprofen Tablets 520
Zydone Tablets 1330

Hydrocodone Polistirex (Co-administration results in enhanced response to CNS depressants). Products include:
Tussionex Pennkinetic Extended-Release Suspension 1174

Hydromorphone Hydrochloride (Co-administration results in enhanced response to CNS depressants). Products include:
Dilaudid 441
Dilaudid Oral Liquid 445
Dilaudid Powder 441
Dilaudid Rectal Suppositories 441
Dilaudid Tablets 441
Dilaudid Tablets - 8 mg 445
Dilaudid-HP 443

Hydroxyzine Hydrochloride (Co-administration results in enhanced response to CNS depressants). Products include:
Atarax Tablets & Syrup 2667
Vistaril Intramuscular Solution 2738

Hyoscyamine (Co-administration may result in hyperpyrexia, particularly during hot weather). Products include:
Urised Tablets 2876

Hyoscyamine Sulfate (Co-administration may result in hyperpyrexia, particularly during hot weather). Products include:
Arco-Lase Plus Tablets 592
Donnatal 2929
Donnatal Extentabs 2930
Levsin/Levsinex/Levbid 3172
NuLev Orally Disintegrating Tablets 3176
Prosed/DS Tablets 3268
Urimax Tablets 1769

Imipramine Hydrochloride (Co-administration with cytochrome P4502D6 inhibitors, such as antidepressants, may make normal metabolizer resemble poor metabolizer leading to higher than expected plasma concentration of TCA with resultant toxicity; lower than usual doses of either drug may be required).
No products indexed under this heading.

Imipramine Pamoate (Co-administration with cytochrome P4502D6 inhibitors, such as antidepressants, may make normal metabolizer resemble poor metabolizer leading to higher than expected plasma concentration of TCA with resultant toxicity; lower than usual doses of either drug may be required).
No products indexed under this heading.

Ipratropium Bromide (Co-administration may result in hyperpyrexia, particularly during hot weather). Products include:
Atrovent Inhalation Aerosol 1030
Atrovent Inhalation Solution 1031
Atrovent Nasal Spray 0.03% 1032
Atrovent Nasal Spray 0.06% 1033
Combivent Inhalation Aerosol 1041
DuoNeb Inhalation Solution 1233

Isocarboxazid (Co-administration of tricyclic antidepressants and MAO inhibitors has resulted in hyperpyretic crises, severe convulsions, and deaths; concurrent and/or sequential use is contraindicated).
No products indexed under this heading.

Isoflurane (Co-administration results in enhanced response to CNS depressants).
No products indexed under this heading.

Isoproterenol Hydrochloride (Effects of concurrent use not specified; careful adjustment of dosage and close supervision are required).
No products indexed under this heading.

Isoproterenol Sulfate (Effects of concurrent use not specified; careful adjustment of dosage and close supervision are required).
No products indexed under this heading.

Ketamine Hydrochloride (Co-administration results in enhanced response to CNS depressants).
No products indexed under this heading.

Levalbuterol Hydrochloride (Effects of concurrent use not specified; careful adjustment of dosage and close supervision are required). Products include:
Xopenex Inhalation Solution 3207

Levomethadyl Acetate Hydrochloride (Co-administration results in enhanced response to CNS depressants).
No products indexed under this heading.

Levorphanol Tartrate (Co-administration results in enhanced response to CNS depressants). Products include:
Levo-Dromoran 1734
Levorphanol Tartrate Tablets 3059

Levothyroxine Sodium (On rare occasions, concurrent use may result in arrhythmias). Products include:
Levothroid Tablets 1373
Levoxyl Tablets 1819
Synthroid 505
Unithroid Tablets 3445

Liothyronine Sodium (On rare occasions, concurrent use may result in arrhythmias). Products include:
Cytomel Tablets 1817
Triostat Injection 1825

Liotrix (On rare occasions, concurrent use may result in arrhythmias).
No products indexed under this heading.

Lorazepam (Co-administration results in enhanced response to CNS depressants). Products include:
Ativan Injection 3478
Ativan Tablets 3482

Loxapine Hydrochloride (Co-administration results in enhanced response to CNS depressants).
No products indexed under this heading.

Loxapine Succinate (Co-administration results in enhanced response to CNS depressants). Products include:
Loxitane Capsules 3398

Maprotiline Hydrochloride (Co-administration with cytochrome P4502D6 inhibitors, such as antidepressants, may make normal metabolizer resemble poor metabolizer leading to higher than expected plasma concentration of TCA with resultant toxicity; lower than usual doses of either drug may be required).
No products indexed under this heading.

Mepenzolate Bromide (Co-administration may result in hyperpyrexia, particularly during hot weather).
No products indexed under this heading.

Meperidine Hydrochloride (Co-administration results in enhanced response to CNS depressants). Products include:
Demerol 3079
Mepergan Injection 3539

Mephobarbital (Co-administration results in enhanced response to CNS depressants).
No products indexed under this heading.

Meprobamate (Co-administration results in enhanced response to CNS depressants). Products include:
Miltown Tablets 3349

Mesoridazine Besylate (Co-administration with cytochrome P4502D6 inhibitors, such as phenothiazines, may make normal metabolizer resemble poor metabolizer leading to higher than expected plasma concentration of TCA with resultant toxicity; lower than usual doses of either drug may be required; co-administration results in enhanced response to CNS depressants). Products include:
Serentil 1057

Metaproterenol Sulfate (Effects of concurrent use not specified; careful adjustment of dosage and close supervision are required). Products include:
Alupent 1029

Metaraminol Bitartrate (Effects of concurrent use not specified; careful adjustment of dosage and close supervision are required). Products include:
Aramine Injection 2043

Methadone Hydrochloride (Co-administration results in enhanced response to CNS depressants). Products include:
Dolophine Hydrochloride Tablets 3056

Methohexital Sodium (Co-administration results in enhanced response to CNS depressants). Products include:
Brevital Sodium for Injection, USP 1815

Methotrimeprazine (Co-administration with cytochrome P4502D6 inhibitors, such as phenothiazines, may make normal metabolizer resemble poor metabolizer leading to higher than expected plasma concentration of TCA with resultant toxicity; lower than usual doses of either drug may be required; co-administration results in enhanced response to CNS depressants).
No products indexed under this heading.

Methoxamine Hydrochloride (Effects of concurrent use not specified; careful adjustment of dosage and close supervision are required).
No products indexed under this heading.

Methoxyflurane (Co-administration results in enhanced response to CNS depressants).
No products indexed under this heading.

Midazolam Hydrochloride (Co-administration results in enhanced response to CNS depressants). Products include:
Versed Injection 3027
Versed Syrup 3033

Mirtazapine (Co-administration with cytochrome P4502D6 inhibitors, such as antidepressants, may make normal metabolizer resemble poor metabolizer leading to higher than expected plasma concentration of TCA with resultant toxicity; lower than usual doses of either drug may be required). Products include:
Remeron Tablets 2483
Remeron SolTab Tablets 2486

Moclobemide (Co-administration of tricyclic antidepressants and MAO inhibitors has resulted in hyperpyretic crises, severe convulsions, and deaths; concurrent and/or sequential use is contraindicated).
No products indexed under this heading.

Molindone Hydrochloride (Co-administration results in enhanced response to CNS depressants). Products include:

Moban 1320

Morphine Sulfate (Co-administration results in enhanced response to CNS depressants). Products include:
Astramorph/PF Injection, USP (Preservative-Free) 594
Duramorph Injection 1312
Infumorph 200 and Infumorph 500 Sterile Solutions 1314
Kadian Capsules 1335
MS Contin Tablets 2896
MSIR 2898
Oramorph SR Tablets 3062
Roxanol 3066

Nefazodone Hydrochloride (Co-administration with cytochrome P4502D6 inhibitors, such as antidepressants, may make normal metabolizer resemble poor metabolizer leading to higher than expected plasma concentration of TCA with resultant toxicity; lower than usual doses of either drug may be required). Products include:
Serzone Tablets 1104

Norepinephrine Bitartrate (Effects of concurrent use not specified; careful adjustment of dosage and close supervision are required).
No products indexed under this heading.

Nortriptyline Hydrochloride (Co-administration with cytochrome P4502D6 inhibitors, such as antidepressants, may make normal metabolizer resemble poor metabolizer leading to higher than expected plasma concentration of TCA with resultant toxicity; lower than usual doses of either drug may be required).
No products indexed under this heading.

Olanzapine (Co-administration results in enhanced response to CNS depressants). Products include:
Zyprexa Tablets 1973
Zyprexa ZYDIS Orally Disintegrating Tablets 1973

Oxazepam (Co-administration results in enhanced response to CNS depressants).
No products indexed under this heading.

Oxybutynin Chloride (Co-administration may result in hyperpyrexia, particularly during hot weather). Products include:
Ditropan XL Extended Release Tablets 564

Oxycodone Hydrochloride (Co-administration results in enhanced response to CNS depressants). Products include:
OxyContin Tablets 2912
OxyFast Oral Concentrate Solution 2916
OxyIR Capsules 2916
Percocet Tablets 1326
Percodan Tablets 1327
Percolone Tablets 1327
Roxicodone 3067
Tylox Capsules 2597

Pargyline Hydrochloride (Co-administration of tricyclic antidepressants and MAO inhibitors has resulted in hyperpyretic crises, severe convulsions, and deaths; concurrent and/or sequential use is contraindicated).
No products indexed under this heading.

Paroxetine Hydrochloride (Co-administration with cytochrome P4502D6 inhibitors, such as antidepressants, may make normal metabolizer resemble poor metabolizer leading to higher than expected plasma concentration of TCA with resultant toxicity; lower than usual doses of either drug may be required). Products include:
Paxil 1609

Pentobarbital Sodium (Co-administration results in enhanced response to CNS depressants). Products include:
Nembutal Sodium Solution 485

Perphenazine (Co-administration with cytochrome P4502D6 inhibitors, such as phenothiazines, may make normal metabolizer resemble poor metabolizer leading to higher than expected plasma concentration of TCA with resultant toxicity; lower than usual doses of either drug may be required; co-administration results in enhanced response to CNS depressants). Products include:
Etrafon 3115
Trilafon 3160

Phenelzine Sulfate (Co-administration of tricyclic antidepressants and MAO inhibitors has resulted in hyperpyretic crises, severe convulsions, and deaths; concurrent and/or sequential use is contraindicated). Products include:
Nardil Tablets 2653

Phenobarbital (Co-administration results in enhanced response to CNS depressants). Products include:
Arco-Lase Plus Tablets 592
Donnatal 2929
Donnatal Extentabs 2930

Phenylephrine Bitartrate (Effects of concurrent use not specified; careful adjustment of dosage and close supervision are required).
No products indexed under this heading.

Phenylephrine Hydrochloride (Effects of concurrent use not specified; careful adjustment of dosage and close supervision are required). Products include:
Afrin Nasal Decongestant Children's Pump Mist 734
Extendryl 1361
Hycomine Compound Tablets 1317
Neo-Synephrine 614
Phenergan VC Syrup 3560
Phenergan VC with Codeine Syrup 3561
Preparation H Cream 778
Preparation H Cooling Gel 778
Preparation H 778
Vicks Sinex Nasal Spray and Ultra Fine Mist 729

Phenylephrine Tannate (Effects of concurrent use not specified; careful adjustment of dosage and close supervision are required). Products include:
Ryna-12 S Suspension 3351
Reformulated Rynatan Pediatric Suspension 3352
Rynatuss Pediatric Suspension 3353
Rynatuss Tablets 3353

Phenylpropanolamine Hydrochloride (Effects of concurrent use not specified; careful adjustment of dosage and close supervision are required).
No products indexed under this heading.

Pirbuterol Acetate (Effects of concurrent use not specified; careful adjustment of dosage and close supervision are required). Products include:
Maxair Autohaler 1981
Maxair Inhaler 1984

Prazepam (Co-administration results in enhanced response to CNS depressants).
No products indexed under this heading.

Procarbazine Hydrochloride (Co-administration of tricyclic antidepressants and MAO inhibitors has resulted in hyperpyretic crises, severe convulsions, and deaths; concurrent and/or sequential use is contraindicated). Products include:
Matulane Capsules 3246

Prochlorperazine (Co-administration with cytochrome P4502D6 inhibitors, such as phenothiazines, may make normal metabolizer resemble poor metabolizer leading to higher than expected plasma concentration of TCA with resultant toxicity; lower than usual doses of either drug may be required; co-administration results in enhanced response to CNS depressants). Products include:
Compazine 1505

Procyclidine Hydrochloride (Co-administration may result in hyperpyrexia, particularly during hot weather).
No products indexed under this heading.

Promethazine Hydrochloride (Co-administration with cytochrome P4502D6 inhibitors, such as phenothiazines, may make normal metabolizer resemble poor metabolizer leading to higher than expected plasma concentration of TCA with resultant toxicity; lower than usual doses of either drug may be required; co-administration results in enhanced response to CNS depressants). Products include:
Mepergan Injection 3539
Phenergan Injection 3553
Phenergan 3556
Phenergan Syrup 3554
Phenergan with Codeine Syrup 3557
Phenergan with Dextromethorphan Syrup 3559
Phenergan VC Syrup 3560
Phenergan VC with Codeine Syrup 3561

Propafenone Hydrochloride (Co-administration with cytochrome P4502D6 inhibitors, such as propafenone, may make normal metabolizer resemble poor metabolizer leading to higher than expected plasma concentration of TCA with resultant toxicity; lower than usual doses of either drug may be required). Products include:
Rythmol Tablets – 150 mg, 225 mg, 300 mg 502

Propantheline Bromide (Co-administration may result in hyperpyrexia, particularly during hot weather).
No products indexed under this heading.

Propofol (Co-administration results in enhanced response to CNS depressants). Products include:
Diprivan Injectable Emulsion 667

Propoxyphene Hydrochloride (Co-administration results in enhanced response to CNS depressants). Products include:
Darvon Pulvules 1909
Darvon Compound-65 Pulvules 1910

Propoxyphene Napsylate (Co-administration results in enhanced response to CNS depressants). Products include:
Darvon-N/Darvocet-N 1907
Darvon-N Tablets 1912

Pseudoephedrine Hydrochloride (Effects of concurrent use not specified; careful adjustment of dosage and close supervision are required). Products include:
Actifed Cold & Allergy Tablets 688
Actifed Cold & Sinus Caplets and Tablets 688
Advil Cold and Sinus Caplets 771
Advil Cold and Sinus Tablets 771
Advil Flu & Body Ache Caplets 772
Aleve Cold & Sinus Caplets 603
Alka-Seltzer Plus Liqui-Gels 604
Alka-Seltzer Plus Cold & Flu Medicine Liqui-Gels 604
Alka-Seltzer Plus Cold & Sinus Medicine Liqui-Gels 604
Allegra-D Extended-Release Tablets 714
BC Cold Powder 619
Benadryl Allergy/Cold Tablets 691
Benadryl Allergy/Congestion Tablets 692
Benadryl Allergy & Sinus Liquid 693
Benadryl Allergy & Sinus Fastmelt Tablets 693
Benadryl Allergy Sinus Headache Caplets & Gelcaps 693
Benadryl Severe Allergy & Sinus Headache Caplets 694
Benadryl Children's Allergy/Cold Fastmelt Tablets 692
Benylin Multi-Symptom Liquid 697
Bromfed Capsules (Extended-Release) 2269
Bromfed-PD Capsules (Extended-Release) 2269
Children's Cēpacol Sore Throat 788
Comtrex Acute Head Cold & Sinus Pressure Relief Tablets 627
Comtrex Deep Chest Cold & Congestion Relief Softgels 627
Comtrex Flu Therapy & Fever Relief Daytime Caplets 628
Comtrex Flu Therapy & Fever Relief Nighttime Tablets 628
Comtrex Maximum Strength Multi-Symptom Cold & Cough Relief Tablets and Caplets 626
Contac Non-Drowsy 12 Hour Cold Caplets 745
Contac Non-Drowsy Timed Release 12 Hour Cold Caplets 746
Contac Severe Cold and Flu Caplets Maximum Strength 746
Contac Severe Cold and Flu Caplets Non-Drowsy 746
Dimetapp Elixir 777
Dimetapp Cold and Fever Suspension 775
Dimetapp DM Cold & Cough Elixir 775
Dimetapp Nighttime Flu Liquid 776
Dimetapp Non-Drowsy Flu Syrup 777
Dimetapp Infant Drops Decongestant 775
Dimetapp Infant Drops Decongestant Plus Cough 776
Guaifed 2272
Kronofed-A 1341
Children's Motrin Cold Oral Suspension 2007
Motrin Sinus Headache Caplets 2005
PediaCare Cough-Cold Liquid 719
PediaCare Infants' Drops Decongestant 719
PediaCare Infants' Drops Decongestant Plus Cough 719
PediaCare NightRest Cough-Cold Liquid 719
Robitussin Cold Caplets Cold & Congestion 780
Robitussin Cold Softgels Cold & Congestion 780
Robitussin Cold Caplets Multi-Symptom Cold & Flu 781
Robitussin Cold Softgels Multi-Symptom Cold & Flu 781
Robitussin Cold Softgels Severe Congestion 782
Robitussin Cough & Cold Infant Drops 782
Robitussin Maximum Strength Cough & Cold Liquid 785
Robitussin Pediatric Cough & Cold Formula Liquid 785
Robitussin Multi Symptom Honey Flu Liquid 785
Robitussin Nighttime Honey Flu Liquid 786
Robitussin-CF Liquid 783
Robitussin-DAC Syrup 2942
Robitussin-PE Liquid 782
Ryna 768
Semprex-D Capsules 1172
Singlet Caplets 761
Sinutab Non-Drying Liquid Caps 706
Sinutab Sinus Allergy Medication, Maximum Strength Formula, Tablets & Caplets 707
Sinutab Sinus Medication, Maximum Strength Without Drowsiness Formula, Tablets & Caplets 707
Sudafed 12 Hour Tablets 708
Sudafed 24 Hour Tablets 708
Children's Sudafed Cold & Cough Liquid 709
Children's Sudafed Nasal Decongestant Chewables 711
Children's Sudafed Nasal Decongestant Liquid Medication 711
Sudafed Cold & Allergy Tablets 708
Sudafed Cold & Cough Liquid Caps 709
Sudafed Cold & Sinus Liquid Caps 710
Sudafed Nasal Decongestant Tablets 710
Sudafed Non-Drying Sinus Liquid Caps 712
Sudafed Severe Cold 711
Sudafed Sinus Headache Caplets 712
Sudafed Sinus Headache Tablets 712

IMPORTANT NOTE: Always consult each drug listing in the patient's regimen for possible interactions.

Tavist Sinus Non-Drowsy Coated Caplets ▣676
TheraFlu Regular Strength Cold & Cough Night Time Hot Liquid ▣676
TheraFlu Regular Strength Cold & Sore Throat Night Time Hot Liquid ▣676
TheraFlu Maximum Strength Flu & Congestion Non-Drowsy Hot Liquid ▣677
TheraFlu Maximum Strength Flu & Cough Night Time Hot Liquid ▣678
TheraFlu Maximum Strength Flu & Sore Throat Night Time Hot Liquid ▣677
TheraFlu Maximum Strength Severe Cold & Congestion Night Time Caplets ▣678
TheraFlu Maximum Strength Severe Cold & Congestion Night Time Hot Liquid ▣678
TheraFlu Maximum Strength Severe Cold & Congestion Non-Drowsy ▣679
Triaminic Allergy Congestion Liquid ▣680
Triaminic Chest Congestion Liquid ▣680
Triaminic Cold & Allergy Liquid ▣681
Triaminic Cold & Allergy Softchews ▣683
Triaminic Cold & Cough Liquid ▣681
Triaminic Cold & Cough Softchews ▣683
Triaminic Cold & Night Time Cough Liquid ▣681
Triaminic Cold, Cough & Fever Liquid ▣681
Triaminic Cough Liquid ▣682
Triaminic Cough & Congestion Liquid ▣682
Triaminic Cough & Sore Throat Liquid ▣682
Triaminic Cough & Sore Throat Softchews ▣684
Children's Tylenol Allergy-D Liquid ... 2014
Children's Tylenol Cold Suspension Liquid and Chewable Tablets ... 2015
Children's Tylenol Cold Plus Cough Suspension Liquid and Chewable Tablets ... 2015
Children's Tylenol Flu Suspension Liquid ... 2015
Children's Tylenol Sinus Suspension Liquid ... 2017
Infants' Tylenol Cold Decongestant and Fever Reducer Concentrated Drops ... 2015
Infants' Tylenol Cold Decongestant and Fever Reducer Concentrated Drops Plus Cough .. 2015
Tylenol Allergy Sinus ... 2010
Multi-Symptom Tylenol Cold Complete Formula Caplets ... 2010
Multi-Symptom Tylenol Cold Non-Drowsy Caplets and Gelcaps ... 2010
Multi-Symptom Tylenol Cold Severe Congestion Non-Drowsy Caplets ... 2011
Maximum Strength Tylenol Flu NightTime Gelcaps ... 2011
Maximum Strength Tylenol Flu NightTime Liquid ... 2011
Maximum Strength Tylenol Flu Non-Drowsy Gelcaps ... 2011
Maximum Strength Tylenol Sinus NightTime Caplets ... 2012
Maximum Strength Tylenol Sinus Non-Drowsy Geltabs, Gelcaps, Caplets, and Tablets ... 2012
Vicks 44D Cough & Head Congestion Relief Liquid ▣724
Vicks 44M Cough, Cold & Flu Relief Liquid ▣725
Pediatric Vicks 44m Cough & Cold Relief ▣728
Vicks DayQuil LiquiCaps/Liquid Multi-Symptom Cold/Flu Relief ▣727
Children's Vicks NyQuil Cold/Cough Relief ▣726
Vicks NyQuil LiquiCaps/Liquid Multi-Symptom Cold/Flu Relief, Original and Cherry Flavors ▣727
Zephrex Tablets ... 3091
Zephrex LA Tablets ... 3092
Zyrtec-D 12 Hour Extended Relief Tablets ... 2758

Pseudoephedrine Sulfate (Effects of concurrent use not specified; careful adjustment of dosage and close supervision are required). Products include:
Chlor-Trimeton Allergy/Decongestant Tablets ▣736
Claritin-D 12 Hour Extended Release Tablets ... 3102
Claritin-D 24 Hour Extended Release Tablets ... 3104
Coricidin 'D' Cold, Flu & Sinus Tablets ▣737
Drixoral Allergy/Sinus Extended-Release Tablets ▣741
Drixoral Cold & Allergy Sustained-Action Tablets ▣740
Drixoral Cold & Flu Extended-Release Tablets ▣740
Drixoral Nasal Decongestant Long-Acting Non-Drowsy Tablets ▣740
Rynatan Tablets ... 3351

Quazepam (Co-administration results in enhanced response to CNS depressants).
No products indexed under this heading.

Quetiapine Fumarate (Co-administration results in enhanced response to CNS depressants). Products include:
Seroquel Tablets ... 684

Quinidine Gluconate (Co-administration with cytochrome P4502D6 inhibitors, such as quinidine, may make normal metabolizer resemble poor metabolizer leading to higher than expected plasma concentration of TCA with resultant toxicity; lower than usual doses of either drug may be required). Products include:
Quinaglute Dura-Tabs Tablets ... 978

Quinidine Polygalacturonate (Co-administration with cytochrome P4502D6 inhibitors, such as quinidine, may make normal metabolizer resemble poor metabolizer leading to higher than expected plasma concentration of TCA with resultant toxicity; lower than usual doses of either drug may be required).
No products indexed under this heading.

Quinidine Sulfate (Co-administration with cytochrome P4502D6 inhibitors, such as quinidine, may make normal metabolizer resemble poor metabolizer leading to higher than expected plasma concentration of TCA with resultant toxicity; lower than usual doses of either drug may be required). Products include:
Quinidex Extentabs ... 2933

Remifentanil Hydrochloride (Co-administration results in enhanced response to CNS depressants).
No products indexed under this heading.

Risperidone (Co-administration results in enhanced response to CNS depressants). Products include:
Risperdal ... 1796

Salmeterol Xinafoate (Effects of concurrent use not specified; careful adjustment of dosage and close supervision are required). Products include:
Advair Diskus 100/50 ... 1448
Advair Diskus 250/50 ... 1448
Advair Diskus 500/50 ... 1448
Serevent Diskus ... 1637
Serevent Inhalation Aerosol ... 1633

Scopolamine (Co-administration may result in hyperpyrexia, particularly during hot weather). Products include:
Transderm Scōp Transdermal Therapeutic System ... 2302

Scopolamine Hydrobromide (Co-administration may result in hyperpyrexia, particularly during hot weather). Products include:
Donnatal ... 2929
Donnatal Extentabs ... 2930

Secobarbital Sodium (Co-administration results in enhanced response to CNS depressants).
No products indexed under this heading.

Selegiline Hydrochloride (Co-administration of tricyclic antidepressants and MAO inhibitors has resulted in hyperpyretic crises, severe convulsions, and deaths; concurrent and/or sequential use is contraindicated). Products include:
Eldepryl Capsules ... 3266

Sertraline Hydrochloride (Co-administration with cytochrome P4502D6 inhibitors, such as antidepressants, may make normal metabolizer resemble poor metabolizer leading to higher than expected plasma concentration of TCA with resultant toxicity; lower than usual doses of either drug may be required). Products include:
Zoloft ... 2751

Sevoflurane (Co-administration results in enhanced response to CNS depressants).
No products indexed under this heading.

Sufentanil Citrate (Co-administration results in enhanced response to CNS depressants).
No products indexed under this heading.

Temazepam (Co-administration results in enhanced response to CNS depressants).
No products indexed under this heading.

Terbutaline Sulfate (Effects of concurrent use not specified; careful adjustment of dosage and close supervision are required). Products include:
Brethine Ampuls ... 2314
Brethine Tablets ... 2313

Thiamylal Sodium (Co-administration results in enhanced response to CNS depressants).
No products indexed under this heading.

Thioridazine Hydrochloride (Co-administration with cytochrome P4502D6 inhibitors, such as phenothiazines, may make normal metabolizer resemble poor metabolizer leading to higher than expected plasma concentration of TCA with resultant toxicity; lower than usual doses of either drug may be required; co-administration results in enhanced response to CNS depressants). Products include:
Thioridazine Hydrochloride Tablets ... 2289

Thiothixene (Co-administration results in enhanced response to CNS depressants). Products include:
Navane Capsules ... 2701
Thiothixene Capsules ... 2290

Thyroglobulin (On rare occasions, concurrent use may result in arrhythmias).
No products indexed under this heading.

Thyroid (On rare occasions, concurrent use may result in arrhythmias).
No products indexed under this heading.

Thyroxine (On rare occasions, concurrent use may result in arrhythmias).
No products indexed under this heading.

Thyroxine Sodium (On rare occasions, concurrent use may result in arrhythmias).
No products indexed under this heading.

Tolterodine Tartrate (Co-administration may result in hyperpyrexia, particularly during hot weather). Products include:
Detrol Tablets ... 3623
Detrol LA Capsules ... 2801

Tramadol Hydrochloride (Tricyclic antidepressants may enhance the seizure risk in patients taking tramadol). Products include:
Ultracet Tablets ... 2597
Ultram Tablets ... 2600

Tranylcypromine Sulfate (Co-administration of tricyclic antidepressants and MAO inhibitors has resulted in hyperpyretic crises, severe convulsions, and deaths; concurrent and/or sequential use is contraindicated). Products include:
Parnate Tablets ... 1607

Trazodone Hydrochloride (Co-administration with cytochrome P4502D6 inhibitors, such as antidepressants, may make normal metabolizer resemble poor metabolizer leading to higher than expected plasma concentration of TCA with resultant toxicity; lower than usual doses of either drug may be required).
No products indexed under this heading.

Triazolam (Co-administration results in enhanced response to CNS depressants). Products include:
Halcion Tablets ... 2823

Tridihexethyl Chloride (Co-administration may result in hyperpyrexia, particularly during hot weather).
No products indexed under this heading.

Trifluoperazine Hydrochloride (Co-administration with cytochrome P4502D6 inhibitors, such as phenothiazines, may make normal metabolizer resemble poor metabolizer leading to higher than expected plasma concentration of TCA with resultant toxicity; lower than usual doses of either drug may be required; co-administration results in enhanced response to CNS depressants). Products include:
Stelazine ... 1640

Trihexyphenidyl Hydrochloride (Co-administration may result in hyperpyrexia, particularly during hot weather). Products include:
Artane ... 1855

Trimipramine Maleate (Co-administration with cytochrome P4502D6 inhibitors, such as antidepressants, may make normal metabolizer resemble poor metabolizer leading to higher than expected plasma concentration of TCA with resultant toxicity; lower than usual doses of either drug may be required). Products include:
Surmontil Capsules ... 3595

Venlafaxine Hydrochloride (Co-administration with cytochrome P4502D6 inhibitors, such as antidepressants, may make normal metabolizer resemble poor metabolizer leading to higher than expected plasma concentration of TCA with resultant toxicity; lower than usual doses of either drug may be required). Products include:
Effexor Tablets ... 3495
Effexor XR Capsules ... 3499

Zaleplon (Co-administration results in enhanced response to CNS depressants). Products include:
Sonata Capsules ... 3591

Ziprasidone Hydrochloride (Co-administration results in enhanced response to CNS depressants). Products include:
Geodon Capsules ... 2688

Zolpidem Tartrate (Co-administration results in enhanced response to CNS depressants). Products include:
Ambien Tablets ... 3191

Food Interactions

Alcohol (Co-administration results in enhanced response to alcohol).

VIVARIN CAPLETS
(Caffeine) ▣763
May interact with:

Beverages, containing medications (Concurrent use may cause

nervousness, irritability, sleeplessness, and occasionally, rapid heartbeat).

Caffeine-containing medications (Concurrent use may cause nervousness, irritability, sleeplessness, and occasionally, rapid heartbeat).

Food, containing medications (Concurrent use may cause nervousness, irritability, sleeplessness, and occasionally, rapid heartbeat).

VIVARIN TABLETS

(Caffeine) 763

See Vivarin Caplets

VIVELLE TRANSDERMAL SYSTEM

(Estradiol) 2412

May interact with progestins. Compounds in these categories include:

Desogestrel (Potential for adverse effects on carbohydrate and lipid metabolism). Products include:

Cyclessa Tablets 2450
Desogen Tablets 2458
Mircette Tablets 2470
Ortho-Cept 21 Tablets 2546
Ortho-Cept 28 Tablets 2546

Medroxyprogesterone Acetate (Potential for adverse effects on carbohydrate and lipid metabolism). Products include:

Depo-Provera Contraceptive Injection 2798
Lunelle Monthly Injection 2827
Premphase Tablets 3572
Prempro Tablets 3572
Provera Tablets 2853

Megestrol Acetate (Potential for adverse effects on carbohydrate and lipid metabolism). Products include:

Megace Oral Suspension 1124

Norgestimate (Potential for adverse effects on carbohydrate and lipid metabolism). Products include:

Ortho-Cyclen/Ortho Tri-Cyclen 2573
Ortho-Prefest Tablets 2570

VIVELLE-DOT TRANSDERMAL SYSTEM

(Estradiol) 2416

See Vivelle Transdermal System

VIVOTIF BERNA

(Typhoid Vaccine Live Oral TY21a) 997

May interact with:

Chloroquine Phosphate (Several antimalarials, such as chloroquine, possess antibacterial activity which may interfere with the immune response rate; in one study, concomitant treatment did not result in significant reduction in the immune response, therefore, these drugs can be administered together). Products include:

Aralen Tablets 3075

Mefloquine Hydrochloride (Several antimalarials, such as mefloquine, possess antibacterial activity which may interfere with the immune response rate; in one study, concomitant treatment did not result in significant reduction in the immune response, therefore, these drugs can be administered together). Products include:

Lariam Tablets 2989

Proguanil (The simultaneous administration of proguanil results in a significant decrease in the immune response rate).

No products indexed under this heading.

VOLMAX EXTENDED-RELEASE TABLETS

(Albuterol Sulfate) 2276

May interact with beta blockers, loop diuretics, monoamine oxidase inhibitors, nonpotassium-sparing diuretics, sympathomimetics, tricyclic antidepressants, and certain other agents. Compounds in these categories include:

Acebutolol Hydrochloride (Co-administration of albuterol with beta-blockers not only blocks the pulmonary effect of beta-agonists, but may produce severe bronchospasm in asthmatic patients). Products include:

Sectral Capsules 3589

Albuterol (Potential for deleterious cardiovascular effects with other oral sympathomimetic agents). Products include:

Proventil Inhalation Aerosol 3142
Ventolin Inhalation Aerosol and Refill 1679

Amitriptyline Hydrochloride (Action of albuterol on the vascular system may be potentiated). Products include:

Etrafon 3115
Limbitrol 1738

Amoxapine (Action of albuterol on the vascular system may be potentiated).

No products indexed under this heading.

Atenolol (Co-administration of albuterol with beta-blockers not only blocks the pulmonary effect of beta-agonists, but may produce severe bronchospasm in asthmatic patients). Products include:

Tenoretic Tablets 690
Tenormin I.V. Injection 692

Bendroflumethiazide (The ECG changes and/or hypokalemia that may result from the administration of nonpotassium-sparing diuretics can be acutely worsened by beta-agonists, especially when the recommended dose of the beta-agonist is exceeded; the clinical significance is not known). Products include:

Corzide 40/5 Tablets 2247
Corzide 80/5 Tablets 2247

Betaxolol Hydrochloride (Co-administration of albuterol with beta-blockers not only blocks the pulmonary effect of beta-agonists, but may produce severe bronchospasm in asthmatic patients). Products include:

Betoptic S Ophthalmic Suspension 537

Bisoprolol Fumarate (Co-administration of albuterol with beta-blockers not only blocks the pulmonary effect of beta-agonists, but may produce severe bronchospasm in asthmatic patients). Products include:

Zebeta Tablets 1885
Ziac Tablets 1887

Bumetanide (The ECG changes and/or hypokalemia that may result from the administration of nonpotassium-sparing diuretics can be acutely worsened by beta-agonists, especially when the recommended dose of the beta-agonist is exceeded; the clinical significance is not known).

No products indexed under this heading.

Carteolol Hydrochloride (Co-administration of albuterol with beta-blockers not only blocks the pulmonary effect of beta-agonists, but may produce severe bronchospasm in asthmatic patients). Products include:

Carteolol Hydrochloride Ophthalmic Solution USP, 1% .... ⊙ 258
Ocupress Ophthalmic Solution, 1% Sterile .... ⊙ 303

Chlorothiazide (The ECG changes and/or hypokalemia that may result from the administration of nonpotassium-sparing diuretics can be acutely worsened by beta-agonists, especially when the recommended dose of the beta-agonist is exceeded; the clinical significance is not known). Products include:

Aldoclor Tablets 2035
Diuril Oral 2087

Chlorothiazide Sodium (The ECG changes and/or hypokalemia that may result from the administration of nonpotassium-sparing diuretics can be acutely worsened by beta-agonists, especially when the recommended dose of the beta-agonist is exceeded; the clinical significance is not known). Products include:

Diuril Sodium Intravenous 2086

Clomipramine Hydrochloride (Action of albuterol on the vascular system may be potentiated).

No products indexed under this heading.

Desipramine Hydrochloride (Action of albuterol on the vascular system may be potentiated). Products include:

Norpramin Tablets 755

Digoxin (Co-administration has resulted in decreased serum digoxin levels; the clinical significance of this finding is unclear). Products include:

Digitek Tablets 1003
Lanoxicaps Capsules 1574
Lanoxin Injection 1581
Lanoxin Tablets 1587
Lanoxin Elixir Pediatric 1578
Lanoxin Injection Pediatric 1584

Dobutamine Hydrochloride (Potential for deleterious cardiovascular effects with other oral sympathomimetic agents). Products include:

Dobutrex Solution Vials 1914

Dopamine Hydrochloride (Potential for deleterious cardiovascular effects with other oral sympathomimetic agents).

No products indexed under this heading.

Doxepin Hydrochloride (Action of albuterol on the vascular system may be potentiated). Products include:

Sinequan 2713

Ephedrine Hydrochloride (Potential for deleterious cardiovascular effects with other oral sympathomimetic agents). Products include:

Primatene Tablets 780

Ephedrine Sulfate (Potential for deleterious cardiovascular effects with other oral sympathomimetic agents).

No products indexed under this heading.

Ephedrine Tannate (Potential for deleterious cardiovascular effects with other oral sympathomimetic agents). Products include:

Rynatuss Pediatric Suspension 3353
Rynatuss Tablets 3353

Epinephrine (Potential for deleterious cardiovascular effects with other oral sympathomimetic agents). Products include:

Epifrin Sterile Ophthalmic Solution .... ⊙ 235
EpiPen 1236
Primatene Mist 779
Xylocaine with Epinephrine Injection 653

Epinephrine Bitartrate (Potential for deleterious cardiovascular effects with other oral sympathomimetic agents). Products include:

Sensorcaine 643

Epinephrine Hydrochloride (Potential for deleterious cardiovascular effects with other oral sympathomimetic agents).

No products indexed under this heading.

Esmolol Hydrochloride (Co-administration of albuterol with beta-blockers not only blocks the pulmonary effect of beta-agonists, but may produce severe bronchospasm in asthmatic patients). Products include:

Brevibloc Injection 858

Ethacrynic Acid (The ECG changes and/or hypokalemia that may result from the administration of nonpotassium-sparing diuretics can be acutely worsened by beta-agonists, especially when the recommended dose of the beta-agonist is exceeded; the clinical significance is not known). Products include:

Edecrin Tablets 2091

Furosemide (The ECG changes and/or hypokalemia that may result from the administration of nonpotassium-sparing diuretics can be acutely worsened by beta-agonists, especially when the recommended dose of the beta-agonist is exceeded; the clinical significance is not known). Products include:

Furosemide Tablets 2284

Hydrochlorothiazide (The ECG changes and/or hypokalemia that may result from the administration of nonpotassium-sparing diuretics can be acutely worsened by beta-agonists, especially when the recommended dose of the beta-agonist is exceeded; the clinical significance is not known). Products include:

Accuretic Tablets 2614
Aldoril Tablets 2039
Atacand HCT Tablets 597
Avalide Tablets 1070
Diovan HCT Tablets 2338
Dyazide Capsules 1515
HydroDIURIL Tablets 2108
Hyzaar 2109
Inderide Tablets 3517
Inderide LA Long-Acting Capsules 3519
Lotensin HCT Tablets 2367
Maxzide 1008
Micardis HCT Tablets 1051
Microzide Capsules 3414
Moduretic Tablets 2138
Monopril HCT 1094
Prinzide Tablets 2168
Timolide Tablets 2187
Uniretic Tablets 3178
Vaseretic Tablets 2204
Zestoretic Tablets 695
Ziac Tablets 1887

Hydroflumethiazide (The ECG changes and/or hypokalemia that may result from the administration of nonpotassium-sparing diuretics can be acutely worsened by beta-agonists, especially when the recommended dose of the beta-agonist is exceeded; the clinical significance is not known). Products include:

Diucardin Tablets 3494

Imipramine Hydrochloride (Action of albuterol on the vascular system may be potentiated).

No products indexed under this heading.

Imipramine Pamoate (Action of albuterol on the vascular system may be potentiated).

No products indexed under this heading.

Isocarboxazid (Action of albuterol on the vascular system may be potentiated).

No products indexed under this heading.

Isoproterenol Hydrochloride (Potential for deleterious cardiovascular effects with other oral sympathomimetic agents).

No products indexed under this heading.

Isoproterenol Sulfate (Potential for deleterious cardiovascular effects with other oral sympathomi-

metic agents).
No products indexed under this heading.

Labetalol Hydrochloride (Co-administration of albuterol with beta-blockers not only blocks the pulmonary effect of beta-agonists, but may produce severe bronchospasm in asthmatic patients). Products include:
Normodyne Injection 3135
Normodyne Tablets 3137

Levalbuterol Hydrochloride (Potential for deleterious cardiovascular effects with other oral sympathomimetic agents). Products include:
Xopenex Inhalation Solution 3207

Levobunolol Hydrochloride (Co-administration of albuterol with beta-blockers not only blocks the pulmonary effect of beta-agonists, but may produce severe bronchospasm in asthmatic patients). Products include:
Betagan .... ⊙228

Maprotiline Hydrochloride (Action of albuterol on the vascular system may be potentiated).
No products indexed under this heading.

Metaproterenol Sulfate (Potential for deleterious cardiovascular effects with other oral sympathomimetic agents). Products include:
Alupent 1029

Metaraminol Bitartrate (Potential for deleterious cardiovascular effects with other oral sympathomimetic agents). Products include:
Aramine Injection 2043

Methoxamine Hydrochloride (Potential for deleterious cardiovascular effects with other oral sympathomimetic agents).
No products indexed under this heading.

Methyclothiazide (The ECG changes and/or hypokalemia that may result from the administration of nonpotassium-sparing diuretics can be acutely worsened by beta-agonists, especially when the recommended dose of the beta-agonist is exceeded; the clinical significance is not known).
No products indexed under this heading.

Metipranolol Hydrochloride (Co-administration of albuterol with beta-blockers not only blocks the pulmonary effect of beta-agonists, but may produce severe bronchospasm in asthmatic patients).
No products indexed under this heading.

Metoprolol Succinate (Co-administration of albuterol with beta-blockers not only blocks the pulmonary effect of beta-agonists, but may produce severe bronchospasm in asthmatic patients). Products include:
Toprol-XL Tablets 651

Metoprolol Tartrate (Co-administration of albuterol with beta-blockers not only blocks the pulmonary effect of beta-agonists, but may produce severe bronchospasm in asthmatic patients).
No products indexed under this heading.

Moclobemide (Action of albuterol on the vascular system may be potentiated).
No products indexed under this heading.

Nadolol (Co-administration of albuterol with beta-blockers not only blocks the pulmonary effect of beta-agonists, but may produce severe bronchospasm in asthmatic patients). Products include:
Corgard Tablets 2245
Corzide 40/5 Tablets 2247
Corzide 80/5 Tablets 2247
Nadolol Tablets 2288

Norepinephrine Bitartrate (Potential for deleterious cardiovascular effects with other oral sympathomimetic agents).
No products indexed under this heading.

Nortriptyline Hydrochloride (Action of albuterol on the vascular system may be potentiated).
No products indexed under this heading.

Pargyline Hydrochloride (Action of albuterol on the vascular system may be potentiated).
No products indexed under this heading.

Penbutolol Sulfate (Co-administration of albuterol with beta-blockers not only blocks the pulmonary effect of beta-agonists, but may produce severe bronchospasm in asthmatic patients).
No products indexed under this heading.

Phenelzine Sulfate (Action of albuterol on the vascular system may be potentiated). Products include:
Nardil Tablets 2653

Phenylephrine Bitartrate (Potential for deleterious cardiovascular effects with other oral sympathomimetic agents).
No products indexed under this heading.

Phenylephrine Hydrochloride (Potential for deleterious cardiovascular effects with other oral sympathomimetic agents). Products include:
Afrin Nasal Decongestant Children's Pump Mist .... ▣734
Extendryl 1361
Hycomine Compound Tablets 1317
Neo-Synephrine .... ▣614
Phenergan VC Syrup 3560
Phenergan VC with Codeine Syrup .. 3561
Preparation H Cream .... ▣778
Preparation H Cooling Gel .... ▣778
Preparation H .... ▣778
Vicks Sinex Nasal Spray and Ultra Fine Mist .... ▣729

Phenylephrine Tannate (Potential for deleterious cardiovascular effects with other oral sympathomimetic agents). Products include:
Ryna-12 S Suspension 3351
Reformulated Rynatan Pediatric Suspension 3352
Rynatuss Pediatric Suspension 3353
Rynatuss Tablets 3353

Phenylpropanolamine Hydrochloride (Potential for deleterious cardiovascular effects with other oral sympathomimetic agents).
No products indexed under this heading.

Pindolol (Co-administration of albuterol with beta-blockers not only blocks the pulmonary effect of beta-agonists, but may produce severe bronchospasm in asthmatic patients).
No products indexed under this heading.

Pirbuterol Acetate (Potential for deleterious cardiovascular effects with other oral sympathomimetic agents). Products include:
Maxair Autohaler 1981
Maxair Inhaler 1984

Polythiazide (The ECG changes and/or hypokalemia that may result from the administration of nonpotassium-sparing diuretics can be acutely worsened by beta-agonists, especially when the recommended dose of the beta-agonist is exceeded; the clinical significance is not known). Products include:
Minizide Capsules 2700
Renese Tablets 2712

Procarbazine Hydrochloride (Action of albuterol on the vascular system may be potentiated). Products include:
Matulane Capsules 3246

Propranolol Hydrochloride (Co-administration of albuterol with beta-blockers not only blocks the pulmonary effect of beta-agonists, but may produce severe bronchospasm in asthmatic patients). Products include:
Inderal 3513
Inderal LA Long-Acting Capsules 3516
Inderide Tablets 3517
Inderide LA Long-Acting Capsules .. 3519

Protriptyline Hydrochloride (Action of albuterol on the vascular system may be potentiated). Products include:
Vivactil Tablets 2446
Vivactil Tablets 2217

Pseudoephedrine Hydrochloride (Potential for deleterious cardiovascular effects with other oral sympathomimetic agents). Products include:
Actifed Cold & Allergy Tablets ...... ▣688
Actifed Cold & Sinus Caplets and Tablets .... ▣688
Advil Cold and Sinus Caplets .... ▣771
Advil Cold and Sinus Tablets .... ▣771
Advil Flu & Body Ache Caplets ...... ▣772
Aleve Cold & Sinus Caplets .... ▣603
Alka-Seltzer Plus Liqui-Gels .... ▣604
Alka-Seltzer Plus Cold & Flu Medicine Liqui-Gels .... ▣604
Alka-Seltzer Plus Cold & Sinus Medicine Liqui-Gels .... ▣604
Allegra-D Extended-Release Tablets 714
BC Cold Powder .... ▣619
Benadryl Allergy/Cold Tablets .... ▣691
Benadryl Allergy/Congestion Tablets .... ▣692
Benadryl Allergy & Sinus Liquid .... ▣693
Benadryl Allergy & Sinus Fastmelt Tablets .... ▣693
Benadryl Allergy Sinus Headache Caplets & Gelcaps .... ▣693
Benadryl Severe Allergy & Sinus Headache Caplets .... ▣694
Benadryl Children's Allergy/Cold Fastmelt Tablets .... ▣692
Benylin Multi-Symptom Liquid .... ▣697
Bromfed Capsules (Extended-Release) 2269
Bromfed-PD Capsules (Extended-Release) 2269
Children's Cēpacol Sore Throat .... ▣788
Comtrex Acute Head Cold & Sinus Pressure Relief Tablets ...... ▣627
Comtrex Deep Chest Cold & Congestion Relief Softgels .... ▣627
Comtrex Flu Therapy & Fever Relief Daytime Caplets .... ▣628
Comtrex Flu Therapy & Fever Relief Nighttime Tablets .... ▣628
Comtrex Maximum Strength Multi-Symptom Cold & Cough Relief Tablets and Caplets .... ▣626
Contac Non-Drowsy 12 Hour Cold Caplets .... ▣745
Contac Non-Drowsy Timed Release 12 Hour Cold Caplets ... ▣746
Contac Severe Cold and Flu Caplets Maximum Strength .... ▣746
Contac Severe Cold and Flu Caplets Non-Drowsy .... ▣746
Dimetapp Elixir .... ▣777
Dimetapp Cold and Fever Suspension .... ▣775
Dimetapp DM Cold & Cough Elixir . ▣775
Dimetapp Nighttime Flu Liquid ...... ▣776
Dimetapp Non-Drowsy Flu Syrup .... ▣777
Dimetapp Infant Drops Decongestant .... ▣775
Dimetapp Infant Drops Decongestant Plus Cough .... ▣776
Guaifed 2272
Kronofed-A 1341
Children's Motrin Cold Oral Suspension 2007
Motrin Sinus Headache Caplets 2005
PediaCare Cough-Cold Liquid .... ▣719
PediaCare Infants' Drops Decongestant .... ▣719
PediaCare Infants' Drops Decongestant Plus Cough .... ▣719
PediaCare NightRest Cough-Cold Liquid .... ▣719
Robitussin Cold Caplets Cold & Congestion .... ▣780
Robitussin Cold Softgels Cold & Congestion .... ▣780
Robitussin Cold Caplets Multi-Symptom Cold & Flu .... ▣781
Robitussin Cold Softgels Multi-Symptom Cold & Flu .... ▣781
Robitussin Cold Softgels Severe Congestion .... ▣782
Robitussin Cough & Cold Infant Drops .... ▣782
Robitussin Maximum Strength Cough & Cold Liquid .... ▣785
Robitussin Pediatric Cough & Cold Formula Liquid .... ▣785
Robitussin Multi Symptom Honey Flu Liquid .... ▣785
Robitussin Nighttime Honey Flu Liquid .... ▣786
Robitussin-CF Liquid .... ▣783
Robitussin-DAC Syrup 2942
Robitussin-PE Liquid .... ▣782
Ryna .... ▣768
Semprex-D Capsules 1172
Singlet Caplets .... ▣761
Sinutab Non-Drying Liquid Caps .... ▣706
Sinutab Sinus Allergy Medication, Maximum Strength Formula, Tablets & Caplets .... ▣707
Sinutab Sinus Medication, Maximum Strength Without Drowsiness Formula, Tablets & Caplets .... ▣707
Sudafed 12 Hour Tablets .... ▣708
Sudafed 24 Hour Tablets .... ▣708
Children's Sudafed Cold & Cough Liquid .... ▣709
Children's Sudafed Nasal Decongestant Chewables .... ▣711
Children's Sudafed Nasal Decongestant Liquid Medication .... ▣711
Sudafed Cold & Allergy Tablets ...... ▣708
Sudafed Cold & Cough Liquid Caps .... ▣709
Sudafed Cold & Sinus Liquid Caps .... ▣710
Sudafed Nasal Decongestant Tablets .... ▣710
Sudafed Non-Drying Sinus Liquid Caps .... ▣712
Sudafed Severe Cold .... ▣711
Sudafed Sinus Headache Caplets .. ▣712
Sudafed Sinus Headache Tablets .. ▣712
Tavist Sinus Non-Drowsy Coated Caplets .... ▣676
TheraFlu Regular Strength Cold & Cough Night Time Hot Liquid ...... ▣676
TheraFlu Regular Strength Cold & Sore Throat Night Time Hot Liquid .... ▣676
TheraFlu Maximum Strength Flu & Congestion Non-Drowsy Hot Liquid .... ▣677
TheraFlu Maximum Strength Flu & Cough Night Time Hot Liquid ... ▣678
TheraFlu Maximum Strength Flu & Sore Throat Night Time Hot Liquid .... ▣677
TheraFlu Maximum Strength Severe Cold & Congestion Night Time Caplets .... ▣678
TheraFlu Maximum Strength Severe Cold & Congestion Night Time Hot Liquid .... ▣678
TheraFlu Maximum Strength Severe Cold & Congestion Non-Drowsy .... ▣679
Triaminic Allergy Congestion Liquid .... ▣680
Triaminic Chest Congestion Liquid .... ▣680
Triaminic Cold & Allergy Liquid ...... ▣681
Triaminic Cold & Allergy Softchews .... ▣683
Triaminic Cold & Cough Liquid ...... ▣681
Triaminic Cold & Cough Softchews .... ▣683
Triaminic Cold & Night Time Cough Liquid .... ▣681
Triaminic Cold, Cough & Fever Liquid .... ▣681
Triaminic Cough Liquid .... ▣682
Triaminic Cough & Congestion Liquid .... ▣682
Triaminic Cough & Sore Throat Liquid .... ▣682
Triaminic Cough & Sore Throat Softchews .... ▣684
Children's Tylenol Allergy-D Liquid ... 2014
Children's Tylenol Cold Suspension Liquid and Chewable Tablets 2015
Children's Tylenol Cold Plus Cough Suspension Liquid and Chewable Tablets 2015
Children's Tylenol Flu Suspension Liquid 2015

Children's Tylenol Sinus Suspension Liquid 2017
Infants' Tylenol Cold Decongestant and Fever Reducer Concentrated Drops 2015
Infants' Tylenol Cold Decongestant and Fever Reducer Concentrated Drops Plus Cough .. 2015
Tylenol Allergy Sinus 2010
Multi-Symptom Tylenol Cold Complete Formula Caplets 2010
Multi-Symptom Tylenol Cold Non-Drowsy Caplets and Gelcaps 2010
Multi-Symptom Tylenol Cold Severe Congestion Non-Drowsy Caplets 2011
Maximum Strength Tylenol Flu NightTime Gelcaps 2011
Maximum Strength Tylenol Flu NightTime Liquid 2011
Maximum Strength Tylenol Flu Non-Drowsy Gelcaps 2011
Maximum Strength Tylenol Sinus NightTime Caplets 2012
Maximum Strength Tylenol Sinus Non-Drowsy Geltabs, Gelcaps, Caplets, and Tablets 2012
Vicks 44D Cough & Head Congestion Relief Liquid 724
Vicks 44M Cough, Cold & Flu Relief Liquid 725
Pediatric Vicks 44m Cough & Cold Relief 728
Vicks DayQuil LiquiCaps/Liquid Multi-Symptom Cold/Flu Relief 727
Children's Vicks NyQuil Cold/Cough Relief 726
Vicks NyQuil LiquiCaps/Liquid Multi-Symptom Cold/Flu Relief, Original and Cherry Flavors 727
Zephrex Tablets 3091
Zephrex LA Tablets 3092
Zyrtec-D 12 Hour Extended Relief Tablets 2758

Pseudoephedrine Sulfate (Potential for deleterious cardiovascular effects with other oral sympathomimetic agents). Products include:
Chlor-Trimeton Allergy/Decongestant Tablets 736
Claritin-D 12 Hour Extended Release Tablets 3102
Claritin-D 24 Hour Extended Release Tablets 3104
Coricidin 'D' Cold, Flu & Sinus Tablets 737
Drixoral Allergy/Sinus Extended-Release Tablets 741
Drixoral Cold & Allergy Sustained-Action Tablets 740
Drixoral Cold & Flu Extended-Release Tablets 740
Drixoral Nasal Decongestant Long-Acting Non-Drowsy Tablets 740
Rynatan Tablets 3351

Salmeterol Xinafoate (Potential for deleterious cardiovascular effects with other oral sympathomimetic agents). Products include:
Advair Diskus 100/50 1448
Advair Diskus 250/50 1448
Advair Diskus 500/50 1448
Serevent Diskus 1637
Serevent Inhalation Aerosol 1633

Selegiline Hydrochloride (Action of albuterol on the vascular system may be potentiated). Products include:
Eldepryl Capsules 3266

Sotalol Hydrochloride (Co-administration of albuterol with beta-blockers not only blocks the pulmonary effect of beta-agonists, but may produce severe bronchospasm in asthmatic patients). Products include:
Betapace Tablets 950
Betapace AF Tablets 954

Terbutaline Sulfate (Potential for deleterious cardiovascular effects with other oral sympathomimetic agents). Products include:
Brethine Ampuls 2314
Brethine Tablets 2313

Timolol Hemihydrate (Co-administration of albuterol with beta-blockers not only blocks the pulmonary effect of beta-agonists, but may produce severe bronchospasm in asthmatic patients). Products include:
Betimol Ophthalmic Solution .... ⊙ 324

Timolol Maleate (Co-administration of albuterol with beta-blockers not only blocks the pulmonary effect of beta-agonists, but may produce severe bronchospasm in asthmatic patients). Products include:
Blocadren Tablets 2046
Cosopt Sterile Ophthalmic Solution 2065
Timolide Tablets 2187
Timolol GFS .... ⊙ 266
Timoptic in Ocudose 2192
Timoptic Sterile Ophthalmic Solution 2190
Timoptic-XE Sterile Ophthalmic Gel Forming Solution 2194

Torsemide (The ECG changes and/or hypokalemia that may result from the administration of nonpotassium-sparing diuretics can be acutely worsened by beta-agonists, especially when the recommended dose of the beta-agonist is exceeded; the clinical significance is not known). Products include:
Demadex Tablets and Injection 2965

Tranylcypromine Sulfate (Action of albuterol on the vascular system may be potentiated). Products include:
Parnate Tablets 1607

Trimipramine Maleate (Action of albuterol on the vascular system may be potentiated). Products include:
Surmontil Capsules 3595

Food Interactions

Food, unspecified (Food may decrease the rate of absorption without altering the extent of bioavailability).

VOLTAREN OPHTHALMIC STERILE OPHTHALMIC SOLUTION

(Diclofenac Sodium) .... ⊙ 312
None cited in PDR database.

VOLTAREN TABLETS

(Diclofenac Sodium) 2315
May interact with oral anticoagulants, diuretics, oral hypoglycemic agents, insulin, lithium preparations, potassium sparing diuretics, and certain other agents. Compounds in these categories include:

Acarbose (Both hypo- and hyperglycemic effects have been reported rarely; possibility exists that diclofenac may alter diabetic patient's response to oral hypoglycemic agents). Products include:
Precose Tablets 906

Amiloride Hydrochloride (Diclofenac can inhibit the activity of diuretics; concomitant treatment may be associated with hyperkalemia). Products include:
Midamor Tablets 2136
Moduretic Tablets 2138

Aspirin (Co-administration is not recommended because diclofenac is displaced from its binding sites resulting in lower peak plasma concentrations, peak plasma levels and AUC values). Products include:
Aggrenox Capsules 1026
Alka-Seltzer 603
Alka-Seltzer Lemon Lime Antacid and Pain Reliever Effervescent Tablets 603
Alka-Seltzer Extra Strength Antacid and Pain Reliever Effervescent Tablets 603
Alka-Seltzer PM Effervescent Tablets 605
Genuine Bayer Tablets, Caplets and Gelcaps 606
Extra Strength Bayer Caplets and Gelcaps 610
Aspirin Regimen Bayer Children's Chewable Tablets (Orange or Cherry Flavored) 607
Bayer, Aspirin Regimen 606
Aspirin Regimen Bayer 81 mg Caplets with Calcium 607
Genuine Bayer Professional Labeling (Aspirin Regimen Bayer) 608
Extra Strength Bayer Arthritis Caplets 610
Extra Strength Bayer Plus Caplets 610
Extra Strength Bayer PM Caplets 611
BC Powder 619
BC Allergy Sinus Cold Powder 619
Arthritis Strength BC Powder 619
BC Sinus Cold Powder 619
Darvon Compound-65 Pulvules 1910
Ecotrin Enteric Coated Aspirin Low, Regular and Maximum Strength Tablets 1715
Excedrin Extra-Strength Tablets, Caplets, and Geltabs 629
Excedrin Migraine 1070
Goody's Body Pain Formula Powder 620
Goody's Extra Strength Headache Powder 620
Goody's Extra Strength Pain Relief Tablets 620
Percodan Tablets 1327
Robaxisal Tablets 2939
Soma Compound Tablets 3354
Soma Compound w/Codeine Tablets 3355
Vanquish Caplets 617

Bendroflumethiazide (Diclofenac can inhibit the activity of diuretics). Products include:
Corzide 40/5 Tablets 2247
Corzide 80/5 Tablets 2247

Bumetanide (Diclofenac can inhibit the activity of diuretics).
No products indexed under this heading.

Chlorothiazide (Diclofenac can inhibit the activity of diuretics). Products include:
Aldoclor Tablets 2035
Diuril Oral 2087

Chlorothiazide Sodium (Diclofenac can inhibit the activity of diuretics). Products include:
Diuril Sodium Intravenous 2086

Chlorpropamide (Both hypo- and hyperglycemic effects have been reported rarely; possibility exists that diclofenac may alter diabetic patient's response to oral hypoglycemic agents). Products include:
Diabinese Tablets 2680

Chlorthalidone (Diclofenac can inhibit the activity of diuretics). Products include:
Clorpres Tablets 1002
Combipres Tablets 1040
Tenoretic Tablets 690

Cyclosporine (Co-administration may increase cyclosporine's nephrotoxicity since diclofenac may affect renal prostaglandins). Products include:
Gengraf Capsules 457
Neoral Soft Gelatin Capsules 2380
Neoral Oral Solution 2380
Sandimmune 2388

Dicumarol (While studies have not shown interactions with oral anticoagulants, concurrent therapy requires close monitoring of patients for potential modification in anticoagulant dosage).
No products indexed under this heading.

Digoxin (Co-administration may increase serum digoxin concentrations resulting in digoxin toxicity since diclofenac may affect renal prostaglandins). Products include:
Digitek Tablets 1003
Lanoxicaps Capsules 1574
Lanoxin Injection 1581
Lanoxin Tablets 1587
Lanoxin Elixir Pediatric 1578
Lanoxin Injection Pediatric 1584

Ethacrynic Acid (Diclofenac can inhibit the activity of diuretics). Products include:
Edecrin Tablets 2091

Furosemide (Diclofenac can inhibit the activity of diuretics). Products include:
Furosemide Tablets 2284

Glimepiride (Both hypo- and hyperglycemic effects have been reported rarely; possibility exists that diclofenac may alter diabetic patient's response to oral hypoglycemic agents). Products include:
Amaryl Tablets 717

Glipizide (Both hypo- and hyperglycemic effects have been reported rarely; possibility exists that diclofenac may alter diabetic patient's response to oral hypoglycemic agents). Products include:
Glucotrol Tablets 2692
Glucotrol XL Extended Release Tablets 2693

Glyburide (Both hypo- and hyperglycemic effects have been reported rarely; possibility exists that diclofenac may alter diabetic patient's response to oral hypoglycemic agents). Products include:
DiaBeta Tablets 741
Glucovance Tablets 1086

Hydrochlorothiazide (Diclofenac can inhibit the activity of diuretics). Products include:
Accuretic Tablets 2614
Aldoril Tablets 2039
Atacand HCT Tablets 597
Avalide Tablets 1070
Diovan HCT Tablets 2338
Dyazide Capsules 1515
HydroDIURIL Tablets 2108
Hyzaar 2109
Inderide Tablets 3517
Inderide LA Long-Acting Capsules .. 3519
Lotensin HCT Tablets 2367
Maxzide 1008
Micardis HCT Tablets 1051
Microzide Capsules 3414
Moduretic Tablets 2138
Monopril HCT 1094
Prinzide Tablets 2168
Timolide Tablets 2187
Uniretic Tablets 3178
Vaseretic Tablets 2204
Zestoretic Tablets 695
Ziac Tablets 1887

Hydroflumethiazide (Diclofenac can inhibit the activity of diuretics). Products include:
Diucardin Tablets 3494

Indapamide (Diclofenac can inhibit the activity of diuretics). Products include:
Indapamide Tablets 2286

Insulin, Human, Zinc Suspension (Both hypo- and hyperglycemic effects have been reported rarely; possibility exists that dicofenac may alter diabetic patient's response to insulin). Products include:
Humulin L, 100 Units 1937
Humulin U, 100 Units 1943
Novolin L Human Insulin 10 ml Vials 2422

Insulin, Human NPH (Both hypo- and hyperglycemic effects have been reported rarely; possibility exists that dicofenac may alter diabetic patient's response to insulin). Products include:
Humulin N, 100 Units 1939
Humulin N NPH Pen 1940
Novolin N Human Insulin 10 ml Vials 2422
Novolin N PenFill 2423
Novolin N Prefilled Syringe Disposable Insulin Delivery System 2425

Insulin, Human Regular (Both hypo- and hyperglycemic effects have been reported rarely; possibility exists that dicofenac may alter diabetic patient's response to insulin). Products include:
Humulin R Regular (U-500) 1943
Humulin R, 100 Units 1941
Novolin R Human Insulin 10 ml Vials 2423
Novolin R PenFill 2423
Novolin R Prefilled Syringe Disposable Insulin Delivery System 2425
Velosulin BR Human Insulin 10 ml Vials 2435

Insulin, Human Regular and Human NPH Mixture (Both hypo- and hyperglycemic effects have been reported rarely; possibility exists that dicofenac may alter diabetic patient's response to insulin). Products include:

Humulin 50/50, 100 Units 1934
Humulin 70/30, 100 Units 1935
Humulin 70/30 Pen 1936
Novolin 70/30 Human Insulin 10 ml Vials 2421
Novolin 70/30 PenFill 2423
Novolin 70/30 Prefilled Disposable Insulin Delivery System 2425

Insulin, NPH (Both hypo- and hyperglycemic effects have been reported rarely; possibility exists that dicofenac may alter diabetic patient's response to insulin). Products include:

Iletin II, NPH (Pork), 100 Units 1946

Insulin, Regular (Both hypo- and hyperglycemic effects have been reported rarely; possibility exists that dicofenac may alter diabetic patient's response to insulin). Products include:

Iletin II, Regular (Pork), 100 Units ... 1947

Insulin, Zinc Crystals (Both hypo- and hyperglycemic effects have been reported rarely; possibility exists that dicofenac may alter diabetic patient's response to insulin).

No products indexed under this heading.

Insulin, Zinc Suspension (Both hypo- and hyperglycemic effects have been reported rarely; possibility exists that dicofenac may alter diabetic patient's response to insulin). Products include:

Iletin II, Lente (Pork), 100 Units 1945

Insulin Aspart, Human Regular (Both hypo- and hyperglycemic effects have been reported rarely; possibility exists that dicofenac may alter diabetic patient's response to insulin).

No products indexed under this heading.

Insulin glargine (Both hypo- and hyperglycemic effects have been reported rarely; possibility exists that dicofenac may alter diabetic patient's response to insulin). Products include:

Lantus Injection 742

Insulin Lispro, Human (Both hypo- and hyperglycemic effects have been reported rarely; possibility exists that dicofenac may alter diabetic patient's response to insulin). Products include:

Humalog 1926
Humalog Mix 75/25 Pen 1928

Insulin Lispro Protamine, Human (Both hypo- and hyperglycemic effects have been reported rarely; possibility exists that dicofenac may alter diabetic patient's response to insulin). Products include:

Humalog Mix 75/25 Pen 1928

Lithium Carbonate (Decreased lithium renal clearance resulting in increased lithium plasma levels; potential for lithium toxicity). Products include:

Eskalith 1527
Lithium Carbonate 3061
Lithobid Slow-Release Tablets 3255

Lithium Citrate (Decreased lithium renal clearance resulting in increased lithium plasma levels; potential for lithium toxicity). Products include:

Lithium Citrate Syrup 3061

Metformin Hydrochloride (Both hypo- and hyperglycemic effects have been reported rarely; possibility exists that diclofenac may alter diabetic patient's response to oral hypoglycemic agents). Products include:

Glucophage Tablets 1080
Glucophage XR Tablets 1080
Glucovance Tablets 1086

Methotrexate Sodium (Coadministration may increase serum methotrexate concentrations resulting in methotrexate toxicity since diclofenac may affect renal prostaglandins).

No products indexed under this heading.

Methyclothiazide (Diclofenac can inhibit the activity of diuretics).

No products indexed under this heading.

Metolazone (Diclofenac can inhibit the activity of diuretics). Products include:

Mykrox Tablets 1168
Zaroxolyn Tablets 1177

Miglitol (Both hypo- and hyperglycemic effects have been reported rarely; possibility exists that diclofenac may alter diabetic patient's response to oral hypoglycemic agents). Products include:

Glyset Tablets 2821

Phenobarbital (Potential for phenobarbital toxicity in patients on chronic phenobarbital treatment following the initiation of diclofenac therapy). Products include:

Arco-Lase Plus Tablets 592
Donnatal 2929
Donnatal Extentabs 2930

Pioglitazone Hydrochloride (Both hypo- and hyperglycemic effects have been reported rarely; possibility exists that diclofenac may alter diabetic patient's response to oral hypoglycemic agents). Products include:

Actos Tablets 3275

Polythiazide (Diclofenac can inhibit the activity of diuretics). Products include:

Minizide Capsules 2700
Renese Tablets 2712

Repaglinide (Both hypo- and hyperglycemic effects have been reported rarely; possibility exists that diclofenac may alter diabetic patient's response to oral hypoglycemic agents). Products include:

Prandin Tablets (0.5, 1, and 2 mg) 2432

Rosiglitazone Maleate (Both hypo- and hyperglycemic effects have been reported rarely; possibility exists that diclofenac may alter diabetic patient's response to oral hypoglycemic agents). Products include:

Avandia Tablets 1490

Spironolactone (Diclofenac can inhibit the activity of diuretics; concomitant treatment may be associated with hyperkalemia).

No products indexed under this heading.

Tolazamide (Both hypo- and hyperglycemic effects have been reported rarely; possibility exists that diclofenac may alter diabetic patient's response to oral hypoglycemic agents).

No products indexed under this heading.

Tolbutamide (Both hypo- and hyperglycemic effects have been reported rarely; possibility exists that diclofenac may alter diabetic patient's response to oral hypoglycemic agents).

No products indexed under this heading.

Torsemide (Diclofenac can inhibit the activity of diuretics). Products include:

Demadex Tablets and Injection 2965

Triamterene (Diclofenac can inhibit the activity of diuretics; concomitant treatment may be associated with hyperkalemia). Products include:

Dyazide Capsules 1515
Dyrenium Capsules 3458
Maxzide 1008

Troglitazone (Both hypo- and hyperglycemic effects have been reported rarely; possibility exists that diclofenac may alter diabetic patient's response to oral hypoglycemic agents).

No products indexed under this heading.

Warfarin Sodium (While studies have not shown interactions with oral anticoagulants, concurrent therapy requires close monitoring of patients for potential modification in anticoagulant dosage). Products include:

Coumadin for Injection 1243
Coumadin Tablets 1243
Warfarin Sodium Tablets, USP 3302

Food Interactions

Food, unspecified (Food significantly alters the absorption pattern of extended-release dosage form as indicated by delay of 1 to 2 hours in Tmax and a two-fold increase in Cmax values; food also delays the onset of absorption of delayed-release and immediate-release formulations).

VOLTAREN-XR TABLETS

(Diclofenac Sodium) 2315
See Voltaren Tablets

VOSOL HC OTIC SOLUTION

(Acetic Acid, Hydrocortisone) 3356
None cited in PDR database.

WARFARIN SODIUM TABLETS, USP

(Warfarin Sodium) 3302
May interact with 5-lipoxygenase inhibitors, oral aminoglycosides, antacids, antihistamines, antiandrogens, barbiturates, chloramphenicol, corticosteroids, diuretics, doxycycline, fluoroquinolone antibiotics, inhalant anesthetics, leukotriene receptor antagonists, macrolide antibiotics, non-steroidal anti-inflammatory agents, oral contraceptives, phenytoin, quinidine, salicylates, selective serotonin reuptake inhibitors, sulfonamides, thyroid preparations, valproate, and certain other agents. Compounds in these categories include:

Acetaminophen (Increased prothrombin time response). Products include:

Actifed Cold & Sinus Caplets and Tablets .... ▣688
Alka-Seltzer Plus Liqui-Gels .... ▣604
Alka-Seltzer Plus Cold & Flu Medicine Liqui-Gels .... ▣604
Alka-Seltzer Plus Cold & Sinus Medicine Liqui-Gels .... ▣604
Benadryl Allergy/Cold Tablets .... ▣691
Benadryl Allergy Sinus Headache Caplets & Gelcaps .... ▣693
Benadryl Severe Allergy & Sinus Headache Caplets .... ▣694
Children's Cēpacol Sore Throat .... ▣788
Comtrex Acute Head Cold & Sinus Pressure Relief Tablets .... ▣627
Comtrex Deep Chest Cold & Congestion Relief Softgels .... ▣627
Comtrex Flu Therapy & Fever Relief Daytime Caplets .... ▣628
Comtrex Flu Therapy & Fever Relief Nighttime Tablets .... ▣628
Comtrex Maximum Strength Multi-Symptom Cold & Cough Relief Tablets and Caplets .... ▣626
Contac Severe Cold and Flu Caplets Maximum Strength .... ▣746
Contac Severe Cold and Flu Caplets Non-Drowsy .... ▣746
Coricidin 'D' Cold, Flu & Sinus Tablets .... ▣737
Coricidin HBP Cold & Flu Tablets .... ▣738
Coricidin HBP Maximum Strength Flu Tablets .... ▣738
Coricidin HBP Night-Time Cold & Flu Tablets .... ▣738
Darvon-N/Darvocet-N 1907
Dimetapp Cold and Fever Suspension .... ▣775
Dimetapp Nighttime Flu Liquid .... ▣776
Dimetapp Non-Drowsy Flu Syrup .... ▣777
Drixoral Allergy/Sinus Extended-Release Tablets .... ▣741
Drixoral Cold & Flu Extended-Release Tablets .... ▣740
Aspirin Free Excedrin Caplets and Geltabs .... ▣628
Excedrin Extra-Strength Tablets, Caplets, and Geltabs .... ▣629
Excedrin Migraine 1070
Excedrin PM Tablets, Caplets, and Geltabs .... ▣631
Goody's Body Pain Formula Powder .... ▣620
Goody's Extra Strength Headache Powder .... ▣620
Goody's Extra Strength Pain Relief Tablets .... ▣620
Goody's PM Powder .... ▣621
Hycomine Compound Tablets 1317
Lortab 3319
Lortab Elixir 3317
Maxidone Tablets CIII 3399
Maximum Strength Midol Menstrual Caplets and Gelcaps .... ▣612
Maximum Strength Midol PMS Caplets and Gelcaps .... ▣613
Maximum Strength Midol Teen Caplets .... ▣612
Midrin Capsules 3464
Norco 5/325 Tablets CIII 3424
Norco 7.5/325 Tablets CIII 3425
Norco 10/325 Tablets CIII 3427
Norco 10/325 Tablets CIII 3425
Percocet Tablets 1326
Percogesic Aspirin-Free Coated Tablets .... ▣667
Extra Strength Percogesic Aspirin-Free Coated Caplets .... ▣665
Phrenilin 578
Robitussin Cold Caplets Multi-Symptom Cold & Flu .... ▣781
Robitussin Cold Softgels Multi-Symptom Cold & Flu .... ▣781
Robitussin Multi Symptom Honey Flu Liquid .... ▣785
Robitussin Nighttime Honey Flu Liquid .... ▣786
Sedapap Tablets 50 mg/650 mg 2225
Singlet Caplets .... ▣761
Sinutab Sinus Allergy Medication, Maximum Strength Formula, Tablets & Caplets .... ▣707
Sinutab Sinus Medication, Maximum Strength Without Drowsiness Formula, Tablets & Caplets .... ▣707
Sudafed Cold & Cough Liquid Caps .... ▣709
Sudafed Cold & Sinus Liquid Caps .... ▣710
Sudafed Severe Cold .... ▣711
Sudafed Sinus Headache Caplets .... ▣712
Sudafed Sinus Headache Tablets .... ▣712
Tavist Sinus Non-Drowsy Coated Caplets .... ▣676
TheraFlu Regular Strength Cold & Cough Night Time Hot Liquid .... ▣676
TheraFlu Regular Strength Cold & Sore Throat Night Time Hot Liquid .... ▣676
TheraFlu Maximum Strength Flu & Congestion Non-Drowsy Hot Liquid .... ▣677
TheraFlu Maximum Strength Flu & Cough Night Time Hot Liquid .... ▣678
TheraFlu Maximum Strength Flu & Sore Throat Night Time Hot Liquid .... ▣677
TheraFlu Maximum Strength Severe Cold & Congestion Night Time Caplets .... ▣678
TheraFlu Maximum Strength Severe Cold & Congestion Night Time Hot Liquid .... ▣678
TheraFlu Maximum Strength Severe Cold & Congestion Non-Drowsy .... ▣679
Triaminic Cold, Cough & Fever Liquid .... ▣681
Triaminic Cough & Sore Throat Liquid .... ▣682
Triaminic Cough & Sore Throat Softchews .... ▣684
Tylenol, Children's 2014
Children's Tylenol Allergy-D Liquid 2014
Children's Tylenol Cold Suspension Liquid and Chewable Tablets 2015
Children's Tylenol Cold Plus Cough Suspension Liquid and Chewable Tablets 2015
Children's Tylenol Flu Suspension Liquid 2015
Children's Tylenol Sinus Suspension Liquid 2017

Infants' Tylenol Cold Decongestant and Fever Reducer Concentrated Drops ... 2015
Infants' Tylenol Cold Decongestant and Fever Reducer Concentrated Drops Plus Cough .. 2015
Junior Strength Tylenol Soft Chews Chewable Tablets ... 2014
Tylenol ... 2009
Tylenol Allergy Sinus ... 2010
Tylenol Severe Allergy Caplets ... 2010
Multi-Symptom Tylenol Cold Complete Formula Caplets ... 2010
Multi-Symptom Tylenol Cold Non-Drowsy Caplets and Gelcaps ... 2010
Multi-Symptom Tylenol Cold Severe Congestion Non-Drowsy Caplets ... 2011
Maximum Strength Tylenol Flu NightTime Gelcaps ... 2011
Maximum Strength Tylenol Flu NightTime Liquid ... 2011
Maximum Strength Tylenol Flu Non-Drowsy Gelcaps ... 2011
Extra Strength Tylenol PM Caplets, Geltabs, and Gelcaps ... 2012
Maximum Strength Tylenol Sinus NightTime Caplets ... 2012
Maximum Strength Tylenol Sinus Non-Drowsy Geltabs, Gelcaps, Caplets, and Tablets ... 2012
Maximum Strength Tylenol Sore Throat Adult Liquid ... 2013
Tylenol with Codeine ... 2595
Women's Tylenol Menstrual Relief Caplets ... 2013
Tylox Capsules ... 2597
Ultracet Tablets ... 2597
Vanquish Caplets ... 617
Vicks 44M Cough, Cold & Flu Relief Liquid ... 725
Vicks DayQuil LiquiCaps/Liquid Multi-Symptom Cold/Flu Relief ... 727
Vicks NyQuil LiquiCaps/Liquid Multi-Symptom Cold/Flu Relief, Original and Cherry Flavors ... 727
Vicodin Tablets ... 516
Vicodin ES Tablets ... 517
Vicodin HP Tablets ... 518
Zydone Tablets ... 1330

Achillea millefolium (Co-administration with botanicals that contain coagulant properties, such as yarrow, may affect the anticoagulant effects of warfarin).
No products indexed under this heading.

Acrivastine (Decreased prothrombin time response). Products include:
Semprex-D Capsules ... 1172

ACTH (Decreased prothrombin time response).
No products indexed under this heading.

Agrimonia eupatoria (Co-administration with botanicals that contain salicylate and/or have antiplatelet properties, such as agrimony, may result in increased anticoagulant effects; agrimony contains salicylate and has coagulant properties).
No products indexed under this heading.

Alatrofloxacin Mesylate (Increased prothrombin time response). Products include:
Trovan I.V. ... 2722

Allium cepa (Co-administration with botanicals that contain salicylate and/or have antiplatelet or fibrinolytic properties, such as onion, may result in increased anticoagulant effects).
No products indexed under this heading.

Allium sativum (Co-administration is associated most often with increased effects of warfarin; garlic may cause bleeding events when taken alone and may have anticoagulant, antiplatelet, and/or fibrinolytic properties). Products include:
Beta-C Tablets ... 811
Centrum Focused Formulas Heart Tablets ... 816
CorePlex Capsules ... 796
One-A-Day Cholesterol Health Tablets ... 805
System 3-4-3 Capsules ... 800

Allopurinol (Increased prothrombin time response).
No products indexed under this heading.

Aloe Gel (Co-administration with botanicals that contain salicylate and/or have antiplatelet properties, such as aloe gel, may result in increased anticoagulant effects).
No products indexed under this heading.

Alteplase, Recombinant (Increased prothrombin time response). Products include:
Activase I.V. ... 1410
Cathflo Activase ... 3611

Aluminum Carbonate (Decreased prothrombin time response).
No products indexed under this heading.

Aluminum Hydroxide (Decreased prothrombin time response). Products include:
Amphojel Suspension (Mint Flavor) ... 789
Gaviscon Extra Strength Liquid ... 751
Gaviscon Extra Strength Tablets ... 751
Gaviscon Regular Strength Liquid . 751
Gaviscon Regular Strength Tablets ... 750
Maalox Antacid/Anti-Gas Oral Suspension ... 673
Maalox Max Maximum Strength Antacid/Anti-Gas Liquid ... 2300
Maalox Regular Strength Antacid/Antigas Liquid ... 2300
Mylanta ... 1813
Vanquish Caplets ... 617

Amiloride Hydrochloride (Increased or decreased prothrombin time response). Products include:
Midamor Tablets ... 2136
Moduretic Tablets ... 2138

Aminoglutethimide (Decreased prothrombin time response).
No products indexed under this heading.

p-Aminosalicylic Acid (Increased prothrombin time response).
No products indexed under this heading.

Amiodarone Hydrochloride (Increased prothrombin time response). Products include:
Cordarone Intravenous ... 3491
Cordarone Tablets ... 3487
Pacerone Tablets ... 3331

Aniseed (Co-administration with botanicals that contain coumarins, such as aniseed, may result in increased anticoagulant effects).
No products indexed under this heading.

Apium graveolens (Co-administration with botanicals that contain coumarins, such as celery, may result in increased anticoagulant effects).
No products indexed under this heading.

Aprobarbital (Decreased prothrombin time response).
No products indexed under this heading.

Armoracia rusticana (Co-administration with botanicals that contain coumarins, such as horseradish, may result in increased anticoagulant effects).
No products indexed under this heading.

Arnica montana (Co-administration with botanicals that contain coumarins, such as arnica, may result in increased anticoagulant effects).
No products indexed under this heading.

Aspen (Co-administration with botanicals that contain salicylate and/or have antiplatelet properties, such as aspen, may result in increased anticoagulant effects).
No products indexed under this heading.

Aspirin (Increased prothrombin time response; caution should be observed when used concurrently). Products include:
Aggrenox Capsules ... 1026
Alka-Seltzer ... 603
Alka-Seltzer Lemon Lime Antacid and Pain Reliever Effervescent Tablets ... 603
Alka-Seltzer Extra Strength Antacid and Pain Reliever Effervescent Tablets ... 603
Alka-Seltzer PM Effervescent Tablets ... 605
Genuine Bayer Tablets, Caplets and Gelcaps ... 606
Extra Strength Bayer Caplets and Gelcaps ... 610
Aspirin Regimen Bayer Children's Chewable Tablets (Orange or Cherry Flavored) ... 607
Bayer, Aspirin Regimen ... 606
Aspirin Regimen Bayer 81 mg Caplets with Calcium ... 607
Genuine Bayer Professional Labeling (Aspirin Regimen Bayer) ... 608
Extra Strength Bayer Arthritis Caplets ... 610
Extra Strength Bayer Plus Caplets ... 610
Extra Strength Bayer PM Caplets .. 611
BC Powder ... 619
BC Allergy Sinus Cold Powder ... 619
Arthritis Strength BC Powder ... 619
BC Sinus Cold Powder ... 619
Darvon Compound-65 Pulvules ... 1910
Ecotrin Enteric Coated Aspirin Low, Regular and Maximum Strength Tablets ... 1715
Excedrin Extra-Strength Tablets, Caplets, and Geltabs ... 629
Excedrin Migraine ... 1070
Goody's Body Pain Formula Powder ... 620
Goody's Extra Strength Headache Powder ... 620
Goody's Extra Strength Pain Relief Tablets ... 620
Percodan Tablets ... 1327
Robaxisal Tablets ... 2939
Soma Compound Tablets ... 3354
Soma Compound w/Codeine Tablets ... 3355
Vanquish Caplets ... 617

Astemizole (Decreased prothrombin time response).
No products indexed under this heading.

Atorvastatin Calcium (Increased or decreased prothrombin time response). Products include:
Lipitor Tablets ... 2639
Lipitor Tablets ... 2696

Azatadine Maleate (Decreased prothrombin time response). Products include:
Rynatan Tablets ... 3351

Azathioprine (Decreased prothrombin time response).
No products indexed under this heading.

Azithromycin Dihydrate (Increased prothrombin time response). Products include:
Zithromax ... 2743
Zithromax for IV Infusion ... 2748
Zithromax for Oral Suspension, 300 mg, 600 mg, 900 mg, 1200 mg ... 2739
Zithromax Tablets, 250 mg ... 2739

Bendroflumethiazide (Increased prothrombin time response). Products include:
Corzide 40/5 Tablets ... 2247
Corzide 80/5 Tablets ... 2247

Betamethasone Acetate (Decreased prothrombin time response). Products include:
Celestone Soluspan Injectable Suspension ... 3097

Betamethasone Sodium Phosphate (Decreased prothrombin time response). Products include:
Celestone Soluspan Injectable Suspension ... 3097

Bicalutamide (Increased prothrombin time response). Products include:
Casodex Tablets ... 662

Black Cohosh (Co-administration with botanicals that contain salicylate and/or have antiplatelet properties, such as black cohosh, may result in increased anticoagulant effects). Products include:
One-A-Day Menopause Health Tablets ... 808
Remifemin Menopause Tablets ... 839

Bromelains (Co-administration is associated most often with increased effects of warfarin).
No products indexed under this heading.

Bromodiphenhydramine Hydrochloride (Decreased prothrombin time response).
No products indexed under this heading.

Brompheniramine Maleate (Decreased prothrombin time response). Products include:
Bromfed Capsules (Extended-Release) ... 2269
Bromfed-PD Capsules (Extended-Release) ... 2269
Comtrex Acute Head Cold & Sinus Pressure Relief Tablets ... 627
Dimetapp Elixir ... 777
Dimetapp Cold and Fever Suspension ... 775
Dimetapp DM Cold & Cough Elixir . 775
Dimetapp Nighttime Flu Liquid ... 776

Buchu (Co-administration with botanicals that contain coumarins, such as buchu, may result in increased anticoagulant effects).
No products indexed under this heading.

Bumetanide (Increased or decreased prothrombin time response).
No products indexed under this heading.

Butabarbital (Decreased prothrombin time response).
No products indexed under this heading.

Butalbital (Decreased prothrombin time response). Products include:
Phrenilin ... 578
Sedapap Tablets 50 mg/650 mg ... 2225

Capecitabine (Increased prothrombin time response). Products include:
Xeloda Tablets ... 3039

Capsicum annuum (Co-administration with botanicals that contain coumarins, such as capsicum may result in increased anticoagulant effects; capsicum also has fibrinolytic properties).
No products indexed under this heading.

Carbamazepine (Decreased prothrombin time response). Products include:
Carbatrol Capsules ... 3234
Tegretol/Tegretol-XR ... 2404

Cassia angustifolia (Co-administration with botanicals that contain coumarins, such as cassia, may result in increased anticoagulant effects).
No products indexed under this heading.

Cassia fistula (Co-administration with botanicals that contain coumarins, such as cassia, may result in increased anticoagulant effects).
No products indexed under this heading.

Cassia senna (Co-administration with botanicals that contain coumarins, such as cassia, may result in increased anticoagulant effects).
No products indexed under this heading.

Cefamandole Nafate (Increased prothrombin time response). Products include:

Mandol Vials 1953

Cefazolin Sodium (Increased prothrombin time response). Products include:
Ancef for Injection 1474
Ancef Injection 1474
Kefzol Vials, ADD-Vantage 1951

Cefoperazone Sodium (Increased prothrombin time response). Products include:
Cefobid Pharmacy Bulk Package - Not for Direct Infusion 2673

Cefotetan (Increased prothrombin time response). Products include:
Cefotan 664

Cefoxitin Sodium (Increased prothrombin time response). Products include:
Mefoxin for Injection 2124
Mefoxin Premixed Intravenous Solution 2127

Ceftriaxone Sodium (Increased prothrombin time response). Products include:
Rocephin Injectable Vials, ADD-Vantage, Galaxy, Bulk 2993

Celecoxib (Increased prothrombin time response; caution should be observed when used concurrently). Products include:
Celebrex Capsules 2676
Celebrex Capsules 2780

Cetirizine Hydrochloride (Decreased prothrombin time response). Products include:
Zyrtec 2756
Zyrtec-D 12 Hour Extended Relief Tablets 2758

Chamaemelum nobile (Co-administration with botanicals that contain coumarins, such as chamomile, may result in increased anticoagulant effects).
No products indexed under this heading.

Chenodiol (Increased prothrombin time response).
No products indexed under this heading.

Chloral Hydrate (Increased or decreased prothrombin time response).
No products indexed under this heading.

Chloramphenicol (Increased prothrombin time response). Products include:
Chloromycetin Ophthalmic Ointment, 1% ⊙296
Chloromycetin Ophthalmic Solution ⊙297
Chloroptic Sterile Ophthalmic Ointment ⊙234
Chloroptic Sterile Ophthalmic Solution ⊙235

Chloramphenicol Palmitate (Increased prothrombin time response).
No products indexed under this heading.

Chloramphenicol Sodium Succinate (Increased prothrombin time response).
No products indexed under this heading.

Chlordiazepoxide (Decreased prothrombin time response). Products include:
Limbitrol 1738

Chlordiazepoxide Hydrochloride (Decreased prothrombin time response). Products include:
Librium Capsules 1736
Librium for Injection 1737

Chlorothiazide (Increased prothrombin time response). Products include:
Aldoclor Tablets 2035
Diuril Oral 2087

Chlorothiazide Sodium (Increased prothrombin time response). Products include:
Diuril Sodium Intravenous 2086

Chlorpheniramine Maleate (Decreased prothrombin time response). Products include:
Actifed Cold & Sinus Caplets and Tablets ■688
Alka-Seltzer Plus Liqui-Gels ■604
BC Allergy Sinus Cold Powder ■619
Chlor-Trimeton Allergy Tablets ■735
Chlor-Trimeton Allergy/Decongestant Tablets ■736
Comtrex Flu Therapy & Fever Relief Nighttime Tablets ■628
Comtrex Maximum Strength Multi-Symptom Cold & Cough Relief Tablets and Caplets ■626
Contac Severe Cold and Flu Caplets Maximum Strength ■746
Coricidin 'D' Cold, Flu & Sinus Tablets ■737
Coricidin/Coricidin D ■738
Coricidin HBP Maximum Strength Flu Tablets ■738
Extendryl 1361
Hycomine Compound Tablets 1317
Kronofed-A 1341
PediaCare Cough-Cold Liquid ■719
PediaCare NightRest Cough-Cold Liquid ■719
Robitussin Nighttime Honey Flu Liquid ■786
Ryna ■768
Singlet Caplets ■761
Sinutab Sinus Allergy Medication, Maximum Strength Formula, Tablets & Caplets ■707
Sudafed Cold & Allergy Tablets ■708
TheraFlu Regular Strength Cold & Cough Night Time Hot Liquid ■676
TheraFlu Regular Strength Cold & Sore Throat Night Time Hot Liquid ■676
TheraFlu Maximum Strength Flu & Cough Night Time Hot Liquid ■678
TheraFlu Maximum Strength Flu & Sore Throat Night Time Hot Liquid ■677
TheraFlu Maximum Strength Severe Cold & Congestion Night Time Caplets ■678
TheraFlu Maximum Strength Severe Cold & Congestion Night Time Hot Liquid ■678
Triaminic Cold & Allergy Liquid ■681
Triaminic Cold & Allergy Softchews ■683
Triaminic Cold & Cough Liquid ■681
Triaminic Cold & Cough Softchews ■683
Triaminic Cold & Night Time Cough Liquid ■681
Triaminic Cold, Cough & Fever Liquid ■681
Children's Tylenol Cold Suspension Liquid and Chewable Tablets 2015
Children's Tylenol Cold Plus Cough Suspension Liquid and Chewable Tablets 2015
Children's Tylenol Flu Suspension Liquid 2015
Maximum Strength Tylenol Allergy Sinus Caplets, Gelcaps, and Geltabs 2010
Multi-Symptom Tylenol Cold Complete Formula Caplets 2010
Vicks 44M Cough, Cold & Flu Relief Liquid ■725
Pediatric Vicks 44m Cough & Cold Relief ■728
Children's Vicks NyQuil Cold/Cough Relief ■726

Chlorpheniramine Polistirex (Decreased prothrombin time response). Products include:
Tussionex Pennkinetic Extended-Release Suspension 1174

Chlorpheniramine Tannate (Decreased prothrombin time response). Products include:
Reformulated Rynatan Pediatric Suspension 3352
Rynatuss Pediatric Suspension 3353
Rynatuss Tablets 3353
Tussi-12 S Suspension 3356
Tussi-12 Tablets 3356

Chlorpropamide (Increased prothrombin time response; chlorpropamide may accumulate in the body as a result of interference with its metabolism or excretion). Products include:
Diabinese Tablets 2680

Chlorthalidone (Increased or decreased prothrombin time response). Products include:
Clorpres Tablets 1002
Combipres Tablets 1040
Tenoretic Tablets 690

Cholestyramine (Increased or decreased prothrombin time response).
No products indexed under this heading.

Choline Magnesium Trisalicylate (Increased prothrombin time response; caution should be observed when used concurrently). Products include:
Trilisate 2901

Cimetidine (Increased prothrombin time response). Products include:
Tagamet HB 200 Suspension ■762
Tagamet HB 200 Tablets ■761
Tagamet Tablets 1644

Cimetidine Hydrochloride (Increased prothrombin time response). Products include:
Tagamet 1644

Ciprofloxacin (Increased prothrombin time response). Products include:
Cipro I.V. 893
Cipro I.V. Pharmacy Bulk Package 897
Cipro Oral Suspension 887

Ciprofloxacin Hydrochloride (Increased prothrombin time response). Products include:
Ciloxan 538
Cipro HC Otic Suspension 540
Cipro Tablets 887

Cisapride (Increased prothrombin time response).
No products indexed under this heading.

Citalopram Hydrobromide (Increased prothrombin time response). Products include:
Celexa 1365

Clarithromycin (Increased prothrombin time response). Products include:
Biaxin/Biaxin XL 403
PREVPAC 3298

Clemastine Fumarate (Decreased prothrombin time response). Products include:
Tavist 12 Hour Allergy Tablets ■676

Clofibrate (Increased prothrombin time response). Products include:
Atromid-S Capsules 3483

Coenzyme Q-10 (Co-administration is associated most often with decreased effects of warfarin). Products include:
Cardio Essentials Capsules 3321
Centrum Focused Formulas Heart Tablets ■816
CoQuinone Capsules 3335

Cortisone Acetate (Decreased or increased prothrombin time response). Products include:
Cortone Acetate Injectable Suspension 2059
Cortone Acetate Tablets 2061

Cyclophosphamide (Increased or decreased prothrombin time response).
No products indexed under this heading.

Cyproheptadine Hydrochloride (Decreased prothrombin time response). Products include:
Periactin Tablets 2155

Danazol (Increased prothrombin time response).
No products indexed under this heading.

Danshen (Increased prothrombin time response).
No products indexed under this heading.

Daucus carota (Co-administration with botanicals that contain coumarins, such as wild carrots, may result in increased anticoagulant effects).
No products indexed under this heading.

Desflurane (Increased prothrombin time response). Products include:
Suprane Liquid for Inhalation 874

Desogestrel (Decreased prothrombin time response). Products include:
Cyclessa Tablets 2450
Desogen Tablets 2458
Mircette Tablets 2470
Ortho-Cept 21 Tablets 2546
Ortho-Cept 28 Tablets 2546

Dexamethasone (Decreased prothrombin time response). Products include:
Decadron Elixir 2078
Decadron Tablets 2079
TobraDex Ophthalmic Ointment 542
TobraDex Ophthalmic Suspension 541

Dexamethasone Acetate (Decreased prothrombin time response).
No products indexed under this heading.

Dexamethasone Sodium Phosphate (Decreased prothrombin time response). Products include:
Decadron Phosphate Injection 2081
Decadron Phosphate Sterile Ophthalmic Ointment 2083
Decadron Phosphate Sterile Ophthalmic Solution 2084
NeoDecadron Sterile Ophthalmic Solution 2144

Dexchlorpheniramine Maleate (Decreased prothrombin time response).
No products indexed under this heading.

Dextrans (Low Molecular Weight) (Increased prothrombin time response).
No products indexed under this heading.

Diazoxide (Increased prothrombin time response).
No products indexed under this heading.

Diclofenac Potassium (Increased prothrombin time response; caution should be observed when used concurrently). Products include:
Cataflam Tablets 2315

Diclofenac Sodium (Increased prothrombin time response; caution should be observed when used concurrently). Products include:
Arthrotec Tablets 3195
Voltaren Ophthalmic Sterile Ophthalmic Solution ⊙312
Voltaren Tablets 2315
Voltaren-XR Tablets 2315

Dicloxacillin Sodium (Decreased prothrombin time response).
No products indexed under this heading.

Dicumarol (Increased prothrombin time response).
No products indexed under this heading.

Diflunisal (Increased prothrombin time response; caution should be observed when used concurrently). Products include:
Dolobid Tablets 2088

Diphenhydramine Citrate (Decreased prothrombin time response). Products include:
Alka-Seltzer PM Effervescent Tablets ■605
Benadryl Allergy & Sinus Fastmelt Tablets ■693
Benadryl Children's Allergy/Cold Fastmelt Tablets ■692
Excedrin PM Tablets, Caplets, and Geltabs ■631
Goody's PM Powder ■621

Diphenhydramine Hydrochloride (Decreased prothrombin time response). Products include:
Extra Strength Bayer PM Caplets ■611
Benadryl Allergy Chewables ■689
Benadryl Allergy ■691

Benadryl Allergy Liquid 690
Benadryl Allergy/Cold Tablets 691
Benadryl Allergy/Congestion Tablets 692
Benadryl Allergy & Sinus Liquid 693
Benadryl Allergy Sinus Headache Caplets & Gelcaps 693
Benadryl Severe Allergy & Sinus Headache Caplets 694
Benadryl Dye-Free Allergy Liquid 690
Benadryl Dye-Free Allergy Liqui-Gels Softgels 690
Benadryl Itch Relief Stick Extra Strength 695
Benadryl Cream 695
Benadryl Gel 695
Benadryl Spray 696
Benadryl Parenteral 2617
Coricidin HBP Night-Time Cold & Flu Tablets 738
Nytol QuickCaps Caplets 622
Maximum Strength Nytol QuickGels Softgels 621
Extra Strength Percogesic Aspirin-Free Coated Caplets 665
Simply Sleep Caplets 2008
Sominex Original Formula Tablets 761
Children's Tylenol Allergy-D Liquid 2014
Maximum Strength Tylenol Allergy Sinus NightTime Caplets 2010
Tylenol Severe Allergy Caplets 2010
Maximum Strength Tylenol Flu NightTime Gelcaps 2011
Extra Strength Tylenol PM Caplets, Geltabs, and Gelcaps 2012
Unisom Maximum Strength SleepGels 713

Diphenylpyraline Hydrochloride (Decreased prothrombin time response).
No products indexed under this heading.

Dipteryx odorata (Co-administration with botanicals that contain coumarins, such as tonka beans, may result in increased anticoagulant effects).
No products indexed under this heading.

Dirithromycin (Increased prothrombin time response). Products include:
Dynabac Tablets 2269

Disulfiram (Increased prothrombin time response). Products include:
Antabuse Tablets 2444
Antabuse Tablets 3474

Divalproex Sodium (Increased prothrombin time response). Products include:
Depakote Sprinkle Capsules 426
Depakote Tablets 430
Depakote ER Tablets 436

Dong Quai (Co-administration with botanicals that contain coumarins, such as dong quai (angelica), may result in increased anticoagulant effects).
No products indexed under this heading.

Doxycycline Calcium (Increased prothrombin time response). Products include:
Vibramycin Calcium Oral Suspension Syrup 2735

Doxycycline Hyclate (Increased prothrombin time response). Products include:
Doryx Coated Pellet Filled Capsules 3357
Periostat Tablets 1208
Vibramycin Hyclate Capsules 2735
Vibramycin Hyclate Intravenous 2737
Vibra-Tabs Film Coated Tablets 2735

Doxycycline Monohydrate (Increased prothrombin time response). Products include:
Monodox Capsules 2442
Vibramycin Monohydrate for Oral Suspension 2735

Enflurane (Increased prothrombin time response).
No products indexed under this heading.

Enoxacin (Increased prothrombin time response).
No products indexed under this heading.

Erythromycin (Increased prothrombin time response). Products include:
Emgel 2% Topical Gel 1285
Ery-Tab Tablets 448
Erythromycin Base Filmtab Tablets 454
Erythromycin Delayed-Release Capsules, USP 455
PCE Dispertab Tablets 498

Erythromycin Estolate (Increased prothrombin time response).
No products indexed under this heading.

Erythromycin Ethylsuccinate (Increased prothrombin time response). Products include:
E.E.S. 450
EryPed 446
Pediazole Suspension 3050

Erythromycin Gluceptate (Increased prothrombin time response).
No products indexed under this heading.

Erythromycin Stearate (Increased prothrombin time response). Products include:
Erythrocin Stearate Filmtab Tablets 452

Ethacrynic Acid (Increased or decreased prothrombin time response). Products include:
Edecrin Tablets 2091

Ethchlorvynol (Decreased prothrombin time response).
No products indexed under this heading.

Ethinyl Estradiol (Decreased prothrombin time response). Products include:
Alesse-21 Tablets 3468
Alesse-28 Tablets 3473
Brevicon 28-Day Tablets 3380
Cyclessa Tablets 2450
Desogen Tablets 2458
Estinyl Tablets 3112
Estrostep 2627
femhrt Tablets 2635
Levlen 962
Levlite 21 Tablets 962
Levlite 28 Tablets 962
Levora Tablets 3389
Loestrin 21 Tablets 2642
Loestrin Fe Tablets 2642
Lo/Ovral Tablets 3532
Lo/Ovral-28 Tablets 3538
Low-Ogestrel-28 Tablets 3392
Microgestin Fe 1.5/30 Tablets 3407
Microgestin Fe 1/20 Tablets 3400
Mircette Tablets 2470
Modicon 2563
Necon 3415
Nordette-28 Tablets 2257
Norinyl 1 +35 28-Day Tablets 3380
Ogestrel 0.5/50-28 Tablets 3428
Ortho-Cept 21 Tablets 2546
Ortho-Cept 28 Tablets 2546
Ortho-Cyclen/Ortho Tri-Cyclen 2573
Ortho-Novum 2563
Ovcon 3364
Ovral Tablets 3551
Ovral-28 Tablets 3552
Tri-Levlen 962
Tri-Norinyl-28 Tablets 3433
Triphasil-21 Tablets 3600
Triphasil-28 Tablets 3605
Trivora Tablets 3439
Yasmin 28 Tablets 980
Zovia 3449

Ethynodiol Diacetate (Decreased prothrombin time response). Products include:
Zovia 3449

Etodolac (Increased prothrombin time response; caution should be observed when used concurrently). Products include:
Lodine 3528
Lodine XL Extended-Release Tablets 3530

Fenofibrate (Increased prothrombin time response). Products include:
Tricor Capsules, Micronized 513

Fenoprofen Calcium (Increased prothrombin time response; caution should be observed when used concurrently).
No products indexed under this heading.

Ferula foetida (Co-administration with botanicals that contain coumarins, such as asa foetida, may result in increased anticoagulant effects).
No products indexed under this heading.

Fexofenadine Hydrochloride (Decreased prothrombin time response). Products include:
Allegra 712
Allegra-D Extended-Release Tablets 714

Filipendula ulmaria (Co-administration with botanicals that contain coumarins and salicylate, such as meadowsweet, may result in increased anticoagulant effects).
No products indexed under this heading.

Fluconazole (Increased prothrombin time response). Products include:
Diflucan Tablets, Injection, and Oral Suspension 2681

Fludrocortisone Acetate (Decreased prothrombin time response). Products include:
Florinef Acetate Tablets 2250

Fluorouracil (Increased prothrombin time response). Products include:
Carac Cream 1222
Efudex 1733
Fluoroplex 552

Fluoxetine Hydrochloride (Increased prothrombin time response). Products include:
Prozac Pulvules, Liquid, and Weekly Capsules 1238
Sarafem Pulvules 1962

Flurbiprofen (Increased prothrombin time response; caution should be observed when used concurrently).
No products indexed under this heading.

Flutamide (Increased prothrombin time response). Products include:
Eulexin Capsules 3118

Fluvastatin Sodium (Increased prothrombin time response). Products include:
Lescol Capsules 2361
Lescol 2925
Lescol XL Tablets 2361

Fluvoxamine Maleate (Increased prothrombin time response). Products include:
Luvox Tablets (25, 50, 100 mg) 3256

Fosphenytoin Sodium (Increased or decreased prothrombin time; phenytoin may accumulate in the body as a result of interference with its metabolism or excretion). Products include:
Cerebyx Injection 2619

Fucus vesiculosus (Concurrent use may result in increased anticoagulant effects).
No products indexed under this heading.

Furosemide (Increased or decreased prothrombin time response). Products include:
Furosemide Tablets 2284

Galium odoratum (Co-administration with botanicals that contain coumarins, such as sweet woodruff, may result in increased anticoagulant effects).
No products indexed under this heading.

Garlic Extract (Co-administration is associated most often with increased effects of warfarin; garlic may cause bleeding events when taken alone and may have anticoagulant, antiplatelet, and/or fibrinolytic properties).
No products indexed under this heading.

Garlic Oil (Co-administration is associated most often with increased effects of warfarin; garlic may cause bleeding events when taken alone and may have anticoagulant, antiplatelet, and/or fibrinolytic properties). Products include:
One-A-Day Garlic Softgels 806

Gaultheria procumbens (Co-administration with botanicals that contain salicylate and/or have antiplatelet properties, such as wintergreen, may result in increased anticoagulant effects).
No products indexed under this heading.

Ginger (Co-administration with botanicals that contain salicylate and/or have antiplatelet properties, such as ginger, may result in increased anticoagulant effects).
No products indexed under this heading.

Ginkgo biloba (Co-administration is associated most often with increased effects of warfarin; Ginko biloba may cause bleeding events when taken alone and may have anticoagulant, antiplatelet, and/or fibrinolytic properties). Products include:
BioLean Free Tablets 843
Centrum Focused Formulas Mental Clarity Tablets 816
Centrum Ginkgo Biloba Softgels 852
CorePlex Capsules 796
DHEA Plus Capsules 844
Ginkoba Tablets 828
Ginkoba M/E Suppli-Cap Capsules 829
IntelleQ Capsules 797
One-A-Day Memory & Concentration Tablets 807
Phyto-Vite Tablets 849
ReSource Wellness EnVigor Caplets 824
ReSource Wellness MemorAble Softgels 825
Satiete Tablets 846
StePHan Clarity Capsules 844
StePHan Elixir Capsules 848

Ginseng (Co-administration with botanicals that contain salicylate and/or have antiplatelet properties, such as ginseng (Panax), may result in increased anticoagulant effects). Products include:
BioLean Free Tablets 843
Centrum Focused Formulas Energy Tablets 816
Centrum Ginseng Softgels 853
Ginkoba M/E Suppli-Cap Capsules 829
Ginsana 830
Metabolic Nutrition System 798
One-A-Day Energy Formula Tablets 806
Performance Gold Caplets 798
Performance Optimizer System 798
ReSource Wellness EnVigor Caplets 824
ReSource Wellness ResistEx Capsules 826
ReSource Wellness 2nd Wind Capsules 826
Vitasana Gelcaps 834

Glipizide (Increased prothrombin time response). Products include:
Glucotrol Tablets 2692
Glucotrol XL Extended Release Tablets 2693

Glucagon (Increased prothrombin time response). Products include:
GlucaGen for Injection Diagnostic Kit 949
Glucagon for Injection Vials and Emergency Kit 1924

Glutethimide (Decreased prothrombin time response).
No products indexed under this heading.

Glyburide (Increased prothrombin time response). Products include:
DiaBeta Tablets 741
Glucovance Tablets 1086

Grepafloxacin Hydrochloride (Increased prothrombin time response).
No products indexed under this heading.

IMPORTANT NOTE: Always consult each drug listing in the patient's regimen for possible interactions.

Griseofulvin (Decreased prothrombin time response). Products include:
Grifulvin V Tablets Microsize and Oral Suspension Microsize ... 2518
Gris-PEG Tablets ... 2661

Haloperidol (Decreased prothrombin time response). Products include:
Haldol Injection, Tablets and Concentrate ... 2533

Haloperidol Decanoate (Decreased prothrombin time response). Products include:
Haldol Decanoate ... 2535

Halothane (Increased prothrombin time response). Products include:
Fluothane Inhalation ... 3508

Heparin Sodium (Co-administration has resulted in cases of venous limb ischemia, necrosis, and gangrene in patients with heparin-induced thrombocytopneia and deep venous thrombosis when heparin treatment was discontinued and warfarin therapy was started or continued; sequelae have included amputation of the involved limb and/or death). Products include:
Heparin Lock Flush Solution ... 3509
Heparin Sodium Injection ... 3511

Horse Chestnut Seed Extract (Co-administration with botanicals that contain coumarins, such as horse chestnut, may result in increased anticoagulant effects). Products include:
Venastat Suppli-Cap Capsules ... ■□833

Hydrastis canadensis (Co-administration with botanicals with coagulant properties, such as goldenseal, may affect the anticoagulant effects of warfarin).
No products indexed under this heading.

Hydrochlorothiazide (Increased prothrombin time response). Products include:
Accuretic Tablets ... 2614
Aldoril Tablets ... 2039
Atacand HCT Tablets ... 597
Avalide Tablets ... 1070
Diovan HCT Tablets ... 2338
Dyazide Capsules ... 1515
HydroDIURIL Tablets ... 2108
Hyzaar ... 2109
Inderide Tablets ... 3517
Inderide LA Long-Acting Capsules ... 3519
Lotensin HCT Tablets ... 2367
Maxzide ... 1008
Micardis HCT Tablets ... 1051
Microzide Capsules ... 3414
Moduretic Tablets ... 2138
Monopril HCT ... 1094
Prinzide Tablets ... 2168
Timolide Tablets ... 2187
Uniretic Tablets ... 3178
Vaseretic Tablets ... 2204
Zestoretic Tablets ... 695
Ziac Tablets ... 1887

Hydrocortisone (Decreased prothrombin time response). Products include:
Anusol-HC Cream 2.5% ... 2237
Cipro HC Otic Suspension ... 540
Cortaid Intensive Therapy Cream ... ■□717
Cortaid Maximum Strength Cream ... ■□717
Cortisporin Ophthalmic Suspension Sterile ... ⊙297
Cortizone•5 ... ■□699
Cortizone•10 ... ■□699
Cortizone•10 Plus Creme ... ■□700
Cortizone for Kids Creme ... ■□699
Hydrocortone Tablets ... 2106
Massengill Medicated Soft Cloth Towelette ... ■□753
VōSoL HC Otic Solution ... 3356

Hydrocortisone Acetate (Decreased prothrombin time response). Products include:
Analpram-HC ... 1338
Anusol HC-1 Hydrocortisone Anti-Itch Cream ... ■□689
Anusol-HC Suppositories ... 2238
Cortaid ... ■□717
Cortifoam Rectal Foam ... 3170
Cortisporin-TC Otic Suspension ... 2246
Hydrocortone Acetate Injectable Suspension ... 2103
Pramosone ... 1343
Proctocort Suppositories ... 2264
ProctoFoam-HC ... 3177
Terra-Cortril Ophthalmic Suspension ... 2716

Hydrocortisone Sodium Phosphate (Decreased prothrombin time response). Products include:
Hydrocortone Phosphate Injection, Sterile ... 2105

Hydrocortisone Sodium Succinate (Decreased prothrombin time response).
No products indexed under this heading.

Hydroflumethiazide (Increased prothrombin time response). Products include:
Diucardin Tablets ... 3494

Hypericum (Co-administration is associated most often with decreased effects of warfarin). Products include:
Brite-Life Caplets ... ■□795
Centrum St. John's Wort Softgels ... ■□853
Metabolic Nutrition System ... ■□798
Movana Tablets ... ■□832
One-A-Day Tension & Mood Softgels ... ■□808
ReSource Wellness StayCalm Caplets ... ■□826
Satiete Tablets ... ■□846

Ibuprofen (Increased prothrombin time response; caution should be observed when used concurrently). Products include:
Advil ... ■□771
Children's Advil Oral Suspension ... ■□773
Children's Advil Chewable Tablets ... ■□773
Advil Cold and Sinus Caplets ... ■□771
Advil Cold and Sinus Tablets ... ■□771
Advil Flu & Body Ache Caplets ... ■□772
Infants' Advil Drops ... ■□773
Junior Strength Advil Tablets ... ■□773
Junior Strength Advil Chewable Tablets ... ■□773
Advil Migraine Liquigels ... ■□772
Children's Motrin Oral Suspension and Chewable Tablets ... 2006
Children's Motrin Cold Oral Suspension ... 2007
Children's Motrin Oral Suspension ... ■□643
Motrin Suspension, Oral Drops, Chewable Tablets, and Caplets ... 2002
Infants' Motrin Concentrated Drops ... 2006
Junior Strength Motrin Caplets and Chewable Tablets ... 2006
Motrin IB Tablets, Caplets, and Gelcaps ... 2002
Motrin Migraine Pain Caplets ... 2005
Motrin Sinus Headache Caplets ... 2005
Vicoprofen Tablets ... 520

Ifosfamide (Increased prothrombin time response). Products include:
Ifex for Injection ... 1123

Indapamide (Increased or decreased prothrombin time response). Products include:
Indapamide Tablets ... 2286

Indomethacin (Increased prothrombin time response; caution should be observed when used concurrently). Products include:
Indocin ... 2112

Indomethacin Sodium Trihydrate (Increased prothrombin time response; caution should be observed when used concurrently). Products include:
Indocin I.V. ... 2115

Influenza Virus Vaccine (Increased prothrombin time response). Products include:
FluShield Influenza Vaccine ... 3521
Fluzone Vaccine ... 802

Inositol Nicotinate (Co-administration with botanicals that contain salicylate and/or have antiplatelet properties, such as inositol nicotinate, may result in increased anticoagulant effects).
No products indexed under this heading.

Isoflurane (Increased prothrombin time response).
No products indexed under this heading.

Itraconazole (Increased prothrombin time response). Products include:
Sporanox Capsules ... 1800
Sporanox Injection ... 1804
Sporanox Injection ... 2509
Sporanox Oral Solution ... 1808
Sporanox Oral Solution ... 2512

Kanamycin Sulfate (Increased prothrombin time response).
No products indexed under this heading.

Ketoprofen (Increased prothrombin time response; caution should be observed when used concurrently). Products include:
Orudis Capsules ... 3548
Orudis KT Tablets ... ■□778
Oruvail Capsules ... 3548

Ketorolac Tromethamine (Increased prothrombin time response; caution should be observed when used concurrently). Products include:
Acular Ophthalmic Solution ... 544
Acular PF Ophthalmic Solution ... 544
Toradol ... 3018

Levamisole Hydrochloride (Increased prothrombin time response). Products include:
Ergamisol Tablets ... 1789

Levonorgestrel (Decreased prothrombin time response). Products include:
Alesse-21 Tablets ... 3468
Alesse-28 Tablets ... 3473
Levlen ... 962
Levlite 21 Tablets ... 962
Levlite 28 Tablets ... 962
Levora Tablets ... 3389
Mirena Intrauterine System ... 974
Nordette-28 Tablets ... 2257
Norplant System ... 3543
Tri-Levlen ... 962
Triphasil-21 Tablets ... 3600
Triphasil-28 Tablets ... 3605
Trivora Tablets ... 3439

Levothyroxine Sodium (Increased prothrombin time response). Products include:
Levothroid Tablets ... 1373
Levoxyl Tablets ... 1819
Synthroid ... 505
Unithroid Tablets ... 3445

Licorice (Co-administration with botanicals that contain coumarins, such as licorice, may result in increased anticoagulant effects; licorice also has antiplatelet properties).

Liothyronine Sodium (Increased prothrombin time response). Products include:
Cytomel Tablets ... 1817
Triostat Injection ... 1825

Liotrix (Increased prothrombin time response).
No products indexed under this heading.

Lomefloxacin Hydrochloride (Increased prothrombin time response).
No products indexed under this heading.

Loratadine (Decreased prothrombin time response). Products include:
Claritin ... 3100
Claritin-D 12 Hour Extended Release Tablets ... 3102
Claritin-D 24 Hour Extended Release Tablets ... 3104

Lovastatin (Increased prothrombin time response). Products include:
Mevacor Tablets ... 2132

Magaldrate (Decreased prothrombin time response).
No products indexed under this heading.

Magnesium Hydroxide (Decreased prothrombin time response). Products include:
Ex•Lax Milk of Magnesia Liquid ... ■□670
Maalox Antacid/Anti-Gas Oral Suspension ... ■□673
Maalox Max Maximum Strength Antacid/Anti-Gas Liquid ... 2300
Maalox Regular Strength Antacid/Antigas Liquid ... 2300
Mylanta Fast-Acting ... 1813
Mylanta ... 1813
Pepcid Complete Chewable Tablets ... 1815
Phillips' Chewable Tablets ... ■□615
Phillips' Milk of Magnesia Liquid (Original, Cherry, & Mint) ... ■□616
Rolaids Tablets ... ■□706
Extra Strength Rolaids Tablets ... ■□706
Vanquish Caplets ... ■□617

Magnesium Oxide (Decreased prothrombin time response). Products include:
Beelith Tablets ... 946
Mag-Ox 400 Tablets ... 1024
Uro-Mag Capsules ... 1024

Magnesium Salicylate (Increased prothrombin time response; caution should be observed when used concurrently). Products include:
Momentum Backache Relief Extra Strength Caplets ... ■□666

Meclofenamate Sodium (Increased prothrombin time response; caution should be observed when used concurrently).
No products indexed under this heading.

Medicago sativa (Co-administration with botanicals that contain coumarins, such as alfalfa, may result in increased anticoagulant effects).
No products indexed under this heading.

Mefenamic Acid (Increased prothrombin time response; caution should be observed when used concurrently). Products include:
Ponstel Capsules ... 1356

Melilotus officinalis (Co-administration with botanicals that contain coumarins, such as sweet clover, may result in increased anticoagulant effects).
No products indexed under this heading.

Meloxicam (Increased prothrombin time response; caution should be observed when used concurrently). Products include:
Mobic Tablets ... 1054

Menyanthes trifoliata (Co-administration with botanicals that contain coumarins, such as bog bean, may result in increased anticoagulant effects).
No products indexed under this heading.

Mephobarbital (Decreased prothrombin time response).
No products indexed under this heading.

Meprobamate (Decreased prothrombin time response). Products include:
Miltown Tablets ... 3349

Mercaptopurine (Decreased prothrombin time response). Products include:
Purinethol Tablets ... 1615

Mestranol (Decreased prothrombin time response). Products include:
Necon 1/50 Tablets ... 3415
Norinyl 1 + 50 28-Day Tablets ... 3380
Ortho-Novum 1/50□28 Tablets ... 2556

Methdilazine Hydrochloride (Decreased prothrombin time response).
No products indexed under this heading.

Methimazole (Increased or decreased prothrombin time response).
No products indexed under this heading.

Methoxyflurane (Increased prothrombin time response).
No products indexed under this heading.

Methyclothiazide (Increased prothrombin time response).
No products indexed under this heading.

Methyl Salicylate (Increased prothrombin time response). Products include:
BenGay External Analgesic Products .... ◙696
Listerine Mouthrinse .... ◙702
Cool Mint Listerine Mouthrinse .... ◙702
FreshBurst Listerine Mouthrinse .... ◙702
Tartar Control Listerine Mouthrinse .... ◙702
Thera-Gesic Creme 2233

Methyldopa (Increased prothrombin time response). Products include:
Aldoclor Tablets 2035
Aldomet Tablets 2037
Aldoril Tablets 2039

Methyldopate Hydrochloride (Increased prothrombin time response).
No products indexed under this heading.

Methylphenidate Hydrochloride (Increased prothrombin time response). Products include:
Concerta Extended-Release Tablets 1998
Concerta Tablets 561
Metadate CD Capsules 1164
Metadate ER Tablets 1167
Methylin Tablets 1995
Methylin ER Tablets 1995
Ritalin 2387

Methylprednisolone Acetate (Decreased prothrombin time response). Products include:
Depo-Medrol Injectable Suspension 2795

Methylprednisolone Sodium Succinate (Decreased prothrombin time response). Products include:
Solu-Medrol Sterile Powder 2855

Metolazone (Increased or decreased prothrombin time response). Products include:
Mykrox Tablets 1168
Zaroxolyn Tablets 1177

Metronidazole (Increased prothrombin time response). Products include:
MetroCream 1404
MetroGel 1405
MetroGel-Vaginal Gel 1986
MetroLotion 1405
Noritate Cream 1224

Metronidazole Hydrochloride (Increased prothrombin time response).
No products indexed under this heading.

Miconazole (Increased prothrombin time response).
No products indexed under this heading.

Mistletoe (Co-administration with botanicals with coagulant properties, such as mistletoe, may affect the anticoagulant effects of warfarin).
No products indexed under this heading.

Montelukast Sodium (May be responsible, alone or in combination, for increased prothrombin time/international normalized ratio (PT/INR) response). Products include:
Singulair 2181

Moricizine Hydrochloride (Increased prothrombin time response).
No products indexed under this heading.

Moxifloxacin Hydrochloride (Increased prothrombin time response). Products include:
Avelox Tablets 879

Nabumetone (Increased prothrombin time response; caution should be observed when used concurrently). Products include:
Relafen Tablets 1617

Nafcillin Sodium (Decreased prothrombin time response).
No products indexed under this heading.

Nalidixic Acid (Increased prothrombin time response).
No products indexed under this heading.

Naproxen (Increased prothrombin time response; caution should be observed when used concurrently). Products include:
EC-Naprosyn Delayed-Release Tablets 2967
Naprosyn Suspension 2967
Naprosyn Tablets 2967

Naproxen Sodium (Increased prothrombin time response; caution should be observed when used concurrently). Products include:
Aleve Tablets, Caplets and Gelcaps .... ◙602
Aleve Cold & Sinus Caplets .... ◙603
Anaprox Tablets 2967
Anaprox DS Tablets 2967
Naprelan Tablets 1293

Neomycin, oral (Increased prothrombin time response).
No products indexed under this heading.

Nettle (Co-administration with botanicals that contain coumarins, such as nettle, may result in increased anticoagulant effects).
No products indexed under this heading.

Nilutamide (Increased prothrombin time response). Products include:
Nilandron Tablets 753

Norethindrone (Decreased prothrombin time response). Products include:
Brevicon 28-Day Tablets 3380
Micronor Tablets 2543
Modicon 2563
Necon 3415
Norinyl 1 +35 28-Day Tablets 3380
Norinyl 1 + 50 28-Day Tablets 3380
Nor-QD Tablets 3423
Ortho-Novum 2563
Ortho-Novum 1/50□28 Tablets 2556
Ovcon 3364
Tri-Norinyl-28 Tablets 3433

Norethynodrel (Decreased prothrombin time response).
No products indexed under this heading.

Norfloxacin (Increased prothrombin time response). Products include:
Chibroxin Sterile Ophthalmic Solution 2051
Noroxin Tablets 2145

Norgestimate (Decreased prothrombin time response). Products include:
Ortho-Cyclen/Ortho Tri-Cyclen 2573
Ortho-Prefest Tablets 2570

Norgestrel (Decreased prothrombin time response). Products include:
Lo/Ovral Tablets 3532
Lo/Ovral-28 Tablets 3538
Low-Ogestrel-28 Tablets 3392
Ogestrel 0.5/50-28 Tablets 3428
Ovral Tablets 3551
Ovral-28 Tablets 3552
Ovrette Tablets 3552

Ofloxacin (Increased prothrombin time response). Products include:
Floxin I.V. 2526
Floxin Otic Solution 1219
Floxin Tablets 2529
Ocuflox Ophthalmic Solution 554

Olsalazine Sodium (Increased prothrombin time response). Products include:
Dipentum Capsules 2803

Omeprazole (Increased prothrombin time response). Products include:
Prilosec Delayed-Release Capsules 628

Oxaprozin (Increased prothrombin time response; caution should be observed when used concurrently).
No products indexed under this heading.

Paraldehyde (Decreased prothrombin time response).
No products indexed under this heading.

Paromomycin Sulfate (Increased prothrombin time response).
No products indexed under this heading.

Paroxetine Hydrochloride (Increased prothrombin time response). Products include:
Paxil 1609

Passiflora incarnata (Co-administration with botanicals that contain coumarins, such as passion flower, may result in increased anticoagulant effects).
No products indexed under this heading.

Pau d'arco (Concurrent use may result in increased anticoagulant effects).
No products indexed under this heading.

Penicillin G Potassium (Increased prothrombin time response). Products include:
Pfizerpen for Injection 2707

Penicillin G Sodium (Increased prothrombin time response).
No products indexed under this heading.

Pentobarbital Sodium (Decreased prothrombin time response). Products include:
Nembutal Sodium Solution 485

Pentoxifylline (Increased prothrombin time response). Products include:
Trental Tablets 784

Petroselinum crispum (Co-administration with botanicals that contain coumarins, such as parsley, may result in increased anticoagulant effects).
No products indexed under this heading.

Peumus boldus (Co-administration with botanicals that contain coumarins, such as boldo, may result in increased anticoagulant effects).
No products indexed under this heading.

Phenobarbital (Increased or decreased prothrombin time; phenobarbital may accumulate in the body as a result of interference with its metabolism or excretion). Products include:
Arco-Lase Plus Tablets 592
Donnatal 2929
Donnatal Extentabs 2930

Phenylbutazone (Increased prothrombin time response; caution should be observed when used concurrently).
No products indexed under this heading.

Phenytoin (Increased or decreased prothrombin time; phenytoin may accumulate in the body as a result of interference with its metabolism or excretion). Products include:
Dilantin Infatabs 2624
Dilantin-125 Oral Suspension 2625

Phenytoin Sodium (Increased or decreased prothrombin time; phenytoin may accumulate in the body as a result of interference with its metabolism or excretion). Products include:
Dilantin Kapseals 2622

Phytonadione (Decreased prothrombin time response).
No products indexed under this heading.

Piperacillin Sodium (Increased prothrombin time response). Products include:
Pipracil 1866
Zosyn 1890
Zosyn in Galaxy Containers 1894

Piroxicam (Increased prothrombin time response; caution should be observed when used concurrently). Products include:
Feldene Capsules 2685

Policosanol (Co-administration with botanicals that contain salicylate and/or have antiplatelet properties, such as policosanol, may result in increased anticoagulant effects).
No products indexed under this heading.

Polythiazide (Increased prothrombin time response). Products include:
Minizide Capsules 2700
Renese Tablets 2712

Populus species (Co-administration with botanicals that contain salicylate and/or have antiplatelet properties, such as poplar, may result in increased anticoagulant effects).
No products indexed under this heading.

Prednisolone Acetate (Decreased prothrombin time response). Products include:
Blephamide Ophthalmic Ointment 547
Blephamide Ophthalmic Suspension 548
Poly-Pred Liquifilm Ophthalmic Suspension .... ⊙245
Pred Forte Ophthalmic Suspension .... ⊙246
Pred Mild Sterile Ophthalmic Suspension .... ⊙249
Pred-G Ophthalmic Suspension .... ⊙247
Pred-G Sterile Ophthalmic Ointment .... ⊙248

Prednisolone Sodium Phosphate (Decreased prothrombin time response). Products include:
Pediapred Oral Solution 1170

Prednisolone Tebutate (Decreased prothrombin time response).
No products indexed under this heading.

Prednisone (Increased or decreased prothrombin time). Products include:
Prednisone 3064

Prickly Ash (Co-administration with botanicals that contain coumarins, such as prickly ash, may result in increased anticoagulant effects).
No products indexed under this heading.

Primidone (Decreased prothrombin time response).
No products indexed under this heading.

Promethazine Hydrochloride (Decreased prothrombin time response). Products include:
Mepergan Injection 3539
Phenergan Injection 3553
Phenergan 3556
Phenergan Syrup 3554
Phenergan with Codeine Syrup 3557
Phenergan with Dextromethorphan Syrup 3559
Phenergan VC Syrup 3560
Phenergan VC with Codeine Syrup 3561

Propafenone Hydrochloride (Increased prothrombin time response). Products include:
Rythmol Tablets – 150 mg, 225 mg, 300 mg 502

Propranolol Hydrochloride (Increased prothrombin time response). Products include:
Inderal 3513
Inderal LA Long-Acting Capsules 3516
Inderide Tablets 3517
Inderide LA Long-Acting Capsules 3519

Propylthiouracil (Increased or decreased prothrombin time response).
No products indexed under this heading.

Pyrilamine Maleate (Decreased prothrombin time response). Products include:
Maximum Strength Midol Menstrual Caplets and Gelcaps .... ◙612
Maximum Strength Midol PMS Caplets and Gelcaps .... ◙613

Pyrilamine Tannate (Decreased prothrombin time response). Products include:
Ryna-12 S Suspension 3351

Quassia amara (Co-administration with botanicals that contain coumarins, such as quassia, may result in increased anticoagulant effects).
No products indexed under this heading.

Quinidine Gluconate (Increased prothrombin time response). Products include:
Quinaglute Dura-Tabs Tablets 978

Quinidine Polygalacturonate (Increased prothrombin time response).
No products indexed under this heading.

Quinidine Sulfate (Increased prothrombin time response). Products include:
Quinidex Extentabs 2933

Quinine Sulfate (Increased prothrombin time response).
No products indexed under this heading.

Ranitidine Hydrochloride (Increased or decreased prothrombin time response). Products include:
Zantac 1690
Zantac Injection 1688
Zantac 75 Tablets .... ▣717

Rifampin (Decreased prothrombin time response). Products include:
Rifadin 765
Rifamate Capsules 767
Rifater Tablets 769

Rofecoxib (Increased prothrombin time response; caution should be observed when used concurrently). Products include:
Vioxx 2213

Salsalate (Increased prothrombin time response; caution should be observed when used concurrently).
No products indexed under this heading.

Sarsaparilla, German (Co-administration with botanicals that contain salicylate and/or have antiplatelet properties, such as German sarsaparilla, may result in increased anticoagulant effects).
No products indexed under this heading.

Secobarbital Sodium (Decreased prothrombin time response).
No products indexed under this heading.

Senega (Co-administration with botanicals that contain salicylate and/or have antiplatelet properties, such as senega, may result in increased anticoagulant effects).
No products indexed under this heading.

Sertraline Hydrochloride (Increased prothrombin time response). Products include:
Zoloft 2751

Simvastatin (Increased prothrombin time response). Products include:
Zocor Tablets 2219

Sodium Bicarbonate (Decreased prothrombin time response). Products include:
Alka-Seltzer .... ▣603
Alka-Seltzer Lemon Lime Antacid and Pain Reliever Effervescent Tablets .... ▣603
Alka-Seltzer Extra Strength Antacid and Pain Reliever Effervescent Tablets .... ▣603
Alka-Seltzer Heartburn Relief Tablets .... ▣604
Ceo-Two Evacuant Suppository .... ▣618
Colyte with Flavor Packs for Oral Solution..................................... 3170
GoLYTELY and Pineapple Flavor GoLYTELY for Oral Solution.......... 1068
NuLYTELY, Cherry Flavor, Lemon-Lime Flavor, and Orange Flavor NuLYTELY for Oral Solution.. 1068

Spironolactone (Increased or decreased prothrombin time response).
No products indexed under this heading.

Streptokinase (Co-administration is not recommended and may be hazardous; increased prothrombin time response). Products include:
Streptase for Infusion 647

Sucralfate (Decreased prothrombin time response). Products include:
Carafate Suspension 731
Carafate Tablets 730

Sulfacytine (Increased prothrombin time response).

Sulfamethizole (Increased prothrombin time response). Products include:
Urobiotic-250 Capsules 2731

Sulfamethoxazole (Increased prothrombin time response). Products include:
Bactrim 2949
Septra Suspension 2265
Septra Tablets 2265
Septra DS Tablets 2265

Sulfasalazine (Increased prothrombin time response). Products include:
Azulfidine EN-tabs Tablets 2775

Sulfinpyrazone (Increased prothrombin time response).
No products indexed under this heading.

Sulfisoxazole (Increased prothrombin time response).
No products indexed under this heading.

Sulfisoxazole Acetyl (Increased prothrombin time response). Products include:
Pediazole Suspension 3050

Sulfisoxazole Diolamine (Increased prothrombin time response).
No products indexed under this heading.

Sulindac (Increased prothrombin time response; caution should be observed when used concurrently). Products include:
Clinoril Tablets 2053

Syzygium aromaticum (Co-administration with botanicals that contain salicylate and/or have antiplatelet properties, such as clove, may result in increased anticoagulant effects).
No products indexed under this heading.

Tamarindus indica (Co-administration with botanicals that contain salicylate and/or have antiplatelet properties, such as tamarind, may result in increased anticoagulant effects).
No products indexed under this heading.

Tamoxifen Citrate (Increased prothrombin time response). Products include:
Nolvadex Tablets 678

Tanacetum parthenium (Co-administration with botanicals that contain salicylate and/or have antiplatelet properties, such as feverfew, may result in increased anticoagulant effects).
No products indexed under this heading.

Taraxacum officinale (Co-administration with botanicals that contain coumarins, such as dandelion, may result in increased anticoagulant effects; dandelion also has antiplatelet properties).
No products indexed under this heading.

Terfenadine (Increased prothrombin time response).
No products indexed under this heading.

Tetracycline Hydrochloride (Increased prothrombin time response).
No products indexed under this heading.

Tetrahydrozoline Hydrochloride (Increased prothrombin time response). Products include:
Murine Tears Plus Lubricant Redness Reliever Eye Drops....... ⊙323
Visine Original Eye Drops .... ⊙315
Visine A.C. Seasonal Relief From Pollen & Dust Eye Drops............ ⊙314
Advanced Relief Visine Eye Drops . ⊙313

Thiamylal Sodium (Decreased prothrombin time response).
No products indexed under this heading.

Thyroglobulin (Increased prothrombin time response).
No products indexed under this heading.

Thyroid (Increased prothrombin time response).
No products indexed under this heading.

Thyroxine (Increased prothrombin time response).
No products indexed under this heading.

Thyroxine Sodium (Increased prothrombin time response).
No products indexed under this heading.

Ticarcillin Disodium (Increased prothrombin time response). Products include:
Timentin Injection- ADD-Vantage Vial.. 1661
Timentin Injection-Galaxy Container 1664
Timentin Injection-Pharmacy Bulk Package...................................... 1666
Timentin for Intravenous Administration 1658

Ticlopidine Hydrochloride (Co-administration may be associated with cholestatic hepatitis; increased prothrombin time response). Products include:
Ticlid Tablets 3015

Tolazamide (Increased prothrombin time response).
No products indexed under this heading.

Tolbutamide (Increased prothrombin time; tolbutamide may accumulate in the body as a result of interference with its metabolism or excretion).
No products indexed under this heading.

Tolmetin Sodium (Increased prothrombin time response; caution should be observed when used concurrently). Products include:
Tolectin 2589

Torsemide (Increased or decreased prothrombin time response). Products include:
Demadex Tablets and Injection 2965

Tramadol Hydrochloride (Increased prothrombin time response). Products include:
Ultracet Tablets 2597
Ultram Tablets 2600

Trazodone Hydrochloride (Decreased prothrombin time response).
No products indexed under this heading.

Triamcinolone (Decreased prothrombin time response).
No products indexed under this heading.

Triamcinolone Acetonide (Decreased prothrombin time response). Products include:
Azmacort Inhalation Aerosol 728
Nasacort Nasal Inhaler 750
Nasacort AQ Nasal Spray 752
Tri-Nasal Spray 2274

Triamcinolone Diacetate (Decreased prothrombin time response).
No products indexed under this heading.

Triamcinolone Hexacetonide (Decreased prothrombin time response).
No products indexed under this heading.

Triamterene (Increased or decreased prothrombin time response). Products include:
Dyazide Capsules 1515
Dyrenium Capsules 3458
Maxzide 1008

Trifolium pratense (Co-administration with botanicals that contain coumarins, such as red clover, may result in increased anticoagulant effects).
No products indexed under this heading.

Trigonella foenum-graecum (Co-administration with botanicals that contain coumarins, such as fenugreek, may result in increased anticoagulant effects).
No products indexed under this heading.

Trimeprazine Tartrate (Decreased prothrombin time response).
No products indexed under this heading.

Trimethoprim (Increased prothrombin time response). Products include:
Bactrim 2949
Septra Suspension 2265
Septra Tablets 2265
Septra DS Tablets 2265

Tripelennamine Hydrochloride (Decreased prothrombin time response).
No products indexed under this heading.

Triprolidine Hydrochloride (Decreased prothrombin time response). Products include:
Actifed Cold & Allergy Tablets .... ▣688

Troleandomycin (Increased prothrombin time response). Products include:
Tao Capsules 2716

Trovafloxacin Mesylate (Increased prothrombin time response). Products include:
Trovan Tablets 2722

Urokinase (Co-administration is not recommended and may be hazardous; increased prothrombin time response).
No products indexed under this heading.

Valproate Sodium (Increased prothrombin time response). Products include:
Depacon Injection 416

Valproic Acid (Increased prothrombin time response). Products include:
Depakene 421

Viburnum prunifolium (Co-administration with botanicals that contain salicylate and/or have antiplatelet properties, such as black haw, may result in increased anticoagulant effects).
No products indexed under this heading.

Vitamin C (Decreased prothrombin time response with concurrent high dose Vitamin C). Products include:
Beta-C Tablets .... ▣811
C-Grams Caplets .... ▣795
Halls Defense Drops .... ▣687
Peridin-C Tablets .... ▣618

Vitamin E (Increased prothrombin time response). Products include:
Nutr-E-Sol Liquid 526
One-A-Day Cholesterol Health Tablets .... ▣805

One-A-Day Menopause Health Tablets .... ▣808
StePHan Bio-Nutritional Daytime Hydrating Creme .... ▣770
StePHan Feminine Capsules .... ▣848
Unique E Vitamin E Capsules 1723

Vitamin K_1 (Decreased prothrombin time response). Products include:
AquaMEPHYTON Injection 2042
Mephyton Tablets 2129

Wild Lettuce (Co-administration with botanicals that contain coumarins, such as wild lettuce, may result in increased anticoagulant effects).
No products indexed under this heading.

Willow (Co-administration with botanicals that contain salicylate and/or have antiplatelet properties, such as willow, may result in increased anticoagulant effects).
No products indexed under this heading.

Zafirlukast (May be responsible, alone or in combination, for increased prothrombin time/international normalized ratio (PT/INR) response). Products include:
Accolate Tablets 657

Zileuton (May be responsible, alone or in combination, for increased prothrombin time/international normalized ratio (PT/INR) response). Products include:
Zyflo Filmtab Tablets 524

Food Interactions

Alcohol (Decreased or increased prothrombin time response).

Diet high in vitamin K (Decreased prothrombin time response).

Vegetables, green leafy (Decreased prothrombin time response).

WARM CREAM
(L-Arginine) .... ▣841
None cited in PDR database.

WART-OFF LIQUID
(Salicylic Acid) .... ▣716
None cited in PDR database.

WELCHOL TABLETS
(Colesevelam Hydrochloride) 3073
May interact with:

Verapamil Hydrochloride (Co-administration of sustained-release verapamil with colesevelam results in decreased Cmax and AUC of sustained-release verapamil by approximately 31% and 11%, respectively; because of high variability in the bioavailability of verapamil, the clinical significance of this finding is unclear). Products include:
Covera-HS Tablets 3199
Isoptin SR Tablets 467
Tarka Tablets 508
Verelan Capsules 3184
Verelan PM Capsules 3186

WELLBUTRIN TABLETS
(Bupropion Hydrochloride) 1680
See Wellbutrin SR Sustained-Release Tablets

WELLBUTRIN SR SUSTAINED-RELEASE TABLETS
(Bupropion Hydrochloride) 1684
May interact with corticosteroids, monoamine oxidase inhibitors, drugs which lower seizure threshold, and certain other agents. Compounds in these categories include:

Alprazolam (Bupropion is associated with a dose-related risk of seizures; co-administration with drugs that lower seizure threshold may increase the risk of seizure with bupropion; concurrent use should be undertaken with extreme caution). Products include:
Xanax Tablets 2865

Amitriptyline Hydrochloride (Bupropion is associated with a dose-related risk of seizures; co-administration with drugs that lower seizure threshold may increase the risk of seizure with bupropion; concurrent use should be undertaken with extreme caution). Products include:
Etrafon 3115
Limbitrol 1738

Amoxapine (Bupropion is associated with a dose-related risk of seizures; co-administration with drugs that lower seizure threshold may increase the risk of seizure with bupropion; concurrent use should be undertaken with extreme caution).
No products indexed under this heading.

Betamethasone Acetate (Bupropion is associated with a dose-related risk of seizures; co-administration with drugs that lower seizure threshold, such as systemic steroids, may increase the risk of seizure with bupropion). Products include:
Celestone Soluspan Injectable Suspension 3097

Betamethasone Sodium Phosphate (Bupropion is associated with a dose-related risk of seizures; co-administration with drugs that lower seizure threshold, such as systemic steroids, may increase the risk of seizure with bupropion). Products include:
Celestone Soluspan Injectable Suspension 3097

Bupropion (Patients should be made aware that both formulations of Wellbutrin contain the same active moiety found in Zyban, an aid to smoking cessation, combination is contraindicated).
No products indexed under this heading.

Carbamazepine (May induce the metabolism of bupropion). Products include:
Carbatrol Capsules 3234
Tegretol/Tegretol-XR 2404

Chlordiazepoxide (Bupropion is associated with a dose-related risk of seizures; co-administration with drugs that lower seizure threshold may increase the risk of seizure with bupropion; concurrent use should be undertaken with extreme caution). Products include:
Limbitrol 1738

Chlordiazepoxide Hydrochloride (Bupropion is associated with a dose-related risk of seizures; co-administration with drugs that lower seizure threshold may increase the risk of seizure with bupropion; concurrent use should be undertaken with extreme caution). Products include:
Librium Capsules 1736
Librium for Injection 1737

Chlorpromazine (Bupropion is associated with a dose-related risk of seizures; co-administration with drugs that lower seizure threshold may increase the risk of seizure with bupropion; concurrent use should be undertaken with extreme caution). Products include:
Thorazine Suppositories 1656

Chlorpromazine Hydrochloride (Bupropion is associated with a dose-related risk of seizures; co-administration with drugs that lower seizure threshold may increase the risk of seizure with bupropion; concurrent use should be undertaken with extreme caution). Products include:
Thorazine 1656

Cimetidine (May inhibit the metabolism of bupropion). Products include:
Tagamet HB 200 Suspension .... ▣762
Tagamet HB 200 Tablets .... ▣761
Tagamet Tablets 1644

Cimetidine Hydrochloride (May induce the metabolism of bupropion). Products include:
Tagamet 1644

Cortisone Acetate (Bupropion is associated with a dose-related risk of seizures; co-administration with drugs that lower seizure threshold, such as systemic steroids, may increase the risk of seizure with bupropion). Products include:
Cortone Acetate Injectable Suspension 2059
Cortone Acetate Tablets 2061

Cyclophosphamide (Bupropion is primarily metabolized, based on *in vitro* studies, to the morpholinol metabolite by cytochrome P450IIB6 isoenzyme, therefore the potential exists for a drug interaction with agents that affect the cytochrome P450IIB6 metabolism, such as cyclophosphamide).
No products indexed under this heading.

Desipramine Hydrochloride (Co-administration in male subjects who were extensive metabolizers of the CYP2D6 isoenzyme daily doses of bupropion followed by a single dose of desipramine increased the Cmax, AUC and t½ of desipramine by an average of approximately two-, five-, and two-fold, respectively; co-administration should be initiated at the lower end of the dose range of desipramine; potential for increased risk of seizures). Products include:
Norpramin Tablets 755

Dexamethasone (Bupropion is associated with a dose-related risk of seizures; co-administration with drugs that lower seizure threshold, such as systemic steroids, may increase the risk of seizure with bupropion). Products include:
Decadron Elixir 2078
Decadron Tablets 2079
TobraDex Ophthalmic Ointment 542
TobraDex Ophthalmic Suspension 541

Dexamethasone Acetate (Bupropion is associated with a dose-related risk of seizures; co-administration with drugs that lower seizure threshold, such as systemic steroids, may increase the risk of seizure with bupropion).
No products indexed under this heading.

Dexamethasone Sodium Phosphate (Bupropion is associated with a dose-related risk of seizures; co-administration with drugs that lower seizure threshold, such as systemic steroids, may increase the risk of seizure with bupropion). Products include:
Decadron Phosphate Injection 2081
Decadron Phosphate Sterile Ophthalmic Ointment 2083
Decadron Phosphate Sterile Ophthalmic Solution 2084
NeoDecadron Sterile Ophthalmic Solution 2144

Diazepam (Bupropion is associated with a dose-related risk of seizures; co-administration with drugs that lower seizure threshold may increase the risk of seizure with bupropion; concurrent use should be undertaken with extreme caution). Products include:
Valium Injectable 3026
Valium Tablets 3047

Doxepin Hydrochloride (Bupropion is associated with a dose-related risk of seizures; co-administration with drugs that lower seizure threshold may increase the risk of seizure with bupropion; concurrent use should be undertaken with extreme caution). Products include:
Sinequan 2713

Flecainide Acetate (Co-administration of bupropion with drugs that are metabolized by CYP2D6 isoenzyme, such as flecainide, may result in, based on data with desipramine, increased Cmax, AUC and t½; co-administration should be initiated at the lower end of the dose range of flecainide). Products include:
Tambocor Tablets 1990

Fludrocortisone Acetate (Bupropion is associated with a dose-related risk of seizures; co-administration with drugs that lower seizure threshold, such as systemic steroids, may increase the risk of seizure with bupropion). Products include:
Florinef Acetate Tablets 2250

Fluoxetine Hydrochloride (Co-administration of bupropion with drugs that are metabolized by CYP2D6 isoenzyme, such as fluoxetine, may result in, based on data with desipramine, increased Cmax, AUC and t½; co-administration should be initiated at the lower end of the dose range of fluoxetine). Products include:
Prozac Pulvules, Liquid, and Weekly Capsules 1238
Sarafem Pulvules 1962

Fluphenazine Decanoate (Bupropion is associated with a dose-related risk of seizures; co-administration with drugs that lower seizure threshold may increase the risk of seizure with bupropion; concurrent use should be undertaken with extreme caution).
No products indexed under this heading.

Fluphenazine Enanthate (Bupropion is associated with a dose-related risk of seizures; co-administration with drugs that lower seizure threshold may increase the risk of seizure with bupropion; concurrent use should be undertaken with extreme caution).
No products indexed under this heading.

Fluphenazine Hydrochloride (Bupropion is associated with a dose-related risk of seizures; co-administration with drugs that lower seizure threshold may increase the risk of seizure with bupropion; concurrent use should be undertaken with extreme caution).
No products indexed under this heading.

Fosphenytoin Sodium (May induce the metabolism of bupropion). Products include:
Cerebyx Injection 2619

Haloperidol (Co-administration of bupropion with drugs that are metabolized by CYP2D6 isoenzyme, such as haloperidol, may result in, based on data with desipramine, increased Cmax, AUC and t½; co-administration should be initiated at the lower end of the dose range of haloperidol; potential for increased risk of seizures). Products include:
Haldol Injection, Tablets and Concentrate 2533

Haloperidol Decanoate (Co-administration of bupropion with drugs that are metabolized by CYP2D6 isoenzyme, such as haloperidol, may result in, based on data with desipramine, increased Cmax, AUC and t½; co-administration should be initiated at the lower end of the dose range of haloperidol; potential for increased risk of seizures). Products include:
Haldol Decanoate 2535

Hydrocortisone (Bupropion is associated with a dose-related risk of seizures; co-administration with drugs that lower seizure threshold, such as systemic steroids, may increase the risk of seizure with bupropion). Products include:
Anusol-HC Cream 2.5% 2237
Cipro HC Otic Suspension 540
Cortaid Intensive Therapy Cream .... ▣717

Cortaid Maximum Strength Cream .... ▣717
Cortisporin Ophthalmic Suspension Sterile .... ⊙297
Cortizone•5 .... ▣699
Cortizone•10 .... ▣699
Cortizone•10 Plus Creme .... ▣700
Cortizone for Kids Creme .... ▣699
Hydrocortone Tablets 2106
Massengill Medicated Soft Cloth Towelette .... ▣753
VōSoL HC Otic Solution 3356

Hydrocortisone Acetate (Bupropion is associated with a dose-related risk of seizures; co-administration with drugs that lower seizure threshold, such as systemic steroids, may increase the risk of seizure with bupropion). Products include:
Analpram-HC 1338
Anusol HC-1 Hydrocortisone Anti-Itch Cream .... ▣689
Anusol-HC Suppositories 2238
Cortaid .... ▣717
Cortifoam Rectal Foam 3170
Cortisporin-TC Otic Suspension 2246
Hydrocortone Acetate Injectable Suspension 2103
Pramosone 1343
Proctocort Suppositories 2264
ProctoFoam-HC 3177
Terra-Cortril Ophthalmic Suspension 2716

Hydrocortisone Sodium Phosphate (Bupropion is associated with a dose-related risk of seizures; co-administration with drugs that lower seizure threshold, such as systemic steroids, may increase the risk of seizure with bupropion). Products include:
Hydrocortone Phosphate Injection, Sterile 2105

Hydrocortisone Sodium Succinate (Bupropion is associated with a dose-related risk of seizures; co-administration with drugs that lower seizure threshold, such as systemic steroids, may increase the risk of seizure with bupropion).
No products indexed under this heading.

Imipramine Hydrochloride (Co-administration of bupropion with drugs that are metabolized by CYP2D6 isoenzyme, such as imipramine, may result in, based on data with desipramine, increased Cmax, AUC and t½; co-administration should be initiated at the lower end of the dose range of imipramine; potential for increased risk of seizures).
No products indexed under this heading.

Imipramine Pamoate (Co-administration of bupropion with drugs that are metabolized by CYP2D6 isoenzyme, such as imipramine, may result in, based on data with desipramine, increased Cmax, AUC and t½; co-administration should be initiated at the lower end of the dose range of imipramine; potential for increased risk of seizures).
No products indexed under this heading.

Isocarboxazid (Concurrent and/or sequential use with MAO inhibitor is contraindicated).
No products indexed under this heading.

Levodopa (Co-administration has resulted in a higher incidence of adverse experiences). Products include:
Sinemet Tablets 1253
Sinemet CR Tablets 1255

Lorazepam (Bupropion is associated with a dose-related risk of seizures; co-administration with drugs that lower seizure threshold may increase the risk of seizure with bupropion; concurrent use should be undertaken with extreme caution). Products include:
Ativan Injection 3478
Ativan Tablets 3482

Maprotiline Hydrochloride (Bupropion is associated with a dose-related risk of seizures; co-administration with drugs that lower seizure threshold may increase the risk of seizure with bupropion; concurrent use should be undertaken with extreme caution).
No products indexed under this heading.

Mesoridazine Besylate (Bupropion is associated with a dose-related risk of seizures; co-administration with drugs that lower seizure threshold may increase the risk of seizure with bupropion; concurrent use should be undertaken with extreme caution). Products include:
Serentil 1057

Methylprednisolone Acetate (Bupropion is associated with a dose-related risk of seizures; co-administration with drugs that lower seizure threshold, such as systemic steroids, may increase the risk of seizure with bupropion). Products include:
Depo-Medrol Injectable Suspension 2795

Methylprednisolone Sodium Succinate (Bupropion is associated with a dose-related risk of seizures; co-administration with drugs that lower seizure threshold, such as systemic steroids, may increase the risk of seizure with bupropion). Products include:
Solu-Medrol Sterile Powder 2855

Metoprolol Succinate (Co-administration of bupropion with drugs that are metabolized by CYP2D6 isoenzyme, such as metoprolol, may result in, based on data with desipramine, increased Cmax, AUC and t½; co-administration should be initiated at the lower end of the dose range of metoprolol). Products include:
Toprol-XL Tablets 651

Metoprolol Tartrate (Co-administration of bupropion with drugs that are metabolized by CYP2D6 isoenzyme, such as metoprolol, may result in, based on data with desipramine, increased Cmax, AUC and t½; co-administration should be initiated at the lower end of the dose range of metoprolol).
No products indexed under this heading.

Moclobemide (Concurrent and/or sequential use with MAO inhibitor is contraindicated).
No products indexed under this heading.

Nicotine (Co-administration has resulted in a higher incidence of treatment-emergent hypertension). Products include:
Nicoderm CQ Patch 1717
Nicotrol Inhaler 2840
Nicotrol Nasal Spray 2843
Nicotrol Patch 2840

Nortriptyline Hydrochloride (Co-administration of bupropion with drugs that are metabolized by CYP2D6 isoenzyme, such as nortriptyline, may result in, based on data with desipramine, increased Cmax, AUC and t½; co-administration should be initiated at the lower end of the dose range of nortriptyline; potential for increased risk of seizures).
No products indexed under this heading.

Orphenadrine Citrate (Bupropion is primarily metabolized, based on *in vitro* studies, to the morpholinol metabolite by cytochrome P450IIB6 isoenzyme, therefore the potential exists for a drug interaction with agents that affect the cytochrome P450IIB6 metabolism, such as orphenadrine). Products include:
Norflex 1987

Oxazepam (Bupropion is associated with a dose-related risk of seizures; co-administration with drugs that lower seizure threshold may increase the risk of seizure with bupropion; concurrent use should be undertaken with extreme caution).
No products indexed under this heading.

Pargyline Hydrochloride (Concurrent and/or sequential use with MAO inhibitor is contraindicated).
No products indexed under this heading.

Paroxetine Hydrochloride (Co-administration of bupropion with drugs that are metabolized by CYP2D6 isoenzyme, such as paroxetine, may result in, based on data with desipramine, increased Cmax, AUC and t½; co-administration should be initiated at the lower end of the dose range of paroxetine). Products include:
Paxil 1609

Perphenazine (Bupropion is associated with a dose-related risk of seizures; co-administration with drugs that lower seizure threshold may increase the risk of seizure with bupropion; concurrent use should be undertaken with extreme caution). Products include:
Etrafon 3115
Trilafon 3160

Phenelzine Sulfate (Concurrent and/or sequential use with MAO inhibitor is contraindicated; acute toxicity of bupropion is enhanced by phenelzine in animal models). Products include:
Nardil Tablets 2653

Phenobarbital (May induce the metabolism of bupropion). Products include:
Arco-Lase Plus Tablets 592
Donnatal 2929
Donnatal Extentabs 2930

Phenytoin (May induce the metabolism of bupropion). Products include:
Dilantin Infatabs 2624
Dilantin-125 Oral Suspension 2625

Phenytoin Sodium (May induce the metabolism of bupropion). Products include:
Dilantin Kapseals 2622

Prazepam (Bupropion is associated with a dose-related risk of seizures; co-administration with drugs that lower seizure threshold may increase the risk of seizure with bupropion; concurrent use should be undertaken with extreme caution).
No products indexed under this heading.

Prednisolone Acetate (Bupropion is associated with a dose-related risk of seizures; co-administration with drugs that lower seizure threshold, such as systemic steroids, may increase the risk of seizure with bupropion). Products include:
Blephamide Ophthalmic Ointment 547
Blephamide Ophthalmic Suspension 548
Poly-Pred Liquifilm Ophthalmic Suspension .... ⊙245
Pred Forte Ophthalmic Suspension .... ⊙246
Pred Mild Sterile Ophthalmic Suspension .... ⊙249
Pred-G Ophthalmic Suspension .... ⊙247
Pred-G Sterile Ophthalmic Ointment .... ⊙248

Prednisolone Sodium Phosphate (Bupropion is associated with a dose-related risk of seizures; co-administration with drugs that lower seizure threshold, such as systemic steroids, may increase the risk of seizure with bupropion). Products include:
Pediapred Oral Solution 1170

Prednisolone Tebutate (Bupropion is associated with a dose-related risk of seizures; co-administration with drugs that lower seizure threshold, such as systemic steroids, may increase the risk of seizure with bupropion).
No products indexed under this heading.

Prednisone (Bupropion is associated with a dose-related risk of seizures; co-administration with drugs that lower seizure threshold, such as systemic steroids, may increase the risk of seizure with bupropion). Products include:
Prednisone 3064

Procarbazine Hydrochloride (Concurrent and/or sequential use with MAO inhibitor is contraindicated). Products include:
Matulane Capsules 3246

Prochlorperazine (Bupropion is associated with a dose-related risk of seizures; co-administration with drugs that lower seizure threshold may increase the risk of seizure with bupropion; concurrent use should be undertaken with extreme caution). Products include:
Compazine 1505

Promethazine Hydrochloride (Bupropion is associated with a dose-related risk of seizures; co-administration with drugs that lower seizure threshold may increase the risk of seizure with bupropion; concurrent use should be undertaken with extreme caution). Products include:
Mepergan Injection 3539
Phenergan Injection 3553
Phenergan 3556
Phenergan Syrup 3554
Phenergan with Codeine Syrup 3557
Phenergan with Dextromethorphan Syrup 3559
Phenergan VC Syrup 3560
Phenergan VC with Codeine Syrup 3561

Propafenone Hydrochloride (Co-administration of bupropion with drugs that are metabolized by CYP2D6 isoenzyme, such as propafenone, may result in, based on data with desipramine, increased Cmax, AUC and t½; co-administration should be initiated at the lower end of the dose range of propafenone). Products include:
Rythmol Tablets – 150 mg, 225 mg, 300 mg 502

Protriptyline Hydrochloride (Bupropion is associated with a dose-related risk of seizures; co-administration with drugs that lower seizure threshold may increase the risk of seizure with bupropion; concurrent use should be undertaken with extreme caution). Products include:
Vivactil Tablets 2446
Vivactil Tablets 2217

Risperidone (Co-administration of bupropion with drugs that are metabolized by CYP2D6 isoenzyme, such as risperidone, may result in, based on data with desipramine, increased Cmax, AUC and t½; co-administration should be initiated at the lower end of the dose range of risperidone; potential for increased risk of seizures). Products include:
Risperdal 1796

Selegiline Hydrochloride (Concurrent and/or sequential use with MAO inhibitor is contraindicated). Products include:
Eldepryl Capsules 3266

Sertraline Hydrochloride (Co-administration of bupropion with drugs that are metabolized by CYP2D6 isoenzyme, such as sertraline, may result in, based on data with desipramine, increased Cmax, AUC and t½; co-administration

should be initiated at the lower end of the dose range of sertraline). Products include:

Zoloft 2751

Thioridazine Hydrochloride (Co-administration of bupropion with drugs that are metabolized by CYP2D6 isoenzyme, such as thioridazine, may result in, based on data with desipramine, increased Cmax, AUC and t½; co-administration should be initiated at the lower end of the dose range of thioridazine; potential for increased risk of seizures). Products include:

Thioridazine Hydrochloride Tablets 2289

Tranylcypromine Sulfate (Concurrent and/or sequential use with MAO inhibitor is contraindicated). Products include:

Parnate Tablets 1607

Trazodone Hydrochloride (Bupropion is associated with a dose-related risk of seizures; co-administration with drugs that lower seizure threshold may increase the risk of seizure with bupropion; concurrent use should be undertaken with extreme caution).

No products indexed under this heading.

Triamcinolone (Bupropion is associated with a dose-related risk of seizures; co-administration with drugs that lower seizure threshold, such as systemic steroids, may increase the risk of seizure with bupropion).

No products indexed under this heading.

Triamcinolone Acetonide (Bupropion is associated with a dose-related risk of seizures; co-administration with drugs that lower seizure threshold, such as systemic steroids, may increase the risk of seizure with bupropion). Products include:

Azmacort Inhalation Aerosol 728
Nasacort Nasal Inhaler 750
Nasacort AQ Nasal Spray 752
Tri-Nasal Spray 2274

Triamcinolone Diacetate (Bupropion is associated with a dose-related risk of seizures; co-administration with drugs that lower seizure threshold, such as systemic steroids, may increase the risk of seizure with bupropion).

No products indexed under this heading.

Triamcinolone Hexacetonide (Bupropion is associated with a dose-related risk of seizures; co-administration with drugs that lower seizure threshold, such as systemic steroids, may increase the risk of seizure with bupropion).

No products indexed under this heading.

Trifluoperazine Hydrochloride (Bupropion is associated with a dose-related risk of seizures; co-administration with drugs that lower seizure threshold may increase the risk of seizure with bupropion; concurrent use should be undertaken with extreme caution). Products include:

Stelazine 1640

Trimipramine Maleate (Bupropion is associated with a dose-related risk of seizures; co-administration with drugs that lower seizure threshold may increase the risk of seizure with bupropion; concurrent use should be undertaken with extreme caution). Products include:

Surmontil Capsules 3595

Food Interactions

Alcohol (Use and cessation of use of alcohol may alter seizure threshold, and, therefore, the consumption of alcohol should be minimized or avoided completely).

Food, unspecified (Food increases Cmax and AUC of bupropion by 11% and 17%, respectively; no clinically significant food effect).

WINRGY DRINK MIX

(Amino Acid Preparations, Vitamins with Minerals) .... ■852
May interact with:

Aluminum Carbonate (Concomitant use with aluminum-containing antacids should be avoided).

No products indexed under this heading.

Aluminum Hydroxide (Concomitant use with aluminum-containing antacids should be avoided). Products include:

Amphojel Suspension (Mint Flavor) .... ■789
Gaviscon Extra Strength Liquid .... ■751
Gaviscon Extra Strength Tablets .... ■751
Gaviscon Regular Strength Liquid .... ■751
Gaviscon Regular Strength Tablets .... ■750
Maalox Antacid/Anti-Gas Oral Suspension .... ■673
Maalox Max Maximum Strength Antacid/Anti-Gas Liquid 2300
Maalox Regular Strength Antacid/Antigas Liquid 2300
Mylanta 1813
Vanquish Caplets .... ■617

WINRHO SDF

(Rh$_o$ (D) Immune Globulin (Human)) 2297
None cited in PDR database.

XALATAN LATANOPROST OPHTHALMIC SOLUTION

(Latanoprost) .... ⊙320
May interact with:

Thimerosal (*in vitro* studies have shown that precipitation occurs when eye drops containing thimerosal are mixed with Xalatan; administer with an interval of at least five minutes between applications).

No products indexed under this heading.

XALATAN STERILE OPHTHALMIC SOLUTION

(Latanoprost) 2864
May interact with:

Thimerosal (In vitro studies have shown that precipitation occurs when eye drops containing thimerosal are mixed with Xalatan; administer with an interval of at least five minutes between applications).

No products indexed under this heading.

XANAX TABLETS

(Alprazolam) 2865
May interact with antihistamines, central nervous system depressants, anticonvulsants, erythromycin, oral contraceptives, and certain other agents. Compounds in these categories include:

Acrivastine (Additive CNS depressant effects). Products include:

Semprex-D Capsules 1172

Alfentanil Hydrochloride (Additive CNS depressant effects).

No products indexed under this heading.

Amiodarone Hydrochloride (Possible interaction based on the data from *in vitro* studies of other benzodiazepines suggest a possible interaction when co-administered; concurrent use requires caution). Products include:

Cordarone Intravenous 3491
Cordarone Tablets 3487
Pacerone Tablets 3331

Aprobarbital (Additive CNS depressant effects).

No products indexed under this heading.

Astemizole (Additive CNS depressant effects).

No products indexed under this heading.

Azatadine Maleate (Additive CNS depressant effects). Products include:

Rynatan Tablets 3351

Bromodiphenhydramine Hydrochloride (Additive CNS depressant effects).

No products indexed under this heading.

Brompheniramine Maleate (Additive CNS depressant effects). Products include:

Bromfed Capsules (Extended-Release) 2269
Bromfed-PD Capsules (Extended-Release) 2269
Comtrex Acute Head Cold & Sinus Pressure Relief Tablets .... ■627
Dimetapp Elixir .... ■777
Dimetapp Cold and Fever Suspension .... ■775
Dimetapp DM Cold & Cough Elixir .... ■775
Dimetapp Nighttime Flu Liquid .... ■776

Buprenorphine Hydrochloride (Additive CNS depressant effects). Products include:

Buprenex Injectable 2918

Buspirone Hydrochloride (Additive CNS depressant effects).

No products indexed under this heading.

Butabarbital (Additive CNS depressant effects).

No products indexed under this heading.

Butalbital (Additive CNS depressant effects). Products include:

Phrenilin 578
Sedapap Tablets 50 mg/650 mg 2225

Carbamazepine (Additive CNS depressant effects). Products include:

Carbatrol Capsules 3234
Tegretol/Tegretol-XR 2404

Cetirizine Hydrochloride (Additive CNS depressant effects). Products include:

Zyrtec 2756
Zyrtec-D 12 Hour Extended Relief Tablets 2758

Chlordiazepoxide (Additive CNS depressant effects). Products include:

Limbitrol 1738

Chlordiazepoxide Hydrochloride (Additive CNS depressant effects). Products include:

Librium Capsules 1736
Librium for Injection 1737

Chlorpheniramine Maleate (Additive CNS depressant effects). Products include:

Actifed Cold & Sinus Caplets and Tablets .... ■688
Alka-Seltzer Plus Liqui-Gels .... ■604
BC Allergy Sinus Cold Powder .... ■619
Chlor-Trimeton Allergy Tablets .... ■735
Chlor-Trimeton Allergy/Decongestant Tablets .... ■736
Comtrex Flu Therapy & Fever Relief Nighttime Tablets .... ■628
Comtrex Maximum Strength Multi-Symptom Cold & Cough Relief Tablets and Caplets .... ■626
Contac Severe Cold and Flu Caplets Maximum Strength .... ■746
Coricidin 'D' Cold, Flu & Sinus Tablets .... ■737
Coricidin/Coricidin D .... ■738
Coricidin HBP Maximum Strength Flu Tablets .... ■738
Extendryl 1361
Hycomine Compound Tablets 1317
Kronofed-A 1341
PediaCare Cough-Cold Liquid .... ■719
PediaCare NightRest Cough-Cold Liquid .... ■719
Robitussin Nighttime Honey Flu Liquid .... ■786
Ryna .... ■768
Singlet Caplets .... ■761
Sinutab Sinus Allergy Medication, Maximum Strength Formula, Tablets & Caplets .... ■707
Sudafed Cold & Allergy Tablets .... ■708
TheraFlu Regular Strength Cold & Cough Night Time Hot Liquid .... ■676
TheraFlu Regular Strength Cold & Sore Throat Night Time Hot Liquid .... ■676
TheraFlu Maximum Strength Flu & Cough Night Time Hot Liquid .... ■678
TheraFlu Maximum Strength Flu & Sore Throat Night Time Hot Liquid .... ■677
TheraFlu Maximum Strength Severe Cold & Congestion Night Time Caplets .... ■678
TheraFlu Maximum Strength Severe Cold & Congestion Night Time Hot Liquid .... ■678
Triaminic Cold & Allergy Liquid .... ■681
Triaminic Cold & Allergy Softchews .... ■683
Triaminic Cold & Cough Liquid .... ■681
Triaminic Cold & Cough Softchews .... ■683
Triaminic Cold & Night Time Cough Liquid .... ■681
Triaminic Cold, Cough & Fever Liquid .... ■681
Children's Tylenol Cold Suspension Liquid and Chewable Tablets 2015
Children's Tylenol Cold Plus Cough Suspension Liquid and Chewable Tablets 2015
Children's Tylenol Flu Suspension Liquid 2015
Maximum Strength Tylenol Allergy Sinus Caplets, Gelcaps, and Geltabs 2010
Multi-Symptom Tylenol Cold Complete Formula Caplets 2010
Vicks 44M Cough, Cold & Flu Relief Liquid .... ■725
Pediatric Vicks 44m Cough & Cold Relief .... ■728
Children's Vicks NyQuil Cold/Cough Relief .... ■726

Chlorpheniramine Polistirex (Additive CNS depressant effects). Products include:

Tussionex Pennkinetic Extended-Release Suspension 1174

Chlorpheniramine Tannate (Additive CNS depressant effects). Products include:

Reformulated Rynatan Pediatric Suspension 3352
Rynatuss Pediatric Suspension 3353
Rynatuss Tablets 3353
Tussi-12 S Suspension 3356
Tussi-12 Tablets 3356

Chlorpromazine (Additive CNS depressant effects). Products include:

Thorazine Suppositories 1656

Chlorpromazine Hydrochloride (Additive CNS depressant effects). Products include:

Thorazine 1656

Chlorprothixene (Additive CNS depressant effects).

No products indexed under this heading.

Chlorprothixene Hydrochloride (Additive CNS depressant effects).

No products indexed under this heading.

Chlorprothixene Lactate (Additive CNS depressant effects).

No products indexed under this heading.

Cimetidine (Co-administration of cimetidine has increased the maximum plasma concentration of alprazolam by 86%, decreased clearance by 42%, and increased half-life by 16%). Products include:

Tagamet HB 200 Suspension .... ■762
Tagamet HB 200 Tablets .... ■761
Tagamet Tablets 1644

Cimetidine Hydrochloride (Co-administration of cimetidine has increased the maximum plasma concentration of alprazolam by 86%, decreased clearance by 42%, and increased half-life by 16%). Products include:

Tagamet 1644

Clarithromycin (Possible interaction based on the clinical studies involving other benzodiazepines

metabolized similarly as alprazolam; co-administration requires caution). Products include:

Biaxin/Biaxin XL 403
PREVPAC 3298

Clemastine Fumarate (Additive CNS depressant effects). Products include:

Tavist 12 Hour Allergy Tablets .... ■676

Clorazepate Dipotassium (Additive CNS depressant effects). Products include:

Tranxene 511

Clozapine (Additive CNS depressant effects). Products include:

Clozaril Tablets 2319

Codeine Phosphate (Additive CNS depressant effects). Products include:

Phenergan with Codeine Syrup 3557
Phenergan VC with Codeine Syrup .. 3561
Robitussin A-C Syrup 2942
Robitussin-DAC Syrup 2942
Ryna-C Liquid .... ■768
Soma Compound w/Codeine Tablets 3355
Tussi-Organidin NR Liquid 3350
Tussi-Organidin-S NR Liquid 3350
Tylenol with Codeine 2595

Cyclosporine (Possible interaction based on the data from *in vitro* studies of other benzodiazepines suggest a possible interaction when co-administered; concurrent use requires caution). Products include:

Gengraf Capsules 457
Neoral Soft Gelatin Capsules 2380
Neoral Oral Solution 2380
Sandimmune 2388

Cyproheptadine Hydrochloride (Additive CNS depressant effects). Products include:

Periactin Tablets 2155

Desflurane (Additive CNS depressant effects). Products include:

Suprane Liquid for Inhalation 874

Desipramine Hydrochloride (Increased steady state-plasma concentrations of desipramine by 20%). Products include:

Norpramin Tablets 755

Desogestrel (Co-administration of oral contraceptives has increased the maximum plasma concentration of alprazolam by 18%, decreased clearance by 2%, and increased half-life by 29%). Products include:

Cyclessa Tablets 2450
Desogen Tablets 2458
Mircette Tablets 2470
Ortho-Cept 21 Tablets 2546
Ortho-Cept 28 Tablets 2546

Dexchlorpheniramine Maleate (Additive CNS depressant effects).

No products indexed under this heading.

Dezocine (Additive CNS depressant effects).

No products indexed under this heading.

Diazepam (Additive CNS depressant effects). Products include:

Valium Injectable 3026
Valium Tablets 3047

Diltiazem Hydrochloride (Possible interaction based on the clinical studies involving other benzodiazepines metabolized similarly as alprazolam; co-administration requires caution). Products include:

Cardizem Injectable 1018
Cardizem Lyo-Ject Syringe 1018
Cardizem Monovial 1018
Cardizem CD Capsules 1016
Tiazac Capsules 1378

Diphenhydramine Citrate (Additive CNS depressant effects). Products include:

Alka-Seltzer PM Effervescent Tablets .... ■605
Benadryl Allergy & Sinus Fastmelt Tablets .... ■693
Benadryl Children's Allergy/Cold Fastmelt Tablets .... ■692
Excedrin PM Tablets, Caplets, and Geltabs .... ■631
Goody's PM Powder .... ■621

Diphenhydramine Hydrochloride (Additive CNS depressant effects). Products include:

Extra Strength Bayer PM Caplets .... ■611
Benadryl Allergy Chewables .... ■689
Benadryl Allergy .... ■691
Benadryl Allergy Liquid .... ■690
Benadryl Allergy/Cold Tablets .... ■691
Benadryl Allergy/Congestion Tablets .... ■692
Benadryl Allergy & Sinus Liquid .... ■693
Benadryl Allergy Sinus Headache Caplets & Gelcaps .... ■693
Benadryl Severe Allergy & Sinus Headache Caplets .... ■694
Benadryl Dye-Free Allergy Liquid ... ■690
Benadryl Dye-Free Allergy Liqui-Gels Softgels .... ■690
Benadryl Itch Relief Stick Extra Strength .... ■695
Benadryl Cream .... ■695
Benadryl Gel .... ■695
Benadryl Spray .... ■696
Benadryl Parenteral 2617
Coricidin HBP Night-Time Cold & Flu Tablets .... ■738
Nytol QuickCaps Caplets .... ■622
Maximum Strength Nytol QuickGels Softgels .... ■621
Extra Strength Percogesic Aspirin-Free Coated Caplets .... ■665
Simply Sleep Caplets 2008
Sominex Original Formula Tablets . ■761
Children's Tylenol Allergy-D Liquid 2014
Maximum Strength Tylenol Allergy Sinus NightTime Caplets 2010
Tylenol Severe Allergy Caplets 2010
Maximum Strength Tylenol Flu NightTime Gelcaps 2011
Extra Strength Tylenol PM Caplets, Geltabs, and Gelcaps 2012
Unisom Maximum Strength SleepGels .... ■713

Diphenylpyraline Hydrochloride (Additive CNS depressant effects).

No products indexed under this heading.

Divalproex Sodium (Additive CNS depressant effects). Products include:

Depakote Sprinkle Capsules 426
Depakote Tablets 430
Depakote ER Tablets 436

Droperidol (Additive CNS depressant effects).

No products indexed under this heading.

Enflurane (Additive CNS depressant effects).

No products indexed under this heading.

Ergotamine Tartrate (Possible interaction based on the data from *in vitro* studies of other benzodiazepines suggest a possible interaction when co-administered; concurrent use requires caution).

No products indexed under this heading.

Erythromycin (Possible interaction based on the clinical studies involving other benzodiazepines metabolized similarly as alprazolam; co-administration requires caution). Products include:

Emgel 2% Topical Gel 1285
Ery-Tab Tablets 448
Erythromycin Base Filmtab Tablets . 454
Erythromycin Delayed-Release Capsules, USP 455
PCE Dispertab Tablets 498

Erythromycin Estolate (Possible interaction based on the clinical studies involving other benzodiazepines metabolized similarly as alprazolam; co-administration requires caution).

No products indexed under this heading.

Erythromycin Ethylsuccinate (Possible interaction based on the clinical studies involving other benzodiazepines metabolized similarly as alprazolam; co-administration requires caution). Products include:

E.E.S. 450
EryPed 446
Pediazole Suspension 3050

Erythromycin Gluceptate (Possible interaction based on the clinical studies involving other benzodiazepines metabolized similarly as alprazolam; co-administration requires caution).

No products indexed under this heading.

Erythromycin Stearate (Possible interaction based on the clinical studies involving other benzodiazepines metabolized similarly as alprazolam; co-administration requires caution). Products include:

Erythrocin Stearate Filmtab Tablets 452

Estazolam (Additive CNS depressant effects). Products include:

ProSom Tablets 500

Ethchlorvynol (Additive CNS depressant effects).

No products indexed under this heading.

Ethinamate (Additive CNS depressant effects).

No products indexed under this heading.

Ethinyl Estradiol (Co-administration of oral contraceptives has increased the maximum plasma concentration of alprazolam by 18%, decreased clearance by 2%, and increased half-life by 29%). Products include:

Alesse-21 Tablets 3468
Alesse-28 Tablets 3473
Brevicon 28-Day Tablets 3380
Cyclessa Tablets 2450
Desogen Tablets 2458
Estinyl Tablets 3112
Estrostep 2627
femhrt Tablets 2635
Levlen 962
Levlite 21 Tablets 962
Levlite 28 Tablets 962
Levora Tablets 3389
Loestrin 21 Tablets 2642
Loestrin Fe Tablets 2642
Lo/Ovral Tablets 3532
Lo/Ovral-28 Tablets 3538
Low-Ogestrel-28 Tablets 3392
Microgestin Fe 1.5/30 Tablets 3407
Microgestin Fe 1/20 Tablets 3400
Mircette Tablets 2470
Modicon 2563
Necon 3415
Nordette-28 Tablets 2257
Norinyl 1 +35 28-Day Tablets 3380
Ogestrel 0.5/50-28 Tablets 3428
Ortho-Cept 21 Tablets 2546
Ortho-Cept 28 Tablets 2546
Ortho-Cyclen/Ortho Tri-Cyclen 2573
Ortho-Novum 2563
Ovcon 3364
Ovral Tablets 3551
[illegible] .... [illegible]
Tri-Levlen 962
Tri-Norinyl-28 Tablets 3433
Triphasil-21 Tablets 3600
Triphasil-28 Tablets 3605
Trivora Tablets 3439
Yasmin 28 Tablets 980
Zovia 3449

Ethosuximide (Additive CNS depressant effects). Products include:

Zarontin Capsules 2659
Zarontin Syrup 2660

Ethotoin (Additive CNS depressant effects).

No products indexed under this heading.

Ethynodiol Diacetate (Co-administration of oral contraceptives has increased the maximum plasma concentration of alprazolam by 18%, decreased clearance by 2%, and increased half-life by 29%). Products include:

Zovia 3449

Felbamate (Additive CNS depressant effects). Products include:

Felbatol 3343

Fentanyl (Additive CNS depressant effects). Products include:

Duragesic Transdermal System 1786

Fentanyl Citrate (Additive CNS depressant effects). Products include:

Actiq 1184

Fexofenadine Hydrochloride (Additive CNS depressant effects). Products include:

Allegra 712
Allegra-D Extended-Release Tablets 714

Fluconazole (Other azole-type antifungal agents should be considered potent CYP 3A inhibitors and they may have an effect on alprazolam clearance; co-administration is not recommended). Products include:

Diflucan Tablets, Injection, and Oral Suspension 2681

Fluoxetine Hydrochloride (Co-administration of fluoxetine has increased the maximum plasma concentration of alprazolam by 46%, decreased clearance by 21%, increased half-life by 17%, and decreased measured psychomotor performance). Products include:

Prozac Pulvules, Liquid, and Weekly Capsules 1238
Sarafem Pulvules 1962

Fluphenazine Decanoate (Additive CNS depressant effects).

No products indexed under this heading.

Fluphenazine Enanthate (Additive CNS depressant effects).

No products indexed under this heading.

Fluphenazine Hydrochloride (Additive CNS depressant effects).

No products indexed under this heading.

Flurazepam Hydrochloride (Additive CNS depressant effects).

No products indexed under this heading.

Fluvoxamine Maleate (Co-administration of fluvoxamine approximately doubled the maximum plasma concentration of alprazolam, decreased clearance by 49%, increased half-life by 71%, and decreased measured psychomotor performance). Products include:

Luvox Tablets (25, 50, 100 mg) 3256

Fosphenytoin Sodium (Additive CNS depressant effects). Products include:

Cerebyx Injection 2619

Glutethimide (Additive CNS depressant effects).

No products indexed under this heading.

Haloperidol (Additive CNS depressant effects). Products include:

Haldol Injection, Tablets and Concentrate 2533

Haloperidol Decanoate (Additive CNS depressant effects). Products include:

Haldol Decanoate 2535

Hydrocodone Bitartrate (Additive CNS depressant effects). Products include:

Hycodan 1316
Hycomine Compound Tablets 1317
Hycotuss Expectorant Syrup 1318
Lortab 3319
Lortab Elixir 3317
Maxidone Tablets CIII 3399
Norco 5/325 Tablets CIII 3424
Norco 7.5/325 Tablets CIII 3425
Norco 10/325 Tablets CIII 3427
Norco 10/325 Tablets CIII 3425
Vicodin Tablets 516
Vicodin ES Tablets 517
Vicodin HP Tablets 518
Vicodin Tuss Expectorant 519
Vicoprofen Tablets 520
Zydone Tablets 1330

Hydrocodone Polistirex (Additive CNS depressant effects). Products include:

Tussionex Pennkinetic Extended-Release Suspension 1174

Hydromorphone Hydrochloride (Additive CNS depressant effects). Products include:
Dilaudid ... 441
Dilaudid Oral Liquid ... 445
Dilaudid Powder ... 441
Dilaudid Rectal Suppositories ... 441
Dilaudid Tablets ... 441
Dilaudid Tablets - 8 mg ... 445
Dilaudid-HP ... 443

Hydroxyzine Hydrochloride (Additive CNS depressant effects). Products include:
Atarax Tablets & Syrup ... 2667
Vistaril Intramuscular Solution ... 2738

Imipramine Hydrochloride (Increased steady state-plasma concentrations of imipramine by 31%).
No products indexed under this heading.

Imipramine Pamoate (Increased steady state-plasma concentrations of imipramine by 31%).
No products indexed under this heading.

Isoflurane (Additive CNS depressant effects).
No products indexed under this heading.

Isoniazid (Possible interaction based on the clinical studies involving other benzodiazepines metabolized similarly as alprazolam; co-administration requires caution). Products include:
Rifamate Capsules ... 767
Rifater Tablets ... 769

Itraconazole (Co-administration with drugs that inhibit metabolism via cytochrome P450 3A, such as itraconazole, may have profound effect on the clearance of alprazolam; concurrent use is contraindicated). Products include:
Sporanox Capsules ... 1800
Sporanox Injection ... 1804
Sporanox Injection ... 2509
Sporanox Oral Solution ... 1808
Sporanox Oral Solution ... 2512

Ketamine Hydrochloride (Additive CNS depressant effects).
No products indexed under this heading.

Ketoconazole (Co-administration with drugs that inhibit metabolism via cytochrome P450 3A, such as ketoconazole, may have profound effect on the clearance of alprazolam; concurrent use is contraindicated). Products include:
Nizoral 2% Cream ... 3620
Nizoral A-D Shampoo ... 2008
Nizoral 2% Shampoo ... 2007
Nizoral Tablets ... 1791

Lamotrigine (Additive CNS depressant effects). Products include:
Lamictal ... 1567

Levetiracetam (Additive CNS depressant effects). Products include:
Keppra Tablets ... 3314

Levomethadyl Acetate Hydrochloride (Additive CNS depressant effects).
No products indexed under this heading.

Levonorgestrel (Co-administration of oral contraceptives has increased the maximum plasma concentration of alprazolam by 18%, decreased clearance by 2%, and increased half-life by 29%). Products include:
Alesse-21 Tablets ... 3468
Alesse-28 Tablets ... 3473
Levlen ... 962
Levlite 21 Tablets ... 962
Levlite 28 Tablets ... 962
Levora Tablets ... 3389
Mirena Intrauterine System ... 974
Nordette-28 Tablets ... 2257
Norplant System ... 3543
Tri-Levlen ... 962
Triphasil-21 Tablets ... 3600
Triphasil-28 Tablets ... 3605
Trivora Tablets ... 3439

Levorphanol Tartrate (Additive CNS depressant effects). Products include:
Levo-Dromoran ... 1734
Levorphanol Tartrate Tablets ... 3059

Loratadine (Additive CNS depressant effects). Products include:
Claritin ... 3100
Claritin-D 12 Hour Extended Release Tablets ... 3102
Claritin-D 24 Hour Extended Release Tablets ... 3104

Lorazepam (Additive CNS depressant effects). Products include:
Ativan Injection ... 3478
Ativan Tablets ... 3482

Loxapine Hydrochloride (Additive CNS depressant effects).
No products indexed under this heading.

Loxapine Succinate (Additive CNS depressant effects). Products include:
Loxitane Capsules ... 3398

Meperidine Hydrochloride (Additive CNS depressant effects). Products include:
Demerol ... 3079
Mepergan Injection ... 3539

Mephenytoin (Additive CNS depressant effects).
No products indexed under this heading.

Mephobarbital (Additive CNS depressant effects).
No products indexed under this heading.

Meprobamate (Additive CNS depressant effects). Products include:
Miltown Tablets ... 3349

Mesoridazine Besylate (Additive CNS depressant effects). Products include:
Serentil ... 1057

Mestranol (Co-administration of oral contraceptives has increased the maximum plasma concentration of alprazolam by 18%, decreased clearance by 2%, and increased half-life by 29%). Products include:
Necon 1/50 Tablets ... 3415
Norinyl 1 + 50 28-Day Tablets ... 3380
Ortho-Novum 1/50□28 Tablets ... 2556

Methadone Hydrochloride (Additive CNS depressant effects). Products include:
Dolophine Hydrochloride Tablets ... 3056

Methdilazine Hydrochloride (Additive CNS depressant effects).
No products indexed under this heading.

Methohexital Sodium (Additive CNS depressant effects). Products include:
Brevital Sodium for Injection, USP ... 1815

Methotrimeprazine (Additive CNS depressant effects).
No products indexed under this heading.

Methoxyflurane (Additive CNS depressant effects).
No products indexed under this heading.

Methsuximide (Additive CNS depressant effects). Products include:
Celontin Capsules ... 2618

Midazolam Hydrochloride (Additive CNS depressant effects). Products include:
Versed Injection ... 3027
Versed Syrup ... 3033

Molindone Hydrochloride (Additive CNS depressant effects). Products include:
Moban ... 1320

Morphine Sulfate (Additive CNS depressant effects). Products include:
Astramorph/PF Injection, USP (Preservative-Free) ... 594
Duramorph Injection ... 1312
Infumorph 200 and Infumorph 500 Sterile Solutions ... 1314
Kadian Capsules ... 1335
MS Contin Tablets ... 2896
MSIR ... 2898
Oramorph SR Tablets ... 3062
Roxanol ... 3066

Nefazodone Hydrochloride (Co-administration has resulted in increased alprazolam concentration two-fold). Products include:
Serzone Tablets ... 1104

Nicardipine Hydrochloride (Possible interaction based on the data from *in vitro* studies of other benzodiazepines suggest a possible interaction when co-administered; concurrent use requires caution). Products include:
Cardene I.V. ... 3485

Nifedipine (Possible interaction based on the data from *in vitro* studies of other benzodiazepines suggest a possible interaction when co-administered; concurrent use requires caution). Products include:
Adalat CC Tablets ... 877
Procardia Capsules ... 2708
Procardia XL Extended Release Tablets ... 2710

Norethindrone (Co-administration of oral contraceptives has increased the maximum plasma concentration of alprazolam by 18%, decreased clearance by 2%, and increased half-life by 29%). Products include:
Brevicon 28-Day Tablets ... 3380
Micronor Tablets ... 2543
Modicon ... 2563
Necon ... 3415
Norinyl 1 +35 28-Day Tablets ... 3380
Norinyl 1 + 50 28-Day Tablets ... 3380
Nor-QD Tablets ... 3423
Ortho-Novum ... 2563
Ortho-Novum 1/50□28 Tablets ... 2556
Ovcon ... 3364
Tri-Norinyl-28 Tablets ... 3433

Norethynodrel (Co-administration of oral contraceptives has increased the maximum plasma concentration of alprazolam by 18%, decreased clearance by 2%, and increased half-life by 29%).
No products indexed under this heading.

Norgestimate (Co-administration of oral contraceptives has increased the maximum plasma concentration of alprazolam by 18%, decreased clearance by 2%, and increased half-life by 29%). Products include:
Ortho-Cyclen/Ortho Tri-Cyclen ... 2573
Ortho-Prefest Tablets ... 2570

Norgestrel (Co-administration of oral contraceptives has increased the maximum plasma concentration of alprazolam by 18%, decreased clearance by 2%, and increased half-life by 29%). Products include:
Lo/Ovral Tablets ... 3532
Lo/Ovral-28 Tablets ... 3538
Low-Ogestrel-28 Tablets ... 3392
Ogestrel 0.5/50-28 Tablets ... 3428
Ovral Tablets ... 3551
Ovral-28 Tablets ... 3552
Ovrette Tablets ... 3552

Olanzapine (Additive CNS depressant effects). Products include:
Zyprexa Tablets ... 1973
Zyprexa ZYDIS Orally Disintegrating Tablets ... 1973

Oxazepam (Additive CNS depressant effects).
No products indexed under this heading.

Oxcarbazepine (Additive CNS depressant effects). Products include:
Trileptal Oral Suspension ... 2407
Trileptal Tablets ... 2407

Oxycodone Hydrochloride (Additive CNS depressant effects). Products include:
OxyContin Tablets ... 2912
OxyFast Oral Concentrate Solution ... 2916
OxyIR Capsules ... 2916
Percocet Tablets ... 1326
Percodan Tablets ... 1327
Percolone Tablets ... 1327
Roxicodone ... 3067
Tylox Capsules ... 2597

Paramethadione (Additive CNS depressant effects).
No products indexed under this heading.

Paroxetine Hydrochloride (Possible interaction based on the data from *in vitro* studies suggest a possible interaction when co-administered; concurrent use requires caution). Products include:
Paxil ... 1609

Pentobarbital Sodium (Additive CNS depressant effects). Products include:
Nembutal Sodium Solution ... 485

Perphenazine (Additive CNS depressant effects). Products include:
Etrafon ... 3115
Trilafon ... 3160

Phenacemide (Additive CNS depressant effects).
No products indexed under this heading.

Phenobarbital (Additive CNS depressant effects). Products include:
Arco-Lase Plus Tablets ... 592
Donnatal ... 2929
Donnatal Extentabs ... 2930

Phensuximide (Additive CNS depressant effects).
No products indexed under this heading.

Phenytoin (Additive CNS depressant effects). Products include:
Dilantin Infatabs ... 2624
Dilantin-125 Oral Suspension ... 2625

Phenytoin Sodium (Additive CNS depressant effects). Products include:
Dilantin Kapseals ... 2622

Prazepam (Additive CNS depressant effects).
No products indexed under this heading.

Primidone (Additive CNS depressant effects).
No products indexed under this heading.

Prochlorperazine (Additive CNS depressant effects). Products include:
Compazine ... 1505

Promethazine Hydrochloride (Additive CNS depressant effects). Products include:
Mepergan Injection ... 3539
Phenergan Injection ... 3553
Phenergan ... 3556
Phenergan Syrup ... 3554
Phenergan with Codeine Syrup ... 3557
Phenergan with Dextromethorphan Syrup ... 3559
Phenergan VC Syrup ... 3560
Phenergan VC with Codeine Syrup ... 3561

Propofol (Additive CNS depressant effects). Products include:
Diprivan Injectable Emulsion ... 667

Propoxyphene Hydrochloride (Co-administration of propoxyphene has decreased the maximum plasma concentration of alprazolam by 6%, decreased clearance by 38%, and increased half-life by 16%). Products include:
Darvon Pulvules ... 1909
Darvon Compound-65 Pulvules ... 1910

Propoxyphene Napsylate (Co-administration of propoxyphene has decreased the maximum plasma concentration of alprazolam by 6%, decreased clearance by 38%, and increased half-life by 16%). Products include:
Darvon-N/Darvocet-N ... 1907
Darvon-N Tablets ... 1912

Pyrilamine Maleate (Additive CNS depressant effects). Products include:

Maximum Strength Midol Menstrual Caplets and Gelcaps ▣612
Maximum Strength Midol PMS Caplets and Gelcaps ▣613

Pyrilamine Tannate (Additive CNS depressant effects). Products include:
Ryna-12 S Suspension 3351

Quazepam (Additive CNS depressant effects).
No products indexed under this heading.

Quetiapine Fumarate (Additive CNS depressant effects). Products include:
Seroquel Tablets 684

Remifentanil Hydrochloride (Additive CNS depressant effects).
No products indexed under this heading.

Risperidone (Additive CNS depressant effects). Products include:
Risperdal 1796

Secobarbital Sodium (Additive CNS depressant effects).
No products indexed under this heading.

Sertraline Hydrochloride (Possible interaction based on the data from *in vitro* studies suggest a possible interaction when co-administered; concurrent use requires caution). Products include:
Zoloft 2751

Sevoflurane (Additive CNS depressant effects).
No products indexed under this heading.

Sufentanil Citrate (Additive CNS depressant effects).
No products indexed under this heading.

Temazepam (Additive CNS depressant effects).
No products indexed under this heading.

Terfenadine (Additive CNS depressant effects).
No products indexed under this heading.

Thiamylal Sodium (Additive CNS depressant effects).
No products indexed under this heading.

Thioridazine Hydrochloride (Additive CNS depressant effects). Products include:
Thioridazine Hydrochloride Tablets 2289

Thiothixene (Additive CNS depressant effects). Products include:
Navane Capsules 2701
Thiothixene Capsules 2290

Tiagabine Hydrochloride (Additive CNS depressant effects). Products include:
Gabitril Tablets 1189

Topiramate (Additive CNS depressant effects). Products include:
Topamax Sprinkle Capsules 2590
Topamax Tablets 2590

Triazolam (Additive CNS depressant effects). Products include:
Halcion Tablets 2823

Trifluoperazine Hydrochloride (Additive CNS depressant effects). Products include:
Stelazine 1640

Trimeprazine Tartrate (Additive CNS depressant effects).
No products indexed under this heading.

Trimethadione (Additive CNS depressant effects).
No products indexed under this heading.

Tripelennamine Hydrochloride (Additive CNS depressant effects).
No products indexed under this heading.

Triprolidine Hydrochloride (Additive CNS depressant effects). Products include:
Actifed Cold & Allergy Tablets ▣688

Valproate Sodium (Additive CNS depressant effects). Products include:
Depacon Injection 416

Valproic Acid (Additive CNS depressant effects). Products include:
Depakene 421

Zaleplon (Additive CNS depressant effects). Products include:
Sonata Capsules 3591

Ziprasidone Hydrochloride (Additive CNS depressant effects). Products include:
Geodon Capsules 2688

Zolpidem Tartrate (Additive CNS depressant effects). Products include:
Ambien Tablets 3191

Zonisamide (Additive CNS depressant effects). Products include:
Zonegran Capsules 1307

Food Interactions

Alcohol (Additive CNS depressant effects).

Grapefruit Juice (Possible interaction based on the clinical studies involving other benzodiazepines metabolized similarly as alprazolam; co-administration requires caution).

XELODA TABLETS

(Capecitabine) 3039
May interact with oral anticoagulants, phenytoin, and certain other agents. Compounds in these categories include:

Aluminum Hydroxide (Co-administration of capecitabine with aluminum hydroxide- and magnesium hydroxide-containing antacid has resulted in a small increase in plasma concentrations of capecitabine and one metabolite (5'DFCR)). Products include:
Amphojel Suspension (Mint Flavor) ▣789
Gaviscon Extra Strength Liquid ▣751
Gaviscon Extra Strength Tablets ▣751
Gaviscon Regular Strength Liquid ▣751
Gaviscon Regular Strength Tablets ▣750
Maalox Antacid/Anti-Gas Oral Suspension ▣673
Maalox Max Maximum Strength Antacid/Anti-Gas Liquid 2300
Maalox Regular Strength Antacid/Antigas Liquid 2300
Mylanta 1813
Vanquish Caplets ▣617

Dicumarol (Co-administration has resulted in altered coagulation parameters and/or bleeding).
No products indexed under this heading.

Fosphenytoin Sodium (Co-administration has resulted in toxicity associated with elevated phenytoin levels). Products include:
Cerebyx Injection 2619

Leucovorin Calcium (The concentrations of 5-fluorouracil, capecitabine is a prodrug and it is converted to 5-FU, is increased and its toxicity may be enhanced by leucovorin; deaths from severe enterocolitis, diarrhea, and dehydration have been reported in elderly patients receiving fluorouracil and leucovorin).
No products indexed under this heading.

Magnesium Hydroxide (Co-administration of capecitabine with aluminum hydroxide- and magnesium hydroxide-containing antacid has resulted in a small increase in plasma concentrations of capecitabine and one metabolite (5'DFCR)). Products include:
Ex•Lax Milk of Magnesia Liquid ▣670
Maalox Antacid/Anti-Gas Oral Suspension ▣673
Maalox Max Maximum Strength Antacid/Anti-Gas Liquid 2300
Maalox Regular Strength Antacid/Antigas Liquid 2300
Mylanta Fast-Acting 1813
Mylanta 1813
Pepcid Complete Chewable Tablets 1815
Phillips' Chewable Tablets ▣615
Phillips' Milk of Magnesia Liquid (Original, Cherry, & Mint) ▣616
Rolaids Tablets ▣706
Extra Strength Rolaids Tablets ▣706
Vanquish Caplets ▣617

Phenytoin (Co-administration has resulted in toxicity associated with elevated phenytoin levels). Products include:
Dilantin Infatabs 2624
Dilantin-125 Oral Suspension 2625

Phenytoin Sodium (Co-administration has resulted in toxicity associated with elevated phenytoin levels). Products include:
Dilantin Kapseals 2622

Warfarin Sodium (Co-administration has resulted in altered coagulation parameters and/or bleeding). Products include:
Coumadin for Injection 1243
Coumadin Tablets 1243
Warfarin Sodium Tablets, USP 3302

Food Interactions

Food, unspecified (Reduces both rate and extent of absorption of capecitabine and delays Tmax of both parent and 5-FU).

XENICAL CAPSULES

(Orlistat) 3043
May interact with:

Beta-Carotene (Orlistat has been shown to reduce the absorption of some fat soluble vitamins; the vitamin supplement should be taken once a day at least 2 hours before or after the administration of orlistat).
No products indexed under this heading.

Cyclosporine (Co-administration has resulted in reduction in cyclosporine plasma levels; concurrent use is not recommended; if used concurrently, cyclosporine should be taken at least 2 hours before or after Xenical). Products include:
Gengraf Capsules 457
Neoral Soft Gelatin Capsules 2380
Neoral Oral Solution 2380
Sandimmune 2388

Pravastatin Sodium (Co-administration results in additive lipid lowering effect of pravastatin; modest increases in pravastatin plasma concentrations were observed during co-administration). Products include:
Pravachol Tablets 1099

Vitamin A (Orlistat has been shown to reduce the absorption of some fat soluble vitamins; the vitamin supplement should be taken once a day at least 2 hours before or after the administration of orlistat). Products include:
Aquasol A Parenteral 593
Beta-C Tablets ▣811
Centrum Focused Formulas Prostate Softgels ▣816

Vitamin D (Orlistat has been shown to reduce the absorption of some fat soluble vitamins; the vitamin supplement should be taken once a day at least 2 hours before or after the administration of orlistat). Products include:
Active Calcium Tablets 3335
Caltrate 600 PLUS ▣815
Caltrate 600 + D Tablets ▣814
Centrum Focused Formulas Bone Health Tablets ▣815
Citracal Caplets + D ▣823
D-Cal Chewable Caplets ▣794
One-A-Day Calcium Plus Chewable Tablets ▣805
Os-Cal 250 + D Tablets ▣838
Os-Cal 500 + D Tablets ▣839

Vitamin E (Orlistat has been shown to reduce the absorption of some fat soluble vitamins; the vitamin supplement should be taken once a day at least 2 hours before or after the administration of orlistat). Products include:
Nutr-E-Sol Liquid 526
One-A-Day Cholesterol Health Tablets ▣805
One-A-Day Menopause Health Tablets ▣808
StePHan Bio-Nutritional Daytime Hydrating Creme ▣770
StePHan Feminine Capsules ▣848
Unique E Vitamin E Capsules 1723

Vitamin K_1 (Absorption of vitamin K may be decreased). Products include:
AquaMEPHYTON Injection 2042
Mephyton Tablets 2129

Warfarin Sodium (Vitamin K absorption may be decreased with orlistat; patients on chronic stable doses of warfarin who are prescribed orlistat should be monitored closely for changes in coagulation parameters). Products include:
Coumadin for Injection 1243
Coumadin Tablets 1243
Warfarin Sodium Tablets, USP 3302

Food Interactions

Food, unspecified (Gastrointestinal events may increase when orlistat is taken with a diet high in fat).

XERAC AC SOLUTION

(Aluminum Chloride) 2663
None cited in PDR database.

XOPENEX INHALATION SOLUTION

(Levalbuterol Hydrochloride) 3207
May interact with beta blockers, monoamine oxidase inhibitors, potassium-depleting diuretics, sympathomimetic aerosol bronchodilators, tricyclic antidepressants, and certain other agents. Compounds in these categories include:

Acebutolol Hydrochloride (Beta-adrenergic receptor blocking agents block the pulmonary effect of beta agonist and may produce severe bronchospasm in asthmatic patients). Products include:
Sectral Capsules 3589

Albuterol (Potential for deleterious cardiovascular effects with concomitant use). Products include:
Proventil Inhalation Aerosol 3142
Ventolin Inhalation Aerosol and Refill 1679

Amitriptyline Hydrochloride (Action of levalbuterol on the vascular system may be potentiated). Products include:
Etrafon 3115
Limbitrol 1738

Amoxapine (Action of levalbuterol on the vascular system may be potentiated).
No products indexed under this heading.

Atenolol (Beta-adrenergic receptor blocking agents block the pulmonary effect of beta agonist and may produce severe bronchospasm in asthmatic patients). Products include:
Tenoretic Tablets 690
Tenormin I.V. Injection 692

Bendroflumethiazide (The ECG changes and/or hypokalemia that may result from the administration of non-potassium sparing diuretics can be acutely worsened by beta-agonists). Products include:
Corzide 40/5 Tablets 2247
Corzide 80/5 Tablets 2247

Betaxolol Hydrochloride (Beta-adrenergic receptor blocking agents block the pulmonary effect of beta agonist and may produce severe bronchospasm in asthmatic patients). Products include:

Betoptic S Ophthalmic Suspension 537

Bisoprolol Fumarate (Beta-adrenergic receptor blocking agents block the pulmonary effect of beta agonist and may produce severe bronchospasm in asthmatic patients). Products include:
Zebeta Tablets 1885
Ziac Tablets 1887

Bitolterol Mesylate (Potential for deleterious cardiovascular effects with concomitant use).
No products indexed under this heading.

Bumetanide (The ECG changes and/or hypokalemia that may result from the administration of non-potassium sparing diuretics can be acutely worsened by beta-agonists).
No products indexed under this heading.

Carteolol Hydrochloride (Beta-adrenergic receptor blocking agents block the pulmonary effect of beta agonist and may produce severe bronchospasm in asthmatic patients). Products include:
Carteolol Hydrochloride Ophthalmic Solution USP, 1% .... ⊙258
Ocupress Ophthalmic Solution, 1% Sterile .... ⊙303

Chlorothiazide (The ECG changes and/or hypokalemia that may result from the administration of non-potassium sparing diuretics can be acutely worsened by beta-agonists). Products include:
Aldoclor Tablets 2035
Diuril Oral 2087

Chlorothiazide Sodium (The ECG changes and/or hypokalemia that may result from the administration of non-potassium sparing diuretics can be acutely worsened by beta-agonists). Products include:
Diuril Sodium Intravenous 2086

Clomipramine Hydrochloride (Action of levalbuterol on the vascular system may be potentiated).
No products indexed under this heading.

Desipramine Hydrochloride (Action of levalbuterol on the vascular system may be potentiated). Products include:
Norpramin Tablets 755

Digoxin (Mean decreases of 16% and 22% in serum digoxin levels were demonstrated after the single-dose intravenous and oral administration of racemic albuterol, respectively; clinical significance of this finding is unclear). Products include:
Digitek Tablets 1003
Lanoxicaps Capsules 1574
Lanoxin Injection 1581
Lanoxin Tablets 1587
Lanoxin Elixir Pediatric 1578
Lanoxin Injection Pediatric 1584

Doxepin Hydrochloride (Action of levalbuterol on the vascular system may be potentiated). Products include:
Sinequan 2713

Esmolol Hydrochloride (Beta-adrenergic receptor blocking agents block the pulmonary effect of beta agonist and may produce severe bronchospasm in asthmatic patients). Products include:
Brevibloc Injection 858

Ethacrynic Acid (The ECG changes and/or hypokalemia that may result from the administration of non-potassium sparing diuretics can be acutely worsened by beta-agonists). Products include:
Edecrin Tablets 2091

Furosemide (The ECG changes and/or hypokalemia that may result from the administration of non-potassium sparing diuretics can be acutely worsened by beta-agonists). Products include:
Furosemide Tablets 2284

Hydrochlorothiazide (The ECG changes and/or hypokalemia that may result from the administration of non-potassium sparing diuretics can be acutely worsened by beta-agonists). Products include:
Accuretic Tablets 2614
Aldoril Tablets 2039
Atacand HCT Tablets 597
Avalide Tablets 1070
Diovan HCT Tablets 2338
Dyazide Capsules 1515
HydroDIURIL Tablets 2108
Hyzaar 2109
Inderide Tablets 3517
Inderide LA Long-Acting Capsules .. 3519
Lotensin HCT Tablets 2367
Maxzide 1008
Micardis HCT Tablets 1051
Microzide Capsules 3414
Moduretic Tablets 2138
Monopril HCT 1094
Prinzide Tablets 2168
Timolide Tablets 2187
Uniretic Tablets 3178
Vaseretic Tablets 2204
Zestoretic Tablets 695
Ziac Tablets 1887

Hydroflumethiazide (The ECG changes and/or hypokalemia that may result from the administration of non-potassium sparing diuretics can be acutely worsened by beta-agonists). Products include:
Diucardin Tablets 3494

Imipramine Hydrochloride (Action of levalbuterol on the vascular system may be potentiated).
No products indexed under this heading.

Imipramine Pamoate (Action of levalbuterol on the vascular system may be potentiated).
No products indexed under this heading.

Isocarboxazid (Action of levalbuterol on the vascular system may be potentiated).
No products indexed under this heading.

Isoetharine (Potential for deleterious cardiovascular effects with concomitant use).
No products indexed under this heading.

Isoproterenol Hydrochloride (Potential for deleterious cardiovascular effects with concomitant use).
No products indexed under this heading.

Labetalol Hydrochloride (Beta-adrenergic receptor blocking agents block the pulmonary effect of beta agonist and may produce severe bronchospasm in asthmatic patients). Products include:
Normodyne Injection 3135
Normodyne Tablets 3137

Levobunolol Hydrochloride (Beta-adrenergic receptor blocking agents block the pulmonary effect of beta agonist and may produce severe bronchospasm in asthmatic patients). Products include:
Betagan .... ⊙228

Maprotiline Hydrochloride (Action of levalbuterol on the vascular system may be potentiated).
No products indexed under this heading.

Metaproterenol Sulfate (Potential for deleterious cardiovascular effects with concomitant use). Products include:
Alupent 1029

Methyclothiazide (The ECG changes and/or hypokalemia that may result from the administration of non-potassium sparing diuretics can be acutely worsened by beta-agonists).
No products indexed under this heading.

Metipranolol Hydrochloride (Beta-adrenergic receptor blocking agents block the pulmonary effect of beta agonist and may produce severe bronchospasm in asthmatic patients).
No products indexed under this heading.

Metoprolol Succinate (Beta-adrenergic receptor blocking agents block the pulmonary effect of beta agonist and may produce severe bronchospasm in asthmatic patients). Products include:
Toprol-XL Tablets 651

Metoprolol Tartrate (Beta-adrenergic receptor blocking agents block the pulmonary effect of beta agonist and may produce severe bronchospasm in asthmatic patients).
No products indexed under this heading.

Moclobemide (Action of levalbuterol on the vascular system may be potentiated).
No products indexed under this heading.

Nadolol (Beta-adrenergic receptor blocking agents block the pulmonary effect of beta agonist and may produce severe bronchospasm in asthmatic patients). Products include:
Corgard Tablets 2245
Corzide 40/5 Tablets 2247
Corzide 80/5 Tablets 2247
Nadolol Tablets 2288

Nortriptyline Hydrochloride (Action of levalbuterol on the vascular system may be potentiated).
No products indexed under this heading.

Pargyline Hydrochloride (Action of levalbuterol on the vascular system may be potentiated).
No products indexed under this heading.

Penbutolol Sulfate (Beta-adrenergic receptor blocking agents block the pulmonary effect of beta agonist and may produce severe bronchospasm in asthmatic patients).
No products indexed under this heading.

Phenelzine Sulfate (Action of levalbuterol on the vascular system may be potentiated). Products include:
Nardil Tablets 2653

Pindolol (Beta-adrenergic receptor blocking agents block the pulmonary effect of beta agonist and may produce severe bronchospasm in asthmatic patients).
No products indexed under this heading.

Pirbuterol Acetate (Potential for deleterious cardiovascular effects with concomitant use). Products include:
Maxair Autohaler 1981
Maxair Inhaler 1984

Polythiazide (The ECG changes and/or hypokalemia that may result from the administration of non-potassium sparing diuretics can be acutely worsened by beta-agonists). Products include:
Minizide Capsules 2700
Renese Tablets 2712

Procarbazine Hydrochloride (Action of levalbuterol on the vascular system may be potentiated). Products include:
Matulane Capsules 3246

Propranolol Hydrochloride (Beta-adrenergic receptor blocking agents block the pulmonary effect of beta agonist and may produce severe bronchospasm in asthmatic patients). Products include:
Inderal 3513
Inderal LA Long-Acting Capsules 3516
Inderide Tablets 3517
Inderide LA Long-Acting Capsules .. 3519

Protriptyline Hydrochloride (Action of levalbuterol on the vascular system may be potentiated). Products include:
Vivactil Tablets 2446
Vivactil Tablets 2217

Salmeterol Xinafoate (Potential for deleterious cardiovascular effects with concomitant use). Products include:
Advair Diskus 100/50 1448
Advair Diskus 250/50 1448
Advair Diskus 500/50 1448
Serevent Diskus 1637
Serevent Inhalation Aerosol 1633

Selegiline Hydrochloride (Action of levalbuterol on the vascular system may be potentiated). Products include:
Eldepryl Capsules 3266

Sotalol Hydrochloride (Beta-adrenergic receptor blocking agents block the pulmonary effect of beta agonist and may produce severe bronchospasm in asthmatic patients). Products include:
Betapace Tablets 950
Betapace AF Tablets 954

Terbutaline Sulfate (Potential for deleterious cardiovascular effects with concomitant use). Products include:
Brethine Ampuls 2314
Brethine Tablets 2313

Timolol Hemihydrate (Beta-adrenergic receptor blocking agents block the pulmonary effect of beta agonist and may produce severe bronchospasm in asthmatic patients). Products include:
Betimol Ophthalmic Solution .... ⊙324

Timolol Maleate (Beta-adrenergic receptor blocking agents block the pulmonary effect of beta agonist and may produce severe bronchospasm in asthmatic patients). Products include:
Blocadren Tablets 2046
Cosopt Sterile Ophthalmic Solution 2065
Timolide Tablets 2187
Timolol GFS .... ⊙266
Timoptic in Ocudose 2192
Timoptic Sterile Ophthalmic Solution 2190
Timoptic-XE Sterile Ophthalmic Gel Forming Solution 2194

Torsemide (The ECG changes and/or hypokalemia that may result from the administration of non-potassium sparing diuretics can be acutely worsened by beta-agonists). Products include:
Demadex Tablets and Injection 2965

Tranylcypromine Sulfate (Action of levalbuterol on the vascular system may be potentiated). Products include:
Parnate Tablets 1607

Trimipramine Maleate (Action of levalbuterol on the vascular system may be potentiated). Products include:
Surmontil Capsules 3595

X-PREP LIQUID
(Senna) 2900
None cited in PDR database.

XYLOCAINE INJECTION
(Lidocaine Hydrochloride) 653
See Xylocaine with Epinephrine Injection

XYLOCAINE WITH EPINEPHRINE INJECTION
(Epinephrine, Lidocaine Hydrochloride) 653
May interact with butyrophenones, ergot-type oxytocic drugs, monoamine oxidase inhibitors, phenothiazines, and tricyclic antidepressants. Compounds in these categories include:

Amitriptyline Hydrochloride (Potential for severe, prolonged hypertension). Products include:
Etrafon 3115
Limbitrol 1738

Amoxapine (Potential for severe, prolonged hypertension).
No products indexed under this heading.

Chlorpromazine (Reduces or reverses the pressor effect of epinephrine). Products include:
Thorazine Suppositories 1656

Chlorpromazine Hydrochloride (Reduces or reverses the pressor effect of epinephrine). Products include:
Thorazine 1656

Clomipramine Hydrochloride (Potential for severe, prolonged hypertension).
No products indexed under this heading.

Desipramine Hydrochloride (Potential for severe, prolonged hypertension). Products include:
Norpramin Tablets 755

Doxepin Hydrochloride (Potential for severe, prolonged hypertension). Products include:
Sinequan 2713

Fluphenazine Decanoate (Reduces or reverses the pressor effect of epinephrine).
No products indexed under this heading.

Fluphenazine Enanthate (Reduces or reverses the pressor effect of epinephrine).
No products indexed under this heading.

Fluphenazine Hydrochloride (Reduces or reverses the pressor effect of epinephrine).
No products indexed under this heading.

Haloperidol (Reduces or reverses the pressor effect of epinephrine). Products include:
Haldol Injection, Tablets and Concentrate 2533

Haloperidol Decanoate (Reduces or reverses the pressor effect of epinephrine). Products include:
Haldol Decanoate 2535

Imipramine Hydrochloride (Potential for severe, prolonged hypertension).
No products indexed under this heading.

Imipramine Pamoate (Potential for severe, prolonged hypertension).
No products indexed under this heading.

Isocarboxazid (Potential for severe, prolonged hypertension).
No products indexed under this heading.

Maprotiline Hydrochloride (Potential for severe, prolonged hypertension).
No products indexed under this heading.

Mesoridazine Besylate (Reduces or reverses the pressor effect of epinephrine). Products include:
Serentil 1057

Methotrimeprazine (Reduces or reverses the pressor effect of epinephrine).
No products indexed under this heading.

Methylergonovine Maleate (Co-administration of vasopressor drugs for the treatment of hypotension related to obstetric blocks and ergot-type oxytocic drugs may cause severe, persistent hypertension or cerebrovascular accidents).
No products indexed under this heading.

Moclobemide (Potential for severe, prolonged hypertension).
No products indexed under this heading.

Nortriptyline Hydrochloride (Potential for severe, prolonged hypertension).
No products indexed under this heading.

Pargyline Hydrochloride (Potential for severe, prolonged hypertension).
No products indexed under this heading.

Perphenazine (Reduces or reverses the pressor effect of epinephrine). Products include:
Etrafon 3115
Trilafon 3160

Phenelzine Sulfate (Potential for severe, prolonged hypertension). Products include:
Nardil Tablets 2653

Procarbazine Hydrochloride (Potential for severe, prolonged hypertension). Products include:
Matulane Capsules 3246

Prochlorperazine (Reduces or reverses the pressor effect of epinephrine). Products include:
Compazine 1505

Promethazine Hydrochloride (Reduces or reverses the pressor effect of epinephrine). Products include:
Mepergan Injection 3539
Phenergan Injection 3553
Phenergan 3556
Phenergan Syrup 3554
Phenergan with Codeine Syrup 3557
Phenergan with Dextromethorphan Syrup 3559
Phenergan VC Syrup 3560
Phenergan VC with Codeine Syrup 3561

Protriptyline Hydrochloride (Potential for severe, prolonged hypertension). Products include:
Vivactil Tablets 2446
Vivactil Tablets 2217

Selegiline Hydrochloride (Potential for severe, prolonged hypertension). Products include:
Eldepryl Capsules 3266

Thioridazine Hydrochloride (Reduces or reverses the pressor effect of epinephrine). Products include:
Thioridazine Hydrochloride Tablets 2289

Tranylcypromine Sulfate (Potential for severe, prolonged hypertension). Products include:
Parnate Tablets 1607

Trifluoperazine Hydrochloride (Reduces or reverses the pressor effect of epinephrine). Products include:
Stelazine 1640

Trimipramine Maleate (Potential for severe, prolonged hypertension). Products include:
Surmontil Capsules 3595

YASMIN 28 TABLETS

(Drospirenone, Ethinyl Estradiol) 980
May interact with ACE inhibitors, aldosterone-inhibiting diuretic agents, angiotensin-II receptor antagonists, non-steroidal anti-inflammatory agents, phenytoin, prednisolone, potassium sparing diuretics, tetracyclines, theophylline, and certain other agents. Compounds in these categories include:

Acetaminophen (May increase plasma levels of ethinyl estradiol possibly by inhibition of conjugation; co-administration may decrease plasma concentrations of acetaminophen). Products include:
Actifed Cold & Sinus Caplets and Tablets ■ 688
Alka-Seltzer Plus Liqui-Gels ■ 604
Alka-Seltzer Plus Cold & Flu Medicine Liqui-Gels ■ 604
Alka-Seltzer Plus Cold & Sinus Medicine Liqui-Gels ■ 604
Benadryl Allergy/Cold Tablets ■ 691
Benadryl Allergy Sinus Headache Caplets & Gelcaps ■ 693
Benadryl Severe Allergy & Sinus Headache Caplets ■ 694
Children's Cēpacol Sore Throat ■ 788
Comtrex Acute Head Cold & Sinus Pressure Relief Tablets ■ 627
Comtrex Deep Chest Cold & Congestion Relief Softgels ■ 627
Comtrex Flu Therapy & Fever Relief Daytime Caplets ■ 628
Comtrex Flu Therapy & Fever Relief Nighttime Tablets ■ 628
Comtrex Maximum Strength Multi-Symptom Cold & Cough Relief Tablets and Caplets ■ 626
Contac Severe Cold and Flu Caplets Maximum Strength ■ 746
Contac Severe Cold and Flu Caplets Non-Drowsy ■ 746
Coricidin 'D' Cold, Flu & Sinus Tablets ■ 737
Coricidin HBP Cold & Flu Tablets ■ 738
Coricidin HBP Maximum Strength Flu Tablets ■ 738
Coricidin HBP Night-Time Cold & Flu Tablets ■ 738
Darvon-N/Darvocet-N 1907
Dimetapp Cold and Fever Suspension ■ 775
Dimetapp Nighttime Flu Liquid ■ 776
Dimetapp Non-Drowsy Flu Syrup ■ 777
Drixoral Allergy/Sinus Extended-Release Tablets ■ 741
Drixoral Cold & Flu Extended-Release Tablets ■ 740
Aspirin Free Excedrin Caplets and Geltabs ■ 628
Excedrin Extra-Strength Tablets, Caplets, and Geltabs ■ 629
Excedrin Migraine 1070
Excedrin PM Tablets, Caplets, and Geltabs ■ 631
Goody's Body Pain Formula Powder ■ 620
Goody's Extra Strength Headache Powder ■ 620
Goody's Extra Strength Pain Relief Tablets ■ 620
Goody's PM Powder ■ 621
Hycomine Compound Tablets 1317
Lortab 3319
Lortab Elixir 3317
Maxidone Tablets CIII 3399
Maximum Strength Midol Menstrual Caplets and Gelcaps ■ 612
Maximum Strength Midol PMS Caplets and Gelcaps ■ 613
Maximum Strength Midol Teen Caplets ■ 612
Midrin Capsules 3464
Norco 5/325 Tablets CIII 3424
Norco 7.5/325 Tablets CIII 3425
Norco 10/325 Tablets CIII 3427
Norco 10/325 Tablets CIII 3425
Percocet Tablets 1326
Percogesic Aspirin-Free Coated Tablets ■ 667
Extra Strength Percogesic Aspirin-Free Coated Caplets ■ 665
Phrenilin 578
Robitussin Cold Caplets Multi-Symptom Cold & Flu ■ 781
Robitussin Cold Softgels Multi-Symptom Cold & Flu ■ 781
Robitussin Multi Symptom Honey Flu Liquid ■ 785
Robitussin Nighttime Honey Flu Liquid ■ 786
Sedapap Tablets 50 mg/650 mg 2225
Singlet Caplets ■ 761
Sinutab Sinus Allergy Medication, Maximum Strength Formula, Tablets & Caplets ■ 707
Sinutab Sinus Medication, Maximum Strength Without Drowsiness Formula, Tablets & Caplets ■ 707
Sudafed Cold & Cough Liquid Caps ■ 709
Sudafed Cold & Sinus Liquid Caps ■ 710
Sudafed Severe Cold ■ 711
Sudafed Sinus Headache Caplets ■ 712
Sudafed Sinus Headache Tablets ■ 712
Tavist Sinus Non-Drowsy Coated Caplets ■ 676
TheraFlu Regular Strength Cold & Cough Night Time Hot Liquid ■ 676
TheraFlu Regular Strength Cold & Sore Throat Night Time Hot Liquid ■ 676
TheraFlu Maximum Strength Flu & Congestion Non-Drowsy Hot Liquid ■ 677
TheraFlu Maximum Strength Flu & Cough Night Time Hot Liquid ■ 678
TheraFlu Maximum Strength Flu & Sore Throat Night Time Hot Liquid ■ 677
TheraFlu Maximum Strength Severe Cold & Congestion Night Time Caplets ■ 678
TheraFlu Maximum Strength Severe Cold & Congestion Night Time Hot Liquid ■ 678
TheraFlu Maximum Strength Severe Cold & Congestion Non-Drowsy ■ 679
Triaminic Cold, Cough & Fever Liquid ■ 681
Triaminic Cough & Sore Throat Liquid ■ 682
Triaminic Cough & Sore Throat Softchews ■ 684
Tylenol, Children's 2014
Children's Tylenol Allergy-D Liquid 2014
Children's Tylenol Cold Suspension Liquid and Chewable Tablets 2015
Children's Tylenol Cold Plus Cough Suspension Liquid and Chewable Tablets 2015
Children's Tylenol Flu Suspension Liquid 2015
Children's Tylenol Sinus Suspension Liquid 2017
Infants' Tylenol Cold Decongestant and Fever Reducer Concentrated Drops 2015
Infants' Tylenol Cold Decongestant and Fever Reducer Concentrated Drops Plus Cough 2015
Junior Strength Tylenol Soft Chews Chewable Tablets 2014
Tylenol 2009
Tylenol Allergy Sinus 2010
Tylenol Severe Allergy Caplets 2010
Multi-Symptom Tylenol Cold Complete Formula Caplets 2010
Multi-Symptom Tylenol Cold Non-Drowsy Caplets and Gelcaps 2010
Multi-Symptom Tylenol Cold Severe Congestion Non-Drowsy Caplets 2011
Maximum Strength Tylenol Flu NightTime Gelcaps 2011
Maximum Strength Tylenol Flu NightTime Liquid 2011
Maximum Strength Tylenol Flu Non-Drowsy Gelcaps 2011
Extra Strength Tylenol PM Caplets, Geltabs, and Gelcaps 2012
Maximum Strength Tylenol Sinus NightTime Caplets 2012
Maximum Strength Tylenol Sinus Non-Drowsy Geltabs, Gelcaps, Caplets, and Tablets 2012
Maximum Strength Tylenol Sore Throat Adult Liquid 2013
Tylenol with Codeine 2595
Women's Tylenol Menstrual Relief Caplets 2013
Tylox Capsules 2597
Ultracet Tablets 2597
Vanquish Caplets ■ 617
Vicks 44M Cough, Cold & Flu Relief Liquid ■ 725
Vicks DayQuil LiquiCaps/Liquid Multi-Symptom Cold/Flu Relief ■ 727
Vicks NyQuil LiquiCaps/Liquid Multi-Symptom Cold/Flu Relief, Original and Cherry Flavors ■ 727
Vicodin Tablets 516
Vicodin ES Tablets 517
Vicodin HP Tablets 518
Zydone Tablets 1330

Amiloride Hydrochloride (Yasmin has the potential to cause hyperkalemia in high-risk patients; co-administration with other drugs that have the potential to increase serum potassium, such as potassium-sparing diuretics, may increase this risk further). Products include:
Midamor Tablets 2136
Moduretic Tablets 2138

Aminophylline (Co-administration of products containing ethinyl estradiol may inhibit the metabolism of other compounds, such as theophylline, resulting in increased plasma concentrations of theophylline).
No products indexed under this heading.

Ampicillin (Co-administration of combined hormonal contraceptives with certain antibiotics may result in pregnancy).
No products indexed under this heading.

Ampicillin Sodium (Co-administration of combined hormon-

al contraceptives with certain antibiotics may result in pregnancy). Products include:
Unasyn for Injection 2728

Atorvastatin Calcium (Co-administration of atorvastatin and an oral contraceptive increased AUC values for ethinyl estradiol by approximately 20%). Products include:
Lipitor Tablets 2639
Lipitor Tablets 2696

Benazepril Hydrochloride (Yasmin has the potential to cause hyperkalemia in high-risk patients; co-administration with other drugs that have the potential to increase serum potassium, such as ACE inhibitors, may increase this risk further). Products include:
Lotensin Tablets 2365
Lotensin HCT Tablets 2367
Lotrel Capsules 2370

Candesartan Cilexetil (Yasmin has the potential to cause hyperkalemia in high-risk patients; co-administration with other drugs that have the potential to increase serum potassium, such as angiotensin-II receptor antagonists, may increase this risk further). Products include:
Atacand Tablets 595
Atacand HCT Tablets 597

Captopril (Yasmin has the potential to cause hyperkalemia in high-risk patients; co-administration with other drugs that have the potential to increase serum potassium, such as ACE inhibitors, may increase this risk further). Products include:
Captopril Tablets 2281

Carbamazepine (Co-administration results in increased metabolism of ethinyl estradiol and/or some progestins which could result in a reduction of contraceptive effectiveness). Products include:
Carbatrol Capsules 3234
Tegretol/Tegretol-XR 2404

Celecoxib (Yasmin has the potential to cause hyperkalemia in high-risk patients; co-administration with other drugs that have the potential to increase serum potassium, such as NSAIDs, may increase this risk further). Products include:
Celebrex Capsules 2676
Celebrex Capsules 2780

Clofibrate (Co-administration of products containing ethinyl estradiol may increase clearance of clofibric acid). Products include:
Atromid-S Capsules 3483

Cyclosporine (Co-administration of products containing ethinyl estradiol may inhibit the metabolism of other compounds, such as cyclosporine, resulting in increased plasma concentrations of cyclosporine). Products include:
Gengraf Capsules 457
Neoral Soft Gelatin Capsules 2380
Neoral Oral Solution 2380
Sandimmune 2388

Demeclocycline Hydrochloride (Co-administration of combined hormonal contraceptives with certain antibiotics may result in pregnancy). Products include:
Declomycin Tablets 1855

Diclofenac Potassium (Yasmin has the potential to cause hyperkalemia in high-risk patients; co-administration with other drugs that have the potential to increase serum potassium, such as NSAIDs, may increase this risk further). Products include:
Cataflam Tablets 2315

Diclofenac Sodium (Yasmin has the potential to cause hyperkalemia in high-risk patients; co-administration with other drugs that have the potential to increase serum potassium, such as NSAIDs, may increase this risk further). Products include:
Arthrotec Tablets 3195
Voltaren Ophthalmic Sterile Ophthalmic Solution .... ⊙312
Voltaren Tablets 2315
Voltaren-XR Tablets 2315

Doxycycline Calcium (Co-administration of combined hormonal contraceptives with certain antibiotics may result in pregnancy). Products include:
Vibramycin Calcium Oral Suspension Syrup 2735

Doxycycline Hyclate (Co-administration of combined hormonal contraceptives with certain antibiotics may result in pregnancy). Products include:
Doryx Coated Pellet Filled Capsules 3357
Periostat Tablets 1208
Vibramycin Hyclate Capsules 2735
Vibramycin Hyclate Intravenous 2737
Vibra-Tabs Film Coated Tablets 2735

Doxycycline Monohydrate (Co-administration of combined hormonal contraceptives with certain antibiotics may result in pregnancy). Products include:
Monodox Capsules 2442
Vibramycin Monohydrate for Oral Suspension 2735

Dyphylline (Co-administration of products containing ethinyl estradiol may inhibit the metabolism of other compounds, such as theophylline, resulting in increased plasma concentrations of theophylline). Products include:
Lufyllin Tablets 3347
Lufyllin-400 Tablets 3347
Lufyllin-GG Elixir 3348
Lufyllin-GG Tablets 3348

Enalapril Maleate (Yasmin has the potential to cause hyperkalemia in high-risk patients; co-administration with other drugs that have the potential to increase serum potassium, such as ACE inhibitors, may increase this risk further). Products include:
Lexxel Tablets 608
Vaseretic Tablets 2204
Vasotec Tablets 2210

Enalaprilat (Yasmin has the potential to cause hyperkalemia in high-risk patients; co-administration with other drugs that have the potential to increase serum potassium, such as ACE inhibitors, may increase this risk further). Products include:
Enalaprilat Injection 863
Vasotec I.V. Injection 2207

Eprosartan Mesylate (Yasmin has the potential to cause hyperkalemia in high-risk patients; co-administration with other drugs that have the potential to increase serum potassium, such as angiotensin-II receptor antagonists, may increase this risk further). Products include:
Teveten Tablets 3327

Etodolac (Yasmin has the potential to cause hyperkalemia in high-risk patients; co-administration with other drugs that have the potential to increase serum potassium, such as NSAIDs, may increase this risk further). Products include:
Lodine 3528
Lodine XL Extended-Release Tablets 3530

Fenoprofen Calcium (Yasmin has the potential to cause hyperkalemia in high-risk patients; co-administration with other drugs that have the potential to increase serum potassium, such as NSAIDs, may increase this risk further).
No products indexed under this heading.

Flurbiprofen (Yasmin has the potential to cause hyperkalemia in high-risk patients; co-administration with other drugs that have the potential to increase serum potassium, such as NSAIDs, may increase this risk further).
No products indexed under this heading.

Fosinopril Sodium (Yasmin has the potential to cause hyperkalemia in high-risk patients; co-administration with other drugs that have the potential to increase serum potassium, such as ACE inhibitors, may increase this risk further). Products include:
Monopril Tablets 1091
Monopril HCT 1094

Fosphenytoin Sodium (Co-administration results in increased metabolism of ethinyl estradiol and/or some progestins which could result in a reduction of contraceptive effectiveness). Products include:
Cerebyx Injection 2619

Griseofulvin (Co-administration of combined hormonal contraceptives with certain antibiotics may result in pregnancy). Products include:
Grifulvin V Tablets Microsize and Oral Suspension Microsize 2518
Gris-PEG Tablets 2661

Heparin Sodium (Yasmin has the potential to cause hyperkalemia in high-risk patients; co-administration with other drugs that have the potential to increase serum potassium, such as heparin, may increase this risk further). Products include:
Heparin Lock Flush Solution 3509
Heparin Sodium Injection 3511

Hypericum (Herbal products containing St. John's Wort may induce hepatic enzyme and p-glycoprotein transport and may reduce the effectiveness of oral contraceptives and emergency contraceptive pills; potential for breakthrough bleeding). Products include:
Brite-Life Caplets .... ▣795
Centrum St. John's Wort Softgels .... ▣853
Metabolic Nutrition System .... ▣798
Movana Tablets .... ▣832
One-A-Day Tension & Mood Softgels .... ▣808
ReSource Wellness StayCalm Caplets .... ▣826
Satiete Tablets .... ▣846

Ibuprofen (Yasmin has the potential to cause hyperkalemia in high-risk patients; co-administration with other drugs that have the potential to increase serum potassium, such as NSAIDs, may increase this risk further). Products include:
Advil .... ▣771
Children's Advil Oral Suspension .... ▣773
Children's Advil Chewable Tablets .... ▣773
Advil Cold and Sinus Caplets .... ▣771
Advil Cold and Sinus Tablets .... ▣771
Advil Flu & Body Ache Caplets .... ▣772
Infants' Advil Drops .... ▣773
Junior Strength Advil Tablets .... ▣773
Junior Strength Advil Chewable Tablets .... ▣773
Advil Migraine Liquigels .... ▣772
Children's Motrin Oral Suspension and Chewable Tablets 2006
Children's Motrin Cold Oral Suspension 2007
Children's Motrin Oral Suspension .... ▣643
Motrin Suspension, Oral Drops, Chewable Tablets, and Caplets 2002
Infants' Motrin Concentrated Drops 2006
Junior Strength Motrin Caplets and Chewable Tablets 2006
Motrin IB Tablets, Caplets, and Gelcaps 2002
Motrin Migraine Pain Caplets 2005
Motrin Sinus Headache Caplets 2005
Vicoprofen Tablets 520

Indomethacin (Yasmin has the potential to cause hyperkalemia in high-risk patients; co-administration with other drugs that have the potential to increase serum potassium, such as NSAIDs, may increase this risk further). Products include:
Indocin 2112

Indomethacin Sodium Trihydrate (Yasmin has the potential to cause hyperkalemia in high-risk patients; co-administration with other drugs that have the potential to increase serum potassium, such as NSAIDs, may increase this risk further). Products include:
Indocin I.V. 2115

Irbesartan (Yasmin has the potential to cause hyperkalemia in high-risk patients; co-administration with other drugs that have the potential to increase serum potassium, such as angiotensin-II receptor antagonists, may increase this risk further). Products include:
Avalide Tablets 1070
Avapro Tablets 1074
Avapro Tablets 3076

Ketoprofen (Yasmin has the potential to cause hyperkalemia in high-risk patients; co-administration with other drugs that have the potential to increase serum potassium, such as NSAIDs, may increase this risk further). Products include:
Orudis Capsules 3548
Orudis KT Tablets .... ▣778
Oruvail Capsules 3548

Ketorolac Tromethamine (Yasmin has the potential to cause hyperkalemia in high-risk patients; co-administration with other drugs that have the potential to increase serum potassium, such as NSAIDs, may increase this risk further). Products include:
Acular Ophthalmic Solution 544
Acular PF Ophthalmic Solution 544
Toradol 3018

Lisinopril (Yasmin has the potential to cause hyperkalemia in high-risk patients; co-administration with other drugs that have the potential to increase serum potassium, such as ACE inhibitors, may increase this risk further). Products include:
Prinivil Tablets 2164
Prinzide Tablets 2168
Zestoretic Tablets 695
Zestril Tablets 698

Losartan Potassium (Yasmin has the potential to cause hyperkalemia in high-risk patients; co-administration with other drugs that have the potential to increase serum potassium, such as angiotensin-II receptor antagonists, may increase this risk further). Products include:
Cozaar Tablets 2067
Hyzaar 2109

Meclofenamate Sodium (Yasmin has the potential to cause hyperkalemia in high-risk patients; co-administration with other drugs that have the potential to increase serum potassium, such as NSAIDs, may increase this risk further).
No products indexed under this heading.

Mefenamic Acid (Yasmin has the potential to cause hyperkalemia in high-risk patients; co-administration with other drugs that have the potential to increase serum potassium, such as NSAIDs, may increase this risk further). Products include:
Ponstel Capsules 1356

Meloxicam (Yasmin has the potential to cause hyperkalemia in high-risk patients; co-administration with other drugs that have the potential to increase serum potassium, such as NSAIDs, may increase this risk further). Products include:
Mobic Tablets 1054

Methacycline Hydrochloride (Co-administration of combined hormonal contraceptives with certain antibiotics may result in pregnancy).
No products indexed under this heading.

Minocycline Hydrochloride (Co-administration of combined hormonal contraceptives with certain antibiotics may result in pregnancy). Products include:
Dynacin Capsules 2019

Minocin Intravenous 1862
Minocin Oral Suspension 1865
Minocin Pellet-Filled Capsules 1863

Moexipril Hydrochloride (Yasmin has the potential to cause hyperkalemia in high-risk patients; co-administration with other drugs that have the potential to increase serum potassium, such as ACE inhibitors, may increase this risk further). Products include:
Uniretic Tablets 3178
Univasc Tablets 3181

Morphine Sulfate (Co-administration of products containing ethinyl estradiol may increase clearance of morphine). Products include:
Astramorph/PF Injection, USP (Preservative-Free) 594
Duramorph Injection 1312
Infumorph 200 and Infumorph 500 Sterile Solutions 1314
Kadian Capsules 1335
MS Contin Tablets 2896
MSIR 2898
Oramorph SR Tablets 3062
Roxanol 3066

Nabumetone (Yasmin has the potential to cause hyperkalemia in high-risk patients; co-administration with other drugs that have the potential to increase serum potassium, such as NSAIDs, may increase this risk further). Products include:
Relafen Tablets 1617

Naproxen (Yasmin has the potential to cause hyperkalemia in high-risk patients; co-administration with other drugs that have the potential to increase serum potassium, such as NSAIDs, may increase this risk further). Products include:
EC-Naprosyn Delayed-Release Tablets 2967
Naprosyn Suspension 2967
Naprosyn Tablets 2967

Naproxen Sodium (Yasmin has the potential to cause hyperkalemia in high-risk patients; co-administration with other drugs that have the potential to increase serum potassium, such as NSAIDs, may increase this risk further). Products include:
Aleve Tablets, Caplets and Gelcaps .... ■602
Aleve Cold & Sinus Caplets .... ■603
Anaprox Tablets 2967
Anaprox DS Tablets 2967
Naprelan Tablets 1293

Oxaprozin (Yasmin has the potential to cause hyperkalemia in high-risk patients; co-administration with other drugs that have the potential to increase serum potassium, such as NSAIDs, may increase this risk further).
No products indexed under this heading.

Oxytetracycline Hydrochloride (Co-administration of combined hormonal contraceptives with certain antibiotics may result in pregnancy). Products include:
Terra-Cortril Ophthalmic Suspension 2716
Urobiotic-250 Capsules 2731

Perindopril Erbumine (Yasmin has the potential to cause hyperkalemia in high-risk patients; co-administration with other drugs that have the potential to increase serum potassium, such as ACE inhibitors, may increase this risk further). Products include:
Aceon Tablets (2 mg, 4 mg, 8 mg) 3249

Phenobarbital (Co-administration results in increased metabolism of ethinyl estradiol and/or some progestins which could result in a reduction of contraceptive effectiveness). Products include:
Arco-Lase Plus Tablets 592
Donnatal 2929
Donnatal Extentabs 2930

Phenylbutazone (A reduction in contraceptive effectiveness and an increased incidence of menstrual irregularities has been suggested with phenylbutazone).
No products indexed under this heading.

Phenytoin (Co-administration results in increased metabolism of ethinyl estradiol and/or some progestins which could result in a reduction of contraceptive effectiveness). Products include:
Dilantin Infatabs 2624
Dilantin-125 Oral Suspension 2625

Phenytoin Sodium (Co-administration results in increased metabolism of ethinyl estradiol and/or some progestins which could result in a reduction of contraceptive effectiveness). Products include:
Dilantin Kapseals 2622

Piroxicam (Yasmin has the potential to cause hyperkalemia in high-risk patients; co-administration with other drugs that have the potential to increase serum potassium, such as NSAIDs, may increase this risk further). Products include:
Feldene Capsules 2685

Prednisolone (Co-administration of products containing ethinyl estradiol may inhibit the metabolism of other compounds, such as prednisolone, resulting in increased plasma concentrations of prednisolone). Products include:
Prelone Syrup 2273

Prednisolone Acetate (Co-administration of products containing ethinyl estradiol may inhibit the metabolism of other compounds, such as prednisolone, resulting in increased plasma concentrations of prednisolone). Products include:
Blephamide Ophthalmic Ointment 547
Blephamide Ophthalmic Suspension 548
Poly-Pred Liquifilm Ophthalmic Suspension .... ⊙245
Pred Forte Ophthalmic Suspension .... ⊙246
Pred Mild Sterile Ophthalmic Suspension .... ⊙249
Pred-G Ophthalmic Suspension .... ⊙247
Pred-G Sterile Ophthalmic Ointment .... ⊙248

Prednisolone Sodium Phosphate (Co-administration of products containing ethinyl estradiol may inhibit the metabolism of other compounds, such as prednisolone, resulting in increased plasma concentrations of prednisolone). Products include:
Pediapred Oral Solution 1170

Prednisolone Tebutate (Co-administration of products containing ethinyl estradiol may inhibit the metabolism of other compounds, such as prednisolone, resulting in increased plasma concentrations of prednisolone).
No products indexed under this heading.

Quinapril Hydrochloride (Yasmin has the potential to cause hyperkalemia in high-risk patients; co-administration with other drugs that have the potential to increase serum potassium, such as ACE inhibitors, may increase this risk further). Products include:
Accupril Tablets 2611
Accuretic Tablets 2614

Ramipril (Yasmin has the potential to cause hyperkalemia in high-risk patients; co-administration with other drugs that have the potential to increase serum potassium, such as ACE inhibitors, may increase this risk further). Products include:
Altace Capsules 2233

Rifampin (Co-administration results in increased metabolism of ethinyl estradiol precipitating a reduction in contraceptive effectiveness and an increase in menstrual irregularities). Products include:
Rifadin 765
Rifamate Capsules 767
Rifater Tablets 769

Rofecoxib (Yasmin has the potential to cause hyperkalemia in high-risk patients; co-administration with other drugs that have the potential to increase serum potassium, such as NSAIDs, may increase this risk further). Products include:
Vioxx 2213

Salicylic Acid (Co-administration of products containing ethinyl estradiol may increase clearance of salicylic acid). Products include:
Clear Away Gel with Aloe Wart Remover System .... ■736
Clear Away Liquid Wart Remover System .... ■736
Clear Away One Step Wart Remover .... ■737
Clear Away One Step Wart Remover for Kids .... ■737
Clear Away One Step Plantar Wart Remover .... ■737
Compound W One Step Pads for Kids .... ■664
Compound W One Step Plantar Pads .... ■664
Compound W One Step Wart Remover Pads .... ■664
Compound W Wart Remover Gel .... ■665
Compound W Wart Remover Liquid .... ■665
Wart-Off Liquid .... ■716

Spirapril Hydrochloride (Yasmin has the potential to cause hyperkalemia in high-risk patients; co-administration with other drugs that have the potential to increase serum potassium, such as ACE inhibitors, may increase this risk further).
No products indexed under this heading.

Spironolactone (Yasmin has the potential to cause hyperkalemia in high-risk patients; co-administration with other drugs that have the potential to increase serum potassium, such as potassium-sparing diuretics, may increase this risk further).
No products indexed under this heading.

Sulindac (Yasmin has the potential to cause hyperkalemia in high-risk patients; co-administration with other drugs that have the potential to increase serum potassium, such as NSAIDs, may increase this risk further). Products include:
Clinoril Tablets 2053

Telmisartan (Yasmin has the potential to cause hyperkalemia in high-risk patients; co-administration with other drugs that have the potential to increase serum potassium, such as angiotensin-II receptor antagonists, may increase this risk further). Products include:
Micardis Tablets 1049
Micardis HCT Tablets 1051

Temazepam (Co-administration of products containing ethinyl estradiol may increase clearance of temazepam).
No products indexed under this heading.

Tetracycline Hydrochloride (Co-administration of combined hormonal contraceptives with certain antibiotics may result in pregnancy).
No products indexed under this heading.

Theophylline (Co-administration of products containing ethinyl estradiol may inhibit the metabolism of other compounds, such as theophylline, resulting in increased plasma concentrations of theophylline). Products include:
Aerolate 1361
Theo-Dur Extended-Release Tablets 1835
Uni-Dur Extended-Release Tablets 1841
Uniphyl 400 mg and 600 mg Tablets 2903

Theophylline Calcium Salicylate (Co-administration of products containing ethinyl estradiol may inhibit the metabolism of other compounds, such as theophylline, resulting in increased plasma concentrations of theophylline).
No products indexed under this heading.

Theophylline Sodium Glycinate (Co-administration of products containing ethinyl estradiol may inhibit the metabolism of other compounds, such as theophylline, resulting in increased plasma concentrations of theophylline).
No products indexed under this heading.

Tolmetin Sodium (Yasmin has the potential to cause hyperkalemia in high-risk patients; co-administration with other drugs that have the potential to increase serum potassium, such as NSAIDs, may increase this risk further). Products include:
Tolectin 2589

Trandolapril (Yasmin has the potential to cause hyperkalemia in high-risk patients; co-administration with other drugs that have the potential to increase serum potassium, such as ACE inhibitors, may increase this risk further). Products include:
Mavik Tablets 478
Tarka Tablets 508

Triamterene (Yasmin has the potential to cause hyperkalemia in high-risk patients; co-administration with other drugs that have the potential to increase serum potassium, such as potassium-sparing diuretics, may increase this risk further). Products include:
Dyazide Capsules 1515
Dyrenium Capsules 3458
Maxzide 1008

Valsartan (Yasmin has the potential to cause hyperkalemia in high-risk patients; co-administration with other drugs that have the potential to increase serum potassium, such as angiotensin-II receptor antagonists, may increase this risk further). Products include:
Diovan Capsules 2337
Diovan HCT Tablets 2338

Vitamin C (May increase plasma levels of ethinyl estradiol possibly by inhibition of conjugation). Products include:
Beta-C Tablets .... ■811
C-Grams Caplets .... ■795
Halls Defense Drops .... ■687
Peridin C Tablets .... ■618

YF-VAX VACCINE
(Yellow Fever Vaccine) 827
May interact with alkylating agents, corticosteroids, and cytotoxic drugs. Compounds in these categories include:

Betamethasone Acetate (Patients whose immunologic responses are suppressed by corticosteroids should not be vaccinated). Products include:
Celestone Soluspan Injectable Suspension 3097

Betamethasone Sodium Phosphate (Patients whose immunologic responses are suppressed by corticosteroids should not be vaccinated). Products include:
Celestone Soluspan Injectable Suspension 3097

Bleomycin Sulfate (Patients whose immunologic responses are suppressed by antimetabolites should not be vaccinated).
No products indexed under this heading.

Busulfan (Patients whose immunologic responses are suppressed by alkylating drugs should not be vaccinated). Products include:

Myleran Tablets 1603

Carmustine (BCNU) (Patients whose immunologic responses are suppressed by alkylating drugs should not be vaccinated). Products include:

Gliadel Wafer 1723

Chlorambucil (Patients whose immunologic responses are suppressed by alkylating drugs should not be vaccinated). Products include:

Leukeran Tablets 1591

Cortisone Acetate (Patients whose immunologic responses are suppressed by corticosteroids should not be vaccinated). Products include:

Cortone Acetate Injectable Suspension 2059
Cortone Acetate Tablets 2061

Cyclophosphamide (Patients whose immunologic responses are suppressed by alkylating drugs should not be vaccinated).

No products indexed under this heading.

Dacarbazine (Patients whose immunologic responses are suppressed by alkylating drugs should not be vaccinated). Products include:

DTIC-Dome 902

Daunorubicin Hydrochloride (Patients whose immunologic responses are suppressed by antimetabolites should not be vaccinated). Products include:

Cerubidine for Injection 947

Dexamethasone (Patients whose immunologic responses are suppressed by corticosteroids should not be vaccinated). Products include:

Decadron Elixir 2078
Decadron Tablets 2079
TobraDex Ophthalmic Ointment 542
TobraDex Ophthalmic Suspension .. 541

Dexamethasone Acetate (Patients whose immunologic responses are suppressed by corticosteroids should not be vaccinated).

No products indexed under this heading.

Dexamethasone Sodium Phosphate (Patients whose immunologic responses are suppressed by corticosteroids should not be vaccinated). Products include:

Decadron Phosphate Injection 2081
Decadron Phosphate Sterile Ophthalmic Ointment 2083
Decadron Phosphate Sterile Ophthalmic Solution 2084
NeoDecadron Sterile Ophthalmic Solution 2144

Doxorubicin Hydrochloride (Patients whose immunologic responses are suppressed by antimetabolites should not be vaccinated). Products include:

Adriamycin PFS/RDF Injection 2767
Doxil Injection 566

Epirubicin Hydrochloride (Patients whose immunologic responses are suppressed by antimetabolites should not be vaccinated). Products include:

Ellence Injection 2806

Fludrocortisone Acetate (Patients whose immunologic responses are suppressed by corticosteroids should not be vaccinated). Products include:

Florinef Acetate Tablets 2250

Fluorouracil (Patients whose immunologic responses are suppressed by antimetabolites should not be vaccinated). Products include:

Carac Cream 1222
Efudex 1733
Fluoroplex 552

Hydrocortisone (Patients whose immunologic responses are suppressed by corticosteroids should not be vaccinated). Products include:

Anusol-HC Cream 2.5% 2237
Cipro HC Otic Suspension 540
Cortaid Intensive Therapy Cream .. ▣717
Cortaid Maximum Strength Cream .... ▣717
Cortisporin Ophthalmic Suspension Sterile .... ⊙297
Cortizone•5 .... ▣699
Cortizone•10 .... ▣699
Cortizone•10 Plus Creme .... ▣700
Cortizone for Kids Creme .... ▣699
Hydrocortone Tablets 2106
Massengill Medicated Soft Cloth Towelette .... ▣753
VōSoL HC Otic Solution 3356

Hydrocortisone Acetate (Patients whose immunologic responses are suppressed by corticosteroids should not be vaccinated). Products include:

Analpram-HC 1338
Anusol HC-1 Hydrocortisone Anti-Itch Cream .... ▣689
Anusol-HC Suppositories 2238
Cortaid .... ▣717
Cortifoam Rectal Foam 3170
Cortisporin-TC Otic Suspension 2246
Hydrocortone Acetate Injectable Suspension 2103
Pramosone 1343
Proctocort Suppositories 2264
ProctoFoam-HC 3177
Terra-Cortril Ophthalmic Suspension 2716

Hydrocortisone Sodium Phosphate (Patients whose immunologic responses are suppressed by corticosteroids should not be vaccinated). Products include:

Hydrocortone Phosphate Injection, Sterile 2105

Hydrocortisone Sodium Succinate (Patients whose immunologic responses are suppressed by corticosteroids should not be vaccinated).

No products indexed under this heading.

Hydroxyurea (Patients whose immunologic responses are suppressed by antimetabolites should not be vaccinated). Products include:

Mylocel Tablets 2227

Lomustine (CCNU) (Patients whose immunologic responses are suppressed by alkylating drugs should not be vaccinated).

No products indexed under this heading.

Mechlorethamine Hydrochloride (Patients whose immunologic responses are suppressed by alkylating drugs should not be vaccinated). Products include:

Mustargen for Injection 2142

Melphalan (Patients whose immunologic responses are suppressed by alkylating drugs should not be vaccinated). Products include:

Alkeran Tablets 1466

Methotrexate Sodium (Patients whose immunologic responses are suppressed by antimetabolites should not be vaccinated).

No products indexed under this heading.

Methylprednisolone Acetate (Patients whose immunologic responses are suppressed by corticosteroids should not be vaccinated). Products include:

Depo-Medrol Injectable Suspension 2795

Methylprednisolone Sodium Succinate (Patients whose immunologic responses are suppressed by corticosteroids should not be vaccinated). Products include:

Solu-Medrol Sterile Powder 2855

Mitotane (Patients whose immunologic responses are suppressed by antimetabolites should not be vaccinated).

No products indexed under this heading.

Mitoxantrone Hydrochloride (Patients whose immunologic responses are suppressed by antimetabolites should not be vaccinated). Products include:

Novantrone for Injection 1760

Prednisolone Acetate (Patients whose immunologic responses are suppressed by corticosteroids should not be vaccinated). Products include:

Blephamide Ophthalmic Ointment ... 547
Blephamide Ophthalmic Suspension 548
Poly-Pred Liquifilm Ophthalmic Suspension .... ⊙245
Pred Forte Ophthalmic Suspension .... ⊙246
Pred Mild Sterile Ophthalmic Suspension .... ⊙249
Pred-G Ophthalmic Suspension .... ⊙247
Pred-G Sterile Ophthalmic Ointment .... ⊙248

Prednisolone Sodium Phosphate (Patients whose immunologic responses are suppressed by corticosteroids should not be vaccinated). Products include:

Pediapred Oral Solution 1170

Prednisolone Tebutate (Patients whose immunologic responses are suppressed by corticosteroids should not be vaccinated).

No products indexed under this heading.

Prednisone (Patients whose immunologic responses are suppressed by corticosteroids should not be vaccinated). Products include:

Prednisone 3064

Procarbazine Hydrochloride (Patients whose immunologic responses are suppressed by antimetabolites should not be vaccinated). Products include:

Matulane Capsules 3246

Tamoxifen Citrate (Patients whose immunologic responses are suppressed by antimetabolites should not be vaccinated). Products include:

Nolvadex Tablets 678

Thiotepa (Patients whose immunologic responses are suppressed by alkylating drugs should not be vaccinated). Products include:

Thioplex for Injection 1765

Triamcinolone (Patients whose immunologic responses are suppressed by corticosteroids should not be vaccinated).

No products indexed under this heading.

Triamcinolone Acetonide (Patients whose immunologic responses are suppressed by corticosteroids should not be vaccinated). Products include:

Azmacort Inhalation Aerosol 728
Nasacort Nasal Inhaler 750
Nasacort AQ Nasal Spray 752
Tri-Nasal Spray 2274

Triamcinolone Diacetate (Patients whose immunologic responses are suppressed by corticosteroids should not be vaccinated).

No products indexed under this heading.

Triamcinolone Hexacetonide (Patients whose immunologic responses are suppressed by corticosteroids should not be vaccinated).

No products indexed under this heading.

Vincristine Sulfate (Patients whose immunologic responses are suppressed by antimetabolites should not be vaccinated).

No products indexed under this heading.

YODOXIN TABLETS

(Iodoquinol) 1722
None cited in PDR database.

ZADITOR OPHTHALMIC SOLUTION

(Ketotifen Fumarate) 2304
None cited in PDR database.

ZANAFLEX TABLETS

(Tizanidine Hydrochloride) 1305
May interact with benzodiazepines, oral contraceptives, and certain other agents. Compounds in these categories include:

Acetaminophen (Co-administration delays the Tmax of acetaminophen by 16 minutes). Products include:

Actifed Cold & Sinus Caplets and Tablets .... ▣688
Alka-Seltzer Plus Liqui-Gels .... ▣604
Alka-Seltzer Plus Cold & Flu Medicine Liqui-Gels .... ▣604
Alka-Seltzer Plus Cold & Sinus Medicine Liqui-Gels .... ▣604
Benadryl Allergy/Cold Tablets .... ▣691
Benadryl Allergy Sinus Headache Caplets & Gelcaps .... ▣693
Benadryl Severe Allergy & Sinus Headache Caplets .... ▣694
Children's Cēpacol Sore Throat .... ▣788
Comtrex Acute Head Cold & Sinus Pressure Relief Tablets .... ▣627
Comtrex Deep Chest Cold & Congestion Relief Softgels .... ▣627
Comtrex Flu Therapy & Fever Relief Daytime Caplets .... ▣628
Comtrex Flu Therapy & Fever Relief Nighttime Tablets .... ▣628
Comtrex Maximum Strength Multi-Symptom Cold & Cough Relief Tablets and Caplets .... ▣626
Contac Severe Cold and Flu Caplets Maximum Strength .... ▣746
Contac Severe Cold and Flu Caplets Non-Drowsy .... ▣746
Coricidin 'D' Cold, Flu & Sinus Tablets .... ▣737
Coricidin HBP Cold & Flu Tablets .. ▣738
Coricidin HBP Maximum Strength Flu Tablets .... ▣738
Coricidin HBP Night-Time Cold & Flu Tablets .... ▣738
Darvon-N/Darvocet-N 1907
Dimetapp Cold and Fever Suspension .... ▣775
Dimetapp Nighttime Flu Liquid .... ▣776
Dimetapp Non-Drowsy Flu Syrup .. ▣777
Drixoral Allergy/Sinus Extended-Release Tablets .... ▣741
Drixoral Cold & Flu Extended-Release Tablets .... ▣740
Aspirin Free Excedrin Caplets and Geltabs .... ▣628
Excedrin Extra-Strength Tablets, Caplets, and Geltabs .... ▣629
Excedrin Migraine 1070
Excedrin PM Tablets, Caplets, and Geltabs .... ▣631
Goody's Body Pain Formula Powder .... ▣620
Goody's Extra Strength Headache Powder .... ▣620
Goody's Extra Strength Pain Relief Tablets .... ▣620
Goody's PM Powder .... ▣621
Hycomine Compound Tablets 1317
Lortab 3319
Lortab Elixir 3317
Maxidone Tablets CIII 3399
Maximum Strength Midol Menstrual Caplets and Gelcaps .. ▣612
Maximum Strength Midol PMS Caplets and Gelcaps .... ▣613
Maximum Strength Midol Teen Caplets .... ▣612
Midrin Capsules 3464
Norco 5/325 Tablets CIII 3424
Norco 7.5/325 Tablets CIII 3425
Norco 10/325 Tablets CIII 3427
Norco 10/325 Tablets CIII 3425
Percocet Tablets 1326
Percogesic Aspirin-Free Coated Tablets .... ▣667
Extra Strength Percogesic Aspirin-Free Coated Caplets .... ▣665
Phrenilin 578
Robitussin Cold Caplets Multi-Symptom Cold & Flu .... ▣781
Robitussin Cold Softgels Multi-Symptom Cold & Flu .... ▣781
Robitussin Multi Symptom Honey Flu Liquid .... ▣785

Robitussin Nighttime Honey Flu Liquid ◘786
Sedapap Tablets 50 mg/650 mg ... 2225
Singlet Caplets ◘761
Sinutab Sinus Allergy Medication, Maximum Strength Formula, Tablets & Caplets ◘707
Sinutab Sinus Medication, Maximum Strength Without Drowsiness Formula, Tablets & Caplets ◘707
Sudafed Cold & Cough Liquid Caps ◘709
Sudafed Cold & Sinus Liquid Caps ◘710
Sudafed Severe Cold ◘711
Sudafed Sinus Headache Caplets ◘712
Sudafed Sinus Headache Tablets ◘712
Tavist Sinus Non-Drowsy Coated Caplets ◘676
TheraFlu Regular Strength Cold & Cough Night Time Hot Liquid ◘676
TheraFlu Regular Strength Cold & Sore Throat Night Time Hot Liquid ◘676
TheraFlu Maximum Strength Flu & Congestion Non-Drowsy Hot Liquid ◘677
TheraFlu Maximum Strength Flu & Cough Night Time Hot Liquid ◘678
TheraFlu Maximum Strength Flu & Sore Throat Night Time Hot Liquid ◘677
TheraFlu Maximum Strength Severe Cold & Congestion Night Time Caplets ◘678
TheraFlu Maximum Strength Severe Cold & Congestion Night Time Hot Liquid ◘678
TheraFlu Maximum Strength Severe Cold & Congestion Non-Drowsy ◘679
Triaminic Cold, Cough & Fever Liquid ◘681
Triaminic Cough & Sore Throat Liquid ◘682
Triaminic Cough & Sore Throat Softchews ◘684
Tylenol, Children's 2014
Children's Tylenol Allergy-D Liquid 2014
Children's Tylenol Cold Suspension Liquid and Chewable Tablets 2015
Children's Tylenol Cold Plus Cough Suspension Liquid and Chewable Tablets 2015
Children's Tylenol Flu Suspension Liquid 2015
Children's Tylenol Sinus Suspension Liquid 2017
Infants' Tylenol Cold Decongestant and Fever Reducer Concentrated Drops 2015
Infants' Tylenol Cold Decongestant and Fever Reducer Concentrated Drops Plus Cough 2015
Junior Strength Tylenol Soft Chews Chewable Tablets 2014
Tylenol 2009
Tylenol Allergy Sinus 2010
Tylenol Severe Allergy Caplets 2010
Multi-Symptom Tylenol Cold Complete Formula Caplets 2010
Multi-Symptom Tylenol Cold Non-Drowsy Caplets and Gelcaps 2010
Multi-Symptom Tylenol Cold Severe Congestion Non-Drowsy Caplets 2011
Maximum Strength Tylenol Flu NightTime Gelcaps 2011
Maximum Strength Tylenol Flu NightTime Liquid 2011
Maximum Strength Tylenol Flu Non-Drowsy Gelcaps 2011
Extra Strength Tylenol PM Caplets, Geltabs, and Gelcaps 2012
Maximum Strength Tylenol Sinus NightTime Caplets 2012
Maximum Strength Tylenol Sinus Non-Drowsy Geltabs, Gelcaps, Caplets, and Tablets 2012
Maximum Strength Tylenol Sore Throat Adult Liquid 2013
Tylenol with Codeine 2595
Women's Tylenol Menstrual Relief Caplets 2013
Tylox Capsules 2597
Ultracet Tablets 2597
Vanquish Caplets ◘617
Vicks 44M Cough, Cold & Flu Relief Liquid ◘725
Vicks DayQuil LiquiCaps/Liquid Multi-Symptom Cold/Flu Relief ◘727
Vicks NyQuil LiquiCaps/Liquid Multi-Symptom Cold/Flu Relief, Original and Cherry Flavors ◘727
Vicodin Tablets 516
Vicodin ES Tablets 517
Vicodin HP Tablets 518
Zydone Tablets 1330

Alprazolam (Co-administration with benzodiazepines may result in additive sedation). Products include:
Xanax Tablets 2865

Baclofen (Co-administration may result in additive sedation).
No products indexed under this heading.

Chlordiazepoxide (Co-administration with benzodiazepines may result in additive sedation). Products include:
Limbitrol 1738

Chlordiazepoxide Hydrochloride (Co-administration with benzodiazepines may result in additive sedation). Products include:
Librium Capsules 1736
Librium for Injection 1737

Clorazepate Dipotassium (Co-administration with benzodiazepines may result in additive sedation). Products include:
Tranxene 511

Desogestrel (Co-administration with oral contraceptives has resulted, based on retrospective analysis, in 50% reduction in clearance of tizanidine). Products include:
Cyclessa Tablets 2450
Desogen Tablets 2458
Mircette Tablets 2470
Ortho-Cept 21 Tablets 2546
Ortho-Cept 28 Tablets 2546

Diazepam (Co-administration with benzodiazepines may result in additive sedation). Products include:
Valium Injectable 3026
Valium Tablets 3047

Estazolam (Co-administration with benzodiazepines may result in additive sedation). Products include:
ProSom Tablets 500

Ethinyl Estradiol (Co-administration with oral contraceptives has resulted, based on retrospective analysis, in 50% reduction in clearance of tizanidine). Products include:
Alesse-21 Tablets 3468
Alesse-28 Tablets 3473
Brevicon 28-Day Tablets 3380
Cyclessa Tablets 2450
Desogen Tablets 2458
Estinyl Tablets 3112
Estrostep 2627
femhrt Tablets 2635
Levlen 962
Levlite 21 Tablets 962
Levlite 28 Tablets 962
Levora Tablets 3389
Loestrin 21 Tablets 2642
Loestrin Fe Tablets 2642
Lo/Ovral Tablets 3532
Lo/Ovral-28 Tablets 3538
Low-Ogestrel-28 Tablets 3392
Microgestin Fe 1.5/30 Tablets 3407
Microgestin Fe 1/20 Tablets 3400
Mircette Tablets 2470
Modicon 2563
Necon 3415
Nordette-28 Tablets 2257
Norinyl 1 +35 28-Day Tablets 3380
Ogestrel 0.5/50-28 Tablets 3428
Ortho-Cept 21 Tablets 2546
Ortho-Cept 28 Tablets 2546
Ortho-Cyclen/Ortho Tri-Cyclen 2573
Ortho-Novum 2563
Ovcon 3364
Ovral Tablets 3551
Ovral-28 Tablets 3552
Tri-Levlen 962
Tri-Norinyl-28 Tablets 3433
Triphasil-21 Tablets 3600
Triphasil-28 Tablets 3605
Trivora Tablets 3439
Yasmin 28 Tablets 980
Zovia 3449

Ethynodiol Diacetate (Co-administration with oral contraceptives has resulted, based on retrospective analysis, in 50% reduction in clearance of tizanidine). Products include:
Zovia 3449

Flurazepam Hydrochloride (Co-administration with benzodiazepines may result in additive sedation).
No products indexed under this heading.

Halazepam (Co-administration with benzodiazepines may result in additive sedation).
No products indexed under this heading.

Levonorgestrel (Co-administration with oral contraceptives has resulted, based on retrospective analysis, in 50% reduction in clearance of tizanidine). Products include:
Alesse-21 Tablets 3468
Alesse-28 Tablets 3473
Levlen 962
Levlite 21 Tablets 962
Levlite 28 Tablets 962
Levora Tablets 3389
Mirena Intrauterine System 974
Nordette-28 Tablets 2257
Norplant System 3543
Tri-Levlen 962
Triphasil-21 Tablets 3600
Triphasil-28 Tablets 3605
Trivora Tablets 3439

Lorazepam (Co-administration with benzodiazepines may result in additive sedation). Products include:
Ativan Injection 3478
Ativan Tablets 3482

Mestranol (Co-administration with oral contraceptives has resulted, based on retrospective analysis, in 50% reduction in clearance of tizanidine). Products include:
Necon 1/50 Tablets 3415
Norinyl 1 + 50 28-Day Tablets 3380
Ortho-Novum 1/50□28 Tablets 2556

Midazolam Hydrochloride (Co-administration with benzodiazepines may result in additive sedation). Products include:
Versed Injection 3027
Versed Syrup 3033

Norethindrone (Co-administration with oral contraceptives has resulted, based on retrospective analysis, in 50% reduction in clearance of tizanidine). Products include:
Brevicon 28-Day Tablets 3380
Micronor Tablets 2543
Modicon 2563
Necon 3415
Norinyl 1 +35 28-Day Tablets 3380
Norinyl 1 + 50 28-Day Tablets 3380
Nor-QD Tablets 3423
Ortho-Novum 2563
Ortho-Novum 1/50□28 Tablets 2556
Ovcon 3364
Tri-Norinyl-28 Tablets 3433

Norethynodrel (Co-administration with oral contraceptives has resulted, based on retrospective analysis, in 50% reduction in clearance of tizanidine).
No products indexed under this heading.

Norgestimate (Co-administration with oral contraceptives has resulted, based on retrospective analysis, in 50% reduction in clearance of tizanidine). Products include:
Ortho-Cyclen/Ortho Tri-Cyclen 2573
Ortho-Prefest Tablets 2570

Norgestrel (Co-administration with oral contraceptives has resulted, based on retrospective analysis, in 50% reduction in clearance of tizanidine). Products include:
Lo/Ovral Tablets 3532
Lo/Ovral-28 Tablets 3538
Low-Ogestrel-28 Tablets 3392
Ogestrel 0.5/50-28 Tablets 3428
Ovral Tablets 3551
Ovral-28 Tablets 3552
Ovrette Tablets 3552

Oxazepam (Co-administration with benzodiazepines may result in additive sedation).
No products indexed under this heading.

Prazepam (Co-administration with benzodiazepines may result in additive sedation).
No products indexed under this heading.

Quazepam (Co-administration with benzodiazepines may result in additive sedation).
No products indexed under this heading.

Temazepam (Co-administration with benzodiazepines may result in additive sedation).
No products indexed under this heading.

Triazolam (Co-administration with benzodiazepines may result in additive sedation). Products include:
Halcion Tablets 2823

Food Interactions

Alcohol (Increases the AUC of tizanidine by approximately 20% and increases its Cmax by approximately 15%; the CNS depressant effects are additive).

Food, unspecified (Increases Cmax by approximately one-third and shortens time to peak concentration by approximately 40 minutes, but the extent of tizanidine absorption is not affected).

ZANTAC 150 TABLETS
(Ranitidine Hydrochloride) 1690
May interact with:

Triazolam (Ranitidine, similar to other agents that lower gastric acidity, has been shown to increase the absorption of triazolam resulting in increased plasma concentrations on average 14% to 28%; the clinical significance of this finding is unknown). Products include:
Halcion Tablets 2823

Warfarin Sodium (Potential for increased or decreased prothrombin time; doses of ranitidine up to 400 mg per day had no effect on prothrombin time or warfarin clearance). Products include:
Coumadin for Injection 1243
Coumadin Tablets 1243
Warfarin Sodium Tablets, USP 3302

ZANTAC 300 TABLETS
(Ranitidine Hydrochloride) 1690
See Zantac 150 Tablets

ZANTAC 150 EFFERDOSE GRANULES
(Ranitidine Hydrochloride) 1690
See Zantac 150 Tablets

ZANTAC 150 EFFERDOSE TABLETS
(Ranitidine Hydrochloride) 1690
See Zantac 150 Tablets

ZANTAC INJECTION
(Ranitidine Hydrochloride) 1688
See Zantac 150 Tablets

ZANTAC INJECTION PREMIXED
(Ranitidine Hydrochloride) 1688
See Zantac 150 Tablets

ZANTAC SYRUP
(Ranitidine Hydrochloride) 1690
See Zantac 150 Tablets

ZANTAC 75 TABLETS
(Ranitidine Hydrochloride) ◘717
None cited in PDR database.

ZARONTIN CAPSULES
(Ethosuximide) 2659
May interact with phenytoin and valproate. Compounds in these categories include:

Divalproex Sodium (Co-administration may lead to both increase and decrease ethosuximide levels). Products include:
Depakote Sprinkle Capsules 426

Depakote Tablets 430
Depakote ER Tablets 436

Fosphenytoin Sodium (Co-administration may lead to elevated phenytoin serum levels). Products include:
Cerebyx Injection 2619

Phenytoin (Co-administration may lead to elevated phenytoin serum levels). Products include:
Dilantin Infatabs 2624
Dilantin-125 Oral Suspension 2625

Phenytoin Sodium (Co-administration may lead to elevated phenytoin serum levels). Products include:
Dilantin Kapseals 2622

Valproate Sodium (Co-administration may lead to both increase and decrease ethosuximide levels). Products include:
Depacon Injection 416

Valproic Acid (Co-administration may lead to both increase and decrease ethosuximide levels). Products include:
Depakene 421

ZARONTIN SYRUP
(Ethosuximide) 2660
See Zarontin Capsules

ZAROXOLYN TABLETS
(Metolazone) 1177
May interact with antihypertensives, barbiturates, corticosteroids, oral anticoagulants, cardiac glycosides, oral hypoglycemic agents, insulin, lithium preparations, loop diuretics, narcotic analgesics, non-steroidal anti-inflammatory agents, salicylates, and certain other agents. Compounds in these categories include:

Acarbose (Metolazone may raise blood glucose concentrations possibly causing hyperglycemia and glycosuria in patients with diabetes; dose adjustment of oral hypoglycemic agents may be required). Products include:
Precose Tablets 906

Acebutolol Hydrochloride (Co-administration with other antihypertensive agents may potentiate orthostatic hypotension). Products include:
Sectral Capsules 3589

ACTH (Co-administration with ACTH may increase the risk of hypokalemia and increase salt and water retention).
No products indexed under this heading.

Alfentanil Hydrochloride (Co-administration with narcotics may potentiate orthostatic hypotension).
No products indexed under this heading.

Amlodipine Besylate (Co-administration with other antihypertensive agents may potentiate orthostatic hypotension). Products include:
Lotrel Capsules 2370
Norvasc Tablets 2704

Aprobarbital (Co-administration with barbiturates may potentiate orthostatic hypotension).
No products indexed under this heading.

Aspirin (Co-administration with salicylates may decrease the antihypertensive effects of metolazone). Products include:
Aggrenox Capsules 1026
Alka-Seltzer 603
Alka-Seltzer Lemon Lime Antacid and Pain Reliever Effervescent Tablets 603
Alka-Seltzer Extra Strength Antacid and Pain Reliever Effervescent Tablets 603
Alka-Seltzer PM Effervescent Tablets 605
Genuine Bayer Tablets, Caplets and Gelcaps 606
Extra Strength Bayer Caplets and Gelcaps 610
Aspirin Regimen Bayer Children's Chewable Tablets (Orange or Cherry Flavored) 607
Bayer, Aspirin Regimen 606
Aspirin Regimen Bayer 81 mg Caplets with Calcium 607
Genuine Bayer Professional Labeling (Aspirin Regimen Bayer) 608
Extra Strength Bayer Arthritis Caplets 610
Extra Strength Bayer Plus Caplets 610
Extra Strength Bayer PM Caplets 611
BC Powder 619
BC Allergy Sinus Cold Powder 619
Arthritis Strength BC Powder 619
BC Sinus Cold Powder 619
Darvon Compound-65 Pulvules 1910
Ecotrin Enteric Coated Aspirin Low, Regular and Maximum Strength Tablets 1715
Excedrin Extra-Strength Tablets, Caplets, and Geltabs 629
Excedrin Migraine 1070
Goody's Body Pain Formula Powder 620
Goody's Extra Strength Headache Powder 620
Goody's Extra Strength Pain Relief Tablets 620
Percodan Tablets 1327
Robaxisal Tablets 2939
Soma Compound Tablets 3354
Soma Compound w/Codeine Tablets 3355
Vanquish Caplets 617

Atenolol (Co-administration with other antihypertensive agents may potentiate orthostatic hypotension). Products include:
Tenoretic Tablets 690
Tenormin I.V. Injection 692

Benazepril Hydrochloride (Co-administration with other antihypertensive agents may potentiate orthostatic hypotension). Products include:
Lotensin Tablets 2365
Lotensin HCT Tablets 2367
Lotrel Capsules 2370

Bendroflumethiazide (Co-administration with other antihypertensive agents may potentiate orthostatic hypotension). Products include:
Corzide 40/5 Tablets 2247
Corzide 80/5 Tablets 2247

Betamethasone Acetate (Co-administration with corticosteroids may increase the risk of hypokalemia and increase salt and water retention). Products include:
Celestone Soluspan Injectable Suspension 3097

Betamethasone Sodium Phosphate (Co-administration with corticosteroids may increase the risk of hypokalemia and increase salt and water retention). Products include:
Celestone Soluspan Injectable Suspension 3097

Betaxolol Hydrochloride (Co-administration with other antihypertensive agents may potentiate orthostatic hypotension). Products include:
Betoptic S Ophthalmic Suspension 537

Bisoprolol Fumarate (Co-administration with other antihypertensive agents may potentiate orthostatic hypotension). Products include:
Zebeta Tablets 1885
Ziac Tablets 1887

Bumetanide (Co-administration with loop diuretics can cause unusually large or prolonged losses of fluid and electrolytes).
No products indexed under this heading.

Buprenorphine Hydrochloride (Co-administration with narcotics may potentiate orthostatic hypotension). Products include:
Buprenex Injectable 2918

Butabarbital (Co-administration with barbiturates may potentiate orthostatic hypotension).
No products indexed under this heading.

Butalbital (Co-administration with barbiturates may potentiate orthostatic hypotension). Products include:
Phrenilin 578
Sedapap Tablets 50 mg/650 mg 2225

Candesartan Cilexetil (Co-administration with other antihypertensive agents may potentiate orthostatic hypotension). Products include:
Atacand Tablets 595
Atacand HCT Tablets 597

Captopril (Co-administration with other antihypertensive agents may potentiate orthostatic hypotension). Products include:
Captopril Tablets 2281

Carteolol Hydrochloride (Co-administration with other antihypertensive agents may potentiate orthostatic hypotension). Products include:
Carteolol Hydrochloride Ophthalmic Solution USP, 1% .... ⊙258
Ocupress Ophthalmic Solution, 1% Sterile .... ⊙303

Celecoxib (Co-administration with non-steroidal anti-inflammatory agents may decrease the antihypertensive effects of metolazone). Products include:
Celebrex Capsules 2676
Celebrex Capsules 2780

Chlorothiazide (Co-administration with other antihypertensive agents may potentiate orthostatic hypotension). Products include:
Aldoclor Tablets 2035
Diuril Oral 2087

Chlorothiazide Sodium (Co-administration with other antihypertensive agents may potentiate orthostatic hypotension). Products include:
Diuril Sodium Intravenous 2086

Chlorpropamide (Metolazone may raise blood glucose concentrations possibly causing hyperglycemia and glycosuria in patients with diabetes; dose adjustment of oral hypoglycemic agents may be required). Products include:
Diabinese Tablets 2680

Chlorthalidone (Co-administration with other antihypertensive agents may potentiate orthostatic hypotension). Products include:
Clorpres Tablets 1002
Combipres Tablets 1040
Tenoretic Tablets 690

Choline Magnesium Trisalicylate (Co-administration with salicylates may decrease the antihypertensive effects of metolazone). Products include:
Trilisate 2901

Clonidine (Co-administration with other antihypertensive agents may potentiate orthostatic hypotension). Products include:
Catapres-TTS 1038

Clonidine Hydrochloride (Co-administration with other antihypertensive agents may potentiate orthostatic hypotension). Products include:
Catapres Tablets 1037
Clorpres Tablets 1002
Combipres Tablets 1040
Duraclon Injection 3057

Codeine Phosphate (Co-administration with narcotics may potentiate orthostatic hypotension). Products include:
Phenergan with Codeine Syrup 3557
Phenergan VC with Codeine Syrup 3561
Robitussin A-C Syrup 2942
Robitussin-DAC Syrup 2942
Ryna-C Liquid 768
Soma Compound w/Codeine Tablets 3355
Tussi-Organidin NR Liquid 3350
Tussi-Organidin-S NR Liquid 3350
Tylenol with Codeine 2595

Cortisone Acetate (Co-administration with corticosteroids may increase the risk of hypokalemia and increase salt and water retention). Products include:
Cortone Acetate Injectable Suspension 2059
Cortone Acetate Tablets 2061

Deserpidine (Co-administration with other antihypertensive agents may potentiate orthostatic hypotension).
No products indexed under this heading.

Deslanoside (Diuretics induced hypokalemia can increase the sensitivity of the myocardium to digitalis resulting in serious arrhythmias).
No products indexed under this heading.

Dexamethasone (Co-administration with corticosteroids may increase the risk of hypokalemia and increase salt and water retention). Products include:
Decadron Elixir 2078
Decadron Tablets 2079
TobraDex Ophthalmic Ointment 542
TobraDex Ophthalmic Suspension 541

Dexamethasone Acetate (Co-administration with corticosteroids may increase the risk of hypokalemia and increase salt and water retention).
No products indexed under this heading.

Dexamethasone Sodium Phosphate (Co-administration with corticosteroids may increase the risk of hypokalemia and increase salt and water retention). Products include:
Decadron Phosphate Injection 2081
Decadron Phosphate Sterile Ophthalmic Ointment 2083
Decadron Phosphate Sterile Ophthalmic Solution 2084
NeoDecadron Sterile Ophthalmic Solution 2144

Dezocine (Co-administration with narcotics may potentiate orthostatic hypotension).
No products indexed under this heading.

Diazoxide (Co-administration with other antihypertensive agents may potentiate orthostatic hypotension).
No products indexed under this heading.

Diclofenac Potassium (Co-administration with non-steroidal anti-inflammatory agents may decrease the antihypertensive effects of metolazone). Products include:
Cataflam Tablets 2315

Diclofenac Sodium (Co-administration with non-steroidal anti-inflammatory agents may decrease the antihypertensive effects of metolazone). Products include:
Arthrotec Tablets 3195
Voltaren Ophthalmic Sterile Ophthalmic Solution .... ⊙312
Voltaren Tablets 2315
Voltaren-XR Tablets 2315

Dicumarol (Metolazone may affect the hypoprothrombinemic response to anticoagulants; dosage adjustments may be necessary).
No products indexed under this heading.

Diflunisal (Co-administration with salicylates may decrease the antihypertensive effects of metolazone). Products include:
Dolobid Tablets 2088

Digitoxin (Diuretics induced hypokalemia can increase the sensitivity of the myocardium to digitalis resulting

in serious arrhythmias).
No products indexed under this heading.

Digoxin (Diuretics induced hypokalemia can increase the sensitivity of the myocardium to digitalis resulting in serious arrhythmias). Products include:
- Digitek Tablets ... 1003
- Lanoxicaps Capsules ... 1574
- Lanoxin Injection ... 1581
- Lanoxin Tablets ... 1587
- Lanoxin Elixir Pediatric ... 1578
- Lanoxin Injection Pediatric ... 1584

Diltiazem Hydrochloride (Co-administration with other antihypertensive agents may potentiate orthostatic hypotension). Products include:
- Cardizem Injectable ... 1018
- Cardizem Lyo-Ject Syringe ... 1018
- Cardizem Monovial ... 1018
- Cardizem CD Capsules ... 1016
- Tiazac Capsules ... 1378

Doxazosin Mesylate (Co-administration with other antihypertensive agents may potentiate orthostatic hypotension). Products include:
- Cardura Tablets ... 2668

Enalapril Maleate (Co-administration with other antihypertensive agents may potentiate orthostatic hypotension). Products include:
- Lexxel Tablets ... 608
- Vaseretic Tablets ... 2204
- Vasotec Tablets ... 2210

Enalaprilat (Co-administration with other antihypertensive agents may potentiate orthostatic hypotension). Products include:
- Enalaprilat Injection ... 863
- Vasotec I.V. Injection ... 2207

Eprosartan Mesylate (Co-administration with other antihypertensive agents may potentiate orthostatic hypotension). Products include:
- Teveten Tablets ... 3327

Esmolol Hydrochloride (Co-administration with other antihypertensive agents may potentiate orthostatic hypotension). Products include:
- Brevibloc Injection ... 858

Ethacrynic Acid (Co-administration with loop diuretics can cause unusually large or prolonged losses of fluid and electrolytes). Products include:
- Edecrin Tablets ... 2091

Etodolac (Co-administration with non-steroidal anti-inflammatory agents may decrease the antihypertensive effects of metolazone). Products include:
- Lodine ... 3528
- Lodine XL Extended Release Tablets ... 3530

Felodipine (Co-administration with other antihypertensive agents may potentiate orthostatic hypotension). Products include:
- Lexxel Tablets ... 608
- Plendil Extended-Release Tablets ... 623

Fenoprofen Calcium (Co-administration with non-steroidal anti-inflammatory agents may decrease the antihypertensive effects of metolazone).
No products indexed under this heading.

Fentanyl (Co-administration with narcotics may potentiate orthostatic hypotension). Products include:
- Duragesic Transdermal System ... 1786

Fentanyl Citrate (Co-administration with narcotics may potentiate orthostatic hypotension). Products include:
- Actiq ... 1184

Fludrocortisone Acetate (Co-administration with corticosteroids may increase the risk of hypokalemia and increase salt and water retention). Products include:
- Florinef Acetate Tablets ... 2250

Flurbiprofen (Co-administration with non-steroidal anti-inflammatory agents may decrease the antihypertensive effects of metolazone).
No products indexed under this heading.

Fosinopril Sodium (Co-administration with other antihypertensive agents may potentiate orthostatic hypotension). Products include:
- Monopril Tablets ... 1091
- Monopril HCT ... 1094

Furosemide (Co-administration with loop diuretics can cause unusually large or prolonged losses of fluid and electrolytes). Products include:
- Furosemide Tablets ... 2284

Glimepiride (Metolazone may raise blood glucose concentrations possibly causing hyperglycemia and glycosuria in patients with diabetes; dose adjustment of oral hypoglycemic agents may be required). Products include:
- Amaryl Tablets ... 717

Glipizide (Metolazone may raise blood glucose concentrations possibly causing hyperglycemia and glycosuria in patients with diabetes; dose adjustment of oral hypoglycemic agents may be required). Products include:
- Glucotrol Tablets ... 2692
- Glucotrol XL Extended Release Tablets ... 2693

Glyburide (Metolazone may raise blood glucose concentrations possibly causing hyperglycemia and glycosuria in patients with diabetes; dose adjustment of oral hypoglycemic agents may be required). Products include:
- DiaBeta Tablets ... 741
- Glucovance Tablets ... 1086

Guanabenz Acetate (Co-administration with other antihypertensive agents may potentiate orthostatic hypotension).
No products indexed under this heading.

Guanethidine Monosulfate (Co-administration with other antihypertensive agents may potentiate orthostatic hypotension).
No products indexed under this heading.

Hydralazine Hydrochloride (Co-administration with other antihypertensive agents may potentiate orthostatic hypotension).
No products indexed under this heading.

Hydrochlorothiazide (Co-administration with other antihypertensive agents may potentiate orthostatic hypotension). Products include:
- Accuretic Tablets ... 2614
- Aldoril Tablets ... 2039
- Atacand HCT Tablets ... 597
- Avalide Tablets ... 1070
- Diovan HCT Tablets ... 2338
- Dyazide Capsules ... 1515
- HydroDIURIL Tablets ... 2108
- Hyzaar ... 2109
- Inderide Tablets ... 3517
- Inderide LA Long-Acting Capsules ... 3519
- Lotensin HCT Tablets ... 2367
- Maxzide ... 1008
- Micardis HCT Tablets ... 1051
- Microzide Capsules ... 3414
- Moduretic Tablets ... 2138
- Monopril HCT ... 1094
- Prinzide Tablets ... 2168
- Timolide Tablets ... 2187
- Uniretic Tablets ... 3178
- Vaseretic Tablets ... 2204
- Zestoretic Tablets ... 695
- Ziac Tablets ... 1887

Hydrocodone Bitartrate (Co-administration with narcotics may potentiate orthostatic hypotension). Products include:
- Hycodan ... 1316
- Hycomine Compound Tablets ... 1317
- Hycotuss Expectorant Syrup ... 1318
- Lortab ... 3319
- Lortab Elixir ... 3317
- Maxidone Tablets CIII ... 3399
- Norco 5/325 Tablets CIII ... 3424
- Norco 7.5/325 Tablets CIII ... 3425
- Norco 10/325 Tablets CIII ... 3427
- Norco 10/325 Tablets CIII ... 3425
- Vicodin Tablets ... 516
- Vicodin ES Tablets ... 517
- Vicodin HP Tablets ... 518
- Vicodin Tuss Expectorant ... 519
- Vicoprofen Tablets ... 520
- Zydone Tablets ... 1330

Hydrocodone Polistirex (Co-administration with narcotics may potentiate orthostatic hypotension). Products include:
- Tussionex Pennkinetic Extended-Release Suspension ... 1174

Hydrocortisone (Co-administration with corticosteroids may increase the risk of hypokalemia and increase salt and water retention). Products include:
- Anusol-HC Cream 2.5% ... 2237
- Cipro HC Otic Suspension ... 540
- Cortaid Intensive Therapy Cream ... ◘717
- Cortaid Maximum Strength Cream ... ◘717
- Cortisporin Ophthalmic Suspension Sterile ... ⊙297
- Cortizone•5 ... ◘699
- Cortizone•10 ... ◘699
- Cortizone•10 Plus Creme ... ◘700
- Cortizone for Kids Creme ... ◘699
- Hydrocortone Tablets ... 2106
- Massengill Medicated Soft Cloth Towelette ... ◘753
- VōSoL HC Otic Solution ... 3356

Hydrocortisone Acetate (Co-administration with corticosteroids may increase the risk of hypokalemia and increase salt and water retention). Products include:
- Analpram-HC ... 1338
- Anusol HC-1 Hydrocortisone Anti-Itch Cream ... ◘689
- Anusol-HC Suppositories ... 2238
- Cortaid ... ◘717
- Cortifoam Rectal Foam ... 3170
- Cortisporin-TC Otic Suspension ... 2246
- Hydrocortone Acetate Injectable Suspension ... 2103
- Pramosone ... 1343
- Proctocort Suppositories ... 2264
- ProctoFoam-HC ... 3177
- Terra-Cortril Ophthalmic Suspension ... 2716

Hydrocortisone Sodium Phosphate (Co-administration with corticosteroids may increase the risk of hypokalemia and increase salt and water retention). Products include:
- Hydrocortone Phosphate Injection, Sterile ... 2105

Hydrocortisone Sodium Succinate (Co-administration with corticosteroids may increase the risk of hypokalemia and increase salt and water retention).
No products indexed under this heading.

Hydroflumethiazide (Co-administration with other antihypertensive agents may potentiate orthostatic hypotension). Products include:
- Diucardin Tablets ... 3494

Hydromorphone Hydrochloride (Co-administration with narcotics may potentiate orthostatic hypotension). Products include:
- Dilaudid ... 441
- Dilaudid Oral Liquid ... 445
- Dilaudid Powder ... 441
- Dilaudid Rectal Suppositories ... 441
- Dilaudid Tablets ... 441
- Dilaudid Tablets - 8 mg ... 445
- Dilaudid-HP ... 443

Ibuprofen (Co-administration with non-steroidal anti-inflammatory agents may decrease the antihypertensive effects of metolazone). Products include:
- Advil ... ◘771
- Children's Advil Oral Suspension ... ◘773
- Children's Advil Chewable Tablets ... ◘773
- Advil Cold and Sinus Caplets ... ◘771
- Advil Cold and Sinus Tablets ... ◘771
- Advil Flu & Body Ache Caplets ... ◘772
- Infants' Advil Drops ... ◘773
- Junior Strength Advil Tablets ... ◘773
- Junior Strength Advil Chewable Tablets ... ◘773
- Advil Migraine Liquigels ... ◘772
- Children's Motrin Oral Suspension and Chewable Tablets ... 2006
- Children's Motrin Cold Oral Suspension ... 2007
- Children's Motrin Oral Suspension ... ◘643
- Motrin Suspension, Oral Drops, Chewable Tablets, and Caplets ... 2002
- Infants' Motrin Concentrated Drops ... 2006
- Junior Strength Motrin Caplets and Chewable Tablets ... 2006
- Motrin IB Tablets, Caplets, and Gelcaps ... 2002
- Motrin Migraine Pain Caplets ... 2005
- Motrin Sinus Headache Caplets ... 2005
- Vicoprofen Tablets ... 520

Indapamide (Co-administration with other antihypertensive agents may potentiate orthostatic hypotension). Products include:
- Indapamide Tablets ... 2286

Indomethacin (Co-administration with non-steroidal anti-inflammatory agents may decrease the antihypertensive effects of metolazone). Products include:
- Indocin ... 2112

Indomethacin Sodium Trihydrate (Co-administration with non-steroidal anti-inflammatory agents may decrease the antihypertensive effects of metolazone). Products include:
- Indocin I.V. ... 2115

Insulin, Human, Zinc Suspension (Metolazone may raise blood glucose concentrations possibly causing hyperglycemia and glycosuria in patients with diabetes; dose adjustment of insulin may be required). Products include:
- Humulin L, 100 Units ... 1937
- Humulin U, 100 Units ... 1943
- Novolin L Human Insulin 10 ml Vials ... 2422

Insulin, Human NPH (Metolazone may raise blood glucose concentrations possibly causing hyperglycemia and glycosuria in patients with diabetes; dose adjustment of insulin may be required). Products include:
- Humulin N, 100 Units ... 1939
- Humulin N NPH Pen ... 1940
- Novolin N Human Insulin 10 ml Vials ... 2422
- Novolin N PenFill ... 2423
- Novolin N Prefilled Syringe Disposable Insulin Delivery System ... 2425

Insulin, Human Regular (Metolazone may raise blood glucose concentrations possibly causing hyperglycemia and glycosuria in patients with diabetes; dose adjustment of insulin may be required). Products include:
- Humulin R Regular (U-500) ... 1943
- Humulin R, 100 Units ... 1941
- Novolin R Human Insulin 10 ml Vials ... 2423
- Novolin R PenFill ... 2423
- Novolin R Prefilled Syringe Disposable Insulin Delivery System ... 2425
- Velosulin BR Human Insulin 10 ml Vials ... 2435

Insulin, Human Regular and Human NPH Mixture (Metolazone may raise blood glucose concentrations possibly causing hyperglycemia and glycosuria in patients with diabetes; dose adjustment of insulin may be required). Products include:
- Humulin 50/50, 100 Units ... 1934
- Humulin 70/30, 100 Units ... 1935

Humulin 70/30 Pen 1936
Novolin 70/30 Human Insulin 10 ml Vials 2421
Novolin 70/30 PenFill 2423
Novolin 70/30 Prefilled Disposable Insulin Delivery System 2425

Insulin, NPH (Metolazone may raise blood glucose concentrations possibly causing hyperglycemia and glycosuria in patients with diabetes; dose adjustment of insulin may be required). Products include:
Iletin II, NPH (Pork), 100 Units 1946

Insulin, Regular (Metolazone may raise blood glucose concentrations possibly causing hyperglycemia and glycosuria in patients with diabetes; dose adjustment of insulin may be required). Products include:
Iletin II, Regular (Pork), 100 Units ... 1947

Insulin, Zinc Crystals (Metolazone may raise blood glucose concentrations possibly causing hyperglycemia and glycosuria in patients with diabetes; dose adjustment of insulin may be required).
No products indexed under this heading.

Insulin, Zinc Suspension (Metolazone may raise blood glucose concentrations possibly causing hyperglycemia and glycosuria in patients with diabetes; dose adjustment of insulin may be required). Products include:
Iletin II, Lente (Pork), 100 Units 1945

Insulin Aspart, Human Regular (Metolazone may raise blood glucose concentrations possibly causing hyperglycemia and glycosuria in patients with diabetes; dose adjustment of insulin may be required).
No products indexed under this heading.

Insulin glargine (Metolazone may raise blood glucose concentrations possibly causing hyperglycemia and glycosuria in patients with diabetes; dose adjustment of insulin may be required). Products include:
Lantus Injection 742

Insulin Lispro, Human (Metolazone may raise blood glucose concentrations possibly causing hyperglycemia and glycosuria in patients with diabetes; dose adjustment of insulin may be required). Products include:
Humalog 1926
Humalog Mix 75/25 Pen 1928

Insulin Lispro Protamine, Human (Metolazone may raise blood glucose concentrations possibly causing hyperglycemia and glycosuria in patients with diabetes; dose adjustment of insulin may be required). Products include:
Humalog Mix 75/25 Pen 1928

Irbesartan (Co-administration with other antihypertensive agents may potentiate orthostatic hypotension). Products include:
Avalide Tablets 1070
Avapro Tablets 1074
Avapro Tablets 3076

Isradipine (Co-administration with other antihypertensive agents may potentiate orthostatic hypotension). Products include:
DynaCirc Capsules 2921
DynaCirc CR Tablets 2923

Ketoprofen (Co-administration with non-steroidal anti-inflammatory agents may decrease the antihypertensive effects of metolazone). Products include:
Orudis Capsules 3548
Orudis KT Tablets 778
Oruvail Capsules 3548

Ketorolac Tromethamine (Co-administration with non-steroidal anti-inflammatory agents may decrease the antihypertensive effects of metolazone). Products include:
Acular Ophthalmic Solution 544
Acular PF Ophthalmic Solution 544
Toradol 3018

Labetalol Hydrochloride (Co-administration with other antihypertensive agents may potentiate orthostatic hypotension). Products include:
Normodyne Injection 3135
Normodyne Tablets 3137

Levorphanol Tartrate (Co-administration with narcotics may potentiate orthostatic hypotension). Products include:
Levo-Dromoran 1734
Levorphanol Tartrate Tablets 3059

Lisinopril (Co-administration with other antihypertensive agents may potentiate orthostatic hypotension). Products include:
Prinivil Tablets 2164
Prinzide Tablets 2168
Zestoretic Tablets 695
Zestril Tablets 698

Lithium Carbonate (Diuretics reduce lithium renal clearance and add a high risk of lithium toxicity; concurrent use should be avoided). Products include:
Eskalith 1527
Lithium Carbonate 3061
Lithobid Slow-Release Tablets 3255

Lithium Citrate (Diuretics reduce lithium renal clearance and add a high risk of lithium toxicity; concurrent use should be avoided). Products include:
Lithium Citrate Syrup 3061

Losartan Potassium (Co-administration with other antihypertensive agents may potentiate orthostatic hypotension). Products include:
Cozaar Tablets 2067
Hyzaar 2109

Magnesium Salicylate (Co-administration with salicylates may decrease the antihypertensive effects of metolazone). Products include:
Momentum Backache Relief Extra Strength Caplets 666

Mecamylamine Hydrochloride (Co-administration with other antihypertensive agents may potentiate orthostatic hypotension). Products include:
Inversine Tablets 1850

Meclofenamate Sodium (Co-administration with non-steroidal anti-inflammatory agents may decrease the antihypertensive effects of metolazone).
No products indexed under this heading.

Mefenamic Acid (Co-administration with non-steroidal anti-inflammatory agents may decrease the antihypertensive effects of metolazone). Products include:
Ponstel Capsules 1356

Meloxicam (Co-administration with non-steroidal anti-inflammatory agents may decrease the antihypertensive effects of metolazone). Products include:
Mobic Tablets 1054

Meperidine Hydrochloride (Co-administration with narcotics may potentiate orthostatic hypotension). Products include:
Demerol 3079
Mepergan Injection 3539

Mephobarbital (Co-administration with barbiturates may potentiate orthostatic hypotension).
No products indexed under this heading.

Metformin Hydrochloride (Metolazone may raise blood glucose concentrations possibly causing hyperglycemia and glycosuria in patients with diabetes; dose adjustment of oral hypoglycemic agents may be required). Products include:
Glucophage Tablets 1080
Glucophage XR Tablets 1080
Glucovance Tablets 1086

Methadone Hydrochloride (Co-administration with narcotics may potentiate orthostatic hypotension). Products include:
Dolophine Hydrochloride Tablets 3056

Methenamine (Efficacy of methenamine may be decreased due to urinary alkalinizing effect of metolazone). Products include:
Prosed/DS Tablets 3268
Urimax Tablets 1769
Urised Tablets 2876

Methenamine Hippurate (Efficacy of methenamine may be decreased due to urinary alkalinizing effect of metolazone).
No products indexed under this heading.

Methenamine Mandelate (Efficacy of methenamine may be decreased due to urinary alkalinizing effect of metolazone). Products include:
Uroqid-Acid No. 2 Tablets 947

Methyclothiazide (Co-administration with other antihypertensive agents may potentiate orthostatic hypotension).
No products indexed under this heading.

Methyldopa (Co-administration with other antihypertensive agents may potentiate orthostatic hypotension). Products include:
Aldoclor Tablets 2035
Aldomet Tablets 2037
Aldoril Tablets 2039

Methyldopate Hydrochloride (Co-administration with other antihypertensive agents may potentiate orthostatic hypotension).
No products indexed under this heading.

Methylprednisolone Acetate (Co-administration with corticosteroids may increase the risk of hypokalemia and increase salt and water retention). Products include:
Depo-Medrol Injectable Suspension 2795

Methylprednisolone Sodium Succinate (Co-administration with corticosteroids may increase the risk of hypokalemia and increase salt and water retention). Products include:
Solu-Medrol Sterile Powder 2855

Metoprolol Succinate (Co-administration with other antihypertensive agents may potentiate orthostatic hypotension). Products include:
Toprol-XL Tablets 651

Metoprolol Tartrate (Co-administration with other antihypertensive agents may potentiate orthostatic hypotension).
No products indexed under this heading.

Metyrosine (Co-administration with other antihypertensive agents may potentiate orthostatic hypotension). Products include:
Demser Capsules 2085

Mibefradil Dihydrochloride (Co-administration with other antihypertensive agents may potentiate orthostatic hypotension).
No products indexed under this heading.

Miglitol (Metolazone may raise blood glucose concentrations possibly causing hyperglycemia and glycosuria in patients with diabetes; dose adjustment of oral hypoglycemic agents may be required). Products include:
Glyset Tablets 2821

Minoxidil (Co-administration with other antihypertensive agents may potentiate orthostatic hypotension). Products include:
Rogaine Extra Strength for Men Topical Solution 721
Rogaine for Women Topical Solution 721

Moexipril Hydrochloride (Co-administration with other antihypertensive agents may potentiate orthostatic hypotension). Products include:
Uniretic Tablets 3178
Univasc Tablets 3181

Morphine Sulfate (Co-administration with narcotics may potentiate orthostatic hypotension). Products include:
Astramorph/PF Injection, USP (Preservative-Free) 594
Duramorph Injection 1312
Infumorph 200 and Infumorph 500 Sterile Solutions 1314
Kadian Capsules 1335
MS Contin Tablets 2896
MSIR 2898
Oramorph SR Tablets 3062
Roxanol 3066

Nabumetone (Co-administration with non-steroidal anti-inflammatory agents may decrease the antihypertensive effects of metolazone). Products include:
Relafen Tablets 1617

Nadolol (Co-administration with other antihypertensive agents may potentiate orthostatic hypotension). Products include:
Corgard Tablets 2245
Corzide 40/5 Tablets 2247
Corzide 80/5 Tablets 2247
Nadolol Tablets 2288

Naproxen (Co-administration with non-steroidal anti-inflammatory agents may decrease the antihypertensive effects of metolazone). Products include:
EC-Naprosyn Delayed-Release Tablets 2967
Naprosyn Suspension 2967
Naprosyn Tablets 2967

Naproxen Sodium (Co-administration with non-steroidal anti-inflammatory agents may decrease the antihypertensive effects of metolazone). Products include:
Aleve Tablets, Caplets and Gelcaps 602
Aleve Cold & Sinus Caplets 603
Anaprox Tablets 2967
Anaprox DS Tablets 2967
Naprelan Tablets 1293

Nicardipine Hydrochloride (Co-administration with other antihypertensive agents may potentiate orthostatic hypotension). Products include:
Cardene I.V. 3485

Nifedipine (Co-administration with other antihypertensive agents may potentiate orthostatic hypotension). Products include:
Adalat CC Tablets 877
Procardia Capsules 2708
Procardia XL Extended Release Tablets 2710

Nisoldipine (Co-administration with other antihypertensive agents may potentiate orthostatic hypotension). Products include:
Sular Tablets 688

Nitroglycerin (Co-administration with other antihypertensive agents may potentiate orthostatic hypotension). Products include:
Nitro-Dur Transdermal Infusion System 3134
Nitro-Dur Transdermal Infusion System 1834
Nitrolingual Pumpspray 1355
Nitrostat Tablets 2658

Norepinephrine Bitartrate (Metolazone may decrease arterial responsiveness to norepinephrine).
No products indexed under this heading.

Oxaprozin (Co-administration with non-steroidal anti-inflammatory agents may decrease the antihypertensive effects of metolazone).
No products indexed under this heading.

Oxycodone Hydrochloride (Co-administration with narcotics may potentiate orthostatic hypotension). Products include:
- OxyContin Tablets 2912
- OxyFast Oral Concentrate Solution . 2916
- OxyIR Capsules 2916
- Percocet Tablets 1326
- Percodan Tablets 1327
- Percolone Tablets 1327
- Roxicodone 3067
- Tylox Capsules 2597

Penbutolol Sulfate (Co-administration with other antihypertensive agents may potentiate orthostatic hypotension).
No products indexed under this heading.

Pentobarbital Sodium (Co-administration with barbiturates may potentiate orthostatic hypotension). Products include:
- Nembutal Sodium Solution 485

Perindopril Erbumine (Co-administration with other antihypertensive agents may potentiate orthostatic hypotension). Products include:
- Aceon Tablets (2 mg, 4 mg, 8 mg) 3249

Phenobarbital (Co-administration with barbiturates may potentiate orthostatic hypotension). Products include:
- Arco-Lase Plus Tablets 592
- Donnatal 2929
- Donnatal Extentabs 2930

Phenoxybenzamine Hydrochloride (Co-administration with other antihypertensive agents may potentiate orthostatic hypotension). Products include:
- Dibenzyline Capsules 3457

Phentolamine Mesylate (Co-administration with other antihypertensive agents may potentiate orthostatic hypotension).
No products indexed under this heading.

Phenylbutazone (Co-administration with non-steroidal anti-inflammatory agents may decrease the antihypertensive effects of metolazone).
No products indexed under this heading.

Pindolol (Co-administration with other antihypertensive agents may potentiate orthostatic hypotension).
No products indexed under this heading.

Pioglitazone Hydrochloride (Metolazone may raise blood glucose concentrations possibly causing hyperglycemia and glycosuria in patients with diabetes; dose adjustment of oral hypoglycemic agents may be required). Products include:
- Actos Tablets 3275

Piroxicam (Co-administration with non-steroidal anti-inflammatory agents may decrease the antihypertensive effects of metolazone). Products include:
- Feldene Capsules 2685

Polythiazide (Co-administration with other antihypertensive agents may potentiate orthostatic hypotension). Products include:
- Minizide Capsules 2700
- Renese Tablets 2712

Prazosin Hydrochloride (Co-administration with other antihypertensive agents may potentiate orthostatic hypotension). Products include:
- Minipress Capsules 2699
- Minizide Capsules 2700

Prednisolone Acetate (Co-administration with corticosteroids may increase the risk of hypokalemia and increase salt and water retention). Products include:
- Blephamide Ophthalmic Ointment ... 547
- Blephamide Ophthalmic Suspension 548
- Poly-Pred Liquifilm Ophthalmic Suspension .... ⊙ 245
- Pred Forte Ophthalmic Suspension .... ⊙ 246
- Pred Mild Sterile Ophthalmic Suspension .... ⊙ 249
- Pred-G Ophthalmic Suspension .... ⊙ 247
- Pred-G Sterile Ophthalmic Ointment .... ⊙ 248

Prednisolone Sodium Phosphate (Co-administration with corticosteroids may increase the risk of hypokalemia and increase salt and water retention). Products include:
- Pediapred Oral Solution 1170

Prednisolone Tebutate (Co-administration with corticosteroids may increase the risk of hypokalemia and increase salt and water retention).
No products indexed under this heading.

Prednisone (Co-administration with corticosteroids may increase the risk of hypokalemia and increase salt and water retention). Products include:
- Prednisone 3064

Propoxyphene Hydrochloride (Co-administration with narcotics may potentiate orthostatic hypotension). Products include:
- Darvon Pulvules 1909
- Darvon Compound-65 Pulvules 1910

Propoxyphene Napsylate (Co-administration with narcotics may potentiate orthostatic hypotension). Products include:
- Darvon-N/Darvocet-N 1907
- Darvon-N Tablets 1912

Propranolol Hydrochloride (Co-administration with other antihypertensive agents may potentiate orthostatic hypotension). Products include:
- Inderal 3513
- Inderal LA Long-Acting Capsules 3516
- Inderide Tablets 3517
- Inderide LA Long-Acting Capsules .. 3519

Quinapril Hydrochloride (Co-administration with other antihypertensive agents may potentiate orthostatic hypotension). Products include:
- Accupril Tablets 2611
- Accuretic Tablets 2614

Ramipril (Co-administration with other antihypertensive agents may potentiate orthostatic hypotension). Products include:
- Altace Capsules 2233

Rauwolfia serpentina (Co-administration with other antihypertensive agents may potentiate orthostatic hypotension).
No products indexed under this heading.

Remifentanil Hydrochloride (Co-administration with narcotics may potentiate orthostatic hypotension).
No products indexed under this heading.

Repaglinide (Metolazone may raise blood glucose concentrations possibly causing hyperglycemia and glycosuria in patients with diabetes; dose adjustment of oral hypoglycemic agents may be required). Products include:
- Prandin Tablets (0.5, 1, and 2 mg) 2432

Rescinnamine (Co-administration with other antihypertensive agents may potentiate orthostatic hypotension).
No products indexed under this heading.

Reserpine (Co-administration with other antihypertensive agents may potentiate orthostatic hypotension).
No products indexed under this heading.

Rofecoxib (Co-administration with non-steroidal anti-inflammatory agents may decrease the antihypertensive effects of metolazone). Products include:
- Vioxx 2213

Rosiglitazone Maleate (Metolazone may raise blood glucose concentrations possibly causing hyperglycemia and glycosuria in patients with diabetes; dose adjustment of oral hypoglycemic agents may be required). Products include:
- Avandia Tablets 1490

Salsalate (Co-administration with salicylates may decrease the antihypertensive effects of metolazone).
No products indexed under this heading.

Secobarbital Sodium (Co-administration with barbiturates may potentiate orthostatic hypotension).
No products indexed under this heading.

Sodium Nitroprusside (Co-administration with other antihypertensive agents may potentiate orthostatic hypotension).
No products indexed under this heading.

Sotalol Hydrochloride (Co-administration with other antihypertensive agents may potentiate orthostatic hypotension). Products include:
- Betapace Tablets 950
- Betapace AF Tablets 954

Spirapril Hydrochloride (Co-administration with other antihypertensive agents may potentiate orthostatic hypotension).
No products indexed under this heading.

Sufentanil Citrate (Co-administration with narcotics may potentiate orthostatic hypotension).
No products indexed under this heading.

Sulindac (Co-administration with non-steroidal anti-inflammatory agents may decrease the antihypertensive effects of metolazone). Products include:
- Clinoril Tablets 2053

Telmisartan (Co-administration with other antihypertensive agents may potentiate orthostatic hypotension). Products include:
- Micardis Tablets 1049
- Micardis HCT Tablets 1051

Terazosin Hydrochloride (Co-administration with other antihypertensive agents may potentiate orthostatic hypotension). Products include:
- Hytrin Capsules 464

Thiamylal Sodium (Co-administration with barbiturates may potentiate orthostatic hypotension).
No products indexed under this heading.

Timolol Maleate (Co-administration with other antihypertensive agents may potentiate orthostatic hypotension). Products include:
- Blocadren Tablets 2046
- Cosopt Sterile Ophthalmic Solution 2065
- Timolide Tablets 2187
- Timolol GFS .... ⊙ 266
- Timoptic in Ocudose 2192
- Timoptic Sterile Ophthalmic Solution 2190
- Timoptic-XE Sterile Ophthalmic Gel Forming Solution 2194

Tolazamide (Metolazone may raise blood glucose concentrations possibly causing hyperglycemia and glycosuria in patients with diabetes; dose adjustment of oral hypoglycemic agents may be required).
No products indexed under this heading.

Tolbutamide (Metolazone may raise blood glucose concentrations possibly causing hyperglycemia and glycosuria in patients with diabetes; dose adjustment of oral hypoglycemic agents may be required).
No products indexed under this heading.

Tolmetin Sodium (Co-administration with non-steroidal anti-inflammatory agents may decrease the antihypertensive effects of metolazone). Products include:
- Tolectin 2589

Torsemide (Co-administration with loop diuretics can cause unusually large or prolonged losses of fluid and electrolytes). Products include:
- Demadex Tablets and Injection 2965

Trandolapril (Co-administration with other antihypertensive agents may potentiate orthostatic hypotension). Products include:
- Mavik Tablets 478
- Tarka Tablets 508

Triamcinolone (Co-administration with corticosteroids may increase the risk of hypokalemia and increase salt and water retention).
No products indexed under this heading.

Triamcinolone Acetonide (Co-administration with corticosteroids may increase the risk of hypokalemia and increase salt and water retention). Products include:
- Azmacort Inhalation Aerosol 728
- Nasacort Nasal Inhaler 750
- Nasacort AQ Nasal Spray 752
- Tri-Nasal Spray 2274

Triamcinolone Diacetate (Co-administration with corticosteroids may increase the risk of hypokalemia and increase salt and water retention).
No products indexed under this heading.

Triamcinolone Hexacetonide (Co-administration with corticosteroids may increase the risk of hypokalemia and increase salt and water retention).
No products indexed under this heading.

Trimethaphan Camsylate (Co-administration with other antihypertensive agents may potentiate orthostatic hypotension).
No products indexed under this heading.

Troglitazone (Metolazone may raise blood glucose concentrations possibly causing hyperglycemia and glycosuria in patients with diabetes; dose adjustment of oral hypoglycemic agents may be required).
No products indexed under this heading.

Tubocurarine Chloride (Diuretics induced hypokalemia may enhance neuromuscular blocking effect of curariform drugs resulting in respiratory depression which could proceed to apnea).
No products indexed under this heading.

Valsartan (Co-administration with other antihypertensive agents may potentiate orthostatic hypotension). Products include:
- Diovan Capsules 2337
- Diovan HCT Tablets 2338

Verapamil Hydrochloride (Co-administration with other antihypertensive agents may potentiate orthostatic hypotension). Products include:
- Covera-HS Tablets 3199
- Isoptin SR Tablets 467
- Tarka Tablets 508
- Verelan Capsules 3184

Verelan PM Capsules 3186

Warfarin Sodium (Metolazone may affect the hypoprothrombinemic response to anticoagulants; dosage adjustments may be necessary). Products include:
- Coumadin for Injection 1243
- Coumadin Tablets 1243
- Warfarin Sodium Tablets, USP 3302

Food Interactions

Alcohol (Concurrent use with alcohol may potentiate orthostatic hypotension).

ZEBETA TABLETS

(Bisoprolol Fumarate) 1885

May interact with beta blockers, catecholamine depleting drugs, oral hypoglycemic agents, and insulin. Compounds in these categories include:

Acarbose (Possible masking of some of the manifestations of hypoglycemia). Products include:
- Precose Tablets 906

Acebutolol Hydrochloride (Zebeta should not be combined with other beta-blocking drugs). Products include:
- Sectral Capsules 3589

Atenolol (Zebeta should not be combined with other beta-blocking drugs). Products include:
- Tenoretic Tablets 690
- Tenormin I.V. Injection 692

Betaxolol Hydrochloride (Zebeta should not be combined with other beta-blocking drugs). Products include:
- Betoptic S Ophthalmic Suspension 537

Carteolol Hydrochloride (Zebeta should not be combined with other beta-blocking drugs). Products include:
- Carteolol Hydrochloride Ophthalmic Solution USP, 1% ..... ⊙258
- Ocupress Ophthalmic Solution, 1% Sterile .... ⊙303

Chlorpropamide (Possible masking of some of the manifestations of hypoglycemia). Products include:
- Diabinese Tablets 2680

Clonidine (In patients receiving concurrent clonidine, Zebeta should be discontinued for several days before the withdrawal of clonidine). Products include:
- Catapres-TTS 1038

Clonidine Hydrochloride (In patients receiving concurrent clonidine, Zebeta should be discontinued for several days before the withdrawal of clonidine). Products include:
- Catapres Tablets 1037
- Clorpres Tablets 1002
- Combipres Tablets 1040
- Duraclon Injection 3057

Cyclopropane (Care should be taken when anesthetic agents which depress myocardial function are used with Zebeta).
- No products indexed under this heading.

Deserpidine (Potential for added beta-adrenergic blocking action of Zebeta resulting in excessive reduction of sympathetic activity).
- No products indexed under this heading.

Diltiazem Hydrochloride (Potential for additional myocardial depression and/or inhibition of AV conduction). Products include:
- Cardizem Injectable 1018
- Cardizem Lyo-Ject Syringe 1018
- Cardizem Monovial 1018
- Cardizem CD Capsules 1016
- Tiazac Capsules 1378

Disopyramide Phosphate (Potential for additional myocardial depression and/or inhibition of AV conduction).
- No products indexed under this heading.

Epinephrine (Patients with a history of anaphylactic reactions to a variety of allergens may be unresponsive to the usual dose of epinephrine used to treat allergic reactions). Products include:
- Epifrin Sterile Ophthalmic Solution .... ⊙235
- EpiPen 1236
- Primatene Mist 779
- Xylocaine with Epinephrine Injection 653

Epinephrine Bitartrate (Patients with a history of anaphylactic reactions to a variety of allergens may be unresponsive to the usual dose of epinephrine used to treat allergic reactions). Products include:
- Sensorcaine 643

Esmolol Hydrochloride (Zebeta should not be combined with other beta-blocking drugs). Products include:
- Brevibloc Injection 858

Ether (Care should be taken when anesthetic agents which depress myocardial function are used with Zebeta).

Glimepiride (Possible masking of some of the manifestations of hypoglycemia). Products include:
- Amaryl Tablets 717

Glipizide (Possible masking of some of the manifestations of hypoglycemia). Products include:
- Glucotrol Tablets 2692
- Glucotrol XL Extended Release Tablets 2693

Glyburide (Possible masking of some of the manifestations of hypoglycemia). Products include:
- DiaBeta Tablets 741
- Glucovance Tablets 1086

Guanethidine Monosulfate (Potential for added beta-adrenergic blocking action of Zebeta resulting in excessive reduction of sympathetic activity).
- No products indexed under this heading.

Insulin, Human, Zinc Suspension (Possible masking of some of the manifestations of hypoglycemia). Products include:
- Humulin L, 100 Units 1937
- Humulin U, 100 Units 1943
- Novolin L Human Insulin 10 ml Vials 2422

Insulin, Human NPH (Possible masking of some of the manifestations of hypoglycemia). Products include:
- Humulin N, 100 Units 1939
- Humulin N NPH Pen 1940
- Novolin N Human Insulin 10 ml Vials 2422
- Novolin N PenFill 2423
- Novolin N Prefilled Syringe Disposable Insulin Delivery System 2425

Insulin, Human Regular (Possible masking of some of the manifestations of hypoglycemia). Products include:
- Humulin R Regular (U-500) 1943
- Humulin R, 100 Units 1941
- Novolin R Human Insulin 10 ml Vials 2423
- Novolin R PenFill 2423
- Novolin R Prefilled Syringe Disposable Insulin Delivery System 2425
- Velosulin BR Human Insulin 10 ml Vials 2435

Insulin, Human Regular and Human NPH Mixture (Possible masking of some of the manifestations of hypoglycemia). Products include:
- Humulin 50/50, 100 Units 1934
- Humulin 70/30, 100 Units 1935
- Humulin 70/30 Pen 1936
- Novolin 70/30 Human Insulin 10 ml Vials 2421
- Novolin 70/30 PenFill 2423
- Novolin 70/30 Prefilled Disposable Insulin Delivery System 2425

Insulin, NPH (Possible masking of some of the manifestations of hypoglycemia). Products include:
- Iletin II, NPH (Pork), 100 Units 1946

Insulin, Regular (Possible masking of some of the manifestations of hypoglycemia). Products include:
- Iletin II, Regular (Pork), 100 Units ... 1947

Insulin, Zinc Crystals (Possible masking of some of the manifestations of hypoglycemia).
- No products indexed under this heading.

Insulin, Zinc Suspension (Possible masking of some of the manifestations of hypoglycemia). Products include:
- Iletin II, Lente (Pork), 100 Units 1945

Insulin Aspart, Human Regular (Possible masking of some of the manifestations of hypoglycemia).
- No products indexed under this heading.

Insulin glargine (Possible masking of some of the manifestations of hypoglycemia). Products include:
- Lantus Injection 742

Insulin Lispro, Human (Possible masking of some of the manifestations of hypoglycemia). Products include:
- Humalog 1926
- Humalog Mix 75/25 Pen 1928

Insulin Lispro Protamine, Human (Possible masking of some of the manifestations of hypoglycemia). Products include:
- Humalog Mix 75/25 Pen 1928

Labetalol Hydrochloride (Zebeta should not be combined with other beta-blocking drugs). Products include:
- Normodyne Injection 3135
- Normodyne Tablets 3137

Levobunolol Hydrochloride (Zebeta should not be combined with other beta-blocking drugs). Products include:
- Betagan .... ⊙228

Metformin Hydrochloride (Possible masking of some of the manifestations of hypoglycemia). Products include:
- Glucophage Tablets 1080
- Glucophage XR Tablets 1080
- Glucovance Tablets 1086

Metipranolol Hydrochloride (Zebeta should not be combined with other beta-blocking drugs).
- No products indexed under this heading.

Metoprolol Succinate (Zebeta should not be combined with other beta-blocking drugs). Products include:
- Toprol-XL Tablets 651

Metoprolol Tartrate (Zebeta should not be combined with other beta-blocking drugs).
- No products indexed under this heading.

Miglitol (Possible masking of some of the manifestations of hypoglycemia). Products include:
- Glyset Tablets 2821

Nadolol (Zebeta should not be combined with other beta-blocking drugs). Products include:
- Corgard Tablets 2245
- Corzide 40/5 Tablets 2247
- Corzide 80/5 Tablets 2247
- Nadolol Tablets 2288

Penbutolol Sulfate (Zebeta should not be combined with other beta-blocking drugs).
- No products indexed under this heading.

Pindolol (Zebeta should not be combined with other beta-blocking drugs).
- No products indexed under this heading.

Pioglitazone Hydrochloride (Possible masking of some of the manifestations of hypoglycemia). Products include:
- Actos Tablets 3275

Propranolol Hydrochloride (Zebeta should not be combined with other beta-blocking drugs). Products include:
- Inderal 3513
- Inderal LA Long-Acting Capsules 3516
- Inderide Tablets 3517
- Inderide LA Long-Acting Capsules .. 3519

Rauwolfia serpentina (Potential for added beta-adrenergic blocking action of Zebeta resulting in excessive reduction of sympathetic activity).
- No products indexed under this heading.

Repaglinide (Possible masking of some of the manifestations of hypoglycemia). Products include:
- Prandin Tablets (0.5, 1, and 2 mg) 2432

Rescinnamine (Potential for added beta-adrenergic blocking action of Zebeta resulting in excessive reduction of sympathetic activity).
- No products indexed under this heading.

Reserpine (Potential for added beta-adrenergic blocking action of Zebeta resulting in excessive reduction of sympathetic activity).
- No products indexed under this heading.

Rifampin (Concurrent use increases the metabolic clearance of Zebeta, resulting in shortened elimination half-life of Zebeta). Products include:
- Rifadin 765
- Rifamate Capsules 767
- Rifater Tablets 769

Rosiglitazone Maleate (Possible masking of some of the manifestations of hypoglycemia). Products include:
- Avandia Tablets 1490

Sotalol Hydrochloride (Zebeta should not be combined with other beta-blocking drugs). Products include:
- Betapace Tablets 950
- Betapace AF Tablets 954

Timolol Hemihydrate (Zebeta should not be combined with other beta-blocking drugs). Products include:
- Betimol Ophthalmic Solution .... ⊙324

Timolol Maleate (Zebeta should not be combined with other beta-blocking drugs). Products include:
- Blocadren Tablets 2046
- Cosopt Sterile Ophthalmic Solution 2065
- Timolide Tablets 2187
- Timolol GFS .... ⊙266
- Timoptic in Ocudose 2192
- Timoptic Sterile Ophthalmic Solution 2190
- Timoptic-XE Sterile Ophthalmic Gel Forming Solution 2194

Tolazamide (Possible masking of some of the manifestations of hypoglycemia).
- No products indexed under this heading.

Tolbutamide (Possible masking of some of the manifestations of hypoglycemia).
- No products indexed under this heading.

Troglitazone (Possible masking of some of the manifestations of hypoglycemia).
- No products indexed under this heading.

Verapamil Hydrochloride (Potential for additional myocardial depression and/or inhibition of AV conduction). Products include:
- Covera-HS Tablets 3199
- Isoptin SR Tablets 467
- Tarka Tablets 508
- Verelan Capsules 3184

Verelan PM Capsules 3186

ZEMPLAR INJECTION

(Paricalcitol) 522

May interact with cardiac glycosides and certain other agents. Compounds in these categories include:

Calcitriol (Vitamin D-related compounds should not be taken concomitantly with paricalcitol). Products include:

Calcijex Injection 411
Rocaltrol 2991

Deslanoside (Digitalis toxicity is potentiated by hypercalcemia of any cause, so caution should be applied when digitalis compounds are prescribed concomitantly with paricalcitol).

No products indexed under this heading.

Digitoxin (Digitalis toxicity is potentiated by hypercalcemia of any cause, so caution should be applied when digitalis compounds are prescribed concomitantly with paricalcitol).

No products indexed under this heading.

Digoxin (Digitalis toxicity is potentiated by hypercalcemia of any cause, so caution should be applied when digitalis compounds are prescribed concomitantly with paricalcitol). Products include:

Digitek Tablets 1003
Lanoxicaps Capsules 1574
Lanoxin Injection 1581
Lanoxin Tablets 1587
Lanoxin Elixir Pediatric 1578
Lanoxin Injection Pediatric 1584

Potassium Acid Phosphate (Phosphate compounds should not be taken concomitantly with paricalcitol). Products include:

K-Phos Original (Sodium Free) Tablets 947

Potassium Phosphate (Phosphate compounds should not be taken concomitantly with paricalcitol). Products include:

K-Phos Neutral Tablets 946

ZEMURON INJECTION

(Rocuronium Bromide) 2491

May interact with aminoglycosides, anticonvulsants, inhalant anesthetics, tetracyclines, and certain other agents. Compounds in these categories include:

Amikacin Sulfate (Possible prolongation of neuromuscular blockade).

No products indexed under this heading.

Bacitracin (Possible prolongation of neuromuscular blockade).

No products indexed under this heading.

Carbamazepine (Potential for apparent resistance to the effects of rocuronium in the form of diminished magnitude of neuromuscular blockade). Products include:

Carbatrol Capsules 3234
Tegretol/Tegretol-XR 2404

Colistimethate Sodium (Possible prolongation of neuromuscular blockade). Products include:

Coly-Mycin M Parenteral 2243

Colistin Sulfate (Possible prolongation of neuromuscular blockade). Products include:

Cortisporin-TC Otic Suspension 2246

Demeclocycline Hydrochloride (Possible prolongation of neuromuscular blockade). Products include:

Declomycin Tablets 1855

Desflurane (Possible enhanced activity of neuromuscular blocking agent). Products include:

Suprane Liquid for Inhalation 874

Divalproex Sodium (Potential for apparent resistance to the effects of rocuronium in the form of diminished magnitude of neuromuscular blockade). Products include:

Depakote Sprinkle Capsules 426
Depakote Tablets 430
Depakote ER Tablets 436

Doxycycline Calcium (Possible prolongation of neuromuscular blockade). Products include:

Vibramycin Calcium Oral Suspension Syrup 2735

Doxycycline Hyclate (Possible prolongation of neuromuscular blockade). Products include:

Doryx Coated Pellet Filled Capsules 3357
Periostat Tablets 1208
Vibramycin Hyclate Capsules 2735
Vibramycin Hyclate Intravenous 2737
Vibra-Tabs Film Coated Tablets 2735

Doxycycline Monohydrate (Possible prolongation of neuromuscular blockade). Products include:

Monodox Capsules 2442
Vibramycin Monohydrate for Oral Suspension 2735

Enflurane (Possible enhanced activity of neuromuscular blocking agent; may prolong the duration of action).

No products indexed under this heading.

Ethosuximide (Potential for apparent resistance to the effects of rocuronium in the form of diminished magnitude of neuromuscular blockade). Products include:

Zarontin Capsules 2659
Zarontin Syrup 2660

Ethotoin (Potential for apparent resistance to the effects of rocuronium in the form of diminished magnitude of neuromuscular blockade).

No products indexed under this heading.

Felbamate (Potential for apparent resistance to the effects of rocuronium in the form of diminished magnitude of neuromuscular blockade). Products include:

Felbatol 3343

Fosphenytoin Sodium (Potential for apparent resistance to the effects of rocuronium in the form of diminished magnitude of neuromuscular blockade). Products include:

Cerebyx Injection 2619

Gentamicin Sulfate (Possible prolongation of neuromuscular blockade). Products include:

Genoptic Ophthalmic Ointment ..... ⊙ 239
Genoptic Sterile Ophthalmic Solution .... ⊙ 239
Pred-G Ophthalmic Suspension ..... ⊙ 247
Pred-G Sterile Ophthalmic Ointment .... ⊙ 248

Halothane (Possible enhanced activity of neuromuscular blocking agent). Products include:

Fluothane Inhalation 3508

Isoflurane (Possible enhanced activity of neuromuscular blocking agent; may prolong the duration of action).

No products indexed under this heading.

Kanamycin Sulfate (Possible prolongation of neuromuscular blockade).

No products indexed under this heading.

Lamotrigine (Potential for apparent resistance to the effects of rocuronium in the form of diminished magnitude of neuromuscular blockade). Products include:

Lamictal 1567

Levetiracetam (Potential for apparent resistance to the effects of rocuronium in the form of diminished magnitude of neuromuscular blockade). Products include:

Keppra Tablets 3314

Lithium Carbonate (May increase the duration of neuromuscular block). Products include:

Eskalith 1527
Lithium Carbonate 3061
Lithobid Slow-Release Tablets 3255

Lithium Citrate (May increase the duration of neuromuscular block). Products include:

Lithium Citrate Syrup 3061

Magnesium Sulfate Injection (May enhance the neuromuscular blockade).

No products indexed under this heading.

Mephenytoin (Potential for apparent resistance to the effects of rocuronium in the form of diminished magnitude of neuromuscular blockade).

No products indexed under this heading.

Methacycline Hydrochloride (Possible prolongation of neuromuscular blockade).

No products indexed under this heading.

Methoxyflurane (Possible enhanced activity of neuromuscular blocking agent).

No products indexed under this heading.

Methsuximide (Potential for apparent resistance to the effects of rocuronium in the form of diminished magnitude of neuromuscular blockade). Products include:

Celontin Capsules 2618

Minocycline Hydrochloride (Possible prolongation of neuromuscular blockade). Products include:

Dynacin Capsules 2019
Minocin Intravenous 1862
Minocin Oral Suspension 1865
Minocin Pellet-Filled Capsules 1863

Oxcarbazepine (Potential for apparent resistance to the effects of rocuronium in the form of diminished magnitude of neuromuscular blockade). Products include:

Trileptal Oral Suspension 2407
Trileptal Tablets 2407

Oxytetracycline Hydrochloride (Possible prolongation of neuromuscular blockade). Products include:

Terra-Cortril Ophthalmic Suspension 2716
Urobiotic-250 Capsules 2731

Paramethadione (Potential for apparent resistance to the effects of rocuronium in the form of diminished magnitude of neuromuscular blockade).

No products indexed under this heading.

Phenacemide (Potential for apparent resistance to the effects of rocuronium in the form of diminished magnitude of neuromuscular blockade).

No products indexed under this heading.

Phenobarbital (Potential for apparent resistance to the effects of rocuronium in the form of diminished magnitude of neuromuscular blockade). Products include:

Arco-Lase Plus Tablets 592
Donnatal 2929
Donnatal Extentabs 2930

Phensuximide (Potential for apparent resistance to the effects of rocuronium in the form of diminished magnitude of neuromuscular blockade).

No products indexed under this heading.

Phenytoin (Potential for apparent resistance to the effects of rocuronium in the form of diminished magnitude of neuromuscular blockade). Products include:

Dilantin Infatabs 2624
Dilantin-125 Oral Suspension 2625

Phenytoin Sodium (Potential for apparent resistance to the effects of rocuronium in the form of diminished magnitude of neuromuscular blockade). Products include:

Dilantin Kapseals 2622

Polymyxin B Sulfate (Possible prolongation of neuromuscular blockade). Products include:

Betadine Brand First Aid Antibiotics & Moisturizer Ointment 2894
Betadine Brand Plus First Aid Antibiotics & Pain Reliever Ointment 2894
Cortisporin Ophthalmic Suspension Sterile .... ⊙ 297
Neosporin G.U. Irrigant Sterile 2256
Neosporin Ointment .... ▣ 704
Neosporin Ophthalmic Ointment Sterile .... ⊙ 299
Neosporin Ophthalmic Solution Sterile .... ⊙ 300
Neosporin + Pain Relief Maximum Strength Cream .... ▣ 704
Neosporin + Pain Relief Maximum Strength Ointment...... ▣ 704
Poly-Pred Liquifilm Ophthalmic Suspension .... ⊙ 245
Polysporin Ointment .... ▣ 706
Polysporin Ophthalmic Ointment Sterile .... ⊙ 301
Polysporin Powder .... ▣ 706
Polytrim Ophthalmic Solution 556

Primidone (Potential for apparent resistance to the effects of rocuronium in the form of diminished magnitude of neuromuscular blockade).

No products indexed under this heading.

Procainamide Hydrochloride (May increase the duration of neuromuscular block). Products include:

Procanbid Extended-Release Tablets 2262

Quinidine Gluconate (Possible recurrent paralysis; increased duration of neuromuscular block). Products include:

Quinaglute Dura-Tabs Tablets 978

Quinidine Polygalacturonate (Possible recurrent paralysis; increased duration of neuromuscular block).

No products indexed under this heading.

Quinidine Sulfate (Possible recurrent paralysis; increased duration of neuromuscular block). Products include:

Quinidex Extentabs 2933

Streptomycin Sulfate (Possible prolongation of neuromuscular blockade). Products include:

Streptomycin Sulfate Injection 2714

Succinylcholine Chloride (Rocuronium should not be given until recovery from succinylcholine has been observed). Products include:

Anectine Injection 1476

Tetracycline Hydrochloride (Possible prolongation of neuromuscular blockade).

No products indexed under this heading.

Tiagabine Hydrochloride (Potential for apparent resistance to the effects of rocuronium in the form of diminished magnitude of neuromuscular blockade). Products include:

Gabitril Tablets 1189

Tobramycin (Possible prolongation of neuromuscular blockade). Products include:

TOBI Solution for Inhalation 1206
TobraDex Ophthalmic Ointment 542
TobraDex Ophthalmic Suspension .. 541
Tobrex Ophthalmic Ointment .... ⊙ 220
Tobrex Ophthalmic Solution .... ⊙ 221

Tobramycin Sulfate (Possible prolongation of neuromuscular blockade). Products include:

Nebcin Vials, Hyporets & ADD-Vantage 1955

Topiramate (Potential for apparent resistance to the effects of rocuronium in the form of diminished magnitude of neuromuscular blockade). Products include:

Topamax Sprinkle Capsules 2590
Topamax Tablets 2590

Trimethadione (Potential for apparent resistance to the effects of rocu-

ronium in the form of diminished magnitude of neuromuscular blockade).
No products indexed under this heading.

Valproate Sodium (Potential for apparent resistance to the effects of rocuronium in the form of diminished magnitude of neuromuscular blockade). Products include:
Depacon Injection 416

Valproic Acid (Potential for apparent resistance to the effects of rocuronium in the form of diminished magnitude of neuromuscular blockade). Products include:
Depakene 421

Vancomycin Hydrochloride (Possible prolongation of neuromuscular blockade). Products include:
Vancocin HCl Capsules & Pulvules .. 1972
Vancocin HCl Oral Solution 1971
Vancocin HCl, Vials & ADD-Vantage 1970

Zonisamide (Potential for apparent resistance to the effects of rocuronium in the form of diminished magnitude of neuromuscular blockade). Products include:
Zonegran Capsules 1307

ZENAPAX FOR INJECTION
(Daclizumab) 3046
None cited in PDR database.

ZEPHREX TABLETS
(Guaifenesin, Pseudoephedrine Hydrochloride) 3091
See Zephrex LA Tablets

ZEPHREX LA TABLETS
(Guaifenesin, Pseudoephedrine Hydrochloride) 3092
May interact with beta blockers, monoamine oxidase inhibitors, veratrum alkaloids, and certain other agents. Compounds in these categories include:

Acebutolol Hydrochloride (Co-administration with beta-blockers results in increased effect of sympathomimetics). Products include:
Sectral Capsules 3589

Atenolol (Co-administration with beta-blockers results in increased effect of sympathomimetics). Products include:
Tenoretic Tablets 690
Tenormin I.V. Injection 692

Betaxolol Hydrochloride (Co-administration with beta-blockers results in increased effect of sympathomimetics). Products include:
Betoptic S Ophthalmic Suspension 537

Bisoprolol Fumarate (Co-administration with beta-blockers results in increased effect of sympathomimetics). Products include:
Zebeta Tablets 1885
Ziac Tablets 1887

Carteolol Hydrochloride (Co-administration with beta-blockers results in increased effect of sympathomimetics). Products include:
Carteolol Hydrochloride Ophthalmic Solution USP, 1% ..... ⊙258
Ocupress Ophthalmic Solution, 1% Sterile .... ⊙303

Cryptenamine Preparations (Reduced antihypertensive effects).
No products indexed under this heading.

Esmolol Hydrochloride (Co-administration with beta-blockers results in increased effect of sympathomimetics). Products include:
Brevibloc Injection 858

Isocarboxazid (Co-administration with MAO inhibitors results in increased effect of sympathomimetics; concurrent and/or sequential use is contraindicated).
No products indexed under this heading.

Labetalol Hydrochloride (Co-administration with beta-blockers results in increased effect of sympathomimetics). Products include:
Normodyne Injection 3135
Normodyne Tablets 3137

Levobunolol Hydrochloride (Co-administration with beta-blockers results in increased effect of sympathomimetics). Products include:
Betagan .... ⊙228

Mecamylamine Hydrochloride (Reduced antihypertensive effects). Products include:
Inversine Tablets 1850

Methyldopa (Reduced antihypertensive effects). Products include:
Aldoclor Tablets 2035
Aldomet Tablets 2037
Aldoril Tablets 2039

Methyldopate Hydrochloride (Reduced antihypertensive effects).
No products indexed under this heading.

Metipranolol Hydrochloride (Co-administration with beta-blockers results in increased effect of sympathomimetics).
No products indexed under this heading.

Metoprolol Succinate (Co-administration with beta-blockers results in increased effect of sympathomimetics). Products include:
Toprol-XL Tablets 651

Metoprolol Tartrate (Co-administration with beta-blockers results in increased effect of sympathomimetics).
No products indexed under this heading.

Moclobemide (Co-administration with MAO inhibitors results in increased effect of sympathomimetics; concurrent and/or sequential use is contraindicated).
No products indexed under this heading.

Nadolol (Co-administration with beta-blockers results in increased effect of sympathomimetics). Products include:
Corgard Tablets 2245
Corzide 40/5 Tablets 2247
Corzide 80/5 Tablets 2247
Nadolol Tablets 2288

Pargyline Hydrochloride (Co-administration with MAO inhibitors results in increased effect of sympathomimetics; concurrent and/or sequential use is contraindicated).
No products indexed under this heading.

Penbutolol Sulfate (Co-administration with beta-blockers results in increased effect of sympathomimetics).
No products indexed under this heading.

Phenelzine Sulfate (Co-administration with MAO inhibitors results in increased effect of sympathomimetics; concurrent and/or sequential use is contraindicated). Products include:
Nardil Tablets 2653

Pindolol (Co-administration with beta-blockers results in increased effect of sympathomimetics).
No products indexed under this heading.

Procarbazine Hydrochloride (Co-administration with MAO inhibitors results in increased effect of sympathomimetics; concurrent and/or sequential use is contraindicated). Products include:
Matulane Capsules 3246

Propranolol Hydrochloride (Co-administration with beta-blockers results in increased effect of sympathomimetics). Products include:
Inderal 3513
Inderal LA Long-Acting Capsules 3516
Inderide Tablets 3517
Inderide LA Long-Acting Capsules .. 3519

Reserpine (Reduced antihypertensive effects).
No products indexed under this heading.

Selegiline Hydrochloride (Co-administration with MAO inhibitors results in increased effect of sympathomimetics; concurrent and/or sequential use is contraindicated). Products include:
Eldepryl Capsules 3266

Sotalol Hydrochloride (Co-administration with beta-blockers results in increased effect of sympathomimetics). Products include:
Betapace Tablets 950
Betapace AF Tablets 954

Timolol Hemihydrate (Co-administration with beta-blockers results in increased effect of sympathomimetics). Products include:
Betimol Ophthalmic Solution .... ⊙324

Timolol Maleate (Co-administration with beta-blockers results in increased effect of sympathomimetics). Products include:
Blocadren Tablets 2046
Cosopt Sterile Ophthalmic Solution 2065
Timolide Tablets 2187
Timolol GFS .... ⊙266
Timoptic in Ocudose 2192
Timoptic Sterile Ophthalmic Solution 2190
Timoptic-XE Sterile Ophthalmic Gel Forming Solution 2194

Tranylcypromine Sulfate (Co-administration with MAO inhibitors results in increased effect of sympathomimetics; concurrent and/or sequential use is contraindicated). Products include:
Parnate Tablets 1607

ZERIT CAPSULES
(Stavudine) 1147
May interact with drugs that may exacerbate peripheral neuropathy (selected) and certain other agents. Compounds in these categories include:

Carboplatin (Concurrent use may exacerbate peripheral neuropathy). Products include:
Paraplatin for Injection 1126

Didanosine (Co-administration of stavudine and didanosine with other antiretroviral agents has resulted in fatal lactic acidosis in pregnant women; pancreatitis, peripheral neuropathy and liver function abnormalities occur more frequently with concurrent use). Products include:
Videx 1138
Videx EC Capsules 1143

Isoniazid (Concurrent use may exacerbate peripheral neuropathy). Products include:
Rifamate Capsules 767
Rifater Tablets 769

Paclitaxel (Concurrent use may exacerbate peripheral neuropathy). Products include:
Taxol Injection 1129

Zalcitabine (Concurrent use may exacerbate peripheral neuropathy). Products include:
Hivid Tablets 2975

Zidovudine (May competitively inhibit the intracellular phosphorylation of stavudine; concurrent use is not recommended). Products include:
Combivir Tablets 1502
Retrovir 1625
Retrovir IV Infusion 1629
Trizivir Tablets 1669

Food Interactions

Meal, unspecified (Co-administration with food decreases Cmax by approximately 45%, however, the systemic availability (AUC) is unchanged; Zerit Capsules can be taken without regard to meals).

ZERIT FOR ORAL SOLUTION
(Stavudine) 1147
See Zerit Capsules

ZESTORETIC TABLETS
(Hydrochlorothiazide, Lisinopril) 695
May interact with antihypertensives, barbiturates, corticosteroids, diuretics, oral hypoglycemic agents, insulin, lithium preparations, narcotic analgesics, nondepolarizing neuromuscular blocking agents, non-steroidal anti-inflammatory agents, potassium preparations, potassium sparing diuretics, and certain other agents. Compounds in these categories include:

Acarbose (Dosage adjustment of the antidiabetic may be required). Products include:
Precose Tablets 906

Acebutolol Hydrochloride (Additive effects). Products include:
Sectral Capsules 3589

ACTH (Intensifies electrolyte depletion).
No products indexed under this heading.

Alfentanil Hydrochloride (Potentiates orthostatic hypotension).
No products indexed under this heading.

Amiloride Hydrochloride (Additive antihypertensive effects; potential for hyperkalemia). Products include:
Midamor Tablets 2136
Moduretic Tablets 2138

Amlodipine Besylate (Additive effects). Products include:
Lotrel Capsules 2370
Norvasc Tablets 2704

Aprobarbital (Potentiates orthostatic hypotension).
No products indexed under this heading.

Atenolol (Additive effects). Products include:
Tenoretic Tablets 690
Tenormin I.V. Injection 692

Atracurium Besylate (Possible increased responsiveness to the muscle relaxant).
No products indexed under this heading.

Benazepril Hydrochloride (Additive effects). Products include:
Lotensin Tablets 2365
Lotensin HCT Tablets 2367
Lotrel Capsules 2370

Bendroflumethiazide (Additive effects). Products include:
Corzide 40/5 Tablets 2247
Corzide 80/5 Tablets 2247

Betamethasone Acetate (Intensifies electrolyte depletion). Products include:
Celestone Soluspan Injectable Suspension 3097

Betamethasone Sodium Phosphate (Intensifies electrolyte depletion). Products include:
Celestone Soluspan Injectable Suspension 3097

Betaxolol Hydrochloride (Additive effects). Products include:
Betoptic S Ophthalmic Suspension 537

Bisoprolol Fumarate (Additive effects). Products include:
Zebeta Tablets 1885
Ziac Tablets 1887

Bumetanide (Additive effects).
No products indexed under this heading.

Buprenorphine Hydrochloride (Potentiates orthostatic hypotension). Products include:
Buprenex Injectable 2918

IMPORTANT NOTE: Always consult each drug listing in the patient's regimen for possible interactions.

Butabarbital (Potentiates orthostatic hypotension).
No products indexed under this heading.

Butalbital (Potentiates orthostatic hypotension). Products include:
Phrenilin 578
Sedapap Tablets 50 mg/650 mg 2225

Candesartan Cilexetil (Additive effects). Products include:
Atacand Tablets 595
Atacand HCT Tablets 597

Captopril (Additive effects). Products include:
Captopril Tablets 2281

Carteolol Hydrochloride (Additive effects). Products include:
Carteolol Hydrochloride Ophthalmic Solution USP, 1% .... ⊙258
Ocupress Ophthalmic Solution, 1% Sterile .... ⊙303

Celecoxib (Reduces antihypertensive effects). Products include:
Celebrex Capsules 2676
Celebrex Capsules 2780

Chlorothiazide (Additive effects). Products include:
Aldoclor Tablets 2035
Diuril Oral 2087

Chlorothiazide Sodium (Additive effects). Products include:
Diuril Sodium Intravenous 2086

Chlorpropamide (Dosage adjustment of the antidiabetic may be required). Products include:
Diabinese Tablets 2680

Chlorthalidone (Additive effects). Products include:
Clorpres Tablets 1002
Combipres Tablets 1040
Tenoretic Tablets 690

Cholestyramine (Absorption of hydrochlorothiazide is impaired in the presence of anionic exchange resins, such as cholestyramine; binds hydrochlorothiazide and reduces its absorption from the GI tract by up to 85%).
No products indexed under this heading.

Cisatracurium Besylate (Possible increased responsiveness to the muscle relaxant).
No products indexed under this heading.

Clonidine (Additive effects). Products include:
Catapres-TTS 1038

Clonidine Hydrochloride (Additive effects). Products include:
Catapres Tablets 1037
Clorpres Tablets 1002
Combipres Tablets 1040
Duraclon Injection 3057

Codeine Phosphate (Potentiates orthostatic hypotension). Products include:
Phenergan with Codeine Syrup 3557
Phenergan VC with Codeine Syrup 3561
Robitussin A-C Syrup 2942
Robitussin-DAC Syrup 2942
Ryna-C Liquid .... ▣768
Soma Compound w/Codeine Tablets 3355
Tussi-Organidin NR Liquid 3350
Tussi-Organidin-S NR Liquid 3350
Tylenol with Codeine 2595

Colestipol Hydrochloride (Absorption of hydrochlorothiazide is impaired in the presence of anionic exchange resins, such as colestipol; binds hydrochlorothiazide and reduces its absorption from the GI tract by up to 43%). Products include:
Colestid Tablets 2791

Cortisone Acetate (Intensifies electrolyte depletion). Products include:
Cortone Acetate Injectable Suspension 2059
Cortone Acetate Tablets 2061

Deserpidine (Additive effects).
No products indexed under this heading.

Dexamethasone (Intensifies electrolyte depletion). Products include:
Decadron Elixir 2078
Decadron Tablets 2079
TobraDex Ophthalmic Ointment 542
TobraDex Ophthalmic Suspension 541

Dexamethasone Acetate (Intensifies electrolyte depletion).
No products indexed under this heading.

Dexamethasone Sodium Phosphate (Intensifies electrolyte depletion). Products include:
Decadron Phosphate Injection 2081
Decadron Phosphate Sterile Ophthalmic Ointment 2083
Decadron Phosphate Sterile Ophthalmic Solution 2084
NeoDecadron Sterile Ophthalmic Solution 2144

Dezocine (Potentiates orthostatic hypotension).
No products indexed under this heading.

Diazoxide (Additive effects).
No products indexed under this heading.

Diclofenac Potassium (Reduces antihypertensive effects). Products include:
Cataflam Tablets 2315

Diclofenac Sodium (Reduces antihypertensive effects). Products include:
Arthrotec Tablets 3195
Voltaren Ophthalmic Sterile Ophthalmic Solution .... ⊙312
Voltaren Tablets 2315
Voltaren-XR Tablets 2315

Diltiazem Hydrochloride (Additive effects). Products include:
Cardizem Injectable 1018
Cardizem Lyo-Ject Syringe 1018
Cardizem Monovial 1018
Cardizem CD Capsules 1016
Tiazac Capsules 1378

Doxazosin Mesylate (Additive effects). Products include:
Cardura Tablets 2668

Enalapril Maleate (Additive effects). Products include:
Lexxel Tablets 608
Vaseretic Tablets 2204
Vasotec Tablets 2210

Enalaprilat (Additive effects). Products include:
Enalaprilat Injection 863
Vasotec I.V. Injection 2207

Eprosartan Mesylate (Additive effects). Products include:
Teveten Tablets 3327

Esmolol Hydrochloride (Additive effects). Products include:
Brevibloc Injection 858

Ethacrynic Acid (Additive effects). Products include:
Edecrin Tablets 2091

Etodolac (Reduces antihypertensive effects). Products include:
Lodine 3528
Lodine XL Extended-Release Tablets 3530

Felodipine (Additive effects). Products include:
Lexxel Tablets 608
Plendil Extended-Release Tablets 623

Fenoprofen Calcium (Reduces antihypertensive effects).
No products indexed under this heading.

Fentanyl (Potentiates orthostatic hypotension). Products include:
Duragesic Transdermal System 1786

Fentanyl Citrate (Potentiates orthostatic hypotension). Products include:
Actiq 1184

Fludrocortisone Acetate (Intensifies electrolyte depletion). Products include:
Florinef Acetate Tablets 2250

Flurbiprofen (Reduces antihypertensive effects).
No products indexed under this heading.

Fosinopril Sodium (Additive effects). Products include:
Monopril Tablets 1091
Monopril HCT 1094

Furosemide (Additive effects). Products include:
Furosemide Tablets 2284

Glimepiride (Dosage adjustment of the antidiabetic may be required). Products include:
Amaryl Tablets 717

Glipizide (Dosage adjustment of the antidiabetic may be required). Products include:
Glucotrol Tablets 2692
Glucotrol XL Extended Release Tablets 2693

Glyburide (Dosage adjustment of the antidiabetic may be required). Products include:
DiaBeta Tablets 741
Glucovance Tablets 1086

Guanabenz Acetate (Additive effects).
No products indexed under this heading.

Guanethidine Monosulfate (Additive effects).
No products indexed under this heading.

Hydralazine Hydrochloride (Additive effects).
No products indexed under this heading.

Hydrocodone Bitartrate (Potentiates orthostatic hypotension). Products include:
Hycodan 1316
Hycomine Compound Tablets 1317
Hycotuss Expectorant Syrup 1318
Lortab 3319
Lortab Elixir 3317
Maxidone Tablets CIII 3399
Norco 5/325 Tablets CIII 3424
Norco 7.5/325 Tablets CIII 3425
Norco 10/325 Tablets CIII 3427
Norco 10/325 Tablets CIII 3425
Vicodin Tablets 516
Vicodin ES Tablets 517
Vicodin HP Tablets 518
Vicodin Tuss Expectorant 519
Vicoprofen Tablets 520
Zydone Tablets 1330

Hydrocodone Polistirex (Potentiates orthostatic hypotension). Products include:
Tussionex Pennkinetic Extended-Release Suspension 1174

Hydrocortisone (Intensifies electrolyte depletion). Products include:
Anusol-HC Cream 2.5% 2237
Cipro HC Otic Suspension 540
Cortaid Intensive Therapy Cream .... ▣717
Cortaid Maximum Strength Cream .... ▣717
Cortisporin Ophthalmic Suspension Sterile .... ⊙297
Cortizone•5 .... ▣699
Cortizone•10 .... ▣699
Cortizone•10 Plus Creme .... ▣700
Cortizone for Kids Creme .... ▣699
Hydrocortone Tablets 2106
Massengill Medicated Soft Cloth Towelette .... ▣753
VōSoL HC Otic Solution 3356

Hydrocortisone Acetate (Intensifies electrolyte depletion). Products include:
Analpram-HC 1338
Anusol HC-1 Hydrocortisone Anti-Itch Cream .... ▣689
Anusol-HC Suppositories 2238
Cortaid .... ▣717
Cortifoam Rectal Foam 3170
Cortisporin-TC Otic Suspension 2246
Hydrocortone Acetate Injectable Suspension 2103
Pramosone 1343
Proctocort Suppositories 2264
ProctoFoam-HC 3177
Terra-Cortril Ophthalmic Suspension 2716

Hydrocortisone Sodium Phosphate (Intensifies electrolyte depletion). Products include:
Hydrocortone Phosphate Injection, Sterile 2105

Hydrocortisone Sodium Succinate (Intensifies electrolyte depletion).
No products indexed under this heading.

Hydroflumethiazide (Additive effects). Products include:
Diucardin Tablets 3494

Hydromorphone Hydrochloride (Potentiates orthostatic hypotension). Products include:
Dilaudid 441
Dilaudid Oral Liquid 445
Dilaudid Powder 441
Dilaudid Rectal Suppositories 441
Dilaudid Tablets 441
Dilaudid Tablets - 8 mg 445
Dilaudid-HP 443

Ibuprofen (Reduces antihypertensive effects). Products include:
Advil .... ▣771
Children's Advil Oral Suspension .... ▣773
Children's Advil Chewable Tablets .... ▣773
Advil Cold and Sinus Caplets .... ▣771
Advil Cold and Sinus Tablets .... ▣771
Advil Flu & Body Ache Caplets .... ▣772
Infants' Advil Drops .... ▣773
Junior Strength Advil Tablets .... ▣773
Junior Strength Advil Chewable Tablets .... ▣773
Advil Migraine Liquigels .... ▣772
Children's Motrin Oral Suspension and Chewable Tablets 2006
Children's Motrin Cold Oral Suspension 2007
Children's Motrin Oral Suspension .... ▣643
Motrin Suspension, Oral Drops, Chewable Tablets, and Caplets 2002
Infants' Motrin Concentrated Drops 2006
Junior Strength Motrin Caplets and Chewable Tablets 2006
Motrin IB Tablets, Caplets, and Gelcaps 2002
Motrin Migraine Pain Caplets 2005
Motrin Sinus Headache Caplets 2005
Vicoprofen Tablets 520

Indapamide (Additive effects). Products include:
Indapamide Tablets 2286

Indomethacin (Reduces antihypertensive effects). Products include:
Indocin 2112

Indomethacin Sodium Trihydrate (Reduces antihypertensive effects). Products include:
Indocin I.V. 2115

Insulin, Human, Zinc Suspension (Dosage adjustment of the antidiabetic may be required). Products include:
Humulin L, 100 Units 1937
Humulin U, 100 Units 1943
Novolin L Human Insulin 10 ml Vials 2422

Insulin, Human NPH (Dosage adjustment of the antidiabetic may be required). Products include:
Humulin N, 100 Units 1939
Humulin N NPH Pen 1940
Novolin N Human Insulin 10 ml Vials 2422
Novolin N PenFill 2423
Novolin N Prefilled Syringe Disposable Insulin Delivery System 2425

Insulin, Human Regular (Dosage adjustment of the antidiabetic may be required). Products include:
Humulin R Regular (U-500) 1943
Humulin R, 100 Units 1941
Novolin R Human Insulin 10 ml Vials 2423
Novolin R PenFill 2423
Novolin R Prefilled Syringe Disposable Insulin Delivery System 2425
Velosulin BR Human Insulin 10 ml Vials 2435

Insulin, Human Regular and Human NPH Mixture (Dosage adjustment of the antidiabetic may be required). Products include:
Humulin 50/50, 100 Units 1934
Humulin 70/30, 100 Units 1935
Humulin 70/30 Pen 1936
Novolin 70/30 Human Insulin 10 ml Vials 2421
Novolin 70/30 PenFill 2423

Novolin 70/30 Prefilled Disposable Insulin Delivery System 2425

Insulin, NPH (Dosage adjustment of the antidiabetic may be required). Products include:
Iletin II, NPH (Pork), 100 Units 1946

Insulin, Regular (Dosage adjustment of the antidiabetic may be required). Products include:
Iletin II, Regular (Pork), 100 Units 1947

Insulin, Zinc Crystals (Dosage adjustment of the antidiabetic may be required).
No products indexed under this heading.

Insulin, Zinc Suspension (Dosage adjustment of the antidiabetic may be required). Products include:
Iletin II, Lente (Pork), 100 Units 1945

Insulin Aspart, Human Regular (Dosage adjustment of the antidiabetic may be required).
No products indexed under this heading.

Insulin glargine (Dosage adjustment of the antidiabetic may be required). Products include:
Lantus Injection 742

Insulin Lispro, Human (Dosage adjustment of the antidiabetic may be required). Products include:
Humalog 1926
Humalog Mix 75/25 Pen 1928

Insulin Lispro Protamine, Human (Dosage adjustment of the antidiabetic may be required). Products include:
Humalog Mix 75/25 Pen 1928

Irbesartan (Additive effects). Products include:
Avalide Tablets 1070
Avapro Tablets 1074
Avapro Tablets 3076

Isradipine (Additive effects). Products include:
DynaCirc Capsules 2921
DynaCirc CR Tablets 2923

Ketoprofen (Reduces antihypertensive effects). Products include:
Orudis Capsules 3548
Orudis KT Tablets .... ⊡778
Oruvail Capsules 3548

Ketorolac Tromethamine (Reduces antihypertensive effects). Products include:
Acular Ophthalmic Solution 544
Acular PF Ophthalmic Solution 544
Toradol 3018

Labetalol Hydrochloride (Additive effects). Products include:
Normodyne Injection 3135
Normodyne Tablets 3137

Levorphanol Tartrate (Potentiates orthostatic hypotension). Products include:
Levo-Dromoran 1734
Levorphanol Tartrate Tablets 3059

Lithium Carbonate (Reduced renal clearance of lithium resulting in lithium toxicity). Products include:
Eskalith 1527
Lithium Carbonate 3061
Lithobid Slow-Release Tablets 3255

Lithium Citrate (Reduced renal clearance of lithium resulting in lithium toxicity). Products include:
Lithium Citrate Syrup 3061

Losartan Potassium (Additive effects). Products include:
Cozaar Tablets 2067
Hyzaar 2109

Mecamylamine Hydrochloride (Additive effects). Products include:
Inversine Tablets 1850

Meclofenamate Sodium (Reduces antihypertensive effects).
No products indexed under this heading.

Mefenamic Acid (Reduces antihypertensive effects). Products include:
Ponstel Capsules 1356

Meloxicam (Reduces antihypertensive effects). Products include:
Mobic Tablets 1054

Meperidine Hydrochloride (Potentiates orthostatic hypotension). Products include:
Demerol 3079
Mepergan Injection 3539

Mephobarbital (Potentiates orthostatic hypotension).
No products indexed under this heading.

Metformin Hydrochloride (Dosage adjustment of the antidiabetic may be required). Products include:
Glucophage Tablets 1080
Glucophage XR Tablets 1080
Glucovance Tablets 1086

Methadone Hydrochloride (Potentiates orthostatic hypotension). Products include:
Dolophine Hydrochloride Tablets 3056

Methyclothiazide (Additive effects).
No products indexed under this heading.

Methyldopa (Additive effects). Products include:
Aldoclor Tablets 2035
Aldomet Tablets 2037
Aldoril Tablets 2039

Methyldopate Hydrochloride (Additive effects).
No products indexed under this heading.

Methylprednisolone Acetate (Intensifies electrolyte depletion). Products include:
Depo-Medrol Injectable Suspension 2795

Methylprednisolone Sodium Succinate (Intensifies electrolyte depletion). Products include:
Solu-Medrol Sterile Powder 2855

Metocurine Iodide (Possible increased responsiveness to the muscle relaxant).
No products indexed under this heading.

Metolazone (Additive effects). Products include:
Mykrox Tablets 1168
Zaroxolyn Tablets 1177

Metoprolol Succinate (Additive effects). Products include:
Toprol-XL Tablets 651

Metoprolol Tartrate (Additive effects).
No products indexed under this heading.

Metyrosine (Additive effects). Products include:
Demser Capsules 2085

Mibefradil Dihydrochloride (Additive effects).
No products indexed under this heading.

Miglitol (Dosage adjustment of the antidiabetic may be required). Products include:
Glyset Tablets 2821

Minoxidil (Additive effects). Products include:
Rogaine Extra Strength for Men Topical Solution .... ⊡721
Rogaine for Women Topical Solution .... ⊡721

Mivacurium Chloride (Possible increased responsiveness to the muscle relaxant).
No products indexed under this heading.

Moexipril Hydrochloride (Additive effects). Products include:
Uniretic Tablets 3178
Univasc Tablets 3181

Morphine Sulfate (Potentiates orthostatic hypotension). Products include:
Astramorph/PF Injection, USP (Preservative-Free) 594
Duramorph Injection 1312
Infumorph 200 and Infumorph 500 Sterile Solutions 1314
Kadian Capsules 1335
MS Contin Tablets 2896
MSIR 2898
Oramorph SR Tablets 3062
Roxanol 3066

Nabumetone (Reduces antihypertensive effects). Products include:
Relafen Tablets 1617

Nadolol (Additive effects). Products include:
Corgard Tablets 2245
Corzide 40/5 Tablets 2247
Corzide 80/5 Tablets 2247
Nadolol Tablets 2288

Naproxen (Reduces antihypertensive effects). Products include:
EC-Naprosyn Delayed-Release Tablets 2967
Naprosyn Suspension 2967
Naprosyn Tablets 2967

Naproxen Sodium (Reduces antihypertensive effects). Products include:
Aleve Tablets, Caplets and Gelcaps .... ⊡602
Aleve Cold & Sinus Caplets .... ⊡603
Anaprox Tablets 2967
Anaprox DS Tablets 2967
Naprelan Tablets 1293

Nicardipine Hydrochloride (Additive effects). Products include:
Cardene I.V. 3485

Nifedipine (Additive effects). Products include:
Adalat CC Tablets 877
Procardia Capsules 2708
Procardia XL Extended Release Tablets 2710

Nisoldipine (Additive effects). Products include:
Sular Tablets 688

Nitroglycerin (Additive effects). Products include:
Nitro-Dur Transdermal Infusion System 3134
Nitro-Dur Transdermal Infusion System 1834
Nitrolingual Pumpspray 1355
Nitrostat Tablets 2658

Norepinephrine Bitartrate (Possible decreased response to pressor amines).
No products indexed under this heading.

Oxaprozin (Reduces antihypertensive effects).
No products indexed under this heading.

Oxycodone Hydrochloride (Potentiates orthostatic hypotension). Products include:
OxyContin Tablets 2912
OxyFast Oral Concentrate Solution 2916
OxyIR Capsules 2916
Percocet Tablets 1326
Percodan Tablets 1327
Percolone Tablets 1327
Roxicodone 3067
Tylox Capsules 2597

Pancuronium Bromide (Possible increased responsiveness to the muscle relaxant).
No products indexed under this heading.

Penbutolol Sulfate (Additive effects).
No products indexed under this heading.

Pentobarbital Sodium (Potentiates orthostatic hypotension). Products include:
Nembutal Sodium Solution 485

Perindopril Erbumine (Additive effects). Products include:
Aceon Tablets (2 mg, 4 mg, 8 mg) 3249

Phenobarbital (Potentiates orthostatic hypotension). Products include:
Arco-Lase Plus Tablets 592
Donnatal 2929
Donnatal Extentabs 2930

Phenoxybenzamine Hydrochloride (Additive effects). Products include:
Dibenzyline Capsules 3457

Phentolamine Mesylate (Additive effects).
No products indexed under this heading.

Phenylbutazone (Reduces antihypertensive effects).
No products indexed under this heading.

Pindolol (Additive effects).
No products indexed under this heading.

Pioglitazone Hydrochloride (Dosage adjustment of the antidiabetic may be required). Products include:
Actos Tablets 3275

Piroxicam (Reduces antihypertensive effects). Products include:
Feldene Capsules 2685

Polythiazide (Additive effects). Products include:
Minizide Capsules 2700
Renese Tablets 2712

Potassium Acid Phosphate (Potential for hyperkalemia). Products include:
K-Phos Original (Sodium Free) Tablets 947

Potassium Bicarbonate (Potential for hyperkalemia).
No products indexed under this heading.

Potassium Chloride (Potential for hyperkalemia). Products include:
Chlor-3 1361
Colyte with Flavor Packs for Oral Solution 3170
GoLYTELY and Pineapple Flavor GoLYTELY for Oral Solution 1068
K-Dur Microburst Release System ER Tablets 1832
Klor-Con M20/Klor-Con M10 Tablets 3329
K-Lor Powder Packets 469
K-Tab Filmtab Tablets 470
Micro-K 3311
NuLYTELY, Cherry Flavor, Lemon-Lime Flavor, and Orange Flavor NuLYTELY for Oral Solution 1068
Rum-K 1363

Potassium Citrate (Potential for hyperkalemia). Products include:
Urocit-K Tablets 2232

Potassium Gluconate (Potential for hyperkalemia).
No products indexed under this heading.

Potassium Phosphate (Potential for hyperkalemia). Products include:
K-Phos Neutral Tablets 946

Prazosin Hydrochloride (Additive effects). Products include:
Minipress Capsules 2699
Minizide Capsules 2700

Prednisolone Acetate (Intensifies electrolyte depletion). Products include:
Blephamide Ophthalmic Ointment 547
Blephamide Ophthalmic Suspension 548
Poly-Pred Liquifilm Ophthalmic Suspension .... ⊙245
Pred Forte Ophthalmic Suspension .... ⊙246
Pred Mild Sterile Ophthalmic Suspension .... ⊙249
Pred-G Ophthalmic Suspension .... ⊙247
Pred-G Sterile Ophthalmic Ointment .... ⊙248

Prednisolone Sodium Phosphate (Intensifies electrolyte depletion). Products include:
Pediapred Oral Solution 1170

Prednisolone Tebutate (Intensifies electrolyte depletion).
No products indexed under this heading.

Prednisone (Intensifies electrolyte depletion). Products include:
Prednisone 3064

Propoxyphene Hydrochloride (Potentiates orthostatic hypotension). Products include:
Darvon Pulvules 1909
Darvon Compound-65 Pulvules 1910

Propoxyphene Napsylate (Potentiates orthostatic hypotension). Products include:
- Darvon-N/Darvocet-N 1907
- Darvon-N Tablets 1912

Propranolol Hydrochloride (Additive effects). Products include:
- Inderal 3513
- Inderal LA Long-Acting Capsules 3516
- Inderide Tablets 3517
- Inderide LA Long-Acting Capsules .. 3519

Quinapril Hydrochloride (Additive effects). Products include:
- Accupril Tablets 2611
- Accuretic Tablets 2614

Ramipril (Additive effects). Products include:
- Altace Capsules 2233

Rapacuronium Bromide (Possible increased responsiveness to the muscle relaxant).
No products indexed under this heading.

Rauwolfia serpentina (Additive effects).
No products indexed under this heading.

Remifentanil Hydrochloride (Potentiates orthostatic hypotension).
No products indexed under this heading.

Repaglinide (Dosage adjustment of the antidiabetic may be required). Products include:
- Prandin Tablets (0.5, 1, and 2 mg) 2432

Rescinnamine (Additive effects).
No products indexed under this heading.

Reserpine (Additive effects).
No products indexed under this heading.

Rocuronium Bromide (Possible increased responsiveness to the muscle relaxant). Products include:
- Zemuron Injection 2491

Rofecoxib (Reduces antihypertensive effects). Products include:
- Vioxx 2213

Rosiglitazone Maleate (Dosage adjustment of the antidiabetic may be required). Products include:
- Avandia Tablets 1490

Secobarbital Sodium (Potentiates orthostatic hypotension).
No products indexed under this heading.

Sodium Nitroprusside (Additive effects).
No products indexed under this heading.

Sotalol Hydrochloride (Additive effects). Products include:
- Betapace Tablets 950
- Betapace AF Tablets 954

Spirapril Hydrochloride (Additive effects).
No products indexed under this heading.

Spironolactone (Additive antihypertensive effects; potential for hyperkalemia).
No products indexed under this heading.

Sufentanil Citrate (Potentiates orthostatic hypotension).
No products indexed under this heading.

Sulindac (Reduces antihypertensive effects). Products include:
- Clinoril Tablets 2053

Telmisartan (Additive effects). Products include:
- Micardis Tablets 1049
- Micardis HCT Tablets 1051

Terazosin Hydrochloride (Additive effects). Products include:
- Hytrin Capsules 464

Thiamylal Sodium (Potentiates orthostatic hypotension).
No products indexed under this heading.

Timolol Maleate (Additive effects). Products include:
- Blocadren Tablets 2046
- Cosopt Sterile Ophthalmic Solution 2065
- Timolide Tablets 2187
- Timolol GFS .... ⊙266
- Timoptic in Ocudose 2192
- Timoptic Sterile Ophthalmic Solution 2190
- Timoptic-XE Sterile Ophthalmic Gel Forming Solution 2194

Tolazamide (Dosage adjustment of the antidiabetic may be required).
No products indexed under this heading.

Tolbutamide (Dosage adjustment of the antidiabetic may be required).
No products indexed under this heading.

Tolmetin Sodium (Reduces antihypertensive effects). Products include:
- Tolectin 2589

Torsemide (Additive effects). Products include:
- Demadex Tablets and Injection 2965

Trandolapril (Additive effects). Products include:
- Mavik Tablets 478
- Tarka Tablets 508

Triamcinolone (Intensifies electrolyte depletion).
No products indexed under this heading.

Triamcinolone Acetonide (Intensifies electrolyte depletion). Products include:
- Azmacort Inhalation Aerosol 728
- Nasacort Nasal Inhaler 750
- Nasacort AQ Nasal Spray 752
- Tri-Nasal Spray 2274

Triamcinolone Diacetate (Intensifies electrolyte depletion).
No products indexed under this heading.

Triamcinolone Hexacetonide (Intensifies electrolyte depletion).
No products indexed under this heading.

Triamterene (Additive antihypertensive effects; potential for hyperkalemia). Products include:
- Dyazide Capsules 1515
- Dyrenium Capsules 3458
- Maxzide 1008

Trimethaphan Camsylate (Additive effects).
No products indexed under this heading.

Troglitazone (Dosage adjustment of the antidiabetic may be required).
No products indexed under this heading.

Tubocurarine Chloride (Possible increased responsiveness to the muscle relaxant).
No products indexed under this heading.

Valsartan (Additive effects). Products include:
- Diovan Capsules 2337
- Diovan HCT Tablets 2338

Vecuronium Bromide (Possible increased responsiveness to the muscle relaxant). Products include:
- Norcuron for Injection 2478

Verapamil Hydrochloride (Additive effects). Products include:
- Covera-HS Tablets 3199
- Isoptin SR Tablets 467
- Tarka Tablets 508
- Verelan Capsules 3184
- Verelan PM Capsules 3186

Food Interactions

Alcohol (Potentiates orthostatic hypotension).

ZESTRIL TABLETS

(Lisinopril) 698

May interact with diuretics, lithium preparations, potassium preparations, potassium sparing diuretics, thiazides, and certain other agents. Compounds in these categories include:

Amiloride Hydrochloride (Potential for significant hyperkalemia; possibility of excessive reduction in blood pressure). Products include:
- Midamor Tablets 2136
- Moduretic Tablets 2138

Bendroflumethiazide (Thiazide-induced potassium loss attenuated; possibility of excessive reduction in blood pressure). Products include:
- Corzide 40/5 Tablets 2247
- Corzide 80/5 Tablets 2247

Bumetanide (Possibility of excessive reduction in blood pressure).
No products indexed under this heading.

Chlorothiazide (Thiazide-induced potassium loss attenuated; possibility of excessive reduction in blood pressure). Products include:
- Aldoclor Tablets 2035
- Diuril Oral 2087

Chlorothiazide Sodium (Thiazide-induced potassium loss attenuated; possibility of excessive reduction in blood pressure). Products include:
- Diuril Sodium Intravenous 2086

Chlorthalidone (Possibility of excessive reduction in blood pressure). Products include:
- Clorpres Tablets 1002
- Combipres Tablets 1040
- Tenoretic Tablets 690

Ethacrynic Acid (Possibility of excessive reduction in blood pressure). Products include:
- Edecrin Tablets 2091

Furosemide (Possibility of excessive reduction in blood pressure). Products include:
- Furosemide Tablets 2284

Hydrochlorothiazide (Thiazide-induced potassium loss attenuated; possibility of excessive reduction in blood pressure). Products include:
- Accuretic Tablets 2614
- Aldoril Tablets 2039
- Atacand HCT Tablets 597
- Avalide Tablets 1070
- Diovan HCT Tablets 2338
- Dyazide Capsules 1515
- HydroDIURIL Tablets 2108
- Hyzaar 2109
- Inderide Tablets 3517
- Inderide LA Long-Acting Capsules .. 3519
- Lotensin HCT Tablets 2367
- Maxzide 1008
- Micardis HCT Tablets 1051
- Microzide Capsules 3414
- Moduretic Tablets 2138
- Monopril HCT 1094
- Prinzide Tablets 2168
- Timolide Tablets 2187
- Uniretic Tablets 3178
- Vaseretic Tablets 2204
- Zestoretic Tablets 695
- Ziac Tablets 1887

Hydroflumethiazide (Thiazide-induced potassium loss attenuated; possibility of excessive reduction in blood pressure). Products include:
- Diucardin Tablets 3494

Indapamide (Possibility of excessive reduction in blood pressure). Products include:
- Indapamide Tablets 2286

Indomethacin (Reduces antihypertensive effect). Products include:
- Indocin 2112

Indomethacin Sodium Trihydrate (Reduces antihypertensive effect). Products include:
- Indocin I.V. 2115

Lithium Carbonate (Possibility of lithium toxicity–serum lithium levels should be monitored frequently). Products include:
- Eskalith 1527
- Lithium Carbonate 3061
- Lithobid Slow-Release Tablets 3255

Lithium Citrate (Possibility of lithium toxicity–serum lithium levels should be monitored frequently). Products include:
- Lithium Citrate Syrup 3061

Methyclothiazide (Thiazide-induced potassium loss attenuated; possibility of excessive reduction in blood pressure).
No products indexed under this heading.

Metolazone (Possibility of excessive reduction in blood pressure). Products include:
- Mykrox Tablets 1168
- Zaroxolyn Tablets 1177

Polythiazide (Thiazide-induced potassium loss attenuated; possibility of excessive reduction in blood pressure). Products include:
- Minizide Capsules 2700
- Renese Tablets 2712

Potassium Acid Phosphate (Potential for significant hyperkalemia). Products include:
- K-Phos Original (Sodium Free) Tablets 947

Potassium Bicarbonate (Potential for significant hyperkalemia).
No products indexed under this heading.

Potassium Chloride (Potential for significant hyperkalemia). Products include:
- Chlor-3 1361
- Colyte with Flavor Packs for Oral Solution 3170
- GoLYTELY and Pineapple Flavor GoLYTELY for Oral Solution 1068
- K-Dur Microburst Release System ER Tablets 1832
- Klor-Con M20/Klor-Con M10 Tablets 3329
- K-Lor Powder Packets 469
- K-Tab Filmtab Tablets 470
- Micro-K 3311
- NuLYTELY, Cherry Flavor, Lemon-Lime Flavor, and Orange Flavor NuLYTELY for Oral Solution 1068
- Rum-K 1363

Potassium Citrate (Potential for significant hyperkalemia). Products include:
- Urocit-K Tablets 2232

Potassium Gluconate (Potential for significant hyperkalemia).
No products indexed under this heading.

Potassium Phosphate (Potential for significant hyperkalemia). Products include:
- K-Phos Neutral Tablets 946

Spironolactone (Potential for significant hyperkalemia; possibility of excessive reduction in blood pressure).
No products indexed under this heading.

Torsemide (Possibility of excessive reduction in blood pressure). Products include:
- Demadex Tablets and Injection 2965

Triamterene (Potential for significant hyperkalemia; possibility of excessive reduction in blood pressure). Products include:
- Dyazide Capsules 1515
- Dyrenium Capsules 3458
- Maxzide 1008

ZIAC TABLETS

(Bisoprolol Fumarate, Hydrochlorothiazide) 1887

May interact with antihypertensives, barbiturates, catecholamine depleting drugs, corticosteroids, oral hypoglycemic agents, insulin, lithium preparations, narcotic analgesics, nondepolarizing neuromuscular blocking agents, non-steroidal anti-inflammatory agents, and certain other agents. Compounds in these categories include:

Acarbose (Beta blockers may mask some of the manifestations of hypo-

glycemia, particularly tachycardia; dosage adjustment of the antidiabetic drug may be required). Products include:
Precose Tablets 906

Acebutolol Hydrochloride (Ziac may potentiate the action of other antihypertensive agents used concomitantly). Products include:
Sectral Capsules 3589

ACTH (Intensifies electrolyte depletion, particularly hypokalemia).
No products indexed under this heading.

Alfentanil Hydrochloride (Potentiation of orthostatic hypotension may occur when thiazide diuretics are used with narcotics).
No products indexed under this heading.

Amlodipine Besylate (Ziac may potentiate the action of other antihypertensive agents used concomitantly). Products include:
Lotrel Capsules 2370
Norvasc Tablets 2704

Aprobarbital (Potentiation of orthostatic hypotension may occur when thiazide diuretics are used with barbiturates).
No products indexed under this heading.

Atenolol (Ziac may potentiate the action of other antihypertensive agents used concomitantly). Products include:
Tenoretic Tablets 690
Tenormin I.V. Injection 692

Atracurium Besylate (Possible increased responsiveness to the muscle relaxant).
No products indexed under this heading.

Benazepril Hydrochloride (Ziac may potentiate the action of other antihypertensive agents used concomitantly). Products include:
Lotensin Tablets 2365
Lotensin HCT Tablets 2367
Lotrel Capsules 2370

Bendroflumethiazide (Ziac may potentiate the action of other antihypertensive agents used concomitantly). Products include:
Corzide 40/5 Tablets 2247
Corzide 80/5 Tablets 2247

Betamethasone Acetate (Intensifies electrolyte depletion, particularly hypokalemia). Products include:
Celestone Soluspan Injectable Suspension 3097

Betamethasone Sodium Phosphate (Intensifies electrolyte depletion, particularly hypokalemia). Products include:
Celestone Soluspan Injectable Suspension 3097

Betaxolol Hydrochloride (Ziac may potentiate the action of other antihypertensive agents used concomitantly). Products include:
Betoptic S Ophthalmic Suspension 537

Buprenorphine Hydrochloride (Potentiation of orthostatic hypotension may occur when thiazide diuretics are used with narcotics). Products include:
Buprenex Injectable 2918

Butabarbital (Potentiation of orthostatic hypotension may occur when thiazide diuretics are used with barbiturates).
No products indexed under this heading.

Butalbital (Potentiation of orthostatic hypotension may occur when thiazide diuretics are used with barbiturates). Products include:
Phrenilin 578
Sedapap Tablets 50 mg/650 mg ... 2225

Candesartan Cilexetil (Ziac may potentiate the action of other antihypertensive agents used concomitantly). Products include:
Atacand Tablets 595
Atacand HCT Tablets 597

Captopril (Ziac may potentiate the action of other antihypertensive agents used concomitantly). Products include:
Captopril Tablets 2281

Carteolol Hydrochloride (Ziac may potentiate the action of other antihypertensive agents used concomitantly). Products include:
Carteolol Hydrochloride Ophthalmic Solution USP, 1% ..... ⊙ 258
Ocupress Ophthalmic Solution, 1% Sterile .... ⊙ 303

Celecoxib (Reduces the diuretic, natriuretic, and antihypertensive effects of thiazides). Products include:
Celebrex Capsules 2676
Celebrex Capsules 2780

Chlorothiazide (Ziac may potentiate the action of other antihypertensive agents used concomitantly). Products include:
Aldoclor Tablets 2035
Diuril Oral 2087

Chlorothiazide Sodium (Ziac may potentiate the action of other antihypertensive agents used concomitantly). Products include:
Diuril Sodium Intravenous 2086

Chlorpropamide (Beta blockers may mask some of the manifestations of hypoglycemia, particularly tachycardia; dosage adjustment of the antidiabetic drug may be required). Products include:
Diabinese Tablets 2680

Chlorthalidone (Ziac may potentiate the action of other antihypertensive agents used concomitantly). Products include:
Clorpres Tablets 1002
Combipres Tablets 1040
Tenoretic Tablets 690

Cholestyramine (Binds the hydrochlorothiazide and reduces its absorption in the GI tract by up to 85%).
No products indexed under this heading.

Cisatracurium Besylate (Possible increased responsiveness to the muscle relaxant).
No products indexed under this heading.

Clonidine (Ziac may potentiate the action of other antihypertensive agents used concomitantly). Products include:
Catapres-TTS 1038

Clonidine Hydrochloride (Ziac may potentiate the action of other antihypertensive agents used concomitantly). Products include:
Catapres Tablets 1037
Clorpres Tablets 1002
Combipres Tablets 1040
Duraclon Injection 3057

Codeine Phosphate (Potentiation of orthostatic hypotension may occur when thiazide diuretics are used with narcotics). Products include:
Phenergan with Codeine Syrup 3557
Phenergan VC with Codeine Syrup . 3561
Robitussin A-C Syrup 2942
Robitussin-DAC Syrup 2942
Ryna-C Liquid .... ▣ 768
Soma Compound w/Codeine Tablets 3355
Tussi-Organidin NR Liquid 3350
Tussi-Organidin-S NR Liquid 3350
Tylenol with Codeine 2595

Colestipol Hydrochloride (Binds the hydrochlorothiazide and reduces its absorption in the GI tract by up to 43%). Products include:
Colestid Tablets 2791

Cortisone Acetate (Intensifies electrolyte depletion, particularly hypokalemia). Products include:
Cortone Acetate Injectable Suspension 2059
Cortone Acetate Tablets 2061

Cyclopropane (Use with caution when administered with anesthetic agent that depresses myocardial function).
No products indexed under this heading.

Deserpidine (Concomitant use may produce excessive reduction of sympathetic activity).
No products indexed under this heading.

Dexamethasone (Intensifies electrolyte depletion, particularly hypokalemia). Products include:
Decadron Elixir 2078
Decadron Tablets 2079
TobraDex Ophthalmic Ointment 542
TobraDex Ophthalmic Suspension .. 541

Dexamethasone Acetate (Intensifies electrolyte depletion, particularly hypokalemia).
No products indexed under this heading.

Dexamethasone Sodium Phosphate (Intensifies electrolyte depletion, particularly hypokalemia). Products include:
Decadron Phosphate Injection 2081
Decadron Phosphate Sterile Ophthalmic Ointment 2083
Decadron Phosphate Sterile Ophthalmic Solution 2084
NeoDecadron Sterile Ophthalmic Solution 2144

Dezocine (Potentiation of orthostatic hypotension may occur when thiazide diuretics are used with narcotics).
No products indexed under this heading.

Diazoxide (Ziac may potentiate the action of other antihypertensive agents used concomitantly).
No products indexed under this heading.

Diclofenac Potassium (Reduces the diuretic, natriuretic, and antihypertensive effects of thiazides). Products include:
Cataflam Tablets 2315

Diclofenac Sodium (Reduces the diuretic, natriuretic, and antihypertensive effects of thiazides). Products include:
Arthrotec Tablets 3195
Voltaren Ophthalmic Sterile Ophthalmic Solution .... ⊙ 312
Voltaren Tablets 2315
Voltaren-XR Tablets 2315

Diltiazem Hydrochloride (Ziac should be used with caution when myocardial depressants or inhibitors of AV conduction are used concurrently). Products include:
Cardizem Injectable 1018
Cardizem Lyo-Ject Syringe 1018
Cardizem Monovial 1018
Cardizem CD Capsules 1016
Tiazac Capsules 1378

Disopyramide Phosphate (Ziac should be used with caution when myocardial depressants or inhibitors of AV conduction are used concurrently).
No products indexed under this heading.

Doxazosin Mesylate (Ziac may potentiate the action of other antihypertensive agents used concomitantly). Products include:
Cardura Tablets 2668

Enalapril Maleate (Ziac may potentiate the action of other antihypertensive agents used concomitantly). Products include:
Lexxel Tablets 608
Vaseretic Tablets 2204
Vasotec Tablets 2210

Enalaprilat (Ziac may potentiate the action of other antihypertensive agents used concomitantly). Products include:
Enalaprilat Injection 863
Vasotec I.V. Injection 2207

Epinephrine Hydrochloride (Patients with history of severe anaphylactic reaction to variety of allergens may be unresponsive to the usual doses of epinephrine used to treat allergic reactions).
No products indexed under this heading.

Eprosartan Mesylate (Ziac may potentiate the action of other antihypertensive agents used concomitantly). Products include:
Teveten Tablets 3327

Esmolol Hydrochloride (Ziac may potentiate the action of other antihypertensive agents used concomitantly). Products include:
Brevibloc Injection 858

Ether (Use with caution when administered with anesthetic agent that depresses myocardial function).
No products indexed under this heading.

Etodolac (Reduces the diuretic, natriuretic, and antihypertensive effects of thiazides). Products include:
Lodine 3528
Lodine XL Extended-Release Tablets 3530

Felodipine (Ziac may potentiate the action of other antihypertensive agents used concomitantly). Products include:
Lexxel Tablets 608
Plendil Extended-Release Tablets ... 623

Fenoprofen Calcium (Reduces the diuretic, natriuretic, and antihypertensive effects of thiazides).
No products indexed under this heading.

Fentanyl (Potentiation of orthostatic hypotension may occur when thiazide diuretics are used with narcotics). Products include:
Duragesic Transdermal System 1786

Fentanyl Citrate (Potentiation of orthostatic hypotension may occur when thiazide diuretics are used with narcotics). Products include:
Actiq 1184

Fludrocortisone Acetate (Intensifies electrolyte depletion, particularly hypokalemia). Products include:
Florinef Acetate Tablets 2250

Flurbiprofen (Reduces the diuretic, natriuretic, and antihypertensive effects of thiazides).
No products indexed under this heading.

Fosinopril Sodium (Ziac may potentiate the action of other antihypertensive agents used concomitantly). Products include:
Monopril Tablets 1091
Monopril HCT 1094

Furosemide (Ziac may potentiate the action of other antihypertensive agents used concomitantly). Products include:
Furosemide Tablets 2284

Glimepiride (Beta blockers may mask some of the manifestations of hypoglycemia, particularly tachycardia; dosage adjustment of the antidiabetic drug may be required). Products include:
Amaryl Tablets 717

Glipizide (Beta blockers may mask some of the manifestations of hypoglycemia, particularly tachycardia; dosage adjustment of the antidiabetic drug may be required). Products include:
Glucotrol Tablets 2692
Glucotrol XL Extended Release Tablets 2693

Glyburide (Beta blockers may mask some of the manifestations of hypoglycemia, particularly tachycardia; dosage adjustment of the antidiabetic drug may be required). Products include:
DiaBeta Tablets 741
Glucovance Tablets 1086

Guanabenz Acetate (Ziac may potentiate the action of other antihypertensive agents used concomitant-

ly).
No products indexed under this heading.

Guanethidine Monosulfate (Concomitant use may produce excessive reduction of sympathetic activity).
No products indexed under this heading.

Hydralazine Hydrochloride (Ziac may potentiate the action of other antihypertensive agents used concomitantly).
No products indexed under this heading.

Hydrocodone Bitartrate (Potentiation of orthostatic hypotension may occur when thiazide diuretics are used with narcotics). Products include:
Hycodan ... 1316
Hycomine Compound Tablets ... 1317
Hycotuss Expectorant Syrup ... 1318
Lortab ... 3319
Lortab Elixir ... 3317
Maxidone Tablets CIII ... 3399
Norco 5/325 Tablets CIII ... 3424
Norco 7.5/325 Tablets CIII ... 3425
Norco 10/325 Tablets CIII ... 3427
Norco 10/325 Tablets CIII ... 3425
Vicodin Tablets ... 516
Vicodin ES Tablets ... 517
Vicodin HP Tablets ... 518
Vicodin Tuss Expectorant ... 519
Vicoprofen Tablets ... 520
Zydone Tablets ... 1330

Hydrocodone Polistirex (Potentiation of orthostatic hypotension may occur when thiazide diuretics are used with narcotics). Products include:
Tussionex Pennkinetic Extended-Release Suspension ... 1174

Hydrocortisone (Intensifies electrolyte depletion, particularly hypokalemia). Products include:
Anusol-HC Cream 2.5% ... 2237
Cipro HC Otic Suspension ... 540
Cortaid Intensive Therapy Cream ... ▣717
Cortaid Maximum Strength Cream ... ▣717
Cortisporin Ophthalmic Suspension Sterile ... ⊙297
Cortizone•5 ... ▣699
Cortizone•10 ... ▣699
Cortizone•10 Plus Creme ... ▣700
Cortizone for Kids Creme ... ▣699
Hydrocortone Tablets ... 2106
Massengill Medicated Soft Cloth Towelette ... ▣753
VōSoL HC Otic Solution ... 3356

Hydrocortisone Acetate (Intensifies electrolyte depletion, particularly hypokalemia). Products include:
Analpram-HC ... 1338
Anusol HC-1 Hydrocortisone Anti-Itch Cream ... ▣689
Anusol-HC Suppositories ... 2238
Cortaid ... ▣717
Cortifoam Rectal Foam ... 3170
Cortisporin-TC Otic Suspension ... 2246
Hydrocortisone Acetate Injectable Suspension ... 2103
Pramosone ... 1343
Proctocort Suppositories ... 2264
ProctoFoam-HC ... 3177
Terra-Cortril Ophthalmic Suspension ... 2716

Hydrocortisone Sodium Phosphate (Intensifies electrolyte depletion, particularly hypokalemia). Products include:
Hydrocortone Phosphate Injection, Sterile ... 2105

Hydrocortisone Sodium Succinate (Intensifies electrolyte depletion, particularly hypokalemia).
No products indexed under this heading.

Hydroflumethiazide (Ziac may potentiate the action of other antihypertensive agents used concomitantly). Products include:
Diucardin Tablets ... 3494

Hydromorphone Hydrochloride (Potentiation of orthostatic hypotension may occur when thiazide diuretics are used with narcotics). Products include:
Dilaudid ... 441
Dilaudid Oral Liquid ... 445
Dilaudid Powder ... 441
Dilaudid Rectal Suppositories ... 441
Dilaudid Tablets ... 441
Dilaudid Tablets - 8 mg ... 445
Dilaudid-HP ... 443

Ibuprofen (Reduces the diuretic, natriuretic, and antihypertensive effects of thiazides). Products include:
Advil ... ▣771
Children's Advil Oral Suspension ... ▣773
Children's Advil Chewable Tablets ... ▣773
Advil Cold and Sinus Caplets ... ▣771
Advil Cold and Sinus Tablets ... ▣771
Advil Flu & Body Ache Caplets ... ▣772
Infants' Advil Drops ... ▣773
Junior Strength Advil Tablets ... ▣773
Junior Strength Advil Chewable Tablets ... ▣773
Advil Migraine Liquigels ... ▣772
Children's Motrin Oral Suspension and Chewable Tablets ... 2006
Children's Motrin Cold Oral Suspension ... 2007
Children's Motrin Oral Suspension ... ▣643
Motrin Suspension, Oral Drops, Chewable Tablets, and Caplets ... 2002
Infants' Motrin Concentrated Drops ... 2006
Junior Strength Motrin Caplets and Chewable Tablets ... 2006
Motrin IB Tablets, Caplets, and Gelcaps ... 2002
Motrin Migraine Pain Caplets ... 2005
Motrin Sinus Headache Caplets ... 2005
Vicoprofen Tablets ... 520

Indapamide (Ziac may potentiate the action of other antihypertensive agents used concomitantly). Products include:
Indapamide Tablets ... 2286

Indomethacin (Reduces the diuretic, natriuretic, and antihypertensive effects of thiazides). Products include:
Indocin ... 2112

Indomethacin Sodium Trihydrate (Reduces the diuretic, natriuretic, and antihypertensive effects of thiazides). Products include:
Indocin I.V. ... 2115

Insulin, Human, Zinc Suspension (Beta blockers may mask some of the manifestations of hypoglycemia, particularly tachycardia; dosage adjustment of the antidiabetic drug may be required). Products include:
Humulin L, 100 Units ... 1937
Humulin U, 100 Units ... 1943
Novolin L Human Insulin 10 ml Vials ... 2422

Insulin, Human NPH (Beta blockers may mask some of the manifestations of hypoglycemia, particularly tachycardia; dosage adjustment of the antidiabetic drug may be required). Products include:
Humulin N, 100 Units ... 1939
Humulin N NPH Pen ... 1940
Novolin N Human Insulin 10 ml Vials ... 2422
Novolin N PenFill ... 2423
Novolin N Prefilled Syringe Disposable Insulin Delivery System ... 2425

Insulin, Human Regular (Beta blockers may mask some of the manifestations of hypoglycemia, particularly tachycardia; dosage adjustment of the antidiabetic drug may be required). Products include:
Humulin R Regular (U-500) ... 1943
Humulin R, 100 Units ... 1941
Novolin R Human Insulin 10 ml Vials ... 2423
Novolin R PenFill ... 2423
Novolin R Prefilled Syringe Disposable Insulin Delivery System ... 2425
Velosulin BR Human Insulin 10 ml Vials ... 2435

Insulin, Human Regular and Human NPH Mixture (Beta blockers may mask some of the manifestations of hypoglycemia, particularly tachycardia; dosage adjustment of the antidiabetic drug may be required). Products include:
Humulin 50/50, 100 Units ... 1934
Humulin 70/30, 100 Units ... 1935
Humulin 70/30 Pen ... 1936
Novolin 70/30 Human Insulin 10 ml Vials ... 2421
Novolin 70/30 PenFill ... 2423
Novolin 70/30 Prefilled Disposable Insulin Delivery System ... 2425

Insulin, NPH (Beta blockers may mask some of the manifestations of hypoglycemia, particularly tachycardia; dosage adjustment of the antidiabetic drug may be required). Products include:
Iletin II, NPH (Pork), 100 Units ... 1946

Insulin, Regular (Beta blockers may mask some of the manifestations of hypoglycemia, particularly tachycardia; dosage adjustment of the antidiabetic drug may be required). Products include:
Iletin II, Regular (Pork), 100 Units ... 1947

Insulin, Zinc Crystals (Beta blockers may mask some of the manifestations of hypoglycemia, particularly tachycardia; dosage adjustment of the antidiabetic drug may be required).
No products indexed under this heading.

Insulin, Zinc Suspension (Beta blockers may mask some of the manifestations of hypoglycemia, particularly tachycardia; dosage adjustment of the antidiabetic drug may be required). Products include:
Iletin II, Lente (Pork), 100 Units ... 1945

Insulin Aspart, Human Regular (Beta blockers may mask some of the manifestations of hypoglycemia, particularly tachycardia; dosage adjustment of the antidiabetic drug may be required).
No products indexed under this heading.

Insulin glargine (Beta blockers may mask some of the manifestations of hypoglycemia, particularly tachycardia; dosage adjustment of the antidiabetic drug may be required). Products include:
Lantus Injection ... 742

Insulin Lispro, Human (Beta blockers may mask some of the manifestations of hypoglycemia, particularly tachycardia; dosage adjustment of the antidiabetic drug may be required). Products include:
Humalog ... 1926
Humalog Mix 75/25 Pen ... 1928

Insulin Lispro Protamine, Human (Beta blockers may mask some of the manifestations of hypoglycemia, particularly tachycardia; dosage adjustment of the antidiabetic drug may be required). Products include:
Humalog Mix 75/25 Pen ... 1928

Irbesartan (Ziac may potentiate the action of other antihypertensive agents used concomitantly). Products include:
Avalide Tablets ... 1070
Avapro Tablets ... 1074
Avapro Tablets ... 3076

Isradipine (Ziac may potentiate the action of other antihypertensive agents used concomitantly). Products include:
DynaCirc Capsules ... 2921
DynaCirc CR Tablets ... 2923

Ketoprofen (Reduces the diuretic, natriuretic, and antihypertensive effects of thiazides). Products include:
Orudis Capsules ... 3548
Orudis KT Tablets ... ▣778
Oruvail Capsules ... 3548

Ketorolac Tromethamine (Reduces the diuretic, natriuretic, and antihypertensive effects of thiazides). Products include:
Acular Ophthalmic Solution ... 544
Acular PF Ophthalmic Solution ... 544
Toradol ... 3018

Labetalol Hydrochloride (Ziac may potentiate the action of other antihypertensive agents used concomitantly). Products include:
Normodyne Injection ... 3135
Normodyne Tablets ... 3137

Levorphanol Tartrate (Potentiation of orthostatic hypotension may occur when thiazide diuretics are used with narcotics). Products include:
Levo-Dromoran ... 1734
Levorphanol Tartrate Tablets ... 3059

Lisinopril (Ziac may potentiate the action of other antihypertensive agents used concomitantly). Products include:
Prinivil Tablets ... 2164
Prinzide Tablets ... 2168
Zestoretic Tablets ... 695
Zestril Tablets ... 698

Lithium Carbonate (Reduced renal clearance of lithium and increased risk of lithium toxicity). Products include:
Eskalith ... 1527
Lithium Carbonate ... 3061
Lithobid Slow-Release Tablets ... 3255

Lithium Citrate (Reduced renal clearance of lithium and increased risk of lithium toxicity). Products include:
Lithium Citrate Syrup ... 3061

Losartan Potassium (Ziac may potentiate the action of other antihypertensive agents used concomitantly). Products include:
Cozaar Tablets ... 2067
Hyzaar ... 2109

Mecamylamine Hydrochloride (Ziac may potentiate the action of other antihypertensive agents used concomitantly). Products include:
Inversine Tablets ... 1850

Meclofenamate Sodium (Reduces the diuretic, natriuretic, and antihypertensive effects of thiazides).
No products indexed under this heading.

Mefenamic Acid (Reduces the diuretic, natriuretic, and antihypertensive effects of thiazides). Products include:
Ponstel Capsules ... 1356

Meloxicam (Reduces the diuretic, natriuretic, and antihypertensive effects of thiazides). Products include:
Mobic Tablets ... 1054

Meperidine Hydrochloride (Potentiation of orthostatic hypotension may occur when thiazide diuretics are used with narcotics). Products include:
Demerol ... 3079
Mepergan Injection ... 3539

Mephobarbital (Potentiation of orthostatic hypotension may occur when thiazide diuretics are used with barbiturates).
No products indexed under this heading.

Metformin Hydrochloride (Beta blockers may mask some of the manifestations of hypoglycemia, particularly tachycardia; dosage adjustment of the antidiabetic drug may be required). Products include:
Glucophage Tablets ... 1080
Glucophage XR Tablets ... 1080
Glucovance Tablets ... 1086

Methadone Hydrochloride (Potentiation of orthostatic hypotension may occur when thiazide diuretics are used with narcotics). Products include:
Dolophine Hydrochloride Tablets ... 3056

Methyclothiazide (Ziac may potentiate the action of other antihypertensive agents used concomitantly).
No products indexed under this heading.

Methyldopa (Ziac may potentiate the action of other antihypertensive agents used concomitantly). Products include:
- Aldoclor Tablets ... 2035
- Aldomet Tablets ... 2037
- Aldoril Tablets ... 2039

Methyldopate Hydrochloride (Ziac may potentiate the action of other antihypertensive agents used concomitantly).
- No products indexed under this heading.

Methylprednisolone Acetate (Intensifies electrolyte depletion, particularly hypokalemia). Products include:
- Depo-Medrol Injectable Suspension ... 2795

Methylprednisolone Sodium Succinate (Intensifies electrolyte depletion, particularly hypokalemia). Products include:
- Solu-Medrol Sterile Powder ... 2855

Metocurine Iodide (Possible increased responsiveness to the muscle relaxant).
- No products indexed under this heading.

Metolazone (Ziac may potentiate the action of other antihypertensive agents used concomitantly). Products include:
- Mykrox Tablets ... 1168
- Zaroxolyn Tablets ... 1177

Metoprolol Succinate (Ziac may potentiate the action of other antihypertensive agents used concomitantly). Products include:
- Toprol-XL Tablets ... 651

Metoprolol Tartrate (Ziac may potentiate the action of other antihypertensive agents used concomitantly).
- No products indexed under this heading.

Metyrosine (Ziac may potentiate the action of other antihypertensive agents used concomitantly). Products include:
- Demser Capsules ... 2085

Mibefradil Dihydrochloride (Ziac may potentiate the action of other antihypertensive agents used concomitantly).
- No products indexed under this heading.

Miglitol (Beta blockers may mask some of the manifestations of hypoglycemia, particularly tachycardia; dosage adjustment of the antidiabetic drug may be required). Products include:
- Glyset Tablets ... 2821

Minoxidil (Ziac may potentiate the action of other antihypertensive agents used concomitantly). Products include:
- Rogaine Extra Strength for Men Topical Solution ... ▣721
- Rogaine for Women Topical Solution ... ▣721

Mivacurium Chloride (Possible increased responsiveness to the muscle relaxant).
- No products indexed under this heading.

Moexipril Hydrochloride (Ziac may potentiate the action of other antihypertensive agents used concomitantly). Products include:
- Uniretic Tablets ... 3178
- Univasc Tablets ... 3181

Morphine Sulfate (Potentiation of orthostatic hypotension may occur when thiazide diuretics are used with narcotics). Products include:
- Astramorph/PF Injection, USP (Preservative-Free) ... 594
- Duramorph Injection ... 1312
- Infumorph 200 and Infumorph 500 Sterile Solutions ... 1314
- Kadian Capsules ... 1335
- MS Contin Tablets ... 2896
- MSIR ... 2898
- Oramorph SR Tablets ... 3062
- Roxanol ... 3066

Nabumetone (Reduces the diuretic, natriuretic, and antihypertensive effects of thiazides). Products include:
- Relafen Tablets ... 1617

Nadolol (Ziac may potentiate the action of other antihypertensive agents used concomitantly). Products include:
- Corgard Tablets ... 2245
- Corzide 40/5 Tablets ... 2247
- Corzide 80/5 Tablets ... 2247
- Nadolol Tablets ... 2288

Naproxen (Reduces the diuretic, natriuretic, and antihypertensive effects of thiazides). Products include:
- EC-Naprosyn Delayed-Release Tablets ... 2967
- Naprosyn Suspension ... 2967
- Naprosyn Tablets ... 2967

Naproxen Sodium (Reduces the diuretic, natriuretic, and antihypertensive effects of thiazides). Products include:
- Aleve Tablets, Caplets and Gelcaps ... ▣602
- Aleve Cold & Sinus Caplets ... ▣603
- Anaprox Tablets ... 2967
- Anaprox DS Tablets ... 2967
- Naprelan Tablets ... 1293

Nicardipine Hydrochloride (Ziac may potentiate the action of other antihypertensive agents used concomitantly). Products include:
- Cardene I.V. ... 3485

Nifedipine (Ziac may potentiate the action of other antihypertensive agents used concomitantly). Products include:
- Adalat CC Tablets ... 877
- Procardia Capsules ... 2708
- Procardia XL Extended Release Tablets ... 2710

Nisoldipine (Ziac may potentiate the action of other antihypertensive agents used concomitantly). Products include:
- Sular Tablets ... 688

Nitroglycerin (Ziac may potentiate the action of other antihypertensive agents used concomitantly). Products include:
- Nitro-Dur Transdermal Infusion System ... 3134
- Nitro-Dur Transdermal Infusion System ... 1834
- Nitrolingual Pumpspray ... 1355
- Nitrostat Tablets ... 2658

Norepinephrine Bitartrate (Possible decreased response to pressor amines).
- No products indexed under this heading.

Norepinephrine Hydrochloride (Possible decreased response to pressor amines).
- No products indexed under this heading.

Oxaprozin (Reduces the diuretic, natriuretic, and antihypertensive effects of thiazides).
- No products indexed under this heading.

Oxycodone Hydrochloride (Potentiation of orthostatic hypotension may occur when thiazide diuretics are used with narcotics). Products include:
- OxyContin Tablets ... 2912
- OxyFast Oral Concentrate Solution ... 2916
- OxyIR Capsules ... 2916
- Percocet Tablets ... 1326
- Percodan Tablets ... 1327
- Percolone Tablets ... 1327
- Roxicodone ... 3067
- Tylox Capsules ... 2597

Pancuronium Bromide (Possible increased responsiveness to the muscle relaxant).
- No products indexed under this heading.

Penbutolol Sulfate (Ziac may potentiate the action of other antihypertensive agents used concomitantly).
- No products indexed under this heading.

Pentobarbital Sodium (Potentiation of orthostatic hypotension may occur when thiazide diuretics are used with barbiturates). Products include:
- Nembutal Sodium Solution ... 485

Perindopril Erbumine (Ziac may potentiate the action of other antihypertensive agents used concomitantly). Products include:
- Aceon Tablets (2 mg, 4 mg, 8 mg) ... 3249

Phenobarbital (Potentiation of orthostatic hypotension may occur when thiazide diuretics are used with barbiturates). Products include:
- Arco-Lase Plus Tablets ... 592
- Donnatal ... 2929
- Donnatal Extentabs ... 2930

Phenoxybenzamine Hydrochloride (Ziac may potentiate the action of other antihypertensive agents used concomitantly). Products include:
- Dibenzyline Capsules ... 3457

Phentolamine Mesylate (Ziac may potentiate the action of other antihypertensive agents used concomitantly).
- No products indexed under this heading.

Phenylbutazone (Reduces the diuretic, natriuretic, and antihypertensive effects of thiazides).
- No products indexed under this heading.

Pindolol (Ziac may potentiate the action of other antihypertensive agents used concomitantly).
- No products indexed under this heading.

Pioglitazone Hydrochloride (Beta blockers may mask some of the manifestations of hypoglycemia, particularly tachycardia; dosage adjustment of the antidiabetic drug may be required). Products include:
- Actos Tablets ... 3275

Piroxicam (Reduces the diuretic, natriuretic, and antihypertensive effects of thiazides). Products include:
- Feldene Capsules ... 2685

Polythiazide (Ziac may potentiate the action of other antihypertensive agents used concomitantly). Products include:
- Minizide Capsules ... 2700
- Renese Tablets ... 2712

Prazosin Hydrochloride (Ziac may potentiate the action of other antihypertensive agents used concomitantly). Products include:
- Minipress Capsules ... 2699
- Minizide Capsules ... 2700

Prednisolone Acetate (Intensifies electrolyte depletion, particularly hypokalemia). Products include:
- Blephamide Ophthalmic Ointment ... 547
- Blephamide Ophthalmic Suspension ... 548
- Poly-Pred Liquifilm Ophthalmic Suspension ... ⊙245
- Pred Forte Ophthalmic Suspension ... ⊙246
- Pred Mild Sterile Ophthalmic Suspension ... ⊙249
- Pred-G Ophthalmic Suspension ... ⊙247
- Pred-G Sterile Ophthalmic Ointment ... ⊙248

Prednisolone Sodium Phosphate (Intensifies electrolyte depletion, particularly hypokalemia). Products include:
- Pediapred Oral Solution ... 1170

Prednisolone Tebutate (Intensifies electrolyte depletion, particularly hypokalemia).
- No products indexed under this heading.

Prednisone (Intensifies electrolyte depletion, particularly hypokalemia). Products include:
- Prednisone ... 3064

Propoxyphene Hydrochloride (Potentiation of orthostatic hypotension may occur when thiazide diuretics are used with narcotics). Products include:
- Darvon Pulvules ... 1909
- Darvon Compound-65 Pulvules ... 1910

Propoxyphene Napsylate (Potentiation of orthostatic hypotension may occur when thiazide diuretics are used with narcotics). Products include:
- Darvon-N/Darvocet-N ... 1907
- Darvon-N Tablets ... 1912

Propranolol Hydrochloride (Ziac may potentiate the action of other antihypertensive agents used concomitantly). Products include:
- Inderal ... 3513
- Inderal LA Long-Acting Capsules ... 3516
- Inderide Tablets ... 3517
- Inderide LA Long-Acting Capsules ... 3519

Quinapril Hydrochloride (Ziac may potentiate the action of other antihypertensive agents used concomitantly). Products include:
- Accupril Tablets ... 2611
- Accuretic Tablets ... 2614

Ramipril (Ziac may potentiate the action of other antihypertensive agents used concomitantly). Products include:
- Altace Capsules ... 2233

Rapacuronium Bromide (Possible increased responsiveness to the muscle relaxant).
- No products indexed under this heading.

Rauwolfia serpentina (Concomitant use may produce excessive reduction of sympathetic activity).
- No products indexed under this heading.

Remifentanil Hydrochloride (Potentiation of orthostatic hypotension may occur when thiazide diuretics are used with narcotics).
- No products indexed under this heading.

Repaglinide (Beta blockers may mask some of the manifestations of hypoglycemia, particularly tachycardia; dosage adjustment of the antidiabetic drug may be required). Products include:
- Prandin Tablets (0.5, 1, and 2 mg) ... 2432

Rescinnamine (Concomitant use may produce excessive reduction of sympathetic activity).
- No products indexed under this heading.

Reserpine (Concomitant use may produce excessive reduction of sympathetic activity).
- No products indexed under this heading.

Rifampin (Increases the metabolic clearance of bisoprolol fumarate and shortening its elimination half-life). Products include:
- Rifadin ... 765
- Rifamate Capsules ... 767
- Rifater Tablets ... 769

Rocuronium Bromide (Possible increased responsiveness to the muscle relaxant). Products include:
- Zemuron Injection ... 2491

Rofecoxib (Reduces the diuretic, natriuretic, and antihypertensive effects of thiazides). Products include:
- Vioxx ... 2213

Rosiglitazone Maleate (Beta blockers may mask some of the manifestations of hypoglycemia, particularly tachycardia; dosage adjustment of the antidiabetic drug may be required). Products include:
- Avandia Tablets ... 1490

Secobarbital Sodium (Potentiation of orthostatic hypotension may occur when thiazide diuretics are used with barbiturates).
No products indexed under this heading.

Sodium Nitroprusside (Ziac may potentiate the action of other antihypertensive agents used concomitantly).
No products indexed under this heading.

Sotalol Hydrochloride (Ziac may potentiate the action of other antihypertensive agents used concomitantly). Products include:
Betapace Tablets 950
Betapace AF Tablets 954

Spirapril Hydrochloride (Ziac may potentiate the action of other antihypertensive agents used concomitantly).
No products indexed under this heading.

Sufentanil Citrate (Potentiation of orthostatic hypotension may occur when thiazide diuretics are used with narcotics).
No products indexed under this heading.

Sulindac (Reduces the diuretic, natriuretic, and antihypertensive effects of thiazides). Products include:
Clinoril Tablets 2053

Telmisartan (Ziac may potentiate the action of other antihypertensive agents used concomitantly). Products include:
Micardis Tablets 1049
Micardis HCT Tablets 1051

Terazosin Hydrochloride (Ziac may potentiate the action of other antihypertensive agents used concomitantly). Products include:
Hytrin Capsules 464

Thiamylal Sodium (Potentiation of orthostatic hypotension may occur when thiazide diuretics are used with barbiturates).
No products indexed under this heading.

Timolol Maleate (Ziac may potentiate the action of other antihypertensive agents used concomitantly). Products include:
Blocadren Tablets 2046
Cosopt Sterile Ophthalmic Solution 2065
Timolide Tablets 2187
Timolol GFS .... ⊙ 266
Timoptic in Ocudose 2192
Timoptic Sterile Ophthalmic Solution 2190
Timoptic-XE Sterile Ophthalmic Gel Forming Solution 2194

Tolazamide (Beta blockers may mask some of the manifestations of hypoglycemia, particularly tachycar dia; dosage adjustment of the antidiabetic drug may be required).
No products indexed under this heading.

Tolbutamide (Beta blockers may mask some of the manifestations of hypoglycemia, particularly tachycardia; dosage adjustment of the antidiabetic drug may be required).
No products indexed under this heading.

Tolmetin Sodium (Reduces the diuretic, natriuretic, and antihypertensive effects of thiazides). Products include:
Tolectin 2589

Torsemide (Ziac may potentiate the action of other antihypertensive agents used concomitantly). Products include:
Demadex Tablets and Injection 2965

Trandolapril (Ziac may potentiate the action of other antihypertensive agents used concomitantly). Products include:
Mavik Tablets 478
Tarka Tablets 508

Triamcinolone (Intensifies electrolyte depletion, particularly hypokalemia).
No products indexed under this heading.

Triamcinolone Acetonide (Intensifies electrolyte depletion, particularly hypokalemia). Products include:
Azmacort Inhalation Aerosol 728
Nasacort Nasal Inhaler 750
Nasacort AQ Nasal Spray 752
Tri-Nasal Spray 2274

Triamcinolone Diacetate (Intensifies electrolyte depletion, particularly hypokalemia).
No products indexed under this heading.

Triamcinolone Hexacetonide (Intensifies electrolyte depletion, particularly hypokalemia).
No products indexed under this heading.

Trichloroethylene (Use with caution when administered with anesthetic agent that depresses myocardial function).
No products indexed under this heading.

Trimethaphan Camsylate (Ziac may potentiate the action of other antihypertensive agents used concomitantly).
No products indexed under this heading.

Troglitazone (Beta blockers may mask some of the manifestations of hypoglycemia, particularly tachycardia; dosage adjustment of the antidiabetic drug may be required).
No products indexed under this heading.

Tubocurarine Chloride (Possible increased responsiveness to the muscle relaxant).
No products indexed under this heading.

Valsartan (Ziac may potentiate the action of other antihypertensive agents used concomitantly). Products include:
Diovan Capsules 2337
Diovan HCT Tablets 2338

Vecuronium Bromide (Possible increased responsiveness to the muscle relaxant). Products include:
Norcuron for Injection 2478

Verapamil Hydrochloride (Ziac should be used with caution when myocardial depressants or inhibitors of AV conduction are used concurrently). Products include:
Covera-HS Tablets 3199
Isoptin SR Tablets 467
Tarka Tablets 508
Verelan Capsules 3184
Verelan PM Capsules 3186

Food Interactions

Alcohol (Potentiation of orthostatic hypotension may occur when thiazide diuretics are used with alcohol).

ZIAGEN ORAL SOLUTION

(Abacavir Sulfate) 1692
See Ziagen Tablets

ZIAGEN TABLETS

(Abacavir Sulfate) 1692
May interact with:

Methadone Hydrochloride (Coadministration in patients on methadone-maintenance therapy has resulted in increased methadone clearance by 22%; this alteration will not result in a methadone dose modification in the majority of patients; however, an increased methadone dose may be required in a small number of patients.). Products include:
Dolophine Hydrochloride Tablets 3056

Food Interactions

Alcohol (Decreases the elimination of abacavir causing an increase in overall exposure).

ZILACTIN GEL

(Benzyl Alcohol) .... ▣ 790
None cited in PDR database.

ZILACTIN BABY GEL

(Benzocaine) .... ▣ 791
None cited in PDR database.

ZILACTIN-B GEL

(Benzocaine) .... ▣ 790
None cited in PDR database.

ZILACTIN-L LIQUID

(Lidocaine) .... ▣ 790
None cited in PDR database.

ZINACEF INJECTION

(Cefuroxime) 1696
May interact with aminoglycosides and certain other agents. Compounds in these categories include:

Amikacin Sulfate (Concomitant administration may produce nephrotoxicity).
No products indexed under this heading.

Gentamicin Sulfate (Concomitant administration may produce nephrotoxicity). Products include:
Genoptic Ophthalmic Ointment .... ⊙ 239
Genoptic Sterile Ophthalmic Solution .... ⊙ 239
Pred-G Ophthalmic Suspension .... ⊙ 247
Pred-G Sterile Ophthalmic Ointment .... ⊙ 248

Kanamycin Sulfate (Concomitant administration may produce nephrotoxicity).
No products indexed under this heading.

Probenecid (Concurrent administration of probenecid decreases renal clearance and increases peak serum levels of cefuroxime).
No products indexed under this heading.

Streptomycin Sulfate (Concomitant administration may produce nephrotoxicity). Products include:
Streptomycin Sulfate Injection 2714

Tobramycin (Concomitant administration may produce nephrotoxicity). Products include:
TOBI Solution for Inhalation 1206
TobraDex Ophthalmic Ointment 542
TobraDex Ophthalmic Suspension 541
Tobrex Ophthalmic Ointment .... ⊙ 220
Tobrex Ophthalmic Solution .... ⊙ 221

Tobramycin Sulfate (Concomitant administration may produce nephrotoxicity). Products include:
Nebcin Vials, Hyporets & ADD-Vantage 1955

ZINACEF FOR INJECTION

(Cefuroxime) 1696
See Zinacef Injection

ZINECARD FOR INJECTION

(Dexrazoxane) 2869
May interact with antineoplastics and certain other agents. Compounds in these categories include:

Altretamine (Dexrazoxane may add to the myelosuppression caused by chemotherapeutic agents). Products include:
Hexalen Capsules 2226

Anastrozole (Dexrazoxane may add to the myelosuppression caused by chemotherapeutic agents). Products include:
Arimidex Tablets 659

Asparaginase (Dexrazoxane may add to the myelosuppression caused by chemotherapeutic agents). Products include:
Elspar for Injection 2092

Bicalutamide (Dexrazoxane may add to the myelosuppression caused by chemotherapeutic agents). Products include:
Casodex Tablets 662

Bleomycin Sulfate (Dexrazoxane may add to the myelosuppression caused by chemotherapeutic agents).
No products indexed under this heading.

Busulfan (Dexrazoxane may add to the myelosuppression caused by chemotherapeutic agents). Products include:
Myleran Tablets 1603

Carboplatin (Dexrazoxane may add to the myelosuppression caused by chemotherapeutic agents). Products include:
Paraplatin for Injection 1126

Carmustine (BCNU) (Dexrazoxane may add to the myelosuppression caused by chemotherapeutic agents). Products include:
Gliadel Wafer 1723

Chlorambucil (Dexrazoxane may add to the myelosuppression caused by chemotherapeutic agents). Products include:
Leukeran Tablets 1591

Cisplatin (Dexrazoxane may add to the myelosuppression caused by chemotherapeutic agents).
No products indexed under this heading.

Cyclophosphamide (Use of dexrazoxane concurrently with the initiation of fluorouracil, doxorubicin and cyclophosphamide (FAC) therapy may interfere with the antitumor efficacy of the regimen).
No products indexed under this heading.

Dacarbazine (Dexrazoxane may add to the myelosuppression caused by chemotherapeutic agents). Products include:
DTIC-Dome 902

Daunorubicin Citrate (Use of dexrazoxane concurrently with the initiation of fluorouracil, doxorubicin and cyclophosphamide (FAC) therapy may interfere with the antitumor efficacy of the regimen). Products include:
DaunoXome Injection 1442

Daunorubicin Hydrochloride (Dexrazoxane may add to the myelosuppression caused by chemotherapeutic agents). Products include:
Cerubidine for Injection 947

Denileukin Diftitox (Dexrazoxane may add to the myelosuppression caused by chemotherapeutic agents).
No products indexed under this heading.

Docetaxel (Dexrazoxane may add to the myelosuppression caused by chemotherapeutic agents). Products include:
Taxotere for Injection Concentrate 778

Doxorubicin Hydrochloride (Use of dexrazoxane concurrently with the initiation of fluorouracil, doxorubicin and cyclophosphamide (FAC) therapy may interfere with the antitumor efficacy of the regimen). Products include:
Adriamycin PFS/RDF Injection 2767
Doxil Injection 566

Epirubicin Hydrochloride (Dexrazoxane may add to the myelosuppression caused by chemotherapeutic agents). Products include:
Ellence Injection 2806

Estramustine Phosphate Sodium (Dexrazoxane may add to the myelosuppression caused by chemotherapeutic agents). Products include:
Emcyt Capsules 2810

Etoposide (Dexrazoxane may add to the myelosuppression caused by chemotherapeutic agents).
No products indexed under this heading.

Exemestane (Dexrazoxane may add to the myelosuppression caused by chemotherapeutic agents). Products include:
Aromasin Tablets 2769

Floxuridine (Dexrazoxane may add to the myelosuppression caused by chemotherapeutic agents). Products include:
Sterile FUDR 2974

Fluorouracil (Use of dexrazoxane concurrently with the initiation of fluorouracil, doxorubicin and cyclophosphamide (FAC) therapy may interfere with the antitumor efficacy of the regimen). Products include:
Carac Cream 1222
Efudex 1733
Fluoroplex 552

Flutamide (Dexrazoxane may add to the myelosuppression caused by chemotherapeutic agents). Products include:
Eulexin Capsules 3118

Gemcitabine Hydrochloride (Dexrazoxane may add to the myelosuppression caused by chemotherapeutic agents). Products include:
Gemzar for Injection 1919

Hydroxyurea (Dexrazoxane may add to the myelosuppression caused by chemotherapeutic agents). Products include:
Mylocel Tablets 2227

Idarubicin Hydrochloride (Dexrazoxane may add to the myelosuppression caused by chemotherapeutic agents). Products include:
Idamycin PFS Injection 2825

Ifosfamide (Dexrazoxane may add to the myelosuppression caused by chemotherapeutic agents). Products include:
Ifex for Injection 1123

Interferon alfa-2A, Recombinant (Dexrazoxane may add to the myelosuppression caused by chemotherapeutic agents). Products include:
Roferon-A Injection 2996

Interferon alfa-2B, Recombinant (Dexrazoxane may add to the myelosuppression caused by chemotherapeutic agents). Products include:
Intron A for Injection 3120
Rebetron Combination Therapy 3153

Irinotecan Hydrochloride (Dexrazoxane may add to the myelosuppression caused by chemotherapeutic agents).
No products indexed under this heading.

Levamisole Hydrochloride (Dexrazoxane may add to the myelosuppression caused by chemotherapeutic agents). Products include:
Ergamisol Tablets 1789

Lomustine (CCNU) (Dexrazoxane may add to the myelosuppression caused by chemotherapeutic agents).
No products indexed under this heading.

Mechlorethamine Hydrochloride (Dexrazoxane may add to the myelosuppression caused by chemotherapeutic agents). Products include:
Mustargen for Injection 2142

Megestrol Acetate (Dexrazoxane may add to the myelosuppression caused by chemotherapeutic agents). Products include:
Megace Oral Suspension 1124

Melphalan (Dexrazoxane may add to the myelosuppression caused by chemotherapeutic agents). Products include:
Alkeran Tablets 1466

Mercaptopurine (Dexrazoxane may add to the myelosuppression caused by chemotherapeutic agents). Products include:
Purinethol Tablets 1615

Methotrexate Sodium (Dexrazoxane may add to the myelosuppression caused by chemotherapeutic agents).
No products indexed under this heading.

Mitomycin (Mitomycin-C) (Dexrazoxane may add to the myelosuppression caused by chemotherapeutic agents).
No products indexed under this heading.

Mitotane (Dexrazoxane may add to the myelosuppression caused by chemotherapeutic agents).
No products indexed under this heading.

Mitoxantrone Hydrochloride (Dexrazoxane may add to the myelosuppression caused by chemotherapeutic agents). Products include:
Novantrone for Injection 1760

Paclitaxel (Dexrazoxane may add to the myelosuppression caused by chemotherapeutic agents). Products include:
Taxol Injection 1129

Procarbazine Hydrochloride (Dexrazoxane may add to the myelosuppression caused by chemotherapeutic agents). Products include:
Matulane Capsules 3246

Streptozocin (Dexrazoxane may add to the myelosuppression caused by chemotherapeutic agents).
No products indexed under this heading.

Tamoxifen Citrate (Dexrazoxane may add to the myelosuppression caused by chemotherapeutic agents). Products include:
Nolvadex Tablets 678

Teniposide (Dexrazoxane may add to the myelosuppression caused by chemotherapeutic agents).
No products indexed under this heading.

Thioguanine (Dexrazoxane may add to the myelosuppression caused by chemotherapeutic agents). Products include:
Tabloid Tablets 1642

Thiotepa (Dexrazoxane may add to the myelosuppression caused by chemotherapeutic agents). Products include:
Thioplex for Injection 1765

Topotecan Hydrochloride (Dexrazoxane may add to the myelosuppression caused by chemotherapeutic agents). Products include:
Hycamtin for Injection 1546

Toremifene Citrate (Dexrazoxane may add to the myelosuppression caused by chemotherapeutic agents). Products include:
Fareston Tablets 3237

Valrubicin (Dexrazoxane may add to the myelosuppression caused by chemotherapeutic agents). Products include:
Valstar Sterile Solution for Intravesical Instillation 1175

Vincristine Sulfate (Dexrazoxane may add to the myelosuppression caused by chemotherapeutic agents).
No products indexed under this heading.

Vinorelbine Tartrate (Dexrazoxane may add to the myelosuppression caused by chemotherapeutic agents). Products include:
Navelbine Injection 1604

ZITHROMAX CAPSULES, 250 MG

(Azithromycin Dihydrate) 2743

May interact with antacids containing aluminum, calcium and magnesium, oral anticoagulants, phenytoin, theophylline, and certain other agents. Compounds in these categories include:

Aluminum Carbonate (Aluminum- and magnesium-containing antacids reduce the peak serum levels (rate) but not the AUC (extent) of azithromycin absorption; simultaneous administration should be avoided).
No products indexed under this heading.

Aluminum Hydroxide (Aluminum- and magnesium-containing antacids reduce the peak serum levels (rate) but not the AUC (extent) of azithromycin absorption; simultaneous administration should be avoided). Products include:
Amphojel Suspension (Mint Flavor) .... ⊞789
Gaviscon Extra Strength Liquid .... ⊞751
Gaviscon Extra Strength Tablets .... ⊞751
Gaviscon Regular Strength Liquid .... ⊞751
Gaviscon Regular Strength Tablets .... ⊞750
Maalox Antacid/Anti-Gas Oral Suspension .... ⊞673
Maalox Max Maximum Strength Antacid/Anti-Gas Liquid 2300
Maalox Regular Strength Antacid/Antigas Liquid 2300
Mylanta 1813
Vanquish Caplets .... ⊞617

Aminophylline (Concurrent use of macrolides and theophylline has been associated with increases in the serum concentrations of theophylline; the effect of azithromycin on the plasma levels of theophylline administered in multiple doses is not known).
No products indexed under this heading.

Carbamazepine (Caution is advised since co-administration of drugs metabolized by cytochrome P450 system and macrolide antibiotics is associated with elevation in carbamazepine serum levels). Products include:
Carbatrol Capsules 3234
Tegretol/Tegretol-XR 2404

Cyclosporine (Caution is advised since co-administration of drugs metabolized by cytochrome P450 system and macrolide antibiotics is associated with elevation in cyclosporine serum levels). Products include:
Gengraf Capsules 457
Neoral Soft Gelatin Capsules 2380
Neoral Oral Solution 2380
Sandimmune 2388

Dicumarol (Concurrent use of macrolides and warfarin in clinical practice has been associated with increased anticoagulant effects).
No products indexed under this heading.

Digoxin (Caution is advised since macrolide antibiotics elevate digoxin serum levels). Products include:
Digitek Tablets 1003
Lanoxicaps Capsules 1574
Lanoxin Injection 1581
Lanoxin Tablets 1587
Lanoxin Elixir Pediatric 1578
Lanoxin Injection Pediatric 1584

Dihydroergotamine Mesylate (Caution is advised since macrolide antibiotics and ergotamine co-administration is associated with acute ergot toxicity). Products include:
D.H.E. 45 Injection 2334
Migranal Nasal Spray 2376

Dyphylline (Concurrent use of macrolides and theophylline has been associated with increases in the serum concentrations of theophylline; the effect of azithromycin on the plasma levels of theophylline administered in multiple doses is not known). Products include:
Lufyllin Tablets 3347
Lufyllin-400 Tablets 3347
Lufyllin-GG Elixir 3348
Lufyllin-GG Tablets 3348

Efavirenz (Co-administration produced a 22% increase in the Cmax of azithromycin). Products include:
Sustiva Capsules 1258

Ergotamine Tartrate (Caution is advised since macrolide antibiotics and ergotamine co-administration is associated with acute ergot toxicity).
No products indexed under this heading.

Fosphenytoin Sodium (Caution is advised since co-administration of drugs metabolized by cytochrome P450 system and macrolide antibiotics is associated with elevation in phenytoin serum levels). Products include:
Cerebyx Injection 2619

Hexobarbital (Caution is advised since co-administration of drugs metabolized by cytochrome P450 system and macrolide antibiotics is associated with elevation in hexobarbital serum levels).

Magaldrate (Aluminum- and magnesium-containing antacids reduce the peak serum levels (rate) but not the AUC (extent) of azithromycin absorption; simultaneous administration should be avoided).
No products indexed under this heading.

Magnesium Hydroxide (Aluminum- and magnesium-containing antacids reduce the peak serum levels (rate) but not the AUC (extent) of azithromycin absorption; simultaneous administration should be avoided). Products include:
Ex•Lax Milk of Magnesia Liquid .... ⊞670
Maalox Antacid/Anti-Gas Oral Suspension .... ⊞673
Maalox Max Maximum Strength Antacid/Anti-Gas Liquid 2300
Maalox Regular Strength Antacid/Antigas Liquid 2300
Mylanta Fast-Acting 1813
Mylanta 1813
Pepcid Complete Chewable Tablets 1815
Phillips' Chewable Tablets .... ⊞615
Phillips' Milk of Magnesia Liquid (Original, Cherry, & Mint) .... ⊞616
Rolaids Tablets .... ⊞706
Extra Strength Rolaids Tablets .... ⊞706
Vanquish Caplets .... ⊞617

Magnesium Oxide (Aluminum- and magnesium-containing antacids reduce the peak serum levels (rate) but not the AUC (extent) of azithromycin absorption; simultaneous administration should be avoided). Products include:
Beelith Tablets 946
Mag-Ox 400 Tablets 1024
Uro-Mag Capsules 1024

Nelfinavir Mesylate (Co-administration produced a decrease of approximately 15% in mean AUC of nelfinavir and its M8 metabolite; no dosage adjustment is necessary). Products include:
Viracept 532

Phenytoin (Caution is advised since co-administration of drugs metabolized by cytochrome P450 system and macrolide antibiotics is associated with elevation in phenytoin serum levels). Products include:
Dilantin Infatabs 2624
Dilantin-125 Oral Suspension 2625

Phenytoin Sodium (Caution is advised since co-administration of drugs metabolized by cytochrome P450 system and macrolide antibiotics is associated with elevation in phenytoin serum levels). Products include:
Dilantin Kapseals 2622

Terfenadine (Caution is advised since co-administration of drugs metabolized by cytochrome P450 system and macrolide antibiotics is associated with elevation in terfenadine serum levels).
No products indexed under this heading.

Theophylline (Concurrent use of macrolides and theophylline has been associated with increases in

the serum concentrations of theophylline; the effect of azithromycin on the plasma levels of theophylline administered in multiple doses is not known). Products include:

- Aerolate 1361
- Theo-Dur Extended-Release Tablets 1835
- Uni-Dur Extended-Release Tablets .. 1841
- Uniphyl 400 mg and 600 mg Tablets 2903

Theophylline Calcium Salicylate (Concurrent use of macrolides and theophylline has been associated with increases in the serum concentrations of theophylline; the effect of azithromycin on the plasma levels of theophylline administered in multiple doses is not known).

No products indexed under this heading.

Theophylline Sodium Glycinate (Concurrent use of macrolides and theophylline has been associated with increases in the serum concentrations of theophylline; the effect of azithromycin on the plasma levels of theophylline administered in multiple doses is not known).

No products indexed under this heading.

Triazolam (Caution is advised since macrolide antibiotics decrease the clearance of triazolam and thereby increasing the pharmacologic effect of triazolam). Products include:

- Halcion Tablets 2823

Warfarin Sodium (Concurrent use of macrolides and warfarin in clinical practice has been associated with increased anticoagulant effects). Products include:

- Coumadin for Injection 1243
- Coumadin Tablets 1243
- Warfarin Sodium Tablets, USP 3302

Food Interactions

Food, unspecified (Zithromax should not be taken with food; reduces the rate of absorption (Cmax) of azithromycin capsules by 52% and the extent of absorption (AUC) by 43%; when oral suspension of azithromycin was administered with food the Cmax increased by 56% and the AUC was unchanged).

ZITHROMAX FOR IV INFUSION

(Azithromycin Dihydrate) 2748
See Zithromax Capsules, 250 mg

ZITHROMAX FOR ORAL SUSPENSION, 1 G

(Azithromycin Dihydrate) 2743
See Zithromax Capsules, 250 mg

ZITHROMAX FOR ORAL SUSPENSION, 300 MG, 600 MG, 900 MG, 1200 MG

(Azithromycin Dihydrate) 2739
See Zithromax Capsules, 250 mg

ZITHROMAX TABLETS, 250 MG

(Azithromycin Dihydrate) 2739
See Zithromax Capsules, 250 mg

ZITHROMAX TABLETS, 600 MG

(Azithromycin Dihydrate) 2743
See Zithromax Capsules, 250 mg

ZOCOR TABLETS

(Simvastatin) 2219

May interact with azole antifungals, oral anticoagulants, erythromycin, fibrates, protease inhibitors, and certain other agents. Compounds in these categories include:

Amprenavir (The risk of myopathy appears to be increased by high levels of HMG-CoA reductase inhibitory activity in plasma; simvastatin is metabolized by CYP3A4 isoenzyme, certain agents, such as HIV protease inhibitors, share this metabolic pathway and can raise the plasma levels of simvastatin and may increase the risk of myopathy). Products include:

- Agenerase Capsules 1454
- Agenerase Oral Solution 1459

Clarithromycin (The risk of myopathy appears to be increased by high levels of HMG-CoA reductase inhibitory activity and the drugs that share the same metabolic pathways as simvastatin, such as clarithromycin, can raise the plasma levels of simvastatin and may increase the risk of myopathy). Products include:

- Biaxin/Biaxin XL 403
- PREVPAC 3298

Clofibrate (The incidence and severity of myopathy are increased by co-administration of HMG-CoA reductase inhibitors with drugs that cause myopathy when given alone, such as fibrates; in patients on concomitant fibrates, the dose of simvastatin should generally not exceed 10 mg/day). Products include:

- Atromid-S Capsules 3483

Clotrimazole (The risk of myopathy appears to be increased by high levels of HMG-CoA reductase inhibitory activity and the drugs that share the same metabolic pathways as simvastatin, such as antifungal azoles, can raise the plasma levels of simvastatin and may increase the risk of myopathy). Products include:

- Gyne-Lotrimin 3, 3-Day Cream ......▣741
- Lotrimin AF Cream, Lotion, Solution, and Jock Itch Cream ....▣742
- Lotrimin 3128
- Lotrisone 3129
- Mycelex Troche 573
- Mycelex-7 Combination-Pack Vaginal Inserts & External Vulvar Cream ....▣614
- Mycelex-7 Vaginal Cream ....▣614
- Mycelex-7 Vaginal Cream with 7 Disposable Applicators ....▣614

Cyclosporine (The risk of myopathy appears to be increased by high levels of HMG-CoA reductase inhibitory activity and the drugs that share the same metabolic pathways as simvastatin, such as cyclosporine, can raise the plasma levels of simvastatin and may increase the risk of myopathy; in patients on concomitant cyclosporine, the dose of simvastatin should begin with 5 mg/day and not exceed 10 mg/day). Products include:

- Gengraf Capsules 457
- Neoral Soft Gelatin Capsules 2380
- Neoral Oral Solution 2380
- Sandimmune 2388

Dicumarol (Simvastatin modestly potentiates the effect of coumarin anticoagulants; the prothrombin time is increased from baseline).

No products indexed under this heading.

Digoxin (Slight elevation in digoxin plasma levels). Products include:

- Digitek Tablets 1003
- Lanoxicaps Capsules 1574
- Lanoxin Injection 1581
- Lanoxin Tablets 1587
- Lanoxin Elixir Pediatric 1578
- Lanoxin Injection Pediatric 1584

Erythromycin (The risk of myopathy appears to be increased by high levels of HMG-CoA reductase inhibitory activity and the drugs that share the same metabolic pathways as simvastatin, such as erythromycin, can raise the plasma levels of simvastatin and may increase the risk of myopathy). Products include:

- Emgel 2% Topical Gel 1285
- Ery-Tab Tablets 448
- Erythromycin Base Filmtab Tablets . 454
- Erythromycin Delayed-Release Capsules, USP 455
- PCE Dispertab Tablets 498

Erythromycin Estolate (The risk of myopathy appears to be increased by high levels of HMG-CoA reductase inhibitory activity and the drugs that share the same metabolic pathways as simvastatin, such as erythromycin, can raise the plasma levels of simvastatin and may increase the risk of myopathy).

No products indexed under this heading.

Erythromycin Ethylsuccinate (The risk of myopathy appears to be increased by high levels of HMG-CoA reductase inhibitory activity and the drugs that share the same metabolic pathways as simvastatin, such as erythromycin, can raise the plasma levels of simvastatin and may increase the risk of myopathy). Products include:

- E.E.S. 450
- EryPed 446
- Pediazole Suspension 3050

Erythromycin Gluceptate (The risk of myopathy appears to be increased by high levels of HMG-CoA reductase inhibitory activity and the drugs that share the same metabolic pathways as simvastatin, such as erythromycin, can raise the plasma levels of simvastatin and may increase the risk of myopathy).

No products indexed under this heading.

Erythromycin Stearate (The risk of myopathy appears to be increased by high levels of HMG-CoA reductase inhibitory activity and the drugs that share the same metabolic pathways as simvastatin, such as erythromycin, can raise the plasma levels of simvastatin and may increase the risk of myopathy). Products include:

- Erythrocin Stearate Filmtab Tablets 452

Fenofibrate (The incidence and severity of myopathy are increased by co-administration of HMG-CoA reductase inhibitors with drugs that cause myopathy when given alone, such as fibrates; in patients on concomitant fibrates, the dose of simvastatin should generally not exceed 10 mg/day). Products include:

- Tricor Capsules, Micronized 513

Fluconazole (The risk of myopathy appears to be increased by high levels of HMG-CoA reductase inhibitory activity and the drugs that share the same metabolic pathways as simvastatin, such as antifungal azoles, can raise the plasma levels of simvastatin and may increase the risk of myopathy). Products include:

- Diflucan Tablets, Injection, and Oral Suspension 2681

Gemfibrozil (The incidence and severity of myopathy are increased by co-administration of HMG-CoA reductase inhibitors with drugs that cause myopathy when given alone, such as fibrates; in patients on concomitant fibrates, the dose of simvastatin should generally not exceed 10 mg/day). Products include:

- Lopid Tablets 2650

Indinavir Sulfate (The risk of myopathy appears to be increased by high levels of HMG-CoA reductase inhibitory activity in plasma; simvastatin is metabolized by CYP3A4 isoenzyme, certain agents, such as HIV protease inhibitors, share this metabolic pathway and can raise the plasma levels of simvastatin and may increase the risk of myopathy). Products include:

- Crixivan Capsules 2070

Itraconazole (The risk of myopathy appears to be increased by high levels of HMG-CoA reductase inhibitory activity and the drugs that share the same metabolic pathways as simvastatin, such as itraconazole, can raise the plasma levels of simvastatin and may increase the risk of myopathy). Products include:

- Sporanox Capsules 1800
- Sporanox Injection 1804
- Sporanox Injection 2509
- Sporanox Oral Solution 1808
- Sporanox Oral Solution 2512

Ketoconazole (The risk of myopathy appears to be increased by high levels of HMG-CoA reductase inhibitory activity and the drugs that share the same metabolic pathways as simvastatin, such as ketoconazole, can raise the plasma levels of simvastatin and may increase the risk of myopathy). Products include:

- Nizoral 2% Cream 3620
- Nizoral A-D Shampoo 2008
- Nizoral 2% Shampoo 2007
- Nizoral Tablets 1791

Lopinavir (The risk of myopathy appears to be increased by high levels of HMG-CoA reductase inhibitory activity in plasma; simvastatin is metabolized by CYP3A4 isoenzyme, certain agents, such as HIV protease inhibitors, share this metabolic pathway and can raise the plasma levels of simvastatin and may increase the risk of myopathy). Products include:

- Kaletra Capsules 471
- Kaletra Oral Solution 471

Miconazole (The risk of myopathy appears to be increased by high levels of HMG-CoA reductase inhibitory activity and the drugs that share the same metabolic pathways as simvastatin, such as antifungal azoles, can raise the plasma levels of simvastatin and may increase the risk of myopathy).

No products indexed under this heading.

Nefazodone Hydrochloride (The risk of myopathy appears to be increased by high levels of HMG-CoA reductase inhibitory activity and the drugs that share the same metabolic pathways as simvastatin, such as nefazodone, can raise the plasma levels of simvastatin and may increase the risk of myopathy). Products include:

- Serzone Tablets 1104

Nelfinavir Mesylate (The risk of myopathy appears to be increased by high levels of HMG-CoA reductase inhibitory activity in plasma; simvastatin is metabolized by CYP3A4 isoenzyme, certain agents, such as HIV protease inhibitors, share this metabolic pathway and can raise the plasma levels of simvastatin and may increase the risk of myopathy). Products include:

- Viracept 532

Niacin (The incidence and severity of myopathy are increased by co-administration of HMG-CoA reductase inhibitors with drugs that cause myopathy when given alone, such as lipid-lowering doses of niacin; in patients on concomitant niacin, the dose of simvastatin should generally not exceed 10 mg). Products include:

- Niaspan Extended-Release Tablets 1846
- Nicotinex Elixir ....▣633

Oxiconazole Nitrate (The risk of myopathy appears to be increased by high levels of HMG-CoA reductase inhibitory activity and the drugs that share the same metabolic pathways as simvastatin, such as antifungal azoles, can raise the plasma levels of simvastatin and may increase the risk of myopathy). Products include:

- Oxistat 1298

Propranolol Hydrochloride (Significant decreases in mean Cmax, but no change in AUC). Products include:

- Inderal 3513
- Inderal LA Long-Acting Capsules 3516
- Inderide Tablets 3517
- Inderide LA Long-Acting Capsules .. 3519

Ritonavir (The risk of myopathy appears to be increased by high levels of HMG-CoA reductase inhibitory activity in plasma; simvastatin is metabolized by CYP3A4 isoenzyme, certain agents, such as HIV protease inhibitors, share this metabolic pathway and can raise the plasma levels of simvastatin and may increase the risk of myopathy). Products include:

Kaletra Capsules 471
Kaletra Oral Solution 471
Norvir Capsules 487
Norvir Oral Solution 487

Saquinavir (The risk of myopathy appears to be increased by high levels of HMG-CoA reductase inhibitory activity in plasma; simvastatin is metabolized by CYP3A4 isoenzyme, certain agents, such as HIV protease inhibitors, share this metabolic pathway and can raise the plasma levels of simvastatin and may increase the risk of myopathy). Products include:

Fortovase Capsules 2970

Saquinavir Mesylate (The risk of myopathy appears to be increased by high levels of HMG-CoA reductase inhibitory activity in plasma; simvastatin is metabolized by CYP3A4 isoenzyme, certain agents, such as HIV protease inhibitors, share this metabolic pathway and can raise the plasma levels of simvastatin and may increase the risk of myopathy). Products include:

Invirase Capsules 2979

Terconazole (The risk of myopathy appears to be increased by high levels of HMG-CoA reductase inhibitory activity and the drugs that share the same metabolic pathways as simvastatin, such as antifungal azoles, can raise the plasma levels of simvastatin and may increase the risk of myopathy). Products include:

Terazol 3 Vaginal Cream 2587
Terazol 3 Vaginal Suppositories 2587
Terazol 7 Vaginal Cream 2587

Verapamil Hydrochloride (Co-administration may increase the risk of myopathy; although the data are insufficient for simvastatin). Products include:

Covera-HS Tablets 3199
Isoptin SR Tablets 467
Tarka Tablets 508
Verelan Capsules 3184
Verelan PM Capsules 3186

Warfarin Sodium (Simvastatin modestly potentiates the effect of coumarin anticoagulants; the prothrombin time is increased from baseline). Products include:

Coumadin for Injection 1243
Coumadin Tablets 1243
Warfarin Sodium Tablets, USP 3302

Food Interactions

Alcohol (Simvastatin causes persistent increases in serum transaminase in 1% of patients, therefore, it should be used with caution in patients who consume substantial quantities of alcohol).

Grapefruit Juice (Simvastatin is a substrate for CYP4503A4 and grapefruit juice contains one or more components that inhibit CYP3A4; co-administration with grapefruit juice can increase the plasma concentrations of simvastatin and its B-hydroxyacid metabolite; large quantity of grapefruit juice (>1 quart daily) significantly increases the serum concentrations and should be avoided).

ZOFRAN INJECTION

(Ondansetron Hydrochloride) 1698
See Zofran Tablets

ZOFRAN INJECTION PREMIXED

(Ondansetron Hydrochloride) 1698
See Zofran Tablets

ZOFRAN ORAL SOLUTION

(Ondansetron Hydrochloride) 1703
See Zofran Tablets

ZOFRAN TABLETS

(Ondansetron Hydrochloride) 1703
May interact with phenytoin, quinidine, and certain other agents. Compounds in these categories include:

Cimetidine (Co-administration with inhibitors of cytochrome P450, such as cimetidine, may change the clearance and, hence, the half-life of ondansetron; based on the limited data, no dosage adjustment is recommended for patients on concomitant therapy). Products include:

Tagamet HB 200 Suspension 762
Tagamet HB 200 Tablets 761
Tagamet Tablets 1644

Cimetidine Hydrochloride (Co-administration with inhibitors of cytochrome P450, such as cimetidine, may change the clearance and, hence, the half-life of ondansetron; based on the limited data, no dosage adjustment is recommended for patients on concomitant therapy). Products include:

Tagamet 1644

Fosphenytoin Sodium (Co-administration with inducers of cytochrome P450, such as phenytoin, may change the clearance and, hence, the half-life of ondansetron; based on the limited data, no dosage adjustment is recommended for patients on concomitant therapy). Products include:

Cerebyx Injection 2619

Phenobarbital (Co-administration with inducers of cytochrome P450, such as phenobarbital, may change the clearance and, hence, the half-life of ondansetron; based on the limited data, no dosage adjustment is recommended for patients on concomitant therapy). Products include:

Arco-Lase Plus Tablets 592
Donnatal 2929
Donnatal Extentabs 2930

Phenytoin (Co-administration with inducers of cytochrome P450, such as phenytoin, may change the clearance and, hence, the half-life of ondansetron; based on the limited data, no dosage adjustment is recommended for patients on concomitant therapy). Products include:

Dilantin Infatabs 2624
Dilantin-125 Oral Suspension 2625

Phenytoin Sodium (Co-administration with inducers of cytochrome P450, such as phenytoin, may change the clearance and, hence, the half-life of ondansetron; based on the limited data, no dosage adjustment is recommended for patients on concomitant therapy). Products include:

Dilantin Kapseals 2622

Quinidine Gluconate (Co-administration with inhibitors of cytochrome P450, such as quinidine, may change the clearance and, hence, the half-life of ondansetron; based on the limited data, no dosage adjustment is recommended for patients on concomitant therapy). Products include:

Quinaglute Dura-Tabs Tablets 978

Quinidine Polygalacturonate (Co-administration with inhibitors of cytochrome P450, such as quinidine, may change the clearance and, hence, the half-life of ondansetron; based on the limited data, no dosage adjustment is recommended for patients on concomitant therapy).

No products indexed under this heading.

Quinidine Sulfate (Co-administration with inhibitors of cytochrome P450, such as quinidine, may change the clearance and, hence, the half-life of ondansetron; based on the limited data, no dosage adjustment is recommended for patients on concomitant therapy). Products include:

Quinidex Extentabs 2933

Rifampin (Co-administration with inducers of cytochrome P450, such as rifampin, may change the clearance and, hence, the half-life of ondansetron; based on the limited data, no dosage adjustment is recommended for patients on concomitant therapy). Products include:

Rifadin 765
Rifamate Capsules 767
Rifater Tablets 769

Food Interactions

Food, unspecified (Increases significantly (about 17%) the extent of absorption of ondansetron).

ZOFRAN ODT ORALLY DISINTEGRATING TABLETS

(Ondansetron) 1703
See Zofran Tablets

ZOLADEX

(Goserelin Acetate) 702
None cited in PDR database.

ZOLADEX 3-MONTH

(Goserelin Acetate) 706
None cited in PDR database.

ZOLOFT ORAL CONCENTRATE

(Sertraline Hydrochloride) 2751
May interact with antidepressant drugs, lithium preparations, monoamine oxidase inhibitors, tricyclic antidepressants, and certain other agents. Compounds in these categories include:

Amitriptyline Hydrochloride (Concurrent use of drugs that inhibit the biochemical activity of P450IID6, such as tricyclic antidepressants, may increase plasma concentrations of co-administered drugs that are metabolized by P450IID6; changes in the dosage may be required; the duration of an appropriate washout period which should intervene before switching has not been established). Products include:

Etrafon 3115
Limbitrol 1738

Amoxapine (Concurrent use of drugs that inhibit the biochemical activity of P450IID6, such as tricyclic antidepressants, may increase plasma concentrations of co-administered drugs that are metabolized by P450IID6; changes in the dosage may be required; the duration of an appropriate washout period which should intervene before switching has not been established).

No products indexed under this heading.

Astemizole (Sertraline has been shown to have some inhibition of P4503A4 *in vitro*, astemizole is metabolized by P4503A4 isoenzyme and inhibition of this enzyme system may result in increased serum levels of astemizole; co-administration requires caution).

No products indexed under this heading.

Bupropion Hydrochloride (Concurrent use of drugs that inhibit the biochemical activity of P450IID6, such as tricyclic antidepressants, may increase plasma concentrations of co-administered drugs that are metabolized by P450IID6; changes in the dosage may be required; the duration of an appropriate washout period which should intervene before switching has not been established). Products include:

Wellbutrin Tablets 1680
Wellbutrin SR Sustained-Release Tablets 1684
Zyban Sustained-Release Tablets 1710

Cimetidine (Potential for increase in Zoloft mean AUC (50%), Cmax (24%) and half-life (26%); clinical significance is unknown). Products include:

Tagamet HB 200 Suspension 762
Tagamet HB 200 Tablets 761
Tagamet Tablets 1644

Cimetidine Hydrochloride (Potential for increase in Zoloft mean AUC (50%), Cmax (24%) and half-life (26%); clinical significance is unknown). Products include:

Tagamet 1644

Cisapride (Sertraline has been shown to have some inhibition of P4503A4 *in vitro*, cisapride is metabolized by P4503A4 isoenzyme and inhibition of this enzyme system may result in increased serum levels of cisapride; co-administration requires caution).

No products indexed under this heading.

Citalopram Hydrobromide (Concurrent use of drugs that inhibit the biochemical activity of P450IID6, such as tricyclic antidepressants, may increase plasma concentrations of co-administered drugs that are metabolized by P450IID6; changes in the dosage may be required; the duration of an appropriate washout period which should intervene before switching has not been established). Products include:

Celexa 1365

Clomipramine Hydrochloride (Concurrent use of drugs that inhibit the biochemical activity of P450IID6, such as tricyclic antidepressants, may increase plasma concentrations of co-administered drugs that are metabolized by P450IID6; changes in the dosage may be required; the duration of an appropriate washout period which should intervene before switching has not been established).

No products indexed under this heading.

CNS-Active Drugs, unspecified (Caution is advised if Zoloft is co-administered with other CNS active drugs).

Desipramine Hydrochloride (Concurrent use of drugs that inhibit the biochemical activity of P450IID6, such as tricyclic antidepressants, may increase plasma concentrations of co-administered drugs that are metabolized by P450IID6; changes in the dosage may be required; the duration of an appropriate washout period which should intervene before switching has not been established). Products include:

Norpramin Tablets 755

Diazepam (Co-administration with intravenous diazepam has resulted in decrease in relative to baseline diazepam clearance and increase in Tmax for desmethyldiazepam; the clinical significance is unknown). Products include:

Valium Injectable 3026
Valium Tablets 3047

Digitoxin (Co-administration with drugs that are highly protein bound, such as digitoxin, may cause a shift in plasma concentrations, potentially resulting in an adverse effect).

No products indexed under this heading.

Disulfiram (Zoloft Oral Concentrate contains 12% alcohol; concurrent use with disulfiram may result in Antabuse-Alcohol reaction; co-administration of Zoloft Oral Concentrate and disulfiram is contraindicated). Products include:

Antabuse Tablets 2444
Antabuse Tablets 3474

Doxepin Hydrochloride (Concurrent use of drugs that inhibit the biochemical activity of P450IID6, such as tricyclic antidepressants, may increase plasma concentrations of

co-administered drugs that are metabolized by P450IID6; changes in the dosage may be required; the duration of an appropriate washout period which should intervene before switching has not been established). Products include:

Sinequan **2713**

Flecainide Acetate (Concurrent use of drugs that inhibit the biochemical activity of P450IID6, such as flecainide, may increase plasma concentrations of co-administered drugs that are metabolized by P450IID6; changes in the dosage may be required). Products include:

Tambocor Tablets **1990**

Fluoxetine Hydrochloride (Concurrent use of drugs that inhibit the biochemical activity of P450IID6, such as SSRIs, may increase plasma concentrations of co-administered drugs that are metabolized by P450IID6; changes in the dosage may be required; the duration of an appropriate washout period which should intervene before switching has not been established). Products include:

Prozac Pulvules, Liquid, and Weekly Capsules **1238**
Sarafem Pulvules **1962**

Fluvoxamine Maleate (Concurrent use of drugs that inhibit the biochemical activity of P450IID6, such as SSRIs, may increase plasma concentrations of co-administered drugs that are metabolized by P450IID6; changes in the dosage may be required; the duration of an appropriate washout period which should intervene before switching has not been established). Products include:

Luvox Tablets (25, 50, 100 mg) **3256**

Imipramine Hydrochloride (Concurrent use of drugs that inhibit the biochemical activity of P450IID6, such as tricyclic antidepressants, may increase plasma concentrations of co-administered drugs that are metabolized by P450IID6; changes in the dosage may be required; the duration of an appropriate washout period which should intervene before switching has not been established).

No products indexed under this heading.

Imipramine Pamoate (Concurrent use of drugs that inhibit the biochemical activity of P450IID6, such as tricyclic antidepressants, may increase plasma concentrations of co-administered drugs that are metabolized by P450IID6; changes in the dosage may be required; the duration of an appropriate washout period which should intervene before switching has not been established).

No products indexed under this heading.

Isocarboxazid (Co-administration has resulted in serious, sometimes fatal, reactions including hyperthermia, rigidity, myoclonus, autonomic instability, extreme agitation progressing to delirium and coma; concurrent and/or sequential use is contraindicated).

No products indexed under this heading.

Lithium Carbonate (No significant alteration in plasma lithium levels or renal clearance, nonetheless, plasma lithium levels should be monitored). Products include:

Eskalith **1527**
Lithium Carbonate **3061**
Lithobid Slow-Release Tablets **3255**

Lithium Citrate (No significant alteration in plasma lithium levels or renal clearance, nonetheless, plasma lithium levels should be monitored). Products include:

Lithium Citrate Syrup **3061**

Maprotiline Hydrochloride (Concurrent use of drugs that inhibit the biochemical activity of P450IID6, such as tricyclic antidepressants, may increase plasma concentrations of co-administered drugs that are metabolized by P450IID6; changes in the dosage may be required; the duration of an appropriate washout period which should intervene before switching has not been established).

No products indexed under this heading.

Mirtazapine (Concurrent use of drugs that inhibit the biochemical activity of P450IID6, such as tricyclic antidepressants, may increase plasma concentrations of co-administered drugs that are metabolized by P450IID6; changes in the dosage may be required; the duration of an appropriate washout period which should intervene before switching has not been established). Products include:

Remeron Tablets **2483**
Remeron SolTab Tablets **2486**

Moclobemide (Concomitant use in patients taking MAO inhibitors and SSRI, such as sertraline, has resulted in cases of serious fatal reactions including hyperthermia, rigidity, myoclonus, autonomic instability, delirium and coma; concurrent and/or sequential use is contraindicated).

No products indexed under this heading.

Nefazodone Hydrochloride (Care and prudent medical judgment should be exercised regarding the optimal timing of switching from another antidepressant to Zoloft; the duration of an appropriate washout period which should intervene before switching has not been established). Products include:

Serzone Tablets **1104**

Nortriptyline Hydrochloride (Concurrent use of drugs that inhibit the biochemical activity of P450IID6, such as tricyclic antidepressants, may increase plasma concentrations of co-administered drugs that are metabolized by P450IID6; changes in the dosage may be required; the duration of an appropriate washout period which should intervene before switching has not been established).

No products indexed under this heading.

Pargyline Hydrochloride (Concomitant use in patients taking MAO inhibitors and SSRI, such as sertraline, has resulted in cases of serious fatal reactions including hyperthermia, rigidity, myoclonus, autonomic instability, delirium and coma; concurrent and/or sequential use is contraindicated).

No products indexed under this heading.

Paroxetine Hydrochloride (Concurrent use of drugs that inhibit the biochemical activity of P450II6, such as SSRIs, may increase plasma concentrations of co-administered drugs that are metabolized by P450IID6; changes in the dosage may be required; the duration of an appropriate washout period which should intervene before switching has not been established). Products include:

Paxil **1609**

Phenelzine Sulfate (Co-administration has resulted in serious, sometimes fatal, reactions including hyperthermia, rigidity, myoclonus, autonomic instability, extreme agitation progressing to delirium and coma; concurrent and/or sequential use is contraindicated). Products include:

Nardil Tablets **2653**

Procarbazine Hydrochloride (Concomitant use in patients taking MAO inhibitors and SSRI, such as sertraline, has resulted in cases of serious fatal reactions including hyperthermia, rigidity, myoclonus, autonomic instability, delirium and coma; concurrent and/or sequential use is contraindicated). Products include:

Matulane Capsules **3246**

Propafenone Hydrochloride (Concurrent use of drugs that inhibit the biochemical activity of P450IID6, such as propafenone, may increase plasma concentrations of co-administered drugs that are metabolized by P450IID6; changes in the dosage may be required). Products include:

Rythmol Tablets – 150 mg, 225 mg, 300 mg **502**

Protriptyline Hydrochloride (Concurrent use of drugs that inhibit the biochemical activity of P450IID6, such as tricyclic antidepressants, may increase plasma concentrations of co-administered drugs that are metabolized by P450IID6; changes in the dosage may be required; the duration of an appropriate washout period which should intervene before switching has not been established). Products include:

Vivactil Tablets **2446**
Vivactil Tablets **2217**

Selegiline Hydrochloride (Concomitant use in patients taking MAO inhibitors and SSRI, such as sertraline, has resulted in cases of serious fatal reactions including hyperthermia, rigidity, myoclonus, autonomic instability, delirium and coma; concurrent and/or sequential use is contraindicated). Products include:

Eldepryl Capsules **3266**

Sumatriptan (Co-administration of SSRI and sumatriptan has resulted in rare reports of weakness, hyperreflexia, and incoordination). Products include:

Imitrex Nasal Spray **1554**

Sumatriptan Succinate (Co-administration of SSRI and sumatriptan has resulted in rare reports of weakness, hyperreflexia, and incoordination). Products include:

Imitrex Injection **1549**
Imitrex Tablets **1558**

Tolbutamide (Co-administration has caused a statistically significant 16% decrease from baseline in the clearance of tolbutamide; the clinical significance of this finding is unknown).

No products indexed under this heading.

Tranylcypromine Sulfate (Concomitant use in patients taking MAO inhibitors and SSRI, such as sertraline, has resulted in cases of serious fatal reactions including hyperthermia, rigidity, myoclonus, autonomic instability, delirium and coma; concurrent and/or sequential use is contraindicated). Products include:

Parnate Tablets **1607**

Trazodone Hydrochloride (Concurrent use of drugs that inhibit the biochemical activity of P450IID6, such as tricyclic antidepressants, may increase plasma concentrations of co-administered drugs that are metabolized by P450IID6; changes in the dosage may be required; the duration of an appropriate washout period which should intervene before switching has not been established).

No products indexed under this heading.

Trimipramine Maleate (Concurrent use of drugs that inhibit the biochemical activity of P450IID6, such as tricyclic antidepressants, may increase plasma concentrations of co-administered drugs that are metabolized by P450IID6; changes in the dosage may be required; the duration of an appropriate washout period which should intervene before switching has not been established). Products include:

Surmontil Capsules **3595**

Venlafaxine Hydrochloride (Concurrent use of drugs that inhibit the biochemical activity of P450IID6, such as SSRIs, may increase plasma concentrations of co-administered drugs that are metabolized by P450IID6; changes in the dosage may be required; the duration of an appropriate washout period which should intervene before switching has not been established). Products include:

Effexor Tablets **3495**
Effexor XR Capsules **3499**

Warfarin Sodium (Co-administration has resulted in a mean increase in prothrombin time of 8% relative to baseline for sertraline; the clinical significance of this change is not known). Products include:

Coumadin for Injection **1243**
Coumadin Tablets **1243**
Warfarin Sodium Tablets, USP **3302**

Food Interactions

Alcohol (Concomitant use of Zoloft and alcohol in depressed patient is not recommended).

Food, unspecified (Co-administration of Zoloft Tablets with food slightly increased AUC but the Cmax was 25% greater, while time to reach peak plasma concentration (Tmax) decreased from 8 hours to 5.5 hours; for oral concentrate, Tmax was slightly prolonged from 5.9 hours to 7 hours with food).

ZOLOFT TABLETS

(Sertraline Hydrochloride) **2751**
See Zoloft Oral Concentrate

ZOMETA FOR INTRAVENOUS INFUSION

(Zoledronic acid) **3621**
May interact with aminoglycosides and loop diuretics. Compounds in these categories include:

Amikacin Sulfate (Co-administration with aminoglycosides may have an additive effect to lower serum calcium for prolonged period).

No products indexed under this heading.

Bumetanide (Increased risk of hypocalcemia).

No products indexed under this heading.

Ethacrynic Acid (Increased risk of hypocalcemia). Products include:

Edecrin Tablets **2091**

Furosemide (Increased risk of hypocalcemia). Products include:

Furosemide Tablets **2284**

Gentamicin Sulfate (Co-administration with aminoglycosides may have an additive effect to lower serum calcium for prolonged period). Products include:

Genoptic Ophthalmic Ointment ..... ⊙ **239**
Genoptic Sterile Ophthalmic Solution .... ⊙ **239**
Pred-G Ophthalmic Suspension ..... ⊙ **247**
Pred-G Sterile Ophthalmic Ointment .... ⊙ **248**

Kanamycin Sulfate (Co-administration with aminoglycosides may have an additive effect to lower serum calcium for prolonged period).

No products indexed under this heading.

Streptomycin Sulfate (Co-administration with aminoglycosides may have an additive effect to lower serum calcium for prolonged period). Products include:

Streptomycin Sulfate Injection **2714**

Tobramycin (Co-administration with aminoglycosides may have an addi-

tive effect to lower serum calcium for prolonged period). Products include:

- TOBI Solution for Inhalation ... 1206
- TobraDex Ophthalmic Ointment ... 542
- TobraDex Ophthalmic Suspension .. 541
- Tobrex Ophthalmic Ointment ... ⊙220
- Tobrex Ophthalmic Solution ... ⊙221

Tobramycin Sulfate (Co-administration with aminoglycosides may have an additive effect to lower serum calcium for prolonged period). Products include:

- Nebcin Vials, Hyporets & ADD-Vantage ... 1955

Torsemide (Increased risk of hypocalcemia). Products include:

- Demadex Tablets and Injection ... 2965

ZOMIG TABLETS

(Zolmitriptan) ... 708

May interact with 5HT1-receptor agonists, ergot-containing drugs, nonselective MAO inhibitors, oral contraceptives, selective serotonin reuptake inhibitors, and certain other agents. Compounds in these categories include:

Acetaminophen (Zolmitriptan delayed the Tmax of acetaminophen by 1 hour in a single dose study). Products include:

- Actifed Cold & Sinus Caplets and Tablets ... ▣688
- Alka-Seltzer Plus Liqui-Gels ... ▣604
- Alka-Seltzer Plus Cold & Flu Medicine Liqui-Gels ... ▣604
- Alka-Seltzer Plus Cold & Sinus Medicine Liqui-Gels ... ▣604
- Benadryl Allergy/Cold Tablets ... ▣691
- Benadryl Allergy Sinus Headache Caplets & Gelcaps ... ▣693
- Benadryl Severe Allergy & Sinus Headache Caplets ... ▣694
- Children's Cēpacol Sore Throat ... ▣788
- Comtrex Acute Head Cold & Sinus Pressure Relief Tablets ... ▣627
- Comtrex Deep Chest Cold & Congestion Relief Softgels ... ▣627
- Comtrex Flu Therapy & Fever Relief Daytime Caplets ... ▣628
- Comtrex Flu Therapy & Fever Relief Nighttime Tablets ... ▣628
- Comtrex Maximum Strength Multi-Symptom Cold & Cough Relief Tablets and Caplets ... ▣626
- Contac Severe Cold and Flu Caplets Maximum Strength ... ▣746
- Contac Severe Cold and Flu Caplets Non-Drowsy ... ▣746
- Coricidin 'D' Cold, Flu & Sinus Tablets ... ▣737
- Coricidin HBP Cold & Flu Tablets .. ▣738
- Coricidin HBP Maximum Strength Flu Tablets ... ▣738
- Coricidin HBP Night-Time Cold & Flu Tablets ... ▣738
- Darvon-N/Darvocet-N ... 1907
- Dimetapp Cold and Fever Suspension ... ▣775
- Dimetapp Nighttime Flu Liquid ... ▣776
- Dimetapp Non-Drowsy Flu Syrup .. ▣777
- Drixoral Allergy/Sinus Extended-Release Tablets ... ▣741
- Drixoral Cold & Flu Extended-Release Tablets ... ▣740
- Aspirin Free Excedrin Caplets and Geltabs ... ▣628
- Excedrin Extra-Strength Tablets, Caplets, and Geltabs ... ▣629
- Excedrin Migraine ... 1070
- Excedrin PM Tablets, Caplets, and Geltabs ... ▣631
- Goody's Body Pain Formula Powder ... ▣620
- Goody's Extra Strength Headache Powder ... ▣620
- Goody's Extra Strength Pain Relief Tablets ... ▣620
- Goody's PM Powder ... ▣621
- Hycomine Compound Tablets ... 1317
- Lortab ... 3319
- Lortab Elixir ... 3317
- Maxidone Tablets CIII ... 3399
- Maximum Strength Midol Menstrual Caplets and Gelcaps .. ▣612
- Maximum Strength Midol PMS Caplets and Gelcaps ... ▣613
- Maximum Strength Midol Teen Caplets ... ▣612
- Midrin Capsules ... 3464
- Norco 5/325 Tablets CIII ... 3424
- Norco 7.5/325 Tablets CIII ... 3425
- Norco 10/325 Tablets CIII ... 3427
- Norco 10/325 Tablets CIII ... 3425
- Percocet Tablets ... 1326
- Percogesic Aspirin-Free Coated Tablets ... ▣667
- Extra Strength Percogesic Aspirin-Free Coated Caplets ... ▣665
- Phrenilin ... 578
- Robitussin Cold Caplets Multi-Symptom Cold & Flu ... ▣781
- Robitussin Cold Softgels Multi-Symptom Cold & Flu ... ▣781
- Robitussin Multi Symptom Honey Flu Liquid ... ▣785
- Robitussin Nighttime Honey Flu Liquid ... ▣786
- Sedapap Tablets 50 mg/650 mg ... 2225
- Singlet Caplets ... ▣761
- Sinutab Sinus Allergy Medication, Maximum Strength Formula, Tablets & Caplets ... ▣707
- Sinutab Sinus Medication, Maximum Strength Without Drowsiness Formula, Tablets & Caplets ... ▣707
- Sudafed Cold & Cough Liquid Caps ... ▣709
- Sudafed Cold & Sinus Liquid Caps ... ▣710
- Sudafed Severe Cold ... ▣711
- Sudafed Sinus Headache Caplets . ▣712
- Sudafed Sinus Headache Tablets . ▣712
- Tavist Sinus Non-Drowsy Coated Caplets ... ▣676
- TheraFlu Regular Strength Cold & Cough Night Time Hot Liquid ... ▣676
- TheraFlu Regular Strength Cold & Sore Throat Night Time Hot Liquid ... ▣676
- TheraFlu Maximum Strength Flu & Congestion Non-Drowsy Hot Liquid ... ▣677
- TheraFlu Maximum Strength Flu & Cough Night Time Hot Liquid ... ▣678
- TheraFlu Maximum Strength Flu & Sore Throat Night Time Hot Liquid ... ▣677
- TheraFlu Maximum Strength Severe Cold & Congestion Night Time Caplets ... ▣678
- TheraFlu Maximum Strength Severe Cold & Congestion Night Time Hot Liquid ... ▣678
- TheraFlu Maximum Strength Severe Cold & Congestion Non-Drowsy ... ▣679
- Triaminic Cold, Cough & Fever Liquid ... ▣681
- Triaminic Cough & Sore Throat Liquid ... ▣682
- Triaminic Cough & Sore Throat Softchews ... ▣684
- Tylenol, Children's ... 2014
- Children's Tylenol Allergy-D Liquid ... 2014
- Children's Tylenol Cold Suspension Liquid and Chewable Tablets ... 2015
- Children's Tylenol Cold Plus Cough Suspension Liquid and Chewable Tablets ... 2015
- Children's Tylenol Flu Suspension Liquid ... 2015
- Children's Tylenol Sinus Suspension Liquid ... 2017
- Infants' Tylenol Cold Decongestant and Fever Reducer Concentrated Drops ... 2015
- Infants' Tylenol Cold Decongestant and Fever Reducer Concentrated Drops Plus Cough .. 2015
- Junior Strength Tylenol Soft Chews Chewable Tablets ... 2014
- Tylenol ... 2009
- Tylenol Allergy Sinus ... 2010
- Tylenol Severe Allergy Caplets ... 2010
- Multi-Symptom Tylenol Cold Complete Formula Caplets ... 2010
- Multi-Symptom Tylenol Cold Non-Drowsy Caplets and Gelcaps ... 2010
- Multi-Symptom Tylenol Cold Severe Congestion Non-Drowsy Caplets ... 2011
- Maximum Strength Tylenol Flu NightTime Gelcaps ... 2011
- Maximum Strength Tylenol Flu NightTime Liquid ... 2011
- Maximum Strength Tylenol Flu Non-Drowsy Gelcaps ... 2011
- Extra Strength Tylenol PM Caplets, Geltabs, and Gelcaps ... 2012
- Maximum Strength Tylenol Sinus NightTime Caplets ... 2012
- Maximum Strength Tylenol Sinus Non-Drowsy Geltabs, Gelcaps, Caplets, and Tablets ... 2012
- Maximum Strength Tylenol Sore Throat Adult Liquid ... 2013
- Tylenol with Codeine ... 2595
- Women's Tylenol Menstrual Relief Caplets ... 2013
- Tylox Capsules ... 2597
- Ultracet Tablets ... 2597
- Vanquish Caplets ... ▣617
- Vicks 44M Cough, Cold & Flu Relief Liquid ... ▣725
- Vicks DayQuil LiquiCaps/Liquid Multi-Symptom Cold/Flu Relief ... ▣727
- Vicks NyQuil LiquiCaps/Liquid Multi-Symptom Cold/Flu Relief, Original and Cherry Flavors ... ▣727
- Vicodin Tablets ... 516
- Vicodin ES Tablets ... 517
- Vicodin HP Tablets ... 518
- Zydone Tablets ... 1330

Cimetidine (Following the administration of cimetidine, the half-life and AUC of a 5 mg dose of zolmitriptan and its active metabolite were approximately doubled). Products include:

- Tagamet HB 200 Suspension ... ▣762
- Tagamet HB 200 Tablets ... ▣761
- Tagamet Tablets ... 1644

Cimetidine Hydrochloride (Following the administration of cimetidine, the half-life and AUC of a 5 mg dose of zolmitriptan and its active metabolite were approximately doubled). Products include:

- Tagamet ... 1644

Citalopram Hydrobromide (Co-administration of 5-HT1 agonists with selective serotonin reuptake inhibitors (SSRIs) has resulted, rarely, in hyperreflexia, weakness, and incoordination). Products include:

- Celexa ... 1365

Desogestrel (Retrospective analysis of pharmacokinetic data indicates that mean plasma concentrations, Cmax and AUC, of zolmitriptan were generally higher in females taking oral contraceptives; Tmax was delayed by one-half hour in these females). Products include:

- Cyclessa Tablets ... 2450
- Desogen Tablets ... 2458
- Mircette Tablets ... 2470
- Ortho-Cept 21 Tablets ... 2546
- Ortho-Cept 28 Tablets ... 2546

Dihydroergotamine Mesylate (Ergot-containing drugs have been reported to cause prolonged vasospastic reactions; because there is a theoretical basis that these effects may be additive, use of ergot-type agents and zolmitriptan within 24 hours is contraindicated). Products include:

- D.H.E. 45 Injection ... 2334
- Migranal Nasal Spray ... 2376

Ergonovine Maleate (Ergot-containing drugs have been reported to cause prolonged vasospastic reactions; because there is a theoretical basis that these effects may be additive, use of ergot-type agents and zolmitriptan within 24 hours is contraindicated).

No products indexed under this heading.

Ergotamine Tartrate (Ergot-containing drugs have been reported to cause prolonged vasospastic reactions; because there is a theoretical basis that these effects may be additive, use of ergot-type agents and zolmitriptan within 24 hours is contraindicated).

No products indexed under this heading.

Ethinyl Estradiol (Retrospective analysis of pharmacokinetic data indicates that mean plasma concentrations, Cmax and AUC, of zolmitriptan were generally higher in females taking oral contraceptives; Tmax was delayed by one-half hour in these females). Products include:

- Alesse-21 Tablets ... 3468
- Alesse-28 Tablets ... 3473
- Brevicon 28-Day Tablets ... 3380
- Cyclessa Tablets ... 2450
- Desogen Tablets ... 2458
- Estinyl Tablets ... 3112
- Estrostep ... 2627
- femhrt Tablets ... 2635
- Levlen ... 962
- Levlite 21 Tablets ... 962
- Levlite 28 Tablets ... 962
- Levora Tablets ... 3389
- Loestrin 21 Tablets ... 2642
- Loestrin Fe Tablets ... 2642
- Lo/Ovral Tablets ... 3532
- Lo/Ovral-28 Tablets ... 3538
- Low-Ogestrel-28 Tablets ... 3392
- Microgestin Fe 1.5/30 Tablets ... 3407
- Microgestin Fe 1/20 Tablets ... 3400
- Mircette Tablets ... 2470
- Modicon ... 2563
- Necon ... 3415
- Nordette-28 Tablets ... 2257
- Norinyl 1 +35 28-Day Tablets ... 3380
- Ogestrel 0.5/50-28 Tablets ... 3428
- Ortho-Cept 21 Tablets ... 2546
- Ortho-Cept 28 Tablets ... 2546
- Ortho-Cyclen/Ortho Tri-Cyclen ... 2573
- Ortho-Novum ... 2563
- Ovcon ... 3364
- Ovral Tablets ... 3551
- Ovral-28 Tablets ... 3552
- Tri-Levlen ... 962
- Tri-Norinyl-28 Tablets ... 3433
- Triphasil-21 Tablets ... 3600
- Triphasil-28 Tablets ... 3605
- Trivora Tablets ... 3439
- Yasmin 28 Tablets ... 980
- Zovia ... 3449

Ethynodiol Diacetate (Retrospective analysis of pharmacokinetic data indicates that mean plasma concentrations, Cmax and AUC, of zolmitriptan were generally higher in females taking oral contraceptives; Tmax was delayed by one-half hour in these females). Products include:

- Zovia ... 3449

Fluoxetine Hydrochloride (Co-administration of 5-HT1 agonists with selective serotonin reuptake inhibitors (SSRIs) has resulted, rarely, in hyperreflexia, weakness, and incoordination). Products include:

- Prozac Pulvules, Liquid, and Weekly Capsules ... 1238
- Sarafem Pulvules ... 1962

Fluvoxamine Maleate (Co-administration of 5-HT1 agonists with selective serotonin reuptake inhibitors (SSRIs) has resulted, rarely, in hyperreflexia, weakness, and incoordination). Products include:

- Luvox Tablets (25, 50, 100 mg) ... 3256

Isocarboxazid (MAO-A inhibitors increase the systemic exposure of zolmitriptan; concurrent and/or sequential use is contraindicated).

No products indexed under this heading.

Levonorgestrel (Retrospective analysis of pharmacokinetic data indicates that mean plasma concentrations, Cmax and AUC, of zolmitriptan were generally higher in females taking oral contraceptives; Tmax was delayed by one-half hour in these females). Products include:

- Alesse-21 Tablets ... 3468
- Alesse-28 Tablets ... 3473
- Levlen ... 962
- Levlite 21 Tablets ... 962
- Levlite 28 Tablets ... 962
- Levora Tablets ... 3389
- Mirena Intrauterine System ... 974
- Nordette-28 Tablets ... 2257
- Norplant System ... 3543
- Tri-Levlen ... 962
- Triphasil-21 Tablets ... 3600
- Triphasil-28 Tablets ... 3605
- Trivora Tablets ... 3439

Mestranol (Retrospective analysis of pharmacokinetic data indicates that mean plasma concentrations, Cmax and AUC, of zolmitriptan were generally higher in females taking oral contraceptives; Tmax was delayed by one-half hour in these females). Products include:

- Necon 1/50 Tablets ... 3415
- Norinyl 1 + 50 28-Day Tablets ... 3380
- Ortho-Novum 1/50□28 Tablets ... 2556

Methylergonovine Maleate (Ergot-containing drugs have been reported to cause prolonged vasospastic reactions; because there is a theoretical basis that these effects may be additive, use of ergot-type agents and zolmitriptan within 24 hours is contraindicated).
No products indexed under this heading.

Methysergide Maleate (Ergot-containing drugs have been reported to cause prolonged vasospastic reactions; because there is a theoretical basis that these effects may be additive, use of ergot-type agents and zolmitriptan within 24 hours is contraindicated).
No products indexed under this heading.

Naratriptan Hydrochloride (Co-administration with other 5-HT1 agonists within 24 hours of each other is contraindicated because the vasospastic effects may be additive). Products include:
Amerge Tablets **1467**

Norethindrone (Retrospective analysis of pharmacokinetic data indicates that mean plasma concentrations, Cmax and AUC, of zolmitriptan were generally higher in females taking oral contraceptives; Tmax was delayed by one-half hour in these females). Products include:
Brevicon 28-Day Tablets **3380**
Micronor Tablets **2543**
Modicon **2563**
Necon **3415**
Norinyl 1 +35 28-Day Tablets **3380**
Norinyl 1 + 50 28-Day Tablets **3380**
Nor-QD Tablets **3423**
Ortho-Novum **2563**
Ortho-Novum 1/50□28 Tablets **2556**
Ovcon **3364**
Tri-Norinyl-28 Tablets **3433**

Norethynodrel (Retrospective analysis of pharmacokinetic data indicates that mean plasma concentrations, Cmax and AUC, of zolmitriptan were generally higher in females taking oral contraceptives; Tmax was delayed by one-half hour in these females).
No products indexed under this heading.

Norgestimate (Retrospective analysis of pharmacokinetic data indicates that mean plasma concentrations, Cmax and AUC, of zolmitriptan were generally higher in females taking oral contraceptives; Tmax was delayed by one-half hour in these females). Products include:
Ortho-Cyclen/Ortho Tri-Cyclen **2573**
Ortho-Prefest Tablets **2570**

Norgestrel (Retrospective analysis of pharmacokinetic data indicates that mean plasma concentrations, Cmax and AUC, of zolmitriptan were generally higher in females taking oral contraceptives; Tmax was delayed by one-half hour in these females). Products include:
Lo/Ovral Tablets **3532**
Lo/Ovral-28 Tablets **3538**
Low-Ogestrel-28 Tablets **3392**
Ogestrel 0.5/50-28 Tablets **3428**
Ovral Tablets **3551**
Ovral-28 Tablets **3552**
Ovrette Tablets **3552**

Pargyline Hydrochloride (MAO-A inhibitors increase the systemic exposure of zolmitriptan; concurrent and/or sequential use is contraindicated).
No products indexed under this heading.

Paroxetine Hydrochloride (Co-administration of 5-HT1 agonists with selective serotonin reuptake inhibitors (SSRIs) has resulted, rarely, in hyperreflexia, weakness, and incoordination). Products include:
Paxil **1609**

Phenelzine Sulfate (MAO-A inhibitors increase the systemic exposure of zolmitriptan; concurrent and/or sequential use is contraindicated). Products include:
Nardil Tablets **2653**

Procarbazine Hydrochloride (MAO-A inhibitors increase the systemic exposure of zolmitriptan; concurrent and/or sequential use is contraindicated). Products include:
Matulane Capsules **3246**

Propranolol Hydrochloride (Co-administration has resulted in increased (1.5-fold) Cmax and AUC of zolmitriptan after one week of propranolol dosing). Products include:
Inderal **3513**
Inderal LA Long-Acting Capsules **3516**
Inderide Tablets **3517**
Inderide LA Long-Acting Capsules **3519**

Rizatriptan Benzoate (Co-administration with other 5-HT1 agonists within 24 hours of each other is contraindicated because the vasospastic effects may be additive). Products include:
Maxalt Tablets **2120**
Maxalt-MLT Orally Disintegrating Tablets **2120**

Sertraline Hydrochloride (Co-administration of 5-HT1 agonists with selective serotonin reuptake inhibitors (SSRIs) has resulted, rarely, in hyperreflexia, weakness, and incoordination). Products include:
Zoloft **2751**

Sumatriptan (Co-administration with other 5-HT1 agonists within 24 hours of each other is contraindicated because the vasospastic effects may be additive). Products include:
Imitrex Nasal Spray **1554**

Sumatriptan Succinate (Co-administration with other 5-HT1 agonists within 24 hours of each other is contraindicated because the vasospastic effects may be additive). Products include:
Imitrex Injection **1549**
Imitrex Tablets **1558**

Tranylcypromine Sulfate (MAO-A inhibitors increase the systemic exposure of zolmitriptan; concurrent and/or sequential use is contraindicated). Products include:
Parnate Tablets **1607**

ZOMIG-ZMT TABLETS
(Zolmitriptan) **708**
See Zomig Tablets

ZONEGRAN CAPSULES
(Zonisamide) **1307**
May interact with phenytoin, valproate, and certain other agents. Compounds in these categories include:

Carbamazepine (Co-administration with drugs that induce liver enzymes increase the metabolism and clearance of zonisamide and decrease half-life; the half-life of zonisamide concurrently on carbamazepine was between 27-38 hours). Products include:
Carbatrol Capsules **3234**
Tegretol/Tegretol-XR **2404**

Divalproex Sodium (The half-life of zonisamide in patients concurrently on the non-enzyme inducing AED, valproate, was 46 hours). Products include:
Depakote Sprinkle Capsules **426**
Depakote Tablets **430**
Depakote ER Tablets **436**

Fosphenytoin Sodium (Co-administration with drugs that induce liver enzymes increase the metabolism and clearance of zonisamide and decrease half-life; the half-life of zonisamide concurrently on phenytoin was between 27-38 hours). Products include:
Cerebyx Injection **2619**

Phenobarbital (Co-administration with drugs that induce liver enzymes increase the metabolism and clearance of zonisamide and decrease half-life; the half-life of zonisamide concurrently on phenobarbital was between 27-38 hours). Products include:
Arco-Lase Plus Tablets **592**
Donnatal **2929**
Donnatal Extentabs **2930**

Phenytoin (Co-administration with drugs that induce liver enzymes increase the metabolism and clearance of zonisamide and decrease half-life; the half-life of zonisamide concurrently on phenytoin was between 27-38 hours). Products include:
Dilantin Infatabs **2624**
Dilantin-125 Oral Suspension **2625**

Phenytoin Sodium (Co-administration with drugs that induce liver enzymes increase the metabolism and clearance of zonisamide and decrease half-life; the half-life of zonisamide concurrently on phenytoin was between 27-38 hours). Products include:
Dilantin Kapseals **2622**

Valproate Sodium (The half-life of zonisamide in patients concurrently on the non-enzyme inducing AED, valproate, was 46 hours). Products include:
Depacon Injection **416**

Valproic Acid (The half-life of zonisamide in patients concurrently on the non-enzyme inducing AED, valproate, was 46 hours). Products include:
Depakene **421**

ZOSYN
(Piperacillin Sodium, Tazobactam Sodium) **1890**
May interact with aminoglycosides, anticoagulants, nondepolarizing neuromuscular blocking agents, and certain other agents. Compounds in these categories include:

Amikacin Sulfate (The mixing of Zosyn with an aminoglycoside *in vitro* can result in substantial inactivation due to penicillin-aminoglycoside complex; this complex is microbiologically inactive and of unknown toxicity).
No products indexed under this heading.

Ardeparin Sodium (Coagulation parameters should be tested more frequently and monitored regularly during simultaneous administration; effect of concurrent use is not specified).
No products indexed under this heading.

Atracurium Besylate (Due to similar mechanism of action as vecuronium, it is expected that the neuromuscular blockade produced by other non-depolarizing muscle relaxants could be prolonged in the presence of piperacillin).
No products indexed under this heading.

Cisatracurium Besylate (Due to similar mechanism of action as vecuronium, it is expected that the neuromuscular blockade produced by other non-depolarizing muscle relaxants could be prolonged in the presence of piperacillin).
No products indexed under this heading.

Dalteparin Sodium (Coagulation parameters should be tested more frequently and monitored regularly during simultaneous administration; effect of concurrent use is not specified). Products include:
Fragmin Injection **2814**

Danaparoid Sodium (Coagulation parameters should be tested more frequently and monitored regularly during simultaneous administration; effect of concurrent use is not specified). Products include:
Orgaran Injection **2480**

Dicumarol (Coagulation parameters should be tested more frequently and monitored regularly during simultaneous administration; effect of concurrent use is not specified).
No products indexed under this heading.

Enoxaparin (Coagulation parameters should be tested more frequently and monitored regularly during simultaneous administration; effect of concurrent use is not specified). Products include:
Lovenox Injection **746**

Gentamicin Sulfate (The mixing of Zosyn with an aminoglycoside *in vitro* can result in substantial inactivation due to penicillin-aminoglycoside complex; this complex is microbiologically inactive and of unknown toxicity). Products include:
Genoptic Ophthalmic Ointment .... ⊙**239**
Genoptic Sterile Ophthalmic Solution .... ⊙**239**
Pred-G Ophthalmic Suspension .... ⊙**247**
Pred-G Sterile Ophthalmic Ointment .... ⊙**248**

Heparin Sodium (Coagulation parameters should be tested more frequently and monitored regularly during simultaneous administration; effect of concurrent use is not specified). Products include:
Heparin Lock Flush Solution **3509**
Heparin Sodium Injection **3511**

Kanamycin Sulfate (The mixing of Zosyn with an aminoglycoside *in vitro* can result in substantial inactivation due to penicillin-aminoglycoside complex; this complex is microbiologically inactive and of unknown toxicity).
No products indexed under this heading.

Metocurine Iodide (Due to similar mechanism of action as vecuronium, it is expected that the neuromuscular blockade produced by other non-depolarizing muscle relaxants could be prolonged in the presence of piperacillin).
No products indexed under this heading.

Mivacurium Chloride (Due to similar mechanism of action as vecuronium, it is expected that the neuromuscular blockade produced by other non-depolarizing muscle relaxants could be prolonged in the presence of piperacillin).
No products indexed under this heading.

Pancuronium Bromide (Due to similar mechanism of action as vecuronium, it is expected that the neuromuscular blockade produced by other non-depolarizing muscle relaxants could be prolonged in the presence of piperacillin).
No products indexed under this heading.

Probenecid (Concomitant administration prolongs half-life of piperacillin by 21% and of tazobactam by 71%).
No products indexed under this heading.

Rapacuronium Bromide (Due to similar mechanism of action as vecuronium, it is expected that the neuromuscular blockade produced by other non-depolarizing muscle relaxants could be prolonged in the presence of piperacillin).
No products indexed under this heading.

Rocuronium Bromide (Due to similar mechanism of action as vecuronium, it is expected that the neuromuscular blockade produced by other non-depolarizing muscle relaxants could be prolonged in the presence of piperacillin). Products include:

Zemuron Injection 2491

Streptomycin Sulfate (The mixing of Zosyn with an aminoglycoside *in vitro* can result in substantial inactivation due to penicillin-aminoglycoside complex; this complex is microbiologically inactive and of unknown toxicity). Products include:

Streptomycin Sulfate Injection 2714

Tinzaparin sodium (Coagulation parameters should be tested more frequently and monitored regularly during simultaneous administration; effect of concurrent use is not specified). Products include:

Innohep Injection 1248

Tobramycin (The mixing of Zosyn with an aminoglycoside *in vitro* can result in substantial inactivation due to penicillin-aminoglycoside complex; this complex is microbiologically inactive and of unknown toxicity). Products include:

TOBI Solution for Inhalation 1206
TobraDex Ophthalmic Ointment 542
TobraDex Ophthalmic Suspension .. 541
Tobrex Ophthalmic Ointment .... ⊙220
Tobrex Ophthalmic Solution .... ⊙221

Tobramycin Sulfate (Co-administration has resulted in the alteration of tobramycin pharmacokinetics which may be due to *in vitro* and *in vivo* inactivation of tobramycin). Products include:

Nebcin Vials, Hyporets & ADD-Vantage 1955

Vecuronium Bromide (Co-administration of piperacillin and vecuronium has been implicated in the prolongation of the neuromuscular blockade). Products include:

Norcuron for Injection 2478

Warfarin Sodium (Coagulation parameters should be tested more frequently and monitored regularly during simultaneous administration; effect of concurrent use is not specified). Products include:

Coumadin for Injection 1243
Coumadin Tablets 1243
Warfarin Sodium Tablets, USP 3302

ZOSYN IN GALAXY CONTAINERS

(Piperacillin Sodium, Tazobactam Sodium) 1894
See Zosyn

ZOVIA 1/35E TABLETS

(Ethinyl Estradiol, Ethynodiol Diacetate) 3449

May interact with barbiturates, phenytoin, tetracyclines, and certain other agents. Compounds in these categories include:

Ampicillin (Potential for reduced efficacy and increased incidence of breakthrough bleeding and menstrual irregularities with concomitant use).

No products indexed under this heading.

Ampicillin Sodium (Potential for reduced efficacy and increased incidence of breakthrough bleeding and menstrual irregularities with concomitant use). Products include:

Unasyn for Injection 2728

Aprobarbital (Potential for reduced efficacy and increased incidence of breakthrough bleeding and menstrual irregularities with concomitant use).

No products indexed under this heading.

Butabarbital (Potential for reduced efficacy and increased incidence of breakthrough bleeding and menstrual irregularities with concomitant use).

No products indexed under this heading.

Butalbital (Potential for reduced efficacy and increased incidence of breakthrough bleeding and menstrual irregularities with concomitant use). Products include:

Phrenilin 578
Sedapap Tablets 50 mg/650 mg ... 2225

Demeclocycline Hydrochloride (Potential for reduced efficacy and increased incidence of breakthrough bleeding and menstrual irregularities with concomitant use). Products include:

Declomycin Tablets 1855

Doxycycline Calcium (Potential for reduced efficacy and increased incidence of breakthrough bleeding and menstrual irregularities with concomitant use). Products include:

Vibramycin Calcium Oral Suspension Syrup 2735

Doxycycline Hyclate (Potential for reduced efficacy and increased incidence of breakthrough bleeding and menstrual irregularities with concomitant use). Products include:

Doryx Coated Pellet Filled Capsules 3357
Periostat Tablets 1208
Vibramycin Hyclate Capsules 2735
Vibramycin Hyclate Intravenous 2737
Vibra-Tabs Film Coated Tablets 2735

Doxycycline Monohydrate (Potential for reduced efficacy and increased incidence of breakthrough bleeding and menstrual irregularities with concomitant use). Products include:

Monodox Capsules 2442
Vibramycin Monohydrate for Oral Suspension 2735

Fosphenytoin Sodium (Potential for reduced efficacy and increased incidence of breakthrough bleeding and menstrual irregularities with concomitant use). Products include:

Cerebyx Injection 2619

Griseofulvin (Potential for reduced efficacy and increased incidence of breakthrough bleeding and menstrual irregularities with concomitant use). Products include:

Grifulvin V Tablets Microsize and Oral Suspension Microsize 2518
Gris-PEG Tablets 2661

Mephobarbital (Potential for reduced efficacy and increased incidence of breakthrough bleeding and menstrual irregularities with concomitant use).

No products indexed under this heading.

Methacycline Hydrochloride (Potential for reduced efficacy and increased incidence of breakthrough bleeding and menstrual irregularities with concomitant use).

No products indexed under this heading.

Minocycline Hydrochloride (Potential for reduced efficacy and increased incidence of breakthrough bleeding and menstrual irregularities with concomitant use). Products include:

Dynacin Capsules 2019
Minocin Intravenous 1862
Minocin Oral Suspension 1865
Minocin Pellet-Filled Capsules 1863

Oxytetracycline Hydrochloride (Potential for reduced efficacy and increased incidence of breakthrough bleeding and menstrual irregularities with concomitant use). Products include:

Terra-Cortril Ophthalmic Suspension 2716
Urobiotic-250 Capsules 2731

Pentobarbital Sodium (Potential for reduced efficacy and increased incidence of breakthrough bleeding and menstrual irregularities with concomitant use). Products include:

Nembutal Sodium Solution 485

Phenobarbital (Potential for reduced efficacy and increased incidence of breakthrough bleeding and menstrual irregularities with concomitant use). Products include:

Arco-Lase Plus Tablets 592
Donnatal 2929
Donnatal Extentabs 2930

Phenylbutazone (Potential for reduced efficacy and increased incidence of breakthrough bleeding and menstrual irregularities with concomitant use).

No products indexed under this heading.

Phenytoin (Potential for reduced efficacy and increased incidence of breakthrough bleeding and menstrual irregularities with concomitant use). Products include:

Dilantin Infatabs 2624
Dilantin-125 Oral Suspension 2625

Phenytoin Sodium (Potential for reduced efficacy and increased incidence of breakthrough bleeding and menstrual irregularities with concomitant use). Products include:

Dilantin Kapseals 2622

Rifampin (Co-administration has been associated with reduced efficacy and increased incidence of breakthrough bleeding and menstrual irregularities). Products include:

Rifadin 765
Rifamate Capsules 767
Rifater Tablets 769

Secobarbital Sodium (Potential for reduced efficacy and increased incidence of breakthrough bleeding and menstrual irregularities with concomitant use).

No products indexed under this heading.

Tetracycline Hydrochloride (Potential for reduced efficacy and increased incidence of breakthrough bleeding and menstrual irregularities with concomitant use).

No products indexed under this heading.

Thiamylal Sodium (Potential for reduced efficacy and increased incidence of breakthrough bleeding and menstrual irregularities with concomitant use).

No products indexed under this heading.

ZOVIA 1/50E TABLETS

(Ethinyl Estradiol, Ethynodiol Diacetate) 3449
See Zovia 1/35E Tablets

ZOVIRAX CAPSULES

(Acyclovir) 1706

May interact with:

Nephrotoxic Drugs (Increased risk of renal dysfunction).

No products indexed under this heading.

Probenecid (Co-administration of probenecid with intravenous acyclovir has been shown to increase acyclovir half-life and systemic exposure; urinary excretion and renal clearance were correspondingly reduced).

No products indexed under this heading.

ZOVIRAX FOR INJECTION

(Acyclovir Sodium) 1708
See Zovirax Capsules

ZOVIRAX OINTMENT

(Acyclovir) 1707
None cited in PDR database.

ZOVIRAX SUSPENSION

(Acyclovir) 1706
See Zovirax Capsules

ZOVIRAX TABLETS

(Acyclovir) 1706
See Zovirax Capsules

ZYBAN SUSTAINED-RELEASE TABLETS

(Bupropion Hydrochloride) 1710

May interact with antidepressant drugs, monoamine oxidase inhibitors, antipsychotic agents, phenytoin, drugs which lower seizure threshold, theophylline, and certain other agents. Compounds in these categories include:

Alprazolam (Bupropion is associated with dose-dependent risk of seizures; co-administration with drugs that lower seizure threshold may increase the risk of seizure with bupropion). Products include:

Xanax Tablets 2865

Aminophylline (Bupropion is associated with dose-dependent risk of seizures; co-administration with drugs that lower seizure threshold, such as theophylline, may increase the risk of seizure with bupropion).

No products indexed under this heading.

Amitriptyline Hydrochloride (Bupropion is associated with dose-dependent risk of seizures; co-administration with drugs that lower seizure threshold, such as antidepressants, may increase the risk of seizure with bupropion). Products include:

Etrafon 3115
Limbitrol 1738

Amoxapine (Bupropion is associated with dose-dependent risk of seizures; co-administration with drugs that lower seizure threshold, such as antidepressants, may increase the risk of seizure with bupropion).

No products indexed under this heading.

Bupropion (Zyban should not be used in combination with any other medications containing bupropion, such as Wellbutrin or Wellbutrin SR).

No products indexed under this heading.

Carbamazepine (May induce the metabolism of bupropion). Products include:

Carbatrol Capsules 3234
Tegretol/Tegretol-XR 2404

Chlordiazepoxide (Bupropion is associated with dose-dependent risk of seizures; co-administration with drugs that lower seizure threshold may increase the risk of seizure with bupropion). Products include:

Limbitrol 1738

Chlordiazepoxide Hydrochloride (Bupropion is associated with dose-dependent risk of seizures; co-administration with drugs that lower seizure threshold may increase the risk of seizure with bupropion). Products include:

Librium Capsules 1736
Librium for Injection 1737

Chlorpromazine (Bupropion is associated with dose-dependent risk of seizures; co-administration with drugs that lower seizure threshold, such as antipsychotics, may increase the risk of seizure with bupropion). Products include:

Thorazine Suppositories 1656

Chlorpromazine Hydrochloride (Bupropion is associated with dose-dependent risk of seizures; co-administration with drugs that lower seizure threshold, such as antipsychotics, may increase the risk of seizure with bupropion). Products include:

Thorazine 1656

Chlorprothixene (Bupropion is associated with dose-dependent risk of seizures; co-administration with drugs that lower seizure threshold, such as antipsychotics, may increase the risk of seizure with bupropion).
No products indexed under this heading.

Chlorprothixene Hydrochloride (Bupropion is associated with dose-dependent risk of seizures; co-administration with drugs that lower seizure threshold, such as antipsychotics, may increase the risk of seizure with bupropion).
No products indexed under this heading.

Cimetidine (May inhibit the metabolism of bupropion). Products include:
Tagamet HB 200 Suspension .... ▣ 762
Tagamet HB 200 Tablets .... ▣ 761
Tagamet Tablets 1644

Cimetidine Hydrochloride (May inhibit the metabolism of bupropion). Products include:
Tagamet 1644

Citalopram Hydrobromide (Bupropion is associated with dose-dependent risk of seizures; co-administration with drugs that lower seizure threshold, such as antidepressants, may increase the risk of seizure with bupropion). Products include:
Celexa 1365

Clozapine (Bupropion is associated with dose-dependent risk of seizures; co-administration with drugs that lower seizure threshold, such as antipsychotics, may increase the risk of seizure with bupropion). Products include:
Clozaril Tablets 2319

Cyclophosphamide (Bupropion is primarily metabolized, based on in vitro studies, to hydroxybupropion by the CYP2B6 isoenzyme, therefore the potential exists for a drug interaction with agents that affect the CYP2B6 isoenzyme metabolism, such as cyclophosphamide).
No products indexed under this heading.

Desipramine Hydrochloride (Co-administration in male subjects who were extensive metabolizers of the CYP2D6 isoenzyme daily doses of bupropion followed by a single dose of desipramine increased the Cmax, AUC and t1/2 of desipramine by an average of approximately two-, five-, and two-fold respectively; co-administration should be initiated at the lower end of the dose range of desipriamine; potential for increased risk of seizures). Products include:
Norpramin Tablets 755

Diazepam (Bupropion is associated with dose-dependent risk of seizures; co-administration with drugs that lower seizure threshold may increase the risk of seizure with bupropion). Products include:
Valium Injectable 3026
Valium Tablets 3047

Doxepin Hydrochloride (Bupropion is associated with dose-dependent risk of seizures; co-administration with drugs that lower seizure threshold, such as antidepressants, may increase the risk of seizure with bupropion). Products include:
Sinequan 2713

Dyphylline (Bupropion is associated with dose-dependent risk of seizures; co-administration with drugs that lower seizure threshold, such as theophylline, may increase the risk of seizure with bupropion). Products include:
Lufyllin Tablets 3347
Lufyllin-400 Tablets 3347
Lufyllin-GG Elixir 3348
Lufyllin-GG Tablets 3348

Flecainide Acetate (Co-administration of bupropion with drugs that are metabolized by CYP2D6 isoenzyme, such as flecainide, may result in, based on data with desipramine, increased Cmax, AUC and t1/2; co-administration should be initiated at the lower end of the dose range of flecainide). Products include:
Tambocor Tablets 1990

Fluoxetine Hydrochloride (Co-administration of bupropion with drugs that are metabolized by CYP2D6 isoenzyme, such as fluoxetine, may result in, based on data with desipramine, increased Cmax, AUC and t1/2; co-administration should be initiated at the lower end of the dose range of fluoxetine). Products include:
Prozac Pulvules, Liquid, and Weekly Capsules 1238
Sarafem Pulvules 1962

Fluphenazine Decanoate (Bupropion is associated with dose-dependent risk of seizures; co-administration with drugs that lower seizure threshold, such as antipsychotics, may increase the risk of seizure with bupropion).
No products indexed under this heading.

Fluphenazine Enanthate (Bupropion is associated with dose-dependent risk of seizures; co-administration with drugs that lower seizure threshold, such as antipsychotics, may increase the risk of seizure with bupropion).
No products indexed under this heading.

Fluphenazine Hydrochloride (Bupropion is associated with dose-dependent risk of seizures; co-administration with drugs that lower seizure threshold, such as antipsychotics, may increase the risk of seizure with bupropion).
No products indexed under this heading.

Fosphenytoin Sodium (May induce the metabolism of bupropion). Products include:
Cerebyx Injection 2619

Haloperidol (Co-administration of bupropion with drugs that are metabolized by CYP2D6 isoenzyme, such as haloperidol, may result in, based on data with desipramine, increased Cmax, AUC and t1/2; co-administration should be initiated at the lower end of the dose range of haloperidol; potential for increased risk of seizures). Products include:
Haldol Injection, Tablets and Concentrate 2533

Haloperidol Decanoate (Co-administration of bupropion with drugs that are metabolized by CYP2D6 isoenzyme, such as haloperidol, may result in, based on data with desipramine, increased Cmax, AUC and t1/2; co-administration should be initiated at the lower end of the dose range of haloperidol; potential for increased risk of seizures). Products include:
Haldol Decanoate 2535

Imipramine Hydrochloride (Co-administration of bupropion with drugs that are metabolized by CYP2D6 isoenzyme, such as imipramine, may result in, based on data with desipramine, increased Cmax, AUC and t1/2; co-administration should be initiated at the lower end of the dose range of imipramine; potential for increased risk of seizures).
No products indexed under this heading.

Imipramine Pamoate (Co-administration of bupropion with drugs that are metabolized by CYP2D6 isoenzyme, such as imipramine, may result in, based on data with desipramine, increased Cmax, AUC and t1/2; co-administration should be initiated at the lower end of the dose range of imipramine; potential for increased risk of seizures).
No products indexed under this heading.

Isocarboxazid (Bupropion is associated with dose-dependent risk of seizures; co-administration with drugs that lower seizure threshold, such as antidepressants, may increase the risk of seizure with bupropion).
No products indexed under this heading.

Levodopa (Co-administration has resulted in a higher incidence of adverse experiences). Products include:
Sinemet Tablets 1253
Sinemet CR Tablets 1255

Lithium Carbonate (Bupropion is associated with dose-dependent risk of seizures; co-administration with drugs that lower seizure threshold, such as antipsychotics, may increase the risk of seizure with bupropion). Products include:
Eskalith 1527
Lithium Carbonate 3061
Lithobid Slow-Release Tablets 3255

Lithium Citrate (Bupropion is associated with dose-dependent risk of seizures; co-administration with drugs that lower seizure threshold, such as antipsychotics, may increase the risk of seizure with bupropion). Products include:
Lithium Citrate Syrup 3061

Lorazepam (Bupropion is associated with dose-dependent risk of seizures; co-administration with drugs that lower seizure threshold may increase the risk of seizure with bupropion). Products include:
Ativan Injection 3478
Ativan Tablets 3482

Loxapine Hydrochloride (Bupropion is associated with dose-dependent risk of seizures; co-administration with drugs that lower seizure threshold, such as antipsychotics, may increase the risk of seizure with bupropion).
No products indexed under this heading.

Loxapine Succinate (Bupropion is associated with dose-dependent risk of seizures; co-administration with drugs that lower seizure threshold, such as antipsychotics, may increase the risk of seizure with bupropion). Products include:
Loxitane Capsules 3398

Maprotiline Hydrochloride (Bupropion is associated with dose-dependent risk of seizures; co-administration with drugs that lower seizure threshold, such as antidepressants, may increase the risk of seizure with bupropion).
No products indexed under this heading.

Mesoridazine Besylate (Bupropion is associated with dose-dependent risk of seizures; co-administration with drugs that lower seizure threshold, such as antipsychotics, may increase the risk of seizure with bupropion). Products include:
Serentil 1057

Methotrimeprazine (Bupropion is associated with dose-dependent risk of seizures; co-administration with drugs that lower seizure threshold, such as antipsychotics, may increase the risk of seizure with bupropion).
No products indexed under this heading.

Metoprolol Succinate (Co-administration of bupropion with drugs that are metabolized by CYP2D6 isoenzyme, such as metoprolol, may result in, based on data with desipramine, increased Cmax, AUC and t1/2; co-administration should be initiated at the lower end of the dose range of metoprolol). Products include:
Toprol-XL Tablets 651

Metoprolol Tartrate (Co-administration of bupropion with drugs that are metabolized by CYP2D6 isoenzyme, such as metoprolol, may result in, based on data with desipramine, increased Cmax, AUC and t1/2; co-administration should be initiated at the lower end of the dose range of metoprolol).
No products indexed under this heading.

Mirtazapine (Bupropion is associated with dose-dependent risk of seizures; co-administration with drugs that lower seizure threshold, such as antidepressants, may increase the risk of seizure with bupropion). Products include:
Remeron Tablets 2483
Remeron SolTab Tablets 2486

Moclobemide (Concurrent and/or sequential use with MAO inhibitor is contraindicated).
No products indexed under this heading.

Molindone Hydrochloride (Bupropion is associated with dose-dependent risk of seizures; co-administration with drugs that lower seizure threshold, such as antipsychotics, may increase the risk of seizure with bupropion). Products include:
Moban 1320

Nefazodone Hydrochloride (Bupropion is associated with dose-dependent risk of seizures; co-administration with drugs that lower seizure threshold, such as antidepressants, may increase the risk of seizure with bupropion). Products include:
Serzone Tablets 1104

Nicotine (Co-administration of bupropion and nicotine transdermal system has resulted in a higher incidence of treatment-emergent hypertension). Products include:
Nicoderm CQ Patch 1717
Nicotrol Inhaler 2840
Nicotrol Nasal Spray 2843
Nicotrol Patch 2840

Nortriptyline Hydrochloride (Co-administration of bupropion with drugs that are metabolized by CYP2D6 isoenzyme, such as nortriptyline, may result in, based on data with desipramine, increased Cmax, AUC and t1/2; co-administration should be initiated at the lower end of the dose range of nortriptyline; potential for increased risk of seizures).
No products indexed under this heading.

Olanzapine (Bupropion is associated with dose-dependent risk of seizures; co-administration with drugs that lower seizure threshold, such as antipsychotics, may increase the risk of seizure with bupropion). Products include:
Zyprexa Tablets 1973
Zyprexa ZYDIS Orally Disintegrating Tablets 1973

Orphenadrine Citrate (Bupropion is primarily metabolized, based on in vitro studies, to hydroxybupropion by the CYP2B6 isoenzyme, therefore the potential exists for a drug interaction with agents that affect the CYP2B6 isoenzyme metabolism, such as orphenadrine). Products include:
Norflex 1987

Oxazepam (Bupropion is associated with dose-dependent risk of seizures; co-administration with drugs that lower seizure threshold may increase the risk of seizure with bupropion).
No products indexed under this heading.

Pargyline Hydrochloride (Concurrent and/or sequential use with MAO inhibitor is contraindicated).
No products indexed under this heading.

Paroxetine Hydrochloride (Co-administration of bupropion with drugs that are metabolized by CYP2D6 isoenzyme, such as paroxetine, may result in, based on data with desipramine, increased Cmax, AUC and t1/2; co-administration should be initiated at the lower end of the dose range of paroxetine). Products include:
Paxil 1609

Perphenazine (Bupropion is associated with dose-dependent risk of seizures; co-administration with drugs that lower seizure threshold, such as antipsychotics, may increase the risk of seizure with bupropion). Products include:
Etrafon 3115
Trilafon 3160

Phenelzine Sulfate (Concurrent and/or sequential use with MAO inhibitor is contraindicated; acute toxicity of bupropion is enhanced by phenelzine in animal models). Products include:
Nardil Tablets 2653

Phenobarbital (May induce the metabolism of bupropion). Products include:
Arco-Lase Plus Tablets 592
Donnatal 2929
Donnatal Extentabs 2930

Phenytoin (May induce the metabolism of bupropion). Products include:
Dilantin Infatabs 2624
Dilantin-125 Oral Suspension 2625

Phenytoin Sodium (May induce the metabolism of bupropion). Products include:
Dilantin Kapseals 2622

Pimozide (Bupropion is associated with dose-dependent risk of seizures; co-administration with drugs that lower seizure threshold, such as antipsychotics, may increase the risk of seizure with bupropion). Products include:
Orap Tablets 1407

Prazepam (Bupropion is associated with dose-dependent risk of seizures; co-administration with drugs that lower seizure threshold may increase the risk of seizure with bupropion).
No products indexed under this heading.

Procarbazine Hydrochloride (Concurrent and/or sequential use with MAO inhibitor is contraindicated). Products include:
Matulane Capsules 3246

Prochlorperazine (Bupropion is associated with dose-dependent risk of seizures; co-administration with drugs that lower seizure threshold, such as antipsychotics, may increase the risk of seizure with bupropion). Products include:
Compazine 1505

Promethazine Hydrochloride (Bupropion is associated with dose-dependent risk of seizures; co-administration with drugs that lower seizure threshold, such as antipsychotics, may increase the risk of seizure with bupropion). Products include:
Mepergan Injection 3539
Phenergan Injection 3553
Phenergan 3556
Phenergan Syrup 3554
Phenergan with Codeine Syrup 3557
Phenergan with Dextromethorphan Syrup 3559
Phenergan VC Syrup 3560
Phenergan VC with Codeine Syrup 3561

Propafenone Hydrochloride (Co-administration of bupropion with drugs that are metabolized by CYP2D6 isoenzyme, such as propafenone, may result in, based on data with desipramine, increased Cmax, AUC and t1/2; co-administration should be initiated at the lower end of the dose range of propafenone). Products include:
Rythmol Tablets – 150 mg, 225 mg, 300 mg 502

Protriptyline Hydrochloride (Bupropion is associated with dose-dependent risk of seizures; co-administration with drugs that lower seizure threshold, such as antidepressants, may increase the risk of seizure with bupropion). Products include:
Vivactil Tablets 2446
Vivactil Tablets 2217

Quetiapine Fumarate (Bupropion is associated with dose-dependent risk of seizures; co-administration with drugs that lower seizure threshold, such as antipsychotics, may increase the risk of seizure with bupropion). Products include:
Seroquel Tablets 684

Risperidone (Co-administration of bupropion with drugs that are metabolized by CYP2D6 isoenzyme, such as risperidone, may result in, based on data with desipramine, increased Cmax, AUC and t1/2; co-administration should be initiated at the lower end of the dose range of risperidone; potential for increased risk of seizures). Products include:
Risperdal 1796

Selegiline Hydrochloride (Concurrent and/or sequential use with MAO inhibitor is contraindicated). Products include:
Eldepryl Capsules 3266

Sertraline Hydrochloride (Co-administration of bupropion with drugs that are metabolized by CYP2D6 isoenzyme, such as sertraline, may result in, based on data with desipramine, increased Cmax, AUC and t1/2; co-administration should be initiated at the lower end of the dose range of sertraline). Products include:
Zoloft 2751

Theophylline (Bupropion is associated with dose-dependent risk of seizures; co-administration with drugs that lower seizure threshold, such as theophylline, may increase the risk of seizure with bupropion). Products include:
Aerolate 1361
Theo-Dur Extended-Release Tablets 1835
Uni-Dur Extended-Release Tablets 1841
Uniphyl 400 mg and 600 mg Tablets 2903

Theophylline Calcium Salicylate (Bupropion is associated with dose-dependent risk of seizures; co-administration with drugs that lower seizure threshold, such as theophylline, may increase the risk of seizure with bupropion).
No products indexed under this heading.

Theophylline Sodium Glycinate (Bupropion is associated with dose-dependent risk of seizures; co-administration with drugs that lower seizure threshold, such as theophylline, may increase the risk of seizure with bupropion).
No products indexed under this heading.

Thioridazine Hydrochloride (Co-administration of bupropion with drugs that are metabolized by CYP2D6 isoenzyme, such as thioridazine, may result in, based on data with desipramine, increased Cmax, AUC and t1/2; co-administration should be initiated at the lower end of the dose range of thioridazine; potential for increased risk of seizures). Products include:
Thioridazine Hydrochloride Tablets 2289

Thiothixene (Bupropion is associated with dose-dependent risk of seizures; co-administration with drugs that lower seizure threshold, such as antipsychotics, may increase the risk of seizure with bupropion). Products include:
Navane Capsules 2701
Thiothixene Capsules 2290

Tranylcypromine Sulfate (Bupropion is associated with dose-dependent risk of seizures; co-administration with drugs that lower seizure threshold, such as antidepressants, may increase the risk of seizure with bupropion). Products include:
Parnate Tablets 1607

Trazodone Hydrochloride (Bupropion is associated with dose-dependent risk of seizures; co-administration with drugs that lower seizure threshold, such as antidepressants, may increase the risk of seizure with bupropion).
No products indexed under this heading.

Trifluoperazine Hydrochloride (Bupropion is associated with dose-dependent risk of seizures; co-administration with drugs that lower seizure threshold, such as antipsychotics, may increase the risk of seizure with bupropion). Products include:
Stelazine 1640

Trimipramine Maleate (Bupropion is associated with dose-dependent risk of seizures; co-administration with drugs that lower seizure threshold, such as antidepressants, may increase the risk of seizure with bupropion). Products include:
Surmontil Capsules 3595

Venlafaxine Hydrochloride (Bupropion is associated with dose-dependent risk of seizures; co-administration with drugs that lower seizure threshold, such as antidepressants, may increase the risk of seizure with bupropion). Products include:
Effexor Tablets 3495
Effexor XR Capsules 3499

Ziprasidone Hydrochloride (Bupropion is associated with dose-dependent risk of seizures; co-administration with drugs that lower seizure threshold, such as antipsychotics, may increase the risk of seizure with bupropion). Products include:
Geodon Capsules 2688

Food Interactions

Alcohol (Bupropion is associated with dose-dependent risk of seizures; excessive use of alcohol or abrupt withdrawal of alcohol is associated with an increased seizure risk).

Food, unspecified (Food increases Cmax and AUC of bupropion by 11% and 17% respectively; the mean time to peak concentration Tmax was prolonged by 1 hour; this effect was of no clinical significance).

ZYDONE TABLETS

(Acetaminophen, Hydrocodone Bitartrate) 1330
May interact with anticholinergics, central nervous system depressants, monoamine oxidase inhibitors, narcotic analgesics, tricyclic antidepressants, and certain other agents. Compounds in these categories include:

Alfentanil Hydrochloride (Co-administration may exhibit additive CNS depression).
No products indexed under this heading.

Alprazolam (Co-administration may exhibit additive CNS depression). Products include:
Xanax Tablets 2865

Amitriptyline Hydrochloride (Co-administration of tricyclic antidepressants with hydrocodone may increase the effect of either hydrocodone or antidepressant). Products include:
Etrafon 3115
Limbitrol 1738

Amoxapine (Co-administration of tricyclic antidepressants with hydrocodone may increase the effect of either hydrocodone or antidepressant).
No products indexed under this heading.

Aprobarbital (Co-administration may exhibit additive CNS depression).
No products indexed under this heading.

Atropine Sulfate (Co-administration may produce paralytic ileus). Products include:
Donnatal 2929
Donnatal Extentabs 2930
Motofen Tablets 577
Prosed/DS Tablets 3268
Urised Tablets 2876

Belladonna Alkaloids (Co-administration may produce paralytic ileus). Products include:
Hyland's Teething Tablets 766
Urimax Tablets 1769

Benztropine Mesylate (Co-administration may produce paralytic ileus). Products include:
Cogentin 2055

Biperiden Hydrochloride (Co-administration may produce paralytic ileus). Products include:
Akineton 402

Buprenorphine Hydrochloride (Co-administration may exhibit additive CNS depression). Products include:
Buprenex Injectable 2918

Buspirone Hydrochloride (Co-administration may exhibit additive CNS depression).
No products indexed under this heading.

Butabarbital (Co-administration may exhibit additive CNS depression).
No products indexed under this heading.

Butalbital (Co-administration may exhibit additive CNS depression). Products include:
Phrenilin 578
Sedapap Tablets 50 mg/650 mg 2225

Chlordiazepoxide (Co-administration may exhibit additive CNS depression). Products include:
Limbitrol 1738

Chlordiazepoxide Hydrochloride (Co-administration may exhibit additive CNS depression). Products include:
Librium Capsules 1736
Librium for Injection 1737

Chlorpromazine (Co-administration may exhibit additive CNS depression). Products include:
Thorazine Suppositories 1656

Chlorpromazine Hydrochloride (Co-administration may exhibit additive CNS depression). Products include:
Thorazine 1656

Chlorprothixene (Co-administration may exhibit additive CNS depression).
No products indexed under this heading.

Chlorprothixene Hydrochloride (Co-administration may exhibit addi-

tive CNS depression).
No products indexed under this heading.

Chlorprothixene Lactate (Co-administration may exhibit additive CNS depression).
No products indexed under this heading.

Clidinium Bromide (Co-administration may produce paralytic ileus).
No products indexed under this heading.

Clomipramine Hydrochloride (Co-administration of tricyclic antidepressants with hydrocodone may increase the effect of either hydrocodone or antidepressant).
No products indexed under this heading.

Clorazepate Dipotassium (Co-administration may exhibit additive CNS depression). Products include:
Tranxene 511

Clozapine (Co-administration may exhibit additive CNS depression). Products include:
Clozaril Tablets 2319

Codeine Phosphate (Co-administration may exhibit additive CNS depression). Products include:
Phenergan with Codeine Syrup 3557
Phenergan VC with Codeine Syrup .. 3561
Robitussin A-C Syrup 2942
Robitussin-DAC Syrup 2942
Ryna-C Liquid .... ▣ 768
Soma Compound w/Codeine Tablets 3355
Tussi-Organidin NR Liquid 3350
Tussi-Organidin-S NR Liquid 3350
Tylenol with Codeine 2595

Desflurane (Co-administration may exhibit additive CNS depression). Products include:
Suprane Liquid for Inhalation 874

Desipramine Hydrochloride (Co-administration of tricyclic antidepressants with hydrocodone may increase the effect of either hydrocodone or antidepressant). Products include:
Norpramin Tablets 755

Dezocine (Co-administration may exhibit additive CNS depression).
No products indexed under this heading.

Diazepam (Co-administration may exhibit additive CNS depression). Products include:
Valium Injectable 3026
Valium Tablets 3047

Dicyclomine Hydrochloride (Co-administration may produce paralytic ileus).
No products indexed under this heading.

Doxepin Hydrochloride (Co-administration of tricyclic antidepressants with hydrocodone may increase the effect of either hydrocodone or antidepressant). Products include:
Sinequan 2713

Droperidol (Co-administration may exhibit additive CNS depression).
No products indexed under this heading.

Enflurane (Co-administration may exhibit additive CNS depression).
No products indexed under this heading.

Estazolam (Co-administration may exhibit additive CNS depression). Products include:
ProSom Tablets 500

Ethchlorvynol (Co-administration may exhibit additive CNS depression).
No products indexed under this heading.

Ethinamate (Co-administration may exhibit additive CNS depression).
No products indexed under this heading.

Fentanyl (Co-administration may exhibit additive CNS depression). Products include:
Duragesic Transdermal System 1786

Fentanyl Citrate (Co-administration may exhibit additive CNS depression). Products include:
Actiq 1184

Fluphenazine Decanoate (Co-administration may exhibit additive CNS depression).
No products indexed under this heading.

Fluphenazine Enanthate (Co-administration may exhibit additive CNS depression).
No products indexed under this heading.

Fluphenazine Hydrochloride (Co-administration may exhibit additive CNS depression).
No products indexed under this heading.

Flurazepam Hydrochloride (Co-administration may exhibit additive CNS depression).
No products indexed under this heading.

Glutethimide (Co-administration may exhibit additive CNS depression).
No products indexed under this heading.

Glycopyrrolate (Co-administration may produce paralytic ileus). Products include:
Robinul Forte Tablets 1358
Robinul Injectable 2940
Robinul Tablets 1358

Haloperidol (Co-administration may exhibit additive CNS depression). Products include:
Haldol Injection, Tablets and Concentrate 2533

Haloperidol Decanoate (Co-administration may exhibit additive CNS depression). Products include:
Haldol Decanoate 2535

Hydrocodone Polistirex (Co-administration may exhibit additive CNS depression). Products include:
Tussionex Pennkinetic Extended-Release Suspension 1174

Hydromorphone Hydrochloride (Co-administration may exhibit additive CNS depression). Products include:
Dilaudid 441
Dilaudid Oral Liquid 445
Dilaudid Powder 441
Dilaudid Rectal Suppositories 441
Dilaudid Tablets 441
Dilaudid Tablets - 8 mg 445
Dilaudid-HP 443

Hydroxyzine Hydrochloride (Co-administration may exhibit additive CNS depression). Products include:
Atarax Tablets & Syrup 2667
Vistaril Intramuscular Solution 2738

Hyoscyamine (Co-administration may produce paralytic ileus). Products include:
Urised Tablets 2876

Hyoscyamine Sulfate (Co-administration may produce paralytic ileus). Products include:
Arco-Lase Plus Tablets 592
Donnatal 2929
Donnatal Extentabs 2930
Levsin/Levsinex/Levbid 3172
NuLev Orally Disintegrating Tablets 3176
Prosed/DS Tablets 3268
Urimax Tablets 1769

Imipramine Hydrochloride (Co-administration of tricyclic antidepressants with hydrocodone may increase the effect of either hydrocodone or antidepressant).
No products indexed under this heading.

Imipramine Pamoate (Co-administration of tricyclic antidepressants with hydrocodone may increase the effect of either hydrocodone or antidepressant).
No products indexed under this heading.

Ipratropium Bromide (Co-administration may produce paralytic ileus). Products include:
Atrovent Inhalation Aerosol 1030
Atrovent Inhalation Solution 1031
Atrovent Nasal Spray 0.03% 1032
Atrovent Nasal Spray 0.06% 1033
Combivent Inhalation Aerosol 1041
DuoNeb Inhalation Solution 1233

Isocarboxazid (Co-administration of MAO inhibitors with hydrocodone may increase the effect of either hydrocodone or MAO inhibitor).
No products indexed under this heading.

Isoflurane (Co-administration may exhibit additive CNS depression).
No products indexed under this heading.

Ketamine Hydrochloride (Co-administration may exhibit additive CNS depression).
No products indexed under this heading.

Levomethadyl Acetate Hydrochloride (Co-administration may exhibit additive CNS depression).
No products indexed under this heading.

Levorphanol Tartrate (Co-administration may exhibit additive CNS depression). Products include:
Levo-Dromoran 1734
Levorphanol Tartrate Tablets 3059

Lorazepam (Co-administration may exhibit additive CNS depression). Products include:
Ativan Injection 3478
Ativan Tablets 3482

Loxapine Hydrochloride (Co-administration may exhibit additive CNS depression).
No products indexed under this heading.

Loxapine Succinate (Co-administration may exhibit additive CNS depression). Products include:
Loxitane Capsules 3398

Maprotiline Hydrochloride (Co-administration of tricyclic antidepressants with hydrocodone may increase the effect of either hydrocodone or antidepressant).
No products indexed under this heading.

Mepenzolate Bromide (Co-administration may produce paralytic ileus).
No products indexed under this heading.

Meperidine Hydrochloride (Co-administration may exhibit additive CNS depression). Products include:
Demerol 3079
Mepergan Injection 3539

Mephobarbital (Co-administration may exhibit additive CNS depression).
No products indexed under this heading.

Meprobamate (Co-administration may exhibit additive CNS depression). Products include:
Miltown Tablets 3349

Mesoridazine Besylate (Co-administration may exhibit additive CNS depression). Products include:
Serentil 1057

Methadone Hydrochloride (Co-administration may exhibit additive CNS depression). Products include:
Dolophine Hydrochloride Tablets 3056

Methohexital Sodium (Co-administration may exhibit additive CNS depression). Products include:
Brevital Sodium for Injection, USP .. 1815

Methotrimeprazine (Co-administration may exhibit additive CNS depression).
No products indexed under this heading.

Methoxyflurane (Co-administration may exhibit additive CNS depression).
No products indexed under this heading.

Midazolam Hydrochloride (Co-administration may exhibit additive CNS depression). Products include:
Versed Injection 3027
Versed Syrup 3033

Moclobemide (Co-administration of MAO inhibitors with hydrocodone may increase the effect of either hydrocodone or MAO inhibitor).
No products indexed under this heading.

Molindone Hydrochloride (Co-administration may exhibit additive CNS depression). Products include:
Moban 1320

Morphine Sulfate (Co-administration may exhibit additive CNS depression). Products include:
Astramorph/PF Injection, USP (Preservative-Free) 594
Duramorph Injection 1312
Infumorph 200 and Infumorph 500 Sterile Solutions 1314
Kadian Capsules 1335
MS Contin Tablets 2896
MSIR 2898
Oramorph SR Tablets 3062
Roxanol 3066

Nortriptyline Hydrochloride (Co-administration of tricyclic antidepressants with hydrocodone may increase the effect of either hydrocodone or antidepressant).
No products indexed under this heading.

Olanzapine (Co-administration may exhibit additive CNS depression). Products include:
Zyprexa Tablets 1973
Zyprexa ZYDIS Orally Disintegrating Tablets 1973

Oxazepam (Co-administration may exhibit additive CNS depression).
No products indexed under this heading.

Oxybutynin Chloride (Co-administration may produce paralytic ileus). Products include:
Ditropan XL Extended Release Tablets 564

Oxycodone Hydrochloride (Co-administration may exhibit additive CNS depression). Products include:
OxyContin Tablets 2912
OxyFast Oral Concentrate Solution . 2916
OxyIR Capsules 2916
Percocet Tablets 1326
Percodan Tablets 1327
Percolone Tablets 1327
Roxicodone 3067
Tylox Capsules 2597

Pargyline Hydrochloride (Co-administration of MAO inhibitors with hydrocodone may increase the effect of either hydrocodone or MAO inhibitor).
No products indexed under this heading.

Pentobarbital Sodium (Co-administration may exhibit additive CNS depression). Products include:
Nembutal Sodium Solution 485

Perphenazine (Co-administration may exhibit additive CNS depression). Products include:
Etrafon 3115
Trilafon 3160

Phenelzine Sulfate (Co-administration of MAO inhibitors with hydrocodone may increase the effect of either hydrocodone or MAO inhibitor). Products include:
Nardil Tablets 2653

Phenobarbital (Co-administration may exhibit additive CNS depression). Products include:
Arco-Lase Plus Tablets 592
Donnatal 2929
Donnatal Extentabs 2930

Prazepam (Co-administration may exhibit additive CNS depression).
No products indexed under this heading.

Procarbazine Hydrochloride (Co-administration of MAO inhibitors with hydrocodone may increase the effect of either hydrocodone or MAO inhibitor). Products include:
Matulane Capsules 3246

Prochlorperazine (Co-administration may exhibit additive CNS depression). Products include:
Compazine 1505

Procyclidine Hydrochloride (Co-administration may produce paralytic ileus).
No products indexed under this heading.

Promethazine Hydrochloride (Co-administration may exhibit additive CNS depression). Products include:
Mepergan Injection 3539
Phenergan Injection 3553
Phenergan 3556
Phenergan Syrup 3554
Phenergan with Codeine Syrup 3557
Phenergan with Dextromethorphan Syrup 3559
Phenergan VC Syrup 3560
Phenergan VC with Codeine Syrup .. 3561

Propantheline Bromide (Co-administration may produce paralytic ileus).
No products indexed under this heading.

Propofol (Co-administration may exhibit additive CNS depression). Products include:
Diprivan Injectable Emulsion 667

Propoxyphene Hydrochloride (Co-administration may exhibit additive CNS depression). Products include:
Darvon Pulvules 1909
Darvon Compound-65 Pulvules 1910

Propoxyphene Napsylate (Co-administration may exhibit additive CNS depression). Products include:
Darvon-N/Darvocet-N 1907
Darvon-N Tablets 1912

Protriptyline Hydrochloride (Co-administration of tricyclic antidepressants with hydrocodone may increase the effect of either hydrocodone or antidepressant). Products include:
Vivactil Tablets 2446
Vivactil Tablets 2217

Quazepam (Co-administration may exhibit additive CNS depression).
No products indexed under this heading.

Quetiapine Fumarate (Co-administration may exhibit additive CNS depression). Products include:
Seroquel Tablets 684

Remifentanil Hydrochloride (Co-administration may exhibit additive CNS depression).
No products indexed under this heading.

Risperidone (Co-administration may exhibit additive CNS depression). Products include:
Risperdal 1796

Scopolamine (Co-administration may produce paralytic ileus). Products include:
Transderm Scōp Transdermal Therapeutic System 2302

Scopolamine Hydrobromide (Co-administration may produce paralytic ileus). Products include:
Donnatal 2929
Donnatal Extentabs 2930

Secobarbital Sodium (Co-administration may exhibit additive CNS depression).
No products indexed under this heading.

Selegiline Hydrochloride (Co-administration of MAO inhibitors with hydrocodone may increase the effect of either hydrocodone or MAO inhibitor). Products include:
Eldepryl Capsules 3266

Sevoflurane (Co-administration may exhibit additive CNS depression).
No products indexed under this heading.

Sufentanil Citrate (Co-administration may exhibit additive CNS depression).
No products indexed under this heading.

Temazepam (Co-administration may exhibit additive CNS depression).
No products indexed under this heading.

Thiamylal Sodium (Co-administration may exhibit additive CNS depression).
No products indexed under this heading.

Thioridazine Hydrochloride (Co-administration may exhibit additive CNS depression). Products include:
Thioridazine Hydrochloride Tablets 2289

Thiothixene (Co-administration may exhibit additive CNS depression). Products include:
Navane Capsules 2701
Thiothixene Capsules 2290

Tolterodine Tartrate (Co-administration may produce paralytic ileus). Products include:
Detrol Tablets 3623
Detrol LA Capsules 2801

Tranylcypromine Sulfate (Co-administration of MAO inhibitors with hydrocodone may increase the effect of either hydrocodone or MAO inhibitor). Products include:
Parnate Tablets 1607

Triazolam (Co-administration may exhibit additive CNS depression). Products include:
Halcion Tablets 2823

Tridihexethyl Chloride (Co-administration may produce paralytic ileus).
No products indexed under this heading.

Trifluoperazine Hydrochloride (Co-administration may exhibit additive CNS depression). Products include:
Stelazine 1640

Trihexyphenidyl Hydrochloride (Co-administration may produce paralytic ileus). Products include:
Artane 1855

Trimipramine Maleate (Co-administration of tricyclic antidepressants with hydrocodone may increase the effect of either hydrocodone or antidepressant). Products include:
Surmontil Capsules 3595

Zaleplon (Co-administration may exhibit additive CNS depression). Products include:
Sonata Capsules 3591

Ziprasidone Hydrochloride (Co-administration may exhibit additive CNS depression). Products include:
Geodon Capsules 2688

Zolpidem Tartrate (Co-administration may exhibit additive CNS depression). Products include:
Ambien Tablets 3191

Food Interactions

Alcohol (Co-administration may exhibit additive CNS depression).

ZYFLO FILMTAB TABLETS

(Zileuton) 524
May interact with theophylline and certain other agents. Compounds in these categories include:

Aminophylline (Co-administration with theophylline results in, on average, an approximate doubling of serum theophylline concentrations; theophylline dosage in these patients should be reduced and serum theophylline concentrations monitored closely).
No products indexed under this heading.

Dyphylline (Co-administration with theophylline results in, on average, an approximate doubling of serum theophylline concentrations; theophylline dosage in these patients should be reduced and serum theophylline concentrations monitored closely). Products include:
Lufyllin Tablets 3347
Lufyllin-400 Tablets 3347
Lufyllin-GG Elixir 3348
Lufyllin-GG Tablets 3348

Propranolol Hydrochloride (Co-administration results in a significant increase in propranolol concentrations and consequent increase in beta-blocker activity). Products include:
Inderal 3513
Inderal LA Long-Acting Capsules 3516
Inderide Tablets 3517
Inderide LA Long-Acting Capsules .. 3519

Terfenadine (Co-administration of multiple doses for 7 days has resulted in a decrease in clearance of terfenadine by 22% leading to a statistically significant increase in mean AUC and Cmax of terfenadine).
No products indexed under this heading.

Theophylline (Co-administration with theophylline results in, on average, an approximate doubling of serum theophylline concentrations; theophylline dosage in these patients should be reduced and serum theophylline concentrations monitored closely). Products include:
Aerolate 1361
Theo-Dur Extended-Release Tablets 1835
Uni-Dur Extended-Release Tablets .. 1841
Uniphyl 400 mg and 600 mg Tablets 2903

Theophylline Calcium Salicylate (Co-administration with theophylline results in, on average, an approximate doubling of serum theophylline concentrations; theophylline dosage in these patients should be reduced and serum theophylline concentrations monitored closely).
No products indexed under this heading.

Theophylline Sodium Glycinate (Co-administration with theophylline results in, on average, an approximate doubling of serum theophylline concentrations; theophylline dosage in these patients should be reduced and serum theophylline concentrations monitored closely).
No products indexed under this heading.

Warfarin Sodium (Co-administration results in a clinically significant increase in prothrombin time). Products include:
Coumadin for Injection 1243
Coumadin Tablets 1243
Warfarin Sodium Tablets, USP 3302

Food Interactions

Food, unspecified (Co-administration has resulted in a small but statistically significant increase (27%) in zileuton Cmax without significant changes in the extent of absorption (AUC) or Tmax; zileuton can be administered with or without food).

ZYPREXA TABLETS

(Olanzapine) 1973
May interact with antihypertensives, dopamine agonists, and certain other agents. Compounds in these categories include:

Acebutolol Hydrochloride (Olanzapine, because of its potential for inducing hypotension, may enhance the effects of certain antihypertensive agents). Products include:
Sectral Capsules 3589

Amlodipine Besylate (Olanzapine, because of its potential for inducing hypotension, may enhance the effects of certain antihypertensive agents). Products include:
Lotrel Capsules 2370
Norvasc Tablets 2704

Atenolol (Olanzapine, because of its potential for inducing hypotension, may enhance the effects of certain antihypertensive agents). Products include:
Tenoretic Tablets 690
Tenormin I.V. Injection 692

Benazepril Hydrochloride (Olanzapine, because of its potential for inducing hypotension, may enhance the effects of certain antihypertensive agents). Products include:
Lotensin Tablets 2365
Lotensin HCT Tablets 2367
Lotrel Capsules 2370

Bendroflumethiazide (Olanzapine, because of its potential for inducing hypotension, may enhance the effects of certain antihypertensive agents). Products include:
Corzide 40/5 Tablets 2247
Corzide 80/5 Tablets 2247

Betaxolol Hydrochloride (Olanzapine, because of its potential for inducing hypotension, may enhance the effects of certain antihypertensive agents). Products include:
Betoptic S Ophthalmic Suspension 537

Bisoprolol Fumarate (Olanzapine, because of its potential for inducing hypotension, may enhance the effects of certain antihypertensive agents). Products include:
Zebeta Tablets 1885
Ziac Tablets 1887

Bromocriptine Mesylate (Olanzapine may antagonize the effects of dopamine agonists).
No products indexed under this heading.

Candesartan Cilexetil (Olanzapine, because of its potential for inducing hypotension, may enhance the effects of certain antihypertensive agents). Products include:
Atacand Tablets 595
Atacand HCT Tablets 597

Captopril (Olanzapine, because of its potential for inducing hypotension, may enhance the effects of certain antihypertensive agents). Products include:
Captopril Tablets 2281

Carbamazepine (Causes an approximately 50% increase in the clearance of olanzapine at 400 mg daily; higher daily doses of carbamazepine may cause an even greater increase in olanzapine clearance). Products include:
Carbatrol Capsules 3234
Tegretol/Tegretol-XR 2404

Carteolol Hydrochloride (Olanzapine, because of its potential for inducing hypotension, may enhance the effects of certain antihypertensive agents). Products include:
Carteolol Hydrochloride Ophthalmic Solution USP, 1% ..... ⊙ 258
Ocupress Ophthalmic Solution, 1% Sterile .... ⊙ 303

Charcoal, Activated (Co-administration with activated charcoal reduces the Cmax and AUC of

olanzapine by about 60%).
No products indexed under this heading.

Chlorothiazide (Olanzapine, because of its potential for inducing hypotension, may enhance the effects of certain antihypertensive agents). Products include:
Aldoclor Tablets ... 2035
Diuril Oral ... 2087

Chlorothiazide Sodium (Olanzapine, because of its potential for inducing hypotension, may enhance the effects of certain antihypertensive agents). Products include:
Diuril Sodium Intravenous ... 2086

Chlorthalidone (Olanzapine, because of its potential for inducing hypotension, may enhance the effects of certain antihypertensive agents). Products include:
Clorpres Tablets ... 1002
Combipres Tablets ... 1040
Tenoretic Tablets ... 690

Clonidine (Olanzapine, because of its potential for inducing hypotension, may enhance the effects of certain antihypertensive agents). Products include:
Catapres-TTS ... 1038

Clonidine Hydrochloride (Olanzapine, because of its potential for inducing hypotension, may enhance the effects of certain antihypertensive agents). Products include:
Catapres Tablets ... 1037
Clorpres Tablets ... 1002
Combipres Tablets ... 1040
Duraclon Injection ... 3057

Deserpidine (Olanzapine, because of its potential for inducing hypotension, may enhance the effects of certain antihypertensive agents).
No products indexed under this heading.

Diazepam (Co-administration of diazepam with olanzapine potentiates orthostatic hypotension). Products include:
Valium Injectable ... 3026
Valium Tablets ... 3047

Diazoxide (Olanzapine, because of its potential for inducing hypotension, may enhance the effects of certain antihypertensive agents).
No products indexed under this heading.

Diltiazem Hydrochloride (Olanzapine, because of its potential for inducing hypotension, may enhance the effects of certain antihypertensive agents). Products include:
Cardizem Injectable ... 1018
Cardizem Lyo-Ject Syringe ... 1018
Cardizem Monovial ... 1018
Cardizem CD Capsules ... 1016
Tiazac Capsules ... 1378

Dopamine Hydrochloride (Olanzapine may antagonize the effects of dopamine agonists).
No products indexed under this heading.

Doxazosin Mesylate (Olanzapine, because of its potential for inducing hypotension, may enhance the effects of certain antihypertensive agents). Products include:
Cardura Tablets ... 2668

Enalapril Maleate (Olanzapine, because of its potential for inducing hypotension, may enhance the effects of certain antihypertensive agents). Products include:
Lexxel Tablets ... 608
Vaseretic Tablets ... 2204
Vasotec Tablets ... 2210

Enalaprilat (Olanzapine, because of its potential for inducing hypotension, may enhance the effects of certain antihypertensive agents). Products include:
Enalaprilat Injection ... 863
Vasotec I.V. Injection ... 2207

Eprosartan Mesylate (Olanzapine, because of its potential for inducing hypotension, may enhance the effects of certain antihypertensive agents). Products include:
Teveten Tablets ... 3327

Esmolol Hydrochloride (Olanzapine, because of its potential for inducing hypotension, may enhance the effects of certain antihypertensive agents). Products include:
Brevibloc Injection ... 858

Felodipine (Olanzapine, because of its potential for inducing hypotension, may enhance the effects of certain antihypertensive agents). Products include:
Lexxel Tablets ... 608
Plendil Extended-Release Tablets ... 623

Fluoxetine Hydrochloride (Co-administration causes a small increase in the maximum concentration of olanzapine and a small decrease in olanzapine clearance; the magnitude of the impact of this factor is small in comparison to the overall variability between individuals and therefore dose modification is not routinely recomended). Products include:
Prozac Pulvules, Liquid, and Weekly Capsules ... 1238
Sarafem Pulvules ... 1962

Fluvoxamine Maleate (Inhibitors of CYP1A2, e.g., fluvoxamine, could potentially inhibit olanzapine elimination). Products include:
Luvox Tablets (25, 50, 100 mg) ... 3256

Fosinopril Sodium (Olanzapine, because of its potential for inducing hypotension, may enhance the effects of certain antihypertensive agents). Products include:
Monopril Tablets ... 1091
Monopril HCT ... 1094

Furosemide (Olanzapine, because of its potential for inducing hypotension, may enhance the effects of certain antihypertensive agents). Products include:
Furosemide Tablets ... 2284

Guanabenz Acetate (Olanzapine, because of its potential for inducing hypotension, may enhance the effects of certain antihypertensive agents).
No products indexed under this heading.

Guanethidine Monosulfate (Olanzapine, because of its potential for inducing hypotension, may enhance the effects of certain antihypertensive agents).
No products indexed under this heading.

Hydralazine Hydrochloride (Olanzapine, because of its potential for inducing hypotension, may enhance the effects of certain antihypertensive agents).
No products indexed under this heading.

Hydrochlorothiazide (Olanzapine, because of its potential for inducing hypotension, may enhance the effects of certain antihypertensive agents). Products include:
Accuretic Tablets ... 2614
Aldoril Tablets ... 2039
Atacand HCT Tablets ... 597
Avalide Tablets ... 1070
Diovan HCT Tablets ... 2338
Dyazide Capsules ... 1515
HydroDIURIL Tablets ... 2108
Hyzaar ... 2109
Inderide Tablets ... 3517
Inderide LA Long-Acting Capsules ... 3519
Lotensin HCT Tablets ... 2367
Maxzide ... 1008
Micardis HCT Tablets ... 1051
Microzide Capsules ... 3414
Moduretic Tablets ... 2138
Monopril HCT ... 1094
Prinzide Tablets ... 2168
Timolide Tablets ... 2187
Uniretic Tablets ... 3178
Vaseretic Tablets ... 2204
Zestoretic Tablets ... 695
Ziac Tablets ... 1887

Hydroflumethiazide (Olanzapine, because of its potential for inducing hypotension, may enhance the effects of certain antihypertensive agents). Products include:
Diucardin Tablets ... 3494

Indapamide (Olanzapine, because of its potential for inducing hypotension, may enhance the effects of certain antihypertensive agents). Products include:
Indapamide Tablets ... 2286

Irbesartan (Olanzapine, because of its potential for inducing hypotension, may enhance the effects of certain antihypertensive agents). Products include:
Avalide Tablets ... 1070
Avapro Tablets ... 1074
Avapro Tablets ... 3076

Isradipine (Olanzapine, because of its potential for inducing hypotension, may enhance the effects of certain antihypertensive agents). Products include:
DynaCirc Capsules ... 2921
DynaCirc CR Tablets ... 2923

Labetalol Hydrochloride (Olanzapine, because of its potential for inducing hypotension, may enhance the effects of certain antihypertensive agents). Products include:
Normodyne Injection ... 3135
Normodyne Tablets ... 3137

Levodopa (Olanzapine may antagonize the effects of levodopa). Products include:
Sinemet Tablets ... 1253
Sinemet CR Tablets ... 1255

Lisinopril (Olanzapine, because of its potential for inducing hypotension, may enhance the effects of certain antihypertensive agents). Products include:
Prinivil Tablets ... 2164
Prinzide Tablets ... 2168
Zestoretic Tablets ... 695
Zestril Tablets ... 698

Losartan Potassium (Olanzapine, because of its potential for inducing hypotension, may enhance the effects of certain antihypertensive agents). Products include:
Cozaar Tablets ... 2067
Hyzaar ... 2109

Mecamylamine Hydrochloride (Olanzapine, because of its potential for inducing hypotension, may enhance the effects of certain antihypertensive agents). Products include:
Inversine Tablets ... 1850

Methyclothiazide (Olanzapine, because of its potential for inducing hypotension, may enhance the effects of certain antihypertensive agents).
No products indexed under this heading.

Methyldopa (Olanzapine, because of its potential for inducing hypotension, may enhance the effects of certain antihypertensive agents). Products include:
Aldoclor Tablets ... 2035
Aldomet Tablets ... 2037
Aldoril Tablets ... 2039

Methyldopate Hydrochloride (Olanzapine, because of its potential for inducing hypotension, may enhance the effects of certain antihypertensive agents).
No products indexed under this heading.

Metolazone (Olanzapine, because of its potential for inducing hypotension, may enhance the effects of certain antihypertensive agents). Products include:
Mykrox Tablets ... 1168
Zaroxolyn Tablets ... 1177

Metoprolol Succinate (Olanzapine, because of its potential for inducing hypotension, may enhance the effects of certain antihypertensive agents). Products include:
Toprol-XL Tablets ... 651

Metoprolol Tartrate (Olanzapine, because of its potential for inducing hypotension, may enhance the effects of certain antihypertensive agents).
No products indexed under this heading.

Metyrosine (Olanzapine, because of its potential for inducing hypotension, may enhance the effects of certain antihypertensive agents). Products include:
Demser Capsules ... 2085

Mibefradil Dihydrochloride (Olanzapine, because of its potential for inducing hypotension, may enhance the effects of certain antihypertensive agents).
No products indexed under this heading.

Minoxidil (Olanzapine, because of its potential for inducing hypotension, may enhance the effects of certain antihypertensive agents). Products include:
Rogaine Extra Strength for Men Topical Solution ... ▣721
Rogaine for Women Topical Solution ... ▣721

Moexipril Hydrochloride (Olanzapine, because of its potential for inducing hypotension, may enhance the effects of certain antihypertensive agents). Products include:
Uniretic Tablets ... 3178
Univasc Tablets ... 3181

Nadolol (Olanzapine, because of its potential for inducing hypotension, may enhance the effects of certain antihypertensive agents). Products include:
Corgard Tablets ... 2245
Corzide 40/5 Tablets ... 2247
Corzide 80/5 Tablets ... 2247
Nadolol Tablets ... 2288

Nicardipine Hydrochloride (Olanzapine, because of its potential for inducing hypotension, may enhance the effects of certain antihypertensive agents). Products include:
Cardene I.V. ... 3485

Nifedipine (Olanzapine, because of its potential for inducing hypotension, may enhance the effects of certain antihypertensive agents). Products include:
Adalat CC Tablets ... 877
Procardia Capsules ... 2708
Procardia XL Extended Release Tablets ... 2710

Nisoldipine (Olanzapine, because of its potential for inducing hypotension, may enhance the effects of certain antihypertensive agents). Products include:
Sular Tablets ... 688

Nitroglycerin (Olanzapine, because of its potential for inducing hypotension, may enhance the effects of certain antihypertensive agents). Products include:
Nitro-Dur Transdermal Infusion System ... 3134
Nitro-Dur Transdermal Infusion System ... 1834
Nitrolingual Pumpspray ... 1355
Nitrostat Tablets ... 2658

Omeprazole (May cause an increase in olanzapine clearance by inducing CYP1A2 or glucuronyl transferase clearance). Products include:
Prilosec Delayed-Release Capsules ... 628

Penbutolol Sulfate (Olanzapine, because of its potential for inducing hypotension, may enhance the effects of certain antihypertensive agents).
No products indexed under this heading.

Pergolide Mesylate (Olanzapine may antagonize the effects of dopamine agonists). Products include:
Permax Tablets 1299

Perindopril Erbumine (Olanzapine, because of its potential for inducing hypotension, may enhance the effects of certain antihypertensive agents). Products include:
Aceon Tablets (2 mg, 4 mg, 8 mg) 3249

Phenoxybenzamine Hydrochloride (Olanzapine, because of its potential for inducing hypotension, may enhance the effects of certain antihypertensive agents). Products include:
Dibenzyline Capsules 3457

Phentolamine Mesylate (Olanzapine, because of its potential for inducing hypotension, may enhance the effects of certain antihypertensive agents).
No products indexed under this heading.

Pindolol (Olanzapine, because of its potential for inducing hypotension, may enhance the effects of certain antihypertensive agents).
No products indexed under this heading.

Polythiazide (Olanzapine, because of its potential for inducing hypotension, may enhance the effects of certain antihypertensive agents). Products include:
Minizide Capsules 2700
Renese Tablets 2712

Pramipexole Dihydrochloride (Olanzapine may antagonize the effects of dopamine agonists). Products include:
Mirapex Tablets 2834

Prazosin Hydrochloride (Olanzapine, because of its potential for inducing hypotension, may enhance the effects of certain antihypertensive agents). Products include:
Minipress Capsules 2699
Minizide Capsules 2700

Propranolol Hydrochloride (Olanzapine, because of its potential for inducing hypotension, may enhance the effects of certain antihypertensive agents). Products include:
Inderal 3513
Inderal LA Long-Acting Capsules 3516
Inderide Tablets 3517
Inderide LA Long-Acting Capsules 3519

Quinapril Hydrochloride (Olanzapine, because of its potential for inducing hypotension, may enhance the effects of certain antihypertensive agents). Products include:
Accupril Tablets 2611
Accuretic Tablets 2614

Ramipril (Olanzapine, because of its potential for inducing hypotension, may enhance the effects of certain antihypertensive agents). Products include:
Altace Capsules 2233

Rauwolfia serpentina (Olanzapine, because of its potential for inducing hypotension, may enhance the effects of certain antihypertensive agents).
No products indexed under this heading.

Rescinnamine (Olanzapine, because of its potential for inducing hypotension, may enhance the effects of certain antihypertensive agents).
No products indexed under this heading.

Reserpine (Olanzapine, because of its potential for inducing hypotension, may enhance the effects of certain antihypertensive agents).
No products indexed under this heading.

Rifampin (May cause an increase in olanzapine clearance by inducing CYP1A2 or glucuronyl tranferase clearance). Products include:
Rifadin 765
Rifamate Capsules 767
Rifater Tablets 769

Ropinirole Hydrochloride (Olanzapine may antagonize the effects of dopamine agonists). Products include:
Requip Tablets 1621

Sodium Nitroprusside (Olanzapine, because of its potential for inducing hypotension, may enhance the effects of certain antihypertensive agents).
No products indexed under this heading.

Sotalol Hydrochloride (Olanzapine, because of its potential for inducing hypotension, may enhance the effects of certain antihypertensive agents). Products include:
Betapace Tablets 950
Betapace AF Tablets 954

Spirapril Hydrochloride (Olanzapine, because of its potential for inducing hypotension, may enhance the effects of certain antihypertensive agents).
No products indexed under this heading.

Telmisartan (Olanzapine, because of its potential for inducing hypotension, may enhance the effects of certain antihypertensive agents). Products include:
Micardis Tablets 1049
Micardis HCT Tablets 1051

Terazosin Hydrochloride (Olanzapine, because of its potential for inducing hypotension, may enhance the effects of certain antihypertensive agents). Products include:
Hytrin Capsules 464

Timolol Maleate (Olanzapine, because of its potential for inducing hypotension, may enhance the effects of certain antihypertensive agents). Products include:
Blocadren Tablets 2046
Cosopt Sterile Ophthalmic Solution 2065
Timolide Tablets 2187
Timolol GFS .... ⊙266
Timoptic in Ocudose 2192
Timoptic Sterile Ophthalmic Solution 2190
Timoptic-XE Sterile Ophthalmic Gel Forming Solution 2194

Torsemide (Olanzapine, because of its potential for inducing hypotension, may enhance the effects of certain antihypertensive agents). Products include:
Demadex Tablets and Injection 2965

Trandolapril (Olanzapine, because of its potential for inducing hypotension, may enhance the effects of certain antihypertensive agents). Products include:
Mavik Tablets 478
Tarka Tablets 508

Trimethaphan Camsylate (Olanzapine, because of its potential for inducing hypotension, may enhance the effects of certain antihypertensive agents).
No products indexed under this heading.

Valsartan (Olanzapine, because of its potential for inducing hypotension, may enhance the effects of certain antihypertensive agents). Products include:
Diovan Capsules 2337
Diovan HCT Tablets 2338

Verapamil Hydrochloride (Olanzapine, because of its potential for inducing hypotension, may enhance the effects of certain antihypertensive agents). Products include:
Covera-HS Tablets 3199
Isoptin SR Tablets 467
Tarka Tablets 508
Verelan Capsules 3184
Verelan PM Capsules 3186

Food Interactions

Alcohol (Co-administration of alcohol with olanzapine potentiates orthostatic hypotension; concurrent use should be avoided).

ZYPREXA ZYDIS ORALLY DISINTEGRATING TABLETS

(Olanzapine) 1973
See Zyprexa Tablets

ZYRTEC SYRUP

(Cetirizine Hydrochloride) 2756
See Zyrtec Tablets

ZYRTEC TABLETS

(Cetirizine Hydrochloride) 2756
May interact with central nervous system depressants, theophylline, and certain other agents. Compounds in these categories include:

Alfentanil Hydrochloride (Concurrent use may result in additional impairment of CNS performance and reduction in mental alertness).
No products indexed under this heading.

Alprazolam (Concurrent use may result in additional impairment of CNS performance and reduction in mental alertness). Products include:
Xanax Tablets 2865

Aminophylline (Small decrease in the clearance of cetirizine caused by a larger dose, e.g., 400 mg dose of theophylline).
No products indexed under this heading.

Aprobarbital (Concurrent use may result in additional impairment of CNS performance and reduction in mental alertness).
No products indexed under this heading.

Buprenorphine Hydrochloride (Concurrent use may result in additional impairment of CNS performance and reduction in mental alertness). Products include:
Buprenex Injectable 2918

Buspirone Hydrochloride (Concurrent use may result in additional impairment of CNS performance and reduction in mental alertness).
No products indexed under this heading.

Butabarbital (Concurrent use may result in additional impairment of CNS performance and reduction in mental alertness).
No products indexed under this heading.

Butalbital (Concurrent use may result in additional impairment of CNS performance and reduction in mental alertness). Products include:
Phrenilin 578
Sedapap Tablets 50 mg/650 mg 2225

Chlordiazepoxide (Concurrent use may result in additional impairment of CNS performance and reduction in mental alertness). Products include:
Limbitrol 1738

Chlordiazepoxide Hydrochloride (Concurrent use may result in additional impairment of CNS performance and reduction in mental alertness). Products include:
Librium Capsules 1736
Librium for Injection 1737

Chlorpromazine (Concurrent use may result in additional impairment of CNS performance and reduction in mental alertness). Products include:
Thorazine Suppositories 1656

Chlorpromazine Hydrochloride (Concurrent use may result in additional impairment of CNS performance and reduction in mental alertness). Products include:
Thorazine 1656

Chlorprothixene (Concurrent use may result in additional impairment of CNS performance and reduction in mental alertness).
No products indexed under this heading.

Chlorprothixene Hydrochloride (Concurrent use may result in additional impairment of CNS performance and reduction in mental alertness).
No products indexed under this heading.

Chlorprothixene Lactate (Concurrent use may result in additional impairment of CNS performance and reduction in mental alertness).
No products indexed under this heading.

Clorazepate Dipotassium (Concurrent use may result in additional impairment of CNS performance and reduction in mental alertness). Products include:
Tranxene 511

Clozapine (Concurrent use may result in additional impairment of CNS performance and reduction in mental alertness). Products include:
Clozaril Tablets 2319

Codeine Phosphate (Concurrent use may result in additional impairment of CNS performance and reduction in mental alertness). Products include:
Phenergan with Codeine Syrup 3557
Phenergan VC with Codeine Syrup 3561
Robitussin A-C Syrup 2942
Robitussin-DAC Syrup 2942
Ryna-C Liquid 768
Soma Compound w/Codeine Tablets 3355
Tussi-Organidin NR Liquid 3350
Tussi-Organidin-S NR Liquid 3350
Tylenol with Codeine 2595

Desflurane (Concurrent use may result in additional impairment of CNS performance and reduction in mental alertness). Products include:
Suprane Liquid for Inhalation 874

Dezocine (Concurrent use may result in additional impairment of CNS performance and reduction in mental alertness).
No products indexed under this heading.

Diazepam (Concurrent use may result in additional impairment of CNS performance and reduction in mental alertness). Products include:
Valium Injectable 3026
Valium Tablets 3047

Droperidol (Concurrent use may result in additional impairment of CNS performance and reduction in mental alertness).
No products indexed under this heading.

Dyphylline (Small decrease in the clearance of cetirizine caused by a larger dose, e.g., 400 mg dose of theophylline). Products include:
Lufyllin Tablets 3347
Lufyllin-400 Tablets 3347
Lufyllin-GG Elixir 3348
Lufyllin-GG Tablets 3348

Enflurane (Concurrent use may result in additional impairment of CNS performance and reduction in mental alertness).
No products indexed under this heading.

Estazolam (Concurrent use may result in additional impairment of CNS performance and reduction in mental alertness). Products include:
ProSom Tablets 500

Ethchlorvynol (Concurrent use may result in additional impairment of CNS performance and reduction in mental alertness).
No products indexed under this heading.

Ethinamate (Concurrent use may result in additional impairment of CNS performance and reduction in mental alertness).
No products indexed under this heading.

Fentanyl (Concurrent use may result in additional impairment of CNS performance and reduction in mental alertness). Products include:
Duragesic Transdermal System 1786

Fentanyl Citrate (Concurrent use may result in additional impairment of CNS performance and reduction in mental alertness). Products include:
Actiq 1184

Fluphenazine Decanoate (Concurrent use may result in additional impairment of CNS performance and reduction in mental alertness).
No products indexed under this heading.

Fluphenazine Enanthate (Concurrent use may result in additional impairment of CNS performance and reduction in mental alertness).
No products indexed under this heading.

Fluphenazine Hydrochloride (Concurrent use may result in additional impairment of CNS performance and reduction in mental alertness).
No products indexed under this heading.

Flurazepam Hydrochloride (Concurrent use may result in additional impairment of CNS performance and reduction in mental alertness).
No products indexed under this heading.

Glutethimide (Concurrent use may result in additional impairment of CNS performance and reduction in mental alertness).
No products indexed under this heading.

Haloperidol (Concurrent use may result in additional impairment of CNS performance and reduction in mental alertness). Products include:
Haldol Injection, Tablets and Concentrate 2533

Haloperidol Decanoate (Concurrent use may result in additional impairment of CNS performance and reduction in mental alertness). Products include:
Haldol Decanoate 2535

Hydrocodone Bitartrate (Concurrent use may result in additional impairment of CNS performance and reduction in mental alertness). Products include:
Hycodan 1316
Hycomine Compound Tablets 1317
Hycotuss Expectorant Syrup 1318
Lortab 3319
Lortab Elixir 3317
Maxidone Tablets CIII 3399
Norco 5/325 Tablets CIII 3424
Norco 7.5/325 Tablets CIII 3425
Norco 10/325 Tablets CIII 3427
Norco 10/325 Tablets CIII 3425
Vicodin Tablets 516
Vicodin ES Tablets 517
Vicodin HP Tablets 518
Vicodin Tuss Expectorant 519
Vicoprofen Tablets 520
Zydone Tablets 1330

Hydrocodone Polistirex (Concurrent use may result in additional impairment of CNS performance and reduction in mental alertness). Products include:
Tussionex Pennkinetic Extended-Release Suspension 1174

Hydromorphone Hydrochloride (Concurrent use may result in additional impairment of CNS performance and reduction in mental alertness). Products include:
Dilaudid 441
Dilaudid Oral Liquid 445
Dilaudid Powder 441
Dilaudid Rectal Suppositories 441
Dilaudid Tablets 441
Dilaudid Tablets - 8 mg 445
Dilaudid-HP 443

Hydroxyzine Hydrochloride (Concurrent use may result in additional impairment of CNS performance and reduction in mental alertness). Products include:
Atarax Tablets & Syrup 2667
Vistaril Intramuscular Solution 2738

Isoflurane (Concurrent use may result in additional impairment of CNS performance and reduction in mental alertness).
No products indexed under this heading.

Ketamine Hydrochloride (Concurrent use may result in additional impairment of CNS performance and reduction in mental alertness).
No products indexed under this heading.

Levomethadyl Acetate Hydrochloride (Concurrent use may result in additional impairment of CNS performance and reduction in mental alertness).
No products indexed under this heading.

Levorphanol Tartrate (Concurrent use may result in additional impairment of CNS performance and reduction in mental alertness). Products include:
Levo-Dromoran 1734
Levorphanol Tartrate Tablets 3059

Lorazepam (Concurrent use may result in additional impairment of CNS performance and reduction in mental alertness). Products include:
Ativan Injection 3478
Ativan Tablets 3482

Loxapine Hydrochloride (Concurrent use may result in additional impairment of CNS performance and reduction in mental alertness).
No products indexed under this heading.

Loxapine Succinate (Concurrent use may result in additional impairment of CNS performance and reduction in mental alertness). Products include:
Loxitane Capsules 3398

Meperidine Hydrochloride (Concurrent use may result in additional impairment of CNS performance and reduction in mental alertness). Products include:
Demerol 3079
Mepergan Injection 3539

Mephobarbital (Concurrent use may result in additional impairment of CNS performance and reduction in mental alertness).
No products indexed under this heading.

Meprobamate (Concurrent use may result in additional impairment of CNS performance and reduction in mental alertness). Products include:
Miltown Tablets 3349

Mesoridazine Besylate (Concurrent use may result in additional impairment of CNS performance and reduction in mental alertness). Products include:
Serentil 1057

Methadone Hydrochloride (Concurrent use may result in additional impairment of CNS performance and reduction in mental alertness). Products include:
Dolophine Hydrochloride Tablets 3056

Methohexital Sodium (Concurrent use may result in additional impairment of CNS performance and reduction in mental alertness). Products include:
Brevital Sodium for Injection, USP 1815

Methotrimeprazine (Concurrent use may result in additional impairment of CNS performance and reduction in mental alertness).
No products indexed under this heading.

Methoxyflurane (Concurrent use may result in additional impairment of CNS performance and reduction in mental alertness).
No products indexed under this heading.

Midazolam Hydrochloride (Concurrent use may result in additional impairment of CNS performance and reduction in mental alertness). Products include:
Versed Injection 3027
Versed Syrup 3033

Molindone Hydrochloride (Concurrent use may result in additional impairment of CNS performance and reduction in mental alertness). Products include:
Moban 1320

Morphine Sulfate (Concurrent use may result in additional impairment of CNS performance and reduction in mental alertness). Products include:
Astramorph/PF Injection, USP (Preservative-Free) 594
Duramorph Injection 1312
Infumorph 200 and Infumorph 500 Sterile Solutions 1314
Kadian Capsules 1335
MS Contin Tablets 2896
MSIR 2898
Oramorph SR Tablets 3062
Roxanol 3066

Olanzapine (Concurrent use may result in additional impairment of CNS performance and reduction in mental alertness). Products include:
Zyprexa Tablets 1973
Zyprexa ZYDIS Orally Disintegrating Tablets 1973

Oxazepam (Concurrent use may result in additional impairment of CNS performance and reduction in mental alertness).
No products indexed under this heading.

Oxycodone Hydrochloride (Concurrent use may result in additional impairment of CNS performance and reduction in mental alertness). Products include:
OxyContin Tablets 2912
OxyFast Oral Concentrate Solution 2916
OxyIR Capsules 2916
Percocet Tablets 1326
Percodan Tablets 1327
Percolone Tablets 1327
Roxicodone 3067
Tylox Capsules 2597

Pentobarbital Sodium (Concurrent use may result in additional impairment of CNS performance and reduction in mental alertness). Products include:
Nembutal Sodium Solution 485

Perphenazine (Concurrent use may result in additional impairment of CNS performance and reduction in mental alertness). Products include:
Etrafon 3115
Trilafon 3160

Phenobarbital (Concurrent use may result in additional impairment of CNS performance and reduction in mental alertness). Products include:
Arco-Lase Plus Tablets 592
Donnatal 2929
Donnatal Extentabs 2930

Prazepam (Concurrent use may result in additional impairment of CNS performance and reduction in mental alertness).
No products indexed under this heading.

Prochlorperazine (Concurrent use may result in additional impairment of CNS performance and reduction in mental alertness). Products include:
Compazine 1505

Promethazine Hydrochloride (Concurrent use may result in additional impairment of CNS performance and reduction in mental alertness). Products include:
Mepergan Injection 3539
Phenergan Injection 3553
Phenergan 3556
Phenergan Syrup 3554
Phenergan with Codeine Syrup 3557
Phenergan with Dextromethorphan Syrup 3559
Phenergan VC Syrup 3560
Phenergan VC with Codeine Syrup 3561

Propofol (Concurrent use may result in additional impairment of CNS performance and reduction in mental alertness). Products include:
Diprivan Injectable Emulsion 667

Propoxyphene Hydrochloride (Concurrent use may result in additional impairment of CNS performance and reduction in mental alertness). Products include:
Darvon Pulvules 1909
Darvon Compound-65 Pulvules 1910

Propoxyphene Napsylate (Concurrent use may result in additional impairment of CNS performance and reduction in mental alertness). Products include:
Darvon-N/Darvocet-N 1907
Darvon-N Tablets 1912

Quazepam (Concurrent use may result in additional impairment of CNS performance and reduction in mental alertness).
No products indexed under this heading.

Quetiapine Fumarate (Concurrent use may result in additional impairment of CNS performance and reduction in mental alertness). Products include:
Seroquel Tablets 684

Remifentanil Hydrochloride (Concurrent use may result in additional impairment of CNS performance and reduction in mental alertness).
No products indexed under this heading.

Risperidone (Concurrent use may result in additional impairment of CNS performance and reduction in mental alertness). Products include:
Risperdal 1796

Secobarbital Sodium (Concurrent use may result in additional impairment of CNS performance and reduction in mental alertness).
No products indexed under this heading.

Sevoflurane (Concurrent use may result in additional impairment of CNS performance and reduction in mental alertness).
No products indexed under this heading.

Sufentanil Citrate (Concurrent use may result in additional impairment of CNS performance and reduction in mental alertness).
No products indexed under this heading.

Temazepam (Concurrent use may result in additional impairment of CNS performance and reduction in mental alertness).
No products indexed under this heading.

Theophylline (Small decrease in the clearance of cetirizine caused by a larger dose, e.g., 400 mg dose of theophylline). Products include:
Aerolate 1361
Theo-Dur Extended-Release Tablets 1835
Uni-Dur Extended-Release Tablets 1841
Uniphyl 400 mg and 600 mg Tablets 2903

Theophylline Calcium Salicylate (Small decrease in the clearance of cetirizine caused by a larger dose,

e.g., 400 mg dose of theophylline).
No products indexed under this heading.

Theophylline Sodium Glycinate (Small decrease in the clearance of cetirizine caused by a larger dose, e.g., 400 mg dose of theophylline).
No products indexed under this heading.

Thiamylal Sodium (Concurrent use may result in additional impairment of CNS performance and reduction in mental alertness).
No products indexed under this heading.

Thioridazine Hydrochloride (Concurrent use may result in additional impairment of CNS performance and reduction in mental alertness). Products include:
Thioridazine Hydrochloride Tablets 2289

Thiothixene (Concurrent use may result in additional impairment of CNS performance and reduction in mental alertness). Products include:
Navane Capsules 2701
Thiothixene Capsules 2290

Triazolam (Concurrent use may result in additional impairment of CNS performance and reduction in mental alertness). Products include:
Halcion Tablets 2823

Trifluoperazine Hydrochloride (Concurrent use may result in additional impairment of CNS performance and reduction in mental alertness). Products include:
Stelazine 1640

Zaleplon (Concurrent use may result in additional impairment of CNS performance and reduction in mental alertness). Products include:
Sonata Capsules 3591

Ziprasidone Hydrochloride (Concurrent use may result in additional impairment of CNS performance and reduction in mental alertness). Products include:
Geodon Capsules 2688

Zolpidem Tartrate (Concurrent use may result in additional impairment of CNS performance and reduction in mental alertness). Products include:
Ambien Tablets 3191

Food Interactions

Alcohol (Concurrent use may result in additional impairment of CNS performance and reduction in mental alertness).

Food, unspecified (Food has no effect on the extent of cetirizine absorption, but Tmax may be delayed and Cmax may be decreased in the presence of food).

ZYRTEC-D 12 HOUR EXTENDED RELIEF TABLETS

(Cetirizine Hydrochloride, Pseudoephedrine Hydrochloride) 2758

May interact with central nervous system depressants, cardiac glycosides, histamine H_2-receptor antagonists, monoamine oxidase inhibitors, proton pump inhibitor, sympathomimetics, theophylline, and certain other agents. Compounds in these categories include:

Albuterol (Co-administration with other sympathomimetic agents may result in harmful cardiovascular effects). Products include:
Proventil Inhalation Aerosol 3142
Ventolin Inhalation Aerosol and Refill 1679

Albuterol Sulfate (Co-administration with other sympathomimetic agents may result in harmful cardiovascular effects). Products include:
AccuNeb Inhalation Solution 1230
Combivent Inhalation Aerosol 1041
DuoNeb Inhalation Solution 1233
Proventil Inhalation Solution 0.083% 3146
Proventil Repetabs Tablets 3148
Proventil Solution for Inhalation 0.5% 3144
Proventil HFA Inhalation Aerosol 3150
Ventolin HFA Inhalation Aerosol 3618
Volmax Extended-Release Tablets 2276

Alfentanil Hydrochloride (Concurrent use may result in additional reduction in alertness impairment of CNS performance).
No products indexed under this heading.

Alprazolam (Concurrent use may result in additional reduction in alertness impairment of CNS performance). Products include:
Xanax Tablets 2865

Aminophylline (Small decrease in the clearance of cetirizine caused by a 400 mg dose of theophylline; it is possible that larger theophylline doses could have a greater effect).
No products indexed under this heading.

Aprobarbital (Concurrent use may result in additional reduction in alertness impairment of CNS performance).
No products indexed under this heading.

Buprenorphine Hydrochloride (Concurrent use may result in additional reduction in alertness impairment of CNS performance). Products include:
Buprenex Injectable 2918

Buspirone Hydrochloride (Concurrent use may result in additional reduction in alertness impairment of CNS performance).
No products indexed under this heading.

Butabarbital (Concurrent use may result in additional reduction in alertness impairment of CNS performance).
No products indexed under this heading.

Butalbital (Concurrent use may result in additional reduction in alertness impairment of CNS performance). Products include:
Phrenilin 578
Sedapap Tablets 50 mg/650 mg 2225

Chlordiazepoxide (Concurrent use may result in additional reduction in alertness impairment of CNS performance). Products include:
Limbitrol 1738

Chlordiazepoxide Hydrochloride (Concurrent use may result in additional reduction in alertness impairment of CNS performance). Products include:
Librium Capsules 1736
Librium for Injection 1737

Chlorpromazine (Concurrent use may result in additional reduction in alertness impairment of CNS performance). Products include:
Thorazine Suppositories 1656

Chlorpromazine Hydrochloride (Concurrent use may result in additional reduction in alertness impairment of CNS performance). Products include:
Thorazine 1656

Chlorprothixene (Concurrent use may result in additional reduction in alertness impairment of CNS performance).
No products indexed under this heading.

Chlorprothixene Hydrochloride (Concurrent use may result in additional reduction in alertness impairment of CNS performance).
No products indexed under this heading.

Chlorprothixene Lactate (Concurrent use may result in additional reduction in alertness impairment of CNS performance).
No products indexed under this heading.

Cimetidine (H2 antagonists increase gastric pH and may reduce the absorption of delavirdine; chronic use of these drugs with delavirdine is not recommended). Products include:
Tagamet HB 200 Suspension 762
Tagamet HB 200 Tablets 761
Tagamet Tablets 1644

Cimetidine Hydrochloride (H2 antagonists increase gastric pH and may reduce the absorption of delavirdine; chronic use of these drugs with delavirdine is not recommended). Products include:
Tagamet 1644

Clorazepate Dipotassium (Concurrent use may result in additional reduction in alertness impairment of CNS performance). Products include:
Tranxene 511

Clozapine (Concurrent use may result in additional reduction in alertness impairment of CNS performance). Products include:
Clozaril Tablets 2319

Codeine Phosphate (Concurrent use may result in additional reduction in alertness impairment of CNS performance). Products include:
Phenergan with Codeine Syrup 3557
Phenergan VC with Codeine Syrup 3561
Robitussin A-C Syrup 2942
Robitussin-DAC Syrup 2942
Ryna-C Liquid 768
Soma Compound w/Codeine Tablets 3355
Tussi-Organidin NR Liquid 3350
Tussi-Organidin-S NR Liquid 3350
Tylenol with Codeine 2595

Desflurane (Concurrent use may result in additional reduction in alertness impairment of CNS performance). Products include:
Suprane Liquid for Inhalation 874

Deslanoside (Co-administration of pseudoephedrine may increase ectopic pacemaker activity).
No products indexed under this heading.

Dezocine (Concurrent use may result in additional reduction in alertness impairment of CNS performance).
No products indexed under this heading.

Diazepam (Concurrent use may result in additional reduction in alertness impairment of CNS performance). Products include:
Valium Injectable 3026
Valium Tablets 3047

Digitoxin (Co-administration of pseudoephedrine may increase ectopic pacemaker activity).
No products indexed under this heading.

Digoxin (Co-administration of pseudoephedrine may increase ectopic pacemaker activity). Products include:
Digitek Tablets 1003
Lanoxicaps Capsules 1574
Lanoxin Injection 1581
Lanoxin Tablets 1587
Lanoxin Elixir Pediatric 1578
Lanoxin Injection Pediatric 1584

Dobutamine Hydrochloride (Co-administration with other sympathomimetic agents may result in harmful cardiovascular effects). Products include:
Dobutrex Solution Vials 1914

Dopamine Hydrochloride (Co-administration with other sympathomimetic agents may result in harmful cardiovascular effects).
No products indexed under this heading.

Droperidol (Concurrent use may result in additional reduction in alertness impairment of CNS performance).
No products indexed under this heading.

Dyphylline (Small decrease in the clearance of cetirizine caused by a 400 mg dose of theophylline; it is possible that larger theophylline doses could have a greater effect). Products include:
Lufyllin Tablets 3347
Lufyllin-400 Tablets 3347
Lufyllin-GG Elixir 3348
Lufyllin-GG Tablets 3348

Enflurane (Concurrent use may result in additional reduction in alertness impairment of CNS performance).
No products indexed under this heading.

Ephedrine Hydrochloride (Co-administration with other sympathomimetic agents may result in harmful cardiovascular effects). Products include:
Primatene Tablets 780

Ephedrine Sulfate (Co-administration with other sympathomimetic agents may result in harmful cardiovascular effects).
No products indexed under this heading.

Ephedrine Tannate (Co-administration with other sympathomimetic agents may result in harmful cardiovascular effects). Products include:
Rynatuss Pediatric Suspension 3353
Rynatuss Tablets 3353

Epinephrine (Co-administration with other sympathomimetic agents may result in harmful cardiovascular effects). Products include:
Epifrin Sterile Ophthalmic Solution .... ⊙235
EpiPen 1236
Primatene Mist 779
Xylocaine with Epinephrine Injection 653

Epinephrine Bitartrate (Co-administration with other sympathomimetic agents may result in harmful cardiovascular effects). Products include:
Sensorcaine 643

Epinephrine Hydrochloride (Co-administration with other sympathomimetic agents may result in harmful cardiovascular effects).
No products indexed under this heading.

Esomeprazole Magnesium (Proton pump inhibitors increase gastric pH and may reduce the absorption of delavirdine chronic use of these drugs with delavirdine is not recommended). Products include:
Nexium Delayed-Release Capsules 619

Estazolam (Concurrent use may result in additional reduction in alertness impairment of CNS performance). Products include:
ProSom Tablets 500

Ethchlorvynol (Concurrent use may result in additional reduction in alertness impairment of CNS performance).
No products indexed under this heading.

Ethinamate (Concurrent use may result in additional reduction in alertness impairment of CNS performance).
No products indexed under this heading.

Famotidine (H2 antagonists increase gastric pH and may reduce the absorption of delavirdine; chronic use of these drugs with delavirdine is not recommended). Products include:
Famotidine Injection 866
Pepcid AC 1814

Pepcid Complete Chewable Tablets **1815**
Pepcid Injection **2153**
Pepcid for Oral Suspension **2150**
Pepcid RPD Orally Disintegrating Tablets **2150**
Pepcid Tablets **2150**

Fentanyl (Concurrent use may result in additional reduction in alertness impairment of CNS performance). Products include:
Duragesic Transdermal System **1786**

Fentanyl Citrate (Concurrent use may result in additional reduction in alertness impairment of CNS performance). Products include:
Actiq **1184**

Fluphenazine Decanoate (Concurrent use may result in additional reduction in alertness impairment of CNS performance).
No products indexed under this heading.

Fluphenazine Enanthate (Concurrent use may result in additional reduction in alertness impairment of CNS performance).
No products indexed under this heading.

Fluphenazine Hydrochloride (Concurrent use may result in additional reduction in alertness impairment of CNS performance).
No products indexed under this heading.

Flurazepam Hydrochloride (Concurrent use may result in additional reduction in alertness impairment of CNS performance).
No products indexed under this heading.

Glutethimide (Concurrent use may result in additional reduction in alertness impairment of CNS performance).
No products indexed under this heading.

Haloperidol (Concurrent use may result in additional reduction in alertness impairment of CNS performance). Products include:
Haldol Injection, Tablets and Concentrate **2533**

Haloperidol Decanoate (Concurrent use may result in additional reduction in alertness impairment of CNS performance). Products include:
Haldol Decanoate **2535**

Hydrocodone Bitartrate (Concurrent use may result in additional reduction in alertness impairment of CNS performance). Products include:
Hycodan **1316**
Hycomine Compound Tablets **1317**
Hycotuss Expectorant Syrup **1318**
Lortab **3319**
Lortab Elixir **3317**
Maxidone Tablets CIII **3399**
Norco 5/325 Tablets CIII **3424**
Norco 7.5/325 Tablets CIII **3425**
Norco 10/325 Tablets CIII **3427**
Norco 10/325 Tablets CIII **3425**
Vicodin Tablets **516**
Vicodin ES Tablets **517**
Vicodin HP Tablets **518**
Vicodin Tuss Expectorant **519**
Vicoprofen Tablets **520**
Zydone Tablets **1330**

Hydrocodone Polistirex (Concurrent use may result in additional reduction in alertness impairment of CNS performance). Products include:
Tussionex Pennkinetic Extended-Release Suspension **1174**

Hydromorphone Hydrochloride (Concurrent use may result in additional reduction in alertness impairment of CNS performance). Products include:
Dilaudid **441**
Dilaudid Oral Liquid **445**
Dilaudid Powder **441**
Dilaudid Rectal Suppositories **441**
Dilaudid Tablets **441**
Dilaudid Tablets - 8 mg **445**
Dilaudid-HP **443**

Hydroxyzine Hydrochloride (Concurrent use may result in additional reduction in alertness impairment of CNS performance). Products include:
Atarax Tablets & Syrup **2667**
Vistaril Intramuscular Solution **2738**

Isocarboxazid (Concurrent and/or sequential use with MAO inhibitors is contraindicated).
No products indexed under this heading.

Isoflurane (Concurrent use may result in additional reduction in alertness impairment of CNS performance).
No products indexed under this heading.

Isoproterenol Hydrochloride (Co-administration with other sympathomimetic agents may result in harmful cardiovascular effects).
No products indexed under this heading.

Isoproterenol Sulfate (Co-administration with other sympathomimetic agents may result in harmful cardiovascular effects).
No products indexed under this heading.

Ketamine Hydrochloride (Concurrent use may result in additional reduction in alertness impairment of CNS performance).
No products indexed under this heading.

Lansoprazole (Proton pump inhibitors increase gastric pH and may reduce the absorption of delavirdine chronic use of these drugs with delavirdine is not recommended). Products include:
Prevacid Delayed-Release Capsules **3292**
PREVPAC **3298**

Levalbuterol Hydrochloride (Co-administration with other sympathomimetic agents may result in harmful cardiovascular effects). Products include:
Xopenex Inhalation Solution **3207**

Levomethadyl Acetate Hydrochloride (Concurrent use may result in additional reduction in alertness impairment of CNS performance).
No products indexed under this heading.

Levorphanol Tartrate (Concurrent use may result in additional reduction in alertness impairment of CNS performance). Products include:
Levo-Dromoran **1734**
Levorphanol Tartrate Tablets **3059**

Lorazepam (Concurrent use may result in additional reduction in alertness impairment of CNS performance). Products include:
Ativan Injection **3478**
Ativan Tablets **3482**

Loxapine Hydrochloride (Concurrent use may result in additional reduction in alertness impairment of CNS performance).
No products indexed under this heading.

Loxapine Succinate (Concurrent use may result in additional reduction in alertness impairment of CNS performance). Products include:
Loxitane Capsules **3398**

Mecamylamine Hydrochloride (Pseudoephedrine may reduce the antihypertensive effect). Products include:
Inversine Tablets **1850**

Meperidine Hydrochloride (Concurrent use may result in additional reduction in alertness impairment of CNS performance). Products include:
Demerol **3079**
Mepergan Injection **3539**

Mephobarbital (Concurrent use may result in additional reduction in alertness impairment of CNS performance).
No products indexed under this heading.

Meprobamate (Concurrent use may result in additional reduction in alertness impairment of CNS performance). Products include:
Miltown Tablets **3349**

Mesoridazine Besylate (Concurrent use may result in additional reduction in alertness impairment of CNS performance). Products include:
Serentil **1057**

Metaproterenol Sulfate (Co-administration with other sympathomimetic agents may result in harmful cardiovascular effects). Products include:
Alupent **1029**

Metaraminol Bitartrate (Co-administration with other sympathomimetic agents may result in harmful cardiovascular effects). Products include:
Aramine Injection **2043**

Methadone Hydrochloride (Concurrent use may result in additional reduction in alertness impairment of CNS performance). Products include:
Dolophine Hydrochloride Tablets **3056**

Methohexital Sodium (Concurrent use may result in additional reduction in alertness impairment of CNS performance). Products include:
Brevital Sodium for Injection, USP **1815**

Methotrimeprazine (Concurrent use may result in additional reduction in alertness impairment of CNS performance).
No products indexed under this heading.

Methoxamine Hydrochloride (Co-administration with other sympathomimetic agents may result in harmful cardiovascular effects).
No products indexed under this heading.

Methoxyflurane (Concurrent use may result in additional reduction in alertness impairment of CNS performance).
No products indexed under this heading.

Methyldopa (Pseudoephedrine may reduce the antihypertensive effect). Products include:
Aldoclor Tablets **2035**
Aldomet Tablets **2037**
Aldoril Tablets .... **[illegible]**

Methyldopate Hydrochloride (Pseudoephedrine may reduce the antihypertensive effect).
No products indexed under this heading.

Midazolam Hydrochloride (Concurrent use may result in additional reduction in alertness impairment of CNS performance). Products include:
Versed Injection **3027**
Versed Syrup **3033**

Moclobemide (Concurrent and/or sequential use with MAO inhibitors is contraindicated).
No products indexed under this heading.

Molindone Hydrochloride (Concurrent use may result in additional reduction in alertness impairment of CNS performance). Products include:
Moban **1320**

Morphine Sulfate (Concurrent use may result in additional reduction in alertness impairment of CNS performance). Products include:
Astramorph/PF Injection, USP (Preservative-Free) **594**
Duramorph Injection **1312**
Infumorph 200 and Infumorph 500 Sterile Solutions **1314**
Kadian Capsules **1335**
MS Contin Tablets **2896**
MSIR **2898**
Oramorph SR Tablets **3062**
Roxanol **3066**

Nizatidine (H2 antagonists increase gastric pH and may reduce the absorption of delavirdine; chronic use of these drugs with delavirdine is not recommended). Products include:
Axid Pulvules **1903**
Axid Pulvules **2919**

Norepinephrine Bitartrate (Co-administration with other sympathomimetic agents may result in harmful cardiovascular effects).
No products indexed under this heading.

Olanzapine (Concurrent use may result in additional reduction in alertness impairment of CNS performance). Products include:
Zyprexa Tablets **1973**
Zyprexa ZYDIS Orally Disintegrating Tablets **1973**

Omeprazole (Proton pump inhibitors increase gastric pH and may reduce the absorption of delavirdine chronic use of these drugs with delavirdine is not recommended). Products include:
Prilosec Delayed-Release Capsules **628**

Oxazepam (Concurrent use may result in additional reduction in alertness impairment of CNS performance).
No products indexed under this heading.

Oxycodone Hydrochloride (Concurrent use may result in additional reduction in alertness impairment of CNS performance). Products include:
OxyContin Tablets **2912**
OxyFast Oral Concentrate Solution **2916**
OxyIR Capsules **2916**
Percocet Tablets **1326**
Percodan Tablets **1327**
Percolone Tablets **1327**
Roxicodone **3067**
Tylox Capsules **2597**

Pantoprazole Sodium (Proton pump inhibitors increase gastric pH and may reduce the absorption of delavirdine chronic use of these drugs with delavirdine is not recommended). Products include:
Protonix I.V. **3580**
Protonix Tablets **3577**

Pargyline Hydrochloride (Concurrent and/or sequential use with MAO inhibitors is contraindicated).
No products indexed under this heading.

Pentobarbital Sodium (Concurrent use may result in additional reduction in alertness impairment of CNS performance). Products include:
Nembutal Sodium Solution **485**

Perphenazine (Concurrent use may result in additional reduction in alertness impairment of CNS performance). Products include:
Etrafon **3115**
Trilafon **3160**

Phenelzine Sulfate (Concurrent and/or sequential use with MAO inhibitors is contraindicated). Products include:
Nardil Tablets **2653**

Phenobarbital (Concurrent use may result in additional reduction in alertness impairment of CNS performance). Products include:
Arco-Lase Plus Tablets **592**
Donnatal **2929**
Donnatal Extentabs **2930**

Phenylephrine Bitartrate (Co-administration with other sympathomimetic agents may result in harmful

cardiovascular effects).
No products indexed under this heading.

Phenylephrine Hydrochloride (Co-administration with other sympathomimetic agents may result in harmful cardiovascular effects).
Products include:
Afrin Nasal Decongestant Children's Pump Mist .... ▣734
Extendryl 1361
Hycomine Compound Tablets 1317
Neo-Synephrine .... ▣614
Phenergan VC Syrup 3560
Phenergan VC with Codeine Syrup .. 3561
Preparation H Cream .... ▣778
Preparation H Cooling Gel .... ▣778
Preparation H .... ▣778
Vicks Sinex Nasal Spray and Ultra Fine Mist .... ▣729

Phenylephrine Tannate (Co-administration with other sympathomimetic agents may result in harmful cardiovascular effects). Products include:
Ryna-12 S Suspension 3351
Reformulated Rynatan Pediatric Suspension 3352
Rynatuss Pediatric Suspension 3353
Rynatuss Tablets 3353

Phenylpropanolamine Hydrochloride (Co-administration with other sympathomimetic agents may result in harmful cardiovascular effects).
No products indexed under this heading.

Pirbuterol Acetate (Co-administration with other sympathomimetic agents may result in harmful cardiovascular effects). Products include:
Maxair Autohaler 1981
Maxair Inhaler 1984

Prazepam (Concurrent use may result in additional reduction in alertness impairment of CNS performance).
No products indexed under this heading.

Procarbazine Hydrochloride (Concurrent and/or sequential use with MAO inhibitors is contraindicated). Products include:
Matulane Capsules 3246

Prochlorperazine (Concurrent use may result in additional reduction in alertness impairment of CNS performance). Products include:
Compazine 1505

Promethazine Hydrochloride (Concurrent use may result in additional reduction in alertness impairment of CNS performance).
Products include:
Mepergan Injection 3539
Phenergan Injection 3553
Phenergan 3556
Phenergan Syrup 3554
Phenergan with Codeine Syrup 3557
Phenergan with Dextromethorphan Syrup 3559
Phenergan VC Syrup 3560
Phenergan VC with Codeine Syrup .. 3561

Propofol (Concurrent use may result in additional reduction in alertness impairment of CNS performance). Products include:
Diprivan Injectable Emulsion 667

Propoxyphene Hydrochloride (Concurrent use may result in additional reduction in alertness impairment of CNS performance).
Products include:
Darvon Pulvules 1909
Darvon Compound-65 Pulvules 1910

Propoxyphene Napsylate (Concurrent use may result in additional reduction in alertness impairment of CNS performance). Products include:
Darvon-N/Darvocet-N 1907
Darvon-N Tablets 1912

Pseudoephedrine Sulfate (Co-administration with other sympathomimetic agents may result in harmful cardiovascular effects). Products include:
Chlor-Trimeton Allergy/Decongestant Tablets .... ▣736
Claritin-D 12 Hour Extended Release Tablets 3102
Claritin-D 24 Hour Extended Release Tablets 3104
Coricidin 'D' Cold, Flu & Sinus Tablets .... ▣737
Drixoral Allergy/Sinus Extended-Release Tablets .... ▣741
Drixoral Cold & Allergy Sustained-Action Tablets .... ▣740
Drixoral Cold & Flu Extended-Release Tablets .... ▣740
Drixoral Nasal Decongestant Long-Acting Non-Drowsy Tablets .... ▣740
Rynatan Tablets 3351

Quazepam (Concurrent use may result in additional reduction in alertness impairment of CNS performance).
No products indexed under this heading.

Quetiapine Fumarate (Concurrent use may result in additional reduction in alertness impairment of CNS performance). Products include:
Seroquel Tablets 684

Rabeprazole Sodium (Proton pump inhibitors increase gastric pH and may reduce the absorption of delavirdine chronic use of these drugs with delavirdine is not recommended). Products include:
Aciphex Tablets 1267
Aciphex Tablets 1783

Ranitidine Bismuth Citrate (H2 antagonists increase gastric pH and may reduce the absorption of delavirdine; chronic use of these drugs with delavirdine is not recommended).
No products indexed under this heading.

Ranitidine Hydrochloride (H2 antagonists increase gastric pH and may reduce the absorption of delavirdine; chronic use of these drugs with delavirdine is not recommended). Products include:
Zantac 1690
Zantac Injection 1688
Zantac 75 Tablets .... ▣717

Remifentanil Hydrochloride (Concurrent use may result in additional reduction in alertness impairment of CNS performance).
No products indexed under this heading.

Reserpine (Pseudoephedrine may reduce the antihypertensive effect).
No products indexed under this heading.

Risperidone (Concurrent use may result in additional reduction in alertness impairment of CNS performance). Products include:
Risperdal 1796

Salmeterol Xinafoate (Co-administration with other sympathomimetic agents may result in harmful cardiovascular effects). Products include:
Advair Diskus 100/50 1448
Advair Diskus 250/50 1448
Advair Diskus 500/50 1448
Serevent Diskus 1637
Serevent Inhalation Aerosol 1633

Secobarbital Sodium (Concurrent use may result in additional reduction in alertness impairment of CNS performance).
No products indexed under this heading.

Selegiline Hydrochloride (Concurrent and/or sequential use with MAO inhibitors is contraindicated).
Products include:
Eldepryl Capsules 3266

Sevoflurane (Concurrent use may result in additional reduction in alertness impairment of CNS performance).
No products indexed under this heading.

Sufentanil Citrate (Concurrent use may result in additional reduction in alertness impairment of CNS performance).
No products indexed under this heading.

Temazepam (Concurrent use may result in additional reduction in alertness impairment of CNS performance).
No products indexed under this heading.

Terbutaline Sulfate (Co-administration with other sympathomimetic agents may result in harmful cardiovascular effects). Products include:
Brethine Ampuls 2314
Brethine Tablets 2313

Theophylline (Small decrease in the clearance of cetirizine caused by a 400 mg dose of theophylline; it is possible that larger theophylline doses could have a greater effect).
Products include:
Aerolate 1361
Theo-Dur Extended-Release Tablets 1835
Uni-Dur Extended-Release Tablets .. 1841
Uniphyl 400 mg and 600 mg Tablets 2903

Theophylline Calcium Salicylate (Small decrease in the clearance of cetirizine caused by a 400 mg dose of theophylline; it is possible that larger theophylline doses could have a greater effect).
No products indexed under this heading.

Theophylline Sodium Glycinate (Small decrease in the clearance of cetirizine caused by a 400 mg dose of theophylline; it is possible that larger theophylline doses could have a greater effect).
No products indexed under this heading.

Thiamylal Sodium (Concurrent use may result in additional reduction in alertness impairment of CNS performance).
No products indexed under this heading.

Thioridazine Hydrochloride (Concurrent use may result in additional reduction in alertness impairment of CNS performance). Products include:
Thioridazine Hydrochloride Tablets 2289

Thiothixene (Concurrent use may result in additional reduction in alertness impairment of CNS performance). Products include:
Navane Capsules 2701
Thiothixene Capsules 2290

Tranylcypromine Sulfate (Concurrent and/or sequential use with MAO inhibitors is contraindicated).
Products include:
Parnate Tablets 1607

Triazolam (Concurrent use may result in additional reduction in alertness impairment of CNS performance). Products include:
Halcion Tablets 2823

Trifluoperazine Hydrochloride (Concurrent use may result in additional reduction in alertness impairment of CNS performance).
Products include:
Stelazine 1640

Zaleplon (Concurrent use may result in additional reduction in alertness impairment of CNS performance). Products include:
Sonata Capsules 3591

Ziprasidone Hydrochloride (Concurrent use may result in additional reduction in alertness impairment of CNS performance). Products include:
Geodon Capsules 2688

Zolpidem Tartrate (Concurrent use may result in additional reduction in alertness impairment of CNS performance). Products include:
Ambien Tablets 3191

Food Interactions

Alcohol (Concurrent use may result in additional reduction in alertness impairment of CNS performance).

ZYVOX INJECTION

(Linezolid) 2871
See Zyvox Tablets

ZYVOX FOR ORAL SUSPENSION

(Linezolid) 2871
See Zyvox Tablets

ZYVOX TABLETS

(Linezolid) 2871
May interact with serotoninergic agents, sympathomimetics, and certain other agents. Compounds in these categories include:

Albuterol (Linezolid is a reversible nonselective inhibitor of MAO; therefore, linezolid has the potential for interaction with adrenergic agents). Products include:
Proventil Inhalation Aerosol 3142
Ventolin Inhalation Aerosol and Refill 1679

Albuterol Sulfate (Linezolid is a reversible nonselective inhibitor of MAO; therefore, linezolid has the potential for interaction with adrenergic agents). Products include:
AccuNeb Inhalation Solution 1230
Combivent Inhalation Aerosol 1041
DuoNeb Inhalation Solution 1233
Proventil Inhalation Solution 0.083% 3146
Proventil Repetabs Tablets 3148
Proventil Solution for Inhalation 0.5% 3144
Proventil HFA Inhalation Aerosol 3150
Ventolin HFA Inhalation Aerosol 3618
Volmax Extended-Release Tablets .. 2276

Citalopram Hydrobromide (Linezolid is a reversible nonselective inhibitor of MAO; therefore, linezolid has the potential for interaction with serotonergic agents). Products include:
Celexa 1365

Dobutamine Hydrochloride (Linezolid is a reversible nonselective inhibitor of MAO; therefore, linezolid has the potential for interaction with adrenergic agents). Products include:
Dobutrex Solution Vials 1914

Dopamine Hydrochloride (Some patients receiving Zyvox with dopaminergic agents may experience a reversible enhancement of pressor response; initial dose of dopamine should be reduced and titrated to achieve the desired response).
No products indexed under this heading.

Ephedrine Hydrochloride (Linezolid is a reversible nonselective inhibitor of MAO; therefore, linezolid has the potential for interaction with adrenergic agents). Products include:
Primatene Tablets .... ▣780

Ephedrine Sulfate (Linezolid is a reversible nonselective inhibitor of MAO; therefore, linezolid has the potential for interaction with adrenergic agents).
No products indexed under this heading.

Ephedrine Tannate (Linezolid is a reversible nonselective inhibitor of

MAO; therefore, linezolid has the potential for interaction with adrenergic agents). Products include:
- Rynatuss Pediatric Suspension 3353
- Rynatuss Tablets 3353

Epinephrine (Linezolid is a reversible nonselective inhibitor of MAO; therefore, linezolid has the potential for interaction with adrenergic agents). Products include:
- Epifrin Sterile Ophthalmic Solution ...... ⊙235
- EpiPen 1236
- Primatene Mist ...... ■779
- Xylocaine with Epinephrine Injection 653

Epinephrine Bitartrate (Linezolid is a reversible nonselective inhibitor of MAO; therefore, linezolid has the potential for interaction with adrenergic agents). Products include:
- Sensorcaine 643

Epinephrine Hydrochloride (Some patients receiving Zyvox with vasopressors may experience a reversible enhancement of pressor response; initial dose of epinephrine should be reduced and titrated to achieve the desired response).
No products indexed under this heading.

Fluoxetine Hydrochloride (Linezolid is a reversible nonselective inhibitor of MAO; therefore, linezolid has the potential for interaction with serotonergic agents). Products include:
- Prozac Pulvules, Liquid, and Weekly Capsules 1238
- Sarafem Pulvules 1962

Fluvoxamine Maleate (Linezolid is a reversible nonselective inhibitor of MAO; therefore, linezolid has the potential for interaction with serotonergic agents). Products include:
- Luvox Tablets (25, 50, 100 mg) 3256

Isoproterenol Hydrochloride (Linezolid is a reversible nonselective inhibitor of MAO; therefore, linezolid has the potential for interaction with adrenergic agents).
No products indexed under this heading.

Isoproterenol Sulfate (Linezolid is a reversible nonselective inhibitor of MAO; therefore, linezolid has the potential for interaction with adrenergic agents).
No products indexed under this heading.

Levalbuterol Hydrochloride (Linezolid is a reversible nonselective inhibitor of MAO; therefore, linezolid has the potential for interaction with adrenergic agents). Products include:
- Xopenex Inhalation Solution 3207

Metaproterenol Sulfate (Linezolid is a reversible nonselective inhibitor of MAO; therefore, linezolid has the potential for interaction with adrenergic agents). Products include:
- Alupent 1029

Metaraminol Bitartrate (Linezolid is a reversible nonselective inhibitor of MAO; therefore, linezolid has the potential for interaction with adrenergic agents). Products include:
- Aramine Injection 2043

Methoxamine Hydrochloride (Linezolid is a reversible nonselective inhibitor of MAO; therefore, linezolid has the potential for interaction with adrenergic agents).
No products indexed under this heading.

Norepinephrine Bitartrate (Linezolid is a reversible nonselective inhibitor of MAO; therefore, linezolid has the potential for interaction with adrenergic agents).
No products indexed under this heading.

Paroxetine Hydrochloride (Linezolid is a reversible nonselective inhibitor of MAO; therefore, linezolid has the potential for interaction with serotonergic agents). Products include:
- Paxil 1609

Phenylephrine Bitartrate (Linezolid is a reversible nonselective inhibitor of MAO; therefore, linezolid has the potential for interaction with adrenergic agents).
No products indexed under this heading.

Phenylephrine Hydrochloride (Linezolid is a reversible nonselective inhibitor of MAO; therefore, linezolid has the potential for interaction with adrenergic agents). Products include:
- Afrin Nasal Decongestant Children's Pump Mist ...... ■734
- Extendryl 1361
- Hycomine Compound Tablets 1317
- Neo-Synephrine ...... ■614
- Phenergan VC Syrup 3560
- Phenergan VC with Codeine Syrup 3561
- Preparation H Cream ...... ■778
- Preparation H Cooling Gel ...... ■778
- Preparation H ...... ■778
- Vicks Sinex Nasal Spray and Ultra Fine Mist ...... ■729

Phenylephrine Tannate (Linezolid is a reversible nonselective inhibitor of MAO; therefore, linezolid has the potential for interaction with adrenergic agents). Products include:
- Ryna-12 S Suspension 3351
- Reformulated Rynatan Pediatric Suspension 3352
- Rynatuss Pediatric Suspension 3353
- Rynatuss Tablets 3353

Phenylpropanolamine Hydrochloride (Co-administration has resulted in a reversible enhancement of pressor response of phenylpropanolamine).
No products indexed under this heading.

Pirbuterol Acetate (Linezolid is a reversible nonselective inhibitor of MAO; therefore, linezolid has the potential for interaction with adrenergic agents). Products include:
- Maxair Autohaler 1981
- Maxair Inhaler 1984

Pseudoephedrine Hydrochloride (Co-administration has resulted in a reversible enhancement of pressor response of pseudoephedrine). Products include:
- Actifed Cold & Allergy Tablets ...... ■688
- Actifed Cold & Sinus Caplets and Tablets ...... ■688
- Advil Cold and Sinus Caplets ...... ■771
- Advil Cold and Sinus Tablets ...... ■771
- Advil Flu & Body Ache Caplets ...... ■772
- Aleve Cold & Sinus Caplets ...... ■603
- Alka-Seltzer Plus Liqui-Gels ...... ■604
- Alka-Seltzer Plus Cold & Flu Medicine Liqui-Gels ...... ■604
- Alka-Seltzer Plus Cold & Sinus Medicine Liqui-Gels ...... ■604
- Allegra-D Extended-Release Tablets 714
- BC Cold Powder ...... ■619
- Benadryl Allergy/Cold Tablets ...... ■691
- Benadryl Allergy/Congestion Tablets ...... ■692
- Benadryl Allergy & Sinus Liquid ...... ■693
- Benadryl Allergy & Sinus Fastmelt Tablets ...... ■693
- Benadryl Allergy Sinus Headache Caplets & Gelcaps ...... ■693
- Benadryl Severe Allergy & Sinus Headache Caplets ...... ■694
- Benadryl Children's Allergy/Cold Fastmelt Tablets ...... ■692
- Benylin Multi-Symptom Liquid ...... ■697
- Bromfed Capsules (Extended-Release) 2269
- Bromfed-PD Capsules (Extended-Release) 2269
- Children's Cēpacol Sore Throat ...... ■788
- Comtrex Acute Head Cold & Sinus Pressure Relief Tablets ...... ■627
- Comtrex Deep Chest Cold & Congestion Relief Softgels ...... ■627
- Comtrex Flu Therapy & Fever Relief Daytime Caplets ...... ■628
- Comtrex Flu Therapy & Fever Relief Nighttime Tablets ...... ■628
- Comtrex Maximum Strength Multi-Symptom Cold & Cough Relief Tablets and Caplets ...... ■626
- Contac Non-Drowsy 12 Hour Cold Caplets ...... ■745
- Contac Non-Drowsy Timed Release 12 Hour Cold Caplets ...... ■746
- Contac Severe Cold and Flu Caplets Maximum Strength ...... ■746
- Contac Severe Cold and Flu Caplets Non-Drowsy ...... ■746
- Dimetapp Elixir ...... ■777
- Dimetapp Cold and Fever Suspension ...... ■775
- Dimetapp DM Cold & Cough Elixir ...... ■775
- Dimetapp Nighttime Flu Liquid ...... ■776
- Dimetapp Non-Drowsy Flu Syrup ...... ■777
- Dimetapp Infant Drops Decongestant ...... ■775
- Dimetapp Infant Drops Decongestant Plus Cough ...... ■776
- Guaifed 2272
- Kronofed-A 1341
- Children's Motrin Cold Oral Suspension 2007
- Motrin Sinus Headache Caplets 2005
- PediaCare Cough-Cold Liquid ...... ■719
- PediaCare Infants' Drops Decongestant ...... ■719
- PediaCare Infants' Drops Decongestant Plus Cough ...... ■719
- PediaCare NightRest Cough-Cold Liquid ...... ■719
- Robitussin Cold Caplets Cold & Congestion ...... ■780
- Robitussin Cold Softgels Cold & Congestion ...... ■780
- Robitussin Cold Caplets Multi-Symptom Cold & Flu ...... ■781
- Robitussin Cold Softgels Multi-Symptom Cold & Flu ...... ■781
- Robitussin Cold Softgels Severe Congestion ...... ■782
- Robitussin Cough & Cold Infant Drops ...... ■782
- Robitussin Maximum Strength Cough & Cold Liquid ...... ■785
- Robitussin Pediatric Cough & Cold Formula Liquid ...... ■785
- Robitussin Multi Symptom Honey Flu Liquid ...... ■785
- Robitussin Nighttime Honey Flu Liquid ...... ■786
- Robitussin-CF Liquid ...... ■783
- Robitussin-DAC Syrup 2942
- Robitussin-PE Liquid ...... ■782
- Ryna ...... ■768
- Semprex-D Capsules 1172
- Singlet Caplets ...... ■761
- Sinutab Non-Drying Liquid Caps ...... ■706
- Sinutab Sinus Allergy Medication, Maximum Strength Formula, Tablets & Caplets ...... ■707
- Sinutab Sinus Medication, Maximum Strength Without Drowsiness Formula, Tablets & Caplets ...... ■707
- Sudafed 12 Hour Tablets ...... ■708
- Sudafed 24 Hour Tablets ...... ■708
- Children's Sudafed Cold & Cough Liquid ...... ■709
- Children's Sudafed Nasal Decongestant Chewables ...... ■711
- Children's Sudafed Nasal Decongestant Liquid Medication ...... ■711
- Sudafed Cold & Allergy Tablets ...... ■708
- Sudafed Cold & Cough Liquid Caps ...... ■709
- Sudafed Cold & Sinus Liquid Caps ...... ■710
- Sudafed Nasal Decongestant Tablets ...... ■710
- Sudafed Non-Drying Sinus Liquid Caps ...... ■712
- Sudafed Severe Cold ...... ■711
- Sudafed Sinus Headache Caplets ...... ■712
- Sudafed Sinus Headache Tablets ...... ■712
- Tavist Sinus Non-Drowsy Coated Caplets ...... ■676
- TheraFlu Regular Strength Cold & Cough Night Time Hot Liquid ...... ■676
- TheraFlu Regular Strength Cold & Sore Throat Night Time Hot Liquid ...... ■676
- TheraFlu Maximum Strength Flu & Congestion Non-Drowsy Hot Liquid ...... ■677
- TheraFlu Maximum Strength Flu & Cough Night Time Hot Liquid ...... ■678
- TheraFlu Maximum Strength Flu & Sore Throat Night Time Hot Liquid ...... ■677
- TheraFlu Maximum Strength Severe Cold & Congestion Night Time Caplets ...... ■678
- TheraFlu Maximum Strength Severe Cold & Congestion Night Time Hot Liquid ...... ■678
- TheraFlu Maximum Strength Severe Cold & Congestion Non-Drowsy ...... ■679
- Triaminic Allergy Congestion Liquid ...... ■680
- Triaminic Chest Congestion Liquid ...... ■680
- Triaminic Cold & Allergy Liquid ...... ■681
- Triaminic Cold & Allergy Softchews ...... ■683
- Triaminic Cold & Cough Liquid ...... ■681
- Triaminic Cold & Cough Softchews ...... ■683
- Triaminic Cold & Night Time Cough Liquid ...... ■681
- Triaminic Cold, Cough & Fever Liquid ...... ■681
- Triaminic Cough Liquid ...... ■682
- Triaminic Cough & Congestion Liquid ...... ■682
- Triaminic Cough & Sore Throat Liquid ...... ■682
- Triaminic Cough & Sore Throat Softchews ...... ■684
- Children's Tylenol Allergy-D Liquid 2014
- Children's Tylenol Cold Suspension Liquid and Chewable Tablets 2015
- Children's Tylenol Cold Plus Cough Suspension Liquid and Chewable Tablets 2015
- Children's Tylenol Flu Suspension Liquid 2015
- Children's Tylenol Sinus Suspension Liquid 2017
- Infants' Tylenol Cold Decongestant and Fever Reducer Concentrated Drops 2015
- Infants' Tylenol Cold Decongestant and Fever Reducer Concentrated Drops Plus Cough 2015
- Tylenol Allergy Sinus 2010
- Multi-Symptom Tylenol Cold Complete Formula Caplets 2010
- Multi-Symptom Tylenol Cold Non-Drowsy Caplets and Gelcaps 2010
- Multi-Symptom Tylenol Cold Severe Congestion Non-Drowsy Caplets 2011
- Maximum Strength Tylenol Flu NightTime Gelcaps 2011
- Maximum Strength Tylenol Flu NightTime Liquid 2011
- Maximum Strength Tylenol Flu Non-Drowsy Gelcaps 2011
- Maximum Strength Tylenol Sinus NightTime Caplets 2012
- Maximum Strength Tylenol Sinus Non-Drowsy Geltabs, Gelcaps, Caplets, and Tablets 2012
- Vicks 44D Cough & Head Congestion Relief Liquid ...... ■724
- Vicks 44M Cough, Cold & Flu Relief Liquid ...... ■725
- Pediatric Vicks 44m Cough & Cold Relief ...... ■728
- Vicks DayQuil LiquiCaps/Liquid Multi-Symptom Cold/Flu Relief ...... ■727
- Children's Vicks NyQuil Cold/Cough Relief ...... ■726
- Vicks NyQuil LiquiCaps/Liquid Multi-Symptom Cold/Flu Relief, Original and Cherry Flavors ...... ■727
- Zephrex Tablets 3091
- Zephrex LA Tablets 3092
- Zyrtec-D 12 Hour Extended Relief Tablets 2758

Pseudoephedrine Sulfate (Linezolid is a reversible nonselective inhibitor of MAO; therefore, linezolid has the potential for interaction with adrenergic agents). Products include:
- Chlor-Trimeton Allergy/Decongestant Tablets ...... ■736
- Claritin-D 12 Hour Extended Release Tablets 3102
- Claritin-D 24 Hour Extended Release Tablets 3104
- Coricidin 'D' Cold, Flu & Sinus Tablets ...... ■737
- Drixoral Allergy/Sinus Extended-Release Tablets ...... ■741
- Drixoral Cold & Allergy Sustained-Action Tablets ...... ■740
- Drixoral Cold & Flu Extended-Release Tablets ...... ■740
- Drixoral Nasal Decongestant Long-Acting Non-Drowsy Tablets ...... ■740
- Rynatan Tablets 3351

Salmeterol Xinafoate (Linezolid is a reversible nonselective inhibitor of MAO; therefore, linezolid has the potential for interaction with adrenergic agents). Products include:
Advair Diskus 100/50 .... **1448**
Advair Diskus 250/50 .... **1448**
Advair Diskus 500/50 .... **1448**
Serevent Diskus **1637**
Serevent Inhalation Aerosol **1633**

Sertraline Hydrochloride (Linezolid is a reversible nonselective inhibitor of MAO; therefore, linezolid has the potential for interaction with serotonergic agents). Products include:
Zoloft **2751**

Terbutaline Sulfate (Linezolid is a reversible nonselective inhibitor of MAO; therefore, linezolid has the potential for interaction with adrenergic agents). Products include:
Brethine Ampuls **2314**
Brethine Tablets **2313**

Tyramine (Co-administration has resulted in a significant pressor response).
No products indexed under this heading.

Venlafaxine Hydrochloride (Linezolid is a reversible nonselective inhibitor of MAO; therefore, linezolid has the potential for interaction with serotonergic agents). Products include:
Effexor Tablets **3495**
Effexor XR Capsules **3499**

Food Interactions

Beverages with high tyramine (Co-administration has resulted in a significant pressor response; patients receiving linezolid should avoid consuming large amounts of beverages containing tyramine).

Food, unspecified (The time to reach maximum concentration is delayed from 1.5 hours to 2.2 hours and Cmax is decreased by about 17% when linezolid is co-administered with high fat food; linezolid may be administered without regard to the timing of meals).

Food high in tyramine (Co-administration has resulted in a significant pressor response; patients receiving linezolid should avoid consuming large amounts of food containing tyramine).

ZZZ SPRAY LIQUID

(5-hydroxytryptophan, Herbals with Vitamins & Minerals, Melatonin)....................................... **801**
None cited in PDR database.

SECTION 2

FOOD INTERACTIONS CROSS-REFERENCE

In this section, drug/food and drug/alcohol interactions listed in the preceding index are cross-referenced by dietary item. Under each entry is an alphabetical list, by brand name, of drugs said to interact with the item. A brief description of the interaction follows each brand, along with the page number of the underlying text. Page numbers refer to the 2002 editions of *PDR®* and *PDR for Ophthalmic Medicines™* and the 2001 edition of *PDR for Nonprescription Drugs and Dietary Supplements™*, which is published later each year. A key to the symbols denoting the companion volumes appears in the bottom margin.

Entries in this section are limited to drug/food and drug/alcohol interactions listed in official prescribing information as published by *PDR®*.

Alcohol

Accuretic Tablets (May potentiate orthostatic hypotension) 2614

Actifed Cold & Allergy Tablets (May increase drowsiness effect) .... ■688

Actifed Cold & Sinus Caplets and Tablets (May increase drowsiness effect; patients consuming 3 or more alcoholic beverages a day should consult a physician for advice on when and how they should take this medication) .... ■688

Actiq (Concurrent use with alcoholic beverages may result in increased depressant effects; hypoventilation, hypotension, and profound sedation may occur) 1184

Adipex-P Tablets (May result in adverse drug interaction) 1406

Advil Tablets (Chronic heavy alcohol users, 3 or more drinks per day, should consult their physicians for advice on when and how they should take pain relievers/fever reducers including ibuprofen) .... ■771

Advil Cold and Sinus Tablets (Chronic heavy alcohol users, 3 or more drinks per day, should consult their physician for advice on when and how they should take pain relievers/fever reducers including ibuprofen) .... ■771

Advil Flu & Body Ache Caplets (Chronic heavy alcohol users, 3 or more drinks per day, should consult their physican for advice on when and how they should take pain relievers/fever reducers including ibuprofen) .... ■772

Advil Migraine Liquigels (Chronic heavy alcohol users, 3 or more drinks per day, should consult their physician for advice on when and how they should take pain relievers/fever reducers including ibuprofen) .... ■772

Agenerase Oral Solution (Concurrent use of Agenerase Oral Solution with alcoholic beverages is not recommended) 1459

Aggrenox Capsules (Patients who consume three or more alcoholic drinks every day should be counseled about the bleeding risks involved with chronic, heavy alcohol use while taking aspirin) 1026

Aldoclor Tablets (Aggravates orthostatic hypotension) 2035

Aldoril Tablets (Aggravates orthostatic hypotension) 2039

Aleve Tablets, Caplets and Gelcaps (Individuals consuming 3 or more alcohol-containing drinks per day should consult their physicians for advice on when and how they should take this product) .... ■602

Aleve Cold & Sinus Caplets (Chronic heavy alcohol users, 3 or more drinks per day, should consult their physician for advice on when and how they should take pain relievers/fever reducers including naproxen) .... ■603

Alka-Seltzer Original Antacid and Pain Reliever Effervescent Tablets (Chronic heavy alcohol users, 3 or more drinks per day, should consult their physicians for advice on when and how they should take pain relievers/fever reducers including aspirin) .... ■603

Alka-Seltzer Plus Night-Time Cold Medicine Liqui-Gels (Chronic heavy alcohol users, 3 or more drinks per day, should consult their physicians for advice on when and how they should take pain relievers/fever reducers including acetaminophen; increases drowsiness effect) .... ■604

Alka-Seltzer PM Effervescent Tablets (Chronic heavy alcohol users, 3 or more drinks per day, should consult their physicians for advice on when and how they should take pain relievers/fever reducers including aspirin; diphenhydramine is an antihistamine, therefore, concurrent use with alcoholic beverages should be avoided) .... ■605

Alphagan Ophthalmic Solution (Possible additive or potentiating effect with CNS depressants) 545

Ambien Tablets (Co-administration produces additive effects on psychomotor performance) 3191

Antabuse Tablets (Disulfiram plus alcohol, even small amounts, produce flushing, throbbing in head and neck, throbbing headache, respiratory difficulty, nausea, vomiting, and confusion; concurrent use with alcohol-containing preparations, such as cough syrups, tonics, sauces, vinegars, and even aftershave lotion and back rubs should be avoided) 2444

Antabuse Tablets (Antabuse plus alcohol, even small amounts, produces flushing, throbbing in head and neck, throbbing headache, respiratory difficulty, nausea, copious vomiting, thirst, dyspnea, chest pain, palpitations, and other serious cardiovascular and respiratory reactions resulting in possible fatality; concurrent use with alcohol or alcohol containing preparations, such as cough syrups, tonics, sauces, and even after shave lotions and back rubs is contraindicated) 3474

Antivert, Antivert/25, & Antivert/50 Tablets (Concurrent use should be avoided) 2664

Astelin Nasal Spray (Concurrent use may result in additional reduction in alertness and impairment of CNS performance; alcohol intake should be avoided) 3339

Astramorph/PF Injection, USP (Preservative-Free) (Potentiation of depressant effects of morphine) 594

Atacand HCT Tablets (May aggravate orthostatic hypotension produced by hydrochlorothiazide) 597

Atarax Tablets & Syrup (Increased effect of alcohol) 2667

Ativan Injection (Concurrent use results in additive CNS depression of the central nervous system) 3478

Avalide Tablets (Potentiation of orthostatic hypotension) 1070

Extra Strength Bayer Plus Caplets (Chronic heavy alcohol users, 3 or more drinks per day, should consult their physicians for advice on when and how they should take pain relievers/fever reducers including aspirin) .... ■610

Extra Strength Bayer PM Caplets (Chronic heavy alcohol users, 3 or more drinks per day, should consult their physicians for advice on when and how they should take pain relievers/fever reducers including aspirin) .... ■611

BC Allergy Sinus Cold Powder (Individuals consuming 3 or more alcohol-containing drinks per day should consult their physician for advice on when and how they should take this product; increases drowsiness; avoid concurrent use) .... ■619

Benadryl Allergy Kapseal Capsules (May increase drowsiness effect) .... ■691

Benadryl Allergy/Cold Tablets (May increase drowsiness effect) .... ■691

Benadryl Allergy/Congestion Tablets (Increases the drowsiness effect; avoid concomitant use) ▣ 692

Benadryl Allergy & Sinus Liquid (May increase drowsiness effect; avoid concurrent use) ▣ 693

Benadryl Allergy Sinus Headache Caplets & Gelcaps (May increase drowsiness effect) ▣ 693

Benadryl Severe Allergy & Sinus Headache Caplets (Chronic heavy alcohol users, 3 or more drinks per day, should consult their physician for advice on when and how they should take pain relievers/fever reducers including acetaminophen; increases drowsiness effect) ▣ 694

Benadryl Children's Allergy/Cold Fastmelt Tablets (May increase drowsiness) ▣ 692

Benadryl Dye-Free Allergy Liquid (May increase the drowsiness effect) ▣ 690

Benadryl Dye-Free Allergy Liqui-Gels Softgels (May increase the drowsiness effect) ▣ 690

Benadryl Parenteral (Additive effects) 2617

Brevital Sodium for Injection, USP (Barbiturates may influence the absorption and elimination of other concomitantly used drugs, such as ethyl alcohol) 1815

Bromfed Capsules (Extended-Release) (Co-administration may have an additive effect) 2269

Buprenex Injectable (Increased CNS depression) 2918

Catapres Tablets (Clonidine may potentiate the CNS-depressive effects) 1037

Catapres-TTS (Clonidine may potentiate the CNS-depressive effects) 1038

Cefobid Pharmacy Bulk Package - Not for Direct Infusion (A disulfiram-like reaction characterized by flushing, sweating, headache, and tachycardia has been reported when alcohol was ingested within 72 hours after Cefobid administration) 2673

Cefotan for Injection (When ingested within 72 hours after Cefotan administration may cause disulfiram-like reactions, including flushing, headache, sweating and tachycardia) 664

Celexa Tablets (Concurrent use is not recommended; although, citalopram did not potentiate cognitive and motor effects of alcohol) 1365

Cerebyx Injection (Acute alcohol intake may increase plasma phenytoin concentration; chronic alcohol abuse may decrease plasma phenytoin concentration) 2619

Chlor-Trimeton Allergy Tablets (May increase drowsiness effect, avoid alcoholic beverages) ▣ 735

Chlor-Trimeton Allergy/Decongestant Tablets (May increase drowsiness effect) ▣ 736

Clorpres Tablets (Clonidine may enhance the CNS-depressive effects of alcohol; orthostatic hypotension may be aggravated by alcohol) 1002

Clozaril Tablets (Caution is advised with concomitant use) 2319

Combipres Tablets (Orthostatic hypotension produced by chlorthalidone may be aggravated by alcohol; potential for enhanced CNS-depressive effects) 1040

Compazine Tablets (Phenothiazines may intensify or prolong the action of other central nervous system depressants) 1505

Comtan Tablets (Possible additive sedative effects) 2328

Comtrex Deep Chest Cold & Congestion Relief Softgels (Chronic heavy alcohol users, 3 or more drinks per day, should consult their physicians for advice on when and how they should take pain relievers/fever reducers including acetaminophen) ▣ 627

Comtrex Flu Therapy & Fever Relief Nighttime Tablets (Chronic heavy alcohol users, 3 or more drinks per day, should consult their physicians for advice on when and how they should take pain relievers/fever reducers including acetaminophen; increases drowsiness effect) ▣ 628

Comtrex Maximum Strength Multi-Symptom Cold & Cough Relief Tablets and Caplets (Chronic heavy alcohol users, 3 or more drinks per day, should consult their physicians for advice on when and how they should take pain relievers/fever reducers; may increase drowsiness) ▣ 626

Contac Severe Cold and Flu Caplets Maximum Strength (May increase drowsiness effect; concurrent use should be avoided) ▣ 746

Coricidin 'D' Cold, Flu & Sinus Tablets (May increase drowsiness effect; patients consuming 3 or more alcoholic drinks per day should consult their physician on when and how they should take this medication) ▣ 737

Coricidin HBP Maximum Strength Flu Tablets (Chronic heavy alcohol users, 3 or more drinks per day, should consult their physician for advice on when and how they should take pain relievers/fever reducers including acetaminophen; increases drowsiness effect) ▣ 738

Corzide 80/5 Tablets (Co-administration may result in potentiation of orthostatic hypotension) 2247

Coumadin Tablets (Decreased or increased prothrombin time response) 1243

Covera-HS Tablets (Verapamil may increase blood alcohol concentrations and prolong its effect) 3199

Dantrium Capsules (Co-administration may result in increased drowsiness; caution should be exercised) 2885

Darvocet-N 50 Tablets (Additive CNS depression) 1907

Darvon Pulvules (The CNS-depressant effect of propoxyphene is additive with that of alcohol) 1909

Darvon Compound-65 Pulvules (Concurrent use can lead to potentially serious CNS depressant effects) 1910

Darvon-N Tablets (Concurrent use can lead to potentially serious CNS depressant effects) 1912

Demerol Tablets (Concurrent use may result in respiratory depression, hypotension, and profound sedation or coma) 3079

Demser Capsules (Additive sedative effects) 2085

Depacon Injection (Co-administration may result in additive CNS depression) 416

Depakene Capsules (Valproate produces CNS depression, especially when combined with another CNS depressant, such as alcohol) 421

Depakote Tablets (Valproate produces CNS depression, especially when combined with another CNS depressant, such as alcohol) 430

DiaBeta Tablets (Potential for hypoglycemia) 741

Diabinese Tablets (In some patients disulfiram-like reaction may be produced by the ingestion of alcohol) 2680

Dilantin Infatabs (Acute alcohol intake increases serum phenytoin levels; chronic alcohol intake decreases serum phenytoin levels) 2624

Dilantin Kapseals (Acute alcohol intake increases serum phenytoin levels; chronic alcohol intake decreases serum phenytoin levels) 2622

Dilantin-125 Oral Suspension (Acute alcohol intake increases serum phenytoin levels; chronic alcohol intake decreases serum phenytoin levels) 2625

Dilaudid Ampules (Additive CNS depression) 441

Dilaudid Oral Liquid (May exhibit an additive CNS depression) 445

Dimetapp Elixir (May increase drowsiness effect) ▣ 777

Dimetapp Cold and Fever Suspension (May increase drowsiness effect) ▣ 775

Dimetapp DM Cold & Cough Elixir (Increases drowsiness effect; avoid concurrent use) ▣ 775

Dimetapp Nighttime Flu Liquid (Chronic heavy alcohol users, 3 or more drinks per day, should consult their physician for advice on when and how they should take pain relievers/fever reducers including acetaminophen; increases drowsiness effect) ▣ 776

Dimetapp Non-Drowsy Flu Syrup (Patients consuming three or more alcohol-containing drinks every day should consult their doctor for advice on when and how they should take acetaminophen-containing products) ▣ 777

Diovan HCT Tablets (Co-administration of thiazide diuretics and alcohol may result in potentiation of orthostatic hypotension) 2338

Ditropan XL Extended Release Tablets (Enhances the drowsiness effect caused by anticholinergic agents such as oxybutynin) 564

Diucardin Tablets (Thiazide-induced orthostatic hypotension may be potentiated) 3494

Diuril Oral Suspension (Potentiation of orthostatic hypotension may occur) 2087

Diuril Sodium Intravenous (Potentiation of orthostatic hypotension may occur) 2086

Dolophine Hydrochloride Tablets (Concurrent use with other CNS depressants may result in respiratory depression, hypotension, and profound sedation or coma) 3056

Dramamine Original Formula Tablets (May increase drowsiness effect) ▣ 718

Dramamine Less Drowsy Tablets (May increase drowsiness effect) ▣ 718

Drixoral Allergy/Sinus Extended-Release Tablets (May increase drowsiness effect; individuals who consume 3 or more alcohol containing drinks per day should consult their doctor on when and how they should take this product) ▣ 741

Drixoral Cold & Allergy Sustained-Action Tablets (May increase drowsiness effect) ▣ 740

Drixoral Cold & Flu Extended-Release Tablets (May increase drowsiness effect; individuals who consume 3 or more alcohol containing drinks per day should consult their doctor on when and how they should take this product) ▣ 740

Duraclon Injection (Clonidine may potentiate the CNS-depressive effects of alcohol) 3057

Duragesic Transdermal System (May produce additive depressant effects) 1786

Duramorph Injection (Potentiation of depressant effect) 1312

Ecotrin Enteric Coated Aspirin Low, Regular and Maximum Strength Tablets (Chronic heavy alcohol users, 3 or more drinks per day, in combination with analgesic/antipyretic drug products containing aspirin increases the risk of adverse GI events, including stomach bleeding) 1715

Effexor XR Capsules (Co-administration of venlafaxine as a stable regimen did not exaggerate the psychomotor and psychometric effects of alcohol; however, patients should be advised to avoid alcohol while taking venlafaxine) 3499

Ergamisol Tablets (May result in Antabuse-like side effects) 1789

Etrafon Tablets (2-25) (Amitriptyline may enhance the response to alcohol; potential for additive effects and hypotension; concurrent use should be avoided) 3115

Aspirin Free Excedrin Caplets and Geltabs (Chronic heavy alcohol users, 3 or more drinks per day, should consult their physicians for advice on when and how they should take pain relievers/fever reducers including acetaminophen) ▣ 628

Excedrin Extra-Strength Tablets, Caplets, and Geltabs (Chronic heavy alcohol users, 3 or more drinks per day, should consult their physicians for advice on when and how they should take pain relievers/fever reducers including acetaminophen) ▣ 629

Excedrin Migraine Caplets (Chronic heavy alcohol users, 3 or more drinks per day, should consult their physicians for advice on when and how they should take pain relievers/fever reducers including acetaminophen and aspirin) 1070

Excedrin PM Tablets, Caplets, and Geltabs (Chronic heavy alcohol users, 3 or more drinks per day, should consult their physicians for advice on when and how they should take pain relievers/fever reducers including acetaminophen; Excedrine P.M. contains diphenhydramine that causes drowsiness, therefore, concomitant use should be avoided) ▣ 631

Extendryl Syrup (Concomitant use of antihistamines with alcohol may have an additive effect) 1361

Flexeril Tablets (Concurrent use results in enhanced effects) 2094

Flexeril Tablets (Concurrent use results in enhanced effects) 572

Fluothane Inhalation (Co-administration with agents known to elevate hepatic levels of CYP450 enzyme, such as alcohol, enhances the metabolism of volatile anesthetics) 3508

Furosemide Tablets (Aggravates orthostatic hypotension) 2284

Gabitril Tablets (Possible additive depressive effects) 1189

Geodon Capsules (Somnolence was a commonly reported adverse event in patients treated with ziprasidone; concurrent use with alcohol or other CNS active drugs, such as depressants, should be undertaken with caution) 2688

Glucophage Tablets (Alcohol potentiates the effect of metformin on lactate metabolism; patients should be warned against excessive alcohol intake, acute or chronic) 1080

Glucotrol Tablets (Co-administration with alcohol may result in hypoglycemia) 2692

Glucotrol XL Extended Release Tablets (Co-administration with alcohol may result in hypoglycemia) 2693

Goody's Body Pain Formula Powder (Individuals consuming 3 or more alcohol-containing drinks per day should consult their physicians for advice on when and how they should take this product) ▣ 620

Goody's Extra Strength Headache Powder (Individuals consuming 3 or more alcohol-containing drinks per day should consult their physicians for advice on when and how they should take this product) ▣ 620

Goody's Extra Strength Pain Relief Tablets (Individuals consuming 3 or more alcohol-containing drinks per day should consult their physicians for advice on when and how they should take this product) ▣ 620

Goody's PM Powder (Individuals consuming 3 or more alcohol-containing drinks per day should consult their physicians for advice on when and how they should take this product; avoid alcoholic beverages since diphenhydramine causes drowsiness) ▣ 621

Gris-PEG Tablets (The effects of alcohol may be potentiated by griseofulvin, producing such effects as tachycardia and flushing) 2661

Halcion Tablets (Concurrent use results in additive CNS depressant effects) 2823

Haldol Injection, Tablets and Concentrate (Potentiation of CNS depressant effects) 2533

Humalog (Co-administration with drugs with hypoglycemic activity may result in decreased insulin requirements) 1926

Hycodan Tablets (Exhibits an additive CNS depression) 1316

Hycomine Compound Tablets (Exhibits an additive CNS depression) 1317

Hycotuss Expectorant Syrup (Exhibits an additive CNS depression) 1318

HydroDIURIL Tablets (Potentiation of orthostatic hypotension) 2108

Hyzaar 50-12.5 Tablets (Potentiation of orthostatic hypotension) 2109

Imdur Tablets (Additive vasodilating effects) 1826

Indapamide Tablets (Aggravates orthostatic hypotension) 2286

Inderal Injectable (Slows the rate of absorption of propranolol) 3513

Inderide Tablets (Slows the rate of absorption of propranolol) 3517

Infumorph 200 and Infumorph 500 Sterile Solutions (Potentiates CNS depressant effects) 1314

Inversine Tablets (The action of mecamylamine may be potentiated by alcohol) 1850

Ionamin Capsules (Possible adverse interactions with alcohol) 1163

Ismo Tablets (Additive vasodilating effects) 3524

Isoptin SR Tablets (Verapamil has been found to significantly inhibit alcohol elimination resulting in elevated blood alcohol concentrations that may prolong the intoxicating effect of alcohol) 467

Isordil Titradose Tablets (Alcohol exhibits additive vasodilating effects) 3526

Kadian Capsules (Co-administration may increase the risk of respiratory depression, hypotension and profound sedation and coma) 1335

Klonopin Tablets (Potentiates CNS-depressant action) 2983

Lantus Injection (May either potentiate or weaken the blood-glucose-lowering effect of insulin) 742

Levo-Dromoran Injectable (Concurrent use may result in additive central nervous system depressant effects, including respiratory depression, hypotension, profound sedation and coma) 1734

Levorphanol Tartrate Tablets (Concurrent use may result in additive CNS depressant effects) 3059

Librium Capsules (Potential for additive effects) 1736

Limbitrol Tablets (Concurrent use may produce additive effects resulting in harmful level of sedation and CNS depression) 1738

Lortab 10/500 Tablets (Co-administration may exhibit additive CNS-depression; concurrent use should be avoided) 3319

Lotensin HCT Tablets (Orthostatic hypotension produced by thiazides may be potentiated by alcohol) 2367

Loxitane Capsules (Loxapine may impair mental and/or physical abilities; concomitant use may result in additive effects; loxapine is contraindicated in severe alcohol-induced depressed state) 3398

Luvox Tablets (25, 50, 100 mg) (Concurrent use should be avoided) 3256

Mandol Vials (Concurrent ingestion of ethanol may result in nausea, vomiting, vasomotor instability with hypotension and peripheral vasodilation) 1953

Marinol Capsules (Co-administration results in additive drowsiness and CNS depression) 3325

Matulane Capsules (Concurrent use may produce an Antabuse-like reaction; concomitant use should be avoided) 3246

Maxidone Tablets CIII (Co-administration may exhibit an additive CNS depression) 3399

Maxzide Tablets (May aggravate orthostatic hypotension) 1008

Mepergan Injection (Respiratory depression, hypotension, profound sedation or coma) 3539

Meridia Capsules (Concurrent use has not resulted in psychomotor reactions of clinical significance, however, concomitant use with excessive alcohol is not recommended) 481

MetroGel-Vaginal Gel (Possibility of a disulfiram-like reaction) 1986

Mevacor Tablets (Lovastatin should be used with caution in patients who have consumed substantial quantity of alcohol and have a past history of liver disease; active liver disease and unexplained elevation in transaminase are contraindications to the use of lovastatin) 2132

Micardis HCT Tablets (Potentiation of orthostatic hypotension) 1051

Microzide Capsules (May potentiate orthostatic hypotension) 3414

Maximum Strength Midol Menstrual Caplets and Gelcaps (Chronic heavy alcohol users, 3 or more drinks per day, should consult their physicians for advice on when and how they should take pain relievers/fever reducers including acetaminophen; increases drowsiness effect) ▣ 612

Maximum Strength Midol PMS Caplets and Gelcaps (Chronic heavy alcohol users, 3 or more drinks per day, should consult their physicians for advice on when and how they should take pain relievers/fever reducers including acetaminophen; increases drowsiness effect) ▣ 613

Maximum Strength Midol Teen Caplets (Chronic heavy alcohol users, 3 or more drinks per day, should consult their physicians for advice on when and how they should take pain relievers/fever reducers including acetaminophen; increases drowsiness effect) ▣ 612

Miltown Tablets (Simultaneous use can lead to additive CNS depressant effects) 3349

Minizide Capsules (Concurrent use may aggravate orthostatic hypotension) 2700

Moduretic Tablets (Potentiation of orthostatic hypotension) 2138

Momentum Backache Relief Extra Strength Caplets (Chronic heavy alcohol users, 3 or more drinks per day, should consult their physician for advice on when and how they should take pain relievers/fever reducers including salicylates) ▣ 666

Motofen Tablets (Effects potentiated) 577

Motrin IB Tablets, Caplets, and Gelcaps (Chronic heavy alcohol users, 3 or more drinks per day, should consult their physicians for advice on when and how they should take pain relievers/fever reducers including ibuprofen) 2002

Motrin Migraine Pain Caplets (Chronic heavy alcohol users, 3 or more drinks per day, should consult their physicians for advice on when and how they should take pain relievers, including ibuprofen) 2005

Motrin Sinus Headache Caplets (Chronic heavy alcohol users, three or more drinks per day, should consult their physicians for advice on when and how they should take pain relievers/fever reducers including ibuprofen) 2005

MS Contin Tablets (Respiratory depression, hypotension and profound sedation or coma may result) 2896

MSIR Oral Solution (Additive depressant effects; potential for respiratory depression, hypotension and profound sedation or coma) 2898

Mykrox Tablets (Potentiates orthostatic hypotensive effects) 1168

Nardil Tablets (Concurrent use should be avoided) 2653

Navane Capsules (Possible additive effects which may include hypotension) 2701

Nembutal Sodium Solution (Concomitant use of other CNS depressants may produce additive depressant effects) 485

Niaspan Extended-Release Tablets (Concomitant alcohol may increase the side effects of flushing and pruritus and should be avoided around the time of Niaspan ingestion) 1846

Nilandron Tablets (Because of possibility of an intolerance to alcohol (facial flushes, malaise, hypotension) following ingestion of Nilandron, it is recommended that intake of alcohol be avoided by patients who experience this reaction) 753

Nitro-Dur Transdermal Infusion System (Enhances sensitivity to the hypotensive effects) 1834

Nitro-Dur Transdermal Infusion System (Enhances sensitivity to the hypotensive effects) 3134

Nitrolingual Pumpspray (Enhanced sensitivity to hypotensive effects) 1355

Nitrostat Tablets (Concomitant use may cause hypotension) 2658

Nizoral Tablets (Potential for disulfiram-like reaction to alcohol resulting in flushing, rash, peripheral edema, nausea and headache) 1791

Norco 7.5/325 Tablets CIII (Concurrent use results in additive CNS depression; alcohol intake should be avoided) 3425

Norpramin Tablets (Concurrent use results in exaggerated response to alcohol; alcohol induces liver enzyme activity and thereby reduces tricyclic antidepressant plasma levels) 755

NovoLog Injection (May either potentiate or weaken the blood-glucose-lowering effect of insulin) 2427

Nubain Injection (Additive CNS depression) 1323

Numorphan Injection (Concomitant use may produce additive CNS depressant effects) 1324

Nytol Natural Tablets (Concurrent use should be avoided while taking this product) ▣ 622

Maximum Strength Nytol QuickGels Softgels (Concurrent use will heighten the depressant effect of Nytol; avoid alcoholic beverages while taking this product) ▣ 621

One-A-Day Bedtime & Rest Tablets (Kava-Kava and Valerian Root may potentiate the effect of alcohol) ▣ 805

One-A-Day Tension & Mood Softgels (May increase drowsiness effect; avoid alcoholic beverages) ▣ 808

Oramorph SR Tablets (CNS depressant effects are potentiated) 3062

Orap Tablets (Pimozide may be capable of potentiating CNS depressants, including alcohol) 1407

Orudis KT Tablets (Patients consuming three or more alcohol-containing drinks should consult their doctor for advice on when and how they should take Orudis KT) ▣ 778

OxyContin Tablets (Concurrent use with the usual dose of OxyContin may result in respiratory depression, profound sedation or coma) 2912

OxyIR Capsules (Concomitant use may exhibit an additive CNS depression) 2916

Parafon Forte DSC Caplets (May produce additive effect) 2582

Parnate Tablets (Concurrent use is contraindicated; a marked potentiating effect on alcohol has been reported) 1607

Paxil Tablets (Concurrent use should be avoided) 1609

Percocet Tablets (Additive CNS depression) 1326

Percodan Tablets (Additive CNS depression) 1327

Extra Strength Percogesic Aspirin-Free Coated Caplets (Chronic heavy alcohol users, 3 or more drinks per day, should consult their physician for advice on when and how they should take pain relievers/fever reducers including acetaminophen; increases drowsiness effect; avoid alcoholic beverages) ▣ 665

Percolone Tablets (Concurrent use may exhibit an additive CNS depression) 1327

Periactin Tablets (Antihistimines may have additive effects with alcohol) 2155

Permax Tablets (Pergolide may cause somnolence and concurrent use with alcohol may result in additive sedative effects) 1299

Phenergan Injection (Co-administration may increase, prolong, or intensify the sedative action of CNS depressants, such as alcohol) 3553

Phenergan Suppositories (Promethazine may increase, prolong, or intensify the sedative action of other CNS depressants, such as alcohol) 3556

Phenergan Syrup Fortis (Additive sedative effects) 3554

Phenergan with Codeine Syrup (Additive sedative effects) 3557

Phenergan with Dextromethorphan Syrup (Additive sedative effects) 3559

Phenergan VC Syrup (Additive sedative effects) 3560

Phenergan VC with Codeine Syrup (Additive sedative effects) 3561

Photofrin for Injection (Compounds that quench active oxygen species or scavenge radicals, such as ethanol, would be expected to decrease photodynamic therapy; no human data available to support or rebut this possibility) 831

Phrenilin Forte Capsules (Potential for increased CNS depression) 578

Prinzide Tablets (Co-administration of thiazide and alcohol may potentiate orthostatic hypotension) 2168

Procanbid Extended-Release Tablets (Alcohol consumption tends to decrease the half-life of procainamide in the blood through induction of its acetylation to NAPA) 2262

ProSom Tablets (Co-administration results in increased CNS depression) 500

Prozac Pulvules, Liquid, and Weekly Capsules (Concurrent use with CNS active agents, such as alcohol, requires caution) 1238

Reglan Injectable (Increased rate and/or extent of absorption from the small bowel; additive sedative effects) 2935

Remeron Tablets (Co-administration has shown to result in an additive impairment of motor skills) ... 2483
Remeron SolTab Tablets (Co-administration has shown to result in an additive impairment of motor skills) ... 2486
Renese Tablets (Orthostatic hypotension may be aggravated by alcohol) ... 2712
Renova 0.05% Cream (Topical products with high concentration of alcohol may increase the irritation when used concurrently) ... 2519
Requip Tablets (Possible additive sedative effects) ... 1621
ReSource Wellness StayCalm Caplets (Resource Wellness StayCalm contains valerian extract which causes drowsiness; concurrent use with alcohol is not recommended) ... ■ 826
Rifamate Capsules (Daily ingestion of alcohol may be associated with a higher incidence of isoniazid hepatitis) ... 767
Rifater Tablets (Daily ingestion of alcohol may be associated with higher incidence of isoniazid hepatitis) ... 769
Rilutek Tablets (Alcohol may increase the risk of hepatotoxicity; patients on riluzole should be discouraged from drinking excessive amounts of alcohol) ... 772
Risperdal Tablets (Effects not specified; concurrent use should be avoided) ... 1796
Robaxin Injectable (Increased depressant effect) ... 2938
Robaxisal Tablets (Increased general CNS depressant effects with concurrent use) ... 2939
Robitussin Cold Softgels Multi-Symptom Cold & Flu (Chronic heavy alcohol users, 3 or more drinks per day, should consult their physicians for advice on when and how they should take pain relievers/fever reducers including acetaminophen) ... ■ 781
Robitussin Multi Symptom Honey Flu Liquid (Chronic heavy alcohol users, 3 or more drinks per day, should consult their physicians for advice on when and how they should take pain relievers/fever reducers including acetaminophen) ... ■ 785
Robitussin Nighttime Honey Flu Liquid (Chronic heavy alcohol users, 3 or more drinks per day, should consult their physician for advice on when and how they should take pain relievers/fever reducers including acetaminophen; increases drowsiness effect; avoid alcoholic beverages) ... ■ 786
Romazicon Injection (Concurrent use should be avoided) ... 3000
Roxanol Concentrated Oral Solution (May enhance the CNS depressant actions of morphine) ... 3066
Roxicodone Intensol (Possible additive CNS depression) ... 3067
Roxicodone Oral Solution (Possible additive CNS depression) ... 3067
Roxicodone Tablets (Concurrent use may exhibit an additive CNS depression) ... 3067
Ryna-C Liquid (May increase the drowsiness effect) ... ■ 768
Ryna-12 S Suspension (Ryan-12 S contains an antihistamine which may cause drowsiness and may have additive central nervous system effects with alcohol) ... 3351
Reformulated Rynatan Pediatric Suspension (Antihistamines cause drowsiness and co-administration may increase drowsiness effect) ... 3352
Rynatan Tablets (May enhance the drowsiness caused by antihistamines) ... 3351
Rynatuss Pediatric Suspension (Antihistamines cause drowsiness and co-administration may increase drowsiness effect) ... 3353
Sarafem Pulvules (Concurrent use with CNS active agents, such as alcohol, requires caution) ... 1962
Sedapap Tablets 50 mg/650 mg (Additive CNS depression) ... 2225
Semprex-D Capsules (Co-administration may result in additional reduction in alertness and impairment of CNS performance and should be avoided) ... 1172
Serentil Ampuls (Potentiation of central nervous system depressant) ... 1057
Seroquel Tablets (The cognitive and motor effect of alcohol is potentiated; alcohol use should be avoided) ... 684
Serzone Tablets (Concomitant use should be avoided) ... 1104
Simply Sleep Caplets (Diphenhydramine is an antihistamine with sedative properties; concurrent use with alcoholic beverages should be avoided) ... 2008
Sinequan Capsules (Doxepin may enhance the response to alcohol) ... 2713
Singlet Caplets (Chronic heavy alcohol users, 3 or more drinks per day, should consult their physicians for advice on when and how they should take pain relievers/fever reducers including acetaminophen; increases drowsiness effect) ... ■ 761
Sinutab Sinus Allergy Medication, Maximum Strength Formula, Tablets & Caplets (May increase drowsiness effect; patients consuming 3 or more alcoholic beverages a day should consult a physician for advice on when and how they should take this medication) ... ■ 707
Sinutab Sinus Medication, Maximum Strength Without Drowsiness Formula, Tablets & Caplets (Patients consuming 3 or more alcohol-containing drinks per day should consult physician for advice on when and how they should take this product) ... ■ 707
Sleep-Tite Caplets (Concurrent use is not recommended) ... ■ 850
Soma Tablets (Carisoprodol causes drowsiness and co-administration may increase drowsiness effect) ... 3353
Soma Compound Tablets (Additive effects including enhanced aspirin-induced fecal blood loss) ... 3354
Soma Compound w/Codeine Tablets (Additive effects including gastrointestinal bleeding) ... 3355
Sominex Original Formula Tablets (Concurrent use of alcoholic beverages is not recommended) ... ■ 761
Sonata Capsules (Concurrent use may produce additive CNS depressant effects) ... 3591
Soriatane Capsules (Concurrent ingestion has been associated with the formation of etretinate, which has a longer elimination half-life than acitretin; longer elimination half-life increases the duration of teratogenic potential for female patients; alcohol must not be ingested during or for 2 months after the cessation of therapy) ... 3003
Stadol NS Nasal Spray (Concurrent use may result in increased CNS depressant effects, such as drowsiness, dizziness, and impaired mental function) ... 1108
Stelazine Injection (Additive depressant effects) ... 1640
Sudafed Cold & Allergy Tablets (May increase drowsiness effect) ... ■ 708
Sudafed Cold & Cough Liquid Caps (Patients consuming 3 or more alcohol-containing drinks per day should consult physician for advice on when and how they should take this product) ... ■ 709
Sudafed Cold & Sinus Liquid Caps (Patients consuming 3 or more alcohol-containing drinks per day should consult physician for advice on when and how they should take this product) ... ■ 710
Sudafed Sinus Headache Caplets (Patients consuming 3 or more alcohol-containing drinks per day should consult physician for advice on when and how they should take this product) ... ■ 712
Surmontil Capsules (Concomitant use of alcoholic beverages and trimipramine may be associated with exaggerated effects) ... 3595
Sustiva Capsules (Potential for additive central nervous system effects when Sustiva is used concomitantly with alcohol) ... 1258
Symmetrel Tablets (May increase the potential for CNS effects such as dizziness, confusion, light-headedness and orthostatic hypotension; avoid excessive alcohol usage) ... 1328
Talacen Caplets (Potential for increased CNS depressant effects) ... 3089
Talwin Nx Tablets (May increase CNS depression) ... 3090
Tasmar Tablets (Possible additive sedative effects when used in combination with CNS depressants, such as alcohol) ... 3010
Tavist 12 Hour Allergy Tablets (May increase drowsiness effect) ... ■ 676
Tavist Sinus Non-Drowsy Coated Caplets (Chronic heavy alcohol users, 3 or more drinks per day, should consult their physicians for advice on when and how they should take pain relievers/fever reducers including acetaminophen) ... ■ 676
Thalomid Capsules (Thalidomide has been reported to enhance the sedative activity of alcohol) ... 1154
Theo-Dur Extended-Release Tablets (Concurrent use with a single dose of alcohol (3mL/kg of whiskey) decreases theophylline clearance for up to 24 hours) ... 1835
TheraFlu Regular Strength Cold & Cough Night Time Hot Liquid (Chronic heavy alcohol users, 3 or more drinks per day, should consult their physicians for advice on when and how they should take pain relievers/fever reducers including acetaminophen; may increase the drowsiness effect) ... ■ 676
TheraFlu Maximum Strength Flu & Congestion Non-Drowsy Hot Liquid (Chronic heavy alcohol users, 3 or more drinks per day, should consult their physicians for advice on when and how they should take pain relievers/fever reducers including acetaminophen) ... ■ 677
TheraFlu Maximum Strength Flu & Sore Throat Night Time Hot Liquid (Chronic heavy alcohol users, 3 or more drinks per day, should consult their physicians for advice on when and how they should take pain relievers/fever reducers including acetaminophen; increases drowsiness effect) ... ■ 677
TheraFlu Maximum Strength Severe Cold & Congestion Night Time Hot Liquid (Chronic heavy alcohol users, 3 or more drinks per day, should consult their physicians for advice on when and how they should take pain relievers/fever reducers including acetaminophen; increases drowsiness effect) ... ■ 678
TheraFlu Maximum Strength Severe Cold & Congestion Non-Drowsy Hot Liquid (Chronic heavy alcohol users, 3 or more drinks per day, should consult their physicians for advice on when and how they should take pain relievers/fever reducers including acetaminophen) ... ■ 679
Thiothixene Capsules (Possible additive effects which may include hypotension) ... 2290
Topamax Tablets (Potential for increased CNS depression) ... 2590
Transderm Scōp Transdermal Therapeutic System (Scopolamine is an anticholinergic agent and causes certain CNS effects, such as drowsiness and dizziness, and hence it should be used with care in patients on concomitant therapy) ... 2302
Tranxene T-TAB Tablets (Actions of benzodiazepines may be potentiated; prolonged sleeping time) ... 511
Trecator-SC Tablets (Excessive ingestion of alcohol should be avoided because a psychotic reaction has been reported) ... 3598
Triaminic Cold & Cough Softchews (May increase drowsiness effect) ... ■ 683
Trilafon Tablets (Concurrent use may result in additive effects and hypotension; the use of alcohol should be avoided) ... 3160
Trileptal Tablets (Oxcarbazepine causes dizziness and somnolence, concurrent use with alcohol could result in possible additive sedative effect) ... 2407
Trilisate Liquid (Chronic heavy alcohol users, 3 or more drinks per day, in combination with analgesic/antipyretic drug products containing NSAID ingredients, including choline and magnesium salicylates increases the risk of adverse GI events, including stomach bleeding) ... 2901
Trizivir Tablets (Concurrent use decreases the elimination of abacavir causing an increase in overall exposure) ... 1669
Tussi-12 S Suspension (Tussi-12 contains antihistamine which may cause drowsiness and co-administration may result in additive CNS effects) ... 3356
Tussionex Pennkinetic Extended-Release Suspension (Combined use may result in additive CNS depression) ... 1174
Tussi-Organidin DM NR Liquid (Potential for additive CNS depressant effects) ... 3350
Regular Strength Tylenol Tablets (Chronic heavy alcohol users, 3 or more drinks per day, should consult their physicians for advice on when and how they should take pain relievers including acetaminophen) ... 2009
Maximum Strength Tylenol Allergy Sinus NightTime Caplets (Concurrent use may increase drowsiness effect; chronic heavy alcohol abusers, 3 or more drinks per day, may be at increased risk of liver toxicity from excessive acetaminophen use) ... 2010
Multi-Symptom Tylenol Cold Severe Congestion Non-Drowsy Caplets (Chronic heavy alcohol abusers, 3 or more drinks per day, may be at increased risk of liver toxicity from acetaminophen use) ... 2011
Maximum Strength Tylenol Flu NightTime Gelcaps (Concurrent use may increase drowsiness effect; chronic heavy alcohol abusers, 3 or more drinks per day, may be at increased risk of liver toxicity from excessive acetaminophen use) ... 2011
Extra Strength Tylenol PM Caplets, Geltabs, and Gelcaps (Avoid concurrent use; chronic heavy alcohol abusers, 3 or more drinks per day, may be at increased risk of liver toxicity from acetaminophen use) ... 2012
Maximum Strength Tylenol Sinus NightTime Caplets (Chronic heavy alcohol users, 3 or more drinks per day, are at increased risk of liver toxicity from excessive acetaminophen use; alcohol increases drowsiness effect and concurrent use of alcoholic beverages should be avoided) ... 2012
Tylenol with Codeine Elixir (Concurrent use with other CNS depressants may exhibit an additive CNS depression) ... 2595

Women's Tylenol Menstrual Relief Caplets (Chronic heavy alcohol users, 3 or more drinks per day, should consult their physicians for advice on when and how they should take pain relievers, including acetaminophen) 2013
Tylox Capsules (Additive CNS depression) 2597
Ultracet Tablets (Tramadol increases the risk of CNS and respiratory depression with concurrent use; alcohol consumption with Ultracet is not recommended) 2597
Ultram Tablets (Concurrent use should be avoided; contraindicated in cases of acute alcohol intoxication) 2600
Uni-Dur Extended-Release Tablets (Concurrent use with a single dose of alcohol (3 mL/kg of whiskey) decreases theophylline clearance for up to 24 hours) 1841
Uniphyl 400 mg and 600 mg Tablets (Concurrent use with a single dose of alcohol (3mL/kg of whiskey) decreases theophylline clearance for up to 24 hours) 2903
Uniretic Tablets (Co-administration of alcohol with thiazide diuretics may result in potentiation of orthostatic hypotension) 3178
Unisom SleepTabs (Use Unisom cautiously) ....■ 713
Unisom Maximum Strength SleepGels (Concurrent use of alcoholic beverages should be avoided) ....■ 713
Valium Injectable (Concomitant use increases central nervous system depression with increased risk of apnea; injectable diazepam should not be administered in acute alcoholic intoxication) 3026
Valium Tablets (May potentiate the actions of diazepam) 3047
Vanquish Caplets (Chronic heavy alcohol users, 3 or more drinks per day, should consult their physicians for advice on when and how they should take pain relievers/fever reducers including acetaminophen and aspirin) ....■ 617
Vaseretic Tablets (Co-administration of thiazide and alcohol may potentiate orthostatic hypotension) 2204
Verelan Capsules (Verapamil has been found to significantly inhibit ethanol elimination resulting in elevated blood ethanol concentration that may prolong the intoxicating effects of alcohol) 3184
Versed Syrup (Concurrent use with alcohol increases effects of alcohol) 3033
Vicks 44M Cough, Cold & Flu Relief Liquid (May increase drowsiness effect; patients consuming 3 or more alcoholic drinks per day should consult their physician for advice on when and how they should take this medication) ....■ 725
Pediatric Vicks 44m Cough & Cold Relief (May increase drowsiness effect) ....■ 728
Vicks DayQuil LiquiCaps/Liquid Multi-Symptom Cold/Flu Relief (Patients consuming 3 or more alcoholic drinks per day should consult their physician for advice on when and how they should take this medication) ....■ 727
Children's Vicks NyQuil Cold/Cough Relief (May increase drowsiness effect) ....■ 726
Vicks NyQuil LiquiCaps/Liquid Multi-Symptom Cold/Flu Relief, Original and Cherry Flavors (May increase drowsiness effect; patients consuming 3 or more alcoholic drinks per day should consult their physician for advice on when and how they should take this medication) ....■ 727
Vicodin Tablets (May exhibit an additive CNS depression) 516
Vicodin ES Tablets (Additive CNS depression) 517
Vicodin HP Tablets (Concurrent use results in an additive CNS depression) 518
Vicodin Tuss Expectorant (Co-administration may exhibit an additive CNS depression) 519
Vicoprofen Tablets (May exhibit additive CNS depression) 520
Vistaril Capsules (Increased effect of alcohol) 2738
Vistaril Intramuscular Solution (May be potentiated) 2738
Visudyne for Injection (Co-administration with compounds that quench active oxygen species or scavenge radicals, such as ethanol, would be expected to decrease verteporfin activity) ....⊙ 308
Vivactil Tablets (Co-administration results in enhanced response to alcohol) 2217
Vivactil Tablets (Co-administration results in enhanced response to alcohol) 2446
Warfarin Sodium Tablets, USP (Decreased or increased prothrombin time response) 3302
Wellbutrin SR Sustained-Release Tablets (Use and cessation of use of alcohol may alter seizure threshold, and, therefore, the consumption of alcohol should be minimized or avoided completely) 1684
Xanax Tablets (Additive CNS depressant effects) 2865
Zanaflex Tablets (Increases the AUC of tizanidine by approximately 20% and increases its Cmax by approximately 15%; the CNS depressant effects are additive) 1305
Zaroxolyn Tablets (Concurrent use with alcohol may potentiate orthostatic hypotension) 1177
Zestoretic Tablets (Potentiates orthostatic hypotension) 695
Ziac Tablets (Potentiation of orthostatic hypotension may occur when thiazide diuretics are used with alcohol) 1887
Ziagen Tablets (Decreases the elimination of abacavir causing an increase in overall exposure) 1692
Zocor Tablets (Simvastatin causes persistent increases in serum transaminase in 1% of patients, therefore, it should be used with caution in patients who consume substantial quantities of alcohol) 2219
Zoloft Oral Concentrate (Concomitant use of Zoloft and alcohol in depressed patient is not recommended) 2751
Zyban Sustained-Release Tablets (Bupropion is associated with dose-dependent risk of seizures; excessive use of alcohol or abrupt withdrawal of alcohol is associated with an increased seizure risk) 1710
Zydone Tablets (Co-administration may exhibit additive CNS depression) 1330
Zyprexa Tablets (Co-administration of alcohol with olanzapine potentiates orthostatic hypotension; concurrent use should be avoided) 1973
Zyrtec Tablets (Concurrent use may result in additional impairment of CNS performance and reduction in mental alertness) 2756
Zyrtec-D 12 Hour Extended Relief Tablets (Concurrent use may result in additional reduction in alertness impairment of CNS performance) 2758

Anchovies
Parnate Tablets (Potential for hypertensive crisis; concurrent use is contraindicated) 1607

Avocados
Parnate Tablets (Potential for hypertensive crisis; concurrent use is contraindicated) 1607

Bananas
Matulane Capsules (Procarbazine exhibits some MAO inhibitory activity: concurrent use should be avoided) 3246
Parnate Tablets (Potential for hypertensive crisis; concurrent use is contraindicated) 1607

Beans, broad
Nardil Tablets (Concurrent and/or sequential intake must be avoided) 2653
Parnate Tablets (Potential for hypertensive crisis; concurrent use is contraindicated) 1607

Beans, Fava
Nardil Tablets (Concurrent and/or sequential intake must be avoided) 2653
Parnate Tablets (Potential for hypertensive crisis; concurrent use is contraindicated) 1607

Beer, alcohol-free
Nardil Tablets (Concurrent and/or sequential intake must be avoided) 2653
Parnate Tablets (Potential for hypertensive crisis; concurrent use is contraindicated) 1607

Beer, reduced-alcohol
Nardil Tablets (Concurrent and/or sequential intake must be avoided) 2653

Beer, unspecified
Nardil Tablets (Concurrent and/or sequential intake must be avoided) 2653
Parnate Tablets (Potential for hypertensive crisis; concurrent use is contraindicated) 1607

Beverages, caffeine-containing
BioLean Free Tablets (Concurrent caffeine intake should be minimized) ....■ 843
Excedrin Migraine Caplets (Concomitant use may cause nervousness, irritability, sleeplessness, and occasionally, rapid heart beat) 1070
Fosamax Tablets (Concomitant administration of alendronate with coffee reduces bioavailability by approximately 60%) 2095
Maximum Strength Midol Menstrual Caplets and Gelcaps (Concomitant use may cause nervousness, irritability, sleeplessness, and occasionally, rapid heartbeat) ....■ 612
Nardil Tablets (Excessive caffeine intake should be avoided) 2653
Parnate Tablets (Potential for hypertensive crisis; concurrent use is contraindicated) 1607

Beverages with high tyramine
Zyvox Tablets (Co-administration has resulted in a significant pressor response; patients receiving linezolid should avoid consuming large amounts of beverages containing tyramine) 2871

Bologna, Lebanon
Nardil Tablets (Concurrent and/or sequential intake must be avoided) 2653

Caviar
Parnate Tablets (Potential for hypertensive crisis; concurrent use is contraindicated) 1607

Cheese, aged
Matulane Capsules (Procarbazine exhibits some MAO inhibitory activity: concurrent use should be avoided) 3246
Nardil Tablets (Concurrent and/or sequential intake must be avoided) 2653
Parnate Tablets (Potential for hypertensive crisis; concurrent use is contraindicated) 1607

Cheese, strong, unpasteurized
Parnate Tablets (Potential for hypertensive crisis; concurrent use is contraindicated) 1607

Cheese, unspecified
Nardil Tablets (Concurrent and/or sequential intake must be avoided) 2653
Parnate Tablets (Potential for hypertensive crisis; concurrent use is contraindicated) 1607
Rifater Tablets (Isoniazid has some MAO inhibiting activity, an interaction with tyramine-containing food may occur) 769

Chocolate
Nardil Tablets (Concurrent and/or sequential intake must be avoided) 2653
Parnate Tablets (Potential for hypertensive crisis; concurrent use is contraindicated) 1607

Cola
Sporanox Capsules (Absorption of oral itraconazole is enhanced when administered with a cola beverage in patients with achlorhydria, such as AIDS or patients taking acid suppressors, e.g., H_2 inhibitors and proton pump inhibitors) 1800

Cream, sour
Parnate Tablets (Potential for hypertensive crisis; concurrent use is contraindicated) 1607

Dairy products
Cipro Tablets (Oral ciprofloxacin should not be taken concurrently with milk or yogurt alone, since absorption of ciprofloxacin may be significantly reduced; dietary calcium as part of a meal, however, does not significantly affect ciprofloxacin absorption) 887
Correctol Laxative Tablets and Caplets (Concurrent use within one hour after taking milk is not recommended) ....■ 739
Declomycin Tablets (Interferes with absorption) 1855
Depen Titratable Tablets (Penicillamine should be given on an empty stomach or at least one hour apart from food or milk because this permits maximum absorption and reduces the likelihood of inactivation by metal binding in the GI tract) 3341
Emcyt Capsules (Calcium-rich foods may impair the absorption of estramustine) 2810
Fleet Prep Kits (Concurrent use within one-hour should be avoided) 1361
Minocin Pellet-Filled Capsules (The peak plasma concentrations were slightly decreased (11.2%) and delayed by 1 hour) 1863
Noroxin Tablets (Avoid simultaneous ingestion; administer norfloxacin at least one hour before or two hours after ingestion of milk and/or other dairy products) 2145
Relafen Tablets (Potential for more rapid absorption, however, the total amount of GMNA in the plasma is unchanged) 1617
Tambocor Tablets (Milk may inhibit absorption in infants; a reduction in Tambocor dosage should be considered when milk is removed from the diet of infants) 1990
Tolectin 200 Tablets (Decreases total tolmetin bioavailability by 16%) 2589
Vibramycin Hyclate Capsules (Absorption of doxycycline is not markedly influenced by simultaneous ingestion of milk) 2735

Diet, high-lipid
Accupril Tablets (Rate and extent of quinapril absorption are diminished moderately) 2611
Adalat CC Tablets (High fat meal increases peak plasma nifedipine concentrations by 60%, a prolongation in the time to peak concentration, but no significant change in the AUC; administer on an empty stomach) 877
Albenza Tablets (Oral bioavailability appears to be enhanced when albendazole is co-administered with a fatty meal) 1463
Allegra-D Extended-Release Tablets (Co-administration with a high-fat meal decreased fexofenadine plasma concentrations Cmax and AUC and Tmax was delayed by 50%; the rate of extent of pseudoephedrine absorption was not affected by food; administration of Allegra-D with food should be avoided) 714

Gengraf Capsules (A high fat meal within one-half hour before cyclosporine administration decreases the AUC by 13% and Cmax by 33%) 457
Mycobutin Capsules (High-fat meals slow the rate without influencing the extent of absorption from the capsule dosage form) 2838
Neoral Soft Gelatin Capsules (A high fat meal consumed within one-half hour before Neoral administration decreased the AUC by 13% and Cmax by 33%) 2380
Rilutek Tablets (Co-administration with high-fat meal decreases absorption, reduces AUC by about 20% and peak blood levels by about 45%) 772
Salagen Tablets (Decrease in the rate of absorption of pilocarpine when taken with high fat meal) 2229
Sular Tablets (Food with a high fat content has a pronounced effect on the release of nisoldipine resulting in a significant increase in peak concentration (Cmax) by up to 300%; concomitant intake of high-fat meal should be avoided) 688
Toradol Tablets (Oral administration of Toradol after a high-fat meal resulted in decreased peak and delayed time-to-peak concentrations of Toradol by about 1 hour) 3018
Uni-Dur Extended-Release Tablets (Co-administration with a high-fat breakfast delays the time to peak concentration, however, the extent of theophylline absorption is similar when administered fasting or immediately after a high-fat breakfast) 1841
Uniphyl 400 mg and 600 mg Tablets (Co-administration with a standardized high-fat meal results in increased peak plasma concentration and bioavailability; however, a precipitous increase in the rate and extent of absorption was not evident; the dosing should be ideally administered consistently either with or without food) 2903

Diet, potassium-rich

Maxzide Tablets (Concurrent use is contraindicated) 1008
Midamor Tablets (Potential for rapid increases in serum potassium levels) 2136
Moduretic Tablets (Potential for rapid increases in serum potassium levels) 2138

Diet high in vitamin K

Coumadin Tablets (Decreased prothrombin time) 1243
Warfarin Sodium Tablets, USP (Decreased prothrombin time response) 3302

Dietary Fiber

Levoxyl Tablets (Concurrent use of dietary fiber may bind and decrease the absorption of levothyroxine sodium from GI tract) 1819
Unithroid Tablets (Concurrent use of dietary fiber may bind and decrease the absorption of levothyroxine sodium from GI tract) 3445

Drinks, hot, unspecified

Niaspan Extended-Release Tablets (Concomitant hot drinks may increase the side effects of flushing and pruritus and should be avoided around the time of Niaspan ingestion) 1846

Figs, canned

Parnate Tablets (Potential for hypertensive crisis; concurrent use is contraindicated) 1607

Fish, smoked

Nardil Tablets (Concurrent and/or sequential intake must be avoided) 2653

Fish, tropical

Rifater Tablets (Isoniazid may inhibit diamine oxidase, causing exaggerated response (headache, sweating, palpitations, flushing, hypotension) to food containing histamine) 769

Food, caffeine-containing

Excedrin Migraine Caplets (Concomitant use may cause nervousness, irritability, sleeplessness, and occasionally, rapid heart beat) 1070
Maximum Strength Midol Menstrual Caplets and Gelcaps (Concomitant use may cause nervousness, irritability, sleeplessness, and occasionally, rapid heartbeat) .... ▣ 612

Food, calcium-rich

Emcyt Capsules (Calcium-rich foods may impair the absorption of estramustine) 2810

Food, charcoal-broiled

Rilutek Tablets (Potential inducers of CYP1A2, such as charcoal-broiled food, could increase the rate of riluzole elimination) 772

Food, unspecified

Accolate Tablets (Co-administration with food reduces mean bioavailability by approximately 40%; patients should be instructed to take Accolate at least 1 hour before or 2 hours after meals) 657
Accuretic Tablets (The rate of quinapril absorption was reduced by 14% and hydrochlorothiazide absorption by 12%, when Accuretic was administered with a high-fat meal compared to fasting, while extent of absorption was not affected; Accuretic can be given without regard to food) 2614
Aceon Tablets (2 mg, 4 mg, 8 mg) (The presence of food in the GI tract does not affect the rate or extent of absorption of perindopril but reduces bioavailability of perindoprilat by about 35%; in clinical trials, perindopril was generally administered in a non-fasting state) 3249
Actonel Tablets (Mean oral bioavailability is decreased when risedronate is administered with food; Actonel is effective when administered at least 30 minutes before breakfast) 2879
Adderall XR Capsules (Concurrent use with food prolongs T_{max} by 2.5 hours, however, food does not affect the extent of absorption) ....
Agenerase Oral Solution (High fat meals may decrease the absorption of Agenerase and should be avoided; Agenerase may be taken with meals of normal fat content) 1459
Altace Capsules (The rate of absorption is reduced, not the extent of absorption) 2233
Aromasin Tablets (Exemestane plasma levels increased approximately 40% after high-fat breakfast) 2769
Biaxin Filmtab Tablets (Food slightly delays both the onset of absorption and the formation of the active metabolite, but does not affect the extent of bioavailability; Biaxin may be administered without regard to food) 403
Captopril Tablets (Reduces absorption by about 30% to 40%; should be given one hour before meals) 2281
Carbatrol Capsules (A high fat meal increased the rat of absorption of a single 400 mg dose but not the AUC; elimination half-life remains unchanged between fasting and fed states) 3234
Ceclor CD Tablets (The extent of absorption (AUC) and the maximum plasma concentration (Cmax) of cefaclor from Ceclor CD are greater when it is taken with food) 1279
Cedax Capsules (Food delays the time of Cmax, decreases the Cmax, and the extent of absorption (AUC); ceftibuten oral suspension should be taken at least 2 hours before meal or at least 1 hour after meal) 1021
Ceftin Tablets (Absorption is greater when taken after food) 1898
Celebrex Capsules (Co-administration with a high-fat meal delayed peak plasma levels for about 1 to 2 hours with an increase in total absorption (AUC) of 10% to 20%; Celebrex can be administered without regard to the timing of meals) 2676
Celebrex Capsules (Co-administration with a high-fat meal delayed peak plasma levels for about 1 to 2 hours with an increase in total absorption (AUC) of 10% to 20%; Celebrex can be administered without regard to the timing of meals) 2780
CellCept Capsules (Food has no effect on MPA AUC, but has been shown to decrease MPA Cmax by 40%; it is recommended that CellCept be administered on an empty stomach) 2951
Cipro Tablets (Delays the oral absorption of the drug resulting in peak concentrations that are closer to 2 hours after dosing) 887
Claritin-D 24 Hour Extended Release Tablets (Increases the AUC of loratadine by approximately 125% and Cmax by approximately 80%, however, food did not significantly affect the pharmacokinetics of pseudoephedrine or descarboethoxyloratadine) 3104
Clinoril Tablets (The peak plasma concentrations of biologically active sulfide metabolite is delayed slightly in the presence of food) 2053
Cognex Capsules (Food reduces tacrine bioavailability by approximately 30% to 40%; no effect if tacrine is administered at least one hour before meals) 1351
Cordarone Tablets (Increases the rate and extent of absorption of amiodarone; because of the food effect on absorption, Cordarone should be administered consistently with regard to meals) 3487
Coreg Tablets (When carvedilol is administered with food, the rate of absorption is slowed, as evidenced by a delay in the time to reach peak plasma levels, with no significant difference in extent of bioavailability; patients should be instructed to take Coreg with food in order to minimize the risk of hypotension) 1508
Crixivan Capsules (Co-administration with a meal high in calories, fat, and protein has resulted in a 77% ±8% reduction in AUC and an 84% ±7% reduction in Cmax; administer without food 1 hour before or 2 hours after a meal) 2070
Cytotec Tablets (Diminishes maximum plasma concentrations) 3202
Declomycin Tablets (Interferes with absorption) 1855
Demadex Tablets and Injection (Simultaneous food intake delays the time to Cmax by about 30 minutes, but overall bioavailability (AUC) and diuretic activity are unchanged) 2965
Depen Titratable Tablets (Penicillamine should be given on an empty stomach or at least one hour apart from food or milk because this permits maximum absorption and reduces the likelihood of inactivation by metal binding in the GI tract) 3341
Diovan Capsules (Decreases the exposure (as measured by AUC) to valsartan about 40% and peak plasma concentration by about 50%) 2337
Dynabac Tablets (Slight increase in the absorption of erythromycyclamine when dirithromycin tablets were administered after food; significant decrease in Cmax (33%) and AUC (31%) occurs when administered one hour before food; administer with food or within an hour of having eaten) 2269
Dynacin Capsules (The peak plasma concentrations were slightly decreased and delayed by one hour when administered with a meal which included dairy products; extent of absorption was not noticeably influenced) 2019
EC-Naprosyn Delayed-Release Tablets (The presence of food prolonged the time the EC-Naprosyn remained in the stomach, time to first detectable serum naproxen levels, and time to maximal naproxen levels (Tmax), but did not affect peak naproxen levels (Cmax)) 2967
Eldepryl Capsules (The bioavailability of selegiline is increased 3 to 4 fold when it is taken with food) 3266
Epivir Tablets (Absorption of lamivudine was slower in the fed state compared with fasted state; there was no significant difference in systemic exposure in the fed state and fasted states; Epivir may be given with or without food) 1520
Erythromycin Delayed-Release Capsules, USP (Lowers the blood levels of systemically available erythromycin) 455
Evista Tablets (Administration of raloxifene with a standardized, high fat meal increases the absorption of raloxifene, but does not lead to clinically meaningful changes in systemic exposure; Evista can be administered without regard to meals) 1915
Evoxac Capsules (Co-administration with food decreases the rate of absorption, with a fasting Tmax of 1.53 hours and a Tmax of 2.86 hours after a meal; the peak concentration is reduced by 17.3%) 1217
Exelon Oral Solution (Co-administration with food delays absorption (tmax) by 90 minutes, lowers Cmax by approximately 30% and increases AUC by approximately 30%) 2345
Feldene Capsules (With food there is a slight delay in the rate but not the extent of absorption) 2685
Flomax Capsules (Tmax is reached by 4 to 5 hours under fasting conditions and by 6 to 7 hours when tamsulosin is administered with food; taking tamsulosin under fasted conditions results in a 30% increase in AUC and 40% to 70% increase in Cmax compared to fed conditions; Flomax should be taken approximately 30 minutes following the meal) 1044
Floxin Tablets (Food does not affect the Cmax and AUC∞ of the drug, but Tmax is prolonged) 2529
Fortovase Capsules (The mean 12-hour AUC is increased in fed condition; Fortovase should be taken with a meal or up to 2 hours after a meal) 2970
Gabitril Tablets (A high fat meal decreases the rate (mean Tmax was prolonged to 2.5 hours, and Cmax was reduced by about 40%) but not the extent (AUC) of tiagabine) 1189
Gengraf Capsules (The administration of food with Gengraf decreases the cyclosporine AUC and Cmax) 457
Glucophage Tablets (Food decreases the extent and slightly delays the absorption of metformin) 1080

Glucotrol Tablets (Delays absorption by 40 minutes; administer 30 minutes prior to meals) 2692
GoLYTELY and Pineapple Flavor GoLYTELY for Oral Solution (For best results, no solid food should be consumed during 3 to 4 hour period before drinking solution) 1068
Hivid Tablets (The absorption rate of a 15mg oral dose of zalactabine was reduced when administered with food) 2975
Hytrin Capsules (Delays the time to peak concentration by about 40 minutes; minimal effect on the extent of absorption) 464
Imdur Tablets (May decrease the rate (increase in Tmax) but not the extent (AUC) of absorption) 1826
Imitrex Tablets (Delays the Tmax slightly by about 0.5 hour with no significant effect on the bioavailability) 1558
Invirase Capsules (Saquinavir 24-hour AUC and Cmax following the administration of a high calorie meal were an average two times higher than after a lower calorie, lower fat meal; the effect of food has been shown to persist for up to 2 hours) 2979
Isoptin SR Tablets (Produces decreased bioavailability (AUC) but a narrower peak to trough ratio) 467
Kadian Capsules (Slows the rate of absorption of Kadian, the extent of absorption is not affected and Kadian can be administered without regard to meals; the pellets in Kadian should not be dissolved) 1335
Kaletra Capsules (Co-administration with moderate fat meal was associated with a mean increase in AUC and Cmax; to enhance bioavailability Kaletra should be taken with food) 471
Keppra Tablets (Decreases Cmax by 20% and delays Tmax by 1.5 hours, does not affect the extent of absorption) 3314
Kytril Tablets (When oral granisetron was administered with food, AUC was decreased by 5% and Cmax increased by 30% in non-fasted individuals) 2988
Lamisil Tablets (Co-administration has resulted in an increase in the AUC of terbinafine of less than 20%) 2360
Lescol Capsules (Administration of regular formulation of fluvastatin with food reduces the rate but not the extent of absorption; administration with evening meal results in a two-fold decrease in Cmax and more than a two-fold increase in tmax as compared to administration 4 hours after the evening meal; administration of Lescol XL with a high fat meal delayed the absorption and increased the bioavailability by 50%) 2361
Lescol Capsules (Administration of regular formulation of fluvastatin with food reduces the rate but not the extent of absorption; administration with evening meal results in a two-fold decrease in Cmax and more than a two-fold increase in tmax as compared to administration 4 hours after the evening meal; administration of Lescol XL with a high fat meal delayed the absorption and increased the bioavailability by 50%) 2925
Levaquin Tablets (Co-administration slightly prolongs the time to peak concentration by approximately 1 hour and slightly decreases the peak concentration by approximately 14%; levofloxacin can be administered without regard to food) 2537
Lexxel Tablets (When Lexxel is taken with food (a substantial meal of 650 Kcal or greater), some of the pharmacokinetics of its components are changed; Lexxel should be regularly taken either without food or with a light meal) 608
Lodine XL Extended-Release Tablets (Food significantly increased Cmax (54%) following 600 mg dose) 3530
Lopid Tablets (Gemfibrozil pharmacokinetics are affected by the timing of meals relative to dosing; the rate and extent of absorption of gemfibrozil were significantly increased when administered 0.5 hours before meals; AUC is decreased when it is after meals) 2650
Lorabid Suspension and Pulvules (Delays the peak plasma concentration with no change in the total absorption) 2251
Macrobid Capsules (Increases bioavailability by approximately 40%) 2889
Macrodantin Capsules (Increases bioavailability of Macrodantin) 2891
Malarone Tablets (Dietary fat intake with atovaquone increases the rate and extent of absorption; Malarone should be taken with food or milky drink) 1596
Mavik Tablets (Slows absorption of trandolapril but does not affect AUC or Cmax) 478
Maxalt Tablets (Delays the time to reach peak concentration by an hour; no significant effect on the bioavailability) 2120
Mepron Suspension (Food enhances absorption by approximately two-fold) 1598
Meridia Capsules (Co-administration with a standard breakfast has resulted in reduced peak M1 and M2 amine concentrations and delayed the time to peak by approximately three hours; the AUCs of M1 and M2 were not significantly altered) 481
Micardis Tablets (Slightly reduces the bioavailability of telmisartan; Micardis tablets may be administered with or without food) 1049
Micardis HCT Tablets (Slightly reduces the bioavailability of telmisartan with reduction in AUC of about 6%) 1051
Mirapex Tablets (Food does not affect the extent of pramipexole absorption, although the time of maximum plasma concentration is increased by about 1 hour when the drug is taken with a meal) 2834
Mobic Tablets (Co-administration with a high fat breakfast did not affect extent of absorption of meloxicam capsules but led to 22% higher Cmax values; mean Cmax values were achieved between 5 to 6 hours; Mobic tablets can be administered without regard to timing of meals) 1054
Monopril Tablets (Rate of absorption may be slowed by the presence of food in the GI tract; the extent of absorption is not affected) 1091
Monurol Sachet (The oral bioavailability of fosfomycin is reduced to 30% under fed conditions compared to 37% under fasting condition; Monurol can be taken with or without food) 1375
Motrin Suspension, Oral Drops, Chewable Tablets, and Caplets (Food affects the rate but not the extent of absorption; Tmax is delayed by approximately 30 to 60 minutes and peak levels are reduced by approximately 30 to 50%) 2002
Naprelan Tablets (Food causes a slight decrease in the rate of naproxen absorption following Naprelan administration) 1293
Nascobal Gel (Hot foods may cause nasal secretions and a resulting loss of medication; therefore, patients should be told to administer Nascobal at least one hour before or one hour after ingestion of hot foods or liquids) 3174
Neoral Soft Gelatin Capsules (Administration of food with Neoral decreases the AUC and Cmax) 2380
Noroxin Tablets (Co-administration may decrease the absorption of norfloxacin; administer at least one hour before or two hours after a meal) 2145
NuLYTELY, Cherry Flavor, Lemon-Lime Flavor, and Orange Flavor NuLYTELY for Oral Solution (Solid food should not be given for at least two hours before the solution is given) 1068
Omnicef Capsules (Although Cmax and AUC of cefdinir absorption from capsules are reduced by 16% and 10% respectively, when given with a high-fat meal, the magnitude of these reduction is not likely to clinically significant, therefore, cefdinir may be taken without regard to food) 493
Ortho-Prefest Tablets (Co-administration with a high fat meal results in increased Cmax values for estrone and estrone sulfate; Cmax values 17- deacetylnorgestimate were decreased; the AUC values for these analytes were not significantly affected by food) 2570
Orudis Capsules (Slows rate of absorption resulting in delayed and reduced peak concentrations) 3548
Paxil Tablets (Co-administration with food resulted in slight increase (6%) in AUC, but Cmax was 29% greater, while time to reach peak plasma concentration decreased from 6.4 hours post-dosing to 4.9 hours) 1609
Pepcid for Oral Suspension (Bioavailability may be slightly increased by antacids) 2150
Plendil Extended-Release Tablets (When Plendil is administered either with high fat or carbohydrate diet, Cmax is increased by approximately 60%, AUC is unchanged; Plendil should regularly be taken either without food or with a light meal) ... 623
Pletal Tablets (Co-administration with high fat meal increases absorption, with an approximately 90% increase in Cmax and a 25% increase in AUC; patients should be advised to take Pletal at least one hour before or two hours after breakfast and dinner) 2605
Pletal Tablets (Co-administration with high fat meal increases absorption, with an approximately 90% increase in Cmax and a 25% increase in AUC; patients should be advised to take Pletal at least one hour before or two hours after breakfast and dinner) 2848
Prandin Tablets (0.5, 1, and 2 mg) (When repaglinide was given with food the mean Cmax and AUC were decreased 20% and 12.4% respectively; Tmax was unchanged) 2432
Premphase Tablets (Administration with a high fat breakfast decreased total estrone Cmax and increased total equilin Cmax compared to fasting state, no other effect on rate or extent of absorption; administration with food doubles MPA Cmax and increases MPA AUC) 3572
Prempro Tablets (Administration with food decreased Cmax of total estrone compared to fasting state, no other effect on rate or extent of absorption; administration with food doubles MPA Cmax and increases MPA AUC) 3572
Prevacid Delayed-Release Capsules (Cmax and AUC are diminished by about 50% if the drug is given 30 minutes after food as opposed to the fasting condition; Prevacid should be taken before eating) 3292
PREVPAC (Both Cmax and AUC are diminished by about 50% if the lansoprazole is given 30 minutes after food as opposed to the fasting condition) 3298
Priftin Tablets (Increases AUC and Cmax by 43% and 44% respectively compared to fasting conditions; administration with food may be useful to avoid gastrointestinal upsest) 758
Prilosec Delayed-Release Capsules (Absorption of Prilosec begins only after the granules leave the stomach; it should be taken before eating) 628
Prograf (The presence and composition of food has decreased both the rate and extent of tacrolimus absorption; this effect was most pronounced with a high-fat meal; the rate and extent of tacrolimus absorption were greatest under fasted conditions) 1393
Prometrium Capsules (100 mg, 200 mg) (Concomitant food ingestion increases the bioavailability of Prometrium Capsules relative to the fasting state) 3261
Provigil Tablets (Delays the absorption (tmax) by approximately one hour; no effect on overall bioavailability) 1193
Prozac Pulvules, Liquid, and Weekly Capsules (May delay absorption of fluoxetine inconsequentially; Prozac may be administered with or without food) 1238
Quinaglute Dura-Tabs Tablets (Increases absorption of quinidine in both rate (27%) and extent (17%)) 978
Quinidex Extentabs (Peak serum quinidine levels obtained from immediate-release quinidine sulfate are known to be delayed by nearly an hour without change in total absorption when these products are taken with food) 2933
Rapamune Oral Solution and Tablets (A fat breakfast altered the bioavailability characteristics of sirolimus compared to fasting; 34% decrease in the peak blood sirolimus concentration, a 3.5 fold increase in the time-to-peak concentration and 35% increase in total exposure; to minimize variability, Rapamune should be taken consistently with or without food) 3584
Rebetron Combination Therapy (Both AUC and Cmax increased by 70% when Rebetrol Capsules were administered with a high-fat meal in a single-dose pharmacokinetic study; there are insufficient data to address the clinical relevance of these results) 3153
Relafen Tablets (Potential for more rapid absorption, however, the total amount of GMNA in the plasma is unchanged) 1617
Remeron Tablets (The presence of food in the stomach has a minimal effect on both the rate and extent of absorption and does not require a dosage adjustment) 2483
Remeron SolTab Tablets (The presence of food in the stomach has a minimal effect on both the rate and extent of absorption and does not require a dosage adjustment) 2486
Requip Tablets (Increases ropinirole Tmax by 2.5 hours; food does not affect the extent of absorption of ropinirole) 1621
Rifadin Capsules (Absorption of rifampin is reduced by about 30% when the drug is ingested with food; patients should be instructed to take 1 hour before or 2 hours after a meal) 765
Rifater Tablets (Ingestion with food may reduce the absorption of isoniazid; daily dose of Rifater should be given on an empty stomach at least one hour before the ingestion of food) 769
Rythmol Tablets – 150 mg, 225 mg, 300 mg (Increased peak blood level and bioavailability in a single dose study) 502

Sarafem Pulvules (May delay fluoxetine's absorption inconsequentially, thus, fluoxetine may be administered with or without food) 1962

Sectral Capsules (Slightly decreases absorption and peak concentration) 3589

Seroquel Tablets (The bioavailability of quetiapine is marginally affected by administration with food, with Cmax and AUC values increased by 25% and 15% respectively) 684

Serzone Tablets (Food delays the absorption of nefazodone and decreases the bioavailability by approximately 20%) 1104

Sinemet CR Tablets (The extent of availability and peak concentrations of levodopa after a single dose of Sinemet CR increased by about 50% and 25% respectively when administered with food; foods that are high in protein may delay the absorption of levodopa and may reduce the amount taken up in the circulation)...........1255

Skelid Tablets (Reduces bioavailability by 90% when an oral dose equivalent to 400 mg tiludronic acid was administered with, or 2 hours after, a standard breakfast compared to the same dose administered after an overnight fast and 4 hours before a standard breakfast; Skelid should not be taken within 2 hours of food).........3088

Sonata Capsules (A high-fat/heavy meal prolongs the absorption of zaleplon compared to fasting state, delays tmax by approximately 2 hours and reduces Cmax approximately 35%; the effect of Sonata on sleep onset may be reduced if it is taken with or immediately after a high-fat/heavy meal)....................3591

Sporanox Capsules (Presence of food increases systemic bioavailability; when taken on an empty stomach the systemic bioavailability is reduced; Sporanox Capsules should be taken with a full meal to ensure maximal absorption) 1800

Starlix Tablets (Administration of nateglinide with liquid meal significantly reduces peak plasma levels) 2401

Suprax Tablets (Increases time to maximal absorption approximately 0.8 hour) 1877

Sustiva Capsules (High fat meal may increase the absorption of Sustiva and should be avoided; it can be taken with or without meals of normal composition) 1258

Tarka Tablets (Co-administration with food decreases verapamil bioavailability and the time to peak plasma concentration is delayed; bioavailability of trandolapril is not altered; Tarka should be administered with food) 508

Tasmar Tablets (Food given within 1 hour before and 2 hours after dosing of tolcapone decreases the relative bioavailability by 10% to 20%; Tasmar may be taken with or without food) 3010

Temodar Capsules (Co-administration with a modified high-fat breakfast has resulted in decrease in mean plasma concentration and AUC by 32% and 9% respectively, and 2-fold increase in Tmax) 3157

Teveten Tablets (Co-administration with food delays absorption, and causes variable changes in Cmax and AUC values which do not appear clinically important) 3327

Thalomid Capsules (Co-administration of Thalomid with a high fat meal causes minor changes in the observed AUC and Cmax values; however, it causes an increase in Tmax to approximately 6 hours) 1154

Theo-Dur Extended-Release Tablets (Available data suggests that co-administration with food may influence the absorption characteristics of controlled-release theophylline formulations)................................1835

Trental Tablets (Co-administration of Trental tablets with meals resulted in an increase in mean Cmax and AUC by about 28% and 13% for pentoxifylline, respectively; Cmax for Metabolite 1 also increased by about 20%)............................ 784

Tricor Capsules, Micronized (The absorption of fenofibrate is increased when administered with food; Tricor should be given with meals)........................... 513

Uniretic Tablets (Bioavailability varies with formulation and food intake which reduces Cmax and AUC of moexiprilat by about 70% and 40% respectively after ingestion of low-fat breakfast or by 80% and 50% respectively after the ingestion of a high-fat breakfast; patients should be advised to take Uniretic one hour before a meal) 3178

Univasc Tablets (Food reduces Cmax and AUC by about 70% and 40% respectively after ingestion of a low-fat breakfast or by 80% and 50% respectively after the ingestion of high-fat breakfast) 3181

Valcyte Tablets (Co-administration with high fat meals has resulted in increased steady-state ganciclovir AUC and Cmax without any prolongation in time to peak plasma concentrations; Valcyte should be administered with food) 3022

Vantin Tablets and Oral Suspension (The extent of absorption and the mean peak plasma concentration increased when film-coated tablets were administered with food) 2860

Vesanoid Capsules (The absorption of retinoids as a class has been shown to be enhanced when taken with food) ...3037

Viagra Tablets (When Viagra is taken with a high fat meal, the rate of absorption is reduced with a mean delay in Tmax of 60 minutes and a mean reduction in Cmax of 29%)..........................2732

Vibramycin Hyclate Capsules (Absorption of doxycycline is not markedly influenced by simultaneous ingestion of food) 2735

Videx EC Capsules (In the presence of food, the Cmax and AUC for Videx EC were reduced by approximately 46% and 19%, respectively; Videx EC should be taken on an empty stomach) 1143

Vioxx Tablets (The time to peak plasma concentration (Tmax) was delayed by 1 to 2 hours when administered with high fat meal; Vioxx tablets can be administered without regard to timing of meals)..........................2213

Viracept Tablets (Maximum plasma concentrations and AUC were 2- to 3-fold higher under fed conditions compared to fasting; Viracept should be taken with a meal or light snack) ... 532

Volmax Extended-Release Tablets (Food may decrease the rate of absorption without altering the extent of bioavailability) 2276

Voltaren Tablets (Food significantly alters the absorption pattern of extended-release dosage form as indicated by delay of 1 to 2 hours in Tmax and a two-fold increase in Cmax values; food also delays the onset of absorption of delayed-release and immediate-release formulations).................................2315

Wellbutrin SR Sustained-Release Tablets (Food increases Cmax and AUC of bupropion by 11% and 17%, respectively; no clinically significant food effect) 1684

Xeloda Tablets (Reduces both rate and extent of absorption of capecitabine and delays Tmax of both parent and 5-FU) 3039

Xenical Capsules (Gastrointestinal events may increase when orlistat is taken with a diet high in fat) 3043

Zanaflex Tablets (Increases Cmax by approximately one-third and shortens time to peak concentration by approximately 40 minutes, but the extent of tizanidine absorption is not affected) 1305

Zithromax Capsules, 250 mg (Zithromax should not be taken with food; reduces the rate of absorption (Cmax) of azithromycin capsules by 52% and the extent of absorption (AUC) by 43%; when oral suspension of azithromycin was administered with food the Cmax increased by 56% and the AUC was unchanged) 2743

Zofran Tablets (Increases significantly (about 17%) the extent of absorption of ondansetron).................................1703

Zoloft Oral Concentrate (Co-administration of Zoloft Tablets with food slightly increased AUC but the Cmax was 25% greater, while time to reach peak plasma concentration (Tmax) decreased from 8 hours to 5.5 hours; for oral concentrate, Tmax was slightly prolonged from 5.9 hours to 7 hours with food) 2751

Zyban Sustained-Release Tablets (Food increases Cmax and AUC of bupropion by 11% and 17% respectively; the mean time to peak concentration Tmax was prolonged by 1 hour; this effect was of no clinical significance) 1710

Zyflo Filmtab Tablets (Co-administration has resulted in a small but statistically significant increase (27%) in zileuton Cmax without significant changes in the extent of absorption (AUC) or Tmax; zileuton can be administered with or without food) 524

Zyrtec Tablets (Food has no effect on the extent of cetirizine absorption, but Tmax may be delayed and Cmax may be decreased in the presence of food) 2756

Zyvox Tablets (The time to reach maximum concentration is delayed from 1.5 hours to 2.2 hours and Cmax is decreased by about 17% when linezolid is co-administered with high fat food; linezolid may be administered without regard to the timing of meals)...........................2871

Food having a pH greater than 5.5

Creon 5 Capsules (Can dissolve the protective coating resulting in early release of enzymes, irritation of oral mucosa, and/or loss of enzyme activity)......3251

Ultrase Capsules (Can dissolve the protective coating resulting in early release of enzymes, irritation of oral mucosa, and/or loss of enzyme activity) 835

Ultrase MT Capsules (Can dissolve the protective enteric shell).. 835

Food high in tyramine

Zyvox Tablets (Co-administration has resulted in a significant pressor response; patients receiving linezolid should avoid consuming large amounts of food containing tyramine).............2871

Food that lowers urinary pH

Trilisate Liquid (Decreases urinary salicylate excretion and increases plasma levels).........2901

Food that raises urinary pH

Trilisate Liquid (Enhances renal salicylate clearance and diminishes plasma salicylate concentration) 2901

Urised Tablets (Methenamine has therapeutic activity in acidic urine; concurrent use with foods which produce an alkaline urine should be restricted).....................2876

Food with high concentration of dopamine

Nardil Tablets (Concurrent and/or sequential intake must be avoided) 2653

Food with high concentration of tyramine

Matulane Capsules (Procarbazine exhibits some MAO inhibitory activity; concurrent use should be avoided) 3246

Nardil Tablets (Concurrent and/or sequential intake must be avoided) 2653

Parnate Tablets (Potential for hypertensive crisis; concurrent use is contraindicated) 1607

Rifater Tablets (Isoniazid has some MAO inhibiting activity, an interaction with tyramine-containing food may occur).. 769

Fruit juices, unspecified

Dexedrine Spansule Capsules (Lowers absorption of amphetamines) 1512

DextroStat Tablets (Lowers absorption of amphetamines by acting as gastrointestinal acidifying agent) 3236

Fruits, dried

Parnate Tablets (Potential for hypertensive crisis; concurrent use is contraindicated) 1607

Fruits, overripe

Parnate Tablets (Potential for hypertensive crisis; concurrent use is contraindicated) 1607

Grapefruit

Gengraf Capsules (Affects the metabolism of cyclosporine by increasing blood concentration of cyclosporine; concurrent use should be avoided)................ 457

Neoral Soft Gelatin Capsules (Affects the metabolism of cyclosporine and should be avoided)...2380

Sandimmune I.V. Ampuls for Infusion (Co-administration results in increased blood concentrations of cyclosporine; concurrent use should be avoided) 2388

Grapefruit Juice

Adalat CC Tablets (Co-administration of nifedipine with grapefruit juice results in up to a 2-fold increase in AUC and Cmax, due to inhibition of CYP3A4 related first pass metabolism; co-administration should be avoided) 877

Crixivan Capsules (Potential for decrease in indinavir AUC) 2070

Evoxac Capsules (Co-administration with drugs which inhibit CYP3A3/4, such as grapefruit juice, may inhibit the metabolism of cevimeline resulting in a higher risk of adverse events) 1217

Gengraf Capsules (Affects the metabolism of cyclosporine by increasing blood concentration of cyclosporine; concurrent use should be avoided) 457

Halcion Tablets (Co-administration of grapefruit juice increased the maximum plasma concentration of triazolam by 25%; increased the AUC by 48%, and increased the half-life by 18%) 2823

Lexxel Tablets (Felodipine is metabolized by CYP3A4; co-administration of CYP3A4 inhibitors, such as grapefruit juice has resulted in more than 2-fold increase in the AUC and Cmax) 608

Mevacor Tablets (Lovastatin is a substrate for CYP4503A4 and grapefruit juice contains one or more components that inhibit CYP3A4; co-administration with grapefruit juice can increase the plasma concentrations of lovastatin and its B-hydroxyacid metabolite; large quantity of grapefruit juice (> 1 quart daily) significantly increase the serum concentrations and should be avoided) 2132

Neoral Soft Gelatin Capsules (Affects the metabolism of cyclosporine and should be avoided) 2380

Plendil Extended-Release Tablets (The bioavailability of felodipine is increased more than two-fold when taken with doubly concentrated grapefruit juice) 623

Pletal Tablets (Co-administration of cilostazol with inhibitors of CYP3A4, such as grapefruit juice, may increase cilostazol plasma concentration; this interaction has not been studied, however, concurrent consumption of grapefruit juice should be avoided) 2605

Pletal Tablets (Co-administration of cilostazol with inhibitors of CYP3A4, such as grapefruit juice, may increase cilostazol plasma concentration; this interaction has not been studied, however, concurrent consumption of grapefruit juice should be avoided) 2848

Procardia Capsules (Co-administration of nifedipine with grapefruit juice has resulted in approximately a 2-fold increase in nifedipine AUC and Cmax and no change in half-life; concurrent use should be avoided) 2708

Prograf (Co-administered grapefruit juice has been reported to increase tacrolimus blood trough concentrations in liver transplant patients; grapefruit juice should be avoided) 1393

Quinaglute Dura-Tabs Tablets (Because grapefruit juice inhibits CYPIIIA4-mediated metabolism of quinidine to 3-hydroxyquinidine, the ingestion of grapefruit juice during treatment with quinidine should be avoided; the clinical significance of this interaction is unknown) 978

Rapamune Oral Solution and Tablets (Induces CYP3A4-mediated metabolism of sirolimus; Rapamune must not be administered or diluted with grapefruit juice) 3584

Sandimmune I.V. Ampuls for Infusion (Co-administration results in increased blood concentrations of cyclosporine; concurrent use should be avoided) 2388

Tikosyn Capsules (Dofetilide is metabolized to a small extent by the CYP4503A4 system; co-administration with inhibitors of this isoenzyme, such as grapefruit juice, could increase systemic dofetilide exposure) 2717

Versed Syrup (Co-administration with agents known to inhibit CYP3A4, such as grapefruit juice, increases oral midazolam Cmax by 56% and AUC by 52%; Versed Syrup should not be taken with grapefruit juice) 3033

Xanax Tablets (Possible interaction based on the clinical studies involving other benzodiazepines metabolized similarly as alprazolam; co-administration requires caution) 2865

Zocor Tablets (Simvastatin is a substrate for CYP4503A4 and grapefruit juice contains one or more components that inhibit CYP3A4; co-administration with grapefruit juice can increase the plasma concentrations of simvastatin and its B-hydroxyacid metabolite; large quantity of grapefruit juice (>1 quart daily) significantly increases the serum concentrations and should be avoided) 2219

Herring, pickled

Nardil Tablets (Concurrent and/or sequential intake must be avoided) 2653

Parnate Tablets (Potential for hypertensive crisis; concurrent use is contraindicated) 1607

Liqueurs

Parnate Tablets (Potential for hypertensive crisis; concurrent use is contraindicated) 1607

Liver

Nardil Tablets (Concurrent and/or sequential intake must be avoided) 2653

Parnate Tablets (Potential for hypertensive crisis; concurrent use is contraindicated) 1607

Meal, high in bran fiber

Digitek Tablets (The amount of digoxin from an oral dose may be reduced when taken with meal high in bran fiber) 1003

Lanoxin Tablets (The amount of digoxin from an oral dose may be reduced) 1587

Meal, unspecified

Amaryl Tablets (When glimepiride is given with meals the mean Tmax is slightly increased (12%) and mean Cmax and AUC are slightly decreased) 717

Ambien Tablets (Mean AUC and Cmax decreased by 15% and 25% respectively, while Tmax was prolonged by 60%; for faster sleep onset, Ambien should not be administered with or immediately after meal) 3191

Claritin Tablets (Food increases the AUC by approximately 73%, the time to peak plasma concentration is delayed by one-hour) 3100

Cozaar Tablets (Meal slows absorption and decreases Cmax, but has minor effects on losartan AUC or on the AUC of the metabolite) 2067

Cytovene Capsules (Meal containing 46.5% fat increases the steady-state AUC of oral Cytovene by 22% ±22% and significant prolongation of time Tmax and a higher Cmax; patients should take Cytovene Capsules with food to maximize bioavailability) 2959

Digitek Tablets (Slows the rate of absorption) 1003

Famvir Tablets (Penciclovir Cmax decreased approximately 50% and Tmax was delayed by 1.5 hours when a capsule formulation of famciclovir was administered with food; there is no effect on the extent of availability (AUC) of penciclovir) 2348

Fosamax Tablets (Standardized breakfast decreases bioavailability by approximately 40% when alendronate is administered either 0.5 or 1 hour before breakfast) 2095

Hyzaar 50-12.5 Tablets (Meal slows absorption and decreases Cmax but has minor effects on losartan AUC or on the AUC of the metabolite) 2109

Lanoxin Tablets (Slows the rate of absorption) 1587

Mevacor Tablets (When lovastatin was given under fasting conditions, plasma concentrations of total inhibitors were on average about two-thirds those found when lovastatin was administered immediately after a standard meal) 2132

Nimotop Capsules (Administration of nimodipine capsules following a standard breakfast resulted in 68% lower peak plasma concentration and 38% lower bioavailability) 904

Norvir Capsules (Relative to fasting conditions, the extent of absorption of ritonavir from capsule formulation was 15% higher when administered with a meal; decreased peak ritonavir concentrations when oral solution was given under non-fasting condition) 487

PCE Dispertab Tablets (Presence of food results in lower blood levels; optimal blood levels are obtained when PCE is given in the fasting state (at least ½ hour and preferably 2 hours before meals)) 498

Ticlid Tablets (Administration after meals results in a 20% increase in the AUC of ticlopidine) 3015

Tolectin 200 Tablets (Decreases total tolmetin bioavailability by 16%; reduces peak plasma concentrations by 50%) 2589

Vascor Tablets (May result in a clinically insignificant delay in time to peak concentration, but neither peak plasma levels nor the extent of absorption was changed) 2602

Zerit Capsules (Co-administration with food decreases Cmax by approximately 45%, however, the systemic availability (AUC) is unchanged; Zerit Capsules can be taken without regard to meals) 1147

Meal with dairy products

Minocin Pellet-Filled Capsules (The peak plasma concentrations were slightly decreased (11.2%) and delayed by 1 hour) 1863

Meat, unspecified

Nardil Tablets (Concurrent and/or sequential intake must be avoided) 2653

Meat extracts

Nardil Tablets (Concurrent and/or sequential intake must be avoided) 2653

Parnate Tablets (Potential for hypertensive crisis; concurrent use is contraindicated) 1607

Meat prepared with tenderizers

Parnate Tablets (Potential for hypertensive crisis; concurrent use is contraindicated) 1607

Milk, low fat

Dyazide Capsules (Concurrent use of low-salt milk with triamterene may result in hyperkalemia, especially in patients with renal insufficiency) 1515

Milk, low salt

Dyrenium Capsules (Co-administration may promote serum potassium accumulation and possibly result in hyperkalemia) 3458

Orange Juice

Fosamax Tablets (Concomitant administration of alendronate with orange juice reduces bioavailability by approximately 60%) 2095

Pepperoni

Nardil Tablets (Concurrent and/or sequential intake must be avoided) 2653

Prunes

Parnate Tablets (Potential for hypertensive crisis; concurrent use is contraindicated) 1607

Raisins

Parnate Tablets (Potential for hypertensive crisis; concurrent use is contraindicated) 1607

Raspberries

Parnate Tablets (Potential for hypertensive crisis; concurrent use is contraindicated) 1607

Salami, Genoa

Nardil Tablets (Concurrent and/or sequential intake must be avoided) 2653

Salami, Hard

Nardil Tablets (Concurrent and/or sequential intake must be avoided) 2653

Salt Substitutes, Potassium-Containing

Altace Capsules (Increases risk of hyperkalemia) 2233

Sauerkraut

Nardil Tablets (Concurrent and/or sequential intake must be avoided) 2653

Parnate Tablets (Potential for hypertensive crisis; concurrent use is contraindicated) 1607

Sausage, Dry

Nardil Tablets (Concurrent and/or sequential intake must be avoided) 2653

Sherry

Parnate Tablets (Potential for hypertensive crisis; concurrent use is contraindicated) 1607

Skipjack fish

Rifater Tablets (Isoniazid may inhibit diamine oxidase, causing exaggerated response (headache, sweating, palpitations, flushing, hypotension) to food containing histamine) 769

Soy Sauce

Parnate Tablets (Potential for hypertensive crisis; concurrent use is contraindicated) 1607

Soybean Formula, Children's

Levoxyl Tablets (Concurrent use of soybean flour may bind and decrease the absorption of levothyroxine sodium from GI tract) 1819

Synthroid Tablets (Binds and decreases absorption of levothyroxine sodium from the gastrointestinal tract) 505

Unithroid Tablets (Concurrent use of soybean flour may bind and decrease the absorption of levothyroxine sodium from GI tract) 3445

Tuna Fish

Rifater Tablets (Isoniazid may inhibit diamine oxidase, causing exaggerated response (headache, sweating, palpitations, flushing, hypotension) to food containing histamine) 769

Vegetables, green leafy

Coumadin Tablets (Large amounts of green leafy vegetables may affect Coumadin therapy) 1243

Warfarin Sodium Tablets, USP (Decreased prothrombin time response) 3302

Wine, Chianti

Parnate Tablets (Potential for hypertensive crisis; concurrent use is contraindicated) 1607

Wine, Red

Rifater Tablets (Isoniazid has some MAO inhibiting activity, an interaction with tyramine-containing food may occur) 769

Wine, unspecified

Matulane Capsules (Procarbazine exhibits some MAO inhibitory activity: concurrent use should be avoided) 3246

Nardil Tablets (Concurrent and/or sequential intake must be avoided) 2653

Wine products

Nardil Tablets (Concurrent and/or sequential intake must be avoided) 2653

Yeast, Brewer's

Nardil Tablets (Concurrent and/or sequential intake must be avoided) 2653

Yeast Extract

Nardil Tablets (Concurrent and/or sequential intake must be avoided) 2653

Parnate Tablets (Potential for hypertensive crisis; concurrent use is contraindicated) 1607

Yogurt

Matulane Capsules (Procarbazine exhibits some MAO inhibitory activity: concurrent use should be avoided) 3246

Nardil Tablets (Concurrent and/or sequential intake must be avoided) 2653

Parnate Tablets (Potential for hypertensive crisis; concurrent use is contraindicated) 1607

SECTION 3

SIDE EFFECTS INDEX

Presented in this section is an alphabetical list of every side effect reported in the "Adverse Reactions" section of the product descriptions in *PDR®* and its companion volumes. Under each side effect is an alphabetical list of brands associated with the reaction.

If noted in the underlying text, incidence is shown in parentheses immediately after the brand name. Products reporting an incidence rate of 3% or more are marked with a ▲ symbol at their left. Because incidence data are sometimes drawn from controlled clinical trials, the rates seen in actual clinical practice may vary from those found in the published reports.

This index lists only side effects noted in official prescribing information as published by *PDR®*. To alert you to the full range of possibilities, the entries include adverse effects shared by an entire class of drugs, but not necessarily reported for the specific drug in question. The index is restricted to reactions that may be expected to occur at recommended dosages in the general patient population. Precautions to be taken under special circumstances are not listed, nor are the effects of overdosage.

The page numbers shown for the products refer to the 2002 editions of *PDR®* and *PDR for Ophthalmic Medicines™*, and the 2001 edition of *PDR for Nonprescription Drugs and Dietary Supplements™*, which is published later in the year. A key to the symbols denoting the companion volumes appears in the bottom margin.

A

Abdomen, redistribution/ accumulation of body fat

Crixivan Capsules 2070

Abdominal adhesion

ParaGard T 380A Intrauterine Copper Contraceptive 2582

Abdominal bloating

Aciphex Tablets (Rare) 1267
Aciphex Tablets (Rare) 1783
Activella Tablets 2764
Aerobid/Aerobid-M (Less than 1%) 1363
Alesse-21 Tablets 3468
Alesse-28 Tablets 3473
Alora Transdermal System 3372
Aricept Tablets (Frequent) 1270
Aricept Tablets (Frequent) 2665
Asacol Delayed-Release Tablets (2% or greater) 2884
Atromid-S Capsules 3483
Brevicon 28-Day Tablets 3380
Cenestin Tablets 1263
Climara Transdermal System 958
▲ Clomid Tablets (5.5%) 735
Colazal Capsules 3069
Colestid Tablets (Less frequent) 2791
▲ Colyte with Flavor Packs for Oral Solution (Up to 50%) 3170
Corgard Tablets (1 to 5 per 1000 patients) 2245
Corlopam Injection (1% to 2%) 412
Corzide 40/5 Tablets (1 to 5 of 1000 patients) 2247
Corzide 80/5 Tablets (1 to 5 of 1000 patients) 2247
Coumadin for Injection (Infrequent) 1243
Coumadin Tablets (Infrequent) 1243
▲ Creon 5 Capsules (Among most frequent) 3251
▲ Creon 10 Capsules (Among most frequent) 3251
▲ Creon 20 Capsules (Among most frequent) 3251
▲ Crinone (13%) 3213
Cyclessa Tablets 2450
Depo-Provera Contraceptive Injection (1% to 5%) 2798
Desogen Tablets 2458
DiaBeta Tablets (1.8%) 741
Dipentum Capsules (1.5%) 2803
Donnatal 2929
Donnatal Extentabs 2930
Donnatal Tablets 2929
▲ Esclim Transdermal System (2.1% to 6.4%) 3460
Estinyl Tablets 3112
Estrace Vaginal Cream 3358
Estrace Tablets 3361
Estratest 3252
Estrostep 2627
femhrt Tablets 2635
▲ GoLYTELY and Pineapple Flavor GoLYTELY for Oral Solution (Up to 50%) 1068
Hivid Tablets (Less than 1%) 2975
Humegon for Injection 2468
Imitrex Nasal Spray 1554
IMUPlus Formula 3274
Indocin Capsules (Less than 1%) 2112
Indocin I.V. (Less than 1%) 2115
Indocin (Less than 1%) 2112
Levbid Extended-Release Tablets 3172
Levlen 962
Levlite 21 Tablets 962
Levlite 28 Tablets 962
Levora Tablets 3389
Levsin/Levsinex/Levbid 3172
▲ Limbitrol (Among most frequent) 1738
Loestrin 21 Tablets 2642
Loestrin Fe Tablets 2642
Lo/Ovral Tablets 3532
Lo/Ovral-28 Tablets 3538
Low-Ogestrel-28 Tablets 3392
Menest Tablets 2254
MetroGel-Vaginal Gel (Less than 1%) 1986
Microgestin Fe 1.5/30 Tablets 3407
Microgestin Fe 1/20 Tablets 3400
Midamor Tablets (Less than or equal to 1%) 2136
MiraLax Powder for Oral Solution 1069
Mircette Tablets 2470
Mitrolan Chewable Tablets (Occasional) .... ◘789
Modicon 2563
Moduretic Tablets (Less than or equal to 1%) 2138
Motrin Suspension, Oral Drops, Chewable Tablets, and Caplets (1% to less than 3%) 2002
Mykrox Tablets (Less than 2%) 1168
Nadolol Tablets (1 to 5 of 1000 patients) 2288
Necon 3415
Nordette-28 Tablets 2257
Norinyl 1 +35 28-Day Tablets 3380
Norinyl 1 + 50 28-Day Tablets 3380
Noroxin Tablets (Less frequent) 2145
Norvir Capsules (Less than 2%) 487
Norvir Oral Solution (Less than 2%) 487
NuLev Orally Disintegrating Tablets 3176
▲ NuLYTELY, Cherry Flavor, Lemon-Lime Flavor, and Orange Flavor NuLYTELY for Oral Solution (Among most common) 1068
Ogen Tablets 2846
Ogestrel 0.5/50-28 Tablets 3428
Ortho Dienestrol Cream 2554
Ortho-Cept 21 Tablets 2546
Ortho-Cept 28 Tablets 2546
Ortho-Cyclen/Ortho Tri-Cyclen 2573
Ortho-Est Tablets 3464
Ortho-Novum 2563
Ortho-Novum 1/50□28 Tablets 2556
Ortho-Prefest Tablets 2570
Ortho-Cyclen/Ortho Tri-Cyclen 2573
Ovcon 3364
Ovral Tablets 3551
Ovral-28 Tablets 3552
Ovrette Tablets 3552
Pergonal for Injection 3223
Premarin Intravenous 3563
Premarin Tablets 3566
Premarin Vaginal Cream 3570
Premphase Tablets 3572
Prempro Tablets 3572
Prilosec Delayed-Release Capsules (Less than 1%) 628
▲ Prometrium Capsules (100 mg, 200 mg) (12%) 3261
Repronex for Intramuscular and Subcutaneous Injection 1347
Robinul Forte Tablets 1358
Robinul Injectable 2940
Robinul Tablets 1358
Roferon-A Injection (Infrequent) 2996
Rowasa Rectal Suspension Enema 4.0 grams/unit (60 mL) (1.47%) 3264
▲ Thrombate III (1 of 17) 944
Ticlid Tablets (0.5% to 1.0%) 3015
Toradol (Greater than 1%) 3018
Trental Tablets (0.6%) 784
Tri-Levlen 962
Tri-Norinyl-28 Tablets 3433
Triphasil-21 Tablets 3600
Triphasil-28 Tablets 3605
Trivora Tablets 3439
Visicol Tablets 1767
Vivelle Transdermal System 2412
Vivelle-Dot Transdermal System 2416
Warfarin Sodium Tablets, USP 3302
Yasmin 28 Tablets 980
Zaroxolyn Tablets 1177
Zovia 3449

Abdominal discomfort
(*see also under* Distress, abdominal; Distress, gastrointestinal)

Aquasol A Parenteral 593
Biaxin/Biaxin XL (2%) 403
Brevibloc Injection (Less than 1%) 858
Carafate Tablets (Less than 0.5%) 730
Centrum Focused Formulas Prostate Softgels .... ◘816
Cipro I.V. (1.7%) 893
Cipro (0.3% to 1.7%) 887
▲ Clomid Tablets (5.5%) 735
▲ Clozaril Tablets (4%) 2319
Colestid Tablets (Less frequent) 2791
Corgard Tablets (1 to 5 per 1000 patients) 2245
Correctol Laxative Tablets and Caplets .... ◘739
Corzide 40/5 Tablets (1 to 5 of 1000 patients) 2247
Corzide 80/5 Tablets (1 to 5 of 1000 patients) 2247
Desferal Vials 2333
Dulcolax Suppositories .... ◘668
Dulcolax Tablets .... ◘668
DynaCirc Capsules (1.7% to 3.3%) 2921
DynaCirc CR Tablets (1.3% to 5.1%) 2923
▲ Epivir-HBV (16%) 1524
Famotidine Injection (Infrequent) 866
Fleet Bisacodyl Laxatives 1359
Fleet Prep Kits 1361
▲ Flovent Diskus (4%) 3614
Flovent Rotadisk (1% to 3%) 1537
Follistim for Injection (2.9%) 2465
Gengraf Capsules (Up to 7%) 457
▲ Glucophage Tablets (6.4%) 1080
Imitrex Nasal Spray (Infrequent) 1554
Imitrex Tablets 1558

K-Dur Microburst Release System ER Tablets 1832
Klonopin Tablets (Infrequent) 2983
▲ Klor-Con M20/Klor-Con M10 Tablets (Among most common) 3329
Children's Motrin Oral Suspension and Chewable Tablets 2006
Children's Motrin Oral Suspension ▣643
Infants' Motrin Concentrated Drops 2006
Mykrox Tablets (Less than 2%) 1168
Nadolol Tablets (1 to 5 of 1000 patients) 2288
Neoral Soft Gelatin Capsules (Up to 7%) 2380
Neoral Oral Solution (Up to 7%) 2380
Pepcid Injection (Infrequent) 2153
Pepcid for Oral Suspension (Infrequent) 2150
Pepcid RPD Orally Disintegrating Tablets (Infrequent) 2150
Pepcid Tablets (Infrequent) 2150
▲ Sandimmune (Less than 1% to 7%) 2388
▲ Sandostatin Injection (34% to 61%) 2394
▲ Serophene Tablets (Approximately 1 in 15 patients) 3226
Tonocard Tablets (Less than 1%) 649
Trental Tablets 784
▲ Trisenox Injection (8%) 1158
Urecholine Tablets 2445
Urocit-K Tablets (Some patients) 2232
▲ Xenical Capsules (25.5%) 3043

Abdominal distention

Actiq (1% or greater) 1184
Aldoclor Tablets 2035
Aldomet Tablets 2037
Aldoril Tablets 2039
Aloprim for Injection (Less than 1%) 2292
AmBisome for Injection (Less common) 1383
▲ Amphotec (5% or more) 1774
Avalide Tablets 1070
Avapro Tablets (Less than 1%) 1074
Avapro Tablets (Less than 1%) 3076
Betapace AF Tablets (0.7% to 2.5%) 954
Cataflam Tablets (1% to 3%) 2315
Celestone Soluspan Injectable Suspension 3097
Celestone Syrup 3099
▲ CellCept Capsules (3%) 2951
▲ CellCept Intravenous (3%) 2951
▲ CellCept Oral Suspension (3%) 2951
▲ CellCept Tablets (3% to 18.8%) 2951
Chirocaine Injection (2.9%) 2909
Claritin-D 12 Hour Extended Release Tablets (Less frequent) 3102
Claritin-D 24 Hour Extended Release Tablets (Fewer than 2%) 3104
▲ Clomid Tablets (5.5%) 735
Clozaril Tablets (Less than 1%) 2319
Cortone Acetate Injectable Suspension 2059
Cortone Acetate Tablets 2061
Crixivan Capsules (Less than 2%) 2070
Cytovene (At least 3 subjects) 2959
Decadron Elixir 2078
Decadron Tablets 2079
Decadron Phosphate Injection 2081
Depo-Medrol Injectable Suspension 2795
Doxil Injection (1% to 5%) 566
Duragesic Transdermal System (Less than 1%) 1786
DynaCirc Capsules (0.5% to 1%) 2921
DynaCirc CR Tablets (1.2%) 2923
Effexor Tablets (Infrequent) 3495
Estring Vaginal Ring (At least 1 report) 2811
Evoxac Capsules 1217
▲ Flolan for Injection (4%) 1528
Florinef Acetate Tablets 2250
Follistim for Injection 2465
Fosamax Tablets (1.0%) 2095
Gengraf Capsules (1% to less than 3%) 457
Glucophage XR Tablets (1% to 5%) 1080
Gonal-F for Injection 3216
Humegon for Injection 2468
Hydrocortone Tablets 2106
Hydrocortone Acetate Injectable Suspension 2103
Hydrocortone Phosphate Injection, Sterile 2105
Imitrex Nasal Spray 1554
Indocin I.V. (1% to 3%) 2115
Intron A for Injection (Less than 5%) 3120
Lamictal (Rare) 1567
▲ Leukine (4%) 1755
Lunelle Monthly Injection 2827
Lupron Depot–3 Month 22.5 mg (Less than 5%) 3288
Mavik Tablets (0.3% to 1.0%) 478
Merrem I.V. (0.1% to 1.0%) 673
Mirapex Tablets (Less than 1%) 2834
Monopril Tablets (0.2% to 1.0%) 1091
Monopril HCT 1094
▲ Mylotarg for Injection (9% to 13%) 3540
Naprelan Tablets (Less than 1%) 1293
Neoral Soft Gelatin Capsules (1% to less than 3%) 2380
Neoral Oral Solution (1% to less than 3%) 2380
Nexium Delayed-Release Capsules (Less than 1%) 619
▲ NuLYTELY, Cherry Flavor, Lemon-Lime Flavor, and Orange Flavor NuLYTELY for Oral Solution (Among most common) 1068
Ovidrel for Injection 3220
Pediapred Oral Solution 1170
Pentasa Capsules (Less than 1%) 3239
Pergonal for Injection 3223
Permax Tablets (Infrequent) 1299
Prednisone 3064
Prelone Syrup 2273
▲ Prograf (3% to 15%) 1393
▲ Proleukin for Injection (10%) 1199
▲ Prometrium Capsules (100 mg, 200 mg) (6% to 8%) 3261
▲ Rapamune Oral Solution and Tablets (3% to 20%) 3584
Remeron Tablets (Infrequent) 2483
Remeron SolTab Tablets (Infrequent) 2486
ReoPro Vials (0.1%) 1958
▲ Repronex for Intramuscular and Subcutaneous Injection (2.1% to 6%) 1347
Requip Tablets (Infrequent) 1621
Rescriptor Tablets (Less than 2%) 526
Rilutek Tablets (Infrequent) 772
Risperdal (Rare) 1796
Rituxan for Infusion (1% to 5%) 1750
Rituxan I.V. (1% to 5%) 1428
▲ Sandostatin Injection (Less than 10%) 2394
Sandostatin LAR Depot (Rare) 2395
Serophene Tablets 3226
Seroquel Tablets (Rare) 684
Serzone Tablets (Infrequent) 1104
▲ Simulect for Injection (3% to 10%) 2399
Solu-Medrol Sterile Powder 2855
▲ Taxotere for Injection Concentrate (6%) 778
Thalomid Capsules 1154
Tiazac Capsules (2%) 1378
Topamax Sprinkle Capsules (Infrequent) 2590
Topamax Tablets (Infrequent) 2590
▲ Trisenox Injection (8%) 1158
Unasyn for Injection (Less than 1%) 2728
Vantin Tablets and Oral Suspension (Less than 1%) 2860
▲ Vesanoid Capsules (11%) 3037
Vioxx (Greater than 0.1% to 1.9%) 2213
Voltaren Tablets (1% to 3%) 2315
Voltaren-XR Tablets (1% to 3%) 2315
▲ Zenapax for Injection (Greater than 5%) 3046
Zyprexa Tablets (Rare) 1973
Zyprexa ZYDIS Orally Disintegrating Tablets (Rare) 1973
Zyrtec (Less than 2%) 2756
Zyrtec-D 12 Hour Extended Relief Tablets (Less than 2%) 2758

Abdominal guarding

Sandostatin LAR Depot (Rare) 2395

Abdominal mass

Estratest 3252

Abdominal pain/cramps

▲ Abelcet Injection (4%) 1273
Accolate Tablets (1.8% to 2.8%) 657
Accupril Tablets (1.0%) 2611
Accuretic Tablets (1.7%) 2614
Aceon Tablets (2 mg, 4 mg, 8 mg) (2.7%) 3249
Aciphex Tablets 1267
Aciphex Tablets 1783
▲ Actimmune (8%) 1772
Actiq (1% or greater) 1184
Activella Tablets 2764
▲ Actonel Tablets (11.5% to 11.6%) 2879
Adalat CC Tablets (Less than 1.0%) 877
▲ Adderall XR Capsules (14%)
▲ Advair Diskus 100/50 (4%) 1448
Advair Diskus 250/50 (2%) 1448
Advair Diskus 500/50 (1% to 4%) 1448
▲ Aerobid/Aerobid-M (3% to 9%) 1363
Agenerase Capsules 1454
Agenerase Oral Solution 1459
▲ Aggrenox Capsules (17.5%) 1026
▲ Agrylin Capsules (16.4%) 3232
▲ Albenza Tablets (Up to 6.0%) 1463
Aldoclor Tablets 2035
Aldoril Tablets 2039
Alesse-21 Tablets 3468
Alesse-28 Tablets 3473
Allegra-D Extended-Release Tablets (1.4%) 714
▲ Alora Transdermal System (3.2% to 5.7%) 3372
Altace Capsules (Less than 1%) 2233
Ambien Tablets (2%) 3191
▲ AmBisome for Injection (9.9% to 19.8%) 1383
Amerge Tablets (Infrequent) 1467
Amicar Injection 3608
Amicar Syrup 3608
Amicar Tablets 3608
Aminohippurate Sodium PAH Injection 2041
▲ Amphotec (5% or more) 1774
▲ Anaprox Tablets (3% to 9%) 2967
▲ Anaprox DS Tablets (3% to 9%) 2967
Ancef for Injection 1474
Ancef Injection 1474
Ancobon Capsules 1730
Antagon Injection (1% to 4.8%) 2447
▲ Anzemet Injection (3.2%) 719
Anzemet Tablets (Rare) 722
Aralen Tablets 3075
▲ Arava Tablets (6%) 724
▲ Aredia for Injection (22.6%) 2309
Argatroban Injection (2.6%) 1478
Aricept Tablets 1270
Aricept Tablets 2665
▲ Arimidex Tablets (5.7% to 7.9%) 659
▲ Aromasin Tablets (6%) 2769
▲ Arthrotec Tablets (21%) 3195
▲ Asacol Delayed-Release Tablets (18%) 2884
Astelin Nasal Spray (Infrequent) 3339
Atacand Tablets (More than 1%) 595
Atacand HCT Tablets (0.5% or greater) 597
Avalide Tablets (2%) 1070
Avapro Tablets (1% or greater) 1074
Avapro Tablets (1% or greater) 3076
Avelox Tablets (2%) 879
▲ Avonex (9%) 1013
Axert Tablets (Infrequent) 2772
▲ Axid Pulvules (7.5%) 1903
▲ Axid Pulvules (7.5%) 2919
Azactam for Injection (Less than 1%) 1276
Azmacort Inhalation Aerosol (1% to 3%) 728
Azulfidine EN-tabs Tablets (Rare) 2775
Bactrim 2949
Bactroban Cream (Less than 1%) 1494
Baycol Tablets (2.5%) 883
Beano ▣809
Betapace Tablets (Less than 1% to 3%) 950
Betapace AF Tablets (2.5% to 3.5%) 954
▲ Betaseron for SC Injection (32%) 988
Biaxin/Biaxin XL (2% to 3%) 403
Blocadren Tablets 2046
Brevicon 28-Day Tablets 3380
Brevital Sodium for Injection, USP 1815
▲ Campath Ampules (2% to 11%) 992
Canasa Rectal Suppositories 829
Cancidas for Injection (2.5% to 3.6%) 2048
Captopril Tablets (About 0.5% to 2%) 2281
Carbatrol Capsules 3234
Cardene I.V. (0.7%) 3485
Cardura Tablets (2.4%) 2668
▲ Carnitor Injection (5% to 21%) 3242
Carnitor Tablets and Oral Solution 3245
▲ Casodex Tablets (8%) 662
▲ Cataflam Tablets (3% to 9%) 2315
Catapres Tablets (Rare) 1037
Ceclor CD Tablets (1.6%) 1279
Ceclor 1905
Cedax (1%) 1021
Cefotan 664
Ceftin (0.1% to 1%) 1898
Cefzil (1%) 1076
▲ Celebrex Capsules (4.1%) 2676
▲ Celebrex Capsules (4.1%) 2780
Celexa (2%) 1365
▲ CellCept Capsules (24.7% to 33.9%) 2951
▲ CellCept Intravenous (24.7% to 33.9%) 2951
▲ CellCept Oral Suspension (24.7% to 33.9%) 2951
▲ CellCept Tablets (24.7% to 62.5%) 2951
Celontin Capsules (Frequent) 2618
▲ Cenestin Tablets (28%) 1263
Ceptaz for Injection (One in 416 patients) 1499
▲ Cerezyme for Injection (5.4%) 1438
Cervidil Vaginal Insert (Less than 1%) 1369
▲ Chemet Capsules (5.2% to 15.7%) 3078
Chirocaine Injection (2.2%) 2909
New Formulation Chromagen OB Capsules 3094
Cipro I.V. (1% or less) 893
Cipro I.V. Pharmacy Bulk Package (Less than 1%) 897
Cipro (1.7%) 887
Claritin (2%) 3100
Claritin-D 12 Hour Extended Release Tablets (Less frequent) 3102
Cleocin HCl Capsules 2784
Cleocin Phosphate Sterile Solution 2785
Cleocin T Topical 2790
Cleocin Vaginal Cream (Less than 1% to 2%) 2788
Cleocin Vaginal Ovules (Less than 1%) 2789
Climara Transdermal System 958
Clindagel 1401
▲ Clinoril Tablets (10%) 2053
Clomid Tablets 735
▲ Cognex Capsules (8%) 1351
▲ Colazal Capsules (6%) 3069
Colestid Tablets (Less frequent) 2791
Colyte with Flavor Packs for Oral Solution (Less frequent) 3170
▲ CombiPatch Transdermal System (12% to 14%) 2323
▲ Combivir Tablets (6% to 9%) 1502
▲ Comtan Tablets (8%) 2328
▲ Concerta Extended-Release Tablets (7%) 1998
▲ Concerta Tablets (7%) 561
Copaxone for Injection (At least 2%) 3306
Cordarone Tablets (1% to 3%) 3487
▲ Coreg Tablets (1.4% to 7.2%) 1508
Corlopam Injection (1% to 2%) 412
Correctol Laxative Tablets and Caplets ▣739
Corzide 40/5 Tablets 2247
Corzide 80/5 Tablets 2247
Cosmegen for Injection 2062
Cosopt Sterile Ophthalmic Solution (1% to 5%) 2065
Coumadin for Injection (Infrequent) 1243
Coumadin Tablets (Infrequent) 1243
Cozaar Tablets (1% or greater) 2067
▲ Creon 5 Capsules (Among most frequent) 3251
▲ Creon 10 Capsules (Among most frequent) 3251
▲ Creon 20 Capsules (Among most frequent) 3251
▲ Crinone (5%) 3213
▲ Crixivan Capsules (8.7%) 2070
Cyclessa Tablets 2450
▲ Cytotec Tablets (13% to 20%) 3202
Cytovene (At least 3 subjects) 2959
Dantrium Capsules (Less frequent) 2885
Dapsone Tablets USP 1780
Darvon-N/Darvocet-N 1907
Darvon Pulvules 1909
Darvon Compound-65 Pulvules 1910
Darvon-N Tablets 1912
▲ DaunoXome Injection (3% to 20%) 1442
DDAVP Injection 4 mcg/mL (Infrequent) 737
DDAVP Nasal Spray (2%) 738
DDAVP Rhinal Tube (2%) 738
DDAVP Tablets 739
Demser Capsules (Infrequent) 2085
▲ Depacon Injection (1.1% to 23%) 416
▲ Depakene (12% to 23%) 421
▲ Depakote Sprinkle Capsules (9% to 23%) 426
▲ Depakote Tablets (9% to 23%) 430
▲ Depakote ER Tablets (7% to 23%) 436
▲ Depo-Provera Contraceptive Injection (More than 5%) 2798
Desmopressin Acetate Injection (Infrequent) 1344
Desmopressin Acetate Rhinal Tube (2%) 1345
Desogen Tablets 2458
▲ Detrol Tablets (7.6%) 3623
▲ Detrol LA Capsules (4%) 2801
▲ Diflucan Tablets, Injection, and Oral Suspension (1.7% to 6%) 2681
Digitek Tablets 1003
Dilaudid-HP (Less frequent) 443
Diovan Capsules (2%) 2337
Diovan HCT Tablets (Greater than 0.2%) 2338
▲ Dipentum Capsules (10.1%) 2803
Diprivan Injectable Emulsion (Less than 1%) 667
Ditropan XL Extended Release Tablets (2% to 5%) 564
Diucardin Tablets 3494
Diuril Sodium Intravenous 2086
▲ Dostinex Tablets (5%) 2804
▲ Doxil Injection (1% to 8%) 566
Duraclon Injection (Rare) 3057
▲ Duragesic Transdermal System (3% to 10%) 1786
Duricef 1079
Dyazide Capsules 1515
▲ Dynabac Tablets (7.1% to 9.7%) 2269
▲ EC-Naprosyn Delayed-Release Tablets (3% to 9%) 2967
Edecrin 2091
▲ E.E.S. (Among most frequent) 450
▲ Effexor Tablets (2.2% to 8.0%) 3495
▲ Effexor XR Capsules (6%) 3499
▲ Eldepryl Capsules (4 of 49 patients) 3266
Elmiron Capsules (2%) 570
Elspar for Injection 2092
Enalaprilat Injection 863
▲ Enbrel for Injection (5% to 19%) 1752
▲ Enbrel for Injection (5% to 19%) 3504
Engerix-B Vaccine (Less than 1%) 1517
▲ Epivir (6% to 9%) 1520
▲ Epivir-HBV (16%) 1524

Epogen for Injection 582
▲ Ergamisol Tablets (2% to 5%) 1789
▲ EryPed (Among most frequent) 446
▲ Ery-Tab Tablets (Among most frequent) 448
▲ Erythrocin Stearate Filmtab Tablets (Among most frequent) 452
▲ Erythromycin Base Filmtab Tablets (Among most frequent) 454
▲ Erythromycin Delayed-Release Capsules, USP (Among most frequent) 455
▲ Esclim Transdermal System (2.1% to 10.6%) 3460
Eskalith 1527
Estinyl Tablets 3112
Estrace Vaginal Cream 3358
Estrace Tablets 3361
Estratest 3252
▲ Estring Vaginal Ring (4%) 2811
Estrostep 2627
Ethiodol Injection 3095
Eulexin Capsules 3118
▲ Evista Tablets (6.6%) 1915
▲ Evoxac Capsules (7.6%) 1217
▲ Exelon Capsules (13%) 2342
▲ Exelon Oral Solution (13%) 2345
▲ Famvir Tablets (1.1% to 7.9%) 2348
▲ Felbatol (5.3%) 3343
▲ Feldene Capsules (1% to 10%) 2685
▲ Femara Tablets (4% to 6%) 2351
▲ femhrt Tablets (8.1%) 2635
▲ Ferrlecit Injection (6%) 3386
Fleet Bisacodyl Laxatives 1359
Fleet Prep Kits 1361
▲ Flolan for Injection (5% to 27%) 1528
Flonase Nasal Spray (1% to 3%) 1533
▲ Flovent Diskus (4%) 3614
Flovent Rotadisk (1% to 3%) 1537
Floxin I.V. (1% to 3%) 2526
Floxin Otic Solution (Single report) 1219
Floxin Tablets (1% to 3%) 2529
Flumadine (1.4%) 1370
Follistim for Injection (1.9% to 2.9%) 2465
Fortaz (1 in 416) 1541
▲ Fortovase Capsules (2.3% to 7.8%) 2970
▲ Fosamax Tablets (1.7% to 6.6%) 2095
▲ Foscavir Injection (5% or greater) 605
Sterile FUDR 2974
Furosemide Tablets 2284
▲ Gabitril Tablets (5% to 7%) 1189
Gamimune N, 5% Solvent/Detergent Treated 925
Gamimune N, 10% Solvent/Detergent Treated 928
Gammar-P I.V. 787
Gastrocrom Oral Concentrate (2 of 87 patients) 1162
▲ Gengraf Capsules (2.7% to 15%) 457
Geocillin Tablets 2687
Geodon Capsules (Frequent) 2688
▲ Gleevec Capsules (20% to 26%) 2357
Glucophage Tablets (1% to 5%) 1080
Glucophage XR Tablets (1% to 5%) 1080
▲ Glucovance Tablets (6.9%) 1086
▲ Glyset Tablets (11.7%) 2821
GoLYTELY and Pineapple Flavor GoLYTELY for Oral Solution (Infrequent) 1068
▲ Gonal-F for Injection (8.9% to 9.3%) 3216
▲ Gynazole-1 Vaginal Cream (5.7%) 3310
Halcion Tablets (0.5% to 0.9%) 2823
Havrix Vaccine (Less than 1%) 1544
▲ Herceptin I.V. (22%) 1414
Hivid Tablets (Less than 1% to 3.0%) 2975
Humegon for Injection 2468
Humorsol Sterile Ophthalmic Solution (Rare) 2102
▲ Hycamtin for Injection (Less than 1% to 33%) 1546
HydroDIURIL Tablets 2108
Hytrin Capsules (At least 1%) 464
Hyzaar (1.2%) 2109
▲ Idamycin PFS Injection (73%) 2825
Imdur Tablets (Less than or equal to 5%) 1826
Imitrex Injection 1549
Imitrex Nasal Spray 1554
▲ Imovax Rabies Vaccine (About 20%) 807
IMUPlus Formula 3274
Indapamide Tablets (Less than 5%) 2286
Inderal 3513
Inderal LA Long-Acting Capsules 3516
Inderide Tablets 3517
Inderide LA Long-Acting Capsules 3519
Indocin (Greater than 1%) 2112
INFeD Injection 3388
▲ Infergen (24% to 41%) 1777
Innohep Injection (0.8%) 1248
▲ Intron A for Injection (1% to 21%) 3120
Invirase Capsules (0.3% to 2.0%) 2979
Iopidine Sterile Ophthalmic Solution ⊙212
Ismo Tablets (Fewer than 1%) 3524
Isopto Carbachol Ophthalmic Solution ⊙215
▲ JE-VAX Vaccine (Approximately 10%) 811
Kadian Capsules (Less than 3%) 1335
Kaletra Capsules (1.1% to 4.8%) 471
Kaletra Oral Solution (1.1% to 4.8%) 471
K-Dur Microburst Release System ER Tablets 1832
Keflex 1237
Kefzol Vials, ADD-Vantage 1951
Keppra Tablets (1% or more) 3314
Klonopin Tablets (1%) 2983
▲ Klor-Con M20/Klor-Con M10 Tablets (Among most common) 3329
▲ K-Lor Powder Packets (Among most common) 469
Kristalose for Oral Solution 1007
▲ Kytril Tablets (4% to 6%) 2988
▲ Lamictal (3% to 5.2%) 1567
Lamisil Tablets (2.4%) 2360
Lanoxicaps Capsules (Rare) 1574
Lanoxin Injection (Rare) 1581
Lanoxin Tablets (Rare) 1587
Lanoxin Elixir Pediatric (Rare) 1578
Lanoxin Injection Pediatric (Rare) 1584
▲ Lariam Tablets (Among most frequent) 2989
▲ Lescol Capsules (4.9%) 2361
▲ Lescol Capsules (4.9%) 2925
▲ Lescol XL Tablets (3.7%) 2361
▲ Lescol XL Tablets (3.7%) 2925
▲ Leukine (38%) 1755
▲ Leustatin Injection (6%) 2495
Levaquin (0.3% to 2.0%) 2537
Levlen 962
Levlite 21 Tablets 962
Levlite 28 Tablets 962
Levo-Dromoran 1734
Levora Tablets 3389
Levorphanol Tartrate Tablets (1% to 3%) 3059
Levoxyl Tablets 1819
Lexxel Tablets (Infrequent) 608
Lipitor Tablets (Up to 3.8%) 2639
Lipitor Tablets (Up to 3.8%) 2696
Lithobid Slow-Release Tablets 3255
▲ Lodine (3% to 9%) 3528
▲ Lodine XL Extended-Release Tablets (1% to 10%) 3530
Lodosyn Tablets 1251
Loestrin 21 Tablets 2642
Loestrin Fe Tablets 2642
Lo/Ovral Tablets 3532
Lo/Ovral-28 Tablets 3538
▲ Lopid Tablets (9.8%) 2650
Lorabid Suspension and Pulvules (1.4%) 2251
Lotensin HCT Tablets (0.3% to 1%) 2367
Lotrel Capsules 2370
Low-Ogestrel-28 Tablets 3392
Lunelle Monthly Injection 2827
Luvox Tablets (25, 50, 100 mg) (1%) 3256
Macrobid Capsules (Less than 1%) 2889
Macrodantin Capsules (Less common) 2891
▲ Malarone (6% to 33%) 1596
▲ Marinol Capsules (3% to 10%) 3325
Massengill Disposable Douches ■752
Massengill Medicated Disposable Douche ■753
Matulane Capsules 3246
Mavik Tablets (0.3% to 1.0%) 478
Maxair Autohaler 1981
Maxair Inhaler (Less than 1%) 1984
Mefoxin for Injection 2124
Mefoxin Premixed Intravenous Solution 2127
Megace Oral Suspension (1% to 3%) 1124
Menest Tablets 2254
▲ Mepron Suspension (4% to 21%) 1598
▲ Meridia Capsules (4.5%) 481
Merrem I.V. (0.1% to 1.0%) 673
Mestinon 1740
▲ Metadate CD Capsules (7%) 1164
Metadate ER Tablets 1167
Methylin Tablets 1995
Methylin ER Tablets 1995
▲ Mevacor Tablets (2.0% to 5.7%) 2132
Mexitil Capsules (1.2%) 1047
Miacalcin Injection 2373
Miacalcin Nasal Spray (1% to 3%) 2375
Micardis Tablets (1%) 1049
Micardis HCT Tablets (Less than 2%) 1051
Micro-K 3311
Microgestin Fe 1.5/30 Tablets 3407
Microgestin Fe 1/20 Tablets 3400
Microzide Capsules 3414
Midamor Tablets (Between 1% and 3%) 2136
Migranal Nasal Spray (Rare) 2376
Minipress Capsules (Less than 1%) 2699
Minizide Capsules (Rare) 2700
Mintezol 2137
MiraLax Powder for Oral Solution 1069
Mirapex Tablets (1% or more) 2834
Mircette Tablets 2470
▲ Mirena Intrauterine System (5% or more) 974
▲ Mobic Tablets (11.8% to 26.6%) 1054
Modicon 2563
Moduretic Tablets (Greater than 1%, less than 3%) 2138
Monopril Tablets (0.2% to 1.0% or more) 1091
Monopril HCT (Less than 2%) 1094
Monurol Sachet (2.2%) 1375
Motrin Suspension, Oral Drops, Chewable Tablets, and Caplets (1% to less than 3%) 2002
MS Contin Tablets (Less frequent) 2896
MSIR (Less frequent) 2898
Myambutol Tablets 1290
▲ Mycobutin Capsules (4%) 2838
Mykrox Tablets (Less than 2%) 1168
▲ Mylotarg for Injection (23% to 52%) 3540
Nabi-HB 2295
▲ Naprelan Tablets (3% to 9%) 1293
▲ Naprosyn Suspension (3% to 9%) 2967
▲ Naprosyn Tablets (3% to 9%) 2967
Natrecor for Injection (1%) 3189
Navelbine Injection 1604
Necon 3415
▲ Neoral Soft Gelatin Capsules (2.7% to 15%) 2380
▲ Neoral Oral Solution (2.7% to 15%) 2380
▲ Neumega for Injection (Greater than or equal to 10%) 1434
Neupogen for Injection (Infrequent) 587
Neurontin Capsules 2655
Neurontin Oral Solution 2655
Neurontin Tablets 2655
Nexium Delayed-Release Capsules (Greater than or equal to 1% to 3.8%) 619
▲ Niaspan Extended-Release Tablets (2% to 5%) 1846
▲ Nicotrol Nasal Spray (3%) 2843
▲ Nilandron Tablets (10%) 753
▲ Nipent for Injection (4% to 16%) 3272
Nizoral Tablets (1.2%) 1791
Nolvadex Tablets (1%) 678
Nordette-28 Tablets 2257
Norinyl 1 +35 28-Day Tablets 3380
Norinyl 1 + 50 28-Day Tablets 3380
Normodyne Tablets 3137
Noroxin Tablets (0.3% to 1.6%) 2145
Norpramin Tablets 755
Norvasc Tablets (1.6%) 2704
▲ Norvir Capsules (3.4% to 7.0%) 487
▲ Norvir Oral Solution (3.4% to 7.0%) 487
▲ Novantrone for Injection (9% to 15%) 1760
Nubain Injection (1% or less) 1323
NuLYTELY, Cherry Flavor, Lemon-Lime Flavor, and Orange Flavor NuLYTELY for Oral Solution (Less frequent) 1068
Numorphan 1324
Ogen Tablets 2846
Ogestrel 0.5/50-28 Tablets 3428
Omnicef (1%) 493
▲ Oncaspar (Greater than 1% but less than 5%) 756
Oramorph SR Tablets (Less frequent) 3062
Ortho Dienestrol Cream 2554
Ortho-Cept 21 Tablets 2546
Ortho-Cept 28 Tablets 2546
Orthoclone OKT3 Sterile Solution 2498
Ortho-Cyclen/Ortho Tri-Cyclen 2573
Ortho-Est Tablets 3464
Ortho-Novum 2563
Ortho-Novum 1/50□28 Tablets 2556
▲ Ortho-Prefest Tablets (12%) 2570
Ortho-Cyclen/Ortho Tri-Cyclen 2573
▲ Orudis Capsules (3% to 9%) 3548
▲ Oruvail Capsules (3% to 9%) 3548
Ovcon 3364
▲ Ovidrel for Injection (3% to 4.2%) 3220
Ovral Tablets 3551
Ovral-28 Tablets 3552
Ovrette Tablets 3552
OxyContin Tablets (Between 1% and 5%) 2912
Pacerone Tablets (1% to 3%) 3331
▲ Pancrease Capsules (Among most frequent) 2580
▲ Pancrease MT Capsules (Among most frequent) 2581
ParaGard T 380A Intrauterine Copper Contraceptive 2582
Parnate Tablets 1607
▲ Paser Granules (Among most common) 1781
▲ Paxil (4%) 1609
▲ PCE Dispertab Tablets (Among most frequent) 498
▲ Pediazole Suspension (Among most frequent) 3050
▲ PEG-Intron Powder for Injection (15%) 3140
Pentasa Capsules (1.1% to 1.7%) 3239
Pergonal for Injection 3223
Peri-Colace Capsules and Syrup 3240
▲ Permax Tablets (5.8%) 1299
▲ Photofrin for Injection (20%) 831
▲ Phrenilin (Among most frequent) 578
Plaquenil Tablets 3082
▲ Plavix Tablets (5.6%) 1097
▲ Plavix Tablets (5.6%) 3084
Plendil Extended-Release Tablets (0.5% to 1.5%) 623
▲ Pletal Tablets (4% to 5%) 2605
▲ Pletal Tablets (4% to 5%) 2848
▲ Ponstel Capsules (1% to 10%) 1356
▲ Pravachol Tablets (2.0% to 5.4%) 1099
▲ Precose Tablets (19%) 906
Premarin Intravenous 3563
Premarin Tablets 3566
Premarin Vaginal Cream 3570
Premphase Tablets 3572
▲ Prempro Tablets (16% to 21%) 3572
Prevacid Delayed-Release Capsules (1.8%) 3292
PREVPAC (1.8% to 3%) 3298
▲ Prilosec Delayed-Release Capsules (2.4% to 5.2%) 628
Primaxin I.M. 2158
Primaxin I.V. (Less than 0.2%) 2160
▲ Prinivil Tablets (0.3% to 4.0%) 2164
Prinzide Tablets (0.3% to 1%) 2168
▲ Procanbid Extended-Release Tablets (3% to 4%) 2262
Procardia Capsules (2% or less) 2708
Procardia XL Extended Release Tablets (Less than 3%) 2710
▲ Prograf (29% to 59%) 1393
▲ Proleukin for Injection (11%) 1199
▲ Prometrium Capsules (100 mg, 200 mg) (10% to 20%) 3261
ProSom Tablets (1%) 500
▲ Prostigmin Injectable (Most common) 1744
Prostigmin Tablets 1744
▲ Protonix I.V. (12%) 3580
Protonix Tablets (1% to 4%) 3577
Protopic Ointment (1% to 5%) 1397
Provigil Tablets (At least 1%) 1193
Prozac Pulvules, Liquid, and Weekly Capsules (Less than 1%) 1238
Pulmicort Respules (2% to 3%) 632
Pulmicort Turbuhaler Inhalation Powder (1% to 3%) 636
Pulmozyme Inhalation Solution 1426
▲ Rapamune Oral Solution and Tablets (28% to 36%) 3584
Recombivax HB (Less than 1%) 2178
ReFacto Vials 1437
▲ Relafen Tablets (12%) 1617
Relenza Rotadisk (Less than 1.5%) 1619
Remeron Tablets (Frequent) 2483
Remeron SolTab Tablets (Frequent) 2486
▲ Remicade for IV Injection (Less than 2% to 12%) 1178
▲ Reminyl Oral Solution (5%) 1792
▲ Reminyl Tablets (5%) 1792
Renese Tablets 2712
▲ Repronex for Intramuscular and Subcutaneous Injection (5.2% to 6.9%) 1347
▲ Requip Tablets (6% to 9%) 1621
Rescriptor Tablets (Less than 2%) 526
▲ Retrovir Capsules (3.2%) 1625
▲ Retrovir IV Infusion (4%) 1629
▲ Retrovir (3.2%) 1625
Rifadin (Some patients) 765
Rifater Tablets 769
▲ Rilutek Tablets (6.8% to 7.8%) 772
Risperdal (1% to 4%) 1796
Ritalin 2387
▲ Rituxan for Infusion (1% to 6%) 1750
▲ Rituxan I.V. (1% to 6%) 1428
Rocephin Injectable Vials, ADD-Vantage, Galaxy, Bulk (Rare) 2993
▲ Roferon-A Injection (12% to 15%) 2996
▲ Rowasa Rectal Suspension Enema 4.0 grams/unit (60 mL) (8.1%) 3264
Roxicodone Tablets (Less than 3%) 3067
Rynatan Tablets 3351
Rythmol Tablets – 150 mg, 225 mg, 300 mg (1.7% to 1.9%) 502
▲ Salagen Tablets (3% to 4%) 2229
▲ Sandostatin LAR Depot (29.1%) 2395
▲ Sarafem Pulvules (6%) 1962
Sectral Capsules (Up to 2%) 3589
▲ Sedapap Tablets 50 mg/650 mg (Among the most frequent) 2225
Septra Suspension 2265
Septra Tablets 2265
Septra DS Tablets 2265
Serevent Inhalation Aerosol (1% to 3%) 1633
Serophene Tablets 3226
▲ Seroquel Tablets (3%) 684
▲ Serostim for Injection (17.1%) 3229
Serzone Tablets 1104
▲ Simulect for Injection (Greater than or equal to 10%) 2399
Sinemet Tablets 1253
Sinemet CR Tablets 1255
Skelid Tablets (More than or equal to 1%) 3088

▲ Sonata Capsules (5% to 6%) 3591
▲ Soriatane Capsules (1% to 10%) 3003
Sporanox Capsules (1.5% to 4%).... 1800
Sporanox Injection (2%)..................... 1804
Sporanox Injection (2%)..................... 2509
▲ Sporanox Oral Solution (4.0% to 5.7%)... 1808
▲ Sporanox Oral Solution (4.0% to 5.7%)... 2512
Stimate Nasal Spray........................ 796
Stromectol Tablets (0.9%)............. 2185
▲ Suprax (3%) 1877
Surmontil Capsules........................... 3595
Sustiva Capsules (1% to 3%)............ 1258
Synercid I.V. (Less than 1%)............ 775
▲ Tambocor Tablets (3.3%) 1990
▲ Tamiflu Capsules (2% to 4.7%) 3008
▲ Tamiflu Oral Suspension (2% to 4.7%)... 3008
▲ Tao Capsules (Most frequent) 2716
▲ Tasmar Tablets (5% to 6%) 3010
Taxotere for Injection Concentrate .. 778
Tazicef for Injection (Less than 2%) 1647
Tazicef Galaxy Container (Less than 2%) 1650
Tazicef Pharmacy Bulk Package (Less than 2%) 1653
Tazidime Vials, Faspak & ADD-Vantage (1 in 416) 1966
Tegretol/Tegretol-XR 2404
▲ Temodar Capsules (9%) 3157
Tenex Tablets (3% or less) 2942
Tensilon Injectable 1745
Tequin Injection (0.1% to 3%) 1110
Tequin Tablets (0.1% to 3%) 1110
▲ Terazol 3 Vaginal Cream (3.4%) 2587
Teveten Tablets (2%)........................ 3327
▲ Thalomid Capsules (4.2%) 1154
▲ TheraCys Injection (3%) 823
Thioplex for Injection 1765
▲ Thymoglobulin for Injection (37.8%)... 3071
▲ Tice BCG, BCG Live (1.5% to 4.0%)... 2489
▲ Tikosyn Capsules (3%) 2717
▲ TOBI Solution for Inhalation (12.8%)... 1206
▲ Tolectin (3% to 9%) 2589
Tonocard Tablets (Less than 1%) 649
▲ Topamax Sprinkle Capsules (5.3% to 7.3%)...................................... 2590
▲ Topamax Tablets (5.3% to 7.3%) 2590
Toprol-XL Tablets (Greater than 1%) 651
▲ Trecator-SC Tablets (Among most common) 3598
▲ Tricor Capsules, Micronized (3%) ... 513
▲ Trileptal Oral Suspension (3% to 13%)... 2407
▲ Trileptal Tablets (3% to 13%) 2407
Tri-Levlen 962
Tri-Norinyl-28 Tablets 3433
Triphasil-21 Tablets (Occasional) 3600
Triphasil-28 Tablets 3605
▲ Trisenox Injection (58%) 1158
Trivora Tablets 3439
▲ Trizivir Tablets (6% to 9%) 1669
Trovan (1%) 2722
Twinrix Vaccine (Less than 1%) 1674
Tylenol with Codeine 2595
TYPHIM Vi Vaccine 825
Ultracet Tablets (At least 1%) 2597
Ultram Tablets (1% to 5%) 2600
Ultrase Capsules 835
▲ Ultrase MT Capsules (5.7%) 835
Uniretic Tablets (More than 1%) 3178
Unithroid Tablets 3445
Univasc Tablets (Less than 1%) 3181
Urecholine 2198
Urecholine Tablets 2445
▲ Vagifem Tablets (7%) 2857
▲ Valcyte Tablets (15%) 3022
▲ Valstar Sterile Solution for Intravesical Instillation (5%) 1175
▲ Valtrex Caplets (2% to 11%) 1676
Vancocin HCl, Vials & ADD-Vantage 1970
Vantin Tablets and Oral Suspension (Less than 1% to 1.6%)... 2860
Vaqta (1.1% to 1.6%) 2199
Varivax (Greater than or equal to 1%) 2202
▲ Vascor Tablets (3.02%) 2602
Vaseretic Tablets (0.5% to 2.0%) 2204
Vasotec I.V. Injection 2207
Vasotec Tablets (1.6%) 2210
Venofer Injection (Greater than 1%) 580
Vermox Chewable Tablets 2017
▲ Vesanoid Capsules (31%) 3037
Viadur Implant (Less than 2%) 912
Viagra Tablets (Less than 2%) 2732
▲ Vicoprofen Tablets (3% to 9%) 520
▲ Videx (7% to 13%) 1138
Videx EC Capsules 1143
▲ Vioxx (4.1%)................................... 2213
Viracept (2% to 4%) 532
Viramune Oral Suspension (1%) 1060
Viramune Tablets (1%) 1060
Visicol Tablets 1767
▲ Vistide Injection (17%) 1445
▲ Vitravene for Injection (5% to 20%).. ⊙310
Vivactil Tablets 2217
Vivactil Tablets 2446
Vivelle Transdermal System............ 2412
Vivelle-Dot Transdermal System...... 2416
Vivotif Berna..................................... 997
Voltaren Ophthalmic Sterile Ophthalmic Solution (Less than 3%)... ⊙312
▲ Voltaren Tablets (3% to 9%) 2315
▲ Voltaren-XR Tablets (3% to 9%) 2315
Warfarin Sodium Tablets, USP 3302
▲ WelChol Tablets (5%) 3073
▲ Wellbutrin SR Sustained-Release Tablets (3% to 9%).......................... 1684
WinRho SDF 2297
▲ Xeloda Tablets (4%) 3039
▲ Xenical Capsules (25.5%) 3043
Yasmin 28 Tablets (Greater than 1%) 980
Yodoxin Tablets 1722
Zanaflex Tablets (Frequent)............. 1305
Zantac 1690
Zantac Injection 1688
Zantac Syrup 1690
Zarontin Capsules (Frequent)........... 2659
Zarontin Syrup (Frequent)................ 2660
Zaroxolyn Tablets 1177
Zebeta Tablets 1885
▲ Zenapax for Injection (Greater than 5%)... 3046
▲ Zerit (34%) 1147
Zestoretic Tablets (0.3% to 1.0%).... 695
Zestril Tablets (0.3% to 2.2%).......... 698
Ziac Tablets 1887
Ziagen (Frequent)............................. 1692
Zinacef Injection 1696
Zinacef for Injection 1696
▲ Zithromax Capsules, 250 mg (2% to 7%)... 2743
Zithromax for IV Infusion (1.9% to 3.7%)... 2748
▲ Zithromax for Oral Suspension, 1 g (3% to 5%)................................ 2743
▲ Zithromax for Oral Suspension, 300 mg, 600 mg, 900 mg, 1200 mg (2% to 7%)...................... 2739
▲ Zithromax Tablets, 250 mg (2% to 7%)... 2739
▲ Zithromax Tablets, 600 mg (3% to 5%)... 2743
▲ Zocor Tablets (3.2%) 2219
Zofran Injection (2%)........................ 1698
Zofran (1% to 3%)............................. 1703
Zofran ODT Orally Disintegrating Tablets (1% to 3%)......................... 1703
▲ Zoladex (7% to 11%) 702
Zoladex 3-month (1% to 5%)............ 706
Zoloft (1 or more)............................. 2751
▲ Zometa for Intravenous Infusion (16.3%)... 3621
▲ Zonegran Capsules (6%) 1307
Zosyn (1.3%).................................... 1890
Zosyn in Galaxy Containers (1.3%)... 1894
Zovia 3449
Zovirax for Injection (Less than 1%) 1708
▲ Zyban Sustained-Release Tablets (3%)... 1710
▲ Zyflo Filmtab Tablets (4.6%) 524
▲ Zyprexa Tablets (4%) 1973
▲ Zyprexa ZYDIS Orally Disintegrating Tablets (4%)............ 1973
Zyrtec (Less than 2% to 5.6%)......... 2756
Zyrtec-D 12 Hour Extended Relief Tablets 2758
Zyvox 2071

Abdominal symptom complex, acute

Clomid Tablets (Fewer than 1%)...... 735
Permax Tablets (Rare).................... 1299
Prozac Pulvules, Liquid, and Weekly Capsules (Rare)............... 1238
Remeron Tablets (Frequent)............ 2483
Remeron SolTab Tablets (Frequent)...................................... 2486
Sarafem Pulvules (Rare).................. 1962

Abortion

Copaxone for Injection (Infrequent).. 3306
Effexor Tablets (Rare)...................... 3495
Effexor XR Capsules (Rare).............. 3499
Gabitril Tablets (Infrequent)............ 1189
Gonal-F for Injection........................ 3216
Imitrex Injection 1549
Imitrex Nasal Spray.......................... 1554
Imitrex Tablets (Rare)...................... 1558
Paxil (Infrequent)............................. 1609
Permax Tablets (Infrequent)............ 1299
Prozac Pulvules, Liquid, and Weekly Capsules (Infrequent)....... 1238
Sarafem Pulvules (Infrequent)......... 1962

Abortion, septic

ParaGard T 380A Intrauterine Copper Contraceptive 2582

Abortion, spontaneous

Celexa (At least 3 patients)............. 1365
Lupron Depot-PED 7.5 mg, 11.25 mg and 15 mg (Possible).. 3291
Nolvadex Tablets 678
Ovidrel for Injection 3220
ParaGard T 380A Intrauterine Copper Contraceptive 2582

Abrasion

Neurontin Oral Solution (1.3%)........ 2655
Vioxx (Greater than 0.1% to 1.9%).. 2213

Abscess

Actiq (Less than 1%)........................ 1184
Ambien Tablets (Rare)...................... 3191
Apligraf (1.3% to 2.7%).................... 2305
Aramine Injection.............................. 2043
Arava Tablets (1% to 3%).................. 724
Aricept Tablets (Infrequent)............. 1270
Aricept Tablets (Infrequent)............. 2665
Avonex.. 1013
Betaseron for SC Injection................ 988
Bicillin C-R 900/300 Injection........... 2240
Bicillin C-R Injection......................... 2238
Campath Ampules 992
Celestone Soluspan Injectable Suspension 3097
▲ CellCept Capsules (3% to 10%) 2951
▲ CellCept Intravenous (3% to 10%) .. 2951
▲ CellCept Oral Suspension (3% to 10%)... 2951
▲ CellCept Tablets (3% to 10%) 2951
Claritin-D 24 Hour Extended Release Tablets (Fewer than 2%) 3104
Colazal Capsules 3069
Cortone Acetate Injectable Suspension 2059
Decadron Phosphate Injection 2081
Doxil Injection (Less than 1%) 566
Evoxac Capsules (1% to 3%) 1217
Ferrlecit Injection 3386
Fortovase Capsules (Less than 2%) 2970
Foscavir Injection (Between 1% and 5%) 605
Sterile FUDR 2974
Gabitril Tablets (Infrequent) 1189
▲ Gengraf Capsules (4.4%) 457
▲ Gliadel Wafer (4%) 1723
▲ Hectorol Capsules (3.3%) 1064
▲ Hectorol Injection (3.3%) 1066
Hydrocortone Acetate Injectable Suspension 2103
Hydrocortone Phosphate Injection, Sterile 2105
INFeD Injection 3388
Intron A for Injection (Less than 5%) 3120
Invirase Capsules (Less than 2%) 2979
Lamictal (Rare) 1567
Lupron Depot-4 Month 30 mg (Less than 5%) 3289
▲ Lupron Depot-PED 7.5 mg, 11.25 mg and 15 mg (5%) 3291
Micardis Tablets (More than 0.3%) .. 1049
Micardis HCT Tablets 1051
Myobloc Injectable Solution (2% or greater) 1291
Naprelan Tablets (Less than 1%) 1293
Neoral Soft Gelatin Capsules (1% to 4.4%) 2380
Nipent for Injection (2%) 3272
Paxil (Rare) 1609
PEG-Intron Powder for Injection (Less than or equal to 1%) 3140
Permax Tablets (Infrequent) 1299
▲ Prograf (3% to 15%) 1393
Prometrium Capsules (100 mg, 200 mg) (Less than 5%) 3261
Protonix I.V. (Less than 1%) 3580
Protonix Tablets (Less than 1%) 3577
▲ Rapamune Oral Solution and Tablets (3% to 20%) 3584
Remicade for IV Injection (Less than 2%) 1178
ReoPro Vials (0.2%) 1958
Requip Tablets (Infrequent) 1621
Rescriptor Tablets 526
Rilutek Tablets (Infrequent) 772
▲ Sandimmune (4.4 to 5.3%) 2388
▲ Serostim for Injection (1% to 10%) . 3229
Solu-Medrol Sterile Powder 2855
Tasmar Tablets (Infrequent) 3010
Tice BCG, BCG Live (1.8%) 2489
Uniretic Tablets (Less than 1%) 3178
Vantin Tablets and Oral Suspension (Less than 1%) 2860
Vioxx (Greater than 0.1% to 1.9%) .. 2213
Zanaflex Tablets (Infrequent) 1305

Abscess, abdominal

Enbrel for Injection 1752
Enbrel for Injection 3504

Abscess, cellulitis

Norplant System (Less than 1%) 3543

Abscess, foot

Enbrel for Injection 1752
Enbrel for Injection 3504

Abscess, periodontal

Actiq (1% or greater) 1184
Aricept Tablets (Infrequent) 1270
Aricept Tablets (Infrequent) 2665
Avonex 1013
Betaseron for SC Injection............... 988
▲ Casodex Tablets (2% to 5%) 662
Copaxone for Injection (At least 2%).. 3306
Depacon Injection (1% to 5%)......... 416
Depakene (1% to 5%)....................... 421
Depakote Sprinkle Capsules (1% to 5%)... 426
Depakote Tablets (1% to 5%)........... 430
Depakote ER Tablets (Greater than 1%)... 436
Doxil Injection (Less than 1%).......... 566
Gabitril Tablets (Infrequent)............ 1189
Hivid Tablets (Less than 1%)............ 2975
Lupron Depot-4 Month 30 mg (Less than 5%).............................. 3289
Naprelan Tablets (Less than 1%)..... 1293
Norvir Capsules (Less than 2%)....... 487
Norvir Oral Solution (Less than 2%).. 487
▲ Periostat Tablets (4%) 1208
Permax Tablets (Infrequent)............ 1299
Pletal Tablets (Less than 2%).......... 2605
Pletal Tablets (Less than 2%).......... 2848
Protonix I.V. (Less than 1%)............ 3580
Protonix Tablets (Less than 1%)...... 3577
Protopic Ointment (Up to 3%).......... 1397
Serzone Tablets (Infrequent)........... 1104
Uniretic Tablets (Less than 1%)....... 3178
Zyprexa Tablets (Infrequent)............ 1973
Zyprexa ZYDIS Orally Disintegrating Tablets (Infrequent)...................................... 1973

Abscess, peritonsillar

Tamiflu Capsules (Less than 1%)..... 3008
Tamiflu Oral Suspension (Less than 1%)... 3008

Abscess, renal

Gengraf Capsules (1% to less than 3%)... 457
Neoral Oral Solution (1% to less than 3%)... 2380
Sandostatin LAR Depot (1% to 4%).. 2395

Abscess, tubo-ovarian

ParaGard T 380A Intrauterine Copper Contraceptive..................... 2582

Abscess at injection site

Bicillin L-A Injection........................ 2242
Cerezyme for Injection (Less than 1%).. 1438
Cleocin Phosphate Sterile Solution... 2785
Copaxone for Injection (Frequent)... 3306
Cytovene-IV...................................... 2959
Diphtheria & Tetanus Toxoids Adsorbed Purogenated for Pediatric Use.............................. 1857
Lupron Depot 3.75 mg...................... 3281
Lupron Depot 7.5 mg........................ 3284
Lupron Depot-3 Month 11.25 mg..... 3285
Lupron Depot-3 Month 22.5 mg...... 3288
Lupron Depot-4 Month 30 mg.......... 3289
Lupron Injection Pediatric................ 3280
Liquid PedvaxHIB.............................. 2148

Abuse

Ambien Tablets (Rare)...................... 3191
Astramorph/PF Injection, USP (Preservative-Free)......................... 594
Miltown Tablets................................ 3349
Prozac Pulvules, Liquid, and Weekly Capsules........................... 1238
Sarafem Pulvules.............................. 1962
Sonata Capsules............................... 3591

Acanthosis nigricans

Niaspan Extended-Release Tablets.. 1846

Accommodation, impaired

Amaryl Tablets................................. 717
Ambien Tablets (Rare)...................... 3191
Aralen Tablets.................................. 3075
Atrovent Inhalation Aerosol (About 1 in 100)....................................... 1030
Blephamide Ophthalmic Ointment (Occasional).................................. 547
Blephamide Ophthalmic Suspension....................................... 548
Celexa (Frequent)............................. 1365
Clomid Tablets.................................. 735
Concerta Extended-Release Tablets.. 1998
Concerta Tablets............................... 561
Crixivan Capsules (Less than 2%).... 2070
▲ Detrol Tablets (4.7%) 3623
DiaBeta Tablets................................ 741
▲ Effexor Tablets (5.6% to 9.1%) 3495
Effexor XR Capsules (Frequent)...... 3499
Etrafon... 3115
FML Ophthalmic Ointment (Occasional).................................. ⊙237
FML Ophthalmic Suspension (Occasional).................................. ⊙236
FML Forte Ophthalmic Suspension (Occasional)........... ⊙235
Imitrex Nasal Spray.......................... 1554
Lamictal (Infrequent)........................ 1567

Limbitrol 1738
Luvox Tablets (25, 50, 100 mg) (Infrequent) 3256
Metadate CD Capsules 1164
Metadate ER Tablets 1167
Methylin Tablets 1995
Methylin ER Tablets 1995
Neurontin Capsules (Rare) 2655
Neurontin Oral Solution (Rare) 2655
Neurontin Tablets (Rare) 2655
Norpramin Tablets 755
Norvasc Tablets (Less than or equal to 0.1%) 2704
▲ Orap Tablets (4 of 20 patients) 1407
Paxil (Infrequent) 1609
Plaquenil Tablets 3082
Pred Forte Ophthalmic Suspension (Occasional) ⊙ 246
Pred Mild Sterile Ophthalmic Suspension (Occasional) ⊙ 249
Protopam Chloride for Injection 3582
Remeron Tablets (Infrequent) 2483
Remeron SolTab Tablets (Infrequent) 2486
Requip Tablets (Infrequent) 1621
Risperdal (Infrequent) 1796
Ritalin 2387
Serophene Tablets 3226
Seroquel Tablets (Rare) 684
Serzone Tablets (Infrequent) 1104
Sonata Capsules (Rare) 3591
Surmontil Capsules 3595
Transderm Scōp Transdermal Therapeutic System 2302
Trileptal Oral Suspension (Up to 2%) 2407
Trileptal Tablets (Up to 2%) 2407
Vivactil Tablets 2217
Vivactil Tablets 2446
Wellbutrin SR Sustained-Release Tablets (Infrequent) 1684
Zantac (Rare) 1690
Zantac Injection (Rare) 1688
Zantac Syrup (Rare) 1690
Zofran Injection 1698
Zoloft (Infrequent) 2751
Zyban Sustained-Release Tablets (Infrequent) 1710
Zyprexa Tablets (Rare) 1973
Zyprexa ZYDIS Orally Disintegrating Tablets (Rare) 1973
Zyrtec (Less than 2%) 2756
Zyrtec-D 12 Hour Extended Relief Tablets (Less than 2%) 2758

Accommodation, spasm
Tensilon Injectable 1745

Accommodation paresis
Diphtheria & Tetanus Toxoids Adsorbed Purogenated for Pediatric Use 1857
Tetanus & Diphtheria Toxoids Adsorbed for Adult Use 1880
Tetanus and Diphtheria Toxoids Adsorbed For Adult Use 815
Tripedia Vaccine 817

Aches
Asacol Delayed-Release Tablets 2884
Cipro I.V. (1% or less) 893
Cipro I.V. Pharmacy Bulk Package (Less than 1%) 897
Cipro (Less than 1%) 887
Corgard Tablets 2245
Cosopt Sterile Ophthalmic Solution 2065
Cytotec Tablets (Infrequent) 3202
Eldepryl Capsules (1 of 49 patients) 3266
Flonase Nasal Spray (1% to 3%) 1533
Flovent (1% to 3%) 1535
Flovent Rotadisk (1% to 3%) 1537
Humegon for Injection 2468
Humorsol Sterile Ophthalmic Solution 2102
Inderal 3513
Inderal LA Long-Acting Capsules 3516
Inderide Tablets 3517
Inderide LA Long-Acting Capsules 3519
LYMErix Vaccine (2.78%) 1592
Midamor Tablets (Less than or equal to 1%) 2136
▲ Nabi-HB (3%) 2295
Nadolol Tablets 2288
Navelbine Injection 1604
Normodyne Tablets 3137
Orthoclone OKT3 Sterile Solution 2498
Pergonal for Injection 3223
Recombivax HB (Less than 1%) 2178
Repronex for Intramuscular and Subcutaneous Injection 1347
Sectral Capsules 3589
Serevent Diskus (1% to 3%) 1637
Tenoretic Tablets 690
Tenormin 692
Timolol GFS ⊙ 266
Timoptic in Ocudose 2192
Timoptic Sterile Ophthalmic Solution 2190
Timoptic-XE Sterile Ophthalmic Gel Forming Solution 2194
Toprol-XL Tablets 651
Trilafon 3160
Ziac Tablets 1887

Aches, joints
(*see under* Arthralgia)

Acid-base disturbances
Demadex Tablets and Injection 2965

Acidosis
▲ Abelcet Injection (3%) 1273
Actiq (Less than 1%) 1184
AmBisome for Injection (Less common) 1383
Amphotec (1% to 5%) 1774
Ativan Injection (Less than 1%) 3478
Cafcit (2.2%) 1035
Campath Ampules 992
▲ CellCept Capsules (3% to 14.2%) 2951
▲ CellCept Intravenous (3% to 14.2%) 2951
▲ CellCept Oral Suspension (3% to 14.2%) 2951
▲ CellCept Tablets (3% to 14.2%) 2951
Cipro I.V. (1% or less) 893
Cipro I.V. Pharmacy Bulk Package (Less than 1%) 897
Cipro (Less than 1%) 887
Cytovene 2959
D.H.E. 45 Injection 2334
Dyazide Capsules 1515
Fleet Enema 1359
Fleet Phospho-soda 1360
Floxin I.V. 2526
Floxin Tablets 2529
Foscavir Injection (Between 1% and 5%) 605
Ifex for Injection (Rare) 1123
Indocin I.V. (Less than 3%) 2115
Minocin Intravenous 1862
Minocin Oral Suspension 1865
Minocin Pellet-Filled Capsules 1863
Motrin Suspension, Oral Drops, Chewable Tablets, and Caplets (Less than 1%) 2002
Permax Tablets (Rare) 1299
▲ Prograf (3% to 15%) 1393
▲ Proleukin for Injection (12%) 1199
▲ Rapamune Oral Solution and Tablets (3% to 20%) 3584
Requip Tablets (Infrequent) 1621
▲ Serostim for Injection (1% to 10%) 3229
▲ Simulect for Injection (3% to 10%) 2399
Topamax Sprinkle Capsules (Infrequent) 2590
Topamax Tablets (Infrequent) 2590
Trasylol Injection (1% to 2%) 909
▲ Trisenox Injection (5%) 1158
▲ Vesanoid Capsules (3%) 3037
Zyprexa Tablets (Frequent) 1973
Zyprexa ZYDIS Orally Disintegrating Tablets (Frequent) 1973

Acidosis, hypochloremic metabolic
Gengraf Capsules 457
Sandimmune (Occasional) 2388

Acidosis, metabolic
Aggrenox Capsules 1026
Aloprim for Injection (Less than 1%) 2292
Aquasol A Parenteral 593
Cerebyx Injection (Infrequent) 2619
Corzide 40/5 Tablets 2247
Corzide 80/5 Tablets 2247
Daranide Tablets 2077
Diamox Intravenous (Occasional) ⊙ 269
Diamox Sequels Sustained Release Capsules ⊙ 270
Diamox Tablets (Occasional) ⊙ 269
Diprivan Injectable Emulsion (Less than 1%) 667
Ecotrin Enteric Coated Aspirin Low, Regular and Maximum Strength Tablets 1715
Fludara for Injection 995
Foradil Aerolizer 2354
▲ Ifex for Injection (31%) 1123
Nardil Tablets (Less frequent) 2653
Neptazane Tablets ⊙ 271
Oncaspar 756
Rifamate Capsules 767
Rifater Tablets 769
Sensorcaine 643
Sensorcaine-MPF Injection 643
Sulfamylon Cream 1011
Sulfamylon Topical Solution 1011
Viracept 532
Vistide Injection (Less than 1%) 1445

Acidosis, renal tubular
Abelcet Injection 1273
Ifex for Injection (1 episode) 1123
Topamax Sprinkle Capsules 2590
Topamax Tablets 2590

Acidosis, respiratory
▲ CellCept Capsules (3% to 10%) 2951
▲ CellCept Intravenous (3% to 10%) 2951
▲ CellCept Oral Suspension (3% to 10%) 2951
▲ CellCept Tablets (3% to 10%) 2951
▲ Diprivan Injectable Emulsion (3% to 10%) 667
Rilutek Tablets (Infrequent) 772
Zanaflex Tablets (Rare) 1305

Acne
(*see under* Acneiform eruptions)

Acne, cystic, flare-up
Parnate Tablets 1607

Acne, flare-up of
Differin Cream (Less than 1%) 1402
Differin Solution/Pledgets (1% or less) 1404
Noritate Cream (One patient) 1224

Acne, transient exacerbation of
Oxandrin Tablets 1153

Acne fulminaris
Accutane Capsules 2944

Acneiform eruptions
Aclovate (Infrequent) 1275
Activella Tablets 2764
Aerobid/Aerobid-M (1% to 3%) 1363
Alesse-21 Tablets 3468
Alesse-28 Tablets 3473
Ambien Tablets (Rare) 3191
Amerge Tablets (Rare) 1467
Amphotec (1% to 5%) 1774
Anadrol-50 Tablets 3321
Analpram-HC 1338
Androderm Transdermal System CIII (Less than 1%) 3377
▲ AndroGel (1% to 8%) 3322
▲ Android Capsules, 10 mg (Among most common) 1731
Antabuse Tablets 2444
Antabuse Tablets (Small number of patients) 3474
Anusol-HC Cream 2.5% (Infrequent to frequent) 2237
Arava Tablets (1% to 3%) 724
Arthrotec Tablets (Rare) 3195
Asacol Delayed-Release Tablets (1% to 2%) 2884
Aygestin Tablets 1333
Brevicon 28-Day Tablets 3380
Canasa Rectal Suppositories (1.2%) 829
Capex Shampoo 1400
Celexa (Infrequent) 1365
▲ CellCept Capsules (3% to 10%) 2951
▲ CellCept Intravenous (3% to 10%) 2951
▲ CellCept Oral Suspension (3% to 10%) 2951
▲ CellCept Tablets (3% to 10%) 2951
Claritin-D 12 Hour Extended Release Tablets (Less frequent) 3102
Claritin-D 24 Hour Extended Release Tablets (Fewer than 2%) 3104
Clobevate Gel 3271
Clomid Tablets 735
Cognex Capsules (Infrequent) 1351
▲ CombiPatch Transdermal System (4% to 5%) 2323
Copaxone for Injection (At least 2%) 3306
Cordran Lotion (Infrequent) 2438
Cordran Tape (Infrequent) 2439
Cormax Cream (Infrequent) 2440
Cormax Ointment (Infrequent) 2440
Cormax Scalp Application (Infrequent) 2441
Cortifoam Rectal Foam 3170
Cosmegen for Injection 2062
Crinone 8% Gel (Less than 5%) 3213
Cutivate Cream (Infrequent) 1282
Cutivate Ointment (Infrequent to more frequent) 1284
Cyclessa Tablets 2450
Dantrium Capsules (Less frequent) 2885
Delatestryl Injection 1151
▲ Depo-Provera Contraceptive Injection (More than 5%) 2798
Dermatop Emollient Cream (Infrequent to frequent) 2517
Desogen Tablets 2458
DesOwen (Infrequent) 1401
Diprolene Gel 0.05% (Infrequent) 3107
Diprolene Lotion 0.05% (1%) 3107
Diprolene Ointment 0.05% (Infrequent) 3108
Diprolene AF Cream 0.05% (Infrequent) 3106
Diprosone 3109
▲ Dostinex Tablets (1% to less than 10%) 2804
Doxil Injection (Less than 1%) 566
Effexor Tablets (Infrequent) 3495
Effexor XR Capsules (Infrequent) 3499
Elocon Cream 0.1% (Infrequent) 3110
Elocon Lotion 0.1% (Infrequent) 3111
Elocon Ointment 0.1% (Infrequent) 3112
Eskalith 1527
Estratest 3252
Estrostep 2627
Evoxac Capsules (Less than 1%) 1217
Famotidine Injection (Infrequent) 866
▲ Felbatol (3.4%) 3343
Flovent Diskus (1% to 3%) 3614
Fortovase Capsules (Less than 2%) 2970
Gabitril Tablets (1% or more) 1189
▲ Gengraf Capsules (1% to 6%) 457
▲ Gonal-F for Injection (59% of men) 3216
Herceptin I.V. (2%) 1414
Hivid Tablets (Less than 1%) 2975
Humatrope Vials and Cartridges (Up to 5.8%) 1930
Imdur Tablets (Less than or equal to 5%) 1826
Intron A for Injection (Less than 5%) 3120
Invirase Capsules (Less than 2%) 2979
Kaletra Capsules (Less than 2%) 471
Kaletra Oral Solution (Less than 2%) 471
Lamictal (1.3%) 1567
Levlen 962
Levlite 21 Tablets 962
Levlite 28 Tablets 962
Levora Tablets 3389
Lidex (Infrequent) 2020
Lipitor Tablets (Less than 2%) 2639
Lipitor Tablets (Less than 2%) 2696
Lithobid Slow-Release Tablets 3255
Locoid Lipocream Cream (Infrequent) 1342
Loestrin 21 Tablets 2642
Loestrin Fe Tablets 2642
Loprox Gel 2022
Lotrisone 3129
Lunelle Monthly Injection 2827
▲ Lupron Depot–3 Month 11.25 mg (Up to 10%) 3285
Lupron Depot-PED 7.5 mg, 11.25 mg and 15 mg (2%) 3291
Lupron Injection Pediatric 3280
Luvox Tablets (25, 50, 100 mg) (Infrequent) 3256
Luxíq Foam (One patient) 1210
Maxalt Tablets (Rare) 2120
Maxalt-MLT Orally Disintegrating Tablets (Rare) 2120
Meridia Capsules (1%) 481
Microgestin Fe 1.5/30 Tablets 3407
Microgestin Fe 1/20 Tablets 3400
Micronor Tablets (Rare) 2543
Mircette Tablets 2470
▲ Mirena Intrauterine System (5% or more) 974
Modicon 2563
Naprelan Tablets (Less than 1%) 1293
Necon 3415
▲ Neoral Soft Gelatin Capsules (1% to 6%) 2380
▲ Neoral Oral Solution (1% to 6%) 2380
Neurontin Capsules 2655
Neurontin Oral Solution 2655
Neurontin Tablets 2655
Nexium Delayed-Release Capsules (Less than 1%) 619
▲ Nicotrol Nasal Spray (3%) 2843
Nimotop Capsules (Up to 1.4%) 904
Nipent for Injection (Less than 3%) 3272
Norinyl 1 +35 28-Day Tablets 3380
Norinyl 1 + 50 28-Day Tablets 3380
Noritate Cream (One patient) 1224
Norplant System 3543
Nor-QD Tablets (Rare) 3423
Norvir Capsules (Less than 2%) 487
Norvir Oral Solution (Less than 2%) 487
Olux Foam 1211
Ortho-Cept 21 Tablets 2546
Ortho-Cept 28 Tablets 2546
Ortho-Cyclen/Ortho Tri-Cyclen 2573
Ortho-Novum 2563
Ortho-Novum 1/50□28 Tablets 2556
Ortho-Cyclen/Ortho Tri-Cyclen 2573
Ovcon 3364
Oxandrin Tablets 1153
Paxil (Infrequent) 1609
Pentasa Capsules (0.2%) 3239
Pepcid Injection (Infrequent) 2153
Pepcid for Oral Suspension (Infrequent) 2150
Pepcid RPD Orally Disintegrating Tablets (Infrequent) 2150
Pepcid Tablets (Infrequent) 2150
Permax Tablets (Infrequent) 1299
Pramosone 1343
Premphase Tablets 3572
Prempro Tablets 3572
Prevacid Delayed-Release Capsules (Less than 1%) 3292
PREVPAC (Less than 1%) 3298
Priftin Tablets (2.2%) 758
ProctoFoam-HC 3177
▲ Prograf (3% to 15%) 1393
Prometrium Capsules (100 mg, 200 mg) (Less than 5%) 3261
ProSom Tablets (Rare) 500
Protonix I.V. (Less than 1%) 3580

- Protonix Tablets (Less than 1%) ... 3577
- ▲ Protopic Ointment (2% to 7%) ... 1397
- Provera Tablets ... 2853
- Prozac Pulvules, Liquid, and Weekly Capsules (Infrequent) ... 1238
- Psorcon E Cream ... 1227
- Psorcon E Ointment ... 1228
- Pyrazinamide Tablets (Rare) ... 1876
- ▲ Rapamune Oral Solution and Tablets (20% to 31%) ... 3584
- ReFacto Vials ... 1437
- Relafen Tablets (Less than 1%) ... 1617
- Retrovir Capsules ... 1625
- Retrovir IV Infusion ... 1629
- Retrovir ... 1625
- Rifater Tablets (Rare) ... 769
- Risperdal (Infrequent) ... 1796
- Rowasa Rectal Suspension Enema 4.0 grams/unit (60 mL) (1.2%) ... 3264
- ▲ Sandimmune (1% to 6%) ... 2388
- Sandostatin LAR Depot (1% to 4%) ... 2395
- Sarafem Pulvules (Infrequent) ... 1962
- Serophene Tablets ... 3226
- Seroquel Tablets (Infrequent) ... 684
- ▲ Serostim for Injection (1% to 10%) ... 3229
- Serzone Tablets (Infrequent) ... 1104
- ▲ Simulect for Injection (Greater than or equal to 10%) ... 2399
- Sonata Capsules (Infrequent) ... 3591
- Soriatane Capsules (Less than 1%) ... 3003
- Sular Tablets (Less than or equal to 1%) ... 688
- Synalar (Infrequent) ... 2020
- ▲ Synarel Nasal Solution for Central Precocious Puberty (10%) ... 3204
- ▲ Synarel Nasal Solution for Endometriosis (13% of patients) ... 3205
- Temovate Cream ... 1301
- Temovate Gel (Infrequent) ... 1303
- Temovate Ointment ... 1301
- Temovate Scalp Application (Infrequent) ... 1304
- Temovate E Emollient (Infrequent) ... 1302
- ▲ Testoderm Transdermal Systems (4%) ... 574
- Testopel Pellets ... 3610
- Testred Capsules, 10 mg ... 1746
- ▲ Thalomid Capsules (3.1% to 11.1%) ... 1154
- Topamax Sprinkle Capsules (Frequent) ... 2590
- Topamax Tablets (Frequent) ... 2590
- Topicort (Infrequent) ... 2025
- Trecator-SC Tablets ... 3598
- Tricor Capsules, Micronized ... 513
- Trileptal Oral Suspension (1% to 2%) ... 2407
- Trileptal Tablets (1% to 2%) ... 2407
- Tri-Levlen ... 962
- Tri-Norinyl-28 Tablets ... 3433
- Trivora Tablets ... 3439
- Ultravate Cream ... 1119
- Ultravate Ointment ... 1120
- Uniretic Tablets (Less than 1%) ... 3178
- ▲ Vaniqa Cream (10.8%) ... 1121
- Vantin Tablets and Oral Suspension (Less than 1%) ... 2860
- Vistide Injection ... 1445
- Wellbutrin Tablets (Rare) ... 1680
- Wellbutrin SR Sustained-Release Tablets (At least 1%) ... 1684
- Yasmin 28 Tablets (Greater than 1%) ... 980
- Yodoxin Tablets ... 1722
- Zanaflex Tablets (Infrequent) ... 1305
- Zebeta Tablets ... 1885
- ▲ Zenapax for Injection (Greater than 5%) ... 3046
- Ziac Tablets ... 1887
- ▲ Zoladex (42%) ... 702
- Zoladex 3-month ... 706
- Zoloft (Infrequent) ... 2751
- Zonegran Capsules (Infrequent) ... 1307
- Zovia ... 3449
- Zyban Sustained-Release Tablets (Infrequent) ... 1710
- Zyrtec (Less than 2%) ... 2756
- Zyrtec-D 12 Hour Extended Relief Tablets (Less than 2%) ... 2758

Acneiform reactions

- Elocon Lotion 0.1% (2 in 209 patients) ... 3111
- Haldol Decanoate ... 2535
- Haldol Injection, Tablets and Concentrate ... 2533

Adenitis

- Clinoril Tablets ... 2053
- Dolobid Tablets (Less than 1 in 100) ... 2088
- Norpramin Tablets (Rare) ... 755
- Pneumovax 23 (Rare) ... 2156
- Pnu-Imune 23 (Rare) ... 1868
- Surmontil Capsules ... 3595
- Vivactil Tablets (Rare) ... 2217
- Vivactil Tablets (Rare) ... 2446

Adenoma, nephrogenic

- Tice BCG, BCG Live (Two cases) ... 2489

Adenomas, benign

- Betaseron for SC Injection ... 988

Adenomas, endocrine system

- Permax Tablets (Infrequent) ... 1299

Adenopathy

- Carbatrol Capsules ... 3234
- Enbrel for Injection ... 1752
- Enbrel for Injection ... 3504
- Helixate Concentrate ... 788
- Kogenate FS ... 936
- Miltown Tablets ... 3349
- Rescriptor Tablets ... 526
- Tegretol/Tegretol-XR ... 2404
- Tetanus Toxoid Adsorbed Purogenated ... 1882

ADH syndrome, inappropriate

- Amaryl Tablets ... 717
- Betaseron for SC Injection ... 988
- Carbatrol Capsules ... 3234
- Celexa (Several cases) ... 1365
- Cytovene ... 2959
- Depacon Injection ... 416
- Depakene ... 421
- Depakote Sprinkle Capsules ... 426
- Depakote Tablets ... 430
- Depakote ER Tablets ... 436
- DiaBeta Tablets ... 741
- Diabinese Tablets (Rare) ... 2680
- Effexor Tablets ... 3495
- Effexor XR Capsules ... 3499
- Etrafon ... 3115
- Felbatol ... 3343
- Flexeril Tablets (Rare) ... 572
- Flexeril Tablets (Rare) ... 2094
- Foscavir Injection (Less than 1%) ... 605
- Glucotrol Tablets ... 2692
- Glucotrol XL Extended Release Tablets ... 2693
- Kadian Capsules (Less than 3%) ... 1335
- Limbitrol ... 1738
- Lufyllin Tablets ... 3347
- Lufyllin-400 Tablets ... 3347
- Lufyllin-GG Elixir ... 3348
- Lufyllin-GG Tablets ... 3348
- Navelbine Injection (Less than 1%) ... 1604
- Norpramin Tablets ... 755
- OxyContin Tablets (Less than 1%) ... 2912
- Parnate Tablets ... 1607
- Paxil ... 1609
- Permax Tablets (Infrequent) ... 1299
- Requip Tablets (Rare) ... 1621
- Roxanol 100 Concentrated Oral Solution ... 3066
- Rythmol Tablets – 150 mg, 225 mg, 300 mg (Less than 1%) ... 502
- Sinequan ... 2713
- Surmontil Capsules ... 3595
- Tegretol/Tegretol-XR ... 2404
- Thalomid Capsules ... 1154
- Theo-Dur Extended-Release Tablets ... 1835
- Trilafon ... 3160
- Uni-Dur Extended-Release Tablets ... 1841
- Vivactil Tablets ... 2217
- Vivactil Tablets ... 2446
- Wellbutrin Tablets ... 1680
- Wellbutrin SR Sustained-Release Tablets ... 1684
- Zyban Sustained-Release Tablets ... 1710

Adnexal enlargement

- Norplant System ... 3543

Adnexal torsion, ovarian

- Follistim for Injection ... 2465
- Gonal-F for Injection ... 3216
- Humegon for Injection ... 2468
- Pergonal for Injection ... 3223
- Repronex for Intramuscular and Subcutaneous Injection ... 1347
- Serophene Tablets ... 3226

Adrenal insufficiency

- Azmacort Inhalation Aerosol ... 728
- Beconase Inhalation Aerosol ... 1497
- Beconase AQ Nasal Spray ... 1498
- Cortifoam Rectal Foam ... 3170
- Heparin Lock Flush Solution ... 3509
- Heparin Sodium Injection ... 3511
- Nasacort Nasal Inhaler ... 750
- Pulmicort Respules (Less than 1%) ... 632
- Pulmicort Turbuhaler Inhalation Powder (Rare) ... 636
- Rifadin (Rare) ... 765
- Sporanox Capsules (Infrequent) ... 1800
- Sporanox Oral Solution (Less than 2%) ... 1808
- Sporanox Oral Solution (Less than 2%) ... 2512
- Vanceril Double Strength Inhalation Aerosol (Rare) ... 3167
- Vistide Injection ... 1445
- Zanaflex Tablets (Rare) ... 1305

Adrenergic syndrome, unspecified

- Paxil (Rare) ... 1609

Adrenocortical suppression

- Dermatop Emollient Cream ... 2517
- Nasacort Nasal Inhaler ... 750

Adrenocortical unresponsiveness, secondary

- Celestone Soluspan Injectable Suspension ... 3097
- Celestone Syrup ... 3099
- Cortone Acetate Injectable Suspension ... 2059
- Cortone Acetate Tablets ... 2061
- Decadron Elixir ... 2078
- Decadron Tablets ... 2079
- Decadron Phosphate Injection ... 2081
- Depo-Medrol Injectable Suspension ... 2795
- Florinef Acetate Tablets ... 2250
- Hydrocortone Tablets ... 2106
- Hydrocortone Acetate Injectable Suspension ... 2103
- Hydrocortone Phosphate Injection, Sterile ... 2105
- Pediapred Oral Solution ... 1170
- Prednisone ... 3064
- Prelone Syrup ... 2273
- Solu-Medrol Sterile Powder ... 2855

Afibrinogenemia

- Depacon Injection (One infant) ... 416
- Depakene (One infant) ... 421
- Depakote Tablets (One infant) ... 430
- Depakote ER Tablets (One infant) ... 436

Aftertaste

- Antabuse Tablets (Small number of patients) ... 3474
- ▲ Nasarel Nasal Solution 0.025% (8% to 17%) ... 1296

Ageusia

- ▲ Aerobid/Aerobid-M (3% to 9%) ... 1363
- Aggrenox Capsules (Less than 1%) ... 1026
- Arthrotec Tablets (Rare) ... 3195
- Astelin Nasal Spray (Infrequent) ... 3339
- Beconase Inhalation Aerosol (Rare) ... 1497
- Beconase AQ Nasal Spray (Rare) ... 1498
- Betaseron for SC Injection ... 988
- Campath Ampules ... 992
- Captopril Tablets (Approximately 2 to 4 of 100 patients) ... 2281
- Celexa (Rare) ... 1365
- Cerebyx Injection (Infrequent) ... 2619
- Cipro ... 887
- Claritin-D 12 Hour Extended Release Tablets (Less frequent) ... 3102
- Clinoril Tablets (Less than 1 in 100) ... 2053
- Copaxone for Injection (Infrequent) ... 3306
- ▲ Depen Titratable Tablets (12%) ... 3341
- Donnatal ... 2929
- Donnatal Extentabs ... 2930
- Donnatal Tablets ... 2929
- Doxil Injection (Less than 1%) ... 566
- Effexor Tablets (Infrequent) ... 3495
- Effexor XR Capsules (Infrequent) ... 3499
- Exelon Capsules (Infrequent) ... 2342
- Exelon Oral Solution (Infrequent) ... 2345
- Flexeril Tablets (Less than 1%) ... 572
- Flexeril Tablets (Less than 1%) ... 2094
- Flonase Nasal Spray ... 1533
- Flumadine (Less than 0.3%) ... 1370
- Gabitril Tablets (Infrequent) ... 1189
- Hivid Tablets (Less than 1%) ... 2975
- Intron A for Injection (Less than 5%) ... 3120
- Klonopin Tablets (Infrequent) ... 2983
- Lamictal (Rare) ... 1567
- Lamisil Tablets (Uncommon) ... 2360
- Levsin/Levsinex/Levbid ... 3172
- Lipitor Tablets (Less than 2%) ... 2639
- Lipitor Tablets (Less than 2%) ... 2696
- Luvox Tablets (25, 50, 100 mg) (Infrequent) ... 3256
- Nasalide Nasal Spray ... 1295
- Neptazane Tablets ... ⊙ 271
- Neurontin Capsules (Infrequent) ... 2655
- Neurontin Oral Solution (Infrequent) ... 2655
- Neurontin Tablets (Infrequent) ... 2655
- Nexium Delayed-Release Capsules (Less than 1%) ... 619
- Nolvadex Tablets (Infrequent) ... 678
- Norvir Capsules (Less than 2%) ... 487
- Norvir Oral Solution (Less than 2%) ... 487
- NuLev Orally Disintegrating Tablets ... 3176
- Paxil (Infrequent) ... 1609
- Prozac Pulvules, Liquid, and Weekly Capsules (Rare) ... 1238
- Remeron Tablets (Rare) ... 2483
- Remeron SolTab Tablets (Rare) ... 2486
- Rilutek Tablets (Rare) ... 772
- Robinul Forte Tablets ... 1358
- Robinul Injectable ... 2940
- Robinul Tablets ... 1358
- Salagen Tablets (Less than 1%) ... 2229
- Sarafem Pulvules (Rare) ... 1962
- Serzone Tablets (Rare) ... 1104
- Sonata Capsules (Rare) ... 3591
- Soriatane Capsules (Less than 1%) ... 3003
- Tapazole Tablets ... 1823
- Tequin Injection (Less than 0.1%) ... 1110
- Tequin Tablets (Less than 0.1%) ... 1110
- Topamax Sprinkle Capsules (Rare) ... 2590
- Topamax Tablets (Rare) ... 2590
- Valstar Sterile Solution for Intravesical Instillation (Less than 1%) ... 1175
- Vantin Tablets and Oral Suspension (Less than 1%) ... 2860
- Zyrtec (Less than 2%) ... 2756
- Zyrtec-D 12 Hour Extended Relief Tablets (Less than 2%) ... 2758

Aggression

- Advair Diskus 100/50 ... 1448
- Advair Diskus 250/50 ... 1448
- Advair Diskus 500/50 ... 1448
- Ambien Tablets (Rare) ... 3191
- Amerge Tablets (Rare) ... 1467
- Aricept Tablets (Frequent) ... 1270
- Aricept Tablets (Frequent) ... 2665
- Celexa (Infrequent) ... 1365
- Celontin Capsules ... 2618
- Claritin-D 12 Hour Extended Release Tablets (Less frequent) ... 3102
- Claritin-D 24 Hour Extended Release Tablets (Fewer than 2%) ... 3104
- Crinone (Less than 5%) ... 3213
- Depacon Injection ... 416
- Depakene ... 421
- Depakote Sprinkle Capsules ... 426
- Depakote Tablets ... 430
- Depakote ER Tablets ... 436
- Evoxac Capsules ... 1217
- ▲ Exelon Capsules (3%) ... 2342
- ▲ Exelon Oral Solution (3%) ... 2345
- Felbatol (Frequent) ... 3343
- Flexeril Tablets ... 572
- Flexeril Tablets ... 2094
- Flovent Diskus ... 3614
- Flovent ... 1535
- Flovent Rotadisk ... 1537
- Floxin I.V. ... 2526
- Floxin Tablets ... 2529
- Foscavir Injection (Between 1% and 5%) ... 605
- Genotropin Lyophilized Powder ... 2818
- Halcion Tablets ... 2823
- Imitrex Injection ... 1549
- Imitrex Tablets (Rare) ... 1558
- Intron A for Injection (Less than 5%) ... 3120
- Klonopin Tablets (Infrequent) ... 2983
- Levaquin (Less than 0.5%) ... 2537
- Neurontin Capsules ... 2655
- Neurontin Oral Solution ... 2655
- Neurontin Tablets ... 2655
- Priftin Tablets (Less than 1%) ... 758
- Prilosec Delayed-Release Capsules (Less than 1%) ... 628
- Pulmicort Respules (Less than 1%) ... 632
- Pulmicort Turbuhaler Inhalation Powder (Rare) ... 636
- Requip Tablets (Infrequent) ... 1621
- Rhinocort Nasal Inhaler (Rare) ... 640
- Risperdal (1% to 3%) ... 1796
- Symmetrel ... 1328
- Topamax Sprinkle Capsules (2.7% to 4%) ... 2590
- Topamax Tablets (2.7% to 4%) ... 2590
- Trileptal Oral Suspension ... 2407
- Trileptal Tablets ... 2407
- Ventolin Inhalation Aerosol and Refill (1%) ... 1679
- Versed Syrup (Less than 1%) ... 3033
- Xanax Tablets (Rare) ... 2865
- Zarontin Capsules ... 2659
- Zarontin Syrup ... 2660
- Zoloft (Infrequent) ... 2751
- Zosyn (1.0% or less) ... 1890
- Zosyn in Galaxy Containers (1.0% or less) ... 1894

Agitation

- Aciphex Tablets (Rare) ... 1267
- Aciphex Tablets (Rare) ... 1783
- Actiq (Less than 1%) ... 1184
- Advair Diskus 100/50 ... 1448
- Advair Diskus 250/50 ... 1448
- Advair Diskus 500/50 ... 1448
- Aggrenox Capsules (Less than 1%) ... 1026
- Akineton ... 402
- Allegra-D Extended-Release Tablets (1.9%) ... 714
- Aloprim for Injection (Less than 1%) ... 2292
- Ambien Tablets (Infrequent) ... 3191
- AmBisome for Injection (Less common) ... 1383
- Amerge Tablets (Rare) ... 1467
- Amoxil Chewable Tablets (Rare) ... 1471
- Amoxil for Oral Suspension (Rare) ... 1471
- Amoxil (Rare) ... 1471

Amphotec (1% to 5%) 1774
Anzemet Injection (Infrequently) 719
Anzemet Tablets (Infrequently) 722
Aricept Tablets 1270
Aricept Tablets 2665
Artane 1855
Ativan Injection (Infrequent) 3478
Ativan Tablets (Less frequent) 3482
Augmentin Chewable Tablets (Rare) 1482
Augmentin Powder for Oral Suspension (Rare) 1482
Augmentin Tablets (Rare) 1485
Augmentin ES-600 Powder for Oral Suspension (Rare) 1487
Betaseron for SC Injection 988
Bicillin L-A Injection 2242
Bontril Slow-Release Capsules 576
Brevibloc Injection (About 2%) 858
Buprenex Injectable (Rare) 2918
Carbatrol Capsules 3234
Cardura Tablets (0.5% to 1%) 2668
Catapres Tablets (About 3 in 100 patients) 1037
Catapres-TTS (0.5% or less) 1038
Cedax Oral Suspension (0.1% to 1%) 1021
▲ Celexa (3%) 1365
▲ CellCept Capsules (3% to 10%) 2951
▲ CellCept Intravenous (3% to 10%) 2951
▲ CellCept Oral Suspension (3% to 10%) 2951
▲ CellCept Tablets (3% to 10%) 2951
▲ Cerebyx Injection (3.3% to 9.5%) 2619
Cipro I.V. 893
Cipro I.V. Pharmacy Bulk Package 897
Cipro 887
Claritin (At least one patient) 3100
Claritin-D 12 Hour Extended Release Tablets (Less frequent) 3102
Claritin-D 24 Hour Extended Release Tablets (Fewer than 2%) 3104
Clorpres Tablets (About 3%) 1002
▲ Clozaril Tablets (4%) 2319
▲ Cognex Capsules (7%) 1351
Combipres Tablets (About 3%) 1040
Compazine 1505
Comtan Tablets (1%) 2328
Comvax 2056
▲ Copaxone for Injection (4%) 3306
Crixivan Capsules (Less than 2%) 2070
Cuprimine Capsules 2075
Demerol 3079
Depacon Injection (1% or more) 416
Depakene (1% or more) 421
Depakote Sprinkle Capsules 426
Depakote Tablets (1% to 5%) 430
Depakote ER Tablets (Greater than 1%) 436
Dexedrine 1512
Dilaudid Oral Liquid (Less frequent) 445
Dilaudid Tablets - 8 mg (Less frequent) 445
Dilaudid-HP (Less frequent) 443
Diprivan Injectable Emulsion (Less than 1%) 667
Dolophine Hydrochloride Tablets 3056
Donnatal (In elderly patients) 2929
Donnatal Extentabs (In elderly patients) 2930
Donnatal Tablets (In elderly patients) 2929
▲ Duraclon Injection (3%) 3057
Duragesic Transdermal System (1% or greater) 1786
Ecotrin Enteric Coated Aspirin Low, Regular and Maximum Strength Tablets 1715
▲ Effexor Tablets (2% to 4.5%) 3495
▲ Effexor XR Capsules (3%) 3499
Eldepryl Capsules 3266
Elspar for Injection 2092
Engerix-B Vaccine (Less than 1%) 1517
Evoxac Capsules (Less than 1%) 1217
Exelon Capsules (2% or more) 2342
Exelon Oral Solution (2% or more) 2345
Famotidine Injection (Infrequent) 866
Felbatol (Frequent) 3343
Ferrlecit Injection (Greater than 1%) 3386
Flexeril Tablets (Less than 1%) 572
Flexeril Tablets (Less than 1%) 2094
▲ Flolan for Injection (11%) 1528
Flovent Diskus 3614
Flovent 1535
Flovent Rotadisk 1537
Floxin I.V. 2526
Floxin Tablets 2529
Fludara for Injection 995
Flumadine (0.3% to 1%) 1370
Fortovase Capsules (Less than 2%) 2970
Foscavir Injection (Between 1% and 5%) 605
Gabitril Tablets (1%) 1189
Geodon Capsules (Frequent) 2688
Halcion Tablets 2823
Haldol Decanoate 2535
Haldol Injection, Tablets and Concentrate 2533
Hivid Tablets (Less than 1%) 2975
Imitrex Injection (Infrequent) 1549
Imitrex Nasal Spray (Infrequent) 1554
Imitrex Tablets (Up to 2%) 1558
▲ Indapamide Tablets (Greater than or equal to 5%) 2286
▲ Infergen (4% to 6%) 1777
Intron A for Injection (Less than 5%) 3120
Invirase Capsules (Less than 2%) 2979
Ismo Tablets (Fewer than 1%) 3524
Kadian Capsules (Less than 3%) 1335
Kaletra Capsules (Less than 2%) 471
Kaletra Oral Solution (Less than 2%) 471
Keflex 1237
Klonopin Tablets 2983
Kytril Injection (Less than 2%) 2986
Lamictal (Infrequent) 1567
Leukeran Tablets (Rare) 1591
Levaquin (0.5% to less than 1.0%) 2537
Levsin/Levsinex/Levbid 3172
Lexxel Tablets 608
Lodosyn Tablets 1251
Loxitane Capsules 3398
Lufyllin Tablets 3347
Lufyllin-400 Tablets 3347
Lufyllin-GG Elixir 3348
Lufyllin-GG Tablets 3348
Lupron Depot 7.5 mg (Less than 5%) 3284
Lupron Depot–3 Month 11.25 mg 3285
Luvox Tablets (25, 50, 100 mg) (2%) 3256
Maxalt Tablets (Infrequent) 2120
Maxalt-MLT Orally Disintegrating Tablets (Infrequent) 2120
Mepergan Injection 3539
Meridia Capsules (Greater than or equal to 1%) 481
Merrem I.V. (0.1% to 1.0%) 673
Miacalcin Nasal Spray (Less than 1%) 2375
Mirapex Tablets (1.1%) 2834
MS Contin Tablets (Less frequent) 2896
MSIR (Less frequent) 2898
Narcan Injection (Infrequent) 1322
Nardil Tablets (Uncommon) 2653
Naropin Injection (Less than 1%) 612
Navane Oral 2701
Navane Intramuscular 2703
Nembutal Sodium Solution (Less than 1%) 485
Neurontin Capsules (Infrequent) 2655
Neurontin Oral Solution (Infrequent) 2655
Neurontin Tablets (Infrequent) 2655
Norflex 1987
Norpramin Tablets 755
Norvasc Tablets (Less than or equal to 0.1%) 2704
Norvir Capsules (Less than 2%) 487
Norvir Oral Solution (Less than 2%) 487
Nubain Injection 1323
Oramorph SR Tablets (Less frequent) 3062
Orthoclone OKT3 Sterile Solution 2498
OxyContin Tablets (Less than 1%) 2912
Parnate Tablets 1607
Paxil (1.1% to 5%) 1609
Pepcid Injection (Infrequent) 2153
Pepcid for Oral Suspension (Infrequent) 2150
Pepcid RPD Orally Disintegrating Tablets (Infrequent) 2150
Pepcid Tablets (Infrequent) 2150
Permax Tablets (Infrequent) 1299
Phrenilin (Infrequent) 578
Prevacid Delayed-Release Capsules (Less than 1%) 3292
PREVPAC (Less than 1%) 3298
▲ Prograf (3% to 15%) 1393
Proleukin for Injection 1199
ProSom Tablets (Infrequent) 500
Prozac Pulvules, Liquid, and Weekly Capsules (Frequent) 1238
Recombivax HB 2178
Reglan 2935
Relafen Tablets (1%) 1617
Remeron Tablets (Frequent) 2483
Remeron SolTab Tablets (Frequent) 2486
Reminyl Oral Solution (Greater than or equal to 2%) 1792
Reminyl Tablets (Greater than or equal to 2%) 1792
ReoPro Vials (0.7%) 1958
Requip Tablets (Infrequent) 1621
Rescriptor Tablets (Less than 2%) 526
Rilutek Tablets (Frequent) 772
▲ Risperdal (22% to 26%) 1796
Rituxan for Infusion (1% to 5%) 1750
Rituxan I.V. (1% to 5%) 1428
Roferon-A Injection 2996
▲ Romazicon Injection (3% to 9%) 3000
Roxanol 3066
Roxicodone Tablets (Less than 3%) 3067
Salagen Tablets (Rare) 2229
Sarafem Pulvules (Frequent) 1962
Sedapap Tablets 50 mg/650 mg (Infrequent) 2225
Serentil 1057
Serzone Tablets 1104
▲ Simulect for Injection (3% to 10%) 2399
Sinemet Tablets 1253
Sinemet CR Tablets 1255
Soma Tablets 3353
Soma Compound Tablets (Very rare to infrequent) 3354
Soma Compound w/Codeine Tablets (Infrequent or rare) 3355
Sonata Capsules (Infrequent) 3591
Stadol NS Nasal Spray (Less than 1%) 1108
Stelazine 1640
Stimate Nasal Spray 796
Suprane Liquid for Inhalation (Less than 1%) 874
Surmontil Capsules 3595
Sustiva Capsules (Less than 2%) 1258
Symmetrel (1% to 5%) 1328
Tagamet 1644
Tasmar Tablets (1%) 3010
Tegretol/Tegretol-XR 2404
Tenex Tablets (Less frequent) 2942
Tequin Injection (Less than 0.1%) 1110
Tequin Tablets (Less than 0.1%) 1110
Thalomid Capsules 1154
Thioridazine Hydrochloride Tablets 2289
Thiothixene Capsules 2290
Thorazine 1656
Tonocard Tablets (Less than 1%) 649
▲ Topamax Sprinkle Capsules (4% to 4.4%) 2590
▲ Topamax Tablets (4% to 4.4%) 2590
Trasylol Injection (1% to 2%) 909
Trental Tablets 784
Trileptal Oral Suspension (1% to 2%) 2407
Trileptal Tablets (1% to 2%) 2407
▲ Trisenox Injection (5%) 1158
Trovan (Less than 1%) 2722
Twinrix Vaccine (Less than 1%) 1674
▲ Ultram Tablets (1% to 14%) 2600
Valcyte Tablets (Less than 5%) 3022
Valtrex Caplets 1676
Ventolin Inhalation Aerosol and Refill (1%) 1679
Versed Injection (Less than 1%) 3027
Versed Syrup (2%) 3033
▲ Vesanoid Capsules (9%) 3037
Vicoprofen Tablets (Less than 1%) 520
Vistide Injection 1445
Vivactil Tablets 2217
Vivactil Tablets 2446
▲ Wellbutrin Tablets (31.9%) 1680
▲ Wellbutrin SR Sustained-Release Tablets (0.3% to 9%) 1684
Xanax Tablets (Rare; 2.9%) 2865
Zanaflex Tablets (Infrequent) 1305
Zantac (Rare) 1690
Zantac Injection 1688
Zantac Syrup (Rare) 1690
Zithromax Capsules, 250 mg (1% or less) 2743
Zithromax for Oral Suspension, 300 mg, 600 mg, 900 mg, 1200 mg (1% or less) 2739
Zithromax Tablets, 250 mg (1% or less) 2739
▲ Zofran Injection (2% to 6%) 1698
▲ Zofran (6%) 1703
▲ Zofran ODT Orally Disintegrating Tablets (6%) 1703
▲ Zoloft (6%) 2751
▲ Zometa for Intravenous Infusion (12.8%) 3621
Zomig Tablets (Infrequent) 708
Zomig-ZMT Tablets (Infrequent) 708
▲ Zonegran Capsules (9%) 1307
▲ Zosyn (2.1% to 7.1%) 1890
▲ Zosyn in Galaxy Containers (2.1% to 7.1%) 1894
Zovirax Capsules 1706
Zovirax for Injection (Approximately 1%) 1708
Zovirax 1706
Zyban Sustained-Release Tablets (Frequent) 1710
▲ Zyprexa Tablets (23%) 1973
▲ Zyprexa ZYDIS Orally Disintegrating Tablets (23%) 1973
Zyrtec (Less than 2%) 2756
Zyrtec-D 12 Hour Extended Relief Tablets (Less than 2%) 2758

Agnosia

▲ Vesanoid Capsules (3%) 3037

Agoraphobia

Luvox Tablets (25, 50, 100 mg) (Infrequent) 3256

Agranulocytopenia

Sterile FUDR (Remote possibility) 2974

Agranulocytosis

Accolate Tablets 657
Accupril Tablets (Rare) 2611
Accuretic Tablets (0.5% to 1%) 2614
Accutane Capsules 2944
Aceon Tablets (2 mg, 4 mg, 8 mg) 3249
Aciphex Tablets 1267
Aciphex Tablets 1783
Albenza Tablets (Rare) 1463
Aldoclor Tablets 2035
Aldoril Tablets 2039
Altace Capsules (Rare) 2233
Amaryl Tablets 717
AmBisome for Injection (Infrequent) 1383
Amicar Injection 3608
Amicar Syrup 3608
Amicar Tablets 3608
Amoxil Chewable Tablets 1471
Amoxil for Oral Suspension 1471
Amoxil 1471
Anaprox Tablets (Less than 1%) 2967
Anaprox DS Tablets (Less than 1%) 2967
Ancobon Capsules 1730
Arthrotec Tablets (Rare) 3195
Asacol Delayed-Release Tablets (Rare) 2884
Atacand Tablets (Very rare) 595
Atacand HCT Tablets 597
Atromid-S Capsules 3483
Augmentin Chewable Tablets 1482
Augmentin Powder for Oral Suspension 1482
Augmentin Tablets 1485
Augmentin ES-600 Powder for Oral Suspension 1487
Avalide Tablets 1070
Azulfidine EN-tabs Tablets (Rare) 2775
Bactrim (Rare) 2949
Benadryl Parenteral 2617
▲ Blephamide Ophthalmic Ointment (Among most often) 547
Blephamide Ophthalmic Suspension 548
Blocadren Tablets 2046
Campath Ampules 992
Captopril Tablets 2281
Carbatrol Capsules 3234
Cataflam Tablets (Rare) 2315
Ceclor 1905
Cedax 1021
Cefizox for Intramuscular or Intravenous Use 1390
Cefotan 664
Ceftin 1898
Cefzil 1076
Ceptaz for Injection (Very rare) 1499
Cipro I.V. 893
Cipro I.V. Pharmacy Bulk Package (Less than 1%) 897
Cipro 887
Claforan Injection (Less than 1%) 732
Cleocin HCl Capsules 2784
Cleocin Phosphate Sterile Solution 2785
Cleocin Vaginal Cream 2788
Cleocin Vaginal Ovules 2789
Clinoril Tablets (Less than 1%) 2053
Clorpres Tablets 1002
Clozaril Tablets (1% to 1.3%) 2319
Combipres Tablets 1040
Compazine 1505
Corgard Tablets 2245
Corzide 40/5 Tablets 2247
Corzide 80/5 Tablets 2247
Cosmegen for Injection 2062
Cosopt Sterile Ophthalmic Solution 2065
Cuprimine Capsules 2075
Dapsone Tablets USP 1780
Daranide Tablets 2077
Depen Titratable Tablets 3341
DiaBeta Tablets 741
Diabinese Tablets 2680
Diamox Intravenous ⊙ 269
Diamox Sequels Sustained Release Capsules ⊙ 270
Diamox Tablets ⊙ 269
Didronel Tablets (Rare) 2888
Diflucan Tablets, Injection, and Oral Suspension 2681
Dilantin Infatabs (Occasional) 2624
Dilantin Kapseals (Occasional) 2622
Dilantin-125 Oral Suspension (Occasional) 2625
Diovan HCT Tablets 2338
Diucardin Tablets 3494
Diuril Oral 2087
Diuril Sodium Intravenous 2086
Dolobid Tablets (Less than 1 in 100) 2088
Duricef 1079
Dyazide Capsules 1515
EC-Naprosyn Delayed-Release Tablets (Less than 1%) 2967
Edecrin 2091
Effexor Tablets 3495
Effexor XR Capsules 3499
Enalaprilat Injection (Several cases) 863
Ergamisol Tablets (One patient) 1789
Etrafon 3115
Famotidine Injection (Rare) 866
Felbatol (Rare) 3343

Feldene Capsules (Rare)........ 2685
Floxin I.V........ 2526
Floxin Tablets........ 2529
FML-S Liquifilm Sterile Ophthalmic Suspension........ ⊙238
Fortaz (Very rare)........ 1541
Furosemide Tablets........ 2284
Glucotrol Tablets........ 2692
Glucotrol XL Extended Release Tablets........ 2693
Haldol Decanoate (Rare)........ 2535
Haldol Injection, Tablets and Concentrate (Rare)........ 2533
HydroDIURIL Tablets........ 2108
Hyzaar........ 2109
Indapamide Tablets........ 2286
Inderal........ 3513
Inderal LA Long-Acting Capsules........ 3516
Inderide Tablets........ 3517
Inderide LA Long-Acting Capsules........ 3519
Indocin Capsules (Less than 1%)........ 2112
Indocin I.V. (Less than 1%)........ 2115
Indocin (Less than 1%)........ 2112
Kefurox Vials, ADD-Vantage........ 1948
Lamictal........ 1567
Lamisil Tablets (Rare)........ 2360
▲ Leukine (6%)........ 1755
Lexxel Tablets (Several cases)........ 608
Librium Capsules (Occasional)........ 1736
Librium for Injection (Occasional)........ 1737
Limbitrol........ 1738
Lodine (Less than 1%)........ 3528
Lodine XL Extended-Release Tablets (Less than 1%)........ 3530
Lodosyn Tablets........ 1251
Lorabid Suspension and Pulvules........ 2251
Lortab........ 3319
Lortab Elixir........ 3317
Lotensin HCT Tablets........ 2367
Lotrel Capsules........ 2370
Loxitane Capsules (Rare)........ 3398
Luvox Tablets (25, 50, 100 mg)........ 3256
Macrobid Capsules........ 2889
Macrodantin Capsules........ 2891
Mavik Tablets (Rare)........ 478
Maxidone Tablets CIII........ 3399
Maxipime for Injection........ 1285
Maxzide........ 1008
Mefoxin for Injection........ 2124
Mefoxin Premixed Intravenous Solution........ 2127
Mepergan Injection (1 instance)........ 3539
Mexitil Capsules (About 1 in 1,000)........ 1047
Micardis HCT Tablets........ 1051
Microzide Capsules........ 3414
Miltown Tablets........ 3349
Minizide Capsules........ 2700
Mobic Tablets (Less than 0.1%)........ 1054
Moduretic Tablets........ 2138
Monopril Tablets........ 1091
Monopril HCT........ 1094
Motrin Suspension, Oral Drops, Chewable Tablets, and Caplets (Less than 1%)........ 2002
Mustargen for Injection (Relatively infrequent)........ 2142
Mykrox Tablets........ 1168
Nadolol Tablets........ 2288
▲ Naprelan Tablets (3% to 9%)........ 1293
Naprosyn Suspension (Less than 1%)........ 2967
Naprosyn Tablets (Less than 1%)........ 2967
Navane Oral........ 2701
Navane Intramuscular........ 2703
Neptazane Tablets........ ⊙271
▲ Nipent for Injection (3% to 10%)........ 3272
Norco 5/325 Tablets CIII........ 3424
Norco 7.5/325 Tablets CIII........ 3425
Norco 10/325 Tablets CIII........ 3425
Norco 10/325 Tablets CIII........ 3427
Normodyne Tablets........ 3137
Noroxin Tablets........ 2145
Norpramin Tablets........ 755
Omnicef........ 493
Oncaspar........ 756
Orudis Capsules (Less than 1%)........ 3548
Oruvail Capsules (Less than 1%)........ 3548
Parnate Tablets........ 1607
Paser Granules........ 1781
Paxil........ 1609
Pediazole Suspension........ 3050
Pentasa Capsules........ 3239
Pepcid Injection (Rare)........ 2153
Pepcid for Oral Suspension (Rare)........ 2150
Pepcid RPD Orally Disintegrating Tablets (Rare)........ 2150
Pepcid Tablets (Rare)........ 2150
Periactin Tablets........ 2155
Phenergan Injection........ 3553
Phenergan Suppositories........ 3556
Phenergan Syrup (1 case)........ 3554
Phenergan Tablets........ 3556
Phenergan with Codeine Syrup (1 case)........ 3557
Phenergan with Dextromethorphan Syrup (1 case)........ 3559
Phenergan VC Syrup (1 case)........ 3560
Phenergan VC with Codeine Syrup (1 case)........ 3561
Phrenilin (Infrequent)........ 578
Plaquenil Tablets........ 3082
Plavix Tablets (Less than 1%)........ 1097
Plavix Tablets (Less than 1%)........ 3084
Ponstel Capsules (Rare)........ 1356
Prevacid Delayed-Release Capsules (Less than 1%)........ 3292
PREVPAC........ 3298
Prilosec Delayed-Release Capsules (Rare)........ 628
Primaxin I.M........ 2158
Primaxin I.V........ 2160
Prinivil Tablets (Rare to frequent)........ 2164
Prinzide Tablets (Rare)........ 2168
Procanbid Extended-Release Tablets (Approximately 0.5%)........ 2262
ProSom Tablets (Rare)........ 500
Quinaglute Dura-Tabs Tablets........ 978
Quinidex Extentabs........ 2933
Reglan (A few cases)........ 2935
Remeron Tablets (Three patients)........ 2483
Remeron SolTab Tablets (Three patients)........ 2486
Renese Tablets........ 2712
Rifamate Capsules........ 767
Rifater Tablets........ 769
Rocephin Injectable Vials, ADD-Vantage, Galaxy, Bulk........ 2993
Rynatan Tablets........ 3351
Rythmol Tablets – 150 mg, 225 mg, 300 mg (Less than 1%)........ 502
Sectral Capsules........ 3589
Sedapap Tablets 50 mg/650 mg........ 2225
Septra Suspension........ 2265
Septra Tablets........ 2265
Septra DS Tablets........ 2265
Serentil........ 1057
Silvadene Cream 1%........ 2267
Sinemet Tablets........ 1253
Sinemet CR Tablets........ 1255
Sinequan (Occasional)........ 2713
Stelazine........ 1640
Sultrin Triple Sulfa Cream (One case)........ 2587
Suprax........ 1877
Surmontil Capsules........ 3595
Tagamet (Approximately 3 per 1,000,000)........ 1644
Talacen Caplets (Rare)........ 3089
Tapazole Tablets........ 1823
Tazicef for Injection (Very rare)........ 1647
Tazicef Galaxy Container (Very rare)........ 1650
Tazicef Pharmacy Bulk Package (Very rare)........ 1653
Tazidime Vials, Faspak & ADD-Vantage (Very rare)........ 1966
Tegretol/Tegretol-XR (Very low incidence)........ 2404
Tenoretic Tablets........ 690
Tenormin........ 692
Thioridazine Hydrochloride Tablets (Infrequent)........ 2289
Thiothixene Capsules........ 2290
Thorazine........ 1656
Ticlid Tablets (Rare)........ 3015
Timolide Tablets........ 2187
Timolol GFS........ ⊙266
Timoptic in Ocudose........ 2192
Timoptic Sterile Ophthalmic Solution........ 2190
Timoptic-XE Sterile Ophthalmic Gel Forming Solution........ 2194
Tolectin (Less than 1%)........ 2589
Tonocard Tablets (Less than 1%)........ 649
Toprol-XL Tablets (Rare)........ 651
Trilafon........ 3160
Trusopt Sterile Ophthalmic Solution (Rare)........ 2196
Unasyn for Injection........ 2728
Uniretic Tablets (More than 1%)........ 3178
Univasc Tablets (More than 1%)........ 3181
Urobiotic-250 Capsules........ 2731
Vancocin HCl, Vials & ADD-Vantage (Rare)........ 1970
Vantin Tablets and Oral Suspension........ 2860
Vascor Tablets........ 2602
Vaseretic Tablets (Rare)........ 2204
Vasotec I.V. Injection (Several cases)........ 2207
Vasotec Tablets (Several cases)........ 2210
Vermox Chewable Tablets........ 2017
Vicodin Tablets........ 516
Vicodin ES Tablets........ 517
Vicodin HP Tablets........ 518
Vioxx........ 2213
Vivactil Tablets........ 2217
Vivactil Tablets........ 2446
Voltaren Tablets (Rare)........ 2315
Voltaren-XR Tablets (Rare)........ 2315
Zantac (Rare)........ 1690
Zantac Injection (Rare)........ 1688
Zantac Syrup (Rare)........ 1690
Zarontin Capsules........ 2659
Zarontin Syrup........ 2660
Zaroxolyn Tablets........ 1177
Zebeta Tablets........ 1885
Zestoretic Tablets........ 695
Zestril Tablets........ 698
Ziac Tablets........ 1887
Zinacef Injection........ 1696
Zinacef for Injection........ 1696
Zoloft........ 2751

AICD discharge
Betapace Tablets (Less than 1% to 3%)........ 950

Airway constriction
Amerge Tablets (Rare)........ 1467

Airway obstruction
Altace Capsules........ 2233
Amerge Tablets (Rare)........ 1467
Ativan Injection (5 patients)........ 3478
Captopril Tablets........ 2281
Diprivan Injectable Emulsion (Less than 1%)........ 667
Enalaprilat Injection........ 863
Floxin I.V........ 2526
Floxin Tablets........ 2529
▲ Infasurf Intratracheal Suspension (39%)........ 1372
Monopril Tablets........ 1091
Orthoclone OKT3 Sterile Solution........ 2498
Prinivil Tablets........ 2164
Prinzide Tablets........ 2168
Vaseretic Tablets........ 2204
Vasotec I.V. Injection........ 2207
Vasotec Tablets........ 2210
Versed Injection (Less than 1%)........ 3027
Versed Syrup (1%)........ 3033
Zestoretic Tablets........ 695
Zestril Tablets........ 698

Airway resistance
Demerol........ 3079

Akathisia
Cerebyx Injection (Infrequent)........ 2619
▲ Clozaril Tablets (3%)........ 2319
Cognex Capsules (Rare)........ 1351
Compazine........ 1505
Effexor Tablets (Rare)........ 3495
Effexor XR Capsules (Rare)........ 3499
Etrafon........ 3115
Feldene Capsules (Rare)........ 2685
▲ Geodon Capsules (8%)........ 2688
Haldol Decanoate (Frequent)........ 2535
Haldol Injection, Tablets and Concentrate........ 2533
Lamictal (Infrequent)........ 1567
Loxitane Capsules........ 3398
Luvox Tablets (25, 50, 100 mg) (Infrequent)........ 3256
▲ Mirapex Tablets (10% to 14%)........ 2834
Moban........ 1320
Navane Oral........ 2701
Navane Intramuscular........ 2703
▲ Orap Tablets (8 of 20 patients)........ 1407
Paxil........ 1609
Permax Tablets (1.6%)........ 1299
Prozac Pulvules, Liquid, and Weekly Capsules (Infrequent)........ 1238
Reglan........ 2935
Remeron Tablets (Rare)........ 2483
Remeron SolTab Tablets (Rare)........ 2486
▲ Risperdal (17% to 34%)........ 1796
Sarafem Pulvules (Infrequent)........ 1962
Serentil........ 1057
Stelazine........ 1640
Thioridazine Hydrochloride Tablets........ 2289
Thiothixene Capsules........ 2290
Trilafon........ 3160
Vascor Tablets (0.5% to 2.0%)........ 2602
Wellbutrin Tablets (1.5%)........ 1680
Xanax Tablets (1.6% to 3.0%)........ 2865
Zomig Tablets (Rare)........ 708
Zomig-ZMT Tablets (Rare)........ 708
▲ Zyprexa Tablets (5% to 27%)........ 1973
▲ Zyprexa ZYDIS Orally Disintegrating Tablets (5% to 27%)........ 1973

Akinesia
Cardura Tablets (1%)........ 2668
▲ Clozaril Tablets (4%)........ 2319
Effexor Tablets (Rare)........ 3495
Effexor XR Capsules (Rare)........ 3499
Geodon Capsules (Frequent)........ 2688
Loxitane Capsules........ 3398
Luvox Tablets (25, 50, 100 mg) (Rare)........ 3256
Maxalt Tablets (Rare)........ 2120
Maxalt-MLT Orally Disintegrating Tablets (Rare)........ 2120
Moban........ 1320
▲ Orap Tablets (8 of 20 patients)........ 1407
Parnate Tablets........ 1607
Paxil (Infrequent)........ 1609
Permax Tablets (1.1%)........ 1299
Serentil........ 1057
Thioridazine Hydrochloride Tablets........ 2289
▲ Wellbutrin Tablets (8.0%)........ 1680
Wellbutrin SR Sustained-Release Tablets........ 1684
Zyban Sustained-Release Tablets........ 1710
▲ Zyprexa Tablets (8% to 20%)........ 1973
▲ Zyprexa ZYDIS Orally Disintegrating Tablets (8% to 20%)........ 1973

Alanine aminotransferase levels, changes in
Cataflam Tablets (About 1% to about 4%)........ 2315
Humegon for Injection (Occasional)........ 2468
Sarafem Pulvules (Rare)........ 1962
Sinemet Tablets........ 1253
Sinemet CR Tablets........ 1255
Voltaren Tablets (About 1% to about 4%)........ 2315
Voltaren-XR Tablets (About 1% to about 4%)........ 2315

Alanine aminotransferase levels, elevation of
Abelcet Injection........ 1273
Accolate Tablets (1.5%)........ 657
Accutane Capsules........ 2944
Aceon Tablets (2 mg, 4 mg, 8 mg) (1.6% to 1.7%)........ 3249
Aciphex Tablets (0.2%)........ 1267
Aciphex Tablets (0.2%)........ 1783
Actos Tablets (0.26%)........ 3275
Adalat CC Tablets (Rare)........ 877
Ambien Tablets (Infrequent)........ 3191
▲ AmBisome for Injection (14.6%)........ 1383
Amoxil Chewable Tablets........ 1471
Amoxil for Oral Suspension........ 1471
Amoxil........ 1471
Amphotec (1% to 5%)........ 1774
Anaprox Tablets (Less than 1%)........ 2967
Anaprox DS Tablets (Less than 1%)........ 2967
Ancef for Injection........ 1474
Ancef Injection........ 1474
Anzemet Injection........ 719
Anzemet Tablets........ 722
Arava Tablets (1.5% to 4.4%)........ 724
Arimidex Tablets (2% to 5%)........ 659
Asacol Delayed-Release Tablets........ 2884
Astelin Nasal Spray (Infrequent)........ 3339
Atromid-S Capsules........ 3483
Augmentin Chewable Tablets (Infrequent)........ 1482
Augmentin Powder for Oral Suspension (Infrequent)........ 1482
Augmentin Tablets (Infrequent)........ 1485
Augmentin ES-600 Powder for Oral Suspension........ 1487
Avandia Tablets (0.2%)........ 1490
Axid Pulvules (Less common)........ 1903
Axid Pulvules (Less common)........ 2919
Aygestin Tablets........ 1333
Azactam for Injection (Less than 1% to 6.5%)........ 1276
Azulfidine EN-tabs Tablets........ 2775
▲ Betaseron for SC Injection (19%)........ 988
Biaxin/Biaxin XL........ 403
Calcijex Injection........ 411
Calcium Disodium Versenate Injection........ 1980
▲ Cancidas for Injection (10.6% to 10.8%)........ 2048
Cardizem Injectable........ 1018
Cardizem Lyo-Ject Syringe........ 1018
Cardizem Monovial........ 1018
Cardizem CD Capsules (Less than 1%)........ 1016
▲ Casodex Tablets (2% to 5%)........ 662
Ceclor CD Tablets (0.3%)........ 1279
Ceclor (1 in 40)........ 1905
Cedax (0.1% to 1%)........ 1021
Cefizox for Intramuscular or Intravenous Use (1% to 5%)........ 1390
Cefotan (1 in 150)........ 664
Ceftin (0.1% to 1%)........ 1898
Cefzil (2%)........ 1076
Celebrex Capsules (0.1% to 1.9%)........ 2676
Celebrex Capsules (0.1% to 1.9%)........ 2780
▲ CellCept Capsules (3% to 15.6%)........ 2951
▲ CellCept Intravenous (3% to 15.6%)........ 2951
▲ CellCept Oral Suspension (3% to 15.6%)........ 2951
▲ CellCept Tablets (3% to 15.6%)........ 2951
▲ Chemet Capsules (4.2% to 10.4%)........ 3078
Chibroxin Sterile Ophthalmic Solution........ 2051
▲ Cipro I.V. (Among most frequent)........ 893
▲ Cipro I.V. Pharmacy Bulk Package (Among most frequent)........ 897
Cipro (1.9%)........ 887
Claforan Injection (Less than 1%)........ 732
Cognex Capsules........ 1351
Colazal Capsules........ 3069
Colestid Tablets (One or more occasions)........ 2791
Combivir Tablets........ 1502
Cordarone Intravenous (Common)........ 3491
Cordarone Tablets........ 3487
Coreg Tablets (1% to 2%)........ 1508
Covera-HS Tablets (1.4%)........ 3199
▲ Crixivan Capsules (5.5%)........ 2070
Cylert Tablets........ 415
Cytovene (At least 3 subjects)........ 2959
Depacon Injection (1% to 5%)........ 416
Depakene (Frequent)........ 421

Depakote Sprinkle Capsules (1% to 5%) 426
Depakote Tablets (Frequent) 430
Depakote ER Tablets (Greater than 1%) 436
Dipentum Capsules (Rare) 2803
Doxil Injection (1% to 5%) 566
Duricef 1079
Dynabac Tablets (0.1% to 1%) 2269
EC-Naprosyn Delayed-Release Tablets (Less than 1%) 2967
Effexor Tablets (Rare) 3495
Effexor XR Capsules (Rare) 3499
Elspar for Injection 2092
▲ Epivir (3.7% to 4%) 1520
▲ Epivir-HBV (11%) 1524
Eulexin Capsules 3118
Evoxac Capsules (Less than 1%) 1217
▲ Famvir Tablets (3.2%) 2348
▲ Felbatol (3.5% to 5.2%) 3343
Feldene Capsules (Approximately 1%) 2685
Femara Tablets 2351
Floxin I.V. (More than or equal to 1%) 2526
Floxin Tablets (More than or equal to 1%) 2529
▲ Fortaz (1 in 15) 1541
Fortovase Capsules (Up to 3%) 2970
Foscavir Injection (Between 1% and 5%) 605
▲ Gemzar for Injection (38% to 72%) 1919
Gleevec Capsules 2357
Hectorol Capsules 1064
Heparin Lock Flush Solution 3509
Heparin Sodium Injection 3511
Hivid Tablets (Less than 1%) 2975
▲ Humatrope Vials and Cartridges (6.25% to 6.67%) 1930
Hycamtin for Injection (Less than 1% to 5%) 1546
Imdur Tablets (Less than or equal to 5%) 1826
▲ Innohep Injection (13%) 1248
▲ Intron A for Injection (Up to 15% of patients) 3120
Invirase Capsules (Up to 3%) 2979
Isoptin SR Tablets 467
▲ Kaletra Capsules (1.1% to 8.3%) 471
▲ Kaletra Oral Solution (1.1% to 8.3%) 471
Keflex 1237
▲ Kefurox Vials, ADD-Vantage (1 in 25) 1948
Kefzol Vials, ADD-Vantage 1951
▲ Kytril Injection (3.3%) 2986
▲ Kytril Tablets (6%) 2988
▲ Leukine (13%) 1755
Lexxel Tablets (Infrequent) 608
Lodosyn Tablets 1251
Lopid Tablets (Occasional) 2650
Lorabid Suspension and Pulvules 2251
Lovenox Injection (Up to 5.5% of patients) 746
Loxitane Capsules 3398
▲ Lupron Depot–4 Month 30 mg (Greater than or equal to 5%) 3289
Macrobid Capsules (1% to 5%) 2889
Macrodantin Capsules 2891
Malarone 1596
Mandol Vials 1953
Marinol Capsules (Less than 1%) 3325
Mavik Tablets (0.3% to 1.0%) 478
Maxipime for Injection (2.8%) 1285
Mefoxin for Injection 2124
Mefoxin Premixed Intravenous Solution 2127
▲ Mepron Suspension (6%) 1598
Meridia Capsules (1.6%) 481
Merrem I.V. (Greater than 0.2%) 673
Mevacor Tablets 2132
Mithracin for Intravenous Use 903
Mobic Tablets (Less than 2%) 1054
Monurol Sachet (Less than 1%) 1375
Motrin Suspension, Oral Drops, Chewable Tablets, and Caplets (Less than 1%) 2002
▲ Mycobutin Capsules (9%) 2838
▲ Mylotarg for Injection (9%) 3540
Naprelan Tablets (Less than 1%) 1293
Naprosyn Suspension (Less than 1%) 2967
Naprosyn Tablets (Less than 1%) 2967
Nebcin Vials, Hyporets & ADD-Vantage 1955
Nexium Delayed-Release Capsules (Less than 1%) 619
Niaspan Extended-Release Tablets 1846
▲ Nilandron Tablets (9.1%) 753
Nimotop Capsules (0.2%; rare) 904
Noroxin Tablets (1.4%) 2145
▲ Novantrone for Injection (5% to 6%) 1760
Omnicef (0.4%) 493
▲ Oncaspar (Greater than 5%) 756
Orthoclone OKT3 Sterile Solution 2498
Orudis Capsules 3548
Oruvail Capsules 3548
Pacerone Tablets 3331
Paxil (Infrequent) 1609
▲ PEG-Intron Powder for Injection (10%) 3140
Pentasa Capsules (Less than 1%) 3239
Pipracil (Less frequent) 1866
Plendil Extended-Release Tablets (0.5% to 1.5%) 623
Pravachol Tablets 1099
Precose Tablets 906
Prevacid Delayed-Release Capsules 3292
PREVPAC (Less than 1%) 3298
▲ Priftin Tablets (5.3%) 758
Prilosec Delayed-Release Capsules (Rare) 628
Primaxin I.M. 2158
Primaxin I.V. 2160
Procardia Capsules (Rare) 2708
Procardia XL Extended Release Tablets (Rare) 2710
▲ Prograf (3% to 15%) 1393
Protonix I.V. (Greater than or equal to 1%) 3580
Protonix Tablets (Greater than or equal to 1%) 3577
Protopic Ointment (Greater than or equal to 1%) 1397
Prozac Pulvules, Liquid, and Weekly Capsules (Rare) 1238
▲ Rapamune Oral Solution and Tablets (3% to 20%) 3584
Remeron Tablets (Rare; 2.0%) 2483
Remeron SolTab Tablets (Rare; 2.0%) 2486
▲ Remicade for IV Injection (37%) 1178
▲ Rescriptor Tablets (2% to 6.7%) 526
Rifamate Capsules 767
Rifater Tablets 769
Risperdal (Infrequent) 1796
Rocaltrol 2991
▲ Rocephin Injectable Vials, ADD-Vantage, Galaxy, Bulk (3.3%) 2993
Sectral Capsules 3589
▲ Serostim for Injection (10.2%) 3229
Serzone Tablets (Infrequent) 1104
Singulair (2.1%) 2181
Solu-Medrol Sterile Powder 2855
Sonata Capsules (Rare) 3591
▲ Soriatane Capsules (Approximately 1 in 3 patients) 3003
Sporanox Injection (2%) 1804
Sporanox Injection (2%) 2509
Stromectol Tablets (2%) 2185
Suprax (Less than 2%) 1877
Sustiva Capsules (2%) 1258
Symmetrel 1328
Synagis Intramuscular (More than 1%) 2028
Synarel Nasal Solution for Endometriosis (One patient) 3205
Synercid I.V. 775
Tarka Tablets 508
Tasmar Tablets (1% to 5%) 3010
▲ Tazicef for Injection (1 in 15 patients) 1647
▲ Tazicef Galaxy Container (1 in 15 patients) 1650
▲ Tazicef Pharmacy Bulk Package (1 in 15 patients) 1653
▲ Tazidime Vials, Faspak & ADD-Vantage (1 in 15) 1966
Tequin Injection (Less than 0.1%) 1110
Tequin Tablets (Less than 0.1%) 1110
Teveten Tablets (Less than 1%) 3327
Thalomid Capsules 1154
Tiazac Capsules (Less than 2%) 1378
Ticlid Tablets (Rare) 3015
Timentin Injection- ADD-Vantage Vial 1661
Timentin Injection-Galaxy Container 1664
Timentin Injection-Pharmacy Bulk Package 1666
Timentin for Intravenous Administration 1658
Topamax Sprinkle Capsules (Infrequent) 2590
Topamax Tablets (Infrequent) 2590
Trasylol Injection 909
Trecator-SC Tablets 3598
Tricor Capsules, Micronized 513
▲ Trisenox Injection (20%) 1158
▲ Trizivir Tablets (3.7%) 1669
Trovan (Greater than or equal to 1%) 2722
Unasyn for Injection 2728
Uniretic Tablets (More than 1%) 3178
Vantin Tablets and Oral Suspension 2860
Vascor Tablets (0.5% to 2.0%) 2602
Verelan Capsules 3184
Verelan PM Capsules 3186
Vermox Chewable Tablets (Rare) 2017
▲ Videx (2% to 9%) 1138
▲ Videx EC Capsules (2% to 39%) 1143
Viracept 532
▲ Viramune Oral Suspension (3.4%) 1060
▲ Viramune Tablets (3.4%) 1060
Vistide Injection 1445
▲ Zanaflex Tablets (3%) 1305
Zantac 1690
Zantac Injection 1688
Zantac Syrup 1690
Zebeta Tablets 1885
▲ Zerit (13%) 1147
▲ Zinacef Injection (1 in 25 patients) 1696
▲ Zinacef for Injection (1 in 25 patients) 1696
Zithromax Capsules, 250 mg (1% to 2%) 2743
▲ Zithromax for IV Infusion (4% to 6%) 2748
Zithromax for Oral Suspension, 1 g (1% to 2%) 2743
Zithromax for Oral Suspension, 300 mg, 600 mg, 900 mg, 1200 mg (1% to 2%) 2739
Zithromax Tablets, 250 mg (1% to 2%) 2739
Zithromax Tablets, 600 mg (1% to 2%) 2743
Zocor Tablets 2219
▲ Zofran Injection (Approximately 5% of patients) 1698
Zofran (Approximately 1% to 2%) 1703
Zofran ODT Orally Disintegrating Tablets (Approximately 1% to 2%) 1703
Zoladex (Less than 1%) 702
Zoladex 3-month 706
Zoloft (Infrequent) 2751
Zonegran Capsules (Rare) 1307
Zosyn 1890
Zosyn in Galaxy Containers 1894
Zyprexa Tablets (2%) 1973
Zyprexa ZYDIS Orally Disintegrating Tablets (2%) 1973
▲ Zyvox (1.7% to 9.6%) 2871

Albuminuria
Accuretic Tablets 2614
Aciphex Tablets 1267
Aciphex Tablets 1783
Amphotec (1% to 5%) 1774
Arava Tablets (1% to 3%) 724
Astelin Nasal Spray (Infrequent) 3339
Atacand Tablets (More than 1%) 595
Atacand HCT Tablets 597
Calcijex Injection 411
Carbatrol Capsules 3234
Ceclor CD Tablets (0.3%) 1279
▲ CellCept Capsules (3%) 2951
▲ CellCept Intravenous (3%) 2951
▲ CellCept Oral Suspension (3%) 2951
▲ CellCept Tablets (3% to 10 %) 2951
Cerebyx Injection (Infrequent) 2619
Chirocaine Injection (2.9%) 2909
Cipro I.V. (1% or less) 893
Cipro I.V. Pharmacy Bulk Package (Less than 1%) 897
Cipro 887
Coreg Tablets (1% to 2%) 1508
Dapsone Tablets USP 1780
Dopram Injectable 2931
Doxil Injection (1% to 5%) 566
Effexor Tablets (Infrequent) 3495
Effexor XR Capsules (Infrequent) 3499
Eskalith 1527
Evoxac Capsules (Less than 1%) 1217
Exelon Capsules (Infrequent) 2342
Exelon Oral Solution (Infrequent) 2345
Floxin I.V. 2526
Floxin Tablets 2529
Foscavir Injection (Between 1% and 5%) 605
Geodon Capsules (Infrequent) 2688
Hectorol Capsules 1064
Hectorol Injection 1066
Hivid Tablets (Less than 1%) 2975
Intron A for Injection (Less than 5%) 3120
Lipitor Tablets (Less than 2%) 2639
Lipitor Tablets (Less than 2%) 2696
Lithium Carbonate 3061
Lithium Citrate Syrup 3061
Lithobid Slow-Release Tablets 3255
Lufyllin Tablets 3347
Lufyllin-400 Tablets 3347
Lufyllin-GG Elixir 3348
Lufyllin-GG Tablets 3348
Megace Oral Suspension (1% to 3%) 1124
Mobic Tablets (Less than 2%) 1054
Naprelan Tablets (Less than 1%) 1293
Nexium Delayed-Release Capsules (Less than 1%) 619
Noroxin Tablets 2145
Ovidrel for Injection (Less than 2%) 3220
Pentasa Capsules (Less than 1%) 3239
Pletal Tablets (Less than 2%) 2605
Pletal Tablets (Less than 2%) 2848
Prevacid Delayed-Release Capsules (Less than 1%) 3292
PREVPAC (Less than 1%) 3298
▲ Prograf (3% to 15%) 1393
Protonix I.V. (Less than 1%) 3580
Protonix Tablets (Less than 1%) 3577
Provigil Tablets (1%) 1193
Prozac Pulvules, Liquid, and Weekly Capsules (Infrequent) 1238
▲ Rapamune Oral Solution and Tablets (3% to 20%) 3584
Relafen Tablets (Less than 1%) 1617
Requip Tablets (Infrequent) 1621
Rocaltrol 2991
Sandostatin LAR Depot (1% to 4%) 2395
Sarafem Pulvules (Infrequent) 1962
▲ Serostim for Injection (15.1%) 3229
▲ Simulect for Injection (3% to 10%) 2399
Sonata Capsules (Rare) 3591
Sporanox Capsules (1.2%) 1800
Sporanox Injection (1%) 1804
Sporanox Injection (1%) 2509
Tegretol/Tegretol-XR 2404
Teveten Tablets (Less than 1%) 3327
▲ Thalomid Capsules (3.1% to 8.3%) 1154
Topamax Sprinkle Capsules (Infrequent) 2590
Topamax Tablets (Infrequent) 2590
Ultracet Tablets (Less than 1%) 2597
Uniretic Tablets (Less than 1%) 3178
Uroqid-Acid No. 2 Tablets 947
▲ Visudyne for Injection (1% to 10%) ⊙ 308
Xanax Tablets (Less than 1%) 2865
Zanaflex Tablets (Rare) 1305
Zonegran Capsules (Rare) 1307
Zyprexa Tablets (Rare) 1973
Zyprexa ZYDIS Orally Disintegrating Tablets (Rare) 1973

Alcohol, increased sensitivity to
Ativan Injection 3478
Betaseron for SC Injection 988
Catapres Tablets 1037
Celexa (Infrequent) 1365
Clorpres Tablets 1002
Combipres Tablets 1040
Copaxone for Injection (Infrequent) 3306
Duraclon Injection 3057
Effexor Tablets (Rare) 3495
Effexor XR Capsules (Rare) 3499
Lamictal (Rare) 1567
Neurontin Capsules (Rare) 2655
Neurontin Oral Solution (Rare) 2655
Neurontin Tablets (Rare) 2655
Nicotinex Elixir ▣ 633
▲ Nilandron Tablets (5%) 753
▲ Protopic Ointment (Up to 7%) 1397
Prozac Pulvules, Liquid, and Weekly Capsules (Rare) 1238
Rescriptor Tablets (Less than 2%) 526
Sarafem Pulvules (Rare) 1962
Seroquel Tablets (Infrequent) 684
Soriatane Capsules (Less than 1%) 3003
Tequin Injection (Less than 0.1%) 1110
Tequin Tablets (Less than 0.1%) 1110
Teveten Tablets (Less than 1%) 3327
Topamax Sprinkle Capsules (Rare) 2590
Topamax Tablets (Rare) 2590
Trovan (Less than 1%) 2722

Alcohol abuse
Effexor Tablets (Rare) 3495
Effexor XR Capsules (Rare) 3499
Paxil (Infrequent) 1609
Zyprexa Tablets (Infrequent) 1973
Zyprexa ZYDIS Orally Disintegrating Tablets (Infrequent) 1973

Aldosterone synthesis, suppression
Heparin Lock Flush Solution 3509
Heparin Sodium Injection 3511

Alkalinuria
Floxin I.V. (More than or equal to 1%) 2526
Floxin Tablets (More than or equal to 1%) 2529

Alkalosis
Ancef for Injection 1474
Ancef Injection 1474
▲ CellCept Capsules (3% to 10%) 2951
▲ CellCept Intravenous (3% to 10%) 2951
▲ CellCept Oral Suspension (3% to 10%) 2951
▲ CellCept Tablets (3% to 10%) 2951
Kefurox Vials, ADD-Vantage (1 in 50) 1948
Naprelan Tablets (Less than 1%) 1293
▲ Prograf (3% to 15%) 1393
▲ Proleukin for Injection (4%) 1199

Alkalosis, metabolic
Cerebyx Injection (Infrequent) 2619
Indocin I.V. (Less than 3%) 2115

Allergic reactions
Abelcet Injection 1273
AccuNeb Inhalation Solution (0.9% to 3.4%) 1230
Accutane Capsules 2944
Aceon Tablets (2 mg, 4 mg, 8 mg) (2.0%) 3249
Aciphex Tablets 1267
Aciphex Tablets 1783
Actiq (Less than 1%) 1184
Activase I.V. (Very rare) 1410

Activella Tablets 2764
▲ Acular Ophthalmic Solution (Approximately 1% to 10%) 544
▲ Acular PF Ophthalmic Solution (Approximately 1% to 10%) 544
Adipex-P 1406
Aggrastat 2031
Aggrenox Capsules (Less than 1%) 1026
Alamast Ophthalmic Solution (Less than 5%) 3092
Albenza Tablets (Rare) 1463
Aleve Tablets, Caplets and Gelcaps ▣602
Alkeran for Injection 1465
Alkeran Tablets 1466
Alphagan P Ophthalmic Solution (1% to 4%) 546
Amaryl Tablets (Less than 1%) 717
Ambien Tablets (Rare) 3191
AmBisome for Injection (Less common) 1383
Amerge Tablets (Rare) 1467
Amicar Injection 3608
Amicar Syrup 3608
Amicar Tablets 3608
Amoxil Chewable Tablets 1471
Amoxil for Oral Suspension 1471
Amoxil 1471
Amphotec (1% to 5%) 1774
Ancef for Injection 1474
Ancef Injection 1474
Ancobon Capsules 1730
Antivenin (Micrurus fulvius) 3477
Antivenin Polyvalent 3475
AquaMEPHYTON Injection 2042
Aquasol A Parenteral (Rare) 593
Arava Tablets (2%) 724
Aredia for Injection (Rare) 2309
Arthrotec Tablets (0.1%) 3195
Astelin Nasal Spray (Infrequent) 3339
Atromid-S Capsules 3483
Atrovent Inhalation Aerosol 1030
Attenuvax (Rare) 2044
Augmentin Chewable Tablets 1482
Augmentin Powder for Oral Suspension 1482
Augmentin Tablets 1485
Autoplex T 2294
Avelox Tablets (0.05% to 1%) 879
Azelex Cream 547
Azopt Ophthalmic Suspension (Less than 1%) 536
▲ Bactrim (Among most common) 2949
Baycol Tablets 883
Beano (Rare) ▣809
Betasept Surgical Scrub 2895
Betimol Ophthalmic Solution (1% to 5%) ⊙324
Betoptic S Ophthalmic Suspension 537
Biaxin/Biaxin XL 403
Bicillin L-A Injection 2242
Campath Ampules 992
Carac Cream (1.2%) 1222
Cardura Tablets 2668
▲ Carnitor Injection (2% to 6%) 3242
Cataflam Tablets 2315
Catapres Tablets 1037
Ceclor CD Tablets 1279
Ceclor 1905
Cedax 1021
Ceftin 1898
Celebrex Capsules (0.1% to 1.9%) 2676
Celebrex Capsules (0.1% to 1.9%) 2780
CellCept Capsules 2951
CellCept Intravenous 2951
CellCept Oral Suspension 2951
CellCept Tablets 2951
▲ Ceptaz for Injection (Among most common) 1499
Cetacaine Topical Anesthetic 1196
Chloromycetin Ophthalmic Ointment, 1% ⊙296
Ciloxan (Less than 1%) 538
Cipro I.V. (1% or less) 893
Cipro I.V. Pharmacy Bulk Package (Less than 1%) 897
Cipro 887
Clomid Tablets 735
Cogentin Injection 2055
Colyte with Flavor Packs for Oral Solution (Isolated cases) 3170
Compazine 1505
Copaxone for Injection (Rare) 3306
Coreg Tablets (1% to 2%) 1508
Cosopt Sterile Ophthalmic Solution 2065
Coumadin for Injection (Infrequent) 1243
Coumadin Tablets (Infrequent) 1243
Creon 5 Capsules (Less frequent) 3251
Creon 10 Capsules (Less frequent) 3251
Creon 20 Capsules (Less frequent) 3251
Crinone (Less than 5%) 3213
CytoGam Intravenous (Rare) 2026
Cytomel Tablets (Rare) 1817
Cytovene 2959
▲ DaunoXome Injection (3% to 21%) 1442
DDAVP Injection 4 mcg/mL (Rare) 737
DDAVP Nasal Spray 738
DDAVP Rhinal Tube 738
DDAVP Tablets (Rare) 739
Depakene 421
Depakote Tablets (1% to 5%) 430
Depakote ER Tablets 436
Depen Titratable Tablets 3341
Depo-Provera Contraceptive Injection (Fewer than 1%) 2798
Desmopressin Acetate Injection (Rare) 1344
D.H.E. 45 Injection 2334
DiaBeta Tablets (1.5%) 741
Digibind Powder (Rare) 1514
Dilantin-125 Oral Suspension 2625
Dilaudid Oral Liquid 445
Dilaudid Tablets - 8 mg 445
Diovan Capsules 2337
Diovan HCT Tablets (Greater than 0.2%) 2338
Donnatal 2929
Donnatal Extentabs 2930
Donnatal Tablets 2929
Doxil Injection (1% to 5%) 566
Duranest Injections 600
Dynabac Tablets (0.1% to 1%) 2269
E.E.S. 450
Effexor Tablets (Infrequent) 3495
Effexor XR Capsules (Infrequent) 3499
8-MOP Capsules 1727
ELA-Max Cream 1340
ELA-Max 5 Cream 1340
Elmiron Capsules (Less than or equal to 1%) 570
Elspar for Injection 2092
Emcyt Capsules 2810
Emla 602
Enbrel for Injection (Less than 0.5%) 1752
Enbrel for Injection (Less than 0.5%) 3504
Epifrin Sterile Ophthalmic Solution ⊙235
Epogen for Injection (Rare) 582
Ergamisol Tablets 1789
EryPed 446
Ery-Tab Tablets 448
Erythrocin Stearate Filmtab Tablets 452
Estrace Vaginal Cream 3358
Estrace Tablets 3361
Estring Vaginal Ring (1%) 2811
Ethyol for Injection 2029
Evoxac Capsules (1% to 3%) 1217
Exelon Capsules (Frequent) 2342
Exelon Oral Solution (Frequent) 2345
Feiba VH 843
Felbatol (Rare) 3343
femhrt Tablets 2635
Flomax Capsules 1044
Florinef Acetate Tablets 2250
FluShield Influenza Vaccine (Rare) 3521
Fluzone Vaccine (Rare) 802
FML Ophthalmic Suspension ⊙236
▲ Fortaz (Among most common) 1541
Fortovase Capsules (Less than 2%) 2970
Fragmin Injection (Rare) 2814
Sterile FUDR (Remote possibility) 2974
Gabitril Tablets (Frequent) 1189
Gamimune N, 5% Solvent/Detergent Treated 925
Gamimune N, 10% Solvent/Detergent Treated 928
Gengraf Capsules (1% to less than 3%) 457
Genoptic Ophthalmic Ointment (Rare) ⊙239
Genoptic Sterile Ophthalmic Solution (Rare) ⊙239
Ginsana Sport Capsules ▣831
Gliadel Wafer (1%) 1723
GlucaGen for Injection Diagnostic Kit 949
Glucagon for Injection Vials and Emergency Kit 1924
Halcion Tablets (Rare) 2823
Haldol Injection, Tablets and Concentrate 2533
Hemofil M (Extremely rare) 847
▲ Herceptin I.V. (3%) 1414
Hivid Tablets (Less than 1%) 2975
Humalog (Less common) 1926
Humalog Mix 75/25 Pen 1928
Humate-P Concentrate (Rare) 790
Humegon for Injection 2468
Humulin 50/50, 100 Units (Less common to occasional) 1934
Humulin 70/30, 100 Units 1935
Humulin 70/30 Pen 1936
Humulin L, 100 Units 1937
Humulin R Regular (U-500) 1943
Humulin N NPH Pen 1940
Hurricaine Topical Anesthetic Gel, 1 oz. Fresh Mint, Wild Cherry, Pina Colada, Watermelon, 1/6 oz. Wild Cherry, Watermelon (Rare) ▣618
Hurricaine Topical Anesthetic Liquid, 1 oz. Wild Cherry, Pina Colada, .25 ml Dry Handle Swab Wild Cherry, 1/6 oz. Wild Cherry (Rare) ▣618
Hurricaine Topical Anesthetic Spray Extension Tubes (200) (Rare) ▣618
Hurricaine Topical Anesthetic Spray Kit, 2 oz. Wild Cherry (Rare) ▣618
Hurricaine Topical Anesthetic Spray, 2 oz. Wild Cherry (Rare) ▣618
Hyalgan Solution (Three cases) 3080
Hycamtin for Injection (Infrequent) 1546
Hytrin Capsules (Rare) 464
Ifex for Injection (Less than 1%) 1123
Iletin II, Regular (Pork), 100 Units 1947
Inderide Tablets 3517
▲ Infergen (3% to 7%) 1777
Innohep Injection 1248
Integrilin Injection 1213
Integrilin Injection 1828
Invirase Capsules (Less than 2%) 2979
Iopidine Sterile Ophthalmic Solution ⊙212
Keflex 1237
Kefzol Vials, ADD-Vantage 1951
Klonopin Tablets (2%) 2983
Koāte-DVI 931
Koāte-HP 932
Kogenate FS 936
Kytril Injection (Rare) 2986
Lamictal (Infrequent) 1567
Lamisil Tablets (Rare) 2360
Lantus Injection 742
Lescol Capsules (2.3%) 2361
Lescol Capsules (2.3%) 2925
Lescol XL Tablets (1%) 2361
Lescol XL Tablets (1%) 2925
Leukeran Tablets 1591
▲ Leukine (12%) 1755
Levaquin 2537
Levsin/Levsinex/Levbid 3172
Lidoderm Patch (Rare) 1319
Lipitor Tablets (Up to 2.8%) 2639
Lipitor Tablets (Up to 2.8%) 2696
Lodine (Less than 1%) 3528
Lodine XL Extended-Release Tablets (Less than 1%) 3530
Lorabid Suspension and Pulvules 2251
Lortab 3319
Lortab Elixir 3317
Lovenox Injection 746
Lupron Depot-4 Month 30 mg (Less than 5%) 3289
Luvox Tablets (25, 50, 100 mg) (Infrequent) 3256
Matulane Capsules 3246
Maxidone Tablets CIII 3399
May-Vita Elixir 2224
Mefoxin for Injection 2124
Mefoxin Premixed Intravenous Solution 2127
Mepron Suspension (0.8% to 1.1%) 1598
Meridia Capsules (1.5%) 481
Merrem I.V. 673
Metamucil 2877
▲ MetroLotion (3%) 1405
Miacalcin Injection (A few cases) 2373
Miacalcin Nasal Spray (Less than 1%) 2375
Micardis Tablets (More than 0.3%) 1049
Micardis HCT Tablets 1051
Miltown Tablets 3349
Minipress Capsules 2699
Minocin Intravenous (Rare) 1862
Minocin Oral Suspension 1865
Mirapex Tablets (1% or more) 2834
Mobic Tablets (Less than 2%) 1054
Monoclate P Concentrate 793
Mononine Concentrate 794
Children's Motrin Oral Suspension and Chewable Tablets 2006
Children's Motrin Cold Oral Suspension 2007
Children's Motrin Oral Suspension ▣643
Infants' Motrin Concentrated Drops 2006
Junior Strength Motrin Caplets and Chewable Tablets 2006
Motrin IB Tablets, Caplets, and Gelcaps 2002
Motrin Sinus Headache Caplets 2005
Movana Tablets (Rare) ▣832
Mumpsvax (Extremely rare) 2141
Myobloc Injectable Solution (2% or greater) 1291
Naprelan Tablets (Less than 1%) 1293
Naropin Injection (Rare) 612
Natacyn Antifungal Ophthalmic Suspension (One case) ⊙216
Navelbine Injection 1604
Nebcin Vials, Hyporets & ADD-Vantage (Rare) 1955
Neoral Soft Gelatin Capsules (1% to less than 3%) 2380
Neoral Oral Solution (1% to less than 3%) 2380
Neosporin G.U. Irrigant Sterile 2256
Nesacaine/Nesacaine MPF (Rare) 617
Neupogen for Injection (Less than 1 in 4000) 587
Neurontin Capsules (Infrequent) 2655
Neurontin Oral Solution 2655
Neurontin Tablets (Infrequent) 2655
Nexium Delayed-Release Capsules (Less than 1%) 619
▲ Nicotrol Inhaler (Greater than 3%) 2840
Nicotrol Nasal Spray (Less than 1%) 2843
▲ Nipent for Injection (2% to 11%) 3272
Nitro-Dur Transdermal Infusion System (Uncommon) 1834
Nitro-Dur Transdermal Infusion System (Uncommon) 3134
▲ Nizoral 2% Cream (5%) 3620
Norco 5/325 Tablets CIII 3424
Norco 7.5/325 Tablets CIII 3425
Norco 10/325 Tablets CIII 3425
Norco 10/325 Tablets CIII 3427
Noroxin Tablets (Less frequent) 2145
Norvasc Tablets (More than 0.1% to 1%) 2704
Norvir Capsules (Less than 2%) 487
Norvir Oral Solution (Less than 2%) 487
Novolin 70/30 PenFill (Rare) 2423
Novolin 70/30 Prefilled Disposable Insulin Delivery System (Rare) 2425
Novolin N PenFill (Rare) 2423
Novolin R PenFill (Rare) 2423
NovoLog Injection 2427
NovoSeven (1%) 2430
Nubain Injection (1% or less) 1323
NuLev Orally Disintegrating Tablets 3176
NuLYTELY, Cherry Flavor, Lemon-Lime Flavor, and Orange Flavor NuLYTELY for Oral Solution (Isolated cases) 1068
Numorphan 1324
Nutropin AQ Injection 1420
Nutropin for Injection 1417
Nystatin Vaginal Tablets, USP (Rare) 2445
Nystop Topical Powder USP (More common) 2608
Obegyn Prenatal Supplement 1362
Omnicef 493
▲ Oncaspar (Greater than 5%) 756
OptiPranolol Metipranolol Ophthalmic Solution 0.3% (A small number of patients) ⊙263
Orgaran Injection 2480
Orudis Capsules (Less than 1%) 3548
Oruvail Capsules (Less than 1%) 3548
Ovidrel for Injection 3220
ParaGard T 380A Intrauterine Copper Contraceptive 2582
▲ Paraplatin for Injection (2% to 12%) 1126
Paxil (Infrequent) 1609
PCE Dispertab Tablets 498
Pediazole Suspension 3050
Pentasa Capsules 3239
Pergonal for Injection 3223
Phenergan Injection 3553
PhosLo 1069
Phrenilin (Infrequent) 578
Plasbumin-5 (Rare) 939
Plasbumin-20 (Rare) 940
Plasbumin-25 (Rare) 941
Plavix Tablets (Less than 1%) 1097
Plavix Tablets (Less than 1%) 3084
Polocaine Injection, USP 625
Polocaine-MPF Injection, USP 625
Polysporin Ophthalmic Ointment Sterile ⊙301
Prandin Tablets (0.5, 1, and 2 mg) (1% to 2%) 2432
Pred Forte Ophthalmic Suspension ⊙246
Pred Mild Sterile Ophthalmic Suspension ⊙249
PREVPAC 3298
Prilosec Delayed-Release Capsules 628
Primaxin I.M. 2158
Procrit for Injection (Rare) 2502
▲ Prograf (3% to 15%) 1393
Prolastin (Occasional) 943
Proleukin for Injection (1%) 1199
Propine Ophthalmic Solution ⊙250
ProSom Tablets (Infrequent) 500
Prostigmin Injectable 1744
Prostigmin Tablets 1744
Protonix I.V. (Less than 1%) 3580
Protonix Tablets (Less than 1%) 3577
▲ Protopic Ointment (6% to 22%) 1397
▲ Proventil HFA Inhalation Aerosol (6%) 3150
Provigil Tablets (At least 1%) 1193
▲ Prozac Pulvules, Liquid, and Weekly Capsules (7%) 1238
Psoriatec Cream (Very few instances) 3247
Pulmicort Respules (1% to 3%) 632

(▣ Described in PDR For Nonprescription Drugs) Incidence data in parenthesis; ▲ 3% or more (⊙ Described in PDR For Ophthalmic Medicines™)

Quixin Ophthalmic Solution (Less than 1%) 3093
Rabies Vaccine RabAvert (Rare) 1203
Recombinate (Extremely rare) 853
ReFacto Vials 1437
▲ Refludan for Injection (3.5%) 761
ReoPro Vials 1958
Repronex for Intramuscular and Subcutaneous Injection 1347
Rescriptor Tablets (Less than 2%) 526
Rescula Ophthalmic Solution (1% to 5%) ⊙ 306
Retavase Vials (3 patients) 1182
Risperdal (Rare) 1796
Robinul Forte Tablets 1358
Robinul Injectable 2940
Robinul Tablets 1358
Rocaltrol (One case) 2991
Roxicodone Tablets (Less than 3%) 3067
Salagen Tablets (1% to 2%) 2229
Sandimmune (2% or less) 2388
Sandostatin Injection (Less than 1%) 2394
▲ Sandostatin LAR Depot (5% to 15%) 2395
Sarafem Pulvules 1962
Sedapap Tablets 50 mg/650 mg (Infrequent) 2225
Selsun Rx 2.5% Lotion, USP 3053
Sensorcaine (Rare) 643
Sensorcaine-MPF Injection (Rare) 643
▲ Septra Suspension (Among most common) 2265
▲ Septra Tablets (Among most common) 2265
▲ Septra DS Tablets (Among most common) 2265
Serophene Tablets 3226
▲ Serostim for Injection (1% to 10%) 3229
Serzone Tablets (Infrequent) 1104
Silvadene Cream 1% 2267
Sinequan (Occasional) 2713
Soma Tablets 3353
Soma Compound Tablets 3354
Soma Compound w/Codeine Tablets 3355
Sporanox Capsules 1800
Sporanox Oral Solution 1808
Sporanox Oral Solution 2512
Stelazine (Occasional) 1640
Stimate Nasal Spray 796
Streptase for Infusion (1% to 4%) 647
Sultrin Triple Sulfa Cream (Frequent) 2587
Suprax 1877
Sustiva Capsules 1258
Symmetrel 1328
Synarel Nasal Solution for Central Precocious Puberty (2.6%) 3204
Synercid I.V. (Less than 1%) 775
Tagamet (Rare) 1644
Talacen Caplets 3089
Tasmar Tablets (Infrequent) 3010
▲ Tazicef for Injection (Among most common) 1647
▲ Tazicef Galaxy Container (Among most common) 1650
▲ Tazicef Pharmacy Bulk Package (Among most common) 1653
Tequin Injection (0.1% to 3%) 1110
Tequin Tablets (0.1% to 3%) 1110
Terra-Cortril Ophthalmic Suspension 2716
Thalomid Capsules 1154
Thioplex for Injection (Rare) 1765
Thiothixene Capsules 2290
Thorazine (Occasional) 1656
Thrombin-JMI 1824
Thyrel TRH for Injection (Less frequent) 3630
Tiazac Capsules (1%) 1378
Tice BCG, BCG Live (2.1%) 2489
Ticlid Tablets 3015
Timolol GFS ⊙ 266
Timoptic in Ocudose 2192
Timoptic Sterile Ophthalmic Solution 2190
Timoptic-XE Sterile Ophthalmic Gel Forming Solution 2194
TNKase I.V. (Rare) 1430
Trasylol Injection (0.3%) 909
Traumeel Injection Solution (Rare) 1726
Tricor Capsules, Micronized 513
Trileptal Oral Suspension (Up to 2%) 2407
Trileptal Tablets (Up to 2%) 2407
Tri-Nasal Spray (2%) 2274
Triostat Injection (Rare) 1825
Trovan (Less than 1%) 2722
Trusopt Sterile Ophthalmic Solution 2196
Twinrix Vaccine 1674
Tylenol with Codeine 2595
Tylox Capsules 2597
TYPHIM Vi Vaccine (Rare) 825
Ultracet Tablets 2597
Ultram Tablets (Less than 1%) 2600
Ultrase Capsules (Less frequent) 835
Ultrase MT Capsules (Less frequent) 835
Uniretic Tablets (Less than 1%) 3178
Urobiotic-250 Capsules (Rare) 2731
▲ Vagifem Tablets (3% to 5%) 2857
Vanceril Double Strength Inhalation Aerosol (Fewer than 2%) 3167
Vantin Tablets and Oral Suspension 2860
Varivax (Greater than or equal to 1%) 2202
Versed Injection (Less than 1%) 3027
Viagra Tablets (Less than 2%) 2732
Vibramycin Hyclate Intravenous 2737
Vicodin Tablets 516
Vicodin ES Tablets 517
Vicodin HP Tablets 518
Vicoprofen Tablets (Less than 1%) 520
Vioxx (Greater than 0.1% to 1.9%) 2213
Viracept 532
Viramune Oral Suspension 1060
Viramune Tablets 1060
Vistide Injection 1445
Vitravene for Injection (2% to 5%) ⊙ 310
Voltaren Tablets 2315
Voltaren-XR Tablets 2315
Warfarin Sodium Tablets, USP 3302
Wellbutrin Tablets 1680
Wellbutrin SR Sustained-Release Tablets 1684
▲ Xanax Tablets (3.8%) 2865
Xylocaine Injections (Extremely rare) 653
Yasmin 28 Tablets 980
Zaditor Ophthalmic Solution (Less than 5%) 2304
Zanaflex Tablets (Infrequent) 1305
Zemuron Injection (Rare) 2491
▲ Zerit (9%) 1147
Zinacef Injection 1696
Zinacef for Injection 1696
Zithromax Capsules, 250 mg (Rare) 2743
Zithromax for IV Infusion (Rare) 2748
Zithromax for Oral Suspension, 1 g (Rare) 2743
Zithromax for Oral Suspension, 300 mg, 600 mg, 900 mg, 1200 mg (Rare) 2739
Zithromax Tablets, 250 mg (Rare) 2739
Zithromax Tablets, 600 mg (Rare) 2743
Zoladex (1% or greater) 702
Zoladex 3-month 706
Zoloft (Rare) 2751
Zomig Tablets (Infrequent) 708
Zomig-ZMT Tablets (Infrequent) 708
Zonegran Capsules (Infrequent) 1307
Zosyn 1890
Zosyn in Galaxy Containers 1894
Zyban Sustained-Release Tablets (1%) 1710

Allergic sensitization

▲ Alferon N Injection (1% to 18%) 1770
▲ Blephamide Ophthalmic Ointment (Among most often) 547
▲ Blephamide Ophthalmic Suspension (Most often) 548
▲ Catapres-TTS (5 of 101 patients) 1038
Chloroptic Sterile Ophthalmic Ointment ⊙ 234
Citracal Prenatal Rx Tablets 2231
Cortisporin Ophthalmic Suspension ⊙ 297
▲ FML-S Liquifilm Sterile Ophthalmic Suspension (Among most often) ⊙ 238
NataChew Tablets (Rare) 3364
▲ NeoDecadron Sterile Ophthalmic Solution (Most often) 2144
Neosporin Ophthalmic Ointment Sterile ⊙ 299
Neosporin Ophthalmic Solution Sterile ⊙ 300
Nestabs RX Tablets 1351
Ovide Lotion 2023
▲ Poly-Pred Liquifilm Ophthalmic Suspension (Most often) ⊙ 245
Polysporin Ophthalmic Ointment ⊙ 301
PreCare Chewable Tablets 3312
PreCare Conceive Tablets 3312
PreCare Prenatal Caplets 3313
▲ Pred-G Ophthalmic Suspension (Most often) ⊙ 247
Pred-G Sterile Ophthalmic Ointment ⊙ 248
PremesisRx Tablets 3313

Allergic vasospastic reactions

Heparin Lock Flush Solution 3509
Heparin Sodium Injection 3511

Allergy
(*see under* Allergic reactions)

Alopecia

Accupril Tablets (0.5% to 1.0%) 2611
Accuretic Tablets (0.5% to 1%) 2614
Accutane Capsules 2944
Aciphex Tablets 1267
Aciphex Tablets 1783
Actiq (Less than 1%) 1184
Activella Tablets 2764
Adalat CC Tablets (Rare) 877
▲ Adriamycin PFS/RDF Injection (Most cases) 2767
Aggrenox Capsules 1026
Agrylin Capsules (1% to 5%) 3232
Albenza Tablets (Less than 1.0% to 1.6%) 1463
Aldoclor Tablets 2035
Aldoril Tablets 2039
Alesse-21 Tablets 3468
Alesse-28 Tablets 3473
Alkeran for Injection 1465
Alkeran Tablets 1466
Aloprim for Injection (Less than 1%) 2292
Alora Transdermal System 3372
AmBisome for Injection (Less common) 1383
Amerge Tablets (Rare) 1467
Amphotec (1% to 5%) 1774
Anadrol-50 Tablets 3321
Anaprox Tablets (Less than 1%) 2967
Anaprox DS Tablets (Less than 1%) 2967
AndroGel (1%) 3322
Aquasol A Parenteral 593
Aralen Tablets 3075
▲ Arava Tablets (10%) 724
Aricept Tablets (Infrequent) 1270
Aricept Tablets (Infrequent) 2665
▲ Aromasin Tablets (2% to 5%) 2769
Arthrotec Tablets (Rare) 3195
Asacol Delayed-Release Tablets 2884
Atacand HCT Tablets 597
Atromid-S Capsules (Less frequent) 3483
Atrovent Inhalation Aerosol (Less frequent) 1030
▲ Avonex (4%) 1013
Azopt Ophthalmic Suspension (Less than 1%) 536
Azulfidine EN-tabs Tablets (Rare) 2775
Baycol Tablets 883
Betagan ⊙ 228
Betapace Tablets (Rare) 950
Betapace AF Tablets (Rare) 954
▲ Betaseron for SC Injection (4%) 988
Betaxon Ophthalmic Suspension (Less than 2%) 537
▲ Betimol Ophthalmic Solution (More than 5%) ⊙ 324
Betoptic S Ophthalmic Suspension (Rare) 537
Blocadren Tablets (Less than 1%) 2046
Brevicon 28-Day Tablets 3380
Canasa Rectal Suppositories 829
Captopril Tablets (About 0.5% to 2%) 2281
Carbatrol Capsules 3234
Cardizem Injectable 1018
Cardizem Lyo-Ject Syringe 1018
Cardizem Monovial 1018
Cardizem CD Capsules (Infrequent) 1016
Cardura Tablets (Less than 0.5%) 2668
▲ Casodex Tablets (2% to 5%) 662
Cataflam Tablets (Less than 1%) 2315
Catapres Tablets 1037
Catapres-TTS 1038
Celebrex Capsules (0.1% to 1.9%) 2676
Celebrex Capsules (0.1% to 1.9%) 2780
Celexa (Infrequent) 1365
▲ CellCept Capsules (3%) 2951
▲ CellCept Intravenous (3%) 2951
▲ CellCept Oral Suspension (3%) 2951
▲ CellCept Tablets (3%) 2951
Cenestin Tablets 1263
▲ Cerubidine for Injection (In most patients) 947
Cipro HC Otic Suspension (One patient) 540
Claritin (Rare) 3100
Claritin-D 12 Hour Extended Release Tablets 3102
Claritin-D 24 Hour Extended Release Tablets 3104
Climara Transdermal System 958
Clinoril Tablets (Less than 1%) 2053
Clomid Tablets (Fewer than 1%) 735
Clorpres Tablets (About 2 in 1,000) 1002
Cognex Capsules (Infrequent) 1351
Colazal Capsules 3069
Combipres Tablets (About 2 in 1,000) 1040
Combivent Inhalation Aerosol 1041
Combivir Tablets 1502
Comvax 2056
Concerta Extended-Release Tablets 1998
Concerta Tablets 561
Copaxone for Injection (At least 2%) 3306
Cordarone Tablets (Less than 1%) 3487
Coreg Tablets (Less than or equal to 0.1%) 1508
Corgard Tablets (Infrequently) 2245
Cormax Scalp Application (Approximately 0.3%) 2441
Corzide 40/5 Tablets (Infrequent) 2247
Corzide 80/5 Tablets (Infrequent) 2247
Cosmegen for Injection 2062
Cosopt Sterile Ophthalmic Solution 2065
Coumadin for Injection (Infrequent) 1243
Coumadin Tablets (Infrequent) 1243
Covera-HS Tablets (Less than 2%) 3199
Cozaar Tablets (Less than 1%) 2067
Crixivan Capsules 2070
Cuprimine Capsules (Rare) 2075
Cyclessa Tablets 2450
Cytotec Tablets (Infrequent) 3202
Cytovene (At least 3 subjects) 2959
▲ DaunoXome Injection (2% to 8%) 1442
Delatestryl Injection 1151
▲ Depacon Injection (6% to 24%) 416
▲ Depakene (6% to 24%) 421
▲ Depakote Sprinkle Capsules (6% to 24%) 426
▲ Depakote Tablets (1% to 24%) 430
▲ Depakote ER Tablets (7%) 436
Depen Titratable Tablets (Rare) 3341
▲ Depo-Provera Contraceptive Injection (More than 5%) 2798
Desogen Tablets 2458
Didronel Tablets 2888
Diflucan Tablets, Injection, and Oral Suspension 2681
Diovan Capsules 2337
Diovan HCT Tablets 2338
Dipentum Capsules (Rare) 2803
Diuril Oral 2087
Diuril Sodium Intravenous 2086
▲ Doxil Injection (8.9% to 15.2%) 566
DTIC-Dome 902
Duraclon Injection (0.2%) 3057
EC-Naprosyn Delayed-Release Tablets (Less than 1%) 2967
Effexor Tablets (Infrequent) 3495
Effexor XR Capsules (Infrequent) 3499
Efudex 1733
Eldepryl Capsules 3266
▲ Ellence Injection (19.3% to 95.5%) 2806
▲ Elmiron Capsules (4%) 570
Emcyt Capsules (1%) 2810
Enalaprilat Injection 863
▲ Enbrel for Injection (6%) 1752
▲ Enbrel for Injection (6%) 3504
Engerix-B Vaccine 1517
Epivir 1520
Epivir-HBV 1524
▲ Ergamisol Tablets (3% to 22%) 1789
Esclim Transdermal System 3460
Eskalith 1527
Estinyl Tablets 3112
Estrace Vaginal Cream 3358
Estrace Tablets 3361
Estratest 3252
Estrostep 2627
Etrafon 3115
Evoxac Capsules (Less than 1%) 1217
Exelon Capsules (Infrequent) 2342
Exelon Oral Solution (Infrequent) 2345
Famotidine Injection (Infrequent) 866
Fareston Tablets 3237
Felbatol 3343
Feldene Capsules (Occasional) 2685
▲ Femara Tablets (5%) 2351
femhrt Tablets 2635
Flexeril Tablets (Rare) 572
Flexeril Tablets (Rare) 2094
Fludara for Injection (Up to 3%) 995
Follistim for Injection 2465
Fortovase Capsules (Less than 2%) 2970
Sterile FUDR 2974
Gabitril Tablets (Frequent) 1189
▲ Gemzar for Injection (15% to 18%) 1919
▲ Gengraf Capsules (4%) 457
Genotropin Lyophilized Powder 2818
Geodon Capsules (Infrequent) 2688
Haldol Decanoate (Isolated cases) 2535
Haldol Injection, Tablets and Concentrate (Isolated cases) 2533
Heparin Lock Flush Solution 3509
Heparin Sodium Injection 3511
Hexalen Capsules (Less than 1%) 2226
Hivid Tablets (Less than 1%) 2975
▲ Hycamtin for Injection (42% to 62%) 1546
HydroDIURIL Tablets 2108
Hyzaar 2109
▲ Idamycin PFS Injection (77%) 2825
▲ Ifex for Injection (83%) 1123
Inderal (Rare) 3513
Inderal LA Long-Acting Capsules (Rare) 3516
Inderide Tablets (Rare) 3517
Inderide LA Long-Acting Capsules (Rare) 3519
Indocin Capsules (Less than 1%) 2112
Indocin I.V. (Less than 1%) 2115
Indocin (Less than 1%) 2112
▲ Infergen (10% to 14%) 1777
▲ Intron A for Injection (Up to 38%) 3120
Invirase Capsules (Less than 2%) 2979
Isoptin SR Tablets (1% or less) 467
Kaletra Capsules (Less than 2%) 471

Kaletra Oral Solution (Less than 2%) 471
Klonopin Tablets (Infrequent) 2983
▲ Kytril Tablets (3%) 2988
Lamictal (1.3%) 1567
Lamisil Tablets 2360
Lariam Tablets (Less than 1%) 2989
Lescol Capsules 2361
Lescol Capsules 2925
Lescol XL Tablets 2361
Lescol XL Tablets 2925
▲ Leukine (37% to 73%) 1755
Levlen 962
Levlite 21 Tablets 962
Levlite 28 Tablets 962
Levora Tablets 3389
Levothroid Tablets 1373
Levoxyl Tablets 1819
Lexxel Tablets 608
Limbitrol 1738
Lipitor Tablets (Less than 2%) 2639
Lipitor Tablets (Less than 2%) 2696
Lithium Carbonate 3061
Lithium Citrate Syrup 3061
Lithobid Slow-Release Tablets 3255
Lodine (Less than 1%) 3528
Lodine XL Extended-Release Tablets (Less than 1%) 3530
Lodosyn Tablets 1251
Loestrin 21 Tablets 2642
Loestrin Fe Tablets 2642
Lo/Ovral Tablets 3532
Lo/Ovral-28 Tablets 3538
Lopid Tablets 2650
Loprox Gel 2022
Lotensin Tablets (Less than 1%) 2365
Lotensin HCT Tablets (0.3% or more) 2367
Lotrel Capsules (Infrequent) 2370
Low-Ogestrel-28 Tablets 3392
Loxitane Capsules 3398
Lunelle Monthly Injection 2827
▲ Lupron Depot 3.75 mg (Among most frequent) 3281
Lupron Depot–3 Month 11.25 mg (Less than 5%) 3285
Lupron Depot-PED 7.5 mg, 11.25 mg and 15 mg (Less than 2%) 3291
Lupron Injection (Less than 5%) 3279
Lupron Injection Pediatric (Less than 2%) 3280
Luvox Tablets (25, 50, 100 mg) (Infrequent) 3256
Luxiq Foam (One patient) 1210
Macrobid Capsules (Less than 1%) 2889
Macrodantin Capsules 2891
Matulane Capsules 3246
Maxair Autohaler 1981
Maxair Inhaler (Less than 1%) 1984
Megace Oral Suspension (1% to 3%) 1124
Menest Tablets 2254
Meridia Capsules 481
Metadate CD Capsules 1164
Metadate ER Tablets 1167
Methylin Tablets 1995
Methylin ER Tablets 1995
Mevacor Tablets (0.5% to 1.0%) 2132
Mexitil Capsules (About 4 in 1,000) 1047
Miacalcin Nasal Spray (Less than 1%) 2375
Microgestin Fe 1.5/30 Tablets 3407
Microgestin Fe 1/20 Tablets 3400
Microzide Capsules 3414
Midamor Tablets (Less than or equal to 1%) 2136
Minipress Capsules (Less than 1%) 2699
Minizide Capsules (Rare) 2700
Mircette Tablets 2470
Mobic Tablets (Less than 2%) 1054
Modicon 2563
Moduretic Tablets 2138
Motrin Suspension, Oral Drops, Chewable Tablets, and Caplets (Less than 1%) 2002
Mustargen for Injection (Infrequent) 2142
Myleran Tablets (Rare) 1603
Mylocel Tablets (Very rare) 2227
Nadolol Tablets (Infrequent) 2288
Naprelan Tablets (Less than 1%) 1293
Naprosyn Suspension (Less than 1%) 2967
Naprosyn Tablets (Less than 1%) 2967
▲ Navelbine Injection (Up to 12%) 1604
Necon 3415
▲ Neoral Soft Gelatin Capsules (4%) 2380
▲ Neoral Oral Solution (4%) 2380
▲ Neumega for Injection (Greater than or equal to 10%) 1434
▲ Neupogen for Injection (18%) 587
Neurontin Capsules (Infrequent) 2655
Neurontin Oral Solution (Infrequent) 2655
Neurontin Tablets (Infrequent) 2655
▲ Nilandron Tablets (5.7%) 753
Nipent for Injection (Less than 3%) 3272
Nizoral 2% Shampoo (Less than 1%) 2007
Nizoral Tablets (Rare) 1791
Nolvadex Tablets (Infrequent) 678
Nordette-28 Tablets 2257
Norinyl 1 +35 28-Day Tablets 3380
Norinyl 1 + 50 28-Day Tablets 3380
Normodyne Tablets (Less common) 3137
Norplant System 3543
Norpramin Tablets 755
Norvasc Tablets (Less than or equal to 0.1%) 2704
▲ Novantrone for Injection (22% to 61%) 1760
Ogen Tablets 2846
Ogestrel 0.5/50-28 Tablets 3428
Oncaspar 756
Ortho Dienestrol Cream 2554
Ortho-Cept 21 Tablets 2546
Ortho-Cept 28 Tablets 2546
Ortho-Cyclen/Ortho Tri-Cyclen 2573
Ortho-Est Tablets 3464
Ortho-Novum 2563
Ortho-Novum 1/50◘28 Tablets 2556
Ortho-Prefest Tablets 2570
Ortho-Cyclen/Ortho Tri-Cyclen 2573
Orudis Capsules (Less than 1%) 3548
Oruvail Capsules (Less than 1%) 3548
Ovcon 3364
Ovral Tablets 3551
Ovral-28 Tablets 3552
Ovrette Tablets 3552
Pacerone Tablets (Less than 1%) 3331
▲ Paraplatin for Injection (2% to 50%) 1126
Paxil (Infrequent) 1609
Pentasa Capsules (Less than 1%) 3239
Pepcid Injection (Infrequent) 2153
Pepcid for Oral Suspension (Infrequent) 2150
Pepcid RPD Orally Disintegrating Tablets (Infrequent) 2150
Pepcid Tablets (Infrequent) 2150
Permax Tablets (Infrequent) 1299
Persantine Tablets (Rare) 1057
Plaquenil Tablets 3082
Ponstel Capsules (Occasional) 1356
Pravachol Tablets 1099
Premarin Intravenous 3563
Premarin Tablets 3566
Premarin Vaginal Cream 3570
Premphase Tablets 3572
Prempro Tablets 3572
Prevacid Delayed-Release Capsules (Less than 1%) 3292
PREVPAC (Less than 1%) 3298
Prilosec Delayed-Release Capsules (Less than 1%) 628
Prinivil Tablets (0.3% to 1.0%) 2164
Prinzide Tablets 2168
Procardia XL Extended Release Tablets (1% or less) 2710
▲ Prograf (3% to 15%) 1393
Proleukin for Injection (1%) 1199
Protonix I.V. (Less than 1%) 3580
Protonix Tablets (Less than 1%) 3577
Provera Tablets 2853
Prozac Pulvules, Liquid, and Weekly Capsules (Infrequent) 1238
▲ Rebetron Combination Therapy (27% to 32%) 3153
Relafen Tablets (Less than 1%) 1617
Remeron Tablets (Infrequent) 2483
Remeron SolTab Tablets (Infrequent) 2486
Requip Tablets (Infrequent) 1621
Rescriptor Tablets (Less than 2%) 526
Rhinocort Nasal Inhaler (Rare) 640
Rilutek Tablets (Up to 1.2%) 772
Risperdal (Infrequent) 1796
Ritalin (A few instances) 2387
▲ Roferon-A Injection (17% to 22%) 2996
Rowasa Rectal Suspension Enema 4.0 grams/unit (60 mL) (0.86%) 3264
Rythmol Tablets – 150 mg, 225 mg, 300 mg (Less than 1%) 502
Salagen Tablets (Less than 1%) 2229
Sandostatin Injection (1% to 4%) 2394
Sandostatin LAR Depot (1% to 4%) 2395
Sarafem Pulvules (Infrequent) 1962
Sectral Capsules 3589
Selsun Rx 2.5% Lotion, USP 3053
Serophene Tablets (Less than 1 in 100 patients) 3226
▲ Serostim for Injection (1% to 10%) 3229
Serzone Tablets (Infrequent) 1104
Sinemet Tablets 1253
Sinemet CR Tablets 1255
Sinequan (Occasional) 2713
Sonata Capsules (Infrequent) 3591
▲ Soriatane Capsules (50% to 75%) 3003
Sporanox Capsules (Rare) 1800
Sporanox Injection (Rare) 1804
Sporanox Injection (Rare) 2509
Sporanox Oral Solution (Rare) 1808
Sporanox Oral Solution (Rare) 2512
Sular Tablets (Less than or equal to 1%) 688
Surmontil Capsules 3595
Sustiva Capsules (Less than 2%) 1258
Synarel Nasal Solution for Endometriosis (Some patients) 3205
Synthroid 505
Tagamet (Very rare) 1644
Tambocor Tablets (Less than 1%) 1990
Tapazole Tablets 1823
Tarka Tablets 508
Tasmar Tablets (1%) 3010
▲ Taxol Injection (87%) 1129
▲ Taxotere for Injection Concentrate (80%) 778
Tegretol/Tegretol-XR 2404
Temovate Scalp Application (1 of 294 patients) 1304
Tenex Tablets (Less frequent) 2942
Tenoretic Tablets 690
Tenormin 692
Thalomid Capsules 1154
Theo-Dur Extended-Release Tablets 1835
Thioplex for Injection 1765
Tiazac Capsules (Infrequent) 1378
Timolide Tablets 2187
Timolol GFS ⊙266
Timoptic in Ocudose (Less frequent) 2192
Timoptic Sterile Ophthalmic Solution (Less frequent) 2190
Timoptic-XE Sterile Ophthalmic Gel Forming Solution 2194
Tonocard Tablets (Less than 1%) 649
Topamax Sprinkle Capsules (Frequent) 2590
Topamax Tablets (Frequent) 2590
Toprol-XL Tablets (Rare) 651
Tricor Capsules, Micronized (Less than 1%) 513
Trileptal Oral Suspension 2407
Trileptal Tablets 2407
Tri-Levlen 962
Tri-Norinyl-28 Tablets 3433
Triphasil-21 Tablets 3600
Triphasil-28 Tablets 3605
Trivora Tablets 3439
Trizivir Tablets 1669
Twinrix Vaccine 1674
Uni-Dur Extended-Release Tablets 1841
Uniretic Tablets (Less than 1%) 3178
Unithroid Tablets 3445
Vaniqa Cream (1.3%) 1121
Vantin Tablets and Oral Suspension (Less than 1%) 2860
Vaseretic Tablets 2204
Vasotec I.V. Injection 2207
Vasotec Tablets (0.5% to 1.0%) 2210
Verelan Capsules (1% or less) 3184
Verelan PM Capsules (2% or less) 3186
▲ Vesanoid Capsules (14%) 3037
Viadur Implant (2.3%) 912
Videx 1138
Videx EC Capsules 1143
Vioxx (Greater than 0.1% to 1.9%) 2213
▲ Vistide Injection (27%) 1445
Vivactil Tablets 2217
Vivactil Tablets 2446
Vivelle Transdermal System 2412
Vivelle-Dot Transdermal System 2416
Voltaren Tablets (Less than 1%) 2315
Voltaren XR Tablets (Less than 1%) 2315
Warfarin Sodium Tablets, USP 3302
Wellbutrin Tablets (Infrequent) 1680
Yasmin 28 Tablets 980
Zanaflex Tablets (Infrequent) 1305
Zantac (Rare) 1690
Zantac Injection (Rare) 1688
Zantac Syrup (Rare) 1690
Zebeta Tablets 1885
Zestoretic Tablets 695
Zestril Tablets (0.3% to 1.0%) 698
Ziac Tablets 1887
▲ Zinecard for Injection (94% to 100%) 2869
Zocor Tablets 2219
Zoladex (1% or greater) 702
Zoladex 3-month 706
Zoloft (Infrequent) 2751
Zonegran Capsules (Infrequent) 1307
Zovia 3449
Zovirax Capsules 1706
Zovirax for Injection 1708
Zovirax 1706
Zyprexa Tablets (Infrequent) 1973
Zyprexa ZYDIS Orally Disintegrating Tablets (Infrequent) 1973
Zyrtec (Less than 2%) 2756
Zyrtec-D 12 Hour Extended Relief Tablets (Less than 2%) 2758

Alopecia hereditaria

Anadrol-50 Tablets 3321
Androderm Transdermal System CIII 3377
▲ Android Capsules, 10 mg (Among most common) 1731
Estratest 3252
Oxandrin Tablets 1153
Testoderm Transdermal Systems 574
Testopel Pellets 3610
Testred Capsules, 10 mg 1746

Alpha-glutamyl transferase, elevation

Eulexin Capsules 3118

ALT elevation

(*see under* Alanine aminotransferase levels, elevation of)

Alveolitis

Cordarone Tablets 3487
Cuprimine Capsules 2075
Pacerone Tablets 3331

Alveolitis, allergic

Depen Titratable Tablets (Rare) 3341
Paxil 1609
Relafen Tablets (Less than 1%) 1617
Tricor Capsules, Micronized (Less than 1%) 513

Alveolitis, fibrosing

Azulfidine EN-tabs Tablets (Rare) 2775
Canasa Rectal Suppositories 829
Rowasa Rectal Suspension Enema 4.0 grams/unit (60 mL) 3264
Tonocard Tablets (Less than 1%) 649

Amaurosis

Zofran Injection (One patient) 1698

Amblyopia

Accupril Tablets (0.5% to 1.0%) 2611
Accuretic Tablets 2614
Aciphex Tablets 1267
Aciphex Tablets 1783
▲ Actonel Tablets (3.3%) 2879
Adalat CC Tablets (Less than 1.0%) 877
Agrylin Capsules (1% to 5%) 3232
Amphotec (1% to 5%) 1774
Arthrotec Tablets (Rare) 3195
Avelox Tablets (0.05% to 1%) 879
Axid Pulvules (1.0%) 1903
Axid Pulvules (1.0%) 2919
Buprenex Injectable (Infrequent) 2918
Cardizem Injectable (Less than 1%) 1018
Cardizem Lyo-Ject Syringe (Less than 1%) 1018
Cardizem Monovial (Less than 1%) 1018
Cardizem CD Capsules (Less than 1%) 1016
▲ Carnitor Injection (3% to 6%) 3242
Cataflam Tablets (Less than 1%) 2315
▲ CellCept Capsules (3% to 14.9%) 2951
▲ CellCept Intravenous (3% to 14.9%) 2951
▲ CellCept Oral Suspension (3% to 14.9%) 2951
▲ CellCept Tablets (3% to 14.9%) 2951
Cerebyx Injection (2.2%) 2619
Cognex Capsules (Infrequent) 1351
Copaxone for Injection (At least 2%) 3306
▲ Depacon Injection (4% to 12%) 416
▲ Depakene (8% to 12%) 421
▲ Depakote Sprinkle Capsules (4% to 12%) 426
▲ Depakote Tablets (1% to 12%) 430
Depakote ER Tablets (Greater than 1%) 436
Diprivan Injectable Emulsion (Less than 1%) 667
Doxil Injection (Less than 1%) 566
Duragesic Transdermal System (Less than 1%) 1786
Dynabac Tablets (0.1% to 1%) 2269
Elmiron Capsules (Less than or equal to 1%) 570
▲ Flolan for Injection (8%) 1528
Flomax Capsules (0.2% to 2.0%) 1044
▲ Gabitril Tablets (1% to 9%) 1189
Herceptin I.V. (At least one of the 958 patients) 1414
Hytrin Capsules (0.6% to 1.3%) 464
Kadian Capsules (Less than 3%) 1335
Keppra Tablets (1% or more) 3314
Lipitor Tablets (Less than 2%) 2639
Lipitor Tablets (Less than 2%) 2696
Lupron Depot–3 Month 22.5 mg (Less than 5%) 3288
▲ Luvox Tablets (25, 50, 100 mg) (3%) 3256
Macrobid Capsules (Less than 1%) 2889
Megace Oral Suspension (1% to 3%) 1124
Meridia Capsules (Greater than or equal to 1%) 481
Motrin Suspension, Oral Drops, Chewable Tablets, and Caplets (Less than 1%) 2002

Myobloc Injectable Solution (2% or greater) 1291
Natrecor for Injection (At least 1%) 3189
Neumega for Injection 1434
▲ Neurontin Capsules (4.2%) 2655
▲ Neurontin Oral Solution (4.2%) 2655
▲ Neurontin Tablets (4.2%) 2655
Niaspan Extended-Release Tablets 1846
Nipent for Injection (Less than 3%) 3272
Norvir Capsules (Less than 2%) 487
Norvir Oral Solution (Less than 2%) 487
Paxil (Rare) 1609
Pletal Tablets (Less than 2%) 2605
Pletal Tablets (Less than 2%) 2848
Prevacid Delayed-Release Capsules (Less than 1%) 3292
PREVPAC (Less than 1%) 3298
▲ Prograf (3% to 15%) 1393
Protonix I.V. (Less than 1%) 3580
Protonix Tablets (Less than 1%) 3577
Provigil Tablets (2%) 1193
Retrovir Capsules 1625
Retrovir IV Infusion 1629
Retrovir 1625
Rilutek Tablets (Infrequent) 772
Roxicodone Tablets (Less than 3%) 3067
▲ Salagen Tablets (4%) 2229
Sular Tablets (Less than or equal to 1%) 688
Thalomid Capsules 1154
Tiazac Capsules (Less than 2%) 1378
Tricor Capsules, Micronized (Less than 1%) 513
Vistide Injection 1445
Voltaren Tablets (Less than 1%) 2315
Voltaren-XR Tablets (Less than 1%) 2315
Wellbutrin SR Sustained-Release Tablets (2% to 3%) 1684
▲ Zanaflex Tablets (3%) 1305
Zoladex (1% or greater) 702
Zoladex 3-month 706
Zonegran Capsules (Frequent) 1307
Zyban Sustained-Release Tablets (Frequent) 1710
▲ Zyprexa Tablets (5%) 1973
▲ Zyprexa ZYDIS Orally Disintegrating Tablets (5%) 1973

Amblyopia scleritis
Naprelan Tablets (Less than 1%) 1293

Amelia
Thalomid Capsules 1154

Amenorrhea
Aldoclor Tablets 2035
Aldomet Tablets 2037
Aldoril Tablets 2039
Alesse-21 Tablets 3468
Alesse-28 Tablets 3473
Alkeran for Injection 1465
Alkeran Tablets (A significant number of patients) 1466
▲ Android Capsules, 10 mg (Among most common) 1731
Astelin Nasal Spray (Infrequent) 3339
Aygestin Tablets 1333
Brevicon 28-Day Tablets 3380
Celexa (Frequent) 1365
Compazine 1505
Cyclessa Tablets 2450
▲ Delatestryl Injection (Among most frequent) 1151
Depacon Injection (1% to 5%) 416
Depakene (1% to 5%) 421
Depakote Sprinkle Capsules (1% to 5%) 426
Depakote Tablets (1% to 5%) 430
Depakote ER Tablets (1% to 5%) 436
▲ Depo-Provera Contraceptive Injection (More than 5%) 2798
Desogen Tablets 2458
Effexor Tablets (Infrequent) 3495
Effexor XR Capsules (Infrequent) 3499
▲ Ellence Injection (Up to 71.8%) 2806
Estinyl Tablets 3112
▲ Estratest (Among most common) 3252
Estrostep 2627
Etrafon 3115
Evoxac Capsules (Less than 1%) 1217
Gabitril Tablets (Infrequent) 1189
Geodon Capsules (Infrequent) 2688
Haldol Decanoate 2535
Haldol Injection, Tablets and Concentrate 2533
Intron A for Injection (Less than 5%) 3120
Kadian Capsules (Less than 3%) 1335
Lamictal (1.9%) 1567
Leukeran Tablets 1591
Levlen 962
Levlite 21 Tablets 962
Levlite 28 Tablets 962
Levora Tablets 3389
Loestrin 21 Tablets 2642
Loestrin Fe Tablets 2642
Lo/Ovral Tablets 3532
Lo/Ovral-28 Tablets 3538
Low-Ogestrel-28 Tablets 3392
Loxitane Capsules (Rare) 3398
Lunelle Monthly Injection 2827
Menest Tablets 2254
Microgestin Fe 1.5/30 Tablets 3407
Microgestin Fe 1/20 Tablets 3400
Micronor Tablets 2543
Mircette Tablets 2470
▲ Mirena Intrauterine System (20%) 974
Moban (Infrequent) 1320
Modicon 2563
Mustargen for Injection 2142
Navane Oral 2701
Navane Intramuscular 2703
Necon 3415
Neurontin Capsules (Infrequent) 2655
Neurontin Oral Solution (Infrequent) 2655
Neurontin Tablets (Infrequent) 2655
Nipent for Injection (Less than 3%) 3272
▲ Nolvadex Tablets (16.3%) 678
Nordette-28 Tablets 2257
Norinyl 1 +35 28-Day Tablets 3380
Norinyl 1 + 50 28-Day Tablets 3380
▲ Norplant System (9.4%) 3543
▲ Novantrone for Injection (28% to 43%) 1760
Ogestrel 0.5/50-28 Tablets 3428
Ortho Dienestrol Cream 2554
Ortho-Cept 21 Tablets 2546
Ortho-Cept 28 Tablets 2546
Ortho-Cyclen/Ortho Tri-Cyclen 2573
Ortho-Est Tablets 3464
Ortho-Novum 2563
Ortho-Novum 1/50□28 Tablets 2556
Ortho-Cyclen/Ortho Tri-Cyclen 2573
Ovcon 3364
Ovral Tablets 3551
Ovral-28 Tablets 3552
Ovrette Tablets 3552
OxyContin Tablets 2912
ParaGard T 380A Intrauterine Copper Contraceptive 2582
Paxil (Infrequent) 1609
Pentasa Capsules (Less than 1%) 3239
Permax Tablets (Rare) 1299
Premarin Intravenous 3563
Premarin Vaginal Cream 3570
Premphase Tablets 3572
Prempro Tablets 3572
Prometrium Capsules (100 mg, 200 mg) 3261
Provera Tablets 2853
Prozac Pulvules, Liquid, and Weekly Capsules (Infrequent) 1238
Reglan 2935
Remeron Tablets (Infrequent) 2483
Remeron SolTab Tablets (Infrequent) 2486
Requip Tablets (Infrequent) 1621
Rescriptor Tablets 526
Rilutek Tablets (Rare) 772
Risperdal (Infrequent) 1796
Sandostatin Injection (Less than 1%) 2394
Sarafem Pulvules (Infrequent) 1962
Serentil 1057
Seroquel Tablets (Infrequent) 684
Serzone Tablets (Infrequent) 1104
Stelazine 1640
Testred Capsules, 10 mg 1746
Thalomid Capsules 1154
Thioplex for Injection 1765
Thioridazine Hydrochloride Tablets 2289
Thiothixene Capsules 2290
Thorazine 1656
Topamax Sprinkle Capsules (Frequent) 2590
Topamax Tablets (Frequent) 2590
Trilafon 3160
Tri-Levlen 962
Tri-Norinyl-28 Tablets 3433
Triphasil-21 Tablets 3600
Triphasil-28 Tablets 3605
Trivora Tablets 3439
Yasmin 28 Tablets 980
Zoladex (Rare) 702
Zoloft (Infrequent) 2751
Zonegran Capsules (Infrequent) 1307
Zovia 3449
Zyprexa Tablets (Infrequent) 1973
Zyprexa ZYDIS Orally Disintegrating Tablets (Infrequent) 1973

Amentia
Clozaril Tablets (Less than 1%) 2319

Amnesia
Accuretic Tablets 2614
Aceon Tablets (2 mg, 4 mg, 8 mg) (0.3% to 1%) 3249
Aciphex Tablets (Rare) 1267
Aciphex Tablets (Rare) 1783
Actiq (Less than 1%) 1184
Aggrenox Capsules (2.4%) 1026
Agrylin Capsules (1% to 5%) 3232
Altace Capsules (Less than 1%) 2233
Ambien Tablets (1%) 3191
AndroGel (Fewer than 1%) 3322
Ativan Tablets 3482
Avonex 1013
Betaseron for SC Injection (2%) 988
Cardizem Injectable 1018
Cardizem Lyo-Ject Syringe 1018
Cardizem Monovial 1018
Cardizem CD Capsules (Less than 1%) 1016
Cardura Tablets (Less than 0.5%) 2668
Celexa (Frequent) 1365
Cerebyx Injection (Infrequent) 2619
Claritin (At least one patient) 3100
Claritin-D 12 Hour Extended Release Tablets 3102
Claritin-D 24 Hour Extended Release Tablets 3104
Clozaril Tablets (Less than 1%) 2319
Cognex Capsules (Infrequent) 1351
Copaxone for Injection (At least 2%) 3306
Coreg Tablets (Less than or equal to 0.1%) 1508
DaunoXome Injection (Less than or equal to 5%) 1442
▲ Depacon Injection (4% to 7%) 416
▲ Depakene (5% to 7%) 421
▲ Depakote Sprinkle Capsules (4% to 7%) 426
▲ Depakote Tablets (1% to 7%) 430
Depakote ER Tablets (Greater than 1%) 436
D.H.E. 45 Injection 2334
Didronel Tablets 2888
Duragesic Transdermal System (1% or greater) 1786
Effexor Tablets 3495
Effexor XR Capsules (Frequent) 3499
Ergamisol Tablets (Up to 1%) 1789
Evoxac Capsules 1217
Exelon Capsules (Infrequent) 2342
Exelon Oral Solution (Infrequent) 2345
Fortovase Capsules (Less than 2%) 2970
Foscavir Injection (Between 1% and 5%) 605
Geodon Capsules (Frequent) 2688
Gliadel Wafer (1%) 1723
Halcion Tablets 2823
Hivid Tablets (Less than 1%) 2975
▲ Infergen (2% to 10%) 1777
▲ Intron A for Injection (Up to 14%) 3120
Invirase Capsules (Less than 2%) 2979
Kadian Capsules (Less than 3%) 1335
Kaletra Capsules (Less than 2%) 471
Kaletra Oral Solution (Less than 2%) 471
Keppra Tablets (2%) 3314
Klonopin Tablets 2983
Lamictal (Frequent) 1567
Levo-Dromoran 1734
Lipitor Tablets (Less than 2%) 2639
Lipitor Tablets (Less than 2%) 2696
Lupron Depot–4 Month 30 mg (Less than 5%) 3289
Luvox Tablets (25, 50, 100 mg) (Frequent) 3256
Marinol Capsules (Greater than 1%) 3325
Meridia Capsules 481
▲ Mirapex Tablets (3% to 6%) 2834
Naprelan Tablets (Less than 1%) 1293
Naropin Injection (Less than 1%) 612
Neurontin Capsules (2.2%) 2655
Neurontin Oral Solution (2.2%) 2655
Neurontin Tablets (2.2%) 2655
Nicotrol Nasal Spray (Less than 1%) 2843
Norvasc Tablets (Less than or equal to 0.1%) 2704
Norvir Capsules (Less than 2%) 487
Norvir Oral Solution (Less than 2%) 487
Orudis Capsules (Less than 1%) 3548
Oruvail Capsules (Less than 1%) 3548
OxyContin Tablets (Less than 1%) 2912
Paxil (2%) 1609
Permax Tablets (Frequent) 1299
Prevacid Delayed-Release Capsules (Less than 1%) 3292
PREVPAC (Less than 1%) 3298
▲ Prograf (3% to 15%) 1393
ProSom Tablets (Infrequent) 500
Provigil Tablets (1%) 1193
Prozac Pulvules, Liquid, and Weekly Capsules (Frequent) 1238
Remeron Tablets (Frequent) 2483
Remeron SolTab Tablets (Frequent) 2486
▲ Requip Tablets (3%) 1621
Rescriptor Tablets (Less than 2%) 526
Rilutek Tablets (Infrequent) 772
Risperdal (Infrequent) 1796
Robaxin Injectable 2938
Robaxin Tablets 2939
Roferon-A Injection (Less than 0.5% to less than 3%) 2996
Sandostatin Injection (Less than 1%) 2394
Sarafem Pulvules (Frequent) 1962
Seroquel Tablets (Infrequent) 684
▲ Serostim for Injection (1% to 10%) 3229
Sonata Capsules (2% to 4%) 3591
Sular Tablets (Less than or equal to 1%) 688
Sustiva Capsules (Less than 2%) 1258
Symmetrel (0.1% to 1%) 1328
Tambocor Tablets (Less than 1%) 1990
Tasmar Tablets (Infrequent) 3010
▲ Temodar Capsules (10%) 3157
Tenex Tablets (3% or less) 2942
Thalomid Capsules 1154
Tiazac Capsules (Less than 2%) 1378
Trileptal Oral Suspension (1% to 5%) 2407
Trileptal Tablets (1% to 5%) 2407
Trovan (Less than 1%) 2722
Ultracet Tablets (Less than 1%) 2597
Ultram Tablets (Less than 1%) 2600
Uniretic Tablets (Less than 1%) 3178
Versed Injection (Less than 1%) 3027
Versed Syrup 3033
Viadur Implant (Less than 2%) 912
Vistide Injection 1445
Wellbutrin SR Sustained-Release Tablets (Rare) 1684
Xanax Tablets 2865
Zoloft (Infrequent) 2751
Zomig Tablets (Rare) 708
Zomig-ZMT Tablets (Rare) 708
Zyban Sustained-Release Tablets (Rare) 1710
Zyprexa Tablets (2%) 1973
Zyprexa ZYDIS Orally Disintegrating Tablets (2%) 1973
Zyrtec (Less than 2%) 2756
Zyrtec-D 12 Hour Extended Relief Tablets (Less than 2%) 2758

Amnesia, traveler's
Halcion Tablets 2823

Amnionitis
▲ Cleocin Vaginal Cream (6%) 2788
Prepidil Gel 2851

Amputation, gangrene of the extremities-induced
Heparin Lock Flush Solution 3509
Heparin Sodium Injection 3511

Amyloidosis
Thalomid Capsules 1154

ANA, positive
Aceon Tablets (2 mg, 4 mg, 8 mg) 3249
Adalat CC Tablets (Rare) 877
Aldoclor Tablets 2035
Aldomet Tablets 2037
Aldoril Tablets 2039
Altace Capsules (Less than 1%) 2233
Baycol Tablets (Rare) 883
Captopril Tablets 2281
Depen Titratable Tablets (Certain patients) 3341
D.H.E. 45 Injection 2334
Enalaprilat Injection 863
▲ Enbrel for Injection (11%) 1752
▲ Enbrel for Injection (11%) 3504
Felbatol (Rare) 3343
Feldene Capsules (Rare) 2685
Lescol Capsules (Rare) 2361
Lescol Capsules (Rare) 2925
Lescol XL Tablets 2361
Lescol XL Tablets 2925
Lexxel Tablets 608
Lopid Tablets 2650
Mevacor Tablets (Rare) 2132
Mexitil Capsules (About 2 in 1,000) 1047
Minipress Capsules 2699
Monopril Tablets 1091
Monopril HCT 1094
Normodyne Tablets (Less common) 3137
Pravachol Tablets (Rare) 1099
Prinivil Tablets (0.3% to 1.0%) 2164
Prinzide Tablets 2168
Procanbid Extended-Release Tablets 2262
Procardia Capsules (Less than 0.5%) 2708
▲ Remicade for IV Injection (49%) 1178
Rythmol Tablets – 150 mg, 225 mg, 300 mg (0.7%) 502
Tenoretic Tablets 690
Tenormin 692
Ticlid Tablets (Rare) 3015
Tonocard Tablets (Less than 1%) 649
Vaseretic Tablets 2204
Vasotec I.V. Injection 2207
Vasotec Tablets (0.5% to 1.0%) 2210
Zestoretic Tablets 695
Zestril Tablets (0.3% to 1.0%) 698
Zocor Tablets (Rare) 2219

Analgesia, reversal
Narcan Injection 1322

Anaphylactic reactions
Acel-Imune (Rare) 1851

Aceon Tablets (2 mg, 4 mg, 8 mg) (0.3% to 1%) 3249
Aggrastat 2031
Aldoclor Tablets 2035
Aldoril Tablets 2039
Amoxil Chewable Tablets 1471
Amoxil for Oral Suspension 1471
Amoxil 1471
Ancef for Injection 1474
Ancef Injection 1474
Antivenin (Black Widow Spider Antivenin) 2042
Anzemet Injection (Rare) 719
Anzemet Tablets (Rare) 722
AquaMEPHYTON Injection 2042
Arava Tablets (One case) 724
Atacand HCT Tablets 597
Atrovent Inhalation Aerosol 1030
Atrovent Nasal Spray 0.06% 1033
Augmentin Chewable Tablets 1482
Augmentin Powder for Oral Suspension 1482
Augmentin Tablets 1485
Augmentin ES-600 Powder for Oral Suspension 1487
Avalide Tablets 1070
Avelox Tablets 879
Aygestin Tablets 1333
BayGam 914
BayHep B (Rare) 915
Bebulin VH (Rare) 840
Bicillin C-R 900/300 Injection 2240
Bicillin C-R Injection 2238
Bicillin L-A Injection 2242
Cefotan 664
Celebrex Capsules (Less than 0.1%) 2676
Celebrex Capsules (Less than 0.1%) 2780
Ceptaz for Injection (Rare) 1499
Cipro I.V. (1% or less) 893
Cipro I.V. Pharmacy Bulk Package (Less than 1%) 897
Cipro 887
Combivent Inhalation Aerosol (Less than 2%) 1041
Coreg Tablets 1508
Corzide 40/5 Tablets 2247
Corzide 80/5 Tablets 2247
Cozaar Tablets 2067
Cytovene 2959
Desferal Vials 2333
Diflucan Tablets, Injection, and Oral Suspension (Rare) 2681
Digibind Powder 1514
Dilaudid Oral Liquid 445
Dilaudid Tablets - 8 mg 445
Diphtheria & Tetanus Toxoids Adsorbed Purogenated for Pediatric Use (Rare) 1857
Diucardin Tablets 3494
Diuril Oral 2087
Diuril Sodium Intravenous 2086
Dobutrex Solution Vials 1914
Dolobid Tablets (Less than 1 in 100) 2088
Elspar for Injection 2092
Factrel (Rare) 3633
Feldene Capsules (Rare) 2685
Floxin I.V. 2526
Floxin Tablets 2529
Foradil Aerolizer (Rare) 2354
Fortaz 1541
Gamimune N, 5% Solvent/Detergent Treated 925
Gamimune N, 10% Solvent/Detergent Treated 928
Gammagard S/D (A remote possibility) 845
Gastrocrom Oral Concentrate (Rare) 1162
Geocillin Tablets 2687
Heparin Lock Flush Solution 3509
Heparin Sodium Injection 3511
Humalog (Less common) 1926
Humalog Mix 75/25 Pen 1928
Humate-P Concentrate 790
HydroDIURIL Tablets 2108
Hyzaar 2109
IC-Green ⊙ 203
Imogam Rabies - HT (Rare) 805
Indapamide Tablets 2286
Inderide Tablets 3517
Inderide LA Long-Acting Capsules 3519
INFeD Injection 3388
Innohep Injection 1248
Iveegam EN 849
Kogenate FS 936
Lodine 3528
Lodine XL Extended-Release Tablets (Rare) 3530
Lotensin HCT Tablets 2367
Lunelle Monthly Injection 2827
Lupron Depot 7.5 mg (One report) 3284
Lupron Injection (One report) 3279
Lupron Injection Pediatric 3280
Luvox Tablets (25, 50, 100 mg) 3256
Mefoxin Premixed Intravenous Solution 2127
Meruvax II 2130
Micardis HCT Tablets 1051
Microzide Capsules 3414
Mintezol 2137
Moduretic Tablets 2138
Monopril HCT 1094
Mykrox Tablets (rare) 1168
Nabi-HB (Rare) 2295
Norflex (Rare) 1987
Normodyne Tablets 3137
Noroxin Tablets (Occasional) 2145
Nubain Injection (1% or less) 1323
▲ Oncaspar (Greater than 1% but less than 5%) 756
Orthoclone OKT3 Sterile Solution 2498
Orudis Capsules (Less than 1%) 3548
Oruvail Capsules (Less than 1%) 3548
Parafon Forte DSC Caplets (Extremely rare) 2582
Paraplatin for Injection 1126
Pergonal for Injection (Some patients) 3223
Pfizerpen for Injection (Occasional) 2707
Phenergan Injection 3553
Pipracil 1866
Pred Mild Sterile Ophthalmic Suspension ⊙ 249
Premarin Tablets 3566
Premarin Vaginal Cream 3570
Prevnar for Injection 1870
PREVPAC 3298
Primaxin I.M. 2158
Primaxin I.V. 2160
Prinzide Tablets 2168
Prograf (A few patients) 1393
Rabies Vaccine RabAvert 1203
Repronex for Intramuscular and Subcutaneous Injection (Some patients) 1347
Risperdal 1796
Robaxin Injectable 2938
Robaxin Tablets 2939
Roferon-A Injection (Rare) 2996
Sandimmune I.V. Ampuls for Infusion (Rare) 2388
Sandoglobulin I.V. 2391
Sensorcaine 643
Sensorcaine-MPF Injection 643
Soma Compound w/Codeine Tablets 3355
Stelazine Injection 1640
Streptase for Infusion (Rare) 647
Streptomycin Sulfate Injection 2714
Symmetrel 1328
Talacen Caplets (One instance) 3089
Tao Capsules 2716
Tetanus & Diphtheria Toxoids Adsorbed for Adult Use (Rare) 1880
Tetanus and Diphtheria Toxoids Adsorbed For Adult Use (Rare) 815
Thorazine 1656
Timentin Injection- ADD-Vantage Vial 1661
Timentin Injection-Galaxy Container 1664
Timentin Injection-Pharmacy Bulk Package 1666
Timentin for Intravenous Administration 1658
Timolide Tablets 2187
Tisseel VH (Rare) 854
Toradol 3018
Trasylol Injection (Less than 0.5%) 909
Trilafon 3160
Tripedia Vaccine (Rare) 817
Trovan (Less than 1%) 2722
TYPHIM Vi Vaccine 825
Unasyn for Injection (Occasional) 2728
Vaseretic Tablets 2204
Vibramycin Hyclate Intravenous 2737
Vibra-Tabs Film Coated Tablets 2735
Zaroxolyn Tablets 1177
Zemuron Injection (Rare) 2491
Zestoretic Tablets 695
Ziac Tablets 1887
Zoladex 3-month (One report) 706
Zosyn (Occasional) 1890
Zosyn in Galaxy Containers (Occasional) 1894

Anaphylactic shock

Ambien Tablets (Rare) 3191
Aquasol A Parenteral 593
Aredia for Injection (Very rare) 2309
Avelox Tablets 879
BayRab (Rare) 917
BayTet (Few isolated cases) 923
Bebulin VH 840
Benadryl Parenteral 2617
Cordarone Intravenous 3491
CytoGam Intravenous (A possibility) 2026
Declomycin Tablets 1855
GlucaGen for Injection Diagnostic Kit (Rare) 949
Levaquin 2537
Lodine 3528
Lodine XL Extended-Release Tablets 3530
Maxipime for Injection 1285
Meridia Capsules 481
Miacalcin Injection (A few cases) 2373
Orthoclone OKT3 Sterile Solution 2498
Periactin Tablets 2155
Protonix I.V. 3580
Rabies Vaccine RabAvert (Two cases) 1203
Rynatan Tablets 3351
Sandostatin Injection 2394
Sandostatin LAR Depot (Rare) 2395
Soma Tablets 3353
Soma Compound Tablets 3354
Soma Compound w/Codeine Tablets 3355
Streptase for Infusion (Very rare) 647
Thioplex for Injection 1765
Toradol 3018
Trasylol Injection 909
Tripedia Vaccine (Rare) 817
Vantin Tablets and Oral Suspension (Less than 1%) 2860
Venofer Injection (8 patients) 580
Wellbutrin Tablets (Rare) 1680
Wellbutrin SR Sustained-Release Tablets (Rare) 1684
Zyban Sustained-Release Tablets (Rare) 1710

Anaphylactoid reactions

Abelcet Injection 1273
Accupril Tablets 2611
Activase I.V. (Very rare) 1410
Altace Capsules (Less than 1%) 2233
Amerge Tablets 1467
Amicar Injection 3608
Amicar Syrup 3608
Amicar Tablets 3608
Amoxil Chewable Tablets (occasional) 1471
Amoxil for Oral Suspension (occasional) 1471
Amoxil (occasional) 1471
Anaprox Tablets (Less than 1%) 2967
Anaprox DS Tablets (Less than 1%) 2967
Androderm Transdermal System CIII (Rare) 3377
Android Capsules, 10 mg (Rare) 1731
Aquasol A Parenteral (One case) 593
Arthrotec Tablets 3195
Astelin Nasal Spray 3339
Attenuvax 2044
Aygestin Tablets 1333
Baycol Tablets 883
Bebulin VH (Rare) 840
Betaseron for SC Injection 988
Campath Ampules 992
Captopril Tablets 2281
Cataflam Tablets (Less than 1%) 2315
Ceclor CD Tablets 1279
Ceclor 1905
Celestone Soluspan Injectable Suspension (Rare) 3097
Ceptaz for Injection (Rare) 1499
Cerezyme for Injection 1438
Cerubidine for Injection (Rare) 947
Chibroxin Sterile Ophthalmic Solution 2051
Cleocin HCl Capsules (A few cases) 2784
Cleocin Phosphate Sterile Solution (A few cases) 2785
Cleocin Vaginal Cream (A few cases) 2788
Cleocin Vaginal Ovules (A few cases) 2789
Compazine 1505
Copaxone for Injection (Rare) 3306
Coreg Tablets (Less than or equal to 0.1%) 1508
Cortone Acetate Injectable Suspension 2059
Crixivan Capsules 2070
Decadron Phosphate Injection 2081
Delatestryl Injection (Rare) 1151
Depo-Provera Contraceptive Injection 2798
Detrol Tablets 3623
Detrol LA Capsules 2801
Digibind Powder 1514
Diprivan Injectable Emulsion (Less than 1%) 667
Doxil Injection (Less than 1%) 566
Duranest Injections 600
EC-Naprosyn Delayed-Release Tablets (Less than 1%) 2967
ELA-Max Cream 1340
ELA-Max 5 Cream 1340
Emla 602
Enalaprilat Injection 863
Engerix-B Vaccine 1517
Epogen for Injection 582
Estratest (Rare) 3252
Ethyol for Injection (Rare) 2029
Etrafon 3115
Feiba VH 843
Felbatol (Rare) 3343
femhrt Tablets 2635
Flonase Nasal Spray 1533
Florinef Acetate Tablets 2250
Floxin I.V. 2526
Floxin Tablets 2529
Fortaz 1541
Fragmin Injection (A few cases) 2814
Gamimune N, 5% Solvent/Detergent Treated (Very rare) 925
Gamimune N, 10% Solvent/Detergent Treated (Very rare) 928
Gemzar for Injection (Rare) 1919
Havrix Vaccine (Rare) 1544
Herceptin I.V. (At least one of the 958 patients) 1414
Hivid Tablets (One patient) 2975
Hyalgan Solution 3080
Hycamtin for Injection (Rare) 1546
Hydrocortone Acetate Injectable Suspension 2103
Hydrocortone Phosphate Injection, Sterile 2105
Imitrex Injection (Rare) 1549
Imitrex Nasal Spray 1554
Imitrex Tablets (Rare) 1558
Imogam Rabies - HT (Rare) 805
Innohep Injection 1248
Kytril Injection (Rare) 2986
Levaquin 2537
Lexxel Tablets 608
Lidoderm Patch (Rare) 1319
Lodine (Less than 1%) 3528
Lodine XL Extended-Release Tablets (Less than 1%) 3530
Lotrel Capsules 2370
Lovenox Injection 746
Lupron Depot 3.75 mg (Rare) 3281
Lupron Depot 7.5 mg (Rare) 3284
Lupron Depot-3 Month 11.25 mg 3285
Lupron Depot-3 Month 22.5 mg (Rare) 3288
Lupron Depot-PED 7.5 mg, 11.25 mg and 15 mg 3291
Mavik Tablets 478
Meridia Capsules 481
Meruvax II 2130
M-M-R II 2118
Mobic Tablets (Less than 0.1%) 1054
Monopril Tablets 1091
Motrin Suspension, Oral Drops, Chewable Tablets, and Caplets (Less than 1%) 2002
Mumpsvax 2141
Myambutol Tablets 1290
▲ Naprelan Tablets (3% to 9%) 1293
Naprosyn Suspension (Less than 1%) 2967
Naprosyn Tablets (Less than 1%) 2967
Naropin Injection 612
Nesacaine/Nesacaine MPF 617
Nitro-Dur Transdermal Infusion System (A few reports) 1834
Nitro-Dur Transdermal Infusion System (A few reports) 3134
Normodyne Injection (Rare) 3135
Normodyne Tablets (Rare) 3137
Noroxin Tablets (Occasional) 2145
Nubain Injection (1% or less) 1323
Orthoclone OKT3 Sterile Solution 2498
Plavix Tablets (Very rare) 1097
Plavix Tablets (Very rare) 3084
Pneumovax 23 (Rare) 2156
Pnu-Imune 23 (Rare) 1868
Polocaine Injection, USP 625
Polocaine-MPF Injection, USP 625
Ponstel Capsules (Rare) 1356
Prandin Tablets (0.5, 1, and 2 mg) (One patient) 2432
Premarin Tablets 3566
Premarin Vaginal Cream 3570
Premphase Tablets 3572
Prempro Tablets 3572
Prevacid Delayed-Release Capsules 3292
Prevnar for Injection 1870
PREVPAC 3298
Prinivil Tablets (0.3% to 1.0%) 2164
Prinzide Tablets 2168
Procrit for Injection 2502
Prometrium Capsules (100 mg, 200 mg) 3261
Protopic Ointment (Greater than or equal to 1%) 1397
Provera Tablets 2853
Relafen Tablets (Less than 1%) 1617
Sandoglobulin I.V. 2391
Sandostatin Injection 2394
Sandostatin LAR Depot (Rare) 2395
Sensorcaine-MPF with Epinephrine Injection 643
Sensorcaine-MPF Injection 643
Solu-Medrol Sterile Powder 2855
Stelazine Injection 1640
Streptase for Infusion (Rare) 647
Suprax 1877
Testoderm Transdermal Systems (Rare) 574
Testopel Pellets (Rare) 3610
Testred Capsules, 10 mg (Rare) 1746
Tetanus Toxoid Adsorbed Purogenated 1882
Tisseel VH (Rare) 854
Tolectin (Less than 1%) 2589
Toradol 3018

Trasylol Injection 909
Trental Tablets (Rare) 784
Twinrix Vaccine 1674
Ultram Tablets 2600
Uniretic Tablets (More than 1%) 3178
Univasc Tablets 3181
Vancocin HCl Oral Solution 1971
Vancocin HCl, Vials & ADD-Vantage 1970
Vaseretic Tablets 2204
Vasotec I.V. Injection 2207
Vasotec Tablets (0.5% to 1.0%) 2210
Venofer Injection (27 patients) 580
Versed Injection (Less than 1%) 3027
Videx 1138
Videx EC Capsules 1143
Vioxx (Greater than 0.1%) 2213
Voltaren Tablets (Less than 1%) 2315
Voltaren-XR Tablets (Less than 1%) 2315
Wellbutrin Tablets 1680
Wellbutrin SR Sustained-Release Tablets 1684
Xylocaine Injections (Extremely rare) 653
Zemuron Injection (Rare) 2491
Zestoretic Tablets 695
Zestril Tablets (0.3% to 1.0%) 698
Zofran Injection 1698
Zofran 1703
Zofran ODT Orally Disintegrating Tablets 1703
Zoloft 2751
Zyban Sustained-Release Tablets 1710

Anaphylaxis

Abelcet Injection (Less than 0.1%) 1273
Aciphex Tablets 1267
Adriamycin PFS/RDF Injection 2767
Aggrastat 2031
Albuminar-5, U.S.P. 785
Albuminar-25, U.S.P. 786
Alferon N Injection 1770
Alkeran for Injection (2.4%) 1465
Alkeran Tablets (Rare) 1466
Allegra (Rare) 712
Allegra-D Extended-Release Tablets (Rare) 714
Amerge Tablets 1467
Amicar Injection 3608
Amicar Syrup 3608
Amicar Tablets 3608
Amoxil Chewable Tablets 1471
Amoxil for Oral Suspension 1471
Amoxil 1471
Amphotec 1774
Ancef for Injection 1474
Ancef Injection 1474
Anectine Injection (Rare) 1476
Antivenin (Micrurus fulvius) 3477
Antivenin Polyvalent 3475
AquaMEPHYTON Injection 2042
Atrovent Inhalation Solution (A single case) 1031
Attenuvax 2044
Axid Pulvules (Rare) 1903
Axid Pulvules (Rare) 2919
Azactam for Injection (Less than 1%) 1276
Azmacort Inhalation Aerosol 728
Azulfidine EN-tabs Tablets (Rare) 2775
Bactrim 2949
Baycol Tablets (Rare) 883
BayGam (Rare) 914
Biaxin/Biaxin XL (Rare) 403
Bicillin C-R 900/300 Injection 2240
Bicillin C-R Injection 2238
Brevital Sodium for Injection, USP (Rare) 1815
Cataflam Tablets (Rare) 2315
Ceclor CD Tablets (Rare) 1279
Ceclor (Rare) 1905
Cedax 1021
Cefizox for Intramuscular or Intravenous Use (Rare) 1390
Ceftin 1898
Cefzil (Rare) 1076
Ceptaz for Injection (Very rare) 1499
Claforan Injection (Less frequent) 732
Claritin (Rare) 3100
Claritin-D 12 Hour Extended Release Tablets 3102
Claritin-D 24 Hour Extended Release Tablets 3104
Clinoril Tablets 2053
Combivent Inhalation Aerosol (Rare) 1041
Combivir Tablets 1502
Comvax 2056
Cortisporin Ophthalmic Suspension (Rare) .... ⊙297
CytoGam Intravenous 2026
Cytotec Tablets (Infrequent) 3202
Dantrium Capsules (Less frequent) 2885
Dantrium Intravenous (One case) 2886
Daraprim Tablets 1511
DDAVP Injection 4 mcg/mL (Rare) 737
Declomycin Tablets 1855
Depakene 421
Depakote Tablets 430
Depakote ER Tablets 436
Depo-Provera Contraceptive Injection 2798
Desmopressin Acetate Injection (Rare) 1344
Diamox .... ⊙269
Diflucan Tablets, Injection, and Oral Suspension (Rare) 2681
Digibind Powder 1514
Diovan HCT Tablets (Greater than 0.2%) 2338
Diphtheria & Tetanus Toxoids Adsorbed Purogenated for Pediatric Use (Rare) 1857
Diprivan Injectable Emulsion (Rare) 667
Donnatal 2929
Donnatal Extentabs 2930
Donnatal Tablets 2929
Doryx Coated Pellet Filled Capsules 3357
Duricef 1079
Dyazide Capsules 1515
Dynabac Tablets 2269
Dynacin Capsules 2019
Dyrenium Capsules 3458
Ecotrin Enteric Coated Aspirin Low, Regular and Maximum Strength Tablets 1715
E.E.S. 450
Effexor Tablets 3495
Effexor XR Capsules 3499
Ellence Injection 2806
Elspar for Injection 2092
Engerix-B Vaccine 1517
Epivir 1520
Epivir-HBV 1524
Ergamisol Tablets (Less frequent) 1789
EryPed 446
Ery-Tab Tablets 448
Erythrocin Stearate Filmtab Tablets 452
Erythromycin Base Filmtab Tablets 454
Erythromycin Delayed-Release Capsules, USP 455
Famotidine Injection (Infrequent) 866
Flexeril Tablets 572
Flexeril Tablets 2094
Flonase Nasal Spray 1533
Fludara for Injection (Up to 1%) 995
Fluorescite Injection .... ⊙211
FluShield Influenza Vaccine (One case) 3521
Fluzone Vaccine (Rare) 802
Fortaz (Very rare) 1541
Sterile FUDR (Remote possibility) 2974
Gamimune N, 5% Solvent/Detergent Treated (Rare) 925
Gammagard S/D 845
Havrix Vaccine (Rare) 1544
Herceptin I.V. 1414
Hytrin Capsules (Rare) 464
Imitrex Injection (Rare) 1549
Imitrex Nasal Spray 1554
Imitrex Tablets (Rare) 1558
Indocin Capsules (Less than 1%) 2112
Indocin I.V. (Less than 1%) 2115
Indocin (Less than 1%) 2112
INFeD Injection 3388
Integrilin Injection (One patient) 1213
Integrilin Injection (One patient) 1828
Intron A for Injection (Rare) 3120
JE-VAX Vaccine (One episode) 811
Keflex 1237
Kefurox Vials, ADD-Vantage (Rare) 1948
Kefzol Vials, ADD-Vantage 1951
Kytril Injection (Rare) 2986
Kytril Tablets (Rare) 2988
Lamisil Tablets (Rare) 2360
Lescol Capsules (Rare) 2361
Lescol Capsules (Rare) 2925
Lescol XL Tablets 2361
Lescol XL Tablets 2925
Lipitor Tablets 2639
Lipitor Tablets 2696
Lopid Tablets 2650
Lorabid Suspension and Pulvules (Rare) 2251
LYMErix Vaccine (Very rare) 1592
Macrobid Capsules 2889
Macrodantin Capsules 2891
Malarone (One case) 1596
Mandol Vials 1953
Maxipime for Injection 1285
Maxzide 1008
Mefoxin for Injection 2124
Mefoxin Premixed Intravenous Solution 2127
Meruvax II 2130
Mevacor Tablets (Rare) 2132
Miacalcin Injection (One case) 2373
Miacalcin Nasal Spray (One case) 2375
Miltown Tablets (Rare) 3349
Minocin Intravenous 1862
Minocin Oral Suspension 1865
Minocin Pellet-Filled Capsules 1863
Mintezol 2137
M-M-R II 2118
Monodox Capsules 2442
Mononine Concentrate 794
Motofen Tablets 577
Motrin Suspension, Oral Drops, Chewable Tablets, and Caplets (Less than 1%) 2002
MS Contin Tablets (Extremely rare) 2896
Mumpsvax 2141
Mustargen for Injection 2142
Mylotarg for Injection 3540
Nasonex Nasal Spray 3131
Navane Oral (Rare) 2701
Navane Intramuscular (Rare) 2703
Navelbine Injection 1604
Nebcin Vials, Hyporets & ADD-Vantage (Rare) 1955
Neosporin Ophthalmic Ointment Sterile (Rare) .... ⊙299
Neosporin Ophthalmic Solution Sterile (Rare) .... ⊙300
Neptazane Tablets .... ⊙271
Nizoral Tablets (Rare) 1791
Norvir Capsules (Rare) 487
Norvir Oral Solution (Rare) 487
Omnicef 493
Oncaspar 756
Orthoclone OKT3 Sterile Solution 2498
Orudis Capsules (Less than 1%) 3548
Oruvail Capsules (Less than 1%) 3548
Paxil 1609
PCE Dispertab Tablets 498
Pediazole Suspension 3050
Pepcid Injection (Infrequent) 2153
Pepcid for Oral Suspension (Infrequent) 2150
Pepcid RPD Orally Disintegrating Tablets (Infrequent) 2150
Pepcid Tablets (Infrequent) 2150
Periostat Tablets 1208
Permapen Isoject 2706
Pfizerpen for Injection (Severe & occasionally fatal (See Warnings)) 2707
Polysporin Ophthalmic Ointment (Rare) .... ⊙301
Pravachol Tablets (Rare) 1099
Premphase Tablets 3572
Prempro Tablets 3572
PREVPAC (Rare) 3298
Prilosec Delayed-Release Capsules (Rare) 628
Prograf (A small percentage of patients) 1393
Proleukin for Injection 1199
Prometrium Capsules (100 mg, 200 mg) 3261
Prostigmin Injectable 1744
Prostigmin Tablets 1744
Protonix I.V. 3580
Protonix Tablets 3577
Provera Tablets 2853
Rebetron Combination Therapy 3153
Recombivax HB (Less than 1%) 2178
ReFacto Vials 1437
Relafen Tablets (Less than 1%) 1617
Remicade for IV Injection (Infrequent) 1178
ReoPro Vials 1958
Retrovir Capsules (One patient) 1625
Retrovir IV Infusion (One patient) 1629
Retrovir (One patient) 1625
Rifadin (Rare) 765
Robinul Forte Tablets 1358
Robinul Injectable 2940
Robinul Tablets 1358
Rocephin Injectable Vials, ADD-Vantage, Galaxy, Bulk (Rare) 2993
Semprex-D Capsules (Rare) 1172
Septra Suspension 2265
Septra Tablets 2265
Septra DS Tablets 2265
Serevent Diskus 1637
Simulect for Injection 2399
Singulair 2181
Sporanox Capsules (Rare) 1800
Sporanox Injection (Rare) 1804
Sporanox Injection (Rare) 2509
Sporanox Oral Solution (Rare) 1808
Sporanox Oral Solution (Rare) 2512
Suprax 1877
Tagamet (Rare) 1644
Tao Capsules 2716
Taxol Injection (2%) 1129
Tazicef for Injection (Very rare) 1647
Tazicef Galaxy Container (Very rare) 1650
Tazicef Pharmacy Bulk Package (Very rare) 1653
Tazidime Vials, Faspak & ADD-Vantage (Very rare) 1966
Tetanus & Diphtheria Toxoids Adsorbed for Adult Use (Rare) 1880
Tetanus and Diphtheria Toxoids Adsorbed For Adult Use (Rare) 815
Tetanus Toxoid Adsorbed Purogenated 1882
Thiothixene Capsules (Rare) 2290
Ticlid Tablets 3015
Timolol GFS .... ⊙266
Timoptic in Ocudose 2192
Timoptic Sterile Ophthalmic Solution 2190
Timoptic-XE Sterile Ophthalmic Gel Forming Solution 2194
TNKase I.V. (Rare) 1430
Toradol 3018
Trasylol Injection 909
Trizivir Tablets 1669
Trovan 2722
Twinrix Vaccine 1674
Ultracet Tablets 2597
Ultram Tablets (Less than 1%) 2600
Valtrex Caplets 1676
Vancocin HCl Capsules & Pulvules 1972
Vancocin HCl Oral Solution (Infrequent) 1971
Vancocin HCl, Vials & ADD-Vantage (Infrequent) 1970
Varivax 2202
Velosulin BR Human Insulin 10 ml Vials 2435
Ventolin Inhalation Aerosol and Refill 1679
Vibramycin Calcium Oral Suspension Syrup 2735
Vibramycin Hyclate Capsules 2735
Vibramycin Monohydrate for Oral Suspension 2735
Viramune Oral Suspension 1060
Viramune Tablets 1060
Vistide Injection 1445
Vivelle Transdermal System (Isolated reports) 2412
Voltaren Tablets (Rare) 2315
Voltaren-XR Tablets (Rare) 2315
Xenical Capsules 3043
YF-VAX Vaccine 827
Zantac (Rare) 1690
Zantac Injection (Rare) 1688
Zantac Syrup (Rare) 1690
Ziagen 1692
Zinacef Injection (Rare) 1696
Zinacef for Injection (Rare) 1696
Zithromax Capsules, 250 mg (Rare) 2743
Zithromax for IV Infusion (Rare) 2748
Zithromax for Oral Suspension, 1 g (Rare) 2743
Zithromax for Oral Suspension, 300 mg, 600 mg, 900 mg, 1200 mg (Rare) 2739
Zithromax Tablets, 250 mg (Rare) 2739
Zithromax Tablets, 600 mg (Rare) 2743
Zocor Tablets (Rare) 2219
Zofran Injection (Rare) 1698
Zofran (Rare) 1703
Zofran ODT Orally Disintegrating Tablets (Rare) 1703
Zoladex (Rare) 702
Zoladex 3-month (Rare) 706
Zosyn (1.0% or less) 1890
Zosyn in Galaxy Containers (1.0% or less) 1894
Zovirax Capsules (Rare) 1706
Zovirax for Injection (Rare) 1708
Zovirax (Rare) 1706
Zyrtec (Rare) 2756
Zyrtec-D 12 Hour Extended Relief Tablets (Rare) 2758

Anasarca

▲ Gleevec Capsules (2% to 16%) 2357

Androgen excess, signs or symptoms of

Lupron Depot 3.75 mg (Less than 5%) 3281
Lupron Depot–3 Month 11.25 mg (Less than 5%) 3285

Anemia

▲ Abelcet Injection (4%) 1273
Accuretic Tablets 2614
Accutane Capsules 2944
Aceon Tablets (2 mg, 4 mg, 8 mg) 3249
Aciphex Tablets 1267
Aciphex Tablets 1783
Actiq (Less than 1%) 1184
Actonel Tablets (2.4%) 2879
Actos Tablets (1%) 3275
Adalat CC Tablets (Rare) 877
Aggrenox Capsules (1.6%) 1026
Agrylin Capsules (1% to 5%) 3232
Alkeran for Injection 1465
Alkeran Tablets 1466
Aloprim for Injection (Less than 1%) 2292
Ambien Tablets (Rare) 3191
AmBisome for Injection (Less common) 1383
Amerge Tablets (Rare) 1467
Amoxil Chewable Tablets 1471
Amoxil for Oral Suspension 1471
Amoxil 1471
▲ Amphotec (5% or more) 1774
Ancobon Capsules 1730
Anzemet Injection (Infrequently) 719
Anzemet Tablets (Infrequently) 722
Apligraf (2.7%) 2305
Arava Tablets (1% to 3%) 724

▲ Aredia for Injection (42.5%) 2309
Aricept Tablets (Infrequent)............ 1270
Aricept Tablets (Infrequent)............ 2665
▲ Arimidex Tablets (2% to 5%) 659
Arthrotec Tablets (Rare).................. 3195
Asacol Delayed-Release Tablets...... 2884
Atacand Tablets............................. 595
Atromid-S Capsules........................ 3483
Augmentin Chewable Tablets.......... 1482
Augmentin Powder for Oral Suspension.............................. 1482
Augmentin Tablets.......................... 1485
Augmentin ES-600 Powder for Oral Suspension......................... 1487
Avandia Tablets (1.9%).................... 1490
▲ Avonex (8%) 1013
▲ Axid Pulvules (More frequent) 1903
▲ Axid Pulvules (More frequent) 2919
Azactam for Injection (Less than 1%).. 1276
Azulfidine EN-tabs Tablets 2775
Baycol Tablets 883
Calcium Disodium Versenate Injection 1980
▲ Campath Ampules (38% to 80%) 992
Cancidas for Injection (Up to 3.8%) 2048
Captopril Tablets 2281
▲ Carnitor Injection (3% to 12%) 3242
▲ Casodex Tablets (7%) 662
Cataflam Tablets (Sometimes) 2315
Cefizox for Intramuscular or Intravenous Use (Rare) 1390
Celebrex Capsules (0.1% to 1.9%) 2676
Celebrex Capsules (0.1% to 1.9%) 2780
Celexa (Infrequent) 1365
▲ CellCept Capsules (25.6% to 42.9%) 2951
▲ CellCept Intravenous (25.6% to 42.9%) 2951
▲ CellCept Oral Suspension (25.6% to 42.9%) 2951
▲ CellCept Tablets (25.6% to 43%) ... 2951
Cerebyx Injection (Infrequent) 2619
▲ Chirocaine Injection (9.6%) 2909
Cipro (Less than 0.1%) 887
Clinoril Tablets (Less than 1%) 2053
Clozaril Tablets (Less than 1%) 2319
Cognex Capsules (Infrequent) 1351
Colazal Capsules 3069
Combivir Tablets (2.9%) 1502
Concerta Extended-Release Tablets 1998
Concerta Tablets 561
Coreg Tablets (0.1% to more than 2%) 1508
Cosmegen for Injection 2062
Cozaar Tablets (Less than 1%) 2067
▲ Crinone (Less than 5%) 3213
Crixivan Capsules (Less than 2%) ... 2070
Cytotec Tablets (Infrequent) 3202
▲ Cytovene (1% to 19%) 2959
Demser Capsules (Rare) 2085
Depacon Injection 416
Depakene 421
Depakote Sprinkle Capsules 426
Depakote Tablets 430
Depakote ER Tablets (Greater than 1%) 436
DepoCyt Injection (1%) 1197
Depo-Provera Contraceptive Injection (Fewer than 1%) 2798
D.H.E. 45 Injection 2334
Dipentum Capsules (Rare) 2803
▲ Doxil Injection (6.5% to 52.6%) 566
DTIC-Dome 902
Effexor Tablets (Infrequent) 3495
Effexor XR Capsules (Infrequent) 3499
Eldepryl Capsules 3266
▲ Ellence Injection (5.8% to 72.2%) ... 2806
Elmiron Capsules (Less than or equal to 1%) 570
Enalaprilat Injection 863
Enbrel for Injection 1752
Enbrel for Injection 3504
Epivir (2% to 2.9%) 1520
Epivir-HBV 1524
▲ Ergamisol Tablets (Up to 6%) 1789
Esclim Transdermal System 3460
▲ Eulexin Capsules (6%) 3118
Evoxac Capsules (1% to 3%) 1217
Exelon Capsules (Frequent) 2342
Exelon Oral Solution (Frequent) 2345
Famvir Tablets (0.1%) 2348
Felbatol 3343
▲ Feldene Capsules (1% to 10%) 2685
Ferrlecit Injection (Greater than 1%) 3386
Flolan for Injection 1528
Floxin I.V. (More than or equal to 1%) 2526
Floxin Tablets (More than or equal to 1%) 2529
▲ Fludara for Injection (Among most common) 995
Fortovase Capsules (Less than 2%) 2970
▲ Foscavir Injection (5% to 33%) 605
▲ Sterile FUDR (Among more common) 2974
Furosemide Tablets 2284
Gabitril Tablets (Infrequent)............. 1189
▲ Gemzar for Injection (45% to 73%) 1919
Gengraf Capsules (1% to less than 3%) 457
Geocillin Tablets 2687
Geodon Capsules (Infrequent)......... 2688
▲ Gleevec Capsules (4% to 31%) 2357
▲ Gliadel Wafer (4% to 9%) 1723
Haldol Decanoate 2535
Haldol Injection, Tablets and Concentrate 2533
Helixate Concentrate 788
▲ Herceptin I.V. (4%) 1414
▲ Hivid Tablets (Less than 1% to 8.4%) 2975
▲ Hycamtin for Injection (40% to 95%) 1546
Hyzaar 2109
Imitrex Injection 1549
Imitrex Nasal Spray 1554
Imitrex Tablets (Rare) 1558
Indocin Capsules (Less than 1%) 2112
Indocin I.V. (Less than 1%) 2115
Indocin (Less than 1%) 2112
Innohep Injection (Greater than or equal to 1%) 1248
▲ Intron A for Injection (Less than 5% to 22%) 3120
Invirase Capsules (Less than 2%) 2979
Kadian Capsules (Less than 3%) 1335
Kaletra Capsules (Less than 2%) 471
Kaletra Oral Solution (Less than 2%) 471
Klonopin Tablets 2983
Kogenate FS 936
▲ Kytril Tablets (4%) 2988
Lamictal (Infrequent) 1567
▲ Leustatin Injection (37%) 2495
Levaquin (Less than 0.3%) 2537
Lexxel Tablets 608
Lipitor Tablets (Less than 2%) 2639
Lipitor Tablets (Less than 2%) 2696
Lodine (Less than 1%) 3528
Lodine XL Extended-Release Tablets (Less than 1%) 3530
Lopid Tablets (Rare) 2650
▲ Lovenox Injection (3%) 746
▲ Lupron Depot—3 Month 22.5 mg (Less than 5%) 3288
▲ Lupron Injection (5% or more) 3279
Luvox Tablets (25, 50, 100 mg) (Infrequent) 3256
Macrobid Capsules 2889
Macrodantin Capsules 2891
Matulane Capsules (Frequent) 3246
Mefoxin for Injection 2124
Mefoxin Premixed Intravenous Solution 2127
▲ Megace Oral Suspension (Up to 5%) 1124
▲ Mepron Suspension (4% to 6%) 1598
Meridia Capsules 481
Merrem I.V. (0.1% to 1.0%) 673
Metadate CD Capsules 1164
Metadate ER Tablets 1167
Methylin Tablets 1995
Methylin ER Tablets 1995
Miacalcin Nasal Spray (Less than 1%) 2375
Mirapex Tablets (1% or more) 2834
Mobic Tablets (0.1% to 4.1%) 1054
Monopril Tablets 1091
▲ Mycobutin Capsules (6%) 2838
Myleran Tablets 1603
Mylocel Tablets .... [illegible]
▲ Mylotarg for Injection (47%) 3540
Naprelan Tablets (Less than 3%) 1293
▲ Naropin Injection (1% to 5%) 612
Natrecor for Injection (At least 1%) 3189
▲ Navelbine Injection (1% to 77%) 1604
Nebcin Vials, Hyporets & ADD-Vantage 1955
Neoral Soft Gelatin Capsules (1% to less than 3%) 2380
Neoral Oral Solution (1% to less than 3%) 2380
▲ Neupogen for Injection (Approximately 10%) 587
Neurontin Capsules (Infrequent) 2655
Neurontin Oral Solution (Infrequent) 2655
Neurontin Tablets (Infrequent) 2655
Nexium Delayed-Release Capsules (Less than 1%) 619
▲ Nilandron Tablets (7.2%) 753
Nimotop Capsules (Less than 1%) .. 904
▲ Nipent for Injection (8% to 35%) 3272
Nolvadex Tablets 678
Norplant System (Rare) 3543
Norvir Capsules (Less than 2%) 487
Norvir Oral Solution (Less than 2%) 487
▲ Novantrone for Injection (6% to 9%) 1760
Oncaspar 756
Orgaran Injection (2.2%) 2480
Orudis Capsules (Less than 1%) 3548
Oruvail Capsules (Less than 1%) 3548
ParaGard T 380A Intrauterine Copper Contraceptive 2582
▲ Paraplatin for Injection (8% to 91%) 1126
Parnate Tablets 1607
Paxil (Infrequent)............................ 1609
Pediazole Suspension 3050
Pentasa Capsules 3239
Permax Tablets (1.1%) 1299
▲ Photofrin for Injection (32%) 831
Plavix Tablets (1% to 2.5%)............. 1097
Plavix Tablets (1% to 2.5%)............. 3084
Plendil Extended-Release Tablets (0.5% to 1.5%) 623
Pletal Tablets (Less than 2%) 2605
Pletal Tablets (Less than 2%) 2848
▲ Ponstel Capsules (1% to 10%) 1356
Pravachol Tablets 1099
Prevacid Delayed-Release Capsules (Less than 1%)............. 3292
PREVPAC (Less than 1%)................ 3298
Priftin Tablets (2.5%) 758
Prilosec Delayed-Release Capsules (Rare)......................... 628
Prinivil Tablets 2164
Procardia Capsules (Less than 0.5%) 2708
▲ Prograf (5% to 47%) 1393
▲ Proleukin for Injection (29%) 1199
Protonix I.V. (Less than 1%) 3580
Protonix Tablets (Less than 1%) 3577
Provigil Tablets (At least 1%) 1193
Prozac Pulvules, Liquid, and Weekly Capsules (Infrequent) 1238
Purinethol Tablets (Frequent) 1615
▲ Rapamune Oral Solution and Tablets (23% to 37%) 3584
▲ Rebetron Combination Therapy (10%) 3153
▲ Refludan for Injection (12.4%) 761
Relafen Tablets (Less than 1%) 1617
Remeron Tablets (Rare) 2483
Remeron SolTab Tablets (Rare) 2486
Remicade for IV Injection (Less than 2%) 1178
▲ Reminyl Oral Solution (3%) 1792
▲ Reminyl Tablets (3%) 1792
ReoPro Vials (1.2%) 1958
Requip Tablets (1% or more) 1621
Rescriptor Tablets (0.7% to 1.0%) .. 526
Retavase Vials (0.9% to 2.6%) 1182
▲ Retrovir Capsules (1.1% to 29%) ... 1625
▲ Retrovir IV Infusion (1.1% to 29%) .. 1629
▲ Retrovir (1.1% to 29%) 1625
Rilutek Tablets (Infrequent) 772
Risperdal (Infrequent) 1796
Ritalin 2387
Rituxan for Infusion (1%) 1750
Rituxan I.V. (1%) 1428
Rocephin Injectable Vials, ADD-Vantage, Galaxy, Bulk (Less than 1%) 2993
Roxicodone Tablets (Less than 3%) 3067
Rythmol Tablets – 150 mg, 225 mg, 300 mg (Less than 1%) 502
Sandimmune (2% or less) 2388
Sandostatin Injection (Less than 1%) 2394
▲ Sandostatin LAR Depot (5% to 15%) 2395
Sarafem Pulvules (Infrequent) 1962
Serentil 1057
Seroquel Tablets (Infrequent) 684
▲ Serostim for Injection (12.2%) 3229
Serzone Tablets (Infrequent) 1104
▲ Simulect for Injection (Greater than or equal to 10%) 2399
Sonata Capsules (Infrequent) 3591
Stelazine 1640
Stromectol Tablets (One patient) 2185
Sular Tablets (Less than or equal to 1%) 688
Synagis Intramuscular (More than 1%) 2028
Tabloid Tablets 1642
Tamiflu Capsules (Less than 1%) 3008
Tamiflu Oral Suspension (Less than 1%) 3008
Tasmar Tablets (Infrequent) 3010
▲ Taxol Injection (16% to 78%) 1129
▲ Taxotere for Injection Concentrate (89.5%) 778
Teveten Tablets (Less than 1%) 3327
▲ Thalomid Capsules (5.6% to 12.5%) 1154
▲ TheraCys Injection (21%) 823
Thioplex for Injection 1765
Thioridazine Hydrochloride Tablets 2289
Tice BCG, BCG Live (1.3%) 2489
Ticlid Tablets 3015
Tonocard Tablets (Less than 1%) 649
Topamax Sprinkle Capsules (Frequent) 2590
Topamax Tablets (Frequent) 2590
Toradol (1% or less) 3018
Trasylol Injection (2%) 909
Tricor Capsules, Micronized 513
▲ Trisenox Injection (20%) 1158
Trizivir Tablets (2.9%) 1669
Trovan (Less than 1%) 2722
Ultracet Tablets (Less than 1%) 2597
Uniretic Tablets (Less than 1%) 3178
▲ Valcyte Tablets (8% to 26%) 3022
Valstar Sterile Solution for Intravesical Instillation (2%)........... 1175
Valtrex Caplets (Up to 0.8%)............ 1676
Vantin Tablets and Oral Suspension (Less than 1%)........... 2860
Vaseretic Tablets 2204
Vasotec I.V. Injection 2207
Vasotec Tablets 2210
Viadur Implant (2.3%) 912
Viagra Tablets (Less than 2%).......... 2732
Videx 1138
Videx EC Capsules 1143
Vioxx 2213
Viracept 532
Virazole for Inhalation Solution 1747
▲ Vistide Injection (24%) 1445
▲ Visudyne for Injection (1% to 10%) .... ⊙308
▲ Vitravene for Injection (5% to 20%) .... ⊙310
Voltaren Tablets (Sometimes) 2315
Voltaren-XR Tablets (Sometimes) 2315
Wellbutrin Tablets (Rare) 1680
Wellbutrin SR Sustained-Release Tablets 1684
Xeloda Tablets (1% to 3%) 3039
Zanaflex Tablets (Infrequent) 1305
Zerit (Fewer than 1%) 1147
Zestoretic Tablets 695
Ziagen 1692
Zoladex (1% to 5%) 702
Zoladex 3-month (1% to 5%) 706
Zoloft (Rare) 2751
▲ Zometa for Intravenous Infusion (22.1%) 3621
Zonegran Capsules (Infrequent) 1307
Zovirax Capsules 1706
Zovirax for Injection (Less than 1%) 1708
Zovirax 1706
Zyban Sustained-Release Tablets 1710
Zyprexa Tablets (Infrequent) 1973
Zyprexa ZYDIS Orally Disintegrating Tablets (Infrequent) 1973

Anemia, aplastic

Accuretic Tablets 2614
Aceon Tablets (2 mg, 4 mg, 8 mg) 3249
Aggrenox Capsules 1026
Aldoclor Tablets 2035
Aldoril Tablets 2039
Amaryl Tablets 717
Anaprox Tablets (Less than 1%) 2967
Anaprox DS Tablets (Less than 1%) 2967
Ancobon Capsules 1730
Arthrotec Tablets (Rare) 3195
Asacol Delayed-Release Tablets (Rare) 2884
Atacand HCT Tablets 597
Avalide Tablets 1070
Azulfidine EN-tabs Tablets (Rare) 2775
Bactrim (Rare) 2949
▲ Blephamide Ophthalmic Ointment (Among most often) 547
Blephamide Ophthalmic Suspension 548
Carbatrol Capsules 3234
Cataflam Tablets (Rare) 2315
Ceclor 1905
Cedax 1021
Cefizox for Intramuscular or Intravenous Use 1390
Cefotan 664
Ceftin 1898
Cefzil 1076
Ceptaz for Injection 1499
Chloromycetin Ophthalmic Ointment, 1% .... ⊙296
Chloromycetin Ophthalmic Solution .... ⊙297
Chloroptic Sterile Ophthalmic Solution (Rare) .... ⊙235
Clinoril Tablets (Less than 1 in 100) 2053
Clorpres Tablets 1002
Combipres Tablets 1040
Compazine 1505
Cordarone Tablets 3487
Coreg Tablets (Rare) 1508
Corzide 40/5 Tablets 2247
Corzide 80/5 Tablets 2247
Cosmegen for Injection 2062
Cuprimine Capsules 2075
Cylert Tablets (Isolated reports) 415
Dantrium Capsules (Less frequent) 2885
Dantrium Intravenous 2886
Dapsone Tablets USP 1780
Depacon Injection 416
Depakene 421
Depakote Sprinkle Capsules 426
Depakote Tablets 430
Depakote ER Tablets 436
Depen Titratable Tablets 3341
DiaBeta Tablets (Occasional) 741
Diabinese Tablets 2680
Diamox Intravenous .... ⊙269

Diamox Sequels Sustained Release Capsules ⊙ 270
Diamox Tablets ⊙ 269
Diovan HCT Tablets 2338
Diucardin Tablets 3494
Diuril Oral 2087
Diuril Sodium Intravenous 2086
Duricef 1079
Dyazide Capsules 1515
EC-Naprosyn Delayed-Release Tablets (Less than 1%) 2967
Effexor Tablets 3495
Effexor XR Capsules 3499
Enbrel for Injection 1752
Enbrel for Injection 3504
Felbatol 3343
Feldene Capsules (Rare) 2685
Floxin I.V. 2526
Floxin Tablets 2529
FML-S Liquifilm Sterile Ophthalmic Suspension ⊙ 238
Fortaz 1541
Furosemide Tablets 2284
Glucotrol Tablets 2692
Glucotrol XL Extended Release Tablets 2693
▲ Hexalen Capsules (13% to 33%) 2226
HydroDIURIL Tablets 2108
Hyzaar 2109
Indapamide Tablets 2286
Inderide Tablets 3517
Inderide LA Long-Acting Capsules 3519
Indocin Capsules (Less than 1%) 2112
Indocin I.V. (Less than 1%) 2115
Indocin (Less than 1%) 2112
Kefurox Vials, ADD-Vantage 1948
Lamictal 1567
Leustatin Injection (Some reports) 2495
Lodine XL Extended-Release Tablets 3530
Lorabid Suspension and Pulvules 2251
Lotensin HCT Tablets 2367
Luvox Tablets (25, 50, 100 mg) 3256
Macrobid Capsules (Rare) 2889
Macrodantin Capsules (Rare) 2891
Maxipime for Injection 1285
Maxzide 1008
Mefoxin for Injection 2124
Mefoxin Premixed Intravenous Solution 2127
Micardis HCT Tablets 1051
Microzide Capsules 3414
Midamor Tablets (Rare) 2136
Miltown Tablets 3349
Minizide Capsules 2700
Moduretic Tablets 2138
Monopril Tablets 1091
Monopril HCT 1094
Monurol Sachet 1375
Motrin Suspension, Oral Drops, Chewable Tablets, and Caplets (Less than 1%) 2002
Mykrox Tablets 1168
Myleran Tablets 1603
▲ Naprelan Tablets (3% to 9%) 1293
Naprosyn Suspension (Less than 1%) 2967
Naprosyn Tablets (Less than 1%) 2967
Neptazane Tablets ⊙ 271
Nipent for Injection (Less than 3%) 3272
Norflex (Very rare) 1987
Omnicef 493
Orthoclone OKT3 Sterile Solution 2498
Paxil 1609
Pediazole Suspension 3050
Pentasa Capsules 3239
Plaquenil Tablets 3082
Plavix Tablets (Less than 1%) 1097
Plavix Tablets (Less than 1%) 3084
Ponstel Capsules (Rare) 1356
Prevacid Delayed-Release Capsules (Less than 1%) 3292
PREVPAC 3298
Prinzide Tablets 2168
Prozac Pulvules, Liquid, and Weekly Capsules 1238
Rebetron Combination Therapy (Very rare) 3153
Renese Tablets 2712
Rifamate Capsules 767
Rifater Tablets (Rare) 769
Rilutek Tablets (Rare) 772
Rituxan for Infusion (One case) 1750
Rituxan I.V. (One case) 1428
Roferon-A Injection (Rare) 2996
Sarafem Pulvules 1962
Septra Suspension 2265
Septra Tablets 2265
Septra DS Tablets 2265
Serentil 1057
Silvadene Cream 1% 2267
Stelazine 1640
Suprax 1877
Tagamet (Very rare) 1644
Tapazole Tablets 1823
Tazicef for Injection 1647
Tazicef Galaxy Container 1650
Tazicef Pharmacy Bulk Package 1653
Tazidime Vials, Faspak & ADD-Vantage 1966
Tegretol/Tegretol-XR (Very low incidence) 2404
Tenoretic Tablets 690
Thalomid Capsules 1154
Thioridazine Hydrochloride Tablets 2289
Thorazine 1656
Ticlid Tablets (Rare) 3015
Timolide Tablets 2187
Trental Tablets (Rare) 784
Trusopt Sterile Ophthalmic Solution (Rare) 2196
Urobiotic-250 Capsules 2731
Valcyte Tablets (Less than 5%) 3022
Valtrex Caplets 1676
Vantin Tablets and Oral Suspension 2860
Vaseretic Tablets 2204
Voltaren Tablets (Rare) 2315
Voltaren-XR Tablets (Rare) 2315
Zantac (Rare) 1690
Zantac Injection (Rare) 1688
Zantac Syrup (Rare) 1690
Zaroxolyn Tablets 1177
Zestoretic Tablets 695
Zinacef Injection 1696
Zinacef for Injection 1696
Zoloft 2751

Anemia, dilutional

Prolastin 943

Anemia, glucose-6-phosphate dehydrogenase deficiency

Chibroxin Sterile Ophthalmic Solution 2051
Macrobid Capsules 2889
Macrodantin Capsules 2891

Anemia, Heinz-body

Azulfidine EN-tabs Tablets (Less frequent) 2775

Anemia, hemolytic

Accupril Tablets 2611
Accuretic Tablets 2614
Aceon Tablets (2 mg, 4 mg, 8 mg) 3249
Aciphex Tablets 1267
Aciphex Tablets 1783
Agenerase Capsules 1454
Agenerase Oral Solution 1459
Aldoclor Tablets 2035
Aldomet Tablets 2037
Aldoril Tablets 2039
Alkeran for Injection 1465
Alkeran Tablets 1466
Altace Capsules (Less than 1%) 2233
Amaryl Tablets 717
Amoxil Chewable Tablets 1471
Amoxil for Oral Suspension 1471
Amoxil 1471
Anaprox Tablets (Less than 1%) 2967
Anaprox DS Tablets (Less than 1%) 2967
Aricept Tablets (Rare) 1270
Aricept Tablets (Rare) 2665
Arthrotec Tablets (Rare) 3195
Atacand HCT Tablets 597
Augmentin Chewable Tablets 1482
Augmentin Powder for Oral Suspension 1482
Augmentin Tablets 1485
Augmentin ES-600 Powder for Oral Suspension 1487
Avalide Tablets 1070
Azulfidine EN-tabs Tablets (One in every 30 patients or less) 2775
Bactrim 2949
Baycol Tablets 883
Benadryl Parenteral 2617
Bicillin C-R 900/300 Injection 2240
Bicillin C-R Injection 2238
Bicillin L-A Injection (Infrequent) 2242
Campath Ampules 992
Captopril Tablets 2281
Cardizem Injectable 1018
Cardizem Lyo-Ject Syringe 1018
Cardizem Monovial 1018
Cardizem CD Capsules (Infrequent) 1016
Cataflam Tablets (Rare) 2315
Ceclor CD Tablets 1279
Ceclor (Rare) 1905
Cedax 1021
Cefizox for Intramuscular or Intravenous Use (Rare) 1390
Cefotan (Uncommon) 664
Ceftin 1898
Cefzil 1076
Ceptaz for Injection (Exceedingly rare cases) 1499
Chibroxin Sterile Ophthalmic Solution 2051
Cipro I.V. (Rare) 893
Cipro I.V. Pharmacy Bulk Package (Rare) 897
Cipro 887
Claforan Injection (Rare) 732
Clinoril Tablets (Less than 1 in 100) 2053
Compazine 1505
Cordarone Tablets 3487
Corzide 40/5 Tablets 2247
Corzide 80/5 Tablets 2247
Crixivan Capsules 2070
Cuprimine Capsules 2075
Cytovene 2959
Declomycin Tablets 1855
Depen Titratable Tablets 3341
D.H.E. 45 Injection 2334
DiaBeta Tablets (Occasional) 741
Diabinese Tablets 2680
Diamox ⊙ 269
Diovan HCT Tablets 2338
Dipentum Capsules (Rare) 2803
Diucardin Tablets 3494
Diuril Oral 2087
Diuril Sodium Intravenous 2086
Dolobid Tablets (Less than 1 in 100) 2088
Doryx Coated Pellet Filled Capsules 3357
Duricef 1079
Dyazide Capsules 1515
Dynacin Capsules 2019
EC-Naprosyn Delayed-Release Tablets (Less than 1%) 2967
Enalaprilat Injection 863
Etrafon 3115
Eulexin Capsules 3118
Felbatol 3343
Feldene Capsules (Rare) 2685
Floxin I.V. 2526
Floxin Tablets 2529
Fludara for Injection (Rare) 995
Fortaz (Rare) 1541
Fortovase Capsules (Rare) 2970
Furosemide Tablets 2284
Gengraf Capsules 457
Glucotrol Tablets 2692
Glucotrol XL Extended Release Tablets 2693
HydroDIURIL Tablets 2108
Hyzaar 2109
Imitrex Injection 1549
Imitrex Tablets 1558
Indocin Capsules (Less than 1%) 2112
Indocin I.V. (Less than 1%) 2115
Indocin (Less than 1%) 2112
Intron A for Injection (Less than 5%) 3120
Invirase Capsules (Rare) 2979
Iveegam EN (0.91%) 849
Lamictal 1567
Lescol Capsules (Rare) 2361
Lescol Capsules (Rare) 2925
Lescol XL Tablets 2361
Lescol XL Tablets 2925
Leustatin Injection (Some reports) 2495
Levaquin 2537
Lodine (Less than 1%) 3528
Lodine XL Extended-Release Tablets (Less than 1%) 3530
Lodosyn Tablets 1251
Lorabid Suspension and Pulvules 2251
Lotensin Tablets (Less than 1%) 2365
Lotensin HCT Tablets (Rare) 2367
Lotrel Capsules (Rare) 2370
Macrobid Capsules 2889
Macrodantin Capsules 2891
Matulane Capsules 3246
Maxipime for Injection 1285
Maxzide 1008
Mefoxin for Injection 2124
Mefoxin Premixed Intravenous Solution 2127
Mevacor Tablets (Rare) 2132
Micardis HCT Tablets 1051
Microzide Capsules 3414
Minocin Intravenous 1862
Minocin Oral Suspension 1865
Minocin Pellet-Filled Capsules 1863
Moduretic Tablets 2138
Monodox Capsules 2442
Monopril Tablets 1091
Monopril HCT 1094
Motrin Suspension, Oral Drops, Chewable Tablets, and Caplets (Less than 1%) 2002
Mustargen for Injection (Rare) 2142
▲ Naprelan Tablets (3% to 9%) 1293
Naprosyn Suspension (Less than 1%) 2967
Naprosyn Tablets (Less than 1%) 2967
Navane Oral 2701
Navane Intramuscular 2703
Neoral Soft Gelatin Capsules 2380
Neoral Oral Solution 2380
Neptazane Tablets ⊙ 271
Nipent for Injection (Less than 3%) 3272
Nizoral Tablets (Less than 1%) 1791
Noroxin Tablets (Rare) 2145
Omnicef 493
Oncaspar (Greater than 1% but less than 5%) 756
Orap Tablets 1407
Orthoclone OKT3 Sterile Solution 2498
Paser Granules 1781
Paxil 1609
Pediazole Suspension 3050
Periactin Tablets 2155
Periostat Tablets 1208
Permapen Isoject 2706
Pfizerpen for Injection (Rare) 2707
Pneumovax 23 (Rare) 2156
Ponstel Capsules (Rare) 1356
Pravachol Tablets (Rare) 1099
Prevacid Delayed-Release Capsules (Less than 1%) 3292
PREVPAC 3298
Prilosec Delayed-Release Capsules (Rare) 628
Primaxin I.M. 2158
Primaxin I.V. 2160
Prinivil Tablets 2164
Prinzide Tablets 2168
Procanbid Extended-Release Tablets (Rare) 2262
Procardia Capsules 2708
Procardia XL Extended Release Tablets 2710
Prozac Pulvules, Liquid, and Weekly Capsules 1238
Quinaglute Dura-Tabs Tablets 978
Quinidex Extentabs 2933
▲ Rebetron Combination Therapy (10%) 3153
ReoPro Vials (0.3%) 1958
Rescriptor Tablets 526
Rifadin 765
Rifamate Capsules 767
Rifater Tablets 769
Rituxan for Infusion (Two cases) 1750
Rituxan I.V. (Two cases) 1428
Rocephin Injectable Vials, ADD-Vantage, Galaxy, Bulk (Less than 1%) 2993
Roferon-A Injection (Rare) 2996
Rynatan Tablets 3351
Sarafem Pulvules 1962
Septra Suspension 2265
Septra Tablets 2265
Septra DS Tablets 2265
Silvadene Cream 1% 2267
Sinemet Tablets 1253
Sinemet CR Tablets 1255
Skelaxin Tablets 1301
Stelazine 1640
Sulfamylon Cream 1011
Sulfamylon Topical Solution 1011
Suprax 1877
Talacen Caplets (Rare) 3089
Tazicef for Injection 1647
Tazicef Galaxy Container 1650
Tazicef Pharmacy Bulk Package 1653
Tazidime Vials, Faspak & ADD-Vantage (Rare) 1966
Thiothixene Capsules 2290
Thorazine 1656
Tiazac Capsules (Infrequent) 1378
Ticlid Tablets (Rare) 3015
Timolide Tablets 2187
Tolectin (Less than 1%) 2589
Tonocard Tablets (Less than 1%) 649
Trilafon 3160
Uniretic Tablets (Less than 1%) 3178
Univasc Tablets (Less than 1%) 3181
Vantin Tablets and Oral Suspension 2860
Vaseretic Tablets 2204
Vasotec I.V. Injection 2207
Vasotec Tablets 2210
Vibramycin Calcium Oral Suspension Syrup 2735
Vibramycin Hyclate Capsules 2735
Vibramycin Hyclate Intravenous 2737
Vibramycin Monohydrate for Oral Suspension 2735
Vibra-Tabs Film Coated Tablets 2735
Virazole for Inhalation Solution 1747
Voltaren Tablets (Rare) 2315
Voltaren-XR Tablets (Rare) 2315
Zestoretic Tablets 695
Zestril Tablets (Rare) 698
Zinacef Injection 1696
Zinacef for Injection 1696
Zocor Tablets (Rare) 2219
Zosyn 1890
Zosyn in Galaxy Containers 1894
Zyrtec (Rare) 2756
Zyrtec-D 12 Hour Extended Relief Tablets (Rare) 2758

Anemia, hemolytic, immune

Campath Ampules 992
Fludara for Injection 995
Tagamet (Extremely rare) 1644
Zantac (Exceedingly rare) 1690
Zantac Injection (Exceedingly rare) 1688
Zantac Syrup (Exceedingly rare) 1690

Anemia, hemolytic, sideroblastic

Rifamate Capsules 767

Anemia, hypochromic

Aciphex Tablets 1267
Aciphex Tablets 1783
Amphotec (1% to 5%) 1774
▲ Casodex Tablets (7%) 662
Celexa (Rare) 1365

▲ CellCept Capsules (7.4% to 24.6%) ... 2951
▲ CellCept Intravenous (7.4% to 24.6%) ... 2951
▲ CellCept Oral Suspension (7.4% to 24.6%) ... 2951
▲ CellCept Tablets (7.4% to 24.6%) ... 2951
Cerebyx Injection (Infrequent) ... 2619
▲ Doxil Injection (5.2% to 9.8%) ... 566
Evoxac Capsules (Less than 1%) ... 1217
Exelon Capsules (Infrequent) ... 2342
Exelon Oral Solution (Infrequent) ... 2345
Felbatol ... 3343
Geodon Capsules (Rare) ... 2688
Imdur Tablets (Less than or equal to 5%) ... 1826
Lovenox Injection (2%) ... 746
Nexium Delayed-Release Capsules (Less than 1%) ... 619
Paxil (Rare) ... 1609
Plavix Tablets (Less than 1%) ... 1097
Plavix Tablets (Less than 1%) ... 3084
▲ Prograf (3% to 15%) ... 1393
Protonix I.V. (Less than 1%) ... 3580
Protonix Tablets (Less than 1%) ... 3577
Prozac Pulvules, Liquid, and Weekly Capsules (Rare) ... 1238
Requip Tablets (Infrequent) ... 1621
Rilutek Tablets (Rare) ... 772
Risperdal (Infrequent) ... 1796
Sarafem Pulvules (Rare) ... 1962
Seroquel Tablets (Infrequent) ... 684
Thalomid Capsules ... 1154
Uniretic Tablets (Less than 1%) ... 3178
Vistide Injection ... 1445

Anemia, hypoplastic
Mykrox Tablets ... 1168
Procanbid Extended-Release Tablets (Approximately 0.5%) ... 2262
Rynatan Tablets ... 3351
Tonocard Tablets (Less than 1%) ... 649
Zaroxolyn Tablets ... 1177

Anemia, iron deficiency
Anadrol-50 Tablets ... 3321
Arava Tablets (1% to 3%) ... 724
▲ Casodex Tablets (7%) ... 662
Lamictal (Rare) ... 1567
Paxil (Rare) ... 1609
Permax Tablets (Infrequent) ... 1299
Pletal Tablets (Less than 2%) ... 2605
Pletal Tablets (Less than 2%) ... 2848
Protonix I.V. (Less than 1%) ... 3580
Protonix Tablets (Less than 1%) ... 3577
Prozac Pulvules, Liquid, and Weekly Capsules (Rare) ... 1238
Rilutek Tablets (Rare) ... 772
Roxicodone Tablets (Less than 3%) ... 3067
Sarafem Pulvules (Rare) ... 1962
Viadur Implant (Less than 2%) ... 912

Anemia, macrocytic
Ambien Tablets (Rare) ... 3191
Depacon Injection ... 416
Depakene ... 421
Depakote Tablets ... 430
Depakote ER Tablets ... 436
Dilantin Infatabs ... 2624
Dilantin-125 Oral Suspension ... 2625
Eulexin Capsules ... 3118
Lamictal (Rare) ... 1567
Thalomid Capsules ... 1154

Anemia, megaloblastic
Azulfidine EN-tabs Tablets (Rare) ... 2775
Bactrim ... 2949
Daraprim Tablets ... 1511
Dilantin Infatabs ... 2624
Dilantin Kapseals ... 2622
Dilantin-125 Oral Suspension ... 2625
Dyazide Capsules ... 1515
Dyrenium Capsules (Rare) ... 3458
Macrobid Capsules ... 2889
Macrodantin Capsules ... 2891
Nembutal Sodium Solution ... 485
Permax Tablets (Infrequent) ... 1299
Septra Suspension ... 2265
Septra Tablets ... 2265
Septra DS Tablets ... 2265
Thalomid Capsules ... 1154
Zovirax for Injection (Less than 1%) ... 1708

Anemia, microangiopathic hemolytic
Gengraf Capsules ... 457
Plavix Tablets ... 1097
Plavix Tablets ... 3084
Sandimmune (Occasional) ... 2388

Anemia, microcytic
Paxil (Rare) ... 1609
Thalomid Capsules ... 1154
Zonegran Capsules (Rare) ... 1307

Anemia, nonhemolytic
Lodosyn Tablets ... 1251
Sinemet Tablets ... 1253
Sinemet CR Tablets ... 1255

Anemia, normocytic
Paxil (Rare) ... 1609
Risperdal (Rare) ... 1796
Zyprexa Tablets (Infrequent) ... 1973
Zyprexa ZYDIS Orally Disintegrating Tablets (Infrequent) ... 1973

Anemia, sideroblastic
Cuprimine Capsules ... 2075
Depen Titratable Tablets ... 3341
Pyrazinamide Tablets (Rare) ... 1876
Rifater Tablets (Rare) ... 769

Anencephaly
Cetrotide for Injection ... 3209
Felbatol ... 3343
Serophene Tablets ... 3226

Anesthesia, local
Chirocaine Injection (1%) ... 2909
Denavir Cream (0.9%) ... 2332
Migranal Nasal Spray (Infrequent) ... 2376

Anesthesia, persistent
Naropin Injection ... 612

Anesthetic effect
Lithium Carbonate ... 3061
Lithium Citrate Syrup ... 3061
Sensorcaine ... 643
Sensorcaine-MPF Injection ... 643
Tonocard Tablets (Less than 1%) ... 649
Versed Injection (Less than 1%) ... 3027

Anetoderma
Cuprimine Capsules (Rare) ... 2075
Depen Titratable Tablets (Rare) ... 3341

Aneurysm
Cognex Capsules (Infrequent) ... 1351
Fludara for Injection (Up to 1%) ... 995
Requip Tablets (Infrequent) ... 1621
Sandostatin LAR Depot (Rare) ... 2395

Aneurysm, abdominal aortic
Imitrex Nasal Spray (Rare) ... 1554

Anger
Meridia Capsules ... 481
Valium Injectable ... 3026

Angiectases, cutaneous
Adalat CC Tablets (Less than 1.0%) ... 877

Angiitis
Indocin Capsules (Less than 1%) ... 2112
Indocin I.V. (Less than 1%) ... 2115
Indocin (Less than 1%) ... 2112
Timolide Tablets ... 2187

Angina
Amerge Tablets ... 1467
Atromid-S Capsules ... 3483
Cardizem CD Capsules (Less than 1%) ... 1016
Clozaril Tablets (1%) ... 2319
Colestid Tablets (Infrequent) ... 2791
Combivent Inhalation Aerosol (Less than 2%) ... 1041
Concerta Extended-Release Tablets ... 1998
Concerta Tablets ... 561
Dobutrex Solution Vials (1% to 3%) ... 1914
Ergamisol Tablets ... 1789
Femara Tablets (Less than or equal to 2%) ... 2351
▲ Fludara for Injection (Up to 6%) ... 995
Foradil Aerolizer ... 2354
Sterile FUDR (Remote possibility) ... 2974
Imitrex Nasal Spray ... 1554
Imitrex Tablets (Rare) ... 1558
Intron A for Injection (Less than 5%) ... 3120
Levoxyl Tablets ... 1819
Lupron Depot 7.5 mg (Less than 5%) ... 3284
Lupron Injection (Less than 5%) ... 3279
Metadate CD Capsules ... 1164
Metadate ER Tablets ... 1167
Methylin Tablets ... 1995
Methylin ER Tablets ... 1995
Mexitil Capsules (1.7% or about 3 in 1,000) ... 1047
Migranal Nasal Spray (Rare) ... 2376
Monopril Tablets (0.2% to 1.0%) ... 1091
Monopril HCT ... 1094
Nilandron Tablets (2%) ... 753
Normodyne Tablets ... 3137
OptiPranolol Metipranolol Ophthalmic Solution 0.3% (A small number of patients) ... ⊙263
Orthoclone OKT3 Sterile Solution (Less than 1%) ... 2498
Prandin Tablets (0.5, 1, and 2 mg) (1.8%) ... 2432
Pravachol Tablets (0.1% to 4.0%) ... 1099
Prevacid Delayed-Release Capsules (Less than 1%) ... 3292
PREVPAC (Less than 1%) ... 3298
Prilosec Delayed-Release Capsules (Less than 1%) ... 628
Primacor Injection (1.2%) ... 3086
Proleukin for Injection ... 1199
Proventil Inhalation Aerosol ... 3142
Proventil Repetabs Tablets ... 3148
Proventil HFA Inhalation Aerosol ... 3150
▲ Quinidex Extentabs (6%) ... 2933
Relafen Tablets (Less than 1%) ... 1617
Rifater Tablets ... 769
Ritalin ... 2387
Rituxan for Infusion (One patient) ... 1750
Rituxan I.V. (One patient) ... 1428
Rynatan Tablets ... 3351
▲ Rythmol Tablets – 150 mg, 225 mg, 300 mg (1.2% to 4.6%) ... 502
Tamiflu Capsules (Less than 1%) ... 3008
Tamiflu Oral Suspension (Less than 1%) ... 3008
Tarka Tablets (0.3% or more) ... 508
Taxotere for Injection Concentrate (Rare) ... 778
Tiazac Capsules (Less than 2%) ... 1378
Tonocard Tablets (Less than 1%) ... 649
Trental Tablets (0.3%) ... 784
Tricor Capsules, Micronized (Less than 1%) ... 513
Triostat Injection (1% or fewer) ... 1825
Unithroid Tablets ... 3445
Univasc Tablets (Less than 1%) ... 3181
Ventolin Inhalation Aerosol and Refill ... 1679
Ventolin HFA Inhalation Aerosol ... 3618
Volmax Extended-Release Tablets ... 2276
Zofran Injection (Rare) ... 1698
Zofran (Rare) ... 1703
Zofran ODT Orally Disintegrating Tablets (Rare) ... 1703
Zosyn (1.0% or less) ... 1890
Zosyn in Galaxy Containers (1.0% or less) ... 1894

Angina, crescendo
Isordil Sublingual Tablets (Uncommon) ... 3525
Isordil Titradose Tablets (Uncommon) ... 3526
Nitro-Dur Transdermal Infusion System (Uncommon) ... 1834
Nitro-Dur Transdermal Infusion System (Uncommon) ... 3134

Angina, increased
Isordil Sublingual Tablets ... 3525
Isordil Titradose Tablets ... 3526
Lotrel Capsules (Rare) ... 2370
Nitro-Dur Transdermal Infusion System (2%) ... 1834
Nitro-Dur Transdermal Infusion System (2%) ... 3134
Nitrostat Tablets ... 2658
Norvasc Tablets (Rare) ... 2704
Procardia Capsules (Very rare) ... 2708
Procardia XL Extended Release Tablets (1% or less) ... 2710
▲ Vascor Tablets (4.5%) ... 2602

Angina, Prinzmetal's, episodes of
Imitrex Injection ... 1549
Imitrex Nasal Spray ... 1554

Angina pectoris
Accupril Tablets (Rare) ... 2611
Accuretic Tablets (0.5% to 1%) ... 2614
Aciphex Tablets ... 1267
Aciphex Tablets ... 1783
Actiq (Less than 1%) ... 1184
Actonel Tablets (2.5%) ... 2879
Aggrenox Capsules ... 1026
Agrylin Capsules (1% to 5%) ... 3232
Altace Capsules (Less than 1% to 3%) ... 2233
Ambien Tablets (Rare) ... 3191
Apligraf (1.8%) ... 2305
Arava Tablets (1% to 3%) ... 724
Aricept Tablets (Infrequent) ... 1270
Aricept Tablets (Infrequent) ... 2665
Arimidex Tablets ... 659
Atacand Tablets (Less frequently) ... 595
Atacand HCT Tablets (Less than 0.5%) ... 597
Avalide Tablets ... 1070
Avapro Tablets (Less than 1%) ... 1074
Avapro Tablets (Less than 1%) ... 3076
Baycol Tablets ... 883
Betapace AF Tablets (1.6% to 2%) ... 954
Betaseron for SC Injection ... 988
Campath Ampules ... 992
Captopril Tablets (2 to 3 of 1000 patients) ... 2281
Cardene I.V. (Rare) ... 3485
Cardura Tablets (Less than 0.5% to 0.6%) ... 2668
▲ Casodex Tablets (2% to 5%) ... 662
Celebrex Capsules (0.1% to 1.9%) ... 2676
Celebrex Capsules (0.1% to 1.9%) ... 2780
Celexa (Infrequent) ... 1365
▲ CellCept Capsules (3%) ... 2951
▲ CellCept Intravenous (3%) ... 2951
▲ CellCept Oral Suspension (3%) ... 2951
▲ CellCept Tablets (3%) ... 2951
Cipro I.V. (1% or less) ... 893
Cipro I.V. Pharmacy Bulk Package (Less than 1%) ... 897
Cipro (Less than 1%) ... 887
Cognex Capsules (Infrequent) ... 1351
Coreg Tablets (More than 2%) ... 1508
Corlopam Injection (0.5% to 5%) ... 412
Cosopt Sterile Ophthalmic Solution ... 2065
Covera-HS Tablets (2% or less) ... 3199
Cozaar Tablets (Less than 1%) ... 2067
Crixivan Capsules ... 2070
Dobutrex Solution Vials (1% to 3%) ... 1914
Doxil Injection (Less than 1%) ... 566
Effexor Tablets (Infrequent) ... 3495
Effexor XR Capsules (Infrequent) ... 3499
Eldepryl Capsules ... 3266
Enalaprilat Injection ... 863
Evoxac Capsules (Less than 1%) ... 1217
Exelon Capsules (Frequent) ... 2342
Exelon Oral Solution (Frequent) ... 2345
Fareston Tablets (Less than 1%) ... 3237
Ferrlecit Injection (Greater than 1%) ... 3386
▲ Flolan for Injection (19%) ... 1528
Gabitril Tablets (Infrequent) ... 1189
Geodon Capsules (Infrequent) ... 2688
Hyzaar ... 2109
Imitrex Injection ... 1549
Imitrex Tablets ... 1558
Innohep Injection (Greater than or equal to 1%) ... 1248
Isoptin SR Tablets (1% or less) ... 467
Kytril Tablets (Rare) ... 2988
Lamictal (Rare) ... 1567
Levaquin (Less than 0.3%) ... 2537
Levlen (Very infrequent) ... 962
Levlite 21 Tablets (Very infrequent) ... 962
Levlite 28 Tablets (Very infrequent) ... 962
Lexxel Tablets ... 608
Lipitor Tablets (Less than 2%) ... 2639
Lipitor Tablets (Less than 2%) ... 2696
Luvox Tablets (25, 50, 100 mg) (Infrequent) ... 3256
Maxalt Tablets (Rare) ... 2120
Maxalt-MLT Orally Disintegrating Tablets (Rare) ... 2120
Meridia Capsules ... 481
Miacalcin Nasal Spray (1% to 3%) ... 2375
Micardis Tablets (More than 0.3%) ... 1049
Micardis HCT Tablets ... 1051
Midamor Tablets (Less than or equal to 1%) ... 2136
Minipress Capsules ... 2699
Mirapex Tablets (1.6%) ... 2834
Mobic Tablets (Less than 2%) ... 1054
Modicon ... 2563
Moduretic Tablets (Less than or equal to 1%) ... 2138
Monopril Tablets (1.0% or more) ... 1091
Naprelan Tablets (Less than 1%) ... 1293
Natrecor for Injection (2%) ... 3189
Neurontin Capsules (Infrequent) ... 2655
Neurontin Oral Solution (Infrequent) ... 2655
Neurontin Tablets (Infrequent) ... 2655
Nipent for Injection (Less than 3%) ... 3272
Ortho-Cyclen/Ortho Tri-Cyclen ... 2573
Ortho-Novum ... 2563
Ortho-Novum 1/50□28 Tablets ... 2556
Ortho-Cyclen/Ortho Tri-Cyclen ... 2573
Paxil (Rare) ... 1609
Permax Tablets (Infrequent) ... 1299
Persantine Tablets (Rare) ... 1057
Photofrin for Injection ... 831
Plendil Extended-Release Tablets (0.5% to 1.5%) ... 623
Pletal Tablets (2% or greater) ... 2605
Pletal Tablets (2% or greater) ... 2848
Prinivil Tablets (Greater than 1%) ... 2164
Prinzide Tablets ... 2168
▲ Prograf (3% to 15%) ... 1393
Prometrium Capsules (100 mg, 200 mg) (Less than 5%) ... 3261
Protonix I.V. (Less than 1%) ... 3580
Protonix Tablets (Less than 1%) ... 3577
Protopic Ointment (Greater than or equal to 1%) ... 1397
Prozac Pulvules, Liquid, and Weekly Capsules (Infrequent) ... 1238
ReFacto Vials ... 1437
Remeron Tablets (Infrequent) ... 2483
Remeron SolTab Tablets (Infrequent) ... 2486
Remicade for IV Injection (Less than 2%) ... 1178
Requip Tablets (Infrequent) ... 1621
Rilutek Tablets (Infrequent) ... 772
Risperdal (Rare) ... 1796
Salagen Tablets (Less than 1%) ... 2229
Sarafem Pulvules (Infrequent) ... 1962
Seroquel Tablets (Infrequent) ... 684
Serzone Tablets (Infrequent) ... 1104
▲ Simulect for Injection (3% to 10%) ... 2399
Sonata Capsules (Infrequent) ... 3591
Tambocor Tablets (Less than 1%) ... 1990
Tasmar Tablets (Infrequent) ... 3010

Teveten Tablets (Less than 1%) 3327
Thalomid Capsules 1154
Tikosyn Capsules (Greater than 2%) 2717
Timolide Tablets 2187
Topamax Sprinkle Capsules (Infrequent) 2590
Topamax Tablets (Infrequent) 2590
Travatan Ophthalmic Solution (1% to 5%) 543
Tricor Capsules, Micronized 513
Tri-Levlen (Very infrequent) 962
Trovan (Less than 1%) 2722
Vaseretic Tablets 2204
Vasotec I.V. Injection 2207
Vasotec Tablets (1.5%) 2210
Verelan Capsules (1% or less) 3184
Verelan PM Capsules (2% or less) 3186
Viagra Tablets (Less than 2%) 2732
Vioxx (Greater than 0.1% to 1.9%) 2213
Xalatan Latanoprost Ophthalmic Solution (1% to 2%) ⊙320
Xalatan Sterile Ophthalmic Solution (1% to 2%) 2864
Xeloda Tablets (Less than 5%) 3039
Zanaflex Tablets (Rare) 1305
Zestoretic Tablets 695
Zestril Tablets (Greater than 1%) 698
Zoladex 3-month (1% to 5%) 706
Zomig Tablets 708
Zomig-ZMT Tablets 708

Angina pectoris, aggravation

Aldoclor Tablets 2035
Aldomet Tablets 2037
Aldoril Tablets 2039
Blocadren Tablets (Less than 1%) 2046
Coreg Tablets (2.0%) 1508
Eldepryl Capsules 3266
Feldene Capsules (Rare) 2685
Imdur Tablets (Less than or equal to 5%) 1826
Ismo Tablets (Fewer than 1%) 3524
Isordil Sublingual Tablets 3525
Isordil Titradose Tablets 3526
Nitrostat Tablets 2658
Sandostatin LAR Depot (Rare) 2395
Timolol GFS ⊙266
Timoptic in Ocudose (Less frequent) 2192
Timoptic Sterile Ophthalmic Solution (Less frequent) 2190
Timoptic-XE Sterile Ophthalmic Gel Forming Solution 2194

Angina pectoris, exacerbation of, post-abrupt discontinuation

Inderal 3513
Inderal LA Long-Acting Capsules 3516
Normodyne Injection 3135
Normodyne Tablets 3137
Tenoretic Tablets 690
Tenormin 692
Toprol-XL Tablets 651

Angina tonsillaris

Fortovase Capsules (Less than 2%) 2970
Invirase Capsules (Less than 2%) 2979

Angioedema

(*see also under* Edema, angioneurotic)

Accuretic Tablets (0.1%) 2614
Aceon Tablets (2 mg, 4 mg, 8 mg) (0.1%) 3249
Aciphex Tablets 1267
Allegra (Rare) 712
Allegra-D Extended-Release Tablets (Rare) 714
AmBisome for Injection (Infrequent) 1383
Aredia for Injection (Rare) 2309
Arthrotec Tablets (Rare) 3195
Atacand Tablets (Less frequently) 595
Atacand HCT Tablets (Less than 0.5%) 597
Avalide Tablets (Rare) 1070
Avapro Tablets (Rare) 1074
Avapro Tablets (Rare) 3076
Bactrim 2949
Baycol Tablets 883
BayGam 914
Beconase Inhalation Aerosol (Rare) 1497
Beconase AQ Nasal Spray (Rare) 1498
Campath Ampules 992
Captopril Tablets (Approximately 1 in 1000 patients) 2281
Cataflam Tablets (Less than 1%) 2315
Catapres Tablets 1037
Ceftin 1898
Celebrex Capsules (Less than 0.1%) 2676
Celebrex Capsules (Less than 0.1%) 2780
Celexa (At least 3 patients) 1365
Ceptaz for Injection (Very rare) 1499
Cipro I.V. (1% or less) 893
Cipro (Less than 1%) 887
Colazal Capsules 3069
Comvax 2056
Copaxone for Injection (Infrequent) 3306
Cordarone Intravenous 3491
Cosopt Sterile Ophthalmic Solution 2065
Cozaar Tablets (Rare) 2067
D.H.E. 45 Injection 2334
Didronel Tablets 2888
Diovan Capsules (Rare) 2337
Diovan HCT Tablets (Rare) 2338
Doryx Coated Pellet Filled Capsules 3357
Ecotrin Enteric Coated Aspirin Low, Regular and Maximum Strength Tablets 1715
ELA-Max Cream 1340
ELA-Max 5 Cream 1340
Emcyt Capsules 2810
Enalaprilat Injection (0.5% to 1%) 863
Enbrel for Injection 1752
Enbrel for Injection 3504
Eskalith 1527
Feldene Capsules (Rare) 2685
Flovent Diskus (Rare) 3614
Foradil Aerolizer (Rare) 2354
Fortaz (Very rare) 1541
Fosamax Tablets (Rare) 2095
Herceptin I.V. 1414
Hycamtin for Injection (Rare) 1546
Hyzaar (Rare) 2109
Indocin (Less than 1%) 2112
Keflex 1237
Levoxyl Tablets 1819
Lidoderm Patch (Rare) 1319
Lodosyn Tablets 1251
Lotensin Tablets (Less than 1%) 2365
Lotensin HCT Tablets (0.3%) 2367
Lotrel Capsules (About 0.5%) 2370
Luvox Tablets (25, 50, 100 mg) 3256
Macrobid Capsules 2889
Macrodantin Capsules 2891
Maxalt Tablets 2120
Maxalt-MLT Orally Disintegrating Tablets 2120
Merrem I.V. 673
Micardis Tablets (Single case) 1049
Micardis HCT Tablets (Single case) 1051
Mintezol 2137
Mobic Tablets (Less than 2%) 1054
Monurol Sachet 1375
Nasonex Nasal Spray 3131
Navelbine Injection 1604
Nembutal Sodium Solution 485
Neurontin Capsules 2655
Neurontin Oral Solution 2655
Neurontin Tablets 2655
Nexium Delayed-Release Capsules (Less than 1%) 619
Noroxin Tablets 2145
Norvasc Tablets (More than 0.1% to 1%) 2704
Pima Syrup 1362
Plavix Tablets (Very rare) 1097
Plavix Tablets (Very rare) 3084
Polocaine Injection, USP 625
Polocaine-MPF Injection, USP 625
Ponstel Capsules (Rare) 1356
Prinivil Tablets (0.3% to 1.0%) 2164
Protonix I.V. 3580
Protonix Tablets 3577
Protopic Ointment (Greater than or equal to 1%) 1397
Proventil Inhalation Aerosol (Rare) 3142
Proventil Repetabs Tablets 3148
Quinaglute Dura-Tabs Tablets 978
Quinidex Extentabs 2933
Qvar Inhalation Aerosol (Rare) 1987
Rebetron Combination Therapy 3153
Recombivax HB (Less than 1%) 2178
Reglan (Rare) 2935
Rhinocort Aqua Nasal Spray (Rare) 642
Rhinocort Nasal Inhaler (Rare) 640
▲ Rituxan for Infusion (0.3% to 13%) 1750
▲ Rituxan I.V. (0.3% to 13%) 1428
Robaxisal Tablets 2939
Septra Suspension 2265
Septra Tablets 2265
Septra DS Tablets 2265
Singulair 2181
Soma Compound Tablets (Less common) 3354
Soma Compound w/Codeine Tablets 3355
Suprax 1877
Thalomid Capsules 1154
Tikosyn Capsules (Less than or equal to 2%) 2717
Timolol GFS ⊙266
Timoptic in Ocudose 2192
Timoptic Sterile Ophthalmic Solution 2190
Timoptic-XE Sterile Ophthalmic Gel Forming Solution 2194
TNKase I.V. (Rare) 1430
Trental Tablets (Less than 1%) 784
Trovan (Less than 1%) 2722
Trusopt Sterile Ophthalmic Solution 2196
Twinrix Vaccine 1674
Uniretic Tablets (Less than 0.5% to more than 1%) 3178
Unithroid Tablets 3445
Valtrex Caplets 1676
Vancenase PocketHaler Nasal Inhaler (Rare) 3162
Vanceril Inhalation Aerosol (Rare) 3165
Vanceril Double Strength Inhalation Aerosol (Rare) 3167
Vaseretic Tablets (0.6%) 2204
Vasotec I.V. Injection (0.5% to 1%) 2207
Vasotec Tablets 2210
Ventolin Inhalation Aerosol and Refill (Rare) 1679
Ventolin HFA Inhalation Aerosol 3618
Vioxx 2213
Viramune Oral Suspension 1060
Viramune Tablets 1060
Vistide Injection 1445
Voltaren Tablets (Less than 1%) 2315
Voltaren-XR Tablets (Less than 1%) 2315
Xenical Capsules 3043
Zestril Tablets (0.1%) 698
Zinacef Injection 1696
Zinacef for Injection 1696
Zithromax Capsules, 250 mg (1% or less; rare) 2743
Zithromax for IV Infusion (Rare) 2748
Zithromax for Oral Suspension, 1 g (1% or less) 2743
Zithromax for Oral Suspension, 300 mg, 600 mg, 900 mg, 1200 mg (1% or less; rare) 2739
Zithromax Tablets, 250 mg (1% or less; rare) 2739
Zithromax Tablets, 600 mg (1% or less) 2743
Zofran Injection 1698
Zofran 1703
Zofran ODT Orally Disintegrating Tablets 1703
Zoloft 2751

Angioedema, extremities

Accupril Tablets (0.1%) 2611
Aceon Tablets (2 mg, 4 mg, 8 mg) (0.1%) 3249
Altace Capsules 2233
Captopril Tablets (Approximately 1 in 1000 patients) 2281
Enalaprilat Injection 863
Lexxel Tablets 608
Lotensin Tablets 2365
Lotrel Capsules 2370
Monopril Tablets 1091
Prinivil Tablets 2164
Prinzide Tablets (Rare) 2168
Uniretic Tablets 3178
Univasc Tablets 3181
Vaseretic Tablets 2204
Vasotec I.V. Injection 2207
Vasotec Tablets 2210
Zestoretic Tablets (Rare) 695
Zestril Tablets 698

Angioedema, eyes

Accupril Tablets 2611
Altace Capsules 2233
Captopril Tablets 2281
Uniretic Tablets 3178
Zestoretic Tablets 695
Zestril Tablets 698

Angioedema, face

Accupril Tablets (0.1%) 2611
Aceon Tablets (2 mg, 4 mg, 8 mg) (0.3% to 1%) 3249
Altace Capsules 2233
Atrovent Inhalation Aerosol 1030
Atrovent Nasal Spray 0.06% 1033
Avalide Tablets (Rare) 1070
Avapro Tablets (Rare) 1074
Avapro Tablets (Rare) 3076
Captopril Tablets (Approximately 1 in 1000 patients) 2281
Catapres-TTS (2 of 3,539 patients) 1038
Cozaar Tablets (Rare) 2067
Enalaprilat Injection 863
Flomax Capsules 1044
Hyzaar (Rare) 2109
Lexxel Tablets 608
Lotensin Tablets 2365
Lotrel Capsules (About 0.5%) 2370
Monopril Tablets 1091
Monopril HCT 1094
Prinivil Tablets 2164
Prinzide Tablets (Rare) 2168
Uniretic Tablets (Less than 0.5%) 3178
Univasc Tablets (Less than 0.5%) 3181
Vaseretic Tablets 2204
Vasotec I.V. Injection 2207
Vasotec Tablets 2210
Zestoretic Tablets (Rare) 695
Zestril Tablets 698

Angioedema, glottis

Accupril Tablets (0.1%) 2611
Aceon Tablets (2 mg, 4 mg, 8 mg) (0.1%) 3249
Altace Capsules 2233
Captopril Tablets (Approximately 1 in 1000 patients) 2281
Cozaar Tablets 2067
Enalaprilat Injection 863
Hyzaar 2109
Lexxel Tablets 608
Lotensin Tablets 2365
Lotrel Capsules (About 0.5%) 2370
Mavik Tablets (0.3% to 1.0%) 478
Monopril Tablets 1091
Monopril HCT 1094
Prinivil Tablets 2164
Prinzide Tablets (Rare) 2168
Tarka Tablets 508
Uniretic Tablets 3178
Univasc Tablets 3181
Vaseretic Tablets 2204
Vasotec I.V. Injection 2207
Vasotec Tablets 2210
Zestoretic Tablets (Rare) 695
Zestril Tablets 698

Angioedema, larynx

Accupril Tablets (0.1%) 2611
Aceon Tablets (2 mg, 4 mg, 8 mg) (0.1%) 3249
Altace Capsules 2233
Captopril Tablets (Approximately 1 in 1000 patients) 2281
Enalaprilat Injection 863
Floxin Tablets 2529
Lexxel Tablets 608
Lotensin Tablets 2365
Monopril Tablets 1091
Monopril HCT 1094
Prinivil Tablets 2164
Prinzide Tablets (Rare) 2168
Uniretic Tablets 3178
Univasc Tablets 3181
Vaseretic Tablets 2204
Vasotec I.V. Injection 2207
Vasotec Tablets 2210
Zestoretic Tablets (Rare) 695
Zestril Tablets 698

Angioedema, lips

Accupril Tablets (0.1%) 2611
Aceon Tablets (2 mg, 4 mg, 8 mg) (0.1%) 3249
Altace Capsules 2233
Atrovent Inhalation Aerosol 1030
Atrovent Nasal Spray 0.06% 1033
Avalide Tablets (Rare) 1070
Avapro Tablets (Rare) 1074
Avapro Tablets (Rare) 3076
Captopril Tablets (Approximately 1 in 1000 patients) 2281
Cozaar Tablets (Rare) 2067
Enalaprilat Injection 863
Flomax Capsules 1044
Hyzaar (Rare) 2109
Lexxel Tablets 608
Lotensin Tablets 2365
Lotrel Capsules 2370
Monopril Tablets 1091
Monopril HCT 1094
Prinivil Tablets 2164
Prinzide Tablets (Rare) 2168
Uniretic Tablets 3178
Univasc Tablets 3181
Vaseretic Tablets 2204
Vasotec I.V. Injection 2207
Vasotec Tablets 2210
Zestoretic Tablets (Rare) 695
Zestril Tablets 698

Angioedema, oropharyngeal

Avalide Tablets (Rare) 1070
Avapro Tablets (Rare) 1074
Avapro Tablets (Rare) 3076
Cozaar Tablets (Rare) 2067
Hyzaar (Rare) 2109

Angioedema of tongue

Accupril Tablets (0.1%) 2611
Aceon Tablets (2 mg, 4 mg, 8 mg) (0.1%) 3249
Altace Capsules 2233
Atrovent Inhalation Aerosol 1030
Atrovent Nasal Spray 0.06% 1033
Avalide Tablets (Rare) 1070
Avapro Tablets (Rare) 1074
Avapro Tablets (Rare) 3076
Captopril Tablets (Approximately 1 in 1000 patients) 2281
Catapres-TTS (One case) 1038
Cozaar Tablets (Rare) 2067
Enalaprilat Injection 863
Flomax Capsules 1044
Floxin I.V. 2526
Floxin Tablets 2529
Hyzaar (Rare) 2109
Lexxel Tablets 608
Lotensin Tablets 2365
Lotrel Capsules (About 0.5%) 2370
Monopril Tablets 1091
Monopril HCT 1094
Prinivil Tablets 2164
Prinzide Tablets (Rare) 2168
Uniretic Tablets 3178
Univasc Tablets 3181
Vaseretic Tablets 2204

Vasotec I.V. Injection ... 2207
Vasotec Tablets ... 2210
Zestoretic Tablets (Rare) ... 695
Zestril Tablets ... 698

Angioma, spider
Avonex ... 1013
Betaseron for SC Injection ... 988

Angiopathy
FluShield Influenza Vaccine ... 3521

Anhidrosis
Cogentin ... 2055

Anisocoria
Betoptic S Ophthalmic Suspension ... 537
Paxil (Rare) ... 1609

Ankylosing spondylosis
Lupron Injection ... 3279

Anophthalmos
Thalomid Capsules ... 1154

Anorexia
Abelcet Injection ... 1273
Accuretic Tablets ... 2614
Aciphex Tablets ... 1267
Aciphex Tablets ... 1783
▲ ActHIB Vaccine (2.2% to 26.1%) ... 798
▲ Actimmune (3%) ... 1772
Actiq (Less than 1%) ... 1184
Adderall Tablets ... 3231
▲ Adderall XR Capsules (2.9% to 22%)
Adriamycin PFS/RDF Injection (Occasional) ... 2767
Aggrenox Capsules (1.2%) ... 1026
▲ Agrylin Capsules (7.7%) ... 3232
Aldoclor Tablets ... 2035
Aldoril Tablets ... 2039
▲ Alferon N Injection (1% to 68%) ... 1770
Altace Capsules (Less than 1%) ... 2233
Ambien Tablets (1%) ... 3191
AmBisome for Injection (Less common) ... 1383
Amphotec (1% to 5%) ... 1774
Ancef for Injection ... 1474
Ancef Injection ... 1474
Ancobon Capsules ... 1730
Antabuse Tablets ... 3474
Anzemet Injection (Rare) ... 719
Anzemet Tablets (Rare) ... 722
Aquasol A Parenteral ... 593
Aralen Tablets ... 3075
▲ Arava Tablets (3%) ... 724
▲ Aredia for Injection (1% to 20.8%) ... 2309
▲ Aricept Tablets (4%) ... 1270
▲ Aricept Tablets (4%) ... 2665
▲ Arimidex Tablets (5.1% to 7.7%) ... 659
▲ Aromasin Tablets (6%) ... 2769
Arthrotec Tablets (Rare) ... 3195
Asacol Delayed-Release Tablets ... 2884
Atacand HCT Tablets ... 597
Avalide Tablets ... 1070
Avelox Tablets (0.05% to 1%) ... 879
▲ Avonex (7%) ... 1013
Axid Pulvules (1.2%) ... 1903
Axid Pulvules (1.2%) ... 2919
▲ Azulfidine EN-tabs Tablets (Among most common) ... 2775
▲ Bactrim (Among most common) ... 2949
Baycol Tablets (Rare) ... 883
Benadryl Parenteral ... 2617
Biaxin/Biaxin XL ... 403
Brevibloc Injection (Less than 1%) ... 858
Buprenex Injectable (Rare) ... 2918
Calcijex Injection ... 411
Calcium Disodium Versenate Injection ... 1980
▲ Campath Ampules (20%) ... 992
Cancidas for Injection (Up to 1.3%) ... 2048
Captopril Tablets (About 0.5% to 2%) ... 2281
Carbatrol Capsules ... 3234
Cardizem Injectable ... 1018
Cardizem Lyo-Ject Syringe ... 1018
Cardizem Monovial ... 1018
Cardizem CD Capsules (Less than 1%) ... 1016
Cardura Tablets (Less than 0.5%) ... 2668
▲ Carnitor Injection (3% to 6%) ... 3242
▲ Casodex Tablets (5%) ... 662
Catapres Tablets (About 1 in 100 patients) ... 1037
Catapres-TTS (0.5% or less) ... 1038
Ceclor CD Tablets (0.1% to 1%) ... 1279
Cedax (0.1% to 1%) ... 1021
Ceftin Tablets (0.1% to 1%) ... 1898
Celebrex Capsules (0.1% to 1.9%) ... 2676
Celebrex Capsules (0.1% to 1.9%) ... 2780
▲ Celexa (3%) ... 1365
▲ CellCept Capsules (3%) ... 2951
▲ CellCept Intravenous (3%) ... 2951
▲ CellCept Oral Suspension (3%) ... 2951
▲ CellCept Tablets (3% to 25.3%) ... 2951
Celontin Capsules (Frequent) ... 2618
Cerebyx Injection (Infrequent) ... 2619
Cipro I.V. (1% or less) ... 893
Cipro I.V. Pharmacy Bulk Package (Less than 1%) ... 897
Cipro (Less than 1%) ... 887
Claritin (At least one patient) ... 3100
Claritin-D 12 Hour Extended Release Tablets (2%) ... 3102
Claritin-D 24 Hour Extended Release Tablets (2%) ... 3104
Clinoril Tablets (Greater than 1%) ... 2053
Clorpres Tablets (About 1%) ... 1002
Clozaril Tablets (1%) ... 2319
▲ Cognex Capsules (9%) ... 1351
Colazal Capsules (2%) ... 3069
Colestid Tablets (Infrequent) ... 2791
Combipres Tablets (About 1%) ... 1040
▲ Combivir Tablets (10%) ... 1502
Comvax (0.8% to 3.9%) ... 2056
▲ Concerta Extended-Release Tablets (4%) ... 1998
▲ Concerta Tablets (4%) ... 561
▲ Copaxone for Injection (8%) ... 3306
▲ Cordarone Tablets (4% to 9%) ... 3487
Coreg Tablets (More than 2%) ... 1508
Corgard Tablets (1 to 5 per 1000 patients) ... 2245
Corzide 40/5 Tablets (1 to 5 of 1000 patients) ... 2247
Corzide 80/5 Tablets (1 to 5 of 1000 patients) ... 2247
Cosmegen for Injection ... 2062
Cosopt Sterile Ophthalmic Solution ... 2065
Cozaar Tablets (Less than 1%) ... 2067
Crixivan Capsules (0.5%) ... 2070
Cuprimine Capsules ... 2075
Cylert Tablets ... 415
▲ Cytovene (15%) ... 2959
Dantrium Capsules (Rare) ... 2885
▲ Daranide Tablets (Among the most common effects) ... 2077
Daraprim Tablets ... 1511
▲ DaunoXome Injection (2% to 21%) ... 1442
Declomycin Tablets ... 1855
▲ Depacon Injection (4% to 12%) ... 416
▲ Depakene (11% to 12%) ... 421
▲ Depakote Sprinkle Capsules (4% to 12%) ... 426
▲ Depakote Tablets (1% to 12%) ... 430
Depakote ER Tablets (Greater than 1%) ... 436
▲ Depen Titratable Tablets (17%) ... 3341
Dexedrine ... 1512
DextroStat Tablets ... 3236
Diabinese Tablets (Less than 2%) ... 2680
Diamox Intravenous ... ⊙269
Diamox Sequels Sustained Release Capsules ... ⊙270
Diamox Tablets ... ⊙269
Digitek Tablets (1%) ... 1003
Dilaudid Oral Liquid ... 445
Dilaudid Tablets - 8 mg ... 445
Dilaudid-HP (Less frequent) ... 443
Diovan Capsules (Less frequent) ... 2337
Diovan HCT Tablets (Less frequent) ... 2338
Dipentum Capsules (1.3%) ... 2803
▲ Diphtheria & Tetanus Toxoids Adsorbed Purogenated for Pediatric Use (7%) ... 1857
Diucardin Tablets ... 3494
Diuril Oral ... 2087
Diuril Sodium Intravenous ... 2086
Dolobid Tablets (Less than 1 in 100) ... 2088
Dolophine Hydrochloride Tablets ... 3056
Doryx Coated Pellet Filled Capsules ... 3357
▲ Dostinex Tablets (1% to less than 10%) ... 2804
▲ Doxil Injection (1% to 11.9%) ... 566
▲ DTIC-Dome (90% with the initial few doses) ... 902
Duraclon Injection (1%) ... 3057
▲ Duragesic Transdermal System (3% to 10%) ... 1786
Dynabac Tablets (0.1% to 1%) ... 2269
Dynacin Capsules ... 2019
Edecrin ... 2091
▲ E.E.S. (Among most frequent) ... 450
▲ Effexor Tablets (11% to 17.0%) ... 3495
▲ Effexor XR Capsules (8% to 13%) ... 3499
Eldepryl Capsules ... 3266
Ellence Injection (Up to 2.9%) ... 2806
Elmiron Capsules (Less than or equal to 1%) ... 570
Elspar for Injection ... 2092
▲ Emcyt Capsules (4%) ... 2810
Enalaprilat Injection ... 863
Enbrel for Injection ... 1752
Enbrel for Injection ... 3504
Engerix-B Vaccine (Less than 1%) ... 1517
▲ Epivir (10%) ... 1520
▲ Ergamisol Tablets (2% to 6%) ... 1789
▲ EryPed (Among most frequent) ... 446
▲ Ery-Tab Tablets (Among most frequent) ... 448
▲ Erythrocin Stearate Filmtab Tablets (Among most frequent) ... 452
▲ Erythromycin Base Filmtab Tablets (Among most frequent) ... 454
▲ Erythromycin Delayed-Release Capsules, USP (Among most frequent) ... 455
Eskalith ... 1527
Etrafon (Occasional) ... 3115
▲ Eulexin Capsules (4%) ... 3118
Evoxac Capsules (1% to 3%) ... 1217
▲ Exelon Capsules (17%) ... 2342
▲ Exelon Oral Solution (17%) ... 2345
Famotidine Injection (Infrequent) ... 866
Famvir Tablets (1.1% to 2.6%) ... 2348
Fareston Tablets ... 3237
▲ Felbatol (19.3% to 54.8%) ... 3343
▲ Feldene Capsules (1% to 10%) ... 2685
▲ Femara Tablets (3% to 5%) ... 2351
Ferrlecit Injection ... 3386
Flexeril Tablets (Less than 1%) ... 572
Flexeril Tablets (Less than 1%) ... 2094
▲ Flolan for Injection (25% to 66%) ... 1528
▲ Fludara for Injection (7% to 34%) ... 995
Flumadine (1.6%) ... 1370
Fortovase Capsules (Less than 2%) ... 2970
▲ Foscavir Injection (5% or greater) ... 605
Sterile FUDR ... 2974
Furosemide Tablets ... 2284
Gabitril Tablets (1% or more) ... 1189
Gemzar for Injection (Common) ... 1919
Gengraf Capsules (Less than 2% to 3%) ... 457
Geocillin Tablets ... 2687
Geodon Capsules (2%) ... 2688
▲ Gleevec Capsules (3% to 14%) ... 2357
Glucotrol XL Extended Release Tablets (Less than 1%) ... 2693
Gonal-F for Injection ... 3216
Halcion Tablets ... 2823
Haldol Decanoate ... 2535
Haldol Injection, Tablets and Concentrate ... 2533
▲ Havrix Vaccine (1% to 10%) ... 1544
▲ Hectorol Capsules (4.9%) ... 1064
▲ Hectorol Injection (4.9%) ... 1066
▲ Herceptin I.V. (14%) ... 1414
Hexalen Capsules (1%) ... 2226
HibTITER ... 1859
Hivid Tablets (Less than 1%) ... 2975
▲ Hycamtin for Injection (Up to 19%) ... 1546
HydroDIURIL Tablets ... 2108
Hyzaar ... 2109
Ifex for Injection (Less than 1%) ... 1123
Indapamide Tablets (Less than 5%) ... 2286
Inderide Tablets ... 3517
Inderide LA Long-Acting Capsules ... 3519
Indocin (Less than 1%) ... 2112
▲ Infergen (21% to 24%) ... 1777
▲ Intron A for Injection (1% to 69%) ... 3120
Inversine Tablets ... 1850
Invirase Capsules (Less than 2%) ... 2979
▲ IPOL Vaccine (1.3% to 16.6%) ... 809
Kadian Capsules (Less than 3%) ... 1335
Kaletra Capsules (Less than 2%) ... 471
Kaletra Oral Solution (Less than 2%) ... 471
Kefzol Vials, ADD-Vantage ... 1951
▲ Keppra Tablets (3%) ... 3314
Klonopin Tablets ... 2983
Lamictal (1.8% to 3%) ... 1567
Lamisil Tablets ... 2360
Lanoxicaps Capsules (Common) ... 1574
Lanoxin Injection (Common) ... 1581
Lanoxin Tablets ... 1587
Lanoxin Elixir Pediatric ... 1578
Lanoxin Injection Pediatric ... 1584
▲ Lariam Tablets (Among most frequent) ... 2989
Lescol Capsules ... 2361
Lescol Capsules ... 2925
Lescol XL Tablets ... 2361
Lescol XL Tablets ... 2925
▲ Leukine (13% to 54%) ... 1755
Levaquin (0.1% to less than 1.0%) ... 2537
Levlen ... 962
Levlite 21 Tablets ... 962
Levlite 28 Tablets ... 962
Lexxel Tablets ... 608
Limbitrol ... 1738
Lipitor Tablets (Less than 2%) ... 2639
Lipitor Tablets (Less than 2%) ... 2696
Lithium Carbonate ... 3061
Lithium Citrate Syrup ... 3061
Lithobid Slow-Release Tablets ... 3255
Lodine (Less than 1%) ... 3528
Lodine XL Extended-Release Tablets (Less than 1%) ... 3530
Lodosyn Tablets ... 1251
Lorabid Suspension and Pulvules (0.3% to 2.3%) ... 2251
Lotensin HCT Tablets (0.3% to 1%) ... 2367
Lupron Depot 7.5 mg (Less than 5%) ... 3284
Lupron Depot–3 Month 22.5 mg (Less than 5%) ... 3288
Lupron Depot–4 Month 30 mg (Less than 5%) ... 3289
▲ Lupron Injection (5% or more) ... 3279
▲ Luvox Tablets (25, 50, 100 mg) (1% to 6%) ... 3256
▲ Macrodantin Capsules (Among most often) ... 2891
▲ Malarone (5%) ... 1596
Marinol Capsules (Less than 1%) ... 3325
Matulane Capsules ... 3246
Maxair Autohaler ... 1981
Maxair Inhaler (Less than 1%) ... 1984
Maxalt Tablets (Rare) ... 2120
Maxalt-MLT Orally Disintegrating Tablets (Rare) ... 2120
Maxzide ... 1008
▲ Mepron Suspension (7%) ... 1598
▲ Meridia Capsules (13%) ... 481
Merrem I.V. (0.1% to 1.0%) ... 673
▲ Metadate CD Capsules (9%) ... 1164
Metadate ER Tablets ... 1167
Methylin Tablets ... 1995
Methylin ER Tablets ... 1995
Mevacor Tablets (Rare) ... 2132
Miacalcin Nasal Spray (Less than 1%) ... 2375
Microzide Capsules ... 3414
▲ Midamor Tablets (3% to 8%) ... 2136
Migranal Nasal Spray (Rare) ... 2376
Minizide Capsules ... 2700
Minocin Intravenous ... 1862
Minocin Oral Suspension ... 1865
Minocin Pellet-Filled Capsules ... 1863
Mintezol ... 2137
▲ Mirapex Tablets (4%) ... 2834
Mithracin for Intravenous Use ... 903
Modicon ... 2563
▲ Moduretic Tablets (3% to 8%) ... 2138
Monodox Capsules ... 2442
Monopril HCT ... 1094
Monurol Sachet (Less than 1%) ... 1375
Motofen Tablets ... 577
Motrin Suspension, Oral Drops, Chewable Tablets, and Caplets ... 2002
MS Contin Tablets (Less frequent) ... 2896
MSIR (Less frequent) ... 2898
Mustargen for Injection ... 2142
Myambutol Tablets ... 1290
Mycobutin Capsules (2%) ... 2838
Mykrox Tablets ... 1168
Myleran Tablets ... 1603
Mylocel Tablets ... 2227
▲ Mylotarg for Injection (25% to 41%) ... 3540
Nadolol Tablets (1 to 5 of 1000 patients) ... 2288
Naprelan Tablets (Less than 1%) ... 1293
Navane Oral ... 2701
Navane Intramuscular ... 2703
▲ Navelbine Injection (Less than 20%) ... 1604
Neoral Soft Gelatin Capsules (2% or less to 3%) ... 2380
Neoral Oral Solution (2% or less to 3%) ... 2380
Neptazane Tablets ... ⊙271
▲ Neumega for Injection (Greater than or equal to 10%) ... 1434
▲ Neupogen for Injection (9%) ... 587
Neurontin Capsules (Frequent) ... 2655
Neurontin Oral Solution (More than 2%) ... 2655
Neurontin Tablets (Frequent) ... 2655
Nexium Delayed-Release Capsules (Less than 1%) ... 619
▲ Nilandron Tablets (11%) ... 753
▲ Nipent for Injection (13% to 16%) ... 3272
Nizoral Tablets ... 1791
Nolvadex Tablets (1%) ... 678
Normodyne Injection ... 3135
Normodyne Tablets ... 3137
Noroxin Tablets (Less frequent) ... 2145
Norpramin Tablets ... 755
Norvasc Tablets (More than 0.1% to 1%) ... 2704
▲ Norvir Capsules (0.9% to 6.1%) ... 487
▲ Norvir Oral Solution (0.9% to 6.1%) ... 487
▲ Novantrone for Injection (25%) ... 1760
Omnicef (0.3%) ... 493
▲ Oncaspar (Greater than 1% but less than 5%) ... 756
Oramorph SR Tablets (Less frequent) ... 3062
Orap Tablets ... 1407
Orthoclone OKT3 Sterile Solution (Less than 1%) ... 2498
Ortho-Cyclen/Ortho Tri-Cyclen ... 2573
Ortho-Novum ... 2563
Ortho-Novum 1/50◻28 Tablets ... 2556
Ortho-Cyclen/Ortho Tri-Cyclen ... 2573
Orudis Capsules (Greater than 1%) ... 3548
Oruvail Capsules (Greater than 1%) ... 3548
OxyContin Tablets (Between 1% and 5%) ... 2912
▲ Pacerone Tablets (4% to 9%) ... 3331
Paraplatin for Injection ... 1126
Parnate Tablets ... 1607
Paser Granules (Less frequent) ... 1781
▲ PCE Dispertab Tablets (Among most frequent) ... 498
▲ Pediazole Suspension (Among most frequent) ... 3050
▲ PEG-Intron Powder for Injection (20%) ... 3140
Pentasa Capsules (Less than 1% to 1.1%) ... 3239
Pepcid Injection (Infrequent) ... 2153
Pepcid for Oral Suspension (Infrequent) ... 2150
Pepcid RPD Orally Disintegrating Tablets (Infrequent) ... 2150

Pepcid Tablets (Infrequent) 2150
Periactin Tablets 2155
Periostat Tablets 1208
▲ Permax Tablets (4.8%) 1299
PhosLo 1069
▲ Photofrin for Injection (8%) 831
Plaquenil Tablets 3082
Pletal Tablets (Less than 2%) 2605
Pletal Tablets (Less than 2%) 2848
Potaba (Infrequent) 1721
Pravachol Tablets (Rare) 1099
Prevacid Delayed-Release Capsules (Less than 1%) 3292
PREVPAC (Less than 1%) 3298
Priftin Tablets (2.2%) 758
Prilosec Delayed-Release Capsules (Less than 1%) 628
Prinivil Tablets (Greater than 1%) 2164
Prinzide Tablets 2168
▲ Procanbid Extended-Release Tablets (3% to 4%) 2262
▲ Prograf (3% to 34%) 1393
▲ Proleukin for Injection (20%) 1199
Prometrium Capsules (100 mg, 200 mg) 3261
Protonix I.V. (Less than 1%) 3580
Protonix Tablets (Less than 1%) 3577
Protopic Ointment (Greater than or equal to 1%) 1397
▲ Provigil Tablets (5%) 1193
▲ Prozac Pulvules, Liquid, and Weekly Capsules (8% to 17%) 1238
Pulmicort Respules (1% to 3%) 632
Purinethol Tablets (Uncommon) 1615
Pyrazinamide Tablets 1876
▲ Rapamune Oral Solution and Tablets (3% to 20%) 3584
▲ Rebetron Combination Therapy (21% to 27%) 3153
ReFacto Vials 1437
Relafen Tablets (Less than 1%) 1617
Remeron Tablets (Frequent) 2483
Remeron SolTab Tablets (Frequent) 2486
▲ Reminyl Oral Solution (Less than 1% to 9%) 1792
▲ Reminyl Tablets (Less than 1% to 9%) 1792
Renese Tablets 2712
▲ Requip Tablets (4%) 1621
Rescriptor Tablets (Less than 2%) 526
▲ Retrovir Capsules (11% to 20.1%) 1625
▲ Retrovir IV Infusion (11% to 20.1%) 1629
▲ Retrovir (11% to 20.1%) 1625
Rifadin (Some patients) 765
Rifamate Capsules (Some patients) 767
Rifater Tablets 769
▲ Rilutek Tablets (3.8% to 8.6%) 772
Risperdal (Frequent) 1796
Ritalin 2387
▲ Rituxan for Infusion (Among most frequent) 1750
▲ Rituxan I.V. (Among most frequent) 1428
Rocaltrol 2991
▲ Roferon-A Injection (43% to 65%) 2996
Roxanol 3066
Roxicodone Tablets (Less than 3%) 3067
Rynatan Tablets 3351
Rythmol Tablets – 150 mg, 225 mg, 300 mg (1.6% to 2%) 502
Salagen Tablets (Less than 1%) 2229
Sandimmune (2% or less) 2388
▲ Sandostatin LAR Depot (5% to 15%) 2395
▲ Sarafem Pulvules (11%) 1962
Sectral Capsules 3589
▲ Septra Suspension (Among most common) 2265
▲ Septra Tablets (Among most common) 2265
▲ Septra DS Tablets (Among most common) 2265
Serentil 1057
Seroquel Tablets (Frequent) 684
▲ Serostim for Injection (12.2%) 3229
Serzone Tablets 1104
Sinemet Tablets 1253
Sinemet CR Tablets (1.2%) 1255
Sinequan 2713
Skelid Tablets (More than or equal to 1%) 3088
Sonata Capsules (Less than 1% to 2%) 3591
▲ Soriatane Capsules (1% to 10%) 3003
Sporanox Capsules 1800
▲ Stadol NS Nasal Spray (3% to 9%) 1108
Stelazine 1640
Stromectol Tablets (0.9%) 2185
Sular Tablets (Less than or equal to 1%) 688
Surmontil Capsules 3595
Sustiva Capsules (1% to 2%) 1258
Symmetrel (1% to 5%) 1328
Tabloid Tablets (Less frequent) 1642
Talacen Caplets (Rare) 3089
Talwin Nx Tablets 3090
Tambocor Tablets (1% to 3%) 1990
▲ Tasmar Tablets (19% to 23%) 3010
Tegretol/Tegretol-XR 2404
▲ Temodar Capsules (9%) 3157
Tenoretic Tablets 690
Tequin Injection (Less than 0.1%) 1110
Tequin Tablets (Less than 0.1%) 1110
▲ Tetanus & Diphtheria Toxoids Adsorbed for Adult Use (7%) 1880
Teveten Tablets (Less than 1%) 3327
▲ Thalomid Capsules (2.8% to 9.4%) 1154
▲ TheraCys Injection (11%) 823
Thioplex for Injection 1765
Thioridazine Hydrochloride Tablets 2289
Thiothixene Capsules 2290
Tiazac Capsules (Less than 2%) 1378
Tice BCG, BCG Live (2.2%) 2489
Ticlid Tablets (1.0%) 3015
Timolide Tablets 2187
Timolol GFS ⊙266
Timoptic in Ocudose (Less frequent) 2192
Timoptic Sterile Ophthalmic Solution (Less frequent) 2190
Timoptic-XE Sterile Ophthalmic Gel Forming Solution 2194
▲ TOBI Solution for Inhalation (18.6%) 1206
▲ Tonocard Tablets (1.2% to 11.3%) 649
▲ Topamax Sprinkle Capsules (4.4% to 11.3%) 2590
▲ Topamax Tablets (4.4% to 11.3%) 2590
Toradol (1% or less) 3018
▲ Trecator-SC Tablets (Among most common) 3598
Trental Tablets (Less than 1%) 784
Trilafon (Occasional) 3160
▲ Trileptal Oral Suspension (3% to 5%) 2407
▲ Trileptal Tablets (3% to 5%) 2407
Tri-Levlen 962
Trilisate (Less than 1%) 2901
▲ Tripedia Vaccine (1% to 6%) 817
▲ Trisenox Injection (23%) 1158
▲ Trizivir Tablets (15%) 1669
Trovan (Less than 1%) 2722
Twinrix Vaccine (Less than 1%) 1674
▲ Ultracet Tablets (3%) 2597
Ultram Tablets (1% to 5%) 2600
Uniretic Tablets (Less than 1%) 3178
Valtrex Caplets (Less than 1% to 2%) 1676
Vaniqa Cream (0.7%) 1121
Vantin Tablets and Oral Suspension (Less than 1%) 2860
▲ Vascor Tablets (3.02% to 6.82%) 2602
Vaseretic Tablets 2204
Vasotec I.V. Injection 2207
Vasotec Tablets (0.5% to 1.0%) 2210
▲ Vesanoid Capsules (17%) 3037
Vibramycin Calcium Oral Suspension Syrup 2735
Vibramycin Hyclate Capsules 2735
Vibramycin Hyclate Intravenous 2737
Vibramycin Monohydrate for Oral Suspension 2735
Vibra-Tabs Film Coated Tablets 2735
Vicoprofen Tablets (Less than 3%) 520
Videx 1138
Videx EC Capsules 1143
Viracept 532
▲ Vistide Injection (23%) 1445
Vitravene for Injection (2% to 5%) ⊙310
Vivactil Tablets 2217
Vivactil Tablets 2446
▲ Wellbutrin Tablets (18.3%) 1680
▲ Wellbutrin SR Sustained-Release Tablets (3% to 5%) 1684
Xanax Tablets 2865
Xeloda Tablets (2% to 3%) 3039
Zarontin Capsules (Frequent) 2659
Zarontin Syrup (Frequent) 2660
Zaroxolyn Tablets 1177
▲ Zerit (19%) 1147
Zestoretic Tablets 695
Zestril Tablets (Greater than 1%) 698
Ziac Tablets 1887
▲ Ziagen (9% to 15%) 1692
▲ Zinecard for Injection (27% to 42%) 2869
Zithromax Capsules, 250 mg (1% or less) 2743
Zithromax for IV Infusion (1.9%) 2748
Zithromax for Oral Suspension, 300 mg, 600 mg, 900 mg, 1200 mg (1% or less) 2739
Zithromax Tablets, 250 mg (1% or less) 2739
Zocor Tablets 2219
Zoladex (1% to 5%) 702
Zoladex 3-month 706
▲ Zoloft (3% to 11%) 2751
▲ Zometa for Intravenous Infusion (9.3%) 3621
Zomig Tablets (Rare) 708
Zomig-ZMT Tablets (Rare) 708
▲ Zonegran Capsules (13%) 1307
Zovirax for Injection (Less than 1%) 1708
Zyban Sustained-Release Tablets (1% to 3%) 1710
Zyprexa Tablets 1973
Zyprexa ZYDIS Orally Disintegrating Tablets 1973
Zyrtec (Less than 2%) 2756
Zyrtec-D 12 Hour Extended Relief Tablets (Less than 2%) 2758

Anorgasmia
Depo-Provera Contraceptive Injection (1% to 5%) 2798
Effexor Tablets 3495
▲ Effexor XR Capsules (3% to 17%) 3499
Eldepryl Capsules 3266
Geodon Capsules (Infrequent) 2688
Luvox Tablets (25, 50, 100 mg) (2%) 3256
Nardil Tablets (Common) 2653
Neurontin Capsules (Infrequent) 2655
Neurontin Oral Solution (Infrequent) 2655
Neurontin Tablets (Infrequent) 2655
▲ Paxil (2% to 10.0%) 1609
Prozac Pulvules, Liquid, and Weekly Capsules (Infrequent) 1238
Risperdal (Frequent) 1796
Sarafem Pulvules 1962
Serzone Tablets (Rare) 1104
Viagra Tablets (Less than 2%) 2732

Anosmia
▲ Aerobid/Aerobid-M (3% to 9%) 1363
Beconase Inhalation Aerosol (Rare) 1497
Beconase AQ Nasal Spray (Rare) 1498
Cipro I.V. (1% or less) 893
Cipro I.V. Pharmacy Bulk Package (Less than 1%) 897
Cipro 887
Cytovene 2959
Enalaprilat Injection 863
Flonase Nasal Spray 1533
Lexxel Tablets 608
Nasalide Nasal Spray 1295
Rhinocort Aqua Nasal Spray (Rare) 642
Vaseretic Tablets 2204
Vasotec I.V. Injection 2207
Vasotec Tablets (0.5% to 1.0%) 2210

Anotia
Thalomid Capsules 1154

Anotia, fetal
Accutane Capsules 2944

Anticholinergic syndrome
Clozaril Tablets 2319
Diprivan Injectable Emulsion (Less than 1%) 667
Serentil 1057

Antidiuretic effect
Demerol 3079
Dilaudid-HP (Less frequent) 443
Dolophine Hydrochloride Tablets 3056
Mepergan Injection 3539
MS Contin Tablets (Less frequent) 2896
MSIR (Less frequent) 2898
Oramorph SR Tablets (Less frequent) 3062
Phenergan with Codeine Syrup 3557
Phenergan VC with Codeine Syrup 3561
Risperdal (Rare) 1796

Antimitochondrial antibodies
Normodyne Tablets (Less common) 3137

Antisocial reaction
Zyprexa Tablets (Infrequent) 1973
Zyprexa ZYDIS Orally Disintegrating Tablets (Infrequent) 1973

Antithrombin, decrease
Brevicon 28-Day Tablets 3380
Estrace Vaginal Cream 3358
Estrace Tablets 3361
Estratest 3252
Norinyl 1 +35 28-Day Tablets 3380
Norinyl 1 + 50 28-Day Tablets 3380
Oncaspar 756
Ortho-Cyclen/Ortho Tri-Cyclen 2573
Tri-Norinyl-28 Tablets 3433

Anuria
Abelcet Injection 1273
Azulfidine EN-tabs Tablets (Rare) 2775
Bactrim 2949
Betaseron for SC Injection 988
Campath Ampules 992
CytoGam Intravenous 2026
Effexor Tablets (Rare) 3495
Effexor XR Capsules (Rare) 3499
Floxin I.V. 2526
Floxin Tablets 2529
Gamimune N, 5% Solvent/Detergent Treated 925
Gamimune N, 10% Solvent/Detergent Treated 928
Gammagard S/D (Some patients) 845
Gammar-P I.V. 787
Luvox Tablets (25, 50, 100 mg) (Infrequent) 3256
Miltown Tablets (Rare) 3349
Neurontin Capsules (Rare) 2655
Neurontin Oral Solution (Rare) 2655
Neurontin Tablets (Rare) 2655
Orthoclone OKT3 Sterile Solution (Less than 1%) 2498
Pediazole Suspension 3050
Primaxin I.M. 2158
Primaxin I.V. (2.2%) 2160
Prinivil Tablets (0.3% to 1.0%) 2164
Prinzide Tablets 2168
▲ Proleukin for Injection (5%) 1199
Sandoglobulin I.V. 2391
Septra Suspension 2265
Septra Tablets 2265
Septra DS Tablets 2265
Zestoretic Tablets 695
Zestril Tablets (0.3% to 1.0%) 698
Zovirax for Injection (Less than 1%) 1708

Anuria, neonatal
Accupril Tablets 2611
Aceon Tablets (2 mg, 4 mg, 8 mg) 3249
Altace Capsules 2233
Avapro Tablets 1074
Avapro Tablets 3076
Captopril Tablets 2281
Cozaar Tablets 2067
Enalaprilat Injection 863
Hyzaar 2109
Lexxel Tablets 608
Lotrel Capsules 2370
Monopril Tablets 1091
Prinivil Tablets 2164
Prinzide Tablets 2168
Univasc Tablets 3181
Vaseretic Tablets 2204
Vasotec I.V. Injection 2207
Vasotec Tablets 2210
Zestoretic Tablets 695
Zestril Tablets 698

Anxiety
▲ Acel-Imune (9% to 18%) 1851
Aceon Tablets (2 mg, 4 mg, 8 mg) (0.3% to 1%) 3249
Aciphex Tablets 1267
Aciphex Tablets 1783
▲ Actonel Tablets (4.3%) 2879
Adalat CC Tablets (Less than 1.0%) 877
Aerobid/Aerobid-M (1% to 3%) 1363
Allegra-D Extended-Release Tablets (1.4%) 714
Alphagan Ophthalmic Solution (Less than 3%) 545
Altace Capsules (Less than 1%) 2233
Ambien Tablets (1%) 3191
▲ AmBisome for Injection (7.4% to 13.7%) 1383
Amerge Tablets (Infrequent) 1467
Amoxil Chewable Tablets (Rare) 1471
Amoxil for Oral Suspension (Rare) 1471
Amoxil (Rare) 1471
Androderm Transdermal System CIII (Less than 1%) 3377
AndroGel (Fewer than 1%) 3322
▲ Android Capsules, 10 mg (Among most common) 1731
Anzemet Injection (Infrequently) 719
Anzemet Tablets (Infrequently) 722
Arava Tablets (1% to 3%) 724
▲ Aredia for Injection (14.3%) 2309
▲ Arimidex Tablets (2% to 5%) 659
▲ Aromasin Tablets (10%) 2769
Arthrotec Tablets (Rare) 3195
Asacol Delayed-Release Tablets (2% or greater) 2884
Astelin Nasal Spray (Infrequent) 3339
Astramorph/PF Injection, USP (Preservative-Free) 594
Atacand Tablets (0.5% or greater) 595
Atacand HCT Tablets (0.5% or greater) 597
Augmentin Chewable Tablets (Rare) 1482
Augmentin Powder for Oral Suspension (Rare) 1482
Augmentin Tablets (Rare) 1485
Augmentin ES-600 Powder for Oral Suspension (Rare) 1487
Avalide Tablets (1% or greater) 1070
Avapro Tablets (Less than 1%) 1074
Avapro Tablets (Less than 1%) 3076
Avelox Tablets (0.05% to 1%) 879
Avonex 1013
Axert Tablets (Infrequent) 2772
Axid Pulvules (1.6%) 1903
Axid Pulvules (1.6%) 2919
Baycol Tablets 883
▲ Betapace Tablets (2% to 4%) 950
▲ Betaseron for SC Injection (15%) 988
Betaxon Ophthalmic Suspension (Less than 2%) 537
Biaxin/Biaxin XL 403
Bicillin C-R 900/300 Injection 2240
Bicillin C-R Injection 2238
Bicillin L-A Injection 2242
Brethine Ampuls (Less than 0.5%) 2314
Brethine Tablets (1%) 2313
Brevibloc Injection (Less than 1%) 858
Brevital Sodium for Injection, USP 1815
Cardura Tablets (1.1%) 2668
Carnitor Injection (1% to 2%) 3242
▲ Casodex Tablets (2% to 5%) 662

Cataflam Tablets (Less than 1%) 2315
Catapres Tablets 1037
Catapres-TTS (0.5% or less) 1038
Ceclor CD Tablets (0.1% to 1%) 1279
Celebrex Capsules (0.1% to 1.9%) 2676
Celebrex Capsules (0.1% to 1.9%) 2780
▲ Celexa (4%) 1365
▲ CellCept Capsules (3% to 28.4%) 2951
▲ CellCept Intravenous (3% to 28.4%) 2951
▲ CellCept Oral Suspension (3% to 28.4%) 2951
▲ CellCept Tablets (3% to 28.4%) 2951
Chirocaine Injection (1%) 2909
Cipro I.V. (1% or less) 893
Cipro I.V. Pharmacy Bulk Package (Less than 1%) 897
Cipro 887
Claritin (At least one patient) 3100
Claritin-D 12 Hour Extended Release Tablets (Less frequent) 3102
Claritin-D 24 Hour Extended Release Tablets (Fewer than 2%) 3104
Clomid Tablets 735
Clorpres Tablets 1002
Clozaril Tablets (1%) 2319
▲ Cognex Capsules (3%) 1351
Colazal Capsules 3069
Combipres Tablets 1040
Comtan Tablets (2%) 2328
▲ Copaxone for Injection (23%) 3306
Corlopam Injection (1% to 2%) 412
Cosopt Sterile Ophthalmic Solution 2065
Cozaar Tablets (Less than 1%) 2067
Crixivan Capsules (Less than 2%) 2070
Cuprimine Capsules 2075
Cytotec Tablets (Infrequent) 3202
Cytovene (At least 3 subjects) 2959
DaunoXome Injection (Less than or equal to 5%) 1442
Delatestryl Injection 1151
Demser Capsules 2085
Depacon Injection (1% to 5%) 416
Depakene (1% to 5%) 421
Depakote Sprinkle Capsules (1% to 5%) 426
Depakote Tablets (1% to 5%) 430
Depakote ER Tablets (1% to 5%) 436
Detrol LA Capsules (1%) 2801
D.H.E. 45 Injection (Occasional) 2334
Digitek Tablets 1003
Dilaudid 441
Dilaudid Powder 441
Dilaudid Rectal Suppositories 441
Dilaudid Tablets 441
Diovan Capsules 2337
Diovan HCT Tablets (Greater than 0.2%) 2338
▲ Diphtheria & Tetanus Toxoids Adsorbed Purogenated for Pediatric Use (22.6%) 1857
Diprivan Injectable Emulsion (Less than 1%) 667
▲ Dostinex Tablets (1% to less than 10%) 2804
Doxil Injection (Less than 1% to 5%) 566
▲ Duraclon Injection (38%) 3057
▲ Duragesic Transdermal System (3% to 10%) 1786
Duramorph Injection 1312
Dynabac Tablets (0.1% to 1%) 2269
▲ Effexor Tablets (2% to 11.2%) 3495
Effexor XR Capsules 3499
Eldepryl Capsules (1 of 49 patients) 3266
Emcyt Capsules (1%) 2810
EpiPen 1236
▲ Epogen for Injection (2% to 7%) 582
Ergamisol Tablets (1%) 1789
▲ Esclim Transdermal System (Up to 8.3%) 3460
Estratest 3252
Estring Vaginal Ring (1% to 3%) 2811
Etrafon 3115
Eulexin Capsules (1%) 3118
Evoxac Capsules (1.3%) 1217
▲ Exelon Capsules (5%) 2342
▲ Exelon Oral Solution (5%) 2345
Famotidine Injection (Infrequent) 866
▲ Felbatol (5.2% to 5.3%) 3343
Feldene Capsules (Occasional) 2685
Femara Tablets (Less frequent) 2351
Flexeril Tablets (Less than 1%) 572
Flexeril Tablets (Less than 1%) 2094
▲ Flolan for Injection (7% to 21%) 1528
Floxin I.V. (Less than 1%) 2526
Floxin Tablets (Less than 1%) 2529
Fortovase Capsules (2.2%) 2970
▲ Foscavir Injection (5% or greater) 605
Gabitril Tablets (1% or more) 1189
Gamimune N, 5% Solvent/Detergent Treated 925
Gamimune N, 10% Solvent/Detergent Treated 928
Gammar-P I.V. 787
Gastrocrom Oral Concentrate (Less common) 1162
Gengraf Capsules (1% to less than 3%) 457
Geodon Capsules 2688
Glucotrol XL Extended Release Tablets (Less than 3%) 2693
Gonal-F for Injection 3216
Haldol Decanoate 2535
Haldol Injection, Tablets and Concentrate 2533
Hivid Tablets (Less than 1%) 2975
Hycodan 1316
Hycomine Compound Tablets 1317
Hycotuss Expectorant Syrup 1318
Hytrin Capsules (At least 1%) 464
Hyzaar 2109
Imdur Tablets (Less than or equal to 5%) 1826
Imitrex Injection (1.1%) 1549
Imitrex Nasal Spray (Infrequent) 1554
Imitrex Tablets 1558
▲ Indapamide Tablets (Greater than or equal to 5%) 2286
Indocin (Less than 1%) 2112
▲ Infanrix Vaccine (3.3% to 9.2%) 1562
▲ Infergen (10% to 19%) 1777
Infumorph 200 and Infumorph 500 Sterile Solutions 1314
▲ Intron A for Injection (Up to 5%) 3120
Invirase Capsules (Less than 2%) 2979
IPOL Vaccine 809
Ismo Tablets (Fewer than 1%) 3524
▲ Kadian Capsules (Less than 3% to 6%) 1335
Kaletra Capsules (Less than 2%) 471
Kaletra Oral Solution (Less than 2%) 471
Keppra Tablets (2%) 3314
Klonopin Tablets (Infrequent) 2983
Kytril Injection (Less than 2%) 2986
Kytril Tablets (2%) 2988
▲ Lamictal (3.8%) 1567
Lanoxicaps Capsules 1574
Lanoxin Injection 1581
Lanoxin Tablets 1587
Lanoxin Elixir Pediatric 1578
Lanoxin Injection Pediatric 1584
Lariam Tablets 2989
Lescol Capsules 2361
Lescol Capsules 2925
Lescol XL Tablets 2361
Lescol XL Tablets 2925
▲ Leukine (11%) 1755
Levaquin (0.1% to less than 1.0%) 2537
Levbid Extended-Release Tablets 3172
Levoxyl Tablets 1819
Levsin/Levsinex/Levbid 3172
Lexxel Tablets 608
Lodine XL Extended-Release Tablets (Less than 1%) 3530
Lodosyn Tablets 1251
Lortab 3319
Lortab Elixir 3317
Lotensin Tablets (Less than 1%) 2365
Lotrel Capsules 2370
Lupron Depot 3.75 mg (Less than 5%) 3281
Lupron Depot–3 Month 11.25 mg (Less than 5%) 3285
Lupron Depot–3 Month 22.5 mg (Less than 5%) 3288
Lupron Injection (Less than 5%) 3279
Luvox Tablets (25, 50, 100 mg) (1% to 5%) 3256
Marinol Capsules (Greater than 1%) 3325
Mavik Tablets (0.3% to 1.0%) 478
Maxair Autohaler 1981
Maxair Inhaler (Less than 1%) 1984
Maxalt Tablets (Infrequent) 2120
Maxalt-MLT Orally Disintegrating Tablets (Infrequent) 2120
Maxidone Tablets CIII 3399
Maxzide 1008
▲ Mepron Suspension (7%) 1598
▲ Meridia Capsules (4.5%) 481
Merrem I.V. (0.1% to 1.0%) 673
Mevacor Tablets (0.5% to 1.0%) 2132
Miacalcin Nasal Spray (Less than 1%) 2375
Micardis Tablets (More than 0.3%) 1049
Micardis HCT Tablets 1051
Migranal Nasal Spray (Rare) 2376
Mirapex Tablets (1% or more) 2834
Mobic Tablets (Less than 2%) 1054
Mykrox Tablets (Less than 2%) 1168
Myobloc Injectable Solution (2% or greater) 1291
Naprelan Tablets (Less than 1%) 1293
Nardil Tablets (Less frequent) 2653
Naropin Injection (1% to 5%) 612
Nascobal Gel 3174
▲ Natrecor for Injection (3%) 3189
Nembutal Sodium Solution (Less than 1%) 485
Neoral Soft Gelatin Capsules (1% to less than 3%) 2380
Neoral Oral Solution (1% to less than 3%) 2380
Nesacaine/Nesacaine MPF 617
Neurontin Capsules (Frequent) 2655
Neurontin Oral Solution (Frequent) 2655
Neurontin Tablets (Frequent) 2655
▲ Nicotrol Nasal Spray (Over 5%) 2843
▲ Nipent for Injection (3% to 10%) 3272
Norco 5/325 Tablets CIII 3424
Norco 7.5/325 Tablets CIII 3425
Norco 10/325 Tablets CIII 3425
Norco 10/325 Tablets CIII 3427
Noroxin Tablets (Less frequent) 2145
Norplant System 3543
Norpramin Tablets 755
Norvasc Tablets (More than 0.1% to 1%) 2704
Norvir Capsules (Less than 2%) 487
Norvir Oral Solution (Less than 2%) 487
▲ Novantrone for Injection (5%) 1760
OptiPranolol Metipranolol Ophthalmic Solution 0.3% (A small number of patients) ⊙263
OxyContin Tablets (Between 1% and 5%) 2912
Parnate Tablets 1607
▲ Paxil (5% to 5.9%) 1609
Pediazole Suspension 3050
▲ PEG-Intron Powder for Injection (28%) 3140
Pepcid Injection (Infrequent) 2153
Pepcid for Oral Suspension (Infrequent) 2150
Pepcid RPD Orally Disintegrating Tablets (Infrequent) 2150
Pepcid Tablets (Infrequent) 2150
▲ Permax Tablets (6.4%) 1299
Phenergan VC Syrup 3560
Phenergan VC with Codeine Syrup 3561
▲ Photofrin for Injection (7%) 831
Plavix Tablets (1% to 2.5%) 1097
Plavix Tablets (1% to 2.5%) 3084
Plendil Extended-Release Tablets (0.5% to 1.5%) 623
Pletal Tablets (Less than 2%) 2605
Pletal Tablets (Less than 2%) 2848
Polocaine Injection, USP 625
Polocaine-MPF Injection, USP 625
Pravachol Tablets 1099
Prevacid Delayed-Release Capsules (Less than 1%) 3292
PREVPAC (Less than 1%) 3298
Prilosec Delayed-Release Capsules (Less than 1%) 628
ProAmatine Tablets (Less frequent) 3241
Procardia XL Extended Release Tablets (1% or less) 2710
▲ Procrit for Injection (2% to 11%) 2502
▲ Prograf (3% to 15%) 1393
▲ Proleukin for Injection (12%) 1199
Prometrium Capsules (100 mg, 200 mg) (Less than 5%) 3261
ProSom Tablets (Frequent) 500
Protonix I.V. (Greater than or equal to 1%) 3580
Protonix Tablets (Greater than or equal to 1%) 3577
Proventil HFA Inhalation Aerosol (Less than 3%) 3150
▲ Provigil Tablets (4%) 1193
▲ Prozac Pulvules, Liquid, and Weekly Capsules (2% to 28%) 1238
Pulmicort Respules (Less than 1%) 632
Pulmicort Turbuhaler Inhalation Powder (Rare) 636
▲ Rapamune Oral Solution and Tablets (3% to 20%) 3584
Reglan 2935
Relafen Tablets (Less than 1%) 1617
Remeron Tablets (Frequent) 2483
Remeron SolTab Tablets (Frequent) 2486
Remicade for IV Injection (Less than 2%) 1178
Reminyl Oral Solution (Greater than or equal to 2%) 1792
Reminyl Tablets (Greater than or equal to 2%) 1792
ReoPro Vials (1.7%) 1958
Requip Tablets (1% or more) 1621
Retrovir Capsules 1625
Retrovir IV Infusion 1629
Retrovir 1625
Rhinocort Nasal Inhaler (Rare) 640
Rifater Tablets 769
▲ Risperdal (12% to 20%) 1796
▲ Roferon-A Injection (5% to 6%) 2996
▲ Romazicon Injection (3% to 9%) 3000
Roxicodone Tablets (Less than 3%) 3067
Rynatan Tablets 3351
Rythmol Tablets – 150 mg, 225 mg, 300 mg (1.5% to 2.0%) 502
Salagen Tablets (Less than 1%) 2229
Sandimmune (Rare) 2388
Sandostatin Injection (Less than 1%) 2394
▲ Sandostatin LAR Depot (5% to 15%) 2395
▲ Sarafem Pulvules (13%) 1962
Sectral Capsules (Up to 2%) 3589
Sensorcaine 643
Sensorcaine-MPF Injection 643
Serophene Tablets 3226
▲ Serostim for Injection (1% to 10%) 3229
Serzone Tablets 1104
▲ Simulect for Injection (3% to 10%) 2399
Sinemet Tablets 1253
Sinemet CR Tablets 1255
Skelid Tablets (More than or equal to 1%) 3088
Sonata Capsules (Less than 1% to 3%) 3591
Soriatane Capsules (Less than 1%) 3003
▲ Sporanox Capsules (3%) 1800
Stadol NS Nasal Spray (1% or greater) 1108
Sular Tablets (Less than or equal to 1%) 688
Surmontil Capsules 3595
Sustiva Capsules (Less than 2%) 1258
Symmetrel (1% to 5%) 1328
Synercid I.V. (Less than 1%) 775
Synvisc 3596
Tagamet 1644
Tambocor Tablets (1% to 3%) 1990
Tarka Tablets (0.3% or more) 508
Tasmar Tablets (1% or more) 3010
▲ Temodar Capsules (7%) 3157
Tenex Tablets (Less frequent) 2942
Tequin Injection (Less than 0.1%) 1110
Tequin Tablets (Less than 0.1%) 1110
Testoderm Transdermal Systems 574
Testopel Pellets 3610
Testred Capsules, 10 mg 1746
Teveten Tablets (Less than 1%) 3327
Thalomid Capsules 1154
Thyrel TRH for Injection (Less frequent) 3630
Tikosyn Capsules (Greater than 2%) 2717
Timolol GFS ⊙266
Timoptic in Ocudose (Less frequent) 2192
Timoptic Sterile Ophthalmic Solution (Less frequent) 2190
Timoptic-XE Sterile Ophthalmic Gel Forming Solution 2194
Tonocard Tablets (1.1% to 1.5%) 649
▲ Topamax Sprinkle Capsules (2.2% to 9.3%) 2590
▲ Topamax Tablets (2.2% to 9.3%) 2590
Trasylol Injection (1% to 2%) 909
Travatan Ophthalmic Solution (1% to 5%) 543
Trental Tablets (Less than 1%) 784
Tricor Capsules, Micronized (Less than 1%) 513
▲ Trileptal Oral Suspension (5% to 7%) 2407
▲ Trileptal Tablets (5% to 7%) 2407
Tripedia Vaccine 817
▲ Trisenox Injection (30%) 1158
Trovan (Less than 1%) 2722
Tussionex Pennkinetic Extended-Release Suspension 1174
Ultracet Tablets (At least 1%) 2597
▲ Ultram Tablets (1% to 14%) 2600
Uniretic Tablets (Less than 1%) 3178
Unithroid Tablets 3445
Univasc Tablets (Less than 1%) 3181
Vantin Tablets and Oral Suspension (Less than 1%) 2860
Vascor Tablets (0.5% to 2.0%) 2602
Versed Injection (Less than 1%) 3027
▲ Vesanoid Capsules (17%) 3037
Viadur Implant (Less than 2%) 912
Viagra Tablets 2732
Vicodin Tablets 516
Vicodin ES Tablets 517
Vicodin HP Tablets 518
Vicodin Tuss Expectorant 519
▲ Vicoprofen Tablets (3% to 9%) 520
Vioxx (Greater than 0.1% to 1.9%) 2213
Viracept 532
Vistide Injection 1445
Vivactil Tablets 2217
Vivactil Tablets 2446
Voltaren Tablets (Less than 1%) 2315
Voltaren-XR Tablets (Less than 1%) 2315
▲ Wellbutrin Tablets (3.1%) 1680
▲ Wellbutrin SR Sustained-Release Tablets (5% to 6%) 1684
▲ Xanax Tablets (16.6%) 2865
▲ Xenical Capsules (2.8% to 4.4%) 3043
Xopenex Inhalation Solution (2.7%) 3207
Xylocaine Injections 653
Zanaflex Tablets (Frequent) 1305
Zebeta Tablets 1885
▲ Zenapax for Injection (2% to 5%) 3046
Ziac Tablets 1887
Zocor Tablets 2219
▲ Zofran Injection (2% to 6%) 1698
▲ Zofran (6%) 1703
▲ Zofran ODT Orally Disintegrating Tablets (6%) 1703
Zoladex (1% to 5%) 702
Zoladex 3-month 706
▲ Zoloft (4%) 2751
▲ Zometa for Intravenous Infusion (14%) 3621
Zomig Tablets (Infrequent) 708
Zomig-ZMT Tablets (Infrequent) 708

▲ Zonegran Capsules (3%) ... 1307
Zosyn (1.2% to 3.2%) ... 1890
Zosyn in Galaxy Containers (1.2% to 3.2%) ... 1894
▲ Zyban Sustained-Release Tablets (8%) ... 1710
Zydone Tablets ... 1330
▲ Zyprexa Tablets (9%) ... 1973
▲ Zyprexa ZYDIS Orally Disintegrating Tablets (9%) ... 1973
Zyrtec (Less than 2%) ... 2756
Zyrtec-D 12 Hour Extended Relief Tablets (Less than 2%) ... 2758

Anxiety, paradoxical
Halcion Tablets ... 2823
Valium Injectable ... 3026
Valium Tablets ... 3047
Vivactil Tablets ... 2217
Vivactil Tablets ... 2446

Apathy
Ambien Tablets (Rare) ... 3191
Bactrim ... 2949
Betaseron for SC Injection ... 988
Bicillin C-R 900/300 Injection ... 2240
Bicillin C-R Injection ... 2238
Campath Ampules ... 992
Celexa (Infrequent) ... 1365
Claritin-D 12 Hour Extended Release Tablets (Less frequent) ... 3102
Claritin-D 24 Hour Extended Release Tablets (Fewer than 2%) ... 3104
Cognex Capsules (Infrequent) ... 1351
D.H.E. 45 Injection ... 2334
Digitek Tablets ... 1003
Effexor Tablets (Infrequent) ... 3495
Effexor XR Capsules (Infrequent) ... 3499
Eldepryl Capsules ... 3266
Evoxac Capsules ... 1217
Exelon Capsules (Infrequent) ... 2342
Exelon Oral Solution (Infrequent) ... 2345
Felbatol ... 3343
Gabitril Tablets (Infrequent) ... 1189
Imitrex Injection ... 1549
Imitrex Nasal Spray (Rare) ... 1554
Imitrex Tablets (Rare) ... 1558
Intron A for Injection (Less than 5%) ... 3120
Kadian Capsules (Less than 3%) ... 1335
Klonopin Tablets (Infrequent) ... 2983
Lamictal (Infrequent) ... 1567
Lanoxicaps Capsules ... 1574
Lanoxin Injection ... 1581
Lanoxin Tablets ... 1587
Lanoxin Elixir Pediatric ... 1578
Lanoxin Injection Pediatric ... 1584
Luvox Tablets (25, 50, 100 mg) (Frequent) ... 3256
Mirapex Tablets (1% or more) ... 2834
Neurontin Capsules (Infrequent) ... 2655
Neurontin Oral Solution (Infrequent) ... 2655
Neurontin Tablets (Infrequent) ... 2655
Nexium Delayed-Release Capsules (Less than 1%) ... 619
Nicotrol Nasal Spray (Under 5%) ... 2843
Norvasc Tablets (Less than or equal to 0.1%) ... 2704
Permax Tablets (Infrequent) ... 1299
Prevacid Delayed-Release Capsules (Less than 1%) ... 3292
PREVPAC (Less than 1%) ... 3298
Prilosec Delayed-Release Capsules (Less than 1%) ... 628
ProSom Tablets (Infrequent) ... 500
Prozac Pulvules, Liquid, and Weekly Capsules (Infrequent) ... 1238
Remeron Tablets (Frequent) ... 2483
Remeron SolTab Tablets (Frequent) ... 2486
Reminyl Oral Solution (Infrequent) ... 1792
Reminyl Tablets (Infrequent) ... 1792
Requip Tablets (Infrequent) ... 1621
Rilutek Tablets (Infrequent) ... 772
Risperdal (Infrequent) ... 1796
Roferon-A Injection (Infrequent) ... 2996
Sarafem Pulvules (Infrequent) ... 1962
Septra Suspension ... 2265
Septra Tablets ... 2265
Septra DS Tablets ... 2265
Seroquel Tablets (Infrequent) ... 684
Serzone Tablets (Infrequent) ... 1104
Sonata Capsules (Frequent) ... 3591
Sustiva Capsules (Less than 2%) ... 1258
Tambocor Tablets (Less than 1%) ... 1990
Tasmar Tablets (Infrequent) ... 3010
Topamax Sprinkle Capsules (1.8% to 4.5%) ... 2590
Topamax Tablets (1.8% to 4.5%) ... 2590
Trileptal Oral Suspension ... 2407
Trileptal Tablets ... 2407
Zoloft (Infrequent) ... 2751
Zomig Tablets (Rare) ... 708
Zomig-ZMT Tablets (Rare) ... 708
Zyprexa Tablets ... 1973
Zyprexa ZYDIS Orally Disintegrating Tablets ... 1973

Aphasia
Amerge Tablets (Rare) ... 1467
Aricept Tablets (Frequent) ... 1270
Aricept Tablets (Frequent) ... 2665
Betaseron for SC Injection ... 988
Campath Ampules ... 992
Cedax ... 1021
Cerebyx Injection (Infrequent) ... 2619
Cognex Capsules (Infrequent) ... 1351
Colazal Capsules ... 3069
Duragesic Transdermal System (Less than 1%) ... 1786
Effexor Tablets (Rare) ... 3495
Effexor XR Capsules (Rare) ... 3499
Evoxac Capsules ... 1217
Exelon Capsules (Infrequent) ... 2342
Exelon Oral Solution (Infrequent) ... 2345
Foscavir Injection (Between 1% and 5%) ... 605
▲ Gliadel Wafer (9%) ... 1723
Hivid Tablets (Less than 1%) ... 2975
Intron A for Injection (Less than 5%) ... 3120
Lamictal (Infrequent) ... 1567
Mycobutin Capsules (More than one patient) ... 2838
Neurontin Capsules (Infrequent) ... 2655
Neurontin Oral Solution (Infrequent) ... 2655
Neurontin Tablets (Infrequent) ... 2655
Nicotrol Nasal Spray (Less than 1%) ... 2843
Norvir Capsules (Less than 2%) ... 487
Norvir Oral Solution (Less than 2%) ... 487
Orthoclone OKT3 Sterile Solution (Less than 1%) ... 2498
Paxil (Rare) ... 1609
Remeron Tablets (Rare) ... 2483
Remeron SolTab Tablets (Rare) ... 2486
Reminyl Oral Solution (Infrequent) ... 1792
Reminyl Tablets (Infrequent) ... 1792
Requip Tablets (Infrequent) ... 1621
Risperdal (Rare) ... 1796
Roferon-A Injection (Less than 0.5%) ... 2996
Salagen Tablets (Less than 1%) ... 2229
Sandostatin LAR Depot (Rare) ... 2395
Seroquel Tablets (Rare) ... 684
Trileptal Oral Suspension ... 2407
Trileptal Tablets ... 2407
▲ Vesanoid Capsules (3%) ... 3037
Wellbutrin Tablets (Rare) ... 1680
Wellbutrin SR Sustained-Release Tablets ... 1684
Zyban Sustained-Release Tablets ... 1710

Aphonia
Advair Diskus 100/50 ... 1448
Advair Diskus 250/50 ... 1448
Advair Diskus 500/50 ... 1448
Flovent Diskus ... 3614
Flovent ... 1535
Flovent Rotadisk ... 1537
Klonopin Tablets ... 2983
Migranal Nasal Spray (Rare) ... 2376
Roferon-A Injection (Less than 0.5%) ... 2996

Aphthous stomatitis
(*see under* Stomatitis, ulcerative)

APL differentiation syndrome
Trisenox Injection ... 1158

Aplasia, bone marrow
Paxil ... 1609

Aplasia, red cell
Cuprimine Capsules ... 2075
Depen Titratable Tablets ... 3341
Lamictal (One case) ... 1567

Aplasia, unspecified
Campath Ampules ... 992

Aplastic anemia
(*see under* Anemia, aplastic)

Apnea
Aciphex Tablets (Rare) ... 1267
Aciphex Tablets (Rare) ... 1783
Actiq ... 1184
Aloprim for Injection (Less than 1%) ... 2292
▲ Amphotec (5% or more) ... 1774
Anectine Injection ... 1476
Aricept Tablets (Infrequent) ... 1270
Aricept Tablets (Infrequent) ... 2665
Ativan Injection (1.2%) ... 3478
Betaseron for SC Injection ... 988
Bicillin C-R 900/300 Injection ... 2240
Bicillin C-R Injection ... 2238
Bicillin L-A Injection ... 2242
Brevital Sodium for Injection, USP ... 1815
Buprenex Injectable (Infrequent) ... 2918
▲ CellCept Capsules (3% to 10%) ... 2951
▲ CellCept Intravenous (3% to 10%) ... 2951
▲ CellCept Oral Suspension (3% to 10%) ... 2951
▲ CellCept Tablets (3% to 10%) ... 2951
Cerebyx Injection (Infrequent) ... 2619
Chirocaine Injection (Less than 1%) ... 2909
Coly-Mycin M Parenteral ... 2243
Demerol ... 3079
D.H.E. 45 Injection ... 2334
Dilaudid Oral Liquid ... 445
Dilaudid Tablets - 8 mg ... 445
Dilaudid-HP ... 443
Diprivan Injectable Emulsion (1% to 3%) ... 667
▲ Duragesic Transdermal System (3% to 10%) ... 1786
Effexor XR Capsules (Rare) ... 3499
Evoxac Capsules ... 1217
Exelon Capsules (Infrequent) ... 2342
Exelon Oral Solution (Infrequent) ... 2345
Gabitril Tablets (Infrequent) ... 1189
Herceptin I.V. (At least one of the 958 patients) ... 1414
Indocin I.V. (Less than 3%) ... 2115
▲ Infasurf Intratracheal Suspension (61% to 76%) ... 1372
Lamictal ... 1567
Levo-Dromoran ... 1734
Luvox Tablets (25, 50, 100 mg) (Rare) ... 3256
Merrem I.V. (1.2%) ... 673
Motrin Suspension, Oral Drops, Chewable Tablets, and Caplets (Less than 1%) ... 2002
MS Contin Tablets ... 2896
MSIR ... 2898
Natrecor for Injection (At least 1%) ... 3189
Nembutal Sodium Solution (Less than 1%) ... 485
Nesacaine/Nesacaine MPF ... 617
Neurontin Capsules (Infrequent) ... 2655
Neurontin Oral Solution (Infrequent) ... 2655
Neurontin Tablets (Infrequent) ... 2655
Norcuron for Injection ... 2478
Oramorph SR Tablets (Less frequent) ... 3062
Orthoclone OKT3 Sterile Solution (Less than 1%) ... 2498
OxyContin Tablets ... 2912
Permax Tablets (Infrequent) ... 1299
Phenergan ... 3556
Polocaine Injection, USP ... 625
Polocaine-MPF Injection, USP ... 625
Proleukin for Injection (1%) ... 1199
Prozac Pulvules, Liquid, and Weekly Capsules (Rare) ... 1238
Pulmozyme Inhalation Solution ... 1426
Rilutek Tablets (More than 2%) ... 772
Risperdal ... 1796
Rythmol Tablets – 150 mg, 225 mg, 300 mg (Less than 1%) ... 502
Sarafem Pulvules (Rare) ... 1962
Sensorcaine ... 643
Sensorcaine-MPF Injection ... 643
Sonata Capsules (Rare) ... 3591
Stadol NS Nasal Spray (Less than 1%) ... 1108
▲ Suprane Liquid for Inhalation (3% to 15%) ... 874
▲ Survanta Intratracheal Suspension (46.1% to 65.4%) ... 3053
Synagis Intramuscular (More than 1%) ... 2028
Tasmar Tablets (Rare) ... 3010
Thalomid Capsules ... 1154
Thioplex for Injection ... 1765
▲ Trasylol Injection (3%) ... 909
▲ Versed Injection (2.8% to 15.4%) ... 3027
Versed Syrup (Less than 1%) ... 3033
Virazole for Inhalation Solution ... 1747
Zomig Tablets (Rare) ... 708
Zomig-ZMT Tablets (Rare) ... 708
Zonegran Capsules (Rare) ... 1307
Zyprexa Tablets (Infrequent) ... 1973
Zyprexa ZYDIS Orally Disintegrating Tablets (Infrequent) ... 1973

Apnea, neonatal
Alphagan Ophthalmic Solution (Rare) ... 545
Sinequan (One case) ... 2713
Survanta Intratracheal Suspension (Less than 1%) ... 3053

Appendicitis
Advair Diskus 100/50 (1% to 3%) ... 1448
Advair Diskus 250/50 (1% to 3%) ... 1448
Advair Diskus 500/50 (1% to 3%) ... 1448
Effexor Tablets (Rare) ... 3495
Effexor XR Capsules (Rare) ... 3499
Evoxac Capsules (Less than 1%) ... 1217
Lopid Tablets (1.2%) ... 2650
Remicade for IV Injection (Less than 2%) ... 1178
Sandostatin Injection (Less than 1%) ... 2394
Sandostatin LAR Depot (Rare) ... 2395

Appetite, changes
Activella Tablets ... 2764
Alesse-21 Tablets ... 3468
Alesse-28 Tablets ... 3473
Arthrotec Tablets (Rare) ... 3195
Ativan Tablets (Less frequent) ... 3482
Betapace Tablets (1% to 3%) ... 950
Brevicon 28-Day Tablets ... 3380
Cataflam Tablets (Less than 1%) ... 2315
Compazine ... 1505
Cortone Acetate Injectable Suspension ... 2059
Cortone Acetate Tablets ... 2061
Cyclessa Tablets ... 2450
Cytotec Tablets (Infrequent) ... 3202
Decadron Elixir ... 2078
Decadron Tablets ... 2079
Decadron Phosphate Injection ... 2081
Depo-Provera Contraceptive Injection (Fewer than 1%) ... 2798
Desogen Tablets ... 2458
▲ Effexor Tablets (1% to 6%) ... 3495
▲ Effexor XR Capsules (1% to 6%) ... 3499
Eldepryl Capsules ... 3266
Estrostep ... 2627
Feldene Capsules (Rare) ... 2685
Fortovase Capsules (Less than 2%) ... 2970
Hydrocortone Tablets ... 2106
Hydrocortone Acetate Injectable Suspension ... 2103
Hydrocortone Phosphate Injection, Sterile ... 2105
Invirase Capsules (Up to 1.0%) ... 2979
Levlen ... 962
Levlite 21 Tablets ... 962
Levlite 28 Tablets ... 962
Levora Tablets ... 3389
Lodine XL Extended-Release Tablets ... 3530
Loestrin 21 Tablets ... 2642
Loestrin Fe Tablets ... 2642
Lo/Ovral Tablets ... 3532
Lo/Ovral-28 Tablets ... 3538
Low-Ogestrel-28 Tablets ... 3392
Lunelle Monthly Injection ... 2827
Lupron Depot 3.75 mg (Less than 5%) ... 3281
Lupron Depot–3 Month 11.25 mg (Less than 5%) ... 3285
Maxzide ... 1008
Mexitil Capsules (2.6%) ... 1047
Microgestin Fe 1.5/30 Tablets ... 3407
Microgestin Fe 1/20 Tablets ... 3400
Midamor Tablets (Between 1% and 3%) ... 2136
Mircette Tablets ... 2470
Modicon ... 2563
Moduretic Tablets (Less than or equal to 1%) ... 2138
Monopril Tablets (0.2% to 1.0%) ... 1091
Monopril HCT ... 1094
Navane Oral ... 2701
Navane Intramuscular ... 2703
Necon ... 3415
Nordette-28 Tablets ... 2257
Norinyl 1 +35 28-Day Tablets ... 3380
Norinyl 1 + 50 28-Day Tablets ... 3380
Norplant System ... 3543
Ogestrel 0.5/50-28 Tablets ... 3428
Ortho-Cept 21 Tablets ... 2546
Ortho-Cept 28 Tablets ... 2546
Ortho-Cyclen/Ortho Tri-Cyclen ... 2573
Ortho-Novum ... 2563
Ortho-Novum 1/50□28 Tablets ... 2556
Ortho-Cyclen/Ortho Tri-Cyclen ... 2573
Ovcon ... 3364
Ovral Tablets ... 3551
Ovral-28 Tablets ... 3552
Ovrette Tablets ... 3552
Ponstel Capsules (Rare) ... 1356
Prednisone ... 3064
Premphase Tablets ... 3572
Prempro Tablets ... 3572
Provera Tablets ... 2853
Stelazine (Occasional) ... 1640
Thorazine (Sometimes) ... 1656
Trilafon ... 3160
Tri-Levlen ... 962
Tri-Norinyl-28 Tablets ... 3433
Triphasil-21 Tablets ... 3600
Triphasil-28 Tablets ... 3605
Trivora Tablets ... 3439
Univasc Tablets (Less than 1%) ... 3181
Vioxx (Greater than 0.1% to 1.9%) ... 2213
Voltaren Tablets (Less than 1%) ... 2315
Voltaren-XR Tablets (Less than 1%) ... 2315
▲ Wellbutrin Tablets (3.7%) ... 1680
Yasmin 28 Tablets ... 980
Zovia ... 3449

Appetite, decreased
▲ Acel-Imune (7% to 10%) ... 1851
▲ Aerobid/Aerobid-M (3% to 9%) ... 1363
Betapace AF Tablets (1.6% to 2%) ... 954
▲ Combivir Tablets (10%) ... 1502
Crinone (Less than 5%) ... 3213
DynaCirc CR Tablets (0.5% to 1%) ... 2923
▲ Epivir (10%) ... 1520
▲ Femara Tablets (4%) ... 2351
Floxin I.V. (1% to 3%) ... 2526
Floxin Tablets (1% to 3%) ... 2529
Fortovase Capsules (Less than 2%) ... 2970
Imitrex Injection (Rare) ... 1549
Imitrex Nasal Spray (Rare) ... 1554

Imitrex Tablets (Rare) 1558
Klonopin Tablets (1%) 2983
▲ Kytril Tablets (5%) 2988
▲ Leustatin Injection (17%) 2495
MetroGel-Vaginal Gel (1%) 1986
Oncaspar 756
▲ Paxil (2.0% to 9%) 1609
▲ Prevnar for Injection (24.7% to 33%) 1870
ProSom Tablets (Infrequent) 500
Recombivax HB (Greater than 1%) 2178
Rescriptor Tablets (Less than 2%) 526
▲ Trisenox Injection (15%) 1158
Vantin Tablets and Oral Suspension (Less than 1%) 2860
▲ Xanax Tablets (27.8%) 2865

Appetite, increased

Aceon Tablets (2 mg, 4 mg, 8 mg) (0.3% to 1%) 3249
Aciphex Tablets 1267
Aciphex Tablets 1783
Aerobid/Aerobid-M (1% to 3%) 1363
Ambien Tablets (Rare) 3191
Androderm Transdermal System CIII (Less than 1%) 3377
Aricept Tablets (Infrequent) 1270
Aricept Tablets (Infrequent) 2665
Arimidex Tablets (Up to 0.4%) 659
▲ Aromasin Tablets (3%) 2769
Asacol Delayed-Release Tablets 2884
Astelin Nasal Spray (Infrequent) 3339
Avonex 1013
Cardura Tablets (Less than 0.5%) 2668
Celebrex Capsules (0.1% to 1.9%) 2676
Celebrex Capsules (0.1% to 1.9%) 2780
Celexa (Frequent) 1365
Claritin (At least one patient) 3100
Claritin-D 12 Hour Extended Release Tablets (Less frequent) 3102
Claritin-D 24 Hour Extended Release Tablets 3104
Clomid Tablets (Fewer than 1%) 735
Clozaril Tablets (Less than 1%) 2319
Cognex Capsules (Infrequent) 1351
Copaxone for Injection (Infrequent) 3306
Cortifoam Rectal Foam 3170
▲ Crinone (5%) 3213
Crixivan Capsules (Less than 2%) 2070
DaunoXome Injection (Less than or equal to 5%) 1442
Depacon Injection (1% to 5%) 416
Depakene (1% to 5%) 421
Depakote Sprinkle Capsules (1% to 5%) 426
▲ Depakote Tablets (1% to 6%) 430
Depakote ER Tablets (1% to 5%) 436
Diovan HCT Tablets (Greater than 0.2%) 2338
Doxil Injection (Less than 1%) 566
DynaCirc CR Tablets (0.5% to 1%) 2923
Etrafon 3115
Evoxac Capsules (Less than 1%) 1217
Felbatol (Infrequent) 3343
Gabitril Tablets (2%) 1189
Gengraf Capsules (1% to less than 3%) 457
Intron A for Injection (Less than 5%) 3120
Ismo Tablets (Fewer than 1%) 3524
Kaletra Capsules (Less than 2%) 471
Kaletra Oral Solution (Less than 2%) 471
Klonopin Tablets (Infrequent) 2983
Lamictal (Infrequent) 1567
Levoxyl Tablets 1819
Lipitor Tablets (Less than 2%) 2639
Lipitor Tablets (Less than 2%) 2696
Lupron Depot–3 Month 22.5 mg (Less than 5%) 3288
Lupron Depot–4 Month 30 mg (Less than 5%) 3289
Luvox Tablets (25, 50, 100 mg) 3256
Maxalt Tablets (Rare) 2120
Maxalt-MLT Orally Disintegrating Tablets (Rare) 2120
▲ Meridia Capsules (8.7%) 481
Miacalcin Nasal Spray (Less than 1%) 2375
Neoral Soft Gelatin Capsules (1% to less than 3%) 2380
Neoral Oral Solution (1% to less than 3%) 2380
Neurontin Capsules (1.1%) 2655
Neurontin Oral Solution (1.1%) 2655
Neurontin Tablets (1.1%) 2655
Nexium Delayed-Release Capsules (Less than 1%) 619
Nicotrol Nasal Spray (Under 5%) 2843
Norvasc Tablets (Less than or equal to 0.1%) 2704
Oncaspar (Less than 1%) 756
▲ Orap Tablets (1 of 20 patients) 1407
Orudis Capsules (Less than 1%) 3548
Oruvail Capsules (Less than 1%) 3548
OxyContin Tablets (Less than 1%) 2912
▲ Paxil (4%) 1609
Periactin Tablets 2155
Permax Tablets (Infrequent) 1299
Prevacid Delayed-Release Capsules (Less than 1%) 3292
PREVPAC (Less than 1%) 3298
▲ Prograf (3% to 15%) 1393
Prometrium Capsules (100 mg, 200 mg) 3261
ProSom Tablets (Infrequent) 500
Protonix I.V. (Less than 1%) 3580
Protonix Tablets (Less than 1%) 3577
Provigil Tablets (At least 1%) 1193
Prozac Pulvules, Liquid, and Weekly Capsules (Frequent) 1238
Relafen Tablets (Less than 1%) 1617
▲ Remeron Tablets (17%) 2483
▲ Remeron SolTab Tablets (17%) 2486
Rescriptor Tablets (Less than 2%) 526
Rilutek Tablets (Infrequent) 772
Risperdal (Infrequent) 1796
Salagen Tablets (Less than 1%) 2229
Sarafem Pulvules (Frequent) 1962
Seroquel Tablets (Infrequent) 684
▲ Serostim for Injection (1% to 10%) 3229
▲ Serzone Tablets (5%) 1104
Sonata Capsules (Infrequent) 3591
▲ Soriatane Capsules (1% to 10%) 3003
Sporanox Capsules (2%) 1800
Sular Tablets (Less than or equal to 1%) 688
Thalomid Capsules 1154
Thiothixene Capsules 2290
Topamax Sprinkle Capsules (Infrequent) 2590
Topamax Tablets (Infrequent) 2590
Toradol (1% or less) 3018
Tricor Capsules, Micronized (1%) 513
Trileptal Oral Suspension 2407
Trileptal Tablets 2407
Trovan (Less than 1%) 2722
Uniretic Tablets (Less than 1%) 3178
Unithroid Tablets 3445
Vascor Tablets (0.5% to 2.0%) 2602
Wellbutrin SR Sustained-Release Tablets (At least 1%) 1684
▲ Xanax Tablets (32.7%) 2865
Zoladex (2%) 702
Zoladex 3-month 706
Zoloft (Frequent) 2751
Zomig Tablets (Infrequent) 708
Zomig-ZMT Tablets (Infrequent) 708
Zyban Sustained-Release Tablets (2%) 1710
Zyprexa Tablets (2%) 1973
Zyprexa ZYDIS Orally Disintegrating Tablets (2%) 1973
Zyrtec (Less than 2%) 2756
Zyrtec-D 12 Hour Extended Relief Tablets (Less than 2%) 2758

Appetite, loss of
(*see also under* Anorexia)

▲ Chemet Capsules (12.0% to 20.9%) 3078
▲ Concerta Extended-Release Tablets (4%) 1998
▲ Concerta Tablets (4%) 561
HibTITER (23 of 1,118 vaccinations) 1859
▲ Infanrix Vaccine (6.0% to 16.5%) 1562
Metadate CD Capsules 1164
Metadate ER Tablets 1167
Methylin Tablets 1995
Methylin ER Tablets 1995
Miacalcin Injection 2373
Numorphan 1324
Priftin Tablets 758
Tasmar Tablets 3010
Varivax (Greater than or equal to 1%) 2202
▲ Ziagen (9% to 15%) 1692

Apprehension

Adenocard Injection (Less than 1%) 1380
Dilaudid Oral Liquid (Less frequent) 445
Dilaudid Tablets - 8 mg (Less frequent) 445
Dilaudid-HP (Less frequent) 443
Dopram Injectable 2931
Duranest Injections 600
Edecrin 2091
ELA-Max Cream 1340
Emla (Unlikely with cream) 602
EpiPen 1236
Lidoderm Patch 1319
Limbitrol 1738
Matulane Capsules 3246
Maxalt Tablets (Rare) 2120
Maxalt-MLT Orally Disintegrating Tablets (Rare) 2120
MS Contin Tablets (Less frequent) 2896
MSIR (Less frequent) 2898
Oramorph SR Tablets (Less frequent) 3062
Quinaglute Dura-Tabs Tablets 978
Quinidex Extentabs 2933
▲ Xylocaine Injections (Among most common) 653

Apraxia

Cognex Capsules (Rare) 1351
Eldepryl Capsules 3266
Exelon Capsules (Infrequent) 2342
Exelon Oral Solution (Infrequent) 2345
Neurontin Capsules (Rare) 2655
Neurontin Oral Solution (Rare) 2655
Neurontin Tablets (Rare) 2655
Reminyl Oral Solution (Infrequent) 1792
Reminyl Tablets (Infrequent) 1792
Topamax Sprinkle Capsules (Infrequent) 2590
Topamax Tablets (Infrequent) 2590

Arachnoiditis

Nesacaine/Nesacaine MPF 617
Streptomycin Sulfate Injection 2714

Areflexia

Cognex Capsules (Infrequent) 1351
Neurontin Capsules (Frequent) 2655
Neurontin Oral Solution 2655
Neurontin Tablets (Frequent) 2655

Argumentativeness

Versed Injection (Less than 1%) 3027

Arm, stiffness of

Engerix-B Vaccine (Less than 1%) 1517

Arrhythmia, exacerbation of

Cordarone Tablets 3487
Corvert Injection 2793
Pacerone Tablets 3331
Toprol-XL Tablets (Greater than 1%) 651

Arrhythmia, nodal

Pletal Tablets (Less than 2%) 2605
Pletal Tablets (Less than 2%) 2848
ReoPro Vials (0.2%) 1958

Arrhythmias

Abelcet Injection (Rare) 1273
Activase I.V. 1410
Adenocard Injection 1380
Adenoscan (1%) 1381
Adriamycin PFS/RDF Injection 2767
Advair Diskus 100/50 1448
Advair Diskus 250/50 1448
Advair Diskus 500/50 1448
Aggrenox Capsules (Less than 1%) 1026
Agrylin Capsules (1% to 5%) 3232
Allegra-D Extended-Release Tablets 714
Alphagan Ophthalmic Solution (Less than 3%) 545
Altace Capsules (Less than 1%) 2233
Ambien Tablets (Rare) 3191
AmBisome for Injection (Less common) 1383
Amicar Injection 3608
Amphotec (1% to 5%) 1774
Anectine Injection 1476
Apligraf (1.3%) 2305
Aramine Injection 2043
Arthrotec Tablets (Rare) 3195
Atromid-S Capsules 3483
Avalide Tablets 1070
Avapro Tablets (Less than 1%) 1074
Avapro Tablets (Less than 1%) 3076
Avonex 1013
Betagan ⊙ 228
Betaseron for SC Injection 988
Betimol Ophthalmic Solution ⊙ 324
Blocadren Tablets (Greater than 1.1%) 2046
Brethine Ampuls 2314
Calcijex Injection 411
Carbatrol Capsules 3234
Cardizem Injectable (1.0%) 1018
Cardizem Lyo-Ject Syringe (1.0%) 1018
Cardizem Monovial (1.0%) 1018
Cardizem CD Capsules (Less than 1%) 1016
Cardura Tablets (1%) 2668
Carnitor Injection (2% to 3%) 3242
Carteolol Hydrochloride Ophthalmic Solution USP, 1% (Occasional) ⊙ 258
Catapres Tablets (Rare) 1037
Catapres-TTS (0.5% or less) 1038
▲ CellCept Capsules (19%) 2951
▲ CellCept Intravenous (19%) 2951
▲ CellCept Oral Suspension (19%) 2951
▲ CellCept Tablets (19%) 2951
Chemet Capsules (Up to 1.8%) 3078
Chirocaine Injection (Less than 1%) 2909
Cipro I.V. (1% or less) 893
Cipro I.V. Pharmacy Bulk Package (Less than 1%) 897
Claforan Injection 732
Claritin-D 12 Hour Extended Release Tablets 3102
Claritin-D 24 Hour Extended Release Tablets 3104
Clinoril Tablets (Rare) 2053
Clomid Tablets 735
Clorpres Tablets (Rare) 1002
Clozaril Tablets (Several patients) 2319
Combipres Tablets (Rare) 1040
Combivent Inhalation Aerosol (Less than 2%) 1041
Compazine 1505
Concerta Extended-Release Tablets 1998
Concerta Tablets 561
Copaxone for Injection 3306
Cordarone Tablets (1% to 3%) 3487
Corvert Injection (1.7%) 2793
Cosopt Sterile Ophthalmic Solution 2065
Cozaar Tablets (Less than 1%) 2067
Cytotec Tablets (Infrequent) 3202
Demadex Tablets and Injection 2965
Depakote ER Tablets (Greater than 1%) 436
Diprivan Injectable Emulsion (1.2%) 667
Dopram Injectable 2931
Doxil Injection (Less than 1%) 566
Duragesic Transdermal System (1% or greater) 1786
Dyazide Capsules 1515
Effexor Tablets (Infrequent) 3495
Effexor XR Capsules (Infrequent) 3499
Eldepryl Capsules 3266
EpiPen 1236
Ery-Tab Tablets (Occasional reports) 448
Erythrocin Stearate Filmtab Tablets (Occasional reports) 452
Erythromycin Base Filmtab Tablets (Occasional reports) 454
Erythromycin Delayed-Release Capsules, USP (Occasional reports) 455
Eskalith 1527
Etrafon 3115
Evoxac Capsules (Less than 1%) 1217
Famotidine Injection (Infrequent) 866
Fareston Tablets (1.5%) 3237
Feldene Capsules (Rare) 2685
Flexeril Tablets (Less than 1%) 572
Flexeril Tablets (Less than 1%) 2094
▲ Flolan for Injection (27%) 1528
Fludara for Injection (Up to 3%) 995
Fluothane Inhalation 3508
Foradil Aerolizer 2354
Furosemide Tablets 2284
Gemzar for Injection (2%) 1919
Gengraf Capsules (2%) 457
Glucotrol XL Extended Release Tablets (Less than 1%) 2693
Haldol Decanoate 2535
Hectorol Capsules 1064
Hectorol Injection 1066
Herceptin I.V. (At least one of the 958 patients) 1414
Hivid Tablets (Less than 1%) 2975
Hytrin Capsules (At least 1%) 464
Hyzaar 2109
Idamycin PFS Injection 2825
Imdur Tablets (Less than or equal to 5%) 1826
Imitrex Injection (Rare) 1549
Imitrex Nasal Spray (Infrequent) 1554
Imitrex Tablets (Rare to infrequent) 1558
Indocin Capsules (Less than 1%) 2112
Indocin I.V. (Less than 1%) 2115
Indocin (Less than 1%) 2112
INFeD Injection 3388
Innohep Injection 1248
Intron A for Injection (Less than 5%) 3120
Iopidine 0.5% Ophthalmic Solution (Less than 1%) ⊙ 213
Ismo Tablets (Fewer than 1%) 3524
Isopto Carbachol Ophthalmic Solution ⊙ 215
Kytril Injection (Rare) 2986
Lanoxicaps Capsules 1574
Lanoxin Injection 1581
Lanoxin Elixir Pediatric 1578
Lanoxin Injection Pediatric 1584
Leukine 1755
Levaquin (Less than 0.3%) 2537
Levo-Dromoran 1734
Levoxyl Tablets 1819
Lexxel Tablets 608
Limbitrol 1738
Lipitor Tablets (Less than 2%) 2639
Lipitor Tablets (Less than 2%) 2696
Lithium Carbonate 3061
Lithium Citrate Syrup 3061
Lithobid Slow-Release Tablets 3255
Lodine (Less than 1%) 3528
Lodine XL Extended-Release Tablets (Less than 1%) 3530
Lupron Depot 7.5 mg (Less than 5%) 3284
Lupron Depot–3 Month 22.5 mg (Less than 5%) 3288
Lupron Injection (Less than 5%) 3279
Maxalt Tablets (Infrequent) 2120
Maxalt-MLT Orally Disintegrating Tablets (Infrequent) 2120
Metadate CD Capsules 1164
Metadate ER Tablets 1167
Methylin Tablets 1995
Methylin ER Tablets 1995
Midamor Tablets (Less than or equal to 1%) 2136
Miltown Tablets 3349

Mirapex Tablets (1% or more) 2834
Moban 1320
Mobic Tablets (Less than 2%) 1054
Moduretic Tablets (Greater than 1%, less than 3%) 2138
Monopril Tablets (0.2% to 1.0%) 1091
Motrin Suspension, Oral Drops, Chewable Tablets, and Caplets (Less than 1%) 2002
Naprelan Tablets (Less than 1%) 1293
Naropin Injection (Less than 1%) 612
Navane Oral 2701
Navane Intramuscular 2703
Neoral Soft Gelatin Capsules (2%) 2380
Neoral Oral Solution (2%) 2380
▲ Neupogen for Injection (11 of 375 cancer patients) 587
Niaspan Extended-Release Tablets 1846
Nipent for Injection (Less than 3%) 3272
Norpramin Tablets 755
Norvasc Tablets (More than 0.1% to 1%) 2704
▲ Novantrone for Injection (3% to 18%) 1760
Ocupress Ophthalmic Solution, 1% Sterile (Occasional) ⊙ 303
Orap Tablets 1407
Orthoclone OKT3 Sterile Solution (Less than 1%) 2498
Orudis Capsules (Rare) 3548
Oruvail Capsules (Rare) 3548
Ovidrel for Injection (Less than 2%) 3220
Pacerone Tablets (1% to 3%) 3331
Paxil (Rare) 1609
Pepcid Injection (Infrequent) 2153
Pepcid for Oral Suspension (Infrequent) 2150
Pepcid RPD Orally Disintegrating Tablets (Infrequent) 2150
Pepcid Tablets (Infrequent) 2150
Permax Tablets (1.1%) 1299
Pfizerpen for Injection 2707
Phenergan 3556
Plendil Extended-Release Tablets (0.5% to 1.5%) 623
Polocaine Injection, USP 625
Polocaine-MPF Injection, USP 625
Ponstel Capsules (Rare) 1356
Prandin Tablets (0.5, 1, and 2 mg) (Less than or equal to 1%) 2432
Prinivil Tablets (0.3% to 1.0%) 2164
Prinzide Tablets 2168
Procardia XL Extended Release Tablets (1% or less) 2710
▲ Proleukin for Injection (10%) 1199
Propine Ophthalmic Solution ⊙ 250
ProSom Tablets (Rare) 500
Prostigmin Injectable 1744
Prostigmin Tablets 1744
Prostin E2 Suppositories 2852
Protonix I.V. (Less than 1%) 3580
Protonix Tablets (Less than 1%) 3577
Protopic Ointment (Greater than or equal to 1%) 1397
Proventil Repetabs Tablets 3148
Provigil Tablets (1%) 1193
Prozac Pulvules, Liquid, and Weekly Capsules (Infrequent) 1238
▲ Quinaglute Dura-Tabs Tablets (3%) 978
Relafen Tablets (Less than 1%) 1617
Remicade for IV Injection (Less than 2%) 1178
Risperdal 1796
Ritalin 2387
Rituxan for Infusion (Four patients) 1750
Rituxan I.V. (Four patients) 1428
Robinul Injectable 2940
Rocaltrol 2991
Roferon-A Injection (1% to 3%) 2996
Romazicon Injection (Less than 1%) 3000
Rum-K 1363
Rynatan Tablets 3351
Salagen Tablets (Less than 1%) 2229
▲ Sandostatin Injection (9%) 2394
Sarafem Pulvules (Infrequent) 1962
Sensorcaine 643
Sensorcaine-MPF Injection 643
Serentil 1057
Serevent Diskus 1637
Serevent Inhalation Aerosol 1633
Serophene Tablets 3226
Seroquel Tablets 684
Solu-Medrol Sterile Powder 2855
Stelazine 1640
Streptase for Infusion 647
Suprane Liquid for Inhalation (Less than 1%) 874
Surmontil Capsules 3595
Symmetrel 1328
Tagamet Injection (Rare) 1644
Tamiflu Capsules 3008
Tamiflu Oral Suspension 3008
Tasmar Tablets (Infrequent) 3010
Taxol Injection (Approximately 1%) 1129
Tegretol/Tegretol-XR 2404
Tensilon Injectable 1745
Thalomid Capsules 1154
Theo-Dur Extended-Release Tablets 1835
Timolide Tablets (Less than 1%) 2187
Timolol GFS ⊙ 266
Timoptic in Ocudose (Less frequent) 2192
Timoptic Sterile Ophthalmic Solution (Less frequent) 2190
Timoptic-XE Sterile Ophthalmic Gel Forming Solution 2194
TNKase I.V. 1430
Topamax Sprinkle Capsules (Rare) 2590
Topamax Tablets (Rare) 2590
▲ Trasylol Injection (4%) 909
Trental Tablets (Rare) 784
Tricor Capsules, Micronized (1%) 513
Trilafon 3160
▲ Triostat Injection (6%) 1825
Uni-Dur Extended-Release Tablets 1841
Uniphyl 400 mg and 600 mg Tablets 2903
Uniretic Tablets (Less than 1%) 3178
Unithroid Tablets 3445
Univasc Tablets (Less than 1%) 3181
Vascor Tablets (About 2.4%) 2602
Vaseretic Tablets 2204
Vasotec Tablets (0.5% to 1.0%) 2210
Ventolin Inhalation Aerosol and Refill 1679
Ventolin HFA Inhalation Aerosol 3618
▲ Vesanoid Capsules (23%) 3037
Vicoprofen Tablets (Less than 1%) 520
Vivactil Tablets 2217
Vivactil Tablets 2446
▲ Wellbutrin Tablets (5.3%) 1680
Zanaflex Tablets (Infrequent) 1305
Zantac (Rare) 1690
Zantac Injection (Rare) 1688
Zantac Syrup (Rare) 1690
Zaroxolyn Tablets 1177
Zemuron Injection (Less than 1%) 2491
Zestoretic Tablets 695
Zestril Tablets (0.3% to 1.0%) 698
Ziac Tablets (Up to 0.4%) 1887
Zithromax Capsules, 250 mg 2743
Zithromax for IV Infusion 2748
Zithromax for Oral Suspension, 300 mg, 600 mg, 900 mg, 1200 mg 2739
Zithromax Tablets, 250 mg 2739
Zofran Injection 1698
Zoladex (1% to 5%) 702
Zoladex 3-month 706
Zomig Tablets (Infrequent) 708
Zomig-ZMT Tablets (Infrequent) 708
Zosyn (1.0% or less) 1890
Zosyn in Galaxy Containers (1.0% or less) 1894
Zyrtec-D 12 Hour Extended Relief Tablets 2758

Arrhythmias, junctional
Proleukin for Injection (1%) 1199

Arrhythmias, malignant
Symmetrel 1328

Arrhythmias, pre-existing, worsening of
Cordarone Intravenous 3491
Corvert Injection 2793
Mexitil Capsules 1047
▲ Rythmol Tablets – 150 mg, 225 mg, 300 mg (4.7%) 502

Arrhythmias, sinus
Anzemet Injection 719
Anzemet Tablets 722
Imitrex Injection (Infrequent) 1549
Imitrex Nasal Spray 1554
Imitrex Tablets 1558

Arrhythmias, supraventricular
Intron A for Injection (Rare) 3120
Leukine (Occasional) 1755
PEG-Intron Powder for Injection (Less than or equal to 1%) 3140
▲ Primacor Injection (3.8%) 3086
▲ Proleukin for Injection (5%) 1199
Rituxan for Infusion (Four patients) 1750
Rituxan I.V. (Four patients) 1428
Tikosyn Capsules (Less than or equal to 2%) 2717

Arterial carbon dioxide, decrease
Sulfamylon Cream 1011

Arterial insufficiency
Blocadren Tablets 2046
Cosopt Sterile Ophthalmic Solution 2065
Inderal 3513
Inderal LA Long-Acting Capsules 3516
Inderide Tablets 3517
Inderide LA Long-Acting Capsules 3519
Timolide Tablets 2187
Timolol GFS ⊙ 266
Timoptic in Ocudose 2192
Timoptic Sterile Ophthalmic Solution 2190
Timoptic-XE Sterile Ophthalmic Gel Forming Solution 2194
Toprol-XL Tablets (About 1 of 100 patients) 651

Arterial occlusion
Humegon for Injection 2468
Serophene Tablets (Rare) 3226

Arteriosclerosis
Apligraf (1.8%) 2305
Tasmar Tablets (Rare) 3010

Arteriospasm
Ceptaz for Injection 1499
Fortaz 1541
Tasmar Tablets (Infrequent) 3010

Arteritis
Ambien Tablets (Rare) 3191
Aricept Tablets (Infrequent) 1270
Aricept Tablets (Infrequent) 2665
Avonex 1013
Effexor Tablets (Rare) 3495
Effexor XR Capsules (Rare) 3499
Pediazole Suspension 3050
Zyprexa Tablets (Rare) 1973
Zyprexa ZYDIS Orally Disintegrating Tablets (Rare) 1973

Arteritis, temporal
Imitrex Nasal Spray 1554
Imitrex Tablets 1558
Orthoclone OKT3 Sterile Solution (Less than 1%) 2498

Arthralgia
Abelcet Injection 1273
Accupril Tablets (0.5% to 1.0%) 2611
Accuretic Tablets (0.5% to 1%) 2614
Accutane Capsules 2944
Acel-Imune (Rare) 1851
Aceon Tablets (2 mg, 4 mg, 8 mg) (0.3% to 1.1%) 3249
Actimmune (2%) 1772
Actiq (1% or greater) 1184
Activella Tablets 2764
▲ Actonel Tablets (23.7% to 32.8%) 2879
Adalat CC Tablets (Less than 1.0%) 877
Advair Diskus 100/50 (1% to 3%) 1448
Advair Diskus 250/50 (1% to 3%) 1448
Advair Diskus 500/50 (1% to 3%) 1448
▲ Aggrenox Capsules (5.5%) 1026
Agrylin Capsules (1% to 5%) 3232
Aldoclor Tablets 2035
Aldomet Tablets 2037
Aldoril Tablets 2039
▲ Alferon N Injection (3% to 10%) 1770
Aloprim for Injection (Less than 1%) 2292
Alora Transdermal System (1.1% to 6.8%) 3372
Altace Capsules (Less than 1%) 2233
▲ Ambien Tablets (4%) 3191
AmBisome for Injection (Less common) 1383
Amerge Tablets (Infrequent) 1467
Amphotec (1% to 5%) 1774
Anzemet Injection (Rare) 719
Anzemet Tablets (Rare) 722
Arava Tablets (1%) 724
▲ Aredia for Injection (11.5% to 26%) 2309
▲ Arimidex Tablets (2% to 5%) 659
▲ Aromasin Tablets (2% to 5%) 2769
Arthrotec Tablets (Rare) 3195
▲ Asacol Delayed-Release Tablets (5%) 2884
Atacand Tablets (More than 1%) 595
Atacand HCT Tablets (0.5% or greater) 597
Atromid-S Capsules 3483
Augmentin Chewable Tablets 1482
Augmentin Powder for Oral Suspension 1482
Augmentin Tablets 1485
Augmentin ES-600 Powder for Oral Suspension 1487
Avalide Tablets 1070
Avapro Tablets (Less than 1%) 1074
Avapro Tablets (Less than 1%) 3076
Avelox Tablets (0.05% to 1%) 879
▲ Avonex (9%) 1013
Axert Tablets (Rare) 2772
Azmacort Inhalation Aerosol 728
Azulfidine EN-tabs Tablets (Rare) 2775
Bactrim 2949
▲ Baycol Tablets (4.3%) 883
Beconase Inhalation Aerosol 1497
Beconase AQ Nasal Spray 1498
Bicillin C-R 900/300 Injection 2240
Bicillin C-R Injection 2238
Bicillin L-A Injection 2242
Blocadren Tablets (Less than 1%) 2046
Calcium Disodium Versenate Injection 1980
▲ Captopril Tablets (About 4 to 7 of 100 patients) 2281
Carbatrol Capsules 3234
Cardura Tablets (1%) 2668
Catapres Tablets (About 6 in 1,000 patients) 1037
Catapres-TTS (0.5% or less) 1038
Ceclor CD Tablets (0.1% to 1%) 1279
Ceclor 1905
Ceftin for Oral Suspension (0.1% to 1%) 1898
Celebrex Capsules (0.1% to 1.9%) 2676
Celebrex Capsules (0.1% to 1.9%) 2780
Celexa (2%) 1365
▲ CellCept Capsules (3%) 2951
▲ CellCept Intravenous (3%) 2951
▲ CellCept Oral Suspension (3%) 2951
▲ CellCept Tablets (3%) 2951
▲ Cenestin Tablets (25%) 1263
Cerebyx Injection (Infrequent) 2619
Chibroxin Sterile Ophthalmic Solution 2051
Cipro I.V. (1% or less) 893
Cipro I.V. Pharmacy Bulk Package (Less than 1%) 897
Cipro (Less than 1%) 887
Claritin (At least one patient) 3100
Claritin-D 12 Hour Extended Release Tablets (Less frequent) 3102
Claritin-D 24 Hour Extended Release Tablets (Fewer than 2%) 3104
Clinoril Tablets (Less than 1 in 100) 2053
Clomid Tablets 735
Clorpres Tablets (About 6 in 1,000) 1002
Clozaril Tablets (Less than 1%) 2319
Cognex Capsules (Frequent) 1351
▲ Colazal Capsules (4%) 3069
Colestid Tablets 2791
▲ CombiPatch Transdermal System (6%) 2323
Combipres Tablets (About 6 in 1,000) 1040
Combivent Inhalation Aerosol (Less than 2%) 1041
▲ Combivir Tablets (5%) 1502
Comvax 2056
Concerta Extended-Release Tablets 1998
Concerta Tablets 561
▲ Copaxone for Injection (24%) 3306
▲ Coreg Tablets (6.4%) 1508
Cosopt Sterile Ophthalmic Solution 2065
Coumadin for Injection 1243
Coumadin Tablets 1243
Covera-HS Tablets (Less than 2%) 3199
Cozaar Tablets (Less than 1%) 2067
▲ Crinone 8% Gel (8%) 3213
Crixivan Capsules (Less than 2%) 2070
Cuprimine Capsules 2075
CytoGam Intravenous (Less than 5.0%) 2026
Cytotec Tablets (Infrequent) 3202
Cytovene (At least 3 subjects) 2959
▲ DaunoXome Injection (Up to 7%) 1442
Demadex Tablets and Injection (1.8%) 2965
Depacon Injection (1% to 5%) 416
Depakene (1% to 5%) 421
Depakote Sprinkle Capsules (1% to 5%) 426
Depakote Tablets (1% to 5%) 430
Depakote ER Tablets (Greater than 1%) 436
Depen Titratable Tablets 3341
▲ Depo-Provera Contraceptive Injection (More than 5%) 2798
Desferal Vials 2333
Detrol Tablets (2.3%) 3623
DiaBeta Tablets 741
Didronel Tablets 2888
Dilantin Infatabs 2624
Dilantin Kapseals 2622
Dilantin-125 Oral Suspension 2625
Diovan Capsules (More than 1%) 2337
Diovan HCT Tablets (Greater than 0.2%) 2338
▲ Dipentum Capsules (4.0%) 2803
Diphtheria & Tetanus Toxoids Adsorbed Purogenated for Pediatric Use 1857
Dolobid Tablets (Less than 1 in 100) 2088
Dostinex Tablets (1%) 2804
Doxil Injection (Less than 1%) 566
Duraclon Injection (About 0.6%) 3057
Duricef (Rare) 1079
DynaCirc CR Tablets (0.5% to 1%) 2923
Effexor Tablets 3495
Effexor XR Capsules (Frequent) 3499
Elspar for Injection 2092
Enalaprilat Injection 863
Enbrel for Injection 1752
Enbrel for Injection 3504
Engerix-B Vaccine (Less than 1%) 1517
▲ Epivir (5%) 1520
▲ Epivir-HBV (7%) 1524
Epogen for Injection (Rare) 582
▲ Ergamisol Tablets (4% to 5%) 1789
▲ Esclim Transdermal System (2.1% to 6.3%) 3460
Eskalith 1527
▲ Estring Vaginal Ring (3%) 2811
▲ Evista Tablets (10.7% to 15.5%) 1915

▲ Evoxac Capsules (3.7%) 1217
Exelon Capsules (2% or more) 2342
Exelon Oral Solution (2% or more) 2345
Famotidine Injection (Infrequent) 866
Famvir Tablets (1.3% to 1.5%) 2348
Felbatol 3343
▲ Femara Tablets (6% to 14%) 2351
▲ femhrt Tablets (5.8%) 2635
Ferrlecit Injection (Greater than 1%) 3386
▲ Flolan for Injection (6% to 84%) 1528
▲ Flovent Diskus (1% to 17%) 3614
▲ Flovent (1% to 19%) 1535
Flovent Rotadisk (1% to 3%) 1537
Floxin I.V. (Less than 1%) 2526
Floxin Tablets (Less than 1%) 2529
Fludara for Injection (Up to 1%) 995
FluShield Influenza Vaccine 3521
Follistim for Injection 2465
Fortovase Capsules (Less than 2%) 2970
▲ Fosamax Tablets (4.1% to approximately 6%) 2095
Foscavir Injection (Between 1% and 5%) 605
Gamimune N, 5% Solvent/Detergent Treated 925
Gamimune N, 10% Solvent/Detergent Treated 928
Gammar-P I.V. 787
Gastrocrom Oral Concentrate (Less common) 1162
Gengraf Capsules (1% to 6%) 457
Genotropin Lyophilized Powder 2818
Geodon Capsules 2688
▲ Gleevec Capsules (21% to 26%) 2357
Glucotrol XL Extended Release Tablets (Less than 3%) 2693
Havrix Vaccine (Less than 1%) 1544
▲ Hectorol Capsules (4.9%) 1064
▲ Hectorol Injection (4.9%) 1066
▲ Herceptin I.V. (6%) 1414
Hivid Tablets (Less than 1%) 2975
▲ Humatrope Vials and Cartridges (13.6% to 17.3%) 1930
Humegon for Injection 2468
Hycamtin for Injection (0.2% to 0.9%) 1546
Hytrin Capsules (At least 1%) 464
Hyzaar 2109
Imdur Tablets (Less than or equal to 5%) 1826
Imitrex Injection (Infrequent) 1549
INFeD Injection 3388
▲ Infergen (43% to 51%) 1777
▲ Intron A for Injection (Up to 19%) 3120
Invirase Capsules (Less than 2%) 2979
Ismo Tablets (Fewer than 1%) 3524
Isoptin SR Tablets (1% or less) 467
Kadian Capsules (Less than 3%) 1335
Kaletra Capsules (Less than 2%) 471
Kaletra Oral Solution (Less than 2%) 471
Keflex 1237
Keppra Tablets (1% or more) 3314
Klonopin Tablets (Infrequent) 2983
K-Phos Neutral Tablets 946
K-Phos Original (Sodium Free) Tablets (Less frequent) 947
Lamictal (2.0%) 1567
Lamisil Tablets 2360
▲ Lescol Capsules (4.0%) 2361
▲ Lescol Capsules (4.0%) 2925
Lescol XL Tablets (1.3%) 2361
Lescol XL Tablets (1.3%) 2925
▲ Leukine (11% to 21%) 1733
▲ Leustatin Injection (5%) 2495
Levaquin (0.5% to less than 1.0%) 2537
Levoxyl Tablets 1819
Lexxel Tablets 608
▲ Lipitor Tablets (Up to 5.1%) 2639
▲ Lipitor Tablets (Up to 5.1%) 2696
Lithobid Slow-Release Tablets 3255
Lopid Tablets 2650
Lotensin Tablets (Less than 1%) 2365
Lotensin HCT Tablets (0.3% to 1%) 2367
Lupron Depot–3 Month 11.25 mg 3285
Lupron Injection (Less than 5%) 3279
Luvox Tablets (25, 50, 100 mg) (Infrequent) 3256
▲ LYMErix Vaccine (6.78% to 13.64%) 1592
Macrobid Capsules 2889
Macrodantin Capsules 2891
Matulane Capsules 3246
Maxalt Tablets (Infrequent) 2120
Maxalt-MLT Orally Disintegrating Tablets (Infrequent) 2120
▲ Meridia Capsules (5.9%) 481
Meruvax II 2130
Metadate CD Capsules 1164
Metadate ER Tablets 1167
Methylin Tablets 1995
Methylin ER Tablets 1995
Mevacor Tablets (0.5% to 1.0%) 2132
Mexitil Capsules (1.7%) 1047
▲ Miacalcin Nasal Spray (3.8%) 2375
Micardis Tablets (More than 0.3%) 1049
Micardis HCT Tablets 1051
Midamor Tablets (Less than or equal to 1%) 2136
Migranal Nasal Spray (Rare) 2376
Minipress Capsules 2699
Mirapex Tablets (Less than 1%) 2834
M-M-R II 2118
Mobic Tablets (0.5% to 5.3%) 1054
Moduretic Tablets (Less than or equal to 1%) 2138
Monopril Tablets (0.2% to 1.0%) 1091
Monopril HCT 1094
Myambutol Tablets 1290
Mycobutin Capsules (Less than 1%) 2838
▲ Mykrox Tablets (3.1%) 1168
▲ Mylotarg for Injection (8% to 12%) 3540
▲ Myobloc Injectable Solution (1% to 7%) 1291
Naprelan Tablets (Less than 3%) 1293
Nasacort Nasal Inhaler 750
Nascobal Gel 3174
Nasonex Nasal Spray (Greater than or equal to 2%) 3131
Navelbine Injection (Less than 5%) 1604
Neoral Soft Gelatin Capsules (1% to 6%) 2380
Neoral Oral Solution (1% to 6%) 2380
Neupogen for Injection (Infrequent) 587
Neurontin Capsules (Frequent) 2655
Neurontin Oral Solution (Frequent) 2655
Neurontin Tablets (Frequent) 2655
Nexium Delayed-Release Capsules (Less than 1%) 619
▲ Nicotrol Nasal Spray (5%) 2843
▲ Nipent for Injection (3% to 10%) 3272
Noroxin Tablets 2145
Norvasc Tablets (More than 0.1% to 1%) 2704
Norvir Capsules (Less than 2%) 487
Norvir Oral Solution (Less than 2%) 487
Nutropin AQ Injection 1420
▲ Nutropin Depot for Injectable Suspension (4%) 1423
Nutropin for Injection 1417
▲ Oncaspar (Greater than 1% but less than 5%) 756
Ortho Diaphragm Kits – All-Flex Arcing Spring; Ortho Coil Spring 2552
Orthoclone OKT3 Sterile Solution (Less than 1%) 2498
▲ Ortho-Prefest Tablets (9%) 2570
Paxil (Frequent) 1609
Pentasa Capsules (Less than 1%) 3239
Pepcid Injection (Infrequent) 2153
Pepcid for Oral Suspension (Infrequent) 2150
Pepcid RPD Orally Disintegrating Tablets (Infrequent) 2150
Pepcid Tablets (Infrequent) 2150
Pergonal for Injection 3223
▲ Periostat Tablets (6%) 1208
Permax Tablets (1.6%) 1299
Pfizerpen for Injection 2707
Pima Syrup 1362
▲ Plavix Tablets (6.3%) 1097
▲ Plavix Tablets (6.3%) 3084
Plendil Extended-Release Tablets (0.5% to 1.5%) 623
Pletal Tablets (Less than 2%) 2605
Pletal Tablets (Less than 2%) 2848
Pneumovax 23 (Rare) 2156
Pnu-Imune 23 (Rare to infrequent) 1868
▲ Prandin Tablets (0.5, 1, and 2 mg) (3% to 6%) 2432
Pravachol Tablets (Rare) 1000
▲ Prempro Tablets (7% to 9%) 3572
Prevacid Delayed-Release Capsules (Less than 1%) 3292
PREVPAC (Less than 1%) 3298
Priftin Tablets (2.5%) 758
Prilosec Delayed-Release Capsules (Less than 1%) 628
Prinivil Tablets (0.3% to 1.0%) 2164
Prinzide Tablets 2168
Procanbid Extended-Release Tablets (Fairly common) 2262
Procardia XL Extended Release Tablets (Less than 3%) 2710
▲ Procrit for Injection (Rare to 11%) 2502
▲ Prograf (3% to 15%) 1393
▲ Proleukin for Injection (6%) 1199
▲ Prometrium Capsules (100 mg, 200 mg) (21%) 3261
ProSom Tablets (Rare) 500
Prostigmin Injectable 1744
Prostigmin Tablets 1744
Prostin E2 Suppositories 2852
Protonix I.V. (Greater than or equal to 1%) 3580
Protonix Tablets (Greater than or equal to 1%) 3577
Protopic Ointment (Greater than or equal to 1%) 1397
Provigil Tablets (At least 1%) 1193
Prozac Pulvules, Liquid, and Weekly Capsules (1.2% to 3%) 1238
▲ Pulmicort Turbuhaler Inhalation Powder (Up to 6%) 636
Pyrazinamide Tablets (Frequent) 1876
Quinaglute Dura-Tabs Tablets 978
Quinidex Extentabs 2933
▲ Rapamune Oral Solution and Tablets (25% to 31%) 3584
▲ Rebetron Combination Therapy (29% to 33%) 3153
Recombivax HB (Less than 1%) 2178
Relenza Rotadisk (Less than 1.5%) 1619
Remeron Tablets (Frequent) 2483
Remeron SolTab Tablets (Frequent) 2486
▲ Remicade for IV Injection (5% to 6%) 1178
Repronex for Intramuscular and Subcutaneous Injection 1347
Requip Tablets (1% or more) 1621
Rescriptor Tablets (Less than 2%) 526
Retrovir Capsules 1625
Retrovir IV Infusion 1629
Retrovir 1625
Rhinocort Nasal Inhaler (Less than 1%) 640
Rifater Tablets (Frequent) 769
Rilutek Tablets (1.6% to 5.1%) 772
Risperdal (2% to 3%) 1796
Ritalin 2387
Rituxan for Infusion (0.3%) 1750
Rituxan I.V. (0.3%) 1428
▲ Roferon-A Injection (24% to 51%) 2996
Rowasa Rectal Suspension Enema 4.0 grams/unit (60 mL) (2.09%) 3264
Roxicodone Tablets (Less than 3%) 3067
Rythmol Tablets – 150 mg, 225 mg, 300 mg (1.0%) 502
Salagen Tablets (Less than 1%) 2229
Sandimmune (Rare) 2388
Sandostatin Injection (1% to 4%) 2394
▲ Sandostatin LAR Depot (5% to 15%) 2395
Sectral Capsules 3589
Septra Suspension 2265
Septra Tablets 2265
Septra DS Tablets 2265
Serevent Diskus (1% to 3%) 1637
Serevent Inhalation Aerosol (1% to 3%) 1633
Serophene Tablets 3226
Seroquel Tablets (Infrequent) 684
Serzone Tablets (1%) 1104
▲ Simulect for Injection (3% to 10%) 2399
Skelid Tablets (2.7%) 3088
Solu-Medrol Sterile Powder 2855
Sonata Capsules (Rare) 3591
▲ Soriatane Capsules (10% to 25%) 3003
▲ Stromectol Tablets (9.3%) 2185
Sular Tablets (Less than or equal to 1%) 688
Sustiva Capsules (Less than 2%) 1258
Synarel Nasal Solution for Endometriosis (Less than 1%) 3205
Synercid I.V. (Less than 1%) 775
Tagamet (Rare) 1644
Tambocor Tablets (Less than 1%) 1990
Tapazole Tablets 1823
Tarka Tablets (0.3% to 1.7%) 508
Tasmar Tablets (1% or more) 3010
▲ Taxol Injection (8% to 60%) 1129
Taxotere for Injection Concentrate 778
Tegretol/Tegretol-XR 2404
Tenex Tablets (Less frequent) 2942
Tequin Injection (Less than 0.1%) 1110
Tequin Tablets (Less than 0.1%) 1110
Tetanus & Diphtheria Toxoids Adsorbed for Adult Use 1880
Tetanus and Diphtheria Toxoids Adsorbed For Adult Use 815
Teveten Tablets (2%) 3327
Thalomid Capsules 1154
TheraCys Injection 823
▲ Tice BCG, BCG Live (3%) 2489
Tikosyn Capsules (Greater than 2%) 2717
Timentin Injection- ADD-Vantage Vial 1661
Timentin Injection-Galaxy Container 1664
Timentin Injection-Pharmacy Bulk Package 1666
Timentin for Intravenous Administration 1658
Timolide Tablets 2187
Timolol GFS .... ⊙ 266
Timoptic in Ocudose 2192
Timoptic Sterile Ophthalmic Solution 2190
Timoptic-XE Sterile Ophthalmic Gel Forming Solution 2194
Tonocard Tablets (Less than 1% to 4.7%) 649
Topamax Sprinkle Capsules (Frequent) 2590
Topamax Tablets (Frequent) 2590
Trasylol Injection (1% to 2%) 909
▲ Tricor Capsules, Micronized (3%) 513
Trileptal Oral Suspension 2407
Trileptal Tablets 2407
▲ Trisenox Injection (33%) 1158
▲ Trizivir Tablets (5%) 1669
Trovan (Less than 1%) 2722
Twinrix Vaccine (Less than 1%) 1674
TYPHIM Vi Vaccine (One report) 825
Uniretic Tablets (Less than 1%) 3178
Unithroid Tablets 3445
Univasc Tablets (Less than 1%) 3181
Uroqid-Acid No. 2 Tablets 947
Valtrex Caplets 1676
Vanceril Double Strength Inhalation Aerosol (Fewer than 2%) 3167
Varivax (Greater than or equal to 1%) 2202
Vaseretic Tablets (0.5% to 2.0%) 2204
Vasotec I.V. Injection 2207
Vasotec Tablets (0.5% to 1.0%) 2210
Verelan Capsules (1% or less) 3184
Verelan PM Capsules (2% or less) 3186
Viagra Tablets (Greater than 2%) 2732
Vicoprofen Tablets (Less than 1%) 520
Videx 1138
Videx EC Capsules 1143
Vioxx (Greater than 0.1% to 1.9%) 2213
Viracept 532
▲ Viramune Oral Suspension (2% to 6%) 1060
▲ Viramune Tablets (2% to 6%) 1060
Vistide Injection 1445
▲ Visudyne for Injection (1% to 10%) .... ⊙ 308
Warfarin Sodium Tablets, USP 3302
Wellbutrin Tablets 1680
Wellbutrin SR Sustained-Release Tablets (1% to 4%) 1684
WinRho SDF 2297
Xalatan Latanoprost Ophthalmic Solution (1% to 2%) .... ⊙ 320
Xalatan Sterile Ophthalmic Solution (1% to 2%) 2864
Zanaflex Tablets (Infrequent) 1305
Zantac (Rare) 1690
Zantac Injection (Rare) 1688
Zantac Syrup (Rare) 1690
Zaroxolyn Tablets 1177
Zebeta Tablets (2.2% to 2.7%) 1885
▲ Zenapax for Injection (2% to 5%) 3046
Zestoretic Tablets 695
Zestril Tablets (0.3% to 1.0%) 698
Ziac Tablets 1887
Ziagen 1692
Zithromax Capsules, 250 mg 2743
Zithromax for IV Infusion 2748
Zithromax for Oral Suspension, 300 mg, 600 mg, 900 mg, 1200 mg 2739
Zithromax Tablets, 250 mg 2739
Zocor Tablets 2219
Zofran Injection (2%) 1698
Zoladex (1% or greater) 702
Zoladex 3-month 706
Zoloft (Infrequent) 2751
▲ Zometa for Intravenous Infusion (5% to 10%) 3621
Zonegran Capsules (Infrequent) 1307
Zosyn (1.0% or less) 1890
Zosyn in Galaxy Containers (1.0% or less) 1894
▲ Zyban Sustained-Release Tablets (4% to 5%) 1710
Zyflo Filmtab Tablets (Less common) 524
▲ Zyprexa Tablets (5%) 1973
▲ Zyprexa ZYDIS Orally Disintegrating Tablets (5%) 1973
Zyrtec (Less than 2%) 2756
Zyrtec-D 12 Hour Extended Relief Tablets (Less than 2%) 2758

Arthralgia, migratory

Aquasol A Parenteral 590

Arthralgia, monoarticular

Recombivax HB (Less than 1%) 2178

Arthritis

Accuretic Tablets 2614
Accutane Capsules 2944
Aceon Tablets (2 mg, 4 mg, 8 mg) (1.0%) 3249
Aciphex Tablets 1267
Aciphex Tablets 1783
Actiq (Less than 1%) 1184
Adalat CC Tablets (Less than 1.0%) 877
Aggrenox Capsules (2.1%) 1026
Altace Capsules (Less than 1%) 2233
Ambien Tablets (Infrequent) 3191
Apligraf (1.3% to 1.8%) 2305
Aricept Tablets (2%) 1270
Aricept Tablets (2%) 2665
Asacol Delayed-Release Tablets (1% to 2%) 2884
Atacand HCT Tablets (0.5% or greater) 597
Atrovent Inhalation Solution (0.9%) 1031
Augmentin Chewable Tablets 1482
Augmentin Powder for Oral Suspension 1482
Augmentin Tablets 1485
Augmentin ES-600 Powder for Oral Suspension 1487
Avalide Tablets 1070
Avapro Tablets (Less than 1%) 1074
Avapro Tablets (Less than 1%) 3076
Avonex 1013

Axert Tablets (Rare) 2772
Baycol Tablets (Rare) 883
Betaseron for SC Injection 988
Betaxon Ophthalmic Suspension (Less than 2%) 537
Campath Ampules 992
Cardura Tablets (1%) 2668
▲ Casodex Tablets (5%) 662
Ceclor CD Tablets 1279
Ceclor 1905
Celexa (Infrequent) 1365
Chibroxin Sterile Ophthalmic Solution 2051
Clinoril Tablets (Less than 1 in 100) 2053
Cognex Capsules (Frequent) 1351
Colazal Capsules 3069
Colestid Tablets 2791
Comvax 2056
Copaxone for Injection (Infrequent) 3306
Coreg Tablets (More than 2%) 1508
Cozaar Tablets (Less than 1%) 2067
Cytovene 2959
Demadex Tablets and Injection 2965
Didronel Tablets 2888
Ditropan XL Extended Release Tablets (2% to 5%) 564
Dolobid Tablets (Less than 1 in 100) 2088
Effexor Tablets (Infrequent) 3495
Effexor XR Capsules (Infrequent) 3499
Enalaprilat Injection 863
Engerix-B Vaccine (Less than 1%) 1517
▲ Estring Vaginal Ring (4%) 2811
Evoxac Capsules (Less than 1%) 1217
Exelon Capsules (Frequent) 2342
Exelon Oral Solution (Frequent) 2345
▲ Flolan for Injection (52%) 1528
Fortovase Capsules (Less than 2%) 2970
Gabitril Tablets (Infrequent) 1189
Hivid Tablets (Less than 1%) 2975
Hytrin Capsules (At least 1%) 464
Hyzaar 2109
Imitrex Nasal Spray (Infrequent) 1554
Imitrex Tablets 1558
INFeD Injection 3388
Intron A for Injection (Less than 5%) 3120
Invirase Capsules (Less than 2%) 2979
Keflex 1237
Lamictal (Rare) 1567
Lescol Capsules (Rare) 2361
Lescol Capsules (Rare) 2925
Lescol XL Tablets (1.3%) 2361
Lescol XL Tablets (1.3%) 2925
Levaquin (Less than 0.3%) 2537
Lexxel Tablets 608
Lipitor Tablets (Greater than or equal to 2%) 2639
Lipitor Tablets (Greater than or equal to 2%) 2696
Lotensin Tablets (Less than 1%) 2365
Lotensin HCT Tablets (0.3% or more) 2367
Luvox Tablets (25, 50, 100 mg) (Infrequent) 3256
LYMErix Vaccine (2.91%) 1592
Meridia Capsules (Greater than or equal to 1%) 481
Meruvax II (Rare) 2130
Mevacor Tablets (Rare) 2132
Miacalcin Nasal Spray (Less than 1%) 2375
Micardis Tablets (More than 0.3%) 1049
Micardis HCT Tablets 1051
Mirapex Tablets (Rare) 2834
M-M-R II 2118
Monopril Tablets 1091
Monopril HCT 1094
Myobloc Injectable Solution (2% or greater) 1291
Neurontin Capsules (Infrequent) 2655
Neurontin Oral Solution (Infrequent) 2655
Neurontin Tablets (Infrequent) 2655
Nilandron Tablets (2%) 753
Nipent for Injection (Less than 3%) 3272
Noroxin Tablets 2145
OptiPranolol Metipranolol Ophthalmic Solution 0.3% (A small number of patients) ⊙263
Orthoclone OKT3 Sterile Solution (Less than 1%) 2498
Paxil (Infrequent) 1609
Permax Tablets (Infrequent) 1299
Persantine Tablets (Rare) 1057
Plavix Tablets (1% to 2.5%) 1097
Plavix Tablets (1% to 2.5%) 3084
Pletal Tablets (2% or greater) 2605
Pletal Tablets (2% or greater) 2848
Pneumovax 23 2156
Pnu-Imune 23 (Rare) 1868
Pravachol Tablets (Rare) 1099
Prevacid Delayed-Release Capsules (Less than 1%) 3292
PREVPAC (Less than 1%) 3298
Prinivil Tablets (0.3% to 1.0%) 2164
Prinzide Tablets 2168
Procanbid Extended-Release Tablets (Fairly common) 2262
Procardia Capsules (Less than 0.5%) 2708
Proleukin for Injection (1%) 1199
Prometrium Capsules (100 mg, 200 mg) (Less than 5%) 3261
ProSom Tablets (Infrequent) 500
Prostin E2 Suppositories 2852
Protonix I.V. (Less than 1%) 3580
Protonix Tablets (Less than 1%) 3577
Protopic Ointment (Greater than or equal to 1%) 1397
Provigil Tablets (At least 1%) 1193
Prozac Pulvules, Liquid, and Weekly Capsules (Infrequent) 1238
Rabies Vaccine RabAvert (Rare) 1203
Recombivax HB (Greater than 1%) 2178
Remeron Tablets (Infrequent) 2483
Remeron SolTab Tablets (Infrequent) 2486
Remicade for IV Injection (Less than 2%) 1178
Requip Tablets (1% or more) 1621
Rescriptor Tablets (Less than 2%) 526
Risperdal (Rare) 1796
Roferon-A Injection (Rare) 2996
Roxicodone Tablets (Less than 3%) 3067
Salagen Tablets (Less than 1%) 2229
Sandostatin Injection (Less than 1%) 2394
Sandostatin LAR Depot (Rare) 2395
Sarafem Pulvules (Infrequent) 1962
Seroquel Tablets (Infrequent) 684
Serzone Tablets (Infrequent) 1104
Sonata Capsules (Frequent) 3591
▲ Soriatane Capsules (1% to 10%) 3003
Sular Tablets (Less than or equal to 1%) 688
Tasmar Tablets (1% to 2%) 3010
Teveten Tablets (Less than 1%) 3327
Thalomid Capsules 1154
TheraCys Injection 823
Tice BCG, BCG Live (2.7%) 2489
▲ Tonocard Tablets (4.7%) 649
Travatan Ophthalmic Solution (1% to 5%) 543
Tricor Capsules, Micronized 513
Twinrix Vaccine 1674
Uniretic Tablets (Less than 1%) 3178
Vascor Tablets (0.5% to 2.0%) 2602
Vaseretic Tablets 2204
Vasotec I.V. Injection 2207
Vasotec Tablets (0.5% to 1.0%) 2210
Viadur Implant (Less than 2%) 912
Viagra Tablets (Less than 2%) 2732
Viracept 532
▲ Wellbutrin Tablets (3.1%) 1680
Wellbutrin SR Sustained-Release Tablets (Up to 2%) 1684
▲ Xenical Capsules (5.4%) 3043
Zanaflex Tablets (Infrequent) 1305
Zestoretic Tablets 695
Zestril Tablets (0.3% to 1.0%) 698
Zocor Tablets (Rare) 2219
Zomig Tablets (Rare) 708
Zomig-ZMT Tablets (Rare) 708
Zonegran Capsules (Infrequent) 1307
Zyban Sustained-Release Tablets 1710
Zyprexa Tablets (Infrequent) 1973
Zyprexa ZYDIS Orally Disintegrating Tablets (Infrequent) 1973
Zyrtec (Less than 2%) 2756
Zyrtec-D 12 Hour Extended Relief Tablets (Less than 2%) 2758

Arthritis, acute gouty, precipitation of
Pyrazinamide Tablets 1876

Arthritis, exacerbation of
Bicillin C-R 900/300 Injection 2240
Bicillin C-R Injection 2238
Bicillin L-A Injection 2242
Campath Ampules 992
Evoxac Capsules (Less than 1%) 1217
Nexium Delayed-Release Capsules (Less than 1%) 619
Teveten Tablets (Less than 1%) 3327

Arthritis, polyarticular
Rituxan for Infusion (Less than 0.1%) 1750
Rituxan I.V. (Less than 0.1%) 1428

Arthritis, tuberculous
Enbrel for Injection 1752
Enbrel for Injection 3504

Arthritis, septic
Enbrel for Injection 1752
Enbrel for Injection 3504

Arthropathy, Charcot-like
Celestone Soluspan Injectable Suspension 3097
Decadron Phosphate Injection 2081
Hydrocortone Acetate Injectable Suspension 2103

Arthropathy, traumatic
Vioxx (Greater than 0.1% to 1.9%) 2213

Arthropathy, unspecified
Campath Ampules 992
Colazal Capsules 3069
Didronel Tablets 2888
Evoxac Capsules (Less than 1%) 1217
▲ Gengraf Capsules (4%) 457
Hivid Tablets (Less than 1%) 2975
▲ Lescol XL Tablets (3.2%) 2361
▲ Lescol XL Tablets (3.2%) 2925
LYMErix Vaccine 1592
▲ Neoral Soft Gelatin Capsules (4%) 2380
▲ Neoral Oral Solution (4%) 2380
Nexium Delayed-Release Capsules (Less than 1%) 619
Remicade for IV Injection (Less than 2%) 1178
▲ Simulect for Injection (3% to 10%) 2399
▲ Starlix Tablets (3.3%) 2401
Ticlid Tablets (Rare) 3015
Trovan (Less than 1%) 2722

Arthrosis
Aciphex Tablets 1267
Aciphex Tablets 1783
Aggrenox Capsules (1.1%) 1026
Ambien Tablets (Rare) 3191
Apligraf (1.8%) 2305
Arava Tablets (1% to 3%) 724
▲ Aredia for Injection (At least 10%) 2309
Atacand HCT Tablets (0.5% or greater) 597
Betaseron for SC Injection 988
Celebrex Capsules (0.1% to 1.9%) 2676
Celebrex Capsules (0.1% to 1.9%) 2780
Depacon Injection (1% or more) 416
Depakene (1% or more) 421
Depakote Sprinkle Capsules 426
Depakote Tablets (1% to 5%) 430
Depakote ER Tablets (Greater than 1%) 436
Effexor Tablets (Infrequent) 3495
Effexor XR Capsules (Infrequent) 3499
Gabitril Tablets (Infrequent) 1189
Hivid Tablets (Less than 1%) 2975
Intron A for Injection (Less than 5%) 3120
Kaletra Capsules (Less than 2%) 471
Kaletra Oral Solution (Less than 2%) 471
Levaquin Injection (Less than 0.5%) 2537
Luvox Tablets (25, 50, 100 mg) (Rare) 3256
LYMErix Vaccine (1.66%) 1592
Meridia Capsules 481
Miacalcin Nasal Spray (1% to 3%) 2375
Norvasc Tablets (More than 0.1% to 1%) 2704
Norvir Capsules (Less than 2%) 487
Norvir Oral Solution (Less than 2%) 487
NovoSeven (1%) 2430
Paxil (Rare) 1609
Plavix Tablets (1% to 2.5%) 1097
Plavix Tablets (1% to 2.5%) 3084
Priftin Tablets (Less than 1%) 758
Protonix I.V. (Less than 1%) 3580
Protonix Tablets (Less than 1%) 3577
Prozac Pulvules, Liquid, and Weekly Capsules (Rare) 1238
▲ Rapamune Oral Solution and Tablets (3% to 20%) 3584
Remeron Tablets (Rare) 2483
Remeron SolTab Tablets (Rare) 2486
Requip Tablets (1% or more) 1621
Rilutek Tablets (Infrequent) 772
Risperdal (Rare) 1796
Sarafem Pulvules (Rare) 1962
Skelid Tablets (2.7%) 3088
Sonata Capsules (Infrequent) 3591
▲ Soriatane Capsules (1% to 10%) 3003
Tasmar Tablets (Infrequent) 3010
Teveten Tablets (Less than 1%) 3327
Topamax Sprinkle Capsules (Infrequent) 2590
Topamax Tablets (Infrequent) 2590
Tricor Capsules, Micronized 513
Uniretic Tablets (Less than 1%) 3178
Viagra Tablets (Less than 2%) 2732
Vistide Injection 1445
▲ Visudyne for Injection (1% to 10%) ⊙308
Zoloft (Infrequent) 2751
Zyprexa Tablets (Infrequent) 1973
Zyprexa ZYDIS Orally Disintegrating Tablets (Infrequent) 1973
Zyrtec (Less than 2%) 2756
Zyrtec-D 12 Hour Extended Relief Tablets (Less than 2%) 2758

Ascaris, appearance in mouth and nose
Mintezol 2137

Ascites
Accuretic Tablets 2614
Actiq (1% or greater) 1184
Aquasol A Parenteral 593
Avonex 1013
Betaseron for SC Injection 988
Campath Ampules 992
▲ CellCept Capsules (24.2%) 2951
▲ CellCept Intravenous (24.2%) 2951
▲ CellCept Oral Suspension (24.2%) 2951
▲ CellCept Tablets (24.2%) 2951
Clomid Tablets 735
Cosmegen for Injection 2062
Doxil Injection (Less than 1%) 566
Ellence Injection 2806
▲ Flolan for Injection (12% to 23%) 1528
Follistim for Injection 2465
▲ Gleevec Capsules (2% to 16%) 2357
Herceptin I.V. (At least one of the 958 patients) 1414
Humegon for Injection 2468
Intron A for Injection (Less than 5%) 3120
Invirase Capsules (Rare) 2979
Oncaspar 756
Ovidrel for Injection 3220
▲ Prograf (7% to 27%) 1393
▲ Proleukin for Injection (4%) 1199
▲ Rapamune Oral Solution and Tablets (3% to 20%) 3584
Requip Tablets (Rare) 1621
Risperdal (Rare) 1796
Sandostatin LAR Depot (1% to 4%) 2395
Serophene Tablets 3226
Taxotere for Injection Concentrate (Less frequent) 778
Thalomid Capsules 1154
▲ Vesanoid Capsules (3%) 3037

Aseptic meningitis syndrome
Clinoril Tablets (Less than 1 in 100) 2053
CytoGam Intravenous (Infrequent) 2026
Gamimune N, 5% Solvent/Detergent Treated (Infrequent) 925
Gamimune N, 10% Solvent/Detergent Treated (Infrequent) 928
Gammar-P I.V. (Infrequently) 787
Orthoclone OKT3 Sterile Solution (Less than 1%) 2498

Aseptic necrosis of femoral/humeral heads
Celestone Soluspan Injectable Suspension 3097
Celestone Syrup 3099
Cortone Acetate Injectable Suspension 2059
Cortone Acetate Tablets 2061
Decadron Elixir 2078
Decadron Tablets 2079
Decadron Phosphate Injection 2081
Depo-Medrol Injectable Suspension 2795
Florinef Acetate Tablets 2250
Hydrocortone Tablets 2106
Hydrocortone Acetate Injectable Suspension 2103
Hydrocortone Phosphate Injection, Sterile 2105
Pediapred Oral Solution 1170
Prednisone 3064
Prelone Syrup 2273
Solu-Medrol Sterile Powder 2855
Vancenase AQ Nasal Spray 0.084% (Single case) 3163

Aspartate aminotransferase levels, changes in
▲ Avonex (3%) 1013
▲ Emcyt Capsules (2% to 34%) 2810
Humegon for Injection (Occasional) 2468
▲ Roferon-A Injection (1% to 46%) 2996
Sinemet Tablets 1253
Sinemet CR Tablets 1255

Aspartate aminotransferase levels, elevation of
Abelcet Injection 1273
Accutane Capsules 2944
Aceon Tablets (2 mg, 4 mg, 8 mg) (0.3% to 1%) 3249
Aciphex Tablets (0.2%) 1267
Aciphex Tablets (0.2%) 1783
Adalat CC Tablets (Rare) 877
Ambien Tablets (Rare) 3191
▲ AmBisome for Injection (12.8%) 1383
Amoxil Chewable Tablets 1471
Amoxil for Oral Suspension 1471
Amoxil 1471
Amphotec (1% to 5%) 1774
Anadrol-50 Tablets 3321
Anaprox Tablets (Less than 1%) 2967
Anaprox DS Tablets (Less than 1%) 2967
Ancef for Injection 1474
Ancef Injection 1474
Anzemet Injection 719
Anzemet Tablets 722
Arava Tablets (1.5% to 2.2%) 724
Arimidex Tablets (2% to 5%) 659

Asacol Delayed-Release Tablets...... 2884
Atromid-S Capsules...... 3483
Augmentin Chewable Tablets (Infrequent)...... 1482
Augmentin Powder for Oral Suspension (Infrequent)...... 1482
Augmentin Tablets (Infrequent)...... 1485
Augmentin ES-600 Powder for Oral Suspension...... 1487
Axid Pulvules (Less common)...... 1903
Axid Pulvules (Less common)...... 2919
Aygestin Tablets...... 1333
Azactam for Injection (Less than 1% to 3.8%)...... 1276
Azulfidine EN-tabs Tablets...... 2775
▲ Betaseron for SC Injection (4%)...... 988
Biaxin/Biaxin XL (Less than 1%)...... 403
Bicillin C-R 900/300 Injection...... 2240
Bicillin C-R Injection...... 2238
Bicillin L-A Injection...... 2242
Calcijex Injection...... 411
Calcium Disodium Versenate Injection...... 1980
▲ Cancidas for Injection (10.8% to 13%)...... 2048
Cardizem Injectable (Less than 1%)...... 1018
Cardizem Lyo-Ject Syringe (Less than 1%)...... 1018
Cardizem Monovial (Less than 1%)...... 1018
Cardizem CD Capsules (Less than 1%)...... 1016
▲ Casodex Tablets (2% to 5%)...... 662
Cataflam Tablets (About 1% to about 4%)...... 2315
Ceclor CD Tablets (0.3%)...... 1279
Ceclor (1 in 40)...... 1905
Cedax (0.1% to 1%)...... 1021
Cefizox for Intramuscular or Intravenous Use (1% to 5%)...... 1390
Cefotan (1 in 300)...... 664
Ceftin (0.1% to 1%)...... 1898
Cefzil (2%)...... 1076
Celebrex Capsules (0.1% to 1.9%)...... 2676
Celebrex Capsules (0.1% to 1.9%)...... 2780
▲ CellCept Capsules (3% to 15.6%)...... 2951
▲ CellCept Intravenous (3% to 15.6%)...... 2951
▲ CellCept Oral Suspension (3% to 15.6%)...... 2951
▲ CellCept Tablets (3% to 15.6%)...... 2951
▲ Chemet Capsules (4.2% to 10.4%)...... 3078
Chibroxin Sterile Ophthalmic Solution...... 2051
▲ Cipro I.V. (Among most frequent)...... 893
▲ Cipro I.V. Pharmacy Bulk Package (Among most frequent)...... 897
Cipro (1.7%)...... 887
Claforan Injection (Less than 1%)...... 732
Colazal Capsules...... 3069
Colestid Tablets (One or more occasions)...... 2791
Combivir Tablets...... 1502
Cordarone Intravenous (Common)...... 3491
Cordarone Tablets...... 3487
Coreg Tablets (1% to 2%)...... 1508
Covera-HS Tablets (1.4%)...... 3199
▲ Crixivan Capsules (4%)...... 2070
Cytovene (At least 3 subjects)...... 2959
DDAVP Tablets...... 739
Demser Capsules (Rare)...... 2085
Depacon Injection (1% to 5%)...... 416
Depakene (Frequent)...... 421
Depakote Sprinkle Capsules (1% to 5%)...... 426
Depakote Tablets (Frequent)...... 430
Depakote ER Tablets (Greater than 1%)...... 436
Diflucan Tablets, Injection, and Oral Suspension...... 2681
Dipentum Capsules (Rare)...... 2803
Duricef...... 1079
Dynabac Tablets (0.1% to 1%)...... 2269
EC-Naprosyn Delayed-Release Tablets (Less than 1%)...... 2967
Effexor Tablets (Infrequent)...... 3495
Effexor XR Capsules (Infrequent)...... 3499
Elspar for Injection...... 2092
Epivir (Up to 1.7%)...... 1520
Eulexin Capsules...... 3118
Evoxac Capsules (Less than 1%)...... 1217
Famvir Tablets (2.3%)...... 2348
▲ Fareston Tablets (5% to 19%)...... 3237
Felbatol (Frequent)...... 3343
Feldene Capsules (Approximately 1%)...... 2685
Femara Tablets...... 2351
Floxin I.V. (More than or equal to 1%)...... 2526
Floxin Tablets (More than or equal to 1%)...... 2529
▲ Fortaz (1 in 16)...... 1541
Fortovase Capsules (2% to 3%)...... 2970
Foscavir Injection (Between 1% and 5%)...... 605
▲ Gemzar for Injection (52% to 78%)...... 1919
Geocillin Tablets...... 2687
Gleevec Capsules (1.1% to 2.1%)...... 2357
Glucotrol Tablets (Occasional)...... 2692
Glucotrol XL Extended Release Tablets (Occasional)...... 2693
Hectorol Capsules...... 1064
Hectorol Injection...... 1066
Heparin Lock Flush Solution...... 3509
Heparin Sodium Injection...... 3511
▲ Hivid Tablets (Less than 1% to 7.6%)...... 2975
▲ Humatrope Vials and Cartridges (6.67% to 12.50%)...... 1930
Hycamtin for Injection (Less than 1% to 5%)...... 1546
Imdur Tablets (Less than or equal to 5%)...... 1826
▲ Innohep Injection (8.8%)...... 1248
▲ Intron A for Injection (Up to 63% of patients)...... 3120
Invirase Capsules (2% to 3%)...... 2979
Isoptin SR Tablets...... 467
▲ Kaletra Capsules (0.3% to 9.5%)...... 471
▲ Kaletra Oral Solution (0.3% to 9.5%)...... 471
Keflex...... 1237
▲ Kefurox Vials, ADD-Vantage (1 in 25)...... 1948
Kefzol Vials, ADD-Vantage...... 1951
Kytril Injection (2.8%)...... 2986
▲ Kytril Tablets (5%)...... 2988
Lexxel Tablets (Infrequent)...... 608
Lodosyn Tablets...... 1251
Lopid Tablets (Occasional)...... 2650
Lorabid Suspension and Pulvules...... 2251
Lovenox Injection (Up to 3.9% of patients)...... 746
Loxitane Capsules...... 3398
Lupron Depot 3.75 mg (One patient)...... 3281
Lupron Depot 7.5 mg (Greater than or equal to 5%)...... 3284
▲ Lupron Depot–4 Month 30 mg (Greater than or equal to 5%)...... 3289
Macrobid Capsules (1% to 5%)...... 2889
Macrodantin Capsules...... 2891
Malarone...... 1596
Mandol Vials...... 1953
Marinol Capsules (Less than 1%)...... 3325
Maxipime for Injection (2.4%)...... 1285
Mefoxin for Injection...... 2124
Mefoxin Premixed Intravenous Solution...... 2127
▲ Mepron Suspension (4%)...... 1598
Meridia Capsules (1.6%)...... 481
Merrem I.V. (Greater than 0.2%)...... 673
Mevacor Tablets...... 2132
Mexitil Capsules (About 1%)...... 1047
Mithracin for Intravenous Use...... 903
Mobic Tablets (Less than 2%)...... 1054
Monurol Sachet...... 1375
Motrin Suspension, Oral Drops, Chewable Tablets, and Caplets (Less than 1%)...... 2002
▲ Mycelex Troche (15%)...... 573
▲ Mycobutin Capsules (7%)...... 2838
▲ Mylotarg for Injection (17%)...... 3540
Naprelan Tablets (Less than 1%)...... 1293
Naprosyn Suspension (Less than 1%)...... 2967
Naprosyn Tablets (Less than 1%)...... 2967
▲ Navelbine Injection (1% to 54%)...... 1604
Nebcin Vials, Hyporets & ADD-Vantage...... 1955
Nexium Delayed-Release Capsules (Less than 1%)...... 619
Niaspan Extended-Release Tablets...... 1846
▲ Nilandron Tablets (12.9%)...... 753
▲ Nolvadex Tablets (4.8%)...... 678
Noroxin Tablets (1.4% to 1.6%)...... 2145
▲ Novantrone for Injection (8% to 9%)...... 1760
Omnicef (0.9%)...... 493
Oncaspar (Greater than 1% but less than 5%)...... 756
Orthoclone OKT3 Sterile Solution (Less than 1%)...... 2498
Orudis Capsules...... 3548
Oruvail Capsules...... 3548
Oxandrin Tablets...... 1153
Pacerone Tablets...... 3331
▲ Paraplatin for Injection (15% to 23%)...... 1126
Paxil (Infrequent)...... 1609
Pentasa Capsules (Less than 1%)...... 3239
Pipracil (Less frequent)...... 1866
Pravachol Tablets...... 1099
Precose Tablets...... 906
Prevacid Delayed-Release Capsules...... 3292
PREVPAC (Less than 1%)...... 3298
▲ Priftin Tablets (4.4%)...... 758
Prilosec Delayed-Release Capsules (Rare)...... 628
Primaxin I.M....... 2158
Primaxin I.V....... 2160
Procardia Capsules (Rare)...... 2708
Procardia XL Extended Release Tablets (Rare)...... 2710
▲ Prograf (3% to 15%)...... 1393
▲ Proleukin for Injection (23%)...... 1199
ProSom Tablets (Rare)...... 500
Protonix I.V. (Greater than or equal to 1%)...... 3580
Protonix Tablets (Less than 1%)...... 3577
Protopic Ointment (Greater than or equal to 1%)...... 1397
Provigil Tablets (At least 1%)...... 1193
▲ Rapamune Oral Solution and Tablets (3% to 20%)...... 3584
Remeron Tablets (Rare)...... 2483
Remeron SolTab Tablets (Rare)...... 2486
▲ Remicade for IV Injection (37%)...... 1178
▲ Rescriptor Tablets (1.7% to 5.6%)...... 526
Rifamate Capsules...... 767
Rifater Tablets...... 769
Risperdal (Infrequent)...... 1796
Rocaltrol...... 2991
▲ Rocephin Injectable Vials, ADD-Vantage, Galaxy, Bulk (3.1%)...... 2993
Sectral Capsules...... 3589
▲ Serostim for Injection (11.7%)...... 3229
Serzone Tablets (Infrequent)...... 1104
Sinemet Tablets...... 1253
Singulair (1.6%)...... 2181
Solu-Medrol Sterile Powder...... 2855
Sonata Capsules (Rare)...... 3591
▲ Soriatane Capsules (Approximately 1 in 3 patients)...... 3003
Sporanox Injection (1%)...... 1804
Sporanox Injection (1%)...... 2509
Stromectol Tablets (2%)...... 2185
Suprax (Less than 2%)...... 1877
Sustiva Capsules (2%)...... 1258
Symmetrel...... 1328
▲ Synagis Intramuscular (4.9%)...... 2028
Synarel Nasal Solution for Endometriosis (One patient)...... 3205
Synercid I.V....... 775
Tarka Tablets...... 508
Tasmar Tablets (1% to 5%)...... 3010
▲ Taxol Injection (19%)...... 1129
▲ Tazicef for Injection (1 in 16 patients)...... 1647
▲ Tazicef Galaxy Container (1 in 16 patients)...... 1650
▲ Tazicef Pharmacy Bulk Package (1 in 16 patients)...... 1653
▲ Tazidime Vials, Faspak & ADD-Vantage (1 in 16)...... 1966
Tequin Injection (Less than 0.1%)...... 1110
Tequin Tablets (Less than 0.1%)...... 1110
Teveten Tablets (Less than 1%)...... 3327
▲ Thalomid Capsules (2.8% to 12.5%)...... 1154
Tiazac Capsules (Less than 2%)...... 1378
Ticlid Tablets (Rare)...... 3015
Timentin Injection- ADD-Vantage Vial...... 1661
Timentin Injection-Galaxy Container...... 1664
Timentin Injection-Pharmacy Bulk Package...... 1666
Timentin for Intravenous Administration...... 1658
Topamax Sprinkle Capsules (Infrequent)...... 2590
Topamax Tablets (Infrequent)...... 2590
Trecator-SC Tablets...... 3598
Tricor Capsules, Micronized...... 513
▲ Trisenox Injection (13%)...... 1158
Trizivir Tablets (1.7%)...... 1669
Trovan (Greater than or equal to 1%)...... 2722
Unasyn for Injection...... 2728
Uniretic Tablets (Less than 1%)...... 3178
Valtrex Caplets...... 1676
Vantin Tablets and Oral Suspension...... 2860
Verelan Capsules...... 3184
Verelan PM Capsules...... 3186
Vermox Chewable Tablets (Rare)...... 2017
▲ Videx (7% to 14%)...... 1138
▲ Videx EC Capsules (4% to 40%)...... 1143
Viracept...... 532
Viramune Oral Suspension (2.0%)...... 1060
Viramune Tablets (2.0%)...... 1060
Vistide Injection...... 1445
Voltaren Tablets (About 1% to about 4%)...... 2315
Voltaren-XR Tablets (About 1% to about 4%)...... 2315
Xanax Tablets (Less than 1% to 3.2%)...... 2865
Zebeta Tablets...... 1885
▲ Zerit (11%)...... 1147
▲ Zinacef Injection (1 in 25 patients)...... 1696
▲ Zinacef for Injection (1 in 25 patients)...... 1696
Zithromax Capsules, 250 mg (1% to 2%)...... 2743
▲ Zithromax for IV Infusion (4% to 6%)...... 2748
Zithromax for Oral Suspension, 1 g (1% to 2%)...... 2743
Zithromax for Oral Suspension, 300 mg, 600 mg, 900 mg, 1200 mg (1% to 2%)...... 2739
Zithromax Tablets, 250 mg (1% to 2%)...... 2739
Zithromax Tablets, 600 mg (1% to 2%)...... 2743
Zocor Tablets...... 2219
▲ Zofran Injection (Approximately 5% of patients)...... 1698
Zofran (Approximately 1% to 2%)...... 1703
Zofran ODT Orally Disintegrating Tablets (Approximately 1% to 2%)...... 1703
Zoladex (Less than 1%)...... 702
Zoladex 3-month...... 706
Zoloft (Infrequent)...... 2751
Zonegran Capsules (Rare)...... 1307
Zosyn...... 1890
Zosyn in Galaxy Containers...... 1894
▲ Zyvox (1.7% to 9.6%)...... 2871

Asphyxia

Compazine...... 1505
Navane Intramuscular...... 2703
Remeron Tablets (Rare)...... 2483
Remeron SolTab Tablets (Rare)...... 2486
Stelazine...... 1640
Thorazine...... 1656

Aspiration

Clozaril Tablets...... 2319
Compazine...... 1505
Risperdal (Rare)...... 1796
Seroquel Tablets...... 684

AST elevation

(*see under* Aspartate aminotransferase levels, elevation of)

Asterixis

Ceptaz for Injection...... 1499
Depacon Injection...... 416
Depakene...... 421
Depakote Sprinkle Capsules...... 426
Depakote Tablets...... 430
Depakote ER Tablets...... 436
Dilantin Infatabs (Rare)...... 2624
Dilantin Kapseals (Rare)...... 2622
Dilantin-125 Oral Suspension (Rare)...... 2625
Fortaz...... 1541
Orthoclone OKT3 Sterile Solution (Less than 1%)...... 2498
Tazidime Vials, Faspak & ADD-Vantage...... 1966
▲ Vesanoid Capsules (3%)...... 3037

Asthenia

Accolate Tablets (1.8%)...... 657
Accuretic Tablets (1.1%)...... 2614
Accutane Capsules...... 2944
▲ Aceon Tablets (2 mg, 4 mg, 8 mg) (7.9%)...... 3249
Aciphex Tablets...... 1267
Aciphex Tablets...... 1783
▲ Actiq (4% to 38%)...... 1184
▲ Actonel Tablets (4.9% to 5.1%)...... 2879
▲ Adalat CC Tablets (4%)...... 877
Adderall XR Capsules (2%)
Adenoscan (Less than 1%)...... 1381
Aerobid/Aerobid-M (1% to 3%)...... 1363
Aggrenox Capsules (1.8%)...... 1026
▲ Agrylin Capsules (23.1%)...... 3232
Albalon Ophthalmic Solution...... ⊙225
Aldoclor Tablets...... 2035
Aldomet Tablets...... 2037
Aldoril Tablets...... 2039
Allegra-D Extended-Release Tablets...... 714
▲ Alphagan Ophthalmic Solution (Approximately 3% to 9%)...... 545
Alphagan P Ophthalmic Solution (1% to 4%)...... 546
Altace Capsules (0.3% to 2.0%)...... 2233
Amaryl Tablets (1.6%)...... 717
Ambien Tablets (Frequent)...... 3191
▲ AmBisome for Injection (6.2% to 13.1%)...... 1383
Amphotec (1% to 5%)...... 1774
Ancobon Capsules...... 1730
AndroGel (0% to 3%)...... 3322
Antabuse Tablets...... 3474
Apligraf (1.3%)...... 2305
▲ Arava Tablets (3%)...... 724
▲ Aredia for Injection (22.2%)...... 2309
▲ Arimidex Tablets (13.4% to 16.4%)...... 659
Aromasin Tablets (Less frequent)...... 2769
Artane...... 1855
Arthrotec Tablets (Rare)...... 3195
▲ Asacol Delayed-Release Tablets (7%)...... 2884
Atacand Tablets (0.5% or greater)...... 595
Atacand HCT Tablets (0.5% or greater)...... 597
Ativan Injection (Infrequent)...... 3478
▲ Ativan Tablets (4.2%)...... 3482
Atromid-S Capsules (Less often)...... 3483
Avalide Tablets...... 1070
Avapro Tablets (1% or greater)...... 1074
Avapro Tablets (1% or greater)...... 3076
Avelox Tablets (0.05% to 1%)...... 879
▲ Avonex (21%)...... 1013
Axert Tablets (Infrequent)...... 2772
▲ Axid Pulvules (3.1%)...... 1903
▲ Axid Pulvules (3.1%)...... 2919
Azactam for Injection (Less than 1%)...... 1276
Bactrim...... 2949

▲ Baycol Tablets (3.4%) 883
Betagan .... ⊙ 228
▲ Betapace Tablets (4% to 13%) 950
▲ Betapace AF Tablets (4.9% to 5.2%) 954
▲ Betaseron for SC Injection (49%) 988
Betimol Ophthalmic Solution (1% to 5%) .... ⊙ 324
Bicillin C-R 900/300 Injection 2240
Bicillin C-R Injection 2238
Bicillin L-A Injection 2242
Blocadren Tablets (0.6%) 2046
▲ Botox Purified Neurotoxin Complex (2% to 10%) 549
Brethine Tablets (2%) 2313
Brevibloc Injection (Less than 1%) 858
Calcijex Injection 411
▲ Campath Ampules (4% to 13%) 992
Captopril Tablets 2281
Cardene I.V. (0.7%) 3485
Cardizem Injectable (Less than 1%) 1018
Cardizem Lyo-Ject Syringe (Less than 1%) 1018
Cardizem Monovial (Less than 1%) 1018
Cardizem CD Capsules (1.8% to 2.6%) 1016
Cardura Tablets (1%) 2668
▲ Carnitor Injection (8% to 12%) 3242
Carteolol Hydrochloride Ophthalmic Solution USP, 1% (Occasional) .... ⊙ 258
▲ Casodex Tablets (15%) 662
▲ Catapres Tablets (About 10 in 100 patients) 1037
Catapres-TTS (0.5% or less) 1038
Caverject Sterile Powder (Less than 1%) 2777
Ceclor 1905
Celebrex Capsules (0.1% to 1.9%) 2676
Celebrex Capsules (0.1% to 1.9%) 2780
Celexa (At least 2%) 1365
▲ CellCept Capsules (13.7% to 43.3%) 2951
▲ CellCept Intravenous (13.7% to 43.3%) 2951
▲ CellCept Oral Suspension (13.7% to 43.3%) 2951
▲ CellCept Tablets (13.7% to 43.3%) 2951
▲ Cenestin Tablets (33%) 1263
▲ Cerebyx Injection (2.2% to 3.9%) 2619
Chirocaine Injection (Less than 1%) 2909
Cipro I.V. (1% or less) 893
Cipro I.V. Pharmacy Bulk Package (Less than 1%) 897
Cipro (Less than 1%) 887
Claritin (At least one patient) 3100
Claritin-D 12 Hour Extended Release Tablets (Less frequent) 3102
Claritin-D 24 Hour Extended Release Tablets (Fewer than 2%) 3104
Clinoril Tablets (Less than 1 in 100) 2053
Clomid Tablets 735
▲ Clorpres Tablets (About 10%) 1002
Clozaril Tablets (1%) 2319
Cogentin 2055
Cognex Capsules (2%) 1351
Colazal Capsules 3069
Colestid Tablets (Infrequent) 2791
▲ CombiPatch Transdermal System (10% to 13%) 2323
▲ Combipres Tablets (About 10%) 1040
Combivent Inhalation Aerosol 1041
Comtan Tablets (2%) 2328
▲ Copaxone for Injection (41%) 3306
Coreg Tablets (More than 2%) 1508
Cortone Acetate Injectable Suspension 2059
Cortone Acetate Tablets 2061
Corzide 40/5 Tablets 2247
Corzide 80/5 Tablets 2247
Cosopt Sterile Ophthalmic Solution 2065
Coumadin for Injection (Infrequent) 1243
Coumadin Tablets (Infrequent) 1243
Cozaar Tablets (1% or greater) 2067
Crinone (Less than 5%) 3213
▲ Crixivan Capsules (3.6%) 2070
Cytotec Tablets (Infrequent) 3202
Cytovene (At least 3 subjects) 2959
▲ Dantrium Capsules (Among most frequent) 2885
Dapsone Tablets USP 1780
Daranide Tablets 2077
Darvon-N/Darvocet-N 1907
Darvon Pulvules 1909
Darvon Compound-65 Pulvules 1910
Darvon-N Tablets 1912
DDAVP Nasal Spray (Up to 2%) 738
DDAVP Rhinal Tube (Up to 2%) 738
Decadron Elixir 2078
Demadex Tablets and Injection (2.0%) 2965
Demerol 3079
▲ Depacon Injection (10% to 27%) 416
▲ Depakene (21% to 27%) 421
▲ Depakote Sprinkle Capsules (10% to 27%) 426
▲ Depakote Tablets (10% to 27%) 430
▲ Depakote ER Tablets (Greater than 5%) 436
▲ DepoCyt Injection (5% to 19%) 1197
▲ Depo-Provera Contraceptive Injection (More than 5%) 2798
Desmopressin Acetate Rhinal Tube (Up to 2%) 1345
Digitek Tablets 1003
Dilaudid Oral Liquid (Less frequent) 445
Dilaudid Tablets - 8 mg (Less frequent) 445
Dilaudid-HP (Less frequent) 443
Diovan Capsules 2337
Diovan HCT Tablets (Greater than 0.2%) 2338
Diprivan Injectable Emulsion (Less than 1%) 667
▲ Ditropan XL Extended Release Tablets (6.8%) 564
Diucardin Tablets 3494
Diuril Oral 2087
Diuril Sodium Intravenous 2086
Dolobid Tablets (Less than 1 in 100) 2088
Dolophine Hydrochloride Tablets 3056
Donnatal 2929
Donnatal Extentabs 2930
Donnatal Tablets 2929
▲ Dostinex Tablets (6% to 9%) 2804
▲ Doxil Injection (6.5% to 33.3%) 566
▲ Duraclon Injection (5% to 10%) 3057
▲ Duragesic Transdermal System (10% or more) 1786
Dyazide Capsules 1515
Dynabac Tablets (1.4% to 2%) 2269
DynaCirc Capsules (Up to 1.2%) 2921
DynaCirc CR Tablets 2923
Dyrenium Capsules (Rare) 3458
▲ Effexor Tablets (2% to 16.9%) 3495
▲ Effexor XR Capsules (3% to 16%) 3499
Eldepryl Capsules 3266
Emadine Ophthalmic Solution (Less than 5%) .... ⊙ 211
Enalaprilat Injection 863
▲ Enbrel for Injection (11%) 1752
▲ Enbrel for Injection (11%) 3504
Engerix-B Vaccine (Less than 1%) 1517
EpiPen 1236
Epivir 1520
Epivir-HBV 1524
▲ Epogen for Injection (7% to 13%) 582
Ergamisol Tablets (10 out of 463 patients) 1789
▲ Esclim Transdermal System (2.1% to 10.6%) 3460
Eskalith 1527
Estrace Vaginal Cream 3358
Estrace Tablets 3361
Etrafon 3115
Evoxac Capsules (0.5%) 1217
▲ Exelon Capsules (6%) 2342
▲ Exelon Oral Solution (6%) 2345
Famotidine Injection (Infrequent) 866
Felbatol (Frequent) 3343
Feldene Capsules (Occasional) 2685
▲ Femara Tablets (4% to 5%) 2351
▲ Ferrlecit Injection (7%) 3386
Flexeril Tablets (Less than 1%) 572
Flexeril Tablets (Less than 1%) 2094
▲ Flolan for Injection (87% to 100%) 1528
▲ Flomax Capsules (7.8% to 8.5%) 1044
Floxin I.V. (Less than 1%) 2526
Floxin Tablets (Less than 1%) 2529
▲ Fludara for Injection (9% to 65%) 995
Flumadine (1.4%) 1370
FluShield Influenza Vaccine 3521
Fortovase Capsules (Less than 2%) 2970
▲ Foscavir Injection (5% or greater) 605
Sterile FUDR 2974
Furosemide Tablets 2284
▲ Gabitril Tablets (18% to 23%) 1189
Gemzar for Injection (Common) 1919
Gengraf Capsules (Rare) 457
▲ Geodon Capsules (5%) 2688
▲ Gleevec Capsules (5% to 10%) 2357
Gliadel Wafer (1%) 1723
▲ Glucophage Tablets (9.2%) 1080
▲ Glucotrol XL Extended Release Tablets (10.1%) 2693
Halcion Tablets (Rare) 2823
Hectorol Capsules 1064
Hectorol Injection 1066
▲ Herceptin I.V. (42%) 1414
Hivid Tablets (Less than 1%) 2975
▲ Humatrope Vials and Cartridges (3.33% to 6.25%) 1930
▲ Hycamtin for Injection (Less than 1% to 21%) 1546
HydroDIURIL Tablets 2108
▲ Hytrin Capsules (1.6% to 11.3%) 464
Hyzaar (1% or greater) 2109
Imdur Tablets (Less than or equal to 5%) 1826
▲ Imitrex Injection (4.9%) 1549
Imitrex Nasal Spray (Infrequent) 1554
Imitrex Tablets (Less than 1% to 2%) 1558
Indapamide Tablets (Less than 5%) 2286
Inderal 3513
Inderal LA Long-Acting Capsules 3516
Inderide Tablets 3517
Inderide LA Long-Acting Capsules 3519
INFeD Injection 3388
▲ Infergen (9% to 10%) 1777
▲ Intron A for Injection (Up to 40%) 3120
Inversine Tablets 1850
▲ Invirase Capsules (0.3% to 9.2%) 2979
Iopidine 0.5% Ophthalmic Solution (Less than 3%) .... ⊙ 213
Ismo Tablets (Fewer than 1%) 3524
Kadian Capsules (Less than 3%) 1335
▲ Kaletra Capsules (3.4% to 7.1%) 471
▲ Kaletra Oral Solution (3.4% to 7.1%) 471
▲ Keppra Tablets (15%) 3314
K-Phos Neutral Tablets 946
▲ Kytril Injection (5%) 2986
▲ Kytril Tablets (5% to 14%) 2988
Lamictal (1% to 3%) 1567
Lanoxicaps Capsules 1574
Lanoxin Injection 1581
Lanoxin Tablets 1587
Lanoxin Elixir Pediatric 1578
Lanoxin Injection Pediatric 1584
Lariam Tablets (Less than 1%) 2989
Lescol Capsules (Rare) 2361
Lescol Capsules (Rare) 2925
Lescol XL Tablets 2361
Lescol XL Tablets 2925
▲ Leukine (17% to 66%) 1755
▲ Leustatin Injection (9%) 2495
Levaquin Injection (Less than 0.5%) 2537
Levbid Extended-Release Tablets 3172
Levlen 962
Levlite 21 Tablets 962
Levlite 28 Tablets 962
Levsin/Levsinex/Levbid 3172
Lexxel Tablets (1.9%) 608
Limbitrol 1738
Lipitor Tablets (Up to 3.8%) 2639
Lipitor Tablets (Up to 3.8%) 2696
Lithobid Slow-Release Tablets 3255
Lodine (1% to 3%) 3528
Lodine XL Extended-Release Tablets (1% to 3%) 3530
Lodosyn Tablets 1251
Lopid Tablets 2650
Lotensin Tablets (Less than 1%) 2365
Lotensin HCT Tablets (0.3% to1%) 2367
Lotrel Capsules 2370
Loxitane Capsules 3398
Lumigan Ophthalmic Solution (1% to 5%) 553
Lunelle Monthly Injection 2827
▲ Lupron Depot 3.75 mg (8.4%) 3281
Lupron Depot 7.5 mg (Less than 5%) 3284
▲ Lupron Depot–3 Month 11.25 mg (3% to 8.4%) 3285
▲ Lupron Depot–3 Month 22.5 mg (7.4%) 3288
▲ Lupron Depot–4 Month 30 mg (4.2% to 12.2%) 3289
▲ Lupron Injection (5% or more) 3279
▲ Luvox Tablets (25, 50, 100 mg) (2% to 14%) 3256
Macrobid Capsules 2889
Macrodantin Capsules 2891
▲ Malarone (3%) 1596
Marinol Capsules (Greater than 1%) 3325
Matulane Capsules 3246
▲ Mavik Tablets (3.3%) 478
Maxair Autohaler 1981
Maxair Inhaler (Less than 1%) 1984
▲ Maxalt Tablets (4% to 7%) 2120
▲ Maxalt-MLT Orally Disintegrating Tablets (4% to 7%) 2120
Maxzide 1008
▲ Megace Oral Suspension (2% to 6%) 1124
Mepergan Injection 3539
▲ Mepron Suspension (8% to 31%) 1598
▲ Meridia Capsules (5.9%) 481
Mestinon 1740
Mevacor Tablets (1.2% to 1.7%) 2132
▲ Mexitil Capsules (1.9% to 5%) 1047
Micardis HCT Tablets 1051
Microzide Capsules 3414
Midamor Tablets (Between 1% and 3%) 2136
Migranal Nasal Spray (1%) 2376
▲ Minipress Capsules (6.5%) 2699
▲ Minizide Capsules (6.5%) 2700
Mintezol 2137
Mirapex Tablets (Infrequent) 2834
Mithracin for Intravenous Use 903
Modicon 2563
▲ Moduretic Tablets (3% to 8%) 2138
Monopril Tablets (0.2% to 1.4%) 1091
Monopril HCT (Less than 2%) 1094
Monurol Sachet (1.1% to 1.7%) 1375
MS Contin Tablets (Less frequent) 2896
MSIR (Less frequent) 2898
Mustargen for Injection 2142
Mycobutin Capsules (1%) 2838
Mykrox Tablets (Less than 2%) 1168
Myleran Tablets 1603
Mylocel Tablets 2227
▲ Mylotarg for Injection (36% to 63%) 3540
▲ Myobloc Injectable Solution (3% to 6%) 1291
Naprelan Tablets (Less than 3%) 1293
Narcan Injection 1322
Nardil Tablets (Common) 2653
Naropin Injection (Less than 1%) 612
Nascobal Gel (One patient) 3174
Navane Oral 2701
Navane Intramuscular 2703
▲ Navelbine Injection (Up to 27%) 1604
Neoral Soft Gelatin Capsules (Rare) 2380
Neoral Oral Solution (Rare) 2380
▲ Neumega for Injection (14%) 1434
▲ Neupogen for Injection (4%) 587
Neurontin Capsules (Frequent) 2655
Neurontin Oral Solution (Frequent) 2655
Neurontin Tablets (Frequent) 2655
Nexium Delayed-Release Capsules (Less than 1%) 619
Niaspan Extended-Release Tablets 1846
▲ Nilandron Tablets (19.1%) 753
▲ Nipent for Injection (10% to 13%) 3272
Nitrolingual Pumpspray 1355
Nitrostat Tablets (Occasional) 2658
Norditropin Cartridges 2420
Norditropin for Injection 2419
Norflex 1987
Normodyne Tablets (1%) 3137
Noroxin Tablets (Less frequent) 2145
Norplant System (Less than 1%) 3543
Norpramin Tablets 755
Norvasc Tablets (Less than 1% to 2%) 2704
▲ Norvir Capsules (9.4% to 14.2%) 487
▲ Norvir Oral Solution (9.4% to 14.2%) 487
▲ Novantrone for Injection (24%) 1760
Nubain Injection (1% or less) 1323
NuLev Orally Disintegrating Tablets 3176
Numorphan 1324
Ocupress Ophthalmic Solution, 1% Sterile (Occasional) .... ⊙ 303
Omnicef (0.2%) 493
OptiPranolol Metipranolol Ophthalmic Solution 0.3% (A small number of patients) .... ⊙ 263
Oramorph SR Tablets (Less frequent) 3062
▲ Orap Tablets (25.0%) 1407
Orgaran Injection (2.3%) 2480
Ortho Diaphragm Kits – All-Flex Arcing Spring; Ortho Coil Spring 2552
Orthoclone OKT3 Sterile Solution (Less than 1%) 2498
Ortho-Cyclen/Ortho Tri-Cyclen 2573
Ortho-Est Tablets 3464
Ortho-Novum 2563
Ortho-Novum 1/50□28 Tablets 2556
Ortho-Cyclen/Ortho Tri-Cyclen 2573
▲ OxyContin Tablets (6%) 2912
▲ Paraplatin for Injection (11% to 43%) 1126
Parnate Tablets 1607
Patanol Ophthalmic Solution (Less than 5%) 540
▲ Paxil (1.6% to 22%) 1609
Pediazole Suspension 3050
Pentasa Capsules (Less than 1%) 3239
Pepcid Injection (Infrequent) 2153
Pepcid for Oral Suspension (Infrequent) 2150
Pepcid RPD Orally Disintegrating Tablets (Infrequent) 2150
Pepcid Tablets (Infrequent) 2150
▲ Permax Tablets (4.2%) 1299
Phenergan with Codeine Syrup 3557
Phenergan VC Syrup 3560
Phenergan VC with Codeine Syrup 3561
▲ Photofrin for Injection (6%) 831
Plaquenil Tablets 3082
Plavix Tablets (1% to 2.5%) 1097
Plavix Tablets (1% to 2.5%) 3084
Plendil Extended-Release Tablets (2.2% to 3.9%) 623
Pletal Tablets (2% or greater) 2605
Pletal Tablets (2% or greater) 2848
Pneumovax 23 2156
Polocaine Injection, USP 625
Polocaine-MPF Injection, USP 625
Ponstel Capsules (Occasional) 1356
Pravachol Tablets (Rare) 1099
▲ Prempro Tablets (6% to 8%) 3572
Prevacid Delayed-Release Capsules (Less than 1%) 3292
PREVPAC (Less than 1%) 3298
Prilosec Delayed-Release Capsules (1.1% to 1.3%) 628
Primaxin I.M. 2158
Primaxin I.V. (Less than 0.2%) 2160
Prinivil Tablets (Greater than 1%) 2164
Prinzide Tablets (1.8%) 2168
ProAmatine Tablets (Rare) 3241
Procanbid Extended-Release Tablets (Occasional) 2262

▲ Procardia Capsules (Approximately 10% to 12%) 2708
▲ Procardia XL Extended Release Tablets (Less than 3% to 12%) 2710
▲ Procrit for Injection (7% to 13%) 2502
▲ Prograf (11% to 52%) 1393
▲ Proleukin for Injection (23%) 1199
Prometrium Capsules (100 mg, 200 mg) 3261
▲ ProSom Tablets (11%) 500
Prostigmin Injectable 1744
Prostigmin Tablets 1744
Prostin E2 Suppositories 2852
Protonix I.V. (Greater than or equal to 1%) 3580
Protonix Tablets (Greater than or equal to 1%) 3577
Protopic Ointment (1% to 3%) 1397
Proventil Repetabs Tablets (2%) 3148
Provigil Tablets (At least 1%) 1193
▲ Prozac Pulvules, Liquid, and Weekly Capsules (9% to 21%) 1238
▲ Pulmicort Turbuhaler Inhalation Powder (2% to 9%) 636
Pulmozyme Inhalation Solution 1426
Quinaglute Dura-Tabs Tablets (2%) 978
▲ Quinidex Extentabs (5%) 2933
▲ Rapamune Oral Solution and Tablets (22% to 40%) 3584
▲ Rebetron Combination Therapy (4% to 9%) 3153
Recombivax HB (Equal to or greater than 1%) 2178
ReFacto Vials 1437
Relafen Tablets (Less than 1%) 1617
▲ Remeron Tablets (8%) 2483
▲ Remeron SolTab Tablets (8%) 2486
Remicade for IV Injection (Less than 2%) 1178
Reminyl Oral Solution (Greater than or equal to 2%) 1792
Reminyl Tablets (Greater than or equal to 2%) 1792
Renese Tablets 2712
ReoPro Vials (0.7%) 1958
Requip Tablets (Infrequent) 1621
Rescriptor Tablets (Less than 2%) 526
▲ Retrovir Capsules (8.6% to 69%) 1625
▲ Retrovir IV Infusion (8.6% to 69%) 1629
▲ Retrovir (8.6% to 69%) 1625
Rifamate Capsules 767
Rifater Tablets 769
▲ Rilutek Tablets (14.8% to 20.1%) 772
Risperdal 1796
▲ Rituxan for Infusion (16%) 1750
▲ Rituxan I.V. (16%) 1428
Robinul Forte Tablets 1358
Robinul Injectable 2940
Robinul Tablets 1358
Rocaltrol 2991
▲ Roferon-A Injection (Less than 0.5% to 88%) 2996
Romazicon Injection (1% to 3%) 3000
Rowasa Rectal Suspension Enema 4.0 grams/unit (60 mL) (0.12%) 3264
Roxanol 3066
Rum-K 1363
Rynatan Tablets 3351
Rythmol Tablets – 150 mg, 225 mg, 300 mg (2.4%) 502
▲ Salagen Tablets (6% to 12%) 2229
Sandimmune (Rare) 2388
Sandostatin Injection (1% to 4%) 2394
▲ Sandostatin LAR Depot (5% to 15%) 2395
▲ Sarafem Pulvules (12% to 14%) 1962
Semprex-D Capsules (2%) 1172
Sensorcaine 643
Sensorcaine-MPF Injection 643
Septra Suspension 2265
Septra Tablets 2265
Septra DS Tablets 2265
Serentil 1057
Serophene Tablets 3226
▲ Seroquel Tablets (4%) 684
▲ Serostim for Injection (1% to 10%) 3229
▲ Serzone Tablets (11%) 1104
▲ Simulect for Injection (3% to 10%) 2399
Sinemet Tablets 1253
Sinemet CR Tablets 1255
Sinequan (Occasional) 2713
Singulair (1.8%) 2181
Skelid Tablets (More than or equal to 1%) 3088
Soma Tablets 3353
Soma Compound Tablets (Very rare) 3354
Soma Compound w/Codeine Tablets (Very rare) 3355
▲ Sonata Capsules (5% to 8%) 3591
Sporanox Capsules (2%) 1800
Sporanox Oral Solution (Less than 2%) 1808
Sporanox Oral Solution (Less than 2%) 2512
Stadol NS Nasal Spray (1% or greater) 1108
Stromectol Tablets (0.9%) 2185
Surmontil Capsules 3595
Sustiva Capsules (Less than 2%) 1258
Symmetrel (0.1% to 1%) 1328
Synarel Nasal Solution for Endometriosis (Less than 1%) 3205
Talacen Caplets (Infrequent) 3089
Talwin Nx Tablets (Infrequent) 3090
▲ Tambocor Tablets (Less than 1% to 4.9%) 1990
Tarka Tablets (0.3% or more) 508
Tasmar Tablets (1% or more) 3010
▲ Taxotere for Injection Concentrate (11.1%) 778
▲ Temodar Capsules (13%) 3157
▲ Tenex Tablets (Up to 10%) 2942
Tenoretic Tablets 690
Tensilon Injectable 1745
Tequin Injection (Less than 0.1%) 1110
Tequin Tablets (Less than 0.1%) 1110
Testoderm Transdermal Systems (1%) 574
Teveten Tablets (Less than 1%) 3327
▲ Thalomid Capsules (8.3%) 1154
Thioplex for Injection 1765
Thiothixene Capsules 2290
▲ Thymoglobulin for Injection (26.8%) 3071
▲ Thyrogen for Injection (3.4%) 1441
Tiazac Capsules (1% to 4%) 1378
Ticlid Tablets (0.5% to 1.0%) 3015
Tikosyn Capsules (Greater than 2%) 2717
Timolide Tablets (1.9%) 2187
Timolol GFS .... ⊙266
Timoptic in Ocudose (Less frequent) 2192
Timoptic Sterile Ophthalmic Solution (Less frequent) 2190
Timoptic-XE Sterile Ophthalmic Gel Forming Solution 2194
▲ TOBI Solution for Inhalation (35.7%) 1206
▲ Tolectin (3% to 9%) 2589
Tonocard Tablets (Less than 1%) 649
▲ Topamax Sprinkle Capsules (4.5% to 8%) 2590
▲ Topamax Tablets (4.5% to 8%) 2590
Toradol (1% or less) 3018
Trasylol Injection (2%) 909
▲ Tricor Capsules, Micronized (5%) 513
▲ Trileptal Oral Suspension (3% to 6%) 2407
▲ Trileptal Tablets (3% to 6%) 2407
Tri-Levlen 962
▲ Trisenox Injection (10%) 1158
Trovan (Less than 1%) 2722
Trusopt Sterile Ophthalmic Solution (Infrequent) 2196
Twinrix Vaccine (Less than 1%) 1674
Ultracet Tablets (At least 1%) 2597
▲ Ultram Tablets (6% to 12%) 2600
Uniretic Tablets (Less than 1%) 3178
Uroqid-Acid No. 2 Tablets 947
▲ Valstar Sterile Solution for Intravesical Instillation (4%) 1175
Valtrex Caplets (1% to 4%) 1676
Vaniqa Cream (0.3%) 1121
Vantin Tablets and Oral Suspension (Less than 1%) 2860
▲ Vaqta (3.9%) 2199
▲ Vascor Tablets (0.5% to 13.95%) 2602
Vaseretic Tablets (2.4%) 2204
Vasotec I.V. Injection 2207
Vasotec Tablets (1.1% to 1.6%) 2210
Venofer Injection (Greater than 1%) 580
Verelan PM Capsules (2%) 3186
Versed Injection (Less than 1%) 3027
Vesanoid Capsules 3037
▲ Viadur Implant (7.6%) 912
Viagra Tablets (Less than 2%) 2732
▲ Vicoprofen Tablets (3% to 9%) 520
▲ Videx (4%) 1138
Videx EC Capsules 1143
Vioxx (1%) 2213
Viracept (1% to 4%) 532
Virazole for Inhalation Solution 1747
▲ Vistide Injection (7% to 43%) 1445
▲ Visudyne for Injection (1% to 10%) .... ⊙308
▲ Vitravene for Injection (5% to 20%) .... ⊙310
Vivactil Tablets 2217
Vivactil Tablets 2446
Volmax Extended-Release Tablets 2276
Voltaren Ophthalmic Sterile Ophthalmic Solution (Less than 3%) .... ⊙312
Warfarin Sodium Tablets, USP 3302
▲ WelChol Tablets (4%) 3073
Wellbutrin SR Sustained-Release Tablets (2% to 4%) 1684
WinRho SDF 2297
▲ Xanax Tablets (7.1%) 2865
Yasmin 28 Tablets (Greater than 1%) 980
▲ Zanaflex Tablets (41% to 78%) 1305
Zaroxolyn Tablets 1177
Zebeta Tablets (0.4% to 1.5%) 1885
▲ Zemplar Injection (3%) 522
▲ Zenapax for Injection (2% to 5%) 3046
Zestoretic Tablets (1.8%) 695
Zestril Tablets (1.3% to greater than 1%) 698
Ziac Tablets 1887
Zithromax Capsules, 250 mg 2743
Zithromax for IV Infusion 2748
Zithromax for Oral Suspension, 1 g 2743
Zithromax for Oral Suspension, 300 mg, 600 mg, 900 mg, 1200 mg 2739
Zithromax Tablets, 250 mg 2739
Zithromax Tablets, 600 mg 2743
Zocor Tablets (1.6%) 2219
Zofran (Up to 2%) 1703
Zofran ODT Orally Disintegrating Tablets (Up to 2%) 1703
▲ Zoladex (11%) 702
Zoloft (Frequent) 2751
▲ Zometa for Intravenous Infusion (5% to 10%) 3621
▲ Zomig Tablets (3% to 9%) 708
▲ Zomig-ZMT Tablets (3% to 9%) 708
Zonegran Capsules (Frequent) 1307
Zosyn (1.0% or less) 1890
Zosyn in Galaxy Containers (1.0% or less) 1894
Zyban Sustained-Release Tablets (Frequent) 1710
▲ Zyflo Filmtab Tablets (3.8%) 524
▲ Zyprexa Tablets (8% to 20%) 1973
▲ Zyprexa ZYDIS Orally Disintegrating Tablets (8% to 20%) 1973
Zyrtec (Less than 2%) 2756
Zyrtec-D 12 Hour Extended Relief Tablets (Less than 2%) 2758

Asthenopia
Lumigan Ophthalmic Solution (1% to 3%) 553

Asthma, allergic
Abelcet Injection 1273
FluShield Influenza Vaccine (Rare) 3521
Fluzone Vaccine (Rare) 802

Asthma, bronchial
Agrylin Capsules (1% to 5%) 3232
Ceclor CD Tablets (0.1% to 1%) 1279
▲ CellCept Capsules (3% to 11%) 2951
▲ CellCept Intravenous (3% to 11%) 2951
▲ CellCept Oral Suspension (3% to 11%) 2951
▲ CellCept Tablets (3% to 11%) 2951
Cerebyx Injection (Infrequent) 2619
Crinone (Less than 5%) 3213
Cuprimine Capsules 2075
Cytovene-IV (One report) 2959
Depen Titratable Tablets 3341
Doxil Injection (Less than 1%) 566
Enalaprilat Injection 863
Felbatol 3343
Fortovase Capsules (Less than 2%) 2970
Haldol Injection, Tablets and Concentrate 2533
Kadian Capsules (Less than 3%) 1335
Levaquin (Less than 0.3%) 2537
Lexxel Tablets 608
Lipitor Tablets (Less than 2%) 2639
Lipitor Tablets (Less than 2%) 2696
Naprelan Tablets (Less than 1%) 1293
Norvir Capsules (Less than 2%) 487
Norvir Oral Solution (Less than 2%) 487
Nubain Injection (1% or less) 1323
Permax Tablets (Infrequent) 1299
Prevacid Delayed-Release Capsules (Less than 1%) 3292
PREVPAC (Less than 1%) 3298
Prinivil Tablets (0.3% to 1.0%) 2164
Prozac Pulvules, Liquid, and Weekly Capsules (Infrequent) 1238
Relafen Tablets (Less than 1%) 1617
Sarafem Pulvules (Infrequent) 1962
Serzone Tablets (Infrequent) 1104
Soma Compound Tablets 3354
Tasmar Tablets (Infrequent) 3010
Toradol 3018
Uniretic Tablets (Less than 1%) 3178
Vaqta (Less than 1%) 2199
Vaseretic Tablets 2204
Vasotec I.V. Injection 2207
Vasotec Tablets (0.5% to 1.0%) 2210
▲ Vesanoid Capsules (3%) 3037
Vicoprofen Tablets (Less than 1%) 520
Vistide Injection 1445
Zanaflex Tablets (Rare) 1305
Zestoretic Tablets 695

Asthma, worsening of
▲ AccuNeb Inhalation Solution (1.3% to 11.1%) 1230
▲ Asacol Delayed-Release Tablets (5% or greater) 2884
Azelex Cream (Rare) 547
D.H.E. 45 Injection 2334
Finevin Cream 962
Flovent Diskus 3614
Flovent 1535
Flovent Rotadisk 1537
Foradil Aerolizer 2354
Gonal-F for Injection 3216
Monurol Sachet 1375
Nexium Delayed-Release Capsules (Less than 1%) 619
Qvar Inhalation Aerosol (Up to 4%) 1987
Sinequan (Occasional) 2713
Stromectol Tablets 2185
▲ Tamiflu Capsules (3.5%) 3008
▲ Tamiflu Oral Suspension (3.5%) 3008
Xalatan Latanoprost Ophthalmic Solution .... ⊙320
Xalatan Sterile Ophthalmic Solution 2864
Xopenex Inhalation Solution 3207

Asthmatic episodes
Accuretic Tablets 2614
Aciphex Tablets 1267
Aciphex Tablets 1783
Actiq (Less than 1%) 1184
Aggrenox Capsules (Less than 1%) 1026
Aleve Tablets, Caplets and Gelcaps .... ▣602
▲ Alocril Ophthalmic Solution (1% to 10%) 545
Alupent (1% to 4%) 1029
AmBisome for Injection (Less common) 1383
Amerge Tablets (Rare) 1467
▲ Amphotec (5% or more) 1774
Arava Tablets (1% to 3%) 724
Arthrotec Tablets (Rare) 3195
Avelox Tablets (0.05% to 1%) 879
Betapace Tablets (1% to 2%) 950
Betaseron for SC Injection 988
Betoptic S Ophthalmic Suspension (Rare) 537
Campath Ampules 992
▲ Casodex Tablets (2% to 5%) 662
Cataflam Tablets (Less than 1%) 2315
Celexa (Rare) 1365
▲ CellCept Capsules (3% to 10%) 2951
▲ CellCept Intravenous (3% to 10%) 2951
▲ CellCept Oral Suspension (3% to 10%) 2951
▲ CellCept Tablets (3% to 10%) 2951
Cognex Capsules (Infrequent) 1351
Compazine 1505
Copaxone for Injection (Infrequent) 3306
Coreg Tablets (0.1% to 1%) 1508
Depo-Provera Contraceptive Injection (Fewer than 1%) 2798
Desferal Vials 2333
Dilaudid Oral Liquid 445
Dilaudid Tablets - 8 mg 445
Dobutrex Solution Vials 1914
Doxil Injection (Less than 1%) 566
Duragesic Transdermal System (Less than 1%) 1786
Ecotrin Enteric Coated Aspirin Low, Regular and Maximum Strength Tablets 1715
Effexor Tablets (Infrequent) 3495
Effexor XR Capsules (Infrequent) 3499
Eldepryl Capsules 3266
Engerix-B Vaccine 1517
Estrace Vaginal Cream 3358
Estrace Tablets 3361
Etrafon 3115
Evoxac Capsules (Less than 1%) 1217
Feldene Capsules (Occasional) 2685
▲ Flonase Nasal Spray (3.3% to 7.2%) 1533
FluShield Influenza Vaccine (One case) 3521
Gabitril Tablets (Infrequent) 1189
Gengraf Capsules (1% to less than 3%) 457
Heparin Lock Flush Solution 3509
Heparin Sodium Injection 3511
Herceptin I.V. (At least one of the 958 patients) 1414
Imitrex Injection 1549
Imitrex Nasal Spray (Rare) 1554
Imitrex Tablets (Infrequent) 1558
Indocin Capsules (Less than 1%) 2112
Indocin I.V. (Less than 1%) 2115
Indocin (Less than 1%) 2112
Iopidine 0.5% Ophthalmic Solution (Less than 3%) .... ⊙213
Isopto Carbachol Ophthalmic Solution .... ⊙215
Klonopin Tablets (Infrequent) 2983
Lodine (Less than 1%) 3528
Lodine XL Extended-Release Tablets (Less than 1%) 3530
Lotensin Tablets (Less than 1%) 2365
Lupron Depot 3.75 mg (Rare) 3281
Lupron Depot 7.5 mg (Rare) 3284
Lupron Depot–3 Month 11.25 mg 3285
Lupron Depot–3 Month 22.5 mg (Rare) 3288
Lupron Depot–4 Month 30 mg (Less than 5%) 3289
Lupron Depot-PED 7.5 mg, 11.25 mg and 15 mg 3291
Luvox Tablets (25, 50, 100 mg) (Infrequent) 3256
Micardis Tablets (More than 0.3%) 1049
Micardis HCT Tablets 1051
Minocin Oral Suspension 1865
Mobic Tablets (Less than 2%) 1054
Children's Motrin Oral Suspension and Chewable Tablets 2006
Children's Motrin Cold Oral Suspension 2007

Children's Motrin Oral Suspension ▣ 643
Infants' Motrin Concentrated Drops 2006
Junior Strength Motrin Caplets and Chewable Tablets 2006
Motrin IB Tablets, Caplets, and Gelcaps 2002
Motrin Sinus Headache Caplets 2005
Nasacort AQ Nasal Spray 752
Nasonex Nasal Spray (Greater than or equal to 2%) 3131
▲ Nipent for Injection (3% to 10%) 3272
Omnicef 493
▲ Optivar Ophthalmic Solution (1% to 10%) 2273
Paxil (Infrequent) 1609
Phenergan Injection 3553
Phenergan 3556
Pletal Tablets (Less than 2%) 2605
Pletal Tablets (Less than 2%) 2848
Ponstel Capsules (Occasional) 1356
Pred Mild Sterile Ophthalmic Suspension ⊙ 249
Prevnar for Injection 1870
Prinzide Tablets 2168
▲ Prograf (3% to 15%) 1393
Proleukin for Injection 1199
ProSom Tablets (Infrequent) 500
Protonix I.V. (Less than 1%) 3580
Protonix Tablets (Less than 1%) 3577
▲ Protopic Ointment (4% to 16%) 1397
Provigil Tablets (1%) 1193
▲ Rapamune Oral Solution and Tablets (3% to 20%) 3584
Relenza Rotadisk (Less than 1%) 1619
Remeron Tablets (Infrequent) 2483
Remeron SolTab Tablets (Infrequent) 2486
Requip Tablets (Infrequent) 1621
Rilutek Tablets (Infrequent) 772
Risperdal (Rare) 1796
Rituxan for Infusion (0.3%) 1750
Rituxan I.V. (0.3%) 1428
Robaxisal Tablets 2939
Sensorcaine 643
Sensorcaine-MPF Injection 643
Serentil 1057
▲ Serevent Diskus (3% to 4%) 1637
Seroquel Tablets (Rare) 684
Soma Tablets 3353
Soma Compound Tablets (Less common) 3354
Soma Compound w/Codeine Tablets (Rare) 3355
Sonata Capsules (Infrequent) 3591
Stelazine 1640
Streptomycin Sulfate Injection 2714
Sular Tablets (Less than or equal to 1%) 688
Suprane Liquid for Inhalation (Less than 1%) 874
Sustiva Capsules (Less than 2%) 1258
Synagis Intramuscular (More than 1%) 2028
▲ Tamiflu Capsules (3.5%) 3008
▲ Tamiflu Oral Suspension (3.5%) 3008
Tequin Injection (Less than 0.1%) 1110
Tequin Tablets (Less than 0.1%) 1110
Teveten Tablets (Less than 1%) 3327
Thioplex for Injection 1765
Thioridazine Hydrochloride Tablets 2289
Thorazine 1656
▲ TOBI Solution for Inhalation (15.9%) 1206
Topamax Sprinkle Capsules (Infrequent) 2590
Topamax Tablets (Infrequent) 2590
Trasylol Injection (2%) 909
Tricor Capsules, Micronized 513
Trilafon 3160
Trileptal Oral Suspension 2407
Trileptal Tablets 2407
Trilisate (Rare) 2901
▲ Tri-Nasal Spray (4.3% to 5.4%) 2274
Trovan (Less than 1%) 2722
Twinrix Vaccine 1674
Urecholine 2198
Urecholine Tablets 2445
Vantin Tablets and Oral Suspension (Less than 1%) 2860
Viagra Tablets (Less than 2%) 2732
Viokase 837
Vioxx (Greater than 0.1% to 1.9%) 2213
Voltaren Tablets (Less than 1%) 2315
Voltaren-XR Tablets (Less than 1%) 2315
Xalatan Latanoprost Ophthalmic Solution ⊙ 320
Xalatan Sterile Ophthalmic Solution 2864
YF-VAX Vaccine (Uncommon) 827
Zebeta Tablets 1885
Zemuron Injection (Less than 1%) 2491
Zestril Tablets (0.3% to 1.0%) 698
Ziac Tablets 1887
Zyprexa Tablets (Infrequent) 1973
Zyprexa ZYDIS Orally Disintegrating Tablets (Infrequent) 1973

Astigmatism

Vitrasert Implant (Less than 1%) ⊙ 254

Astrocytoma

Serophene Tablets 3226

Asystole

Acthrel for Injection (One patient) 3629
Adenocard Injection 1380
Brevibloc Injection (2 Patients) 858
Digitek Tablets 1003
Diprivan Injectable Emulsion 667
Fluothane Inhalation 3508
GoLYTELY and Pineapple Flavor GoLYTELY for Oral Solution 1068
Lanoxicaps Capsules 1574
Lanoxin Injection 1581
Lanoxin Tablets 1587
Lanoxin Elixir Pediatric 1578
Lanoxin Injection Pediatric 1584
NuLYTELY, Cherry Flavor, Lemon-Lime Flavor, and Orange Flavor NuLYTELY for Oral Solution 1068
Zantac Injection (Rare) 1688

Asystole, ventricular

Procanbid Extended-Release Tablets 2262

Ataxia

Actiq (Less than 1%) 1184
Ambien Tablets (Frequent) 3191
Ancobon Capsules 1730
Anzemet Injection (Rare) 719
Anzemet Tablets (Rare) 722
Aricept Tablets (Frequent) 1270
Aricept Tablets (Frequent) 2665
Ativan Injection (Infrequent) 3478
Attenuvax (Rare) 2044
Avelox Tablets (0.05% to 1%) 879
Avonex (2%) 1013
Axert Tablets (Rare) 2772
Azulfidine EN-tabs Tablets (Rare) 2775
Bactrim 2949
Betagan (Rare) ⊙ 228
Betapace Tablets (Rare) 950
Betaseron for SC Injection 988
Buprenex Injectable (Rare) 2918
Captopril Tablets 2281
Cardura Tablets (1%) 2668
Celebrex Capsules (Less than 0.1%) 2676
Celebrex Capsules (Less than 0.1%) 2780
Celexa (Infrequent) 1365
Celontin Capsules (Frequent) 2618
▲ Cerebyx Injection (4.4% to 11.1%) 2619
Chibroxin Sterile Ophthalmic Solution 2051
Cipro I.V. (1% or less) 893
Cipro I.V. Pharmacy Bulk Package (Less than 1%) 897
Cipro (Less than 1%) 887
Clozaril Tablets (1%) 2319
▲ Cognex Capsules (6%) 1351
Copaxone for Injection (At least 2%) 3306
▲ Cordarone Tablets (4% to 9%) 3487
Cozaar Tablets (Less than 1%) 2067
Daranide Tablets 2077
DaunoXome Injection (Less than or equal to 5%) 1442
Demerol 3079
▲ Depacon Injection (8%) 416
▲ Depakene (8%) 421
▲ Depakote Sprinkle Capsules (1% to 8%) 426
▲ Depakote Tablets (1% to 8%) 430
▲ Depakote ER Tablets (Greater than 1%) 436
▲ Dilantin Infatabs (Among most common) 2624
▲ Dilantin Kapseals (Among most common) 2622
▲ Dilantin-125 Oral Suspension (Among most common) 2625
Doxil Injection (Less than 1%) 566
Effexor Tablets (Infrequent) 3495
Effexor XR Capsules (Infrequent) 3499
Enalaprilat Injection 863
Ergamisol Tablets (Up to 2%) 1789
Eskalith 1527
Etrafon 3115
Exelon Capsules (Frequent) 2342
Exelon Oral Solution (Frequent) 2345
▲ Felbatol (3.5% to 6.5%) 3343
Flexeril Tablets (Less than 1%) 572
Flexeril Tablets (Less than 1%) 2094
Floxin I.V. 2526
Floxin Tablets 2529
Flumadine (0.3% to 1%) 1370
Fortovase Capsules (Less than 2%) 2970
Foscavir Injection (Between 1% and 5%) 605
▲ Gabitril Tablets (5%) 1189
Geodon Capsules (Frequent) 2688
Gliadel Wafer (2%) 1723
▲ Halcion Tablets (4.6%) 2823
Herceptin I.V. (At least one of the 958 patients) 1414
Hexalen Capsules 2226
Hivid Tablets (Less than 1%) 2975
Hyzaar 2109
Imitrex Tablets (Infrequent) 1558
Intron A for Injection (Less than 5%) 3120
Invirase Capsules (Less than 2%) 2979
Kadian Capsules (Less than 3%) 1335
Kaletra Capsules (Less than 2%) 471
Kaletra Oral Solution (Less than 2%) 471
Keppra Tablets (3%) 3314
▲ Klonopin Tablets (30%) 2983
▲ Lamictal (4% to 28%) 1567
Leukeran Tablets (Rare) 1591
Levsin/Levsinex/Levbid 3172
Lexxel Tablets 608
Librium Capsules (Some patients) 1736
Librium for Injection 1737
Limbitrol 1738
Lithium Carbonate 3061
Lithium Citrate Syrup 3061
Lithobid Slow-Release Tablets 3255
Lodosyn Tablets 1251
Luvox Tablets (25, 50, 100 mg) (Infrequent) 3256
LYMErix Vaccine (Greater than 1%) 1592
Marinol Capsules (Greater than 1%) 3325
Matulane Capsules 3246
Maxalt Tablets (Infrequent) 2120
Maxalt-MLT Orally Disintegrating Tablets (Infrequent) 2120
Mepergan Injection 3539
Miltown Tablets 3349
Mintezol 2137
Mirapex Tablets (1% or more) 2834
M-M-R II (Rare) 2118
Nardil Tablets (Less frequent) 2653
Nascobal Gel 3174
Nembutal Sodium Solution (Less than 1%) 485
▲ Neurontin Capsules (12.5%) 2655
▲ Neurontin Oral Solution (12.5%) 2655
▲ Neurontin Tablets (12.5%) 2655
Nipent for Injection (Less than 3%) 3272
Noroxin Tablets 2145
Norpramin Tablets 755
Norvasc Tablets (Less than or equal to 0.1%) 2704
Norvir Capsules (Less than 2%) 487
Norvir Oral Solution (Less than 2%) 487
NuLev Orally Disintegrating Tablets 3176
▲ Pacerone Tablets (4% to 9%) 3331
Parnate Tablets 1607
Paxil (Rare to infrequent) 1609
Pediazole Suspension 3050
Permax Tablets (1.6%) 1299
Phenergan Injection 3553
Phenergan 3556
Plaquenil Tablets 3082
Prinivil Tablets (0.3% to 1.0%) 2164
Prinzide Tablets 2168
Procardia XL Extended Release Tablets (1% or less) 2710
▲ Prograf (3% to 15%) 1393
ProSom Tablets (Rare) 500
Proventil HFA Inhalation Aerosol (Less than 3%) 3150
Provigil Tablets (1%) 1193
Prozac Pulvules, Liquid, and Weekly Capsules (Infrequent) 1238
Quinaglute Dura-Tabs Tablets 978
Quinidex Extentabs (1%) 2933
Remeron Tablets (Infrequent) 2483
Remeron SolTab Tablets (Infrequent) 2486
Reminyl Oral Solution (Infrequent) 1792
Reminyl Tablets (Infrequent) 1792
Rifadin 765
Rifamate Capsules 767
Rifater Tablets 769
Rilutek Tablets (Infrequent) 772
▲ Risperdal (17% to 34%) 1796
Robaxin Injectable 2938
Robaxin Tablets 2939
Roferon-A Injection (Less than 1%) 2996
▲ Romazicon Injection (10%) 3000
Rythmol Tablets – 150 mg, 225 mg, 300 mg (2%) 502
Sarafem Pulvules (Infrequent) 1962
Septra Suspension 2265
Septra Tablets 2265
Septra DS Tablets 2265
Serentil 1057
Seroquel Tablets (Infrequent) 684
Serzone Tablets (2%) 1104
Sinemet Tablets 1253
Sinemet CR Tablets 1255
Sinequan (Infrequent) 2713
Soma Tablets 3353
Soma Compound Tablets (Very rare to less frequent) 3354
Soma Compound w/Codeine Tablets 3355
Sonata Capsules (Infrequent) 3591
Sular Tablets (Less than or equal to 1%) 688
Surmontil Capsules 3595
Sustiva Capsules 1258
Symmetrel (1% to 5%) 1328
Tambocor Tablets (1% to 3%) 1990
Taxol Injection (Rare) 1129
▲ Temodar Capsules (8%) 3157
Tequin Injection (Less than 0.1%) 1110
Tequin Tablets (Less than 0.1%) 1110
Teveten Tablets (Less than 1%) 3327
Thalomid Capsules 1154
▲ Tonocard Tablets (0.2% to 10.8%) 649
▲ Topamax Sprinkle Capsules (17% to 21.2%) 2590
▲ Topamax Tablets (17% to 21.2%) 2590
Tranxene 511
Trilafon 3160
▲ Trileptal Oral Suspension (5% to 31%) 2407
▲ Trileptal Tablets (5% to 31%) 2407
Trovan (Less than 1%) 2722
Ultracet Tablets (Less than 1%) 2597
Uniretic Tablets (Less than 1%) 3178
Valcyte Tablets 3022
▲ Valium Injectable (Among most common) 3026
▲ Valium Tablets (Among most common) 3047
Varivax 2202
Vaseretic Tablets 2204
Vasotec I.V. Injection 2207
Vasotec Tablets (0.5% to 1.0%) 2210
Versed Injection (Less than 1%) 3027
Versed Syrup (Less than 1%) 3033
Viagra Tablets (Less than 2%) 2732
Vistide Injection 1445
Vivactil Tablets 2217
Vivactil Tablets 2446
Wellbutrin Tablets (Frequent) 1680
Wellbutrin SR Sustained-Release Tablets (Rare) 1684
Xanax Tablets 2865
Xeloda Tablets (Less than 5%) 3039
Zarontin Capsules 2659
Zarontin Syrup 2660
Zestoretic Tablets 695
Zestril Tablets (0.3% to 1.0%) 698
Zoloft (Infrequent) 2751
Zomig Tablets (Rare) 708
Zomig-ZMT Tablets (Rare) 708
▲ Zonegran Capsules (6%) 1307
Zovirax 1706
Zyban Sustained-Release Tablets (Rare) 1710
Zyprexa Tablets (Infrequent) 1973
Zyprexa ZYDIS Orally Disintegrating Tablets (Infrequent) 1973
Zyrtec (Less than 2%) 2756
Zyrtec-D 12 Hour Extended Relief Tablets (Less than 2%) 2758

Ataxia, cerebellar

JE-VAX Vaccine (One case) 811

Atelectasis

AmBisome for Injection (Less common) 1383
Betaseron for SC Injection 988
▲ CellCept Capsules (13.7%) 2951
▲ CellCept Intravenous (13.7%) 2951
▲ CellCept Oral Suspension (13.7%) 2951
▲ CellCept Tablets (13.7%) 2951
Cerebyx Injection (Infrequent) 2619
Effexor Tablets (Rare) 3495
Effexor XR Capsules (Rare) 3499
Evoxac Capsules 1217
Gonal-F for Injection 3216
Humegon for Injection 2468
Kadian Capsules (Less than 3%) 1335
Numorphan 1324
Pergonal for Injection 3223
▲ Prograf (5% to 28%) 1393
Prozac Pulvules, Liquid, and Weekly Capsules (Rare) 1238
▲ Rapamune Oral Solution and Tablets (3% to 20%) 3584
Repronex for Intramuscular and Subcutaneous Injection 1347
Sarafem Pulvules (Rare) 1962
▲ Trasylol Injection (5%) 909
Virazole for Inhalation Solution (Infrequent) 1747
▲ Zenapax for Injection (2% to 5%) 3046
Zosyn (1.0% or less) 1890
Zosyn in Galaxy Containers (1.0% or less) 1894
Zyprexa Tablets (Infrequent) 1973
Zyprexa ZYDIS Orally Disintegrating Tablets (Infrequent) 1973

Atherosclerosis

Imitrex Injection 1549
Imitrex Nasal Spray 1554

Athetosis

Versed Injection (Less than 1%) 3027

Atrial arrhythmias

Diprivan Injectable Emulsion (Less than 1%) 667

Felbatol 3343
Imdur Tablets (Less than or equal to 5%) 1826
Mexitil Capsules (1 in 1,000) 1047
Mirapex Tablets (Less than 1%) 2834
Monopril Tablets (0.4% to 1.0%) 1091
▲ Neumega for Injection (Approximately 10%) 1434
Proleukin for Injection (Less than 1%) 1199
Remeron Tablets (Rare) 2483
Remeron SolTab Tablets (Rare) 2486
Romazicon Injection (Less than 1%) 3000
Topamax Sprinkle Capsules (Rare) 2590
Topamax Tablets (Rare) 2590
▲ Trasylol Injection (3%) 909
Zoloft 2751

Atrial contractions, premature

Adenocard Injection 1380
Cognex Capsules (Rare) 1351
Diprivan Injectable Emulsion (Less than 1%) 667
Neurontin Capsules (Rare) 2655
Neurontin Oral Solution (Rare) 2655
Neurontin Tablets (Rare) 2655
▲ Proleukin for Injection (4%) 1199
Risperdal (Rare) 1796

Atrial fibrillations

Adalat CC Tablets (Less than 1.0%) 877
Advair Diskus 100/50 1448
Advair Diskus 250/50 1448
Advair Diskus 500/50 1448
Agrylin Capsules 3232
AmBisome for Injection (Less common) 1383
Amerge Tablets (Infrequent) 1467
Amphotec (1% to 5%) 1774
Anzemet Injection 719
Anzemet Tablets 722
Aredia for Injection (Up to 6%) 2309
▲ Argatroban Injection (3%) 1478
Aricept Tablets (Frequent) 1270
Aricept Tablets (Frequent) 2665
Arthrotec Tablets (Rare) 3195
Betaseron for SC Injection 988
Campath Ampules 992
▲ Carnitor Injection (2% to 6%) 3242
Celexa (Rare) 1365
▲ CellCept Capsules (3%) 2951
▲ CellCept Intravenous (3%) 2951
▲ CellCept Oral Suspension (3%) 2951
▲ CellCept Tablets (3%) 2951
Chirocaine Injection (Less than 1%) 2909
Clozaril Tablets 2319
Cognex Capsules (Infrequent) 1351
Copaxone for Injection (Infrequent) 3306
Cordarone Intravenous (Less than 2%) 3491
Cozaar Tablets (Less than 1%) 2067
Demadex Tablets and Injection 2965
Diprivan Injectable Emulsion (Less than 1%) 667
DynaCirc Capsules (0.5% to 1%) 2921
DynaCirc CR Tablets (0.5% to 1%) 2923
Effexor Tablets 3495
Effexor XR Capsules 3499
Enalaprilat Injection 863
Exelon Capsules (Frequent) 2342
Exelon Oral Solution (Frequent) 2345
Felbatol 3343
Geodon Capsules (Infrequent) 2688
Hivid Tablets (Less than 1%) 2975
Hyzaar 2109
Idamycin PFS Injection 2825
Imdur Tablets (Less than or equal to 5%) 1826
Imitrex Injection (Extremely rare) 1549
Imitrex Nasal Spray 1554
Imitrex Tablets (Rare) 1558
Intron A for Injection (Less than 5%) 3120
Ismo Tablets (Fewer than 1%) 3524
Kadian Capsules (Less than 3%) 1335
Kytril Injection (Rare) 2986
Kytril Tablets (Rare) 2988
Lamictal (Rare) 1567
Levaquin Injection (Less than 0.5%) 2537
Lexxel Tablets 608
Lopid Tablets (0.7%) 2650
Lovenox Injection (0.7%) 746
Lupron Depot–4 Month 30 mg (Less than 5%) 3289
Meridia Capsules 481
Mirapex Tablets (1% or more) 2834
Naropin Injection (Less than 1%) 612
Natrecor for Injection (At least 1%) 3189
▲ Neumega for Injection (12%) 1434
Neurontin Capsules (Rare) 2655
Neurontin Oral Solution (Rare) 2655
Neurontin Tablets (Rare) 2655
Niaspan Extended-Release Tablets 1846
Norvasc Tablets (More than 0.1% to 1%) 2704
OptiPranolol Metipranolol Ophthalmic Solution 0.3% (A small number of patients) ⊙263
Paxil (Rare) 1609
Permax Tablets (Infrequent) 1299
▲ Photofrin for Injection (10%) 831
Plavix Tablets (1% to 2.5%) 1097
Plavix Tablets (1% to 2.5%) 3084
Pletal Tablets (Less than 2%) 2605
Pletal Tablets (Less than 2%) 2848
Prinivil Tablets (0.3% to 1.0%) 2164
Prinzide Tablets 2168
Proventil Repetabs Tablets 3148
Prozac Pulvules, Liquid, and Weekly Capsules (Rare) 1238
▲ Rapamune Oral Solution and Tablets (3% to 20%) 3584
Reminyl Oral Solution (Infrequent) 1792
Reminyl Tablets (Infrequent) 1792
▲ ReoPro Vials (3.5%) 1958
Requip Tablets (2%) 1621
Rilutek Tablets (Infrequent) 772
Risperdal 1796
Rythmol Tablets – 150 mg, 225 mg, 300 mg (1.2%) 502
Sandostatin LAR Depot (Rare) 2395
Sarafem Pulvules 1962
Serevent Diskus 1637
Serevent Inhalation Aerosol 1633
Seroquel Tablets (Rare) 684
▲ Simulect for Injection (3% to 10%) 2399
Sular Tablets (Less than or equal to 1%) 688
Tasmar Tablets (Infrequent) 3010
Taxol Injection (Rare) 1129
Taxotere for Injection Concentrate 778
▲ Tenormin (5%) 692
Teveten Tablets (Less than 1%) 3327
Thalomid Capsules 1154
Tikosyn Capsules (Greater than 2%) 2717
Topamax Sprinkle Capsules (Rare) 2590
Topamax Tablets (Rare) 2590
▲ Trasylol Injection (21%) 909
Tricor Capsules, Micronized 513
Uniretic Tablets (Less than 1%) 3178
Vaseretic Tablets 2204
Vasotec I.V. Injection 2207
Vasotec Tablets (0.5% to 1.0%) 2210
Ventolin Inhalation Aerosol and Refill 1679
Ventolin HFA Inhalation Aerosol 3618
Vioxx (Greater than 0.1% to 1.9%) 2213
Visicol Tablets (One patient) 1767
▲ Visudyne for Injection (1% to 10%) ⊙308
Zestril Tablets (0.3% to 1.0%) 698
Zofran Injection 1698
Zonegran Capsules (Rare) 1307
Zosyn (1.0% or less) 1890
Zosyn in Galaxy Containers (1.0% or less) 1894
Zyprexa Tablets 1973
Zyprexa ZYDIS Orally Disintegrating Tablets 1973

Atrial flutter

Amerge Tablets (Infrequent) 1467
Anzemet Injection 719
Anzemet Tablets 722
Aredia for Injection (Up to 1%) 2309
Cardizem Injectable (Less than 1%) 1018
Cardizem Lyo-Ject Syringe (Less than 1%) 1018
Cardizem Monovial (Less than 1%) 1018
▲ CellCept Capsules (3% to 10%) 2951
▲ CellCept Intravenous (3% to 10%) 2951
▲ CellCept Oral Suspension (3% to 10%) 2951
▲ CellCept Tablets (3% to 10%) 2951
Cerebyx Injection (Infrequent) 2619
Cipro (Less than 1%) 887
Cognex Capsules (Infrequent) 1351
▲ Neumega for Injection (12%) 1434
Pletal Tablets (Less than 2%) 2605
Pletal Tablets (Less than 2%) 2848
▲ ReoPro Vials (3.5%) 1958
Rythmol Tablets – 150 mg, 225 mg, 300 mg (Less than 1%) 502
Taxotere for Injection Concentrate (Rare) 778
Tenormin (1.6%) 692
Theo-Dur Extended-Release Tablets 1835
▲ Trasylol Injection (6%) 909
Uni-Dur Extended-Release Tablets 1841
Uniphyl 400 mg and 600 mg Tablets 2903

Atrial tachycardia

Digitek Tablets 1003
Enalaprilat Injection 863
Lanoxicaps Capsules 1574
Lanoxin Injection 1581
Lanoxin Tablets 1587
Lanoxin Elixir Pediatric 1578
Lanoxin Injection Pediatric 1584
Lexxel Tablets 608
Prinivil Tablets (0.3% to 1.0%) 2164
Prinzide Tablets 2168
Theo-Dur Extended-Release Tablets 1835
Uni-Dur Extended-Release Tablets 1841
Uniphyl 400 mg and 600 mg Tablets 2903
Vaseretic Tablets 2204
Vasotec I.V. Injection 2207
Vasotec Tablets (0.5% to 1.0%) 2210
Zestril Tablets (0.3% to 1.0%) 698

Atrioventricular dissociation

Covera-HS Tablets (Less than 2%) 3199
Digitek Tablets 1003
Isoptin SR Tablets (1% or less) 467
Lanoxicaps Capsules (Common) 1574
Lanoxin Injection (Common) 1581
Lanoxin Tablets (Common) 1587
Rythmol Tablets – 150 mg, 225 mg, 300 mg (Less than 1%) 502
Tarka Tablets 508
Verelan Capsules (1% or less) 3184
Verelan PM Capsules (2% or less) 3186

Atrophy

Bicillin C-R 900/300 Injection 2240
Bicillin C-R Injection 2238
Bicillin L-A Injection 2242
Cuprimine Capsules 2075
Norcuron for Injection 2478

Atrophy, cutaneous

Anusol-HC Cream 2.5% (Infrequent to frequent) 2237
Celestone Soluspan Injectable Suspension 3097
▲ Cordran Lotion (More frequent) 2438
▲ Cordran Tape (More frequent) 2439
Cortone Acetate Injectable Suspension 2059
Decadron Phosphate Injection 2081
Depen Titratable Tablets (Rare) 3341
Hydrocortone Acetate Injectable Suspension 2103
Hydrocortone Phosphate Injection, Sterile 2105
Solu-Medrol Sterile Powder 2855

Atrophy, iris

Healon GV ⊙320

Atrophy, subcutaneous

Celestone Soluspan Injectable Suspension 3097
Cortone Acetate Injectable Suspension 2059
Decadron Phosphate Injection 2081
Diphtheria & Tetanus Toxoids Adsorbed Purogenated for Pediatric Use 1857
Florinef Acetate Tablets 2250
Hydrocortone Acetate Injectable Suspension 2103
Hydrocortone Phosphate Injection, Sterile 2105
Lidex 2020
Synalar 2020

Atrophy, proximal muscle group

Plaquenil Tablets 3082

Atypical measles

Attenuvax 2044

Auditory acuity, decrease

Desferal Vials 2333

Auditory canals, small or absent, fetal

Accutane Capsules 2944

Auditory disturbances

Aralen Tablets 3075
Navelbine Injection 1604
▲ Wellbutrin Tablets (5.3%) 1680

Aura disappeared

Neurontin Capsules 2655
Neurontin Oral Solution 2655
Neurontin Tablets 2655

Autoimmune disorders, life-threatening, aggravation of

Roferon-A Injection 2996

Autonomic deficit, persistent

Duranest Injections 600
Nesacaine/Nesacaine MPF 617
Stelazine 1640
Symmetrel (Uncommon) 1328
Xylocaine Injections (Rare) 653

A-V block

Activase I.V. 1410
Adenocard Injection 1380
Anzemet Injection 719
Anzemet Tablets 722
Blocadren Tablets (Less than 1%) 2046
Carbatrol Capsules 3234
Cardene I.V. (Rare) 3485
Catapres Tablets (Rare) 1037
Catapres-TTS (0.5% or less) 1038
Clorpres Tablets (Rare) 1002
Cognex Capsules (Rare) 1351
Combipres Tablets (Rare) 1040
Cordarone Intravenous 3491
Coreg Tablets (0.1% to 2.9%) 1508
Corvert Injection (1.5%) 2793
Covera-HS Tablets (0.8% to 2%) 3199
Digitek Tablets 1003
Diprivan Injectable Emulsion (Less than 1%) 667
Duraclon Injection (Rare) 3057
Ellence Injection 2806
Exelon Capsules (Infrequent) 2342
Exelon Oral Solution (Infrequent) 2345
Famotidine Injection (Infrequent) 866
Inderide Tablets 3517
Inderide LA Long-Acting Capsules 3519
Isoptin SR Tablets (0.8% to 1.2%) 467
Kytril Injection (Rare) 2986
Lanoxicaps Capsules 1574
Lanoxin Injection 1581
Lanoxin Tablets 1587
Lanoxin Elixir Pediatric (Common) 1578
Lanoxin Injection Pediatric (Common) 1584
Luvox Tablets (25, 50, 100 mg) (Rare) 3256
Mexitil Capsules (About 2 in 1,000) 1047
Nipent for Injection (Less than 3%) 3272
Normodyne Tablets 3137
Pepcid Injection (Infrequent) 2153
Pepcid for Oral Suspension (Infrequent) 2150
Pepcid RPD Orally Disintegrating Tablets (Infrequent) 2150
Pepcid Tablets (Infrequent) 2150
Permax Tablets (Infrequent) 1299
Prostigmin Injectable 1744
Prostigmin Tablets 1744
Reglan 2935
Remicade for IV Injection (Less than 2%) 1178
Reminyl Oral Solution (Infrequent) 1792
Reminyl Tablets (Infrequent) 1792
ReoPro Vials (1.3%) 1958
Retavase Vials 1182
Risperdal (Infrequent) 1796
▲ Rythmol Tablets – 150 mg, 225 mg, 300 mg (2% to 5%) 502
Salagen Tablets (Rare) 2229
Sectral Capsules 3589
Serzone Tablets (Rare) 1104
Tagamet (Rare) 1644
Tambocor Tablets 1990
Taxol Injection 1129
Tegretol/Tegretol-XR 2404
▲ Tiazac Capsules (4%) 1378
Tikosyn Capsules (Up to 1.5%) 2717
Timolide Tablets 2187
TNKase I.V. 1430
Tonocard Tablets (Less than 1%) 649
Topamax Sprinkle Capsules (Infrequent) 2590
Topamax Tablets (Infrequent) 2590
Verelan Capsules (0.8% to 1.2%) 3184
Verelan PM Capsules (0.8% to 1.2%) 3186
Viagra Tablets (Less than 2%) 2732
Wellbutrin SR Sustained-Release Tablets 1684
Zantac (Rare) 1690
Zantac Injection (Rare) 1688
Zantac Syrup (Rare) 1690
Zoloft 2751
Zyban Sustained-Release Tablets 1710

A-V block, first-degree

Adenocard Injection 1380
Adenoscan (2.9% to 3%) 1381
Aricept Tablets (Infrequent) 1270
Aricept Tablets (Infrequent) 2665
Cardizem Injectable (Less than 1%) 1018
Cardizem Lyo-Ject Syringe (Less than 1%) 1018
Cardizem Monovial (Less than 1%) 1018
Cardizem CD Capsules (2.4% to 3.3%) 1016
Corgard Tablets (Single instance) 2245
Corzide 40/5 Tablets (One instance) 2247
Corzide 80/5 Tablets (One instance) 2247
Covera-HS Tablets (1.2% to 1.7%) 3199
Digitek Tablets 1003
Effexor Tablets (Rare) 3495
Effexor XR Capsules (Rare) 3499
Foscavir Injection (Between 1% and 5%) 605
Geodon Capsules (Rare) 2688
Isoptin SR Tablets (1.2%) 467
Lanoxicaps Capsules 1574
Lanoxin Injection 1581

Lanoxin Tablets 1587
Lanoxin Elixir Pediatric 1578
Lanoxin Injection Pediatric 1584
Mavik Tablets (0.3% to 1.0%) 478
Rythmol Tablets – 150 mg, 225 mg, 300 mg (1.9% to 4.5%) 502
Seroquel Tablets (Infrequent) 684
Sular Tablets (Less than or equal to 1%) 688
▲ Tarka Tablets (3.9%) 508
Uniretic Tablets (Less than 1%) 3178
Verelan Capsules (1.2%) 3184
Verelan PM Capsules (1.2%) 3186

A-V block, intensification of
Blocadren Tablets 2046
Duraclon Injection (Rare) 3057
Inderal 3513
Inderal LA Long-Acting Capsules 3516
Inderide Tablets 3517
Inderide LA Long-Acting Capsules 3519
Nadolol Tablets (Single instance) 2288
Sectral Capsules 3589
Tenoretic Tablets 690
Toprol-XL Tablets 651

A-V block, second-degree
Adenocard Injection 1380
Adenoscan (2.6% to 3%) 1381
Blocadren Tablets (Less than 1%) 2046
Cardizem Injectable (Less than 1%) 1018
Cardizem Lyo-Ject Syringe (Less than 1%) 1018
Cardizem Monovial (Less than 1%) 1018
Cardizem CD Capsules (Less than 1%) 1016
Covera-HS Tablets (0.8% to 2%) 3199
Cozaar Tablets (Less than 1%) 2067
Digitek Tablets 1003
Hyzaar 2109
Isoptin SR Tablets (0.8%) 467
Lanoxicaps Capsules 1574
Lanoxin Injection 1581
Lanoxin Tablets 1587
Lanoxin Elixir Pediatric 1578
Lanoxin Injection Pediatric 1584
Proleukin for Injection (Less than 1%) 1199
Rythmol Tablets – 150 mg, 225 mg, 300 mg (1.2%) 502
Tambocor Tablets (Less than 1%) 1990
Tarka Tablets (Less frequent) 508
Verelan Capsules (0.8% to 1.2%) 3184
Verelan PM Capsules (0.8% to 1.2%) 3186

A-V block, third-degree
Adenocard Injection 1380
Adenoscan (0.8%; less than 1%) 1381
Blocadren Tablets (Less than 1%) 2046
Cardizem Injectable 1018
Cardizem Lyo-Ject Syringe 1018
Cardizem Monovial 1018
Cardizem CD Capsules (Less than 1%) 1016
Corzide 40/5 Tablets (One instance) 2247
Corzide 80/5 Tablets (One instance) 2247
Covera-HS Tablets (0.8% to 2%) 3199
Digitek Tablets 1003
Isoptin SR Tablets (0.8%) 467
Lanoxicaps Capsules 1574
Lanoxin Injection 1581
Lanoxin Tablets 1587
Lanoxin Elixir Pediatric 1578
Lanoxin Injection Pediatric 1584
Tambocor Tablets (Less than 1%) 1990
Tarka Tablets 508
Verelan Capsules (0.8% to 1.2%) 3184
Verelan PM Capsules (0.8% to 1.2%) 3186
Wellbutrin Tablets 1680

A-V conduction, prolongation
Sensorcaine 643
Sensorcaine-MPF Injection 643

A-V conduction changes, unspecified
Natrecor for Injection (At least 1%) 3189
Nimotop Capsules 904

A-V shunt, thrombosis of
(*see under* Thrombosis of vascular access)

Avitaminosis
Kaletra Capsules (Less than 2%) 471
Kaletra Oral Solution (Less than 2%) 471
Norvir Capsules (Less than 2%) 487
Norvir Oral Solution (Less than 2%) 487
Thalomid Capsules 1154

Awareness, altered
Diprivan Injectable Emulsion (Less than 1%) 667
Halcion Tablets 2823
▲ Tonocard Tablets (1.5% to 11.0%) 649
Wellbutrin SR Sustained-Release Tablets (Rare) 1684

Awareness, heightened
Demser Capsules 2085
Imitrex Tablets (Rare) 1558
▲ Marinol Capsules (8% to 24%) 3325

Azoospermia
Mustargen for Injection 2142

Azotemia
Altace Capsules 2233
Ancobon Capsules 1730
Aredia for Injection (Up to 4%) 2309
Avalide Tablets 1070
Carbatrol Capsules 3234
Cataflam Tablets (Less than 1%) 2315
Cleocin HCl Capsules (Rare) 2784
Cleocin Phosphate Sterile Solution (Rare) 2785
Cleocin Vaginal Cream (Rare) 2788
Cleocin Vaginal Ovules (Rare) 2789
Demadex Tablets and Injection 2965
Diuril Sodium Intravenous 2086
Dyrenium Capsules (Rare) 3458
Effexor Tablets (Rare) 3495
Effexor XR Capsules (Rare) 3499
Elspar for Injection (Frequent) 2092
Enalaprilat Injection 863
Furosemide Tablets 2284
HydroDIURIL Tablets 2108
Hyzaar 2109
▲ Indocin I.V. (41% of infants) 2115
Lotrel Capsules 2370
Minocin Intravenous 1862
Minocin Oral Suspension 1865
Minocin Pellet-Filled Capsules 1863
Monopril Tablets 1091
Monopril HCT 1094
Motrin Suspension, Oral Drops, Chewable Tablets, and Caplets (Less than 1%) 2002
Mykrox Tablets 1168
Prinivil Tablets (0.3% to 1.0%) 2164
Prinzide Tablets 2168
Relafen Tablets (Less than 1%) 1617
Remicade for IV Injection (Less than 2%) 1178
Renese Tablets 2712
Requip Tablets (Rare) 1621
Tegretol/Tegretol-XR 2404
Tenoretic Tablets 690
Toradol 3018
Vancocin HCl Capsules & Pulvules 1972
Vancocin HCl Oral Solution 1971
Vancocin HCl, Vials & ADD-Vantage 1970
Vaseretic Tablets 2204
Vasotec I.V. Injection 2207
Vasotec Tablets 2210
Voltaren Tablets (Less than 1%) 2315
Voltaren-XR Tablets (Less than 1%) 2315
Zaroxolyn Tablets 1177
Zestoretic Tablets 695
Zestril Tablets (0.3% to 1.0%) 698

B

Babinski's phenomenon, bilateral
Cerebyx Injection (Infrequent) 2619
Dopram Injectable 2931
Neurontin Capsules (Infrequent) 2655
Neurontin Oral Solution (Infrequent) 2655
Neurontin Tablets (Infrequent) 2655

Back strain
Prinzide Tablets (0.3% to 1%) 2168
Zestoretic Tablets (0.3% to 1.0%) 695

Backache
Accolate Tablets (1.5%) 657
Accupril Tablets (0.5% to 1.2%) 2611
Accuretic Tablets (1.5%) 2614
Aceon Tablets (2 mg, 4 mg, 8 mg) (Up to 5.8%) 3249
Actimmune (2%) 1772
Actiq (1% or greater) 1184
▲ Activella Tablets (3% to 6%) 2764
▲ Actonel Tablets (26.1%) 2879
Adenocard Injection (Less than 1%) 1380
Adenoscan (Less than 1%) 1381
Advair Diskus 100/50 1448
Advair Diskus 250/50 1448
Advair Diskus 500/50 1448
▲ Aggrenox Capsules (4.6%) 1026
▲ Agrylin Capsules (5.9%) 3232
Alamast Ophthalmic Solution (Less than 5%) 3092
Alferon N Injection (Up to 4%) 1770
Allegra (2.2% to 2.8%) 712
Allegra-D Extended-Release Tablets (1.9%) 714
▲ Alora Transdermal System (3.4% to 7.4%) 3372
▲ Ambien Tablets (3%) 3191
▲ AmBisome for Injection (12%) 1383
▲ Amphotec (5% or more) 1774
Apligraf (1.8%) 2305
▲ Arava Tablets (5%) 724
▲ Aredia for Injection (At least 5%) 2309
▲ Arimidex Tablets (10.6% to 11.9%) 659
▲ Aromasin Tablets (2% to 5%) 2769
▲ Asacol Delayed-Release Tablets (7%) 2884
Astelin Nasal Spray (Infrequent) 3339
▲ Atacand Tablets (3%) 595
▲ Atacand HCT Tablets (3.3%) 597
▲ Atrovent Inhalation Solution (3.2%) 1031
▲ Avandia Tablets (4% to 5%) 1490
Avelox Tablets (0.05% to 1%) 879
Axert Tablets (Infrequent) 2772
Axid Pulvules (2.4%) 1903
Axid Pulvules (2.4%) 2919
▲ Azmacort Inhalation Aerosol (2% to 4%) 728
▲ Baycol Tablets (3.4%) 883
Betapace Tablets (1% to 3%) 950
▲ Botox Purified Neurotoxin Complex (2% to 10%) 549
▲ Campath Ampules (3% to 10%) 992
Carafate Suspension (Less than 0.5%) 731
Carafate Tablets (Less than 0.5%) 730
Cardura Tablets (1.8%) 2668
▲ Carnitor Injection (6% to 9%) 3242
▲ Casodex Tablets (15%) 662
Caverject Sterile Powder (1%) 2777
Ceclor CD Tablets (1.0%) 1279
Celebrex Capsules (2.8%) 2676
Celebrex Capsules (2.8%) 2780
Celexa (At least 2%) 1365
▲ CellCept Capsules (11.6% to 12.1%) 2951
▲ CellCept Intravenous (11.6% to 12.1%) 2951
▲ CellCept Oral Suspension (11.6% to 12.1%) 2951
▲ CellCept Tablets (11.6% to 46.6%) 2951
▲ Cenestin Tablets (14%) 1263
Cerebyx Injection (2.2%) 2619
Cerezyme for Injection 1438
▲ Chemet Capsules (5.2% to 15.7%) 3078
▲ Chirocaine Injection (5.7%) 2909
Cipro I.V. (1% or less) 893
Cipro I.V. Pharmacy Bulk Package (Less than 1%) 897
Cipro (Less than 1%) 887
Claritin (At least one patient) 3100
Claritin-D 12 Hour Extended Release Tablets (Less frequent) 3102
Claritin-D 24 Hour Extended Release Tablets (Fewer than 2%) 3104
Clomid Tablets 735
Clozaril Tablets (1%) 2319
Cognex Capsules (2%) 1351
Colazal Capsules (2%) 3069
Colestid Tablets 2791
▲ CombiPatch Transdermal System (14% to 15%) 2323
Comtan Tablets (2%) 2328
▲ Copaxone for Injection (16%) 3306
▲ Coreg Tablets (2.3% to 6.9%) 1508
Corlopam Injection (1% to 2%) 412
Cosopt Sterile Ophthalmic Solution (1% to 5%) 2065
Cozaar Tablets (1.8%) 2067
▲ Crinone (8%) 3213
Crixivan Capsules (2%) 2070
CytoGam Intravenous (Less than 5.0%) 2026
Cytotec Tablets (Infrequent) 3202
Dantrium Capsules (Less frequent) 2885
▲ DaunoXome Injection (13.8% to 16%) 1442
Depacon Injection (1% to 5%) 416
Depakene (1% to 5%) 421
Depakote Sprinkle Capsules (1% to 5%) 426
▲ Depakote Tablets (1% to 8%) 430
▲ Depakote ER Tablets (8%) 436
▲ DepoCyt Injection (7%) 1197
▲ Depo-Provera Contraceptive Injection (More than 5%) 2798
Detrol Tablets (2.7%) 3623
Diovan Capsules 2337
Diovan HCT Tablets (More than 2%) 2338
Ditropan XL Extended Release Tablets (2% to 5%) 564
▲ Doxil Injection (Approximately 6.8%) 566
DuoNeb Inhalation Solution 1233
Duranest Injections 600
DynaCirc CR Tablets (0.5% to 1%) 2923
Effexor Tablets 3495
Effexor XR Capsules 3499
Eldepryl Capsules (1 of 49 patients) 3266
Engerix-B Vaccine (Less than 1%) 1517
▲ Esclim Transdermal System (2.1% to 6.4%) 3460
▲ Estring Vaginal Ring (6%) 2811
▲ Evoxac Capsules (4.5%) 1217
Exelon Capsules (2% or more) 2342
Exelon Oral Solution (2% or more) 2345
Famvir Tablets (1.5% to 1.9%) 2348
▲ Femara Tablets (17% to 22%) 2351
▲ femhrt Tablets (4.7%) 2635
Ferrlecit Injection (Greater than 1%) 3386
▲ Flolan for Injection (2% to 13%) 1528
▲ Flomax Capsules (7.0% to 8.3%) 1044
Flovent Rotadisk (Less than 1% to 4%) 1537
Fortovase Capsules (Less than 2%) 2970
Foscavir Injection (Between 1% and 5%) 605
Gabitril Tablets (1% or more) 1189
Gamimune N, 5% Solvent/Detergent Treated 925
Gamimune N, 10% Solvent/Detergent Treated 928
Gammagard S/D (Occasional) 845
▲ Gammar-P I.V. (3.6%) 787
Gliadel Wafer (1%) 1723
▲ Gonal-F for Injection (5.1%) 3216
▲ Herceptin I.V. (22%) 1414
Hivid Tablets (Less than 1%) 2975
▲ Humatrope Vials and Cartridges (9.1% to 9.8%) 1930
Hycamtin for Injection (2%) 1546
Hytrin Capsules (2.4%) 464
Hyzaar (2.1%) 2109
Imdur Tablets (Less than or equal to 5%) 1826
Imitrex Injection (Rare) 1549
Imitrex Nasal Spray (Infrequent) 1554
▲ Indapamide Tablets (Greater than or equal to 5%) 2286
INFeD Injection 3388
▲ Infergen (29% to 42%) 1777
Innohep Injection (1.5%) 1248
▲ Intron A for Injection (Up to 19%) 3120
Invirase Capsules (Less than 2%) 2979
Kadian Capsules (Less than 3%) 1335
Kaletra Capsules (Less than 2%) 471
Kaletra Oral Solution (Less than 2%) 471
Keppra Tablets (1% or more) 3314
Klonopin Tablets (Infrequent) 2983
Lamictal (More than 1%) 1567
▲ Lescol Capsules (5.7%) 2361
▲ Lescol Capsules (5.7%) 2925
▲ Lescol XL Tablets (4.7%) 2361
▲ Lescol XL Tablets (4.7%) 2925
▲ Leukine (9%) 1755
Levaquin (1.0%) 2537
Lexxel Tablets (Infrequent) 608
▲ Lipitor Tablets (Up to 3.8%) 2639
▲ Lipitor Tablets (Up to 3.8%) 2696
Lodosyn Tablets 1251
Lotensin HCT Tablets (More than 1%) 2367
Lotrel Capsules 2370
Luvox Tablets (25, 50, 100 mg) 3256
LYMErix Vaccine (1.90% to 3.58%) 1592
▲ Malarone (4% to 8%) 1596
▲ Meridia Capsules (8.2%) 481
Merrem I.V. (0.1% to 1.0%) 673
▲ Miacalcin Nasal Spray (5.0%) 2375
▲ Micardis Tablets (3%) 1049
Micardis HCT Tablets (Less than 2%) 1051
Midamor Tablets (Less than or equal to 1%) 2136
Mirapex Tablets (Less than 1%) 2834
▲ Mirena Intrauterine System (5% or more) 974
Mobic Tablets (0.5% to 3%) 1054
Moduretic Tablets (Less than or equal to 1%) 2138
▲ Monurol Sachet (3.0%) 1375
MUSE Urethral Suppository (2%) 3335
Mykrox Tablets (Less than 2%) 1168
▲ Mylotarg for Injection (14% to 22%) 3540
▲ Myobloc Injectable Solution (3% to 7%) 1291
▲ Naprelan Tablets (3% to 9%) 1293
▲ Naropin Injection (More than 5% to 16.4%) 612
Nascobal Gel 3174
▲ Natrecor for Injection (4%) 3189
Navelbine Injection 1604
Nesacaine/Nesacaine MPF 617
Neurontin Capsules (1.8%) 2655
Neurontin Oral Solution (1.8%) 2655
Neurontin Tablets (1.8%) 2655
Nexium Delayed-Release Capsules (Less than 1%) 619
▲ Nicotrol Inhaler (Greater than 3%) 2840
▲ Nicotrol Nasal Spray (6%) 2843
▲ Nilandron Tablets (11.5%) 753
Noroxin Tablets (0.3% to 1.0%) 2145
Norvasc Tablets (More than 0.1% to 1%) 2704
Norvir Capsules (Less than 2%) 487
Norvir Oral Solution (Less than 2%) 487
▲ Novantrone for Injection (6% to 8%) 1760
▲ Ortho-Prefest Tablets (12%) 2570
ParaGard T 380A Intrauterine Copper Contraceptive 2582
▲ Paxil (3%) 1609
Periostat Tablets (2% to 3%) 1208

Permax Tablets (1.6%) 1299
▲ Photofrin for Injection (11%) 831
Plasmanate (Occasional) 942
▲ Plavix Tablets (5.8%) 1097
▲ Plavix Tablets (5.8%) 3084
Plendil Extended-Release Tablets (0.5% to 1.5%) 623
▲ Pletal Tablets (6% to 7%) 2605
▲ Pletal Tablets (6% to 7%) 2848
▲ Prandin Tablets (0.5, 1, and 2 mg) (5% to 6%) 2432
Premphase Tablets 3572
▲ Prempro Tablets (13% to 14%) 3572
▲ Prepidil Gel (3.1%) 2851
Prilosec Delayed-Release Capsules (1.1%) 628
Prinivil Tablets (0.3% to greater than 1.0%) 2164
Prinzide Tablets (0.3% to 1%) 2168
ProAmatine Tablets (Rare) 3241
Procardia XL Extended Release Tablets (1% or less) 2710
▲ Prograf (17% to 30%) 1393
▲ Proleukin for Injection (9%) 1199
▲ Prometrium Capsules (100 mg, 200 mg) (8%) 3261
ProSom Tablets (2%) 500
Prostin E2 Suppositories 2852
Protonix I.V. (Greater than or equal to 1%) 3580
Protonix Tablets (Greater than or equal to 1%) 3577
Protopic Ointment (1% to 3%) 1397
▲ Proventil HFA Inhalation Aerosol (4%) 3150
Provera Tablets 2853
Provigil Tablets (At least 1%) 1193
Prozac Pulvules, Liquid, and Weekly Capsules (Less than 1%) 1238
▲ Pulmicort Turbuhaler Inhalation Powder (2% to 6%) 636
Qvar Inhalation Aerosol (Less than 1% to 4%) 1987
▲ Rapamune Oral Solution and Tablets (16% to 26%) 3584
Recombivax HB (Less than 1%) 2178
Remeron Tablets (2%) 2483
Remeron SolTab Tablets (2%) 2486
▲ Remicade for IV Injection (5% to 6%) 1178
Reminyl Oral Solution (Greater than or equal to 2%) 1792
Reminyl Tablets (Greater than or equal to 2%) 1792
Requip Tablets (1% or more) 1621
Rescriptor Tablets (Less than 2%) 526
Retrovir Capsules 1625
Retrovir IV Infusion 1629
Retrovir 1625
▲ Rilutek Tablets (1.7% to 4.1%) 772
Risperdal (Up to 2%) 1796
Rituxan for Infusion (1% to 5%) 1750
Rituxan I.V. (1% to 5%) 1428
▲ Roferon-A Injection (16%) 2996
Rowasa Rectal Suspension Enema 4.0 grams/unit (60 mL) (1.35%) 3264
Roxicodone Tablets (Less than 3%) 3067
Salagen Tablets (1% to 2%) 2229
Sandostatin Injection (1% to 4%) 2394
Sectral Capsules (Up to 2%) 3589
Sensorcaine 643
Sensorcaine-MPF Injection 643
Serevent Inhalation Aerosol (1% to 4%) 1633
Serophene Tablets 3226
Seroquel Tablets (2%) 684
▲ Serostim for Injection (1% to 10%) 3229
Serzone Tablets 1104
▲ Simulect for Injection (3% to 10%) 2399
Sinemet Tablets 1253
Sinemet CR Tablets (1.6%) 1255
▲ Skelid Tablets (8.0%) 3088
Sonata Capsules (Frequent) 3591
▲ Soriatane Capsules (1% to 10%) 3003
Sporanox Oral Solution (Less than 2%) 1808
Sporanox Oral Solution (Less than 2%) 2512
▲ Starlix Tablets (4%) 2401
Streptase for Infusion 647
Synvisc 3596
Tarka Tablets (2.2%) 508
Taxol Injection (Rare) 1129
Taxotere for Injection Concentrate 778
▲ Temodar Capsules (8%) 3157
Tequin Injection (0.1% to 3%) 1110
Tequin Tablets (0.1% to 3%) 1110
Teveten Tablets (Less than 1%) 3327
Thalomid Capsules (4.2%) 1154
▲ Tikosyn Capsules (3%) 2717
▲ TOBI Solution for Inhalation (7%) 1206
▲ Topamax Sprinkle Capsules (2% to 6.2%) 2590
▲ Topamax Tablets (2% to 6.2%) 2590
Travatan Ophthalmic Solution (1% to 5%) 543
▲ Tricor Capsules, Micronized (3.4%) 513
Trileptal Oral Suspension (2% to 4%) 2407
Trileptal Tablets (2% to 4%) 2407
▲ Tri-Nasal Spray (4.7% to 7.8%) 2274
▲ Trisenox Injection (18%) 1158
Trovan (Less than 1%) 2722
Twinrix Vaccine (Less than 1%) 1674
Uniretic Tablets (More than 1%) 3178
▲ Vagifem Tablets (7%) 2857
▲ Valstar Sterile Solution for Intravesical Instillation (3%) 1175
Vancocin HCl Capsules & Pulvules 1972
Vancocin HCl Oral Solution 1971
Vancocin HCl, Vials & ADD-Vantage 1970
Vantin Tablets and Oral Suspension (Less than 1%) 2860
Vaqta (1.1%) 2199
Vaseretic Tablets (0.5% to 2.0%) 2204
Viagra Tablets (Greater than 2%) 2732
Vioxx (1.9%) 2213
Viracept 532
Vistide Injection 1445
▲ Visudyne for Injection (1% to 10%) ⊙308
Vitravene for Injection (2% to 5%) ⊙310
▲ WelChol Tablets (3%) 3073
Wellbutrin SR Sustained-Release Tablets (At least 1%) 1684
WinRho SDF 2297
Xalatan Latanoprost Ophthalmic Solution (1% to 2%) ⊙320
Xalatan Sterile Ophthalmic Solution (1% to 2%) 2864
▲ Xenical Capsules (13.90%) 3043
▲ Xylocaine Injections (3%) 653
Yasmin 28 Tablets (Greater than 1%) 980
Zanaflex Tablets (Frequent) 1305
Zebeta Tablets 1885
▲ Zenapax for Injection (Greater than 5%) 3046
Zestoretic Tablets (0.3% to 1%) 695
Zestril Tablets (0.3% to 1.0%) 698
Ziac Tablets 1887
▲ Zoladex (4% to 7%) 702
Zoladex 3-month (1% to 5%) 706
Zoloft (Frequent) 2751
Zomig Tablets (Infrequent) 708
Zomig-ZMT Tablets (Infrequent) 708
Zosyn (1.0% or less) 1890
Zosyn in Galaxy Containers (1.0% or less) 1894
Zyban Sustained-Release Tablets (Infrequent) 1710
▲ Zyprexa Tablets (4%) 1973
▲ Zyprexa ZYDIS Orally Disintegrating Tablets (4%) 1973
Zyrtec (Less than 2%) 2756
Zyrtec-D 12 Hour Extended Relief Tablets (Less than 2%) 2758

Bacteremia

Enbrel for Injection 1752
Enbrel for Injection 3504
Retrovir Capsules (1.6%) 1625
Retrovir IV Infusion (2%) 1629
Retrovir (1.6%) 1625
Zenapax for Injection 3046

Bacteriuria

Primaxin I.M. 2158
Sinemet Tablets 1253
Sinemet CR Tablets (1% or greater) 1255

Bad breath
(see under Halitosis)

Balance, loss of
(see also under Equilibrium dysfunction)

Eldepryl Capsules 3266
Rythmol Tablets – 150 mg, 225 mg, 300 mg (1.2%) 502
Tarka Tablets (Less frequent) 508
Tasmar Tablets (2% to 3%) 3010
Versed Injection (Less than 1%) 3027

Balanitis

Betaseron for SC Injection 988
Declomycin Tablets 1855
Doxil Injection (Less than 1%) 566
Dynacin Capsules (Rare) 2019
Lupron Depot 7.5 mg (Less than 5%) 3284
Minocin Intravenous (Rare) 1862
Minocin Oral Suspension (Rare) 1865
Minocin Pellet-Filled Capsules (Rare) 1863
Protonix I.V. (Less than 1%) 3580
Protonix Tablets (Less than 1%) 3577
Stimate Nasal Spray 796

Balanoposthitis

Requip Tablets (Infrequent) 1621
Trovan (Less than 1%) 2722
Zoloft (Rare) 2751
Zosyn (1.0% or less) 1890
Zosyn in Galaxy Containers (1.0% or less) 1894

Baldness, male pattern
(see under Alopecia hereditaria)

Barrett's esophagus

Nexium Delayed-Release Capsules (Less than 1%) 619

Basophils, increase

Dynabac Tablets (0.1% to 1%) 2269
Effexor Tablets (Rare) 3495
Effexor XR Capsules (Rare) 3499
Geodon Capsules (Rare) 2688
Paxil (Rare) 1609
Primaxin I.M. 2158
Primaxin I.V. 2160
Rocephin Injectable Vials, ADD-Vantage, Galaxy, Bulk (Rare) 2993
Unasyn for Injection 2728
Vantin Tablets and Oral Suspension 2860
Vesanoid Capsules (Isolated cases) 3037

BBB + Major Axis Deviation

▲ Tenormin (6.6%) 692

BCG infection, disseminated

Tice BCG, BCG Live (Very rare) 2489

Beckwith-Wiedemann syndrome

Antagon Injection 2447

Behavior, hypochondriacal

Celontin Capsules 2618

Behavior, inappropriate

Artane 1855
Ativan Injection (Occasional) 3478
Diprivan Injectable Emulsion (Less than 1%) 667
Halcion Tablets 2823
ProSom Tablets 500
Ritalin 2387
Serentil 1057
Symmetrel 1328
Tessalon Capsules (Isolated instances) 1377
Xanax Tablets (Rare) 2865

Behavior, schizophrenic

Zonegran Capsules (2%) 1307

Behavior, violent

Prozac Pulvules, Liquid, and Weekly Capsules 1238
Sarafem Pulvules 1962
Tenex Tablets 2942
Zovirax 1706

Behavioral changes

Akineton 402
Ambien Tablets 3191
Amoxil Chewable Tablets (Rare) 1471
Amoxil for Oral Suspension (Rare) 1471
Amoxil (Rare) 1471
Augmentin Chewable Tablets (Rare) 1482
Augmentin Powder for Oral Suspension (Rare) 1482
Augmentin Tablets (Rare) 1485
Augmentin ES-600 Powder for Oral Suspension (Rare) 1487
Biaxin/Biaxin XL 403
Catapres Tablets 1037
Catapres-TTS (0.5% or less) 1038
Clorpres Tablets 1002
Combipres Tablets 1040
Corgard Tablets (6 of 1000 patients) 2245
Cosopt Sterile Ophthalmic Solution 2065
Cytotec Tablets (Infrequent) 3202
Duraclon Injection (Rare) 3057
Eldepryl Capsules 3266
Fortovase Capsules (Less than 2%) 2970
Gastrocrom Oral Concentrate (Less common) 1162
JE-VAX Vaccine (One case) 811
▲ Klonopin Tablets (5% to 25%) 2983
Monopril Tablets (0.4% to 1.0%) 1091
Nadolol Tablets (6 of 1000 patients) 2288
Neurontin Capsules 2655
Neurontin Oral Solution 2655
Neurontin Tablets 2655
▲ Orap Tablets (27.7%) 1407
PREVPAC 3298
Priftin Tablets 758
Rifadin 765
Rifater Tablets 769
▲ Roferon-A Injection (3%) 2996
Thioridazine Hydrochloride Tablets 2289
Timolol GFS ⊙266
Timoptic in Ocudose (Less frequent) 2192
Timoptic Sterile Ophthalmic Solution (Less frequent) 2190
Timoptic-XE Sterile Ophthalmic Gel Forming Solution 2194
Uniphyl 400 mg and 600 mg Tablets 2903
Valtrex Caplets 1676
Vascor Tablets (0.5% to 2.0%) 2602
Ventolin Inhalation Aerosol and Refill (1%) 1679
Versed Syrup (Less than 1%) 3033
Zyprexa Tablets 1973
Zyprexa ZYDIS Orally Disintegrating Tablets 1973

Behavioral deterioration

Depacon Injection 416
Depakene 421
Depakote Sprinkle Capsules 426
Depakote Tablets 430
Depakote ER Tablets 436

BEI, increase

Aygestin Tablets 1333

Belching

▲ Actonel Tablets (3.3%) 2879
Urecholine Tablets 2445

Bell's palsy

Aldoclor Tablets 2035
Aldomet Tablets 2037
Aldoril Tablets 2039
Avonex 1013
Cognex Capsules (Rare) 1351
Comvax 2056
Cytovene 2959
Engerix-B Vaccine 1517
Flexeril Tablets (Rare) 572
Flexeril Tablets (Rare) 2094
Hivid Tablets (Less than 1%) 2975
Intron A for Injection (Less than 5%) 3120
JE-VAX Vaccine (One case) 811
Mevacor Tablets (0.5% to 1.0%) 2132
Permax Tablets (Rare) 1299
Pravachol Tablets 1099
Recombivax HB 2178
Sandostatin Injection (Less than 1%) 2394
Sandostatin LAR Depot (Rare) 2395
Soriatane Capsules (Less than 5%) 3003
Thalomid Capsules 1154
Twinrix Vaccine 1674
Varivax 2202
Zocor Tablets 2219

Benzyl alcohol, sensitivity to

Amicar Injection 3608
AquaMEPHYTON Injection 2042
Cardizem Lyo-Ject Syringe 1018
Cleocin Phosphate Sterile Solution 2785
Depo-Medrol Injectable Suspension 2795
Dopram Injectable 2931
Epogen for Injection 582
Fragmin Injection 2814
Heparin Lock Flush Solution 3509
Herceptin I.V. 1414
Innohep Injection 1248
Leukine 1755
Leustatin Injection 2495
Lupron Injection 3279
Lupron Injection Pediatric 3280
Norditropin Cartridges 2420
Norditropin for Injection 2419
Nutropin for Injection 1417
Procrit for Injection 2502
Roferon-A Injection 2996
Saizen for Injection 3225
Solu-Medrol Sterile Powder 2855
Versed Injection 3027

Bezoar

Carafate Suspension 731
Carafate Tablets 730
Ecotrin Enteric Coated Aspirin Low, Regular and Maximum Strength Tablets 1715
Prevacid Delayed-Release Capsules (Less than 1%) 3292
PREVPAC (Less than 1%) 3298

Bigeminy

Digitek Tablets 1003
Diprivan Injectable Emulsion (Less than 1%) 667
Effexor Tablets (Rare) 3495
Effexor XR Capsules (Rare) 3499
Lanoxicaps Capsules 1574
Lanoxin Injection 1581
Lanoxin Tablets 1587
Lanoxin Elixir Pediatric 1578
Lanoxin Injection Pediatric 1584
Remeron Tablets (Rare) 2483
Remeron SolTab Tablets (Rare) 2486
Sonata Capsules (Rare) 3591
Suprane Liquid for Inhalation (Less than 1%) 874
Taxol Injection (Approximately 1%) 1129
Uniretic Tablets (Less than 1%) 3178
Versed Injection (Less than 1%) 3027
Versed Syrup (Less than 1%) 3033
Virazole for Inhalation Solution (Infrequent) 1747

Bile duct obstruction
Thalomid Capsules 1154

Bile duct sludge, presence of metabolites
Clinoril Tablets (Rare) 2053

Biliary lithiasis
Rocephin Injectable Vials, ADD-Vantage, Galaxy, Bulk 2993

Biliary sclerosis
Sterile FUDR 2974

Biliary sludge
Rocephin Injectable Vials, ADD-Vantage, Galaxy, Bulk (Rare) 2993
Sandostatin Injection (Frequent) 2394

Biliary stasis
Compazine 1505
Serentil 1057
Stelazine 1640
Thioridazine Hydrochloride Tablets 2289
Trilafon 3160

Biliary tract spasm
Levo-Dromoran 1734
Mepergan Injection 3539

Bilirubinemia
▲ Abelcet Injection (4%) 1273
Ambien Tablets (Rare) 3191
▲ AmBisome for Injection (11.1% to 18.1%) 1383
Arthrotec Tablets (Rare) 3195
Asacol Delayed-Release Tablets 2884
Cancidas for Injection (0.6%) 2048
Ceclor 1905
Celexa (Rare) 1365
▲ CellCept Capsules (18%) 2951
▲ CellCept Intravenous (18%) 2951
▲ CellCept Oral Suspension (18%) 2951
▲ CellCept Tablets (14.4% to 18%) 2951
Chirocaine Injection (Less than 1%) 2909
Coreg Tablets (0.1% to 1%) 1508
Doxil Injection (Less than 1%) 566
Effexor Tablets (Rare) 3495
Effexor XR Capsules (Rare) 3499
Gengraf Capsules (1% to less than 3%) 457
Hivid Tablets (Less than 1%) 2975
Intron A for Injection (Less than 5%) 3120
Lamictal (Rare) 1567
Mefoxin for Injection 2124
Mefoxin Premixed Intravenous Solution 2127
Mobic Tablets (Less than 2%) 1054
Neoral Soft Gelatin Capsules (1% to less than 3%) 2380
Neoral Oral Solution (1% to less than 3%) 2380
Nexium Delayed-Release Capsules (Less than 1%) 619
Niaspan Extended-Release Tablets 1846
Oncaspar (Greater than 1% but less than 5%) 756
Paxil (Rare) 1609
Plavix Tablets (Less than 1%) 1097
Plavix Tablets (Less than 1%) 3084
Prevacid Delayed-Release Capsules 3292
PREVPAC 3298
Priftin Tablets (Less than 1%) 758
▲ Prograf (3% to 15%) 1393
▲ Proleukin for Injection (40%) 1199
Protonix I.V. (Less than 1%) 3580
Protonix Tablets (Less than 1%) 3577
Protopic Ointment (Greater than or equal to 1%) 1397
ReFacto Vials 1437
Requip Tablets (Infrequent) 1621
Rescriptor Tablets (Less than 2%) 526
Rifater Tablets 769
Salagen Tablets (Less than 1%) 2229
Sonata Capsules (Rare) 3591
▲ Sporanox Injection (4%) 1804
▲ Sporanox Injection (4%) 2509
Thalomid Capsules 1154
Trovan (Less than 1%) 2722
Uniretic Tablets (Less than 1%) 3178
Viracept 532
Zyprexa Tablets (Infrequent) 1973
Zyprexa ZYDIS Orally Disintegrating Tablets (Infrequent) 1973

Bilirubinuria
Primaxin I.M. 2158
Primaxin I.V. 2160
Relafen Tablets (Less than 1%) 1617
Rifamate Capsules 767
Rifater Tablets 769

Birth, premature
Accutane Capsules 2944
Sandimmune 2388

Birth defects, increased risk of
Activella Tablets 2764
Alora Transdermal System 3372
Arava Tablets 724
Aygestin Tablets 1333
Celontin Capsules 2618
Coumadin for Injection 1243
Coumadin Tablets 1243
Cuprimine Capsules 2075
Depacon Injection (Multiple reports) 416
Depakene (Multiple reports) 421
Depakote Tablets (Multiple reports) 430
Depakote ER Tablets (Multiple reports) 436
Depen Titratable Tablets 3341
Dilantin Infatabs 2624
Dilantin Kapseals 2622
Dilantin-125 Oral Suspension 2625
Efudex 1733
Humegon for Injection (1.7%) 2468
Klonopin Tablets 2983
Lo/Ovral Tablets 3532
Lo/Ovral-28 Tablets 3538
Low-Ogestrel-28 Tablets 3392
Nolvadex Tablets 678
Nordette-28 Tablets 2257
Ogestrel 0.5/50-28 Tablets 3428
Ortho Dienestrol Cream 2554
Ortho-Est Tablets 3464
Ovral Tablets 3551
Ovral-28 Tablets 3552
Ovrette Tablets 3552
Pergonal for Injection (1.7%) 3223
Podocon-25 Liquid 2608
Premarin Intravenous 3563
Premarin Vaginal Cream 3570
Premphase Tablets 3572
Prempro Tablets 3572
Rebetron Combination Therapy 3153
Repronex for Intramuscular and Subcutaneous Injection (1.7%) 1347
Serophene Tablets (2.5%) 3226
Soriatane Capsules 3003
Thalomid Capsules 1154
Triphasil-21 Tablets 3600
Triphasil-28 Tablets 3605
Vivelle Transdermal System 2412
Vivelle-Dot Transdermal System 2416
Warfarin Sodium Tablets, USP 3302
Zarontin Capsules 2659
Zarontin Syrup 2660

Birth weight, low
Adderall Tablets 3231
Adderall XR Capsules
Aggrenox Capsules 1026
Betapace Tablets 950
Dexedrine 1512
Ecotrin Enteric Coated Aspirin Low, Regular and Maximum Strength Tablets 1715
Sandimmune 2388
Sectral Capsules 3589

Births, multiple
Follistim for Injection 2465
Gonal-F for Injection 3216
▲ Humegon for Injection (20%) 2468
Ovidrel for Injection 3220
▲ Pergonal for Injection (20%) 3223
▲ Repronex for Intramuscular and Subcutaneous Injection (20%) 1347
▲ Serophene Tablets (Less than 1% to 10%) 3226

Blackout spells
Eskalith 1527
Lithium Carbonate 3061
Lithium Citrate Syrup 3061
Lithobid Slow-Release Tablets 3255
Lupron Injection (Less than 5%) 3279

Bladder, irritability
Anadrol-50 Tablets 3321
Ifex for Injection 1123
Oxandrin Tablets 1153

Bladder, loss of control
Duranest Injections 600
Nesacaine/Nesacaine MPF 617
Trilafon 3160
Xylocaine Injections 653

Bladder, neurogenic
Bicillin C-R 900/300 Injection 2240
Bicillin C-R Injection 2238
Bicillin L-A Injection 2242

Bladder, spasms
Furosemide Tablets 2284
Lupron Injection (Less than 5%) 3279
Midamor Tablets (Less than or equal to 1%) 2136
Moduretic Tablets 2138
▲ Valstar Sterile Solution for Intravesical Instillation (3% to 31%) 1175

Bladder dysfunction
Aricept Tablets (Infrequent) 1270
Aricept Tablets (Infrequent) 2665

Blanching
Catapres-TTS (1 of 101 patients) 1038
▲ Emla (37%) 602
Iopidine 0.5% Ophthalmic Solution (Less than 3%) ⊙213

Blebs, filtering (ocular)
Blephamide Ophthalmic Ointment (Increased incidence) 547
Decadron Phosphate Sterile Ophthalmic Ointment (Rare) 2083
Decadron Phosphate Sterile Ophthalmic Solution (Rare) 2084
FML Ophthalmic Ointment ⊙237
FML Ophthalmic Suspension ⊙236
FML Forte Ophthalmic Suspension ⊙235
Pred Forte Ophthalmic Suspension ⊙246
Pred Mild Sterile Ophthalmic Suspension ⊙249

Bleeding
Accolate Tablets 657
▲ Activase I.V. (Most common complication) 1410
Adriamycin PFS/RDF Injection 2767
▲ Aggrastat (Among most common) 2031
▲ Aggrenox Capsules (3.2%) 1026
Agrylin Capsules (1% to 5%) 3232
Aldara Cream, 5% (More than 1%) 1978
Alkeran for Injection 1465
Alkeran Tablets 1466
Aloprim for Injection (Less than 1%) 2292
AmBisome for Injection (Less common) 1383
▲ Amphotec (5% or more) 1774
Avonex 1013
Betapace Tablets (1% to 2%) 950
▲ Betaseron for SC Injection (3%) 988
Cafcit (2.2%) 1035
▲ Carnitor Injection (2% to 9%) 3242
▲ Cathflo Activase (Among most frequent) 3611
Ceclor 1905
Cedax 1021
Cefizox for Intramuscular or Intravenous Use 1390
Cefotan 664
Ceftin 1898
Cefzil 1076
▲ CellCept Capsules (3% to 34.6%) 2951
▲ CellCept Intravenous (3% to 34.6%) 2951
▲ CellCept Oral Suspension (3% to 34.6%) 2951
▲ CellCept Tablets (3% to 34.6%) 2951
Ceptaz for Injection 1499
Colazal Capsules 3069
Condylox Topical Solution (Less than 5%) 2437
Corlopam Injection (0.5% to 5%) 412
Coumadin for Injection 1243
Coumadin Tablets 1243
Crixivan Capsules 2070
Cytovene-IV (1% or less) 2959
Demadex Tablets and Injection 2965
Depacon Injection 416
Depakene 421
Depakote Sprinkle Capsules 426
Depakote Tablets 430
Depakote ER Tablets 436
Depen Titratable Tablets 3341
Diprivan Injectable Emulsion (Less than 1%) 667
Doxil Injection (1% to 5%) 566
Duricef 1079
Effexor Tablets 3495
Effexor XR Capsules 3499
Elspar for Injection 2092
Felbatol 3343
Ferrlecit Injection (Two or more patients) 3386
▲ Flolan for Injection (11%) 1528
Floxin I.V. 2526
Floxin Tablets 2529
Fludara for Injection (Up to 1%) 995
Fortaz 1541
Fortovase Capsules (Less than 2%) 2970
Fragmin Injection 2814
Sterile FUDR 2974
Gabitril Tablets (Infrequent) 1189
▲ Gemzar for Injection (Up to 17%) 1919
▲ Gleevec Capsules (13% to 48%) 2357
Heparin Lock Flush Solution 3509
Heparin Sodium Injection 3511
Herceptin I.V. (At least one of the 958 patients) 1414
Hycamtin for Injection (Rare) 1546
▲ Idamycin PFS Injection (63%) 2825
▲ Innohep Injection (Among most common) 1248
▲ Integrilin Injection (10.5% to 14.2%) 1213
▲ Integrilin Injection (10.5% to 14.2%) 1828
▲ Intron A for Injection (8%) 3120
Lamictal (Rare to 3%) 1567
Leukeran Tablets 1591
▲ Leukine (23% to 29%) 1755
Levulan Kerastick (Up to 4%) 971
Lorabid Suspension and Pulvules 2251
▲ Lovenox Injection (4% to 7%) 746
Maxipime for Injection 1285
Mefoxin for Injection 2124
Mefoxin Premixed Intravenous Solution 2127
Motrin Suspension, Oral Drops, Chewable Tablets, and Caplets (Less than 1%) 2002
Mustargen for Injection 2142
▲ Mylotarg for Injection (15%) 3540
Naprelan Tablets (Less than 1%) 1293
▲ Nipent for Injection (3% to 10%) 3272
Norvir Capsules (Less than 2%) 487
Norvir Oral Solution (Less than 2%) 487
▲ Novantrone for Injection (20% to 37%) 1760
NovoSeven (Greater than or equal to 2%) 2430
Omnicef 493
Oncaspar 756
▲ Paraplatin for Injection (5% to 10%) 1126
Pletal Tablets (Less than 2%) 2605
Pletal Tablets (Less than 2%) 2848
▲ Prograf (3% to 15%) 1393
Proleukin for Injection (Less than 1%) 1199
Protonix I.V. (Less than 1%) 3580
Protonix Tablets (Less than 1%) 3577
Prozac Pulvules, Liquid, and Weekly Capsules (Infrequent) 1238
▲ Rapamune Oral Solution and Tablets (3% to 20%) 3584
ReFacto Vials 1437
▲ ReoPro Vials (10.6% to 16.8%) 1958
▲ Retavase Vials (21.1%) 1182
Rilutek Tablets (Rare) 772
Risperdal (Rare) 1796
Roxicodone Tablets (Less than 3%) 3067
Sarafem Pulvules (Frequent) 1962
Serzone Tablets (Rare) 1104
▲ Simulect for Injection (3% to 10%) 2399
Soma Compound w/Codeine Tablets 3355
Soriatane Capsules (Less than 1%) 3003
Streptase for Infusion 647
Suprane Liquid for Inhalation (Less than 1%) 874
Suprax 1877
Tasmar Tablets (1%) 3010
▲ Taxol Injection (14%) 1129
Tazicef for Injection 1647
Tazicef Galaxy Container 1650
Tazicef Pharmacy Bulk Package 1653
Tazidime Vials, Faspak & ADD-Vantage 1966
Testred Capsules, 10 mg 1746
Thioplex for Injection 1765
Thrombin-JMI 1824
Ticlid Tablets 3015
Tine Test, Tuberculin, Old 3631
▲ TNKase I.V. (4.7% to 21.8%) 1430
Tonocard Tablets 649
Trasylol Injection (1% to 2%) 909
▲ Trisenox Injection (8%) 1158
Uniretic Tablets (Less than 1%) 3178
Valcyte Tablets (Less than 5%) 3022
Vantin Tablets and Oral Suspension 2860
▲ Vesanoid Capsules (60%) 3037
Warfarin Sodium Tablets, USP 3302
▲ Zenapax for Injection (Greater than 5%) 3046
Zinacef Injection 1696
Zinacef for Injection 1696
Zinecard for Injection (2% to 3%) 2869
Zoladex (1% or greater) 702
Zoladex 3-month 706
Zosyn (1.0% or less) 1890
Zosyn in Galaxy Containers (1.0% or less) 1894
Zyprexa Tablets (Infrequent) 1973
Zyprexa ZYDIS Orally Disintegrating Tablets (Infrequent) 1973

Bleeding, antepartum
Aggrenox Capsules 1026
Ecotrin Enteric Coated Aspirin Low, Regular and Maximum Strength Tablets 1715

Bleeding, at invaded sites
Streptase for Infusion 647

Bleeding, at site of administration
Avonex 1013
Bicillin L-A Injection 2242
Cerebyx Injection (Infrequent) 2619
▲ Condylox Gel (0.6% to 19.2%) 2436
▲ Copaxone for Injection (5%) 3306
Doxil Injection (Less than 1%) 566
Enbrel for Injection 1752
Enbrel for Injection 3504
▲ Flolan for Injection (11%) 1528

Genotropin Lyophilized Powder (Infrequent) ... 2818
Innohep Injection ... 1248
Intron A for Injection (Less than 5%) ... 3120
ReoPro Vials (1 to 50 events) ... 1958
▲ Retavase Vials (4.6% to 48.6%) ... 1182
Streptase for Infusion ... 647

Bleeding, breakthrough

Activella Tablets ... 2764
Alesse-21 Tablets ... 3468
Alesse-28 Tablets ... 3473
Alora Transdermal System ... 3372
Aygestin Tablets ... 1333
Brevicon 28-Day Tablets ... 3380
Cenestin Tablets ... 1263
Climara Transdermal System ... 958
Cyclessa Tablets ... 2450
Desogen Tablets ... 2458
Esclim Transdermal System ... 3460
Estinyl Tablets ... 3112
Estrace Vaginal Cream ... 3358
Estrace Tablets ... 3361
Estratest ... 3252
Estrostep ... 2627
femhrt Tablets ... 2635
Levlen (Sometimes) ... 962
Levlite 21 Tablets (Sometimes) ... 962
Levlite 28 Tablets (Sometimes) ... 962
Levora Tablets ... 3389
Loestrin 21 Tablets ... 2642
Loestrin Fe Tablets ... 2642
Lo/Ovral Tablets ... 3532
Lo/Ovral-28 Tablets ... 3538
Low-Ogestrel-28 Tablets ... 3392
Megace Oral Suspension ... 1124
Menest Tablets ... 2254
Microgestin Fe 1.5/30 Tablets ... 3407
Microgestin Fe 1/20 Tablets ... 3400
Mircette Tablets ... 2470
Modicon (Sometimes) ... 2563
Necon ... 3415
Nordette-28 Tablets ... 2257
Norinyl 1 +35 28-Day Tablets ... 3380
Norinyl 1 + 50 28-Day Tablets ... 3380
Ogen Tablets ... 2846
Ogestrel 0.5/50-28 Tablets ... 3428
Ortho Dienestrol Cream ... 2554
Ortho-Cept 21 Tablets ... 2546
Ortho-Cept 28 Tablets ... 2546
Ortho-Cyclen/Ortho Tri-Cyclen ... 2573
Ortho-Est Tablets ... 3464
Ortho-Novum (Sometimes) ... 2563
Ortho-Novum 1/50▫28 Tablets (Sometimes) ... 2556
Ortho-Prefest Tablets ... 2570
Ortho-Cyclen/Ortho Tri-Cyclen ... 2573
Ovcon (Sometimes) ... 3364
Ovral Tablets ... 3551
Ovral-28 Tablets ... 3552
Ovrette Tablets ... 3552
Premarin Intravenous ... 3563
Premarin Tablets ... 3566
Premarin Vaginal Cream ... 3570
Premphase Tablets ... 3572
Prempro Tablets ... 3572
Prometrium Capsules (100 mg, 200 mg) ... 3261
Provera Tablets ... 2853
Tri-Levlen (Sometimes) ... 962
Tri-Norinyl-28 Tablets (Sometimes) ... 3433
Triphasil-21 Tablets ... 3600
Triphasil-28 Tablets ... 3605
Trivora Tablets ... 3439
Vivelle Transdermal System ... 2412
Vivelle-Dot Transdermal System ... 2416
Yasmin 28 Tablets ... 980
Zovia ... 3449

Bleeding, dental

Accutane Capsules ... 2944
Actiq (Less than 1%) ... 1184
Activase I.V. (Less than 1%) ... 1410
Aggrenox Capsules (Less than 1%) ... 1026
AmBisome for Injection (Less common) ... 1383
Avonex ... 1013
Celexa (Rare) ... 1365
Claritin-D 12 Hour Extended Release Tablets (Less frequent) ... 3102
Copaxone for Injection (Infrequent) ... 3306
Coumadin for Injection ... 1243
Coumadin Tablets ... 1243
Crixivan Capsules (Less than 2%) ... 2070
DaunoXome Injection (Less than or equal to 5%) ... 1442
Depakote ER Tablets (Greater than 1%) ... 436
Doxil Injection (Less than 1%) ... 566
Effexor Tablets (Rare) ... 3495
Effexor XR Capsules (Rare) ... 3499
Elmiron Capsules (Less than or equal to 1%) ... 570
Felbatol ... 3343
Gengraf Capsules (1% to less than 3%) ... 457
Geodon Capsules (Rare) ... 2688
Hivid Tablets (Less than 1%) ... 2975
Intron A for Injection (Less than 5%) ... 3120
Lamictal (Rare) ... 1567
Lipitor Tablets (Less than 2%) ... 2639
Lipitor Tablets (Less than 2%) ... 2696
Lupron Depot–4 Month 30 mg (Less than 5%) ... 3289
Mustargen for Injection ... 2142
Neoral Soft Gelatin Capsules (1% to less than 3%) ... 2380
Neoral Oral Solution (1% to less than 3%) ... 2380
Neurontin Capsules (Infrequent) ... 2655
Neurontin Oral Solution (Infrequent) ... 2655
Neurontin Tablets (Infrequent) ... 2655
Pletal Tablets (Less than 2%) ... 2605
Pletal Tablets (Less than 2%) ... 2848
Prozac Pulvules, Liquid, and Weekly Capsules (Infrequent) ... 1238
Remeron Tablets (Infrequent) ... 2483
Remeron SolTab Tablets (Infrequent) ... 2486
Rescriptor Tablets (Less than 2%) ... 526
Retrovir Capsules ... 1625
Retrovir IV Infusion ... 1629
Retrovir ... 1625
Rilutek Tablets (Infrequent) ... 772
Roferon-A Injection (Rare) ... 2996
Sarafem Pulvules (Infrequent) ... 1962
Seroquel Tablets (Infrequent) ... 684
Sonata Capsules (Rare) ... 3591
▲ Soriatane Capsules (1% to 10%) ... 3003
Topamax Sprinkle Capsules (Infrequent) ... 2590
Topamax Tablets (Infrequent) ... 2590
Trileptal Oral Suspension ... 2407
Trileptal Tablets ... 2407
Warfarin Sodium Tablets, USP ... 3302
Wellbutrin SR Sustained-Release Tablets ... 1684
Zonegran Capsules (Infrequent) ... 1307
Zyban Sustained-Release Tablets ... 1710

Bleeding, gastrointestinal

▲ Abelcet Injection (4%) ... 1273
Accupril Tablets (Rare) ... 2611
Accuretic Tablets (0.5% to 1%) ... 2614
Aciphex Tablets (Rare) ... 1267
Aciphex Tablets (Rare) ... 1783
Actimmune (Rare) ... 1772
Actiq (1% or greater) ... 1184
▲ Activase I.V. (5%) ... 1410
Adalat CC Tablets (Less than 1.0%) ... 877
Advil ... ▣771
Advil Cold and Sinus Caplets ... ▣771
Advil Cold and Sinus Tablets ... ▣771
Advil Flu & Body Ache Caplets ... ▣772
Advil Migraine Liquigels ... ▣772
Aggrastat (0.1%) ... 2031
Aggrenox Capsules (1.2%) ... 1026
Agrylin Capsules (1% to 5%) ... 3232
Aleve Tablets, Caplets and Gelcaps ... ▣602
Aleve Cold & Sinus Caplets ... ▣603
Alka-Seltzer ... ▣603
Alka-Seltzer Lemon Lime Antacid and Pain Reliever Effervescent Tablets ... ▣603
Alka-Seltzer Extra Strength Antacid and Pain Reliever Effervescent Tablets ... ▣603
Alka-Seltzer PM Effervescent Tablets ... ▣605
Aloprim for Injection (Less than 1%) ... 2292
▲ AmBisome for Injection (9.9%) ... 1383
Anaprox Tablets (Approximately 1% to 4%) ... 2967
Anaprox DS Tablets (Approximately 1% to 4%) ... 2967
Ancobon Capsules ... 1730
Androderm Transdermal System CIII (2%) ... 3377
▲ Aredia for Injection (Up to 6%) ... 2309
▲ Argatroban Injection (2.3% to 14.4%) ... 1478
Aricept Tablets (Frequent) ... 1270
Aricept Tablets (Frequent) ... 2665
Arthrotec Tablets (Rare) ... 3195
Asacol Delayed-Release Tablets (2% to 5%) ... 2884
Atromid-S Capsules ... 3483
Avonex ... 1013
Azactam for Injection (Less than 1%) ... 1276
Baycol Tablets ... 883
Genuine Bayer Tablets, Caplets and Gelcaps ... ▣606
Extra Strength Bayer Caplets and Gelcaps ... ▣610
Aspirin Regimen Bayer Children's Chewable Tablets (Orange or Cherry Flavored) ... ▣607
Aspirin Regimen Bayer Adult Low Strength 81 mg Tablets ... ▣606
Aspirin Regimen Bayer 81 mg Caplets with Calcium ... ▣607
Aspirin Regimen Bayer Regular Strength 325 mg Caplets ... ▣606
Genuine Bayer Professional Labeling (Aspirin Regimen Bayer) ... ▣608
Extra Strength Bayer Arthritis Caplets ... ▣610
Extra Strength Bayer Plus Caplets ... ▣610
Extra Strength Bayer PM Caplets ... ▣611
Betaseron for SC Injection ... 988
Cafcit (2.2%) ... 1035
Campath Ampules ... 992
Cataflam Tablets (0.6% to 4%) ... 2315
Cathflo Activase ... 3611
Celebrex Capsules (Less than 0.1%) ... 2676
Celebrex Capsules (Less than 0.1%) ... 2780
▲ CellCept Capsules (3%) ... 2951
▲ CellCept Intravenous (3%) ... 2951
▲ CellCept Oral Suspension (3%) ... 2951
▲ CellCept Tablets (3%) ... 2951
Cerebyx Injection (Infrequent) ... 2619
Cipro I.V. (Less than 1%) ... 893
Cipro I.V. Pharmacy Bulk Package (Less than 1%) ... 897
Cipro (Less than 1%) ... 887
Clinoril Tablets (Less than 1%) ... 2053
Cognex Capsules (Infrequent) ... 1351
Coreg Tablets (Less than or equal to 0.1%) ... 1508
Cortone Acetate Injectable Suspension ... 2059
Cortone Acetate Tablets ... 2061
Corzide 40/5 Tablets ... 2247
Corzide 80/5 Tablets ... 2247
Cytotec Tablets (Infrequent) ... 3202
Dantrium Capsules (Rare) ... 2885
DaunoXome Injection (Less than or equal to 5%) ... 1442
Demadex Tablets and Injection ... 2965
Dolobid Tablets (Less than 1 in 100) ... 2088
Doxil Injection (Less than 1%) ... 566
EC-Naprosyn Delayed-Release Tablets (Approximately 1% to 4%) ... 2967
Ecotrin Enteric Coated Aspirin Low, Regular and Maximum Strength Tablets ... 1715
Edecrin ... 2091
Effexor Tablets (Rare) ... 3495
Effexor XR Capsules (Rare) ... 3499
Eldepryl Capsules ... 3266
Emcyt Capsules (1%) ... 2810
Enbrel for Injection (Infrequent) ... 1752
Enbrel for Injection (Infrequent) ... 3504
Ergamisol Tablets ... 1789
Evoxac Capsules (Less than 1%) ... 1217
Excedrin Extra-Strength Tablets, Caplets, and Geltabs ... ▣629
Excedrin Migraine ... 1070
Exelon Capsules (Infrequent) ... 2342
Exelon Oral Solution (Infrequent) ... 2345
Felbatol ... 3343
▲ Feldene Capsules (1% to 10%) ... 2685
Floxin I.V. ... 2526
Floxin Tablets ... 2529
▲ Fludara for Injection (3% to 13%) ... 995
Fosamax Tablets (Occasional) ... 2095
Sterile FUDR ... 2974
Gabitril Tablets (Infrequent) ... 1189
Gengraf Capsules (1% to less than 3%) ... 457
Gleevec Capsules (0.2% to 5%) ... 2357
Gliadel Wafer (1%) ... 1723
Glucotrol XL Extended Release Tablets (Rare) ... 2693
GoLYTELY and Pineapple Flavor GoLYTELY for Oral Solution ... 1068
Goody's Body Pain Formula Powder ... ▣620
Heparin Lock Flush Solution ... 3509
Heparin Sodium Injection ... 3511
Hivid Tablets (Less than 1%) ... 2975
Imitrex Injection ... 1549
Imitrex Nasal Spray (Rare) ... 1554
Imitrex Tablets (Rare) ... 1558
Indocin Capsules (Less than 1%) ... 2112
▲ Indocin I.V. (3% to 9%) ... 2115
Indocin (Less than 1%) ... 2112
Innohep Injection ... 1248
Integrilin Injection ... 1213
Integrilin Injection ... 1828
Intron A for Injection (Less than 5%) ... 3120
K-Dur Microburst Release System ER Tablets ... 1832
Klor-Con M20/Klor-Con M10 Tablets ... 3329
K-Tab Filmtab Tablets ... 470
Lamictal (Rare) ... 1567
▲ Leukine (11% to 27%) ... 1755
Levaquin (Less than 0.3%) ... 2537
Lodine ... 3528
Lodine XL Extended-Release Tablets ... 3530
Lodosyn Tablets ... 1251
Lupron Depot–4 Month 30 mg (Less than 5%) ... 3289
Lupron Injection (Less than 5%) ... 3279
Luvox Tablets (25, 50, 100 mg) (Infrequent) ... 3256
Meridia Capsules ... 481
Merrem I.V. (0.7%) ... 673
Mexitil Capsules (About 7 in 10,000) ... 1047
Micro-K ... 3311
Midamor Tablets (Less than or equal to 1%) ... 2136
Mobic Tablets (Less than 2%) ... 1054
Moduretic Tablets (Less than or equal to 1%) ... 2138
Momentum Backache Relief Extra Strength Caplets ... ▣666
Motrin Suspension, Oral Drops, Chewable Tablets, and Caplets (Less than 1% to 4%) ... 2002
Motrin IB Tablets, Caplets, and Gelcaps ... 2002
Motrin Migraine Pain Caplets ... 2005
Motrin Sinus Headache Caplets ... 2005
Mustargen for Injection ... 2142
Naprelan Tablets (Less than 1% to 4%) ... 1293
Naprosyn Suspension (Approximately 1% to 4%) ... 2967
Naprosyn Tablets (Approximately 1% to 4%) ... 2967
Neoral Soft Gelatin Capsules (1% to less than 3%) ... 2380
Neoral Oral Solution (1% to less than 3%) ... 2380
Nexium Delayed-Release Capsules (Less than 1%) ... 619
Nilandron Tablets (2%) ... 753
Nimotop Capsules (Less than 1%) ... 904
Norvir Capsules (Less than 2%) ... 487
Norvir Oral Solution (Less than 2%) ... 487
▲ Novantrone for Injection (2% to 16%) ... 1760
NovoSeven ... 2430
NuLYTELY, Cherry Flavor, Lemon-Lime Flavor, and Orange Flavor NuLYTELY for Oral Solution ... 1068
Omnicef ... 493
Orthoclone OKT3 Sterile Solution (Less than 1%) ... 2498
Orudis Capsules (Less than 1%) ... 3548
Orudis KT Tablets ... ▣778
Oruvail Capsules (Less than 1%) ... 3548
Parafon Forte DSC Caplets (Rare) ... 2582
Pediazole Suspension ... 3050
Pentasa Capsules (Less than 1%) ... 3239
Plavix Tablets (1% to 2.5%) ... 1097
Plavix Tablets (1% to 2.5%) ... 3084
▲ Ponstel Capsules (1% to 10%) ... 1356
Prevacid Delayed-Release Capsules (Less than 1%) ... 3292
PREVPAC (Less than 1%) ... 3298
Procardia XL Extended Release Tablets (Less than 1%) ... 2710
▲ Prograf (3% to 15%) ... 1393
▲ Proleukin for Injection (13%) ... 1199
Protonix I.V. (Less than 1%) ... 3580
Protonix Tablets (Less than 1%) ... 3577
Prozac Pulvules, Liquid, and Weekly Capsules (Rare) ... 1238
▲ Refludan for Injection (5.3%) ... 761
Relafen Tablets (Less than 1%) ... 1617
Remicade for IV Injection (Less than 2%) ... 1178
ReoPro Vials (11 events) ... 1958
Requip Tablets (Infrequent) ... 1621
Rescriptor Tablets (Less than 2%) ... 526
▲ Retavase Vials (1.8% to 9%) ... 1182
Rilutek Tablets (Infrequent) ... 772
Risperdal (Rare) ... 1796
Roferon-A Injection (Infrequent) ... 2996
Sandimmune (Rare) ... 2388
Sandostatin Injection (Less than 1%) ... 2394
Sandostatin LAR Depot (Rare) ... 2395
Sarafem Pulvules (Rare) ... 1962
Serzone Tablets (Rare) ... 1104
▲ Simulect for Injection (3% to 10%) ... 2399
Sinemet Tablets ... 1253
Sinemet CR Tablets ... 1255
Soma Compound Tablets ... 3354
Streptase for Infusion ... 647
Sular Tablets (Less than or equal to 1%) ... 688
Tasmar Tablets (Infrequent) ... 3010
Taxotere for Injection Concentrate (One patient) ... 778
Tequin Injection (Less than 0.1%) ... 1110
Tequin Tablets (Less than 0.1%) ... 1110
Thalomid Capsules ... 1154
Ticlid Tablets ... 3015
TNKase I.V. (1%) ... 1430
Tolectin (Less than 1%) ... 2589
Toradol ... 3018
Trasylol Injection (1% to 2%) ... 909
▲ Trisenox Injection (8%) ... 1158
Ultracet Tablets ... 2597
Ultram Tablets (Infrequent) ... 2600
Uniretic Tablets (Less than 1%) ... 3178
Vanquish Caplets ... ▣617
▲ Vesanoid Capsules (34%) ... 3037
Vioxx (Less than 0.1%) ... 2213

Viracept 532
Vistide Injection 1445
Voltaren Tablets (0.6% to 4%) 2315
Voltaren-XR Tablets (0.6% to 4%) 2315
Wellbutrin Tablets (Rare) 1680
Wellbutrin SR Sustained-Release Tablets 1684
Xeloda Tablets (Less than 5%) 3039
Zanaflex Tablets (Infrequent) 1305
▲ Zemplar Injection (5%) 522
Zyban Sustained-Release Tablets 1710

Bleeding, genitourinary tract
▲ Activase I.V. (4%) 1410
Activella Tablets 2764
Aggrastat (0.1%) 2031
Argatroban Injection (0.9%) 1478
Premphase Tablets 3572
Prempro Tablets 3572
ReoPro Vials (5 to 8 events) 1958
▲ Retavase Vials (0.9% to 9.5%) 1182
Streptase for Infusion 647

Bleeding, gingival
(*see under* Bleeding, dental)

Bleeding, hemorrhoidal
Colestid Tablets (Infrequent) 2791

Bleeding, intermenstrual
Arthrotec Tablets (Rare) 3195
Estring Vaginal Ring (At least 1 report) 2811
Evoxac Capsules (Less than 1%) 1217
▲ Felbatol (3.4%) 3343
▲ Gonal-F for Injection (3.6% to 9.3%) 3216
Imitrex Injection 1549
Imitrex Nasal Spray 1554
Imitrex Tablets (Infrequent) 1558
Levlen 962
Levlite 21 Tablets 962
Levlite 28 Tablets 962
Risperdal (Infrequent) 1796
Topamax Sprinkle Capsules (Frequent) 2590
Topamax Tablets (Frequent) 2590
Trileptal Oral Suspension 2407
Trileptal Tablets 2407
Tri-Levlen 962
▲ Trisenox Injection (8%) 1158
Yasmin 28 Tablets (Greater than 1%) 980
Zoloft (Infrequent) 2751
Zyrtec (Less than 2%) 2756
Zyrtec-D 12 Hour Extended Relief Tablets (Less than 2%) 2758

Bleeding, internal
Activase I.V. 1410
Streptase for Infusion 647

Bleeding, intracerebral
▲ Lopid Tablets (More common) 2650
Streptase for Infusion 647
Ticlid Tablets (Rare) 3015

Bleeding, intracranial
Activase I.V. (0.4% to 1.3%) 1410
Aggrastat (0.1%) 2031
Aggrenox Capsules (Less than 1%) 1026
Argatroban Injection 1478
Aricept Tablets (Infrequent) 1270
Aricept Tablets (Infrequent) 2665
Campath Ampules 992
Cardene I.V. (0.7%) 3485
▲ Curosurf Intratracheal Suspension (51%) 1232
Ecotrin Enteric Coated Aspirin Low, Regular and Maximum Strength Tablets 1715
Elspar for Injection 2092
Exelon Capsules (Infrequent) 2342
Exelon Oral Solution (Infrequent) 2345
Fortovase Capsules (Rare) 2970
▲ Indocin I.V. (3% to 9%) 2115
▲ Infasurf Intratracheal Suspension (29% to 36%) 1372
Innohep Injection (0.8%) 1248
Integrilin Injection (Rare) 1213
Integrilin Injection (Rare) 1828
Invirase Capsules (Rare) 2979
Lovenox Injection 746
Mylotarg for Injection (2%) 3540
Neurontin Capsules (Infrequent) 2655
Neurontin Oral Solution (Infrequent) 2655
Neurontin Tablets (Infrequent) 2655
Plavix Tablets (Less than 1%) 1097
Plavix Tablets (Less than 1%) 3084
Refludan for Injection 761
ReoPro Vials (1 to 3 events) 1958
Retavase Vials (0.8%) 1182
Salagen Tablets (Less than 1%) 2229
Sandostatin LAR Depot (Rare) 2395
▲ Survanta Intratracheal Suspension (24.1% to 48.1%) 3053

Bleeding, lip
Neurontin Capsules (Rare) 2655
Neurontin Oral Solution (Rare) 2655
Neurontin Tablets (Rare) 2655

Bleeding, menstrual
▲ Norplant System (7.0%) 3543

Bleeding, mouth
Evoxac Capsules (Less than 1%) 1217
Intron A for Injection (Less than 5%) 3120
ReoPro Vials (4 events) 1958

Bleeding, mucosal
Effexor Tablets (Rare) 3495
Unasyn for Injection (Less than 1%) 2728
Visicol Tablets 1767

Bleeding, nasal
(*see under* Epistaxis)

Bleeding, oropharyngeal
Integrilin Injection 1213
Integrilin Injection 1828

Bleeding, otic
Relenza Rotadisk (Less than 1%) 1619
ReoPro Vials (9 to 11 events) 1958

Bleeding, pericardial
Activase I.V. 1410

Bleeding, perioperative
Ticlid Tablets 3015

Bleeding, pharyngeal
▲ TNKase I.V. (3.1%) 1430

Bleeding, postmenopausal
▲ Activella Tablets (5% to 11%) 2764
Avonex 1013

Bleeding, puncture site
TNKase I.V. (Less than 1%) 1430

Bleeding, renal-pelvic
Cipro I.V. (1% or less) 893

Bleeding, respiratory tract
TNKase I.V. (Less than 1%) 1430

Bleeding, retroperitoneal
Activase I.V. (Less than 1%) 1410
Aggrastat (0.6%) 2031
Heparin Lock Flush Solution 3509
Heparin Sodium Injection 3511
Innohep Injection (0.8%) 1248
Integrilin Injection 1213
Integrilin Injection 1828
Lovenox Injection 746
Plavix Tablets (Less than 1%) 1097
Plavix Tablets (Less than 1%) 3084
Pletal Tablets (Less than 2%) 2605
Pletal Tablets (Less than 2%) 2848
Proleukin for Injection 1199
ReoPro Vials (2 to 12 events) 1958
Streptase for Infusion 647
TNKase I.V. (Less than 1%) 1430

Bleeding, subcutaneous
Imitrex Injection 1549

Bleeding, superficial
Activase I.V. 1410

Bleeding, upper GI
(*see under* Bleeding, gastrointestinal)

Bleeding, urethral
Ceftin Tablets (0.1% to 1%) 1898
Cipro (Less than 1%) 887
Klonopin Tablets (Infrequent) 2983
▲ MUSE Urethral Suppository (5%) 3335

Bleeding, urinary tract
Amerge Tablets (Rare) 1467
TNKase I.V. (Less than 1% to 3.7%) 1430
▲ Zenapax for Injection (2% to 5%) 3046

Bleeding, uterine
Activella Tablets 2764
Aggrenox Capsules (Less than 1%) 1026
Climara Transdermal System 958
Clomid Tablets 735
Cytotec Tablets 3202
Effexor Tablets (Rare) 3495
Effexor XR Capsules (Infrequent) 3499
Estrace Vaginal Cream 3358
Estrace Tablets 3361
Estratest 3252
Evoxac Capsules (Less than 1%) 1217
Gengraf Capsules (1% to less than 3%) 457
Geodon Capsules (Rare) 2688
Intron A for Injection (Less than 5%) 3120
Lipitor Tablets (Less than 2%) 2639
Lipitor Tablets (Less than 2%) 2696
Menest Tablets 2254
Neoral Soft Gelatin Capsules (1% to less than 3%) 2380
Neoral Oral Solution (1% to less than 3%) 2380
Ogen Tablets 2846
Ortho-Est Tablets 3464
Permax Tablets (Infrequent) 1299
Premarin Intravenous 3563
Premarin Tablets 3566
Premarin Vaginal Cream 3570
Premphase Tablets 3572
Prempro Tablets 3572
Prozac Pulvules, Liquid, and Weekly Capsules (Rare) 1238
Requip Tablets (Rare) 1621
Rilutek Tablets (Rare) 772
Sarafem Pulvules (Rare) 1962
Serophene Tablets (Less than 1 in 100 patients) 3226
Serzone Tablets (Rare) 1104
Tasmar Tablets (Rare) 3010
▲ Zoladex (6%) 702

Bleeding, uterine, irregularities
Clomid Tablets (1.3%) 735
Depo-Provera Contraceptive Injection 2798
Estring Vaginal Ring (Uncommon) 2811
Lodine (Less than 1%) 3528
Lodine XL Extended-Release Tablets (Less than 1%) 3530

Bleeding, vaginal
Actiq (Less than 1%) 1184
Activella Tablets 2764
▲ Alora Transdermal System (3.4% to 20.2%) 3372
AmBisome for Injection (Less common) 1383
Antagon Injection (1.8%) 2447
Arimidex Tablets (1%) 659
Arthrotec Tablets (Rare) 3195
Avonex 1013
Betaseron for SC Injection 988
Brevicon 28-Day Tablets 3380
Cataflam Tablets (Less than 1%) 2315
Celebrex Capsules (0.1% to 1.9%) 2676
Celebrex Capsules (0.1% to 1.9%) 2780
Celexa (Infrequent) 1365
Cenestin Tablets 1263
Climara Transdermal System 958
Clinoril Tablets (Less than 1%) 2053
Cognex Capsules (Infrequent) 1351
▲ CombiPatch Transdermal System (3% to 6%) 2323
Coumadin for Injection 1243
Coumadin Tablets 1243
Depacon Injection (1% or more) 416
Depakene (1% or more) 421
Depakote Sprinkle Capsules 426
Depakote Tablets (1% to 5%) 430
Depakote ER Tablets (1% or more) 436
▲ Depo-Provera Contraceptive Injection (More than 5%) 2798
Doxil Injection (Less than 1%) 566
Effexor Tablets (Infrequent) 3495
Effexor XR Capsules (Infrequent) 3499
Ergamisol Tablets (Less frequent) 1789
Esclim Transdermal System 3460
Estrace Vaginal Cream 3358
Estrace Tablets 3361
Estratest 3252
▲ Estring Vaginal Ring (4%) 2811
▲ Evista Tablets (2.5% to 6.2%) 1915
Evoxac Capsules (Less than 1%) 1217
Fareston Tablets (2%) 3237
Felbatol 3343
femhrt Tablets 2635
Follistim for Injection (1.5%) 2465
Gabitril Tablets (Infrequent) 1189
Geodon Capsules (Rare) 2688
▲ Gonal-F for Injection (3.6%) 3216
Indocin Capsules (Less than 1%) 2112
Indocin I.V. (Less than 1%) 2115
Indocin (Less than 1%) 2112
Innohep Injection 1248
Levlen 962
Levlite 21 Tablets 962
Levlite 28 Tablets 962
Lipitor Tablets (Less than 2%) 2639
Lipitor Tablets (Less than 2%) 2696
Lo/Ovral Tablets 3532
Lo/Ovral-28 Tablets 3538
Low-Ogestrel-28 Tablets 3392
Lupron Depot-PED 7.5 mg, 11.25 mg and 15 mg (2%) 3291
Lupron Injection Pediatric 3280
Luvox Tablets (25, 50, 100 mg) (Infrequent) 3256
Massengill Disposable Douches ▣ 752
Modicon 2563
▲ Mylotarg for Injection (2% to 7%) 3540
Neurontin Capsules (Infrequent) 2655
Neurontin Oral Solution (Infrequent) 2655
Neurontin Tablets (Infrequent) 2655
Nolvadex Tablets (Less frequent; 2%) 678
Norinyl 1 +35 28-Day Tablets 3380
Norinyl 1 + 50 28-Day Tablets 3380
Ogen Tablets 2846
Ogestrel 0.5/50-28 Tablets 3428
Ortho-Cyclen/Ortho Tri-Cyclen 2573
Ortho-Novum 2563
Ortho-Novum 1/50▫28 Tablets 2556
▲ Ortho-Prefest Tablets (9%) 2570
Ortho-Cyclen/Ortho Tri-Cyclen 2573
Ovral Tablets 3551
Ovral-28 Tablets 3552
Ovrette Tablets 3552
Paxil (Rare) 1609
Permax Tablets (Infrequent) 1299
Pletal Tablets (Less than 2%) 2605
Pletal Tablets (Less than 2%) 2848
Premarin Tablets 3566
Prempro Tablets (1% to 2%) 3572
Prozac Pulvules, Liquid, and Weekly Capsules (Infrequent) 1238
Refludan for Injection (1.8%) 761
Relafen Tablets (Less than 1%) 1617
▲ Repronex for Intramuscular and Subcutaneous Injection (3.1% to 7.9%) 1347
Requip Tablets (Infrequent) 1621
Risperdal (Infrequent) 1796
Salagen Tablets (Less than 1%) 2229
Sarafem Pulvules (Infrequent) 1962
Seroquel Tablets (Infrequent) 684
Serzone Tablets (Infrequent) 1104
Sonata Capsules (Rare) 3591
Sular Tablets (Less than or equal to 1%) 688
▲ Synarel Nasal Solution for Central Precocious Puberty (8%) 3204
Synarel Nasal Solution for Endometriosis 3205
Tri-Levlen 962
Tri-Norinyl-28 Tablets 3433
Triphasil-21 Tablets 3600
Triphasil-28 Tablets 3605
▲ Trisenox Injection (13%) 1158
Uniretic Tablets (Less than 1%) 3178
Vivelle Transdermal System 2412
Vivelle-Dot Transdermal System 2416
Voltaren Tablets (Less than 1%) 2315
Voltaren-XR Tablets (Less than 1%) 2315
Warfarin Sodium Tablets, USP 3302
Wellbutrin SR Sustained-Release Tablets (Up to 2%) 1684
Zarontin Capsules 2659
Zarontin Syrup 2660
Zoladex (1% or greater) 702
Zoloft (Infrequent) 2751

Bleeding diathesis
Cipro I.V. (Rare) 893
Cipro (Less than 0.1%) 887

Bleeding irregularities
Activella Tablets 2764
Climara Transdermal System 958
Estrace Vaginal Cream 3358
Estrace Tablets 3361
Levlen 962
Levlite 21 Tablets 962
Levlite 28 Tablets 962
Micronor Tablets 2543
Mirena Intrauterine System 974
Modicon (Sometimes) 2563
▲ Norplant System (7.6%) 3543
Nor-QD Tablets (common) 3423
Ogen Tablets 2846
Ortho-Est Tablets 3464
Ortho-Novum (Sometimes) 2563
Ortho-Novum 1/50▫28 Tablets (Sometimes) 2556
Ovcon 3364
Plavix Tablets (1% to 2.5%) 1097
Plavix Tablets (1% to 2.5%) 3084
Premarin Tablets 3566
Premphase Tablets 3572
Prempro Tablets 3572
Tri-Levlen 962

Bleeding secondary to eczema
Bactroban Cream (One report) 1494

Bleeding syndrome
Mithracin for Intravenous Use 903

Bleeding tendency, increased
Singulair 2181

Bleeding time, prolongation
Actiq (Less than 1%) 1184
Cardizem Injectable 1018
Cardizem Lyo-Ject Syringe 1018
Cardizem Monovial 1018
Cardizem CD Capsules (Infrequent) 1016
Depakote ER Tablets (Greater than 1%) 436
Elmiron Capsules 570
▲ Feldene Capsules (1% to 10%) 2685
Lodine (Less than 1%) 3528
Lodine XL Extended-Release Tablets (Less than 1%) 3530
Mithracin for Intravenous Use 903
Naprelan Tablets (Less than 1%) 1293
Neurontin Capsules (Rare) 2655
Neurontin Oral Solution (Rare) 2655
Neurontin Tablets (Rare) 2655
Paxil (Rare) 1609
▲ Ponstel Capsules (1% to 10%) 1356
Procardia Capsules 2708
Procardia XL Extended Release Tablets (Some patients) 2710

Rythmol Tablets – 150 mg, 225 mg, 300 mg (Less than 1%) 502
Soriatane Capsules (Less than 1%) 3003
Tiazac Capsules (Infrequent) 1378
Timentin Injection- ADD-Vantage Vial 1661
Timentin Injection-Galaxy Container 1664
Timentin Injection-Pharmacy Bulk Package 1666
Timentin for Intravenous Administration 1658
Tolectin 2589
Toradol 3018

Blepharitis
Alomide Ophthalmic Solution (Less than 1%) ⊙204
▲ Alphagan Ophthalmic Solution (Approximately 3% to 9%) 545
Alphagan P Ophthalmic Solution (1% to 4%) 546
Aricept Tablets (Infrequent) 1270
Aricept Tablets (Infrequent) 2665
Azopt Ophthalmic Suspension (1% to 5%) 536
Bactroban Nasal (Less than 1%) 1495
Betaseron for SC Injection 988
Betimol Ophthalmic Solution (1% to 5%) ⊙324
Cognex Capsules (Rare) 1351
Cosopt Sterile Ophthalmic Solution (1% to 5%) 2065
Doxil Injection (Less than 1%) 566
Effexor Tablets (Rare) 3495
Effexor XR Capsules (Rare) 3499
Evoxac Capsules (Less than 1%) 1217
Exelon Capsules (Infrequent) 2342
Exelon Oral Solution (Infrequent) 2345
Fortovase Capsules (Less than 2%) 2970
Gabitril Tablets (Infrequent) 1189
Geodon Capsules (Infrequent) 2688
Invirase Capsules (Less than 2%) 2979
Iopidine 0.5% Ophthalmic Solution (Less than 3%) ⊙213
▲ Lumigan Ophthalmic Solution (3% to 10%) 553
Norvir Capsules (Less than 2%) 487
Norvir Oral Solution (Less than 2%) 487
OptiPranolol Metipranolol Ophthalmic Solution 0.3% (A small number of patients) ⊙263
Paxil (Rare) 1609
Prozac Pulvules, Liquid, and Weekly Capsules (Rare) 1238
Remeron Tablets (Rare) 2483
Remeron SolTab Tablets (Rare) 2486
Requip Tablets (Infrequent) 1621
Rescriptor Tablets (Less than 2%) 526
Rescula Ophthalmic Solution (1% to 5%) ⊙306
Rilutek Tablets (Rare) 772
Risperdal (Rare) 1796
Sarafem Pulvules (Rare) 1962
Seroquel Tablets (Infrequent) 684
Sonata Capsules (Rare) 3591
Soriatane Capsules (Less than 5%) 3003
Sular Tablets (Less than or equal to 1%) 688
Timolol GFS (1% to 5%) ⊙266
Timoptic in Ocudose (Less frequent) 2192
Timoptic Sterile Ophthalmic Solution (Less frequent) 2190
Timoptic-XE Sterile Ophthalmic Gel Forming Solution 2194
Travatan Ophthalmic Solution (1% to 4%) 543
Zyprexa Tablets (2%) 1973
Zyprexa ZYDIS Orally Disintegrating Tablets (2%) 1973

Blepharoconjunctivitis
▲ Betagan (About 1 in 20 patients) ⊙228
Carteolol Hydrochloride Ophthalmic Solution USP, 1% (Occasional) ⊙258
Flovent Diskus (1% to 3%) 3614
Iopidine 0.5% Ophthalmic Solution (Less than 3%) ⊙213
Ocupress Ophthalmic Solution, 1% Sterile (Occasional) ⊙303

Blepharoptosis
(*see also under* Ptosis, eyelids)
Betagan ⊙228
Betimol Ophthalmic Solution ⊙324

Blepharospasm
Claritin (At least one patient) 3100
Claritin-D 12 Hour Extended Release Tablets 3102
Claritin-D 24 Hour Extended Release Tablets 3104
Eldepryl Capsules 3266
Lodosyn Tablets 1251
Requip Tablets (Infrequent) 1621
Sinemet Tablets 1253
Sinemet CR Tablets 1255

Blind spot, enlargement
Eskalith 1527

Blindness
Betaseron for SC Injection 988
Bicillin C-R 900/300 Injection 2240
Bicillin C-R Injection 2238
Bicillin L-A Injection 2242
Celestone Soluspan Injectable Suspension (Rare) 3097
Cordarone Tablets 3487
Cortone Acetate Injectable Suspension 2059
Decadron Phosphate Injection (Rare) 2081
Doxil Injection (Less than 1%) 566
Eskalith 1527
Gabitril Tablets (Infrequent) 1189
Hydrocortone Acetate Injectable Suspension (Rare) 2103
Hydrocortone Phosphate Injection, Sterile (Rare) 2105
Imitrex Nasal Spray 1554
Levlen (Rare) 962
Levlite 21 Tablets (Rare) 962
Levlite 28 Tablets (Rare) 962
Modicon (Rare) 2563
Neoral Soft Gelatin Capsules 2380
Neoral Oral Solution 2380
Neurontin Capsules (Rare) 2655
Neurontin Oral Solution (Rare) 2655
Neurontin Tablets (Rare) 2655
Orthoclone OKT3 Sterile Solution (Less than 1%) 2498
Ortho-Cyclen/Ortho Tri-Cyclen (Rare) 2573
Ortho-Novum (Rare) 2563
Ortho-Novum 1/50□28 Tablets (Rare) 2556
Ortho-Cyclen/Ortho Tri-Cyclen (Rare) 2573
Pacerone Tablets 3331
Permax Tablets (Rare) 1299
Pletal Tablets (Less than 2%) 2605
Pletal Tablets (Less than 2%) 2848
Proleukin for Injection (Less than 1%) 1199
Sandimmune 2388
Tri-Levlen (Rare) 962
Vistide Injection 1445
Zoloft 2751
Zyrtec (Less than 2%) 2756
Zyrtec-D 12 Hour Extended Relief Tablets (Less than 2%) 2758

Blindness, color
Rescula Ophthalmic Solution (Less than 1%) ⊙306
Topamax Sprinkle Capsules (Infrequent) 2590
Topamax Tablets (Infrequent) 2590

Blindness, night
(*see under* Nyctalopia)

Blindness, sudden
Factrel 3633

Blindness, transient
Adalat CC Tablets (Rare) 877
Procardia Capsules (Less than 0.5%) 2708
Proleukin for Injection (Less than 1%) 1199
Thyrel TRH for Injection 3630

Blistering
Accolate Tablets 657
▲ Androderm Transdermal System CIII (12%) 3377
Avita Cream 999
Avita Gel 1000
Avonex 1013
Condylox Gel (Less common) 2436
Cutivate Cream (0.8%) 1282
Efudex (Infrequent) 1733
Lotrimin 3128
Lotrisone 3129
Navelbine Injection 1604
Norplant System 3543
Retin-A Micro 0.1% 2522
Sulfamylon Cream 1011
Sulfamylon Topical Solution 1011
▲ Trisenox Injection (8%) 1158
Viramune Oral Suspension 1060
Viramune Tablets 1060
Xeloda Tablets 3039

Blistering, foreskin
Emla (Two reports) 602

Bloating
(*see under* Abdominal bloating)

Blood clotting, mechanisms, disorders of
Estrace Vaginal Cream 3358
Estrace Tablets 3361
Ortho-Est Tablets 3464
Plavix Tablets (Less than 1%) 1097
Plavix Tablets (Less than 1%) 3084
Pyrazinamide Tablets (Rare) 1876
Rifater Tablets (Rare) 769

Blood dyscrasias
Abelcet Injection 1273
Aralen Tablets 3075
Asacol Delayed-Release Tablets 2884
Azulfidine EN-tabs Tablets 2775
Bactrim (Rare) 2949
▲ Blephamide Ophthalmic Ointment (Among most often) 547
Blephamide Ophthalmic Suspension 548
Campath Ampules 992
Celontin Capsules 2618
Chloromycetin Ophthalmic Ointment, 1% ⊙296
Chloromycetin Ophthalmic Solution ⊙297
Chloroptic Sterile Ophthalmic Solution (Rare) ⊙235
Compazine 1505
Dapsone Tablets USP 1780
Depo-Provera Contraceptive Injection (Fewer than 1%) 2798
Diamox Intravenous ⊙269
Diamox Sequels Sustained Release Capsules ⊙270
Diamox Tablets ⊙269
Etrafon (Less frequent) 3115
Furosemide Tablets 2284
▲ Leukine (25%) 1755
Librium Capsules (Occasional) 1736
Mexitil Capsules 1047
Neptazane Tablets ⊙271
Plaquenil Tablets 3082
Procanbid Extended-Release Tablets (Approximately 0.5%) 2262
Prozac Pulvules, Liquid, and Weekly Capsules (Rare) 1238
Sarafem Pulvules (Rare) 1962
Septra Suspension 2265
Septra Tablets 2265
Septra DS Tablets 2265
Silvadene Cream 1% 2267
Stelazine 1640
Tambocor Tablets (Extremely rare) 1990
Tonocard Tablets 649
Trusopt Sterile Ophthalmic Solution (Rare) 2196
Urobiotic-250 Capsules 2731
Zarontin Capsules 2659
Zarontin Syrup 2660

Blood glucose, elevation
(*see under* Hyperglycinemia)

Blood glucose, reduction
(*see under* Hypoglycemia)

Blood loss, increase
(*see under* Bleeding)

Blood pressure, changes
Activella Tablets 2764
Autoplex T 2294
Clozaril Tablets 2319
Dantrium Capsules (Less frequent) 2885
DDAVP Injection 4 mcg/mL (Infrequent) 737
Desmopressin Acetate Injection (Infrequent) 1344
Desoxyn Tablets 440
Evoxac Capsules 1217
femhrt Tablets 2635
Gammar-P I.V. 787
Haldol Decanoate 2535
Isordil Sublingual Tablets 3525
Isordil Titradose Tablets 3526
Loxitane Capsules 3398
Moban 1320
Orap Tablets 1407
Ortho-Prefest Tablets 2570
Plasbumin-5 (Rare) 939
Plasbumin-20 (Rare) 940
Plasbumin-25 (Rare) 941
Premphase Tablets (Occasional) 3572
Prempro Tablets (Occasional) 3572
Proplex T 851
Risperdal 1796
Ritalin 2387
Sandimmune 2388
Sensorcaine 643
Sensorcaine-MPF Injection 643
Serentil 1057
Stelazine 1640
Stimate Nasal Spray 796
Trilafon 3160
Zemuron Injection 2491

Blood pressure, elevation
(*see under* Hypertension)

Blood pressure, reduction
(*see under* Hypotension)

Blood urea levels, increase
Ceptaz for Injection (Occasional) 1499
Fortaz (Occasional) 1541
Inderide Tablets 3517
Normodyne Tablets (Rare) 3137
▲ Paraplatin for Injection (Up to 17%) 1126
Tazidime Vials, Faspak & ADD-Vantage (Occasional) 1966

Blood urea nitrogen levels, increase
(*see under* BUN levels, elevation)

Blurred vision
(*see under* Vision, blurred)

Body odor
Carnitor Injection (Less frequent) 3242
Carnitor Tablets and Oral Solution 3245
Crixivan Capsules (Less than 2%) 2070
Depo-Provera Contraceptive Injection (Fewer than 1%) 2798
Effexor Tablets (Rare) 3495
Felbatol 3343
Lupron Depot 3.75 mg (Less than 5%) 3281
Lupron Depot-PED 7.5 mg, 11.25 mg and 15 mg (Less than 2%) 3291
Lupron Injection Pediatric (Less than 2%) 3280
Retrovir Capsules 1625
Retrovir IV Infusion 1629
Retrovir 1625
Rimso-50 Solution 1267
Salagen Tablets (Less than 1%) 2229
▲ Synarel Nasal Solution for Central Precocious Puberty (4%) 3204
Topamax Sprinkle Capsules (1.8%) 2590
Topamax Tablets (1.8%) 2590
Wellbutrin Tablets (Rare) 1680

Bone density, changes
Depo-Provera Contraceptive Injection 2798
Lupron Depot 3.75 mg 3281
Lupron Depot–3 Month 11.25 mg 3285
Lupron Depot–4 Month 30 mg 3289
Viadur Implant (Less than 2%) 912
▲ Zoladex (4.3% decrease) 702

Bone dislocation
▲ Apligraf (4.5%) 2305

Bone disorders
Accutane Capsules 2944
▲ Actonel Tablets (4%) 2879
Advair Diskus 100/50 (1% to 3%) 1448
Advair Diskus 250/50 (1% to 3%) 1448
Advair Diskus 500/50 (1% to 3%) 1448
Celebrex Capsules (0.1% to 1.9%) 2676
Celebrex Capsules (0.1% to 1.9%) 2780
Clomid Tablets 735
Desferal Vials 2333
Effexor Tablets (Infrequent) 3495
Evoxac Capsules (Less than 1%) 1217
▲ Humatrope Vials and Cartridges (9.6%) 1930
Naprelan Tablets (Less than 1%) 1293
Protonix I.V. (Less than 1%) 3580
Protonix Tablets (Less than 1%) 3577
Rescriptor Tablets (Less than 2%) 526
Risperdal (Rare) 1796
Salagen Tablets (Less than 1%) 2229
Soriatane Capsules (Less than 1%) 3003
Thalomid Capsules 1154
▲ Vesanoid Capsules (3%) 3037

Bone fractures
Apligraf (1.8%) 2305
Aricept Tablets (Frequent) 1270
Aricept Tablets (Frequent) 2665
Campath Ampules 992
Didronel Tablets 2888
Gengraf Capsules (1% to less than 3%) 457
Naprelan Tablets (Less than 1%) 1293
Neoral Soft Gelatin Capsules (1% to less than 3%) 2380
Neoral Oral Solution (1% to less than 3%) 2380
Remicade for IV Injection (Less than 2%) 1178
Salagen Tablets (Less than 1%) 2229
Zoladex 3-month 706

Bone marrow depression
Accupril Tablets (Rare) 2611
Adriamycin PFS/RDF Injection (High incidence) 2767
Aldoclor Tablets 2035
Aldomet Tablets 2037
Aldoril Tablets 2039
Altace Capsules (Rare) 2233
Calcium Disodium Versenate Injection 1980
Campath Ampules 992
Carbatrol Capsules 3234

Chloroptic Sterile Ophthalmic Solution (Three cases) ⊙235
Clinoril Tablets (Less than 1%) 2053
Cuprimine Capsules 2075
Depen Titratable Tablets 3341
Diamox ⊙269
Doxil Injection 566
Elspar for Injection (Rare) 2092
Enalaprilat Injection (Rare) 863
Felbatol 3343
Flexeril Tablets (Rare) 572
Flexeril Tablets (Rare) 2094
Floxin I.V. 2526
Floxin Tablets 2529
FML-S Liquifilm Sterile Ophthalmic Suspension ⊙238
Indocin Capsules (Less than 1%) 2112
Indocin I.V. (Less than 1%) 2115
Indocin (Less than 1%) 2112
Lexxel Tablets (Rare) 608
Limbitrol 1738
Lotrel Capsules 2370
Mavik Tablets (Rare) 478
Mefoxin for Injection 2124
Mefoxin Premixed Intravenous Solution 2127
Mylocel Tablets (Less frequently) 2227
Neptazane Tablets ⊙271
Norpramin Tablets 755
Primaxin I.M. 2158
Primaxin I.V. 2160
Prinivil Tablets (Rare) 2164
Prinzide Tablets (Rare) 2168
Procanbid Extended-Release Tablets (Approximately 0.5%) 2262
Sinequan (Occasional) 2713
Sulfamylon Cream (A single case) 1011
Sulfamylon Topical Solution 1011
Surmontil Capsules 3595
Tegretol/Tegretol-XR 2404
Thioplex for Injection 1765
Ticlid Tablets 3015
Tonocard Tablets (Less than 1%) 649
Topamax Sprinkle Capsules (Rare) 2590
Topamax Tablets (Rare) 2590
Valcyte Tablets (Less than 5%) 3022
Vaseretic Tablets (Rare) 2204
Vasotec I.V. Injection (Rare) 2207
Vasotec Tablets (Rare) 2210
Vivactil Tablets 2217
Vivactil Tablets 2446
Zestoretic Tablets (Rare) 695
Zestril Tablets (Rare) 698

Bone marrow fibrosis

Fludara for Injection (One patient) 995

Bone marrow hypoplasia

Campath Ampules 992
Captopril Tablets 2281
Chloromycetin Ophthalmic Ointment, 1% ⊙296
Chloromycetin Ophthalmic Solution ⊙297
Lopid Tablets (Rare) 2650
Rituxan for Infusion 1750
Rituxan I.V. 1428
Zantac (Rare) 1690
Zantac Injection (Sometimes) 1688
Zantac Syrup (Rare) 1690

Bone marrow suppression

▲ Alkeran for Injection (Most common) 1465
▲ Alkeran Tablets (Most common) 1466
Aloprim for Injection (Less than 1%) 2292
Celontin Capsules 2618
▲ Cerubidine for Injection (All patients) 947
Chloroptic Sterile Ophthalmic Ointment ⊙234
Clozaril Tablets 2319
Depacon Injection 416
Depakene 421
Depakote Sprinkle Capsules 426
Depakote Tablets 430
Depakote ER Tablets 436
Dilantin Infatabs 2624
Dilantin Kapseals 2622
Dilantin-125 Oral Suspension 2625
Doxil Injection 566
Etrafon 3115
Fludara for Injection 995
▲ Foscavir Injection (10%) 605
Hycamtin for Injection 1546
Leukeran Tablets (Frequent) 1591
Leustatin Injection (Common) 2495
Mylocel Tablets 2227
Paraplatin for Injection 1126
Purinethol Tablets (Frequent) 1615
Tabloid Tablets 1642
Taxol Injection 1129
Taxotere for Injection Concentrate 778
Zarontin Capsules 2659
Zarontin Syrup 2660

Bone mineral density, decreased

Zoladex 3-month 706

Borborygmi

Urecholine 2198
Urecholine Tablets 2445

Bowel, loss of control

Duranest Injections 600
Nesacaine/Nesacaine MPF 617
Xylocaine Injections 653

Bowel disease, inflammatory, exacerbation of

Accutane Capsules 2944
Asacol Delayed-Release Tablets 2884

Bowel frequency, increase

Fortovase Capsules (Less than 2%) 2970
Sterile FUDR 2974
HeartBar 1212
Invirase Capsules (Less than 2%) 2979
Klonopin Tablets (Infrequent) 2983

Bowel habits, changes

Evoxac Capsules 1217
Nexium Delayed-Release Capsules (Less than 1%) 619
Trovan (Less than 1%) 2722

Bowel infarction

Activase I.V. 1410
Orthoclone OKT3 Sterile Solution (Less than 1%) 2498
Proleukin for Injection 1199
Retavase Vials 1182
Streptase for Infusion 647

Bowel strictures, fibrotic

Pancrease MT Capsules 2581

Bowel syndrome, irritable

Evoxac Capsules (Less than 1%) 1217
Neurontin Capsules (Rare) 2655
Neurontin Oral Solution (Rare) 2655
Neurontin Tablets (Rare) 2655

Bowel urgency

Copaxone for Injection (Frequent) 3306

Bowels, perforation

Cortone Acetate Injectable Suspension 2059
Cortone Acetate Tablets 2061
Decadron Elixir 2078
Decadron Tablets 2079
Decadron Phosphate Injection 2081
Hydrocortone Tablets 2106
Hydrocortone Acetate Injectable Suspension 2103
Hydrocortone Phosphate Injection, Sterile 2105
Indocin I.V. (1% to 3%) 2115
Prednisone 3064
Proleukin for Injection 1199

Brachial plexus neuropathies

Botox Purified Neurotoxin Complex 549
Diphtheria & Tetanus Toxoids Adsorbed Purogenated for Pediatric Use 1857
Fluzone Vaccine 802
Tetanus & Diphtheria Toxoids Adsorbed for Adult Use 1880
Tetanus and Diphtheria Toxoids Adsorbed For Adult Use 815
Tripedia Vaccine 817

Bradycardia

Accuretic Tablets 2614
Aciphex Tablets (Rare) 1267
Aciphex Tablets (Rare) 1783
Adalat CC Tablets (Less than 1.0%) 877
Adenoscan (Less than 1%) 1381
▲ Aggrastat (4%) 2031
Akineton 402
Aldoclor Tablets 2035
Aldomet Tablets 2037
Aldoril Tablets 2039
Aloprim for Injection (Less than 1%) 2292
AmBisome for Injection (Less common) 1383
Amerge Tablets (Rare) 1467
Amicar Injection 3608
Amicar Syrup 3608
Amicar Tablets 3608
Amphotec (1% to 5%) 1774
Anectine Injection 1476
▲ Anzemet Injection (5.1%) 719
▲ Anzemet Tablets (5.1%) 722
Aricept Tablets (Infrequent) 1270
Aricept Tablets (Infrequent) 2665
Atacand HCT Tablets (0.5% or greater) 597
Betagan ⊙228
▲ Betapace Tablets (8% to 16%) 950
▲ Betapace AF Tablets (12.3% to 13.1%) 954
Betaxon Ophthalmic Suspension (Less than 2%) 537
Betimol Ophthalmic Solution ⊙324
Betoptic S Ophthalmic Suspension (Rare) 537
▲ Blocadren Tablets (5% to 9.1%) 2046
Brevibloc Injection (Less than 1%) 858
Buprenex Injectable (Less than 1%) 2918
Cardizem Injectable (Less than 1%) 1018
Cardizem Lyo-Ject Syringe (Less than 1%) 1018
Cardizem Monovial (Less than 1%) 1018
Cardizem CD Capsules (1.7% to 3.3%) 1016
Cardura Tablets 2668
Carteolol Hydrochloride Ophthalmic Solution USP, 1% ⊙258
Catapres Tablets (About 5 in 1,000 patients) 1037
Catapres-TTS (0.5% or less) 1038
Celexa (Infrequent) 1365
▲ CellCept Capsules (17.3%) 2951
▲ CellCept Intravenous (17.3%) 2951
▲ CellCept Oral Suspension (17.3%) 2951
▲ CellCept Tablets (17.3%) 2951
Chirocaine Injection (2.2%) 2909
Clorpres Tablets (About 5 in 1,000) 1002
Clozaril Tablets (Less than 1%) 2319
Cognex Capsules (Infrequent) 1351
Colazal Capsules 3069
Combipres Tablets (About 5 in 1,000) 1040
Copaxone for Injection (Infrequent) 3306
▲ Cordarone Intravenous (4.9%) 3491
Cordarone Tablets (Uncommon) 3487
▲ Coreg Tablets (2.1% to 8.8%) 1508
Corgard Tablets (2 of 100 patients) 2245
Corlopam Injection (0.5% to 5%) 412
Cortrosyn for Injection 2449
Corvert Injection (1.2%) 2793
Corzide 40/5 Tablets (Common) 2247
Corzide 80/5 Tablets (Common) 2247
Cosopt Sterile Ophthalmic Solution (Less than 1%) 2065
Covera-HS Tablets (1.4%) 3199
Demerol 3079
Depacon Injection 416
Depakene 421
Depakote Sprinkle Capsules 426
Depakote Tablets 430
Depakote ER Tablets 436
D.H.E. 45 Injection 2334
Dilaudid Oral Liquid 445
Dilaudid Tablets - 8 mg 445
Dilaudid-HP (Less frequent) 443
Diprivan Injectable Emulsion (1% to 3%) 667
Dolophine Hydrochloride Tablets 3056
Doxil Injection (Less than 1%) 566
Duraclon Injection (0.5%) 3057
Duragesic Transdermal System (Less than 1%) 1786
Duranest Injections 600
Effexor Tablets (Rare) 3495
Effexor XR Capsules (Rare) 3499
Ellence Injection 2806
Emla (Unlikely with cream) 602
Enalaprilat Injection 863
Eskalith 1527
Etrafon 3115
Exelon Capsules (Frequent) 2342
Exelon Oral Solution (Frequent) 2345
Extendryl 1361
Felbatol 3343
Ferrlecit Injection (Greater than 1%) 3386
▲ Flolan for Injection (5% to 15%) 1528
Fluothane Inhalation 3508
Geodon Capsules (Infrequent) 2688
▲ Hectorol Capsules (6.6%) 1064
▲ Hectorol Injection (6.6%) 1066
Humorsol Sterile Ophthalmic Solution (Rare) 2102
Imdur Tablets (Less than or equal to 5%) 1826
Imitrex Injection (Infrequent) 1549
Imitrex Nasal Spray (Rare) 1554
Imitrex Tablets (Rare) 1558
Inderal 3513
Inderal LA Long-Acting Capsules 3516
Inderide Tablets 3517
Inderide LA Long-Acting Capsules 3519
Indocin I.V. (Less than 3%) 2115
▲ Infasurf Intratracheal Suspension (34%) 1372
INFeD Injection 3388
Intron A for Injection (Less than 5%) 3120
Iopidine Sterile Ophthalmic Solution ⊙212
Isoptin SR Tablets (1.4%) 467
Kadian Capsules (Less than 3%) 1335
Lariam Tablets (Less than 1%) 2989
Levaquin (Less than 0.3%) 2537
Levo-Dromoran 1734
Levorphanol Tartrate Tablets (1% to 3%) 3059
Lexxel Tablets 608
Lidoderm Patch 1319
Lithobid Slow-Release Tablets 3255
Lupron Depot-3 Month 22.5 mg (Less than 5%) 3288
Luvox Tablets (25, 50, 100 mg) (Infrequent) 3256
Mavik Tablets (0.3% to 4.7%) 478
Maxalt Tablets (Infrequent) 2120
Maxalt-MLT Orally Disintegrating Tablets (Infrequent) 2120
Mepergan Injection 3539
Merrem I.V. (0.1% to 1.0%) 673
Mexitil Capsules (About 4 in 1,000) 1047
Midamor Tablets 2136
Minipress Capsules 2699
Miochol-E System Pak (Rare) ⊙305
Miochol-E with Steri-Tags (Rare) ⊙305
Mirena Intrauterine System 974
Monopril Tablets (0.4% to 1.0%) 1091
MS Contin Tablets (Less frequent) 2896
MSIR (Less frequent) 2898
Nadolol Tablets (Common) 2288
▲ Naropin Injection (More than 5% to 19.5%) 612
Natrecor for Injection (1%) 3189
Nembutal Sodium Solution (Less than 1%) 485
Nesacaine/Nesacaine MPF 617
Neurontin Capsules (Rare) 2655
Neurontin Oral Solution (Rare) 2655
Neurontin Tablets (Rare) 2655
Nimotop Capsules (Up to 1.0%) 904
Nipent for Injection (Less than 3%) 3272
Normodyne Injection (Rare) 3135
Normodyne Tablets (Rare) 3137
Norvasc Tablets (More than 0.1% to 1%) 2704
NovoSeven (1%) 2430
Nubain Injection (1% or less) 1323
Numorphan 1324
Ocupress Ophthalmic Solution, 1% Sterile ⊙303
OptiPranolol Metipranolol Ophthalmic Solution 0.3% (A small number of patients) ⊙263
Oramorph SR Tablets (Less frequent) 3062
Orthoclone OKT3 Sterile Solution (Less than 1%) 2498
Pacerone Tablets (Uncommon) 3331
ParaGard T 380A Intrauterine Copper Contraceptive 2582
Paxil (Infrequent) 1609
Permax Tablets (Infrequent) 1299
Phenergan Injection 3553
Phenergan 3556
Phenergan with Codeine Syrup 3557
Phenergan VC with Codeine Syrup 3561
Photofrin for Injection 831
Polocaine Injection, USP 625
Polocaine-MPF Injection, USP 625
Prilosec Delayed-Release Capsules (Less than 1%) 628
Prinivil Tablets (0.3% to 1.0%) 2164
Prinzide Tablets 2168
▲ Proleukin for Injection (7%) 1199
Prostigmin Injectable 1744
Prostigmin Tablets 1744
Provigil Tablets (At least 1%) 1193
Prozac Pulvules, Liquid, and Weekly Capsules (Rare) 1238
Reglan 2935
Remeron Tablets (Infrequent) 2483
Remeron SolTab Tablets (Infrequent) 2486
Remicade for IV Injection (Less than 2%) 1178
Reminyl Oral Solution (2%) 1792
Reminyl Tablets (2%) 1792
▲ ReoPro Vials (5.2%) 1958
Requip Tablets (Infrequent) 1621
Rescriptor Tablets (Less than 2%) 526
Rilutek Tablets (Rare) 772
Risperdal 1796
Rituxan for Infusion (1% to 5%) 1750
Rituxan I.V. (1% to 5%) 1428
Robaxin Injectable 2938
Robaxin Tablets 2939
Robinul Injectable 2940
Romazicon Injection (Less than 1%) 3000
Roxanol 3066
Rythmol Tablets - 150 mg, 225 mg, 300 mg (2%) 502
Salagen Tablets (Less than 1%) 2229
Sarafem Pulvules (Rare) 1962
Sectral Capsules (Up to 2%) 3589
Sensorcaine 643
Sensorcaine-MPF Injection 643
Seroquel Tablets (Infrequent) 684
Streptase for Infusion (Occasional) 647
Suprane Liquid for Inhalation (Greater than 1%) 874
Tagamet (Rare) 1644
Tambocor Tablets (Less than 1%) 1990
Tarka Tablets (1.8%) 508
Tasmar Tablets (Infrequent) 3010

▲ Taxol Injection (3%) 1129
Tenex Tablets (3% or less) 2942
▲ Tenoretic Tablets (3%) 690
▲ Tenormin (3% to 18%) 692
Tensilon Injectable 1745
Tequin Injection (Less than 0.1%) 1110
Tequin Tablets (Less than 0.1%) 1110
Teveten Tablets (Less than 1%) 3327
Thalomid Capsules 1154
Tikosyn Capsules (Less than or equal to 2%) 2717
Timolide Tablets (1.2%) 2187
Timolol GFS .... ⊙266
Timoptic in Ocudose (Less frequent) 2192
Timoptic Sterile Ophthalmic Solution (Less frequent) 2190
Timoptic-XE Sterile Ophthalmic Gel Forming Solution 2194
Tonocard Tablets (0.4% to 1.8%) 649
Topamax Sprinkle Capsules (Infrequent) 2590
Topamax Tablets (Infrequent) 2590
Toprol-XL Tablets (1.5% to approximately 3 of 100 patients) 651
Trasylol Injection (1% to 2%) 909
Travatan Ophthalmic Solution (1% to 5%) 543
Trilafon 3160
Trileptal Oral Suspension 2407
Trileptal Tablets 2407
Trovan (Less than 1%) 2722
Uniretic Tablets (Less than 1%) 3178
Valium Injectable 3026
Vancocin HCl, Vials & ADD-Vantage (Infrequent) 1970
Vascor Tablets 2602
Vaseretic Tablets 2204
Vasotec I.V. Injection 2207
Vasotec Tablets (0.5% to 1.0%) 2210
Verelan Capsules (1.4%) 3184
Verelan PM Capsules (1.4%) 3186
Versed Injection (Less than 1%) 3027
Versed Syrup (1%) 3033
Vioxx (Greater than 0.1% to 1.9%) 2213
Virazole for Inhalation Solution (Infrequent) 1747
Xylocaine Injections 653
▲ Zanaflex Tablets (2% to 10%) 1305
Zantac (Rare) 1690
Zantac Injection (Rare) 1688
Zantac Syrup (Rare) 1690
Zebeta Tablets (0.4% to 0.5%) 1885
Zestril Tablets (0.3% to 1.0%) 698
Ziac Tablets (0.9% to 1.1%) 1887
Zofran Injection (Rare) 1698
▲ Zofran (6%) 1703
▲ Zofran ODT Orally Disintegrating Tablets (6%) 1703
Zoloft 2751
Zomig Tablets (Rare) 708
Zomig-ZMT Tablets (Rare) 708
Zonegran Capsules (Infrequent) 1307
Zosyn (1.0% or less) 1890
Zosyn in Galaxy Containers (1.0% or less) 1894
Zyprexa Tablets (Infrequent) 1973
Zyprexa ZYDIS Orally Disintegrating Tablets (Infrequent) 1973

Bradycardia, fetal

Duranest Injections 600
▲ Naropin Injection (More than 5% to 17.2%) 612
Nesacaine/Nesacaine MPF 617
▲ Prepidil Gel (4.1%) 2851
Sensorcaine 643
▲ Xylocaine Injections (20% to 30%) 653

Bradycardia, neonatal

Alphagan Ophthalmic Solution (Rare) 545
Normodyne Injection 3135
Normodyne Tablets (Rare) 3137
Tenoretic Tablets 690
Tenormin 692

Bradycardia, paradoxical

Ismo Tablets 3524
Isordil Sublingual Tablets 3525
Isordil Titradose Tablets 3526
Nitrostat Tablets 2658

Bradycardia, severe

Brevibloc Injection 858
Eskalith 1527
Lithium Carbonate 3061
Lithium Citrate Syrup 3061

Bradycardia, symptomatic

Corgard Tablets (2 of 100 patients) 2245
Corzide 40/5 Tablets (2 of 100 patients) 2247
Corzide 80/5 Tablets (2 of 100 patients) 2247
Nadolol Tablets (2 of 100 patients) 2288

Bradycardia, transient

Covera-HS Tablets (1.4%) 3199
▲ Survanta Intratracheal Suspension (11.9%) 3053

Bradycardia with nodal escape rhythms

Isoptin SR Tablets 467
Verelan Capsules 3184

Bradykinesia

Cognex Capsules (Infrequent) 1351
Effexor Tablets (Rare) 3495
Effexor XR Capsules (Rare) 3499
Eldepryl Capsules 3266
Maxalt Tablets (Rare) 2120
Maxalt-MLT Orally Disintegrating Tablets (Rare) 2120
Paxil 1609
Reglan 2935
▲ Wellbutrin Tablets (8.0%) 1680

Bradykinetic episodes

Lodosyn Tablets 1251
Sinemet Tablets 1253
Sinemet CR Tablets 1255

Bradylogia

Imitrex Tablets (Rare) 1558

Bradypnea

Zoloft (Rare) 2751

Brain abscess

Serophene Tablets 3226

Brain syndrome, acute

Actiq (Less than 1%) 1184
Betaseron for SC Injection 988
Cerebyx Injection (Infrequent) 2619
Diphtheria & Tetanus Toxoids Adsorbed Purogenated for Pediatric Use 1857
Doxil Injection (Less than 1%) 566
Permax Tablets (Infrequent) 1299
Prozac Pulvules, Liquid, and Weekly Capsules (Infrequent) 1238
Rilutek Tablets (Rare) 772
Sarafem Pulvules (Infrequent) 1962
Tetanus & Diphtheria Toxoids Adsorbed for Adult Use 1880
Virazole for Inhalation Solution 1747
Vistide Injection 1445

Brain syndrome, chronic

Betaseron for SC Injection 988

Breast, redistribution/accumulation of body fat

Crixivan Capsules 2070

Breast abscess

Betaxon Ophthalmic Suspension (Less than 2%) 537
Lamictal (Rare) 1567
Rilutek Tablets (Rare) 772

Breast atrophy

Paxil (Rare) 1609
▲ Zoladex (33%) 702

Breast carcinoma

Actiq (1% or greater) 1184
Activella Tablets 2764
Ambien Tablets (Rare) 3191
Betaseron for SC Injection (2%) 988
Celebrex Capsules (0.1% to 1.9%) 2676
Celebrex Capsules (0.1% to 1.9%) 2780
Climara Transdermal System 958
Clomid Tablets 735
Cognex Capsules (Rare) 1351
Depo-Provera Contraceptive Injection (Fewer than 1%) 2798
Estratest 3252
Eulexin Capsules (Two reports) 3118
Imitrex Nasal Spray 1554
Lamictal (Rare) 1567
Levlen 962
Levlite 21 Tablets 962
Levlite 28 Tablets 962
Naprelan Tablets (Less than 1%) 1293
Ogen Tablets 2846
Ortho-Cyclen/Ortho Tri-Cyclen 2573
Ortho-Est Tablets 3464
Ortho-Cyclen/Ortho Tri-Cyclen 2573
Paxil (Rare) 1609
Permax Tablets (Infrequent) 1299
Premphase Tablets 3572
Prempro Tablets 3572
Prometrium Capsules (100 mg, 200 mg) (2%) 3261
Remicade for IV Injection 1178
Requip Tablets (Infrequent) 1621
Sandostatin LAR Depot (Rare) 2395
Serophene Tablets 3226
Tasmar Tablets (Infrequent) 3010
Tri-Levlen 962
Uniretic Tablets (Less than 1%) 3178

Breast changes, unspecified

Brevicon 28-Day Tablets 3380
Desogen Tablets 2458
▲ Emcyt Capsules (Up to 66%) 2810
Lo/Ovral Tablets 3532
Lo/Ovral-28 Tablets 3538
Low-Ogestrel-28 Tablets 3392
Lupron Depot 3.75 mg (Less than 5%) 3281
Lupron Depot–3 Month 11.25 mg (1.8% to 6%) 3285
Lupron Depot-PED 7.5 mg, 11.25 mg and 15 mg (Less than 2%) 3291
Lupron Injection Pediatric (Less than 2%) 3280
Modicon 2563
Nordette-28 Tablets 2257
Norinyl 1 +35 28-Day Tablets 3380
Norinyl 1 + 50 28-Day Tablets 3380
Ogestrel 0.5/50-28 Tablets 3428
Ortho-Cept 21 Tablets 2546
Ortho-Cept 28 Tablets 2546
Ortho-Cyclen/Ortho Tri-Cyclen 2573
Ortho-Novum 2563
Ortho-Novum 1/50▫28 Tablets 2556
Ortho-Cyclen/Ortho Tri-Cyclen 2573
Ovral Tablets 3551
Ovral-28 Tablets 3552
Ovrette Tablets 3552
Tri-Norinyl-28 Tablets 3433
Triphasil-21 Tablets 3600
Triphasil-28 Tablets 3605

Breast engorgement

Adalat CC Tablets (Less than 1.0%) 877
Betaseron for SC Injection 988
Copaxone for Injection (Infrequent) 3306
Effexor Tablets (Rare) 3495
Effexor XR Capsules (Rare) 3499
Estring Vaginal Ring (At least 1 report) 2811
Haldol Decanoate 2535
Haldol Injection, Tablets and Concentrate 2533
Permax Tablets (Rare) 1299
Prozac Pulvules, Liquid, and Weekly Capsules (Rare) 1238
Remeron Tablets (Rare) 2483
Remeron SolTab Tablets (Rare) 2486
Sarafem Pulvules (Rare) 1962
Synarel Nasal Solution for Endometriosis (Less than 1%) 3205
Thioridazine Hydrochloride Tablets 2289
Zoladex (1% to 5%) 702

Breast enlargement

Aciphex Tablets (Rare) 1267
Aciphex Tablets (Rare) 1783
Activella Tablets 2764
Aldoclor Tablets 2035
Aldomet Tablets 2037
Aldoril Tablets 2039
Alesse-21 Tablets 3468
Alesse-28 Tablets 3473
Alora Transdermal System 3372
Aygestin Tablets 1333
Brevicon 28-Day Tablets 3380
Catapres-TTS (0.5% or less) 1038
Celexa (Infrequent) 1365
Cenestin Tablets 1263
Claritin (Rare) 3100
Claritin-D 12 Hour Extended Release Tablets 3102
Claritin-D 24 Hour Extended Release Tablets 3104
Climara Transdermal System 958
▲ CombiPatch Transdermal System (2% to 7%) 2323
Copaxone for Injection (Infrequent) 3306
▲ Crinone 8% Gel (40%) 3213
Cyclessa Tablets 2450
Demser Capsules (Infrequent) 2085
Depacon Injection 416
Depakene 421
Depakote Sprinkle Capsules 426
Depakote Tablets 430
Depakote ER Tablets 436
Desogen Tablets 2458
D.H.E. 45 Injection 2334
Effexor Tablets (Rare) 3495
Effexor XR Capsules (Rare) 3499
▲ Emcyt Capsules (60%) 2810
▲ Esclim Transdermal System (2.1% to 8.5%) 3460
Estinyl Tablets 3112
Estrace Vaginal Cream 3358
Estrace Tablets 3361
Estratest 3252
Estring Vaginal Ring (At least 1 report) 2811
Estrostep 2627
Etrafon 3115
femhrt Tablets 2635
Flexeril Tablets (Rare) 572
Flexeril Tablets (Rare) 2094
Fortovase Capsules 2970
Gabitril Tablets (Infrequent) 1189
Imitrex Nasal Spray 1554
Indocin Capsules (Less than 1%) 2112
Indocin I.V. (Less than 1%) 2115
Indocin (Less than 1%) 2112
Levlen 962
Levlite 21 Tablets 962
Levlite 28 Tablets 962
Levora Tablets 3389
Limbitrol 1738
Lipitor Tablets (Less than 2%) 2639
Lipitor Tablets (Less than 2%) 2696
Loestrin 21 Tablets 2642
Loestrin Fe Tablets 2642
Lunelle Monthly Injection 2827
Lupron Depot 7.5 mg (Less than 5%) 3284
Menest Tablets 2254
Microgestin Fe 1.5/30 Tablets 3407
Microgestin Fe 1/20 Tablets 3400
Mircette Tablets 2470
Modicon 2563
Navane Oral 2701
Navane Intramuscular 2703
Necon 3415
Norinyl 1 +35 28-Day Tablets 3380
Norinyl 1 + 50 28-Day Tablets 3380
Norpramin Tablets 755
Ogen Tablets 2846
Ortho Dienestrol Cream 2554
Ortho-Cept 21 Tablets 2546
Ortho-Cept 28 Tablets 2546
Ortho-Cyclen/Ortho Tri-Cyclen 2573
Ortho-Est Tablets 3464
Ortho-Novum 2563
Ortho-Novum 1/50▫28 Tablets 2556
Ortho-Prefest Tablets 2570
Ortho-Cyclen/Ortho Tri-Cyclen 2573
Ovcon 3364
Paxil (Rare) 1609
Premarin Intravenous 3563
Premarin Tablets 3566
Premarin Vaginal Cream 3570
Premphase Tablets 3572
Prempro Tablets 3572
Prevacid Delayed-Release Capsules (Less than 1%) 3292
PREVPAC (Less than 1%) 3298
Prometrium Capsules (100 mg, 200 mg) 3261
Propecia Tablets 2172
Proscar Tablets 2175
ProSom Tablets (Rare) 500
Prozac Pulvules, Liquid, and Weekly Capsules (Infrequent) 1238
Remeron Tablets (Rare) 2483
Remeron SolTab Tablets (Rare) 2486
Requip Tablets (Rare) 1621
Rescriptor Tablets (Less than 2%) 526
Sarafem Pulvules (Infrequent) 1962
Serzone Tablets (Infrequent) 1104
Sinequan 2713
Surmontil Capsules 3595
▲ Synarel Nasal Solution for Central Precocious Puberty (8%) 3204
Thiothixene Capsules 2290
Thorazine 1656
Thyrel TRH for Injection 3630
Trilafon 3160
Tri-Levlen 962
Tri-Norinyl-28 Tablets 3433
Triphasil-21 Tablets 3600
Triphasil-28 Tablets 3605
Trivora Tablets 3439
Uniretic Tablets (Less than 1%) 3178
▲ Viadur Implant (6.9%) 912
Viagra Tablets (Less than 2%) 2732
Vivactil Tablets 2217
Vivactil Tablets 2446
Vivelle Transdermal System 2412
Vivelle-Dot Transdermal System 2416
Yasmin 28 Tablets 980
▲ Zoladex (18%) 702
Zoloft (Rare) 2751
Zovia 3449

Breast fibroadenosis

Ambien Tablets (Rare) 3191
Aricept Tablets (Infrequent) 1270
Aricept Tablets (Infrequent) 2665
Avonex 1013
Celebrex Capsules (0.1% to 1.9%) 2676
Celebrex Capsules (0.1% to 1.9%) 2780
Gengraf Capsules (1% to less than 3%) 457
Neoral Soft Gelatin Capsules (1% to less than 3%) 2380
Neoral Oral Solution (1% to less than 3%) 2380

Breast fibrocystic

Alora Transdermal System (1.1% to 5.3%) 3372
Aricept Tablets (Infrequent) 1270
Aricept Tablets (Infrequent) 2665
Avonex 1013
▲ Betaseron for SC Injection (3%) 988
Clomid Tablets 735
Copaxone for Injection (Infrequent) 3306
Effexor Tablets (Rare) 3495
Effexor XR Capsules (Rare) 3499
Gabitril Tablets (Infrequent) 1189

Levlen 962
Levlite 21 Tablets 962
Levlite 28 Tablets 962
Lipitor Tablets (Less than 2%) 2639
Lipitor Tablets (Less than 2%) 2696
Modicon 2563
Ortho-Cyclen/Ortho Tri-Cyclen 2573
Ortho-Novum 2563
Ortho-Novum 1/50□28 Tablets 2556
Ortho-Cyclen/Ortho Tri-Cyclen 2573
Paxil (Rare) 1609
Permax Tablets (Infrequent) 1299
Prozac Pulvules, Liquid, and Weekly Capsules (Infrequent) 1238
Tri-Levlen 962

Breast lumps

Amerge Tablets (Rare) 1467
Avonex 1013
Depo-Provera Contraceptive Injection (Fewer than 1%) 2798
Imitrex Nasal Spray 1554
Levlen 962
Levlite 21 Tablets 962
Levlite 28 Tablets 962
Nipent for Injection (Less than 3%) 3272
Ortho-Cyclen/Ortho Tri-Cyclen 2573
Ortho-Est Tablets 3464
Ortho-Cyclen/Ortho Tri-Cyclen 2573
Tri-Levlen 962
Vioxx (Greater than 0.1% to 1.9%) 2213

Breast milk, maternal, excreted in

Accolate Tablets 657
Accuretic Tablets 2614
Activella Tablets 2764
Adalat CC Tablets 877
Adderall Tablets 3231
Adderall XR Capsules
Advair Diskus 100/50 1448
Advair Diskus 250/50 1448
Advair Diskus 500/50 1448
Aggrenox Capsules 1026
Aldoclor Tablets 2035
Aldomet Tablets 2037
Aldoril Tablets 2039
Alesse-21 Tablets 3468
Alesse-28 Tablets 3473
Aloprim for Injection 2292
Altace Capsules 2233
Ambien Tablets 3191
Anaprox Tablets 2967
Anaprox DS Tablets 2967
Androderm Transdermal System CIII 3377
Arthrotec Tablets 3195
Asacol Delayed-Release Tablets 2884
Astramorph/PF Injection, USP (Preservative-Free) 594
Ativan Injection 3478
Atromid-S Capsules 3483
Augmentin Chewable Tablets 1482
Augmentin Powder for Oral Suspension 1482
Augmentin Tablets 1485
Augmentin ES-600 Powder for Oral Suspension 1487
Avalide Tablets 1070
AVC 1350
Axid Pulvules 1903
Axid Pulvules 2919
Azactam for Injection 1276
Azulfidine EN-tabs Tablets 2775
Bactrim 2949
Baycol Tablets 883
Betapace Tablets 950
Bicillin C-R 900/300 Injection 2240
Bicillin C-R Injection 2238
Bicillin L-A Injection 2242
Biltricide Tablets 887
Blocadren Tablets 2046
Brevicon 28-Day Tablets 3380
Captopril Tablets 2281
Carbatrol Capsules 3234
Cardizem Injectable 1018
Cardizem Lyo-Ject Syringe 1018
Cardizem Monovial 1018
Cardizem CD Capsules 1016
Cataflam Tablets 2315
Catapres Tablets 1037
Catapres-TTS 1038
Ceclor 1905
Cefizox for Intramuscular or Intravenous Use 1390
Cefotan 664
Ceftin Tablets 1898
Celexa 1365
Ceptaz for Injection 1499
Cerebyx Injection 2619
Cipro HC Otic Suspension 540
Cipro I.V. 893
Cipro 887
Claforan Injection 732
Claritin 3100
Claritin-D 24 Hour Extended Release Tablets 3104
Cleocin HCl Capsules 2784
Cleocin Phosphate Sterile Solution 2785
Clorpres Tablets 1002
Clozaril Tablets 2319
CombiPatch Transdermal System 2323
Combipres Tablets 1040
Compazine 1505
Cordarone Intravenous 3491
Cordarone Tablets 3487
Corgard Tablets 2245
Cortone Acetate Injectable Suspension 2059
Cortone Acetate Tablets 2061
Corzide 40/5 Tablets 2247
Corzide 80/5 Tablets 2247
Cosopt Sterile Ophthalmic Solution 2065
Coumadin for Injection 1243
Coumadin Tablets 1243
Covera-HS Tablets 3199
Crinone 3213
Cyclessa Tablets 2450
Cytotec Tablets 3202
Dapsone Tablets USP 1780
Daraprim Tablets 1511
Darvon Compound-65 Pulvules 1910
Darvon-N Tablets 1912
Decadron Elixir 2078
Decadron Tablets 2079
Decadron Phosphate Injection 2081
Declomycin Tablets 1855
Demerol 3079
Depacon Injection 416
Depakene 421
Depakote Sprinkle Capsules 426
Depakote Tablets 430
Depakote ER Tablets 436
Desogen Tablets 2458
Desoxyn Tablets 440
Dexedrine 1512
DextroStat Tablets 3236
Diabinese Tablets 2680
Diflucan Tablets, Injection, and Oral Suspension 2681
Digitek Tablets 1003
Dilantin Infatabs 2624
Dilantin Kapseals 2622
Dilantin-125 Oral Suspension 2625
Dilaudid Oral Liquid 445
Dilaudid Tablets - 8 mg 445
Dilaudid-HP 443
Diovan HCT Tablets 2338
Diprivan Injectable Emulsion 667
Diucardin Tablets 3494
Diuril Oral 2087
Diuril Sodium Intravenous 2086
Dolobid Tablets 2088
Doryx Coated Pellet Filled Capsules 3357
Duraclon Injection 3057
Duragesic Transdermal System 1786
Duramorph Injection 1312
Dyazide Capsules 1515
Dyrenium Capsules 3458
EC-Naprosyn Delayed-Release Tablets 2967
Ecotrin Enteric Coated Aspirin Low, Regular and Maximum Strength Tablets 1715
E.E.S. 450
Effexor Tablets 3495
Effexor XR Capsules 3499
Emla 602
EryPed 446
Ery-Tab Tablets 448
Erythrocin Stearate Filmtab Tablets 452
Eskalith 1527
Estrostep 2627
Famotidine Injection 866
Felbatol 3343
Florinef Acetate Tablets 2250
Floxin I.V. 2526
Floxin Tablets 2529
Fluorescite Injection ⊙ 211
Fortaz 1541
Furosemide Tablets 2284
Gengraf Capsules 457
Glyset Tablets 2821
Guaifed 2272
Halcion Tablets 2823
Haldol Decanoate 2535
Haldol Injection, Tablets and Concentrate 2533
Hydrocortone Tablets 2106
Hydrocortone Acetate Injectable Suspension 2103
Hydrocortone Phosphate Injection, Sterile 2105
HydroDIURIL Tablets 2108
Ifex for Injection 1123
Imitrex Injection 1549
Imitrex Nasal Spray 1554
Imitrex Tablets 1558
Inderal 3513
Inderal LA Long-Acting Capsules 3516
Inderide Tablets 3517
Inderide LA Long-Acting Capsules 3519
Indocin 2112
INFeD Injection 3388
Inversine Tablets 1850
Isoptin SR Tablets 467
Kadian Capsules 1335
Keflex 1237
Kefurox Vials, ADD-Vantage 1948
Kefzol Vials, ADD-Vantage 1951
Lamictal 1567
Lamisil Tablets 2360
Lanoxicaps Capsules 1574
Lanoxin Injection 1581
Lanoxin Tablets 1587
Lanoxin Elixir Pediatric 1578
Lanoxin Injection Pediatric 1584
Lariam Tablets 2989
Lescol Capsules 2361
Lescol Capsules 2925
Lescol XL Tablets 2361
Lescol XL Tablets 2925
Levbid Extended-Release Tablets 3172
Levlen 962
Levlite 21 Tablets 962
Levlite 28 Tablets 962
Levora Tablets 3389
Levothroid Tablets 1373
Levoxyl Tablets 1819
Levsin/Levsinex/Levbid 3172
Lexxel Tablets 608
Lindane Lotion USP 1% 559
Lindane Shampoo USP 1% 560
Lithium Carbonate 3061
Lithium Citrate Syrup 3061
Lithobid Slow-Release Tablets 3255
Loestrin 21 Tablets 2642
Loestrin Fe Tablets 2642
Lo/Ovral Tablets 3532
Lo/Ovral-28 Tablets 3538
Lortab 3319
Lortab Elixir 3317
Lotensin Tablets 2365
Lotensin HCT Tablets 2367
Lotrel Capsules 2370
Low-Ogestrel-28 Tablets 3392
Lufyllin Tablets 3347
Lufyllin-400 Tablets 3347
Lufyllin-GG Elixir 3348
Lufyllin-GG Tablets 3348
Lunelle Monthly Injection 2827
Luvox Tablets (25, 50, 100 mg) 3256
Macrobid Capsules 2889
Macrodantin Capsules 2891
Marinol Capsules 3325
Maxidone Tablets CIII 3399
Maxipime for Injection 1285
Maxzide 1008
Mefoxin for Injection 2124
Mefoxin Premixed Intravenous Solution 2127
Mepergan Injection 3539
Meruvax II 2130
MetroCream 1404
MetroGel 1405
MetroLotion 1405
Mexitil Capsules 1047
Microgestin Fe 1.5/30 Tablets 3407
Microgestin Fe 1/20 Tablets 3400
Micronor Tablets 2543
Microzide Capsules 3414
Midamor Tablets 2136
Migranal Nasal Spray 2376
Miltown Tablets 3349
Minizide Capsules 2700
Minocin Intravenous 1862
Minocin Oral Suspension 1865
Minocin Pellet-Filled Capsules 1863
Mircette Tablets 2470
Modicon 2563
Moduretic Tablets 2138
Monodox Capsules 2442
Monopril Tablets 1091
Monopril HCT 1094
MS Contin Tablets 2896
MSIR 2898
Mykrox Tablets 1168
Naprelan Tablets 1293
Naprosyn Suspension 2967
Naprosyn Tablets 2967
Necon 3415
Nembutal Sodium Solution 485
Neoral Soft Gelatin Capsules 2380
Neoral Oral Solution 2380
Neurontin Capsules 2655
Neurontin Oral Solution 2655
Neurontin Tablets 2655
Niaspan Extended-Release Tablets 1846
Nicotrol Inhaler 2840
Nicotrol Nasal Spray 2843
Nizoral Tablets 1791
Norco 5/325 Tablets CIII 3424
Norco 7.5/325 Tablets CIII 3425
Norco 10/325 Tablets CIII 3425
Norco 10/325 Tablets CIII 3427
Nordette-28 Tablets 2257
Norinyl 1 +35 28-Day Tablets 3380
Norinyl 1 + 50 28-Day Tablets 3380
Noritate Cream 1224
Normodyne Injection 3135
Normodyne Tablets 3137
Norplant System 3543
Novantrone for Injection 1760
Nubain Injection 1323
Ogestrel 0.5/50-28 Tablets 3428
Oramorph SR Tablets 3062
Ortho-Cept 21 Tablets 2546
Ortho-Cept 28 Tablets 2546
Ortho-Cyclen/Ortho Tri-Cyclen 2573
Ortho-Novum 2563
Ortho-Novum 1/50□28 Tablets 2556
Ortho-Cyclen/Ortho Tri-Cyclen 2573
Ovcon 3364
Ovral Tablets 3551
Ovral-28 Tablets 3552
Ovrette Tablets 3552
Oxistat 1298
OxyContin Tablets 2912
OxyFast Oral Concentrate Solution 2916
OxyIR Capsules 2916
Pacerone Tablets 3331
Paxil 1609
PCE Dispertab Tablets 498
Pediapred Oral Solution 1170
Pediazole Suspension 3050
Pentasa Capsules 3239
Pepcid Injection 2153
Pepcid for Oral Suspension 2150
Pepcid RPD Orally Disintegrating Tablets 2150
Pepcid Tablets 2150
Periostat Tablets 1208
Permapen Isoject 2706
Persantine Tablets 1057
Pfizerpen for Injection 2707
Phenergan with Codeine Syrup 3557
Phenergan VC with Codeine Syrup 3561
Phrenilin 578
Pravachol Tablets 1099
Prednisone 3064
Premphase Tablets 3572
Prempro Tablets 3572
Prevacid Delayed-Release Capsules 3292
PREVPAC 3298
Prinzide Tablets 2168
Procanbid Extended-Release Tablets 2262
Prograf 1393
Protopic Ointment 1397
Provera Tablets 2853
Prozac Pulvules, Liquid, and Weekly Capsules 1238
Pulmicort Respules 632
Pulmicort Turbuhaler Inhalation Powder 636
Pyrazinamide Tablets 1876
Quinaglute Dura-Tabs Tablets 978
Quinidex Extentabs 2933
Qvar Inhalation Aerosol 1987
Reglan 2935
Renese Tablets 2712
Retrovir Capsules 1625
Retrovir IV Infusion 1629
Retrovir 1625
Rifamate Capsules 767
Rifater Tablets 769
Robaxisal Tablets 2939
Rocaltrol 2991
Rocephin Injectable Vials, ADD-Vantage, Galaxy, Bulk 2993
Roxanol 3066
Sandimmune 2388
Sarafem Pulvules 1962
Sectral Capsules 3589
Sedapap Tablets 50 mg/650 mg 2225
Semprex-D Capsules 1172
Septra Suspension 2265
Septra Tablets 2265
Septra DS Tablets 2265
Soma Tablets 3353
Soma Compound Tablets 3354
Soma Compound w/Codeine Tablets 3355
Sonata Capsules 3591
Sporanox Capsules 1800
Sporanox Injection 1804
Sporanox Injection 2509
Sporanox Oral Solution 1808
Sporanox Oral Solution 2512
Stadol NS Nasal Spray 1108
Stelazine 1640
Stromectol Tablets 2185
Symmetrel 1328
Synthroid 505
Tagamet 1644
Tambocor Tablets 1990
Tapazole Tablets 1823
Tarka Tablets 508
Tazicef for Injection 1647
Tazicef Galaxy Container 1650
Tazicef Pharmacy Bulk Package 1653
Tazidime Vials, Faspak & ADD-Vantage 1966
Tegretol/Tegretol-XR 2404
Tenoretic Tablets 690
Tenormin 692
Testoderm Transdermal Systems 574
Theo-Dur Extended-Release Tablets 1835
Thorazine 1656
Tiazac Capsules 1378
Timolide Tablets 2187
Timolol GFS ⊙ 266

Timoptic in Ocudose ... 2192
Timoptic Sterile Ophthalmic Solution ... 2190
Timoptic-XE Sterile Ophthalmic Gel Forming Solution ... 2194
Tolectin ... 2589
Toprol-XL Tablets ... 651
Toradol ... 3018
Tranxene ... 511
Trental Tablets ... 784
Trileptal Oral Suspension ... 2407
Trileptal Tablets ... 2407
Tri-Levlen ... 962
Trilisate ... 2901
Tri-Norinyl-28 Tablets ... 3433
Triphasil-21 Tablets ... 3600
Triphasil-28 Tablets ... 3605
Trisenox Injection ... 1158
Trivora Tablets ... 3439
Trovan ... 2722
Tylenol with Codeine ... 2595
Ultracet Tablets ... 2597
Ultram Tablets ... 2600
Unasyn for Injection ... 2728
Uni-Dur Extended-Release Tablets ... 1841
Uniphyl 400 mg and 600 mg Tablets ... 2903
Uniretic Tablets ... 3178
Unithroid Tablets ... 3445
Uroqid-Acid No. 2 Tablets ... 947
Vanceril Inhalation Aerosol ... 3165
Vanceril Double Strength Inhalation Aerosol ... 3167
Vancocin HCl Capsules & Pulvules ... 1972
Vancocin HCl Oral Solution ... 1971
Vancocin HCl, Vials & ADD-Vantage ... 1970
Vantin Tablets and Oral Suspension ... 2860
Vascor Tablets ... 2602
Vaseretic Tablets ... 2204
Vasotec Tablets ... 2210
Verelan Capsules ... 3184
Verelan PM Capsules ... 3186
Versed Injection ... 3027
Versed Syrup ... 3033
Vibramycin Calcium Oral Suspension Syrup ... 2735
Vibramycin Hyclate Capsules ... 2735
Vibramycin Hyclate Intravenous ... 2737
Vibramycin Monohydrate for Oral Suspension ... 2735
Vibra-Tabs Film Coated Tablets ... 2735
Vicodin Tablets ... 516
Vicodin ES Tablets ... 517
Vicodin HP Tablets ... 518
Viramune Oral Suspension ... 1060
Viramune Tablets ... 1060
Voltaren Tablets ... 2315
Voltaren-XR Tablets ... 2315
Warfarin Sodium Tablets, USP ... 3302
Wellbutrin SR Sustained-Release Tablets ... 1684
Xanax Tablets ... 2865
Yasmin 28 Tablets ... 980
Zantac ... 1690
Zantac Injection ... 1688
Zantac Syrup ... 1690
Zaroxolyn Tablets ... 1177
Zestoretic Tablets ... 695
Ziac Tablets ... 1887
Zinacef Injection ... 1696
Zinacef for Injection ... 1696
Zosyn ... 1890
Zosyn in Galaxy Containers ... 1894
Zovia ... 3449
Zovirax Capsules ... 1706
Zovirax for Injection ... 1708
Zovirax ... 1706
Zyban Sustained-Release Tablets ... 1710
Zyrtec ... 2756
Zyrtec-D 12 Hour Extended Relief Tablets ... 2758

Breast nipple bleeding

Depo-Provera Contraceptive Injection (Fewer than 1%) ... 2798

Breast pain

Actiq (1% or greater) ... 1184
▲ Activella Tablets (17% to 24%) ... 2764
▲ Alora Transdermal System (4.5% to 5.3%) ... 3372
Ambien Tablets (Rare) ... 3191
AndroGel (1% to 3%) ... 3322
▲ Arimidex Tablets (2% to 5%) ... 659
Arthrotec Tablets (Rare) ... 3195
Astelin Nasal Spray (Infrequent) ... 3339
▲ Betaseron for SC Injection (7%) ... 988
Cardura Tablets (Less than 0.5%) ... 2668
▲ Casodex Tablets (6%) ... 662
Celebrex Capsules (0.1% to 1.9%) ... 2676
Celebrex Capsules (0.1% to 1.9%) ... 2780
Celexa (Infrequent) ... 1365
▲ Cenestin Tablets (29%) ... 1263
Chirocaine Injection (1%) ... 2909
Cipro (0.3% to 1%) ... 887
Claritin (At least one patient) ... 3100
Claritin-D 12 Hour Extended Release Tablets ... 3102
Claritin-D 24 Hour Extended Release Tablets ... 3104
Clomid Tablets (1.5%) ... 735
Clozaril Tablets (Less than 1%) ... 2319
Cognex Capsules (Infrequent) ... 1351
▲ CombiPatch Transdermal System (34% to 48%) ... 2323
Copaxone for Injection (At least 2%) ... 3306
▲ Crinone 8% Gel (13%) ... 3213
Cytotec Tablets (Infrequent) ... 3202
▲ Depo-Provera Contraceptive Injection (More than 5%) ... 2798
Dostinex Tablets (1% to 2%) ... 2804
Doxil Injection (Less than 1%) ... 566
Effexor Tablets (Infrequent) ... 3495
Effexor XR Capsules (Infrequent) ... 3499
▲ Esclim Transdermal System (25% to 46.8%) ... 3460
Estring Vaginal Ring (1%) ... 2811
▲ Evista Tablets (4.4%) ... 1915
Evoxac Capsules (Less than 1%) ... 1217
Exelon Capsules (Infrequent) ... 2342
Exelon Oral Solution (Infrequent) ... 2345
▲ Femara Tablets (5%) ... 2351
▲ femhrt Tablets (8.1%) ... 2635
Gabitril Tablets (Infrequent) ... 1189
Gengraf Capsules (1% to less than 3%) ... 457
▲ Gonal-F for Injection (13.6% of men) ... 3216
Humegon for Injection (Occasional) ... 2468
Imdur Tablets (Less than or equal to 5%) ... 1826
Infergen (2%) ... 1777
Klonopin Tablets (Infrequent) ... 2983
Lamictal (Infrequent) ... 1567
Lunelle Monthly Injection ... 2827
▲ Lupron Depot–3 Month 11.25 mg (1.8% to 6%) ... 3285
▲ Lupron Injection (5% or more) ... 3279
Luvox Tablets (25, 50, 100 mg) (Infrequent) ... 3256
▲ Mirena Intrauterine System (5% or more) ... 974
Neoral Soft Gelatin Capsules (1% to less than 3%) ... 2380
Neoral Oral Solution (1% to less than 3%) ... 2380
Neurontin Capsules (Rare) ... 2655
Neurontin Oral Solution (Rare) ... 2655
Neurontin Tablets (Rare) ... 2655
▲ Ortho-Prefest Tablets (16%) ... 2570
Ovidrel for Injection (Less than 2%) ... 3220
Paxil (Infrequent) ... 1609
Pentasa Capsules (Less than 1%) ... 3239
Permax Tablets (Infrequent) ... 1299
▲ Premphase Tablets (Approximately one-third of subjects) ... 3572
▲ Prempro Tablets (33% to 38%) ... 3572
Prinivil Tablets (0.3% to 1.0%) ... 2164
Prinzide Tablets ... 2168
Procardia XL Extended Release Tablets (1% or less) ... 2710
▲ Prometrium Capsules (100 mg, 200 mg) (6% to 16%) ... 3261
Protonix I.V. (Less than 1%) ... 3580
Protonix Tablets (Less than 1%) ... 3577
Protopic Ointment (Greater than or equal to 1%) ... 1397
Prozac Pulvules, Liquid, and Weekly Capsules (Infrequent) ... 1238
Remeron Tablets (Infrequent) ... 2483
Remeron SolTab Tablets (Infrequent) ... 2486
Rilutek Tablets (Rare) ... 772
Risperdal (Rare to infrequent) ... 1796
Salagen Tablets (Less than 1%) ... 2229
Sandostatin LAR Depot (1% to 4%) ... 2395
Sarafem Pulvules (Infrequent) ... 1962
Serzone Tablets (1%) ... 1104
Sonata Capsules (Infrequent) ... 3591
Soriatane Capsules (Less than 1%) ... 3003
Sporanox Capsules (Infrequent) ... 1800
Sporanox Oral Solution (Less than 2%) ... 1808
Sporanox Oral Solution (Less than 2%) ... 2512
▲ Temodar Capsules (6%) ... 3157
▲ Topamax Sprinkle Capsules (8.3%) ... 2590
▲ Topamax Tablets (8.3%) ... 2590
Uniretic Tablets (Less than 1%) ... 3178
▲ Viadur Implant (3.1%) ... 912
Yasmin 28 Tablets (Greater than 1%) ... 980
Zestril Tablets (0.3% to 1.0%) ... 698
▲ Zoladex (7%) ... 702
Zoladex 3-month (1% to 5%) ... 706
Zoloft (Rare) ... 2751
Zyprexa Tablets (Infrequent) ... 1973
Zyprexa ZYDIS Orally Disintegrating Tablets (Infrequent) ... 1973
Zyrtec (Less than 2%) ... 2756
Zyrtec-D 12 Hour Extended Relief Tablets (Less than 2%) ... 2758

Breast pain, male

▲ Serostim for Injection (1% to 10%) ... 3229

Breast secretion

Alesse-21 Tablets ... 3468
Alesse-28 Tablets ... 3473
Amerge Tablets (Rare) ... 1467
Brevicon 28-Day Tablets ... 3380
Cyclessa Tablets ... 2450
Desogen Tablets ... 2458
Estinyl Tablets ... 3112
Estratest ... 3252
Estrostep ... 2627
Imitrex Nasal Spray ... 1554
Imitrex Tablets (Rare) ... 1558
Levlen ... 962
Levlite 21 Tablets ... 962
Levlite 28 Tablets ... 962
Levora Tablets ... 3389
Loestrin 21 Tablets ... 2642
Loestrin Fe Tablets ... 2642
Lunelle Monthly Injection ... 2827
Menest Tablets ... 2254
Microgestin Fe 1.5/30 Tablets ... 3407
Microgestin Fe 1/20 Tablets ... 3400
Mircette Tablets ... 2470
Modicon ... 2563
Necon ... 3415
Norinyl 1 +35 28-Day Tablets ... 3380
Norinyl 1 + 50 28-Day Tablets ... 3380
▲ Norplant System (5% or greater) ... 3543
Ortho Dienestrol Cream ... 2554
Ortho-Cept 21 Tablets ... 2546
Ortho-Cept 28 Tablets ... 2546
Ortho-Cyclen/Ortho Tri-Cyclen ... 2573
Ortho-Novum ... 2563
Ortho-Novum 1/50◘28 Tablets ... 2556
Ortho-Cyclen/Ortho Tri-Cyclen ... 2573
Ovcon ... 3364
Premarin Intravenous ... 3563
Premarin Vaginal Cream ... 3570
Topamax Sprinkle Capsules (Infrequent) ... 2590
Topamax Tablets (Infrequent) ... 2590
Tri-Levlen ... 962
Tri-Norinyl-28 Tablets ... 3433
Trivora Tablets ... 3439
Yasmin 28 Tablets ... 980
Zovia ... 3449

Breast size, changes

Depo-Provera Contraceptive Injection (Fewer than 1%) ... 2798

Breast size reduction

▲ Synarel Nasal Solution for Endometriosis (10% of patients) ... 3205

Breast tenderness

Activella Tablets ... 2764
Alesse-21 Tablets ... 3468
Alesse-28 Tablets ... 3473
Alora Transdermal System ... 3372
Aygestin Tablets ... 1333
Azactam for Injection (Less than 1%) ... 1276
Brevicon 28-Day Tablets ... 3380
Cenestin Tablets ... 1263
Climara Transdermal System ... 958
Cyclessa Tablets ... 2450
Desogen Tablets ... 2458
▲ Emcyt Capsules (66%) ... 2810
Esclim Transdermal System ... 3460
Estinyl Tablets ... 3112
Estrace Vaginal Cream ... 3358
Estrace Tablets ... 3361
Estratest ... 3252
Estrostep ... 2627
femhrt Tablets ... 2635
Follistim for Injection ... 2465
Imitrex Nasal Spray ... 1554
Imitrex Tablets (Infrequent) ... 1558
Indocin Capsules (Less than 1%) ... 2112
Indocin I.V. (Less than 1%) ... 2115
Indocin (Less than 1%) ... 2112
Levlen ... 962
Levlite 21 Tablets ... 962
Levlite 28 Tablets ... 962
Levora Tablets ... 3389
Loestrin 21 Tablets ... 2642
Loestrin Fe Tablets ... 2642
Lo/Ovral Tablets ... 3532
Lo/Ovral-28 Tablets ... 3538
Low-Ogestrel-28 Tablets ... 3392
Lunelle Monthly Injection ... 2827
▲ Lupron Depot–3 Month 11.25 mg (1.8% to 6%) ... 3285
▲ Lupron Injection (5% or more) ... 3279
Menest Tablets ... 2254
Microgestin Fe 1.5/30 Tablets ... 3407
Microgestin Fe 1/20 Tablets ... 3400
Micronor Tablets ... 2543
Mircette Tablets ... 2470
Modicon ... 2563
Necon ... 3415
Norinyl 1 +35 28-Day Tablets ... 3380
Norinyl 1 + 50 28-Day Tablets ... 3380
Nor-QD Tablets ... 3423
Ogen Tablets ... 2846
Ogestrel 0.5/50-28 Tablets ... 3428
Ortho Dienestrol Cream ... 2554
Ortho-Cept 21 Tablets ... 2546
Ortho-Cept 28 Tablets ... 2546
Ortho-Cyclen/Ortho Tri-Cyclen ... 2573
Ortho-Est Tablets ... 3464
Ortho-Novum ... 2563
Ortho-Novum 1/50◘28 Tablets ... 2556
Ortho-Prefest Tablets ... 2570
Ortho-Cyclen/Ortho Tri-Cyclen ... 2573
Ovcon ... 3364
Ovral Tablets ... 3551
Ovral-28 Tablets ... 3552
Ovrette Tablets ... 3552
Premarin Intravenous ... 3563
Premarin Tablets ... 3566
Premarin Vaginal Cream ... 3570
Premphase Tablets ... 3572
Prempro Tablets ... 3572
Prevacid Delayed-Release Capsules (Less than 1%) ... 3292
PREVPAC (Less than 1%) ... 3298
▲ Prometrium Capsules (100 mg, 200 mg) (27%) ... 3261
Propecia Tablets ... 2172
Proscar Tablets ... 2175
Prostin E2 Suppositories ... 2852
Provera Tablets ... 2853
Repronex for Intramuscular and Subcutaneous Injection (2%) ... 1347
Serophene Tablets (Approximately 1 in 50) ... 3226
▲ Testoderm Transdermal Systems (3%) ... 574
Tri-Levlen ... 962
Tri-Norinyl-28 Tablets ... 3433
Triphasil-21 Tablets ... 3600
Triphasil-28 Tablets ... 3605
Trivora Tablets ... 3439
Vivelle Transdermal System ... 2412
Vivelle-Dot Transdermal System ... 2416
Yasmin 28 Tablets ... 980
Zoladex (1% to 5%) ... 702
Zoladex 3-month ... 706
Zovia ... 3449

Breath, shortness of

▲ Adenocard Injection (12%) ... 1380
Aerobid/Aerobid-M (Less than 1%) ... 1363
Bactrim ... 2949
Ceftin Tablets (0.1% to 1%) ... 1898
Clomid Tablets ... 735
Clozaril Tablets (1%) ... 2319
Colestid Tablets (Infrequent) ... 2791
Coumadin for Injection ... 1243
Coumadin Tablets ... 1243
Dipentum Capsules (Rare) ... 2803
Dobutrex Solution Vials (1% to 3%) ... 1914
▲ Doxil Injection (Approximately 6.8%) ... 566
DynaCirc Capsules (0.5% to 1%) ... 2921
DynaCirc CR Tablets (0.5% to 1%) ... 2923
Eldepryl Capsules ... 3266
▲ Epogen for Injection (0.14% to 14%) ... 582
Estrace Vaginal Cream ... 3358
Estrace Tablets ... 3361
Floxin I.V. ... 2526
Floxin Tablets ... 2529
Gamimune N, 5% Solvent/Detergent Treated ... 925
Gamimune N, 10% Solvent/Detergent Treated ... 928
Guaifed ... 2272
Humalog (Less common) ... 1926
Humalog Mix 75/25 Pen (Less common) ... 1928
Humulin 50/50, 100 Units ... 1934
Humulin 70/30, 100 Units (Less common) ... 1935
Humulin 70/30 Pen (Less common) ... 1936
Humulin L, 100 Units (Less common) ... 1937
Humulin R Regular (U-500) (Less common) ... 1943
Humulin N NPH Pen (Less common) ... 1940
Iletin II, Regular (Pork), 100 Units (Less common) ... 1947
Imitrex Injection ... 1549
Imitrex Nasal Spray ... 1554
Imitrex Tablets ... 1558
Iopidine Sterile Ophthalmic Solution ... ⊙212
Klonopin Tablets ... 2983
K-Phos Neutral Tablets ... 946
K-Phos Original (Sodium Free) Tablets (Less frequent) ... 947
Kytril Injection (Rare) ... 2986
Kytril Tablets (Rare) ... 2988
▲ Leustatin Injection (7%) ... 2495
Levlen ... 962
Levlite 21 Tablets ... 962
Levlite 28 Tablets ... 962
Lupron Depot–3 Month 11.25 mg ... 3285
Maxzide ... 1008
Midamor Tablets (Less than or equal to 1%) ... 2136
Modicon ... 2563

Moduretic Tablets 2138
Children's Motrin Oral Suspension and Chewable Tablets 2006
Children's Motrin Oral Suspension .... ▣ 643
Infants' Motrin Concentrated Drops 2006
Junior Strength Motrin Caplets and Chewable Tablets 2006
▲ Navelbine Injection (3%; infrequent) 1604
Niaspan Extended-Release Tablets 1846
Novolin 70/30 PenFill (Rare) 2423
Novolin 70/30 Prefilled Disposable Insulin Delivery System (Rare) 2425
Novolin N PenFill (Rare) 2423
Novolin R PenFill (Rare) 2423
NovoLog Injection 2427
One-A-Day Tension & Mood Softgels .... ▣ 808
Orthoclone OKT3 Sterile Solution (Less than 1%) 2498
Ortho-Cyclen/Ortho Tri-Cyclen 2573
Ortho-Est Tablets 3464
Ortho-Novum 2563
Ortho-Novum 1/50▫28 Tablets 2556
Ortho-Cyclen/Ortho Tri-Cyclen 2573
Pediazole Suspension 3050
▲ Phrenilin (Among most frequent) 578
Procardia Capsules (2% or less) 2708
▲ Procrit for Injection (0.14% to 14%) 2502
Prosed/DS Tablets 3268
Retrovir Capsules 1625
Retrovir IV Infusion 1629
Retrovir 1625
Rifadin 765
Rifater Tablets 769
Sandostatin Injection (Less than 1%) 2394
▲ Sedapap Tablets 50 mg/650 mg (Among the most frequent) 2225
Septra Suspension (Rare) 2265
Septra Tablets (Rare) 2265
Septra DS Tablets (Rare) 2265
Serevent Inhalation Aerosol (1% to 3%) 1633
Serophene Tablets 3226
Soma Compound Tablets 3354
Sular Tablets (Very rare) 688
Synarel Nasal Solution for Central Precocious Puberty (2.6%) 3204
▲ Thrombate III (1 of 17) 944
▲ Toprol-XL Tablets (Approximately 3 of 100 patients) 651
Tri-Levlen 962
▲ Tylenol with Codeine (Among most frequent) 2595
Urimax Tablets 1769
Uroqid-Acid No. 2 Tablets 947
Velosulin BR Human Insulin 10 ml Vials 2435
Vivelle Transdermal System 2412
Vivelle-Dot Transdermal System 2416
Warfarin Sodium Tablets, USP 3302
Wellbutrin Tablets (Infrequent) 1680
Ziagen 1692
Zofran Injection (Rare) 1698
Zofran 1703
Zofran ODT Orally Disintegrating Tablets 1703

Breath sounds, abnormal
Epivir 1520
Epivir-HBV 1524
▲ Trisenox Injection (10%) 1158
▲ Zenapax for Injection (2% to 5%) 3046

Breathholding
▲ Suprane Liquid for Inhalation (30% to 68%) 874

Breathing, difficult
(*see under* Dyspnea)

Breathing, irregular
Dilaudid 441
Dilaudid Powder 441
Dilaudid Rectal Suppositories 441
Dilaudid Tablets 441
Dilaudid-HP 443
Imitrex Nasal Spray 1554
Lodosyn Tablets 1251
Lortab 3319
Lortab Elixir 3317
Monopril Tablets (0.4% to 1.0%) 1091
Sinemet Tablets 1253
Sinemet CR Tablets 1255
Vicodin Tablets 516
Vicodin ES Tablets 517
Vicoprofen Tablets 520
Zydone Tablets 1330

Breathing, labored
(*see under* Dyspnea)

Breathing, shallow
(*see under* Hypopnea)

Breathing, stertorous
Duragesic Transdermal System (Less than 1%) 1786
Neurontin Capsules (Rare) 2655
Neurontin Oral Solution (3.4%) 2655
Neurontin Tablets (Rare) 2655

Bromsulphalein retention, increase
(*see under* BSP retention, increase)

Bronchial constriction
Vaqta (Less than 1%) 2199

Bronchial obstruction
Blocadren Tablets 2046
Cosopt Sterile Ophthalmic Solution 2065
Timolol GFS .... ⊙ 266
Timoptic in Ocudose 2192
Timoptic Sterile Ophthalmic Solution 2190
Timoptic-XE Sterile Ophthalmic Gel Forming Solution 2194

Bronchial secretion, decreased
Atrovent Inhalation Aerosol (About 1 in 100) 1030

Bronchial secretions, increase
Mestinon 1740
Prostigmin Injectable 1744
Prostigmin Tablets 1744
Tensilon Injectable 1745

Bronchial secretions, thickening
▲ Benadryl Parenteral (Among most frequent) 2617
Betoptic S Ophthalmic Suspension (Rare) 537
Periactin Tablets 2155
▲ Rynatan Tablets (Among most common) 3351

Bronchiectasis
Pulmozyme Inhalation Solution 1426

Bronchiolitis
Comvax (Two vaccinees) 2056
Cuprimine Capsules 2075
Haldol Decanoate 2535
Prevnar for Injection 1870
Proventil Solution for Inhalation 0.5% (1.5% to 4%) 3144
Synagis Intramuscular (More than 1%) 2028

Bronchiolitis, obliterative
Depen Titratable Tablets (Rare) 3341
Pentasa Capsules (One case) 3239
Rituxan for Infusion (0.3%) 1750
Rituxan I.V. (0.3%) 1428

Bronchiolitis obliterans organizing pneumonia
Pacerone Tablets 3331

Bronchitis
AccuNeb Inhalation Solution (0.9% to 1.7%) 1230
Accuretic Tablets (1.2%) 2614
Aceon Tablets (2 mg, 4 mg, 8 mg) (0.3% to 1%) 3249
Actiq (1% or greater) 1184
▲ Actonel Tablets (3.3%) 2879
Advair Diskus 100/50 (2%) 1448
▲ Advair Diskus 250/50 (8%) 1448
▲ Advair Diskus 500/50 (2% to 8%) 1448
Aerobid/Aerobid-M (1% to 3%) 1363
Agrylin Capsules (1% to 5%) 3232
Alamast Ophthalmic Solution (Less than 5%) 3092
Alphagan P Ophthalmic Solution (1% to 4%) 546
Ambien Tablets (Infrequent) 3191
Amerge Tablets (Infrequent) 1467
▲ Apligraf (3.6%) 2305
Arava Tablets (7%) 724
Aricept Tablets (Frequent) 1270
Aricept Tablets (Frequent) 2665
▲ Arimidex Tablets (2% to 5%) 659
Aromasin Tablets (Less frequent) 2769
Asacol Delayed-Release Tablets (2% or greater) 2884
Atacand Tablets (More than 1%) 595
Atacand HCT Tablets (0.5% or greater) 597
▲ Atrovent Inhalation Solution (14.6%) 1031
Axert Tablets (Infrequent) 2772
Baycol Tablets (1.3%) 883
Betaxon Ophthalmic Suspension (Less than 2%) 537
▲ Campath Ampules (13% to 21%) 992
▲ Carnitor Injection (3% to 5%) 3242
▲ Casodex Tablets (6%) 662
Ceclor CD Tablets (0.1% to 1%) 1279
Celebrex Capsules (0.1% to 1.9%) 2676
Celebrex Capsules (0.1% to 1.9%) 2780
Celexa (Infrequent) 1365
▲ CellCept Capsules (8.5% to 11.9%) 2951
▲ CellCept Intravenous (8.5% to 11.9%) 2951
▲ CellCept Oral Suspension (8.5% to 11.9%) 2951
▲ CellCept Tablets (8.5% to 11.9%) 2951
Cerebyx Injection (Infrequent) 2619
Claritin (At least one patient) 3100
Claritin-D 12 Hour Extended Release Tablets (Less frequent) 3102
Claritin-D 24 Hour Extended Release Tablets 3104
Clozaril Tablets (Less than 1%) 2319
Cognex Capsules (Frequent) 1351
▲ CombiPatch Transdermal System (3% to 5%) 2323
▲ Combivent Inhalation Aerosol (12.3%) 1041
▲ Copaxone for Injection (9%) 3306
▲ Coreg Tablets (5.4%) 1508
Cosopt Sterile Ophthalmic Solution (1% to 5%) 2065
Cozaar Tablets (Less than 1%) 2067
Cytotec Tablets (Infrequent) 3202
▲ Depacon Injection (5%) 416
▲ Depakene (5%) 421
▲ Depakote Sprinkle Capsules (5%) 426
▲ Depakote Tablets (5%) 430
Depakote ER Tablets (Greater than %) 436
Detrol Tablets (2.1%) 3623
Ditropan XL Extended Release Tablets (2% to 5%) 564
Doxil Injection (Less than 1%) 566
DuoNeb Inhalation Solution (1.7%) 1233
Effexor Tablets (Frequent) 3495
Enalaprilat Injection 863
Enbrel for Injection 1752
Enbrel for Injection 3504
Estring Vaginal Ring (1% to 3%) 2811
▲ Evoxac Capsules (4.1%) 1217
Exelon Capsules (2% or more) 2342
Exelon Oral Solution (2% or more) 2345
Flonase Nasal Spray (1% to 3%) 1533
Flovent Diskus (2%) 3614
Flovent (1% to 3%) 1535
Flovent Rotadisk (1% to 4%) 1537
Fludara for Injection (Up to 1%) 995
▲ Foradil Aerolizer (4.6%) 2354
Fortovase Capsules (Less than 2%) 2970
Gabitril Tablets (Frequent) 1189
Gengraf Capsules (1%) 457
Hytrin Capsules (At least 1%) 464
Hyzaar (1% or greater) 2109
Imdur Tablets (Less than or equal to 5%) 1826
Imitrex Nasal Spray 1554
▲ Infergen (2% to 6%) 1777
Intron A for Injection (Less than or equal to 5%) 3120
Invirase Capsules (Less than 2%) 2979
Ismo Tablets (Fewer than 1%) 3524
Kaletra Capsules (Less than 2%) 471
Kaletra Oral Solution (Less than 2%) 471
Keppra Tablets (1% or more) 3314
Klonopin Tablets (1%) 2983
Lescol Capsules (1.8%) 2361
Lescol Capsules (1.8%) 2925
Lescol XL Tablets (2.6%) 2361
Lescol XL Tablets (2.6%) 2925
Lexxel Tablets (Infrequent) 608
Lipitor Tablets (Greater than or equal to 2%) 2639
Lipitor Tablets (Greater than or equal to 2%) 2696
Lodine (Less than 1%) 3528
Lodine XL Extended-Release Tablets (Less than 1%) 3530
Lotensin Tablets (Less than 1%) 2365
Lotensin HCT Tablets (0.3% or more) 2367
Lupron Depot–4 Month 30 mg (Less than 5%) 3289
Luvox Tablets (25, 50, 100 mg) (Infrequent) 3256
LYMErix Vaccine (1.1% to 1.32%) 1592
Meridia Capsules (Greater than or equal to 1%) 481
Miacalcin Nasal Spray (Less than 1%) 2375
Micardis Tablets (More than 0.3%) 1049
Micardis HCT Tablets (Less than 2%) 1051
Migranal Nasal Spray (Rare) 2376
Naprelan Tablets (Less than 3%) 1293
Nasonex Nasal Spray (Greater than or equal to 2%) 3131
Neoral Soft Gelatin Capsules (1%) 2380
Neoral Oral Solution (1%) 2380
▲ Neurontin Oral Solution (3.4%) 2655
▲ Nicotrol Inhaler (Greater than 3%) 2840
Nicotrol Nasal Spray (Less than 1%) 2843
▲ Nipent for Injection (3%) 3272
OptiPranolol Metipranolol Ophthalmic Solution 0.3% (A small number of patients) .... ⊙ 263
Paxil (Infrequent) 1609
▲ Periostat Tablets (3%) 1208
Permax Tablets (Infrequent) 1299
Photofrin for Injection 831
▲ Plavix Tablets (3.7%) 1097
▲ Plavix Tablets (3.7%) 3084
Plendil Extended-Release Tablets (0.5% to 1.5%) 623
Pletal Tablets (2% or greater) 2605
Pletal Tablets (2% or greater) 2848
▲ Prandin Tablets (0.5, 1, and 2 mg) (2% to 6%) 2432
Prevacid Delayed-Release Capsules (Less than 1%) 3292
PREVPAC (Less than 1%) 3298
Prinivil Tablets (0.3% to 1.0%) 2164
Prinzide Tablets (0.3% to 1%) 2168
▲ Prograf (3% to 15%) 1393
Prometrium Capsules (100 mg, 200 mg) (Less than 5%) 3261
Protonix I.V. (Greater than or equal to 1%) 3580
Protonix Tablets (Greater than or equal to 1%) 3577
▲ Protopic Ointment (2% to 6%) 1397
Proventil Inhalation Solution 0.083% (1.5% to 4%) 3146
Provigil Tablets (At least 1%) 1193
Pulmozyme Inhalation Solution 1426
▲ Rapamune Oral Solution and Tablets (3% to 20%) 3584
Relenza Rotadisk (2%) 1619
Remeron Tablets (Infrequent) 2483
Remeron SolTab Tablets (Infrequent) 2486
▲ Remicade for IV Injection (6% to 26%) 1178
Reminyl Oral Solution (Greater than or equal to 2%) 1792
Reminyl Tablets (Greater than or equal to 2%) 1792
ReoPro Vials (0.3%) 1958
▲ Requip Tablets (3%) 1621
Rilutek Tablets (More than 2%) 772
Rituxan for Infusion (1% to 5%) 1750
Rituxan I.V. (1% to 5%) 1428
Roxicodone Tablets (Less than 3%) 3067
Salagen Tablets (Less than 1%) 2229
Sandostatin LAR Depot (1% to 4%) 2395
▲ Serevent Diskus (4% to 7%) 1637
Serevent Inhalation Aerosol (1% to 3%) 1633
▲ Serostim for Injection (1% to 10%) 3229
Serzone Tablets (Frequent) 1104
▲ Simulect for Injection (3% to 10%) 2399
Singulair (Greater than or equal to 2%) 2181
Skelid Tablets (More than or equal to 1%) 3088
Sonata Capsules (Frequent) 3591
Stadol NS Nasal Spray (1% or greater) 1108
Starlix Tablets (2.7%) 2401
Synagis Intramuscular (More than 1%) 2028
Tamiflu Capsules (0.7% to 2.3%) 3008
Tamiflu Oral Suspension (0.7% to 2.3%) 3008
Tarka Tablets (1.5%) 508
Tasmar Tablets (Frequent) 3010
Teveten Tablets (1% or greater) 3327
Tiazac Capsules (1% to 4%) 1378
Topamax Sprinkle Capsules (Frequent; More than 1%) 2590
Topamax Tablets (Frequent; More than 1%) 2590
Travatan Ophthalmic Solution (1% to 5%) 543
Tricor Capsules, Micronized 513
Trileptal Oral Suspension (Up to 3%) 2407
Trileptal Tablets (Up to 3%) 2407
Uniretic Tablets (More than 1%) 3178
▲ Vagifem Tablets (3% to 5%) 2857
Vanceril Double Strength Inhalation Aerosol (Fewer than 2%) 3167
Vantin Tablets and Oral Suspension (Less than 1%) 2860
Vaseretic Tablets 2204
Vasotec I.V. Injection 2207
Vasotec Tablets (0.5% to 1.0%) 2210
Viagra Tablets (Less than 2%) 2732
Vicoprofen Tablets (Less than 1%) 520
Vioxx (0.8%) 2213
Vistide Injection 1445
Vitravene for Injection (2% to 5%) .... ⊙ 310
Wellbutrin Tablets (Infrequent) 1680
Wellbutrin SR Sustained-Release Tablets 1684
Xeloda Tablets (Less than 5%) 3039
Yasmin 28 Tablets (Greater than 1%) 980
Zanaflex Tablets (Infrequent) 1305

Zebeta Tablets ... 1885
Zestoretic Tablets (0.3% to 1%) ... 695
Zestril Tablets (0.3% to 1.0%) ... 698
Ziac Tablets ... 1887
Zoladex (1% or greater) ... 702
Zoladex 3-month ... 706
Zoloft (Rare) ... 2751
Zomig Tablets (Infrequent) ... 708
Zomig-ZMT Tablets (Infrequent) ... 708
Zyban Sustained-Release Tablets (2%) ... 1710
Zyrtec (Less than 2%) ... 2756
Zyrtec-D 12 Hour Extended Relief Tablets (Less than 2%) ... 2758

Bronchoconstriction

Intron A for Injection (Rare) ... 3120
Rebetron Combination Therapy ... 3153
Tensilon Injectable ... 1745
Urecholine ... 2198
Urecholine Tablets ... 2445

Bronchoconstriction, paradoxical

Maxair Inhaler ... 1984

Bronchopneumonia

Xeloda Tablets (Less than 5%) ... 3039

Bronchopulmonary dysplasia

▲ Curosurf Intratracheal Suspension (18%) ... 1232
Myleran Tablets ... 1603

Bronchospasm

Abelcet Injection (Rare) ... 1273
Accutane Capsules ... 2944
Actimmune (Rare) ... 1772
Adenocard Injection ... 1380
Aggrenox Capsules (Less than 1%) ... 1026
AK-Fluor Injection 10% and 25% ... ⊙ 202
Albuminar-5, U.S.P. ... 785
Albuminar-25, U.S.P. ... 786
Alkeran for Injection (In some patients) ... 1465
Ambien Tablets (Rare) ... 3191
Anzemet Injection (Rare) ... 719
Anzemet Tablets (Rare) ... 722
Astelin Nasal Spray (Infrequent) ... 3339
Atrovent Inhalation Solution (2.3%) ... 1031
Atrovent Nasal Spray 0.06% (Rare) ... 1033
Attenuvax ... 2044
Avonex ... 1013
Axid Pulvules (Rare) ... 1903
Axid Pulvules (Rare) ... 2919
Azactam for Injection (Less than 1%) ... 1276
Beconase Inhalation Aerosol (Rare) ... 1497
Beconase AQ Nasal Spray (Rare) ... 1498
Betagan ... ⊙ 228
▲ Betimol Ophthalmic Solution (More than 5%) ... ⊙ 324
Betoptic S Ophthalmic Suspension (Rare) ... 537
Blocadren Tablets (0.6%) ... 2046
Brevibloc Injection (Less than 1%) ... 858
Brevital Sodium for Injection, USP ... 1815
▲ Campath Ampules (2% to 9%) ... 992
Captopril Tablets ... 2281
Cardura Tablets (Less than 0.5%) ... 2668
Carteolol Hydrochloride Ophthalmic Solution USP, 1% ... ⊙ 258
Cataflam Tablets ... 2315
Celebrex Capsules (0.1% to 1.9%) ... 2676
Celebrex Capsules (0.1% to 1.9%) ... 2780
Celexa (Rare) ... 1365
Ceptaz for Injection (Very rare) ... 1499
Chirocaine Injection (Less than 1%) ... 2909
Cipro (Less than 1%) ... 887
Claritin (At least one patient) ... 3100
Claritin-D 12 Hour Extended Release Tablets (Less frequent) ... 3102
Claritin-D 24 Hour Extended Release Tablets (Fewer than 2%) ... 3104
Clinoril Tablets (Less than 1 in 100) ... 2053
Colazal Capsules ... 3069
Combivent Inhalation Aerosol (0.3%; rare) ... 1041
Coreg Tablets (Less than or equal to 0.1%) ... 1508
Corgard Tablets (1 of 1000 patients) ... 2245
Corzide 40/5 Tablets (1 of 1000 patients) ... 2247
Corzide 80/5 Tablets (1 of 1000 patients) ... 2247
Cosopt Sterile Ophthalmic Solution ... 2065
Cytotec Tablets (Infrequent) ... 3202
Cytovene ... 2959
D.H.E. 45 Injection ... 2334
Dilaudid Oral Liquid ... 445
Dilaudid Tablets - 8 mg ... 445
Dilaudid-HP (Less frequent) ... 443
Diovan HCT Tablets (Greater than 0.2%) ... 2338
Dipentum Capsules (Rare) ... 2803
Diprivan Injectable Emulsion (Rare) ... 667
Dobutrex Solution Vials (Occasional) ... 1914
Dolobid Tablets (Less than 1 in 100) ... 2088
Dopram Injectable ... 2931
Ecotrin Enteric Coated Aspirin Low, Regular and Maximum Strength Tablets ... 1715
ELA-Max Cream ... 1340
ELA-Max 5 Cream ... 1340
Emla ... 602
Enalaprilat Injection ... 863
Engerix-B Vaccine ... 1517
Evoxac Capsules (Less than 1%) ... 1217
Exelon Capsules (Infrequent) ... 2342
Exelon Oral Solution (Infrequent) ... 2345
Factrel (Rare) ... 3633
Famotidine Injection (Infrequent) ... 866
Flonase Nasal Spray ... 1533
Flovent (Rare) ... 1535
Floxin I.V. ... 2526
Floxin Tablets ... 2529
Flumadine (Less than 0.3%) ... 1370
Fluorescite Injection ... ⊙ 211
Fortaz (Very rare) ... 1541
Foscavir Injection (Between 1% and 5%) ... 605
Gammagard S/D ... 845
Gemzar for Injection (Less than 2%) ... 1919
Gengraf Capsules (1% to 5.0%) ... 457
Haldol Decanoate ... 2535
Haldol Injection, Tablets and Concentrate ... 2533
Herceptin I.V. ... 1414
Imdur Tablets (Less than or equal to 5%) ... 1826
Imitrex Injection ... 1549
Imitrex Nasal Spray ... 1554
Inderal ... 3513
Inderal LA Long-Acting Capsules ... 3516
Inderide Tablets ... 3517
Inderide LA Long-Acting Capsules ... 3519
INFeD Injection ... 3388
Intron A for Injection (Less than or equal to 5%) ... 3120
Lamictal (Rare) ... 1567
Lexxel Tablets ... 608
Lidoderm Patch (Rare) ... 1319
Meruvax II ... 2130
Miacalcin Injection (A few cases) ... 2373
Miacalcin Nasal Spray (1% to 3%) ... 2375
Migranal Nasal Spray (Rare) ... 2376
Miltown Tablets (Rare) ... 3349
M-M-R II ... 2118
Mobic Tablets (Less than 2%) ... 1054
Monopril Tablets (0.2% to 1.0%) ... 1091
Monopril HCT ... 1094
Motrin Suspension, Oral Drops, Chewable Tablets, and Caplets (Less than 1%) ... 2002
Mumpsvax ... 2141
Mykrox Tablets ... 1168
Nadolol Tablets (1 of 1000 patients) ... 2288
Naropin Injection (Less than 1%) ... 612
Navelbine Injection (Infrequent) ... 1604
Neoral Soft Gelatin Capsules (1% to 5.0%) ... 2380
Neoral Oral Solution (1% to 5.0%) ... 2380
Neurontin Capsules (Rare) ... 2655
Neurontin Oral Solution (Rare) ... 2655
Neurontin Tablets (Rare) ... 2655
Nicotrol Nasal Spray (Less than 1%) ... 2843
Nipent for Injection (Less than 3%) ... 3272
Norcuron for Injection (Rare) ... 2478
Normodyne Tablets (Less common) ... 3137
Norvir Capsules ... 487
Norvir Oral Solution ... 487
Nubain Injection (1% or less) ... 1323
Numorphan ... 1324
Ocupress Ophthalmic Solution, 1% Sterile ... ⊙ 303
▲ Oncaspar (Less than 1% to greater than 5%) ... 756
Orthoclone OKT3 Sterile Solution (Less than 1%) ... 2498
Orudis Capsules (Less than 1%) ... 3548
Oruvail Capsules (Less than 1%) ... 3548
Paraplatin for Injection (Rare) ... 1126
Pepcid Injection (Infrequent) ... 2153
Pepcid for Oral Suspension (Infrequent) ... 2150
Pepcid RPD Orally Disintegrating Tablets (Infrequent) ... 2150
Pepcid Tablets (Infrequent) ... 2150
Photofrin for Injection ... 831
Plavix Tablets (Very rare) ... 1097
Plavix Tablets (Very rare) ... 3084
Prevnar for Injection ... 1870
Prinivil Tablets (0.3% to 1.0%) ... 2164
Prinzide Tablets ... 2168
Prostigmin Injectable ... 1744
Prostigmin Tablets ... 1744
Proventil Inhalation Aerosol (Rare) ... 3142
▲ Proventil Inhalation Solution 0.083% (8% to 15.4%) ... 3146
▲ Proventil Solution for Inhalation 0.5% (8% to 15.4%) ... 3144
Proventil HFA Inhalation Aerosol (Rare) ... 3150
Pulmicort Respules (Less than 1%) ... 632
Pulmicort Turbuhaler Inhalation Powder (Rare) ... 636
Quinaglute Dura-Tabs Tablets ... 978
Quinidex Extentabs ... 2933
Qvar Inhalation Aerosol (Rare) ... 1987
Recombivax HB (Less than 1%) ... 2178
Refludan for Injection (Common) ... 761
Reglan (A few cases) ... 2935
Relenza Rotadisk (Less than 1%) ... 1619
ReoPro Vials (0.3%) ... 1958
Rhinocort Aqua Nasal Spray (2%) ... 642
Rhinocort Nasal Inhaler (Rare) ... 640
Risperdal (Infrequent) ... 1796
▲ Rituxan for Infusion (1% to 8%) ... 1750
▲ Rituxan I.V. (1% to 8%) ... 1428
Rocephin Injectable Vials, ADD-Vantage, Galaxy, Bulk (Rare) ... 2993
Roferon-A Injection (Less than 1%) ... 2996
Semprex-D Capsules (Rare) ... 1172
Serevent Inhalation Aerosol (Rare) ... 1633
▲ Serostim for Injection (1% to 10%) ... 3229
▲ Simulect for Injection (3% to 10%) ... 2399
Streptase for Infusion (Rare) ... 647
▲ Suprane Liquid for Inhalation (3% to 10%) ... 874
Tambocor Tablets (Less than 1%) ... 1990
Taxotere for Injection Concentrate (0.9%) ... 778
Tazicef for Injection (Very rare) ... 1647
Tazicef Galaxy Container (Very rare) ... 1650
Tazicef Pharmacy Bulk Package (Very rare) ... 1653
Tazidime Vials, Faspak & ADD-Vantage (Very rare) ... 1966
Tenormin (1.2%) ... 692
Tequin Injection (Less than 0.1%) ... 1110
Tequin Tablets (Less than 0.1%) ... 1110
Tessalon Capsules ... 1377
Timolide Tablets (1.6%) ... 2187
Timolol GFS ... ⊙ 266
Timoptic in Ocudose (Less frequent) ... 2192
Timoptic Sterile Ophthalmic Solution (Less frequent) ... 2190
Timoptic-XE Sterile Ophthalmic Gel Forming Solution ... 2194
TOBI Solution for Inhalation ... 1206
Topamax Sprinkle Capsules (Infrequent) ... 2590
Topamax Tablets (Infrequent) ... 2590
Toprol-XL Tablets (About 1 of 100 patients) ... 651
Toradol ... 3018
Trovan (Less than 1%) ... 2722
Trusopt Sterile Ophthalmic Solution ... 2196
Twinrix Vaccine ... 1674
Ultram Tablets ... 2600
Univasc Tablets (Less than 1%) ... 3181
Vancenase PocketHaler Nasal Inhaler (Rare) ... 3162
Vanceril Inhalation Aerosol (Rare) ... 3165
Vanceril Double Strength Inhalation Aerosol (Rare) ... 3167
Vaseretic Tablets ... 2204
Vasotec I.V. Injection ... 2207
Vasotec Tablets (0.5% to 1.0%) ... 2210
Ventolin Inhalation Aerosol and Refill (Rare) ... 1679
Ventolin HFA Inhalation Aerosol ... 3618
Versed Injection (Less than 1%) ... 3027
Viracept ... 532
Virazole for Inhalation Solution (Infrequent) ... 1747
Volmax Extended-Release Tablets (Rare) ... 2276
Voltaren Tablets ... 2315
Voltaren-XR Tablets ... 2315
Wellbutrin SR Sustained-Release Tablets (Rare) ... 1684
Xeloda Tablets (Less than 5%) ... 3039
Zantac (Rare) ... 1690
Zantac Injection ... 1688
Zantac Syrup (Rare) ... 1690
Zaroxolyn Tablets ... 1177
Zebeta Tablets ... 1885
Zemuron Injection (Less than 1%) ... 2491
Zestoretic Tablets ... 695
Zestril Tablets (0.3% to 1.0%) ... 698
Ziac Tablets (Rare) ... 1887
Zithromax for IV Infusion (1% or less) ... 2748
Zofran Injection (Rare) ... 1698
Zofran (Rare) ... 1703
Zofran ODT Orally Disintegrating Tablets (Rare) ... 1703
Zoloft (Infrequent) ... 2751
Zomig Tablets (Infrequent) ... 708
Zomig-ZMT Tablets (Infrequent) ... 708
Zosyn (1.0% or less) ... 1890
Zosyn in Galaxy Containers (1.0% or less) ... 1894
Zyban Sustained-Release Tablets (Rare) ... 1710
Zyrtec (1.9% to 3.1%) ... 2756

Bronchospasm, exacerbation of

AccuNeb Inhalation Solution ... 1230
Brethine Ampuls ... 2314
Brethine Tablets ... 2313
Cardura Tablets ... 2668
Celebrex Capsules (0.1% to 1.9%) ... 2676
Celebrex Capsules (0.1% to 1.9%) ... 2780
Didronel Tablets (Rare) ... 2888
Nicotrol Nasal Spray ... 2843
Proventil Repetabs Tablets ... 3148
Serevent Diskus ... 1637
Serevent Inhalation Aerosol ... 1633

Bronchospasm, paradoxical

AccuNeb Inhalation Solution ... 1230
Advair Diskus 100/50 ... 1448
Advair Diskus 250/50 ... 1448
Advair Diskus 500/50 ... 1448
Alupent Inhalation Solution ... 1029
Combivent Inhalation Aerosol (Less than 2%) ... 1041
DuoNeb Inhalation Solution ... 1233
Flovent Diskus ... 3614
Flovent Rotadisk ... 1537
Proventil Repetabs Tablets ... 3148
Proventil Solution for Inhalation 0.5% ... 3144
Proventil HFA Inhalation Aerosol ... 3150
Serevent Diskus ... 1637
Serevent Inhalation Aerosol ... 1633
Ventolin Inhalation Aerosol and Refill ... 1679
Ventolin HFA Inhalation Aerosol ... 3618
Xopenex Inhalation Solution ... 3207

Browache

Epifrin Sterile Ophthalmic Solution ... ⊙ 235
Humorsol Sterile Ophthalmic Solution ... 2102
OptiPranolol Metipranolol Ophthalmic Solution 0.3% (A small number of patients) ... ⊙ 263
▲ Rēv-Eyes Sterile Ophthalmic Eyedrops 0.5% (10% to 40%) ... ⊙ 265
Vexol 1% Ophthalmic Suspension (Less than 1%) ... ⊙ 222

Bruising

Accolate Tablets ... 657
Accutane Capsules ... 2944
Arthrotec Tablets (Rare) ... 3195
Azmacort Inhalation Aerosol ... 728
Carbatrol Capsules ... 3234
Cataflam Tablets (Rare) ... 2315
Cetrotide for Injection ... 3209
Clozaril Tablets (Less than 1%) ... 2319
Coumadin for Injection ... 1243
Coumadin Tablets ... 1243
Covera-HS Tablets (Less than 2%) ... 3199
Depacon Injection ... 416
Depakene ... 421
Depakote Sprinkle Capsules ... 426
Depakote Tablets ... 430
Depakote ER Tablets ... 436
Depen Titratable Tablets ... 0041
▲ Emcyt Capsules (3%) ... 2810
Enbrel for Injection ... 1752
Enbrel for Injection ... 3504
Felbatol ... 3343
Feldene Capsules (Occasional) ... 2685
Florinef Acetate Tablets ... 2250
Floxin I.V. ... 2526
Floxin Tablets ... 2529
Hycamtin for Injection ... 1546
Imitrex Injection ... 1549
Isoptin SR Tablets (1% or less) ... 467
Lexxel Tablets ... 608
Maxair Autohaler (0.6%) ... 1981
Maxair Inhaler (Less than 1%) ... 1984
Neurontin Capsules (Frequent) ... 2655
Neurontin Oral Solution (Frequent) ... 2655
Neurontin Tablets (Frequent) ... 2655
Norplant System (Less than 1%) ... 3543
▲ Nutropin Depot for Injectable Suspension (20%) ... 1423
Oncaspar ... 756
▲ Ovidrel for Injection (3% to 4.7%) ... 3220
Plendil Extended-Release Tablets (0.5% to 1.5%) ... 623
ReFacto Vials ... 1437
Rescriptor Tablets (Less than 2%) ... 526
Roferon-A Injection (Less than 4%) ... 2996
Rythmol Tablets – 150 mg, 225 mg, 300 mg (Less than 1%) ... 502
Sandostatin Injection (1% to 4%) ... 2394
Singulair ... 2181
Tarka Tablets ... 508
Tegretol/Tegretol-XR ... 2404
Tonocard Tablets ... 649
Trileptal Oral Suspension ... 2407

Trileptal Tablets 2407
Verelan Capsules (1% or less) 3184
Verelan PM Capsules (2% or less) 3186
Voltaren Tablets (Rare) 2315
Voltaren-XR Tablets (Rare) 2315
Warfarin Sodium Tablets, USP 3302

Bruxism
Crixivan Capsules (Less than 2%) 2070
Effexor Tablets (Infrequent) 3495
Effexor XR Capsules (Infrequent) 3499
Eldepryl Capsules 3266
Lodosyn Tablets 1251
Paxil (Infrequent) 1609
Seroquel Tablets (Infrequent) 684
Sinemet Tablets 1253
Sinemet CR Tablets 1255
Sonata Capsules (Rare) 3591
Wellbutrin Tablets (Infrequent) 1680
Wellbutrin SR Sustained-Release Tablets (Infrequent) 1684
Zyban Sustained-Release Tablets (Infrequent) 1710

BSP retention
Atromid-S Capsules 3483
Sterile FUDR 2974
Mylocel Tablets 2227

BSP retention, increase
Anadrol-50 Tablets 3321
Estratest 3252
Mithracin for Intravenous Use 903
Oxandrin Tablets 1153
Rifamate Capsules 767
▲ Serophene Tablets (Approximately 10% to 20% of patients) 3226

Buccal-lingual-masticatory syndrome
Prozac Pulvules, Liquid, and Weekly Capsules (One case) 1238
Sarafem Pulvules (One case) 1962

Buccoglossal syndrome
Effexor Tablets (Rare) 3495
Effexor XR Capsules (Rare) 3499
Geodon Capsules (Frequent) 2688
Prozac Pulvules, Liquid, and Weekly Capsules (Infrequent) 1238
Sarafem Pulvules (Infrequent) 1962
Seroquel Tablets (Rare) 684
Zyprexa Tablets (Up to 2%) 1973
Zyprexa ZYDIS Orally Disintegrating Tablets (Up to 2%) 1973

Bucking
Diprivan Injectable Emulsion (Less than 1%) 667

Budd-Chiari syndrome
Alesse-21 Tablets 3468
Alesse-28 Tablets 3473
Brevicon 28-Day Tablets 3380
Cyclessa Tablets 2450
Desogen Tablets 2458
Estrostep 2627
Levlen 962
Levlite 21 Tablets 962
Levlite 28 Tablets 962
Levora Tablets 3389
Loestrin 21 Tablets 2642
Loestrin Fe Tablets 2642
Lunelle Monthly Injection 2827
Microgestin Fe 1.5/30 Tablets 3407
Microgestin Fe 1/20 Tablets 3400
Mircette Tablets 2470
Modicon 2563
Necon 3415
Norinyl 1 +35 28-Day Tablets 3380
Norinyl 1 + 50 28-Day Tablets 3380
Ortho-Cept 21 Tablets 2546
Ortho-Cept 28 Tablets 2546
Ortho-Cyclen/Ortho Tri-Cyclen 2573
Ortho-Novum 2563
Ortho-Novum 1/50□28 Tablets 2556
Ortho-Cyclen/Ortho Tri-Cyclen 2573
Ovcon 3364
Tri-Levlen 962
Tri-Norinyl-28 Tablets 3433
Trivora Tablets 3439
Yasmin 28 Tablets 980
Zovia 3449

Bulbus oculi, perforation
Alrex Sterile Ophthalmic Suspension 0.2% ⊙256
Blephamide Ophthalmic Ointment 547
Blephamide Ophthalmic Suspension 548
FML Ophthalmic Ointment ⊙237
FML Ophthalmic Suspension ⊙236
FML Forte Ophthalmic Suspension ⊙235
FML-S Liquifilm Sterile Ophthalmic Suspension ⊙238
Lotemax Sterile Ophthalmic Suspension 0.5% ⊙261
Pred Forte Ophthalmic Suspension ⊙246
Pred Mild Sterile Ophthalmic Suspension ⊙249
TobraDex Ophthalmic Ointment 542
TobraDex Ophthalmic Suspension 541
Vexol 1% Ophthalmic Suspension ⊙222

Bulimia
Paxil (Rare) 1609

Bullae
▲ Androderm Transdermal System CIII (Less than 1% to 12%) 3377
8-MOP Capsules 1727

BUN levels, changes
Celestone Soluspan Injectable Suspension 3097
Celestone Syrup 3099
Cortifoam Rectal Foam 3170
Cortone Acetate Injectable Suspension 2059
Cortone Acetate Tablets 2061
Decadron Elixir 2078
Decadron Tablets 2079
Decadron Phosphate Injection 2081
Depo-Medrol Injectable Suspension 2795
▲ Enalaprilat Injection (About 0.2% to 20%) 863
Etrafon 3115
▲ Intron A for Injection (Up to 12%) 3120
Lodosyn Tablets 1251
Moban 1320
▲ Paraplatin for Injection (14% to 22%) 1126
Pediapred Oral Solution 1170
Prelone Syrup 2273
Sinemet Tablets 1253
▲ Vasotec I.V. Injection (About 0.2% to 20%) 2207
▲ Vasotec Tablets (About 0.2% to 20%) 2210

BUN levels, decrease
Cipro I.V. (Infrequent) 893
Cipro I.V. Pharmacy Bulk Package (Less than 1%) 897

BUN levels, elevation
Accupril Tablets (2%) 2611
▲ Accuretic Tablets (4%) 2614
Aceon Tablets (2 mg, 4 mg, 8 mg) 3249
Aldoclor Tablets 2035
Aldomet Tablets 2037
Aldoril Tablets 2039
Altace Capsules (0.5% to 3%) 2233
Ambien Tablets (Rare) 3191
▲ AmBisome for Injection (21%) 1383
Amicar Injection 3608
Amicar Syrup 3608
Amicar Tablets 3608
Amphotec (1% to 5%) 1774
Ancef for Injection 1474
Ancef Injection 1474
Ancobon Capsules 1730
Arthrotec Tablets (Rare) 3195
Asacol Delayed-Release Tablets 2884
Atacand Tablets (Infrequent) 595
Atacand HCT Tablets (0.5% or greater) 597
Avalide Tablets 1070
Avapro Tablets (Less than 0.7%) 1074
Avapro Tablets (Less than 0.7%) 3076
Bactrim 2949
Genuine Bayer Professional Labeling (Aspirin Regimen Bayer) ▣608
Betaseron for SC Injection 988
▲ Biaxin/Biaxin XL (4%) 403
Bicillin C-R 900/300 Injection 2240
Bicillin C-R Injection 2238
Bicillin L-A Injection 2242
Blocadren Tablets 2046
Calcijex Injection 411
Captopril Tablets 2281
Carbatrol Capsules 3234
▲ Casodex Tablets (2% to 5%) 662
Ceclor CD Tablets (0.2%) 1279
Ceclor (Less than 1 in 500) 1905
▲ Cedax (4%) 1021
Cefizox for Intramuscular or Intravenous Use (Occasional) 1390
▲ Cefobid Intravenous/Intramuscular (1 in 16) 2671
▲ Cefobid Pharmacy Bulk Package - Not for Direct Infusion (1 in 16) 2673
Cefotan 664
Ceftin 1898
Cefzil (0.1%) 1076
Celebrex Capsules (0.1% to 1.9%) 2676
Celebrex Capsules (0.1% to 1.9%) 2780
▲ CellCept Capsules (34.6%) 2951
▲ CellCept Intravenous (34.6%) 2951
▲ CellCept Oral Suspension (34.6%) 2951
▲ CellCept Tablets (34.6%) 2951
Ceptaz for Injection (Occasional) 1499
Chibroxin Sterile Ophthalmic Solution 2051
Cipro I.V. 893
▲ Cipro I.V. Pharmacy Bulk Package (Among most frequent) 897
Cipro (0.9%) 887
Claforan Injection (Occasional) 732
Coly-Mycin M Parenteral 2243
Coreg Tablets (Less than 0.1% to 6.0%) 1508
Corlopam Injection (0.5% to 5%) 412
Cozaar Tablets (Less than 0.1%) 2067
CytoGam Intravenous 2026
Cytotec Tablets (Infrequent) 3202
Declomycin Tablets 1855
Demadex Tablets and Injection 2965
Diprivan Injectable Emulsion (Less than 1%) 667
Dopram Injectable 2931
Doryx Coated Pellet Filled Capsules 3357
Doxil Injection (Less than 1%) 566
Duricef 1079
Dyazide Capsules 1515
Dynacin Capsules 2019
Dyrenium Capsules (Rare) 3458
Ecotrin Enteric Coated Aspirin Low, Regular and Maximum Strength Tablets 1715
Effexor Tablets (Rare) 3495
Effexor XR Capsules (Rare) 3499
Eulexin Capsules 3118
Evoxac Capsules (Less than 1%) 1217
Floxin I.V. (More than or equal to 1%) 2526
Floxin Tablets (More than or equal to 1%) 2529
Fortaz (Occasional) 1541
Foscavir Injection (Between 1% and 5%) 605
Gamimune N, 5% Solvent/Detergent Treated 925
Gamimune N, 10% Solvent/Detergent Treated 928
Gammagard S/D 845
Gammar-P I.V. 787
▲ Gemzar for Injection (8% to 16%) 1919
Gengraf Capsules (1% to less than 3%) 457
Geodon Capsules (Rare) 2688
Glucotrol Tablets 2692
Glucotrol XL Extended Release Tablets 2693
Hectorol Capsules 1064
Hectorol Injection 1066
▲ Hexalen Capsules (1% to 9%) 2226
Hivid Tablets (Less than 1%) 2975
Hyzaar (0.6%) 2109
Ifex for Injection 1123
Indapamide Tablets (Less than 5%) 2286
Indocin Capsules (Less than 1%) 2112
▲ Indocin I.V. (41% of infants) 2115
Indocin (Less than 1%) 2112
Intron A for Injection (Less than 5%) 3120
Kefurox Vials, ADD-Vantage 1948
Kefzol Vials, ADD-Vantage 1951
▲ Leukine (23%) 1755
Lithobid Slow-Release Tablets 3255
Lodine (Less than 1%) 3528
Lodine XL Extended-Release Tablets (Less than 1%) 3530
Lorabid Suspension and Pulvules 2251
Lotensin HCT Tablets 2367
Lotrel Capsules 2370
Lupron Depot 7.5 mg (Greater than or equal to 5%) 3284
Lupron Depot–3 Month 22.5 mg 3288
▲ Lupron Depot–4 Month 30 mg (Greater than or equal to 5%) 3289
Lupron Injection (Less than 5%) 3279
Mandol Vials 1953
▲ Mavik Tablets (0.6% to 9%) 478
Maxipime for Injection (0.1% to 1%) 1285
Maxzide 1008
Mefoxin for Injection 2124
Mefoxin Premixed Intravenous Solution 2127
Mepron Suspension (1%) 1598
Merrem I.V. (Greater than 0.2%) 673
Micardis HCT Tablets 1051
Minocin Intravenous 1862
Minocin Oral Suspension 1865
Minocin Pellet-Filled Capsules 1863
Mithracin for Intravenous Use 903
Mobic Tablets (Less than 2%) 1054
Monodox Capsules 2442
Monopril Tablets 1091
Monopril HCT 1094
Motrin Suspension, Oral Drops, Chewable Tablets, and Caplets 2002
Mykrox Tablets 1168
Mylocel Tablets 2227
Naprelan Tablets (Less than 1%) 1293
Nebcin Vials, Hyporets & ADD-Vantage 1955
Neoral Soft Gelatin Capsules (1% to less than 3%) 2380
Neoral Oral Solution (1% to less than 3%) 2380
▲ Nilandron Tablets (3%) 753
▲ Nolvadex Tablets (18.1%) 678
▲ Normodyne Injection (8%) 3135
Noroxin Tablets (Less frequent) 2145
Omnicef (0.2%) 493
▲ Orudis Capsules (3% to 9%) 3548
▲ Oruvail Capsules (3% to 9%) 3548
Paxil (Rare) 1609
Pediazole Suspension 3050
Periostat Tablets 1208
Pipracil 1866
▲ PREVPAC (4%) 3298
Primaxin I.M. 2158
Primaxin I.V. 2160
▲ Prinivil Tablets (2.0% to 11.6%) 2164
Prinzide Tablets 2168
Procardia Capsules (Rare) 2708
Procardia XL Extended Release Tablets (Rare) 2710
▲ Prograf (3% to 15%) 1393
▲ Proleukin for Injection (63%) 1199
Prozac Pulvules, Liquid, and Weekly Capsules (Rare) 1238
▲ Rapamune Oral Solution and Tablets (3% to 20%) 3584
Requip Tablets (Frequent) 1621
Rifadin 765
Rifamate Capsules 767
Rifater Tablets 769
Rocaltrol 2991
Rocephin Injectable Vials, ADD-Vantage, Galaxy, Bulk (1.2%) 2993
Sandimmune 2388
Sandoglobulin I.V. 2391
Sarafem Pulvules (Rare) 1962
Septra Suspension 2265
Septra Tablets 2265
Septra DS Tablets 2265
Sinemet CR Tablets 1255
Sular Tablets (Less than or equal to 1%) 688
Suprax (Less than 2%) 1877
Symmetrel 1328
Tazicef for Injection (Occasional) 1647
Tazicef Galaxy Container (Occasional) 1650
Tazicef Pharmacy Bulk Package (Occasional) 1653
Tazidime Vials, Faspak & ADD-Vantage (Occasional) 1966
Tegretol/Tegretol-XR 2404
Teveten Tablets (0.6%) 3327
Thalomid Capsules 1154
Timentin Injection- ADD-Vantage Vial 1661
Timentin Injection-Galaxy Container 1664
Timentin Injection-Pharmacy Bulk Package 1666
Timentin for Intravenous Administration 1658
Tolectin (1% to 3%) 2589
Toradol 3018
Trilisate (Less than 1%) 2901
Trovan (Greater than or equal to 1%) 2722
Unasyn for Injection 2728
Uniretic Tablets (Less than 1%) 3178
Univasc Tablets (Approximately 1%) 3181
Vancocin HCl Capsules & Pulvules (Rare) 1972
Vancocin HCl Oral Solution (Rare) 1971
Vancocin HCl, Vials & ADD-Vantage (Rare) 1970
Vantin Tablets and Oral Suspension 2860
▲ Vaseretic Tablets (About 0.6% to 20%) 2204
Vibramycin Calcium Oral Suspension Syrup 2735
Vibramycin Hyclate Capsules 2735
Vibramycin Hyclate Intravenous 2737
Vibramycin Monohydrate for Oral Suspension 2735
Vibra-Tabs Film Coated Tablets 2735
Vistide Injection 1445
Zaroxolyn Tablets 1177
Zebeta Tablets 1885
Zestoretic Tablets 695
Zestril Tablets (About 2.0%) 698
Zinacef Injection 1696
Zinacef for Injection 1696
Zithromax (Less than 1%) 2743
Zithromax for Oral Suspension, 300 mg, 600 mg, 900 mg, 1200 mg (Less than 1%) 2739
Zithromax Tablets, 250 mg (Less than 1%) 2739
Zithromax Tablets, 600 mg (Less than 1%) 2743
Zosyn 1890
Zosyn in Galaxy Containers 1894
Zovirax Capsules 1706
▲ Zovirax for Injection (5% to 10%) 1708
Zovirax 1706
Zyvox (0.2% to 2.1%) 2871

Bundle branch block
Aciphex Tablets 1267
Aciphex Tablets 1783
Anzemet Injection 719

Anzemet Tablets ... 722
Cardizem Injectable ... 1018
Cardizem Lyo-Ject Syringe ... 1018
Cardizem Monovial ... 1018
Cardizem CD Capsules (Less than 1%) ... 1016
Celexa (Rare) ... 1365
Cerebyx Injection (Infrequent) ... 2619
Cognex Capsules (Rare) ... 1351
Coreg Tablets (Less than or equal to 0.1%) ... 1508
Corvert Injection (1.9%) ... 2793
Diprivan Injectable Emulsion (Less than 1%) ... 667
Doxil Injection (Less than 1%) ... 566
Effexor Tablets (Rare) ... 3495
Effexor XR Capsules (Infrequent) ... 3499
Ellence Injection ... 2806
Evoxac Capsules ... 1217
Exelon Capsules (Infrequent) ... 2342
Exelon Oral Solution (Infrequent) ... 2345
Geodon Capsules (Rare) ... 2688
Imdur Tablets (Less than or equal to 5%) ... 1826
Macrobid Capsules ... 2889
Macrodantin Capsules ... 2891
Miacalcin Nasal Spray (Less than 1%) ... 2375
Naprelan Tablets (Less than 1%) ... 1293
Paxil (Rare) ... 1609
Reminyl Oral Solution (Infrequent) ... 1792
Reminyl Tablets (Infrequent) ... 1792
Rilutek Tablets (Infrequent) ... 772
Rythmol Tablets – 150 mg, 225 mg, 300 mg (1.2% to 1.9%) ... 502
Seroquel Tablets (Infrequent) ... 684
Sonata Capsules (Infrequent) ... 3591
Tarka Tablets (Less frequent) ... 508
▲ Tenormin (6.6%) ... 692
Tiazac Capsules (Less than 2%) ... 1378
Tikosyn Capsules (Up to 0.5%) ... 2717
Tonocard Tablets (Less than 1%) ... 649
Topamax Sprinkle Capsules (Infrequent) ... 2590
Topamax Tablets (Infrequent) ... 2590
Trasylol Injection (1% to 2%) ... 909
Uniretic Tablets (Less than 1%) ... 3178

Burning
Aclovate (Approximately 2%) ... 1275
▲ Acular Ophthalmic Solution (Up to 40%) ... 544
Afrin Severe Congestion Nasal Spray ... ▣733
Afrin Original Pump Mist ... ▣733
▲ Alomide Ophthalmic Solution (Among most frequent) ... ⊙204
Americaine Anesthetic Lubricant ... 1162
Americaine Otic Topical Anesthetic Ear Drops ... 1162
Analpram-HC ... 1338
Anusol-HC Cream 2.5% (Infrequent to frequent) ... 2237
Anusol-HC Suppositories ... 2238
Azelex Cream (Approximately 1% to 5%) ... 547
Bactroban Nasal (2%) ... 1495
Bactroban Ointment (1.5%) ... 1496
Capex Shampoo ... 1400
Catapres-TTS (3 of 101 patients) ... 1038
▲ Cerebyx Injection (7 of 16 volunteers) ... 2619
Cipro I.V. Pharmacy Bulk Package (Less than 1%) ... 897
Clobevate Gel (Less than 2%) ... 3271
▲ Condylox Topical Solution (64% to 78%) ... 2437
Cordran Lotion (Infrequent) ... 2438
Cordran Tape (Infrequent) ... 2439
Cormax Cream (Infrequent) ... 2440
Cormax Ointment (Infrequent) ... 2440
Cormax Scalp Application (Infrequent) ... 2441
Cutivate Cream (0.6% to 1.6%) ... 1282
Cutivate Ointment (Less than 1%) ... 1284
Decadron Phosphate Injection ... 2081
Dermatop Emollient Cream (Less than 1%) ... 2517
DesOwen (Approximately 3%) ... 1401
▲ Diprolene Gel 0.05% (6%) ... 3107
▲ Elimite Cream (10%) ... 552
Elocon Cream 0.1% (1.6%) ... 3110
Elocon Lotion 0.1% (4 in 209 patients) ... 3111
▲ Elocon Ointment 0.1% (4.8%) ... 3112
Evoxac Capsules (Less than 1%) ... 1217
Finevin Cream (1% to 5%) ... 962
Fleet Bisacodyl Laxatives ... 1359
Fleet Prep Kits ... 1361
Fluoroplex ... 552
Heparin Lock Flush Solution ... 3509
Heparin Sodium Injection ... 3511
Humorsol Sterile Ophthalmic Solution ... 2102
Hydrocortone Phosphate Injection, Sterile ... 2105
Iopidine Sterile Ophthalmic Solution ... ⊙212
▲ Lac-Hydrin Cream (Approximately 3% to 15%) ... 1118
▲ Lac-Hydrin Lotion (1 in 10 to 30 patients) ... 1119
Lidex (Infrequent) ... 2020
Locoid (Infrequent) ... 1341
Loprox Lotion (1 patient) ... 2021
Lotrimin ... 3128
Lotrisone Cream ... 3129
▲ Naftin Gel (5.0%) ... 2224
Nystop Topical Powder USP (More common) ... 2608
Olux Foam (Less than 2%) ... 1211
Ophthetic Ophthalmic Solution (Occasional) ... ⊙244
Panafil Ointment (Occasional) ... 1726
Pramosone ... 1343
Pred-G Ophthalmic Suspension ... ⊙247
▲ Renova 0.02% Cream (Almost all subjects) ... 2520
▲ Renova 0.05% Cream (Almost all subjects) ... 2519
▲ Rēv-Eyes Sterile Ophthalmic Eyedrops 0.5% (Approximately 50%) ... ⊙265
Synalar (Infrequent) ... 2020
Tasmar Tablets (1% to 2%) ... 3010
Taxol Injection ... 1129
Temovate Cream (1%) ... 1301
▲ Temovate Gel (Among most frequent) ... 1303
Temovate Scalp Application (Infrequent) ... 1304
▲ Temovate E Emollient (5%) ... 1302
Terazol 3 Vaginal Suppositories ... 2587
Testoderm Transdermal Systems (1%) ... 574
Topicort (0.8%) ... 2025
VōSoL HC Otic Solution (Occasional) ... 3356
Zantac Injection ... 1688
▲ Zovirax Ointment (28.3%) ... 1707

Burning, extremities
Zerit ... 1147

Burning, local
Aci-Jel Therapeutic Vaginal Jelly (Occasional cases) ... 2525
Acticin Cream ... 998
Afrin Nasal Decongestant Children's Pump Mist ... ▣734
Afrin Original Nasal Spray ... ▣733
Afrin No Drip Original Nasal Spray ... ▣735
Afrin No Drip Extra Moisturizing Nasal Spray ... ▣735
Afrin No Drip Severe Congestion Nasal Spray ... ▣735
Afrin No Drip Sinus Nasal Spray ... ▣735
▲ Aldara Cream, 5% (More than 1% to 26%) ... 1978
▲ Alphagan Ophthalmic Solution (Approximately 10% to 30%) ... 545
▲ Alphagan P Ophthalmic Solution (Approximately 5% to 9%) ... 546
Americaine Anesthetic Lubricant ... 1162
▲ Androderm Transdermal System CIII (3%) ... 3377
Aphthasol Oral Paste (1% to 2%) ... 1025
Bactroban Cream (Less than 1% to 3.6%) ... 1494
▲ Chibroxin Sterile Ophthalmic Solution (One of the two most frequent) ... 2051
▲ Condylox Gel (11.5% to 37.1%) ... 2436
▲ Condylox Topical Solution (64% to 78%) ... 2437
▲ Dovonex Scalp Solution (Approximately 23%) ... 1110
▲ Efudex (Among most frequent) ... 1733
▲ Elimite Cream (10%) ... 552
Klaron Lotion 10% ... 1224
Locoid Lipocream Cream (Infrequent) ... 1342
Loprox Cream (1 out of 514 patients) ... 2021
Mentax Cream (Approximately 1%) ... 1009
Mumpsvax ... 2141
▲ MUSE Urethral Suppository (12%) ... 3335
▲ Naftin Cream (6%) ... 2224
Proctocort Suppositories ... 2264
Psorcon E Cream ... 1227
Psorcon E Ointment ... 1228
Selsun Rx 2.5% Lotion, USP ... 3053
Sulfamylon Topical Solution ... 1011
▲ Valstar Sterile Solution for Intravesical Instillation (5%) ... 1175

Burning, vaginal
(*see under* Vaginal burning)

Burning, vulvovaginal
(*see under* Vaginal burning)

Burning at injection site
Anzemet Injection ... 719
▲ Ativan Injection (17%) ... 3478
Attenuvax ... 2044
Brevibloc Injection (Less than 1%) ... 858
▲ Cardizem Injectable (3.9%) ... 1018
▲ Cardizem Lyo-Ject Syringe (3.9%) ... 1018
▲ Cardizem Monovial (3.9%) ... 1018
Cefizox for Intramuscular or Intravenous Use (1% to 5%) ... 1390
Cerezyme for Injection (Less than 1%) ... 1438
Cipro I.V. (1% or less) ... 893
DDAVP Injection 4 mcg/mL (Occasional) ... 737
Desferal Vials ... 2333
Desmopressin Acetate Injection (Occasional) ... 1344
▲ Diprivan Injectable Emulsion (10% to 17.6%) ... 667
Genotropin Lyophilized Powder (Infrequent) ... 2818
Helixate Concentrate ... 788
Intron A for Injection (Less than 5%) ... 3120
Kogenate ... 934
Meruvax II ... 2130
M-M-R II ... 2118
Mononine Concentrate ... 794
Mumpsvax ... 2141
Novantrone for Injection ... 1760
Nubain Injection ... 1323
Timentin Injection- ADD-Vantage Vial ... 1661
Timentin Injection-Galaxy Container ... 1664
Timentin Injection-Pharmacy Bulk Package ... 1666
Timentin for Intravenous Administration ... 1658
Versed Injection (Less than 1%) ... 3027
▲ Zofran Injection (4%) ... 1698

Burning sensation
Accuzyme Debriding Ointment (A small percentage) ... 1725
Adenocard Injection (Less than 1%) ... 1380
Adriamycin PFS/RDF Injection ... 2767
Amerge Tablets (Infrequent) ... 1467
AVC (Occasional) ... 1350
BeneFix for Injection ... 1432
Benoquin Cream 20% ... 1732
Chloromycetin Ophthalmic Solution ... ⊙297
Clobevate Gel (1.8%) ... 3271
Copaxone for Injection (Infrequent) ... 3306
Cormax Cream (0.5%) ... 2440
Cormax Ointment (0.5%) ... 2440
▲ Cormax Scalp Application (Approximately 10%) ... 2441
Decadron Phosphate Sterile Ophthalmic Ointment (Rare) ... 2083
Decadron Phosphate Sterile Ophthalmic Solution (Rare) ... 2084
Dopram Injectable ... 2931
Doxil Injection ... 566
▲ Emla (17%) ... 602
Fleet Glycerin Laxatives ... 1359
Gamimune N, 5% Solvent/Detergent Treated ... 925
Gamimune N, 10% Solvent/Detergent Treated ... 928
Idamycin PFS Injection ... 2825
▲ Imitrex Injection (7.5%) ... 1549
Imitrex Nasal Spray (0.4% to 1.4%) ... 1554
Imitrex Tablets (Frequent) ... 1558
Olux Foam ... 1211
Silvadene Cream 1% (Infrequent) ... 2267
▲ Sulfamylon Cream (One of two most frequent) ... 1011
Temovate Cream (1%) ... 1301
Temovate Gel (1.8%) ... 1303
Temovate Ointment (0.5%) ... 1301
▲ Temovate Scalp Application (29 of 294 patients) ... 1304
Topicort LP Cream (0.8%) ... 2025
Zilactin Gel ... ▣790

Bursitis
Aciphex Tablets ... 1267
Aciphex Tablets ... 1783
▲ Actonel Tablets (3%) ... 2879
Arava Tablets (1% to 3%) ... 724
Avalide Tablets ... 1070
Avapro Tablets (Less than 1%) ... 1074
Avapro Tablets (Less than 1%) ... 3076
Azmacort Inhalation Aerosol (1% to 3%) ... 728
Betaseron for SC Injection ... 988
Celexa (Rare) ... 1365
Cognex Capsules (Infrequent) ... 1351
Copaxone for Injection (Infrequent) ... 3306
Effexor Tablets (Infrequent) ... 3495
Effexor XR Capsules (Infrequent) ... 3499
Enbrel for Injection (Infrequent) ... 1752
Enbrel for Injection (Infrequent) ... 3504
Evoxac Capsules (Less than 1%) ... 1217
Gabitril Tablets (Infrequent) ... 1189
Gengraf Capsules (1% to less than 3%) ... 457
Hivid Tablets (Less than 1%) ... 2975
Lamictal (Rare) ... 1567
Lipitor Tablets (Less than 2%) ... 2639
Lipitor Tablets (Less than 2%) ... 2696
Luvox Tablets (25, 50, 100 mg) (Infrequent) ... 3256
LYMErix Vaccine ... 1592
Meridia Capsules ... 481
Naprelan Tablets (Less than 1%) ... 1293
Neoral Soft Gelatin Capsules (1% to less than 3%) ... 2380
Neoral Oral Solution (1% to less than 3%) ... 2380
Neurontin Capsules (Rare) ... 2655
Neurontin Oral Solution (Rare) ... 2655
Neurontin Tablets (Rare) ... 2655
Noroxin Tablets (Less frequent) ... 2145
Paxil (Rare) ... 1609
Permax Tablets (1.6%) ... 1299
Pletal Tablets (Less than 2%) ... 2605
Pletal Tablets (Less than 2%) ... 2848
Protonix I.V. (Less than 1%) ... 3580
Protonix Tablets (Less than 1%) ... 3577
Prozac Pulvules, Liquid, and Weekly Capsules (Infrequent) ... 1238
Remeron Tablets (Rare) ... 2483
Remeron SolTab Tablets (Rare) ... 2486
Requip Tablets (Infrequent) ... 1621
Risperdal (Rare) ... 1796
Sarafem Pulvules (Infrequent) ... 1962
Serzone Tablets (Infrequent) ... 1104
Sonata Capsules (Infrequent) ... 3591
▲ Sporanox Capsules (3%) ... 1800
Tricor Capsules, Micronized ... 513
Uniretic Tablets (Less than 1%) ... 3178
Vioxx (Greater than 0.1% to 1.9%) ... 2213
Zanaflex Tablets (Infrequent) ... 1305
Zyprexa Tablets (Infrequent) ... 1973
Zyprexa ZYDIS Orally Disintegrating Tablets (Infrequent) ... 1973

C

Cachexia
Actiq (1% or greater) ... 1184
Cerebyx Injection (Infrequent) ... 2619
Cognex Capsules (Infrequent) ... 1351
Cytovene-IV (One report) ... 2959
Doxil Injection (Less than 1%) ... 566
Exelon Capsules (Infrequent) ... 2342
Exelon Oral Solution (Infrequent) ... 2345
Foscavir Injection (Between 1% and 5%) ... 605
Hivid Tablets (Less than 1%) ... 2975
Intron A for Injection (Less than or equal to 5%) ... 3120
Norvir Capsules (Less than 2%) ... 487
Norvir Oral Solution (Less than 2%) ... 487
Permax Tablets (Rare) ... 1299
Risperdal (Rare) ... 1796
Sandostatin LAR Depot (1% to 4%) ... 2395
▲ Serostim for Injection (1% to 10%) ... 3229
Vistide Injection ... 1445
Vitravene for Injection (2% to 5%) ... ⊙310
Xeloda Tablets (Less than 5%) ... 3039

Calcification, ectopic
Calcijex Injection ... 411
Hectorol Capsules ... 1064
Hectorol Injection ... 1066
Rocaltrol ... 2991

Calcium retention
Estratest ... 3252
Inderide Tablets ... 3517
Lupron Injection (Less than 5%) ... 3279
Oxandrin Tablets ... 1153
Testred Capsules, 10 mg ... 1746

Calf muscles, need to flex
Imitrex Injection (Rare) ... 1549

Cancer, breast
Estrace Vaginal Cream ... 3358
Estrace Tablets ... 3361
Modicon ... 2563
Neurontin Capsules (Infrequent) ... 2655
Neurontin Oral Solution (Infrequent) ... 2655
Neurontin Tablets (Infrequent) ... 2655
Ortho-Novum ... 2563
Ortho-Novum 1/50□28 Tablets ... 2556
Ovcon ... 3364

Cancer, cervical
Depo-Provera Contraceptive Injection (Fewer than 1%) ... 2798
Estratest ... 3252
Levlen ... 962
Levlite 21 Tablets ... 962
Levlite 28 Tablets ... 962
Modicon ... 2563
Ortho-Cyclen/Ortho Tri-Cyclen ... 2573
Ortho-Novum ... 2563
Ortho-Novum 1/50□28 Tablets ... 2556
Ortho-Cyclen/Ortho Tri-Cyclen ... 2573
Ovcon ... 3364
Permax Tablets (Infrequent) ... 1299
Premarin Intravenous ... 3563
Premarin Vaginal Cream ... 3570
Tri-Levlen ... 962

Cancer, vaginal
Estratest ... 3252
Ortho-Est Tablets ... 3464
Premarin Intravenous ... 3563

Premarin Vaginal Cream 3570
Vivelle Transdermal System 2412
Vivelle-Dot Transdermal System 2416

Candidiasis
▲ Advair Diskus 100/50 (3%) 1448
Advair Diskus 500/50 (Up to 3%) 1448
▲ Aerobid/Aerobid-M (3% to 9%) 1363
Aredia for Injection (Up to 6%) 2309
Augmentin Chewable Tablets 1482
Augmentin Powder for Oral Suspension 1482
Augmentin Tablets 1485
Augmentin ES-600 Powder for Oral Suspension (1.4%) 1487
Avelox Tablets (0.05% to 1%) 879
Beconase Inhalation Aerosol (Rare) 1497
Biaxin/Biaxin XL 403
▲ Campath Ampules (1% to 8%) 992
Cedax Capsules (0.1% to 1%) 1021
Ceftin for Oral Suspension (0.1% to 1%) 1898
Celebrex Capsules (0.1% to 1.9%) 2676
Celebrex Capsules (0.1% to 1.9%) 2780
CellCept Capsules (Up to 0.6%) 2951
CellCept Intravenous (Up to 0.6%) 2951
CellCept Oral Suspension (Up to 0.6%) 2951
CellCept Tablets (Up to 0.6%) 2951
Ceptaz for Injection (Fewer than 1%) 1499
▲ Chemet Capsules (5.2% to 15.7%) 3078
Cipro I.V. (1% or less) 893
Cipro I.V. Pharmacy Bulk Package (Less than 1%) 897
Cipro (Less than 1%) 887
Cleocin Vaginal Ovules (Less than 1%) 2789
Colazal Capsules 3069
Doryx Coated Pellet Filled Capsules 3357
▲ Doxil Injection (23.5%) 566
Effexor Tablets (Infrequent) 3495
Evoxac Capsules (1% to 3%) 1217
Fortaz (Less than 1%) 1541
Fortovase Capsules (Less than 2%) 2970
Foscavir Injection (Between 1% and 5%) 605
Hivid Tablets (Less than 1%) 2975
Imdur Tablets (Less than or equal to 5%) 1826
▲ Intron A for Injection (Up to 17%) 3120
Invirase Capsules (Less than 2%) 2979
Klonopin Tablets (Infrequent) 2983
Macrobid Capsules 2889
Megace Oral Suspension (1% to 3%) 1124
Merrem I.V. (0.1% to 2.0%) 673
Monodox Capsules 2442
Nipent for Injection (2%) 3272
Norvir Capsules (Less than 2%) 487
Norvir Oral Solution (Less than 2%) 487
Omnicef 493
Paxil (Infrequent) 1609
Pentasa Capsules (Less than 1%) 3239
Permax Tablets (Infrequent) 1299
▲ Photofrin for Injection (9%) 831
Pipracil 1866
Prevacid Delayed-Release Capsules (Less than 1%) 3292
PREVPAC (Less than 1%) 3298
Primaxin I.M. 2158
Primaxin I.V. (Less than 0.2%) 2160
Protonix I.V. (Less than 1%) 3580
Protonix Tablets (Less than 1%) 3577
▲ Pulmicort Respules (3% to 4%) 632
Remeron Tablets (Rare) 2483
Remeron SolTab Tablets (Rare) 2486
▲ Remicade for IV Injection (3% to 5%) 1178
Rhinocort Nasal Inhaler (Less than 1%) 640
Rilutek Tablets (0.4% to 1.2%) 772
Salagen Tablets (Less than 1%) 2229
Sandostatin LAR Depot (1% to 4%) 2395
Seroquel Tablets (Infrequent) 684
▲ Serostim for Injection (1% to 10%) 3229
Serzone Tablets (Rare) 1104
▲ Simulect for Injection (3% to 10%) 2399
Soriatane Capsules (Less than 1%) 3003
Suprax (Less than 2%) 1877
Tazicef for Injection (Less than 1%) 1647
Tazicef Galaxy Container (Less than %) 1650
Tazicef Pharmacy Bulk Package (Less than 1%) 1653
Thalomid Capsules 1154
Trovan (Less than 1%) 2722
Unasyn for Injection (Less than 1%) 2728
Uniretic Tablets (Less than 1%) 3178
Vantin Tablets and Oral Suspension (Less than 1%) 2860
Vibramycin Calcium Oral Suspension Syrup 2735
Vibramycin Hyclate Capsules 2735
Vibramycin Monohydrate for Oral Suspension 2735
Vibra-Tabs Film Coated Tablets 2735
Vistide Injection 1445
Zanaflex Tablets (Infrequent) 1305
Zithromax for IV Infusion (1% or less) 2748
▲ Zometa for Intravenous Infusion (11.6%) 3621
Zosyn (1.6%) 1890
Zosyn in Galaxy Containers (1.6%) 1894
Zyprexa Tablets (Infrequent) 1973
Zyprexa ZYDIS Orally Disintegrating Tablets (Infrequent) 1973

Candidiasis, esophageal
Prilosec Delayed-Release Capsules (Less than 1%) 628
▲ Taxol Injection (7% to 9%) 1129
Xeloda Tablets (Less than 5%) 3039

Candidiasis, gastrointestinal
▲ CellCept Capsules (3% to 10%) 2951
▲ CellCept Intravenous (3% to 10%) 2951
▲ CellCept Oral Suspension (3% to 10%) 2951
▲ CellCept Tablets (3% to 10%) 2951
Protonix I.V. (Less than 1%) 3580
Protonix Tablets (Less than 1%) 3577
Rescriptor Tablets 526
▲ Thymoglobulin for Injection (4.9%) 3071
Xeloda Tablets (Less than 5%) 3039
Zyrtec-D 12 Hour Extended Relief Tablets 2758

Candidiasis, genital
(*see also under* Vaginal candidiasis)
Activella Tablets (0% to 6%) 2764
Ancef for Injection 1474
Ancef Injection 1474
Azmacort Inhalation Aerosol (1% to 3%) 728
Ceclor CD Tablets (2.2%) 1279
Celebrex Capsules (0.1% to 1.9%) 2676
Celebrex Capsules (0.1% to 1.9%) 2780
Cerebyx Injection (Infrequent) 2619
Claforan Injection (Less than 1%) 732
▲ Crinone 8% Gel (7%) 3213
Declomycin Tablets 1855
Dynabac Tablets (0.1% to 1%) 2269
Dynacin Capsules 2019
Effexor Tablets (Infrequent) 3495
Effexor XR Capsules 3499
▲ Estring Vaginal Ring (6%) 2811
Evoxac Capsules (Less than 1%) 1217
Gonal-F for Injection (2.5%) 3216
Infergen (2%) 1777
Keflex 1237
Lamictal (Infrequent) 1567
Levaquin (0.3%) 2537
Lorabid Suspension and Pulvules (1.1%) 2251
Mefoxin for Injection 2124
Mefoxin Premixed Intravenous Solution 2127
Minocin Intravenous 1862
Minocin Oral Suspension 1865
Minocin Pellet-Filled Capsules 1863
Nexium Delayed-Release Capsules (Less than 1%) 619
Ovidrel for Injection (Less than 2%) 3220
Paxil (Rare) 1609
PREVPAC (Less than 3%) 3298
Requip Tablets (Infrequent) 1621
Rescriptor Tablets (Less than 2%) 526
Rilutek Tablets (Rare) 772
Rocephin Injectable Vials, ADD-Vantage, Galaxy, Bulk (Occasional) 2993
▲ Vagifem Tablets (5%) 2857
Zanaflex Tablets (Infrequent) 1305

Candidiasis, mouth
(*see under* Candidiasis, oral)

Candidiasis, nasal
Nasacort Nasal Inhaler (Rare) 750
Nasonex Nasal Spray (Rare) 3131
Vancenase PocketHaler Nasal Inhaler (Rare) 3162

Candidiasis, oral
Actiq (Less than 1%) 1184
Advair Diskus 100/50 (1%) 1448
▲ Advair Diskus 250/50 (4%) 1448
Advair Diskus 500/50 (1% to 4%) 1448
Amphotec (1% to 5%) 1774
Ancef for Injection 1474
Ancef Injection 1474
Arava Tablets (1% to 3%) 724
Augmentin ES-600 Powder for Oral Suspension 1487
Avelox Tablets (0.05% to 1%) 879
Azmacort Inhalation Aerosol (A few cases) 728
Betaseron for SC Injection 988
▲ CellCept Capsules (10.1% to 12.1%) 2951
▲ CellCept Intravenous (10.1% to 12.1%) 2951
▲ CellCept Oral Suspension (10.1% to 12.1%) 2951
▲ CellCept Tablets (10.1% to 12.1%) 2951
Ceptaz for Injection 1499
Cipro I.V. (1% or less) 893
Cipro I.V. Pharmacy Bulk Package (Less than 1%) 897
Cipro (Less than 1%) 887
Comvax (0.2% to 0.8%) 2056
Copaxone for Injection (Frequent) 3306
Doxil Injection (1% to 5%) 566
Effexor Tablets (Rare) 3495
Effexor XR Capsules (Infrequent) 3499
▲ Flovent Diskus (Less than 1% to 31%) 3614
▲ Flovent (2% to 5%) 1535
▲ Flovent Rotadisk (3% to 11%) 1537
Fortaz (Less than 1%) 1541
▲ Gliadel Wafer (4% to 9%) 1723
Grifulvin V Tablets Microsize and Oral Suspension Microsize (Occasional) 2518
Gris-PEG Tablets (Occasional) 2661
Kefzol Vials, ADD-Vantage 1951
Maxipime for Injection (0.1% to 1%) 1285
Megace Oral Suspension (1% to 3%) 1124
▲ Mepron Suspension (5% to 10%) 1598
Nasonex Nasal Spray (Rare) 3131
▲ Neumega for Injection (14%) 1434
Prevnar for Injection 1870
▲ Prograf (3% to 15%) 1393
Protonix I.V. (Less than 1%) 3580
Protonix Tablets (Less than 1%) 3577
▲ Pulmicort Turbuhaler Inhalation Powder (Up to 10%) 636
▲ Rapamune Oral Solution and Tablets (3% to 20%) 3584
Rescriptor Tablets 526
Serevent Inhalation Aerosol (1% to 3%) 1633
Synagis Intramuscular (More than 1%) 2028
Synercid I.V. (Less than 1%) 775
Tazidime Vials, Faspak & ADD-Vantage (Less than 1%) 1966
Tequin Injection (0.1% to 3%) 1110
Tequin Tablets (0.1% to 3%) 1110
▲ Thalomid Capsules (4.2%) 1154
▲ Thymoglobulin for Injection (3.7%) 3071
▲ Trisenox Injection (5%) 1158
Vantin Tablets and Oral Suspension (Less than 1%) 2860
▲ Vistide Injection (18%) 1445
Xeloda Tablets (Less than 5%) 3039
Zithromax (1% or less) 2743
Zithromax for Oral Suspension, 300 mg, 600 mg, 900 mg, 1200 mg (1% or less) 2739
Zithromax Tablets, 250 mg (1% or less) 2739
Zithromax Tablets, 600 mg 2743
▲ Zosyn (3.9%) 1890
▲ Zosyn in Galaxy Containers (3.9%) 1894
Zyprexa Tablets (Infrequent) 1973
Zyprexa ZYDIS Orally Disintegrating Tablets (Infrequent) 1973
Zyvox (0.4% to 1.1%) 2871

Candidiasis, pharynx
Azmacort Inhalation Aerosol 728
▲ Flovent (19% to 25%) 1535
Flovent Rotadisk 1537
Nasacort Nasal Inhaler (Rare) 750
Vancenase PocketHaler Nasal Inhaler (Rare) 3162

Candidiasis, urinary tract
Nexium Delayed-Release Capsules (Less than 1%) 619

Candidiasis, vaginal
(*see under* Vaginal candidiasis)

Candiduria
Cipro I.V. (1% or less) 893
Cipro I.V. Pharmacy Bulk Package (Less than 1%) 897
Cipro 887
Floxin I.V. 2526
Floxin Tablets 2529
Noroxin Tablets 2145
Zosyn (1.0% or less) 1890
Zosyn in Galaxy Containers (1.0% or less) 1894

Capillary fragility
Aerobid/Aerobid-M (1% to 3%) 1363
Campath Ampules 992

Capillary leak syndrome
Leukine 1755
Neupogen for Injection (One event) 587
Orthoclone OKT3 Sterile Solution (Less than 1%) 2498
Proleukin for Injection 1199
Simulect for Injection 2399

Carbohydrate tolerance, decrease
Activella Tablets 2764
Alesse-21 Tablets 3468
Alesse-28 Tablets 3473
Alora Transdermal System 3372
Brevicon 28-Day Tablets 3380
Celestone Soluspan Injectable Suspension 3097
Celestone Syrup 3099
Cenestin Tablets 1263
Climara Transdermal System 958
Cortone Acetate Injectable Suspension 2059
Cortone Acetate Tablets 2061
Cyclessa Tablets 2450
Decadron Elixir 2078
Decadron Tablets 2079
Decadron Phosphate Injection 2081
Depo-Medrol Injectable Suspension 2795
Desogen Tablets 2458
Esclim Transdermal System 3460
Estinyl Tablets 3112
Estrace Vaginal Cream 3358
Estrace Tablets 3361
Estratest 3252
Estrostep 2627
femhrt Tablets 2635
Florinef Acetate Tablets 2250
Hydrocortone Tablets 2106
Hydrocortone Acetate Injectable Suspension 2103
Hydrocortone Phosphate Injection, Sterile 2105
Levlen 962
Levlite 21 Tablets 962
Levlite 28 Tablets 962
Levora Tablets 3389
Loestrin 21 Tablets 2642
Loestrin Fe Tablets 2642
Lo/Ovral Tablets 3532
Lo/Ovral-28 Tablets 3538
Low-Ogestrel-28 Tablets 3392
Lunelle Monthly Injection 2827
Menest Tablets 2254
Microgestin Fe 1.5/30 Tablets 3407
Microgestin Fe 1/20 Tablets 3400
Mircette Tablets 2470
Modicon 2563
Necon 3415
Nordette-28 Tablets 2257
Norinyl 1 +35 28-Day Tablets 3380
Norinyl 1 + 50 28-Day Tablets 3380
Ogen Tablets 2846
Ogestrel 0.5/50-28 Tablets 3428
Ortho Dienestrol Cream 2554
Ortho-Cept 21 Tablets 2546
Ortho-Cept 28 Tablets 2546
Ortho-Cyclen/Ortho Tri-Cyclen 2573
Ortho-Est Tablets 3464
Ortho-Novum 2563
Ortho-Novum 1/50□28 Tablets 2556
Ortho-Prefest Tablets 2570
Ortho-Cyclen/Ortho Tri-Cyclen 2573
Ovcon 3364
Ovral Tablets 3551
Ovral-28 Tablets 3552
Ovrette Tablets 3552
Prednisone 3064
Prelone Syrup 2273
Premarin Intravenous 3563
Premarin Tablets 3566
Premarin Vaginal Cream 3570
Premphase Tablets 3572
Prempro Tablets 3572
Solu-Medrol Sterile Powder 2855
Tri-Levlen 962
Tri-Norinyl-28 Tablets 3433
Triphasil-21 Tablets 3600
Triphasil-28 Tablets 3605
Trivora Tablets 3439
Vivelle Transdermal System 2412
Vivelle-Dot Transdermal System 2416
Yasmin 28 Tablets 980
Zovia 3449

Carcinoma, basal cell
Evoxac Capsules (Less than 1%) 1217
Neoral Soft Gelatin Capsules (0.4%) 2380
Neoral Oral Solution (0.4%) 2380
Remicade for IV Injection (Less than 2%) 1178
Requip Tablets (1% or more) 1621
Sandostatin Injection (Less than 1%) 2394
Sandostatin LAR Depot (Rare) 2395
Topamax Sprinkle Capsules (Infrequent) 2590
Topamax Tablets (Infrequent) 2590
Vioxx (Greater than 0.1% to 1.9%) 2213

Carcinoma, bladder
Clomid Tablets 735
Lupron Depot–4 Month 30 mg (Less than 5%) 3289
Requip Tablets (Infrequent) 1621
Serophene Tablets 3226
Testoderm Transdermal Systems (1%) 574
Zoladex 3-month (1% to 5%) 706

Carcinoma, cervix
Copaxone for Injection (Infrequent) 3306
Ovidrel for Injection (Less than 2%) 3220

Carcinoma, ear
Lupron Injection (Less than 5%) 3279

Carcinoma, endometrial
Activella Tablets 2764
Climara Transdermal System 958
Clomid Tablets 735
Estrace Vaginal Cream 3358
Estrace Tablets 3361
Estratest 3252
Levlen 962
Levlite 21 Tablets 962
Levlite 28 Tablets 962
Menest Tablets 2254
Nolvadex Tablets 678
Ogen Tablets 2846
Ortho Dienestrol Cream 2554
Ortho-Est Tablets 3464
Premarin Intravenous 3563
Premarin Tablets 3566
Premarin Vaginal Cream 3570
Premphase Tablets 3572
Prempro Tablets 3572
Serophene Tablets 3226
Tri-Levlen 962
Vivelle Transdermal System 2412
Vivelle-Dot Transdermal System 2416

Carcinoma, esophageal
Requip Tablets (Infrequent) 1621

Carcinoma, gastrointestinal
Accuretic Tablets 2614
Apligraf (1.8%) 2305
▲ Casodex Tablets (2% to 5%) 662
Copaxone for Injection (Infrequent) 3306
Protonix I.V. (Less than 1%) 3580
Protonix Tablets (Less than 1%) 3577
Tasmar Tablets (Rare) 3010
▲ Visudyne for Injection (1% to 10%) ⊙308

Carcinoma, hepatocellular
Anadrol-50 Tablets (Rare) 3321
Androderm Transdermal System CIII 3377
Android Capsules, 10 mg (Rare) 1731
Brevicon 28-Day Tablets (Extremely rare) 3380
Clomid Tablets 735
Delatestryl Injection 1151
Levlen (Extremely rare) 962
Levlite 21 Tablets (Extremely rare) 962
Levlite 28 Tablets (Extremely rare) 962
Modicon (Rare) 2563
Nolvadex Tablets (3 cases) 678
Norinyl 1 + 35 28-Day Tablets (Extremely rare) 3380
Norinyl 1 + 50 28-Day Tablets (Extremely rare) 3380
Ortho-Cyclen/Ortho Tri-Cyclen (Rare) 2573
Ortho-Novum (Rare) 2563
Ortho-Novum 1/50▢28 Tablets (Rare) 2556
Ortho-Cyclen/Ortho Tri-Cyclen (Rare) 2573
Serophene Tablets 3226
Testoderm Transdermal Systems (Rare) 574
Testopel Pellets 3610
Tri-Levlen (Extremely rare) 962
Tri-Norinyl-28 Tablets (Extremely rare) 3433

Carcinoma, lung
Betaseron for SC Injection 988
Cognex Capsules (Rare) 1351
Permax Tablets (Rare) 1299
Prinivil Tablets (0.3% to 1.0%) 2164
Rilutek Tablets (Infrequent) 772
Uniretic Tablets (Less than 1%) 3178

Carcinoma, ovarian
Clomid Tablets 735
Follistim for Injection 2465
Humegon for Injection (Infrequent) 2468
Pergonal for Injection 3223
Repronex for Intramuscular and Subcutaneous Injection (Infrequent) 1347
Serophene Tablets 3226
Tasmar Tablets (Rare) 3010

Carcinoma, prostate
Androderm Transdermal System CIII (Less than 1%) 3377
Android Capsules, 10 mg 1731
Campath Ampules 992
Cognex Capsules (Infrequent) 1351
Mirapex Tablets (Less than 1%) 2834
Paxil (Rare) 1609
Rilutek Tablets (Infrequent) 772
Tasmar Tablets (Infrequent) 3010
Testoderm Transdermal Systems 574

Carcinoma, rectal
Requip Tablets (Infrequent) 1621

Carcinoma, renal cell
Serophene Tablets 3226

Carcinoma, skin
Actonel Tablets (2%) 2879
Avonex 1013
Betaseron for SC Injection 988
▲ Casodex Tablets (2% to 5%) 662
Cognex Capsules (Infrequent) 1351
Copaxone for Injection (Infrequent) 3306
8-MOP Capsules 1727
Gabitril Tablets (Infrequent) 1189
Lupron Injection (Less than 5%) 3279
Orthoclone OKT3 Sterile Solution 2498
Permax Tablets (Infrequent) 1299
▲ Prograf (One of the two most common forms) 1393
Remicade for IV Injection 1178
Sandimmune 2388
Uniretic Tablets (Less than 1%) 3178
Zanaflex Tablets (Rare) 1305

Carcinoma, skin, benign
Betaseron for SC Injection 988
CellCept Capsules (1.6% to 4.0%) 2951
CellCept Intravenous (1.6% to 4.0%) 2951
CellCept Oral Suspension (1.6% to 4.0%) 2951
CellCept Tablets (1.6% to 4.0%) 2951
Copaxone for Injection (Infrequent) 3306
Gabitril Tablets (Infrequent) 1189
Kaletra Capsules (Less than 2%) 471
Kaletra Oral Solution (Less than 2%) 471
Permax Tablets (Rare) 1299
Protopic Ointment (1% to 3%) 1397
Thalomid Capsules 1154
Virazole for Inhalation Solution 1747

Carcinoma, squamous
Campath Ampules 992
Evoxac Capsules (Less than 1%) 1217
Remicade for IV Injection 1178

Carcinoma, tongue
Serophene Tablets 3226

Carcinoma, unspecified
Accuretic Tablets 2614
▲ Actonel Tablets (3.3%) 2879
Aggrenox Capsules (1.7%) 1026
Avonex 1013
▲ Casodex Tablets (2% to 5%) 662
▲ CellCept Capsules (3% to 10%) 2951
▲ CellCept Intravenous (3% to 10%) 2951
▲ CellCept Oral Suspension (3% to 10%) 2951
▲ CellCept Tablets (3% to 10%) 2951
Colazal Capsules 2069
Effexor Tablets (Rare) 3495
Effexor XR Capsules (Rare) 3499
Felbatol 3343
Ferrlecit Injection (Greater than 1%) 3386
Gabitril Tablets (Infrequent) 1189
Gengraf Capsules 457
Innohep Injection 1248
Levaquin Injection (Less than 0.5%) 2537
Lupron Depot 7.5 mg (Less than 5%) 3284
Lupron Depot–4 Month 30 mg (Less than 5%) 3289
Myobloc Injectable Solution (2% or greater) 1291
Naprelan Tablets (Less than 1%) 1293
Neoral Soft Gelatin Capsules (1% to less than 3%) 2380
Neoral Oral Solution (1% to less than 3%) 2380
Nipent for Injection (Less than 3%) 3272
Paxil (Infrequent) 1609
Permax Tablets (Infrequent) 1299
Protonix I.V. (Less than 1%) 3580
Protonix Tablets (Less than 1%) 3577
Rilutek Tablets (Infrequent) 772
Tasmar Tablets (Infrequent) 3010
Zanaflex Tablets (Rare) 1305

Carcinoma, uterine
Nolvadex Tablets 678
Requip Tablets (Rare) 1621

Carcinoma, testicular
Campath Ampules 992

Cardiac abnormalities
Accolate Tablets (Rare) 657
Albalon Ophthalmic Solution ⊙225
Clozaril Tablets (1%) 2319
Cordarone Tablets (Infrequent) 3487
Flovent Diskus 3614
Flovent 1535
Flovent Rotadisk 1537
Hivid Tablets (Less than 1%) 2975
Humorsol Sterile Ophthalmic Solution 2102
▲ Leukine (23%) 1755
Lodosyn Tablets 1251
Novantrone for Injection 1760
Pacerone Tablets (Infrequent) 3331
Pergonal for Injection (One report) 3223
Sinemet Tablets 1253
Sinemet CR Tablets 1255

Cardiac anomalies
Eskalith 1527
Lithium Carbonate 3061
Lithium Citrate Syrup 3061
Repronex for Intramuscular and Subcutaneous Injection (One report) 1347

Cardiac arrest
▲ Abelcet Injection (6%) 1273
Aceon Tablets (2 mg, 4 mg, 8 mg) 3249
Activase I.V. 1410
Adalat CC Tablets (Less than 1.0%) 877
Adenoscan 1381
AK-Fluor Injection 10% and 25% ⊙202
Alupent Inhalation Aerosol (Several cases) 1029
AmBisome for Injection (Less common) 1383
Amphotec (1% to 5%) 1774
Ancobon Capsules 1730
Anectine Injection (Rare) 1476
Antivenin Polyvalent (Isolated cases) 3475
AquaMEPHYTON Injection 2042
▲ Argatroban Injection (5.8%) 1478
Avonex 1013
Betagan ⊙228
Betaseron for SC Injection 988
Betimol Ophthalmic Solution ⊙324
Bicillin C-R 900/300 Injection 2240
Bicillin C-R Injection 2238
Bicillin L-A Injection 2242
Blocadren Tablets (Less than 1%) 2046
Captopril Tablets 2281
▲ Casodex Tablets (2% to 5%) 662
Celexa (Rare) 1365
▲ CellCept Capsules (3% to 10%) 2951
▲ CellCept Intravenous (3% to 10%) 2951
▲ CellCept Oral Suspension (3% to 10%) 2951
▲ CellCept Tablets (3% to 10%) 2951
Cerebyx Injection (Infrequent) 2619
Chirocaine Injection (Less than 1%) 2909
Clozaril Tablets (Rare) 2319
Cognex Capsules (Rare) 1351
Compazine 1505
Cordarone Intravenous (2.9%) 3491
Cosopt Sterile Ophthalmic Solution 2065
Cytovene 2959
Demerol 3079
Digitek Tablets (1%) 1003
Dilaudid 441
Dilaudid Oral Liquid 445
Dilaudid Tablets - 8 mg 445
Dilaudid-HP 443
Diprivan Injectable Emulsion (Rare) 667
Doxil Injection (Less than 1%) 566
Duranest Injections 600
Effexor Tablets (Rare) 3495
Effexor XR Capsules (Rare) 3499
Emla (Unlikely with cream) 602
Enalaprilat Injection 863
Ethyol for Injection (Rare) 2029
Etrafon 3115
Exelon Capsules (Infrequent) 2342
Exelon Oral Solution (Infrequent) 2345
Felbatol 3343
Floxin I.V. (Less than 1%) 2526
Floxin Tablets (Less than 1%) 2529
Fluorescite Injection ⊙211
Fluothane Inhalation 3508
Foscavir Injection (Less than 1%) 605
Herceptin I.V. (At least one of the 958 patients) 1414
Imitrex Injection 1549
Imitrex Tablets 1558
INFeD Injection 3388
Kadian Capsules 1335
K-Lor Powder Packets 469
K-Tab Filmtab Tablets 470
Lanoxicaps Capsules 1574
Lanoxin Injection 1581
Lanoxin Tablets 1587
Lanoxin Elixir Pediatric 1578
Lanoxin Injection Pediatric 1584
Levaquin (Less than 0.3%) 2537
Levo-Dromoran 1734
Levoxyl Tablets 1819
Lexxel Tablets 608
Lidoderm Patch 1319
Mepergan Injection 3539
Meridia Capsules 481
Merrem I.V. (0.1% to 1.0%) 673
Micro-K 3311
Monopril Tablets 1091
Monopril HCT 1094
MS Contin Tablets 2896
MSIR 2898
Narcan Injection 1322
Naropin Injection 612
Navane Intramuscular 2703
Nesacaine/Nesacaine MPF 617
Nipent for Injection (Less than 3%) 3272
Nubain Injection (1% or less) 1323
Oramorph SR Tablets (Less frequent) 3062
Orthoclone OKT3 Sterile Solution (Less than 1%) 2498
Permax Tablets (Infrequent) 1299
Pfizerpen for Injection 2707
Pletal Tablets (Less than 2%) 2605
Pletal Tablets (Less than 2%) 2848
Polocaine Injection, USP 625
Polocaine-MPF Injection, USP 625
Prinivil Tablets (0.3% to 1.0%) 2164
Prinzide Tablets 2168
Proleukin for Injection (Less than 1% to 2%) 1199
Prostigmin Injectable 1744
Prostigmin Tablets 1744
Proventil Inhalation Aerosol 3142
Prozac Pulvules, Liquid, and Weekly Capsules (Rare) 1238
Pulmozyme Inhalation Solution 1426
Remicade for IV Injection (Less than 2%) 1178
Requip Tablets (Infrequent) 1621
Retavase Vials 1182
Rilutek Tablets (More than 2%) 772
Robinul Injectable 2940
Roxanol 3066
Roxicodone Tablets 3067
Rythmol Tablets – 150 mg, 225 mg, 300 mg (Less than 1%) 502
Sandostatin LAR Depot (Rare) 2395
Sarafem Pulvules (Rare) 1962
Sensorcaine 643
Sensorcaine-MPF Injection 643
Serentil (Rare) 1057
Solu-Medrol Sterile Powder 2855
Stelazine 1640
Symmetrel 1328
▲ Tambocor Tablets (5.1%) 1990
Tasmar Tablets (Infrequent) 3010
Tenormin (1.6%) 692
Thalomid Capsules 1154
Thioridazine Hydrochloride Tablets 2289
Thorazine 1656
Tikosyn Capsules (Less than or equal to 2%) 2717
Timolide Tablets 2187
Timolol GFS ⊙266
Timoptic in Ocudose (Less frequent) 2192
Timoptic Sterile Ophthalmic Solution (Less frequent) 2190
Timoptic-XE Sterile Ophthalmic Gel Forming Solution 2194
TNKase I.V. 1430
Tonocard Tablets 649
Trasylol Injection (1% to 2%) 909
Trilafon 3160
Uniretic Tablets (Less than 1%) 3178
Unithroid Tablets 3445
Vancocin HCl, Vials & ADD-Vantage (Rare) 1970
Vaseretic Tablets 2204
Vasotec I.V. Injection 2207
Vasotec Tablets (0.5% to 1.0%) 2210
▲ Vesanoid Capsules (3%) 3037
Viagra Tablets (Less than 2%) 2732
Virazole for Inhalation Solution 1747
Xylocaine Injections 653
Zestoretic Tablets 695
Zestril Tablets (0.3% to 1.0%) 698
Zosyn (1.0% or less) 1890
Zosyn in Galaxy Containers (1.0% or less) 1894
Zyprexa Tablets (Rare) 1973
Zyprexa ZYDIS Orally Disintegrating Tablets (Rare) 1973

Cardiac arrhythmias
(*see under* Arrhythmias)

Cardiac asystole
(*see under* Asystole)

Cardiac collapse
Botox Purified Neurotoxin Complex (2 patients) 549

Cardiac death
Viagra Tablets ... 2732

Cardiac dysrhythmias
(*see under* Arrhythmias)

Cardiac enlargement
Florinef Acetate Tablets ... 2250

Cardiac enzymes, elevation
Cytotec Tablets (Infrequent) ... 3202

Cardiac failure
(*see under* Heart failure)

Cardiac insufficiency
Rescriptor Tablets ... 526

Cardiac murmur
Aceon Tablets (2 mg, 4 mg, 8 mg) (0.3% to 1%) ... 3249
Amerge Tablets (Rare) ... 1467
Avalide Tablets ... 1070
Avapro Tablets (Less than 1%) ... 1074
Avapro Tablets (Less than 1%) ... 3076
Cipro I.V. (1% or less) ... 893
Cipro I.V. Pharmacy Bulk Package (Less than 1%) ... 897
Copaxone for Injection (Infrequent) ... 3306
Evoxac Capsules (Less than 1%) ... 1217
Fortovase Capsules (Less than 2%) ... 2970
Imdur Tablets (Less than or equal to 5%) ... 1826
Invirase Capsules (Less than 2%) ... 2979
▲ Lupron Injection (5% or more) ... 3279
Neurontin Capsules (Infrequent) ... 2655
Neurontin Oral Solution (Infrequent) ... 2655
Neurontin Tablets (Infrequent) ... 2655
Ovidrel for Injection (Less than 2%) ... 3220
Roferon-A Injection (Rare) ... 2996
▲ Serostim for Injection (1% to 10%) ... 3229
Thalomid Capsules ... 1154
▲ Vesanoid Capsules (3%) ... 3037

Cardiac output, decrease
Digibind Powder (Few instances) ... 1514
Diprivan Injectable Emulsion (1% to 3%) ... 667
Naropin Injection ... 612
Paxil (Rare) ... 1609
Sensorcaine ... 643
Sensorcaine-MPF Injection ... 643
Tensilon Injectable ... 1745

Cardiac rhythms, disturbances
Accupril Tablets (Rare) ... 2611
Accuretic Tablets (0.5% to 1%) ... 2614
Betapace AF Tablets (1.6% to 2%) ... 954
Calcium Disodium Versenate Injection ... 1980
Captopril Tablets ... 2281
Corgard Tablets (1 of 100 patients) ... 2245
Corzide 40/5 Tablets (1 of 100 patients) ... 2247
Corzide 80/5 Tablets (1 of 100 patients) ... 2247
Daraprim Tablets ... 1511
Digitek Tablets ... 1003
Enalaprilat Injection ... 863
Lanoxicaps Capsules ... 1574
Lanoxin Injection ... 1581
Lanoxin Tablets ... 1587
Lanoxin Elixir Pediatric ... 1578
Lanoxin Injection Pediatric ... 1584
Monopril Tablets (0.2% to 1.4%) ... 1091
Monopril HCT ... 1094
Nadolol Tablets (1 of 100 patients) ... 2288
Prinzide Tablets ... 2168
Rescriptor Tablets ... 526
Vaseretic Tablets ... 2204
Vasotec I.V. Injection ... 2207
Vasotec Tablets (0.5% to 1.0%) ... 2210
Zebeta Tablets ... 1885
Zestoretic Tablets ... 695

Cardiac stimulation, unspecified
Sensorcaine ... 643
Sensorcaine-MPF Injection ... 643

Cardiac tamponade
Activase I.V. ... 1410
Myleran Tablets (A small number of patients) ... 1603
Retavase Vials ... 1182
▲ Taxotere for Injection Concentrate (6%) ... 778
TNKase I.V. ... 1430
Zovirax for Injection (Less than 1%) ... 1708

Cardiac toxicity, unspecified
Adriamycin PFS/RDF Injection ... 2767
Ancobon Capsules ... 1730
Cerubidine for Injection ... 947
DaunoXome Injection ... 1442
Digitek Tablets ... 1003
Doxil Injection ... 566
Ellence Injection (1.4% to 1.8%) ... 2806
▲ Idamycin PFS Injection (16%) ... 2825
Ifex for Injection (Less than 1%) ... 1123
Lanoxicaps Capsules ... 1574
Lanoxin Injection ... 1581
Lanoxin Tablets ... 1587
Lanoxin Elixir Pediatric ... 1578
Lanoxin Injection Pediatric ... 1584
TheraCys Injection ... 823
Tice BCG, BCG Live (1.9%) ... 2489

Cardiac valve disorder, unspecified
Adipex-P ... 1406
Fortovase Capsules (Less than 2%) ... 2970

Cardialgia
(*see under* Heartburn)

Cardiodynia
(*see under* Heartburn)

Cardiogenic shock
Accupril Tablets (Rare) ... 2611
Activase I.V. ... 1410
▲ Mavik Tablets (3.8%) ... 478
Mexitil Capsules (1 in 1,000) ... 1047
Rituxan I.V. ... 1428
Tenormin (0.4%) ... 692
TNKase I.V. ... 1430
Tonocard Tablets (Less than 1%) ... 649

Cardiomegaly
Agrylin Capsules ... 3232
AmBisome for Injection (Less common) ... 1383
Apligraf (1.8%) ... 2305
Betaseron for SC Injection ... 988
Cerebyx Injection (Infrequent) ... 2619
Doxil Injection (Less than 1%) ... 566
Evoxac Capsules ... 1217
Geodon Capsules (Rare) ... 2688
Remeron Tablets (Rare) ... 2483
Remeron SolTab Tablets (Rare) ... 2486
Requip Tablets (Infrequent) ... 1621
Tonocard Tablets (Less than 1%) ... 649

Cardiomyopathy
Abelcet Injection ... 1273
Adderall Tablets (Isolated reports) ... 3231
Adderall XR Capsules (Isolated cases) ...
Adriamycin PFS/RDF Injection ... 2767
Agrylin Capsules ... 3232
Avonex ... 1013
DaunoXome Injection ... 1442
Dexedrine (Isolated reports) ... 1512
DextroStat Tablets (Isolated reports) ... 3236
Doxil Injection (1% to 5%) ... 566
Ellence Injection ... 2806
Herceptin I.V. ... 1414
Hivid Tablets (Less than 1%) ... 2975
Idamycin PFS Injection ... 2825
Imitrex Injection ... 1549
Imitrex Nasal Spray ... 1554
Imitrex Tablets ... 1558
Intron A for Injection (Less than 5%) ... 3120
Luvox Tablets (25, 50, 100 mg) (Infrequent) ... 3256
Megace Oral Suspension (1% to 3%) ... 1124
PEG-Intron Powder for Injection (Less than or equal to 1%) ... 3140
Plaquenil Tablets (Rare) ... 3082
Proleukin for Injection ... 1199
Rescriptor Tablets ... 526
Retrovir Capsules (0.8%) ... 1625
Retrovir IV Infusion (1%) ... 1629
Retrovir (0.8%) ... 1625
Roferon-A Injection (Rare) ... 2996
Viagra Tablets (Less than 2%) ... 2732
Vistide Injection ... 1445
Xeloda Tablets (Less than 5%) ... 3039

Cardiomyopathy, hypertrophic
Decadron Phosphate Injection ... 2081

Cardiopulmonary arrest
Brevital Sodium for Injection, USP ... 1815
Ceptaz for Injection ... 1499
Cipro I.V. (1% or less) ... 893
Cipro I.V. Pharmacy Bulk Package (Less than 1%) ... 897
Cipro (Less than 1%) ... 887
Cleocin Phosphate Sterile Solution (Rare) ... 2785
Fortaz ... 1541
Lariam Tablets (One patient) ... 2989
Pulmozyme Inhalation Solution ... 1426
Risperdal ... 1796
Triostat Injection (2%) ... 1825
Zofran Injection ... 1698
Zofran ... 1703
Zofran ODT Orally Disintegrating Tablets ... 1703

Cardiorespiratory arrest
Aloprim for Injection (Less than 1%) ... 2292
Avalide Tablets ... 1070
Avapro Tablets (Less than 1%) ... 1074
Avapro Tablets (Less than 1%) ... 3076
Brevital Sodium for Injection, USP ... 1815
Monopril Tablets (0.4% to 1.0%) ... 1091
Orthoclone OKT3 Sterile Solution ... 2498

Cardiospasm
Betaseron for SC Injection ... 988
Lodine (Less than 1%) ... 3528
Lodine XL Extended-Release Tablets (Less than 1%) ... 3530
Naprelan Tablets (Less than 1%) ... 1293
Prevacid Delayed-Release Capsules (Less than 1%) ... 3292
PREVPAC (Less than 1%) ... 3298
Protonix I.V. (Less than 1%) ... 3580
Protonix Tablets (Less than 1%) ... 3577
Sonata Capsules (Rare) ... 3591

Cardiovascular abnormalities, fetal
Accutane Capsules ... 2944
Cataflam Tablets ... 2315
Clinoril Tablets ... 2053
Dolobid Tablets ... 2088
Voltaren Tablets ... 2315
Voltaren-XR Tablets ... 2315

Cardiovascular collapse
Allegra-D Extended-Release Tablets ... 714
Carbatrol Capsules ... 3234
Cipro I.V. (1% or less) ... 893
Cipro I.V. Pharmacy Bulk Package (Less than 1%) ... 897
Cipro ... 887
Claritin-D 12 Hour Extended Release Tablets ... 3102
Claritin-D 24 Hour Extended Release Tablets ... 3104
Duranest Injections ... 600
Emla (Unlikely with cream) ... 602
Floxin I.V. ... 2526
Floxin Tablets ... 2529
INFeD Injection ... 3388
Lidoderm Patch ... 1319
Nesacaine/Nesacaine MPF ... 617
Noroxin Tablets ... 2145
Orthoclone OKT3 Sterile Solution ... 2498
Rynatan Tablets ... 3351
Tegretol/Tegretol-XR ... 2404
Tessalon Capsules ... 1377
Tetanus and Diphtheria Toxoids Adsorbed For Adult Use ... 815
Trovan ... 2722
Valium Injectable ... 3026
Xylocaine Injections ... 653
Zyrtec-D 12 Hour Extended Relief Tablets ... 2758

Cardiovascular depression
Nardil Tablets (Less frequent) ... 2653

Cardiovascular disorders
Actonel Tablets (2.5%) ... 2879
Agrylin Capsules (1% to 5%) ... 3232
Allegra-D Extended-Release Tablets (Rare) ... 714
Aloprim for Injection (Less than 1%) ... 2292
Alora Transdermal System ... 3372
▲ Amphotec (5% or more) ... 1774
Argatroban Injection (2.3%) ... 1478
Betapace Tablets (1% to 3%) ... 950
▲ Carnitor Injection (3% to 6%) ... 3242
▲ CellCept Capsules (3% to 25.6%) ... 2951
▲ CellCept Intravenous (3% to 25.6%) ... 2951
▲ CellCept Oral Suspension (3% to 25.6%) ... 2951
▲ CellCept Tablets (3% to 25.6%) ... 2951
▲ Cleocin Vaginal Cream (4%) ... 2788
▲ Clozaril Tablets (Greater than 5%) ... 2319
Crixivan Capsules (Less than 2%) ... 2070
Estrace Vaginal Cream ... 3358
Estrace Tablets ... 3361
Evoxac Capsules (Less than 1%) ... 1217
Foscavir Injection (Less than 1%) ... 605
Luvox Tablets (25, 50, 100 mg) (Infrequent) ... 3256
▲ Neoral Soft Gelatin Capsules (28.0%) ... 2380
▲ Neoral Oral Solution (28.0%) ... 2380
▲ Novantrone for Injection (11% to 26%) ... 1760
▲ Paraplatin for Injection (6% to 23%) ... 1126
Protonix I.V. (Less than 1%) ... 3580
Protonix Tablets (Less than 1%) ... 3577
Salagen Tablets (Two patients) ... 2229
Sinequan (Occasional) ... 2713
Singulair ... 2181
Tasmar Tablets (Rare) ... 3010
Taxol Injection (Approximately 1%) ... 1129
Tricor Capsules, Micronized ... 513
Vistide Injection ... 1445
Zyban Sustained-Release Tablets ... 1710

Carnitine concentrations, decreased
Depacon Injection ... 416
Depakene ... 421
Depakote Sprinkle Capsules ... 426
Depakote Tablets ... 430
Depakote ER Tablets ... 436

Carotid sinus hypersensitivity
Aldoclor Tablets ... 2035
Aldomet Tablets ... 2037
Aldoril Tablets ... 2039

Carpal tunnel syndrome
Evoxac Capsules (Less than 1%) ... 1217
Humatrope Vials and Cartridges (Rare) ... 1930
Intron A for Injection (Less than 5%) ... 3120
LYMErix Vaccine (Greater than 1%) ... 1592
Nutropin AQ Injection (Rare) ... 1420
Nutropin Depot for Injectable Suspension ... 1423
Nutropin for Injection (Rare) ... 1417
▲ Serostim for Injection (1% to 10%) ... 3229
Thalomid Capsules ... 1154

Carpopedal spasm
Compazine ... 1505
Stelazine ... 1640
Thorazine ... 1656

Cartilage trauma
Vioxx (Greater than 0.1% to 1.9%) ... 2213

Cataplexy
Clozaril Tablets ... 2319
▲ Provigil Tablets (3%) ... 1193

Cataracts
Accutane Capsules ... 2944
Aciphex Tablets ... 1267
Aciphex Tablets ... 1783
▲ Actonel Tablets (5.9%) ... 2879
Alesse-21 Tablets ... 3468
Alesse-28 Tablets ... 3473
Apligraf (2.7%) ... 2305
Arava Tablets (1% to 3%) ... 724
Aricept Tablets (Frequent) ... 1270
Aricept Tablets (Frequent) ... 2665
Baycol Tablets ... 883
Beconase Inhalation Aerosol (Rare) ... 1497
Beconase AQ Nasal Spray (Rare) ... 1498
Betaxon Ophthalmic Suspension (Less than 2%) ... 537
Betimol Ophthalmic Solution (1% to 5%) ... ⊙ 324
Brevicon 28-Day Tablets ... 3380
▲ Casodex Tablets (2% to 5%) ... 662
Celebrex Capsules (0.1% to 1.9%) ... 2676
Celebrex Capsules (0.1% to 1.9%) ... 2780
Celexa (Rare) ... 1365
▲ CellCept Capsules (3%) ... 2951
▲ CellCept Intravenous (3%) ... 2951
▲ CellCept Oral Suspension (3%) ... 2951
▲ CellCept Tablets (3%) ... 2951
Clomid Tablets ... 735
Cognex Capsules (Infrequent) ... 1351
Copaxone for Injection (Infrequent) ... 3306
Cyclessa Tablets ... 2450
Cytovene ... 2959
Desferal Vials ... 2333
Desogen Tablets ... 2458
Effexor Tablets (Infrequent) ... 3495
Effexor XR Capsules (Infrequent) ... 3499
Estrostep ... 2627
Evoxac Capsules (Less than 1%) ... 1217
Exelon Capsules (Frequent) ... 2342
Exelon Oral Solution (Frequent) ... 2345
▲ Fareston Tablets (10%) ... 3237
Flonase Nasal Spray ... 1533
Flovent Diskus ... 3614
Floxin I.V. ... 2526
Floxin Tablets ... 2529
Gengraf Capsules (1% to less than 3%) ... 457
Geodon Capsules (Infrequent) ... 2688
Haldol Decanoate ... 2535
Haldol Injection, Tablets and Concentrate ... 2533
Lescol Capsules ... 2361
Lescol Capsules ... 2925
Lescol XL Tablets ... 2361
Lescol XL Tablets ... 2925
Levlen ... 962
Levlite 21 Tablets ... 962
Levlite 28 Tablets ... 962
Levora Tablets ... 3389
Loestrin 21 Tablets ... 2642
Loestrin Fe Tablets ... 2642
Lo/Ovral Tablets ... 3532
Lo/Ovral-28 Tablets ... 3538
▲ Lopid Tablets (More common) ... 2650
Low-Ogestrel-28 Tablets ... 3392

▲ Lumigan Ophthalmic Solution (3% to 10%) ... 553
Lunelle Monthly Injection ... 2827
Microgestin Fe 1.5/30 Tablets ... 3407
Microgestin Fe 1/20 Tablets ... 3400
Minipress Capsules (A few reports) ... 2699
Minizide Capsules (Rare) ... 2700
Mirapex Tablets (Less than 1%) ... 2834
Mircette Tablets ... 2470
Modicon ... 2563
Motrin Suspension, Oral Drops, Chewable Tablets, and Caplets (Less than 1%) ... 2002
Myleran Tablets (Rare) ... 1603
Naprelan Tablets (Less than 1%) ... 1293
Necon ... 3415
Neoral Soft Gelatin Capsules (1% to less than 3%) ... 2380
Neoral Oral Solution (1% to less than 3%) ... 2380
Neurontin Capsules (Infrequent) ... 2655
Neurontin Oral Solution (Infrequent) ... 2655
Neurontin Tablets (Infrequent) ... 2655
Nilandron Tablets (2%) ... 753
Nolvadex Tablets ... 678
Nordette-28 Tablets ... 2257
Norinyl 1 +35 28-Day Tablets ... 3380
Norinyl 1 + 50 28-Day Tablets ... 3380
Ogestrel 0.5/50-28 Tablets ... 3428
Orap Tablets ... 1407
Ortho-Cept 21 Tablets ... 2546
Ortho-Cept 28 Tablets ... 2546
Ortho-Cyclen/Ortho Tri-Cyclen ... 2573
Ortho-Novum ... 2563
Ortho-Novum 1/50□28 Tablets ... 2556
Ortho-Cyclen/Ortho Tri-Cyclen ... 2573
Ovcon ... 3364
Ovral Tablets ... 3551
Ovral-28 Tablets ... 3552
Ovrette Tablets ... 3552
Paxil (Rare) ... 1609
Permax Tablets (Rare) ... 1299
Plavix Tablets (1% to 2.5%) ... 1097
Plavix Tablets (1% to 2.5%) ... 3084
Pravachol Tablets ... 1099
Protonix I.V. (Less than 1%) ... 3580
Protonix Tablets (Less than 1%) ... 3577
Prozac Pulvules, Liquid, and Weekly Capsules ... 1238
Pulmicort Turbuhaler Inhalation Powder (Rare) ... 636
▲ Rapamune Oral Solution and Tablets (3% to 20%) ... 3584
Rescula Ophthalmic Solution (1% to 5%) ... ⊙306
Rilutek Tablets (Rare) ... 772
Salagen Tablets (Less than 1%) ... 2229
Sarafem Pulvules ... 1962
Serophene Tablets ... 3226
Skelid Tablets (2.7%) ... 3088
Sonata Capsules (Rare) ... 3591
Tasmar Tablets (Rare) ... 3010
Topamax Sprinkle Capsules (Rare) ... 2590
Topamax Tablets (Rare) ... 2590
Travatan Ophthalmic Solution (1% to 4%) ... 543
Tricor Capsules, Micronized ... 513
Trileptal Oral Suspension ... 2407
Trileptal Tablets ... 2407
Tri-Levlen ... 962
Tri-Norinyl-28 Tablets ... 3433
Triphasil-21 Tablets ... 3600
Triphasil-28 Tablets ... 3605
Trivora Tablets ... 3439
Ultram Tablets (Infrequent) ... 2600
Uniretic Tablets (Less than 1%) ... 3178
Vanceril Double Strength Inhalation Aerosol (Rare) ... 3167
Viagra Tablets (Less than 2%) ... 2732
Vistide Injection ... 1445
▲ Visudyne for Injection (1% to 10%) ... ⊙308
Vitrasert Implant (Approximately 1% to 5%) ... ⊙254
▲ Vitravene for Injection (5% to 20%) ... ⊙310
Yasmin 28 Tablets ... 980
Zoloft ... 2751
Zovia ... 3449
Zyprexa Tablets (Infrequent) ... 1973
Zyprexa ZYDIS Orally Disintegrating Tablets (Infrequent) ... 1973

Cataracts, posterior subcapsular
Alrex Sterile Ophthalmic Suspension 0.2% ... ⊙256
Blephamide Ophthalmic Ointment (Infrequent) ... 547
Blephamide Ophthalmic Suspension ... 548
Celestone Soluspan Injectable Suspension ... 3097
Celestone Syrup ... 3099
Cortisporin Ophthalmic Suspension ... ⊙297
Cortone Acetate Injectable Suspension ... 2059
Cortone Acetate Tablets ... 2061
Cosopt Sterile Ophthalmic Solution (1% to 5%) ... 2065
Decadron Elixir ... 2078
Decadron Tablets ... 2079
Decadron Phosphate Injection ... 2081
Decadron Phosphate Sterile Ophthalmic Ointment ... 2083
Decadron Phosphate Sterile Ophthalmic Solution ... 2084
Depo-Medrol Injectable Suspension ... 2795
Florinef Acetate Tablets ... 2250
FML Ophthalmic Ointment (Infrequent) ... ⊙237
FML Ophthalmic Suspension ... ⊙236
FML Forte Ophthalmic Suspension (Infrequent) ... ⊙235
FML-S Liquifilm Sterile Ophthalmic Suspension ... ⊙238
HMS Sterile Ophthalmic Suspension (Rare) ... ⊙240
Hydrocortone Tablets ... 2106
Hydrocortone Acetate Injectable Suspension ... 2103
Hydrocortone Phosphate Injection, Sterile ... 2105
Lotemax Sterile Ophthalmic Suspension 0.5% ... ⊙261
NeoDecadron Sterile Ophthalmic Solution ... 2144
Pediapred Oral Solution ... 1170
Poly-Pred Liquifilm Ophthalmic Suspension ... ⊙245
Pred Forte Ophthalmic Suspension ... ⊙246
Pred Mild Sterile Ophthalmic Suspension (Infrequent) ... ⊙249
Pred-G Ophthalmic Suspension ... ⊙247
Pred-G Sterile Ophthalmic Ointment ... ⊙248
Prednisone ... 3064
Prelone Syrup ... 2273
Solu-Medrol Sterile Powder ... 2855
Soriatane Capsules (1% to 5%) ... 3003
Terra-Cortril Ophthalmic Suspension ... 2716
TobraDex Ophthalmic Ointment ... 542
TobraDex Ophthalmic Suspension ... 541
Vexol 1% Ophthalmic Suspension ... ⊙222

Catatonia
Blocadren Tablets ... 2046
Celexa (Rare) ... 1365
Compazine ... 1505
Corgard Tablets ... 2245
Corzide 40/5 Tablets ... 2247
Corzide 80/5 Tablets ... 2247
Cosopt Sterile Ophthalmic Solution ... 2065
Depacon Injection (1% or more) ... 416
Depakene (1% or more) ... 421
Depakote Sprinkle Capsules ... 426
Depakote Tablets (1% to 5%) ... 430
Depakote ER Tablets (Greater than 1%) ... 436
Effexor Tablets ... 3495
Effexor XR Capsules ... 3499
Etrafon ... 3115
Haldol Decanoate ... 2535
Haldol Injection, Tablets and Concentrate ... 2533
Inderal ... 3513
Inderal LA Long-Acting Capsules ... 3516
Inderide Tablets ... 3517
Inderide LA Long-Acting Capsules ... 3519
Nadolol Tablets ... 2288
Normodyne Tablets ... 3137
Phenergan Injection ... 3553
Phenergan ... 3556
Risperdal (Infrequent) ... 1796
Sectral Capsules ... 3589
Seroquel Tablets (Infrequent) ... 684
Stelazine ... 1640
Tenoretic Tablets ... 690
Tenormin ... 692
Thorazine (Rare) ... 1656
Timolide Tablets ... 2187
Timolol GFS ... ⊙266
Timoptic in Ocudose ... 2192
Timoptic Sterile Ophthalmic Solution ... 2190
Timoptic-XE Sterile Ophthalmic Gel Forming Solution ... 2194
Toprol-XL Tablets ... 651
Trilafon ... 3160
Zebeta Tablets ... 1885
Ziac Tablets ... 1887

Cauda equina syndrome
Azulfidine EN-tabs Tablets (Rare) ... 2775

Causalgia
Thalomid ... 1154

Cellulitis
Accuretic Tablets ... 2614
Actiq (1% or greater) ... 1184
Adalat CC Tablets (Less than 1.0%) ... 877
Adriamycin PFS/RDF Injection ... 2767
Aloprim for Injection (Less than 1%) ... 2292
AmBisome for Injection (Less common) ... 1383
▲ Apligraf (7.5% to 9.8%) ... 2305
Aricept Tablets (Infrequent) ... 1270
Aricept Tablets (Infrequent) ... 2665
Avonex ... 1013
Bactroban Cream (Less than 1%) ... 1494
BeneFix for Injection ... 1432
Betaseron for SC Injection ... 988
Bicillin C-R 900/300 Injection ... 2240
Bicillin C-R Injection ... 2238
Bicillin L-A Injection ... 2242
Campath Ampules ... 992
Celebrex Capsules (0.1% to 1.9%) ... 2676
Celebrex Capsules (0.1% to 1.9%) ... 2780
Celexa (Rare) ... 1365
▲ CellCept Capsules (3% to 10%) ... 2951
▲ CellCept Intravenous (3% to 10%) ... 2951
▲ CellCept Oral Suspension (3% to 10%) ... 2951
▲ CellCept Tablets (3% to 10%) ... 2951
Cognex Capsules (Infrequent) ... 1351
Copaxone for Injection (Infrequent) ... 3306
Diphtheria & Tetanus Toxoids Adsorbed Purogenated for Pediatric Use ... 1857
Doxil Injection (Less than 1%) ... 566
Effexor Tablets (Rare) ... 3495
Effexor XR Capsules (Rare) ... 3499
Enbrel for Injection ... 1752
Enbrel for Injection ... 3504
Evoxac Capsules (Less than 1%) ... 1217
Exelon Capsules (Infrequent) ... 2342
Exelon Oral Solution (Infrequent) ... 2345
Fortovase Capsules (Less than 2%) ... 2970
Gabitril Tablets (Infrequent) ... 1189
Gengraf Capsules (1% to less than 3%) ... 457
Herceptin I.V. (At least one of the 958 patients) ... 1414
Hivid Tablets (Less than 1%) ... 2975
Innohep Injection ... 1248
Intron A for Injection (Less than 5%) ... 3120
Invirase Capsules (Less than 2%) ... 2979
Klonopin Tablets (Infrequent) ... 2983
Lupron Depot 7.5 mg (Less than 5%) ... 3284
Naprelan Tablets (Less than 1%) ... 1293
Neoral Soft Gelatin Capsules (1% to less than 3%) ... 2380
Neoral Oral Solution (1% to less than 3%) ... 2380
▲ Nipent for Injection (6%) ... 3272
Norplant System (Uncommon) ... 3543
Paxil (Rare) ... 1609
Permax Tablets (Infrequent) ... 1299
▲ Prograf (3% to 15%) ... 1393
Proleukin for Injection ... 1199
Protopic Ointment (Greater than or equal to 1%) ... 1397
▲ Rapamune Oral Solution and Tablets (3% to 20%) ... 3584
Regranex Gel ... 2586
Remeron Tablets (Rare) ... 2483
Remeron SolTab Tablets (Rare) ... 2486
▲ Remicade for IV Injection (Less than 2% to 26%) ... 1178
ReoPro Vials (0.3%) ... 1958
Requip Tablets (Infrequent) ... 1621
Rilutek Tablets (Infrequent) ... 772
Sandostatin Injection (Less than 1%) ... 2394
Sandostatin LAR Depot (1% to 4%) ... 2395
Serzone Tablets (Rare) ... 1104
Sular Tablets (Less than or equal to 1%) ... 688
Tasmar Tablets (Infrequent) ... 3010
Taxol Injection (Rare) ... 1129
Tetanus & Diphtheria Toxoids Adsorbed for Adult Use ... 1880
Thalomid Capsules ... 1154
Uniretic Tablets (Less than 1%) ... 3178
Varivax ... 2202
▲ Vesanoid Capsules (8%) ... 3037
Vioxx (Greater than 0.1% to 1.9%) ... 2213
Vistide Injection ... 1445
Zanaflex Tablets (Infrequent) ... 1305

Cellulitis, at injection site
Cefizox for Intramuscular or Intravenous Use (1% to 5%) ... 1390
INFeD Injection ... 3388

Cellulitis, scrotal
Testoderm Transdermal Systems (1%) ... 574

Centrilobular sinusoidal fibrosis
Myleran Tablets ... 1603

Cephalin flocculation test, positive
Cuprimine Capsules ... 2075
Depen Titratable Tablets (Few reports) ... 3341

Cerebellar dysfunction
Cerebyx Injection (Rare) ... 2619
▲ Idamycin PFS Injection (4%) ... 2825
Neurontin Capsules (Infrequent) ... 2655
Neurontin Oral Solution (Infrequent) ... 2655
Neurontin Tablets (Infrequent) ... 2655

Cerebellar malformation, fetal
Accutane Capsules ... 2944

Cerebellar syndrome, acute
Ergamisol Tablets ... 1789
Fludara for Injection (Up to 1%) ... 995
Sterile FUDR (Remote possibility) ... 2974
Lamictal (Rare) ... 1567
Topamax Sprinkle Capsules (Rare) ... 2590
Topamax Tablets (Rare) ... 2590

Cerebral abnormalities, fetal
Accutane Capsules ... 2944

Cerebral arterial insufficiency, symptoms
Carbatrol Capsules ... 3234
Tegretol/Tegretol-XR ... 2404

Cerebral arteritis
Concerta Extended-Release Tablets (Isolated cases) ... 1998
Concerta Tablets (Isolated cases) ... 561
Metadate CD Capsules (Isolated cases) ... 1164
Metadate ER Tablets (Isolated cases) ... 1167
Methylin Tablets (Isolated cases) ... 1995
Methylin ER Tablets (Isolated cases) ... 1995
Ritalin (Isolated cases) ... 2387

Cerebral atrophy
Depacon Injection (Several cases) ... 416
Depakene (Several reports) ... 421
Depakote Sprinkle Capsules (Several reports) ... 426
Depakote Tablets (Several reports) ... 430
Depakote ER Tablets (Several reports) ... 436

Cerebral bleeding
(*see under* Cerebral hemorrhage)

Cerebral embolism
Aygestin Tablets ... 1333
Prozac Pulvules, Liquid, and Weekly Capsules (Rare) ... 1238
Rilutek Tablets (Rare) ... 772
Sarafem Pulvules (Rare) ... 1962
Trasylol Injection (1% to 2%) ... 909

Cerebral hemorrhage
Alesse-21 Tablets ... 3468
Alesse-28 Tablets ... 3473
Betaseron for SC Injection ... 988
Brevicon 28-Day Tablets ... 3380
Cafcit (2.2%) ... 1035
Campath Ampules ... 992
Cerebyx Injection (Infrequent) ... 2619
Cyclessa Tablets ... 2450
Desogen Tablets ... 2458
Estrostep ... 2627
Fortovase Capsules (Less than 2%) ... 2970
Gliadel Wafer (Less than 1%) ... 1723
Imitrex Injection ... 1549
Imitrex Tablets ... 1558
Innohep Injection ... 1248
Levlen ... 962
Levlite 21 Tablets ... 962
Levlite 28 Tablets ... 962
Levora Tablets ... 3389
Loestrin 21 Tablets ... 2642
Loestrin Fe Tablets ... 2642
Lo/Ovral Tablets ... 3532
Lo/Ovral-28 Tablets ... 3538
Low-Ogestrel-28 Tablets ... 3392
Lunelle Monthly Injection ... 2827
Microgestin Fe 1.5/30 Tablets ... 3407
Microgestin Fe 1/20 Tablets ... 3400
Mircette Tablets ... 2470
Modicon ... 2563
Mylotarg for Injection (2%) ... 3540
Necon ... 3415
Nordette-28 Tablets ... 2257
Norinyl 1 +35 28-Day Tablets ... 3380
Norinyl 1 + 50 28-Day Tablets ... 3380
Ogestrel 0.5/50-28 Tablets ... 3428
Ortho-Cept 21 Tablets ... 2546
Ortho-Cept 28 Tablets ... 2546
Ortho-Cyclen/Ortho Tri-Cyclen ... 2573
Ortho-Novum ... 2563
Ortho-Novum 1/50□28 Tablets ... 2556

Ortho-Cyclen/Ortho Tri-Cyclen 2573
Ovcon 3364
Ovral Tablets 3551
Ovral-28 Tablets 3552
Ovrette Tablets 3552
Permax Tablets (Rare) 1299
Proleukin for Injection 1199
Rifadin 765
Rilutek Tablets (Infrequent) 772
Tasmar Tablets (Infrequent) 3010
Trileptal Oral Suspension 2407
Trileptal Tablets 2407
Tri-Levlen 962
Tri-Norinyl-28 Tablets 3433
Triphasil-21 Tablets 3600
Triphasil-28 Tablets 3605
Trivora Tablets 3439
▲ Vesanoid Capsules (9%) 3037
Yasmin 28 Tablets 980
Zovia 3449

Cerebral herniation
Activase 1410

Cerebral infarction
Aloprim for Injection (Less than 1%) 2292
Amerge Tablets 1467
Arimidex Tablets 659
Cerebyx Injection (Infrequent) 2619
Geodon Capsules (Rare) 2688
Gliadel Wafer (Less than 1%) 1723
Monopril Tablets (0.4% to 1.0%) 1091
Pletal Tablets (Less than 2%) 2605
Pletal Tablets (Less than 2%) 2848
Remicade for IV Injection (Less than 2%) 1178
Retavase Vials 1182
Streptase for Infusion 647
Uniretic Tablets (Less than 1%) 3178

Cerebral ischemia
(*see under* Ischemia, cerebral)

Cerebral lesions
Proleukin for Injection 1199

Cerebral occlusion
Concerta Extended-Release Tablets (Isolated cases) 1998
Concerta Tablets (Isolated cases) 561
Humegon for Injection 2468
Metadate CD Capsules (Isolated cases) 1164
Metadate ER Tablets (Isolated cases) 1167
Methylin Tablets (Isolated cases) 1995
Methylin ER Tablets (Isolated cases) 1995
Ritalin (Isolated cases) 2387

Cerebral thrombosis
Activella Tablets 2764
Alesse-21 Tablets 3468
Alesse-28 Tablets 3473
Aygestin Tablets 1333
Brevicon 28-Day Tablets 3380
Cipro I.V. (1% or less) 893
Cipro I.V. Pharmacy Bulk Package (Less than 1%) 897
Cipro (Less than 1%) 887
Cyclessa Tablets 2450
DDAVP Injection 4 mcg/mL (Rare) 737
Desmopressin Acetate Injection (Rare) 1344
Desogen Tablets 2458
Estrostep 2627
Floxin I.V. 2526
Floxin Tablets 2529
Lamictal (Rare) 1567
Levlen 962
Levlite 21 Tablets 962
Levlite 28 Tablets 962
Levora Tablets 3389
Loestrin 21 Tablets 2642
Loestrin Fe Tablets 2642
Lo/Ovral Tablets 3532
Lo/Ovral-28 Tablets 3538
Low-Ogestrel-28 Tablets 3392
Lunelle Monthly Injection 2827
Microgestin Fe 1.5/30 Tablets 3407
Microgestin Fe 1/20 Tablets 3400
Mircette Tablets 2470
Modicon 2563
Necon 3415
Nordette-28 Tablets 2257
Norinyl 1 +35 28-Day Tablets 3380
Norinyl 1 + 50 28-Day Tablets 3380
Ogestrel 0.5/50-28 Tablets 3428
Ortho-Cept 21 Tablets 2546
Ortho-Cept 28 Tablets 2546
Ortho-Cyclen/Ortho Tri-Cyclen 2573
Ortho-Novum 2563
Ortho-Novum 1/50□28 Tablets 2556
Ortho-Cyclen/Ortho Tri-Cyclen 2573
Ovcon 3364
Ovral Tablets 3551
Ovral-28 Tablets 3552
Ovrette Tablets 3552
Premphase Tablets 3572
Prempro Tablets 3572
Provera Tablets 2853
Trasylol Injection (0.5%) 909
Tri-Levlen 962
Tri-Norinyl-28 Tablets 3433
Triphasil-21 Tablets 3600
Triphasil-28 Tablets 3605
Trivora Tablets 3439
Viagra Tablets (Less than 2%) 2732
Yasmin 28 Tablets 980
Zovia 3449

Cerebrospinal fluid, sterilization of
Kefurox Vials, ADD-Vantage 1948

Cerebrospinal fluid proteins, changes
Compazine 1505
Etrafon 3115
Navane Oral 2701
Navane Intramuscular 2703
Stelazine 1640
Thiothixene Capsules 2290
Thorazine 1656
Trilafon 3160

Cerebrovascular accident
Abelcet Injection 1273
Accupril Tablets (Rare) 2611
Accuretic Tablets (0.5% to 1%) 2614
Aceon Tablets (2 mg, 4 mg, 8 mg) (0.2%) 3249
Agrylin Capsules (1% to 5%) 3232
Amerge Tablets 1467
Aricept Tablets (Infrequent) 1270
Aricept Tablets (Infrequent) 2665
Arimidex Tablets 659
Avalide Tablets 1070
Avapro Tablets (Less than 1%) 1074
Avapro Tablets (Less than 1%) 3076
Betagan .... ⊙228
Betimol Ophthalmic Solution .... ⊙324
Bicillin C-R 900/300 Injection 2240
Bicillin C-R Injection 2238
Bicillin L-A Injection 2242
Blocadren Tablets (Less than 1%) 2046
Captopril Tablets 2281
Cardura Tablets (Less than 0.5%) 2668
Carteolol Hydrochloride Ophthalmic Solution USP, 1% .... ⊙258
Catapres-TTS (0.5% or less) 1038
Celebrex Capsules (Less than 0.1%) 2676
Celebrex Capsules (Less than 0.1%) 2780
Celexa (Infrequent) 1365
Cognex Capsules (Infrequent) 1351
Cosopt Sterile Ophthalmic Solution (Less than 1%) 2065
Covera-HS Tablets (Less than 2%) 3199
Cozaar Tablets (Less than 1%) 2067
D.H.E. 45 Injection (Extremely rare) 2334
Duraclon Injection (Rare) 3057
Effexor Tablets (Rare) 3495
Effexor XR Capsules (Rare) 3499
Emcyt Capsules (2%) 2810
Enalaprilat Injection 863
Epogen for Injection (0.4%) 582
Fareston Tablets (Less than 1% to 2%) 3237
femhrt Tablets 2635
▲ Flolan for Injection (4%) 1528
Fludara for Injection (Up to 3%) 995
Gemzar for Injection (2%) 1919
Geodon Capsules (Rare) 2688
Hyzaar 2109
Imitrex Injection 1549
Imitrex Nasal Spray 1554
Imitrex Tablets 1558
Isoptin SR Tablets (1% or less) 467
Lamictal (Rare) 1567
Lexxel Tablets 608
Lodine (Less than 1%) 3528
Lodine XL Extended-Release Tablets (Less than 1%) 3530
Luvox Tablets (25, 50, 100 mg) (Rare) 3256
Maxalt Tablets (Very rare) 2120
Maxalt-MLT Orally Disintegrating Tablets (Very rare) 2120
Meridia Capsules 481
Miacalcin Nasal Spray (Less than 1%) 2375
Monopril Tablets (0.2% to 1.0%) 1091
Monopril HCT 1094
Motrin Suspension, Oral Drops, Chewable Tablets, and Caplets (Less than 1%) 2002
Neurontin Capsules (Rare) 2655
Neurontin Oral Solution (Rare) 2655
Neurontin Tablets (Rare) 2655
Ocupress Ophthalmic Solution, 1% Sterile .... ⊙303
Orthoclone OKT3 Sterile Solution 2498
Paraplatin for Injection 1126
Paxil (Rare) 1609
Permax Tablets (Infrequent) 1299
Prevacid Delayed-Release Capsules (Less than 1%) 3292
PREVPAC (Less than 1%) 3298
Prinivil Tablets (0.3% to 1.0%) 2164
Prinzide Tablets 2168
Procrit for Injection (0.4% to 3.2%) 2502
Protopic Ointment (Greater than or equal to 1%) 1397
Prozac Pulvules, Liquid, and Weekly Capsules (Rare) 1238
Sarafem Pulvules (Rare) 1962
Seroquel Tablets (Infrequent) 684
Serzone Tablets (Rare) 1104
Sular Tablets (Less than or equal to 1%) 688
Tarka Tablets 508
Tasmar Tablets (Infrequent) 3010
Tenex Tablets (Rare) 2942
Thalomid Capsules 1154
Tikosyn Capsules (Less than or equal to 2%) 2717
Timolide Tablets 2187
Timolol GFS .... ⊙266
Timoptic in Ocudose (Less frequent) 2192
Timoptic Sterile Ophthalmic Solution (Less frequent) 2190
Timoptic-XE Sterile Ophthalmic Gel Forming Solution 2194
Tonocard Tablets 649
Trasylol Injection (1% to 2%) 909
Vaseretic Tablets 2204
Vasotec I.V. Injection 2207
Vasotec Tablets (0.5% to 1.0%) 2210
Verelan Capsules (1% or less) 3184
Verelan PM Capsules (2% or less) 3186
Vioxx (Less than 0.1%) 2213
Xeloda Tablets (Less than 5%) 3039
Zestoretic Tablets 695
Zestril Tablets (0.3% to 1.0%) 698
Zoladex (1% to 5%) 702
Zoladex 3-month (1% to 5%) 706
Zonegran Capsules (Infrequent) 1307
Zosyn (1.0% or less) 1890
Zosyn in Galaxy Containers (1.0% or less) 1894
Zyprexa Tablets (Infrequent) 1973
Zyprexa ZYDIS Orally Disintegrating Tablets (Infrequent) 1973

Cerebrovascular disorders
Activella Tablets 2764
Aldoclor Tablets 2035
Aldomet Tablets 2037
Aldoril Tablets 2039
Altace Capsules (Less than 1%) 2233
Ambien Tablets (Infrequent) 3191
Brevicon 28-Day Tablets 3380
Campath Ampules 992
Coreg Tablets (Less than or equal to 0.1%) 1508
Crixivan Capsules 2070
Depo-Provera Contraceptive Injection 2798
Felbatol 3343
Flumadine (Less than 0.3%) 1370
Foscavir Injection (Between 1% and 5%) 605
Levaquin (Less than 0.3%) 2537
Micardis Tablets (More than 0.3%) 1049
Micardis HCT Tablets (More than 0.3%) 1051
Modicon 2563
Norinyl 1 +35 28-Day Tablets 3380
Norinyl 1 + 50 28-Day Tablets 3380
Norplant System 3543
Ortho-Cyclen/Ortho Tri-Cyclen 2573
Ortho-Novum 2563
Ortho-Novum 1/50□28 Tablets 2556
Ortho-Cyclen/Ortho Tri-Cyclen 2573
Ovcon 3364
Premphase Tablets 3572
Prempro Tablets 3572
Provera Tablets 2853
Risperdal 1796
Toprol-XL Tablets (Greater than 1%) 651
Tri-Norinyl-28 Tablets 3433
Vistide Injection 1445
Zoloft (Rare) 2751

Cerebrovascular insufficiency
Captopril Tablets 2281

Cerumen, increased
Norvir Capsules (Less than 2%) 487
Norvir Oral Solution (Less than 2%) 487

Cerumen impaction
Vioxx (Greater than 0.1% to 1.9%) 2213

Ceruminosis
Remicade for IV Injection (Less than 2%) 1178

Cervical disorders
(*see under* Cervical irregularities)

Cervical dysplasia
Campath Ampules 992

Cervical erosion, changes
Activella Tablets 2764
Alesse-21 Tablets 3468
Alesse-28 Tablets 3473
Aygestin Tablets 1333
Brevicon 28-Day Tablets 3380
Cyclessa Tablets 2450
Desogen Tablets 2458
Estinyl Tablets 3112
Estratest 3252
Estrostep 2627
Levlen 962
Levlite 21 Tablets 962
Levlite 28 Tablets 962
Levora Tablets 3389
Loestrin 21 Tablets 2642
Loestrin Fe Tablets 2642
Lo/Ovral Tablets 3532
Lo/Ovral-28 Tablets 3538
Low-Ogestrel-28 Tablets 3392
Menest Tablets 2254
Microgestin Fe 1.5/30 Tablets 3407
Microgestin Fe 1/20 Tablets 3400
Mircette Tablets 2470
Modicon 2563
Necon 3415
Nordette-28 Tablets 2257
Norinyl 1 +35 28-Day Tablets 3380
Norinyl 1 + 50 28-Day Tablets 3380
Ogestrel 0.5/50-28 Tablets 3428
Ortho-Cept 21 Tablets 2546
Ortho-Cept 28 Tablets 2546
Ortho-Cyclen/Ortho Tri-Cyclen 2573
Ortho-Novum 2563
Ortho-Novum 1/50□28 Tablets 2556
Ortho-Cyclen/Ortho Tri-Cyclen 2573
Ovcon 3364
Ovral Tablets 3551
Ovral-28 Tablets 3552
Ovrette Tablets 3552
ParaGard T 380A Intrauterine Copper Contraceptive 2582
Premarin Intravenous 3563
Premarin Vaginal Cream 3570
Premphase Tablets 3572
Prempro Tablets 3572
Provera Tablets 2853
Tri-Levlen 962
Tri-Norinyl-28 Tablets 3433
Triphasil-21 Tablets 3600
Triphasil-28 Tablets 3605
Trivora Tablets 3439
Yasmin 28 Tablets 980
Zovia 3449

Cervical eversion, changes in
Ortho Dienestrol Cream 2554

Cervical irregularities
Gonal-F for Injection (2.5%) 3216
Hivid Tablets (Less than 1%) 2975
Lunelle Monthly Injection 2827
Lupron Depot-PED 7.5 mg, 11.25 mg and 15 mg (Less than 2%) 3291
Lupron Injection Pediatric (Less than 2%) 3280

Cervical secretion, changes
Activella Tablets 2764
Alesse-21 Tablets 3468
Alesse-28 Tablets 3473
Alora Transdermal System 3372
Aygestin Tablets 1333
Brevicon 28-Day Tablets 3380
Cenestin Tablets 1263
Climara Transdermal System 958
Cyclessa Tablets 2450
Desogen Tablets 2458
Esclim Transdermal System 3460
Estinyl Tablets 3112
Estrace Vaginal Cream 3358
Estrace Tablets 3361
Estratest 3252
Estrostep 2627
femhrt Tablets 2635
Levlen 962
Levlite 21 Tablets 962
Levlite 28 Tablets 962
Levora Tablets 3389
Loestrin 21 Tablets 2642
Loestrin Fe Tablets 2642
Lo/Ovral Tablets 3532
Lo/Ovral-28 Tablets 3538
Low-Ogestrel-28 Tablets 3392
Menest Tablets 2254
Microgestin Fe 1.5/30 Tablets 3407
Microgestin Fe 1/20 Tablets 3400
Mircette Tablets 2470
Modicon 2563
Necon 3415
Nordette-28 Tablets 2257
Norinyl 1 +35 28-Day Tablets 3380
Norinyl 1 + 50 28-Day Tablets 3380
Ogen Tablets 2846
Ogestrel 0.5/50-28 Tablets 3428
Ortho Dienestrol Cream 2554
Ortho-Cept 21 Tablets 2546
Ortho-Cept 28 Tablets 2546
Ortho-Cyclen/Ortho Tri-Cyclen 2573
Ortho-Est Tablets 3464

- Ortho-Novum ... 2563
- Ortho-Novum 1/50□28 Tablets ... 2556
- Ortho-Prefest Tablets ... 2570
- Ortho-Cyclen/Ortho Tri-Cyclen ... 2573
- Ovcon ... 3364
- Ovral Tablets ... 3551
- Ovral-28 Tablets ... 3552
- Ovrette Tablets ... 3552
- Premarin Intravenous ... 3563
- Premarin Tablets ... 3566
- Premarin Vaginal Cream ... 3570
- Premphase Tablets ... 3572
- Prempro Tablets ... 3572
- Prometrium Capsules (100 mg, 200 mg) ... 3261
- Provera Tablets ... 2853
- Tri-Levlen ... 962
- Tri-Norinyl-28 Tablets ... 3433
- Triphasil-21 Tablets ... 3600
- Triphasil-28 Tablets ... 3605
- Trivora Tablets ... 3439
- Vivelle Transdermal System ... 2412
- Vivelle-Dot Transdermal System ... 2416
- Yasmin 28 Tablets ... 980
- Zovia ... 3449

Cervical smear test, positive
- Evoxac Capsules (Less than 1%) ... 1217

Cervicitis
- Betaseron for SC Injection ... 988
- ▲ Cleocin Vaginal Cream (16% to 33%) ... 2788
- Effexor Tablets (Rare) ... 3495
- Effexor XR Capsules (Rare) ... 3499
- ▲ Norplant System (5% or greater) ... 3543

Chafing, genital
- Condylox Topical Solution (Less than 5%) ... 2437

Chalazion
- Fortovase Capsules (Less than 2%) ... 2970
- Invirase Capsules (Less than 2%) ... 2979
- Soriatane Capsules (Less than 1%) ... 3003

Change in blood glucose levels
(see under Insulin reaction)

Charcot's syndrome
- Atromid-S Capsules ... 3483
- Imdur Tablets (Less than or equal to 5%) ... 1826
- ▲ Mavik Tablets (3.8%) ... 478
- ReoPro Vials (0.4%) ... 1958
- Soriatane Capsules (Less than 1%) ... 3003
- Timolide Tablets ... 2187
- Tonocard Tablets (Less than 1%) ... 649

Cheek puffing
- Compazine ... 1505
- Etrafon ... 3115
- Haldol Decanoate ... 2535
- Haldol Injection, Tablets and Concentrate ... 2533
- Moban ... 1320
- Navane Intramuscular ... 2703
- Orap Tablets ... 1407
- Stelazine ... 1640
- Thiothixene Capsules ... 2290
- Thorazine ... 1656

Cheilitis
- Accutane Capsules ... 2944
- Actiq (Less than 1%) ... 1184
- Betaseron for SC Injection ... 988
- Cosmegen for Injection ... 2062
- Crixivan Capsules (Less than 2%) ... 2070
- Effexor Tablets (Rare) ... 3495
- Effexor XR Capsules (Rare) ... 3499
- Fortovase Capsules (Less than 2%) ... 2970
- Invirase Capsules (Less than 2%) ... 2979
- Lipitor Tablets (Less than 2%) ... 2639
- Lipitor Tablets (Less than 2%) ... 2696
- Norvir Capsules (Less than 2%) ... 487
- Norvir Oral Solution (Less than 2%) ... 487
- Protopic Ointment (Greater than or equal to 1%) ... 1397
- Rilutek Tablets (Rare) ... 772
- Sonata Capsules (Rare) ... 3591
- ▲ Soriatane Capsules (More than 75%) ... 3003
- Tequin Injection (Less than 0.1%) ... 1110
- Tequin Tablets (Less than 0.1%) ... 1110
- Trovan (Less than 1%) ... 2722
- Uniretic Tablets (Less than 1%) ... 3178
- Vaniqa Cream (Less than 1%) ... 1121

Cheilosis
- Calcium Disodium Versenate Injection ... 1980
- Cuprimine Capsules (Rare) ... 2075
- Depen Titratable Tablets (Rare) ... 3341

Chemosis
- Alomide Ophthalmic Solution (Less than 1%) ... ⊙204
- ▲ Alrex Sterile Ophthalmic Suspension 0.2% (5% to 15%) ... ⊙256
- Chibroxin Sterile Ophthalmic Solution ... 2051
- ▲ Lotemax Sterile Ophthalmic Suspension 0.5% (5% to 15%) ... ⊙261
- ▲ Rēv-Eyes Sterile Ophthalmic Eyedrops 0.5% (10% to 40%) ... ⊙265
- Vitrasert Implant (Less than 1%) ... ⊙254

Chest congestion
- Aerobid/Aerobid-M (3% to 9%) ... 1363
- Azmacort Inhalation Aerosol (1% to 3%) ... 728
- Claritin-D 12 Hour Extended Release Tablets (Less frequent) ... 3102
- Cognex Capsules (Infrequent) ... 1351
- Effexor Tablets (Infrequent) ... 3495
- Effexor XR Capsules (Infrequent) ... 3499
- Flovent (1% to 3%) ... 1535
- Flovent Rotadisk (1% to 3%) ... 1537
- Hivid Tablets (Less than 1%) ... 2975
- Klonopin Tablets ... 2983
- Rescriptor Tablets (Less than 2%) ... 526
- Roferon-A Injection (Less than 3%) ... 2996
- ▲ Serevent Inhalation Aerosol (4%) ... 1633
- Vanceril Double Strength Inhalation Aerosol (Fewer than 2%) ... 3167

Chest numbness
- Tessalon Capsules ... 1377

Chest pain
- ▲ Abelcet Injection (3%) ... 1273
- AccuNeb Inhalation Solution (0.9% to 1.7%) ... 1230
- Accupril Tablets (2.4%) ... 2611
- Accuretic Tablets (1%) ... 2614
- Accutane Capsules (Less frequent) ... 2944
- Aceon Tablets (2 mg, 4 mg, 8 mg) (2.4%) ... 3249
- Actiq (1% or greater) ... 1184
- ▲ Actonel Tablets (5% to 6.6%) ... 2879
- Adalat CC Tablets (3% or less) ... 877
- Adenocard Injection (Less than 1%) ... 1380
- ▲ Aerobid/Aerobid-M (3% to 9%) ... 1363
- Aggrenox Capsules ... 1026
- ▲ Agrylin Capsules (7.8%) ... 3232
- ▲ Alferon N Injection (6% to 10%) ... 1770
- Altace Capsules (Less than 1% to 1.1%) ... 2233
- Ambien Tablets (1%) ... 3191
- ▲ AmBisome for Injection (8.2% to 12%) ... 1383
- ▲ Amphotec (5% or more) ... 1774
- Ancobon Capsules ... 1730
- Anzemet Injection (Rare) ... 719
- Anzemet Tablets (Rare) ... 722
- ▲ Apligraf (3.6%) ... 2305
- Arava Tablets (2%) ... 724
- Aricept Tablets (Frequent) ... 1270
- Aricept Tablets (Frequent) ... 2665
- ▲ Arimidex Tablets (5.0% to 7.3%) ... 659
- ▲ Aromasin Tablets (2% to 5%) ... 2769
- ▲ Asacol Delayed-Release Tablets (3%) ... 2884
- Astelin Nasal Spray ... 3339
- Atacand Tablets (More than 1%) ... 595
- Atacand HCT Tablets (0.5% or greater) ... 597
- ▲ Atrovent Inhalation Solution (3.2%) ... 1031
- Avalide Tablets (2%) ... 1070
- Avapro Tablets (1% or greater) ... 1074
- Avapro Tablets (1% or greater) ... 3076
- Avelox Tablets (0.05% to 1%) ... 879
- ▲ Avonex (6%) ... 1013
- Axert Tablets (Infrequent) ... 2772
- Axid Pulvules (2.3%) ... 1903
- Axid Pulvules (2.3%) ... 2919
- Azactam for Injection (Less than 1%) ... 1276
- Azopt Ophthalmic Suspension (Less than 1%) ... 536
- Baycol Tablets (2%) ... 883
- Betagan ... ⊙228
- ▲ Betapace Tablets (4% to 16%) ... 950
- Betapace AF Tablets (2.5% to 4.6%) ... 954
- Betimol Ophthalmic Solution ... ⊙324
- Blocadren Tablets (0.6%) ... 2046
- Brevibloc Injection (Less than 1%) ... 858
- ▲ Campath Ampules (1% to 10%) ... 992
- Captopril Tablets (Approximately 1 in 100 patients) ... 2281
- Cardene I.V. (0.7%) ... 3485
- Cardizem Injectable (Less than 1%) ... 1018
- Cardizem Lyo-Ject Syringe (Less than 1%) ... 1018
- Cardizem Monovial (Less than 1%) ... 1018
- Cardura Tablets (1.2% to 2%) ... 2668
- ▲ Carnitor Injection (6% to 15%) ... 3242
- ▲ Casodex Tablets (6%) ... 662
- Cataflam Tablets (Less than 1%) ... 2315
- Catapres-TTS (0.5% or less) ... 1038
- Ceclor CD Tablets (0.1% to 1%) ... 1279
- Ceftin Tablets (0.1% to 1%) ... 1898
- Celebrex Capsules (0.1% to 1.9%) ... 2676
- Celebrex Capsules (0.1% to 1.9%) ... 2780
- ▲ CellCept Capsules (13.3% to 26.3%) ... 2951
- ▲ CellCept Intravenous (13.3% to 26.3%) ... 2951
- ▲ CellCept Oral Suspension (13.3% to 26.3%) ... 2951
- ▲ CellCept Tablets (13.3% to 26.3%) ... 2951
- Cipro I.V. (1% or less) ... 893
- Cipro I.V. Pharmacy Bulk Package (Less than 1%) ... 897
- Cipro (Less than 1%) ... 887
- Claritin (At least one patient) ... 3100
- Claritin-D 12 Hour Extended Release Tablets (Less frequent) ... 3102
- Claritin-D 24 Hour Extended Release Tablets (Fewer than 2%) ... 3104
- Clinoril Tablets (Less than 1 in 100) ... 2053
- Clomid Tablets ... 735
- Clozaril Tablets (1%) ... 2319
- ▲ Cognex Capsules (4%) ... 1351
- Colazal Capsules ... 3069
- Colestid Tablets (Infrequent) ... 2791
- Combivent Inhalation Aerosol (0.3%) ... 1041
- ▲ Copaxone for Injection (21%) ... 3306
- ▲ Coreg Tablets (14.4%) ... 1508
- Corlopam Injection (0.5% to 5%) ... 412
- Cosopt Sterile Ophthalmic Solution (Less than 1%) ... 2065
- Coumadin for Injection ... 1243
- Coumadin Tablets ... 1243
- Covera-HS Tablets (Less than 2%) ... 3199
- Cozaar Tablets (1% or greater) ... 2067
- Crixivan Capsules (Less than 2%) ... 2070
- Cytotec Tablets (Infrequent) ... 3202
- Cytovene (At least 3 subjects) ... 2959
- ▲ DaunoXome Injection (1% to 9%) ... 1442
- Demadex Tablets and Injection (1.2%) ... 2965
- Depacon Injection (1% to 5%) ... 416
- Depakene (1% to 5%) ... 421
- Depakote Sprinkle Capsules (1% to 5%) ... 426
- Depakote Tablets (1% to 5%) ... 430
- Depakote ER Tablets (1% to 5%) ... 436
- Depo-Provera Contraceptive Injection (Fewer than 1%) ... 2798
- ▲ Detrol Tablets (3.4%) ... 3623
- D.H.E. 45 Injection ... 2334
- Diovan Capsules (Less frequent) ... 2337
- Diovan HCT Tablets (More than 2%) ... 2338
- Dipentum Capsules (Rare) ... 2803
- Diprivan Injectable Emulsion (Less than 1%) ... 667
- Dobutrex Solution Vials (1% to 3%) ... 1914
- Dolobid Tablets (Rare) ... 2088
- Dopram Injectable ... 2931
- Doxil Injection (1% to 5%) ... 566
- DuoNeb Inhalation Solution (2.6%) ... 1233
- ▲ Duraclon Injection (5.3%) ... 3057
- Duragesic Transdermal System (1% or greater) ... 1786
- DynaCirc Capsules (1.7% to 2.7%) ... 2921
- DynaCirc CR Tablets (0.5% to 1%) ... 2923
- Effexor Tablets (2%) ... 3495
- Effexor XR Capsules (Frequent) ... 3499
- Emcyt Capsules (1%) ... 2810
- Enalaprilat Injection ... 863
- Enbrel for Injection ... 1752
- Enbrel for Injection ... 3504
- ▲ Epogen for Injection (7%) ... 582
- Ergamisol Tablets (Less than 1% to 1%) ... 1789
- Ery-Tab Tablets (Isolated reports) ... 448
- Erythrocin Stearate Filmtab Tablets (Isolated reports) ... 452
- Erythromycin Base Filmtab Tablets (Isolated reports) ... 454
- Erythromycin Delayed-Release Capsules, USP (Isolated reports) ... 455
- Estrace Vaginal Cream ... 3358
- Estrace Tablets ... 3361
- Estring Vaginal Ring (1% to 3%) ... 2811
- ▲ Evista Tablets (4%) ... 1915
- Evoxac Capsules (1% to 3%) ... 1217
- Exelon Capsules (2% or more) ... 2342
- Exelon Oral Solution (2% or more) ... 2345
- Felbatol (2.6%) ... 3343
- ▲ Femara Tablets (3% to 8%) ... 2351
- ▲ Ferrlecit Injection (10%) ... 3386
- Flexeril Tablets (Rare) ... 572
- Flexeril Tablets (Rare) ... 2094
- ▲ Flolan for Injection (11% to 67%) ... 1528
- ▲ Flomax Capsules (4.0% to 4.1%) ... 1044
- Floxin I.V. (1% to 3%) ... 2526
- Floxin Tablets (1% to 3%) ... 2529
- Fortovase Capsules (Less than 2%) ... 2970
- Foscavir Injection (Between 1% and 5%) ... 605
- Gabitril Tablets (1% or more) ... 1189
- Gamimune N, 5% Solvent/Detergent Treated ... 925
- Gamimune N, 10% Solvent/Detergent Treated ... 928
- Gastrocrom Oral Concentrate (Less common) ... 1162
- ▲ Gengraf Capsules (6%) ... 457
- Gliadel Wafer (1%) ... 1723
- Gonal-F for Injection ... 3216
- Halcion Tablets ... 2823
- Hivid Tablets (Less than 1%) ... 2975
- Hytrin Capsules (At least 1%) ... 464
- Hyzaar ... 2109
- Idamycin PFS Injection ... 2825
- Imdur Tablets (Less than or equal to 5%) ... 1826
- Imitrex Injection ... 1549
- Imitrex Nasal Spray ... 1554
- Imitrex Tablets (Frequent) ... 1558
- Indapamide Tablets (Less than 5%) ... 2286
- Indocin (Less than 1%) ... 2112
- INFeD Injection ... 3388
- ▲ Infergen (5% to 13%) ... 1777
- Innohep Injection (2.3%) ... 1248
- ▲ Intron A for Injection (Up to 28%) ... 3120
- Invirase Capsules (Less than 2%) ... 2979
- Iopidine 0.5% Ophthalmic Solution (Less than 3%) ... ⊙213
- Isoptin SR Tablets (1% or less) ... 467
- Kadian Capsules (Less than 3%) ... 1335
- Kaletra Capsules (Less than 2%) ... 471
- Kaletra Oral Solution (Less than 2%) ... 471
- Keppra Tablets (1% or more) ... 3314
- Klonopin Tablets (Infrequent) ... 2983
- Lamictal (More than 1%) ... 1567
- ▲ Leukine (15%) ... 1755
- Levaquin (1.1%) ... 2537
- Levlen ... 962
- Levlite 21 Tablets ... 962
- Levlite 28 Tablets ... 962
- Lexxel Tablets ... 608
- Lipitor Tablets (Greater than or equal to 2%) ... 2639
- Lipitor Tablets (Greater than or equal to 2%) ... 2696
- Lodosyn Tablets ... 1251
- Lotensin HCT Tablets (0.3% to 1%) ... 2367
- Lotrel Capsules (Infrequent) ... 2370
- Luvox Tablets (25, 50, 100 mg) ... 3256
- Macrobid Capsules ... 2889
- Macrodantin Capsules ... 2891
- Mavik Tablets (0.3% to 1.0%) ... 478
- Maxair Autohaler (1.3%) ... 1981
- Maxair Inhaler (Less than 1% to 1.3%) ... 1984
- Maxalt Tablets (Less than 2% to 3%) ... 2120
- Maxalt-MLT Orally Disintegrating Tablets (Less than 2% to 3%) ... 2120
- Maxzide ... 1008
- Megace Oral Suspension (1% to 3%) ... 1124
- ▲ Meridia Capsules (1.8%) ... 481
- Merrem I.V. (0.1% to 1.0%) ... 673
- Mevacor Tablets (0.5% to 1.0%) ... 2132
- ▲ Mexitil Capsules (2.6% to 7.5%) ... 1047
- Micardis Tablets (1%) ... 1049
- Micardis HCT Tablets ... 1051
- Midamor Tablets (Less than or equal to 1%) ... 2136
- Mirapex Tablets (1% or more) ... 2834
- Modicon ... 2563
- Moduretic Tablets (Less than or equal to 1%) ... 2138
- Monopril Tablets (0.2% to 2.2%) ... 1091
- Mycobutin Capsules (1%) ... 2838
- Mykrox Tablets (2.7%) ... 1168
- Myobloc Injectable Solution (2% or greater) ... 1291
- Naprelan Tablets (Less than 3%) ... 1293
- Naropin Injection (1% to 5%) ... 612
- Nasonex Nasal Spray (Greater than or equal to 2%) ... 3131
- ▲ Navelbine Injection (5%) ... 1604
- ▲ Neoral Soft Gelatin Capsules (6%) ... 2380
- ▲ Neoral Oral Solution (6%) ... 2380
- ▲ Neupogen for Injection (5%) ... 587
- ▲ Nilandron Tablets (7.2%) ... 753
- ▲ Nipent for Injection (3% to 10%) ... 3272
- Noroxin Tablets (Less frequent) ... 2145
- Norvasc Tablets (More than 0.1% to 1%) ... 2704
- Norvir Capsules (Less than 2%) ... 487
- Norvir Oral Solution (Less than 2%) ... 487
- Novantrone for Injection ... 1760
- Omnicef ... 493
- Oncaspar (Less than 1%) ... 756
- Orap Tablets ... 1407
- ▲ Orthoclone OKT3 Sterile Solution (14%) ... 2498
- Ortho-Cyclen/Ortho Tri-Cyclen ... 2573
- Ortho-Est Tablets ... 3464
- Ortho-Novum ... 2563
- Ortho-Novum 1/50□28 Tablets ... 2556
- Ortho-Cyclen/Ortho Tri-Cyclen ... 2573
- OxyContin Tablets (Less than 1%) ... 2912
- ▲ Paxil (3%) ... 1609
- Pentasa Capsules (Infrequent) ... 3239
- ▲ Permax Tablets (3.7%) ... 1299

▲ Photofrin for Injection (22%) 831
▲ Plavix Tablets (8.3%) 1097
▲ Plavix Tablets (8.3%) 3084
Plendil Extended-Release Tablets (0.5% to 1.5%) 623
Prandin Tablets (0.5, 1, and 2 mg) (1.8% to 3%) 2432
Pravachol Tablets (0.3% to 3.7%) 1099
Prevacid Delayed-Release Capsules (Less than 1%) 3292
PREVPAC (Less than 1%) 3298
Prilosec Delayed-Release Capsules (Less than 1%) 628
Primacor Injection (1.2%) 3086
▲ Prinivil Tablets (3.4%) 2164
Prinzide Tablets (0.3% to 1%) 2168
Procardia XL Extended Release Tablets (Less than 3%) 2710
▲ Procrit for Injection (7%) 2502
▲ Prograf (3% to 19%) 1393
▲ Proleukin for Injection (12%) 1199
▲ Prometrium Capsules (100 mg, 200 mg) (Less than 5% to 7%) 3261
ProSom Tablets (1%) 500
Prostin E2 Suppositories 2852
▲ Protonix I.V. (6%) 3580
Protonix Tablets (Greater than or equal to 1%) 3577
Proventil HFA Inhalation Aerosol (Less than 3%) 3150
Provigil Tablets (2%) 1193
Prozac Pulvules, Liquid, and Weekly Capsules (Less than 1%) 1238
Pulmicort Respules (1% to 3%) 632
▲ Pulmozyme Inhalation Solution (18% to 25%) 1426
▲ Rapamune Oral Solution and Tablets (16% to 24%) 3584
▲ Rebetron Combination Therapy (5% to 9%) 3153
▲ Remicade for IV Injection (5% to 6%) 1178
Reminyl Oral Solution (Frequent) 1792
Reminyl Tablets (Frequent) 1792
▲ Requip Tablets (4%) 1621
Rescriptor Tablets (Less than 2%) 526
Retrovir Capsules 1625
Retrovir IV Infusion 1629
Retrovir 1625
Rifater Tablets 769
Risperdal (2% to 3%) 1796
Rituxan for Infusion (1% to 5%) 1750
Rituxan I.V. (1% to 5%) 1428
▲ Roferon-A Injection (Less than 4% to 11%) 2996
Romazicon Injection (Less than 1%) 3000
Rythmol Tablets – 150 mg, 225 mg, 300 mg (1.8%) 502
Salagen Tablets (Less than 1%) 2229
Sandimmune (Rare) 2388
Sandostatin Injection (Less than 1%) 2394
Sarafem Pulvules (Frequent) 1962
Sectral Capsules (2%) 3589
Serophene Tablets 3226
▲ Serostim for Injection (1% to 10%) 3229
Serzone Tablets 1104
▲ Simulect for Injection (3% to 10%) 2399
Sinemet Tablets 1253
Sinemet CR Tablets (1.0%) 1255
Skelid Tablets (2.7%) 3088
Sonata Capsules (Frequent) 3591
Soriatane Capsules (Less than 1%) 3003
Sporanox Oral Solution (2.6% to 2.9%) 1808
Sporanox Oral Solution (2.6% to 2.9%) 2512
Stadol NS Nasal Spray (Infrequent) 1108
Stimate Nasal Spray 796
Sular Tablets (2%) 688
Synarel Nasal Solution for Central Precocious Puberty (2.6%) 3204
Synercid I.V. (Less than 1%) 775
▲ Tambocor Tablets (5.4%) 1990
Tarka Tablets (0.3% to 2.2%) 508
Tasmar Tablets (1% to 3%) 3010
Taxol Injection 1129
Taxotere for Injection Concentrate 778
Tenex Tablets (Less frequent) 2942
Tequin Injection (0.1% to 3%) 1110
Tequin Tablets (0.1% to 3%) 1110
Teveten Tablets (1% or greater) 3327
Thalomid Capsules 1154
▲ Thrombate III (1 of 17) 944
▲ Tikosyn Capsules (10%) 2717
Timolide Tablets (Less than 1%) 2187
Timolol GFS ⊙266
Timoptic in Ocudose (Less frequent) 2192
Timoptic Sterile Ophthalmic Solution (Less frequent) 2190
Timoptic-XE Sterile Ophthalmic Gel Forming Solution 2194
▲ TOBI Solution for Inhalation (26%) 1206
Tolectin (1% to 3%) 2589
Tonocard Tablets (0.4% to 1.6%) 649
Topamax Sprinkle Capsules (2% to 4.4%) 2590
Topamax Tablets (2% to 4.4%) 2590
Toprol-XL Tablets (Greater than 1%) 651
Trasylol Injection (2%) 909
Travatan Ophthalmic Solution (1% to 5%) 543
Trental Tablets (0.3%) 784
Tricor Capsules, Micronized 513
Trileptal Oral Suspension (Up to 2%) 2407
Trileptal Tablets (Up to 2%) 2407
Tri-Levlen 962
▲ Trisenox Injection (25%) 1158
Trovan (Less than 1%) 2722
Ultracet Tablets (Less than 1%) 2597
Unasyn for Injection (Less than 1%) 2728
Uniretic Tablets (More than 1%) 3178
Univasc Tablets (More than 1%) 3181
Valium Injectable 3026
▲ Valstar Sterile Solution for Intravesical Instillation (3%) 1175
Vanceril Double Strength Inhalation Aerosol (Fewer than 2%) 3167
Vancocin HCl Capsules & Pulvules 1972
Vancocin HCl Oral Solution 1971
Vancocin HCl, Vials & ADD-Vantage 1970
Vantin Tablets and Oral Suspension (Less than 1%) 2860
Vaseretic Tablets (0.5% to 2.0%) 2204
Vasotec I.V. Injection 2207
Vasotec Tablets (0.5% to 2.1%) 2210
Venofer Injection (Greater than 1%) 580
Verelan Capsules (1% or less) 3184
Verelan PM Capsules (2% or less) 3186
Viagra Tablets (Less than 2%) 2732
Vioxx (Greater than 0.1% to 1.9%) 2213
Virazole for Inhalation Solution 1747
Vistide Injection 1445
Vitravene for Injection (2% to 5%) ⊙310
Vivelle Transdermal System 2412
Vivelle-Dot Transdermal System 2416
Voltaren Tablets (Less than 1%) 2315
Voltaren-XR Tablets (Less than 1%) 2315
Warfarin Sodium Tablets, USP 3302
Wellbutrin Tablets (Infrequent) 1680
▲ Wellbutrin SR Sustained-Release Tablets (3% to 4%) 1684
Xalatan Latanoprost Ophthalmic Solution (1% to 2%) ⊙320
Xalatan Sterile Ophthalmic Solution (1% to 2%) 2864
▲ Xanax Tablets (10.6%) 2865
Xeloda Tablets (Less than 5%) 3039
Xopenex Inhalation Solution 3207
Zaroxolyn Tablets 1177
Zebeta Tablets (1.1% to 1.5%) 1885
▲ Zenapax for Injection (Greater than 5%) 3046
Zestoretic Tablets (0.3% to 1.0%) 695
▲ Zestril Tablets (3.4%) 698
Ziac Tablets (0.9% to 1.8%) 1887
Zithromax (1% or less) 2743
Zithromax for Oral Suspension, 300 mg, 600 mg, 900 mg, 1200 mg (1% or less) 2739
Zithromax Tablets, 250 mg (1% or less) 2739
Zithromax Tablets, 600 mg (1% or less) 2743
Zofran Injection (Rare) 1698
Zofran (Rare) 1703
Zofran ODT Orally Disintegrating Tablets (Rare) 1703
Zoladex (1% or greater) 702
Zoladex 3-month 706
Zoloft (Frequent) 2751
▲ Zometa for Intravenous Infusion (5% to 10%) 3621
Zomig Tablets (2% to 4%) 708
Zomig-ZMT Tablets (2% to 4%) 708
Zonegran Capsules (Infrequent) 1307
Zosyn (1.0% or less to 1.3%) 1890
Zosyn in Galaxy Containers (1.0% or less to 1.3%) 1894
Zovirax for Injection (Less than 1%) 1708
Zyban Sustained-Release Tablets (Less than 1%) 1710
Zyflo Filmtab Tablets (Less common) 524
▲ Zyprexa Tablets (4%) 1973
▲ Zyprexa ZYDIS Orally Disintegrating Tablets (4%) 1973
Zyrtec (Less than 2%) 2756
Zyrtec-D 12 Hour Extended Relief Tablets (Less than 2%) 2758

Chest pain, substernal

Aciphex Tablets 1267
Aciphex Tablets 1783
Coreg Tablets (0.1% to 1%) 1508
Effexor Tablets (Frequent) 3495
Effexor XR Capsules (Frequent) 3499
Felbatol (Rare) 3343
Intron A for Injection (Less than 5%) 3120
Kaletra Capsules (Less than 2%) 471
Kaletra Oral Solution (Less than 2%) 471
Nexium Delayed-Release Capsules (Less than 1%) 619
Norvir Capsules (Less than 2%) 487
Norvir Oral Solution (Less than 2%) 487
▲ Photofrin for Injection (5%) 831
Protonix I.V. (Less than 1%) 3580
Protonix Tablets (Less than 1%) 3577
Remeron Tablets (Rare) 2483
Remeron SolTab Tablets (Rare) 2486
Tequin Injection (Less than 0.1%) 1110
Tequin Tablets (Less than 0.1%) 1110
Zoloft (Rare) 2751

Chest sound, abnormalities

Gengraf Capsules (1% to less than 3%) 457
Imdur Tablets (Less than or equal to 5%) 1826
▲ Leustatin Injection (9%) 2495
Neoral Soft Gelatin Capsules (1% to less than 3%) 2380
Neoral Oral Solution (1% to less than 3%) 2380
Orthoclone OKT3 Sterile Solution 2498
Prinivil Tablets (Greater than 1%) 2164
Prinzide Tablets 2168
▲ Simulect for Injection (3% to 10%) 2399
Zestoretic Tablets 695
Zestril Tablets (Greater than 1%) 698

Chest tightness

Acthrel for Injection 3629
▲ Adenocard Injection (7%) 1380
Advair Diskus 100/50 1448
Advair Diskus 250/50 1448
Advair Diskus 500/50 1448
Aerobid/Aerobid-M (1% to 3%) 1363
Alferon N Injection 1770
Allegra (Rare) 712
Allegra-D Extended-Release Tablets (Rare) 714
Benadryl Parenteral 2617
BeneFix for Injection 1432
Ceftin Tablets (0.1% to 1%) 1898
▲ DaunoXome Injection (13.8% to 16%) 1442
Dopram Injectable 2931
▲ Doxil Injection (Approximately 6.8%) 566
Eskalith 1527
Ethyol for Injection (Rare) 2029
Flovent Diskus 3614
Flovent 1535
Flovent Rotadisk 1537
Gamimune N, 5% Solvent/Detergent Treated 925
Gamimune N, 10% Solvent/Detergent Treated 928
Gammar-P I.V. 787
Hivid Tablets (Less than 1%) 2975
Humate-P Concentrate 790
Imitrex Injection (2.7%) 1549
Imitrex Nasal Spray (Infrequent) 1554
Imitrex Tablets (Frequent) 1558
INFeD Injection 3388
Levlen 962
Levlite 21 Tablets 962
Levlite 28 Tablets 962
Lithobid Slow-Release Tablets 3255
Maxair Autohaler (1.3%) 1981
Maxalt Tablets (Less than 2% to 3%) 2120
Maxalt-MLT Orally Disintegrating Tablets (Less than 2% to 3%) 2120
Meridia Capsules 481
Modicon 2563
Nicotrol Nasal Spray (Common) 2843
Orthoclone OKT3 Sterile Solution 2498
Ortho-Cyclen/Ortho Tri-Cyclen 2573
Ortho-Novum 2563
Ortho-Novum 1/50□28 Tablets 2556
Ortho-Cyclen/Ortho Tri-Cyclen 2573
Periactin Tablets 2155
Prostin E2 Suppositories 2852
Rifater Tablets 769
Rynatan Tablets 3351
Sandoglobulin I.V. 2391
Sular Tablets (Very rare) 688
Taxotere for Injection Concentrate 778
▲ Thrombate III (3 of 17) 944
Thyrel TRH for Injection (Less frequent) 3630
Tri-Levlen 962
Tussionex Pennkinetic Extended-Release Suspension (Occasional) 1174
Zomig Tablets (2% to 4%) 708
Zomig-ZMT Tablets (2% to 4%) 708

Chewing movements

Compazine 1505
Etrafon 3115
Haldol Decanoate 2535
Haldol Injection, Tablets and Concentrate 2533
Moban 1320
Navane Oral 2701
Navane Intramuscular 2703
Orap Tablets 1407
Serentil 1057
Stelazine 1640
Thioridazine Hydrochloride Tablets 2289
Thiothixene Capsules 2290
Thorazine 1656
Trilafon 3160

CHF

(*see under* Congestive heart failure)

Chills

▲ Abelcet Injection (18%) 1273
Aceon Tablets (2 mg, 4 mg, 8 mg) (0.3% to 1%) 3249
Aciphex Tablets 1267
Aciphex Tablets 1783
▲ Actimmune (14%) 1772
Actiq (1% or greater) 1184
Adalat CC Tablets (Less than 1.0%) 877
Adriamycin PFS/RDF Injection (Occasional) 2767
Aerobid/Aerobid-M (1% to 3%) 1363
Aggrastat 2031
▲ Agrylin Capsules (1% to 5%) 3232
Albumin (Human) 5% (Very rare) 838
Albumin (Human) 25% (Very rare) 839
Albuminar-5, U.S.P. 785
Albuminar-25, U.S.P. 786
▲ Alferon N Injection (14% to 87%) 1770
Aloprim for Injection (Less than 1%) 2292
▲ AmBisome for Injection (40% to 48.1%) 1383
Amerge Tablets (Infrequent) 1467
▲ Amphotec (50% to 77%) 1774
Anadrol-50 Tablets 3321
Anaprox Tablets (Less than 1%) 2967
Anaprox DS Tablets (Less than 1%) 2967
Anzemet Injection (2%) 719
Anzemet Tablets (1.3%) 722
Aricept Tablets (Infrequent) 1270
Aricept Tablets (Infrequent) 2665
▲ Asacol Delayed-Release Tablets (3%) 2884
Ativan Injection (Infrequent) 3478
Autoplex T 2294
Avalide Tablets (2%) 1070
Avapro Tablets (Less than 1%) 1074
Avapro Tablets (Less than 1%) 3076
Avelox Tablets (0.05% to 1%) 879
▲ Avonex (21%) 1013
Axert Tablets (Infrequent) 2772
Bactrim 2949
Baycol Tablets (Rare) 883
Benadryl Parenteral 2617
BeneFix for Injection 1432
▲ Betaseron for SC Injection (46%) 988
Bicillin C-R 900/300 Injection 2240
Bicillin C-R Injection 2238
Bicillin L-A Injection 2242
Buminate 5% Solution, USP (Occasional) 841
Buminate 25% Solution, USP (Occasional) 842
Buprenex Injectable (Less than 1%) 2918
Calcium Disodium Versenate Injection 1980
Cancidas for Injection (1.5% to 2.5%) 2048
Carbatrol Capsules 3234
▲ Casodex Tablets (2% to 5%) 662
Ceclor CD Tablets (0.1% to 1%) 1279
Ceftin Tablets (0.1% to 1%) 1898
▲ CellCept Capsules (3% to 11.4%) 2951
▲ CellCept Intravenous (3% to 11.4%) 2951
▲ CellCept Oral Suspension (3% to 11.4%) 2951
▲ CellCept Tablets (3% to 11.4%) 2951
Cerebyx Injection (Frequent) 2619
Cerezyme for Injection 1438
Cerubidine for Injection (Rare) 947
▲ Chemet Capsules (5.2% to 15.7%) 3078
Cipro I.V. (1% or less) 893
Cipro I.V. Pharmacy Bulk Package (Less than 1%) 897
Cipro (Less than 1%) 887
Clinoril Tablets (Less than 1 in 100) 2053
Clozaril Tablets (Less than 1%) 2319
Cognex Capsules (Frequent) 1351
Colazal Capsules 3069
▲ Combivir Tablets (10%) 1502
▲ Copaxone for Injection (4%) 3306
Coumadin for Injection (Infrequent) 1243
Coumadin Tablets (Infrequent) 1243
Crixivan Capsules (Less than 2%) 2070
CytoGam Intravenous (Less than 5.0%) 2026
▲ Cytovene (7%) 2959
Dantrium Capsules (Less frequent) 2885
DDAVP Nasal Spray (Up to 2%) 738
DDAVP Rhinal Tube (Up to 2%) 738
Depacon Injection (1% or more) 416
Depakene (1% or more) 421

Depakote Sprinkle Capsules 426
Depakote Tablets (1% to 5%) 430
Depakote ER Tablets (Greater than 1%) 436
Depen Titratable Tablets 3341
Depo-Provera Contraceptive Injection (Fewer than 1%) 2798
Desmopressin Acetate Rhinal Tube (Up to 2%) 1345
Dilaudid Oral Liquid 445
Dilaudid Tablets - 8 mg 445
Dilaudid-HP (Less frequent) 443
Dipentum Capsules (Rare) 2803
Diprivan Injectable Emulsion (Less than 1%) 667
Dolobid Tablets (Less than 1 in 100) 2088
Doxil Injection (1% to 5%) 566
EC-Naprosyn Delayed-Release Tablets (Less than 1%) 2967
Edecrin 2091
▲ Effexor Tablets (2.2% to 6.8%) 3495
▲ Effexor XR Capsules (3%) 3499
Eldepryl Capsules 3266
Ellence Injection 2806
Elspar for Injection 2092
Engerix-B Vaccine (Less than 1%) 1517
▲ Epivir (10%) 1520
▲ Epivir-HBV (7%) 1524
Ergamisol Tablets (5 patients) 1789
Ethyol for Injection 2029
Ferrlecit Injection (Greater than 1%) 3386
▲ Flolan for Injection (13% to 25%) 1528
Floxin I.V. (Less than 1%) 2526
Floxin Tablets (Less than 1%) 2529
▲ Fludara for Injection (11% to 19%) 995
FluShield Influenza Vaccine 3521
Follistim for Injection 2465
Gabitril Tablets (Frequent) 1189
▲ Gamimune N, 5% Solvent/Detergent Treated (Among most common) 925
▲ Gamimune N, 10% Solvent/Detergent Treated (Among most common) 928
Gammagard S/D (Occasional) 845
▲ Gammar-P I.V. (8.9%) 787
Gemzar for Injection (Common) 1919
Geodon Capsules (Frequent) 2688
Glucophage Tablets (1% to 5%) 1080
Glucotrol XL Extended Release Tablets (Less than 1%) 2693
Hemofil M (Extremely rare) 847
Heparin Lock Flush Solution 3509
Heparin Sodium Injection 3511
▲ Herceptin I.V. (32%) 1414
Hivid Tablets (Less than 1%) 2975
Humate-P Concentrate (2%) 790
Humegon for Injection 2468
Imitrex Injection (Infrequent) 1549
Imitrex Nasal Spray (Infrequent) 1554
Imitrex Tablets 1558
INFeD Injection 3388
▲ Intron A for Injection (Up to 54%) 3120
Iscar Mali Injection 3456
Iscar Mali Special Injection 3456
Iscar Pini Injection 3456
Iscar Quercus Injection 3456
Iscar Quercus Special Injection 3456
Iveegam EN (One case) 849
▲ JE-VAX Vaccine (Approximately 10%) 811
Kadian Capsules (Less than 3%) 1335
Kaletra Capsules (Less than 2%) 471
Kaletra Oral Solution (Less than 2%) 471
Konÿne 80 937
Lamictal (1.3%) 1567
▲ Lariam Tablets (Among most frequent) 2989
Lescol Capsules (Rare) 2361
Lescol Capsules (Rare) 2925
Lescol XL Tablets 2361
Lescol XL Tablets 2925
▲ Leukine (19% to 25%) 1755
▲ Leustatin Injection (9%) 2495
Lodine (Greater than or equal to 1%) 3528
Lodine XL Extended-Release Tablets (Less than 1%) 3530
Lotensin HCT Tablets (0.3% or more) 2367
Lupron Depot 7.5 mg (Less than 5%) 3284
Lupron Injection (Less than 5%) 3279
Luvox Tablets (25, 50, 100 mg) (2%) 3256
LYMErix Vaccine (1.74% to 2.78%) 1592
Macrobid Capsules (Less than 1%) 2889
Macrodantin Capsules 2891
Marinol Capsules (Less than 1%) 3325
Matulane Capsules 3246
Maxalt Tablets (Infrequent) 2120
Maxalt-MLT Orally Disintegrating Tablets (Infrequent) 2120
Menomune-A/C/Y/W-135 Vaccine (2.5%) 813
Mevacor Tablets (Rare) 2132
Miltown Tablets (Rare) 3349
Mintezol 2137
Monoclate-P Concentrate 793
Mononine Concentrate 794
MS Contin Tablets (Less frequent) 2896
MSIR (Less frequent) 2898
Mykrox Tablets 1168
Mylocel Tablets 2227
▲ Mylotarg for Injection (11% to 62%) 3540
Myobloc Injectable Solution (2% or greater) 1291
Nabi-HB 2295
▲ Naprelan Tablets (3% to 9%) 1293
Naprosyn Suspension (Less than 1%) 2967
Naprosyn Tablets (Less than 1%) 2967
Naropin Injection (2.2% to 4.4%) 612
Navelbine Injection 1604
▲ Neumega for Injection (Greater than or equal to 10%) 1434
Neurontin Capsules (Infrequent) 2655
Neurontin Oral Solution (Infrequent) 2655
Neurontin Tablets (Infrequent) 2655
Niaspan Extended-Release Tablets 1846
▲ Nipent for Injection (11% to 19%) 3272
Nizoral Tablets (Less than 1%) 1791
Noroxin Tablets (Less frequent) 2145
Norvir Capsules (Less than 2%) 487
Norvir Oral Solution (Less than 2%) 487
▲ Novantrone for Injection (5%) 1760
▲ Oncaspar (Greater than 5%) 756
Oramorph SR Tablets (Less frequent) 3062
▲ Orthoclone OKT3 Sterile Solution (59%) 2498
Orudis Capsules (Less than 1%) 3548
Oruvail Capsules (Less than 1%) 3548
OxyContin Tablets (Between 1% and 5%) 2912
Parnate Tablets 1607
Paxil (2%) 1609
Pergonal for Injection 3223
Periactin Tablets 2155
Permax Tablets (1.1%) 1299
Pfizerpen for Injection 2707
Plasbumin-5 (Rare) 939
Plasbumin-20 (Rare) 940
Plasbumin-25 (Rare) 941
Pletal Tablets (Less than 2%) 2605
Pletal Tablets (Less than 2%) 2848
Polocaine Injection, USP 625
Polocaine-MPF Injection, USP 625
Pravachol Tablets (Rare) 1099
Prinivil Tablets (0.3% to 1.0%) 2164
Prinzide Tablets 2168
▲ ProAmatine Tablets (4.9%) 3241
Procanbid Extended-Release Tablets (Fairly common) 2262
Procardia Capsules (2% or less) 2708
▲ Prograf (3% to 15%) 1393
Prolastin (Occasional) 943
▲ Proleukin for Injection (52%) 1199
Proplex T (Occasional) 851
ProSom Tablets (Infrequent) 500
▲ Prostin E2 Suppositories (Approximately one-tenth) 2852
Protonix I.V. (Less than 1%) 3580
Protonix Tablets (Less than 1%) 3577
Protopic Ointment (Greater than or equal to 1%) 1397
Provigil Tablets (1%) 1193
Prozac Pulvules, Liquid, and Weekly Capsules (Frequent) 1238
Rabies Vaccine RabAvert (Rare) 1203
▲ Rapamune Oral Solution and Tablets (3% to 20%) 3584
Recombinate (Extremely rare) 853
Recombivax HB (Less than 1%) 2178
ReFacto Vials 1437
Refludan for Injection (Uncommon) 761
Relafen Tablets (Less than 1%) 1617
Remeron Tablets (Infrequent) 2483
Remeron SolTab Tablets (Infrequent) 2486
Remicade for IV Injection 1178
Repronex for Intramuscular and Subcutaneous Injection 1347
Rescriptor Tablets (Less than 2%) 526
Retrovir Capsules 1625
Retrovir IV Infusion 1629
Retrovir 1625
Rifadin 765
Rifater Tablets 769
Rilutek Tablets (Infrequent) 772
▲ Rituxan for Infusion (32%) 1750
▲ Rituxan I.V. (32%) 1428
Rocephin Injectable Vials, ADD-Vantage, Galaxy, Bulk (Less than 1%) 2993
▲ Roferon-A Injection (23% to 64%) 2996
Roxicodone Tablets (Less than 3%) 3067
Rynatan Tablets 3351
Rythmol Tablets – 150 mg, 225 mg, 300 mg 502
▲ Salagen Tablets (3% to 14%) 2229
Sandoglobulin I.V. 2391
Sarafem Pulvules (Frequent) 1962
Sensorcaine 643
Sensorcaine-MPF Injection 643
Septra Suspension 2265
Septra Tablets 2265
Septra DS Tablets 2265
Seroquel Tablets (Infrequent) 684
Serzone Tablets (2%) 1104
Sinequan (Occasional) 2713
Sonata Capsules (Infrequent) 3591
Stimate Nasal Spray 796
Sular Tablets (Less than or equal to 1%) 688
Synvisc 3596
Talacen Caplets (Rare) 3089
Talwin Nx Tablets (Rare) 3090
Tasmar Tablets (Infrequent) 3010
Taxol Injection (Rare) 1129
Taxotere for Injection Concentrate 778
Tegretol/Tegretol-XR 2404
Tequin Injection (0.1% to 3%) 1110
Tequin Tablets (0.1% to 3%) 1110
Terazol 3 Vaginal Suppositories (1.8% of 284 patients) 2587
Terazol 7 Vaginal Cream (0.4% of 521 patients) 2587
Tessalon Capsules 1377
Tetanus Toxoid Adsorbed Purogenated 1882
▲ Thalomid Capsules (4.2%) 1154
▲ TheraCys Injection (34%) 823
▲ Thrombate III (2 of 17) 944
▲ Thymoglobulin for Injection (57.3%) 3071
Thyrogen for Injection (1%) 1441
▲ Tice BCG, BCG Live (3.3%) 2489
Ticlid Tablets 3015
Timentin Injection- ADD-Vantage Vial 1661
Timentin Injection-Galaxy Container 1664
Timentin Injection-Pharmacy Bulk Package 1666
Timentin for Intravenous Administration 1658
Tonocard Tablets (Less than 1%) 649
▲ Trizivir Tablets (20%) 1669
Trovan (Less than 1%) 2722
Unasyn for Injection (Less than 1%) 2728
Uniretic Tablets (Less than 1%) 3178
Vancocin HCl Capsules & Pulvules (Infrequent) 1972
Vancocin HCl Oral Solution (Infrequent) 1971
Vancocin HCl, Vials & ADD-Vantage (Infrequent) 1970
Vantin Tablets and Oral Suspension (Less than 1%) 2860
Varivax (Greater than or equal to 1%) 2202
Versed Injection (Less than 1%) 3027
Viadur Implant (Less than 2%) 912
Viagra Tablets (Less than 2%) 2732
▲ Videx (9% to 12%) 1138
Videx EC Capsules 1143
Vioxx (Greater than 0.1% to 1.9%) 2213
▲ Vistide Injection (22%) 1445
Voltaren Ophthalmic Sterile Ophthalmic Solution (Less than 3%) .... ⊙312
Warfarin Sodium Tablets, USP 3302
Wellbutrin Tablets (1.2%) 1680
Wellbutrin SR Sustained-Release Tablets (Infrequent) 1684
WinRho SDF (Less than 2%) 2297
Xopenex Inhalation Solution (Less than 2%) 3207
Yodoxin Tablets 1722
Zaroxolyn Tablets 1177
▲ Zemplar Injection (5%) 522
▲ Zerit (50%) 1147
Zestoretic Tablets 695
Zestril Tablets (0.3% to 1.0%) 698
▲ Ziagen (20%) 1692
Zocor Tablets (Rare) 2219
Zoladex (1% to 5%) 702
Zoladex 3-month 706
Zometa for Intravenous Infusion 3621
Zomig Tablets (Infrequent) 708
Zomig-ZMT Tablets (Infrequent) 708
Zyban Sustained-Release Tablets (Infrequent) 1710
Zyprexa Tablets (Infrequent) 1973
Zyprexa ZYDIS Orally Disintegrating Tablets (Infrequent) 1973

Chloasma

Activella Tablets 2764
Alesse-21 Tablets 3468
Alesse-28 Tablets 3473
Alora Transdermal System 3372
Aygestin Tablets 1333
Brevicon 28-Day Tablets 3380
Cenestin Tablets 1263
Climara Transdermal System 958
Depo-Provera Contraceptive Injection (Fewer than 1%) 2798
Desogen Tablets 2458
Esclim Transdermal System 3460
Estinyl Tablets 3112
Estrace Vaginal Cream 3358
Estrace Tablets 3361
Estratest 3252
Estrostep 2627
femhrt Tablets 2635
Levlen 962
Levlite 21 Tablets 962
Levlite 28 Tablets 962
Levora Tablets 3389
Loestrin 21 Tablets 2642
Loestrin Fe Tablets 2642
Lo/Ovral Tablets 3532
Lo/Ovral-28 Tablets 3538
Low-Ogestrel-28 Tablets 3392
Menest Tablets 2254
Mircette Tablets 2470
Modicon 2563
Necon 3415
Nordette-28 Tablets 2257
Norinyl 1 +35 28-Day Tablets 3380
Norinyl 1 + 50 28-Day Tablets 3380
Ogen Tablets 2846
Ogestrel 0.5/50-28 Tablets 3428
Ortho Dienestrol Cream 2554
Ortho-Cept 21 Tablets 2546
Ortho-Cept 28 Tablets 2546
Ortho-Cyclen/Ortho Tri-Cyclen 2573
Ortho-Est Tablets 3464
Ortho-Novum 2563
Ortho-Novum 1/50▫28 Tablets 2556
Ortho-Prefest Tablets 2570
Ortho-Cyclen/Ortho Tri-Cyclen 2573
Ovcon 3364
Ovral Tablets 3551
Ovral-28 Tablets 3552
Ovrette Tablets 3552
Premarin Intravenous 3563
Premarin Tablets 3566
Premarin Vaginal Cream 3570
Premphase Tablets 3572
Prempro Tablets 3572
Prometrium Capsules (100 mg, 200 mg) 3261
Synarel Nasal Solution for Endometriosis (Less than 1%) 3205
Topamax Sprinkle Capsules (Rare) 2590
Topamax Tablets (Rare) 2590
Tri-Levlen 962
Tri-Norinyl-28 Tablets 3433
Triphasil-21 Tablets 3600
Triphasil-28 Tablets 3605
Trivora Tablets 3439
Vivelle Transdermal System 2412
Vivelle-Dot Transdermal System 2416
Zovia 3449

Chloride retention

Estratest 3252
Oxandrin Tablets 1153
Testred Capsules, 10 mg 1746

Choking sensation

Advair Diskus 100/50 1448
Advair Diskus 250/50 1448
Advair Diskus 500/50 1448
Dantrium Intravenous 2886
Evoxac Capsules (Less than 1%) 1217
Serevent Diskus (Rare) 1637
Serevent Inhalation Aerosol (Rare) 1633

Cholangitis

Abelcet Injection 1273
Aciphex Tablets (Rare) 1267
Aciphex Tablets (Rare) 1783
▲ CellCept Capsules (11.9%) 2951
▲ CellCept Intravenous (11.9%) 2951
▲ CellCept Oral Suspension (11.9%) 2951
▲ CellCept Tablets (11.9%) 2951
Norvir Capsules (Less than 2%) 487
Norvir Oral Solution (Less than 2%) 487
▲ Prograf (3% to 15%) 1393
Thalomid Capsules 1154
Vistide Injection 1445
Zonegran Capsules (Rare) 1307

Cholangitis, sclerosing

Doxil Injection (Less than 1%) 566
Fortovase Capsules (Less than 2%) 2970

Cholecystectomy

Prometrium Capsules (100 mg, 200 mg) (2%) 3261

Cholecystitis

Abelcet Injection 1273
Aciphex Tablets 1267
Aciphex Tablets 1783
Aricept Tablets 1270
Aricept Tablets 2665
Asacol Delayed-Release Tablets 2884
Betaseron for SC Injection 988
Celexa (Rare) 1365
Cognex Capsules (Infrequent) 1351
Colestid Tablets (Rare) 2791
Copaxone for Injection (Infrequent) 3306
Crixivan Capsules (Less than 2%) 2070
Effexor Tablets (Rare) 3495
Effexor XR Capsules (Rare) 3499
Enbrel for Injection (Infrequent) 1752

Enbrel for Injection (Infrequent) 3504
Exelon Capsules (Infrequent) 2342
Exelon Oral Solution (Infrequent) 2345
Flovent Diskus (1% to 3%) 3614
Gabitril Tablets (Infrequent) 1189
Hivid Tablets (Less than 1%) 2975
Kaletra Capsules (Less than 2%) 471
Kaletra Oral Solution (Less than 2%) 471
Lopid Tablets 2650
Luvox Tablets (25, 50, 100 mg) (Rare) 3256
Meridia Capsules 481
Naprelan Tablets (Less than 1%) 1293
Permax Tablets (Rare) 1299
Premphase Tablets 3572
Prempro Tablets 3572
Proleukin for Injection 1199
Protonix I.V. (Less than 1%) 3580
Protonix Tablets (Less than 1%) 3577
Prozac Pulvules, Liquid, and Weekly Capsules (Rare) 1238
Remeron Tablets (Infrequent) 2483
Remeron SolTab Tablets (Infrequent) 2486
Remicade for IV Injection (Less than 2%) 1178
Requip Tablets (Infrequent) 1621
Rilutek Tablets (Rare) 772
Risperdal (Rare) 1796
Sarafem Pulvules (Rare) 1962
Tasmar Tablets (Rare) 3010
Trental Tablets (Less than 1%) 784
Tricor Capsules, Micronized (Less than 1%) 513
Vioxx (Less than 0.1%) 2213
Ziac Tablets 1887
Zonegran Capsules (Rare) 1307

Cholecystitis, acalculus
Sterile FUDR 2974

Cholelithiasis
Aciphex Tablets 1267
Aciphex Tablets 1783
Aggrenox Capsules (Less than 1%) 1026
Arava Tablets (1% to 3%) 724
Aricept Tablets (Infrequent) 1270
Aricept Tablets (Infrequent) 2665
Atromid-S Capsules 3483
Betaseron for SC Injection 988
Celebrex Capsules (Less than 0.1%) 2676
Celebrex Capsules (Less than 0.1%) 2780
Celexa (Rare) 1365
Claritin-D 24 Hour Extended Release Tablets (Fewer than 2%) 3104
Cognex Capsules (Infrequent) 1351
Colestid Tablets (Rare) 2791
Cytovene 2959
Effexor Tablets (Rare) 3495
Effexor XR Capsules (Rare) 3499
Evoxac Capsules (Less than 1%) 1217
Fludara for Injection (Up to 3%) 995
Fortovase Capsules (Less than 2%) 2970
Gabitril Tablets (Infrequent) 1189
Levaquin Injection (Less than 0.5%) 2537
Lopid Tablets 2650
Luvox Tablets (25, 50, 100 mg) (Rare) 3256
Meridia Capsules 481
Miacalcin Nasal Spray (Less than 1%) 2375
Naprelan Tablets (Less than 1%) 1293
Paxil (Rare) 1609
Permax Tablets (Infrequent) 1299
Persantine Tablets (Rare) 1057
Pletal Tablets (Less than 2%) 2605
Pletal Tablets (Less than 2%) 2848
Premphase Tablets 3572
Prempro Tablets 3572
Prevacid Delayed-Release Capsules (Less than 1%) 3292
PREVPAC (Less than 1%) 3298
Protonix I.V. (Less than 1%) 3580
Protonix Tablets (Less than 1%) 3577
Prozac Pulvules, Liquid, and Weekly Capsules (Infrequent) 1238
Remicade for IV Injection (Less than 2%) 1178
Requip Tablets (Infrequent) 1621
Risperdal (Rare) 1796
Salagen Tablets (Less than 1%) 2229
Sarafem Pulvules (Infrequent) 1962
Sonata Capsules (Rare) 3591
Tasmar Tablets (Infrequent) 3010
Tricor Capsules, Micronized (Less than 1%) 513
Trileptal Oral Suspension 2407
Trileptal Tablets 2407
Uniretic Tablets (Less than 1%) 3178
Zanaflex Tablets (Infrequent) 1305
Zonegran Capsules (Infrequent) 1307

Cholestasis
Amaryl Tablets (Isolated cases) 717
Aquasol A Parenteral 593
Captopril Tablets (Rare) 2281
Ceclor CD Tablets 1279
Cefotan 664
Ceftin 1898
Ceptaz for Injection 1499
Clinoril Tablets (Less than 1%) 2053
Clozaril Tablets 2319
Crixivan Capsules (Less than 2%) 2070
Cytovene 2959
Diflucan Tablets, Injection, and Oral Suspension (Rare) 2681
Dolobid Tablets (Less than 1 in 100) 2088
Duricef 1079
Flexeril Tablets (Less than 1%) 572
Flexeril Tablets (Less than 1%) 2094
Fortaz 1541
Lorabid Suspension and Pulvules (Rare) 2251
Maxipime for Injection 1285
Mefoxin for Injection 2124
Mefoxin Premixed Intravenous Solution 2127
Mintezol 2137
Nolvadex Tablets (Rare) 678
Norvasc Tablets 2704
Omnicef 493
Periactin Tablets 2155
Procardia Capsules 2708
Procardia XL Extended Release Tablets 2710
Rythmol Tablets – 150 mg, 225 mg, 300 mg (0.1%) 502
Suprax 1877
Tagamet (Rare) 1644
Tambocor Tablets (Rare) 1990
Tazicef for Injection 1647
Tazicef Galaxy Container 1650
Tazicef Pharmacy Bulk Package 1653
Tazidime Vials, Faspak & ADD-Vantage 1966
Ticlid Tablets 3015
Vantin Tablets and Oral Suspension 2860
Zinacef Injection 1696
Zinacef for Injection 1696
Zyrtec (Rare) 2756
Zyrtec-D 12 Hour Extended Relief Tablets (Rare) 2758

Cholestasis, intrahepatic
Amoxil Chewable Tablets 1471
Amoxil for Oral Suspension 1471
Amoxil 1471
Cedax 1021
Cuprimine Capsules (Rare) 2075
Depen Titratable Tablets (Rare) 3341

Cholestatic hepatic injury
Axid Pulvules (Rare) 1903
Axid Pulvules (Rare) 2919
Coumadin for Injection (Infrequent) 1243
Coumadin Tablets (Infrequent) 1243
Warfarin Sodium Tablets, USP 3302

Cholesterol, systemic, microembolism
Coumadin for Injection (Infrequent) 1243
Coumadin Tablets (Infrequent) 1243
Warfarin Sodium Tablets, USP 3302

Cholinergic reactions
Cognex Capsules (Rare) 1351
Evoxac Capsules 1217
Risperdal (Rare) 1796
Tensilon Injectable 1745

Chondrodystrophy
Prozac Pulvules, Liquid, and Weekly Capsules (Rare) 1238
Sarafem Pulvules (Rare) 1962

Chorea
Activella Tablets 2764
Alora Transdermal System 3372
Cenestin Tablets 1263
Climara Transdermal System 958
Dilantin Infatabs (Rare) 2624
Dilantin Kapseals (Rare) 2622
Dilantin-125 Oral Suspension (Rare) 2625
Dilaudid-HP 443
Eldepryl Capsules 3266
Esclim Transdermal System 3460
Estinyl Tablets 3112
Estrace Vaginal Cream 3358
Estrace Tablets 3361
Estratest 3252
femhrt Tablets 2635
Inversine Tablets 1850
Klonopin Tablets 2983
▲ Lodosyn Tablets (Among most common) 1251
Lo/Ovral Tablets 3532
Lo/Ovral-28 Tablets 3538
Low-Ogestrel-28 Tablets 3392
Menest Tablets 2254
Nordette-28 Tablets 2257
Ogen Tablets 2846
Ogestrel 0.5/50-28 Tablets 3428
Ortho Dienestrol Cream 2554
Ortho-Est Tablets 3464
Ortho-Prefest Tablets 2570
Ovral Tablets 3551
Ovral-28 Tablets 3552
Ovrette Tablets 3552
Premarin Intravenous 3563
Premarin Tablets 3566
Premarin Vaginal Cream 3570
Premphase Tablets 3572
Prempro Tablets 3572
▲ Sinemet Tablets (Among most common) 1253
Sinemet CR Tablets 1255
Triphasil-21 Tablets 3600
Triphasil-28 Tablets 3605
Vivelle Transdermal System 2412
Vivelle-Dot Transdermal System 2416

Choreoathetosis
Celexa (At least 3 patients) 1365
Gabitril Tablets (Infrequent) 1189
Geodon Capsules (Frequent) 2688
Neurontin Capsules (Rare) 2655
Neurontin Oral Solution (Rare) 2655
Neurontin Tablets (Rare) 2655
Requip Tablets (Infrequent) 1621
Seroquel Tablets (Rare) 684

Choreoathetotic movements
Aldoclor Tablets 2035
Aldomet Tablets 2037
Aldoril Tablets 2039
Eskalith 1527
Felbatol 3343
Lamictal (Rare) 1567
Lithium Carbonate 3061
Lithium Citrate Syrup 3061
Lithobid Slow-Release Tablets 3255
Loxitane Capsules 3398
Neurontin Capsules (Rare) 2655
Neurontin Oral Solution (Rare) 2655
Neurontin Tablets (Rare) 2655
Paxil (Rare) 1609
Permax Tablets (Frequent) 1299
Reglan 2935
Risperdal (Rare) 1796
Serentil 1057
Tasmar Tablets (Infrequent) 3010
Thioridazine Hydrochloride Tablets 2289
Zoloft (Rare) 2751
Zyprexa Tablets (Up to 2%) 1973
Zyprexa ZYDIS Orally Disintegrating Tablets (Up to 2%) 1973

Choreoretinitis, granulomatous
TheraCys Injection 823

Choriocarcinoma
Serophene Tablets 3226

Chorioretinitis
Neurontin Capsules (Rare) 2655
Neurontin Oral Solution (Rare) 2655
Neurontin Tablets (Rare) 2655
Stromectol Tablets 2185

Choroidal detachment, post-filtration procedures
Cosopt Sterile Ophthalmic Solution 2065
Timolol GFS .... ⊙266
Timoptic in Ocudose 2192
Timoptic Sterile Ophthalmic Solution 2190
Timoptic-XE Sterile Ophthalmic Gel Forming Solution 2194
Trusopt Sterile Ophthalmic Solution 2196

Choroidal folds
Vitrasert Implant (Less than 1%) .... ⊙254

Choroiditis
Stromectol Tablets 2185
Vitrasert Implant (Less than 1%) .... ⊙254

Chromatopsia
Effexor Tablets (Rare) 3495
Effexor XR Capsules (Rare) 3499
▲ Nilandron Tablets (8.6%) 753

Chromaturia
Rescriptor Tablets 526

Chromosomal abnormalities
Clomid Tablets 735
Depo-Provera Contraceptive Injection 2798
Mustargen for Injection 2142
Roferon-A Injection (One case) 2996

Churg-Strauss syndrome
Accolate Tablets (Rare) 657
Advair Diskus 100/50 (Rare) 1448
Advair Diskus 250/50 (Rare) 1448
Advair Diskus 500/50 (Rare) 1448
Flovent Diskus (Rare) 3614
Singulair 2181

Ciliary injection
Isopto Carbachol Ophthalmic Solution .... ⊙215

Ciliary redness
Humorsol Sterile Ophthalmic Solution 2102

Ciliary spasm
Isopto Carbachol Ophthalmic Solution .... ⊙215
Isopto Carpine Ophthalmic Solution .... ⊙215
Pilopine HS Ophthalmic Gel .... ⊙217

Cinchonism
Quinaglute Dura-Tabs Tablets 978
Quinidex Extentabs 2933
Tonocard Tablets (Less than 1%) 649

Circulatory collapse
Amerge Tablets 1467
Etrafon (Extremely rare) 3115
Furosemide Tablets 2284
Solu-Medrol Sterile Powder 2855

Circulatory collapse, peripheral
Eskalith 1527
Intron A for Injection (Less than or equal to 5%) 3120
Lithium Carbonate 3061
Lithium Citrate Syrup 3061
Lithobid Slow-Release Tablets 3255
Tenormin 692

Circulatory depression
Actiq 1184
Brevital Sodium for Injection, USP ... 1815
Demerol 3079
Dilaudid 441
Dilaudid Oral Liquid 445
Dilaudid Tablets - 8 mg 445
Dilaudid-HP 443
Mepergan Injection 3539
MS Contin Tablets 2896
MSIR 2898
OxyContin Tablets 2912
Phenergan with Codeine Syrup 3557
Phenergan VC with Codeine Syrup .. 3561
Roxicodone Tablets 3067

Circulatory failure
Ambien Tablets (Rare) 3191
Dilaudid 441
Levaquin (Less than 0.3%) 2537
Lufyllin Tablets 3347
Lufyllin-400 Tablets 3347
Lufyllin-GG Elixir 3348
Lufyllin-GG Tablets 3348
Prevacid Delayed-Release Capsules (Less than 1%) 3292
PREVPAC (Less than 1%) 3298
Theo-Dur Extended-Release Tablets 1835
Trasylol Injection 909
Trilafon (Extremely rare) 3160
Uni-Dur Extended-Release Tablets ... 1841
Zosyn (1.0% or less) 1890
Zosyn in Galaxy Containers (1.0% or less) 1894

Cirrhosis, hepatic
(*see under* Cirrhosis of liver)

Cirrhosis of liver
Azulfidine EN-tabs Tablets 2775
Baycol Tablets (Rare) 883
Cataflam Tablets (Rare) 2315
Colazal Capsules 3069
Cordarone Tablets (Rare) 3487
Crixivan Capsules (Less than 2%) 2070
Lescol Capsules (Rare) 2361
Lescol Capsules (Rare) 2925
Lescol XL Tablets (Rare) 2361
Lescol XL Tablets (Rare) 2925
Mevacor Tablets (Rare) 2132
Pacerone Tablets (Rare) 3331
Pentasa Capsules 3239
Pravachol Tablets (Rare) 1099
Remeron Tablets (Rare) 2483
Remeron SolTab Tablets (Rare) 2486
Voltaren Tablets (Rare) 2315
Voltaren-XR Tablets (Rare) 2315
Zocor Tablets (Rare) 2219

Clamminess
Avonex 1013
Evoxac Capsules (Less than 1%) 1217
Exelon Capsules (Infrequent) 2342
Exelon Oral Solution (Infrequent) 2345
Intron A for Injection (Less than 5%) 3120
Iopidine Sterile Ophthalmic Solution .... ⊙212
Migranal Nasal Spray (Infrequent) ... 2376
Norvasc Tablets (Less than or equal to 0.1%) 2704
▲ Nubain Injection (9%) 1323
▲ Stadol NS Nasal Spray (3% to 9%) . 1108
Trovan (Less than 1%) 2722

Zoloft (Infrequent) 2751

Claudication
Blocadren Tablets 2046
Cosopt Sterile Ophthalmic Solution 2065
Covera-HS Tablets (Less than 2%) 3199
Isoptin SR Tablets (1% or less) 467
Monopril Tablets (0.2% to 1.0%) 1091
Monopril HCT 1094
Tarka Tablets 508
Timolide Tablets 2187
Timolol GFS ⊙266
Timoptic in Ocudose 2192
Timoptic Sterile Ophthalmic Solution 2190
Timoptic-XE Sterile Ophthalmic Gel Forming Solution 2194
Tonocard Tablets (Less than 1%) 649
Verelan Capsules (1% or less) 3184
Verelan PM Capsules (2% or less) 3186
Zebeta Tablets 1885
Ziac Tablets 1887

Claudication, intermittent
(*see under* Charcot's syndrome)

Claustrophobia
Roferon-A Injection (Infrequent) 2996

Cleft palate, neonatal
Accutane Capsules 2944
Proventil Inhalation Aerosol 3142
Proventil Inhalation Solution 0.083% 3146
Proventil Solution for Inhalation 0.5% 3144
Ventolin Inhalation Aerosol and Refill 1679

Clitoris, enlargement
(*see under* Clitoromegaly)

Clitoromegaly
Anadrol-50 Tablets 3321
▲ Android Capsules, 10 mg (Among most common) 1731
▲ Delatestryl Injection (Among most frequent) 1151
Estratest 3252
Oxandrin Tablets 1153
Provera Tablets (Rare) 2853
Testred Capsules, 10 mg 1746

Clonic movements of whole limbs
Diprivan Injectable Emulsion (Less than 1%) 667
Eskalith 1527
Lithium Carbonate 3061
Lithium Citrate Syrup 3061
Lithobid Slow-Release Tablets 3255

Clonus
Dopram Injectable 2931

Clotting time, prolongation
Anadrol-50 Tablets 3321
Mithracin for Intravenous Use 903
Oncaspar (Less than 1%) 756
Zosyn 1890
Zosyn in Galaxy Containers 1894

CNS, unresponsiveness, unspecified
Cipro I.V. 893

CNS abnormalities, fetal
Accutane Capsules 2944
Sensorcaine 643

CNS depression
Anaprox Tablets (Less than 1%) 2967
Anaprox DS Tablets (Less than 1%) 2967
Ativan Injection 3478
Cerebyx Injection (Infrequent) 2619
Depacon Injection 416
Depakene 421
Depakote Tablets 430
Depakote ER Tablets 436
Duranest Injections 600
EC-Naprosyn Delayed-Release Tablets (Less than 1%) 2967
ELA-Max Cream 1340
Emla (Unlikely with cream) 602
▲ Klonopin Tablets (Most frequent) 2983
Lamictal (Infrequent) 1567
Luvox Tablets (25, 50, 100 mg) (Infrequent) 3256
Naprosyn Suspension (Less than 1%) 2967
Naprosyn Tablets (Less than 1%) 2967
Nembutal Sodium Solution (Less than 1%) 485
Neurontin Capsules 2655
Neurontin Oral Solution 2655
Neurontin Tablets 2655
Phenergan with Codeine Syrup 3557
Phenergan VC with Codeine Syrup 3561
Prozac Pulvules, Liquid, and Weekly Capsules (Infrequent) 1238
Rilutek Tablets (Rare) 772
Rynatan Tablets 3351
Sarafem Pulvules (Infrequent) 1962
▲ Vesanoid Capsules (3%) 3037
▲ Xanax Tablets (13.8% to 13.9%) 2865
▲ Xylocaine Injections (Among most common) 653

CNS depression, neonatal
Halcion Tablets 2823
Streptomycin Sulfate Injection 2714
Versed Injection 3027

CNS reactions
Attenuvax 2044
Azulfidine EN-tabs Tablets 2775
Chibroxin Sterile Ophthalmic Solution 2051
▲ Cipro I.V. Pharmacy Bulk Package (Among most frequent) 897
Clozaril Tablets 2319
Compazine 1505
Digitek Tablets 1003
Hexalen Capsules 2226
Intron A for Injection (Less than 5%) 3120
Lanoxicaps Capsules (Rare) 1574
Lanoxin Injection 1581
Lanoxin Tablets 1587
Lanoxin Elixir Pediatric 1578
Lanoxin Injection Pediatric 1584
Lariam Tablets 2989
▲ Leukine (11%) 1755
Levsin/Levsinex/Levbid 3172
▲ Nipent for Injection (1% to 11%) 3272
Noroxin Tablets 2145
▲ Novantrone for Injection (30% to 34%) 1760
Orap Tablets 1407
Orthoclone OKT3 Sterile Solution 2498
Orudis Capsules (Less than 1%) 3548
Oruvail Capsules (Less than 1%) 3548
▲ Paraplatin for Injection (5%) 1126
Roferon-A Injection (Less than 5%) 2996
Serentil 1057
Silvadene Cream 1% 2267
Stelazine 1640

CNS stimulation
Adipex-P 1406
Avelox Tablets 879
Axert Tablets (Infrequent) 2772
Cafcit 1035
Chibroxin Sterile Ophthalmic Solution 2051
Cipro I.V. 893
Cipro 887
Claritin-D 12 Hour Extended Release Tablets 3102
Claritin-D 24 Hour Extended Release Tablets 3104
Combivent Inhalation Aerosol 1041
Duranest Injections 600
Effexor Tablets (Infrequent) 3495
Effexor XR Capsules (Infrequent) 3499
ELA-Max Cream 1340
Emla (Unlikely with cream) 602
Floxin Tablets 2529
Kytril Injection (Less than 2%) 2986
Lamictal (Rare) 1567
Levaquin 2537
Levo-Dromoran 1734
Lidoderm Patch 1319
Lindane Lotion USP 1% 559
Lindane Shampoo USP 1% 560
Lufyllin-GG Elixir 3348
Lufyllin-GG Tablets 3348
Luvox Tablets (25, 50, 100 mg) (2%) 3256
Meridia Capsules (1.5%) 481
Noroxin Tablets 2145
Paxil (Frequent) 1609
Proventil Inhalation Aerosol 3142
Proventil Repetabs Tablets 3148
Proventil HFA Inhalation Aerosol 3150
Prozac Pulvules, Liquid, and Weekly Capsules (Infrequent) 1238
Sarafem Pulvules (Infrequent) 1962
Serzone Tablets 1104
Tequin Injection 1110
Tequin Tablets 1110
Trovan 2722
▲ Ultram Tablets (7% to 14%) 2600
Ventolin Inhalation Aerosol and Refill 1679
Ventolin HFA Inhalation Aerosol 3618
Volmax Extended-Release Tablets 2276
Wellbutrin SR Sustained-Release Tablets (1% to 2%) 1684
▲ Xylocaine Injections (Among most common) 653
Zyban Sustained-Release Tablets (Infrequent) 1710
Zyprexa Tablets (Infrequent) 1973
Zyprexa ZYDIS Orally Disintegrating Tablets (Infrequent) 1973
Zyrtec-D 12 Hour Extended Relief Tablets 2758

CNS stimulation, paradoxical
Halcion Tablets 2823
Librium Capsules 1736
Numorphan 1324

CNS toxicity
Duranest Injections 600
▲ Ifex for Injection (12%) 1123
Lindane Lotion USP 1% 559
Lindane Shampoo USP 1% 560
▲ Nipent for Injection (1% to 11%) 3272

Coagulation defects, neonatal
Dilantin Infatabs 2624
Dilantin Kapseals 2622
Dilantin-125 Oral Suspension 2625

Coagulation dysfunction
Abelcet Injection 1273
AmBisome for Injection (Less common) 1383
Amicar Injection 3608
Amicar Syrup 3608
Amicar Tablets 3608
▲ Amphotec (5% or more) 1774
Avonex 1013
Campath Ampules 992
Celexa (Rare) 1365
Cordarone Tablets (1% to 3%) 3487
Depacon Injection 416
Depakene 421
Depakote Tablets 430
Depakote ER Tablets 436
Diprivan Injectable Emulsion (Less than 1%) 667
Elspar for Injection 2092
Estratest 3252
Felbatol 3343
Herceptin I.V. (At least one of the 958 patients) 1414
Ifex for Injection (Less than 1%) 1123
▲ Leukine (19%) 1755
Lo/Ovral Tablets 3532
Lo/Ovral-28 Tablets 3538
Low-Ogestrel-28 Tablets 3392
Neurontin Capsules 2655
Neurontin Oral Solution 2655
Neurontin Tablets 2655
Nimotop Capsules (Less than 1%) 904
NovoSeven (1%) 2430
Ogestrel 0.5/50-28 Tablets 3428
Omnicef 493
Oncaspar (Less than 1%) 756
Orthoclone OKT3 Sterile Solution 2498
Ovral Tablets 3551
Ovral-28 Tablets 3552
Ovrette Tablets 3552
Pacerone Tablets (1% to 3%) 3331
Pediazole Suspension 3050
Plavix Tablets (1% to 2.5%) 1097
Plavix Tablets (1% to 2.5%) 3084
Premarin Intravenous 3563
Premarin Tablets 3566
Premarin Vaginal Cream 3570
▲ Prograf (3% to 15%) 1393
▲ Proleukin for Injection (10%) 1199
Rifadin (Rare) 765
Rituxan for Infusion (0.3%) 1750
Rituxan I.V. (0.3%) 1428
Roferon-A Injection (Less than 4%) 2996
Tice BCG, BCG Live (0.3%) 2489
Xeloda Tablets (Less than 5%) 3039

Coagulation tests, altered results
Provera Tablets 2853
Zosyn 1890
Zosyn in Galaxy Containers 1894

Coagulation time, increase in
Arthrotec Tablets (Rare) 3195
Zoloft 2751

Coagulopathy
Aggrenox Capsules 1026
Ecotrin Enteric Coated Aspirin Low, Regular and Maximum Strength Tablets 1715
Enbrel for Injection 1752
Enbrel for Injection 3504
▲ TheraCys Injection (3%) 823

Coccidioidomycosis, disseminated
Remicade for IV Injection (One patient) 1178

Cochlear damage
Nebcin Vials, Hyporets & ADD-Vantage 1955
Streptomycin Sulfate Injection 2714
Tripedia Vaccine 817

Cochlear lesion
Diphtheria & Tetanus Toxoids Adsorbed Purogenated for Pediatric Use 1857
Tetanus & Diphtheria Toxoids Adsorbed for Adult Use 1880
Tetanus and Diphtheria Toxoids Adsorbed For Adult Use 815

Cognitive dysfunction
Ambien Tablets (Infrequent) 3191
Amerge Tablets (Infrequent) 1467
Anaprox Tablets (Less than 1%) 2967
Anaprox DS Tablets (Less than 1%) 2967
EC-Naprosyn Delayed-Release Tablets (Rare) 2967
Floxin I.V. (Less than 1%) 2526
Floxin Tablets (Less than 1%) 2529
▲ Naprelan Tablets (3% to 9%) 1293
Naprosyn Suspension (Less than 1%) 2967
Naprosyn Tablets (Less than 1%) 2967
Orthoclone OKT3 Sterile Solution 2498
Rescriptor Tablets (Less than 2%) 526
Risperdal 1796
Ultracet Tablets 2597
Ultram Tablets (Less than 1%) 2600
▲ Xanax Tablets (28.8%) 2865

Cogwheel rigidity
Cognex Capsules (Infrequent) 1351
Compazine 1505
Eskalith 1527
Geodon Capsules (Frequent) 2688
Lithobid Slow-Release Tablets 3255
Paxil 1609
Reglan 2935
Stelazine 1640
Thioridazine Hydrochloride Tablets 2289
Thiothixene Capsules 2290
Thorazine 1656
▲ Zyprexa Tablets (8% to 20%) 1973
▲ Zyprexa ZYDIS Orally Disintegrating Tablets (8% to 20%) 1973

Cold, reduced tolerance
Coumadin for Injection (Infrequent) 1243
Coumadin Tablets (Infrequent) 1243
Warfarin Sodium Tablets, USP 3302

Cold sensations
Aceon Tablets (2 mg, 4 mg, 8 mg) (0.3% to 1%) 3249
Aricept Tablets (Infrequent) 1270
Aricept Tablets (Infrequent) 2665
Betapace AF Tablets (2% to 2.5%) 954
Buprenex Injectable (Less than 1%) 2918
Coumadin for Injection (Infrequent) 1243
Coumadin Tablets (Infrequent) 1243
Diphtheria & Tetanus Toxoids Adsorbed Purogenated for Pediatric Use 1857
Duranest Injections 600
Emla (Unlikely with cream) 602
Ethyol for Injection 2029
Imitrex Injection (1.1%) 1549
Imitrex Nasal Spray (Rare) 1554
Imitrex Tablets (Rare) 1558
Migranal Nasal Spray (Infrequent) 2376
Monopril Tablets (0.4% to 1.0%) 1091
Roferon-A Injection (Infrequent) 2996
Tetanus & Diphtheria Toxoids Adsorbed for Adult Use 1880
Versed Injection (Less than 1%) 3027
Warfarin Sodium Tablets, USP 3302
▲ Xylocaine Injections (Among most common) 653
Zofran Injection (2%) 1698
▲ Zomig Tablets (5% to 7%) 708
▲ Zomig-ZMT Tablets (5% to 7%) 708

Cold sore, non-herpetic
Hivid Tablets (Less than 1%) 2975
Intron A for Injection (Less than 5%) 3120
Varivax (Greater than or equal to 1%) 2202

Cold symptoms, unspecified
AccuNeb Inhalation Solution (Up to 3.4%) 1230
▲ Aerobid/Aerobid-M (15%) 1363
▲ Alamast Ophthalmic Solution (10% to 25%) 3092
Carac Cream (2.3%) 1222
▲ Geodon Capsules (8%) 2688
Nascobal Gel (Three patients) 3174
Patanol Ophthalmic Solution (Less than 5%) 540
Paxil 1609
▲ Periostat Tablets (22%) 1208
Prinivil Tablets (1.1%) 2164
▲ ProSom Tablets (3%) 500
Rowasa Rectal Suspension Enema 4.0 grams/unit (60 mL) (2.33%) 3264
Sandostatin Injection (1% to 4%) 2394
▲ Xalatan Latanoprost Ophthalmic Solution (Approximately 4%) ⊙320
▲ Xalatan Sterile Ophthalmic Solution (Approximately 4%) 2864
Zestril Tablets (1.1%) 698

Coldness of extremities
▲ Blocadren Tablets (8%) 2046
Cosopt Sterile Ophthalmic Solution 2065
Effexor Tablets (Infrequent) 3495
Effexor XR Capsules (Infrequent) 3499
Eskalith (A few reports) 1527

Hivid Tablets (Less than 1%) 2975
Lithium Carbonate (A single report) 3061
Lithium Citrate Syrup 3061
Lithobid Slow-Release Tablets (A few reports) 3255
Luvox Tablets (25, 50, 100 mg) (Infrequent) 3256
Maxalt Tablets (Infrequent) 2120
Maxalt-MLT Orally Disintegrating Tablets (Infrequent) 2120
Mykrox Tablets (Less than 2%) 1168
ReoPro Vials (0.2%) 1958
▲ Tenoretic Tablets (Up to 12%) 690
▲ Tenormin (Up to 12%) 692
Timolide Tablets 2187
Timolol GFS ⊙266
Timoptic in Ocudose 2192
Timoptic Sterile Ophthalmic Solution 2190
Timoptic-XE Sterile Ophthalmic Gel Forming Solution 2194
Tonocard Tablets (Less than 1%) 649
Toprol-XL Tablets (About 1 of 100 patients) 651
Zebeta Tablets 1885
Ziac Tablets 1887

Colds, susceptibility
Betimol Ophthalmic Solution (1% to 5%) ⊙324
Hytrin Capsules (At least 1%) 464
Lopid Tablets 2650
▲ Pravachol Tablets (Up to 7.0%) 1099
Prinzide Tablets (0.3% to 1%) 2168
Sinemet CR Tablets 1255
Zestoretic Tablets (0.3% to 1%) 695

Colic
Feldene Capsules (Rare) 2685
Fortovase Capsules (Less than 2%) 2970
Glucotrol Tablets (1 in 100) 2692
Invirase Capsules (Less than 2%) 2979
Prevnar for Injection 1870
Urecholine 2198
Urecholine Tablets 2445

Colic, biliary
Kadian Capsules (Less than 3%) 1335

Colitis
Accutane Capsules 2944
Aciphex Tablets 1267
Aciphex Tablets 1783
▲ Actonel Tablets (3.3%) 2879
Aldoclor Tablets 2035
Aldomet Tablets 2037
Aldoril Tablets 2039
Alesse-21 Tablets 3468
Alesse-28 Tablets 3473
Anaprox Tablets (Less than 1%) 2967
Anaprox DS Tablets (Less than 1%) 2967
Ancef for Injection 1474
Ancef Injection 1474
Apligraf (1.8%) 2305
Arava Tablets (1% to 3%) 724
Avonex 1013
Baycol Tablets 883
Benzaclin Topical Gel 1220
Brevicon 28-Day Tablets 3380
Campath Ampules 992
Canasa Rectal Suppositories (1.2%) 829
Cataflam Tablets (Rare; less than 1%) 2315
Cefotan 664
Cefzil (Rare) 1076
Celebrex Capsules (Less than 0.1%) 2676
Celebrex Capsules (Less than 0.1%) 2780
Celexa (Rare) 1365
CellCept Capsules 2951
CellCept Intravenous 2951
CellCept Oral Suspension 2951
CellCept Tablets 2951
Ceptaz for Injection 1499
Claforan Injection (1.4%) 732
Cleocin HCl Capsules 2784
Cleocin Phosphate Sterile Solution 2785
Cleocin T Topical (Rare) 2790
Cleocin Vaginal Cream 2788
Clindagel 1401
Clinoril Tablets (Less than 1%) 2053
Copaxone for Injection (Infrequent) 3306
Cyclessa Tablets 2450
Desogen Tablets 2458
Doxil Injection (Less than 1%) 566
EC-Naprosyn Delayed-Release Tablets (Less than 1%) 2967
Effexor Tablets (Infrequent) 3495
Effexor XR Capsules (Infrequent) 3499
Elmiron Capsules (Less than or equal to 1%) 570
Estrostep 2627
Exelon Capsules (Infrequent) 2342
Exelon Oral Solution (Infrequent) 2345
Flovent Rotadisk (1% to 3%) 1537
Fortaz 1541
Herceptin I.V. (At least one of the 958 patients) 1414
Hivid Tablets (Less than 1%) 2975
Imitrex Nasal Spray (Rare) 1554
Imitrex Tablets 1558
Kefurox Vials, ADD-Vantage 1948
Levlen 962
Levlite 21 Tablets 962
Levlite 28 Tablets 962
Levora Tablets 3389
Lipitor Tablets (Less than 2%) 2639
Lipitor Tablets (Less than 2%) 2696
Lodine (Less than 1%) 3528
Lodine XL Extended-Release Tablets (Less than 1%) 3530
Loestrin 21 Tablets 2642
Loestrin Fe Tablets 2642
Lopid Tablets 2650
Lunelle Monthly Injection 2827
Luvox Tablets (25, 50, 100 mg) (Infrequent) 3256
Maxipime for Injection (0.1% to 1%) 1285
Mefoxin for Injection 2124
Mefoxin Premixed Intravenous Solution 2127
Microgestin Fe 1.5/30 Tablets 3407
Microgestin Fe 1/20 Tablets 3400
Mircette Tablets 2470
Mobic Tablets (Less than 2%) 1054
Modicon 2563
Naprelan Tablets (Less than 1%) 1293
Naprosyn Suspension (Less than 1%) 2967
Naprosyn Tablets (Less than 1%) 2967
Necon 3415
Neurontin Capsules (Rare) 2655
Neurontin Oral Solution (Rare) 2655
Neurontin Tablets (Rare) 2655
Norinyl 1 +35 28-Day Tablets 3380
Norinyl 1 + 50 28-Day Tablets 3380
Norvir Capsules (Less than 2%) 487
Norvir Oral Solution (Less than 2%) 487
Oncaspar 756
Ortho-Cept 21 Tablets 2546
Ortho-Cept 28 Tablets 2546
Ortho-Cyclen/Ortho Tri-Cyclen 2573
Ortho-Novum 2563
Ortho-Novum 1/50□28 Tablets 2556
Ortho-Cyclen/Ortho Tri-Cyclen 2573
Ovcon 3364
Paxil (Rare) 1609
Permax Tablets (Rare) 1299
Pletal Tablets (Less than 2%) 2605
Pletal Tablets (Less than 2%) 2848
Prevnar for Injection 1870
Proleukin for Injection 1199
Protonix I.V. (Less than 1%) 3580
Protonix Tablets (Less than 1%) 3577
Prozac Pulvules, Liquid, and Weekly Capsules (Infrequent) 1238
Remeron Tablets (Infrequent) 2483
Remeron SolTab Tablets (Infrequent) 2486
Requip Tablets (Infrequent) 1621
Rescriptor Tablets (Less than 2%) 526
Rocephin Injectable Vials, ADD-Vantage, Galaxy, Bulk (Rare) 2993
Roferon-A Injection (Infrequent) 2996
Salagen Tablets (Less than 1%) 2229
Sandostatin LAR Depot (1% to 4%) 2395
Sarafem Pulvules (Infrequent) 1962
▲ Serostim for Injection (1% to 10%) 3229
Serzone Tablets (Infrequent) 1104
Sonata Capsules (Less than 1%) 3591
Sular Tablets (Less than or equal to 1%) 688
Suprax 1877
Tasmar Tablets (Infrequent) 3010
Tazicef for Injection 1647
Tazicef Galaxy Container 1650
Tazicef Pharmacy Bulk Package 1653
Tazidime Vials, Faspak & ADD-Vantage 1966
Tequin Injection (Less than 0.1%) 1110
Tequin Tablets (Less than 0.1%) 1110
Thalomid Capsules 1154
Ticlid Tablets 3015
Tricor Capsules, Micronized 513
Trileptal Oral Suspension 2407
Trileptal Tablets 2407
Tri-Levlen 962
Tri-Norinyl-28 Tablets 3433
Trivora Tablets 3439
Trovan (Less than 1%) 2722
Uniretic Tablets (Less than 1%) 3178
Vioxx (Less than 0.1%) 2213
Vistide Injection 1445
Voltaren Tablets (Rare; less than 1%) 2315
Voltaren-XR Tablets (Rare; less than 1%) 2315
Wellbutrin Tablets (Rare) 1680
Wellbutrin SR Sustained-Release Tablets 1684
Xeloda Tablets (Less than 5%) 3039
Yasmin 28 Tablets 980
Zinacef Injection 1696
Zinacef for Injection 1696
Zoloft (Rare) 2751
Zonegran Capsules (Rare) 1307
Zovia 3449
Zyban Sustained-Release Tablets 1710

Colitis, hemorrhagic
Augmentin ES-600 Powder for Oral Suspension 1487

Colitis, ischemic
Blocadren Tablets 2046
Corgard Tablets 2245
Corzide 40/5 Tablets 2247
Corzide 80/5 Tablets 2247
Cosopt Sterile Ophthalmic Solution 2065
Imitrex Injection 1549
Imitrex Nasal Spray 1554
Imitrex Tablets 1558
Nadolol Tablets 2288
Taxol Injection (Rare) 1129
Tenoretic Tablets 690
Tenormin 692
Timolol GFS ⊙266
Timoptic-XE Sterile Ophthalmic Gel Forming Solution 2194
Zebeta Tablets 1885
Ziac Tablets 1887

Colitis, necrotizing
Adriamycin PFS/RDF Injection 2767

Colitis, pseudomembranous
(*see under* Pseudomembranous colitis)

Colitis, ulcerative
Ancobon Capsules 1730
Evoxac Capsules (Less than 1%) 1217
Indocin (Less than 1%) 2112
Orudis Capsules (Rare) 3548
Oruvail Capsules (Rare) 3548
Prevacid Delayed-Release Capsules (Less than 1%) 3292
PREVPAC (Less than 1%) 3298
Protonix I.V. (Less than 1%) 3580
Protonix Tablets (Less than 1%) 3577
Serzone Tablets (Rare) 1104
Vantin Tablets and Oral Suspension 2860

Colitis, ulcerative, worsening of
▲ Asacol Delayed-Release Tablets (3%) 2884
Colazal Capsules 3069
Pentasa Capsules (0.4%) 3239

Collagen disease, unspecified
▲ Flolan for Injection (82%) 1528

Collapse
Carbatrol Capsules 3234
Clozaril Tablets (Rare) 2319
Mintezol 2137
Nitrolingual Pumpspray 1355
Nitrostat Tablets 2658
Norpramin Tablets (One report) 755
Tegretol/Tegretol-XR 2404
Venofer Injection (8 patients) 580

Colon, dilatation
Artane (Rare) 1855
Phenergan with Codeine Syrup 3557
Phenergan VC with Codeine Syrup 3561

Colon, irritable
Aricept Tablets (Infrequent) 1270
Aricept Tablets (Infrequent) 2665
Compazine 1505
Prilosec Delayed-Release Capsules (Less than 1%) 628

Colon motility, increased
Phenergan with Codeine Syrup 3557
Phenergan VC with Codeine Syrup 3561

Colon problem, unspecified
Betapace Tablets (2% to 3%) 950

Colonic strictures
Creon 5 Capsules 3251
Creon 10 Capsules 3251
Creon 20 Capsules 3251
Ultrase Capsules 835
Ultrase MT Capsules 835

Color perception, disturbed
Cataflam Tablets 2315
Cipro (Less than 1%) 887
Quinaglute Dura-Tabs Tablets (Occasional) 978
Quinidex Extentabs (Occasional) 2933
Voltaren Tablets 2315
Voltaren-XR Tablets 2315

Coma
Aciphex Tablets 1267
Aciphex Tablets 1783
Aggrenox Capsules (Less than 1%) 1026
Aloprim for Injection (Less than 1%) 2292
AmBisome for Injection (Less common) 1383
Arthrotec Tablets (Rare) 3195
Ativan Injection (Less than 1%) 3478
Betaseron for SC Injection 988
Bicillin C-R 900/300 Injection 2240
Bicillin C-R Injection 2238
Bicillin L-A Injection 2242
Buprenex Injectable (Infrequent) 2918
Campath Ampules 992
Cataflam Tablets (Rare) 2315
Cerebyx Injection (Infrequent) 2619
Cognex Capsules (Rare) 1351
Compazine 1505
Copaxone for Injection (Infrequent) 3306
DDAVP Injection 4 mcg/mL (Rare) 737
DDAVP Nasal Spray (Rare) 738
DDAVP Rhinal Tube (Rare) 738
Depacon Injection (Rare) 416
Depakene (Rare) 421
Depakote Sprinkle Capsules (Rare) 426
Depakote Tablets (Rare) 430
Depakote ER Tablets (Rare) 436
Desmopressin Acetate Injection (Rare) 1344
Ecotrin Enteric Coated Aspirin Low, Regular and Maximum Strength Tablets 1715
Elspar for Injection 2092
Ergamisol Tablets 1789
Eskalith 1527
Evoxac Capsules (Less than 1%) 1217
Felbatol 3343
Feldene Capsules (Rare) 2685
Fludara for Injection 995
Foscavir Injection (Less than 1%) 605
Gabitril Tablets (Infrequent) 1189
Gliadel Wafer (1%) 1723
Ifex for Injection (Occasional) 1123
Indocin Capsules (Less than 1%) 2112
Indocin I.V. (Less than 1%) 2115
Indocin (Less than 1%) 2112
Intron A for Injection (Less than 5%) 3120
Klonopin Tablets 2983
Levaquin (Less than 0.3%) 2537
Levbid Extended-Release Tablets 3172
Levo-Dromoran 1734
Levsin/Levsinex/Levbid 3172
Lithium Carbonate 3061
Lithium Citrate Syrup 3061
Lithobid Slow-Release Tablets 3255
Lodine XL Extended-Release Tablets 3530
Luvox Tablets (25, 50, 100 mg) (Rare) 3256
LYMErix Vaccine (Greater than 1%) 1592
Matulane Capsules 3246
Motrin Suspension, Oral Drops, Chewable Tablets, and Caplets (Rare; less than 1%) 2002
Nardil Tablets (Less frequent) 2653
Naropin Injection (Less than 1%) 612
Oncaspar 756
Orthoclone OKT3 Sterile Solution 2498
Permax Tablets (Infrequent) 1299
Pfizerpen for Injection 2707
PhosLo 1069
Podocon-25 Liquid 2608
Ponstel Capsules (Rare) 1356
Prograf 1393
Proleukin for Injection (1%) 1199
Prozac Pulvules, Liquid, and Weekly Capsules (Rare) 1238
ReoPro Vials (0.4%) 1958
Requip Tablets (Infrequent) 1621
Rilutek Tablets (Infrequent) 772
Risperdal (Rare) 1796
Roferon-A Injection (Rare to infrequent) 2996
Rythmol Tablets – 150 mg, 225 mg, 300 mg (Less than 1%) 502
Sarafem Pulvules (Rare) 1962
Stimate Nasal Spray 796
Streptomycin Sulfate Injection (Occasional) 2714
Symmetrel 1328
Tonocard Tablets (Less than 1%) 649
Topamax Sprinkle Capsules (Infrequent) 2590
Topamax Tablets (Infrequent) 2590
▲ Trisenox Injection (5%) 1158
Valtrex Caplets 1676
▲ Vesanoid Capsules (3%) 3037
Voltaren Tablets (Rare) 2315
Voltaren-XR Tablets (Rare) 2315
Wellbutrin Tablets 1680
Wellbutrin SR Sustained-Release Tablets 1684
Zoloft (Rare) 2751
Zovirax Capsules 1706
Zovirax for Injection (Approximately 1%) 1708
Zovirax 1706
Zyban Sustained-Release Tablets 1710

Zyprexa Tablets (Infrequent) 1973
Zyprexa ZYDIS Orally Disintegrating Tablets (Infrequent) 1973

Coma, hepatic
(*see under* Hepatic coma)

Coma, hypoglycemic
Tapazole Tablets 1823

Combativeness
Diprivan Injectable Emulsion (Less than 1%) 667
Orthoclone OKT3 Sterile Solution 2498
Versed Injection 3027
Zosyn (1.0% or less) 1890
Zosyn in Galaxy Containers (1.0% or less) 1894

Conduction delay, intraventricular
Rythmol Tablets – 150 mg, 225 mg, 300 mg (1.1% to 4.0%) 502

Conduction disturbances
Aceon Tablets (2 mg, 4 mg, 8 mg) (0.3% to 1%) 3249
Avalide Tablets 1070
Avapro Tablets (Less than 1%) 1074
Avapro Tablets (Less than 1%) 3076
Blocadren Tablets 2046
Catapres-TTS 1038
Clorpres Tablets (Rare) 1002
Combipres Tablets (Rare) 1040
Corgard Tablets (1 of 100 patients) 2245
Corzide 40/5 Tablets (1 of 100 patients) 2247
Corzide 80/5 Tablets (1 of 100 patients) 2247
Cytovene 2959
Digitek Tablets 1003
Etrafon 3115
▲ Lanoxicaps Capsules (Among most common) 1574
▲ Lanoxin Injection (Among most common) 1581
▲ Lanoxin Tablets (Among most common) 1587
▲ Lanoxin Elixir Pediatric (Among most common) 1578
▲ Lanoxin Injection Pediatric (Among most common) 1584
Luvox Tablets (25, 50, 100 mg) (Infrequent) 3256
Mexitil Capsules (2 in 1,000) 1047
Monopril Tablets (0.4% to 1.0%) 1091
Nadolol Tablets (1 of 100 patients) 2288
Paxil (Infrequent) 1609
Procardia Capsules (Fewer than 0.5%) 2708
Procardia XL Extended Release Tablets (Fewer than 0.5%) 2710
▲ Rythmol Tablets – 150 mg, 225 mg, 300 mg (1.1% to 4.0%) 502
Taxol Injection 1129
Tonocard Tablets 649

Confusion
Aciphex Tablets (Rare) 1267
Aciphex Tablets (Rare) 1783
Actimmune (Rare) 1772
▲ Actiq (1% to 6%) 1184
Adalat CC Tablets (Less than 1.0%) 877
Aggrenox Capsules (1.1%) 1026
Agrylin Capsules (1% to 5%) 3232
Aldoclor Tablets 2035
Aldomet Tablets 2037
Aldoril Tablets 2039
Alferon N Injection (One patient to 3%) 1770
Ambien Tablets (Frequent) 3191
▲ AmBisome for Injection (8.6% to 12.9%) 1383
Amerge Tablets (Rare) 1467
Amicar Injection 3608
Amicar Syrup 3608
Amicar Tablets 3608
Amoxil Chewable Tablets (Rare) 1471
Amoxil for Oral Suspension (Rare) 1471
Amoxil (Rare) 1471
▲ Amphotec (5% or more) 1774
Ancobon Capsules 1730
Androderm Transdermal System CIII (Less than 1%) 3377
Anzemet Injection (Infrequently) 719
Anzemet Tablets (Infrequently) 722
Apligraf (1.8%) 2305
Aricept Tablets 1270
Aricept Tablets 2665
Arimidex Tablets (2% to 5%) 659
▲ Aromasin Tablets (2% to 5%) 2769
Artane 1855
Arthrotec Tablets (Rare) 3195
Asacol Delayed-Release Tablets 2884
Astelin Nasal Spray 3339
Ativan Injection (1.3%) 3478
Augmentin Chewable Tablets (Rare) 1482
Augmentin Powder for Oral Suspension (Rare) 1482
Augmentin Tablets (Rare) 1485
Augmentin ES-600 Powder for Oral Suspension (Rare) 1487
Avalide Tablets 1070
Avelox Tablets (0.05% to 1%) 879
Avonex 1013
Axid Pulvules (Rare) 1903
Axid Pulvules (Rare) 2919
Azactam for Injection (Less than 1%) 1276
Benadryl Parenteral 2617
Betagan ⊙ 228
▲ Betaseron for SC Injection (4%) 988
Biaxin/Biaxin XL 403
Bicillin C-R 900/300 Injection 2240
Bicillin C-R Injection 2238
Bicillin L-A Injection 2242
Brevibloc Injection (About 2%) 858
Campath Ampules 992
Captopril Tablets 2281
Carbatrol Capsules 3234
Cardene I.V. (Rare) 3485
Cardura Tablets (Less than 0.5%) 2668
▲ Casodex Tablets (2% to 5%) 662
Ceclor CD Tablets 1279
Ceclor (Rare) 1905
Cefzil (Less than 1%) 1076
Celexa (Frequent) 1365
▲ CellCept Capsules (13.5%) 2951
▲ CellCept Intravenous (13.5%) 2951
▲ CellCept Oral Suspension (13.5%) 2951
▲ CellCept Tablets (13.5% to 17.3%) 2951
Celontin Capsules 2618
Cerebyx Injection (Infrequent) 2619
Chibroxin Sterile Ophthalmic Solution 2051
Chirocaine Injection (Less than 1%) 2909
Cipro I.V. (1% or less) 893
Cipro I.V. Pharmacy Bulk Package (Less than 1%) 897
Cipro 887
Claritin (At least one patient) 3100
Claritin-D 12 Hour Extended Release Tablets (Less frequent) 3102
Claritin-D 24 Hour Extended Release Tablets (Fewer than 2%) 3104
▲ Clozaril Tablets (3%) 2319
Cogentin 2055
▲ Cognex Capsules (7%) 1351
Copaxone for Injection (2%) 3306
Cosopt Sterile Ophthalmic Solution 2065
Covera-HS Tablets (Less than 2%) 3199
Cozaar Tablets (Less than 1%) 2067
Cytotec Tablets 3202
Cytovene (At least 3 subjects) 2959
Dantrium Capsules (Less frequent) 2885
Daranide Tablets 2077
DaunoXome Injection (Less than or equal to 5%) 1442
Demser Capsules 2085
Depacon Injection (1% to 5%) 416
Depakene (1% to 5%) 421
Depakote Sprinkle Capsules (1% to 5%) 426
Depakote Tablets (1% to 5%) 430
Depakote ER Tablets (1% to 5%) 436
▲ DepoCyt Injection (4% to 14%) 1197
D.H.E. 45 Injection 2334
Diamox Intravenous (Occasional) ⊙ 269
Diamox Sequels Sustained Release Capsules (Occasional) ⊙ 270
Diamox Tablets (Occasional) ⊙ 269
Didronel Tablets 2888
Digitek Tablets 1003
▲ Dilantin Infatabs (Among most common) 2624
▲ Dilantin Kapseals (Among most common) 2622
▲ Dilantin-125 Oral Suspension (Among most common) 2625
Diovan HCT Tablets 2338
Diprivan Injectable Emulsion (Less than 1%) 667
Ditropan XL Extended Release Tablets (2% to 5%) 564
Diuril Oral 2087
Diuril Sodium Intravenous 2086
Dolobid Tablets (Less than 1 in 100) 2088
Dostinex Tablets 2804
Doxil Injection (Less than 1%) 566
▲ Duraclon Injection (13.2% to 38%) 3057
▲ Duragesic Transdermal System (10% or more) 1786
Duranest Injections 600
Dyazide Capsules 1515
Ecotrin Enteric Coated Aspirin Low, Regular and Maximum Strength Tablets 1715
Edecrin 2091
Effexor Tablets (2%) 3495
Effexor XR Capsules (Frequent) 3499
ELA-Max Cream 1340
▲ Eldepryl Capsules (3 of 49 patients) 3266
Elspar for Injection 2092
Emla (Unlikely with cream) 602
Enalaprilat Injection 863
Ergamisol Tablets (Less frequent) 1789
Ery-Tab Tablets (Isolated reports) 448
Erythrocin Stearate Filmtab Tablets (Isolated reports) 452
Erythromycin Base Filmtab Tablets (Isolated reports) 454
Erythromycin Delayed-Release Capsules, USP (Isolated reports) 455
Eskalith 1527
Etrafon 3115
Eulexin Capsules (1%) 3118
Evoxac Capsules (Less than 1%) 1217
▲ Exelon Capsules (8%) 2342
▲ Exelon Oral Solution (8%) 2345
Famotidine Injection (Infrequent) 866
Famvir Tablets (Infrequent) 2348
Felbatol 3343
Feldene Capsules (Occasional) 2685
▲ Flolan for Injection (6%) 1528
Floxin I.V. (Less than 1%) 2526
Floxin Tablets (Less than 1%) 2529
Fludara for Injection 995
Flumadine (Less than 0.3%) 1370
Fortovase Capsules (Less than 2%) 2970
▲ Foscavir Injection (5% or greater) 605
Sterile FUDR (Remote possibility) 2974
▲ Gabitril Tablets (5%) 1189
Gengraf Capsules (1% to less than 3%) 457
Geodon Capsules (Frequent) 2688
▲ Gliadel Wafer (10%) 1723
Glucotrol XL Extended Release Tablets (Less than 1%) 2693
Grifulvin V Tablets Microsize and Oral Suspension Microsize (Occasional) 2518
Gris-PEG Tablets (Occasional) 2661
Halcion Tablets (0.5% to 0.9%) 2823
Haldol Decanoate 2535
Haldol Injection, Tablets and Concentrate 2533
Herceptin I.V. (At least one of the 958 patients) 1414
Hivid Tablets (Less than 1%) 2975
HydroDIURIL Tablets 2108
Hyzaar 2109
▲ Ifex for Injection (Among most common) 1123
Imdur Tablets (Less than or equal to 5%) 1826
Imitrex Injection (Infrequent) 1549
Imitrex Nasal Spray (Infrequent) 1554
Imitrex Tablets (Infrequent) 1558
Indocin (Less than 1%) 2112
▲ Infergen (4%) 1777
Innohep Injection (Greater than or equal to 1%) 1248
▲ Intron A for Injection (Up to 12%) 3120
Invirase Capsules (Less than 2%) 2979
Ismo Tablets (Fewer than 1%) 3524
Isoptin SR Tablets (1% or less) 467
Kadian Capsules (Less than 3%) 1335
Kaletra Capsules (Less than 2%) 471
Kaletra Oral Solution (Less than 2%) 471
Keflex 1237
Keppra Tablets (1% or more) 3314
Klonopin Tablets (1%) 2983
K-Phos Neutral Tablets 946
K-Phos Original (Sodium Free) Tablets (Less frequent) 947
Lamictal (1.8%) 1567
Lanoxicaps Capsules 1574
Lanoxin Injection 1581
Lanoxin Tablets 1587
Lanoxin Elixir Pediatric 1578
Lanoxin Injection Pediatric 1584
Lariam Tablets 2989
Leukeran Tablets (Rare) 1591
Levaquin (Less than 0.3%) 2537
Levbid Extended-Release Tablets 3172
Levo-Dromoran 1734
▲ Levorphanol Tartrate Tablets (3% to 9%) 3059
Levsin/Levsinex/Levbid 3172
Lexxel Tablets 608
Librium Capsules (Some patients) 1736
Librium for Injection 1737
Lidoderm Patch 1319
Limbitrol (Less common) 1738
Lithium Carbonate 3061
Lithium Citrate Syrup 3061
Lithobid Slow-Release Tablets 3255
Lodine (Less than 1%) 3528
Lodine XL Extended-Release Tablets (Less than 1%) 3530
Lodosyn Tablets 1251
Lopid Tablets 2650
Loxitane Capsules 3398
Lupron Depot 3.75 mg 3281
Lupron Depot–4 Month 30 mg (Less than 5%) 3289
Luvox Tablets (25, 50, 100 mg) 3256
Macrobid Capsules (Rare) 2889
Macrodantin Capsules (Rare) 2891
Marinol Capsules (Greater than 1%) 3325
Matulane Capsules 3246
Maxair Autohaler 1981
Maxair Inhaler (Less than 1%) 1984
Maxalt Tablets (Infrequent) 2120
Maxalt-MLT Orally Disintegrating Tablets (Infrequent) 2120
Megace Oral Suspension (1% to 3%) 1124
Meridia Capsules 481
Merrem I.V. (0.1% to 1.0%) 673
Mexitil Capsules (1.9% to 2.6%) 1047
Midamor Tablets (Less than or equal to 1%) 2136
Migranal Nasal Spray (Infrequent) 2376
Mintezol 2137
▲ Mirapex Tablets (4% to 10%) 2834
Mobic Tablets (Less than 2%) 1054
Moduretic Tablets (Less than or equal to 1%) 2138
Monopril Tablets (0.2% to 1.0%) 1091
Monopril HCT 1094
Motofen Tablets (1 in 200 to 1 in 600) 577
Motrin Suspension, Oral Drops, Chewable Tablets, and Caplets (Less than 1%) 2002
Myambutol Tablets 1290
Mycobutin Capsules (More than one patient) 2838
Myobloc Injectable Solution (2% or greater) 1291
Naprelan Tablets (Less than 1%) 1293
Naropin Injection (Less than 1%) 612
Natrecor for Injection (At least 1%) 3189
Nebcin Vials, Hyporets & ADD-Vantage 1955
Nembutal Sodium Solution (Less than 1%) 485
Neoral Soft Gelatin Capsules (1% to less than 3%) 2380
Neoral Oral Solution (1% to less than 3%) 2380
Neptazane Tablets (Occasional) ⊙ 271
Neurontin Capsules 2655
Neurontin Oral Solution 2655
Neurontin Tablets 2655
Nexium Delayed-Release Capsules (Less than 1%) 619
▲ Nicotrol Nasal Spray (3%) 2843
Norflex (Infrequent) 1987
Noroxin Tablets 2145
Norpramin Tablets 755
Norvir Capsules (Less than 2%) 487
Norvir Oral Solution (Less than 2%) 487
Nubain Injection (1% or less) 1323
NuLev Orally Disintegrating Tablets 3176
Numorphan 1324
Oncaspar (Less than 1%) 756
Oramorph SR Tablets 3062
Orthoclone OKT3 Sterile Solution 2498
Orudis Capsules (Less than 1%) 3548
Oruvail Capsules (Less than 1%) 3548
OxyContin Tablets (Between 1% and 5%) 2912
Parnate Tablets 1607
Paxil (1%) 1609
Pepcid Injection (Infrequent) 2153
Pepcid for Oral Suspension (Infrequent) 2150
Pepcid RPD Orally Disintegrating Tablets (Infrequent) 2150
Pepcid Tablets (Infrequent) 2150
Periactin Tablets 2155
▲ Permax Tablets (11.1%) 1299
Phenergan Suppositories 3556
Phenergan Syrup (Rare) 3554
Phenergan with Codeine Syrup (Rare) 3557
Phenergan with Dextromethorphan Syrup (Rare) 3559
Phenergan VC Syrup (Rare) 3560
Phenergan VC with Codeine Syrup (Rare) 3561
PhosLo 1069
▲ Photofrin for Injection (8%) 831
Phrenilin 578
Ponstel Capsules (Occasional) 1356
Prevacid Delayed-Release Capsules (Less than 1%) 3292
PREVPAC (Less than 1% to 3%) 3298
Prilosec Delayed-Release Capsules (Less than 1%) 628
Primaxin I.M. 2158
Primaxin I.V. (Less than 0.2%) 2160
Prinivil Tablets (0.3% to 1.0%) 2164
Prinzide Tablets 2168
ProAmatine Tablets (Less frequent) 3241
▲ Prograf (3% to 15%) 1393
▲ Proleukin for Injection (34%) 1199
Prometrium Capsules (100 mg, 200 mg) (Less than 5%) 3261
ProSom Tablets (2%) 500
Protonix I.V. (Less than 1%) 3580
Protonix Tablets (Less than 1%) 3577
Provigil Tablets (1%) 1193

Prozac Pulvules, Liquid, and Weekly Capsules (Frequent) ... 1238
Quinaglute Dura-Tabs Tablets ... 978
Quinidex Extentabs ... 2933
▲ Rapamune Oral Solution and Tablets (3% to 20%) ... 3584
Reglan (Less frequent) ... 2935
Relafen Tablets (Less than 1%) ... 1617
Remeron Tablets (2%) ... 2483
Remeron SolTab Tablets (2%) ... 2486
Remicade for IV Injection (Less than 2%) ... 1178
Reminyl Oral Solution (Greater than or equal to 2%) ... 1792
Reminyl Tablets (Greater than or equal to 2%) ... 1792
ReoPro Vials (0.6%) ... 1958
▲ Requip Tablets (5%) ... 1621
Rescriptor Tablets (Less than 2%) ... 526
Retrovir Capsules ... 1625
Retrovir IV Infusion ... 1629
Retrovir ... 1625
Rifadin ... 765
Rifamate Capsules ... 767
Rifater Tablets ... 769
Rilutek Tablets (Infrequent) ... 772
Risperdal (Infrequent) ... 1796
Robaxin Injectable ... 2938
Robaxin Tablets ... 2939
Robinul Forte Tablets ... 1358
Robinul Injectable ... 2940
Robinul Tablets ... 1358
▲ Roferon-A Injection (Less than 4% to 8%) ... 2996
Romazicon Injection (Less than 1%) ... 3000
Roxanol ... 3066
Roxicodone ... 3067
Rynatan Tablets ... 3351
Rythmol Tablets – 150 mg, 225 mg, 300 mg (Less than 1%) ... 502
Salagen Tablets (Less than 1%) ... 2229
Sandimmune (2% or less) ... 2388
▲ Sandostatin LAR Depot (5% to 15%) ... 2395
Sarafem Pulvules (Frequent) ... 1962
Sedapap Tablets 50 mg/650 mg (Infrequent) ... 2225
Sensorcaine ... 643
Sensorcaine-MPF Injection ... 643
Serentil ... 1057
Seroquel Tablets (Infrequent) ... 684
▲ Serzone Tablets (7% to 8%) ... 1104
Sinemet Tablets ... 1253
▲ Sinemet CR Tablets (3.7%) ... 1255
Sinequan (Infrequent) ... 2713
Soma Tablets ... 3353
Soma Compound Tablets (Very rare) ... 3354
Soma Compound w/Codeine Tablets (Very rare) ... 3355
Sonata Capsules (Infrequent) ... 3591
▲ Stadol NS Nasal Spray (3% to 9%) ... 1108
Sular Tablets (Less than or equal to 1%) ... 688
Surmontil Capsules ... 3595
Sustiva Capsules (Less than 2%) ... 1258
Symmetrel (0.1% to 5%) ... 1328
Synercid I.V. (Less then 1%) ... 775
Tagamet (Occasional) ... 1644
Talacen Caplets ... 3089
Talwin Nx Tablets ... 3090
Tambocor Tablets (Less than 1%) ... 1990
Tamiflu Capsules ... 3008
Tamiflu Oral Suspension ... 3008
Tarka Tablets ... 508
▲ Tasmar Tablets (10% to 11%) ... 3010
Taxotere for Injection Concentrate ... 778
Tegretol/Tegretol-XR ... 2404
▲ Temodar Capsules (5%) ... 3157
Tenex Tablets (3% or less) ... 2942
Tequin Injection (Less than 0.1%) ... 1110
Tequin Tablets (Less than 0.1%) ... 1110
Tessalon Capsules ... 1377
Thalomid Capsules ... 1154
Timolide Tablets (Less than 1%) ... 2187
Timolol GFS ... ⊙ 266
Timoptic in Ocudose (Less frequent) ... 2192
Timoptic Sterile Ophthalmic Solution (Less frequent) ... 2190
Timoptic-XE Sterile Ophthalmic Gel Forming Solution ... 2194
▲ Tonocard Tablets (2.1% to 11.2%) ... 649
▲ Topamax Sprinkle Capsules (8.9% to 15%) ... 2590
▲ Topamax Tablets (8.9% to 15%) ... 2590
Toprol-XL Tablets ... 651
Transderm Scōp Transdermal Therapeutic System (Infrequent) ... 2302
Tranxene (Less common) ... 511
▲ Trasylol Injection (4%) ... 909
Trental Tablets (Less than 1%) ... 784
Tricor Capsules, Micronized (Less than 1%) ... 513
Trileptal Oral Suspension (1% to 2%) ... 2407
Trileptal Tablets (1% to 2%) ... 2407
Trilisate (Rare) ... 2901
▲ Trisenox Injection (5%) ... 1158
Trovan (Less than 1%) ... 2722
Ultracet Tablets (At least 1%) ... 2597
Ultram Tablets (1% to 5%) ... 2600
Uroqid-Acid No. 2 Tablets ... 947
Valcyte Tablets (Less than 5%) ... 3022
Valium Injectable ... 3026
Valium Tablets (Infrequent) ... 3047
Valtrex Caplets ... 1676
Vantin Tablets and Oral Suspension (Less than 1%) ... 2860
Vaseretic Tablets ... 2204
Vasotec I.V. Injection ... 2207
Vasotec Tablets (0.5% to 1%) ... 2210
Verelan Capsules (1% or less) ... 3184
Verelan PM Capsules (2% or less) ... 3186
Versed Injection (Less than 1%) ... 3027
Versed Syrup (Less than 1%) ... 3033
▲ Vesanoid Capsules (14%) ... 3037
Vicoprofen Tablets (Less than 3%) ... 520
Vioxx ... 2213
Vistide Injection ... 1445
Vivactil Tablets ... 2217
Vivactil Tablets ... 2446
▲ Wellbutrin Tablets (8.4%) ... 1680
Wellbutrin SR Sustained-Release Tablets ... 1684
▲ Xanax Tablets (9.9% to 10.4%) ... 2865
Xeloda Tablets (Less than 5%) ... 3039
▲ Xylocaine Injections (Among most common) ... 653
Zantac (Rare) ... 1690
Zantac Injection (Rare) ... 1688
Zantac Syrup (Rare) ... 1690
Zestoretic Tablets ... 695
Zestril Tablets (0.3% to 1.0%) ... 698
Zoloft (Infrequent) ... 2751
▲ Zometa for Intravenous Infusion (12.8%) ... 3621
▲ Zonegran Capsules (6%) ... 1307
Zosyn (1.0% or less) ... 1890
Zosyn in Galaxy Containers (1.0% or less) ... 1894
Zovirax Capsules ... 1706
Zovirax for Injection (Approximately 1%) ... 1708
Zovirax ... 1706
Zyban Sustained-Release Tablets (Infrequent) ... 1710
Zyprexa Tablets ... 1973
Zyprexa ZYDIS Orally Disintegrating Tablets ... 1973
Zyrtec (Less than 2%) ... 2756
Zyrtec-D 12 Hour Extended Relief Tablets (Less than 2%) ... 2758

Confusion, mental
(*see under* Confusion)

Confusion, nocturnal
Etrafon ... 3115
Thioridazine Hydrochloride Tablets (Extremely rare) ... 2289
Trilafon ... 3160

Confusional state
(*see under* Confusion)

Congelation
Eldepryl Capsules ... 3266
Gebauer's Ethyl Chloride ... 1409

Congenital anomalies
Antagon Injection ... 2447
Arthrotec Tablets ... 3195
Aygestin Tablets ... 1333
Cetrotide for Injection ... 3209
Cordarone Intravenous ... 3491
Cytotec Tablets ... 3202
Cytovene ... 2959
Depacon Injection ... 416
Depakene ... 421
Depakote Tablets ... 430
Depakote ER Tablets ... 436
Diabinese Tablets ... 2680
Effexor Tablets ... 3495
Effexor XR Capsules ... 3499
Estrace Vaginal Cream ... 3358
Estrace Tablets ... 3361
Gonal-F for Injection ... 3216
Havrix Vaccine (Rare) ... 1544
Humegon for Injection ... 2468
Innohep Injection ... 1248
Lescol Capsules (Rare) ... 2361
Lescol Capsules (Rare) ... 2925
Lescol XL Tablets ... 2361
Lescol XL Tablets ... 2925
Lo/Ovral Tablets ... 3532
Lo/Ovral-28 Tablets ... 3538
Low-Ogestrel-28 Tablets ... 3392
Mevacor Tablets (Rare) ... 2132
Nordette-28 Tablets ... 2257
Norplant System (Rare) ... 3543
Ogen Tablets ... 2846
Ogestrel 0.5/50-28 Tablets ... 3428
Ortho Dienestrol Cream ... 2554
Ortho-Est Tablets ... 3464
Ovidrel for Injection ... 3220
Ovral Tablets ... 3551
Ovral-28 Tablets ... 3552
Ovrette Tablets ... 3552
Pergonal for Injection ... 3223
Permax Tablets ... 1299
Premarin Intravenous ... 3563
Premarin Tablets ... 3566
Proventil Inhalation Aerosol ... 3142
Proventil Inhalation Solution 0.083% ... 3146
Proventil Repetabs Tablets ... 3148
Proventil Solution for Inhalation 0.5% ... 3144
Provera Tablets ... 2853
Repronex for Intramuscular and Subcutaneous Injection ... 1347
Retrovir Capsules ... 1625
Retrovir IV Infusion ... 1629
Retrovir ... 1625
Robaxin Injectable (Very rare) ... 2938
Robaxin Tablets (Very rare) ... 2939
Serophene Tablets ... 3226
Triphasil-21 Tablets ... 3600
Triphasil-28 Tablets ... 3605
Twinrix Vaccine ... 1674
Ventolin Inhalation Aerosol and Refill ... 1679
Vivelle Transdermal System ... 2412
Vivelle-Dot Transdermal System ... 2416
Xanax Tablets ... 2865
Zanaflex Tablets (Rare) ... 1305

Congenital malformation
Activella Tablets ... 2764
Ativan Injection ... 3478
Ativan Tablets ... 3482
Carbatrol Capsules ... 3234
Cerebyx Injection ... 2619
Dilantin Infatabs ... 2624
Dilantin Kapseals ... 2622
Dilantin-125 Oral Suspension ... 2625
Halcion Tablets ... 2823
Librium Capsules ... 1736
Librium for Injection ... 1737
Limbitrol ... 1738
Miltown Tablets ... 3349
Pravachol Tablets (One case) ... 1099
Premphase Tablets ... 3572
Prempro Tablets ... 3572
Tegretol/Tegretol-XR ... 2404
Tranxene ... 511
Valium Injectable ... 3026
Valium Tablets ... 3047

Congenital nevi
Cetrotide for Injection ... 3209

Congestion
Advair Diskus 100/50 (1% to 3%) ... 1448
Advair Diskus 250/50 (1% to 3%) ... 1448
Advair Diskus 500/50 (1% to 3%) ... 1448
Avalide Tablets ... 1070
Avapro Tablets (Less than 1%) ... 1074
Avapro Tablets (Less than 1%) ... 3076
Halcion Tablets (Rare) ... 2823
▲ Infergen (5% to 12%) ... 1777
Procardia Capsules (2% or less) ... 2708
Tricor Capsules, Micronized (Less than 1%) ... 513
▲ Zenapax for Injection (2% to 5%) ... 3046

Congestion, nasal
(*see under* Nasal congestion)

Congestive heart failure
Adriamycin PFS/RDF Injection ... 2767
Agrylin Capsules ... 3232
Aldoclor Tablets ... 2035
Aldomet Tablets ... 2037
Aldoril Tablets ... 2039
Aminohippurate Sodium PAH Injection ... 2041
Anaprox Tablets (Less than 1%) ... 2967
Anaprox DS Tablets (Less than 1%) ... 2967
Apligraf (1.8%) ... 2305
Aricept Tablets (Infrequent) ... 1270
Aricept Tablets (Infrequent) ... 2665
Arthrotec Tablets (Rare) ... 3195
Avonex ... 1013
Betagan ... ⊙ 228
Betoptic S Ophthalmic Suspension (Rare) ... 537
Captopril Tablets (2 to 3 of 1000 patients) ... 2281
Carbatrol Capsules ... 3234
Cardizem Injectable (Less than 1%) ... 1018
Cardizem Lyo-Ject Syringe (Less than 1%) ... 1018
Cardizem Monovial (Less than 1%) ... 1018
Cardizem CD Capsules (Less than 1%) ... 1016
Carteolol Hydrochloride Ophthalmic Solution USP, 1% ... ⊙ 258
▲ Casodex Tablets (2% to 5%) ... 662
Cataflam Tablets (Less than 1%) ... 2315
Catapres Tablets (Rare) ... 1037
Catapres-TTS (0.5% or less) ... 1038
Ceclor CD Tablets (0.1% to 1%) ... 1279
Celebrex Capsules (Less than 0.1%) ... 2676
Celebrex Capsules (Less than 0.1%) ... 2780
Celestone Soluspan Injectable Suspension ... 3097
Celestone Syrup ... 3099
▲ CellCept Capsules (3% to 10%) ... 2951
▲ CellCept Intravenous (3% to 10%) ... 2951
▲ CellCept Oral Suspension (3% to 10%) ... 2951
▲ CellCept Tablets (3% to 10%) ... 2951
Cerebyx Injection (Infrequent) ... 2619
Cerubidine for Injection ... 947
Clinoril Tablets (Less than 1%) ... 2053
Clorpres Tablets (Rare) ... 1002
Clozaril Tablets ... 2319
Combipres Tablets (Rare) ... 1040
Cordarone Intravenous (2.1%) ... 3491
Cordarone Tablets (1% to 3%) ... 3487
Cortone Acetate Injectable Suspension ... 2059
Cortone Acetate Tablets ... 2061
Corvert Injection (0.5%) ... 2793
Covera-HS Tablets (1.8% to 2%) ... 3199
DaunoXome Injection ... 1442
Decadron Elixir ... 2078
Decadron Tablets ... 2079
Decadron Phosphate Injection ... 2081
Depo-Medrol Injectable Suspension ... 2795
Digibind Powder (Few instances) ... 1514
Doxil Injection (1% to 5%) ... 566
Duraclon Injection (Rare) ... 3057
EC-Naprosyn Delayed-Release Tablets (Less than 1%) ... 2967
Effexor Tablets (Rare) ... 3495
Effexor XR Capsules (Infrequent) ... 3499
Ellence Injection (0.4% to 1.5%) ... 2806
▲ Emcyt Capsules (3%) ... 2810
Enalaprilat Injection (1.8%) ... 863
Feldene Capsules (Occasional) ... 2685
Florinef Acetate Tablets ... 2250
Fludara for Injection (Up to 3%) ... 995
▲ Herceptin I.V. (7%) ... 1414
Hivid Tablets (Infrequent) ... 2975
Hydrocortone Tablets ... 2106
Hydrocortone Acetate Injectable Suspension ... 2103
Hydrocortone Phosphate Injection, Sterile ... 2105
Idamycin PFS Injection ... 2825
Inderal ... 3513
Inderal LA Long-Acting Capsules ... 3516
Inderide Tablets ... 3517
Inderide LA Long-Acting Capsules ... 3519
Indocin Capsules (Less than 1%) ... 2112
Indocin I.V. (Less than 1%) ... 2115
Indocin (Less than 1%) ... 2112
Isoptin SR Tablets (1.8%) ... 467
Iveegam EN ... 849
Lodine (Less than 1%) ... 3528
Lodine XL Extended-Release Tablets (Less than 1%) ... 3530
Lupron Depot 7.5 mg (Less than 5%) ... 3284
Lupron Depot–3 Month 22.5 mg (Less than 5%) ... 3288
▲ Lupron Injection (5% or more) ... 3279
Luvox Tablets (25, 50, 100 mg) (Infrequent) ... 3256
Meridia Capsules ... 481
Mexitil Capsules (Less than 1%) ... 1047
Motrin Suspension, Oral Drops, Chewable Tablets, and Caplets (Less than 1%) ... 2002
▲ Naprelan Tablets (3% to 9%) ... 1293
Naprosyn Suspension (Less than 1%) ... 2967
Naprosyn Tablets (Less than 1%) ... 2967
Nimotop Capsules (Less than 1%) ... 904
Normodyne Injection ... 3135
Normodyne Tablets ... 3137
Novantrone for Injection (Up to 5%) ... 1760
Ocupress Ophthalmic Solution, 1% Sterile ... ⊙ 303
Orudis Capsules (Less than 1%) ... 3548
Oruvail Capsules (Less than 1%) ... 3548
Pacerone Tablets (1% to 3%) ... 3331
Paxil (Rare) ... 1609
Pediapred Oral Solution ... 1170
Permax Tablets (Frequent) ... 1299
Pletal Tablets (Less than 2%) ... 2605
Pletal Tablets (Less than 2%) ... 2848
Ponstel Capsules (Occasional) ... 1356
Prednisone ... 3064
Prelone Syrup ... 2273
Prevnar for Injection ... 1870
Procardia Capsules (About 2%) ... 2708
Procardia XL Extended Release Tablets (About 2%) ... 2710
Proleukin for Injection (1%) ... 1199
Protonix I.V. (Less than 1%) ... 3580
Protonix Tablets (Less than 1%) ... 3577
Prozac Pulvules, Liquid, and Weekly Capsules (Infrequent) ... 1238
▲ Rapamune Oral Solution and Tablets (3% to 20%) ... 3584
Reglan ... 2935
Retrovir Capsules (0.8%) ... 1625
Retrovir IV Infusion ... 1629
Retrovir (0.8%) ... 1625
Rilutek Tablets (Infrequent) ... 772
Roferon-A Injection (Infrequent) ... 2996
▲ Rythmol Tablets – 150 mg, 225 mg, 300 mg (1.9% to 3.7%) ... 502

Sandostatin Injection (Less than 1%) 2394
Sarafem Pulvules (Infrequent) 1962
Seroquel Tablets (Infrequent) 684
Serzone Tablets (Rare) 1104
Solu-Medrol Sterile Powder 2855
Sporanox Capsules (Rare) 1800
Sporanox Injection (Rare) 1804
Sporanox Injection (Rare) 2509
Sporanox Oral Solution (Rare) 1808
Sporanox Oral Solution (Rare) 2512
Sular Tablets (Less than or equal to 1%) 688
Symmetrel (0.1% to 1%) 1328
Tambocor Tablets 1990
Tarka Tablets 508
Taxol Injection 1129
Tegretol/Tegretol-XR 2404
Tenex Tablets (Rare) 2942
Testoderm Transdermal Systems (1%) 574
Thalomid Capsules 1154
Tiazac Capsules (Less than 2%) 1378
Tolectin (Less than 1%) 2589
▲ Tonocard Tablets (4.0%) 649
Toprol-XL Tablets (About 1 of 100 patients) 651
Trasylol Injection (1% to 2%) 909
Triostat Injection (1% or fewer) 1825
Vantin Tablets and Oral Suspension (Less than 1%) 2860
Vascor Tablets (About 1%) 2602
Vasotec I.V. Injection (1.8%) 2207
Verelan Capsules (1.8%) 3184
Verelan PM Capsules (1.8%) 3186
Vioxx (Less than 0.1%) 2213
Vistide Injection 1445
Voltaren Tablets (Less than 1%) 2315
Voltaren-XR Tablets (Less than 1%) 2315
Zebeta Tablets 1885
Ziac Tablets 1887
▲ Zoladex (5%) 702
Zoladex 3-month (1% to 5%) 706
Zyprexa Tablets (Infrequent) 1973
Zyprexa ZYDIS Orally Disintegrating Tablets (Infrequent) 1973

Conjunctiva, progressive pigmentation
Serentil 1057

Conjunctiva, sensitization
Polysporin Ophthalmic Ointment Sterile .... ⊙301

Conjunctiva, thickening
Humorsol Sterile Ophthalmic Solution 2102

Conjunctival blanching
▲ Alphagan Ophthalmic Solution (Approximately 3% to 9%) 545
Iopidine Sterile Ophthalmic Solution (Less than 2%) .... ⊙212

Conjunctival chemosis
Natacyn Antifungal Ophthalmic Suspension (One case) .... ⊙216

Conjunctival deposits
Epifrin Sterile Ophthalmic Solution .... ⊙235
Propine Ophthalmic Solution .... ⊙250

Conjunctival epithelial defects, unspecified
▲ Genoptic Ophthalmic Ointment (Among most frequent) .... ⊙239
▲ Genoptic Sterile Ophthalmic Solution (Among most frequent) .... ⊙239

Conjunctival erythema
Cortisporin Ophthalmic Suspension .... ⊙297

Conjunctival follicles
Cosopt Sterile Ophthalmic Solution (1% to 5%) 2065

Conjunctival hyperemia
▲ Ciloxan (Less than 10%) 538
▲ Cosopt Sterile Ophthalmic Solution (5% to 30%) 2065
Epifrin Sterile Ophthalmic Solution .... ⊙235
▲ Lumigan Ophthalmic Solution (15% to 45%) 553
Natacyn Antifungal Ophthalmic Suspension (One case) .... ⊙216
Ophthetic Ophthalmic Solution .... ⊙244
Pred Forte Ophthalmic Suspension (Occasional) .... ⊙246
Pred Mild Sterile Ophthalmic Suspension (Occasional) .... ⊙249
Suprane Liquid for Inhalation (Greater than 1%) 874
▲ Travatan Ophthalmic Solution (15% to 45%) 543
Vitravene for Injection (2% to 5%) .. ⊙310

Conjunctival injection
Azulfidine EN-tabs Tablets (Rare) 2775
Bactrim 2949
▲ Betimol Ophthalmic Solution (More than 5%) .... ⊙324
Cosopt Sterile Ophthalmic Solution (1% to 5%) 2065
Crolom Sterile Ophthalmic Solution USP 4% (Infrequent) .... ⊙259
Famotidine Injection (Infrequent) 866
Isopto Carbachol Ophthalmic Solution .... ⊙215
Mintezol 2137
▲ Neumega for Injection (19%) 1434
Opticrom Ophthalmic Solution (Infrequent) 555
Pediazole Suspension 3050
Pepcid Injection (Infrequent) 2153
Pepcid for Oral Suspension (Infrequent) 2150
Pepcid RPD Orally Disintegrating Tablets (Infrequent) 2150
Pepcid Tablets (Infrequent) 2150
▲ Rēv-Eyes Sterile Ophthalmic Eyedrops 0.5% (80%) .... ⊙265
Septra Suspension 2265
Septra Tablets 2265
Septra DS Tablets 2265
▲ Visudyne for Injection (1% to 10%) .... ⊙308
▲ Zaditor Ophthalmic Solution (10% to 25%) 2304

Conjunctival irritation
Efudex (Infrequent) 1733

Conjunctival microhemorrhage
Iopidine Sterile Ophthalmic Solution .... ⊙212

Conjunctival vascular congestion
Isopto Carpine Ophthalmic Solution .... ⊙215
Pilopine HS Ophthalmic Gel .... ⊙217

Conjunctivitis
Accutane Capsules 2944
Aceon Tablets (2 mg, 4 mg, 8 mg) (0.3% to 1%) 3249
Actiq (1% or greater) 1184
▲ Actonel Tablets (3.1%) 2879
Adalat CC Tablets (Less than 1.0%) 877
Adriamycin PFS/RDF Injection (Rare) 2767
Advair Diskus 100/50 (1% to 3%) 1448
Advair Diskus 250/50 (1% to 3%) 1448
Advair Diskus 500/50 (1% to 3%) 1448
▲ Alocril Ophthalmic Solution (1% to 10%) 545
Alphagan P Ophthalmic Solution (1% to 4%) 546
Alrex Sterile Ophthalmic Suspension 0.2% (Less than 5%) .... ⊙256
Ambien Tablets (Rare) 3191
AmBisome for Injection (Less common) 1383
Arava Tablets (1% to 3%) 724
Arthrotec Tablets (Rare) 3195
Asacol Delayed-Release Tablets (1% to 2%) 2884
Astelin Nasal Spray (Infrequent) 3339
Atacand HCT Tablets (0.5% or greater) 597
Atrovent Nasal Spray 0.03% (Less than 2%) 1032
Atrovent Nasal Spray 0.06% (Less than 1%) 1033
Attenuvax 2044
Avalide Tablets 1070
Avapro Tablets (Less than 1%) 1074
Avapro Tablets (Less than 1%) 3076
Avonex 1013
Axert Tablets (Rare) 2772
Azopt Ophthalmic Suspension (Less than 1%) 536
▲ Betaseron for SC Injection (12%) 988
Betimol Ophthalmic Solution .... ⊙324
Buprenex Injectable (Less than 1%) 2918
Carbatrol Capsules 3234
Cardene I.V. (Rare) 3485
Cardura Tablets (1%) 2668
Ceclor CD Tablets (0.1% to 1%) 1279
Celebrex Capsules (0.1% to 1.9%) 2676
Celebrex Capsules (0.1% to 1.9%) 2780
Celexa (Infrequent) 1365
▲ CellCept Capsules (3%) 2951
▲ CellCept Intravenous (3%) 2951
▲ CellCept Oral Suspension (3%) 2951
▲ CellCept Tablets (3%) 2951
Cerebyx Injection (Infrequent) 2619
Claritin (2%) 3100
Claritin-D 12 Hour Extended Release Tablets (Less frequent) 3102
Claritin-D 24 Hour Extended Release Tablets (Fewer than 2%) 3104
Clinoril Tablets (Less than 1 in 100) 2053
Cognex Capsules (Frequent) 1351
Colazal Capsules 3069
Comvax 2056
Copaxone for Injection (At least 2%) 3306
Cosopt Sterile Ophthalmic Solution (1% to 5%) 2065
Cozaar Tablets (Less than 1%) 2067
Crinone (Less than 5%) 3213
Cytotec Tablets (Infrequent) 3202
DaunoXome Injection (Less than or equal to 5%) 1442
DDAVP Nasal Spray (Up to 2%) 738
DDAVP Rhinal Tube (Up to 2%) 738
Depacon Injection (1% or more) 416
Depakene (1% or more) 421
Depakote Sprinkle Capsules 426
Depakote Tablets (1% to 5%) 430
Depakote ER Tablets (Greater than 1%) 436
Desmopressin Acetate Rhinal Tube (Up to 2%) 1345
Differin Cream (Less than 1%) 1402
Doxil Injection (1% to 5%) 566
Effexor Tablets (Infrequent) 3495
Effexor XR Capsules (Infrequent) 3499
Ellence Injection 2806
Elmiron Capsules (Less than or equal to 1%) 570
Enalaprilat Injection 863
Engerix-B Vaccine 1517
Ergamisol Tablets (Less than 1% to 2%) 1789
▲ Evoxac Capsules (4.3%) 1217
Felbatol 3343
Feldene Capsules (Rare) 2685
Flonase Nasal Spray 1533
Flovent Diskus (1% to 3%) 3614
Flovent Rotadisk (1% to 3%) 1537
Floxin I.V. 2526
Floxin Tablets 2529
FML Ophthalmic Ointment (Occasional) .... ⊙237
FML Ophthalmic Suspension (Occasional) .... ⊙236
FML Forte Ophthalmic Suspension (Occasional) .... ⊙235
Fortovase Capsules (Less than 2%) 2970
Foscavir Injection (Between 1% and 5%) 605
Gabitril Tablets (1% or more) 1189
Gengraf Capsules (1% to less than 3%) 457
▲ Genoptic Ophthalmic Ointment (Among most frequent) .... ⊙239
▲ Genoptic Sterile Ophthalmic Solution (Among most frequent) .... ⊙239
Geodon Capsules (Infrequent) 2688
Glucotrol XL Extended Release Tablets (Less than 1%) 2693
Hectorol Capsules 1064
Hectorol Injection 1066
Hytrin Capsules (At least 1%) 464
Hyzaar 2109
Imdur Tablets (Less than or equal to 5%) 1826
Imitrex Injection 1549
Imitrex Nasal Spray 1554
Indapamide Tablets (Less than 5%) 2286
▲ Infergen (4% to 8%) 1777
Intron A for Injection (Less than 5%) 3120
Iopidine 0.5% Ophthalmic Solution (Less than 3%) .... ⊙213
Kadian Capsules (Less than 3%) 1335
Lamictal (Infrequent) 1567
Levaquin Injection (Less than 0.5%) 2537
Loxxel Tablets (Infrequent) 608
Lodine (Less than 1%) 3528
Lodine XL Extended-Release Tablets (Less than 1%) 3530
Lotemax Sterile Ophthalmic Suspension 0.5% (Less than 5%) .... ⊙261
Lotensin HCT Tablets (0.3% or more) 2367
Lupron Depot 3.75 mg (Less than 5%) 3281
Lupron Depot–3 Month 11.25 mg (Less than 5%) 3285
Luvox Tablets (25, 50, 100 mg) (Infrequent) 3256
Luxiq Foam (One patient) 1210
Marinol Capsules (0.3% to 1%) 3325
Meruvax II 2130
Miacalcin Nasal Spray (1% to 3%) 2375
Micardis Tablets (More than 0.3%) .. 1049
Micardis HCT Tablets 1051
Migranal Nasal Spray (Infrequent) 2376
Mirapex Tablets (1% or more) 2834
M-M-R II 2118
Mobic Tablets (Less than 2%) 1054
Motrin Suspension, Oral Drops, Chewable Tablets, and Caplets (Less than 1%) 2002
Mumpsvax 2141
Naprelan Tablets (Less than 1%) 1293
Nasonex Nasal Spray (Greater than or equal to 2%) 3131
Neoral Soft Gelatin Capsules (1% to less than 3%) 2380
Neoral Oral Solution (1% to less than 3%) 2380
Neurontin Capsules (Infrequent) 2655
Neurontin Oral Solution (Infrequent) 2655
Neurontin Tablets (Infrequent) 2655
Nexium Delayed-Release Capsules (Less than 1%) 619
▲ Nipent for Injection (4%) 3272
Norvasc Tablets (More than 0.1% to 1%) 2704
Novantrone for Injection (Up to 5%) 1760
Ocuflox Ophthalmic Solution 554
Omnicef 493
OptiPranolol Metipranolol Ophthalmic Solution 0.3% (A small number of patients) .... ⊙263
▲ Optivar Ophthalmic Solution (1% to 10%) 2273
Orthoclone OKT3 Sterile Solution 2498
Orudis Capsules (Less than 1%) 3548
Oruvail Capsules (Less than 1%) 3548
Ovide Lotion 2023
Paxil (Infrequent) 1609
Pentasa Capsules (Less than 1%) 3239
Permax Tablets (Infrequent) 1299
Plavix Tablets (1% to 2.5%) 1097
Plavix Tablets (1% to 2.5%) 3084
Pletal Tablets (Less than 2%) 2605
Pletal Tablets (Less than 2%) 2848
Ponstel Capsules (Rare) 1356
Pred Forte Ophthalmic Suspension (Occasional) .... ⊙246
Pred Mild Sterile Ophthalmic Suspension (Occasional) .... ⊙249
Prevnar for Injection 1870
▲ Proleukin for Injection (4%) 1199
Protopic Ointment (2% to 4%) 1397
Prozac Pulvules, Liquid, and Weekly Capsules (Infrequent) 1238
Pulmicort Respules (Less than 1% to 4%) 632
Pulmozyme Inhalation Solution (1% to 5%) 1426
▲ Rapamune Oral Solution and Tablets (3% to 20%) 3584
Recombivax HB 2178
Remeron Tablets (Infrequent) 2483
Remeron SolTab Tablets (Infrequent) 2486
Requip Tablets (Infrequent) 1621
Rescriptor Tablets (Less than 2%) 526
Rescula Ophthalmic Solution (1% to 5%) .... ⊙306
Rifadin (Occasional) 765
Rifater Tablets (Occasional) 769
Rituxan for Infusion (1% to 5%) 1750
Rituxan I.V. (1% to 5%) 1428
Robaxin Injectable 2938
Robaxin Tablets 2939
Rocaltrol 2991
▲ Roferon-A Injection (4%) 2996
Salagen Tablets (2%) 2229
Sandimmune (2% or less) 2388
Sarafem Pulvules (Infrequent) 1962
Sectral Capsules (Up to 2%) 3589
Seroquel Tablets (Infrequent) 684
Serzone Tablets (Infrequent) 1104
▲ Simulect for Injection (3% to 10%) .. 2399
Skelid Tablets (2.7%) 3088
Sonata Capsules (Frequent) 3591
▲ Soriatane Capsules (1% to 10%) 3003
Stromectol Tablets 2185
Sular Tablets (Less than or equal to 1%) 688
Suprane Liquid for Inhalation (Greater than 1%) 874
Synagis Intramuscular (More than 1%) 2028
Tamiflu Capsules (1%) 3008
Tamiflu Oral Suspension (1%) 3008
Tegretol/Tegretol-XR 2404
Tenex Tablets (3% or less) 2942
Teveten Tablets (Less than 1%) 3327
TheraCys Injection 823
Thioplex for Injection 1765
Tiazac Capsules (2%) 1378
Timolol GFS (1% to 5%) .... ⊙266
Timoptic in Ocudose (Less frequent) 2192
Timoptic Sterile Ophthalmic Solution (Less frequent) 2190
Timoptic-XE Sterile Ophthalmic Gel Forming Solution (1% to 5%) .. 2194
Topamax Sprinkle Capsules (Frequent) 2590
Topamax Tablets (Frequent) 2590
Travatan Ophthalmic Solution (1% to 4%) 543
Trental Tablets (Less than 1%) 784
Tricor Capsules, Micronized (1%) 513
Tri-Nasal Spray (1.3% to 4.4%) 2274
Trizivir Tablets 1669
Trovan (Less than 1%) 2722

Trusopt Sterile Ophthalmic Solution (Approximately 1% to 5%) 2196
Twinrix Vaccine 1674
Uniretic Tablets (Less than 1%) 3178
Vancenase AQ Nasal Spray 0.084% (2%) 3163
Vaseretic Tablets 2204
Vasotec I.V. Injection 2207
Vasotec Tablets (0.5% to 1.0%) 2210
Viagra Tablets (Less than 2%) 2732
Vioxx (Greater than 0.1% to 1.9%) 2213
Viramune Oral Suspension 1060
Viramune Tablets 1060
Virazole for Inhalation Solution 1747
Vistide Injection 1445
▲ Visudyne for Injection (1% to 10%) ⊙ 308
Vitravene for Injection (2% to 5%) ⊙ 310
Voltaren Ophthalmic Sterile Ophthalmic Solution (Less than 5%) ⊙ 312
Xalatan Latanoprost Ophthalmic Solution (Less than 1%) ⊙ 320
Xalatan Sterile Ophthalmic Solution (Less than 1%) 2864
Zaditor Ophthalmic Solution (Less than 5%) 2304
Zanaflex Tablets (Infrequent) 1305
Ziagen 1692
Zithromax Capsules, 250 mg (1% or less) 2743
Zithromax for Oral Suspension, 300 mg, 600 mg, 900 mg, 1200 mg (1% or less) 2739
Zithromax Tablets, 250 mg (1% or less) 2739
Zoloft (Infrequent) 2751
Zonegran Capsules (Infrequent) 1307
Zosyn (1.0% or less) 1890
Zosyn in Galaxy Containers (1.0% or less) 1894
Zyflo Filmtab Tablets (Less common) 524
Zyprexa Tablets 1973
Zyprexa ZYDIS Orally Disintegrating Tablets 1973
Zyrtec (Less than 2%) 2756
Zyrtec-D 12 Hour Extended Relief Tablets (Less than 2%) 2758

Conjunctivitis, allergic
▲ Alphagan P Ophthalmic Solution (Approximately 10% to 20%) 546
Lumigan Ophthalmic Solution (1% to 3%) 553

Conjunctivitis, calcific
Calcijex Injection 411

Conjunctivitis, exudative
Rifamate Capsules (Occasional) 767

Conjunctivitis, follicular
▲ Alphagan Ophthalmic Solution (Approximately 10% to 30%) 545
▲ Alphagan P Ophthalmic Solution (Approximately 5% to 9%) 546
Propine Ophthalmic Solution ⊙ 250

Conjunctivitis, hemorrhagic
Alphagan Ophthalmic Solution (Less than 3%) 545
Alphagan P Ophthalmic Solution (1% to 4%) 546

Conjunctivitis, mucopurulent
Hivid Tablets (Less than 1%) 2975

Conjunctivitis sicca
Orudis Capsules (Less than 1%) 3548
Oruvail Capsules (Less than 1%) 3548

Consciousness, disorders of
Amerge Tablets (Rare) 1467
▲ Betapace Tablets (2% to 4%) 950
Comtan Tablets 2328
Hexalen Capsules 2226
Intron A for Injection (Less than 5%) 3120
Neoral Soft Gelatin Capsules 2380
Neoral Oral Solution 2380
Permax Tablets 1299
Reglan 2935
Sandimmune 2388
Symmetrel (Uncommon) 1328
Tasmar Tablets (Four cases) 3010
Valtrex Caplets 1676
Zovirax 1706

Consciousness, loss of
Acthrel for Injection (Two patients) 3629
Cipro I.V. (1% or less) 893
Cipro 887
Duranest Injections 600
Effexor Tablets (Rare) 3495
Effexor XR Capsules (Rare) 3499
Emla (Unlikely with cream) 602
Floxin I.V. 2526
Floxin Tablets 2529
Fortovase Capsules (Less than 2%) 2970
INFeD Injection 3388
Invirase Capsules (Less than 2%) 2979
Lidoderm Patch 1319
Mexitil Capsules (Less than 1% or about 6 in 10,000) 1047
Naropin Injection 612
Nesacaine/Nesacaine MPF 617
Noroxin Tablets 2145
Omnicef 493
Orthoclone OKT3 Sterile Solution 2498
PEG-Intron Powder for Injection (Less than or equal to 1%) 3140
Polocaine Injection, USP 625
Polocaine-MPF Injection, USP 625
Prostigmin Injectable 1744
Prostigmin Tablets 1744
Sensorcaine 643
Sensorcaine-MPF Injection 643
Stelazine Tablets 1640
TYPHIM Vi Vaccine 825
Venofer Injection (8 patients) 580
▲ Vesanoid Capsules (3%) 3037
Xeloda Tablets (Less than 5%) 3039
▲ Xylocaine Injections (Among most common) 653

Constipation
Accupril Tablets (0.5% to 1.0%) 2611
Accuretic Tablets (Greater than 0.5%) 2614
Aceon Tablets (2 mg, 4 mg, 8 mg) (0.3% to 1%) 3249
Aciphex Tablets 1267
Aciphex Tablets 1783
Actiq (1% to 4%) 1184
▲ Actonel Tablets (6.6%) 2879
Adalat CC Tablets (1% to 3% or less) 877
Adderall Tablets 3231
Adderall XR Capsules
Adipex-P 1406
Advair Diskus 100/50 (1% to 3%) 1448
Advair Diskus 250/50 (1% to 3%) 1448
Advair Diskus 500/50 (1% to 3%) 1448
Aerobid/Aerobid-M (1% to 3%) 1363
Agrylin Capsules (1% to 5%) 3232
Akineton 402
Aldoclor Tablets 2035
Aldomet Tablets 2037
Aldoril Tablets 2039
Alferon N Injection (One patient) 1770
Aloprim for Injection (Less than 1%) 2292
Altace Capsules (Less than 1%) 2233
Ambien Tablets (Infrequent) 3191
AmBisome for Injection (Less common) 1383
Amerge Tablets (Infrequent) 1467
Amphojel Suspension (Mint Flavor) ▣ 789
Amphotec (1% to 5%) 1774
▲ Anaprox Tablets (3% to 9%) 2967
▲ Anaprox DS Tablets (3% to 9%) 2967
Anzemet Injection (Rare) 719
Anzemet Tablets (Rare) 722
Arava Tablets (1% to 3%) 724
▲ Aredia for Injection (33.2%) 2309
▲ Arimidex Tablets (6.9% to 9.3%) 659
▲ Aromasin Tablets (5%) 2769
Artane 1855
Arthrotec Tablets (Rare) 3195
▲ Asacol Delayed-Release Tablets (5%) 2884
Astelin Nasal Spray (Infrequent) 3339
Astramorph/PF Injection, USP (Preservative-Free) 594
Atacand HCT Tablets 597
Atrovent Inhalation Aerosol (Less frequent) 1030
Atrovent Inhalation Solution (0.9%) 1031
Atrovent Nasal Spray 0.03% 1032
Atrovent Nasal Spray 0.06% 1033
Avalide Tablets 1070
Avapro Tablets (Less than 1%) 1074
Avapro Tablets (Less than 1%) 3076
Avelox Tablets (0.05% to 1%) 879
Avonex 1013
Axid Pulvules (2.5%) 1903
Axid Pulvules (2.5%) 2919
Baycol Tablets (2.2%) 883
Benadryl Parenteral 2617
▲ Betaseron for SC Injection (24%) 988
Betaxon Ophthalmic Suspension (Less than 2%) 537
Bontril Slow-Release Capsules 576
Brevibloc Injection (Less than 1%) 858
Buprenex Injectable (Less than 1%) 2918
Calcijex Injection 411
▲ Campath Ampules (1% to 9%) 992
Captopril Tablets (About 0.5% to 2%) 2281
Carafate Suspension (2%) 731
Carafate Tablets (2%) 730
Carbatrol Capsules 3234
Cardizem Injectable (Less than 1%) 1018
Cardizem Lyo-Ject Syringe (Less than 1%) 1018
Cardizem Monovial (Less than 1%) 1018
Cardizem CD Capsules (Less than 1%) 1016
Cardura Tablets (1%) 2668
▲ Carnitor Injection (3%) 3242
▲ Casodex Tablets (17%) 662
▲ Cataflam Tablets (3% to 9%) 2315
▲ Catapres Tablets (About 10 in 100 patients) 1037
Catapres-TTS (1 of 101 patients) 1038
Ceclor CD Tablets (0.1% to 1%) 1279
Cedax Capsules (0.1% to 1%) 1021
Celebrex Capsules (0.1% to 1.9%) 2676
Celebrex Capsules (0.1% to 1.9%) 2780
Celexa (At least 2%) 1365
▲ CellCept Capsules (18.5% to 41.2%) 2951
▲ CellCept Intravenous (18.5% to 41.2%) 2951
▲ CellCept Oral Suspension (18.5% to 41.2%) 2951
▲ CellCept Tablets (18.5% to 41.2%) 2951
Celontin Capsules (Frequent) 2618
▲ Cenestin Tablets (6%) 1263
Cerebyx Injection (Frequent) 2619
Chirocaine Injection (2.8%) 2909
New Formulation Chromagen OB Capsules 3094
Cipro I.V. (1% or less) 893
Cipro I.V. Pharmacy Bulk Package (Less than 1%) 897
Cipro 887
Claritin (At least one patient) 3100
Claritin-D 12 Hour Extended Release Tablets (Less frequent) 3102
Claritin-D 24 Hour Extended Release Tablets (Fewer than 2%) 3104
Cleocin Vaginal Cream (Less than 1%) 2788
▲ Clinoril Tablets (3% to 9%) 2053
Clomid Tablets (Fewer than 1%) 735
▲ Clorpres Tablets (About 10%) 1002
▲ Clozaril Tablets (More than 5% to 14%) 2319
Cogentin 2055
▲ Cognex Capsules (4%) 1351
Colazal Capsules (1%) 3069
▲ Colestid Tablets (Among most common) 2791
CombiPatch Transdermal System (2% to 5%) 2323
▲ Combipres Tablets (About 10%) 1040
Combivent Inhalation Aerosol 1041
Compazine 1505
▲ Comtan Tablets (6%) 2328
Copaxone for Injection (At least 2%) 3306
▲ Cordarone Tablets (4% to 9%) 3487
Corgard Tablets (1 to 5 per 1000 patients) 2245
Corlopam Injection (2%) 412
Corzide 40/5 Tablets (1 to 5 of 1000 patients) 2247
Corzide 80/5 Tablets (1 to 5 of 1000 patients) 2247
▲ Covera-HS Tablets (7.2% to 11.7%) 3199
Cozaar Tablets (Less than 1%) 2067
▲ Creon 5 Capsules (Among most frequent) 3251
▲ Creon 10 Capsules (Among most frequent) 3251
▲ Creon 20 Capsules (Among most frequent) 3251
▲ Crinone 8% Gel (27%) 3213
Crixivan Capsules (Less than 2%) 2070
Cytotec Tablets (1.1%) 3202
Cytovene (At least 3 subjects) 2959
Dantrium Capsules (Less frequent) 2885
Daranide Tablets 2077
Darvon-N/Darvocet-N 1907
Darvon Pulvules 1909
Darvon Compound-65 Pulvules 1910
Darvon-N Tablets 1912
▲ DaunoXome Injection (Up to 7%) 1442
Demadex Tablets and Injection (1.8%) 2965
Demerol 3079
Depacon Injection (Up to 5%) 416
▲ Depakene (5%) 421
▲ Depakote Sprinkle Capsules (5%) 426
Depakote Tablets (1% to 5%) 430
Depakote ER Tablets (1% to 5%) 436
▲ DepoCyt Injection (7%) 1197
Desoxyn Tablets 440
▲ Detrol Tablets (6.5%) 3623
▲ Detrol LA Capsules (6%) 2801
Dexedrine 1512
DextroStat Tablets 3236
Dilantin Infatabs 2624
Dilantin Kapseals 2622
Dilantin-125 Oral Suspension 2625
Dilaudid 441
Dilaudid Oral Liquid 445
Dilaudid Powder 441
Dilaudid Rectal Suppositories 441
Dilaudid Tablets 441
Dilaudid Tablets - 8 mg 445
Dilaudid-HP (Less frequent) 443
Diovan Capsules 2337
Diovan HCT Tablets (Greater than 0.2%) 2338
▲ Ditropan XL Extended Release Tablets (13.1%) 564
Diucardin Tablets 3494
Diuril Oral 2087
Diuril Sodium Intravenous 2086
Dolobid Tablets (Greater than 1 in 100) 2088
Dolophine Hydrochloride Tablets 3056
Donnatal 2929
Donnatal Extentabs 2930
Donnatal Tablets 2929
▲ Dostinex Tablets (7% to 10%) 2804
▲ Doxil Injection (1% to 12.7%) 566
DuoNeb Inhalation Solution (More than 1%) 1233
▲ Duraclon Injection (2.6% to 6%) 3057
▲ Duragesic Transdermal System (10% or more) 1786
Duramorph Injection (Frequent) 1312
Dyazide Capsules 1515
Dynabac Tablets (0.1% to 1%) 2269
DynaCirc Capsules (0.5% to 1%) 2921
DynaCirc CR Tablets (1.2% to 3.8%) 2923
▲ EC-Naprosyn Delayed-Release Tablets (3% to 9%) 2967
▲ Effexor Tablets (15%) 3495
▲ Effexor XR Capsules (8% to 12%) 3499
Eldepryl Capsules 3266
Elmiron Capsules (Less than or equal to 1%) 570
Enalaprilat Injection (0.5% to 1%) 863
Engerix-B Vaccine (Less than 1%) 1517
▲ Epogen for Injection (42% to 43%) 582
Ergamisol Tablets (2% to 3%) 1789
Etrafon (Occasional) 3115
Evoxac Capsules (1% to 3%) 1217
▲ Exelon Capsules (5%) 2342
▲ Exelon Oral Solution (5%) 2345
Extendryl 1361
Famotidine Injection (1.2%) 866
Famvir Tablets (1.4% to 4.4%) 2348
Fareston Tablets 3237
▲ Felbatol (6.9% to 12.9%) 3343
▲ Feldene Capsules (1% to 10%) 2685
▲ Femara Tablets (5% to 9%) 2351
▲ femhrt Tablets (3.1%) 2635
Feosol Caplets (Occasional) 1717
Feosol Tablets (Occasional) 1717
Flexeril Tablets (1% to 3%) 572
Flexeril Tablets (1% to 3%) 2094
▲ Flolan for Injection (4% to 6%) 1528
Flomax Capsules (Infrequent) 1044
Floxin I.V. (1% to 3%) 2526
Floxin Tablets (1% to 3%) 2529
Fludara for Injection (1% to 3%) 995
Flumadine 1370
▲ Fortovase Capsules (3.3%) 2970
Fosamax Tablets (0.6% to 3.1%) 2095
Foscavir Injection (Between 1% and 5%) 605
Furosemide Tablets 2284
Gabitril Tablets (1% or more) 1189
Gastrocrom Oral Concentrate 1162
▲ Gemzar for Injection (10% to 31%) 1919
Gengraf Capsules (1% to less than 3%) 457
▲ Geodon Capsules (9%) 2688
▲ Gleevec Capsules (4% to 13%) 2357
Gliadel Wafer (2%) 1723
Glucophage Tablets (1% to 5%) 1080
Glucophage XR Tablets (1% to 5%) 1080
Glucotrol Tablets (1 in 100) 2692
Glucotrol XL Extended Release Tablets (Less than 3%) 2693
Halcion Tablets (Rare) 2823
Haldol Decanoate 2535
Haldol Injection, Tablets and Concentrate 2533
▲ Hectorol Capsules (3.3%) 1064
▲ Hectorol Injection (3.3%) 1066
Helixate Concentrate 788
Hivid Tablets (Less than 1% to 2.5%) 2975
▲ Hycamtin for Injection (Less than 1% to 39%) 1546
Hycodan 1316
HydroDIURIL Tablets 2108
Hytrin Capsules (At least 1%) 464
Hyzaar 2109
Ifex for Injection (Less than 1%) 1123
Imdur Tablets (Less than or equal to 5%) 1826
Imitrex Nasal Spray (Infrequent) 1554
Imitrex Tablets (Infrequent) 1558
Indapamide Tablets (Less than 5%) 2286
Inderal 3513
Inderal LA Long-Acting Capsules 3516
Inderide Tablets 3517
Inderide LA Long-Acting Capsules 3519
Indocin Capsules (Greater than 1%) 2112
Indocin I.V. (1% to 3%) 2115
Indocin (Greater than 1%) 2112
▲ Infergen (5% to 9%) 1777
Infumorph 200 and Infumorph 500 Sterile Solutions (Frequent) 1314

Innohep Injection (1.3%)........ 1248
▲ Intron A for Injection (Up to 10%) 3120
Inversine Tablets........ 1850
Invirase Capsules (Less than 2%).... 2979
Ionamin Capsules........ 1163
Iopidine 0.5% Ophthalmic Solution (Less than 3%)........ ⊙213
▲ Isoptin SR Tablets (7.3%) 467
▲ Kadian Capsules (Virtually all patients)........ 1335
Kaletra Capsules (Less than 2%)..... 471
Kaletra Oral Solution (Less than 2%)........ 471
Keppra Tablets (1% or more)........ 3314
Klonopin Tablets (2%)........ 2983
Kogenate FS........ 936
▲ Kytril Injection (3%) 2986
▲ Kytril Tablets (3% to 18%) 2988
▲ Lamictal (4.1% to 5%) 1567
▲ Lescol Capsules (3.1%) 2361
▲ Lescol Capsules (3.1%) 2925
Lescol XL Tablets (2.3%) 2361
Lescol XL Tablets (2.3%) 2925
▲ Leukine (8%)........ 1755
▲ Leustatin Injection (9%) 2495
Levaquin (0.1% to 3.1%)........ 2537
Levsin/Levsinex/Levbid 3172
Lexxel Tablets 608
Librium Capsules (Isolated cases) .. 1736
Librium for Injection (Isolated instances)........ 1737
▲ Limbitrol (Among most frequent) 1738
Lipitor Tablets (Up to 2.5%) 2639
Lipitor Tablets (Up to 2.5%) 2696
Lodine (1% to 3%) 3528
▲ Lodine XL Extended-Release Tablets (1% to 10%) 3530
Lodosyn Tablets 1251
Lopid Tablets (1.4%) 2650
Lortab 3319
Lortab Elixir 3317
Lotensin Tablets (Less than 1%) 2365
Lotensin HCT Tablets (0.3% to 1%)........ 2367
Lotrel Capsules 2370
Loxitane Capsules 3398
▲ Lupron Injection (5% or more) 3279
▲ Luvox Tablets (25, 50, 100 mg) (10%) 3256
Macrobid Capsules (Less than 1%) 2889
Matulane Capsules 3246
Mavik Tablets (0.3% to 1.0%) 478
Maxalt Tablets (Infrequent) 2120
Maxalt-MLT Orally Disintegrating Tablets (Infrequent) 2120
Maxidone Tablets CIII 3399
Maxzide 1008
Megace Oral Suspension (1% to 3%) 1124
Mepergan Injection 3539
▲ Mepron Suspension (3%) 1598
▲ Meridia Capsules (11.5%) 481
Merrem I.V. (1.2%) 673
▲ Mevacor Tablets (2.0% to 4.9%) 2132
▲ Mexitil Capsules (4%) 1047
Miacalcin Nasal Spray (1% to 3%) 2375
Micardis Tablets (More than 0.3%) .. 1049
Micardis HCT Tablets 1051
Microzide Capsules 3414
Midamor Tablets (Between 1% and 3%) 2136
Minipress Capsules (1% to 4%) 2699
Minizide Capsules (Rare) 2700
▲ Mirapex Tablets (10% to 14%) 2834
Moban 1320
Mobic Tablets (0.8% to 1.8%) 1054
Moduretic Tablets (Less than or equal to 1%) 2138
Monopril Tablets (0.2% to 1.0%) 1091
Monopril HCT 1094
Monurol Sachet (Less than 1%) 1375
Motofen Tablets (1 in 300) 577
Motrin Suspension, Oral Drops, Chewable Tablets, and Caplets (1% to less than 3%) 2002
▲ MS Contin Tablets (Less frequent to among most frequent) 2896
▲ MSIR (Among most frequent) 2898
Mykrox Tablets (Less than 2%) 1168
Mylocel Tablets (Less frequently) 2227
▲ Mylotarg for Injection (22% to 36%) 3540
Nadolol Tablets (1 to 5 of 1000 patients) 2288
▲ Naprelan Tablets (3% to 9%) 1293
▲ Naprosyn Suspension (3% to 9%) .. 2967
▲ Naprosyn Tablets (3% to 9%) 2967
Nardil Tablets (Common) 2653
Navane Oral 2701
Navane Intramuscular 2703
▲ Navelbine Injection (Up to 29%) 1604
Nembutal Sodium Solution (Less than 1%) 485
Neoral Soft Gelatin Capsules (1% to less than 3%) 2380
Neoral Oral Solution (1% to less than 3%) 2380
▲ Neumega for Injection (Greater than or equal to 10%) 1434
▲ Neupogen for Injection (5%) 587
Neurontin Capsules (1.5%) 2655
Neurontin Oral Solution (1.5%) 2655
Neurontin Tablets (1.5%)........ 2655
Nexium Delayed-Release Capsules (Greater than or equal to 1%)........ 619
Nicotrol Nasal Spray (Common)...... 2843
▲ Nilandron Tablets (19.6%) 753
Nipent for Injection (Less than 3%)........ 3272
Norco 5/325 Tablets CIII........ 3424
Norco 7.5/325 Tablets CIII........ 3425
Norco 10/325 Tablets CIII........ 3425
Norco 10/325 Tablets CIII........ 3427
Norflex........ 1987
Noroxin Tablets (0.3% to 1.0%)....... 2145
Norpramin Tablets........ 755
Norvasc Tablets (More than 0.1% to 1%)........ 2704
▲ Novantrone for Injection (10% to 14%)........ 1760
NuLev Orally Disintegrating Tablets........ 3176
Numorphan........ 1324
Omnicef (0.3%)........ 493
Oncaspar (Less than 1%)........ 756
▲ Oramorph SR Tablets (Among most frequent)........ 3062
▲ Orap Tablets (4 of 20 patients) 1407
▲ Orgaran Injection (3.5% to 11.3%) . 2480
▲ Orudis Capsules (3% to 9%) 3548
▲ Oruvail Capsules (3% to 9%) 3548
▲ OxyContin Tablets (23%) 2912
OxyFast Oral Concentrate Solution........ 2916
OxyIR Capsules 2916
▲ Pacerone Tablets (4% to 9%) 3331
▲ Pancrease Capsules (Among most frequent)........ 2580
▲ Pancrease MT Capsules (Among most frequent)........ 2581
▲ Paraplatin for Injection (6%) 1126
Parnate Tablets 1607
▲ Paxil (1.1% to 16%) 1609
Pentasa Capsules (Less than 1%)... 3239
Pepcid Injection (1.2%)........ 2153
Pepcid for Oral Suspension (1.2%)........ 2150
Pepcid RPD Orally Disintegrating Tablets (1.2%)........ 2150
Pepcid Tablets (1.2%)........ 2150
Percocet Tablets........ 1326
Percodan Tablets........ 1327
Percolone Tablets........ 1327
Periactin Tablets........ 2155
▲ Permax Tablets (10.6%; frequent) .. 1299
Phenergan with Codeine Syrup 3557
Phenergan VC with Codeine Syrup .. 3561
PhosLo 1069
▲ Photofrin for Injection (24%) 831
Phrenilin (Infrequent)........ 578
Plavix Tablets (1% to 2.5%)........ 1097
Plavix Tablets (1% to 2.5%)........ 3084
Plendil Extended-Release Tablets (0.3% to 1.5%)........ 623
▲ Ponstel Capsules (1% to 10%) 1356
Prandin Tablets (0.5, 1, and 2 mg) (2% to 3%)........ 2432
▲ Pravachol Tablets (2.4% to 4.0%) .. 1099
Prevacid Delayed-Release Capsules (Less than 1%)........ 3292
PREVPAC (Less than 1%)........ 3298
Priftin Tablets (Less than 1%)........ 758
Prilosec Delayed-Release Capsules (1.1% to 1.5%)........ 628
Prinivil Tablets (0.3% to 1.0%)........ 2164
Prinzide Tablets (0.3% to 1%)........ 2168
Procardia Capsules (2% or less)...... 2708
▲ Procardia XL Extended Release Tablets (3.3%)........ 2710
▲ Procrit for Injection (42% to 53%) .. 2502
▲ Prograf (23% to 35%) 1393
▲ Proleukin for Injection (5%) 1199
Prometrium Capsules (100 mg, 200 mg) (Less than 5%)........ 3261
ProSom Tablets (Frequent) 500
Protonix I.V. (Greater than or equal to 1%)........ 3580
Protonix Tablets (Greater than or equal to 1%)........ 3577
Protopic Ointment (Greater than or equal to 1%)........ 1397
Provigil Tablets (At least 1%)........ 1193
Prozac Pulvules, Liquid, and Weekly Capsules (Less than 1%)........ 1238
▲ Rapamune Oral Solution and Tablets (28% to 38%)........ 3584
Recombivax HB........ 2178
ReFacto Vials........ 1437
▲ Relafen Tablets (3% to 9%) 1617
▲ Remeron Tablets (13%) 2483
▲ Remeron SolTab Tablets (13%) 2486
Reminyl Oral Solution (Greater than or equal to 2%)........ 1792
Reminyl Tablets (Greater than or equal to 2%)........ 1792
Renagel Capsules (2%)........ 1439
Renagel Tablets (2%)........ 1439
Renese Tablets........ 2712
ReoPro Vials (0.3%)........ 1958
▲ Requip Tablets (6%) 1621
Rescriptor Tablets (Less than 2%).... 526
▲ Retrovir Capsules (6.4%) 1625
▲ Retrovir IV Infusion (6.4%) 1629
▲ Retrovir (6.4%) 1625
Rilutek Tablets (More than 2%)........ 772
▲ Risperdal (7% to 13%) 1796
Robaxisal Tablets 2939
Robinul Forte Tablets........ 1358
Robinul Injectable........ 2940
Robinul Tablets........ 1358
Robitussin A-C Syrup........ 2942
Robitussin-DAC Syrup........ 2942
Rocaltrol........ 2991
Roferon-A Injection (Less than 3%).. 2996
Rowasa Rectal Suspension Enema 4.0 grams/unit (60 mL) (0.98%)........ 3264
Roxanol........ 3066
Roxicodone........ 3067
Ryna-C Liquid........ ▣ 768
Rynatan Tablets........ 3351
▲ Rythmol Tablets – 150 mg, 225 mg, 300 mg (4.0% to 8%).... 502
Salagen Tablets (1% to 2%)........ 2229
Sandimmune (Rare)........ 2388
▲ Sandostatin Injection (Less than 10%)........ 2394
▲ Sandostatin LAR Depot (18.8%) 2395
▲ Sarafem Pulvules (5%) 1962
▲ Sectral Capsules (4%) 3589
Sedapap Tablets 50 mg/650 mg (Infrequent)........ 2225
Serentil........ 1057
Serevent Inhalation Aerosol (1% to 3%)........ 1633
▲ Seroquel Tablets (9%) 684
▲ Serostim for Injection (1% to 10%) . 3229
▲ Serzone Tablets (10% to 17%) 1104
▲ Simulect for Injection (Greater than or equal to 10%)........ 2399
Sinemet Tablets........ 1253
Sinemet CR Tablets (0.2%)........ 1255
Sinequan........ 2713
Skelid Tablets (More than or equal to 1%)........ 3088
▲ Soma Compound Tablets (Among most common)........ 3354
Soma Compound w/Codeine Tablets........ 3355
Sonata Capsules (Frequent)........ 3591
Soriatane Capsules (Less than 1%)........ 3003
Sporanox Capsules (Infrequent; 2%)........ 1800
Sporanox Injection (Less than 1%).. 1804
Sporanox Injection (Less than 1%).. 2509
Sporanox Oral Solution (2.0% to 2.2%)........ 1808
Sporanox Oral Solution (2.0% to 2.2%)........ 2512
▲ Stadol NS Nasal Spray (3% to 9%) . 1108
Stelazine........ 1640
Stromectol Tablets (0.9%)........ 2185
Surmontil Capsules........ 3595
Sustiva Capsules........ 1258
Symmetrel (1% to 5%)........ 1328
Synercid I.V. (Less than 1%)........ 775
Talacen Caplets (Infrequent)........ 3089
Talwin Nx Tablets........ 3090
▲ Tambocor Tablets (4.4%) 1990
▲ Tarka Tablets (3.3%) 508
▲ Tasmar Tablets (6% to 8%) 3010
Taxotere for Injection Concentrate.. 778
Tegretol/Tegretol-XR........ 2404
▲ Temodar Capsules (33%) 3157
▲ Tenex Tablets (Up to 16%) 2942
Tenoretic Tablets........ 690
Tequin Injection (0.1% to 3%)........ 1110
Tequin Tablets (0.1% to 3%)........ 1110
Tessalon Capsules........ 1377
Teveten Tablets (Less than 1%)........ 3327
▲ Thalomid Capsules (4.2%) 1154
TheraCys Injection (1%)........ 823
Thioridazine Hydrochloride Tablets........ 2289
Thiothixene Capsules (Infrequently)........ 2290
Thorazine........ 1656
Tiazac Capsules (Less than 2%)........ 1378
Timolide Tablets (Less than 1%)...... 2187
Tolectin (1% to 3%)........ 2589
Tonocard Tablets (Less than 1%)...... 649
▲ Topamax Sprinkle Capsules (3.2% to 5.3%)........ 2590
▲ Topamax Tablets (3.2% to 5.3%) 2590
Toprol-XL Tablets (About 1 of 100 patients)........ 651
Toradol (Greater than 1%)........ 3018
▲ Trasylol Injection (4%) 909
Trental Tablets (Less than 1%)........ 784
▲ Tricor Capsules, Micronized (3%) 513
Trilafon (Occasional)........ 3160
▲ Trileptal Oral Suspension (2% to 6%)........ 2407
▲ Trileptal Tablets (2% to 6%) 2407
▲ Trilisate (Less than 20%) 2901
▲ Trisenox Injection (28%) 1158
Trovan (Less than 1%)........ 2722
Tussionex Pennkinetic Extended-Release Suspension..... 1174
Tussi-Organidin NR Liquid........ 3350
Tussi-Organidin-S NR Liquid........ 3350
Twinrix Vaccine (Less than 1%)........ 1674
Tylenol with Codeine........ 2595
Tylox Capsules........ 2597
▲ Ultracet Tablets (6%) 2597
▲ Ultram Tablets (24% to 46%) 2600
Uniretic Tablets (Less than 1%)........ 3178
Univasc Tablets (Less than 1%)........ 3181
Valium Injectable 3026
Valium Tablets (Infrequent)........ 3047
Valtrex Caplets (Less than 1% to 4%)........ 1676
Varivax (Greater than or equal to 1%)........ 2202
Vascor Tablets (0.5% to 2.84%)........ 2602
Vaseretic Tablets (0.5% to 2.0%)........ 2204
Vasotec I.V. Injection (0.5% to 1%).. 2207
Vasotec Tablets (0.5% to 1.0%)........ 2210
▲ Verelan Capsules (7.3% to 7.4%) 3184
▲ Verelan PM Capsules (7.3% to 8.8%)........ 3186
▲ Vesanoid Capsules (17%) 3037
Viadur Implant (Less than 2%)........ 912
Vicodin Tablets........ 516
Vicodin ES Tablets........ 517
Vicodin HP Tablets........ 518
▲ Vicoprofen Tablets (22%) 520
Vioxx (Greater than 0.1% to 1.9%).. 2213
Vistide Injection........ 1445
▲ Visudyne for Injection (1% to 10%)........ ⊙308
Vivactil Tablets........ 2217
Vivactil Tablets........ 2446
▲ Voltaren Tablets (3% to 9%) 2315
▲ Voltaren-XR Tablets (3% to 9%) 2315
▲ WelChol Tablets (11%) 3073
▲ Wellbutrin Tablets (26.0%) 1680
▲ Wellbutrin SR Sustained-Release Tablets (5% to 10%)........ 1684
▲ Xanax Tablets (10.4% to 26.2%) 2865
Xeloda Tablets (1%)........ 3039
▲ Zanaflex Tablets (4%) 1305
Zantac........ 1690
Zantac Injection........ 1688
Zantac Syrup........ 1690
Zaroxolyn Tablets........ 1177
Zebeta Tablets........ 1885
▲ Zenapax for Injection (Greater than 5%)........ 3046
Zestoretic Tablets (0.3% to 1%)........ 695
Zestril Tablets (0.3% to 1.0%)........ 698
Ziac Tablets........ 1887
Zithromax Capsules, 250 mg (1% or less)........ 2743
Zithromax for IV Infusion........ 2748
Zithromax for Oral Suspension, 300 mg, 600 mg, 900 mg, 1200 mg (1% or less)........ 2739
Zithromax Tablets, 250 mg (1% or less)........ 2739
Zocor Tablets (2.3%)........ 2219
▲ Zofran Injection (11%) 1698
▲ Zofran (6% to 9%) 1703
▲ Zofran ODT Orally Disintegrating Tablets (6% to 9%)........ 1703
Zoladex (1% to 5%)........ 702
Zoladex 3-month 706
▲ Zoloft (6% to 8%) 2751
▲ Zometa for Intravenous Infusion (26.7%)........ 3621
Zomig Tablets (Rare)........ 708
Zomig-ZMT Tablets (Rare)........ 708
Zonegran Capsules (2%)........ 1307
▲ Zosyn (7.7% to 8.4%) 1890
▲ Zosyn in Galaxy Containers (7.7% to 8.4%)........ 1894
▲ Zyban Sustained-Release Tablets (8%)........ 1710
Zydone Tablets........ 1330
Zyflo Filmtab Tablets (Less common)........ 524
▲ Zyprexa Tablets (9% to 11%) 1973
▲ Zyprexa ZYDIS Orally Disintegrating Tablets (9% to 11%)........ 1973
Zyrtec (Less than 2%)........ 2756
Zyrtec-D 12 Hour Extended Relief Tablets (Less than 2%)........ 2758
Zyvox (2.2%)........ 2871

Constipation, aggravation of
Nexium Delayed-Release Capsules (Less than 1%)........ 619

Constriction, pupillary
(*see under* Miosis)

Constriction, pupils
(*see under* Miosis)

Contact lens staining
Rifadin........ 765
Rifater Tablets........ 769

Contact lenses, intolerance
Accutane Capsules........ 2944
Activella Tablets........ 2764
Alesse-21 Tablets........ 3468
Alesse-28 Tablets........ 3473
Alora Transdermal System........ 3372
Brevicon 28-Day Tablets........ 3380
Cenestin Tablets........ 1263
Climara Transdermal System........ 958
Cyclessa Tablets........ 2450
Desogen Tablets........ 2458
Esclim Transdermal System........ 3460
Estinyl Tablets........ 3112
Estrace Vaginal Cream........ 3358
Estrace Tablets........ 3361

Estratest 3252
Estrostep 2627
femhrt Tablets 2635
Levlen 962
Levlite 21 Tablets 962
Levlite 28 Tablets 962
Levora Tablets 3389
Loestrin 21 Tablets 2642
Loestrin Fe Tablets 2642
Lo/Ovral Tablets 3532
Lo/Ovral-28 Tablets 3538
Low-Ogestrel-28 Tablets 3392
Lunelle Monthly Injection 2827
Menest Tablets 2254
Microgestin Fe 1.5/30 Tablets 3407
Microgestin Fe 1/20 Tablets 3400
Mircette Tablets 2470
Modicon 2563
Necon 3415
Nordette-28 Tablets 2257
Norinyl 1 +35 28-Day Tablets 3380
Norinyl 1 + 50 28-Day Tablets 3380
Ogen Tablets 2846
Ogestrel 0.5/50-28 Tablets 3428
Ortho Dienestrol Cream 2554
Ortho-Cept 21 Tablets 2546
Ortho-Cept 28 Tablets 2546
Ortho-Cyclen/Ortho Tri-Cyclen 2573
Ortho-Est Tablets 3464
Ortho-Novum 2563
Ortho-Novum 1/50□28 Tablets 2556
Ortho-Prefest Tablets 2570
Ortho-Cyclen/Ortho Tri-Cyclen 2573
Ovcon 3364
Ovral Tablets 3551
Ovral-28 Tablets 3552
Ovrette Tablets 3552
Premarin Intravenous 3563
Premarin Tablets 3566
Premarin Vaginal Cream 3570
Premphase Tablets 3572
Prempro Tablets 3572
Tri-Levlen 962
Tri-Norinyl-28 Tablets 3433
Trivora Tablets 3439
Vivelle Transdermal System 2412
Vivelle-Dot Transdermal System 2416
Yasmin 28 Tablets 980
Zovia 3449

Contusions
Advair Diskus 100/50 (1% to 3%) 1448
Advair Diskus 250/50 (1% to 3%) 1448
Advair Diskus 500/50 (1% to 3%) 1448
Flovent Diskus (1% to 3%) 3614
Flovent 1535
Flovent Rotadisk 1537
Vioxx (Greater than 0.1% to 1.9%) 2213

Convulsions
Abelcet Injection 1273
Aciphex Tablets 1267
Aciphex Tablets 1783
ActHIB Vaccine (2 definite; 3 possible) 798
Aggrenox Capsules (1.7%) 1026
AK-Fluor Injection 10% and 25% ⊙202
Aldoclor Tablets 2035
Aldoril Tablets 2039
Altace Capsules (Less than 1%) 2233
Ambien Tablets 3191
AmBisome for Injection (Less common) 1383
Amerge Tablets (Rare) 1467
Amicar Injection 3608
Amicar Syrup 3608
Amicar Tablets 3608
Amphotec (1% to 5%) 1774
Ancobon Capsules 1730
Aricept Tablets 1270
Aricept Tablets 2665
Arthrotec Tablets (Rare) 3195
Astramorph/PF Injection, USP (Preservative-Free) 594
Atarax Tablets & Syrup (Rare) 2667
Ativan Injection (Less than 1%) 3478
Attenuvax (Rare) 2044
Augmentin Chewable Tablets (Rare) 1482
Augmentin Powder for Oral Suspension (Rare) 1482
Augmentin Tablets (Rare) 1485
Augmentin ES-600 Powder for Oral Suspension (Rare) 1487
Avelox Tablets 879
Azulfidine EN-tabs Tablets (Rare) 2775
Bactrim 2949
Benadryl Parenteral 2617
Betaseron for SC Injection (2%) 988
Brevibloc Injection (Less than 1%) 858
Brevital Sodium for Injection, USP 1815
Buprenex Injectable (Rare) 2918
Cataflam Tablets (Rare) 2315
Cefotan 664
Ceftin for Oral Suspension 1898
Celestone Soluspan Injectable Suspension 3097
Celestone Syrup 3099
▲ CellCept Capsules (3% to 10%) 2951
▲ CellCept Intravenous (3% to 10%) 2951
▲ CellCept Oral Suspension (3% to 10%) 2951
▲ CellCept Tablets (3% to 10%) 2951
Cerebyx Injection (Infrequent) 2619
Chibroxin Sterile Ophthalmic Solution 2051
Cipro I.V. 893
Cipro I.V. Pharmacy Bulk Package (Less than 1%) 897
Cipro 887
Claritin-D 12 Hour Extended Release Tablets 3102
Claritin-D 24 Hour Extended Release Tablets (Fewer than 2%) 3104
Clinoril Tablets (Less than 1%) 2053
▲ Clozaril Tablets (3%) 2319
Cognex Capsules (Frequent) 1351
Compazine 1505
Coreg Tablets (Less than or equal to 0.1%) 1508
Cortone Acetate Injectable Suspension 2059
Cortone Acetate Tablets 2061
Cytovene (At least 3 subjects) 2959
DaunoXome Injection (Less than or equal to 5%) 1442
Decadron Elixir 2078
Decadron Tablets 2079
Decadron Phosphate Injection 2081
Demerol 3079
Depo-Medrol Injectable Suspension 2795
Depo-Provera Contraceptive Injection (Fewer than 1%) 2798
Diamox Intravenous (Occasional) ⊙269
Diamox Sequels Sustained Release Capsules ⊙270
Diamox Tablets (Occasional) ⊙269
Diphtheria & Tetanus Toxoids Adsorbed Purogenated for Pediatric Use 1857
Diprivan Injectable Emulsion (Rare) 667
Diuril Oral 2087
Diuril Sodium Intravenous 2086
Dopram Injectable 2931
Doxil Injection (Less than 1%) 566
Duramorph Injection (May accompany high doses) 1312
Duranest Injections 600
Effexor Tablets (Infrequent) 3495
Effexor XR Capsules (Infrequent) 3499
ELA-Max Cream 1340
Emla (Unlikely with cream) 602
Ergamisol Tablets (Less frequent) 1789
Evoxac Capsules 1217
Exelon Capsules (Frequent) 2342
Exelon Oral Solution (Frequent) 2345
Feldene Capsules (Rare) 2685
Flexeril Tablets (Less than 1%) 572
Flexeril Tablets (Less than 1%) 2094
▲ Flolan for Injection (4%) 1528
Florinef Acetate Tablets 2250
Floxin I.V. 2526
Floxin Tablets 2529
Flumadine (Less than 0.3%) 1370
Fluorescite Injection ⊙211
Fortovase Capsules (Less than 2%) 2970
Gastrocrom Oral Concentrate (Less common) 1162
Gengraf Capsules 457
▲ Gliadel Wafer (19%) 1723
Havrix Vaccine (Rare) 1544
Herceptin I.V. (At least one of the 958 patients) 1414
HibTITER 1859
Hydrocortone Tablets 2106
Hydrocortone Acetate Injectable Suspension 2103
Hydrocortone Phosphate Injection, Sterile 2105
HydroDIURIL Tablets 2108
Imitrex Injection (Rare) 1549
Imitrex Tablets (Rare) 1558
Indocin Capsules (Less than 1%) 2112
Indocin I.V. (Less than 1%) 2115
Indocin (Less than 1%) 2112
INFeD Injection 3388
Infumorph 200 and Infumorph 500 Sterile Solutions 1314
Intron A for Injection (Less than 5%) 3120
Inversine Tablets 1850
Invirase Capsules (Less than 2%) 2979
Keppra Tablets (1% or more) 3314
▲ Lamictal (3.2% to 4%) 1567
Levaquin (Less than 0.3%) 2537
Levo-Dromoran 1734
Lidoderm Patch 1319
Lindane Lotion USP 1% 559
Lindane Shampoo USP 1% 560
Lodine XL Extended-Release Tablets 3530
Lodosyn Tablets 1251
Lopid Tablets 2650
Lufyllin-GG Elixir 3348
Lufyllin-GG Tablets 3348
Lupron Depot–4 Month 30 mg (Less than 5%) 3289
Luvox Tablets (25, 50, 100 mg) (0.2%) 3256
Matulane Capsules 3246
Megace Oral Suspension (1% to 3%) 1124
Meridia Capsules (0.1%) 481
Mexitil Capsules (About 2 in 1,000) 1047
Mintezol 2137
Mirapex Tablets (Rare) 2834
Mobic Tablets (Less than 2%) 1054
Motrin Suspension, Oral Drops, Chewable Tablets, and Caplets (Less than 1%) 2002
Mycobutin Capsules (More than one patient) 2838
Mylocel Tablets (Extremely rare) 2227
Narcan Injection 1322
Nardil Tablets (Less frequent) 2653
Naropin Injection (Less than 1%) 612
Nebcin Vials, Hyporets & ADD-Vantage 1955
Neoral Soft Gelatin Capsules (1% to 5%) 2380
Neoral Oral Solution (1% to 5%) 2380
Neptazane Tablets ⊙271
Nesacaine/Nesacaine MPF 617
Neurontin Capsules (More than 1%) 2655
Neurontin Oral Solution 2655
Neurontin Tablets (More than 1%) 2655
Nipent for Injection (Less than 3%) 3272
Noroxin Tablets 2145
Norvir Capsules (Less than 2%) 487
Norvir Oral Solution (Less than 2%) 487
Oncaspar (Greater than 1% but less than 5%) 756
One-A-Day Tension & Mood Softgels ▣808
Paxil (0.1%) 1609
Pediapred Oral Solution 1170
Pediazole Suspension 3050
Periactin Tablets 2155
Permax Tablets (Infrequent) 1299
Pfizerpen for Injection 2707
Phenergan with Codeine Syrup 3557
Phenergan VC with Codeine Syrup 3561
Phrenilin (Infrequent) 578
Plaquenil Tablets 3082
Polocaine Injection, USP 625
Polocaine-MPF Injection, USP 625
Ponstel Capsules (Rare) 1356
Prednisone 3064
Prelone Syrup 2273
▲ Primaxin I.V. (5.9%) 2160
▲ Prograf (3% to 15%) 1393
Prostigmin Injectable 1744
Prostigmin Tablets 1744
Protonix I.V. (Less than 1%) 3580
Protonix Tablets (Less than 1%) 3577
Prozac Pulvules, Liquid, and Weekly Capsules (0.2%) 1238
Quinaglute Dura-Tabs Tablets 978
Quinidex Extentabs 2933
Reminyl Oral Solution (Infrequent) 1792
Reminyl Tablets (Infrequent) 1792
Requip Tablets (Infrequent) 1621
Rifamate Capsules (Uncommon) 767
Rifater Tablets (Uncommon) 769
Rilutek Tablets (Infrequent) 772
Romazicon Injection 3000
Rynatan Tablets 3351
Sandimmune (1% to 5%) 2388
Sandostatin LAR Depot (Rare) 2395
Sedapap Tablets 50 mg/650 mg (Infrequent) 2225
Sensorcaine (0.1%) 643
Sensorcaine-MPF Injection (Approximately 0.1%) 643
Septra Suspension 2265
Septra Tablets 2265
Septra DS Tablets 2265
▲ Serostim for Injection (1% to 10%) 3229
Sinemet Tablets 1253
Sinemet CR Tablets 1255
Solu-Medrol Sterile Powder 2855
Stadol NS Nasal Spray (Less than 1%) 1108
Stelazine 1640
Sustiva Capsules (Less than 2%) 1258
Symmetrel (Less than 0.1%) 1328
Tambocor Tablets (Less than 1%) 1990
Tazicef for Injection 1647
Tazicef Galaxy Container 1650
Tazicef Pharmacy Bulk Package 1653
▲ Temodar Capsules (23%) 3157
Tensilon Injectable 1745
Tequin Injection (Less than 0.1%) 1110
Tequin Tablets (Less than 0.1%) 1110
Tetanus & Diphtheria Toxoids Adsorbed for Adult Use 1880
Thyrel TRH for Injection (Rare) 3630
Timolide Tablets 2187
Tonocard Tablets (Less than 1%) 649
Toradol 3018
Trasylol Injection (1% to 2%) 909
Trental Tablets (Less than 1%) 784
▲ Trisenox Injection (8%) 1158
Trovan (Less than 1%) 2722
Twinrix Vaccine 1674
Ultracet Tablets (Less than 1%) 2597
Ultram Tablets 2600
Urecholine 2198
Valcyte Tablets (Less than 5%) 3022
Vantin Tablets and Oral Suspension 2860
Venofer Injection (8 patients) 580
Vermox Chewable Tablets (Very rare) 2017
▲ Vesanoid Capsules (3%) 3037
Virazole for Inhalation Solution 1747
Vistaril Capsules (Rare) 2738
Vistaril Intramuscular Solution (Rare) 2738
Vistaril Oral Suspension (Rare) 2738
Vistide Injection 1445
Voltaren Tablets (Rare) 2315
Voltaren-XR Tablets (Rare) 2315
▲ Xylocaine Injections (Among most common) 653
Zanaflex Tablets (Infrequent) 1305
Zestoretic Tablets 695
Zithromax Capsules, 250 mg 2743
Zithromax for IV Infusion 2748
Zithromax for Oral Suspension, 300 mg, 600 mg, 900 mg, 1200 mg 2739
Zithromax Tablets, 250 mg 2739
Zoloft 2751
Zonegran Capsules (Frequent) 1307
Zosyn (1.0% or less) 1890
Zosyn in Galaxy Containers (1.0% or less) 1894
Zovirax for Injection 1708

Convulsions, aggravated
Trileptal Oral Suspension (1% to 2%) 2407
Trileptal Tablets (1% to 2%) 2407

Convulsions, clonic
Lufyllin Tablets 3347
Lufyllin-400 Tablets 3347
Lufyllin-GG Elixir 3348
Lufyllin-GG Tablets 3348
Uniphyl 400 mg and 600 mg Tablets (A few isolated reports) 2903

Convulsions, grand mal
Campath Ampules 992
Compazine 1505
Keppra Tablets (1% or more) 3314
Lamictal (Rare) 1567
Norvir Capsules (Less than 2%) 487
Norvir Oral Solution (Less than 2%) 487
Paxil (Rare) 1609
Remeron Tablets (Rare) 2483
Remeron SolTab Tablets (Rare) 2486
Requip Tablets (Rare) 1621
Stelazine 1640

Convulsions, tonic generalized
Lufyllin Tablets 3347
Lufyllin-400 Tablets 3347
Lufyllin-GG Elixir 3348
Lufyllin-GG Tablets 3348
Uniphyl 400 mg and 600 mg Tablets (A few isolated reports) 2903

Coombs' test, positive
Adalat CC Tablets 877
Aldoclor Tablets 2035
Aldomet Tablets 2037
Aldoril Tablets 2039
Azactam for Injection 1276
Catapres Tablets 1037
Ceclor CD Tablets 1279
Ceclor (Less than 1 in 200) 1905
Cefizox for Intramuscular or Intravenous Use (1% to 5%) 1390
Cefobid Intravenous/Intramuscular (1 in 60) 2671
Cefobid Pharmacy Bulk Package - Not for Direct Infusion (1 in 60) 2673
Cefotan (1 in 250) 664
Ceftin (0.1% to 1%) 1898
Cefzil 1076
Ceptaz for Injection (One in 23) 1499
Claforan Injection (Less than 1%) 732
Clorpres Tablets 1002
Combipres Tablets 1040
Duraclon Injection 3057
Duricef 1079
▲ Fortaz (1 in 23) 1541
Keflex 1237
Kefurox Vials, ADD-Vantage (Less than 1 in 250) 1948
Lodosyn Tablets 1251
Lorabid Suspension and Pulvules 2251
Mandol Vials 1953
▲ Maxipime for Injection (16.2%) 1285
Mefoxin for Injection 2124
Mefoxin Premixed Intravenous Solution 2127
Merrem I.V. (Greater than 0.2%) 673
Motrin Suspension, Oral Drops, Chewable Tablets, and Caplets (Sometimes) 2002
Paser Granules 1781
Pipracil (Less frequent) 1866

Primaxin I.M. 2158
Primaxin I.V. 2160
Procardia Capsules 2708
Procardia XL Extended Release Tablets 2710
Rilutek Tablets (Infrequent) 772
Roferon-A Injection (Rare) 2996
Sinemet Tablets 1253
Sinemet CR Tablets 1255
Suprax 1877
▲ Tazicef for Injection (1 in 23 patients) 1647
▲ Tazicef Galaxy Container (1 in 23 patients) 1650
▲ Tazicef Pharmacy Bulk Package (1 in 23 patients) 1653
▲ Tazidime Vials, Faspak & ADD-Vantage (1 in 23) 1966
Unasyn for Injection (Some individuals) 2728
Vantin Tablets and Oral Suspension (Occasional) 2860
Zinacef Injection (Fewer than 1 in 250 patients) 1696
Zinacef for Injection (Fewer than 1 in 250 patients) 1696
Zosyn 1890
Zosyn in Galaxy Containers 1894

Coordination, disturbed
(*see under* Coordination, impaired)

Coordination, impaired
Amerge Tablets (Rare) 1467
Arthrotec Tablets (Rare) 3195
Atrovent Inhalation Aerosol (Less frequent) 1030
▲ Benadryl Parenteral (Among most frequent) 2617
Carbatrol Capsules 3234
Cataflam Tablets (Rare) 2315
Celexa (Rare) 1365
Clozaril Tablets (Less than 1%) 2319
Combivent Inhalation Aerosol 1041
▲ Cordarone Tablets (4% to 9%) 3487
Depacon Injection (1% to 5%) 416
Dilantin Infatabs 2624
▲ Dilantin Kapseals (Among most common) 2622
Dilantin-125 Oral Suspension 2625
Duragesic Transdermal System (1% or greater) 1786
Evoxac Capsules (Less than 1%) 1217
Foscavir Injection (Between 1% and 5%) 605
▲ Halcion Tablets (4.6%) 2823
Hivid Tablets (Less than 1%) 2975
Intron A for Injection (Less than 5%) 3120
Iopidine 0.5% Ophthalmic Solution (Less than 3%) .... ⊙213
Ismo Tablets (Fewer than 1%) 3524
▲ Klonopin Tablets (6%) 2983
▲ Lamictal (6.0%) 1567
Levaquin (Less than 0.5%) 2537
Lithium Carbonate 3061
Lithium Citrate Syrup 3061
Luvox Tablets (25, 50, 100 mg) (Infrequent) 3256
Marinol Capsules 3325
▲ Mexitil Capsules (9.4% to 10.2%) 1047
Naprelan Tablets (Less than 1%) 1293
Neurontin Capsules (1.1%) 2655
Neurontin Oral Solution (1.1%) 2655
Neurontin Tablets (1.1%) 2655
▲ Nicotrol Nasal Spray (Under 5%) 2843
▲ Pacerone Tablets (4% to 9%) 3331
Periactin Tablets 2155
▲ ProSom Tablets (4%) 500
Remeron Tablets (Infrequent) 2483
Remeron SolTab Tablets (Infrequent) 2486
Requip Tablets (Infrequent) 1621
Rescriptor Tablets (Less than 2%) 526
Rilutek Tablets (Infrequent) 772
Roferon-A Injection (Less than 0.5%) 2996
▲ Rynatan Tablets (Among most common) 3351
Tegretol/Tegretol-XR 2404
▲ Temodar Capsules (11%) 3157
Tonocard Tablets (Up to 1.2%) 649
▲ Topamax Sprinkle Capsules (3.6% to 5.3%) 2590
▲ Topamax Tablets (3.6% to 5.3%) 2590
Trileptal Oral Suspension (1% to 3%) 2407
Trileptal Tablets (1% to 3%) 2407
Trovan (Less than 1%) 2722
Ultram Tablets (1% to 5%) 2600
Voltaren Tablets (Rare) 2315
Voltaren-XR Tablets (Rare) 2315
Wellbutrin SR Sustained-Release Tablets (Infrequent) 1684
▲ Xanax Tablets (40.1%) 2865
Zoloft (Infrequent) 2751
Zyban Sustained-Release Tablets (Infrequent) 1710
Zyrtec (Less than 2%) 2756
Zyrtec-D 12 Hour Extended Relief Tablets (Less than 2%) 2758

Coordination, lack of
(*see under* Ataxia)

Coordination difficulty
(*see under* Coordination, impaired)

Cor pulmonale
Accuretic Tablets 2614
Pulmozyme Inhalation Solution 1426

Cornea, discoloration
Serentil 1057
Xalatan Latanoprost Ophthalmic Solution .... ⊙320
Xalatan Sterile Ophthalmic Solution 2864

Cornea, fungal infections
Blephamide Ophthalmic Ointment 547
NeoDecadron Sterile Ophthalmic Solution 2144
Polysporin Ophthalmic Ointment Sterile .... ⊙301
Pred Forte Ophthalmic Suspension .... ⊙246
Pred Mild Sterile Ophthalmic Suspension .... ⊙249
Pred-G Ophthalmic Suspension .... ⊙247
Terra-Cortril Ophthalmic Suspension 2716
TobraDex Ophthalmic Ointment 542
TobraDex Ophthalmic Suspension 541

Cornea, gray, ground-glass appearance
Ophthetic Ophthalmic Solution .... ⊙244

Cornea, opacities
Accutane Capsules 2944
Imitrex Injection 1549
Imitrex Tablets 1558
Plaquenil Tablets 3082
Serentil 1057
Symmetrel (0.1% to 1%) 1328
Topamax Sprinkle Capsules (Rare) 2590
Topamax Tablets (Rare) 2590

Cornea, white crystalline precipitates, presence of
▲ Ciloxan (Approximately 17%) 538

Corneal abrasion
Alomide (Less than 1%) .... ⊙204

Corneal changes
Aralen Tablets 3075
Azulfidine EN-tabs Tablets (Rare) 2775
Efudex (Infrequent) 1733
Fareston Tablets 3237
Neurontin Capsules (Rare) 2655
Neurontin Oral Solution (Rare) 2655
Neurontin Tablets (Rare) 2655
Nolvadex Tablets 678
Plaquenil Tablets 3082
Vitrasert Implant (Less than 1%) .... ⊙254

Corneal clouding
Chemet Capsules (1.0% to 3.7%) 3078
Miochol-E System Pak (Infrequent) .... ⊙305
Miochol-E with Steri-Tags (Infrequent) .... ⊙306
Voltaren Ophthalmic Sterile Ophthalmic Solution (Less than 5%) .... ⊙312

Corneal curvature, steepening
Activella Tablets 2764
Alesse-21 Tablets 3468
Alesse-28 Tablets 3473
Alora Transdermal System 3372
Brevicon 28-Day Tablets 3380
Cenestin Tablets 1263
Climara Transdermal System 958
Cyclessa Tablets 2450
Desogen Tablets 2458
Esclim Transdermal System 3460
Estinyl Tablets 3112
Estrace Vaginal Cream 3358
Estrace Tablets 3361
Estratest 3252
Estrostep 2627
Levlen 962
Levlite 21 Tablets 962
Levlite 28 Tablets 962
Levora Tablets 3389
Loestrin 21 Tablets 2642
Loestrin Fe Tablets 2642
Lo/Ovral Tablets 3532
Lo/Ovral-28 Tablets 3538
Low-Ogestrel-28 Tablets 3392
Menest Tablets 2254
Microgestin Fe 1.5/30 Tablets 3407
Microgestin Fe 1/20 Tablets 3400
Mircette Tablets 2470
Modicon 2563
Necon 3415
Nordette-28 Tablets 2257
Norinyl 1 +35 28-Day Tablets 3380
Norinyl 1 + 50 28-Day Tablets 3380
Ogen Tablets 2846
Ogestrel 0.5/50-28 Tablets 3428
Ortho Dienestrol Cream 2554
Ortho-Cept 21 Tablets 2546
Ortho-Cept 28 Tablets 2546
Ortho-Cyclen/Ortho Tri-Cyclen 2573
Ortho-Est Tablets 3464
Ortho-Novum 2563
Ortho-Novum 1/50□28 Tablets 2556
Ortho-Prefest Tablets 2570
Ortho-Cyclen/Ortho Tri-Cyclen 2573
Ovcon 3364
Ovral Tablets 3551
Ovral-28 Tablets 3552
Ovrette Tablets 3552
Premarin Intravenous 3563
Premarin Tablets 3566
Premarin Vaginal Cream 3570
Premphase Tablets 3572
Prempro Tablets 3572
Tri-Levlen 962
Tri-Norinyl-28 Tablets 3433
Triphasil-21 Tablets 3600
Triphasil-28 Tablets 3605
Trivora Tablets 3439
Vivelle Transdermal System 2412
Vivelle-Dot Transdermal System 2416
Yasmin 28 Tablets 980
Zovia 3449

Corneal decompensation
Amvisc Plus .... ⊙329
Cytovene-IV (One report) 2959
Healon (Rare) .... ⊙316
Healon GV .... ⊙320
Miochol-E System Pak (Infrequent) .... ⊙305
Miochol-E with Steri-Tags (Infrequent) .... ⊙305
Ocucoat .... ⊙330

Corneal degeneration
Cordarone Tablets 3487
Pacerone Tablets 3331

Corneal deposits
Chibroxin Sterile Ophthalmic Solution 2051
Compazine 1505
▲ Cordarone Tablets (Majority of adults) 3487
Epifrin Sterile Ophthalmic Solution .... ⊙235
Etrafon 3115
Indocin (Less than 1%) 2112
▲ Pacerone Tablets (Majority of adults) 3331
Plaquenil Tablets 3082
Propine Ophthalmic Solution .... ⊙250
Rescula Ophthalmic Solution (Less than 1%) .... ⊙306
Stelazine 1640
Thioridazine Hydrochloride Tablets 2289
Thorazine 1656
Trilafon 3160
Voltaren Ophthalmic Sterile Ophthalmic Solution (Less than 5%) .... ⊙312

Corneal erosion
Sonata Capsules (Rare) 3591

Corneal infiltrate
Acular Ophthalmic Solution (Rare) 544
Ciloxan (Less than 1%) 538
Emadine Ophthalmic Solution (Less than 5%) .... ⊙211
Iopidine 0.5% Ophthalmic Solution (Less than 3%) .... ⊙213
Vexol 1% Ophthalmic Suspension (Less than 1%) .... ⊙222

Corneal keratopathy
Fareston Tablets (2%) 3237

Corneal opacity
Aciphex Tablets 1267
Aciphex Tablets 1783
Evoxac Capsules (Less than 1%) 1217
Rescula Ophthalmic Solution (Less than 1%) .... ⊙306
Vistide Injection 1445

Corneal punctate, defects
Symmetrel (0.1% to 1%) 1328

Corneal punctate keratitis
Betoptic S Ophthalmic Suspension (Small number of patients) 537

Corneal sensitivity, decrease
Betagan (A small number of patients) .... ⊙228
Betimol Ophthalmic Solution .... ⊙324
Betoptic S Ophthalmic Suspension 537
Cosopt Sterile Ophthalmic Solution 2065
Plaquenil Tablets 3082
Timolol GFS .... ⊙266
Timoptic in Ocudose (Less frequent) 2192
Timoptic Sterile Ophthalmic Solution (Less frequent) 2190
Timoptic-XE Sterile Ophthalmic Gel Forming Solution 2194

Corneal sensitivity, unspecified
Carteolol Hydrochloride Ophthalmic Solution USP, 1% (Occasional) .... ⊙258
Ocupress Ophthalmic Solution, 1% Sterile (Occasional) .... ⊙303

Corneal staining
▲ Alphagan Ophthalmic Solution (Approximately 3% to 9%) 545
Betimol Ophthalmic Solution (1% to 5%) .... ⊙324
Carteolol Hydrochloride Ophthalmic Solution USP, 1% (Occasional) .... ⊙258
Ciloxan (Less than 1%) 538
Emadine Ophthalmic Solution (Less than 5%) .... ⊙211
Iopidine 0.5% Ophthalmic Solution (Less than 3%) .... ⊙213
Ocupress Ophthalmic Solution, 1% Sterile (Occasional) .... ⊙303
Vexol 1% Ophthalmic Suspension (Less than 1%) .... ⊙222

Corneal thinning
Myleran Tablets 1603

Corneal ulceration
Acular Ophthalmic Solution (Rare) 544
Alomide Ophthalmic Solution (Less than 1%) .... ⊙204
Ambien Tablets (Rare) 3191
Botox Purified Neurotoxin Complex 549
Evoxac Capsules (Less than 1%) 1217
Paxil (Rare) 1609
Pred Forte Ophthalmic Suspension (Occasional) .... ⊙246
Pred Mild Sterile Ophthalmic Suspension (Occasional) .... ⊙249
Soriatane Capsules (Less than 1%) 3003
Vexol 1% Ophthalmic Suspension (Less than 1%) .... ⊙222

Corneal verticulata
Fareston Tablets 3237

Coronary artery disease, aggravation
Carbatrol Capsules 3234
Enalaprilat Injection (One case) 863
Tegretol/Tegretol-XR 2404
Tenoretic Tablets 690
Vasotec I.V. Injection (One case) 2207

Coronary artery disease, unspecified
Campath Ampules 992
▲ Casodex Tablets (2% to 5%) 662
Celebrex Capsules (0.1% to 1.9%) 2676
Celebrex Capsules (0.1% to 1.9%) 2780
Effexor Tablets (Rare) 3495
Effexor XR Capsules (Rare) 3499
Intron A for Injection (Less than 5%) 3120
Luvox Tablets (25, 50, 100 mg) (Rare) 3256
Naprelan Tablets (Less than 1%) 1293
Proleukin for Injection (Less than 1%) 1199
Tasmar Tablets (Infrequent) 3010
Toprol-XL Tablets (Greater than 1%) 651
Tricor Capsules, Micronized 513
Zanaflex Tablets (Rare) 1305

Coronary occlusion
Trasylol Injection (1% to 2%) 909

Coronary thrombosis
Innohep Injection 1248
Levaquin (Less than 0.5%) 2537
Lo/Ovral Tablets 3532
Lo/Ovral-28 Tablets 3538
Low-Ogestrel-28 Tablets 3392
Modicon 2563
Nordette-28 Tablets 2257
Ogestrel 0.5/50-28 Tablets 3428
Ortho-Novum 2563
Ortho-Novum 1/50□28 Tablets 2556
Ovral Tablets 3551
Ovral-28 Tablets 3552
Ovrette Tablets 3552
Triphasil-21 Tablets 3600
Triphasil-28 Tablets 3605

Corpuscular volume, mean, elevation
Thalomid Capsules 1154

Cortical lens opacities, scattered punctate
Carbatrol Capsules 3234
Tegretol/Tegretol-XR 2404

Costochondritis
Evoxac Capsules (Less than 1%) 1217
Neurontin Capsules (Rare) 2655
Neurontin Oral Solution (Rare) 2655
Neurontin Tablets (Rare) 2655

Cough
Accupril Tablets (2.0% to 4.3%) 2611
▲ Accuretic Tablets (3.2%) 2614
▲ Aceon Tablets (2 mg, 4 mg, 8 mg) (6.0% to 12.0%) 3249
Actiq (1% or greater) 1184
Adalat CC Tablets (Less than 1.0%) 877
Adenoscan (Less than 1%) 1381
▲ Advair Diskus 100/50 (3%) 1448
▲ Advair Diskus 250/50 (6%) 1448
▲ Advair Diskus 500/50 (3% to 6%) 1448
▲ Aerobid/Aerobid-M (3% to 9%) 1363
Aggrenox Capsules (1.5%) 1026
▲ Agrylin Capsules (6.3%) 3232
Alamast Ophthalmic Solution (Less than 5%) 3092
Alferon N Injection (One patient to 1%) 1770
Alkeran for Injection 1465
Alkeran Tablets 1466
▲ Allegra (3.8%) 712
Alphagan P Ophthalmic Solution (1% to 4%) 546
▲ Altace Capsules (7.6% to 12%) 2233
Alupent (1% to 4%) 1029
Ambien Tablets (Infrequent) 3191
▲ AmBisome for Injection (17.8%) 1383
Amerge Tablets (Infrequent) 1467
▲ Amphotec (5% or more) 1774
Apligraf (1.3%) 2305
▲ Arava Tablets (3%) 724
▲ Aredia for Injection (25.7%) 2309
Argatroban Injection (2.8%) 1478
▲ Arimidex Tablets (7.3% to 8.4%) 659
▲ Aromasin Tablets (6%) 2769
Arthrotec Tablets (Rare) 3195
Asacol Delayed-Release Tablets (1% to 2%) 2884
Astelin Nasal Spray (Infrequent) 3339
Atacand Tablets (More than 1%) 595
Atacand HCT Tablets (0.5% or greater) 597
▲ Atrovent Inhalation Aerosol (5.9%) 1030
▲ Atrovent Inhalation Solution (4.6%) 1031
Atrovent Nasal Spray 0.03% (Less than 2%) 1032
Atrovent Nasal Spray 0.06% (Less than 1%) 1033
Attenuvax 2044
Avalide Tablets (1% or greater) 1070
Avapro Tablets (2.8%) 1074
Avapro Tablets (2.8%) 3076
Avelox Tablets (0.05% to 1%) 879
Axid Pulvules (2.0%) 1903
Axid Pulvules (2.0%) 2919
Azmacort Inhalation Aerosol 728
Bactrim 2949
Bactroban Nasal (2%) 1495
Baycol Tablets (2.4%) 883
BeneFix for Injection (One case) 1432
Betapace AF Tablets (2.5% to 3.3%) 954
Blocadren Tablets 2046
▲ Botox Purified Neurotoxin Complex (2% to 10%) 549
▲ Campath Ampules (2% to 25%) 992
Captopril Tablets (0.5% to 2%) 2281
Cardura Tablets (Less than 0.5%) 2668
▲ Carnitor Injection (9% to 18%) 3242
▲ Casodex Tablets (2% to 5%) 662
Caverject Sterile Powder (1%) 2777
Ceclor CD Tablets (1.5%) 1279
Ceftin for Oral Suspension (0.1% to 1%) 1898
Celebrex Capsules (0.1% to 1.9%) 2676
Celebrex Capsules (0.1% to 1.9%) 2780
Celexa (Frequent) 1365
▲ CellCept Capsules (13.3% to 31.1%) 2951
▲ CellCept Intravenous (13.3% to 31.1%) 2951
▲ CellCept Oral Suspension (13.3% to 31.1%) 2951
▲ CellCept Tablets (13.3% to 31.1%) 2951
▲ Cenestin Tablets (6%) 1263
Cerebyx Injection (Infrequent) 2619
Chemet Capsules (0.7% to 3.7%) 3078
Chirocaine Injection (1.4%) 2909
Cipro HC Otic Suspension (One patient) 540
Claritin (At least one patient) 3100
Claritin-D 12 Hour Extended Release Tablets (Less frequent) 3102
▲ Claritin-D 24 Hour Extended Release Tablets (3%) 3104
Clozaril Tablets (Less than 1%) 2319
▲ Cognex Capsules (3%) 1351
Colazal Capsules (2%) 3069
▲ Combivent Inhalation Aerosol (4.2%) 1041
▲ Combivir Tablets (18%) 1502
Comvax (0.2% to 0.9%) 2056
▲ Concerta Extended-Release Tablets (4%) 1998
▲ Concerta Tablets (4%) 561
Copaxone for Injection (At least 2%) 3306
▲ Cordarone Tablets (2% to 7%) 3487
Coreg Tablets (More than 2%) 1508
Corgard Tablets (1 to 5 per 1000 patients) 2245
Corzide 40/5 Tablets (1 to 5 of 1000 patients) 2247
Corzide 80/5 Tablets (1 to 5 of 1000 patients) 2247
Cosopt Sterile Ophthalmic Solution (1% to 5%) 2065
▲ Cozaar Tablets (3.4%) 2067
Crixivan Capsules (Less than 2%) 2070
Cytovene (At least 3 subjects) 2959
▲ DaunoXome Injection (2% to 26%) 1442
DDAVP Nasal Spray 738
DDAVP Rhinal Tube 738
Demadex Tablets and Injection (2.0%) 2965
Depacon Injection (1% to 5%) 416
Depakene (1% to 5%) 421
Depakote Sprinkle Capsules (1% to 5%) 426
Depakote Tablets (1% to 5%) 430
Depakote ER Tablets (1% to 5%) 436
Depen Titratable Tablets 3341
Desmopressin Acetate Rhinal Tube 1345
Detrol Tablets (2.1%) 3623
Diovan Capsules (More than 1% to 2.6%) 2337
▲ Diovan HCT Tablets (3%) 2338
Diprivan Injectable Emulsion (Less than 1%) 667
Ditropan XL Extended Release Tablets (2% to 5%) 564
Dopram Injectable 2931
Doxil Injection (Less than 1% to 5%) 566
Dynabac Tablets (0.2% to 1.5%) 2269
DynaCirc Capsules (0.5% to 1%) 2921
DynaCirc CR Tablets (0.5% to 1%) 2923
Effexor Tablets 3495
▲ Effexor XR Capsules (3%) 3499
Enalaprilat Injection 863
▲ Enbrel for Injection (6%) 1752
▲ Enbrel for Injection (6%) 3504
▲ Epivir (18%) 1520
▲ Epogen for Injection (18%) 582
Ergamisol Tablets (1 out of 463 patients) 1789
▲ Evista Tablets (6% to 9.3%) 1915
▲ Evoxac Capsules (6.1%) 1217
Exelon Capsules (2% or more) 2342
Exelon Oral Solution (2% or more) 2345
▲ Felbatol (6.5%) 3343
▲ Femara Tablets (5% to 11%) 2351
▲ Ferrlecit Injection (6%) 3386
▲ Flolan for Injection (38% to 82%) 1528
▲ Flomax Capsules (3.4% to 4.5%) 1044
▲ Flonase Nasal Spray (3.6% to 3.8%) 1533
▲ Flovent Diskus (3% to 9%) 3614
Flovent 1535
Flovent Rotadisk 1537
Floxin I.V. (Less than 1%) 2526
Floxin Otic Solution (Single report) 1219
Floxin Tablets (Less than 1%) 2529
▲ Fludara for Injection (10% to 44%) 995
Flumadine (Less than 0.3%) 1370
Fortovase Capsules (Less than 2%) 2970
▲ Foscavir Injection (5% or greater) 605
▲ Gabitril Tablets (4%) 1189
Gemzar for Injection (Common) 1919
▲ Gengraf Capsules (4% to 5%) 457
▲ Geodon Capsules (3%) 2688
▲ Gleevec Capsules (9% to 22%) 2357
Gonal-F for Injection (1.7%) 3216
▲ Herceptin I.V. (26%) 1414
Hivid Tablets (Less than 1%) 2975
▲ Humatrope Vials and Cartridges (Up to 6.25%) 1930
Hycamtin for Injection (1%) 1546
Hytrin Capsules (At least 1%) 464
Hyzaar (2.6%) 2109
▲ Imdur Tablets (Less than or equal to 5%) 1826
Imitrex Nasal Spray (Infrequent) 1554
Imitrex Tablets (Infrequent) 1558
Indapamide Tablets (Less than 5%) 2286
▲ Intron A for Injection (Up to 31%) 3120
Invirase Capsules (Less than 2%) 2979
Iveegam EN (0.91%) 849
Keppra Tablets (2%) 3314
Klonopin Tablets (2%) 2983
▲ Lamictal (7.5%) 1567
Lescol Capsules (2.4%) 2361
Lescol Capsules (2.4%) 2925
Lescol XL Tablets (1.9%) 2361
Lescol XL Tablets (1.9%) 2925
Leukeran Tablets 1591
▲ Leustatin Injection (7% to 10%) 2495
Lexxel Tablets (2.2%) 608
Livostin (Approximately 1% to 3%) .... ⊙ 305
Lodosyn Tablets 1251
▲ Lopid Tablets (More common) 2650
Lotensin Tablets (1.2%) 2365
Lotensin HCT Tablets (2.1%) 2367
▲ Lotrel Capsules (3.3%) 2370
Lupron Injection (Less than 5%) 3279
Luvox Tablets (25, 50, 100 mg) (Frequent) 3256
LYMErix Vaccine (1.5%) 1592
Macrobid Capsules (Common) 2889
Macrodantin Capsules (Common) 2891
▲ Malarone (4% to 9%) 1596
Marinol Capsules (Less than 1%) 3325
Matulane Capsules 3246
▲ Mavik Tablets (0.3% to 35%) 478
Maxair Autohaler (1.2%) 1981
Maxair Inhaler (1.2%) 1984
Maxalt Tablets (Rare) 2120
Maxalt-MLT Orally Disintegrating Tablets (Rare) 2120
Megace Oral Suspension (1% to 3%) 1124
▲ Mepron Suspension (25%) 1598
▲ Meridia Capsules (3.8%) 481
Meruvax II 2130
Miacalcin Nasal Spray (Less than 1%) 2375
Micardis Tablets (1%) 1049
Micardis HCT Tablets (2% or greater) 1051
Midamor Tablets (Between 1% and 3%) 2136
Mirapex Tablets (1% or more) 2834
M-M-R II 2118
Mobic Tablets (0.2% to 2.4%) 1054
Moduretic Tablets 2138
▲ Monopril Tablets (2.2% to 9.7%) 1091
▲ Monopril HCT (5.6%) 1094
Mumpsvax 2141
Mykrox Tablets (Less than 2%) 1168
▲ Mylotarg for Injection (15% to 28%) 3540
▲ Myobloc Injectable Solution (3% to 7%) 1291
Nadolol Tablets (1 to 5 of 1000 patients) 2288
Naprelan Tablets (Less than 3%) 1293
Naropin Injection (Less than 1%) 612
Nasacort AQ Nasal Spray (2.1%) 752
Nasarel Nasal Solution 0.025% (Greater than 1%) 1296
▲ Nasonex Nasal Spray (7% to 13%) 3131
Natrecor for Injection (At least 1%) 3189
Navelbine Injection 1604
▲ Neoral Soft Gelatin Capsules (4% to 5%) 2380
▲ Neoral Oral Solution (4% to 5%) 2380
▲ Neumega for Injection (29%) 1434
▲ Neupogen for Injection (6%) 587
Neurontin Capsules (1.8%) 2655
Neurontin Oral Solution (1.8%) 2655
Neurontin Tablets (1.8%) 2655
Nexium Delayed-Release Capsules (Less than 1%) 619
▲ Nicotrol Inhaler (32%) 2840
Nicotrol Nasal Spray (Common) 2843
Nilandron Tablets (2%) 753
▲ Nipent for Injection (17% to 20%) 3272
▲ Nolvadex Tablets (3.8%) 678
Norvasc Tablets (Less than or equal to 0.1%) 2704
Norvir Capsules (Less than 2%) 487
Norvir Oral Solution (Less than 2%) 487
▲ Novantrone for Injection (9% to 13%) 1760
Oncaspar (Less than 1%) 756
OptiPranolol Metipranolol Ophthalmic Solution 0.3% (A small number of patients) .... ⊙ 263
▲ Ortho-Prefest Tablets (5%) 2570
Ovidrel for Injection (Less than 2%) 3220
OxyContin Tablets (Less than 1%) 2912
▲ Pacerone Tablets (2% to 7%) 3331
Paxil (Frequent) 1609
Pediazole Suspension 3050
▲ Periostat Tablets (4%) 1208
▲ Photofrin for Injection (7% to 9%) 831
▲ Plavix Tablets (3.1%) 1097
▲ Plavix Tablets (3.1%) 3084
Plendil Extended-Release Tablets (0.8% to 1.7%) 623
▲ Pletal Tablets (3% to 4%) 2605
▲ Pletal Tablets (3% to 4%) 2848
Pravachol Tablets (0.1% to 2.6%) 1099
Prevacid Delayed-Release Capsules (Less than 1%) 3292
PREVPAC (Less than 1%) 3298
Prilosec Delayed-Release Capsules (1.1%) 628
Prinivil Tablets (1% to 3.5%) 2164
▲ Prinzide Tablets (3.9%) 2168
▲ Procardia Capsules (6%) 2708
Procardia XL Extended Release Tablets (1% or less to 6%) 2710
▲ Procrit for Injection (18%) 2502
▲ Prograf (3% to 18%) 1393
▲ Proleukin for Injection (11%) 1199
▲ Prometrium Capsules (100 mg, 200 mg) (8%) 3261
ProSom Tablets (Infrequent) 500
Prostin E2 Suppositories 2852
Protonix I.V. (Greater than or equal to 1%) 3580
Protonix Tablets (Greater than or equal to 1%) 3577
▲ Protopic Ointment (1% to 15%) 1397
▲ Proventil Inhalation Solution 0.083% (3.1% to 4%) 3146
▲ Proventil Solution for Inhalation 0.5% (3.1% to 4%) 3144
Provigil Tablets (At least 1%) 1193
Prozac Pulvules, Liquid, and Weekly Capsules (1.6% to 3%) 1238
▲ Pulmicort Respules (5% to 9%) 632
▲ Pulmicort Turbuhaler Inhalation Powder (2% to 6%) 636
Pulmozyme Inhalation Solution 1426
▲ Rapamune Oral Solution and Tablets (3% to 20%) 3584
Recombivax HB (Less than 1%) 2178
ReFacto Vials 1437
Refludan for Injection (Common) 761
Relafen Tablets (Less than 1%) 1617
Relenza Rotadisk (Less than 2%) 1619
Remeron Tablets (Frequent) 2483
Remeron SolTab Tablets (Frequent) 2486
▲ Remicade for IV Injection (5% to 13%) 1178
Reminyl Oral Solution (Greater than or equal to 2%) 1792
Reminyl Tablets (Greater than or equal to 2%) 1792
▲ Renagel Capsules (4%) 1439
▲ Renagel Tablets (4%) 1439
Requip Tablets (1% or more) 1621
Rescriptor Tablets (Less than 2%) 526
Rescula Ophthalmic Solution (1% to 5%) .... ⊙ 306
Retrovir Capsules 1625
Retrovir IV Infusion 1629
Retrovir 1625
▲ Rhinocort Aqua Nasal Spray (2%) 642
▲ Rhinocort Nasal Inhaler (3% to 9%) 640
Rifater Tablets 769
Rilutek Tablets (2.1% to 3.7%) 772
▲ Risperdal (3%) 1796
Rituxan for Infusion (0.3%) 1750
Rituxan I.V. (0.3%) 1428
▲ Roferon-A Injection (1% to 27%) 2996
Roxicodone Tablets (Less than 3%) 3067
Salagen Tablets (1% to 2%) 2229
Sarafem Pulvules 1962
Sectral Capsules (1%) 3589
Semprex-D Capsules (2%) 1172
Septra Suspension (Rare) 2265
Septra Tablets (Rare) 2265
Septra DS Tablets (Rare) 2265
▲ Serevent Diskus (Greater than 3%) 1637
▲ Serevent Inhalation Aerosol (7%) 1633
Seroquel Tablets (Infrequent) 684
▲ Serostim for Injection (1% to 10%) 3229
▲ Serzone Tablets (3%) 1104
▲ Simulect for Injection (Greater than or equal to 10%) 2399
Sinemet Tablets 1253
Sinemet CR Tablets 1255
Singulair (2.7%) 2181
Skelid Tablets (2.7%) 3088
Soriatane Capsules (Less than 1%) 3003
▲ Sporanox Oral Solution (4.0% to 4.4%) 1808
▲ Sporanox Oral Solution (4.0% to 4.4%) 2512
Stadol NS Nasal Spray (1% or greater) 1108
Starlix Tablets (2.4%) 2401
Stimate Nasal Spray 796
Sular Tablets (Less than or equal to 1%) 688
▲ Suprane Liquid for Inhalation (34% to 72%) 874
▲ Sustiva Capsules (25%) 1258
Synagis Intramuscular (More than 1%) 2028
▲ Tamiflu Capsules (1.2% to 5.6%) 3008
▲ Tamiflu Oral Suspension (1.2% to 5.6%) 3008
▲ Tarka Tablets (4.6%) 508
Tasmar Tablets (Infrequent) 3010
▲ Temodar Capsules (5%) 3157
▲ Teveten Tablets (4%) 3327
Thalomid Capsules 1154
TheraCys Injection 823
Tiazac Capsules (1% to 2%) 1378
Tice BCG, BCG Live 2489
Tikosyn Capsules (Less than or equal to 2%) 2717
Timolide Tablets 2187
Timolol GFS .... ⊙ 266
Timoptic in Ocudose (Less frequent) 2192

Timoptic Sterile Ophthalmic Solution (Less frequent)............. 2190
Timoptic-XE Sterile Ophthalmic Gel Forming Solution................. 2194
▲ TOBI Solution for Inhalation (46.1%)... 1206
Topamax Sprinkle Capsules (Frequent; More than 1%)............ 2590
Topamax Tablets (Frequent; More than 1%)....................................... 2590
Toradol (1% or less)....................... 3018
Tricor Capsules, Micronized (1%).... 513
Trileptal Oral Suspension (Up to 5%)... 2407
Trileptal Tablets (Up to 5%)............ 2407
Tri-Nasal Spray (2% to 2.7%)......... 2274
▲ Trisenox Injection (65%) 1158
▲ Trizivir Tablets (18%) 1669
Trovan (Less than 1%).................... 2722
Uniretic Tablets (Less than 1% to 3%)... 3178
▲ Univasc Tablets (6.1%) 3181
Valium Injectable 3026
▲ Vancenase AQ Nasal Spray 0.084% (6%)................................. 3163
▲ Vanceril Double Strength Inhalation Aerosol (9%)................ 3167
Vantin Tablets and Oral Suspension (Less than 1%).......... 2860
Vaqta (1.0%)................................... 2199
Varivax (Greater than or equal to 1%)... 2202
Vascor Tablets (0.5% to 2.0%)........ 2602
▲ Vaseretic Tablets (3.5%) 2204
Vasotec I.V. Injection 2207
Vasotec Tablets (1.3% to 2.2%)....... 2210
Venofer Injection (Greater than 1%)... 580
Ventolin Inhalation Aerosol and Refill (2%)...................................... 1679
▲ Ventolin HFA Inhalation Aerosol (5%)... 3618
Versed Injection (1.3%)................... 3027
▲ Versed Syrup (8%) 3033
Viagra Tablets (Less than 2%)......... 2732
Vicoprofen Tablets (Less than 1%).. 520
Vioxx (Greater than 0.1% to 1.9%).. 2213
▲ Vistide Injection (19%) 1445
Vitravene for Injection (2% to 5%).. ⊙310
WelChol Tablets (2%)..................... 3073
Wellbutrin SR Sustained-Release Tablets (1% to 2%)...................... 1684
Xopenex Inhalation Solution (1.4% to 4.1%)....................................... 3207
Zebeta Tablets (2.5% to 2.6%)........ 1885
▲ Zenapax for Injection (Greater than 5%)...................................... 3046
▲ Zestoretic Tablets (3.9%) 695
Zestril Tablets (Greater than 1% to 3.5%).. 698
Ziac Tablets (1.5% to 2.2%)........... 1887
Ziagen... 1692
Zoladex (1% or greater).................. 702
Zoladex 3-month (1% to 5%)........... 706
Zoloft (Infrequent).......................... 2751
▲ Zometa for Intravenous Infusion (11.6%)... 3621
Zosyn (1.0% or less)....................... 1890
Zosyn in Galaxy Containers (1.0% or less).. 1894
▲ Zyban Sustained-Release Tablets (3%).. 1710
▲ Zyprexa Tablets (5%) 1973
▲ Zyprexa ZYDIS Orally Disintegrating Tablets (5%).......... 1973
Zyrtec (2.8% to 4.4%)..................... 2756

Cough, productive

Permax Tablets (Frequent).............. 1299

Cough reflex, depression

Astramorph/PF Injection, USP (Preservative-Free)....................... 594
Compazine....................................... 1505
Duramorph Injection....................... 1312
Infumorph 200 and Infumorph 500 Sterile Solutions.................. 1314
Kadian Capsules (Less than 3%)..... 1335
Stelazine.. 1640
Thorazine... 1656

CPK, elevation

(see under Creatine kinase, increase)

Cramping

Advair Diskus 100/50...................... 1448
Advair Diskus 250/50...................... 1448
Advair Diskus 500/50...................... 1448
Aldoclor Tablets............................. 2035
Aldoril Tablets................................ 2039
Alferon N Injection (One patient)...... 1770
Aminohippurate Sodium PAH Injection....................................... 2041
Asacol Delayed-Release Tablets...... 2884
Atacand HCT Tablets...................... 597
Avalide Tablets............................... 1070
Clinoril Tablets (Greater than 1%).... 2053
Clorpres Tablets.............................. 1002
Colazal Capsules (1%)..................... 3069
Combipres Tablets........................... 1040
Coumadin for Injection (Infrequent)................................... 1243
Coumadin Tablets (Infrequent)......... 1243
▲ Crinone (19%) 3213
Cytotec Tablets (0.6%).................... 3202
Dilaudid Oral Liquid........................ 445
Dilaudid Tablets - 8 mg................... 445
Diovan HCT Tablets........................ 2338
Diucardin Tablets............................ 3494
Diuril Oral....................................... 2087
Diuril Sodium Intravenous............... 2086
Exelon Capsules (Infrequent).......... 2342
Exelon Oral Solution (Infrequent)..... 2345
▲ Ferrlecit Injection (25%) 3386
Sterile FUDR.................................... 2974
Gengraf Capsules (1% to 4%)......... 457
HydroDIURIL Tablets...................... 2108
Hyzaar... 2109
Inderide Tablets.............................. 3517
Inderide LA Long-Acting Capsules... 3519
Lotensin HCT Tablets...................... 2367
Maxzide... 1008
MetroGel-Vaginal Gel (1%).............. 1986
Moduretic Tablets........................... 2138
Neoral Soft Gelatin Capsules (1% to 4%)... 2380
Neoral Oral Solution (1% to 4%)...... 2380
Nexium Delayed-Release Capsules (Less than 1%)............. 619
Oramorph SR Tablets (Less frequent)..................................... 3062
ParaGard T 380A Intrauterine Copper Contraceptive................. 2582
Prinzide Tablets.............................. 2168
Renese Tablets................................ 2712
Rifamate Capsules.......................... 767
Sandimmune (Up to 4%)................. 2388
Serzone Tablets.............................. 1104
Tenoretic Tablets............................ 690
▲ Thrombate III (2 of 17) 944
Timolide Tablets............................. 2187
Uniretic Tablets............................... 3178
Vaseretic Tablets............................ 2204
Warfarin Sodium Tablets, USP........ 3302
Zarontin Capsules (Frequent).......... 2659
Zarontin Syrup (Frequent)............... 2660
Zestoretic Tablets (0.3% to 1%)...... 695
Ziac Tablets.................................... 1887

Cramping, abdominal

(see under Abdominal pain/cramps)

Cramping, muscular

Adalat CC Tablets (Rare)................ 877
Alferon N Injection (1%).................. 1770
Amerge Tablets (Infrequent)............ 1467
Anadrol-50 Tablets.......................... 3321
Arava Tablets (1% to 3%)................ 724
▲ Aricept Tablets (3% to 8%) 1270
▲ Aricept Tablets (3% to 8%) 2665
Asacol Delayed-Release Tablets...... 2884
Atromid-S Capsules (Less often)..... 3483
Avalide Tablets (1% or greater)....... 1070
Avapro Tablets (Less than 1%)....... 1074
Avapro Tablets (Less than 1%)....... 3076
Baycol Tablets................................. 883
Brethine Ampuls (Less than 0.5%).... 2314
Brethine Tablets (Less than 1%)..... 2313
Cardizem Injectable......................... 1018
Cardizem Lyo-Ject Syringe.............. 1018
Cardizem Monovial.......................... 1018
Cardizem CD Capsules (Less than 1%)... 1016
Cardura Tablets (1%)...................... 2668
Ceftin Tablets (0.1% to 1%)............ 1898
Covera-HS Tablets (Less than 2%)... 3199
Cozaar Tablets (1.1%)..................... 2067
Crixivan Capsules (Less than 2%)..... 2070
CytoGam Intravenous (Less than 5.0%).. 2026
Cytotec Tablets (Infrequent)............ 3202
Demadex Tablets and Injection....... 2965
Diovan Capsules.............................. 2337
Diovan HCT Tablets (Greater than 0.2%).. 2338
Dipentum Capsules (Rare).............. 2803
Diucardin Tablets............................ 3494
Diuril Sodium Intravenous............... 2086
Dolobid Tablets (Rare).................... 2088
Dyazide Capsules............................ 1515
Eldepryl Capsules........................... 3266
Enalaprilat Injection......................... 863
Famotidine Injection (Infrequent)..... 866
Foradil Aerolizer.............................. 2354
Fortovase Capsules (Less than 2%)... 2970
Furosemide Tablets......................... 2284
▲ Gleevec Capsules (25% to 46%) 2357
Hivid Tablets (Less than 1%)........... 2975
Hyzaar... 2109
Imitrex Injection (1.1%)................... 1549
Imitrex Nasal Spray (Rare).............. 1554
Imitrex Tablets (Infrequent)............. 1558
▲ Indapamide Tablets (Greater than or equal to 5%)............................ 2286
Invirase Capsules (Less than 2%).... 2979
Isoptin SR Tablets (1% or less)....... 467
Klonopin Tablets (Infrequent)........... 2983
K-Phos Neutral Tablets.................... 946
K-Phos Original (Sodium Free) Tablets (Less frequent)............... 947
Lescol Capsules.............................. 2361
Lescol Capsules.............................. 2925
Lescol XL Tablets............................ 2361
Lescol XL Tablets............................ 2925
Lexxel Tablets................................. 608
Lodosyn Tablets.............................. 1251
Lotrel Capsules............................... 2370
Mavik Tablets (0.3% to 1.0%)......... 478
Maxalt Tablets (Infrequent).............. 2120
Maxalt-MLT Orally Disintegrating Tablets (Infrequent)..................... 2120
Maxzide... 1008
Mestinon... 1740
Mevacor Tablets (0.6% to 1.1%)..... 2132
Midamor Tablets (Between 1% and 3%)... 2136
Migranal Nasal Spray (Infrequent)... 2376
Moduretic Tablets (Less than or equal to 1%)................................. 2138
Monopril Tablets (0.2% to 1.0% or more)... 1091
Monopril HCT (Less than 2%)......... 1094
▲ Mykrox Tablets (5.8%) 1168
Naropin Injection (Less than 1%) 612
Nimotop Capsules (Up to 1.4%) 904
Normodyne Tablets (Less common)....................................... 3137
Norvasc Tablets (Less than 1% to 2%)... 2704
Norvir Capsules (Less than 2%) 487
Norvir Oral Solution (Less than 2%) 487
Oncaspar 756
Pepcid Injection (Infrequent) 2153
Pepcid for Oral Suspension (Infrequent).................................... 2150
Pepcid RPD Orally Disintegrating Tablets (Infrequent) 2150
Pepcid Tablets (Infrequent) 2150
Plendil Extended-Release Tablets (0.5% to 1.5%) 623
Prilosec Delayed-Release Capsules (Less than 1%) 628
Prinivil Tablets (Greater than 1%) 2164
Prinzide Tablets (2%) 2168
▲ Procardia Capsules (2% or less to 8%) 2708
▲ Procardia XL Extended Release Tablets (8%)................................. 2710
▲ Prograf (3% to 15%) 1393
Prostigmin Injectable 1744
Prostigmin Tablets 1744
Prostin E2 Suppositories 2852
▲ Proventil Repetabs Tablets (3%) 3148
Rescriptor Tablets (Less than 2%) ... 526
Roferon-A Injection (Infrequent) 2996
Rythmol Tablets – 150 mg, 225 mg, 300 mg (Less than 1%) 502
Serevent Inhalation Aerosol (1% to 3%) 1633
▲ Simulect for Injection (3% to 10%) . 2399
Sinemet Tablets 1253
Sinemet CR Tablets (0.8%) 1255
Synvisc 3596
▲ Tasmar Tablets (17% to 18%) 3010
Tenoretic Tablets 690
Teveten Tablets (Less than 1%) 3327
Tiazac Capsules (Less than 2%) 1378
Timolide Tablets 2187
Tonocard Tablets (Less than 1%) 649
Trovan (Less than 1%) 2722
Uroqid-Acid No. 2 Tablets 947
Vaseretic Tablets (2.7%) 2204
Vasotec I.V. Injection 2207
Vasotec Tablets (0.5% to 1.0%) 2210
Ventolin Inhalation Aerosol and Refill (1%) 1679
Verelan Capsules (1% or less) 3184
Verelan PM Capsules (2% or less) ... 3186
Vioxx (Greater than 0.1% to 1.9%) .. 2213
Viracept 532
Volmax Extended-Release Tablets (2.7%) 2276
Xanax Tablets (2.4%) 2865
Zaroxolyn Tablets 1177
Zebeta Tablets 1885
Zestoretic Tablets (2.0%) 695
Zestril Tablets (0.5% to greater than 1%) 698
Ziac Tablets (1.1% to 1.2%) 1887
Zocor Tablets 2219
Zoloft (Infrequent) 2751

Cramps, abdominal

(see under Abdominal pain/cramps)

Cramps, lower limbs

Aciphex Tablets 1267
Aciphex Tablets 1783
Actiq (1% or greater) 1184
▲ Actonel Tablets (3.3% to 3.5%) 2879
Adalat CC Tablets (3% or less) 877
Agrylin Capsules (1% to 5%) 3232
Ambien Tablets (Infrequent) 3191
Arava Tablets (1%) 724
Atacand HCT Tablets (0.5% or greater) 597
Betaseron for SC Injection 988
Carbatrol Capsules 3234
▲ Carnitor Injection (4% to 8%) 3242
▲ Casodex Tablets (2% to 5%) 662
Catapres Tablets (About 3 in 1,000) 1037
Catapres-TTS (0.5% or less)........... 1038
Caverject Sterile Powder (Less than 1%)....................................... 2777
Celebrex Capsules (0.1% to 1.9%)... 2676
Celebrex Capsules (0.1% to 1.9%)... 2780
Celexa (Infrequent).......................... 1365
▲ CellCept Capsules (3% to 16.6%) ... 2951
▲ CellCept Intravenous (3% to 16.6%)... 2951
▲ CellCept Oral Suspension (3% to 16.6%)... 2951
▲ CellCept Tablets (3% to 16.6%) 2951
▲ Cenestin Tablets (10%) 1263
Cerebyx Injection (Infrequent).......... 2619
Claritin (At least one patient)........... 3100
Claritin-D 12 Hour Extended Release Tablets (Less frequent)... 3102
Claritin-D 24 Hour Extended Release Tablets (Fewer than 2%) 3104
Clorpres Tablets (About 3 in 1,000)... 1002
Combipres Tablets (About 3 in 1,000) 1040
Coreg Tablets (More than 2%)......... 1508
Corlopam Injection (0.5% to 5%) 412
Crinone (Less than 5%) 3213
Cytovene (At least 3 subjects) 2959
Depacon Injection (1% to 5%) 416
Depakene (1% to 5%) 421
Depakote Sprinkle Capsules (1% to 5%) 426
Depakote Tablets (1% to 5%) 430
Depakote ER Tablets (1% to 5%) 436
▲ Depo-Provera Contraceptive Injection (More than 5%) 2798
Desferal Vials 2333
Didronel Tablets 2888
DuoNeb Inhalation Solution (1.4%) .. 1233
Duraclon Injection (0.3%) 3057
DynaCirc Capsules (0.5% to 1%) 2921
DynaCirc CR Tablets (0.5% to 1%) .. 2923
Effexor Tablets (Infrequent) 3495
Effexor XR Capsules (Infrequent) 3499
8-MOP Capsules 1727
▲ Emcyt Capsules (8%) 2810
▲ Evista Tablets (5.9% to 7%) 1915
Evoxac Capsules (1% to 3%) 1217
Exelon Capsules (Frequent) 2342
Exelon Oral Solution (Frequent) 2345
▲ Ferrlecit Injection (10%) 3386
Fortovase Capsules (Less than 2%) 2970
Foscavir Injection (Between 1% and 5%) 605
Gabitril Tablets (Infrequent) 1189
Gammagard S/D (Occasional) 845
▲ Gengraf Capsules (12%) 457
Glucotrol XL Extended Release Tablets (Less than 3%)................. 2693
Hivid Tablets (Less than 1%) 2975
Intron A for Injection (Less than 5%) 3120
Invirase Capsules (Less than 2%) 2979
Klonopin Tablets (Infrequent) 2983
Lamictal (Rare) 1567
Lipitor Tablets (Less than 2%) 2639
Lipitor Tablets (Less than 2%) 2696
Lupron Depot–4 Month 30 mg (Less than 5%) 3289
Luvox Tablets (25, 50, 100 mg) 3256
Meridia Capsules (Greater than or equal to 1%) 481
Micardis Tablets (More than 0.3%) .. 1049
Micardis HCT Tablets 1051
Mirapex Tablets (1% or more) 2834
Naprelan Tablets (Less than 3%) 1293
Natrecor for Injection (At least 1%) 3189
▲ Neoral Soft Gelatin Capsules (12%) 2380
▲ Neoral Oral Solution (12%) 2380
Oxsoralen-Ultra Capsules 1741
Pentasa Capsules (Less than 1%) ... 3239
Plavix Tablets (1% to 2.5%) 1097
Plavix Tablets (1% to 2.5%) 3084
Pletal Tablets (2% or greater) 2605
Pletal Tablets (2% or greater) 2848
ProAmatine Tablets (Rare) 3241
Procardia XL Extended Release Tablets (Less than 3%) 2710
▲ Prograf (3% to 15%) 1393
Prometrium Capsules (100 mg, 200 mg) (Less than 5%) 3261
Protonix I.V. (Less than 1%) 3580
Protonix Tablets (Less than 1%) 3577
Proventil HFA Inhalation Aerosol (Less than 3%) 3150
Provigil Tablets (At least 1%) 1193
Prozac Pulvules, Liquid, and Weekly Capsules (Infrequent) 1238
▲ Rapamune Oral Solution and Tablets (3% to 20%) 3584
Requip Tablets (1% or more) 1621
Rescriptor Tablets (Less than 2%) ... 526
Rilutek Tablets (Infrequent) 772
Risperdal (Rare) 1796
▲ Roferon-A Injection (3%) 2996
Salagen Tablets 2229

▲ Sandostatin LAR Depot (5% to 15%) 2395
Sarafem Pulvules (Infrequent) 1962
Serevent Inhalation Aerosol (1% to 3%) 1633
Seroquel Tablets (Infrequent) 684
Sular Tablets (Less than or equal to 1%) 688
Synvisc 3596
Tegretol/Tegretol-XR 2404
Tenex Tablets (3% or less) 2942
Tequin Injection (Less than 0.1%) 1110
Tequin Tablets (Less than 0.1%) 1110
Thalomid Capsules 1154
Topamax Sprinkle Capsules (Infrequent) 2590
Topamax Tablets (Infrequent) 2590
Tricor Capsules, Micronized 513
▲ Venofer Injection (23%) 580
Vistide Injection 1445
Wellbutrin SR Sustained-Release Tablets (Infrequent) 1684
Xopenex Inhalation Solution (2.7%) 3207
▲ Zenapax for Injection (2% to 5%) 3046
Zoladex (2%) 702
Zoladex 3-month 706
Zoloft (Infrequent) 2751
Zomig Tablets (Infrequent) 708
Zomig-ZMT Tablets (Infrequent) 708
Zonegran Capsules (Infrequent) 1307
Zyban Sustained-Release Tablets (Infrequent) 1710
Zyprexa Tablets (Infrequent) 1973
Zyprexa ZYDIS Orally Disintegrating Tablets (Infrequent) 1973
Zyrtec (Less than 2%) 2756
Zyrtec-D 12 Hour Extended Relief Tablets (Less than 2%) 2758

Cramps, pelvic
Cytotec Tablets (0.6%) 3202

Cranial nerve, dysfunction
Baycol Tablets 883
Ifex for Injection (Less frequent) 1123
JE-VAX Vaccine (One case) 811
Lescol Capsules 2361
Lescol Capsules 2925
Lescol XL Tablets 2361
Lescol XL Tablets 2925
Pravachol Tablets 1099
Zocor Tablets 2219

Cranial nerve, paralysis of
Amerge Tablets (Rare) 1467

Cranial nerve deficit, fetal
Accutane Capsules 2944

Craniofacial deformities
Accupril Tablets 2611
Altace Capsules 2233
Captopril Tablets 2281
Cozaar Tablets 2067
Enalaprilat Injection 863
Hyzaar 2109
Lexxel Tablets 608
Lotrel Capsules 2370
Monopril Tablets 1091
Prinivil Tablets 2164
Prinzide Tablets 2168
Univasc Tablets 3181
Vaseretic Tablets 2204
Vasotec I.V. Injection 2207
Vasotec Tablets 2210
Zestoretic Tablets 695
Zestril Tablets 698

Craniosynostosis
Synthroid 505

Creatine kinase, increase
Accutane Capsules 2944
Aciphex Tablets 1267
Aciphex Tablets 1783
Actos Tablets 3275
Adalat CC Tablets (Rare) 877
Amicar Injection 3608
Amicar Syrup 3608
Amicar Tablets 3608
Anadrol-50 Tablets 3321
Arava Tablets (1% to 3%) 724
Atacand Tablets (0.5% or greater) 595
Atacand HCT Tablets (0.5% or greater) 597
Atromid-S Capsules 3483
Axert Tablets (Infrequent) 2772
Cardizem Injectable 1018
Cardizem Lyo-Ject Syringe 1018
Cardizem Monovial 1018
Cardizem CD Capsules (Less than 1%) 1016
Clozaril Tablets 2319
Colazal Capsules 3069
Combivir Tablets 1502
Comtan Tablets 2328
Dynabac Tablets (1.2%) 2269
Effexor Tablets 3495
Effexor XR Capsules 3499
Epivir 1520
▲ Epivir-HBV (9%) 1524
Evoxac Capsules 1217
Felbatol (Rare) 3343
Lopid Tablets 2650
▲ Mevacor Tablets (11%) 2132
Nardil Tablets 2653
Orap Tablets 1407
Oxandrin Tablets 1153
Paxil (Rare) 1609
Pravachol Tablets (Rare) 1099
Procardia Capsules (Rare) 2708
Procardia XL Extended Release Tablets (Rare) 2710
▲ Rapamune Oral Solution and Tablets (3% to 20%) 3584
ReFacto Vials 1437
Sandostatin Injection (Less than 1%) 2394
Sandostatin LAR Depot (Rare) 2395
Seroquel Tablets 684
Sinemet Tablets 1253
Symmetrel 1328
Tasmar Tablets (Three cases) 3010
Teveten Tablets (Less than 1%) 3327
Tiazac Capsules (Less than 2%) 1378
▲ Tricor Capsules, Micronized (3%) 513
Trizivir Tablets 1669
Twinrix Vaccine 1674
Uniretic Tablets (Less than 1%) 3178
▲ Videx (6% to 8%) 1138
Videx EC Capsules 1143
Ziagen 1692
Zocor Tablets 2219

Creatinine, increase
(*see under* Serum creatinine, elevation)

Creatinine clearance, decrease
Coly-Mycin M Parenteral 2243
Cytovene (At least 3 subjects) 2959
Eskalith 1527
▲ Foscavir Injection (5% or greater) 605
Ifex for Injection 1123
Kefurox Vials, ADD-Vantage 1948
Lithobid Slow-Release Tablets 3255
Macrobid Capsules 2889
Macrodantin Capsules 2891
Mandol Vials 1953
Motrin Suspension, Oral Drops, Chewable Tablets, and Caplets (Less than 1%) 2002
Paraplatin for Injection 1126
Valcyte Tablets (Less than 5%) 3022
▲ Vistide Injection (Up to 53%) 1445
Zinacef Injection 1696
Zinacef for Injection 1696

Crepitations
▲ Trisenox Injection (10%) 1158

Crohn's disease
Remicade for IV Injection (Less than 2%) 1178

Crohn's disease, exacerbation
Proleukin for Injection (Two patients) 1199

Croup
(*see under* Laryngotracheobronchitis)

Crying
ActHIB Vaccine (Up to 1.6%) 798
Ambien Tablets 3191
Aricept Tablets (Frequent) 1270
Aricept Tablets (Frequent) 2665
Ativan Injection (1.3%) 3478
▲ Comvax (0.2% to 10.6%) 2056
Crinone (Less than 5%) 3213
Diphtheria & Tetanus Toxoids Adsorbed Purogenated for Pediatric Use (0.7%) 1857
HibTITER (38 of 1,118 vaccinations) 1859
Infanrix Vaccine (2.2% to 3.9%) 1562
IPOL Vaccine (Up to 1.4%) 809
Nubain Injection (1% or less) 1323
Recombivax HB (Greater than 1%) 2178
Romazicon Injection (1% to 3%) 3000
Tripedia Vaccine 817

Cryptococcosis
Cerebyx Injection (Infrequent) 2619
Doxil Injection (Less than 1%) 566
Vistide Injection 1445

Cryptorchidism
Gonal-F for Injection 3216

Cryptosporidiosis
▲ Taxol Injection (7%) 1129

Crystalluria
Ancobon Capsules 1730
Azulfidine EN-tabs Tablets (Rare) 2775
Bactrim 2949
Cipro I.V. (1% or less) 893
Cipro I.V. Pharmacy Bulk Package (Less than 1%) 897
Cipro (Rare) 887
Clinoril Tablets (Less than 1 in 100) 2053
Crixivan Capsules 2070
Dantrium Capsules (Less frequent) 2885
Demser Capsules (A few patients) 2085
Diamox ⊙269
Effexor Tablets (Rare) 3495
Effexor XR Capsules (Rare) 3499
Floxin I.V. 2526
Floxin Tablets 2529
Fludara for Injection 995
Levaquin 2537
Mintezol 2137
Neptazane Tablets (Rare) ⊙271
Noroxin Tablets 2145
Paser Granules 1781
Pediazole Suspension 3050
Septra Suspension 2265
Septra Tablets 2265
Septra DS Tablets 2265
Uniretic Tablets (Less than 1%) 3178
Urobiotic-250 Capsules 2731

Cushingoid state
(*see under* Cushing's syndrome)

Cushing's syndrome
Aclovate 1275
Advair Diskus 100/50 1448
Advair Diskus 250/50 1448
Advair Diskus 500/50 1448
Beconase Inhalation Aerosol 1497
Betaseron for SC Injection 988
Celestone Soluspan Injectable Suspension 3097
Celestone Syrup 3099
▲ CellCept Capsules (3% to 10%) 2951
▲ CellCept Intravenous (3% to 10%) 2951
▲ CellCept Oral Suspension (3% to 10%) 2951
▲ CellCept Tablets (3% to 10%) 2951
Clobevate Gel 3271
Copaxone for Injection (Infrequent) 3306
Cormax Cream 2440
Cormax Ointment 2440
Cormax Scalp Application 2441
Cortone Acetate Injectable Suspension 2059
Cortone Acetate Tablets 2061
Cutivate Cream 1282
Cutivate Ointment 1284
Decadron Elixir 2078
Decadron Tablets 2079
Decadron Phosphate Injection 2081
Depo-Medrol Injectable Suspension 2795
Dermatop Emollient Cream 2517
Diprolene Ointment 0.05% (Some patients) 3108
Diprolene AF Cream 0.05% (Some patients) 3106
Elocon Cream 0.1% 3110
Florinef Acetate Tablets 2250
Flovent Diskus 3614
Flovent 1535
Flovent Rotadisk 1537
Hydrocortone Tablets 2106
Hydrocortone Acetate Injectable Suspension 2103
Hydrocortone Phosphate Injection, Sterile 2105
Kaletra Capsules (Less than 2%) 471
Kaletra Oral Solution (Less than 2%) 471
Neurontin Capsules (Rare) 2655
Neurontin Oral Solution (Rare) 2655
Neurontin Tablets (Rare) 2655
Olux Foam 1211
Pediapred Oral Solution 1170
Prednisone 3064
Prelone Syrup 2273
▲ Prograf (3% to 15%) 1393
▲ Rapamune Oral Solution and Tablets (3% to 20%) 3584
Solu-Medrol Sterile Powder 2855
Temovate Cream 1301
Temovate Gel 1303
Temovate Ointment 1301
Temovate Scalp Application 1304
Temovate E Emollient 1302
Vancenase PocketHaler Nasal Inhaler 3162

Cutaneous tenderness
8-MOP Capsules 1727
Oxsoralen-Ultra Capsules 1741

Cyanosis
AmBisome for Injection (Infrequent) 1383
Americaine Anesthetic Lubricant 1162
Americaine Otic Topical Anesthetic Ear Drops 1162
AquaMEPHYTON Injection 2042
Azulfidine EN-tabs Tablets (One in every 30 patients or less) 2775
Betaseron for SC Injection 988
Bicillin C-R 900/300 Injection 2240
Bicillin C-R Injection 2238
Bicillin L-A Injection 2242
Buprenex Injectable (Less than 1%) 2918
Campath Ampules 992
Cerebyx Injection (Infrequent) 2619
▲ Cerezyme for Injection (Approximately 4%) 1438
Clozaril Tablets (Less than 1%) 2319
Copaxone for Injection (Infrequent) 3306
Cytovene-IV (One report) 2959
Effexor Tablets (Rare) 3495
Effexor XR Capsules (Rare) 3499
▲ Flolan for Injection (31% to 54%) 1528
Fortovase Capsules (Less than 2%) 2970
Gammar-P I.V. 787
Hivid Tablets (Less than 1%) 2975
Imitrex Injection 1549
Imitrex Nasal Spray 1554
Imitrex Tablets 1558
▲ Infasurf Intratracheal Suspension (65%) 1372
INFeD Injection 3388
Intron A for Injection (Less than or equal to 5%) 3120
Invirase Capsules (Less than 2%) 2979
Levo-Dromoran 1734
Macrobid Capsules (Rare) 2889
Macrodantin Capsules (Rare) 2891
Mephyton Tablets (Rare) 2129
Pediazole Suspension 3050
Permax Tablets (Infrequent) 1299
Primaxin I.M. 2158
Primaxin I.V. (Less than 0.2%) 2160
Rilutek Tablets (Rare) 772
Roferon-A Injection (Less than 1%) 2996
Seroquel Tablets (Rare) 684
Sonata Capsules (Rare) 3591
Soriatane Capsules (Less than 1%) 3003
Tequin Injection (Less than 0.1%) 1110
Tequin Tablets (Less than 0.1%) 1110
Thalomid Capsules 1154
Virazole for Inhalation Solution (Infrequent) 1747
Zomig Tablets (Rare) 708
Zomig-ZMT Tablets (Rare) 708
Zyprexa Tablets (Infrequent) 1973
Zyprexa ZYDIS Orally Disintegrating Tablets (Infrequent) 1973

Cyanosis, hand
Intron A for Injection (Less than 5%) 3120

Cycloplegia
Donnatal 2929
Donnatal Extentabs 2930
Donnatal Tablets 2929
Levsin/Levsinex/Levbid 3172
NuLev Orally Disintegrating Tablets 3176
Robinul Forte Tablets 1358
Robinul Injectable 2940
Robinul Tablets 1358

Cylindruria
Cipro I.V. (1% or less) 893
Cipro I.V. Pharmacy Bulk Package (Less than 1%) 897
Cipro 887
Floxin I.V. 2526
Floxin Tablets 2529
Levaquin 2537
Nebcin Vials, Hyporets & ADD-Vantage 1955
Noroxin Tablets 2145

Cyst, renal
Hivid Tablets (Less than 1%) 2975

Cyst, sebaceous
Rescriptor Tablets (Less than 2%) 526

Cyst, synovial
Gengraf Capsules (1% to less than 3%) 457
Neoral Soft Gelatin Capsules (1% to less than 3%) 2380
Neoral Oral Solution (1% to less than 3%) 2380

Cyst, unspecified
Actiq (Less than 1%) 1184
Arava Tablets (1% to 3%) 724
▲ Betaseron for SC Injection (4%) 988
▲ Casodex Tablets (2% to 5%) 662
▲ CellCept Capsules (3%) 2951
▲ CellCept Intravenous (3%) 2951
▲ CellCept Oral Suspension (3%) 2951
▲ CellCept Tablets (3%) 2951
Cognex Capsules (Infrequent) 1351
Copaxone for Injection (2%) 3306
Crinone (Less than 5%) 3213
Gabitril Tablets (Frequent) 1189
Imitrex Injection 1549
Lupron Depot–4 Month 30 mg (Less than 5%) 3289
Luvox Tablets (25, 50, 100 mg) (Rare) 3256
Myobloc Injectable Solution (2% or greater) 1291

Neurontin Capsules (Infrequent)...... 2655
Neurontin Oral Solution (Infrequent)........ 2655
Neurontin Tablets (Infrequent)........ 2655
Protonix I.V. (Less than 1%)........ 3580
Protonix Tablets (Less than 1%)........ 3577
Protopic Ointment (Up to 3%)........ 1397
Rescriptor Tablets (Less than 2%)... 526
Salagen Tablets (Less than 1%)...... 2229
▲ Simulect for Injection (3% to 10%) .. 2399
Soriatane Capsules (Less than 1%)........ 3003
Thalomid Capsules........ 1154
Tricor Capsules, Micronized........ 513
Uniretic Tablets (Less than 1%)....... 3178
Vioxx (Greater than 0.1% to 1.9%).. 2213
Vistide Injection........ 1445

Cystic masses in the pelvis

ParaGard T 380A Intrauterine Copper Contraceptive........ 2582

Cystitis

Aciphex Tablets........ 1267
Aciphex Tablets........ 1783
Activella Tablets........ 2764
▲ Actonel Tablets (4.1%)........ 2879
Alesse-21 Tablets........ 3468
Alesse-28 Tablets........ 3473
Ambien Tablets (Infrequent)........ 3191
Arava Tablets (1% to 3%)........ 724
Aricept Tablets (Infrequent)........ 1270
Aricept Tablets (Infrequent)........ 2665
Atacand HCT Tablets (0.5% or greater)........ 597
Ativan Injection (Less than 1%)........ 3478
Avelox Tablets (0.05% to 1%)........ 879
Azmacort Inhalation Aerosol (1% to 3%)........ 728
▲ Betaseron for SC Injection (8%)........ 988
Betaxon Ophthalmic Suspension (Less than 2%)........ 537
Brevicon 28-Day Tablets........ 3380
Cognex Capsules (Infrequent)........ 1351
Copaxone for Injection (At least 2%)........ 3306
Crinone (Less than 5%)........ 3213
Cyclessa Tablets........ 2450
Depacon Injection (1% or more)........ 416
Depakene (1% or more)........ 421
Depakote Sprinkle Capsules........ 426
Depakote Tablets (1% to 5%)........ 430
Depakote ER Tablets (Greater than 1%)........ 436
Desogen Tablets........ 2458
Ditropan XL Extended Release Tablets (2% to 5%)........ 564
Doxil Injection (Less than 1% to 5%)........ 566
Effexor Tablets (Infrequent)........ 3495
Effexor XR Capsules (Infrequent)........ 3499
Estinyl Tablets........ 3112
Estratest........ 3252
Estring Vaginal Ring (1% to 3%)........ 2811
Estrostep........ 2627
▲ Eulexin Capsules (16%)........ 3118
▲ Evista Tablets (3.3% to 4.6%)........ 1915
Evoxac Capsules (1% to 3%)........ 1217
Exelon Capsules (Infrequent)........ 2342
Exelon Oral Solution (Infrequent)........ 2345
Feldene Capsules (Occasional)........ 2685
femhrt Tablets........ 2635
Gabitril Tablets (Infrequent)........ 1189
Intron A for Injection (Less than 5%)........ 3120
Klonopin Tablets (Infrequent)........ 2983
Lamictal (Rare)........ 1567
Leukeran Tablets........ 1591
Levlen........ 962
Levlite 21 Tablets........ 962
Levlite 28 Tablets........ 962
Levora Tablets........ 3389
Lipitor Tablets (Less than 2%)........ 2639
Lipitor Tablets (Less than 2%)........ 2696
Lodine (Less than 1%)........ 3528
Lodine XL Extended-Release Tablets (Less than 1%)........ 3530
Loestrin 21 Tablets........ 2642
Loestrin Fe Tablets........ 2642
Lo/Ovral Tablets........ 3532
Lo/Ovral-28 Tablets........ 3538
Low-Ogestrel-28 Tablets........ 3392
Lunelle Monthly Injection........ 2827
Luvox Tablets (25, 50, 100 mg) (Infrequent)........ 3256
Menest Tablets........ 2254
Miacalcin Nasal Spray (1% to 3%)........ 2375
Micardis Tablets (More than 0.3%)........ 1049
Micardis HCT Tablets........ 1051
Microgestin Fe 1.5/30 Tablets........ 3407
Microgestin Fe 1/20 Tablets........ 3400
Migranal Nasal Spray (Infrequent)........ 2376
Mircette Tablets........ 2470
Modicon........ 2563
Motrin Suspension, Oral Drops, Chewable Tablets, and Caplets (Less than 1%)........ 2002
Myobloc Injectable Solution (2% or greater)........ 1291
Naprelan Tablets (Less than 3%)........ 1293
Necon........ 3415
Neurontin Capsules (Infrequent)........ 2655
Neurontin Oral Solution (Infrequent)........ 2655
Neurontin Tablets (Infrequent)........ 2655
Nexium Delayed-Release Capsules (Less than 1%)........ 619
Nordette-28 Tablets........ 2257
Norinyl 1 +35 28-Day Tablets........ 3380
Norinyl 1 + 50 28-Day Tablets........ 3380
Ogestrel 0.5/50-28 Tablets........ 3428
Ortho Dienestrol Cream........ 2554
Ortho-Cept 21 Tablets........ 2546
Ortho-Cept 28 Tablets........ 2546
Ortho-Cyclen/Ortho Tri-Cyclen........ 2573
Ortho-Novum........ 2563
Ortho-Novum 1/50▢28 Tablets........ 2556
Ortho-Cyclen/Ortho Tri-Cyclen........ 2573
Ovcon........ 3364
Ovral Tablets........ 3551
Ovral-28 Tablets........ 3552
Ovrette Tablets........ 3552
Paxil (Infrequent)........ 1609
Permax Tablets (Infrequent)........ 1299
Plavix Tablets (1% to 2.5%)........ 1097
Plavix Tablets (1% to 2.5%)........ 3084
Pletal Tablets (Less than 2%)........ 2605
Pletal Tablets (Less than 2%)........ 2848
Premarin Intravenous........ 3563
Premarin Vaginal Cream........ 3570
Premphase Tablets........ 3572
Prempro Tablets........ 3572
▲ Prograf (3% to 15%)........ 1393
Protonix I.V. (Less than 1%)........ 3580
Protonix Tablets (Less than 1%)........ 3577
Provera Tablets........ 2853
Provigil Tablets (At least 1%)........ 1193
Prozac Pulvules, Liquid, and Weekly Capsules (Infrequent)........ 1238
Remeron Tablets (Infrequent)........ 2483
Remeron SolTab Tablets (Infrequent)........ 2486
Reminyl Oral Solution (Infrequent)........ 1792
Reminyl Tablets (Infrequent)........ 1792
Risperdal (Rare)........ 1796
Sarafem Pulvules (Infrequent)........ 1962
Seroquel Tablets (Infrequent)........ 684
Serzone Tablets (Infrequent)........ 1104
Sonata Capsules (Infrequent)........ 3591
▲ Sporanox Capsules (3%)........ 1800
Teveten Tablets (Less than 1%)........ 3327
▲ TheraCys Injection (29%)........ 823
Thioplex for Injection (Rare)........ 1765
▲ Tice BCG, BCG Live (5.9%)........ 2489
Tricor Capsules, Micronized........ 513
Tri-Levlen........ 962
Tri-Norinyl-28 Tablets........ 3433
Triphasil-21 Tablets........ 3600
Triphasil-28 Tablets........ 3605
Trivora Tablets........ 3439
Uniretic Tablets (Less than 1%)........ 3178
▲ Valstar Sterile Solution for Intravesical Instillation (4% to 15%)........ 1175
Viagra Tablets (Less than 2%)........ 2732
Vicoprofen Tablets (Less than 1%)........ 520
Vioxx (Greater than 0.1% to 1.9%)........ 2213
Wellbutrin Tablets (Rare)........ 1680
Wellbutrin SR Sustained-Release Tablets........ 1684
Yasmin 28 Tablets (Greater than 1%)........ 980
Zanaflex Tablets (Infrequent)........ 1305
Zebeta Tablets........ 1885
Ziac Tablets........ 1887
▲ Zoladex (16%)........ 702
▲ Zoladex 3-month (16%)........ 706
Zoloft (Rare)........ 2751
Zomig Tablets (Infrequent)........ 708
Zomig-ZMT Tablets (Infrequent)........ 708
Zovia........ 3449
Zyban Sustained-Release Tablets........ 1710
Zyprexa Tablets (Infrequent)........ 1973
Zyprexa ZYDIS Orally Disintegrating Tablets (Infrequent)........ 1973
Zyrtec (Less than 2%)........ 2756
Zyrtec-D 12 Hour Extended Relief Tablets (Less than 2%)........ 2758

Cystitis, chemical

Rimso-50 Solution........ 1267

Cystitis, hemorrhagic

Adriamycin PFS/RDF Injection........ 2767
AmBisome for Injection (Infrequent)........ 1383
Cipro I.V. (1% or less)........ 893
Cipro I.V. Pharmacy Bulk Package (Less than 1%)........ 897
Fludara for Injection (Rare)........ 995
Herceptin I.V. (At least one of the 958 patients)........ 1414
Ifex for Injection........ 1123
Navelbine Injection (Less than 1%)........ 1604
Oncaspar........ 756
Thioplex for Injection (Rare)........ 1765

Cystitis, viral

Retrovir Capsules (0.8%)........ 1625
Retrovir IV Infusion (1%)........ 1629
Retrovir (0.8%)........ 1625

Cystitis-like syndrome

(see under Cystitis)

Cysts, vaginal

Depo-Provera Contraceptive Injection (Fewer than 1%)........ 2798

Cytokine Released Syndrome

Orthoclone OKT3 Sterile Solution (Occasional)........ 2498
Simulect for Injection........ 2399

D

Deafness

Abelcet Injection........ 1273
Aciphex Tablets........ 1267
Aciphex Tablets........ 1783
Actiq (Less than 1%)........ 1184
Aggrenox Capsules (Less than 1%)........ 1026
Amphotec (1% to 5%)........ 1774
Aralen Tablets (A few cases)........ 3075
Betasept Surgical Scrub........ 2895
Betaseron for SC Injection........ 988
Celebrex Capsules (0.1% to 1.9%)........ 2676
Celebrex Capsules (0.1% to 1.9%)........ 2780
▲ CellCept Capsules (3% to 10%)........ 2951
▲ CellCept Intravenous (3% to 10%)........ 2951
▲ CellCept Oral Suspension (3% to 10%)........ 2951
▲ CellCept Tablets (3% to 10%)........ 2951
Cerebyx Injection (2.2%; infrequent)........ 2619
Clomid Tablets........ 735
Cognex Capsules (Infrequent)........ 1351
Copaxone for Injection (At least 2%)........ 3306
Cytotec Tablets (Infrequent)........ 3202
DaunoXome Injection (Less than or equal to 5%)........ 1442
Depacon Injection (1% to 5%)........ 416
Depakene (1% to 5%)........ 421
Depakote Sprinkle Capsules (1% to 5%)........ 426
Depakote Tablets (1% to 5%)........ 430
Depakote ER Tablets (Greater than 1%)........ 436
Edecrin........ 2091
Effexor Tablets (Rare)........ 3495
Effexor XR Capsules (Rare)........ 3499
Evoxac Capsules (Less than 1%)........ 1217
Gabitril Tablets (Infrequent)........ 1189
Gengraf Capsules (1% to less than 3%)........ 457
Herceptin I.V. (At least one of the 958 patients)........ 1414
Imitrex Injection........ 1549
Imitrex Nasal Spray........ 1554
Imitrex Tablets........ 1558
Indocin Capsules (Less than 1%)........ 2112
Indocin I.V. (Less than 1%)........ 2115
Indocin (Less than 1%)........ 2112
Lamictal (Rare)........ 1567
Lipitor Tablets (Less than 2%)........ 2639
Lipitor Tablets (Less than 2%)........ 2696
Lodine (Less than 1%)........ 3528
Lodine XL Extended-Release Tablets (Less than 1%)........ 3530
Luvox Tablets (25, 50, 100 mg) (Infrequent)........ 3256
Naprelan Tablets (Less than 1%)........ 1293
Nebcin Vials, Hyporets & ADD-Vantage........ 1955
Neoral Soft Gelatin Capsules (1% to less than 3%)........ 2380
Neoral Oral Solution (1% to less than 3%)........ 2380
Nipent for Injection (Less than 3%)........ 3272
Paxil (Rare)........ 1609
Permax Tablets (Infrequent)........ 1299
Prevacid Delayed-Release Capsules (Less than 1%)........ 3292
PREVPAC (Less than 1%)........ 3298
Protonix I.V. (Less than 1%)........ 3580
Protonix Tablets (Less than 1%)........ 3577
Prozac Pulvules, Liquid, and Weekly Capsules (Rare)........ 1238
Quinaglute Dura-Tabs Tablets........ 978
Quinidex Extentabs........ 2933
▲ Rapamune Oral Solution and Tablets (3% to 20%)........ 3584
Remeron Tablets (Infrequent)........ 2483
Remeron SolTab Tablets (Infrequent)........ 2486
Rilutek Tablets (Rare)........ 772
Salagen Tablets (Less than 1%)........ 2229
Sandostatin LAR Depot (Rare)........ 2395
Sarafem Pulvules (Rare)........ 1962
Seroquel Tablets (Infrequent)........ 684
Serzone Tablets (Rare)........ 1104
Sonata Capsules (Rare)........ 3591
Soriatane Capsules (Less than 1%)........ 3003
Ultram Tablets (Infrequent)........ 2600
Uniretic Tablets (Less than 1%)........ 3178
Viagra Tablets (Less than 2%)........ 2732
Wellbutrin SR Sustained-Release Tablets........ 1684
Zanaflex Tablets (Infrequent)........ 1305
Zithromax Capsules, 250 mg........ 2743
Zithromax for IV Infusion........ 2748
Zithromax for Oral Suspension, 300 mg, 600 mg, 900 mg, 1200 mg........ 2739
Zithromax Tablets, 250 mg........ 2739
Zonegran Capsules (Infrequent)........ 1307
Zosyn (1.0% or less)........ 1890
Zosyn in Galaxy Containers (1.0% or less)........ 1894
Zyban Sustained-Release Tablets........ 1710
Zyprexa Tablets (Infrequent)........ 1973
Zyprexa ZYDIS Orally Disintegrating Tablets (Infrequent)........ 1973
Zyrtec (Less than 2%)........ 2756
Zyrtec-D 12 Hour Extended Relief Tablets (Less than 2%)........ 2758

Deafness, transient

Actiq (Less than 1%)........ 1184
Dynabac Tablets (A few cases)........ 2269
Remeron Tablets (Rare)........ 2483
Remeron SolTab Tablets (Rare)........ 2486

Death, fetal

Accupril Tablets........ 2611
Aceon Tablets (2 mg, 4 mg, 8 mg)........ 3249
Altace Capsules........ 2233
▲ Antagon Injection (3.7%)........ 2447
Arthrotec Tablets........ 3195
Atacand Tablets........ 595
Atacand HCT Tablets........ 597
Avalide Tablets........ 1070
Avapro Tablets........ 1074
Avapro Tablets........ 3076
Captopril Tablets........ 2281
Cozaar Tablets........ 2067
Cytotec Tablets........ 3202
Enalaprilat Injection........ 863
Felbatol........ 3343
Hyzaar........ 2109
Innohep Injection........ 1248
Lotrel Capsules........ 2370
Monopril Tablets........ 1091
Nolvadex Tablets........ 678
Podocon-25 Liquid........ 2608
Prinivil Tablets........ 2164
Prinzide Tablets........ 2168
Prometrium Capsules (100 mg, 200 mg) (Rare)........ 3261
Sensorcaine........ 643
Thalomid Capsules........ 1154
Uniretic Tablets (More than 1%)........ 3178
Univasc Tablets........ 3181
Vaseretic Tablets........ 2204
Vasotec I.V. Injection........ 2207
Vasotec Tablets........ 2210
Zestoretic Tablets........ 695
Zestril Tablets........ 698
Zyrtec (Rare)........ 2756

Death, infants

Virazole for Inhalation Solution (20 cases)........ 1747

Death, sudden

Aciphex Tablets........ 1267
Aciphex Tablets........ 1783
Celebrex Capsules (Less than 0.1%)........ 2676
Celebrex Capsules (Less than 0.1%)........ 2780
Clozaril Tablets (Rare)........ 2319
Coreg Tablets (1% to 2%)........ 1508
Felbatol........ 3343
Gabitril Tablets (Infrequent)........ 1189
Haldol Decanoate........ 2535
Imitrex Tablets........ 1558
JE-VAX Vaccine (One case)........ 811
Luvox Tablets (25, 50, 100 mg) (Rare)........ 3256
Meridia Capsules........ 481
Monopril Tablets (0.4% to 1.0%)........ 1091
Neumega for Injection (Two patients)........ 1434
Norpramin Tablets (One report)........ 755
Orap Tablets........ 1407
Phenergan........ 3556
Prozac Pulvules, Liquid, and Weekly Capsules........ 1238
Risperdal (Rare)........ 1796
Sarafem Pulvules........ 1962
Serentil........ 1057
Thorazine........ 1656
Tikosyn Capsules (Less than or equal to 2%)........ 2717
Topamax Sprinkle Capsules (Rare)........ 2590
Topamax Tablets (Rare)........ 2590
Vascor Tablets (1.6%)........ 2602
Zyprexa Tablets (Rare)........ 1973
Zyprexa ZYDIS Orally Disintegrating Tablets (Rare)........ 1973

Deep tendon reflexes, loss

Plaquenil Tablets........ 3082

Defecate, desire to
- Aminohippurate Sodium PAH Injection 2041
- Dopram Injectable 2931

Defecation, increased
- ▲ Xenical Capsules (2.8% to 10.8%) 3043

Defecation, painful
- Fortovase Capsules (Less than 2%) 2970
- Invirase Capsules (Less than 2%) 2979

Dehydration
- Aciphex Tablets 1267
- Aciphex Tablets 1783
- Actiq (1% or greater) 1184
- Aggrenox Capsules 1026
- Agrylin Capsules (1% to 5%) 3232
- Amerge Tablets (Infrequent) 1467
- Amphotec (1% to 5%) 1774
- Aricept Tablets (Frequent) 1270
- Aricept Tablets (Frequent) 2665
- Arthrotec Tablets (Rare) 3195
- Avonex 1013
- Campath Ampules 992
- Captopril Tablets 2281
- ▲ Casodex Tablets (2% to 5%) 662
- Cedax Oral Suspension (0.1% to 1%) 1021
- Celexa (Rare) 1365
- ▲ CellCept Capsules (3%) 2951
- ▲ CellCept Intravenous (3%) 2951
- ▲ CellCept Oral Suspension (3%) 2951
- ▲ CellCept Tablets (3%) 2951
- Cerebyx Injection (Infrequent) 2619
- Claritin-D 12 Hour Extended Release Tablets (Less frequent) 3102
- Cognex Capsules (Infrequent) 1351
- Coreg Tablets (2.1%) 1508
- Cytotec Tablets (Rare) 3202
- DaunoXome Injection (Less than or equal to 5%) 1442
- Demadex Tablets and Injection 2965
- Diovan HCT Tablets (Greater than 0.2%) 2338
- Dipentum Capsules (Rare) 2803
- Diprivan Injectable Emulsion (Less than 1%) 667
- Doxil Injection (Less than 1%) 566
- Dynabac Tablets (0.1% to 1%) 2269
- Ecotrin Enteric Coated Aspirin Low, Regular and Maximum Strength Tablets 1715
- Effexor Tablets (Rare) 3495
- Effexor XR Capsules (Rare) 3499
- Ellence Injection 2806
- Eskalith 1527
- Evoxac Capsules (Less than 1%) 1217
- Exelon Capsules (Frequent) 2342
- Exelon Oral Solution (Frequent) 2345
- Felbatol 3343
- Fleet Enema 1359
- Fludara for Injection (Up to 1%) 995
- Fortovase Capsules (Less than 2%) 2970
- Foscavir Injection (Less than 1%) 605
- Furosemide Tablets 2284
- Gabitril Tablets (Infrequent) 1189
- Geodon Capsules (Infrequent) 2688
- Glucophage Tablets 1080
- Glucophage XR Tablets 1080
- Haldol Decanoate 2535
- Imitrex Injection (Rare) 1549
- Imitrex Nasal Spray 1554
- Imitrex Tablets 1558
- Intron A for Injection (Less than or equal to 5%) 3120
- Invirase Capsules (Less than 2%) 2979
- Kaletra Capsules (Less than 2%) 471
- Kaletra Oral Solution (Less than 2%) 471
- Klonopin Tablets 2983
- Levaquin Injection (Less than 0.5%) 2537
- Lithium Carbonate 3061
- Lithium Citrate Syrup 3061
- Lithobid Slow-Release Tablets 3255
- Lupron Depot–3 Month 22.5 mg (Less than 5%) 3288
- ▲ Lupron Depot–4 Month 30 mg (Up to 8.2%) 3289
- Luvox Tablets (25, 50, 100 mg) (Infrequent) 3256
- Maxalt Tablets (Infrequent) 2120
- Maxalt-MLT Orally Disintegrating Tablets (Infrequent) 2120
- Mobic Tablets (Less than 2%) 1054
- Moduretic Tablets (Less than or equal to 1%) 2138
- Naprelan Tablets (Less than 1%) 1293
- Neumega for Injection 1434
- Neurontin Capsules 2655
- Neurontin Oral Solution 2655
- Neurontin Tablets 2655
- Norvir Capsules (Less than 2%) 487
- Norvir Oral Solution (Less than 2%) 487
- OxyContin Tablets (Less than 1%) 2912
- Paxil (Rare) 1609
- Permax Tablets (Infrequent) 1299
- ▲ Photofrin for Injection (7%) 831
- Prinivil Tablets (0.3% to 1.0%) 2164
- Prinzide Tablets 2168
- ▲ Prograf (3% to 15%) 1393
- Prostin E2 Suppositories 2852
- Protonix I.V. 3580
- Protonix Tablets 3577
- Protopic Ointment (Greater than or equal to 1%) 1397
- Prozac Pulvules, Liquid, and Weekly Capsules (Infrequent) 1238
- ▲ Rapamune Oral Solution and Tablets (3% to 20%) 3584
- Remeron Tablets (Infrequent) 2483
- Remeron SolTab Tablets (Infrequent) 2486
- Remicade for IV Injection (Less than 2%) 1178
- Requip Tablets (Infrequent) 1621
- Risperdal (Rare) 1796
- ▲ Sandostatin LAR Depot (5% to 15%) 2395
- Sarafem Pulvules (Infrequent) 1962
- Seroquel Tablets (Infrequent) 684
- ▲ Serostim for Injection (1% to 10%) 3229
- Serzone Tablets (Infrequent) 1104
- ▲ Simulect for Injection (3% to 10%) 2399
- Sporanox Oral Solution (Less than 2%) 1808
- Sporanox Oral Solution (Less than 2%) 2512
- Tasmar Tablets (Infrequent) 3010
- Taxol Injection (Rare) 1129
- Thalomid Capsules 1154
- Topamax Sprinkle Capsules (Infrequent) 2590
- Topamax Tablets (Infrequent) 2590
- Uniretic Tablets (Less than 1%) 3178
- Univasc Tablets 3181
- Vantin Tablets and Oral Suspension (Less than 1%) 2860
- Vaseretic Tablets 2204
- Vasotec Tablets 2210
- Viracept 532
- Vistide Injection 1445
- Vitravene for Injection (2% to 5%) .. ⊙ 310
- Xeloda Tablets (1% to 4%) 3039
- ▲ Zenapax for Injection (2% to 5%) 3046
- Zestoretic Tablets 695
- Zestril Tablets (0.3% to 1.0%) 698
- Zithromax Capsules, 250 mg (Rare) 2743
- Zithromax for IV Infusion (Rare) 2748
- Zithromax for Oral Suspension, 300 mg, 600 mg, 900 mg, 1200 mg (Rare) 2739
- Zithromax Tablets, 250 mg (Rare) .. 2739
- Zoloft (Rare) 2751
- ▲ Zometa for Intravenous Infusion (5% to 10%) 3621
- Zonegran Capsules (Infrequent) 1307
- Zyprexa Tablets (Infrequent) 1973
- Zyprexa ZYDIS Orally Disintegrating Tablets (Infrequent) 1973
- Zyrtec (Less than 2%) 2756
- Zyrtec-D 12 Hour Extended Relief Tablets (Less than 2%) 2758

Delirium
- Aciphex Tablets 1267
- Aciphex Tablets 1783
- Amicar Injection 3608
- Amicar Syrup 3608
- Amicar Tablets 3608
- Ativan Injection (1.3%) 3478
- Betaseron for SC Injection 988
- Brevital Sodium for Injection, USP .. 1815
- Catapres Tablets 1037
- Catapres-TTS (0.5% or less) 1038
- ▲ CellCept Capsules (3% to 10%) 2951
- ▲ CellCept Intravenous (3% to 10%) .. 2951
- ▲ CellCept Oral Suspension (3% to 10%) 2951
- ▲ CellCept Tablets (3% to 10%) 2951
- Cerebyx Injection 2619
- Cipro I.V. 893
- Cipro I.V. Pharmacy Bulk Package .. 897
- Cipro 887
- Clorpres Tablets 1002
- Clozaril Tablets 2319
- Cognex Capsules (Infrequent) 1351
- Combipres Tablets 1040
- Digitek Tablets 1003
- Diprivan Injectable Emulsion (Less than 1%) 667
- Duraclon Injection (Rare) 3057
- Effexor Tablets 3495
- Effexor XR Capsules 3499
- Evoxac Capsules 1217
- Exelon Capsules (Infrequent) 2342
- Exelon Oral Solution (Infrequent) 2345
- Famvir Tablets (Infrequent) 2348
- Geodon Capsules (Frequent) 2688
- Lamictal (Rare) 1567
- Lanoxicaps Capsules 1574
- Lanoxin Injection 1581
- Lanoxin Tablets 1587
- Lanoxin Elixir Pediatric 1578
- Lanoxin Injection Pediatric 1584
- Levaquin (Less than 0.3%) 2537
- Luvox Tablets (25, 50, 100 mg) (Infrequent) 3256
- Merrem I.V. (0.1% to 1.0%) 673
- Nardil Tablets (Less frequent) 2653
- Orthoclone OKT3 Sterile Solution (Less than 1%) 2498
- Paxil (Rare) 1609
- PhosLo 1069
- Prograf 1393
- Quinaglute Dura-Tabs Tablets 978
- Quinidex Extentabs 2933
- Remeron Tablets (Infrequent) 2483
- Remeron SolTab Tablets (Infrequent) 2486
- Remicade for IV Injection (Less than 2%) 1178
- Reminyl Oral Solution (Infrequent) ... 1792
- Reminyl Tablets (Infrequent) 1792
- Requip Tablets (Infrequent) 1621
- Rilutek Tablets (Infrequent) 772
- Risperdal (Rare) 1796
- Romazicon Injection (Less than 1%) 3000
- Seroquel Tablets (Rare) 684
- Symmetrel 1328
- Tasmar Tablets (Rare) 3010
- Topamax Sprinkle Capsules (Infrequent) 2590
- Topamax Tablets (Infrequent) 2590
- Trileptal Oral Suspension 2407
- Trileptal Tablets 2407
- Vistide Injection 1445
- Wellbutrin Tablets 1680
- Wellbutrin SR Sustained-Release Tablets 1684
- Zovirax Capsules 1706
- Zovirax for Injection 1708
- Zovirax 1706
- Zyban Sustained-Release Tablets 1710
- Zyprexa Tablets (Infrequent) 1973
- Zyprexa ZYDIS Orally Disintegrating Tablets (Infrequent) 1973

Delivery complications, unspecified
- Advil .... ▣ 771
- Advil Cold and Sinus Caplets .... ▣ 771
- Advil Cold and Sinus Tablets .... ▣ 771
- Advil Flu & Body Ache Caplets .... ▣ 772
- Aleve Tablets, Caplets and Gelcaps .... ▣ 602
- Alka-Seltzer .... ▣ 603
- Alka-Seltzer Lemon Lime Antacid and Pain Reliever Effervescent Tablets .... ▣ 603
- Alka-Seltzer Extra Strength Antacid and Pain Reliever Effervescent Tablets .... ▣ 603
- Alka-Seltzer PM Effervescent Tablets .... ▣ 605
- Genuine Bayer Tablets, Caplets and Gelcaps .... ▣ 606
- Extra Strength Bayer Caplets and Gelcaps .... ▣ 610
- Aspirin Regimen Bayer Children's Chewable Tablets (Orange or Cherry Flavored) .... ▣ 607
- Aspirin Regimen Bayer Adult Low Strength 81 mg Tablets .... ▣ 606
- Aspirin Regimen Bayer 81 mg Caplets with Calcium .... ▣ 607
- Aspirin Regimen Bayer Regular Strength 325 mg Caplets .... ▣ 606
- Genuine Bayer Professional Labeling (Aspirin Regimen Bayer) .... ▣ 608
- Extra Strength Bayer Arthritis Caplets .... ▣ 610
- Extra Strength Bayer Plus Caplets .... ▣ 610
- Extra Strength Bayer PM Caplets .. ▣ 611
- BC Powder .... ▣ 619
- BC Cold Powder .... ▣ 619
- Ecotrin Enteric Coated Aspirin Low, Regular and Maximum Strength Tablets 1715
- Excedrin Migraine 1070
- Goody's Body Pain Formula Powder .... ▣ 620
- Goody's Extra Strength Headache Powder .... ▣ 620
- Goody's Extra Strength Pain Relief Tablets .... ▣ 620
- Motrin IB Tablets, Caplets, and Gelcaps 2002
- Motrin Sinus Headache Caplets 2005
- Orudis KT Tablets .... ▣ 778
- Sensorcaine 643
- Soma Compound Tablets 3354
- Soma Compound w/Codeine Tablets 3355
- Vanquish Caplets .... ▣ 617

Delusions
- Ambien Tablets (Rare) 3191
- Aricept Tablets (Frequent) 1270
- Aricept Tablets (Frequent) 2665
- Artane (Rare) 1855
- Betaseron for SC Injection 988
- Celexa (Rare) 1365
- Clozaril Tablets (Less than 1%) 2319
- Effexor Tablets (Rare) 3495
- Effexor XR Capsules (Rare) 3499
- Eldepryl Capsules 3266
- Etrafon 3115
- Evoxac Capsules 1217
- Exelon Capsules (2% or more) 2342
- Exelon Oral Solution (2% or more) ... 2345
- Felbatol 3343
- Flexeril Tablets (Rare) 572
- Flexeril Tablets (Rare) 2094
- Gabitril Tablets (Infrequent) 1189
- Halcion Tablets 2823
- Lamictal (Rare) 1567
- Limbitrol 1738
- Lodosyn Tablets 1251
- ▲ Lupron Depot 3.75 mg (Among most frequent) 3281
- Lupron Depot–3 Month 11.25 mg (Less than 5%) 3285
- Lupron Depot–3 Month 22.5 mg (Less than 5%) 3288
- Luvox Tablets (25, 50, 100 mg) (Infrequent) 3256
- Mirapex Tablets (1%) 2834
- Norpramin Tablets 755
- Nubain Injection (1% or less) 1323
- Paxil (Rare) 1609
- Permax Tablets (Infrequent) 1299
- Prozac Pulvules, Liquid, and Weekly Capsules (Rare) 1238
- Remeron Tablets (Infrequent) 2483
- Remeron SolTab Tablets (Infrequent) 2486
- Requip Tablets (Infrequent) 1621
- Rilutek Tablets (Infrequent) 772
- Salagen Tablets (Rare) 2229
- Sarafem Pulvules (Rare) 1962
- Seroquel Tablets (Infrequent) 684
- Sinemet Tablets 1253
- Sinemet CR Tablets 1255
- Sonata Capsules (Rare) 3591
- Stadol NS Nasal Spray (Less than 1%) 1108
- Surmontil Capsules 3595
- Sustiva Capsules 1258
- Symmetrel 1328
- Tasmar Tablets (Infrequent) 3010
- Topamax Sprinkle Capsules (Infrequent) 2590
- Topamax Tablets (Infrequent) 2590
- Trileptal Oral Suspension 2407
- Trileptal Tablets 2407
- Vivactil Tablets 2217
- Vivactil Tablets 2446
- Wellbutrin Tablets (1.2%) 1680
- Wellbutrin SR Sustained-Release Tablets 1684
- Zoloft (Infrequent) 2751
- Zyban Sustained-Release Tablets 1710

Dementia
- Ambien Tablets (Rare) 3191
- Betaseron for SC Injection 988
- Depacon Injection (Several reports) 416
- Depakene (Several reports) 421
- Depakote Sprinkle Capsules (Several reports) 426
- Depakote Tablets (Several reports) 430
- Depakote ER Tablets (Several reports) 436
- Effexor Tablets (Rare) 3495
- Effexor XR Capsules (Rare) 3499
- Evoxac Capsules 1217
- Exelon Capsules (Infrequent) 2342
- Exelon Oral Solution (Infrequent) 2345
- Foscavir Injection (Between 1% and 5%) 605
- Hivid Tablets (Less than 1%) 2975
- Lodosyn Tablets 1251
- Lupron Depot–4 Month 30 mg (Less than 5%) 3289
- Remeron Tablets (Rare) 2483
- Remeron SolTab Tablets (Rare) 2486
- Requip Tablets (Infrequent) 1621
- Rilutek Tablets (Rare) 772
- Sinemet Tablets 1253
- Sinemet CR Tablets 1255
- ▲ Vesanoid Capsules (3%) 3037
- Vistide Injection 1445
- Zanaflex Tablets (Rare) 1305

Demyelination
- Proleukin for Injection 1199

Dental caries
- Actiq (Less than 1%) 1184
- Ambien Tablets (Rare) 3191
- Claritin (At least one patient) 3100
- Copaxone for Injection (Frequent) ... 3306
- DaunoXome Injection (Less than or equal to 5%) 1442
- Eskalith 1527
- Gabitril Tablets (Infrequent) 1189
- Lithobid Slow-Release Tablets 3255
- ▲ Luvox Tablets (25, 50, 100 mg) (3%) 3256
- Paxil (Rare) 1609
- Permax Tablets (Infrequent) 1299
- Seroquel Tablets (Infrequent) 684

Topamax Sprinkle Capsules (Infrequent) 2590
Topamax Tablets (Infrequent) 2590
Uniretic Tablets (Less than 1%) 3178
Vioxx (Greater than 0.1% to 1.9%) 2213
Vistide Injection 1445
Zoloft (Infrequent) 2751

Dependence, drug

Actiq 1184
Adderall Tablets 3231
Adderall XR Capsules
Adipex-P 1406
Ambien Tablets (Rare) 3191
Astramorph/PF Injection, USP (Preservative-Free) 594
Avonex 1013
▲ Carnitor Injection (2% to 6%) 3242
Celexa (Infrequent) 1365
Darvon-N/Darvocet-N 1907
Darvon Pulvules 1909
Darvon Compound-65 Pulvules 1910
Darvon-N Tablets 1912
Demerol 3079
Dexedrine 1512
DextroStat Tablets 3236
Dilaudid 441
Dilaudid Oral Liquid 445
Dilaudid Powder 441
Dilaudid Rectal Suppositories 441
Dilaudid Tablets 441
Dilaudid Tablets - 8 mg 445
Dolophine Hydrochloride Tablets 3056
Duragesic Transdermal System 1786
Duramorph Injection 1312
Halcion Tablets 2823
Ionamin Capsules 1163
Librium Capsules 1736
Librium for Injection 1737
Limbitrol 1738
Lortab 3319
Lortab Elixir 3317
Luvox Tablets (25, 50, 100 mg) (Infrequent) 3256
Mepergan Injection 3539
MS Contin Tablets 2896
MSIR 2898
Nembutal Sodium Solution 485
Oramorph SR Tablets 3062
OxyFast Oral Concentrate Solution 2916
OxyIR Capsules 2916
Paxil (Rare) 1609
Percocet Tablets 1326
Percodan Tablets 1327
Percolone Tablets 1327
Peri-Colace Capsules and Syrup 3240
Phenergan with Codeine Syrup 3557
Phenergan VC with Codeine Syrup 3561
Remeron Tablets (Rare) 2483
Remeron SolTab Tablets (Rare) 2486
Ritalin 2387
Roxanol 3066
Roxicodone 3067
Sonata Capsules 3591
Stadol NS Nasal Spray (Less than 1%) 1108
Talwin Nx Tablets 3090
Tranxene 511
Tussi-Organidin NR Liquid 3350
Tussi-Organidin-S NR Liquid 3350
Tylenol with Codeine 2595
Tylox Capsules 2597
Valium Injectable 3026
Valium Tablets 3047
Vicodin Tuss Expectorant 519
Vicoprofen Tablets 520
Vistide Injection 1445

Dependence, physical

Demerol 3079
Dexedrine 1512
Dilaudid Ampules 441
Dilaudid Oral Liquid 445
Dilaudid Powder 441
Dilaudid Rectal Suppositories 441
Dilaudid Tablets 441
Dilaudid Tablets - 8 mg 445
Duragesic Transdermal System 1786
Duramorph Injection 1312
Hycodan 1316
Hycomine Compound Tablets 1317
Hycotuss Expectorant Syrup 1318
Infumorph 200 and Infumorph 500 Sterile Solutions 1314
Isordil Titradose Tablets 3526
Klonopin Tablets 2983
Levo-Dromoran 1734
Lortab 3319
Lortab Elixir 3317
Marinol Capsules (Uncommon) 3325
Miltown Tablets 3349
MS Contin Tablets 2896
MSIR 2898
Oramorph SR Tablets 3062
OxyContin Tablets 2912
Percocet Tablets 1326
Percodan Tablets 1327
Percolone Tablets 1327
Phrenilin 578
ProSom Tablets 500
Roxanol 3066
Sedapap Tablets 50 mg/650 mg 2225
Talacen Caplets 3089
Talwin Nx Tablets 3090
Tranxene 511
Tylenol with Codeine 2595
Tylox Capsules 2597
Ultram Tablets 2600
Versed Injection 3027
Vicodin HP Tablets 518
Vicodin Tuss Expectorant 519
Vicoprofen Tablets 520
Xanax Tablets 2865

Dependence, psychic

(*see under* Dependence, psychological)

Dependence, psychological

Adderall Tablets 3231
Adderall XR Capsules
Darvon-N/Darvocet-N 1907
Darvon Pulvules 1909
Darvon Compound-65 Pulvules 1910
Darvon-N Tablets 1912
Demerol 3079
Desoxyn Tablets 440
Dexedrine 1512
DextroStat Tablets 3236
Dilaudid 441
Dilaudid Oral Liquid 445
Dilaudid Powder 441
Dilaudid Rectal Suppositories 441
Dilaudid Tablets 441
Dilaudid Tablets - 8 mg 445
Dolophine Hydrochloride Tablets 3056
Duragesic Transdermal System 1786
Duramorph Injection 1312
Etrafon 3115
Hycodan 1316
Hycomine Compound Tablets 1317
Hycotuss Expectorant Syrup 1318
Infumorph 200 and Infumorph 500 Sterile Solutions 1314
Ionamin Capsules 1163
Kadian Capsules (Very rare) 1335
Klonopin Tablets 2983
Levo-Dromoran 1734
Lortab 3319
Lortab Elixir 3317
Marinol Capsules (Uncommon) 3325
Maxidone Tablets CIII 3399
Miltown Tablets 3349
MS Contin Tablets (Very rare) 2896
MSIR 2898
Nembutal Sodium Solution 485
Norco 5/325 Tablets CIII 3424
Norco 7.5/325 Tablets CIII 3425
Norco 10/325 Tablets CIII 3425
Norco 10/325 Tablets CIII 3427
Numorphan 1324
Oramorph SR Tablets 3062
OxyContin Tablets 2912
OxyFast Oral Concentrate Solution 2916
OxyIR Capsules 2916
Percocet Tablets 1326
Percodan Tablets 1327
Percolone Tablets 1327
Phrenilin 578
ProSom Tablets 500
Ritalin 2387
Roxanol 3066
Roxicodone 3067
Sedapap Tablets 50 mg/650 mg 2225
Talacen Caplets 3089
Talwin Nx Tablets 3090
Tranxene 511
Tussionex Pennkinetic Extended-Release Suspension 1174
Tylenol with Codeine 2595
Tylox Capsules 2597
Ultram Tablets 2600
Vicodin Tablets 516
Vicodin ES Tablets 517
Vicodin HP Tablets 518
Vicodin Tuss Expectorant 519
Vicoprofen Tablets 520
Zydone Tablets 1330

Depersonalization

Ambien Tablets (Rare) 3191
Anzemet Injection (Infrequently) 719
Anzemet Tablets (Infrequently) 722
Astelin Nasal Spray (Infrequent) 3339
Avelox Tablets (0.05% to 1%) 879
Avonex 1013
Betaseron for SC Injection 988
Biaxin/Biaxin XL 403
Buprenex Injectable (Infrequent) 2918
Cardura Tablets (Less than 0.5%) 2668
Celexa (Infrequent) 1365
Cerebyx Injection (Infrequent) 2619
Cipro I.V. (1% or less) 893
Cipro I.V. Pharmacy Bulk Package (Less than 1%) 897
Cipro (Less than 1%) 887
Copaxone for Injection (Infrequent) 3306
Duragesic Transdermal System (Less than 1%) 1786
Effexor Tablets (1%) 3495
Effexor XR Capsules (Frequent) 3499
Evoxac Capsules (Less than 1%) 1217
Exelon Capsules (Infrequent) 2342
Exelon Oral Solution (Infrequent) 2345
Gabitril Tablets (Frequent) 1189
Halcion Tablets 2823
Helixate Concentrate 788
Hivid Tablets (Less than 1%) 2975
Indocin (Less than 1%) 2112
Klonopin Tablets (Infrequent) 2983
Kogenate FS 936
Lamictal (Infrequent) 1567
Luvox Tablets (25, 50, 100 mg) (Infrequent) 3256
Marinol Capsules (Greater than 1%) 3325
Maxalt Tablets (Rare) 2120
Maxalt-MLT Orally Disintegrating Tablets (Rare) 2120
Neurontin Capsules (Infrequent) 2655
Neurontin Oral Solution (Infrequent) 2655
Neurontin Tablets (Infrequent) 2655
Norvasc Tablets (More than 0.1% to 1%) 2704
Nubain Injection (1% or less) 1323
OxyContin Tablets (Less than 1%) 2912
Paxil (Infrequent) 1609
PREVPAC 3298
Prozac Pulvules, Liquid, and Weekly Capsules (Infrequent) 1238
Remeron Tablets (Infrequent) 2483
Remeron SolTab Tablets (Infrequent) 2486
Requip Tablets (Infrequent) 1621
Rilutek Tablets (Infrequent) 772
Romazicon Injection (1% to 3%) 3000
Sarafem Pulvules (Infrequent) 1962
Seroquel Tablets (Infrequent) 684
Serzone Tablets (Infrequent) 1104
Sonata Capsules (Less than 1% to 2%) 3591
Tambocor Tablets (Less than 1%) 1990
Tequin Injection (Less than 0.1%) 1110
Tequin Tablets (Less than 0.1%) 1110
Topamax Sprinkle Capsules (1.6% to 1.8%) 2590
Topamax Tablets (1.6% to 1.8%) 2590
Trovan (Less than 1%) 2722
Ultracet Tablets (Less than 1%) 2597
Wellbutrin Tablets (Infrequent) 1680
Wellbutrin SR Sustained-Release Tablets (Infrequent) 1684
Xanax Tablets 2865
Zanaflex Tablets (Infrequent) 1305
Zoloft (Infrequent) 2751
Zyban Sustained-Release Tablets (Infrequent) 1710
Zyprexa Tablets (Infrequent) 1973
Zyprexa ZYDIS Orally Disintegrating Tablets (Infrequent) 1973
Zyrtec (Less than 2%) 2756
Zyrtec-D 12 Hour Extended Relief Tablets (Less than 2%) 2758

Depigmentation

Azelex Cream (Rare) 547
Finevin Cream 962
Intron A for Injection (Less than 5%) 3120
Thioplex for Injection 1765

Depression

Accupril Tablets (0.5% to 1.0%) 2611
Accuretic Tablets (Greater than 0.5%) 2614
Accutane Capsules 2944
Aceon Tablets (2 mg, 4 mg, 8 mg) (2.0%) 3249
Aciphex Tablets 1267
Aciphex Tablets 1783
▲ Actimmune (3%) 1772
Activella Tablets 2764
▲ Actonel Tablets (6.8%) 2879
Adalat CC Tablets (Less than 1.0%) 877
Adderall XR Capsules (0.7%)
Advair Diskus 100/50 1448
Advair Diskus 250/50 1448
Advair Diskus 500/50 1448
Aerobid/Aerobid-M (1% to 3%) 1363
▲ Agenerase Capsules (9% to 16%) 1454
▲ Agenerase Oral Solution (9% to 16%) 1459
Agrylin Capsules (1% to 5%) 3232
Aldoclor Tablets 2035
Aldomet Tablets 2037
Aldoril Tablets 2039
Alesse-21 Tablets 3468
Alesse-28 Tablets 3473
Alferon N Injection (One patient to 3%) 1770
Alora Transdermal System 3372
Alphagan Ophthalmic Solution (Less than 3%) 545
Altace Capsules (Less than 1%) 2233
Ambien Tablets (2%) 3191
AmBisome for Injection (Less common) 1383
Amerge Tablets (Infrequent) 1467
Amphotec (1% to 5%) 1774
▲ Androderm Transdermal System CIII (3%) 3377
AndroGel (Up to 1%) 3322
▲ Android Capsules, 10 mg (Among most common) 1731
Arava Tablets (1% to 3%) 724
▲ Aricept Tablets (3%) 1270
▲ Aricept Tablets (3%) 2665
▲ Arimidex Tablets (2.4% to 5.3%) 659
▲ Aromasin Tablets (13%) 2769
Arthrotec Tablets (Rare) 3195
Asacol Delayed-Release Tablets 2884
Astelin Nasal Spray (Infrequent) 3339
Atacand Tablets (0.5% or greater) 595
Atacand HCT Tablets (0.5% or greater) 597
Ativan Injection (1.3%) 3478
Ativan Tablets (Less frequent) 3482
Avalide Tablets 1070
Avapro Tablets (Less than 1%) 1074
Avapro Tablets (Less than 1%) 3076
Avelox Tablets 879
Avonex 1013
Axert Tablets (Rare) 2772
Aygestin Tablets 1333
Azmacort Inhalation Aerosol 728
Azulfidine EN-tabs Tablets (Rare) 2775
Bactrim 2949
Baycol Tablets 883
Beconase Inhalation Aerosol 1497
Beconase AQ Nasal Spray 1498
Betagan ⊙ 228
Betapace Tablets (1% to 4%) 950
Betaseron for SC Injection 988
Betimol Ophthalmic Solution ⊙ 324
Betoptic S Ophthalmic Suspension (Rare) 537
Blocadren Tablets 2046
Brevibloc Injection (Less than 1%) 858
Brevicon 28-Day Tablets 3380
▲ Campath Ampules (1% to 7%) 992
Captopril Tablets 2281
Carbatrol Capsules 3234
Cardizem Injectable 1018
Cardizem Lyo-Ject Syringe 1018
Cardizem Monovial 1018
Cardizem CD Capsules (Less than 1%) 1016
Cardura Tablets (1%) 2668
▲ Carnitor Injection (5% to 6%) 3242
Carteolol Hydrochloride Ophthalmic Solution USP, 1% ⊙ 258
▲ Casodex Tablets (4%) 662
Cataflam Tablets (Less than 1%) 2315
Catapres Tablets (About 1 in 100 patients) 1037
Catapres-TTS (0.5% or less) 1038
Celebrex Capsules (0.1% to 1.9%) 2676
Celebrex Capsules (0.1% to 1.9%) 2780
Celestone Soluspan Injectable Suspension 3097
Celexa (Frequent) 1365
▲ CellCept Capsules (3% to 15.6%) 2951
▲ CellCept Intravenous (3% to 15.6%) 2951
▲ CellCept Oral Suspension (3% to 15.6%) 2951
▲ CellCept Tablets (3% to 17.3%) 2951
Celontin Capsules 2618
▲ Cenestin Tablets (28%) 1263
Cerebyx Injection (Infrequent) 2619
Chibroxin Sterile Ophthalmic Solution 2051
Cipro I.V. (1% or less) 893
Cipro I.V. Pharmacy Bulk Package (Less than 1%) 897
Cipro (Less than 1%) 887
Claritin (At least one patient) 3100
Claritin-D 12 Hour Extended Release Tablets (Less frequent) 3102
Claritin-D 24 Hour Extended Release Tablets (Fewer than 2%) 3104
Climara Transdermal System 958
Clinoril Tablets (Less than 1%) 2053
Clomid Tablets (Fewer than 1%) 735
Clorpres Tablets (About 1%) 1002
Clozaril Tablets (1%) 2319
Cogentin 2055
▲ Cognex Capsules (4%) 1351
Colazal Capsules 3069
▲ CombiPatch Transdermal System (8% to 9%) 2323
Combipres Tablets (About 1%) 1040
Concerta Extended-Release Tablets 1998
Concerta Tablets 561
Copaxone for Injection (At least 2%) 3306
Coreg Tablets (More than 2%) 1508
Corgard Tablets 2245
Cortone Acetate Injectable Suspension 2059
Cortone Acetate Tablets 2061
Corzide 40/5 Tablets 2247
Corzide 80/5 Tablets 2247
Cosopt Sterile Ophthalmic Solution (Less than 1%) 2065
Cozaar Tablets (Less than 1%) 2067
▲ Crinone (19%) 3213

Crixivan Capsules (Less than 2%).... 2070
Cyclessa Tablets 2450
Cylert Tablets 415
Cytovene (At least 3 subjects) 2959
Dantrium Capsules (Less frequent) 2885
Daranide Tablets 2077
▲ DaunoXome Injection (3% to 7%) 1442
DDAVP Nasal Spray 738
DDAVP Rhinal Tube 738
Decadron Elixir 2078
Decadron Tablets 2079
Decadron Phosphate Injection 2081
Delatestryl Injection 1151
Demser Capsules 2085
▲ Depacon Injection (4% to 5%) 416
▲ Depakene (5%) 421
▲ Depakote Sprinkle Capsules (4% to 5%) 426
Depakote Tablets (1% to 5%) 430
Depakote ER Tablets (Greater than 1%) 436
Depo-Provera Contraceptive Injection (1% to 5%) 2798
Desmopressin Acetate Rhinal Tube 1345
Desogen Tablets 2458
Didronel Tablets 2888
Digitek Tablets 1003
Dilaudid Oral Liquid (Less frequent) 445
Dilaudid Tablets - 8 mg (Less frequent) 445
Dilaudid-HP (Less frequent) 443
Diovan HCT Tablets (Greater than 0.2%) 2338
Dipentum Capsules (1.5%) 2803
Diprivan Injectable Emulsion (Less than 1%) 667
Dolobid Tablets (Less than 1 in 100) 2088
▲ Dostinex Tablets (3%) 2804
Doxil Injection (Less than 1% to 5%) 566
Duraclon Injection (1%) 3057
▲ Duragesic Transdermal System (3% to 10%) 1786
Duranest Injections 600
Dynabac Tablets (0.1% to 1%) 2269
DynaCirc Capsules (0.5% to 1%) 2921
DynaCirc CR Tablets (0.5% to 1%) .. 2923
Effexor Tablets (1%) 3495
▲ Effexor XR Capsules (3%) 3499
8-MOP Capsules 1727
Eldepryl Capsules 3266
Elmiron Capsules 570
Elspar for Injection 2092
Enalaprilat Injection 863
Enbrel for Injection (Infrequent) 1752
Enbrel for Injection (Infrequent) 3504
Ergamisol Tablets (1% to 2%) 1789
Esclim Transdermal System 3460
Estinyl Tablets 3112
Estrace Vaginal Cream 3358
Estrace Tablets 3361
Estratest 3252
Estring Vaginal Ring (At least 1 report) 2811
Estrostep 2627
Eulexin Capsules (1%) 3118
▲ Evista Tablets (6.4%) 1915
Evoxac Capsules (1% to 3%) 1217
▲ Exelon Capsules (6%) 2342
▲ Exelon Oral Solution (6%) 2345
Famotidine Injection (Infrequent) 866
Fareston Tablets 3237
▲ Felbatol (5.3%) 3343
Feldene Capsules (Occasional) 2685
Femara Tablets (Less frequent) 2351
▲ femhrt Tablets (5.8%) 2635
Flexeril Tablets (Less than 1%) 572
Flexeril Tablets (Less than 1%) 2094
▲ Flolan for Injection (13% to 37%) 1528
Florinef Acetate Tablets 2250
Flovent Diskus 3614
Flovent 1535
Flovent Rotadisk 1537
Floxin I.V. (Less than 1%) 2526
Floxin Tablets (Less than 1%) 2529
Fludara for Injection (Up to 1%) 995
Flumadine (0.3% to 1%) 1370
Fortovase Capsules (2.7%) 2970
▲ Foscavir Injection (5% or greater) .. 605
▲ Gabitril Tablets (3%) 1189
Gastrocrom Oral Concentrate (Less common) 1162
Gengraf Capsules (Rare) 457
▲ Gliadel Wafer (3%) 1723
Glucotrol XL Extended Release Tablets (Less than 3%) 2693
Halcion Tablets (0.5% to 0.9%) 2823
Haldol Decanoate 2535
Haldol Injection, Tablets and Concentrate 2533
▲ Herceptin I.V. (6%) 1414
Hivid Tablets (0.4%) 2975
Hydrocortone Tablets 2106
Hydrocortone Acetate Injectable Suspension 2103
Hydrocortone Phosphate Injection, Sterile 2105
Hytrin Capsules (0.3%) 464
Hyzaar 2109
Imdur Tablets (Less than or equal to 5%) 1826
Imitrex Injection (Rare) 1549
Imitrex Nasal Spray (Infrequent) 1554
Imitrex Tablets (Infrequent) 1558
Indapamide Tablets (Less than 5%) 2286
Inderal 3513
Inderal LA Long-Acting Capsules 3516
Inderide Tablets 3517
Inderide LA Long-Acting Capsules ... 3519
Indocin (Greater than 1%) 2112
▲ Infergen (18% to 26%) 1777
▲ Intron A for Injection (2% to 40%) ... 3120
Invirase Capsules (Less than 2%) 2979
Iopidine 0.5% Ophthalmic Solution (Less than 3%) .... ⊙213
Kadian Capsules (Less than 3%) 1335
Kaletra Capsules (Less than 2%) 471
Kaletra Oral Solution (Less than 2%) 471
▲ Keppra Tablets (4%) 3314
▲ Klonopin Tablets (4% to 7%) 2983
▲ Lamictal (4.2%) 1567
Lanoxicaps Capsules 1574
Lanoxin Injection 1581
Lanoxin Tablets 1587
Lanoxin Elixir Pediatric 1578
Lanoxin Injection Pediatric 1584
Lariam Tablets 2989
Lescol Capsules 2361
Lescol Capsules 2925
Lescol XL Tablets 2361
Lescol XL Tablets 2925
Levaquin (Less than 0.3%) 2537
Levlen 962
Levlite 21 Tablets 962
Levlite 28 Tablets 962
Levo-Dromoran 1734
Levora Tablets 3389
Lexxel Tablets 608
Lidoderm Patch 1319
Lipitor Tablets (Less than 2%) 2639
Lipitor Tablets (Less than 2%) 2696
Lodine (1% to 3%) 3528
Lodine XL Extended-Release Tablets (1% to 3%) 3530
Loestrin 21 Tablets 2642
Loestrin Fe Tablets 2642
Lo/Ovral Tablets 3532
Lo/Ovral-28 Tablets 3538
Lopid Tablets 2650
Low-Ogestrel-28 Tablets 3392
Lunelle Monthly Injection 2827
▲ Lupron Depot 3.75 mg (10.8%) 3281
▲ Lupron Depot–3 Month 11.25 mg (10.8% to 22%) 3285
Lupron Depot–3 Month 22.5 mg (Less than 5%) 3288
Lupron Depot–4 Month 30 mg (Less than 5%) 3289
Lupron Injection (Less than 5%) 3279
Luvox Tablets (25, 50, 100 mg) (2%) 3256
LYMErix Vaccine (1.02%) 1592
Macrobid Capsules (Rare) 2889
Macrodantin Capsules (Rare) 2891
Marinol Capsules (Less than 1%) 3325
Matulane Capsules 3246
Maxair Autohaler 1981
Maxair Inhaler (Less than 1%) 1984
Maxalt Tablets (Infrequent) 2120
Maxalt-MLT Orally Disintegrating Tablets (Infrequent) 2120
Maxzide 1008
Megace Oral Suspension (1% to 3%) 1124
Menest Tablets 2254
▲ Meridia Capsules (4.3%) 481
Merrem I.V. (0.1% to 1.0%) 673
Metadate CD Capsules 1164
Metadate ER Tablets 1167
Methylin Tablets 1995
Methylin ER Tablets 1995
MetroGel-Vaginal Gel (Less than 1%) 1986
Mevacor Tablets (0.5% to 1.0%) 2132
Mexitil Capsules (2.4%) 1047
Miacalcin Nasal Spray (1% to 3%) 2375
Micardis Tablets (More than 0.3%) .. 1049
Micardis HCT Tablets 1051
Microgestin Fe 1.5/30 Tablets 3407
Microgestin Fe 1/20 Tablets 3400
Midamor Tablets (Less than or equal to 1%) 2136
Migranal Nasal Spray (Rare) 2376
Minipress Capsules (1% to 4%) 2699
Minizide Capsules (Rare) 2700
Mintezol 2137
Mirapex Tablets (1% or more) 2834
▲ Mirena Intrauterine System (5% or more) 974
Mithracin for Intravenous Use 903
Moban (Less frequent) 1320
Mobic Tablets (Less than 2%) 1054
Modicon 2563
Moduretic Tablets (Less than or equal to 1%) 2138
Monopril Tablets (0.4% to 1.0%) 1091
Monopril HCT (Less than 2%) 1094
Motofen Tablets 577
Motrin Suspension, Oral Drops, Chewable Tablets, and Caplets (Less than 1%) 2002
MS Contin Tablets (Less frequent) ... 2896
MSIR (Less frequent) 2898
Mykrox Tablets (Less than 2%) 1168
▲ Mylotarg for Injection (8% to 13%) .. 3540
Nadolol Tablets 2288
Naprelan Tablets (Less than 1%) 1293
Naropin Injection 612
Nasacort Nasal Inhaler 750
Necon 3415
Neoral Soft Gelatin Capsules (Rare) 2380
Neoral Oral Solution (Rare) 2380
Nesacaine/Nesacaine MPF 617
Neurontin Capsules (1.8%) 2655
Neurontin Oral Solution (1.8%) 2655
Neurontin Tablets (1.8%) 2655
Nicotrol Nasal Spray (Under 5%) 2843
▲ Nilandron Tablets (8.6%) 753
Nimotop Capsules (Up to 1.4%) 904
▲ Nipent for Injection (3% to 10%) 3272
Nizoral Tablets (Rare) 1791
Nolvadex Tablets (Infrequent) 678
Nordette-28 Tablets 2257
Norinyl 1 +35 28-Day Tablets 3380
Norinyl 1 + 50 28-Day Tablets 3380
Normodyne Tablets 3137
Noroxin Tablets (Less frequent) 2145
Norvasc Tablets (More than 0.1% to 1%) 2704
Norvir Capsules (Less than 2%) 487
Norvir Oral Solution (Less than 2%) 487
Novarel for Injection 1347
Nubain Injection (1% or less) 1323
Numorphan 1324
Ocupress Ophthalmic Solution, 1% Sterile .... ⊙303
Ogen Tablets 2846
Ogestrel 0.5/50-28 Tablets 3428
OptiPranolol Metipranolol Ophthalmic Solution 0.3% (A small number of patients) .... ⊙263
Oramorph SR Tablets (Less frequent) 3062
▲ Orap Tablets (2 of 20 patients) 1407
Ortho Dienestrol Cream 2554
Ortho-Cept 21 Tablets 2546
Ortho-Cept 28 Tablets 2546
Ortho-Cyclen/Ortho Tri-Cyclen 2573
Ortho-Est Tablets 3464
Ortho-Novum 2563
Ortho-Novum 1/50□28 Tablets 2556
▲ Ortho-Prefest Tablets (5%) 2570
Ortho-Cyclen/Ortho Tri-Cyclen 2573
Orudis Capsules (Greater than 1%) 3548
Oruvail Capsules (Greater than 1%) 3548
Ovcon 3364
Ovral Tablets 3551
Ovral-28 Tablets 3552
Ovrette Tablets 3552
Oxandrin Tablets 1153
Oxsoralen-Ultra Capsules 1741
OxyContin Tablets (Less than 1%) ... 2912
Paxil (Frequent) 1609
Pediazole Suspension 3050
▲ PEG-Intron Powder for Injection (29%) 3140
Pentasa Capsules (Less than 1%) 3239
Pepcid Injection (Infrequent) 2153
Pepcid for Oral Suspension (Infrequent) 2150
Pepcid RPD Orally Disintegrating Tablets (Infrequent) 2150
Pepcid Tablets (Infrequent) 2150
▲ Permax Tablets (3.2%) 1299
Phrenilin 578
▲ Plavix Tablets (3.6%) 1097
▲ Plavix Tablets (3.6%) 3084
Plendil Extended-Release Tablets (0.5% to 1.5%) 623
Polocaine Injection, USP 625
Polocaine-MPF Injection, USP 625
Ponstel Capsules (Occasional) 1356
Pravachol Tablets 1099
Prednisone 3064
Pregnyl for Injection 2482
Prelone Syrup 2273
Premarin Intravenous 3563
Premarin Tablets 3566
Premarin Vaginal Cream 3570
Premphase Tablets 3572
▲ Prempro Tablets (6% to 11%) 3572
Prevacid Delayed-Release Capsules (Less than 1%) 3292
PREVPAC (Less than 1%) 3298
Prilosec Delayed-Release Capsules (Less than 1%) 628
Prinivil Tablets (Greater than 1%) 2164
Prinzide Tablets (0.3% to 1%) 2168
Procanbid Extended-Release Tablets (Occasional) 2262
Procardia Capsules (Less than 0.5%) 2708
Procardia XL Extended Release Tablets (1% or less) 2710
▲ Prograf (3% to 15%) 1393
Proleukin for Injection (Less than 1%) 1199
▲ Prometrium Capsules (100 mg, 200 mg) (Less than 5% to 19%) ... 3261
ProSom Tablets (2%) 500
Protonix I.V. (Less than 1%) 3580
Protonix Tablets (Less than 1%) 3577
Protopic Ointment (Greater than or equal to 1%) 1397
Proventil HFA Inhalation Aerosol (Less than 3%) 3150
Provera Tablets 2853
▲ Provigil Tablets (4%) 1193
Prozac Pulvules, Liquid, and Weekly Capsules (Less than 1%) 1238
Pulmicort Respules (Less than 1%) 632
Pulmicort Turbuhaler Inhalation Powder (Rare) 636
Quinaglute Dura-Tabs Tablets 978
Quinidex Extentabs (Occasional) 2933
▲ Rapamune Oral Solution and Tablets (3% to 20%) 3584
▲ Rebetron Combination Therapy (23% to 36%) 3153
Reglan (Less frequent) 2935
Relafen Tablets (Less than 1%) 1617
Remeron Tablets (Frequent) 2483
Remeron SolTab Tablets (Frequent) 2486
Remicade for IV Injection (Less than 2%) 1178
▲ Reminyl Oral Solution (7%) 1792
▲ Reminyl Tablets (7%) 1792
Requip Tablets (1% or more) 1621
Retrovir Capsules 1625
Retrovir IV Infusion 1629
Retrovir 1625
Rhinocort Nasal Inhaler (Rare) 640
▲ Rilutek Tablets (4.2% to 6.1%) 772
Risperdal (Infrequent) 1796
Ritalin 2387
▲ Rituxan for Infusion (Among most frequent) 1750
▲ Rituxan I.V. (Among most frequent) 1428
▲ Roferon-A Injection (16% to 28%) ... 2996
Romazicon Injection (1% to 3%) 3000
Rythmol Tablets – 150 mg, 225 mg, 300 mg (Less than 1%) 502
Salagen Tablets (Less than 1%) 2229
Sandimmune (Rare) 2388
Sandostatin Injection (1% to 4%) 2394
▲ Sandostatin LAR Depot (5% to 15%) 2395
Sectral Capsules (2%) 3589
Sedapap Tablets 50 mg/650 mg (Infrequent) 2225
Sensorcaine 643
Sensorcaine-MPF Injection 643
Septra Suspension 2265
Septra Tablets 2265
Septra DS Tablets 2265
Serophene Tablets (Less than 1 in 100 patients) 3226
▲ Serostim for Injection (1% to 10%) . 3229
Serzone Tablets 1104
▲ Simulect for Injection (3% to 10%) . 2399
Sinemet Tablets 1253
Sinemet CR Tablets (2.2%) 1255
Solu-Medrol Sterile Powder 2855
Sonata Capsules (Frequent) 3591
▲ Soriatane Capsules (1% to 10%) 3003
Sporanox Capsules (Infrequent) 1800
Sporanox Oral Solution (1.1% to 2.0%) 1808
Sporanox Oral Solution (1.1% to 2.0%) 2512
Stadol NS Nasal Spray (Less than 1%) 1108
Sular Tablets (Less than or equal to 1%) 688
Sustiva Capsules (2% to 3%) 1258
Symmetrel (1% to 5%) 1328
▲ Synarel Nasal Solution for Endometriosis (3% of patients) 3205
Tagamet 1644
Talacen Caplets (Infrequent) 3089
Talwin Nx Tablets 3090
Tambocor Tablets (1% to 3%) 1990
Tasmar Tablets (Frequent) 3010
Tegretol/Tegretol-XR 2404
▲ Temodar Capsules (6%) 3157
Tenex Tablets (3% or less) 2942
▲ Tenoretic Tablets (0.6% to 12%) 690
▲ Tenormin (0.6% to 12%) 692
Tequin Injection (Less than 0.1%) 1110
Tequin Tablets (Less than 0.1%) 1110
Testoderm Transdermal Systems ... 574
Testopel Pellets 3610
Testred Capsules, 10 mg 1746
Teveten Tablets (1%) 3327
Thalomid Capsules 1154
Tiazac Capsules (Less than 2%) 1378
Timolide Tablets 2187
Timolol GFS .... ⊙266

Timoptic in Ocudose (Less frequent) 2192
Timoptic Sterile Ophthalmic Solution (Less frequent) 2190
Timoptic-XE Sterile Ophthalmic Gel Forming Solution 2194
Tolectin (1% to 3%) 2589
Tonocard Tablets (Less than 1%) 649
▲ Topamax Sprinkle Capsules (8% to 13.4%) 2590
▲ Topamax Tablets (8% to 13.4%) 2590
▲ Toprol-XL Tablets (About 5 of 100 patients) 651
Toradol (1% or less) 3018
Tranxene 511
Travatan Ophthalmic Solution (1% to 5%) 543
Trecator-SC Tablets 3598
Trental Tablets (Less than 1%) 784
Tricor Capsules, Micronized 513
Tri-Levlen 962
Tri-Norinyl-28 Tablets 3433
Triphasil-21 Tablets 3600
Triphasil-28 Tablets 3605
▲ Trisenox Injection (20%) 1158
Trivora Tablets 3439
▲ Trizivir Tablets (9%) 1669
Trovan (Less than 1%) 2722
Ultracet Tablets (Less than 1%) 2597
Ultram Tablets (Less than 1%) 2600
Uniretic Tablets (Less than 1%) 3178
Valium Injectable 3026
Valium Tablets (Infrequent) 3047
▲ Valtrex Caplets (Less than 1% to 7%) 1676
Vanceril Double Strength Inhalation Aerosol (Fewer than 2%) 3167
Vascor Tablets (0.5% to 2.0%) 2602
Vaseretic Tablets 2204
Vasotec I.V. Injection 2207
Vasotec Tablets (0.5% to 1%) 2210
▲ Vesanoid Capsules (14%) 3037
▲ Viadur Implant (5.3%) 912
Viagra Tablets (Less than 2%) 2732
Vicoprofen Tablets (Less than 1%) 520
Vioxx (Greater than 0.1% to 1.9%) 2213
Viracept 532
Vistide Injection 1445
Vivelle Transdermal System 2412
Vivelle-Dot Transdermal System 2416
Voltaren Tablets (Less than 1%) 2315
Voltaren-XR Tablets (Less than 1%) 2315
Wellbutrin Tablets (Frequent) 1680
▲ Xanax Tablets (13.8% to 13.9%) 2865
▲ Xenical Capsules (3.4%) 3043
Yasmin 28 Tablets (Greater than 1%) 980
Zanaflex Tablets (Frequent) 1305
Zantac (Rare) 1690
Zantac Injection (Rare) 1688
Zantac Syrup (Rare) 1690
Zarontin Capsules (Rare) 2659
Zarontin Syrup (Rare) 2660
Zaroxolyn Tablets 1177
Zebeta Tablets (Up to 0.2%) 1885
▲ Zenapax for Injection (2% to 5%) 3046
Zestoretic Tablets (0.3% to 1%) 695
Zestril Tablets (Greater than 1%) 698
Ziac Tablets 1887
Zocor Tablets 2219
▲ Zoladex (1% to 54%) 702
Zoladex 3-month 706
Zoloft (Infrequent) 2751
Zomig Tablets (Infrequent) 708
Zomig-ZMT Tablets (Infrequent) 708
▲ Zonegran Capsules (6%) 1307
Zosyn (1.0% or less) 1890
Zosyn in Galaxy Containers (1.0% or less) 1894
Zovia 3449
Zyban Sustained-Release Tablets (Frequent) 1710
Zyprexa Tablets 1973
Zyprexa ZYDIS Orally Disintegrating Tablets 1973
Zyrtec (Less than 2%) 2756
Zyrtec-D 12 Hour Extended Relief Tablets (Less than 2%) 2758

Depression, aggravation of
Celexa (Frequent) 1365
Coreg Tablets (0.1% to 1%) 1508
Evoxac Capsules (Less than 1%) 1217
Halcion Tablets 2823
Intron A for Injection (Less than 5%) 3120
Lupron Depot 3.75 mg (A possibility) 3281
Lupron Depot–3 Month 11.25 mg (Possible) 3285
Meridia Capsules 481
Nexium Delayed-Release Capsules (Less than 1%) 619
Sustiva Capsules (Less than 2%) 1258
Tegretol-XR Tablets 2404
Zoloft (Infrequent) 2751

Depression, circulatory
Kadian Capsules 1335
Oramorph SR Tablets 3062
Roxanol 3066

Depression, mood
(see *under* Depression)

Depression, psychotic
Celexa (Infrequent) 1365
Copaxone for Injection (Infrequent) 3306
Effexor Tablets (Rare) 3495
Effexor XR Capsules (Infrequent) 3499
8-MOP Capsules 1727
▲ Ifex for Injection (Among most common) 1123
Paxil (Rare) 1609
Remeron Tablets (Rare) 2483
Remeron SolTab Tablets (Rare) 2486
Rilutek Tablets (Rare) 772

Depression, respiratory, neonatal
Astramorph/PF Injection, USP (Preservative-Free) 594
Demerol 3079
Dilaudid 441
Dilaudid Powder 441
Dilaudid Rectal Suppositories 441
Dilaudid Tablets 441
Duramorph Injection 1312
Kadian Capsules 1335
Lortab 3319
Lortab Elixir 3317
Mepergan Injection 3539
MS Contin Tablets 2896
MSIR 2898
Normodyne Injection 3135
Oramorph SR Tablets 3062
Percocet Tablets 1326
Roxanol 3066
Streptomycin Sulfate Injection (Occasional) 2714
Tussionex Pennkinetic Extended-Release Suspension 1174
Tylenol with Codeine 2595
Tylox Capsules 2597
Vicodin Tablets 516
Vicodin ES Tablets 517

Depressive reactions
▲ Combivir Tablets (9%) 1502
▲ Epivir (9%) 1520
Rescriptor Tablets (Less than 2%) 526
Soma Tablets 3353
Soma Compound Tablets (Infrequent or rare) 3354
Soma Compound w/Codeine Tablets (Infrequent or rare) 3355
Xanax Tablets 2865

Dermatitis
Ambien Tablets (Rare) 3191
Amerge Tablets (Rare) 1467
▲ Apligraf (2.5% to 6.2%) 2305
Aricept Tablets (Infrequent) 1270
Aricept Tablets (Infrequent) 2665
Atacand HCT Tablets (0.5% or greater) 597
Avalide Tablets 1070
Avapro Tablets (Less than 1%) 1074
Avapro Tablets (Less than 1%) 3076
Axert Tablets (Rare) 2772
Azelex Cream (Less than 1%) 547
Azopt Ophthalmic Suspension (1% to 5%) 536
Bactroban Cream (Less than 1%) 1494
Benoquin Cream 20% 1732
Betaxon Ophthalmic Suspension (Less than 2%) 537
Cataflam Tablets (Less than 1%) 2315
Celebrex Capsules (0.1% to 1.9%) 2676
Celebrex Capsules (0.1% to 1.9%) 2780
Celexa (Infrequent) 1365
Cerumenex Eardrops (1% of 2,700 patients) 2895
Ciloxan (Less than 1%) 538
Claritin (At least one patient) 3100
Claritin-D 12 Hour Extended Release Tablets 3102
Claritin-D 24 Hour Extended Release Tablets 3104
Clindagel 1401
Clomid Tablets (Fewer than 1%) 735
Clozaril Tablets (Less than 1%) 2319
Cognex Capsules (Infrequent) 1351
Colazal Capsules 3069
Colestid Tablets (Rare) 2791
Colyte with Flavor Packs for Oral Solution (Isolated cases) 3170
Copaxone for Injection (Infrequent) 3306
Cormax Scalp Application (Approximately 0.3%) 2441
Cosopt Sterile Ophthalmic Solution 2065
Coumadin for Injection (Infrequent) 1243
Coumadin Tablets (Infrequent) 1243
Cozaar Tablets (Less than 1%) 2067
Crixivan Capsules (Less than 2%) 2070
Cytotec Tablets (Infrequent) 3202
Differin Cream (Less than 1%) 1402
Dilantin Infatabs 2624
Dilantin Kapseals (Rare) 2622
Dilantin-125 Oral Suspension (Rare) 2625
▲ Dovonex Cream (1% to 10%) 1116
▲ Dovonex Ointment (1% to 10%) 1117
Emadine Ophthalmic Solution (Less than 5%) ⊙211
▲ Ergamisol Tablets (8% to 23%) 1789
Estring Vaginal Ring (1% to 3%) 2811
Evoxac Capsules (Less than 1%) 1217
Fareston Tablets 3237
Finevin Cream (Less than 1%) 962
Flovent Diskus (1% to 3%) 3614
Flovent (1% to 3%) 1535
Flovent Rotadisk (1% to 3%) 1537
Floxin Otic Solution (Single report) 1219
Fortovase Capsules (Less than 2%) 2970
Sterile FUDR 2974
Gengraf Capsules (1% to less than 3%) 457
GoLYTELY and Pineapple Flavor GoLYTELY for Oral Solution (Isolated cases) 1068
Halcion Tablets (Rare) 2823
Hivid Tablets (Less than 1%) 2975
Hycamtin for Injection (Rare) 1546
Hyzaar 2109
Ifex for Injection (Less than 1%) 1123
▲ Intron A for Injection (Up to 8%) 3120
Invirase Capsules (Less than 2%) 2979
Iopidine 0.5% Ophthalmic Solution (Less than 3%) ⊙213
Lopid Tablets 2650
Lotensin Tablets (Less than 1%) 2365
Lotrel Capsules 2370
Loxitane Capsules 3398
Lupron Depot 7.5 mg (Less than 5%) 3284
▲ Lupron Injection (5% or more) 3279
Maxair Autohaler 1981
Maxair Inhaler (Less than 1%) 1984
Meridia Capsules 481
Micardis Tablets (More than 0.3%) 1049
Micardis HCT Tablets 1051
Myambutol Tablets 1290
Mykrox Tablets 1168
Neoral Soft Gelatin Capsules (1% to less than 3%) 2380
Neoral Oral Solution (1% to less than 3%) 2380
Nexium Delayed-Release Capsules (Less than 1%) 619
Norplant System 3543
Norvasc Tablets (Less than or equal to 0.1%) 2704
NuLYTELY, Cherry Flavor, Lemon-Lime Flavor, and Orange Flavor NuLYTELY for Oral Solution (Isolated cases) 1068
Pancrease Capsules (Frequent) 2580
Pancrease MT Capsules (Frequent) 2581
Phenergan Injection 3553
Phenergan 3556
Prevnar for Injection 1870
Prilosec Delayed-Release Capsules 628
Prinzide Tablets (0.3% to 1%) 2168
Procardia Capsules (2% or less) 2708
Requip Tablets (Infrequent) 1621
Rescriptor Tablets (Less than 2%) 526
Salagen Tablets (Rare) 2229
▲ Serostim for Injection (1% to 10%) 3229
▲ Soriatane Capsules (1% to 10%) 3003
Talwin Nx Tablets 3090
Tamiflu Capsules (1%) 3008
Tamiflu Oral Suspension (1%) 3008
Temovate Scalp Application (1 of 294 patients) 1304
Tenex Tablets (3% or less) 2942
Thioplex for Injection 1765
Thioridazine Hydrochloride Tablets (Infrequent) 2289
Topamax Sprinkle Capsules (Infrequent) 2590
Topamax Tablets (Infrequent) 2590
▲ Trisenox Injection (43%) 1158
Trovan (Less than 1%) 2722
Urobiotic-250 Capsules (Rare) 2731
Vaqta (Less than 1%) 2199
Varivax (Greater than or equal to 1%) 2202
Viracept 532
Voltaren Tablets (Less than 1%) 2315
Voltaren-XR Tablets (Less than 1%) 2315
Warfarin Sodium Tablets, USP 3302
▲ Xanax Tablets (3.8%) 2865
Xeloda Tablets (1%) 3039
Zaroxolyn Tablets 1177
Ziac Tablets 1887
Zoloft (Rare) 2751
Zyrtec (Less than 2%) 2756
Zyrtec-D 12 Hour Extended Relief Tablets (Less than 2%) 2758

Dermatitis, allergic
Antabuse Tablets 2444
Antabuse Tablets (Small number of patients) 3474
Cortone Acetate Injectable Suspension 2059
Cortone Acetate Tablets 2061
Decadron Elixir 2078
Decadron Tablets 2079
Decadron Phosphate Injection 2081
Hydrocortone Tablets 2106
Hydrocortone Acetate Injectable Suspension 2103
Hydrocortone Phosphate Injection, Sterile 2105
Prednisone 3064
ProctoFoam-HC 3177
Serophene Tablets (Less than 1 in 100 patients) 3226

Dermatitis, allergic contact
Aclovate (Infrequent) 1275
Analpram-HC 1338
▲ Androderm Transdermal System CIII (4%) 3377
Anusol-HC Cream 2.5% (Infrequent to frequent) 2237
Anusol-HC Suppositories 2238
Capex Shampoo 1400
▲ Catapres-TTS (About 19 in 100) 1038
Cerumenex Eardrops 2895
Clinac BPO Gel USP 1339
Clobevate Gel 3271
Cordran Lotion (Infrequent) 2438
Cordran Tape (Infrequent) 2439
Cormax Cream (Infrequent) 2440
Cormax Ointment (Infrequent) 2440
Cormax Scalp Application (Infrequent) 2441
Cutivate Cream (Infrequent) 1282
Cutivate Ointment (Infrequent to more frequent) 1284
Dermatop Emollient Cream (Less than 1%) 2517
DesOwen (Less than 2%) 1401
Diprolene Gel 0.05% (Less frequent) 3107
Diprolene Lotion 0.05% (Infrequent) 3107
Diprolene Ointment 0.05% (Infrequent) 3108
Diprolene AF Cream 0.05% (Infrequent) 3106
Diprosone 3109
▲ Efudex (Among most frequent) 1733
Elocon Cream 0.1% (Infrequent) 3110
Elocon Lotion 0.1% (Infrequent) 3111
Elocon Ointment 0.1% (Infrequent) 3112
Fluoroplex 552
Lidex (Infrequent) 2020
Locoid Cream (Infrequent) 1341
Locoid Lipocream Cream (Infrequent) 1342
Locoid (Infrequent) 1341
Lotrisone 3129
Luxiq Foam 1210
Olux Foam 1211
Ophthetic Ophthalmic Solution ⊙244
Oxistat Cream 1298
Pramosone 1343
Proctocort Suppositories 2264
Psorcon E Cream 1227
Psorcon E Ointment 1228
Retin-A Micro 0.1% (Rare) 2522
Synalar (Infrequent) 2020
Temovate Cream 1301
Temovate Gel (Infrequent) 1303
Temovate Ointment 1301
Temovate Scalp Application (Infrequent) 1304
Temovate E Emollient (Infrequent) 1302
Topicort (Infrequent) 2025
Triaz Cleanser 2026
Triaz Gel 2026
Ultravate Cream 1119
Ultravate Ointment 1120

Dermatitis, atopic
Cutivate Cream (0.8%) 1282
Vioxx (Greater than 0.1% to 1.9%) 2213

Dermatitis, bullous
Chloroptic Sterile Ophthalmic Solution ⊙235
Dilantin Infatabs 2624
Dilantin Kapseals 2622
Dilantin-125 Oral Suspension 2625
Miltown Tablets (Rare) 3349

Dermatitis, contact
Advair Diskus 100/50 1448
Advair Diskus 250/50 1448
Advair Diskus 500/50 1448
Alustra Cream 2018
Americaine Anesthetic Lubricant 1162
Americaine Otic Topical Anesthetic Ear Drops 1162
Arava Tablets (1% to 3%) 724
Astelin Nasal Spray (Infrequent) 3339
▲ Augmentin ES-600 Powder for Oral Suspension (3.5%) 1487
Avonex 1013
Azelex Cream (Less than 1%) 547
Bactroban Ointment (Less than 1%) 1496
Betaseron for SC Injection 988

- ▲ Catapres-TTS (About 8 to 34 in 100 patients) 1038
- Celebrex Capsules (0.1% to 1.9%) 2676
- Celebrex Capsules (0.1% to 1.9%) 2780
- Cerebyx Injection (Infrequent) 2619
- Cleocin Vaginal Cream 2788
- Clindagel 1401
- Compazine 1505
- Copaxone for Injection (Infrequent) 3306
- Cosopt Sterile Ophthalmic Solution 2065
- Crixivan Capsules (Less than 2%) 2070
- Doxil Injection (Less than 1%) 566
- Effexor Tablets (Infrequent) 3495
- Effexor XR Capsules (Infrequent) 3499
- Eldopaque Forte 4% Cream (Occasional) 1734
- Eldoquin Forte 4% Cream (Occasional) 1734
- Etrafon 3115
- Evoxac Capsules (Less than 1%) 1217
- Exelon Capsules (Infrequent) 2342
- Exelon Oral Solution (Infrequent) 2345
- Finevin Cream (Less than 1%) 962
- Gabitril Tablets (Infrequent) 1189
- Geodon Capsules (Infrequent) 2688
- Iopidine 0.5% Ophthalmic Solution (Less than 3%) ⊙213
- Klonopin Tablets (Infrequent) 2983
- Lipitor Tablets (Less than 2%) 2639
- Lipitor Tablets (Less than 2%) 2696
- Loprox Gel (1% to 5%) 2022
- Lustra Cream 2023
- Lustra-AF Cream 2023
- LYMErix Vaccine (1.68%) 1592
- Mentax Cream (Less than 2%) 1009
- ▲ MetroLotion (3%) 1405
- Naprelan Tablets (Less than 1%) 1293
- Navane Oral 2701
- Navane Intramuscular 2703
- Nitro-Dur Transdermal Infusion System (Uncommon) 1834
- Nitro-Dur Transdermal Infusion System (Uncommon) 3134
- Nizoral 2% Cream (Rare) 3620
- Norvir Capsules (Less than 2%) 487
- Norvir Oral Solution (Less than 2%) 487
- Paxil (Rare) 1609
- Protonix I.V. (Less than 1%) 3580
- Protonix Tablets (Less than 1%) 3577
- Protopic Ointment (1% to 3%) 1397
- Prozac Pulvules, Liquid, and Weekly Capsules (Infrequent) 1238
- Pulmicort Respules (1% to 3%) 632
- Pulmicort Turbuhaler Inhalation Powder (Rare) 636
- Rhinocort Nasal Inhaler (Rare) 640
- Rilutek Tablets (Rare) 772
- Salagen Tablets (Less than 1%) 2229
- Sarafem Pulvules (Infrequent) 1962
- Serentil 1057
- Serevent Diskus (1% to 3%) 1637
- Seroquel Tablets (Infrequent) 684
- Solaquin Forte (Occasional) 1734
- Sonata Capsules (Infrequent) 3591
- ▲ Tazorac Gel (1% to 10%) 556
- Thioplex for Injection 1765
- Thioridazine Hydrochloride Tablets 2289
- Thiothixene Capsules 2290
- Thorazine 1656
- Tricor Capsules, Micronized 513
- Trileptal Oral Suspension 2407
- Trileptal Tablets 2407
- Trusopt Sterile Ophthalmic Solution 2196
- Uniretic Tablets (Less than 1%) 3178
- Vaniqa Cream (Less than 1%) 1121
- Varivax (Greater than or equal to 1%) 2202
- Viagra Tablets (Less than 2%) 2732
- Vioxx (Greater than 0.1% to 1.9%) 2213
- Zoloft (Rare) 2751
- Zyprexa Tablets (Infrequent) 1973
- Zyprexa ZYDIS Orally Disintegrating Tablets (Infrequent) 1973

Dermatitis, eczematoid

- Symmetrel (Less than 0.1%) 1328

Dermatitis, exfoliative

- Abelcet Injection 1273
- Accupril Tablets (Rare) 2611
- Accuretic Tablets (0.5% to 1%) 2614
- Aceon Tablets (2 mg, 4 mg, 8 mg) 3249
- Actiq (Less than 1%) 1184
- Adalat CC Tablets (Rare) 877
- Aldoclor Tablets 2035
- Aldoril Tablets 2039
- Amoxil Chewable Tablets 1471
- Amoxil for Oral Suspension 1471
- Amoxil 1471
- Arthrotec Tablets (Rare) 3195
- Atacand HCT Tablets 597
- Augmentin Chewable Tablets (Occasional case) 1482
- Augmentin Powder for Oral Suspension (Occasional case) 1482
- Augmentin Tablets (Occasional) 1485
- Augmentin ES-600 Powder for Oral Suspension (Occasional) 1487
- Avalide Tablets 1070
- Axid Pulvules 1903
- Axid Pulvules 2919
- Azactam for Injection (Less than 1%) 1276
- Azulfidine EN-tabs Tablets (Rare) 2775
- Bactrim 2949
- Betaseron for SC Injection 988
- Bicillin C-R 900/300 Injection 2240
- Bicillin C-R Injection 2238
- Bicillin L-A Injection 2242
- Captopril Tablets 2281
- Carbatrol Capsules 3234
- Cardizem Injectable 1018
- Cardizem Lyo-Ject Syringe 1018
- Cardizem Monovial 1018
- Cardizem CD Capsules (Infrequent) 1016
- Cataflam Tablets (Rare) 2315
- Celebrex Capsules (Less than 0.1%) 2676
- Celebrex Capsules (Less than 0.1%) 2780
- Chibroxin Sterile Ophthalmic Solution 2051
- Cipro I.V. (1% or less) 893
- Cipro I.V. Pharmacy Bulk Package (Less than 1%) 897
- Cipro 887
- Cleocin Phosphate Sterile Solution (Rare) 2785
- Clinoril Tablets 2053
- Compazine 1505
- Concerta Extended-Release Tablets 1998
- Concerta Tablets 561
- Coreg Tablets (Less than or equal to 0.1%) 1508
- Corzide 40/5 Tablets 2247
- Corzide 80/5 Tablets 2247
- Cuprimine Capsules 2075
- Cytovene 2959
- Declomycin Tablets (Uncommon) 1855
- Depen Titratable Tablets 3341
- Diabinese Tablets 2680
- Diflucan Tablets, Injection, and Oral Suspension (Rare) 2681
- Dilantin Infatabs 2624
- Dilantin Kapseals 2622
- Dilantin-125 Oral Suspension 2625
- Diovan HCT Tablets 2338
- Diuril Oral 2087
- Diuril Sodium Intravenous 2086
- Dolobid Tablets (Less than 1 in 100) 2088
- Doryx Coated Pellet Filled Capsules 3357
- Doxil Injection (Less than 1% to 5%) 566
- Duragesic Transdermal System (Less than 1%) 1786
- Dynacin Capsules (Uncommon) 2019
- Effexor Tablets (Rare) 3495
- Effexor XR Capsules (Rare) 3499
- Enalaprilat Injection 863
- Ergamisol Tablets (Less frequent) 1789
- Etrafon 3115
- Feldene Capsules (Rare) 2685
- Floxin I.V. 2526
- Floxin Tablets 2529
- Furosemide Tablets 2284
- Gabitril Tablets (Infrequent) 1189
- Geodon Capsules (Infrequent) 2688
- Hivid Tablets (Less than 1%) 2975
- HydroDIURIL Tablets 2108
- Hyzaar 2109
- Imitrex Tablets (Rare) 1558
- Indocin Capsules (Less than 1%) 2112
- Indocin I.V. (Less than 1%) 2115
- Indocin (Less than 1%) 2112
- Kaletra Capsules (Less than 2%) 471
- Kaletra Oral Solution (Less than 2%) 471
- Lexxel Tablets 608
- Lodine XL Extended-Release Tablets 3530
- Lopid Tablets 2650
- Luvox Tablets (25, 50, 100 mg) (Infrequent) 3256
- Macrobid Capsules (Rare) 2889
- Macrodantin Capsules (Rare) 2891
- Mefoxin for Injection 2124
- Mefoxin Premixed Intravenous Solution 2127
- Metadate CD Capsules 1164
- Metadate ER Tablets 1167
- Methylin Tablets 1995
- Methylin ER Tablets 1995
- Mexitil Capsules (Rare) 1047
- Micardis HCT Tablets 1051
- Microzide Capsules 3414
- Miltown Tablets (Rare) 3349
- Minocin Intravenous (Uncommon) 1862
- Minocin Oral Suspension (Uncommon) 1865
- Minocin Pellet-Filled Capsules (Uncommon) 1863
- Moduretic Tablets 2138
- Monodox Capsules (Uncommon) 2442
- Monopril Tablets 1091
- Monopril HCT 1094
- Motrin Suspension, Oral Drops, Chewable Tablets, and Caplets (Less than 1%) 2002
- Navane Oral 2701
- Navane Intramuscular 2703
- Nebcin Vials, Hyporets & ADD-Vantage (Rare) 1955
- Nembutal Sodium Solution 485
- Neumega for Injection 1434
- Nitrolingual Pumpspray 1355
- Nitrostat Tablets 2658
- Noroxin Tablets 2145
- Omnicef 493
- Orudis Capsules (Less than 1%) 3548
- Oruvail Capsules (Less than 1%) 3548
- OxyContin Tablets (Less than 1%) 2912
- Paser Granules 1781
- Paxil (Rare) 1609
- Pediazole Suspension 3050
- Periostat Tablets 1208
- Permapen Isoject 2706
- Pfizerpen for Injection 2707
- Plaquenil Tablets 3082
- Ponstel Capsules (Rare) 1356
- Prinzide Tablets 2168
- Procardia Capsules (Rare) 2708
- Procardia XL Extended Release Tablets (Rare) 2710
- ▲ Prograf (3% to 15%) 1393
- ▲ Proleukin for Injection (18%) 1199
- Protopic Ointment (Up to 3%) 1397
- Prozac Pulvules, Liquid, and Weekly Capsules 1238
- Remeron Tablets (Infrequent) 2483
- Remeron SolTab Tablets (Infrequent) 2486
- Rifamate Capsules 767
- Rifater Tablets 769
- Rilutek Tablets (Up to 1.2%) 772
- Risperdal (Infrequent) 1796
- Ritalin 2387
- Salagen Tablets (Less than 1%) 2229
- Sarafem Pulvules 1962
- Septra Suspension 2265
- Septra Tablets 2265
- Septra DS Tablets 2265
- Serentil 1057
- Seroquel Tablets (Rare) 684
- Silvadene Cream 1% 2267
- Stelazine (Occasional) 1640
- Sular Tablets (Less than or equal to 1%) 688
- Sustiva Capsules (Up to 3.5%) 1258
- Tagamet (Very rare) 1644
- Tambocor Tablets (Less than 1%) 1990
- Taxol Injection (Rare) 1129
- Tegretol/Tegretol-XR 2404
- Tenex Tablets (Less frequent) 2942
- Thalomid Capsules 1154
- Thioridazine Hydrochloride Tablets 2289
- Thiothixene Capsules 2290
- Thorazine 1656
- Tiazac Capsules (Infrequent) 1378
- Ticlid Tablets (Rare) 3015
- Timolide Tablets 2187
- Tonocard Tablets (Less than 1%) 649
- Toradol 3018
- Trilafon 3160
- Unasyn for Injection (Occasional) 2728
- Vancocin HCl Capsules & Pulvules (Infrequent) 1972
- Vancocin HCl Oral Solution (Infrequent) 1971
- Vancocin HCl, Vials & ADD-Vantage (Infrequent) 1970
- Vantin Tablets and Oral Suspension (Less than 1%) 2860
- Vaseretic Tablets 2204
- Vasotec I.V. Injection 2207
- Vasotec Tablets (0.5% to 1.0%) 2210
- Viagra Tablets (Less than 2%) 2732
- Vibramycin Calcium Oral Suspension Syrup (Uncommon) 2735
- Vibramycin Hyclate Capsules (Uncommon) 2735
- Vibramycin Hyclate Intravenous (Uncommon) 2737
- Vibramycin Monohydrate for Oral Suspension (Uncommon) 2735
- Vibra-Tabs Film Coated Tablets (Uncommon) 2735
- Vistide Injection 1445
- Voltaren Tablets (Rare) 2315
- Voltaren-XR Tablets (Rare) 2315
- Wellbutrin Tablets 1680
- Wellbutrin SR Sustained-Release Tablets 1684
- Zanaflex Tablets (Rare) 1305
- Zebeta Tablets 1885
- Zestoretic Tablets 695
- Ziac Tablets (Very rare) 1887
- Zyban Sustained-Release Tablets 1710

Dermatitis, eyelid

- OptiPranolol Metipranolol Ophthalmic Solution 0.3% (A small number of patients) ⊙263
- Vantin Tablets and Oral Suspension 2860

Dermatitis, fungal

- Arava Tablets (1% to 3%) 724
- Aricept Tablets (Infrequent) 1270
- Aricept Tablets (Infrequent) 2665
- ▲ CellCept Capsules (3%) 2951
- ▲ CellCept Intravenous (3%) 2951
- ▲ CellCept Oral Suspension (3%) 2951
- ▲ CellCept Tablets (3%) 2951
- Cipro HC Otic Suspension (One patient) 540
- Clindagel 1401
- Copaxone for Injection (Infrequent) 3306
- Doxil Injection (Less than 1%) 566
- Effexor Tablets (Rare) 3495
- Geodon Capsules (2%) 2688
- Lamictal (Rare) 1567
- Paxil (Rare) 1609
- Permax Tablets (Infrequent) 1299
- ▲ Prograf (3% to 15%) 1393
- Protonix I.V. (Less than 1%) 3580
- Protonix Tablets (Less than 1%) 3577
- ▲ Protopic Ointment (1% to 6%) 1397
- ▲ Rapamune Oral Solution and Tablets (3% to 20%) 3584
- Requip Tablets (Infrequent) 1621
- Rescriptor Tablets (Less than 2%) 526
- Rilutek Tablets (Infrequent) 772
- Sular Tablets (Less than or equal to 1%) 688
- Synagis Intramuscular (More than 1%) 2028
- ▲ Thalomid Capsules (4.2%) 1154
- Tricor Capsules, Micronized 513
- Trovan (Less than 1%) 2722
- Uniretic Tablets (Less than 1%) 3178
- Vantin Tablets and Oral Suspension (Less than 1%) 2860
- Viracept 532

Dermatitis, lichenoides

- Betaseron for SC Injection 988
- Effexor Tablets (Rare) 3495
- Effexor XR Capsules (Rare) 3499
- Evoxac Capsules (Less than 1%) 1217
- Intron A for Injection (Less than 5%) 3120
- Permax Tablets (Rare) 1299
- Protonix I.V. (Less than 1%) 3580
- Protonix Tablets (Less than 1%) 3577
- Risperdal (Rare) 1796

Dermatitis, maculopapular

- Chloroptic Sterile Ophthalmic Ointment ⊙234
- Chloroptic Sterile Ophthalmic Solution ⊙235
- Permapen Isoject 2706

Dermatitis, perioral

- Aclovate (Infrequent) 1275
- Analpram-HC 1338
- Anusol-HC Cream 2.5% (Infrequent to frequent) 2237
- Capex Shampoo 1400
- Clobevate Gel 3271
- Cordran Lotion (Infrequent) 2438
- Cordran Tape (Infrequent) 2439
- Cormax Cream (Infrequent) 2440
- Cormax Ointment (Infrequent) 2440
- Cormax Scalp Application (Infrequent) 2441
- Cutivate Cream (Infrequent) 1282
- Cutivate Ointment (Infrequent to more frequent) 1284
- Dermatop Emollient Cream (Infrequent to frequent) 2517
- DesOwen (Infrequent) 1401
- Diprolene Gel 0.05% (Infrequent) 3107
- Diprolene Lotion 0.05% (Infrequent) 3107
- Diprolene Ointment 0.05% (Infrequent) 3108
- Diprolene AF Cream 0.05% (Infrequent) 3106
- Diprosone 3109
- Elocon Cream 0.1% (Infrequent) 3110
- Elocon Lotion 0.1% (Infrequent) 3111
- Elocon Ointment 0.1% (Infrequent) 3112
- Lidex (Infrequent) 2020
- Locoid Cream (Infrequent) 1341
- Locoid Lipocream Cream (Infrequent) 1342
- Locoid (Infrequent) 1341
- Lotrisone 3129
- Luxíq Foam 1210
- Olux Foam 1211
- Pramosone 1343
- ProctoFoam-HC 3177
- Psorcon E Cream 1227
- Psorcon E Ointment 1228
- Synalar (Infrequent) 2020
- Temovate Cream 1301
- Temovate Gel (Infrequent) 1303
- Temovate Ointment 1301

Temovate Scalp Application (Infrequent) 1304
Temovate E Emollient (Infrequent) 1302
Topicort (Infrequent) 2025
Ultravate Cream 1119
Ultravate Ointment 1120

Dermatitis, photosensitive
Advair Diskus 100/50 1448
Advair Diskus 250/50 1448
Advair Diskus 500/50 1448
Amerge Tablets (Rare) 1467
Anaprox Tablets (Less than 1%) 2967
Anaprox DS Tablets (Less than 1%) 2967
▲ Cordarone Tablets (4% to 9%) 3487
EC-Naprosyn Delayed-Release Tablets (Less than 1%) 2967
Flovent Diskus (1% to 3%) 3614
▲ Naprelan Tablets (3% to 9%) 1293
Naprosyn Suspension (Less than 1%) 2967
Naprosyn Tablets (Less than 1%) 2967
▲ Pacerone Tablets (4% to 9%) 3331

Dermatitis, purpuric
Dilantin Infatabs 2624
Dilantin Kapseals 2622
Dilantin-125 Oral Suspension 2625

Dermatitis, radiation recall
Navelbine Injection 1604
Taxol Injection (Rare) 1129

Dermatitis, vesicular bullous
(*see under* Dermatitis, bullous)

Dermatitis seborrhic
Fortovase Capsules (Less than 2%) 2970
Imitrex Injection 1549
Imitrex Nasal Spray 1554

Dermatologic reactions, unspecified
Aceon Tablets (2 mg, 4 mg, 8 mg) 3249
Altace Capsules (Less than 1%) 2233
Ativan Tablets (Less frequent) 3482
Captopril Tablets 2281
Clinoril Tablets (Less than 1 in 100) 2053
Depen Titratable Tablets (Rare) 3341
Enalaprilat Injection 863
Floxin I.V. 2526
Floxin Tablets 2529
▲ Idamycin PFS Injection (46%) 2825
Levsin/Levsinex/Levbid 3172
Lexxel Tablets 608
Monopril Tablets 1091
Mylocel Tablets 2227
Norflex (Rare) 1987
Phrenilin (Several cases) 578
Prinivil Tablets (0.3% to 1.0%) 2164
Prinzide Tablets 2168
Protonix I.V. 3580
Protonix Tablets 3577
Sedapap Tablets 50 mg/650 mg (Several cases) 2225
Silvadene Cream 1% 2267
Tasmar Tablets (Infrequent) 3010
Vaseretic Tablets 2204
Vasotec I.V. Injection 2207
Vasotec Tablets (0.5% to 1.0%) 2210
Zestoretic Tablets 695
Zestril Tablets (0.3% to 1.0%) 698
Zithromax Capsules, 250 mg (Rare) 2743
Zithromax for IV Infusion (Rare) 2748
Zithromax for Oral Suspension, 300 mg, 600 mg, 900 mg, 1200 mg (Rare) 2739
Zithromax Tablets, 250 mg (Rare) 2739

Dermatomyositis
Baycol Tablets 883
Cuprimine Capsules (Rare) 2075
Depen Titratable Tablets (Rare) 3341
Mevacor Tablets 2132
Mylocel Tablets (Less frequently) 2227
Pravachol Tablets (Rare) 1099
Zocor Tablets 2219

Dermatomyositis, exacerbation of
Actimmune (Rare) 1772

Dermatopolymycositis
Accupril Tablets (Rare) 2611

Dermatosis
Amerge Tablets (Rare) 1467
Flovent Diskus (1% to 3%) 3614

Descemetitis
Ophthetic Ophthalmic Solution ⊙244

Desquamation
Aquasol A Parenteral 593
Cognex Capsules (Rare) 1351
Condylox Gel (Less common) 2436
Doxil Injection (Some patients) 566
Feldene Capsules (Occasional) 2685
Hivid Tablets (Less than 1%) 2975
Neurontin Capsules (Rare) 2655
Neurontin Oral Solution (Rare) 2655
Neurontin Tablets (Rare) 2655
Oxistat Lotion (0.4%) 1298
Rescriptor Tablets (Less than 2%) 526
▲ Sustiva Capsules (16.7% to 24.5%) 1258
▲ Taxotere for Injection Concentrate (5.6%) 778
▲ Tazorac Gel (1% to 30%) 556
Vantin Tablets and Oral Suspension (Less than 1%) 2860
Xeloda Tablets 3039

Diabetes
(*see under* Diabetes mellitus)

Diabetes, aggravation of
Campath Ampules 992
Serostim for Injection 3229
Tamiflu Capsules 3008
Tamiflu Oral Suspension 3008

Diabetes, unstable
Viagra Tablets (Less than 2%) 2732

Diabetes insipidus
Betaseron for SC Injection 988
Sandostatin LAR Depot (Rare) 2395

Diabetes insipidus, nephrogenic
Declomycin Tablets 1855
Eskalith (Some reports) 1527
Foscavir Injection (Rare) 605
Lithobid Slow-Release Tablets (Some reports) 3255

Diabetes mellitus
Accutane Capsules 2944
Arava Tablets (1% to 3%) 724
Aricept Tablets (Infrequent) 1270
Aricept Tablets (Infrequent) 2665
Betaseron for SC Injection 988
Betaxon Ophthalmic Suspension (Less than 2%) 537
Celebrex Capsules (0.1% to 1.9%) 2676
Celebrex Capsules (0.1% to 1.9%) 2780
▲ CellCept Capsules (3%) 2951
▲ CellCept Intravenous (3%) 2951
▲ CellCept Oral Suspension (3%) 2951
▲ CellCept Tablets (3%) 2951
Cognex Capsules (Infrequent) 1351
Coreg Tablets (0.1% to 1%) 1508
Crixivan Capsules 2070
Doxil Injection (Less than 1%) 566
Dyazide Capsules 1515
Effexor Tablets (Rare) 3495
Effexor XR Capsules (Infrequent) 3499
Evoxac Capsules (Less than 1%) 1217
Exelon Capsules (Infrequent) 2342
Exelon Oral Solution (Infrequent) 2345
Fortovase Capsules (Less than 2%) 2970
Gengraf Capsules (1% to less than 3%) 457
Hivid Tablets (Less than 1%) 2975
Invirase Capsules (Less than 2%) 2979
Lupron Depot 7.5 mg (Less than 5%) 3284
Lupron Injection (Less than 5%) 3279
Luvox Tablets (25, 50, 100 mg) (Rare) 3256
Macrobid Capsules 2889
Macrodantin Capsules 2891
Maxzide 1008
Micardis Tablets (More than 0.3%) 1049
Micardis HCT Tablets 1051
M-M-R II 2118
Mumpsvax 2141
Neoral Soft Gelatin Capsules (1% to less than 3%) 2380
Neoral Oral Solution (1% to less than 3%) 2380
Norvir Capsules (Less than 2%) 487
Norvir Oral Solution (Less than 2%) 487
Paxil (Rare) 1609
Permax Tablets (Infrequent) 1299
Pletal Tablets (Less than 2%) 2605
Pletal Tablets (Less than 2%) 2848
Prevacid Delayed-Release Capsules (Less than 1%) 3292
PREVPAC (Less than 1%) 3298
Prinivil Tablets (0.3% to 1.0%) 2164
Prinzide Tablets 2168
▲ Prograf (3% to 24%) 1393
Protonix I.V. (Less than 1%) 3580
Protonix Tablets (Less than 1%) 3577
Proventil HFA Inhalation Aerosol (Less than 3%) 3150
Prozac Pulvules, Liquid, and Weekly Capsules (Rare) 1238
Pulmozyme Inhalation Solution 1426
▲ Rapamune Oral Solution and Tablets (3% to 20%) 3584
Rebetron Combination Therapy 3153
Remeron Tablets (Rare) 2483
Remeron SolTab Tablets (Rare) 2486
ReoPro Vials (0.1%) 1958
Requip Tablets (Infrequent) 1621
Rescula Ophthalmic Solution (1% to 5%) ⊙306
Rilutek Tablets (Infrequent) 772
Risperdal (Infrequent) 1796
Roferon-A Injection (Infrequent) 2996
Sandostatin Injection (Less than 1%) 2394
Sandostatin LAR Depot (Rare) 2395
Sarafem Pulvules (Rare) 1962
Seroquel Tablets (Infrequent) 684
Serostim for Injection 3229
▲ Simulect for Injection (3% to 10%) 2399
Sonata Capsules (Rare) 3591
Sular Tablets (Less than or equal to 1%) 688
Tasmar Tablets (Infrequent) 3010
Tequin Injection (Less than 0.1%) 1110
Tequin Tablets (Less than 0.1%) 1110
Teveten Tablets (Less than 1%) 3327
Thalomid Capsules 1154
Topamax Sprinkle Capsules (Rare) 2590
Topamax Tablets (Rare) 2590
Toprol-XL Tablets (Greater than 1%) 651
Tricor Capsules, Micronized 513
Uniretic Tablets (Less than 1%) 3178
Videx 1138
Videx EC Capsules 1143
Viracept 532
▲ Zenapax for Injection (2% to 5%) 3046
Zestoretic Tablets 695
Zestril Tablets (0.3% to 1.0%) 698
Zoladex 3-month (1% to 5%) 706
Zyprexa Tablets (Infrequent) 1973
Zyprexa ZYDIS Orally Disintegrating Tablets (Infrequent) 1973
Zyrtec (Less than 2%) 2756
Zyrtec-D 12 Hour Extended Relief Tablets (Less than 2%) 2758

Diabetes mellitus, increase
▲ Actos Tablets (5.1%) 3275
Agenerase Capsules 1454
Agenerase Oral Solution 1459
Florinef Acetate Tablets 2250
Hydrocortone Phosphate Injection, Sterile 2105
Levaquin Injection (Less than 0.5%) 2537
Solu-Medrol Sterile Powder 2855
Toprol-XL Tablets (Greater than 1%) 651

Diabetes mellitus, insulin-dependent, post-transplant
▲ Prograf (20%) 1393

Diabetes mellitus, precipitation of latent
Celestone Soluspan Injectable Suspension 3097
Celestone Syrup 3099
Cortone Acetate Injectable Suspension 2059
Cortone Acetate Tablets 2061
Decadron Elixir 2078
Decadron Tablets 2079
Decadron Phosphate Injection 2081
Depo-Medrol Injectable Suspension 2795
Furosemide Tablets 2284
Hydrocortone Tablets 2106
Hydrocortone Acetate Injectable Suspension 2103
Intron A for Injection (Less than 5%) 3120
Levaquin (Less than 0.3%) 2537
Maxzide 1008
Orudis Capsules (Rare) 3548
Oruvail Capsules (Rare) 3548
Pediapred Oral Solution 1170
Prednisone 3064
Prelone Syrup 2273
Prinzide Tablets 2168
Risperdal 1796
Tenoretic Tablets 690
Vaseretic Tablets 2204
Viracept 532
Zestoretic Tablets 695

Diabetes mellitus, type I
Enbrel for Injection 1752
Enbrel for Injection 3504

Diabetes mellitus de novo
Agenerase Capsules (2 patients) 1454
Agenerase Oral Solution (1 patient) 1459

Diabetic acidosis
Prozac Pulvules, Liquid, and Weekly Capsules (Rare) 1238
Sarafem Pulvules (Rare) 1962
Zyprexa Tablets (Rare) 1973
Zyprexa ZYDIS Orally Disintegrating Tablets (Rare) 1973

Diabetic ketoacidosis
Agenerase Capsules 1454
Agenerase Oral Solution 1459
Risperdal 1796
Viracept (Some cases) 532

Dialysis encephalopathy
Amphojel Suspension (Mint Flavor) ▣789
Maalox Antacid/Anti-Gas Oral Suspension ▣673
Maalox Max Maximum Strength Antacid/Anti-Gas Liquid 2300
Maalox Regular Strength Antacid/Antigas Liquid 2300
Mylanta 1813

Dialysis osteomalacia, results in, or worsening of
Amphojel Suspension (Mint Flavor) ▣789
Maalox Antacid/Anti-Gas Oral Suspension ▣673
Maalox Max Maximum Strength Antacid/Anti-Gas Liquid 2300
Maalox Regular Strength Antacid/Antigas Liquid 2300
Mylanta 1813

Diaphoresis
Accupril Tablets (0.5% to 1.0%) 2611
Accuretic Tablets (0.5% to 1%) 2614
Accutane Capsules 2944
Aceon Tablets (2 mg, 4 mg, 8 mg) (0.3% to 1%) 3249
Aciphex Tablets 1267
Aciphex Tablets 1783
Actiq (1% to 2%) 1184
Adalat CC Tablets (Less than 1.0%) 877
Adenocard Injection (Less than 1%) 1380
Adenoscan (Less than 1%) 1381
Advair Diskus 100/50 (1% to 3%) 1448
Advair Diskus 250/50 (1% to 3%) 1448
Advair Diskus 500/50 (1% to 3%) 1448
Aerobid/Aerobid-M (1% to 3%) 1363
Aggrastat (2%) 2031
Albalon Ophthalmic Solution ⊙225
Alferon N Injection (One patient to 3%) 1770
Aloprim for Injection (Less than 1%) 2292
Altace Capsules (Less than 1%) 2233
Ambien Tablets (Infrequent) 3191
▲ AmBisome for Injection (7%) 1383
Amerge Tablets (Infrequent) 1467
▲ Amphotec (5% or more) 1774
Anaprox Tablets (Less than 3%) 2967
Anaprox DS Tablets (Less than 3%) 2967
AndroGel (Fewer than 1%) 3322
Anzemet Injection (Rare) 719
Anzemet Tablets (Rare) 722
AquaMEPHYTON Injection 2042
Arava Tablets (1% to 3%) 724
Aredia for Injection 2309
Aricept Tablets (Frequent) 1270
Aricept Tablets (Frequent) 2665
Arimidex Tablets (1.2% to 1.5%) 659
▲ Aromasin Tablets (6%) 2769
Arthrotec Tablets (Rare) 3195
▲ Asacol Delayed-Release Tablets (3%) 2884
Atacand Tablets (0.5% or greater) 595
Atacand HCT Tablets (0.5% or greater) 597
Atromid-S Capsules 3483
Avelox Tablets (0.05% to 1%) 879
Axert Tablets (Rare) 2772
▲ Axid Pulvules (More frequent) 1903
▲ Axid Pulvules (More frequent) 2919
Azactam for Injection (Less than 1%) 1276
Benadryl Parenteral 2617
▲ Betapace Tablets (1% to 6%) 950
▲ Betaseron for SC Injection (23%) 988
Bicillin L-A Injection 2242
Blocadren Tablets (Less than 1%) 2046
Bontril Slow-Release Capsules 576
Brethine Ampuls (0.0% to 2.4%) 2314
Brethine Tablets (1%) 2313
▲ Brevibloc Injection (12%) 858
Buprenex Injectable (1% to 5%) 2918
▲ Campath Ampules (1% to 19%) 992
Cancidas for Injection (Up to 1.3%) 2048
Captopril Tablets 2281
Carbatrol Capsules 3234
Cardene I.V. (1.4%) 3485
Cardizem Injectable (Less than 1%) 1018
Cardizem Lyo-Ject Syringe (Less than 1%) 1018
Cardizem Monovial (Less than 1%) 1018
Cardura Tablets (0.5% to 1.1%) 2668
▲ Casodex Tablets (5%) 662
Cataflam Tablets (Less than 1%) 2315
Caverject Sterile Powder (Less than 1%) 2777
Ceclor CD Tablets (0.1% to 1%) 1279
Celebrex Capsules (0.1% to 1.9%) 2676

Celebrex Capsules (0.1% to 1.9%) 2780
Celestone Soluspan Injectable Suspension 3097
Celestone Syrup 3099
▲ Celexa (11%) 1365
▲ CellCept Capsules (3%) 2951
▲ CellCept Intravenous (3%) 2951
▲ CellCept Oral Suspension (3%) 2951
▲ CellCept Tablets (3% to 10.8%) 2951
Cerebyx Injection (Infrequent) 2619
Chirocaine Injection (Less than 1%) 2909
Cipro I.V. (1% or less) 893
Cipro I.V. Pharmacy Bulk Package (Less than 1%) 897
Claritin (At least one patient) 3100
Claritin-D 12 Hour Extended Release Tablets (Less frequent) 3102
Claritin-D 24 Hour Extended Release Tablets (Fewer than 2%) 3104
Clinoril Tablets (Less than 1 in 100) 2053
▲ Clozaril Tablets (More than 5% to 6%) 2319
Cognex Capsules (Frequent) 1351
Compazine 1505
Comtan Tablets (2%) 2328
▲ Copaxone for Injection (15%) 3306
Coreg Tablets (0.1% to 2.9%) 1508
Corgard Tablets (1 to 5 per 1000 patients) 2245
Corlopam Injection (1% to 2%) 412
Cortifoam Rectal Foam 3170
Cortone Acetate Injectable Suspension 2059
Cortone Acetate Tablets 2061
Corzide 40/5 Tablets (1 to 5 of 1000 patients) 2247
Corzide 80/5 Tablets (1 to 5 of 1000 patients) 2247
Cosopt Sterile Ophthalmic Solution 2065
Covera-HS Tablets (Less than 2%) 3199
Cozaar Tablets (Less than 1%) 2067
Crinone (Less than 5%) 3213
Crixivan Capsules (Less than 2%) 2070
Cytotec Tablets (Infrequent) 3202
▲ Cytovene (11%) 2959
Dantrium Capsules (Less frequent) 2885
▲ DaunoXome Injection (2% to 12%) 1442
Decadron Elixir 2078
Decadron Tablets 2079
Decadron Phosphate Injection 2081
▲ Demerol (Among most frequent) 3079
Depacon Injection (0.9%) 416
Depakote ER Tablets (Greater than 1%) 436
Depo-Medrol Injectable Suspension 2795
Depo-Provera Contraceptive Injection (Fewer than 1%) 2798
D.H.E. 45 Injection (Occasional) 2334
Dilaudid Oral Liquid 445
Dilaudid Tablets - 8 mg 445
▲ Dilaudid-HP (Among most frequent) 443
Diovan HCT Tablets (Greater than 0.2%) 2338
Diphtheria & Tetanus Toxoids Adsorbed Purogenated for Pediatric Use 1857
Diprivan Injectable Emulsion (Less than 1%) 667
Dolobid Tablets (Less than 1 in 100) 2088
▲ Dolophine Hydrochloride Tablets (Among most frequent) 3056
Dopram Injectable 2931
Doxil Injection (1% to 5%) 566
▲ Duraclon Injection (5.3%) 3057
▲ Duragesic Transdermal System (10% or more) 1786
Dyazide Capsules 1515
Dynabac Tablets (0.1% to 1%) 2269
EC-Naprosyn Delayed-Release Tablets (Less than 3%) 2967
▲ Effexor Tablets (2% to 19.3%) 3495
▲ Effexor XR Capsules (11% to 14%) 3499
Eldepryl Capsules 3266
Enalaprilat Injection 863
Engerix-B Vaccine (Less than 1%) 1517
Etrafon (Occasional) 3115
Evista Tablets (2.5% to 3.1%) 1915
▲ Evoxac Capsules (18.7%) 1217
▲ Exelon Capsules (4%) 2342
▲ Exelon Oral Solution (4%) 2345
Felbatol 3343
Feldene Capsules (Occasional) 2685
Femara Tablets (Less frequent) 2351
Ferrlecit Injection (Greater than 1%) 3386
Flexeril Tablets (Less than 1%) 572
Flexeril Tablets (Less than 1%) 2094
▲ Flolan for Injection (1% to 41%) 1528
Florinef Acetate Tablets 2250
Floxin I.V. (Less than 1%) 2526
Floxin Tablets (Less than 1%) 2529
▲ Fludara for Injection (1% to 13%) 995
Flumadine 1370
Fortovase Capsules (Less than 2%) 2970
▲ Foscavir Injection (5% or greater) 605
Gabitril Tablets (Frequent) 1189
Gammar-P I.V. 787
Gemzar for Injection (Infrequent) 1919
Gengraf Capsules (1% to less than 3%) 457
Glucophage Tablets (1% to 5%) 1080
Glucotrol XL Extended Release Tablets (Less than 3%) 2693
Haldol Decanoate 2535
Haldol Injection, Tablets and Concentrate 2533
Hivid Tablets (Less than 1%) 2975
Humalog (Less common) 1926
Humalog Mix 75/25 Pen (Less common) 1928
Humorsol Sterile Ophthalmic Solution (Rare) 2102
Humulin 50/50, 100 Units 1934
Humulin 70/30, 100 Units 1935
Humulin 70/30 Pen 1936
Humulin L, 100 Units (Less common) 1937
Humulin R Regular (U-500) (Less common) 1943
Humulin N NPH Pen 1940
Hydrocortone Tablets 2106
Hydrocortone Acetate Injectable Suspension 2103
Hydrocortone Phosphate Injection, Sterile 2105
Hytrin Capsules (At least 1%) 464
Hyzaar 2109
Iletin II, Regular (Pork), 100 Units (Less common) 1947
Imdur Tablets (Less than or equal to 5%) 1826
Imitrex Injection (1.6%) 1549
Imitrex Nasal Spray (Infrequent) 1554
Imitrex Tablets (Infrequent) 1558
Indocin (Less than 1%) 2112
INFeD Injection 3388
▲ Infergen (12% to 13%) 1777
▲ Intron A for Injection (1% to 21%) 3120
Invirase Capsules (Less than 2%) 2979
Isoptin SR Tablets (1% or less) 467
Isopto Carbachol Ophthalmic Solution ⊙ 215
Kadian Capsules (Less than 3%) 1335
Kaletra Capsules (Less than 2%) 471
Kaletra Oral Solution (Less than 2%) 471
Lamictal (Infrequent) 1567
▲ Leukine (6%) 1755
▲ Leustatin Injection (9%) 2495
Levaquin (0.1% to less than 1.0%) 2537
Levo-Dromoran 1734
Levoxyl Tablets 1819
Lexxel Tablets 608
Limbitrol 1738
Lipitor Tablets (Less than 2%) 2639
Lipitor Tablets (Less than 2%) 2696
Lithobid Slow-Release Tablets 3255
Lodine (Less than 1%) 3528
Lodine XL Extended-Release Tablets (Less than 1%) 3530
Lodosyn Tablets 1251
Lotensin Tablets (Less than 1%) 2365
Lotensin HCT Tablets (0.3% to 1%) 2367
Loxitane Capsules 3398
▲ Lupron Depot 3.75 mg (72.9%) 3281
▲ Lupron Depot 7.5 mg (57.1%) 3284
▲ Lupron Depot–3 Month 11.25 mg (72.9% to 84%) 3285
▲ Lupron Depot–3 Month 22.5 mg (58.5%) 3288
▲ Lupron Depot–4 Month 30 mg (8.3% to 46.9%) 3289
▲ Luvox Tablets (25, 50, 100 mg) (7%) 3256
Marinol Capsules (Less than 1%) 3325
Matulane Capsules 3246
Maxalt Tablets (Infrequent) 2120
Maxalt-MLT Orally Disintegrating Tablets (Infrequent) 2120
Megace Oral Suspension (1% to 3%) 1124
▲ Mepergan Injection (Among most frequent) 3539
Mephyton Tablets (Rare) 2129
▲ Mepron Suspension (10%) 1598
Meridia Capsules (2.5%) 481
Merrem I.V. (0.1% to 1.0%) 673
Mestinon 1740
Mexitil Capsules (Less than 1% or about 6 in 1,000) 1047
Micardis Tablets (More than 0.3%) 1049
Micardis HCT Tablets 1051
Migranal Nasal Spray (Infrequent) 2376
Minipress Capsules 2699
Minizide Capsules 2700
Miochol-E System Pak (Rare) ⊙ 305
Miochol-E with Steri-Tags (Rare) ⊙ 305
Mirapex Tablets (1% or more) 2834
Moban 1320
Mobic Tablets (Less than 2%) 1054
Moduretic Tablets (Less than or equal to 1%) 2138
Monopril Tablets (0.2% to 1.0%) 1091
▲ MS Contin Tablets (Less frequent to among most frequent) 2896
▲ MSIR (Among most frequent) 2898
Nadolol Tablets (1 to 5 of 1000 patients) 2288
Naprelan Tablets (Less than 1%) 1293
Naprosyn Suspension (Less than 3%) 2967
Naprosyn Tablets (Less than 3%) 2967
Narcan Injection 1322
Nardil Tablets (Less common) 2653
Naropin Injection 612
Natrecor for Injection (At least 1%) 3189
Navane Oral 2701
Navane Intramuscular 2703
Neoral Soft Gelatin Capsules (1% to less than 3%) 2380
Neoral Oral Solution (1% to less than 3%) 2380
Nesacaine/Nesacaine MPF 617
Neurontin Capsules (Infrequent) 2655
Neurontin Oral Solution (Infrequent) 2655
Neurontin Tablets (Infrequent) 2655
Nexium Delayed-Release Capsules (Less than 1%) 619
Niaspan Extended-Release Tablets 1846
▲ Nicotrol Nasal Spray (Over 5%) 2843
▲ Nilandron Tablets (6.2%) 753
Nimotop Capsules (Less than 1%) 904
▲ Nipent for Injection (8% to 10%) 3272
Nitrolingual Pumpspray 1355
Nitrostat Tablets 2658
▲ Normodyne Injection (4%) 3135
Normodyne Tablets (Less than 1%) 3137
Norpramin Tablets 755
Norvasc Tablets (More than 0.1% to 1%) 2704
Norvir Capsules (1.3% to 2.6%) 487
Norvir Oral Solution (1.3% to 2.6%) 487
▲ Novantrone for Injection (9%) 1760
Novolin 70/30 PenFill (Rare) 2423
Novolin 70/30 Prefilled Disposable Insulin Delivery System (Rare) 2425
Novolin N PenFill (Rare) 2423
Novolin R PenFill (Rare) 2423
▲ Nubain Injection (9%) 1323
NuLev Orally Disintegrating Tablets 3176
Numorphan 1324
▲ Oramorph SR Tablets (Among most frequent) 3062
Orap Tablets 1407
Orthoclone OKT3 Sterile Solution (Less than 1%) 2498
Orudis Capsules (Less than 1%) 3548
Oruvail Capsules (Less than 1%) 3548
▲ OxyContin Tablets (5%) 2912
▲ Paxil (1.1% to 19.2%) 1609
Pediapred Oral Solution 1170
▲ PEG-Intron Powder for Injection (6%) 3140
Pentasa Capsules (Less than 1%) 3239
Periactin Tablets 2155
Permax Tablets (2.1%) 1299
Phenergan 3556
Phenergan with Codeine Syrup 3557
Phenergan VC with Codeine Syrup 3561
Pilopine HS Ophthalmic Gel (Occasional) ⊙ 217
Polocaine Injection, USP 625
Polocaine-MPF Injection, USP 625
Ponstel Capsules (Occasional) 1356
Prednisone 3064
Prelone Syrup 2273
Prinivil Tablets (0.3% to 1.0%) 2164
Prinzide Tablets (0.3% to 1%) 2168
Procardia Capsules (2% or less) 2708
Procardia XL Extended Release Tablets (1% or less) 2710
▲ Prograf (3% to 15%) 1393
Prometrium Capsules (100 mg, 200 mg) 3261
ProSom Tablets (Infrequent) 500
Prostigmin Injectable 1744
Prostigmin Tablets 1744
Prostin E2 Suppositories 2852
Protonix I.V. (Less than 1%) 3580
Protonix Tablets (Less than 1%) 3577
Protopic Ointment (Greater than or equal to 1%) 1397
Proventil HFA Inhalation Aerosol (Less than 3%) 3150
Provigil Tablets (At least 1%) 1193
▲ Prozac Pulvules, Liquid, and Weekly Capsules (7% to 8%) 1238
Rabies Vaccine RabAvert (Rare) 1203
▲ Rapamune Oral Solution and Tablets (3% to 20%) 3584
Recombivax HB (Less than 1%) 2178
ReFacto Vials 1437
Relafen Tablets (1% to 3%) 1617
Remicade for IV Injection (Less than 2%) 1178
ReoPro Vials (1%) 1958
▲ Requip Tablets (6% to 7%) 1621
Rescriptor Tablets (Less than 2%) 526
▲ Retrovir Capsules (5%) 1625
▲ Retrovir IV Infusion (5%) 1629
▲ Retrovir (5%) 1625
Rifater Tablets 769
Risperdal (Infrequent) 1796
Rocephin Injectable Vials, ADD-Vantage, Galaxy, Bulk (Occasional) 2993
▲ Roferon-A Injection (More than 1% to 22%) 2996
▲ Romazicon Injection (1% to 9%) 3000
▲ Roxanol (Among most frequent) 3066
Roxicodone Tablets (Less than 3%) 3067
Rynatan Tablets 3351
Rythmol Tablets – 150 mg, 225 mg, 300 mg (1.4%) 502
▲ Salagen Tablets (29% to 68%) 2229
Sandoglobulin I.V. 2391
▲ Sandostatin LAR Depot (5% to 15%) 2395
▲ Sarafem Pulvules (8%) 1962
Sensorcaine (Rare) 643
Sensorcaine-MPF Injection (Rare) 643
Serentil 1057
Seroquel Tablets (Frequent) 684
▲ Serostim for Injection (14.1%) 3229
Serzone Tablets 1104
Sinemet Tablets 1253
Sinemet CR Tablets 1255
Sinequan (Occasional) 2713
Skelid Tablets (More than or equal to 1%) 3088
Solu-Medrol Sterile Powder 2855
Sonata Capsules (Infrequent) 3591
▲ Soriatane Capsules (1% to 10%) 3003
Sporanox Injection (1%) 1804
Sporanox Injection (1%) 2509
▲ Sporanox Oral Solution (3.4% to 3.7%) 1808
▲ Sporanox Oral Solution (3.4% to 3.7%) 2512
Stadol NS Nasal Spray (1% or greater) 1108
Stelazine 1640
Sular Tablets (Less than or equal to 1%) 688
Surmontil Capsules 3595
Sustiva Capsules (1% to 2%) 1258
Symmetrel 1328
Synercid I.V. (Less than 1%) 775
Talacen Caplets 3089
Talwin Nx Tablets 3090
Tambocor Tablets (1% to 3%) 1990
Tarka Tablets 508
▲ Tasmar Tablets (4% to 7%) 3010
Tegretol/Tegretol-XR 2404
Tenex Tablets (3% or less) 2942
Tensilon Injectable 1745
Tequin Injection (0.1% to 3%) 1110
Tequin Tablets (0.1% to 3%) 1110
Tetanus & Diphtheria Toxoids Adsorbed for Adult Use 1880
Teveten Tablets (Less than 1%) 3327
Thalomid Capsules 1154
Thiothixene Capsules (Infrequently) 2290
Thorazine 1656
Thyrel TRH for Injection (Less frequent) 3630
Tikosyn Capsules (Greater than 2%) 2717
Timolide Tablets 2187
Timolol GFS ⊙ 266
Timoptic in Ocudose 2192
Timoptic Sterile Ophthalmic Solution 2190
Timoptic-XE Sterile Ophthalmic Gel Forming Solution 2194
▲ Tonocard Tablets (2.3% to 5.1%) 649
Topamax Sprinkle Capsules (0.4% to 1.8%) 2590
Topamax Tablets (0.4% to 1.8%) 2590
Toradol (Greater than 1%) 3018
Tricor Capsules, Micronized 513
Trilafon 3160
Trileptal Oral Suspension (Up to 3%) 2407
Trileptal Tablets (Up to 3%) 2407
▲ Trisenox Injection (13%) 1158
Trovan (Less than 1%) 2722
Twinrix Vaccine (Less than 1%) 1674
▲ Ultracet Tablets (4%) 2597
▲ Ultram Tablets (6% to 9%) 2600
Uniretic Tablets (Less than 1%) 3178
Unithroid Tablets 3445
Univasc Tablets (Less than 1%) 3181
Urecholine 2198
Urecholine Tablets 2445
Vascor Tablets (0.5% to 2.0%) 2602
Vaseretic Tablets (0.5% to 2.0%) 2204
Vasotec I.V. Injection 2207
Vasotec Tablets (0.5% to 1.0%) 2210
Velosulin BR Human Insulin 10 ml Vials 2435
Verelan Capsules (1% or less) 3184
Verelan PM Capsules (2% or less) 3186
▲ Vesanoid Capsules (20%) 3037
▲ Viadur Implant (5.3%) 912
Viagra Tablets (Less than 2%) 2732
▲ Vicoprofen Tablets (3% to 9%) 520

Vioxx (Greater than 0.1% to 1.9%) 2213
Viracept 532
Vistide Injection 1445
Vitravene for Injection (2% to 5%) ⊙310
Vivactil Tablets 2217
Vivactil Tablets 2446
Voltaren Tablets (Less than 1%) 2315
Voltaren-XR Tablets (Less than 1%) 2315
▲ Wellbutrin Tablets (22.3%) 1680
▲ Wellbutrin SR Sustained-Release Tablets (5% to 6%) 1684
WinRho SDF 2297
▲ Xanax Tablets (15.1%) 2865
Xeloda Tablets (Less than 5%) 3039
Xopenex Inhalation Solution 3207
Zanaflex Tablets (Frequent) 1305
Zebeta Tablets (0.7% to 1.0%) 1885
▲ Zenapax for Injection (2% to 5%) 3046
Zestoretic Tablets (0.3% to 1%) 695
Zestril Tablets (0.3% to 1.0%) 698
Ziac Tablets 1887
▲ Zoladex (6% to 45%) 702
Zoladex 3-month 706
▲ Zoloft (5% to 8%) 2751
Zomig Tablets (2% to 3%) 708
Zomig-ZMT Tablets (2% to 3%) 708
Zonegran Capsules (Infrequent) 1307
Zosyn (1.0% or less) 1890
Zosyn in Galaxy Containers (1.0% or less) 1894
Zovirax for Injection (Less than 1%) 1708
Zyban Sustained-Release Tablets (Frequent) 1710
Zyprexa Tablets 1973
Zyprexa ZYDIS Orally Disintegrating Tablets 1973
Zyrtec (Less than 2%) 2756
Zyrtec-D 12 Hour Extended Relief Tablets (Less than 2%) 2758

Diaphoresis, nocturnal

Sandimmune (Rare) 2388

Diaphragm, paralyzed

Survanta Intratracheal Suspension 3053

Diaphragmatic hernia

(*see under* Hernia, hiatal)

Diarrhea

▲ Abelcet Injection (6%) 1273
Accolate Tablets (2.8%) 657
Accupril Tablets (1.7%) 2611
Accuretic Tablets (1.4%) 2614
Accutane Capsules 2944
▲ Aceon Tablets (2 mg, 4 mg, 8 mg) (4.3%) 3249
Aciphex Tablets 1267
Aciphex Tablets 1783
▲ ActHIB Vaccine (1.5% to 9.0%) 798
▲ Actimmune (14%) 1772
Actiq (1% or greater) 1184
▲ Actonel Tablets (10.6% to 19.7%) 2879
Adalat CC Tablets (Less than 1.0%) 877
Adderall Tablets 3231
Adderall XR Capsules (2%)
Adipex-P 1406
Adriamycin PFS/RDF Injection (Occasional) 2767
▲ Advair Diskus 100/50 (4%) 1448
Advair Diskus 250/50 (2%) 1448
Advair Diskus 500/50 (2% to 4%) 1448
▲ Aerobid/Aerobid M (10%) 1363
▲ Agenerase Capsules (39% to 60%) 1454
▲ Agenerase Oral Solution (39% to 60%) 1459
▲ Aggrenox Capsules (12.7%) 1026
▲ Agrylin Capsules (25.7%) 3232
Aldara Cream, 5% (More than 1%) 1978
Aldoclor Tablets 2035
Aldomet Tablets 2037
Aldoril Tablets 2039
▲ Alferon N Injection (2% to 6%) 1770
Alkeran for Injection (Infrequent) 1465
Alkeran Tablets (Infrequent) 1466
Aloprim for Injection (Less than 1%) 2292
Altace Capsules (Less than 1% to 1.1%) 2233
Amaryl Tablets (Less than 1%) 717
Ambien Tablets (1% to 3%) 3191
▲ AmBisome for Injection (15.3% to 30.3%) 1383
Amerge Tablets (Infrequent) 1467
Amicar Injection 3608
Amicar Syrup 3608
Amicar Tablets 3608
▲ Amoxil Chewable Tablets (8%) 1471
▲ Amoxil for Oral Suspension (8%) 1471
▲ Amoxil (8%) 1471
▲ Amphotec (5% or more) 1774
Anadrol-50 Tablets 3321
Anaprox Tablets (Less than 3%) 2967
Anaprox DS Tablets (Less than 3%) 2967
Ancef for Injection 1474
Ancef Injection 1474
Ancobon Capsules 1730
▲ Anzemet Injection (12.4%) 719
Anzemet Tablets (2.1%) 722
Aphthasol Oral Paste (Infrequent) 1025
Apligraf (1.8%) 2305
Aralen Tablets 3075
▲ Arava Tablets (17%) 724
▲ Aredia for Injection (28.5%) 2309
▲ Argatroban Injection (6.2%) 1478
▲ Aricept Tablets (10%) 1270
▲ Aricept Tablets (10%) 2665
▲ Arimidex Tablets (7.3% to 8.4%) 659
▲ Aromasin Tablets (4%) 2769
▲ Arthrotec Tablets (19%) 3195
▲ Asacol Delayed-Release Tablets (7%) 2884
Astelin Nasal Spray 3339
Atacand Tablets (More than 1%) 595
Atacand HCT Tablets (0.5% or greater) 597
Atromid-S Capsules 3483
Attenuvax (Rare) 2044
▲ Augmentin Chewable Tablets (9%) 1482
▲ Augmentin Powder for Oral Suspension (9%) 1482
▲ Augmentin Tablets (9%) 1485
Augmentin ES-600 Powder for Oral Suspension (2.9%) 1487
Avalide Tablets (1% or greater) 1070
▲ Avandia Tablets (2.3% to 15.6%) 1490
▲ Avapro Tablets (3%) 1074
▲ Avapro Tablets (3%) 3076
▲ Avelox Tablets (6%) 879
▲ Avonex (16%) 1013
Axert Tablets (Infrequent) 2772
▲ Axid Pulvules (7.2%) 1903
▲ Axid Pulvules (7.2%) 2919
Azactam for Injection (1% to 1.4%) 1276
Azmacort Inhalation Aerosol (1% to 3%) 728
Azopt Ophthalmic Suspension (Less than 1%) 536
Azulfidine EN-tabs Tablets (Rare) 2775
Bactrim 2949
Bactroban Nasal (Less than 1%) 1495
▲ Baycol Tablets (3.3%) 883
Beano ▣809
Benadryl Parenteral 2617
Benzaclin Topical Gel 1220
Betagan ⊙228
▲ Betapace Tablets (2% to 7%) 950
▲ Betapace AF Tablets (5.2% to 5.7%) 954
▲ Betaseron for SC Injection (35%) 988
Betimol Ophthalmic Solution ⊙324
▲ Biaxin/Biaxin XL (3% to 6%) 403
Blocadren Tablets (Less than 1%) 2046
Bontril Slow-Release Capsules 576
Buprenex Injectable (Rare) 2918
▲ Campath Ampules (1% to 22%) 992
▲ Canasa Rectal Suppositories (Among most common) 829
Cancidas for Injection (1.3% to 3.6%) 2048
Captopril Tablets (About 0.5% to 2%) 2281
Carafate Suspension (Less than 0.5%) 731
Carafate Tablets (Less than 0.5%) 730
Carbatrol Capsules 3234
Cardizem Injectable 1018
Cardizem Lyo-Ject Syringe 1018
Cardizem Monovial 1018
Cardizem CD Capsules (Less than 1%) 1016
Cardura Tablets (2% to 2.3%) 2668
▲ Carnitor Injection (9% to 35%) 3242
Carnitor Tablets and Oral Solution 3245
▲ Casodex Tablets (10%) 662
▲ Cataflam Tablets (3% to 9%) 2315
▲ Ceclor CD Tablets (3.8%) 1279
Ceclor (1 in 70) 1905
▲ Cedax (3%) 1021
Cefizox for Intramuscular or Intravenous Use (Occasional) 1390
▲ Cefobid Intravenous/Intramuscular (1 in 30) 2671
▲ Cefobid Pharmacy Bulk Package - Not for Direct Infusion (1 in 30) 2673
Cefotan (1 in 80) 664
▲ Ceftin (8.6%) 1898
Cefzil (2.9%) 1076
▲ Celebrex Capsules (5.6%) 2676
▲ Celebrex Capsules (5.6%) 2780
▲ Celexa (5%) 1365
▲ CellCept Capsules (16.4% to 45.3%) 2951
▲ CellCept Intravenous (16.4% to 45.3%) 2951
▲ CellCept Oral Suspension (16.4% to 45.3%) 2951
▲ CellCept Tablets (16.4% to 51.3%) 2951
Celontin Capsules (Frequent) 2618
▲ Cenestin Tablets (6%) 1263
Ceptaz for Injection (One in 78 patients) 1499
Cerebyx Injection (Infrequent) 2619
▲ Cerezyme for Injection (5.4%) 1438
Cerubidine for Injection (Occasional) 947
Cervidil Vaginal Insert (Less than 1%) 1369
▲ Chemet Capsules (12.0% to 20.9%) 3078
Chirocaine Injection (1%) 2909
New Formulation Chromagen OB Capsules 3094
▲ Cipro I.V. (Among most frequent) 893
▲ Cipro I.V. Pharmacy Bulk Package (Among most frequent) 897
Cipro (2.3%) 887
Claforan Injection (1.4%) 732
Claritin (At least one patient) 3100
Claritin-D 12 Hour Extended Release Tablets (Less frequent) 3102
Claritin-D 24 Hour Extended Release Tablets (Fewer than 2%) 3104
Cleocin HCl Capsules 2784
Cleocin Phosphate Sterile Solution 2785
Cleocin T Topical (Rare) 2790
Cleocin Vaginal Cream (Less than 1%) 2788
Cleocin Vaginal Ovules (Less than 1%) 2789
Clindagel 1401
▲ Clinoril Tablets (3% to 9%) 2053
Clomid Tablets (Fewer than 1%) 735
Clorpres Tablets 1002
Clozaril Tablets (2%) 2319
▲ Cognex Capsules (16%) 1351
▲ Colazal Capsules (5%) 3069
Colestid Tablets (Infrequent) 2791
▲ CombiPatch Transdermal System (9% to 14%) 2323
Combipres Tablets 1040
Combivent Inhalation Aerosol (Less than 2%) 1041
▲ Combivir Tablets (18%) 1502
▲ Comtan Tablets (10%) 2328
Comvax (0.8% to 2.2%) 2056
▲ Copaxone for Injection (12%) 3306
Cordarone Intravenous (Less than 2%) 3491
▲ Coreg Tablets (2.2% to 11.8%) 1508
Corgard Tablets (1 to 5 per 1000 patients) 2245
Corlopam Injection (2%) 412
Corzide 40/5 Tablets (1 to 5 of 1000 patients) 2247
Corzide 80/5 Tablets (1 to 5 of 1000 patients) 2247
Cosmegen for Injection 2062
Cosopt Sterile Ophthalmic Solution (Less than 1%) 2065
Coumadin for Injection (Infrequent) 1243
Coumadin Tablets (Infrequent) 1243
Covera-HS Tablets (Less than 2%) 3199
Cozaar Tablets (2.4%) 2067
▲ Creon 5 Capsules (Among most frequent) 3251
▲ Creon 10 Capsules (Among most frequent) 3251
▲ Creon 20 Capsules (Among most frequent) 3251
▲ Crinone 8% Gel (8%) 3213
▲ Crixivan Capsules (4.6%) 2070
Cuprimine Capsules 2075
▲ Cytotec Tablets (14% to 40%) 3202
▲ Cytovene (41%) 2959
▲ Dantrium Capsules (Among most frequent) 2885
▲ DaunoXome Injection (4% to 34%) 1442
DDAVP Tablets 739
Declomycin Tablets 1855
Demadex Tablets and Injection (2.0%) 2965
▲ Demser Capsules (10%) 2085
▲ Depacon Injection (0.9% to 23%) 416
▲ Depakene (13% to 23%) 421
▲ Depakote Sprinkle Capsules (13% to 23%) 426
▲ Depakote Tablets (12% to 23%) 430
▲ Depakote ER Tablets (7% to 23%) 436
▲ Depen Titratable Tablets (17%) 3341
Desferal Vials 2333
Desoxyn Tablets 440
▲ Detrol Tablets (4%) 3623
Dexedrine 1512
DextroStat Tablets 3236
D.H.E. 45 Injection (Occasional) 2334
Diabinese Tablets (Less than 2%) 2680
Diamox Intravenous ⊙269
Diamox Sequels Sustained Release Capsules ⊙270
Diamox Tablets ⊙269
▲ Didronel Tablets (About 1 patient in 15; possibly 2 or 3 in 10) 2888
Diflucan Tablets, Injection, and Oral Suspension (1.5% to 3%) 2681
▲ Digitek Tablets (4%) 1003
Dilaudid Oral Liquid 445
Dilaudid Tablets - 8 mg 445
Dilaudid-HP (Less frequent) 443
Diovan Capsules (More than 1%) 2337
▲ Diovan HCT Tablets (3%) 2338
▲ Dipentum Capsules (11.1% to about 17%) 2803
Diprivan Injectable Emulsion (Less than 1%) 667
▲ Ditropan XL Extended Release Tablets (9.1%) 564
Diucardin Tablets 3494
Diuril Oral 2087
Diuril Sodium Intravenous 2086
▲ Dolobid Tablets (3% to 9%) 2088
Dopram Injectable 2931
Doryx Coated Pellet Filled Capsules 3357
▲ Dostinex Tablets (2% to less than 10%) 2804
▲ Doxil Injection (5.2% to 10%) 566
DTIC-Dome (Rare) 902
DuoNeb Inhalation Solution (1.8%) 1233
▲ Duragesic Transdermal System (3% to 10%) 1786
Duricef 1079
Dyazide Capsules 1515
▲ Dynabac Tablets (6.7% to 7.7%) 2269
Dynacin Capsules (Infrequent) 2019
DynaCirc Capsules (1.1%) 2921
DynaCirc CR Tablets (0.5% to 1%) 2923
Dyrenium Capsules (Rare) 3458
EC-Naprosyn Delayed-Release Tablets (Less than 3%) 2967
Edecrin 2091
▲ E.E.S. (Among most frequent) 450
▲ Effexor Tablets (8%) 3495
▲ Effexor XR Capsules (12%) 3499
Eldepryl Capsules (1 of 49 patients) 3266
▲ Ellence Injection (0.8% to 24.8%) 2806
▲ Elmiron Capsules (4%) 570
▲ Emcyt Capsules (12%) 2810
Enalaprilat Injection 863
Enbrel for Injection 1752
Enbrel for Injection 3504
Engerix-B Vaccine (Less than 1%) 1517
▲ Epivir (18%) 1520
▲ Epivir-HBV (14%) 1524
▲ Epogen for Injection (0.11 to 21%) 582
▲ Ergamisol Tablets (13% to 52%) 1789
▲ EryPed (Among most frequent) 446
▲ Ery-Tab Tablets (Among most frequent) 448
▲ Erythrocin Stearate Filmtab Tablets (Among most frequent) 452
▲ Erythromycin Base Filmtab Tablets (Among most frequent) 454
▲ Erythromycin Delayed-Release Capsules, USP (Among most frequent) 455
▲ Esclim Transdermal System (Up to 8.5%) 3460
Eskalith 1527
Estring Vaginal Ring (1% to 3%) 2811
Etrafon (Occasional) 3115
▲ Eulexin Capsules (12% to 40%) 3118
▲ Evoxac Capsules (10.3%) 1217
▲ Exelon Capsules (19%) 2342
▲ Exelon Oral Solution (19%) 2345
Famotidine Injection (1.7%) 866
▲ Famvir Tablets (4.5% to 9%) 2348
▲ Felbatol (5.2% to 5.3%) 3343
▲ Feldene Capsules (1% to 10%) 2685
▲ Femara Tablets (5% to 7%) 2351
Feosol Caplets (Occasional) 1717
Feosol Tablets (Occasional) 1717
▲ Ferrlecit Injection (35%) 3386
Flexeril Tablets (Less than 1%) 572
Flexeril Tablets (Less than 1%) 2094
▲ Flolan for Injection (37% to 50%) 1528
▲ Flomax Capsules (4.3% to 6.2%) 1044
Flonase Nasal Spray (1% to 3%) 1533
Flovent Diskus (1% to 3%) 3614
Flovent (1% to 3%) 1535
Flovent Rotadisk (2% to 4%) 1537
Floxin I.V. (1% to 4%) 2526
Floxin Otic Solution (0.6%) 1219
Floxin Tablets (1% to 4%) 2529
▲ Fludara for Injection (13% to 15%) 995
Flumadine (0.3% to 1%) 1370
FluShield Influenza Vaccine 3521
Follistim for Injection 2465
Fortaz (1 in 78 patients) 1541
▲ Fortovase Capsules (15.6% to 19.9%) 2970
Fosamax Tablets (1.1% to 3.1%) 2095
▲ Foscavir Injection (5% to 30%) 605
▲ Sterile FUDR (Among more common) 2974
Furosemide Tablets 2284
▲ Gabitril Tablets (2% to 10%) 1189
▲ Gastrocrom Oral Concentrate (4 of 87 patients) 1162
▲ Gemzar for Injection (19% to 31%) 1919
▲ Gengraf Capsules (3% to 13%) 457
Geocillin Tablets 2687
▲ Geodon Capsules (5%) 2688
Ginsana Sport Capsules ▣831
▲ Gleevec Capsules (33% to 49%) 2357
Gliadel Wafer (2%) 1723
▲ Glucophage Tablets (53.2%) 1080
▲ Glucophage XR Tablets (9.6%) 1080
Glucotrol Tablets (1 in 70) 2692
▲ Glucotrol XL Extended Release Tablets (5.4%) 2693
▲ Glucovance Tablets (17%) 1086
▲ Glyset Tablets (28.7%) 2821
▲ Gonal-F for Injection (7.6%) 3216
Grifulvin V Tablets Microsize and Oral Suspension Microsize (Occasional) 2518
Gris-PEG Tablets (Occasional) 2661
Guaifed 2272
Halcion Tablets (Rare) 2823
Haldol Decanoate 2535
Haldol Injection, Tablets and Concentrate 2533
Havrix Vaccine (Less than 1%) 1544

▲ Herceptin I.V. (25%) 1414
HibTITER (2 of 1,118 vaccinations) 1859
Hivid Tablets (2.5%) 2975
Humegon for Injection 2468
Humorsol Sterile Ophthalmic Solution (Rare) 2102
▲ Hycamtin for Injection (Less than 1% to 42%) 1546
HydroDIURIL Tablets 2108
Hytrin Capsules (At least 1%) 464
Hyzaar (1% or greater) 2109
▲ Idamycin PFS Injection (73%) 2825
Ifex for Injection (Less than 1%) 1123
Imdur Tablets (Less than or equal to 5%) 1826
Imitrex Injection (Infrequent) 1549
Imitrex Nasal Spray (Infrequent) 1554
Imitrex Tablets (Frequent) 1558
Indapamide Tablets (Less than 5%) 2286
Inderal 3513
Inderal LA Long-Acting Capsules 3516
Inderide Tablets 3517
Inderide LA Long-Acting Capsules 3519
Indocin Capsules (Greater than 1%) 2112
Indocin I.V. (1% to 3%) 2115
Indocin (Greater than 1%) 2112
INFeD Injection 3388
▲ Infergen (24% to 29%) 1777
Innohep Injection (0.6%) 1248
▲ Intron A for Injection (2% to 45%) 3120
Invirase Capsules (1.0% to 4.9%) 2979
Ionamin Capsules 1163
Iopidine Sterile Ophthalmic Solution ⊙212
Ismo Tablets (Fewer than 1%) 3524
Isoptin SR Tablets (1% or less) 467
Isopto Carbachol Ophthalmic Solution ⊙215
Kadian Capsules (Less than 3%) 1335
▲ Kaletra Capsules (13.8% to 23.8%) 471
▲ Kaletra Oral Solution (13.8% to 23.8%) 471
K-Dur Microburst Release System ER Tablets 1832
▲ Keflex (Most frequent) 1237
Kefurox Vials, ADD-Vantage (1 in 220) 1948
Kefzol Vials, ADD-Vantage 1951
Keppra Tablets (1% or more) 3314
Klonopin Tablets 2983
▲ Klor-Con M20/Klor-Con M10 Tablets (Among most common) 3329
▲ K-Lor Powder Packets (Among most common) 469
Kogenate (One report) 934
K-Phos Neutral Tablets 946
K-Phos Original (Sodium Free) Tablets 947
Kristalose for Oral Solution 1007
▲ K-Tab Filmtab Tablets (Most common) 470
▲ Kytril Injection (4%) 2986
▲ Kytril Tablets (4% to 9%) 2988
▲ Lamictal (4% to 6.3%) 1567
▲ Lamisil Tablets (5.6%) 2360
Lanoxicaps Capsules (Less common) 1574
Lanoxin Injection (Less common) 1581
Lanoxin Tablets (Less common) 1587
Lanoxin Elixir Pediatric (Less common) 1578
Lanoxin Injection Pediatric 1584
▲ Lariam Tablets (Among most frequent) 2989
▲ Lescol Capsules (4.9%) 2361
▲ Lescol Capsules (4.9%) 2925
▲ Lescol XL Tablets (3.3%) 2361
▲ Lescol XL Tablets (3.3%) 2925
Leukeran Tablets (Infrequent) 1591
▲ Leukine (52% to 89%) 1755
▲ Leustatin Injection (10%) 2495
Levaquin (1.2% to 5.4%) 2537
Levbid Extended-Release Tablets 3172
Levoxyl Tablets 1819
Levsin/Levsinex/Levbid 3172
Lexxel Tablets 608
Limbitrol 1738
Lipitor Tablets (Up to 5.3%) 2639
Lipitor Tablets (Up to 5.3%) 2696
Lithium Carbonate 3061
Lithium Citrate Syrup 3061
Lithobid Slow-Release Tablets 3255
▲ Lodine (3% to 9%) 3528
▲ Lodine XL Extended-Release Tablets (1% to 10%) 3530
Lodosyn Tablets 1251
▲ Lopid Tablets (7.2%) 2650
▲ Lorabid Suspension and Pulvules (3.6% to 5.8%) 2251
Lotensin HCT Tablets (0.3% to 1%) 2367
Lotrel Capsules 2370
Lufyllin Tablets 3347
Lufyllin-400 Tablets 3347
Lufyllin-GG Elixir 3348
Lufyllin-GG Tablets 3348
Lupron Depot 7.5 mg (Less than 5%) 3284
Lupron Injection (Less than 5%) 3279
▲ Luvox Tablets (25, 50, 100 mg) (1% to 11%) 3256
LYMErix Vaccine (1.01%) 1592
Macrobid Capsules (Less than 1%) 2889
Macrodantin Capsules (Less common) 2891
▲ Malarone (2% to 6%) 1596
Marinol Capsules (0.3% to 1%) 3325
Matulane Capsules 3246
Mavik Tablets (0.3% to 1.6%) 478
Maxair Autohaler (1.3%) 1981
Maxair Inhaler (Less than 1%) 1984
Maxalt Tablets (Frequent) 2120
Maxalt-MLT Orally Disintegrating Tablets (Frequent) 2120
Maxipime for Injection (0.1% to 3%) 1285
Maxzide 1008
Mefoxin for Injection 2124
Mefoxin Premixed Intravenous Solution 2127
▲ Megace Oral Suspension (6% to 15%) 1124
▲ Mepron Suspension (2.1% to 42%) 1598
Meridia Capsules (Greater than or equal to 1%) 481
▲ Merrem I.V. (3.5% to 5.0%) 673
Meruvax II 2130
Mestinon 1740
MetroGel-Vaginal Gel (1%) 1986
▲ Mevacor Tablets (2.2% to 5.5%) 2132
▲ Mexitil Capsules (5.2%) 1047
Miacalcin Nasal Spray (1% to 3%) 2375
▲ Micardis Tablets (3%) 1049
▲ Micardis HCT Tablets (3%) 1051
▲ Micro-K (Among most common) 3311
Microzide Capsules 3414
▲ Midamor Tablets (3% to 8%) 2136
Migranal Nasal Spray (2%) 2376
Miltown Tablets 3349
▲ Minipress Capsules (1% to 4%) 2699
Minizide Capsules (Rare) 2700
Minocin Intravenous 1862
Minocin Oral Suspension 1865
Minocin Pellet-Filled Capsules (Infrequent) 1863
Mintezol 2137
MiraLax Powder for Oral Solution 1069
Mirapex Tablets (Rare) 2834
Mithracin for Intravenous Use 903
M-M-R II 2118
Mobic Tablets (1.9% to 5.9%) 1054
Moduretic Tablets (Greater than 1%, less than 3%) 2138
Monodox Capsules (Infrequent) 2442
▲ Monopril Tablets (Less than 1% to 11.9%) 1091
Monopril HCT (Less than 2%) 1094
▲ Monurol Sachet (9.0% to 10.4%) 1375
Motrin Suspension, Oral Drops, Chewable Tablets, and Caplets (1% to less than 3%) 2002
MS Contin Tablets (Less frequent) 2896
MSIR (Less frequent) 2898
Mumpsvax 2141
Mustargen for Injection 2142
▲ Mycobutin Capsules (3%) 2838
Mykrox Tablets (Less than 2%) 1168
Mylanta (Occasional) 1813
Mylocel Tablets (Less frequently) 2227
▲ Mylotarg for Injection (30% to 50%) 3540
▲ Nabi-HB (3%) 2295
Nadolol Tablets (1 to 5 of 1000 patients) 2288
▲ Naprelan Tablets (3% to 9%) 1293
Naprosyn Suspension (Less than 3%) 2967
Naprosyn Tablets (Less than 3%) 2967
Narcan Injection 1322
Nasonex Nasal Spray (Greater than or equal to 2%) 3131
Navane Oral 2701
Navane Intramuscular 2703
▲ Navelbine Injection (Up to 13% but less than 20%) 1604
Nebcin Vials, Hyporets & ADD-Vantage 1955
▲ Neoral Soft Gelatin Capsules (3% to 13%) 2380
▲ Neoral Oral Solution (3% to 13%) 2380
Neptazane Tablets ⊙271
▲ Neumega for Injection (43%) 1434
▲ Neupogen for Injection (14%) 587
Neurontin Capsules (More than 1%) 2655
Neurontin Oral Solution (More than 2%) 2655
Neurontin Tablets (More than 1%) 2655
▲ Nexium Delayed-Release Capsules (Greater than or equal to 1% to 9.2%) 619
▲ Niaspan Extended-Release Tablets (6% to 8%) 1846
▲ Nicotrol Inhaler (Greater than 3%) 2840
Nicotrol Nasal Spray (Less than 1%) 2843
Nilandron Tablets (2%) 753
▲ Nimotop Capsules (Up to 4.2%) 904
▲ Nipent for Injection (15% to 17%) 3272
Nizoral Tablets (Less than 1%) 1791
▲ Nolvadex Tablets (11.2%) 678
Normodyne Tablets (Less than 1%) 3137
Noroxin Tablets (0.3% to 1.0%) 2145
Norpramin Tablets 755
Norvasc Tablets (More than 0.1% to 1%) 2704
▲ Norvir Capsules (12.8% to 18.3%) 487
▲ Norvir Oral Solution (12.8% to 18.3%) 487
▲ Novantrone for Injection (18% to 47%) 1760
Omnicef 493
▲ Oncaspar (Greater than 1% but less than 5%) 756
Oramorph SR Tablets (Less frequent) 3062
▲ Orap Tablets (1 of 20 patients) 1407
Ortho Diaphragm Kits – All-Flex Arcing Spring; Ortho Coil Spring 2552
▲ Orthoclone OKT3 Sterile Solution (14%) 2498
▲ Orudis Capsules (3% to 9%) 3548
▲ Oruvail Capsules (3% to 9%) 3548
Ovcon 3364
Ovidrel for Injection (Less than 2%) 3220
OxyContin Tablets (Between 1% and 5%) 2912
▲ Pancrease Capsules (Among most frequent) 2580
▲ Pancrease MT Capsules (Among most frequent) 2581
▲ Paraplatin for Injection (6%) 1126
Parnate Tablets 1607
▲ Paser Granules (Among most common) 1781
▲ Paxil (1.0% to 12%) 1609
▲ PCE Dispertab Tablets (Among most frequent) 498
▲ Pediazole Suspension (Among most frequent) 3050
Liquid PedvaxHIB (One case) 2148
▲ PEG-Intron Powder for Injection (18%) 3140
▲ Pentasa Capsules (3.4% to 3.5%) 3239
Pepcid Injection (1.7%) 2153
Pepcid for Oral Suspension (1.7%) 2150
Pepcid RPD Orally Disintegrating Tablets (1.7%) 2150
Pepcid Tablets (1.7%) 2150
Pergonal for Injection 3223
Periactin Tablets 2155
Peri-Colace Capsules and Syrup 3240
▲ Periostat Tablets (6%) 1208
▲ Permax Tablets (6.4%) 1299
Persantine Tablets 1057
▲ Photofrin for Injection (5%) 831
Pima Syrup (Less frequent) 1362
Pipracil (2%) 1866
Plaquenil Tablets 3082
▲ Plavix Tablets (4.5%) 1097
▲ Plavix Tablets (4.5%) 3084
Plendil Extended-Release Tablets (0.5% to 1.5%) 623
▲ Pletal Tablets (12% to 19%) 2605
▲ Pletal Tablets (12% to 19%) 2848
▲ Ponstel Capsules (1% to 10%) 1356
▲ Prandin Tablets (0.5, 1, and 2 mg) (4% to 5%) 2432
▲ Pravachol Tablets (2.0% to 6.2%) 1099
▲ Precose Tablets (31%) 906
▲ Prempro Tablets (6%) 3572
▲ Prevacid Delayed-Release Capsules (1.4% to 7.4%) 3292
▲ Prevnar for Injection (10.9% to 12.1%) 1870
▲ PREVPAC (3% to 7.4%) 3298
Priftin Tablets (1.1%) 758
▲ Prilosec Delayed-Release Capsules (3.0% to 14%) 628
Primaxin I.M. (0.6%) 2158
Primaxin I.V. (1.8% to 3.9%) 2160
▲ Prinivil Tablets (3.7%) 2164
Prinzide Tablets (2.5%) 2168
▲ Procanbid Extended-Release Tablets (3% to 4%) 2262
Procardia Capsules (2% or less) 2708
Procardia XL Extended Release Tablets (Less than 3%) 2710
▲ Procrit for Injection (0.11% to 21%) 2502
▲ Prograf (37% to 72%) 1393
▲ Proleukin for Injection (67%) 1199
▲ Prometrium Capsules (100 mg, 200 mg) (8%) 3261
Prostigmin Injectable 1744
Prostigmin Tablets 1744
▲ Prostin E2 Suppositories (Approximately two-fifths) 2852
Protonix I.V. (Greater than 1%) 3580
▲ Protonix Tablets (4% to 6%) 3577
▲ Protopic Ointment (3% to 6%) 1397
▲ Provigil Tablets (8%) 1193
▲ Prozac Pulvules, Liquid, and Weekly Capsules (12%) 1238
Pulmicort Respules (2% to 4%) 632
Purinethol Tablets (Occasional) 1615
▲ Quinaglute Dura-Tabs Tablets (24%) 978
▲ Quinidex Extentabs (35%) 2933
▲ Rapamune Oral Solution and Tablets (25% to 42%) 3584
Recombivax HB (Greater than 1%) 2178
ReFacto Vials 1437
Reglan 2935
▲ Relafen Tablets (14%) 1617
▲ Relenza Rotadisk (2% to 3%) 1619
▲ Remicade for IV Injection (3% to 13%) 1178
▲ Reminyl Oral Solution (6% to 12%) 1792
▲ Reminyl Tablets (6% to 12%) 1792
▲ Renagel Capsules (4% to 16%) 1439
▲ Renagel Tablets (4% to 16%) 1439
Renese Tablets 2712
ReoPro Vials (1.1%) 1958
Repronex for Intramuscular and Subcutaneous Injection (Up to 2.1%) 1347
Requip Tablets (1% or more) 1621
Rescriptor Tablets (Less than 2% to 4.5%) 526
▲ Retrovir Capsules (0.8% to 12%) 1625
▲ Retrovir IV Infusion (1% to 12%) 1629
▲ Retrovir (0.8% to 12%) 1625
Rifadin (Some patients) 765
Rifamate Capsules (Some patients) 767
Rifater Tablets 769
▲ Rilutek Tablets (5.5% to 9.0%) 772
Risperdal (Infrequent) 1796
Rituxan for Infusion (1% to 5%) 1750
Rituxan I.V. (1% to 5%) 1428
Robaxisal Tablets 2939
Rocephin Injectable Vials, ADD-Vantage, Galaxy, Bulk (2.7%) 2993
▲ Roferon-A Injection (20% to 42%) 2996
Rowasa Rectal Suspension Enema 4.0 grams/unit (60 mL) (2.33%) 3264
Roxicodone Tablets (Less than 3%) 3067
Rum-K 1363
Rynatan Tablets 3351
▲ Rythmol Tablets – 150 mg, 225 mg, 300 mg (1.2% to 5.7%) 502
▲ Salagen Tablets (6%) 2229
▲ Sandimmune (3% to 8%) 2388
▲ Sandostatin Injection (34% to 61%) 2394
▲ Sandostatin LAR Depot (36%) 2395
▲ Sarafem Pulvules (10%) 1962
▲ Sectral Capsules (4%) 3589
Septra Suspension 2265
Septra Tablets 2265
Septra DS Tablets 2265
Serevent Inhalation Aerosol (1% to 5%) 1633
Serophene Tablets 3226
▲ Serostim for Injection (25.9%) 3229
▲ Serzone Tablets (8%) 1104
▲ Simulect for Injection (Greater than or equal to 10%) 2399
Sinemet Tablets 1253
Sinemet CR Tablets (1.2%) 1255
Sinequan 2713
Singulair (Greater than or equal to 2%) 2181
▲ Skelid Tablets (9.3%) 3088
▲ Soma Compound Tablets (Among most common) 3354
Soma Compound w/Codeine Tablets 3355
▲ Soriatane Capsules (1% to 10%) 3003
▲ Sporanox Capsules (3.3% to 4%) 1800
▲ Sporanox Injection (8%) 1804
▲ Sporanox Injection (8%) 2509
▲ Sporanox Oral Solution (10.3% to 10.9%) 1808
▲ Sporanox Oral Solution (10.3% to 10.9%) 2512
▲ Starlix Tablets (3.2%) 2401
Stromectol Tablets (1.8%) 2185
Sular Tablets (Less than or equal to 1%) 688
▲ Suprax (16%) 1877
Surmontil Capsules 3595
▲ Sustiva Capsules (2% to 39%) 1258
Symmetrel (1% to 5%) 1328
Synagis Intramuscular (More than 1%) 2028
Synercid I.V. (2.7%) 775
Tagamet (Approximately 1 in 100) 1644
Talacen Caplets (Rare) 3089
Talwin Nx Tablets 3090
Tambocor Tablets (1% to 3%) 1990
▲ Tamiflu Capsules (3.2% to 9.5%) 3008
▲ Tamiflu Oral Suspension (3.2% to 9.5%) 3008
Tao Capsules (Infrequent) 2716
Tarka Tablets (1.5%) 508
▲ Tasmar Tablets (16% to 18%) 3010
▲ Taxol Injection (38% to 90%) 1129
Taxotere for Injection Concentrate 778
Tazicef for Injection (Less than 2%) 1647
Tazicef Galaxy Container (Less than 2%) 1650
Tazicef Pharmacy Bulk Package (Less than 2%) 1653
Tazidime Vials, Faspak & ADD-Vantage (1 in 78) 1966
Tegretol/Tegretol-XR 2404
▲ Temodar Capsules (16%) 3157
Tenex Tablets (3% or less) 2942

Tenoretic Tablets (2% to 3%) 690
Tenormin (2% to 3%) 692
Tensilon Injectable 1745
▲ Tequin Injection (4%) 1110
▲ Tequin Tablets (4%) 1110
Teveten Tablets (1% or greater) 3327
▲ Thalomid Capsules (4.2%) 1154
Theo-Dur Extended-Release Tablets 1835
▲ TheraCys Injection (6%) 823
Thioridazine Hydrochloride Tablets 2289
Thiothixene Capsules 2290
▲ Thymoglobulin for Injection (36.6%) 3071
Tiazac Capsules (Less than 2%) 1378
Tice BCG, BCG Live (1.2%) 2489
▲ Ticlid Tablets (12.5%) 3015
▲ Tikosyn Capsules (3%) 2717
Timentin Injection- ADD-Vantage Vial 1661
Timentin Injection-Galaxy Container 1664
Timentin Injection-Pharmacy Bulk Package 1666
Timentin for Intravenous Administration 1658
Timolide Tablets (Less than 1%) 2187
Timolol GFS ⊙266
Timoptic in Ocudose (Less frequent) 2192
Timoptic Sterile Ophthalmic Solution (Less frequent) 2190
Timoptic-XE Sterile Ophthalmic Gel Forming Solution 2194
▲ TOBI Solution for Inhalation (6.2%) 1206
▲ Tolectin (3% to 9%) 2589
▲ Tonocard Tablets (Up to 6.8%) 649
Topamax Sprinkle Capsules (Frequent) 2590
Topamax Tablets (Frequent) 2590
▲ Toprol-XL Tablets (About 5 of 100 patients) 651
▲ Toradol (7%) 3018
▲ Trasylol Injection (3%) 909
▲ Trecator-SC Tablets (Among most common) 3598
Trental Tablets 784
▲ Tricor Capsules, Micronized (3%) 513
Trilafon (Occasional) 3160
▲ Trileptal Oral Suspension (5% to 7%) 2407
▲ Trileptal Tablets (5% to 7%) 2407
▲ Trilisate (Less than 20%) 2901
Tripedia Vaccine (Up to 3%) 817
▲ Trisenox Injection (53%) 1158
▲ Trizivir Tablets (12% to 26%) 1669
Trovan (2%) 2722
▲ Twinrix Vaccine (4% to 6%) 1674
TYPHIM Vi Vaccine (Up to 3.1%) 825
▲ Ultracet Tablets (3%) 2597
▲ Ultram Tablets (5% to 10%) 2600
Ultrase Capsules 835
▲ Ultrase MT Capsules (3.7%; among most frequent) 835
▲ Unasyn for Injection (3%) 2728
Uni-Dur Extended-Release Tablets 1841
Uniphyl 400 mg and 600 mg Tablets 2903
Uniretic Tablets (More than 1%) 3178
Unithroid Tablets 3445
▲ Univasc Tablets (3.1%) 3181
Urecholine 2198
Urecholine Tablets 2445
Urobiotic-250 Capsules (Rare) 2731
Urocit-K Tablets (Some patients) 2232
Uroqid-Acid No. 2 Tablets 947
Urso Tablets 836
▲ Valcyte Tablets (16% to 41%) 3022
▲ Valstar Sterile Solution for Intravesical Instillation (3%) 1175
Valtrex Caplets 1676
Vanceril Double Strength Inhalation Aerosol (Fewer than 2%) 3167
Vancocin HCl, Vials & ADD-Vantage 1970
▲ Vantin Tablets and Oral Suspension (1.2% to 7.2%) 2860
Vaqta (1.0% to 2.5%) 2199
Varivax (Greater than or equal to 1%) 2202
▲ Vascor Tablets (6.82% to 10.87%) 2602
Vaseretic Tablets (2.1%) 2204
Vasotec I.V. Injection 2207
Vasotec Tablets (1.4% to 2.1%) 2210
▲ Venofer Injection (Greater than 5%) 580
Ventolin Inhalation Aerosol and Refill (1%) 1679
Ventolin HFA Inhalation Aerosol (Less than 3%) 3618
Verelan Capsules (1% or less) 3184
Verelan PM Capsules (2.4%) 3186
Vermox Chewable Tablets 2017
▲ Vesanoid Capsules (23%) 3037
Viadur Implant (2.3%) 912
▲ Viagra Tablets (3%) 2732
Vibramycin Calcium Oral Suspension Syrup (Infrequent) 2735
Vibramycin Hyclate Capsules (Infrequent) 2735
Vibramycin Hyclate Intravenous 2737
Vibramycin Monohydrate for Oral Suspension (Infrequent) 2735
Vibra-Tabs Film Coated Tablets (Infrequent) 2735
▲ Vicoprofen Tablets (3% to 9%) 520
▲ Videx (19% to 34%) 1138
▲ Videx EC Capsules (54%) 1143
Viokase 837
▲ Vioxx (6.8%) 2213
▲ Viracept (3% to 32%) 532
Viramune Oral Suspension (2%) 1060
Viramune Tablets (2%) 1060
▲ Vistide Injection (7% to 26%) 1445
▲ Vitravene for Injection (5% to 20%) ⊙310
Vivactil Tablets 2217
Vivactil Tablets 2446
Vivotif Berna 997
▲ Voltaren Tablets (3% to 9%) 2315
▲ Voltaren-XR Tablets (3% to 9%) 2315
Warfarin Sodium Tablets, USP 3302
▲ WelChol Tablets (5%) 3073
▲ Wellbutrin Tablets (6.8%) 1680
▲ Wellbutrin SR Sustained-Release Tablets (5% to 7%) 1684
WinRho SDF 2297
▲ Xanax Tablets (10.1% to 20.6%) 2865
▲ Xeloda Tablets (2% to 12%) 3039
Xopenex Inhalation Solution 3207
Yodoxin Tablets 1722
Zanaflex Tablets (Frequent) 1305
Zantac 1690
Zantac Injection 1688
Zantac Syrup 1690
Zarontin Capsules (Frequent) 2659
Zarontin Syrup (Frequent) 2660
Zaroxolyn Tablets 1177
Zebeta Tablets (2.6% to 3.5%) 1885
▲ Zenapax for Injection (Greater than 5%) 3046
▲ Zerit (50%) 1147
Zestoretic Tablets (2.5%) 695
▲ Zestril Tablets (3.7%) 698
Ziac Tablets (1.1% to 4.3%) 1887
▲ Ziagen (12% to 26%) 1692
Zinacef Injection (1 in 220 patients) 1696
Zinacef for Injection (1 in 220 patients) 1696
▲ Zinecard for Injection (14% to 21%) 2869
▲ Zithromax Capsules, 250 mg (2% to 14%) 2743
▲ Zithromax for IV Infusion (Up to 8.5%) 2748
▲ Zithromax for Oral Suspension, 1 g (5% to 7%) 2743
▲ Zithromax for Oral Suspension, 300 mg, 600 mg, 900 mg, 1200 mg (2% to 14%) 2739
▲ Zithromax Tablets, 250 mg (2% to 14%) 2739
▲ Zithromax Tablets, 600 mg (5% to 7%) 2743
Zocor Tablets (1.9%) 2219
▲ Zofran Injection (8% to 16%) 1698
▲ Zofran (4% to 6%) 1703
▲ Zofran ODT Orally Disintegrating Tablets (4% to 6%) 1703
▲ Zoladex (1% to 36%) 702
▲ Zoladex 3-month (1% to 40%) 706
▲ Zoloft (18% to 24%) 2751
▲ Zometa for Intravenous Infusion (17.4%) 3621
▲ Zonegran Capsules (5%) 1307
▲ Zosyn (11.3% to 20%) 1890
▲ Zosyn in Galaxy Containers (11.3% to 20%) 1894
Zovirax (2.4% to 3.2%) 1706
▲ Zyban Sustained-Release Tablets (4%) 1710
Zyprexa Tablets 1973
Zyprexa ZYDIS Orally Disintegrating Tablets 1973
Zyrtec (1.9% to 3.1%) 2756
Zyrtec-D 12 Hour Extended Relief Tablets 2758
▲ Zyvox (4% to 8.3%) 2871

Diarrhea, bloody

Aciphex Tablets (Rare) 1267
Aciphex Tablets (Rare) 1783
Amphotec (1% to 5%) 1774
Asacol Delayed-Release Tablets 2884
Azulfidine EN-tabs Tablets (Rare) 2775
Benzaclin Topical Gel 1220
Canasa Rectal Suppositories 829
Cataflam Tablets (Less than 1%) 2315
Cleocin HCl Capsules 2784
Cleocin T Topical (Rare) 2790
Clindagel 1401
Colazal Capsules 3069
Norvir Capsules (Less than 2%) 487
Norvir Oral Solution (Less than 2%) 487
Omnicef 493
Paxil (Rare) 1609
Pentasa Capsules (0.9%) 3239
Pipracil (Less frequent) 1866
Proleukin for Injection (Less than 1%) 1199
Prozac Pulvules, Liquid, and Weekly Capsules (Rare) 1238
Rowasa Rectal Suspension Enema 4.0 grams/unit (60 mL) 3264
Sarafem Pulvules (Rare) 1962
Ticlid Tablets 3015
Vantin Tablets and Oral Suspension 2860
Voltaren Tablets (Less than 1%) 2315
Voltaren-XR Tablets (Less than 1%) 2315

Diarrhea, infectious

Fortovase Capsules (Less than 2%) 2970
▲ Xenical Capsules (5.3%) 3043

Digitalis toxicity

Demadex Tablets and Injection 2965
Lanoxicaps Capsules 1574
Virazole for Inhalation Solution 1747

Diplegia

Imitrex Injection (Rare) 1549
Imitrex Nasal Spray (Rare) 1554
Imitrex Tablets 1558

Diplopia

Abelcet Injection 1273
Aciphex Tablets 1267
Aciphex Tablets 1783
Adalat CC Tablets (Less than 1.0%) 877
Agrylin Capsules (1% to 5%) 3232
Ambien Tablets (Frequent) 3191
Arthrotec Tablets (Rare) 3195
Ativan Injection (Occasional) 3478
Axert Tablets (Rare) 2772
Azactam for Injection (Less than 1%) 1276
Azopt Ophthalmic Suspension (Less than 1%) 536
Benadryl Parenteral 2617
Betagan ⊙228
Betaseron for SC Injection 988
Betimol Ophthalmic Solution ⊙324
Blocadren Tablets 2046
Botox Purified Neurotoxin Complex (Rare) 549
Brevicon 28-Day Tablets (Rare) 3380
Buprenex Injectable (Less than 1%) 2918
Carbatrol Capsules 3234
Carteolol Hydrochloride Ophthalmic Solution USP, 1% ⊙258
Cataflam Tablets (Less than 1%) 2315
Celexa (Rare) 1365
▲ Cerebyx Injection (3.3%) 2619
Chibroxin Sterile Ophthalmic Solution 2051
Chirocaine Injection (2.5%) 2909
Cipro I.V. (1% or less) 893
Cipro I.V. Pharmacy Bulk Package (Less than 1%) 897
Cipro (Less than 1%) 887
Clomid Tablets (1.5%) 735
Cognex Capsules (Infrequent) 1351
Copaxone for Injection (At least 2%) 3306
Cosopt Sterile Ophthalmic Solution 2065
Dantrium Capsules (Less frequent) 2885
▲ Depacon Injection (16%) 416
▲ Depakene (16%) 421
▲ Depakote Sprinkle Capsules (16%) 426
▲ Depakote Tablets (1% to 16%) 430
Depakote ER Tablets (Greater than 1%) 436
Depen Titratable Tablets 3341
Depo-Provera Contraceptive Injection 2798
Dilaudid Oral Liquid (Less frequent) 445
Dilaudid Tablets - 8 mg (Less frequent) 445
Dilaudid-HP (Less frequent) 443
Diprivan Injectable Emulsion (Less than 1%) 667
Duranest Injections 600
Effexor Tablets (Infrequent) 3495
Effexor XR Capsules (Infrequent) 3499
ELA-Max Cream 1340
Eldepryl Capsules 3266
Emla (Unlikely with cream) 602
Evoxac Capsules (Less than 1%) 1217
Exelon Capsules (Infrequent) 2342
Exelon Oral Solution (Infrequent) 2345
Fareston Tablets 3237
▲ Felbatol (3.4% to 6.1%) 3343
femhrt Tablets 2635
Flexeril Tablets (Less than 1%) 572
Flexeril Tablets (Less than 1%) 2094
Floxin I.V. 2526
Floxin Tablets 2529
Gabitril Tablets (1% or more) 1189
Geodon Capsules (Frequent) 2688
Gliadel Wafer (1%) 1723
Indocin (Less than 1%) 2112
Intron A for Injection (Less than 5%) 3120
Ismo Tablets (Fewer than 1%) 3524
Kadian Capsules (Less than 3%) 1335
Keppra Tablets (2%) 3314
Klonopin Tablets (Infrequent) 2983
▲ Lamictal (24% to 49%) 1567
Levaquin (Less than 0.3%) 2537
Levlen (Rare) 962
Levlite 21 Tablets (Rare) 962
Levlite 28 Tablets (Rare) 962
Levo-Dromoran 1734
Lidoderm Patch 1319
Lodosyn Tablets 1251
Luvox Tablets (25, 50, 100 mg) (Infrequent) 3256
Matulane Capsules 3246
Mirapex Tablets (1% or more) 2834
Modicon (Rare) 2563
Motrin Suspension, Oral Drops, Chewable Tablets, and Caplets (Less than 1%) 2002
MS Contin Tablets (Less frequent) 2896
MSIR (Less frequent) 2898
Naprelan Tablets (Less than 1%) 1293
▲ Neurontin Capsules (5.9%) 2655
▲ Neurontin Oral Solution (5.9%) 2655
▲ Neurontin Tablets (5.9%) 2655
Norinyl 1 +35 28-Day Tablets 3380
Norinyl 1 + 50 28-Day Tablets 3380
Noroxin Tablets 2145
Norvasc Tablets (More than 0.1% to 1%) 2704
Norvir Capsules (Less than 2%) 487
Norvir Oral Solution (Less than 2%) 487
Numorphan 1324
Ocupress Ophthalmic Solution, 1% Sterile ⊙303
Oramorph SR Tablets (Less frequent) 3062
Orthoclone OKT3 Sterile Solution 2498
Ortho-Cyclen/Ortho Tri-Cyclen (Rare) 2573
Ortho-Novum (Rare) 2563
Ortho-Novum 1/50□28 Tablets (Rare) 2556
Ortho-Cyclen/Ortho Tri-Cyclen (Rare) 2573
Ovcon 3364
Paxil (Rare) 1609
Periactin Tablets 2155
Permax Tablets (2.1%) 1299
Phenergan Injection 3553
Phenergan 3556
Photofrin for Injection 831
Pletal Tablets (Less than 2%) 2605
Pletal Tablets (Less than 2%) 2848
Premphase Tablets 3572
Prempro Tablets 3572
Prinivil Tablets (0.3% to 1.0%) 2164
Prinzide Tablets 2168
ProSom Tablets (Rare) 500
Protonix I.V. (Less than 1%) 3580
Protonix Tablets (Less than 1%) 3577
Protopam Chloride for Injection 3582
Provera Tablets 2853
Prozac Pulvules, Liquid, and Weekly Capsules (Rare) 1238
Quinaglute Dura-Tabs Tablets 978
Quinidex Extentabs 2933
Remeron Tablets (Rare) 2483
Remeron SolTab Tablets (Rare) 2486
ReoPro Vials (0.1%) 1958
Requip Tablets (2%) 1621
Rescriptor Tablets (Less than 2%) 526
Rescula Ophthalmic Solution (Less than 1%) ⊙306
Rilutek Tablets (Rare) 772
Risperdal (Rare) 1796
Robaxin Injectable 2938
Robaxin Tablets 2939
Romazicon Injection (1% to 3%) 3000
Sarafem Pulvules (Rare) 1962
Serophene Tablets 3226
Serzone Tablets (Infrequent) 1104
Sinemet Tablets 1253
Sinemet CR Tablets 1255
Soma Tablets 3353
Soma Compound Tablets (Very rare) 3354
Soma Compound w/Codeine Tablets (Very rare) 3355
Sonata Capsules (Infrequent) 3591
Soriatane Capsules (1% to 5%) 3003
Sustiva Capsules (Less than 2%) 1258
Tambocor Tablets (1% to 3%) 1990
Tasmar Tablets (Infrequent) 3010
Tegretol/Tegretol-XR 2404
▲ Temodar Capsules (5%) 3157
Tensilon Injectable 1745
Thalomid Capsules 1154
Timolide Tablets 2187
Timolol GFS ⊙266
Timoptic in Ocudose (Less frequent) 2192
Timoptic Sterile Ophthalmic Solution (Less frequent) 2190
Timoptic-XE Sterile Ophthalmic Gel Forming Solution 2194
Tonocard Tablets (Less than 1%) 649
▲ Topamax Sprinkle Capsules (14.2% to 14.6%) 2590
▲ Topamax Tablets (14.2% to 14.6%) 2590
Tranxene 511
Trecator-SC Tablets (Rare) 3598

▲ Trileptal Oral Suspension (5% to 40%) 2407
▲ Trileptal Tablets (5% to 40%) 2407
Tri-Levlen (Rare) 962
Tri-Norinyl-28 Tablets 3433
Valium Injectable 3026
Valium Tablets (Infrequent) 3047
Versed Injection (Less than 1%) 3027
Versed Syrup (Less than 1%) 3033
Viagra Tablets 2732
Vistide Injection 1445
▲ Visudyne for Injection (1% to 10%) ⊙ 308
Voltaren Tablets (Less than 1%) 2315
Voltaren-XR Tablets (Less than 1%) 2315
Wellbutrin Tablets (Rare) 1680
Wellbutrin SR Sustained-Release Tablets 1684
Xalatan Latanoprost Ophthalmic Solution (Less than 1%) ⊙ 320
Xalatan Sterile Ophthalmic Solution (Less than 1%) 2864
Xanax Tablets 2865
Xylocaine Injections (Less than 1%) 653
Zestoretic Tablets 695
Zestril Tablets (0.3% to 1.0%) 698
Zoloft (Rare) 2751
Zomig Tablets (Rare) 708
Zomig-ZMT Tablets (Rare) 708
▲ Zonegran Capsules (6%) 1307
Zyban Sustained-Release Tablets 1710
Zyprexa Tablets (Infrequent) 1973
Zyprexa ZYDIS Orally Disintegrating Tablets (Infrequent) 1973

Dipsesis

Aciphex Tablets (Rare) 1267
Aciphex Tablets (Rare) 1783
Actiq (Less than 1%) 1184
Aggrenox Capsules (Less than 1%) 1026
Alferon N Injection (1%) 1770
Ambien Tablets (Infrequent) 3191
Amerge Tablets (Infrequent) 1467
Anaprox Tablets (Less than 3%) 2967
Anaprox DS Tablets (Less than 3%) 2967
Aricept Tablets (Infrequent) 1270
Aricept Tablets (Infrequent) 2665
Atrovent Nasal Spray 0.06% (Less than 1%) 1033
Avonex 1013
Axert Tablets (Rare) 2772
Betaseron for SC Injection 988
Calcium Disodium Versenate Injection 1980
Cardizem Injectable 1018
Cardizem Lyo-Ject Syringe 1018
Cardizem Monovial 1018
Cardizem CD Capsules (Less than 1%) 1016
Cardura Tablets (Less than 0.5%) 2668
Ceftin Tablets (0.1% to 1%) 1898
Celexa (Infrequent) 1365
▲ CellCept Capsules (3% to 10%) 2951
▲ CellCept Intravenous (3% to 10%) 2951
▲ CellCept Oral Suspension (3% to 10%) 2951
▲ CellCept Tablets (3% to 10%) 2951
Claritin (At least one patient) 3100
Claritin-D 12 Hour Extended Release Tablets (2%) 3102
Claritin-D 24 Hour Extended Release Tablets (Fewer than 2%) 3104
Crinone (Less than 5%) 3213
Cytotec Tablets (Infrequent) 3202
DaunoXome Injection (Less than or equal to 5%) 1442
Demadex Tablets and Injection 2965
Depo-Provera Contraceptive Injection (Fewer than 1%) 2798
Dyazide Capsules 1515
Dynabac Tablets (0.1% to 1%) 2269
EC-Naprosyn Delayed-Release Tablets (Less than 3%) 2967
Ecotrin Enteric Coated Aspirin Low, Regular and Maximum Strength Tablets 1715
Effexor Tablets (Infrequent) 3495
Effexor XR Capsules (Infrequent) 3499
Emcyt Capsules (1%) 2810
Eskalith 1527
Evoxac Capsules (Less than 1%) 1217
Exelon Capsules (Infrequent) 2342
Exelon Oral Solution (Infrequent) 2345
Flexeril Tablets (Less than 1%) 572
Flexeril Tablets (Less than 1%) 2094
Floxin I.V. (Less than 1%) 2526
Floxin Tablets (Less than 1%) 2529
Fortovase Capsules (Less than 2%) 2970
Foscavir Injection (Between 1% and 5%) 605
Furosemide Tablets 2284
Gabitril Tablets (Infrequent) 1189
Geodon Capsules (Infrequent) 2688
Glucotrol XL Extended Release Tablets (Less than 1%) 2693
Gonal-F for Injection 3216
Imitrex Injection (Infrequent) 1549
Imitrex Nasal Spray (Infrequent) 1554
Imitrex Tablets (Infrequent) 1558
Intron A for Injection (Less than or equal to 5%) 3120
Klonopin Tablets (Infrequent) 2983
K-Phos Neutral Tablets 946
Lamictal (Infrequent) 1567
Lithium Carbonate 3061
Lithium Citrate Syrup 3061
Lithobid Slow-Release Tablets 3255
Lodine (Less than 1%) 3528
Lodine XL Extended-Release Tablets (Less than 1%) 3530
▲ Lupron Depot 3.75 mg (Among most frequent) 3281
Lupron Depot–3 Month 11.25 mg (Less than 5%) 3285
Lupron Depot–3 Month 22.5 mg (Less than 5%) 3288
Luvox Tablets (25, 50, 100 mg) 3256
Maxalt Tablets (Infrequent) 2120
Maxalt-MLT Orally Disintegrating Tablets (Infrequent) 2120
Maxzide 1008
Meridia Capsules (1.7%) 481
MetroGel-Vaginal Gel (Less than 1%) 1986
Miacalcin Nasal Spray (Less than 1%) 2375
Midamor Tablets (Less than or equal to 1%) 2136
Mirapex Tablets (Less than 1%) 2834
Moduretic Tablets (Less than or equal to 1%) 2138
Naprelan Tablets (Less than 3%) 1293
Naprosyn Suspension (Less than 3%) 2967
Naprosyn Tablets (Less than 3%) 2967
Neurontin Capsules (Infrequent) 2655
Neurontin Oral Solution (Infrequent) 2655
Neurontin Tablets (Infrequent) 2655
Nexium Delayed-Release Capsules (Less than 1%) 619
Norvasc Tablets (More than 0.1% to 1%) 2704
Norvir Capsules (Less than 2%) 487
Norvir Oral Solution (Less than 2%) 487
Oncaspar (Less than 1%) 756
▲ Orap Tablets (1 of 20 patients) 1407
Orudis Capsules (Less than 1%) 3548
Oruvail Capsules (Less than 1%) 3548
OxyContin Tablets (Less than 1%) 2912
Paxil (Infrequent) 1609
Pentasa Capsules (Less than 1%) 3239
Permax Tablets (Infrequent) 1299
Prevacid Delayed-Release Capsules (Less than 1%) 3292
PREVPAC (Less than 1% to 3%) 3298
Prinzide Tablets 2168
ProSom Tablets (Infrequent) 500
Protonix I.V. (Less than 1%) 3580
Protonix Tablets (Less than 1%) 3577
Provigil Tablets (At least 1%) 1193
Prozac Pulvules, Liquid, and Weekly Capsules (Infrequent) 1238
Remeron Tablets (Frequent) 2483
Remeron SolTab Tablets (Frequent) 2486
Requip Tablets (Infrequent) 1621
Rescriptor Tablets (Less than 2%) 526
Rilutek Tablets (Infrequent) 772
Risperdal (Infrequent) 1796
Sarafem Pulvules (Infrequent) 1962
Seroquel Tablets (Infrequent) 684
▲ Serostim for Injection (1% to 10%) 3229
Serzone Tablets (1%) 1104
Singulair (Greater than or equal to 2%) 2181
Sonata Capsules (Infrequent) 3591
▲ Soriatane Capsules (1% to 10%) 3003
Tasmar Tablets (Infrequent) 3010
Tenoretic Tablets 690
Tequin Injection (Less than 0.1%) 1110
Tequin Tablets (Less than 0.1%) 1110
Tiazac Capsules (Less than 2%) 1378
Tonocard Tablets (Less than 1%) 649
Topamax Sprinkle Capsules (Infrequent) 2590
Topamax Tablets (Infrequent) 2590
Toradol (1% or less) 3018
Trental Tablets (Less than 1%) 784
Trileptal Oral Suspension (Up to 2%) 2407
Trileptal Tablets (Up to 2%) 2407
Uniretic Tablets (Less than 1%) 3178
Uroqid-Acid No. 2 Tablets 947
Vantin Tablets and Oral Suspension (Less than 1%) 2860
Vaseretic Tablets 2204
Viagra Tablets (Less than 2%) 2732
Vicoprofen Tablets (Less than 3%) 520
Vistide Injection 1445
Wellbutrin SR Sustained-Release Tablets (Infrequent) 1684
Zaroxolyn Tablets 1177
Zestoretic Tablets 695
Zoloft (Infrequent) 2751
Zomig Tablets (Infrequent) 708
Zomig-ZMT Tablets (Infrequent) 708
Zonegran Capsules (Infrequent) 1307
Zosyn (1.0% or less) 1890
Zosyn in Galaxy Containers (1.0% or less) 1894
Zovirax for Injection (Less than 1%) 1708
Zyban Sustained-Release Tablets (Less than 1%) 1710
Zyprexa Tablets (Frequent) 1973
Zyprexa ZYDIS Orally Disintegrating Tablets (Frequent) 1973
Zyrtec (Less than 2%) 2756
Zyrtec-D 12 Hour Extended Relief Tablets (Less than 2%) 2758

Discoloration, injection site

Diprivan Injectable Emulsion (Less than 1%) 667
▲ Navelbine Injection (Approximately 1/3 of patients) 1604

Discomfort, arm

▲ Adenoscan (4%) 1381
Imitrex Injection 1549

Discomfort, chest

▲ Adenoscan (40%) 1381
Amerge Tablets (Frequent) 1467
Brethine Ampuls (1.3% to 1.5%) 2314
▲ Cerezyme for Injection (Approximately 4%) 1438
Glucophage Tablets (1% to 5%) 1080
Imitrex Injection (Rare) 1549
Imitrex Nasal Spray (Infrequent) 1554
Imitrex Tablets (Frequent) 1558
Kogenate 934
▲ Nicotrol Inhaler (Greater than 3%) 2840
Primaxin I.M. 2158
Primaxin I.V. (Less than 0.2%) 2160
Prinivil Tablets (0.3% to 1.0%) 2164
Prinzide Tablets (0.3% to 1%) 2168
Proventil Repetabs Tablets (Less than 1%) 3148
Recombivax HB (Less than 1%) 2178
Serevent Inhalation Aerosol (1% to 3%) 1633
Tasmar Tablets (1% to 2%) 3010
Timentin Injection- ADD-Vantage Vial 1661
Timentin Injection-Galaxy Container 1664
Timentin Injection-Pharmacy Bulk Package 1666
Timentin for Intravenous Administration 1658
▲ Vesanoid Capsules (32%) 3037
Volmax Extended-Release Tablets (Less frequent) 2276
Zaroxolyn Tablets 1177
Zestoretic Tablets (0.3% to 1.0%) 695
Zestril Tablets (0.3% to 1.0%) 698

Discomfort, general

AVC (Occasional) 1350
Coumadin for Injection 1243
Coumadin Tablets 1243
Emadine Ophthalmic Solution (Less than 5%) ⊙ 211
Epifrin Sterile Ophthalmic Solution ⊙ 235
Eskalith 1527
Iopidine Sterile Ophthalmic Solution ⊙ 212
Lithium Carbonate 3061
Lithium Citrate Syrup 3061
Lithobid Slow-Release Tablets 3255
Pilopine HS Ophthalmic Gel ⊙ 217
Warfarin Sodium Tablets, USP 3302
Zovirax Ointment 1707

Discomfort, jaw

▲ Adenoscan (15%) 1381
Imitrex Injection (1.8%) 1549

Discomfort, local

Albalon Ophthalmic Solution ⊙ 225
▲ Betimol Ophthalmic Solution (More than 5%) ⊙ 324
▲ Chibroxin Sterile Ophthalmic Solution (One of the two most frequent) 2051
▲ Ciloxan (Among most frequent) 538
Efudex (Infrequent) 1733
OptiPranolol Metipranolol Ophthalmic Solution 0.3% (A small number of patients) ⊙ 263
▲ Testoderm Transdermal Systems (4%) 574

Discomfort, lower extremities

Adenoscan (Less than 1%) 1381

Discomfort, nasal

Amerge Tablets (Frequent) 1467
Imitrex Injection (2.2%) 1549
Imitrex Nasal Spray (Infrequent) 1554
▲ Imitrex Tablets (5% to 7%) 1558

Discomfort at injection site

Azactam for Injection (2.4%) 1276
BeneFix for Injection 1432
Cefotan (1 in 500) 664
Cerezyme for Injection 1438
MICRhoGAM Injection 2524
Nutropin AQ Injection 1420
RhoGAM Injection 2524
Rimso-50 Solution 1267
Tine Test, Tuberculin, Old 3631
Tubersol Diagnostic Antigen 3628

Discontinuation syndrome

Catapres-TTS 1038
Clorpres Tablets (About 1%) 1002
Combipres Tablets (About 1%) 1040

Disinhibition

Versed Syrup (Less than 1%) 3033

Disorientation

Aciphex Tablets 1267
Aciphex Tablets 1783
Actimmune (Rare) 1772
Akineton 402
Alferon N Injection (1%) 1770
Arthrotec Tablets (Rare) 3195
Asacol Delayed-Release Tablets 2884
Ativan Tablets (Less frequent) 3482
Biaxin/Biaxin XL 403
Botox Purified Neurotoxin Complex 549
Cataflam Tablets (Rare) 2315
Cosopt Sterile Ophthalmic Solution 2065
Daranide Tablets 2077
Demerol 3079
Demser Capsules 2085
Dilaudid Oral Liquid (Less frequent) 445
Dilaudid Tablets - 8 mg (Less frequent) 445
Dilaudid-HP (Less frequent) 443
Dolobid Tablets (Less than 1 in 100) 2088
Dolophine Hydrochloride Tablets 3056
Dopram Injectable 2931
Eldepryl Capsules 3266
Etrafon 3115
Famvir Tablets (Infrequent) 2348
Flexeril Tablets (Less than 1%) 572
Flexeril Tablets (Less than 1%) 2094
Floxin I.V. 2526
Floxin Tablets 2529
Sterile FUDR (Remote possibility) 2974
Halcion Tablets 2823
Ifex for Injection (Less frequent) 1123
INFeD Injection 3388
Levsin/Levsinex/Levbid 3172
Lodosyn Tablets 1251
Maxalt Tablets (Infrequent) 2120
Maxalt-MLT Orally Disintegrating Tablets (Infrequent) 2120
Mepergan Injection 3539
MS Contin Tablets (Less frequent) 2896
MSIR (Less frequent) 2898
Myambutol Tablets 1290
Mylocel Tablets (Extremely rare) 2227
Nebcin Vials, Hyporets & ADD-Vantage 1955
Norpramin Tablets 755
Oncaspar 756
Oramorph SR Tablets (Less frequent) 3062
Orthoclone OKT3 Sterile Solution 2498
Parnate Tablets 1607
Pediazole Suspension 3050
Phenergan Suppositories 3556
Phenergan Syrup 3554
Phenergan with Codeine Syrup 3557
Phenergan with Dextromethorphan Syrup 3559
Phenergan VC Syrup 3560
Phenergan VC with Codeine Syrup 3561
PREVPAC 3298
Rescriptor Tablets (Less than 2%) 526
Roxanol 3066
Sinemet Tablets 1253
Sinemet CR Tablets 1255
Sinequan (Infrequent) 2713
Soma Tablets 3353
Soma Compound Tablets (Very rare) 3354
Soma Compound w/Codeine Tablets (Very rare) 3355
Surmontil Capsules 3595
Tagamet 1644
Talacen Caplets 3089
Talwin Nx Tablets 3090
Timolol GFS ⊙ 266
Timoptic in Ocudose (Less frequent) 2192
Timoptic Sterile Ophthalmic Solution (Less frequent) 2190
Timoptic-XE Sterile Ophthalmic Gel Forming Solution 2194
▲ Tonocard Tablets (2.1% to 11.2%) 649
Transderm Scōp Transdermal Therapeutic System (Infrequent) 2302
Vivactil Tablets 2217
Vivactil Tablets 2446
Voltaren Tablets (Rare) 2315
Voltaren-XR Tablets (Rare) 2315

Disorientation, place

Blocadren Tablets 2046

Corgard Tablets ... 2245
Corzide 40/5 Tablets ... 2247
Corzide 80/5 Tablets ... 2247
Cosopt Sterile Ophthalmic Solution ... 2065
Inderal ... 3513
Inderal LA Long-Acting Capsules ... 3516
Inderide Tablets ... 3517
Inderide LA Long-Acting Capsules ... 3519
Nadolol Tablets ... 2288
Normodyne Tablets ... 3137
Sectral Capsules ... 3589
Tenoretic Tablets ... 690
Tenormin ... 692
Timolide Tablets ... 2187
Timolol GFS ... ⊙266
Timoptic in Ocudose ... 2192
Timoptic Sterile Ophthalmic Solution ... 2190
Timoptic-XE Sterile Ophthalmic Gel Forming Solution ... 2194
Toprol-XL Tablets ... 651
Zebeta Tablets ... 1885
Ziac Tablets ... 1887

Disorientation, time

Blocadren Tablets ... 2046
Corgard Tablets ... 2245
Corzide 40/5 Tablets ... 2247
Corzide 80/5 Tablets ... 2247
Cosopt Sterile Ophthalmic Solution ... 2065
Inderal ... 3513
Inderal LA Long-Acting Capsules ... 3516
Inderide Tablets ... 3517
Inderide LA Long-Acting Capsules ... 3519
Nadolol Tablets ... 2288
Normodyne Tablets ... 3137
Sectral Capsules ... 3589
Tenoretic Tablets ... 690
Tenormin ... 692
Timolide Tablets ... 2187
Timolol GFS ... ⊙266
Timoptic in Ocudose ... 2192
Timoptic Sterile Ophthalmic Solution ... 2190
Timoptic-XE Sterile Ophthalmic Gel Forming Solution ... 2194
Toprol-XL Tablets ... 651
Zebeta Tablets ... 1885
Ziac Tablets ... 1887

Distention, abdominal

(*see under* Abdominal distention)

Distress, abdominal

Ambien Tablets (Rare) ... 3191
Atromid-S Capsules (Less frequent) ... 3483
Augmentin Chewable Tablets (Less frequent) ... 1482
Augmentin Powder for Oral Suspension (Less frequent) ... 1482
Augmentin Tablets (Less frequent) ... 1485
Claritin-D 12 Hour Extended Release Tablets (Less frequent) ... 3102
Claritin-D 24 Hour Extended Release Tablets ... 3104
▲ Depo-Provera Contraceptive Injection (More than 5%) ... 2798
Ery-Tab Tablets ... 448
Erythrocin Stearate Filmtab Tablets ... 452
Estrace Vaginal Cream ... 3358
Estrace Tablets ... 3361
Factrel (Rare) ... [illegible]
Fortovase Capsules (Less than 2%) ... 2970
Glucovance Tablets ... 1086
Imitrex Injection (1.3%) ... 1549
Imitrex Tablets ... 1558
Indocin (Greater than 1%) ... 2112
▲ Invirase Capsules (0.9% to 3.1%) ... 2979
Iopidine Sterile Ophthalmic Solution ... ⊙212
▲ K-Lor Powder Packets (Among most common) ... 469
▲ K-Tab Filmtab Tablets (Most common) ... 470
Lodosyn Tablets ... 1251
Mexitil Capsules (1.2%) ... 1047
Motrin Suspension, Oral Drops, Chewable Tablets, and Caplets (1% to less than 3%) ... 2002
▲ Norplant System (5% or greater) ... 3543
▲ Persantine Tablets (6.1%) ... 1057
Rum-K ... 1363
Sinemet Tablets ... 1253
Talacen Caplets (Rare) ... 3089
Talwin Nx Tablets (Rare) ... 3090
Thyrel TRH for Injection ... 3630
▲ Ultrase MT Capsules (Among most frequent) ... 835
▲ Xanax Tablets (18.3%) ... 2865
X-Prep Liquid ... 2900
Zantac Injection ... 1688

Distress, epigastric

Abelcet Injection ... 1273
Aerolate ... 1361
Amaryl Tablets (Less than 1%) ... 717
Aricept Tablets (Frequent) ... 1270
Aricept Tablets (Frequent) ... 2665
▲ Benadryl Parenteral (Among most frequent) ... 2617
Celontin Capsules (Frequent) ... 2618
Cipro I.V. (1% or less) ... 893
Cipro I.V. Pharmacy Bulk Package (Less than 1%) ... 897
Clorpres Tablets ... 1002
Colazal Capsules ... 3069
Combipres Tablets ... 1040
Cuprimine Capsules ... 2075
▲ Depen Titratable Tablets (17%) ... 3341
D.H.E. 45 Injection ... 2334
DiaBeta Tablets (1.8%) ... 741
Dipentum Capsules (Rare) ... 2803
Etrafon ... 3115
Ferrlecit Injection ... 3386
Geocillin Tablets ... 2687
Grifulvin V Tablets Microsize and Oral Suspension Microsize (Occasional) ... 2518
Gris-PEG Tablets (Occasional) ... 2661
Hivid Tablets (Less than 1%) ... 2975
Inderal ... 3513
Inderal LA Long-Acting Capsules ... 3516
Inderide Tablets ... 3517
Inderide LA Long-Acting Capsules ... 3519
▲ Indocin (3% to 9%) ... 2112
Limbitrol ... 1738
Lufyllin Tablets ... 3347
Lufyllin-400 Tablets ... 3347
Lufyllin-GG Elixir ... 3348
Lufyllin-GG Tablets ... 3348
▲ MetroGel-Vaginal Gel (7%) ... 1986
▲ Mexitil Capsules (41%) ... 1047
Mintezol ... 2137
Motofen Tablets (1 in 100) ... 577
▲ Motrin Suspension, Oral Drops, Chewable Tablets, and Caplets (3% to 9%) ... 2002
Nexium Delayed-Release Capsules (Less than 1%) ... 619
Norpramin Tablets ... 755
Oncaspar (Less than 1%) ... 756
Periactin Tablets ... 2155
Phenergan VC Syrup ... 3560
Phenergan VC with Codeine Syrup ... 3561
Pima Syrup ... 1362
Rifadin (Some patients) ... 765
Rifamate Capsules (Some patients) ... 767
Rifater Tablets ... 769
▲ Rynatan Tablets (Among most common) ... 3351
Sandostatin LAR Depot (Rare) ... 2395
Sinemet Tablets ... 1253
Soma Tablets ... 3353
Soma Compound Tablets ... 3354
Soma Compound w/Codeine Tablets ... 3355
Surmontil Capsules ... 3595
Tapazole Tablets ... 1823
Theo-Dur Extended-Release Tablets ... 1835
▲ Ticlid Tablets (3.7%) ... 3015
Timentin Injection- ADD-Vantage Vial ... 1661
Timentin Injection-Galaxy Container ... 1664
Timentin Injection-Pharmacy Bulk Package ... 1666
Timentin for Intravenous Administration ... 1658
Toprol-XL Tablets (About 1 of 100 patients) ... 651
▲ Toradol (13%) ... 3018
▲ Trilisate (Less than 20%) ... [illegible]
Uni-Dur Extended-Release Tablets ... 1841
Vioxx (2.8%) ... 2213
Viracept ... 532
Vivactil Tablets ... 2217
Vivactil Tablets ... 2446
Zarontin Capsules (Frequent) ... 2659
Zarontin Syrup (Frequent) ... 2660
Zaroxolyn Tablets ... 1177
Zebeta Tablets ... 1885
▲ Zenapax for Injection (Greater than 5%) ... 3046
Ziac Tablets ... 1887

Distress, gastric

(*see under* Distress, gastrointestinal)

Distress, gastrointestinal

Agrylin Capsules (1% to 5%) ... 3232
AK-Fluor Injection 10% and 25% ... ⊙202
Alferon N Injection (One patient) ... 1770
Alupent (1% to 4%) ... 1029
Atrovent Inhalation Aerosol (2.4%) ... 1030
▲ Azulfidine EN-tabs Tablets (Among most common) ... 2775
Biltricide Tablets ... 887
Carafate Suspension (Less than 0.5%) ... 731
Carafate Tablets (Less than 0.5%) ... 730
Carbatrol Capsules ... 3234
Celontin Capsules (Frequent) ... 2618
Claritin (At least one patient) ... 3100
▲ Clinoril Tablets (10%) ... 2053
Combivent Inhalation Aerosol ... 1041
Covera-HS Tablets (Less than 2%) ... 3199
Cuprimine Capsules ... 2075
▲ Dolobid Tablets (3% to 9%) ... 2088
▲ Emcyt Capsules (11%) ... 2810
Feosol Caplets ... 1717
Feosol Tablets (Occasional) ... 1717
Flexeril Tablets (Less than 1%) ... 572
Flexeril Tablets (Less than 1%) ... 2094
Floxin I.V. (1% to 3%) ... 2526
Floxin Tablets (1% to 3%) ... 2529
Fluorescite Injection ... ⊙211
Imitrex Tablets (Frequent) ... 1558
Isoptin SR Tablets (1% or less) ... 467
Kadian Capsules (Less than 3%) ... 1335
K-Dur Microburst Release System ER Tablets ... 1832
Klor-Con M20/Klor-Con M10 Tablets ... 3329
Lopid Tablets ... 2650
▲ Lupron Depot–3 Month 11.25 mg (3% to 7%) ... 3285
Lupron Depot–3 Month 22.5 mg ... 3288
▲ Lupron Depot–4 Month 30 mg (10.2% to 12.5%) ... 3289
Midamor Tablets (Between 1% and 3%) ... 2136
Minipress Capsules (Less than 1%) ... 2699
Minizide Capsules (Rare) ... 2700
Moduretic Tablets (Greater than 1%, less than 3%) ... 2138
Nardil Tablets (Common) ... 2653
Orap Tablets ... 1407
▲ Ponstel Capsules (1% to 10%) ... 1356
ProAmatine Tablets (Rare) ... 3241
▲ Quinidex Extentabs (22%) ... 2933
Robaxisal Tablets ... 2939
Roferon-A Injection (Less than 1%) ... 2996
▲ Sandostatin LAR Depot (29.1%) ... 2395
Sedapap Tablets 50 mg/650 mg (Less frequent) ... 2225
Tegretol/Tegretol-XR ... 2404
Timolide Tablets (Less than 1%) ... 2187
Timoptic in Ocudose ... 2192
Timoptic Sterile Ophthalmic Solution ... 2190
▲ Tolectin (3% to 9%) ... 2589
▲ Vascor Tablets (4.35% to about 22%) ... 2602
Verelan Capsules (1% or less) ... 3184
Verelan PM Capsules (2% or less) ... 3186
Zarontin Capsules (Frequent) ... 2659
Zarontin Syrup (Frequent) ... 2660
Zebeta Tablets ... 1885
Ziac Tablets ... 1887
Zovirax ... 1706

Distress, precordial

(*see under* Distress, epigastric)

Distress, stomach

(*see under* Distress, gastrointestinal)

Distress, upper GI

(*see under* Distress, epigastric)

Disturbances, emotional

(*see under* Emotional disturbances)

Disturbances, gastrointestinal

(*see under* Distress, gastrointestinal)

Disulfiram-like reactions

Amaryl Tablets ... 717
DiaBeta Tablets (Very rare) ... 741
Diabinese Tablets ... 2680
Glucotrol Tablets ... 2692
Glucotrol XL Extended Release Tablets ... 2693
Glucovance Tablets (Very rare) ... 1086

Diuresis

Amerge Tablets (Infrequent) ... 1467
Azulfidine EN-tabs Tablets (Rare) ... 2775
Bactrim (Rare) ... 2949
Lufyllin Tablets ... 3347
Lufyllin-400 Tablets ... 3347
Lufyllin-GG Elixir ... 3348
Lufyllin-GG Tablets ... 3348
Pediazole Suspension (Rare) ... 3050
Phrenilin (Infrequent) ... 578
Sedapap Tablets 50 mg/650 mg (Infrequent) ... 2225
Septra Suspension (Rare) ... 2265
Septra Tablets (Rare) ... 2265
Septra DS Tablets (Rare) ... 2265
Theo-Dur Extended-Release Tablets ... 1835
Tonocard Tablets (Less than 1%) ... 649
Uni-Dur Extended-Release Tablets ... 1841

Diuresis, potentiation of

Uniphyl 400 mg and 600 mg Tablets ... 2903

Diverticulitis

Aricept Tablets (Infrequent) ... 1270
Aricept Tablets (Infrequent) ... 2665
Avonex ... 1013
Celebrex Capsules (0.1% to 1.9%) ... 2676
Celebrex Capsules (0.1% to 1.9%) ... 2780
Celexa (Rare) ... 1365
Cognex Capsules (Infrequent) ... 1351
Colazal Capsules ... 3069
Evoxac Capsules (Less than 1%) ... 1217
Reminyl Oral Solution (Infrequent) ... 1792
Reminyl Tablets (Infrequent) ... 1792
Requip Tablets (Infrequent) ... 1621
Rescriptor Tablets (Less than 2%) ... 526
Risperdal (Rare) ... 1796
Sandostatin LAR Depot (1% to 4%) ... 2395
Zoloft (Rare) ... 2751

Dizziness

Accolate Tablets (1.6%) ... 657
▲ Accupril Tablets (3.9% to 7.7%) ... 2611
▲ Accuretic Tablets (4.8%) ... 2614
Accutane Capsules ... 2944
Aciphex Tablets ... 1267
Aciphex Tablets ... 1783
Actifed Cold & Allergy Tablets ... ◘688
▲ Actiq (6% to 17%) ... 1184
Activella Tablets ... 2764
▲ Actonel Tablets (6.4% to 6.6%) ... 2879
▲ Adalat CC Tablets (4%) ... 877
Adderall Tablets ... 3231
Adderall XR Capsules (2%)
Adenocard Injection (1%) ... 1380
▲ Adenoscan (12%) ... 1381
Adipex-P ... 1406
Advil Cold and Sinus Caplets ... ◘771
Advil Cold and Sinus Tablets ... ◘771
▲ Aerobid/Aerobid-M (3% to 9%) ... 1363
Aerolate ... 1361
▲ Aggrastat (3%) ... 2031
Aggrenox Capsules (Less than 1%) ... 1026
▲ Agrylin Capsules (15.4%) ... 3232
Albalon Ophthalmic Solution ... ⊙225
Albenza Tablets (Less than 1.0% to 1.2%) ... 1463
Aldoclor Tablets ... 2035
Aldomet Tablets ... 2037
Aldoril Tablets ... 2039
Alesse-21 Tablets ... 3468
Alesse-28 Tablets ... 3473
▲ Alferon N Injection (9%) ... 1770
Allegra (2.2%) ... 712
Allegra-D Extended-Release Tablets (1.9%) ... 714
Alomide Ophthalmic Solution (Less than 1%) ... ⊙204
Alora Transdermal System ... 3372
▲ Alphagan Ophthalmic Solution (Approximately 3% to 9%) ... 545
Alphagan P Ophthalmic Solution (1% to 4%) ... 546
▲ Altace Capsules (2.2% to 4.1%) ... 2233
Alupent (1% to 4%) ... 1029
Amaryl Tablets (1.7%) ... 717
Ambien Tablets (1% to 5%) ... 3191
AmBisome for Injection (Less common) ... 1383
Amerge Tablets (1% to 2%) ... 1467
Amicar Injection ... 3608
Amicar Syrup ... 3608
Amicar Tablets ... 3608
Amoxil Chewable Tablets (Rare) ... 1471
Amoxil for Oral Suspension (Rare) ... 1471
Amoxil (Rare) ... 1471
▲ Amphotec (5% or more) ... 1774
▲ Anaprox Tablets (3% to 9%) ... 2967
▲ Anaprox DS Tablets (3% to 9%) ... 2967
AndroGel (Fewer than 1%) ... 3322
▲ Anzemet Injection (2.4% to 5.5%) ... 719
Anzemet Tablets (1.3% to 4.4%) ... 722
AquaMEPHYTON Injection ... 2042
▲ Arava Tablets (4%) ... 724
Aredia for Injection ... 2309
▲ Aricept Tablets (8%) ... 1270
▲ Aricept Tablets (8%) ... 2665
▲ Arimidex Tablets (4.9% to 6.1%) ... 659
▲ Aromasin Tablets (8%) ... 2769
▲ Artane (30% to 50%) ... 1855
Arthrotec Tablets (Rare) ... 3195
▲ Asacol Delayed-Release Tablets (8%) ... 2884
Astelin Nasal Spray (2.0%) ... 3339
▲ Atacand Tablets (4%) ... 595
Atacand HCT Tablets (2.9%) ... 597
Ativan Injection (Occasional) ... 3478
▲ Ativan Tablets (6.9%) ... 3482
Atromid-S Capsules (Less often) ... 3483
Atrovent Inhalation Aerosol (2.4%) ... 1030
Atrovent Inhalation Solution (2.3%) ... 1031
Atrovent Nasal Spray 0.03% (Less than 2%) ... 1032
Atrovent Nasal Spray 0.06% (Less than 1%) ... 1033
Attenuvax ... 2044
Augmentin Chewable Tablets (Rare) ... 1482
Augmentin Powder for Oral Suspension (Rare) ... 1482
Augmentin Tablets (Rare) ... 1485
Augmentin ES-600 Powder for Oral Suspension ... 1487
▲ Avalide Tablets (8%) ... 1070
Avapro Tablets (1% or greater) ... 1074
Avapro Tablets (1% or greater) ... 3076

(◘ Described in PDR For Nonprescription Drugs) Incidence data in parenthesis; ▲ 3% or more (⊙ Described in PDR For Ophthalmic Medicines™)

▲ Avelox Tablets (3%) 879
▲ Avonex (15%) 1013
Axert Tablets (Frequent) 2772
▲ Axid Pulvules (4.6%) 1903
▲ Axid Pulvules (4.6%) 2919
Azactam for Injection (Less than 1%) 1276
Azopt Ophthalmic Suspension (Less than 1%) 536
Azulfidine EN-tabs Tablets (Less frequent) 2775
Bactroban Cream (Less than 1%) 1494
Baycol Tablets (2.1%) 883
Benadryl Allergy/Congestion Tablets ▣692
Benadryl Allergy & Sinus Liquid ▣693
Benadryl Allergy Sinus Headache Caplets & Gelcaps ▣693
▲ Benadryl Parenteral (Among most frequent) 2617
BeneFix for Injection 1432
Benylin Multi-Symptom Liquid ▣697
Betagan (Rare) ⊙228
▲ Betapace Tablets (7% to 20%) 950
▲ Betapace AF Tablets (13.1% to 16.3%) 954
▲ Betaseron for SC Injection (35%) 988
Betaxon Ophthalmic Suspension (Less than 2%) 537
Betimol Ophthalmic Solution (1% to 5%) ⊙324
Betoptic S Ophthalmic Suspension (Rare) 537
Biaxin/Biaxin XL 403
Bicillin C-R 900/300 Injection 2240
Bicillin C-R Injection 2238
Bicillin L-A Injection 2242
Biltricide Tablets 887
Blocadren Tablets (2.3%) 2046
Bontril Slow-Release Capsules 576
▲ Botox Purified Neurotoxin Complex (2% to 10%) 549
▲ Brethine Ampuls (1.3% to 10.2%) 2314
▲ Brethine Tablets (3.5%) 2313
▲ Brevibloc Injection (3% to 12%) 858
Brevicon 28-Day Tablets 3380
Bromfed Capsules (Extended-Release) 2269
Bromfed-PD Capsules (Extended-Release) 2269
▲ Buprenex Injectable (5% to 10%) 2918
▲ Campath Ampules (1% to 12%) 992
▲ Canasa Rectal Suppositories (3%) 829
Captopril Tablets (About 0.5% to 2%) 2281
Carafate Suspension (Less than 0.5%) 731
Carafate Tablets (Less than 0.5%) 730
▲ Carbatrol Capsules (Among most frequent) 3234
Cardene I.V. (1.4%) 3485
Cardizem Injectable (Less than 1%) 1018
Cardizem Lyo-Ject Syringe (Less than 1%) 1018
Cardizem Monovial (Less than 1%) 1018
▲ Cardizem CD Capsules (3.0% to 3.5%) 1016
▲ Cardura Tablets (Up to 23%) 2668
▲ Carnitor Injection (5% to 6%) 3242
Carteolol Hydrochloride Ophthalmic Solution USP, 1% (Occasional) ⊙258
▲ Casodex Tablets (7%) 662
Cataflam Tablets (1% to 3%) 2315
▲ Catapres Tablets (About 16 in 100 patients) 1037
Catapres-TTS (2 of 101 patients) 1038
Caverject Sterile Powder (1%) 2777
Ceclor CD Tablets (0.1% to 1%) 1279
Ceclor (Rare) 1905
Cedax (1%) 1021
Ceftin Tablets (0.1% to 1%) 1898
Cefzil (1%) 1076
Celebrex Capsules (2%) 2676
Celebrex Capsules (2%) 2780
▲ Celexa (At least 2%) 1365
▲ CellCept Capsules (5.7% to 28.7%) 2951
▲ CellCept Intravenous (5.7% to 28.7%) 2951
▲ CellCept Oral Suspension (5.7% to 28.7%) 2951
▲ CellCept Tablets (5.7% to 28.7%) 2951
Celontin Capsules (Frequent) 2618
▲ Cenestin Tablets (11%) 1263
Ceptaz for Injection (Fewer than 1%) 1499
▲ Cerebyx Injection (5.0% to 31.1%) 2619
▲ Cerezyme for Injection (5.4%) 1438
▲ Chemet Capsules (1.0% to 12.7%) 3078
▲ Chirocaine Injection (5.1%) 2909
Chlor-Trimeton Allergy/Decongestant Tablets ▣736
Cipro I.V. (1% or less) 893
Cipro I.V. Pharmacy Bulk Package (Less than 1%) 897
Cipro (0.3% to 1%) 887
Claritin (At least one patient) 3100
▲ Claritin-D 12 Hour Extended Release Tablets (4%) 3102
▲ Claritin-D 24 Hour Extended Release Tablets (4%) 3104
Cleocin Vaginal Cream (Less than 1%) 2788
Climara Transdermal System 958
▲ Clinoril Tablets (3% to 9%) 2053
Clomid Tablets (Fewer than 1%) 735
▲ Clorpres Tablets (About 16%) 1002
▲ Clozaril Tablets (More than 5% to 19%) 2319
▲ Cognex Capsules (12%) 1351
Colazal Capsules (1%) 3069
Colestid Tablets (Less frequent) 2791
Coly-Mycin M Parenteral 2243
▲ CombiPatch Transdermal System (6% to 7%) 2323
▲ Combipres Tablets (About 16%) 1040
Combivent Inhalation Aerosol (Less than 2%) 1041
▲ Combivir Tablets (10%) 1502
Compazine 1505
▲ Comtan Tablets (8%) 2328
Concerta Extended-Release Tablets (2%) 1998
Concerta Tablets (2%) 561
Condylox Topical Solution (Less than 5%) 2437
Contac Non-Drowsy 12 Hour Cold Caplets ▣745
Contac Non-Drowsy Timed Release 12 Hour Cold Caplets ▣746
Contac Severe Cold and Flu Caplets Maximum Strength ▣746
Copaxone for Injection (At least 2%) 3306
▲ Cordarone Tablets (4% to 9%) 3487
▲ Coreg Tablets (6.2% to 32.4%) 1508
Corgard Tablets (2 of 100 patients) 2245
Coricidin 'D' Cold, Flu & Sinus Tablets ▣737
Coricidin HBP Cough & Cold Tablets ▣738
Corlopam Injection (1% to 2%) 412
Corzide 40/5 Tablets (2 of 100 patients) 2247
Corzide 80/5 Tablets (2 of 100 patients) 2247
Cosopt Sterile Ophthalmic Solution (1% to 5%) 2065
Coumadin for Injection (Infrequent) 1243
Coumadin Tablets (Infrequent) 1243
▲ Covera-HS Tablets (3.3% to 4.7%) 3199
▲ Cozaar Tablets (3.5%) 2067
▲ Crinone 8% Gel (5%) 3213
Crixivan Capsules (1.0%) 2070
Cyclessa Tablets 2450
Cylert Tablets 415
Cytotec Tablets (Infrequent) 3202
Cytovene (At least 3 subjects) 2959
▲ Dantrium Capsules (Among most frequent) 2885
Daranide Tablets 2077
▲ Darvon-N/Darvocet-N (Among most frequent) 1907
▲ Darvon Pulvules (Among most frequent) 1909
▲ Darvon Compound-65 Pulvules (Among most frequent) 1910
▲ Darvon-N Tablets (Among most frequent) 1912
▲ DaunoXome Injection (Up to 8%) 1442
DDAVP Nasal Spray (Up to 3%) 738
DDAVP Rhinal Tube (Up to 3%) 738
Declomycin Tablets 1855
▲ Demadex Tablets and Injection (3.2%) 2965
▲ Demerol (Among most frequent) 3079
▲ Depacon Injection (5.2% to 25%) 416
▲ Depakene (18% to 25%) 421
▲ Depakote Sprinkle Capsules (13% to 25%) 426
▲ Depakote Tablets (12% to 25%) 430
▲ Depakote ER Tablets (1% to 25%) 436
▲ Depo-Provera Contraceptive Injection (More than 5%) 2798
Desferal Vials 2333
Desmopressin Acetate Rhinal Tube (Up to 3%) 1345
Desogen Tablets 2458
Desoxyn Tablets (Rare) 440
▲ Detrol Tablets (8.6%) 3623
Detrol LA Capsules (2%) 2801
Dexedrine 1512
DextroStat Tablets 3236
D.H.E. 45 Injection (Occasional) 2334
Diflucan Tablets, Injection, and Oral Suspension (1%) 2681
▲ Digitek Tablets (6%) 1003
Dilantin Infatabs 2624
Dilantin Kapseals 2622
Dilantin-125 Oral Suspension 2625
Dilaudid 441
Dilaudid Oral Liquid 445
Dilaudid Powder 441
Dilaudid Rectal Suppositories 441
Dilaudid Tablets 441
Dilaudid Tablets - 8 mg 445
▲ Dilaudid-HP (Among most frequent) 443
Diovan Capsules (More than 1%) 2337
▲ Diovan HCT Tablets (9%) 2338
Dipentum Capsules (1.0%) 2803
Diphtheria & Tetanus Toxoids Adsorbed Purogenated for Pediatric Use 1857
Diprivan Injectable Emulsion (Less than 1%) 667
▲ Ditropan XL Extended Release Tablets (6.3%) 564
Diucardin Tablets 3494
Diuril Oral 2087
Diuril Sodium Intravenous 2086
Dolobid Tablets (Greater than 1 in 100) 2088
▲ Dolophine Hydrochloride Tablets (Among most frequent) 3056
Donnagel Liquid (Rare) ▣789
Donnatal 2929
Donnatal Extentabs 2930
Donnatal Tablets 2929
Dopram Injectable 2931
▲ Dostinex Tablets (15% to 17%) 2804
Doxil Injection (1% to 5%) 566
Drixoral Allergy/Sinus Extended-Release Tablets ▣741
Drixoral Cold & Allergy Sustained-Action Tablets ▣740
Drixoral Cold & Flu Extended-Release Tablets ▣740
▲ Duraclon Injection (13.2%) 3057
▲ Duragesic Transdermal System (3% to 10%) 1786
Duramorph Injection 1312
Duranest Injections 600
Dyazide Capsules 1515
Dynabac Tablets (2.1% to 2.6%) 2269
Dynacin Capsules 2019
▲ DynaCirc Capsules (3.4% to 8%) 2921
▲ DynaCirc CR Tablets (3.7% to 6.4%) 2923
Dyrenium Capsules (Rare) 3458
▲ EC-Naprosyn Delayed-Release Tablets (3% to 9%) 2967
Ecotrin Enteric Coated Aspirin Low, Regular and Maximum Strength Tablets 1715
▲ Effexor Tablets (3% to 23.9%) 3495
▲ Effexor XR Capsules (20%) 3499
8-MOP Capsules 1727
ELA-Max Cream 1340
▲ Eldepryl Capsules (7 of 49 patients) 3266
Elmiron Capsules (1%) 570
Emla (Unlikely with cream) 602
Enalaprilat Injection (0.5% to 1%) 863
▲ Enbrel for Injection (8%) 1752
▲ Enbrel for Injection (8%) 3504
▲ Engerix-B Vaccine (1% to 10%) 1517
EpiPen 1236
▲ Epivir (10%) 1520
▲ Epogen for Injection (5% to 12%) 582
▲ Ergamisol Tablets (3% to 4%) 1789
Ery-Tab Tablets (Isolated reports) 448
Erythrocin Stearate Filmtab Tablets (Isolated reports) 452
Erythromycin Base Filmtab Tablets (Isolated reports) 454
Erythromycin Delayed-Release Capsules, USP (Isolated reports) 455
Esclim Transdermal System 3460
Eskalith 1527
Estinyl Tablets 3112
Estrace Vaginal Cream 3358
Estrace Tablets 3361
Estratest 3252
Estring Vaginal Ring (At least 1 report) 2811
Estrostep 2627
Ethyol for Injection 2029
Etrafon 3115
▲ Evoxac Capsules (4.1%) 1217
▲ Exelon Capsules (21%) 2342
▲ Exelon Oral Solution (21%) 2345
Extendryl 1361
Famotidine Injection (1.3%) 866
▲ Famvir Tablets (3.3% to 5.5%) 2348
▲ Fareston Tablets (9%) 3237
▲ Felbatol (18.4%) 3343
▲ Feldene Capsules (1% to 10%) 2685
▲ Femara Tablets (3% to 5%) 2351
femhrt Tablets 2635
▲ Ferrlecit Injection (13%) 3386
▲ Flexeril Tablets (3% to 11%) 572
▲ Flexeril Tablets (3% to 11%) 2094
▲ Flolan for Injection (8% to 83%) 1528
▲ Flomax Capsules (14.9% to 17.1%) 1044
Flonase Nasal Spray (1% to 3%) 1533
Flovent Diskus (1% to 3%) 3614
Flovent (1% to 3%) 1535
Floxin I.V. (1% to 5%) 2526
Floxin Otic Solution (1%) 1219
Floxin Tablets (1% to 5%) 2529
Flumadine (0.7% to 1.9%) 1370
FluShield Influenza Vaccine 3521
Follistim for Injection 2465
Foradil Aerolizer (1.6%) 2354
Fortaz (Less than 1%) 1541
Fortovase Capsules (Less than 2%) 2970
▲ Foscavir Injection (5% or greater) 605
Furosemide Tablets 2284
▲ Gabitril Tablets (27% to 31%) 1189
Gamimune N, 5% Solvent/Detergent Treated 925
Gamimune N, 10% Solvent/Detergent Treated 928
Gammar-P I.V. 787
Gastrocrom Oral Concentrate (Less common) 1162
▲ Gengraf Capsules (1% to 8%) 457
▲ Geodon Capsules (8%) 2688
▲ Geref for Injection (1 patient in 6) 3215
Gliadel Wafer (2%) 1723
Glucophage XR Tablets (1% to 5%) 1080
Glucotrol Tablets (About 1 in 50) 2692
▲ Glucotrol XL Extended Release Tablets (6.8%) 2693
▲ Glucovance Tablets (5.5%) 1086
Gonal-F for Injection (2.5%) 3216
Grifulvin V Tablets Microsize and Oral Suspension Microsize (Occasional) 2518
Gris-PEG Tablets (Occasional) 2661
Guaifed 2272
▲ Halcion Tablets (7.8%) 2823
Havrix Vaccine (Rare) 1544
▲ Hectorol Capsules (11.5%) 1064
▲ Hectorol Injection (11.5%) 1066
Helixate Concentrate 788
▲ Herceptin I.V. (13%) 1414
Hexalen Capsules 2226
Hivid Tablets (Less than 1%) 2975
Humegon for Injection 2468
Hycodan 1316
Hycomine Compound Tablets 1317
Hycotuss Expectorant Syrup 1318
HydroDIURIL Tablets 2108
▲ Hytrin Capsules (2.0% to 28%) 464
▲ Hyzaar (5.7%) 2109
Ifex for Injection (Less frequent) 1123
▲ Imdur Tablets (8% to 11%) 1826
▲ Imitrex Injection (11.9%) 1549
Imitrex Nasal Spray (1% to 1.7%) 1554
Imitrex Tablets 1558
▲ Imovax Rabies Vaccine (About 20%) 807
▲ Indapamide Tablets (Greater than or equal to 5%) 2286
Inderide Tablets 3517
Inderide LA Long-Acting Capsules 3519
▲ Indocin (3% to 9%) 2112
INFeD Injection 3388
▲ Infergen (18% to 22%) 1777
Infumorph 200 and Infumorph 500 Sterile Solutions 1314
Innohep Injection (Greater than or equal to 1%) 1248
▲ Intron A for Injection (7% to 24%) 3120
Inversine Tablets 1850
Invirase Capsules (0.3% to 2.0%) 2979
Ionamin Capsules 1163
Iopidine 0.5% Ophthalmic Solution (Less than 3%) ⊙213
▲ Ismo Tablets (3% to 5%) 3524
▲ Isoptin SR Tablets (3.3%) 467
▲ JE-VAX Vaccine (Approximately 10%) 811
▲ Kadian Capsules (Among most frequent) 1335
Kaletra Capsules (Less than 2%) 471
Kaletra Oral Solution (Less than 2%) 471
Keflex 1237
▲ Keppra Tablets (9%) 3314
▲ Klonopin Tablets (1% to 8%) 2983
Kogenate 934
Kogenate FS 936
K-Phos Neutral Tablets 946
K-Phos Original (Sodium Free) Tablets (Less frequent) 947
▲ Kytril Tablets (3% to 5%) 2988
▲ Lamictal (31% to 54%) 1567
Lanoxicaps Capsules 1574
Lanoxin Injection 1581
Lanoxin Tablets 1587
Lanoxin Elixir Pediatric 1578
Lanoxin Injection Pediatric 1584
▲ Lariam Tablets (Among most frequent) 2989
Lescol Capsules (2.2%) 2361
Lescol Capsules (2.2%) 2925
Lescol XL Tablets (1.9%) 2361
Lescol XL Tablets (1.9%) 2925
▲ Leustatin Injection (9%) 2495
Levaquin (0.3% to 2.5%) 2537
Levbid Extended-Release Tablets 3172
Levlen 962
Levlite 21 Tablets 962
Levlite 28 Tablets 962
Levo-Dromoran 1734
Levora Tablets 3389
▲ Levorphanol Tartrate Tablets (Greater than 10%) 3059
Levsin/Levsinex/Levbid 3172
▲ Lexxel Tablets (4.4%) 608
Lidoderm Patch 1319
▲ Limbitrol (Among most frequent) 1738
Lindane Lotion USP 1% 559
Lindane Shampoo USP 1% 560
Lithium Carbonate 3061
Lithium Citrate Syrup 3061
Lithobid Slow-Release Tablets 3255
▲ Lodine (3% to 9%) 3528
▲ Lodine XL Extended-Release Tablets (3% to 9%) 3530

Lodosyn Tablets 1251
Loestrin 21 Tablets 2642
Loestrin Fe Tablets 2642
Lo/Ovral Tablets 3532
Lo/Ovral-28 Tablets 3538
Lopid Tablets 2650
Lorabid Suspension and Pulvules 2251
▲ Lortab (Among most frequent) 3319
▲ Lortab Elixir (Among most frequent) 3317
▲ Lotensin Tablets (3.6%) 2365
▲ Lotensin HCT Tablets (6.3%) 2367
Lotrel Capsules (1.3%) 2370
Low-Ogestrel-28 Tablets 3392
Loxitane Capsules 3398
Lunelle Monthly Injection 2827
Lupron Depot 3.75 mg (Less than 5%) 3281
▲ Lupron Depot–3 Month 11.25 mg (1.8% to 11%) 3285
▲ Lupron Depot–3 Month 22.5 mg (6.4%) 3288
▲ Lupron Depot–4 Month 30 mg (6.1% to 8.3%) 3289
▲ Lupron Injection (5% or more) 3279
▲ Luvox Tablets (25, 50, 100 mg) (2% to 11%) 3256
LYMErix Vaccine (1.02% to 1.1%) 1592
Macrobid Capsules (Less than 1%) 2889
▲ Malarone (5%) 1596
▲ Marinol Capsules (3% to 10%) 3325
Matulane Capsules 3246
▲ Mavik Tablets (1.3% to 23%) 478
Maxair Autohaler (0.6% to 1.2%) 1981
Maxair Inhaler (0.6% to 1.2%) 1984
▲ Maxalt Tablets (4% to 9%) 2120
▲ Maxalt-MLT Orally Disintegrating Tablets (4% to 9%) 2120
▲ Maxidone Tablets CIII (Among most frequent) 3399
Maxzide 1008
Menest Tablets 2254
▲ Mepergan Injection (Among most frequent) 3539
Mephyton Tablets (Rare) 2129
▲ Mepron Suspension (3% to 8%) 1598
▲ Meridia Capsules (7%) 481
Merrem I.V. (0.1% to 1.0%) 673
Meruvax II 2130
Metadate CD Capsules 1164
Metadate ER Tablets 1167
Methylin Tablets 1995
Methylin ER Tablets 1995
MetroGel-Vaginal Gel (2%) 1986
Mevacor Tablets (0.5% to 2.0%) 2132
▲ Mexitil Capsules (18.9% to 26.4%) 1047
Miacalcin Nasal Spray (1% to 3%) 2375
Micardis Tablets (1%) 1049
▲ Micardis HCT Tablets (5%) 1051
Microgestin Fe 1.5/30 Tablets 3407
Microgestin Fe 1/20 Tablets 3400
Micronor Tablets 2543
Microzide Capsules 3414
Midamor Tablets (Between 1% and 3%) 2136
Midrin Capsules 3464
▲ Migranal Nasal Spray (4%) 2376
Miltown Tablets 3349
▲ Minipress Capsules (10.3%) 2699
▲ Minizide Capsules (10.3%) 2700
Minocin Intravenous 1862
Minocin Oral Suspension 1865
Minocin Pellet-Filled Capsules 1863
Mintezol 2137
▲ Mirapex Tablets (25% to 26%) 2834
Mircette Tablets 2470
M-M-R II 2118
Mobic Tablets (1.1% to 3.8%) 1054
Modicon 2563
▲ Moduretic Tablets (3% to 8%) 2138
▲ Monopril Tablets (1.6% to 11.9%) 1091
▲ Monopril HCT (3.2%) 1094
Monurol Sachet (1.3% to 2.3%) 1375
▲ Motofen Tablets (1 in 20) 577
▲ Motrin Suspension, Oral Drops, Chewable Tablets, and Caplets (3% to 9%) 2002
Motrin Sinus Headache Caplets 2005
▲ MS Contin Tablets (Among most frequent) 2896
▲ MSIR (Among most frequent) 2898
MUSE Urethral Suppository (2%) 3335
Myambutol Tablets 1290
▲ Mykrox Tablets (10.2%) 1168
Mylocel Tablets (Extremely rate) 2227
▲ Mylotarg for Injection (9% to 22%) 3540
▲ Myobloc Injectable Solution (3% to 6%) 1291
Nadolol Tablets (2 of 100 patients) 2288
Naprelan Tablets (Less than 3%) 1293
▲ Naprosyn Suspension (3% to 9%) 2967
▲ Naprosyn Tablets (3% to 9%) 2967
Nardil Tablets (Common) 2653
Naropin Injection (1% to 5%) 612
Nascobal Gel 3174
▲ Natrecor for Injection (3%) 3189
Nebcin Vials, Hyporets & ADD-Vantage 1955
Necon 3415
Nembutal Sodium Solution (Less than 1%) 485
▲ Neoral Soft Gelatin Capsules (1% to 8%) 2380
▲ Neoral Oral Solution (1% to 8%) 2380
Nesacaine/Nesacaine MPF 617
▲ Neumega for Injection (38%) 1434
▲ Neurontin Capsules (17.1%) 2655
▲ Neurontin Oral Solution (2.4% to 17.1%) 2655
▲ Neurontin Tablets (17.1%) 2655
Nexium Delayed-Release Capsules (Less than 1%) 619
Niaspan Extended-Release Tablets 1846
▲ Nicotrol Nasal Spray (Over 5%) 2843
▲ Nilandron Tablets (10%) 753
Nimotop Capsules (Less than 1%) 904
▲ Nipent for Injection (3% to 10%) 3272
Nitrolingual Pumpspray (Occasional) 1355
Nizoral Tablets (Less than 1%) 1791
Nolvadex Tablets (Infrequent) 678
▲ Norco 5/325 Tablets CIII (Among most frequent) 3424
▲ Norco 7.5/325 Tablets CIII (Among most frequent) 3425
▲ Norco 10/325 Tablets CIII (Among most frequent) 3425
▲ Norco 10/325 Tablets CIII (Among most frequent) 3427
Nordette-28 Tablets 2257
Norflex 1987
Norinyl 1 +35 28-Day Tablets 3380
Norinyl 1 + 50 28-Day Tablets 3380
▲ Normodyne Injection (9%) 3135
▲ Normodyne Tablets (1% to 16%) 3137
Noroxin Tablets (1.7% to 2.6%) 2145
Norplant System 3543
Norpramin Tablets 755
Nor-QD Tablets 3423
Norvasc Tablets (0.1% to 3.4%) 2704
Norvir Capsules (2.6% to 3.3%) 487
Norvir Oral Solution (2.6% to 3.3%) 487
▲ Nubain Injection (5%) 1323
NuLev Orally Disintegrating Tablets 3176
Ocuflox Ophthalmic Solution (Rare) 554
Ocupress Ophthalmic Solution, 1% Sterile (Occasional) .... ⊙303
Ogen Tablets 2846
Ogestrel 0.5/50-28 Tablets 3428
Omnicef (0.2%) 493
Oncaspar (Less than 1%) 756
OptiPranolol Metipranolol Ophthalmic Solution 0.3% (A small number of patients) .... ⊙263
▲ Oramorph SR Tablets (Among most frequent) 3062
Orap Tablets 1407
Organidin NR Liquid (Rare) 3350
Organidin NR Tablets (Rare) 3350
Orgaran Injection (2.3%) 2480
Ortho Diaphragm Kits – All-Flex Arcing Spring; Ortho Coil Spring 2552
Ortho Dienestrol Cream 2554
Ortho-Cept 21 Tablets 2546
Ortho-Cept 28 Tablets 2546
Orthoclone OKT3 Sterile Solution 2498
Ortho-Cyclen/Ortho Tri-Cyclen 2573
Ortho-Est Tablets 3464
Ortho-Novum 2563
Ortho-Novum 1/50□28 Tablets 2556
▲ Ortho-Prefest Tablets (5%) 2570
Ortho-Cyclen/Ortho Tri-Cyclen 2573
Orudis Capsules (Greater than 1%) 3548
Oruvail Capsules (Greater than 1%) 3548
Ovcon 3364
Ovidrel for Injection (Less than 2%) 3220
Ovral Tablets 3551
Ovral-28 Tablets 3552
Ovrette Tablets 3552
Oxsoralen-Ultra Capsules 1741
▲ OxyContin Tablets (13%) 2912
▲ OxyFast Oral Concentrate Solution (Among most frequent) 2916
▲ OxyIR Capsules (Among most frequent) 2916
▲ Pacerone Tablets (4% to 9%) 3331
Parafon Forte DSC Caplets (Occasional) 2582
Parnate Tablets 1607
▲ Paxil (1% to 14%) 1609
Pediazole Suspension 3050
▲ PEG-Intron Powder for Injection (12%) 3140
Pentasa Capsules (Less than 1%) 3239
Pepcid Injection (1.3%) 2153
Pepcid for Oral Suspension (1.3%) 2150
Pepcid RPD Orally Disintegrating Tablets (1.3%) 2150
Pepcid Tablets (1.3%) 2150
▲ Percocet Tablets (Among most frequent) 1326
▲ Percodan Tablets (Among most frequent) 1327
▲ Percolone Tablets (Among most frequent) 1327
Pergonal for Injection 3223
Periactin Tablets 2155
▲ Permax Tablets (19.1%) 1299
▲ Persantine Tablets (13.6%) 1057
Phenergan Injection 3553
Phenergan Suppositories 3556
Phenergan Syrup 3554
Phenergan Tablets 3556
Phenergan with Codeine Syrup 3557
Phenergan with Dextromethorphan Syrup 3559
Phenergan VC Syrup 3560
Phenergan VC with Codeine Syrup 3561
▲ Phrenilin (Among most frequent) 578
Pipracil 1866
Plaquenil Tablets 3082
▲ Plavix Tablets (6.2%) 1097
▲ Plavix Tablets (6.2%) 3084
Plendil Extended-Release Tablets (2.7% to 3.7%) 623
▲ Pletal Tablets (9% to 10%) 2605
▲ Pletal Tablets (9% to 10%) 2848
Polocaine Injection, USP 625
Polocaine-MPF Injection, USP 625
▲ Ponstel Capsules (1% to 10%) 1356
Pravachol Tablets (1.0% to 3.3%) 1099
Premarin Intravenous 3563
Premarin Tablets 3566
Premarin Vaginal Cream 3570
Premphase Tablets 3572
▲ Prempro Tablets (3% to 5%) 3572
Prevacid Delayed-Release Capsules (Less than 1%) 3292
PREVPAC (Less than 1% to 3%) 3298
Priftin Tablets (1.1%) 758
Prilosec Delayed-Release Capsules (1.5%) 628
Primaxin I.M. 2158
Primaxin I.V. (0.3%) 2160
▲ Prinivil Tablets (5.4% to 11.8%) 2164
▲ Prinzide Tablets (7.5%) 2168
ProAmatine Tablets (Rare) 3241
Procanbid Extended-Release Tablets (Occasional) 2262
▲ Procardia Capsules (Approximately 10% to 27%) 2708
▲ Procardia XL Extended Release Tablets (4.1% to 27%) 2710
▲ Procrit for Injection (5% to 21%) 2502
▲ Prograf (3% to 19%) 1393
Prolastin (0.19%) 943
▲ Proleukin for Injection (11%) 1199
▲ Prometrium Capsules (100 mg, 200 mg) (16% to 24%) 3261
Prosed/DS Tablets 3268
▲ ProSom Tablets (7%) 500
Prostigmin Injectable 1744
Prostigmin Tablets 1744
Prostin E2 Suppositories 2852
Protonix I.V. (Greater than 1%) 3580
Protonix Tablets (Greater than or equal to 1%) 3577
Protopam Chloride for Injection 3582
Protopic Ointment (Greater than or equal to 1%) 1397
Proventil Inhalation Aerosol (Less than 5%) 3142
▲ Proventil Inhalation Solution 0.083% (7%) 3146
Proventil Repetabs Tablets (2%) 3148
▲ Proventil Solution for Inhalation 0.5% (7%) 3144
Proventil HFA Inhalation Aerosol (Less than 3%) 3150
Provera Tablets 2953
▲ Prozac Pulvules, Liquid, and Weekly Capsules (10%) 1238
▲ Quinaglute Dura-Tabs Tablets (3%) 978
▲ Rabies Vaccine RabAvert (15%) 1203
▲ Rapamune Oral Solution and Tablets (3% to 20%) 3584
▲ Rebetron Combination Therapy (6% to 17%) 3153
ReFacto Vials 1437
Reglan (Less frequent) 2935
▲ Relafen Tablets (3% to 9%) 1617
Relenza Rotadisk (1% to 2%) 1619
▲ Remeron Tablets (7%) 2483
▲ Remeron SolTab Tablets (7%) 2486
▲ Remicade for IV Injection (8% to 10%) 1178
▲ Reminyl Oral Solution (1% to 9%) 1792
▲ Reminyl Tablets (1% to 9%) 1792
Renese Tablets 2712
ReoPro Vials (2.9%) 1958
Repronex for Intramuscular and Subcutaneous Injection 1347
▲ Requip Tablets (26% to 40%) 1621
Rescriptor Tablets (Less than 2%) 526
Rescula Ophthalmic Solution (1% to 5%) .... ⊙306
▲ Retrovir Capsules (6% to 17.9%) 1625
▲ Retrovir IV Infusion (6% to 17.9%) 1629
▲ Retrovir (6% to 17.9%) 1625
Rifadin 765
Rifamate Capsules 767
Rifater Tablets 769
▲ Rilutek Tablets (5.1% to 12.7%) 772
▲ Risperdal (4% to 7%) 1796
Ritalin 2387
▲ Rituxan for Infusion (7%) 1750
▲ Rituxan I.V. (7%) 1428
Robaxin Injectable 2938
Robaxin Tablets 2939
▲ Robaxisal Tablets (One in 20 to 25) 2939
Robinul Forte Tablets 1358
Robinul Injectable 2940
Robinul Tablets 1358
Robitussin Maximum Strength Cough & Cold Liquid .... ■785
Robitussin Pediatric Cough & Cold Formula Liquid .... ■785
Robitussin-CF Liquid .... ■783
Robitussin-DAC Syrup 2942
Robitussin-PE Liquid .... ■782
Rocephin Injectable Vials, ADD-Vantage, Galaxy, Bulk (Occasional) 2993
▲ Roferon-A Injection (11% to 40%) 2996
▲ Romazicon Injection (1% to 9%) 3000
Rowasa Rectal Suspension Enema 4.0 grams/unit (60 mL) (1.84%) 3264
▲ Roxanol (Among most frequent) 3066
▲ Roxicodone (Among most frequent) 3067
Ryna .... ■768
Ryna-12 S Suspension 3351
Reformulated Rynatan Pediatric Suspension 3352
▲ Rynatan Tablets (Among most common) 3351
▲ Rythmol Tablets – 150 mg, 225 mg, 300 mg (6.5% to 15.1%) 502
▲ Salagen Tablets (5% to 12%) 2229
Sandoglobulin I.V. 2391
▲ Sandostatin Injection (5%) 2394
▲ Sarafem Pulvules (7% to 11%) 1962
▲ Sectral Capsules (6%) 3589
▲ Sedapap Tablets 50 mg/650 mg (Among the most frequent) 2225
▲ Semprex-D Capsules (3%) 1172
Sensorcaine (Rare) 643
Sensorcaine-MPF Injection (Rare) 643
Serentil 1057
Serophene Tablets (Less than 1 in 100 patients) 3226
▲ Seroquel Tablets (10%) 684
▲ Serostim for Injection (1% to 10%) 3229
▲ Serzone Tablets (11% to 22%) 1104
▲ Simulect for Injection (Greater than or equal to 10%) 2399
Sinemet Tablets 1253
Sinemet CR Tablets (2.9%) 1255
Sinequan (Occasional) 2713
Singulair (1.9%) 2181
Sinutab Non-Drying Liquid Caps .... ■706
Skelaxin Tablets 1301
▲ Skelid Tablets (4.0%) 3088
Soma Tablets 3353
Soma Compound Tablets (Very rare to less frequent) 3354
Soma Compound w/Codeine Tablets 3355
▲ Sonata Capsules (7% to 8%) 3591
Soriatane Capsules (Less than 1%) 3003
Sporanox Capsules (1.7% to 4%) 1800
Sporanox Injection (1%) 1804
Sporanox Injection (1%) 2509
Sporanox Oral Solution (1.5% to 2.0%) 1808
Sporanox Oral Solution (1.5% to 2.0%) 2512
▲ Stadol NS Nasal Spray (19%) 1108
Starlix Tablets (2.2%) 2401
Stelazine 1640
Stimate Nasal Spray 796
Stromectol Tablets (2.8%) 2185
Sudafed 12 Hour Tablets .... ■708
Sudafed 24 Hour Tablets .... ■708
Children's Sudafed Cold & Cough Liquid .... ■709
Sudafed Cold & Allergy Tablets .... ■708
Sudafed Nasal Decongestant Tablets .... ■710
Sudafed Sinus Headache Caplets .... ■712
Sudafed Sinus Headache Tablets .... ■712
▲ Sular Tablets (5%) 688
Suprane Liquid for Inhalation (Less than 1%) 874
Suprax (Less than 2%) 1877
Surmontil Capsules 3595
▲ Sustiva Capsules (2% to 10%) 1258
▲ Symmetrel (5% to 10%) 1328
Synercid I.V. (Less than 1%) 775
Synvisc 3596
Tagamet (Approximately 1 in 100) 1644
Talacen Caplets 3089
Talwin Nx Tablets 3090
▲ Tambocor Tablets (18.9%) 1990
▲ Tamiflu Capsules (1.6% to 2.1%) 3008
▲ Tamiflu Oral Suspension (1.6% to 2.1%) 3008
▲ Tarka Tablets (3.1%) 508
▲ Tasmar Tablets (6% to 13%) 3010
Tazicef for Injection (Less than 1%) 1647
Tazicef Galaxy Container (Less than 1%) 1650
Tazicef Pharmacy Bulk Package (Less than 1%) 1653

Tazidime Vials, Faspak & ADD-Vantage (Less than 1%)........ 1966
▲ Tegretol/Tegretol-XR (Among most frequent)........ 2404
▲ Temodar Capsules (12%)........ 3157
▲ Tenex Tablets (1% to 15%)........ 2942
▲ Tenoretic Tablets (4% to 13%)........ 690
▲ Tenormin (4% to 13%)........ 692
▲ Tequin Injection (3%)........ 1110
▲ Tequin Tablets (3%)........ 1110
Tessalon Capsules........ 1377
Tetanus & Diphtheria Toxoids Adsorbed for Adult Use........ 1880
Teveten Tablets (1% or greater)........ 3327
▲ Thalomid Capsules (4.2%)........ 1154
TheraCys Injection (1%)........ 823
TheraFlu Regular Strength Cold & Cough Night Time Hot Liquid........ ▣676
TheraFlu Regular Strength Cold & Sore Throat Night Time Hot Liquid........ ▣676
TheraFlu Maximum Strength Flu & Cough Night Time Hot Liquid........ ▣678
TheraFlu Maximum Strength Severe Cold & Congestion Night Time Caplets........ ▣678
TheraFlu Maximum Strength Severe Cold & Congestion Night Time Hot Liquid........ ▣678
Thioplex for Injection........ 1765
Thorazine........ 1656
▲ Thrombate III (7 of 17)........ 944
▲ Thymoglobulin for Injection (8.5%)........ 3071
Thyrogen for Injection (1.6%)........ 1441
▲ Tiazac Capsules (5%)........ 1378
Tice BCG, BCG Live (2.4%)........ 2489
Ticlid Tablets (1.1%)........ 3015
▲ Tikosyn Capsules (8%)........ 2717
Timentin Injection- ADD-Vantage Vial........ 1661
Timentin Injection-Galaxy Container........ 1664
Timentin Injection-Pharmacy Bulk Package........ 1666
Timentin for Intravenous Administration........ 1658
Timolide Tablets (1.2%)........ 2187
Timolol GFS (1% to 5%)........ ⊙266
Timoptic in Ocudose (Less frequent)........ 2192
Timoptic Sterile Ophthalmic Solution (Less frequent)........ 2190
Timoptic-XE Sterile Ophthalmic Gel Forming Solution (1% to 5%)........ 2194
▲ TOBI Solution for Inhalation (5.8%)........ 1206
▲ Tolectin (3% to 9%)........ 2589
▲ Tonocard Tablets (8.0% to 25.3%)........ 649
▲ Topamax Sprinkle Capsules (28.3% to 32.4%)........ 2590
▲ Topamax Tablets (28.3% to 32.4%)........ 2590
▲ Toprol-XL Tablets (1.8% to about 10 of 100 patients)........ 651
▲ Toradol (7%)........ 3018
Transderm Scōp Transdermal Therapeutic System (Infrequent)........ 2302
Tranxene (Less common)........ 511
Trasylol Injection (1% to 2%)........ 909
Trecator-SC Tablets........ 3598
Trental Tablets (1.9%)........ 784
Triaminic Allergy Congestion Liquid........ ▣680
Triaminic Chest Congestion Liquid........ ▣680
Triaminic Cold & Allergy Liquid........ ▣681
Triaminic Cold & Allergy Softchews........ ▣683
Triaminic Cold & Cough Liquid........ ▣681
Triaminic Cold & Night Time Cough Liquid........ ▣681
Triaminic Cold, Cough & Fever Liquid........ ▣681
Triaminic Cough Liquid........ ▣682
Triaminic Cough & Congestion Liquid........ ▣682
Triaminic Cough & Sore Throat Liquid........ ▣682
Triaminic Cough & Sore Throat Softchews........ ▣684
Tricor Capsules, Micronized (2%)........ 513
Trilafon (Rare)........ 3160
▲ Trileptal Oral Suspension (8% to 49%)........ 2407
▲ Trileptal Tablets (8% to 49%)........ 2407
Tri-Levlen........ 962
Trilisate (Less than 2%)........ 2901
Tri-Norinyl-28 Tablets........ 3433
Triphasil-21 Tablets........ 3600
Triphasil-28 Tablets........ 3605
▲ Trisenox Injection (23%)........ 1158
Trivora Tablets........ 3439
▲ Trizivir Tablets (10%)........ 1669
Trovan (2%)........ 2722
Trusopt Sterile Ophthalmic Solution........ 2196
Tussionex Pennkinetic Extended-Release Suspension........ 1174
Tussi-Organidin NR Liquid........ 3350
Tussi-Organidin DM NR Liquid (Rare)........ 3350
Tussi-Organidin DM-S NR Liquid (Rare)........ 3350
Tussi-Organidin-S NR Liquid........ 3350
Twinrix Vaccine (Less than 1%)........ 1674
Children's Tylenol Cold Suspension Liquid and Chewable Tablets........ 2015
Multi-Symptom Tylenol Cold Complete Formula Caplets........ 2010
Multi-Symptom Tylenol Cold Non-Drowsy Caplets and Gelcaps........ 2010
Maximum Strength Tylenol Flu NightTime Liquid........ 2011
Maximum Strength Tylenol Sinus NightTime Caplets........ 2012
Maximum Strength Tylenol Sinus Non-Drowsy Geltabs, Gelcaps, Caplets, and Tablets........ 2012
▲ Tylenol with Codeine (Among most frequent)........ 2595
▲ Tylox Capsules (Among most frequent)........ 2597
Ultracet Tablets (At least 1%)........ 2597
▲ Ultram Tablets (26% to 33%)........ 2600
Uniretic Tablets (Less than 1% to 1.4%)........ 3178
▲ Univasc Tablets (4.3%)........ 3181
Urecholine........ 2198
Urimax Tablets........ 1769
Urised Tablets........ 2876
Uroqid-Acid No. 2 Tablets........ 947
Valcyte Tablets........ 3022
▲ Valstar Sterile Solution for Intravesical Instillation (3%)........ 1175
Valtrex Caplets (2% to 3%)........ 1676
Vancocin HCl Capsules & Pulvules (Rare)........ 1972
Vancocin HCl Oral Solution (Rare)........ 1971
Vancocin HCl, Vials & ADD-Vantage (Rare)........ 1970
Vaniqa Cream (1.3%)........ 1121
Vantin Tablets and Oral Suspension (Less than 1%)........ 2860
▲ Vascor Tablets (11.63% to 27.27%)........ 2602
▲ Vaseretic Tablets (8.6%)........ 2204
Vasotec I.V. Injection (0.5% to 1%)........ 2207
▲ Vasotec Tablets (4.3% to 7.9%)........ 2210
Venofer Injection (Greater than 1%)........ 580
Ventolin Inhalation Aerosol and Refill (Less than 5%)........ 1679
Ventolin HFA Inhalation Aerosol (Less than 3%)........ 3618
▲ Verelan Capsules (3.3% to 4.2%)........ 3184
▲ Verelan PM Capsules (3% to 3.3%)........ 3186
Versed Injection (Less than 1%)........ 3027
▲ Vesanoid Capsules (20%)........ 3037
Viadur Implant (Less than 2%)........ 912
Viagra Tablets (2%)........ 2732
Vicks 44D Cough & Head Congestion Relief Liquid........ ▣724
Vicks 44M Cough, Cold & Flu Relief Liquid........ ▣725
Pediatric Vicks 44m Cough & Cold Relief........ ▣728
Vicks DayQuil LiquiCaps/Liquid Multi-Symptom Cold/Flu Relief........ ▣727
Children's Vicks NyQuil Cold/Cough Relief........ ▣726
Vicks NyQuil LiquiCaps/Liquid Multi-Symptom Cold/Flu Relief, Original and Cherry Flavors........ ▣727
Vicodin Tablets........ 516
▲ Vicodin ES Tablets (Among most frequent)........ 517
▲ Vicodin HP Tablets (Among most frequent)........ 518
Vicodin Tuss Expectorant........ 519
▲ Vicoprofen Tablets (14%)........ 520
Vioxx (2.2%)........ 2213
Viracept........ 532
Visicol Tablets........ 1767
Vistide Injection........ 1445
Vitravene for Injection (2% to 5%)........ ⊙310
Vivactil Tablets........ 2217
Vivactil Tablets........ 2446
Vivelle Transdermal System........ 2412
Vivelle-Dot Transdermal System........ 2416
Volmax Extended-Release Tablets (1.5%)........ 2276
Voltaren Ophthalmic Sterile Ophthalmic Solution (Less than 3%)........ ⊙312
Voltaren Tablets (1% to 3%)........ 2315
Voltaren-XR Tablets (1% to 3%)........ 2315
Warfarin Sodium Tablets, USP........ 3302
▲ Wellbutrin Tablets (22.3%)........ 1680
▲ Wellbutrin SR Sustained-Release Tablets (7% to 11%)........ 1684
WinRho SDF........ 2297
▲ Xanax Tablets (1.8% to 29.8%)........ 2865
Xeloda Tablets........ 3039
▲ Xenical Capsules (5.2%)........ 3043
Xopenex Inhalation Solution (1.4% to 2.7%)........ 3207
▲ Xylocaine Injections (Among most common)........ 653
Yasmin 28 Tablets (Greater than 1%)........ 980
▲ Zanaflex Tablets (16% to 45%)........ 1305
Zantac (Rare)........ 1690
Zantac Injection (Rare)........ 1688
Zantac Syrup (Rare)........ 1690
Zarontin Capsules........ 2659
Zarontin Syrup........ 2660
Zaroxolyn Tablets........ 1177
▲ Zebeta Tablets (2.9% to 3.5%)........ 1885
▲ Zenapax for Injection (Greater than 5%)........ 3046
Zephrex Tablets........ 3091
Zephrex LA Tablets........ 3092
▲ Zestoretic Tablets (7.5%)........ 695
▲ Zestril Tablets (5.4% to 11.8%)........ 698
▲ Ziac Tablets (3.2% to 5.1%)........ 1887
Zithromax Capsules, 250 mg (1% or less)........ 2743
Zithromax for IV Infusion (1.9%)........ 2748
Zithromax for Oral Suspension, 1 g (1% or less)........ 2743
Zithromax for Oral Suspension, 300 mg, 600 mg, 900 mg, 1200 mg (1% or less)........ 2739
Zithromax Tablets, 250 mg (1% or less)........ 2739
Zithromax Tablets, 600 mg (1% or less)........ 2743
Zocor Tablets........ 2219
▲ Zofran Injection (12%)........ 1698
▲ Zofran (4% to 7%)........ 1703
▲ Zofran ODT Orally Disintegrating Tablets (4% to 7%)........ 1703
▲ Zoladex (5% to 6%)........ 702
Zoladex 3-month (1% to 5%)........ 706
▲ Zoloft (Infrequent to 13%)........ 2751
▲ Zomig Tablets (6% to 10%)........ 708
▲ Zomig-ZMT Tablets (6% to 10%)........ 708
▲ Zonegran Capsules (13%)........ 1307
Zosyn (1.4%)........ 1890
Zosyn in Galaxy Containers (1.4%)........ 1894
Zovia........ 3449
Zovirax Capsules........ 1706
Zovirax for Injection........ 1708
Zovirax........ 1706
▲ Zyban Sustained-Release Tablets (8% to 10%)........ 1710
▲ Zydone Tablets (Among most frequent)........ 1330
Zyflo Filmtab Tablets (Less common)........ 524
▲ Zyprexa Tablets (11% to 18%)........ 1973
▲ Zyprexa ZYDIS Orally Disintegrating Tablets (11% to 18%)........ 1973
Zyrtec (2%)........ 2756
Zyrtec-D 12 Hour Extended Relief Tablets........ 2758
Zyvox (2%)........ 2871

Dorsocervical fat enlargement

Agenerase Capsules (1 patient)........ 1454
Agenerase Oral Solution (1 patient)........ 1459
Crixivan Capsules........ 2070
Fortovase Capsules........ 2970

Down's syndrome

Pergonal for Injection........ 3223
Repronex for Intramuscular and Subcutaneous Injection........ 1347
Serophene Tablets (Six cases)........ 3226

Dreaming

Amerge Tablets (Rare)........ 1467
Dilaudid Oral Liquid (Less frequent)........ 445
Dilaudid Tablets - 8 mg (Less frequent)........ 445
Limbitrol (Less common)........ 1738
MS Contin Tablets (Less frequent)........ 2896
MSIR (Less frequent)........ 2898
Nicotrol Nasal Spray (Under 5%)........ 2843
▲ Orudis Capsules (3% to 9%)........ 3548
▲ Oruvail Capsules (3% to 9%)........ 3548
Tenoretic Tablets (Up to 3%)........ 690
Tenormin (Up to 3%)........ 692
Versed Injection (Less than 1%)........ 3027

Dreaming abnormalities

Aciphex Tablets........ 1267
Aciphex Tablets........ 1783
Actiq (Less than 1%)........ 1184
Ambien Tablets (1%)........ 3191
Anaprox Tablets (Less than 1%)........ 2967
Anaprox DS Tablets (Less than 1%)........ 2967
Anzemet Injection (Infrequently)........ 719
Anzemet Tablets (Infrequently)........ 722
▲ Aricept Tablets (3%)........ 1270
▲ Aricept Tablets (3%)........ 2665
Arthrotec Tablets (Rare)........ 3195
Axert Tablets (Rare)........ 2772
Axid Pulvules (1.9%)........ 1903
Axid Pulvules (1.9%)........ 2919
Blocadren Tablets (Less than 1%)........ 2046
Buprenex Injectable (Less than 1%)........ 2918
Cardizem Injectable........ 1018
Cardizem Lyo-Ject Syringe........ 1018
Cardizem Monovial........ 1018
Cardizem CD Capsules (Less than 1%)........ 1016
Catapres Tablets........ 1037
Catapres-TTS (0.5% or less)........ 1038
Clorpres Tablets........ 1002
Cognex Capsules (Infrequent)........ 1351
Combipres Tablets........ 1040
Copaxone for Injection (Frequent)........ 3306
Cozaar Tablets (Less than 1%)........ 2067
Crixivan Capsules (Less than 2%)........ 2070
Cytovene (At least 3 subjects)........ 2959
Depacon Injection (1% to 5%)........ 416
Depakene (1% to 5%)........ 421
Depakote Sprinkle Capsules (1% to 5%)........ 426
Depakote Tablets (1% to 5%)........ 430
Depakote ER Tablets (1% to 5%)........ 436
Dilaudid-HP (Less frequent)........ 443
Diprivan Injectable Emulsion (Less than 1%)........ 667
Duraclon Injection (Rare)........ 3057
Duragesic Transdermal System (1% or greater)........ 1786
EC-Naprosyn Delayed-Release Tablets (Less than 1%)........ 2967
▲ Effexor Tablets (4%)........ 3495
▲ Effexor XR Capsules (4% to 7%)........ 3499
▲ Eldepryl Capsules (2 of 49 patients)........ 3266
Emadine Ophthalmic Solution (Less than 5%)........ ⊙211
Enalaprilat Injection........ 863
Etrafon........ 3115
Evoxac Capsules (Less than 1%)........ 1217
Exelon Capsules (Infrequent)........ 2342
Exelon Oral Solution (Infrequent)........ 2345
Feldene Capsules (Occasional)........ 2685
Flexeril Tablets (Less than 1%)........ 572
Flexeril Tablets (Less than 1%)........ 2094
Floxin I.V. (Less than 1%)........ 2526
Floxin Tablets (Less than 1%)........ 2529
Fortovase Capsules (Less than 2%)........ 2970
Gabitril Tablets (Infrequent)........ 1189
Halcion Tablets (Rare)........ 2823
Hyzaar........ 2109
Inderal........ 3513
Inderal LA Long-Acting Capsules........ 3516
Inderide Tablets........ 3517
Intron A for Injection (Less than 5%)........ 3120
Invirase Capsules (Less than 2%)........ 2979
Iopidine Sterile Ophthalmic Solution........ ⊙212
Kadian Capsules (Less than 3%)........ 1335
Kaletra Capsules (Less than 2%)........ 471
Kaletra Oral Solution (Less than 2%)........ 471
Klonopin Tablets (Infrequent)........ 2983
Lamictal (Infrequent)........ 1567
Levaquin (Less than 0.3%)........ 2537
Levo-Dromoran........ 1734
Levorphanol Tartrate Tablets (1% to 3%)........ 3059
Lipitor Tablets (Less than 2%)........ 2639
Lipitor Tablets (Less than 2%)........ 2696
Lodine XL Extended-Release Tablets (Less than 1%)........ 3530
Lodosyn Tablets........ 1251
Lotensin HCT Tablets (0.3% or more)........ 2367
Luvox Tablets (25, 50, 100 mg)........ 3256
Maxalt Tablets (Infrequent)........ 2120
Maxalt-MLT Orally Disintegrating Tablets (Infrequent)........ 2120
Meridia Capsules........ 481
▲ Mirapex Tablets (11%)........ 2834
Motrin Suspension, Oral Drops, Chewable Tablets, and Caplets (Less than 1%)........ 2002
▲ Naprelan Tablets (3% to 9%)........ 1293
Naprosyn Suspension (Less than 1%)........ 2967
Naprosyn Tablets (Less than 1%)........ 2967
Neurontin Capsules (Infrequent)........ 2655
Neurontin Oral Solution (Infrequent)........ 2655
Neurontin Tablets (Infrequent)........ 2655
Nipent for Injection (Less than 3%)........ 3272
Norvasc Tablets (More than 0.1% to 1%)........ 2704
Norvir Capsules (Less than 2%)........ 487
Norvir Oral Solution (Less than 2%)........ 487
Nubain Injection (1% or less)........ 1323
Oramorph SR Tablets (Less frequent)........ 3062
Orap Tablets (2.7%)........ 1407
OxyContin Tablets (Between 1% and 5%)........ 2912
▲ Paxil (4%)........ 1609
Permax Tablets (2.7%)........ 1299
Ponstel Capsules (Occasional)........ 1356
Prilosec Delayed-Release Capsules (Less than 1%)........ 628
▲ Prograf (3% to 15%)........ 1393
ProSom Tablets (2%)........ 500
Protonix I.V. (Less than 1%)........ 3580
Protonix Tablets (Less than 1%)........ 3577
▲ Prozac Pulvules, Liquid, and Weekly Capsules (Less than 1% to 5%)........ 1238
▲ Remeron Tablets (4%)........ 2483
▲ Remeron SolTab Tablets (4%)........ 2486
▲ Requip Tablets (11%)........ 1621
Rescriptor Tablets (Less than 2%)........ 526
Rilutek Tablets (Rare)........ 772
Risperdal (Frequent)........ 1796

Rythmol Tablets – 150 mg, 225 mg, 300 mg (Less than 1%) 502
Salagen Tablets (Less than 1%) 2229
▲ Sarafem Pulvules (3%) 1962
Sectral Capsules (2%) 3589
Serentil 1057
Seroquel Tablets (Infrequent) 684
▲ Serzone Tablets (3%) 1104
Sinemet Tablets 1253
Sinemet CR Tablets (1.8%) 1255
Singulair (Very rare) 2181
Sporanox Capsules (2%) 1800
Stadol NS Nasal Spray (Less than 1%) 1108
Sular Tablets (Less than or equal to 1%) 688
Sustiva Capsules (1% to 4%) 1258
Symmetrel (1% to 5%) 1328
Talacen Caplets (Infrequent) 3089
Talwin Nx Tablets 3090
Tambocor Tablets (Less than 1%) 1990
▲ Tasmar Tablets (16% to 21%) 3010
Tequin Injection (0.1% to 3%) 1110
Tequin Tablets (0.1% to 3%) 1110
Thioridazine Hydrochloride Tablets 2289
Tiazac Capsules (Less than 2%) 1378
Tonocard Tablets (Less than 1%) 649
Topamax Sprinkle Capsules (Infrequent) 2590
Topamax Tablets (Infrequent) 2590
Toradol (1% or less) 3018
Trilafon 3160
Trovan (Less than 1%) 2722
Vantin Tablets and Oral Suspension (Less than 1%) 2860
Vaseretic Tablets 2204
Vasotec I.V. Injection 2207
Vasotec Tablets (0.5% to 1.0%) 2210
Viagra Tablets (Less than 2%) 2732
Vicoprofen Tablets (Less than 1%) 520
Vistide Injection 1445
Wellbutrin Tablets 1680
Wellbutrin SR Sustained-Release Tablets (At least 1%) 1684
Xanax Tablets (1.8%) 2865
Zanaflex Tablets (Infrequent) 1305
Zebeta Tablets 1885
Ziac Tablets 1887
Zoloft (Infrequent) 2751
Zonegran Capsules (Infrequent) 1307
▲ Zyban Sustained-Release Tablets (5%) 1710
Zyprexa Tablets 1973
Zyprexa ZYDIS Orally Disintegrating Tablets 1973

Drooling

Aricept Tablets 1270
Aricept Tablets 2665
Compazine 1505
Dantrium Capsules (Less frequent) 2885
Demser Capsules 2085
Stelazine 1640
Thioridazine Hydrochloride Tablets 2289
Thiothixene Capsules 2290
Thorazine 1656
Versed Syrup (Less than 1%) 3033

Drowsiness

Accupril Tablets (0.5% to 1.0%) 2611
Accuretic Tablets (1.2%) 2614
Accutane Capsules 2944
▲ Acel-Imune (6% to 23%) 1851
Aceon Tablets (2 mg, 4 mg, 8 mg) (1.3%) 3249
Aciphex Tablets 1267
Aciphex Tablets 1783
▲ Act HIB Vaccine (2.5% to 63.7%) 798
Actifed Cold & Allergy Tablets ■ 688
Actifed Cold & Sinus Caplets and Tablets ■ 688
▲ Actiq (9% to 20%) 1184
Adalat CC Tablets (Less than 1.0%) 877
Adenoscan (Less than 1%) 1381
Aggrenox Capsules (1.2%) 1026
Agrylin Capsules (1% to 5%) 3232
Akineton 402
Albalon Ophthalmic Solution ⊙ 225
▲ Alferon N Injection (3% to 10%) 1770
Alka-Seltzer Plus Liqui-Gels ■ 604
Allegra (1.3% to 2.2%) 712
Allegra-D Extended-Release Tablets 714
Alomide Ophthalmic Solution (Less than 1%) ⊙ 204
▲ Alphagan Ophthalmic Solution (Approximately 10% to 30%) 545
Alphagan P Ophthalmic Solution (Less than 1%) 546
Altace Capsules (Less than 1%) 2233
▲ Ambien Tablets (2% to 8%) 3191
AmBisome for Injection (Less common) 1383
Amerge Tablets (1% to 2%) 1467
▲ Amphotec (5% or more) 1774
▲ Anaprox Tablets (3% to 9%) 2967
▲ Anaprox DS Tablets (3% to 9%) 2967
Antabuse Tablets 2444
Antabuse Tablets (Small number of patients) 3474
Antivert, Antivert/25, & Antivert/50 Tablets 2664
Anzemet Injection (2.4%) 719
▲ Aredia for Injection (Up to 6%) 2309
Aricept Tablets (2%) 1270
Aricept Tablets (2%) 2665
Arimidex Tablets (2% to 5%) 659
Artane 1855
Arthrotec Tablets (Rare) 3195
Asacol Delayed-Release Tablets 2884
▲ Astelin Nasal Spray (3.2%) 3339
Atacand Tablets (0.5% or greater) 595
Atacand HCT Tablets 597
Atarax Tablets & Syrup 2667
▲ Ativan Injection (6%) 3478
Atromid-S Capsules 3483
Atrovent Inhalation Aerosol (Less frequent) 1030
Avalide Tablets 1070
Avapro Tablets (Less than 1%) 1074
Avapro Tablets (Less than 1%) 3076
Avelox Tablets (0.05% to 1%) 879
Axert Tablets (Frequent) 2772
Axid Pulvules (1.9%) 1903
Axid Pulvules (1.9%) 2919
Azulfidine EN-tabs Tablets (Rare) 2775
Baycol Tablets 883
BC Allergy Sinus Cold Powder ■ 619
Benadryl Allergy Chewables ■ 689
Benadryl Allergy Kapseal Capsules ■ 691
Benadryl Allergy Liquid ■ 690
Benadryl Allergy Ultratab Tablets ■ 691
Benadryl Allergy/Cold Tablets ■ 691
Benadryl Allergy/Congestion Tablets ■ 692
Benadryl Allergy & Sinus Liquid ■ 693
Benadryl Allergy & Sinus Fastmelt Tablets ■ 693
Benadryl Severe Allergy & Sinus Headache Caplets ■ 694
Benadryl Children's Allergy/Cold Fastmelt Tablets ■ 692
Benadryl Dye-Free Allergy Liquid ■ 690
Benadryl Dye-Free Allergy Liqui-Gels Softgels ■ 690
▲ Benadryl Parenteral (Among most frequent) 2617
BeneFix for Injection 1432
▲ Betaseron for SC Injection (6%) 988
Bicillin C-R 900/300 Injection 2240
Bicillin C-R Injection 2238
Bicillin L-A Injection 2242
Blocadren Tablets (Less than 1%) 2046
▲ Botox Purified Neurotoxin Complex (2% to 10%) 549
▲ Brethine Ampuls (9.8 to 11.7%) 2314
▲ Brethine Tablets (5.5%) 2313
▲ Brevibloc Injection (3%) 858
Bromfed Capsules (Extended-Release) 2269
Bromfed-PD Capsules (Extended-Release) 2269
Calcijex Injection 411
Campath Ampules (1% to 5%) 992
Captopril Tablets 2281
Carafate Suspension (Less than 0.5%) 731
Carafate Tablets (Less than 0.5%) 730
▲ Carbatrol Capsules (Among most frequent) 3234
Cardizem Injectable 1018
Cardizem Lyo-Ject Syringe 1018
Cardizem Monovial 1018
Cardizem CD Capsules (Less than 1%) 1016
▲ Cardura Tablets (3% to 5%) 2668
▲ Casodex Tablets (2% to 5%) 662
Cataflam Tablets (Less than 1%) 2315
▲ Catapres Tablets (About 33 in 100 patients) 1037
▲ Catapres-TTS (12 of 101 patients) 1038
Ceclor CD Tablets (0.1% to 1%) 1279
Ceclor (Rare) 1905
Cedax Capsules (0.1% to 1%) 1021
Ceftin Tablets (0.1% to 1%) 1898
Cefzil (Less than 1%) 1076
Celebrex Capsules (0.1% to 1.9%) 2676
Celebrex Capsules (0.1% to 1.9%) 2780
▲ Celexa (18%) 1365
▲ CellCept Capsules (3% to 11.1%) 2951
▲ CellCept Intravenous (3% to 11.1%) 2951
▲ CellCept Oral Suspension (3% to 11.1%) 2951
▲ CellCept Tablets (3% to 11.1%) 2951
Celontin Capsules (Frequent) 2618
▲ Cerebyx Injection (6.7% to 20.0%) 2619
▲ Chemet Capsules (1.0% to 12.7%) 3078
Chirocaine Injection (1.2%) 2909
Chlor-Trimeton Allergy Tablets ■ 735
Chlor-Trimeton Allergy/Decongestant Tablets ■ 736
Cipro I.V. (1% or less) 893
Cipro I.V. Pharmacy Bulk Package (Less than 1%) 897
Cipro (Less than 1%) 887
▲ Claritin (8%) 3100
▲ Claritin-D 12 Hour Extended Release Tablets (7%) 3102
▲ Claritin-D 24 Hour Extended Release Tablets (6%) 3104
Clinoril Tablets (Less than 1%) 2053
▲ Clorpres Tablets (About 33%) 1002
▲ Clozaril Tablets (More than 5% to 39%) 2319
▲ Cognex Capsules (4%) 1351
Colazal Capsules 3069
▲ Combipres Tablets (About 33%) 1040
Combivent Inhalation Aerosol 1041
Compazine 1505
Comtan Tablets (2%) 2328
Comtrex Acute Head Cold & Sinus Pressure Relief Tablets ■ 627
Comtrex Flu Therapy & Fever Relief Nighttime Tablets ■ 628
Comtrex Maximum Strength Multi-Symptom Cold & Cough Relief Tablets and Caplets ■ 626
▲ Comvax (21.1% to 49.5%) 2056
Concerta Extended-Release Tablets 1998
Concerta Tablets 561
Contac Severe Cold and Flu Caplets Maximum Strength ■ 746
Copaxone for Injection (At least 2%) 3306
Coreg Tablets (1% to 2%) 1508
Coricidin 'D' Cold, Flu & Sinus Tablets ■ 737
Coricidin/Coricidin D ■ 738
Coricidin HBP Maximum Strength Flu Tablets ■ 738
Coricidin HBP Night-Time Cold & Flu Tablets ■ 738
Covera-HS Tablets (Less than 2%) 3199
Cozaar Tablets (Less than 1%) 2067
▲ Crinone 8% Gel (27%) 3213
Crixivan Capsules (1.0%) 2070
Cylert Tablets 415
CytoGam Intravenous (Infrequent) 2026
Cytotec Tablets (Infrequent) 3202
Cytovene (At least 3 subjects) 2959
▲ Dantrium Capsules (Among most frequent) 2885
▲ Daranide Tablets (Among the most common effects) 2077
DaunoXome Injection (Less than or equal to 5%) 1442
Demadex Tablets and Injection 2965
▲ Depacon Injection (1.7% to 30%) 416
▲ Depakene (27% to 30%) 421
▲ Depakote Sprinkle Capsules (18% to 30%) 426
▲ Depakote Tablets (17% to 30%) 430
▲ Depakote ER Tablets (7% to 30%) 436
▲ DepoCyt Injection (4% to 12%) 1197
Depo-Provera Contraceptive Injection (Fewer than 1%) 2798
▲ Detrol Tablets (3%) 3623
▲ Detrol LA Capsules (3%) 2801
Diamox Intravenous (Occasional) ⊙ 269
Diamox Sequels Sustained Release Capsules (Occasional) ⊙ 270
Diamox Tablets (Occasional) ⊙ 269
Dibenzyline Capsules 3457
Dilaudid 441
Dilaudid Powder 441
Dilaudid Rectal Suppositories 441
Dilaudid Tablets 441
Dimetapp Elixir ■ 777
Dimetapp Cold and Fever Suspension ■ 775
Dimetapp Nighttime Flu Liquid ■ 776
Diovan Capsules 2337
Diovan HCT Tablets (Greater than 0.2%) 2338
Dipentum Capsules (1.8%) 2803
▲ Diphtheria & Tetanus Toxoids Adsorbed Purogenated for Pediatric Use (14.9%) 1857
Diprivan Injectable Emulsion (Less than 1%) 667
▲ Ditropan XL Extended Release Tablets (11.9%) 564
Diuril Sodium Intravenous 2086
Dolobid Tablets (Greater than 1 in 100) 2088
Donnatal (In elderly patients) 2929
Donnatal Extentabs (In elderly patients) 2930
Donnatal Tablets (In elderly patients) 2929
▲ Dostinex Tablets (2% to less than 10%) 2804
Doxil Injection (1% to 5%) 566
Dramamine ■ 718
Dramamine Less Drowsy Tablets ■ 718
Drixoral Allergy/Sinus Extended-Release Tablets ■ 741
Drixoral Cold & Allergy Sustained-Action Tablets ■ 740
Drixoral Cold & Flu Extended-Release Tablets ■ 740
DuoNeb Inhalation Solution 1233
▲ Duraclon Injection (13.2% to 25%) 3057
▲ Duragesic Transdermal System (10% or more) 1786
Duranest Injections 600
Dyazide Capsules 1515
Dynabac Tablets (0.1% to 1%) 2269
DynaCirc Capsules (0.5% to 1%) 2921
DynaCirc CR Tablets (0.5% to 1%) 2923
▲ EC-Naprosyn Delayed-Release Tablets (3% to 9%) 2967
▲ Effexor Tablets (3% to 26.1%) 3495
▲ Effexor XR Capsules (17% to 20%) 3499
ELA-Max Cream 1340
Eldepryl Capsules 3266
Elspar for Injection 2092
Emla (Unlikely with cream) 602
Enalaprilat Injection 863
Engerix-B Vaccine (Less than 1%) 1517
Ergamisol Tablets (2% to 3%) 1789
Eskalith 1527
Ethyol for Injection 2029
Etrafon 3115
Eulexin Capsules (1%) 3118
Evoxac Capsules (Less than 1%) 1217
▲ Exelon Capsules (5%) 2342
▲ Exelon Oral Solution (5%) 2345
Extendryl 1361
Famotidine Injection (Infrequent) 866
Famvir Tablets (1.6% to 2.6%) 2348
▲ Felbatol (19.3% to 48.4%) 3343
Feldene Capsules (Occasional) 2685
▲ Femara Tablets (2% to 4%) 2351
Ferrlecit Injection (Greater than 1%) 3386
▲ Flexeril Tablets (16% to 39%) 572
▲ Flexeril Tablets (16% to 39%) 2094
▲ Flolan for Injection (4%) 1528
▲ Flomax Capsules (3.0% to 4.3%) 1044
Floxin I.V. (1% to 3%) 2526
Floxin Tablets (1% to 3%) 2529
Flumadine (0.3% to 1%) 1370
Fortovase Capsules (Less than 2%) 2970
Foscavir Injection (Between 1% and 5%) 605
Furosemide Tablets 2284
▲ Gabitril Tablets (18%) 1189
Gamimune N, 5% Solvent/Detergent Treated (Infrequent) 925
Gamimune N, 10% Solvent/Detergent Treated (Infrequent) 928
▲ Gemzar for Injection (5% to 11%) 1919
Gengraf Capsules (1% to less than 3%) 457
▲ Geodon Capsules (14%) 2688
▲ Geref for Injection (1 patient in 6) 3215
▲ Gliadel Wafer (14%) 1723
Glucophage Tablets 1080
Glucophage XR Tablets 1080
Glucotrol Tablets (About 1 in 50) 2692
Glucotrol XL Extended Release Tablets (Less than 1%) 2693
Glucovance Tablets 1086
Gonal-F for Injection 3216
Goody's PM Powder ■ 621
Guaifed 2272
▲ Halcion Tablets (14.0%) 2823
Haldol Decanoate 2535
Haldol Injection, Tablets and Concentrate 2533
Havrix Vaccine (Rare) 1544
Hectorol Capsules 1064
Hectorol Injection 1066
HibTITER (91 of 1,118 vaccinations) 1859
Hivid Tablets (Less than 1%) 2975
Hycodan 1316
Hycomine Compound Tablets 1317
Hycotuss Expectorant Syrup 1318
▲ Hytrin Capsules (0.6% to 5.4%) 464
Hyzaar 2109
▲ Ifex for Injection (Among most common) 1123
Imdur Tablets (Less than or equal to 5%) 1826
Imitrex Injection (2.7%) 1549
Imitrex Nasal Spray (Infrequent) 1554
Imitrex Tablets 1558
Indapamide Tablets (Less than 5%) 2286
Indocin (Less than 1%) 2112
▲ Infanrix Vaccine (6.6% to 37.5%) 1562
▲ Infergen (4% to 5%) 1777
▲ Intron A for Injection (Up to 14%) 3120
Invirase Capsules (Less than 2%) 2979
Iopidine 0.5% Ophthalmic Solution (Less than 3%) ⊙ 213
IPOL Vaccine 809
Isoptin SR Tablets (1% or less) 467
▲ Kadian Capsules (Among most frequent) 1335
Kaletra Capsules (Less than 2%) 471
Kaletra Oral Solution (Less than 2%) 471
▲ Keppra Tablets (15%) 3314
▲ Klonopin Tablets (7% to 50%) 2983
▲ Kytril Injection (4%) 2986
Kytril Tablets (1% to 4%) 2988
▲ Lamictal (14.2%) 1567
Levaquin (0.5% to less than 1.0%) 2537
Levsin/Levsinex/Levbid 3172
Lexxel Tablets 608
Librium Capsules (Some patients) 1736
Librium for Injection 1737
Lidoderm Patch 1319

▲ Limbitrol (Among most frequent) 1738
Lipitor Tablets (Less than 2%)......... 2639
Lipitor Tablets (Less than 2%)......... 2696
Lithium Carbonate........................... 3061
Lithium Citrate Syrup........................ 3061
Lithobid Slow-Release Tablets......... 3255
Livostin (Approximately 1% to 3%)... ⊙305
Lodine (Less than 1%)..................... 3528
Lodine XL Extended-Release Tablets (Less than 1%)................. 3530
Lodosyn Tablets............................... 1251
Lopid Tablets.................................... 2650
Lorabid Suspension and Pulvules (0.4% to 2.1%)............................ 2251
Lortab.. 3319
Lortab Elixir....................................... 3317
Lotensin Tablets (1.6%).................. 2365
Lotensin HCT Tablets (1.2%).......... 2367
Lotrel Capsules (Up to 0.3%)........... 2370
Loxitane Capsules............................ 3398
Lupron Depot-PED 7.5 mg, 11.25 mg and 15 mg (Less than 2%) 3291
Lupron Injection Pediatric (Less than 2%) 3280
▲ Luvox Tablets (25, 50, 100 mg) (4% to 22%) 3256
Macrobid Capsules (Less than 1%) 2889
▲ Marinol Capsules (3% to 10%) 3325
Matulane Capsules 3246
Mavik Tablets (0.3% to 1.0%) 478
▲ Maxalt Tablets (4% to 8%) 2120
▲ Maxalt-MLT Orally Disintegrating Tablets (4% to 8%) 2120
Maxidone Tablets CIII 3399
Maxzide 1008
Meridia Capsules (1.7%) 481
Merrem I.V. (0.1% to 1.0%) 673
Metadate CD Capsules 1164
Metadate ER Tablets 1167
Methylin Tablets 1995
Methylin ER Tablets 1995
Micardis Tablets (More than 0.3%) .. 1049
Micardis HCT Tablets 1051
Midamor Tablets (Less than or equal to 1%) 2136
Maximum Strength Midol Menstrual Caplets and Gelcaps .... ▣612
Maximum Strength Midol PMS Caplets and Gelcaps .... ▣613
▲ Migranal Nasal Spray (3%) 2376
Miltown Tablets 3349
▲ Minipress Capsules (7.6%) 2699
▲ Minizide Capsules (7.6%) 2700
Mintezol 2137
▲ Mirapex Tablets (9% to 22%) 2834
Mithracin for Intravenous Use 903
▲ Moban (Most frequent) 1320
Mobic Tablets (Less than 2%) 1054
Moduretic Tablets (Less than or equal to 1%) 2138
Monopril Tablets (0.2% to 1.0%) 1091
Monopril HCT (Less than 2%) 1094
Monurol Sachet (Less than 1%) 1375
▲ Motofen Tablets (1 in 25) 577
Motrin Suspension, Oral Drops, Chewable Tablets, and Caplets (Less than 1%) 2002
Mykrox Tablets 1168
Mylocel Tablets 2227
Myobloc Injectable Solution (2% or greater) 1291
▲ Naprelan Tablets (3% to 9%) 1293
▲ Naprosyn Suspension (3% to 9%) .. 2967
▲ Naprosyn Tablets (3% to 9%) 2967
Nardil Tablets (Common) 2653
Naropin Injection (Less than 1%) 612
Natrecor for Injection (At least 1%) 3189
Navane Oral 2701
Navane Intramuscular 2703
Nembutal Sodium Solution (1% to 3%) 485
Neoral Soft Gelatin Capsules (1% to less than 3%) 2380
Neoral Oral Solution (1% to less than 3%) 2380
Neptazane Tablets (Occasional) ..... ⊙271
Nesacaine/Nesacaine MPF 617
▲ Neurontin Capsules (19.3%) 2655
▲ Neurontin Oral Solution (8.4% to 19.3%) 2655
▲ Neurontin Tablets (19.3%) 2655
Nexium Delayed-Release Capsules (Less than 1%) 619
▲ Nicotrol Nasal Spray (Over 5%) 2843
▲ Nipent for Injection (3% to 10%) 3272
Nizoral Tablets (Less than 1%) 1791
Norco 5/325 Tablets CIII 3424
Norco 7.5/325 Tablets CIII 3425
Norco 10/325 Tablets CIII 3425
Norco 10/325 Tablets CIII 3427
Norflex 1987
▲ Normodyne Injection (3%) 3135
Normodyne Tablets (Less than 1%) 3137
Noroxin Tablets (0.3% to 1.0%) 2145
Norpramin Tablets 755
Norvasc Tablets (1.3% to 1.6%) 2704
Norvir Capsules (2.0% to 2.6%)...... 487
Norvir Oral Solution (2.0% to 2.6%)... 487
NuLev Orally Disintegrating Tablets 3176
Numorphan 1324
Maximum Strength Nytol QuickGels Softgels .... ▣621
Omnicef (0.2%)................................. 493
Oncaspar (Less than 1%)................. 756
One-A-Day Bedtime & Rest Tablets .... ▣805
One-A-Day Tension & Mood Softgels.. ▣808
OptiPranolol Metipranolol Ophthalmic Solution 0.3% (A small number of patients)........... ⊙263
▲ Orap Tablets (27.7%) 1407
Orudis Capsules (Greater than 1%) 3548
Oruvail Capsules (Greater than 1%) 3548
▲ OxyContin Tablets (23%) 2912
Parafon Forte DSC Caplets (Occasional) 2582
Parnate Tablets 1607
▲ Paxil (1.9% to 24%) 1609
PediaCare Cough-Cold Liquid......... ▣719
PediaCare NightRest Cough-Cold Liquid .... ▣719
Pediazole Suspension 3050
▲ Liquid PedvaxHIB (Among most frequent) 2148
Pentasa Capsules (Less than 1%)... 3239
Pepcid Injection (Infrequent)........... 2153
Pepcid for Oral Suspension (Infrequent) 2150
Pepcid RPD Orally Disintegrating Tablets (Infrequent)..................... 2150
Pepcid Tablets (Infrequent)............. 2150
Percogesic Aspirin-Free Coated Tablets .... ▣667
Extra Strength Percogesic Aspirin-Free Coated Caplets....... ▣665
Periactin Tablets............................... 2155
▲ Permax Tablets (10.1%) 1299
Phenergan Injection.......................... 3553
Phenergan Suppositories................. 3556
Phenergan Syrup.............................. 3554
Phenergan Tablets............................ 3556
Phenergan with Codeine Syrup 3557
Phenergan with Dextromethorphan Syrup 3559
Phenergan VC Syrup........................ 3560
Phenergan VC with Codeine Syrup .. 3561
▲ Phrenilin (Among most frequent) 578
Plendil Extended-Release Tablets (0.5% to 1.5%)............................... 623
Polocaine Injection, USP.................. 625
Polocaine-MPF Injection, USP.......... 625
Ponstel Capsules (Occasional)........ 1356
Premphase Tablets........................... 3572
Prempro Tablets................................ 3572
▲ Prevnar for Injection (21.3% to 49.2%)... 1870
Prilosec Delayed-Release Capsules (Less than 1%)............. 628
Primaxin I.M. 2158
Primaxin I.V. (0.2%).......................... 2160
Prinivil Tablets (0.3% to 1.0%)......... 2164
Prinzide Tablets (0.3% to 1%)......... 2168
ProAmatine Tablets (Rare).............. 3241
Procardia XL Extended Release Tablets (Less than 3%).................. 2710
▲ Prograf (3% to 15%) 1393
▲ Proleukin for Injection (22%) 1199
Prometrium Capsules (100 mg, 200 mg) (Less than 5%) 3261
▲ ProSom Tablets (42%) 500
Prostigmin Injectable........................ 1744
Prostigmin Tablets............................ 1744
Protonix I.V. (Less than 1%)............ 3580
Protonix Tablets (Less than 1%)...... 3577
Protopam Chloride for Injection 3582
Proventil Repetabs Tablets (Less than 1% to 2%)............................... 3148
Proventil HFA Inhalation Aerosol (Less than 3%)............................... 3150
Provera Tablets................................. 2853
Provigil Tablets (At least 1%)........... 1193
▲ Prozac Pulvules, Liquid, and Weekly Capsules (13% to 17%).... 1238
▲ Rapamune Oral Solution and Tablets (3% to 20%)...................... 3584
Recombivax HB................................ 2178
ReFacto Vials 1437
▲ Reglan (Approximately 10%) 2935
Relafen Tablets (1% to 3%).............. 1617
▲ Remeron Tablets (10.4% to 54%) .. 2483
▲ Remeron SolTab Tablets (10.4% to 54%).. 2486
Remicade for IV Injection (Less than 2%).. 1178
▲ Reminyl Oral Solution (4%) 1792
▲ Reminyl Tablets (4%) 1792
▲ Requip Tablets (20% to 40%) 1621
Rescriptor Tablets (Less than 2%).... 526
ReSource Wellness StayCalm Caplets... ▣826
▲ Retrovir Capsules (8%) 1625
▲ Retrovir IV Infusion (8%) 1629
▲ Retrovir (8%) 1625
Rifadin... 765
Rifamate Capsules 767
Rifater Tablets.................................. 769
Rilutek Tablets (0.8% to 4.1%)......... 772
▲ Risperdal (3% to 41%) 1796
Ritalin.. 2387
Robaxin Injectable............................ 2938
Robaxin Tablets................................ 2939
Robaxisal Tablets.............................. 2939
Robinul Forte Tablets........................ 1358
Robinul Injectable.............................. 2940
Robinul Tablets.................................. 1358
Robitussin Nighttime Honey Flu Liquid.. ▣786
Rocaltrol.. 2991
Romazicon Injection (Less than 1%).. 3000
▲ Roxicodone Tablets (Greater than or equal to 3%).............................. 3067
Ryna.. ▣768
▲ Ryna-12 S Suspension (Among most common) 3351
▲ Reformulated Rynatan Pediatric Suspension (Among most common) 3352
▲ Rynatan Tablets (Among most common) 3351
▲ Rynatuss Pediatric Suspension (Among most common) 3353
▲ Rynatuss Tablets (Among most common) 3353
Rythmol Tablets – 150 mg, 225 mg, 300 mg (1.2%) 502
Salagen Tablets (1% to 2%) 2229
Sandoglobulin I.V. 2391
Sandostatin LAR Depot (1% to 4%) 2395
▲ Sarafem Pulvules (13%) 1962
▲ Sedapap Tablets 50 mg/650 mg (Among the most frequent) 2225
▲ Semprex-D Capsules (12%) 1172
Sensorcaine 643
Sensorcaine-MPF Injection 643
▲ Serentil (One of the two most prevalent) 1057
▲ Seroquel Tablets (18%) 684
▲ Serostim for Injection (1% to 10%) . 3229
▲ Serzone Tablets (16% to 28%) 1104
Sinemet Tablets 1253
Sinemet CR Tablets 1255
▲ Sinequan (Most common) 2713
Singlet Caplets .... ▣761
Singulair (Very rare) 2181
Sinutab Sinus Allergy Medication, Maximum Strength Formula, Tablets & Caplets .... ▣707
Skelaxin Tablets 1301
Skelid Tablets (More than or equal to 1%) 3088
Sleep-Tite Caplets .... ▣850
Soma Tablets 3353
▲ Soma Compound Tablets (Most frequent) 3354
▲ Soma Compound w/Codeine Tablets (Most frequent) 3355
▲ Sonata Capsules (5%) 3591
▲ Soriatane Capsules (1% to 10%) ... 3003
Sporanox Capsules (1.2%) 1800
▲ Stadol NS Nasal Spray (43%) 1108
Stelazine 1640
Stimate Nasal Spray 796
Stromectol Tablets (0.9%) 2185
Sudafed Cold & Allergy Tablets ..... ▣708
Sular Tablets (Less than or equal to 1%) 688
Surmontil Capsules 3595
Sustiva Capsules (2% to 3%) 1258
Symmetrel (1% to 5%) 1328
Tagamet (Approximately 1 in 100) .. 1644
Tambocor Tablets (1% to 3%) 1990
Tapazole Tablets 1823
Tarka Tablets (0.3% or more) 508
▲ Tasmar Tablets (14% to 18%) 3010
Tavist 12 Hour Allergy Tablets .... ▣676
▲ Tegretol/Tegretol-XR (Among most frequent) 2404
▲ Temodar Capsules (9%) 3157
▲ Tenex Tablets (Up to 39%) 2942
Tenoretic Tablets (0.6% to 2%) 690
Tenormin (0.6% to 2%) 692
Tequin Injection (Less than 0.1%) 1110
Tequin Tablets (Less than 0.1%) 1110
▲ Tetanus & Diphtheria Toxoids Adsorbed for Adult Use (14.9%) .. 1880
Teveten Tablets (Less than 1%) 3327
▲ Thalomid Capsules (37.5%) 1154
TheraFlu Regular Strength Cold & Cough Night Time Hot Liquid .. ▣676
TheraFlu Regular Strength Cold & Sore Throat Night Time Hot Liquid .... ▣676
TheraFlu Maximum Strength Flu & Cough Night Time Hot Liquid .. ▣678
TheraFlu Maximum Strength Flu & Sore Throat Night Time Hot Liquid .... ▣677
TheraFlu Maximum Strength Severe Cold & Congestion Night Time Caplets .... ▣678
TheraFlu Maximum Strength Severe Cold & Congestion Night Time Hot Liquid .... ▣678
Thioridazine Hydrochloride Tablets (Occasional)...................... 2289
Thiothixene Capsules 2290
Thorazine.. 1656
Thyrel TRH for Injection (Less frequent).. 3630
Tiazac Capsules (Less than 2%)...... 1378
Timolide Tablets (Less than 1%)...... 2187
Timolol GFS .... ⊙266
Timoptic in Ocudose (Less frequent).. 2192
Timoptic Sterile Ophthalmic Solution (Less frequent)............... 2190
Timoptic-XE Sterile Ophthalmic Gel Forming Solution.................... 2194
Tolectin (1% to 3%).......................... 2589
Tonocard Tablets (0.8% to 1.6%).... 649
▲ Topamax Sprinkle Capsules (25.9% to 30.1%)........................... 2590
▲ Topamax Tablets (25.9% to 30.1%)... 2590
Toprol-XL Tablets 651
▲ Toradol (6%) 3018
▲ Transderm Scōp Transdermal Therapeutic System (Less than one-sixth) 2302
▲ Tranxene (Most frequent) 511
Trecator-SC Tablets 3598
Trental Tablets 784
Triaminic Cold & Allergy Liquid ...... ▣681
Triaminic Cold & Allergy Softchews .... ▣683
Triaminic Cold & Cough Liquid ...... ▣681
Triaminic Cold & Cough Softchews .... ▣683
Triaminic Cold & Night Time Cough Liquid .... ▣681
Triaminic Cold, Cough & Fever Liquid .... ▣681
Tricor Capsules, Micronized 513
Trilafon 3160
▲ Trileptal Oral Suspension (5% to 36%) 2407
▲ Trileptal Tablets (5% to 36%) 2407
Trilisate (Less than 2%) 2901
▲ Tripedia Vaccine (1% to 13%) 817
▲ Trisenox Injection (8%) 1158
Tussi-12 S Suspension 3356
Tussi-12 Tablets 3356
Tussionex Pennkinetic Extended-Release Suspension 1174
Tussi-Organidin NR Liquid 3350
Tussi-Organidin DM NR Liquid (Rare) 3350
Tussi-Organidin DM-S NR Liquid (Rare) 3350
Tussi-Organidin-S NR Liquid 3350
Twinrix Vaccine (Less than 1%) 1674
Children's Tylenol Allergy-D Liquid .. 2014
Children's Tylenol Cold Suspension Liquid and Chewable Tablets 2015
Children's Tylenol Cold Plus Cough Suspension Liquid and Chewable Tablets 2015
Children's Tylenol Flu Suspension Liquid 2015
Tylenol Allergy Sinus 2010
Tylenol Severe Allergy Caplets 2010
Multi-Symptom Tylenol Cold Complete Formula Caplets 2010
Maximum Strength Tylenol Flu NightTime Gelcaps 2011
Maximum Strength Tylenol Flu NightTime Liquid 2011
Extra Strength Tylenol PM Caplets, Geltabs, and Gelcaps 2012
Maximum Strength Tylenol Sinus NightTime Caplets 2012
▲ Ultracet Tablets (6%) 2597
▲ Ultram Tablets (16% to 25%) 2600
Uniretic Tablets (Less than 1%) 3178
Unisom SleepTabs .... ▣713
Univasc Tablets (Less than 1%) 3181
▲ Valium Injectable (Among most common) 3026
▲ Valium Tablets (Among most common) 3047
Vantin Tablets and Oral Suspension (Less than 1%) 2860
▲ Vascor Tablets (0.5% to 6.98%) 2602
Vaseretic Tablets (0.5% to 2.0%) 2204
Vasotec I.V. Injection 2207
Vasotec Tablets (0.5% to 1.0%) 2210
Verelan Capsules (1% or less) 3184
Verelan PM Capsules (2% or less) ... 3186
Versed Injection (1.2%) 3027
▲ Vesanoid Capsules (3%) 3037
Viagra Tablets (Less than 2%) 2732
Vicks 44M Cough, Cold & Flu Relief Liquid .... ▣725
Pediatric Vicks 44m Cough & Cold Relief .... ▣728
Children's Vicks NyQuil Cold/Cough Relief .... ▣726
Vicks NyQuil LiquiCaps/Liquid Multi-Symptom Cold/Flu Relief, Original and Cherry Flavors .... ▣727
Vicodin Tablets 516
Vicodin ES Tablets 517
Vicodin HP Tablets 518
Vicodin Tuss Expectorant 519

▲ Vicoprofen Tablets (22%) ... 520
Vioxx (Greater than 0.1% to 1.9%) .. 2213
Viracept ... 532
▲ Viramune Oral Suspension (3% to 8%) ... 1060
▲ Viramune Tablets (3% to 8%) ... 1060
Vistaril Capsules ... 2738
Vistaril Intramuscular Solution ... 2738
Vistaril Oral Suspension ... 2738
Vistide Injection ... 1445
Vivactil Tablets ... 2217
Vivactil Tablets ... 2446
Volmax Extended-Release Tablets (0.3%) ... 2276
Voltaren Tablets (Less than 1%) ... 2315
Voltaren-XR Tablets (Less than 1%) ... 2315
Wellbutrin SR Sustained-Release Tablets (2% to 3%) ... 1684
WinRho SDF ... 2297
▲ Xanax Tablets (41% to 76.8%) ... 2865
▲ Xylocaine Injections (Among most common) ... 653
▲ Zanaflex Tablets (48% to 92%) ... 1305
Zantac (Rare) ... 1690
Zantac Injection ... 1688
Zantac Syrup (Rare) ... 1690
Zarontin Capsules ... 2659
Zarontin Syrup ... 2660
Zaroxolyn Tablets ... 1177
Zebeta Tablets ... 1885
Zestoretic Tablets (0.3% to 1%) ... 695
Zestril Tablets (0.3% to 1.0%) ... 698
Ziac Tablets (0.9% to 1.1%) ... 1887
Zithromax Capsules, 250 mg (1% or less) ... 2743
Zithromax for IV Infusion (1% or less) ... 2748
Zithromax for Oral Suspension, 1 g (1% or less) ... 2743
Zithromax for Oral Suspension, 300 mg, 600 mg, 900 mg, 1200 mg (1% or less) ... 2739
Zithromax Tablets, 250 mg (1% or less) ... 2739
Zithromax Tablets, 600 mg (1% or less) ... 2743
▲ Zofran Injection (5% to 8%) ... 1698
▲ Zofran (20%) ... 1703
▲ Zofran ODT Orally Disintegrating Tablets (20%) ... 1703
Zoladex (1% or greater) ... 702
Zoladex 3-month ... 706
▲ Zoloft (13% to 15%) ... 2751
▲ Zometa for Intravenous Infusion (5% to 10%) ... 3621
▲ Zomig Tablets (5% to 8%) ... 708
▲ Zomig-ZMT Tablets (5% to 8%) ... 708
▲ Zonegran Capsules (17%) ... 1307
Zovirax ... 1706
Zyban Sustained-Release Tablets (2%) ... 1710
Zydone Tablets ... 1330
Zyflo Filmtab Tablets (Less common) ... 524
▲ Zyprexa Tablets (20% to 39%) ... 1973
▲ Zyprexa ZYDIS Orally Disintegrating Tablets (20% to 39%) ... 1973
▲ Zyrtec (1.9% to 14%) ... 2756
▲ Zyrtec-D 12 Hour Extended Relief Tablets (13.7%) ... 2758

Drug administration site reactions, unspecified
Abelcet Injection ... 1273
Aloprim for Injection (Less than 1%) ... 2292
▲ AndroGel (3% to 5%) ... 3322
▲ Avonex (4%) ... 1013
▲ Betaseron for SC Injection (85%) ... 988
Cardene I.V. (1.4%) ... 3485
▲ Ceptaz for Injection (Among most common) ... 1499
Cerebyx Injection (Frequent) ... 2619
▲ CombiPatch Transdermal System (2% to 23%) ... 2323
▲ Cytovene-IV (22%) ... 2959
Denavir Cream (1.3%) ... 2332
Depacon Injection (2.4%) ... 416
D.H.E. 45 Injection ... 2334
Doxil Injection ... 566
Duragesic Transdermal System (1% or greater) ... 1786
Engerix-B Vaccine ... 1517
▲ Epogen for Injection (7% to 25%) ... 582
▲ Floxin Otic Solution (3%) ... 1219
▲ Fortaz (Among most common) ... 1541
Fragmin Injection (Rare) ... 2814
▲ Imitrex Injection (58.7%) ... 1549
Intron A for Injection (Less than 5%) ... 3120
Leukine ... 1755
▲ Leustatin Injection (9% to 19%) ... 2495
▲ Levaquin Injection (5.6%) ... 2537
Levo-Dromoran ... 1734
Lupron Depot 3.75 mg (Less than 5%) ... 3281
Lupron Depot–3 Month 11.25 mg (Less than 5%) ... 3285
▲ Lupron Depot–3 Month 22.5 mg (13.8%) ... 3288
▲ Lupron Depot–4 Month 30 mg (8.2% to 37.5%) ... 3289
▲ Lupron Depot-PED 7.5 mg, 11.25 mg and 15 mg (5%) ... 3291
Lupron Injection Pediatric ... 3280
▲ Maxipime for Injection (3.0%) ... 1285
Merrem I.V. (1.1%) ... 673
▲ Migranal Nasal Spray (6%) ... 2376
▲ Navelbine Injection (Up to 38%) ... 1604
Neupogen for Injection (Infrequent) ... 587
Oncaspar (Greater than 1% but less than 5%) ... 756
▲ Procrit for Injection (7% to 29%) ... 2502
▲ Proleukin for Injection (3%) ... 1199
Retrovir IV Infusion (Infrequent) ... 1629
Rilutek Tablets (Infrequent) ... 772
▲ Rocephin Injectable Vials, ADD-Vantage, Galaxy, Bulk (5% to 17%) ... 2993
▲ Roferon-A Injection (29%) ... 2996
▲ Serostim for Injection (1% to 10%) . 3229
▲ Sporanox Injection (4%) ... 1804
▲ Sporanox Injection (4%) ... 2509
▲ Taxol Injection (13%) ... 1129
Taxotere for Injection Concentrate .. 778
▲ Tazicef for Injection (Among most common) ... 1647
▲ Tazicef Galaxy Container (Among most common) ... 1650
▲ Tazicef Pharmacy Bulk Package (Among most common) ... 1653
▲ Trovan I.V. (2% to 5%) ... 2722
Venofer Injection (Greater than 1%) ... 580
▲ Vesanoid Capsules (17%) ... 3037
Zithromax for IV Infusion (1.9%) ... 2748
▲ Zoladex (6%) ... 702
Zoladex 3-month ... 706
Zosyn (0.5%) ... 1890
Zosyn in Galaxy Containers (0.5%) ... 1894
▲ Zyban Sustained-Release Tablets (11%) ... 1710

Drug effect, unspecified, prolonged
Diprivan Injectable Emulsion (Less than 1%) ... 667

Drug fever
Aldoclor Tablets ... 2035
Aldomet Tablets ... 2037
Aldoril Tablets ... 2039
Ancef for Injection ... 1474
Ancef Injection ... 1474
Bactrim ... 2949
Cedax ... 1021
Cefobid Intravenous/Intramuscular (1 in 260) ... 2671
Cefobid Pharmacy Bulk Package - Not for Direct Infusion (1 in 260) ... 2673
Clozaril Tablets ... 2319
Compazine ... 1505
Depen Titratable Tablets ... 3341
DynaCirc CR Tablets (0.5% to 1%) .. 2923
Fortovase Capsules (Rare) ... 2970
Invirase Capsules (Rare) ... 2979
Kefurox Vials, ADD-Vantage ... 1948
Kefzol Vials, ADD-Vantage ... 1951
Leukeran Tablets ... 1591
Macrobid Capsules ... 2889
Macrodantin Capsules ... 2891
Mandol Vials ... 1953
Norpramin Tablets ... 755
Orap Tablets ... 1407
Primaxin I.M. ... 2158
Primaxin I.V. (Less than 0.2%) ... 2160
Purinethol Tablets (Very rare) ... 1615
Septra Suspension ... 2265
Septra Tablets ... 2265
Septra DS Tablets ... 2265
Serentil ... 1057
Stelazine ... 1640
Suprax (Less than 2%) ... 1877
Taxotere for Injection Concentrate .. 778
Timentin Injection- ADD-Vantage Vial ... 1661
Timentin Injection-Galaxy Container ... 1664
Timentin Injection-Pharmacy Bulk Package ... 1666
Timentin for Intravenous Administration ... 1658
Urobiotic-250 Capsules ... 2731
Vancocin HCl Capsules & Pulvules (Infrequent) ... 1972
Vancocin HCl Oral Solution (Infrequent) ... 1971
Vancocin HCl, Vials & ADD-Vantage (Infrequent) ... 1970
Vivactil Tablets ... 2217
Vivactil Tablets ... 2446
Zinacef Injection (Rare) ... 1696
Zinacef for Injection (Rare) ... 1696

Drug idiosyncrasies
(*see under* Allergic reactions)

Dry mouth
(*see under* Xerostomia)

Dry skin
(*see under* Xerosis cutis)

Dry sockets
Vioxx (At least 2%) ... 2213

Dryness
Aclovate Cream (Approximately 2%) ... 1275
Analpram-HC ... 1338
Anusol-HC Cream 2.5% (Infrequent to frequent) ... 2237
Anusol-HC Suppositories ... 2238
Azelex Cream (Less than 1%) ... 547
Condylox Gel (Less common) ... 2436
Condylox Topical Solution (Less than 5%) ... 2437
Cordran Lotion (Infrequent) ... 2438
Cordran Tape (Infrequent) ... 2439
Cormax Cream (Infrequent) ... 2440
Cormax Ointment (Infrequent) ... 2440
Cormax Scalp Application (Infrequent) ... 2441
Cutivate Cream (1.2%) ... 1282
Cutivate Ointment (Infrequent to more frequent) ... 1284
Elocon Lotion 0.1% (Infrequent) ... 3111
Lidex (Infrequent) ... 2020
Locoid Cream (Infrequent) ... 1341
Locoid Lipocream Cream (Infrequent) ... 1342
Locoid (Infrequent) ... 1341
Melanex Topical Solution ... 2300
▲ Naftin Cream (3%) ... 2224
Olux Foam ... 1211
Ophthetic Ophthalmic Solution ... ⊙ 244
Pramosone ... 1343
Proctocort Suppositories ... 2264
Synalar (Infrequent) ... 2020
Temovate Cream ... 1301
Temovate Gel (Infrequent) ... 1303
Temovate Ointment ... 1301
Temovate Scalp Application (Infrequent) ... 1304
Temovate E Emollient (Infrequent) ... 1302
Topicort (Infrequent) ... 2025
Triaz Cleanser ... 2026
Triaz Gel ... 2026

Dryness, mucous membrane
Cataflam Tablets (Less than 1%) ... 2315
Dolobid Tablets (Less than 1 in 100) ... 2088
Mintezol Chewable Tablets ... 2137
Myleran Tablets (Rare) ... 1603
Nasacort Nasal Inhaler (Fewer than 5%) ... 750
Pravachol Tablets ... 1099
▲ Ryna-12 S Suspension (Among most common) ... 3351
▲ Reformulated Rynatan Pediatric Suspension (Among most common) ... 3352
▲ Rynatuss Pediatric Suspension (Among most common) ... 3353
▲ Rynatuss Tablets (Among most common) ... 3353
Timolide Tablets (Less than 1%) ... 2187
Tussi-12 S Suspension ... 3356
Tussi-12 Tablets ... 3356
▲ Vesanoid Capsules (77%) ... 3037
Voltaren Tablets (Less than 1%) ... 2315
Voltaren-XR Tablets (Less than 1%) ... 2315

Dryness, nose
(*see under* Xeromycteria)

Duodenitis
Aciphex Tablets (Rare) ... 1267
Aciphex Tablets (Rare) ... 1783
Evoxac Capsules (Less than 1%) ... 1217
Sterile FUDR ... 2974
Lodine (Less than 1%) ... 3528
Lodine XL Extended-Release Tablets (Less than 1%) ... 3530
Motrin Suspension, Oral Drops, Chewable Tablets, and Caplets (Less than 1%) ... 2002
Nexium Delayed-Release Capsules (Less than 1%) ... 619
Paxil (Rare) ... 1609
Permax Tablets (Rare) ... 1299
Pletal Tablets (Less than 2%) ... 2605
Pletal Tablets (Less than 2%) ... 2848
Protonix I.V. (Less than 1%) ... 3580
Protonix Tablets (Less than 1%) ... 3577
Relafen Tablets (Less than 1%) ... 1617
Requip Tablets (Infrequent) ... 1621
Rescriptor Tablets (Less than 2%) ... 526
Xeloda Tablets (Less than 5%) ... 3039
Zonegran Capsules (Rare) ... 1307

Dupuytren's contracture
Requip Tablets (Rare) ... 1621

Dypnea
Brevital Sodium for Injection, USP ... 1815

Dysarthria
Ambien Tablets (Infrequent) ... 3191
Aricept Tablets (Infrequent) ... 1270
Aricept Tablets (Infrequent) ... 2665
Cerebyx Injection (2.2%; frequent) .. 2619
Clozaril Tablets (Less than 1%) ... 2319
Cognex Capsules (Infrequent) ... 1351
Depacon Injection ... 416
Depakene ... 421
Depakote Sprinkle Capsules ... 426
Depakote Tablets (1% to 5%) ... 430
Depakote ER Tablets (Greater than 1%) ... 436
Felbatol ... 3343
Flexeril Tablets (Less than 1%) ... 572
Flexeril Tablets (Less than 1%) ... 2094
Fortovase Capsules (Less than 2%) ... 2970
Gabitril Tablets (Frequent) ... 1189
Geodon Capsules (Frequent) ... 2688
Halcion Tablets ... 2823
Imitrex Injection (Rare) ... 1549
Imitrex Nasal Spray (Infrequent) ... 1554
Imitrex Tablets (Infrequent) ... 1558
Indocin Capsules (Less than 1%) ... 2112
Indocin I.V. (Less than 1%) ... 2115
Indocin (Less than 1%) ... 2112
Invirase Capsules (Less than 2%) ... 2979
Klonopin Tablets (2%) ... 2983
Lamictal (1.0%) ... 1567
Levsin/Levsinex/Levbid ... 3172
Maxalt Tablets (Infrequent) ... 2120
Maxalt-MLT Orally Disintegrating Tablets (Infrequent) ... 2120
Neurontin Capsules (2.4%) ... 2655
Neurontin Oral Solution (2.4%) ... 2655
Neurontin Tablets (2.4%) ... 2655
Nipent for Injection (Less than 3%) ... 3272
Paxil (Rare) ... 1609
Prostigmin Injectable ... 1744
Prostigmin Tablets ... 1744
Protonix I.V. (Less than 1%) ... 3580
Protonix Tablets (Less than 1%) ... 3577
Prozac Pulvules, Liquid, and Weekly Capsules (Rare) ... 1238
Remeron Tablets (Infrequent) ... 2483
Remeron SolTab Tablets (Infrequent) ... 2486
Rilutek Tablets (Infrequent) ... 772
Risperdal (Infrequent) ... 1796
Roferon-A Injection (Less than 0.5%) ... 2996
Sarafem Pulvules (Rare) ... 1962
Seroquel Tablets (Frequent) ... 684
Serzone Tablets (Infrequent) ... 1104
Soma Tablets ... 3353
Soma Compound Tablets (Very rare) ... 3354
Soma Compound w/Codeine Tablets (Very rare) ... 3355
Sonata Capsules (Rare) ... 3591
Tensilon Injectable ... 1745
Tonocard Tablets (Less than 1%) ... 649
Valium Injectable ... 3026
Valium Tablets (Infrequent) ... 3047
Versed Syrup (Less than 1%) ... 3033
▲ Vesanoid Capsules (3%) ... 3037
Wellbutrin Tablets (Infrequent) ... 1680
Wellbutrin SR Sustained-Release Tablets ... 1684
▲ Xanax Tablets (23.3%) ... 2865
Zonegran Capsules (Infrequent) ... 1307
Zyban Sustained-Release Tablets ... 1710
Zyprexa Tablets (Infrequent) ... 1973
Zyprexa ZYDIS Orally Disintegrating Tablets (Infrequent) ... 1973

Dysautonomia
Zanaflex Tablets (Infrequent) ... 1305

Dyschromatopsia
Desferal Vials ... 2333

Dyscrasias, blood
(*see under* Blood dyscrasias)

Dysdiadochokinesia
Klonopin Tablets ... 2983

Dysesthesia
AmBisome for Injection (Less common) ... 1383
▲ Astelin Nasal Spray (7.9%) ... 3339
Cognex Capsules (Rare) ... 1351
Copaxone for Injection (At least 2%) ... 3306
Crixivan Capsules (Less than 2%) ... 2070
Cytovene ... 2959
Enalaprilat Injection ... 863
Evoxac Capsules (Less than 1%) ... 1217
Floxin Otic Solution (Single report) ... 1219
Fortovase Capsules (Less than 2%) ... 2970
Halcion Tablets (Rare) ... 2823
Hivid Tablets ... 2975
Imitrex Injection (Rare) ... 1549

Imitrex Nasal Spray (Rare) 1554
Imitrex Tablets (Rare) 1558
Invirase Capsules (Less than 2%) 2979
Levulan Kerastick (Up to 2%) 971
Lexxel Tablets 608
Maxalt Tablets (Rare) 2120
Maxalt-MLT Orally Disintegrating Tablets (Rare) 2120
Neurontin Capsules (Infrequent) 2655
Neurontin Oral Solution (Infrequent) 2655
Neurontin Tablets (Infrequent) 2655
Prinivil Tablets (0.3% to 1.0%) 2164
Prinzide Tablets 2168
▲ Taxotere for Injection Concentrate (7 of 134 patients) 778
Thalomid Capsules 1154
Vaseretic Tablets 2204
Vasotec I.V. Injection 2207
Vasotec Tablets (0.5% to 1.0%) 2210
Xeloda Tablets 3039
Zestril Tablets (0.3% to 1.0%) 698

Dysesthesia, hemifacial
Prilosec Delayed-Release Capsules (Less than 1%) 628

Dysgeusia
Captopril Tablets (Approximately 2 to 4 of 100 patients) 2281
Cardizem Injectable 1018
Cardizem Lyo-Ject Syringe 1018
Cardizem Monovial 1018
Cardizem CD Capsules (Less than 1%) 1016
Eskalith 1527
Floxin I.V. (1% to 3%) 2526
Floxin Tablets (1% to 3%) 2529
Havrix Vaccine (Less than 1%) 1544
Lithobid Slow-Release Tablets 3255
Maxalt Tablets 2120
Maxalt-MLT Orally Disintegrating Tablets 2120
Mevacor Tablets (0.8%) 2132
Noroxin Tablets 2145
Rocephin Injectable Vials, ADD-Vantage, Galaxy, Bulk (Less than 1%) 2993
Tiazac Capsules (Less than 1%) 1378
Trilisate (Less than 1%) 2901
Twinrix Vaccine (Less than 1%) 1674
Ultram Tablets (Less than 1%) 2600
Vioxx (Greater than 0.1% to 1.9%) 2213

Dyskinesia
Adderall Tablets 3231
Adderall XR Capsules
Cognex Capsules (Rare) 1351
Compazine 1505
▲ Comtan Tablets (25%) 2328
Concerta Extended-Release Tablets 1998
Concerta Tablets 561
Cylert Tablets 415
Dexedrine 1512
DextroStat Tablets 3236
Dilantin Infatabs (Rare) 2624
Dilantin Kapseals (Rare) 2622
Dilantin-125 Oral Suspension (Rare) 2625
Dostinex Tablets 2804
▲ Eldepryl Capsules (2 of 49 patients) 3266
Etrafon 3115
Evoxac Capsules (Less than 1%) 1217
Felbatol 3343
Geodon Capsules (Frequent) 2688
Haldol Decanoate 2535
Haldol Injection, Tablets and Concentrate 2533
Kaletra Capsules (Less than 2%) 471
Kaletra Oral Solution (Less than 2%) 471
Lamictal (Infrequent) 1567
Levo-Dromoran 1734
Levorphanol Tartrate Tablets (Less than 1%) 3059
▲ Lodosyn Tablets (Among most common) 1251
Loxitane Capsules (Less frequent) 3398
Luvox Tablets (25, 50, 100 mg) (Infrequent) 3256
Metadate CD Capsules 1164
Metadate ER Tablets 1167
Methylin Tablets 1995
Methylin ER Tablets 1995
▲ Mirapex Tablets (47%) 2834
MSIR (Less frequent) 2898
Naropin Injection (Less than 1%) 612
Orap Tablets 1407
Paxil (Rare) 1609
▲ Permax Tablets (62.4%) 1299
Provigil Tablets (2%) 1193
Prozac Pulvules, Liquid, and Weekly Capsules 1238
Remeron Tablets (Infrequent) 2483
Remeron SolTab Tablets (Infrequent) 2486
Requip Tablets (1% or more) 1621
Ritalin 2387
Sarafem Pulvules 1962
Seroquel Tablets (Infrequent) 684
▲ Sinemet Tablets (Among most common) 1253
▲ Sinemet CR Tablets (16.5%) 1255
Stelazine 1640
▲ Tasmar Tablets (42% to 51%) 3010
Thalomid Capsules 1154
Topamax Sprinkle Capsules (Infrequent) 2590
Topamax Tablets (Infrequent) 2590
Trilafon 3160
Trovan (Less than 1%) 2722
Vistaril 2738
Wellbutrin Tablets (Frequent) 1680
Wellbutrin SR Sustained-Release Tablets 1684
▲ Zanaflex Tablets (3%) 1305
Zoloft (Rare) 2751
Zonegran Capsules 1307
Zyban Sustained-Release Tablets 1710
Zyprexa Tablets (Up to 2%) 1973
Zyprexa ZYDIS Orally Disintegrating Tablets (Up to 2%) 1973

Dyskinesia, orofacial
Neurontin Capsules (Rare) 2655
Neurontin Oral Solution (Rare) 2655
Neurontin Tablets (Rare) 2655
Provigil Tablets (At least 1%) 1193
Zyrtec (Rare) 2756
Zyrtec-D 12 Hour Extended Relief Tablets (Rare) 2758

Dyskinesia, tardive
(*see under* Tardive dyskinesia)

Dyskinesia, transient
Orap Tablets 1407

Dysmenorrhea
Aciphex Tablets 1267
Aciphex Tablets 1783
Advair Diskus 100/50 1448
Advair Diskus 250/50 1448
Advair Diskus 500/50 1448
Alamast Ophthalmic Solution (Less than 5%) 3092
Allegra (1.5%) 712
Arthrotec Tablets (Rare) 3195
▲ Asacol Delayed-Release Tablets (3%) 2884
Axert Tablets (Infrequent) 2772
▲ Betaseron for SC Injection (18%) 988
Ceclor CD Tablets (0.1% to 1%) 1279
Celebrex Capsules (0.1% to 1.9%) 2676
Celebrex Capsules (0.1% to 1.9%) 2780
▲ Celexa (3%) 1365
▲ Cenestin Tablets (6%) 1263
Claritin (At least one patient) 3100
Claritin-D 12 Hour Extended Release Tablets (Less frequent) 3102
Claritin-D 24 Hour Extended Release Tablets (2%) 3104
Clozaril Tablets (Less than 1%) 2319
▲ CombiPatch Transdermal System (30% to 31%) 2323
▲ Copaxone for Injection (6%) 3306
Crinone (Less than 5%) 3213
Cytotec Tablets (0.1%) 3202
Depacon Injection (1% to 5%) 416
Depakene (1% to 5%) 421
Depakote Sprinkle Capsules (1% to 5%) 426
Depakote Tablets (1% to 5%) 430
Depakote ER Tablets (Greater than 1%) 436
Depo-Provera Contraceptive Injection (Fewer than 1%) 2798
▲ Dostinex Tablets (1% to less than 10%) 2804
Dynabac Tablets (0.1% to 1%) 2269
Effexor Tablets 3495
▲ Effexor XR Capsules (6%) 3499
▲ Esclim Transdermal System (2.1% to 6.4%) 3460
Estinyl Tablets 3112
Estratest 3252
Evoxac Capsules (Less than 1%) 1217
▲ Famvir Tablets (2.2% to 7.6%) 2348
Flovent (1% to 3%) 1535
Flovent Rotadisk (1% to 3%) 1537
Floxin I.V. (Less than 1%) 2526
Floxin Tablets (Less than 1%) 2529
Gabitril Tablets (Frequent) 1189
Gonal-F for Injection (2.5%) 3216
Imitrex Injection (Rare) 1549
Imitrex Nasal Spray (Infrequent) 1554
Imitrex Tablets (Infrequent) 1558
▲ Infergen (2% to 9%) 1777
Intron A for Injection (Less than 5%) 3120
▲ Klonopin Tablets (3%) 2983
▲ Lamictal (6.6%) 1567
Lo/Ovral Tablets 3532
Lo/Ovral-28 Tablets 3538
Low-Ogestrel-28 Tablets 3392
Lunelle Monthly Injection 2827
Luvox Tablets (25, 50, 100 mg) 3256
Menest Tablets 2254
▲ Meridia Capsules (3.5%) 481
▲ Mirena Intrauterine System (5% or more) 974
Monurol Sachet (2.6%) 1375
Naprelan Tablets (Less than 1%) 1293
Nasonex Nasal Spray (1% to 5%) 3131
Neurontin Capsules (Infrequent) 2655
Neurontin Oral Solution (Infrequent) 2655
Neurontin Tablets (Infrequent) 2655
Nexium Delayed-Release Capsules (Less than 1%) 619
▲ Nicotrol Nasal Spray (3%) 2843
Nordette-28 Tablets 2257
Noroxin Tablets (Less frequent) 2145
Norplant System 3543
Ogestrel 0.5/50-28 Tablets 3428
Ortho Dienestrol Cream 2554
▲ Ortho-Prefest Tablets (8%) 2570
Ovral Tablets 3551
Ovral-28 Tablets 3552
Ovrette Tablets 3552
ParaGard T 380A Intrauterine Copper Contraceptive 2582
Paxil (Infrequent) 1609
Permax Tablets (Frequent) 1299
Premarin Intravenous 3563
Premarin Vaginal Cream 3570
▲ Prempro Tablets (5% to 8%) 3572
Protonix I.V. (Less than 1%) 3580
Protonix Tablets (Less than 1%) 3577
Protopic Ointment (Up to 4%) 1397
Provigil Tablets (At least 1%) 1193
Prozac Pulvules, Liquid, and Weekly Capsules (Less than 1%) 1238
Qvar Inhalation Aerosol (1% to 3%) 1987
Remeron Tablets (Infrequent) 2483
Remeron SolTab Tablets (Infrequent) 2486
Risperdal (Infrequent) 1796
Semprex-D Capsules (2%) 1172
Serevent Inhalation Aerosol (1% to 3%) 1633
Seroquel Tablets (Infrequent) 684
Serzone Tablets 1104
Sonata Capsules (2% to 4%) 3591
▲ Terazol 3 Vaginal Cream (6%) 2587
▲ Topamax Sprinkle Capsules (8.3%) 2590
▲ Topamax Tablets (8.3%) 2590
Tri-Nasal Spray (2%) 2274
Triphasil-21 Tablets 3600
Triphasil-28 Tablets 3605
Uniretic Tablets (Less than 1%) 3178
▲ Valtrex Caplets (Less than 1% to 8%) 1676
▲ Vanceril Double Strength Inhalation Aerosol (4%) 3167
Wellbutrin SR Sustained-Release Tablets (At least 1%) 1684
Yasmin 28 Tablets (Greater than 1%) 980
▲ Zoladex (1% to 7%) 702
Zoloft (Infrequent) 2751
Zomig Tablets (Rare) 708
Zomig-ZMT Tablets (Rare) 708
Zyprexa Tablets 1973
Zyprexa ZYDIS Orally Disintegrating Tablets 1973
Zyrtec (Less than 2%) 2756
Zyrtec-D 12 Hour Extended Relief Tablets (Less than 2%) 2758

Dysmetria
Trileptal Oral Suspension 2407
Trileptal Tablets 2407

Dyspareunia
▲ Crinone 8% Gel (6%) 3213
Depo-Provera Contraceptive Injection (Fewer than 1%) 2798
ParaGard T 380A Intrauterine Copper Contraceptive 2582
Wellbutrin Tablets (Rare) 1680
Wellbutrin SR Sustained-Release Tablets 1684
▲ Zoladex (14%) 702
Zyban Sustained-Release Tablets 1710

Dyspepsia
Abelcet Injection 1273
Accolate Tablets (1.5%) 657
Accuretic Tablets (1.2%) 2614
Aceon Tablets (2 mg, 4 mg, 8 mg) (0.3% to 1.9%) 3249
Aciphex Tablets 1267
Aciphex Tablets 1783
Actiq (1% or greater) 1184
Adalat CC Tablets (Less than 1.0%) 877
Adderall XR Capsules (2%)
Advair Diskus 100/50 1448
Advair Diskus 250/50 1448
Advair Diskus 500/50 1448
Aerobid/Aerobid-M (1% to 3%) 1363
▲ Aggrenox Capsules (18.4%) 1026
▲ Agrylin Capsules (5.2%) 3232
▲ Alferon N Injection (3%) 1770
Allegra (1.3%) 712
Allegra-D Extended-Release Tablets (2.8%) 714
Alphagan P Ophthalmic Solution (1% to 4%) 546
Altace Capsules (Less than 1%) 2233
▲ Ambien Tablets (5%) 3191
AmBisome for Injection (Less common) 1383
Amerge Tablets (Infrequent) 1467
Amphotec (1% to 5%) 1774
Anaprox Tablets (Less than 3%) 2967
Anaprox DS Tablets (Less than 3%) 2967
▲ Anzemet Injection (3%) 719
▲ Anzemet Tablets (3%) 722
Apligraf (1.8%) 2305
▲ Arava Tablets (5%) 724
▲ Aredia for Injection (22.6%) 2309
▲ Aromasin Tablets (2% to 5%) 2769
▲ Arthrotec Tablets (14%) 3195
▲ Asacol Delayed-Release Tablets (6%) 2884
Atacand Tablets (0.5% or greater) 595
Atacand HCT Tablets (0.5% or greater) 597
Atromid-S Capsules 3483
Avalide Tablets (2%) 1070
Avapro Tablets (2%) 1074
Avapro Tablets (2%) 3076
Avelox Tablets (1%) 879
▲ Avonex (11%) 1013
Axert Tablets (Infrequent) 2772
▲ Axid Pulvules (3.6%) 1903
▲ Axid Pulvules (3.6%) 2919
Azopt Ophthalmic Suspension (Less than 1%) 536
▲ Azulfidine EN-tabs Tablets (15%) 2775
▲ Baycol Tablets (3.8%) 883
▲ Betapace Tablets (2% to 6%) 950
Betapace AF Tablets (2% to 2.5%) 954
Betaxon Ophthalmic Suspension (Less than 2%) 537
Biaxin/Biaxin XL (2%) 403
Blocadren Tablets (0.6%) 2046
Brevibloc Injection (Less than 1%) 858
Buprenex Injectable (Infrequent) 2918
▲ Campath Ampules (10%) 992
Captopril Tablets 2281
Cardene I.V. (Rare) 3485
Cardizem Injectable 1018
Cardizem Lyo-Ject Syringe 1018
Cardizem Monovial 1018
Cardizem CD Capsules (Less than 1%) 1016
Cardura Tablets (1% to 1.7%) 2668
▲ Carnitor Injection (5% to 9%) 3242
Casodex Tablets (2% to 5%) 662
Cataflam Tablets (Common) 2315
Ceclor CD Tablets (0.1% to 1%) 1279
Cedax (2%) 1021
Ceftin Tablets (0.1% to 1%) 1898
▲ Celebrex Capsules (8.8%) 2676
▲ Celebrex Capsules (8.8%) 2780
▲ Celexa (4%) 1365
▲ CellCept Capsules (13.6% to 18.7%) 2951
▲ CellCept Intravenous (13.6% to 18.7%) 2951
▲ CellCept Oral Suspension (13.6% to 18.7%) 2951
▲ CellCept Tablets (13.6% to 22.4%) 2951
▲ Cenestin Tablets (10%) 1263
Cerebyx Injection (Infrequent) 2619
Chirocaine Injection (2%) 2909
Cipro I.V. 893
Cipro 887
Claritin (At least one patient) 3100
▲ Claritin-D 12 Hour Extended Release Tablets (3%) 3102
Claritin-D 24 Hour Extended Release Tablets (Fewer than 2%) 3104
▲ Clinoril Tablets (3% to 9%) 2053
▲ Cognex Capsules (9%) 1351
Colazal Capsules (2%) 3069
▲ CombiPatch Transdermal System (6% to 8%) 2323
Combivent Inhalation Aerosol (Less than 2%) 1041
▲ Combivir Tablets (5%) 1502
Comtan Tablets (2%) 2328
Copaxone for Injection (At least 2%) 3306
Coreg Tablets (More than 2%) 1508
Cosopt Sterile Ophthalmic Solution (1% to 5%) 2065
Cozaar Tablets (1.3%) 2067
Crinone (Less than 5%) 3213
Crixivan Capsules (Less than 2%) 2070
Cytotec Tablets (2.0%) 3202
Cytovene (At least 3 subjects) 2959
Demadex Tablets and Injection (1.6%) 2965
▲ Depacon Injection (8% to 11%) 416
▲ Depakene (8% to 11%) 421
▲ Depakote Sprinkle Capsules (8% to 11%) 426
▲ Depakote Tablets (8% to 13%) 430
▲ Depakote ER Tablets (7% to 11%) 436
▲ Detrol Tablets (5.9%) 3623
▲ Detrol LA Capsules (3%) 2801
Diflucan Tablets, Injection, and Oral Suspension (1%) 2681
Diovan Capsules 2337
Diovan HCT Tablets (Greater than 0.2%) 2338
▲ Dipentum Capsules (4.0%) 2803

▲ Ditropan XL Extended Release Tablets (6.8%) 564
▲ Dolobid Tablets (3% to 9%) 2088
▲ Dostinex Tablets (2% to 5%) 2804
Doxil Injection (Less than 1% to 5%) 566
DuoNeb Inhalation Solution (1.3%) 1233
▲ Duragesic Transdermal System (3% to 10%) 1786
Duricef (Rare) 1079
Dynabac Tablets (2.6% to 4.1%) 2269
EC-Naprosyn Delayed-Release Tablets (Less than 3%) 2967
Ecotrin Enteric Coated Aspirin Low, Regular and Maximum Strength Tablets 1715
▲ Effexor Tablets (4.5% to 5%) 3495
Effexor XR Capsules (At least 2%) 3499
Elmiron Capsules (2%) 570
Enalaprilat Injection 863
▲ Enbrel for Injection (11%) 1752
▲ Enbrel for Injection (11%) 3504
Engerix-B Vaccine 1517
▲ Epivir (5%) 1520
▲ Epogen for Injection (9% to 11%) 582
Ergamisol Tablets (Less than 1% to 1%) 1789
Estring Vaginal Ring (1% to 3%) 2811
▲ Evista Tablets (5.9%) 1915
▲ Evoxac Capsules (7.8%) 1217
▲ Exelon Capsules (9%) 2342
▲ Exelon Oral Solution (9%) 2345
Famvir Tablets (1.1% to 3.4%) 2348
▲ Felbatol (6.5% to 12.3%) 3343
▲ Feldene Capsules (1% to 10%) 2685
▲ Femara Tablets (3% to 4%) 2351
Ferrlecit Injection (Greater than 1%) 3386
Flexeril Tablets (1% to 3%) 572
Flexeril Tablets (1% to 3%) 2094
Flolan for Injection (1%) 1528
Flovent (1% to 3%) 1535
Floxin I.V. (Less than 1%) 2526
Floxin Otic Solution (Single report) 1219
Floxin Tablets (Less than 1%) 2529
Flumadine (0.3% to 1%) 1370
▲ Fortovase Capsules (8.4% to 8.9%) 2970
Fosamax Tablets (1.9% to 3.6%) 2095
Foscavir Injection (Between 1% and 5%) 605
Gabitril Tablets (1% or more) 1189
Gastrocrom Oral Concentrate 1162
▲ Gengraf Capsules (2.2% to 8%) 457
▲ Geodon Capsules (8%) 2688
▲ Gleevec Capsules (9% to 18%) 2357
Glucophage Tablets (1% to 5%) 1080
Glucophage XR Tablets (1% to 5%) 1080
Glucotrol XL Extended Release Tablets (Less than 3%) 2693
Gonal-F for Injection (1.7%) 3216
Haldol Decanoate 2535
Haldol Injection, Tablets and Concentrate 2533
▲ Hectorol Capsules (4.9%) 1064
▲ Hectorol Injection (4.9%) 1066
Hivid Tablets (Less than 1%) 2975
Hytrin Capsules (At least 1%) 464
Hyzaar 2109
Imdur Tablets (Less than or equal to 5%) 1826
Imitrex Nasal Spray 1554
Indapamide Tablets (Less than 5%) 2286
▲ Indocin (3% to 9%) 2112
▲ Infergen (12% to 21%) 1777
Innohep Injection (Greater than or equal to 1%) 1248
▲ Intron A for Injection (Up to 8%) 3120
Invirase Capsules (0.9% to 2%) 2979
Ismo Tablets (Fewer than 1%) 3524
Kadian Capsules (Less than 3%) 1335
Kaletra Capsules (Less than 2%) 471
Kaletra Oral Solution (Less than 2%) 471
Keflex 1237
Keppra Tablets (1% or more) 3314
Klonopin Tablets (Infrequent) 2983
▲ Kytril Tablets (4% to 6%) 2988
▲ Lamictal (5.3%) 1567
▲ Lamisil Tablets (4.3%) 2360
▲ Lescol Capsules (7.9%) 2361
▲ Lescol Capsules (7.9%) 2925
▲ Lescol XL Tablets (3.5%) 2361
▲ Lescol XL Tablets (3.5%) 2925
▲ Leukine (17%) 1755
Levaquin (0.3% to 2.0%) 2537
Levo-Dromoran 1734
Lexxel Tablets 608
Lipitor Tablets (1.3% to 2.8%) 2639
Lipitor Tablets (1.3% to 2.8%) 2696
▲ Lodine (10%) 3528
▲ Lodine XL Extended-Release Tablets (1% to 10%) 3530
Lodosyn Tablets 1251
▲ Lopid Tablets (19.6%) 2650
Lotensin HCT Tablets (0.3% to 1%) 2367
Lotrel Capsules 2370
▲ Luvox Tablets (25, 50, 100 mg) (1% to 10%) 3256
Macrobid Capsules (Less than 1%) 2889
Malarone (2% to 3%) 1596
▲ Mavik Tablets (0.3% to 6.4%) 478
Maxalt Tablets (Infrequent) 2120
Maxalt-MLT Orally Disintegrating Tablets (Infrequent) 2120
Megace Oral Suspension (Up to 4%) 1124
▲ Mepron Suspension (5%) 1598
▲ Meridia Capsules (5%) 481
▲ Mevacor Tablets (1.0% to 3.9%) 2132
Miacalcin Nasal Spray (1% to 3%) 2375
Micardis Tablets (1%) 1049
Micardis HCT Tablets (Less than 2%) 1051
Midamor Tablets (Less than or equal to 1%) 2136
Migranal Nasal Spray (Infrequent) 2376
Mirapex Tablets (Rare) 2834
▲ Mobic Tablets (3.8% to 8.9%) 1054
Moduretic Tablets 2138
Monopril HCT (Less than 2%) 1094
Monurol Sachet (1.1% to 1.8%) 1375
Motrin Suspension, Oral Drops, Chewable Tablets, and Caplets (Common) 2002
▲ Mycobutin Capsules (3%) 2838
▲ Mylotarg for Injection (9% to 16%) 3540
▲ Myobloc Injectable Solution (3% to 10%) 1291
▲ Naprelan Tablets (14%) 1293
Naprosyn Suspension (Less than 3%) 2967
Naprosyn Tablets (Less than 3%) 2967
Nascobal Gel 3174
Nasonex Nasal Spray (Greater than or equal to 2%) 3131
▲ Neoral Soft Gelatin Capsules (2.2% to 8%) 2380
▲ Neoral Oral Solution (2.2% to 8%) 2380
▲ Neumega for Injection (Greater than or equal to 10%) 1434
Neurontin Capsules (2.2%) 2655
Neurontin Oral Solution (2.2%) 2655
Neurontin Tablets (2.2%) 2655
Nexium Delayed-Release Capsules (Less than 1%) 619
▲ Nicotrol Inhaler (18%) 2840
Nicotrol Nasal Spray (Common) 2843
▲ Nilandron Tablets (6.7%) 753
▲ Nipent for Injection (3% to 10%) 3272
Normodyne Injection (1%) 3135
▲ Normodyne Tablets (Up to 4%) 3137
Noroxin Tablets (0.3% to 1.0%) 2145
Norvasc Tablets (Less than 1% to 2%) 2704
Norvir Capsules (Up to 4.8%) 487
Norvir Oral Solution (Up to 4.8%) 487
▲ Novantrone for Injection (5%) 1760
Nubain Injection (1% or less) 1323
Omnicef (0.8%) 493
▲ Orudis Capsules (11%) 3548
▲ Oruvail Capsules (11%) 3548
OxyContin Tablets (Between 1% and 5%) 2912
Paxil (2%) 1609
▲ PEG-Intron Powder for Injection (6%) 3140
Pentasa Capsules (1.6%) 3239
▲ Periostat Tablets (4% to 6%) 1208
▲ Permax Tablets (6.4%) 1299
Persantine Tablets (Rare) 1057
▲ Photofrin for Injection (6%) 831
▲ Plavix Tablets (5.2%) 1097
▲ Plavix Tablets (5.2%) 3084
▲ Plendil Extended-Release Tablets (0.5% to 3.9%) 623
▲ Pletal Tablets (6%) 2605
▲ Pletal Tablets (6%) 2848
▲ Ponstel Capsules (1% to 10%) 1356
Prandin Tablets (0.5, 1, and 2 mg) (2% to 3%) 2432
▲ Prempro Tablets (6%) 3572
Prevacid Delayed-Release Capsules (Less than 1%) 3292
PREVPAC (Less than 1% to 3%) 3298
Priftin Tablets (1.1%) 758
Prinivil Tablets (0.3% to 1.0%) 2164
Prinzide Tablets (1.3%) 2168
Procardia XL Extended Release Tablets (Less than 3%) 2710
▲ Procrit for Injection (7% to 11%) 2502
▲ Prograf (3% to 28%) 1393
▲ Proleukin for Injection (7%) 1199
Prometrium Capsules (100 mg, 200 mg) (Less than 5%) 3261
ProSom Tablets (2%) 500
Protonix I.V. (Greater than 1%) 3580
Protonix Tablets (Greater than or equal to 1%) 3577
Protopic Ointment (1% to 4%) 1397
Proventil Inhalation Solution 0.083% (1% to 1.5%) 3146
Proventil Repetabs Tablets (2%) 3148
Proventil Solution for Inhalation 0.5% (1% to 1.5%) 3144
Provigil Tablets (At least 1%) 1193
▲ Prozac Pulvules, Liquid, and Weekly Capsules (7% to 10%) 1238
▲ Pulmicort Turbuhaler Inhalation Powder (Up to 8%) 636
▲ Pulmozyme Inhalation Solution (3%) 1426
▲ Rapamune Oral Solution and Tablets (17% to 25%) 3584
▲ Rebetron Combination Therapy (14% to 16%) 3153
Recombivax HB (Less than 1%) 2178
ReFacto Vials 1437
▲ Relafen Tablets (13%) 1617
▲ Remicade for IV Injection (5% to 6%) 1178
▲ Reminyl Oral Solution (5%) 1792
▲ Reminyl Tablets (5%) 1792
▲ Renagel Capsules (5% to 11%) 1439
▲ Renagel Tablets (5% to 11%) 1439
ReoPro Vials (2.1%) 1958
▲ Requip Tablets (10%) 1621
Rescriptor Tablets (Less than 2%) 526
▲ Retrovir Capsules (5% to 6%) 1625
▲ Retrovir IV Infusion (5% to 6%) 1629
▲ Retrovir (5% to 6%) 1625
Rhinocort Nasal Inhaler (1% to 3%) 640
▲ Rilutek Tablets (2.5% to 6.1%) 772
▲ Risperdal (5% to 10%) 1796
Rituxan for Infusion (1% to 5%) 1750
Rituxan I.V. (1% to 5%) 1428
Robaxin Injectable 2938
Robaxin Tablets 2939
Rocephin Injectable Vials, ADD-Vantage, Galaxy, Bulk (Rare) 2993
Roxicodone Tablets (Less than 3%) 3067
▲ Rythmol Tablets – 150 mg, 225 mg, 300 mg (1.9% to 3.4%) 502
▲ Salagen Tablets (7%) 2229
▲ Sandostatin LAR Depot (5% to 15%) 2395
▲ Sarafem Pulvules (7%) 1962
▲ Sectral Capsules (4%) 3589
Semprex-D Capsules (2%) 1172
Serevent Inhalation Aerosol (1% to 3%) 1633
▲ Seroquel Tablets (6%) 684
▲ Serostim for Injection (1% to 10%) 3229
▲ Serzone Tablets (9%) 1104
▲ Simulect for Injection (Greater than or equal to 10%) 2399
Sinemet Tablets 1253
Sinemet CR Tablets (0.6%) 1255
Singulair (2.1%) 2181
▲ Skelid Tablets (5.3%) 3088
▲ Sonata Capsules (4% to 7%) 3591
Soriatane Capsules (Less than 1%) 3003
▲ Sporanox Capsules (4%) 1800
Sporanox Oral Solution (Less than 2%) 1808
Sporanox Oral Solution (Less than 2%) 2512
Stimate Nasal Spray 796
Sular Tablets (Less than or equal to 1%) 688
▲ Suprax (3%) 1877
Sustiva Capsules (1% to 4%) 1258
Synercid I.V. (Less than 1%) 775
Tambocor Tablets (1% to 3%) 1990
Tarka Tablets (0.3% or more) 508
▲ Tasmar Tablets (3% to 4%) 3010
Tenex Tablets (3% or less) 2942
Tequin Injection (0.1% to 3%) 1110
Tequin Tablets (0.1% to 3%) 1110
Teveten Tablets (1% or greater) 3327
Thalomid Capsules 1154
▲ Tiazac Capsules (4%) 1378
▲ Ticlid Tablets (7.0%) 3015
Timolide Tablets (Less than 1%) 2187
Timolol GFS ⊙266
Timoptic in Ocudose (Less frequent) 2192
Timoptic Sterile Ophthalmic Solution 2190
Timoptic-XE Sterile Ophthalmic Gel Forming Solution 2194
▲ Tolectin (3% to 9%) 2589
Tonocard Tablets (Less than 1%) 649
▲ Topamax Sprinkle Capsules (5.7% to 8%) 2590
▲ Topamax Tablets (5.7% to 8%) 2590
▲ Toradol (12%) 3018
Trasylol Injection (1% to 2%) 909
Travatan Ophthalmic Solution (1% to 5%) 543
Trental Tablets (2.8%) 784
▲ Tricor Capsules, Micronized (5%) 513
▲ Trileptal Oral Suspension (2% to 6%) 2407
▲ Trileptal Tablets (2% to 6%) 2407
Tri-Nasal Spray (2.7% to 4.9%) 2274
▲ Trisenox Injection (10%) 1158
▲ Trizivir Tablets (5%) 1669
Trovan (Less than 1%) 2722
Twinrix Vaccine 1674
Ultracet Tablets (At least 1%) 2597
▲ Ultram Tablets (5% to 13%) 2600
Uniretic Tablets (More than 1%) 3178
Univasc Tablets (More than 1%) 3181
▲ Vagifem Tablets (3% to 5%) 2857
▲ Vanceril Double Strength Inhalation Aerosol (3%) 3167
Vantin Tablets and Oral Suspension (Less than 1%) 2860
▲ Vascor Tablets (6.81% to about 22%) 2602
Vaseretic Tablets (0.5% to 2.0%) 2204
Vasotec I.V. Injection 2207
Vasotec Tablets (0.5% to 1.0%) 2210
Verelan Capsules (2.5%) 3184
Verelan PM Capsules (2.7%) 3186
▲ Vesanoid Capsules (14%) 3037
▲ Viagra Tablets (7%) 2732
▲ Vicoprofen Tablets (12%) 520
Videx 1138
Videx EC Capsules 1143
Vioxx (2.7%) 2213
Viracept 532
Vistide Injection 1445
Voltaren Tablets (Common) 2315
Voltaren-XR Tablets (Common) 2315
▲ WelChol Tablets (8%) 3073
▲ Wellbutrin Tablets (3.1%) 1680
Wellbutrin SR Sustained-Release Tablets (At least 1%) 1684
Xopenex Inhalation Solution (1.4% to 2.7%) 3207
Zanaflex Tablets (Frequent) 1305
Zebeta Tablets 1885
▲ Zenapax for Injection (Greater than 5%) 3046
Zestoretic Tablets (1.3%) 695
Zestril Tablets (0.3% to 1.0%) 698
Ziac Tablets (0.9% to 1.2%) 1887
Zithromax Capsules, 250 mg (1% or less) 2743
Zithromax for IV Infusion (1% or less) 2748
Zithromax for Oral Suspension, 1 g (1% or less to 1%) 2743
Zithromax for Oral Suspension, 300 mg, 600 mg, 900 mg, 1200 mg (1% or less) 2739
Zithromax Tablets, 250 mg (1% or less) 2739
Zithromax Tablets, 600 mg (1% or less to 1%) 2743
Zocor Tablets (1.1%) 2219
Zoladex (1% or greater) 702
Zoladex 3-month 706
▲ Zoloft (6% to 10%) 2751
Zomig Tablets (1% to 3%) 708
Zomig-ZMT Tablets (1% to 3%) 708
▲ Zonegran Capsules (3%) 1307
▲ Zosyn (1.9% to 3.3%) 1890
▲ Zosyn in Galaxy Containers (1.9% to 3.3%) 1894
Zyban Sustained-Release Tablets (Frequent) 1710
▲ Zyflo Filmtab Tablets (8.2%) 524
▲ Zyprexa Tablets (11%) 1973
▲ Zyprexa ZYDIS Orally Disintegrating Tablets (11%) 1973
Zyrtec (Less than 2%) 2756
Zyrtec-D 12 Hour Extended Relief Tablets (Less than 2%) 2758
Zyvox 2871

Dysphagia

Aciphex Tablets 1267
Aciphex Tablets 1783
Actiq (1% or greater) 1184
Actonel Tablets 2879
Altace Capsules (Less than 1%) 2233
Ambien Tablets (Infrequent) 3191
AmBisome for Injection (Less common) 1383
Arthrotec Tablets (Rare) 3195
▲ Botox Purified Neurotoxin Complex (19%) 549
▲ Casodex Tablets (2% to 5%) 662
Celebrex Capsules (0.1% to 1.9%) 2676
Celebrex Capsules (0.1% to 1.9%) 2780
Celexa (Infrequent) 1365
▲ CellCept Capsules (3% to 10%) 2951
▲ CellCept Intravenous (3% to 10%) 2951
▲ CellCept Oral Suspension (3% to 10%) 2951
▲ CellCept Tablets (3% to 10%) 2951
Cerebyx Injection (Infrequent) 2619
Cipro I.V. (1% or less) 893
Cipro I.V. Pharmacy Bulk Package (Less than 1%) 897
Cipro (Less than 1%) 887
Clozaril Tablets 2319
Cognex Capsules (Infrequent) 1351
Copaxone for Injection (At least 2%) 3306
Cosmegen for Injection 2062
Cytotec Tablets (Infrequent) 3202
DaunoXome Injection (Less than or equal to 5%) 1442
Declomycin Tablets 1855
Depakote ER Tablets (Greater than 1%) 436
Doryx Coated Pellet Filled Capsules 3357
Doxil Injection (1% to 5%) 566
Dynacin Capsules 2019
Edecrin 2091
Effexor Tablets (Infrequent) 3495
Effexor XR Capsules (Infrequent) 3499
Eldepryl Capsules 3266
Etrafon 3115
Evoxac Capsules (Less than 1%) 1217
Exelon Capsules (Infrequent) 2342
Exelon Oral Solution (Infrequent) 2345
Extendryl 1361
Felbatol 3343

Fludara for Injection (Up to 1%) 995
Flumadine 1370
Fortovase Capsules (Less than 2%) 2970
Fosamax Tablets (1.0%) 2095
Foscavir Injection (Between 1% and 5%) 605
Gabitril Tablets (Infrequent) 1189
Gastrocrom Oral Concentrate 1162
Gengraf Capsules (1% to less than 3%) 457
Geodon Capsules (Infrequent) 2688
▲ Geref for Injection (1 patient in 6) 3215
Gliadel Wafer (1%) 1723
Hivid Tablets (Less than 1%) 2975
Imitrex Injection (1.1%) 1549
Imitrex Nasal Spray (Infrequent) 1554
Imitrex Tablets (Infrequent) 1558
Intron A for Injection (Less than 5%) 3120
Invirase Capsules (Less than 2%) 2979
Kadian Capsules (Less than 3%) 1335
Kaletra Capsules (Less than 2%) 471
Kaletra Oral Solution (Less than 2%) 471
Lamictal (Infrequent) 1567
▲ Leukine (11%) 1755
Levaquin Injection (Less than 0.5%) 2537
Lipitor Tablets (Less than 2%) 2639
Lipitor Tablets (Less than 2%) 2696
Lodosyn Tablets 1251
Lupron Depot 7.5 mg (Less than 5%) 3284
Lupron Depot-PED 7.5 mg, 11.25 mg and 15 mg (Less than 2%) 3291
Lupron Injection (Less than 5%) 3279
Lupron Injection Pediatric (Less than 2%) 3280
Luvox Tablets (25, 50, 100 mg) (2%) 3256
Matulane Capsules 3246
Maxalt Tablets (Infrequent) 2120
Maxalt-MLT Orally Disintegrating Tablets (Infrequent) 2120
Mexitil Capsules (About 2 in 1,000) 1047
Migranal Nasal Spray (Infrequent) 2376
Minocin Intravenous 1862
Minocin Oral Suspension 1865
Minocin Pellet-Filled Capsules 1863
Mirapex Tablets (2%) 2834
Monodox Capsules 2442
Monopril Tablets (0.2% to 1.0%) 1091
Monopril HCT 1094
▲ Myobloc Injectable Solution (10% to 25%) 1291
Naprelan Tablets (Less than 3%) 1293
Navelbine Injection 1604
Neoral Soft Gelatin Capsules (1% to less than 3%) 2380
Neoral Oral Solution (1% to less than 3%) 2380
Neurontin Capsules (Rare) 2655
Neurontin Oral Solution (Rare) 2655
Neurontin Tablets (Rare) 2655
Nexium Delayed-Release Capsules (Less than 1%) 619
Nipent for Injection (Less than 3%) 3272
Noroxin Tablets 2145
Norvasc Tablets (More than 0.1% to 1%) 2704
Norvir Capsules (Less than 2%) 487
Norvir Oral Solution (Less than 2%) 487
Orap Tablets (2.7%) 1407
OxyContin Tablets (Less than 1%) 2912
Paxil (Infrequent) 1609
Pentasa Capsules (Less than 1%) 3239
Periostat Tablets 1208
Permax Tablets (Frequent) 1299
▲ Photofrin for Injection (10%) 831
Prevacid Delayed-Release Capsules (Less than 1%) 3292
PREVPAC (Less than 1%) 3298
▲ Prograf (3% to 15%) 1393
Protonix I.V. (Less than 1%) 3580
Protonix Tablets (Less than 1%) 3577
Prozac Pulvules, Liquid, and Weekly Capsules (Infrequent) 1238
▲ Rapamune Oral Solution and Tablets (3% to 20%) 3584
Relafen Tablets (Less than 1%) 1617
Remicade for IV Injection 1178
Reminyl Oral Solution (Infrequent) 1792
Reminyl Tablets (Infrequent) 1792
Requip Tablets (Infrequent) 1621
Rescriptor Tablets (Less than 2%) 526
Retrovir Capsules 1625
Retrovir IV Infusion 1629
Retrovir 1625
Rilutek Tablets (More than 2%) 772
Risperdal (Infrequent) 1796
Roxicodone Tablets (Less than 3%) 3067
Salagen Tablets (2%) 2229
Sandostatin LAR Depot (1% to 4%) 2395
Sarafem Pulvules (Infrequent) 1962
Seroquel Tablets (Infrequent) 684
▲ Serostim for Injection (1% to 10%) 3229
Serzone Tablets (Rare) 1104
Sinemet Tablets 1253
Sinemet CR Tablets 1255
Skelid Tablets 3088
Sonata Capsules (Rare) 3591
Sporanox Oral Solution (Less than 2%) 1808
Sporanox Oral Solution (Less than 2%) 2512
Sular Tablets (Less than or equal to 1%) 688
Symmetrel 1328
Tasmar Tablets (Infrequent) 3010
Tenex Tablets (3% or less) 2942
Tensilon Injectable 1745
Tequin Injection (Less than 0.1%) 1110
Tequin Tablets (Less than 0.1%) 1110
Thalomid Capsules 1154
Tonocard Tablets (Less than 1%) 649
Topamax Sprinkle Capsules (Infrequent) 2590
Topamax Tablets (Infrequent) 2590
Trilafon 3160
Trileptal Oral Suspension 2407
Trileptal Tablets 2407
Trovan (Less than 1%) 2722
Ultracet Tablets (Less than 1%) 2597
Uniretic Tablets (Less than 1%) 3178
Viagra Tablets (Less than 2%) 2732
Vibramycin Calcium Oral Suspension Syrup 2735
Vibramycin Hyclate Capsules 2735
Vibramycin Hyclate Intravenous 2737
Vibramycin Monohydrate for Oral Suspension 2735
Vibra-Tabs Film Coated Tablets 2735
Vicoprofen Tablets (Less than 1%) 520
Vistide Injection 1445
Wellbutrin Tablets (Infrequent) 1680
Wellbutrin SR Sustained-Release Tablets (Up to 2%) 1684
Zanaflex Tablets (Infrequent) 1305
▲ Zinecard for Injection (Up to 8%) 2869
Zoloft (Infrequent) 2751
▲ Zometa for Intravenous Infusion (5% to 10%) 3621
Zomig Tablets (2%) 708
Zomig-ZMT Tablets (2%) 708
Zonegran Capsules (Infrequent) 1307
Zyban Sustained-Release Tablets (Infrequent) 1710
Zyprexa Tablets (Infrequent) 1973
Zyprexa ZYDIS Orally Disintegrating Tablets (Infrequent) 1973

Dysphasia

Ambien Tablets (Rare) 3191
Aricept Tablets (Infrequent) 1270
Aricept Tablets (Infrequent) 2665
Cipro I.V. (1% or less) 893
Cipro I.V. Pharmacy Bulk Package (Less than 1%) 897
Cipro 887
Cytovene 2959
Floxin I.V. 2526
Floxin Tablets 2529
Imitrex Injection 1549
Imitrex Nasal Spray 1554
Roferon-A Injection (Infrequent) 2996
▲ Temodar Capsules (7%) 3157

Dysphonia

▲ Advair Diskus 100/50 (5%) 1448
Advair Diskus 250/50 (2%) 1448
▲ Advair Diskus 500/50 (2% to 5%) 1448
Claritin (Up to 2%) 3100
Claritin-D 12 Hour Extended Release Tablets (Less frequent) 3102
Claritin-D 24 Hour Extended Release Tablets (Fewer than 2%) 3104
Colazal Capsules 3069
Combivent Inhalation Aerosol (Less than 2%) 1041
Evoxac Capsules (Less than 1%) 1217
Exelon Capsules (Infrequent) 2342
Exelon Oral Solution (Infrequent) 2345
▲ Flovent Diskus (1% to 9%) 3614
▲ Flovent (3% to 19%) 1535
▲ Flovent Rotadisk (Less than 1% to 6%) 1537
Foradil Aerolizer (1%) 2354
Hivid Tablets (Less than 1%) 2975
Intron A for Injection (Less than 5%) 3120
Levaquin 2537
LYMErix Vaccine (Greater than 1%) 1592
Proventil HFA Inhalation Aerosol (Less than 3%) 3150
Pulmicort Respules (1% to 3%) 632
Qvar Inhalation Aerosol (Up to 4%) 1987
ReoPro Vials (0.3%) 1958
Requip Tablets (Infrequent) 1621
Romazicon Injection (Less than 1%) 3000
Sandostatin LAR Depot (1% to 4%) 2395
Soriatane Capsules (Less than 1%) 3003
Tensilon Injectable 1745
Topamax Sprinkle Capsules (Infrequent) 2590
Topamax Tablets (Infrequent) 2590
Trileptal Oral Suspension 2407
Trileptal Tablets 2407
Vanceril Double Strength Inhalation Aerosol (Fewer than 2%) 3167
Versed Injection (Less than 1%) 3027
Zoloft (Rare) 2751
Zyrtec (Less than 2%) 2756
Zyrtec-D 12 Hour Extended Relief Tablets (Less than 2%) 2758

Dysphoria

Accuretic Tablets 2614
Actiq 1184
Adderall Tablets 3231
Adderall XR Capsules
Adipex-P 1406
Advair Diskus 100/50 1448
Advair Diskus 250/50 1448
Advair Diskus 500/50 1448
Aldoclor Tablets 2035
Aldoril Tablets 2039
Allegra-D Extended-Release Tablets 714
Ambien Tablets 3191
Amerge Tablets (Rare) 1467
Aricept Tablets (Infrequent) 1270
Aricept Tablets (Infrequent) 2665
Astramorph/PF Injection, USP (Preservative-Free) 594
Atacand HCT Tablets 597
Ativan Injection (1.3%) 3478
Avalide Tablets 1070
Axert Tablets (Infrequent) 2772
Benadryl Parenteral 2617
Bontril Slow-Release Capsules 576
Brevital Sodium for Injection, USP 1815
Buprenex Injectable (Rare) 2918
Cafcit 1035
Catapres Tablets 1037
Catapres-TTS (0.5% or less) 1038
Chibroxin Sterile Ophthalmic Solution 2051
Cipro I.V. (Greater than 1%) 893
Cipro I.V. Pharmacy Bulk Package (Greater than 1%) 897
Cipro (1.1%) 887
Claritin-D 12 Hour Extended Release Tablets 3102
Claritin-D 24 Hour Extended Release Tablets 3104
Clorpres Tablets 1002
▲ Clozaril Tablets (4%) 2319
Combipres Tablets 1040
Darvon-N/Darvocet-N 1907
Darvon Pulvules 1909
Darvon Compound-65 Pulvules 1910
Darvon-N Tablets 1912
Demadex Tablets and Injection 2965
Demerol 3079
Desoxyn Tablets (Rare) 440
Dexedrine 1512
DextroStat Tablets 3236
Dilaudid 441
Dilaudid Oral Liquid 445
Dilaudid Powder 441
Dilaudid Rectal Suppositories 441
Dilaudid Tablets 441
Dilaudid Tablets - 8 mg 445
Dilaudid-HP (Less frequent) 443
Diovan HCT Tablets 2338
Diucardin Tablets 3494
Diuril Oral 2087
Diuril Sodium Intravenous 2086
Dolophine Hydrochloride Tablets 3056
Duraclon Injection (Rare) 3057
Duramorph Injection 1312
Duranest Injections 600
Eldepryl Capsules 3266
Eskalith 1527
Etrafon 3115
Flovent Diskus 3614
Flovent 1535
Flovent Rotadisk 1537
Floxin I.V. 2526
Floxin Tablets 2529
Furosemide Tablets 2284
Halcion Tablets 2823
Haldol Decanoate 2535
Haldol Injection, Tablets and Concentrate 2533
Hycodan 1316
Hycomine Compound Tablets 1317
Hycotuss Expectorant Syrup 1318
HydroDIURIL Tablets 2108
Hyzaar 2109
Inderide LA Long-Acting Capsules 3519
Infanrix Vaccine 1562
Infumorph 200 and Infumorph 500 Sterile Solutions 1314
Ionamin Capsules 1163
Lamictal (Infrequent) 1567
Lariam Tablets 2989
Levaquin (0.1% to less than 0.5%) 2537
Limbitrol 1738
Lithium Carbonate 3061
Lithium Citrate Syrup 3061
Lithobid Slow-Release Tablets 3255
Lortab 3319
Lortab Elixir 3317
Lotensin HCT Tablets 2367
Lufyllin Tablets 3347
Lufyllin-400 Tablets 3347
Lufyllin-GG Elixir 3348
Lufyllin-GG Tablets 3348
Maxidone Tablets CIII 3399
Maxzide 1008
Mepergan Injection 3539
Micardis HCT Tablets 1051
Microzide Capsules 3414
Minizide Capsules 2700
Moduretic Tablets 2138
Monopril HCT 1094
▲ MS Contin Tablets (Among most frequent) 2896
▲ MSIR (Among most frequent) 2898
Mykrox Tablets 1168
Narcan Injection 1322
Naropin Injection 612
Navane Oral 2701
Navane Intramuscular 2703
Nesacaine/Nesacaine MPF 617
▲ Nicotrol Nasal Spray (Over 5%) 2843
Nitrolingual Pumpspray 1355
Norco 5/325 Tablets CIII 3424
Norco 7.5/325 Tablets CIII 3425
Norco 10/325 Tablets CIII 3425
Norco 10/325 Tablets CIII 3427
Noroxin Tablets 2145
Norpramin Tablets 755
Novarel for Injection 1347
Nubain Injection (1% or less) 1323
Numorphan 1324
▲ Oramorph SR Tablets (Among most frequent) 3062
Orudis Capsules (Rare) 3548
Oruvail Capsules (Rare) 3548
Oxsoralen-Ultra Capsules 1741
OxyFast Oral Concentrate Solution 2916
OxyIR Capsules 2916
Parnate Tablets 1607
Percocet Tablets 1326
Percodan Tablets 1327
Percolone Tablets 1327
Periactin Tablets 2155
Phenergan with Codeine Syrup 3557
Phenergan VC Syrup 3560
Phenergan VC with Codeine Syrup 3561
Pregnyl for Injection 2482
Prinzide Tablets 2168
Proventil Repetabs Tablets (Less than 1%) 3148
▲ Reglan (Approximately 10%) 2935
Renese Tablets 2712
Rescriptor Tablets (Less than 2%) 526
Romazicon Injection (1% to 3%) 3000
Roxanol 3066
Roxicodone 3067
Rynatan Tablets 3351
Sensorcaine 643
Sensorcaine-MPF Injection 643
Serentil 1057
Serzone Tablets 1104
Singulair (Very rare) 2181
Stadol NS Nasal Spray (Less than 1%) 1108
Surmontil Capsules 3595
Tenoretic Tablets 690
Tequin Injection 1110
Tequin Tablets 1110
Theo-Dur Extended-Release Tablets 1835
Thioridazine Hydrochloride Tablets (Extremely rare) 2289
Thiothixene Capsules 2290
Timolide Tablets 2187
Transderm Scōp Transdermal Therapeutic System (Infrequent) 2302
Trecator-SC Tablets 3598
Trilafon 3160
Trovan (Less than 1%) 2722
Tussionex Pennkinetic Extended-Release Suspension 1174
Tylenol with Codeine 2595
Tylox Capsules 2597
Uni-Dur Extended-Release Tablets 1841
Uniphyl 400 mg and 600 mg Tablets 2903
Uniretic Tablets 3178
Vaseretic Tablets 2204
Versed Injection (Less than 1%) 3027
Versed Syrup (Less than 1%) 3033
Vicodin Tablets 516
Vicodin ES Tablets 517
Vicodin HP Tablets 518
Vicodin Tuss Expectorant 519
Vivactil Tablets 2217
Vivactil Tablets 2446
Volmax Extended-Release Tablets (Less frequent) 2276
Wellbutrin Tablets (Infrequent) 1680
Wellbutrin SR Sustained-Release Tablets (Infrequent) 1684
Xylocaine Injections 653
Zaroxolyn Tablets 1177

Zebeta Tablets 1885
Zestoretic Tablets 695
Ziac Tablets 1887
Zyban Sustained-Release Tablets (Less than 1%) 1710
Zydone Tablets 1330

Dysplasia, cervical

Vivelle Transdermal System 2412
Vivelle-Dot Transdermal System 2416

Dysplasia, gastrointestinal

Nexium Delayed-Release Capsules (Less than 1%) 619

Dyspnea

▲ Abelcet Injection (7%) 1273
Accupril Tablets (1.9%) 2611
Accuretic Tablets (0.5% to 1%) 2614
Acel-Imune (Rare) 1851
Aceon Tablets (2 mg, 4 mg, 8 mg) (0.3% to 1%) 3249
Aciphex Tablets 1267
Aciphex Tablets 1783
Acthrel for Injection 3629
▲ Actiq (2% to 6%) 1184
▲ Actonel Tablets (3.8%) 2879
Adalat CC Tablets (Less than 1.0%) 877
▲ Adenocard Injection (12%) 1380
▲ Adenoscan (Approximately 28%) 1381
Aerobid/Aerobid-M (1% to 3%) 1363
Aggrenox Capsules 1026
▲ Agrylin Capsules (11.9%) 3232
Alkeran for Injection (In some patients) 1465
Allegra (Rare) 712
Allegra-D Extended-Release Tablets (Rare) 714
Alphagan P Ophthalmic Solution (1% to 4%) 546
Altace Capsules (Less than 1%) 2233
Ambien Tablets (Infrequent) 3191
▲ AmBisome for Injection (17.6% to 23%) 1383
Amerge Tablets 1467
Amicar Injection 3608
Amicar Syrup 3608
Amicar Tablets 3608
▲ Amphotec (4% to 9%) 1774
▲ Anaprox Tablets (3% to 9%) 2967
▲ Anaprox DS Tablets (3% to 9%) 2967
Ancobon Capsules 1730
Anzemet Injection (Rare) 719
Anzemet Tablets (Rare) 722
Apligraf (1.8%) 2305
AquaMEPHYTON Injection 2042
Arava Tablets (1% to 3%) 724
▲ Aredia for Injection (Up to 23.3%) 2309
▲ Argatroban Injection (8.1%) 1478
Aricept Tablets (Frequent) 1270
Aricept Tablets (Frequent) 2665
▲ Arimidex Tablets (9.2% to 11.0%) 659
▲ Aromasin Tablets (10%) 2769
Arthrotec Tablets (Rare) 3195
Astelin Nasal Spray 3339
Atacand Tablets (0.5% or greater) 595
Atacand HCT Tablets (0.5% or greater) 597
▲ Atrovent Inhalation Solution (9.6%) 1031
Avalide Tablets 1070
Avapro Tablets (Less than 1%) 1074
Avapro Tablets (Less than 1%) 3076
Avelox Tablets (0.05% to 1%) 879
▲ Avonex (6%) 1013
Axert Tablets (Infrequent) 2772
Azactam for Injection (Less than 1%) 1276
Azopt Ophthalmic Suspension (Less than 1%) 536
Baycol Tablets (Rare) 883
Bebulin VH 840
Betagan .... ⊙ 228
▲ Betapace Tablets (5% to 21%) 950
▲ Betapace AF Tablets (9.2% to 9.8%) 954
▲ Betaseron for SC Injection (8%) 988
Betaxon Ophthalmic Suspension (Less than 2%) 537
Betimol Ophthalmic Solution .... ⊙ 324
Betoptic S Ophthalmic Suspension (Rare) 537
Bicillin C-R 900/300 Injection 2240
Bicillin C-R Injection 2238
Bicillin L-A Injection 2242
Blocadren Tablets (1.7%) 2046
Botox Purified Neurotoxin Complex (Rare) 549
Brethine Ampuls (0.0% to 2.0%) 2314
Brevibloc Injection (Less than 1%) 858
Buprenex Injectable (Less than 1%) 2918
Cafcit (2.2%) 1035
▲ Campath Ampules (9% to 26%) 992
Captopril Tablets (About 0.5% to 2%) 2281
Carbatrol Capsules 3234
Cardene I.V. (0.7%) 3485
Cardizem Injectable (Less than 1%) 1018
Cardizem Lyo-Ject Syringe (Less than 1%) 1018
Cardizem Monovial (Less than 1%) 1018
Cardizem CD Capsules (Less than 1%) 1016
Cardura Tablets (1% to 2.6%) 2668
▲ Carnitor Injection (3% to 11%) 3242
Carteolol Hydrochloride Ophthalmic Solution USP, 1% (Occasional) .... ⊙ 258
▲ Casodex Tablets (7%) 662
Cataflam Tablets (Less than 1%) 2315
Ceclor 1905
Cedax Capsules (0.1% to 1%) 1021
Celebrex Capsules (0.1% to 1.9%) 2676
Celebrex Capsules (0.1% to 1.9%) 2780
Celexa (Infrequent) 1365
▲ CellCept Capsules (15.5% to 36.7%) 2951
▲ CellCept Intravenous (15.5% to 36.7%) 2951
▲ CellCept Oral Suspension (15.5% to 36.7%) 2951
▲ CellCept Tablets (15.5% to 36.7%) 2951
Cerebyx Injection (Infrequent) 2619
Chibroxin Sterile Ophthalmic Solution 2051
Chirocaine Injection (Less than 1%) 2909
Cipro I.V. (1% or less) 893
Cipro I.V. Pharmacy Bulk Package (Less than 1%) 897
Cipro (Less than 1%) 887
Claritin (At least one patient) 3100
Claritin-D 12 Hour Extended Release Tablets (Less frequent) 3102
Claritin-D 24 Hour Extended Release Tablets (Fewer than 2%) 3104
Clinoril Tablets (Less than 1%) 2053
Clomid Tablets 735
Clozaril Tablets (1%) 2319
Cognex Capsules (Frequent) 1351
Colazal Capsules 3069
▲ Combivent Inhalation Aerosol (4.5%) 1041
▲ Comtan Tablets (3%) 2328
Comvax 2056
▲ Copaxone for Injection (19%) 3306
▲ Cordarone Tablets (2% to 7%) 3487
Coreg Tablets (1.4% to more than 2%) 1508
Cosopt Sterile Ophthalmic Solution (Less than 1%) 2065
Coumadin for Injection 1243
Coumadin Tablets 1243
Covera-HS Tablets (1.4% to 2%) 3199
Cozaar Tablets (Less than 1%) 2067
Crinone (Less than 5%) 3213
Crixivan Capsules (Less than 2%) 2070
Crolom Sterile Ophthalmic Solution USP 4% .... ⊙ 259
Cytotec Tablets (Infrequent) 3202
Cytovene (At least 3 subjects) 2959
▲ DaunoXome Injection (3% to 23%) 1442
Depacon Injection (1% to 5%) 416
▲ Depakene (5%) 421
Depakote Sprinkle Capsules (1% to 5%) 426
▲ Depakote Tablets (1% to 5%) 430
Depakote ER Tablets (1% to 5%) 436
Depen Titratable Tablets 3341
Depo-Provera Contraceptive Injection (Fewer than 1%) 2798
D.H.E. 45 Injection (Occasional) 2334
Diovan Capsules 2337
Diovan HCT Tablets (Greater than 0.2%) 2338
Diphtheria & Tetanus Toxoids Adsorbed Purogenated for Pediatric Use (Rare) 1857
Diprivan Injectable Emulsion (Less than 1%) 667
Dolobid Tablets (Rare) 2088
Dopram Injectable 2931
Doxil Injection (1% to 5%) 566
▲ Duraclon Injection (6%) 3057
▲ Duragesic Transdermal System (3% to 10%) 1786
Dynabac Tablets (1.2% to 1.8%) 2269
DynaCirc Capsules (0.5% to 3.4%) 2921
DynaCirc CR Tablets (0.5% to 1%) 2923
▲ EC-Naprosyn Delayed-Release Tablets (3% to 9%) 2967
Effexor Tablets (Frequent) 3495
Effexor XR Capsules (Frequent) 3499
Ellence Injection 2806
Elmiron Capsules (Less than or equal to 1%) 570
▲ Emcyt Capsules (11%) 2810
Enalaprilat Injection 863
Enbrel for Injection (Infrequent) 1752
Enbrel for Injection (Infrequent) 3504
Ethyol for Injection 2029
Evoxac Capsules (Less than 1%) 1217
Fareston Tablets 3237
Felbatol 3343
Feldene Capsules (Occasional) 2685
▲ Femara Tablets (7% to 14%) 2351
▲ Ferrlecit Injection (11%) 3386
Flexeril Tablets (Rare) 572
Flexeril Tablets (Rare) 2094
▲ Flolan for Injection (2% to 100%) 1528
Flonase Nasal Spray (1% to 3%) 1533
Flovent Diskus 3614
Flovent 1535
Flovent Rotadisk (1% to 3%) 1537
Floxin I.V. 2526
Floxin Tablets 2529
▲ Fludara for Injection (9% to 22%) 995
Flumadine (0.3% to 1%) 1370
Follistim for Injection 2465
Foradil Aerolizer (2.1%) 2354
Fortovase Capsules (Less than 2%) 2970
▲ Foscavir Injection (5% or greater) 605
Gabitril Tablets (Frequent) 1189
Gamimune N, 5% Solvent/Detergent Treated 925
Gamimune N, 10% Solvent/Detergent Treated 928
Gastrocrom Oral Concentrate (Less common) 1162
▲ Gemzar for Injection (3% to 23%) 1919
Gengraf Capsules (1% to 5.0%) 457
Geodon Capsules (Frequent) 2688
▲ Gleevec Capsules (5% to 16%) 2357
GlucaGen for Injection Diagnostic Kit (Rare) 949
Glucophage Tablets (1% to 5%) 1080
Glucotrol XL Extended Release Tablets (Less than 1%) 2693
GoLYTELY and Pineapple Flavor GoLYTELY for Oral Solution 1068
Gonal-F for Injection 3216
Guaifed 2272
Havrix Vaccine (Rare) 1544
▲ Hectorol Capsules (11.5%) 1064
▲ Hectorol Injection (11.5%) 1066
▲ Herceptin I.V. (22%) 1414
Hivid Tablets (Less than 1%) 2975
Humegon for Injection 2468
Humorsol Sterile Ophthalmic Solution 2102
▲ Hycamtin for Injection (1.8% to 20%) 1546
▲ Hytrin Capsules (0.5% to 3.1%) 464
Hyzaar 2109
Imdur Tablets (Less than or equal to 5%) 1826
Imitrex Injection (Infrequent) 1549
Imitrex Nasal Spray (Infrequent) 1554
Imitrex Tablets (Frequent) 1558
Indocin Capsules (Less than 1%) 2112
Indocin I.V. (Less than 1%) 2115
Indocin (Less than 1%) 2112
INFeD Injection 3388
▲ Infergen (7% to 8%) 1777
Innohep Injection (1.2%) 1248
▲ Intron A for Injection (Up to 34%) 3120
Invirase Capsules (Less than 2%) 2979
Iopidine 0.5% Ophthalmic Solution (Less than 3%) .... ⊙ 213
Isoptin SR Tablets (1.4%) 467
Kadian Capsules (Less than 3%) 1335
Kaletra Capsules (Less than 2%) 471
Kaletra Oral Solution (Less than 2%) 471
Klonopin Tablets (Infrequent) 2983
K-Phos Neutral Tablets 946
K-Phos Original (Sodium Free) Tablets (Less frequent) 947
Lamictal (1.1%) 1567
Lescol Capsules (Rare) 2361
Lescol Capsules (Rare) 2925
Lescol XL Tablets 2361
Lescol XL Tablets 2925
▲ Leukine (15% to 28%) 1755
▲ Leustatin Injection (11%) 2495
Levaquin 2537
Levoxyl Tablets 1819
Lexxel Tablets 608
Lipitor Tablets (Less than 2%) 2639
Lipitor Tablets (Less than 2%) 2696
Livostin (Approximately 1% to 3%) .... ⊙ 305
Lodine (Less than 1%) 3528
Lodine XL Extended-Release Tablets (Less than 1%) 3530
Lodosyn Tablets 1251
Lortab 3319
Lortab Elixir 3317
Lotensin Tablets (Less than 1%) 2365
Loxitane Capsules 3398
▲ Lupron Depot 7.5 mg (5.4%) 3284
▲ Lupron Injection (5% or more) 3279
Luvox Tablets (25, 50, 100 mg) (2%) 3256
LYMErix Vaccine (Very rare) 1592
Macrobid Capsules (Common) 2889
Macrodantin Capsules (Common) 2891
Mavik Tablets (0.3% to 1.0%) 478
Maxalt Tablets (Frequent) 2120
Maxalt-MLT Orally Disintegrating Tablets (Frequent) 2120
Mefoxin for Injection 2124
Mefoxin Premixed Intravenous Solution 2127
Megace Oral Suspension (1% to 3%) 1124
Mephyton Tablets (Rare) 2129
▲ Mepron Suspension (15% to 21%) 1598
Meridia Capsules (Greater than or equal to 1%) 481
Merrem I.V. (0.1% to 1.0%) 673
Mevacor Tablets (Rare) 2132
▲ Mexitil Capsules (3.3% to 5.7%) 1047
Miacalcin Nasal Spray (Less than 1%) 2375
Micardis Tablets (More than 0.3%) 1049
Micardis HCT Tablets 1051
Midamor Tablets (Between 1% and 3%) 2136
Migranal Nasal Spray (Infrequent) 2376
▲ Minipress Capsules (1% to 4%) 2699
Minizide Capsules 2700
Miochol-E System Pak (Rare) .... ⊙ 305
Miochol-E with Steri-Tags (Rare) .... ⊙ 305
Mirapex Tablets (Infrequent) 2834
Mobic Tablets (Less than 2%) 1054
Moduretic Tablets (Greater than 1%, less than 3%) 2138
Monopril Tablets (1.0% or more) 1091
Motrin Suspension, Oral Drops, Chewable Tablets, and Caplets (Less than 1%) 2002
Mycobutin Capsules (Less than 1%) 2838
Mylocel Tablets (Rare) 2227
▲ Mylotarg for Injection (4% to 46%) 3540
Myobloc Injectable Solution (2% or greater) 1291
▲ Naprelan Tablets (Less than 1% to 9%) 1293
▲ Naprosyn Suspension (3% to 9%) 2967
▲ Naprosyn Tablets (3% to 9%) 2967
Naropin Injection (Less than 1%) 612
Nascobal Gel 3174
Navelbine Injection (Up to 3%) 1604
Neoral Soft Gelatin Capsules (1% to 5.0%) 2380
Neoral Oral Solution (1% to 5.0%) 2380
▲ Neumega for Injection (48%) 1434
▲ Neupogen for Injection (9%) 587
Neurontin Capsules (Infrequent) 2655
Neurontin Oral Solution (Infrequent) 2655
Neurontin Tablets (Infrequent) 2655
Nexium Delayed-Release Capsules (Less than 1%) 619
▲ Nicotrol Nasal Spray (5%) 2843
▲ Nilandron Tablets (10.5%) 753
Nimotop Capsules (Up to 1.2%) 904
▲ Nipent for Injection (8% to 11%) 3272
Nolvadex Tablets 678
Normodyne Injection (Rare) 3135
Normodyne Tablets (Rare; 2%) 3137
Noroxin Tablets 2145
Norvasc Tablets (Less than 1% to 2%) 2704
Norvir Capsules (Less than 2%) 487
Norvir Oral Solution (Less than 2%) 487
▲ Novantrone for Injection (6% to 18%) 1760
Nubain Injection (1% or less) 1323
NuLYTELY, Cherry Flavor, Lemon-Lime Flavor, and Orange Flavor NuLYTELY for Oral Solution 1068
Ocupress Ophthalmic Solution, 1% Sterile (Occasional) .... ⊙ 303
▲ Oncaspar (Greater than 5%) 756
Opticrom Ophthalmic Solution (Rare) 555
OptiPranolol Metipranolol Ophthalmic Solution 0.3% (A small number of patients) .... ⊙ 263
▲ Orthoclone OKT3 Sterile Solution (21%) 2498
Orudis Capsules (Less than 1%) 3548
Oruvail Capsules (Less than 1%) 3548
OxyContin Tablets (Between 1% and 5%) 2912
▲ Pacerone Tablets (2% to 7%) 3331
Paxil (Infrequent) 1609
Pentasa Capsules (One case) 3239
Pergonal for Injection 3223
▲ Permax Tablets (4.8%) 1299
▲ Photofrin for Injection (7% to 20%) 831
▲ Plavix Tablets (4.5%) 1097
▲ Plavix Tablets (4.5%) 3084
Plendil Extended-Release Tablets (0.5% to 1.5%) 623
Pletal Tablets (2% or greater) 2605
Pletal Tablets (2% or greater) 2848
Ponstel Capsules (Occasional) 1356
Pravachol Tablets (Rare) 1099
Prevacid Delayed-Release Capsules (Less than 1%) 3292
PREVPAC (Less than 1%) 3298
Primaxin I.M. 2158
Primaxin I.V. (Less than 0.2%) 2160
Prinivil Tablets (Greater than 1%) 2164
Prinzide Tablets (0.3% to 1%) 2168
▲ Procardia Capsules (A few patients to 6%) 2708
▲ Procardia XL Extended Release Tablets (Less than 3% to 6%) 2710
▲ Prograf (5% to 29%) 1393
Prolastin (Occasional) 943
▲ Proleukin for Injection (43%) 1199
Prosed/DS Tablets 3268
ProSom Tablets (Infrequent) 500

Prostigmin Injectable 1744
Prostigmin Tablets 1744
Prostin E2 Suppositories 2852
Protonix I.V. (Greater than or equal to 1%) 3580
Protonix Tablets (Greater than or equal to 1%) 3577
Protopic Ointment (Greater than or equal to 1%) 1397
Proventil Inhalation Solution 0.083% (1.5%) 3146
Proventil Solution for Inhalation 0.5% (1.5%) 3144
Provigil Tablets (2%) 1193
Prozac Pulvules, Liquid, and Weekly Capsules 1238
▲ Pulmozyme Inhalation Solution (17%) 1426
▲ Rapamune Oral Solution and Tablets (22% to 30%) 3584
▲ Rebetron Combination Therapy (17% to 19%) 3153
Recombivax HB (Less than 1%) 2178
ReFacto Vials 1437
Refludan for Injection (Common) 761
Reglan (Rare) 2935
Relafen Tablets (1%) 1617
Relenza Rotadisk (Less than 1%) 1619
Remeron Tablets (1%) 2483
Remeron SolTab Tablets (1%) 2486
Remicade for IV Injection (Less than 2%) 1178
Repronex for Intramuscular and Subcutaneous Injection (1% to 2.1%) 1347
▲ Requip Tablets (3%) 1621
Rescriptor Tablets (Less than 2%) 526
Retavase Vials (One patient) 1182
▲ Retrovir Capsules (5%) 1625
▲ Retrovir IV Infusion (5%) 1629
▲ Retrovir (5%) 1625
Rhinocort Nasal Inhaler (Less than 1%) 640
Rilutek Tablets (More than 2%) 772
Risperdal (Up to 1%) 1796
Rituxan for Infusion (0.3%) 1750
Rituxan I.V. (0.3%) 1428
▲ Roferon-A Injection (More than 1% to 12%) 2996
▲ Romazicon Injection (3% to 9%) 3000
Roxicodone Tablets (Less than 3%) 3067
▲ Rythmol Tablets – 150 mg, 225 mg, 300 mg (2.0% to 5.3%) 502
Salagen Tablets (Less than 1%) 2229
Sandimmune 2388
▲ Sectral Capsules (4%) 3589
Serevent Inhalation Aerosol (1% to 3%) 1633
Serophene Tablets 3226
Seroquel Tablets (Infrequent) 684
▲ Serostim for Injection (1% to 10%) 3229
Serzone Tablets (Frequent) 1104
▲ Simulect for Injection (Greater than or equal to 10%) 2399
Sinemet Tablets 1253
Sinemet CR Tablets (1.6%) 1255
Sonata Capsules (Infrequent) 3591
Sporanox Injection (Less than 1%) 1804
Sporanox Injection (Less than 1%) 2509
Sporanox Oral Solution (2.3% to 2.6%) 1808
Sporanox Oral Solution (2.3% to 2.6%) 2512
▲ Stadol NS Nasal Spray (3% to 9%) 1108
Streptase for Infusion (Rare) 647
Sular Tablets (Less than or equal to 1%) 688
Suprane Liquid for Inhalation (Less than 1%) 874
Sustiva Capsules 1258
Symmetrel (0.1% to 1%) 1328
Synagis Intramuscular (More than 1%) 2028
Synercid I.V. (Less than 1%) 775
▲ Tambocor Tablets (10.3%) 1990
Tarka Tablets (1.3%) 508
▲ Tasmar Tablets (3%) 3010
Taxol Injection (2%) 1129
▲ Taxotere for Injection Concentrate (6%) 778
Tegretol/Tegretol-XR 2404
▲ Tenex Tablets (3% or less) 2942
▲ Tenoretic Tablets (0.6% to 6%) 690
▲ Tenormin (0.6% to 6%) 692
Tequin Injection (0.1% to 3%) 1110
Tequin Tablets (0.1% to 3%) 1110
Tetanus & Diphtheria Toxoids Adsorbed for Adult Use (Rare) 1880
Thalomid Capsules 1154
▲ Thymoglobulin for Injection (28%) 3071
Tiazac Capsules (Less than 2%) 1378
▲ Tikosyn Capsules (6%) 2717
Timolide Tablets (1.2%) 2187
Timolol GFS ⊙ 266
Timoptic in Ocudose (Less frequent) 2192
Timoptic Sterile Ophthalmic Solution (Less frequent) 2190
Timoptic-XE Sterile Ophthalmic Gel Forming Solution 2194
▲ TOBI Solution for Inhalation (33.7%) 1206
Tonocard Tablets (Less than 1%) 649
Topamax Sprinkle Capsules (1.8% to 3.2%) 2590
Topamax Tablets (1.8% to 3.2%) 2590
Toprol-XL Tablets (Greater than 1%) 651
Toradol (1% or less) 3018
▲ Trasylol Injection (4%) 909
Trental Tablets (Less than 1%) 784
Tricor Capsules, Micronized 513
Tripedia Vaccine (Rare) 817
▲ Trisenox Injection (53%) 1158
Trizivir Tablets 1669
Trovan (Less than 1%) 2722
Trusopt Sterile Ophthalmic Solution 2196
Twinrix Vaccine 1674
Ultracet Tablets (Less than 1%) 2597
Ultram Tablets (Less than 1%) 2600
Uniretic Tablets (Less than 1%) 3178
Unithroid Tablets 3445
Univasc Tablets (Less than 1%) 3181
Urimax Tablets 1769
Uroqid-Acid No. 2 Tablets 947
Valium Injectable 3026
Valtrex Caplets 1676
Vancocin HCl Capsules & Pulvules 1972
Vancocin HCl Oral Solution 1971
Vancocin HCl, Vials & ADD-Vantage 1970
Vantin Tablets and Oral Suspension (Less than 1%) 2860
▲ Vascor Tablets (3.59% to 8.70%) 2602
Vaseretic Tablets (0.5% to 2.0%) 2204
Vasotec I.V. Injection 2207
Vasotec Tablets (0.5% to 1.3%) 2210
Venofer Injection (Greater than 1%) 580
Verelan Capsules (1% or less) 3184
Verelan PM Capsules (2% or less) 3186
Versed Injection (Less than 1%) 3027
▲ Vesanoid Capsules (60%) 3037
Viadur Implant (2.3%) 912
Viagra Tablets (Less than 2%) 2732
Vicoprofen Tablets (Less than 3%) 520
Vioxx (Greater than 0.1% to 1.9%) 2213
Viracept 532
Virazole for Inhalation Solution 1747
▲ Vistide Injection (10% to 23%) 1445
Vitravene for Injection (2% to 5%) ⊙ 310
Voltaren Tablets (Less than 1%) 2315
Voltaren-XR Tablets (Less than 1%) 2315
Warfarin Sodium Tablets, USP 3302
Wellbutrin Tablets (Infrequent) 1680
Wellbutrin SR Sustained-Release Tablets 1684
Xalatan Latanoprost Ophthalmic Solution ⊙ 320
Xalatan Sterile Ophthalmic Solution 2864
Xeloda Tablets (Less than 5%) 3039
Zebeta Tablets (1.1% to 1.5%) 1885
▲ Zenapax for Injection (Greater than 5%) 3046
Zestoretic Tablets (0.3% to 1%) 695
▲ Zestril Tablets (Greater than 1%) 698
Ziac Tablets 1887
Ziagen 1692
Zithromax for IV Infusion (1.9%) 2748
Zocor Tablets (Rare) 2219
▲ Zoladex 3-month (1% to 5%) 706
Zoloft (Infrequent) 2751
▲ Zometa for Intravenous Infusion (22.1%) 3621
Zonegran Capsules (Infrequent) 1307
Zosyn (0.1% or less to 1.1%) 1890
Zosyn in Galaxy Containers (0.1% or less to 1.1%) 1894
Zyban Sustained-Release Tablets (1%) 1710
Zyprexa Tablets (Frequent) 1973
Zyprexa ZYDIS Orally Disintegrating Tablets (Frequent) 1973
Zyrtec (Less than 2%) 2756
Zyrtec-D 12 Hour Extended Relief Tablets (Less than 2%) 2758

Dyspnea, aggravation of
Toprol-XL Tablets (Greater than 1%) 651

Dyspnea, nocturnal
Prinivil Tablets (0.3% to 1.0%) 2164
Prinzide Tablets 2168
Zestoretic Tablets 695
Zestril Tablets (0.3% to 1.0%) 698

Dyspnea, nocturnal, paroxysmal
Herceptin I.V. 1414

Dysrhythmia
Anectine Injection (Rare) 1476
Ecotrin Enteric Coated Aspirin Low, Regular and Maximum Strength Tablets 1715
Loxitane Capsules 3398
Procardia Capsules 2708
Procardia XL Extended Release Tablets (About 1 patient in 150) 2710
▲ Roferon-A Injection (7%) 2996
Taxotere for Injection Concentrate (Rare) 778

Dysthesias
▲ Campath Ampules (15%) 992

Dystonia
Aloprim for Injection (Less than 1%) 2292
AmBisome for Injection (Less common) 1383
Betaseron for SC Injection 988
Celexa (Infrequent) 1365
Clozaril Tablets 2319
Cognex Capsules (Rare) 1351
Compazine 1505
Cuprimine Capsules 2075
Dilantin Infatabs (Rare) 2624
Dilantin Kapseals (Rare) 2622
Dilantin-125 Oral Suspension (Rare) 2625
Diprivan Injectable Emulsion (Less than 1%) 667
Effexor Tablets (Rare) 3495
Effexor XR Capsules (Rare) 3499
Eldepryl Capsules 3266
Eskalith (One report in a child) 1527
Etrafon 3115
Felbatol (Infrequent) 3343
Gabitril Tablets (Infrequent) 1189
▲ Geodon Capsules (4%) 2688
Halcion Tablets 2823
Haldol Decanoate (Frequent) 2535
Haldol Injection, Tablets and Concentrate 2533
Imitrex Injection (Rare) 1549
Imitrex Tablets (Rare) 1558
Lamictal (Rare) 1567
Lithium Carbonate 3061
Lithium Citrate Syrup 3061
Lithobid Slow-Release Tablets 3255
▲ Lodosyn Tablets (Among most common) 1251
Loxitane Capsules 3398
Luvox Tablets (25, 50, 100 mg) (Infrequent) 3256
Migranal Nasal Spray (Infrequent) 2376
▲ Mirapex Tablets (2% to 7%) 2834
Moban (Infrequent) 1320
Navane Oral 2701
Navane Intramuscular 2703
Neurontin Capsules (Infrequent) 2655
Neurontin Oral Solution (Infrequent) 2655
Neurontin Tablets (Infrequent) 2655
Orap Tablets (Less frequent) 1407
Paxil (Infrequent) 1609
▲ Permax Tablets (11.6%) 1299
Prozac Pulvules, Liquid, and Weekly Capsules (Rare) 1238
Reglan (Approximately 0.2%) 2935
Remeron Tablets (Infrequent) 2483
Remeron SolTab Tablets (Infrequent) 2486
Requip Tablets (1% or more) 1621
▲ Risperdal (17% to 34%) 1796
Sarafem Pulvules (Rare) 1962
Serentil 1057
▲ Sinemet Tablets (Among most common) 1253
Sinemet CR Tablets (1.8%) 1255
Stelazine 1640
Syprine Capsules 2186
▲ Tasmar Tablets (19% to 22%) 3010
Thioridazine Hydrochloride Tablets 2289
Thiothixene Capsules 2290
Thorazine 1656
Topamax Sprinkle Capsules (Infrequent) 2590
Topamax Tablets (Infrequent) 2590
Trilafon 3160
Trileptal Oral Suspension 2407
Trileptal Tablets 2407
Wellbutrin Tablets (Frequent) 1680
Wellbutrin SR Sustained-Release Tablets 1684
Xanax Tablets 2865
Zofran Injection 1698
Zofran 1703
Zofran ODT Orally Disintegrating Tablets 1703
Zoloft (Infrequent) 2751
Zomig Tablets (Rare) 708
Zomig-ZMT Tablets (Rare) 708
Zonegran Capsules (Rare) 1307
Zyban Sustained-Release Tablets 1710
Zyprexa Tablets (2% to 3%) 1973
Zyprexa ZYDIS Orally Disintegrating Tablets (2% to 3%) 1973

Dystonia, tardive
Compazine 1505
Haldol Decanoate 2535
Haldol Injection, Tablets and Concentrate 2533
Thioridazine Hydrochloride Tablets 2289
Thiothixene Capsules 2290
Thorazine 1656

Dystonic reactions
(*see under* Dystonia)

Dysuria
Abelcet Injection 1273
Aciphex Tablets 1267
Aciphex Tablets 1783
Actiq (Less than 1%) 1184
Agrylin Capsules (1% to 5%) 3232
Alferon N Injection (1%) 1770
Allegra-D Extended-Release Tablets 714
Ambien Tablets (Rare) 3191
AmBisome for Injection (Less common) 1383
Amphotec (1% to 5%) 1774
Androderm Transdermal System CIII (Less than 1%) 3377
Anzemet Injection (Rare) 719
Anzemet Tablets (Rare) 722
Aricept Tablets (Infrequent) 1270
Aricept Tablets (Infrequent) 2665
Arthrotec Tablets (Rare) 3195
Asacol Delayed-Release Tablets 2884
Atromid-S Capsules 3483
Avonex 1013
Bontril Slow-Release Capsules 576
Cardura Tablets (0.5%) 2668
▲ Casodex Tablets (2% to 5%) 662
Ceclor CD Tablets (0.1% to 1%) 1279
Cedax Capsules (0.1% to 1%) 1021
Ceftin Tablets (0.1% to 1%) 1898
Celexa (Infrequent) 1365
▲ CellCept Capsules (3%) 2951
▲ CellCept Intravenous (3%) 2951
▲ CellCept Oral Suspension (3%) 2951
▲ CellCept Tablets (3%) 2951
Cerebyx Injection (Infrequent) 2619
Claritin-D 12 Hour Extended Release Tablets (Less frequent) 3102
Claritin-D 24 Hour Extended Release Tablets 3104
Cleocin Vaginal Cream (Less than 1%) 2788
Cleocin Vaginal Ovules (Less than 1%) 2789
Clinoril Tablets 2053
Clorpres Tablets (Rare) 1002
Cogentin 2055
Cognex Capsules (Infrequent) 1351
Combipres Tablets (Rare) 1040
Combivent Inhalation Aerosol (Less than 2%) 1041
Copaxone for Injection (At least 2%) 3306
▲ Crinone (Less than 5%) 3213
Crixivan Capsules (Less than 2%) 2070
Cytotec Tablets (Infrequent) 3202
▲ DaunoXome Injection (Less than or equal to 5%) 1442
Demser Capsules (A few patients) 2085
Depacon Injection (1% or more) 416
Depakene (1% or more) 421
Depakote Sprinkle Capsules 426
▲ Depakote Tablets (1% to 5%) 430
Depakote ER Tablets (1% or more) 436
Desferal Vials 2333
Detrol Tablets (2.5%) 3623
Detrol LA Capsules (1%) 2801
Diovan HCT Tablets (Greater than 0.2%) 2338
Dipentum Capsules (Rare) 2803
Dolobid Tablets (Less than 1 in 100) 2088
Doxil Injection (Less than 1%) 566
DynaCirc CR Tablets (0.5% to 1%) 2923
Effexor Tablets (Infrequent) 3495
Effexor XR Capsules (Infrequent) 3499
Estring Vaginal Ring (1% to 3%) 2811
Evoxac Capsules (Less than 1%) 1217
Exelon Capsules (Infrequent) 2342
Exelon Oral Solution (Infrequent) 2345
Felbatol 3343
Feldene Capsules (Occasional) 2685
Floxin I.V. (Less than 1%) 2526
Floxin Tablets (Less than 1%) 2529
▲ Fludara for Injection (3% to 4%) 995
Foscavir Injection (Between 1% and 5%) 605
Gabitril Tablets (Frequent) 1189
Gastrocrom Oral Concentrate (Less common) 1162
Gengraf Capsules (1%) 457
Glucotrol XL Extended Release Tablets (Less than 1%) 2693
Hivid Tablets (Less than 1%) 2975
Ifex for Injection 1123
Imitrex Injection (Rare) 1549
Imitrex Nasal Spray (Infrequent) 1554
Imitrex Tablets (Up to 2%) 1558
Innohep Injection (Greater than or equal to 1%) 1248
Intron A for Injection (Less than 5%) 3120
Ismo Tablets (Fewer than 1%) 3524
Klonopin Tablets (Infrequent) 2983
Lamictal (Rare) 1567
Lexxel Tablets 608
Lipitor Tablets (Less than 2%) 2639

Lipitor Tablets (Less than 2%)......... 2696
Lodine (1% to 3%)......................... 3528
Lodine XL Extended-Release Tablets (1% to 3%)......................... 3530
▲ Lupron Depot 3.75 mg (Among most frequent)......................... 3281
Lupron Depot 7.5 mg (Less than 5%)......................... 3284
Lupron Depot–3 Month 11.25 mg (Less than 5%)......................... 3285
Lupron Injection (Less than 5%)...... 3279
Luvox Tablets (25, 50, 100 mg) (Infrequent)......................... 3256
Maxalt Tablets (Rare)......................... 2120
Maxalt-MLT Orally Disintegrating Tablets (Rare)......................... 2120
Merrem I.V. (0.1% to 1.0%)............ 673
Midamor Tablets (Less than or equal to 1%)......................... 2136
Mirapex Tablets (Infrequent)............ 2834
Moduretic Tablets (Less than or equal to 1%)......................... 2138
Monopril HCT (Less than 2%)......... 1094
Monurol Sachet (Less than 1%)....... 1375
Mylocel Tablets (Very rare)............ 2227
Naprelan Tablets (Less than 1%)...... 1293
Neoral Soft Gelatin Capsules (1%)... 2380
Neoral Oral Solution (1%)............... 2380
Neurontin Capsules (Infrequent)...... 2655
Neurontin Oral Solution (Infrequent)......................... 2655
Neurontin Tablets (Infrequent)......... 2655
Nexium Delayed-Release Capsules (Less than 1%)............ 619
Norvasc Tablets (Less than or equal to 0.1%)......................... 2704
Norvir Capsules (Less than 2%)...... 487
Norvir Oral Solution (Less than 2%)......................... 487
Ovidrel for Injection (Less than 2%)......................... 3220
OxyContin Tablets (Less than 1%)... 2912
Paxil (Infrequent)......................... 1609
Permax Tablets (Infrequent)............ 1299
Plendil Extended-Release Tablets (0.5% to 1.5%)......................... 623
Ponstel Capsules (Occasional)......... 1356
Prinivil Tablets (0.3% to 1.0%)......... 2164
Prinzide Tablets......................... 2168
▲ ProAmatine Tablets (13.4%)......... 3241
Procardia XL Extended Release Tablets (1% or less)......................... 2710
▲ Prograf (3% to 15%) 1393
▲ Proleukin for Injection (3%) 1199
Protonix I.V. (Less than 1%)............ 3580
Protonix Tablets (Less than 1%)......... 3577
Prozac Pulvules, Liquid, and Weekly Capsules (Infrequent)....... 1238
Pyrazinamide Tablets (Rare)............ 1876
▲ Rapamune Oral Solution and Tablets (3% to 20%)......................... 3584
Recombivax HB (Less than 1%)....... 2178
Relafen Tablets (Less than 1%)....... 1617
Remeron Tablets (Infrequent)......... 2483
Remeron SolTab Tablets (Infrequent)......................... 2486
Remicade for IV Injection (Less than 2%)......................... 1178
ReoPro Vials (0.4%)......................... 1958
Requip Tablets (Infrequent)............ 1621
Retrovir Capsules......................... 1625
Retrovir IV Infusion......................... 1629
Retrovir......................... 1625
Rifater Tablets (Rare)......................... 769
Rilutek Tablets (Up to 1.2%)............ 772
Risperdal (Infrequent)......................... 1796
Rynatan Tablets......................... 3351
Salagen Tablets (Less than 1%)...... 2229
Sarafem Pulvules (Infrequent)......... 1962
Sectral Capsules (Up to 2%)........... 3589
Seroquel Tablets (Infrequent).......... 684
Serzone Tablets......................... 1104
▲ Simulect for Injection (3% to 10%) .. 2399
Sonata Capsules (Infrequent).......... 3591
Soriatane Capsules (Less than 1%)......................... 3003
Sular Tablets (Less than or equal to 1%)......................... 688
Tasmar Tablets (Infrequent)............ 3010
Tequin Injection (0.1% to 3%)......... 1110
Tequin Tablets (0.1% to 3%)........... 1110
▲ TheraCys Injection (4% to 52%) 823
Thioplex for Injection......................... 1765
▲ Tice BCG, BCG Live (59.5%) 2489
Tolectin (Less than 1%)......................... 2589
Topamax Sprinkle Capsules (Frequent)......................... 2590
Topamax Tablets (Frequent)............ 2590
Trileptal Oral Suspension......................... 2407
Trileptal Tablets......................... 2407
Trovan (Less than 1%)......................... 2722
Ultram Tablets (Less than 1%)......... 2600
Unasyn for Injection (Less than 1%)......................... 2728
Uniretic Tablets (Less than 1%)....... 3178
Uroqid-Acid No. 2 Tablets (Occasional)......................... 947
▲ Valstar Sterile Solution for Intravesical Instillation (11% to 56%)......................... 1175
Vantin Tablets and Oral Suspension (Less than 1%)......... 2860
▲ Vesanoid Capsules (9%) 3037
Viadur Implant (Less than 2%)......... 912
Vioxx (Greater than 0.1% to 1.9%).. 2213
Vistide Injection......................... 1445
Wellbutrin Tablets (Rare)......................... 1680
Wellbutrin SR Sustained-Release Tablets......................... 1684
▲ Zenapax for Injection (Greater than 5%)......................... 3046
Zestril Tablets (0.3% to 1.0%)......... 698
Zofran Injection (2%)......................... 1698
Zoloft (Infrequent)......................... 2751
Zonegran Capsules (Infrequent)...... 1307
Zosyn (1.0% or less)......................... 1890
Zosyn in Galaxy Containers (1.0% or less)......................... 1894
Zyban Sustained-Release Tablets.... 1710
Zyprexa Tablets (Infrequent)............ 1973
Zyprexa ZYDIS Orally Disintegrating Tablets (Infrequent)......................... 1973
Zyrtec (Less than 2%) 2756
Zyrtec-D 12 Hour Extended Relief Tablets (Less than 2%) 2758

Dyuria

Tricor Capsules, Micronized 513

E

Ear, discomfort

Aerobid/Aerobid-M (1% to 3%) 1363
Cytotec Tablets (Infrequent) 3202
Fortovase Capsules (Less than 2%)......................... 2970
Invirase Capsules (Less than 2%) 2979
Versed Injection (Less than 1%) 3027

Ear, drainage

Hivid Tablets (Less than 1%) 2975

Ear, external abnormalities, fetal

Accutane Capsules 2944
Depen Titratable Tablets 3341

Ear disease, unspecified

Actiq (1% or greater) 1184
Asacol Delayed-Release Tablets (2% or greater)......................... 2884
Avapro Tablets (Less than 1%) 1074
Avapro Tablets (Less than 1%) 3076
Cardene I.V. (Rare) 3485
Celebrex Capsules (0.1% to 1.9%)......................... 2676
Celebrex Capsules (0.1% to 1.9%)......................... 2780
▲ CellCept Capsules (3% to 10%) 2951
▲ CellCept Intravenous (3% to 10%) .. 2951
▲ CellCept Oral Suspension (3% to 10%)......................... 2951
▲ CellCept Tablets (3% to 10%) 2951
Clozaril Tablets (Less than 1%) 2319
Depakote Tablets (1% to 5%) 430
Ferrlecit Injection 3386
Gengraf Capsules (1%) 457
▲ Humatrope Vials and Cartridges (11.8%)......................... 1930
Monurol Sachet (Less than 1%) 1375
Naprelan Tablets (Less than 1%) 1293
Neoral Soft Gelatin Capsules (1%) .. 2380
Neoral Oral Solution (1%) 2380
Provigil Tablets (At least 1%) 1193
Salagen Tablets (Rare) 2229
▲ Serostim for Injection (1% to 10%) ... [illegible]
Tamiflu Capsules (1.7%) 3008
Tamiflu Oral Suspension (1.7%) 3008
▲ Vesanoid Capsules (6%) 3037
Vistide Injection 1445

Ear drum, perforated

Neurontin Capsules (Rare) 2655
Neurontin Oral Solution (Rare) 2655
Neurontin Tablets (Rare) 2655

Ears, blocked

Asacol Delayed-Release Tablets 2884
Chemet Capsules (1.0% to 3.7%) 3078
Hivid Tablets (Less than 1%) 2975
Neurontin Capsules (Infrequent) 2655
Neurontin Oral Solution (Infrequent)......................... 2655
Neurontin Tablets (Infrequent) 2655
Orthoclone OKT3 Sterile Solution 2498
Versed Injection (Less than 1%) 3027

Ears, ringing

(*see under* Tinnitus)

Ears, roaring in

Nebcin Vials, Hyporets & ADD-Vantage 1955

Ebriety, feeling of

Intron A for Injection (Less than 5%)......................... 3120

Ebstein's anomaly

Eskalith 1527
Lithium Carbonate 3061
Lithium Citrate Syrup 3061

Ecchymoses

Aceon Tablets (2 mg, 4 mg, 8 mg) (0.3% to 1%)......................... 3249
Aciphex Tablets......................... 1267
Aciphex Tablets......................... 1783
Actiq (1% or greater)......................... 1184
Activase I.V. (Less than 1% to 1%).. 1410
▲ Actonel Tablets (4.3%)......................... 2879
Advair Diskus 100/50......................... 1448
Advair Diskus 250/50......................... 1448
Advair Diskus 500/50......................... 1448
Agrylin Capsules (1% to 5%)............ 3232
Aloprim for Injection (Less than 1%)......................... 2292
Amphotec (1% to 5%)......................... 1774
▲ Anaprox Tablets (3% to 9%) 2967
▲ Anaprox DS Tablets (3% to 9%) 2967
Arava Tablets (1% to 3%)......................... 724
▲ Aricept Tablets (4%) 1270
▲ Aricept Tablets (4%) 2665
Arthrotec Tablets (Rare)......................... 3195
Avalide Tablets......................... 1070
Avapro Tablets (Less than 1%) 1074
Avapro Tablets (Less than 1%) 3076
Avonex (2%) 1013
Bicillin C-R 900/300 Injection 2240
Bicillin C-R Injection 2238
Bicillin L-A Injection 2242
Caverject Sterile Powder (2%) 2777
Celebrex Capsules (0.1% to 1.9%)......................... 2676
Celebrex Capsules (0.1% to 1.9%)......................... 2780
Celestone Syrup 3099
▲ CellCept Capsules (3% to 16.6%) .. 2951
▲ CellCept Intravenous (3% to 16.6%)......................... 2951
▲ CellCept Oral Suspension (3% to 16.6%)......................... 2951
▲ CellCept Tablets (3% to 16.6%) 2951
▲ Cerebyx Injection (7.3%) 2619
Clinoril Tablets (Less than 1%) 2053
Comvax 2056
▲ Copaxone for Injection (8%) 3306
Cordarone Tablets (Less than 1%) .. 3487
Cortifoam Rectal Foam 3170
Cortone Acetate Injectable Suspension......................... 2059
Cortone Acetate Tablets 2061
Corzide 40/5 Tablets 2247
Corzide 80/5 Tablets 2247
Covera-HS Tablets (Less than 2%) .. 3199
Cozaar Tablets (Less than 1%) 2067
Decadron Elixir 2078
Decadron Phosphate Injection 2081
▲ Depacon Injection (4% to 5%) 416
▲ Depakene (5%) 421
▲ Depakote Sprinkle Capsules (4% to 5%)......................... 426
Depakote Tablets (1% to 5%) 430
Depakote ER Tablets (1% to 5%) 436
Depo-Medrol Injectable Suspension......................... 2795
Doxil Injection (Less than 1%) 566
▲ EC-Naprosyn Delayed-Release Tablets (3% to 9%) 2967
Effexor Tablets (Frequent) 3495
Effexor XR Capsules (Frequent) 3499
Elmiron Capsules (Less than or equal to 1%) 570
Engerix-B Vaccine (Less than 1%) ... 1517
Feldene Capsules (Occasional) 2685
Florinef Acetate Tablets 2250
Flovent Diskus 3614
Flovent 1535
Flovent Rotadisk 1537
Floxin I.V. 2526
Floxin Tablets 2529
▲ Gabitril Tablets (1% to 6%) 1189
Geodon Capsules (Infrequent) 2688
▲ Hyalgan Solution (14%) 3080
Hydrocortone Tablets 2106
Hydrocortone Acetate Injectable Suspension......................... 2103
Hydrocortone Phosphate Injection, Sterile 2105
Hyzaar 2109
Indocin Capsules (Less than 1%) 2112
Indocin I.V. (Less than 1%) 2115
Indocin (Less than 1%) 2112
▲ Infergen (4% to 6%) 1777
Innohep Injection 1248
Isoptin SR Tablets (1% or less) 467
Keppra Tablets (1% or more) 3314
Lamictal (Infrequent) 1567
Lipitor Tablets (Less than 2%) 2639
Lipitor Tablets (Less than 2%) 2696
Lodine (Less than 1%) 3528
Lodine XL Extended-Release Tablets (Less than 1%) 3530
Lovenox Injection (Up to 3%) 746
▲ Lupron Depot 3.75 mg (Among most frequent) 3281
Lupron Depot 7.5 mg (Less than 5%)......................... 3284
Lupron Depot–3 Month 11.25 mg (Less than 5%) 3285
Lupron Injection (Less than 5%) 3279
Luvox Tablets (25, 50, 100 mg) (Infrequent) 3256
Meridia Capsules (0.7%) 481
Miltown Tablets 3349
▲ Mylotarg for Injection (12% to 18%)......................... 3540
Myobloc Injectable Solution (2% or greater)......................... 1291
▲ Naprelan Tablets (Less than 3% to 9%)......................... 1293
▲ Naprosyn Suspension (3% to 9%) ... 2967
▲ Naprosyn Tablets (3% to 9%) 2967
▲ Neumega for Injection (Greater than or equal to 10%)......................... 1434
Norvir Capsules (Less than 2%)...... 487
Norvir Oral Solution (Less than 2%)......................... 487
▲ Novantrone for Injection (7% to 11%)......................... 1760
Oncaspar......................... 756
Pacerone Tablets (Less than 1%).... 3331
Parafon Forte DSC Caplets (Rare)... 2582
Paxil (Infrequent)......................... 1609
Pentasa Capsules (Less than 1%)... 3239
Pipracil (Less frequent)......................... 1866
Pletal Tablets (Less than 2%) 2605
Pletal Tablets (Less than 2%) 2848
Ponstel Capsules (Occasional) 1356
Prednisone 3064
▲ Prograf (3% to 15%) 1393
Protonix I.V. (Less than 1%) 3580
Protonix Tablets (Less than 1%) 3577
Protopic Ointment (Greater than or equal to 1%)......................... 1397
Provigil Tablets (At least 1%)......................... 1193
Prozac Pulvules, Liquid, and Weekly Capsules (Infrequent) 1238
Pulmicort Turbuhaler Inhalation Powder (1% to 3%) 636
▲ Rapamune Oral Solution and Tablets (3% to 20%)......................... 3584
Rilutek Tablets (Infrequent) 772
Roferon-A Injection (Rare) 2996
Sarafem Pulvules (Infrequent) 1962
Seroquel Tablets (Infrequent) 684
Serzone Tablets (Infrequent) 1104
Solu-Medrol Sterile Powder 2855
Sonata Capsules (Infrequent) 3591
Sular Tablets (Less than or equal to 1%)......................... 688
Tarka Tablets 508
Tequin Injection (Less than 0.1%) 1110
Tequin Tablets (Less than 0.1%) 1110
Ticlid Tablets 3015
Tricor Capsules, Micronized 513
Trilisate (Rare)......................... 2901
▲ Trisenox Injection (20%) 1158
Twinrix Vaccine (Less than 1%) 1674
Uniretic Tablets (Less than 1%) 3178
Vaqta (1.3%) 2199
Verelan Capsules (1% or less) 3184
Verelan PM Capsules (2% or less) ... 3186
▲ Viadur Implant (4.6%) 912
Wellbutrin Tablets 1680
Wellbutrin SR Sustained-Release Tablets (Infrequent)......................... 1684
Zanaflex Tablets (Infrequent) 1305
Zoladex (1% or greater) 702
Zoladex 3-month 706
Zomig Tablets (Infrequent) 708
Zomig-ZMT Tablets (Infrequent) 708
Zonegran Capsules (2%) 1307
Zosyn (1.0% or less) 1890
Zosyn in Galaxy Containers (1.0% or less) 1894
Zyban Sustained-Release Tablets (Infrequent) 1710
Zyprexa Tablets 1973
Zyprexa ZYDIS Orally Disintegrating Tablets 1973

Ecchymosis, soft eyelid tissue

Botox Purified Neurotoxin Complex 549

ECG changes

(*see under* EKG changes)

Eclampsia

Paxil 1609

Ectropion

Botox Purified Neurotoxin Complex (Less than 1%) 549
Soriatane Capsules (Less than 1%) 3003

Eczema

Accutane Capsules 2944
▲ Aerobid/Aerobid-M (3% to 9%) 1363
Arava Tablets (2%) 724
Arthrotec Tablets (Rare) 3195
Astelin Nasal Spray (Infrequent) 3339
Atacand HCT Tablets (0.5% or greater) 597
Benoquin Cream 20% 1732
Cardura Tablets (Less than 0.5%) ... 2668
Cataflam Tablets (Less than 1%) 2315
Celexa (Infrequent) 1365
Cerumenex Eardrops (1% of 2,700 patients) 2895
Claritin-D 12 Hour Extended Release Tablets (Less frequent) ... 3102
Clozaril Tablets (Less than 1%) 2319
Cognex Capsules (Infrequent) 1351
Compazine 1505
Copaxone for Injection (Frequent) ... 3306

Cutivate Cream (0.8%) 1282
Dantrium Capsules (Less frequent) 2885
Differin Cream (Less than 1%) 1402
Effexor Tablets (Infrequent) 3495
Effexor XR Capsules (Infrequent) 3499
Engerix-B Vaccine 1517
Etrafon 3115
Evoxac Capsules (Less than 1%) 1217
Exelon Capsules (Frequent) 2342
Exelon Oral Solution (Frequent) 2345
▲ Flolan for Injection (25%) 1528
Flovent Diskus (1% to 3%) 3614
Floxin Otic Solution (Single report) 1219
Fortovase Capsules (Less than 2%) 2970
Gabitril Tablets (Infrequent) 1189
Gengraf Capsules (1% to less than 3%) 457
Geodon Capsules (Infrequent) 2688
Glucotrol Tablets (About 1 in 70) 2692
Imitrex Injection 1549
Imitrex Nasal Spray 1554
Intron A for Injection (Less than 5%) 3120
Invirase Capsules (Less than 2%) 2979
Lac-Hydrin Lotion (Less frequent) 1119
▲ Lamictal (4%) 1567
Lindane Lotion USP 1% (Relatively infrequent) 559
Lindane Shampoo USP 1% (Relatively infrequent) 560
Lipitor Tablets (Less than 2%) 2639
Lipitor Tablets (Less than 2%) 2696
Lopid Tablets (1.9%) 2650
Luvox Tablets (25, 50, 100 mg) (Infrequent) 3256
Macrobid Capsules 2889
Macrodantin Capsules 2891
Miacalcin Nasal Spray (Less than 1%) 2375
Micardis Tablets (More than 0.3%) 1049
Micardis HCT Tablets 1051
Naprelan Tablets (Less than 1%) 1293
Neoral Soft Gelatin Capsules (1% to less than 3%) 2380
Neoral Oral Solution (1% to less than 3%) 2380
Neurontin Capsules (Infrequent) 2655
Neurontin Oral Solution (Infrequent) 2655
Neurontin Tablets (Infrequent) 2655
Nipent for Injection (Less than 3%) 3272
Norvir Capsules (Less than 2%) 487
Norvir Oral Solution (Less than 2%) 487
Nystop Topical Powder USP (More common) 2608
Olux Foam (One case) 1211
Orudis Capsules (Less than 1%) 3548
Oruvail Capsules (Less than 1%) 3548
Paxil (Infrequent) 1609
Pentasa Capsules (Less than 1%) 3239
Permax Tablets (Infrequent) 1299
Plavix Tablets (1% to 2.5%) 1097
Plavix Tablets (1% to 2.5%) 3084
Protonix I.V. (Less than 1%) 3580
Protonix Tablets (Less than 1%) 3577
Protopic Ointment (Up to 3%) 1397
Prozac Pulvules, Liquid, and Weekly Capsules (Infrequent) 1238
Pulmicort Respules (1% to 3%) 632
Requip Tablets (Infrequent) 1621
Rilutek Tablets (0.8% to 1.6%) 772
Roferon-A Injection (Less than 1%) 2996
Salagen Tablets (Less than 1%) 2229
Sarafem Pulvules (Infrequent) 1962
Serevent Diskus (1% to 3%) 1637
Seroquel Tablets (Infrequent) 684
Serzone Tablets (Infrequent) 1104
Sonata Capsules (Infrequent) 3591
Soriatane Capsules (Less than 1%) 3003
Stelazine 1640
Sustiva Capsules (Less than 2%) 1258
Synagis Intramuscular (More than 1%) 2028
Tasmar Tablets (Infrequent) 3010
Teveten Tablets (Less than 1%) 3327
Thalomid Capsules 1154
Topamax Sprinkle Capsules (Infrequent) 2590
Topamax Tablets (Infrequent) 2590
Tricor Capsules, Micronized (Less than 1%) 513
Trilafon 3160
Uniretic Tablets (Less than 1%) 3178
Vanceril Double Strength Inhalation Aerosol (2%) 3167
Varivax (Greater than or equal to 1%) 2202
Vistide Injection 1445
▲ Visudyne for Injection (1% to 10%) ⊙ 308
Voltaren Tablets (Less than 1%) 2315
Voltaren-XR Tablets (Less than 1%) 2315
Zebeta Tablets 1885
Ziac Tablets 1887
Zoloft (Rare) 2751
Zonegran Capsules (Infrequent) 1307
▲ Zosyn (4.2%) 1890
▲ Zosyn in Galaxy Containers (4.2%) 1894
Zyprexa Tablets (Infrequent) 1973
Zyprexa ZYDIS Orally Disintegrating Tablets (Infrequent) 1973
Zyrtec (Less than 2%) 2756
Zyrtec-D 12 Hour Extended Relief Tablets (Less than 2%) 2758

Eczema, dyshidrotic
Oxistat Lotion (0.4%) 1298

Eczema, exacerbation of
Cutivate (0.8% to 3.0%) 1282

Eczema herpecticum
Protopic Ointment (Up to 2%) 1397

Eczematous reactions
(*see under* Eczema)

Edema
Accolate Tablets 657
Accupril Tablets (0.5% to 1%) 2611
Accuretic Tablets 2614
Accutane Capsules 2944
▲ Aceon Tablets (2 mg, 4 mg, 8 mg) (0.3% to 3.9%) 3249
Aciphex Tablets 1267
Aciphex Tablets 1783
Actiq (Less than 1%) 1184
Activella Tablets 2764
▲ Actos Tablets (4.8% to 15.3%) 3275
Advair Diskus 100/50 (1% to 3%) 1448
Advair Diskus 250/50 (1% to 3%) 1448
Advair Diskus 500/50 (1% to 3%) 1448
▲ Aerobid/Aerobid-M (3% to 9%) 1363
Aggrastat (2%) 2031
▲ Agrylin Capsules (20.6%) 3232
Albuminar-5, U.S.P. 785
Albuminar-25, U.S.P. 786
▲ Aldara Cream, 5% (Up to 17%) 1978
Aldoclor Tablets 2035
Aldomet Tablets 2037
Aldoril Tablets 2039
Alesse-21 Tablets 3468
Alesse-28 Tablets 3473
Alferon N Injection (One patient) 1770
Alkeran for Injection 1465
Aloprim for Injection (Less than 1%) 2292
Alora Transdermal System 3372
Altace Capsules (Less than 1%) 2233
Ambien Tablets (Infrequent) 3191
▲ AmBisome for Injection (12.3% to 14.3%) 1383
Amerge Tablets (Infrequent) 1467
Americaine Anesthetic Lubricant 1162
Americaine Otic Topical Anesthetic Ear Drops 1162
Amicar Injection 3608
Amicar Syrup 3608
Amicar Tablets 3608
Anadrol-50 Tablets 3321
▲ Anaprox Tablets (3% to 9%) 2967
▲ Anaprox DS Tablets (3% to 9%) 2967
Androderm Transdermal System CIII 3377
▲ Android Capsules, 10 mg (Among most common) 1731
Anzemet Injection (Rare) 719
Anzemet Tablets (Rare) 722
Aredia for Injection (Up to 1%) 2309
▲ Arimidex Tablets (7.3% to 11.4%) 659
▲ Aromasin Tablets (7%) 2769
Arthrotec Tablets (Rare) 3195
Asacol Delayed-Release Tablets 2884
▲ Avalide Tablets (3%) 1070
▲ Avandia Tablets (4.8%) 1490
Avapro Tablets (1% or greater) 1074
Avapro Tablets (1% or greater) 3076
Aygestin Tablets 1333
Baycol Tablets 883
▲ Betapace Tablets (2% to 8%) 950
▲ Betaseron for SC Injection (8%) 988
Bicillin C-R 900/300 Injection 2240
Bicillin C-R Injection 2238
Bicillin L-A Injection 2242
Blocadren Tablets (0.6%) 2046
Brevibloc Injection (Less than 1%) 858
Brevicon 28-Day Tablets 3380
▲ Campath Ampules (1% to 13%) 992
Captopril Tablets 2281
Carbatrol Capsules 3234
Cardizem Injectable (Less than 1%) 1018
Cardizem Lyo-Ject Syringe (Less than 1%) 1018
Cardizem Monovial (Less than 1%) 1018
▲ Cardizem CD Capsules (2.6% to 4.6%) 1016
▲ Cardura Tablets (About 0.7% to 4%) 2668
▲ Casodex Tablets (2% to 5%) 662
Cataflam Tablets (1% to 3%) 2315
Catapres-TTS (3 of 101 patients) 1038
Ceclor CD Tablets (0.1% to 1%) 1279
Ceclor 1905
Celebrex Capsules (0.1% to 1.9%) 2676
Celebrex Capsules (0.1% to 1.9%) 2780
Celestone Soluspan Injectable Suspension 3097
Celestone Syrup 3099
▲ CellCept Capsules (11.8% to 26.6%) 2951
▲ CellCept Intravenous (11.8% to 26.6%) 2951
▲ CellCept Oral Suspension (11.8% to 26.6%) 2951
▲ CellCept Tablets (11.8% to 28.2%) 2951
Cenestin Tablets 1263
Cerebyx Injection (Infrequent) 2619
Chirocaine Injection (Less than 1%) 2909
Claritin-D 12 Hour Extended Release Tablets (Less frequent) 3102
Cleocin Vaginal Ovules (Less than 1%) 2789
Climara Transdermal System 958
Clinoril Tablets (Greater than 1%) 2053
Clomid Tablets 735
Clozaril Tablets (Less than 1%) 2319
Cognex Capsules (Infrequent) 1351
Colazal Capsules 3069
Combivent Inhalation Aerosol (Less than 2%) 1041
Comvax 2056
Condylox Topical Solution (Less than 5%) 2437
▲ Copaxone for Injection (3%) 3306
Cordarone Tablets (1% to 3%) 3487
Coreg Tablets (0.1% to 5.1%) 1508
Cortifoam Rectal Foam 3170
Cortone Acetate Injectable Suspension 2059
Cortone Acetate Tablets 2061
Coumadin for Injection (Infrequent) 1243
Coumadin Tablets (Infrequent) 1243
Covera-HS Tablets (1.9% to 3.0%) 3199
Cozaar Tablets (1% or greater) 2067
Crinone (Less than 5%) 3213
Crolom Sterile Ophthalmic Solution USP 4% ⊙ 259
Cyclessa Tablets 2450
Cytotec Tablets (Infrequent) 3202
Cytovene (At least 3 subjects) 2959
▲ DaunoXome Injection (2% to 9%) 1442
DDAVP Tablets 739
Decadron Elixir 2078
Decadron Tablets 2079
Decadron Phosphate Injection 2081
Delatestryl Injection 1151
Demadex Tablets and Injection (1.1%) 2965
Depakote Tablets (1% to 5%) 430
Depakote ER Tablets (1% to 5%) 436
Depo-Medrol Injectable Suspension 2795
▲ Depo-Provera Contraceptive Injection (More than 5%) 2798
Dermatop Emollient Cream (Less than 1%) 2517
Desogen Tablets 2458
Diovan Capsules (More than 1%) 2337
Diprivan Injectable Emulsion (Less than 1%) 667
Dolobid Tablets (Less than 1 in 100) 2088
Dolophine Hydrochloride Tablets 3056
Doxil Injection (Less than 1%) 566
Duragesic Transdermal System (1% or greater) 1786
Duranest Injections 600
Dynabac Tablets (0.1% to 1%) 2269
▲ DynaCirc Capsules (3.5% to 8.7%) 2921
▲ DynaCirc CR Tablets (8.9% to 35.9%) 2923
▲ EC-Naprosyn Delayed-Release Tablets (3% to 9%) 2967
Effexor Tablets (Infrequent) 3495
Effexor XR Capsules (Frequent) 3499
8-MOP Capsules 1727
▲ Emcyt Capsules (19%) 2810
▲ Epogen for Injection (6% to 17%) 582
Ergamisol Tablets (1%) 1789
Esclim Transdermal System (4.2% to 6.4%) 3460
Estinyl Tablets 3112
Estrace Vaginal Cream 3358
Estrace Tablets 3361
Estratest 3252
Estrostep 2627
▲ Eulexin Capsules (4%) 3118
Evoxac Capsules (1% to 3%) 1217
Exelon Capsules (Frequent) 2342
Exelon Oral Solution (Frequent) 2345
▲ Fareston Tablets (5%) 3237
Felbatol 3343
▲ Feldene Capsules (1% to 10%) 2685
▲ Femara Tablets (5%) 2351
▲ femhrt Tablets (4.7%) 2635
▲ Ferrlecit Injection (5%) 3386
Flexeril Tablets (Rare) 572
Flexeril Tablets (Rare) 2094
▲ Flolan for Injection (60% to 79%) 1528
Florinef Acetate Tablets 2250
Flovent Diskus (1% to 3%) 3614
Floxin I.V. (Less than 1%) 2526
Floxin Tablets (Less than 1%) 2529
▲ Fludara for Injection (8% to 19%) 995
Fortovase Capsules (Less than 2%) 2970
Foscavir Injection (Between 1% and 5%) 605
Gabitril Tablets (Frequent) 1189
Gammar-P I.V. 787
Gastrocrom Oral Concentrate (Less common) 1162
▲ Gemzar for Injection (Less than 1% to 13%) 1919
▲ Gengraf Capsules (10%) 457
Genotropin Lyophilized Powder 2818
▲ Gleevec Capsules (52% to 68%) 2357
Glucotrol XL Extended Release Tablets (Less than 1%) 2693
▲ Hectorol Capsules (34.4%) 1064
▲ Hectorol Injection (34.4%) 1066
▲ Herceptin I.V. (8%) 1414
Hivid Tablets (Less than 1%) 2975
Humate-P Concentrate 790
▲ Humatrope Vials and Cartridges (2.5% to 21.2%) 1930
Hydrocortone Tablets 2106
Hydrocortone Acetate Injectable Suspension 2103
Hydrocortone Phosphate Injection, Sterile 2105
Hytrin Capsules (0.9%) 464
Hyzaar (1.3%) 2109
Imdur Tablets (Less than or equal to 5%) 1826
Imitrex Nasal Spray (Infrequent) 1554
Imitrex Tablets (Rare to infrequent) 1558
Indocin Capsules (Less than 1%) 2112
Indocin I.V. (Less than 1%) 2115
Indocin (Less than 1%) 2112
▲ Intron A for Injection (Less than or equal to 5%) 3120
Invirase Capsules (Less than 2%) 2979
Iopidine 0.5% Ophthalmic Solution (Less than 1%) ⊙ 213
Ismo Tablets (Fewer than 1%) 3524
Isoptin SR Tablets (1.9%) 467
Iveegam EN 849
Kadian Capsules (Less than 3%) 1335
Kaletra Capsules (Less than 2%) 471
Kaletra Oral Solution (Less than 2%) 471
Klaron Lotion 10% (One of 105 patients) 1224
Klonopin Tablets (Infrequent) 2983
Lamictal (Rare) 1567
▲ Leukine (13% to 34%) 1755
▲ Leustatin Injection (6%) 2495
Levaquin (0.1% to less than 1.0%) 2537
Levlen 962
Levlite 21 Tablets 962
Levlite 28 Tablets 962
Levora Tablets 3389
Levulan Kerastick (Up to 1%) 971
▲ Lexxel Tablets (4.1%) 608
Librium Capsules (Isolated cases) 1736
Librium for Injection (Isolated cases) 1737
Lidoderm Patch 1319
Lipitor Tablets (Less than 2%) 2639
Lipitor Tablets (Less than 2%) 2696
Lodine (Less than 1%) 3528
Lodine XL Extended-Release Tablets (Less than 1%) 3530
Lodosyn Tablets 1251
Loestrin 21 Tablets 2642
Loestrin Fe Tablets 2642
Lo/Ovral Tablets 3532
Lo/Ovral-28 Tablets 3538
Lotrel Capsules (0.6% to 3.2%) 2370
Lotrimin 3128
Lotrisone (Less than 1%) 3129
Lovenox Injection (2%) 746
Low-Ogestrel-28 Tablets 3392
Lunelle Monthly Injection 2827
▲ Lupron Depot 3.75 mg (5.4%) 3281
▲ Lupron Depot 7.5 mg (14.3%) 3284
▲ Lupron Depot-3 Month 11.25 mg (5.4% to 7%) 3285
Lupron Depot-3 Month 22.5 mg (Less than 5%) 3288
▲ Lupron Depot-4 Month 30 mg (Less than 5% to 20.8%) 3289
Luvox Tablets (25, 50, 100 mg) (Frequent) 3256
Matulane Capsules 3246
Mavik Tablets (0.3% to 1.0%) 478
Maxair Autohaler 1981
Maxair Inhaler (Less than 1%) 1984
Maxalt Tablets (Rare) 2120
Maxalt-MLT Orally Disintegrating Tablets (Rare) 2120
Megace Oral Suspension (1% to 3%) 1124
Menest Tablets 2254
Meridia Capsules (1.2%) 481
Mexitil Capsules (Less than 1% to 3.8%) 1047
Microgestin Fe 1.5/30 Tablets 3407
Microgestin Fe 1/20 Tablets 3400
Migranal Nasal Spray (Infrequent) 2376
Minipress Capsules (1% to 4%) 2699
Minizide Capsules 2700

▲ Mirapex Tablets (4% to 5%) 2834
Mircette Tablets 2470
Mobic Tablets (0.6% to 4.5%) 1054
Modicon 2563
Monopril Tablets (0.2% to 1.0% or more) 1091
Monopril HCT (Less than 2%) 1094
Motrin Suspension, Oral Drops, Chewable Tablets, and Caplets (1% to less than 3%) 2002
MS Contin Tablets (Less frequent) ... 2896
MSIR (Less frequent) 2898
Mykrox Tablets (Less than 2%) 1168
Myobloc Injectable Solution (2% or greater) 1291
▲ Naprelan Tablets (Less than 3% to 9%) 1293
▲ Naprosyn Suspension (3% to 9%) ... 2967
▲ Naprosyn Tablets (3% to 9%) 2967
Nardil Tablets (Common) 2653
Necon 3415
▲ Neoral Soft Gelatin Capsules (2% to 10%) 2380
▲ Neoral Oral Solution (2% to 10%) ... 2380
▲ Neumega for Injection (59%) 1434
Neurontin Capsules (Infrequent) 2655
Neurontin Oral Solution (Infrequent) 2655
Neurontin Tablets (Infrequent) 2655
Nexium Delayed-Release Capsules (Less than 1%) 619
Niaspan Extended-Release Tablets 1846
Nilandron Tablets (2%) 753
Nimotop Capsules (Up to 1.2%) 904
▲ Nolvadex Tablets (3.8% to 32.4%) . 678
Nordette-28 Tablets 2257
Norinyl 1 +35 28-Day Tablets 3380
Norinyl 1 + 50 28-Day Tablets 3380
Normodyne Tablets (Up to 2%) 3137
Noroxin Tablets (Less frequent) 2145
Norpramin Tablets 755
▲ Norvasc Tablets (1.8% to 14.6%) ... 2704
Norvir Capsules (Less than 2%) 487
Norvir Oral Solution (Less than 2%) 487
▲ Novantrone for Injection (10%) 1760
Novarel for Injection 1347
NovoSeven (1%) 2430
Nubain Injection (1% or less) 1323
▲ Nutropin AQ Injection (41%) 1420
Nutropin Depot for Injectable Suspension (Less than 1%) 1423
▲ Nutropin for Injection (41%) 1417
Ogen Tablets 2846
Ogestrel 0.5/50-28 Tablets 3428
▲ Oncaspar (Greater than 5%) 756
Opticrom Ophthalmic Solution (Rare) 555
OptiPranolol Metipranolol Ophthalmic Solution 0.3% (A small number of patients) .... ⊙263
Oramorph SR Tablets (Less frequent) 3062
Orgaran Injection (2.6%) 2480
Ortho Dienestrol Cream 2554
Ortho-Cept 21 Tablets 2546
Ortho-Cept 28 Tablets 2546
Ortho-Cyclen/Ortho Tri-Cyclen 2573
Ortho-Est Tablets 3464
Ortho-Novum 2563
Ortho-Novum 1/50□28 Tablets 2556
Ortho-Prefest Tablets 2570
Ortho-Cyclen/Ortho Tri-Cyclen 2573
▲ Orudis Capsules (3% to 9%) 3548
▲ Oruvail Capsules (3% to 9%) 3548
Ovcon 3364
Ovral Tablets 3551
Ovral-28 Tablets 3552
Ovrette Tablets 3552
Oxandrin Tablets 1153
Oxsoralen-Ultra Capsules 1741
OxyContin Tablets (Less than 1%) ... 2912
Pacerone Tablets (1% to 3%) 3331
Parnate Tablets 1607
Paxil (Frequent) 1609
Pediapred Oral Solution 1170
Pediazole Suspension 3050
Pentasa Capsules (Less than 1%) ... 3239
Permax Tablets (1.6%) 1299
Pfizerpen for Injection 2707
▲ Photofrin for Injection (5% to 18%) . 831
▲ Plavix Tablets (4.1%) 1097
▲ Plavix Tablets (4.1%) 3084
Pletal Tablets (Less than 2%) 2605
Pletal Tablets (Less than 2%) 2848
▲ Ponstel Capsules (1% to 10%) 1356
Precose Tablets (Rare) 906
Prednisone 3064
Pregnyl for Injection 2482
Prelone Syrup 2273
Premarin Intravenous 3563
Premarin Tablets 3566
Premarin Vaginal Cream 3570
Premphase Tablets 3572
Prevacid Delayed-Release Capsules (Less than 1%) 3292
PREVPAC (Less than 1%) 3298
Prinivil Tablets (0.3% to 1.0%) 2164
Prinzide Tablets 2168
▲ Procardia XL Extended Release Tablets (Approximately 10% to about 30%) 2710
▲ Procrit for Injection (6% to 17%) 2502
▲ Prograf (3% to 18%) 1393
▲ Proleukin for Injection (15%) 1199
Prometrium Capsules (100 mg, 200 mg) (Less than 5%) 3261
ProSom Tablets (Rare) 500
Protonix I.V. (Less than 1%) 3580
Protonix Tablets (Less than 1%) 3577
Protopic Ointment (Greater than or equal to 1%) 1397
Proventil HFA Inhalation Aerosol (Less than 3%) 3150
Provera Tablets 2853
Provigil Tablets (At least 1%) 1193
Prozac Pulvules, Liquid, and Weekly Capsules (Infrequent) 1238
▲ Rapamune Oral Solution and Tablets (16% to 24%) 3584
Recombivax HB (Less than 1%) 2178
Reglan 2935
▲ Relafen Tablets (3% to 9%) 1617
Remeron Tablets (1%) 2483
Remeron SolTab Tablets (1%) 2486
Remicade for IV Injection (Less than 2%) 1178
ReoPro Vials (0.3%) 1958
▲ Requip Tablets (Infrequent) 1621
Rescriptor Tablets (Less than 2%) 526
Retrovir Capsules (0.8%) 1625
Retrovir IV Infusion (1%) 1629
Retrovir (0.8%) 1625
Rilutek Tablets (Rare to frequent) 772
Risperdal (Infrequent) 1796
▲ Roferon-A Injection (More than 1% to 11%) 2996
Rowasa Rectal Suspension Enema 4.0 grams/unit (60 mL) (1.2%) 3264
Roxanol 3066
Roxicodone Tablets (Less than 3%) 3067
Rythmol Tablets – 150 mg, 225 mg, 300 mg (1.4%) 502
▲ Salagen Tablets (5%) 2229
Sandimmune (2% or less) 2388
Sandostatin Injection (1% to 4%) 2394
Sandostatin LAR Depot (Rare) 2395
Sarafem Pulvules (Infrequent) 1962
Sectral Capsules (2%) 3589
Serentil 1057
Serophene Tablets 3226
Serzone Tablets 1104
▲ Simulect for Injection (Greater than or equal to 10%) 2399
Sinemet Tablets 1253
Sinemet CR Tablets 1255
Sinequan (Occasional) 2713
Singulair 2181
Solu-Medrol Sterile Powder 2855
Soma Compound Tablets 3354
Soma Compound w/Codeine Tablets 3355
Sonata Capsules (Infrequent) 3591
▲ Soriatane Capsules (1% to 10%) 3003
▲ Sporanox Capsules (3.5%) 1800
Sporanox Injection (1%) 1804
Sporanox Injection (1%) 2509
Sporanox Oral Solution 1808
Sporanox Oral Solution 2512
Stadol NS Nasal Spray (Less than 1%) 1108
Stimate Nasal Spray 796
Symmetrel 1328
▲ Synarel Nasal Solution for Endometriosis (8% of patients) ... 3205
▲ Tambocor Tablets (3.5%) 1990
Tapazole Tablets 1823
Tarka Tablets (0.3% to 1.3%) 508
Tasmar Tablets (Infrequent) 3010
▲ Taxol Injection (21%) 1129
▲ Taxotere for Injection Concentrate (6%) 778
Tegretol/Tegretol-XR 2404
Tenex Tablets (Less frequent) 2942
Tequin Injection (Less than 0.1%) 1110
Tequin Tablets (Less than 0.1%) 1110
Testoderm Transdermal Systems ... 574
Testopel Pellets 3610
Tetanus Toxoid Adsorbed Purogenated 1882
Thalomid Capsules 1154
Thioridazine Hydrochloride Tablets 2289
Thyrogen for Injection (Four patients) 1441
Tiazac Capsules (2%) 1378
Tikosyn Capsules (Less than or equal to 2%) 2717
Timolide Tablets 2187
Timolol GFS .... ⊙266
Timoptic in Ocudose 2192
Timoptic Sterile Ophthalmic Solution 2190
Timoptic-XE Sterile Ophthalmic Gel Forming Solution 2194
▲ Tolectin (3% to 9%) 2589
Tonocard Tablets (Less than 1%) 649
Topamax Sprinkle Capsules (1.2% to 1.8%) 2590
Topamax Tablets (1.2% to 1.8%) 2590
▲ Toradol (4%) 3018
Trental Tablets (Less than 1%) 784
Tricor Capsules, Micronized 513
Trileptal Oral Suspension (1% to 2%) 2407
Trileptal Tablets (1% to 2%) 2407
Tri-Levlen 962
Trilisate (Less than 1%) 2901
Tri-Norinyl-28 Tablets 3433
Triphasil-21 Tablets 3600
Triphasil-28 Tablets 3605
▲ Trisenox Injection (40%) 1158
Trivora Tablets 3439
Trovan (Less than 1%) 2722
Unasyn for Injection (Less than 1%) 2728
Uniretic Tablets (Less than 1%) 3178
Vaqta (Less than 1%) 2199
Vascor Tablets (0.5% to 2.0%) 2602
Verelan Capsules (1.9%) 3184
Verelan PM Capsules (1.7% to 1.9%) 3186
▲ Vesanoid Capsules (29% to 32%) ... 3037
Viadur Implant (Less than 2%) 912
Viagra Tablets (Less than 2%) 2732
▲ Vicoprofen Tablets (3% to 9%) 520
Vioxx (Greater than 0.1% to 1.9%) .. 2213
Viracept 532
Vistide Injection 1445
Vivactil Tablets 2217
Vivactil Tablets 2446
Vivelle Transdermal System 2412
Vivelle-Dot Transdermal System 2416
Voltaren Tablets (1% to 3%) 2315
Voltaren-XR Tablets (1% to 3%) 2315
Warfarin Sodium Tablets, USP 3302
Wellbutrin Tablets (Frequent) 1680
Wellbutrin SR Sustained-Release Tablets (Infrequent) 1684
▲ Xanax Tablets (4.9%) 2865
Xeloda Tablets (1%) 3039
Xylocaine Injections (Extremely rare) 653
Yasmin 28 Tablets 980
Zanaflex Tablets (Infrequent) 1305
Zebeta Tablets 1885
▲ Zemplar Injection (7%) 522
▲ Zenapax for Injection (Greater than 5%) 3046
Zestoretic Tablets 695
Zestril Tablets (0.3% to 1.0%) 698
Ziac Tablets 1887
Ziagen 1692
Zithromax Capsules, 250 mg 2743
Zithromax for IV Infusion 2748
Zithromax for Oral Suspension, 300 mg, 600 mg, 900 mg, 1200 mg 2739
Zithromax Tablets, 250 mg 2739
▲ Zoladex (1% to 7%) 702
Zoladex 3-month 706
Zoloft (Infrequent) 2751
Zomig Tablets (Infrequent) 708
Zomig-ZMT Tablets (Infrequent) 708
Zonegran Capsules (Infrequent) 1307
Zosyn (0.1% to 1.9%) 1890
Zosyn in Galaxy Containers (0.1% to 1.9%) 1894
Zovia 3449
Zovirax for Injection (Less than 1%) 1708
Zyban Sustained-Release Tablets (Infrequent) 1710
Zyrtec (Less than 2%) 2756
Zyrtec-D 12 Hour Extended Relief Tablets (Less than 2%) 2758

Edema, aggravated

▲ Gleevec Capsules (2% to 16%) 2357

Edema, allergic

Periactin Tablets 2155

Edema, angioneurotic

Accolate Tablets 657
Accupril Tablets 2611
Altace Capsules (0.3%) 2233
Anaprox Tablets (Less than 1%) 2967
Anaprox DS Tablets (Less than 1%) 2967
Atrovent Nasal Spray 0.06% (Rare) 1033
Augmentin Chewable Tablets 1482
Augmentin Powder for Oral Suspension 1482
Augmentin Tablets 1485
Azactam for Injection (Less than 1%) 1276
Baycol Tablets 883
BayHep B 915
BayRab (Rare) 917
BayTet (Few isolated cases) 923
Carafate Suspension 731
Carafate Tablets 730
Catapres Tablets (About 5 in 1,000 patients) 1037
Catapres-TTS (0.5% or less) 1038
Ceclor CD Tablets 1279
Ceclor 1905
Ceftin 1898
Cefzil 1076
Ceptaz for Injection (Very rare) 1499
▲ Cerezyme for Injection (Approximately 4%) 1438
Chibroxin Sterile Ophthalmic Solution 2051
Chloroptic Sterile Ophthalmic Ointment .... ⊙234
Chloroptic Sterile Ophthalmic Solution .... ⊙235
Cipro I.V. Pharmacy Bulk Package (Less than 1%) 897
Claritin (At least one patient) 3100
Claritin-D 12 Hour Extended Release Tablets 3102
Claritin-D 24 Hour Extended Release Tablets 3104
Clinoril Tablets (Less than 1 in 100) 2053
Clorpres Tablets (About 5 in 1,000) 1002
Combipres Tablets (About 5 in 1,000) 1040
Combivent Inhalation Aerosol (Rare) 1041
Compazine 1505
Comvax (Rare) 2056
Cordarone Tablets 3487
Cortone Acetate Injectable Suspension 2059
Cortone Acetate Tablets 2061
Cozaar Tablets (Rare) 2067
CytoGam Intravenous (A possibility) 2026
Decadron Elixir 2078
Decadron Tablets 2079
Decadron Phosphate Injection 2081
Declomycin Tablets 1855
Demadex Tablets and Injection (One patient) 2965
DiaBeta Tablets 741
Diflucan Tablets, Injection, and Oral Suspension (Rare) 2681
Diovan Capsules (Less frequent) 2337
Diovan HCT Tablets (Less frequent) 2338
Diprivan Injectable Emulsion (Rare) 667
Dolobid Tablets (Less than 1 in 100) 2088
Duraclon Injection (0.5%) 3057
Duricef 1079
Dynacin Capsules 2019
EC-Naprosyn Delayed-Release Tablets (Less than 1%) 2967
Emla 602
Engerix-B Vaccine 1517
Etrafon 3115
Famotidine Injection (Infrequent) 866
Flexeril Tablets 572
Flexeril Tablets 2094
Flonase Nasal Spray 1533
Flovent (Rare) 1535
Floxin I.V. (Less than 1%) 2526
Floxin Tablets (Less than 1%) 2529
FluShield Influenza Vaccine (Rare) ... 3521
Fluzone Vaccine (Rare) 802
Gastrocrom Oral Concentrate (Less common) 1162
Gengraf Capsules (1% to less than 3%) 457
Grifulvin V Tablets Microsize and Oral Suspension Microsize (Rare) 2518
Gris-PEG Tablets (Rare) 2661
Havrix Vaccine (Rare) 1544
Hydrocortone Tablets 2106
Hydrocortone Acetate Injectable Suspension 2103
Hydrocortone Phosphate Injection, Sterile 2105
Imitrex Injection 1549
Imitrex Nasal Spray 1554
Imitrex Tablets 1558
Imogam Rabies - HT 805
Intron A for Injection (Rare) 3120
JE-VAX Vaccine 811
Lamictal (Rare) 1567
Lescol Capsules (Rare) 2361
Lescol Capsules (Rare) 2925
Lescol XL Tablets 2361
Lescol XL Tablets 2925
Leukeran Tablets 1591
Levaquin 2537
Lexxel Tablets 608
Lipitor Tablets 2639
Lipitor Tablets 2696
Lithobid Slow-Release Tablets 3255
Lodine (Less than 1%) 3528
Lodine XL Extended-Release Tablets (Less than 1%) 3530
Lopid Tablets 2650
Mavik Tablets (0.13%) 478
Mefoxin for Injection 2124
Mefoxin Premixed Intravenous Solution 2127
Mevacor Tablets (Rare) 2132
Miltown Tablets (Rare) 3349
Minocin Intravenous 1862
Minocin Oral Suspension 1865
Minocin Pellet-Filled Capsules 1863
M-M-R II 2118
Monodox Capsules 2442

Monopril Tablets (0.2% to 1.0%) 1091
Monopril HCT (Less than 2%) 1094
Monurol Sachet 1375
Motofen Tablets 577
Motrin Suspension, Oral Drops, Chewable Tablets, and Caplets (Less than 1%) 2002
Mykrox Tablets 1168
▲ Naprelan Tablets (3% to 9%) 1293
Naprosyn Suspension (Less than 1%) 2967
Naprosyn Tablets (Less than 1%) 2967
Naropin Injection 612
Navelbine Injection 1604
Neoral Soft Gelatin Capsules (1% to less than 3%) 2380
Neoral Oral Solution (1% to less than 3%) 2380
Nesacaine/Nesacaine MPF 617
Normodyne Injection (Rare) 3135
Normodyne Tablets (Rare) 3137
Noroxin Tablets 2145
Norvir Capsules 487
Norvir Oral Solution 487
Orthoclone OKT3 Sterile Solution 2498
Pacerone Tablets 3331
Parafon Forte DSC Caplets (Extremely rare) 2582
Paxil (Rare) 1609
Pediazole Suspension 3050
Liquid PedvaxHIB (Rare) 2148
Pepcid Injection (Infrequent) 2153
Pepcid for Oral Suspension (Infrequent) 2150
Pepcid RPD Orally Disintegrating Tablets (Infrequent) 2150
Pepcid Tablets (Infrequent) 2150
Pergonal for Injection 3223
Periostat Tablets 1208
Phenergan Injection 3553
Phenergan Tablets 3556
Phenergan with Codeine Syrup (Infrequent) 3557
Phenergan VC with Codeine Syrup 3561
Pravachol Tablets (Rare) 1099
Prednisone 3064
Prevnar for Injection 1870
Prilosec Delayed-Release Capsules (Less than 1%) 628
Primaxin I.M. 2158
Primaxin I.V. (Less than 0.2%) 2160
Prinzide Tablets (Rare) 2168
Procanbid Extended-Release Tablets (Occasional) 2262
Procardia Capsules (Less than 0.5%) 2708
Proventil Inhalation Solution 0.083% (Rare) 3146
Proventil Solution for Inhalation 0.5% (Rare) 3144
Proventil HFA Inhalation Aerosol (Rare) 3150
Pulmicort Respules (Less than 1%) 632
Pulmicort Turbuhaler Inhalation Powder (Rare) 636
Relafen Tablets (1%) 1617
Repronex for Intramuscular and Subcutaneous Injection 1347
Rescriptor Tablets (Less than 2%) 526
Retin-A Micro 0.1% 2522
Rilutek Tablets (Rare) 772
Risperdal 1796
Robaxisal Tablets 2939
Semprex-D Capsules (Rare) 1172
Sensorcaine (Rare) 643
Sensorcaine-MPF Injection (Rare) 643
Serentil 1057
Serevent Inhalation Aerosol (Rare) 1633
Soma Tablets 3353
Soma Compound Tablets 3354
Soma Compound w/Codeine Tablets 3355
Sporanox Capsules 1800
Sporanox Injection 1804
Sporanox Injection 2509
Sporanox Oral Solution 1808
Sporanox Oral Solution 2512
Stelazine 1640
Streptase for Infusion (Rare) 647
▲ Stromectol Tablets (22.7%) 2185
Sular Tablets (Very rare) 688
Tarka Tablets (0.15%) 508
Taxol Injection (2%) 1129
Tazicef for Injection (Very rare) 1647
Tazicef Galaxy Container (Very rare) 1650
Tazicef Pharmacy Bulk Package (Very rare) 1653
Tazidime Vials, Faspak & ADD-Vantage (Very rare) 1966
Thioridazine Hydrochloride Tablets 2289
Thorazine 1656
Trilafon 3160
Trusopt Sterile Ophthalmic Solution 2196
Ultram Tablets 2600
Univasc Tablets (Less than 0.5%) 3181
Velosulin BR Human Insulin 10 ml Vials 2435
Vermox Chewable Tablets (Rare) 2017
Vibramycin Calcium Oral Suspension Syrup 2735
Vibramycin Hyclate Capsules 2735
Vibramycin Hyclate Intravenous 2737
Vibramycin Monohydrate for Oral Suspension 2735
Vibra-Tabs Film Coated Tablets 2735
Volmax Extended-Release Tablets (Rare) 2276
Wellbutrin Tablets 1680
Wellbutrin SR Sustained-Release Tablets 1684
Zantac (Rare) 1690
Zantac Injection (Rare) 1688
Zantac Syrup (Rare) 1690
Zaroxolyn Tablets 1177
Zebeta Tablets 1885
Zestoretic Tablets 695
Ziac Tablets 1887
Zocor Tablets (Rare) 2219
Zofran Injection (Rare) 1698
Zyban Sustained-Release Tablets 1710
Zyrtec (Less than 2%) 2756
Zyrtec-D 12 Hour Extended Relief Tablets (Less than 2%) 2758

Edema, ankle

Synvisc 3596
Verelan Capsules (1.4%) 3184

Edema, aphakic cystoid macular

Cosopt Sterile Ophthalmic Solution 2065
Timolol GFS ..... ⊙266
Timoptic in Ocudose (Less frequent) 2192
Timoptic Sterile Ophthalmic Solution (Less frequent) 2190
Timoptic-XE Sterile Ophthalmic Gel Forming Solution 2194

Edema, cerebral

Activase I.V. 1410
Aggrenox Capsules 1026
Ativan Injection (Less than 1%) 3478
Betaseron for SC Injection 988
Cerebyx Injection (2.2%) 2619
Compazine 1505
Ecotrin Enteric Coated Aspirin Low, Regular and Maximum Strength Tablets 1715
Etrafon (Extremely rare) 3115
Felbatol 3343
▲ Gliadel Wafer (4%) 1723
Navane Oral 2701
Navane Intramuscular 2703
Orthoclone OKT3 Sterile Solution 2498
Permax Tablets (Rare) 1299
Proleukin for Injection (Less than 1%) 1199
Stelazine 1640
Thiothixene Capsules 2290
Thorazine 1656
Trilafon (Extremely rare) 3160
▲ Vesanoid Capsules (3%) 3037

Edema, conjunctival

▲ Alphagan Ophthalmic Solution (Approximately 3% to 9%) 545
Alphagan P Ophthalmic Solution (1% to 4%) 546
Cipro 887
Cosopt Sterile Ophthalmic Solution (1% to 5%) 2065
Differin Cream (Less than 1%) 1402
Effexor Tablets (Rare) 3495
Effexor XR Capsules (Rare) 3499
Lumigan Ophthalmic Solution (1% to 3%) 553
Ocuflox Ophthalmic Solution 554
Patanol Ophthalmic Solution (Less than 5%) 540
Paxil (Rare) 1609
Trileptal Oral Suspension 2407
Trileptal Tablets 2407
Vexol 1% Ophthalmic Suspension (Less than 1%) ..... ⊙222

Edema, corneal

▲ Acular Ophthalmic Solution (1% to 10%) 544
Amvisc Plus ..... ⊙329
Healon (Rare) ..... ⊙316
Healon GV ..... ⊙320
Miochol-E System Pak (Infrequent) ..... ⊙305
Miochol-E with Steri-Tags (Infrequent) ..... ⊙305
Ocucoat ..... ⊙330
Plaquenil Tablets 3082
Rescula Ophthalmic Solution (Less than 1%) ..... ⊙306
▲ Rēv-Eyes Sterile Ophthalmic Eyedrops 0.5% (10% to 40%) ..... ⊙265
Symmetrel (0.1% to 1%) 1328
Vexol 1% Ophthalmic Suspension (Less than 1%) ..... ⊙222
Vitravene for Injection (2% to 5%) ..... ⊙310
Voltaren Ophthalmic Sterile Ophthalmic Solution (Less than 5%) ..... ⊙312

Edema, cystoid macular

Lumigan Ophthalmic Solution 553
Niaspan Extended-Release Tablets 1846
Travatan Ophthalmic Solution 543
Xalatan Latanoprost Ophthalmic Solution ..... ⊙320
Xalatan Sterile Ophthalmic Solution 2864

Edema, dependent

Coreg Tablets (1.7% to 3.7%) 1508
Diovan HCT Tablets (Greater than 0.2%) 2338
Ellence Injection 2806
Innohep Injection 1248
Micardis Tablets (More than 0.3%) 1049
Micardis HCT Tablets 1051
Mobic Tablets (0.6% to 4.5%) 1054
Reminyl Oral Solution (Infrequent) 1792
Reminyl Tablets (Infrequent) 1792
▲ Requip Tablets (6%) 1621
▲ Simulect for Injection (3% to 10%) 2399
Skelid Tablets (2.7%) 3088
Teveten Tablets (1% or greater) 3327
Zoloft (Infrequent) 2751

Edema, esophageal

▲ Photofrin for Injection (8%) 831

Edema, extremities

Ceclor CD Tablets 1279
Ceclor 1905
Celexa (Infrequent) 1365
Cipro I.V. (1% or less) 893
Cipro (Less than 1%) 887
Depacon Injection 416
Depakene 421
Depakote Sprinkle Capsules 426
Depakote Tablets 430
Depakote ER Tablets 436
Mavik Tablets (0.13%) 478
Rifadin 765
Rifater Tablets 769
Tarka Tablets 508
Taxotere for Injection Concentrate 778
▲ Zenapax for Injection (Greater than 5%) 3046

Edema, facial

Aciphex Tablets (Rare) 1267
Aciphex Tablets (Rare) 1783
Actiq (Less than 1%) 1184
Adalat CC Tablets (Less than 1.0%) 877
Ambien Tablets (Rare) 3191
AmBisome for Injection (Less common) 1383
▲ Amphotec (5% or more) 1774
Anzemet Injection (Rare) 719
Anzemet Tablets (Rare) 722
Aricept Tablets (Infrequent) 1270
Aricept Tablets (Infrequent) 2665
Asacol Delayed-Release Tablets 2884
Astelin Nasal Spray 3339
Attenuvax 2044
Avalide Tablets 1070
Avapro Tablets (Less than 1%) 1074
Avapro Tablets (Less than 1%) 3076
Avonex 1013
Azmacort Inhalation Aerosol (1% to 3%) 728
Campath Ampules 992
Cancidas for Injection (Up to 3.1%) 2048
▲ Carac Cream (35.4%) 1222
Cardura Tablets (1%) 2668
Ceclor CD Tablets 1279
Ceclor 1905
Celebrex Capsules (0.1% to 1.9%) 2676
Celebrex Capsules (0.1% to 1.9%) 2780
Celexa (Rare) 1365
▲ CellCept Capsules (3%) 2951
▲ CellCept Intravenous (3%) 2951
▲ CellCept Oral Suspension (3%) 2951
▲ CellCept Tablets (3%) 2951
Cerebyx Injection (Frequent) 2619
Cipro I.V. (1% or less) 893
Cipro I.V. Pharmacy Bulk Package (Less than 1%) 897
Cipro (Less than 1%) 887
Claritin-D 24 Hour Extended Release Tablets (Fewer than 2%) 3104
Cognex Capsules (Infrequent) 1351
Combivent Inhalation Aerosol (Less than 2%) 1041
▲ Copaxone for Injection (6%) 3306
Cozaar Tablets (Rare) 2067
Crinone (Less than 5%) 3213
Depacon Injection (1% or more) 416
Depakene (1% or more) 421
Depakote Sprinkle Capsules 426
Depakote Tablets (1% to 5%) 430
Depakote ER Tablets (1% or more) 436
▲ Dostinex Tablets (Less than 10%) 2804
Doxil Injection (Less than 1%) 566
Effexor Tablets (Infrequent) 3495
Effexor XR Capsules (Infrequent) 3499
Etrafon 3115
Evoxac Capsules (Less than 1%) 1217
Exelon Capsules (Infrequent) 2342
Exelon Oral Solution (Infrequent) 2345
Famotidine Injection (Infrequent) 866
▲ Felbatol (3.4%) 3343
Flexeril Tablets (Less than 1%) 572
Flexeril Tablets (Less than 1%) 2094
Flonase Nasal Spray 1533
Floxin I.V. 2526
Floxin Tablets 2529
Foscavir Injection (Between 1% and 5%) 605
Gabitril Tablets (Infrequent) 1189
Geodon Capsules (Frequent) 2688
Hytrin Capsules (At least 1%) 464
Imitrex Nasal Spray 1554
Imitrex Tablets 1558
▲ Intron A for Injection (Up to 10%) 3120
Iopidine 0.5% Ophthalmic Solution (Less than 3%) ..... ⊙213
Kaletra Capsules (Less than 2%) 471
Kaletra Oral Solution (Less than 2%) 471
Klonopin Tablets 2983
Lamictal (Infrequent) 1567
Levaquin Injection (Less than 0.5%) 2537
Limbitrol 1738
Lipitor Tablets (Less than 2%) 2639
Lipitor Tablets (Less than 2%) 2696
Loprox Gel 2022
Loxitane Capsules 3398
Lupron Depot-3 Month 11.25 mg 3285
Mavik Tablets (0.13%) 478
Maxalt Tablets (Infrequent) 2120
Maxalt-MLT Orally Disintegrating Tablets (Infrequent) 2120
Meridia Capsules 481
Meruvax II 2130
M-M-R II 2118
Mobic Tablets (Less than 2%) 1054
Mumpsvax 2141
Neupogen for Injection 587
Neurontin Capsules (Frequent) 2655
Neurontin Oral Solution (Frequent) 2655
Neurontin Tablets (Frequent) 2655
Nexium Delayed-Release Capsules (Less than 1%) 619
▲ Nipent for Injection (3% to 10%) 3272
Noroxin Tablets 2145
Norpramin Tablets 755
Norvir Capsules (Less than 2%) 487
Norvir Oral Solution (Less than 2%) 487
Numorphan 1324
Ocuflox Ophthalmic Solution 554
Omnicef 493
Oncaspar (Less than 1%) 756
Orudis Capsules (Less than 1%) 3548
Oruvail Capsules (Less than 1%) 3548
OxyContin Tablets (Less than 1%) 2912
Paxil (Infrequent) 1609
Pepcid Injection (Infrequent) 2153
Pepcid for Oral Suspension (Infrequent) 2150
Pepcid RPD Orally Disintegrating Tablets (Infrequent) 2150
Pepcid Tablets (Infrequent) 2150
Pergonal for Injection 3223
Permax Tablets (1.1%) 1299
Plendil Extended-Release Tablets (0.5% to 1.5%) 623
Pletal Tablets (Less than 2%) 2605
Pletal Tablets (Less than 2%) 2848
Prevnar for Injection 1870
Primaxin I.V. (Less than 0.2%) 2160
Prinivil Tablets (0.3% to 1.0%) 2164
Prinzide Tablets 2168
Procardia XL Extended Release Tablets (1% or less) 2710
Propecia Tablets 2172
Protonix I.V. (Less than 1%) 3580
Protonix Tablets (Less than 1%) 3577
Protopic Ointment (1% to 3%) 1397
Prozac Pulvules, Liquid, and Weekly Capsules (Infrequent) 1238
▲ Rapamune Oral Solution and Tablets (3% to 20%) 3584
Relenza Rotadisk 1619
Remeron Tablets (Infrequent) 2483
Remeron SolTab Tablets (Infrequent) 2486
Remicade for IV Injection 1178
Repronex for Intramuscular and Subcutaneous Injection 1347
Rhinocort Nasal Inhaler (Less than 1%) 640
Rifadin 765
Rifater Tablets 769
Rilutek Tablets (Infrequent) 772
Salagen Tablets (1% to 2%) 2229
Sandostatin LAR Depot (Rare) 2395
Sarafem Pulvules (Infrequent) 1962
Seroquel Tablets (Infrequent) 684
Serzone Tablets (Infrequent) 1104
▲ Simulect for Injection (3% to 10%) 2399
Sonata Capsules (Infrequent) 3591
Stromectol Tablets (1.2%) 2185
Sular Tablets (Less than or equal to 1%) 688
Sulfamylon Cream 1011

Sulfamylon Topical Solution 1011
Suprax 1877
Surmontil Capsules 3595
Talacen Caplets (Rare) 3089
Talwin Nx Tablets 3090
Tarka Tablets 508
Tasmar Tablets (Infrequent) 3010
Tequin Injection (Less than 0.1%) 1110
Tequin Tablets (Less than 0.1%) 1110
▲ Thalomid Capsules (4.2%) 1154
Topamax Sprinkle Capsules (Infrequent) 2590
Topamax Tablets (Infrequent) 2590
Tricor Capsules, Micronized (Less than 1%) 513
▲ Trisenox Injection (8%) 1158
Trovan (Less than 1%) 2722
Valtrex Caplets 1676
Vaniqa Cream (0.9%) 1121
Vantin Tablets and Oral Suspension (Less than 1%) 2860
▲ Vesanoid Capsules (6%) 3037
Viagra Tablets (Less than 2%) 2732
Viramune Oral Suspension 1060
Viramune Tablets 1060
Vistide Injection 1445
Voltaren Ophthalmic Sterile Ophthalmic Solution (Less than 3%) ⊙312
Wellbutrin SR Sustained-Release Tablets (Infrequent) 1684
Zestoretic Tablets 695
Zestril Tablets (0.3% to 1.0%) 698
Zoloft (Infrequent) 2751
Zomig Tablets (Infrequent) 708
Zomig-ZMT Tablets (Infrequent) 708
Zonegran Capsules (Infrequent) 1307
Zyban Sustained-Release Tablets (Less than 1%) 1710
Zyprexa Tablets (Infrequent) 1973
Zyprexa ZYDIS Orally Disintegrating Tablets (Infrequent) 1973
Zyrtec (Less than 2%) 2756
Zyrtec-D 12 Hour Extended Relief Tablets (Less than 2%) 2758

Edema, genital

Cerebyx Injection (Infrequent) 2619
Doxil Injection (Less than 1%) 566
Estring Vaginal Ring (At least 1 report) 2811
▲ Simulect for Injection (3% to 10%) 2399
Viagra Tablets (Less than 2%) 2732

Edema, hand

Remicade for IV Injection 1178
Seroquel Tablets (Rare) 684

Edema, heart failure

(*see under* Congestive heart failure)

Edema, independent

Dostinex Tablets (1%) 2804

Edema, laryngeal

Activase I.V. (Very rare) 1410
Arthrotec Tablets (Rare) 3195
Axid Pulvules (Rare) 1903
Axid Pulvules (Rare) 2919
Bicillin C-R 900/300 Injection 2240
Bicillin C-R Injection 2238
Bicillin L-A Injection 2242
Cataflam Tablets (Less than 1%) 2315
Ceptaz for Injection 1499
Cipro I.V. (1% or less) 893
Cipro (Less than 1%) 887
Compazine 1505
Ecotrin Enteric Coated Aspirin Low, Regular and Maximum Strength Tablets 1715
Enalaprilat Injection 863
Ethyol for Injection (Rare) 2029
Etrafon 3115
Floxin I.V. 2526
Fortaz 1541
Lopid Tablets 2650
Lotrel Capsules (About 0.5%) 2370
Mavik Tablets (0.13%) 478
Nardil Tablets 2653
Naropin Injection 612
Nesacaine/Nesacaine MPF 617
Nexium Delayed-Release Capsules (Less than 1%) 619
Nipent for Injection (Less than 3%) 3272
Nubain Injection (1% or less) 1323
Numorphan 1324
Omnicef 493
Orthoclone OKT3 Sterile Solution 2498
Orudis Capsules (Less than 1%) 3548
Oruvail Capsules (Less than 1%) 3548
Pergonal for Injection 3223
Permapen Isoject 2706
Permax Tablets (Rare) 1299
Persantine Tablets (Rare) 1057
Phenergan with Codeine Syrup (Infrequent) 3557
Phenergan VC with Codeine Syrup 3561
Polocaine Injection, USP 625
Polocaine-MPF Injection, USP 625
Prinivil Tablets (0.3% to 1.0%) 2164
Prinzide Tablets (Rare) 2168
Prozac Pulvules, Liquid, and Weekly Capsules (Rare) 1238
Reglan (Rare) 2935
Repronex for Intramuscular and Subcutaneous Injection 1347
Sarafem Pulvules (Rare) 1962
Sensorcaine 643
Sensorcaine-MPF Injection (Rare) 643
Serentil 1057
Stelazine 1640
Tarka Tablets 508
Thioplex for Injection 1765
Thioridazine Hydrochloride Tablets 2289
Thorazine 1656
TNKase I.V. (Rare) 1430
Toradol 3018
Trilafon 3160
Vaseretic Tablets 2204
Vasotec I.V. Injection 2207
Vasotec Tablets 2210
▲ Vesanoid Capsules (3%) 3037
Voltaren Tablets (Less than 1%) 2315
Voltaren-XR Tablets (Less than 1%) 2315
Zestoretic Tablets 695
Zestril Tablets (0.3% to 1.0%) 698
Zofran Injection 1698
Zofran 1703
Zofran ODT Orally Disintegrating Tablets 1703

Edema, laryngotracheal

Photofrin for Injection 831

Edema, lesional

Oncaspar (Less than 1%) 756

Edema, lips

Cipro I.V. (1% or less) 893
Cipro I.V. Pharmacy Bulk Package (Less than 1%) 897
Cipro (Less than 1%) 887
Combivent Inhalation Aerosol (Less than 2%) 1041
Cozaar Tablets (Rare) 2067
Imitrex Tablets 1558
Mavik Tablets (0.13%) 478
▲ Oncaspar (Greater than 1% but less than 5%) 756
Orthoclone OKT3 Sterile Solution 2498
Propecia Tablets 2172
Remicade for IV Injection 1178
Rescriptor Tablets (Less than 2%) 526
Retrovir Capsules 1625
Retrovir IV Infusion 1629
Retrovir 1625
Tarka Tablets 508

Edema, local

Avita Gel 1000
Bicillin L-A Injection 2242
Celestone Soluspan Injectable Suspension 3097
Condylox Gel (Less common) 2436
Desferal Vials 2333
D.H.E. 45 Injection 2334
Diphtheria & Tetanus Toxoids Adsorbed Purogenated for Pediatric Use 1857
ELA-Max Cream 1340
ELA-Max 5 Cream 1340
▲ Emla (6% to 56%) 602
FluShield Influenza Vaccine 3521
Havrix Vaccine (Rare) 1544
Oncaspar 756
Rescriptor Tablets (Less than 2%) 526
▲ Tazorac Gel (1% to 10%) 556
Tetanus & Diphtheria Toxoids Adsorbed for Adult Use 1880
Tetanus and Diphtheria Toxoids Adsorbed For Adult Use 815
Vantin Tablets and Oral Suspension (Less than 1%) 2860
Zovirax Ointment 1707

Edema, lower extremities

▲ Aromasin Tablets (7%) 2769
Cipro I.V. Pharmacy Bulk Package (Less than 1%) 897
Coreg Tablets (2.2%) 1508
Eldepryl Capsules 3266
Estring Vaginal Ring (1% to 3%) 2811
▲ Femara Tablets (5%) 2351
Ferrlecit Injection (Greater than 1%) 3386
Miacalcin Injection 2373
Micardis Tablets (More than 0.3%) 1049
Micardis HCT Tablets 1051
Mobic Tablets (0.6% to 4.5%) 1054
Monopril Tablets (0.4% to 1.0%) 1091
Nexium Delayed-Release Capsules (Less than 1%) 619
▲ Procardia Capsules (About 1 in 10 patients) 2708
▲ Requip Tablets (6%) 1621
▲ Simulect for Injection (Greater than or equal to 10%) 2399
Taxotere for Injection Concentrate 778
Trileptal Oral Suspension (1% to 2%) 2407
Trileptal Tablets (1% to 2%) 2407
Vioxx (1.1%) 2213
Xenical Capsules (2.8%) 3043
▲ Zometa for Intravenous Infusion (5% to 10%) 3621
Zyprexa Tablets (1%) 1973
Zyprexa ZYDIS Orally Disintegrating Tablets (1%) 1973
Zyrtec (Less than 2%) 2756
Zyrtec-D 12 Hour Extended Relief Tablets (Less than 2%) 2758

Edema, macular

Clomid Tablets 735
Lumigan Ophthalmic Solution 553
Retrovir Capsules (A single case) 1625
Retrovir IV Infusion (A single case) 1629
Retrovir (A single case) 1625
Serophene Tablets 3226
Travatan Ophthalmic Solution 543
Xalatan Latanoprost Ophthalmic Solution ⊙320
Xalatan Sterile Ophthalmic Solution 2864

Edema, mouth

Campath Ampules 992
Evoxac Capsules (Less than 1%) 1217
Tequin Injection (Less than 0.1%) 1110
Tequin Tablets (Less than 0.1%) 1110

Edema, nasal

▲ Atrovent Nasal Spray 0.03% (3.1%) 1032

Edema, non-specific

(*see under* Edema)

Edema, oropharyngeal

Arthrotec Tablets (Rare) 3195
Atrovent Nasal Spray 0.06% (Rare) 1033
Cataflam Tablets (Less than 1%) 2315
Cipro I.V. (1% or less) 893
Cipro (Less than 1%) 887
Combivent Inhalation Aerosol (Rare) 1041
Procardia Capsules (A few patients) 2708
Proventil Inhalation Aerosol (Rare) 3142
Proventil Inhalation Solution 0.083% (Rare) 3146
Proventil Repetabs Tablets 3148
Proventil Solution for Inhalation 0.5% (Rare) 3144
Proventil HFA Inhalation Aerosol (Rare) 3150
Relenza Rotadisk (Less than 1%) 1619
Ventolin Inhalation Aerosol and Refill (Rare) 1679
Ventolin HFA Inhalation Aerosol (Less than 3%) 3618
Volmax Extended-Release Tablets (Rare) 2276
Voltaren Tablets (Less than 1%) 2315
Voltaren-XR Tablets (Less than 1%) 2315

Edema, palpebral

Alomide Ophthalmic Solution (Less than 1%) ⊙204
Aralen Tablets 3075
Aredia for Injection (One patient) 2309
Betoptic S Ophthalmic Suspension 537
▲ Carteolol Hydrochloride Ophthalmic Solution USP, 1% (About 1 of 4 patients) ⊙258
Cipro I.V. (1% or less) 893
Cipro I.V. Pharmacy Bulk Package (Less than 1%) 897
Crixivan Capsules (Less than 2%) 2070
Crolom Sterile Ophthalmic Solution USP 4% (Infrequent) ⊙259
DDAVP Nasal Spray (Up to 2%) 738
DDAVP Rhinal Tube (Up to 2%) 738
Desmopressin Acetate Rhinal Tube (Up to 2%) 1345
Feldene Capsules (Rare) 2685
Imitrex Nasal Spray 1554
Imitrex Tablets 1558
Iopidine 0.5% Ophthalmic Solution (Less than 3%) ⊙213
Livostin (Approximately 1% to 3%) ⊙305
Mavik Tablets 478
Maxalt Tablets (Infrequent) 2120
Maxalt-MLT Orally Disintegrating Tablets (Infrequent) 2120
Monopril Tablets 1091
▲ Ocupress Ophthalmic Solution, 1% Sterile (About 1 of 4 patients) ⊙303
Opticrom Ophthalmic Solution (Infrequent) 555
Orthoclone OKT3 Sterile Solution 2498
▲ Polysporin Ophthalmic Ointment Sterile (Among those occurring most often) ⊙301
Prinzide Tablets 2168
ProSom Tablets (Infrequent) 500
Vaseretic Tablets 2204
Vasotec Tablets 2210
Viagra Tablets 2732
Viroptic Ophthalmic Solution Sterile (2.8%) ⊙301

Edema, paramacular

Viagra Tablets 2732

Edema, penile

Caverject Sterile Powder (1%) 2777

Edema, periorbital

(*see under* Edema, peripheral)

Edema, peripheral

Aciphex Tablets 1267
Aciphex Tablets 1783
Actiq (1% or greater) 1184
▲ Actonel Tablets (8.2%) 2879
▲ Adalat CC Tablets (18% to 29%) 877
Aerobid/Aerobid-M (1% to 3%) 1363
▲ Agrylin Capsules (8.9%) 3232
Ambien Tablets (Rare) 3191
▲ AmBisome for Injection (14.6%) 1383
▲ Amphotec (5% or more) 1774
Anaprox Tablets (Some patients) 2967
Anaprox DS Tablets (Some patients) 2967
AndroGel (Fewer than 1%) 3322
Anzemet Injection (Rare) 719
Anzemet Tablets (Rare) 722
▲ Apligraf (4.5% to 5%) 2305
Arava Tablets (1% to 3%) 724
Aricept Tablets (Infrequent) 1270
Aricept Tablets (Infrequent) 2665
▲ Arimidex Tablets (5.3% to 10.1%) 659
▲ Aromasin Tablets (7%) 2769
Arthrotec Tablets (Rare) 3195
▲ Asacol Delayed-Release Tablets (3%) 2884
Atacand HCT Tablets (0.5% or greater) 597
Attenuvax 2044
Avelox Tablets (0.05% to 1%) 879
Azulfidine EN-tabs Tablets (Rare) 2775
Baycol Tablets (2.0%) 883
Betimol Ophthalmic Solution (1% to 5%) ⊙324
▲ Campath Ampules (1% to 13%) 992
Cardene I.V. (Rare) 3485
▲ Carnitor Injection (3% to 6%) 3242
▲ Casodex Tablets (8%) 662
Ceclor CD Tablets (0.1% to 1%) 1279
Celebrex Capsules (2.1%) 2676
Celebrex Capsules (2.1%) 2780
▲ CellCept Capsules (27.0% to 64%) 2951
▲ CellCept Intravenous (27.0% to 64%) 2951
▲ CellCept Oral Suspension (27.0% to 64%) 2951
▲ CellCept Tablets (27.0% to 64%) 2951
Celontin Capsules 2618
▲ Cenestin Tablets (10%) 1263
Cerezyme for Injection 1438
Claritin (Rare) 3100
Claritin-D 12 Hour Extended Release Tablets (Less frequent) 3102
Claritin-D 24 Hour Extended Release Tablets 3104
Clozaril Tablets 2319
Cognex Capsules (Frequent) 1351
▲ CombiPatch Transdermal System (6%) 2323
Compazine 1505
▲ Copaxone for Injection (7%) 3306
Coreg Tablets (1% to 2%) 1508
Cortrosyn for Injection 2449
Crixivan Capsules (Less than 2%) 2070
Demser Capsules (Rare) 2085
▲ Depacon Injection (3% to 8%) 416
▲ Depakene (8%) 421
▲ Depakote Sprinkle Capsules (3% to 8%) 426
▲ Depakote Tablets (1% to 8%) 430
Depakote ER Tablets (1% to 5%) 436
▲ DepoCyt Injection (7%) 1197
Detrol Tablets 3623
Detrol LA Capsules 2801
Dipentum Capsules (Rare) 2803
Dostinex Tablets (1%) 2804
Doxil Injection (1% to 5%) 566
Dynabac Tablets (0.1% to 1%) 2269
EC-Naprosyn Delayed-Release Tablets (Some patients) 2967
Effexor Tablets (Frequent) 3495
Eldepryl Capsules 3266
Emcyt Capsules 2810
▲ Enbrel for Injection (8%) 1752
▲ Enbrel for Injection (8%) 3504
Ergamisol Tablets (Less frequent) 1789
▲ Esclim Transdermal System (2.1% to 6.4%) 3460
Etrafon 3115
▲ Evista Tablets (3.3% to 5.2%) 1915
Evoxac Capsules (Less than 1% to 3%) 1217
Exelon Capsules (2% or more) 2342
Exelon Oral Solution (2% or more) 2345
Famotidine Injection (Infrequent) 866
▲ Femara Tablets (5%) 2351
Ferrlecit Injection 3386
▲ Flolan for Injection (79%) 1528
Gabitril Tablets (Frequent) 1189
▲ Gemzar for Injection (20%) 1919
Geodon Capsules (Infrequent) 2688

Gliadel Wafer (2%) 1723
▲ Herceptin I.V. (10%) 1414
▲ Humatrope Vials and Cartridges (11.5% to 18.2%) 1930
▲ Hytrin Capsules (0.6% to 5.5%) 464
Imitrex Nasal Spray 1554
Imitrex Tablets 1558
Indapamide Tablets (Less than 5%) 2286
▲ Infergen (4% to 9%) 1777
Infumorph 200 and Infumorph 500 Sterile Solutions (Several reports) 1314
Intron A for Injection (Less than or equal to 5%) 3120
Iopidine 0.5% Ophthalmic Solution (Less than 3%) .... ⊙ 213
Kadian Capsules (Less than 3%) 1335
Kaletra Capsules (Less than 2%) 471
Kaletra Oral Solution (Less than 2%) 471
Klonopin Tablets (Infrequent) 2983
Lamictal (Infrequent) 1567
▲ Leukine (11% to 15%) 1755
Lipitor Tablets (Greater than or equal to 2%) 2639
Lipitor Tablets (Greater than or equal to 2%) 2696
▲ Lovenox Injection (3%) 746
Lupron Depot-PED 7.5 mg, 11.25 mg and 15 mg (Less than 2%) 3291
▲ Lupron Injection (5% or more) 3279
Lupron Injection Pediatric (Less than 2%) 3280
Megace Oral Suspension (1% to 3%) 1124
Meridia Capsules (Greater than or equal to 1%) 481
Merrem I.V. (0.1% to 1.0%) 673
Meruvax II 2130
Miacalcin Nasal Spray (Less than 1%) 2375
Micardis Tablets (1%) 1049
Micardis HCT Tablets (1%) 1051
Migranal Nasal Spray (Rare) 2376
Miltown Tablets 3349
M-M-R II 2118
Mobic Tablets (0.6% to 4.5%) 1054
Mumpsvax 2141
▲ Mylotarg for Injection (17% to 23%) 3540
Myobloc Injectable Solution (2% or greater) 1291
Naprelan Tablets (Less than 3%) 1293
Naprosyn Suspension (Some patients) 2967
Naprosyn Tablets (Some patients) 2967
Navane Oral 2701
Navane Intramuscular 2703
Neurontin Capsules (1.7%) 2655
Neurontin Oral Solution (1.7%) 2655
Neurontin Tablets (1.7%) 2655
Nexium Delayed-Release Capsules (Less than 1%) 619
Nicotrol Nasal Spray (Less than 1%) 2843
▲ Nilandron Tablets (12.4%) 753
▲ Nipent for Injection (3% to 10%) 3272
Nolvadex Tablets (Infrequent) 678
Norvir Capsules (Less than 2%) 487
Norvir Oral Solution (Less than 2%) 487
▲ Nutropin AQ Injection (41%) 1420
Nutropin Depot for Injectable Suspension 1423
▲ Nutropin for Injection (41%) 1417
▲ Oncaspar (Greater than 1% but less than 5%) 756
Orap Tablets 1407
▲ Orgaran Injection (3.3%) 2480
Orudis Capsules (Approximately 2%) 3548
Oruvail Capsules (Approximately 2%) 3548
OxyContin Tablets (Less than 1%) 2912
Paxil (Infrequent) 1609
Pediazole Suspension 3050
Pepcid Injection (Infrequent) 2153
Pepcid for Oral Suspension (Infrequent) 2150
Pepcid RPD Orally Disintegrating Tablets (Infrequent) 2150
Pepcid Tablets (Infrequent) 2150
▲ Permax Tablets (7.4%) 1299
▲ Photofrin for Injection (7%) 831
▲ Plendil Extended-Release Tablets (2.0% to 17.4%) 623
▲ Pletal Tablets (7% to 9%) 2605
▲ Pletal Tablets (7% to 9%) 2848
▲ Prempro Tablets (4%) 3572
Priftin Tablets (Less than 1%) 758
Prilosec Delayed-Release Capsules (Less than 1%) 628
Prinivil Tablets (0.3% to 1.0%) 2164
Prinzide Tablets 2168
▲ Procardia Capsules (7% to 10%) 2708
▲ Procardia XL Extended Release Tablets (1% or less to about 30%) 2710
▲ Prograf (12% to 36%) 1393
▲ Proleukin for Injection (28%) 1199
Prometrium Capsules (100 mg, 200 mg) (Less than 5%) 3261
Protonix I.V. (Less than 1%) 3580
Protonix Tablets (Less than 1%) 3577
Protopic Ointment (1% to 4%) 1397
Provigil Tablets (At least 1%) 1193
Prozac Pulvules, Liquid, and Weekly Capsules (Infrequent) 1238
▲ Rapamune Oral Solution and Tablets (54% to 64%) 3584
Remeron Tablets (2%) 2483
Remeron SolTab Tablets (2%) 2486
Reminyl Oral Solution (Greater than or equal to 2%) 1792
Reminyl Tablets (Greater than or equal to 2%) 1792
ReoPro Vials (1.6%) 1958
Requip Tablets (Infrequent) 1621
▲ Rilutek Tablets (3.3% to 4.2%) 772
▲ Rituxan for Infusion (Among most frequent) 1750
▲ Rituxan I.V. (Among most frequent) 1428
Rowasa Rectal Suspension Enema 4.0 grams/unit (60 mL) (0.61%) 3264
Roxicodone Tablets (Less than 3%) 3067
Salagen Tablets (Less than 1%) 2229
▲ Sandostatin LAR Depot (5% to 15%) 2395
Sarafem Pulvules (Infrequent) 1962
Seroquel Tablets (Infrequent) 684
▲ Serzone Tablets (3%) 1104
▲ Simulect for Injection (Greater than or equal to 10%) 2399
Skelid Tablets (2.7%) 3088
Sonata Capsules (Less than 1%) 3591
Sporanox Capsules 1800
Sporanox Injection 1804
Sporanox Injection 2509
Sporanox Oral Solution 1808
Sporanox Oral Solution 2512
Stelazine 1640
▲ Stromectol Tablets (3.2%) 2185
▲ Sular Tablets (22%) 688
Sustiva Capsules (Less than 2%) 1258
Symmetrel (1% to 5%) 1328
Synercid I.V. (Less than 1%) 775
Synvisc 3596
Tasmar Tablets (1% or more) 3010
▲ Taxotere for Injection Concentrate (6%) 778
▲ Temodar Capsules (11%) 3157
Tequin Injection (0.1% to 3%) 1110
Tequin Tablets (0.1% to 3%) 1110
Teveten Tablets (Less than 1%) 3327
▲ Thalomid Capsules (4.2%) 1154
Thioridazine Hydrochloride Tablets 2289
Thiothixene Capsules 2290
Thorazine 1656
▲ Thymoglobulin for Injection (34.1%) 3071
▲ Tiazac Capsules (3% to 5%) 1378
Tikosyn Capsules (Greater than 2%) 2717
Tolectin (Some patients) 2589
Toprol-XL Tablets (About 1 of 100 patients) 651
▲ Trasylol Injection (5%) 909
Tricor Capsules, Micronized (Less than 1%) 513
Trilafon 3160
Trovan (Less than 1%) 2722
Uniretic Tablets (More than 1%) 3178
Univasc Tablets (More than 1%) 3181
Valstar Sterile Solution for Intravesical Instillation (1%) 1175
Vantin Tablets and Oral Suspension (Less than 1%) 2860
▲ Verelan PM Capsules (3.7%) 3186
▲ Vesanoid Capsules (52%) 3037
▲ Viadur Implant (3.1%) 912
Viagra Tablets (Less than 2%) 2732
Vioxx (Greater than 0.1% to 1.9%) 2213
Vistide Injection 1445
Wellbutrin SR Sustained-Release Tablets (Infrequent) 1684
▲ Zebeta Tablets (3.0% to 3.7%) 1885
Zestoretic Tablets 695
Zestril Tablets (0.3% to 1.0%) 698
Ziac Tablets (0.9% to 1.1%) 1887
▲ Zoladex (21%) 702
Zoladex 3-month (1% to 5%) 706
Zoloft (Infrequent) 2751
Zonegran Capsules (Infrequent) 1307
Zovirax Capsules 1706
Zovirax for Injection 1708
Zovirax 1706
Zyban Sustained-Release Tablets (Infrequent) 1710
Zyprexa Tablets (2%) 1973
Zyprexa ZYDIS Orally Disintegrating Tablets (2%) 1973
Zyrtec (Less than 2%) 2756
Zyrtec-D 12 Hour Extended Relief Tablets (Less than 2%) 2758

Edema, pharyngeal

Atacand Tablets (More than 1%) 595
Avonex 1013
Cipro 887
Cozaar Tablets (Rare) 2067
Maxalt Tablets (Rare) 2120
Maxalt-MLT Orally Disintegrating Tablets (Rare) 2120
Noroxin Tablets 2145

Edema, pulmonary

Abelcet Injection 1273
Accuretic Tablets 2614
Activase I.V. 1410
Aggrenox Capsules (Less than 1%) 1026
Aldoclor Tablets 2035
Aldoril Tablets 2039
Ambien Tablets (Rare) 3191
AmBisome for Injection (Less common) 1383
Atacand HCT Tablets 597
Avalide Tablets 1070
Betapace Tablets (Rare) 950
Betapace AF Tablets (Rare) 954
Betaseron for SC Injection 988
Blocadren Tablets 2046
Brethine Ampuls 2314
Brevibloc Injection (Less than 1%) 858
Cafcit (2.2%) 1035
Campath Ampules 992
▲ CellCept Capsules (3%) 2951
▲ CellCept Intravenous (3%) 2951
▲ CellCept Oral Suspension (3%) 2951
▲ CellCept Tablets (3%) 2951
Chirocaine Injection (Less than 1%) 2909
Cipro I.V. (1% or less) 893
Cipro I.V. Pharmacy Bulk Package (Less than 1%) 897
Cipro (Less than 1%) 887
Clomid Tablets 735
Cognex Capsules (Rare) 1351
Cordarone Intravenous (Less than 2%) 3491
Coreg Tablets (Less than or equal to 0.1%) 1508
Cosopt Sterile Ophthalmic Solution 2065
Covera-HS Tablets (1.8% to 2%) 3199
Dantrium Intravenous (Rare) 2886
Diovan HCT Tablets 2338
Diprivan Injectable Emulsion (Rare) 667
Diuril Oral 2087
Diuril Sodium Intravenous 2086
Dyazide Capsules 1515
Ellence Injection 2806
Enalaprilat Injection 863
Ferrlecit Injection (Greater than 1%) 3386
▲ Flolan for Injection (4%) 1528
Floxin I.V. 2526
Floxin Tablets 2529
Fluothane Inhalation 3508
▲ Gleevec Capsules (2% to 16%) 2357
GoLYTELY and Pineapple Flavor GoLYTELY for Oral Solution 1068
Herceptin I.V. 1414
HydroDIURIL Tablets 2108
Hyzaar 2109
Indocin Capsules (Less than 1%) 2112
Indocin I.V. (Less than 1%) 2115
Indocin (Less than 1%) 2112
Inversine Tablets 1850
Isoptin SR Tablets (1.8%) 467
Kaletra Capsules (Less than 2%) 471
Kaletra Oral Solution (Less than 2%) 471
Lexxel Tablets 608
Lotensin HCT Tablets 2367
Lovenox Injection (0.7%) 746
Lupron Depot 7.5 mg (Less than 5%) 3284
Micardis HCT Tablets 1051
Microzide Capsules 3414
Moduretic Tablets 2138
Monopril HCT 1094
Naprelan Tablets (Less than 1%) 1293
Narcan Injection (Several instances) 1322
Navelbine Injection 1604
Neurontin Capsules (Rare) 2655
Neurontin Oral Solution (Rare) 2655
Neurontin Tablets (Rare) 2655
Nubain Injection 1323
NuLYTELY, Cherry Flavor, Lemon-Lime Flavor, and Orange Flavor NuLYTELY for Oral Solution 1068
Orthoclone OKT3 Sterile Solution (Less than 2%) 2498
Paxil (Rare) 1609
Permax Tablets (Infrequent) 1299
Photofrin for Injection 831
Prinivil Tablets (Greater than 1%) 2164
Prinzide Tablets 2168
Procardia Capsules (About 2%) 2708
Procardia XL Extended Release Tablets (About 2%) 2710
▲ Prograf (3% to 15%) 1393
▲ Proleukin for Injection (Less than 1% to 10%) 1199
Prozac Pulvules, Liquid, and Weekly Capsules (Rare) 1238
▲ Rapamune Oral Solution and Tablets (3% to 20%) 3584
Remicade for IV Injection (Less than 2%) 1178
ReoPro Vials (1.5%) 1958
Requip Tablets (Infrequent) 1621
Retavase Vials 1182
Rilutek Tablets (Infrequent) 772
▲ Roferon-A Injection (9%) 2996
Sarafem Pulvules (Rare) 1962
▲ Simulect for Injection (3% to 10%) 2399
Sporanox Capsules 1800
Sporanox Injection 1804
Sporanox Injection 2509
Sporanox Oral Solution 1808
Sporanox Oral Solution 2512
Symmetrel 1328
Tarka Tablets 508
Tasmar Tablets (Rare) 3010
Taxotere for Injection Concentrate (Rare) 778
Thalomid Capsules 1154
Timolide Tablets 2187
Timolol GFS .... ⊙ 266
Timoptic in Ocudose (Less frequent) 2192
Timoptic Sterile Ophthalmic Solution (Less frequent) 2190
Timoptic-XE Sterile Ophthalmic Gel Forming Solution 2194
TNKase I.V. 1430
Tonocard Tablets (Less than 1%) 649
Toradol (1% or less) 3018
Trasylol Injection (1.2%) 909
Ultracet Tablets 2597
Ultram Tablets 2600
Uniretic Tablets 3178
Vaseretic Tablets 2204
Vasotec I.V. Injection 2207
Vasotec Tablets (0.5% to 1.0%) 2210
Verelan Capsules (1.8%) 3184
Verelan PM Capsules (1.8%) 3186
▲ Vesanoid Capsules (3%) 3037
Virazole for Inhalation Solution (Infrequent) 1747
▲ Zenapax for Injection (Greater than 5%) 3046
Zestoretic Tablets 695
Zestril Tablets (Greater than 1%) 698
Ziac Tablets 1887
Zosyn (1.0% or less) 1890
Zosyn in Galaxy Containers (1.0% or less) 1894
Zovirax for Injection (Less than 1%) 1708

Edema, pulmonary, non-cardiogenic

Kadian Capsules (Less than 3%) 1335
Streptase for Infusion (Rare) 647

Edema, retinal

Aralen Tablets 3075
Lopid Tablets 2650
Plaquenil Tablets 3082
▲ Vitravene for Injection (5% to 20%) .... ⊙ 310

Edema, scrotal

Actiq (1% or greater) 1184
Caverject Sterile Powder (Less than 1%) 2777
▲ CellCept Capsules (3% to 10%) 2951
▲ CellCept Intravenous (3% to 10%) 2951
▲ CellCept Oral Suspension (3% to 10%) 2951
▲ CellCept Tablets (3% to 10%) 2951
Intron A for Injection (Less than or equal to 5%) 3120
Protonix I.V. (Less than 1%) 3580
Protonix Tablets (Less than 1%) 3577
▲ Rapamune Oral Solution and Tablets (3% to 20%) 3584
Uniretic Tablets (Less than 1%) 3178

Edema, skin

(*see under* Edema, angioneurotic)

Edema, stromal

Viroptic Ophthalmic Solution Sterile .... ⊙ 301

Edema, tongue

Aricept Tablets (Infrequent) 1270
Aricept Tablets (Infrequent) 2665
Cataflam Tablets (Less than 1%) 2315
Cerebyx Injection (Infrequent) 2619
Combivent Inhalation Aerosol (Less than 2%) 1041
Cozaar Tablets (Rare) 2067
Effexor Tablets (Infrequent) 3495
Effexor XR Capsules (Infrequent) 3499
Etrafon 3115
Flexeril Tablets (Less than 1%) 572
Flexeril Tablets (Less than 1%) 2094
Flonase Nasal Spray 1533
Geodon Capsules (Infrequent) 2688
Lamictal (Rare) 1567
Levaquin Injection (Less than 0.5%) 2537
Limbitrol 1738
Mavik Tablets (0.13%) 478

- Maxalt Tablets (Infrequent) 2120
- Maxalt-MLT Orally Disintegrating Tablets (Infrequent) 2120
- Meridia Capsules 481
- Nexium Delayed-Release Capsules (Less than 1%) 619
- Norpramin Tablets 755
- Paxil (Rare) 1609
- Pletal Tablets (Less than 2%) 2605
- Pletal Tablets (Less than 2%) 2848
- Prozac Pulvules, Liquid, and Weekly Capsules (Rare) 1238
- Reglan 2935
- Remeron Tablets (Rare) 2483
- Remeron SolTab Tablets (Rare) 2486
- Requip Tablets (Infrequent) 1621
- Retrovir Capsules 1625
- Retrovir IV Infusion 1629
- Retrovir 1625
- Risperdal (Rare) 1796
- Sarafem Pulvules (Rare) 1962
- Seroquel Tablets (Infrequent) 684
- Sonata Capsules (Rare) 3591
- Surmontil Capsules 3595
- Tarka Tablets 508
- Tequin Injection (Less than 0.1%) 1110
- Tequin Tablets (Less than 0.1%) 1110
- Topamax Sprinkle Capsules (Infrequent) 2590
- Topamax Tablets (Infrequent) 2590
- Toradol 3018
- Ultracet Tablets (Less than 1%) 2597
- Uniretic Tablets (Less than 1%) 3178
- Voltaren Tablets (Less than 1%) 2315
- Voltaren-XR Tablets (Less than 1%) 2315
- Wellbutrin SR Sustained-Release Tablets (Rare) 1684
- Zoloft (Rare) 2751
- Zomig Tablets (Infrequent) 708
- Zomig-ZMT Tablets (Infrequent) 708
- Zyban Sustained-Release Tablets (Rare) 1710
- Zyprexa Tablets (Infrequent) 1973
- Zyprexa ZYDIS Orally Disintegrating Tablets (Infrequent) 1973
- Zyrtec (Less than 2%) 2756
- Zyrtec-D 12 Hour Extended Relief Tablets (Less than 2%) 2758

Edema, turbinate

- Xopenex Inhalation Solution (1.4% to 2.8%) 3207

Edema, upper extremities

- Avalide Tablets 1070
- Avapro Tablets (Less than 1%) 1074
- Avapro Tablets (Less than 1%) 3076
- Vioxx (Greater than 0.1% to 1.9%) 2213
- Zyprexa Tablets (Infrequent) 1973
- Zyprexa ZYDIS Orally Disintegrating Tablets (Infrequent) 1973

EEG changes

- Clozaril Tablets 2319
- Compazine 1505
- Diphtheria & Tetanus Toxoids Adsorbed Purogenated for Pediatric Use 1857
- Eskalith 1527
- Etrafon 3115
- Flexeril Tablets (Rare) 572
- Flexeril Tablets (Rare) 2001
- Foscavir Injection (Between 1% and 5%) 605
- Gabitril Tablets 1189
- Levaquin 2537
- Librium Capsules (Isolated cases) 1736
- Librium for Injection 1737
- Limbitrol 1738
- Lithium Carbonate 3061
- Lithium Citrate Syrup 3061
- Lithobid Slow-Release Tablets 3255
- Miltown Tablets 3349
- Norpramin Tablets 755
- Paxil (Rare) 1609
- ProSom Tablets 500
- Prozac Pulvules, Liquid, and Weekly Capsules (Rare) 1238
- Sarafem Pulvules (Rare) 1962
- Surmontil Capsules 3595
- Tetanus & Diphtheria Toxoids Adsorbed for Adult Use 1880
- Tetanus and Diphtheria Toxoids Adsorbed For Adult Use 815
- Topamax Sprinkle Capsules (Rare) 2590
- Topamax Tablets (Rare) 2590
- Trileptal Oral Suspension (Up to 2%) 2407
- Trileptal Tablets (Up to 2%) 2407
- Tripedia Vaccine 817
- Valium Injectable 3026
- Valium Tablets (Infrequent) 3047
- Vivactil Tablets 2217
- Vivactil Tablets 2446
- Wellbutrin Tablets (Rare) 1680
- Wellbutrin SR Sustained-Release Tablets 1684
- Zyban Sustained-Release Tablets 1710

E-Ferol syndrome

- Aquasol A Parenteral 593

Efficacy, lack of

- Neoral Soft Gelatin Capsules (1.4%) 2380
- Neoral Oral Solution (1.4%) 2380

Ejaculation, delayed

- ▲ Effexor XR Capsules (17%) 3499
- ▲ Zoloft (14%) 2751

Ejaculation, dry

- Amicar Injection 3608
- Amicar Syrup 3608
- Amicar Tablets 3608

Ejaculation, inhibition

- Demser Capsules (Infrequent) 2085
- Dibenzyline Capsules 3457
- Etrafon 3115
- Levaquin Injection (Less than 0.5%) 2537
- ▲ Luvox Tablets (25, 50, 100 mg) (8%) 3256
- Normodyne Injection (Up to 5%) 3135
- ▲ Normodyne Tablets (Up to 5%) 3137
- Parnate Tablets 1607
- ▲ Paxil (3.7% to 10.0%) 1609
- Serentil 1057
- Trilafon 3160
- Wellbutrin Tablets (Infrequent) 1680

Ejaculation, retrograde

- Flomax 1044

Ejaculation disturbances

- ▲ Celexa (6%) 1365
- Clozaril Tablets (1%) 2319
- Compazine 1505
- ▲ Effexor Tablets (3% to 12.5%) 3495
- ▲ Effexor XR Capsules (16% to 17%) 3499
- ▲ Flomax Capsules (8.4% to 18.1%) 1044
- Geodon Capsules (Infrequent) 2688
- Kaletra Capsules (Less than 2%) 471
- Kaletra Oral Solution (Less than 2%) 471
- Klonopin Tablets (1%) 2983
- Lamictal (Rare) 1567
- Lipitor Tablets (Less than 2%) 2639
- Lipitor Tablets (Less than 2%) 2696
- ▲ Luvox Tablets (25, 50, 100 mg) (8%) 3256
- Meridia Capsules 481
- Mirapex Tablets (Less than 1%) 2834
- Nardil Tablets 2653
- Neurontin Capsules (Infrequent) 2655
- Neurontin Oral Solution (Infrequent) 2655
- Neurontin Tablets (Infrequent) 2655
- Norpramin Tablets 755
- ▲ Paxil (1.6% to 25%) 1609
- Propecia Tablets (1.2%) 2172
- Proscar Tablets (2.8%) 2175
- Provigil Tablets (1%) 1193
- ▲ Prozac Pulvules, Liquid, and Weekly Capsules (7%) 1238
- Remeron Tablets (Rare) 2483
- Remeron SolTab Tablets (Rare) 2486
- Requip Tablets (Rare) 1621
- Risperdal (Infrequent) 1796
- Seroquel Tablets (Infrequent) 684
- Serzone Tablets (Infrequent) 1104
- Stelazine 1640
- Surmontil Capsules 3595
- Thioridazine Hydrochloride Tablets 2289
- Thorazine 1656
- Topamax Sprinkle Capsules (Infrequent) 2590
- Topamax Tablets (Infrequent) 2590
- Viagra Tablets (Less than 2%) 2732
- Wellbutrin Tablets (Rare) 1680
- Wellbutrin SR Sustained-Release Tablets 1684
- ▲ Zoloft (7% to 19%) 2751
- Zyban Sustained-Release Tablets 1710
- Zyprexa Tablets (Infrequent) 1973
- Zyprexa ZYDIS Orally Disintegrating Tablets (Infrequent) 1973

Ejaculation failure

- Flomax Capsules 1044

Ejection fraction reduction

- Adriamycin PFS/RDF Injection 2767
- Herceptin I.V. 1414
- Novantrone for Injection 1760

EKG changes

- Aceon Tablets (2 mg, 4 mg, 8 mg) (1.8%) 3249
- Aciphex Tablets 1267
- Aciphex Tablets 1783
- Aloprim for Injection (Less than 1%) 2292
- Amerge Tablets (Infrequent) 1467
- Anzemet Injection (Rare) 719
- Anzemet Tablets (Rare) 722
- Aralen Tablets (Rare) 3075
- Atacand HCT Tablets (0.5% or greater) 597
- Azactam for Injection (Less than 1%) 1276
- ▲ Betapace Tablets (4% to 7%) 950
- Betapace AF Tablets (2.5% to 3.3%) 954
- Cardene I.V. (1.4%) 3485
- Cardizem Injectable 1018
- Cardizem Lyo-Ject Syringe 1018
- Cardizem Monovial 1018
- Cardizem CD Capsules (Less than 1% to 1.6%) 1016
- ▲ Carnitor Injection (2% to 6%) 3242
- Catapres Tablets (Rare) 1037
- Catapres-TTS (0.5% or less) 1038
- ▲ Chirocaine Injection (3.1%) 2909
- Clorpres Tablets (Rare) 1002
- Clozaril Tablets (1%) 2319
- Combipres Tablets (Rare) 1040
- Compazine 1505
- Demadex Tablets and Injection (2.0%) 2965
- Digitek Tablets 1003
- Diprivan Injectable Emulsion (Less than 1%) 667
- Duraclon Injection (Rare) 3057
- Effexor Tablets 3495
- Effexor XR Capsules 3499
- Eskalith 1527
- Etrafon (Occasional) 3115
- Evoxac Capsules (Less than 1%) 1217
- Foscavir Injection (Between 1% and 5%) 605
- Gabitril Tablets (Infrequent) 1189
- Haldol Decanoate 2535
- Haldol Injection, Tablets and Concentrate 2533
- Imitrex Nasal Spray (Infrequent) 1554
- Imitrex Tablets (Infreqent) 1558
- Kytril Injection (Rare) 2986
- Lanoxicaps Capsules 1574
- Lanoxin Injection 1581
- Lanoxin Tablets 1587
- Lanoxin Elixir Pediatric 1578
- Lanoxin Injection Pediatric 1584
- Lithium Carbonate 3061
- Lithium Citrate Syrup 3061
- Lithobid Slow-Release Tablets 3255
- Lotensin HCT Tablets 2367
- Loxitane Capsules (A few cases) 3398
- ▲ Lupron Injection (5% or more) 3279
- Macrobid Capsules 2889
- Macrodantin Capsules 2891
- Micardis Tablets (More than 0.3%) 1049
- Micardis HCT Tablets 1051
- Midamor Tablets 2136
- Miltown Tablets 3349
- Naprelan Tablets (Less than 1%) 1293
- Naropin Injection (Less than 1%) 612
- Navane Oral 2701
- Navane Intramuscular 2703
- Nimotop Capsules (Up to 1.4%) 904
- ▲ Novantrone for Injection (5% to 11%) 1760
- Orap Tablets (2.7%) 1407
- Paxil (Infrequent) 1609
- Permax Tablets (Infrequent) 1299
- Prandin Tablets (0.5, 1, and 2 mg) (Less than or equal to 1%) 2432
- ▲ Prograf (3% to 15%) 1393
- Prostigmin Injectable 1744
- Prostigmin Tablets 1744
- Protonix I.V. (Less than 1%) 3580
- Protonix Tablets (Less than 1%) 3577
- ▲ Quinaglute Dura-Tabs Tablets (3%) 978
- Quinidex Extentabs 2933
- Remeron Tablets 2483
- Remeron SolTab Tablets 2486
- Retrovir Capsules (2.4%) 1625
- ▲ Retrovir IV Infusion (3%) 1629
- Retrovir (2.4%) 1625
- Salagen Tablets (Less than 1%) 2229
- Seroquel Tablets (Rare) 684
- ▲ Serostim for Injection (1% to 10%) 3229
- Stelazine 1640
- Suprane Liquid for Inhalation (Less than 1%) 874
- ▲ Taxol Injection (14% to 23%) 1129
- Taxotere for Injection Concentrate 778
- Teveten Tablets (Less than 1%) 3327
- Thioridazine Hydrochloride Tablets 2289
- Thorazine 1656
- Tiazac Capsules (Less than 2%) 1378
- Tricor Capsules, Micronized 513
- Trilafon (Occasional) 3160
- Ultram Tablets (Infrequent) 2600
- Uniretic Tablets (More than 1%) 3178
- Verelan PM Capsules (2%) 3186
- Viagra Tablets (Less than 2%) 2732
- Wellbutrin Tablets (Infrequent) 1680
- Xopenex Inhalation Solution 3207
- Zemuron Injection (Less than 1%) 2491
- Zofran Injection (Rare) 1698
- Zofran (Rare) 1703
- Zofran ODT Orally Disintegrating Tablets (Rare) 1703
- Zomig Tablets (Rare) 708
- Zomig-ZMT Tablets (Rare) 708

EKG changes, PR prolongation

- Amerge Tablets (Infrequent) 1467
- Digitek Tablets 1003
- Imitrex Injection (Infrequent) 1549
- Imitrex Tablets 1558
- Lanoxicaps Capsules 1574
- Lanoxin Injection 1581
- Lanoxin Tablets 1587
- Lanoxin Elixir Pediatric 1578
- Lanoxin Injection Pediatric 1584

EKG changes, Q wave disturbances

- Compazine 1505
- ▲ Imdur Tablets (Less than or equal to 5%) 1826
- Stelazine 1640
- Thorazine 1656

EKG changes, QRS interval prolonged

- Aralen Tablets (Rare) 3075
- Haldol Injection, Tablets and Concentrate 2533
- Quinaglute Dura-Tabs Tablets 978
- Rum-K 1363
- Rythmol Tablets – 150 mg, 225 mg, 300 mg (1.9%) 502
- Seroquel Tablets (Infrequent) 684
- Tonocard Tablets (Less than 1%) 649

EKG changes, QT interval prolonged

- Aciphex Tablets (Rare) 1267
- Aciphex Tablets (Rare) 1783
- Amerge Tablets (Infrequent) 1467
- Betapace AF Tablets 954
- Cerebyx Injection (Infrequent) 2619
- Cordarone Intravenous (Less than 2%) 3491
- Corvert Injection (1.2%) 2793
- Erythrocin Stearate Filmtab Tablets (Rare) 452
- Erythromycin Base Filmtab Tablets (Rare) 454
- Fluothane Inhalation 3508
- Foscavir Injection (Rare) 605
- Geodon Capsules 2688
- Haldol Decanoate 2535
- Imitrex Injection (Infrequent) 1549
- Orap Tablets 1407
- Prozac Pulvules, Liquid, and Weekly Capsules 1238
- Quinidex Extentabs 2933
- Reminyl Oral Solution (Infrequent) 1792
- Reminyl Tablets (Infrequent) 1792
- Risperdal 1796
- Sarafem Pulvules 1962
- Serentil 1057
- Seroquel Tablets (Infrequent) 684
- Thioridazine Hydrochloride Tablets 2289
- Tonocard Tablets (Less than 1%) 649
- ▲ Trisenox Injection (8%) 1158
- Uniretic Tablets (Less than 1%) 3178
- Vascor Tablets (0.5% to 2.0%) 2602
- Zoloft 2751
- Zomig Tablets (Rare) 708
- Zomig-ZMT Tablets (Rare) 708

EKG changes, reversible flattening

- Eskalith 1527
- Lithium Carbonate 3061
- Lithium Citrate Syrup 3061
- Lithobid Slow-Release Tablets 3255

EKG changes, sinus pause

- Tambocor Tablets (1% to 3%) 1990

EKG changes, ST section

- AccuNeb Inhalation Solution (One case) 1230
- ▲ Adenoscan (3%) 1381
- Amerge Tablets (Infrequent) 1467
- Anzemet Injection 719
- Anzemet Tablets 722
- Cardene I.V. (Rare) 3485
- Clozaril Tablets 2319
- Corlopam Injection (1% to 2%) 412
- Digitek Tablets 1003
- Diprivan Injectable Emulsion (Less than 1%) 667
- Ellence Injection 2806
- Foscavir Injection (Between 1% and 5%) 605
- Imitrex Injection (Infrequent) 1549
- Imitrex Tablets 1558
- Lanoxicaps Capsules 1574
- Lanoxin Injection 1581
- Lanoxin Tablets 1587
- Lanoxin Elixir Pediatric 1578
- Lanoxin Injection Pediatric 1584
- Luvox Tablets (25, 50, 100 mg) (Infrequent) 3256
- Macrobid Capsules 2889
- Macrodantin Capsules 2891
- Naropin Injection (Less than 1%) 612
- OxyContin Tablets (Less than 1%) 2912
- Risperdal (Rare) 1796
- Rum-K 1363
- Seroquel Tablets (Rare) 684
- Tarka Tablets (0.3% or more) 508

EKG changes, T-wave
Adenoscan (Less than 1%)............ 1381
Amerge Tablets (Infrequent)............ 1467
Anzemet Injection............ 719
Anzemet Tablets............ 722
Aralen Tablets (Rare)............ 3075
Cardene I.V. (Rare)............ 3485
Clozaril Tablets............ 2319
Compazine............ 1505
Corlopam Injection (1% to 2%)............ 412
Dopram Injectable............ 2931
Eskalith............ 1527
Evoxac Capsules (Less than 1%)..... 1217
Imitrex Injection (Infrequent)............ 1549
Imitrex Tablets............ 1558
Lithium Carbonate............ 3061
Lithium Citrate Syrup............ 3061
Lithobid Slow-Release Tablets......... 3255
Macrobid Capsules............ 2889
Macrodantin Capsules............ 2891
Moban (Rare)............ 1320
Mycobutin Capsules (More than one patient)............ 2838
Orap Tablets............ 1407
Pentasa Capsules (Infrequent)............ 3239
Reminyl Oral Solution (Infrequent)... 1792
Reminyl Tablets (Infrequent)............ 1792
Risperdal (Rare)............ 1796
Rum-K............ 1363
Serentil............ 1057
Stelazine............ 1640
Sular Tablets (Less than or equal to 1%)............ 688
Tarka Tablets (0.3% or more)............ 508
Thorazine............ 1656
Uniretic Tablets (less than 1%)............ 3178

Elastosis perforans, serpiginosa
Cuprimine Capsules (Rare)............ 2075
Depen Titratable Tablets (Rare)............ 3341

Elation
▲ Marinol Capsules (8% to 24%)............ 3325

Electrocardiographic changes
(*see under* EKG changes)

Electroencephalographic changes
(*see under* EEG changes)

Electrolyte disturbances
(*see under* Electrolyte imbalance)

Electrolyte imbalance
Aldoclor Tablets............ 2035
Aldoril Tablets............ 2039
Aloprim for Injection (Less than 1%)............ 2292
Anadrol-50 Tablets............ 3321
Atromid-S Capsules............ 3483
Avalide Tablets............ 1070
Celestone Soluspan Injectable Suspension............ 3097
Daranide Tablets............ 2077
Decadron Elixir............ 2078
Decadron Phosphate Injection............ 2081
Demadex Tablets and Injection............ 2965
Diamox Intravenous............ ⊙ 269
Diamox Sequels Sustained Release Capsules............ ⊙ 270
Diamox Tablets............ ⊙ 269
Diovan HCT Tablets............ 2338
Diuril Oral............ 2087
Diuril Sodium Intravenous............ 2086
Dyazide Capsules............ 1515
Follistim for Injection............ 2465
▲ Foscavir Injection (5% or greater)............ 605
Humegon for Injection............ 2468
HydroDIURIL Tablets............ 2108
Indapamide Tablets............ 2286
Macrobid Capsules............ 2889
Macrodantin Capsules............ 2891
Maxzide............ 1008
Microzide Capsules............ 3414
Moduretic Tablets............ 2138
Navelbine Injection............ 1604
Neptazane Tablets............ ⊙ 271
Permax Tablets (Rare)............ 1299
Pravachol Tablets............ 1099
Prevacid Delayed-Release Capsules............ 3292
PREVPAC............ 3298
Prinzide Tablets............ 2168
Renese Tablets............ 2712
Risperdal............ 1796
Serophene Tablets............ 3226
Tenoretic Tablets............ 690
Tequin Injection (Less than 0.1%)............ 1110
Tequin Tablets (Less than 0.1%)............ 1110
Thalomid Capsules............ 1154
Timolide Tablets............ 2187
Uniretic Tablets (More than 1%)............ 3178
Vaseretic Tablets............ 2204
Zaroxolyn Tablets............ 1177
Zestoretic Tablets............ 695
Zosyn............ 1890
Zosyn in Galaxy Containers............ 1894

Electro-oculogram, abnormal
Norvir Capsules (Less than 2%)............ 487
Norvir Oral Solution (Less than 2%)............ 487

Electroretinogram, abnormal
Norvir Capsules (Less than 2%)............ 487
Norvir Oral Solution (Less than 2%)............ 487

Elevated bilirubin levels
(*see under* Hyperbilirubinemia)

Embolism
Activase I.V.............. 1410
Activella Tablets............ 2764
Demadex Tablets and Injection............ 2965
Desogen Tablets............ 2458
Sterile FUDR............ 2974
Furosemide Tablets............ 2284
Levaquin (Less than 0.3%)............ 2537
Luvox Tablets (25, 50, 100 mg) (Rare)............ 3256
Ortho-Cept 21 Tablets............ 2546
Ortho-Cept 28 Tablets............ 2546
Ortho-Cyclen/Ortho Tri-Cyclen............ 2573
Paraplatin for Injection............ 1126
Premphase Tablets............ 3572
Prempro Tablets............ 3572
Provera Tablets............ 2853
TNKase I.V.............. 1430
Trasylol Injection (1% to 2%)............ 909
Zosyn (1.0% or less)............ 1890
Zosyn in Galaxy Containers (1.0% or less)............ 1894

Embolism, cholesterol
Activase I.V. (Rare)............ 1410
Retavase Vials (Rare)............ 1182
Streptase for Infusion (Rare)............ 647
TNKase I.V.............. 1430

Embolism, limb
Felbatol............ 3343
ReoPro Vials (0.3%)............ 1958
Requip Tablets (Rare)............ 1621

Embolism, lower extremities
Rilutek Tablets (Infrequent)............ 772

Embolism, pulmonary
Abelcet Injection............ 1273
Aciphex Tablets (Rare)............ 1267
Aciphex Tablets (Rare)............ 1783
Actimmune (Rare)............ 1772
Activella Tablets............ 2764
Alesse-21 Tablets............ 3468
Alesse-28 Tablets............ 3473
Aloprim for Injection (Less than 1%)............ 2292
Ambien Tablets (Rare)............ 3191
Amicar Injection............ 3608
Amicar Syrup............ 3608
Amicar Tablets............ 3608
Arthrotec Tablets (Rare)............ 3195
Avonex............ 1013
Betaseron for SC Injection............ 988
Bicillin C-R 900/300 Injection............ 2240
Bicillin C-R Injection............ 2238
Bicillin L-A Injection............ 2242
Brevicon 28-Day Tablets............ 3380
Campath Ampules............ 992
Celebrex Capsules (Less than 0.1%)............ 2676
Celebrex Capsules (Less than 0.1%)............ 2780
Celexa (Rare)............ 1365
Cerebyx Injection (Infrequent)............ 2619
Cipro I.V. (1% or less)............ 893
Cipro I.V. Pharmacy Bulk Package (Less than 1%)............ 897
Cipro (Less than 1%)............ 887
Climara Transdermal System............ 958
Clomid Tablets............ 735
Clozaril Tablets............ 2319
Cognex Capsules (Infrequent)............ 1351
Cyclessa Tablets............ 2450
Depo-Provera Contraceptive Injection (Fewer than 1%)............ 2798
Desogen Tablets............ 2458
Effexor Tablets (Rare)............ 3495
Effexor XR Capsules (Rare)............ 3499
Emcyt Capsules (2%)............ 2810
Enalaprilat Injection............ 863
Enbrel for Injection (Infrequent)............ 1752
Enbrel for Injection (Infrequent)............ 3504
Epogen for Injection (Rare)............ 582
Estrace Vaginal Cream............ 3358
Estrace Tablets............ 3361
Estratest............ 3252
Estrostep............ 2627
Evoxac Capsules (Less than 1%)..... 1217
Exelon Capsules (Infrequent)............ 2342
Exelon Oral Solution (Infrequent)..... 2345
Fareston Tablets (Less than 1% to 2%)............ 3237
Femara Tablets (Less than or equal to 2%)............ 2351
femhrt Tablets............ 2635
Geodon Capsules (Rare)............ 2688
▲ Gliadel Wafer (4% to 9%)............ 1723
Heparin Lock Flush Solution............ 3509
Heparin Sodium Injection............ 3511
Humegon for Injection............ 2468
Imitrex Nasal Spray............ 1554
Imitrex Tablets............ 1558
Innohep Injection (2.3%)............ 1248
Levlen............ 962
Levlite 21 Tablets............ 962
Levlite 28 Tablets............ 962
Levora Tablets............ 3389
Lexxel Tablets............ 608
Loestrin 21 Tablets............ 2642
Loestrin Fe Tablets............ 2642
Lo/Ovral Tablets............ 3532
Lo/Ovral-28 Tablets............ 3538
Low-Ogestrel-28 Tablets............ 3392
Lunelle Monthly Injection............ 2827
Lupron Depot–3 Month 11.25 mg.... 3285
Lupron Injection (Less than 5%)............ 3279
Megace Oral Suspension (1% to 3%)............ 1124
Menest Tablets............ 2254
Merrem I.V. (0.1% to 1.0%)............ 673
Microgestin Fe 1.5/30 Tablets............ 3407
Microgestin Fe 1/20 Tablets............ 3400
Mircette Tablets............ 2470
Modicon............ 2563
Naropin Injection (Less than 1%)............ 612
Navelbine Injection............ 1604
Necon............ 3415
Neurontin Capsules (Rare)............ 2655
Neurontin Oral Solution (Rare)............ 2655
Neurontin Tablets (Rare)............ 2655
Nipent for Injection (Less than 3%)............ 3272
Nolvadex Tablets (0.4%)............ 678
Nordette-28 Tablets............ 2257
Norinyl 1 +35 28-Day Tablets............ 3380
Norinyl 1 + 50 28-Day Tablets............ 3380
Norplant System............ 3543
Ogen Tablets............ 2846
Ogestrel 0.5/50-28 Tablets............ 3428
Ortho Dienestrol Cream............ 2554
Ortho-Cept 21 Tablets............ 2546
Ortho-Cept 28 Tablets............ 2546
Ortho-Cyclen/Ortho Tri-Cyclen............ 2573
Ortho-Est Tablets............ 3464
Ortho-Novum............ 2563
Ortho-Novum 1/50▫28 Tablets............ 2556
Ortho-Cyclen/Ortho Tri-Cyclen............ 2573
Ovcon............ 3364
Ovral Tablets............ 3551
Ovral-28 Tablets............ 3552
Ovrette Tablets............ 3552
Paxil (Rare)............ 1609
Permax Tablets (Infrequent)............ 1299
Premarin Intravenous............ 3563
Premarin Tablets............ 3566
Premarin Vaginal Cream............ 3570
Premphase Tablets............ 3572
Prempro Tablets............ 3572
Prinivil Tablets (0.3% to 1.0%)............ 2164
Prinzide Tablets............ 2168
▲ Procrit for Injection (3.2%)............ 2502
Proleukin for Injection (Less than 1%)............ 1199
Provera Tablets............ 2853
Prozac Pulvules, Liquid, and Weekly Capsules............ 1238
Remeron Tablets (Rare)............ 2483
Remeron SolTab Tablets (Rare)............ 2486
Remicade for IV Injection (Less than 2%)............ 1178
ReoPro Vials (0.3%)............ 1958
Requip Tablets (Rare)............ 1621
Risperdal............ 1796
Sandostatin LAR Depot (1% to 4%)............ 2395
Sarafem Pulvules............ 1962
Serophene Tablets............ 3226
Sonata Capsules (Rare)............ 3591
Tasmar Tablets (Infrequent)............ 3010
Taxol Injection (Rare)............ 1129
Taxotere for Injection Concentrate.. 778
Tenormin (1.2%)............ 692
Thalomid Capsules............ 1154
Tonocard Tablets (Less than 1%)............ 649
Topamax Sprinkle Capsules (Infrequent)............ 2590
Topamax Tablets (Infrequent)............ 2590
Trasylol Injection (1% to 2%)............ 909
Tri-Levlen............ 962
Tri-Norinyl-28 Tablets............ 3433
Triphasil-21 Tablets............ 3600
Triphasil-28 Tablets............ 3605
Trivora Tablets............ 3439
Vaseretic Tablets............ 2204
Vasotec I.V. Injection............ 2207
Vasotec Tablets (0.5% to 1.0%)............ 2210
Vioxx (Less than 0.1%)............ 2213
Vivelle Transdermal System............ 2412
Vivelle-Dot Transdermal System............ 2416
Wellbutrin Tablets (Rare)............ 1680
Wellbutrin SR Sustained-Release Tablets............ 1684
Xeloda Tablets (Less than 5%)............ 3039
Yasmin 28 Tablets............ 980
Zanaflex Tablets (Rare)............ 1305
Zestoretic Tablets............ 695
Zestril Tablets (0.3% to 1.0%)............ 698
Zoladex 3-month (1% to 5%)............ 706
Zonegran Capsules (Rare)............ 1307
Zosyn (1.0% or less)............ 1890
Zosyn in Galaxy Containers (1.0% or less)............ 1894
Zovia............ 3449
Zyban Sustained-Release Tablets.... 1710
Zyprexa Tablets............ 1973
Zyprexa ZYDIS Orally Disintegrating Tablets............ 1973

Embolism, retinal artery
Xalatan Latanoprost Ophthalmic Solution (Extremely rare)............ ⊙ 320
Xalatan Sterile Ophthalmic Solution (Extremely rare)............ 2864

Embolism, venous
Retavase Vials............ 1182

Emergence delirium
Versed Injection (Less than 1%)............ 3027

Emesis
(*see under* Vomiting)

Emotional disturbances
Accutane Capsules............ 2944
Avalide Tablets............ 1070
Avapro Tablets (Less than 1%)............ 1074
Avapro Tablets (Less than 1%)............ 3076
Depacon Injection............ 416
Depakene............ 421
Depakote Sprinkle Capsules............ 426
Depakote Tablets............ 430
Depakote ER Tablets............ 436
Efudex (Infrequent)............ 1733
Imitrex Nasal Spray (Rare)............ 1554
Lariam Tablets (Less than 1%)............ 2989
Paxil (Infrequent)............ 1609
Plaquenil Tablets............ 3082
Prelone Syrup............ 2273

Emotional lability
Accutane Capsules............ 2944
Actiq (Less than 1%)............ 1184
Activella Tablets (0% to 6%)............ 2764
▲ Adderall XR Capsules (1% to 9%)
Adenoscan (Less than 1%)............ 1381
Ambien Tablets (Infrequent)............ 3191
AndroGel (Up to 3%)............ 3322
Aricept Tablets (Infrequent)............ 1270
Aricept Tablets (Infrequent)............ 2665
Asacol Delayed-Release Tablets............ 2884
Avonex............ 1013
Betapace Tablets (Rare)............ 950
Betapace AF Tablets (Rare)............ 954
Blocadren Tablets............ 2046
Cardura Tablets (Less than 0.5%)... 2668
Celexa (Infrequent)............ 1365
▲ CellCept Capsules (3% to 10%)............ 2951
▲ CellCept Intravenous (3% to 10%) . 2951
▲ CellCept Oral Suspension (3% to 10%)............ 2951
▲ CellCept Tablets (3% to 10%)............ 2951
Cerebyx Injection (Infrequent)............ 2619
Claritin-D 12 Hour Extended Release Tablets (Less frequent)... 3102
Claritin-D 24 Hour Extended Release Tablets (Fewer than 2%)............ 3104
Copaxone for Injection (At least 2%)............ 3306
Coreg Tablets (0.1% to 1%)............ 1508
Corgard Tablets............ 2245
Corzide 40/5 Tablets............ 2247
Corzide 80/5 Tablets............ 2247
Cosopt Sterile Ophthalmic Solution............ 2065
▲ Crinone (23%)............ 3213
DaunoXome Injection (Less than or equal to 5%)............ 1442
▲ Depacon Injection (6%)............ 416
▲ Depakene (6%)............ 421
▲ Depakote Sprinkle Capsules (6%) .. 426
▲ Depakote Tablets (1% to 6%)............ 430
Depakote ER Tablets (Greater than 1%)............ 436
Diprivan Injectable Emulsion (Less than 1%)............ 667
Doxil Injection (1% to 5%)............ 566
Effexor Tablets (Frequent)............ 3495
Effexor XR Capsules (Frequent)............ 3499
Elmiron Capsules............ 570
Emcyt Capsules (2%)............ 2810
▲ Esclim Transdermal System (2.1% to 8.3%)............ 3460
Evoxac Capsules (Less than 1%)..... 1217
Exelon Capsules (Infrequent)............ 2342
Exelon Oral Solution (Infrequent)..... 2345
▲ Felbatol (6.5%)............ 3343
Floxin I.V.............. 2526
Floxin Tablets............ 2529
▲ Gabitril Tablets (3%)............ 1189
Gengraf Capsules (1% to less than 3%)............ 457
▲ Gonal-F for Injection (5.1%)............ 3216
Hivid Tablets (Less than 1%)............ 2975
Inderal............ 3513
Inderal LA Long-Acting Capsules..... 3516
Inderide Tablets............ 3517

Inderide LA Long-Acting Capsules ... 3519
▲ Infergen (6% to 12%) ... 1777
Intron A for Injection (Less than 5%) ... 3120
Kaletra Capsules (Less than 2%) ... 471
Kaletra Oral Solution (Less than 2%) ... 471
Keppra Tablets (2%) ... 3314
Klonopin Tablets (1%) ... 2983
Lamictal (1.3%) ... 1567
Levaquin (Less than 0.3%) ... 2537
Levoxyl Tablets ... 1819
Lipitor Tablets (Less than 2%) ... 2639
Lipitor Tablets (Less than 2%) ... 2696
Lunelle Monthly Injection ... 2827
▲ Lupron Depot 3.75 mg (10.8%) ... 3281
▲ Lupron Depot–3 Month 11.25 mg (10.8% to 22%) ... 3285
Lupron Depot-PED 7.5 mg, 11.25 mg and 15 mg (Less than 2%) ... 3291
Lupron Injection Pediatric (Less than 2%) ... 3280
Luvox Tablets (25, 50, 100 mg) (Infrequent) ... 3256
Meridia Capsules (1.3%) ... 481
Motrin Suspension, Oral Drops, Chewable Tablets, and Caplets (Less than 1%) ... 2002
Nadolol Tablets ... 2288
Naprelan Tablets (Less than 1%) ... 1293
Naropin Injection (Less than 1%) ... 612
Neoral Soft Gelatin Capsules (1% to less than 3%) ... 2380
Neoral Oral Solution (1% to less than 3%) ... 2380
▲ Neurontin Capsules (4.2% to 6%) ... 2655
▲ Neurontin Oral Solution (4.2% to 6%) ... 2655
▲ Neurontin Tablets (4.2% to 6%) ... 2655
▲ Nicotrol Nasal Spray (Over 5%) ... 2843
Nipent for Injection (Less than 3%) ... 3272
Normodyne Tablets ... 3137
Norplant System (Less than 1%) ... 3543
Norvir Capsules (Less than 2%) ... 487
Norvir Oral Solution (Less than 2%) ... 487
Oncaspar (Less than 1%) ... 756
Ovidrel for Injection (Less than 2%) ... 3220
OxyContin Tablets (Less than 1%) ... 2912
Paxil (Frequent) ... 1609
Pediapred Oral Solution ... 1170
▲ PEG-Intron Powder for Injection (28%) ... 3140
Permax Tablets (Infrequent) ... 1299
▲ Prograf (3% to 15%) ... 1393
▲ Prometrium Capsules (100 mg, 200 mg) (6%) ... 3261
ProSom Tablets (Infrequent) ... 500
Protonix I.V. (Less than 1%) ... 3580
Protonix Tablets (Less than 1%) ... 3577
Provigil Tablets (1%) ... 1193
Prozac Pulvules, Liquid, and Weekly Capsules (Frequent) ... 1238
Pulmicort Respules (1% to 3%) ... 632
▲ Rapamune Oral Solution and Tablets (3% to 20%) ... 3584
▲ Rebetron Combination Therapy (7% to 12%) ... 3153
Remeron Tablets (Infrequent) ... 2483
Remeron SolTab Tablets (Infrequent) ... 2486
Requip Tablets (Infrequent) ... 1621
Rescriptor Tablets (Less than 2%) ... 520
Retrovir Capsules ... 1625
Retrovir IV Infusion ... 1629
Retrovir ... 1625
Rilutek Tablets (Infrequent) ... 772
Risperdal (Rare) ... 1796
Roferon-A Injection (Less than 3%) ... 2996
Romazicon Injection (1% to 3%) ... 3000
Salagen Tablets (Less than 1%) ... 2229
Sarafem Pulvules (Frequent) ... 1962
Sectral Capsules ... 3589
Seroquel Tablets (Rare) ... 684
Serzone Tablets ... 1104
Sonata Capsules (Frequent) ... 3591
Sustiva Capsules (Less than 2%) ... 1258
▲ Synarel Nasal Solution for Central Precocious Puberty (6%) ... 3204
▲ Synarel Nasal Solution for Endometriosis (15% of patients) ... 3205
Tasmar Tablets (Frequent) ... 3010
Tenoretic Tablets ... 690
Tenormin ... 692
Thalomid Capsules ... 1154
Timolide Tablets ... 2187
Timolol GFS ... ⊙266
Timoptic in Ocudose ... 2192
Timoptic Sterile Ophthalmic Solution ... 2190
Timoptic-XE Sterile Ophthalmic Gel Forming Solution ... 2194
Topamax Sprinkle Capsules (1.8% to 2.4%) ... 2590
Topamax Tablets (1.8% to 2.4%) ... 2590
Toprol-XL Tablets ... 651
Trileptal Oral Suspension (2% to 3%) ... 2407
Trileptal Tablets (2% to 3%) ... 2407
Trovan (Less than 1%) ... 2722
Ultracet Tablets (Less than 1%) ... 2597
▲ Ultram Tablets (7% to 14%) ... 2600
Uniretic Tablets (Less than 1%) ... 3178
Unithroid Tablets ... 3445
Viracept ... 532
Wellbutrin SR Sustained-Release Tablets (Infrequent) ... 1684
Yasmin 28 Tablets ... 980
Zanaflex Tablets (Infrequent) ... 1305
Zebeta Tablets ... 1885
Ziac Tablets ... 1887
▲ Zoladex (60%) ... 702
Zoladex 3-month ... 706
Zoloft (Infrequent to 2%) ... 2751
Zomig Tablets (Infrequent) ... 708
Zomig-ZMT Tablets (Infrequent) ... 708
Zyban Sustained-Release Tablets (Infrequent) ... 1710
Zyprexa Tablets ... 1973
Zyprexa ZYDIS Orally Disintegrating Tablets ... 1973
Zyrtec (Less than 2%) ... 2756
Zyrtec-D 12 Hour Extended Relief Tablets (Less than 2%) ... 2758

Emphysema
Avonex ... 1013
Lupron Depot 7.5 mg (Less than 5%) ... 3284
Paxil (Rare) ... 1609
Permax Tablets (Infrequent) ... 1299
Prozac Pulvules, Liquid, and Weekly Capsules (Rare) ... 1238
Sarafem Pulvules (Rare) ... 1962
Thalomid Capsules ... 1154

Enanthema
Gengraf Capsules (1% to less than 3%) ... 457
Neoral Soft Gelatin Capsules (1% to less than 3%) ... 2380
Neoral Oral Solution (1% to less than 3%) ... 2380

Encephalitis
Attenuvax ... 2044
Cerebyx Injection (Infrequent) ... 2619
Cognex Capsules (Rare) ... 1351
JE-VAX Vaccine (1 to 2.3 per million vaccines) ... 811
M-M-R II (Very rare) ... 2118
Mumpsvax (Very rare) ... 2141
Nipent for Injection (Less than 3%) ... 3272
Orthoclone OKT3 Sterile Solution (Less than 1%) ... 2498
Rabies Vaccine RabAvert (Ten cases) ... 1203
Recombivax HB ... 2178
Varivax ... 2202
YF-VAX Vaccine (Two cases) ... 827

Encephalitis, measles inclusion body
Attenuvax ... 2044
M-M-R II ... 2118

Encephalocele
Felbatol ... 3343

Encephalomyelitis
JE-VAX Vaccine (Two cases.) ... 811

Encephalopathy
Abelcet Injection ... 1273
Acel-Imune ... 1851
Attenuvax ... 2044
Betaseron for SC Injection ... 988
Ceptaz for Injection ... 1499
Cerebyx Injection (Infrequent) ... 2619
Cytovene ... 2959
Depacon Injection (Rare) ... 416
Depakene (Rare instances) ... 421
Depakote Sprinkle Capsules (Rare) ... 426
Depakote Tablets (Rare instances) ... 430
Depakote ER Tablets (Rare instances) ... 436
Diphtheria & Tetanus Toxoids Adsorbed Purogenated for Pediatric Use ... 1857
Ergamisol Tablets ... 1789
Felbatol ... 3343
FluShield Influenza Vaccine ... 3521
Fluzone Vaccine ... 802
Fortaz ... 1541
Gabitril Tablets (Infrequent) ... 1189
Gengraf Capsules ... 457
Havrix Vaccine (Rare) ... 1544
JE-VAX Vaccine (1 to 2.3 per million vaccines) ... 811
Kaletra Capsules (Less than 2%) ... 471
Kaletra Oral Solution (Less than 2%) ... 471
Lariam Tablets ... 2989
Levaquin ... 2537
Lithobid Slow-Release Tablets ... 3255
Maxipime for Injection ... 1285
Midamor Tablets (Between 1% and 3%) ... 2136
M-M-R II (Very rare) ... 2118
Moduretic Tablets ... 2138
Neoral Soft Gelatin Capsules ... 2380
Neoral Oral Solution ... 2380
Neurontin Capsules (Rare) ... 2655
Neurontin Oral Solution (Rare) ... 2655
Neurontin Tablets (Rare) ... 2655
Orthoclone OKT3 Sterile Solution (Less than 1%) ... 2498
Paser Granules ... 1781
Primaxin I.M. ... 2158
Primaxin I.V. (Less than 0.2%) ... 2160
▲ Prograf (3% to 15%) ... 1393
Proleukin for Injection ... 1199
Remicade for IV Injection (Less than 2%) ... 1178
Roferon-A Injection (Infrequent) ... 2996
Sandimmune ... 2388
▲ Serostim for Injection (1% to 10%) ... 3229
Streptomycin Sulfate Injection ... 2714
Stromectol Tablets ... 2185
Tasmar Tablets (Rare) ... 3010
Tazidime Vials, Faspak & ADD-Vantage ... 1966
Tetanus & Diphtheria Toxoids Adsorbed for Adult Use ... 1880
Tetanus and Diphtheria Toxoids Adsorbed For Adult Use ... 815
Topamax Sprinkle Capsules (Infrequent) ... 2590
Topamax Tablets (Infrequent) ... 2590
Tripedia Vaccine ... 817
Trovan (Less than 1%) ... 2722
Twinrix Vaccine ... 1674
Valtrex Caplets ... 1676
▲ Vesanoid Capsules (3%) ... 3037
Vistide Injection ... 1445
Xeloda Tablets (Less than 5%) ... 3039
Zonegran Capsules (Rare) ... 1307
Zovirax Capsules ... 1706
Zovirax for Injection (Approximately 1%) ... 1708
Zovirax ... 1706
Zyprexa Tablets (Rare) ... 1973
Zyprexa ZYDIS Orally Disintegrating Tablets (Rare) ... 1973

Encephalopathy, hepatic
Aciphex Tablets (Rare) ... 1267
Aciphex Tablets (Rare) ... 1783
Eulexin Capsules ... 3118
Intron A for Injection (Very rare) ... 3120
Prilosec Delayed-Release Capsules (Rare) ... 628
Taxol Injection (Rare) ... 1129

Encephalopathy, hypertensive
Catapres-TTS (Rare) ... 1038
Clorpres Tablets ... 1002
Combipres Tablets ... 1040
Epogen for Injection (On occasion) ... 582
Procrit for Injection (Occasional) ... 2502

Encephalopathy, toxic
Rifamate Capsules (Uncommon) ... 767
Rifater Tablets (Uncommon) ... 769

Endocardial fibrosis
Myleran Tablets (One case) ... 1603

Endocarditis
Betaseron for SC Injection ... 988
Oncaspar (Less than 1%) ... 756
Proleukin for Injection (1%) ... 1199

Endocarditis, infectious
CellCept Capsules (Occasional) ... 2951
CellCept Intravenous (Occasional) ... 2951
CellCept Oral Suspension (Occasional) ... 2951
CellCept Tablets (Occasional) ... 2951

Endocrine disturbances
▲ Cleocin Vaginal Cream (4%) ... 2788
Compazine ... 1505
Imitrex Nasal Spray ... 1554
Norplant System ... 3543
Permax Tablets (Rare) ... 1299
Pravachol Tablets ... 1099
Stelazine ... 1640

Endometrial carcinoma
(*see under* Carcinoma, endometrial)

Endometrial disorder, unspecified
Evoxac Capsules (Less than 1%) ... 1217

Endometrial hyperplasia
Nolvadex Tablets ... 678

Endometriosis
Clomid Tablets ... 735
femhrt Tablets ... 2635
Imitrex Injection ... 1549
Imitrex Nasal Spray (Rare) ... 1554
Imitrex Tablets ... 1558
Nolvadex Tablets (A few reports) ... 678
Remicade for IV Injection (Less than 2%) ... 1178
Serophene Tablets ... 3226
Tarka Tablets (Less frequent) ... 508

Endometritis
▲ Cleocin Vaginal Cream (5%) ... 2788
ParaGard T 380A Intrauterine Copper Contraceptive ... 2582
Prostin E2 Suppositories ... 2852

Endometrium disorders, unspecified
Amerge Tablets (Rare) ... 1467

Endophthalmitis
Campath Ampules ... 992
Healon 5 (Rare) ... ⊙317
Healon GV ... ⊙320
Vitrasert Implant (Less than 1%) ... ⊙254

Endotracheal tube, reflux into
▲ Infasurf Intratracheal Suspension (21%) ... 1372
Survanta (Less than 1%) ... 3053

Energy, high
Eldepryl Capsules ... 3266
Phrenilin (Infrequent) ... 578
Sedapap Tablets 50 mg/650 mg (Infrequent) ... 2225

Energy, loss of
▲ Gabitril Tablets (20%) ... 1189
Levlen ... 962
Levlite 21 Tablets ... 962
Levlite 28 Tablets ... 962
▲ Minipress Capsules (6.9%) ... 2699
▲ Minizide Capsules (6.9%) ... 2700
Modicon ... 2563
Ortho-Cyclen/Ortho Tri-Cyclen ... 2573
Ortho-Novum ... 2563
Ortho-Novum 1/50□28 Tablets ... 2556
Ortho-Cyclen/Ortho Tri-Cyclen ... 2573
Tri-Levlen ... 962

Enteritis
Ambien Tablets (Rare) ... 3191
Arthrotec Tablets (Rare) ... 3195
Betaseron for SC Injection ... 988
Felbatol ... 3343
▲ Sterile FUDR (Among more common) ... 2974
Lipitor Tablets (Less than 2%) ... 2639
Lipitor Tablets (Less than 2%) ... 2696
Micardis HCT Tablets ... 1051
Paxil (Rare) ... 1609
Protonix I.V. (Less than 1%) ... 3580
Protonix Tablets (Less than 1%) ... 3577
Prozac Pulvules, Liquid, and Weekly Capsules (Rare) ... 1238
Rescriptor Tablets (Less than 2%) ... 526
Sarafem Pulvules (Rare) ... 1962
Sonata Capsules (Rare) ... 3591
Trileptal Oral Suspension ... 2407
Trileptal Tablets ... 2407
Trovan (Less than 1%) ... 2722
Uniretic Tablets (Less than 1%) ... 3178
Zyprexa Tablets (Rare) ... 1973
Zyprexa ZYDIS Orally Disintegrating Tablets (Rare) ... 1973

Enterocolitis
Augmentin Chewable Tablets ... 1482
Augmentin Powder for Oral Suspension ... 1482
Augmentin Tablets ... 1485
Augmentin ES-600 Powder for Oral Suspension ... 1487
Declomycin Tablets ... 1855
Doryx Coated Pellet Filled Capsules ... 3357
Dynacin Capsules ... 2019
Evoxac Capsules (Less than 1%) ... 1217
Indocin I.V. (Less than 3%) ... 2115
Kaletra Capsules (Less than 2%) ... 471
Kaletra Oral Solution (Less than 2%) ... 471
Minocin Intravenous ... 1862
Minocin Oral Suspension ... 1865
Minocin Pellet-Filled Capsules ... 1863
Monodox Capsules ... 2442
Omnicef ... 493
Periostat Tablets ... 1208
ProSom Tablets (Rare) ... 500
Unasyn for Injection ... 2728
Vibramycin Calcium Oral Suspension Syrup ... 2735
Vibramycin Hyclate Capsules ... 2735
Vibramycin Hyclate Intravenous ... 2737
Vibramycin Monohydrate for Oral Suspension ... 2735
Vibra-Tabs Film Coated Tablets ... 2735

Enterocolitis, necrotizing
▲ Cafcit (4.3%) ... 1035
▲ Infasurf Intratracheal Suspension (5% to 17%) ... 1372
▲ Survanta Intratracheal Suspension (6.1%) ... 3053
Xeloda Tablets (Less than 5%) ... 3039

Enterocolitis, neutropenic
Azulfidine EN-tabs Tablets (Rare) ... 2775
Taxol Injection (Rare) ... 1129

Enterocolitis with perforation
Idamycin PFS Injection (Rare) ... 2825

Entropion
Botox Purified Neurotoxin Complex (Less than 1%)... 549

Enuresis
Aricept Tablets... 1270
Aricept Tablets... 2665
Depacon Injection... 416
Depakene... 421
Depakote Sprinkle Capsules... 426
Depakote Tablets... 430
Depakote ER Tablets... 436
Klonopin Tablets (Infrequent)... 2983
Mintezol... 2137
Serentil... 1057
Thalomid Capsules... 1154
Wellbutrin Tablets (Rare)... 1680
Zonegran Capsules (Rare)... 1307

Eosinophilia
Abelcet Injection... 1273
Accolate Tablets (Rare)... 657
Aceon Tablets (2 mg, 4 mg, 8 mg)... 3249
Advair Diskus 100/50 (Rare)... 1448
Advair Diskus 250/50 (Rare)... 1448
Advair Diskus 500/50 (Rare)... 1448
Aldoclor Tablets... 2035
Aldomet Tablets... 2037
Aldoril Tablets... 2039
Aloprim for Injection (Less than 1%)... 2292
Altace Capsules (Less than 1%)... 2233
Amoxil Chewable Tablets... 1471
Amoxil for Oral Suspension... 1471
Amoxil... 1471
Anaprox Tablets (Less than 1%)... 2967
Anaprox DS Tablets (Less than 1%)... 2967
Ancef for Injection... 1474
Ancef Injection... 1474
Ancobon Capsules... 1730
Arava Tablets (Rare)... 724
Aricept Tablets (Infrequent)... 1270
Aricept Tablets (Infrequent)... 2665
Arthrotec Tablets (Rare)... 3195
Asacol Delayed-Release Tablets... 2884
Atromid-S Capsules... 3483
Augmentin Chewable Tablets... 1482
Augmentin Powder for Oral Suspension... 1482
Augmentin Tablets... 1485
Augmentin ES-600 Powder for Oral Suspension... 1487
Avelox Tablets (0.05% to 1%)... 879
▲ Avonex (5%)... 1013
Axid Pulvules (Rare)... 1903
Axid Pulvules (Rare)... 2919
▲ Azactam for Injection (6.3%)... 1276
Azulfidine EN-tabs Tablets (Rare)... 2775
Bactrim... 2949
Baycol Tablets (Rare)... 883
Betapace Tablets (Rare)... 950
Betapace AF Tablets (Rare)... 954
Bicillin C-R 900/300 Injection... 2240
Bicillin C-R Injection... 2238
Bicillin L-A Injection... 2242
▲ Cancidas for Injection (3.2%)... 2048
▲ Captopril Tablets (About 4 to 7 of 100 patients)... 2281
Carbatrol Capsules... 3234
Cataflam Tablets (Rare)... 2315
Ceclor CD Tablets (0.3%)... 1279
Ceclor (1 in 50)... 1905
▲ Cedax (3%)... 1021
Cefizox for Intramuscular or Intravenous Use (1% to 5%)... 1390
▲ Cefobid Intravenous/Intramuscular (1 in 10)... 2671
▲ Cefobid Pharmacy Bulk Package - Not for Direct Infusion (1 in 10)... 2673
Cefotan (1 in 200)... 664
Ceftin (0.1% to 1%)... 1898
Cefzil (2.3%)... 1076
Celontin Capsules... 2618
▲ Ceptaz for Injection (One in 13)... 1499
Chemet Capsules (0.5% to 1.5%)... 3078
Cipro I.V.... 893
▲ Cipro I.V. Pharmacy Bulk Package (Among most frequent)... 897
Cipro (0.6%)... 887
Claforan Injection (Less than 1% to 2.4%)... 732
Cleocin HCl Capsules... 2784
Cleocin Phosphate Sterile Solution... 2785
Cleocin Vaginal Cream... 2788
Cleocin Vaginal Ovules... 2789
Clinoril Tablets (Less than 1 in 100)... 2053
Clozaril Tablets (1%)... 2319
Colazal Capsules... 3069
Compazine... 1505
Copaxone for Injection (Infrequent)... 3306
Cuprimine Capsules... 2075
Declomycin Tablets... 1855
Demser Capsules (Rare)... 2085
Depacon Injection... 416
Depakene... 421
Depakote Sprinkle Capsules... 426
Depakote Tablets... 430
Depakote ER Tablets... 436
Depen Titratable Tablets... 3341
Diabinese Tablets... 2680
Dilantin Infatabs... 2624
Dilantin Kapseals... 2622
Dilantin-125 Oral Suspension... 2625
Dipentum Capsules (Rare)... 2803
Dobutrex Solution Vials (Occasional)... 1914
Dolobid Tablets (Less than 1 in 100)... 2088
Doryx Coated Pellet Filled Capsules... 3357
Doxil Injection (Less than 1%)... 566
Duricef... 1079
Dynabac Tablets (1.2%)... 2269
Dynacin Capsules... 2019
EC-Naprosyn Delayed-Release Tablets (Less than 1%)... 2967
Effexor Tablets (Rare)... 3495
Effexor XR Capsules (Rare)... 3499
Efudex... 1733
Enalaprilat Injection... 863
Etrafon... 3115
Evoxac Capsules (Less than 1%)... 1217
Felbatol... 3343
Feldene Capsules (Occasional)... 2685
Flexeril Tablets (Rare)... 572
Flexeril Tablets (Rare)... 2094
Flovent Diskus... 3614
Flovent... 1535
Flovent Rotadisk... 1537
Floxin I.V. (More than or equal to 1%)... 2526
Floxin Tablets (More than or equal to 1%)... 2529
▲ Fortaz (1 in 13)... 1541
Geocillin Tablets... 2687
Geodon Capsules (Infrequent)... 2688
Hivid Tablets (2.5%)... 2975
Iscar Mali Injection... 3456
Iscar Mali Special Injection... 3456
Iscar Pini Injection... 3456
Iscar Quercus Injection... 3456
Iscar Quercus Special Injection... 3456
Keflex... 1237
▲ Kefurox Vials, ADD-Vantage (1 in 14)... 1948
Kefzol Vials, ADD-Vantage... 1951
Klonopin Tablets... 2983
Lamictal (Infrequent)... 1567
Lescol Capsules (Rare)... 2361
Lescol Capsules (Rare)... 2925
Lescol XL Tablets... 2361
Lescol XL Tablets... 2925
Leukine... 1755
Levaquin... 2537
Lexxel Tablets... 608
Limbitrol... 1738
Lodine... 3528
Lodine XL Extended-Release Tablets... 3530
Lopid Tablets... 2650
Lorabid Suspension and Pulvules... 2251
Lotensin HCT Tablets... 2367
▲ Lupron Depot–4 Month 30 mg (Greater than or equal to 5%)... 3289
Macrobid Capsules (1% to 5%)... 2889
Macrodantin Capsules (Less often)... 2891
Mandol Vials... 1953
Matulane Capsules... 3246
Maxipime for Injection (1.7%)... 1285
Mefoxin for Injection... 2124
Mefoxin Premixed Intravenous Solution... 2127
Merrem I.V. (Greater than 0.2%)... 673
Mevacor Tablets... 2132
Miltown Tablets... 3349
Minocin Intravenous... 1862
Minocin Oral Suspension... 1865
Minocin Pellet-Filled Capsules... 1863
Monodox Capsules... 2442
Monopril Tablets (2 patients)... 1091
Monopril HCT... 1094
Monurol Sachet... 1375
Motrin Suspension, Oral Drops, Chewable Tablets, and Caplets (Less than 1%)... 2002
Myambutol Tablets... 1290
Mycobutin Capsules (1%)... 2838
Naprelan Tablets (Less than 1%)... 1293
Naprosyn Suspension (Less than 1%)... 2967
Naprosyn Tablets (Less than 1%)... 2967
Navane Oral... 2701
Navane Intramuscular... 2703
Nebcin Vials, Hyporets & ADD-Vantage... 1955
Noroxin Tablets (0.6% to 1.5%)... 2145
Norpramin Tablets... 755
Omnicef (0.6%)... 493
Orthoclone OKT3 Sterile Solution (Less than 1%)... 2498
▲ Paser Granules (55% of 38 patients with drug-induced hepatitis)... 1781
Paxil (Rare)... 1609
Pediazole Suspension... 3050
Pentasa Capsules... 3239
Periostat Tablets... 1208
Permapen Isoject... 2706
Permax Tablets (Rare)... 1299
Pima Syrup... 1362
Pipracil... 1866
Ponstel Capsules (Occasional)... 1356
Pravachol Tablets (Rare)... 1099
Prevacid Delayed-Release Capsules (Less than 1%)... 3292
PREVPAC (Less than 1%)... 3298
Primaxin I.M.... 2158
Primaxin I.V.... 2160
Prinivil Tablets (0.3% to 1.0%)... 2164
Prinzide Tablets... 2168
▲ Proleukin for Injection (6%)... 1199
Protonix I.V. (Less than 1%)... 3580
Protonix Tablets (Less than 1%)... 3577
Provigil Tablets (2%)... 1193
Requip Tablets (Infrequent)... 1621
Rescriptor Tablets (Less than 2%)... 526
Rifadin (Occasional)... 765
Rifamate Capsules... 767
Rifater Tablets (Occasional)... 769
▲ Rocephin Injectable Vials, ADD-Vantage, Galaxy, Bulk (6%)... 2993
Septra Suspension... 2265
Septra Tablets... 2265
Septra DS Tablets... 2265
Serentil... 1057
Seroquel Tablets (Infrequent)... 684
▲ Serostim for Injection (1% to 10%)... 3229
Sinequan (A few patients)... 2713
Singulair... 2181
Soma Tablets... 3353
Soma Compound Tablets... 3354
Soma Compound w/Codeine Tablets... 3355
Sonata Capsules (Rare)... 3591
Stelazine... 1640
▲ Stromectol Tablets (3%)... 2185
Sulfamylon Cream... 1011
Sulfamylon Topical Solution... 1011
Suprax (Less than 2%)... 1877
Surmontil Capsules... 3595
▲ Synarel Nasal Solution for Endometriosis (10% to 15%)... 3205
Talacen Caplets (Rare)... 3089
Talwin Nx Tablets (Rare)... 3090
Tao Capsules... 2716
▲ Tazicef for Injection (1 in 13 patients)... 1647
▲ Tazicef Galaxy Container (1 in 13 patients)... 1650
▲ Tazicef Pharmacy Bulk Package (1 in 13 patients)... 1653
▲ Tazidime Vials, Faspak & ADD-Vantage (1 in 13)... 1966
Tegretol/Tegretol-XR... 2404
Thalomid Capsules... 1154
Thioridazine Hydrochloride Tablets... 2289
Thiothixene Capsules... 2290
Thorazine... 1656
Ticlid Tablets... 3015
Timentin Injection- ADD-Vantage Vial... 1661
Timentin Injection-Galaxy Container... 1664
Timentin Injection-Pharmacy Bulk Package... 1666
Timentin for Intravenous Administration... 1658
Tonocard Tablets (Less than 1%)... 649
Topamax Sprinkle Capsules (Infrequent)... 2590
Topamax Tablets (Infrequent)... 2590
Toradol (1% or less)... 3018
Tricor Capsules, Micronized... 513
Trilafon... 3160
Trileptal Oral Suspension... 2407
Trileptal Tablets... 2407
Trovan (Greater than or equal to 1%)... 2722
Unasyn for Injection... 2728
Uniretic Tablets (Less than 1%)... 3178
Vancocin HCl Capsules & Pulvules (Infrequent)... 1972
Vancocin HCl Oral Solution (Infrequent)... 1971
Vancocin HCl, Vials & ADD-Vantage (Infrequent)... 1970
Vantin Tablets and Oral Suspension... 2860
Vaqta (Isolated reports)... 2199
Vascor Tablets... 2602
Vaseretic Tablets... 2204
Vasotec I.V. Injection... 2207
Vasotec Tablets (0.5% to 1.0%)... 2210
Vibramycin Calcium Oral Suspension Syrup... 2735
Vibramycin Hyclate Capsules... 2735
Vibramycin Hyclate Intravenous... 2737
Vibramycin Monohydrate for Oral Suspension... 2735
Vibra-Tabs Film Coated Tablets... 2735
Viramune Oral Suspension... 1060
Viramune Tablets... 1060
Vivactil Tablets... 2217
Vivactil Tablets... 2446
Voltaren Tablets (Rare)... 2315
Voltaren-XR Tablets (Rare)... 2315
▲ Xanax Tablets (3.2% to 9.5%)... 2865
Zantac (Rare)... 1690
Zantac Injection... 1688
Zantac Syrup (Rare)... 1690
Zarontin Capsules... 2659
Zarontin Syrup... 2660
Zestoretic Tablets... 695
Zestril Tablets (0.3% to 1.0%)... 698
▲ Zinacef Injection (1 in 14 patients)... 1696
▲ Zinacef for Injection (1 in 14 patients)... 1696
Zocor Tablets... 2219
Zomig Tablets (Rare)... 708
Zomig-ZMT Tablets (Rare)... 708
Zosyn... 1890
Zosyn in Galaxy Containers... 1894

Eosinophilia, myoclonus
Carbatrol Capsules (One case)... 3234
Tegretol/Tegretol-XR (One case)... 2404

Eosinophilia, peripheral
Carbatrol Capsules (One case)... 3234
Tegretol/Tegretol-XR (One case)... 2404
Trovan... 2722

Eosinophilia, pulmonary
Dapsone Tablets USP... 1780
Daraprim Tablets (Rare)... 1511
Dynacin Capsules (Rare)... 2019

Eosinophilic infiltration
Trovan... 2722

Eosinophilic pneumonitis
(*see under* Pneumonitis, eosinophilic)

Epidermolysis bullosa
Anaprox Tablets (Less than 1%)... 2967
Anaprox DS Tablets (Less than 1%)... 2967
EC-Naprosyn Delayed-Release Tablets (Less than 1%)... 2967
▲ Naprelan Tablets (3% to 9%)... 1293
Naprosyn Suspension (Less than 1%)... 2967
Naprosyn Tablets (Less than 1%)... 2967

Epididymitis
Anadrol-50 Tablets... 3321
Asacol Delayed-Release Tablets... 2884
Avonex... 1013
Betaseron for SC Injection... 988
Cognex Capsules (Rare)... 1351
Cordarone Tablets (Rare)... 3487
Evoxac Capsules (Less than 1%)... 1217
Fortovase Capsules (Less than 2%)... 2970
Lamictal (Rare)... 1567
Lipitor Tablets (Less than 2%)... 2639
Lipitor Tablets (Less than 2%)... 2696
Lupron Depot–4 Month 30 mg (Less than 5%)... 3289
Neurontin Capsules (Rare)... 2655
Neurontin Oral Solution (Rare)... 2655
Neurontin Tablets (Rare)... 2655
Oxandrin Tablets... 1153
Pacerone Tablets (Rare)... 3331
Paxil (Rare)... 1609
Permax Tablets (Rare)... 1299
Protonix I.V. (Less than 1%)... 3580
Protonix Tablets (Less than 1%)... 3577
Requip Tablets (Infrequent)... 1621
Rescriptor Tablets (Less than 2%)... 526
▲ Serostim for Injection (1% to 10%)... 3229
TheraCys Injection... 823
Tice BCG, BCG Live (0.3%)... 2489

Epigastric pain
(*see under* Distress, epigastric)

Epilepsy, aggravation
Estrace Vaginal Cream... 3358
Estrace Tablets... 3361
Indocin Capsules (Less than 1%)... 2112
Indocin I.V. (Less than 1%)... 2115
Indocin (Less than 1%)... 2112

Epileptic ictal phenomenon
Trileptal Oral Suspension... 2407
Trileptal Tablets... 2407

Epileptiform movements, unspecified
Clozaril Tablets (1%)... 2319

Epinephrine effect, reversal
Compazine... 1505
Etrafon... 3115
Stelazine... 1640

Epiphora
Alphagan P Ophthalmic Solution (1% to 4%)... 546
▲ Alrex Sterile Ophthalmic Suspension 0.2% (5% to 15%)... ⊙ 256
Betimol Ophthalmic Solution (1% to 5%)... ⊙ 324
▲ Lotemax Sterile Ophthalmic Suspension 0.5% (5% to 15%)... ⊙ 261

Epiphyseal closure
Accutane Capsules... 2944

Anadrol-50 Tablets 3321
Aquasol A Parenteral 593
Estratest 3252
Oxandrin Tablets 1153

Episcleritis
Aredia for Injection (Rare) 2309

Epistaxis
Accutane Capsules 2944
Aceon Tablets (2 mg, 4 mg, 8 mg) (0.3% to 1%) 3249
Aciphex Tablets 1267
Aciphex Tablets 1783
Actiq (1% or greater) 1184
Activase I.V. (Less than 1%) 1410
Adalat CC Tablets (3% or less) 877
Advair Diskus 100/50 (1% to 3%) ... 1448
Advair Diskus 250/50 (1% to 3%) ... 1448
Advair Diskus 500/50 (1% to 3%) ... 1448
Aerobid/Aerobid-M (1% to 3%) 1363
Aggrenox Capsules (2.4%) 1026
Agrylin Capsules (1% to 5%) 3232
Alferon N Injection (1%) 1770
Altace Capsules (Less than 1%) 2233
Ambien Tablets (Rare) 3191
▲ AmBisome for Injection (8.6% to 14.9%) 1383
Amerge Tablets (Rare) 1467
▲ Amphotec (5% or more) 1774
Anzemet Injection (Rare) 719
Anzemet Tablets (Rare) 722
Arava Tablets (1% to 3%) 724
Aricept Tablets (Infrequent) 1270
Aricept Tablets (Infrequent) 2665
Arthrotec Tablets (Rare) 3195
Astelin Nasal Spray (2.0% to 3.2%) 3339
Atacand Tablets (0.5% or greater) .. 595
Atacand HCT Tablets (0.5% or greater) 597
▲ Atrovent Nasal Spray 0.03% (7.0% to 9.0%) 1032
▲ Atrovent Nasal Spray 0.06% (8.2%) 1033
Avalide Tablets 1070
Avapro Tablets (Less than 1%) 1074
Avapro Tablets (Less than 1%) 3076
Axert Tablets (Infrequent) 2772
Bactroban Nasal (Less than 1%) 1495
Baycol Tablets 883
Beconase Inhalation Aerosol (Two in 100 patients) 1497
Beconase AQ Nasal Spray (Fewer than 3 per 100 patients) 1498
▲ Campath Ampules (1% to 7%) 992
Cardizem Injectable 1018
Cardizem Lyo-Ject Syringe 1018
Cardizem Monovial 1018
Cardizem CD Capsules (Less than 1%) 1016
Cardura Tablets (1%) 2668
▲ Casodex Tablets (2% to 5%) 662
Cataflam Tablets (Less than 1%) 2315
Celebrex Capsules (0.1% to 1.9%) 2676
Celebrex Capsules (0.1% to 1.9%) 2780
Celexa (Infrequent) 1365
Cerebyx Injection (Infrequent) 2619
Cipro I.V. (1% or less) 893
Cipro I.V. Pharmacy Bulk Package (Less than 1%) 897
Cipro (Less than 1%) 887
Claritin (At least one patient) 3100
Claritin-D 12 Hour Extended Release Tablets (Less frequent) ... 3102
Claritin-D 24 Hour Extended Release Tablets (Fewer than 2%) 3104
Clinoril Tablets (Less than 1%) 2053
Clozaril Tablets (Less than 1%) 2319
Cognex Capsules (Infrequent) 1351
Colazal Capsules 3069
Copaxone for Injection (Infrequent) 3306
Coumadin for Injection 1243
Coumadin Tablets 1243
Cozaar Tablets (Less than 1%) 2067
Cytotec Tablets (Infrequent) 3202
DDAVP Nasal Spray (Up to 3%) 738
DDAVP Rhinal Tube (Up to 3%) 738
Depacon Injection (1% to 5%) 416
Depakene (1% to 5%) 421
Depakote Sprinkle Capsules (1% to 5%) 426
Depakote Tablets (1% to 5%) 430
Depakote ER Tablets (1% to 5%) 436
Desmopressin Acetate Rhinal Tube (Up to 3%) 1345
Diovan HCT Tablets (Greater than 0.2%) 2338
▲ Dostinex Tablets (Less than 10%) .. 2804
Doxil Injection (Less than 1%) 566
Dynabac Tablets (0.1% to 1%) 2269
DynaCirc CR Tablets (0.5% to 1%) .. 2923
Effexor Tablets (Infrequent) 3495
Effexor XR Capsules (Infrequent) 3499
Elmiron Capsules (Less than or equal to 1%) 570
Ergamisol Tablets (Up to 1%) 1789
Evoxac Capsules (1% to 3%) 1217
Exelon Capsules (Frequent) 2342
Exelon Oral Solution (Frequent) 2345
Felbatol 3343
Feldene Capsules (Occasional) 2685
▲ Flolan for Injection (4% to 9%) 1528
▲ Flonase Nasal Spray (6% to 6.9%) . 1533
Flovent Diskus (1% to 3%) 3614
Flovent Rotadisk (1% to 3%) 1537
Floxin I.V. (Less than 1%) 2526
Floxin Tablets (Less than 1%) 2529
Fludara for Injection (Up to 1%) 995
Fortovase Capsules (Less than 2%) 2970
Sterile FUDR (Remote possibility) 2974
Gabitril Tablets (Frequent) 1189
Gengraf Capsules (1% to less than 3%) 457
Geodon Capsules (Infrequent) 2688
▲ Gleevec Capsules (3% to 12%) 2357
Hivid Tablets (Less than 1%) 2975
Hytrin Capsules (At least 1%) 464
Hyzaar 2109
Imitrex Nasal Spray 1554
Indocin Capsules (Less than 1%) 2112
Indocin I.V. (Less than 1%) 2115
Indocin (Less than 1%) 2112
▲ Infergen (6% to 8%) 1777
Innohep Injection (1.9%) 1248
Intron A for Injection (Less than or equal to 5%) 3120
Invirase Capsules (Less than 2%) 2979
Klonopin Tablets (Infrequent) 2983
Lamictal (Infrequent) 1567
▲ Leukine (17%) 1755
▲ Leustatin Injection (5%) 2495
Levaquin Injection (Less than 0.5%) 2537
Lexxel Tablets 608
Lipitor Tablets (Less than 2%) 2639
Lipitor Tablets (Less than 2%) 2696
Lotensin HCT Tablets (0.3% or more) 2367
Lupron Depot–3 Month 22.5 mg (Less than 5%) 3288
Lupron Depot-PED 7.5 mg, 11.25 mg and 15 mg (Less than 2%) 3291
Lupron Injection Pediatric (Less than 2%) 3280
Luvox Tablets (25, 50, 100 mg) (Infrequent) 3256
Matulane Capsules 3246
Mavik Tablets (0.3% to 1.0%) 478
Maxalt Tablets (Infrequent) 2120
Maxalt-MLT Orally Disintegrating Tablets (Infrequent) 2120
Meridia Capsules 481
Merrem I.V. (0.7%) 673
▲ Miacalcin Nasal Spray (3.5%) 2375
Micardis Tablets (More than 0.3%) .. 1049
Micardis HCT Tablets 1051
Migranal Nasal Spray (Rare) 2376
Minipress Capsules (1% to 4%) 2699
Minizide Capsules 2700
Mithracin for Intravenous Use 903
Monopril Tablets (0.2% to 1.0%) 1091
Monopril HCT 1094
Motrin Suspension, Oral Drops, Chewable Tablets, and Caplets (Less than 1%) 2002
Mykrox Tablets (Less than 2%) 1168
▲ Mylotarg for Injection (23% to 44%) 3540
Naprelan Tablets (Less than 1%) 1293
Nasacort Nasal Inhaler (Fewer than 5%) 750
Nasacort AQ Nasal Spray (2.7%) 752
Nasalide Nasal Spray (5% or less) .. 1295
▲ Nasarel Nasal Solution 0.025% (3% to 9%) 1296
▲ Nasonex Nasal Spray (8% to 11%) 3131
Neoral Soft Gelatin Capsules (1% to less than 3%) 2380
Neoral Oral Solution (1% to less than 3%) 2380
▲ Neupogen for Injection (9% to 15%) 587
Neurontin Capsules (Infrequent) 2655
Neurontin Oral Solution (Infrequent) 2655
Neurontin Tablets (Infrequent) 2655
Nexium Delayed-Release Capsules (Less than 1%) 619
▲ Nicotrol Nasal Spray (More common) 2843
Norvasc Tablets (More than 0.1% to 1%) 2704
Norvir Capsules (Less than 2%) 487
Norvir Oral Solution (Less than 2%) 487
Oncaspar (Less than 1%) 756
OptiPranolol Metipranolol Ophthalmic Solution 0.3% (A small number of patients) .... ⊙ 263
Orudis Capsules (Less than 1%) 3548
Oruvail Capsules (Less than 1%) 3548
Paxil (Infrequent) 1609
Permax Tablets (1.6%) 1299
Plavix Tablets (2.9%) 1097
Plavix Tablets (2.9%) 3084
Plendil Extended-Release Tablets (0.5% to 1.5%) 623
Pletal Tablets (Less than 2%) 2605
Pletal Tablets (Less than 2%) 2848
Prevacid Delayed-Release Capsules (Less than 1%) 3292
PREVPAC (Less than 1%) 3298
Prilosec Delayed-Release Capsules (Less than 1%) 628
Prinivil Tablets (0.3% to 1.0%) 2164
Prinzide Tablets 2168
Procardia XL Extended Release Tablets (1% or less) 2710
ProSom Tablets (Rare) 500
Protonix I.V. (Less than 1%) 3580
Protonix Tablets (Less than 1%) 3577
Protopic Ointment (Greater than or equal to 1%) 1397
Provigil Tablets (1%) 1193
Prozac Pulvules, Liquid, and Weekly Capsules (Infrequent) 1238
Pulmicort Respules (2% to 4%) 632
▲ Rapamune Oral Solution and Tablets (3% to 20%) 3584
Recombinate 853
▲ Refludan for Injection (4.4%) 761
Relenza Rotadisk (Less than 1%) 1619
Remeron Tablets (Infrequent) 2483
Remeron SolTab Tablets (Infrequent) 2486
Reminyl Oral Solution (Infrequent) ... 1792
Reminyl Tablets (Infrequent) 1792
ReoPro Vials (9 to 11 events) 1958
Requip Tablets (Infrequent) 1621
Rescriptor Tablets (Less than 2%) ... 526
Retrovir Capsules 1625
Retrovir IV Infusion 1629
Retrovir 1625
▲ Rhinocort Aqua Nasal Spray (8%) ... 642
▲ Rhinocort Nasal Inhaler (3% to 9%) 640
Rilutek Tablets (Infrequent) 772
Risperdal (Infrequent) 1796
Rocephin Injectable Vials, ADD-Vantage, Galaxy, Bulk (Rare) 2993
Roferon-A Injection (Rare) 2996
Roxicodone Tablets (Less than 3%) 3067
Salagen Tablets (2%) 2229
Sandostatin Injection (Less than 1%) 2394
Sandostatin LAR Depot (1% to 4%) 2395
Sarafem Pulvules (Infrequent) 1962
Serevent Inhalation Aerosol (1% to 3%) 1633
Seroquel Tablets (Infrequent) 684
Serzone Tablets (Infrequent) 1104
Sonata Capsules (Less than 1%) 3591
▲ Stadol NS Nasal Spray (3% to 9%) . 1108
Stimate Nasal Spray 796
Sular Tablets (Less than or equal to 1%) 688
▲ Tamiflu Capsules (3.1%) 3008
▲ Tamiflu Oral Suspension (3.1%) 3008
Tarka Tablets (Less frequent) 508
Tasmar Tablets (Infrequent) 3010
Tequin Injection (Less than 0.1%) 1110
Tequin Tablets (Less than 0.1%) 1110
Teveten Tablets (Less than 1%) 3327
Thalomid Capsules 1154
Tiazac Capsules (Less than 2%) 1378
Ticlid Tablets (0.5% to 1.0%) 3015
TNKase I.V. (1.5%) 1430
▲ TOBI Solution for Inhalation (7%) 1206
Tolectin (Less than 1%) 2589
Topamax Sprinkle Capsules (0.8% to 1.8%) 2590
Topamax Tablets (0.8% to 1.8%) 2590
Toradol (1% or less) 3018
Trental Tablets (Less than 1%) 784
Tricor Capsules, Micronized (Less than 1%) 513
Trileptal Oral Suspension (2% to 4%) 2407
Trileptal Tablets (2% to 4%) 2407
Trilisate (Less than 1%) 2901
▲ Trisenox Injection (25%) 1158
Trovan (Less than 1%) 2722
Unasyn for Injection (Less than 1%) 2728
Uniretic Tablets (Less than 1%) 3178
Vancenase PocketHaler Nasal Inhaler (2 per 100 patients) 3162
▲ Vancenase AQ Nasal Spray 0.084% (5%) 3163
Vantin Tablets and Oral Suspension (Less than 1%) 2860
▲ Ventolin Inhalation Aerosol and Refill (3%) 1679
Vioxx (Greater than 0.1% to 1.9%) .. 2213
Vistide Injection 1445
Voltaren Tablets (Less than 1%) 2315
Voltaren-XR Tablets (Less than 1%) 2315
Warfarin Sodium Tablets, USP 3302
Wellbutrin Tablets (Rare) 1680
Xeloda Tablets (Less than 5%) 3039
Zestoretic Tablets 695
Zestril Tablets (0.3% to 1.0%) 698
Zoladex (1% or greater) 702
Zoladex 3-month 706
Zoloft (Infrequent to 2%) 2751
Zomig Tablets (Infrequent) 708
Zomig-ZMT Tablets (Infrequent) 708
Zosyn (1.0% or less) 1890
Zosyn in Galaxy Containers (1.0% or less) 1894
Zyban Sustained-Release Tablets (2%) 1710
Zyprexa Tablets (Infrequent) 1973
Zyprexa ZYDIS Orally Disintegrating Tablets (Infrequent) 1973
Zyrtec (1.9% to 3.7%) 2756

Epitheliopathy
Alomide Ophthalmic Solution .... ⊙ 204
Ciloxan (Less than 1%) 538

Equilibrium dysfunction
Amerge Tablets (Infrequent) 1467
Covera-HS Tablets (Less than 2%) ... 3199
Floxin I.V. 2526
Floxin Tablets 2529
Hivid Tablets (Less than 1%) 2975
Isoptin SR Tablets (1% or less) 467
Lariam Tablets 2989
Procardia Capsules (2% or less) 2708
Rifater Tablets 769
Streptomycin Sulfate Injection 2714
Transderm Scōp Transdermal Therapeutic System (Few patients) 2302
Verelan Capsules (1% or less) 3184
Verelan PM Capsules (2% or less) ... 3186

Erection disturbances, unspecified
(*see also under* Impotence)
Anadrol-50 Tablets 3321
Baycol Tablets 883
Dantrium Capsules (Less frequent) 2885
Effexor Tablets (Rare) 3495
Effexor XR Capsules (Rare) 3499
Fortovase Capsules (Less than 2%) 2970
Lescol Capsules 2361
Lescol Capsules 2925
Lescol XL Tablets 2361
Lescol XL Tablets 2925
Mevacor Tablets (0.5% to 1.0%) 2132
MUSE Urethral Suppository (0.3%) 3335
▲ Paxil (3.7% to 10.0%) 1609
Pravachol Tablets 1099
Propecia Tablets (1.3%) 2172
Risperdal (Frequent) 1796
Wellbutrin Tablets (Infrequent) 1680
Wellbutrin SR Sustained-Release Tablets 1684
Zocor Tablets 2219
▲ Zoladex (18%) 702
Zoladex 3-month 706
Zyban Sustained-Release Tablets 1710

Erosion, genital
▲ Aldara Cream, 5% (1% to 30%) 1978
▲ Condylox Gel (8.9% to 27.0%) 2436
▲ Condylox Topical Solution (67%) 2437

Eructation
Aciphex Tablets 1267
Aciphex Tablets 1783
Actiq (Less than 1%) 1184
Agrylin Capsules (1% to 5%) 3232
Ambien Tablets (Rare) 3191
AmBisome for Injection (Less common) 1383
Aricept Tablets (Infrequent) 1270
Aricept Tablets (Infrequent) 2665
Arthrotec Tablets (Rare) 3195
▲ Asacol Delayed-Release Tablets (16%) 2884
Cedax Capsules (0.1% to 1%) 1021
Celebrex Capsules (0.1% to 1.9%) 2676
Celebrex Capsules (0.1% to 1.9%) 2780
Celexa (Infrequent) 1365
Claritin-D 12 Hour Extended Release Tablets (Less frequent) ... 3102
Clozaril Tablets (Less than 1%) 2319
Colazal Capsules 3069
Crinone (Less than 5%) 3213
Crixivan Capsules (Less than 2%) 2070
Cytovene (At least 3 subjects) 2959
Depacon Injection (1% to 5%) 416
Depakene (1% to 5%) 421
Depakote Sprinkle Capsules (1% to 5%) 426
Depakote Tablets (1% to 5%) 430
Depakote ER Tablets (Greater than 1%) 436
Dolobid Tablets (Less than 1 in 100) 2088
Doxil Injection (Less than 1%) 566
Effexor Tablets (Frequent) 3495
Effexor XR Capsules (Frequent) 3499
Evoxac Capsules (1% to 3%) 1217
Exelon Capsules (2%) 2342
Exelon Oral Solution (2%) 2345
Feldene Capsules (Rare) 2685

- Ferrlecit Injection (Greater than 1%) 3386
- Fortovase Capsules (Less than 2%) 2970
- Gabitril Tablets (Infrequent) 1189
- Gengraf Capsules (1% to less than 3%) 457
- Hivid Tablets (Less than 1%) 2975
- Imitrex Injection (Rare) 1549
- Imitrex Nasal Spray (Rare) 1554
- Imitrex Tablets 1558
- Intron A for Injection (Less than 5%) 3120
- Invirase Capsules (Less than 2%) 2979
- Kaletra Capsules (Less than 2%) 471
- Kaletra Oral Solution (Less than 2%) 471
- Lamictal (Rare) 1567
- Lipitor Tablets (Less than 2%) 2639
- Lipitor Tablets (Less than 2%) 2696
- Lodine (Less than 1%) 3528
- Lodine XL Extended-Release Tablets (Less than 1%) 3530
- Lupron Depot 7.5 mg (Less than 5%) 3284
- Lupron Depot–4 Month 30 mg (Less than 5%) 3289
- Luvox Tablets (25, 50, 100 mg) (Infrequent) 3256
- Maxalt Tablets (Rare) 2120
- Maxalt-MLT Orally Disintegrating Tablets (Rare) 2120
- Meridia Capsules 481
- Mobic Tablets (Less than 2%) 1054
- ▲ Mycobutin Capsules (3%) 2838
- Naprelan Tablets (Less than 1%) 1293
- Neoral Soft Gelatin Capsules (1% to less than 3%) 2380
- Neoral Oral Solution (1% to less than 3%) 2380
- Neurontin Capsules (Rare) 2655
- Neurontin Oral Solution (Rare) 2655
- Neurontin Tablets (Rare) 2655
- Nexium Delayed-Release Capsules (Less than 1%) 619
- Norvir Capsules (Less than 2%) 487
- Norvir Oral Solution (Less than 2%) 487
- Orap Tablets 1407
- Orudis Capsules (Less than 1%) 3548
- Oruvail Capsules (Less than 1%) 3548
- OxyContin Tablets (Less than 1%) 2912
- Paxil (Infrequent) 1609
- Pentasa Capsules (Less than 1%) 3239
- Permax Tablets (Infrequent) 1299
- ▲ Photofrin for Injection (5%) 831
- Ponstel Capsules (Rare) 1356
- Prevacid Delayed-Release Capsules (Less than 1%) 3292
- PREVPAC (Less than 1%) 3298
- Procardia XL Extended Release Tablets (1% or less) 2710
- Protonix I.V. (Greater than or equal to 1%) 3580
- Protonix Tablets (1%) 3577
- Proventil HFA Inhalation Aerosol (Less than 3%) 3150
- Prozac Pulvules, Liquid, and Weekly Capsules (Infrequent) 1238
- ▲ Rapamune Oral Solution and Tablets (3% to 20%) 3584
- Relafen Tablets (Less than 1%) 1617
- Remeron Tablets (Infrequent) 2483
- Remeron SolTab Tablets (Infrequent) 2486
- Requip Tablets (Infrequent) 1621
- Rescriptor Tablets 526
- Retrovir Capsules 1625
- Retrovir IV Infusion 1629
- Retrovir 1625
- Risperdal (Rare) 1796
- Salagen Tablets (Less than 1%) 2229
- Sarafem Pulvules (Infrequent) 1962
- Serzone Tablets (Infrequent) 1104
- Sonata Capsules (Infrequent) 3591
- Thalomid Capsules 1154
- Topamax Sprinkle Capsules (Rare) 2590
- Topamax Tablets (Rare) 2590
- Toradol (1% or less) 3018
- Trental Tablets (0.6%) 784
- Tricor Capsules, Micronized (1%) 513
- Trileptal Oral Suspension 2407
- Trileptal Tablets 2407
- Trovan (Less than 1%) 2722
- Uniretic Tablets (Less than 1%) 3178
- Vantin Tablets and Oral Suspension (Less than 1%) 2860
- Zoloft (Infrequent) 2751
- Zyprexa Tablets (Infrequent) 1973
- Zyprexa ZYDIS Orally Disintegrating Tablets (Infrequent) 1973
- Zyrtec (Less than 2%) 2756
- Zyrtec-D 12 Hour Extended Relief Tablets (Less than 2%) 2758

Eruptions

- Cuprimine Capsules 2075
- Diabinese Tablets (Approximately 1% or less) 2680

Eruptions, acneiform

(*see under* Acneiform eruptions)

Eruptions, bullous

- Aciphex Tablets 1267
- Aciphex Tablets 1783
- Ambien Tablets (Rare) 3191
- ▲ Argatroban Injection (1% to 10%) 1478
- Campath Ampules 992
- Cataflam Tablets (Rare) 2315
- Coumadin for Injection (Infrequent) 1243
- Coumadin Tablets (Infrequent) 1243
- Dynabac Tablets 2269
- Eulexin Capsules 3118
- Evoxac Capsules (Less than 1%) 1217
- Felbatol (Infrequent) 3343
- Fortovase Capsules (Rare) 2970
- Fragmin Injection (Rare) 2814
- Gengraf Capsules (1%) 457
- Hivid Tablets (Less than 1%) 2975
- Hycamtin for Injection (Less than 1%) 1546
- Indapamide Tablets 2286
- Innohep Injection (Greater than or equal to 1%) 1248
- Invirase Capsules (Rare) 2979
- Luvox Tablets (25, 50, 100 mg) 3256
- Mobic Tablets (Less than 2%) 1054
- Neoral Soft Gelatin Capsules (1%) 2380
- Neoral Oral Solution (1%) 2380
- Plavix Tablets (Less than 1%) 1097
- Plavix Tablets (Less than 1%) 3084
- Relafen Tablets (Less than 1%) 1617
- ReoPro Vials (0.1%) 1958
- Risperdal (Rare) 1796
- ▲ Soriatane Capsules (1% to 10%) 3003
- Viramune Oral Suspension 1060
- Viramune Tablets 1060
- Voltaren Tablets (Rare) 2315
- Voltaren-XR Tablets (Rare) 2315
- Warfarin Sodium Tablets, USP 3302
- Yodoxin Tablets 1722
- Zoloft (Rare) 2751
- Zyrtec (Less than 2%) 2756
- Zyrtec-D 12 Hour Extended Relief Tablets (Less than 2%) 2758

Eruptions, cutaneous

- Rifater Tablets (Rare) 769
- Roferon-A Injection (Less than 1%) 2996
- Taxotere for Injection Concentrate 778

Eruptions, eczematoid

(*see under* Eczema)

Eruptions, erythema annulare centrifugum

- Plaquenil Tablets 3082

Eruptions, erythematous

- Benoquin Cream 20% 1732
- Macrobid Capsules 2889
- Macrodantin Capsules 2891

Eruptions, exfoliative

- Quinidex Extentabs 2933
- Rifater Tablets 769

Eruptions, fixed drug

- Declomycin Tablets 1855
- Depen Titratable Tablets 3341
- Dynacin Capsules (Rare) 2019
- Ergamisol Tablets (Less frequent) 1789
- Miltown Tablets 3349
- Minocin Intravenous (Rare) 1862
- Minocin Oral Suspension (Rare) 1865
- Minocin Pellet-Filled Capsules (Rare) 1863
- Nitro-Dur Transdermal Infusion System (Uncommon) 1834
- Nitro-Dur Transdermal Infusion System (Uncommon) 3134
- Soma Tablets 3353
- Soma Compound Tablets 3354
- Soma Compound w/Codeine Tablets 3355

Eruptions, hemorrhagic

- Activella Tablets 2764
- Alesse-21 Tablets 3468
- Alesse-28 Tablets 3473
- Alora Transdermal System 3372
- Brevicon 28-Day Tablets 3380
- Cenestin Tablets 1263
- Climara Transdermal System 958
- Cyclessa Tablets 2450
- Desogen Tablets 2458
- Esclim Transdermal System 3460
- Estinyl Tablets 3112
- Estrace Vaginal Cream 3358
- Estrace Tablets 3361
- Estratest 3252
- Estrostep 2627
- femhrt Tablets 2635
- Levlen 962
- Levlite 21 Tablets 962
- Levlite 28 Tablets 962
- Levora Tablets 3389
- Loestrin 21 Tablets 2642
- Loestrin Fe Tablets 2642
- Lo/Ovral Tablets 3532
- Lo/Ovral-28 Tablets 3538
- Low-Ogestrel-28 Tablets 3392
- Lunelle Monthly Injection 2827
- Menest Tablets 2254
- Microgestin Fe 1.5/30 Tablets 3407
- Microgestin Fe 1/20 Tablets 3400
- Mircette Tablets 2470
- Modicon 2563
- Necon 3415
- Nolvadex Tablets (Rare) 678
- Nordette-28 Tablets 2257
- Norinyl 1 +35 28-Day Tablets 3380
- Norinyl 1 + 50 28-Day Tablets 3380
- Ogen Tablets 2846
- Ogestrel 0.5/50-28 Tablets 3428
- Ortho Dienestrol Cream 2554
- Ortho-Cept 21 Tablets 2546
- Ortho-Cept 28 Tablets 2546
- Ortho-Cyclen/Ortho Tri-Cyclen 2573
- Ortho-Est Tablets 3464
- Ortho-Novum 2563
- Ortho-Novum 1/50◻28 Tablets 2556
- Ortho-Prefest Tablets 2570
- Ortho-Cyclen/Ortho Tri-Cyclen 2573
- Ovcon 3364
- Ovral Tablets 3551
- Ovral-28 Tablets 3552
- Ovrette Tablets 3552
- Premarin Intravenous 3563
- Premarin Tablets 3566
- Premarin Vaginal Cream 3570
- Premphase Tablets 3572
- Prempro Tablets 3572
- Provera Tablets 2853
- Tri-Levlen 962
- Tri-Norinyl-28 Tablets 3433
- Triphasil-21 Tablets 3600
- Triphasil-28 Tablets 3605
- Trivora Tablets 3439
- Vivelle Transdermal System 2412
- Vivelle-Dot Transdermal System 2416
- Yasmin 28 Tablets 980
- Zovia 3449

Eruptions, herpetic

- ▲ Chemet Capsules (2.6% to 11.2%) 3078

Eruptions, lichenoid

- Plaquenil Tablets 3082

Eruptions, maculopapular

- Amaryl Tablets (Less than 1%) 717
- Bicillin C-R 900/300 Injection 2240
- Bicillin C-R Injection 2238
- Bicillin L-A Injection 2242
- DiaBeta Tablets (1.5%) 741
- Glucotrol Tablets (About 1 in 70) 2692
- Macrobid Capsules 2889
- Macrodantin Capsules 2891
- Mustargen for Injection (Occasional) 2142
- Pfizerpen for Injection 2707
- Plaquenil Tablets 3082
- Rifater Tablets 769

Eruptions, morbilliform

- Amaryl Tablets (Less than 1%) 717
- Ceclor (1 in 100) 1905
- DiaBeta Tablets (1.5%) 741
- Glucotrol Tablets (About 1 in 70) 2692
- Plaquenil Tablets 3082
- Rifater Tablets 769

Eruptions, mucocutaneous

- ▲ Chemet Capsules (2.6% to 11.2%) 3078

Eruptions, purpuric

- Plaquenil Tablets 3082
- Rifater Tablets 769

Eruptions, vascular

- Pipracil (Less frequent) 1866

Erythema

- Accutane Capsules 2944
- ▲ Acel-Imune (2% to 35%) 1851
- Aceon Tablets (2 mg, 4 mg, 8 mg) (0.3% to 1%) 3249
- Aclovate (Approximately 2%) 1275
- Acticin Cream (1% to 2%) 998
- Albuminar-5, U.S.P. 785
- Albuminar-25, U.S.P. 786
- ▲ Aldara Cream, 5% (1% to 61%) 1978
- Amaryl Tablets (Less than 1%) 717
- AmBisome for Injection (Infrequent) 1383
- Amerge Tablets (Infrequent) 1467
- Americaine Anesthetic Lubricant 1162
- Americaine Otic Topical Anesthetic Ear Drops 1162
- Apligraf (1.3%) 2305
- Aricept Tablets (Infrequent) 1270
- Aricept Tablets (Infrequent) 2665
- Ativan Injection 3478
- Avita Cream 999
- Avita Gel 1000
- Avonex 1013
- Axert Tablets (Rare) 2772
- Azelex Cream (Less than 1%) 547
- Bactroban Ointment (Less than 1%) 1496
- Benzaclin Topical Gel (2%) 1220
- Betoptic S Ophthalmic Suspension (Small number of patients) 537
- Brevibloc Injection (Less than 1%) 858
- Brevital Sodium for Injection, USP 1815
- Brevoxyl 3269
- ▲ Brevoxyl Cleansing (5 of 100 patients) 3269
- Brevoxyl 3270
- Cancidas for Injection (1.3% to 1.5%) 2048
- ▲ Carac Cream (93.4%) 1222
- ▲ Catapres-TTS (26 of 101 patients) 1038
- Ceftin Tablets (0.1% to 1%) 1898
- Cerumenex Eardrops (1% of 2,700 patients) 2895
- Cipro I.V. (1% or less) 893
- Cipro I.V. Pharmacy Bulk Package (Less than 1%) 897
- Claritin-D 12 Hour Extended Release Tablets (Less frequent) 3102
- ▲ Cleocin T Topical (7% to 16%) 2790
- Cleocin Vaginal Cream (Less than 1%) 2788
- ▲ Climara Transdermal System (9%) 958
- ▲ Clindets Pledgets (7% to 16%) 3270
- Clobevate Gel (Less than 2%) 3271
- Clomid Tablets 735
- Clozaril Tablets (Less than 1%) 2319
- Collagenase Santyl Ointment 3248
- Compazine 1505
- ▲ Condylox Gel (5%) 2436
- ▲ Copaxone for Injection (4%) 3306
- Cormax Cream (Approximately 0.3%) 2440
- Cormax Ointment (Approximately 0.3%) 2440
- Cortone Acetate Injectable Suspension 2059
- Cortone Acetate Tablets 2061
- Cosmegen for Injection 2062
- Cozaar Tablets (Less than 1%) 2067
- Cutivate Cream (1.6%) 1282
- Cutivate Ointment (Less than 1%) 1284
- Dantrium Intravenous (Rare) 2886
- Decadron Elixir 2078
- Decadron Tablets 2079
- Decadron Phosphate Injection 2081
- Desferal Vials 2333
- DesOwen (Less than 2%) 1401
- Detrol Tablets (1.9%) 3623
- DiaBeta Tablets (1.5%) 741
- ▲ Differin Cream (Less than 1% to 38%) 1402
- ▲ Differin Gel (10% to 40%) 1403
- Differin Solution/Pledgets (1% or less) 1404
- Digibind Powder (One patient) 1514
- Dipentum Capsules (Rare) 2803
- Diprivan Injectable Emulsion (Rare) 667
- Diprolene Gel 0.05% (Less frequent) 3107
- Diprolene Ointment 0.05% (3 per 767 patients) 3108
- ▲ Dovonex Ointment (1% to 10%) 1117
- ▲ Doxil Injection (3.4%) 566
- Duragesic Transdermal System (1% or greater) 1786
- Dynacin Capsules (Rare) 2019
- ▲ Efudex (Among most frequent) 1733
- 8-MOP Capsules 1727
- ELA-Max Cream 1340
- ELA-Max 5 Cream 1340
- Elimite Cream (1 to 2% or less) 552
- Emgel 2% Topical Gel (Occasional) 1285
- ▲ Emla (30% to 56%) 602
- Engerix-B Vaccine (Less than 1%) 1517
- Etrafon 3115
- Eulexin Capsules 3118
- Feldene Capsules (Occasional) 2685
- Finevin Cream (Less than 1%) 962
- Fortovase Capsules (Less than 2%) 2970
- Fosamax Tablets (Rare) 2095
- ▲ Sterile FUDR (Among more common) 2974
- Gammar-P I.V. 787
- Gastrocrom Oral Concentrate (Less common) 1162
- Glucotrol Tablets (About 1 in 70) 2692
- Heparin Lock Flush Solution 3509
- Heparin Sodium Injection 3511
- Hycamtin for Injection 1546
- Hydrocortone Tablets 2106
- Hydrocortone Acetate Injectable Suspension 2103
- Hydrocortone Phosphate Injection, Sterile 2105
- Hyzaar 2109
- Imitrex Injection (Infrequent) 1549
- Imitrex Nasal Spray 1554
- Imitrex Tablets (Infrequent) 1558
- ▲ Infergen (6%) 1777
- Intron A for Injection (Less than 5%) 3120
- Invirase Capsules (Less than 2%) 2979
- IPOL Vaccine (Up to 3.2%) 809
- Iscar Mali Injection 3456

Iscar Mali Special Injection 3456
Iscar Pini Injection 3456
Iscar Quercus Injection 3456
Iscar Quercus Special Injection 3456
Klaron Lotion 10% (One of 105 patients) 1224
▲ Lac-Hydrin Cream (Approximately 10% to 15%) 1118
▲ Lac-Hydrin Lotion (1 in 10 to 50 patients) 1119
Lamictal (Infrequent) 1567
▲ Leustatin Injection (6%) 2495
Levulan Kerastick 971
Lexxel Tablets 608
Lidoderm Patch 1319
Livostin (Approximately 1% to 3%) ⊙305
Lotrimin 3128
Lotrisone 3129
Lovenox Injection 746
Lupron Injection 3279
Maxalt Tablets (Infrequent) 2120
Maxalt-MLT Orally Disintegrating Tablets (Infrequent) 2120
Melanex Topical Solution 2300
▲ Menomune-A/C/Y/W-135 Vaccine (1.8% to 89%) 813
Mentax Cream (Less than 2%) 1009
Meruvax II 2130
MetroCream (Less than 3%) 1404
MetroGel 1405
MetroLotion 1405
▲ Miacalcin Nasal Spray (10.6%) 2375
Minocin Intravenous 1862
Minocin Oral Suspension 1865
Minocin Pellet-Filled Capsules 1863
M-M-R II 2118
Monodox Capsules 2442
Mylocel Tablets (Less frequently) 2227
▲ Nabi-HB (3%) 2295
Naftin Cream (2%) 2224
Naftin Gel (0.5%) 2224
Naropin Injection 612
Nesacaine/Nesacaine MPF 617
Nolvadex Tablets 678
Noroxin Tablets (Less frequent) 2145
Novantrone for Injection 1760
Olux Foam (Less than 2%) 1211
▲ Oncaspar (Greater than 5%) 756
Orthoclone OKT3 Sterile Solution (Less than 1%) 2498
Ovidrel for Injection 3220
Oxistat Cream (0.2%) 1298
Oxsoralen-Ultra Capsules 1741
Paraplatin for Injection 1126
▲ Photofrin for Injection (Approximately 20%) 831
Pipracil (2%) 1866
Plaquenil Tablets 3082
Plendil Extended-Release Tablets (0.5% to 1.5%) 623
Polocaine Injection, USP 625
Polocaine-MPF Injection, USP 625
Prednisone 3064
▲ Prevnar for Injection (12.4% to 15.2%) 1870
Prinivil Tablets (0.3% to 1.0%) 2164
Prinzide Tablets 2168
▲ Proleukin for Injection (41%) 1199
▲ Protopic Ointment (9% to 28%) 1397
Recombivax HB (Equal to or greater than 1%) 2178
▲ Renova 0.02% Cream (Almost all subjects) 2520
▲ Renova 0.05% Cream (Almost all subjects) 2519
Rescriptor Tablets (Less than 2%) 526
Retin-A Micro 0.1% 2522
Rifater Tablets 769
Robinul Injectable 2940
Sensorcaine (Rare) 643
Sensorcaine-MPF Injection (Rare) 643
Serentil 1057
Serophene Tablets 3226
Stelazine 1640
Sulfamylon Cream 1011
Sulfamylon Topical Solution 1011
▲ Sustiva Capsules (8.8% to 9.9%) 1258
Taxol Injection 1129
Taxotere for Injection Concentrate (0.9%) 778
▲ Tazorac Gel (10% to 30%) 556
▲ Temovate Gel (Among most frequent) 1303
Temovate Ointment (Less frequent) 1301
Temovate E Emollient (Less than 2%) 1302
▲ Testoderm Transdermal Systems (3%) 574
Tetanus Toxoid Adsorbed Purogenated 1882
Thioridazine Hydrochloride Tablets 2289
Topicort LP Cream (0.8%) 2025
Transderm Scōp Transdermal Therapeutic System (Infrequent) 2302
Trilafon 3160
▲ Tripedia Vaccine (3% to 25%) 817
▲ Trisenox Injection (13%) 1158
Twinrix Vaccine (Less than 1%) 1674
Ultravate Cream (Less frequent) 1119
Ultravate Ointment (Less frequent) 1120
Unasyn for Injection (Less than 1%) 2728
Vaniqa Cream (2.5%) 1121
Vaqta (Less than 1%) 2199
Vibramycin Hyclate Intravenous 2737
Vioxx (Greater than 0.1% to 1.9%) 2213
▲ Vivelle Transdermal System (One of the two most common) 2412
▲ Vivelle-Dot Transdermal System (One of the two most common) 2416
Xeloda Tablets 3039
Zestoretic Tablets 695
Zestril Tablets (0.3% to 1.0%) 698
▲ Zinecard for Injection (4% to 5%) 2869

Erythema, conjunctival

Neosporin Ophthalmic Ointment Sterile ⊙299
Neosporin Ophthalmic Solution Sterile ⊙300
▲ Polysporin Ophthalmic Ointment (Among those occurring most often) ⊙301
▲ Rēv-Eyes Sterile Ophthalmic Eyedrops 0.5% (10% to 40%) ⊙265
TobraDex Ophthalmic Ointment (Less than 4%) 542
TobraDex Ophthalmic Suspension (Less than 4%) 541
Tobrex Ophthalmic Ointment (Less than 3 of 100 patients) ⊙220
Tobrex Ophthalmic Solution (Less than 3 of 100 patients) ⊙221

Erythema, facial

Avalide Tablets 1070
Avapro Tablets (Less than 1%) 1074
Avapro Tablets (Less than 1%) 3076
▲ Carac Cream (89.4% to 96.5%) 1222
Celestone Soluspan Injectable Suspension 3097
Celestone Syrup 3099
Depo-Medrol Injectable Suspension 2795
Florinef Acetate Tablets 2250
Mylocel Tablets (Less frequently) 2227
Normodyne Tablets (Less common) 3137
Pediapred Oral Solution 1170
Prelone Syrup 2273
Solu-Medrol Sterile Powder 2855

Erythema, hemorrhagic exudative

(*see under* Henoch-Schönlein purpura)

Erythema, oral

Advair Diskus 100/50 (1% to 3%) 1448
Advair Diskus 250/50 (1% to 3%) 1448
Advair Diskus 500/50 (1% to 3%) 1448

Erythema, penile

▲ Caverject Sterile Powder (3%) 2777

Erythema, periungual

▲ Penlac (5%) 1225

Erythema at injection site

▲ ActHIB Vaccine (Up to 14.3%) 798
▲ Actimmune (14%) 1772
Aplisol Injection 2609
Attenuvax 2044
Azactam for Injection (0.5% to 2.9%) 1276
Cetrotide for Injection 3209
▲ Comvax (22.4% to 27.2%) 2056
Cortrosyn for Injection (Single instance) 2449
DDAVP Injection 4 mcg/mL (Occasional) 737
Desmopressin Acetate Injection (Occasional) 1344
▲ Diphtheria & Tetanus Toxoids Adsorbed Purogenated for Pediatric Use (7.6%) 1857
▲ Enbrel for Injection (37%) 1752
▲ Enbrel for Injection (37%) 3504
▲ Engerix-B Vaccine (1% to 10%) 1517
Floxin I.V. (Approximately 2%) 2526
FluShield Influenza Vaccine 3521
Gamimune N, 5% Solvent/Detergent Treated (Some cases) 925
Gamimune N, 10% Solvent/Detergent Treated (Some cases) 928
Gonal-F for Injection 3216
HibTITER (Less than 1% to 2.0%) 1859
▲ Imovax Rabies Vaccine (About 25%) 807
▲ Infergen (17% to 23%) 1777
Kogenate 934
▲ Leustatin Injection (9%) 2495
▲ Navelbine Injection (Approximately 1/3 of patients) 1604
Novantrone for Injection 1760
Liquid PedvaxHIB (0.4% to 2.2%) 2148
Pneumovax 23 (Common) 2156
Primaxin I.V. (0.4%) 2160
Saizen for Injection (Infrequent) 3225
Taxol Injection 1129
Taxotere for Injection Concentrate 778
▲ Tetanus & Diphtheria Toxoids Adsorbed for Adult Use (7.6%) 1880
▲ Tetanus and Diphtheria Toxoids Adsorbed For Adult Use (19%) 815
Tubersol Diagnostic Antigen (Infrequent) 3628
▲ TYPHIM Vi Vaccine (Up to 11%) 825
▲ Vaqta (0.8% to 13.1%) 2199
▲ Varivax (19.3% to 32.5%) 2202
Velosulin BR Human Insulin 10 ml Vials 2435

Erythema multiforme

Abelcet Injection 1273
Accuretic Tablets (0.5% to 1%) 2614
Acel-Imune 1851
Activella Tablets 2764
Aldoclor Tablets 2035
Aldoril Tablets 2039
Alesse-21 Tablets 3468
Alesse-28 Tablets 3473
Alora Transdermal System 3372
Altace Capsules (Less than 1%) 2233
Amoxil Chewable Tablets 1471
Amoxil for Oral Suspension 1471
Amoxil 1471
Anaprox Tablets (Less than 1%) 2967
Anaprox DS Tablets (Less than 1%) 2967
Arava Tablets (Rare) 724
Arthrotec Tablets (Rare) 3195
Atacand HCT Tablets 597
Atromid-S Capsules 3483
Attenuvax (Rare) 2044
Augmentin Chewable Tablets 1482
Augmentin Powder for Oral Suspension 1482
Augmentin Tablets 1485
Augmentin ES-600 Powder for Oral Suspension 1487
Avalide Tablets 1070
Azactam for Injection (Less than 1%) 1276
Azulfidine EN-tabs Tablets (Rare) 2775
Bactrim 2949
Baycol Tablets (Rare) 883
Brevicon 28-Day Tablets 3380
Captopril Tablets 2281
Carbatrol Capsules 3234
Cardizem Injectable 1018
Cardizem Lyo-Ject Syringe 1018
Cardizem Monovial 1018
Cardizem CD Capsules (Infrequent) 1016
Cataflam Tablets (Rare) 2315
Ceclor CD Tablets 1279
Ceclor 1905
Cefizox for Intramuscular or Intravenous Use 1390
Cefotan 664
Ceftin 1898
Cefzil (Rare) 1076
Celebrex Capsules (Less than 0.1%) 2676
Celebrex Capsules (Less than 0.1%) 2780
Celexa (At least 3 patients) 1365
Cenestin Tablets 1263
Ceptaz for Injection 1499
Chibroxin Sterile Ophthalmic Solution 2051
Cipro I.V. (1% or less) 893
Cipro I.V. Pharmacy Bulk Package (Less than 1%) 897
Cipro 887
Claritin (Rare) 3100
Claritin-D 12 Hour Extended Release Tablets 3102
Claritin-D 24 Hour Extended Release Tablets 3104
Cleocin HCl Capsules (Rare) 2784
Cleocin Phosphate Sterile Solution (Rare) 2785
Cleocin Vaginal Cream (Rare) 2788
Cleocin Vaginal Ovules (Rare) 2789
Climara Transdermal System 958
Clinoril Tablets (Less than 1%) 2053
Clomid Tablets 735
Clozaril Tablets 2319
Combivir Tablets 1502
Comvax 2056
Concerta Extended-Release Tablets 1998
Concerta Tablets 561
Covera-HS Tablets (Less than 2%) 3199
Crixivan Capsules 2070
Cyclessa Tablets 2450
Daraprim Tablets 1511
Depacon Injection 416
Depakene 421
Depakote Sprinkle Capsules 426
Depakote Tablets 430
Depakote ER Tablets 436
Desogen Tablets 2458
Diabinese Tablets 2680
Diamox ⊙269
Diovan HCT Tablets 2338
Diuril Oral 2087
Diuril Sodium Intravenous 2086
Dolobid Tablets (Less than 1 in 100) 2088
Doxil Injection (Less than 1%) 566
Duricef 1079
Dynacin Capsules 2019
EC-Naprosyn Delayed-Release Tablets (Less than 1%) 2967
E.E.S. (Rare) 450
Effexor Tablets 3495
Effexor XR Capsules 3499
Enalaprilat Injection 863
Engerix-B Vaccine (Less than 1%) 1517
EryPed (Rare) 446
Esclim Transdermal System 3460
Estinyl Tablets 3112
Estrace Vaginal Cream 3358
Estrace Tablets 3361
Estratest 3252
Estrostep 2627
Ethyol for Injection 2029
Feldene Capsules (Rare) 2685
femhrt Tablets 2635
Floxin I.V. 2526
Floxin Tablets 2529
Fortaz 1541
Foscavir Injection (Rare) 605
Furosemide Tablets 2284
Grifulvin V Tablets Microsize and Oral Suspension Microsize 2518
Gris-PEG Tablets (Occasional) 2661
Havrix Vaccine (Rare) 1544
HibTITER 1859
HydroDIURIL Tablets 2108
Hyzaar 2109
Indocin Capsules (Less than 1%) 2112
Indocin I.V. (Less than 1%) 2115
Indocin (Less than 1%) 2112
Isoptin SR Tablets (1% or less) 467
Keflex (Rare) 1237
Kefurox Vials, ADD-Vantage 1948
Lamictal 1567
Lariam Tablets 2989
Lescol Capsules (Rare) 2361
Lescol Capsules (Rare) 2925
Lescol XL Tablets 2361
Lescol XL Tablets 2925
Leukeran Tablets (Rare) 1591
Levaquin 2537
Levlen 962
Levlite 21 Tablets 962
Levlite 28 Tablets 962
Levora Tablets 3389
Lexxel Tablets 608
Lipitor Tablets 2639
Lipitor Tablets 2696
Lodine (Less than 1%) 3528
Lodine XL Extended-Release Tablets (Less than 1%) 3530
Loestrin 21 Tablets 2642
Loestrin Fe Tablets 2642
Lo/Ovral Tablets 3532
Lo/Ovral-28 Tablets 3538
Lorabid Suspension and Pulvules 2251
Low-Ogestrel-28 Tablets 3392
Lunelle Monthly Injection 2827
Lupron Depot-PED 7.5 mg, 11.25 mg and 15 mg (2%) 3291
Lupron Injection Pediatric 3280
Macrobid Capsules (Rare) 2889
Macrodantin Capsules (Rare) 2891
Maxipime for Injection 1285
Mefoxin for Injection 2124
Mefoxin Premixed Intravenous Solution 2127
Menest Tablets 2254
Mepron Suspension 1598
Merrem I.V. 673
Meruvax II (Rare) 2130
Metadate CD Capsules 1164
Metadate ER Tablets 1167
Methylin Tablets 1995
Methylin ER Tablets 1995
Mevacor Tablets (Rare) 2132
Micardis HCT Tablets 1051
Microgestin Fe 1.5/30 Tablets 3407
Microgestin Fe 1/20 Tablets 3400
Microzide Capsules 3414
Miltown Tablets (Rare) 3349
Minocin Intravenous 1862
Minocin Oral Suspension 1865
Minocin Pellet-Filled Capsules 1863
Mintezol 2137
Mircette Tablets 2470
M-M-R II (Rare) 2118
Mobic Tablets (Less than 0.1%) 1054
Modicon 2563
Moduretic Tablets 2138
Motrin Suspension, Oral Drops, Chewable Tablets, and Caplets (Less than 1%) 2002
Mumpsvax (Rare) 2141
Mustargen for Injection 2142
Myleran Tablets (Rare) 1603
▲ Naprelan Tablets (3% to 9%) 1293
Naprosyn Suspension (Less than 1%) 2967
Naprosyn Tablets (Less than 1%) 2967
Necon 3415
Neptazane Tablets ⊙271
Neurontin Capsules 2655
Neurontin Oral Solution 2655

Neurontin Tablets 2655
Nolvadex Tablets (Very rare) 678
Nordette-28 Tablets 2257
Norinyl 1 +35 28-Day Tablets 3380
Norinyl 1 + 50 28-Day Tablets 3380
Noroxin Tablets 2145
Norvasc Tablets (More than 0.1% to 1%) 2704
Ogen Tablets 2846
Ogestrel 0.5/50-28 Tablets 3428
Omnicef 493
Ortho Dienestrol Cream 2554
Ortho-Cept 21 Tablets 2546
Ortho-Cept 28 Tablets 2546
Ortho-Cyclen/Ortho Tri-Cyclen 2573
Ortho-Est Tablets 3464
Ortho-Novum 2563
Ortho-Novum 1/50▫28 Tablets 2556
Ortho-Prefest Tablets 2570
Ortho-Cyclen/Ortho Tri-Cyclen 2573
Orudis Capsules (Less than 1%) 3548
Oruvail Capsules (Less than 1%) 3548
Ovcon 3364
Ovral Tablets 3551
Ovral-28 Tablets 3552
Ovrette Tablets 3552
Paxil (Rare) 1609
PCE Dispertab Tablets (Rare) 498
Pediazole Suspension 3050
Phrenilin (Several cases) 578
Pipracil (Rare) 1866
Ponstel Capsules (Rare) 1356
Pravachol Tablets (Rare) 1099
Premarin Intravenous 3563
Premarin Tablets 3566
Premarin Vaginal Cream 3570
Premphase Tablets 3572
Prempro Tablets 3572
Prevnar for Injection 1870
PREVPAC 3298
Prilosec Delayed-Release Capsules (Very rare) 628
Primaxin I.M. 2158
Primaxin I.V. (Less than 0.2%) 2160
Prinzide Tablets 2168
ProAmatine Tablets (Rare) 3241
Procardia Capsules (Rare) 2708
Procardia XL Extended Release Tablets (Rare) 2710
Protonix I.V. 3580
Protonix Tablets 3577
Provera Tablets 2853
Relafen Tablets (Less than 1%) 1617
Rescriptor Tablets (Less than 2%) 526
Rifadin (Occasional) 765
Rilutek Tablets (Rare) 772
Ritalin 2387
Rocaltrol (One case) 2991
Sedapap Tablets 50 mg/650 mg (Several cases) 2225
Semprex-D Capsules (Rare) 1172
Septra Suspension 2265
Septra Tablets 2265
Septra DS Tablets 2265
Serophene Tablets 3226
Silvadene Cream 1% (Infrequent) 2267
Soma Tablets 3353
Soma Compound Tablets 3354
Soma Compound w/Codeine Tablets 3355
Suprax (Less than 2%) 1877
Sustiva Capsules (Up to 3.3%) 1258
Tagamet (Very rare) 1644
Talacen Caplets 3089
Talwin Nx Tablets 3090
Tarka Tablets 508
Tasmar Tablets (Infrequent) 3010
Tazicef for Injection 1647
Tazicef Galaxy Container 1650
Tazicef Pharmacy Bulk Package 1653
Tazidime Vials, Faspak & ADD-Vantage 1966
Tegretol/Tegretol-XR 2404
Tiazac Capsules (Infrequent) 1378
Ticlid Tablets (Rare) 3015
Timentin Injection- ADD-Vantage Vial 1661
Timentin Injection-Galaxy Container 1664
Timentin Injection-Pharmacy Bulk Package 1666
Timentin for Intravenous Administration 1658
Timolide Tablets 2187
Tolectin (Less than 1%) 2589
Tonocard Tablets (Less than 1%) 649
Trileptal Oral Suspension 2407
Trileptal Tablets 2407
Tri-Levlen 962
Trilisate (Rare) 2901
Tri-Norinyl-28 Tablets 3433
Triphasil-21 Tablets 3600
Triphasil-28 Tablets 3605
Trivora Tablets 3439
Trizivir Tablets 1669
Twinrix Vaccine 1674
Unasyn for Injection 2728
Valtrex Caplets 1676
Vantin Tablets and Oral Suspension 2860
Varivax 2202
Vaseretic Tablets 2204
Vasotec I.V. Injection 2207
Vasotec Tablets (0.5% to 1.0%) 2210
Verelan Capsules (1% or less) 3184
Verelan PM Capsules (2% or less) 3186
Vivelle Transdermal System 2412
Vivelle-Dot Transdermal System 2416
Voltaren Tablets (Rare) 2315
Voltaren-XR Tablets (Rare) 2315
Wellbutrin Tablets (Rare) 1680
Wellbutrin SR Sustained-Release Tablets (Rare) 1684
Yasmin 28 Tablets 980
Zantac (Rare) 1690
Zantac Injection (Rare) 1688
Zantac Syrup (Rare) 1690
Zestoretic Tablets 695
Zinacef Injection (Rare) 1696
Zinacef for Injection (Rare) 1696
Zithromax Capsules, 250 mg (Rare) 2743
Zithromax for IV Infusion (Rare) 2748
Zithromax for Oral Suspension, 300 mg, 600 mg, 900 mg, 1200 mg (Rare) 2739
Zithromax Tablets, 250 mg (Rare) 2739
Zocor Tablets (Rare) 2219
Zosyn (Rare) 1890
Zosyn in Galaxy Containers (Rare) 1894
Zovia 3449
Zovirax Capsules 1706
Zovirax for Injection 1708
Zovirax 1706
Zyban Sustained-Release Tablets (Rare) 1710

Erythema nodosum
Accutane Capsules 2944
Activella Tablets 2764
Alesse-21 Tablets 3468
Alesse-28 Tablets 3473
Alora Transdermal System 3372
Asacol Delayed-Release Tablets 2884
Betaseron for SC Injection 988
Brevicon 28-Day Tablets 3380
Carbatrol Capsules 3234
Cenestin Tablets 1263
Cipro I.V. (1% or less) 893
Cipro I.V. Pharmacy Bulk Package (Less than 1%) 897
Cipro (Less than 1%) 887
Climara Transdermal System 958
Clomid Tablets 735
Colazal Capsules 3069
Copaxone for Injection (Infrequent) 3306
Cyclessa Tablets 2450
Depakote ER Tablets (Greater than 1%) 436
Desogen Tablets 2458
Dipentum Capsules (Rare) 2803
Doxil Injection (Less than 1%) 566
Effexor Tablets (Rare) 3495
Effexor XR Capsules (Rare) 3499
Engerix-B Vaccine (Less than 1%) 1517
Esclim Transdermal System 3460
Estinyl Tablets 3112
Estrace Vaginal Cream 3358
Estrace Tablets 3361
Estratest 3252
Estrostep 2627
femhrt Tablets 2635
Floxin I.V. 2526
Floxin Tablets 2529
Indocin Capsules (Less than 1%) 2112
Indocin I.V. (Less than 1%) 2115
Indocin (Less than 1%) 2112
Intron A for Injection (Less than 5%) 3120
Levaquin (Less than 0.3%) 2537
Levlen 962
Levlite 21 Tablets 962
Levlite 28 Tablets 962
Levora Tablets 3389
Loestrin 21 Tablets 2642
Loestrin Fe Tablets 2642
Lo/Ovral Tablets 3532
Lo/Ovral-28 Tablets 3538
Low-Ogestrel-28 Tablets 3392
Lunelle Monthly Injection 2827
Menest Tablets 2254
Microgestin Fe 1.5/30 Tablets 3407
Microgestin Fe 1/20 Tablets 3400
Mircette Tablets 2470
Modicon 2563
Myleran Tablets (Rare) 1603
Necon 3415
Neupogen for Injection (One event) 587
Nordette-28 Tablets 2257
Norinyl 1 +35 28-Day Tablets 3380
Norinyl 1 + 50 28-Day Tablets 3380
Ogen Tablets 2846
Ogestrel 0.5/50-28 Tablets 3428
Omnicef 493
Ortho Dienestrol Cream 2554
Ortho-Cept 21 Tablets 2546
Ortho-Cept 28 Tablets 2546
Ortho-Cyclen/Ortho Tri-Cyclen 2573
Ortho-Est Tablets 3464
Ortho-Novum 2563
Ortho-Novum 1/50▫28 Tablets 2556
Ortho-Prefest Tablets 2570
Ortho-Cyclen/Ortho Tri-Cyclen 2573
Ovcon 3364
Ovral Tablets 3551
Ovral-28 Tablets 3552
Ovrette Tablets 3552
Paxil (Rare) 1609
Pentasa Capsules (Less than 1%) 3239
Premarin Intravenous 3563
Premarin Tablets 3566
Premarin Vaginal Cream 3570
Premphase Tablets 3572
Prempro Tablets 3572
Provera Tablets 2853
Prozac Pulvules, Liquid, and Weekly Capsules 1238
Recombivax HB (Less than 1%) 2178
Salagen Tablets (Less than 1%) 2229
Sarafem Pulvules 1962
Serophene Tablets 3226
Tegretol/Tegretol-XR 2404
Thalomid Capsules 1154
Tri-Levlen 962
Tri-Norinyl-28 Tablets 3433
Triphasil-21 Tablets 3600
Triphasil-28 Tablets 3605
Trivora Tablets 3439
Twinrix Vaccine 1674
Uniretic Tablets (Less than 1%) 3178
Vesanoid Capsules (Isolated cases) 3037
Vivelle Transdermal System 2412
Vivelle-Dot Transdermal System 2416
Yasmin 28 Tablets 980
Zovia 3449

Erythema simplex
Oncaspar (Less than 1%) 756

Erythematous streaking
Adriamycin PFS/RDF Injection 2767
▲ Zinecard for Injection (4% to 5%) 2869

Erythrocytes, abnormal
Ceclor CD Tablets (0.3%) 1279
▲ Ferrlecit Injection (11%) 3386
Gabitril Tablets (Infrequent) 1189
Paxil (Rare) 1609
Uniretic Tablets (Less than 1%) 3178

Erythrocytes, vacuolation of
Pyrazinamide Tablets (Rare) 1876
Rifater Tablets (Rare) 769

Erythrocytosis
Moban 1320
Pergonal for Injection (One patient) 3223
Repronex for Intramuscular and Subcutaneous Injection (One patient) 1347

Erythroderma, exfoliative
Tagamet 1644

Erythroid hyperplasia
Pyrazinamide Tablets (Rare) 1876
Rifater Tablets (Rare) 769

Erythroleukemia
Thalomid Capsules 1154

Erythromelalgia
Adalat CC Tablets (Rare) 877
Procardia Capsules (Approximately 0.5%) 2708

Erythropenia
Accutane Capsules 2944
Aricept Tablets (Infrequent) 1270
Aricept Tablets (Infrequent) 2665
Dopram Injectable 2931
Haldol Decanoate 2535
Moban 1320
Mustargen for Injection 2142
Primaxin I.M. 2158
Unasyn for Injection 2728

Escharotic effect
Cetacaine Topical Anesthetic 1196

Esophageal disease, unspecified
Myleran Tablets 1603
Nexium Delayed-Release Capsules (Less than 1%) 619

Esophageal erosions
Fosamax Tablets 2095

Esophageal perforation
Celebrex Capsules (Less than 0.1%) 2676
Celebrex Capsules (Less than 0.1%) 2780
Fosamax Tablets 2095
GoLYTELY and Pineapple Flavor GoLYTELY for Oral Solution 1068
NuLYTELY, Cherry Flavor, Lemon-Lime Flavor, and Orange Flavor NuLYTELY for Oral Solution 1068
Reminyl Oral Solution (Rare) 1792
Reminyl Tablets (Rare) 1792

Esophageal rupture
Exelon Capsules (One case) 2342
Exelon Oral Solution (One case) 2345

Esophageal stenosis
Actiq (Less than 1%) 1184
Rilutek Tablets (Infrequent) 772

Esophageal stricture
Evoxac Capsules (Less than 1%) 1217
Fosamax Tablets (Rare) 2095
Lodine (Less than 1%) 3528
Lodine XL Extended-Release Tablets (Less than 1%) 3530
Nexium Delayed-Release Capsules (Less than 1%) 619
▲ Photofrin for Injection (6%) 831
Prevacid Delayed-Release Capsules (Less than 1%) 3292
PREVPAC (Less than 1%) 3298

Esophageal ulceration
Arthrotec Tablets (Rare) 3195
Mexitil Capsules (About 1 in 10,000) 1047
Micro-K 3311
Minocin Pellet-Filled Capsules (Rare) 1863
Pediapred Oral Solution 1170
Prevacid Delayed-Release Capsules (Less than 1%) 3292
PREVPAC (Less than 1%) 3298

Esophagitis
Accuretic Tablets 2614
Aciphex Tablets 1267
Aciphex Tablets 1783
Actiq (Less than 1%) 1184
Adalat CC Tablets (Less than 1.0%) 877
Adriamycin PFS/RDF Injection 2767
Amerge Tablets (Rare) 1467
Arava Tablets (1% to 3%) 724
Arthrotec Tablets (Rare) 3195
Betaseron for SC Injection 988
Campath Ampules 992
Celebrex Capsules (0.1% to 1.9%) 2676
Celebrex Capsules (0.1% to 1.9%) 2780
Celexa (Infrequent) 1365
▲ CellCept Capsules (3%) 2951
▲ CellCept Intravenous (3%) 2951
▲ CellCept Oral Suspension (3%) 2951
▲ CellCept Tablets (3%) 2951
Cleocin Vaginal Cream 2788
Cleocin Vaginal Ovules 2789
Cognex Capsules (Infrequent) 1351
Copaxone for Injection (Infrequent) 3306
Cosmegen for Injection 2062
Didronel Tablets 2888
Doryx Coated Pellet Filled Capsules 3357
Doxil Injection (1% to 5%) 566
Dynacin Capsules (Rare) 2019
Effexor Tablets (Infrequent) 3495
Effexor XR Capsules (Infrequent) 3499
Elmiron Capsules (Less than or equal to 1%) 570
Enbrel for Injection 1752
Enbrel for Injection 3504
Evoxac Capsules (Less than 1%) 1217
Exelon Capsules (Infrequent) 2342
Exelon Oral Solution (Infrequent) 2345
Felbatol (Infrequent) 3343
Feldene Capsules (Occasional) 2685
Fludara for Injection (Up to 3%) 995
Fortovase Capsules (Less than 2%) 2970
Fosamax Tablets 2095
Gabitril Tablets (Infrequent) 1189
Gengraf Capsules (1% to less than 3%) 457
Hivid Tablets (Less than 1%) 2975
Intron A for Injection (Less than 5%) 3120
Invirase Capsules (Less than 2%) 2979
Kaletra Capsules (Less than 2%) 471
Kaletra Oral Solution (Less than 2%) 471
Lamictal 1567
Lipitor Tablets (Less than 2%) 2639
Lipitor Tablets (Less than 2%) 2696
Lodine (Less than 1%) 3528
Lodine XL Extended-Release Tablets (Less than 1%) 3530
Lotrel Capsules 2370
Luvox Tablets (25, 50, 100 mg) (Infrequent) 3256
Minocin Pellet-Filled Capsules (Rare) 1863
Mobic Tablets (Less than 2%) 1054
Monodox Capsules (Rare) 2442
Monopril HCT (Less than 2%) 1094

Motrin Suspension, Oral Drops, Chewable Tablets, and Caplets (Less than 1%)........ 2002
Naprelan Tablets (Less than 1%)..... 1293
Navelbine Injection........ 1604
Neoral Soft Gelatin Capsules (1% to less than 3%)........ 2380
Neoral Oral Solution (1% to less than 3%)........ 2380
Neurontin Capsules (Rare)........ 2655
Neurontin Oral Solution (Rare)........ 2655
Neurontin Tablets (Rare)........ 2655
Nexium Delayed-Release Capsules (Less than 1%)........ 619
Norvir Capsules (Less than 2%)...... 487
Norvir Oral Solution (Less than 2%)........ 487
Paxil (Rare)........ 1609
Periostat Tablets (Rare)........ 1208
Permax Tablets (Infrequent)........ 1299
▲ Photofrin for Injection (5%)........ 831
Pletal Tablets (Less than 2%)........ 2605
Pletal Tablets (Less than 2%)........ 2848
Ponstel Capsules (Occasional)........ 1356
Prevacid Delayed-Release Capsules (Less than 1%)........ 3292
PREVPAC (Less than 1%)........ 3298
Priftin Tablets (Less than 1%)........ 758
▲ Prograf (3% to 15%)........ 1393
Protonix I.V. (Less than 1%)........ 3580
Protonix Tablets (Less than 1%)........ 3577
Prozac Pulvules, Liquid, and Weekly Capsules (Infrequent)........ 1238
▲ Quinaglute Dura-Tabs Tablets (Among most frequent)........ 978
▲ Quinidex Extentabs (Among most frequent)........ 2933
▲ Rapamune Oral Solution and Tablets (3% to 20%)........ 3584
Requip Tablets (Infrequent)........ 1621
Rescriptor Tablets (Less than 2%)... 526
Risperdal (Rare)........ 1796
Rythmol Tablets – 150 mg, 225 mg, 300 mg (1.9%)........ 502
Salagen Tablets (Less than 1%)........ 2229
Sarafem Pulvules (Infrequent)........ 1962
▲ Serostim for Injection (1% to 10%).. 3229
Serzone Tablets (Infrequent)........ 1104
▲ Simulect for Injection (3% to 10%).. 2399
Skelid Tablets........ 3088
Sonata Capsules (Infrequent)........ 3591
Soriatane Capsules (Less than 1%)........ 3003
Tasmar Tablets (Infrequent)........ 3010
Taxotere for Injection Concentrate .. 778
Teveten Tablets (Less than 1%)........ 3327
Thalomid Capsules........ 1154
Topamax Sprinkle Capsules (Infrequent)........ 2590
Topamax Tablets (Infrequent)........ 2590
Tricor Capsules, Micronized........ 513
Trileptal Oral Suspension........ 2407
Trileptal Tablets........ 2407
Trilisate (Rare)........ 2901
Uniretic Tablets (Less than 1%)........ 3178
Urobiotic-250 Capsules (Rare)........ 2731
Viagra Tablets (Less than 2%)........ 2732
Vibramycin Hyclate Capsules (Rare)........ 2735
Vibra-Tabs Film Coated Tablets (Rare)........ 2735
Vicoprofen Tablets (Less than 1%).. 520
Vioxx (Greater than 0.1% to 1.9%).. 2213
Vistide Injection........ 1445
Wellbutrin Tablets........ 1680
Wellbutrin SR Sustained-Release Tablets........ 1684
Xeloda Tablets (Less than 5%)........ 3039
▲ Zinecard for Injection (3% to 6%)........ 2869
Zoloft (Infrequent)........ 2751
Zomig Tablets (Infrequent)........ 708
Zomig-ZMT Tablets (Infrequent)........ 708
Zonegran Capsules (Rare)........ 1307
Zyban Sustained-Release Tablets........ 1710
Zyprexa Tablets (Infrequent)........ 1973
Zyprexa ZYDIS Orally Disintegrating Tablets (Infrequent)........ 1973

Esophagitis, ulcerative

Celestone Soluspan Injectable Suspension........ 3097
Celestone Syrup........ 3099
Cortone Acetate Injectable Suspension........ 2059
Cortone Acetate Tablets........ 2061
Decadron Elixir........ 2078
Decadron Tablets........ 2079
Decadron Phosphate Injection........ 2081
Depo-Medrol Injectable Suspension........ 2795
Doryx Coated Pellet Filled Capsules........ 3357
Dynacin Capsules (Rare)........ 2019
Florinef Acetate Tablets........ 2250
Hydrocortone Tablets........ 2106
Hydrocortone Acetate Injectable Suspension........ 2103
Hydrocortone Phosphate Injection, Sterile........ 2105
Indocin I.V. (Less than 1%)........ 2115
Monodox Capsules (Rare)........ 2442
Prednisone........ 3064
Prelone Syrup........ 2273
Solu-Medrol Sterile Powder........ 2855
Vibramycin Calcium Oral Suspension Syrup (Rare)........ 2735
Vibramycin Hyclate Capsules (Rare)........ 2735
Vibramycin Monohydrate for Oral Suspension (Rare)........ 2735
Vibra-Tabs Film Coated Tablets (Rare)........ 2735

Esophagopharyngitis

Ergamisol Tablets........ 1789
Sterile FUDR........ 2974

Esophagospasm

Ambien Tablets (Rare)........ 3191
Gastrocrom Oral Concentrate........ 1162
Migranal Nasal Spray (Rare)........ 2376
Neurontin Capsules (Rare)........ 2655
Neurontin Oral Solution (Rare)........ 2655
Neurontin Tablets (Rare)........ 2655

ESR, elevation

Accutane Capsules........ 2944
Aceon Tablets (2 mg, 4 mg, 8 mg)........ 3249
Altace Capsules (Less than 1%)........ 2233
Ambien Tablets (Rare)........ 3191
Baycol Tablets (Rare)........ 883
Captopril Tablets........ 2281
Cipro I.V. (Rare)........ 893
Cipro I.V. Pharmacy Bulk Package (Rare)........ 897
Clozaril Tablets........ 2319
Comvax........ 2056
Cytotec Tablets (Infrequent)........ 3202
Enalaprilat Injection........ 863
Floxin I.V. (More than or equal to 1%)........ 2526
Floxin Tablets (More than or equal to 1%)........ 2529
Lescol Capsules (Rare)........ 2361
Lescol Capsules (Rare)........ 2925
Lescol XL Tablets........ 2361
Lescol XL Tablets........ 2925
Lexxel Tablets........ 608
Mevacor Tablets (Rare)........ 2132
Monopril Tablets........ 1091
Monopril HCT........ 1094
Pravachol Tablets (Rare)........ 1099
Prinivil Tablets (0.3% to 1.0%)........ 2164
Prinzide Tablets........ 2168
Recombivax HB........ 2178
Vaseretic Tablets........ 2204
Vasotec I.V. Injection........ 2207
Vasotec Tablets (0.5% to 1.0%)........ 2210
Zestoretic Tablets........ 695
Zestril Tablets (0.3% to 1.0%)........ 698
Zocor Tablets (Rare)........ 2219

ESR decrease

Thalomid Capsules........ 1154

Euphoria

Actiq (Less than 1%)........ 1184
Adderall Tablets........ 3231
Adderall XR Capsules
Adipex-P........ 1406
Akineton........ 402
Ambien Tablets (Frequent)........ 3191
Artane........ 1855
Axert Tablets (Rare)........ 2772
Benadryl Parenteral........ 2617
Betaseron for SC Injection........ 988
Bicillin C-R 900/300 Injection........ 2240
Bicillin C-R Injection........ 2238
Bicillin L-A Injection........ 2242
Celestone Soluspan Injectable Suspension........ 3097
Celexa (Infrequent)........ 1365
Claritin-D 12 Hour Extended Release Tablets (Less frequent)... 3102
Claritin-D 24 Hour Extended Release Tablets (Fewer than 2%)........ 3104
Copaxone for Injection (At least 2%)........ 3306
Cortone Acetate Injectable Suspension........ 2059
Cortone Acetate Tablets........ 2061
Darvon-N/Darvocet-N........ 1907
Darvon Pulvules........ 1909
Darvon Compound-65 Pulvules........ 1910
Darvon-N Tablets........ 1912
Decadron Elixir........ 2078
Decadron Tablets........ 2079
Decadron Phosphate Injection........ 2081
Demerol........ 3079
Depacon Injection (0.9%)........ 416
Desoxyn Tablets........ 440
Dexedrine........ 1512
DextroStat Tablets........ 3236
Dilaudid Oral Liquid........ 445
Dilaudid Tablets - 8 mg........ 445
Dilaudid-HP (Less frequent)........ 443
Diprivan Injectable Emulsion (Less than 1%)........ 667
Dolophine Hydrochloride Tablets........ 3056
▲ Duragesic Transdermal System (3% to 10%)........ 1786
Duramorph Injection........ 1312
Duranest Injections........ 600
Effexor Tablets (Infrequent)........ 3495
Effexor XR Capsules (Infrequent)........ 3499
ELA-Max Cream........ 1340
Eldepryl Capsules........ 3266
Emla (Unlikely with cream)........ 602
Ergamisol Tablets........ 1789
Felbatol (Infrequent)........ 3343
Floxin I.V. (Less than 1%)........ 2526
Floxin Tablets (Less than 1%)........ 2529
Flumadine (Less than 0.3%)........ 1370
Fortovase Capsules (Less than 2%)........ 2970
Sterile FUDR (Remote possibility)........ 2974
Gabitril Tablets (Frequent)........ 1189
Halcion Tablets (0.5% to 0.9%)........ 2823
Haldol Decanoate........ 2535
Haldol Injection, Tablets and Concentrate........ 2533
Hivid Tablets (Less than 1%)........ 2975
Hydrocortone Tablets........ 2106
Hydrocortone Acetate Injectable Suspension........ 2103
Hydrocortone Phosphate Injection, Sterile........ 2105
Imitrex Injection (Infrequent)........ 1549
Imitrex Nasal Spray (Infrequent)........ 1554
Imitrex Tablets (Infrequent)........ 1558
Infumorph 200 and Infumorph 500 Sterile Solutions........ 1314
Invirase Capsules (Less than 2%)........ 2979
Ionamin Capsules........ 1163
Kadian Capsules (Less than 3%)........ 1335
Lamictal (Infrequent)........ 1567
Levsin/Levsinex/Levbid........ 3172
Lidoderm Patch........ 1319
Limbitrol........ 1738
Lodosyn Tablets........ 1251
Luvox Tablets (25, 50, 100 mg) (Infrequent)........ 3256
▲ Marinol Capsules (3% to 10%)........ 3325
Maxalt Tablets (Frequent)........ 2120
Maxalt-MLT Orally Disintegrating Tablets (Frequent)........ 2120
Mepergan Injection........ 3539
Migranal Nasal Spray (Infrequent)........ 2376
Miltown Tablets........ 3349
Moban (Less frequent)........ 1320
Motofen Tablets........ 577
▲ MS Contin Tablets (Among most frequent)........ 2896
▲ MSIR (Among most frequent)........ 2898
Nardil Tablets (Less common)........ 2653
Neurontin Capsules (Infrequent)........ 2655
Neurontin Oral Solution (Infrequent)........ 2655
Neurontin Tablets (Infrequent)........ 2655
Norvir Capsules (Less than 2%)........ 487
Norvir Oral Solution (Less than 2%)........ 487
Nubain Injection (1% or less)........ 1323
Numorphan........ 1324
▲ Oramorph SR Tablets (Among most frequent)........ 3062
OxyContin Tablets (Between 1% and 5%)........ 2912
OxyFast Oral Concentrate Solution........ 2916
OxyIR Capsules........ 2916
Paxil (Rare)........ 1609
Percocet Tablets........ 1326
Percodan Tablets........ 1327
Percolone Tablets........ 1327
Periactin Tablets........ 2155
Permax Tablets (Infrequent)........ 1299
Phenergan Injection........ 3553
Phenergan........ 3556
Phenergan with Codeine Syrup........ 3557
Phenergan VC with Codeine Syrup.. 3561
Phrenilin (Infrequent)........ 578
Prednisone........ 3064
Prelone Syrup........ 2273
ProSom Tablets (Infrequent)........ 500
Prozac Pulvules, Liquid, and Weekly Capsules (Infrequent)........ 1238
Remeron Tablets (Infrequent)........ 2483
Remeron SolTab Tablets (Infrequent)........ 2486
Requip Tablets (Infrequent)........ 1621
Rescriptor Tablets........ 526
Rilutek Tablets (Rare)........ 772
Risperdal (Infrequent)........ 1796
Romazicon Injection (1% to 3%)........ 3000
Roxanol........ 3066
Roxicodone........ 3067
Rynatan Tablets........ 3351
Sarafem Pulvules (Infrequent)........ 1962
Sedapap Tablets 50 mg/650 mg (Infrequent)........ 2225
Seroquel Tablets (Rare)........ 684
Serzone Tablets (Infrequent)........ 1104
Sinemet Tablets........ 1253
Sinemet CR Tablets........ 1255
Solu-Medrol Sterile Powder........ 2855
Soma Tablets........ 3353
Soma Compound Tablets (Very rare)........ 3354
Soma Compound w/Codeine Tablets........ 3355
Sonata Capsules (Frequent)........ 3591
Stadol NS Nasal Spray (1% or greater)........ 1108
Sustiva Capsules (Less than 2%)........ 1258
Symmetrel (0.1% to 1%)........ 1328
Talacen Caplets........ 3089
Talwin Nx Tablets........ 3090
Tambocor Tablets (Less than 1%)........ 1990
Tasmar Tablets (1%)........ 3010
Tequin Injection (Less than 0.1%)........ 1110
Tequin Tablets (Less than 0.1%)........ 1110
Thalomid Capsules........ 1154
Topamax Sprinkle Capsules (Frequent)........ 2590
Topamax Tablets (Frequent)........ 2590
Toradol (1% or less)........ 3018
Trileptal Oral Suspension........ 2407
Trileptal Tablets........ 2407
Trovan (Less than 1%)........ 2722
Tussionex Pennkinetic Extended-Release Suspension........ 1174
Tussi-Organidin NR Liquid........ 3350
Tussi-Organidin-S NR Liquid........ 3350
Tylenol with Codeine........ 2595
Tylox Capsules........ 2597
Ultracet Tablets (At least 1%)........ 2597
▲ Ultram Tablets (1% to 14%)........ 2600
Versed Injection (Less than 1%)........ 3027
Vicoprofen Tablets (Less than 1%).. 520
Wellbutrin Tablets (1.2%)........ 1680
Wellbutrin SR Sustained-Release Tablets........ 1684
▲ Xylocaine Injections (Among most common)........ 653
Zanaflex Tablets (Infrequent)........ 1305
Zarontin Capsules........ 2659
Zarontin Syrup........ 2660
Zoloft (Infrequent)........ 2751
Zomig Tablets (Rare)........ 708
Zomig-ZMT Tablets (Rare)........ 708
Zonegran Capsules (Infrequent)........ 1307
Zyban Sustained-Release Tablets........ 1710
Zyprexa Tablets (2%)........ 1973
Zyprexa ZYDIS Orally Disintegrating Tablets (2%)........ 1973
Zyrtec (Less than 2%)........ 2756
Zyrtec-D 12 Hour Extended Relief Tablets (Less than 2%)........ 2758

Eustachian tube dysfunction

Neurontin Capsules (Rare)........ 2655
Neurontin Oral Solution (Rare)........ 2655
Neurontin Tablets (Rare)........ 2655

Exanthema

Copaxone for Injection (Infrequent)........ 3306
Covera-HS Tablets (Less than 2%).. 3199
Isoptin SR Tablets (1% or less)........ 467
Tarka Tablets........ 508
Verelan Capsules (1% or less)........ 3184
Verelan PM Capsules (2% or less)... 3186

Excitability

Actifed Cold & Allergy Tablets........ ■688
Actifed Cold & Sinus Caplets and Tablets........ ■688
Alka-Seltzer Plus Liqui-Gels........ ■604
Anadrol-50 Tablets........ 3321
Astramorph/PF Injection, USP (Preservative-Free)........ 594
Benadryl Allergy Chewables........ ■689
Benadryl Allergy Kapseal Capsules........ ■691
Benadryl Allergy Liquid........ ■690
Benadryl Allergy Ultratab Tablets... ■691
Benadryl Allergy/Congestion Tablets........ ■692
Benadryl Allergy & Sinus Liquid........ ■693
Benadryl Dye-Free Allergy Liquid... ■690
Benadryl Dye-Free Allergy Liqui-Gels Softgels........ ■690
Benadryl Parenteral........ 2617
Bromfed Capsules (Extended-Release)........ 2269
Bromfed-PD Capsules (Extended-Release)........ 2269
Chlor-Trimeton Allergy Tablets........ ■735
Claritin-D 12 Hour Extended Release Tablets........ 3102
Claritin-D 24 Hour Extended Release Tablets........ 3104
Cogentin........ 2055
Comtrex Acute Head Cold & Sinus Pressure Relief Tablets........ ■627
Comtrex Flu Therapy & Fever Relief Nighttime Tablets........ ■628
Contac Severe Cold and Flu Caplets Maximum Strength........ ■746
Coricidin 'D' Cold, Flu & Sinus Tablets........ ■737
Coricidin/Coricidin D........ ■738
Crixivan Capsules (Less than 2%)... 2070
Dimetapp Elixir........ ■777
Dimetapp Cold and Fever Suspension........ ■775
Donnatal (In elderly patients)........ 2929
Donnatal Extentabs (In elderly patients)........ 2930

Donnatal Tablets (In elderly patients).... 2929
Drixoral Allergy/Sinus Extended-Release Tablets.... ■741
Drixoral Cold & Allergy Sustained-Action Tablets.... ■740
Drixoral Cold & Flu Extended-Release Tablets.... ■740
Duramorph Injection.... 1312
Etrafon.... 3115
Extendryl.... 1361
Flexeril Tablets (Less than 1%).... 572
Flexeril Tablets (Less than 1%).... 2094
Guaifed.... 2272
Infumorph 200 and Infumorph 500 Sterile Solutions.... 1314
Klonopin Tablets (Infrequent).... 2983
Levsin/Levsinex/Levbid.... 3172
Narcan Injection.... 1322
Naropin Injection.... 612
Nesacaine/Nesacaine MPF.... 617
NuLev Orally Disintegrating Tablets.... 3176
Orap Tablets.... 1407
Orudis Capsules (Greater than 1%).... 3548
Oruvail Capsules (Greater than 1%).... 3548
Oxandrin Tablets.... 1153
PediaCare Cough-Cold Liquid.... ■719
PediaCare NightRest Cough-Cold Liquid.... ■719
Periactin Tablets.... 2155
Phenergan Injection.... 3553
Phenergan.... 3556
Phrenilin (Infrequent).... 578
Polocaine Injection, USP.... 625
Polocaine-MPF Injection, USP.... 625
Protopam Chloride for Injection (Several cases).... 3582
Robinul Injectable.... 2940
Robitussin Nighttime Honey Flu Liquid.... ■786
Ryna.... ■768
Ryna-12 S Suspension.... 3351
Reformulated Rynatan Pediatric Suspension.... 3352
Rynatan Tablets.... 3351
Rynatuss Pediatric Suspension.... 3353
Rynatuss Tablets.... 3353
Sedapap Tablets 50 mg/650 mg (Infrequent).... 2225
Sensorcaine.... 643
Sensorcaine-MPF Injection.... 643
Serentil.... 1057
Serevent Inhalation Aerosol.... 1633
Singlet Caplets.... ■761
Sudafed Cold & Allergy Tablets.... ■708
Talacen Caplets (Rare).... 3089
Talwin Nx Tablets.... 3090
TheraFlu Regular Strength Cold & Cough Night Time Hot Liquid.... ■676
TheraFlu Regular Strength Cold & Sore Throat Night Time Hot Liquid.... ■676
TheraFlu Maximum Strength Severe Cold & Congestion Night Time Caplets.... ■678
Triaminic Cold & Allergy Softchews.... ■683
Triaminic Cold & Cough Softchews.... ■683
Children's Tylenol Cold Suspension Liquid and Chewable Tablets.... 2015
Children's Tylenol Cold Plus Cough Suspension Liquid and Chewable Tablets.... 2015
Maximum Strength Tylenol Allergy Sinus Caplets, Gelcaps, and Geltabs.... 2010
Multi-Symptom Tylenol Cold Complete Formula Caplets.... 2010
Maximum Strength Tylenol Flu NightTime Gelcaps.... 2011
Maximum Strength Tylenol Flu NightTime Liquid.... 2011
Pediatric Vicks 44m Cough & Cold Relief.... ■728
Children's Vicks NyQuil Cold/Cough Relief.... ■726
Vicks NyQuil LiquiCaps/Liquid Multi-Symptom Cold/Flu Relief, Original and Cherry Flavors.... ■727
Zephrex Tablets.... 3091
Zephrex LA Tablets.... 3092
Zyrtec-D 12 Hour Extended Relief Tablets.... 2758

Excitement, paradoxical
Etrafon.... 3115
Halcion Tablets.... 2823
Librium Capsules.... 1736
Miltown Tablets.... 3349
ProSom Tablets.... 500
Valium Injectable.... 3026
Valium Tablets.... 3047
Versed Syrup (Less than 1%).... 3033

Excoriation
▲ Aldara Cream, 5% (Up to 25%).... 1978
Catapres-TTS (3 of 101 patients).... 1038
Levulan Kerastick (Up to 1%).... 971
Sulfamylon Cream (Rare).... 1011

Exercise tolerance, decreased
Blocadren Tablets.... 2046
Cosopt Sterile Ophthalmic Solution.... 2065
Timolol GFS.... ⊙266
Timoptic in Ocudose (Less frequent).... 2192
Timoptic Sterile Ophthalmic Solution (Less frequent).... 2190
Timoptic-XE Sterile Ophthalmic Gel Forming Solution.... 2194

Exophthalmos
Aquasol A Parenteral.... 593
Celestone Soluspan Injectable Suspension.... 3097
Celestone Syrup.... 3099
Cortone Acetate Injectable Suspension.... 2059
Cortone Acetate Tablets.... 2061
Decadron Elixir.... 2078
Decadron Tablets.... 2079
Decadron Phosphate Injection.... 2081
Depo-Medrol Injectable Suspension.... 2795
Effexor Tablets (Infrequent).... 3495
Effexor XR Capsules (Infrequent).... 3499
Eskalith.... 1527
Florinef Acetate Tablets.... 2250
Hydrocortone Tablets.... 2106
Hydrocortone Acetate Injectable Suspension.... 2103
Hydrocortone Phosphate Injection, Sterile.... 2105
Lithobid Slow-Release Tablets.... 3255
Paxil (Rare).... 1609
Pediapred Oral Solution.... 1170
Prednisone.... 3064
Prelone Syrup.... 2273
Prozac Pulvules, Liquid, and Weekly Capsules (Rare).... 1238
Sarafem Pulvules (Rare).... 1962
Solu-Medrol Sterile Powder.... 2855
Zoloft (Rare).... 2751

Extraocular movement, impairment of
Lescol Capsules.... 2361
Lescol Capsules.... 2925
Lescol XL Tablets.... 2361
Lescol XL Tablets.... 2925

Extraocular muscles, permanent injury to
Duranest Injections.... 600
Xylocaine Injections.... 653

Extrapyramidal symptoms
Abelcet Injection.... 1273
Aciphex Tablets (Rare).... 1267
Aciphex Tablets (Rare).... 1783
Cardizem Injectable.... 1018
Cardizem Lyo-Ject Syringe.... 1018
Cardizem Monovial.... 1018
Cardizem CD Capsules (Infrequent).... 1016
Celexa (Infrequent).... 1365
▲ Cerebyx Injection (4.4%).... 2619
Clozaril Tablets.... 2319
Cognex Capsules (Infrequent).... 1351
Compazine.... 1505
Cytovene.... 2959
▲ Demser Capsules (10%).... 2085
Effexor Tablets.... 3495
Effexor XR Capsules.... 3499
Eskalith.... 1527
Etrafon (More common).... 3115
Felbatol.... 3343
Flexeril Tablets (Rare).... 572
Flexeril Tablets (Rare).... 2094
Floxin I.V..... 2526
Floxin Tablets.... 2529
▲ Geodon Capsules (5%).... 2688
Haldol Decanoate (Frequent).... 2535
Haldol Injection, Tablets and Concentrate (Frequent).... 2533
Intron A for Injection (Less than 5%).... 3120
Kytril Injection (Rare).... 2986
Kytril Tablets (One case).... 2988
Librium Capsules (Isolated cases).... 1736
Librium for Injection (Isolated cases).... 1737
Limbitrol.... 1738
Lithobid Slow-Release Tablets.... 3255
Lodosyn Tablets.... 1251
▲ Loxitane Capsules (Frequent).... 3398
Luvox Tablets (25, 50, 100 mg) (Infrequent).... 3256
Mepergan Injection (Rare).... 3539
▲ Mirapex Tablets (28%).... 2834
Moban.... 1320
Navane Oral.... 2701
Navane Intramuscular.... 2703
Norpramin Tablets.... 755
Orap Tablets (Frequent).... 1407
Paxil (Rare).... 1609
Permax Tablets (1.6%).... 1299
Phenergan Injection.... 3553
Phenergan Suppositories.... 3556
Phenergan Syrup.... 3554
Phenergan Tablets.... 3556
Phenergan with Codeine Syrup.... 3557
Proleukin for Injection.... 1199
Prozac Pulvules, Liquid, and Weekly Capsules (Rare).... 1238
Reglan (Approximately 0.2%).... 2935
Remeron Tablets (Infrequent).... 2483
Remeron SolTab Tablets (Infrequent).... 2486
Requip Tablets (Infrequent).... 1621
Rilutek Tablets (Infrequent).... 772
▲ Risperdal (17% to 34%).... 1796
Sarafem Pulvules (Rare).... 1962
Serentil.... 1057
Seroquel Tablets.... 684
Sinemet Tablets.... 1253
Sinemet CR Tablets.... 1255
Sinequan (Infrequent).... 2713
Stelazine.... 1640
Surmontil Capsules.... 3595
Tasmar Tablets (Infrequent).... 3010
Thioridazine Hydrochloride Tablets (Infrequent).... 2289
Thiothixene Capsules.... 2290
Thorazine.... 1656
Tiazac Capsules (Infrequent).... 1378
Toradol (1% or less).... 3018
Trilafon.... 3160
Trileptal Oral Suspension.... 2407
Trileptal Tablets.... 2407
Vivactil Tablets.... 2217
Vivactil Tablets.... 2446
Wellbutrin SR Sustained-Release Tablets.... 1684
Zofran Injection (Rare).... 1698
Zofran (Rare).... 1703
Zofran ODT Orally Disintegrating Tablets (Rare).... 1703
Zoloft.... 2751
Zyban Sustained-Release Tablets.... 1710
▲ Zyprexa Tablets (8% to 32%).... 1973
▲ Zyprexa ZYDIS Orally Disintegrating Tablets (8% to 32%).... 1973

Extrasystoles
Adalat CC Tablets (Less than 1.0%).... 877
Advair Diskus 100/50.... 1448
Advair Diskus 250/50.... 1448
Advair Diskus 500/50.... 1448
Ambien Tablets (Rare).... 3191
Anzemet Injection.... 719
Anzemet Tablets.... 722
Atacand HCT Tablets (0.5% or greater).... 597
Benadryl Parenteral.... 2617
Cardene I.V. (0.7%).... 3485
Celexa (Infrequent).... 1365
▲ CellCept Capsules (3% to 10%).... 2951
▲ CellCept Intravenous (3% to 10%).... 2951
▲ CellCept Oral Suspension (3% to 10%).... 2951
▲ CellCept Tablets (3% to 10%).... 2951
Chirocaine Injection (Less than 1%).... 2909
Coreg Tablets (More than 2%).... 1508
Corlopam Injection (0.5% to 5%).... 412
Diprivan Injectable Emulsion (Less than 1%).... 667
Effexor Tablets (Infrequent).... 3495
Effexor XR Capsules (Infrequent).... 3499
Evoxac Capsules (Less than 1%).... 1217
Exelon Capsules (Infrequent).... 2342
Exelon Oral Solution (Infrequent).... 2345
Imdur Tablets (Less than or equal to 5%).... 1826
Intron A for Injection (Less than 5%).... 3120
Lariam Tablets (Less than 1%).... 2989
Levo-Dromoran.... 1734
Lopid Tablets.... 2650
Lufyllin Tablets.... 3347
Lufyllin-400 Tablets.... 3347
Lufyllin-GG Elixir.... 3348
Lufyllin-GG Tablets.... 3348
Meridia Capsules.... 481
Naropin Injection (Less than 1%).... 612
Norvasc Tablets (Less than or equal to 0.1%).... 2704
Periactin Tablets.... 2155
Proventil Repetabs Tablets.... 3148
Prozac Pulvules, Liquid, and Weekly Capsules (Rare).... 1238
Quinidex Extentabs.... 2933
Requip Tablets (2%).... 1621
Rynatan Tablets.... 3351
Sarafem Pulvules (Rare).... 1962
Serevent Diskus.... 1637
Serevent Inhalation Aerosol.... 1633
Teveten Tablets (Less than 1%).... 3327
Theo-Dur Extended-Release Tablets.... 1835
Tiazac Capsules (2%).... 1378
Tricor Capsules, Micronized.... 513
Uni-Dur Extended-Release Tablets.... 1841
Ventolin Inhalation Aerosol and Refill.... 1679
Ventolin HFA Inhalation Aerosol (Less than 3%).... 3618
Wellbutrin SR Sustained-Release Tablets.... 1684
Zomig Tablets (Rare).... 708
Zomig-ZMT Tablets (Rare).... 708
Zyban Sustained-Release Tablets.... 1710

Extrasystoles, supraventricular
Caverject Sterile Powder (Less than 1%).... 2777
▲ CellCept Capsules (3% to 10%).... 2951
▲ CellCept Intravenous (3% to 10%).... 2951
▲ CellCept Oral Suspension (3% to 10%).... 2951
▲ CellCept Tablets (3% to 10%).... 2951
Corvert Injection (0.9% to 5.1%).... 2793
Luvox Tablets (25, 50, 100 mg) (Rare).... 3256

Extravasation
Adriamycin PFS/RDF Injection.... 2767
Brevibloc Injection (Less than 1%).... 858
Cerubidine for Injection.... 947
Claforan Injection (Rare).... 732
Cosmegen for Injection.... 2062
DaunoXome Injection.... 1442
Doxil Injection.... 566
Fluorescite Injection.... ⊙211
Gemzar for Injection (Infrequent).... 1919
Idamycin PFS Injection.... 2825
Novantrone for Injection.... 1760
Romazicon Injection.... 3000
Taxol Injection.... 1129
Taxotere for Injection Concentrate.... 778
▲ Visudyne for Injection (10% to 20%).... ⊙308
Zinecard for Injection (1% to 3%).... 2869

Extroversion
Ambien Tablets.... 3191
Halcion Tablets.... 2823

Exudate, increased
▲ Apligraf (5.6%).... 2305
Bactroban Ointment (Less than 1%).... 1496
▲ Thrombate III (1 of 17).... 944
Xalatan Latanoprost Ophthalmic Solution (Less than 1%).... ⊙320
Xalatan Sterile Ophthalmic Solution (Less than 1%).... 2864

Eye abnormalities, fetal
Accutane Capsules.... 2944
Clomid Tablets.... 735

Eye globe, perforation
(*see under* Bulbus oculi, perforation)

Eye movements, abnormal
Klonopin Tablets.... 2983
Mevacor Tablets (0.5% to 1.0%).... 2132
Zocor Tablets.... 2219

Eyeball, perforation
(*see under* Bulbus oculi, perforation)

Eyelash changes
Xalatan Latanoprost Ophthalmic Solution.... ⊙320
Xalatan Sterile Ophthalmic Solution.... 2864

Eyelash darkening
▲ Lumigan Ophthalmic Solution (3% to 10%).... 553
▲ Travatan Ophthalmic Solution (Among most frequent).... 543

Eyelashes, increase in growth
▲ Lumigan Ophthalmic Solution (15% to 45%).... 553
▲ Rescula Ophthalmic Solution (10% to 25%).... ⊙306
▲ Travatan Ophthalmic Solution (Among most frequent).... 543

Eyelashes, increase in number
Rescula Ophthalmic Solution (Less than 1%).... ⊙306

Eyelashes, matting of
Alomide Ophthalmic Solution (Less than 1%).... ⊙204
Betoptic S Ophthalmic Suspension (Small number of patients).... 537
Iopidine 0.5% Ophthalmic Solution (Less than 1%).... ⊙213
Lacrisert Sterile Ophthalmic Insert.... 2117

Eyelid crusting
Cosopt Sterile Ophthalmic Solution.... 2065
Travatan Ophthalmic Solution (1% to 4%).... 543
Trusopt Sterile Ophthalmic Solution.... 2196

Eyelid skin darkening
▲ Lumigan Ophthalmic Solution (3% to 10%) 553
▲ Travatan Ophthalmic Solution (Among most frequent) 543
Xalatan Latanoprost Ophthalmic Solution ⊙320
Xalatan Sterile Ophthalmic Solution 2864

Eyelids, cyclic, movement of
Versed Injection (Less than 1%) 3027

Eyelids, deposits in
Alomide Ophthalmic Solution (Less than 1%) ⊙204
Iopidine 0.5% Ophthalmic Solution (Less than 3%) ⊙213
Soriatane Capsules (Less than 5%) 3003
Xalatan Latanoprost Ophthalmic Solution (1% to 4%) ⊙320
Xalatan Sterile Ophthalmic Solution (1% to 4%) 2864

Eyelids, edema of
▲ Alphagan Ophthalmic Solution (Approximately 3% to 9%) 545
Alphagan P Ophthalmic Solution (1% to 4%) 546
Botox Purified Neurotoxin Complex (2 cases) 549
Ciloxan (Less than 1%) 538
Hyzaar 2109
Lacrisert Sterile Ophthalmic Insert 2117
Polytrim Ophthalmic Solution (Multiple reports) 556
Quixin Ophthalmic Solution (Less than 1%) 3093
▲ Rēv-Eyes Sterile Ophthalmic Eyedrops 0.5% (10% to 40%) ⊙265
Stromectol Tablets 2185
Tobrex Ophthalmic Ointment (Less than 3 of 100 patients) ⊙220
Tobrex Ophthalmic Solution (Less than 3 of 100 patients) ⊙221
▲ Trisenox Injection (5%) 1158
Voltaren Ophthalmic Sterile Ophthalmic Solution (Less than 5%) ⊙312
Xalatan Latanoprost Ophthalmic Solution (1% to 4%) ⊙320
Xalatan Sterile Ophthalmic Solution (1% to 4%) 2864

Eyelids, erythema
▲ Alphagan Ophthalmic Solution (Approximately 3% to 9%) 545
Alphagan P Ophthalmic Solution (1% to 4%) 546
Alrex Sterile Ophthalmic Suspension 0.2% (Less than 5%) ⊙256
▲ Betimol Ophthalmic Solution (More than 5%) ⊙324
Lotemax Sterile Ophthalmic Suspension 0.5% (Less than 5%) ⊙261
▲ Lumigan Ophthalmic Solution (3% to 10%) 553
Xalatan Latanoprost Ophthalmic Solution (1% to 4%) ⊙320
Xalatan Sterile Ophthalmic Solution (1% to 4%) 2864

Eyelids, heavy
Phrenilin (Infrequent) 578
Sedapap Tablets 50 mg/650 mg (Infrequent) 2225

Eyes, burning of
▲ Acular PF Ophthalmic Solution (Approximately 20%) 544
Alamast Ophthalmic Solution (Less than 5%) 3092
▲ Alocril Ophthalmic Solution (10% to 30%) 545
▲ Alrex Sterile Ophthalmic Suspension 0.2% (5% to 15%) ⊙256
▲ Betagan (About 1 in 3 patients) ⊙228
▲ Betimol Ophthalmic Solution (1 in 8 patients) ⊙324
Bleph-10 ⊙230
▲ Carac Cream (5.4%) 1222
▲ Carteolol Hydrochloride Ophthalmic Solution USP, 1% (About 1 of 4 patients) ⊙258
Catapres Tablets 1037
Catapres-TTS (0.5% or less) 1038
Chloromycetin Ophthalmic Ointment, 1% (Occasional) ⊙296
▲ Ciloxan (Among most frequent) 538
Cleocin T Topical 2790
Clorpres Tablets 1002
Combipres Tablets 1040
▲ Cosopt Sterile Ophthalmic Solution (Up to 30%) 2065
Cozaar Tablets (Less than 1%) 2067
Duraclon Injection (Rare) 3057
Emadine Ophthalmic Solution (Less than 5%) ⊙211
FML Ophthalmic Suspension ⊙236
FML Forte Ophthalmic Suspension ⊙235
▲ Genoptic Ophthalmic Ointment (Among most frequent) ⊙239
▲ Genoptic Sterile Ophthalmic Solution (Among most frequent) ⊙239
Hivid Tablets (Less than 1%) 2975
HMS Sterile Ophthalmic Suspension ⊙240
Hyzaar 2109
Iopidine Sterile Ophthalmic Solution ⊙212
Isopto Carpine Ophthalmic Solution ⊙215
▲ Livostin (29%) ⊙305
▲ Lotemax Sterile Ophthalmic Suspension 0.5% (5% to 15%) ⊙261
▲ Lumigan Ophthalmic Solution (3% to 10%) 553
Maxalt Tablets (Infrequent) 2120
Maxalt-MLT Orally Disintegrating Tablets (Infrequent) 2120
Motofen Tablets (Less frequent) 577
Muro 128 Sterile Ophthalmic Ointment ⊙262
Muro 128 Sterile Ophthalmic Solution 2% and 5% ⊙262
Nicotrol Nasal Spray (More common) 2843
Ocufen Ophthalmic Solution ⊙242
▲ Ocuflox Ophthalmic Solution (Among most frequent) 554
▲ Ocupress Ophthalmic Solution, 1% Sterile (About 1 of 4 patients) ⊙303
Ophthetic Ophthalmic Solution ⊙244
▲ Optivar Ophthalmic Solution (Approximately 30%) 2273
Patanol Ophthalmic Solution (Less than 5%) 540
Pilopine HS Ophthalmic Gel ⊙217
▲ Polytrim Ophthalmic Solution (Among most frequent) 556
Pred Forte Ophthalmic Suspension ⊙246
Pred Mild Sterile Ophthalmic Suspension ⊙249
▲ Propine Ophthalmic Solution (6%) ⊙250
Quixin Ophthalmic Solution (1% to 3%) 3093
▲ Rescula Ophthalmic Solution (10% to 25%) ⊙306
Soma Compound Tablets 3354
Soma Compound w/Codeine Tablets 3355
Taxol Injection 1129
Tessalon Capsules 1377
▲ Timolol GFS (1 in 8 patients) ⊙266
▲ Timoptic in Ocudose (Approximately 1 in 8 patients) 2192
▲ Timoptic Sterile Ophthalmic Solution (Approximately 1 in 8 patients) 2190
▲ Timoptic-XE Sterile Ophthalmic Gel Forming Solution (1 in 8 patients) 2194
▲ Trusopt Sterile Ophthalmic Solution (Approximately one-third of patients) 2196
Viagra Tablets 2732
▲ Viroptic Ophthalmic Solution Sterile (4.6%) ⊙301
▲ Voltaren Ophthalmic Sterile Ophthalmic Solution (15%) ⊙312
▲ Xalatan Latanoprost Ophthalmic Solution (5% to 15%) ⊙320
▲ Xalatan Sterile Ophthalmic Solution (5% to 15%) 2864
Zaditor Ophthalmic Solution (Less than 5%) 2304

Eyes, cotton wood spots
Vitrasert Implant (Less than 1%) ⊙254

Eyes, dilatation of pupil
(*see under* Mydriasis)

Eyes, disorders of
Aerobid/Aerobid-M (1% to 3%) 1363
Alphagan P Ophthalmic Solution (1% to 4%) 546
Arava Tablets (1% to 3%) 724
Astelin Nasal Spray (Infrequent) 3339
Ativan Tablets (Less frequent) 3482
Avapro Tablets (Less than 1%) 1074
Avapro Tablets (Less than 1%) 3076
Carbatrol Capsules 3234
▲ Carnitor Injection (3% to 6%) 3242
Clinoril Tablets (Less than 1%) 2053
▲ Copaxone for Injection (4%) 3306
Cordarone Tablets 3487
Depakote ER Tablets (Greater than 1%) 436
Desferal Vials 2333
Dynabac Tablets (0.1% to 1%) 2269
Foscavir Injection (Between 1% and 5%) 605
Hivid Tablets (Less than 1%) 2975
Kaletra Capsules (Less than 2%) 471
Kaletra Oral Solution (Less than 2%) 471
Loxitane Capsules 3398
▲ Lupron Depot 3.75 mg (Among most frequent) 3281
Lupron Injection (Less than 5%) 3279
Mintezol 2137
Mirapex Tablets (Less than 1%) 2834
Nasalide Nasal Spray (5% or less) 1295
Neurontin Capsules (Rare) 2655
Neurontin Oral Solution (Rare) 2655
Neurontin Tablets (Rare) 2655
▲ Novantrone for Injection (2% to 7%) 1760
Pacerone Tablets 3331
Permax Tablets (1.1%) 1299
Protopic Ointment (Greater than or equal to 1%) 1397
▲ Requip Tablets (3%) 1621
▲ Rescula Ophthalmic Solution (5% to 10%) ⊙306
Salagen Tablets (Less than 1%) 2229
▲ Soriatane Capsules (1% to 10%) 3003
Stromectol Tablets 2185
Tambocor Tablets 1990
Tegretol/Tegretol-XR 2404
▲ Thrombate III (1 of 17) 944
Travatan Ophthalmic Solution (1% to 4%) 543
Tricor Capsules, Micronized 513
Varivax (Greater than or equal to 1%) 2202
Versed Injection (Less than 1%) 3027
▲ Vesanoid Capsules (17%) 3037
Viracept 532
Vistide Injection 1445

Eyes, dry
(*see under* Xerophthalmia)

Eyes, irritation of
▲ Acular Ophthalmic Solution (Approximately 1% to 10%) 544
▲ Acular PF Ophthalmic Solution (Approximately 1% to 10%) 544
Albalon Ophthalmic Solution ⊙225
▲ Alocril Ophthalmic Solution (10% to 30%) 545
▲ Alphagan Ophthalmic Solution (Approximately 3% to 9%) 545
Alphagan P Ophthalmic Solution (1% to 4%) 546
Alrex Sterile Ophthalmic Suspension 0.2% (Less than 5%) ⊙256
Ambien Tablets (Infrequent) 3191
Aricept Tablets (Frequent) 1270
Aricept Tablets (Frequent) 2665
Atrovent Nasal Spray 0.03% (Less than 2%) 1032
Bleph-10 ⊙230
Blocadren Tablets (1.1%) 2046
▲ Botox Purified Neurotoxin Complex (10.0%) 549
▲ Carac Cream (5.4%) 1222
Cardizem Injectable 1018
Cardizem Lyo-Ject Syringe 1018
Cardizem Monovial 1018
Cardizem CD Capsules (Less than 1%) 1016
▲ Carteolol Hydrochloride Ophthalmic Solution USP, 1% (About 1 of 4 patients) ⊙258
Cleocin T Topical 2790
Cormax Scalp Application (Approximately 0.3%) 2441
Crolom Sterile Ophthalmic Solution USP 4% (Infrequent) ⊙259
Emgel 2% Topical Gel 1285
Flonase Nasal Spray 1533
Flovent (1% to 3%) 1535
FML Ophthalmic Suspension ⊙236
FML Forte Ophthalmic Suspension ⊙235
Fortovase Capsules (Less than 2%) 2970
▲ Genoptic Ophthalmic Ointment (Among most frequent) ⊙239
▲ Genoptic Sterile Ophthalmic Solution (Among most frequent) ⊙239
Hivid Tablets (Less than 1%) 2975
Imitrex Injection (Infrequent) 1549
Imitrex Nasal Spray (Infrequent) 1554
Imitrex Tablets (Up to 2%) 1558
Invirase Capsules (Less than 2%) 2979
Iopidine 0.5% Ophthalmic Solution (Less than 3%) ⊙213
Isopto Carbachol Ophthalmic Solution ⊙215
Klonopin Tablets (Infrequent) 2983
Lacrisert Sterile Ophthalmic Insert 2117
Lotemax Sterile Ophthalmic Suspension 0.5% (Less than 5%) ⊙261
▲ Lumigan Ophthalmic Solution (3% to 10%) 553
Maxalt Tablets (Infrequent) 2120
Maxalt-MLT Orally Disintegrating Tablets (Infrequent) 2120
Mevacor Tablets (0.5% to 1.0%) 2132
Monopril Tablets (0.2% to 1.0%) 1091
Monopril HCT 1094
Muro 128 Sterile Ophthalmic Ointment ⊙262
Muro 128 Sterile Ophthalmic Solution 2% and 5% ⊙262
Neosporin Ophthalmic Ointment Sterile ⊙299
Neosporin Ophthalmic Solution Sterile ⊙300
Nicotrol Nasal Spray (More common) 2843
Ocufen Ophthalmic Solution ⊙242
▲ Ocupress Ophthalmic Solution, 1% Sterile (About 1 of 4 patients) ⊙303
Opticrom Ophthalmic Solution (Infrequent) 555
Polysporin Ophthalmic Ointment Sterile ⊙301
▲ Polytrim Ophthalmic Solution (Among most frequent) 556
Pred Forte Ophthalmic Suspension ⊙246
Pred Mild Sterile Ophthalmic Suspension ⊙249
ProSom Tablets (Infrequent) 500
Roferon-A Injection (Less than 1%) 2996
Rogaine Extra Strength for Men Topical Solution ▣721
Rogaine for Women Topical Solution ▣721
Rythmol Tablets – 150 mg, 225 mg, 300 mg (Less than 1%) 502
▲ Soriatane Capsules (1% to 10%) 3003
Tambocor Tablets (Less than 1%) 1990
Temovate Scalp Application (1 of 294 patients) 1304
Tiazac Capsules (Less than 2%) 1378
Timolide Tablets 2187
Timolol GFS ⊙266
Timoptic in Ocudose (Less frequent) 2192
Timoptic Sterile Ophthalmic Solution (Less frequent) 2190
Timoptic-XE Sterile Ophthalmic Gel Forming Solution 2194
Tricor Capsules, Micronized (2%) 513
▲ Trisenox Injection (10%) 1158
Vaqta (Less than 1%) 2199
Vexol 1% Ophthalmic Suspension (Less than 1%) ⊙222
Viroptic Ophthalmic Solution Sterile ⊙301
Vitravene for Injection (2% to 5%) ⊙310
Voltaren Ophthalmic Sterile Ophthalmic Solution (Less than 5%) ⊙312
Xeloda Tablets 3039
Zaditor Ophthalmic Solution (Less than 5%) 2304

Eyes, nonreactive
Nipent for Injection (Less than 3%) 3272

Eyes, redness of
Advair Diskus 100/50 (1% to 3%) 1448
Advair Diskus 250/50 (1% to 3%) 1448
Advair Diskus 500/50 (1% to 3%) 1448
Albalon Ophthalmic Solution ⊙225
▲ Alocril Ophthalmic Solution (1% to 10%) 545
Clozaril Tablets (Less than 1%) 2319
Hivid Tablets (Less than 1%) 2975
Humorsol Sterile Ophthalmic Solution 2102
Livostin (Approximately 1% to 3%) ⊙305
Ocuflox Ophthalmic Solution 554
Ortho Diaphragm Kits – All-Flex Arcing Spring; Ortho Coil Spring 2552
▲ Polytrim Ophthalmic Solution (Among most frequent) 556
Transderm Scōp Transdermal Therapeutic System (Infrequent) 2302
▲ Travatan Ophthalmic Solution (35% to 50%) 543
Trusopt Sterile Ophthalmic Solution 2196
Viagra Tablets 2732

Eyes, spots before the
Aricept Tablets (Infrequent) 1270
Aricept Tablets (Infrequent) 2665
Clomid Tablets (Occasional) 735
Depacon Injection 416
Depakene 421
Depakote Sprinkle Capsules 426
Depakote Tablets 430
Depakote ER Tablets 436
Tambocor Tablets 1990

Eyes, swollen
(*see under* Edema, palpebral)

Eyes, tearing
▲ Alomide Ophthalmic Solution (1% to 5%) ⊙204
▲ Alphagan Ophthalmic Solution (Approximately 3% to 9%) 545
Amicar Injection 3608
Amicar Syrup 3608
Amicar Tablets 3608

Astelin Nasal Spray (Infrequent)...... 3339
Beconase AQ Nasal Spray (Fewer than 3 per 100 patients).............. 1498
Betoptic S Ophthalmic Suspension (Small number of patients)...................................... 537
▲ Carac Cream (5.4%) 1222
▲ Carteolol Hydrochloride Ophthalmic Solution USP, 1% (About 1 of 4 patients)............... ⊙258
Chemet Capsules (1.0% to 3.7%)... 3078
Ciloxan (Less than 1%).................. 538
Cosopt Sterile Ophthalmic Solution.. 2065
Dantrium Capsules (Less frequent).. 2885
Dipentum Capsules (Rare).............. 2803
Emcyt Capsules (1%)..................... 2810
▲ Iopidine 0.5% Ophthalmic Solution (4%)................................ ⊙213
Lexxel Tablets 608
Lumigan Ophthalmic Solution (1% to 3%)... 553
Nasalide Nasal Spray.................... 1295
Nipent for Injection (Less than 3%).. 3272
Ocuflox Ophthalmic Solution............ 554
▲ Ocupress Ophthalmic Solution, 1% Sterile (About 1 of 4 patients)...................................... ⊙303
Polytrim Ophthalmic Solution (Multiple reports)......................... 556
▲ Rescula Ophthalmic Solution (5% to 10%).. ⊙306
Rēv-Eyes Sterile Ophthalmic Eyedrops 0.5% (Less frequently)................................... ⊙265
Sonata Capsules (Infrequent).......... 3591
Timolol GFS (1% to 5%)............... ⊙266
Timoptic in Ocudose (Less frequent).. 2192
Timoptic Sterile Ophthalmic Solution (Less frequent)............... 2190
Timoptic-XE Sterile Ophthalmic Gel Forming Solution (1% to 5%).. 2194
Travatan Ophthalmic Solution (1% to 4%)... 543
Xalatan Latanoprost Ophthalmic Solution (1% to 4%).................. ⊙320
Xalatan Sterile Ophthalmic Solution (1% to 4%).................. 2864

F

Face, rhythmical involuntary movements
Compazine....................................... 1505
Etrafon.. 3115
Haldol Decanoate............................ 2535
Lithobid Slow-Release Tablets......... 3255
Moban... 1320
Orap Tablets.................................... 1407
Reglan... 2935
Stelazine... 1640
Thiothixene Capsules...................... 2290
Thorazine.. 1656

Facial dysmorphia, fetal
Accutane Capsules.......................... 2944

Facial features, coarsening
Dilantin Infatabs............................ 2624
Dilantin Kapseals........................... 2622
Dilantin-125 Oral Suspension.......... 2625

Facial paresis
(*see also under* Bell's palsy)
Baycol Tablets................................ 883

Facial swelling
Aleve Tablets, Caplets and Gelcaps.. ▣602
Altace Capsules.............................. 2233
Carafate Suspension....................... 731
Carafate Tablets............................. 730
Corgard Tablets (1 to 5 per 1000 patients).. 2245
Cortifoam Rectal Foam.................... 3170
Corzide 40/5 Tablets (1 to 5 of 1000 patients)............................. 2247
Corzide 80/5 Tablets (1 to 5 of 1000 patients)............................. 2247
▲ Doxil Injection (Approximately 6.8%).. 566
Hivid Tablets (Less than 1%).......... 2975
Imitrex Nasal Spray (Rare).............. 1554
JE-VAX Vaccine (0.1%)................... 811
Levaquin... 2537
Nadolol Tablets (1 to 5 of 1000 patients)... 2288
Proscar Tablets.............................. 2175
Stelazine Tablets............................ 1640
Synvisc... 3596
Unasyn for Injection (Less than 1%).. 2728

Facies, mask-like
Compazine...................................... 1505
Loxitane Capsules........................... 3398
Reglan.. 2935
Stelazine.. 1640

Thiothixene Capsules..................... 2290
Thorazine....................................... 1656
▲ Zyprexa Tablets (8% to 20%) 1973
▲ Zyprexa ZYDIS Orally Disintegrating Tablets (8% to 20%)... 1973

Factors II, V, VII, X, decrease
Anadrol-50 Tablets......................... 3321
Androderm Transdermal System CIII.. 3377
▲ Android Capsules, 10 mg (Among most common)............................ 1731
Estratest... 3252
Oxandrin Tablets............................ 1153
Testoderm Transdermal Systems... 574
Testopel Pellets.............................. 3610
Testred Capsules, 10 mg................ 1746

Factors VII, VIII, IX, X, increase
Aygestin Tablets............................. 1333
Brevicon 28-Day Tablets................. 3380
Estratest... 3252
Norinyl 1 +35 28-Day Tablets......... 3380
Norinyl 1 + 50 28-Day Tablets........ 3380
Ortho-Cyclen/Ortho Tri-Cyclen........ 2573
Tri-Norinyl-28 Tablets..................... 3433

Fainting
(*see under* Syncope)

Falling
Ambien Tablets (Infrequent)............ 3191
Cognex Capsules............................ 1351
Detrol Tablets (1.5%)...................... 3623
Eldepryl Capsules........................... 3266
Evoxac Capsules (Less than 1%)..... 1217
Geodon Capsules (Frequent)........... 2688
Halcion Tablets............................... 2823
Klonopin Tablets (Infrequent).......... 2983
Lodosyn Tablets............................. 1251
Matulane Capsules......................... 3246
Mobic Tablets (Up to 2.6%)............ 1054
Monopril Tablets (0.4% to 1.0%)..... 1091
Remicade for IV Injection (Less than 2%).................................... 1178
Reminyl Oral Solution (Greater than or equal to 2%).................. 1792
Reminyl Tablets (Greater than or equal to 2%)............................... 1792
Requip Tablets (1% or more)........... 1621
Sinemet Tablets.............................. 1253
Sinemet CR Tablets........................ 1255
▲ Tasmar Tablets (4% to 6%) 3010
Trileptal Oral Suspension (Up to 4%).. 2407
Trileptal Tablets (Up to 4%)............ 2407
Viagra Tablets (Less than 2%)......... 2732

Fanconi syndrome
Depacon Injection (Rare)................. 416
Depakene (Rare)............................. 421
Depakote Sprinkle Capsules (Rare)... 426
Depakote Tablets (Rare)................. 430
Depakote ER Tablets (Rare)............ 436
Ifex for Injection............................. 1123
Vistide Injection (2%)...................... 1445

Fasciculations
Amerge Tablets (Rare)..................... 1467
Anectine Injection........................... 1476
Aricept Tablets (Infrequent)............ 1270
Aricept Tablets (Infrequent)............ 2665
Clozaril Tablets (Less than 1%)....... 2319
Crixivan Capsules (Less than 2%).... 2070
Depakote Sprinkle Capsules (1% to 5%)... 426
Dilaudid Oral Liquid (Less frequent)... 445
Dilaudid Tablets - 8 mg (Less frequent)... 445
Dilaudid-HP.................................... 443
Dopram Injectable.......................... 2931
Eldepryl Capsules........................... 3266
Eskalith.. 1527
Flexeril Tablets (Less than 1%)....... 572
Flexeril Tablets (Less than 1%)....... 2094
Humorsol Sterile Ophthalmic Solution.. 2102
Leukeran Tablets (Rare).................. 1591
Lithium Carbonate.......................... 3061
Lithium Citrate Syrup...................... 3061
Lithobid Slow-Release Tablets......... 3255
Lodosyn Tablets............................. 1251
Loxitane Capsules.......................... 3398
Lufyllin Tablets............................... 3347
Lufyllin-400 Tablets........................ 3347
Lufyllin-GG Elixir............................ 3348
Lufyllin-GG Tablets......................... 3348
Mestinon.. 1740
Migranal Nasal Spray (Rare)............ 2376
MS Contin Tablets (Less frequent)... 2896
Nebcin Vials, Hyporets & ADD-Vantage................................... 1955
Parnate Tablets.............................. 1607
Paxil (Rare).................................... 1609
▲ Prostigmin Injectable (Among most common)............................. 1744
▲ Prostigmin Tablets (Among most common)....................................... 1744
ReoPro Vials (0.4%)....................... 1958
Retrovir.. 1625

Sinemet Tablets.............................. 1253
Sinemet CR Tablets........................ 1255
Tensilon Injectable......................... 1745
Theo-Dur Extended-Release Tablets... 1835
Tonocard Tablets (Less than 1%)..... 649
Uni-Dur Extended-Release Tablets... 1841
Uniphyl 400 mg and 600 mg Tablets... 2903
▲ Xanax Tablets (7.9%) 2865

Fasciitis, necrotizing fulminant
Clinoril Tablets (Rare)..................... 2053
Dolobid Tablets.............................. 2088
Indocin (Rare)................................. 2112

Fatality, hepatic related
Eulexin Capsules............................ 3118
Macrobid Capsules......................... 2889
Macrodantin Capsules..................... 2891

Fatality, non-cardiovascular related
Atromid-S Capsules........................ 3483

Fatigue
Accupril Tablets (2.6%).................. 2611
Accuretic Tablets (2.9%)................. 2614
Accutane Capsules.......................... 2944
▲ Actimmune (14%) 1772
Activella Tablets............................. 2764
▲ Adalat CC Tablets (4%) 877
Aerobid/Aerobid-M (1% to 3%)....... 1363
▲ Aggrenox Capsules (5.8%) 1026
Aldara Cream, 5% (More than 1%)... 1978
▲ Alferon N Injection (6% to 14%) 1770
Allegra (1.3%)................................ 712
▲ Alphagan Ophthalmic Solution (Approximately 10% to 30%)....... 545
Altace Capsules (2.0%)................... 2233
Ambien Tablets (1%)....................... 3191
Amerge Tablets (2%)....................... 1467
Ancobon Capsules.......................... 1730
Androderm Transdermal System CIII (Less than 1%)...................... 3377
Antabuse Tablets............................ 2444
Antabuse Tablets (Small number of patients).................................... 3474
▲ Anzemet Injection (3.6%) 719
Anzemet Tablets (2.6%)................... 722
Aquasol A Parenteral...................... 593
▲ Aredia for Injection (37.2%) 2309
▲ Aricept Tablets (5%) 1270
▲ Aricept Tablets (5%) 2665
▲ Aromasin Tablets (22%) 2769
Arthrotec Tablets (Rare).................. 3195
Astelin Nasal Spray (2.3%)............... 3339
Atacand Tablets (More than 1%)...... 595
Atacand HCT Tablets (0.5% or greater).. 597
Atromid-S Capsules (Less often)..... 3483
Atrovent Inhalation Aerosol (Less than 1%)....................................... 1030
▲ Avalide Tablets (7%) 1070
Avandia Tablets (1.9% to 4%)......... 1490
▲ Avapro Tablets (4%) 1074
▲ Avapro Tablets (4%) 3076
Axert Tablets (Infrequent)................ 2772
Azmacort Inhalation Aerosol............ 728
Azopt Ophthalmic Suspension (Less than 1%)............................. 536
Bactrim... 2949
Benadryl Parenteral......................... 2617
▲ Betapace Tablets (5% to 20%) 950
▲ Betapace AF Tablets (18.9% to 19.6%).. 954
Bicillin C-R 900/300 Injection.......... 2240
Bicillin C-R Injection........................ 2238
Bicillin L-A Injection........................ 2242
▲ Blocadren Tablets (3.4% to 5%) 2046
Brevibloc Injection (About 1%)......... 858
Calcium Disodium Versenate Injection.. 1980
▲ Campath Ampules (5% to 34%) 992
Captopril Tablets (About 0.5% to 2%).. 2281
Carbatrol Capsules......................... 3234
▲ Cardura Tablets (8% to 12%) 2668
Casodex Tablets............................. 662
Cataflam Tablets............................ 2315
▲ Catapres Tablets (About 4 in 100 patients)...................................... 1037
▲ Catapres-TTS (6 of 101 patients) 1038
Cedax Capsules (0.1% to 1%)......... 1021
Celebrex Capsules (0.1% to 1.9%).. 2676
Celebrex Capsules (0.1% to 1.9%).. 2780
▲ Celexa (5%) 1365
▲ Cerezyme for Injection (5.4%) 1438
▲ Chemet Capsules (5.2% to 15.7%).. 3078
▲ Claritin (3% to 4%) 3100
▲ Claritin-D 12 Hour Extended Release Tablets (4%)................... 3102
▲ Claritin-D 24 Hour Extended Release Tablets (3%)................... 3104
Clinoril Tablets (Less than 1 in 100)... 2053
Clomid Tablets (Fewer than 1%)...... 735
▲ Clorpres Tablets (About 4%) 1002
Clozaril Tablets (2%)....................... 2319
▲ Cognex Capsules (4%) 1351
Colazal Capsules (2%)..................... 3069
Colestid Tablets (Infrequent)........... 2791

▲ Combipres Tablets (About 4%) 1040
Combivent Inhalation Aerosol (Less than 2%).............................. 1041
▲ Combivir Tablets (10%) 1502
▲ Comtan Tablets (6%) 2328
▲ Cordarone Tablets (4% to 9%) 3487
▲ Coreg Tablets (4.3% to 23.9%) 1508
Corgard Tablets (2 of 100 patients)... 2245
Cortifoam Rectal Foam................... 3170
Corzide 40/5 Tablets (2 of 100 patients)... 2247
Corzide 80/5 Tablets (2 of 100 patients)... 2247
Cosmegen for Injection.................... 2062
Cosopt Sterile Ophthalmic Solution.. 2065
Coumadin for Injection (Infrequent)................................... 1243
Coumadin Tablets (Infrequent)........ 1243
Covera-HS Tablets (1.7% to 4.5%).. 3199
Cozaar Tablets (1% or greater)....... 2067
▲ Crinone (21%) 3213
▲ Crixivan Capsules (3.6%) 2070
Cytotec Tablets (Infrequent)............ 3202
▲ Dantrium Capsules (Among most frequent).. 2885
▲ DaunoXome Injection (6% to 43%) . 1442
▲ Depo-Provera Contraceptive Injection (More than 5%).............. 2798
▲ Detrol Tablets (6.8%) 3623
Detrol LA Capsules (2%)................. 2801
Dibenzyline Capsules...................... 3457
Diovan Capsules (2%)...................... 2337
▲ Diovan HCT Tablets (5%) 2338
Dipentum Capsules (1.8%)............... 2803
Diphtheria & Tetanus Toxoids Adsorbed Purogenated for Pediatric Use.................................. 1857
Diprivan Injectable Emulsion (Less than 1%)....................................... 667
Dolobid Tablets (Greater than 1 in 100).. 2088
▲ Dostinex Tablets (5% to 7%) 2804
Doxil Injection................................. 566
▲ Duraclon Injection (4%) 3057
Dyazide Capsules........................... 1515
▲ DynaCirc Capsules (2% to 8.5%) 2921
▲ DynaCirc CR Tablets (2.5% to 7.6%).. 2923
Dyrenium Capsules (Rare)............... 3458
Edecrin... 2091
Effexor XR Capsules....................... 3499
Eldepryl Capsules........................... 3266
Elspar for Injection......................... 2092
Enalaprilat Injection (0.5% to 1%)..... 863
Enbrel for Injection......................... 1752
Enbrel for Injection......................... 3504
▲ Engerix-B Vaccine (14%) 1517
▲ Epivir (27%) 1520
▲ Epivir-HBV (24%) 1524
▲ Epogen for Injection (9% to 25%) ... 582
▲ Ergamisol Tablets (6% to 11%) 1789
Eskalith.. 1527
Etrafon... 3115
Eulexin Capsules............................ 3118
▲ Evoxac Capsules (3.3%) 1217
▲ Exelon Capsules (9%) 2342
▲ Exelon Oral Solution (9%) 2345
Famotidine Injection (Infrequent)..... 866
▲ Famvir Tablets (4% to 6.3%) 2348
▲ Felbatol (6.9% to 16.8%) 3343
▲ Femara Tablets (6% to 11%) 2351
femhrt Tablets................................ 2635
▲ Ferrlecit Injection (6%) 3386
Flexeril Tablets (1% to 3%)............. 572
Flexeril Tablets (1% to 3%)............. 2094
Flolan for Injection.......................... 1528
▲ Flovent Diskus (1% to 16%) 3614
▲ Flovent (22% to 28%) 1535
Flovent Rotadisk............................. 1537
Floxin I.V. (1% to 3%)..................... 2526
Floxin Tablets (1% to 3%)............... 2529
▲ Fludara for Injection (10% to 38%) . 995
Flumadine (1.0%)............................ 1370
Foradil Aerolizer.............................. 2354
▲ Fortovase Capsules (4.8% to 6.7%).. 2970
▲ Foscavir Injection (5% or greater) ... 605
Gabitril Tablets............................... 1189
Gammagard S/D (Occasional)......... 845
Gammar-P I.V. 787
Gastrocrom Oral Concentrate (Less common)............................. 1162
▲ Gengraf Capsules (3%) 457
▲ Gleevec Capsules (24% to 33%) 2357
Gonal-F for Injection....................... 3216
Grifulvin V Tablets Microsize and Oral Suspension Microsize (Occasional)................................. 2518
Gris-PEG Tablets............................ 2661
Halcion Tablets (0.5% to 0.9%)...... 2823
▲ Havrix Vaccine (1% to 10%) 1544
Hexalen Capsules (1%)................... 2226
Hivid Tablets (Less than 1% to 3.8%).. 2975
▲ Hycamtin for Injection (Up to 37%) . 1546
▲ Hytrin Capsules (7.4% to 11.3%) ... 464
Hyzaar (1% or greater).................... 2109
Ifex for Injection (Less than 1%)...... 1123
Imdur Tablets (Less than or equal to 5%)... 1826
Imitrex Injection (1.1%)................... 1549
Imitrex Tablets................................ 1558

▲ Indapamide Tablets (Greater than or equal to 5%) 2286
Inderal 3513
Inderal LA Long-Acting Capsules 3516
Inderide Tablets 3517
Inderide LA Long-Acting Capsules 3519
Indocin (Greater than 1%) 2112
▲ Infergen (65% to 69%) 1777
▲ Intron A for Injection (4% to 96%) 3120
Inversine Tablets 1850
Invirase Capsules (Less than 2%) 2979
Iopidine Sterile Ophthalmic Solution ⊙212
▲ IPOL Vaccine (4.0% to 60.7%) 809
Isoptin SR Tablets (1.7%) 467
Keflex 1237
▲ Klonopin Tablets (7%) 2983
K-Phos Neutral Tablets 946
K-Phos Original (Sodium Free) Tablets (Less frequent) 947
Lamisil Tablets 2360
▲ Lariam Tablets (Among most frequent) 2989
Lescol Capsules (2.7%) 2361
Lescol Capsules (2.7%) 2925
Lescol XL Tablets (1.6%) 2361
Lescol XL Tablets (1.6%) 2925
▲ Leustatin Injection (11% to 45%) 2495
Levaquin (0.1% to less than 1.0%) 2537
Levbid Extended-Release Tablets 3172
Levlen 962
Levlite 21 Tablets 962
Levlite 28 Tablets 962
Levoxyl Tablets 1819
Levsin/Levsinex/Levbid 3172
Lexxel Tablets (1.9%) 608
Limbitrol 1738
Lithium Carbonate 3061
Lithium Citrate Syrup 3061
Lithobid Slow-Release Tablets 3255
Livostin (Approximately 1% to 3%) ⊙305
Lodosyn Tablets 1251
▲ Lopid Tablets (3.8%) 2650
Lotensin Tablets (2.4%) 2365
▲ Lotensin HCT Tablets (5.2%) 2367
Lotrel Capsules 2370
Lupron Injection (Less than 5%) 3279
▲ LYMErix Vaccine (3.68% to 5.01%) 1592
Mavik Tablets (More than 1%) 478
Maxair Autohaler 1981
Maxair Inhaler (Less than 1%) 1984
▲ Maxalt Tablets (4% to 7%) 2120
▲ Maxalt-MLT Orally Disintegrating Tablets (4% to 7%) 2120
Maxzide 1008
MetroGel-Vaginal Gel (Less than 1%) 1986
▲ Mexitil Capsules (1.9% to 3.8%) 1047
Miacalcin Nasal Spray (1% to 3%) 2375
Micardis Tablets (1%) 1049
▲ Micardis HCT Tablets (3%) 1051
Midamor Tablets (Between 1% and 3%) 2136
Migranal Nasal Spray (1%) 2376
Mintezol 2137
Mobic Tablets (Less than 2%) 1054
Modicon 2563
Moduretic Tablets (Greater than 1%, less than 3%) 2138
Monopril Tablets (Less than 1.0% to 1.0% or more) 1091
▲ Monopril HCT (3.9%) 1094
Motofen Tablets (1 in 200 to 1 in 600) 577
Motrin Suspension, Oral Drops, Chewable Tablets, and Caplets 2002
Movana Tablets (Rare) ▣832
▲ Mykrox Tablets (4.4%) 1168
Myleran Tablets 1603
Nabi-HB 2295
Nadolol Tablets (2 of 100 patients) 2288
Nardil Tablets (Common) 2653
Navane Oral 2701
Navane Intramuscular 2703
▲ Navelbine Injection (27%) 1604
▲ Neoral Soft Gelatin Capsules (3%) 2380
▲ Neoral Oral Solution (3%) 2380
Neptazane Tablets ⊙271
▲ Neupogen for Injection (11%) 587
▲ Neurontin Capsules (11%) 2655
▲ Neurontin Oral Solution (3.4% to 11%) 2655
▲ Neurontin Tablets (11%) 2655
Nexium Delayed-Release Capsules (Less than 1%) 619
▲ Nicotrol Nasal Spray (Over 5%) 2843
Nilandron Tablets 753
▲ Nipent for Injection (29% to 42%) 3272
Nizoral Tablets 1791
▲ Nolvadex Tablets (3.8%) 678
▲ Normodyne Tablets (1% to 10%) 3137
Norplant System (Less than 1%) 3543
Norpramin Tablets 755
▲ Norvasc Tablets (4.5%) 2704
▲ Novantrone for Injection (39%) 1760
Novarel for Injection 1347
Numorphan 1324
Oncaspar 756
▲ Optivar Ophthalmic Solution (1% to 10%) 2273
Orthoclone OKT3 Sterile Solution 2498
Ortho-Cyclen/Ortho Tri-Cyclen 2573
Ortho-Novum 2563
Ortho-Novum 1/50▫28 Tablets 2556
▲ Ortho-Prefest Tablets (6%) 2570
Ortho-Cyclen/Ortho Tri-Cyclen 2573
Ovidrel for Injection 3220
▲ Pacerone Tablets (4% to 9%) 3331
Pediazole Suspension 3050
▲ PEG-Intron Powder for Injection (52%) 3140
Pepcid Injection (Infrequent) 2153
Pepcid for Oral Suspension (Infrequent) 2150
Pepcid RPD Orally Disintegrating Tablets (Infrequent) 2150
Pepcid Tablets (Infrequent) 2150
Periactin Tablets 2155
Persantine Tablets (Rare) 1057
Phenergan Injection 3553
Phenergan 3556
Phrenilin (Infrequent) 578
Pipracil 1866
▲ Plavix Tablets (3.3%) 1097
▲ Plavix Tablets (3.3%) 3084
▲ Pravachol Tablets (1.9% to 3.8%) 1099
Pregnyl for Injection 2482
Premphase Tablets 3572
Prempro Tablets 3572
Priftin Tablets (Less than 1%) 758
Prilosec Delayed-Release Capsules (Less than 1%) 628
Prinivil Tablets (2.5%) 2164
▲ Prinzide Tablets (3.7%) 2168
▲ Procardia XL Extended Release Tablets (5.9%) 2710
▲ Procrit for Injection (9% to 25%) 2502
▲ Proleukin for Injection (53%) 1199
▲ Prometrium Capsules (100 mg, 200 mg) (8% to 9%) 3261
Provera Tablets 2853
Prozac Pulvules, Liquid, and Weekly Capsules 1238
Pulmicort Respules (1% to 3%) 632
▲ Quinidex Extentabs (7%) 2933
Rabies Vaccine RabAvert (Rare) 1203
▲ Rebetron Combination Therapy (62% to 70%) 3153
Recombinate 853
Recombivax HB (Greater than 1%) 2178
▲ Reglan (Approximately 10%) 2935
Relafen Tablets (1% to 3%) 1617
Relenza Rotadisk (Less than 1.5%) 1619
▲ Remicade for IV Injection (8% to 11%) 1178
▲ Reminyl Oral Solution (5%) 1792
▲ Reminyl Tablets (5%) 1792
▲ Requip Tablets (11%) 1621
▲ Rescriptor Tablets (2.9% to 5.2%) 526
RhoGAM Injection 2524
Rifadin 765
Rifamate Capsules 767
Rifater Tablets 769
Risperdal (Frequent) 1796
▲ Roferon-A Injection (58% to 95%) 2996
Romazicon Injection (1% to 3%) 3000
▲ Rowasa Rectal Suspension Enema 4.0 grams/unit (60 mL) (3.44%) 3264
Rynatan Tablets 3351
▲ Rythmol Tablets – 150 mg, 225 mg, 300 mg (3.8% to 6.0%) 502
Sandostatin Injection (1% to 4%) 2394
▲ Sectral Capsules (11%) 3589
Sedapap Tablets 50 mg/650 mg (Infrequent) 2225
Septra Suspension 2265
Septra Tablets 2265
Septra DS Tablets 2265
Serevent Inhalation Aerosol (1% to 3%) 1633
Serophene Tablets (Less than 1 in 100 patients) 3226
▲ Serostim for Injection (17.1%) 3229
▲ Simulect for Injection (3% to 10%) 2399
Sinemet Tablets 1253
Sinemet CR Tablets 1255
Sinequan (Occasional) 2713
Singulair (1.8%) 2181
Skelid Tablets (More than or equal to 1%) 3088
▲ Soriatane Capsules (1% to 10%) 3003
Sporanox Capsules (2.8% to 3%) 1800
Sporanox Oral Solution (1.1% to 2.0%) 1808
Sporanox Oral Solution (1.1% to 2.0%) 2512
Stelazine 1640
Stromectol Tablets (0.9%) 2185
Surmontil Capsules 3595
▲ Sustiva Capsules (2% to 7%) 1258
Symmetrel (0.1% to 5%) 1328
▲ Tambocor Tablets (7.7%) 1990
▲ Tamiflu Capsules (1% to 7.9%) 3008
▲ Tamiflu Oral Suspension (1% to 7.9%) 3008
Tarka Tablets (2.8%) 508
▲ Tasmar Tablets (3% to 8%) 3010
Tegretol/Tegretol-XR 2404
▲ Temodar Capsules (34%) 3157
▲ Tenex Tablets (2% to 12%) 2942
▲ Tenoretic Tablets (0.6% to 26%) 690
▲ Tenormin (0.6% to 26%) 692
Tetanus & Diphtheria Toxoids Adsorbed for Adult Use 1880
Teveten Tablets (2%) 3327
TheraCys Injection (1%) 823
Thioplex for Injection 1765
Thiothixene Capsules 2290
▲ Tice BCG, BCG Live (7.4%) 2489
Timolide Tablets (1.9%) 2187
Timolol GFS ⊙266
Timoptic in Ocudose (Less frequent) 2192
Timoptic Sterile Ophthalmic Solution (Less frequent) 2190
Timoptic-XE Sterile Ophthalmic Gel Forming Solution 2194
Tonocard Tablets (0.8% to 1.6%) 649
▲ Topamax Sprinkle Capsules (11.1% to 30.8%) 2590
▲ Topamax Tablets (11.1% to 30.8%) 2590
▲ Toprol-XL Tablets (About 10 of 100 patients) 651
Tranxene 511
▲ Tricor Capsules, Micronized (5%) 513
▲ Trileptal Oral Suspension (7% to 21%) 2407
▲ Trileptal Tablets (7% to 21%) 2407
Tri-Levlen 962
▲ Trisenox Injection (63%) 1158
▲ Trizivir Tablets (44%) 1669
Trovan (Less than 1%) 2722
Trusopt Sterile Ophthalmic Solution (Infrequent) 2196
▲ Twinrix Vaccine (11% to 14%) 1674
Ultracet Tablets (At least 1%) 2597
Unasyn for Injection (Less than 1%) 2728
Uniretic Tablets (1%) 3178
Unithroid Tablets 3445
Univasc Tablets (2.4%) 3181
Uroqid-Acid No. 2 Tablets 947
▲ Valium Injectable (Among most common) 3026
▲ Valium Tablets (Among most common) 3047
▲ Vanceril Double Strength Inhalation Aerosol (3%) 3167
Vantin Tablets and Oral Suspension (Less than 1%) 2860
▲ Vaqta (3.9%) 2199
Varivax (Greater than or equal to 1%) 2202
▲ Vaseretic Tablets (3.9%) 2204
Vasotec I.V. Injection (0.5% to 1%) 2207
Vasotec Tablets (1.8% to 3.0%) 2210
Verelan Capsules (1.7%) 3184
Verelan PM Capsules (1.7%) 3186
Vesanoid Capsules 3037
▲ Viramune Oral Suspension (7% to 19%) 1060
▲ Viramune Tablets (7% to 19%) 1060
Vivactil Tablets 2217
Vivactil Tablets 2446
Voltaren Tablets 2315
Voltaren-XR Tablets 2315
Warfarin Sodium Tablets, USP 3302
▲ Wellbutrin Tablets (5.0%) 1680
▲ Xanax Tablets (48.6%) 2865
▲ Xeloda Tablets (5% to 8%) 3039
▲ Xenical Capsules (3.1% to 7.2%) 3043
▲ Zanaflex Tablets (41% to 78%) 1305
Zarontin Capsules 2659
Zarontin Syrup 2660
Zaroxolyn Tablets 1177
▲ Zebeta Tablets (6.6% to 8.2%) 1885
▲ Zenapax for Injection (Greater than 5%) 3046
▲ Zestoretic Tablets (3.7%) 695
Zestril Tablets (2.5%) 698
▲ Ziac Tablets (3.0% to 4.6%) 1887
▲ Ziagen (44%) 1692
▲ Zinecard for Injection (48% to 61%) 2869
Zithromax (1% or less) 2743
Zithromax for Oral Suspension, 300 mg, 600 mg, 900 mg, 1200 mg (1% or less) 2739
Zithromax Tablets, 250 mg (1% or less) 2739
Zithromax Tablets, 600 mg (1% or less) 2743
▲ Zofran Injection (5%) 1698
▲ Zofran (9% to 13%) 1703
▲ Zofran ODT Orally Disintegrating Tablets (9% to 13%) 1703
▲ Zoladex (5%) 702
▲ Zoloft (12%) 2751
▲ Zonegran Capsules (8%) 1307
▲ Zyrtec (5.9%) 2756
▲ Zyrtec-D 12 Hour Extended Relief Tablets (5.9%) 2758

Fatigue, muscular

Demadex Tablets and Injection 2965
Dyazide Capsules 1515
Furosemide Tablets 2284
Imitrex Injection (Rare) 1549
Maxzide 1008
Phrenilin (Infrequent) 578
Prinzide Tablets 2168
Sedapap Tablets 50 mg/650 mg (Infrequent) 2225
▲ Tenoretic Tablets (3% to 6%) 690
▲ Tenormin (3% to 6%) 692
Vaseretic Tablets 2204
Zaroxolyn Tablets 1177
Zestoretic Tablets 695

Fear

Bicillin L-A Injection 2242
Claritin-D 12 Hour Extended Release Tablets 3102
Claritin-D 24 Hour Extended Release Tablets 3104
Dilaudid 441
Dilaudid Powder 441
Dilaudid Rectal Suppositories 441
Dilaudid Tablets 441
Hycodan 1316
Hycomine Compound Tablets 1317
Hycotuss Expectorant Syrup 1318
Lortab 3319
Lortab Elixir 3317
Maxidone Tablets CIII 3399
Norco 5/325 Tablets CIII 3424
Norco 7.5/325 Tablets CIII 3425
Norco 10/325 Tablets CIII 3425
Norco 10/325 Tablets CIII 3427
Rynatan Tablets 3351
Tussionex Pennkinetic Extended-Release Suspension 1174
Vicodin Tablets 516
Vicodin ES Tablets 517
Vicodin HP Tablets 518
Vicodin Tuss Expectorant 519
Xanax Tablets (1.4%) 2865
Zydone Tablets 1330
Zyrtec-D 12 Hour Extended Relief Tablets 2758

Febrile reactions

Albuminar-5, U.S.P. 785
Albuminar-25, U.S.P. 786
Digibind Powder 1514
Follistim for Injection 2465
Humegon for Injection 2468
INFeD Injection 3388
▲ JE-VAX Vaccine (5.5%) 811
▲ Leustatin Injection (11%) 2495
Liquid PedvaxHIB 2148
Pergonal for Injection 3223
Repronex for Intramuscular and Subcutaneous Injection 1347
Thioplex for Injection 1765
Varivax (Less than 0.1%) 2202

Fecal fat, increase

(*see under* Steatorrhea)

Fecal impaction

Actiq (Less than 1%) 1184
Betaseron for SC Injection 988
Clozaril Tablets 2319
Cognex Capsules (Infrequent) 1351
Doxil Injection (Less than 1%) 566
Etrafon (Occasional) 3115
Geodon Capsules (Rare) 2688
Paxil (Rare) 1609
Rilutek Tablets (Infrequent) 772
Trilafon (Occasional) 3160
Zanaflex Tablets (Infrequent) 1305
Zyprexa Tablets (Infrequent) 1973
Zyprexa ZYDIS Orally Disintegrating Tablets (Infrequent) 1973

Fecal urgency

▲ Xenical Capsules (2.8% to 22.1%) 3043

Feces, color change

Prilosec Delayed-Release Capsules (Less than 1%) 628
Rifadin 765
Trovan (Less than 1%) 2722

Feces, discoloration

Fortovase Capsules (Less than 2%) 2970
Invirase Capsules (Less than 2%) 2979
Mycobutin Capsules 2838
Prevacid Delayed-Release Capsules (Less than 1%) 3292
PREVPAC (Less than 1%) 3298
Risperdal (Rare) 1796
Urimax Tablets 1769
Urised Tablets 2876

Feces abnormal

Colazal Capsules 3069

Feeling, drugged

▲ Ambien Tablets (3%) 3191
Neurontin Capsules (Infrequent) 2655
Neurontin Oral Solution (Infrequent) 2655
Neurontin Tablets (Infrequent) 2655
Paxil (2%) 1609

Feeling, high

Neurontin Capsules (Rare) 2655
Neurontin Oral Solution (Rare) 2655
Neurontin Tablets (Rare) 2655

Feeling, intoxicated

Ambien Tablets (Rare) 3191
Imitrex Injection (Rare) 1549

▲ Phrenilin (Among most frequent) 578
▲ Sedapap Tablets 50 mg/650 mg (Among the most frequent) 2225
Trileptal Oral Suspension 2407
Trileptal Tablets 2407

Feeling, shaky
Koāte-DVI (0.7%) 931
Phrenilin (Infrequent) 578

Feeling, strange
Ambien Tablets (Rare) 3191
Amerge Tablets (Infrequent) 1467
Imitrex Injection (2.2%) 1549
Imitrex Nasal Spray (Infrequent) 1554
Imitrex Tablets 1558
MS Contin Tablets (Less frequent) ... 2896
Neurontin Capsules (Rare) 2655
Neurontin Oral Solution (Rare) 2655
Neurontin Tablets (Rare) 2655
Trileptal Oral Suspension (1% to 2%) 2407
Trileptal Tablets (1% to 2%) 2407

Feet, cold
Hivid Tablets (Less than 1%) 2975
Kogenate 934

Fertility, impairment of
Depo-Provera Contraceptive Injection (Fewer than 1%) 2798
Intron A for Injection 3120

Fertility, male, decrease
Lopid Tablets 2650
Tricor Capsules, Micronized (Less than 1%) 513

Festination
Eldepryl Capsules 3266

Fetal acidosis
Prepidil Gel 2851

Fetal death
(*see under* Death, fetal)

Fetal defects
Accupril Tablets 2611
Accutane Capsules 2944
Climara Transdermal System 958
Clomid Tablets (Less than 1%) 735
Depo-Provera Contraceptive Injection 2798
Halcion Tablets 2823
Lexxel Tablets 608
Lotrel Capsules 2370
Naropin Injection (1% to 5%) 612
Nembutal Sodium Solution 485
Serophene Tablets 3226

Fetal depression
Prepidil Gel 2851

Fetal harm
Accupril Tablets 2611
Accutane Capsules 2944
Activella Tablets 2764
Advil Cold and Sinus Caplets .... ▣ 771
Advil Cold and Sinus Tablets .... ▣ 771
Albenza Tablets 1463
Alkeran for Injection 1465
Alkeran Tablets 1466
Aquasol A Parenteral 593
Arava Tablets 724
Arimidex Tablets 659
Aromasin Tablets 2769
Arthrotec Tablets 3195
Atacand Tablets 595
Atacand HCT Tablets 597
Ativan Injection 3478
Avalide Tablets 1070
Avapro Tablets 1074
Avapro Tablets 3076
Aygestin Tablets 1333
Captopril Tablets 2281
Carac Cream 1222
Carbatrol Capsules 3234
Casodex Tablets 662
Cerubidine for Injection 947
Clomid Tablets 735
CombiPatch Transdermal System 2323
Cosmegen for Injection 2062
Cozaar Tablets 2067
Cytotec Tablets 3202
DaunoXome Injection 1442
Declomycin Tablets 1855
Depen Titratable Tablets 3341
Diucardin Tablets 3494
Dynacin Capsules 2019
Efudex 1733
Enalaprilat Injection 863
Eskalith 1527
Estrace Vaginal Cream 3358
Estrace Tablets 3361
Estratest 3252
Eulexin Capsules 3118
Evista Tablets 1915
Fareston Tablets 3237
Femara Tablets 2351
femhrt Tablets 2635
Fludara for Injection 995
Fluoroplex 552
Follistim for Injection 2465
Sterile FUDR 2974
Gemzar for Injection 1919
Gonal-F for Injection 3216
Humegon for Injection 2468
Hycamtin for Injection 1546
Hyzaar 2109
Ifex for Injection 1123
Lescol Capsules 2361
Lescol Capsules 2925
Lescol XL Tablets 2361
Lescol XL Tablets 2925
Leukeran Tablets 1591
Lithium Carbonate 3061
Lithium Citrate Syrup 3061
Lithobid Slow-Release Tablets 3255
Lotensin Tablets 2365
Lotrel Capsules 2370
Lupron Depot 7.5 mg 3284
Mavik Tablets 478
Maxzide 1008
Megace Oral Suspension 1124
Menest Tablets 2254
Mevacor Tablets 2132
Micardis Tablets 1049
Micardis HCT Tablets 1051
Migranal Nasal Spray 2376
Minocin Oral Suspension 1865
Minocin Pellet-Filled Capsules 1863
Mithracin for Intravenous Use 903
Monopril Tablets 1091
Monopril HCT 1094
Motrin Sinus Headache Caplets 2005
Mustargen for Injection 2142
Myleran Tablets 1603
Mylotarg for Injection 3540
Navelbine Injection 1604
Nebcin Vials, Hyporets & ADD-Vantage 1955
Nembutal Sodium Solution 485
Neosporin G.U. Irrigant Sterile 2256
Nicotrol Inhaler 2840
Nicotrol Nasal Spray 2843
Nolvadex Tablets 678
Novantrone for Injection 1760
Ortho Dienestrol Cream 2554
Ovidrel for Injection 3220
ParaGard T 380A Intrauterine Copper Contraceptive 2582
Paraplatin for Injection 1126
Pergonal for Injection 3223
Periostat Tablets 1208
Pravachol Tablets 1099
Premarin Intravenous 3563
Premarin Tablets 3566
Prinivil Tablets 2164
Prinzide Tablets 2168
ProSom Tablets 500
Purinethol Tablets 1615
ReoPro Vials 1958
Repronex for Intramuscular and Subcutaneous Injection 1347
Soma Compound Tablets 3354
Soma Compound w/Codeine Tablets 3355
Streptomycin Sulfate Injection 2714
Synarel Nasal Solution for Endometriosis 3205
Tabloid Tablets 1642
Taxol Injection 1129
Taxotere for Injection Concentrate ... 778
Tazorac Gel 556
Tegretol/Tegretol-XR 2404
Temodar Capsules 3157
Tenoretic Tablets 690
Tenormin 692
Testoderm Transdermal Systems 574
Testred Capsules, 10 mg 1746
Thalomid Capsules 1154
Thioplex for Injection 1765
TOBI Solution for Inhalation 1206
Trisenox Injection 1158
Univasc Tablets 3181
Vaseretic Tablets 2204
Vasotec I.V. Injection 2207
Vasotec Tablets 2210
Vesanoid Capsules 3037
Viadur Implant 912
Virazole for Inhalation Solution 1747
Vivelle Transdermal System 2412
Vivelle-Dot Transdermal System 2416
Xanax Tablets 2865
Xeloda Tablets 3039
Zestoretic Tablets 695
Zestril Tablets 698
Zocor Tablets 2219
Zoladex 702

Fetal heart rate, deceleration
Prepidil Gel (2.1% to 4.3%) 2851

Fetal hemorrhage
Coumadin for Injection 1243
Coumadin Tablets 1243
Soma Compound Tablets 3354
Soma Compound w/Codeine Tablets 3355
Warfarin Sodium Tablets, USP 3302

Fetal hydantoin syndrome
Dilantin Infatabs 2624
Dilantin Kapseals 2622
Dilantin-125 Oral Suspension 2625

Fetal problems, unspecified
Aleve Tablets, Caplets and Gelcaps .... ▣ 602
Alka-Seltzer PM Effervescent Tablets .... ▣ 605
Genuine Bayer Tablets, Caplets and Gelcaps .... ▣ 606
Extra Strength Bayer Caplets and Gelcaps .... ▣ 610
Aspirin Regimen Bayer Children's Chewable Tablets (Orange or Cherry Flavored) .... ▣ 607
Aspirin Regimen Bayer Regular Strength 325 mg Caplets .... ▣ 606
Genuine Bayer Professional Labeling (Aspirin Regimen Bayer) .... ▣ 608
Extra Strength Bayer Arthritis Caplets .... ▣ 610
Extra Strength Bayer Plus Caplets .... ▣ 610
Extra Strength Bayer PM Caplets .. ▣ 611
BC Powder .... ▣ 619
▲ Chirocaine Injection (9.6%) 2909
Cipro I.V. 893
Enalaprilat Injection 863
Humorsol Sterile Ophthalmic Solution 2102
Orudis KT Tablets .... ▣ 778
Polytrim Ophthalmic Solution 556
Vaseretic Tablets 2204
Vasotec I.V. Injection 2207
Vasotec Tablets 2210

Fetal sepsis, intrauterine
Prepidil Gel 2851

Fever
▲ Abelcet Injection (14%) 1273
Accolate Tablets (1.6%) 657
▲ Acel-Imune (0.3% to 26%) 1851
Aceon Tablets (2 mg, 4 mg, 8 mg) (0.3% to 1.5%) 3249
Aciphex Tablets 1267
Aciphex Tablets 1783
▲ ActHIB Vaccine (Up to 24.6%) 798
▲ Actimmune (52%) 1772
Actiq (1% or greater) 1184
Activase I.V. 1410
Adalat CC Tablets (Rare) 877
▲ Adderall XR Capsules (5%)
Adriamycin PFS/RDF Injection (Occasional) 2767
▲ Aerobid/Aerobid-M (3% to 9%) 1363
Aggrastat (Less than 1%) 2031
Aggrenox Capsules (Less than 1%) 1026
▲ Agrylin Capsules (8.9%) 3232
Alamast Ophthalmic Solution (Less than 5%) 3092
Albenza Tablets (Up to 1.0%) 1463
Albumin (Human) 5% (Very rare) 838
Albumin (Human) 25% (Very rare) 839
Aldara Cream, 5% (More than 1%) ... 1978
Aldomet Tablets 2037
Aldoril Tablets 2039
▲ Alferon N Injection (18% to 81%) 1770
Alkeran for Injection 1465
Alkeran Tablets 1466
Allegra (2.4%) 712
Aloprim for Injection (Less than 1%) 2292
Altace Capsules (Less than 1%) 2233
Ambien Tablets (Infrequent) 3191
Amerge Tablets (Infrequent) 1467
▲ Amphotec (33% to 55%) 1774
Anaprox Tablets (Less than 1%) 2967
Anaprox DS Tablets (Less than 1%) 2967
Ancobon Capsules 1730
▲ Anzemet Injection (4.3%) 719
▲ Anzemet Tablets (3.5%) 722
▲ Apligraf (3.6%) 2305
Arava Tablets (1% to 3%) 724
▲ Aredia for Injection (38.5%) 2309
▲ Argatroban Injection (6.9%) 1478
Aricept Tablets (Infrequent) 1270
Aricept Tablets (Infrequent) 2665
Arimidex Tablets (2% to 5%) 659
Aromasin Tablets (Less frequent) 2769
Arthrotec Tablets (Rare) 3195
▲ Asacol Delayed-Release Tablets (6%) 2884
Atacand Tablets (0.5% or greater) .. 595
Attenuvax (Occasional) 2044
Augmentin Chewable Tablets (Frequent) 1482
Augmentin Powder for Oral Suspension (Frequent) 1482
Augmentin Tablets (Frequent) 1485
Augmentin ES-600 Powder for Oral Suspension 1487
Autoplex T 2294
Avalide Tablets 1070
Avapro Tablets (Less than 1%) 1074
Avapro Tablets (Less than 1%) 3076
▲ Avonex (23%) 1013
Axert Tablets (Rare) 2772
Axid Pulvules (1.6%) 1903
Axid Pulvules (1.6%) 2919
Azactam for Injection (Less than 1% to 1.0%) 1276
▲ Azulfidine EN-tabs Tablets (5%) 2775
Baycol Tablets (Rare) 883
Bebulin VH 840
BeneFix for Injection 1432
Betapace Tablets (Rare; 1% to 4%) 950
Betapace AF Tablets (0.7% to 3.3%) 954
▲ Betaseron for SC Injection (59%) ... 988
Bicillin C-R 900/300 Injection 2240
Bicillin C-R Injection 2238
Bicillin L-A Injection 2242
Blocadren Tablets 2046
▲ Botox Purified Neurotoxin Complex (2% to 10%) 549
Brevibloc Injection (Less than 1%) ... 858
Buminate 5% Solution, USP (Occasional) 841
Buminate 25% Solution, USP (Occasional) 842
Calcium Disodium Versenate Injection 1980
▲ Campath Ampules (19% to 86%) 992
Canasa Rectal Suppositories (1.2%) 829
▲ Cancidas for Injection (2.9% to 26.2%) 2048
▲ Captopril Tablets (About 4 to 7 of 100) 2281
Carbatrol Capsules 3234
Cardene I.V. (Rare) 3485
Cardura Tablets (Less than 0.5%) ... 2668
▲ Carnitor Injection (5% to 12%) 3242
▲ Casodex Tablets (2% to 5%) 662
Cataflam Tablets (Rare) 2315
Catapres Tablets 1037
Catapres-TTS (0.5% or less) 1038
Ceclor CD Tablets (0.1% to 1%) 1279
Ceclor (Frequently) 1905
Cedax Oral Suspension (0.1% to 1%) 1021
Cefizox for Intramuscular or Intravenous Use (1% to 5%) 1390
Cefotan 664
Ceftin for Oral Suspension (0.1% to 1%) 1898
Cefzil (Rare) 1076
Celebrex Capsules (0.1% to 1.9%) 2676
Celebrex Capsules (0.1% to 1.9%) 2780
Celestone Soluspan Injectable Suspension 3097
Celexa (2%) 1365
▲ CellCept Capsules (3% to 47.4%) .. 2951
▲ CellCept Intravenous (3% to 47.4%) 2951
▲ CellCept Oral Suspension (3% to 47.4%) 2951
▲ CellCept Tablets (3% to 52.3%) 2951
Cenestin Tablets (1%) 1263
Ceptaz for Injection (2% of patients) 1499
Cerebyx Injection (Frequent) 2619
▲ Cerezyme for Injection (5.4%) 1438
Cerubidine for Injection (Rare) 947
Cervidil Vaginal Insert (Less than 1%) 1369
▲ Chemet Capsules (5.2% to 15.7%) 3078
▲ Chirocaine Injection (8.5%) 2909
Cipro I.V. (1% or less) 893
Cipro I.V. Pharmacy Bulk Package (Less than 1%) 897
Cipro (Less than 1%) 887
Claforan Injection (2.4%) 732
Claritin (At least one patient) 3100
Claritin-D 12 Hour Extended Release Tablets (Less frequent) ... 3102
Claritin-D 24 Hour Extended Release Tablets (Fewer than 2%) 3104
Cleocin Vaginal Ovules (Less than 1%) 2789
Clinoril Tablets (Less than 1%) 2053
Clomid Tablets 735
Clorpres Tablets 1002
▲ Clozaril Tablets (1% to 5% or more) 2319
Cogentin 2055
Cognex Capsules (Frequent) 1351
Colazal Capsules (2%) 3069
Coly-Mycin M Parenteral 2243
Combipres Tablets 1040
▲ Combivir Tablets (10%) 1502
Compazine 1505
Comtan Tablets 2328
▲ Comvax (0.8% to 14.2%) 2056
Concerta Extended-Release Tablets 1998
Concerta Tablets 561
▲ Copaxone for Injection (8%) 3306
Cordarone Intravenous (2.0%) 3491
▲ Coreg Tablets (3.1%) 1508
Corgard Tablets 2245
Corlopam Injection (0.5% to 5%) 412
Corzide 40/5 Tablets 2247
Corzide 80/5 Tablets 2247
Cosmegen for Injection 2062
Cosopt Sterile Ophthalmic Solution 2065

Coumadin for Injection (Infrequent) 1243
Coumadin Tablets (Infrequent) 1243
Cozaar Tablets (Less than 1%) 2067
Crinone (Less than 5%) 3213
Crixivan Capsules (0.5%) 2070
Cuprimine Capsules (Rare) 2075
CytoGam Intravenous (Less than 5.0%) 2026
Cytotec Tablets (Infrequent) 3202
▲ Cytovene (38%) 2959
Dantrium Capsules (Less frequent) 2885
Dapsone Tablets USP 1780
Daranide Tablets 2077
▲ DaunoXome Injection (5% to 42%) 1442
Depacon Injection (Rare to 6%) 416
▲ Depakene (6%) 421
▲ Depakote Sprinkle Capsules (6%) 426
Depakote Tablets (1% to 6%) 430
Depakote ER Tablets (Greater than 1%) 436
Depen Titratable Tablets (Rare) 3341
▲ DepoCyt Injection (4% to 11%) 1197
Depo-Provera Contraceptive Injection (Fewer than 1%) 2798
Desferal Vials 2333
Diamox ⊙269
Dilantin Infatabs 2624
Dilantin Kapseals 2622
Dilantin-125 Oral Suspension 2625
Diovan HCT Tablets 2338
Dipentum Capsules (Rare) 2803
▲ Diphtheria & Tetanus Toxoids Adsorbed Purogenated for Pediatric Use (0.7% to 9.3%) 1857
Diprivan Injectable Emulsion (Less than 1%) 667
Diucardin Tablets 3494
Diuril Oral 2087
Diuril Sodium Intravenous 2086
Dobutrex Solution Vials (Occasional) 1914
Dolobid Tablets (Less than 1 in 100) 2088
Dopram Injectable 2931
▲ Doxil Injection (6.9% to 9.1%) 566
DTIC-Dome (Infrequent) 902
▲ Duraclon Injection (6%) 3057
Duricef 1079
Dynabac Tablets (0.1% to 1%) 2269
EC-Naprosyn Delayed-Release Tablets (Less than 1%) 2967
Ecotrin Enteric Coated Aspirin Low, Regular and Maximum Strength Tablets 1715
Edecrin 2091
Effexor Tablets 3495
▲ Effexor XR Capsules (3%) 3499
▲ Ellence Injection (1.4% to 5.2%) 2806
Elspar for Injection 2092
Enalaprilat Injection (0.5% to 1%) 863
Enbrel for Injection 1752
Enbrel for Injection 3504
▲ Engerix-B Vaccine (1% to 10%) 1517
▲ Epivir (10%) 1520
▲ Epivir-HBV (7%) 1524
▲ Epogen for Injection (29% to 51%) 582
▲ Ergamisol Tablets (3% to 5%) 1789
Eskalith 1527
Ethyol for Injection 2029
Etrafon 3115
▲ Evista Tablets (3.1% to 3.9%) 1915
Evoxac Capsules (1% to 3%) 1217
Exelon Capsules (Frequent) 2342
Exelon Oral Solution (Frequent) 2345
Famotidine Injection (Infrequent) 866
Famvir Tablets (0.8% to 3.3%) 2348
▲ Felbatol (2.6% to 22.6%) 3343
Feldene Capsules (Occasional) 2685
▲ Ferrlecit Injection (5%) 3386
▲ Flolan for Injection (13% to 25%) 1528
Flonase Nasal Spray (1% to 3%) 1533
▲ Flovent Diskus (7%) 3614
Flovent (1% to 3%) 1535
Flovent Rotadisk (2% to 4%) 1537
Floxin I.V. (1% to 3%) 2526
Floxin Otic Solution (0.3%) 1219
Floxin Tablets (1% to 3%) 2529
▲ Fludara for Injection (60% to 69%) 995
Flumadine 1370
Fluothane Inhalation 3508
FluShield Influenza Vaccine 3521
Fluzone Vaccine 802
Follistim for Injection 2465
Fortaz (2%) 1541
Fortovase Capsules (Less than 2%) 2970
▲ Foscavir Injection (5% to 65%) 605
Fragmin Injection (Rare) 2814
Sterile FUDR 2974
Furosemide Tablets 2284
Gabitril Tablets (1% or more) 1189
▲ Gamimune N, 5% Solvent/Detergent Treated (Among most common) 925
▲ Gamimune N, 10% Solvent/Detergent Treated (Among most common) 928
Gammagard S/D (Occasional) 845
Gammar-P I.V. 787
▲ Gemzar for Injection (16% to 41%) 1919
▲ Gengraf Capsules (3%) 457
Geodon Capsules (Frequent) 2688
▲ Gleevec Capsules (14% to 38%) 2357
▲ Gliadel Wafer (12%) 1723
▲ Gonal-F for Injection (4.2%) 3216
Haldol Decanoate 2535
Haldol Injection, Tablets and Concentrate 2533
▲ Havrix Vaccine (1% to 10%) 1544
Hemofil M (Extremely rare) 847
Heparin Lock Flush Solution 3509
Heparin Sodium Injection 3511
▲ Herceptin I.V. (36%) 1414
HibTITER (0.6% to 1.4%) 1859
Hivid Tablets (Less than 1% to 1.7%) 2975
Humate-P Concentrate (Rare) 790
Humegon for Injection 2468
Hyalgan Solution (Seven cases) 3080
▲ Hycamtin for Injection (Less than 1% to 34%) 1546
HydroDIURIL Tablets 2108
Hytrin Capsules (0.5% to at least 1%) 464
Hyzaar 2109
▲ Idamycin PFS Injection (26%) 2825
Ifex for Injection (1%) 1123
Imdur Tablets (Less than or equal to 5%) 1826
Imitrex Injection (Rare) 1549
Imitrex Nasal Spray (Infrequent) 1554
Imitrex Tablets (Infrequent) 1558
Indapamide Tablets 2286
Inderal 3513
Inderal LA Long-Acting Capsules 3516
Inderide Tablets 3517
Inderide LA Long-Acting Capsules 3519
▲ Infanrix Vaccine (Up to 9.0%) 1562
INFeD Injection 3388
▲ Infergen (58% to 61%) 1777
Innohep Injection (1.5%) 1248
▲ Intron A for Injection (3% to 86%) 3120
Invirase Capsules (Less than 2%) 2979
▲ IPOL Vaccine (Up to 38%) 809
Iscar Mali Injection 3456
Iscar Mali Special Injection 3456
Iscar Pini Injection 3456
Iscar Quercus Injection 3456
Iscar Quercus Special Injection 3456
Isoptin SR Tablets 467
Iveegam EN (0.3% to 0.8%) 849
▲ JE-VAX Vaccine (Less than 3% to approximately 10%) 811
Kadian Capsules (Less than 3%) 1335
Kaletra Capsules (Less than 2%) 471
Kaletra Oral Solution (Less than 2%) 471
Kefurox Vials, ADD-Vantage 1948
Keppra Tablets (1% or more) 3314
Klonopin Tablets (Infrequent) 2983
Kogenate (Two reports) 934
Konyne 80 937
▲ Kytril Injection (3%) 2986
▲ Kytril Tablets (5%) 2988
▲ Lamictal (5.5%) 1567
▲ Lariam Tablets (Among most frequent) 2989
Lescol Capsules (Rare) 2361
Lescol Capsules (Rare) 2925
Lescol XL Tablets 2361
Lescol XL Tablets 2925
Leukeran Tablets 1591
▲ Leukine (77% to 95%) 1755
▲ Leustatin Injection (11% to 69%) 2495
Levaquin (0.5% to less than 1.0%) 2537
Levbid Extended-Release Tablets 3172
Levlen 962
Levlite 21 Tablets 962
Levlite 28 Tablets 962
Levoxyl Tablets 1819
Levsin/Levsinex/Levbid 3172
Lexxel Tablets (Infrequent) 608
Lipitor Tablets (Less than 2%) 2639
Lipitor Tablets (Less than 2%) 2696
Lithobid Slow-Release Tablets 3255
Lodine (Greater than or equal to 1%) 3528
Lodine XL Extended-Release Tablets (Less than 1%) 3530
Lotensin HCT Tablets (0.3% or more) 2367
▲ Lovenox Injection (5%) 746
Loxitane Capsules 3398
Lupron Depot 7.5 mg (Less than 5%) 3284
Lupron Depot–3 Month 22.5 mg (Less than 5%) 3288
Lupron Depot–4 Month 30 mg (Less than 5%) 3289
Lupron Depot-PED 7.5 mg, 11.25 mg and 15 mg (Less than 2%) 3291
Lupron Injection (Less than 5%) 3279
Lupron Injection Pediatric (Less than 2%) 3280
Luvox Tablets (25, 50, 100 mg) 3256
▲ LYMErix Vaccine (2.58% to 3.58%) 1592
Macrobid Capsules (Rare) 2889
Macrodantin Capsules (Rare) 2891
▲ Malarone (3% to 6%) 1596
Massengill Disposable Douches ▣752
Massengill Medicated Disposable Douche ▣753
Matulane Capsules 3246
Maxalt Tablets (Rare) 2120
Maxalt-MLT Orally Disintegrating Tablets (Rare) 2120
Maxipime for Injection (0.1% to 1%) 1285
Maxzide 1008
Mefoxin for Injection 2124
Mefoxin Premixed Intravenous Solution 2127
▲ Megace Oral Suspension (1% to 6%) 1124
Menomune-A/C/Y/W-135 Vaccine 813
▲ Mepron Suspension (0.6% to 40%) 1598
Meridia Capsules (Greater than or equal to 1%) 481
Merrem I.V. (0.1% to 1.0%) 673
Meruvax II 2130
Metadate CD Capsules 1164
Metadate ER Tablets 1167
Methylin Tablets 1995
Methylin ER Tablets 1995
Mevacor Tablets (Rare) 2132
Mexitil Capsules (1.2%) 1047
Miacalcin Nasal Spray (Less than 1%) 2375
Micardis Tablets (More than 0.3%) 1049
Micardis HCT Tablets 1051
Microzide Capsules 3414
Migranal Nasal Spray (Infrequent) 2376
Miltown Tablets (Rare) 3349
Minipress Capsules 2699
Minizide Capsules 2700
Mintezol 2137
Mirapex Tablets (1% or more) 2834
Mithracin for Intravenous Use 903
M-M-R II 2118
Moban 1320
Mobic Tablets (Less than 2%) 1054
Modicon 2563
Moduretic Tablets 2138
Mononine Concentrate 794
Monopril Tablets (0.4% to 1.0%) 1091
Monopril HCT (Less than 2%) 1094
Monurol Sachet (Less than 1%) 1375
Motrin Suspension, Oral Drops, Chewable Tablets, and Caplets (Rare; less than 1%) 2002
Mumpsvax (Uncommon) 2141
Myambutol Tablets 1290
Mycobutin Capsules (2%) 2838
Mylocel Tablets 2227
▲ Mylotarg for Injection (7% to 61%) 3540
Myobloc Injectable Solution (2% or greater) 1291
Nadolol Tablets 2288
Naprelan Tablets (Less than 3%) 1293
Naprosyn Suspension (Less than 1%) 2967
Naprosyn Tablets (Less than 1%) 2967
Narcan Injection 1322
Nardil Tablets (Less frequent) 2653
Naropin Injection (1% to 5%) 612
Natrecor for Injection (At least 1%) 3189
Navane Oral 2701
Navane Intramuscular 2703
Navelbine Injection 1604
Nebcin Vials, Hyporets & ADD-Vantage 1955
Nembutal Sodium Solution 485
Neoral Soft Gelatin Capsules (1% to less than 3%) 2380
Neoral Oral Solution (1% to less than 3%) 2380
Neptazane Tablets ⊙271
▲ Neumega for Injection (36%) 1434
▲ Neupogen for Injection (12%) 587
Neurontin Capsules (More than 1%) 2655
▲ Neurontin Oral Solution (10.1%) 2655
Neurontin Tablets (More than 1%) 2655
Nexium Delayed-Release Capsules (Less than 1%) 619
▲ Nicotrol Inhaler (Greater than 3%) 2840
▲ Nilandron Tablets (5.3%) 753
▲ Nipent for Injection (42% to 46%) 3272
Nizoral Tablets (Less than 1%) 1791
Normodyne Tablets 3137
Noroxin Tablets (0.3% to 1.0%) 2145
Norpramin Tablets 755
▲ Norvir Capsules (0.9% to 4.4%) 487
▲ Norvir Oral Solution (0.9% to 4.4%) 487
▲ Novantrone for Injection (24% to 78%) 1760
NovoSeven (Greater than or equal to 2%) 2430
▲ Nutropin Depot for Injectable Suspension (7%) 1423
Omnicef 493
▲ Oncaspar (Greater than 5%) 756
Orap Tablets 1407
▲ Organan Injection (7.3% to 22.2%) 2480
Ortho Diaphragm Kits – All-Flex Arcing Spring; Ortho Coil Spring 2552
▲ Orthoclone OKT3 Sterile Solution (89% to 90%) 2498
Ortho-Cyclen/Ortho Tri-Cyclen 2573
Ortho-Novum 2563
Ortho-Novum 1/50▢28 Tablets 2556
Ortho-Cyclen/Ortho Tri-Cyclen 2573
Ovidrel for Injection (Less than 2%) 3220
OxyContin Tablets (Between 1% and 5%) 2912
Panhematin for Injection 497
ParaGard T 380A Intrauterine Copper Contraceptive 2582
Paraplatin for Injection 1126
Paser Granules 1781
Paxil (2%) 1609
Pediazole Suspension 3050
▲ Liquid PedvaxHIB (0.5% to 18.1%) 2148
▲ PEG-Intron Powder for Injection (22%) 3140
Pentasa Capsules (0.9%) 3239
Pepcid Injection (Infrequent) 2153
Pepcid for Oral Suspension (Infrequent) 2150
Pepcid RPD Orally Disintegrating Tablets (Infrequent) 2150
Pepcid Tablets (Infrequent) 2150
Pergonal for Injection 3223
Permapen Isoject 2706
Permax Tablets (Frequent) 1299
Pfizerpen for Injection 2707
Phenergan 3556
▲ Photofrin for Injection (31%) 831
Phrenilin (Infrequent) 578
Plasbumin-5 (Rare) 939
Plasbumin-20 (Rare) 940
Plasbumin-25 (Rare) 941
Plavix Tablets 1097
Plavix Tablets 3084
Pletal Tablets (Less than 2%) 2605
Pletal Tablets (Less than 2%) 2848
Pneumovax 23 (Rare) 2156
Pnu-Imune 23 (Occasional) 1868
Podocon-25 Liquid 2608
Polocaine Injection, USP 625
Polocaine-MPF Injection, USP 625
Ponstel Capsules (Occasional) 1356
Potaba (Infrequent) 1721
Pravachol Tablets (Rare) 1099
Premphase Tablets 3572
Prempro Tablets 3572
Prepidil Gel (1.4%) 2851
Prevacid Delayed-Release Capsules (Less than 1%) 3292
▲ Prevnar for Injection (33.4% to 41.9%) 1870
PREVPAC (Less than 1%) 3298
Priftin Tablets 758
Prilosec Delayed-Release Capsules (Less than 1%) 628
Primaxin I.M. 2158
Primaxin I.V. (0.5%) 2160
Prinivil Tablets (0.3% to 1.1%) 2164
Prinzide Tablets (0.3% to 1%) 2168
Procanbid Extended-Release Tablets (Fairly common) 2262
Procardia Capsules (2% or less) 2708
Procardia XL Extended Release Tablets (1% or less) 2710
▲ Procrit for Injection (29% to 51%) 2502
▲ Prograf (19% to 48%) 1393
Prolastin (0.77%) 943
▲ Proleukin for Injection (29%) 1199
Prometrium Capsules (100 mg, 200 mg) (Less than 5%) 3261
Proplex T (Occasional) 851
ProSom Tablets (Infrequent) 500
▲ Prostin E2 Suppositories (Approximately one-half) 2852
Protonix I.V. (Less than 1%) 3580
Protonix Tablets (Less than 1%) 3577
▲ Protopic Ointment (1% to 18%) 1397
▲ Proventil HFA Inhalation Aerosol (6%) 3150
Provera Tablets 2853
Provigil Tablets (1%; at least 1%) 1193
Prozac Pulvules, Liquid, and Weekly Capsules (1.4% to 2%) 1238
Pulmicort Turbuhaler Inhalation Powder (Up to 4%) 636
▲ Pulmozyme Inhalation Solution (32%) 1426
Pyrazinamide Tablets (Rare) 1876
▲ Quinaglute Dura-Tabs Tablets (6%) 978
Quinidex Extentabs 2933
Quixin Ophthalmic Solution (1% to 3%) 3093
Rabies Vaccine RabAvert (Uncommon) 1203
▲ Rapamune Oral Solution and Tablets (27% to 34%) 3584
▲ Rebetron Combination Therapy (35% to 41%) 3153
Recombinate (Extremely rare) 853
Recombivax HB (Greater than 1%) 2178
ReFacto Vials 1437
▲ Refludan for Injection (4.4%) 761
Relafen Tablets (Less than 1%) 1617
Relenza Rotadisk (Less than 1.5%) 1619
Remeron Tablets (Infrequent) 2483
Remeron SolTab Tablets (Infrequent) 2486

▲ Remicade for IV Injection (8% to 10%) 1178
Repronex for Intramuscular and Subcutaneous Injection 1347
Requip Tablets (Infrequent) 1621
Rescriptor Tablets (Less than 2%) 526
Retavase Vials 1182
▲ Retrovir Capsules (3.2% to 16%) 1625
▲ Retrovir IV Infusion (4% to 16%) 1629
▲ Retrovir (3.2% to 16%) 1625
RhoGAM Injection 2524
Rifadin 765
Rifamate Capsules 767
Rifater Tablets 769
Risperdal (2% to 3%) 1796
Ritalin 2387
▲ Rituxan for Infusion (49%) 1750
▲ Rituxan I.V. (49%) 1428
Robaxin Injectable 2938
Robaxin Tablets 2939
Robaxisal Tablets 2939
Rocephin Injectable Vials, ADD-Vantage, Galaxy, Bulk (Less than 1%) 2993
▲ Roferon-A Injection (28% to 92%) 2996
▲ Rowasa Rectal Suspension Enema 4.0 grams/unit (60 mL) (3.19%) 3264
Roxicodone Tablets (Less than 3%) 3067
Rythmol Tablets – 150 mg, 225 mg, 300 mg (1.9%) 502
Salagen Tablets (1% to 2%) 2229
Sandimmune (2% or less) 2388
Sandoglobulin I.V. 2391
▲ Sarafem Pulvules (3%) 1962
Sectral Capsules 3589
Sedapap Tablets 50 mg/650 mg (Infrequent) 2225
Septra Suspension 2265
Septra Tablets 2265
Septra DS Tablets 2265
Serentil 1057
Serevent Diskus (1% to 3%) 1637
Serevent Inhalation Aerosol (1% to 3%) 1633
Serophene Tablets 3226
Seroquel Tablets (2%) 684
▲ Serostim for Injection (31.2%) 3229
Serzone Tablets (2%) 1104
Sinequan (Occasional) 2713
Singulair (1.5%) 2181
Soma Tablets 3353
Soma Compound Tablets 3354
Soma Compound w/Codeine Tablets 3355
Sonata Capsules (2%) 3591
Soriatane Capsules (Less than 1%) 3003
Sporanox Capsules (2% to 2.5%) 1800
Sporanox Injection (Less than 1%) 1804
Sporanox Injection (Less than 1%) 2509
▲ Sporanox Oral Solution (6.3% to 6.6.%) 1808
▲ Sporanox Oral Solution (6.3% to 6.6.%) 2512
Stelazine 1640
Streptase for Infusion (1% to 4%) 647
▲ Stromectol Tablets (22.6%) 2185
Sular Tablets (Less than or equal to 1%) 688
Suprane Liquid for Inhalation (Less than 1%) 874
▲ Sustiva Capsules (26%) 1258
Symmetrel 1328
Synagis Intramuscular (More than 1%) 2028
Synercid I.V. (Less than 1%) 775
Synvisc 3596
Tagamet (Rare) 1644
Tambocor Tablets (1% to 3%) 1990
Tamiflu Capsules (Less than 1%) 3008
Tamiflu Oral Suspension (Less than 1%) 3008
Tao Capsules 2716
Tapazole Tablets 1823
Tarka Tablets (Several cases) 508
Tasmar Tablets (1%) 3010
▲ Taxol Injection (12%) 1129
Taxotere for Injection Concentrate 778
Tazicef for Injection (2%) 1647
Tazicef Galaxy Container (2%) 1650
Tazicef Pharmacy Bulk Package (2%) 1653
Tazidime Vials, Faspak & ADD-Vantage (2%) 1966
Tegretol/Tegretol-XR 2404
▲ Temodar Capsules (13%) 3157
Tenoretic Tablets 690
Tenormin 692
Tequin Injection (0.1% to 3%) 1110
Tequin Tablets (0.1% to 3%) 1110
Terazol 3 Vaginal Cream (1%) 2587
Terazol 3 Vaginal Suppositories (2.8% of 284 patients) 2587
Terazol 7 Vaginal Cream (1.7% of 521 patients) 2587
Tetanus & Diphtheria Toxoids Adsorbed for Adult Use 1880
Tetanus and Diphtheria Toxoids Adsorbed For Adult Use (2%) 815
Tetanus Toxoid Adsorbed Purogenated 1882
Teveten Tablets (Less than 1%) 3327
▲ Thalomid Capsules (19.4% to 21.9%) 1154
▲ TheraCys Injection (38%) 823
Thioplex for Injection 1765
Thioridazine Hydrochloride Tablets 2289
Thiothixene Capsules 2290
Thorazine (Occasional) 1656
▲ Thrombate III (1 of 17) 944
▲ Thymoglobulin for Injection (63.4%) 3071
Thyrogen for Injection (1%) 1441
▲ Tice BCG, BCG Live (19.9%) 2489
Ticlid Tablets 3015
Timolide Tablets 2187
Timolol GFS ⊙ 266
Timoptic in Ocudose 2192
Timoptic Sterile Ophthalmic Solution 2190
Timoptic-XE Sterile Ophthalmic Gel Forming Solution 2194
TNKase I.V. 1430
▲ TOBI Solution for Inhalation (32.9%) 1206
Tolectin (Less than 1%) 2589
Tonocard Tablets (Less than 1%) 649
Topamax Sprinkle Capsules (Frequent) 2590
Topamax Tablets (Frequent) 2590
Toprol-XL Tablets 651
Toradol (1% or less) 3018
▲ Trasylol Injection (15%) 909
Tricor Capsules, Micronized (Less than 1%) 513
Trilafon 3160
Trileptal Oral Suspension (Up to 3%) 2407
Trileptal Tablets (Up to 3%) 2407
Tri-Levlen 962
Triostat Injection (1% or fewer) 1825
Tripedia Vaccine (1% to 4%) 817
▲ Trisenox Injection (63%) 1158
▲ Trizivir Tablets (20%) 1669
Trovan (Less than 1%) 2722
Twinrix Vaccine (2% to 4%) 1674
TYPHIM Vi Vaccine (Up to 2%) 825
Uniretic Tablets (More than 1%) 3178
Unithroid Tablets 3445
Univasc Tablets 3181
Urso Tablets 836
▲ Valcyte Tablets (31%) 3022
Valstar Sterile Solution for Intravesical Instillation (2%) 1175
Vanceril Double Strength Inhalation Aerosol (Fewer than 2%) 3167
Vancocin HCl, Vials & ADD-Vantage 1970
Vantin Tablets and Oral Suspension (Less than 1%) 2860
Vaqta (2.7% to 3.1%) 2199
Vascor Tablets (0.5% to 2.0%) 2602
Vaseretic Tablets 2204
Vasotec I.V. Injection (0.5% to 1%) 2207
Vasotec Tablets (0.5% to 1.0%) 2210
Venofer Injection (Greater than 1%) 580
Verelan Capsules 3184
Verelan PM Capsules 3186
▲ Vesanoid Capsules (83%) 3037
Vicoprofen Tablets (Rare; less than 3%) 520
▲ Videx (9% to 12%) 1138
Videx EC Capsules 1143
Vioxx (Greater than 0.1% to 1.9%) 2213
Viracept 532
▲ Viramune Oral Suspension (3%) 1060
▲ Viramune Tablets (3%) 1060
▲ Vistide Injection (15% to 58%) 1445
▲ Visudyne for Injection (1% to 10%) ⊙ 308
▲ Vitravene for Injection (5% to 20%) ⊙ 310
Vivactil Tablets 2217
Vivactil Tablets 2446
Vivotif Berna 997
Voltaren Ophthalmic Sterile Ophthalmic Solution (Less than 3%) ⊙ 312
Voltaren Tablets (Rare) 2315
Voltaren-XR Tablets (Rare) 2315
Warfarin Sodium Tablets, USP 3302
Wellbutrin Tablets (1.2%) 1680
Wellbutrin SR Sustained-Release Tablets (1% to 2%) 1684
WinRho SDF (1%) 2297
Xeloda Tablets (1%) 3039
▲ YF-VAX Vaccine (2% to 5%) 827
Yodoxin Tablets 1722
Zanaflex Tablets (Frequent) 1305
Zantac (Rare) 1690
Zantac Injection 1688
Zantac Syrup (Rare) 1690
Zebeta Tablets 1885
▲ Zemplar Injection (5%) 522
▲ Zenapax for Injection (Greater than 5%) 3046
▲ Zerit (50%) 1147
Zestoretic Tablets (0.3% to 1%) 695
Zestril Tablets (0.3% to 1.0%) 698
Ziac Tablets 1887
▲ Ziagen (19% to 20%) 1692
▲ Zinecard for Injection (22% to 34%) 2869
Zithromax Capsules, 250 mg (1% or less) 2743
Zithromax for Oral Suspension, 300 mg, 600 mg, 900 mg, 1200 mg (1% or less) 2739
Zithromax Tablets, 250 mg (1% or less) 2739
Zocor Tablets (Rare) 2219
▲ Zofran Injection (2% to 8%) 1698
▲ Zofran (8%) 1703
▲ Zofran ODT Orally Disintegrating Tablets (8%) 1703
Zoladex (1% to 5%) 702
Zoladex 3-month 706
Zoloft (Infrequent to 2%) 2751
▲ Zometa for Intravenous Infusion (44.2%) 3621
Zomig Tablets (Infrequent) 708
Zomig-ZMT Tablets (Infrequent) 708
Zosyn (2.4% to 3.2%) 1890
Zosyn in Galaxy Containers (2.4% to 3.2%) 1894
Zovirax Capsules 1706
Zovirax for Injection (Less than 1%) 1708
Zovirax 1706
Zyban Sustained-Release Tablets (Frequent) 1710
Zyflo Filmtab Tablets (Less common) 524
▲ Zyprexa Tablets (5%) 1973
▲ Zyprexa ZYDIS Orally Disintegrating Tablets (5%) 1973
Zyrtec (Less than 2%) 2756
Zyrtec-D 12 Hour Extended Relief Tablets (Less than 2%) 2758
Zyvox (1.6%) 2871

Fever, neutropenic
Campath Ampules 992
▲ Mylotarg for Injection (16% to 30%) 3540
▲ Neumega for Injection (48%) 1434
▲ Neupogen for Injection (13%) 587

Fibrillations
Luvox Tablets (25, 50, 100 mg) (Rare) 3256
Tambocor Tablets 1990
Tenex Tablets (Rare) 2942

Fibrinolysis increased
NovoSeven (1%) 2430

Fibromyalgia
Cozaar Tablets (Less than 1%) 2067
Hyzaar 2109
Lupron Depot 7.5 mg 3284
Lupron Depot–3 Month 11.25 mg 3285
Nexium Delayed-Release Capsules (Less than 1%) 619

Fibrosing colonopathy
Creon 5 Capsules 3251
Creon 10 Capsules 3251
Creon 20 Capsules 3251
Pancrease Capsules 2580
Ultrase Capsules 835
Ultrase MT Capsules 835

Fibrosis
Copaxone for Injection (Infrequent) 3306
Genotropin Lyophilized Powder (Infrequent) 2818
Inversine Tablets 1850
Ocufen Ophthalmic Solution ⊙ 242
Permax Tablets 1299
Taxol Injection (Rare) 1129

Fibrosis, hepatic
Xeloda Tablets (Less than 5%) 3039

Fibrosis, interstitial pulmonary
(*see under* Pulmonary fibrosis)

Fibrosis, pelvic
Lupron Injection 3279

Fibrosis, periportal
Tagamet (A single case) 1644

Fibrosis, pleural
D.H.E. 45 Injection (Occasional) 2334
Intron A for Injection (Less than or equal to 5%) 3120
Migranal Nasal Spray 2376
Permax Tablets (Rare) 1299
Taxol Injection (Rare) 1129

Fibrosis, retroperitoneal
Migranal Nasal Spray 2376
Permax Tablets (Rare) 1299
Tasmar Tablets 3010

Fibrotendinitis
Naprelan Tablets (Less than 1%) 1293

Fingernails, brittle
Gengraf Capsules (2% or less) 457
Neoral Soft Gelatin Capsules (2% or less) 2380
Neoral Oral Solution (2% or less) 2380
Sandimmune (2% or less) 2388
Trental Tablets (Less than 1%) 784

Fingers, discoloration
Eskalith 1527
Lithium Carbonate (A single report) 3061
Lithium Citrate Syrup 3061
Lithobid Slow-Release Tablets (A few reports) 3255

Fissures, lips
Aquasol A Parenteral 593

Fissuring, fingertips
Ophthetic Ophthalmic Solution ⊙ 244

Fissuring, unspecified
Clobevate Gel (Less than 2%) 3271
Condylox Gel (Less common) 2436
Ergamisol Tablets 1789
Sterile FUDR (Remote possibility) 2974
Melanex Topical Solution 2300
Olux Foam (Less than 2%) 1211
Oxistat Cream (0.1%) 1298
▲ Soriatane Capsules (1% to 10%) 3003
▲ Tazorac Gel (1% to 10%) 556
Temovate Cream (1 of 421 patients) 1301
▲ Temovate Gel (Among most frequent) 1303
Temovate E Emollient (Less than 2%) 1302

Fistula, arteriovenous
ReoPro Vials (0.4%) 1958

Fistula, regional lymph node
Tice BCG, BCG Live (Rare) 2489

Fistula, tracheo-esophageal
▲ Photofrin for Injection (6%) 831
Proleukin for Injection (Less than 1%) 1199

Flaccidity
Streptomycin Sulfate Injection 2714

Flare
Dipentum Capsules (Rare) 2803
Nolvadex Tablets 678
Travatan Ophthalmic Solution (1% to 4%) 543

Flare, postinjection
Attenuvax (Rare) 2044
Celestone Soluspan Injectable Suspension 3097
Decadron Phosphate Injection 2081
Demerol 3079
Dilaudid-HP (Less frequent) 443
Hydrocortone Acetate Injectable Suspension 2103
Mepergan Injection 3539
Meruvax II 2130
M-M-R II 2118
Mumpsvax (Rare) 2141

Flatulence
Accupril Tablets (0.5% to 1%) 2611
Aceon Tablets (2 mg, 4 mg, 8 mg) (1.0%) 3249
Aciphex Tablets 1267
Aciphex Tablets 1783
Actiq (1% or greater) 1184
Activella Tablets 2764
▲ Actonel Tablets (4.6%) 2879
Adalat CC Tablets (Less than 1.0%) 877
Aerobid/Aerobid-M (1% to 3%) 1363
▲ Agrylin Capsules (10.2%) 3232
Aldoclor Tablets 2035
Aldomet Tablets 2037
Aldoril Tablets 2039
Aloprim for Injection (Less than 1%) 2292
Alora Transdermal System (2.3% to 5.3%) 3372
Ambien Tablets (Infrequent) 3191
AmBisome for Injection (Less common) 1383
Arava Tablets (1% to 3%) 724
Aricept Tablets (Infrequent) 1270
Aricept Tablets (Infrequent) 2665
▲ Arthrotec Tablets (9%) 3195
▲ Asacol Delayed-Release Tablets (3% to 5%) 2884
Atromid-S Capsules (Less frequent) 3483
Augmentin Chewable Tablets (Less frequent) 1482
Augmentin Powder for Oral Suspension (Less frequent) 1482
Augmentin Tablets (Less frequent) 1485
Avalide Tablets 1070
Avapro Tablets (Less than 1%) 1074
Avapro Tablets (Less than 1%) 3076
▲ Axid Pulvules (4.9%) 1903
▲ Axid Pulvules (4.9%) 2919
Baycol Tablets (2.1%) 883

Betapace Tablets (1% to 2%) ... 950
Betaseron for SC Injection ... 988
Buprenex Injectable (Infrequent) ... 2918
▲ Canasa Rectal Suppositories (Among most common) ... 829
Carafate Suspension (Less than 0.5%) ... 731
Carafate Tablets (Less than 0.5%) ... 730
Cardura Tablets (1%) ... 2668
▲ Casodex Tablets (5%) ... 662
Cataflam Tablets (1% to 3%) ... 2315
Ceclor CD Tablets (0.1% to 1%) ... 1279
Cedax Capsules (0.1% to 1%) ... 1021
Ceftin (0.1% to 1%) ... 1898
Celebrex Capsules (2.2%) ... 2676
Celebrex Capsules (2.2%) ... 2780
Celexa (Frequent) ... 1365
▲ CellCept Capsules (3% to 13.8%) ... 2951
▲ CellCept Intravenous (3% to 13.8%) ... 2951
▲ CellCept Oral Suspension (3% to 13.8%) ... 2951
▲ CellCept Tablets (3% to 13.8%) ... 2951
▲ Cenestin Tablets (29%) ... 1263
Cerebyx Injection (Infrequent) ... 2619
Chirocaine Injection (2.4%) ... 2909
Cipro I.V. (1% or less) ... 893
Cipro I.V. Pharmacy Bulk Package (Less than 1%) ... 897
Cipro ... 887
Claritin (At least one patient) ... 3100
Claritin-D 12 Hour Extended Release Tablets (Less frequent) ... 3102
Claritin-D 24 Hour Extended Release Tablets (Fewer than 2%) ... 3104
Clinoril Tablets (1% to 3%) ... 2053
▲ Cognex Capsules (4%) ... 1351
Colazal Capsules (2%) ... 3069
Colestid Tablets (Less frequent) ... 2791
▲ CombiPatch Transdermal System (5% to 7%) ... 2323
Comtan Tablets (2%) ... 2328
Copaxone for Injection (At least 2%) ... 3306
Coreg Tablets (More than 2%) ... 1508
Corgard Tablets (1 to 5 per 1000 patients) ... 2245
Corzide 40/5 Tablets (1 to 5 of 1000 patients) ... 2247
Corzide 80/5 Tablets (1 to 5 of 1000 patients) ... 2247
Coumadin for Injection (Infrequent) ... 1243
Coumadin Tablets (Infrequent) ... 1243
Cozaar Tablets (Less than 1%) ... 2067
Crinone (Less than 5%) ... 3213
Crixivan Capsules (Less than 2%) ... 2070
Cytotec Tablets (2.9%) ... 3202
Cytovene ... 2959
Depacon Injection (1% to 5%) ... 416
Depakene (1% to 5%) ... 421
Depakote Sprinkle Capsules (1% to 5%) ... 426
Depakote Tablets (1% to 5%) ... 430
Depakote ER Tablets (1% to 5%) ... 436
Detrol Tablets (1.3%) ... 3623
Diovan Capsules ... 2337
Diovan HCT Tablets (Greater than 0.2%) ... 2338
Dipentum Capsules (Rare) ... 2803
Ditropan XL Extended Release Tablets (2% to 5%) ... 564
Dolobid Tablets (Greater than 1 in 100) ... 2088
▲ Dostinex Tablets (2% to less than 10%) ... 2804
Doxil Injection (Less than 1%) ... 566
Duragesic Transdermal System (1% or greater) ... 1786
Dynabac Tablets (1% to 1.5%) ... 2269
▲ Effexor Tablets (3%) ... 3495
▲ Effexor XR Capsules (3% to 4%) ... 3499
Elmiron Capsules (Less than or equal to 1%) ... 570
Emcyt Capsules (2%) ... 2810
Ergamisol Tablets (Less than 1% to 2%) ... 1789
Eskalith ... 1527
Estring Vaginal Ring (1% to 3%) ... 2811
▲ Evista Tablets (3.1%) ... 1915
Evoxac Capsules (1% to 3%) ... 1217
▲ Exelon Capsules (4%) ... 2342
▲ Exelon Oral Solution (4%) ... 2345
Famvir Tablets (1.5% to 1.9%) ... 2348
Felbatol ... 3343
▲ Feldene Capsules (1% to 10%) ... 2685
femhrt Tablets ... 2635
Ferrlecit Injection (Greater than 1%) ... 3386
Flexeril Tablets (Less than 1%) ... 572
Flexeril Tablets (Less than 1%) ... 2094
▲ Flolan for Injection (5%) ... 1528
Floxin I.V. (1% to 3%) ... 2526
Floxin Tablets (1% to 3%) ... 2529
▲ Fortovase Capsules (5.7% to 12.2%) ... 2970
Fosamax Tablets (2.6%) ... 2095
Foscavir Injection (Between 1% and 5%) ... 605
Gabitril Tablets (1% or more) ... 1189
Gastrocrom Oral Concentrate (Infrequent) ... 1162
▲ Gengraf Capsules (4%) ... 457
Geocillin Tablets ... 2687
Ginsana Sport Capsules ... ▣ 831
▲ Glucophage Tablets (12.1%) ... 1080
Glucophage XR Tablets (1% to 5%) ... 1080
▲ Glucotrol XL Extended Release Tablets (3.2%) ... 2693
▲ Glyset Tablets (41.5%) ... 2821
▲ Gonal-F for Injection (3.6% to 6.8%) ... 3216
▲ HeartBar (4 of 41 individuals) ... 1212
Hivid Tablets (Less than 1%) ... 2975
Hytrin Capsules (At least 1%) ... 464
Hyzaar ... 2109
Imdur Tablets (Less than or equal to 5%) ... 1826
Imitrex Injection (Rare) ... 1549
Imitrex Nasal Spray (Rare) ... 1554
Imitrex Tablets ... 1558
Indocin Capsules (Less than 1%) ... 2112
Indocin I.V. (Less than 1%) ... 2115
Indocin (Less than 1%) ... 2112
▲ Infergen (6% to 8%) ... 1777
Innohep Injection (Greater than or equal to 1%) ... 1248
Intron A for Injection (Less than 5%) ... 3120
Invirase Capsules (Less than 2%) ... 2979
Kaletra Capsules (Less than 2%) ... 471
Kaletra Oral Solution (Less than 2%) ... 471
K-Dur Microburst Release System ER Tablets ... 1832
Klonopin Tablets (Infrequent) ... 2983
▲ Klor-Con M20/Klor-Con M10 Tablets (Among most common) ... 3329
▲ K-Lor Powder Packets (Among most common) ... 469
Kristalose for Oral Solution ... 1007
▲ K-Tab Filmtab Tablets (Most common) ... 470
Lamictal (More than 1%) ... 1567
Lamisil Tablets (2.2%) ... 2360
Lescol Capsules (2.6%) ... 2361
Lescol Capsules (2.6%) ... 2925
Lescol XL Tablets (1.4%) ... 2361
Lescol XL Tablets (1.4%) ... 2925
Levaquin (0.5% to 1.6%) ... 2537
Lexxel Tablets ... 608
Lipitor Tablets (1.1% to 2.8%) ... 2639
Lipitor Tablets (1.1% to 2.8%) ... 2696
Lithobid Slow-Release Tablets ... 3255
▲ Lodine (3% to 9%) ... 3528
▲ Lodine XL Extended-Release Tablets (1% to 10%) ... 3530
Lodosyn Tablets ... 1251
Lotensin HCT Tablets (0.3% or more) ... 2367
▲ Luvox Tablets (25, 50, 100 mg) (4%) ... 3256
Macrobid Capsules (1.5%) ... 2889
Maxalt Tablets (Infrequent) ... 2120
Maxalt-MLT Orally Disintegrating Tablets (Infrequent) ... 2120
▲ Megace Oral Suspension (Up to 10%) ... 1124
Meridia Capsules (Greater than or equal to 1%) ... 481
Merrem I.V. (0.1% to 1.0%) ... 673
MetroGel-Vaginal Gel (Less than 1%) ... 1986
▲ Mevacor Tablets (3.7% to 6.4%) ... 2132
Miacalcin Nasal Spray (Less than 1%) ... 2375
Micardis Tablets (More than 0.3%) ... 1049
Micardis HCT Tablets ... 1051
Micro-K ... 3311
Midamor Tablets (Less than or equal to 1%) ... 2136
MiraLax Powder for Oral Solution ... 1069
Mirapex Tablets (Less than 1%) ... 2834
Mobic Tablets (0.4% to 3.2%) ... 1054
Moduretic Tablets (Less than or equal to 1%) ... 2138
Monopril Tablets (0.2% to 1.0%) ... 1091
Monopril HCT ... 1094
Monurol Sachet (Less than 1%) ... 1375
Motrin Suspension, Oral Drops, Chewable Tablets, and Caplets (1% to less than 3%) ... 2002
Mycobutin Capsules (2%) ... 2838
Nadolol Tablets (1 to 5 of 1000 patients) ... 2288
Naprelan Tablets (Less than 3%) ... 1293
▲ Neoral Soft Gelatin Capsules (4%) ... 2380
▲ Neoral Oral Solution (4%) ... 2380
Neurontin Capsules (Frequent) ... 2655
Neurontin Oral Solution (Frequent) ... 2655
Neurontin Tablets (Frequent) ... 2655
Nexium Delayed-Release Capsules (Greater than or equal to 1%) ... 619
▲ Nicotrol Inhaler (Greater than 3%) ... 2840
▲ Nipent for Injection (3% to 10%) ... 3272
Noroxin Tablets (0.3% to 1.0%) ... 2145
Norvasc Tablets (More than 0.1% to 1%) ... 2704
Norvir Capsules (0.9%) ... 487
Norvir Oral Solution (0.9%) ... 487
Omnicef (0.6%) ... 493
Oncaspar (Less than 1%) ... 756
▲ Ortho-Prefest Tablets (5%) ... 2570
▲ Orudis Capsules (3% to 9%) ... 3548
▲ Oruvail Capsules (3% to 9%) ... 3548
Ovidrel for Injection (Less than 2%) ... 3220
OxyContin Tablets (Less than 1%) ... 2912
▲ Pancrease Capsules (Among most frequent) ... 2580
▲ Paxil (4.0%) ... 1609
Pediazole Suspension ... 3050
Permax Tablets (Infrequent) ... 1299
Phrenilin (Less frequent) ... 578
Plendil Extended-Release Tablets (0.5% to 1.5%) ... 623
Pletal Tablets (2% to 3%) ... 2605
Pletal Tablets (2% to 3%) ... 2848
▲ Ponstel Capsules (1% to 10%) ... 1356
Pravachol Tablets (2.7% to 3.3%) ... 1099
▲ Precose Tablets (74%) ... 906
▲ Prempro Tablets (8% to 9%) ... 3572
Prevacid Delayed-Release Capsules (Less than 1%) ... 3292
PREVPAC (Less than 1%) ... 3298
Prilosec Delayed-Release Capsules (Less than 1 to 2.7%) ... 628
Prinivil Tablets (0.3% to 1.0%) ... 2164
Prinzide Tablets ... 2168
ProAmatine Tablets (Rare) ... 3241
Procardia Capsules (2% or less) ... 2708
Procardia XL Extended Release Tablets (Less than 3%) ... 2710
▲ Prograf (3% to 15%) ... 1393
ProSom Tablets (Infrequent) ... 500
Prostigmin Injectable ... 1744
Prostigmin Tablets ... 1744
Protonix I.V. (Greater than or equal to 1%) ... 3580
Protonix Tablets (2% to 4%) ... 3577
Proventil HFA Inhalation Aerosol (Less than 3%) ... 3150
Provigil Tablets (At least 1%) ... 1193
▲ Prozac Pulvules, Liquid, and Weekly Capsules (3%) ... 1238
▲ Rapamune Oral Solution and Tablets (3% to 20%) ... 3584
▲ Relafen Tablets (3% to 9%) ... 1617
Reminyl Oral Solution (Frequent) ... 1792
Reminyl Tablets (Frequent) ... 1792
▲ Renagel Capsules (4%) ... 1439
▲ Renagel Tablets (4%) ... 1439
Requip Tablets (2% to 3%) ... 1621
Rescriptor Tablets (Less than 2%) ... 526
Retrovir Capsules ... 1625
Retrovir IV Infusion ... 1629
Retrovir ... 1625
Rifadin (Some patients) ... 765
Rifamate Capsules (Some patients) ... 767
Rifater Tablets ... 769
Rilutek Tablets (2.0% to 2.5%) ... 772
Risperdal (Infrequent) ... 1796
Rocephin Injectable Vials, ADD-Vantage, Galaxy, Bulk (Rare) ... 2993
Roferon-A Injection (Less than 3% to 3%) ... 2996
▲ Rowasa Rectal Suspension Enema 4.0 grams/unit (60 mL) (6.13%) ... 3264
Rythmol Tablets – 150 mg, 225 mg, 300 mg (1.2% to 1.9%) ... 502
Salagen Tablets (1% to 2%) ... 2229
▲ Sandostatin Injection (Less than 10%) ... 2394
▲ Sandostatin LAR Depot (25.7%) ... 2395
▲ Sectral Capsules (3%) ... 3589
Sedapap Tablets 50 mg/650 mg (Infrequent) ... 2225
Seroquel Tablets (Infrequent) ... 684
▲ Serostim for Injection (1% to 10%) ... 3229
Serzone Tablets ... 1104
▲ Simulect for Injection (3% to 10%) ... 2399
Sinemet Tablets ... 1253
Sinemet CR Tablets ... 1255
Skelid Tablets (2.7%) ... 3088
Sonata Capsules (Infrequent) ... 3591
▲ Sporanox Capsules (4%) ... 1800
Sporanox Oral Solution (Less than 2%) ... 1808
Sporanox Oral Solution (Less than 2%) ... 2512
Sular Tablets (Less than or equal to 1%) ... 688
▲ Suprax (4%) ... 1877
Sustiva Capsules (1% to 2%) ... 1258
Tambocor Tablets (Less than 1%) ... 1990
Tasmar Tablets (2% to 4%) ... 3010
Tequin Injection (Less than 0.1%) ... 1110
Tequin Tablets (Less than 0.1%) ... 1110
Teveten Tablets (Less than 1%) ... 3327
▲ Thalomid Capsules (8.3%) ... 1154
Ticlid Tablets (1.5%) ... 3015
Timentin Injection- ADD-Vantage Vial ... 1661
Timentin Injection-Galaxy Container ... 1664
Timentin Injection-Pharmacy Bulk Package ... 1666
Timentin for Intravenous Administration ... 1658
▲ Tolectin (3% to 9%) ... 2589
Topamax Sprinkle Capsules (Frequent) ... 2590
Topamax Tablets (Frequent) ... 2590
Toprol-XL Tablets (About 1 of 100 patients) ... 651
Toradol (Greater than 1%) ... 3018
Trental Tablets (0.6%) ... 784
▲ Tricor Capsules, Micronized (3%) ... 513
Trileptal Oral Suspension ... 2407
Trileptal Tablets ... 2407
Trovan (Less than 1%) ... 2722
Ultracet Tablets (At least 1%) ... 2597
Ultram Tablets (1% to 5%) ... 2600
Ultrase MT Capsules (1.5%) ... 835
Unasyn for Injection (Less than 1%) ... 2728
Uniretic Tablets (Less than 1%) ... 3178
Urecholine ... 2198
Valstar Sterile Solution for Intravesical Instillation (1%) ... 1175
Vantin Tablets and Oral Suspension (Less than 1%) ... 2860
Vascor Tablets (0.5% to 2.0%) ... 2602
Vaseretic Tablets (0.5% to 2.0%) ... 2204
▲ Vicoprofen Tablets (3% to 9%) ... 520
Videx ... 1138
Videx EC Capsules ... 1143
Vioxx (Greater than 0.1% to 1.9%) ... 2213
▲ Viracept (Up to 8%) ... 532
Vistide Injection ... 1445
Voltaren Tablets (1% to 3%) ... 2315
Voltaren-XR Tablets (1% to 3%) ... 2315
Warfarin Sodium Tablets, USP ... 3302
▲ WelChol Tablets (12%) ... 3073
Wellbutrin SR Sustained-Release Tablets (At least 1%) ... 1684
Zanaflex Tablets (Infrequent) ... 1305
▲ Zenapax for Injection (2% to 5%) ... 3046
Zestoretic Tablets ... 695
Zestril Tablets (0.3% to 1.0%) ... 698
Zithromax Capsules, 250 mg (1% or less) ... 2743
Zithromax for IV Infusion (1% or less) ... 2748
Zithromax for Oral Suspension, 1 g (1% or less) ... 2743
Zithromax for Oral Suspension, 300 mg, 600 mg, 900 mg, 1200 mg (1% or less) ... 2739
Zithromax Tablets, 250 mg (1% or less) ... 2739
Zithromax Tablets, 600 mg (1% or less) ... 2743
Zocor Tablets (1.9%) ... 2219
Zoladex (1% or greater) ... 702
Zoladex 3-month ... 706
▲ Zoloft (3%) ... 2751
Zonegran Capsules (Infrequent) ... 1307
Zosyn (1.0% or less to 1.3%) ... 1890
Zosyn in Galaxy Containers (1.0% or less to 1.3%) ... 1894
Zyban Sustained-Release Tablets (Frequent) ... 1710
Zyflo Filmtab Tablets (Less common) ... 524
Zyprexa Tablets (Infrequent) ... 1973
Zyprexa ZYDIS Orally Disintegrating Tablets (Infrequent) ... 1973
Zyrtec (Less than 2%) ... 2756
Zyrtec-D 12 Hour Extended Relief Tablets (Less than 2%) ... 2758

Flatus with discharge

▲ Xenical Capsules (2.1% to 27.9%) ... 3043

Floating feeling

Dilaudid Oral Liquid (Less frequent) ... 445
Dilaudid Tablets - 8 mg (Less frequent) ... 445
Dilaudid-HP (Less frequent) ... 443
Mintezol ... 2137
MS Contin Tablets (Less frequent) ... 2896
MSIR (Less frequent) ... 2898
Nubain Injection (1% or less) ... 1323
Oramorph SR Tablets (Less frequent) ... 3062
Stadol NS Nasal Spray (1% or greater) ... 1108

Fluid depletion

Captopril Tablets ... 2281
Kristalose for Oral Solution ... 1007

Fluid imbalance

Demadex Tablets and Injection ... 2965
Imitrex Nasal Spray ... 1554
Prinzide Tablets ... 2168
Saizen for Injection (Infrequent) ... 3225
Tenoretic Tablets ... 690
Vaseretic Tablets ... 2204
▲ Vesanoid Capsules (6%) ... 3037
Zestoretic Tablets ... 695

Fluid overload

AmBisome for Injection (Less common) ... 1383
▲ Aredia for Injection (Up to at least 15%) ... 2309
Campath Ampules ... 992
Coreg Tablets (1% to 2%) ... 1508

Orthoclone OKT3 Sterile Solution... 2498
Prinivil Tablets (0.3% to 1.0%)........ 2164
▲ Simulect for Injection (3% to 10%) .. 2399
▲ Zenapax for Injection (2% to 5%) 3046
Zestoretic Tablets........................ 695
Zestril Tablets (0.3% to 1.0%)......... 698
Zosyn (1.9%)................................ 1890
Zosyn in Galaxy Containers (1.9%)................................ 1894

Fluid retention
(*see under* Edema)

Flu-like symptoms
AccuNeb Inhalation Solution (2.6%)................................ 1230
▲ Actimmune (Most common) 1772
Actiq (Less than 1%)...................... 1184
▲ Actonel Tablets (9.8%).................. 2879
Advair Diskus 100/50..................... 1448
Advair Diskus 250/50..................... 1448
Advair Diskus 500/50..................... 1448
▲ Aerobid/Aerobid-M (10%) 1363
Agrylin Capsules (1% to 5%)........... 3232
▲ Alamast Ophthalmic Solution (10% to 25%)............................. 3092
Aldara Cream, 5% (1% to 3%)......... 1978
▲ Alferon N Injection (30%) 1770
Allegra (2.5%)................................. 712
Alphagan P Ophthalmic Solution (1% to 4%)................................. 546
Altace Capsules 2233
Ambien Tablets (2%)........................ 3191
AmBisome for Injection (Less common)....................................... 1383
Arava Tablets (2%)........................... 724
Aricept Tablets (Frequent)............... 1270
Aricept Tablets (Frequent)............... 2665
▲ Arimidex Tablets (2% to 6.9%) 659
▲ Aromasin Tablets (6%) 2769
▲ Asacol Delayed-Release Tablets (3% to 5%)................................. 2884
Atacand HCT Tablets (2.5%)........... 597
Atromid-S Capsules......................... 3483
▲ Atrovent Inhalation Solution (3.7%)... 1031
▲ Avalide Tablets (3%) 1070
Avapro Tablets (1% or greater)....... 1074
Avapro Tablets (1% or greater)....... 3076
▲ Avonex (61%) 1013
▲ Azmacort Inhalation Aerosol (2% to 5%).. 728
▲ Baycol Tablets (3.7%) 883
Betapace AF Tablets (0.8% to 2%).. 954
▲ Betaseron for SC Injection (Up to 76%).. 988
▲ Botox Purified Neurotoxin Complex (2% to 10%)................. 549
Campath Ampules.......................... 992
Cancidas for Injection (Up to 3.1%).. 2048
Cardura Tablets (Less than 0.5% to 1.1%)..................................... 2668
▲ Carnitor Injection (15% to 29%) 3242
▲ Casodex Tablets (4%) 662
Cataflam Tablets............................ 2315
Caverject Sterile Powder (2%)......... 2777
Ceclor CD Tablets (0.1% to 1%)...... 1279
Celebrex Capsules (0.1% to 1.9%).. 2676
Celebrex Capsules (0.1% to 1.9%).. 2780
Celexa (Infrequent)........................ 1365
▲ CellCept Capsules (3%) 2951
▲ CellCept Intravenous (3%) 2951
▲ CellCept Oral Suspension (3%) 2951
▲ CellCept Tablets (3%) 2951
Cerebyx Injection (Infrequent).......... 2619
▲ Chemet Capsules (5.2% to 15.7%)...................................... 3078
Claritin-D 12 Hour Extended Release Tablets (Less frequent)... 3102
Claritin-D 24 Hour Extended Release Tablets (Fewer than 2%)... 3104
Clozaril Tablets............................. 2319
Colazal Capsules (1%).................... 3069
▲ CombiPatch Transdermal System (10% to 14%).............................. 2323
Combivent Inhalation Aerosol (1.4%).. 1041
▲ Copaxone for Injection (19%) 3306
Crinone (Less than 5%).................. 3213
Crixivan Capsules (Less than 2%).... 2070
▲ DaunoXome Injection (Up to 5%) 1442
▲ Depacon Injection (12%) 416
▲ Depakene (12%) 421
▲ Depakote Sprinkle Capsules (12%)... 426
▲ Depakote Tablets (At least 5% to 12%)... 430
▲ Depakote ER Tablets (Greater than 5%)...................................... 436
▲ Detrol Tablets (4.4%) 3623
Ditropan XL Extended Release Tablets (2% to 5%)..................... 564
▲ Dostinex Tablets (1% to less than 10%)... 2804
Doxil Injection (Less than 1%)......... 566
DTIC-Dome.................................... 902
Dynabac Tablets (0.1% to 1%)........ 2269
Effexor Tablets.............................. 3495
Effexor XR Capsules...................... 3499
Enbrel for Injection......................... 1752
Enbrel for Injection......................... 3504
Engerix-B Vaccine (Less than 1%)... 1517
Epogen for Injection (Rare)............. 582
Ergamisol Tablets (5 out of 463 patients)...................................... 1789
▲ Esclim Transdermal System (6.3% to 8.5%)............................ 3460
▲ Estring Vaginal Ring (3%) 2811
Eulexin Capsules 3118
▲ Evista Tablets (13.5% to 14.6%) 1915
Evoxac Capsules (1% to 3%)......... 1217
▲ Exelon Capsules (3%) 2342
▲ Exelon Oral Solution (3%) 2345
Felbatol (Frequent)......................... 3343
Feldene Capsules (Rare)................. 2685
▲ Femara Tablets (5%) 2351
Ferrlecit Injection (Greater than 1%)... 3386
▲ Flolan for Injection (13% to 25%) ... 1528
Flonase Nasal Spray (1% to 3%)..... 1533
▲ Flovent (Up to 13%) 1535
▲ Flovent Rotadisk (3% to 4%) 1537
Follistim for Injection 2465
Fortovase Capsules (Less than 2%)... 2970
Foscavir Injection (Between 1% and 5%) 605
▲ Gabitril Tablets (1% to 9%) 1189
▲ Gemzar for Injection (19%) 1919
Gengraf Capsules (2%) 457
Geodon Capsules (Frequent) 2688
Glucophage Tablets (1% to 5%) 1080
▲ Gonal-F for Injection (4.2%) 3216
▲ Herceptin I.V. (10%) 1414
Hivid Tablets (Less than 1%) 2975
▲ Humatrope Vials and Cartridges (3.9% to 15.6%) 1930
Humegon for Injection 2468
Hytrin Capsules (At least 1% to 2.4%) 464
Imdur Tablets (Less than or equal to 5%) 1826
Imitrex Injection (Rare) 1549
Imitrex Nasal Spray 1554
Imitrex Tablets 1558
Indapamide Tablets (Less than 5%)... 2286
▲ Infergen (8% to 15%) 1777
▲ Intron A for Injection (Up to 79%) ... 3120
Invirase Capsules (Less than 2%) 2979
Iscar Mali Injection 3456
Iscar Mali Special Injection 3456
Iscar Pini Injection 3456
Iscar Quercus Injection 3456
Iscar Quercus Special Injection 3456
JE-VAX Vaccine (Less than 3%) 811
Kadian Capsules (Less than 3%) 1335
Kaletra Capsules (Less than 2%) 471
Kaletra Oral Solution (Less than 2%) 471
Keppra Tablets (1% or more) 3314
▲ Klonopin Tablets (4%) 2983
▲ Lamictal (5% to 7.0%) 1567
▲ Lescol Capsules (5.1%) 2361
▲ Lescol Capsules (5.1%) 2925
▲ Lescol XL Tablets (7.1%) 2361
▲ Lescol XL Tablets (7.1%) 2925
Lexxel Tablets (Infrequent) 608
Lipitor Tablets (Up to 3.2%) 2639
Lipitor Tablets (Up to 3.2%) 2696
Lotensin HCT Tablets (More than 1%) 2367
Lupron Depot 3.75 mg (Less than 5%) 3281
Lupron Depot–3 Month 11.25 mg (Less than 5%) 3285
▲ Lupron Depot–4 Month 30 mg (Up to 12.2%)..................................... 3289
▲ Luvox Tablets (25, 50, 100 mg) (3%) 3256
LYMErix Vaccine (2.54% to 2.87%)... 1592
▲ Malarone (2% to 9%) 1596
▲ Meridia Capsules (8.2%) 481
Miacalcin Nasal Spray (1% to 3%) ... 2375
Micardis Tablets (1%) 1049
Micardis HCT Tablets (2%) 1051
Migranal Nasal Spray (Rare) 2376
Mirapex Tablets (Less than 1%) 2834
▲ Mobic Tablets (4.5% to 5.8%) 1054
Monopril Tablets (0.4% to 1.0%) 1091
Monurol Sachet (Less than 1%) 1375
▲ MUSE Urethral Suppository (4%) 3335
Mycobutin Capsules (Less than 1%) 2838
▲ Myobloc Injectable Solution (6% to 9%) 1291
▲ Naprelan Tablets (10%) 1293
Nasonex Nasal Spray (Greater than or equal to 2%) 3131
▲ Neoral Soft Gelatin Capsules (3% to 9.9%) 2380
▲ Neoral Oral Solution (3% to 9.9%) .. 2380
Neumega for Injection 1434
Nexium Delayed-Release Capsules (Less than 1%) 619
▲ Nicotrol Inhaler (Greater than 3%) .. 2840
▲ Nilandron Tablets (7.2%) 753
Nipent for Injection (Less than 3%) 3272
Normodyne Injection 3135
Normodyne Tablets 3137
Norvir Capsules (Less than 2%) 487
Norvir Oral Solution (Less than 2%)... 487
▲ Optivar Ophthalmic Solution (1% to 10%).. 2273
Orthoclone OKT3 Sterile Solution... 2498
▲ Ortho-Prefest Tablets (11%) 2570
ParaGard T 380A Intrauterine Copper Contraceptive 2582
Paxil (Infrequent)............................ 1609
▲ PEG-Intron Powder for Injection (46%)... 3140
Pergonal for Injection...................... 3223
▲ Periostat Tablets (11%) 1208
▲ Permax Tablets (3.2%) 1299
▲ Plavix Tablets (7.9%) 1097
▲ Plavix Tablets (7.9%) 3084
Plendil Extended-Release Tablets (0.5% to 1.5%)........................... 623
Pletal Tablets (2% or greater)......... 2605
Pletal Tablets (2% or greater)......... 2848
Pravachol Tablets (Up to 2.4%)....... 1099
▲ Prempro Tablets (10% to 13%) 3572
Prevacid Delayed-Release Capsules (Less than 1%)............. 3292
Prevnar for Injection....................... 1870
PREVPAC (Less than 1%)............... 3298
Priftin Tablets 758
Prilosec Delayed-Release Capsules (1%).............................. 628
Prinivil Tablets (0.3%).................... 2164
Prinzide Tablets (0.3% to 1%)......... 2168
Procrit for Injection (Rare).............. 2502
▲ Prograf (3% to 15%) 1393
Prolastin (Occasional)..................... 943
Protonix I.V. (Greater than or equal to 1%)................................. 3580
Protonix Tablets (Greater than or equal to 1%)................................. 3577
▲ Protopic Ointment (22% to 35%) 1397
Provigil Tablets (At least 1%).......... 1193
▲ Prozac Pulvules, Liquid, and Weekly Capsules (3% to 10%)...... 1238
Pulmicort Respules (1% to 3%)....... 632
▲ Pulmicort Turbuhaler Inhalation Powder (6% to 14%).................... 636
Pulmozyme Inhalation Solution 1426
▲ Rapamune Oral Solution and Tablets (3% to 20%)..................... 3584
▲ Rebetron Combination Therapy (14% to 18%)............................... 3153
Recombivax HB (Less than 1%)....... 2178
▲ Remeron Tablets (5%) 2483
▲ Remeron SolTab Tablets (5%) 2486
Repronex for Intramuscular and Subcutaneous Injection.............. 1347
Requip Tablets (Infrequent)............. 1621
Rescriptor Tablets (Less than 2%)... 526
▲ Rescula Ophthalmic Solution (6%)... ⊙ 306
Retrovir Capsules 1625
Retrovir IV Infusion......................... 1629
Retrovir... 1625
Rifadin.. 765
Rifater Tablets................................ 769
Rilutek Tablets (More than 2%)........ 772
Risperdal (Infrequent)...................... 1796
▲ Roferon-A Injection (16% to 33%) .. 2996
▲ Rowasa Rectal Suspension Enema 4.0 grams/unit (60 mL) (5.28%).. 3264
Roxicodone Tablets (Less than 3%)... 3067
Sandostatin Injection (1% to 4%)..... 2394
▲ Sarafem Pulvules (7%) 1962
▲ Serevent Diskus (5%) 1637
Seroquel Tablets (Frequent)............ 684
▲ Serostim for Injection (1% to 10%) . 3229
▲ Serzone Tablets (3%) 1104
▲ Singulair (4.2%)............................. 2181
▲ Skelid Tablets (4.0%) 3088
Soriatane Capsules (Less than 1%)... 3003
▲ Starlix Tablets (3.6%) 2401
Sular Tablets (Less than or equal to 1%).. 688
Synagis Intramuscular (More than 1%)... 2028
▲ Tasmar Tablets (3% to 4%) 3010
Testoderm Transdermal Systems (1%)... 574
Teveten Tablets (Less than 1%)....... 3327
Thalomid Capsules.......................... 1154
TheraCys Injection.......................... 823
Thyrogen for Injection (1%).............. 1441
Tiazac Capsules (2%)...................... 1378
▲ Tice BCG, BCG Live (33.2%) 2489
▲ Tikosyn Capsules (4%) 2717
▲ Topamax Sprinkle Capsules (3.2% to 3.5%)..................................... 2590
▲ Topamax Tablets (3.2% to 3.5%) 2590
Trental Tablets (Less than 1%)......... 784
▲ Tricor Capsules, Micronized (5%) ... 513
Twinrix Vaccine (Less than 1%)....... 1674
TYPHIM Vi Vaccine.......................... 825
Uniretic Tablets (More than 1%)....... 3178
▲ Univasc Tablets (3.1%) 3181
▲ Vanceril Double Strength Inhalation Aerosol (3%)............... 3167
Vascor Tablets (0.5% to 2.08%)...... 2602
▲ Verelan PM Capsules (3.7%) 3186
Viagra Tablets (Greater than 2%)..... 2732
Vicoprofen Tablets (Less than 3%).. 520
▲ Vioxx (3.1%) 2213
Vistide Injection.............................. 1445
▲ Visudyne for Injection (1% to 10%)... ⊙ 308
Vitravene for Injection (2% to 5%).. ⊙ 310
Voltaren Tablets 2315
Voltaren-XR Tablets........................ 2315
▲ WelChol Tablets (3%) 3073
Wellbutrin Tablets (Frequent)........... 1680
Wellbutrin SR Sustained-Release Tablets (At least 1%)................. 1684
▲ Xalatan Latanoprost Ophthalmic Solution (Approximately 4%)....... ⊙ 320
▲ Xalatan Sterile Ophthalmic Solution (Approximately 4%)........ 2864
▲ Xenical Capsules (39.7%) 3043
Xopenex Inhalation Solution (1.4% to 4.2%)..................................... 3207
Yasmin 28 Tablets (Greater than 1%)... 980
Zaditor Ophthalmic Solution (Less than 5%).................................... 2304
▲ Zanaflex Tablets (3%) 1305
▲ Zemplar Injection (5%) 522
Zestoretic Tablets (0.3% to 1%)...... 695
Zestril Tablets (0.3%)..................... 698
▲ Zoladex (5%) 702
Zoladex 3-month (1% to 5%)........... 706
Zometa for Intravenous Infusion...... 3621
▲ Zonegran Capsules (4%) 1307
Zyprexa Tablets (Frequent).............. 1973
Zyprexa ZYDIS Orally Disintegrating Tablets (Frequent).................................. 1973

Flushing
Accutane Capsules.......................... 2944
▲ Acthrel for Injection (16%) 3629
▲ Adalat CC Tablets (4%) 877
▲ Adenoscan (44%) 1381
Aggrenox Capsules (Less than 1%)... 1026
Allegra (Rare)................................. 712
Allegra-D Extended-Release Tablets (Rare).............................. 714
Aloprim for Injection (Less than 1%)... 2292
Ambien Tablets (Rare)..................... 3191
AmBisome for Injection (Less common)...................................... 1383
Aminohippurate Sodium PAH Injection.. 2041
Anzemet Injection (Infrequently)...... 719
Anzemet Tablets (Infrequently)........ 722
AquaMEPHYTON Injection................ 2042
Astelin Nasal Spray (Infrequent)...... 3339
Atrovent Inhalation Aerosol (Less frequent).................................... 1030
Autoplex T...................................... 2294
Avalide Tablets............................... 1070
Avapro Tablets (Less than 1%)........ 1074
Avapro Tablets (Less than 1%)........ 3076
Azactam for Injection (Less than 1%)... 1276
Baycol Tablets (Rare)....................... 883
BeneFix for Injection....................... 1432
Bontril Slow-Release Capsules........ 576
Brethine Ampuls (0.0% to 2.4%)..... 2314
Brevibloc Injection (Less than 1%)... 858
Bromfed Capsules (Extended-Release)...................... 2269
Bromfed-PD Capsules (Extended-Release)...................... 2269
Buprenex Injectable (Less than 1%)... 2918
Cancidas for Injection (2.9%).......... 2048
Captopril Tablets (2 to 5 of 1000 patients)...................................... 2281
Cardizem Injectable (1.7%)............. 1018
Cardizem Lyo-Ject Syringe (1.7%).. 1018
Cardizem Monovial (1.7%).............. 1018
Cardizem CD Capsules (1.4%)......... 1016
Cardura Tablets (Less than 0.5% to 1%)... 2668
Cataflam Tablets (Rare).................. 2315
Celexa (Infrequent)......................... 1365
▲ Cerezyme for Injection (Approximately 4%).................... 1438
Cipro I.V. (1% or less)..................... 893
Cipro I.V. Pharmacy Bulk Package (Less than 1%)........................... 897
Cipro (Less than 1%)...................... 887
Claritin (At least one patient).......... 3100
Claritin-D 12 Hour Extended Release Tablets (Less frequent)... 3102
Claritin-D 24 Hour Extended Release Tablets (Fewer than 2%)... 3104
Clinoril Tablets (Less than 1 in 100).. 2053
▲ Cognex Capsules (3%) 1351
Combivent Inhalation Aerosol.......... 1041
Cordarone Tablets (1% to 3%)......... 3487
▲ Corlopam Injection (More than 5%)... 412
Covera-HS Tablets (0.6% to 0.8%).. 3199
Cozaar Tablets (Less than 1%)........ 2067
Crixivan Capsules (Less than 2%).... 2070
CytoGam Intravenous (Less than 5.0%).. 2026
▲ DaunoXome Injection (13.8% to 16%)... 1442
DDAVP Nasal Spray (Occasional).... 738
DDAVP Rhinal Tube (Occasional).... 738
DDAVP Tablets................................ 739

Desmopressin Acetate Rhinal Tube (Occasional) 1345
D.H.E. 45 Injection (Occasional) 2334
Dilaudid Oral Liquid 445
Dilaudid Tablets - 8 mg 445
Diovan HCT Tablets (Greater than 0.2%) 2338
Diphtheria & Tetanus Toxoids Adsorbed Purogenated for Pediatric Use 1857
Diprivan Injectable Emulsion (Less than 1%) 667
Dolobid Tablets 2088
Donnagel Liquid (Rare) ▣789
Dopram Injectable 2931
▲ Doxil Injection (Approximately 6.8%) 566
DuoNeb Inhalation Solution 1233
DynaCirc Capsules (2.6%) 2921
DynaCirc CR Tablets (1.2% to 3.8%) 2923
Effexor Tablets 3495
Emcyt Capsules (1%) 2810
Enalaprilat Injection 863
Enbrel for Injection 1752
Enbrel for Injection 3504
Engerix-B Vaccine (Less than 1%) 1517
Ethyol for Injection 2029
Evoxac Capsules (0.3%) 1217
Exelon Capsules (Infrequent) 2342
Exelon Oral Solution (Infrequent) 2345
Extendryl 1361
Factrel (Rare) 3633
Famotidine Injection (Infrequent) 866
Felbatol 3343
Ferrlecit Injection (Two cases) 3386
▲ Flolan for Injection (23% to 58%) 1528
Floxin Otic Solution (Single report) 1219
Foscavir Injection (Between 1% and 5%) 605
Gamimune N, 5% Solvent/Detergent Treated 925
Gamimune N, 10% Solvent/Detergent Treated 928
Gammagard S/D (Occasional) 845
Gastrocrom Oral Concentrate (Less common) 1162
Gengraf Capsules (Less than 1% to 5%) 457
▲ Geref for Injection (1 patient in 6) 3215
Glucophage Tablets (1% to 5%) 1080
Glucotrol XL Extended Release Tablets (Less than 1%) 2693
Hivid Tablets (Less than 1%) 2975
Hyzaar 2109
Imdur Tablets (Less than or equal to 5%) 1826
▲ Imitrex Injection (6.6%) 1549
Imitrex Nasal Spray (Infrequent) 1554
Imitrex Tablets (Up to 4%) 1558
Indapamide Tablets (Less than 5%) 2286
Indocin Capsules (Less than 1%) 2112
Indocin I.V. (Less than 1%) 2115
Indocin (Less than 1%) 2112
INFeD Injection 3388
Intron A for Injection (Less than 5%) 3120
Isoptin SR Tablets (0.6%) 467
Iveegam EN (0.3% to 0.8%) 849
Klonopin Tablets (Infrequent) 2983
Konÿne 80 937
Lamictal (Infrequent) 1567
Lescol Capsules (Rare) 2361
Lescol Capsules (Rare) 2925
Lescol XL Tablets 2361
Lescol XL Tablets 2925
Leukine 1755
Levorphanol Tartrate Tablets 3059
Levoxyl Tablets 1819
Lexxel Tablets (1.6%) 608
Lodine (Less than 1%) 3528
Lodine XL Extended-Release Tablets (Less than 1%) 3530
Lotensin Tablets (Less than 1%) 2365
Lotensin HCT Tablets (0.3% to 1%) 2367
Lotrel Capsules (Up to 0.3%) 2370
Lufyllin Tablets 3347
Lufyllin-400 Tablets 3347
Lufyllin-GG Elixir 3348
Lufyllin-GG Tablets 3348
▲ Luvox Tablets (25, 50, 100 mg) (3%) 3256
Marinol Capsules (0.3% to 1%) 3325
Matulane Capsules 3246
Mavik Tablets (0.3% to 1.0%) 478
Maxair Autohaler 1981
Maxair Inhaler (Less than 1%) 1984
Maxalt Tablets (Frequent) 2120
Maxalt-MLT Orally Disintegrating Tablets (Frequent) 2120
Mephyton Tablets 2129
Mevacor Tablets (Rare) 2132
Miacalcin Nasal Spray (Less than 1%) 2375
Micardis Tablets (More than 0.3%) 1049
Micardis HCT Tablets 1051
Minipress Capsules 2699
Miochol-E System Pak (Rare) ⊙305
Miochol-E with Steri-Tags (Rare) ⊙305
Moduretic Tablets (Less than or equal to 1%) 2138
Mononine Concentrate 794
Monopril Tablets (0.2% to 1.0%) 1091
Monopril HCT (Less than 2%) 1094
Motofen Tablets 577
Navelbine Injection 1604
Neoral Soft Gelatin Capsules (1% to 5%) 2380
Neoral Oral Solution (1% to 5%) 2380
Nexium Delayed-Release Capsules (Less than 1%) 619
▲ Niaspan Extended-Release Tablets (Among most common) 1846
Nimotop Capsules (Less than 1% to 2.1%) 904
Nitrolingual Pumpspray 1355
Nitrostat Tablets 2658
▲ Nolvadex Tablets (32.7%) 678
Normodyne Injection (1%) 3135
Norpramin Tablets 755
Norvasc Tablets (0.7% to 4.5%) 2704
Nubain Injection (1% or less) 1323
Numorphan 1324
Orthoclone OKT3 Sterile Solution 2498
Pacerone Tablets (1% to 3%) 3331
Pediazole Suspension 3050
▲ PEG-Intron Powder for Injection (6%) 3140
Pepcid Injection (Infrequent) 2153
Pepcid for Oral Suspension (Infrequent) 2150
Pepcid RPD Orally Disintegrating Tablets (Infrequent) 2150
Pepcid Tablets (Infrequent) 2150
Persantine Tablets 1057
Plasmanate (Occasional) 942
▲ Plendil Extended-Release Tablets (3.9% to 6.9%) 623
Pravachol Tablets (Rare) 1099
Primaxin I.M. 2158
Primaxin I.V. (Less than 0.2%) 2160
Prinivil Tablets (0.3% to 1.0%) 2164
Prinzide Tablets (0.3% to 1%) 2168
Procanbid Extended-Release Tablets (Occasional) 2262
▲ Procardia Capsules (Approximately 10% to 25%) 2708
▲ Procardia XL Extended Release Tablets (Less than 3% to 25%) 2710
Proplex T 851
Prosed/DS Tablets 3268
ProSom Tablets (Infrequent) 500
Prostigmin Injectable 1744
Prostigmin Tablets 1744
Prostin E2 Suppositories 2852
Proventil Repetabs Tablets (Less than 1%) 3148
Quinaglute Dura-Tabs Tablets 978
Recombinate 853
Recombivax HB (Less than 1%) 2178
ReFacto Vials 1437
Refludan for Injection (Uncommon) 761
Reglan 2935
▲ Requip Tablets (3%) 1621
Rifadin 765
Rifater Tablets 769
Risperdal (Rare) 1796
▲ Rituxan for Infusion (Among most frequent) 1750
▲ Rituxan I.V. (Among most frequent) 1428
Robaxin Injectable 2938
Robaxin Tablets 2939
Rocephin Injectable Vials, ADD-Vantage, Galaxy, Bulk (Occasional) 2993
Romazicon Injection (1% to 3%) 3000
Rythmol Tablets – 150 mg, 225 mg, 300 mg (Less than 1%) 502
▲ Salagen Tablets (8% to 13%) 2229
Sandimmune (Less than 1% to 4%) 2388
Sandostatin Injection (1% to 4%) 2394
Sinemet Tablets 1253
Sinemet CR Tablets 1255
Sinequan (Occasional) 2713
Skelid Tablets (More than or equal to 1%) 3088
▲ Soriatane Capsules (1% to 10%) 3003
Stimate Nasal Spray (Occasional) 796
Streptase for Infusion 647
Surmontil Capsules 3595
Sustiva Capsules (Less than 2%) 1258
Talacen Caplets (Infrequent) 3089
Talwin Nx Tablets (Infrequent) 3090
Tambocor Tablets (1% to 3%) 1990
Tarka Tablets (0.3% or more) 508
▲ Taxol Injection (28%) 1129
Taxotere for Injection Concentrate 778
Tetanus & Diphtheria Toxoids Adsorbed for Adult Use 1880
Theo-Dur Extended-Release Tablets 1835
Thyrel TRH for Injection 3630
Topamax Sprinkle Capsules (Infrequent) 2590
Topamax Tablets (Infrequent) 2590
Toradol 3018
Trental Tablets 784
Trileptal Oral Suspension 2407
Trileptal Tablets 2407
▲ Trisenox Injection (10%) 1158
Trovan (Less than 1%) 2722
Twinrix Vaccine (Less than 1%) 1674
Uni-Dur Extended-Release Tablets 1841
Uniretic Tablets (Less than 1%) 3178
Unithroid Tablets 3445
Univasc Tablets (1.6%) 3181
Urised Tablets 2876
Vancocin HCl, Vials & ADD-Vantage 1970
Vantin Tablets and Oral Suspension (Less than 1%) 2860
Vaseretic Tablets 2204
Vasotec I.V. Injection 2207
Vasotec Tablets (0.5% to 1.0%) 2210
Verelan Capsules (0.6%) 3184
Verelan PM Capsules (0.6%) 3186
▲ Vesanoid Capsules (23%) 3037
▲ Viagra Tablets (10%) 2732
Vioxx (Greater than 0.1% to 1.9%) 2213
Vivactil Tablets 2217
Vivactil Tablets 2446
Volmax Extended-Release Tablets (Less frequent) 2276
Voltaren Tablets (Rare) 2315
Voltaren-XR Tablets (Rare) 2315
Wellbutrin Tablets (Rare) 1680
Wellbutrin SR Sustained-Release Tablets (1% to 4%) 1684
Zebeta Tablets 1885
Zestoretic Tablets (0.3% to 1%) 695
Zestril Tablets (0.3% to 1.0%) 698
Ziac Tablets 1887
Zocor Tablets (Rare) 2219
Zofran Injection 1698
Zofran 1703
Zofran ODT Orally Disintegrating Tablets 1703
Zoloft (Infrequent) 2751
Zosyn (1.0% or less) 1890
Zosyn in Galaxy Containers (1.0% or less) 1894
Zyban Sustained-Release Tablets (Infrequent) 1710
Zyrtec (Less than 2%) 2756
Zyrtec-D 12 Hour Extended Relief Tablets (Less than 2%) 2758

Flushing, cutaneous

Kadian Capsules (Less than 3%) 1335
Nicotinex Elixir ▣633
Nitrolingual Pumpspray 1355
Quinidex Extentabs 2933
Roferon-A Injection (Less than 0.5%) 2996
Talwin Nx Tablets 3090
Urecholine 2198

Flushing, facial

▲ Acthrel for Injection (16%) 3629
▲ Adenocard Injection (18%) 1380
Adriamycin PFS/RDF Injection 2767
Alferon N Injection (One patient) 1770
▲ Cognex Capsules (3%) 1351
DDAVP Injection 4 mcg/mL (Occasional) 737
Demerol 3079
Desmopressin Acetate Injection (Occasional) 1344
Dilaudid-HP (Less frequent) 443
Dolophine Hydrochloride Tablets 3056
Doxil Injection 566
DTIC-Dome 902
Ferrlecit Injection 3386
Fortovase Capsules (Less than 2%) 2970
Imitrex Nasal Spray 1554
Imitrex Tablets 1558
Kadian Capsules (Less than 3%) 1335
Kogenate (One report) 934
Loxitane Capsules 3398
Marinol Capsules (Greater than 1%) 3325
Mepergan Injection 3539
Miacalcin Injection (About 2% to 5%) 2373
Mintezol 2137
Mithracin for Intravenous Use 903
MS Contin Tablets (Less frequent) 2896
MSIR (Less frequent) 2898
Nicotrol Nasal Spray (More common) 2843
Oramorph SR Tablets (Less frequent) 3062
Phenergan with Codeine Syrup 3557
Phenergan VC with Codeine Syrup 3561
ProAmatine Tablets (Less frequent) 3241
Roxanol 3066
Sandimmune 2388
Sandoglobulin I.V. 2391
Soma Compound Tablets 3354
Soma Compound w/Codeine Tablets 3355
Stimate Nasal Spray (Occasional) 796
Synvisc 3596
Tonocard Tablets (Less than 1%) 649
Urecholine 2198
Urecholine Tablets 2445

Flushing, hands

Miacalcin Injection (About 2% to 5%) 2373

Flushing, upper thorax

▲ Acthrel for Injection (16%) 3629
Sandimmune 2388

Folic acid absorption, impaired

Azulfidine EN-tabs Tablets (Rare) 2775

Follicular atresia, delayed

Norplant System 3543

Folliculitis

Aclovate (Infrequent) 1275
Amerge Tablets (Rare) 1467
Analpram-HC 1338
Anusol-HC Cream 2.5% (Infrequent to frequent) 2237
Anusol-HC Suppositories 2238
Capex Shampoo 1400
Cleocin T Topical 2790
Cleocin Vaginal Cream 2788
Clindagel 1401
Clobevate Gel (Less than 2%) 3271
Cordran Lotion (Infrequent) 2438
Cordran Tape (Infrequent) 2439
Cormax Cream (Approximately 0.3%) 2440
Cormax Ointment (Approximately 0.3%) 2440
Cormax Scalp Application (Approximately 0.6%) 2441
Crixivan Capsules (Less than 2%) 2070
Cutivate Cream (0.8%) 1282
Cutivate Ointment (Infrequent to more frequent) 1284
DaunoXome Injection (Less than or equal to 5%) 1442
Dermatop Emollient Cream (Infrequent to frequent) 2517
DesOwen (Infrequent) 1401
Didronel Tablets 2888
Diprolene Gel 0.05% (Less frequent) 3107
Diprolene Lotion 0.05% (2%) 3107
Diprolene Ointment 0.05% (2 per 767 patients) 3108
Diprolene AF Cream 0.05% (Infrequent) 3106
Diprosone 3109
Dovonex Ointment (Less than 1%) 1117
Dovonex Scalp Solution 1118
8-MOP Capsules 1727
Elocon Cream 0.1% (Infrequent) 3110
Elocon Lotion 0.1% (4 in 156 subjects) 3111
Elocon Ointment 0.1% (Infrequent) 3112
Eskalith 1527
Flovent Diskus (1% to 3%) 3614
Fortovase Capsules (Less than 2%) 2970
Gengraf Capsules (1% to less than 3%) 457
Intron A for Injection (Less than 5%) 3120
Invirase Capsules (Less than 2%) 2979
Lidex (Infrequent) 2020
Lithium Carbonate 3061
Lithium Citrate Syrup 3061
Lithobid Slow-Release Tablets 3255
Locoid Cream (Infrequent) 1341
Locoid Lipocream Cream (Infrequent) 1342
Locoid (Infrequent) 1341
Lotrisone 3129
Luxiq Foam 1210
Neoral Soft Gelatin Capsules (1% to less than 3%) 2380
Neoral Oral Solution (1% to less than 3%) 2380
Norvir Capsules (Less than 2%) 487
Norvir Oral Solution (Less than 2%) 487
Olux Foam (Less than 2%) 1211
Oxistat Cream (0.3%) 1298
Oxsoralen-Ultra Capsules 1741
Pramosone 1343
Proctocort Suppositories 2264
ProctoFoam-HC 3177
▲ Protopic Ointment (4% to 11%) 1397
Psorcon E Cream 1227
Psorcon E Ointment 1228
Rescriptor Tablets (Less than 2%) 526
▲ Serostim for Injection (1% to 10%) 3229
Sustiva Capsules (Less than 2%) 1258
Synalar (Infrequent) 2020
▲ Temovate Gel (Among most frequent) 1303
Temovate Ointment (Less frequent) 1301
Temovate Scalp Application (2 of 294 patients; infrequent) 1304
Temovate E Emollient (Less than 2%) 1302
Topamax Sprinkle Capsules (Infrequent) 2590
Topamax Tablets (Infrequent) 2590
Topicort (0.8%) 2025
Ultravate Cream 1119

Ultravate Ointment 1120
Vaniqa Cream (1%) 1121
Viracept 532

Fontanels, bulging
Acel-Imune (One case) 1851
Aquasol A Parenteral 593
Declomycin Tablets 1855
Doryx Coated Pellet Filled Capsules 3357
Dynacin Capsules 2019
Macrobid Capsules (Rare) 2889
Macrodantin Capsules 2891
Minocin Intravenous 1862
Minocin Oral Suspension 1865
Minocin Pellet-Filled Capsules 1863
Monodox Capsules 2442
Nizoral Tablets (Less than 1%) 1791
Tripedia Vaccine 817
Urobiotic-250 Capsules 2731
Vibramycin Calcium Oral Suspension Syrup 2735
Vibramycin Hyclate Capsules 2735
Vibramycin Hyclate Intravenous 2737
Vibramycin Monohydrate for Oral Suspension 2735
Vibra-Tabs Film Coated Tablets 2735

Foot drop
Actiq (Less than 1%) 1184
Betaseron for SC Injection 988
▲ Copaxone for Injection 3306
Kadian Capsules (Less than 3%) 1335
Matulane Capsules 3246
Prozac Pulvules, Liquid, and Weekly Capsules (Rare) 1238
Sarafem Pulvules (Rare) 1962
Thalomid Capsules 1154

Forceps delivery, increased incidence
Naropin Injection 612
Sensorcaine 643
Sensorcaine-MPF Injection 643

Foreign body reaction
Alamast Ophthalmic Solution (Less than 5%) 3092
Alphagan P Ophthalmic Solution (1% to 4%) 546
▲ Alrex Sterile Ophthalmic Suspension 0.2% (5% to 15%) .... ⊙256
▲ Ciloxan (Less than 10%) 538
Emadine Ophthalmic Solution (Less than 5%) .... ⊙211
Ethiodol Injection (Infrequent) 3095
▲ Lotemax Sterile Ophthalmic Suspension 0.5% (5% to 15%) .... ⊙261
▲ Lumigan Ophthalmic Solution (3% to 10%) 553
▲ Rescula Ophthalmic Solution (5% to 10%) .... ⊙306
▲ Travatan Ophthalmic Solution (5% to 10%) 543
Vexol 1% Ophthalmic Suspension (1% to 5%) .... ⊙222
▲ Xalatan Latanoprost Ophthalmic Solution (5% to 15%) .... ⊙320
▲ Xalatan Sterile Ophthalmic Solution (5% to 15%) 2864

Foreskin irretraction
(*see under* Preputium, irretraction of)

Formication, extremities
Coly-Mycin M Parenteral 2243

Foveal reflex, loss of
Aralen Tablets 3075
Plaquenil Tablets 3082

Fracture, humerus
Tamiflu Capsules (Less than 1%) 3008
Tamiflu Oral Suspension (Less than 1%) 3008

Fracture, pathological
Actiq (Less than 1%) 1184
Arimidex Tablets (2% to 5%) 659
Aromasin Tablets (Less frequent) 2769
▲ Casodex Tablets (2% to 5%) 662
Celestone Syrup 3099
Depo-Medrol Injectable Suspension 2795
Effexor Tablets (Rare) 3495
Effexor XR Capsules (Rare) 3499
Herceptin I.V. (At least one of the 958 patients) 1414
Lamictal (Rare) 1567
Lupron Depot–4 Month 30 mg (Less than 5%) 3289
Luvox Tablets (25, 50, 100 mg) (Rare) 3256
Remeron Tablets (Rare) 2483
Remeron SolTab Tablets (Rare) 2486
Roxicodone Tablets (Less than 3%) 3067
Seroquel Tablets (Infrequent) 684
Skelid Tablets (More than or equal to 1%) 3088
Vistide Injection 1445
Zanaflex Tablets (Infrequent) 1305

Fractures, long bones
Celestone Soluspan Injectable Suspension 3097
Celestone Syrup 3099
Cortifoam Rectal Foam 3170
Cortone Acetate Injectable Suspension 2059
Cortone Acetate Tablets 2061
Decadron Tablets 2079
Decadron Phosphate Injection 2081
Depo-Medrol Injectable Suspension 2795
Florinef Acetate Tablets 2250
Hydrocortone Tablets 2106
Hydrocortone Acetate Injectable Suspension 2103
Hydrocortone Phosphate Injection, Sterile 2105
Pediapred Oral Solution 1170
Prednisone 3064
Prelone Syrup 2273
Solu-Medrol Sterile Powder 2855

Fractures, unspecified
Celebrex Capsules (0.1% to 1.9%) 2676
Celebrex Capsules (0.1% to 1.9%) 2780
Cognex Capsules (Frequent) 1351
Exelon Capsules (2% or more) 2342
Exelon Oral Solution (2% or more) 2345
Femara Tablets 2351
Klonopin Tablets (Infrequent) 2983
Neurontin Capsules (1.1%) 2655
Neurontin Oral Solution (1.1%) 2655
Neurontin Tablets (1.1%) 2655
Pulmicort Respules (1% to 3%) 632
Pulmicort Turbuhaler Inhalation Powder (1% to 3%) 636
▲ Simulect for Injection (3% to 10%) 2399
Tasmar Tablets (1% or more) 3010

Fractures, vertebral compression
Celestone Soluspan Injectable Suspension 3097
Decadron Tablets 2079
Florinef Acetate Tablets 2250
Hydrocortone Tablets 2106
Hydrocortone Acetate Injectable Suspension 2103
Hydrocortone Phosphate Injection, Sterile 2105
Prednisone 3064
Prelone Syrup 2273
Solu-Medrol Sterile Powder 2855

Free T3 resin uptake, decrease
(*see under* T3, decrease)

Fretfulness
(*see under* Anxiety)

Frigidity, unspecified
Wellbutrin Tablets (Infrequent) 1680

Fullness, abdominal
(*see under* Abdominal bloating)

Fungal invasion
Blephamide Ophthalmic Ointment 547
Blephamide Ophthalmic Suspension 548
Cortisporin Ophthalmic Suspension (Possible) .... ⊙297
FML Ophthalmic Ointment (Possibility) .... ⊙237
FML Ophthalmic Suspension (Possibility) .... ⊙236
FML Forte Ophthalmic Suspension (Possibility) .... ⊙235
FML-S Liquifilm Sterile Ophthalmic Suspension .... ⊙238
Pred Mild Sterile Ophthalmic Suspension .... ⊙249
Pred-G Ophthalmic Suspension .... ⊙247
Pred-G Sterile Ophthalmic Ointment .... ⊙248
TobraDex Ophthalmic Ointment 542
TobraDex Ophthalmic Suspension 541

Furunculosis
Ambien Tablets (Rare) 3191
Astelin Nasal Spray (Infrequent) 3339
Avonex 1013
Betaseron for SC Injection 988
Cognex Capsules (Infrequent) 1351
Copaxone for Injection (Infrequent) 3306
Depacon Injection (1% or more) 416
Depakene (1% or more) 421
Depakote Sprinkle Capsules 426
Depakote Tablets (1% to 5%) 430
Depakote ER Tablets (Greater than 1%) 436
Doxil Injection (Less than 1%) 566
Effexor Tablets (Rare) 3495
Effexor XR Capsules (Rare) 3499
▲ Elocon Cream 0.1% (Approximately 7%) 3110
▲ Elocon Ointment 0.1% (4.8% to approximately 7%) 3112
Evoxac Capsules (Less than 1%) 1217
Fortovase Capsules (Less than 2%) 2970
Gabitril Tablets (Infrequent) 1189
Hivid Tablets (Less than 1%) 2975
Intron A for Injection (Less than 5%) 3120
Invirase Capsules (Less than 2%) 2979
Kaletra Capsules (Less than 2%) 471
Kaletra Oral Solution (Less than 2%) 471
Luvox Tablets (25, 50, 100 mg) (Infrequent) 3256
▲ Nipent for Injection (4%) 3272
Paxil (Infrequent) 1609
Pletal Tablets (Less than 2%) 2605
Pletal Tablets (Less than 2%) 2848
Protopic Ointment (Greater than or equal to 1%) 1397
Prozac Pulvules, Liquid, and Weekly Capsules (Rare) 1238
Remicade for IV Injection (Less than 2%) 1178
Requip Tablets (Infrequent) 1621
Rilutek Tablets (Rare) 772
Risperdal (Rare) 1796
Sarafem Pulvules (Rare) 1962
Soriatane Capsules (Less than 1%) 3003
Tasmar Tablets (Infrequent) 3010
Teveten Tablets (Less than 1%) 3327
Uniretic Tablets (Less than 1%) 3178
Vistide Injection 1445
Zyrtec (Less than 2%) 2756
Zyrtec-D 12 Hour Extended Relief Tablets (Less than 2%) 2758

G

Gagging
Versed Syrup (Less than 1%) 3033

Gait, abnormal
Accuretic Tablets 2614
Actimmune (Rare) 1772
Actiq (1% to 4%) 1184
Ambien Tablets (Rare) 3191
Aricept Tablets (Infrequent) 1270
Aricept Tablets (Infrequent) 2665
Ativan Injection 3478
Avonex 1013
Betaseron for SC Injection 988
Campath Ampules 992
Cardizem Injectable 1018
Cardizem Lyo-Ject Syringe 1018
Cardizem Monovial 1018
Cardizem CD Capsules (Less than 1%) 1016
Celexa (Infrequent) 1365
Colazal Capsules 3069
Compazine 1505
Copaxone for Injection (At least 2%) 3306
▲ Cordarone Tablets (4% to 9%) 3487
DaunoXome Injection (Less than or equal to 5%) 1442
Depacon Injection (1% to 5%) 416
Depakene (1% to 5%) 421
Depakote Sprinkle Capsules (1% to 5%) 426
Depakote Tablets (1% to 5%) 430
Depakote ER Tablets (1% to 5%) 436
DepoCyt Injection (1% to 4%) 1197
Duragesic Transdermal System (1% or greater) 1786
Effexor Tablets (Rare) 3495
Effexor XR Capsules (Rare) 3499
Evoxac Capsules 1217
Exelon Capsules (Frequent) 2342
Exelon Oral Solution (Frequent) 2345
▲ Felbatol (5.3% to 9.7%) 3343
Flexeril Tablets (Rare) 572
Flexeril Tablets (Rare) 2094
Flumadine (Less than 0.3%) 1370
▲ Gabitril Tablets (3%) 1189
Geodon Capsules (Frequent) 2688
Glucotrol XL Extended Release Tablets (Less than 1%) 2693
Intron A for Injection (Less than 5%) 3120
Lamictal (Infrequent) 1567
Lodosyn Tablets 1251
Loxitane Capsules 3398
Luvox Tablets (25, 50, 100 mg) (Infrequent) 3256
Maxalt Tablets (Infrequent) 2120
Maxalt-MLT Orally Disintegrating Tablets (Infrequent) 2120
Meridia Capsules 481
Migranal Nasal Spray (Rare) 2376
▲ Mirapex Tablets (7%) 2834
Nascobal Gel 3174
Navelbine Injection 1604
Norvir Capsules (Less than 2%) 487
Norvir Oral Solution (Less than 2%) 487
OxyContin Tablets (Less than 1%) 2912
▲ Pacerone Tablets (4% to 9%) 3331
Paxil (Rare) 1609
Permax Tablets (1.6%) 1299
Prozac Pulvules, Liquid, and Weekly Capsules (Infrequent) 1238
Requip Tablets (Infrequent) 1621
Rilutek Tablets (Infrequent) 772
▲ Risperdal (17% to 34%) 1796
Roferon-A Injection (Infrequent) 2996
Sandostatin LAR Depot (1% to 4%) 2395
Sarafem Pulvules (Infrequent) 1962
Seroquel Tablets (Infrequent) 684
Serzone Tablets (Infrequent) 1104
Sinemet Tablets 1253
Sinemet CR Tablets 1255
Sonata Capsules (Infrequent) 3591
Soriatane Capsules (Less than 1%) 3003
Stelazine 1640
Symmetrel 1328
Tasmar Tablets (1% or more) 3010
▲ Temodar Capsules (6%) 3157
Thalomid Capsules 1154
Thorazine 1656
Tiazac Capsules (Less than 2%) 1378
Topamax Sprinkle Capsules (More than 1%) 2590
Topamax Tablets (More than 1%) 2590
▲ Trileptal Oral Suspension (5% to 17%) 2407
▲ Trileptal Tablets (5% to 17%) 2407
Trovan (Less than 1%) 2722
Ultram Tablets (Less than 1%) 2600
▲ Vesanoid Capsules (3%) 3037
Vistide Injection 1445
Zantac 150 Tablets 1690
Zantac Injection 1688
Zoloft (Infrequent) 2751
Zonegran Capsules (Frequent) 1307
Zyprexa Tablets (Infrequent) 1973
Zyprexa ZYDIS Orally Disintegrating Tablets (Infrequent) 1973

Galactorrhea
Celexa (Infrequent) 1365
Compazine 1505
Covera-HS Tablets (Less than 2%) 3199
Demser Capsules (Infrequent) 2085
Depacon Injection 416
Depakene 421
Depakote Sprinkle Capsules 426
Depakote Tablets 430
Depakote ER Tablets 436
Depo-Provera Contraceptive Injection (Fewer than 1%) 2798
D.H.E. 45 Injection 2334
Etrafon 3115
Flexeril Tablets (Rare) 572
Flexeril Tablets (Rare) 2094
Haldol Decanoate 2535
Haldol Injection, Tablets and Concentrate 2533
Imitrex Injection 1549
Imitrex Nasal Spray (Rare) 1554
Imitrex Tablets (Rare) 1558
Isoptin SR Tablets (1% or less) 467
Limbitrol 1738
Loxitane Capsules (Rare) 3398
Moban (Infrequent) 1320
Norpramin Tablets 755
Ortho-Prefest Tablets 2570
Paxil 1609
Premphase Tablets 3572
Prempro Tablets 3572
Provera Tablets 2853
Reglan 2935
Sandostatin Injection (Less than 1%) 2394
Sandostatin LAR Depot (Rare) 2395
Serentil 1057
Sinequan 2713
Stelazine 1640
Surmontil Capsules 3595
Tarka Tablets 508
Thalomid Capsules 1154
Thioridazine Hydrochloride Tablets 2289
Trilafon 3160
Verelan PM Capsules (2% or less) 3186
Vivactil Tablets 2217
Vivactil Tablets 2446
Xanax Tablets 2865
Zoloft 2751

Gallbladder, sonographic abnormalities
Rocephin Injectable Vials, ADD-Vantage, Galaxy, Bulk 2993

Gallbladder disease
Activella Tablets 2764
Alesse-21 Tablets 3468
Alesse-28 Tablets 3473
Alora Transdermal System (Increased incidence) 3372
Avonex 1013
Brevicon 28-Day Tablets 3380
Cenestin Tablets 1263
Climara Transdermal System 958
CombiPatch Transdermal System 2323
Cyclessa Tablets 2450
Desogen Tablets 2458
Esclim Transdermal System 3460

Estrace Vaginal Cream 3358
Estrace Tablets 3361
Estratest 3252
Estrostep 2627
femhrt Tablets 2635
Levlen 962
Levlite 21 Tablets 962
Levlite 28 Tablets 962
Levora Tablets 3389
Loestrin 21 Tablets 2642
Loestrin Fe Tablets 2642
Lo/Ovral Tablets 3532
Lo/Ovral-28 Tablets 3538
Lopid Tablets (0.9%) 2650
Low-Ogestrel-28 Tablets 3392
Lunelle Monthly Injection 2827
Menest Tablets 2254
Microgestin Fe 1.5/30 Tablets 3407
Microgestin Fe 1/20 Tablets 3400
Mircette Tablets 2470
Modicon 2563
Necon 3415
Nordette-28 Tablets 2257
Norinyl 1 +35 28-Day Tablets 3380
Norinyl 1 + 50 28-Day Tablets 3380
Ogen Tablets 2846
Ogestrel 0.5/50-28 Tablets 3428
Ortho Dienestrol Cream 2554
Ortho-Cept 21 Tablets 2546
Ortho-Cept 28 Tablets 2546
Ortho-Cyclen/Ortho Tri-Cyclen 2573
Ortho-Est Tablets 3464
Ortho-Novum 2563
Ortho-Novum 1/50◻28 Tablets 2556
Ortho-Prefest Tablets 2570
Ortho-Cyclen/Ortho Tri-Cyclen 2573
Ovcon 3364
Ovral Tablets 3551
Ovral-28 Tablets 3552
Ovrette Tablets 3552
Premarin Intravenous 3563
Premarin Tablets 3566
Premarin Vaginal Cream 3570
Premphase Tablets 3572
Prempro Tablets 3572
Pulmozyme Inhalation Solution 1426
Rocephin Injectable Vials, ADD-Vantage, Galaxy, Bulk 2993
Sandostatin Injection (Frequent) 2394
Sandostatin LAR Depot (Rare) 2395
Topamax Sprinkle Capsules (Infrequent) 2590
Topamax Tablets (Infrequent) 2590
Tri-Levlen 962
Tri-Norinyl-28 Tablets 3433
Triphasil-21 Tablets 3600
Triphasil-28 Tablets 3605
Trivora Tablets 3439
Vivelle Transdermal System 2412
Vivelle-Dot Transdermal System 2416
Yasmin 28 Tablets 980
Zovia 3449

Gallstones
Atromid-S Capsules 3483
Imitrex Injection (Rare) 1549
Imitrex Nasal Spray 1554
Imitrex Tablets 1558
Intron A for Injection (Less than 5%) 3120
Relafen Tablets (Less than 1%) 1617
Sandostatin Injection (Frequent) 2394

Gamma-glutamyl transpeptidase, elevation
Accutane Capsules 2944
Amphotec (1% to 5%) 1774
Arimidex Tablets (2% to 5%) 659
Asacol Delayed-Release Tablets 2884
Avelox Tablets (0.05% to 1%) 879
Axert Tablets (Rare) 2772
Baycol Tablets 883
Biaxin/Biaxin XL (Less than 1%) 403
Ceclor CD Tablets (0.2%) 1279
▲ CellCept Capsules (3%) 2951
▲ CellCept Intravenous (3%) 2951
▲ CellCept Oral Suspension (3%) 2951
▲ CellCept Tablets (3%) 2951
Cipro I.V. (Infrequent) 893
▲ Cipro I.V. Pharmacy Bulk Package (Among most frequent) 897
Cipro (Less than 0.1%) 887
Cordarone Intravenous (Two cases) 3491
Dynabac Tablets (0.1% to 1%) 2269
Effexor Tablets 3495
Effexor XR Capsules 3499
Evoxac Capsules (Less than 1%) 1217
Felbatol (Rare) 3343
Floxin I.V. 2526
Floxin Tablets 2529
▲ Fortaz (1 in 19) 1541
Geodon Capsules (Rare) 2688
Hivid Tablets (Less than 1%) 2975
Lescol Capsules 2361
Lescol Capsules 2925
Lescol XL Tablets 2361
Lescol XL Tablets 2925
▲ Lupron Depot–4 Month 30 mg (Greater than or equal to 5%) 3289
Mevacor Tablets 2132
Mobic Tablets (Less than 2%) 1054
▲ Novantrone for Injection (3% to 15%) 1760
Oncaspar 756
Pentasa Capsules (Less than 1%) 3239
Prevacid Delayed-Release Capsules 3292
PREVPAC (Less than 1%) 3298
Prilosec Delayed-Release Capsules (Rare) 628
▲ Prograf (3% to 15%) 1393
Protonix I.V. (Less than 1%) 3580
Protonix Tablets (Less than 1%) 3577
Provigil Tablets (At least 1%) 1193
Rescriptor Tablets (Less than 2%) 526
Rilutek Tablets (Infrequent) 772
Seroquel Tablets (Infrequent) 684
▲ Soriatane Capsules (Approximately 1 in 3 patients) 3003
Symmetrel 1328
▲ Tazicef for Injection (1 in 19 patients) 1647
▲ Tazicef Galaxy Container (1 in 19 patients) 1650
▲ Tazicef Pharmacy Bulk Package (1 in 19 patients) 1653
▲ Tazidime Vials, Faspak & ADD-Vantage (1 in 19) 1966
Ticlid Tablets (Rare) 3015
Topamax Sprinkle Capsules (Rare) 2590
Topamax Tablets (Rare) 2590
Tricor Capsules, Micronized 513
Trileptal Oral Suspension 2407
Trileptal Tablets 2407
Vantin Tablets and Oral Suspension 2860
Vermox Chewable Tablets (Rare) 2017
Videx EC Capsules 1143
Viracept 532
Viramune Oral Suspension (2.4%) 1060
Viramune Tablets (2.4%) 1060
Vitravene for Injection (2% to 5%) ⊙ 310
Ziagen 1692
Zithromax (1% to 2%) 2743
Zithromax for Oral Suspension, 300 mg, 600 mg, 900 mg, 1200 mg (1% to 2%) 2739
Zithromax Tablets, 250 mg (1% to 2%) 2739
Zithromax Tablets, 600 mg (1% to 2%) 2743
Zocor Tablets 2219

Gangrene
Apligraf (1.8%) 2305
Bicillin C-R 900/300 Injection 2240
Bicillin C-R Injection 2238
Bicillin L-A Injection 2242
Felbatol 3343
Heparin Lock Flush Solution 3509
Heparin Sodium Injection 3511
Mepergan Injection 3539
Phenergan Injection 3553
Proleukin for Injection (1%) 1199
Requip Tablets (Rare) 1621

Gangrene, cutaneous
Retavase Vials 1182

Gangrene, peripheral
Celebrex Capsules (Less than 0.1%) 2676
Celebrex Capsules (Less than 0.1%) 2780
Requip Tablets (Infrequent) 1621

Gastric acid, regurgitation
Prilosec Delayed-Release Capsules (1.9%) 628

Gastric dilation
Felbatol 3343

Gastric discomfort
(see under Distress, gastrointestinal)

Gastric disorder
(see under Distress, gastrointestinal)

Gastric erosion
Robaxisal Tablets 2939
Soma Compound Tablets (Less common) 3354
Soma Compound w/Codeine Tablets (Rare) 3355

Gastric regurgitation
Wellbutrin SR Sustained-Release Tablets (Infrequent) 1684

Gastric secretions, increase
Tensilon Injectable 1745

Gastritis
Actonel Tablets (2.5%) 2879
Aggrenox Capsules (Less than 1%) 1026
Agrylin Capsules (1% to 5%) 3232
Ambien Tablets (Rare) 3191
Amerge Tablets (Rare) 1467
Apligraf (2.7%) 2305
Arava Tablets (1% to 3%) 724
Aricept Tablets (Infrequent) 1270
Aricept Tablets (Infrequent) 2665
Arthrotec Tablets (Rare) 3195
Asacol Delayed-Release Tablets 2884
Atacand HCT Tablets (0.5% or greater) 597
Atromid-S Capsules 3483
Augmentin Chewable Tablets 1482
Augmentin Powder for Oral Suspension 1482
Augmentin Tablets 1485
Augmentin ES-600 Powder for Oral Suspension 1487
Avelox Tablets (0.05% to 1%) 879
Avonex 1013
Axert Tablets (Rare) 2772
Betaseron for SC Injection 988
Cafcit (2.2%) 1035
Carnitor Injection (Less frequent) 3242
Ceclor CD Tablets (0.1% to 1%) 1279
Celebrex Capsules (0.1% to 1.9%) 2676
Celebrex Capsules (0.1% to 1.9%) 2780
Celexa (Infrequent) 1365
▲ CellCept Capsules (3%) 2951
▲ CellCept Intravenous (3%) 2951
▲ CellCept Oral Suspension (3%) 2951
▲ CellCept Tablets (3%) 2951
Cerebyx Injection (Infrequent) 2619
Claritin (At least one patient) 3100
Claritin-D 12 Hour Extended Release Tablets (Less frequent) 3102
Claritin-D 24 Hour Extended Release Tablets (Fewer than 2%) 3104
Clinoril Tablets (Less than 1%) 2053
Cognex Capsules (Infrequent) 1351
Comtan Tablets (1%) 2328
Copaxone for Injection (At least 2%) 3306
Cozaar Tablets (Less than 1%) 2067
Crinone (Less than 5%) 3213
Crixivan Capsules (Less than 2%) 2070
DaunoXome Injection (Less than or equal to 5%) 1442
Didronel Tablets 2888
Dolobid Tablets (Less than 1 in 100) 2088
Doxil Injection (Less than 1%) 566
Dynabac Tablets (0.1% to 1%) 2269
Effexor Tablets (Infrequent) 3495
Effexor XR Capsules (Infrequent) 3499
Elmiron Capsules (Less than or equal to 1%) 570
Enbrel for Injection 1752
Enbrel for Injection 3504
Eskalith 1527
Estring Vaginal Ring (1% to 3%) 2811
Etrafon 3115
Evoxac Capsules (Less than 1%) 1217
Exelon Capsules (Frequent) 2342
Exelon Oral Solution (Frequent) 2345
Felbatol 3343
Feldene Capsules (Occasional) 2685
Flexeril Tablets (Less than 1%) 572
Flexeril Tablets (Less than 1%) 2094
▲ Flolan for Injection (61%) 1528
Fortovase Capsules (Less than 2%) 2970
Fosamax Tablets (0.5%) 2095
Sterile FUDR 2974
Gabitril Tablets (Infrequent) 1189
Gengraf Capsules (1% to less than 3%) 457
Hivid Tablets (Less than 1%) 2975
▲ Humatrope Vials and Cartridges (Up to 6.67%) 1930
Hyzaar 2109
Imdur Tablets (Less than or equal to 5%) 1826
Imitrex Injection 1549
Imitrex Nasal Spray 1554
Intron A for Injection (Less than 5%) 3120
Invirase Capsules (Less than 2%) 2979
Kaletra Capsules (Less than 2%) 471
Kaletra Oral Solution (Less than 2%) 471
Keflex 1237
Klonopin Tablets 2983
Lamictal (Rare) 1567
Lipitor Tablets (Less than 2%) 2639
Lipitor Tablets (Less than 2%) 2696
Lithobid Slow-Release Tablets 3255
Lodine (1% to 3%) 3528
Lodine XL Extended-Release Tablets (1% to 3%) 3530
Lotensin Tablets (Less than 1%) 2365
Luvox Tablets (25, 50, 100 mg) (Infrequent) 3256
Malarone (2% to 3%) 1596
▲ Mavik Tablets (4.2%) 478
Maxalt Tablets (Rare) 2120
Maxalt-MLT Orally Disintegrating Tablets (Rare) 2120
Meridia Capsules (1.7%) 481
Miacalcin Nasal Spray (Less than 1%) 2375
Micardis Tablets (More than 0.3%) 1049
Micardis HCT Tablets 1051
Mobic Tablets (Less than 2%) 1054
Monopril HCT (Less than 2%) 1094
Motrin Suspension, Oral Drops, Chewable Tablets, and Caplets (Less than 1%) 2002
Naprelan Tablets (Less than 3%) 1293
Neoral Soft Gelatin Capsules (1% to less than 3%) 2380
Neoral Oral Solution (1% to less than 3%) 2380
Norvasc Tablets (Less than or equal to 0.1%) 2704
Norvir Capsules (Less than 2%) 487
Norvir Oral Solution (Less than 2%) 487
Orudis Capsules (Less than 1%) 3548
Oruvail Capsules (Less than 1%) 3548
OxyContin Tablets (Between 1% and 5%) 2912
Permax Tablets (Infrequent) 1299
Pletal Tablets (Less than 2%) 2605
Pletal Tablets (Less than 2%) 2848
Ponstel Capsules (Occasional) 1356
Priftin Tablets (Less than 1%) 758
Prinivil Tablets (0.3% to 1.0%) 2164
Prinzide Tablets 2168
▲ Prograf (3% to 15%) 1393
Proleukin for Injection 1199
ProSom Tablets (Infrequent) 500
Protopic Ointment (Greater than or equal to 1%) 1397
Prozac Pulvules, Liquid, and Weekly Capsules (Infrequent) 1238
▲ Rapamune Oral Solution and Tablets (3% to 20%) 3584
ReFacto Vials 1437
Relafen Tablets (1% to 3%) 1617
Remeron Tablets (Rare) 2483
Remeron SolTab Tablets (Rare) 2486
Reminyl Oral Solution (Infrequent) 1792
Reminyl Tablets (Infrequent) 1792
Requip Tablets (Infrequent) 1621
Rescriptor Tablets (Less than 2%) 526
Rilutek Tablets (Infrequent) 772
Risperdal (Infrequent) 1796
Robaxisal Tablets 2939
Salagen Tablets (Less than 1%) 2229
Sandimmune (2% or less) 2388
Sandostatin LAR Depot (1% to 4%) 2395
Sarafem Pulvules (Infrequent) 1962
Seroquel Tablets (Infrequent) 684
▲ Serostim for Injection (1% to 10%) 3229
Serzone Tablets (Infrequent) 1104
Skelid Tablets (More than or equal to 1%) 3088
▲ Soma Compound Tablets (Among most common) 3354
Soma Compound w/Codeine Tablets 3355
Sonata Capsules (Infrequent) 3591
Soriatane Capsules (Less than 1%) 3003
Sporanox Capsules (2%) 1800
Sular Tablets (Less than or equal to 1%) 688
Tequin Injection (Less than 0.1%) 1110
Tequin Tablets (Less than 0.1%) 1110
Teveten Tablets (Less than 1%) 3327
Thymoglobulin for Injection (1.2%) 3071
Tolectin (1% to 3%) 2589
Topamax Sprinkle Capsules (Infrequent) 2590
Topamax Tablets (Infrequent) 2590
Toradol (1% or less) 3010
Tricor Capsules, Micronized 513
Trileptal Oral Suspension (1% to 2%) 2407
Trileptal Tablets (1% to 2%) 2407
Trovan (Less than 1%) 2722
Unasyn for Injection 2728
Uniretic Tablets (Less than 1%) 3178
Vantin Tablets and Oral Suspension (Less than 1%) 2860
Vascor Tablets (0.5% to 2.0%) 2602
Viagra Tablets (Less than 2%) 2732
Vicoprofen Tablets (Less than 3%) 520
Vioxx (Greater than 0.1% to 1.9%) 2213
Vistide Injection 1445
Xeloda Tablets (Less than 5%) 3039
Zebeta Tablets 1885
▲ Zenapax for Injection (2% to 5%) 3046
Zestoretic Tablets 695
Zestril Tablets (0.3% to 1.0%) 698
Ziac Tablets 1887
Zithromax Capsules, 250 mg (1% or less) 2743
Zithromax for IV Infusion (1% or less) 2748
Zithromax for Oral Suspension, 300 mg, 600 mg, 900 mg, 1200 mg (1% or less) 2739
Zithromax Tablets, 250 mg (1% or less) 2739
Zoloft (Rare) 2751
Zomig Tablets (Rare) 708
Zomig-ZMT Tablets (Rare) 708
Zonegran Capsules (Infrequent) 1307
Zosyn (1.0% or less) 1890

Zosyn in Galaxy Containers (1.0% or less) 1894
Zyprexa Tablets (Infrequent) 1973
Zyprexa ZYDIS Orally Disintegrating Tablets (Infrequent) 1973
Zyrtec (Less than 2%) 2756
Zyrtec-D 12 Hour Extended Relief Tablets (Less than 2%) 2758

Gastritis, hemorrhagic

Plavix Tablets (Less than 1%) 1097
Plavix Tablets (Less than 1%) 3084
Requip Tablets (Rare) 1621

Gastroenteritis

AccuNeb Inhalation Solution (0.9% to 3.4%) 1230
Aceon Tablets (2 mg, 4 mg, 8 mg) (0.3% to 1%) 3249
Aciphex Tablets 1267
Aciphex Tablets 1783
Actiq (Less than 1%) 1184
Activella Tablets (0% to 6%) 2764
Advair Diskus 100/50 (1% to 3%) 1448
Advair Diskus 250/50 (1% to 3%) 1448
Advair Diskus 500/50 (1% to 3%) 1448
Altace Capsules (Less than 1%) 2233
Ambien Tablets (Infrequent) 3191
Amerge Tablets (Infrequent) 1467
Apligraf (2.7%) 2305
▲ Arava Tablets (3%) 724
Aricept Tablets (Infrequent) 1270
Aricept Tablets (Infrequent) 2665
Asacol Delayed-Release Tablets (2% or greater) 2884
Astelin Nasal Spray (Infrequent) 3339
Atacand Tablets (0.5% or greater) 595
Atacand HCT Tablets (0.5% or greater) 597
Avalide Tablets 1070
Avapro Tablets (Less than 1%) 1074
Avapro Tablets (Less than 1%) 3076
Axert Tablets (Rare) 2772
Campath Ampules 992
Cardura Tablets (Less than 0.5%) 2668
Celebrex Capsules (0.1% to 1.9%) 2676
Celebrex Capsules (0.1% to 1.9%) 2780
Celexa (Infrequent) 1365
▲ CellCept Capsules (3%) 2951
▲ CellCept Intravenous (3%) 2951
▲ CellCept Oral Suspension (3%) 2951
▲ CellCept Tablets (3%) 2951
Clinoril Tablets (Less than 1%) 2053
Clozaril Tablets (Less than 1%) 2319
Cognex Capsules (Infrequent) 1351
Colazal Capsules 3069
▲ Copaxone for Injection (3%) 3306
Depacon Injection (1% or more) 416
Depakene (1% or more) 421
Depakote Sprinkle Capsules 426
Depakote Tablets (1% to 5%) 430
Depakote ER Tablets (Greater than 1%) 436
Dynabac Tablets (0.1% to 1%) 2269
Effexor Tablets (Infrequent) 3495
Effexor XR Capsules (Infrequent) 3499
Enbrel for Injection 1752
Enbrel for Injection 3504
Esclim Transdermal System 3460
Evista Tablets (2.6%) 1915
Evoxac Capsules (Less than 1%) 1217
Exelon Capsules (Infrequent) 2342
Exelon Oral Solution (Infrequent) 2345
Flovent Diskus (1% to 3%) 3614
Flovent Rotadisk (1% to 3%) 1537
Fortovase Capsules (Less than 2%) 2970
Sterile FUDR 2974
Gabitril Tablets (1% or more) 1189
Gengraf Capsules (1% to less than 3%) 457
Helixate Concentrate 788
Herceptin I.V. (At least one of the 958 patients) 1414
Imitrex Injection 1549
Imitrex Nasal Spray (Rare) 1554
Indocin Capsules (Less than 1%) 2112
Indocin I.V. (Less than 1%) 2115
Indocin (Less than 1%) 2112
Intron A for Injection (Less than 5%) 3120
Invirase Capsules (Less than 2%) 2979
Kaletra Capsules (Less than 2%) 471
Kaletra Oral Solution (Less than 2%) 471
Keppra Tablets (1% or more) 3314
Kogenate FS 936
Levaquin Injection (Less than 0.5%) 2537
Lipitor Tablets (Less than 2%) 2639
Lipitor Tablets (Less than 2%) 2696
Lotensin HCT Tablets (0.3% or more) 2367
Luvox Tablets (25, 50, 100 mg) (Infrequent) 3256
Meridia Capsules (Greater than or equal to 1%) 481
Micardis Tablets (More than 0.3%) 1049
Micardis HCT Tablets 1051
Naprelan Tablets (Less than 1%) 1293
Neoral Soft Gelatin Capsules (1% to less than 3%) 2380
Neoral Oral Solution (1% to less than 3%) 2380
Neurontin Capsules (Infrequent) 2655
Neurontin Oral Solution (Infrequent) 2655
Neurontin Tablets (Infrequent) 2655
Nexium Delayed-Release Capsules (Less than 1%) 619
Norvir Capsules (Less than 2%) 487
Norvir Oral Solution (Less than 2%) 487
Paxil (Rare) 1609
Permax Tablets (Infrequent) 1299
Pletal Tablets (Less than 2%) 2605
Pletal Tablets (Less than 2%) 2848
Prevacid Delayed-Release Capsules (Less than 1%) 3292
Prevnar for Injection 1870
PREVPAC (Less than 1%) 3298
Primaxin I.M. 2158
Primaxin I.V. (Less than 0.2%) 2160
Prometrium Capsules (100 mg, 200 mg) (Less than 5%) 3261
Protonix I.V. (Greater than or equal to 1%) 3580
Protonix Tablets (Greater than or equal to 1%) 3577
Protopic Ointment (2% to 4%) 1397
Provigil Tablets (At least 1%) 1193
Prozac Pulvules, Liquid, and Weekly Capsules (Infrequent) 1238
▲ Pulmicort Respules (5%) 632
Pulmicort Turbuhaler Inhalation Powder (1% to 3%) 636
▲ Rapamune Oral Solution and Tablets (3% to 20%) 3584
ReFacto Vials 1437
Relafen Tablets (Less than 1%) 1617
Remeron Tablets (Rare) 2483
Remeron SolTab Tablets (Rare) 2486
Reminyl Oral Solution (Infrequent) 1792
Reminyl Tablets (Infrequent) 1792
Rescriptor Tablets 526
Risperdal (Rare) 1796
Rythmol Tablets – 150 mg, 225 mg, 300 mg (0.03% to 1.9%) 502
Salagen Tablets (Less than 1%) 2229
Sandostatin LAR Depot (1% to 4%) 2395
Sarafem Pulvules (Infrequent) 1962
Seroquel Tablets (Infrequent) 684
Serzone Tablets (Frequent) 1104
▲ Simulect for Injection (3% to 10%) 2399
Sonata Capsules (Infrequent) 3591
Soriatane Capsules (Less than 1%) 3003
Sporanox Capsules (2%) 1800
Synagis Intramuscular (More than 1%) 2028
Tasmar Tablets (Infrequent) 3010
Teveten Tablets (Less than 1%) 3327
Thalomid Capsules 1154
Topamax Sprinkle Capsules (More than 1%) 2590
Topamax Tablets (More than 1%) 2590
Tricor Capsules, Micronized 513
Trizivir Tablets 1669
Trovan (Less than 1%) 2722
Uniretic Tablets (Less than 1%) 3178
Viagra Tablets (Less than 2%) 2732
Vicoprofen Tablets (Less than 1%) 520
Vioxx (Greater than 0.1% to 1.9%) 2213
Xeloda Tablets (Less than 5%) 3039
Xopenex Inhalation Solution 3207
Yasmin 28 Tablets (Greater than 1%) 980
Zanaflex Tablets (Rare) 1305
Zoloft (Infrequent) 2751
Zomig Tablets (Infrequent) 708
Zomig-ZMT Tablets (Infrequent) 708
Zonegran Capsules (Infrequent) 1307
Zyprexa Tablets (Infrequent) 1973
Zyprexa ZYDIS Orally Disintegrating Tablets (Infrequent) 1973

Gastroenteritis, infectious

Singulair (2.1%) 2181
Vioxx (Greater than 0.1% to 1.9%) 2213

Gastroenteritis, viral

▲ Flovent Diskus (4%) 3614
Flovent Rotadisk (1% to 3%) 1537

Gastroesophageal reflux

Amerge Tablets (Rare) 1467
Axert Tablets (Rare) 2772
Celebrex Capsules (0.1% to 1.9%) 2676
Celebrex Capsules (0.1% to 1.9%) 2780
Celexa (Rare) 1365
Ditropan XL Extended Release Tablets (2% to 5%) 564
Evoxac Capsules (1% to 3%) 1217
Exelon Capsules (Infrequent) 2342
Exelon Oral Solution (Infrequent) 2345
Felbatol 3343
▲ Flolan for Injection (61%) 1528
Fortovase Capsules (Less than 2%) 2970
Imitrex Injection (Infrequent) 1549
Imitrex Nasal Spray (Infrequent) 1554
Imitrex Tablets (Infrequent) 1558
Kadian Capsules (Less than 3%) 1335
Micardis Tablets (More than 0.3%) 1049
Micardis HCT Tablets 1051
Mobic Tablets (Less than 2%) 1054
Procardia XL Extended Release Tablets (1% or less) 2710
ReoPro Vials (0.1%) 1958
Requip Tablets (Infrequent) 1621
Rescriptor Tablets (Less than 2%) 526
Risperdal (Rare) 1796
Seroquel Tablets (Infrequent) 684
Topamax Sprinkle Capsules (Infrequent) 2590
Topamax Tablets (Infrequent) 2590
Vioxx (Greater than 0.1% to 1.9%) 2213

Gastrointestinal bleeding

(*see under* Bleeding, gastrointestinal)

Gastrointestinal disorders

Accutane Capsules 2944
Actonel Tablets (2.3%) 2879
Adderall Tablets 3231
Adderall XR Capsules
▲ Adenoscan (13%) 1381
Adipex-P 1406
▲ Advair Diskus 100/50 (4%) 1448
Advair Diskus 250/50 (1%) 1448
Advair Diskus 500/50 (1% to 4%) 1448
▲ Aerobid/Aerobid-M (1% to 10%) 1363
Aldoclor Tablets 2035
Alkeran for Injection (Infrequent) 1465
Alkeran Tablets (Infrequent) 1466
▲ Alphagan Ophthalmic Solution (Approximately 3% to 9%) 545
Amerge Tablets (Infrequent) 1467
Anaprox Tablets 2967
Anaprox DS Tablets 2967
Aralen Tablets 3075
▲ Arimidex Tablets (33.6%) 659
Ativan Tablets 3482
Atromid-S Capsules (Less frequent) 3483
Avelox Tablets (0.05% to 1%) 879
Axid Pulvules (1.1%) 1903
Axid Pulvules (1.1%) 2919
Baycol Tablets 883
▲ Betaseron for SC Injection (6%) 988
Brevicon 28-Day Tablets 3380
Captopril Tablets 2281
▲ Carnitor Injection (2% to 6%) 3242
Carnitor Tablets and Oral Solution 3245
▲ Cataflam Tablets (About 20%) 2315
Ceclor (About 2.5%) 1905
Cefotan (1.5%) 664
▲ CellCept Capsules (3% to 10%) 2951
▲ CellCept Intravenous (3% to 10%) 2951
▲ CellCept Oral Suspension (3% to 10%) 2951
▲ CellCept Tablets (3% to 10%) 2951
▲ Ceptaz for Injection (Among most common) 1499
▲ Chemet Capsules (About 10%) 3078
Cleocin T Topical 2790
Cleocin Vaginal Cream 2788
Clindagel 1401
▲ Clinoril Tablets (3% to 9%) 2053
▲ Clozaril Tablets (Greater than 5%) 2319
▲ Colestid Tablets (Among most common) 2791
Coly-Mycin M Parenteral 2243
Comtan Tablets (1%) 2328
▲ Copaxone for Injection (5%) 3306
Cosopt Sterile Ophthalmic Solution 2065
▲ Creon 5 Capsules (Among most frequent) 3251
▲ Cuprimine Capsules (17%) 2075
▲ Daranide Tablets (Among the most common effects) 2077
DDAVP Nasal Spray (Up to 2%) 738
DDAVP Rhinal Tube (Up to 2%) 738
Decadron Elixir 2078
Decadron Phosphate Injection 2081
Depacon Injection 416
Depakene 421
Depakote Tablets (1% to 5%) 430
Depakote ER Tablets 436
Depo-Provera Contraceptive Injection (Fewer than 1%) 2798
Desmopressin Acetate Rhinal Tube (Up to 2%) 1345
Dexedrine 1512
DextroStat Tablets 3236
Diamox Intravenous ⊙269
Diamox Sequels Sustained Release Capsules ⊙270
Diamox Tablets ⊙269
Didronel Tablets 2888
Duricef 1079
Dyazide Capsules 1515
Dynabac Tablets (1.6%) 2269
EC-Naprosyn Delayed-Release Tablets 2967
Ecotrin Enteric Coated Aspirin Low, Regular and Maximum Strength Tablets 1715
8-MOP Capsules 1727
▲ Eulexin Capsules (6%) 3118
▲ Evista Tablets (3.3%) 1915
Ferrlecit Injection 3386
▲ Flovent Diskus (4%) 3614
Flovent (1% to 3%) 1535
Flovent Rotadisk (1% to 3%) 1537
▲ Fortaz (Among most common) 1541
Fosamax Tablets 2095
Furosemide Tablets 2284
▲ Gengraf Capsules (4% to 19.8%) 457
Ginkoba Tablets (Very rare) ▣828
Humegon for Injection 2468
▲ Hyalgan Solution (29%) 3080
Ionamin Capsules 1163
Kaletra Capsules (Less than 2%) 471
Kaletra Oral Solution (Less than 2%) 471
K-Dur Microburst Release System ER Tablets 1832
Kefurox Vials, ADD-Vantage (1 in 150) 1948
Klonopin Tablets (Infrequent) 2983
Klor-Con M20/Klor-Con M10 Tablets 3329
K-Phos Neutral Tablets 946
Lanoxicaps Capsules 1574
Leukeran Tablets (Infrequent) 1591
▲ Leukine (37%) 1755
▲ Lopid Tablets (34.2%) 2650
▲ Lorabid Suspension and Pulvules (Most common) 2251
Lupron Depot 3.75 mg (Less than 5%) 3281
▲ Lupron Depot 7.5 mg (14.3%) 3284
▲ Lupron Depot-3 Month 22.5 mg (16%) 3288
Lupron Injection (Less than 5%) 3279
Maxzide 1008
Micardis Tablets (More than 0.3%) 1049
Micardis HCT Tablets 1051
Midamor Tablets (Less than or equal to 1%) 2136
Modicon 2563
Moduretic Tablets (Less than or equal to 1%) 2138
▲ Motrin Suspension, Oral Drops, Chewable Tablets, and Caplets (Most frequent; 4% to 16%) 2002
Movana Tablets (Rare) ▣832
Myambutol Tablets 1290
Mylocel Tablets 2227
Myobloc Injectable Solution (2% or greater) 1291
Naprelan Tablets (Less than 1%) 1293
Naprosyn Suspension 2967
Naprosyn Tablets 2967
▲ Neoral Soft Gelatin Capsules (4% to 19.8%) 2380
▲ Neoral Oral Solution (4% to 19.8%) 2380
Neptazane Tablets ⊙271
Nexium Delayed-Release Capsules (Less than 1%) 619
Nilandron Tablets (2%) 753
Nimotop Capsules (Up to 2.4%) 904
Nipent for Injection 3272
Norinyl 1 +35 28-Day Tablets 3380
Norinyl 1 + 50 28-Day Tablets 3380
Norvir Capsules (Less than 2%) 487
Norvir Oral Solution (Less than 2%) 487
▲ Novantrone for Injection (58% to 88%) 1760
Omnicef 493
Orap Tablets 1407
Ortho-Cyclen/Ortho Tri-Cyclen 2573
Ortho-Novum 2563
Ortho-Novum 1/50▫28 Tablets 2556
Ortho-Cyclen/Ortho Tri-Cyclen 2573
Ovcon 3364
Ovidrel for Injection 3220
Oxsoralen-Ultra Capsules 1741
OxyContin Tablets (Less than 1%) 2912
▲ Pancrease Capsules (Among most frequent) 2580
▲ Pancrease MT Capsules (Among most frequent) 2581
▲ Paraplatin for Injection (21% to 50%) 1126
Phenergan with Dextromethorphan Syrup 3559
Pilopine HS Ophthalmic Gel (Occasional) ⊙217
Pima Syrup 1362
Plaquenil Tablets 3082
▲ Plavix Tablets (About 27.1%) 1097
▲ Plavix Tablets (About 27.1%) 3084
▲ Precose Tablets (Among most common) 906
▲ Prepidil Gel (5.7%) 2851
Priftin Tablets 758
Prinzide Tablets (0.3% to 1%) 2168
Proleukin for Injection (Less than 1%) 1199
Protonix I.V. (Greater than or equal to 1%) 3580
Protonix Tablets (Greater than or equal to 1%) 3577

Provigil Tablets (At least 1%) 1193
Prozac Pulvules, Liquid, and Weekly Capsules (Less than 1%) 1238
Pyrazinamide Tablets 1876
Rabies Vaccine RabAvert (Uncommon) 1203
Rescriptor Tablets (Less than 2%) 526
▲ Retrovir Capsules (20%) 1625
▲ Retrovir IV Infusion (20%) 1629
▲ Retrovir (20%) 1625
Rifadin 765
Rifater Tablets 769
Robaxin Injectable 2938
▲ Ryna-12 S Suspension (Among most common) 3351
▲ Reformulated Rynatan Pediatric Suspension (Among most common) 3352
▲ Rynatuss Pediatric Suspension (Among most common) 3353
▲ Rynatuss Tablets (Among most common) 3353
Salagen Tablets (Less than 1%) 2229
Serophene Tablets 3226
Silvadene Cream 1% 2267
▲ Simulect for Injection (3% to 10%) 2399
Skelaxin Tablets 1301
Soma Compound Tablets 3354
▲ Sporanox Capsules (4%) 1800
▲ Suprax (30%) 1877
Taxotere for Injection Concentrate 778
▲ Tazicef for Injection (Among most common) 1647
▲ Tazicef Galaxy Container (Among most common) 1650
▲ Tazicef Pharmacy Bulk Package (Among most common) 1653
Tenoretic Tablets 690
Tessalon Capsules 1377
Thalomid Capsules 1154
Tice BCG, BCG Live (1.0%) 2489
▲ Ticlid Tablets (30% to 40%) 3015
Timolol GFS ⊙266
Timoptic-XE Sterile Ophthalmic Gel Forming Solution 2194
▲ Tolectin (10%) 2589
Tonocard Tablets (Less than 1%) 649
Toprol-XL Tablets 651
Tranxene (Less common) 511
Travatan Ophthalmic Solution (1% to 5%) 543
▲ Trecator-SC Tablets (Among most common) 3598
▲ Trilisate (Less than 20%) 2901
Tri-Norinyl-28 Tablets 3433
Trovan (Less than 1%) 2722
Tussi-12 S Suspension 3356
Tussi-12 Tablets 3356
Tussi-Organidin DM NR Liquid (Rare) 3350
Tussi-Organidin DM-S NR Liquid (Rare) 3350
▲ Ultrase Capsules (Most frequent) 835
▲ Ultrase MT Capsules (Among most frequent) 835
Uroqid-Acid No. 2 Tablets 947
Vantin Tablets and Oral Suspension 2860
▲ Vascor Tablets (4.35% to 6.98%) 2602
Vaseretic Tablets 2204
▲ Vesanoid Capsules (26%) 3037
Viokase 837
▲ Voltaren Tablets (About 20%) 2315
▲ Voltaren-XR Tablets (About 20%) 2315
▲ Xenical Capsules (Among most frequent) 3043
▲ Zenapax for Injection (Greater than 5%) 3046
Zestoretic Tablets (0.3% to 1.0%) 695
Zinacef Injection (1 in 150 patients) 1696
Zinacef for Injection (1 in 150 patients) 1696
Zosyn 1890
Zosyn in Galaxy Containers 1894

Gastrointestinal neoplasm, benign
Arthrotec Tablets (Rare) 3195

Gastrointestinal obstruction
Claritin-D 24 Hour Extended Release Tablets (Rare) 3104
K-Dur Microburst Release System ER Tablets 1832
Klor-Con M20/Klor-Con M10 Tablets 3329
K-Tab Filmtab Tablets 470
Micro-K 3311

Gastrointestinal perforation
Aggrenox Capsules (Less than 1%) 1026
Anaprox Tablets (Approximately 1% to 4%) 2967
Anaprox DS Tablets (Approximately 1% to 4%) 2967
Cataflam Tablets (Approximately 1% to about 4%) 2315
Clinoril Tablets (Rare) 2053
Cortone Acetate Injectable Suspension 2059
Cortone Acetate Tablets 2061
Cytovene (At least 3 subjects) 2959
Dolobid Tablets (Less than 1 in 100) 2088
EC-Naprosyn Delayed-Release Tablets (Approximately 1% to 4%) 2967
Ecotrin Enteric Coated Aspirin Low, Regular and Maximum Strength Tablets 1715
▲ Feldene Capsules (1% to 10%) 2685
Indocin (Approximately 1%) 2112
K-Dur Microburst Release System ER Tablets 1832
Klor-Con M20/Klor-Con M10 Tablets 3329
K-Tab Filmtab Tablets 470
Lodine 3528
Lodine XL Extended-Release Tablets 3530
Micro-K 3311
Motrin Suspension, Oral Drops, Chewable Tablets, and Caplets (Less than 1% to 4%) 2002
Naprelan Tablets (Approximately 1% to 4%) 1293
Naprosyn Suspension (Approximately 1% to 4%) 2967
Naprosyn Tablets (Approximately 1% to 4%) 2967
Orudis Capsules (Less than 1%) 3548
Oruvail Capsules (Less than 1%) 3548
▲ Ponstel Capsules (1% to 10%) 1356
▲ Prograf (3%) 1393
Relafen Tablets 1617
Tolectin (Less than 1%) 2589
Toradol 3018
Voltaren Tablets (Approximately 1% to about 4%) 2315
Voltaren-XR Tablets (Approximately 1% to about 4%) 2315

Gastrointestinal reactions
(*see under* Gastrointestinal disorders)

Gastrointestinal reflux
Arthrotec Tablets (Rare) 3195
Cytotec Tablets (Infrequent) 3202

Gastrointestinal symptoms
(*see under* Gastrointestinal disorders)

Gastrointestinal toxicity
Alkeran for Injection 1465
Alkeran Tablets 1466
Anaprox Tablets 2967
Anaprox DS Tablets 2967
EC-Naprosyn Delayed-Release Tablets 2967
Naprelan Tablets 1293
Naprosyn Suspension 2967
Naprosyn Tablets 2967
Toradol 3018

Gastrointestinal upset
(*see under* Gastrointestinal disorders)

Genital abnormalities
Clomid Tablets 735
Felbatol 3343
Hivid Tablets (Less than 1%) 2975
Megace Oral Suspension (Several reports) 1124

Genital eruptions
Estring Vaginal Ring (1% to 3%) 2811

Genital malformation
Thalomid Capsules 1154

Genital moniliasis
Duricef 1079

Genitalia, male, external, abnormalities of
Propecia Tablets 2172
Proscar Tablets 2175

Genitourinary disturbances
Betapace Tablets (1% to 3%) 950
Eulexin Capsules (2%) 3118
▲ Leukine (50%) 1755
▲ Nipent for Injection (Up to 15%) 3272
▲ Paraplatin for Injection (2% to 11%) 1126
▲ Paxil (3%) 1609
Tranxene 511

Germinal aplasia
Mustargen for Injection 2142

GGTP, elevation
(*see under* Gamma-glutamyl transpeptidase, elevation)

Giardiasis
Colazal Capsules 3069

Giddiness
(*see under* Dizziness)

Gingival disorder, unspecified
Xenical Capsules (2%) 3043

Gingival hyperplasia
Adalat CC Tablets (Rare) 877
Cardizem Injectable 1018
Cardizem Lyo-Ject Syringe 1018
Cardizem Monovial 1018
Cardizem CD Capsules (Infrequent) 1016
▲ CellCept Capsules (3%) 2951
▲ CellCept Intravenous (3%) 2951
▲ CellCept Oral Suspension (3%) 2951
▲ CellCept Tablets (3%) 2951
Covera-HS Tablets (Less than 2%) 3199
Dilantin Infatabs 2624
Dilantin Kapseals 2622
Dilantin-125 Oral Suspension 2625
Evoxac Capsules 1217
Gabitril Tablets (Infrequent) 1189
▲ Gengraf Capsules (4% to 16%) 457
Intron A for Injection (Less than 5%) 3120
Isoptin SR Tablets (1% or less) 467
Lamictal (Infrequent) 1567
Lexxel Tablets 608
▲ Neoral Soft Gelatin Capsules (3.8% to 16%) 2380
▲ Neoral Oral Solution (3.8% to 16%) 2380
Norvasc Tablets (More than 0.1% to 1%) 2704
Orap Tablets (One patient) 1407
Plendil Extended-Release Tablets (Less than 0.5%) 623
Procardia Capsules (Less than 0.5%) 2708
Procardia XL Extended Release Tablets (1% or less) 2710
▲ Rapamune Oral Solution and Tablets (3% to 20%) 3584
▲ Sandimmune (4% to 16%) 2388
▲ Simulect for Injection (3% to 10%) 2399
Soriatane Capsules (Less than 1%) 3003
Sular Tablets (Less than or equal to 1%) 688
Tarka Tablets 508
Tiazac Capsules (Infrequent) 1378
Topamax Sprinkle Capsules (Infrequent) 2590
Topamax Tablets (Infrequent) 2590
Trileptal Oral Suspension 2407
Trileptal Tablets 2407
Verelan Capsules (1% or less) 3184
Verelan PM Capsules (2% or less) 3186
Zoloft (Rare) 2751
Zonegran Capsules (Infrequent) 1307

Gingival swelling
Motofen Tablets 577

Gingival ulcer
Motrin Suspension, Oral Drops, Chewable Tablets, and Caplets (Less than 1%) 2002

Gingivitis
Accutane Capsules 2944
Aciphex Tablets 1267
Aciphex Tablets 1783
Actiq (1% or greater) 1184
Amphotec (1% to 5%) 1774
Arava Tablets (1% to 3%) 724
Aricept Tablets (Infrequent) 1270
Aricept Tablets (Infrequent) 2665
Avonex 1013
Betaseron for SC Injection 988
Campath Ampules 992
Celexa (Infrequent) 1365
▲ CellCept Capsules (3%) 2951
▲ CellCept Intravenous (3%) 2951
▲ CellCept Oral Suspension (3%) 2951
▲ CellCept Tablets (3%) 2951
Cognex Capsules (Infrequent) 1351
Copaxone for Injection (At least 2%) 3306
Crixivan Capsules (Less than 2%) 2070
Cytotec Tablets (Infrequent) 3202
Doxil Injection (Less than 1%) 566
Effexor Tablets (Infrequent) 3495
Effexor XR Capsules (Infrequent) 3499
Evoxac Capsules (Less than 1%) 1217
Exelon Capsules (Infrequent) 2342
Exelon Oral Solution (Infrequent) 2345
Fortovase Capsules (Less than 2%) 2970
Gabitril Tablets (Frequent) 1189
Gengraf Capsules 457
Hivid Tablets (Less than 1%) 2975
▲ Intron A for Injection (Up to 14%) 3120
Invirase Capsules (Less than 2%) 2979
Iscar Mali Injection 3456
Iscar Mali Special Injection 3456
Iscar Pini Injection 3456
Iscar Quercus Injection 3456
Iscar Quercus Special Injection 3456
Keppra Tablets (1% or more) 3314
Klonopin Tablets 2983
Lamictal (Infrequent) 1567
Lupron Depot-4 Month 30 mg (Less than 5%) 3289
Lupron Depot-PED 7.5 mg, 11.25 mg and 15 mg (Less than 2%) 3291
Lupron Injection Pediatric (Less than 2%) 3280
Luvox Tablets (25, 50, 100 mg) (Infrequent) 3256
Neoral Soft Gelatin Capsules 2380
Neoral Oral Solution 2380
Neurontin Capsules (Frequent) 2655
Neurontin Oral Solution (Frequent) 2655
Neurontin Tablets (Frequent) 2655
▲ Nipent for Injection (3% to 10%) 3272
Norvir Capsules (Less than 2%) 487
Norvir Oral Solution (Less than 2%) 487
Paxil (Rare) 1609
Permax Tablets (Infrequent) 1299
Protonix I.V. (Less than 1%) 3580
Protonix Tablets (Less than 1%) 3577
Provigil Tablets (1%) 1193
▲ Rapamune Oral Solution and Tablets (3% to 20%) 3584
Relafen Tablets (Less than 1%) 1617
Requip Tablets (1% or more) 1621
Rescriptor Tablets (Less than 2%) 526
Risperdal (Rare) 1796
Roxicodone Tablets (Less than 3%) 3067
Salagen Tablets (Less than 1%) 2229
Sandostatin LAR Depot (1% to 4%) 2395
Seroquel Tablets (Infrequent) 684
▲ Serostim for Injection (1% to 10%) 3229
Serzone Tablets (Infrequent) 1104
Sonata Capsules (Infrequent) 3591
▲ Soriatane Capsules (1% to 10%) 3003
Tequin Injection (Less than 0.1%) 1110
Tequin Tablets (Less than 0.1%) 1110
Teveten Tablets (Less than 1%) 3327
Topamax Sprinkle Capsules (0.8% to 1.8%) 2590
Topamax Tablets (0.8% to 1.8%) 2590
Trovan (Less than 1%) 2722
Uniretic Tablets (Less than 1%) 3178
Viagra Tablets (Less than 2%) 2732
Vistide Injection 1445
Wellbutrin SR Sustained-Release Tablets (Infrequent) 1684
Zonegran Capsules (Infrequent) 1307
Zyban Sustained-Release Tablets (Infrequent) 1710
Zyprexa Tablets (Infrequent) 1973
Zyprexa ZYDIS Orally Disintegrating Tablets (Infrequent) 1973

Gingivostomatitis
Cuprimine Capsules (Rare) 2075
Depen Titratable Tablets (Rare) 3341

Glassy-eyed appearance
Klonopin Tablets 2983

Glaucoma
(*see also under* IOP, elevation of)
Aciphex Tablets 1267
Aciphex Tablets 1783
Ambien Tablets (Rare) 3191
Anectine Injection 1476
Aricept Tablets (Infrequent) 1270
Aricept Tablets (Infrequent) 2665
Artane 1855
Arthrotec Tablets (Rare) 3195
Beconase Inhalation Aerosol (Rare) 1497
Beconase AQ Nasal Spray (Rare) 1498
Blephamide Ophthalmic Ointment (A possibility) 547
Blephamide Ophthalmic Suspension 548
Celebrex Capsules (0.1% to 1.9%) 2676
Celebrex Capsules (0.1% to 1.9%) 2780
Celestone Soluspan Injectable Suspension 3097
Celestone Syrup 3099
Cortifoam Rectal Foam 3170
Cortisporin Ophthalmic Suspension ⊙297
Cortone Acetate Injectable Suspension 2059
Cortone Acetate Tablets 2061
Decadron Elixir 2078
Decadron Tablets 2079
Decadron Phosphate Injection 2081
Decadron Phosphate Sterile Ophthalmic Ointment 2083
Decadron Phosphate Sterile Ophthalmic Solution 2084
Depo-Medrol Injectable Suspension 2795
Effexor XR Capsules (Rare) 3499
Etrafon (Occasional) 3115
Evoxac Capsules (Less than 1%) 1217
Exelon Capsules (Infrequent) 2342
Exelon Oral Solution (Infrequent) 2345
Fareston Tablets (Less than 1%) 3237
Flonase Nasal Spray 1533

Florinef Acetate Tablets 2250
FML Forte Ophthalmic Suspension ⊙235
Healon ⊙316
HMS Sterile Ophthalmic Suspension (Rare) ⊙240
Humorsol Sterile Ophthalmic Solution 2102
Hydrocortone Tablets 2106
Hydrocortone Acetate Injectable Suspension 2103
Hydrocortone Phosphate Injection, Sterile 2105
Lexxel Tablets 608
Lipitor Tablets (Less than 2%) 2639
Lipitor Tablets (Less than 2%) 2696
Midamor Tablets (Less than or equal to 1%) 2136
Mirapex Tablets (Less than 1%) 2834
Moduretic Tablets 2138
Nardil Tablets (Less common) 2653
NeoDecadron Sterile Ophthalmic Solution 2144
Neurontin Capsules (Rare) 2655
Neurontin Oral Solution (Rare) 2655
Neurontin Tablets (Rare) 2655
Norpramin Tablets 755
Pediapred Oral Solution 1170
Poly-Pred Liquifilm Ophthalmic Suspension ⊙245
Pred-G Ophthalmic Suspension ⊙247
Pred-G Sterile Ophthalmic Ointment ⊙248
Prednisone 3064
Prelone Syrup 2273
Protonix I.V. (Less than 1%) 3580
Protonix Tablets (Less than 1%) 3577
Prozac Pulvules, Liquid, and Weekly Capsules (Rare) 1238
Pulmicort Turbuhaler Inhalation Powder (Rare) 636
Remeron Tablets (Infrequent) 2483
Remeron SolTab Tablets (Infrequent) 2486
Requip Tablets (Infrequent) 1621
Rhinocort Nasal Inhaler (Rare) 640
Rilutek Tablets (Rare) 772
Salagen Tablets (Less than 1%) 2229
Sandostatin LAR Depot (Rare) 2395
Sarafem Pulvules (Rare) 1962
Seroquel Tablets (Rare) 684
Skelid Tablets (2.7%) 3088
Solu-Medrol Sterile Powder 2855
Sonata Capsules (Rare) 3591
Sular Tablets (Less than or equal to 1%) 688
Tasmar Tablets (Rare) 3010
Terra-Cortril Ophthalmic Suspension 2716
TobraDex Ophthalmic Ointment 542
TobraDex Ophthalmic Suspension 541
Trilafon (Occasional) 3160
Uniretic Tablets (Less than 1%) 3178
Vanceril Double Strength Inhalation Aerosol (Rare) 3167
Vexol 1% Ophthalmic Suspension (1% to 5%) ⊙222
Vitrasert Implant (Approximately 1% to 5%) ⊙254
Vivactil Tablets 2217
Vivactil Tablets 2446
Zanaflex Tablets (Infrequent) 1305
Zoloft (Rare) 2751
Zonegran Capsules (Infrequent) 1307
Zyprexa Tablets (Rare) 1973
Zyprexa ZYDIS Orally Disintegrating Tablets (Rare) 1973
Zyrtec (Less than 2%) 2756

Glaucoma, angle closure precipitation
Atrovent Nasal Spray 0.03% 1032
Atrovent Nasal Spray 0.06% 1033
Botox Purified Neurotoxin Complex (One report) 549
Combivent Inhalation Aerosol 1041
DuoNeb Inhalation Solution 1233
Transderm Scōp Transdermal Therapeutic System (Infrequent) 2302
Vitrasert Implant (Less than 1%) ⊙254

Glaucoma, corticosteroid-induced
Blephamide Ophthalmic Suspension 548
FML Ophthalmic Ointment ⊙237
FML Ophthalmic Suspension ⊙236
FML Forte Ophthalmic Suspension ⊙235
FML-S Liquifilm Sterile Ophthalmic Suspension ⊙238
HMS Sterile Ophthalmic Suspension ⊙240
Poly-Pred Liquifilm Ophthalmic Suspension ⊙245
Pred Forte Ophthalmic Suspension ⊙246
Pred Mild Sterile Ophthalmic Suspension ⊙249
Pred-G Ophthalmic Suspension ⊙247
TobraDex Ophthalmic Ointment 542
TobraDex Ophthalmic Suspension 541

Glaucoma, worsening of narrow angle
Atrovent Inhalation Aerosol 1030
Atrovent Inhalation Solution 1031
Atrovent Nasal Spray 0.03% 1032
Atrovent Nasal Spray 0.06% 1033
Combivent Inhalation Aerosol 1041
DuoNeb Inhalation Solution 1233

Glioblastoma multiforme
Serophene Tablets 3226

Gliosis
Vitrasert Implant (Less than 1%) ⊙254

Globus hystericus
Daranide Tablets 2077
Imitrex Injection (Rare) 1549

Glomerular filtration rate, decrease
Captopril Tablets 2281
Monopril Tablets 1091

Glomerulitis
Motrin Suspension, Oral Drops, Chewable Tablets, and Caplets (Less than 1%) 2002

Glomerulonephritis
Accutane Capsules 2944
Anaprox Tablets (Less than 1%) 2967
Anaprox DS Tablets (Less than 1%) 2967
Cuprimine Capsules 2075
Depen Titratable Tablets (Rare) 3341
EC-Naprosyn Delayed-Release Tablets (Less than 1%) 2967
▲ Naprelan Tablets (3% to 9%) 1293
Naprosyn Suspension (Less than 1%) 2967
Naprosyn Tablets (Less than 1%) 2967
Orthoclone OKT3 Sterile Solution 2498
Zyrtec (Rare) 2756
Zyrtec-D 12 Hour Extended Relief Tablets (Rare) 2758

Glomerulonephritis, allergic
Corzide 40/5 Tablets 2247
Corzide 80/5 Tablets 2247

Glomerulonephropathy, membranous
Enbrel for Injection (Infrequent) 1752
Enbrel for Injection (Infrequent) 3504

Glossitis
Aciphex Tablets 1267
Aciphex Tablets 1783
Actiq (1% or greater) 1184
Aerobid/Aerobid-M (1% to 3%) 1363
Amphotec (1% to 5%) 1774
Arthrotec Tablets (Rare) 3195
Astelin Nasal Spray (Infrequent) 3339
Augmentin Chewable Tablets 1482
Augmentin Powder for Oral Suspension 1482
Augmentin Tablets 1485
Augmentin ES-600 Powder for Oral Suspension 1487
Avelox Tablets (0.05% to 1%) 879
Bactrim 2949
Betaseron for SC Injection 988
Betoptic S Ophthalmic Suspension (Rare) 537
Biaxin/Biaxin XL 403
Captopril Tablets 2281
Carbatrol Capsules 3234
Celexa (Rare) 1365
Clinoril Tablets (Less than 1%) 2053
Cognex Capsules (Infrequent) 1351
Colazal Capsules 3069
Cuprimine Capsules 2075
Daraprim Tablets 1511
Declomycin Tablets 1855
Depacon Injection (1% or more) 416
Depakene (1% or more) 421
Depakote Sprinkle Capsules 426
Depakote Tablets (1% to 5%) 430
Depakote ER Tablets (Greater than 1%) 436
Depen Titratable Tablets (Rare) 3341
Didronel Tablets 2888
Doryx Coated Pellet Filled Capsules 3357
Doxil Injection (1% to 5%) 566
Dynacin Capsules 2019
Effexor Tablets (Infrequent) 3495
Effexor XR Capsules (Infrequent) 3499
Enalaprilat Injection 863
Evoxac Capsules (Less than 1%) 1217
Exelon Capsules (Infrequent) 2342
Exelon Oral Solution (Infrequent) 2345
Felbatol 3343
Feldene Capsules (Occasional) 2685
Fortovase Capsules (Less than 2%) 2970
Sterile FUDR 2974
Gabitril Tablets (Infrequent) 1189
Gastrocrom Oral Concentrate 1162
Gengraf Capsules (1% to less than 3%) 457
Geocillin Tablets 2687
Halcion Tablets 2823
Hivid Tablets (Less than 1%) 2975
Imdur Tablets (Less than or equal to 5%) 1826
Inversine Tablets 1850
Invirase Capsules (Less than 2%) 2979
Lamictal (Infrequent) 1567
Lexxel Tablets 608
Lipitor Tablets (Less than 2%) 2639
Lipitor Tablets (Less than 2%) 2696
Lupron Depot 3.75 mg 3281
Lupron Depot–3 Month 11.25 mg 3285
Luvox Tablets (25, 50, 100 mg) (Infrequent) 3256
Maxair Autohaler 1981
Maxair Inhaler (Less than 1%) 1984
Merrem I.V. (1.0%) 673
Minocin Intravenous 1862
Minocin Oral Suspension 1865
Minocin Pellet-Filled Capsules 1863
Monodox Capsules 2442
Myobloc Injectable Solution (2% or greater) 1291
Nascobal Gel (One patient) 3174
Neoral Soft Gelatin Capsules (1% to less than 3%) 2380
Neoral Oral Solution (1% to less than 3%) 2380
Neurontin Capsules (Infrequent) 2655
Neurontin Oral Solution (Infrequent) 2655
Neurontin Tablets (Infrequent) 2655
Nipent for Injection (Less than 3%) 3272
Paxil (Infrequent) 1609
Pediazole Suspension 3050
Periostat Tablets 1208
Permax Tablets (Rare) 1299
Ponstel Capsules (Occasional) 1356
PREVPAC (Less than 3%) 3298
Primaxin I.M. 2158
Primaxin I.V. (Less than 0.2%) 2160
Protonix I.V. (Less than 1%) 3580
Protonix Tablets (Less than 1%) 3577
Prozac Pulvules, Liquid, and Weekly Capsules (Infrequent) 1238
Relafen Tablets (Less than 1%) 1617
Remeron Tablets (Infrequent) 2483
Remeron SolTab Tablets (Infrequent) 2486
Requip Tablets (Infrequent) 1621
Rilutek Tablets (Infrequent) 772
Roxicodone Tablets (Less than 3%) 3067
Salagen Tablets (1% to 2%) 2229
Sandostatin LAR Depot (1% to 4%) 2395
Sarafem Pulvules (Infrequent) 1962
Septra Suspension 2265
Septra Tablets 2265
Septra DS Tablets 2265
Seroquel Tablets (Infrequent) 684
Serzone Tablets (Rare) 1104
Sonata Capsules (Infrequent) 3591
Soriatane Capsules (Less than 1%) 3003
Sular Tablets (Less than or equal to 1%) 688
Tegretol/Tegretol-XR 2404
Tequin Injection (0.1% to 3%) 1110
Tequin Tablets (0.1% to 3%) 1110
Tolectin (Less than 1%) 2589
Unasyn for Injection (Less than 1%) 2728
Uniretic Tablets (Less than 1%) 3178
Urobiotic-250 Capsules (Rare) 2731
Vaseretic Tablets 2204
Vasotec I.V. Injection 2207
Vasotec Tablets (0.5% to 1.0%) 2210
Viagra Tablets (Less than 2%) 2732
Vibramycin Calcium Oral Suspension Syrup 2735
Vibramycin Hyclate Capsules 2735
Vibramycin Hyclate Intravenous 2737
Vibramycin Monohydrate for Oral Suspension 2735
Vibra-Tabs Film Coated Tablets 2735
Vicoprofen Tablets (Less than 1%) 520
Wellbutrin Tablets (Rare) 1680
Zoloft (Rare) 2751
Zonegran Capsules (Infrequent) 1307
Zyban Sustained-Release Tablets (Infrequent) 1710
Zyprexa Tablets (Infrequent) 1973
Zyprexa ZYDIS Orally Disintegrating Tablets (Infrequent) 1973

Glossodynia
Adenoscan (Less than 1%) 1381
Aldoclor Tablets 2035
Aldomet Tablets 2037
Aldoril Tablets 2039
Clozaril Tablets (1%) 2319
Crixivan Capsules (Less than 2%) 2070
Etrafon 3115
Hivid Tablets (Less than 1%) 2975
▲ Imitrex Injection (4.9%) 1549
Imitrex Tablets 1558
Rifadin (Occasional) 765
Rifamate Capsules (Occasional) 767
Rifater Tablets (Occasional) 769
Trilafon Tablets 3160

Glossoncus
Altace Capsules 2233
Cataflam Tablets (Less than 1%) 2315
Ceftin Tablets (0.1% to 1%) 1898
Levaquin 2537
Maxalt Tablets 2120
Maxalt-MLT Orally Disintegrating Tablets 2120
Miacalcin Injection (A few cases) 2373
Miacalcin Nasal Spray (Few reports) 2375
Romazicon Injection (Less than 1%) 3000
Tambocor Tablets (Less than 1%) 1990
Trovan (Less than 1%) 2722
Voltaren Tablets (Less than 1%) 2315
Voltaren-XR Tablets (Less than 1%) 2315
Zarontin Capsules 2659
Zarontin Syrup 2660

Glossoplegia
Risperdal (Rare) 1796

Glossotrichia
Augmentin Chewable Tablets 1482
Augmentin Powder for Oral Suspension 1482
Augmentin Tablets 1485
Augmentin ES-600 Powder for Oral Suspension 1487
Etrafon 3115
Klonopin Tablets (Infrequent) 2983
Limbitrol 1738
Norpramin Tablets 755
PREVPAC 3298
Surmontil Capsules 3595
Unasyn for Injection 2728
Vivactil Tablets 2217
Vivactil Tablets 2446

Glucocorticoids, increased
Evoxac Capsules (Less than 1%) 1217

Glucose tolerance, changes
Brevicon 28-Day Tablets 3380
Celexa (Infrequent) 1365
Cortifoam Rectal Foam 3170
Estrace Vaginal Cream 3358
Estrace Tablets 3361
Estratest 3252
Furosemide Tablets 2284
Levlen 962
Levlite 21 Tablets 962
Levlite 28 Tablets 962
Modicon 2563
Norinyl 1 + 50 28-Day Tablets 3380
Ortho Dienestrol Cream 2554
Ortho-Novum 2563
Ortho-Novum 1/50▫28 Tablets 2556
Ovcon 3364
Phenergan Injection 3553
Premarin Intravenous 3563
Tri-Levlen 962
Tri-Norinyl-28 Tablets 3433

Glucose tolerance, decreased
Activella Tablets 2764
Anadrol-50 Tablets 3321
Depo-Provera Contraceptive Injection (Some patients) 2798
Emcyt Capsules 2810
Kaletra Capsules (Less than 2%) 471
Kaletra Oral Solution (Less than 2%) 471
Lo/Ovral Tablets 3532
Lo/Ovral-28 Tablets 3538
Low-Ogestrel-28 Tablets 3392
Megace Oral Suspension (1% to 3%) 1124
Menest Tablets 2254
Naprelan Tablets (Less than 1%) 1293
Niaspan Extended-Release Tablets 1846
Nordette-28 Tablets 2257
Norditropin Cartridges 2420
Norditropin for Injection 2419
Nutropin AQ Injection 1420
Nutropin for Injection 1417
Ogen Tablets 2846
Ogestrel 0.5/50-28 Tablets 3428
Ortho-Cyclen/Ortho Tri-Cyclen 2573
Ovral Tablets 3551
Ovral-28 Tablets 3552
Ovrette Tablets 3552
Oxandrin Tablets 1153
Premarin Intravenous 3563
Premarin Vaginal Cream 3570
Premphase Tablets 3572
Prempro Tablets 3572
Provera Tablets 2853
Triphasil-21 Tablets 3600
Triphasil-28 Tablets 3605
Uniretic Tablets (Less than 1%) 3178
Vivelle Transdermal System 2412
Vivelle-Dot Transdermal System 2416

Glucosuria
Aclovate ... 1275
▲ Cipro I.V. Pharmacy Bulk Package (Among most frequent) ... 897
Clorpres Tablets (Rare) ... 1002
Combipres Tablets (Rare) ... 1040
Cormax Cream ... 2440
Cormax Ointment ... 2440
Cormax Scalp Application ... 2441
Dermatop Emollient Cream ... 2517
Diprolene Ointment 0.05% (Some patients) ... 3108
Diprolene AF Cream 0.05% (Some patients) ... 3106
Elspar for Injection (Low) ... 2092
Floxin I.V. (More than or equal to 1%) ... 2526
Floxin Tablets (More than or equal to 1%) ... 2529
Hivid Tablets (Less than 1%) ... 2975
Humatrope Vials and Cartridges (Infrequent) ... 1930
Lodosyn Tablets ... 1251
Naprelan Tablets (Less than 1%) ... 1293
Norditropin Cartridges ... 2420
Norditropin for Injection ... 2419
Olux Foam ... 1211
Rythmol Tablets – 150 mg, 225 mg, 300 mg (Less than 1%) ... 502
Sinemet Tablets ... 1253
Sinemet CR Tablets ... 1255
Temovate Cream ... 1301
Temovate Gel ... 1303
Temovate Ointment ... 1301
Temovate Scalp Application ... 1304

Glycosuria
Accuretic Tablets ... 2614
Aldoclor Tablets ... 2035
Aldoril Tablets ... 2039
Aloprim for Injection (Less than 1%) ... 2292
Amerge Tablets (Rare) ... 1467
Amphotec (1% to 5%) ... 1774
Arthrotec Tablets (Rare) ... 3195
Avalide Tablets ... 1070
Betaseron for SC Injection ... 988
Calcium Disodium Versenate Injection ... 1980
Carbatrol Capsules ... 3234
Clorpres Tablets ... 1002
Cognex Capsules (Infrequent) ... 1351
Combipres Tablets ... 1040
Compazine ... 1505
Coreg Tablets (1% to 2%) ... 1508
Corzide 40/5 Tablets ... 2247
Corzide 80/5 Tablets ... 2247
Cytotec Tablets (Infrequent) ... 3202
Diamox Intravenous (Occasional) ... ⊙269
Diamox Sequels Sustained Release Capsules ... ⊙270
Diamox Tablets (Occasional) ... ⊙269
Diovan HCT Tablets ... 2338
Diucardin Tablets ... 3494
Diuril Oral ... 2087
Diuril Sodium Intravenous ... 2086
Doxil Injection (Less than 1%) ... 566
Dyazide Capsules ... 1515
Effexor Tablets (Infrequent) ... 3495
Effexor XR Capsules (Infrequent) ... 3499
Eskalith ... 1527
Etrafon ... 3115
Evoxac Capsules ... 1217
Florinef Acetate Tablets ... 2250
Furosemide Tablets ... 2284
Geodon Capsules (Infrequent) ... 2688
Hivid Tablets (Less than 1%) ... 2975
HydroDIURIL Tablets ... 2108
Hyzaar ... 2109
Indapamide Tablets (Less than 5%) ... 2286
Inderide Tablets ... 3517
Inderide LA Long-Acting Capsules ... 3519
Indocin Capsules (Less than 1%) ... 2112
Indocin I.V. (Less than 1%) ... 2115
Indocin (Less than 1%) ... 2112
Lithium Carbonate ... 3061
Lithium Citrate Syrup ... 3061
Lithobid Slow-Release Tablets ... 3255
Lotensin HCT Tablets ... 2367
Maxzide ... 1008
Micardis HCT Tablets ... 1051
Microzide Capsules ... 3414
Minizide Capsules ... 2700
Moduretic Tablets ... 2138
Monopril HCT ... 1094
Mykrox Tablets ... 1168
Navane Oral ... 2701
Navane Intramuscular ... 2703
Neptazane Tablets ... ⊙271
Neurontin Capsules (Rare) ... 2655
Neurontin Oral Solution (Rare) ... 2655
Neurontin Tablets (Rare) ... 2655
Nexium Delayed-Release Capsules (Less than 1%) ... 619
Noroxin Tablets (Less frequent) ... 2145
Norvir Capsules (Less than 2%) ... 487
Norvir Oral Solution (Less than 2%) ... 487
Prevacid Delayed-Release Capsules (Less than 1%) ... 3292
PREVPAC (Less than 1%) ... 3298
Prilosec Delayed-Release Capsules (Less than 1%) ... 628
Protonix I.V. (Less than 1%) ... 3580
Protonix Tablets (Less than 1%) ... 3577
Prozac Pulvules, Liquid, and Weekly Capsules (Rare) ... 1238
▲ Rapamune Oral Solution and Tablets (3% to 20%) ... 3584
Renese Tablets ... 2712
Requip Tablets (Infrequent) ... 1621
Rocephin Injectable Vials, ADD-Vantage, Galaxy, Bulk (Rare) ... 2993
Sarafem Pulvules (Rare) ... 1962
Seroquel Tablets (Infrequent) ... 684
▲ Serostim for Injection (1% to 10%) ... 3229
Stelazine ... 1640
Tegretol/Tegretol-XR ... 2404
Tenoretic Tablets ... 690
Teveten Tablets (Less than 1%) ... 3327
Thiothixene Capsules ... 2290
Thorazine ... 1656
Timolide Tablets ... 2187
Trilafon ... 3160
Uniretic Tablets (Less than 1%) ... 3178
Vicoprofen Tablets (Less than 1%) ... 520
Vistide Injection ... 1445
Wellbutrin Tablets (Rare) ... 1680
Wellbutrin SR Sustained-Release Tablets ... 1684
Zanaflex Tablets (Rare) ... 1305
Zaroxolyn Tablets ... 1177
Zyban Sustained-Release Tablets ... 1710

Goiter
Aricept Tablets (Infrequent) ... 1270
Aricept Tablets (Infrequent) ... 2665
Azulfidine EN-tabs Tablets (Rare) ... 2775
Betaseron for SC Injection (2%) ... 988
Celexa (Rare) ... 1365
Copaxone for Injection (Infrequent) ... 3306
Effexor Tablets (Rare) ... 3495
Effexor XR Capsules (Rare) ... 3499
Evoxac Capsules (Less than 1%) ... 1217
Exelon Capsules (Infrequent) ... 2342
Exelon Oral Solution (Infrequent) ... 2345
Gabitril Tablets (Infrequent) ... 1189
Gengraf Capsules (1% to less than 3%) ... 457
Lamictal (Rare) ... 1567
Luvox Tablets (25, 50, 100 mg) (Rare) ... 3256
Meridia Capsules ... 481
Miacalcin Nasal Spray (Less than 1%) ... 2375
Neoral Soft Gelatin Capsules (1% to less than 3%) ... 2380
Neoral Oral Solution (1% to less than 3%) ... 2380
Neurontin Capsules (Rare) ... 2655
Neurontin Oral Solution (Rare) ... 2655
Neurontin Tablets (Rare) ... 2655
Nexium Delayed-Release Capsules (Less than 1%) ... 619
Paxil (Rare) ... 1609
Pediazole Suspension (Rare) ... 3050
Pima Syrup (Rare) ... 1362
Prevacid Delayed-Release Capsules (Less than 1%) ... 3292
PREVPAC (Less than 1%) ... 3298
Protonix I.V. (Less than 1%) ... 3580
Protonix Tablets (Less than 1%) ... 3577
Remeron Tablets (Rare) ... 2483
Remeron SolTab Tablets (Rare) ... 2486
▲ Sandostatin Injection (6%) ... 2394
▲ Sandostatin LAR Depot (8%) ... 2395
Sonata Capsules (Rare) ... 3591
Topamax Sprinkle Capsules (Infrequent) ... 2590
Topamax Tablets (Infrequent) ... 2590
Uniretic Tablets (Less than 1%) ... 3178
Zyprexa Tablets (Infrequent) ... 1973
Zyprexa ZYDIS Orally Disintegrating Tablets (Infrequent) ... 1973

Goiter, diffuse
Lithium Carbonate ... 3061
Lithium Citrate Syrup ... 3061

Goiter, euthyroid
Eskalith ... 1527
Lithium Carbonate ... 3061
Lithium Citrate Syrup ... 3061
Lithobid Slow-Release Tablets ... 3255

Goiter production
(*see under* Goiter)

Gonadotropin secretion, inhibition
▲ Android Capsules, 10 mg (Among most common) ... 1731
▲ Delatestryl Injection (Among most frequent) ... 1151
▲ Estratest (Among most common) ... 3252
Oxandrin Tablets ... 1153
Testred Capsules, 10 mg ... 1746

Goodpasture's syndrome
Cuprimine Capsules ... 2075
Depen Titratable Tablets (Rare) ... 3341

Goosebumps
(*see under* Piloerection)

Gout
Aceon Tablets (2 mg, 4 mg, 8 mg) (0.3% to 1%) ... 3249
Aciphex Tablets ... 1267
Aciphex Tablets ... 1783
Adalat CC Tablets (Less than 1.0%) ... 877
Ambien Tablets (Rare) ... 3191
Aricept Tablets (Infrequent) ... 1270
Aricept Tablets (Infrequent) ... 2665
Arthrotec Tablets (Rare) ... 3195
Asacol Delayed-Release Tablets ... 2884
Avalide Tablets ... 1070
Avapro Tablets (Less than 1%) ... 1074
Avapro Tablets (Less than 1%) ... 3076
Betaxon Ophthalmic Suspension (Less than 2%) ... 537
Cardura Tablets (Less than 0.5%) ... 2668
▲ Casodex Tablets (2% to 5%) ... 662
▲ CellCept Capsules (3% to 10%) ... 2951
▲ CellCept Intravenous (3% to 10%) ... 2951
▲ CellCept Oral Suspension (3% to 10%) ... 2951
▲ CellCept Tablets (3% to 10%) ... 2951
Cipro I.V. (1% or less) ... 893
Cipro I.V. Pharmacy Bulk Package (Less than 1%) ... 897
Cipro (Less than 1%) ... 887
Clorpres Tablets ... 1002
Cognex Capsules (Infrequent) ... 1351
Combipres Tablets ... 1040
Copaxone for Injection (Infrequent) ... 3306
▲ Coreg Tablets (6.3%) ... 1508
Cozaar Tablets (Less than 1%) ... 2067
Cytotec Tablets (Infrequent) ... 3202
Demadex Tablets and Injection ... 2965
Diovan HCT Tablets (Greater than 0.2%) ... 2338
Edecrin ... 2091
Effexor Tablets (Rare) ... 3495
Effexor XR Capsules (Rare) ... 3499
Evoxac Capsules ... 1217
Exelon Capsules (Infrequent) ... 2342
Exelon Oral Solution (Infrequent) ... 2345
Furosemide Tablets ... 2284
Geodon Capsules (Rare) ... 2688
Hivid Tablets (Less than 1%) ... 2975
Hytrin Capsules (At least 1%) ... 464
Hyzaar ... 2109
Klonopin Tablets (Infrequent) ... 2983
Lexxel Tablets ... 608
Lipitor Tablets (Less than 2%) ... 2639
Lipitor Tablets (Less than 2%) ... 2696
Lotensin HCT Tablets (0.3% to 1%) ... 2367
Lotrel Capsules (Infrequent) ... 2370
Mavik Tablets (0.3% to 1.0%) ... 478
Maxzide ... 1008
Micardis Tablets (More than 0.3%) ... 1049
Micardis HCT Tablets ... 1051
Microzide Capsules ... 3414
Mirapex Tablets (Less than 1%) ... 2834
Moduretic Tablets (Less than or equal to 1%) ... 2138
Monopril Tablets (0.2% to 1.0%) ... 1091
Monopril HCT ... 1094
Myambutol Tablets ... 1290
Mykrox Tablets ... 1168
Niaspan Extended-Release Tablets ... 1846
Nipent for Injection (Less than 3%) ... 3272
Norvir Capsules (Less than 2%) ... 487
Norvir Oral Solution (Less than 2%) ... 487
Paxil (Rare) ... 1609
Permax Tablets (Infrequent) ... 1299
Plavix Tablets (1% to 2.5%) ... 1097
Plavix Tablets (1% to 2.5%) ... 3084
Pletal Tablets (Less than 2%) ... 2605
Pletal Tablets (Less than 2%) ... 2848
Prevacid Delayed-Release Capsules (Less than 1%) ... 3292
PREVPAC (Less than 1%) ... 3298
Priftin Tablets (Less than 1%) ... 758
Prinivil Tablets (0.3% to 1.0%) ... 2164
Prinzide Tablets ... 2168
Procardia XL Extended Release Tablets (1% or less) ... 2710
Protonix I.V. (Less than 1%) ... 3580
Protonix Tablets (Less than 1%) ... 3577
Prozac Pulvules, Liquid, and Weekly Capsules (Infrequent) ... 1238
Pyrazinamide Tablets ... 1876
Remeron Tablets (Rare) ... 2483
Remeron SolTab Tablets (Rare) ... 2486
Requip Tablets (1% or more) ... 1621
Rifater Tablets ... 769
Rilutek Tablets (Infrequent) ... 772
Roxicodone Tablets (Less than 3%) ... 3067
Sandostatin LAR Depot (1% to 4%) ... 2395
Sarafem Pulvules (Infrequent) ... 1962
Seroquel Tablets (Infrequent) ... 684
Serzone Tablets (Infrequent) ... 1104
Sonata Capsules (Infrequent) ... 3591
Sular Tablets (Less than or equal to 1%) ... 688
Synercid I.V. (Less than 1%) ... 775
Tarka Tablets (Less frequent) ... 508
Tenoretic Tablets ... 690
Teveten Tablets (Less than 1%) ... 3327
Tiazac Capsules (1% to 2%) ... 1378
Timolide Tablets ... 2187
Tricor Capsules, Micronized ... 513
Uniretic Tablets (Less than 1%) ... 3178
Vantin Tablets and Oral Suspension (Less than 1%) ... 2860
Vaseretic Tablets (0.5% to 2.0%) ... 2204
Viagra Tablets (Less than 2%) ... 2732
Zaroxolyn Tablets ... 1177
Zebeta Tablets ... 1885
Zestoretic Tablets ... 695
Zestril Tablets (0.3% to 1.0%) ... 698
Ziac Tablets ... 1887
Zoladex (1% to 5%) ... 702
Zoladex 3-month ... 706
Zosyn (1.0% or less) ... 1890
Zosyn in Galaxy Containers (1.0% or less) ... 1894
Zyprexa Tablets (Rare) ... 1973
Zyprexa ZYDIS Orally Disintegrating Tablets (Rare) ... 1973

Granulocytopenia
Albenza Tablets (Rare) ... 1463
Aldoclor Tablets ... 2035
Aldomet Tablets ... 2037
Aldoril Tablets ... 2039
Anaprox Tablets (Less than 1%) ... 2967
Anaprox DS Tablets (Less than 1%) ... 2967
▲ Aredia for Injection (19.8%) ... 2309
Celexa (Rare) ... 1365
Claforan Injection (Rare) ... 732
Colazal Capsules ... 3069
▲ Cytovene (6%) ... 2959
Dilantin Infatabs (Occasional) ... 2624
Dilantin Kapseals (Occasional) ... 2622
Dilantin-125 Oral Suspension (Occasional) ... 2625
EC-Naprosyn Delayed-Release Tablets (Less than 1%) ... 2967
Ergamisol Tablets (Less than 1% to 2%) ... 1789
Evoxac Capsules (Less than 1%) ... 1217
Felbatol (Infrequent) ... 3343
▲ Foscavir Injection (5% to 17%) ... 605
Grifulvin V Tablets Microsize and Oral Suspension Microsize ... 2518
Gris-PEG Tablets ... 2661
▲ Infergen (23% to 42%) ... 1777
Innohep Injection ... 1248
Intron A for Injection (Less than 5%) ... 3120
Levaquin (Less than 0.3%) ... 2537
Limbitrol (Rare) ... 1738
Macrobid Capsules ... 2889
Macrodantin Capsules ... 2891
Mefoxin for Injection ... 2124
Mefoxin Premixed Intravenous Solution ... 2127
Mustargen for Injection ... 2142
▲ Naprelan Tablets (3% to 9%) ... 1293
Naprosyn Suspension (Less than 1%) ... 2967
Naprosyn Tablets (Less than 1%) ... 2967
▲ Navelbine Injection (29% to 80%) ... 1604
Nebcin Vials, Hyporets & ADD-Vantage ... 1955
▲ Novantrone for Injection (6%) ... 1760
Omnicef ... 493
Plavix Tablets (Less than 1%) ... 1097
Plavix Tablets (Less than 1%) ... 3084
Relafen Tablets (Less than 1%) ... 1617
▲ Retrovir Capsules (1.8% to 47%) ... 1625
▲ Retrovir IV Infusion (1.8% to 47%) ... 1629
▲ Retrovir (1.8% to 47%) ... 1625
Rythmol Tablets – 150 mg, 225 mg, 300 mg (Less than 1%) ... 502
Serentil (A single case) ... 1057
▲ Serostim for Injection (14.1%) ... 3229
Talacen Caplets ... 3089
Talwin Nx Tablets ... 3090
Tapazole Tablets ... 1823
Thalomid Capsules ... 1154
Tolectin (Less than 1%) ... 2589
Topamax Sprinkle Capsules (Infrequent) ... 2590
Topamax Tablets (Infrequent) ... 2590
Trovan (Less than 1%) ... 2722
▲ Videx (6% to 16%) ... 1138
Viramune Oral Suspension ... 1060
Viramune Tablets ... 1060
Vistide Injection ... 1445
Zantac (A few patients) ... 1690
Zantac Injection (Few patients) ... 1688
Zantac Syrup (A few patients) ... 1690
Zinecard for Injection ... 2869
▲ Zometa for Intravenous Infusion (5% to 10%) ... 3621

Granulocytosis
Hivid Tablets (Less than 1%) ... 2975
Rescriptor Tablets (Less than 2%) ... 526

Vantin Tablets and Oral Suspension 2860

Granuloma, unspecified
Actiq (Less than 1%) 1184
Fluorescite Injection ⊙ 211

Granulomatosis, Wegener's
Accutane Capsules 2944

Grogginess
Versed Injection (Less than 1%) 3027

Groin, itch
Miltown 3349

Growth, suppression in children
Azmacort Inhalation Aerosol 728
Celestone Soluspan Injectable Suspension 3097
Celestone Syrup 3099
Cortifoam Rectal Foam 3170
Cortone Acetate Injectable Suspension 2059
Cortone Acetate Tablets 2061
Cylert Tablets 415
Decadron Elixir 2078
Decadron Tablets 2079
Decadron Phosphate Injection 2081
Depo-Medrol Injectable Suspension 2795
Desoxyn Tablets 440
Florinef Acetate Tablets 2250
Flovent Diskus 3614
Flovent 1535
Flovent Rotadisk 1537
Hydrocortone Tablets 2106
Hydrocortone Acetate Injectable Suspension 2103
Hydrocortone Phosphate Injection, Sterile 2105
Nasacort Nasal Inhaler 750
Pediapred Oral Solution 1170
Prednisone 3064
Prelone Syrup 2273
Rhinocort Aqua Nasal Spray 642
Solu-Medrol Sterile Powder 2855

Growth retardation
Clomid Tablets 735
Cosmegen for Injection 2062
Depen Titratable Tablets (One infant) 3341
Desferal Vials 2333
Herceptin I.V. (At least one of the 958 patients) 1414

Growth retardation, intrauterine
Accupril Tablets 2611
Altace Capsules 2233
Captopril Tablets 2281
Cozaar Tablets 2067
Dilantin Kapseals 2622
Dilantin-125 Oral Suspension 2625
Enalaprilat Injection 863
Hyzaar 2109
Monopril Tablets 1091
Prinivil Tablets 2164
Prinzide Tablets 2168
Tenoretic Tablets 690
Tenormin 692
Univasc Tablets 3181
Vaseretic Tablets 2204
Vasotec I.V. Injection 2207
Vasotec Tablets 2210
Zestoretic Tablets 695
Zestril Tablets 698

Guillain-Barré syndrome
Acel-Imune 1851
ActHIB Vaccine 798
Asacol Delayed-Release Tablets (Rare) 2884
Attenuvax (Rare) 2044
Azulfidine EN-tabs Tablets (Rare) 2775
Chibroxin Sterile Ophthalmic Solution 2051
Comvax 2056
Cuprimine Capsules 2075
Depen Titratable Tablets 3341
Diphtheria & Tetanus Toxoids Adsorbed Purogenated for Pediatric Use 1857
Effexor Tablets (Rare) 3495
Effexor XR Capsules (Rare) 3499
Engerix-B Vaccine (Less than 1%) 1517
FluShield Influenza Vaccine (Rare) 3521
Fluzone Vaccine 802
Havrix Vaccine (Rare) 1544
HibTITER 1859
IPOL Vaccine 809
Meruvax II (Isolated reports) 2130
M-M-R II (Rare) 2118
Mumpsvax 2141
Noroxin Tablets 2145
Paxil 1609
Liquid PedvaxHIB 2148
Pneumovax 23 (Rare) 2156
Pnu-Imune 23 1868
Rabies Vaccine RabAvert (Two cases) 1203
Recombivax HB 2178
Streptase for Infusion 647
Tetanus & Diphtheria Toxoids Adsorbed for Adult Use 1880
Tetanus and Diphtheria Toxoids Adsorbed For Adult Use 815
Tripedia Vaccine 817
Twinrix Vaccine 1674
Varivax 2202

Gums, sore
Hivid Tablets (Less than 1%) 2975
Wellbutrin (Infrequent) 1680

Gynecological disorders, unspecified
▲ Zofran (7%) 1703
▲ Zofran ODT Orally Disintegrating Tablets (7%) 1703

Gynecomastia
Adalat CC Tablets (Rare) 877
Aldoclor Tablets 2035
Aldomet Tablets 2037
Aldoril Tablets 2039
Anadrol-50 Tablets 3321
Androderm Transdermal System CIII 3377
AndroGel (Up to 3%) 3322
▲ Android Capsules, 10 mg (Among most common) 1731
Atromid-S Capsules 3483
Avonex 1013
Axid Pulvules (Rare) 1903
Axid Pulvules (Rare) 2919
Baycol Tablets 883
Betaseron for SC Injection 988
Captopril Tablets 2281
Cardura Tablets 2668
▲ Casodex Tablets (5%) 662
Catapres Tablets (About 1 in 1,000 patients) 1037
Catapres-TTS (0.5% or less) 1038
Celexa (Rare) 1365
Cipro I.V. (1% or less) 893
Cipro I.V. Pharmacy Bulk Package (Less than 1%) 897
Clinoril Tablets (Rare) 2053
Clorpres Tablets (About 1 in 1,000) 1002
Combipres Tablets (About 1 in 1,000) 1040
Compazine 1505
Covera-HS Tablets (Less than 2%) 3199
Delatestryl Injection 1151
Digitek Tablets (Occasional) 1003
Duraclon Injection (1%) 3057
Effexor Tablets (Rare) 3495
Effexor XR Capsules (Rare) 3499
Enalaprilat Injection 863
Etrafon 3115
▲ Eulexin Capsules (9%) 3118
Famotidine Injection (Rare) 866
Flexeril Tablets (Rare) 572
Flexeril Tablets (Rare) 2094
Gengraf Capsules (Less than 1% to 4%) 457
Geodon Capsules (Rare) 2688
Gonal-F for Injection 3216
Haldol Decanoate 2535
Haldol Injection, Tablets and Concentrate 2533
Humatrope Vials and Cartridges (Rare) 1930
Humegon for Injection (Occasional) 2468
Indocin Capsules (Less than 1%) 2112
Indocin I.V. (Less than 1%) 2115
Indocin (Less than 1%) 2112
Intron A for Injection (Less than 5%) 3120
Isoptin SR Tablets (1% or less) 467
Kadian Capsules (Less than 3%) 1335
Kaletra Capsules (Less than 2%) 471
Kaletra Oral Solution (Less than 2%) 471
Lanoxicaps Capsules (Occasional) 1574
Lanoxin Injection (Occasional) 1581
Lanoxin Tablets (Occasional) 1587
Lanoxin Elixir Pediatric (Occasional) 1578
Lanoxin Injection Pediatric (Occasional) 1584
Lescol Capsules 2361
Lescol Capsules 2925
Lescol XL Tablets 2361
Lescol XL Tablets 2925
Lexxel Tablets 608
Limbitrol 1738
Lotrel Capsules 2370
Loxitane Capsules (Rare) 3398
Lupron Depot 7.5 mg (Less than 5%) 3284
Lupron Depot–3 Month 22.5 mg (Less than 5%) 3288
Lupron Depot-PED 7.5 mg, 11.25 mg and 15 mg (Less than 2%) 3291
▲ Lupron Injection (5% or more) 3279
Lupron Injection Pediatric (Less than 2%) 3280
Matulane Capsules 3246
Megace Oral Suspension (1% to 3%) 1124
Mevacor Tablets (0.5% to 1.0%) 2132
Midamor Tablets 2136
Minipress Capsules 2699
Moban (Infrequent) 1320
Moduretic Tablets 2138
Motrin Suspension, Oral Drops, Chewable Tablets, and Caplets (Less than 1%) 2002
Myleran Tablets (Rare) 1603
Navane Oral 2701
Navane Intramuscular 2703
Neoral Soft Gelatin Capsules (Less than 1% to 4%) 2380
Neoral Oral Solution (Less than 1% to 4%) 2380
▲ Nilandron Tablets (10.5%) 753
Nizoral Tablets (Less than 1%) 1791
Norpramin Tablets 755
Norvasc Tablets (Infrequent) 2704
Novarel for Injection 1347
Nutropin AQ Injection (Rare) 1420
Nutropin for Injection (Rare) 1417
Orudis Capsules (Rare) 3548
Oruvail Capsules (Rare) 3548
Oxandrin Tablets 1153
Pepcid Injection (Rare) 2153
Pepcid for Oral Suspension (Rare) 2150
Pepcid RPD Orally Disintegrating Tablets (Rare) 2150
Pepcid Tablets (Rare) 2150
Pergonal for Injection (Occasional) 3223
Plendil Extended-Release Tablets (0.5% to 1.5%) 623
Pravachol Tablets 1099
Pregnyl for Injection 2482
Prevacid Delayed-Release Capsules (Less than 1%) 3292
PREVPAC (Less than 1%) 3298
Prilosec Delayed-Release Capsules (Less than 1%) 628
Procardia Capsules (Less than 0.5%) 2708
Procardia XL Extended Release Tablets (Less than 1%) 2710
Prozac Pulvules, Liquid, and Weekly Capsules 1238
Reglan 2935
Repronex for Intramuscular and Subcutaneous Injection (Occasional) 1347
Requip Tablets (Infrequent) 1621
Rifamate Capsules 767
Rifater Tablets 769
Risperdal (Rare) 1796
Sandimmune (Less than 1% to 4%) 2388
Sandostatin Injection (Less than 1%) 2394
Sandostatin LAR Depot (Rare) 2395
Sarafem Pulvules 1962
Serentil 1057
Seroquel Tablets (Rare) 684
▲ Serostim for Injection (1% to 10%) 3229
Sinequan 2713
Sporanox Capsules (Infrequent) 1800
Sporanox Oral Solution (Less than 2%) 1808
Sporanox Oral Solution (Less than 2%) 2512
Stelazine 1640
Sular Tablets 688
Surmontil Capsules 3595
Sustiva Capsules 1258
▲ Tagamet (4%; 0.3% to 1%) 1644
Tarka Tablets 508
▲ Testoderm Transdermal Systems (5%) 574
Testopel Pellets 3610
Testred Capsules, 10 mg 1746
Thalomid Capsules 1154
Thioridazine Hydrochloride Tablets 2289
Thiothixene Capsules 2290
Thorazine 1656
Tiazac Capsules (Less than 2%) 1378
Trecator-SC Tablets 3598
Tricor Capsules, Micronized 513
Trilafon 3160
Vascor Tablets (Rare) 2602
Vaseretic Tablets 2204
Vasotec I.V. Injection 2207
Vasotec Tablets (0.5% to 1.0%) 2210
Verelan Capsules (1% or less) 3184
Verelan PM Capsules (2% or less) 3186
▲ Viadur Implant (6.9%) 912
Vivactil Tablets 2217
Vivactil Tablets 2446
Wellbutrin Tablets (Infrequent) 1680
Wellbutrin SR Sustained-Release Tablets 1684
Xanax Tablets 2865
Zantac (Occasional) 1690
Zantac Injection 1688
Zantac Syrup (Occasional) 1690
Zocor Tablets 2219
▲ Zoladex 3-month (8%) 706
Zoloft (Rare) 2751
Zonegran Capsules (Rare) 1307
Zyban Sustained-Release Tablets 1710

H

Haemophilus B disease
Liquid PedvaxHIB 2148

Hair, abnormal growth
(*see under* Hirsutism)

Hair, dry brittle
Atromid-S Capsules (Less often) 3483
Claritin (At least one patient) 3100
Claritin-D 12 Hour Extended Release Tablets 3102
Claritin-D 24 Hour Extended Release Tablets 3104
Clomid Tablets (Fewer than 1%) 735
Eskalith 1527
Gengraf Capsules (Rare) 457
Lithium Carbonate 3061
Lithium Citrate Syrup 3061
Lithobid Slow-Release Tablets 3255
Neoral Soft Gelatin Capsules (Rare) 2380
Neoral Oral Solution (Rare) 2380
Nizoral 2% Shampoo 2007
Sandimmune (Rare) 2388
Selsun Rx 2.5% Lotion, USP 3053

Hair, oily
Nizoral 2% Shampoo 2007
Selsun Rx 2.5% Lotion, USP 3053

Hair discoloration
Arava Tablets (1% to 3%) 724
Effexor Tablets (Rare) 3495
Effexor XR Capsules (Rare) 3499
Plaquenil Tablets 3082
Psoriatec Cream 3247
Selsun Rx 2.5% Lotion, USP 3053
Soriatane Capsules (Less than 1%) 3003
Wellbutrin Tablets (Rare) 1680

Hair growth, unwanted
Rogaine for Women Topical Solution (Infrequent) 721

Hair ingrown
Vaniqa Cream (0.9%) 1121

Hair loss
(*see under* Alopecia)

Hair problems, unspecified
Accutane Capsules 2944
Baycol Tablets 883
Emcyt Capsules (1%) 2810
Fortovase Capsules (Less than 2%) 2970
Invirase Capsules (Less than 2%) 2979
Lescol Capsules 2361
Lescol Capsules 2925
Lescol XL Tablets 2361
Lescol XL Tablets 2925
▲ Lupron Depot 3.75 mg (Among most frequent) 3281
Lupron Depot 7.5 mg (Less than 5%) 3284
Lupron Depot–3 Month 11.25 mg (Less than 5%) 3285
Mevacor Tablets 2132
Pravachol Tablets 1099
Zocor Tablets 2219
▲ Zoladex (4%) 702
Zoladex 3-month 706

Hair texture, abnormal
Imdur Tablets (Less than or equal to 5%) 1826
Intron A for Injection (Less than 5%) 3120
Nizoral 2% Shampoo (One occurrence in 41 patients) 2007
▲ Soriatane Capsules (1% to 10%) 3003
Topamax Sprinkle Capsules (Infrequent) 2590
Topamax Tablets (Infrequent) 2590
Zoloft (Rare) 2751

Hair thinning
Accutane Capsules 2944
Arimidex Tablets (2% to 5%) 659
Clorpres Tablets 1002
Combipres Tablets 1040
Cortifoam Rectal Foam 3170
Eskalith 1527
Intron A for Injection 3120
Lithium Carbonate 3061
Lithium Citrate Syrup 3061
Lithobid Slow-Release Tablets 3255
Nolvadex Tablets (Infrequent) 678
Trilafon Tablets 3160

Halitosis
Azactam for Injection (Less than 1%) ... 1276
Claritin-D 12 Hour Extended Release Tablets (Less frequent) ... 3102
Crixivan Capsules (Less than 2%) ... 2070
Effexor Tablets (Rare) ... 3495
Exelon Capsules (Infrequent) ... 2342
Exelon Oral Solution (Infrequent) ... 2345
Floxin Otic Solution (Single report) ... 1219
Gabitril Tablets (Infrequent) ... 1189
Intron A for Injection (Less than 5%) ... 3120
Lamictal (Infrequent) ... 1567
Prevacid Delayed-Release Capsules (Less than 1%) ... 3292
PREVPAC (Less than 1%) ... 3298
Protonix I.V. (Less than 1%) ... 3580
Protonix Tablets (Less than 1%) ... 3577
Serzone Tablets (Infrequent) ... 1104
Tequin Injection (Less than 0.1%) ... 1110
Tequin Tablets (Less than 0.1%) ... 1110
Topamax Sprinkle Capsules (Infrequent) ... 2590
Topamax Tablets (Infrequent) ... 2590
Trovan (Less than 1%) ... 2722

Hallucinations
Actimmune (Rare) ... 1772
Actiq (1% to 2%) ... 1184
Allegra-D Extended-Release Tablets ... 714
Ambien Tablets (Infrequent) ... 3191
AmBisome for Injection (Less common) ... 1383
Amerge Tablets (Rare) ... 1467
Amicar Injection ... 3608
Amicar Syrup ... 3608
Amicar Tablets ... 3608
Amphotec (1% to 5%) ... 1774
Ancobon Capsules ... 1730
Aricept Tablets ... 1270
Aricept Tablets ... 2665
Artane (Rare) ... 1855
Arthrotec Tablets (Rare) ... 3195
Ativan Injection (1%) ... 3478
Avelox Tablets (0.05% to 1%) ... 879
Azulfidine EN-tabs Tablets (Rare) ... 2775
Bactrim ... 2949
Betaseron for SC Injection ... 988
Biaxin/Biaxin XL ... 403
Blocadren Tablets (Less than 1%) ... 2046
Brethine Tablets (Less than 1%) ... 2313
Buprenex Injectable (Infrequent) ... 2918
Campath Ampules ... 992
Cardizem Injectable ... 1018
Cardizem Lyo-Ject Syringe ... 1018
Cardizem Monovial ... 1018
Cardizem CD Capsules (Less than 1%) ... 1016
Catapres Tablets ... 1037
Ceclor (Rare) ... 1905
Celexa (Infrequent) ... 1365
▲ CellCept Capsules (3% to 10%) ... 2951
▲ CellCept Intravenous (3% to 10%) ... 2951
▲ CellCept Oral Suspension (3% to 10%) ... 2951
▲ CellCept Tablets (3% to 10%) ... 2951
Celontin Capsules (Rare) ... 2618
Chibroxin Sterile Ophthalmic Solution ... 2051
Cipro I.V. (1% or less) ... 893
Cipro I.V. Pharmacy Bulk Package (Less than 1%) ... 897
Cipro (Less than 1%) ... 887
Claritin-D 12 Hour Extended Release Tablets ... 3102
Claritin-D 24 Hour Extended Release Tablets ... 3104
Clozaril Tablets (Less than 1%) ... 2319
Cogentin ... 2055
Cognex Capsules (2%) ... 1351
Comtan Tablets ... 2328
Copaxone for Injection (Infrequent) ... 3306
Corgard Tablets ... 2245
Corzide 40/5 Tablets ... 2247
Corzide 80/5 Tablets ... 2247
Cosopt Sterile Ophthalmic Solution ... 2065
Cylert Tablets ... 415
Cytovene ... 2959
Darvon-N/Darvocet-N ... 1907
Darvon Pulvules ... 1909
Darvon Compound-65 Pulvules ... 1910
Darvon-N Tablets ... 1912
DaunoXome Injection (Less than or equal to 5%) ... 1442
Demerol ... 3079
Demser Capsules ... 2085
Depacon Injection ... 416
Depakene ... 421
Depakote Sprinkle Capsules ... 426
Depakote Tablets (1% to 5%) ... 430
Depakote ER Tablets (Greater than 1%) ... 436
D.H.E. 45 Injection ... 2334
Didronel Tablets ... 2888
Digitek Tablets ... 1003
Dilaudid Oral Liquid (Less frequent) ... 445
Dilaudid Tablets - 8 mg (Less frequent) ... 445
Dilaudid-HP (Less frequent) ... 443
Diprivan Injectable Emulsion (Less than 1%) ... 667
Dolobid Tablets (Less than 1 in 100) ... 2088
Dostinex Tablets ... 2804
▲ Duraclon Injection (5.3%) ... 3057
▲ Duragesic Transdermal System (3% to 10%) ... 1786
Effexor Tablets (Infrequent) ... 3495
Effexor XR Capsules (Infrequent) ... 3499
▲ Eldepryl Capsules (3 of 49 patients) ... 3266
Elspar for Injection ... 2092
Ergamisol Tablets (Less frequent) ... 1789
Ery-Tab Tablets (Isolated reports) ... 448
Erythrocin Stearate Filmtab Tablets (Isolated reports) ... 452
Erythromycin Base Filmtab Tablets (Isolated reports) ... 454
Erythromycin Delayed-Release Capsules, USP (Isolated reports) ... 455
Eskalith ... 1527
Etrafon ... 3115
Evoxac Capsules (Less than 1%) ... 1217
▲ Exelon Capsules (4%) ... 2342
▲ Exelon Oral Solution (4%) ... 2345
Famotidine Injection (Infrequent) ... 866
Famvir Tablets (Infrequent) ... 2348
Felbatol (Infrequent) ... 3343
Feldene Capsules (Rare) ... 2685
Flexeril Tablets (Less than 1%) ... 572
Flexeril Tablets (Less than 1%) ... 2094
Floxin I.V. (Less than 1%) ... 2526
Floxin Tablets (Less than 1%) ... 2529
Flumadine (Less than 0.3%) ... 1370
Fortovase Capsules (Less than 2%) ... 2970
Foscavir Injection (Between 1% and 5%) ... 605
Gabitril Tablets (Frequent) ... 1189
Gastrocrom Oral Concentrate (Less common) ... 1162
Genoptic Ophthalmic Ointment (Rare) ... ⊙239
Genoptic Sterile Ophthalmic Solution (Rare) ... ⊙239
Halcion Tablets ... 2823
Haldol Decanoate ... 2535
Haldol Injection, Tablets and Concentrate ... 2533
Hivid Tablets (Less than 1%) ... 2975
▲ Ifex for Injection (Among most common) ... 1123
Imitrex Injection ... 1549
Imitrex Tablets (Rare) ... 1558
Inderal ... 3513
Inderal LA Long-Acting Capsules ... 3516
Inderide Tablets ... 3517
Inderide LA Long-Acting Capsules ... 3519
Invirase Capsules (Less than 2%) ... 2979
Kadian Capsules (Less than 3%) ... 1335
Keflex ... 1237
Klonopin Tablets ... 2983
Lamictal (Infrequent) ... 1567
Lanoxicaps Capsules ... 1574
Lanoxin Injection ... 1581
Lanoxin Tablets ... 1587
Lanoxin Elixir Pediatric ... 1578
Lanoxin Injection Pediatric ... 1584
Lariam Tablets ... 2989
Leukeran Tablets (Rare) ... 1591
Levaquin (Less than 0.3%) ... 2537
Levsin/Levsinex/Levbid ... 3172
Limbitrol ... 1738
Lithobid Slow-Release Tablets ... 3255
Lodine XL Extended-Release Tablets ... 3530
Lodosyn Tablets ... 1251
Luvox Tablets (25, 50, 100 mg) (Infrequent) ... 3256
Marinol Capsules (Greater than 1%) ... 3325
Matulane Capsules ... 3246
Mepergan Injection ... 3539
Merrem I.V. (0.1% to 1.0%) ... 673
Mexitil Capsules (About 3 in 1,000) ... 1047
Minipress Capsules (Less than 1%) ... 2699
Minizide Capsules (Rare) ... 2700
▲ Mirapex Tablets (9% to 17%) ... 2834
Motrin Suspension, Oral Drops, Chewable Tablets, and Caplets (Less than 1%) ... 2002
MS Contin Tablets (Less frequent) ... 2896
MSIR (Less frequent) ... 2898
Myambutol Tablets ... 1290
Mylocel Tablets (Extremely rare) ... 2227
Nadolol Tablets ... 2288
Naropin Injection (Less than 1%) ... 612
Nembutal Sodium Solution (Less than 1%) ... 485
Neurontin Capsules (Infrequent) ... 2655
Neurontin Oral Solution (Infrequent) ... 2655
Neurontin Tablets (Infrequent) ... 2655
Nipent for Injection (Less than 3%) ... 3272
Norflex ... 1987
Noroxin Tablets ... 2145
Norpramin Tablets ... 755
Norvir Capsules (Less than 2%) ... 487
Norvir Oral Solution (Less than 2%) ... 487
Nubain Injection (1% or less) ... 1323
Numorphan ... 1324
Oramorph SR Tablets (Less frequent) ... 3062
Orudis Capsules (Rare) ... 3548
Oruvail Capsules (Rare) ... 3548
OxyContin Tablets (Less than 1%) ... 2912
Paxil (Infrequent) ... 1609
Pediazole Suspension ... 3050
Pepcid Injection (Infrequent) ... 2153
Pepcid for Oral Suspension (Infrequent) ... 2150
Pepcid RPD Orally Disintegrating Tablets (Infrequent) ... 2150
Pepcid Tablets (Infrequent) ... 2150
Periactin Tablets ... 2155
▲ Permax Tablets (13.8%) ... 1299
Phenergan ... 3556
Phenergan with Codeine Syrup ... 3557
Phenergan VC with Codeine Syrup ... 3561
Ponstel Capsules (Rare) ... 1356
Prevacid Delayed-Release Capsules (Less than 1%) ... 3292
PREVPAC (Less than 1%) ... 3298
Prilosec Delayed-Release Capsules (Less than 1%) ... 628
Primaxin I.M. ... 2158
Primaxin I.V. ... 2160
Procanbid Extended-Release Tablets (Occasional) ... 2262
▲ Prograf (3% to 15%) ... 1393
ProSom Tablets (Rare) ... 500
Protonix I.V. (Less than 1%) ... 3580
Protonix Tablets (Less than 1%) ... 3577
Provigil Tablets (At least 1%) ... 1193
Prozac Pulvules, Liquid, and Weekly Capsules (Infrequent) ... 1238
Reglan (Rare) ... 2935
Remeron Tablets (Infrequent) ... 2483
Remeron SolTab Tablets (Infrequent) ... 2486
Reminyl Oral Solution (Greater than or equal to 2%) ... 1792
Reminyl Tablets (Greater than or equal to 2%) ... 1792
▲ Requip Tablets (5% to 10%) ... 1621
Rescriptor Tablets (Less than 2%) ... 526
Rilutek Tablets (Infrequent) ... 772
Roferon-A Injection (Infrequent) ... 2996
Rynatan Tablets ... 3351
Sandostatin LAR Depot (1% to 4%) ... 2395
Sarafem Pulvules (Infrequent) ... 1962
Septra Suspension ... 2265
Septra Tablets ... 2265
Septra DS Tablets ... 2265
Seroquel Tablets (Infrequent) ... 684
Serzone Tablets (Infrequent) ... 1104
Sinemet Tablets ... 1253
▲ Sinemet CR Tablets (3.9%) ... 1255
Sinequan (Infrequent) ... 2713
Sonata Capsules (Less than 1%) ... 3591
Stadol NS Nasal Spray (Less than 1%) ... 1108
Surmontil Capsules ... 3595
Sustiva Capsules (Less than 2%) ... 1258
Symmetrel (1% to 5%) ... 1328
Tagamet ... 1644
Talacen Caplets ... 3089
Talwin Nx Tablets ... 3090
▲ Tasmar Tablets (8% to 10%) ... 3010
Tenoretic Tablets ... 690
Tenormin ... 692
Tequin Injection (Less than 0.1%) ... 1110
Tequin Tablets (Less than 0.1%) ... 1110
Tiazac Capsules (Less than 2%) ... 1378
Timolide Tablets ... 2187
Timolol GFS ... ⊙266
Timoptic in Ocudose (Less frequent) ... 2192
Timoptic Sterile Ophthalmic Solution (Less frequent) ... 2190
Timoptic-XE Sterile Ophthalmic Gel Forming Solution ... 2194
▲ Tonocard Tablets (2.1% to 11.2%) ... 649
Topamax Sprinkle Capsules (Frequent) ... 2590
Topamax Tablets (Frequent) ... 2590
Toradol (1% or less) ... 3018
Transderm Scōp Transdermal Therapeutic System (Infrequent) ... 2302
Trilisate (Rare) ... 2901
Trovan (Less than 1%) ... 2722
Ultracet Tablets (Less than 1%) ... 2597
▲ Ultram Tablets (Less than 1% to 14%) ... 2600
Valcyte Tablets (Less than 5%) ... 3022
Valium Injectable ... 3026
Valium Tablets ... 3047
Vantin Tablets and Oral Suspension (Less than 1%) ... 2860
Versed Injection (Less than 1%) ... 3027
Versed Syrup (Less than 1%) ... 3033
▲ Vesanoid Capsules (6%) ... 3037
Vioxx (Less than 0.1%) ... 2213
Vistide Injection ... 1445
Vivactil Tablets ... 2217
Vivactil Tablets ... 2446
Wellbutrin Tablets (Frequent) ... 1680
Wellbutrin SR Sustained-Release Tablets ... 1684
Xanax Tablets (Rare) ... 2865
Zantac (Rare) ... 1690
Zantac Injection ... 1688
Zantac Syrup (Rare) ... 1690
Zebeta Tablets ... 1885
Ziac Tablets ... 1887
Zoloft (Infrequent) ... 2751
Zomig Tablets (Rare) ... 708
Zomig-ZMT Tablets (Rare) ... 708
Zosyn (1.0% or less) ... 1890
Zosyn in Galaxy Containers (1.0% or less) ... 1894
Zovirax Capsules ... 1706
Zovirax for Injection (Approximately 1%) ... 1708
Zovirax ... 1706
Zyban Sustained-Release Tablets ... 1710
Zyprexa Tablets ... 1973
Zyprexa ZYDIS Orally Disintegrating Tablets ... 1973
Zyrtec-D 12 Hour Extended Relief Tablets ... 2758

Hallucinations, auditory
Bicillin C-R 900/300 Injection ... 2240
Bicillin C-R Injection ... 2238
Bicillin L-A Injection ... 2242
Catapres Tablets (Rare) ... 1037
Catapres-TTS (0.5% or less) ... 1038
Clorpres Tablets ... 1002
Combipres Tablets ... 1040
Orthoclone OKT3 Sterile Solution ... 2498
Valtrex Caplets ... 1676

Hallucinations, visual
Bicillin C-R 900/300 Injection ... 2240
Bicillin C-R Injection ... 2238
Bicillin L-A Injection ... 2242
Carbatrol Capsules ... 3234
Catapres Tablets (Rare) ... 1037
Catapres-TTS (0.5% or less) ... 1038
Clorpres Tablets ... 1002
Cogentin ... 2055
Combipres Tablets ... 1040
Orthoclone OKT3 Sterile Solution ... 2498
Salagen Tablets (Rare) ... 2229
Talwin Nx Tablets ... 3090
Tegretol/Tegretol-XR ... 2404
Tessalon Capsules ... 1377
Valtrex Caplets ... 1676

Halos
Cordarone Tablets ... 3487
Pacerone Tablets ... 3331
Plaquenil Tablets (Fairly common) ... 3082

Hand-foot syndrome
(*see under* Palmar-plantar erythrodysesthesia syndrome)

Hangover
Aciphex Tablets (Rare) ... 1267
Aciphex Tablets (Rare) ... 1783
Effexor Tablets (Infrequent) ... 3495
Effexor XR Capsules (Infrequent) ... 3499
Maxalt Tablets (Infrequent) ... 2120
Maxalt-MLT Orally Disintegrating Tablets (Infrequent) ... 2120
Neurontin Capsules (Rare) ... 2655
Neurontin Oral Solution (Rare) ... 2655
Neurontin Tablets (Rare) ... 2655
Nipent for Injection (Less than 3%) ... 3272
▲ ProSom Tablets (3%) ... 500
Serzone Tablets (Infrequent) ... 1104
Sonata Capsules (Infrequent) ... 3591
Thalomid Capsules ... 1154
Zyprexa Tablets (Infrequent) ... 1973
Zyprexa ZYDIS Orally Disintegrating Tablets (Infrequent) ... 1973

HDL, decrease
Anadrol-50 Tablets ... 3321
▲ AndroGel (3% to 6%) ... 3322
Coreg Tablets (Less than or equal to 0.1%) ... 1508

Head, tight feeling
Adenocard Injection (Less than 1%) ... 1380
Aricept Tablets (Infrequent) ... 1270
Aricept Tablets (Infrequent) ... 2665
Imitrex Injection (2.2%) ... 1549
Imitrex Tablets (Infrequent) ... 1558
Klonopin Tablets (Infrequent) ... 2983
ProAmatine Tablets (Less frequent) ... 3241

Headache
▲ Abelcet Injection (6%) ... 1273
▲ Accolate Tablets (4.5% to 12.9%) ... 657
▲ Accupril Tablets (1.7% to 5.6%) ... 2611
▲ Accuretic Tablets (6.7%) ... 2614
Accutane Capsules ... 2944

▲ Aceon Tablets (2 mg, 4 mg, 8 mg) (23.8%) 3249
Aciphex Tablets (2.4%) 1267
Aciphex Tablets (2.4%) 1783
▲ Actimmune (33%) 1772
▲ Actiq (3% to 6%) 1184
▲ Activella Tablets (11% to 16%) 2764
▲ Actonel Tablets (18%) 2879
▲ Actos Tablets (9.1%) 3275
Acular Ophthalmic Solution (Rare) 544
Acular PF Ophthalmic Solution 544
Adagen Injection (One patient) 1331
▲ Adalat CC Tablets (19%) 877
Adderall Tablets 3231
Adderall XR Capsules
Adenocard Injection (2%) 1380
▲ Adenoscan (18%) 1381
Adipex-P 1406
▲ Advair Diskus 100/50 (12%) 1448
▲ Advair Diskus 250/50 (13%) 1448
▲ Advair Diskus 500/50 (12% to 13%) 1448
▲ Aerobid/Aerobid-M (25%) 1363
Aerolate 1361
Aggrastat (Less than 1%) 2031
▲ Aggrenox Capsules (39.2%) 1026
▲ Agrylin Capsules (43.5%) 3232
AK-Fluor Injection 10% and 25% ⊙ 202
▲ Alamast Ophthalmic Solution (10% to 25%) 3092
Albalon Ophthalmic Solution ⊙ 225
▲ Albenza Tablets (1.3% to 11.0%) 1463
Aldara Cream, 5% (More than 1% to 5%) 1978
Aldoclor Tablets 2035
Aldomet Tablets 2037
Aldoril Tablets 2039
Alesse-21 Tablets 3468
Alesse-28 Tablets 3473
▲ Alferon N Injection (3% to 31%) 1770
▲ Allegra (7.2% to 10.6%) 712
▲ Allegra-D Extended-Release Tablets (13.8%) 714
▲ Alocril Ophthalmic Solution (Approximately 40%) 545
Alomide Ophthalmic Solution (1.5%) ⊙ 204
Aloprim for Injection (Less than 1%) 2292
▲ Alora Transdermal System (12.5% to 21.3%) 3372
▲ Alphagan Ophthalmic Solution (Approximately 10% to 30%) 545
Alphagan P Ophthalmic Solution (1% to 4%) 546
Altace Capsules (1.2% to 5.4%) 2233
Alupent (1% to 4%) 1029
Amaryl Tablets (1.5%) 717
▲ Ambien Tablets (7% to 19%) 3191
▲ AmBisome for Injection (9.4% to 19.8%) 1383
Amicar Injection 3608
Amicar Syrup 3608
Amicar Tablets 3608
▲ Amoxil Chewable Tablets (7%) 1471
▲ Amoxil for Oral Suspension (7%) 1471
▲ Amoxil (7%) 1471
▲ Amphotec (4% to 8%) 1774
▲ Anaprox Tablets (3% to 9%) 2967
▲ Anaprox DS Tablets (3% to 9%) 2967
Ancobon Capsules 1730
▲ Androderm Transdermal System CIII (4%) 3377
AndroGel (Up to 3%) 3322
▲ Android Capsules, 10 mg (Among most common) 1731
Antabuse Tablets 2444
Antabuse Tablets (Small number of patients) 3474
▲ Antagon Injection (3%) 2447
▲ Anzemet Injection (9.4% to 24.3%) 719
▲ Anzemet Tablets (7% to 17.9%) 722
Aquasol A Parenteral 593
Aralen Tablets 3075
▲ Arava Tablets (7%) 724
▲ Aredia for Injection (10% to 26.2%) 2309
▲ Aricept Tablets (10%) 1270
▲ Aricept Tablets (10%) 2665
▲ Arimidex Tablets (9.3% to 17.9%) 659
▲ Aromasin Tablets (8%) 2769
Artane 1855
Arthrotec Tablets (Rare) 3195
▲ Asacol Delayed-Release Tablets (35%) 2884
▲ Astelin Nasal Spray (7.9%) 3339
Astramorph/PF Injection, USP (Preservative-Free) 594
Atacand Tablets (More than 1%) 595
Ativan Injection (1.2%) 3478
Ativan Tablets (Less frequent) 3482
Atromid-S Capsules (Less often) 3483
Atrovent Inhalation Aerosol (2.4%) 1030
▲ Atrovent Inhalation Solution (6.4%) 1031
▲ Atrovent Nasal Spray 0.03% (9.8%) 1032
Attenuvax 2044
Augmentin Chewable Tablets (Less frequent) 1482
Augmentin Powder for Oral Suspension (Less frequent) 1482
Augmentin Tablets (Less frequent) 1485
Autoplex T 2294
Avalide Tablets (1% or greater) 1070
▲ Avandia Tablets (5.4% to 8.9%) 1490
Avapro Tablets (1% or greater) 1074
Avapro Tablets (1% or greater) 3076
Avelox Tablets (2%) 879
▲ Avonex (67%) 1013
Axert Tablets (Frequent) 2772
▲ Axid Pulvules (16.6%) 1903
▲ Axid Pulvules (16.6%) 2919
Aygestin Tablets 1333
Azactam for Injection (Less than 1%) 1276
▲ Azmacort Inhalation Aerosol (7% to 21%) 728
Azopt Ophthalmic Suspension (1% to 5%) 536
▲ Azulfidine EN-tabs Tablets (Among most common) 2775
Bactrim 2949
Bactroban Cream (1.7% to 3.6%) 1494
▲ Bactroban Nasal (9%) 1495
▲ Baycol Tablets (8.5%) 883
Beconase Inhalation Aerosol 1497
Beconase AQ Nasal Spray (Fewer than 5 per 100 patients) 1498
Benadryl Parenteral 2617
BeneFix for Injection 1432
Betagan (Rare) ⊙ 228
▲ Betapace Tablets (3% to 8%) 950
▲ Betapace AF Tablets (3.3% to 11.5%) 954
▲ Betaseron for SC Injection (84%) 988
Betaxon Ophthalmic Suspension (Less than 2%) 537
▲ Betimol Ophthalmic Solution (More than 5%) ⊙ 324
Betoptic S Ophthalmic Suspension (Rare) 537
Biaxin/Biaxin XL (2%) 403
Bicillin C-R 900/300 Injection 2240
Bicillin C-R Injection 2238
Bicillin L-A Injection 2242
Biltricide Tablets 887
Blocadren Tablets (Greater than 1%) 2046
Bontril Slow-Release Capsules 576
▲ Botox Purified Neurotoxin Complex (11%) 549
Brethine Ampuls 2314
▲ Brethine Tablets (7.5%) 2313
Brevibloc Injection (About 2%) 858
Brevicon 28-Day Tablets 3380
Brevital Sodium for Injection, USP 1815
Buprenex Injectable (1% to 5%) 2918
Calcijex Injection 411
Calcium Disodium Versenate Injection 1980
▲ Campath Ampules (1% to 24%) 992
▲ Canasa Rectal Suppositories (Among most common) 829
▲ Cancidas for Injection (6% to 11.3%) 2048
Captopril Tablets (About 0.5% to 2%) 2281
▲ Carac Cream (3.1%) 1222
Carafate Suspension (Less than 0.5%) 731
Carafate Tablets (Less than 0.5%) 730
Carbatrol Capsules 3234
▲ Cardene I.V. (14.6%) 3485
Cardizem Injectable (Less than 1%) 1018
Cardizem Lyo-Ject Syringe (Less than 1%) 1018
Cardizem Monovial (Less than 1%) 1018
▲ Cardizem CD Capsules (4.6% to 5.4%) 1016
▲ Cardura Tablets (9.9% to 14%) 2668
▲ Carnitor Injection (3% to 37%) 3242
Carteolol Hydrochloride Ophthalmic Solution USP, 1% (Occasional) ⊙ 258
▲ Casodex Tablets (4%) 662
▲ Cataflam Tablets (3% to 9%) 2315
Catapres Tablets (About 1 in 100 patients) 1037
▲ Catapres-TTS (5 of 101 patients) 1038
Caverject Sterile Powder (2%) 2777
▲ Ceclor CD Tablets (4.9%) 1279
Cedax (0.1% to 3%) 1021
Ceftin Tablets (0.1% to 1%) 1898
Cefzil (Less than 1%) 1076
▲ Celebrex Capsules (15.8%) 2676
▲ Celebrex Capsules (15.8%) 2780
Celestone Soluspan Injectable Suspension 3097
Celestone Syrup 3099
Celexa (At least 2%) 1365
▲ CellCept Capsules (16.1% to 54.3%) 2951
▲ CellCept Intravenous (16.1% to 54.3%) 2951
▲ CellCept Oral Suspension (16.1% to 54.3%) 2951
▲ CellCept Tablets (16.1% to 54.3%) 2951
Celontin Capsules 2618
▲ Cenestin Tablets (68%) 1263
Ceptaz for Injection (Fewer than 1%) 1499
▲ Cerebyx Injection (2.2% to 8.9%) 2619
▲ Cerezyme for Injection (5.4%) 1438
Cetrotide for Injection (1.1%) 3209
▲ Chemet Capsules (5.2% to 15.7%) 3078
▲ Chirocaine Injection (4.5%) 2909
Cipro HC Otic Suspension (1.2%) 540
Cipro I.V. (Greater than 1%) 893
Cipro I.V. Pharmacy Bulk Package (Greater than 1%) 897
Cipro (1% to 1.2%) 887
Claforan Injection (Less than 1%) 732
▲ Claritin (12%) 3100
▲ Claritin-D 12 Hour Extended Release Tablets (19%) 3102
Claritin-D 24 Hour Extended Release Tablets 3104
Cleocin Vaginal Cream (Less than 1% to 2%) 2788
Cleocin Vaginal Ovules (Less than 1%) 2789
Climara Transdermal System 958
▲ Clinoril Tablets (3% to 9%) 2053
Clomid Tablets (1.3%) 735
Clorpres Tablets (About 1 in 100) 1002
▲ Clozaril Tablets (More than 5% to 7%) 2319
▲ Cognex Capsules (11%) 1351
▲ Colazal Capsules (8%) 3069
Colestid Tablets 2791
▲ CombiPatch Transdermal System (17% to 25%) 2323
Combipres Tablets (About 1 in 100) 1040
▲ Combivent Inhalation Aerosol (5.6%) 1041
▲ Combivir Tablets (35%) 1502
Compazine 1505
▲ Concerta Extended-Release Tablets (14%) 1998
▲ Concerta Tablets (14%) 561
▲ Condylox Gel (7%) 2436
Copaxone for Injection (At least 2%) 3306
Cordarone Tablets (1% to 3%) 3487
▲ Coreg Tablets (8.1%) 1508
Corgard Tablets (1 to 5 per 1000 patients) 2245
▲ Corlopam Injection (More than 5%) 412
Cormax Scalp Application (Approximately 0.3%) 2441
Cortifoam Rectal Foam 3170
Cortone Acetate Injectable Suspension 2059
Cortone Acetate Tablets 2061
▲ Corvert Injection (3.6%) 2793
Corzide 40/5 Tablets (1 to 5 of 1000 patients) 2247
Corzide 80/5 Tablets (1 to 5 of 1000 patients) 2247
Cosopt Sterile Ophthalmic Solution (1% to 5%) 2065
Coumadin for Injection (Infrequent) 1243
Coumadin Tablets (Infrequent) 1243
▲ Covera-HS Tablets (2.2% to 6.6%) 3199
Cozaar Tablets (1% or greater) 2067
▲ Crinone (19%) 3213
▲ Crixivan Capsules (5.6%) 2070
Cyclessa Tablets 2450
Cylert Tablets 415
CytoGam Intravenous (Infrequent) 2026
Cytotec Tablets (2.4%) 3202
Cytovene (At least 3 subjects) 2959
Dantrium Capsules (Less frequent) 2885
Dapsone Tablets USP 1780
Daranide Tablets 2077
Darvon-N/Darvocet-N 1907
Darvon Pulvules 1909
Darvon Compound-65 Pulvules 1910
Darvon-N Tablets 1912
▲ DaunoXome Injection (3% to 22%) 1442
DDAVP Injection 4 mcg/mL (Infrequent) 737
▲ DDAVP Nasal Spray (2 to 5%) 738
▲ DDAVP Rhinal Tube (2 to 5%) 738
▲ DDAVP Tablets (4%) 739
Decadron Elixir 2078
Decadron Tablets 2079
Decadron Phosphate Injection 2081
Declomycin Tablets 1855
Delatestryl Injection 1151
▲ Demadex Tablets and Injection (7.3%) 2965
Demerol 3079
Demser Capsules (Infrequent) 2085
▲ Depacon Injection (4.3% to 31%) 416
▲ Depakene (31%) 421
▲ Depakote Sprinkle Capsules (31%) 426
▲ Depakote Tablets (31%) 430
Depakote ER Tablets (Greater than 1%) 436
▲ DepoCyt Injection (18% to 53%) 1197
Depo-Medrol Injectable Suspension 2795
▲ Depo-Provera Contraceptive Injection (More than 5%) 2798
Desferal Vials 2333
▲ Desmopressin Acetate Rhinal Tube (2% to 5%) 1345
Desogen Tablets 2458
Desoxyn Tablets 440
▲ Detrol Tablets (11%) 3623
▲ Detrol LA Capsules (6%) 2801
Dexedrine 1512
DextroStat Tablets 3236
D.H.E. 45 Injection (Occasional) 2334
Didronel Tablets 2888
▲ Diflucan Tablets, Injection, and Oral Suspension (1.9% to 13%) 2681
▲ Digitek Tablets (4%) 1003
Dilantin Infatabs 2624
Dilantin Kapseals 2622
Dilantin-125 Oral Suspension 2625
Dilaudid Oral Liquid (Less frequent) 445
Dilaudid Tablets - 8 mg (Less frequent) 445
Dilaudid-HP (Less frequent) 443
Diovan Capsules (More than 1%) 2337
Diovan HCT Tablets (More than 2%) 2338
▲ Dipentum Capsules (5.0%) 2803
Diphtheria & Tetanus Toxoids Adsorbed Purogenated for Pediatric Use 1857
Diprivan Injectable Emulsion (Less than 1%) 667
▲ Ditropan XL Extended Release Tablets (9.8%) 564
Diucardin Tablets 3494
Diuril Oral 2087
Diuril Sodium Intravenous 2086
Dobutrex Solution Vials (1% to 3%) 1914
▲ Dolobid Tablets (3% to 9%) 2088
Dolophine Hydrochloride Tablets 3056
Donnatal 2929
Donnatal Extentabs 2930
Donnatal Tablets 2929
Dopram Injectable 2931
▲ Dostinex Tablets (26%) 2804
▲ Doxil Injection (Approximately 5.3% to 6.8%) 566
Duraclon Injection (1%) 3057
▲ Duragesic Transdermal System (3% to 10%) 1786
Duramorph Injection (A significant minority of cases) 1312
Duranest Injections 600
Dyazide Capsules 1515
▲ Dynabac Tablets (7.7% to 8.6%) 2269
Dynacin Capsules 2019
▲ DynaCirc Capsules (10.7% to 22%) 2921
▲ DynaCirc CR Tablets (10.3% to 18.3%) 2923
Dyrenium Capsules (Rare) 3458
▲ EC-Naprosyn Delayed-Release Tablets (3% to 9%) 2967
Ecotrin Enteric Coated Aspirin Low, Regular and Maximum Strength Tablets 1715
Edecrin 2091
▲ Effexor Tablets (3% to 25%) 3495
▲ Effexor XR Capsules (4%) 3499
8-MOP Capsules 1727
▲ Eldepryl Capsules (2 of 49 patients) 3266
▲ Elmiron Capsules (3%) 570
Elspar for Injection 2092
▲ Emadine Ophthalmic Solution (11%) ⊙ 211
Emcyt Capsules (1%) 2810
Enalaprilat Injection (2.9%) 863
▲ Enbrel for Injection (24%) 1752
▲ Enbrel for Injection (24%) 3504
▲ Engerix-B Vaccine (1% to 10%) 1517
Epifrin Sterile Ophthalmic Solution ⊙ 235
EpiPen 1236
▲ Epivir (35%) 1520
▲ Epivir-HBV (21%) 1524
▲ Epogen for Injection (0.4% to 19%) 582
▲ Ergamisol Tablets (3% to 4%) 1789
▲ Esclim Transdermal System (6.4% to 18.8%) 3460
Eskalith 1527
Estinyl Tablets 3112
Estrace Vaginal Cream 3358
Estrace Tablets 3361
Estratest 3252
▲ Estring Vaginal Ring (13%) 2811
Estrostep 2627
Etrafon 3115
▲ Evoxac Capsules (14.4%) 1217
▲ Exelon Capsules (17%) 2342
▲ Exelon Oral Solution (17%) 2345
Factrel (Rare) 3633
▲ Famotidine Injection (4.7%) 866
▲ Famvir Tablets (16% to 39.3%) 2348
▲ Felbatol (6.5% to 36.8%) 3343
▲ Feldene Capsules (1% to 10%) 2685
▲ Femara Tablets (8% to 12%) 2351
▲ femhrt Tablets (39.5%) 2635
▲ Ferrlecit Injection (7%) 3386
Flexeril Tablets (1% to 3%) 572
Flexeril Tablets (1% to 3%) 2094
▲ Flolan for Injection (49% to 83%) 1528
▲ Flomax Capsules (19.3% to 21.1%) 1044
▲ Flonase Nasal Spray (6.6% to 16.1%) 1533
Florinef Acetate Tablets 2250
▲ Flovent Diskus (12%) 3614
▲ Flovent (17% to 34%) 1535
▲ Flovent Rotadisk (9% to 15%) 1537
▲ Floxin I.V. (1% to 9%) 2526

Floxin Otic Solution (0.3%) 1219
▲ Floxin Tablets (1% to 9%) 2529
Fludara for Injection (Up to 3%) 995
Flumadine (1.4%) 1370
Fluorescite Injection ⊙211
Fluothane Inhalation (Rare) 3508
FluShield Influenza Vaccine 3521
Follistim for Injection 2465
Foradil Aerolizer 2354
Fortaz (Less than 1%) 1541
▲ Fortovase Capsules (5% to 8.9%) 2970
Fosamax Tablets (0.6% to 2.6%) 2095
▲ Foscavir Injection (5% to 26%) 605
Sterile FUDR (Remote possibility) 2974
Furosemide Tablets 2284
Gabitril Tablets (1% or more) 1189
Gamimune N, 5% Solvent/Detergent Treated 925
Gamimune N, 10% Solvent/Detergent Treated 928
Gammagard S/D (Occasional) 845
▲ Gammar-P I.V. (5.4%) 787
▲ Gastrocrom Oral Concentrate (4 of 87 patients) 1162
Gemzar for Injection (Common) 1919
▲ Gengraf Capsules (2% to 25%) 457
Genotropin Lyophilized Powder 2818
Geocillin Tablets 2687
▲ Geref for Injection (Less than 6%) 3215
Ginkoba Tablets (Very rare) ▣828
Ginsana Sport Capsules ▣831
▲ Gleevec Capsules (24% to 28%) 2357
▲ Gliadel Wafer (15%) 1723
▲ Glucophage Tablets (5.7%) 1080
Glucophage XR Tablets (1% to 5%) 1080
Glucotrol Tablets (About 1 in 50) 2692
▲ Glucotrol XL Extended Release Tablets (8.6%) 2693
▲ Glucovance Tablets (8.9%) 1086
▲ Gonal-F for Injection (12.5% to 22%) 3216
Grifulvin V Tablets Microsize and Oral Suspension Microsize (Occasional) 2518
Gris-PEG Tablets (Occasional) 2661
Guaifed 2272
▲ Halcion Tablets (9.7%) 2823
Haldol Decanoate 2535
Haldol Injection, Tablets and Concentrate 2533
▲ Havrix Vaccine (9% to 14%) 1544
Hectorol Capsules 1064
▲ Hectorol Injection (27.9%) 1066
Heparin Lock Flush Solution 3509
Heparin Sodium Injection 3511
▲ Herceptin I.V. (26%) 1414
Hivid Tablets (Less than 1% to 2.1%) 2975
▲ Humatrope Vials and Cartridges (6.07% to 9.38%) 1930
Humegon for Injection 2468
Humorsol Sterile Ophthalmic Solution 2102
▲ Hyalgan Solution (18%) 3080
▲ Hycamtin for Injection (0.2% to 21%) 1546
Hydrocortone Tablets 2106
Hydrocortone Acetate Injectable Suspension 2103
Hydrocortone Phosphate Injection, Sterile 2105
HydroDIURIL Tablets 2108
▲ Hytrin Capsules (1.1% to 16.2%) 464
Hyzaar (1% or greater) 2109
▲ Idamycin PFS Injection (20%) 2825
▲ Imdur Tablets (38% to 57%) 1826
Imitrex Injection (2.2%) 1549
Imitrex Tablets 1558
▲ Imovax Rabies Vaccine (About 20%) 807
▲ Indapamide Tablets (Greater than or equal to 5%) 2286
Inderide Tablets 3517
Inderide LA Long-Acting Capsules 3519
▲ Indocin (11.7%) 2112
INFeD Injection 3388
▲ Infergen (78% to 82%) 1777
Infumorph 200 and Infumorph 500 Sterile Solutions (A significant minority of cases) 1314
Innohep Injection (1.7%) 1248
▲ Intron A for Injection (4% to 62%) 3120
Invirase Capsules (Rare) 2979
Ionamin Capsules 1163
Iopidine 0.5% Ophthalmic Solution (Less than 3%) ⊙213
Iopidine Sterile Ophthalmic Solution ⊙212
Iscar Mali Injection 3456
Iscar Mali Special Injection 3456
Iscar Pini Injection 3456
Iscar Quercus Injection 3456
Iscar Quercus Special Injection 3456
▲ Ismo Tablets (19% to 38%) 3524
Isoptin SR Tablets (2.2%) 467
Isopto Carbachol Ophthalmic Solution ⊙215
▲ Isordil Sublingual Tablets (Most common) 3525
▲ Isordil Titradose Tablets (Most common) 3526
Iveegam EN (0.3% to 0.8%) 849
▲ JE-VAX Vaccine (Less than 3% to approximately 15.2%) 811
Kadian Capsules (Less than 3%) 1335
▲ Kaletra Capsules (1.6% to 7.1%) 471
▲ Kaletra Oral Solution (1.6% to 7.1%) 471
Keflex 1237
▲ Keppra Tablets (14%) 3314
Klonopin Tablets 2983
Koāte-DVI (0.7%) 931
Konÿne 80 937
K-Phos Neutral Tablets 946
▲ Kytril Injection (14%) 2986
▲ Kytril Tablets (14% to 21%) 2988
▲ Lamictal (29.1%) 1567
▲ Lamisil Tablets (12.9%) 2360
Lanoxicaps Capsules 1574
Lanoxin Injection 1581
Lanoxin Tablets 1587
Lanoxin Elixir Pediatric 1578
Lanoxin Injection Pediatric 1584
▲ Lariam Tablets (Among most frequent) 2989
▲ Lescol Capsules (8.9%) 2361
▲ Lescol Capsules (8.9%) 2925
▲ Lescol XL Tablets (4.7%) 2361
▲ Lescol XL Tablets (4.7%) 2925
▲ Leukine (26% to 36%) 1755
▲ Leustatin Injection (7% to 22%) 2495
Levaquin (0.1% to 5.4%) 2537
Levbid Extended-Release Tablets 3172
Levlen 962
Levlite 21 Tablets 962
Levlite 28 Tablets 962
Levora Tablets 3389
Levoxyl Tablets 1819
Levsin/Levsinex/Levbid 3172
▲ Lexxel Tablets (10.3%) 608
Limbitrol 1738
▲ Lipitor Tablets (2.5% to 16.7%) 2639
▲ Lipitor Tablets (2.5% to 16.7%) 2696
Lithium Carbonate 3061
Lithium Citrate Syrup 3061
Lithobid Slow-Release Tablets 3255
▲ Livostin (5%) ⊙305
Lodine (Less than 1%) 3528
Lodine XL Extended-Release Tablets (Less than 1%) 3530
Lodosyn Tablets 1251
Loestrin 21 Tablets 2642
Loestrin Fe Tablets 2642
Lo/Ovral Tablets 3532
Lo/Ovral-28 Tablets 3538
Lopid Tablets (1.2%) 2650
Lorabid Suspension and Pulvules (0.9% to 3.2%) 2251
▲ Lotemax Sterile Ophthalmic Suspension 0.5% (Less than 15%) ⊙261
▲ Lotensin Tablets (6.2%) 2365
▲ Lotensin HCT Tablets (3.1%) 2367
Lotrel Capsules (2.2%) 2370
Low-Ogestrel-28 Tablets 3392
Loxitane Capsules 3398
Lufyllin Tablets 3347
Lufyllin-400 Tablets 3347
Lufyllin-GG Elixir 3348
Lufyllin-GG Tablets 3348
Lumigan Ophthalmic Solution (1% to 5%) 553
Lunelle Monthly Injection 2827
▲ Lupron Depot 3.75 mg (25.9%) 3281
Lupron Depot 7.5 mg (Less than 5%) 3284
▲ Lupron Depot–3 Month 11.25 mg (25.9% to 32%) 3285
▲ Lupron Depot–3 Month 22.5 mg (6.4%) 3288
▲ Lupron Depot–4 Month 30 mg (4.2% to 10.2%) 3289
Lupron Depot-PED 7.5 mg, 11.25 mg and 15 mg (Less than 2%) 3291
▲ Lupron Injection (5% or more) 3279
Lupron Injection Pediatric (Less than 2%) 3280
▲ Luvox Tablets (25, 50, 100 mg) (3% to 22%) 3256
▲ LYMErix Vaccine (5.06% to 5.61%) 1592
▲ Macrobid Capsules (6%) 2889
▲ Malarone (17% to 22%) 1596
Marinol Capsules (Less than 1%) 3325
Matulane Capsules 3246
Mavik Tablets (More than 1%) 478
Maxair Autohaler (1.3% to 2.0%) 1981
Maxair Inhaler (1.3% to 2%) 1984
Maxalt Tablets (Less than 2%) 2120
Maxalt-MLT Orally Disintegrating Tablets (Less than 2%) 2120
Maxipime for Injection (0.1% to 1%) 1285
Maxzide 1008
▲ Megace Oral Suspension (Up to 10%) 1124
Menest Tablets 2254
Menomune-A/C/Y/W-135 Vaccine (1.8% to 5.2%) 813
Mepergan Injection 3539
▲ Mepron Suspension (16% to 31%) 1598
▲ Meridia Capsules (30.3%) 481
Merrem I.V. (2.3%) 673
Meruvax II 2130
▲ Metadate CD Capsules (12%) 1164
Metadate ER Tablets 1167
Methylin Tablets 1995
Methylin ER Tablets 1995
▲ MetroGel-Vaginal Gel (5%) 1986
▲ Mevacor Tablets (2.1% to 9.3%) 2132
▲ Mexitil Capsules (5.7% to 7.5%) 1047
▲ Miacalcin Nasal Spray (3.2%) 2375
Micardis Tablets (1%) 1049
Micardis HCT Tablets (2% or greater) 1051
Microgestin Fe 1.5/30 Tablets 3407
Microgestin Fe 1/20 Tablets 3400
Micronor Tablets 2543
Microzide Capsules 3414
▲ Midamor Tablets (3% to 8%) 2136
Miltown Tablets 3349
▲ Minipress Capsules (7.8%) 2699
▲ Minizide Capsules (7.8%) 2700
Minocin Intravenous 1862
Minocin Oral Suspension 1865
Minocin Pellet-Filled Capsules 1863
Mintezol 2137
Mirapex Tablets (1% or more) 2834
Mircette Tablets 2470
▲ Mirena Intrauterine System (5% or more) 974
Mithracin for Intravenous Use 903
M-M-R II 2118
▲ Mobic Tablets (2.4% to 8.3%) 1054
Modicon 2563
▲ Moduretic Tablets (3% to 8%) 2138
Mononine Concentrate 794
Monopril Tablets (Less than 1.0% to 1.0% or more) 1091
▲ Monopril HCT (7%) 1094
▲ Monurol Sachet (3.9% to 10.3%) 1375
Motofen Tablets (1 in 40) 577
Motrin Suspension, Oral Drops, Chewable Tablets, and Caplets (1% to less than 3%) 2002
MS Contin Tablets (Less frequent) 2896
MSIR (Less frequent) 2898
▲ MUSE Urethral Suppository (3%) 3335
Myambutol Tablets 1290
▲ Mycobutin Capsules (3%) 2838
▲ Mykrox Tablets (9.3%) 1168
Mylocel Tablets (Extremely rare) 2227
▲ Mylotarg for Injection (12% to 50%) 3540
▲ Myobloc Injectable Solution (10% to 16%) 1291
▲ Nabi-HB (26%) 2295
Nadolol Tablets (1 to 5 of 1000 patients) 2288
▲ Naprelan Tablets (15%) 1293
▲ Naprosyn Suspension (3% to 9%) 2967
▲ Naprosyn Tablets (3% to 9%) 2967
Nardil Tablets (Common) 2653
▲ Naropin Injection (1% to 7.7%) 612
▲ Nasacort Nasal Inhaler (Approximately 18%) 750
Nasacort AQ Nasal Spray (2% or greater) 752
Nasalide Nasal Spray (5% or less) 1295
Nascobal Gel (One patient) 3174
▲ Nasonex Nasal Spray (17% to 26%) 3131
▲ Natrecor for Injection (8%) 3189
Navelbine Injection 1604
Nebcin Vials, Hyporets & ADD-Vantage 1955
Necon 3415
Nembutal Sodium Solution 485
▲ Neoral Soft Gelatin Capsules (2% to 25%) 2380
▲ Neoral Oral Solution (2% to 25%) 2380
Nesacaine/Nesacaine MPF 617
▲ Neumega for Injection (41%) 1434
▲ Neupogen for Injection (7%) 587
Neurontin Capsules 2655
Neurontin Oral Solution (More than 2%) 2655
Neurontin Tablets 2655
▲ Nexium Delayed-Release Capsules (3.8% to 5.5%) 619
▲ Niaspan Extended-Release Tablets (5% to 11%) 1846
▲ Nicotrol Inhaler (26%) 2840
▲ Nicotrol Nasal Spray (18%) 2843
▲ Nilandron Tablets (13.9%) 753
Nimotop Capsules (Up to 4.1%) 904
▲ Nipent for Injection (13% to 17%) 3272
▲ Nitro-Dur Transdermal Infusion System (63%) 1834
▲ Nitro-Dur Transdermal Infusion System (63%) 3134
▲ Nitrolingual Pumpspray (50%) 1355
Nitrostat Tablets 2658
Nizoral Tablets (Less than 1%) 1791
Nolvadex Tablets (Infrequent) 678
Nordette-28 Tablets 2257
Norditropin Cartridges (Small number of patients) 2420
Norditropin for Injection (Small number of patients) 2419
Norflex 1987
Norinyl 1 +35 28-Day Tablets 3380
Norinyl 1 + 50 28-Day Tablets 3380
Normodyne Tablets (2%) 3137
Noroxin Tablets (2.0% to 2.8%) 2145
Norplant System 3543
Norpramin Tablets 755
Nor-QD Tablets 3423
▲ Norvasc Tablets (7.3%) 2704
▲ Norvir Capsules (5.1% to 6.3%) 487
▲ Norvir Oral Solution (5.1% to 6.3%) 487
▲ Novantrone for Injection (5% to 13%) 1760
Novarel for Injection 1347
NovoSeven (1%) 2430
▲ Nubain Injection (3%) 1323
NuLev Orally Disintegrating Tablets 3176
Numorphan 1324
Nutropin AQ Injection (A small number of patients) 1420
▲ Nutropin Depot for Injectable Suspension (13%) 1423
Nutropin for Injection (A small number of patients) 1417
Ocupress Ophthalmic Solution, 1% Sterile (Occasional) ⊙303
Ogen Tablets 2846
Ogestrel 0.5/50-28 Tablets 3428
Omnicef (2%) 493
Oncaspar (Greater than 1% but less than 5%) 756
OptiPranolol Metipranolol Ophthalmic Solution 0.3% (A small number of patients) ⊙263
▲ Optivar Ophthalmic Solution (Approximately 15%) 2273
Oramorph SR Tablets (Less frequent) 3062
▲ Orap Tablets (22.2%) 1407
Organidin NR Liquid (Rare) 3350
Organidin NR Tablets (Rare) 3350
Orgaran Injection (2.6%) 2480
Ortho Dienestrol Cream 2554
Ortho-Cept 21 Tablets 2546
Ortho-Cept 28 Tablets 2546
▲ Orthoclone OKT3 Sterile Solution (11% to 44%) 2498
Ortho-Cyclen/Ortho Tri-Cyclen 2573
Ortho-Est Tablets 3464
Ortho-Novum 2563
Ortho-Novum 1/50▫28 Tablets 2556
▲ Ortho-Prefest Tablets (23%) 2570
Ortho-Cyclen/Ortho Tri-Cyclen 2573
▲ Orudis Capsules (3% to 9%) 3548
▲ Oruvail Capsules (3% to 9%) 3548
Ovcon 3364
Ovidrel for Injection (Less than 2%) 3220
Ovral Tablets 3551
Ovral-28 Tablets 3552
Ovrette Tablets 3552
Oxsoralen-Ultra Capsules 1741
▲ OxyContin Tablets (7%) 2912
Pacerone Tablets (1% to 3%) 3331
Parnate Tablets 1607
▲ Patanol Ophthalmic Solution (7%) 540
▲ Paxil (17% to 18%) 1609
Pediapred Oral Solution 1170
Pediazole Suspension 3050
▲ PEG-Intron Powder for Injection (56%) 3140
Pentasa Capsules (2.0% to 2.2%) 3239
▲ Pepcid Injection (4.7%) 2153
▲ Pepcid for Oral Suspension (4.7%) 2150
▲ Pepcid RPD Orally Disintegrating Tablets (4.7%) 2150
▲ Pepcid Tablets (4.7%) 2150
Pergonal for Injection 3223
Periactin Tablets 2155
▲ Periostat Tablets (26%) 1208
▲ Permax Tablets (5.3%) 1299
Persantine Tablets (2.3%) 1057
Phenergan with Codeine Syrup 3557
Phenergan VC with Codeine Syrup 3561
Phrenilin (Infrequent) 578
Pipracil 1866
Plaquenil Tablets 3082
Plasmanate (Occasional) 942
▲ Plavix Tablets (7.6%) 1097
▲ Plavix Tablets (7.6%) 3084
▲ Plendil Extended-Release Tablets (10.6% to 14.7%) 623
▲ Pletal Tablets (27% to 34%) 2605
▲ Pletal Tablets (27% to 34%) 2848
Pneumovax 23 2156
▲ Ponstel Capsules (1% to 10%) 1356
▲ Prandin Tablets (0.5, 1, and 2 mg) (9% to 11%) 2432
▲ Pravachol Tablets (1.7% to 6.2%) 1099
Prednisone 3064
Pregnyl for Injection 2482
Prelone Syrup 2273
Premarin Intravenous 3563
Premarin Tablets 3566
Premarin Vaginal Cream 3570
Premphase Tablets 3572
▲ Prempro Tablets (28% to 36%) 3572
Prevacid Delayed-Release Capsules (Greater than 1%) 3292
▲ PREVPAC (1% to 6%) 3298
Priftin Tablets (1.1%) 758
▲ Prilosec Delayed-Release Capsules (2.9% to 7%) 628
Primacor Injection (2.9%) 3086
Primaxin I.M. 2158
Primaxin I.V. (Less than 0.2%) 2160
▲ Prinivil Tablets (4.4% to 5.7%) 2164
▲ Prinzide Tablets (5.2%) 2168

ProAmatine Tablets (Less frequent) 3241
▲ Procardia Capsules (Approximately 10% to 23%) 2708
▲ Procardia XL Extended Release Tablets (15.8% to 23%) 2710
▲ Procrit for Injection (0.40% to 19%) 2502
▲ Prograf (37% to 64%) 1393
▲ Proleukin for Injection (12%) 1199
▲ Prometrium Capsules (100 mg, 200 mg) (10% to 31%) 3261
Propine Ophthalmic Solution ⊙ 250
Proplex T 851
▲ ProSom Tablets (16%) 500
Prostigmin Injectable 1744
Prostigmin Tablets 1744
▲ Prostin E2 Suppositories (Approximately one-tenth) 2852
Protonix I.V. (Greater than 1%) 3580
▲ Protonix Tablets (6% to 9%) 3577
Protopam Chloride for Injection 3582
▲ Protopic Ointment (10% to 20%) 1397
Proventil Inhalation Aerosol 3142
▲ Proventil Inhalation Solution 0.083% (3% to 3.1%) 3146
▲ Proventil Repetabs Tablets (7% to 22%) 3148
▲ Proventil Solution for Inhalation 0.5% (3% to 3.1%) 3144
Proventil HFA Inhalation Aerosol 3150
Provera Tablets 2853
▲ Provigil Tablets (50%) 1193
▲ Prozac Pulvules, Liquid, and Weekly Capsules (21%) 1238
▲ Pulmicort Turbuhaler Inhalation Powder (2% to 14%) 636
▲ Quinaglute Dura-Tabs Tablets (3%) 978
▲ Quinidex Extentabs (7%) 2933
Quixin Ophthalmic Solution (1% to 3%) 3093
▲ Qvar Inhalation Aerosol (8% to 25%) 1987
▲ Rabies Vaccine RabAvert (10% to 52%) 1203
▲ Rapamune Oral Solution and Tablets (23% to 34%) 3584
▲ Rebetron Combination Therapy (63% to 67%) 3153
Recombivax HB (Equal to or greater than 1%) 2178
ReFacto Vials 1437
Reglan (Less frequent) 2935
▲ Relafen Tablets (3% to 9%) 1617
Relenza Rotadisk (2%) 1619
▲ Remicade for IV Injection (20% to 23%) 1178
▲ Reminyl Oral Solution (8%) 1792
▲ Reminyl Tablets (8%) 1792
▲ Renagel Capsules (10%) 1439
▲ Renagel Tablets (10%) 1439
Renese Tablets 2712
▲ Repronex for Intramuscular and Subcutaneous Injection (5.2% to 6%) 1347
Requip Tablets (1% or more) 1621
▲ Rescriptor Tablets (5.6%) 526
Rescula Ophthalmic Solution (1% to 5%) ⊙ 306
▲ Retrovir Capsules (1.6% to 62.5%) 1625
▲ Retrovir IV Infusion (2% to 62.5%) 1629
▲ Retrovir (1.6% to 62.5%) 1625
▲ Rēv-Eyes Sterile Ophthalmic Eyedrops 0.5% (10% to 40%) ⊙ 265
Rifadin 765
Rifamate Capsules 767
Rifater Tablets 769
▲ Rilutek Tablets (7.0% to 8.0%) 772
▲ Risperdal (12% to 14%) 1796
Ritalin 2387
▲ Rituxan for Infusion (14%) 1750
▲ Rituxan I.V. (14%) 1428
Robaxin Injectable 2938
Robaxin Tablets 2939
Robaxisal Tablets 2939
Robinul Forte Tablets 1358
Robinul Injectable 2940
Robinul Tablets 1358
Rocaltrol 2991
Rocephin Injectable Vials, ADD-Vantage, Galaxy, Bulk (Occasional) 2993
▲ Roferon-A Injection (44% to 66%) 2996
▲ Romazicon Injection (1% to 9%) 3000
▲ Rowasa Rectal Suspension Enema 4.0 grams/unit (60 mL) (6.5%) 3264
Roxanol 3066
▲ Roxicodone Tablets (Greater than or equal to 3%) 3067
Rynatan Tablets 3351
▲ Rythmol Tablets – 150 mg, 225 mg, 300 mg (1.9% to 6%) 502
Saizen for Injection (A small number of patients) 3225
▲ Salagen Tablets (11%) 2229
▲ Sandimmune (2 to 15%) 2388
Sandoglobulin I.V. 2391
▲ Sandostatin Injection (6%) 2394
▲ Sarafem Pulvules (13% to 24%) 1962
▲ Sectral Capsules (6%) 3589
Sedapap Tablets 50 mg/650 mg (Infrequent) 2225
▲ Semprex-D Capsules (19%) 1172
Sensorcaine 643
Sensorcaine-MPF Injection 643
Septra Suspension 2265
Septra Tablets 2265
Septra DS Tablets 2265
▲ Serevent Diskus (13% to 17%) 1637
▲ Serevent Inhalation Aerosol (12% to 28%) 1633
Serophene Tablets (Less than 1 in 100 patients) 3226
▲ Seroquel Tablets (19%) 684
▲ Serostim for Injection (19.0%) 3229
▲ Serzone Tablets (36%) 1104
▲ Simulect for Injection (Greater than or equal to 10%) 2399
Sinemet Tablets 1253
Sinemet CR Tablets (2.0%) 1255
Sinequan (Occasional) 2713
▲ Singulair (18.4%) 2181
Skelaxin Tablets 1301
▲ Skelid Tablets (6.7%) 3088
Solu-Medrol Sterile Powder 2855
Soma Tablets 3353
Soma Compound Tablets (Infrequent or rare) 3354
Soma Compound w/Codeine Tablets (Infrequent or rare) 3355
▲ Sonata Capsules (28% to 38%) 3591
▲ Soriatane Capsules (1% to 10%) 3003
▲ Sporanox Capsules (1% to 10%) 1800
Sporanox Injection (2%) 1804
Sporanox Injection (2%) 2509
▲ Sporanox Oral Solution (4.3% to 4.4%) 1808
▲ Sporanox Oral Solution (4.3% to 4.4%) 2512
▲ Stadol NS Nasal Spray (3% to 9%) 1108
Stelazine 1640
Stimate Nasal Spray 796
Streptase for Infusion 647
Streptomycin Sulfate Injection 2714
Stromectol Tablets (0.2%) 2185
▲ Sular Tablets (22%) 688
Suprane Liquid for Inhalation (Greater than 1%) 874
Suprax (Less than 2%) 1877
Surmontil Capsules 3595
▲ Sustiva Capsules (5% to 6%) 1258
Symmetrel (1% to 5%) 1328
▲ Synarel Nasal Solution for Endometriosis (19% of patients) 3205
Synercid I.V. (1.6%) 775
Synvisc 3596
Tagamet (2.1% to 3.5%) 1644
Talacen Caplets 3089
Talwin Nx Tablets 3090
▲ Tambocor Tablets (9.6%) 1990
▲ Tamiflu Capsules (1.8% to 20.1%) 3008
▲ Tamiflu Oral Suspension (1.8% to 20.1%) 3008
Tapazole Tablets 1823
▲ Tarka Tablets (8.9%) 508
▲ Tasmar Tablets (10% to 11%) 3010
Tazicef for Injection (Less than 1%) 1647
Tazicef Galaxy Container (Less than 1%) 1650
Tazicef Pharmacy Bulk Package (Less than 1%) 1653
Tazidime Vials, Faspak & ADD-Vantage (Less than 1%) 1966
Tegretol/Tegretol-XR 2404
▲ Temodar Capsules (41%) 3157
Temovate Scalp Application (1 of 294 patients) 1304
▲ Tenex Tablets (1% to 13%) 2942
Tenoretic Tablets 690
Tenormin 692
▲ Tequin Injection (3%) 1110
▲ Tequin Tablets (3%) 1110
▲ Terazol 3 Vaginal Cream (21%) 2587
▲ Terazol 3 Vaginal Suppositories (30.3% of 284 patients) 2587
▲ Terazol 7 Vaginal Cream (26% of 521 patients) 2587
Tessalon Capsules 1377
▲ Testoderm Transdermal Systems (5%) 574
Testopel Pellets 3610
Testred Capsules, 10 mg 1746
Tetanus & Diphtheria Toxoids Adsorbed for Adult Use 1880
Tetanus and Diphtheria Toxoids Adsorbed For Adult Use (2%) 815
Teveten Tablets (1% or greater) 3327
▲ Thalomid Capsules (12.5%) 1154
Theo-Dur Extended-Release Tablets 1835
TheraCys Injection (2%) 823
Thioplex for Injection 1765
Thioridazine Hydrochloride Tablets (Extremely rare) 2289
▲ Thymoglobulin for Injection (40.2%) 3071
Thyrel TRH for Injection 3630
▲ Thyrogen for Injection (7.3%) 1441
▲ Tiazac Capsules (8%) 1378
Tice BCG, BCG Live (2.4%) 2489
Ticlid Tablets (0.5% to 1.0%) 3015
▲ Tikosyn Capsules (11%) 2717
Timentin Injection- ADD-Vantage Vial 1661
Timentin Injection-Galaxy Container 1664
Timentin Injection-Pharmacy Bulk Package 1666
Timentin for Intravenous Administration 1658
Timolide Tablets (Less than 1%) 2187
Timolol GFS (1% to 5%) ⊙ 266
Timoptic in Ocudose (Less frequent) 2192
Timoptic Sterile Ophthalmic Solution (Less frequent) 2190
Timoptic-XE Sterile Ophthalmic Gel Forming Solution (1% to 5%) 2194
▲ TOBI Solution for Inhalation (26.7%) 1206
▲ Tolectin (3% to 9%) 2589
Tonocard Tablets (2.1% to 4.6%) 649
Topamax Sprinkle Capsules (More than 1%) 2590
Topamax Tablets (More than 1%) 2590
Toprol-XL Tablets 651
▲ Toradol (17%) 3018
Transderm Scōp Transdermal Therapeutic System (Few patients) 2302
Tranxene (Less common) 511
Travatan Ophthalmic Solution (1% to 5%) 543
Trecator-SC Tablets 3598
Trental Tablets (1.2%) 784
▲ Tricor Capsules, Micronized (5%) 513
Trilafon 3160
▲ Trileptal Oral Suspension (15% to 32%) 2407
▲ Trileptal Tablets (15% to 32%) 2407
Tri-Levlen 962
Trilisate (Less than 2%) 2901
▲ Tri-Nasal Spray (44.3% to 51%) 2274
Tri-Norinyl-28 Tablets 3433
Triphasil-21 Tablets 3600
Triphasil-28 Tablets 3605
▲ Trisenox Injection (60%) 1158
Trivora Tablets 3439
▲ Trizivir Tablets (28%) 1669
Trovan (1% to 5%) 2722
Trusopt Sterile Ophthalmic Solution (Infrequent) 2196
Tussi-Organidin NR Liquid 3350
Tussi-Organidin DM NR Liquid (Rare) 3350
Tussi-Organidin DM-S NR Liquid (Rare) 3350
Tussi-Organidin-S NR Liquid 3350
▲ Twinrix Vaccine (13% to 22%) 1674
▲ TYPHIM Vi Vaccine (Up to 27%) 825
Ultracet Tablets (At least 1%) 2597
▲ Ultram Tablets (18% to 32%) 2600
Unasyn for Injection (Less than 1%) 2728
Uni-Dur Extended-Release Tablets 1841
Uniphyl 400 mg and 600 mg Tablets 2903
Uniretic Tablets (More than 1%) 3178
Unithroid Tablets 3445
Univasc Tablets (More than 1%) 3181
Urecholine 2198
Urecholine Tablets 2445
Uroqid-Acid No. 2 Tablets 947
▲ Vagifem Tablets (9% to 10%) 2857
▲ Valcyte Tablets (9% to 22%) 3022
Valium Injectable 3026
Valium Tablets (Infrequent) 3047
▲ Valstar Sterile Solution for Intravesical Instillation (4%) 1175
▲ Valtrex Caplets (14% to 38%) 1676
▲ Vancenase AQ Nasal Spray 0.084% (34%) 3163
▲ Vanceril Double Strength Inhalation Aerosol (22%) 3167
▲ Vaniqa Cream (4%) 1121
Vantin Tablets and Oral Suspension (Less than 1% to 1.1%) 2860
▲ Vaqta (0.4% to 16%) 2199
Varivax (Greater than or equal to 1%) 2202
▲ Vascor Tablets (6.98% to 13.64%) 2602
▲ Vaseretic Tablets (5.5%) 2204
Vasotec I.V. Injection (2.9%) 2207
Vasotec Tablets (1.8% to 5.2%) 2210
▲ Venofer Injection (Greater than 5%) 580
▲ Ventolin Inhalation Aerosol and Refill (3%) 1679
Ventolin HFA Inhalation Aerosol 3618
Verelan Capsules (2.2% to 5.3%) 3184
▲ Verelan PM Capsules (2.2% to 12.1%) 3186
Versed Injection (1.3% to 1.5%) 3027
▲ Vesanoid Capsules (86%) 3037
Vexol 1% Ophthalmic Suspension (Less than 2%) ⊙ 222
▲ Viadur Implant (4.6%) 912
▲ Viagra Tablets (16%) 2732
▲ Vicoprofen Tablets (27%) 520
▲ Videx (6% to 7%) 1138
▲ Videx EC Capsules (21%) 1143
▲ Vioxx (7.5%) 2213
Viracept 532
▲ Viramune Oral Suspension (3%) 1060
▲ Viramune Tablets (3%) 1060
Visicol Tablets 1767
▲ Vistide Injection (30%) 1445
▲ Visudyne for Injection (10% to 20%) ⊙ 308
▲ Vitravene for Injection (5% to 20%) ⊙ 310
Vivactil Tablets 2217
Vivactil Tablets 2446
Vivelle Transdermal System 2412
Vivelle-Dot Transdermal System 2416
Vivotif Berna 997
▲ Volmax Extended-Release Tablets (18.8%) 2276
Voltaren Ophthalmic Sterile Ophthalmic Solution (Less than 3%) ⊙ 312
▲ Voltaren Tablets (3% to 9%) 2315
▲ Voltaren-XR Tablets (3% to 9%) 2315
Warfarin Sodium Tablets, USP 3302
▲ WelChol Tablets (6%) 3073
▲ Wellbutrin SR Sustained-Release Tablets (25% to 26%) 1684
WinRho SDF (2%) 2297
▲ Xanax Tablets (12.9% to 29.2%) 2865
Xeloda Tablets (1%) 3039
▲ Xenical Capsules (30.6%) 3043
Xylocaine Injections 653
Yasmin 28 Tablets (Greater than 1%) 980
▲ YF-VAX Vaccine (2% to 5%) 827
Yodoxin Tablets 1722
▲ Zaditor Ophthalmic Solution (10% to 25%) 2304
Zantac 1690
Zantac Injection 1688
Zantac Syrup 1690
Zarontin Capsules 2659
Zarontin Syrup 2660
Zaroxolyn Tablets 1177
▲ Zebeta Tablets (8.8% to 10.9%) 1885
▲ Zenapax for Injection (Greater than 5%) 3046
Zephrex Tablets 3091
Zephrex LA Tablets 3092
▲ Zerit (54%) 1147
▲ Zestoretic Tablets (5.2%) 695
▲ Zestril Tablets (4.4% to 5.7%) 698
Ziac Tablets (0.4% to 4.5%) 1887
▲ Ziagen (16%) 1692
Zithromax Capsules, 250 mg (1% or less) 2743
Zithromax for IV Infusion (1% or less) 2748
Zithromax for Oral Suspension, 1 g (1% or less) 2743
Zithromax for Oral Suspension, 300 mg, 600 mg, 900 mg, 1200 mg (1% or less) 2739
Zithromax Tablets, 250 mg (1% or less) 2739
Zithromax Tablets, 600 mg (1% or less) 2743
▲ Zocor Tablets (3.5%) 2219
▲ Zofran Injection (17% to 25%) 1698
▲ Zofran (9% to 27%) 1703
▲ Zofran ODT Orally Disintegrating Tablets (9% to 27%) 1703
▲ Zoladex (1% to 75%) 702
Zoladex 3-month (1% to 5%) 706
▲ Zoloft (26%) 2751
▲ Zometa for Intravenous Infusion (5% to 10%) 3621
▲ Zonegran Capsules (10%) 1307
▲ Zosyn (4.5% to 7.7%) 1890
▲ Zosyn in Galaxy Containers (4.5% to 7.7%) 1894
Zovia 3449
Zovirax Capsules (2.2%) 1706
Zovirax for Injection (Less than 1%) 1708
Zovirax (2.2%) 1706
Zyban Sustained-Release Tablets (Frequent) 1710
▲ Zyflo Filmtab Tablets (24.6%) 524
▲ Zyprexa Tablets (17%) 1973
▲ Zyprexa ZYDIS Orally Disintegrating Tablets (17%) 1973
▲ Zyrtec (11.0% to 14.0%) 2756
▲ Zyrtec-D 12 Hour Extended Relief Tablets 2758
▲ Zyvox (1.9% to 6.5%) 2871

Headache, migraine
Meridia Capsules 481
Norvasc Tablets (Less than or equal to 0.1%) 2704
Paxil (Rare) 1609
Prozac Pulvules, Liquid, and Weekly Capsules (Infrequent) 1238
Sarafem Pulvules (Infrequent) 1962
Serophene Tablets 3226
Sustiva Capsules (Less than 2%) 1258
▲ Wellbutrin Tablets (25.7%) 1680
Wellbutrin SR Sustained-Release Tablets (Up to 4%) 1684
Zyban Sustained-Release Tablets (Infrequent) 1710

Headache, periorbital
Pilopine HS Ophthalmic Gel ⊙ 217

Headache, positional
▲ Xylocaine Injections (3%) 653

Headache, sinus
Avonex 1013
Colestid Tablets 2791
▲ Periostat Tablets (5%) 1208
Serevent Diskus (1% to 3%) 1637

▲ Serevent Inhalation Aerosol (4%) 1633

Headache, supraorbital

Isopto Carpine .... ⊙215

Headache, temporal

Pilopine HS Ophthalmic Gel .... ⊙217

Headache, transient

Aralen Tablets 3075
DDAVP Injection 4 mcg/mL (Infrequent) 737
DDAVP Nasal Spray (Infrequent) 738
DDAVP Rhinal Tube (Infrequent) 738
Desmopressin Acetate Injection (Infrequent) 1344
Plaquenil Tablets 3082

Healing, abnormal

Cafcit (2.2%) 1035
▲ Gliadel Wafer (14%) 1723
Lupron Depot–4 Month 30 mg (Less than 5%) 3289
▲ Prograf (3% to 15%) 1393
Soriatane Capsules (Less than 1%) 3003

Hearing, impaired

Accutane Capsules 2944
Anaprox Tablets (Less than 1%) 2967
Anaprox DS Tablets (Less than 1%) 2967
Arthrotec Tablets (Rare) 3195
Desferal Vials 2333
Diamox Sequels Sustained Release Capsules .... ⊙270
EC-Naprosyn Delayed-Release Tablets (Less than 1%) 2967
Feldene Capsules (Rare) 2685
Kefurox Vials, ADD-Vantage 1948
Mustargen for Injection 2142
Naprosyn Suspension (Less than 1%) 2967
Naprosyn Tablets (Less than 1%) 2967
Naropin Injection (Less than 1%) 612
Norvir Capsules (Less than 2%) 487
Norvir Oral Solution (Less than 2%) 487
Orudis Capsules (Less than 1%) 3548
Oruvail Capsules (Less than 1%) 3548
Ponstel Capsules (Rare) 1356
Prostin E2 Suppositories 2852
Requip Tablets (Infrequent) 1621
Streptomycin Sulfate Injection 2714
Trilisate (Less than 2%) 2901
Vesanoid Capsules (Less than 1%) 3037
Vicodin Tablets (Very rare) 516
Vicodin ES Tablets (Very rare) 517
Vicodin HP Tablets (Very rare) 518

Hearing, loss of

Abelcet Injection 1273
Aggrenox Capsules 1026
Alka-Seltzer .... ▣603
Alka-Seltzer Lemon Lime Antacid and Pain Reliever Effervescent Tablets .... ▣603
Alka-Seltzer Extra Strength Antacid and Pain Reliever Effervescent Tablets .... ▣603
Alka-Seltzer PM Effervescent Tablets .... ▣605
Altace Capsules (Less than 1%) 2233
Ancobon Capsules 1730
Azulfidine EN-tabs Tablets (Rare) 2775
Genuine Bayer Tablets, Caplets and Gelcaps .... ▣606
Extra Strength Bayer Caplets and Gelcaps .... ▣610
Aspirin Regimen Bayer Children's Chewable Tablets (Orange or Cherry Flavored) .... ▣607
Aspirin Regimen Bayer Regular Strength 325 mg Caplets .... ▣606
Extra Strength Bayer Arthritis Caplets .... ▣610
Extra Strength Bayer PM Caplets .. ▣611
Cataflam Tablets (Less than 1%) 2315
Cipro I.V. (1% or less) 893
Cipro I.V. Pharmacy Bulk Package (Less than 1%) 897
Cipro (Less than 1%) 887
Demadex Tablets and Injection 2965
Depacon Injection 416
Depakene 421
Depakote Sprinkle Capsules 426
Depakote Tablets 430
Depakote ER Tablets 436
Desferal Vials 2333
Dolobid Tablets (Rare) 2088
Ecotrin Enteric Coated Aspirin Low, Regular and Maximum Strength Tablets 1715
▲ Fludara for Injection (2% to 6%) 995
Furosemide Tablets 2284
Gengraf Capsules (2% or less) 457
Hivid Tablets (Less than 1%) 2975
Imitrex Nasal Spray 1554
Matulane Capsules 3246
Miacalcin Nasal Spray (Less than 1%) 2375
Momentum Backache Relief Extra Strength Caplets .... ▣666
Motrin Suspension, Oral Drops, Chewable Tablets, and Caplets (Less than 1%) 2002
Nebcin Vials, Hyporets & ADD-Vantage 1955
Neoral Soft Gelatin Capsules (2% or less) 2380
Neoral Oral Solution (2% or less) 2380
Neurontin Capsules (Infrequent) 2655
Neurontin Oral Solution (Infrequent) 2655
Neurontin Tablets (Infrequent) 2655
Orthoclone OKT3 Sterile Solution 2498
Pediazole Suspension 3050
PREVPAC 3298
Primaxin I.M. 2158
Primaxin I.V. (Less than 0.2%) 2160
Quinidex Extentabs 2933
Retrovir Capsules 1625
Retrovir IV Infusion 1629
Retrovir 1625
Sandimmune (2% or less) 2388
Sandostatin Injection (Less than 1%) 2394
TOBI Solution for Inhalation 1206
Tonocard Tablets (0.4% to 1.5%) 649
Toradol (1% or less) 3018
Trilisate (Rare) 2901
Vancocin HCl Capsules & Pulvules (A few dozen cases) 1972
Vancocin HCl Oral Solution (A few dozen cases) 1971
Vancocin HCl, Vials & ADD-Vantage (Few dozen cases) 1970
▲ Vesanoid Capsules (6%) 3037
Vistide Injection 1445
Voltaren Tablets (Less than 1%) 2315
Voltaren-XR Tablets (Less than 1%) 2315
Zinacef Injection (A few pediatric patients) 1696
Zinacef for Injection (A few pediatric patients) 1696
Zithromax Capsules, 250 mg 2743
Zithromax for IV Infusion 2748
Zithromax for Oral Suspension, 300 mg, 600 mg, 900 mg, 1200 mg 2739
Zithromax Tablets, 250 mg 2739

Hearing decreased

Aralen Tablets 3075
Aricept Tablets (Infrequent) 1270
Aricept Tablets (Infrequent) 2665
Ativan Injection (Infrequent) 3478
▲ Avonex (3%) 1013
Campath Ampules 992
Clinoril Tablets (Less than 1%) 2053
Coreg Tablets (Less than or equal to 0.1%) 1508
Dynacin Capsules (Rare) 2019
Evoxac Capsules (Less than 1%) 1217
Felbatol 3343
Floxin I.V. (Less than 1%) 2526
Floxin Tablets (Less than 1%) 2529
Fortovase Capsules (Less than 2%) 2970
Invirase Capsules (Less than 2%) 2979
Minocin Intravenous (Rare) 1862
Minocin Oral Suspension (Rare) 1865
Minocin Pellet-Filled Capsules (Rare) 1863
ProSom Tablets (Rare) 500
Risperdal (Rare) 1796
▲ Serostim for Injection (1% to 10%) 3229
Topamax Sprinkle Capsules (1.6% to 1.8%) 2590
Topamax Tablets (1.6% to 1.8%) 2590
▲ Visudyne for Injection (1% to 10%) .... ⊙308
Ziac Tablets 1887

Hearing disturbances

Amerge Tablets (Infrequent) 1467
Anaprox Tablets (Less than 3%) 2967
Anaprox DS Tablets (Less than 3%) 2967
Avalide Tablets 1070
Avapro Tablets (Less than 1%) 1074
Avapro Tablets (Less than 1%) 3076
Diamox .... ⊙269
EC-Naprosyn Delayed-Release Tablets (Less than 3%) 2967
Floxin I.V. 2526
Floxin Tablets 2529
Imitrex Nasal Spray (Infrequent) 1554
Imitrex Tablets (Infrequent) 1558
Indocin Capsules (Less than 1%) 2112
Indocin I.V. (Less than 1%) 2115
Indocin (Less than 1%) 2112
Intron A for Injection (Less than 5%) 3120
Lupron Injection 3279
Naprelan Tablets (Less than 3%) 1293
Naprosyn Suspension (Less than 3%) 2967
Naprosyn Tablets (Less than 3%) 2967
Roferon-A Injection (Less than 4%) 2996
Zithromax Capsules, 250 mg 2743
Zithromax for IV Infusion 2748
Zithromax for Oral Suspension, 300 mg, 600 mg, 900 mg, 1200 mg 2739
Zithromax Tablets, 250 mg 2739

Hearing loss, reversible

Cataflam Tablets (Less than 1%) 2315
Chibroxin Sterile Ophthalmic Solution 2051
Depacon Injection 416
Depakene 421
Depakote Tablets 430
Depakote ER Tablets 436
E.E.S. (Isolated reports) 450
EryPed (Isolated reports) 446
Ery-Tab Tablets (Isolated reports) 448
Erythrocin Stearate Filmtab Tablets (Isolated reports) 452
Erythromycin Base Filmtab Tablets (Isolated reports) 454
Erythromycin Delayed-Release Capsules, USP (Isolated reports) 455
Noroxin Tablets (Rare) 2145
PCE Dispertab Tablets (Isolated reports) 498
Pediazole Suspension (Isolated reports) 3050
Quinaglute Dura-Tabs Tablets 978
Romazicon Injection (Less than 1%) 3000
Voltaren Tablets (Less than 1%) 2315
Voltaren-XR Tablets (Less than 1%) 2315

Heart beat, irregular

Adenocard Injection 1380
Indapamide Tablets (Less than 5%) 2286
Iopidine Sterile Ophthalmic Solution (Less than 2%) .... ⊙212
K-Phos Neutral Tablets 946
K-Phos Original (Sodium Free) Tablets (Less frequent) 947
Maxair Inhaler (Less than 1%) 1984
Children's Motrin Oral Suspension and Chewable Tablets 2006
Children's Motrin Oral Suspension .... ▣643
Infants' Motrin Concentrated Drops 2006
Junior Strength Motrin Caplets and Chewable Tablets 2006
Uroqid-Acid No. 2 Tablets 947
Vioxx (Greater than 0.1% to 1.9%) 2213

Heart beats, ectopic

Imitrex Injection (Infrequent) 1549
Imitrex Nasal Spray 1554
Imitrex Tablets 1558

Heart beats, premature

Plendil Extended-Release Tablets (0.5% to 1.5%) 623
▲ Taxol Injection (23%) 1129

Heart block

(*see also under* Sinoatrial block)

Actimmune (Rare) 1772
Adenocard Injection 1380
Agrylin Capsules 3232
Aricept Tablets 1270
Aricept Tablets 2665
Betagan .... ⊙228
Betaxon Ophthalmic Suspension (Less than 2%) 537
Betimol Ophthalmic Solution .... ⊙324
Betoptic S Ophthalmic Suspension (Rare) 537
Brevibloc Injection (Less than 1%) 858
Carteolol Hydrochloride Ophthalmic Solution USP, 1% .... ⊙258
Cordarone Tablets (2% to 5%) 3487
Digitek Tablets 1003
Diprivan Injectable Emulsion (Less than 1%) 667
Etrafon 3115
Flexeril Tablets (Rare) 572
Flexeril Tablets (Rare) 2094
Imitrex Nasal Spray 1554
Imitrex Tablets (Rare) 1558
Lanoxicaps Capsules 1574
Lanoxin Injection 1581
Lanoxin Tablets 1587
Lanoxin Elixir Pediatric 1578
Lanoxin Injection Pediatric 1584
Levaquin (Less than 0.3%) 2537
Limbitrol 1738
Naropin Injection 612
Normodyne Injection (Rare) 3135
Normodyne Tablets (Less common) 3137
Norpramin Tablets 755
Ocupress Ophthalmic Solution, 1% Sterile .... ⊙303
Pacerone Tablets (2% to 5%) 3331
Paxil (Rare) 1609
Permax Tablets (Rare) 1299
Polocaine Injection, USP 625
Polocaine-MPF Injection, USP 625
Prozac Pulvules, Liquid, and Weekly Capsules (Rare) 1238
Rum-K 1363
Sarafem Pulvules (Rare) 1962
Sensorcaine 643
Sensorcaine-MPF Injection 643
Surmontil Capsules 3595
Tenex Tablets (Rare) 2942
▲ Tenormin (4.5%) 692
Tikosyn Capsules (1.2%) 2717
Timoptic in Ocudose (Less frequent) 2192
Timoptic Sterile Ophthalmic Solution (Less frequent) 2190
Trasylol Injection (1% to 2%) 909
Vascor Tablets 2602
Vivactil Tablets 2217
Vivactil Tablets 2446

Heart block, second degree

Dipentum Capsules (Rare) 2803
Procanbid Extended-Release Tablets (Two of almost 500 patients) 2262
Zofran Injection (Rare) 1698

Heart block, third degree

Corgard Tablets (Single instance) 2245
Nadolol Tablets (Single instance) 2288
Wellbutrin Tablets 1680

Heart defects, congenital

Clomid Tablets 735
Thalomid Capsules 1154

Heart failure

Abelcet Injection 1273
Accupril Tablets (Rare) 2611
Accuretic Tablets (0.5% to 1%) 2614
Actimmune (Rare) 1772
Activase I.V. 1410
Aggrenox Capsules (1.6%) 1026
Agrylin Capsules (1% to 5%) 3232
Aloprim for Injection (Less than 1%) 2292
Altace Capsules (2.0%) 2233
Apligraf (2.7%) 2305
Aredia for Injection (Up to 1%) 2309
Avalide Tablets 1070
Avapro Tablets (Less than 1%) 1074
Avapro Tablets (Less than 1%) 3076
Betapace Tablets (2% to 5%) 950
Betaseron for SC Injection 988
Betimol Ophthalmic Solution .... ⊙324
Blocadren Tablets 2046
Brevibloc Injection 858
Campath Ampules 992
Carteolol Hydrochloride Ophthalmic Solution USP, 1% (In some cases) .... ⊙258
Celexa (Infrequent) 1365
▲ CellCept Capsules (11.8%) 2951
▲ CellCept Intravenous (11.8%) 2951
▲ CellCept Oral Suspension (11.8%) 2951
▲ CellCept Tablets (11.8%) 2951
Cognex Capsules (Infrequent) 1351
Coreg Tablets (More than 2%) 1508
Corgard Tablets (1 of 100 patients) 2245
Corlopam Injection (0.5% to 5%) 412
Corzide 40/5 Tablets (1 of 100 patients) 2247
Corzide 80/5 Tablets (1 of 100 patients) 2247
Cosopt Sterile Ophthalmic Solution (Less than 1%) 2065
Dantrium Capsules (Less frequent) 2885
Dantrium Intravenous 2886
Diprivan Injectable Emulsion (Less than 1%) 667
Dostinex Tablets (Rare) 2804
Doxil Injection (Less than 1%) 566
DynaCirc Capsules (0.5% to 1%) 2921
DynaCirc CR Tablets (0.5% to 1%) 2923
Enbrel for Injection (Infrequent) 1752
Enbrel for Injection (Infrequent) 3504
Exelon Capsules (Frequent) 2342
Exelon Oral Solution (Frequent) 2345
Fareston Tablets (1%) 3237
Felbatol 3343
▲ Flolan for Injection (11%) 1528
Flumadine (Less than 0.3%) 1370
Gengraf Capsules (1% to less than 3%) 457
Herceptin I.V. 1414
Hivid Tablets (Less than 1%) 2975
Imdur Tablets (Less than or equal to 5%) 1826
Intron A for Injection (Less than 5%) 3120
Isoptin SR Tablets 467
Levaquin (0.3% to less than 0.5%) 2537
Levoxyl Tablets 1819
Lovenox Injection (0.95%) 746
Merrem I.V. (0.1% to 1.0%) 673
Mirapex Tablets (Less than 1%) 2834
Mobic Tablets (Less than 2%) 1054
Nadolol Tablets (1 of 100 patients) 2288
Neoral Soft Gelatin Capsules (1% to less than 3%) 2380

(▣ Described in PDR For Nonprescription Drugs) Incidence data in parenthesis; ▲ 3% or more (⊙ Described in PDR For Ophthalmic Medicines™)

Neoral Oral Solution (1% to less than 3%) 2380
Neurontin Capsules (Rare) 2655
Neurontin Oral Solution (Rare) 2655
Neurontin Tablets (Rare) 2655
▲ Nilandron Tablets (3%) 753
Nipent for Injection (Less than 3%) 3272
Normodyne Tablets 3137
Norvasc Tablets (Less than or equal to 0.1%) 2704
Ocupress Ophthalmic Solution, 1% Sterile (In some cases) ⊙ 303
Omnicef 493
Orthoclone OKT3 Sterile Solution 2498
Paraplatin for Injection 1126
▲ Photofrin for Injection (7%) 831
Plavix Tablets (1% to 2.5%) 1097
Plavix Tablets (1% to 2.5%) 3084
Procardia XL Extended Release Tablets (Rare) 2710
Pulmozyme Inhalation Solution 1426
▲ Refludan for Injection (3%) 761
Remeron Tablets (Rare) 2483
Remeron SolTab Tablets (Rare) 2486
Remicade for IV Injection (Less than 2%) 1178
Reminyl Oral Solution (Infrequent) 1792
Reminyl Tablets (Infrequent) 1792
Requip Tablets (Infrequent) 1621
Retavase Vials 1182
Rilutek Tablets (Infrequent) 772
Rituxan for Infusion (Rare) 1750
Rituxan I.V. (Rare) 1428
Roxicodone Tablets (Less than 3%) 3067
Sandostatin LAR Depot (1% to 4%) 2395
Sectral Capsules (Up to 2%) 3589
▲ Simulect for Injection (3% to 10%) 2399
Tasmar Tablets (Infrequent) 3010
Taxotere for Injection Concentrate (Rare) 778
Tenoretic Tablets 690
▲ Tenormin (19%) 692
Thalomid Capsules 1154
Timolide Tablets (Less than 1%) 2187
Timolol GFS ⊙ 266
Timoptic in Ocudose (Less frequent) 2192
Timoptic Sterile Ophthalmic Solution (Less frequent) 2190
Timoptic-XE Sterile Ophthalmic Gel Forming Solution 2194
TNKase I.V. 1430
Toprol-XL Tablets 651
▲ Trasylol Injection (5%) 909
Trileptal Oral Suspension 2407
Trileptal Tablets 2407
Unithroid Tablets 3445
Verelan Capsules 3184
Verelan PM Capsules 3186
▲ Vesanoid Capsules (6%) 3037
Viagra Tablets (Less than 2%) 2732
Zanaflex Tablets (Rare) 1305
Zebeta Tablets 1885
Zonegran Capsules (Rare) 1307
Zosyn (1.0% or less) 1890
Zosyn in Galaxy Containers (1.0% or less) 1894
Zyprexa Tablets 1973
Zyprexa ZYDIS Orally Disintegrating Tablets 1973
Zyrtec (Less than 2%) 2756
Zyrtec-D 12 Hour Extended Relief Tablets (Less than 2%) 2758

Heart failure, congestive
(*see under* Congestive heart failure)

Heart failure, worsening of
Avandia Tablets 1490
Prinivil Tablets (Greater than 1%) 2164
Prinzide Tablets 2168
Toprol-XL Tablets 651
Vascor Tablets (1.9%) 2602
Zestoretic Tablets 695
Zestril Tablets (Greater than 1%) 698

Heart rate, changes
▲ Blocadren Tablets (5%) 2046
Cardura Tablets (About 0.7%) 2668
D.H.E. 45 Injection 2334
Dopram Injectable 2931
Fortovase Capsules (Less than 2%) 2970
Invirase Capsules (Less than 2%) 2979
Zemuron Injection 2491

Heart rate, changes fetal
Brethine Ampuls 2314
▲ Prepidil Gel (17.0%) 2851
Sectral Capsules 3589

Heart rate, decrease
Betagan ⊙ 228
▲ Duraclon Injection (Among most frequent) 3057
Guaifed 2272
ProAmatine Tablets 3241

Heart rate, increased
Brethine Ampuls 2314
DDAVP Injection 4 mcg/mL (Infrequent) 737
Desmopressin Acetate Injection (Infrequent) 1344
▲ Dobutrex Solution Vials (7.5% to approximately 10%) 1914
Effexor Tablets 3495
Hivid Tablets (Less than 1%) 2975
Levaquin 2537
Meridia Capsules 481
One-A-Day Tension & Mood Softgels ▣ 808
Serevent Inhalation Aerosol 1633
Versed Syrup (Less than 1%) 3033

Heart sounds, abnormal
Gengraf Capsules (1% to less than 3%) 457
Neoral Soft Gelatin Capsules (1% to less than 3%) 2380
Neoral Oral Solution (1% to less than 3%) 2380
▲ Simulect for Injection (3% to 10%) 2399

Heart spasms
(*see under* Cardiospasm)

Heartburn
▲ Aerobid/Aerobid-M (3% to 9%) 1363
Aleve Tablets, Caplets and Gelcaps ▣ 602
▲ Alferon N Injection (3%) 1770
▲ Anaprox Tablets (3% to 9%) 2967
▲ Anaprox DS Tablets (3% to 9%) 2967
Arthrotec Tablets (Rare) 3195
Avalide Tablets (2%) 1070
Avapro Tablets (2%) 1074
Avapro Tablets (2%) 3076
Genuine Bayer Professional Labeling (Aspirin Regimen Bayer) ▣ 608
Betapace AF Tablets (2% to 2.5%) 954
Cleocin Vaginal Cream (Less than 1%) 2788
▲ Clozaril Tablets (4%) 2319
Colestid Tablets (Less frequent) 2791
Combivent Inhalation Aerosol 1041
DiaBeta Tablets (1.8%) 741
Dipentum Capsules 2803
▲ EC-Naprosyn Delayed-Release Tablets (3% to 9%) 2967
Ecotrin Enteric Coated Aspirin Low, Regular and Maximum Strength Tablets 1715
Eldepryl Capsules 3266
Etrafon 3115
▲ Feldene Capsules (1% to 10%) 2685
Floxin I.V. 2526
Floxin Tablets 2529
Glucophage XR Tablets (1% to 5%) 1080
Hivid Tablets (Less than 1%) 2975
▲ Indocin (3% to 9%) 2112
Klonopin Tablets (Infrequent) 2983
Lodosyn Tablets 1251
Mevacor Tablets (1.6%) 2132
▲ Mexitil Capsules (39.3% to 39.6%) 1047
Midamor Tablets (Less than or equal to 1%) 2136
Moduretic Tablets 2138
Monopril Tablets (0.2% to 1.0%) 1091
Monopril HCT (Less than 2%) 1094
▲ Motrin Suspension, Oral Drops, Chewable Tablets, and Caplets (3% to 9%) 2002
▲ Naprelan Tablets (3% to 9%) 1293
▲ Naprosyn Suspension (3% to 9%) 2967
▲ Naprosyn Tablets (3% to 9%) 2967
Noroxin Tablets (0.3% to 1.0%) 2145
Phrenilin (Infrequent) 578
▲ Ponstel Capsules (1% to 10%) 1356
Pravachol Tablets (2.0% to 2.9%) 1099
Primaxin I.M. 2158
Primaxin I.V. (Less than 0.2%) 2160
Prinivil Tablets (0.3% to 1.0%) 2164
Prinzide Tablets (0.3% to 1%) 2168
ProAmatine Tablets (Rare) 3241
▲ Procardia Capsules (11%) 2708
▲ Procardia XL Extended Release Tablets (11%) 2710
Proventil Inhalation Aerosol (Less than 5%) 3142
▲ Quinaglute Dura-Tabs Tablets (Among most frequent) 978
▲ Quinidex Extentabs (Among most frequent) 2933
Rifadin (Some patients) 765
Rifamate Capsules (Some patients) 767
Rifater Tablets 769
Sedapap Tablets 50 mg/650 mg (Infrequent) 2225
Serevent Inhalation Aerosol (1% to 3%) 1633
Sinemet Tablets 1253
Sinemet CR Tablets 1255
Syprine Capsules 2186
Toprol-XL Tablets (About 1 of 100 patients) 651
▲ Trilisate (Less than 20%) 2901
Ventolin Inhalation Aerosol and Refill (Less than 5%) 1679
▲ Vioxx (3.6%) 2213
▲ Zenapax for Injection (Greater than 5%) 3046
Zestoretic Tablets (0.3% to 1%) 695
Zestril Tablets (0.3% to 1.0%) 698

Heat intolerance
Alferon N Injection (1%) 1770
Imitrex Tablets 1558
Levoxyl Tablets 1819
Unithroid Tablets 3445

Heat stroke
Clozaril Tablets 2319
Cogentin 2055
Compazine 1505
Evoxac Capsules (Less than 1%) 1217
Haldol Decanoate 2535
Haldol Injection, Tablets and Concentrate 2533
Levsin/Levsinex/Levbid 3172
Loxitane Capsules 3398
Orap Tablets 1407
Protonix I.V. (Less than 1%) 3580
Protonix Tablets (Less than 1%) 3577
Serentil 1057
Stelazine 1640

Heavy sensation, arms
Adenocard Injection (Less than 1%) 1380

Heavy sensation, legs
Eldepryl Capsules 3266
K-Phos Neutral Tablets 946
K-Phos Original (Sodium Free) Tablets (Less frequent) 947

Hemangiomata
Antagon Injection 2447
Cetrotide for Injection 3209

Hemarthrosis
Innohep Injection 1248
Kaletra Capsules 471
Kaletra Oral Solution 471
NovoSeven (Greater than or equal to 2%) 2430
Remicade for IV Injection (Less than 2%) 1178

Hematemesis
Aggrenox Capsules 1026
AmBisome for Injection (Less common) 1383
▲ Amphotec (5% or more) 1774
Anaprox Tablets (Less than 1%) 2967
Anaprox DS Tablets (Less than 1%) 2967
Arthrotec Tablets (Rare) 3195
Betaseron for SC Injection 988
Campath Ampules 992
Clozaril Tablets (Less than 1%) 2319
Copaxone for Injection (Infrequent) 3306
Depacon Injection (1% to 5%) 416
Depakene (1% to 5%) 421
Depakote Sprinkle Capsules (1% to 5%) 426
Depakote Tablets (1% to 5%) 430
Depakote ER Tablets (Greater than 1%) 436
EC-Naprosyn Delayed-Release Tablets (Less than 1%) 2967
Effexor Tablets (Rare) 3495
Effexor XR Capsules (Rare) 3499
Exelon Capsules (Infrequent) 2342
Exelon Oral Solution (Infrequent) 2345
Felbatol 3343
Feldene Capsules (Occasional) 2685
Geodon Capsules (Rare) 2688
Herceptin I.V. (At least one of the 958 patients) 1414
Imitrex Injection 1549
Imitrex Nasal Spray (Rare) 1554
Imitrex Tablets (Rare) 1558
Innohep Injection 1248
Lamictal 1567
▲ Leukine (13%) 1755
Lufyllin Tablets 3347
Lufyllin-400 Tablets 3347
Lufyllin-GG Elixir 3348
Lufyllin-GG Tablets 3348
Luvox Tablets (25, 50, 100 mg) (Rare) 3256
Matulane Capsules 3246
Mithracin for Intravenous Use 903
Mobic Tablets (Less than 2%) 1054
Motrin Suspension, Oral Drops, Chewable Tablets, and Caplets (Less than 1%) 2002
▲ Naprelan Tablets (3% to 9%) 1293
Naprosyn Suspension (Less than 1%) 2967
Naprosyn Tablets (Less than 1%) 2967
Neurontin Capsules (Rare) 2655
Neurontin Oral Solution (Rare) 2655
Neurontin Tablets (Rare) 2655
Orudis Capsules (Less than 1%) 3548
Oruvail Capsules (Less than 1%) 3548
Paxil (Rare) 1609
Permax Tablets (Infrequent) 1299
▲ Photofrin for Injection (8%) 831
Pletal Tablets (Less than 2%) 2605
Pletal Tablets (Less than 2%) 2848
Ponstel Capsules (Occasional) 1356
Prevacid Delayed-Release Capsules (Less than 1%) 3292
PREVPAC (Less than 1%) 3298
Proleukin for Injection (Less than 1%) 1199
Protonix I.V. (Less than 1%) 3580
Protonix Tablets (Less than 1%) 3577
Prozac Pulvules, Liquid, and Weekly Capsules (Rare) 1238
ReoPro Vials (5 to 11 events) 1958
Requip Tablets (Rare) 1621
Rilutek Tablets (Rare) 772
Risperdal (Rare) 1796
Sarafem Pulvules (Rare) 1962
Seroquel Tablets (Infrequent) 684
Tequin Injection (Less than 0.1%) 1110
Tequin Tablets (Less than 0.1%) 1110
Theo-Dur Extended-Release Tablets 1835
Tricor Capsules, Micronized (Less than 1%) 513
Trileptal Oral Suspension 2407
Trileptal Tablets 2407
Uni-Dur Extended-Release Tablets 1841
Xeloda Tablets (Less than 5%) 3039
Zanaflex Tablets (Rare) 1305
Zoladex 3-month (1% to 5%) 706
Zomig Tablets (Rare) 708
Zomig-ZMT Tablets (Rare) 708
Zonegran Capsules (Rare) 1307

Hematochezia
Adriamycin PFS/RDF Injection 2767
Avonex 1013
Bicillin C-R 900/300 Injection 2240
Bicillin C-R Injection 2238
Bicillin L-A Injection 2242
Cataflam Tablets (Less than 1%) 2315
Cognex Capsules (Infrequent) 1351
Colestid Tablets (Infrequent) 2791
Coumadin for Injection 1243
Coumadin Tablets 1243
Dipentum Capsules (Rare) 2803
Fortovase Capsules (Less than 2%) 2970
Glucotrol XL Extended Release Tablets (Less than 1%) 2693
Hivid Tablets (Less than 1%) 2975
Invirase Capsules (Less than 2%) 2979
Neurontin Capsules (Infrequent) 2655
Neurontin Oral Solution (Infrequent) 2655
Neurontin Tablets (Infrequent) 2655
Orudis Capsules (Less than 1%) 3548
Oruvail Capsules (Less than 1%) 3548
Rescriptor Tablets (Less than 2%) 526
Trileptal Oral Suspension 2407
Trileptal Tablets 2407
Vioxx (Greater than 0.1% to 1.9%) 2213
Voltaren Tablets (Less than 1%) 2315
Voltaren-XR Tablets (Less than 1%) 2315
Warfarin Sodium Tablets, USP 3302

Hematocrit, decrease
Aceon Tablets (2 mg, 4 mg, 8 mg) 3249
Actos Tablets 3275
Aggrastat (2.2%) 2031
Aggrenox Capsules 1026
Altace Capsules (Rare) 2233
▲ Argatroban Injection (10.4%) 1478
Atacand Tablets 595
Atacand HCT Tablets 597
Avandia Tablets 1490
Blocadren Tablets 2046
▲ Cancidas for Injection (1.5% to 11.1%) 2048
Cefobid Pharmacy Bulk Package - Not for Direct Infusion (1 in 20) 2673
▲ Cipro I.V. (Among most frequent) 893
▲ Cipro I.V. Pharmacy Bulk Package (Among most frequent) 897
Diovan Capsules (0.8%) 2337
Diovan HCT Tablets 2338
Dopram Injectable 2931
Dynabac Tablets (0.1% to 1%) 2269
Enalaprilat Injection (Frequent) 863
Hivid Tablets (Less than 1%) 2975
Hyzaar 2109
Infergen (1% or less) 1777
▲ Kefurox Vials, ADD-Vantage (1 in 10) 1948
▲ Lariam Tablets (Among most frequent) 2989
Lodosyn Tablets 1251
Lopid Tablets (Occasional) 2650
Lupron Depot 7.5 mg (Greater than or equal to 5%) 3284
▲ Lupron Depot–4 Month 30 mg (Greater than or equal to 5%) 3289
Merrem I.V. (Greater than 0.2%) 673
Micardis HCT Tablets (0.6%) 1051
Monopril Tablets 1091
Monurol Sachet 1375
Motrin Suspension, Oral Drops, Chewable Tablets, and Caplets (Less than 1%) 2002
Noroxin Tablets (Less frequent) 2145

Omnicef for Oral Suspension (0.2%) ... 493
Panhematin for Injection ... 497
Precose Tablets ... 906
Primaxin I.M. ... 2158
Primaxin I.V. ... 2160
Prinivil Tablets (Frequent) ... 2164
Prinzide Tablets (Frequent) ... 2168
ReoPro Vials (7 to 11 events) ... 1958
Serzone Tablets (2.8%) ... 1104
Sinemet Tablets ... 1253
Sinemet CR Tablets (1% or greater) ... 1255
Timentin Injection- ADD-Vantage Vial ... 1661
Timentin Injection-Galaxy Container ... 1664
Timentin Injection-Pharmacy Bulk Package ... 1666
Timentin for Intravenous Administration ... 1658
Tolectin (1% to 3%) ... 2589
Tranxene ... 511
Trovan (Greater than or equal to 1%) ... 2722
Unasyn for Injection ... 2728
Vantin Tablets and Oral Suspension ... 2860
Vaseretic Tablets (0.5% to 2.0%) ... 2204
Vasotec I.V. Injection (Frequent) ... 2207
Vasotec Tablets (Frequent) ... 2210
Xanax Tablets (Less than 1%) ... 2865
Zestoretic Tablets (Frequent) ... 695
Zestril Tablets (Frequent) ... 698
▲ Zinacef Injection (1 in 10 patients) . 1696
▲ Zinacef for Injection (1 in 10 patients) ... 1696
Zosyn ... 1890
Zosyn in Galaxy Containers ... 1894

Hematocrit, increase
▲ AndroGel (3% to 6%) ... 3322
Clozaril Tablets ... 2319
Epogen for Injection ... 582
Maxipime for Injection (0.1% to 1%) ... 1285
Procrit for Injection ... 2502
Synarel Nasal Solution for Endometriosis ... 3205

Hematocrit content, deviation
▲ Avonex (3%) ... 1013

Hematologic reactions
Cefotan (1.4%) ... 664
Dapsone Tablets USP ... 1780
Daraprim Tablets ... 1511
Floxin I.V. ... 2526
Floxin Tablets ... 2529
Lamictal ... 1567
Lopid Tablets ... 2650
Procanbid Extended-Release Tablets (Fairly common) ... 2262

Hematologic toxicity
Adriamycin PFS/RDF Injection ... 2767
Depen Titratable Tablets ... 3341
Doxil Injection ... 566
Sterile FUDR ... 2974
Hivid Tablets (Less than 1%) ... 2975
Retrovir IV Infusion ... 1629

Hematoma
Aceon Tablets (2 mg, 4 mg, 8 mg) (0.3% to 1%) ... 3249
Advair Diskus 100/50 (1% to 3%) ... 1448
Advair Diskus 250/50 (1% to 3%) ... 1440
Advair Diskus 500/50 (1% to 3%) ... 1448
Aggrenox Capsules (Less than 1%) ... 1026
Anzemet Injection (Infrequently) ... 719
Anzemet Tablets (Infrequently) ... 722
Apligraf (1.8%) ... 2305
Arava Tablets (1% to 3%) ... 724
Campath Ampules ... 992
Caverject Sterile Powder ... 2777
Claritin-D 12 Hour Extended Release Tablets (Less frequent) ... 3102
Copaxone for Injection (Infrequent) ... 3306
Depacon Injection ... 416
Depakene ... 421
Depakote Sprinkle Capsules ... 426
Depakote Tablets ... 430
Depakote ER Tablets ... 436
Eldepryl Capsules ... 3266
Evoxac Capsules (Less than 1%) ... 1217
Exelon Capsules (Infrequent) ... 2342
Exelon Oral Solution (Infrequent) ... 2345
Flovent Diskus (1% to 3%) ... 3614
▲ Fragmin Injection (0.2% to 7.1%) ... 2814
Havrix Vaccine (Less than 1%) ... 1544
Heparin Lock Flush Solution ... 3509
Heparin Sodium Injection ... 3511
Imitrex Injection ... 1549
Imitrex Tablets (Rare) ... 1558
Innohep Injection (Greater than or equal to 1%) ... 1248
Lovenox Injection ... 746
Nimotop Capsules (Less than 1%) .. 904
Orgaran Injection ... 2480
Paxil (Infrequent) ... 1609
Pipracil ... 1866
Plavix Tablets (1% to 2.5%) ... 1097
Plavix Tablets (1% to 2.5%) ... 3084
Priftin Tablets (Less than 1%) ... 758
ReFacto Vials ... 1437
▲ Refludan for Injection (10.6%) ... 761
ReoPro Vials ... 1958
Roferon-A Injection (1%) ... 2996
Sandostatin Injection (1% to 4%) ... 2394
Sandostatin LAR Depot (1% to 4%) ... 2395
▲ Simulect for Injection (3% to 10%) .. 2399
▲ Thrombate III (1 of 17) ... 944
▲ TNKase I.V. (1.7% to 12.3%) ... 1430
Toradol ... 3018
Vantin Tablets and Oral Suspension (Less than 1%) ... 2860
▲ Varivax (24.4% to 32.5%) ... 2202
Versed Injection (Less than 1%) ... 3027
Vioxx (Greater than 0.1% to 1.9%).. 2213

Hematoma, splenic
NovoSeven ... 2430

Hematoma, subdermal
Neurontin Oral Solution (Infrequent) ... 2655
Seroquel Tablets (Rare) ... 684

Hematoma, subdural
Actiq (Less than 1%) ... 1184
Betaseron for SC Injection ... 988
Cerebyx Injection (Infrequent) ... 2619
Naprelan Tablets (Less than 1%) ... 1293
Neurontin ... 2655
Rilutek Tablets (Infrequent) ... 772

Hematopoietic depression
Cosmegen for Injection ... 2062
▲ DTIC-Dome (Among most common) ... 902
Mustargen for Injection (Occasional) ... 2142

Hematospermia
Luvox Tablets (25, 50, 100 mg) (Rare) ... 3256

Hematuria
Accuretic Tablets ... 2614
Accutane Capsules ... 2944
Aceon Tablets (2 mg, 4 mg, 8 mg) (0.3% to 1%) ... 3249
Aciphex Tablets (Rare) ... 1267
Aciphex Tablets (Rare) ... 1783
Actiq (Less than 1%) ... 1184
Aggrenox Capsules (Less than 1%) ... 1026
Agrylin Capsules (1% to 5%) ... 3232
Aloprim for Injection (Less than 1%) ... 2292
▲ AmBisome for Injection (14%) ... 1383
▲ Amphotec (5% or more) ... 1774
Anaprox Tablets (Less than 1%) ... 2967
Anaprox DS Tablets (Less than 1%) ... 2967
Androderm Transdermal System CIII (Less than 1%) ... 3377
Anzemet Injection (Rare) ... 719
Anzemet Tablets (Rare) ... 722
Arava Tablets (1% to 3%) ... 724
▲ Argatroban Injection (0.9% to 11.8%) ... 1478
Aricept Tablets (Infrequent) ... 1270
Aricept Tablets (Infrequent) ... 2665
Arthrotec Tablets (Rare) ... 3195
Asacol Delayed-Release Tablets ... 2884
Astelin Nasal Spray (Infrequent) ... 3339
Atacand Tablets (0.5% or greater) .. 595
Atacand HCT Tablets (0.5% or greater) ... 597
Atromid-S Capsules ... 3483
Augmentin Chewable Tablets (Rare) ... 1482
Augmentin Powder for Oral Suspension (Rare) ... 1482
Augmentin Tablets (Rare) ... 1485
Augmentin ES-600 Powder for Oral Suspension (Rare) ... 1487
Avonex ... 1013
Azulfidine EN-tabs Tablets (Rare) ... 2775
Betaseron for SC Injection ... 988
Bicillin C-R 900/300 Injection ... 2240
Bicillin C-R Injection ... 2238
Bicillin L-A Injection ... 2242
Campath Ampules ... 992
Cancidas for Injection (2.2%) ... 2048
Cardene I.V. (0.7%) ... 3485
Cardura Tablets ... 2668
▲ Casodex Tablets (7%) ... 662
Cataflam Tablets (Less than 1%) ... 2315
Caverject Sterile Powder (Less than 1%) ... 2777
Cedax Oral Suspension (0.1% to 1%) ... 1021
Celebrex Capsules (0.1% to 1.9%) ... 2676
Celebrex Capsules (0.1% to 1.9%) ... 2780
Celexa (Rare) ... 1365
▲ CellCept Capsules (12.1% to 14.0%) ... 2951
▲ CellCept Intravenous (12.1% to 14.0%) ... 2951
▲ CellCept Oral Suspension (12.1% to 14.0%) ... 2951
▲ CellCept Tablets (12.1% to 14.0%) ... 2951
Chirocaine Injection (2%) ... 2909
Cipro I.V. (1% or less) ... 893
Cipro I.V. Pharmacy Bulk Package (Less than 1%) ... 897
Cipro ... 887
Clinoril Tablets (Less than 1%) ... 2053
Cognex Capsules (Infrequent) ... 1351
Colazal Capsules ... 3069
Condylox Topical Solution (Less than 5%) ... 2437
Coreg Tablets (2.9%) ... 1508
Coumadin for Injection ... 1243
Coumadin Tablets ... 1243
Crixivan Capsules (Less than 2%) ... 2070
Cuprimine Capsules ... 2075
Cytotec Tablets (Infrequent) ... 3202
Dantrium Capsules (Less frequent) ... 2885
Daraprim Tablets ... 1511
Demser Capsules (A few patients) .. 2085
Depen Titratable Tablets ... 3341
Diamox Intravenous (Occasional) ... ⊙269
Diamox Sequels Sustained Release Capsules ... ⊙270
Diamox Tablets (Occasional) ... ⊙269
Dipentum Capsules (Rare) ... 2803
Diuril Sodium Intravenous (1 case) ... 2086
Dolobid Tablets (Less than 1 in 100) ... 2088
Doxil Injection (Less than 1%) ... 566
EC-Naprosyn Delayed-Release Tablets (Less than 1%) ... 2967
Edecrin ... 2091
Effexor Tablets (Infrequent) ... 3495
Effexor XR Capsules (Infrequent) ... 3499
▲ Eulexin Capsules (7%) ... 3118
Evoxac Capsules (Less than 1%) ... 1217
Exelon Capsules (Frequent) ... 2342
Exelon Oral Solution (Frequent) ... 2345
Felbatol ... 3343
Feldene Capsules (Occasional) ... 2685
▲ Flolan for Injection (5%) ... 1528
Floxin I.V. (More than or equal to 1%) ... 2526
Floxin Tablets (More than or equal to 1%) ... 2529
Fludara for Injection (2% to 3%) ... 995
Foscavir Injection (Less than 1%) ... 605
Gabitril Tablets (Infrequent) ... 1189
▲ Gemzar for Injection (Up to 35%) ... 1919
Gengraf Capsules (1% to less than 3%) ... 457
Genotropin Lyophilized Powder (Infrequent) ... 2818
Geodon Capsules (Infrequent) ... 2688
Herceptin I.V. (At least one of the 958 patients) ... 1414
▲ Ifex for Injection (6% to 92%) ... 1123
Imitrex Nasal Spray ... 1554
Imitrex Tablets (Rare) ... 1558
Indocin Capsules (Less than 1%) ... 2112
Indocin I.V. (Less than 1%) ... 2115
Indocin (Less than 1%) ... 2112
INFeD Injection ... 3388
Innohep Injection (1%) ... 1248
Intron A for Injection (Less than 5%) ... 3120
Lamictal (Infrequent) ... 1567
▲ Leukine (9%) ... 1755
Levaquin Injection (Less than 0.5%) ... 2537
Lipitor Tablets (Less than 2%) ... 2639
Lipitor Tablets (Less than 2%) ... 2696
Lodine (Less than 1%) ... 3528
Lodine XL Extended-Release Tablets (Less than 1%) ... 3530
Lovenox Injection (Less than 1% to 2%) ... 746
Lufyllin Tablets ... 3347
Lufyllin-400 Tablets ... 3347
Lufyllin-GG Elixir ... 3348
Lufyllin-GG Tablets ... 3348
Lupron Depot 7.5 mg (Less than 5%) ... 3284
▲ Lupron Injection (5% or more) ... 3279
Luvox Tablets (25, 50, 100 mg) (Infrequent) ... 3256
Matulane Capsules ... 3246
Meridia Capsules ... 481
Miacalcin Nasal Spray (Less than 1%) ... 2375
Mintezol ... 2137
Mirapex Tablets (Less than 1%) ... 2834
Mobic Tablets (Less than 2%) ... 1054
Monurol Sachet (Less than 1%) ... 1375
Motrin Suspension, Oral Drops, Chewable Tablets, and Caplets (Less than 1%) ... 2002
▲ Mylotarg for Injection (8% to 14%) . 3540
Naprelan Tablets (Less than 1%) ... 1293
Naprosyn Suspension (Less than 1%) ... 2967
Naprosyn Tablets (Less than 1%) ... 2967
Neoral Soft Gelatin Capsules (1% to less than 3%) ... 2380
Neoral Oral Solution (1% to less than 3%) ... 2380
Neptazane Tablets ... ⊙271
Neupogen for Injection (Infrequent) ... 587
Neurontin Capsules (Infrequent) ... 2655
Neurontin Oral Solution (Infrequent) ... 2655
Neurontin Tablets (Infrequent) ... 2655
Nexium Delayed-Release Capsules (Less than 1%) ... 619
▲ Nilandron Tablets (8.1%) ... 753
Noroxin Tablets ... 2145
Norvir Capsules (Less than 2%) ... 487
Norvir Oral Solution (Less than 2%) ... 487
▲ Novantrone for Injection (11%) ... 1760
Oncaspar (Less than 1%) ... 756
Orudis Capsules (Less than 1%) ... 3548
Oruvail Capsules (Less than 1%) ... 3548
OxyContin Tablets (Less than 1%) ... 2912
Paxil (Infrequent) ... 1609
Pediazole Suspension ... 3050
Pentasa Capsules (Less than 1%) ... 3239
Permax Tablets (1.1%) ... 1299
Plavix Tablets (Less than 1%) ... 1097
Plavix Tablets (Less than 1%) ... 3084
Pletal Tablets (2% or greater) ... 2605
Pletal Tablets (2% or greater) ... 2848
Ponstel Capsules (Occasional) ... 1356
Prevacid Delayed-Release Capsules (Less than 1%) ... 3292
PREVPAC (Less than 1%) ... 3298
Prilosec Delayed-Release Capsules (Less than 1%) ... 628
Primaxin I.M. ... 2158
Primaxin I.V. ... 2160
Procardia XL Extended Release Tablets (1% or less) ... 2710
▲ Prograf (3% to 15%) ... 1393
▲ Proleukin for Injection (9%) ... 1199
ProSom Tablets (Rare) ... 500
Protonix I.V. (Less than 1%) ... 3580
Protonix Tablets (Less than 1%) ... 3577
Provigil Tablets (At least 1%) ... 1193
Prozac Pulvules, Liquid, and Weekly Capsules (Infrequent) ... 1238
▲ Rapamune Oral Solution and Tablets (3% to 20%) ... 3584
▲ Refludan for Injection (4.4%) ... 761
Relafen Tablets (Less than 1%) ... 1617
Remeron Tablets (Infrequent) ... 2483
Remeron SolTab Tablets (Infrequent) ... 2486
▲ Reminyl Oral Solution (3%) ... 1792
▲ Reminyl Tablets (3%) ... 1792
ReoPro Vials (4 events) ... 1958
Requip Tablets (Infrequent) ... 1621
Rescriptor Tablets (Less than 2%) ... 526
Retrovir Capsules (0.8%) ... 1625
Retrovir IV Infusion (1%) ... 1629
Retrovir (0.8%) ... 1625
Rifadin (Rare) ... 765
Rifamate Capsules (Rare) ... 767
Rifater Tablets (Rare) ... 769
Rilutek Tablets (Infrequent) ... 772
Risperdal (Infrequent) ... 1796
Rocephin Injectable Vials, ADD-Vantage, Galaxy, Bulk (Rare) ... 2993
Salagen Tablets (Less than 1%) ... 2229
Sandimmune (Rare) ... 2388
Sandostatin Injection (Less than 1%) ... 2394
Sandostatin LAR Depot (Rare) ... 2395
▲ Serostim for Injection (1% to 10%) . 3229
Serzone Tablets (Infrequent) ... 1104
▲ Simulect for Injection (3% to 10%) . 2399
Sinemet Tablets ... 1253
Sinemet CR Tablets (1% or greater) ... 1255
Sonata Capsules (Infrequent) ... 3591
Sporanox Oral Solution (Less than 2%) ... 1808
Sporanox Oral Solution (Less than 2%) ... 2512
Sular Tablets (Less than or equal to 1%) ... 688
Sustiva Capsules (Up to 1%) ... 1258
Synercid I.V. (Less than 1%) ... 775
Tarka Tablets (Less frequent) ... 508
Tasmar Tablets (Infrequent) ... 3010
Tazicef for Injection (Occasional) ... 1647
Tazicef Galaxy Container (Occasional) ... 1650
Tazicef Pharmacy Bulk Package (Occasional) ... 1653
Tequin Injection (0.1% to 3%) ... 1110
Tequin Tablets (0.1% to 3%) ... 1110
Testoderm Transdermal Systems (1%) ... 574
Teveten Tablets (Less than 1%) ... 3327
Thalomid Capsules ... 1154
▲ TheraCys Injection (39%) ... 823
▲ Tice BCG, BCG Live (26.0%) ... 2489
Ticlid Tablets ... 3015
Tolectin (Less than 1%) ... 2589
Topamax Sprinkle Capsules (0.8% to 1.4%) ... 2590
Topamax Tablets (0.8% to 1.4%) ... 2590
Toradol (1% or less) ... 3018
Trileptal Oral Suspension ... 2407

Trileptal Tablets 2407
Unasyn for Injection 2728
Uniretic Tablets (Less than 1%) 3178
Urobiotic-250 Capsules 2731
Uroqid-Acid No. 2 Tablets (Rare) 947
▲ Vagifem Tablets (3% to 5%) 2857
▲ Valstar Sterile Solution for Intravesical Instillation (11% to 29%) 1175
Vantin Tablets and Oral Suspension (Less than 1%) 2860
Viagra Tablets 2732
Vistide Injection 1445
Voltaren Tablets (Less than 1%) 2315
Voltaren-XR Tablets (Less than 1%) 2315
Warfarin Sodium Tablets, USP 3302
Zanaflex Tablets (Rare) 1305
Zarontin Capsules 2659
Zarontin Syrup 2660
▲ Zoladex (7%) 702
▲ Zoladex 3-month (1% to 7%) 706
Zoloft (Rare) 2751
Zomig Tablets (Infrequent) 708
Zomig-ZMT Tablets (Infrequent) 708
Zonegran Capsules (Infrequent) 1307
Zosyn (1.0% or less) 1890
Zosyn in Galaxy Containers (1.0% or less) 1894
Zovirax Capsules 1706
Zovirax for Injection (Less than 1%) 1708
Zovirax 1706
Zyprexa Tablets (Frequent) 1973
Zyprexa ZYDIS Orally Disintegrating Tablets (Frequent) 1973
Zyrtec (Less than 2%) 2756
Zyrtec-D 12 Hour Extended Relief Tablets (Less than 2%) 2758

Hematuria, microscopic
Calcium Disodium Versenate Injection 1980
Celontin Capsules 2618
▲ Crixivan Capsules (Approximately 4%) 2070

Hemianopsia
Felbatol 3343
Trileptal Oral Suspension 2407
Trileptal Tablets 2407

Hemiparesis
Femara Tablets (Less than or equal to 2%) 2351
Klonopin Tablets 2983
Orthoclone OKT3 Sterile Solution 2498
Requip Tablets (Rare) 1621
Sandostatin LAR Depot (Rare) 2395
▲ Temodar Capsules (18%) 3157
Thyrogen for Injection (Four patients) 1441

Hemiplegia
Accuretic Tablets 2614
Actiq (Less than 1%) 1184
Betaseron for SC Injection 988
Cerebyx Injection (Infrequent) 2619
Cognex Capsules (Infrequent) 1351
Doxil Injection (Less than 1%) 566
Gabitril Tablets (Infrequent) 1189
▲ Gliadel Wafer (19%) 1723
Imitrex Injection (Rare) 1549
Imitrex Tablets 1558
Lamictal (Rare) 1567
Luvox Tablets (25, 50, 100 mg) (Infrequent) 3256
Neurontin Capsules (Infrequent) 2655
Neurontin Oral Solution (Infrequent) 2655
Neurontin Tablets (Infrequent) 2655
Orthoclone OKT3 Sterile Solution 2498
Permax Tablets (Rare) 1299
Prevacid Delayed-Release Capsules (Less than 1%) 3292
PREVPAC (Less than 1%) 3298
Requip Tablets (Rare) 1621
Rilutek Tablets (Infrequent) 772
Seroquel Tablets (Infrequent) 684
Tasmar Tablets (Rare) 3010
Thyrogen for Injection (Four patients) 1441
Trileptal Oral Suspension 2407
Trileptal Tablets 2407
▲ Vesanoid Capsules (3%) 3037
Vistide Injection 1445
Zanaflex Tablets (Rare) 1305

Hemochromatosis
Effexor Tablets (Rare) 3495
Effexor XR Capsules (Rare) 3499

Hemoconcentration
Follistim for Injection 2465
Haldol Decanoate 2535
Humegon for Injection 2468
Mykrox Tablets 1168
Serophene Tablets 3226
Zaroxolyn Tablets 1177

Hemoglobin, decrease
Aceon Tablets (2 mg, 4 mg, 8 mg) 3249
Actos Tablets 3275
Aggrastat (2.1%) 2031
Aggrenox Capsules 1026
Altace Capsules (Rare) 2233
▲ Argatroban Injection (10.4%) 1478
Atacand Tablets 595
Atacand HCT Tablets 597
Avalide Tablets 1070
Avandia Tablets 1490
Avapro Tablets (Less than 0.2%) 1074
Avapro Tablets (Less than 0.2%) 3076
Betaseron for SC Injection 988
Blocadren Tablets 2046
▲ Cancidas for Injection (3.1% to 12.3%) 2048
▲ Casodex Tablets (2% to 5%) 662
Cataflam Tablets (Less than 1%) 2315
Ceclor CD Tablets (0.2%) 1279
Cedax (1% to 2%) 1021
▲ Cefobid Intravenous/Intramuscular (1 in 20) 2671
▲ Cefobid Pharmacy Bulk Package - Not for Direct Infusion (1 in 20) 2673
▲ Cipro I.V. (Among most frequent) 893
▲ Cipro I.V. Pharmacy Bulk Package (Among most frequent) 897
Cipro (Less than 0.1%) 887
Crixivan Capsules (0.5%) 2070
▲ Dapsone Tablets USP (Almost all patients) 1780
Dopram Injectable 2931
Dynabac Tablets (0.1% to 1%) 2269
Enalaprilat Injection (Frequent) 863
Fortovase Capsules (Up to 1%) 2970
Hyzaar 2109
Infergen (1% or less) 1777
Invirase Capsules (Up to 1%) 2979
▲ Kefurox Vials, ADD-Vantage (1 in 10) 1948
Lodosyn Tablets 1251
Lopid Tablets (Occasional) 2650
Lupron Depot 7.5 mg (Greater than or equal to 5%) 3284
▲ Lupron Depot–4 Month 30 mg (Greater than or equal to 5%) 3289
Macrobid Capsules (1% to 5%) 2889
Macrodantin Capsules 2891
Merrem I.V. (Greater than 0.2%) 673
Micardis HCT Tablets (1.2%) 1051
Mithracin for Intravenous Use 903
Monopril Tablets 1091
Monurol Sachet 1375
▲ Motrin Suspension, Oral Drops, Chewable Tablets, and Caplets (Less than 1% to 22.8%) 2002
Mustargen for Injection 2142
Noroxin Tablets (0.6%) 2145
Omnicef (0.3%) 493
Primaxin I.M. 2158
Primaxin I.V. 2160
Prinivil Tablets (Frequent) 2164
Prinzide Tablets (Frequent) 2168
Rebetron Combination Therapy 3153
ReoPro Vials (7 to 11 events) 1958
Rifadin 765
Rifamate Capsules 767
Rifater Tablets 769
▲ Roferon-A Injection (Up to 31%) 2996
Sinemet Tablets 1253
Sinemet CR Tablets (1% or greater) 1255
Teveten Tablets (0.1%) 3327
Timentin Injection- ADD-Vantage Vial 1661
Timentin Injection-Galaxy Container 1664
Timentin Injection-Pharmacy Bulk Package 1666
Timentin for Intravenous Administration 1658
Tolectin (1% to 3%) 2589
Trovan (Greater than or equal to 1%) 2722
Ultram Tablets (Infrequent) 2600
Unasyn for Injection 2728
Vantin Tablets and Oral Suspension 2860
Vaseretic Tablets (0.5% to 2.0%) 2204
Vasotec I.V. Injection (Frequent) 2207
Vasotec Tablets (Frequent) 2210
▲ Videx (3% to 7%) 1138
Viramune Oral Suspension (1.2%) 1060
Viramune Tablets (1.2%) 1060
Voltaren Tablets (Less than 1%) 2315
Voltaren-XR Tablets (Less than 1%) 2315
WinRho SDF 2297
Zestoretic Tablets (Frequent) 695
Zestril Tablets (Frequent) 698
▲ Zinacef Injection (1 in 10 patients) 1696
▲ Zinacef for Injection (1 in 10 patients) 1696
Zosyn 1890
Zosyn in Galaxy Containers 1894

Hemoglobin content, deviation
Amerge Tablets (Rare) 1467
Diovan Capsules (0.4%) 2337
Diovan HCT Tablets (0.004%) 2338
▲ Intron A for Injection (Up to 32%) 3120
Xanax Tablets (Less than 1%) 2865

Hemoglobinemia
▲ AndroGel (3% to 6%) 3322
Clozaril Tablets 2319
Hivid Tablets (Less than 1%) 2975
Stromectol Tablets (1%) 2185
Zovirax for Injection (Less than 1%) 1708

Hemoglobinuria
Rifadin (Rare) 765
Rifamate Capsules 767
Rifater Tablets (Rare) 769
WinRho SDF 2297

Hemolysis
Campath Ampules 992
Cognex Capsules (Rare) 1351
Cozaar Tablets 2067
▲ Dapsone Tablets USP (Most common) 1780
Doxil Injection (1% to 5%) 566
Enalaprilat Injection (A few cases) 863
Hyzaar (One subject) 2109
Kefurox Vials, ADD-Vantage 1948
Macrobid Capsules 2889
Macrodantin Capsules 2891
Mycobutin Capsules (Less than 1%) 2838
Orudis Capsules (Less than 1%) 3548
Oruvail Capsules (Less than 1%) 3548
Plaquenil Tablets 3082
Prevacid Delayed-Release Capsules (Less than 1%) 3292
PREVPAC (Less than 1%) 3298
Rebetron Combination Therapy 3153
Rifadin (Rare) 765
Rifamate Capsules (Rare) 767
Rifater Tablets (Rare) 769
Sandoglobulin I.V. (A few cases) 2391
Seroquel Tablets (Rare) 684
Trasylol Injection (0.3%) 909
Uniretic Tablets (Less than 1%) 3178
Vaseretic Tablets (A few cases) 2204
Vasotec I.V. Injection (A few cases) 2207
Vasotec Tablets (A few cases) 2210
Zovirax for Injection 1708

Hemolysis, neonatal
AquaMEPHYTON Injection 2042
Dapsone Tablets USP 1780
Mephyton Tablets 2129

Hemolytic icterus
(*see under* Jaundice)

Hemolytic sideroblastic anemia
(*see under* Anemia, hemolytic, sideroblastic)

Hemolytic-uremic syndrome
Alesse-21 Tablets 3468
Alesse-28 Tablets 3473
Azulfidine EN-tabs Tablets (Rare) 2775
Brevicon 28-Day Tablets 3380
Cyclessa Tablets 2450
Cytovene 2959
Desogen Tablets 2458
Estrostep 2627
Felbatol 3343
Gemzar for Injection (0.25%) 1919
Gengraf Capsules 457
Levlen 962
Levlite 21 Tablets 962
Levlite 28 Tablets 962
Levora Tablets 3389
Loestrin 21 Tablets 2642
Loestrin Fe Tablets 2642
Lo/Ovral Tablets 3532
Lo/Ovral-28 Tablets 3538
Low-Ogestrel-28 Tablets 3392
Lunelle Monthly Injection 2827
Microgestin Fe 1.5/30 Tablets 3407
Microgestin Fe 1/20 Tablets 3400
Mircette Tablets 2470
Modicon 2563
Necon 3415
Neoral Soft Gelatin Capsules 2380
Neoral Oral Solution 2380
Nordette-28 Tablets 2257
Norinyl 1 +35 28-Day Tablets 3380
Norinyl 1 + 50 28-Day Tablets 3380
Ogestrel 0.5/50-28 Tablets 3428
Ortho-Cept 21 Tablets 2546
Ortho-Cept 28 Tablets 2546
Ortho-Cyclen/Ortho Tri-Cyclen 2573
Ortho-Novum 2563
Ortho-Novum 1/50□28 Tablets 2556
Ortho-Cyclen/Ortho Tri-Cyclen 2573
Ovcon 3364
Ovral Tablets 3551
Ovral-28 Tablets 3552
Ovrette Tablets 3552
Paraplatin for Injection (Rare) 1126
▲ Rapamune Oral Solution and Tablets (3% to 20%) 3584
Toradol 3018
Tri-Levlen 962
Tri-Norinyl-28 Tablets 3433
Trivora Tablets 3439
Valtrex Caplets 1676
Yasmin 28 Tablets 980
Zovia 3449

Hemopericardium
Aggrastat 2031
Cardene I.V. (0.7%) 3485

Hemoperitoneum
Follistim for Injection 2465
Gonal-F for Injection 3216
Humegon for Injection 2468
Merrem I.V. (0.7%) 673
Ovidrel for Injection 3220
Pergonal for Injection 3223
Repronex for Intramuscular and Subcutaneous Injection 1347
Serophene Tablets 3226
Trasylol Injection (1% to 2%) 909

Hemophilus
Intron A for Injection (Less than 5%) 3120

Hemoptysis
Abelcet Injection 1273
Actiq (Less than 1%) 1184
Aggrenox Capsules (Less than 1%) 1026
AmBisome for Injection (Less common) 1383
Argatroban Injection (2.9%) 1478
Avonex 1013
Betaseron for SC Injection 988
Campath Ampules 992
▲ CellCept Capsules (3% to 10%) 2951
▲ CellCept Intravenous (3% to 10%) 2951
▲ CellCept Oral Suspension (3% to 10%) 2951
▲ CellCept Tablets (3% to 10%) 2951
Cerebyx Injection (Infrequent) 2619
Cipro I.V. (1% or less) 893
Cipro I.V. Pharmacy Bulk Package (Less than 1%) 897
Cipro (Less than 1%) 887
Claritin (At least one patient) 3100
Claritin-D 12 Hour Extended Release Tablets 3102
Claritin-D 24 Hour Extended Release Tablets (Fewer than 2%) 3104
Cognex Capsules (Rare) 1351
Colazal Capsules 3069
DaunoXome Injection (Less than or equal to 5%) 1442
Duragesic Transdermal System (1% or greater) 1786
Dynabac Tablets (0.1% to 1%) 2269
Effexor Tablets (Rare) 3495
Effexor XR Capsules (Rare) 3499
Evoxac Capsules (Less than 1%) 1217
▲ Fludara for Injection (1% to 6%) 995
Fortovase Capsules (Less than 2%) 2970
Foscavir Injection (Between 1% and 5%) 605
Gabitril Tablets (Infrequent) 1189
Gonal-F for Injection 3216
Hivid Tablets (Less than 1%) 2975
Intron A for Injection (Less than or equal to 5%) 3120
Invirase Capsules (Less than 2%) 2979
Levaquin Injection (Less than 0.5%) 2537
Lupron Depot 7.5 mg (Less than 5%) 3284
Lupron Injection 3279
Luvox Tablets (25, 50, 100 mg) (Rare) 3256
Matulane Capsules 3246
Natrecor for Injection (At least 1%) 3189
Orudis Capsules (Less than 1%) 3548
Oruvail Capsules (Less than 1%) 3548
Paxil (Rare) 1609
Permax Tablets (Infrequent) 1299
Photofrin for Injection (One patient) 831
Plavix Tablets (Less than 1%) 1097
Plavix Tablets (Less than 1%) 3084
Pletal Tablets (Less than 2%) 2605
Pletal Tablets (Less than 2%) 2848
Prevacid Delayed-Release Capsules (Less than 1%) 3292
PREVPAC (Less than 1%) 3298
Priftin Tablets (1.1%) 758
Prinivil Tablets (0.3% to 1.0%) 2164
Prinzide Tablets 2168
Proleukin for Injection (1%) 1199
Prozac Pulvules, Liquid, and Weekly Capsules (Rare) 1238
Pulmozyme Inhalation Solution 1426
ReoPro Vials (9 to 11 events) 1958
Rifater Tablets 769
Rilutek Tablets (Infrequent) 772
Sarafem Pulvules (Rare) 1962
▲ TOBI Solution for Inhalation (19.4%) 1206
▲ Trisenox Injection (8%) 1158
Trovan (Less than 1%) 2722
Uniretic Tablets (Less than 1%) 3178
Vistide Injection 1445
Zestoretic Tablets 695

Zestril Tablets (0.3% to 1.0%)......... 698
Zoloft (Rare)........................ 2751
Zonegran Capsules (Rare)............. 1307
Zosyn (1.0% or less)................. 1890
Zosyn in Galaxy Containers (1.0% or less)........................... 1894
Zyprexa Tablets (Infrequent)........... 1973
Zyprexa ZYDIS Orally Disintegrating Tablets (Infrequent)........................... 1973

Hemorrhage
(*see under* Bleeding)

Hemorrhage, adrenal
Heparin Lock Flush Solution........... 3509
Heparin Sodium Injection.............. 3511

Hemorrhage, cerebral
(*see under* Cerebral hemorrhage)

Hemorrhage, cerebrovascular
Viagra Tablets........................ 2732

Hemorrhage, colon
Actiq (Less than 1%) 1184

Hemorrhage, conjunctival
Exelon Capsules (Infrequent) 2342
Exelon Oral Solution (Infrequent) 2345
Trileptal Oral Suspension 2407
Trileptal Tablets 2407
▲ Vitravene for Injection (5% to 20%) .... ⊙ 310

Hemorrhage, ear
Imitrex Nasal Spray 1554

Hemorrhage, esophageal
Pletal Tablets (Less than 2%) 2605
Pletal Tablets (Less than 2%) 2848
Protonix I.V. (Less than 1%) 3580
Protonix Tablets (Less than 1%) 3577

Hemorrhage, eye, anterior chamber
Evoxac Capsules (Less than 1%) 1217
Zoloft (Rare) 2751

Hemorrhage, eyes
Actiq (Less than 1%) 1184
AmBisome for Injection (Less common) 1383
Amerge Tablets (Rare) 1467
▲ Amphotec (5% or more) 1774
▲ CellCept Capsules (3% to 10%) 2951
▲ CellCept Intravenous (3% to 10%) .. 2951
▲ CellCept Oral Suspension (3% to 10%) 2951
▲ CellCept Tablets (3% to 10%) 2951
Effexor Tablets 3495
Effexor XR Capsules 3499
Hivid Tablets (Less than 1%) 2975
Imitrex Nasal Spray 1554
▲ Leukine (11%) 1755
Lipitor Tablets (Less than 2%) 2639
Lipitor Tablets (Less than 2%) 2696
Neumega for Injection 1434
Neurontin Capsules (Infrequent) 2655
Neurontin Oral Solution (Infrequent) 2655
Neurontin Tablets (Infrequent) 2655
Ocufen Ophthalmic Solution .... ⊙ 242
Paxil (Rare) 1609
Permax Tablets (Infrequent) 1299
Pletal Tablets (Less than 2%) 2605
Pletal Tablets (Less than 2%) 2848
Prozac Pulvules, Liquid, and Weekly Capsules (Rare) 1238
ReoPro Vials (9 to 11 events) 1958
Rescula Ophthalmic Solution (1% to 5%) .... ⊙ 306
Salagen Tablets (Less than 1%) 2229
Sarafem Pulvules (Rare) 1962
Sonata Capsules (Rare) 3591
Soriatane Capsules (Less than 1%) 3003
Tasmar Tablets (Infrequent) 3010
Ticlid Tablets 3015
Uniretic Tablets (Less than 1%) 3178
Viagra Tablets (Less than 2%) 2732
Vitrasert Implant (Less than 1%) .... ⊙ 254
Zyprexa Tablets (Infrequent) 1973
Zyprexa ZYDIS Orally Disintegrating Tablets (Infrequent) 1973
Zyrtec (Less than 2%) 2756
Zyrtec-D 12 Hour Extended Relief Tablets (Less than 2%) 2758

Hemorrhage, focal
Thyrogen for Injection (Four patients) 1441

Hemorrhage, gastrointestinal
(*see under* Bleeding, gastrointestinal)

Hemorrhage, intra-alveolar
Depen Titratable Tablets 3341

Hemorrhage, neonatal
Rifadin 765
Rifater Tablets.............................. 769
Soma Compound Tablets................ 3354

Hemorrhage, ovarian
Clomid Tablets.............................. 735
Heparin Lock Flush Solution........... 3509
Heparin Sodium Injection.............. 3511

Hemorrhage, postpartum
Aggrenox Capsules........................ 1026
Ecotrin Enteric Coated Aspirin Low, Regular and Maximum Strength Tablets........................ 1715
Rifadin.. 765
Rifater Tablets.............................. 769

Hemorrhage, pulmonary
Aggrastat...................................... 2031
Felbatol.. 3343
Photofrin for Injection.................... 831
Plavix Tablets (Less than 1%).......... 1097
Plavix Tablets (Less than 1%).......... 3084
ReoPro Vials (9 to 11 events)......... 1958
▲ Survanta Intratracheal Suspension (7.2%) 3053

Hemorrhage, purpuric
Carbatrol Capsules 3234
Tegretol/Tegretol-XR 2404

Hemorrhage, retinal
Aricept Tablets (Infrequent) 1270
Aricept Tablets (Infrequent) 2665
Clomid Tablets 735
Effexor Tablets (Rare) 3495
Effexor XR Capsules (Rare) 3499
Elmiron Capsules (Less than or equal to 1%) 570
Glucotrol XL Extended Release Tablets (Less than 1%) 2693
Intron A for Injection (Rare) 3120
Matulane Capsules 3246
Orudis Capsules (Less than 1%) 3548
Oruvail Capsules (Less than 1%) 3548
Paxil (Rare) 1609
Pletal Tablets (Less than 2%) 2605
Pletal Tablets (Less than 2%) 2848
Rescula Ophthalmic Solution (Less than 1%) .... ⊙ 306
Serophene Tablets 3226
Viagra Tablets 2732
▲ Visudyne for Injection (1% to 10%) .... ⊙ 308
▲ Vitravene for Injection (5% to 20%) .... ⊙ 310
Zanaflex Tablets (Infrequent) 1305

Hemorrhage, subarachnoid
Aggrenox Capsules (Less than 1%) 1026
Amerge Tablets 1467
Betaseron for SC Injection 988
Brevicon 28-Day Tablets 3380
Campath Ampules 992
Hivid Tablets (Less than 1%) 2975
Imitrex Injection 1549
Imitrex Nasal Spray 1554
Imitrex Tablets 1558
Norinyl 1 +35 28-Day Tablets 3380
Norinyl 1 + 50 28-Day Tablets 3380
Orthoclone OKT3 Sterile Solution ... 2498
Requip Tablets (Rare) 1621
Rilutek Tablets (Rare) 772
Tri-Norinyl-28 Tablets 3433
Zyprexa Tablets (Rare) 1973
Zyprexa ZYDIS Orally Disintegrating Tablets (Rare) 1973

Hemorrhage, subconjunctival
Effexor Tablets (Rare) 3495
Effexor XR Capsules (Rare) 3499
Travatan Ophthalmic Solution (1% to 4%) 543
▲ Visudyne for Injection (1% to 10%) .... ⊙ 308

Hemorrhage, subcutaneous
Mustargen for Injection 2142
Ticlid Tablets 3015

Hemorrhage, throat
Imitrex Nasal Spray 1554

Hemorrhage, vitreous
▲ Visudyne for Injection (1% to 10%) .... ⊙ 308
▲ Vitrasert Implant (Approximately 10% to 20%) .... ⊙ 254
Vitravene for Injection (2% to 5%) .. ⊙ 310
Xalatan Latanoprost Ophthalmic Solution (Extremely rare) .... ⊙ 320
Xalatan Sterile Ophthalmic Solution (Extremely rare) 2864

Hemorrhagic colitis
Amoxil Chewable Tablets 1471
Amoxil for Oral Suspension 1471
Amoxil 1471
Augmentin Chewable Tablets 1482
Augmentin Powder for Oral Suspension 1482
Augmentin Tablets 1485
Kaletra Capsules (Less than 2%) 471
Kaletra Oral Solution (Less than 2%) 471
Lamictal (Rare)............................. 1567
Omnicef.. 493
Primaxin I.M.................................. 2158
Primaxin I.V. (Less than 0.2%)......... 2160

Hemorrhagic complications
Coumadin for Injection.................. 1243
Coumadin Tablets......................... 1243
Fragmin Injection (Low incidence)... 2814
Lovenox Injection (Low incidence).... 746
▲ Paraplatin for Injection (5%) 1126
Warfarin Sodium Tablets, USP 3302

Hemorrhagic diathesis
▲ Mithracin for Intravenous Use (5.4 to 11.9%)......................... 903

Hemorrhagic eruptions
(*see under* Eruptions, hemorrhagic)

Hemorrhagic syndrome
(*see under* Bleeding syndrome)

Hemorrhagic tendency
Mithracin for Intravenous Use 903
Mustargen for Injection 2142

Hemorrhoids
Aggrenox Capsules (1%) 1026
Ambien Tablets (Rare) 3191
AmBisome for Injection (Less common) 1383
Amerge Tablets (Rare) 1467
Aricept Tablets (Infrequent) 1270
Aricept Tablets (Infrequent) 2665
Arthrotec Tablets (Rare) 3195
Campath Ampules 992
Celebrex Capsules (0.1% to 1.9%) 2676
Celebrex Capsules (0.1% to 1.9%) 2780
Celexa (Infrequent) 1365
▲ Chemet Capsules (12.0% to 20.9%) 3078
Claritin-D 12 Hour Extended Release Tablets (Less frequent) ... 3102
Cognex Capsules (Infrequent) 1351
Colazal Capsules 3069
DaunoXome Injection (Less than or equal to 5%) 1442
Effexor Tablets (Infrequent) 3495
Effexor XR Capsules (Infrequent) 3499
Estring Vaginal Ring (1% to 3%) 2811
Evoxac Capsules (Less than 1%) 1217
Exelon Capsules (Infrequent) 2342
Exelon Oral Solution (Infrequent) 2345
Fortovase Capsules (Less than 2%) 2970
Hivid Tablets (Less than 1%) 2975
Imdur Tablets (Less than or equal to 5%) 1826
▲ Infergen (1% to 6%) 1777
Invirase Capsules (Less than 2%) 2979
Klonopin Tablets (Infrequent) 2983
Luvox Tablets (25, 50, 100 mg) (Infrequent) 3256
Micardis Tablets (More than 0.3%) .. 1049
Micardis HCT Tablets 1051
Neurontin Capsules (Infrequent) 2655
Neurontin Oral Solution (Infrequent) 2655
Neurontin Tablets (Infrequent) 2655
Requip Tablets (Infrequent) 1621
Risperdal (Infrequent) 1796
Rowasa Rectal Suspension Enema 4.0 grams/unit (60 mL) (1.35%) 3264
Sandostatin Injection (Less than 1%) 2394
▲ Sandostatin LAR Depot (5% to 15%) 2395
Seroquel Tablets (Infrequent) 684
Soriatane Capsules (Less than 1%) 3003
Sporanox Oral Solution (Less than 2%) 1808
Sporanox Oral Solution (Less than 2%) 2512
Synvisc 3596
Topamax Sprinkle Capsules (Infrequent) 2590
Topamax Tablets (Infrequent) 2590
Trileptal Oral Suspension 2407
Trileptal Tablets 2407
Vioxx (Greater than 0.1% to 1.9%) .. 2213
▲ Zenapax for Injection (2% to 5%) 3046
Zyrtec (Less than 2%) 2756
Zyrtec-D 12 Hour Extended Relief Tablets (Less than 2%) 2758

Hemorrhoids, aggravation
Colestid Tablets 2791

Hemospermia
Rescriptor Tablets (Less than 2%) 526

Hemostasis, interference
Depacon Injection 416
Depakote Tablets 430

Hemothorax
Permax Tablets (Rare) 1299
Plavix Tablets (Less than 1%).......... 1097
Plavix Tablets (Less than 1%).......... 3084
Refludan for Injection..................... 761

Henoch-Schönlein purpura
Bactrim... 2949
Felbatol.. 3343
Lodosyn Tablets............................ 1251
Luvox Tablets (25, 50, 100 mg)....... 3256
Septra Suspension......................... 2265
Septra Tablets............................... 2265
Septra DS Tablets.......................... 2265
Sinemet Tablets............................. 1253
Sinemet CR Tablets....................... 1255
Varivax... 2202

Henoch-Schönlein vasculitis
Motrin Suspension, Oral Drops, Chewable Tablets, and Caplets (Less than 1%)................ 2002

Hepatic adenoma
Alesse-21 Tablets.......................... 3468
Alesse-28 Tablets.......................... 3473
Brevicon 28-Day Tablets 3380
Cyclessa Tablets 2450
Desogen Tablets 2458
Estratest (Rare) 3252
Estrostep 2627
Levora Tablets 3389
Loestrin 21 Tablets 2642
Loestrin Fe Tablets 2642
Lo/Ovral Tablets 3532
Lo/Ovral-28 Tablets 3538
Low-Ogestrel-28 Tablets 3392
Lunelle Monthly Injection 2827
Menest Tablets 2254
Microgestin Fe 1.5/30 Tablets 3407
Microgestin Fe 1/20 Tablets 3400
Mircette Tablets 2470
Necon 3415
Nordette-28 Tablets 2257
Norinyl 1 +35 28-Day Tablets 3380
Norinyl 1 + 50 28-Day Tablets 3380
Ogestrel 0.5/50-28 Tablets 3428
Ortho-Cept 21 Tablets 2546
Ortho-Cept 28 Tablets 2546
Ortho-Cyclen/Ortho Tri-Cyclen 2573
Ovcon (Rare) 3364
Ovral Tablets 3551
Ovral-28 Tablets 3552
Ovrette Tablets 3552
Premarin Intravenous 3563
Premarin Vaginal Cream 3570
Tri-Norinyl-28 Tablets 3433
Triphasil-21 Tablets 3600
Triphasil-28 Tablets 3605
Trivora Tablets 3439
Yasmin 28 Tablets 980
Zovia 3449

Hepatic coma
Concerta Extended-Release Tablets 1998
Concerta Tablets 561
Levaquin (Less than 0.3%) 2537
Maxzide 1008
Metadate CD Capsules 1164
Metadate ER Tablets 1167
Methylin Tablets 1995
Methylin ER Tablets 1995
Prinzide Tablets 2168
Ritalin (Some instances) 2387
Tenoretic Tablets 690
Vaseretic Tablets 2204
Zestoretic Tablets 695

Hepatic dysfunction
Accupril Tablets (Rare) 2611
Accuretic Tablets (0.5% to 1%) 2614
Actimmune (Rare) 1772
Advair Diskus 100/50 (1% to 3%) ... 1448
Advair Diskus 250/50 (1% to 3%) ... 1448
Advair Diskus 500/50 (1% to 3%) ... 1448
Aggrenox Capsules (Less than 1%) 1026
▲ Albenza Tablets (Less than 1.0% to 15.6%) 1463
Aldoclor Tablets 2035
Aldomet Tablets 2037
Aldoril Tablets 2039
Amaryl Tablets (Isolated cases) 717
Ambien Tablets (Infrequent) 3191
AmBisome for Injection (Less common) 1383
Amerge Tablets (Rare) 1467
Amoxil Chewable Tablets 1471
Amoxil for Oral Suspension 1471
Amoxil 1471
Anadrol-50 Tablets 3321
Anaprox Tablets (Less than 1%) 2967
Anaprox DS Tablets (Less than 1%) 2967
Ancobon Capsules 1730
Androderm Transdermal System CIII 3377
▲ Android Capsules, 10 mg (Among most common) 1731
▲ Anzemet Injection (3.6%) 719
▲ Arava Tablets (5%) 724
Arthrotec Tablets (Rare) 3195
Ativan Injection (Less than 1%) 3478
Atromid-S Capsules 3483

Augmentin Chewable Tablets (Infrequent)...... 1482
Augmentin Powder for Oral Suspension (Infrequent)...... 1482
Augmentin Tablets (Infrequent)...... 1485
Augmentin ES-600 Powder for Oral Suspension (Infrequently)...... 1487
Avelox Tablets (1%)...... 879
Avonex...... 1013
Aygestin Tablets...... 1333
Biaxin/Biaxin XL (Infrequent)...... 403
Blocadren Tablets...... 2046
Brevital Sodium for Injection, USP...... 1815
Captopril Tablets...... 2281
Carbatrol Capsules...... 3234
▲ Cataflam Tablets (3% to 9%)...... 2315
Catapres Tablets...... 1037
Ceclor CD Tablets...... 1279
Cefobid Intravenous/Intramuscular (1 patient in 1285)...... 2671
Cefotan...... 664
Celebrex Capsules (0.1% to 1.9%)...... 2676
Celebrex Capsules (0.1% to 1.9%)...... 2780
▲ CellCept Capsules (3%)...... 2951
▲ CellCept Intravenous (3%)...... 2951
▲ CellCept Oral Suspension (3%)...... 2951
▲ CellCept Tablets (3%)...... 2951
Ceptaz for Injection...... 1499
Cerebyx Injection (Infrequent)...... 2619
▲ Cipro I.V. (Among most frequent)...... 893
Claritin (Rare)...... 3100
Claritin-D 12 Hour Extended Release Tablets (Less frequent)...... 3102
Claritin-D 24 Hour Extended Release Tablets (Fewer than 2%)...... 3104
Cleocin HCl Capsules...... 2784
Cleocin Phosphate Sterile Solution...... 2785
Cleocin Vaginal Cream...... 2788
Cleocin Vaginal Ovules...... 2789
Clinoril Tablets (Less than 1 in 100)...... 2053
Clomid Tablets...... 735
Concerta Extended-Release Tablets...... 1998
Concerta Tablets...... 561
▲ Cordarone Intravenous (3.4%)...... 3491
▲ Cordarone Tablets (4% to 9%)...... 3487
Cosmegen for Injection...... 2062
Crixivan Capsules...... 2070
Cuprimine Capsules...... 2075
Cylert Tablets...... 415
Cytotec Tablets (Infrequent)...... 3202
Cytovene...... 2959
Dantrium Capsules...... 2885
Daranide Tablets...... 2077
Darvon-N/Darvocet-N...... 1907
Darvon Pulvules...... 1909
Darvon Compound-65 Pulvules...... 1910
Darvon-N Tablets...... 1912
Delatestryl Injection...... 1151
Depacon Injection...... 416
Depakene...... 421
Depakote Sprinkle Capsules (Occasional)...... 426
Depakote Tablets...... 430
Depakote ER Tablets...... 436
Depen Titratable Tablets (Isolated cases)...... 3341
DiaBeta Tablets (Isolated cases)...... 741
Diamox Intravenous (Occasional)...... ⊙269
Diamox Sequels Sustained Release Capsules...... ⊙270
Diamox Tablets (Occasional)...... ⊙269
Diflucan Tablets, Injection, and Oral Suspension...... 2681
Dilantin Infatabs...... 2624
Dilantin Kapseals...... 2622
Dilantin-125 Oral Suspension...... 2625
Diovan Capsules (Occasional)...... 2337
Diprivan Injectable Emulsion (Less than 1%)...... 667
Dolobid Tablets (Less than 1 in 100)...... 2088
DTIC-Dome (Few reports)...... 902
Duraclon Injection (1%)...... 3057
Duricef...... 1079
Dyazide Capsules...... 1515
EC-Naprosyn Delayed-Release Tablets (Less than 1%)...... 2967
Edecrin (Rare)...... 2091
E.E.S....... 450
Effexor Tablets...... 3495
Effexor XR Capsules...... 3499
Elmiron Capsules (1%)...... 570
Emcyt Capsules...... 2810
Engerix-B Vaccine...... 1517
EryPed...... 446
Ery-Tab Tablets...... 448
Erythrocin Stearate Filmtab Tablets...... 452
Erythromycin Base Filmtab Tablets...... 454
Erythromycin Delayed-Release Capsules, USP...... 455
Estratest...... 3252
Etrafon (Rare)...... 3115
Eulexin Capsules...... 3118
Evoxac Capsules (Less than 1%)...... 1217
Exelon Capsules (Infrequent)...... 2342
Exelon Oral Solution (Infrequent)...... 2345
Felbatol...... 3343
Flexeril Tablets (Less than 1%)...... 572
Flexeril Tablets (Less than 1%)...... 2094
Floxin I.V....... 2526
Floxin Tablets...... 2529
Fludara for Injection (1% to 3%)...... 995
Fluothane Inhalation...... 3508
Fortaz...... 1541
Fortovase Capsules (Rare)...... 2970
Foscavir Injection (Between 1% and 5%)...... 605
Gabitril Tablets (Infrequent)...... 1189
Gastrocrom Oral Concentrate (Less common)...... 1162
Halcion Tablets (Rare)...... 2823
Haldol Decanoate...... 2535
Haldol Injection, Tablets and Concentrate...... 2533
▲ Hivid Tablets (Less than 1% to 8.9%)...... 2975
Idamycin PFS Injection (Less than 5%)...... 2825
▲ Ifex for Injection (3%)...... 1123
Imitrex Injection (Infrequent)...... 1549
Imitrex Nasal Spray...... 1554
Imitrex Tablets...... 1558
Intron A for Injection (Less than 5%)...... 3120
Invirase Capsules (Rare)...... 2979
Lamictal (Infrequent)...... 1567
▲ Lamisil Tablets (3.3%)...... 2360
Leukine...... 1755
Levaquin (Less than 0.3%)...... 2537
Librium Capsules (Occasional)...... 1736
Librium for Injection (Occasional)...... 1737
Limbitrol (Rare)...... 1738
Lipitor Tablets (Less than 2%)...... 2639
Lipitor Tablets (Less than 2%)...... 2696
Lopid Tablets (Occasional)...... 2650
Lorabid Suspension and Pulvules (Rare)...... 2251
Lumigan Ophthalmic Solution (1% to 5%)...... 553
▲ Lupron Depot–3 Month 22.5 mg (More than or equal to 5%)...... 3288
Lupron Injection...... 3279
Matulane Capsules...... 3246
Maxipime for Injection...... 1285
Mefoxin for Injection...... 2124
Mefoxin Premixed Intravenous Solution...... 2127
Metadate CD Capsules...... 1164
Metadate ER Tablets...... 1167
Methylin Tablets...... 1995
Methylin ER Tablets...... 1995
Mevacor Tablets...... 2132
Mexitil Capsules (About 5 in 1,000)...... 1047
Midamor Tablets (Rare)...... 2136
Minipress Capsules (Less than 1%)...... 2699
Minizide Capsules (Rare)...... 2700
Mintezol (Rare)...... 2137
Mithracin for Intravenous Use...... 903
Moban (Rare)...... 1320
Modicon...... 2563
Moduretic Tablets...... 2138
Motrin Suspension, Oral Drops, Chewable Tablets, and Caplets (Less than 1%)...... 2002
Myambutol Tablets...... 1290
Mycelex Troche...... 573
Naprelan Tablets (Less than 1%)...... 1293
Naprosyn Suspension (Less than 1%)...... 2967
Naprosyn Tablets (Less than 1%)...... 2967
Neurontin Capsules...... 2655
Neurontin Oral Solution...... 2655
Neurontin Tablets...... 2655
Nexium Delayed-Release Capsules (Less than 1%)...... 619
Niaspan Extended-Release Tablets...... 1846
Nilandron Tablets...... 753
Nimotop Capsules (Up to 1.2%)...... 904
▲ Nipent for Injection (2% to 19%)...... 3272
Nizoral Tablets (Rare)...... 1791
Normodyne Injection...... 3135
Normodyne Tablets...... 3137
Norpramin Tablets...... 755
Norvir Capsules (Less than 2%)...... 487
Norvir Oral Solution (Less than 2%)...... 487
▲ Novantrone for Injection (10% to 14%)...... 1760
Omnicef...... 493
Oncaspar (Greater than 1% but less than 5%)...... 756
Ortho-Novum...... 2563
Ortho-Novum 1/50▫28 Tablets...... 2556
Orudis Capsules (Less than 1%)...... 3548
Oruvail Capsules (Less than 1%)...... 3548
Oxandrin Tablets...... 1153
▲ Pacerone Tablets (4% to 9%)...... 3331
Paxil...... 1609
PCE Dispertab Tablets...... 498
Pediazole Suspension...... 3050
Pergonal for Injection...... 3223
Periactin Tablets...... 2155
Permax Tablets (Infrequent)...... 1299
Persantine Tablets (Rare)...... 1057
Pipracil (Less than 2%)...... 1866
Plaquenil Tablets...... 3082
Premarin Vaginal Cream...... 3570
Prevacid Delayed-Release Capsules...... 3292
PREVPAC (Infrequent)...... 3298
Priftin Tablets...... 758
Primacor Injection...... 3086
▲ Prograf (5% to 36%)...... 1393
Proleukin for Injection...... 1199
Protopic Ointment (Greater than or equal to 1%)...... 1397
Provera Tablets...... 2853
▲ Provigil Tablets (3%)...... 1193
Prozac Pulvules, Liquid, and Weekly Capsules (Infrequent)...... 1238
▲ Rapamune Oral Solution and Tablets (3% to 20%)...... 3584
▲ Refludan for Injection (5.3%)...... 761
Reglan (Rare)...... 2935
▲ Relafen Tablets (Up to 15%)...... 1617
Remeron Tablets (Infrequent)...... 2483
Remeron SolTab Tablets (Infrequent)...... 2486
Repronex for Intramuscular and Subcutaneous Injection...... 1347
Rifadin (Rare)...... 765
Rifamate Capsules...... 767
Rifater Tablets (Rare)...... 769
Rilutek Tablets (Infrequent)...... 772
Ritalin (Some instances)...... 2387
Salagen Tablets (Less than 1%)...... 2229
Sarafem Pulvules (Infrequent)...... 1962
Serophene Tablets...... 3226
▲ Serostim for Injection (1% to 10%)...... 3229
Serzone Tablets (Infrequent)...... 1104
Sinemet Tablets...... 1253
Sonata Capsules (Rare)...... 3591
Soriatane Capsules (Less than 1%)...... 3003
Sporanox Capsules (2.7% to 3%)...... 1800
Sporanox Injection (2.7% to 3%)...... 1804
Sporanox Injection (2.7% to 3%)...... 2509
Sular Tablets (Less than or equal to 1%)...... 688
Suprax...... 1877
Surmontil Capsules...... 3595
Synagis Intramuscular (More than 1%)...... 2028
Tabloid Tablets (Occasional)...... 1642
Tambocor Tablets (Rare)...... 1990
Tamiflu Capsules...... 3008
Tamiflu Oral Suspension...... 3008
Tasmar Tablets...... 3010
Tazicef for Injection...... 1647
Tazicef Galaxy Container...... 1650
Tazicef Pharmacy Bulk Package...... 1653
Tazidime Vials, Faspak & ADD-Vantage...... 1966
Tegretol/Tegretol-XR...... 2404
Tenex Tablets (Less frequent)...... 2942
Testoderm Transdermal Systems...... 574
Testopel Pellets...... 3610
Thalomid Capsules...... 1154
Ticlid Tablets (1.0%)...... 3015
Timolide Tablets...... 2187
Tolectin (Less than 1%)...... 2589
Tonocard Tablets (Less than 1%)...... 649
Toradol...... 3018
Tranxene...... 511
▲ Trasylol Injection (3%)...... 909
Trileptal Oral Suspension...... 2407
Trileptal Tablets...... 2407
Trovan (Less than 1%)...... 2722
Ultracet Tablets (Less than 1%)...... 2597
Valtrex Caplets...... 1676
Vantin Tablets and Oral Suspension...... 2860
Vaqta (Isolated reports)...... 2199
Vascor Tablets (0.5% to 2.0%)...... 2602
▲ Vesanoid Capsules (50% to 60%)...... 3037
Viagra Tablets (Less than 2%)...... 2732
Viracept...... 532
Viramune Oral Suspension...... 1060
Viramune Tablets...... 1060
Vistide Injection...... 1445
Vivactil Tablets...... 2217
Vivactil Tablets...... 2446
Vivelle Transdermal System (Rare)...... 2412
▲ Voltaren Tablets (3% to 9%)...... 2315
▲ Voltaren-XR Tablets (3% to 9%)...... 2315
Wellbutrin SR Sustained-Release Tablets (Infrequent)...... 1684
▲ Zanaflex Tablets (3%)...... 1305
Zestril Tablets (Rare)...... 698
Zinacef Injection...... 1696
Zinacef for Injection...... 1696
Zithromax Capsules, 250 mg...... 2743
Zithromax for IV Infusion...... 2748
Zithromax for Oral Suspension, 300 mg, 600 mg, 900 mg, 1200 mg...... 2739
Zithromax Tablets, 250 mg...... 2739
Zofran Injection...... 1698
Zofran...... 1703
Zofran ODT Orally Disintegrating Tablets...... 1703
Zoloft (Rare)...... 2751
Zomig Tablets (Infrequent)...... 708
Zomig-ZMT Tablets (Infrequent)...... 708
Zovirax Capsules...... 1706
Zovirax for Injection...... 1708
Zovirax...... 1706
Zyban Sustained-Release Tablets (Infrequent)...... 1710
Zyflo Filmtab Tablets...... 524
Zyrtec (Less than 2%)...... 2756
Zyrtec-D 12 Hour Extended Relief Tablets (Less than 2%)...... 2758
Zyvox (0.4% to 1.3%)...... 2871

Hepatic enzymes, elevation

(*see also under* Serum transaminase, elevation)
Accolate Tablets (Rare)...... 657
Accutane Capsules...... 2944
Agrylin Capsules (2 of 551 patients)...... 3232
Altace Capsules (Rare)...... 2233
Amaryl Tablets (Rare)...... 717
▲ Amphotec (4% to 11%)...... 1774
▲ Anaprox Tablets (Up to 15%)...... 2967
▲ Anaprox DS Tablets (Up to 15%)...... 2967
Asacol Delayed-Release Tablets...... 2884
Atacand Tablets (Infrequent)...... 595
Atacand HCT Tablets...... 597
Avandia Tablets...... 1490
Avapro Tablets...... 1074
Avapro Tablets (Very rare)...... 3076
Biaxin/Biaxin XL (Infrequent)...... 403
Biltricide Tablets...... 887
Brethine Ampuls...... 2314
Brethine Tablets (Rare)...... 2313
Canasa Rectal Suppositories...... 829
Captopril Tablets...... 2281
▲ Casodex Tablets (6%)...... 662
Cataflam Tablets (Rare)...... 2315
Cefobid Pharmacy Bulk Package - Not for Direct Infusion (1 patient in 1285)...... 2673
Cefotan (1.2%)...... 664
Ceftin for Oral Suspension (0.1% to 1%)...... 1898
Celexa (Infrequent)...... 1365
Ceptaz for Injection...... 1499
▲ Cipro I.V. Pharmacy Bulk Package (Among most frequent)...... 897
Colazal Capsules...... 3069
Comvax...... 2056
Cordarone Intravenous (Common)...... 3491
Coreg Tablets (0.1% to 1%)...... 1508
Corgard Tablets...... 2245
Coumadin for Injection (Infrequent)...... 1243
Coumadin Tablets (Infrequent)...... 1243
Covera-HS Tablets (1.4%)...... 3199
Cylert Tablets...... 415
Dantrium Capsules...... 2885
Declomycin Tablets (Rare)...... 1855
Depacon Injection...... 416
Depakene...... 421
Depakote Tablets...... 430
Depakote ER Tablets...... 436
Diovan Capsules...... 2337
Diovan HCT Tablets...... 2338
Dyazide Capsules...... 1515
Dynacin Capsules...... 2019
DynaCirc Capsules (0.5% to 1%)...... 2921
DynaCirc CR Tablets (0.5% to 1%)...... 2923
Dyrenium Capsules (Rare)...... 3458
▲ EC-Naprosyn Delayed-Release Tablets (Up to 15%)...... 2967
Ecotrin Enteric Coated Aspirin Low, Regular and Maximum Strength Tablets...... 1715
Enalaprilat Injection...... 863
Ergamisol Tablets (Rare)...... 1789
EryPed...... 446
Evoxac Capsules (Less than 1%)...... 1217
Fareston Tablets...... 3237
▲ Feldene Capsules (1% to 10%)...... 2685
Hycamtin for Injection (Less than 1%)...... 1546
Hyzaar (Occasional)...... 2109
▲ Ifex for Injection (3%)...... 1123
Imitrex Nasal Spray...... 1554
Imitrex Tablets...... 1558
Isoptin SR Tablets...... 467
Lescol Capsules...... 2361
Lescol Capsules...... 2925
Lescol XL Tablets...... 2361
Lescol XL Tablets...... 2925
Lithobid Slow-Release Tablets...... 3255
Lodine (Less than 1%)...... 3528
Lodine XL Extended-Release Tablets (Less than 1%)...... 3530
Lotrel Capsules (Scattered incidents)...... 2370
Maxzide...... 1008
Micardis HCT Tablets...... 1051
Minocin Intravenous...... 1862
Minocin Oral Suspension...... 1865
Minocin Pellet-Filled Capsules...... 1863
Monopril Tablets...... 1091
Monopril HCT...... 1094
Mylocel Tablets...... 2227

Nadolol Tablets 2288
▲ Naprosyn Suspension (Up to 15%) 2967
▲ Naprosyn Tablets (Up to 15%) 2967
Navelbine Injection 1604
Niaspan Extended-Release Tablets 1846
Nicomide Tablets (Rare) 3247
Nolvadex Tablets 678
Noroxin Tablets 2145
Norvasc Tablets (Infrequent) 2704
Paxil 1609
Pediazole Suspension 3050
Pipracil (Less frequent) 1866
Plavix Tablets (1% to 2.5%) 1097
Plavix Tablets (1% to 2.5%) 3084
▲ Ponstel Capsules (1% to 10%) 1356
Prandin Tablets (0.5, 1, and 2 mg) (Less than 1%) 2432
PREVPAC (Infrequent) 3298
Prinivil Tablets (Rare) 2164
Prinzide Tablets (Rare) 2168
Provigil Tablets (At least 1%) 1193
Recombivax HB 2178
Relafen Tablets (Less than 1%) 1617
Roferon-A Injection (Frequent) 2996
Rowasa Rectal Suspension Enema 4.0 grams/unit (60 mL) 3264
Rythmol Tablets – 150 mg, 225 mg, 300 mg (Less than 1%) 502
Sandostatin Injection (Less than 1%) 2394
Sandostatin LAR Depot (Rare) 2395
Sinemet Tablets 1253
▲ Sporanox Capsules (4%) 1800
Sporanox Injection (Rare) 1804
Sporanox Injection (Rare) 2509
Sporanox Oral Solution 1808
Sporanox Oral Solution 2512
Sustiva Capsules 1258
Tabloid Tablets (Occasional) 1642
Tarka Tablets (2.8%) 508
Tasmar Tablets 3010
Tegretol/Tegretol-XR 2404
Tenoretic Tablets 690
Tenormin 692
Testoderm Transdermal Systems (1%) 574
Thalomid Capsules 1154
Toradol 3018
Trental Tablets (Rare) 784
Trileptal Oral Suspension 2407
Trileptal Tablets 2407
Trizivir Tablets 1669
Trovan (Less than 1%) 2722
Ultracet Tablets 2597
Ultram Tablets (Infrequent) 2600
Univasc Tablets 3181
Vascor Tablets (Approximately 1%) 2602
Vaseretic Tablets (Rare) 2204
Vasotec I.V. Injection 2207
Vasotec Tablets 2210
Venofer Injection (Greater than 1%) 580
Verelan Capsules 3184
Verelan PM Capsules 3186
Vermox Chewable Tablets (Rare) 2017
▲ Vicoprofen Tablets (Up to 15%) 520
▲ Visudyne for Injection (1% to 10%) ⊙308
Voltaren Tablets (Rare) 2315
Voltaren-XR Tablets (Rare) 2315
Warfarin Sodium Tablets, USP 3302
Xanax Tablets 2865
Zestoretic Tablets (Rare) 695
Zestril Tablets (Rare) 698
Zoloft (One or more patients) 2751
Zovirax 1706

Hepatic eosinophilic infiltration

Singulair (Very rare) 2181

Hepatic failure

Abelcet Injection 1273
Accolate Tablets (Rare) 657
Aceon Tablets (2 mg, 4 mg, 8 mg) 3249
Aloprim for Injection (Less than 1%) 2292
Amaryl Tablets 717
Amphotec (1% to 5%) 1774
Antabuse Tablets 2444
Antabuse Tablets 3474
Arthrotec Tablets (Rare) 3195
Asacol Delayed-Release Tablets (Rare) 2884
Azulfidine EN-tabs Tablets 2775
Biaxin/Biaxin XL (Very rare) 403
Campath Ampules 992
Captopril Tablets (Rare) 2281
Celebrex Capsules (Less than 0.1%) 2676
Celebrex Capsules (Less than 0.1%) 2780
Clinoril Tablets (Less than 1 in 100) 2053
Colazal Capsules 3069
Crixivan Capsules 2070
Cylert Tablets 415
Cytovene 2959
Declomycin Tablets (Rare) 1855
Depacon Injection 416
Depakene 421
Depakote Sprinkle Capsules 426
Depakote Tablets 430
Depakote ER Tablets 436
Diflucan Tablets, Injection, and Oral Suspension (Rare) 2681
Doxil Injection (Less than 1%) 566
Dynacin Capsules (Rare) 2019
Effexor Tablets 3495
Effexor XR Capsules 3499
Enalaprilat Injection (Rare) 863
Eulexin Capsules (Rare) 3118
Felbatol 3343
Feldene Capsules (Rare) 2685
Flolan for Injection 1528
Floxin I.V. 2526
Floxin Tablets 2529
Fludara for Injection (Up to 1%) 995
Fluothane Inhalation 3508
Herceptin I.V. (At least one of the 958 patients) 1414
Hivid Tablets (Rare) 2975
Intron A for Injection (Very rare) 3120
Lamisil Tablets (Rare) 2360
Lexxel Tablets 608
Lodine (Rare; less than 1%) 3528
Lodine XL Extended-Release Tablets (Rare; less than 1%) 3530
Mavik Tablets (Rare) 478
Merrem I.V. (0.1% to 1.0%) 673
Minocin Intravenous (Rare) 1862
Minocin Oral Suspension (Rare) 1865
Minocin Pellet-Filled Capsules (Rare) 1863
Mintezol (Rare) 2137
Mobic Tablets (Less than 0.1%) 1054
Monopril Tablets 1091
Motrin Suspension, Oral Drops, Chewable Tablets, and Caplets (Less than 1%) 2002
Mylotarg for Injection 3540
Omnicef 493
Oncaspar 756
Pentasa Capsules 3239
Periactin Tablets 2155
Plaquenil Tablets 3082
Ponstel Capsules (Rare) 1356
PREVPAC (Very rare) 3298
Prilosec Delayed-Release Capsules (Rare) 628
Prinivil Tablets (Rare) 2164
Prinzide Tablets (Rare) 2168
Proleukin for Injection (Less than 1%) 1199
Protonix I.V. 3580
Prozac Pulvules, Liquid, and Weekly Capsules 1238
Relafen Tablets (Less than 1%) 1617
Rescriptor Tablets 526
Risperdal (Rare) 1796
Sarafem Pulvules 1962
Serzone Tablets 1104
Sporanox Capsules (Rare) 1800
Sporanox Injection (Rare) 1804
Sporanox Injection (Rare) 2509
Sporanox Oral Solution (Rare) 1808
Sporanox Oral Solution (Rare) 2512
Sustiva Capsules 1258
Tambocor Tablets (Rare) 1990
Tasmar Tablets 3010
Tegretol/Tegretol-XR (Very rare) 2404
Topamax Sprinkle Capsules 2590
Topamax Tablets 2590
Toradol 3018
Trasylol Injection (1% to 2%) 909
Trizivir Tablets 1669
Trovan 2722
Ultracet Tablets 2597
Univasc Tablets (Rare) 3181
Vaseretic Tablets (Rare) 2204
Vasotec I.V. Injection (Rare) 2207
Vasotec Tablets (0.5% to 1.0%) 2210
Videx 1138
Videx EC Capsules 1143
Viramune Oral Suspension 1060
Viramune Tablets 1060
Vistide Injection (Less than 1%) 1445
Xanax Tablets 2865
Zantac (Rare) 1690
Zantac Injection (Rare) 1688
Zantac Syrup (Rare) 1690
Zerit 1147
Zestoretic Tablets (Rare) 695
Zestril Tablets (Rare) 698
Ziagen 1692
Zofran Injection 1698
Zofran 1703
Zofran ODT Orally Disintegrating Tablets 1703
Zoloft (One or more patients) 2751

Hepatic failure, fulminant

Tasmar Tablets (Three cases) 3010

Hepatic function tests, impaired

(*see under* Hepatic dysfunction)

Hepatic necrosis

Accupril Tablets (Rare) 2611
Aceon Tablets (2 mg, 4 mg, 8 mg) (Rare) 3249
Altace Capsules (Rare) 2233
Asacol Delayed-Release Tablets (Rare) 2884
Azulfidine EN-tabs Tablets (Rare) 2775
Bactrim (Rare) 2949
Baycol Tablets (Rare) 883
▲ Blephamide Ophthalmic Ointment (Among most often) 547
Blephamide Ophthalmic Suspension 548
Captopril Tablets (Rare) 2281
Cataflam Tablets (Rare) 2315
Celebrex Capsules (Rare) 2676
Celebrex Capsules (Rare) 2780
Celexa (2 cases) 1365
Cipro I.V. (1% or less) 893
Cipro I.V. Pharmacy Bulk Package (Less than 1%) 897
Cipro (Rare) 887
Claritin (Rare) 3100
Claritin-D 12 Hour Extended Release Tablets 3102
Colazal Capsules 3069
Cordarone Intravenous 3491
Darvon-N/Darvocet-N 1907
Diamox Intravenous (Occasional) ⊙269
Diamox Sequels Sustained Release Capsules ⊙270
Diamox Tablets (Occasional) ⊙269
DTIC-Dome 902
Effexor Tablets 3495
Effexor XR Capsules 3499
Enalaprilat Injection (Rare) 863
Eulexin Capsules 3118
Floxin I.V. 2526
Floxin Tablets 2529
Fluothane Inhalation 3508
FML-S Liquifilm Sterile Ophthalmic Suspension ⊙238
Sterile FUDR 2974
Lescol Capsules (Rare) 2361
Lescol Capsules (Rare) 2925
Lescol XL Tablets 2361
Lescol XL Tablets 2925
Lodine (Rare; less than 1%) 3528
Lodine XL Extended-Release Tablets (Rare; less than 1%) 3530
Lotrel Capsules (Rare) 2370
Macrobid Capsules (Rare) 2889
Macrodantin Capsules (Rare) 2891
Mavik Tablets (Rare) 478
Mevacor Tablets (Rare) 2132
Mexitil Capsules (Rare) 1047
Monopril Tablets 1091
Monurol Sachet 1375
Motrin Suspension, Oral Drops, Chewable Tablets, and Caplets (Less than 1%) 2002
Myleran Tablets 1603
Nardil Tablets (Less frequent) 2653
Neptazane Tablets ⊙271
Niaspan Extended-Release Tablets 1846
Nolvadex Tablets (Rare) 678
Normodyne Injection 3135
Normodyne Tablets (Less common) 3137
Noroxin Tablets 2145
Oxandrin Tablets (Rare) 1153
Paxil 1609
Pediazole Suspension 3050
Pentasa Capsules 3239
Pravachol Tablets (Rare) 1099
Prilosec Delayed-Release Capsules (Rare) 628
Prinivil Tablets (Rare) 2164
Prinzide Tablets (Rare) 2168
Prozac Pulvules, Liquid, and Weekly Capsules 1238
Sarafem Pulvules 1962
Septra Suspension 2265
Septra Tablets 2265
Septra DS Tablets 2265
Serzone Tablets 1104
Silvadene Cream 1% 2267
Tarka Tablets (Rare) 508
Taxol Injection (Rare) 1129
Ticlid Tablets (Rare) 3015
Trovan 2722
Trusopt Sterile Ophthalmic Solution (Rare) 2196
Uniretic Tablets (Rare) 3178
Univasc Tablets (Rare) 3181
Vaseretic Tablets (Rare) 2204
Vasotec I.V. Injection (Rare) 2207
Vasotec Tablets (Rare) 2210
Viramune Oral Suspension 1060
Viramune Tablets 1060
Voltaren Tablets (Rare) 2315
Voltaren-XR Tablets (Rare) 2315
Zestoretic Tablets (Rare) 695
Zestril Tablets (Rare) 698
Zocor Tablets (Rare) 2219

Hepatic veno-occlusive disease

Abelcet Injection 1273
Alkeran for Injection 1465
AmBisome for Injection (Less common) 1383
Amphotec (1% to 5%) 1774
Cosmegen for Injection 2062
Myleran Tablets 1603
Mylotarg for Injection 3540
Tabloid Tablets 1642

Hepatitis

Abelcet Injection 1273
Accupril Tablets (0.5% to 1.0%) 2611
Accuretic Tablets 2614
Accutane Capsules 2944
Aciphex Tablets (Rare) 1267
Aciphex Tablets (Rare) 1783
Aldoclor Tablets 2035
Aldomet Tablets 2037
Aldoril Tablets 2039
Altace Capsules (Less than 1%) 2233
Amaryl Tablets (Isolated cases) 717
Anaprox Tablets (Rare) 2967
Anaprox DS Tablets (Rare) 2967
Antabuse Tablets 2444
Antabuse Tablets (Multiple cases) 3474
Aricept Tablets 1270
Aricept Tablets 2665
Arthrotec Tablets (Rare) 3195
Asacol Delayed-Release Tablets (Rare) 2884
Augmentin Chewable Tablets (Rare) 1482
Augmentin Powder for Oral Suspension (Rare) 1482
Augmentin Tablets (Rare) 1485
Avandia Tablets 1490
Avonex 1013
Axid Pulvules 1903
Axid Pulvules 2919
Azactam for Injection (Less than 1%) 1276
Azulfidine EN-tabs Tablets (Rare) 2775
Bactrim 2949
Baycol Tablets 883
Betaseron for SC Injection 988
Captopril Tablets 2281
Carbatrol Capsules 3234
Cardura Tablets 2668
Casodex Tablets 662
Cataflam Tablets (Less than 1%) 2315
Catapres Tablets (Rare) 1037
Ceclor (Rare) 1905
Ceftin 1898
Celebrex Capsules (Less than 0.1%) 2676
Celebrex Capsules (Less than 0.1%) 2780
Celexa (Rare) 1365
▲ CellCept Capsules (3%) 2951
▲ CellCept Intravenous (3%) 2951
▲ CellCept Oral Suspension (3%) 2951
▲ CellCept Tablets (3% to 13%) 2951
Chibroxin Sterile Ophthalmic Solution 2051
Claritin (Rare) 3100
Claritin-D 12 Hour Extended Release Tablets 3102
Clinoril Tablets (Less than 1%) 2053
Clomid Tablets 735
Clorpres Tablets (Rare) 1002
Clozaril Tablets 2319
Combipres Tablets (Rare) 1040
Cordarone Tablets 3487
Cosmegen for Injection 2062
Coumadin for Injection (Infrequent) 1243
Coumadin Tablets (Infrequent) 1243
Cozaar Tablets (Rare) 2067
Crixivan Capsules 2070
Cylert Tablets 415
Cytovene 2959
Dantrium Capsules (Less frequent) 2885
Declomycin Tablets (Rare) 1855
DiaBeta Tablets (Rare) 741
Diflucan Tablets, Injection, and Oral Suspension (Rare) 2681
Diovan Capsules (Very rare) 2337
Diovan HCT Tablets (Very rare) 2338
Dipentum Capsules (Rare) 2803
Dolobid Tablets (Less than 1 in 100) 2088
Doxil Injection (Less than 1%) 566
Duraclon Injection (Rare) 3057
Dynacin Capsules (Rare) 2019
EC-Naprosyn Delayed-Release Tablets (Rare) 2967
Ecotrin Enteric Coated Aspirin Low, Regular and Maximum Strength Tablets 1715
E.E.S. 450
Effexor Tablets (Rare) 3495
Effexor XR Capsules (Rare) 3499
Enalaprilat Injection 863
EryPed 446
Etrafon (Rare) 3115
Eulexin Capsules (Less than 1%) 3118
Felbatol 3343
Feldene Capsules (Occasional) 2685
Flexeril Tablets (Rare) 572
Flexeril Tablets (Rare) 2094
Floxin I.V. 2526
Floxin Tablets 2529
Fluothane Inhalation 3508

Fortovase Capsules (Less than 2%) 2970
Havrix Vaccine (Rare) 1544
Herceptin I.V. (At least one of the 958 patients) 1414
Hivid Tablets (Less than 1%) 2975
Hyzaar (Rare) 2109
Invirase Capsules (Less than 2%) 2979
Keflex (Rare) 1237
Konyne 80 937
Lamictal (Rare) 1567
Lescol Capsules 2361
Lescol Capsules 2925
Lescol XL Tablets 2361
Lescol XL Tablets 2925
Lexxel Tablets 608
Lipitor Tablets (Less than 2%) 2639
Lipitor Tablets (Less than 2%) 2696
Lodine (Less than 1%) 3528
Lodine XL Extended-Release Tablets (Less than 1%) 3530
Loxitane Capsules (Rare) 3398
Luvox Tablets (25, 50, 100 mg) 3256
Macrobid Capsules (Rare) 2889
Macrodantin Capsules (Rare) 2891
Mandol Vials (Rare) 1953
Mevacor Tablets 2132
Mexitil Capsules (Rare) 1047
Miacalcin Nasal Spray (Less than 1%) 2375
Minocin Intravenous (Rare) 1862
Minocin Oral Suspension (Rare) 1865
Minocin Pellet-Filled Capsules (Rare) 1863
Mobic Tablets (Less than 2%) 1054
Monopril Tablets (0.2% to 1.0%) 1091
Monopril HCT 1094
Motrin Suspension, Oral Drops, Chewable Tablets, and Caplets (Rare; less than 1%) 2002
Mycobutin Capsules (Less than 1%) 2838
Naprosyn Suspension (Rare) 2967
Naprosyn Tablets (Rare) 2967
Neurontin Capsules 2655
Neurontin Oral Solution 2655
Neurontin Tablets 2655
Nilandron Tablets 753
Nimotop Capsules (Less than 1%) 904
Nizoral Tablets (Several cases) 1791
Nolvadex Tablets (Rare) 678
Normodyne Injection 3135
Normodyne Tablets (Less common) 3137
Noroxin Tablets 2145
Norpramin Tablets 755
Norvasc Tablets (Less than or equal to 0.1%) 2704
Norvir Capsules (Less than 2%) 487
Norvir Oral Solution (Less than 2%) 487
Omnicef 493
Orthoclone OKT3 Sterile Solution 2498
Orudis Capsules (Less than 1%) 3548
Oruvail Capsules (Less than 1%) 3548
Pacerone Tablets 3331
Parnate Tablets (Rare) 1607
Paser Granules 1781
Paxil (Rare) 1609
PCE Dispertab Tablets 498
Pediazole Suspension 3050
Pentasa Capsules (Infrequent) 3239
Periactin Tablets 2155
Permax Tablets (Infrequent) 1299
Persantine Tablets (Rare) 1057
Ponstel Capsules (Occasional) 1356
Pravachol Tablets 1099
Priftin Tablets (Less than 1%) 758
Prilosec Delayed-Release Capsules (Rare) 628
Primaxin I.M. 2158
Primaxin I.V. (Less than 0.2%) 2160
Prinivil Tablets (0.3% to 1.0%) 2164
Prinzide Tablets 2168
▲ Prograf (3% to 15%) 1393
Proleukin for Injection 1199
Prometrium Capsules (100 mg, 200 mg) 3261
Protonix I.V. (Less than 1%) 3580
Protonix Tablets (Less than 1%) 3577
Prozac Pulvules, Liquid, and Weekly Capsules (Rare) 1238
Rescriptor Tablets (Less than 2%) 526
Retrovir Capsules (Rare) 1625
Retrovir IV Infusion (Rare) 1629
Retrovir (Rare) 1625
Rifadin (Rare) 765
Rifamate Capsules (Rare) 767
Rifater Tablets (Rare; occasional) 769
Rilutek Tablets (Infrequent) 772
Risperdal (Rare) 1796
Roferon-A Injection (Infrequent) 2996
Rythmol Tablets – 150 mg, 225 mg, 300 mg (0.03%) 502
Salagen Tablets (Less than 1%) 2229
Sandostatin Injection (Less than 1%) 2394
Sandostatin LAR Depot (Rare) 2395
Sarafem Pulvules (Rare) 1962
Septra Suspension 2265
Septra Tablets 2265
Septra DS Tablets 2265
Serophene Tablets 3226
▲ Serostim for Injection (1% to 10%) 3229
Serzone Tablets (Rare) 1104
Silvadene Cream 1% 2267
Soriatane Capsules (Less than 1%) 3003
Sporanox Capsules (Rare) 1800
Sporanox Injection (Less than 1%) 1804
Sporanox Injection (Less than 1%) 2509
Sporanox Oral Solution (Rare) 1808
Sporanox Oral Solution (Rare) 2512
Stelazine 1640
Suprane Liquid for Inhalation 874
Suprax 1877
Sustiva Capsules (Less than 2%) 1258
Tamiflu Capsules 3008
Tamiflu Oral Suspension 3008
Tapazole Tablets 1823
Tegretol/Tegretol-XR 2404
Thalomid Capsules 1154
Tice BCG, BCG Live (0.2%) 2489
Ticlid Tablets (Rare) 3015
Timentin Injection- ADD-Vantage Vial (Rare) 1661
Timentin Injection-Galaxy Container (Rare) 1664
Timentin Injection-Pharmacy Bulk Package (Rare) 1666
Timentin for Intravenous Administration (Rare) 1658
Tolectin (Less than 1%) 2589
Tonocard Tablets (Less than 1%) 649
Topamax Sprinkle Capsules 2590
Topamax Tablets 2590
Toradol 3018
Trecator-SC Tablets 3598
Trental Tablets (Rare) 784
Tricor Capsules, Micronized (Less than 1%) 513
Trilisate (Rare) 2901
Trovan 2722
Twinrix Vaccine 1674
Ultracet Tablets 2597
Ultram Tablets (Infrequent) 2600
Univasc Tablets (Less than 1%) 3181
Urobiotic-250 Capsules 2731
Valtrex Caplets 1676
Vaseretic Tablets 2204
Vasotec I.V. Injection 2207
Vasotec Tablets (0.5% to 1.0%) 2210
Vermox Chewable Tablets (Rare) 2017
▲ Vesanoid Capsules (3%) 3037
Videx 1138
Videx EC Capsules 1143
Vioxx 2213
Viracept 532
Viramune Oral Suspension (1%) 1060
Viramune Tablets (1%) 1060
Vistide Injection 1445
Voltaren Tablets (Less than 1%) 2315
Voltaren-XR Tablets (Less than 1%) 2315
Warfarin Sodium Tablets, USP 3302
Wellbutrin Tablets 1680
Wellbutrin SR Sustained-Release Tablets 1684
Xanax Tablets 2865
Xeloda Tablets (Less than 5%) 3039
Zanaflex Tablets (Infrequent) 1305
Zantac (Occasional) 1690
Zantac Injection 1688
Zantac Syrup (Occasional) 1690
Zaroxolyn Tablets 1177
Zerit 1147
Zestoretic Tablets 695
Zestril Tablets (0.3% to 1.0%) 698
Zithromax Capsules, 250 mg 2743
Zithromax for IV Infusion 2748
Zithromax for Oral Suspension, 300 mg, 600 mg, 900 mg, 1200 mg 2739
Zithromax Tablets, 250 mg 2739
Zocor Tablets 2219
Zoloft (One or more patients) 2751
Zosyn 1890
Zosyn in Galaxy Containers 1894
Zovirax 1706
Zyban Sustained-Release Tablets 1710
Zyprexa Tablets (Infrequent) 1973
Zyprexa ZYDIS Orally Disintegrating Tablets (Infrequent) 1973
Zyrtec (Rare; a single case) 2756
Zyrtec-D 12 Hour Extended Relief Tablets (Rare; a single case) 2758

Hepatitis, allergic
Adalat CC Tablets (Rare) 877
Procardia Capsules (Less than 0.5%) 2708
Procardia XL Extended Release Tablets (Rare instances) 2710

Hepatitis, cholestatic
Anadrol-50 Tablets 3321
Android Capsules, 10 mg 1731
Antabuse Tablets 2444
Antabuse Tablets (Multiple cases) 3474
Biaxin/Biaxin XL (Infrequent) 403
Cardura Tablets 2668
Ceptaz for Injection 1499
Cordarone Tablets (Rare) 3487
Dipentum Capsules (One case) 2803
Dynabac Tablets (Rare) 2269
EryPed 446
Estratest 3252
Lamisil Tablets (Rare) 2360
Lodine (Less than 1%) 3528
Lodine XL Extended-Release Tablets (Less than 1%) 3530
Orudis Capsules (Less than 1%) 3548
Oruvail Capsules (Less than 1%) 3548
Oxandrin Tablets 1153
Pacerone Tablets (Rare) 3331
Pipracil (Less frequent) 1866
PREVPAC (Infrequent) 3298
Prilosec Delayed-Release Capsules (Rare) 628
Remicade for IV Injection (Less than 2%) 1178
Risperdal (Rare) 1796
Tao Capsules 2716
Testoderm Transdermal Systems 574
Viramune Oral Suspension 1060
Viramune Tablets 1060
Xeloda Tablets (Less than 5%) 3039
Zantac (Occasional) 1690
Zantac Injection (Occasional) 1688
Zantac Syrup (Occasional) 1690
Zosyn 1890
Zosyn in Galaxy Containers 1894

Hepatitis, cytolytic
Amoxil Chewable Tablets 1471
Amoxil for Oral Suspension 1471
Amoxil 1471

Hepatitis, fulminant
Antabuse Tablets 2444
Antabuse Tablets (Multiple cases) 3474
Cataflam Tablets (Rare) 2315
Celebrex Capsules (Less than 0.1%) 2676
Celebrex Capsules (Less than 0.1%) 2780
Omnicef 493
Precose Tablets (Few cases) 906
Rythmol Tablets – 150 mg, 225 mg, 300 mg 502
Viramune Oral Suspension 1060
Viramune Tablets 1060
Voltaren Tablets (Rare) 2315
Voltaren-XR Tablets (Rare) 2315

Hepatitis, granulomatous
Dipentum Capsules (Rare) 2803
Quinaglute Dura-Tabs Tablets 978
Quinidex Extentabs 2933

Hepatitis, idiosyncratic, reversible
Sporanox Capsules (Rare) 1800
Sporanox Oral Solution (Rare) 1808
Sporanox Oral Solution (Rare) 2512

Hepatitis, infectious
Plavix Tablets (Less than 1%) 1097
Plavix Tablets (Less than 1%) 3084

Hepatitis, overt
Prilosec Delayed-Release Capsules (Rare) 628

Hepatitis, post-treatment exacerbations of
Epivir 1520
Epivir-HBV 1524

Hepatitis, reactive
Dipentum Capsules (Rare) 2803
Macrobid Capsules (Rare) 2889
Macrodantin Capsules (Rare) 2891

Hepatitis, symptomatic
Accolate Tablets (Rare) 657
Trovan 2722
Zyflo Filmtab Tablets (One patient) 524

Hepatitis, toxic
Alkeran for Injection 1465
Cuprimine Capsules (Rare) 2075
Dapsone Tablets USP 1780
Depen Titratable Tablets (Rare) 3341
Dilantin Infatabs 2624
Dilantin Kapseals 2622
Dilantin-125 Oral Suspension 2625
Fareston Tablets (One case) 3237
Indocin Capsules (Less than 1%) 2112
Indocin I.V. (Less than 1%) 2115
Indocin (Less than 1%) 2112
Rifamate Capsules 767

Hepatitis, viral
Evoxac Capsules (Less than 1%) 1217
Koāte-HP 932
Prolastin 943

Hepatobiliary dysfunction
Azactam for Injection (Less than 1%) 1276
Lamisil Tablets (Rare) 2360

Hepatocellular atrophy
Myleran Tablets 1603

Hepatomas
Aciphex Tablets (Rare) 1267
Aciphex Tablets (Rare) 1783
Avonex 1013
Baycol Tablets (Rare) 883
Brevicon 28-Day Tablets 3380
Lescol Capsules (Rare) 2361
Lescol Capsules (Rare) 2925
Lescol XL Tablets 2361
Lescol XL Tablets 2925
Lopid Tablets 2650
Mevacor Tablets (Rare) 2132
Norinyl 1 +35 28-Day Tablets 3380
Norinyl 1 + 50 28-Day Tablets 3380
Ovcon 3364
Pravachol Tablets (Rare) 1099
Premarin Intravenous 3563
Premarin Vaginal Cream 3570
Tri-Norinyl-28 Tablets 3433
Zanaflex Tablets (Rare) 1305
Zocor Tablets (Rare) 2219

Hepatomas, benign
Desogen Tablets 2458
Levlen (Rare) 962
Levlite 21 Tablets (Rare) 962
Levlite 28 Tablets (Rare) 962
Lo/Ovral Tablets 3532
Lo/Ovral-28 Tablets 3538
Low-Ogestrel-28 Tablets 3392
Modicon 2563
Nordette-28 Tablets 2257
Ogestrel 0.5/50-28 Tablets 3428
Ortho-Cept 21 Tablets 2546
Ortho-Cept 28 Tablets 2546
Ortho-Cyclen/Ortho Tri-Cyclen (Rare) 2573
Ortho-Novum 2563
Ortho-Novum 1/50□28 Tablets 2556
Ortho-Cyclen/Ortho Tri-Cyclen (Rare) 2573
Ovral Tablets 3551
Ovral-28 Tablets 3552
Ovrette Tablets 3552
Tri-Levlen (Rare) 962
Triphasil-21 Tablets 3600
Triphasil-28 Tablets 3605

Hepatomegaly
Abelcet Injection 1273
Aloprim for Injection (Less than 1%) 2292
AmBisome for Injection (Less common) 1383
Aquasol A Parenteral 593
Atromid-S Capsules 3483
Avonex 1013
Betaseron for SC Injection 988
Blocadren Tablets 2046
Combivir Tablets 1502
Copaxone for Injection (Infrequent) 3306
Cosmegen for Injection 2062
Cosopt Sterile Ophthalmic Solution 2065
DaunoXome Injection (Less than or equal to 5%) 1442
Ellence Injection 2806
Epivir 1520
Epivir-HBV 1524
Fortovase Capsules (Less than 2%) 2970
Gabitril Tablets (Infrequent) 1189
Geodon Capsules (Rare) 2688
Hivid Tablets (Rare) 2975
▲ Infergen (3% to 5%) 1777
Invirase Capsules (Less than 2%) 2979
Klonopin Tablets 2983
Lupron Depot–4 Month 30 mg (Less than 5%) 3289
Megace Oral Suspension (1% to 3%) 1124
Monopril Tablets (0.4% to 1.0%) 1091
Neupogen for Injection (Infrequent) 587
Neurontin Capsules (Infrequent) 2655
Neurontin Oral Solution (Infrequent) 2655
Neurontin Tablets (Infrequent) 2655
Norvir Capsules (Less than 2%) 487
Norvir Oral Solution (Less than 2%) 487
Oncaspar (Less than 1%) 756
Orthoclone OKT3 Sterile Solution 2498
Paser Granules 1781
▲ PEG-Intron Powder for Injection (6%) 3140
Permax Tablets (Infrequent) 1299
Proleukin for Injection (1%) 1199
Rescriptor Tablets 526
Retrovir Capsules (Rare) 1625
Retrovir IV Infusion (Rare) 1629
Retrovir (Rare) 1625
▲ Serostim for Injection (1% to 10%) 3229
Sular Tablets (Less than or equal to 1%) 688
Tabloid Tablets 1642
Thalomid Capsules 1154
Timolide Tablets 2187
Timolol GFS ⊙ 266
Timoptic in Ocudose 2192
Timoptic Sterile Ophthalmic Solution 2190

Timoptic-XE Sterile Ophthalmic Gel Forming Solution 2194
Tricor Capsules, Micronized (Less than 1%) 513
Trizivir Tablets 1669
Vistide Injection 1445
Zerit 1147
Zoloft (One or more patients) 2751

Hepatorenal syndrome, unspecified

Actiq (Less than 1%) 1184
Cataflam Tablets (Less than 1%) 2315
Felbatol 3343
Motrin Suspension, Oral Drops, Chewable Tablets, and Caplets (Less than 1%) 2002
Voltaren Tablets (Less than 1%) 2315
Voltaren-XR Tablets (Less than 1%) 2315

Hepatosplenomegaly

Aquasol A Parenteral 593
Doxil Injection (Less than 1%) 566
Fortovase Capsules (Less than 2%) 2970
Invirase Capsules (Less than 2%) 2979
Mylotarg for Injection 3540
Naprelan Tablets (Less than 1%) 1293
Proleukin for Injection 1199
Tegretol/Tegretol-XR 2404
▲ Vesanoid Capsules (9%) 3037
Vistide Injection 1445

Hepatotoxicity

Accutane Capsules 2944
Actifed Cold & Sinus Caplets and Tablets .... ▣688
Adriamycin PFS/RDF Injection 2767
Alka-Seltzer Plus Night-Time Cold Medicine Liqui-Gels .... ▣604
Alkeran Tablets (Rare) 1466
Anadrol-50 Tablets 3321
Android Capsules, 10 mg 1731
Antabuse Tablets 2444
Antabuse Tablets 3474
Asacol Delayed-Release Tablets (Rare) 2884
Azulfidine EN-tabs Tablets 2775
Benadryl Severe Allergy & Sinus Headache Caplets .... ▣694
Campath Ampules 992
Carbatrol Capsules 3234
Casodex Tablets 662
Cataflam Tablets 2315
▲ CellCept Capsules (3% to 10%) 2951
▲ CellCept Intravenous (3% to 10%) 2951
▲ CellCept Oral Suspension (3% to 10%) 2951
▲ CellCept Tablets (3% to 10%) 2951
Cognex Capsules 1351
Combivir Tablets 1502
Compazine 1505
Comtrex Acute Head Cold & Sinus Pressure Relief Tablets .... ▣627
Comtrex Deep Chest Cold & Congestion Relief Softgels .... ▣627
Comtrex Flu Therapy & Fever Relief Daytime Caplets .... ▣628
Comtrex Flu Therapy & Fever Relief Nighttime Tablets .... ▣628
Comtrex Maximum Strength Multi-Symptom Cold & Cough Relief Tablets and Caplets .... ▣626
Contac Severe Cold and Flu Caplets Maximum Strength .... ▣746
Contac Severe Cold and Flu Caplets Non-Drowsy .... ▣746
Coricidin 'D' Cold, Flu & Sinus Tablets .... ▣737
Coricidin HBP Cold & Flu Tablets .... ▣738
Coricidin HBP Maximum Strength Flu Tablets .... ▣738
Coricidin HBP Night-Time Cold & Flu Tablets .... ▣738
Cosmegen for Injection 2062
Dantrium Capsules 2885
Declomycin Tablets (Rare) 1855
Depacon Injection 416
Depakene 421
Depakote Sprinkle Capsules 426
Depakote Tablets 430
Depakote ER Tablets 436
Diflucan Tablets, Injection, and Oral Suspension (Rare) 2681
Dilantin Infatabs 2624
Dilantin Kapseals 2622
Dilantin-125 Oral Suspension 2625
Dimetapp Nighttime Flu Liquid .... ▣776
Dimetapp Non-Drowsy Flu Syrup .... ▣777
Doryx Coated Pellet Filled Capsules 3357
Effexor Tablets 3495
Effexor XR Capsules 3499
Estratest 3252
Etrafon 3115
Aspirin Free Excedrin Caplets and Geltabs .... ▣628
Excedrin Extra-Strength Tablets, Caplets, and Geltabs .... ▣629
Excedrin Migraine 1070
Excedrin PM Tablets, Caplets, and Geltabs .... ▣631
Furosemide Tablets 2284
▲ Gengraf Capsules (Less than 1% to 7%) 457
Gleevec Capsules 2357
Goody's Body Pain Formula Powder .... ▣620
Hivid Tablets 2975
Intron A for Injection (Rare) 3120
Lamisil Tablets 2360
Leukeran Tablets 1591
▲ Leukine (13%) 1755
Loxitane Capsules 3398
Maximum Strength Midol Menstrual Caplets and Gelcaps .... ▣612
Maximum Strength Midol PMS Caplets and Gelcaps .... ▣613
Maximum Strength Midol Teen Caplets .... ▣612
Minocin Intravenous 1862
Minocin Oral Suspension 1865
Mintezol 2137
Motrin Suspension, Oral Drops, Chewable Tablets, and Caplets 2002
Mylotarg for Injection 3540
Nardil Tablets (Very few patients) 2653
Nembutal Sodium Solution 485
▲ Neoral Soft Gelatin Capsules (Less than 1% to 7%) 2380
▲ Neoral Oral Solution (Less than 1% to 7%) 2380
Nizoral Tablets 1791
Norvir Capsules (Less than 2%) 487
Norvir Oral Solution (Less than 2%) 487
Pentasa Capsules 3239
Percogesic Aspirin-Free Coated Tablets .... ▣667
Extra Strength Percogesic Aspirin-Free Coated Caplets .... ▣665
Periostat Tablets 1208
Prevacid Delayed-Release Capsules 3292
PREVPAC 3298
▲ Prograf (3% to 15%) 1393
Purinethol Tablets (Frequent) 1615
Pyrazinamide Tablets 1876
Quinaglute Dura-Tabs Tablets 978
Quinidex Extentabs (A few cases) 2933
Reglan (Rare) 2935
Rifater Tablets 769
Risperdal (Rare) 1796
Robitussin Cold Caplets Multi-Symptom Cold & Flu .... ▣781
Robitussin Cold Softgels Multi-Symptom Cold & Flu .... ▣781
Robitussin Multi Symptom Honey Flu Liquid .... ▣785
Robitussin Nighttime Honey Flu Liquid .... ▣786
Roferon-A Injection (Unusual) 2996
▲ Sandimmune (Less than 1% to 7%) 2388
Singlet Caplets .... ▣761
Soriatane Capsules 3003
Sporanox Capsules (Rare) 1800
Sporanox Oral Solution (Rare) 1808
Sporanox Oral Solution (Rare) 2512
Stelazine 1640
Tavist Sinus Non-Drowsy Coated Caplets .... ▣676
Tegretol/Tegretol-XR 2404
Testopel Pellets 3610
TheraFlu Regular Strength Cold & Cough Night Time Hot Liquid .... ▣676
TheraFlu Regular Strength Cold & Sore Throat Night Time Hot Liquid .... ▣676
TheraFlu Maximum Strength Flu & Congestion Non-Drowsy Hot Liquid .... ▣677
TheraFlu Maximum Strength Flu & Cough Night Time Hot Liquid .... ▣678
TheraFlu Maximum Strength Flu & Sore Throat Night Time Hot Liquid .... ▣677
TheraFlu Maximum Strength Severe Cold & Congestion Night Time Hot Liquid .... ▣678
TheraFlu Maximum Strength Severe Cold & Congestion Non-Drowsy Hot Liquid .... ▣679
Tikosyn Capsules (Less than or equal to 2%) 2717
Trasylol Injection (0.5%) 909
Trilafon 3160
Maximum Strength Tylenol Sinus NightTime Caplets 2012
Maximum Strength Tylenol Sinus Non-Drowsy Geltabs, Gelcaps, Caplets, and Tablets 2012
Women's Tylenol Menstrual Relief Caplets 2013
Vanquish Caplets .... ▣617
Vibramycin Calcium Oral Suspension Syrup (Rare) 2735
Vibramycin Hyclate Capsules (Rare) 2735
Vibramycin Hyclate Intravenous (Rare) 2737
Vibramycin Monohydrate for Oral Suspension (Rare) 2735
Vibra-Tabs Film Coated Tablets (Rare) 2735
Vicks 44M Cough, Cold & Flu Relief Liquid .... ▣725
Vicks DayQuil LiquiCaps/Liquid Multi-Symptom Cold/Flu Relief .... ▣727
Vicks NyQuil LiquiCaps/Liquid Multi-Symptom Cold/Flu Relief, Original and Cherry Flavors .... ▣727
Viramune Oral Suspension 1060
Viramune Tablets 1060
Voltaren Tablets 2315
Voltaren-XR Tablets 2315
Wellbutrin Tablets (Infrequent) 1680
Wellbutrin SR Sustained-Release Tablets 1684
Zanaflex Tablets (Rare) 1305
Zerit 1147
Zyban Sustained-Release Tablets 1710

Hernia, hiatal

Aricept Tablets (Infrequent) 1270
Aricept Tablets (Infrequent) 2665
Celebrex Capsules (0.1% to 1.9%) 2676
Celebrex Capsules (0.1% to 1.9%) 2780
Cognex Capsules (Infrequent) 1351
Neurontin Capsules (Rare) 2655
Neurontin Oral Solution (Rare) 2655
Neurontin Tablets (Rare) 2655
Prometrium Capsules (100 mg, 200 mg) (Less than 5%) 3261
Remicade for IV Injection (Less than 2%) 1178
Vioxx (Greater than 0.1% to 1.9%) 2213

Hernia, inguinal

Antagon Injection 2447
Prevnar for Injection 1870
▲ Serostim for Injection (1% to 10%) 3229
Zyban Sustained-Release Tablets (Infrequent) 1710

Hernia, unspecified

Accuretic Tablets 2614
Actonel Tablets (2.9%) 2879
Arava Tablets (1% to 3%) 724
Avonex 1013
Betaseron for SC Injection 988
▲ Casodex Tablets (2% to 5%) 662
▲ CellCept Capsules (3%) 2951
▲ CellCept Intravenous (3%) 2951
▲ CellCept Oral Suspension (3%) 2951
▲ CellCept Tablets (3% to 11.6%) 2951
Effexor XR Capsules 3499
Exelon Capsules (Infrequent) 2342
Exelon Oral Solution (Infrequent) 2345
Gabitril Tablets (Infrequent) 1189
Lupron Depot-4 Month 30 mg (Less than 5%) 3289
Myobloc Injectable Solution (2% or greater) 1291
Nexium Delayed-Release Capsules (Less than 1%) 619
Permax Tablets (Infrequent) 1299
Plavix Tablets (1% to 2.5%) 1097
Plavix Tablets (1% to 2.5%) 3084
▲ Prograf (3% to 15%) 1393
Protonix I.V. (Less than 1%) 3580
Protonix Tablets (Less than 1%) 3577
Protopic Ointment (Greater than or equal to 1%) 1397
▲ Rapamune Oral Solution and Tablets (3% to 20%) 3584
Rilutek Tablets (Infrequent) 772
Serzone Tablets (Infrequent) 1104
▲ Simulect for Injection (3% to 10%) 2399
▲ Synagis Intramuscular (6.3%) 2028
Tasmar Tablets (Infrequent) 3010
Thalomid Capsules 1154
Tricor Capsules, Micronized 513
Uniretic Tablets (Less than 1%) 3178

Herpes, precipitation

Oxsoralen-Ultra Capsules 1741

Herpes, unspecified

Imitrex Nasal Spray (Rare) 1554
Matulane Capsules 3246
Megace Oral Suspension (1% to 3%) 1124

Herpes labialis

Alferon N Injection (1%) 1770
Ovidrel for Injection (Less than 2%) 3220

Herpes labialis, recurrent, exacerbation of

Azelex Cream (Rare) 547
Finevin Cream 962

Herpes simplex

Aceon Tablets (2 mg, 4 mg, 8 mg) (0.3% to 1%) 3249
Alrex Sterile Ophthalmic Suspension 0.2% .... ⊙256
Ambien Tablets (Rare) 3191
AmBisome for Injection (Less common) 1383
Arava Tablets (1% to 3%) 724
Aricept Tablets (Infrequent) 1270
Aricept Tablets (Infrequent) 2665
Astelin Nasal Spray (Infrequent) 3339
Avonex (2%) 1013
Blephamide Ophthalmic Ointment 547
▲ Campath Ampules (1% to 11%) 992
Celebrex Capsules (0.1% to 1.9%) 2676
Celebrex Capsules (0.1% to 1.9%) 2780
▲ CellCept Capsules (12.5% to 20.0%) 2951
▲ CellCept Intravenous (12.5% to 20.0%) 2951
▲ CellCept Oral Suspension (12.5% to 20.0%) 2951
▲ CellCept Tablets (12.5% to 20.0%) 2951
Cognex Capsules (Infrequent) 1351
▲ Copaxone for Injection (4%) 3306
Crixivan Capsules (Less than 2%) 2070
Cutivate Cream (0.8%) 1282
Doxil Injection (1% to 5%) 566
Effexor XR Capsules 3499
Efudex (Infrequent) 1733
8-MOP Capsules 1727
Evoxac Capsules (Less than 1%) 1217
Exelon Capsules (Infrequent) 2342
Exelon Oral Solution (Infrequent) 2345
FML Ophthalmic Ointment .... ⊙237
Fortovase Capsules (Less than 2%) 2970
Gabitril Tablets (Infrequent) 1189
Gengraf Capsules (1% to less than 3%) 457
Herceptin I.V. (2%) 1414
Intron A for Injection (Up to 5%) 3120
Invirase Capsules (Less than 2%) 2979
Klonopin Tablets (Infrequent) 2983
Lotemax Sterile Ophthalmic Suspension 0.5% .... ⊙261
Meridia Capsules (1.3%) 481
Migranal Nasal Spray (Rare) 2376
▲ Mylotarg for Injection (12% to 31%) 3540
Naprelan Tablets (Less than 1%) 1293
Neoral Soft Gelatin Capsules (1% to less than 3%) 2380
Neoral Oral Solution (1% to less than 3%) 2380
Neurontin Capsules (Infrequent) 2655
Neurontin Oral Solution (Infrequent) 2655
Neurontin Tablets (Infrequent) 2655
▲ Nipent for Injection (4%) 3272
Oncaspar 756
Paxil (Rare) 1609
Permax Tablets (Infrequent) 1299
▲ Prograf (3% to 15%) 1393
Prometrium Capsules (100 mg, 200 mg) (Less than 5%) 3261
Protonix I.V. (Less than 1%) 3580
Protonix Tablets (Less than 1%) 3577
▲ Protopic Ointment (4% to 12%) 1397
Provigil Tablets (1%) 1193
Pulmicort Respules (1% to 3%) 632
Remeron Tablets (Infrequent) 2483
Remeron SolTab Tablets (Infrequent) 2486
Requip Tablets (Infrequent) 1621
Rescriptor Tablets 526
Rhinocort Nasal Inhaler (Less than 1%) 640
Roxicodone Tablets (Less than 3%) 3067
Salagen Tablets (Less than 1%) .... [illegible]
▲ Serostim for Injection (1% to 10%) 3229
▲ Simulect for Injection (3% to 10%) 2399
Soriatane Capsules (Less than 1%) 3003
Sular Tablets (Less than or equal to 1%) 688
Tasmar Tablets (Infrequent) 3010
▲ Taxol Injection (11% to 38%) 1129
Teveten Tablets (Less than 1%) 3327
Thalomid Capsules 1154
▲ Thymoglobulin for Injection (4.9%) 3071
Tricor Capsules, Micronized 513
▲ Trisenox Injection (13%) 1158
Uniretic Tablets (Less than 1%) 3178
Vaniqa Cream (Less than 1%) 1121
Vexol 1% Ophthalmic Suspension .... ⊙222
Viagra Tablets (Less than 2%) 2732
Vioxx (Greater than 0.1% to 1.9%) 2213
Vistide Injection 1445
Zanaflex Tablets (Rare) 1305
Zoladex 3-month (1% to 5%) 706

Herpes simplex, disseminated

Accutane Capsules 2944

Herpes zoster

Aciphex Tablets (Rare) 1267
Aciphex Tablets (Rare) 1783
Actiq (Less than 1%) 1184
Ambien Tablets (Rare) 3191
Arava Tablets (1% to 3%) 724
Aricept Tablets (Infrequent) 1270
Aricept Tablets (Infrequent) 2665
▲ Avonex (3%) 1013
Campath Ampules 992
▲ Casodex Tablets (2% to 5%) 662

Celebrex Capsules (0.1% to 1.9%) 2676
Celebrex Capsules (0.1% to 1.9%) 2780
▲ CellCept Capsules (6.0% to 7.6%) 2951
▲ CellCept Intravenous (6.0% to 7.6%) 2951
▲ CellCept Oral Suspension (6.0% to 7.6%) 2951
▲ CellCept Tablets (6.0% to 7.6%) 2951
Cognex Capsules (Infrequent) 1351
Copaxone for Injection (Frequent) 3306
Crixivan Capsules (Less than 2%) 2070
Doxil Injection (Less than 1% to 5%) 566
Effexor XR Capsules 3499
Enalaprilat Injection 863
Engerix-B Vaccine 1517
Evoxac Capsules (Less than 1%) 1217
Fortovase Capsules (Less than 2%) 2970
Gabitril Tablets (Infrequent) 1189
Gengraf Capsules (1% to less than 3%) 457
Herceptin I.V. (At least one of the 958 patients) 1414
Intron A for Injection (Less than 5%) 3120
Invirase Capsules (Less than 2%) 2979
Lamictal (Rare) 1567
Leustatin Injection (8 episodes) 2495
Lexxel Tablets 608
Lupron Depot–4 Month 30 mg (Less than 5%) 3289
Mustargen for Injection 2142
Naprelan Tablets (Less than 1%) 1293
Neoral Soft Gelatin Capsules (1% to less than 3%) 2380
Neoral Oral Solution (1% to less than 3%) 2380
Neurontin Capsules (Rare) 2655
Neurontin Oral Solution (Rare) 2655
Neurontin Tablets (Rare) 2655
▲ Nipent for Injection (8%) 3272
Paxil (Rare) 1609
Permax Tablets (Infrequent) 1299
Prinivil Tablets (0.3% to 1.0%) 2164
Prinzide Tablets 2168
Protonix I.V. (Less than 1%) 3580
Protonix Tablets (Less than 1%) 3577
Protopic Ointment (Up to 3%) 1397
Prozac Pulvules, Liquid, and Weekly Capsules (Rare) 1238
▲ Rapamune Oral Solution and Tablets (3% to 20%) 3584
Recombivax HB 2178
Remeron Tablets (Rare) 2483
Remeron SolTab Tablets (Rare) 2486
Remicade for IV Injection (Less than 2%) 1178
Requip Tablets (Infrequent) 1621
Rescriptor Tablets 526
Sarafem Pulvules (Rare) 1962
▲ Serostim for Injection (1% to 10%) 3229
▲ Simulect for Injection (3% to 10%) 2399
Sporanox Capsules (2%) 1800
Sular Tablets (Less than or equal to 1%) 688
Tasmar Tablets (Infrequent) 3010
Tricor Capsules, Micronized 513
▲ Trisenox Injection (8%) 1158
Twinrix Vaccine 1674
Uniretic Tablets (Less than 1%) 3178
Varivax 2202
Vaseretic Tablets 2204
Vasotec I.V. Injection 2207
Vasotec Tablets (0.5% to 1.0%) 2210
Vioxx (Greater than 0.1% to 1.9%) 2213
Zanaflex Tablets (Rare) 1305
Zestoretic Tablets 695
Zestril Tablets (0.3% to 1.0%) 698

Herxheimer's reaction
Bicillin L-A Injection 2242
▲ Ceftin Tablets (5.6%) 1898
Pfizerpen for Injection 2707

Hiccups
Aciphex Tablets 1267
Aciphex Tablets 1783
Actiq (Less than 1%) 1184
Ambien Tablets (Frequent) 3191
AmBisome for Injection (Less common) 1383
Avonex 1013
Betaseron for SC Injection 988
Brevital Sodium for Injection, USP 1815
Celexa (Rare) 1365
▲ CellCept Capsules (3% to 10%) 2951
▲ CellCept Intravenous (3% to 10%) 2951
▲ CellCept Oral Suspension (3% to 10%) 2951
▲ CellCept Tablets (3% to 10%) 2951
Celontin Capsules 2618
Cipro I.V. (1% or less) 893
Cipro I.V. Pharmacy Bulk Package (Less than 1%) 897
Cipro (Less than 1%) 887
Claritin (At least one patient) 3100
DaunoXome Injection (Less than or equal to 5%) 1442
Decadron Elixir 2078
Decadron Tablets 2079
Decadron Phosphate Injection 2081
Depakote ER Tablets (Greater than 1%) 436
Diprivan Injectable Emulsion (Less than 1%) 667
Dopram Injectable 2931
Doxil Injection (Less than 1%) 566
Duragesic Transdermal System (1% or greater) 1786
Ethyol for Injection 2029
Evoxac Capsules (1% to 3%) 1217
▲ Felbatol (9.7%) 3343
Floxin I.V. 2526
Floxin Tablets 2529
Gabitril Tablets (Infrequent) 1189
Gengraf Capsules (2% or less) 457
Imitrex Injection (Rare) 1549
Imitrex Nasal Spray 1554
Imitrex Tablets (Rare) 1558
Kadian Capsules (Less than 3%) 1335
Lamictal (Rare) 1567
Lodosyn Tablets 1251
Lupron Depot–4 Month 30 mg (Less than 5%) 3289
Luvox Tablets (25, 50, 100 mg) (Rare) 3256
Maxalt Tablets (Rare) 2120
Maxalt-MLT Orally Disintegrating Tablets (Rare) 2120
Mexitil Capsules (About 1 in 1,000) 1047
Migranal Nasal Spray (Infrequent) 2376
Moduretic Tablets (Less than or equal to 1%) 2138
Neoral Soft Gelatin Capsules (2% or less) 2380
Neoral Oral Solution (2% or less) 2380
Neurontin Capsules (Rare) 2655
Neurontin Oral Solution (Rare) 2655
Neurontin Tablets (Rare) 2655
Nexium Delayed-Release Capsules (Less than 1%) 619
▲ Nicotrol Inhaler (Greater than 3%) 2840
Nicotrol Nasal Spray (Less than 1%) 2843
Norvir Capsules (Less than 2%) 487
Norvir Oral Solution (Less than 2%) 487
OxyContin Tablets (Between 1% and 5%) 2912
Paxil (Rare) 1609
Permax Tablets (1.1%) 1299
Prevacid Delayed-Release Capsules (Less than 1%) 3292
PREVPAC (Less than 1%) 3298
Protonix I.V. (Less than 1%) 3580
Protonix Tablets (Less than 1%) 3577
Prozac Pulvules, Liquid, and Weekly Capsules (Infrequent) 1238
Remeron Tablets (Rare) 2483
Remeron SolTab Tablets (Rare) 2486
Reminyl Oral Solution (Infrequent) 1792
Reminyl Tablets (Infrequent) 1792
Requip Tablets (Infrequent) 1621
Rescriptor Tablets 526
Rilutek Tablets (Infrequent) 772
Romazicon Injection (Less than 1%) 3000
Salagen Tablets (Less than 1%) 2229
Sandimmune (2% or less) 2388
Sarafem Pulvules (Infrequent) 1962
Seroquel Tablets (Rare) 684
Serzone Tablets (Infrequent) 1104
Sinemet Tablets 1253
Sinemet CR Tablets 1255
Soma Tablets 3353
Soma Compound Tablets 3354
Soma Compound w/Codeine Tablets 3355
Sonata Capsules (Rare) 3591
Tasmar Tablets (Infrequent) 3010
Tonocard Tablets (Less than 1%) 649
Topamax Sprinkle Capsules (Infrequent) 2590
Topamax Tablets (Infrequent) 2590
Trileptal Oral Suspension 2407
Trileptal Tablets 2407
Trovan (Less than 1%) 2722
Valium Injectable 3026
Versed Injection (1.2% to 3.9%) 3027
Versed Syrup (Less than 1%) 3033
Vicoprofen Tablets (Less than 3%) 520
Vistide Injection 1445
Zarontin Capsules 2659
Zarontin Syrup 2660
Zemuron Injection (Less than 1%) 2491
Zofran Injection 1698
Zofran 1703
Zofran ODT Orally Disintegrating Tablets 1703
Zoloft (Rare) 2751
Zomig Tablets (Infrequent) 708
Zomig-ZMT Tablets (Infrequent) 708
Zosyn (1.0% or less to 2.6%) 1890
Zosyn in Galaxy Containers (1.0% or less to 2.6%) 1894
Zyprexa Tablets (Rare) 1973
Zyprexa ZYDIS Orally Disintegrating Tablets (Rare) 1973

Hirsutism
Accutane Capsules 2944
Activella Tablets 2764
Alesse-21 Tablets 3468
Alesse-28 Tablets 3473
Alora Transdermal System 3372
Anadrol-50 Tablets 3321
Androderm Transdermal System CIII 3377
AndroGel (Fewer than 1%) 3322
▲ Android Capsules, 10 mg (Among most common) 1731
Aricept Tablets (Infrequent) 1270
Aricept Tablets (Infrequent) 2665
Betaseron for SC Injection 988
Brevicon 28-Day Tablets 3380
Carbatrol Capsules (Isolated cases) 3234
▲ CellCept Capsules (3%) 2951
▲ CellCept Intravenous (3%) 2951
▲ CellCept Oral Suspension (3%) 2951
▲ CellCept Tablets (3%) 2951
Cenestin Tablets 1263
Climara Transdermal System 958
Cortone Acetate Injectable Suspension 2059
Cortone Acetate Tablets 2061
Cyclessa Tablets 2450
Dantrium Capsules (Less frequent) 2885
Decadron Elixir 2078
Decadron Tablets 2079
Decadron Phosphate Injection 2081
Delatestryl Injection 1151
Depo-Provera Contraceptive Injection (Fewer than 1%) 2798
Desogen Tablets 2458
Effexor Tablets (Rare) 3495
Effexor XR Capsules (Rare) 3499
Eldepryl Capsules 3266
Esclim Transdermal System 3460
Estinyl Tablets 3112
Estrace Vaginal Cream 3358
Estrace Tablets 3361
Estratest 3252
Estrostep 2627
femhrt Tablets 2635
Florinef Acetate Tablets 2250
Gabitril Tablets (Infrequent) 1189
▲ Gengraf Capsules (21% to 45%) 457
Hydrocortone Tablets 2106
Hydrocortone Acetate Injectable Suspension 2103
Hydrocortone Phosphate Injection, Sterile 2105
Intron A for Injection (Less than 5%) 3120
Klonopin Tablets 2983
Lamictal (Infrequent) 1567
Levlen 962
Levlite 21 Tablets 962
Levlite 28 Tablets 962
Levora Tablets 3389
Loestrin 21 Tablets 2642
Loestrin Fe Tablets 2642
Lo/Ovral Tablets 3532
Lo/Ovral-28 Tablets 3538
Low-Ogestrel-28 Tablets 3392
Lumigan Ophthalmic Solution (1% to 5%) 553
Lunelle Monthly Injection 2827
Lupron Depot 7.5 mg (Less than 5%) 3284
Lupron Depot–3 Month 11.25 mg (0.6% to 1%) 3285
Lupron Injection 3279
Menest Tablets 2254
Microgestin Fe 1.5/30 Tablets 3407
Microgestin Fe 1/20 Tablets 3400
Micronor Tablets (Rare) 2543
Mircette Tablets 2470
Modicon 2563
Necon 3415
▲ Neoral Soft Gelatin Capsules (21% to 45%) 2380
▲ Neoral Oral Solution (21% to 45%) 2380
Neurontin Capsules (Infrequent) 2655
Neurontin Oral Solution (Infrequent) 2655
Neurontin Tablets (Infrequent) 2655
Nordette-28 Tablets 2257
Norinyl 1 +35 28-Day Tablets 3380
Norinyl 1 + 50 28-Day Tablets 3380
Norplant System 3543
Nor-QD Tablets (Rare) 3423
Ogen Tablets 2846
Ogestrel 0.5/50-28 Tablets 3428
Ortho Dienestrol Cream 2554
Ortho-Cept 21 Tablets 2546
Ortho-Cept 28 Tablets 2546
Ortho-Cyclen/Ortho Tri-Cyclen 2573
Ortho-Est Tablets 3464
Ortho-Novum 2563
Ortho-Novum 1/50▫28 Tablets 2556
Ortho-Prefest Tablets 2570
Ortho-Cyclen/Ortho Tri-Cyclen 2573
Ovcon 3364
Ovral Tablets 3551
Ovral-28 Tablets 3552
Ovrette Tablets 3552
Oxandrin Tablets 1153
Paxil (Rare) 1609
Permax Tablets (Infrequent) 1299
Photofrin for Injection 831
Prednisone 3064
Premarin Intravenous 3563
Premarin Tablets 3566
Premarin Vaginal Cream 3570
Premphase Tablets 3572
Prempro Tablets 3572
▲ Prograf (3% to 15%) 1393
Provera Tablets 2853
Prozac Pulvules, Liquid, and Weekly Capsules (Rare) 1238
▲ Rapamune Oral Solution and Tablets (3% to 20%) 3584
▲ Sandimmune (21 to 45%) 2388
Sarafem Pulvules (Rare) 1962
Synarel Nasal Solution for Endometriosis (2.5% of patients) 3205
Tegretol/Tegretol-XR (Isolated cases) 2404
Testoderm Transdermal Systems 574
Testopel Pellets 3610
Testred Capsules, 10 mg 1746
Tri-Levlen 962
Tri-Norinyl-28 Tablets 3433
Triphasil-21 Tablets 3600
Triphasil-28 Tablets 3605
Trivora Tablets 3439
Viadur Implant (Less than 2%) 912
Vivelle Transdermal System 2412
Vivelle-Dot Transdermal System 2416
Wellbutrin Tablets (Rare) 1680
Wellbutrin SR Sustained-Release Tablets 1684
Yasmin 28 Tablets 980
Zarontin Capsules 2659
Zarontin Syrup 2660
▲ Zenapax for Injection (2% to 5%) 3046
▲ Zoladex (7%) 702
Zonegran Capsules (Infrequent) 1307
Zovia 3449
Zyban Sustained-Release Tablets 1710
Zyprexa Tablets (Infrequent) 1973
Zyprexa ZYDIS Orally Disintegrating Tablets (Infrequent) 1973

HIV viral load increase
Thalomid Capsules 1154

Hives
(*see under* Urticaria)

Hives at injection site
Diprivan Injectable Emulsion (Less than 1%) 667
Idamycin PFS Injection 2825

Hoarseness
Aceon Tablets (2 mg, 4 mg, 8 mg) (0.3% to 1%) 3249
▲ Advair Diskus 100/50 (5%) 1448
Advair Diskus 250/50 (2%) 1448
▲ Advair Diskus 500/50 (2% to 5%) 1448
▲ Aerobid/Aerobid-M (3% to 9%) 1363
Android Capsules, 10 mg 1731
Atrovent Inhalation Aerosol (Less than 1%) 1030
Atrovent Nasal Spray 0.03% (Less than 2%) 1032
Atrovent Nasal Spray 0.06% (Less than 1%) 1033
Azmacort Inhalation Aerosol 728
Captopril Tablets 2281
Depo-Provera Contraceptive Injection (Fewer than 1%) 2798
Emcyt Capsules (1%) 2810
Enalaprilat Injection 863
Flonase Nasal Spray 1533
▲ Flovent Diskus (1% to 9%) 3614
Flovent 1535
Flovent Rotadisk 1537
Klonopin Tablets (Infrequent) 2983
Levaquin 2537
Lexxel Tablets 608
Lodosyn Tablets 1251
Luvox Tablets (25, 50, 100 mg) (Infrequent) 3256
Matulane Capsules 3246
Maxalt Tablets (Rare) 2120
Maxalt-MLT Orally Disintegrating Tablets (Rare) 2120
Monopril Tablets (0.2% to 1.0%) 1091
Nasarel Nasal Solution 0.025% (1% or less) 1296
Neurontin Capsules 2655
Neurontin Oral Solution 2655
Neurontin Tablets 2655
Nicotrol Nasal Spray (More common) 2843
Oxandrin Tablets 1153
Retrovir Capsules 1625
Retrovir IV Infusion 1629
Retrovir 1625
Rhinocort Nasal Inhaler (Less than 1%) 640
Sinemet Tablets 1253
Sinemet CR Tablets 1255

Vanceril Inhalation Aerosol (Few patients) 3165
Vanceril Double Strength Inhalation Aerosol (Some patients) 3167
Vaseretic Tablets 2204
Vasotec I.V. Injection 2207
Vasotec Tablets (0.5% to 1.0%) 2210
Ventolin Inhalation Aerosol and Refill (Rare) 1679
Ventolin HFA Inhalation Aerosol 3618
Vicoprofen Tablets (Less than 1%) 520

Hodgkin's disease
Clomid Tablets 735
Dilantin Infatabs 2624
Dilantin Kapseals 2622
Dilantin-125 Oral Suspension 2625

Hodgkin's disease, nodular sclerosing
Thalomid Capsules 1154

Hoigne's syndrome
Bicillin C-R 900/300 Injection 2240
Bicillin C-R Injection 2238
Bicillin L-A Injection 2242

Hormonal imbalance
Norvir Capsules (Less than 2%) 487
Norvir Oral Solution (Less than 2%) 487
ParaGard T 380A Intrauterine Copper Contraceptive 2582
Wellbutrin Tablets (Rare) 1680

Horner's syndrome
Lodosyn Tablets 1251
Naropin Injection (Less than 1%) 612
Sinemet Tablets 1253
Sinemet CR Tablets 1255

Hostility
Amerge Tablets (Rare) 1467
Aricept Tablets (Infrequent) 1270
Aricept Tablets (Infrequent) 2665
Cerebyx Injection (Infrequent) 2619
Cognex Capsules (2%) 1351
Copaxone for Injection (Infrequent) 3306
Depacon Injection 416
Depakene 421
Depakote Sprinkle Capsules 426
Depakote Tablets 430
Depakote ER Tablets 436
Duragesic Transdermal System (Less than 1%) 1786
Effexor Tablets (Infrequent) 3495
Effexor XR Capsules (Infrequent) 3499
Floxin I.V. 2526
Floxin Tablets 2529
Gabitril Tablets (2%) 1189
Geodon Capsules (Frequent) 2688
Keppra Tablets (2%) 3314
Klonopin Tablets 2983
Lamictal (Frequent) 1567
Luvox Tablets (25, 50, 100 mg) (Infrequent) 3256
▲ Neurontin Capsules (5.2% to 7.6%) 2655
▲ Neurontin Oral Solution (5.2% to 7.6%) 2655
▲ Neurontin Tablets (5.2% to 7.6%) 2655
Nipent for Injection (Less than 3%) 3272
Nubain Injection (1% or less) 1323
Paxil (Infrequent) 1609
Permax Tablets (Infrequent) 1299
Prevacid Delayed-Release Capsules (Less than 1%) 3292
PREVPAC (Less than 1%) 3298
ProSom Tablets (Infrequent) 500
Prozac Pulvules, Liquid, and Weekly Capsules (Infrequent) 1238
Remeron Tablets (Infrequent) 2483
Remeron SolTab Tablets (Infrequent) 2486
Rilutek Tablets (Frequent) 772
Sarafem Pulvules (Infrequent) 1962
Serzone Tablets (Infrequent) 1104
Sonata Capsules (Rare) 3591
Stadol NS Nasal Spray (Less than 1%) 1108
Tasmar Tablets (Infrequent) 3010
Tequin Injection (Less than 0.1%) 1110
Tequin Tablets (Less than 0.1%) 1110
Thalomid Capsules 1154
▲ Wellbutrin Tablets (5.6%) 1680
Wellbutrin SR Sustained-Release Tablets (Infrequent) 1684
Xanax Tablets (Rare) 2865
Zyban Sustained-Release Tablets (Infrequent) 1710
▲ Zyprexa Tablets (15%) 1973
▲ Zyprexa ZYDIS Orally Disintegrating Tablets (15%) 1973

Hot flashes
Alferon N Injection (1%) 1770
Ambien Tablets (Rare) 3191
Aricept Tablets (Frequent) 1270
Aricept Tablets (Frequent) 2665
▲ Arimidex Tablets (11.8% to 26.5%) 659
▲ Aromasin Tablets (13%) 2769
▲ Casodex Tablets (49%) 662
Celebrex Capsules (0.1% to 1.9%) 2676
Celebrex Capsules (0.1% to 1.9%) 2780
Celexa (Infrequent) 1365
Clozaril Tablets (Less than 1%) 2319
Colazal Capsules 3069
Crinone (Less than 5%) 3213
DaunoXome Injection (Less than or equal to 5%) 1442
▲ Depo-Provera Contraceptive Injection (More than 5%) 2798
Dipentum Capsules (Rare) 2803
Dostinex Tablets (1% to 3%) 2804
▲ Effexor XR Capsules (4%) 3499
▲ Ellence Injection (4% to 38.9%) 2806
Estring Vaginal Ring (2%) 2811
▲ Eulexin Capsules (46% to 61%) 3118
▲ Evista Tablets (9.7% to 24.6%) 1915
Evoxac Capsules (2.4%) 1217
Exelon Capsules (Frequent) 2342
Exelon Oral Solution (Frequent) 2345
▲ Fareston Tablets (35%) 3237
▲ Femara Tablets (5% to 18%) 2351
Floxin Otic Solution (Single report) 1219
Fortovase Capsules (Less than 2%) 2970
Gengraf Capsules (1% to less than 3%) 457
Hivid Tablets (Less than 1%) 2975
Imdur Tablets (Less than or equal to 5%) 1826
▲ Infergen (7% to 13%) 1777
Intron A for Injection (Less than 5%) 3120
Invirase Capsules (Less than 2%) 2979
Lamictal (1.3%) 1567
Lexxel Tablets 608
Lodosyn Tablets 1251
Lotrel Capsules 2370
▲ Lupron Depot 3.75 mg (72.9%) 3281
▲ Lupron Depot 7.5 mg (57.1%) 3284
▲ Lupron Depot–3 Month 11.25 mg (72.9% to 84%) 3285
▲ Lupron Depot–3 Month 22.5 mg (58.5%) 3288
▲ Lupron Depot–4 Month 30 mg (8.3% to 46.9%) 3289
▲ Lupron Injection (5% or more) 3279
Maxalt Tablets (Frequent) 2120
Maxalt-MLT Orally Disintegrating Tablets (Frequent) 2120
Mexitil Capsules (Less than 1% or about 2 in 1,000) 1047
Migranal Nasal Spray (1%) 2376
Mobic Tablets (Less than 2%) 1054
Neoral Soft Gelatin Capsules (1% to less than 3%) 2380
Neoral Oral Solution (1% to less than 3%) 2380
Nexium Delayed-Release Capsules (Less than 1%) 619
▲ Nilandron Tablets (66.5%) 753
▲ Nolvadex Tablets (2.8% to 63.9%) 678
Norvasc Tablets (More than 0.1% to 1%) 2704
Ovidrel for Injection (Less than 2%) 3220
Phrenilin (Infrequent) 578
Procardia XL Extended Release Tablets (1% or less) 2710
▲ Prometrium Capsules (100 mg, 200 mg) (11%) 3261
Prostin E2 Suppositories 2852
Requip Tablets (1% or more) 1621
Roferon-A Injection (Rare to infrequent) 2996
Romazicon Injection (1% to 3%) 3000
Rythmol Tablets – 150 mg, 225 mg, 300 mg (Less than 1%) 502
Sandostatin LAR Depot (1% to 4%) 2395
Sedapap Tablets 50 mg/650 mg (Infrequent) 2225
▲ Serostim for Injection (1% to 10%) 3229
Sinemet Tablets 1253
Sinemet CR Tablets 1255
▲ Soriatane Capsules (1% to 10%) 3003
Sporanox Oral Solution (Less than 2%) 1808
Sporanox Oral Solution (Less than 2%) 2512
Sustiva Capsules (Less than 2%) 1258
▲ Synarel Nasal Solution for Central Precocious Puberty (3%) 3204
▲ Synarel Nasal Solution for Endometriosis (90% of patients) 3205
Teveten Tablets (Less than 1%) 3327
Topamax Sprinkle Capsules (0.8% to 2.7%) 2590
Topamax Tablets (0.8% to 2.7%) 2590
Trileptal Oral Suspension (1% to 2%) 2407
Trileptal Tablets (1% to 2%) 2407
Trovan (Less than 1%) 2722
Ultracet Tablets (At least 1%) 2597
▲ Vagifem Tablets (3% to 5%) 2857
Wellbutrin SR Sustained-Release Tablets (1% to 3%) 1684
▲ Zoladex (62% to 96%) 702
▲ Zoladex 3-month (46% to 64%) 706
Zoloft (2%) 2751
Zyban Sustained-Release Tablets (1%) 1710
Zyrtec (Less than 2%) 2756
Zyrtec-D 12 Hour Extended Relief Tablets (Less than 2%) 2758

HPA axis suppression
Aclovate 1275
Cormax Cream 2440
Cormax Ointment 2440
Cormax Scalp Application 2441
Cutivate Cream 1282
Cutivate Ointment 1284
Dermatop Emollient Cream 2517
Diprolene Ointment 0.05% (Some patients) 3108
Diprolene AF Cream 0.05% (Some patients) 3106
Elocon Cream 0.1% 3110
Olux Foam 1211
Temovate Cream 1301
Temovate Gel 1303
Temovate Ointment 1301
Temovate Scalp Application 1304
Temovate E Emollient 1302

HPA function suppression
Azmacort Inhalation Aerosol 728
Vanceril Inhalation Aerosol 3165
Vanceril Double Strength Inhalation Aerosol 3167

Hunger
Diabinese Tablets (Less than 2%) 2680
Imitrex Injection (Rare) 1549
Imitrex Nasal Spray (Rare) 1554
Imitrex Tablets (Rare) 1558
Klonopin Tablets (Infrequent) 2983

Hydatidiform mole
Serophene Tablets 3226

Hydrocephalus
Betaseron for SC Injection 988
▲ Gliadel Wafer (3%) 1723
Herceptin I.V. (At least one of the 958 patients) 1414
Pergonal for Injection (One report) 3223
Repronex for Intramuscular and Subcutaneous Injection (One report) 1347

Hydrocephalus, fetal
Accutane Capsules 2944
Antagon Injection 2447

Hydronephrosis
Actiq (1% or greater) 1184
▲ Casodex Tablets (2% to 5%) 662
▲ CellCept Capsules (3%) 2951
▲ CellCept Intravenous (3%) 2951
▲ CellCept Oral Suspension (3%) 2951
▲ CellCept Tablets (3%) 2951
▲ Crixivan Capsules (3.1%) 2070
Doxil Injection (Less than 1%) 566
Herceptin I.V. (At least one of the 958 patients) 1414
▲ Prograf (3% to 15%) 1393
▲ Rapamune Oral Solution and Tablets (3% to 20%) 3584
Remicade for IV Injection (Less than 2%) 1178
▲ Zenapax for Injection (2% to 5%) 3046

Hydrothorax
Clomid Tablets 735
Follistim for Injection 2465
Humegon for Injection 2468
Serophene Tablets 3226

Hymen, imperforate
Cetrotide for Injection 3209

Hyperactive deep tendon reflexes
Eskalith 1527
Lithium Carbonate 3061
Lithium Citrate Syrup 3061
Lithobid Slow-Release Tablets 3255

Hyperactivity
Aerobid/Aerobid-M (1% to 3%) 1363
Amerge Tablets (Rare) 1467
Amoxil Chewable Tablets (Rare) 1471
Amoxil for Oral Suspension (Rare) 1471
Amoxil (Rare) 1471
Augmentin Chewable Tablets (Rare) 1482
Augmentin Powder for Oral Suspension (Rare) 1482
Augmentin Tablets (Rare) 1485
Augmentin ES-600 Powder for Oral Suspension (Rare) 1487
Ceclor CD Tablets 1279
Ceclor (Rare) 1905
Ceftin for Oral Suspension (0.1% to 1%) 1898
Cefzil (Less than 1%) 1076
Depacon Injection 416
Depakene 421
Depakote Sprinkle Capsules 426
Depakote Tablets 430
Depakote ER Tablets 436
Dopram Injectable 2931
Etrafon 3115
▲ Geref for Injection (1 patient in 6) 3215
Infumorph 200 and Infumorph 500 Sterile Solutions 1314
Klonopin Tablets (Infrequent) 2983
Levoxyl Tablets 1819
Moban (Less frequent) 1320
Neurontin Capsules 2655
Neurontin Oral Solution 2655
Neurontin Tablets 2655
Roferon-A Injection (Infrequent) 2996
Tasmar Tablets (1%) 3010
Thioridazine Hydrochloride Tablets (Extremely rare) 2289
Trilafon 3160
Unithroid Tablets 3445
Ventolin Inhalation Aerosol and Refill (1%) 1679
Versed Injection 3027
Zarontin Capsules 2659
Zarontin Syrup 2660

Hyperacusis
Axert Tablets (Infrequent) 2772
Carbatrol Capsules 3234
Cerebyx Injection (Infrequent) 2619
Effexor Tablets (Infrequent) 3495
Effexor XR Capsules (Infrequent) 3499
Gabitril Tablets (Infrequent) 1189
Maxalt Tablets (Rare) 2120
Maxalt-MLT Orally Disintegrating Tablets (Rare) 2120
Paxil (Rare) 1609
Prozac Pulvules, Liquid, and Weekly Capsules (Rare) 1238
Remeron Tablets (Infrequent) 2483
Remeron SolTab Tablets (Infrequent) 2486
Rilutek Tablets (Rare) 772
Risperdal (Rare) 1796
Romazicon Injection (Less than 1%) 3000
Sarafem Pulvules (Rare) 1962
Serzone Tablets (Infrequent) 1104
Sonata Capsules (2%) 3591
Tegretol/Tegretol-XR 2404
Topamax Sprinkle Capsules (Rare) 2590
Topamax Tablets (Rare) 2590
Trovan (Less than 1%) 2722
Vistide Injection 1445
Zoloft (Rare) 2751
Zomig Tablets (Infrequent) 708
Zomig-ZMT Tablets (Infrequent) 708

Hyperalgesia
Betaseron for SC Injection 988
Lamictal (Rare) 1567
Paxil (Rare) 1609
Retrovir Capsules 1625
Retrovir IV Infusion 1629
Retrovir 1625
Thalomid Capsules 1154

Hyperammonemia
Aciphex Tablets 1267
Aciphex Tablets 1783
Depacon Injection 416
Depakene 421
Depakote Sprinkle Capsules 426
Depakote Tablets 430
Depakote ER Tablets 436
Felbatol 3343
Haldol Decanoate 2535
Oncaspar (Less than 1%) 756

Hyperbilirubinemia
Abelcet Injection 1273
Accolate Tablets (Rare) 657
Aloprim for Injection (Less than 1%) 2292
Altace Capsules 2233
▲ Amphotec (2% to 19%) 1774
Anadrol-50 Tablets 3321
Ancobon Capsules 1730
▲ AndroGel (3% to 6%) 3322
Anzemet Injection (Less than 1%) 719
Anzemet Tablets (Less than 1%) 722
AquaMEPHYTON Injection 2042
Atacand Tablets (Infrequent) 595
Atacand HCT Tablets 597
Augmentin Chewable Tablets (Infrequent) 1482
Augmentin Powder for Oral Suspension (Infrequent) 1482
Augmentin Tablets (Infrequent) 1485
Augmentin ES-600 Powder for Oral Suspension (Infrequently) 1487
Avelox Tablets (Greater than or equal to 2%) 879
Bactrim 2949
Baycol Tablets 883
BayRho-D Full Dose 921
▲ Betaseron for SC Injection (6%) 988

Biaxin/Biaxin XL (Less than 1%) 403
Campath Ampules 992
Captopril Tablets 2281
▲ Casodex Tablets (2% to 5%) 662
Cedax (Greater than or equal to 1%) 1021
Cefizox for Intramuscular or Intravenous Use (Rare) 1390
Cefotan 664
Ceftin 1898
Ceptaz for Injection 1499
▲ Cipro I.V. (Among most frequent) 893
▲ Cipro I.V. Pharmacy Bulk Package (Among most frequent) 897
Cipro (0.3%) 887
Colazal Capsules 3069
Covera-HS Tablets 3199
▲ Crixivan Capsules (Approximately 10%) 2070
Dapsone Tablets USP 1780
Depacon Injection (Occasional) 416
Depakene 421
Depakote Sprinkle Capsules (Occasional) 426
Depakote Tablets (Occasional) 430
Depakote ER Tablets 436
Doxil Injection (1% to 5%) 566
Duricef 1079
Dynabac Tablets (0.1% to 1%) 2269
Elspar for Injection 2092
Enalaprilat Injection 863
Epivir (0.8%) 1520
Ergamisol Tablets (Less than 1% to 1%) 1789
Eulexin Capsules 3118
Fareston Tablets (Less than 1.5%) 3237
Floxin I.V. 2526
Floxin Tablets 2529
Fortaz 1541
Fortovase Capsules (Up to 1%) 2970
▲ Sterile FUDR (Among more common) 2974
▲ Gemzar for Injection (13% to 26%) 1919
Gengraf Capsules (1% to less than 3%) 457
Gleevec Capsules (1.1% to 3.5%) 2357
Hycamtin for Injection (Less than 3%) 1546
Hyzaar (Occasional) 2109
▲ Ifex for Injection (3%) 1123
Invirase Capsules (Up to 1%) 2979
Isoptin SR Tablets 467
Lescol Capsules 2361
Lescol Capsules 2925
Lescol XL Tablets 2361
Lescol XL Tablets 2925
▲ Leukine (30%) 1755
Leustatin Injection 2495
Lopid Tablets (Occasional) 2650
Lotrel Capsules (Rare) 2370
Mavik Tablets (0.2% of patients) 478
Maxipime for Injection (0.1% to 1%) 1285
Mephyton Tablets (Rare) 2129
Meridia Capsules (1.6%) 481
Merrem I.V. (Greater than 0.2%) 673
Mevacor Tablets 2132
Micardis HCT Tablets (Occasional) 1051
Mithracin for Intravenous Use 903
Monopril Tablets 1091
Monopril HCT 1094
Monurol Sachet 1375
Myleran Tablets 1603
▲ Mylotarg for Injection (23%) 3540
▲ Navelbine Injection (2% to 9%) 1604
Nebcin Vials, Hyporets & ADD-Vantage 1955
Neoral Soft Gelatin Capsules (1% to less than 3%) 2380
Neoral Oral Solution (1% to less than 3%) 2380
Nolvadex Tablets (1.8%) 678
Omnicef (0.2%) 493
Oncaspar 756
Oxandrin Tablets 1153
▲ Paraplatin for Injection (5%) 1126
Pentasa Capsules 3239
Pipracil (Less frequent) 1866
Pravachol Tablets 1099
PREVPAC (Less than 1%) 3298
Prilosec Delayed-Release Capsules (Rare) 628
Primaxin I.M. 2158
Primaxin I.V. 2160
Prinivil Tablets (Rare) 2164
Prinzide Tablets (Rare) 2168
Procanbid Extended-Release Tablets 2262
▲ Prograf (12% to 30%) 1393
▲ Proleukin for Injection (64%) 1199
Rebetron Combination Therapy 3153
Rescriptor Tablets (0.5% to 1.0%) 526
Retrovir Capsules (Rare) 1625
Retrovir IV Infusion (Rare) 1629
Retrovir (Rare) 1625
RhoGAM Injection 2524
Rifadin (Some cases) 765
Rifamate Capsules 767
Rifater Tablets (Some cases) 769
Rocephin Injectable Vials, ADD-Vantage, Galaxy, Bulk (Less than 1%) 2993
Sectral Capsules 3589
Septra Suspension 2265
Septra Tablets 2265
Septra DS Tablets 2265
Sinemet Tablets 1253
Suprax 1877
Symmetrel 1328
▲ Synercid I.V. (Approximately 25%) 775
Tarka Tablets 508
▲ Taxol Injection (7%) 1129
Tazicef for Injection 1647
Tazicef Galaxy Container 1650
Tazicef Pharmacy Bulk Package 1653
Tazidime Vials, Faspak & ADD-Vantage 1966
Tenoretic Tablets 690
Tenormin 692
Tequin Injection (Less than 0.1%) 1110
Tequin Tablets (Less than 0.1%) 1110
Ticlid Tablets (Rare) 3015
Timentin Injection- ADD-Vantage Vial 1661
Timentin Injection-Galaxy Container 1664
Timentin Injection-Pharmacy Bulk Package 1666
Timentin for Intravenous Administration 1658
Trecator-SC Tablets 3598
Trizivir Tablets (0.8%) 1669
Vantin Tablets and Oral Suspension 2860
Vaseretic Tablets (Rare) 2204
Vasotec I.V. Injection 2207
Vasotec Tablets 2210
Verelan Capsules 3184
Verelan PM Capsules 3186
▲ Videx (1% to 6%) 1138
▲ Videx EC Capsules (1% to 7%) 1143
Viramune Oral Suspension (0.4%) 1060
Viramune Tablets (0.4%) 1060
Xanax Tablets 2865
▲ Xeloda Tablets (2% to 14%) 3039
Zerit (2%) 1147
Zestoretic Tablets (Rare) 695
Zestril Tablets (Rare) 698
Zinacef Injection (1 in 500 patients) 1696
Zinacef for Injection (1 in 500 patients) 1696
Zithromax Capsules, 250 mg (Less than 1%) 2743
Zithromax for IV Infusion (1% to 3%) 2748
Zithromax for Oral Suspension, 1 g (Less than 1%) 2743
Zithromax for Oral Suspension, 300 mg, 600 mg, 900 mg, 1200 mg (Less than 1%) 2739
Zithromax Tablets, 250 mg (Less than 1%) 2739
Zithromax Tablets, 600 mg (Less than 1%) 2743
Zocor Tablets 2219
Zoloft (One or more patients) 2751
Zosyn 1890
Zosyn in Galaxy Containers 1894
Zovirax 1706
Zyflo Filmtab Tablets (Three patients) 524
Zyrtec (A single case) 2756
Zyrtec-D 12 Hour Extended Relief Tablets (A single case) 2758

Hypercalcemia

Abelcet Injection 1273
Accuretic Tablets (Rare) 2614
Actiq (Less than 1%) 1184
Activella Tablets 2764
Aloprim for Injection (Less than 1%) 2292
Alora Transdermal System 3372
Anadrol-50 Tablets 3321
Androderm Transdermal System CIII 3377
▲ Android Capsules, 10 mg (Among most common) 1731
Avelox Tablets (Greater than or equal to 2%) 879
Betaseron for SC Injection 988
Calcijex Injection 411
Calcium Disodium Versenate Injection 1980
▲ Carnitor Injection (6% to 15%) 3242
▲ CellCept Capsules (3%) 2951
▲ CellCept Intravenous (3%) 2951
▲ CellCept Oral Suspension (3%) 2951
▲ CellCept Tablets (3%) 2951
Cipro I.V. (Infrequent) 893
▲ Cipro I.V. Pharmacy Bulk Package (Among most frequent) 897
Climara Transdermal System 958
CombiPatch Transdermal System 2323
Cytovene 2959
Delatestryl Injection 1151
Dovonex Ointment (Less than 1%) 1117
Dovonex Scalp Solution 1118
Doxil Injection (Less than 1%) 566
Eskalith 1527
Estrace Vaginal Cream 3358
Estrace Tablets 3361
Estratest 3252
Evoxac Capsules (Less than 1%) 1217
Fareston Tablets (Less than 1% to 3%) 3237
Femara Tablets (Less frequent) 2351
▲ Flolan for Injection (48%) 1528
Fortovase Capsules (0.2%) 2970
Foscavir Injection (Between 1% and 5%) 605
Hectorol Capsules 1064
Hectorol Injection 1066
Herceptin I.V. (At least one of the 958 patients) 1414
Hivid Tablets (Less than 1%) 2975
Hyzaar 2109
Intron A for Injection (Less than or equal to 5%) 3120
Invirase Capsules (Up to 1%) 2979
Lithobid Slow-Release Tablets 3255
Lupron Depot 7.5 mg (Less than 5%) 3284
Maxipime for Injection (0.1% to 1%) 1285
Maxzide 1008
Menest Tablets 2254
Micardis HCT Tablets 1051
Mykrox Tablets (A few patients) 1168
Nipent for Injection (Less than 3%) 3272
Nolvadex Tablets (Infrequent) 678
Ogen Tablets 2846
Ortho Dienestrol Cream 2554
Ortho-Est Tablets 3464
Ortho-Prefest Tablets 2570
Oxandrin Tablets 1153
Paxil (Rare) 1609
PhosLo 1069
Premarin Intravenous 3563
Premarin Tablets 3566
Premarin Vaginal Cream 3570
Premphase Tablets 3572
Prempro Tablets 3572
Prinzide Tablets 2168
▲ Prograf (3% to 15%) 1393
Proleukin for Injection (1%) 1199
▲ Rapamune Oral Solution and Tablets (3% to 20%) 3584
Rilutek Tablets (Rare) 772
▲ Rocaltrol (1 in 3) 2991
▲ Simulect for Injection (3% to 10%) 2399
Tenoretic Tablets 690
Testoderm Transdermal Systems 574
Testopel Pellets 3610
Uniretic Tablets (Less than 1%) 3178
Vaseretic Tablets 2204
Vesanoid Capsules (Isolated cases) 3037
Vistide Injection 1445
Vivelle Transdermal System 2412
Vivelle-Dot Transdermal System 2416
Zaroxolyn Tablets (Infrequent) 1177
Zemplar Injection 522
Zestoretic Tablets 695
Zoladex 702
Zoladex 3-month (Rare) 706
Zosyn 1890
Zosyn in Galaxy Containers 1894

Hypercalciuria

Calcijex Injection (Some instances) 411
Effexor XR Capsules (Rare) 3499
Prelone Syrup 2273
▲ Rocaltrol (1 in 7) 2991

Hypercarbia

Survanta Intratracheal Suspension (Less than 1%) 3053
Versed Syrup (Less than 1%) 3033

Hyperchloremia

Anadrol-50 Tablets 3321
Androderm Transdermal System CIII 3377
▲ Android Capsules, 10 mg (Among most common) 1731
Avelox Tablets (Greater than or equal to 2%) 879
Daranide Tablets 2077
Delatestryl Injection 1151
Demadex Tablets and Injection 2965
Geodon Capsules (Rare) 2688
Primaxin I.M. 2158
Primaxin I.V. 2160
Sulfamylon Cream 1011
Sulfamylon Topical Solution 1011
Testoderm Transdermal Systems 574
Testopel Pellets 3610
Topamax Sprinkle Capsules (Infrequent) 2590
Topamax Tablets (Infrequent) 2590

Hyperchlorhydria

Prozac Pulvules, Liquid, and Weekly Capsules (Infrequent) 1238
Sarafem Pulvules (Infrequent) 1962

Hypercholesterolemia

Accuretic Tablets (Rare) 2614
Accutane Capsules 2944
Aceon Tablets (2 mg, 4 mg, 8 mg) (0.3% to 1%) 3249
Aciphex Tablets 1267
Aciphex Tablets 1783
▲ Agenerase Capsules (7% to 13%) 1454
▲ Agenerase Oral Solution (7% to 13%) 1459
Ambien Tablets (Rare) 3191
Amerge Tablets (Rare) 1467
Androderm Transdermal System CIII 3377
▲ Android Capsules, 10 mg (Among most common) 1731
Arimidex Tablets (2% to 5%) 659
Arthrotec Tablets (Rare) 3195
Axert Tablets (Rare) 2772
Betaxon Ophthalmic Suspension (Less than 2%) 537
Calcijex Injection 411
Carbatrol Capsules (Occasional) 3234
▲ Casodex Tablets (2% to 5%) 662
Celebrex Capsules (0.1% to 1.9%) 2676
Celebrex Capsules (0.1% to 1.9%) 2780
▲ CellCept Capsules (8.5% to 41.2%) 2951
▲ CellCept Intravenous (8.5% to 41.2%) 2951
▲ CellCept Oral Suspension (8.5% to 41.2%) 2951
▲ CellCept Tablets (8.5% to 41.2%) 2951
▲ Chemet Capsules (4.2% to 10.4%) 3078
Cipro I.V. (Infrequent) 893
Cipro I.V. Pharmacy Bulk Package (Less than 1%) 897
Cipro 887
Cognex Capsules (Infrequent) 1351
▲ Coreg Tablets (4.1%) 1508
Crixivan Capsules 2070
Delatestryl Injection 1151
Diflucan Tablets, Injection, and Oral Suspension 2681
Effexor Tablets (Infrequent) 3495
Effexor XR Capsules (Infrequent) 3499
Ergamisol Tablets 1789
Estratest 3252
Evoxac Capsules (Less than 1%) 1217
Exelon Capsules (Infrequent) 2342
Exelon Oral Solution (Infrequent) 2345
▲ Femara Tablets (3%) 2351
Floxin I.V. 2526
Floxin Tablets 2529
Gabitril Tablets (Infrequent) 1189
Gengraf Capsules (Less than 3%) 457
Geodon Capsules (Infrequent) 2688
Hectorol Capsules 1064
Hectorol Injection 1066
Hyzaar 2109
▲ Kaletra Capsules (6.7% to 25.7%) 471
▲ Kaletra Oral Solution (6.7% to 25.7%) 471
▲ Leukine (17%) 1755
▲ Lupron Depot 3.75 mg (7%) 3281
Lupron Depot 7.5 mg (Greater than or equal to 5%) 3284
Luvox Tablets (25, 50, 100 mg) (Infrequent) 3256
Micardis Tablets (More than 0.3%) 1049
Micardis HCT Tablets 1051
Myobloc Injectable Solution (2% or greater) 1291
Naprelan Tablets (Less than 1%) 1293
Neoral Soft Gelatin Capsules (Less than 3%) 2380
Neoral Oral Solution (Less than 3%) 2380
Neurontin Capsules (Rare) 2655
Neurontin Oral Solution (Rare) 2655
Neurontin Tablets (Rare) 2655
Noroxin Tablets 2145
Norvir Capsules (Less than 2%) 487
Norvir Oral Solution (Less than 2%) 487
Oxandrin Tablets 1153
Paxil (Rare) 1609
Permax Tablets (Infrequent) 1299
▲ Plavix Tablets (4%) 1097
▲ Plavix Tablets (4%) 3084
Prevacid Delayed-Release Capsules 3292
PREVPAC 3298
Prinzide Tablets 2168
▲ Prograf (3% to 15%) 1393
Prozac Pulvules, Liquid, and Weekly Capsules (Infrequent) 1238
▲ Rapamune Oral Solution and Tablets (38% to 46%) 3584
Requip Tablets (Infrequent) 1621
Rilutek Tablets (Rare) 772
Rocaltrol 2991
Sarafem Pulvules (Infrequent) 1962
Serzone Tablets (Rare) 1104
Sonata Capsules (Infrequent) 3591
Sustiva Capsules 1258
Synarel Nasal Solution for Endometriosis 3205
Tasmar Tablets (Infrequent) 3010
Tegretol/Tegretol-XR (Occasional) 2404
Testoderm Transdermal Systems 574
Testopel Pellets 3610
Testred Capsules, 10 mg 1746

Teveten Tablets (Less than 1%) 3327
Thalomid Capsules 1154
Ticlid Tablets 3015
Timolide Tablets 2187
Travatan Ophthalmic Solution (1% to 5%) 543
Uniretic Tablets (Less than 1%) 3178
Vaseretic Tablets 2204
▲ Vesanoid Capsules (Up to 60%) 3037
Vioxx (Greater than 0.1% to 1.9%) 2213
Zanaflex Tablets (Infrequent) 1305
Zestoretic Tablets 695
Zoladex 702
Zoladex 3-month 706
▲ Zoloft (Approximately 3%) 2751
Zyprexa Tablets (Rare) 1973
Zyprexa ZYDIS Orally Disintegrating Tablets (Rare) 1973

Hypercorticism

Advair Diskus 100/50 1448
Advair Diskus 250/50 1448
Advair Diskus 500/50 1448
Beconase Inhalation Aerosol 1497
Beconase AQ Nasal Spray 1498
Blephamide Ophthalmic Ointment (Rare) 547
Blephamide Ophthalmic Suspension (Rare) 548
FML Ophthalmic Ointment (Rare) .... ⊙ 237
FML Ophthalmic Suspension (Rare) .... ⊙ 236
FML Forte Ophthalmic Suspension (Rare) .... ⊙ 235
Nasacort Nasal Inhaler 750
Pred Forte Ophthalmic Suspension (Rare) .... ⊙ 246
Pred Mild Sterile Ophthalmic Suspension (Rare) .... ⊙ 249
Pulmicort Respules (Less than 1%) 632
Pulmicort Turbuhaler Inhalation Powder (Rare) 636
Rhinocort Nasal Inhaler (Rare) 640
Vancenase PocketHaler Nasal Inhaler 3162
Vanceril Double Strength Inhalation Aerosol (Rare) 3167

Hyperdipsia
(*see under* Dipsesis)

Hyperemia

▲ Alomide Ophthalmic Solution (1% to 5%) .... ⊙ 204
Azopt Ophthalmic Suspension (1% to 5%) 536
Celontin Capsules 2618
Emadine Ophthalmic Solution (Less than 5%) .... ⊙ 211
▲ Iopidine 0.5% Ophthalmic Solution (13%) .... ⊙ 213
Lacrisert Sterile Ophthalmic Insert 2117
Patanol Ophthalmic Solution (Less than 5%) 540
Timolol GFS (1% to 5%) .... ⊙ 266
Vexol 1% Ophthalmic Suspension (1% to 5%) .... ⊙ 222

Hyperemia, conjunctival

▲ Alphagan Ophthalmic Solution (Approximately 10% to 30%) 545
▲ Alphagan P Ophthalmic Solution (Approximately 10% to 20%) 546
▲ Carteolol Hydrochloride Ophthalmic Solution USP, 1% (About 1 of 4 patients) .... ⊙ 258
Chibroxin Sterile Ophthalmic Solution 2051
Diprivan Injectable Emulsion (Less than 1%) 667
FML Ophthalmic Ointment (Occasional) .... ⊙ 237
FML Ophthalmic Suspension (Occasional) .... ⊙ 236
FML Forte Ophthalmic Suspension (Occasional) .... ⊙ 235
▲ Genoptic Ophthalmic Ointment (Among most frequent) .... ⊙ 239
▲ Genoptic Sterile Ophthalmic Solution (Among most frequent) .... ⊙ 239
▲ Ocupress Ophthalmic Solution, 1% Sterile (About 1 of 4 patients) .... ⊙ 303
Tensilon Injectable 1745
▲ Xalatan Latanoprost Ophthalmic Solution (5% to 15%) .... ⊙ 320
▲ Xalatan Sterile Ophthalmic Solution (5% to 15%) 2864

Hypereosinophilia

Leustatin Injection 2495

Hyperesthesia

Amerge Tablets (Rare) 1467
Arthrotec Tablets (Rare) 3195
Asacol Delayed-Release Tablets 2884
Avonex 1013
Axert Tablets (Infrequent) 2772
Betaseron for SC Injection 988
Celexa (Rare) 1365
Cerebyx Injection (Infrequent) 2619
Doxil Injection (Less than 1%) 566
▲ Duraclon Injection (5%) 3057
Effexor Tablets (Infrequent) 3495
Effexor XR Capsules (Frequent) 3499
Evoxac Capsules 1217
▲ Flolan for Injection (5% to 12%) 1528
Fortovase Capsules (Less than 2%) 2970
Gengraf Capsules 457
Imitrex Injection (Rare) 1549
Imitrex Tablets (Rare) 1558
Intron A for Injection (Less than 5%) 3120
Invirase Capsules (Less than 2%) 2979
Lamictal (Rare) 1567
LYMErix Vaccine (Greater than 1%) 1592
Maxalt Tablets (Infrequent) 2120
Maxalt-MLT Orally Disintegrating Tablets (Infrequent) 2120
Myobloc Injectable Solution (2% or greater) 1291
Neoral Soft Gelatin Capsules 2380
Neoral Oral Solution 2380
Neurontin Capsules (Rare) 2655
Neurontin Oral Solution (Rare) 2655
Neurontin Tablets (Rare) 2655
Norvir Capsules (Less than 2%) 487
Norvir Oral Solution (Less than 2%) 487
Pletal Tablets (2% or greater) 2605
Pletal Tablets (2% or greater) 2848
ProAmatine Tablets (Rare) 3241
▲ Protopic Ointment (Up to 7%) 1397
Prozac Pulvules, Liquid, and Weekly Capsules (Rare) 1238
▲ Requip Tablets (4%) 1621
Rescriptor Tablets (Less than 2%) 526
Salagen Tablets (Less than 1%) 2229
Sarafem Pulvules (Rare) 1962
Sectral Capsules (Up to 2%) 3589
Serzone Tablets (Rare) 1104
Sonata Capsules (Infrequent) 3591
▲ Soriatane Capsules (10% to 25%) 3003
Tequin Injection (Less than 0.1%) 1110
Tequin Tablets (Less than 0.1%) 1110
Thalomid Capsules 1154
Topamax Sprinkle Capsules (Infrequent) 2590
Topamax Tablets (Infrequent) 2590
Vistide Injection 1445
Ziac Tablets 1887
Zoloft (Infrequent) 2751
Zomig Tablets (Infrequent) 708
Zomig-ZMT Tablets (Infrequent) 708
Zonegran Capsules (Rare) 1307
Zyrtec (Less than 2%) 2756
Zyrtec-D 12 Hour Extended Relief Tablets (Less than 2%) 2758

Hyperesthesia, tongue

Alferon N Injection (1%) 1770

Hyperexcitability

Lufyllin Tablets 3347
Lufyllin-400 Tablets 3347
Lufyllin-GG Elixir 3348
Lufyllin-GG Tablets 3348

Hyperexcitability, reflex

Theo-Dur Extended-Release Tablets 1835
Uni-Dur Extended-Release Tablets 1841

Hyperferremia

Pyrazinamide Tablets (Rare) 1876

Hyperfibrinogenemia

Amphotec (1% to 5%) 1774
Colazal Capsules 3069
Neumega for Injection 1434

Hypergammaglobulinemia

Prevacid Delayed-Release Capsules 3292
PREVPAC 3298

Hyperglycemia

Abelcet Injection 1273
Accuretic Tablets 2614
Accutane Capsules 2944
Aceon Tablets (2 mg, 4 mg, 8 mg) (0.3% to 1%) 3249
Aciphex Tablets 1267
Aciphex Tablets 1783
Aclovate 1275
Actimmune (Rare) 1772
Actiq (1% or greater) 1184
Advair Diskus 100/50 1448
Advair Diskus 250/50 1448
Advair Diskus 500/50 1448
▲ Agenerase Capsules (45% to 53%) 1454
▲ Agenerase Oral Solution (45% to 53%) 1459
Aggrenox Capsules (Less than 1%) 1026
Albalon Ophthalmic Solution .... ⊙ 225
Aldoclor Tablets 2035
Aldoril Tablets 2039
Aloprim for Injection (Less than 1%) 2292
Altace Capsules 2233
Ambien Tablets (Infrequent) 3191
▲ AmBisome for Injection (8.2% to 23%) 1383
Amerge Tablets (Rare) 1467
Amphotec (1% to 6%) 1774
Anaprox Tablets (Less than 1%) 2967
Anaprox DS Tablets (Less than 1%) 2967
▲ AndroGel (3% to 6%) 3322
▲ Apligraf (3.6%) 2305
Arava Tablets (1% to 3%) 724
Aricept Tablets (Infrequent) 1270
Aricept Tablets (Infrequent) 2665
Arthrotec Tablets (Rare) 3195
Atacand Tablets (0.5% or greater) 595
Atacand HCT Tablets (0.5% or greater) 597
Avalide Tablets 1070
▲ Avandia Tablets (3.9% to 8.1%) 1490
Avelox Tablets (0.05% to 1%) 879
Axert Tablets (Infrequent) 2772
▲ Betaseron for SC Injection (15%) 988
Blocadren Tablets 2046
Brethine Ampuls 2314
Cafcit 1035
Campath Ampules 992
Cardizem Injectable 1018
Cardizem Lyo-Ject Syringe 1018
Cardizem Monovial 1018
Cardizem CD Capsules (Less than 1%) 1016
▲ Casodex Tablets (6%) 662
Catapres Tablets (Rare) 1037
Celebrex Capsules (0.1% to 1.9%) 2676
Celebrex Capsules (0.1% to 1.9%) 2780
▲ CellCept Capsules (8.6% to 46.7%) 2951
▲ CellCept Intravenous (8.6% to 46.7%) 2951
▲ CellCept Oral Suspension (8.6% to 46.7%) 2951
▲ CellCept Tablets (8.6% to 46.7%) 2951
Cerebyx Injection (Infrequent) 2619
▲ Cipro I.V. (Among most frequent) 893
Cipro I.V. Pharmacy Bulk Package 897
Cipro 887
Clinoril Tablets (Rare) 2053
Clorpres Tablets 1002
Clozaril Tablets 2319
Combipres Tablets 1040
Combivir Tablets 1502
Compazine 1505
▲ Coreg Tablets (12.2%) 1508
Corlopam Injection (0.5% to 5%) 412
Cormax Cream 2440
Cormax Ointment 2440
Cormax Scalp Application 2441
Corzide 40/5 Tablets 2247
Corzide 80/5 Tablets 2247
Cosopt Sterile Ophthalmic Solution 2065
Crixivan Capsules 2070
Demadex Tablets and Injection (Uncommon) 2965
Dermatop Emollient Cream 2517
D.H.E. 45 Injection 2334
Dilantin Kapseals 2622
Dilantin-125 Oral Suspension 2625
Diovan HCT Tablets 2338
Diprivan Injectable Emulsion (Less than 1%) 667
Diprolene Ointment 0.05% (Some patients) 3108
Diprolene AF Cream 0.05% (Some patients) 3106
Diucardin Tablets 3494
Diuril Oral 2087
Diuril Sodium Intravenous 2086
Doxil Injection (1% to 5%) 566
Dyazide Capsules 1515
EC-Naprosyn Delayed-Release Tablets (Less than 1%) 2967
Ecotrin Enteric Coated Aspirin Low, Regular and Maximum Strength Tablets 1715
Edecrin 2091
Effexor Tablets (Infrequent) 3495
Effexor XR Capsules (Infrequent) 3499
Elspar for Injection (Low) 2092
Epivir 1520
Epivir-HBV 1524
Etrafon 3115
Evoxac Capsules (Less than 1%) 1217
Exelon Capsules (Infrequent) 2342
Exelon Oral Solution (Infrequent) 2345
Felbatol 3343
Feldene Capsules (Rare) 2685
Flexeril Tablets (Rare) 572
Flexeril Tablets (Rare) 2094
Florinef Acetate Tablets 2250
Flovent Diskus 3614
Flovent 1535
Flovent Rotadisk 1537
Floxin I.V. (More than or equal to 1%) 2526
Floxin Tablets (More than or equal to 1%) 2529
▲ Fludara for Injection (1% to 6%) 995
Foradil Aerolizer 2354
Fortovase Capsules (Less than 2%) 2970
Furosemide Tablets 2284
Gabitril Tablets (Infrequent) 1189
Gengraf Capsules (2% or less) 457
Genotropin Lyophilized Powder (Infrequent) 2818
Geodon Capsules (Infrequent) 2688
▲ Gliadel Wafer (3%) 1723
Haldol Decanoate 2535
Haldol Injection, Tablets and Concentrate 2533
Hivid Tablets (Less than 1%) 2975
Humatrope Vials and Cartridges (Infrequent) 1930
HydroDIURIL Tablets 2108
Hyzaar 2109
Imitrex Injection 1549
Imitrex Nasal Spray 1554
Imitrex Tablets (Rare) 1558
Indapamide Tablets (Less than 5%) 2286
Inderide LA Long-Acting Capsules 3519
Indocin Capsules (Less than 1%) 2112
Indocin I.V. (1% to 3%) 2115
Indocin (Less than 1%) 2112
Intron A for Injection (Less than or equal to 5%) 3120
Invirase Capsules (Less than 1% to 2%) 2979
Kaletra Capsules (1.6% to 4.4%) 471
Kaletra Oral Solution (1.6% to 4.4%) 471
Lamictal (Rare) 1567
▲ Leukine (25% to 41%) 1755
Levaquin Injection (Less than 0.5%) 2537
Lexxel Tablets (Infrequent) 608
Limbitrol 1738
Lipitor Tablets (Less than 2%) 2639
Lipitor Tablets (Less than 2%) 2696
Lodine (Less than 1%) 3528
Lodine XL Extended-Release Tablets (Less than 1%) 3530
Lodosyn Tablets 1251
Lo/Ovral Tablets 3532
Lo/Ovral-28 Tablets 3538
Lotensin HCT Tablets 2367
Low-Ogestrel-28 Tablets 3392
Lufyllin Tablets 3347
Lufyllin-400 Tablets 3347
Lufyllin-GG Elixir 3348
Lufyllin-GG Tablets 3348
Lupron Depot 7.5 mg (Greater than or equal to 5%) 3284
▲ Lupron Depot–3 Month 22.5 mg (More than or equal to 5%) 3288
▲ Lupron Depot–4 Month 30 mg (Greater than or equal to 5%) 3289
Luvox Tablets (25, 50, 100 mg) (Rare) 3256
Maxzide 1008
▲ Megace Oral Suspension (Up to 6%) 1124
▲ Mepron Suspension (9%) 1598
Meridia Capsules 481
Micardis HCT Tablets 1051
Microzide Capsules 3414
Minizide Capsules 2700
Mintezol 2137
Moduretic Tablets 2138
Monopril HCT 1094
Mykrox Tablets 1168
Mylotarg for Injection (2%) 3540
Naprelan Tablets (Less than 3%) 1293
Naprosyn Suspension (Less than 1%) 2967
Naprosyn Tablets (Less than 1%) 2967
Navane Oral 2701
Navane Intramuscular 2703
Neoral Soft Gelatin Capsules (2% or less) 2380
Neoral Oral Solution (2% or less) 2380
Neurontin Capsules 2655
Neurontin Oral Solution 2655
Neurontin Tablets 2655
Niaspan Extended-Release Tablets 1846
▲ Nilandron Tablets (4%) 753
Nimotop Capsules (0.8%; rare) 904
Norditropin Cartridges 2420
Norditropin for Injection 2419
Noroxin Tablets 2145
Norpramin Tablets 755
Norvasc Tablets (More than 0.1% to 1%) 2704
Norvir Capsules 487
Norvir Oral Solution 487
▲ Novantrone for Injection (31%) 1760
Ogestrel 0.5/50-28 Tablets 3428
Olux Foam 1211
Omnicef (0.9%) 493
▲ Oncaspar (Greater than 1% but less than 5%) 756
Ovral Tablets 3551
Ovral-28 Tablets 3552
Ovrette Tablets 3552
Paxil (Infrequent) 1609
Permax Tablets (Infrequent) 1299
Ponstel Capsules (Rare) 1356
Prevacid Delayed-Release Capsules (Less than 1%) 3292
PREVPAC (Less than 1%) 3298
Prinzide Tablets 2168

▲ Prograf (Many patients; 13% to 47%) 1393
Proleukin for Injection (2%) 1199
Protonix I.V. (Less than or equal to 1%) 3580
Protonix Tablets (Less than or equal to 1%) 3577
Protopic Ointment (Greater than or equal to 1%) 1397
Provigil Tablets (1%) 1193
▲ Rapamune Oral Solution and Tablets (3% to 20%) 3584
Rebetron Combination Therapy 3153
Relafen Tablets (Less than 1%) 1617
Reminyl Oral Solution (Infrequent) 1792
Reminyl Tablets (Infrequent) 1792
Renese Tablets 2712
Requip Tablets (1% or more) 1621
Rescriptor Tablets 526
Rifamate Capsules 767
Rifater Tablets 769
Rituxan I.V. (1% to 5%) 1428
Roferon-A Injection (Rare) 2996
Roxicodone Tablets (Less than 3%) 3067
Sandimmune (2% or less) 2388
▲ Sandostatin Injection (3% to 16%) 2394
▲ Sandostatin LAR Depot (15% to 27%) 2395
Seroquel Tablets (Infrequent) 684
▲ Serostim for Injection (10.2%) 3229
▲ Simulect for Injection (Greater than or equal to 10%) 2399
Sinemet Tablets 1253
Sinemet CR Tablets (1% or greater) 1255
Sinequan 2713
Sonata Capsules (Rare) 3591
Sporanox Injection (Less than 1%) 1804
Sporanox Injection (Less than 1%) 2509
Stelazine 1640
Suprane Liquid for Inhalation 874
Surmontil Capsules 3595
Temovate Cream 1301
Temovate Gel 1303
Temovate Ointment 1301
Temovate Scalp Application 1304
Tenoretic Tablets 690
Tequin Injection (Less than 0.1%) 1110
Tequin Tablets (Less than 0.1%) 1110
Teveten Tablets (Less than 1%) 3327
Thalomid Capsules 1154
Theo-Dur Extended-Release Tablets 1835
Thiothixene Capsules 2290
Thorazine 1656
Tiazac Capsules (Less than 2%) 1378
Timolide Tablets 2187
Timolol GFS ⊙266
Timoptic in Ocudose 2192
Timoptic Sterile Ophthalmic Solution 2190
Timoptic-XE Sterile Ophthalmic Gel Forming Solution 2194
Topamax Sprinkle Capsules (Infrequent) 2590
Topamax Tablets (Infrequent) 2590
Trasylol Injection (1% to 2%) 909
Trilafon 3160
Trileptal Oral Suspension 2407
Trileptal Tablets 2407
Triphasil-21 Tablets 3600
Triphasil-28 Tablets 3605
▲ Trisenox Injection (45%) 1158
Trizivir Tablets 1669
Trovan (Less than 1%) 2722
Uni-Dur Extended-Release Tablets 1841
Uniretic Tablets (More than 1%) 3178
Valstar Sterile Solution for Intravesical Instillation (1%) 1175
Vanceril Double Strength Inhalation Aerosol (Rare) 3167
Vantin Tablets and Oral Suspension 2860
Vaseretic Tablets 2204
Viagra Tablets (Less than 2%) 2732
Videx 1138
Videx EC Capsules 1143
Viracept 532
Vistide Injection 1445
Vivactil Tablets 2217
Vivactil Tablets 2446
Wellbutrin Tablets 1680
Zanaflex Tablets (Rare) 1305
Zaroxolyn Tablets 1177
Zebeta Tablets 1885
Zenapax for Injection 3046
Zestoretic Tablets 695
Ziagen 1692
Zithromax (Less than 1%) 2743
Zithromax for Oral Suspension, 300 mg, 600 mg, 900 mg, 1200 mg (Less than 1%) 2739
Zithromax Tablets, 250 mg (Less than 1%) 2739
Zithromax Tablets, 600 mg (Less than 1%) 2743
Zoladex (1% to 5%) 702
Zoladex 3-month 706
Zoloft 2751
Zomig Tablets (Rare) 708
Zomig-ZMT Tablets (Rare) 708
Zosyn 1890
Zosyn in Galaxy Containers 1894
Zyprexa Tablets (Infrequent) 1973
Zyprexa ZYDIS Orally Disintegrating Tablets (Infrequent) 1973

Hyperglycemia, transient

Duraclon Injection (Rare) 3057
Eskalith 1527
Lithium Carbonate 3061
Lithium Citrate Syrup 3061
Lithobid Slow-Release Tablets 3255
Rituxan for Infusion (1% to 5%) 1750

Hyperglycinemia

Depacon Injection 416
Depakene 421
Depakote Sprinkle Capsules 426
Depakote Tablets 430
Depakote ER Tablets 436
Moban 1320
Urso Tablets 836

Hyperhemoglobinemia

Ambien Tablets (Rare) 3191
Evoxac Capsules 1217

Hyperheparinemia

Mustargen for Injection (Rare) 2142

Hyperhidrosis

Accutane Capsules 2944
▲ Betapace AF Tablets (4.9% to 5.2%) 954
DynaCirc Capsules (0.5% to 1%) 2921
DynaCirc CR Tablets (0.5% to 1%) 2923
Havrix Vaccine (Rare) 1544
Miacalcin Nasal Spray (Less than 1%) 2375
Monopril Tablets (0.4% to 1.0%) 1091
Noroxin Tablets (0.3% to 1.0%) 2145
Phrenilin (Infrequent) 578
Prilosec Delayed-Release Capsules (Less than 1%) 628
Primaxin I.M. 2158
Primaxin I.V. (Less than 0.2%) 2160
Prinivil Tablets 2164
Prinzide Tablets (0.3% to 1%) 2168
Sedapap Tablets 50 mg/650 mg (Infrequent) 2225
Vaseretic Tablets 2204
Vasotec Tablets 2210
Zestoretic Tablets 695

Hyperhistaminemia

▲ Vesanoid Capsules (3%) 3037

Hyperirritability

Mintezol 2137

Hyperirritability, muscle

Eskalith 1527
Lithium Carbonate 3061
Lithium Citrate Syrup 3061
Lithobid Slow-Release Tablets 3255

Hyperirritability, neuromuscular

Timentin Injection- ADD-Vantage Vial 1661
Timentin Injection-Galaxy Container 1664
Timentin Injection-Pharmacy Bulk Package 1666
Timentin for Intravenous Administration 1658

Hyperkalemia

Abelcet Injection 1273
Accupril Tablets (Rare) 2611
Accuretic Tablets (0.5% to 1%) 2614
Aceon Tablets (2 mg, 4 mg, 8 mg) (1.4%) 3249
Aggrenox Capsules 1026
Aloprim for Injection (Less than 1%) 2292
Altace Capsules (Approximately 1%) 2233
AmBisome for Injection (Less common) 1383
Amphotec (1% to 5%) 1774
Anadrol-50 Tablets 3321
Anaprox Tablets (Less than 1%) 2967
Anaprox DS Tablets (Less than 1%) 2967
Androderm Transdermal System CIII 3377
▲ Android Capsules, 10 mg (Among most common) 1731
Anectine Injection (Rare) 1476
Atacand Tablets 595
Atromid-S Capsules 3483
Avalide Tablets 1070
Avapro Tablets (Rare) 1074
Avapro Tablets 3076
Blocadren Tablets 2046
Campath Ampules 992
Captopril Tablets 2281
▲ Carnitor Injection (6%) 3242
▲ CellCept Capsules (8.9% to 14.5%) 2951
▲ CellCept Intravenous (8.9% to 14.5%) 2951
▲ CellCept Oral Suspension (8.9% to 14.5%) 2951
▲ CellCept Tablets (8.9% to 22%) 2951
Ceptaz for Injection 1499
Cerebyx Injection (Infrequent) 2619
Cipro I.V. (Infrequent) 893
Cipro I.V. Pharmacy Bulk Package (Less than 1%) 897
Cipro 887
Clinoril Tablets (Less than 1 in 100) 2053
Coreg Tablets (More than 2%) 1508
Cozaar Tablets 2067
Delatestryl Injection 1151
Demadex Tablets and Injection 2965
▲ Diovan Capsules (4.4%) 2337
Diovan HCT Tablets (0.3%) 2338
Diprivan Injectable Emulsion (Less than 1%) 667
Doxil Injection (Less than 1%) 566
Dyazide Capsules 1515
Dynabac Tablets (2.6%) 2269
Dyrenium Capsules (Rare) 3458
EC-Naprosyn Delayed-Release Tablets (Less than 1%) 2967
Ecotrin Enteric Coated Aspirin Low, Regular and Maximum Strength Tablets 1715
Effexor Tablets (Rare) 3495
Effexor XR Capsules (Rare) 3499
Enalaprilat Injection (Approximately 1%) 863
Epogen for Injection (Approximately 0.11%) 582
Estratest 3252
Evoxac Capsules 1217
Feldene Capsules (Occasional) 2685
▲ Ferrlecit Injection (6%) 3386
▲ Flolan for Injection (4%) 1528
Floxin I.V. 2526
Floxin Tablets 2529
Fludara for Injection 995
Fortovase Capsules (1.2% to 2.7%) 2970
Gengraf Capsules (1% to less than 3%) 457
Geodon Capsules (Rare) 2688
Hivid Tablets (Less than 1%) 2975
Hyzaar (0.4%) 2109
Indocin Capsules (Less than 1%) 2112
Indocin I.V. (Less than 1%) 2115
Indocin (Less than 1%) 2112
Invirase Capsules (Up to 3%) 2979
K-Dur Microburst Release System ER Tablets 1832
Klor-Con M20/Klor-Con M10 Tablets 3329
▲ K-Lor Powder Packets (Among most severe) 469
▲ K-Tab Filmtab Tablets (Most common) 470
Levaquin Injection (Less than 0.5%) 2537
Lexxel Tablets (Infrequent) 608
Lotensin Tablets 2365
Lotrel Capsules (Approximately 1.5%) 2370
Mavik Tablets (0.3% to 5.3%) 478
Maxipime for Injection (0.1% to 1%) 1285
Maxzide 1008
Micro-K 3311
Midamor Tablets (Between 1% and 3%) 2136
Moduretic Tablets (Greater than 1%, less than 3%) 2138
Monopril Tablets (Approximately 2.6%) 1091
▲ Naprelan Tablets (3% to 9%) 1293
Naprosyn Suspension (Less than 1%) 2967
Naprosyn Tablets (Less than 1%) 2967
Neoral Soft Gelatin Capsules (1% to less than 3%) 2380
Neoral Oral Solution (1% to less than 3%) 2380
Noroxin Tablets 2145
Omnicef (0.2%) 493
Oxandrin Tablets 1153
Paxil (Rare) 1609
Priftin Tablets (Less than 1%) 758
Primaxin I.M. 2158
Primaxin I.V. 2160
▲ Prinivil Tablets (Approximately 2.2% to 4.8%) 2164
Prinzide Tablets (Approximately 1.4%) 2168
Procrit for Injection (0.11%) 2502
▲ Prograf (13% to 45%) 1393
▲ Proleukin for Injection (4%) 1199
Prozac Pulvules, Liquid, and Weekly Capsules (Rare) 1238
▲ Rapamune Oral Solution and Tablets (12% to 17%) 3584
ReoPro Vials (0.1%) 1958
Requip Tablets (Infrequent) 1621
Rescriptor Tablets (Less than 2%) 526
Rum-K 1363
Sandimmune (Occasional) 2388
Sarafem Pulvules (Rare) 1962
Septra Suspension 2265
Septra Tablets 2265
Septra DS Tablets 2265
▲ Simulect for Injection (Greater than or equal to 10%) 2399
Tarka Tablets 508
Testoderm Transdermal Systems 574
Testopel Pellets 3610
Testred Capsules, 10 mg 1746
Teveten Tablets (Less than 1%) 3327
Thalomid Capsules 1154
▲ Thymoglobulin for Injection (26.8%) 3071
Toradol 3018
▲ Trisenox Injection (18%) 1158
Uniretic Tablets (Less than 1%) 3178
Univasc Tablets (Approximately 1.3%) 3181
Vaseretic Tablets 2204
Vasotec I.V. Injection (Approximately 1%) 2207
Vasotec Tablets (Approximately 1%) 2210
Vioxx 2213
Zebeta Tablets 1885
Zestoretic Tablets (Approximately 1.4%) 695
▲ Zestril Tablets (Approximately 2.2% to 4.8%) 698
Zithromax (1% to 2%) 2743
Zithromax for Oral Suspension, 300 mg, 600 mg, 900 mg, 1200 mg (1% to 2%) 2739
Zithromax Tablets, 250 mg (1% to 2%) 2739
Zithromax Tablets, 600 mg (1% to 2%) 2743
Zosyn 1890
Zosyn in Galaxy Containers 1894
Zyprexa Tablets (Infrequent) 1973
Zyprexa ZYDIS Orally Disintegrating Tablets (Infrequent) 1973

Hyperkalemia, neonatal

Altace Capsules 2233
Monopril Tablets 1091
Prograf 1393
Zestril Tablets 698

Hyperkeratosis

Aricept Tablets (Infrequent) 1270
Aricept Tablets (Infrequent) 2665
Cognex Capsules (Infrequent) 1351
Covera-HS Tablets (Less than 2%) 3199
Evoxac Capsules (Less than 1%) 1217
Isoptin SR Tablets (1% or less) 467
Requip Tablets (Infrequent) 1621
Risperdal (Infrequent) 1796
Soriatane Capsules (Less than 1%) 3003
Tarka Tablets 508
Verelan Capsules (1% or less) 3184
Zyrtec (Less than 2%) 2756
Zyrtec-D 12 Hour Extended Relief Tablets (Less than 2%) 2758

Hyperkinesia

Aciphex Tablets (Rare) 1267
Aciphex Tablets (Rare) 1783
AndroGel (One patient) 3322
Astelin Nasal Spray (Infrequent) 3339
Baycol Tablets 883
Betaseron for SC Injection (2%) 988
Cedax Oral Suspension (0.1% to 1%) 1021
Celexa (Infrequent) 1365
Cerebyx Injection (Infrequent) 2619
▲ Claritin (3%) 3100
Claritin-D 12 Hour Extended Release Tablets (Less frequent) 3102
Claritin-D 24 Hour Extended Release Tablets (Fewer than 2%) 3104
Clozaril Tablets (1%) 2319
Cognex Capsules (Frequent) 1351
▲ Comtan Tablets (10%) 2328
DaunoXome Injection (Less than or equal to 5%) 1442
Effexor Tablets (Infrequent) 3495
Effexor XR Capsules (Infrequent) 3499
Evoxac Capsules (Less than 1%) 1217
Exelon Capsules (Infrequent) 2342
Exelon Oral Solution (Infrequent) 2345
▲ Flolan for Injection (7%) 1528
Floxin Otic Solution (Single report) 1219
Flumadine (Less than 0.3%) 1370
Gabitril Tablets (Frequent) 1189
Geodon Capsules (Frequent) 2688
Hivid Tablets (Less than 1%) 2975
Intron A for Injection (Less than 5%) 3120
Lamictal (Infrequent) 1567
Levaquin Injection (Less than 0.5%) 2537
Levo-Dromoran 1734
Lipitor Tablets (Less than 2%) 2639
Lipitor Tablets (Less than 2%) 2696
Luvox Tablets (25, 50, 100 mg) (Frequent) 3256
LYMErix Vaccine (Greater than 1%) 1592
Maxair Autohaler 1981

- Maxair Inhaler (Less than 1%) 1984
- Maxalt Tablets (Rare) 2120
- Maxalt-MLT Orally Disintegrating Tablets (Rare) 2120
- Mirapex Tablets 2834
- Nembutal Sodium Solution (Less than 1%) 485
- ▲ Neurontin Capsules (2.5% to 4.7%) 2655
- ▲ Neurontin Oral Solution (2.5% to 4.7%) 2655
- ▲ Neurontin Tablets (2.5% to 4.7%) 2655
- Nipent for Injection (Less than 3%) 3272
- ▲ Orap Tablets (5.5%) 1407
- OxyContin Tablets (Less than 1%) 2912
- Paxil (Infrequent) 1609
- Permax Tablets (Infrequent) 1299
- Protonix I.V. (Less than 1%) 3580
- Protonix Tablets (Less than 1%) 3577
- Proventil HFA Inhalation Aerosol (Less than 3%) 3150
- Provigil Tablets (At least 1%) 1193
- Prozac Pulvules, Liquid, and Weekly Capsules (Infrequent) 1238
- Pulmicort Respules (1% to 3%) 632
- Remeron Tablets (Frequent) 2483
- Remeron SolTab Tablets (Frequent) 2486
- Reminyl Oral Solution (Infrequent) 1792
- Reminyl Tablets (Infrequent) 1792
- Requip Tablets (2%) 1621
- ▲ Risperdal (17% to 34%) 1796
- Salagen Tablets (Less than 1%) 2229
- Sandostatin LAR Depot (1% to 4%) 2395
- Sarafem Pulvules (Infrequent) 1962
- Seroquel Tablets (Infrequent) 684
- Serzone Tablets (Rare) 1104
- Sonata Capsules (Infrequent) 3591
- Symmetrel (0.1% to 1%) 1328
- Tasmar Tablets (2% to 3%) 3010
- Topamax Sprinkle Capsules (Frequent) 2590
- Topamax Tablets (Frequent) 2590
- Toradol (1% or less) 3018
- Trileptal Oral Suspension 2407
- Trileptal Tablets 2407
- Trovan (Less than 1%) 2722
- Vantin Tablets and Oral Suspension (Less than 1%) 2860
- Viracept 532
- Wellbutrin SR Sustained-Release Tablets (Infrequent) 1684
- WinRho SDF 2297
- Zithromax Capsules, 250 mg (1% or less) 2743
- Zithromax for Oral Suspension, 300 mg, 600 mg, 900 mg, 1200 mg (1% or less) 2739
- Zithromax Tablets, 250 mg (1% or less) 2739
- Zoloft (Infrequent to 2%) 2751
- Zomig Tablets (Rare) 708
- Zomig-ZMT Tablets (Rare) 708
- Zonegran Capsules (Infrequent) 1307
- Zyban Sustained-Release Tablets (Infrequent) 1710
- ▲ Zyprexa Tablets (5% to 11%) 1973
- ▲ Zyprexa ZYDIS Orally Disintegrating Tablets (5% to 11%) 1973
- Zyrtec (Less than 2%) 2756
- Zyrtec-D 12 Hour Extended Relief Tablets (Less than 2%) 2758

Hyperlipidemia

- Aciphex Tablets 1267
- Aciphex Tablets 1783
- Ambien Tablets (Rare) 3191
- Amerge Tablets (Rare) 1467
- ▲ AndroGel (3% to 6%) 3322
- Arava Tablets (1% to 3%) 724
- Avelox Tablets (0.05% to 1%) 879
- Betapace Tablets (Rare) 950
- Betapace AF Tablets (Rare) 954
- Betaxon Ophthalmic Suspension (Less than 2%) 537
- ▲ CellCept Capsules (3% to 10.7%) 2951
- ▲ CellCept Intravenous (3% to 10.7%) 2951
- ▲ CellCept Oral Suspension (3% to 10.7%) 2951
- ▲ CellCept Tablets (3% to 10.7%) 2951
- ▲ Diprivan Injectable Emulsion (Less than 1% to 10%) 667
- Doxil Injection (Less than 1%) 566
- Effexor Tablets (Infrequent) 3495
- Effexor XR Capsules (Infrequent) 3499
- Ergamisol Tablets 1789
- Esclim Transdermal System 3460
- Estrace Vaginal Cream 3358
- Estrace Tablets 3361
- Evoxac Capsules (Less than 1%) 1217
- Exelon Capsules (Infrequent) 2342
- Exelon Oral Solution (Infrequent) 2345
- Gabitril Tablets (Infrequent) 1189
- Geodon Capsules (Rare) 2688
- Heparin Lock Flush Solution 3509
- Heparin Sodium Injection 3511
- Hivid Tablets (Less than 1%) 2975
- Lovenox Injection (Rare) 746
- ▲ Lupron Depot–3 Month 22.5 mg (More than or equal to 5%) 3288
- ▲ Lupron Depot–4 Month 30 mg (Greater than or equal to 5%) 3289
- Luvox Tablets (25, 50, 100 mg) (Rare) 3256
- Neurontin Capsules (Rare) 2655
- Neurontin Oral Solution (Rare) 2655
- Neurontin Tablets (Rare) 2655
- Nolvadex Tablets (Infrequent) 678
- Norvir Capsules (1.7% to 4.1%) 487
- Norvir Oral Solution (1.7% to 4.1%) 487
- Ogen Tablets 2846
- Pletal Tablets (Less than 2%) 2605
- Pletal Tablets (Less than 2%) 2848
- Prevacid Delayed-Release Capsules 3292
- PREVPAC 3298
- ▲ Prograf (3% to 15%) 1393
- Protonix I.V. (Greater than or equal to 1%) 3580
- Protonix Tablets (Greater than or equal to 1%) 3577
- Prozac Pulvules, Liquid, and Weekly Capsules (Infrequent) 1238
- ▲ Rapamune Oral Solution and Tablets (38% to 57%) 3584
- Sandimmune 2388
- Sarafem Pulvules (Infrequent) 1962
- Seroquel Tablets (Infrequent) 684
- ▲ Thalomid Capsules (5.6% to 9.4%) 1154
- Topamax Sprinkle Capsules (Infrequent) 2590
- Topamax Tablets (Infrequent) 2590
- Uniretic Tablets (Less than 1%) 3178
- Viracept 532
- Vistide Injection 1445
- Zanaflex Tablets (Infrequent) 1305
- Zyprexa Tablets (Rare) 1973
- Zyprexa ZYDIS Orally Disintegrating Tablets (Rare) 1973

Hypermagnesemia

- Accuretic Tablets (Rare) 2614
- Doxil Injection (Less than 1%) 566

Hypermenorrhea

- Cytotec Tablets (0.5%) 3202

Hypermetabolic syndrome

- Nardil Tablets (Less frequent) 2653

Hypermotility, gastrointestinal

- Roferon-A Injection (Infrequent) 2996

Hypernatremia

- Aloprim for Injection (Less than 1%) 2292
- ▲ AmBisome for Injection (4.1%) 1383
- Anadrol-50 Tablets 3321
- Androderm Transdermal System CIII 3377
- ▲ Android Capsules, 10 mg (Among most common) 1731
- Demadex Tablets and Injection 2965
- Doxil Injection (Less than 1%) 566
- Felbatol 3343
- Fleet Enema 1359
- Fleet Phospho-soda 1360
- Fortovase Capsules 2970
- Hivid Tablets (Less than 1%) 2975
- Invirase Capsules (Less than 1%) 2979
- Kristalose for Oral Solution 1007
- Nardil Tablets (Less common) 2653
- Proleukin for Injection (1%) 1199
- Testoderm Transdermal Systems 574
- Testopel Pellets 3610
- Timentin Injection- ADD-Vantage Vial 1661
- Timentin Injection-Galaxy Container 1664
- Timentin Injection-Pharmacy Bulk Package 1666
- Timentin for Intravenous Administration 1658
- Topamax Sprinkle Capsules (Rare) 2590
- Topamax Tablets (Rare) 2590
- Toradol 3018
- Viagra Tablets (Less than 2%) 2732
- Zosyn 1890
- Zosyn in Galaxy Containers 1894
- Zyprexa Tablets (Rare) 1973
- Zyprexa ZYDIS Orally Disintegrating Tablets (Rare) 1973

Hyperosmolarity

- Diprivan Injectable Emulsion (Less than 1%) 667

Hyperostosis, skeletal

- Accutane Capsules 2944
- ▲ Soriatane Capsules (Less than 1% to 25%) 3003

Hyperparathyroidism

- Eskalith 1527
- Lithobid Slow-Release Tablets 3255
- Maxzide 1008
- Prinzide Tablets 2168
- Skelid Tablets (2.7%) 3088
- Vaseretic Tablets 2204

Hyperphenylalaninemia

- Daraprim Tablets (Rare) 1511

Hyperphosphatemia

- Aloprim for Injection (Less than 1%) 2292
- AmBisome for Injection (Less common) 1383
- Anadrol-50 Tablets 3321
- Androderm Transdermal System CIII 3377
- ▲ Android Capsules, 10 mg (Among most common) 1731
- Delatestryl Injection 1151
- Didronel Tablets 2888
- Effexor Tablets (Rare) 3495
- Effexor XR Capsules (Rare) 3499
- Estratest 3252
- Fleet Enema 1359
- Fleet Phospho-soda 1360
- Fludara for Injection 995
- ▲ Foscavir Injection (5% to 6%) 605
- Hectorol Capsules 1064
- Hectorol Injection 1066
- ▲ Lupron Depot–3 Month 22.5 mg (More than or equal to 5%) 3288
- Minocin Intravenous 1862
- Minocin Oral Suspension 1865
- Minocin Pellet-Filled Capsules 1863
- Oxandrin Tablets 1153
- Paxil (Rare) 1609
- ▲ Prograf (3% to 15%) 1393
- Proleukin for Injection (1%) 1199
- ▲ Rapamune Oral Solution and Tablets (3% to 20%) 3584
- Requip Tablets (Infrequent) 1621
- Risperdal (Rare) 1796
- ▲ Roferon-A Injection (9%) 2996
- ▲ Synarel Nasal Solution for Endometriosis (10% to 15%) 3205
- Testoderm Transdermal Systems 574
- Testopel Pellets 3610
- Testred Capsules, 10 mg 1746
- Zithromax (Less than 1%) 2743
- Zithromax for Oral Suspension, 300 mg, 600 mg, 900 mg, 1200 mg (Less than 1%) 2739
- Zithromax Tablets, 250 mg (Less than 1%) 2739
- Zithromax Tablets, 600 mg (Less than 1%) 2743

Hyperpigmentation

- Accutane Capsules 2944
- Aldara Cream, 5% 1978
- Avita Cream 999
- Avita Gel 1000
- Blocadren Tablets 2046
- ▲ Catapres-TTS (5 of 101 patients) 1038
- Celestone Soluspan Injectable Suspension 3097
- Cipro I.V. (1% or less) 893
- Cipro I.V. Pharmacy Bulk Package (Less than 1%) 897
- Cipro (Less than 1%) 887
- Cortone Acetate Injectable Suspension 2059
- Crixivan Capsules 2070
- Decadron Phosphate Injection 2081
- Dovonex Ointment (Less than 1%) 1117
- Dovonex Scalp Solution 1118
- ▲ Efudex (Among most frequent) 1733
- Ellence Injection 2806
- Emla (Rare) 602
- Florinef Acetate Tablets 2250
- Floxin I.V. 2526
- Floxin Tablets 2529
- Fluoroplex (Occasional) 552
- Hydrocortone Acetate Injectable Suspension 2103
- Hydrocortone Phosphate Injection, Sterile 2105
- Lac-Hydrin Lotion (Less frequent) 1119
- ▲ Levulan Kerastick (20% to 36%) 971
- Lodine (Less than 1%) 3528
- Lodine XL Extended-Release Tablets (Less than 1%) 3530
- Matulane Capsules 3246
- ▲ Myleran Tablets (5% to 10%) 1603
- Mylocel Tablets 2227
- Niaspan Extended-Release Tablets 1846
- Norplant System 3543
- Purinethol Tablets 1615
- Retin-A Micro 0.1% 2522
- Solu-Medrol Sterile Powder 2855
- Taxotere for Injection Concentrate 778
- ▲ Trisenox Injection (8%) 1158

Hyperpigmentation, dermal creases

- Adriamycin PFS/RDF (A few cases primarily in children) 2767

Hyperplasia, endocervical

- Depo-Provera Contraceptive Injection (Fewer than 1%) 2798

Hyperplasia, gingival

(*see under* Gingival hyperplasia)

Hyperplasia, mammary

- Cuprimine Capsules (Rare) 2075
- Depen Titratable Tablets (Rare) 3341

Hyperpnea

- Aggrenox Capsules (Less than 1%) 1026

Hyperprolactinemia

- Aldoclor Tablets 2035
- Aldomet Tablets 2037
- Aldoril Tablets 2039
- Compazine 1505
- Covera-HS Tablets (Less than 2%) 3199
- D.H.E. 45 Injection 2334
- Effexor Tablets 3495
- Effexor XR Capsules 3499
- Haldol Decanoate 2535
- Haldol Injection, Tablets and Concentrate 2533
- Isoptin SR Tablets (1% or less) 467
- Moban 1320
- Paxil 1609
- Prozac Pulvules, Liquid, and Weekly Capsules 1238
- Reglan 2935
- Risperdal 1796
- Sarafem Pulvules 1962
- Stelazine 1640
- Tarka Tablets 508
- Thorazine 1656
- Trilafon 3160
- Verelan PM Capsules (2% or less) 3186
- Xanax Tablets 2865
- Zoloft 2751
- Zyprexa Tablets 1973
- Zyprexa ZYDIS Orally Disintegrating Tablets 1973

Hyperproteinemia

- Evoxac Capsules 1217

Hyperprothrombinemia

- AmBisome for Injection (Less common) 1383
- Brevicon 28-Day Tablets 3380
- Doxil Injection (1% to 5%) 566
- Estratest 3252
- Maxipime for Injection (1.4%) 1285
- Norinyl 1 +35 28-Day Tablets 3380
- Norinyl 1 + 50 28-Day Tablets 3380
- Tri-Norinyl-28 Tablets 3433

Hyperpyrexia

(*see under* Fever)

Hyperreflexia

- Cerebyx Injection (Frequent) 2619
- Compazine 1505
- Depacon Injection (1% or more) 416
- Depakene (1% or more) 421
- Depakote Sprinkle Capsules 426
- Depakote Tablets (1% to 5%) 430
- Depakote ER Tablets (Greater than 1%) 436
- Effexor Tablets (Rare) 3495
- Effexor XR Capsules (Rare) 3499
- Etrafon (Less frequent) 3115
- Exelon Capsules (Infrequent) 2342
- Exelon Oral Solution (Infrequent) 2345
- Fortovase Capsules (Less than 2%) 2970
- Gabitril Tablets (Infrequent) 1189
- Geodon Capsules (Rare) 2688
- Haldol Injection, Tablets and Concentrate 2533
- Invirase Capsules (Less than 2%) 2979
- Lithobid Slow-Release Tablets (One report) 3255
- Nardil Tablets (Common) 2653
- Navane Oral 2701
- Navane Intramuscular 2703
- Neurontin Capsules (Frequent) 2655
- Neurontin Oral Solution (Frequent) 2655
- Neurontin Tablets (Frequent) 2655
- Orap Tablets (Less frequent) 1407
- Orthoclone OKT3 Sterile Solution 2498
- Paxil (Rare) 1609
- Pfizerpen for Injection 2707
- Prozac Pulvules, Liquid, and Weekly Capsules (Rare) 1238
- Remeron Tablets (Infrequent) 2483
- Remeron SolTab Tablets (Infrequent) 2486
- Rescriptor Tablets (Less than 2%) 526
- Risperdal (Rare) 1796
- Sarafem Pulvules (Rare) 1962
- Sonata Capsules (Rare) 3591
- Stelazine 1640
- Topamax Sprinkle Capsules (Infrequent) 2590
- Topamax Tablets (Infrequent) 2590
- Trilafon 3160
- Trileptal Oral Suspension 2407
- Trileptal Tablets 2407
- Zonegran Capsules (Infrequent) 1307

Hyperreflexia, neonatal

- Compazine 1505
- Etrafon 3115
- Stelazine 1640
- Thorazine 1656

Hypersalivation
(*see under* Sialism)

Hypersecretion
Klonopin Tablets 2983

Hypersensitivity
AK-Fluor Injection 10% and 25% (Rare) ⊙202
Alkeran for Injection 1465
Americaine Otic Topical Anesthetic Ear Drops 1162
Amoxil Chewable Tablets 1471
Amoxil for Oral Suspension 1471
Amoxil 1471
Anectine Injection (Rare) 1476
Azulfidine EN-tabs Tablets 2775
Beconase Inhalation Aerosol (Rare) 1497
Betagan ⊙228
Bicillin C-R 900/300 Injection 2240
Bicillin C-R Injection 2238
Bicillin L-A Injection 2242
Bleph-10 ⊙230
Carteolol Hydrochloride Ophthalmic Solution USP, 1% ⊙258
Cefizox for Intramuscular or Intravenous Use (Less than 1%) 1390
Cefobid Intravenous/Intramuscular 2671
Cefobid Pharmacy Bulk Package - Not for Direct Infusion 2673
Cefotan (1.2%) 664
Clinoril Tablets (Less than 1%) 2053
Collagenase Santyl Ointment (One case) 3248
Cortisporin Ophthalmic Suspension ⊙297
Cortone Acetate Injectable Suspension 2059
Cortone Acetate Tablets 2061
Daranide Tablets 2077
Decadron Elixir 2078
Decadron Tablets 2079
Decadron Phosphate Injection 2081
Demser Capsules (Rare) 2085
Dolobid Tablets (Less than 1 in 100) 2088
Elspar for Injection 2092
Estratest (Rare) 3252
Flexeril Tablets 572
Flexeril Tablets 2094
Floxin I.V. 2526
Floxin Tablets (Less than 1%) 2529
Fluorescite Injection ⊙211
FML-S Liquifilm Sterile Ophthalmic Suspension ⊙238
Fortaz (Immediate in 1 in 285 patients) 1541
Geocillin Tablets 2687
Hydrocortone Tablets 2106
Hydrocortone Acetate Injectable Suspension 2103
Hydrocortone Phosphate Injection, Sterile 2105
Imitrex Injection (Infrequent) 1549
Imitrex Nasal Spray (Rare) 1554
Imitrex Tablets (Frequent) 1558
Inderide Tablets 3517
Indocin (Less than 1%) 2112
Kefurox Vials, ADD-Vantage (Less than 1%) 1948
Lacrisert Sterile Ophthalmic Insert 2117
Leukeran Tablets 1591
Lupron Injection 3279
Miltown Tablets 3349
Mustargen for Injection 2142
Nembutal Sodium Solution 485
Nizoral Tablets (Several cases) 1791
Norflex 1987
Normodyne Injection (Rare) 3135
Normodyne Tablets (Rare) 3137
Noroxin Tablets (A few patients) 2145
Ocupress Ophthalmic Solution, 1% Sterile ⊙303
Paraplatin for Injection (2%) 1126
Prednisone 3064
Prinzide Tablets 2168
Recombivax HB 2178
Rifadin (Uncommon) 765
Ritalin 2387
Sandoglobulin I.V. 2391
Synarel Nasal Solution for Endometriosis (0.2%) 3205
Talacen Caplets (A few cases) 3089
Tenoretic Tablets 690
Tetanus Toxoid Adsorbed Purogenated 1882
Timoptic in Ocudose (Less frequent) 2192
Timoptic Sterile Ophthalmic Solution (Less frequent) 2190
TobraDex Ophthalmic Ointment (Less than 4%) 542
TobraDex Ophthalmic Suspension (Less than 4%) 541
Tobrex Ophthalmic Ointment (Less than 3 of 100 patients) ⊙220
Tobrex Ophthalmic Solution (Less than 3 of 100 patients) ⊙221
Tonocard Tablets (Less than 1%) 649
Toradol (1% or less) 3018
Urobiotic-250 Capsules 2731
Vanceril Double Strength Inhalation Aerosol (Rare) 3167
Xylocaine Injections 653
Zantac (Rare) 1690
Zantac Injection (Rare) 1688
Zantac Syrup (Rare) 1690
Zinacef Injection (Fewer than 1%) 1696
Zinacef for Injection (Fewer than 1%) 1696

Hypersensitivity pneumonitis
Pentasa Capsules (Infrequent) 3239
Relafen Tablets (Rarer) 1617

Hypersensitivity reactions, Arthus-type
Acel-Imune 1851
Diphtheria & Tetanus Toxoids Adsorbed Purogenated for Pediatric Use 1857
Tetanus & Diphtheria Toxoids Adsorbed for Adult Use 1880
Tetanus and Diphtheria Toxoids Adsorbed For Adult Use 815
Tripedia Vaccine 817

Hypersensitivity reactions, general
Accolate Tablets 657
Alferon N Injection 1770
Alkeran Tablets 1466
Altace Capsules (Less than 1%) 2233
Aminohippurate Sodium PAH Injection 2041
Ancef for Injection 1474
Ancef Injection 1474
Asacol Delayed-Release Tablets (Some patients) 2884
Augmentin Chewable Tablets 1482
Augmentin Powder for Oral Suspension 1482
Augmentin Tablets 1485
Augmentin ES-600 Powder for Oral Suspension 1487
▲ Avonex (3%) 1013
Axid Pulvules (Rare) 1903
Axid Pulvules (Rare) 2919
Beconase AQ Nasal Spray (Rare) 1498
Betaseron for SC Injection 988
▲ Betimol Ophthalmic Solution (More than 5%) ⊙324
Brethine Ampuls 2314
Carafate Suspension 731
Carafate Tablets 730
Ceclor CD Tablets (Rare) 1279
Ceclor (About 1.5%) 1905
Ceftin 1898
Ceptaz for Injection (2% of patients) 1499
Chibroxin Sterile Ophthalmic Solution 2051
Cipro 887
Cleocin HCl Capsules 2784
Cleocin Phosphate Sterile Solution 2785
Cleocin Vaginal Cream 2788
Clozaril Tablets 2319
Comvax 2056
Cortrosyn for Injection (Rare) 2449
Coumadin for Injection (Infrequent) 1243
Coumadin Tablets (Infrequent) 1243
Didronel Tablets 2888
Digibind Powder 1514
Dilantin-125 Oral Suspension 2625
Dobutrex Solution Vials (Occasional) 1914
Duranest Injections 600
Ethiodol Injection (Infrequent) 3095
Etrafon (Extremely rare) 3115
Factrel (Rare) 3633
Ferrlecit Injection 3386
Flovent (Rare) 1535
FluShield Influenza Vaccine (One case) 3521
Fosamax Tablets 2095
Furosemide Tablets 2284
Gamimune N, 5% Solvent/Detergent Treated (One patient) 925
Gamimune N, 10% Solvent/Detergent Treated (One patient) 928
Grifulvin V Tablets Microsize and Oral Suspension Microsize 2518
Heparin Lock Flush Solution 3509
Heparin Sodium Injection 3511
Hyzaar 2109
INFeD Injection 3388
Keflex 1237
Kytril Injection (Rare) 2986
Kytril Tablets (Rare) 2988
Lescol Capsules (Rare) 2361
Lescol Capsules (Rare) 2925
Lescol XL Tablets (Rare) 2361
Lescol XL Tablets (Rare) 2925
Lorabid Suspension and Pulvules 2251
Maxzide 1008
Mevacor Tablets (Rare) 2132
Minocin Pellet-Filled Capsules 1863
Norcuron for Injection 2478
Nubain Injection (1% or less) 1323
Oncaspar (Greater than 1% but less than 5%) 756
Orthoclone OKT3 Sterile Solution 2498
Pergonal for Injection (Some patients) 3223
Polytrim Ophthalmic Solution (Multiple reports) 556
Propecia Tablets 2172
Proscar Tablets 2175
Pulmicort Turbuhaler Inhalation Powder (Rare) 636
ReoPro Vials 1958
Repronex for Intramuscular and Subcutaneous Injection (Some patients) 1347
Rifater Tablets 769
Semprex-D Capsules (Rare) 1172
Serevent Inhalation Aerosol (Rare) 1633
Skelaxin Tablets 1301
Streptase for Infusion 647
Sular Tablets (Very rare) 688
▲ Taxol Injection (2% to 41%) 1129
Taxotere for Injection Concentrate (0.9%) 778
Tessalon Capsules 1377
Timolol GFS ⊙266
Timoptic-XE Sterile Ophthalmic Gel Forming Solution 2194
Trasylol Injection 909
Unasyn for Injection 2728
Univasc Tablets (Less than 1%) 3181
Valcyte Tablets (Less than 5%) 3022
Viroptic Ophthalmic Solution Sterile ⊙301
Vistide Injection 1445
Warfarin Sodium Tablets, USP 3302
Xeloda Tablets (Less than 5%) 3039
Zenapax for Injection 3046
▲ Ziagen (Approximately 5%) 1692
Zocor Tablets (Rare) 2219
Zofran Injection (Rare) 1698
Zoladex (Rare) 702
Zoladex 3-month (Rare) 706

Hypersensitivity reactions, multi-organ
Tegretol/Tegretol-XR 2404

Hypersensitivity vasculitis
Aldoclor Tablets 2035
Aldoril Tablets 2039
Brethine Ampuls (Rare) 2314
Brethine Tablets (Rare) 2313
Clinoril Tablets (Less than 1 in 100) 2053
Dolobid Tablets (Less than 1 in 100) 2088
Streptase for Infusion 647
Tagamet (Rare) 1644

Hypersomnia
Luvox Tablets (25, 50, 100 mg) (Infrequent) 3256
Maxalt Tablets (Rare) 2120
Maxalt-MLT Orally Disintegrating Tablets (Rare) 2120
Nardil Tablets (Common) 2653
Prinivil Tablets (0.3% to 1.0%) 2164
Prinzide Tablets 2168
Zestoretic Tablets 695
Zestril Tablets (0.3% to 1.0%) 698

Hypersplenism
Flolan for Injection 1528

Hypertension
▲ Abelcet Injection (5%) 1273
Aciphex Tablets 1267
Aciphex Tablets 1783
Actiq (Less than 1%) 1184
Activase I.V. 1410
Activella Tablets 2764
▲ Actonel Tablets (10%) 2879
Adderall Tablets 3231
Adderall XR Capsules
Adenocard Injection 1380
Adenoscan (Less than 1%) 1381
Adipex-P 1406
Aerobid/Aerobid-M (1% to 3%) 1363
Agrylin Capsules (1% to 5%) 3232
Albalon Ophthalmic Solution ⊙225
Alesse-21 Tablets 3468
Alesse-28 Tablets 3473
Aloprim for Injection (Less than 1%) 2292
Alora Transdermal System (Occasional) 3372
Alphagan Ophthalmic Solution (Less than 3%) 545
▲ Alphagan P Ophthalmic Solution (Approximately 5% to 9%) 546
Alupent 1029
Ambien Tablets (Infrequent) 3191
▲ AmBisome for Injection (7.9% to 19.8%) 1383
Amerge Tablets (Infrequent) 1467
▲ Amphotec (7% to 9%) 1774
Androderm Transdermal System CIII (Less than 1%) 3377
Anectine Injection 1476
Anzemet Injection (2.9%) 719
Anzemet Tablets (2.2%) 722
▲ Arava Tablets (10%) 724
▲ Aredia for Injection (Up to at least 15%) 2309
Aricept Tablets (Frequent) 1270
Aricept Tablets (Frequent) 2665
Arimidex Tablets (2% to 5%) 659
▲ Aromasin Tablets (5%) 2769
Arthrotec Tablets (Rare) 3195
Astelin Nasal Spray (Infrequent) 3339
Ativan Injection (0.1%) 3478
Atrovent Inhalation Solution (0.9%) 1031
Avalide Tablets 1070
Avapro Tablets (Less than 1%) 1074
Avapro Tablets (Less than 1%) 3076
Avelox Tablets (0.05% to 1%) 879
Axert Tablets (Rare) 2772
Baycol Tablets 883
Betapace Tablets (Less than 1% to 2%) 950
▲ Betaseron for SC Injection (7%) 988
Betaxon Ophthalmic Suspension (Less than 2%) 537
Betimol Ophthalmic Solution (1% to 5%) ⊙324
Bontril Slow-Release Capsules 576
Brevicon 28-Day Tablets 3380
Buprenex Injectable (Less than 1%) 2918
Calcijex Injection 411
▲ Campath Ampules (2% to 11%) 992
Carbatrol Capsules 3234
Cardene I.V. (0.7%) 3485
▲ Carnitor Injection (18% to 12%) 3242
▲ Casodex Tablets (5%) 662
Cataflam Tablets (Less than 1%) 2315
Catapres-TTS (0.5% or less) 1038
Caverject Sterile Powder (2%) 2777
Celestone Soluspan Injectable Suspension 3097
Celestone Syrup 3099
Celexa (Infrequent) 1365
▲ CellCept Capsules (16.9% to 77.5%) 2951
▲ CellCept Intravenous (16.9% to 77.5%) 2951
▲ CellCept Oral Suspension (16.9% to 77.5%) 2951
▲ CellCept Tablets (16.9% to 77.5%) 2951
Cenestin Tablets 1263
Cerebyx Injection (Frequent) 2619
Chirocaine Injection (1%) 2909
Cipro I.V. (1% or less) 893
Cipro I.V. Pharmacy Bulk Package (Less than 1%) 897
Cipro (Less than 1%) 887
Claritin (At least one patient) 3100
Claritin-D 12 Hour Extended Release Tablets (Less frequent) 3102
Claritin-D 24 Hour Extended Release Tablets (Fewer than 2%) 3104
Climara Transdermal System (Occasional) 958
Clinoril Tablets (Less than 1%) 2053
Clomid Tablets 735
▲ Clozaril Tablets (4%) 2319
Cognex Capsules (Frequent) 1351
Colazal Capsules 3069
CombiPatch Transdermal System 2323
Combivent Inhalation Aerosol (Less than 2%) 1041
Concerta Extended-Release Tablets 1998
Concerta Tablets 561
Copaxone for Injection (Frequent) 3306
Coreg Tablets (2.9%) 1508
Cortifoam Rectal Foam 3170
Cortone Acetate Injectable Suspension 2059
Cortone Acetate Tablets 2061
Cortrosyn for Injection 2449
Corvert Injection (1.2%) 2793
Cosopt Sterile Ophthalmic Solution (1% to 5%) 2065
Cyclessa Tablets 2450
Cytotec Tablets (Infrequent) 3202
Cytovene (1% or less) 2959
DaunoXome Injection (Less than or equal to 5%) 1442
DDAVP Injection 4 mcg/mL (Infrequent) 737
Decadron Elixir 2078
Decadron Tablets 2079
Decadron Phosphate Injection 2081
Depacon Injection (1% to 5%) 416
Depakene (1% or more) 421
Depakote Sprinkle Capsules (1% to 5%) 426
Depakote Tablets (1% to 5%) 430
Depakote ER Tablets (Greater than 1%) 436
Depo-Medrol Injectable Suspension 2795
Desmopressin Acetate Injection (Infrequent) 1344
Desmopressin Acetate Rhinal Tube (Infrequent) 1345
Desogen Tablets 2458

Desoxyn Tablets 440
Detrol Tablets (1.5%) 3623
Dexedrine 1512
DextroStat Tablets 3236
D.H.E. 45 Injection (Occasional) 2334
Dilaudid Oral Liquid 445
Dilaudid Tablets - 8 mg 445
Dilaudid-HP (Less frequent) 443
Dipentum Capsules (Rare) 2803
▲ Diprivan Injectable Emulsion (Less than 1% to 8%) 667
Ditropan XL Extended Release Tablets (2% to 5%) 564
▲ Dobutrex Solution Vials (Most patients) 1914
Dopram Injectable 2931
Doxil Injection (Less than 1%) 566
Duraclon Injection 3057
Duragesic Transdermal System (1% to 3%) 1786
Ecotrin Enteric Coated Aspirin Low, Regular and Maximum Strength Tablets 1715
▲ Effexor Tablets (1.1% to 4.5%) 3495
▲ Effexor XR Capsules (4%) 3499
Eldepryl Capsules 3266
Emcyt Capsules 2810
Enalaprilat Injection 863
Enbrel for Injection (Infrequent) 1752
Enbrel for Injection (Infrequent) 3504
▲ Epogen for Injection (0.75% to 24%) 582
Esclim Transdermal System 3460
Estinyl Tablets 3112
Estrace Vaginal Cream (Occasional) 3358
Estrace Tablets 3361
Estratest (Common) 3252
Estrostep 2627
Etrafon (Occasional) 3115
Eulexin Capsules (1%) 3118
Evoxac Capsules (Less than 1%) 1217
▲ Exelon Capsules (3%) 2342
▲ Exelon Oral Solution (3%) 2345
Felbatol 3343
Feldene Capsules (Occasional) 2685
▲ Femara Tablets (5% to 7%) 2351
femhrt Tablets 2635
▲ Ferrlecit Injection (13%) 3386
Flexeril Tablets (Rare) 572
Flexeril Tablets (Rare) 2094
Florinef Acetate Tablets 2250
Floxin I.V. (Less than 1%) 2526
Floxin Tablets (Less than 1%) 2529
Flumadine (Less than 0.3%) 1370
Fluothane Inhalation (Rare) 3508
Foradil Aerolizer 2354
Fortovase Capsules (Less than 2%) 2970
Foscavir Injection (Between 1% and 5%) 605
Gabitril Tablets (Frequent) 1189
Gammagard S/D (Occasional) 845
Gemzar for Injection (2%) 1919
▲ Gengraf Capsules (25% to 50%) 457
Geodon Capsules (Frequent) 2688
▲ Gliadel Wafer (3%) 1723
GlucaGen for Injection Diagnostic Kit 949
Glucotrol XL Extended Release Tablets (Less than 1%) 2693
Haldol Decanoate 2535
Haldol Injection, Tablets and Concentrate 2533
Hectorol Capsules 1064
Hectorol Injection 1066
Helixate Concentrate 788
Hivid Tablets (Less than 1%) 2975
▲ Humatrope Vials and Cartridges (4.6% to 7.7%) 1930
Hycomine Compound Tablets 1317
Hycotuss Expectorant Syrup 1318
Hydrocortone Tablets 2106
Hydrocortone Acetate Injectable Suspension 2103
Hydrocortone Phosphate Injection, Sterile 2105
Ifex for Injection (Less than 1%) 1123
Imdur Tablets (Less than or equal to 5%) 1826
Imitrex Injection (Infrequent) 1549
Imitrex Nasal Spray (Infrequent) 1554
Imitrex Tablets (Infrequent) 1558
Indocin Capsules (Less than 1%) 2112
Indocin I.V. (Less than 1%) 2115
Indocin (Less than 1%) 2112
INFeD Injection 3388
▲ Infergen (2% to 5%) 1777
Innohep Injection (Greater than or equal to 1%) 1248
▲ Intron A for Injection (Less than 5% to 9%) 3120
Invirase Capsules (Less than 2%) 2979
Ionamin Capsules 1163
Iveegam EN (0.3% to 0.8%) 849
Kadian Capsules (Less than 3%) 1335
Kaletra Capsules (Less than 2%) 471
Kaletra Oral Solution (Less than 2%) 471
Kogenate FS 936
Kytril Injection (2%) 2986
Kytril Tablets (1%) 2988
Lamictal (Rare) 1567
▲ Leukine (25% to 34%) 1755
Levaquin (0.3% to less than 0.5%) 2537
Levlen 962
Levlite 21 Tablets 962
Levlite 28 Tablets 962
Levora Tablets 3389
Levoxyl Tablets 1819
Lexxel Tablets 608
Limbitrol 1738
Lipitor Tablets (Less than 2%) 2639
Lipitor Tablets (Less than 2%) 2696
Lodine (Less than 1%) 3528
Lodine XL Extended-Release Tablets (Less than 1%) 3530
Lodosyn Tablets 1251
Loestrin 21 Tablets 2642
Loestrin Fe Tablets 2642
Lo/Ovral Tablets 3532
Lo/Ovral-28 Tablets 3538
Low-Ogestrel-28 Tablets 3392
Loxitane Capsules 3398
Lunelle Monthly Injection 2827
Lupron Depot–3 Month 22.5 mg (Less than 5%) 3288
Lupron Depot–4 Month 30 mg (Less than 5%) 3289
▲ Lupron Injection (5% or more) 3279
Luvox Tablets (25, 50, 100 mg) (Frequent) 3256
LYMErix Vaccine (0.93%) 1592
Maxalt Tablets (Infrequent) 2120
Maxalt-MLT Orally Disintegrating Tablets (Infrequent) 2120
▲ Megace Oral Suspension (Up to 8%) 1124
Menest Tablets 2254
Mepergan Injection (Rare) 3539
Meridia Capsules (2.1%) 481
Merrem I.V. (0.1% to 1.0%) 673
Metadate CD Capsules 1164
Metadate ER Tablets 1167
Methylin Tablets 1995
Methylin ER Tablets 1995
Mexitil Capsules (Less than 1% or about 1 in 1,000) 1047
Miacalcin Nasal Spray (1% to 3%) 2375
Micardis Tablets (1%) 1049
Micardis HCT Tablets 1051
Microgestin Fe 1.5/30 Tablets 3407
Microgestin Fe 1/20 Tablets 3400
Migranal Nasal Spray (Rare) 2376
Mirapex Tablets (1% or more) 2834
Mircette Tablets 2470
▲ Mirena Intrauterine System (5% or more) 974
Mobic Tablets (Less than 2%) 1054
Modicon 2563
Monopril Tablets (0.4% to 1.0%) 1091
Monopril HCT 1094
Motrin Suspension, Oral Drops, Chewable Tablets, and Caplets (Less than 1%) 2002
MS Contin Tablets (Less frequent) 2896
MSIR (Less frequent) 2898
▲ Mylotarg for Injection (6% to 29%) 3540
Naprelan Tablets (Less than 3%) 1293
Narcan Injection (Several instances) 1322
Naropin Injection (1% to 5%) 612
Navelbine Injection 1604
Necon 3415
▲ Neoral Soft Gelatin Capsules (Approximately 50% to most patients) 2380
▲ Neoral Oral Solution (Approximately 50% to most patients) 2380
▲ Neupogen for Injection (4%) 587
Neurontin Capsules (Frequent) 2655
Neurontin Oral Solution (Frequent) 2655
Neurontin Tablets (Frequent) 2655
Nexium Delayed-Release Capsules (Less than 1%) 619
Nicoderm CQ Patch 1717
▲ Nicotrol Inhaler (Greater than 3%) 2840
Nicotrol Patch 2840
▲ Nilandron Tablets (9.1%) 753
Nimotop Capsules (Less than 1%) 904
Nipent for Injection (Less than 3%) 3272
Nordette-28 Tablets 2257
Norinyl 1 +35 28-Day Tablets 3380
Norinyl 1 + 50 28-Day Tablets 3380
Norpramin Tablets 755
▲ Novantrone for Injection (4%) 1760
NovoSeven (Greater than or equal to 2%) 2430
Nubain Injection (1% or less) 1323
Ogen Tablets (Occasional) 2846
Ogestrel 0.5/50-28 Tablets 3428
Omnicef 493
Oncaspar (Less than 1%) 756
OptiPranolol Metipranolol Ophthalmic Solution 0.3% (A small number of patients) ⊙ 263
Oramorph SR Tablets (Less frequent) 3062
Orap Tablets 1407
Ortho Dienestrol Cream 2554
Ortho-Cept 21 Tablets 2546
Ortho-Cept 28 Tablets 2546
▲ Orthoclone OKT3 Sterile Solution (8%) 2498
Ortho-Cyclen/Ortho Tri-Cyclen 2573
Ortho-Est Tablets (Occasional) 3464
Ortho-Novum 2563
Ortho-Novum 1/50□28 Tablets 2556
Ortho-Prefest Tablets 2570
Ortho-Cyclen/Ortho Tri-Cyclen 2573
Orudis Capsules (Less than 1%) 3548
Oruvail Capsules (Less than 1%) 3548
Ovcon 3364
Ovral Tablets 3551
Ovral-28 Tablets 3552
Ovrette Tablets 3552
Paraplatin for Injection 1126
Paxil (Frequent) 1609
Pediapred Oral Solution 1170
Permax Tablets (1.6%) 1299
Phenergan Injection 3553
Phenergan Suppositories 3556
Phenergan Syrup 3554
Phenergan Tablets 3556
Phenergan with Codeine Syrup 3557
Phenergan with Dextromethorphan Syrup 3559
Phenergan VC Syrup 3560
Phenergan VC with Codeine Syrup 3561
▲ Photofrin for Injection (6%) 831
▲ Plavix Tablets (4.3%) 1097
▲ Plavix Tablets (4.3%) 3084
Pletal Tablets (2% or greater) 2605
Pletal Tablets (2% or greater) 2848
Polocaine Injection, USP 625
Polocaine-MPF Injection, USP 625
Ponstel Capsules (Occasional) 1356
Prandin Tablets (0.5, 1, and 2 mg) (Less than or equal to 1%) 2432
Prednisone 3064
Prelone Syrup 2273
Premarin Intravenous 3563
Premarin Tablets 3566
Premarin Vaginal Cream 3570
Prempro Tablets 3572
Prevacid Delayed-Release Capsules (Less than 1%) 3292
PREVPAC (Less than 1%) 3298
Priftin Tablets (1.1%) 758
Prilosec Delayed-Release Capsules (Less than 1%) 628
▲ Procrit for Injection (0.75% to 24%) 2502
▲ Prograf (Common; 38% to 47%) 1393
Prometrium Capsules (100 mg, 200 mg) (Less than 5%) 3261
Propine Ophthalmic Solution ⊙ 250
Protonix I.V. (Less than 1%) 3580
Protonix Tablets (Less than 1%) 3577
Protopam Chloride for Injection 3582
Protopic Ointment (Greater than or equal to 1%) 1397
Proventil Inhalation Aerosol (Less than 5%) 3142
Proventil Inhalation Solution 0.083% (1% to 3.1%) 3146
Proventil Repetabs Tablets 3148
Proventil Solution for Inhalation 0.5% (1% to 3.1%) 3144
Proventil HFA Inhalation Aerosol 3150
Provera Tablets 2853
Provigil Tablets (2%) 1193
Prozac Pulvules, Liquid, and Weekly Capsules (Frequent) 1238
▲ Rapamune Oral Solution and Tablets (39% to 49%) 3584
Reglan 2935
Relafen Tablets (Less than 1%) 1617
Remeron Tablets (Frequent) 2483
Remeron SolTab Tablets (Frequent) 2486
Remicade for IV Injection (Less than 2%) 1178
Reminyl Oral Solution (Greater than or equal to 2%) 1792
Reminyl Tablets (Greater than or equal to 2%) 1792
▲ Renagel Capsules (9%) 1439
▲ Renagel Tablets (9%) 1439
▲ Requip Tablets (5%) 1621
Rescriptor Tablets 526
Rescula Ophthalmic Solution (1% to 5%) ⊙ 306
Retavase Vials 1182
▲ Rilutek Tablets (3.3% to 6.8%) 772
Risperdal (Infrequent) 1796
Rituxan for Infusion (0.3%) 1750
Rituxan I.V. (0.3%) 1428
Robinul Injectable 2940
Rocaltrol 2991
▲ Roferon-A Injection (11%) 2996
Romazicon Injection (Less than 1%) 3000
Rynatan Tablets 3351
▲ Salagen Tablets (3%) 2229
▲ Sandimmune (13% to 53%) 2388
Sandostatin Injection (Less than 1%) 2394
▲ Sandostatin LAR Depot (5% to 15%) 2395
Sarafem Pulvules (Frequent) 1962
Serevent Diskus 1637
Serevent Inhalation Aerosol 1633
Serophene Tablets 3226
▲ Serostim for Injection (1% to 10%) 3229
Serzone Tablets (Infrequent) 1104
▲ Simulect for Injection (Greater than or equal to 10%) 2399
Sinemet Tablets 1253
Sinemet CR Tablets 1255
Sinequan (Occasional) 2713
Skelid Tablets (More than or equal to 1%) 3088
Solu-Medrol Sterile Powder 2855
Sonata Capsules (Infrequent) 3591
Sporanox Capsules (2% to 3.2%) 1800
Stadol NS Nasal Spray (Less than 1%) 1108
Streptase for Infusion 647
Sular Tablets (Less than or equal to 1%) 688
Suprane Liquid for Inhalation (Greater than 1%) 874
Surmontil Capsules 3595
Survanta Intratracheal Suspension (Less than 1%) 3053
Symmetrel (0.1% to 1%) 1328
Tambocor Tablets (Less than 1%) 1990
Tasmar Tablets (Infrequent) 3010
Taxol Injection (1%) 1129
Taxotere for Injection Concentrate (Rare) 778
Tegretol/Tegretol-XR 2404
Tequin Injection (Less than 0.1%) 1110
Tequin Tablets (Less than 0.1%) 1110
Thalomid Capsules 1154
▲ Thymoglobulin for Injection (36.6%) 3071
Thyrel TRH for Injection (A small number of patients) 3630
Tikosyn Capsules (Greater than 2%) 2717
Timolol GFS (1% to 5%) ⊙ 266
Timoptic in Ocudose (Less frequent) 2192
Timoptic Sterile Ophthalmic Solution (Less frequent) 2190
Timoptic-XE Sterile Ophthalmic Gel Forming Solution 2194
▲ Tolectin (3% to 9%) 2589
Tonocard Tablets (Less than 1%) 649
Topamax Sprinkle Capsules (Infrequent) 2590
Topamax Tablets (Infrequent) 2590
Toradol (Greater than 1%) 3018
▲ Trasylol Injection (4%) 909
Travatan Ophthalmic Solution (1% to 5%) 543
Tricor Capsules, Micronized 513
Trilafon (Occasional) 3160
Trileptal Oral Suspension 2407
Trileptal Tablets 2407
Tri-Levlen 962
Tri-Norinyl-28 Tablets 3433
Triostat Injection (1% or fewer) 1825
Triphasil-21 Tablets 3600
Triphasil-28 Tablets 3605
▲ Trisenox Injection (10%) 1158
Trivora Tablets 3439
Trovan (Less than 1%) 2722
Ultracet Tablets (Less than 1%) 2597
Ultram Tablets (Infrequent) 2600
Unithroid Tablets 3445
Valtrex Caplets 1676
Vantin Tablets and Oral Suspension (Less than 1%) 2860
Vascor Tablets (0.5% to 2.0%) 2602
Vasotec I.V. Injection 2207
Venofer Injection (Greater than 1%) 580
Ventolin Inhalation Aerosol and Refill (Less than 5%) 1679
Ventolin HFA Inhalation Aerosol 3618
Verelan PM Capsules (1.7%) 3186
Versed Injection 3027
▲ Vesanoid Capsules (11%) 3037
Viagra Tablets 2732
Vicodin Tuss Expectorant 519
Vioxx (1.3%) 2213
Vistide Injection 1445
▲ Visudyne for Injection (1% to 10%) ⊙ 308
Vivactil Tablets 2217
Vivactil Tablets 2446
Vivelle Transdermal System 2412
Vivelle-Dot Transdermal System 2416
Volmax Extended-Release Tablets 2276
Voltaren Tablets (Less than 1%) 2315
Voltaren-XR Tablets (Less than 1%) 2315
▲ Wellbutrin Tablets (4.3%) 1680
Wellbutrin SR Sustained-Release Tablets (At least 1%) 1684
Xeloda Tablets (Less than 5%) 3039
Xopenex Inhalation Solution 3207
Yasmin 28 Tablets 980
Zemuron Injection (0.1%; 2%) 2491
▲ Zenapax for Injection (Greater than 5%) 3046
▲ Zestril Tablets (5.7%) 698
▲ Zoladex (Occasional) 702
Zoladex 3-month (Occasional) 706
Zoloft (Infrequent) 2751
Zomig Tablets (Infrequent) 708

Zomig-ZMT Tablets (Infrequent) 708
Zonegran Capsules (Infrequent) 1307
Zosyn (1.3% to 1.6%) 1890
Zosyn in Galaxy Containers (1.3% to 1.6%) 1894
Zovia 3449
Zyban Sustained-Release Tablets (1% to 2.5%) 1710
Zyprexa Tablets 1973
Zyprexa ZYDIS Orally Disintegrating Tablets 1973
Zyrtec (Less than 2%) 2756
Zyrtec-D 12 Hour Extended Relief Tablets (Less than 2%) 2758
Zyvox 2871

Hypertension, aggravation
Ambien Tablets (Rare) 3191
Atrovent Inhalation Solution (0.9%) 1031
Carbatrol Capsules 3234
Celebrex Capsules (0.1% to 1.9%) 2676
Celebrex Capsules (0.1% to 1.9%) 2780
Evoxac Capsules (Less than 1%) 1217
Sandostatin LAR Depot (1% to 4%) 2395
Tegretol/Tegretol-XR 2404
Ultracet Tablets (Less than 1%) 2597
▲ Zenapax for Injection (Greater than 5%) 3046
Zoloft (Rare) 2751

Hypertension, intracranial
Aclovate 1275
Amicar Injection 3608
Amicar Syrup 3608
Amicar Tablets 3608
Betaseron for SC Injection 988
Cerebyx Injection (Frequent) 2619
Cutivate Cream 1282
Cutivate Ointment 1284
Cytovene 2959
Dermatop Emollient Cream 2517
Diprivan Injectable Emulsion (Less than 1%) 667
Doryx Coated Pellet Filled Capsules 3357
Dynacin Capsules 2019
Genotropin Lyophilized Powder (A small number of patients) 2818
▲ Gliadel Wafer (4%) 1723
Humatrope Vials and Cartridges 1930
LYMErix Vaccine (Greater than 1%) 1592
Macrobid Capsules (Rare) 2889
Macrodantin Capsules (Rare) 2891
Minocin Intravenous 1862
Minocin Oral Suspension 1865
Minocin Pellet-Filled Capsules 1863
Monodox Capsules 2442
Norplant System (Less than 1%) 3543
Pediazole Suspension 3050
Permax Tablets (Rare) 1299
Saizen for Injection (A small number of patients) 3225
Urobiotic-250 Capsules 2731
▲ Vesanoid Capsules (9%) 3037
Vibramycin Calcium Oral Suspension Syrup 2735
Vibramycin Hyclate Capsules 2735
Vibramycin Hyclate Intravenous 2737
Vibramycin Monohydrate for Oral Suspension 2735
Vibra-Tabs Film Coated Tablets 2735

Hypertension, portal
Fortovase Capsules (Rare) 2970
Invirase Capsules (Rare) 2979

Hypertension, rebound
▲ Duraclon Injection (Among most frequent) 3057
Isordil Sublingual Tablets (Uncommon) 3525
Isordil Titradose Tablets (Uncommon) 3526
Nitro-Dur Transdermal Infusion System (Uncommon) 1834
Nitro-Dur Transdermal Infusion System (Uncommon) 3134
Tenex Tablets (Less common) 2942

Hypertension, supine
▲ ProAmatine Tablets (7.3%) 3241

Hypertensive crises
Accupril Tablets (Rare) 2611
Accuretic Tablets (0.5% to 1%) 2614
Avalide Tablets 1070
Avapro Tablets (Less than 1%) 1074
Avapro Tablets (Less than 1%) 3076
Imitrex Injection (Rare) 1549
Monopril Tablets (0.2% to 1.0%) 1091
Monopril HCT 1094

Hyperthermia
BayRab 917
BayRho-D Full Dose 921
BayRho-D Mini-Dose 919
BayTet 923
Biltricide Tablets 887
Calcijex Injection 411
Cogentin 2055
Effexor Tablets 3495
Elspar for Injection 2092
Geocillin Tablets 2687
Hectorol Capsules 1064
Hectorol Injection 1066
MICRhoGAM Injection 2524
Motofen Tablets 577
Nesacaine/Nesacaine MPF 617
Reglan 2935
Risperdal 1796
Rocaltrol 2991
Sensorcaine (Rare) 643
Sensorcaine-MPF Injection (Rare) 643
Stelazine Tablets 1640

Hyperthyroidism
Aciphex Tablets 1267
Aciphex Tablets 1783
Arava Tablets (1% to 3%) 724
Avonex 1013
Campath Ampules 992
Cognex Capsules (Rare) 1351
Copaxone for Injection (Infrequent) 3306
Cordarone Tablets (1% to 3%) 3487
Cytomel Tablets 1817
Effexor Tablets (Rare) 3495
Effexor XR Capsules (Rare) 3499
Eskalith (Rare) 1527
Flolan for Injection 1528
Intron A for Injection (Less than 5%) 3120
Levothroid Tablets (Rare) 1373
Levoxyl Tablets 1819
Lithium Carbonate (Rare cases) 3061
Lithium Citrate Syrup 3061
Lithobid Slow-Release Tablets (Rare) 3255
Meridia Capsules 481
Miacalcin Nasal Spray (Less than 1%) 2375
Neurontin Capsules (Rare) 2655
Neurontin Oral Solution (Rare) 2655
Neurontin Tablets (Rare) 2655
Pacerone Tablets (1% to 3%) 3331
Paxil (Rare) 1609
PEG-Intron Powder for Injection (Less than or equal to 1%) 3140
Proleukin for Injection 1199
Requip Tablets (Infrequent) 1621
Roferon-A Injection (Infrequent) 2996
Seroquel Tablets (Rare) 684
Synthroid (Rare) 505
Tenoretic Tablets 690
Tenormin 692
Unithroid Tablets 3445

Hypertonia
Aceon Tablets (2 mg, 4 mg, 8 mg) (0.2% to 2.7%) 3249
Aciphex Tablets 1267
Aciphex Tablets 1783
Actonel Tablets (2.2%) 2879
Adalat CC Tablets (Less than 1.0%) 877
Amphotec (1% to 5%) 1774
Aricept Tablets (Infrequent) 1270
Aricept Tablets (Infrequent) 2665
▲ Arimidex Tablets (3.2%) 659
Arthrotec Tablets (Rare) 3195
▲ Asacol Delayed-Release Tablets (5%) 2884
Avelox Tablets (0.05% to 1%) 879
Avonex 1013
Axert Tablets (Rare) 2772
Azopt Ophthalmic Suspension (Less than 1%) 536
Baycol Tablets 883
▲ Betaseron for SC Injection (26%) 988
Betaxon Ophthalmic Suspension (Less than 2%) 537
▲ Botox Purified Neurotoxin Complex (2% to 10%) 549
Brethine Tablets (Less than 1%) 2313
Cardene I.V. (Rare) 3485
Cardura Tablets (1%) 2668
Carnitor Injection (1% to 3%) 3242
▲ Casodex Tablets (2% to 5%) 662
Ceclor CD Tablets 1279
Ceclor (Rare) 1905
Celebrex Capsules (0.1% to 1.9%) 2676
Celebrex Capsules (0.1% to 1.9%) 2780
Celexa (Infrequent) 1365
▲ CellCept Capsules (3% to 15.6%) 2951
▲ CellCept Intravenous (3% to 15.6%) 2951
▲ CellCept Oral Suspension (3% to 15.6%) 2951
▲ CellCept Tablets (3% to 15.6%) 2951
▲ Cenestin Tablets (6%) 1263
Claritin (At least one patient) 3100
Claritin-D 12 Hour Extended Release Tablets (Less frequent) 3102
Claritin-D 24 Hour Extended Release Tablets (Fewer than 2%) 3104
Cognex Capsules (Frequent) 1351
Colazal Capsules 3069
▲ Copaxone for Injection (22%) 3306
DaunoXome Injection (Less than or equal to 5%) 1442
Depacon Injection (1% to 5%) 416
Depakene (1% to 5%) 421
Depakote Sprinkle Capsules (1% to 5%) 426
Depakote Tablets (1% to 5%) 430
Depakote ER Tablets (1% to 5%) 436
Diprivan Injectable Emulsion (Less than 1%) 667
Doxil Injection (Less than 1%) 566
Duragesic Transdermal System (Less than 1%) 1786
▲ Effexor Tablets (3%; infrequent) 3495
Effexor XR Capsules (Infrequent) 3499
Eskalith 1527
Evoxac Capsules (1% to 3%) 1217
Exelon Capsules (Infrequent) 2342
Exelon Oral Solution (Infrequent) 2345
Ferrlecit Injection (Two or more patients) 3386
Flexeril Tablets (Less than 1%) 572
Flexeril Tablets (Less than 1%) 2094
Gabitril Tablets (Frequent) 1189
▲ Geodon Capsules (3%) 2688
Glucotrol XL Extended Release Tablets (Less than 1%) 2693
Havrix Vaccine (Less than 1%) 1544
Hivid Tablets (Less than 1%) 2975
Indapamide Tablets (Less than 5%) 2286
▲ Infergen (6% to 7%) 1777
Intron A for Injection (Less than 5%) 3120
Kaletra Capsules (Less than 2%) 471
Kaletra Oral Solution (Less than 2%) 471
Klonopin Tablets (Infrequent) 2983
Lamictal (Rare) 1567
Levaquin Injection (Less than 0.5%) 2537
Lipitor Tablets (Less than 2%) 2639
Lipitor Tablets (Less than 2%) 2696
Lithobid Slow-Release Tablets 3255
Lotensin Tablets (Less than 1%) 2365
Lotensin HCT Tablets (1.5%) 2367
Luvox Tablets (25, 50, 100 mg) (2%) 3256
Meridia Capsules (Greater than or equal to 1%) 481
▲ Mirapex Tablets (7%) 2834
Naprelan Tablets (Less than 1%) 1293
Nexium Delayed-Release Capsules (Less than 1%) 619
Norvasc Tablets (Less than or equal to 0.1%) 2704
Paxil (Infrequent) 1609
▲ PEG-Intron Powder for Injection (5%) 3140
Permax Tablets (1.1%) 1299
▲ Prempro Tablets (3% to 4%) 3572
Procardia XL Extended Release Tablets (1% or less) 2710
▲ Prograf (3% to 15%) 1393
Prometrium Capsules (100 mg, 200 mg) (Less than 5%) 3261
Protonix I.V. (Greater than or equal to 1%) 3580
Protonix Tablets (Greater than or equal to 1%) 3577
Provigil Tablets (2%) 1193
Prozac Pulvules, Liquid, and Weekly Capsules (Infrequent) 1238
Pulmicort Turbuhaler Inhalation Powder (1% to 3%) 636
▲ Rapamune Oral Solution and Tablets (3% to 20%) 3584
Reminyl Oral Solution (Infrequent) 1792
Reminyl Tablets (Infrequent) 1792
ReoPro Vials (0.2%) 1958
Requip Tablets (Infrequent) 1621
Rescriptor Tablets 526
▲ Rilutek Tablets (5.3% to 5.9%) 772
▲ Risperdal (17% to 34%) 1796
Rituxan for Infusion (1% to 5%) 1750
Rituxan I.V. (1% to 5%) 1428
Roxicodone Tablets (Less than 3%) 3067
Sandostatin LAR Depot (1% to 4%) 2395
Sarafem Pulvules (Infrequent) 1962
Seroquel Tablets (Frequent) 684
▲ Serostim for Injection (1% to 10%) 3229
Serzone Tablets (1%) 1104
Sonata Capsules (Frequent) 3591
▲ Soriatane Capsules (1% to 10%) 3003
Sular Tablets (Less than or equal to 1%) 688
Symmetrel 1328
Synercid I.V. (Less than 1%) 775
Tasmar Tablets (1%) 3010
Tequin Injection (Less than 0.1%) 1110
Tequin Tablets (Less than 0.1%) 1110
Thalomid Capsules 1154
Topamax Sprinkle Capsules (Frequent) 2590
Topamax Tablets (Frequent) 2590
Tricor Capsules, Micronized 513
Trovan (Less than 1%) 2722
Ultracet Tablets (Less than 1%) 2597
Ultram Tablets (1% to 5%) 2600
Uniretic Tablets (More than 1%) 3178
Viagra Tablets (Less than 2%) 2732
Vicoprofen Tablets (Less than 3%) 520
Vistide Injection 1445
Wellbutrin SR Sustained-Release Tablets (Infrequent) 1684
Zoladex (1%) 702
Zoladex 3-month 706
Zoloft (Frequent) 2751
Zomig Tablets (Rare) 708
Zomig-ZMT Tablets (Rare) 708
Zonegran Capsules (Infrequent) 1307
Zyban Sustained-Release Tablets (Infrequent) 1710
Zyflo Filmtab Tablets (Less common) 524
▲ Zyprexa Tablets (4% to 20%) 1973
▲ Zyprexa ZYDIS Orally Disintegrating Tablets (4% to 20%) 1973
Zyrtec (Less than 2%) 2756
Zyrtec-D 12 Hour Extended Relief Tablets (Less than 2%) 2758

Hypertrichosis
Analpram-HC 1338
Anusol-HC Cream 2.5% (Infrequent to frequent) 2237
Azelex Cream (Rare) 547
Celexa (Rare) 1365
Clobevate Gel 3271
Clomid Tablets 735
Cordran Lotion (Infrequent) 2438
Cordran Tape (Infrequent) 2439
Cormax Cream (Infrequent) 2440
Cormax Ointment (Infrequent) 2440
Cormax Scalp Application (Infrequent) 2441
Cortifoam Rectal Foam 3170
Cutivate Ointment (Less than 1%) 1284
Dilantin Infatabs 2624
Dilantin Kapseals 2622
Dilantin-125 Oral Suspension 2625
Diprolene Lotion 0.05% (Infrequent) 3107
Diprolene Ointment 0.05% (Infrequent) 3108
Diprolene AF Cream 0.05% (Infrequent) 3106
Diprosone 3109
Elocon Cream 0.1% (Infrequent) 3110
Elocon Lotion 0.1% (Infrequent) 3111
Elocon Ointment 0.1% (Infrequent) 3112
Finevin Cream 962
▲ Gengraf Capsules (6.6% to 15%) 457
Lidex (Infrequent) 2020
Locoid Cream (Infrequent) 1341
Locoid Lipocream Cream (Infrequent) 1342
Locoid (Infrequent) 1341
Lotrisone 3129
▲ Neoral Soft Gelatin Capsules (6.6% to 15%) 2380
▲ Neoral Oral Solution (6.6% to 15%) 2380
Norplant System 3543
Olux Foam 1211
Pramosone 1343
ProctoFoam-HC 3177
Psorcon E Cream 1227
Psorcon E Ointment 1228
Risperdal (Rare) 1796
Serophene Tablets 3226
▲ Simulect for Injection (3% to 10%) 2399
Soriatane Capsules (Less than 1%) 3003
Synalar (Infrequent) 2020
Temovate Gel (Infrequent) 1303
Temovate Scalp Application (Infrequent) 1304
Temovate E Emollient (Infrequent) 1302
Topicort (Infrequent) 2025
Ultravate Cream 1119
Ultravate Ointment 1120
Zoloft (Rare) 2751
Zyrtec (Less than 2%) 2756
Zyrtec-D 12 Hour Extended Relief Tablets (Less than 2%) 2758

Hypertriglyceridemia
Accuretic Tablets (Rare) 2614
Accutane Capsules 2944
Aceon Tablets (2 mg, 4 mg, 8 mg) (1.3%) 3249
▲ Agenerase Capsules (41% to 56%) 1454
▲ Agenerase Oral Solution (41% to 56%) 1459
▲ AndroGel (3% to 6%) 3322
Atacand Tablets (0.5% or greater) 595
Atacand HCT Tablets 597
Blocadren Tablets 2046
Brevicon 28-Day Tablets 3380
Carbatrol Capsules (Occasional) 3234
▲ Cipro I.V. (Among most frequent) 893
▲ Cipro I.V. Pharmacy Bulk Package (Among most frequent) 897
Cipro 887
Coreg Tablets (0.1% to 1.2%) 1508
Crixivan Capsules 2070

Cytovene 2959
Diflucan Tablets, Injection, and Oral Suspension 2681
Ergamisol Tablets 1789
Estratest 3252
Evoxac Capsules (Less than 1%) 1217
Floxin I.V. 2526
Floxin Tablets 2529
Fortovase Capsules (Less than 2%) 2970
▲ Gengraf Capsules (About 15%) 457
Hivid Tablets (Less than 1%) 2975
Hyzaar 2109
▲ Infergen (5% to 6%) 1777
Intron A for Injection (Less than 5%) 3120
▲ Kaletra Capsules (5.1% to 26.2%) 471
▲ Kaletra Oral Solution (5.1% to 26.2%) 471
Levlen (A small portion of women) 962
Levlite 21 Tablets (A small portion of women) 962
Levlite 28 Tablets (A small portion of women) 962
Lo/Ovral Tablets 3532
Lo/Ovral-28 Tablets 3538
Lovenox Injection 746
Low-Ogestrel-28 Tablets 3392
▲ Lupron Depot 3.75 mg (12%) 3281
▲ Lupron Depot–3 Month 11.25 mg (32%) 3285
▲ Lupron Depot–4 Month 30 mg (Greater than or equal to 5%) 3289
Modicon 2563
▲ Neoral Soft Gelatin Capsules (About 15%) 2380
▲ Neoral Oral Solution (About 15%) 2380
Nizoral Tablets 1791
Nolvadex Tablets (Rare) 678
Nordette-28 Tablets 2257
Norinyl 1 +35 28-Day Tablets 3380
Norinyl 1 + 50 28-Day Tablets 3380
Noroxin Tablets 2145
Ogestrel 0.5/50-28 Tablets 3428
Ortho-Cyclen/Ortho Tri-Cyclen 2573
Ortho-Novum 2563
Ortho-Novum 1/50□28 Tablets 2556
Ortho-Novum 2563
Ortho-Cyclen/Ortho Tri-Cyclen 2573
Ovcon 3364
Ovral Tablets 3551
Ovral-28 Tablets 3552
Ovrette Tablets 3552
Premarin Tablets 3566
Premarin Vaginal Cream 3570
Prinzide Tablets 2168
Rapamune Oral Solution and Tablets 3584
Rescriptor Tablets 526
Risperdal (Rare) 1796
Roferon-A Injection (Rare) 2996
▲ Serostim for Injection (1% to 10%) 3229
▲ Simulect for Injection (3% to 10%) 2399
Soriatane Capsules (Less common) 3003
Sporanox Capsules (Rare) 1800
Sporanox Injection (Rare) 1804
Sporanox Injection (Rare) 2509
Sporanox Oral Solution (Rare) 1808
Sporanox Oral Solution (Rare) 2512
Sustiva Capsules 1258
▲ Synarel Nasal Solution for Endometriosis (12%) 3205
Tegretol/Tegretol-XR (Occasional) 2404
Teveten Tablets (1%) 3327
Ticlid Tablets 3015
Timolide Tablets 2187
Tri-Levlen (A small portion of women) 962
Tri-Norinyl-28 Tablets 3433
Triphasil-21 Tablets 3600
Triphasil-28 Tablets 3605
Trizivir Tablets 1669
Vaseretic Tablets 2204
▲ Vesanoid Capsules (Up to 60%) 3037
Xeloda Tablets (Less than 5%) 3039
Zebeta Tablets 1885
Zestoretic Tablets 695
Zoladex 702
Zoladex 3-month 706
▲ Zoloft (Approximately 5%) 2751

Hypertrophic papillae of the tongue
Primaxin I.M. 2158
Primaxin I.V. (Less than 0.2%) 2160
Serentil 1057

Hypertrophy, gum
Zarontin Capsules 2659
Zarontin Syrup 2660

Hyperuricemia
Abelcet Injection 1273
Accuretic Tablets 2614
Accutane Capsules 2944
Aceon Tablets (2 mg, 4 mg, 8 mg) (0.3% to 1%) 3249
Aldoclor Tablets 2035
Aldoril Tablets 2039
Aloprim for Injection (Less than 1%) 2292
Altace Capsules 2233
Arthrotec Tablets (Rare) 3195
Atacand Tablets (0.6%) 595
Atacand HCT Tablets (0.5% or greater) 597
Avalide Tablets 1070
Axid Pulvules 1903
Axid Pulvules 2919
Blocadren Tablets 2046
Cardizem Injectable (Less than 1%) 1018
Cardizem Lyo-Ject Syringe (Less than 1%) 1018
Cardizem Monovial (Less than 1%) 1018
Cardizem CD Capsules (Less than 1%) 1016
▲ CellCept Capsules (3% to 16.3%) 2951
▲ CellCept Intravenous (3% to 16.3%) 2951
▲ CellCept Oral Suspension (3% to 16.3%) 2951
▲ CellCept Tablets (3% to 16.3%) 2951
Cerubidine for Injection 947
▲ Cipro I.V. (Among most frequent) 893
▲ Cipro I.V. Pharmacy Bulk Package (Among most frequent) 897
Cipro (Less than 0.1%) 887
Clorpres Tablets 1002
Clozaril Tablets 2319
Combipres Tablets 1040
Coreg Tablets (1% to 2%) 1508
Corzide 40/5 Tablets 2247
Corzide 80/5 Tablets 2247
Creon 5 Capsules 3251
Creon 10 Capsules 3251
Creon 20 Capsules 3251
Daranide Tablets 2077
Demadex Tablets and Injection 2965
Diovan HCT Tablets 2338
Diucardin Tablets 3494
Diuril Oral 2087
Diuril Sodium Intravenous 2086
Doxil Injection (1% to 5%) 566
Dyazide Capsules 1515
Dynabac Tablets (0.1% to 1%) 2269
Ecotrin Enteric Coated Aspirin Low, Regular and Maximum Strength Tablets 1715
Edecrin 2091
Effexor Tablets (Infrequent) 3495
Effexor XR Capsules (Infrequent) 3499
Ellence Injection 2806
Evoxac Capsules (Less than 1%) 1217
Fludara for Injection 995
Furosemide Tablets 2284
Gengraf Capsules (1% to less than 3%) 457
Geodon Capsules (Rare) 2688
Hivid Tablets (Less than 1%) 2975
HydroDIURIL Tablets 2108
Hyzaar 2109
Imdur Tablets (Less than or equal to 5%) 1826
Indapamide Tablets (Less than 5%) 2286
Inderide Tablets 3517
Inderide LA Long-Acting Capsules 3519
Kaletra Capsules (0.5% to 3.6%) 471
Kaletra Oral Solution (0.5% to 3.6%) 471
Lodosyn Tablets 1251
Lotensin HCT Tablets 2367
Lotrel Capsules (Rare) 2370
Lupron Depot 7.5 mg (Greater than or equal to 5%) 3284
Lupron Injection 3279
▲ Mavik Tablets (15%) 478
Maxzide 1008
Micardis HCT Tablets 1051
Microzide Capsules 3414
Minizide Capsules 2700
Moduretic Tablets 2138
Monopril HCT 1094
Myambutol Tablets 1290
Mykrox Tablets 1168
Myleran Tablets 1603
Mylocel Tablets 2227
Naprelan Tablets (Less than 1%) 1293
Neoral Soft Gelatin Capsules (1% to less than 3%) 2380
Neoral Oral Solution (1% to less than 3%) 2380
▲ Neupogen for Injection (27% to 58%) 587
Nexium Delayed-Release Capsules (Less than 1%) 619
Novantrone for Injection 1760
Oncaspar (Greater than 1% but less than 5%) 756
Pancrease MT Capsules 2581
Permax Tablets (Rare) 1299
Plavix Tablets (1% to 2.5%) 1097
Plavix Tablets (1% to 2.5%) 3084
Pletal Tablets (Less than 2%) 2605
Pletal Tablets (Less than 2%) 2848
▲ Priftin Tablets (15.2% to 21.3%) 758
Prinzide Tablets 2168
▲ Prograf (3% to 15%) 1393
▲ Proleukin for Injection (9%) 1199
Prozac Pulvules, Liquid, and Weekly Capsules (Rare) 1238
Purinethol Tablets 1615
Pyrazinamide Tablets 1876
Rebetron Combination Therapy 3153
Relafen Tablets (Less than 1%) 1617
Renese Tablets 2712
Requip Tablets (Infrequent) 1621
Rescriptor Tablets (Less than 2%) 526
Rifadin 765
Rifamate Capsules 767
Rifater Tablets 769
Risperdal (Rare) 1796
▲ Roferon-A Injection (10%) 2996
Sandimmune (Occasional) 2388
Sarafem Pulvules (Rare) 1962
▲ Simulect for Injection (Greater than or equal to 10%) 2399
Sinemet Tablets 1253
Sonata Capsules (Rare) 3591
Starlix Tablets 2401
Tabloid Tablets (Frequent) 1642
Tenoretic Tablets 690
Thalomid Capsules 1154
Tiazac Capsules (Less than 2%) 1378
Timolide Tablets 2187
Tricor Capsules, Micronized 513
Ultrase Capsules 835
Ultrase MT Capsules 835
Uniretic Tablets (More than 1%) 3178
Univasc Tablets 3181
Vaseretic Tablets 2204
Viagra Tablets (Less than 2%) 2732
Videx (Less than 1% to 3%) 1138
Videx EC Capsules 1143
Viokase 837
Viracept 532
Zaroxolyn Tablets 1177
Zebeta Tablets 1885
Zestoretic Tablets 695
Ziac Tablets 1887
Zyprexa Tablets (Infrequent) 1973
Zyprexa ZYDIS Orally Disintegrating Tablets (Infrequent) 1973

Hyperuricosuria
Creon 5 Capsules 3251
Creon 10 Capsules 3251
Creon 20 Capsules 3251
Myleran Tablets 1603
Pancrease Capsules 2580
Pancrease MT Capsules 2581
Ultrase Capsules 835
Ultrase MT Capsules 835

Hyperuricuria
Pancrease Capsules 2580
Viokase 837

Hyperventilation
Aciphex Tablets 1267
Aciphex Tablets 1783
Actiq (Less than 1%) 1184
Adenocard Injection (Less than 1%) 1380
AmBisome for Injection (Less common) 1383
▲ Amphotec (5% or more) 1774
Aricept Tablets (Infrequent) 1270
Aricept Tablets (Infrequent) 2665
Arthrotec Tablets (Rare) 3195
Ativan Injection (Less than 1%) 3478
Avonex 1013
Axert Tablets (Rare) 2772
Betaseron for SC Injection 988
Cataflam Tablets (Less than 1%) 2315
Cerebyx Injection (Infrequent) 2619
Clozaril Tablets (Less than 1%) 2319
Cognex Capsules (Infrequent) 1351
Copaxone for Injection (Frequent) 3306
Crinone (Less than 5%) 3213
Diprivan Injectable Emulsion (Less than 1%) 667
Doxil Injection (Less than 1%) 566
Dynabac Tablets (0.1% to 1%) 2269
Effexor Tablets (Infrequent) 3495
Effexor XR Capsules (Infrequent) 3499
Gabitril Tablets (Infrequent) 1189
Lamictal (Infrequent) 1567
Luvox Tablets (25, 50, 100 mg) (Infrequent) 3256
Neurontin Capsules (Rare) 2655
Neurontin Oral Solution (Rare) 2655
Neurontin Tablets (Rare) 2655
Orthoclone OKT3 Sterile Solution 2498
Paxil (Infrequent) 1609
Permax Tablets (Infrequent) 1299
Primaxin I.M. 2158
Primaxin I.V. (Less than 0.2%) 2160
ProSom Tablets (Rare) 500
Protopam Chloride for Injection 3582
Prozac Pulvules, Liquid, and Weekly Capsules (Infrequent) 1238
Rilutek Tablets (Infrequent) 772
Risperdal (Infrequent) 1796
▲ Romazicon Injection (3% to 9%) 3000
Sarafem Pulvules (Infrequent) 1962
Seroquel Tablets (Rare) 684
Serzone Tablets (Rare) 1104
Sonata Capsules (Rare) 3591
Sulfamylon Cream 1011
Sulfamylon Topical Solution 1011
Tasmar Tablets (Infrequent) 3010
Tequin Injection (Less than 0.1%) 1110
Tequin Tablets (Less than 0.1%) 1110
▲ TOBI Solution for Inhalation (5.4%) 1206
Valium Injectable 3026
Versed Injection (Less than 1%) 3027
Vistide Injection 1445
Voltaren Tablets (Less than 1%) 2315
Voltaren-XR Tablets (Less than 1%) 2315
▲ Xanax Tablets (9.7%) 2865
Zoloft (Rare) 2751
Zyprexa Tablets (Infrequent) 1973
Zyprexa ZYDIS Orally Disintegrating Tablets (Infrequent) 1973
Zyrtec (Less than 2%) 2756
Zyrtec-D 12 Hour Extended Relief Tablets (Less than 2%) 2758

Hypervitaminosis A syndrome
Aquasol A Parenteral 593

Hypervolemia
Aloprim for Injection (Less than 1%) 2292
▲ AmBisome for Injection (8.2% to 12.2%) 1383
Amphotec (1% to 5%) 1774
▲ Carnitor Injection (3% to 12%) 3242
▲ CellCept Capsules (3% to 16.6%) 2951
▲ CellCept Intravenous (3% to 16.6%) 2951
▲ CellCept Oral Suspension (3% to 16.6%) 2951
▲ CellCept Tablets (3% to 16.6%) 2951
Coreg Tablets (2.0%) 1508
Ferrlecit Injection (Greater than 1%) 3386
▲ Prograf (3% to 15%) 1393
▲ Rapamune Oral Solution and Tablets (3% to 20%) 3584
Trasylol Injection (1% to 2%) 909
Venofer Injection (Greater than 1%) 580

Hypesthesia
(*see under* Hypoesthesia)

Hyphema
Viroptic Ophthalmic Solution Sterile ⊙301

Hypnagogic effects
Advair Diskus 100/50 (1% to 3%) 1448
Advair Diskus 250/50 (1% to 3%) 1448
Advair Diskus 500/50 (1% to 3%) 1448

Hypnotic effects
Trilafon 3160

Hypoactivity
Aerobid/Aerobid-M (1% to 3%) 1363
Valium Injectable 3026

Hypoadrenalism
Sandostatin Injection (Less than 1%) 2394
Sandostatin LAR Depot (Rare) 2395

Hypoadrenalism, neonatal
Azmacort Inhalation Aerosol 728
Celestone Soluspan Injectable Suspension 3097
Cortone Acetate Tablets 2061
Decadron Elixir 2078
Decadron Tablets 2079
Decadron Phosphate Injection 2081
Hydrocortone Tablets 2106
Hydrocortone Acetate Injectable Suspension 2103
Hydrocortone Phosphate Injection, Sterile 2105
Nasacort Nasal Inhaler 750
Prednisone 3064
Prelone Syrup 2273
Rhinocort Nasal Inhaler 640

Hypoalbuminemia
Campath Ampules 992
▲ Cancidas for Injection (4.6% to 8.6%) 2048
Cipro I.V. Pharmacy Bulk Package (Less than 1%) 897
Dapsone Tablets USP 1780
Dynabac Tablets (0.1% to 1%) 2269
Evista Tablets 1915
▲ Leukine (27%) 1755
Lupron Depot 7.5 mg (Greater than or equal to 5%) 3284
Oncaspar 756
▲ Proleukin for Injection (8%) 1199
Vantin Tablets and Oral Suspension 2860
Zosyn 1890
Zosyn in Galaxy Containers 1894

Hypoalbuminuria
Elspar for Injection 2092
Unasyn for Injection 2728

Hypocalcemia
Abelcet Injection 1273
Actiq (Less than 1%) 1184
Actonel Tablets (0.8%) 2879

Aloprim for Injection (Less than 1%) ... 2292
▲ AmBisome for Injection (4.9% to 18.4%) ... 1383
▲ Amphotec (5% or more) ... 1774
▲ Aredia for Injection (Up to 12%) ... 2309
Ceclor CD Tablets (0.7%) ... 1279
▲ CellCept Capsules (3%) ... 2951
▲ CellCept Intravenous (3%) ... 2951
▲ CellCept Oral Suspension (3%) ... 2951
▲ CellCept Tablets (3% to 30%) ... 2951
Colazal Capsules ... 3069
Cortifoam Rectal Foam ... 3170
Cosmegen for Injection ... 2062
Doxil Injection (1% to 5%) ... 566
Ethyol for Injection (Rare) ... 2029
Evista Tablets ... 1915
Felbatol ... 3343
Fleet Enema ... 1359
Fleet Phospho-soda ... 1360
Fludara for Injection ... 995
Fortovase Capsules (Up to less than 1%) ... 2970
▲ Fosamax Tablets (Approximately 18%) ... 2095
▲ Foscavir Injection (5% to 15%) ... 605
Furosemide Tablets ... 2284
Geodon Capsules (Rare) ... 2688
Hivid Tablets (Less than 1%) ... 2975
Invirase Capsules (Up to less than 1%) ... 2979
Leukine (2%) ... 1755
▲ Mavik Tablets (4.7%) ... 478
Maxipime for Injection (0.1% to 1%) ... 1285
Mithracin for Intravenous Use ... 903
Nebcin Vials, Hyporets & ADD-Vantage ... 1955
Omnicef for Oral Suspension (0.5%) ... 493
▲ Paraplatin for Injection (16% to 31%) ... 1126
Paxil (Rare) ... 1609
Precose Tablets ... 906
▲ Prograf (3% to 15%) ... 1393
▲ Proleukin for Injection (11%) ... 1199
Prozac Pulvules, Liquid, and Weekly Capsules (Rare) ... 1238
▲ Rapamune Oral Solution and Tablets (3% to 20%) ... 3584
Rescriptor Tablets (Less than 2%) ... 526
▲ Roferon-A Injection (28%) ... 2996
Sarafem Pulvules (Rare) ... 1962
▲ Simulect for Injection (3% to 10%) ... 2399
Synarel Nasal Solution for Endometriosis ... 3205
Tegretol-XR Tablets ... 2404
Thalomid Capsules ... 1154
Topamax Sprinkle Capsules (Infrequent) ... 2590
Topamax Tablets (Infrequent) ... 2590
Trileptal Oral Suspension ... 2407
Trileptal Tablets ... 2407
▲ Trisenox Injection (10%) ... 1158
Uniretic Tablets (Less than 1%) ... 3178
Vistide Injection ... 1445
▲ Zometa for Intravenous Infusion (5% to 10%) ... 3621
Zosyn ... 1890
Zosyn in Galaxy Containers ... 1894

Hypocarbia
Survanta Intratracheal Suspension (Less than 1%) ... 3053

Hypochloremia
▲ CellCept Capsules (3% to 10%) ... 2951
▲ CellCept Intravenous (3% to 10%) ... 2951
▲ CellCept Oral Suspension (3% to 10%) ... 2951
▲ CellCept Tablets (3% to 10%) ... 2951
Demadex Tablets and Injection ... 2965
Doxil Injection (Less than 1%) ... 566
Dyazide Capsules ... 1515
Dynabac Tablets (0.1% to 1%) ... 2269
Geodon Capsules (Rare) ... 2688
Indapamide Tablets (Less than 5%) ... 2286
Maxzide ... 1008
Mykrox Tablets ... 1168
Requip Tablets (Rare) ... 1621
Uniretic Tablets (Less than 1%) ... 3178
Zaroxolyn Tablets ... 1177

Hypochloremic alkalosis
Diuril Sodium Intravenous ... 2086
Furosemide Tablets ... 2284
Maxzide ... 1008
Mykrox Tablets ... 1168
Prinzide Tablets ... 2168
Tenoretic Tablets ... 690
Vaseretic Tablets ... 2204
Zaroxolyn Tablets ... 1177
Zestoretic Tablets ... 695

Hypocholesterolemia
Evista Tablets ... 1915
Geodon Capsules (Rare) ... 2688
▲ Lupron Depot–4 Month 30 mg (Greater than or equal to 5%) ... 3289
Prevacid Delayed-Release Capsules ... 3292
PREVPAC ... 3298
Proleukin for Injection (1%) ... 1199
▲ Simulect for Injection (Greater than or equal to 10%) ... 2399
Topamax Sprinkle Capsules (Rare) ... 2590
Topamax Tablets (Rare) ... 2590

Hypochondriasis
Luvox Tablets (25, 50, 100 mg) (Infrequent) ... 3256

Hypocoagulability
Orudis Capsules (Less than 1%) ... 3548
Oruvail Capsules (Less than 1%) ... 3548

Hypoesthesia (0.9%)
Actiq (1% or greater) ... 1184
Ambien Tablets (Infrequent) ... 3191
Amerge Tablets (Rare) ... 1467
▲ Aromasin Tablets (2% to 5%) ... 2769
Arthrotec Tablets (Rare) ... 3195
Astelin Nasal Spray (Infrequent) ... 3339
Atacand HCT Tablets (0.5% or greater) ... 597
Cardene I.V. (0.7%) ... 3485
Cardura Tablets (0.5% to 1%) ... 2668
Caverject Sterile Powder (Less than 1%) ... 2777
Celebrex Capsules (0.1% to 1.9%) ... 2676
Celebrex Capsules (0.1% to 1.9%) ... 2780
Celexa (Infrequent) ... 1365
Cerebyx Injection (2.2%) ... 2619
Chirocaine Injection (2.8%) ... 2909
Cipro HC Otic Suspension (One patient) ... 540
Claritin (At least one patient) ... 3100
Claritin-D 12 Hour Extended Release Tablets (Less frequent) ... 3102
Claritin-D 24 Hour Extended Release Tablets ... 3104
Cognex Capsules (Infrequent) ... 1351
Colazal Capsules ... 3069
Copaxone for Injection (At least 2%) ... 3306
Coreg Tablets (1% to 2%) ... 1508
Cozaar Tablets (Less than 1%) ... 2067
Crixivan Capsules (Less than 2%) ... 2070
Denavir Cream (0.9%) ... 2332
Depacon Injection (0.6%) ... 416
Depakene ... 421
Depakote Sprinkle Capsules ... 426
Depakote Tablets ... 430
Depakote ER Tablets ... 436
Effexor Tablets ... 3495
Engerix-B Vaccine ... 1517
Evoxac Capsules (1% to 3%) ... 1217
Exelon Capsules (Infrequent) ... 2342
Exelon Oral Solution (Infrequent) ... 2345
▲ Flolan for Injection (1% to 12%) ... 1528
Floxin Otic Solution (Single report) ... 1219
Flumadine ... 1370
▲ Foscavir Injection (5% or greater) ... 605
Gabitril Tablets (Frequent) ... 1189
Gastrocrom Oral Concentrate (Less common) ... 1162
Gengraf Capsules (1% to less than 3%) ... 457
Geodon Capsules (Frequent) ... 2688
Glucotrol XL Extended Release Tablets (Less than 3%) ... 2693
▲ Humatrope Vials and Cartridges (Up to 6.25%) ... 1930
Hyzaar ... 2109
Imdur Tablets (Less than or equal to 5%) ... 1826
▲ Infergen (8% to 10%) ... 1777
▲ Intron A for Injection (Up to 10%) ... 3120
Ismo Tablets (Fewer than 1%) ... 3524
Kadian Capsules (Less than 3%) ... 1335
Klonopin Tablets (Infrequent) ... 2983
Lamictal (Infrequent) ... 1567
Levaquin Injection (Less than 0.5%) ... 2537
Lipitor Tablets (Less than 2%) ... 2639
Lipitor Tablets (Less than 2%) ... 2696
Lopid Tablets (More common) ... 2650
Lotensin HCT Tablets (0.3% or more) ... 2367
Lupron Depot 3.75 mg ... 3281
Lupron Depot–3 Month 11.25 mg ... 3285
Lupron Depot–3 Month 22.5 mg (Less than 5%) ... 3288
LYMErix Vaccine (2.96%) ... 1592
Maxalt Tablets (Frequent) ... 2120
Maxalt-MLT Orally Disintegrating Tablets (Frequent) ... 2120
Megace Oral Suspension (1% to 3%) ... 1124
Meridia Capsules ... 481
Micardis Tablets (More than 0.3%) ... 1049
Micardis HCT Tablets ... 1051
Migranal Nasal Spray (Infrequent) ... 2376
▲ Mirapex Tablets (3%) ... 2834
Naropin Injection (1% to 5%) ... 612
Nascobal Gel ... 3174
▲ Navelbine Injection (Among most frequent) ... 1604
Neoral Soft Gelatin Capsules (1% to less than 3%) ... 2380
Neoral Oral Solution (1% to less than 3%) ... 2380
Neurontin Capsules (Infrequent) ... 2655
Neurontin Oral Solution (Infrequent) ... 2655
Neurontin Tablets (Infrequent) ... 2655
Nexium Delayed-Release Capsules (Less than 1%) ... 619
▲ Nilandron Tablets (5.3%) ... 753
Normodyne Injection (1%) ... 3135
Norvasc Tablets (More than 0.1% to 1%) ... 2704
OxyContin Tablets (Less than 1%) ... 2912
Paxil (Infrequent) ... 1609
Plavix Tablets (1% to 2.5%) ... 1097
Plavix Tablets (1% to 2.5%) ... 3084
Procardia XL Extended Release Tablets (1% or less) ... 2710
Protonix I.V. (Less than 1%) ... 3580
Protonix Tablets (Less than 1%) ... 3577
Prozac Pulvules, Liquid, and Weekly Capsules (Infrequent) ... 1238
▲ Rapamune Oral Solution and Tablets (3% to 20%) ... 3584
Recombivax HB ... 2178
Remeron Tablets (Frequent) ... 2483
Remeron SolTab Tablets (Frequent) ... 2486
ReoPro Vials (0.3%) ... 1958
Requip Tablets (Infrequent) ... 1621
Rescriptor Tablets (Less than 2%) ... 526
Rilutek Tablets (Infrequent) ... 772
Risperdal (Rare) ... 1796
Rituxan for Infusion (1% to 5%) ... 1750
Rituxan I.V. (1% to 5%) ... 1428
Romazicon Injection (1% to 3%) ... 3000
Roxicodone Tablets (Less than 3%) ... 3067
Salagen Tablets (Less than 1%) ... 2229
▲ Sandostatin LAR Depot (5% to 15%) ... 2395
Sarafem Pulvules (Infrequent) ... 1962
Sectral Capsules (Up to 2%) ... 3589
Serzone Tablets ... 1104
▲ Simulect for Injection (3% to 10%) ... 2399
Sonata Capsules (Less than 1% to 2%) ... 3591
Soriatane Capsules (Less than 1%) ... 3003
Sular Tablets (Less than or equal to 1%) ... 688
Sustiva Capsules (1% to 2%) ... 1258
Tambocor Tablets (1% to 3%) ... 1990
Tarka Tablets (Less frequent) ... 508
Tasmar Tablets (Frequent) ... 3010
Topamax Sprinkle Capsules (0.8% to 2.7%) ... 2590
Topamax Tablets (0.8% to 2.7%) ... 2590
Trileptal Oral Suspension (1% to 3%) ... 2407
Trileptal Tablets (1% to 3%) ... 2407
Trovan (Less than 1%) ... 2722
Uniretic Tablets (Less than 1%) ... 3178
Viagra Tablets (Less than 2%) ... 2732
Vioxx (Greater than 0.1% to 1.9%) ... 2213
▲ Visudyne for Injection (1% to 10%) ... ⊙ 308
Wellbutrin SR Sustained-Release Tablets (Infrequent) ... 1684
Xopenex Inhalation Solution ... 3207
Zebeta Tablets (1.1% to 1.5%) ... 1885
Zoloft (Frequent) ... 2751
Zomig Tablets (1% to 2%) ... 708
Zomig-ZMT Tablets (1% to 2%) ... 708
Zyban Sustained-Release Tablets (Infrequent) ... 1710
Zyprexa Tablets (Infrequent) ... 1973
Zyprexa ZYDIS Orally Disintegrating Tablets (Infrequent) ... 1973
Zyrtec (Less than 2%) ... 2756
Zyrtec-D 12 Hour Extended Relief Tablets (Less than 2%) ... 2758

Hypoestrogeneism
▲ Lupron Depot 3.75 mg (Among most frequent) ... 3281
Lupron Depot–3 Month 11.25 mg ... 3285
Neurontin Capsules (Rare) ... 2655
Neurontin Oral Solution (Rare) ... 2655
Neurontin Tablets (Rare) ... 2655
▲ Synarel Nasal Solution for Endometriosis (Most frequent) ... 3205

Hypofibrinogenemia
Depacon Injection ... 416
Depakene ... 421
Depakote Sprinkle Capsules ... 426
Depakote Tablets ... 430
Depakote ER Tablets ... 436
Elspar for Injection ... 2092
Lamictal (Rare) ... 1567
NovoSeven (Greater than or equal to 2%) ... 2430
Oncaspar ... 756
Panhematin for Injection ... 497
Pediazole Suspension ... 3050

Hypogeusia
Cuprimine Capsules (Some patients) ... 2075
Depen Titratable Tablets (Some patients) ... 3341

Hypoglycemia
Abelcet Injection ... 1273
Actiq (Less than 1%) ... 1184
Actos Tablets (2%) ... 3275
Aggrenox Capsules ... 1026
Amaryl Tablets (0.9% to 1.7%) ... 717
Amphotec (1% to 5%) ... 1774
Anaprox Tablets (Less than 1%) ... 2967
Anaprox DS Tablets (Less than 1%) ... 2967
Ancobon Capsules ... 1730
▲ Apligraf (6.3%) ... 2305
Arthrotec Tablets (Rare) ... 3195
Avandia Tablets (0.6% to 5.9%) ... 1490
Avonex ... 1013
Azulfidine EN-tabs Tablets (Rare) ... 2775
Bactrim (Rare) ... 2949
Betaseron for SC Injection ... 988
Biaxin/Biaxin XL (Rare) ... 403
Blocadren Tablets ... 2046
Cafcit ... 1035
Campath Ampules ... 992
Cataflam Tablets (Less than 1%) ... 2315
Celebrex Capsules (Less than 0.1%) ... 2676
Celebrex Capsules (Less than 0.1%) ... 2780
Celexa (Rare) ... 1365
▲ CellCept Capsules (3%) ... 2951
▲ CellCept Intravenous (3%) ... 2951
▲ CellCept Oral Suspension (3%) ... 2951
▲ CellCept Tablets (3% to 10 .5%) ... 2951
Cipro I.V. (Rare) ... 893
Cipro I.V. Pharmacy Bulk Package (Rare) ... 897
Cipro (Less than 0.1%) ... 887
Compazine ... 1505
Coreg Tablets (1% to 2%) ... 1508
Cosopt Sterile Ophthalmic Solution ... 2065
Cuprimine Capsules ... 2075
Depen Titratable Tablets (Extremely rare) ... 3341
D.H.E. 45 Injection ... 2334
DiaBeta Tablets ... 741
Diabinese Tablets ... 2680
Doxil Injection (Less than 1%) ... 566
EC-Naprosyn Delayed-Release Tablets (Less than 1%) ... 2967
Ecotrin Enteric Coated Aspirin Low, Regular and Maximum Strength Tablets ... 1715
Edecrin (In 2 uremic patients) ... 2091
Effexor Tablets (Infrequent) ... 3495
Effexor XR Capsules (Infrequent) ... 3499
Etrafon ... 3115
Evoxac Capsules (Less than 1%) ... 1217
Exelon Capsules (Infrequent) ... 2342
Exelon Oral Solution (Infrequent) ... 2345
Felbatol ... 3343
Feldene Capsules (Rare) ... 2685
Ferrlecit Injection (Greater than 1%) ... 3386
Flexeril Tablets (Rare) ... 572
Flexeril Tablets (Rare) ... 2094
Floxin I.V. (More than or equal to 1%) ... 2526
Floxin Tablets (More than or equal to 1%) ... 2529
Fortovase Capsules (Less than 2%) ... 2970
Gabitril Tablets (Infrequent) ... 1189
Gengraf Capsules (1% to less than 3%) ... 457
Geodon Capsules (Rare) ... 2688
Glucophage Tablets (1% to 5%) ... 1080
Glucotrol Tablets ... 2692
Glucotrol XL Extended Release Tablets (Less than 3%) ... 2693
Glucovance Tablets ... 1086
Haldol Decanoate ... 2535
Haldol Injection, Tablets and Concentrate ... 2533
Herceptin I.V. (At least one of the 958 patients) ... 1414
Hivid Tablets (Less than 1%) ... 2975
▲ Humalog (Most common) ... 1926
Humalog Mix 75/25 Pen ... 1928
Humulin 50/50, 100 Units ... 1934
Humulin 70/30, 100 Units ... 1935
Humulin 70/30 Pen ... 1936
Humulin L, 100 Units ... 1937
Humulin R Regular (U-500) ... 1943
Humulin N NPH Pen ... 1940
Iletin II, Regular (Pork), 100 Units ... 1947
Imitrex Nasal Spray ... 1554
Imitrex Tablets (Rare) ... 1558
Indocin I.V. (1% to 3%) ... 2115
Invirase Capsules (Up to 5%) ... 2979
Lantus Injection ... 742
Levaquin (2.1% to 2.3%) ... 2537
Limbitrol ... 1738
Lipitor Tablets (Less than 2%) ... 2639
Lipitor Tablets (Less than 2%) ... 2696
Lupron Injection (Less than 5%) ... 3279
Luvox Tablets (25, 50, 100 mg) (Rare) ... 3256
Mepron Suspension (1%) ... 1598
Meridia Capsules ... 481
Mithracin for Intravenous Use ... 903
Moban ... 1320

Motrin Suspension, Oral Drops, Chewable Tablets, and Caplets (Less than 1%) 2002
▲ Naprelan Tablets (3% to 9%) 1293
Naprosyn Suspension (Less than 1%) 2967
Naprosyn Tablets (Less than 1%) 2967
Navane Oral 2701
Navane Intramuscular 2703
Neoral Soft Gelatin Capsules (1% to less than 3%) 2380
Neoral Oral Solution (1% to less than 3%) 2380
Neurontin Capsules 2655
Neurontin Oral Solution 2655
Neurontin Tablets 2655
Normodyne Injection 3135
Normodyne Tablets 3137
Noroxin Tablets 2145
Norpramin Tablets 755
NovoLog Injection 2427
Omnicef (0.2%) 493
Oncaspar (Greater than 1% but less than 5%) 756
Paser Granules 1781
Paxil (Rare) 1609
Pediazole Suspension (Rare) 3050
Permax Tablets (Infrequent) 1299
▲ Prandin Tablets (0.5, 1, and 2 mg) (16% to 31%) 2432
Precose Tablets 906
Prevacid Delayed-Release Capsules (Less than 1%) 3292
PREVPAC (Less than 1%) 3298
Prilosec Delayed-Release Capsules (Less than 1%) 628
▲ Prograf (3% to 15%) 1393
Proleukin for Injection (2%) 1199
Protopic Ointment (Greater than or equal to 1%) 1397
Prozac Pulvules, Liquid, and Weekly Capsules (Infrequent) 1238
▲ Rapamune Oral Solution and Tablets (3% to 20%) 3584
Requip Tablets (Infrequent) 1621
Risperdal (Rare) 1796
Saizen for Injection (Infrequent) 3225
Salagen Tablets (Less than 1%) 2229
▲ Sandostatin Injection (3% to 16%) 2394
Sandostatin LAR Depot (2% to 4%) 2395
Sarafem Pulvules 1962
Septra Suspension (Rare) 2265
Septra Tablets (Rare) 2265
Septra DS Tablets (Rare) 2265
Seroquel Tablets (Infrequent) 684
Serzone Tablets (Rare) 1104
Sinequan 2713
Sonata Capsules (Rare) 3591
Starlix Tablets (2.4%) 2401
Stelazine 1640
Surmontil Capsules 3595
Tenoretic Tablets 690
Tenormin 692
Tequin Injection (Less than 0.1%) 1110
Tequin Tablets (Less than 0.1%) 1110
Thiothixene Capsules 2290
Thorazine 1656
Timolide Tablets 2187
Timolol GFS ⊙ 266
Timoptic-XE Sterile Ophthalmic Gel Forming Solution 2194
Topamax Sprinkle Capsules (Rare) 2590
Topamax Tablets (Rare) 2590
Trocator SC Tablets 3598
Tricor Capsules, Micronized 513
Trilafon 3160
Trileptal Oral Suspension 2407
Trileptal Tablets 2407
▲ Trisenox Injection (8%) 1158
Vantin Tablets and Oral Suspension 2860
Viagra Tablets (Less than 2%) 2732
Videx 1138
Videx EC Capsules 1143
Viracept 532
Vistide Injection 1445
Vivactil Tablets 2217
Vivactil Tablets 2446
Voltaren Tablets (Less than 1%) 2315
Voltaren-XR Tablets (Less than 1%) 2315
Wellbutrin Tablets 1680
Zoloft (Rare) 2751
Zonegran Capsules (Rare) 1307
Zosyn (1.0% or less) 1890
Zosyn in Galaxy Containers (1.0% or less) 1894
Zyprexa Tablets (Infrequent) 1973
Zyprexa ZYDIS Orally Disintegrating Tablets (Infrequent) 1973

Hypoglycemia, masked symptoms of

Betagan ⊙ 228
Betimol Ophthalmic Solution ⊙ 324
Timolol GFS ⊙ 266
Timoptic in Ocudose (Less frequent) 2192
Timoptic-XE Sterile Ophthalmic Gel Forming Solution 2194

Hypoglycemia, neonatal

Brethine Ampuls 2314
DiaBeta Tablets 741
Normodyne Injection 3135
Normodyne Tablets (Rare) 3137

Hypogonadism

Permax Tablets (Rare) 1299
Virazole for Inhalation Solution 1747

Hypogonadism, male

Kaletra Capsules (Less than 2%) 471
Kaletra Oral Solution (Less than 2%) 471

Hypohidrosis

Celexa (Rare) 1365
Donnatal 2929
Donnatal Extentabs 2930
Donnatal Tablets 2929
Levsin/Levsinex/Levbid 3172
Paxil (Rare) 1609
Risperdal (Infrequent) 1796
Robinul Forte Tablets 1358
Robinul Injectable 2940
Robinul Tablets 1358
Topamax Sprinkle Capsules (Infrequent) 2590
Topamax Tablets (Infrequent) 2590

Hypokalemia

▲ Abelcet Injection (5%) 1273
Aceon Tablets (2 mg, 4 mg, 8 mg) (0.3% to 1%) 3249
Aciphex Tablets 1267
Aciphex Tablets 1783
Actiq (1% or greater) 1184
Aggrenox Capsules 1026
Aldoclor Tablets 2035
Aldoril Tablets 2039
Aloprim for Injection (Less than 1%) 2292
▲ AmBisome for Injection (37.6% to 43.2%) 1383
▲ Amphotec (7% to 26%) 1774
Ancobon Capsules 1730
▲ AndroGel (3% to 6%) 3322
Arava Tablets (1%) 724
▲ Aredia for Injection (4% to 18%) 2309
Aricept Tablets (Infrequent) 1270
Aricept Tablets (Infrequent) 2665
Atacand HCT Tablets (0.5% or greater) 597
Avalide Tablets 1070
Avonex 1013
Brethine Ampuls 2314
Campath Ampules 992
Cancidas for Injection (2.9%) 2048
Cardene I.V. (0.7%) 3485
Cardura Tablets (Less than 0.5%) 2668
Celebrex Capsules (0.1% to 1.9%) 2676
Celebrex Capsules (0.1% to 1.9%) 2780
Celestone Soluspan Injectable Suspension 3097
Celestone Syrup 3099
Celexa (Rare) 1365
▲ CellCept Capsules (10.0% to 31.8%) 2951
▲ CellCept Intravenous (10.0% to 31.8%) 2951
▲ CellCept Oral Suspension (10.0% to 31.8%) 2951
▲ CellCept Tablets (10.0% to 31.8%) 2951
Cerebyx Injection (Frequent) 2619
Cipro I.V. (Infrequent) 893
Clorpres Tablets 1002
Colazal Capsules 3069
Combipres Tablets 1040
Coreg Tablets (0.1% to 1%) 1508
Corlopam Injection (1% to 2%) 412
Cortifoam Rectal Foam 3170
Cortone Acetate Injectable Suspension 2059
Cortone Acetate Tablets 2061
Corzide 40/5 Tablets 2247
Corzide 80/5 Tablets 2247
▲ Cytovene (25%) 2959
Daranide Tablets 2077
Decadron Elixir 2078
Decadron Tablets 2079
Decadron Phosphate Injection 2081
Demadex Tablets and Injection 2965
Depo-Medrol Injectable Suspension 2795
Diflucan Tablets, Injection, and Oral Suspension 2681
Digibind Powder 1514
▲ Diovan HCT Tablets (4.5%) 2338
Diuril Sodium Intravenous 2086
Dobutrex Solution Vials (Rare) 1914
Doxil Injection (Less than 1%) 566
Dyazide Capsules (Uncommon) 1515
Dyrenium Capsules (Rare) 3458
Effexor Tablets (Infrequent) 3495
Effexor XR Capsules (Infrequent) 3499
Evoxac Capsules (Less than 1%) 1217
Exelon Capsules (Frequent) 2342
Exelon Oral Solution (Frequent) 2345
Felbatol (Infrequent) 3343
Ferrlecit Injection (Greater than 1%) 3386
Fleet Phospho-soda 1360
▲ Flolan for Injection (6%) 1528
Florinef Acetate Tablets 2250
Foradil Aerolizer 2354
▲ Foscavir Injection (5% to 16%) 605
Furosemide Tablets 2284
Gabitril Tablets (Infrequent) 1189
Geodon Capsules (Infrequent) 2688
▲ Gleevec Capsules (2% to 12%) 2357
Gliadel Wafer (1%) 1723
Hivid Tablets (Less than 1%) 2975
Humalog 1926
Humalog Mix 75/25 Pen 1928
Hydrocortone Tablets 2106
Hydrocortone Acetate Injectable Suspension 2103
Hydrocortone Phosphate Injection, Sterile 2105
HydroDIURIL Tablets 2108
▲ Hyzaar (6.7%) 2109
Imdur Tablets (Less than or equal to 5%) 1826
▲ Indapamide Tablets (3% to 7%) 2286
Invirase Capsules (Up to 1%) 2979
Kristalose for Oral Solution 1007
Lanoxicaps Capsules 1574
Levaquin Injection (Less than 0.5%) 2537
Lexxel Tablets (Infrequent) 608
Lodosyn Tablets 1251
Lotrel Capsules 2370
▲ Lupron Depot-3 Month 22.5 mg (More than or equal to 5%) 3288
Luvox Tablets (25, 50, 100 mg) (Rare) 3256
Maxzide 1008
Micardis HCT Tablets (Less than 2%) 1051
Microzide Capsules 3414
Mithracin for Intravenous Use 903
Mykrox Tablets 1168
▲ Mylotarg for Injection (24% to 44%) 3540
Naprelan Tablets (Less than 1%) 1293
Naropin Injection (Less than 1%) 612
Nebcin Vials, Hyporets & ADD-Vantage 1955
▲ Novantrone for Injection (7%) 1760
NovoLog Injection 2427
▲ Paraplatin for Injection (16% to 28%) 1126
Paxil (Rare) 1609
Pediapred Oral Solution 1170
Permax Tablets (Infrequent) 1299
Pipracil (Rare with high doses) 1866
Prednisone 3064
Prelone Syrup 2273
Primacor Injection (0.6%) 3086
Prinzide Tablets 2168
▲ Prograf (13% to 29%) 1393
▲ Proleukin for Injection (9%) 1199
Proventil HFA Inhalation Aerosol (Some patients) 3150
Prozac Pulvules, Liquid, and Weekly Capsules (Infrequent) 1238
▲ Rapamune Oral Solution and Tablets (11% to 21%) 3584
Relafen Tablets (Less than 1%) 1617
Renese Tablets 2712
Requip Tablets (Infrequent) 1621
Rilutek Tablets (Infrequent) 772
Risperdal (Rare) 1796
Sandostatin LAR Depot (1% to 4%) 2395
Sarafem Pulvules (Infrequent) 1962
Septra Suspension 2265
Septra Tablets 2265
Septra DS Tablets 2265
Seroquel Tablets (Rare) 684
▲ Serostim for Injection (1% to 10%) 3229
▲ Simulect for Injection (Greater than or equal to 10%) 2399
Sinemet Tablets 1253
Sinemet CR Tablets 1255
Solu-Medrol Sterile Powder 2855
Sporanox Capsules (2.0%) 1800
▲ Sporanox Injection (5%) 1804
▲ Sporanox Injection (5%) 2509
Sporanox Oral Solution 1808
Sporanox Oral Solution 2512
Sular Tablets (Less than or equal to 1%) 688
Tenoretic Tablets 690
Teveten Tablets (Less than 1%) 3327
Timentin Injection- ADD-Vantage Vial (Rare) 1661
Timentin Injection-Galaxy Container 1664
Timentin Injection-Pharmacy Bulk Package (Rare) 1666
Timentin for Intravenous Administration (Rare) 1658
Timolide Tablets 2187
Topamax Sprinkle Capsules (Infrequent) 2590
Topamax Tablets (Infrequent) 2590
Trasylol Injection (1% to 2%) 909
Trileptal Oral Suspension 2407
Trileptal Tablets 2407
▲ Trisenox Injection (50%) 1158
Uniretic Tablets (More than 1%) 3178
Vaseretic Tablets 2204
Ventolin Inhalation Aerosol and Refill 1679
Vistide Injection 1445
Zanaflex Tablets (Rare) 1305
Zaroxolyn Tablets 1177
Zestoretic Tablets 695
Ziac Tablets 1887
Zofran Injection (Rare) 1698
Zofran (Rare) 1703
Zofran ODT Orally Disintegrating Tablets (Rare) 1703
▲ Zometa for Intravenous Infusion (11.6%) 3621
Zosyn 1890
Zosyn in Galaxy Containers 1894
Zovirax for Injection (Less than 1%) 1708
Zyprexa Tablets (Infrequent) 1973
Zyprexa ZYDIS Orally Disintegrating Tablets (Infrequent) 1973

Hypokalemic alkalosis

Celestone Soluspan Injectable Suspension 3097
Celestone Syrup 3099
Cortone Acetate Injectable Suspension 2059
Cortone Acetate Tablets 2061
Decadron Elixir 2078
Decadron Tablets 2079
Decadron Phosphate Injection 2081
Depo-Medrol Injectable Suspension 2795
Florinef Acetate Tablets 2250
Hydrocortone Tablets 2106
Hydrocortone Acetate Injectable Suspension 2103
Hydrocortone Phosphate Injection, Sterile 2105
Pediapred Oral Solution 1170
Prednisone 3064
Prelone Syrup 2273
Solu-Medrol Sterile Powder 2855

Hypokinesia

Actiq (1% or greater) 1184
Ambien Tablets (Rare) 3191
Aricept Tablets (Infrequent) 1270
Aricept Tablets (Infrequent) 2665
Celexa (Infrequent) 1365
Cerebyx Injection (Infrequent) 2619
Chirocaine Injection (Less than 1%) 2909
▲ Clozaril Tablets (4%) 2319
▲ Comtan Tablets (9%) 2328
Copaxone for Injection (Infrequent) 3306
Coreg Tablets (0.1% to 1%) 1508
Depacon Injection (1% or more) 416
Depakene (1% or more) 421
Depakote Sprinkle Capsules 426
Depakote Tablets (1% to 5%) 430
Depakote ER Tablets (Greater than 1%) 436
Doxil Injection (Less than 1%) 566
Effexor Tablets (Rare) 3495
Effexor XR Capsules (Rare) 3499
Exelon Capsules (Infrequent) 2342
Exelon Oral Solution (Infrequent) 2345
Gabitril Tablets (Frequent) 1189
Geodon Capsules (Frequent) 2688
Hivid Tablets (Less than 1%) 2975
Intron A for Injection (Less than 5%) 3120
Ismo Tablets (Fewer than 1%) 3524
Lamictal (Rare) 1567
Levo-Dromoran 1734
Levorphanol Tartrate Tablets (Less than 1%) 3059
Luvox Tablets (25, 50, 100 mg) (Frequent) 3256
Mirapex Tablets (1% or more) 2834
Naropin Injection (Less than 1%) 612
Neurontin Capsules (Rare) 2655
Neurontin Oral Solution (Rare) 2655
Neurontin Tablets (Rare) 2655
Paxil (Rare) 1609
Permax Tablets (Infrequent) 1299
▲ ProSom Tablets (8%) 500
Protonix I.V. 3580
Remeron Tablets (Frequent) 2483
Remeron SolTab Tablets (Frequent) 2486
Reminyl Oral Solution (Infrequent) 1792
Reminyl Tablets (Infrequent) 1792
Rilutek Tablets (Infrequent) 772
▲ Risperdal (17% to 34%) 1796
Sonata Capsules (Rare) 3591
Symmetrel 1328
Tasmar Tablets (1% to 3%) 3010
Tenex Tablets (3% or less) 2942
Topamax Sprinkle Capsules (Frequent) 2590
Topamax Tablets (Frequent) 2590
Trileptal Oral Suspension 2407
Trileptal Tablets 2407
Trovan (Less than 1%) 2722
Uniretic Tablets (Less than 1%) 3178

Wellbutrin SR Sustained-Release Tablets 1684
Zoloft (Infrequent) 2751
Zonegran Capsules (Rare) 1307
Zyban Sustained-Release Tablets 1710
▲ Zyprexa Tablets (8% to 20%) 1973
▲ Zyprexa ZYDIS Orally Disintegrating Tablets (8% to 20%) 1973

Hypomagnesemia
Abelcet Injection 1273
Actiq (1% or greater) 1184
Aloprim for Injection (Less than 1%) 2292
▲ AmBisome for Injection (15.3% to 25.9%) 1383
▲ Amphotec (4% to 7%) 1774
▲ Aredia for Injection (3.8% to at least 15%) 2309
Avalide Tablets 1070
Avonex 1013
▲ CellCept Capsules (18.3%) 2951
▲ CellCept Intravenous (18.3%) 2951
▲ CellCept Oral Suspension (18.3%) 2951
▲ CellCept Tablets (18.3% to 39%) 2951
Corzide 40/5 Tablets 2247
Corzide 80/5 Tablets 2247
Demadex Tablets and Injection (One case) 2965
Diovan HCT Tablets 2338
Diucardin Tablets 3494
Diuril Sodium Intravenous 2086
Doxil Injection (Less than 1%) 566
Felbatol 3343
▲ Foscavir Injection (5% to 15%) 605
Furosemide Tablets 2284
Gengraf Capsules 457
Geodon Capsules (Rare) 2688
Herceptin I.V. (At least one of the 958 patients) 1414
Hivid Tablets (Less than 1%) 2975
HydroDIURIL Tablets 2108
Hyzaar 2109
Lanoxicaps Capsules 1574
▲ Leukine (15%) 1755
Maxzide 1008
Micardis HCT Tablets 1051
Mykrox Tablets 1168
▲ Mylotarg for Injection (3% to 14%) 3540
Naropin Injection (Less than 1%) 612
Nebcin Vials, Hyporets & ADD-Vantage 1955
▲ Neoral Soft Gelatin Capsules (6%) 2380
▲ Neoral Oral Solution (6%) 2380
▲ Paraplatin for Injection (29% to 63%) 1126
Prinzide Tablets 2168
▲ Prograf (16% to 48%) 1393
▲ Proleukin for Injection (12%) 1199
▲ Rapamune Oral Solution and Tablets (3% to 20%) 3584
Sandimmune (In some patients) 2388
▲ Simulect for Injection (3% to 10%) 2399
Sporanox Injection (1%) 1804
Sporanox Injection (1%) 2509
Thalomid Capsules 1154
▲ Trisenox Injection (45%) 1158
Uniretic Tablets 3178
Vaseretic Tablets 2204
Vistide Injection 1445
Zaroxolyn Tablets 1177
Zestoretic Tablets 695
▲ Zometa for Intravenous Infusion (10.5%) 3621

Hypomania
Celexa 1365
Effexor Tablets (0.5%) 3495
Effexor XR Capsules (0.3%) 3499
Lamictal (Rare) 1567
Limbitrol 1738
Luvox Tablets (25, 50, 100 mg) (Approximately 1%) 3256
▲ Nardil Tablets (Most common) 2653
Norpramin Tablets 755
Paxil (Approximately 1.0%) 1609
Prozac Pulvules, Liquid, and Weekly Capsules (0.1% to 0.8%) 1238
Remeron Tablets (Approximately 0.2%) 2483
Remeron SolTab Tablets (Approximately 0.2%) 2486
Sarafem Pulvules 1962
Serzone Tablets (0.3% to 1.6%) 1104
Surmontil Capsules 3595
Vivactil Tablets 2217
Vivactil Tablets 2446
Wellbutrin Tablets (Frequent) 1680
Wellbutrin SR Sustained-Release Tablets (Rare) 1684
Xanax Tablets 2865
Zoloft (Approximately 0.4%) 2751
Zyban Sustained-Release Tablets (Rare) 1710

Hypomenorrhea
Aquasol A Parenteral 593
Effexor Tablets (Rare) 3495
Effexor XR Capsules (Rare) 3499
Pentasa Capsules (Less than 1%) 3239
Prozac Pulvules, Liquid, and Weekly Capsules (Rare) 1238
Sarafem Pulvules (Rare) 1962

Hyponatremia
Aceon Tablets (2 mg, 4 mg, 8 mg) 3249
Aciphex Tablets 1267
Aciphex Tablets 1783
Actimmune (Rare) 1772
Actiq (Less than 1%) 1184
Aloprim for Injection (Less than 1%) 2292
Altace Capsules 2233
Amaryl Tablets 717
AmBisome for Injection (Less common) 1383
Amphotec (1% to 5%) 1774
Aricept Tablets 1270
Aricept Tablets 2665
Arthrotec Tablets (Rare) 3195
Campath Ampules 992
Captopril Tablets 2281
Carbatrol Capsules 3234
Celexa (Several cases) 1365
▲ CellCept Capsules (11.4%) 2951
▲ CellCept Intravenous (11.4%) 2951
▲ CellCept Oral Suspension (11.4%) 2951
▲ CellCept Tablets (11.4%) 2951
Clozaril Tablets 2319
Coreg Tablets (1% to 2%) 1508
Cytovene 2959
DDAVP Injection 4 mcg/mL 737
DDAVP Nasal Spray 738
DDAVP Rhinal Tube 738
DDAVP Tablets 739
Demadex Tablets and Injection 2965
Depacon Injection 416
Depakene 421
Depakote Sprinkle Capsules 426
Depakote Tablets 430
Depakote ER Tablets 436
Desmopressin Acetate Injection 1344
DiaBeta Tablets 741
Diuril Sodium Intravenous 2086
Doxil Injection (Less than 1%) 566
Dyazide Capsules 1515
Effexor Tablets (Rare) 3495
Effexor XR Capsules 3499
Enalaprilat Injection 863
Evoxac Capsules (Less than 1%) 1217
Exelon Capsules (Infrequent) 2342
Exelon Oral Solution (Infrequent) 2345
Felbatol (Infrequent) 3343
Foscavir Injection (Between 1% and 5%) 605
Furosemide Tablets 2284
Gabitril Tablets (Infrequent) 1189
Geodon Capsules (Rare) 2688
▲ Gliadel Wafer (3% to 9%) 1723
Glucotrol Tablets 2692
Glucotrol XL Extended Release Tablets 2693
Haldol Decanoate 2535
Haldol Injection, Tablets and Concentrate 2533
Herceptin I.V. (At least one of the 958 patients) 1414
Hivid Tablets (Less than 1%) 2975
Hyzaar 2109
Indapamide Tablets (Less than 5%) 2286
▲ Indocin I.V. (3% to 9%) 2115
Invirase Capsules (Up to less than 1%) 2979
Kadian Capsules (Less than 3%) 1335
Lotensin HCT Tablets 2367
Luvox Tablets (25, 50, 100 mg) 3256
Mavik Tablets (0.3% to 1.0%) 478
Maxzide 1008
▲ Mepron Suspension (7% to 10%) 1598
Moduretic Tablets 2138
Monopril Tablets 1091
Mykrox Tablets 1168
Navelbine Injection 1604
Nebcin Vials, Hyporets & ADD-Vantage 1955
Neurontin Capsules 2655
Neurontin Oral Solution 2655
Neurontin Tablets 2655
Nexium Delayed-Release Capsules (Less than 1%) 619
Nimotop Capsules (Less than 1%) 904
Nipent for Injection (Less than 3%) 3272
▲ Novantrone for Injection (9%) 1760
Oncaspar (Less than 1%) 756
Orap Tablets 1407
Orudis Capsules (Less than 1%) 3548
Oruvail Capsules (Less than 1%) 3548
OxyContin Tablets (Less than 1%) 2912
▲ Paraplatin for Injection (10% to 47%) 1126
Paxil (Rare) 1609
Prilosec Delayed-Release Capsules (Less than 1%) 628
Primaxin I.M. 2158
Primaxin I.V. 2160
Prinivil Tablets 2164
Prinzide Tablets 2168
▲ Prograf (3% to 15%) 1393
▲ Proleukin for Injection (4%) 1199
Prozac Pulvules, Liquid, and Weekly Capsules (Several cases) 1238
▲ Rapamune Oral Solution and Tablets (3% to 20%) 3584
Requip Tablets (Infrequent) 1621
Rilutek Tablets (Infrequent) 772
Risperdal (Infrequent) 1796
Rythmol Tablets – 150 mg, 225 mg, 300 mg (Less than 1%) 502
Septra Suspension 2265
Septra Tablets 2265
Septra DS Tablets 2265
Stimate Nasal Spray 796
Tarka Tablets 508
Tegretol/Tegretol-XR 2404
Tenoretic Tablets 690
Teveten Tablets (Less than 1%) 3327
Ticlid Tablets (Rare) 3015
Topamax Sprinkle Capsules (Rare) 2590
Topamax Tablets (Rare) 2590
Toradol 3018
Trileptal Oral Suspension (2.5%) 2407
Trileptal Tablets (2.5%) 2407
Uniretic Tablets (Less than 1%) 3178
Vaseretic Tablets 2204
Vasotec I.V. Injection 2207
Vasotec Tablets 2210
Vistide Injection 1445
Zanaflex Tablets (Rare) 1305
Zaroxolyn Tablets 1177
Zestoretic Tablets 695
Zestril Tablets 698
Zoloft (Several cases) 2751
Zonegran Capsules (Rare) 1307
Zosyn 1890
Zosyn in Galaxy Containers 1894
Zyprexa Tablets (Infrequent) 1973
Zyprexa ZYDIS Orally Disintegrating Tablets (Infrequent) 1973

Hyponatremia, dilutional
Diuril Sodium Intravenous 2086
Hyzaar 2109
Maxzide 1008
Prinzide Tablets 2168
Tenoretic Tablets 690
Vaseretic Tablets 2204
Zestoretic Tablets 695

Hypoparathyroidism
▲ Rocaltrol (1 in 3) 2991

Hypophosphatemia
Abelcet Injection 1273
Actonel Tablets (2.7%) 2879
AmBisome for Injection (Less common) 1383
▲ Amphotec (5% or more) 1774
▲ Aredia for Injection (Up to 18%) 2309
Cardene I.V. (Rare) 3485
▲ CellCept Capsules (12.5% to 15.8%) 2951
▲ CellCept Intravenous (12.5% to 15.8%) 2951
▲ CellCept Oral Suspension (12.5% to 15.8%) 2951
▲ CellCept Tablets (12.5% to 15.8%) 2951
Cerebyx Injection (Frequent) 2619
Doxil Injection (Less than 1%) 566
Effexor Tablets (Rare) 3495
Evista Tablets 1915
▲ Felbatol (3.4%) 3343
▲ Fosamax Tablets (Approximately 10%) 2095
▲ Foscavir Injection (5% to 8%) 605
Hivid Tablets (Less than 1%) 2975
Maalox Antacid/Anti-Gas Oral Suspension ▣673
Maalox Max Maximum Strength Antacid/Anti-Gas Liquid 2300
Maalox Regular Strength Antacid/Antigas Liquid 2300
Maxzide 1008
Mithracin for Intravenous Use 903
Mykrox Tablets 1168
Mylanta 1813
Niaspan Extended-Release Tablets 1846
▲ Prograf (3% to 49%) 1393
▲ Proleukin for Injection (11%) 1199
▲ Rapamune Oral Solution and Tablets (15% to 23%) 3584
Rescriptor Tablets (Less than 2%) 526
▲ Roferon-A Injection (22%) 2996
▲ Simulect for Injection (Greater than or equal to 10%) 2399
Tenoretic Tablets 690
Topamax Sprinkle Capsules (Rare) 2590
Topamax Tablets (Rare) 2590
Vistide Injection 1445
Zaroxolyn Tablets 1177
▲ Zometa for Intravenous Infusion (12.8%) 3621

Hypopigmentation
Accutane Capsules 2944
Aclovate (Infrequent) 1275
Aldara Cream, 5% (More than 1%) 1978
Analpram-HC 1338
Anusol-HC Cream 2.5% (Infrequent to frequent) 2237
Anusol-HC Suppositories 2238
Avita Cream 999
Avita Gel 1000
Capex Shampoo 1400
Catapres-TTS (0.5% or less) 1038
Celestone Soluspan Injectable Suspension 3097
Clobevate Gel 3271
Cordran Lotion (Infrequent) 2438
Cordran Tape (Infrequent) 2439
Cormax Cream (Infrequent) 2440
Cormax Ointment (Infrequent) 2440
Cormax Scalp Application (Infrequent) 2441
Cortone Acetate Injectable Suspension 2059
Cutivate Cream (Infrequent) 1282
Cutivate Ointment (Infrequent to more frequent) 1284
Decadron Phosphate Injection 2081
Dermatop Emollient Cream (Infrequent to frequent) 2517
DesOwen (Infrequent) 1401
Diprolene Gel 0.05% (Infrequent) 3107
Diprolene Lotion 0.05% (Infrequent) 3107
Diprolene Ointment 0.05% (Infrequent) 3108
Diprolene AF Cream 0.05% (Infrequent) 3106
Diprosone 3109
8-MOP Capsules 1727
Elocon Cream 0.1% (Infrequent) 3110
Elocon Lotion 0.1% (Infrequent) 3111
Elocon Ointment 0.1% (Infrequent) 3112
Hydrocortone Acetate Injectable Suspension 2103
Hydrocortone Phosphate Injection, Sterile 2105
▲ Levulan Kerastick (20% to 36%) 971
Lidex (Infrequent) 2020
Locoid Cream (Infrequent) 1341
Locoid Lipocream Cream (Infrequent) 1342
Locoid (Infrequent) 1341
Lotrisone 3129
Luxiq Foam 1210
Olux Foam 1211
Oxsoralen-Ultra Capsules 1741
Pramosone 1343
Proctocort Suppositories 2264
ProctoFoam-HC 3177
Psorcon E Cream 1227
Psorcon E Ointment 1228
Rescula Ophthalmic Solution (Less than 1%) ⊙306
Retin-A Micro 0.1% 2522
Solu-Medrol Sterile Powder 2855
Synalar (Infrequent) 2020
Taxotere for Injection Concentrate 778
Temovate Cream 1301
Temovate Gel (Infrequent) 1303
Temovate Ointment 1301
Temovate Scalp Application (Infrequent) 1304
Temovate E Emollient (Infrequent) 1302
Topicort (Infrequent) 2025
Ultravate Cream 1119
Ultravate Ointment 1120

Hypoplasia, enamel
Declomycin Tablets 1855
Doryx Coated Pellet Filled Capsules 3357
Dynacin Capsules 2019
Minocin Intravenous 1862
Minocin Oral Suspension 1865
Minocin Pellet-Filled Capsules 1863
Monodox Capsules 2442
Vibramycin Calcium Oral Suspension Syrup 2735
Vibramycin Hyclate Capsules 2735
Vibramycin Hyclate Intravenous 2737
Vibramycin Monohydrate for Oral Suspension 2735
Vibra-Tabs Film Coated Tablets 2735

Hypoplasia, erythroid
Captopril Tablets 2281

Hypoplasia, myeloid
(*see under* Bone marrow hypoplasia)

Hypoplastic anemia
(*see under* Anemia, hypoplastic)

Hypopnea
Stadol NS Nasal Spray (Less than 1%) 1108
Vicoprofen Tablets (Less than 1%) 520

Hypoproteinemia
Actiq (Less than 1%) 1184
AmBisome for Injection (Less common) 1383
Amphotec (1% to 5%) 1774
▲ CellCept Capsules (3%) 2951

▲ CellCept Intravenous (3%) 2951
▲ CellCept Oral Suspension (3%) 2951
▲ CellCept Tablets (3%) 2951
Cipro I.V. 893
Cipro I.V. Pharmacy Bulk Package (Less than 1%)........................... 897
Colazal Capsules.......................... 3069
Cortifoam Rectal Foam.................. 3170
Depakote ER Tablets (Greater than 1%)...................................... 436
Doxil Injection (Less than 1%).......... 566
Effexor Tablets (Rare)...................... 3495
Effexor XR Capsules (Rare).............. 3499
Evista Tablets................................ 1915
Foscavir Injection (Less than 1%).... 605
Geodon Capsules (Rare)................. 2688
Lupron Depot 7.5 mg (Greater than or equal to 5%).................... 3284
Lupron Injection.............................. 3279
Oncaspar (Greater than 1% but less than 5%)........................... 756
▲ Prograf (3% to 15%) 1393
▲ Proleukin for Injection (7%) 1199
Risperdal (Rare) 1796
Sandostatin LAR Depot (1% to 4%) 2395
▲ Simulect for Injection (3% to 10%) . 2399
Thalomid Capsules 1154
Unasyn for Injection 2728
Uniretic Tablets (Less than 1%) 3178
Vantin Tablets and Oral Suspension 2860
Vistide Injection 1445
Zanaflex Tablets (Rare) 1305
Zosyn 1890
Zosyn in Galaxy Containers 1894
Zyprexa Tablets (Rare) 1973
Zyprexa ZYDIS Orally Disintegrating Tablets (Rare) 1973

Hypoprothrombinemia

AmBisome for Injection (Less common) 1383
Azulfidine EN-tabs Tablets (Rare) 2775
Bactrim 2949
Cipro I.V. (Rare) 893
Colazal Capsules 3069
Coreg Tablets (1% to 2%) 1508
Felbatol 3343
Limbitrol (Rare) 1738
Merrem I.V. (Greater than 0.2%) 673
Mithracin for Intravenous Use 903
NovoSeven (1%) 2430
Paser Granules 1781
Pediazole Suspension 3050
▲ Prograf (3% to 15%) 1393
Rocephin Injectable Vials, ADD-Vantage, Galaxy, Bulk (Rare) 2993
Septra Suspension 2265
Septra Tablets 2265
Septra DS Tablets 2265
Tapazole Tablets 1823
Trovan (Less than 1%) 2722

Hypoptyalism

Amerge Tablets (Frequent) 1467
Demser Capsules 2085
Imitrex Injection 1549
Imitrex Nasal Spray 1554
▲ Infergen (4% to 6%) 1777
Risperdal (Frequent) 1796
Vantin Tablets and Oral Suspension (Less than 1%) 2860
▲ Xanax Tablets (32.8%) 2865

Hypopyon

Healon (Rare) .... ⊙ 316
Healon 5 (Rare) .... ⊙ 317
Healon GV (Rare) .... ⊙ 320
Ocucoat (Rare) .... ⊙ 330

Hyporeflexia

Axert Tablets (Rare) 2772
Betaseron for SC Injection 988
Cerebyx Injection (2.8%) 2619
Cognex Capsules (Infrequent) 1351
Compazine 1505
Effexor Tablets (Rare) 3495
Evoxac Capsules (1% to 3%) 1217
Fortovase Capsules (Less than 2%) 2970
Gabitril Tablets (Frequent) 1189
Invirase Capsules (Less than 2%) 2979
Luvox Tablets (25, 50, 100 mg) (Rare) 3256
Matulane Capsules 3246
Maxalt Tablets (Rare) 2120
Maxalt-MLT Orally Disintegrating Tablets (Rare) 2120
Navelbine Injection (Less than 5%) .. 1604
Neurontin Capsules (Frequent) 2655
Neurontin Oral Solution (Frequent) .. 2655
Neurontin Tablets (Frequent) 2655
Paxil (Rare) 1609
ProSom Tablets (Rare) 500
Protonix I.V. (Less than 1%) 3580
Protonix Tablets (Less than 1%) 3577
Prozac Pulvules, Liquid, and Weekly Capsules (Rare) 1238
▲ Retrovir Capsules (5.6%) 1625
▲ Retrovir IV Infusion (7%) 1629
▲ Retrovir (5.6%) 1625
▲ Risperdal (17% to 34%) 1796
Sarafem Pulvules (Rare).................. 1962
Sonata Capsules (Rare).................. 3591
Stelazine Tablets............................ 1640
Thalomid Capsules......................... 1154
Thiothixene Capsules 2290
Thorazine....................................... 1656
Topamax Sprinkle Capsules (Infrequent)................................. 2590
Topamax Tablets (Infrequent).......... 2590
Trileptal Oral Suspension................ 2407
Trileptal Tablets.............................. 2407
▲ Vesanoid Capsules (3%) 3037
Viagra Tablets (Less than 2%).......... 2732
Xanax Tablets (2.7%)...................... 2865
Zoloft (Rare).................................... 2751

Hyporeflexia, neonatal

Compazine..................................... 1505
Stelazine Injection 1640
Thorazine....................................... 1656

Hyporesponsive episode, unspecified

Diphtheria & Tetanus Toxoids Adsorbed Purogenated for Pediatric Use............................... 1857
HibTITER (One case)....................... 1859
Tetanus & Diphtheria Toxoids Adsorbed for Adult Use.............. 1880

Hyposalivation

(*see under* Hypoptyalism)

Hypospadias

Depo-Provera Contraceptive Injection (5 to 8 per 1,000 male births)............................... 2798
Megace Oral Suspension.................. 1124
Provera Tablets............................... 2853
Topamax Sprinkle Capsules............ 2590
Topamax Tablets............................. 2590

Hyposthenuria

Floxin I.V. (More than or equal to 1%)... 2526
Floxin Tablets (More than or equal to 1%)...................................... 2529

Hypotaxia

▲ Vesanoid Capsules (3%) 3037

Hypotension

▲ Abelcet Injection (8%) 1273
Accupril Tablets (2.9%)................... 2611
Acel-Imune (Rare)........................... 1851
Aceon Tablets (2 mg, 4 mg, 8 mg) (0.3% to 1%)...................... 3249
Acthrel for Injection........................ 3629
Actimmune (Rare)........................... 1772
Actiq (Less than 1%)....................... 1184
Activase I.V. 1410
Adalat CC Tablets (Less than 1.0%).. 877
Adenocard Injection (Less than 1%)... 1380
Adenoscan (2%).............................. 1381
Aggrenox Capsules (Less than 1%)... 1026
AK-Fluor Injection 10% and 25%.... ⊙ 202
Albumin (Human) 5% (Very rare)...... 838
Albumin (Human) 25% (Very rare).... 839
Albuminar-5, U.S.P.......................... 785
Albuminar-25, U.S.P. 786
Aldoclor Tablets.............................. 2035
Aldomet Tablets.............................. 2037
Aldoril Tablets................................. 2039
▲ Alferon N Injection (6%) 1770
Alkeran for Injection (In some patients).. 1465
Allegra-D Extended-Release Tablets... 714
Aloprim for Injection (Less than 1%)... 2292
▲ Altace Capsules (11%) 2233
Ambien Tablets (Rare)..................... 3191
▲ AmBisome for Injection (7.4% to 14.3%).. 1383
Amerge Tablets (Infrequent)............ 1467
Amicar Injection.............................. 3608
Amicar Syrup.................................. 3608
Amicar Tablets................................ 3608
▲ Amphotec (9% to 12%) 1774
Anectine Injection........................... 1476
Anzemet Injection (Infrequently)....... 719
▲ Anzemet Tablets (5.3%) 722
AquaMEPHYTON Injection............... 2042
Aquasol A Parenteral....................... 593
Aralen Tablets (Rare)....................... 3075
Aredia for Injection (Rare)................ 2309
▲ Argatroban Injection (7.2%) 1478
Aricept Tablets (Frequent)................ 1270
Aricept Tablets (Frequent)................ 2665
Arthrotec Tablets (Rare)................... 3195
Atacand HCT Tablets....................... 597
Ativan Injection (1.5% to 2.4%)........ 3478
Ativan Tablets (Rare)....................... 3482
Atrovent Inhalation Aerosol............. 1030
Autoplex T....................................... 2294
Avalide Tablets................................ 1070
Avapro Tablets (0.4%)..................... 1074
Avapro Tablets (0.4%)..................... 3076
Avelox Tablets (0.05% to 1%).......... 879
Avonex... 1013
Azactam for Injection (Less than 1%)... 1276
Benadryl Parenteral......................... 2617
Betagan.. ⊙ 228
▲ Betapace Tablets (3% to 6%) 950
Betapace AF Tablets....................... 954
Betaseron for SC Injection............... 988
Betaxon Ophthalmic Suspension (Less than 2%)............................ 537
Betimol Ophthalmic Solution.......... ⊙ 324
Bicillin C-R 900/300 Injection.......... 2240
Bicillin C-R Injection........................ 2238
Bicillin L-A Injection........................ 2242
▲ Blocadren Tablets (3%) 2046
▲ Brevibloc Injection (20% to 50%) 858
Brevital Sodium for Injection, USP... 1815
Buprenex Injectable (1% to 5%)....... 2918
Calcium Disodium Versenate Injection...................................... 1980
▲ Campath Ampules (5% to 32%) 992
Captopril Tablets (Rare) 2281
Carbatrol Capsules 3234
▲ Cardene I.V. (5.6%) 3485
Cardizem CD Capsules (Less than 1%) 1016
Cardura Tablets (1% to 1.7%) 2668
▲ Carnitor Injection (3% to 19%) 3242
Carteolol Hydrochloride Ophthalmic Solution USP, 1% ..... ⊙ 258
Cataflam Tablets (Rare) 2315
Caverject Sterile Powder (Less than 1%) 2777
Ceclor CD Tablets 1279
Ceclor 1905
Celexa (Frequent) 1365
▲ CellCept Capsules (3% to 32.5%) .. 2951
▲ CellCept Intravenous (3% to 32.5%) 2951
▲ CellCept Oral Suspension (3% to 32.5%) 2951
▲ CellCept Tablets (3% to 32.5%) 2951
Ceptaz for Injection (Very rare) 1499
▲ Cerebyx Injection (7.7%) 2619
▲ Cerezyme for Injection (Approximately 4%) 1438
▲ Chirocaine Injection (19.6%) 2909
Cipro I.V. (1% or less) 893
Cipro I.V. Pharmacy Bulk Package (Less than 1%) 897
Claritin (At least one patient) 3100
Claritin-D 12 Hour Extended Release Tablets (Less frequent) ... 3102
Cleocin Phosphate Sterile Solution (Rare) 2785
Clinoril Tablets (Less than 1 in 100) 2053
Clomid Tablets 735
▲ Clozaril Tablets (More than 5% to 9%) 2319
Cognex Capsules (Frequent) 1351
Combivent Inhalation Aerosol 1041
Compazine 1505
Comtan Tablets 2328
Comvax 2056
Concerta Extended-Release Tablets 1998
Concerta Tablets 561
Copaxone for Injection (Infrequent) 3306
▲ Cordarone Intravenous (15.6% to 16%) 3491
Cordarone Tablets (Less than 1%) .. 3487
▲ Coreg Tablets (8.5% to 9.7%) 1508
Corgard Tablets (1 of 100 patients) 2245
▲ Corlopam Injection (More than 5%) 412
Corvert Injection (2.0%) 2793
Cosopt Sterile Ophthalmic Solution (Less than 1%) 2065
Coumadin for Injection 1243
Coumadin Tablets 1243
Covera-HS Tablets (0.7% to 2.5%) .. 3199
Cozaar Tablets (Less than 1%) 2067
CytoGam Intravenous 2026
Cytotec Tablets (Infrequent) 3202
DDAVP Injection 4 mcg/mL (Infrequent) 737
DDAVP Nasal Spray (Infrequent) 738
DDAVP Rhinal Tube (Infrequent) 738
Demadex Tablets and Injection 2965
Demerol 3079
Depacon Injection (1% or more) 416
Depakene (1% or more) 421
Depakote Sprinkle Capsules 426
Depakote Tablets (1% to 5%) 430
Depakote ER Tablets (Greater than 1%) 436
Desferal Vials 2333
Desmopressin Acetate Injection (Infrequent) 1344
Dilaudid 441
Dilaudid Oral Liquid 445
Dilaudid Tablets - 8 mg 445
Dilaudid-HP (Less frequent) 443
Diovan HCT Tablets 2338
Diphtheria & Tetanus Toxoids Adsorbed Purogenated for Pediatric Use (Rare) 1857
Diprivan Injectable Emulsion (Rare) 667
Diuril Oral....................................... 2087
Diuril Sodium Intravenous............... 2086
Dobutrex Solution Vials (Occasional)................................ 1914
Dolophine Hydrochloride Tablets.... 3056
▲ Dostinex Tablets (1% to less than 10%)... 2804
▲ Doxil Injection (Approximately 6.8%)... 566
▲ Duraclon Injection (44.8% to 47%) . 3057
Duragesic Transdermal System (1% to 3%).................................. 1786
Duranest Injections......................... 600
Dyazide Capsules........................... 1515
DynaCirc Capsules (0.5% to 1%)..... 2921
DynaCirc CR Tablets (0.5% to 1%)... 2923
Ecotrin Enteric Coated Aspirin Low, Regular and Maximum Strength Tablets........................ 1715
Effexor Tablets (Infrequent)............. 3495
Effexor XR Capsules (Infrequent)..... 3499
8-MOP Capsules 1727
Eldepryl Capsules 3266
Emla (Unlikely with cream) 602
Enalaprilat Injection (Rare) 863
Enbrel for Injection (Infrequent) 1752
Enbrel for Injection (Infrequent) 3504
Engerix-B Vaccine (Less than 1%) ... 1517
Eskalith 1527
▲ Ethyol for Injection (62%) 2029
Etrafon (Occasional) 3115
Evoxac Capsules (Less than 1%) 1217
Exelon Capsules (Frequent) 2342
Exelon Oral Solution (Frequent) 2345
Felbatol 3343
Feldene Capsules (Rare) 2685
▲ Ferrlecit Injection (29%) 3386
Flexeril Tablets (Less than 1%) 572
Flexeril Tablets (Less than 1%) 2094
▲ Flolan for Injection (13% to 27%) 1528
Floxin I.V. (Less than 1%) 2526
Floxin Tablets (Less than 1%) 2529
Fluorescite Injection .... ⊙ 211
Fluothane Inhalation 3508
Foradil Aerolizer (Rare) 2354
Fortaz (Very rare) 1541
Fortovase Capsules (Less than 2%) 2970
Foscavir Injection (Between 1% and 5%) 605
Furosemide Tablets 2284
Gabitril Tablets (Infrequent) 1189
Gamimune N, 5% Solvent/Detergent Treated (Rare) 925
Gliadel Wafer (1%) 1723
GlucaGen for Injection Diagnostic Kit (Rare) 949
Glucagon for Injection Vials and Emergency Kit 1924
Glucophage Tablets 1080
Glucophage XR Tablets 1080
Glucovance Tablets 1086
Haldol Decanoate 2535
Haldol Injection, Tablets and Concentrate 2533
Herceptin I.V. (At least one of the 958 patients) 1414
Humalog (Less common) 1926
Humalog Mix 75/25 Pen (Less common) 1928
Humulin 50/50, 100 Units 1934
Humulin 70/30, 100 Units (Less common) 1935
Humulin 70/30 Pen (Less common) 1930
Humulin L, 100 Units (Less common) 1937
Humulin R Regular (U-500) (Less common) 1943
Humulin N NPH Pen (Less common) 1940
HydroDIURIL Tablets 2108
▲ Hytrin Capsules (0.6%; 21%) 464
Hyzaar 2109
Ifex for Injection (Less than 1%) 1123
Iletin II, Regular (Pork), 100 Units (Less common) 1947
Imdur Tablets (Less than or equal to 5%) 1826
Imitrex Injection (Infrequent) 1549
Imitrex Nasal Spray (Rare) 1554
Imitrex Tablets (Infrequent) 1558
Inderal 3513
Inderal LA Long-Acting Capsules 3516
Inderide Tablets 3517
Inderide LA Long-Acting Capsules ... 3519
Indocin Capsules (Less than 1%) 2112
Indocin I.V. (Less than 1%) 2115
Indocin (Less than 1%) 2112
INFeD Injection 3388
Innohep Injection (Greater than or equal to 1%) 1248
▲ Integrilin Injection (7%) 1213
▲ Integrilin Injection (7%) 1828
Intron A for Injection (Less than 5%) 3120
Invirase Capsules (Less than 2%) 2979
Ismo Tablets (Fewer than 1%) 3524
Isoptin SR Tablets (2.5%) 467

Isopto Carbachol Ophthalmic Solution ⊙215
Isordil Sublingual Tablets (Infrequent) 3525
Isordil Titradose Tablets (Infrequent) 3526
Iveegam EN (Two cases) 849
Kadian Capsules (Less than 3%) 1335
Kogenate 934
Kytril Injection (Rare) 2986
Kytril Tablets (Rare) 2988
▲ Leukine (13%) 1755
Levaquin (Less than 0.3%) 2537
Levo-Dromoran 1734
▲ Levorphanol Tartrate Tablets (3% to 9%) 3059
Lexxel Tablets 608
Librium for Injection (Isolated cases) 1737
Lidoderm Patch 1319
Limbitrol 1738
Lithium Carbonate 3061
Lithium Citrate Syrup 3061
Lithobid Slow-Release Tablets 3255
Lodine XL Extended-Release Tablets 3530
Lodosyn Tablets 1251
Lotensin HCT Tablets (0.6%) 2367
Lotrel Capsules (Rare) 2370
Loxitane Capsules 3398
Lufyllin Tablets 3347
Lufyllin-400 Tablets 3347
Lufyllin-GG Elixir 3348
Lufyllin-GG Tablets 3348
Lupron Depot 3.75 mg 3281
Lupron Depot 7.5 mg 3284
Lupron Depot–3 Month 11.25 mg 3285
Lupron Depot–3 Month 22.5 mg (Less than 5%) 3288
Lupron Depot–4 Month 30 mg 3289
Lupron Depot-PED 7.5 mg, 11.25 mg and 15 mg 3291
Lupron Injection 3279
Luvox Tablets (25, 50, 100 mg) (Frequent) 3256
Marinol Capsules (0.3 to 1%) 3325
Matulane Capsules 3246
▲ Mavik Tablets (0.3% to 11%) 478
Maxair Autohaler 1981
Maxair Inhaler (Less than 1%) 1984
Maxzide 1008
Mefoxin for Injection 2124
Mefoxin Premixed Intravenous Solution 2127
Mepergan Injection (Rare) 3539
Mephyton Tablets (Rare) 2129
Mepron Suspension (1%) 1598
Merrem I.V. (0.1% to 1.0%) 673
Metadate CD Capsules 1164
Metadate ER Tablets 1167
Methylin Tablets 1995
Methylin ER Tablets 1995
Mexitil Capsules (About 6 in 1,000) 1047
Microzide Capsules 3414
Migranal Nasal Spray (Rare) 2376
Minipress Capsules 2699
Mintezol 2137
Miochol-E System Pak (Rare) ⊙305
Miochol-E with Steri-Tags (Rare) ⊙305
Mirapex Tablets (Rare) 2834
Moban (Rare) 1320
Mobic Tablets (Less than 2%) 1054
Monopril Tablets (0.2% to 4.4%) 1091
Monopril HCT 1094
Motrin Suspension, Oral Drops, Chewable Tablets, and Caplets (Less than 1%) 2002
MS Contin Tablets (Less frequent) 2896
MSIR (Less frequent) 2898
▲ Mylotarg for Injection (4% to 28%) 3540
Nadolol Tablets (2 of 100 patients) 2288
Narcan Injection (Several instances) 1322
▲ Naropin Injection (More than 5% to 54.6%) 612
▲ Natrecor for Injection (11%) 3189
Navane Oral 2701
Navane Intramuscular 2703
Navelbine Injection 1604
Nembutal Sodium Solution (Less than 1%) 485
Nesacaine/Nesacaine MPF 617
Neupogen for Injection (7 of 176 patients) 587
Neurontin Capsules (Infrequent) 2655
Neurontin Oral Solution (Infrequent) 2655
Neurontin Tablets (Infrequent) 2655
Niaspan Extended-Release Tablets 1846
▲ Nimotop Capsules (1.2% to 50.0%) 904
▲ Nipent for Injection (3% to 10%) 3272
▲ Nitro-Dur Transdermal Infusion System (4%) 1834
▲ Nitro-Dur Transdermal Infusion System (4%) 3134
Nitrolingual Pumpspray 1355
Norcuron for Injection (Rare) 2478
Normodyne Injection (1%) 3135
Normodyne Tablets 3137
Norpramin Tablets 755
Norvasc Tablets (0.1% to 1%; rare) 2704
Norvir Capsules (Less than 2%) 487
Norvir Oral Solution (Less than 2%) 487
Novantrone for Injection (Occasional) 1760
Novolin 70/30 PenFill (Rare) 2423
Novolin 70/30 Prefilled Disposable Insulin Delivery System (Rare) 2425
Novolin N PenFill (Rare) 2423
Novolin R PenFill (Rare) 2423
NovoLog Injection 2427
NovoSeven (1%) 2430
Nubain Injection (1% or less) 1323
Numorphan 1324
Ocupress Ophthalmic Solution, 1% Sterile ⊙303
Ogen Tablets 2846
Oncaspar (Greater than 1% but less than 5%) 756
Oramorph SR Tablets (Less frequent) 3062
Orap Tablets 1407
Orthoclone OKT3 Sterile Solution 2498
Oxsoralen-Ultra Capsules 1741
OxyContin Tablets 2912
OxyFast Oral Concentrate Solution 2916
OxyIR Capsules 2916
Pacerone Tablets (Less than 1%) 3331
Paraplatin for Injection (Rare) 1126
Paxil (Infrequent) 1609
Periactin Tablets 2155
Permax Tablets (2.1%) 1299
Phenergan Injection 3553
Phenergan Suppositories 3556
Phenergan Syrup 3554
Phenergan Tablets 3556
Phenergan with Codeine Syrup 3557
Phenergan with Dextromethorphan Syrup 3559
Phenergan VC Syrup 3560
Phenergan VC with Codeine Syrup 3561
▲ Photofrin for Injection (7%) 831
Plasmanate 942
Plendil Extended-Release Tablets (0.5% to 1.5%) 623
Pletal Tablets (Less than 2%) 2605
Pletal Tablets (Less than 2%) 2848
Polocaine Injection, USP 625
Polocaine-MPF Injection, USP 625
Ponstel Capsules (Rare) 1356
Pravachol Tablets 1099
Prevacid Delayed-Release Capsules (Less than 1%) 3292
PREVPAC (Less than 1%) 3298
Primacor Injection (2.9%) 3086
Primaxin I.M. 2158
Primaxin I.V. (0.4%) 2160
Prinivil Tablets (0.3% to 4.4%; rare) 2164
Prinzide Tablets (1.4%) 2168
Procanbid Extended-Release Tablets (Rare) 2262
▲ Procardia Capsules (Approximately 5%) 2708
Procardia XL Extended Release Tablets (1% or less) 2710
▲ Prograf (3% to 15%) 1393
Prolastin (Rare) 943
▲ Proleukin for Injection (3% to 71%) 1199
Prometrium Capsules (100 mg, 200 mg) (Rare) 3261
Prostigmin Injectable 1744
Prostigmin Tablets 1744
Prostin E2 Suppositories 2852
Protonix I.V. (Less than 1%) 3580
Protonix Tablets (Less than 1%) 3577
Provigil Tablets (2%) 1193
Prozac Pulvules, Liquid, and Weekly Capsules (Infrequent) 1238
▲ Rapamune Oral Solution and Tablets (3% to 20%) 3584
Recombivax HB (Less than 1%) 2178
ReFacto Vials 1437
Reglan 2935
Remeron Tablets (Infrequent) 2483
Remeron SolTab Tablets (Infrequent) 2486
Remicade for IV Injection (Less than 2%) 1178
Reminyl Oral Solution (Infrequent) 1792
Reminyl Tablets (Infrequent) 1792
▲ Renagel Capsules (11%) 1439
▲ Renagel Tablets (11%) 1439
Renese Tablets 2712
▲ ReoPro Vials (21.1%) 1958
Requip Tablets (2%) 1621
Retavase Vials (One patient) 1182
Rifadin 765
Rifater Tablets 769
Rilutek Tablets (Infrequent) 772
Risperdal (Infrequent) 1796
▲ Rituxan for Infusion (1% to 10%) 1750
▲ Rituxan I.V. (1% to 10%) 1428
Robaxin Injectable 2938
Robaxin Tablets 2939
Robinul Injectable 2940
Roferon-A Injection (Less than 4% to less than 5%) 2996
Roxanol 3066
Roxicodone Tablets (Less than 3%) 3067
Rum-K 1363
Rynatan Tablets 3351
Rythmol Tablets – 150 mg, 225 mg, 300 mg (1.1%) 502
Salagen Tablets (Less than 1%) 2229
Sandoglobulin I.V. 2391
Sarafem Pulvules (Infrequent) 1962
Sectral Capsules (Up to 2%) 3589
Sensorcaine (Rare) 643
Sensorcaine-MPF Injection 643
▲ Serentil (One of the two most prevalent) 1057
▲ Serostim for Injection (1% to 10%) 3229
Serzone Tablets (2%) 1104
▲ Simulect for Injection (3% to 10%) 2399
Sinemet Tablets 1253
Sinemet CR Tablets 1255
Sinequan (Occasional) 2713
Solu-Medrol Sterile Powder 2855
Soma Tablets 3353
Soma Compound Tablets 3354
Soma Compound w/Codeine Tablets 3355
Sonata Capsules (Infrequent) 3591
Sporanox Injection (Less than 1%) 1804
Sporanox Injection (Less than 1%) 2509
Stadol NS Nasal Spray (Less than 1%) 1108
Stelazine 1640
▲ Streptase for Infusion (1% to 10%) 647
Sular Tablets (Less than or equal to 1%; very rare) 688
Surmontil Capsules 3595
Survanta Intratracheal Suspension (Less than 1%) 3053
Symmetrel 1328
Tagamet Injection (Rare) 1644
Talacen Caplets (Infrequent) 3089
Talwin Nx Tablets 3090
Tambocor Tablets (Less than 1%) 1990
Tarka Tablets (0.3% to 0.6%) 508
Tasmar Tablets (2%) 3010
▲ Taxol Injection (2% to 17%) 1129
Taxotere for Injection Concentrate (0.9% to 3.6%) 778
Tazicef for Injection (Very rare) 1647
Tazicef Galaxy Container (Very rare) 1650
Tazicef Pharmacy Bulk Package (Very rare) 1653
Tazidime Vials, Faspak & ADD-Vantage (Very rare) 1966
Tegretol/Tegretol-XR 2404
Tenoretic Tablets 690
▲ Tenormin (25%) 692
Tensilon Injectable 1745
Tetanus & Diphtheria Toxoids Adsorbed for Adult Use (Rare) 1880
Tetanus and Diphtheria Toxoids Adsorbed For Adult Use 815
Teveten Tablets (Less than 1%) 3327
Thalomid Capsules 1154
Theo-Dur Extended-Release Tablets 1835
Thioridazine Hydrochloride Tablets 2289
Thiothixene Capsules 2290
Thyrel TRH for Injection (A small number of patients) 3630
Tiazac Capsules (Less than 2%) 1378
Timolide Tablets (1.6%) 2187
Timolol GFS ⊙266
Timoptic in Ocudose (Less frequent) 2192
Timoptic Sterile Ophthalmic Solution (Less frequent) 2190
Timoptic-XE Sterile Ophthalmic Gel Forming Solution 2194
TNKase I.V. 1430
Tonocard Tablets (1.8% to 3.4%) 649
Topamax Sprinkle Capsules (Infrequent) 2590
Topamax Tablets (Infrequent) 2590
Toprol-XL Tablets (About 1 of 100 patients) 651
Toradol 3018
Tranxene 511
▲ Trasylol Injection (8%) 909
Travatan Ophthalmic Solution (1% to 5%) 543
Trental Tablets (Less than 1%) 784
Tricor Capsules, Micronized 513
Trilafon (Rare) 3160
Trileptal Oral Suspension (1% to 2%) 2407
Trileptal Tablets (1% to 2%) 2407
Triostat Injection (2%) 1825
Tripedia Vaccine (Rare) 817
▲ Trisenox Injection (25%) 1158
Trizivir Tablets 1669
Trovan (Less than 1%) 2722
Twinrix Vaccine (Less than 1%) 1674
TYPHIM Vi Vaccine 825
Ultracet Tablets (Less than 1%) 2597
Ultram Tablets (Infrequent) 2600
Uni-Dur Extended-Release Tablets 1841
Uniretic Tablets (More than 1%) 3178
Urecholine 2198
Urecholine Tablets 2445
Valium Injectable 3026
Valium Tablets (Infrequent) 3047
Vancocin HCl Capsules & Pulvules 1972
Vancocin HCl Oral Solution 1971
Vancocin HCl, Vials & ADD-Vantage (Infrequent) 1970
Vantin Tablets and Oral Suspension (Less than 1%) 2860
Vaseretic Tablets (Rare; 0.9%) 2204
Vasotec I.V. Injection (Rare) 2207
▲ Vasotec Tablets (0.5% to 6.7%) 2210
Velosulin BR Human Insulin 10 ml Vials 2435
▲ Venofer Injection (36%) 580
Verelan Capsules (2.5%) 3184
Verelan PM Capsules (2.5%) 3186
Versed Injection (2.7%) 3027
Versed Syrup (Less than 1%) 3033
▲ Vesanoid Capsules (14%; occasional) 3037
Vexol 1% Ophthalmic Suspension (Less than 2%) ⊙222
Viagra Tablets (Less than 2%) 2732
Vicoprofen Tablets (Less than 1%) 520
Virazole for Inhalation Solution 1747
Vistide Injection 1445
Vivactil Tablets 2217
Vivactil Tablets 2446
Voltaren Tablets (Rare) 2315
Voltaren-XR Tablets (Rare) 2315
Warfarin Sodium Tablets, USP 3302
Wellbutrin Tablets (2.5%) 1680
Wellbutrin SR Sustained-Release Tablets 1684
WinRho SDF 2297
▲ Xanax Tablets (4.7%) 2865
Xeloda Tablets (Less than 5%) 3039
Xopenex Inhalation Solution 3207
▲ Xylocaine Injections (3%) 653
▲ Zanaflex Tablets (16% to 33%) 1305
Zantac Injection 1688
Zaroxolyn Tablets 1177
Zebeta Tablets 1885
Zemuron Injection (0.1%; 2%) 2491
▲ Zenapax for Injection (Greater than 5%) 3046
Zestoretic Tablets (1.4%; rare) 695
▲ Zestril Tablets (Rare; 0.3% to 9.7%) 698
Ziac Tablets 1887
Ziagen 1692
Zofran Injection (Rare) 1698
▲ Zofran (5%) 1703
▲ Zofran ODT Orally Disintegrating Tablets (5%) 1703
Zoladex (Occasional) 702
Zoladex 3-month (Occasional) 706
Zoloft (Infrequent) 2751
▲ Zometa for Intravenous Infusion (10.5%) 3621
Zonegran Capsules (Infrequent) 1307
Zosyn (1.0% or less to 1.3%) 1890
Zosyn in Galaxy Containers (1.0% or less to 1.3%) 1894
Zovirax for Injection (Less than 1%) 1708
Zyban Sustained-Release Tablets 1710
Zyprexa Tablets (2%) 1973
Zyprexa ZYDIS Orally Disintegrating Tablets (2%) 1973
Zyrtec (Rare) 2756
Zyrtec-D 12 Hour Extended Relief Tablets (Rare) 2758

Hypotension, asymptomatic

▲ Brevibloc Injection (About 25%) 858
▲ Cardizem Injectable (4.3%) 1018
▲ Cardizem Lyo-Ject Syringe (4.3%) 1018
▲ Cardizem Monovial (4.3%) 1018
▲ Isoptin SR Tablets (5%) 467
▲ Natrecor for Injection (8%) 3189
▲ Verelan Capsules (5%) 3184

Hypotension, neonatal

Accupril Tablets 2611
Aceon Tablets (2 mg, 4 mg, 8 mg) 3249
Alphagan Ophthalmic Solution (Rare) 545
Altace Capsules 2233
Captopril Tablets 2281
Cozaar Tablets 2067
Enalaprilat Injection 863
Hyzaar 2109
Lexxel Tablets 608
Lotrel Capsules 2370
Monopril Tablets 1091
Normodyne Injection 3135
Normodyne Tablets (Rare) 3137
Prinivil Tablets 2164
Prinzide Tablets 2168
Sectral Capsules 3589
Univasc Tablets 3181
Vaseretic Tablets 2204
Vasotec I.V. Injection 2207
Vasotec Tablets 2210
Versed Injection 3027
Zestoretic Tablets 695

Zestril Tablets ... 698

Hypotension, orthostatic

Accupril Tablets (Rare) ... 2611
Accuretic Tablets (0.5% to 1%) ... 2614
Aceon Tablets (2 mg, 4 mg, 8 mg) (0.3% to 1%) ... 3249
Actiq (Less than 1%) ... 1184
Adalat CC Tablets (Less than 1.0%) ... 877
Agrylin Capsules (1% to 5%) ... 3232
Akineton ... 402
Aldoclor Tablets ... 2035
Aldomet Tablets ... 2037
Aldoril Tablets ... 2039
Altace Capsules (2%) ... 2233
Ambien Tablets (Infrequent) ... 3191
AmBisome for Injection (Less common) ... 1383
▲ Amphotec (5% or more) ... 1774
Anzemet Injection (Rare) ... 719
Anzemet Tablets (Rare) ... 722
Aricept Tablets (Infrequent) ... 1270
Aricept Tablets (Infrequent) ... 2665
Atacand HCT Tablets ... 597
Avalide Tablets ... 1070
Avapro Tablets (0.4%) ... 1074
Avapro Tablets (0.4%) ... 3076
Avonex ... 1013
Betaseron for SC Injection ... 988
Captopril Tablets ... 2281
Cardene I.V. (1.4%) ... 3485
▲ Cardura Tablets (Up to 23%) ... 2668
Catapres-TTS (0.5% or less) ... 1038
Celexa (Frequent) ... 1365
▲ CellCept Capsules (3%) ... 2951
▲ CellCept Intravenous (3%) ... 2951
▲ CellCept Oral Suspension (3%) ... 2951
▲ CellCept Tablets (3%) ... 2951
Cerebyx Injection (Infrequent) ... 2619
Chirocaine Injection (Less than 1%) ... 2909
Cipro I.V. ... 893
Cipro I.V. Pharmacy Bulk Package ... 897
Cipro ... 887
Claritin-D 24 Hour Extended Release Tablets (Fewer than 2%) ... 3104
▲ Clorpres Tablets (About 3 in 100) ... 1002
Clozaril Tablets ... 2319
▲ Combipres Tablets (About 3 in 100) ... 1040
Comtan Tablets ... 2328
Copaxone for Injection (Infrequent) ... 3306
▲ Coreg Tablets (Less than 1% to 9.7%) ... 1508
Corlopam Injection (2%) ... 412
Corvert Injection (2.0%) ... 2793
Corzide 40/5 Tablets ... 2247
Corzide 80/5 Tablets ... 2247
Covera-HS Tablets (0.4%) ... 3199
Depacon Injection (1% or more) ... 416
Depakene (1% or more) ... 421
Depakote Sprinkle Capsules ... 426
Depakote Tablets (1% to 5%) ... 430
Depakote ER Tablets (Greater than 1%) ... 436
Dibenzyline Capsules ... 3457
Dilaudid ... 441
Diovan HCT Tablets ... 2338
Dipentum Capsules (Rare) ... 2803
Diucardin Tablets ... 3494
Diuril Oral ... 2087
Diuril Sodium Intravenous ... 2086
▲ Dostinex Tablets (4%) ... 2804
Doxil Injection (Less than 1%) ... 566
▲ Duraclon Injection (31.6% to 47%) ... 3057
Dyazide Capsules ... 1515
Effexor Tablets (1%) ... 3495
Effexor XR Capsules (Frequent) ... 3499
Eldepryl Capsules ... 3266
Enalaprilat Injection ... 863
Etrafon ... 3115
Evoxac Capsules ... 1217
Exelon Capsules (Frequent) ... 2342
Exelon Oral Solution (Frequent) ... 2345
Flomax Capsules (0.2% to 0.4%) ... 1044
Furosemide Tablets ... 2284
Gabitril Tablets (Infrequent) ... 1189
Geodon Capsules (1%) ... 2688
Hycomine Compound Tablets ... 1317
Hycotuss Expectorant Syrup ... 1318
HydroDIURIL Tablets ... 2108
Hytrin Capsules ... 464
Indapamide Tablets (Less than 5%) ... 2286
Inderide Tablets ... 3517
Inderide LA Long-Acting Capsules ... 3519
Intron A for Injection (Less than 5%) ... 3120
Inversine Tablets ... 1850
Iopidine Sterile Ophthalmic Solution ... ⊙212
Ismo Tablets (Fewer than 1%) ... 3524
Isordil Titradose Tablets ... 3526
Kadian Capsules ... 1335
Klonopin Tablets (Infrequent) ... 2983
Lamictal (Infrequent) ... 1567
Levaquin (Less than 0.3%) ... 2537
Lexxel Tablets ... 608
Lipitor Tablets (Less than 2%) ... 2639
Lipitor Tablets (Less than 2%) ... 2696
Lodosyn Tablets ... 1251
Lotensin Tablets (0.4%) ... 2365
Lotensin HCT Tablets (0.3%) ... 2367
Loxitane Capsules ... 3398
Luvox Tablets (25, 50, 100 mg) ... 3256
Maxzide ... 1008
Micardis HCT Tablets (Less than 2%) ... 1051
Microzide Capsules ... 3414
Midamor Tablets (Less than or equal to 1%) ... 2136
Minipress Capsules (1% to 4%) ... 2699
Minizide Capsules ... 2700
Mirapex Tablets ... 2834
Moduretic Tablets (Less than or equal to 1%) ... 2138
Monopril Tablets (1.4% to 1.9%) ... 1091
Monopril HCT (1.8%) ... 1094
MS Contin Tablets ... 2896
Mykrox Tablets (Less than 2%) ... 1168
Nardil Tablets (Common) ... 2653
Naropin Injection (Less than 1%) ... 612
Niaspan Extended-Release Tablets ... 1846
Nitrolingual Pumpspray (Occasional) ... 1355
Nitrostat Tablets (Occasional) ... 2658
▲ Normodyne Injection (58%) ... 3135
Normodyne Tablets (1%) ... 3137
Noroxin Tablets ... 2145
Norvasc Tablets (More than 0.1% to 1%) ... 2704
Norvir Capsules (Less than 2%) ... 487
Norvir Oral Solution (Less than 2%) ... 487
Numorphan ... 1324
Orap Tablets ... 1407
OxyContin Tablets (Between 1% and 5%) ... 2912
Paxil (1.2%) ... 1609
▲ Permax Tablets (9.0%) ... 1299
Phenergan with Codeine Syrup ... 3557
Phenergan VC with Codeine Syrup ... 3561
Pletal Tablets (Less than 2%) ... 2605
Pletal Tablets (Less than 2%) ... 2848
Prinivil Tablets (0.3% to 1.2%) ... 2164
Prinzide Tablets (0.5% to 1.0%) ... 2168
▲ Prograf (3% to 15%) ... 1393
Prometrium Capsules (100 mg, 200 mg) (Rare) ... 3261
Prozac Pulvules, Liquid, and Weekly Capsules (Infrequent) ... 1238
▲ Rapamune Oral Solution and Tablets (3% to 20%) ... 3584
Reminyl Oral Solution (Infrequent) ... 1792
Reminyl Tablets (Infrequent) ... 1792
Renese Tablets ... 2712
▲ Requip Tablets (6%) ... 1621
Rescriptor Tablets (Less than 2%) ... 526
Rilutek Tablets (0.8% to 1.6%) ... 772
Risperdal ... 1796
Rituxan for Infusion (1% to 5%) ... 1750
Rituxan I.V. (1% to 5%) ... 1428
Roxanol ... 3066
Sandostatin Injection (Less than 1%) ... 2394
Sandostatin LAR Depot (Rare) ... 2395
Sarafem Pulvules (Infrequent) ... 1962
▲ Seroquel Tablets (7%) ... 684
Serzone Tablets (2.8% to 4%) ... 1104
Sinemet Tablets ... 1253
Sinemet CR Tablets (1.0%) ... 1255
Soma Tablets ... 3353
Soma Compound Tablets ... 3354
Soma Compound w/Codeine Tablets ... 3355
Sonata Capsules (Rare) ... 3591
Sporanox Capsules (1%) ... 1800
Stromectol Tablets (1.1%) ... 2185
Sular Tablets (Less than or equal to 1%) ... 688
Symmetrel (1% to 5%) ... 1328
▲ Tasmar Tablets (13% to 14%) ... 3010
Tenoretic Tablets ... 690
Tenormin (2% to 4%) ... 692
Thalomid Capsules ... 1154
Thorazine ... 1656
Timolide Tablets ... 2187
Tonocard Tablets (Less than 1%) ... 649
Topamax Sprinkle Capsules (Infrequent) ... 2590
Topamax Tablets (Infrequent) ... 2590
Trecator-SC Tablets ... 3598
Trilafon ... 3160
Trileptal Oral Suspension ... 2407
Trileptal Tablets ... 2407
Ultracet Tablets ... 2597
Ultram Tablets (Less than 1%) ... 2600
Uniretic Tablets ... 3178
Univasc Tablets (0.51%) ... 3181
Vaseretic Tablets (0.5% to 2.0%) ... 2204
Vasotec I.V. Injection ... 2207
Vasotec Tablets (0.5% to 1.6%) ... 2210
Viagra Tablets (Less than 2%) ... 2732
Vicodin Tuss Expectorant ... 519
Vistide Injection ... 1445
Vivactil Tablets ... 2217
Vivactil Tablets ... 2446
Wellbutrin Tablets ... 1680
Wellbutrin SR Sustained-Release Tablets (Infrequent) ... 1684
Zanaflex Tablets (Infrequent) ... 1305
Zaroxolyn Tablets ... 1177
Zebeta Tablets ... 1885
Zestoretic Tablets (0.3% to 1%) ... 695
Zestril Tablets (0.3% to 1.2%) ... 698
Ziac Tablets ... 1887
Zoloft (Infrequent) ... 2751
Zomig Tablets (Rare) ... 708
Zomig-ZMT Tablets (Rare) ... 708
Zyban Sustained-Release Tablets (Infrequent) ... 1710
Zyprexa Tablets ... 1973
Zyprexa ZYDIS Orally Disintegrating Tablets ... 1973

Hypotension, postural

(*see under* Hypotension, orthostatic)

Hypotension, secondary to spinal block

Duranest Injections ... 600
Naropin Injection ... 612
Sensorcaine ... 643
Sensorcaine-MPF Injection ... 643
Xylocaine Injections ... 653

Hypotension, symptomatic

Accupril Tablets ... 2611
Aceon Tablets (2 mg, 4 mg, 8 mg) ... 3249
Altace Capsules (0.5%) ... 2233
▲ Brevibloc Injection (12%) ... 858
▲ Cardizem Injectable (3.2%) ... 1018
▲ Cardizem Lyo-Ject Syringe (3.2%) ... 1018
▲ Cardizem Monovial (3.2%) ... 1018
Cardizem CD Capsules (Occasional) ... 1016
Covera-HS Tablets ... 3199
Cozaar Tablets ... 2067
Hyzaar ... 2109
Lexxel Tablets (Occasional) ... 608
Lotensin Tablets (0.3%) ... 2365
Lotrel Capsules ... 2370
Mavik Tablets (Rare; 0.6%) ... 478
Monopril Tablets ... 1091
▲ MUSE Urethral Suppository (3%) ... 3335
▲ Natrecor for Injection (4%) ... 3189
Prinivil Tablets ... 2164
Tarka Tablets ... 508
Uniretic Tablets ... 3178
Univasc Tablets (0.5%) ... 3181

Hypotensive crisis

Acthrel for Injection (One patient) ... 3629
Hyalgan Solution (One case) ... 3080
Miltown Tablets ... 3349

Hypothermia

Aggrenox Capsules ... 1026
Alphagan Ophthalmic Solution (Rare) ... 545
Amphotec (1% to 5%) ... 1774
Betaseron for SC Injection ... 988
Chirocaine Injection (2.2%) ... 2909
Clozaril Tablets (Less than 1%) ... 2319
Doxil Injection (Less than 1%) ... 566
Ecotrin Enteric Coated Aspirin Low, Regular and Maximum Strength Tablets ... 1715
Exelon Capsules (Infrequent) ... 2342
Exelon Oral Solution (Infrequent) ... 2345
Felbatol ... 3343
Geodon Capsules (Frequent) ... 2688
Glucophage Tablets ... 1080
Glucophage XR Tablets ... 1080
Glucovance Tablets ... 1086
Naropin Injection (Less than 1%) ... 612
Norvir Capsules (Less than 2%) ... 487
Norvir Oral Solution (Less than 2%) ... 487
Permax Tablets (Infrequent) ... 1299
Proleukin for Injection (Less than 1%) ... 1199
Provigil Tablets (At least 1%) ... 1193
Prozac Pulvules, Liquid, and Weekly Capsules (Rare) ... 1238
Rilutek Tablets (Rare) ... 772
Risperdal ... 1796
Salagen Tablets (Less than 1%) ... 2229
Sarafem Pulvules (Rare) ... 1962
Urecholine ... 2198
▲ Vesanoid Capsules (3%) ... 3037
Vistide Injection ... 1445

Hypothyroidism

Aciphex Tablets ... 1267
Aciphex Tablets ... 1783
Amerge Tablets (Rare) ... 1467
▲ Aredia for Injection (Up to 6%) ... 2309
Avonex ... 1013
Betaseron for SC Injection ... 988
Betaxon Ophthalmic Suspension (Less than 2%) ... 537
Celexa (Rare) ... 1365
▲ CellCept Capsules (3% to 10%) ... 2951
▲ CellCept Intravenous (3% to 10%) ... 2951
▲ CellCept Oral Suspension (3% to 10%) ... 2951
▲ CellCept Tablets (3% to 10%) ... 2951
Cognex Capsules (Rare) ... 1351
Copaxone for Injection (Infrequent) ... 3306
Cordarone Tablets (1% to 3%) ... 3487
Effexor Tablets (Rare) ... 3495
Effexor XR Capsules (Rare) ... 3499
Eskalith ... 1527
Evoxac Capsules (Less than 1%) ... 1217
Exelon Capsules (Infrequent) ... 2342
Exelon Oral Solution (Infrequent) ... 2345
Fortovase Capsules (Less than 2%) ... 2970
Gabitril Tablets (Infrequent) ... 1189
Genotropin Lyophilized Powder (Infrequent) ... 2818
Herceptin I.V. (At least one of the 958 patients) ... 1414
▲ Humatrope Vials and Cartridges (11%) ... 1930
Imitrex Injection ... 1549
Imitrex Nasal Spray (Rare) ... 1554
Imitrex Tablets (Rare) ... 1558
Intron A for Injection (Less than 5%) ... 3120
Kaletra Capsules (Less than 2%) ... 471
Kaletra Oral Solution (Less than 2%) ... 471
Lamictal (Rare) ... 1567
Lithium Carbonate ... 3061
Lithium Citrate Syrup ... 3061
Lithobid Slow-Release Tablets ... 3255
Luvox Tablets (25, 50, 100 mg) (Infrequent) ... 3256
Meridia Capsules ... 481
Neurontin Capsules (Rare) ... 2655
Neurontin Oral Solution (Rare) ... 2655
Neurontin Tablets (Rare) ... 2655
Pacerone Tablets (1% to 3%) ... 3331
Paxil (Rare) ... 1609
▲ PEG-Intron Powder for Injection (5%) ... 3140
Permax Tablets (Infrequent) ... 1299
Proleukin for Injection (Less than 1%) ... 1199
Prozac Pulvules, Liquid, and Weekly Capsules (Infrequent) ... 1238
Remeron Tablets (Rare) ... 2483
Remeron SolTab Tablets (Rare) ... 2486
Requip Tablets (Infrequent) ... 1621
Roferon-A Injection (Rare to infrequent) ... 2996
Saizen for Injection (Infrequent) ... 3225
▲ Sandostatin Injection (12%) ... 2394
▲ Sandostatin LAR Depot (12%) ... 2395
Sarafem Pulvules (Infrequent) ... 1962
Seroquel Tablets (Infrequent) ... 684
Sonata Capsules (Rare) ... 3591
Thalomid Capsules ... 1154
Zanaflex Tablets (Infrequent) ... 1305
Zoloft ... 2751

Hypotonia

Aloprim for Injection (Less than 1%) ... 2292
Alphagan Ophthalmic Solution (Rare) ... 545
Ambien Tablets (Rare) ... 3191
Cerebyx Injection (Infrequent) ... 2619
Diprivan Injectable Emulsion (Less than 1%) ... 667
Doxil Injection (Less than 1%) ... 566
Duragesic Transdermal System (Less than 1%) ... 1786
Effexor Tablets (Infrequent) ... 3495
Effexor XR Capsules (Infrequent) ... 3499
Gabitril Tablets (Frequent) ... 1189
Geodon Capsules (Frequent) ... 2688
Klonopin Tablets ... 2983
Lamictal (Rare) ... 1567
Luvox Tablets (25, 50, 100 mg) (Infrequent) ... 3256
Naropin Injection (Less than 1%) ... 612
Neurontin Capsules (Infrequent) ... 2655
Neurontin Oral Solution (Infrequent) ... 2655
Neurontin Tablets (Infrequent) ... 2655
Orthoclone OKT3 Sterile Solution (Less than 1%) ... 2498
OxyContin Tablets (Less than 1%) ... 2912
Permax Tablets (Infrequent) ... 1299
▲ Rapamune Oral Solution and Tablets (3% to 20%) ... 3584
Remeron Tablets (Rare) ... 2483
Remeron SolTab Tablets (Rare) ... 2486
Requip Tablets (Infrequent) ... 1621
Rilutek Tablets (Rare) ... 772
Risperdal (Rare) ... 1796
Serzone Tablets (Rare) ... 1104
Sonata Capsules (Infrequent) ... 3591
Trileptal Oral Suspension ... 2407
Trileptal Tablets ... 2407
Vistide Injection (1 patient) ... 1445
Zoloft (Rare) ... 2751
Zomig Tablets (Rare) ... 708
Zomig-ZMT Tablets (Rare) ... 708
Zonegran Capsules (Infrequent) ... 1307
Zyprexa Tablets (Infrequent) ... 1973
Zyprexa ZYDIS Orally Disintegrating Tablets (Infrequent) ... 1973

Hypouresis
Atromid-S Capsules 3483
Chemet Capsules (Up to 3.7%) 3078
Coly-Mycin M Parenteral 2243
Dilaudid-HP 443
▲ Indocin I.V. (41% of infants) 2115
K-Phos Neutral Tablets 946
Prograf 1393
Uroqid-Acid No. 2 Tablets 947

Hypouricemia
Cipro I.V. (Infrequent) 893
Cipro I.V. Pharmacy Bulk Package (Less than 1%) 897
Timentin Injection- ADD-Vantage Vial 1661
Timentin Injection-Galaxy Container 1664
Timentin Injection-Pharmacy Bulk Package 1666
Timentin for Intravenous Administration 1658
Vistide Injection 1445
▲ Zoloft (Approximately 7%) 2751

Hypoventilation
Aciphex Tablets (Rare) 1267
Aciphex Tablets (Rare) 1783
Ativan Injection (Less than 1%) 3478
Betaseron for SC Injection 988
Buprenex Injectable (1% to 5%) 2918
Copaxone for Injection (Infrequent) 3306
Diprivan Injectable Emulsion (Less than 1%) 667
Dopram Injectable 2931
Duraclon Injection (2.6%) 3057
▲ Duragesic Transdermal System (2% to 10%) 1786
Effexor XR Capsules (Rare) 3499
Levo-Dromoran 1734
▲ Levorphanol Tartrate Tablets (Greater than 10%) 3059
Nembutal Sodium Solution (Less than 1%) 485
Nesacaine/Nesacaine MPF 617
Neurontin Capsules (Rare) 2655
Neurontin Oral Solution (Rare) 2655
Neurontin Tablets (Rare) 2655
Norvir Capsules (Less than 2%) 487
Norvir Oral Solution (Less than 2%) 487
Permax Tablets (Rare) 1299
Prozac Pulvules, Liquid, and Weekly Capsules (Rare) 1238
Rilutek Tablets (Infrequent) 772
Sarafem Pulvules (Rare) 1962
Sensorcaine-MPF with Epinephrine Injection 643
Sensorcaine-MPF Injection 643
Versed Injection 3027
Virazole for Inhalation Solution (Infrequent) 1747
Zyprexa Tablets (Rare) 1973
Zyprexa ZYDIS Orally Disintegrating Tablets (Rare) 1973

Hypovolemia
Campath Ampules 992
▲ CellCept Capsules (3% to 10%) 2951
▲ CellCept Intravenous (3% to 10%) 2951
▲ CellCept Oral Suspension (3% to 10%) 2951
▲ CellCept Tablets (3% to 10%) 2951
Coreg Tablets (1% to 2%) 1508
Demadex Tablets and Injection 2965
Estratest 3252
Follistim for Injection 2465
Humegon for Injection 2468
Mykrox Tablets 1168
Priftin Tablets (Less than 1%) 758
Serophene Tablets 3226
Zaroxolyn Tablets 1177

Hypoxemia
Glucophage Tablets 1080
Glucophage XR Tablets 1080
Orthoclone OKT3 Sterile Solution 2498

Hypoxia
Ambien Tablets (Rare) 3191
▲ AmBisome for Injection (6.2% to 7.5%) 1383
▲ Amphotec (5% to 9%) 1774
Aricept Tablets (Infrequent) 1270
Aricept Tablets (Infrequent) 2665
Betaseron for SC Injection 988
Bicillin C-R 900/300 Injection 2240
Bicillin C-R Injection 2238
Bicillin L-A Injection 2242
Campath Ampules 992
Carbatrol Capsules 3234
▲ CellCept Capsules (3% to 10%) 2951
▲ CellCept Intravenous (3% to 10%) 2951
▲ CellCept Oral Suspension (3% to 10%) 2951
▲ CellCept Tablets (3% to 10%) 2951
Cerebyx Injection (Infrequent) 2619
Dilantin-125 Oral Suspension 2625
Diprivan Injectable Emulsion (Less than 1%) 667
Effexor Tablets (Rare) 3495
Effexor XR Capsules (Rare) 3499
Ethyol for Injection (Rare) 2029
Felbatol 3343
▲ Flolan for Injection (55%) 1528
Fludara for Injection (Up to 1%) 995
Herceptin I.V. (At least one of the 958 patients) 1414
Kadian Capsules (Less than 3%) 1335
Leukine 1755
Levaquin Injection (Less than 0.5%) 2537
Lupron Depot–4 Month 30 mg (Less than 5%) 3289
Merrem I.V. (0.1% to 1.0%) 673
▲ Mylotarg for Injection (2% to 6%) 3540
Nardil Tablets (Less frequent) 2653
Orthoclone OKT3 Sterile Solution 2498
Permax Tablets (Rare) 1299
Protopic Ointment (Greater than or equal to 1%) 1397
Prozac Pulvules, Liquid, and Weekly Capsules (Rare) 1238
Pulmozyme Inhalation Solution 1426
▲ Rapamune Oral Solution and Tablets (3% to 20%) 3584
Rilutek Tablets (Infrequent) 772
Rituxan for Infusion (0.3%) 1750
Rituxan I.V. (0.3%) 1428
Sarafem Pulvules (Rare) 1962
Suprane Liquid for Inhalation (Less than 1%) 874
Tasmar Tablets (Rare) 3010
Tegretol/Tegretol-XR 2404
Trasylol Injection (2%) 909
▲ Trisenox Injection (23%) 1158
Trovan (Less than 1%) 2722
Versed Syrup (2%) 3033
Vistide Injection 1445
▲ Zenapax for Injection (2% to 5%) 3046
▲ Zofran (9%) 1703
▲ Zofran ODT Orally Disintegrating Tablets (9%) 1703
Zosyn (1.0% or less) 1890
Zosyn in Galaxy Containers (1.0% or less) 1894
Zyprexa Tablets (Rare) 1973
Zyprexa ZYDIS Orally Disintegrating Tablets (Rare) 1973

Hysteria
Ambien Tablets (Rare) 3191
Cognex Capsules (Rare) 1351
Diprivan Injectable Emulsion (Less than 1%) 667
Imitrex Injection (Rare) 1549
Imitrex Tablets (Rare) 1558
Klonopin Tablets 2983
Luvox Tablets (25, 50, 100 mg) (Infrequent) 3256
Neurontin Capsules (Rare) 2655
Neurontin Oral Solution (Rare) 2655
Neurontin Tablets (Rare) 2655
Paxil (Rare) 1609
Periactin Tablets 2155
Phenergan Injection 3553
Phenergan 3556
Rynatan Tablets 3351
Trileptal Oral Suspension 2407
Trileptal Tablets 2407

I

Ichthyosis
Advair Diskus 100/50 (1% to 3%) 1448
Advair Diskus 250/50 (1% to 3%) 1448
Advair Diskus 500/50 (1% to 3%) 1448
Efudex (Infrequent) 1733
Thalomid Capsules 1154
Tricor Capsules, Micronized (Less than 1%) 513

Icterus
(*see under* Jaundice)

Idiosyncrasy
Donnatal 2929
Donnatal Extentabs 2930
Donnatal Tablets 2929
Duranest Injections 600
Etrafon (Extremely rare) 3115
Furosemide Tablets 2284
Miltown Tablets 3349
Robinul Forte Tablets 1358
Robinul Injectable 2940
Robinul Tablets 1358
Soma Tablets (Occasional) 3353
Soma Compound Tablets (Very rare) 3354
Soma Compound w/Codeine Tablets (Very rare) 3355
Xylocaine Injections 653

Idiosyncratic reactions
(*see under* Idiosyncrasy)

Idioventricular rhythms
Activase I.V. 1410
Corvert Injection (0.2%) 2793

Ileitis, regional
Accutane Capsules 2944
Effexor XR Capsules (Rare) 3499
Indocin (Less than 1%) 2112
Norvir Capsules (Less than 2%) 487
Norvir Oral Solution (Less than 2%) 487

Ileus
Aricept Tablets (Infrequent) 1270
Aricept Tablets (Infrequent) 2665
Betaseron for SC Injection 988
Celebrex Capsules (Less than 0.1%) 2676
Celebrex Capsules (Less than 0.1%) 2780
▲ CellCept Capsules (3%) 2951
▲ CellCept Intravenous (3%) 2951
▲ CellCept Oral Suspension (3%) 2951
▲ CellCept Tablets (3%) 2951
Cerebyx Injection (Infrequent) 2619
Chirocaine Injection (Less than 1%) 2909
Cipro I.V. (1% or less) 893
Cipro I.V. Pharmacy Bulk Package (Less than 1%) 897
Cogentin 2055
Dilaudid Oral Liquid 445
Dilaudid Tablets - 8 mg 445
Diprivan Injectable Emulsion (Less than 1%) 667
Doxil Injection (Less than 1%) 566
Duraclon Injection (Rare) 3057
Effexor Tablets (Rare) 3495
Effexor XR Capsules 3499
Enalaprilat Injection 863
Evoxac Capsules (Less than 1%) 1217
Felbatol 3343
Herceptin I.V. (At least one of the 958 patients) 1414
Indocin I.V. (1% to 3%) 2115
Inversine Tablets 1850
Lexxel Tablets 608
Merrem I.V. (0.1% to 1.0%) 673
MS Contin Tablets (Less frequent) 2896
Nimotop Capsules (Rare) 904
Nipent for Injection (Less than 3%) 3272
Omnicef 493
OxyContin Tablets (Less than 1%) 2912
Paxil (Rare) 1609
Photofrin for Injection (Less than 5%) 831
▲ Prograf (3% to 15%) 1393
Proleukin for Injection (2%) 1199
▲ Rapamune Oral Solution and Tablets (3% to 20%) 3584
ReoPro Vials (0.3%) 1958
Rilutek Tablets (Rare) 772
Taxotere for Injection Concentrate 778
Vaseretic Tablets 2204
Vasotec I.V. Injection 2207
Vasotec Tablets (0.5% to 1.0%) 2210
Zosyn (1.0% or less) 1890
Zosyn in Galaxy Containers (1.0% or less) 1894
Zyprexa Tablets (Rare) 1973
Zyprexa ZYDIS Orally Disintegrating Tablets (Rare) 1973

Ileus, adynamic
Compazine 1505
Etrafon (Occasional) 3115
Navane Oral 2701
Navane Intramuscular 2703
Stelazine 1640
Thiothixene Capsules 2290
Thorazine 1656
Trilafon (Occasional) 3160

Ileus, paralytic
Artane (Rare) 1855
Campath Ampules 992
Clozaril Tablets 2319
Cogentin 2055
Covera-HS Tablets (Infrequent) 3199
Etrafon 3115
Flexeril Tablets (Rare) 572
Flexeril Tablets (Rare) 2094
Isoptin SR Tablets (Infrequent) 467
Limbitrol 1738
Loxitane Capsules 3398
Motofen Tablets 577
Navelbine Injection (1%) 1604
Norpramin Tablets 755
Numorphan 1324
Podocon-25 Liquid 2608
Serentil 1057
Surmontil Capsules 3595
Tarka Tablets (Infrequent) 508
Taxol Injection (Rare) 1129
Thioridazine Hydrochloride Tablets 2289
Verelan Capsules (Infrequent) 3184
Vivactil Tablets 2217
Vivactil Tablets 2446

Illusion, unspecified
Ambien Tablets (Infrequent) 3191
Evoxac Capsules 1217
Klonopin Tablets (Infrequent) 2983
Zoloft (Rare) 2751

Immobility
Moban 1320

Immunoglobulin, abnormalities
Dilantin Infatabs 2624
Dilantin Kapseals 2622
Dilantin-125 Oral Suspension 2625
Rilutek Tablets (Infrequent) 772

Immunosuppression
Purinethol Tablets 1615
Rifamate Capsules 767

Immunosuppression, progressive
Lamictal 1567

Impetigo
Cutivate Cream (0.8%) 1282
Hivid Tablets (Less than 1%) 2975
Varivax 2202

Impotence
(*see also under* Sexual dysfunction)
Abelcet Injection 1273
Accupril Tablets (0.5% to 1.0%) 2611
Accuretic Tablets (0.5% to 1%) 2614
Aciphex Tablets (Rare) 1267
Aciphex Tablets (Rare) 1783
Adalat CC Tablets (3% or less) 877
Adderall Tablets 3231
Adderall XR Capsules
Adipex-P 1406
Aldoclor Tablets 2035
Aldomet Tablets 2037
Aldoril Tablets 2039
Altace Capsules (Less than 1%) 2233
Ambien Tablets (Rare) 3191
Anadrol-50 Tablets 3321
Androderm Transdermal System CIII (Less than 1%) 3377
Antabuse Tablets 2444
Antabuse Tablets (Small number of patients) 3474
Arthrotec Tablets (Rare) 3195
Atacand HCT Tablets 597
Atromid-S Capsules 3483
Axid Pulvules 1903
Axid Pulvules 2919
Betagan ⊙228
Betaseron for SC Injection 988
Betimol Ophthalmic Solution ⊙324
Bicillin C-R 900/300 Injection 2240
Bicillin C-R Injection 2238
Bicillin L-A Injection 2242
Blocadren Tablets (Less than 1%) 2046
Captopril Tablets 2281
Carbatrol Capsules 3234
Cardizem Injectable 1018
Cardizem Lyo-Ject Syringe 1018
Cardizem Monovial 1018
Cardizem CD Capsules (Less than 1%) 1016
Cardura Tablets (1.1%) 2668
▲ Casodex Tablets (5%) 662
Cataflam Tablets (Less than 1%) 2315
▲ Catapres Tablets (About 3 in 100 patients) 1037
Catapres-TTS (2 of 101 patients) 1038
▲ Celexa (3%) 1365
▲ CellCept Capsules (3%) 2951
▲ CellCept Intravenous (3%) 2951
▲ CellCept Oral Suspension (3%) 2951
▲ CellCept Tablets (3%) 2951
Claritin (At least one patient) 3100
Claritin-D 12 Hour Extended Release Tablets (Less frequent) 3102
Claritin-D 24 Hour Extended Release Tablets 3104
▲ Clorpres Tablets (About 3%) 1002
Clozaril Tablets (Less than 1%) 2319
Cognex Capsules (Infrequent) 1351
▲ Combipres Tablets (About 3%) 1040
Compazine 1505
Coreg Tablets (1% to 2%) 1508
Corgard Tablets (1 to 5 per 1000 patients) 2245
Corzide 40/5 Tablets (1 to 5 of 1000 patients) 2247
Corzide 80/5 Tablets (1 to 5 of 1000 patients) 2247
Cosopt Sterile Ophthalmic Solution 2065
Covera-HS Tablets (Less than 2%) 3199
Cozaar Tablets (Less than 1%) 2067
Cytotec Tablets (Infrequent) 3202
Demadex Tablets and Injection 2965
Demser Capsules (Infrequent) 2085
Desoxyn Tablets 440
Dexedrine 1512
DextroStat Tablets 3236
Diovan Capsules 2337
Diovan HCT Tablets (Greater than 0.2%) 2338
Dipentum Capsules (Rare) 2803
Diuril Oral 2087
Diuril Sodium Intravenous 2086
Donnatal 2929
Donnatal Extentabs 2930
Donnatal Tablets 2929
▲ Duraclon Injection (3%) 3057
Dyazide Capsules 1515
DynaCirc Capsules (0.5% to 1%) 2921
DynaCirc CR Tablets (0.5% to 1%) 2923
▲ Effexor Tablets (2.1% to 6%) 3495
▲ Effexor XR Capsules (4% to 6%) 3499
Enalaprilat Injection 863

Eskalith ... 1527
Etrafon ... 3115
▲ Eulexin Capsules (33%) ... 3118
Evoxac Capsules ... 1217
Exelon Capsules (Infrequent) ... 2342
Exelon Oral Solution (Infrequent) ... 2345
Famotidine Injection (Rare) ... 866
Flexeril Tablets (Rare) ... 572
Flexeril Tablets (Rare) ... 2094
Fortovase Capsules (Less than 2%) ... 2970
Gabitril Tablets (Infrequent) ... 1189
Geodon Capsules (Infrequent) ... 2688
Haldol Decanoate ... 2535
Haldol Injection, Tablets and Concentrate ... 2533
HydroDIURIL Tablets ... 2108
Hytrin Capsules (1.2% to 1.6%) ... 464
Hyzaar ... 2109
Imdur Tablets (Less than or equal to 5%) ... 1826
Indapamide Tablets (Less than 5%) ... 2286
Inderal (Rare) ... 3513
Inderal LA Long-Acting Capsules (Rare) ... 3516
Inderide Tablets (Rare) ... 3517
Inderide LA Long-Acting Capsules (Rare) ... 3519
Intron A for Injection (Less than 5%) ... 3120
Inversine Tablets ... 1850
Invirase Capsules (Less than 2%) ... 2979
Ionamin Capsules ... 1163
Ismo Tablets (Fewer than 1%) ... 3524
Isoptin SR Tablets (1% or less) ... 467
Klonopin Tablets (1%) ... 2983
▲ Lamictal (13%) ... 1567
Levaquin Injection (Less than 0.5%) ... 2537
Levsin/Levsinex/Levbid ... 3172
Lexxel Tablets ... 608
Limbitrol (Less common) ... 1738
Lipitor Tablets (Less than 2%) ... 2639
Lipitor Tablets (Less than 2%) ... 2696
Lithobid Slow-Release Tablets ... 3255
Lopid Tablets ... 2650
Lotensin Tablets (Less than 1%) ... 2365
Lotensin HCT Tablets (1.2%) ... 2367
Lotrel Capsules ... 2370
▲ Lupron Depot 7.5 mg (5.4%) ... 3284
Lupron Depot–3 Month 22.5 mg (Less than 5%) ... 3288
Lupron Depot–4 Month 30 mg (Less than 5%) ... 3289
▲ Lupron Injection (5% or more) ... 3279
Luvox Tablets (25, 50, 100 mg) (2%) ... 3256
Mavik Tablets (0.3% to 1.0%) ... 478
▲ Megace Oral Suspension (4% to 14%) ... 1124
Meridia Capsules ... 481
Mexitil Capsules (Less than 1% or about 4 in 1,000) ... 1047
Micardis Tablets (More than 0.3%) ... 1049
Micardis HCT Tablets ... 1051
Microzide Capsules ... 3414
Midamor Tablets (Between 1% and 3%) ... 2136
Minipress Capsules (Less than 1%) ... 2699
Minizide Capsules (Rare) ... 2700
Mirapex Tablets (2%) ... 2834
Moduretic Tablets (Less than or equal to 1%) ... 2138
MS Contin Tablets (Less frequent) ... [illegible]
MSIR (Less frequent) ... 2898
Mykrox Tablets (Less than 2%) ... 1168
Nadolol Tablets (1 to 5 of 1000 patients) ... 2288
Nardil Tablets ... 2653
Navane Oral ... 2701
Navane Intramuscular ... 2703
Neurontin Capsules (1.5%) ... 2655
Neurontin Oral Solution (1.5%) ... 2655
Neurontin Tablets (1.5%) ... 2655
Nexium Delayed-Release Capsules (Less than 1%) ... 619
▲ Nilandron Tablets (11%) ... 753
Nipent for Injection (Less than 3%) ... 3272
Nizoral Tablets (Less than 1%) ... 1791
Nolvadex Tablets ... 678
Normodyne Tablets (1% to 4%) ... 3137
Norpramin Tablets ... 755
Norvir Capsules (Less than 2%) ... 487
Norvir Oral Solution (Less than 2%) ... 487
▲ Novantrone for Injection (7%) ... 1760
NuLev Orally Disintegrating Tablets ... 3176
Oramorph SR Tablets (Less frequent) ... 3062
▲ Orap Tablets (3 of 20 patients) ... 1407
Orudis Capsules (Less than 1%) ... 3548
Oruvail Capsules (Less than 1%) ... 3548
Oxandrin Tablets ... 1153
OxyContin Tablets (Less than 1%) ... 2912
Parnate Tablets ... 1607
▲ Paxil (4% to 10.0%) ... 1609
Pepcid Injection (Rare) ... 2153
Pepcid for Oral Suspension (Rare) ... 2150
Pepcid RPD Orally Disintegrating Tablets (Rare) ... 2150
Pepcid Tablets (Rare) ... 2150
Permax Tablets (Infrequent) ... 1299
Plendil Extended-Release Tablets (0.5% to 1.5%) ... 623
Prevacid Delayed-Release Capsules (Less than 1%) ... 3292
PREVPAC (Less than 1%) ... 3298
Prinivil Tablets (1.0%) ... 2164
Prinzide Tablets (1.2%) ... 2168
Procardia XL Extended Release Tablets (Less than 3%) ... 2710
Propecia Tablets (1.3%) ... 2172
▲ Proscar Tablets (3.7%) ... 2175
Protonix I.V. (Less than 1%) ... 3580
Protonix Tablets (Less than 1%) ... 3577
▲ Prozac Pulvules, Liquid, and Weekly Capsules (2% to 7%) ... 1238
▲ Rapamune Oral Solution and Tablets (3% to 20%) ... 3584
Reglan ... 2935
Relafen Tablets (Less than 1%) ... 1617
Remeron Tablets (Infrequent) ... 2483
Remeron SolTab Tablets (Infrequent) ... 2486
▲ Requip Tablets (3%) ... 1621
Rescriptor Tablets (Less than 2%) ... 526
Rilutek Tablets (Infrequent) ... 772
Robinul Forte Tablets ... 1358
Robinul Injectable ... 2940
Robinul Tablets ... 1358
Roferon-A Injection (Less than 4%) ... 2996
Rythmol Tablets – 150 mg, 225 mg, 300 mg (Less than 1%) ... 502
Sandostatin LAR Depot (1% to 4%) ... 2395
Sectral Capsules (Up to 2%) ... 3589
Sensorcaine-MPF with Epinephrine Injection ... 643
Sensorcaine-MPF Injection ... 643
Serentil ... 1057
Seroquel Tablets (Infrequent) ... 684
Serzone Tablets (Frequent) ... 1104
▲ Simulect for Injection (3% to 10%) ... 2399
Sonata Capsules (Infrequent) ... 3591
Sporanox Capsules (0.2% to 1.2%) ... 1800
Stelazine ... 1640
Sular Tablets (Less than or equal to 1%) ... 688
Surmontil Capsules ... 3595
Tagamet ... 1644
Tambocor Tablets (Less than 1%) ... 1990
Tarka Tablets (0.3% or more) ... 508
Tasmar Tablets (Frequent) ... 3010
Tegretol/Tegretol-XR ... 2404
▲ Tenex Tablets (Up to 7%) ... 2942
Tenoretic Tablets ... 690
Tenormin ... 692
▲ Thalomid Capsules (8.3%) ... 1154
Thiothixene Capsules (Infrequently) ... 2290
Thorazine ... 1656
Tiazac Capsules (Less than 2%) ... 1378
Timolide Tablets ... 2187
Timolol GFS ... ⊙266
Timoptic in Ocudose (Less frequent) ... 2192
Timoptic Sterile Ophthalmic Solution (Less frequent) ... 2190
Timoptic-XE Sterile Ophthalmic Gel Forming Solution ... 2194
[illegible] (Frequent) ... 2590
Topamax Tablets (Frequent) ... 2590
Trecator-SC Tablets ... 3598
Trilafon ... 3160
Trovan (Less than 1%) ... 2722
Ultracet Tablets (Less than 1%) ... 2597
Uniretic Tablets (More than 1%) ... 3178
Vascor Tablets (0.5% to 2.0%) ... 2602
Vaseretic Tablets (2.2%) ... 2204
Vasotec I.V. Injection ... 2207
Vasotec Tablets (0.5% to 1.0%) ... 2210
Verelan Capsules (1% or less) ... 3184
Verelan PM Capsules (2% or less) ... 3186
Viadur Implant (2.3%) ... 912
Vicoprofen Tablets (Less than 1%) ... 520
Vivactil Tablets ... 2217
Vivactil Tablets ... 2446
Voltaren Tablets (Less than 1%) ... 2315
Voltaren-XR Tablets (Less than 1%) ... 2315
▲ Wellbutrin Tablets (3.4%) ... 1680
Wellbutrin SR Sustained-Release Tablets (Infrequent) ... 1684
Zantac (Occasional) ... 1690
Zantac Injection ... 1688
Zantac Syrup (Occasional) ... 1690
Zaroxolyn Tablets ... 1177
Zebeta Tablets ... 1885
Zestoretic Tablets (1.2%) ... 695
Zestril Tablets (1.0%) ... 698
Ziac Tablets (1.1%) ... 1887
Zoladex 3-month (1% to 5%) ... 706
Zoloft (Frequent) ... 2751
Zonegran Capsules (Infrequent) ... 1307
Zyban Sustained-Release Tablets (Infrequent) ... 1710
Zyprexa Tablets (Infrequent) ... 1973
Zyprexa ZYDIS Orally Disintegrating Tablets (Infrequent) ... 1973

Incontinence

Halcion Tablets ... 2823
Minipress Capsules (Less than 1%) ... 2699
Minizide Capsules (Rare) ... 2700
Moduretic Tablets (Less than or equal to 1%) ... 2138
Reminyl Oral Solution (Frequent) ... 1792
Reminyl Tablets (Frequent) ... 1792
Sandostatin LAR Depot (1% to 4%) ... 2395
Serentil ... 1057
Tensilon Injectable ... 1745
Valium Injectable ... 3026
Valium Tablets (Infrequent) ... 3047
Xanax Tablets (1.5%) ... 2865

Incontinence, fecal

Actiq (Less than 1%) ... 1184
AmBisome for Injection (Less common) ... 1383
Amphotec (1% to 5%) ... 1774
Aricept Tablets (Frequent) ... 1270
Aricept Tablets (Frequent) ... 2665
Betaseron for SC Injection ... 988
Cardura Tablets (Less than 0.5%) ... 2668
Cognex Capsules (Infrequent) ... 1351
Colazal Capsules ... 3069
Copaxone for Injection (At least 2%) ... 3306
Depacon Injection (1% or more) ... 416
Depakene (1% or more) ... 421
Depakote Sprinkle Capsules ... 426
Depakote Tablets (1% to 5%) ... 430
Depakote ER Tablets (Greater than 1%) ... 436
Eskalith ... 1527
Exelon Capsules (Frequent) ... 2342
Exelon Oral Solution (Frequent) ... 2345
Fortovase Capsules (Less than 2%) ... 2970
Gabitril Tablets (Infrequent) ... 1189
Gliadel Wafer (1%) ... 1723
Kaletra Capsules (Less than 2%) ... 471
Kaletra Oral Solution (Less than 2%) ... 471
Klonopin Tablets ... 2983
Lithium Carbonate ... 3061
Lithium Citrate Syrup ... 3061
Lithobid Slow-Release Tablets ... 3255
Luvox Tablets (25, 50, 100 mg) (Rare) ... 3256
Marinol Capsules (Less than 1%) ... 3325
Naropin Injection (Less than 1%) ... 612
Neurontin Capsules (Infrequent) ... 2655
Neurontin Oral Solution (Infrequent) ... 2655
Neurontin Tablets (Infrequent) ... 2655
Paxil (Rare) ... 1609
Pentasa Capsules (Less than 1%) ... 3239
Permax Tablets (Rare) ... 1299
Prozac Pulvules, Liquid, and Weekly Capsules (Rare) ... 1238
Requip Tablets (Infrequent) ... 1621
Rescriptor Tablets (Less than 2%) ... 526
Rilutek Tablets (Infrequent) ... 772
Risperdal (Rare) ... 1796
Sarafem Pulvules (Rare) ... 1962
Sensorcaine ... 643
Sensorcaine-MPF Injection ... 643
Seroquel Tablets (Infrequent) ... 684
Topamax Sprinkle Capsules (Infrequent) ... 2590
Topamax Tablets (Infrequent) ... 2590
▲ Trisenox Injection (8%) ... 1158
Vistide Injection ... 1445
▲ Xenical Capsules (1.8% to 7.7%) ... 3043
Zoloft (Rare) ... 2751
Zonegran Capsules (Rare) ... 1307
Zosyn (1.0% or less) ... 1890
Zosyn in Galaxy Containers (1.0% or less) ... 1894
Zyprexa Tablets (Infrequent) ... 1973
Zyprexa ZYDIS Orally Disintegrating Tablets (Infrequent) ... 1973

Incoordination

(*see under* Ataxia)

Indigestion

Asacol Delayed-Release Tablets ... 2884
Augmentin Chewable Tablets ... 1482
Augmentin Powder for Oral Suspension ... 1482
Augmentin Tablets ... 1485
Augmentin ES-600 Powder for Oral Suspension ... 1487
Carafate Suspension (Less than 0.5%) ... 731
Carafate Tablets (Less than 0.5%) ... 730
▲ Cataflam Tablets (3% to 9%) ... 2315
Ceftin Tablets (0.1% to 1%) ... 1898
Colestid Tablets (Less frequent) ... 2791
Corgard Tablets (1 to 5 per 1000 patients) ... 2245
Corzide 40/5 Tablets (1 to 5 of 1000 patients) ... 2247
Corzide 80/5 Tablets (1 to 5 of 1000 patients) ... 2247
▲ Depacon Injection (Among most common) ... 416
Depakote Sprinkle Capsules ... 426
▲ Depakote Tablets (Among most common) ... 430
Eskalith ... 1527
▲ Glucophage Tablets (7.1%) ... 1080
▲ Indocin (3% to 9%) ... 2112
Lithobid Slow-Release Tablets ... 3255
Motrin Suspension, Oral Drops, Chewable Tablets, and Caplets (1% to less than 3%) ... 2002
Nadolol Tablets (1 to 5 of 1000 patients) ... 2288
Oncaspar ... 756
Sinequan ... 2713
▲ Trilisate (Less than 20%) ... 2901
▲ Voltaren Tablets (3% to 9%) ... 2315
▲ Voltaren-XR Tablets (3% to 9%) ... 2315

Induration at injection site

▲ Acel-Imune (2% to 30%) ... 1851
▲ ActHIB Vaccine (0.8% to 38.2%) ... 798
Ancef for Injection ... 1474
Ancef Injection ... 1474
▲ Aredia for Injection (Up to 41%) ... 2309
Azactam for Injection (0.5% to 0.9%) ... 1276
▲ Brevibloc Injection (About 8%) ... 858
Cancidas for Injection (Up to 3.1%) ... 2048
Cefizox for Intramuscular or Intravenous Use (1% to 5%) ... 1390
▲ Claforan Injection (4.3%) ... 732
Cleocin Phosphate Sterile Solution ... 2785
▲ Comvax (27.2% to 27.6%) ... 2056
▲ Copaxone for Injection (13%) ... 3306
Demerol ... 3079
Desferal Vials ... 2333
Diphtheria & Tetanus Toxoids Adsorbed Purogenated for Pediatric Use ... 1857
▲ Engerix-B Vaccine (1% to 10 %) ... 1517
Factrel (Rare) ... 3633
FluShield Influenza Vaccine ... 3521
▲ Havrix Vaccine (1% to 10%) ... 1544
Imitrex Injection ... 1549
IPOL Vaccine (1%) ... 809
Kefzol Vials, ADD-Vantage ... 1951
Lupron Depot 3.75 mg ... 3281
Lupron Depot 7.5 mg ... 3284
Lupron Depot–3 Month 11.25 mg ... 3285
Lupron Depot–3 Month 22.5 mg ... 3288
Lupron Depot–4 Month 30 mg ... 3289
Lupron Depot-PED 7.5 mg, 11.25 mg and 15 mg ... 3291
Lupron Injection ... 3279
Menomune-A/C/Y/W-135 Vaccine (1.2% to 4.4%) ... 813
Mepergan Injection ... 3539
Meruvax II ... 2130
M-M-R II ... 2118
Oncaspar ... 756
Liquid PedvaxHIB ... 2148
Pipracil (2%) ... 1866
Pneumovax 23 ... 2156
▲ Prevnar for Injection (10.9% to 12.8%) ... 1870
Primaxin I.V. (0.2%) ... 2160
Rocephin Injectable Vials, ADD-Vantage, Galaxy, Bulk (1%) ... 2993
Taxol Injection (Rare) ... 1129
Tetanus & Diphtheria Toxoids Adsorbed for Adult Use ... 1880
▲ Tetanus and Diphtheria Toxoids Adsorbed For Adult Use (19%) ... 815
Timentin Injection- ADD-Vantage Vial ... 1661
Timentin Injection-Galaxy Container ... 1664
Timentin Injection-Pharmacy Bulk Package ... 1666
Timentin for Intravenous Administration ... 1658
Tripedia Vaccine ... 817
▲ Twinrix Vaccine (1% to 10%) ... 1674
▲ TYPHIM Vi Vaccine (Up to 18%) ... 825
▲ Varivax (19.35% to 32.5%) ... 2202
Versed Injection (0.5% to 1.7%) ... 3027

Inebriated feeling

Klonopin Tablets (Infrequent) ... 2983

Infantile spasms

Acel-Imune ... 1851
Tripedia Vaccine ... 817

Infection, acquired immunodeficiency syndrome

Thalomid Capsules ... 1154
Vistide Injection ... 1445

Infection, bacterial

Actiq (Less than 1%) ... 1184
Advair Diskus 100/50 (1% to 3%) ... 1448
Advair Diskus 250/50 (1% to 3%) ... 1448
Advair Diskus 500/50 (1% to 3%) ... 1448

Campath Ampules 992
Celebrex Capsules (0.1% to 1.9%) 2676
Celebrex Capsules (0.1% to 1.9%) 2780
▲ CellCept Capsules (3%) 2951
▲ CellCept Intravenous (3%) 2951
▲ CellCept Oral Suspension (3%) 2951
▲ CellCept Tablets (3%) 2951
Claritin-D 12 Hour Extended Release Tablets (Less frequent) ... 3102
Comtan Tablets (1%) 2328
▲ Copaxone for Injection (5%) 3306
Enbrel for Injection 1752
Enbrel for Injection 3504
Evoxac Capsules (Less than 1%) 1217
Flovent Diskus (1% to 3%) 3614
Fortovase Capsules (Less than 2%) 2970
Foscavir Injection (Between 1% and 5%) 605
Gengraf Capsules (1% to less than 3%) 457
Imdur Tablets (Less than or equal to 5%) 1826
Intron A for Injection (Less than 5%) 3120
Invirase Capsules (Less than 2%) 2979
▲ Leustatin Injection (42%) 2495
▲ Lopid Tablets (More common) 2650
Neoral Soft Gelatin Capsules (1% to less than 3%) 2380
Neoral Oral Solution (1% to less than 3%) 2380
▲ Nipent for Injection (5%) 3272
Orthoclone OKT3 Sterile Solution ... 2498
▲ Paraplatin for Injection (14% to 18%) 1126
Remicade for IV Injection (Less than 2%) 1178
Rituxan for Infusion 1750
Rituxan I.V. 1428
Sandostatin LAR Depot (1% to 4%) 2395
▲ Serostim for Injection (1% to 10%) . 3229
Tasmar Tablets (Infrequent) 3010
▲ Trisenox Injection (8%) 1158
Trovan (Less than 1%) 2722
Vantin Tablets and Oral Suspension (Less than 1%) 2860
Varivax 2202

Infection, candida albicans
Aerobid/Aerobid-M 1363
▲ Cleocin Vaginal Cream (11% to 26%) 2788
Rhinocort Nasal Inhaler (Rare) 640
Vanceril Inhalation Aerosol 3165

Infection, conjunctiva
Urobiotic-250 Capsules 2731

Infection, cryptococcus
Orthoclone OKT3 Sterile Solution (1.6%) 2498

Infection, cytomegalovirus
▲ CellCept Capsules (3.6% to 15.2%) 2951
▲ CellCept Intravenous (3.6% to 15.2%) 2951
▲ CellCept Oral Suspension (3.6% to 15.2%) 2951
▲ CellCept Tablets (3.6% to 15.2%) .. 2951
▲ Doxil Injection (20.1%) 566
▲ Gengraf Capsules (4.8%) 457
▲ Neoral Soft Gelatin Capsules (4.8%) 2380
▲ Neoral Oral Solution (4.8%) 2380
▲ Orthoclone OKT3 Sterile Solution (3% to 19%) 2498
▲ Sandimmune (4.8% to 12.3%) 2388
▲ Simulect for Injection (14%) 2399
▲ Taxol Injection (27% to 45%) 1129
▲ Thymoglobulin for Injection (12.2%) 3071
▲ Vitravene for Injection (5% to 20%) .... ⊙310

Infection, decreased resistance
Cortifoam Rectal Foam 3170
Orthoclone OKT3 Sterile Solution ... 2498
Prelone Syrup 2273
Prograf 1393
Sandimmune 2388

Infection, ears
Aceon Tablets (2 mg, 4 mg, 8 mg) (Up to 1.3%) 3249
Advair Diskus 100/50 (1% to 3%) ... 1448
Advair Diskus 250/50 (1% to 3%) ... 1448
Advair Diskus 500/50 (1% to 3%) ... 1448
▲ Aerobid/Aerobid-M (3% to 9%) 1363
Amerge Tablets (Frequent) 1467
Avalide Tablets 1070
Avapro Tablets (Less than 1%) 1074
Avapro Tablets (Less than 1%) 3076
Claritin-D 12 Hour Extended Release Tablets (Less frequent) ... 3102
Cognex Capsules (Infrequent) 1351
Colazal Capsules 3069
▲ Epivir-HBV (25%) 1524
Imitrex Nasal Spray (Infrequent) 1554
Neurontin Capsules (Infrequent) 2655
Neurontin Oral Solution (Infrequent) 2655
Neurontin Tablets (Infrequent) 2655
▲ Liquid PedvaxHIB (Among most frequent) 2148
▲ Pulmicort Respules (2% to 5%) 632

Infection, Epstein-Barr virus
Gonal-F for Injection 3216
Rapamune Oral Solution and Tablets (Less frequent) 3584

Infection, eyes
▲ Acular Ophthalmic Solution (Approximately 1% to 10%) 544
▲ Acular PF Ophthalmic Solution (Approximately 1% to 10%) 544
Aerobid/Aerobid-M (1% to 3%) 1363
Decadron Phosphate Sterile Ophthalmic Ointment 2083
Decadron Phosphate Sterile Ophthalmic Solution 2084
Evoxac Capsules (1% to 3%) 1217
Humorsol Sterile Ophthalmic Solution 2102
Pulmicort Respules (1% to 3%) 632

Infection, eyes, fungal
Blephamide Ophthalmic Suspension 548
Cortisporin Ophthalmic Suspension .... ⊙297
Pred-G Sterile Ophthalmic Ointment .... ⊙248

Infection, fungal
Actiq (1% or greater) 1184
▲ Apligraf (6.3%) 2305
Blephamide Ophthalmic Suspension 548
Campath Ampules 992
Celebrex Capsules (0.1% to 1.9%) 2676
Celebrex Capsules (0.1% to 1.9%) 2780
Cleocin Vaginal Ovules (1%) 2789
Crixivan Capsules (Less than 2%) 2070
Detrol Tablets (1.1%) 3623
Enbrel for Injection 1752
Enbrel for Injection 3504
Evoxac Capsules (1% to 3%) 1217
FML Ophthalmic Ointment .... ⊙237
FML Ophthalmic Suspension .... ⊙236
FML Forte Ophthalmic Suspension .... ⊙235
FML-S Liquifilm Sterile Ophthalmic Suspension .... ⊙238
Fortovase Capsules (Less than 2%) 2970
Foscavir Injection (Between 1% and 5%) 605
Gengraf Capsules (1% to less than 3%) 457
Intron A for Injection (Less than 5%) 3120
Invirase Capsules (Less than 2%) 2979
Keppra Tablets (1% or more) 3314
Klonopin Tablets (Infrequent) 2983
▲ Leustatin Injection (20%) 2495
Micardis Tablets (More than 0.3%) .. 1049
Micardis HCT Tablets 1051
Neoral Soft Gelatin Capsules (1% to less than 3%) 2380
Neoral Oral Solution (1% to less than 3%) 2380
▲ Novantrone for Injection (9% to 15%) 1760
▲ Orthoclone OKT3 Sterile Solution (4% to 34%) 2498
Poly-Pred Liquifilm Ophthalmic Suspension .... ⊙245
Remicade for IV Injection (Less than 2%) 1178
Requip Tablets (Infrequent) 1621
▲ Serostim for Injection (1% to 10%) . 3229
Soriatane Capsules (Less than 1%) 3003
Tasmar Tablets (Infrequent) 3010
Trovan (Less than 1%) 2722
Vioxx (Greater than 0.1% to 1.9%) .. 2213
Zenapax for Injection 3046
Zyvox (0.1% to 1.5%) 2871

Infection, fungal, local
Aceon Tablets (2 mg, 4 mg, 8 mg) (0.3% to 1%) 3249
▲ Aldara Cream, 5% (2% to 11%) 1978
Doxil Injection (Less than 1%) 566
▲ Gengraf Capsules (7.5%) 457
▲ Neoral Soft Gelatin Capsules (7.5%) 2380
▲ Neoral Oral Solution (7.5%) 2380
▲ Sandimmune (7.5 to 9.6%) 2388
Vancenase AQ Nasal Spray 0.084% (Single cases) 3163
Vantin Tablets and Oral Suspension (Less than 1% to 3.1%) 2860

Infection, fungal, systemic
Gengraf Capsules (2.2%) 457
Neoral Soft Gelatin Capsules (2.2%) 2380
Neoral Oral Solution (2.2%) 2380
Sandimmune (2.2 to 3.9%) 2388

Infection, gastrointestinal
Adriamycin PFS/RDF Injection 2767
▲ Advair Diskus 100/50 (3%) 1448
Advair Diskus 250/50 1448
Advair Diskus 500/50 (Up to 3%) ... 1448
Ceftin for Oral Suspension (0.1% to 1%) 1898
Cytotec Tablets (Infrequent) 3202
Flovent Diskus (1% to 3%) 3614

Infection, gram-negative bacteria
▲ Orthoclone OKT3 (1.6% to 7.5%) 2498

Infection, localized
Dermatop Emollient Cream 2517
▲ Flolan for Injection (21%) 1528
Norplant System (0.7%) 3543
▲ Proleukin for Injection (23%) 1199
▲ TheraCys Injection (3%) 823
Valcyte Tablets (Less than 5%) 3022
Vanceril Inhalation Aerosol (Frequent) 3165

Infection, lower respiratory tract
Advair Diskus 100/50 (1% to 3%) 1448
Advair Diskus 250/50 (1% to 3%) ... 1448
Advair Diskus 500/50 (1% to 3%) ... 1448
Flovent Diskus (1% to 3%) 3614
Foradil Aerolizer (2.1%) 2354
Imitrex Injection 1549
Imitrex Tablets 1558
▲ Xenical Capsules (7.8%) 3043

Infection, masking signs of
Blephamide Ophthalmic Ointment 547
Blephamide Ophthalmic Suspension 548
FML Ophthalmic Ointment .... ⊙237
FML Ophthalmic Suspension .... ⊙236
FML Forte Ophthalmic Suspension .... ⊙235
FML-S Liquifilm Sterile Ophthalmic Suspension .... ⊙238
Pred Forte Ophthalmic Suspension .... ⊙246
Pred Mild Sterile Ophthalmic Suspension .... ⊙249
Prelone Syrup 2273
TobraDex Ophthalmic Ointment 542
TobraDex Ophthalmic Suspension .. 541

Infection, mononucleosis-like syndrome
Klonopin Tablets (Infrequent) 2983
Neurontin Capsules 2655
Neurontin Oral Solution 2655
Neurontin Tablets 2655
Paser Granules 1781

Infection, mycobacterial
CellCept Capsules 2951
CellCept Intravenous 2951
CellCept Oral Suspension 2951
CellCept Tablets 2951
Rapamune Oral Solution and Tablets (Less frequent) 3584

Infection, mycobacterium tuberculosis
Rescriptor Tablets 526

Infection, nasal
Advair Diskus 100/50 (1% to 3%) 1448
Advair Diskus 250/50 (1% to 3%) ... 1448
Advair Diskus 500/50 (1% to 3%) ... 1448
Amerge Tablets (Frequent) 1467
Beconase Inhalation Aerosol (Rare) 1497
▲ Epivir-HBV (25%) 1524
▲ Miacalcin Nasal Spray (1% to 10.6%) 2375

Infection, opportunistic
Campath Ampules 992
▲ Doxil Injection (50.4%) 566
Leustatin Injection 2495

Infection, parasitic
Fortovase Capsules (Less than 2%) 2970
Intron A for Injection (Less than 5%) 3120
Vantin Tablets and Oral Suspension (Less than 1%) 2860

Infection, pelvis
ParaGard T 380A Intrauterine Copper Contraceptive 2582
Wellbutrin Tablets (Rare) 1680

Infection, pharyngeal
Beconase Inhalation Aerosol (Rare) 1497
▲ Epivir-HBV (25%) 1524

Infection, Pneumocystis carinii
(*see under* Pneumocystis carinii, susceptibility)

Infection, post-treatment, unspecified
▲ Survanta Intratracheal Suspension (10.2% to 20.7%) 3053

Infection, protozoan
Campath Ampules 992
Enbrel for Injection 1752
Enbrel for Injection 3504
Orthoclone OKT3 Sterile Solution ... 2498

Infection, respiratory
Accutane Capsules 2944
▲ Arava Tablets (15%) 724
▲ Aromasin Tablets (2% to 5%) 2769
Betimol Ophthalmic Solution (1% to 5%) .... ⊙324
▲ CellCept Capsules (13.1% to 37%) 2951
▲ CellCept Intravenous (13.1% to 37%) 2951
▲ CellCept Oral Suspension (13.1% to 37%) 2951
▲ CellCept Tablets (13.1% to 37%) ... 2951
Cognex Capsules (Infrequent) 1351
DDAVP Nasal Spray 738
DDAVP Rhinal Tube 738
▲ Depacon Injection (12% to 20%) 416
▲ Depakene (12% to 20%) 421
▲ Depakote Sprinkle Capsules (12% to 20%) 426
▲ Depakote Tablets (12% to 20%) 430
▲ Depakote ER Tablets (12% to 20%) 436
Desmopressin Acetate Rhinal Tube 1345
▲ Flovent Diskus (4%) 3614
Gliadel Wafer (2%) 1723
Imitrex Nasal Spray (Infrequent) 1554
Lexxel Tablets 608
▲ MUSE Urethral Suppository (3%) 3335
Neurontin Oral Solution (2.5%) 2655
Plendil Extended-Release Tablets (0.5% to 1.5%) 623
▲ Pulmicort Respules (34% to 38%) .. 632
▲ Pulmicort Turbuhaler Inhalation Powder (13% to 32%) 636
▲ Serevent Inhalation Aerosol (4%) 1633
▲ TheraCys Injection (3%) 823
▲ Tikosyn Capsules (7%) 2717
▲ TOBI Solution for Inhalation (5.8%) . 1206
Vascor Tablets (2.84%) 2602
▲ Ventolin HFA Inhalation Aerosol (7%) 3618
Viagra Tablets (Greater than 2%) 2732
Vioxx (Greater than 0.1% to 1.9%) .. 2213

Infection, secondary
Aclovate (Infrequent) 1275
Alrex Sterile Ophthalmic Suspension 0.2% .... ⊙256
Analpram-HC 1338
Anusol-HC Cream 2.5% (Infrequent to frequent) 2237
Anusol-HC Suppositories 2238
Bactroban Cream (Less than 1%) 1494
Blephamide Ophthalmic Ointment ... 547
Blephamide Ophthalmic Suspension 548
Capex Shampoo 1400
Clobevate Gel 3271
Cordran Lotion (More frequent) 2438
Cordran Tape (More frequent) 2439
Cormax Cream (Infrequent) 2440
Cormax Ointment (Infrequent) 2440
Cormax Scalp Application (Infrequent) 2441
Cortisporin Ophthalmic Suspension .... ⊙297
Cutivate Cream (Infrequent) 1282
Cutivate Ointment (Infrequent to more frequent) 1284
Decadron Phosphate Sterile Ophthalmic Ointment 2083
Decadron Phosphate Sterile Ophthalmic Solution 2084
Dermatop Emollient Cream (Infrequent to frequent) 2517
DesOwen (Infrequent) 1401
Diprolene Gel 0.05% (Infrequent) 3107
Diprolene Lotion 0.05% (Infrequent) 3107
Diprolene Ointment 0.05% (Infrequent) 3108
Diprolene AF Cream 0.05% (Infrequent) 3106
Diprosone 3109
Elocon Cream 0.1% (Infrequent) 3110
Elocon Lotion 0.1% (Infrequent) 3111
Elocon Ointment 0.1% (Infrequent) 3112
EryPed 200 & EryPed 400 446
Ery-Tab Tablets 448
Erythrocin Stearate Filmtab Tablets 452
FML Ophthalmic Ointment .... ⊙237
FML Ophthalmic Suspension .... ⊙236
FML Forte Ophthalmic Suspension .... ⊙235

FML-S Liquifilm Sterile Ophthalmic Suspension ⊙ 238
Lidex (Infrequent) 2020
Locoid Cream (Infrequent) 1341
Locoid Lipocream Cream (Infrequent) 1342
Locoid (Infrequent) 1341
Lotemax Sterile Ophthalmic Suspension 0.5% ⊙ 261
Lotrisone 3129
Luxíq Foam 1210
Olux Foam 1211
Pipracil 1866
Poly-Pred Liquifilm Ophthalmic Suspension ⊙ 245
Pramosone 1343
Pred Forte Ophthalmic Suspension ⊙ 246
Pred Mild Sterile Ophthalmic Suspension ⊙ 249
Pred-G Ophthalmic Suspension ⊙ 247
Pred-G Sterile Ophthalmic Ointment ⊙ 248
Prelone Syrup 2273
Proctocort Suppositories 2264
ProctoFoam-HC 3177
Psorcon E Cream 1227
Psorcon E Ointment 1228
Synalar (Infrequent) 2020
Temovate Cream 1301
Temovate Gel (Infrequent) 1303
Temovate Ointment 1301
Temovate Scalp Application (Infrequent) 1304
Temovate E Emollient (Infrequent) 1302
TobraDex Ophthalmic Ointment 542
TobraDex Ophthalmic Suspension 541
Topicort (Infrequent) 2025
Ultravate Cream 1119
Ultravate Ointment 1120
Varivax 2202
Vexol 1% Ophthalmic Suspension ⊙ 222

Infection, Serratia
Alkeran Tablets 1466
Orthoclone OKT3 Sterile Solution (1.6%) 2498

Infection, sinus
Alphagan P Ophthalmic Solution (1% to 4%) 546
▲ Flovent Diskus (9% to 33%) 3614

Infection, skin and soft tissue
AccuNeb Inhalation Solution (Up to 1.7%) 1230
Celebrex Capsules (0.1% to 1.9%) 2676
Celebrex Capsules (0.1% to 1.9%) 2780
Enbrel for Injection 1752
Enbrel for Injection 3504
Flovent Diskus (1% to 3%) 3614
▲ Gengraf Capsules (7%) 457
▲ Protopic Ointment (5% to 12%) 1397
Varivax 2202

Infection, Staphylococcus epidermidis
▲ Orthoclone OKT3 Sterile Solution (4.8%) 2498

Infection, trichomonas vaginalis
Cleocin Vaginal Cream (1%) 2788
Zosyn (1.0% or less) 1890
Zosyn in Galaxy Containers (1.0% or less) 1894

Infection, unspecified
▲ Abelcet Injection (5%) 1273
▲ Accolate Tablets (3.5%) 657
Actiq (1% or greater) 1184
▲ Actonel Tablets (29.9%) 2879
▲ Adderall XR Capsules (4%)
Alkeran for Injection 1465
Aloprim for Injection (Less than 1%) 2292
▲ Alora Transdermal System (17.0% to 18.1%) 3372
Ambien Tablets (1%) 3191
▲ AmBisome for Injection (11.1%) 1383
Amphotec (1% to 5%) 1774
▲ Apligraf (5.4%) 2305
▲ Arava Tablets (4%) 724
▲ Argatroban Injection (3.7%) 1478
Arimidex Tablets (2% to 5%) 659
Arthrotec Tablets (Rare) 3195
Asacol Delayed-Release Tablets (2% or greater) 2884
Atacand HCT Tablets (0.5% or greater) 597
Ativan Injection (Less than 1%) 3478
Avelox Tablets (0.05% to 1%) 879
▲ Avonex (11%) 1013
Axid Pulvules (1.7%) 1903
Axid Pulvules (1.7%) 2919
Betadine Ointment 2894
Betapace Tablets (1% to 4%) 950
Betaseron for SC Injection 988
Betaxon Ophthalmic Suspension (Less than 2%) 537
▲ Campath Ampules (1% to 7%) 992
Cardura Tablets (Less than 0.5%) 2668
▲ Carnitor Injection (10% to 24%) 3242
▲ Casodex Tablets (10%) 662
Ceclor CD Tablets (0.1% to 1%) 1279
▲ CellCept Capsules (12.7% to 25.6%) 2951
▲ CellCept Intravenous (12.7% to 25.6%) 2951
▲ CellCept Oral Suspension (12.7% to 25.6%) 2951
▲ CellCept Tablets (12.7% to 27.1%) 2951
▲ Cenestin Tablets (14%) 1263
Cerebyx Injection (Frequent) 2619
Clozaril Tablets 2319
Colazal Capsules 3069
▲ CombiPatch Transdermal System (3% to 5%) 2323
Compazine 1505
▲ Copaxone for Injection (50%) 3306
Coreg Tablets (2.2%) 1508
Cosmegen for Injection 2062
Coumadin for Injection 1243
Coumadin Tablets 1243
Crinone (Less than 5%) 3213
▲ Cytovene (9%) 2959
▲ Depakote ER Tablets (15%) 436
Detrol Tablets (2.1%) 3623
Doxil Injection (1% to 5%) 566
▲ Duraclon Injection (6%) 3057
▲ Effexor Tablets (2.2% to 6%) 3495
▲ Effexor XR Capsules (10%) 3499
▲ Ellence Injection (1.6% to 21.5%) 2806
▲ Enbrel for Injection (35%) 1752
▲ Enbrel for Injection (35%) 3504
▲ Ergamisol Tablets (5% to 12%) 1789
▲ Esclim Transdermal System (8.5% to 10.4%) 3460
Etrafon 3115
▲ Evista Tablets (15.1%) 1915
Evoxac Capsules (1% to 3%) 1217
Exelon Capsules (2% or more) 2342
Exelon Oral Solution (2% or more) 2345
Felbatol 3343
Feldene Capsules (Occasional) 2685
Ferrlecit Injection (Greater than 1%) 3386
▲ Flolan for Injection (21%) 1528
▲ Flomax Capsules (9.0% to 10.8%) 1044
▲ Fludara for Injection (33% to 44%) 995
▲ Foscavir Injection (5% or greater) 605
▲ Gabitril Tablets (1% to 19%) 1189
▲ Gemzar for Injection (3% to 16%) 1919
▲ Gengraf Capsules (1% to 24.7%) 457
▲ Gliadel Wafer (4% to 9%) 1723
▲ Herceptin I.V. (20%) 1414
Hivid Tablets (Less than 1%) 2975
▲ Hycamtin for Injection (26%) 1546
▲ Idamycin PFS Injection (95%) 2825
▲ Ifex for Injection (8%) 1123
▲ Indapamide Tablets (Greater than or equal to 5%) 2286
Infergen (2% to 3%) 1777
Innohep Injection (Greater than or equal to 1%) 1248
Intron A for Injection (Less than 5%) 3120
▲ Keppra Tablets (13%) 3314
▲ Lamictal (4.4%) 1567
▲ Leukine (65%) 1755
▲ Leustatin Injection (28%) 2495
▲ Lipitor Tablets (2.8% to 10.3%) 2639
▲ Lipitor Tablets (2.8% to 10.3%) 2696
Lodine (Less than 1%) 3528
Lodine XL Extended-Release Tablets (Less than 1%) 3530
Lotensin Tablets (Less than 1%) 2365
Lotensin HCT Tablets (0.3% or more) 2367
▲ Lupron Depot 7.5 mg (5.4%) 3284
Lupron Depot-PED 7.5 mg, 11.25 mg and 15 mg (Less than 2%) 3291
Lupron Injection (Less than 5%) 3279
Lupron Injection Pediatric (Less than 2%) 3280
Luvox Tablets (25, 50, 100 mg) 3256
Megace Oral Suspension (1% to 3%) 1124
▲ Mepron Suspension (18% to 22%) 1598
Miacalcin Nasal Spray (1% to 3%) 2375
Micardis Tablets (More than 0.3%) 1049
Micardis HCT Tablets 1051
Monurol Sachet (Less than 1%) 1375
Myleran Tablets 1603
▲ Mylotarg for Injection (28%) 3540
▲ Myobloc Injectable Solution (13% to 19%) 1291
▲ Naprelan Tablets (3% to 9%) 1293
Nasacort AQ Nasal Spray 752
Nascobal Gel (Three patients) 3174
▲ Neoral Soft Gelatin Capsules (1% to 24.7%) 2380
▲ Neoral Oral Solution (1% to 24.7%) 2380
▲ Neumega for Injection (Greater than or equal to 10%) 1434
▲ Nipent for Injection (7% to 36%) 3272
▲ Novantrone for Injection (60% to 66%) 1760
Orgaran Injection (2.1%) 2480
Orudis Capsules (Less than 1%) 3548
Oruvail Capsules (Less than 1%) 3548
▲ Paraplatin for Injection (5% to 16%) 1126
▲ Paxil (6%) 1609
PEG-Intron Powder for Injection (Less than or equal to 1%) 3140
Periostat Tablets (2%) 1208
Permax Tablets (1.1%) 1299
▲ Pletal Tablets (10% to 14%) 2605
▲ Pletal Tablets (10% to 14%) 2848
Ponstel Capsules (Occasional) 1356
Prelone Syrup 2273
▲ Prempro Tablets (16%) 3572
Prevacid Delayed-Release Capsules (Less than 1%) 3292
PREVPAC (Less than 1%) 3298
▲ Prograf (45%) 1393
▲ Proleukin for Injection (13%) 1199
Protonix I.V. (Greater than or equal to 1%) 3580
Protonix Tablets (Greater than or equal to 1%) 3577
▲ Protopic Ointment (1% to 14%) 1397
Provigil Tablets (At least 1%) 1193
Prozac Pulvules, Liquid, and Weekly Capsules (Less than 1%) 1238
Pulmicort Respules (1% to 3%) 632
Pulmicort Turbuhaler Inhalation Powder (1% to 3%) 636
▲ Rapamune Oral Solution and Tablets (3% to 20%) 3584
Refludan for Injection (1.8%) 761
Regranex Gel 2586
Remicade for IV Injection (Less than 2%) 1178
▲ Renagel Capsules (15%) 1439
▲ Renagel Tablets (15%) 1439
Repronex for Intramuscular and Subcutaneous Injection (1%) 1347
Rescriptor Tablets 526
Roxicodone Tablets (Less than 3%) 3067
Salagen Tablets (2%) 2229
▲ Sarafem Pulvules (7%) 1962
Serentil 1057
▲ Serostim for Injection (1% to 10%) 3229
▲ Serzone Tablets (8%) 1104
▲ Simulect for Injection (3% to 10%) 2399
Skelid Tablets (2.7%) 3088
▲ Soriatane Capsules (1% to 10%) 3003
Sporanox Oral Solution (Less than 2%) 1808
Sporanox Oral Solution (Less than 2%) 2512
Stelazine 1640
Synercid I.V. (Less than 1%) 775
Tasmar Tablets (Frequent) 3010
▲ Taxol Injection (30%) 1129
Taxotere for Injection Concentrate 778
▲ Thalomid Capsules (6.3% to 8.3%) 1154
▲ TheraCys Injection (3%) 823
▲ Thymoglobulin for Injection (17.1%) 3071
Tiazac Capsules (2%) 1378
Toradol (1% or less) 3018
▲ Trasylol Injection (6%) 909
Travatan Ophthalmic Solution (1% to 5%) 543
▲ Tricor Capsules, Micronized (18%) 513
Trileptal Oral Suspension (Up to 2%) 2407
Trileptal Tablets (Up to 2%) 2407
Uniretic Tablets (More than 1%) 3178
Valcyte Tablets (Less than 5%) 3022
▲ Verelan PM Capsules (12.1%) 3186
▲ Vesanoid Capsules (58%) 3037
▲ Vicoprofen Tablets (3% to 9%) 520
Vioxx (Greater than 0.1% to 1.9%) 2213
▲ Vistide Injection (12% to 28%) 1445
▲ Vitravene for Injection (5% to 20%) ⊙ 310
Warfarin Sodium Tablets, USP 3302
▲ WelChol Tablets (10%) 3073
Wellbutrin Tablets (Rare) 1680
▲ Wellbutrin SR Sustained-Release Tablets (8% to 9%) 1684
Xanax Tablets (1.3%) 2865
Yasmin 28 Tablets (Greater than 1%) 980
▲ Zanaflex Tablets (6%) 1305
▲ Zinecard for Injection (19% to 23%) 2869
▲ Zoladex (13%) 702
Zoladex 3-month 706
▲ Zometa for Intravenous Infusion (5% to 10%) 3621

Infection, upper respiratory tract
Accuretic Tablets (1.3%) 2614
▲ Aceon Tablets (2 mg, 4 mg, 8 mg) (8.6%) 3249
▲ Activella Tablets (10% to 18%) 2764
▲ Actos Tablets (13.2%) 3275
▲ Advair Diskus 100/50 (27%) 1448
▲ Advair Diskus 250/50 (21%) 1448
▲ Advair Diskus 500/50 (21% to 27%) 1448
▲ Aerobid/Aerobid-M (25%) 1363
Aggrenox Capsules (1%) 1026
▲ Allegra (3.2% to 4.3%) 712
Allegra-D Extended-Release Tablets (1.4%) 714
Altace Capsules 2233
▲ Ambien Tablets (5%) 3191
▲ Aredia for Injection (24.1%) 2309
▲ Atacand Tablets (6%) 595
▲ Atacand HCT Tablets (3.6%) 597
▲ Atrovent Inhalation Solution (13.2%) 1031
▲ Atrovent Nasal Spray 0.03% (9.8%) 1032
Avalide Tablets (1% or greater) 1070
▲ Avandia Tablets (7.3% to 9.9%) 1490
▲ Avapro Tablets (9%) 1074
▲ Avapro Tablets (9%) 3076
▲ Avonex (31%) 1013
Betapace AF Tablets (2.6% to 3.3%) 954
▲ Botox Purified Neurotoxin Complex (12%) 549
▲ Caverject Sterile Powder (4%) 2777
Ceftin for Oral Suspension (0.1% to 1%) 1898
▲ Celebrex Capsules (8.1%) 2676
▲ Celebrex Capsules (8.1%) 2780
▲ Celexa (5%) 1365
Claritin (2%) 3100
Claritin-D 12 Hour Extended Release Tablets (Less frequent) 3102
Claritin-D 24 Hour Extended Release Tablets 3104
▲ Cleocin Vaginal Cream (3%) 2788
▲ Cognex Capsules (3%) 1351
▲ Combivent Inhalation Aerosol (10.9%) 1041
Comvax (0.5% to 1.3%) 2056
▲ Concerta Extended-Release Tablets (8%) 1998
▲ Concerta Tablets (8%) 561
▲ Coreg Tablets (18.3%) 1508
Cosopt Sterile Ophthalmic Solution (1% to 5%) 2065
▲ Covera-HS Tablets (5.4%) 3199
▲ Cozaar Tablets (7.9%) 2067
▲ Crinone (5%) 3213
Crixivan Capsules (Less than 2%) 2070
Cytotec Tablets (Infrequent) 3202
DDAVP Nasal Spray 738
DDAVP Rhinal Tube 738
▲ Detrol Tablets (5.9%) 3623
Diovan Capsules (More than 1%) 2337
Diovan HCT Tablets (More than 2%) 2338
Dipentum Capsules (1.5%) 2803
Ditropan XL Extended Release Tablets (2% to 5%) 564
DuoNeb Inhalation Solution 1233
Enalaprilat Injection 863
▲ Enbrel for Injection (31%) 1752
▲ Enbrel for Injection (31%) 3504
▲ Epogen for Injection (11%) 582
▲ Estring Vaginal Ring (5%) 2811
▲ Evoxac Capsules (11.4%) 1217
Exelon Capsules (2% or more) 2342
Exelon Oral Solution (2% or more) 2345
Famvir Tablets (0.7% to 3.3%) 2348
▲ Felbatol (5.3% to 45.2%) 3343
▲ femhrt Tablets (3.9%) 2635
▲ Ferrlecit Injection (6%) 3386
▲ Flovent Diskus (20% to 31%) 3614
▲ Flovent (15% to 31%) 1535
▲ Flovent Rotadisk (16% to 22%) 1537
▲ Fludara for Injection (2% to 16%) 995
Fortovase Capsules (Less than 2%) 2970
▲ Gengraf Capsules (7.7%) 457
▲ Geodon Capsules (8%) 2688
Glucophage XR Tablets (1% to 5%) 1080
▲ Glucovance Tablets (17.3%) 1086
▲ Gonal-F for Injection (11.9%) 3216
Havrix Vaccine (Less than 1%) 1544
Herceptin I.V. 1414
▲ Hyzaar (6.1%) 2109
▲ Infergen (16% to 31%) 1777
Invirase Capsules (Less than 2%) 2979
Ismo Tablets (Fewer than 1%) 3524
▲ Klonopin Tablets (8%) 2983
▲ Lescol Capsules (16.2%) 2361
▲ Lescol Capsules (16.2%) 2925
▲ Lescol XL Tablets (12.5%) 2361
▲ Lescol XL Tablets (12.5%) 2925
Lexxel Tablets (Infrequent) 608
Lodosyn Tablets 1251
Lotensin HCT Tablets (More than 1%) 2367
▲ Lumigan Ophthalmic Solution (Approximately 10%) 553
▲ Luvox Tablets (25, 50, 100 mg) (9%) 3256
▲ LYMErix Vaccine (2.8% to 4.35%) 1592
Malarone (Less than 1% to 5%) 1596
Mavik Tablets (0.3% to 1.0%) 478
Maxalt Tablets (Infrequent) 2120
Maxalt-MLT Orally Disintegrating Tablets (Infrequent) 2120
Miacalcin Nasal Spray (1% to 3%) 2375
▲ Micardis Tablets (7%) 1049
▲ Micardis HCT Tablets (8%) 1051
Migranal Nasal Spray (Infrequent) 2376
▲ Mirena Intrauterine System (5% or more) 974
Mobic Tablets (0.2% to 8.3%) 1054
Monopril Tablets (2.2%) 1091
Monopril HCT (2.3%) 1094
▲ Nasonex Nasal Spray (5% to 6%) 3131
▲ Neoral Soft Gelatin Capsules (7.7%) 2380
▲ Neoral Oral Solution (7.7%) 2380

Neurontin Oral Solution (More than 2%)....2655
▲ Nilandron Tablets (8.1%)....753
▲ Nipent for Injection (13% to 16%)....3272
▲ Novantrone for Injection (51% to 53%)....1760
Oncaspar (Less than 1%)....756
▲ Ortho-Prefest Tablets (21%)....2570
Ovidrel for Injection (Less than 2%)....3220
▲ Liquid PedvaxHIB (Among most frequent)....2148
▲ Plavix Tablets (8.7%)....1097
▲ Plavix Tablets (8.7%)....3084
Plendil Extended-Release Tablets (0.7% to 3.9%)....623
▲ Prandin Tablets (0.5, 1, and 2 mg) (10% to 16%)....2432
Prevacid Delayed-Release Capsules (Less than 1%)....3292
PREVPAC (Less than 1%)....3298
Prilosec Delayed-Release Capsules (1.9%)....628
Prinivil Tablets (1.2% to 1.5%)....2164
Prinzide Tablets (2.2%)....2168
Procardia XL Extended Release Tablets (1% or less)....2710
▲ Procrit for Injection (11%)....2502
▲ Prometrium Capsules (100 mg, 200 mg) (5%)....3261
Protonix I.V. (Greater than or equal to 1%)....3580
Protonix Tablets (Greater than or equal to 1%)....3577
▲ Proventil HFA Inhalation Aerosol (21%)....3150
▲ Qvar Inhalation Aerosol (5% to 11%)....1987
▲ Rapamune Oral Solution and Tablets (23% to 26%)....3584
Recombivax HB (Equal to or greater than 1%)....2178
ReFacto Vials....1437
▲ Relenza Rotadisk (1% to 5%)....1619
▲ Remicade for IV Injection (16% to 26%)....1178
Reminyl Oral Solution (Greater than or equal to 2%)....1792
Reminyl Tablets (Greater than or equal to 2%)....1792
Requip Tablets (1% or more)....1621
Rescriptor Tablets (Less than 2%)....526
▲ Risperdal (3%)....1796
Rowasa Rectal Suspension Enema 4.0 grams/unit (60 mL) (1.8%)....3264
▲ Serevent Diskus (Greater than 3%)....1637
▲ Serevent Inhalation Aerosol (9% to 14%)....1633
▲ Serostim for Injection (1% to 10%)....3229
▲ Simulect for Injection (Greater than or equal to 10%)....2399
Sinemet Tablets....1253
Sinemet CR Tablets (1.8%)....1255
▲ Skelid Tablets (5.3%)....3088
▲ Sporanox Capsules (8%)....1800
Sporanox Oral Solution (Less than 2%)....1808
Sporanox Oral Solution (Less than 2%)....2512
▲ Stadol NS Nasal Spray (3% to 9%)....1108
▲ Starlix Tablets (10.5%)....2401
Stimate Nasal Spray....796
▲ Synagis Intramuscular (52.6%)....2028
Tarka Tablets (0.3% to 5.4%)....508
▲ Tasmar Tablets (5% to 7%)....3010
Taxol Injection....1129
▲ Temodar Capsules (8%)....3157
▲ Teveten Tablets (8%)....3327
Thalomid Capsules....1154
Timolol GFS (1% to 5%)....⊙266
Timoptic in Ocudose (Less frequent)....2192
Timoptic Sterile Ophthalmic Solution (Less frequent)....2190
Timoptic-XE Sterile Ophthalmic Gel Forming Solution (1% to 5%)....2194
▲ Topamax Sprinkle Capsules (12.1% to 12.4%)....2590
▲ Topamax Tablets (12.1% to 12.4%)....2590
▲ Trileptal Oral Suspension (5% to 10%)....2407
▲ Trileptal Tablets (5% to 10%)....2407
▲ Trisenox Injection (13%)....1158
Trovan (Less than 1%)....2722
▲ Twinrix Vaccine (1% to 10%)....1674
Uniretic Tablets (More than 1%)....3178
Univasc Tablets (More than 1%)....3181
▲ Vagifem Tablets (5% to 11%)....2857
Vanceril Double Strength Inhalation Aerosol (Fewer than 2%)....3167
Vaqta (1.1% to 2.7%)....2199
Vaseretic Tablets....2204
Vasotec I.V. Injection....2207
Vasotec Tablets (0.5% to 1.0%)....2210
▲ Verelan PM Capsules (12.1%)....3186
▲ Vioxx (7.8%)....2213
▲ Xalatan Latanoprost Ophthalmic Solution (Approximately 4%)....⊙320
▲ Xalatan Sterile Ophthalmic Solution (Approximately 4%)....2864
▲ Xanax Tablets (4.3%)....2865
Xeloda Tablets (Less than 5%)....3039
▲ Xenical Capsules (26.1% to 38.1%)....3043
Yasmin 28 Tablets....980
▲ Zebeta Tablets (4.8% to 5.0%)....1885
Zestoretic Tablets (2.2%)....695
Zestril Tablets (1.5% to 2.0%)....698
Ziac Tablets (Up to 2.1%)....1887
Zocor Tablets (2.1%)....2219
▲ Zoladex (7%)....702
Zoladex 3-month....706
Zoloft (Infrequent)....2751
Zyrtec (Less than 2%)....2756
Zyrtec-D 12 Hour Extended Relief Tablets (Less than 2%)....2758

Infection, urinary tract

Accupril Tablets (0.5% to 1%)....2611
Aceon Tablets (2 mg, 4 mg, 8 mg) (2.8%)....3249
Actiq (Less than 1%)....1184
▲ Actonel Tablets (10.9%)....2879
Aloprim for Injection (Less than 1%)....2292
Ambien Tablets (2%)....3191
Androderm Transdermal System CIII (Less than 1%)....3377
Apligraf (1.3% to 2.7%)....2305
▲ Arava Tablets (5%)....724
▲ Aredia for Injection (18.5%)....2309
▲ Argatroban Injection (4.6%)....1478
Arimidex Tablets (2% to 5%)....659
Aromasin Tablets (Less frequent)....2769
Arthrotec Tablets (Rare)....3195
Atacand HCT Tablets (0.5% or greater)....597
Atrovent Inhalation Solution (Less than 3%)....1031
Avalide Tablets (1% or greater)....1070
Avapro Tablets (1% or greater)....1074
Avapro Tablets (1% or greater)....3076
Azmacort Inhalation Aerosol (1% to 3%)....728
Azulfidine EN-tabs Tablets....2775
Baycol Tablets (1.6%)....883
Campath Ampules....992
Cardura Tablets (1.4%)....2668
Carnitor Injection (2% to 3%)....3242
▲ Casodex Tablets (6%)....662
Ceftin for Oral Suspension (0.1% to 1%)....1898
Celebrex Capsules (0.1% to 1.9%)....2676
Celebrex Capsules (0.1% to 1.9%)....2780
▲ CellCept Capsules (13.1% to 45.5%)....2951
▲ CellCept Intravenous (13.1% to 45.5%)....2951
▲ CellCept Oral Suspension (13.1% to 45.5%)....2951
▲ CellCept Tablets (13.1% to 45.5%)....2951
Chirocaine Injection (1%)....2909
Claritin-D 24 Hour Extended Release Tablets (Fewer than 2%)....3104
▲ Cleocin Vaginal Cream (8%)....2788
▲ Cognex Capsules (3%)....1351
Combivent Inhalation Aerosol (Less than 2%)....1041
Coreg Tablets (1.8% to 3.1%)....1508
Corlopam Injection (1% to 2%)....412
Cosopt Sterile Ophthalmic Solution (1% to 5%)....2065
Cozaar Tablets (Less than 1%)....2067
▲ Crinone (5%)....3213
Crixivan Capsules (Less than 2%)....2070
Cytotec Tablets (Infrequent)....3202
Depacon Injection....416
Depakene....421
Depakote Sprinkle Capsules....426
Depakote Tablets....430
Depakote ER Tablets....436
Depo-Provera Contraceptive Injection (Fewer than 1%)....2798
▲ Detrol Tablets (5.5%)....3623
Diovan HCT Tablets (Greater than 0.2%)....2338
▲ Ditropan XL Extended Release Tablets (5.1%)....564
Doxil Injection (Less than 1%)....566
DuoNeb Inhalation Solution (1.6%)....1233
▲ Duraclon Injection (22%)....3057
Effexor Tablets....3495
Enalaprilat Injection....863
Enbrel for Injection....1752
Enbrel for Injection....3504
▲ Epogen for Injection (3% to 12%)....582
Ergamisol Tablets (1 out of 463 patients)....1789
Estring Vaginal Ring (2%)....2811
▲ Evista Tablets (4%)....1915
▲ Evoxac Capsules (6.1%)....1217
▲ Exelon Capsules (7%)....2342
▲ Exelon Oral Solution (7%)....2345
▲ Felbatol (3.4%)....3343
▲ femhrt Tablets (6.2%)....2635
Ferrlecit Injection (Greater than 1%)....3386
▲ Flolan for Injection (7%)....1528
Flovent Diskus (1% to 3%)....3614
▲ Fludara for Injection (2% to 15%)....995
Fortovase Capsules (Less than 2%)....2970
Foscavir Injection (Between 1% and 5%)....605
Gabitril Tablets (1% or more)....1189
▲ Gengraf Capsules (3% to 21.1%)....457
Gliadel Wafer (2%)....1723
Gonal-F for Injection (1.7%)....3216
▲ Herceptin I.V. (5%)....1414
Hytrin Capsules (0.5% to 1.3%)....464
Hyzaar....2109
Imdur Tablets (Less than or equal to 5%)....1826
Imitrex Injection....1549
Imitrex Nasal Spray....1554
▲ Innohep Injection (3.7%)....1248
Intron A for Injection (Less than 5% to 5%)....3120
Invirase Capsules (Less than 2%)....2979
Keppra Tablets (1% or more)....3314
Klonopin Tablets (1%)....2983
Lamictal (More than 1%)....1567
Lescol Capsules (1.6%)....2361
Lescol Capsules (1.6%)....2925
Lescol XL Tablets (2.7%)....2361
Lescol XL Tablets (2.7%)....2925
Lexxel Tablets (Infrequent)....608
Lipitor Tablets (Greater than or equal to 2%)....2639
Lipitor Tablets (Greater than or equal to 2%)....2696
Lodosyn Tablets....1251
Lopid Tablets (More common)....2650
Lotensin Tablets (Less than 1%)....2365
Lotensin HCT Tablets (0.3% or more)....2367
Lupron Depot 7.5 mg (Less than 5%)....3284
Lupron Depot–4 Month 30 mg (Less than 5%)....3289
▲ Lupron Injection (5% or more)....3279
Luvox Tablets (25, 50, 100 mg) (Infrequent)....3256
Megace Oral Suspension (1% to 3%)....1124
Meridia Capsules (2.3%)....481
Micardis Tablets (1%)....1049
Micardis HCT Tablets (2% or greater)....1051
Mirapex Tablets (1% or more)....2834
Mobic Tablets (0.3% to 4.7%)....1054
Monopril HCT (Less than 2%)....1094
Myobloc Injectable Solution (2% or greater)....1291
▲ Naprelan Tablets (3% to 9%)....1293
Naropin Injection (Less than 1%)....612
▲ Neoral Soft Gelatin Capsules (3% to 21.1%)....2380
▲ Neoral Oral Solution (3% to 21.1%)....2380
▲ Nilandron Tablets (8.6%)....753
▲ Nipent for Injection (3%)....3272
▲ Novantrone for Injection (7% to 32%)....1760
Orgaran Injection (2.6% to 4.0%)....2480
Ortho Diaphragm Kits – All-Flex Arcing Spring; Ortho Coil Spring....2552
Ovidrel for Injection (Less than 2%)....3220
Paxil (2%)....1609
Permax Tablets (2.7%)....1299
▲ Photofrin for Injection (7%)....831
▲ Plavix Tablets (3.1%)....1097
▲ Plavix Tablets (3.1%)....3084
Pletal Tablets (2% or greater)....2605
Pletal Tablets (2% or greater)....2848
Prandin Tablets (0.5, 1, and 2 mg) (2% to 3%)....2432
Prevnar for Injection....1870
Prilosec Delayed-Release Capsules (Less than 1%)....628
Prinivil Tablets (0.3% to 1.0%)....2164
Prinzide Tablets (0.3% to 1%)....2168
▲ Procrit for Injection (3% to 12%)....2502
▲ Prograf (16% to 34%)....1393
▲ Proleukin for Injection (23%)....1199
Prometrium Capsules (100 mg, 200 mg) (Less than 5%)....3261
Protonix I.V. (Greater than or equal to 1%)....3580
Protonix Tablets (Greater than or equal to 1%)....3577
▲ Proventil HFA Inhalation Aerosol (3%)....3150
Provigil Tablets (At least 1%)....1193
▲ Rapamune Oral Solution and Tablets (23% to 33%)....3584
Remeron Tablets (Frequent)....2483
Remeron SolTab Tablets (Frequent)....2486
▲ Remicade for IV Injection (3% to 26%)....1178
▲ Reminyl Oral Solution (8%)....1792
▲ Reminyl Tablets (8%)....1792
ReoPro Vials (1.9%)....1958
▲ Requip Tablets (5%)....1621
Rescriptor Tablets....526
Rilutek Tablets (2.5% to 4.5%)....772
Roferon-A Injection (Infrequent)....2996
Rowasa Rectal Suspension Enema 4.0 grams/unit (60 mL) (0.61%)....3264
Roxicodone Tablets (Less than 3%)....3067
Salagen Tablets (1% to 2%)....2229
▲ Sandimmune (20.2% to 21.1%)....2388
Sandostatin Injection (1% to 4%)....2394
▲ Sandostatin LAR Depot (5% to 15%)....2395
Serevent Inhalation Aerosol (1% to 3%)....1633
▲ Serostim for Injection (1% to 10%)....3229
Serzone Tablets (2%)....1104
▲ Simulect for Injection (Greater than or equal to 10%)....2399
Sinemet Tablets....1253
Sinemet CR Tablets (2.2%)....1255
Skelid Tablets (More than or equal to 1%)....3088
▲ Sporanox Capsules (3%)....1800
▲ Tasmar Tablets (5%)....3010
Taxol Injection....1129
▲ Temodar Capsules (8%)....3157
▲ Testoderm Transdermal Systems (4%)....574
Teveten Tablets (1%)....3327
▲ TheraCys Injection (18%)....823
▲ Thymoglobulin for Injection (18.3%)....3071
Tice BCG, BCG Live (1.5%)....2489
Tikosyn Capsules (Greater than 2%)....2717
Tolectin (1% to 3%)....2589
Topamax Sprinkle Capsules (Frequent)....2590
Topamax Tablets (Frequent)....2590
Trasylol Injection (2%)....909
Travatan Ophthalmic Solution (1% to 5%)....543
Trileptal Oral Suspension (1% to 5%)....2407
Trileptal Tablets (1% to 5%)....2407
Uniretic Tablets (More than 1%)....3178
▲ Valstar Sterile Solution for Intravesical Instillation (15%)....1175
Vanceril Double Strength Inhalation Aerosol (Fewer than 2%)....3167
Vaseretic Tablets (0.5% to 2.0%)....2204
Vasotec I.V. Injection....2207
Vasotec Tablets (1.3%)....2210
Viadur Implant (Less than 2%)....912
▲ Viagra Tablets (3%)....2732
Vioxx (2.7%)....2213
Vistide Injection....1445
Wellbutrin Tablets (Infrequent)....1680
Wellbutrin SR Sustained-Release Tablets (Up to 1%)....1684
Xeloda Tablets (Less than 5%)....3039
▲ Xenical Capsules (5.9% to 7.5%)....3043
Yasmin 28 Tablets....980
▲ Zanaflex Tablets (10%)....1305
Zestoretic Tablets (0.3% to 1%)....695
Zestril Tablets (0.3% to 1.0%)....698
Zoladex (1% to 5%)....702
Zoladex 3-month (1% to 5%)....706
▲ Zometa for Intravenous Infusion (14.1%)....3621
Zyflo Filmtab Tablets (Less common)....524
Zyprexa Tablets (Frequent)....1973
Zyprexa ZYDIS Orally Disintegrating Tablets (Frequent)....1973
Zyrtec (Less than 2%)....2756
Zyrtec-D 12 Hour Extended Relief Tablets (Less than 2%)....2758

Infection, urinary tract, fungal

Nexium Delayed-Release Capsules (Less than 1%)....619

Infection, vagina

Cleocin Vaginal Ovules (Less than 1%)....2789
Clozaril Tablets (Less than 1%)....2319
Modicon....2563
Norplant System (Uncommon)....3543
Ortho-Cyclen/Ortho Tri-Cyclen....2573
Ortho-Novum....2563
Ortho-Novum 1/50□28 Tablets....2556
Ortho-Novum....2563
Ortho-Cyclen/Ortho Tri-Cyclen....2573

Infection, viral

Accupril Tablets (0.5% to 1.0%)....2611
Accuretic Tablets (1.9%)....2614
Aceon Tablets (2 mg, 4 mg, 8 mg) (0.3% to 3.4%)....3249
Actiq (1% or greater)....1184
Activella Tablets (0% to 6%)....2764
Adderall XR Capsules (2%)
▲ Advair Diskus 100/50 (4%)....1448
▲ Advair Diskus 250/50 (4%)....1448
▲ Advair Diskus 500/50 (4%)....1448
Allegra (2.5%)....712
Apligraf (1.8%)....2305
Astelin Nasal Spray (Infrequent)....3339
Atacand HCT Tablets (0.5% or greater)....597
Blephamide Ophthalmic Ointment....547
Blephamide Ophthalmic Suspension....548
Campath Ampules....992
Celebrex Capsules (0.1% to 1.9%)....2676

Celebrex Capsules (0.1% to 1.9%) ... 2780
Claritin (At least one patient) ... 3100
Claritin-D 12 Hour Extended Release Tablets (Less frequent) ... 3102
Claritin-D 24 Hour Extended Release Tablets (Fewer than 2%) ... 3104
Colazal Capsules ... 3069
Coreg Tablets (1.8% to more than 2%) ... 1508
Cortisporin Ophthalmic Suspension ... ⊙297
Depakote ER Tablets (1% to 5%) ... 436
▲ Diovan Capsules (3%) ... 2337
▲ Diovan HCT Tablets (3%) ... 2338
Enbrel for Injection ... 1752
Enbrel for Injection ... 3504
Evoxac Capsules (Less than 1%) ... 1217
▲ Femara Tablets (5% to 6%) ... 2351
▲ femhrt Tablets (7%) ... 2635
Flovent Diskus (2%) ... 3614
FML Ophthalmic Ointment ... ⊙237
FML Ophthalmic Suspension ... ⊙236
FML Forte Ophthalmic Suspension ... ⊙235
▲ Foradil Aerolizer (17.2%) ... 2354
▲ Gengraf Capsules (1% to 15.9%) ... 457
Imdur Tablets (Less than or equal to 5%) ... 1826
▲ Intron A for Injection (Less than 5% to 7%) ... 3120
Kaletra Capsules (Less than 2%) ... 471
Kaletra Oral Solution (Less than 2%) ... 471
Klonopin Tablets (Infrequent) ... 2983
Koāte-HP ... 932
Konÿne 80 ... 937
▲ Leustatin Injection (20%) ... 2495
Lopid Tablets (More common) ... 2650
LYMErix Vaccine (2.19% to 2.83%) ... 1592
Monopril HCT (Less than 2%) ... 1094
Myobloc Injectable Solution (2% or greater) ... 1291
▲ Nasonex Nasal Spray (8% to 14%) ... 3131
▲ Neoral Soft Gelatin Capsules (1% to 15.9%) ... 2380
▲ Neoral Oral Solution (1% to 15.9%) ... 2380
▲ Neurontin Capsules (1% to 10.9%) ... 2655
▲ Neurontin Oral Solution (1% to 10.9%) ... 2655
▲ Neurontin Tablets (1% to 10.9%) ... 2655
▲ Nipent for Injection (Up to 8%) ... 3272
Orthoclone OKT3 Sterile Solution (1.5%) ... 2498
▲ Ortho-Prefest Tablets (6%) ... 2570
▲ PEG-Intron Powder for Injection (11%) ... 3140
Prinivil Tablets (0.3% to 1.0%) ... 2164
Prinzide Tablets (0.3% to 1%) ... 2168
Prolastin ... 943
▲ Prometrium Capsules (100 mg, 200 mg) (7% to 12%) ... 3261
▲ Pulmicort Respules (3% to 5%) ... 632
▲ Requip Tablets (11%) ... 1621
Rescriptor Tablets ... 526
Rituxan for Infusion ... 1750
Rituxan I.V. ... 1428
Salagen Tablets (Less than 1%) ... 2229
▲ Sandimmune (15.9% to 18.4%) ... 2388
▲ Sandostatin LAR Depot (5% to 15%) ... 2395
▲ Serostim for Injection (1% to 10%) ... 3229
▲ Simulect for Injection (Greater than or equal to 10%) ... 2399
Singulair (Greater than or equal to 2%) ... 2181
Synagis Intramuscular (More than 1%) ... 2028
Tasmar Tablets (Infrequent) ... 3010
▲ Temodar Capsules (11%) ... 3157
Teveten Tablets (2%) ... 3327
Thalomid Capsules ... 1154
▲ Trileptal Oral Suspension (5% to 7%) ... 2407
▲ Trileptal Tablets (5% to 7%) ... 2407
▲ Vanceril Double Strength Inhalation Aerosol (8%) ... 3167
▲ Ventolin HFA Inhalation Aerosol (7%) ... 3618
Vioxx (Greater than 0.1% to 1.9%) ... 2213
Voltaren Ophthalmic Sterile Ophthalmic Solution (Less than 3%) ... ⊙312
▲ Xopenex Inhalation Solution (6.9% to 12.3%) ... 3207
Zenapax for Injection ... 3046
Zestoretic Tablets (0.3% to 1%) ... 695
Zestril Tablets (0.3% to 1.0%) ... 698

Infection, wound
▲ Apligraf (13.4%) ... 2305

Infection, yersinia
Desferal Vials (Rare) ... 2333

Infection at injection site
▲ Cytovene-IV (9%) ... 2959
▲ Valcyte Tablets (3%) ... 3022

Infectious disorders, life-threatening, aggravation of
Roferon-A Injection ... 2996

Infectious-mononucleosis-like syndrome
Dapsone Tablets USP ... 1780

Infertility
Cytovene ... 2959
Leukeran Tablets ... 1591
Levoxyl Tablets ... 1819
Lo/Ovral Tablets ... 3532
Lo/Ovral-28 Tablets ... 3538
Low-Ogestrel-28 Tablets ... 3392
Nordette-28 Tablets ... 2257
Ogestrel 0.5/50-28 Tablets ... 3428
Ovral Tablets ... 3551
Ovral-28 Tablets ... 3552
Ovrette Tablets ... 3552
ParaGard T 380A Intrauterine Copper Contraceptive ... 2582
Unithroid Tablets ... 3445

Infertility, male
Azulfidine EN-tabs Tablets ... 2775
Dapsone Tablets USP ... 1780

Infertility, temporary
Alesse-21 Tablets ... 3468
Alesse-28 Tablets ... 3473
Brevicon 28-Day Tablets ... 3380
Cyclessa Tablets ... 2450
Desogen Tablets ... 2458
Estrostep ... 2627
Levlen ... 962
Levlite 21 Tablets ... 962
Levlite 28 Tablets ... 962
Levora Tablets ... 3389
Loestrin 21 Tablets ... 2642
Loestrin Fe Tablets ... 2642
Lunelle Monthly Injection ... 2827
Microgestin Fe 1.5/30 Tablets ... 3407
Microgestin Fe 1/20 Tablets ... 3400
Mircette Tablets ... 2470
Modicon ... 2563
Necon ... 3415
Norinyl 1 +35 28-Day Tablets ... 3380
Norinyl 1 + 50 28-Day Tablets ... 3380
Ortho-Cept 21 Tablets ... 2546
Ortho-Cept 28 Tablets ... 2546
Ortho-Cyclen/Ortho Tri-Cyclen ... 2573
Ortho-Novum ... 2563
Ortho-Novum 1/50□28 Tablets ... 2556
Ortho-Novum ... 2563
Ortho-Cyclen/Ortho Tri-Cyclen ... 2573
Ovcon ... 3364
Tri-Levlen ... 962
Tri-Norinyl-28 Tablets ... 3433
Triphasil-21 Tablets ... 3600
Triphasil-28 Tablets ... 3605
Trivora Tablets ... 3439
Yasmin 28 Tablets ... 980
Zovia ... 3449

Inflammation, genital
▲ Condylox Topical Solution (71% to 63%) ... 2437
Tice BCG, BCG Live (1.8%) ... 2489

Inflammation, nasal
Imitrex Nasal Spray ... 1554

Inflammation, ocular
▲ Acular Ophthalmic Solution (1% to 10%) ... 544
▲ Acular PF Ophthalmic Solution (Approximately 1% to 10%) ... 544
Betoptic S Ophthalmic Suspension (Small number of patients) ... 537
Enbrel for Injection ... 1752
Enbrel for Injection ... 3504
Iopidine Sterile Ophthalmic Solution (Less than 2%) ... ⊙212
Rilutek Tablets (Infrequent) ... 772
Tasmar Tablets (1%) ... 3010
▲ Vitravene for Injection (1 in 4 patients) ... ⊙310
Zyprexa Tablets (Infrequent) ... 1973
Zyprexa ZYDIS Orally Disintegrating Tablets (Infrequent) ... 1973

Inflammation, oral
(*see under* Stomatitis)

Inflammation, unspecified
Amvisc Plus (Rare) ... ⊙329
Ceptaz for Injection (1 in 69 patients) ... 1499
Floxin Otic Solution (Single report) ... 1219
Fluoroplex ... 552
Klonopin Tablets (Infrequent) ... 2983
Lupron Injection (Less than 5%) ... 3279
ParaGard T 380A Intrauterine Copper Contraceptive ... 2582
Permax Tablets ... 1299
Prilosec Delayed-Release Capsules (Less than 1%) ... 628
Procardia Capsules (2% or less) ... 2708
ReoPro Vials (0.1%) ... 1958
Zestoretic Tablets (0.3% to 1%) ... 695

Inflammation, upper respiratory tract
▲ Advair Diskus 100/50 (7%) ... 1448
▲ Advair Diskus 250/50 (6%) ... 1448
▲ Advair Diskus 500/50 (6% to 7%) ... 1448
Amerge Tablets (Infrequent) ... 1467
▲ Flovent Diskus (5%) ... 3614
Imitrex Nasal Spray ... 1554
Prevacid Delayed-Release Capsules (Less than 1%) ... 3292
PREVPAC (Less than 1%) ... 3298
▲ Ventolin HFA Inhalation Aerosol (5%) ... 3618

Inflammation at application site
▲ Androderm Transdermal System CIII (7%) ... 3377
▲ Condylox Gel (9.3% to 32.2%) ... 2436
Vivelle Transdermal System ... 2412
Vivelle-Dot Transdermal System ... 2416

Inflammation at injection site
Abelcet Injection ... 1273
Ambien Tablets (Rare) ... 3191
AmBisome for Injection (Less common) ... 1383
▲ Amphotec (5% or more) ... 1774
▲ Aredia for Injection (Up to 41%) ... 2309
▲ Avonex (3%) ... 1013
Betaseron for SC Injection ... 988
Bicillin C-R 900/300 Injection ... 2240
Bicillin C-R Injection ... 2238
Bicillin L-A Injection ... 2242
▲ Brevibloc Injection (About 8%) ... 858
Ceptaz for Injection (One in 69 patients) ... 1499
Cerebyx Injection (Infrequent) ... 2619
▲ Claforan Injection (4.3%) ... 732
▲ Copaxone for Injection (49%) ... 3306
Cytovene-IV (At least 3 subjects) ... 2959
DaunoXome Injection (Two patients) ... 1442
Delatestryl Injection (Rare) ... 1151
Depacon Injection (0.6%) ... 416
Diphtheria & Tetanus Toxoids Adsorbed Purogenated for Pediatric Use ... 1857
Diprivan Injectable Emulsion (Less than 1%) ... 667
Dobutrex Solution Vials ... 1914
Doxil Injection (Less than 1%) ... 566
Estratest ... 3252
FluShield Influenza Vaccine ... 3521
Fortaz (1 in 69 patients) ... 1541
Foscavir Injection (Between 1% and 5%) ... 605
Genotropin Lyophilized Powder (Infrequent) ... 2818
Gonal-F for Injection ... 3216
▲ Havrix Vaccine (1% to 10%) ... 1544
Humalog ... 1926
Humulin 50/50, 100 Units ... 1934
Humulin 70/30, 100 Units ... 1935
Humulin 70/30 Pen ... 1936
Humulin L, 100 Units ... 1937
Humulin R Regular (U-500) ... 1943
Humulin N NPH Pen ... 1940
Iletin II, Regular (Pork), 100 Units ... 1947
Imitrex Injection ... 1549
▲ Infanrix Vaccine (1.0% to 39.5%) ... 1562
INFeD Injection ... 3388
Intron A for Injection (Up to 5%) ... 3120
▲ JE-VAX Vaccine (2.9% to approximately 20%) ... 811
Levaquin Injection (1.5%) ... 2537
Maxipime for Injection (0.6%) ... 1285
Merrem I.V. (2.4%) ... 673
▲ Miacalcin Injection (About 10%) ... 2373
Nubain Injection ... 1323
Ovidrel for Injection (Less than 2%) ... 3220
▲ PEG-Intron Powder for Injection (47%) ... 3140
▲ Rebetron Combination Therapy (5%) ... 3153
Rifadin IV ... 765
Roferon-A Injection (Rare) ... 2996
Romazicon Injection ... 3000
Sandostatin LAR Depot (1% to 4%) ... 2395
Synercid I.V. ... 775
Taxotere for Injection Concentrate ... 778
Tazicef for Injection (Less than 2%) ... 1647
Tazicef Galaxy Container (Less than 2%) ... 1650
Tazicef Pharmacy Bulk Package (Less than 2%) ... 1653
Tazidime Vials, Faspak & ADD-Vantage (1 in 69) ... 1966
Testopel Pellets ... 3610
Testred Capsules, 10 mg ... 1746
Tetanus & Diphtheria Toxoids Adsorbed for Adult Use ... 1880
Vancocin HCl, Vials & ADD-Vantage ... 1970
Varivax (Less than 0.05%) ... 2202
Versed Injection (0.5% to 2.6%) ... 3027
▲ Zithromax for IV Infusion (3.1%) ... 2748
▲ Zofran Injection (4%) ... 1698
Zosyn (0.2% to 1.3%) ... 1890
Zosyn in Galaxy Containers (0.2% to 1.3%) ... 1894
▲ Zovirax for Injection (Approximately 9%) ... 1708

Infused vein complications
Cancidas for Injection (2.9%) ... 2048

Insomnia (14%)
Accupril Tablets (0.5% to 1.0%) ... 2611
Accuretic Tablets (1.2%) ... 2614
Accutane Capsules ... 2944
Aciphex Tablets ... 1267
Aciphex Tablets ... 1783
Actifed Cold & Allergy Tablets ... ⊡688
Actiq (1% to 2%) ... 1184
Activella Tablets (0% to 6%) ... 2764
▲ Actonel Tablets (4.7%) ... 2879
Adalat CC Tablets (Less than 1.0%) ... 877
Adderall Tablets ... 3231
▲ Adderall XR Capsules (1.5% to 17%)
Adipex-P ... 1406
Advil Cold and Sinus Caplets ... ⊡771
Advil Cold and Sinus Tablets ... ⊡771
Aerobid/Aerobid-M (1% to 3%) ... 1363
Agrylin Capsules (1% to 5%) ... 3232
Alferon N Injection (2%) ... 1770
Allegra (Less than 1%) ... 712
▲ Allegra-D Extended-Release Tablets (12.6%) ... 714
Alphagan Ophthalmic Solution (Less than 3%) ... 545
Alphagan P Ophthalmic Solution (Less than 1%) ... 546
Altace Capsules (Less than 1%) ... 2233
Ambien Tablets (Frequent) ... 3191
Amoxil Chewable Tablets (Rare) ... 1471
Amoxil for Oral Suspension (Rare) ... 1471
Amoxil (Rare) ... 1471
▲ Amphotec (5% or more) ... 1774
Anadrol-50 Tablets ... 3321
Anaprox Tablets (Less than 1%) ... 2967
Anaprox DS Tablets (Less than 1%) ... 2967
Arava Tablets (1% to 3%) ... 724
▲ Aredia for Injection (22.2%) ... 2309
▲ Aricept Tablets (9%) ... 1270
▲ Aricept Tablets (9%) ... 2665
Arimidex Tablets (2% to 5.9%) ... 659
▲ Aromasin Tablets (11%) ... 2769
Arthrotec Tablets (Rare) ... 3195
Asacol Delayed-Release Tablets (2%) ... 2884
Atacand HCT Tablets (0.5% or greater) ... 597
Atrovent Inhalation Aerosol (Less than 1%) ... 1030
Atrovent Inhalation Solution (0.9%) ... 1031
Augmentin Chewable Tablets (Rare) ... 1482
Augmentin Powder for Oral Suspension (Rare) ... 1482
Augmentin Tablets (Rare) ... 1485
Augmentin ES-600 Powder for Oral Suspension (Rare) ... 1487
Avelox Tablets (0.05% to 1%) ... 879
Axert Tablets (Infrequent) ... 2772
Axid Pulvules (2.7%) ... 1903
Axid Pulvules (2.7%) ... 2919
Aygestin Tablets ... 1333
Azactam for Injection (Less than 1%) ... 1276
Azulfidine EN-tabs Tablets (Rare) ... 2775
Bactrim ... 2949
Baycol Tablets (2.0%) ... 883
Benadryl Allergy/Congestion Tablets ... ⊡692
Benadryl Allergy & Sinus Liquid ... ⊡693
Benadryl Allergy Sinus Headache Caplets & Gelcaps ... ⊡693
Benadryl Parenteral ... 2617
Benylin Multi-Symptom Liquid ... ⊡697
Betapace AF Tablets (2.6% to 4.1%) ... 954
Betoptic S Ophthalmic Suspension (Rare) ... 537
Biaxin/Biaxin XL ... 403
Blocadren Tablets (Less than 1%) ... 2046
Bontril Slow-Release Capsules ... 576
Brethine Tablets (1.5%) ... 2313
Bromfed Capsules (Extended-Release) ... 2269
Bromfed-PD Capsules (Extended-Release) ... 2269
▲ Campath Ampules (10%) ... 992
Captopril Tablets (About 0.5% to 2%) ... 2281
Carafate Suspension (Less than 0.5%) ... 731
Carafate Tablets (Less than 0.5%) ... 730
Cardizem Injectable ... 1018
Cardizem Lyo-Ject Syringe ... 1018
Cardizem Monovial ... 1018
Cardizem CD Capsules (Less than 1%) ... 1016
Cardura Tablets (1% to 1.2%) ... 2668
Carnitor Injection (1% to 3%) ... 3242
Carteolol Hydrochloride Ophthalmic Solution USP, 1% (Occasional) ... ⊙258

▲ Casodex Tablets (5%) 662
Cataflam Tablets (Less than 1%) 2315
Catapres Tablets (About 5 in 1,000 patients) 1037
Catapres-TTS (2 of 101 patients) 1038
Ceclor CD Tablets (0.1% to 1%) 1279
Ceclor (Rare) 1905
Cedax Oral Suspension (0.1% to 1%) 1021
Cefzil (Less than 1%) 1076
Celebrex Capsules (2.3%) 2676
Celebrex Capsules (2.3%) 2780
Celestone Soluspan Injectable Suspension 3097
▲ Celexa (15%) 1365
▲ CellCept Capsules (8.9% to 40.8%) 2951
▲ CellCept Intravenous (8.9% to 40.8%) 2951
▲ CellCept Oral Suspension (8.9% to 40.8%) 2951
▲ CellCept Tablets (8.9% to 52.3%) 2951
Celontin Capsules 2618
▲ Cenestin Tablets (42%) 1263
Cerebyx Injection (Infrequent) 2619
Cipro I.V. (1% or less) 893
Cipro I.V. Pharmacy Bulk Package (Less than 1%) 897
Cipro (Less than 1%) 887
Claritin (At least one patient) 3100
▲ Claritin-D 12 Hour Extended Release Tablets (16%) 3102
▲ Claritin-D 24 Hour Extended Release Tablets (5%) 3104
Clinoril Tablets (Less than 1%) 2053
Clomid Tablets (Fewer than 1%) 735
Clorpres Tablets (About 5 in 1,000) 1002
Clozaril Tablets (2%) 2319
▲ Cognex Capsules (6%) 1351
Colazal Capsules (2%) 3069
Colestid Tablets (Infrequent) 2791
▲ CombiPatch Transdermal System (8% to 6%) 2323
Combipres Tablets (About 5 in 1,000) 1040
Combivent Inhalation Aerosol (Less than 2%) 1041
▲ Combivir Tablets (11%) 1502
Compazine (Sometimes) 1505
▲ Concerta Extended-Release Tablets (4%) 1998
▲ Concerta Tablets (4%) 561
Condylox Topical Solution (Less than 5%) 2437
Contac Non-Drowsy 12 Hour Cold Caplets ■745
Contac Non-Drowsy Timed Release 12 Hour Cold Caplets ■746
Contac Severe Cold and Flu Caplets Maximum Strength ■746
Copaxone for Injection (At least 2%) 3306
Cordarone Tablets (1% to 3%) 3487
Coreg Tablets (1.6% to more than 2%) 1508
Coricidin 'D' Cold, Flu & Sinus Tablets ■737
Corlopam Injection (2%) 412
Cortifoam Rectal Foam 3170
Cortone Acetate Injectable Suspension 2059
Cortone Acetate Tablets 2061
Cosopt Sterile Ophthalmic Solution 2065
Covera-HS Tablets (Less than 2%) 3199
Cozaar Tablets (1.4%) 2067
Crinone (Less than 5%) 3213
▲ Crixivan Capsules (3.1%) 2070
▲ Cylert Tablets (Most frequent) 415
Cytovene (At least 3 subjects) 2959
Dantrium Capsules (Less frequent) 2885
Dapsone Tablets USP 1780
▲ DaunoXome Injection (Up to 6%) 1442
Decadron Elixir 2078
Decadron Tablets 2079
Decadron Phosphate Injection 2081
Demadex Tablets and Injection (1.2%) 2965
Demser Capsules 2085
▲ Depacon Injection (9% to 15%) 416
▲ Depakene (15%) 421
▲ Depakote Sprinkle Capsules (9% to 15%) 426
▲ Depakote Tablets (1% to 15%) 430
Depakote ER Tablets (1% to 5%) 436
▲ Depo-Provera Contraceptive Injection (More than 5%) 2798
Desoxyn Tablets 440
Dexedrine 1512
DextroStat Tablets 3236
Dilantin Infatabs 2624
Dilantin Kapseals 2622
Dilantin-125 Oral Suspension 2625
Dilaudid Oral Liquid (Less frequent) 445
Dilaudid Tablets - 8 mg (Less frequent) 445
Dilaudid-HP (Less frequent) 443
Diovan Capsules 2337
Diovan HCT Tablets (Greater than 0.2%) 2338
Dipentum Capsules (Rare) 2803
Diprivan Injectable Emulsion (Less than 1%) 667
Ditropan XL Extended Release Tablets (2% to 5%) 564
Dolobid Tablets (Greater than 1 in 100) 2088
Dolophine Hydrochloride Tablets 3056
Donnatal 2929
Donnatal Extentabs 2930
Donnatal Tablets 2929
▲ Dostinex Tablets (1% to less than 10%) 2804
Doxil Injection (Less than 1% to 5%) 566
Drixoral Cold & Allergy Sustained-Action Tablets ■740
Drixoral Cold & Flu Extended-Release Tablets ■740
Duraclon Injection (0.5%) 3057
Dynabac Tablets (0.9% to 1%) 2269
DynaCirc Capsules (0.5% to 1%) 2921
DynaCirc CR Tablets (0.5% to 1%) 2923
EC-Naprosyn Delayed-Release Tablets (Less than 1%) 2967
▲ Effexor Tablets (3% to 22.5%) 3495
▲ Effexor XR Capsules (17% to 22%) 3499
Efudex 1733
8-MOP Capsules 1727
Eldepryl Capsules (1 of 49 patients) 3266
Elmiron Capsules 570
▲ Emcyt Capsules (3%) 2810
Enalaprilat Injection 863
Engerix-B Vaccine (Less than 1%) 1517
▲ Epivir (11%) 1520
▲ Epogen for Injection (13% to 16%) 582
Ergamisol Tablets (1%) 1789
▲ Estring Vaginal Ring (4%) 2811
Etrafon 3115
▲ Evista Tablets (5.5%) 1915
Evoxac Capsules (2.4%) 1217
▲ Exelon Capsules (9%) 2342
▲ Exelon Oral Solution (9%) 2345
Famotidine Injection (Infrequent) 866
Famvir Tablets (1.5% to 2.5%) 2348
▲ Felbatol (8.6% to 17.5%) 3343
Feldene Capsules (Occasional) 2685
▲ Femara Tablets (6%) 2351
femhrt Tablets 2635
Ferrlecit Injection (Greater than 1%) 3386
Flexeril Tablets (Less than 1%) 572
Flexeril Tablets (Less than 1%) 2094
▲ Flolan for Injection (4% to 9%) 1528
Flomax Capsules (1.4% to 2.4%) 1044
Florinef Acetate Tablets 2250
▲ Flovent (3% to 13%) 1535
Flovent Rotadisk 1537
▲ Floxin I.V. (3% to 7%) 2526
Floxin Otic Solution (Single report) 1219
▲ Floxin Tablets (3% to 7%) 2529
Flumadine (2.1% to 3.4%) 1370
Foradil Aerolizer (1.5%) 2354
▲ Fortovase Capsules (5.6%) 2970
Foscavir Injection (Between 1% and 5%) 605
▲ Gabitril Tablets (6%) 1189
Gastrocrom Oral Concentrate (Less common) 1162
Gemzar for Injection (Infrequent) 1919
Gengraf Capsules (1% to less than 3%) 457
Gliadel Wafer (2%) 1723
Glucotrol XL Extended Release Tablets (Less than 3%) 2693
Grifulvin V Tablets Microsize and Oral Suspension Microsize (Occasional) 2518
Gris-PEG Tablets (Occasional) 2661
Halcion Tablets (Rare) 2823
Haldol Decanoate 2535
Haldol Injection, Tablets and Concentrate 2533
Havrix Vaccine (Less than 1%) 1544
▲ Herceptin I.V. (14%) 1414
Hivid Tablets (Less than 1%) 2975
Hydrocortone Tablets 2106
Hydrocortone Acetate Injectable Suspension 2103
Hydrocortone Phosphate Injection, Sterile 2105
Hytrin Capsules (At least 1%) 464
Hyzaar 2109
Imdur Tablets (Less than or equal to 5%) 1826
Indapamide Tablets (Less than 5%) 2286
Inderal 3513
Inderal LA Long-Acting Capsules 3516
Inderide Tablets 3517
Inderide LA Long-Acting Capsules 3519
Indocin (Less than 1%) 2112
▲ Infergen (24% to 39%) 1777
Innohep Injection (Greater than or equal to 1%) 1248
▲ Intron A for Injection (Up to 12%) 3120
Invirase Capsules (Less than 2%) 2979
Ionamin Capsules 1163
Iopidine 0.5% Ophthalmic Solution (Less than 3%) ⊙213
Iopidine Sterile Ophthalmic Solution ⊙212
Ismo Tablets (Fewer than 1%) 3524
Isoptin SR Tablets (1% or less) 467
Kadian Capsules (Less than 3%) 1335
Kaletra Capsules (1.1% to 2.4%) 471
Kaletra Oral Solution (1.1% to 2.4%) 471
Keppra Tablets (1% or more) 3314
Klonopin Tablets (Infrequent) 2983
Kytril Injection (Less than 2%) 2986
▲ Kytril Tablets (3% to 5%) 2988
▲ Lamictal (5.6%) 1567
Lescol Capsules (2.7%) 2361
Lescol Capsules (2.7%) 2925
Lescol XL Tablets (1.8%) 2361
Lescol XL Tablets (1.8%) 2925
▲ Leukine (11%) 1755
▲ Leustatin Injection (7%) 2495
Levaquin (0.3% to 2.9%) 2537
Levbid Extended-Release Tablets 3172
Levlen 962
Levlite 21 Tablets 962
Levlite 28 Tablets 962
Levo-Dromoran 1734
Levoxyl Tablets 1819
Levsin/Levsinex/Levbid 3172
Lexxel Tablets 608
Lipitor Tablets (Greater than or equal to 2%) 2639
Lipitor Tablets (Greater than or equal to 2%) 2696
Lodine (Less than 1%) 3528
Lodine XL Extended-Release Tablets (Less than 1%) 3530
Lodosyn Tablets 1251
Lorabid Suspension and Pulvules 2251
Lotensin Tablets (Less than 1%) 2365
Lotensin HCT Tablets (0.3% to 1%) 2367
Lotrel Capsules 2370
Loxitane Capsules 3398
Lufyllin Tablets 3347
Lufyllin-400 Tablets 3347
Lufyllin-GG Elixir 3348
Lufyllin-GG Tablets 3348
Lupron Depot 3.75 mg (Less than 5%) 3281
Lupron Depot 7.5 mg (Less than 5%) 3284
Lupron Depot–3 Month 11.25 mg (Less than 5%) 3285
▲ Lupron Depot–3 Month 22.5 mg (8.5%) 3288
Lupron Depot–4 Month 30 mg (Less than 5%) 3289
▲ Lupron Injection (5% or more) 3279
▲ Luvox Tablets (25, 50, 100 mg) (4% to 21%) 3256
Matulane Capsules 3246
Mavik Tablets (0.3% to 1.0%) 478
Maxair Autohaler 1981
Maxair Inhaler (Less than 1%) 1984
Maxalt Tablets (Infrequent) 2120
Maxalt-MLT Orally Disintegrating Tablets (Infrequent) 2120
Maxzide 1008
▲ Megace Oral Suspension (Up to 6%) 1124
▲ Mepron Suspension (10% to 19%) 1598
▲ Meridia Capsules (10.7%) 481
Merrem I.V. (0.1% to 1.0%) 673
▲ Metadate CD Capsules (5%) 1164
▲ Metadate ER Tablets (Amongst most common) 1167
▲ Methylin Tablets (Among most common) 1995
▲ Methylin ER Tablets (Among most common) 1995
Mevacor Tablets (0.5% to 1.0%) 2132
Miacalcin Nasal Spray (Less than 1%) 2375
Micardis Tablets (More than 0.3%) 1049
Micardis HCT Tablets 1051
Midamor Tablets (Less than or equal to 1%) 2136
Migranal Nasal Spray (Infrequent) 2376
Minipress Capsules 2699
▲ Mirapex Tablets (17% to 27%) 2834
Mobic Tablets (0.4% to 3.6%) 1054
Modicon 2563
Moduretic Tablets (Less than or equal to 1%) 2138
Monopril Tablets (1.0% or more) 1091
Monurol Sachet (Less than 1%) 1375
Motofen Tablets (1 in 200 to 1 in 600) 577
Motrin Suspension, Oral Drops, Chewable Tablets, and Caplets (Less than 1%) 2002
Motrin Sinus Headache Caplets 2005
MS Contin Tablets (Less frequent) 2896
MSIR (Less frequent) 2898
Mycobutin Capsules (1%) 2838
Mykrox Tablets 1168
▲ Mylotarg for Injection (14% to 22%) 3540
Naprelan Tablets (Less than 3%) 1293
Naprosyn Suspension (Less than 1%) 2967
Naprosyn Tablets (Less than 1%) 2967
Nardil Tablets (Common) 2653
Naropin Injection (Less than 1%) 612
Natrecor for Injection (2%) 3189
Navane Oral 2701
Navane Intramuscular 2703
Nembutal Sodium Solution (Less than 1%) 485
Neoral Soft Gelatin Capsules (1% to less than 3%) 2380
Neoral Oral Solution (1% to less than 3%) 2380
▲ Neumega for Injection (33%) 1434
Nexium Delayed-Release Capsules (Less than 1%) 619
Niaspan Extended-Release Tablets 1846
Nicotrol Nasal Spray 2843
▲ Nilandron Tablets (16.3%) 753
▲ Nipent for Injection (3% to 10%) 3272
Noroxin Tablets (Less frequent) 2145
Norpramin Tablets 755
Norvasc Tablets (More than 0.1% to 1%) 2704
Norvir Capsules (1.3% to 2.6%) 487
Norvir Oral Solution (1.3% to 2.6%) 487
NuLev Orally Disintegrating Tablets 3176
Ocupress Ophthalmic Solution, 1% Sterile (Occasional) ⊙303
Omnicef (0.2%) 493
Oramorph SR Tablets (Less frequent) 3062
▲ Orap Tablets (2 of 20 patients) 1407
▲ Orgaran Injection (3.1%) 2480
Ortho-Cyclen/Ortho Tri-Cyclen 2573
Ortho-Novum 2563
Ortho-Novum 1/50□28 Tablets 2556
Ortho-Novum 2563
Ortho-Cyclen/Ortho Tri-Cyclen 2573
▲ Orudis Capsules (3% to 9%) 3548
▲ Oruvail Capsules (3% to 9%) 3548
Ovidrel for Injection (Less than 2%) 3220
Oxandrin Tablets 1153
Oxsoralen-Ultra Capsules 1741
OxyContin Tablets (Between 1% and 5%) 2912
Pacerone Tablets (1% to 3%) 3331
Parnate Tablets 1607
▲ Paxil (1.3 to 24%) 1609
Pediazole Suspension 3050
▲ PEG-Intron Powder for Injection (23%) 3140
Pentasa Capsules (Less than 1%) 3239
Pepcid Injection (Infrequent) 2153
Pepcid for Oral Suspension (Infrequent) 2150
Pepcid RPD Orally Disintegrating Tablets (Infrequent) 2150
Pepcid Tablets (Infrequent) 2150
Periactin Tablets 2155
▲ Permax Tablets (7.9%) 1299
Phenergan Injection 3553
Phenergan 3556
Phenergan with Dextromethorphan Syrup 3559
Phenergan VC Syrup 3560
▲ Photofrin for Injection (14%) 831
Plavix Tablets (1% to 2.5%) 1097
Plavix Tablets (1% to 2.5%) 3084
Plendil Extended-Release Tablets (0.5% to 1.5%) 623
Pletal Tablets (Less than 2%) 2605
Pletal Tablets (Less than 2%) 2848
Ponstel Capsules (Occasional) 1356
Pravachol Tablets 1099
Prednisone 3064
Prelone Syrup 2273
Premphase Tablets 3572
Prempro Tablets 3572
PREVPAC 3298
Prilosec Delayed-Release Capsules (Less than 1%) 628
Primatene Tablets ■780
Prinivil Tablets (0.3% to 1.0%) 2164
Prinzide Tablets 2168
ProAmatine Tablets (Rare) 3241
Procardia XL Extended Release Tablets (Less than 3%) 2710
▲ Procrit for Injection (13% to 21%) 2502
▲ Prograf (32% to 64%) 1393
Proleukin for Injection 1199
Prometrium Capsules (100 mg, 200 mg) (Less than 5%) 3261
Protonix I.V. (Greater than or equal to 1%) 3580
Protonix Tablets (Less than or equal to 1%) 3577
Protopic Ointment (Up to 4%) 1397
Proventil Inhalation Aerosol 3142
Proventil Inhalation Solution 0.083% (1% to 3.1%) 3146
▲ Proventil Repetabs Tablets (2% to 11%) 3148
Proventil Solution for Inhalation 0.5% (1% to 3.1%) 3144
Proventil HFA Inhalation Aerosol 3150
Provera Tablets 2853
▲ Provigil Tablets (3%) 1193
▲ Prozac Pulvules, Liquid, and Weekly Capsules (1% to 33%) 1238

(■ Described in PDR For Nonprescription Drugs) Incidence data in parenthesis; ▲ 3% or more (⊙ Described in PDR For Ophthalmic Medicines™)

Pulmicort Turbuhaler Inhalation Powder (1% to 3%).................... 636
▲ Rapamune Oral Solution and Tablets (13% to 22%)........................ 3584
▲ Rebetron Combination Therapy (26% to 39%).................................. 3153
Recombivax HB (Less to greater than 1%).. 2178
ReFacto Vials.. 1437
Reglan (Less frequent)............................ 2935
Relafen Tablets (1% to 3%)..................... 1617
▲ Reminyl Oral Solution (5%) 1792
▲ Reminyl Tablets (5%) 1792
ReoPro Vials (0.3%)................................. 1958
Requip Tablets (1% or more).................. 1621
Rescriptor Tablets (Less than 2%)........ 526
Rescula Ophthalmic Solution (1% to 5%).. ⊙ 306
▲ Retrovir Capsules (2.4% to 5%) 1625
▲ Retrovir IV Infusion (3% to 5%) 1629
▲ Retrovir (2.4% to 5%) 1625
Rifater Tablets.. 769
Rilutek Tablets (2.1% to 2.9%) 772
▲ Risperdal (23% to 26%) 1796
▲ Ritalin (One of the two most common) 2387
Rituxan for Infusion (1% to 5%) 1750
Rituxan I.V. (1% to 5%) 1428
Robaxin Tablets 2939
Robinul Forte Tablets 1358
Robinul Injectable 2940
Robinul Tablets 1358
Robitussin Maximum Strength Cough & Cold Liquid .... ■ 785
Robitussin Pediatric Cough & Cold Formula Liquid .... ■ 785
Robitussin-CF Liquid .... ■ 783
Robitussin-DAC Syrup 2942
Robitussin-PE Liquid .... ■ 782
▲ Roferon-A Injection (14%) 2996
▲ Romazicon Injection (3% to 9%) 3000
Rowasa Rectal Suspension Enema 4.0 grams/unit (60 mL) (0.12%) 3264
Roxanol 3066
▲ Roxicodone Tablets (Greater than or equal to 3%) 3067
Ryna .... ■ 768
Rynatan Tablets 3351
Rythmol Tablets – 150 mg, 225 mg, 300 mg (1.5%) 502
Salagen Tablets (Less than 1%) 2229
▲ Sandostatin LAR Depot (5% to 15%) 2395
▲ Sarafem Pulvules (9% to 24%) 1962
▲ Sectral Capsules (3%) 3589
▲ Semprex-D Capsules (4%) 1172
Septra Suspension 2265
Septra Tablets 2265
Septra DS Tablets 2265
Serevent Inhalation Aerosol (1% to 3%) 1633
Serophene Tablets (Approximately 1 in 50 patients) .. 3226
▲ Serostim for Injection (11.2%) 3229
▲ Serzone Tablets (11%) 1104
▲ Simulect for Injection (Greater than or equal to 10%) 2399
Sinemet Tablets 1253
Sinemet CR Tablets (1.2%) 1255
Singulair 2181
Sinutab Non-Drying Liquid Caps .... ■ 706
Skelid Tablets (More than or equal to 1%) 3088
Solu-Medrol Sterile Powder 2855
Soma Tablets 3353
Soma Compound Tablets (Infrequent or rare) 3354
Soma Compound w/Codeine Tablets (Infrequent or rare) 3355
Sonata Capsules (Infrequent) 3591
▲ Soriatane Capsules (1% to 10%) 3003
Sporanox Capsules (Infrequent) 1800
Sporanox Oral Solution (Less than 2%) 1808
Sporanox Oral Solution (Less than 2%) 2512
▲ Stadol NS Nasal Spray (11%) 1108
Stelazine (Sometimes) 1640
Stimate Nasal Spray 796
Sudafed 12 Hour Tablets .... ■ 708
Sudafed 24 Hour Tablets .... ■ 708
Children's Sudafed Cold & Cough Liquid .... ■ 709
Sudafed Cold & Allergy Tablets .... ■ 708
Sudafed Nasal Decongestant Tablets .... ■ 710
Sudafed Sinus Headache Caplets .... ■ 712
Sudafed Sinus Headache Tablets .. ■ 712
Sular Tablets (Less than or equal to 1%) 688
Surmontil Capsules 3595
▲ Sustiva Capsules (1% to 7%) 1258
▲ Symmetrel (5% to 10%) 1328
▲ Synarel Nasal Solution for Endometriosis (8% of patients) 3205
Synercid I.V. (Less than 1%) 775
Talacen Caplets (Infrequent) 3089
Talwin Nx Tablets 3090
Tambocor Tablets (1% to 3%) 1990
Tamiflu Capsules (1.1% to 1.2%) 3008
Tamiflu Oral Suspension (1.1% to 1.2%)... 3008
Tarka Tablets (Less frequent).............. 508
▲ Temodar Capsules (10%) 3157
Tenex Tablets (Less than 3% to 4%)... 2942
Tequin Injection (0.1% to 3%)............ 1110
Tequin Tablets (0.1% to 3%).............. 1110
Teveten Tablets (Less than 1%).......... 3327
Thalomid Capsules 1154
Theo-Dur Extended-Release Tablets.. 1835
TheraFlu Regular Strength Cold & Cough Night Time Hot Liquid .. ■ 676
TheraFlu Regular Strength Cold & Sore Throat Night Time Hot Liquid .... ■ 676
TheraFlu Maximum Strength Severe Cold & Congestion Night Time Caplets .... ■ 678
Thiothixene Capsules 2290
Thorazine 1656
Tiazac Capsules (Less than 2%)......... 1378
▲ Tikosyn Capsules (4%) 2717
Timolide Tablets (Less than 1%)........ 2187
Timolol GFS .... ⊙ 266
Timoptic in Ocudose (Less frequent).. 2192
Timoptic Sterile Ophthalmic Solution... 2190
Timoptic-XE Sterile Ophthalmic Gel Forming Solution.......................... 2194
Tonocard Tablets (Less than 1%)....... 649
Topamax Sprinkle Capsules (Frequent)... 2590
Topamax Tablets (Frequent)............... 2590
Toprol-XL Tablets 651
Toradol (1% or less).............................. 3018
Tranxene.. 511
▲ Trasylol Injection (3%) 909
Trental Tablets 784
Triaminic Allergy Congestion Liquid .... ■ 680
Triaminic Chest Congestion Liquid .... ■ 680
Triaminic Cold & Allergy Liquid .... ■ 681
Triaminic Cold & Allergy Softchews .... ■ 683
Triaminic Cold & Cough Liquid.......... ■ 681
Triaminic Cold & Night Time Cough Liquid .... ■ 681
Triaminic Cold, Cough & Fever Liquid .... ■ 681
Triaminic Cough Liquid .... ■ 682
Triaminic Cough & Congestion Liquid .... ■ 682
Triaminic Cough & Sore Throat Liquid .... ■ 682
Triaminic Cough & Sore Throat Softchews .... ■ 684
Tricor Capsules, Micronized (1%).... 513
Trilafon.. 3160
Trileptal Oral Suspension (2% to 4%)... 2407
Trileptal Tablets (2% to 4%)................ 2407
Tri-Levlen.. 962
▲ Trisenox Injection (43%) 1158
▲ Trizivir Tablets (7% to 13%) 1669
Trovan (Less than 1%).......................... 2722
Twinrix Vaccine (Less than 1%)......... 1674
Children's Tylenol Cold Suspension Liquid and Chewable Tablets.............................. 2015
Multi-Symptom Tylenol Cold Complete Formula Caplets............ 2010
Multi-Symptom Tylenol Cold Non-Drowsy Caplets and Gelcaps.. 2010
Maximum Strength Tylenol Flu NightTime Liquid............................ 2011
Maximum Strength Tylenol Sinus NightTime Caplets.......................... 2012
Maximum Strength Tylenol Sinus Non-Drowsy Geltabs, Gelcaps, Caplets, and Tablets.......................... 2012
Ultracet Tablets (2%)............................ 2597
Uni-Dur Extended-Release Tablets.... 1841
Uniphyl 400 mg and 600 mg Tablets.. 2903
Uniretic Tablets (Less than 1%).......... 3178
Unithroid Tablets 3445
▲ Vagifem Tablets (3% to 5%) 2857
▲ Valcyte Tablets (16%) 3022
Valium Injectable 3026
Valium Tablets 3047
Vanceril Double Strength Inhalation Aerosol (Fewer than 2%)... 3167
Vantin Tablets and Oral Suspension (Less than 1%)............. 2860
Vascor Tablets (0.5% to 2.65%)....... 2602
Vaseretic Tablets (0.5% to 2.0%)..... 2204
Vasotec I.V. Injection 2207
Vasotec Tablets (0.5% to 1.0%)........ 2210
Ventolin Inhalation Aerosol and Refill... 1679
Ventolin HFA Inhalation Aerosol 3618
Verelan Capsules (1% or less)........... 3184
Verelan PM Capsules (2% or less).... 3186
Versed Injection (Less than 1%)......... 3027
▲ Vesanoid Capsules (14%) 3037
Viagra Tablets (Less than 2%)........... 2732
Vicks 44D Cough & Head Congestion Relief Liquid .... ■ 724
Pediatric Vicks 44m Cough & Cold Relief.. ■ 728
Vicks DayQuil LiquiCaps/Liquid Multi-Symptom Cold/Flu Relief ... ■ 727
Children's Vicks NyQuil Cold/Cough Relief.............................. ■ 726
▲ Vicoprofen Tablets (3% to 9%) 520
Vioxx (Greater than 0.1% to 1.9%).. 2213
Viracept 532
Vistide Injection 1445
Vivactil Tablets 2217
Vivactil Tablets 2446
Volmax Extended-Release Tablets (2.4%).. 2276
Voltaren Ophthalmic Sterile Ophthalmic Solution (Less than 3%)... ⊙ 312
Voltaren Tablets (Less than 1%)........ 2315
Voltaren-XR Tablets (Less than 1%)... 2315
▲ Wellbutrin Tablets (18.6%) 1680
▲ Wellbutrin SR Sustained-Release Tablets (11% to 16%)........................ 1684
▲ Xanax Tablets (8.9% to 29.4%) 2865
Xeloda Tablets 3039
Xopenex Inhalation Solution............... 3207
Zantac (Rare)... 1690
Zantac Injection...................................... 1688
Zantac Syrup (Rare)............................... 1690
Zaroxolyn Tablets 1177
Zebeta Tablets (1.5% to 2.5%)........... 1885
▲ Zenapax for Injection (Greater than 5%).. 3046
Zephrex Tablets 3091
Zephrex LA Tablets 3092
▲ Zerit (29%) 1147
Zestoretic Tablets................................... 695
Zestril Tablets (0.3% to 1.0%)............ 698
Ziac Tablets (1.1% to 1.2%)................ 1887
▲ Ziagen (7% to 13%) 1692
Zithromax Capsules, 250 mg (1% or less)... 2743
Zithromax for IV Infusion (1% or less).. 2748
Zithromax for Oral Suspension, 300 mg, 600 mg, 900 mg, 1200 mg (1% or less).................. 2739
Zithromax Tablets, 250 mg (1% or less)... 2739
Zocor Tablets 2219
▲ Zoladex (5% to 11%) 702
Zoladex 3-month 706
▲ Zoloft (16% to 28%) 2751
▲ Zometa for Intravenous Infusion (15.1%).. 3621
Zomig Tablets (Infrequent)................... 708
Zomig-ZMT Tablets (Infrequent)........ 708
▲ Zonegran Capsules (6%) 1307
▲ Zosyn (4.5% to 6.6%) 1890
▲ Zosyn in Galaxy Containers (4.5% to 6.6%).. 1894
▲ Zyban Sustained-Release Tablets (31% to 40%)....................................... 1710
Zyflo Filmtab Tablets (Less common).. 524
▲ Zyprexa Tablets (20%) 1973
▲ Zyprexa ZYDIS Orally Disintegrating Tablets (20%)......... 1973
Zyrtec (Less than 2%)............................ 2756
Zyrtec-D 12 Hour Extended Relief Tablets (Less than 2%)................ 2758
Zyvox (2.5%).. 2871

Inculin allergy

Novolin 70/30 PenFill (Rare)............ 2423
Novolin N PenFill (Rare)...................... 2423
Novolin R PenFill (Rare)...................... 2423
Velosulin BR Human Insulin 10 ml Vials (Very rare).......................... 2435

Insulin autoimmune syndrome

Tapazole Tablets.................................... 1823

Insulin reaction

Modicon.. 2563
Ortho-Cyclen/Ortho Tri-Cyclen......... 2573
Ortho-Novum.. 2563
Ortho-Novum 1/50□28 Tablets......... 2556
Ortho-Cyclen/Ortho Tri-Cyclen......... 2573
Velosulin BR Human Insulin 10 ml Vials.. 2435

Insulin requirement, changes

Celestone Soluspan Injectable Suspension... 3097
Cortone Acetate Injectable Suspension... 2059
Cortone Acetate Tablets...................... 2061
Decadron Elixir....................................... 2078
Decadron Tablets 2079
Decadron Phosphate Injection.......... 2081
Florinef Acetate Tablets....................... 2250
Hydrocortone Tablets........................... 2106
Hydrocortone Phosphate Injection, Sterile.................................. 2105
Maxzide... 1008
Pediapred Oral Solution....................... 1170
Prednisone.. 3064
Prelone Syrup... 2273
Prinzide Tablets..................................... 2168
Solu-Medrol Sterile Powder............... 2855
Tenoretic Tablets 690
Vaseretic Tablets................................... 2204

Insulin resistance

Intercourse, sexual, painful

(*see under* Pain with coitus)

Intervertebral disk disorder, unspecified

Imitrex Nasal Spray (Rare)................ 1554

Intervertebral disk herniation

Remicade for IV Injection (Less than 2%).. 1178

Intestinal obstruction

Aloprim for Injection (Less than 1%)... 2292
Ambien Tablets (Rare)......................... 3191
Avonex... 1013
Betaseron for SC Injection.................. 988
Campath Ampules................................. 992
Celebrex Capsules (Less than 0.1%).. 2676
Celebrex Capsules (Less than 0.1%).. 2780
Clozaril Tablets 2319
Dantrium Capsules (Rare) 2885
Effexor Tablets (Rare) 3495
Effexor XR Capsules (Rare) 3499
Evoxac Capsules 1217
Exelon Capsules (Infrequent) 2342
Exelon Oral Solution (Infrequent) 2345
Felbatol 3343
Fortovase Capsules (Rare) 2970
Herceptin I.V. (At least one of the 958 patients)... 1414
Hycamtin for Injection (1.1% to 4.5%) 1546
Imitrex Injection 1549
Imitrex Nasal Spray (Rare) 1554
Imitrex Tablets 1558
Invirase Capsules (Rare) 2979
Levsin/Levsinex/Levbid 3172
Lupron Depot–4 Month 30 mg (Less than 5%)...................................... 3289
Luvox Tablets (25, 50, 100 mg) (Rare) 3256
Meridia Capsules 481
MS Contin Tablets (Less frequent) .. 2896
Navelbine Injection 1604
▲ Pancrease Capsules (Among most frequent) 2580
▲ Pancrease MT Capsules (Among most frequent) 2581
ParaGard T 380A Intrauterine Copper Contraceptive 2582
Paxil (Rare) 1609
Permax Tablets (Infrequent) 1299
Proleukin for Injection 1199
Pulmozyme Inhalation Solution 1426
Remeron Tablets (Rare) 2483
Remeron SolTab Tablets (Rare) 2486
Remicade for IV Injection (Less than 2%).. 1178
Rilutek Tablets (Infrequent) 772
Risperdal 1796
Sandostatin LAR Depot (Rare) 2395
Sarafem Pulvules (Rare) 1962
Seroquel Tablets (Rare) 684
Sonata Capsules (Rare) 3591
Taxol Injection (Rare) 1129
Taxotere for Injection Concentrate .. 778
Thalomid Capsules 1154
Vioxx (Less than 0.1%) 2213
Xeloda Tablets (Less than 5%) 3039
Zanaflex Tablets (Rare) 1305
Zyprexa Tablets (Rare) 1973
Zyprexa ZYDIS Orally Disintegrating Tablets (Rare) 1973

Intestinal obstruction, pseudo

Catapres Tablets (Rare) 1037
Nimotop Capsules (Rare) 904

Intestinal penetration

ParaGard T 380A Intrauterine Copper Contraceptive 2582

Intestinal perforation

Arthrotec Tablets (Rare) 3195
Avonex 1013
Campath Ampules 992
Cataflam Tablets (Rare) 2315
Celebrex Capsules (Less than 0.1%) 2676
Celebrex Capsules (Less than 0.1%) 2780
Cipro I.V. (Less than 1%) 893
Cipro I.V. Pharmacy Bulk Package (Less than 1%) 897
Cipro (Less than 1%) 887
Enbrel for Injection 1752
Enbrel for Injection 3504
Floxin I.V. 2526
Floxin Tablets 2529
Hydrocortone Tablets 2106
Mobic Tablets (Less than 2%) 1054
Navelbine Injection 1604
Prednisone 3064

Proleukin for Injection (Less than 1%) ... 1199
Remicade for IV Injection (Less than 2%) ... 1178
Tabloid Tablets ... 1642
Taxol Injection (Rare) ... 1129
Vioxx (Less than 0.1%) ... 2213
Voltaren Tablets (Rare) ... 2315
Voltaren-XR Tablets (Rare) ... 2315
Wellbutrin Tablets (Rare) ... 1680
Wellbutrin SR Sustained-Release Tablets ... 1684
Zyban Sustained-Release Tablets ... 1710

Intestinal strictures
Clinoril Tablets (Rare) ... 2053
Indocin Capsules (Less than 1%) ... 2112
Indocin I.V. (Less than 1%) ... 2115
▲ Pancrease Capsules (Among most frequent) ... 2580
▲ Pancrease MT Capsules (Among most frequent) ... 2581
Remicade for IV Injection (Less than 2%) ... 1178

Intestines, hemorrhagic necrosis of
Digitek Tablets ... 1003
Lanoxicaps Capsules ... 1574
Lanoxin Injection ... 1581
Lanoxin Tablets ... 1587
Lanoxin Elixir Pediatric ... 1578
Lanoxin Injection Pediatric ... 1584

Intoxication, chronic
Miltown Tablets ... 3349

Intracranial pressure, increase
Acel-Imune (One case) ... 1851
Albenza Tablets (Up to 1.5%) ... 1463
Anectine Injection ... 1476
Celestone Soluspan Injectable Suspension ... 3097
Celestone Syrup ... 3099
Chibroxin Sterile Ophthalmic Solution ... 2051
Cipro I.V. ... 893
Cipro ... 887
Cortifoam Rectal Foam ... 3170
Cortone Acetate Injectable Suspension ... 2059
Cortone Acetate Tablets ... 2061
Decadron Elixir ... 2078
Decadron Tablets ... 2079
Decadron Phosphate Injection ... 2081
Depo-Medrol Injectable Suspension ... 2795
Dilaudid ... 441
Dilaudid Oral Liquid (Less frequent) ... 445
Dilaudid Powder ... 441
Dilaudid Rectal Suppositories ... 441
Dilaudid Tablets ... 441
Dilaudid Tablets - 8 mg (Less frequent) ... 445
Dilaudid-HP (Less frequent) ... 443
Eskalith ... 1527
Floxin I.V. ... 2526
Floxin Tablets ... 2529
Hydrocortone Tablets ... 2106
Hydrocortone Acetate Injectable Suspension ... 2103
Hydrocortone Phosphate Injection, Sterile ... 2105
Levaquin ... 2537
Lithium Carbonate ... 3061
Lithium Citrate Syrup ... 3061
MS Contin Tablets (Less frequent) ... 2896
MSIR (Less frequent) ... 2898
Nizoral Tablets (Rare) ... 1791
Noroxin Tablets ... 2145
Oramorph SR Tablets (Less frequent) ... 3062
Prednisone ... 3064
Solu-Medrol Sterile Powder ... 2855
Tequin Injection ... 1110
Tequin Tablets ... 1110
Tripedia Vaccine ... 817
Trovan ... 2722

Intracranial pressure with papilledema
Lithobid Slow-Release Tablets ... 3255
Norditropin Cartridges (Small number of patients) ... 2420
Norditropin for Injection (Small number of patients) ... 2419
Nutropin AQ Injection (A small number of patients) ... 1420
Nutropin Depot for Injectable Suspension ... 1423
Nutropin for Injection (A small number of patients) ... 1417
Prelone Syrup ... 2273

Intraocular disorders
Amerge Tablets (Rare) ... 1467
Imitrex Tablets ... 1558

Intraocular pressure, increase
(*see under* Glaucoma)

Intraocular pressure, paradoxical increase
Humorsol Sterile Ophthalmic Solution ... 2102

Intravascular coagulation, disseminated
Aggrenox Capsules ... 1026
Aloprim for Injection (Less than 1%) ... 2292
Cafcit (2.2%) ... 1035
Campath Ampules ... 992
Clinoril Tablets (Less than 1 in 100) ... 2053
Dolobid Tablets (Less than 1 in 100) ... 2088
Ecotrin Enteric Coated Aspirin Low, Regular and Maximum Strength Tablets ... 1715
Felbatol ... 3343
Indocin Capsules (Less than 1%) ... 2112
Indocin I.V. ... 2115
Indocin (Less than 1%) ... 2112
Lamictal ... 1567
Mylotarg for Injection (2%) ... 3540
NovoSeven ... 2430
Omnicef ... 493
Oncaspar (Greater than 1% but less than 5%) ... 756
Sulfamylon Cream ... 1011
Sulfamylon Topical Solution ... 1011
Trasylol Injection (1% to 2%) ... 909
▲ Trisenox Injection (8%) ... 1158
Vantin Tablets and Oral Suspension ... 2860
▲ Vesanoid Capsules (26%) ... 3037
Zovirax for Injection ... 1708

Involuntary movements, abnormal
Carbatrol Capsules ... 3234
Clozaril Tablets (Less than 1%) ... 2319
Cordarone Tablets ... 3487
Dopram Injectable ... 2931
Effexor Tablets ... 3495
Eldepryl Capsules ... 3266
Haldol Decanoate ... 2535
Moban ... 1320
Omnicef ... 493
Orap Tablets ... 1407
Pacerone Tablets ... 3331
▲ Roferon-A Injection (Less than 0.5% to 7%) ... 2996
Seroquel Tablets (Infrequent) ... 684
▲ Sinemet Tablets (Among most common) ... 1253
Symmetrel (Uncommon) ... 1328
Tegretol/Tegretol-XR ... 2404
Versed Injection ... 3027
▲ Xanax Tablets (14.8%) ... 2865

Involuntary movements, extremities
Compazine ... 1505
Etrafon ... 3115
Haldol Decanoate ... 2535
Haldol Injection, Tablets and Concentrate ... 2533
Moban ... 1320
Navane Oral ... 2701
Navane Intramuscular ... 2703
Orap Tablets ... 1407
Reglan ... 2935
Serentil ... 1057
Stelazine ... 1640
Thorazine ... 1656

Involuntary movements, trunk
Haldol Decanoate ... 2535
Orap Tablets ... 1407
Reglan ... 2935
Serentil ... 1057

Iodine uptake, elevated
Lithobid Slow-Release Tablets ... 3255

IOP, elevation of
Albalon Ophthalmic Solution ... ⊙ 225
Alrex Sterile Ophthalmic Suspension 0.2% (2%) ... ⊙ 256
Amvisc Plus ... ⊙ 329
Beconase Inhalation Aerosol (Rare) ... 1497
Beconase AQ Nasal Spray (Rare) ... 1498
Blephamide Ophthalmic Ointment ... 547
Blephamide Ophthalmic Suspension ... 548
Celestone Soluspan Injectable Suspension ... 3097
Celestone Syrup ... 3099
Cognex Capsules (Infrequent) ... 1351
Cortisporin Ophthalmic Suspension Sterile ... ⊙ 297
Depo-Medrol Injectable Suspension ... 2795
Effexor Tablets (Rare) ... 3495
Flonase Nasal Spray ... 1533
FML Ophthalmic Ointment ... ⊙ 237
FML Ophthalmic Suspension ... ⊙ 236
FML Forte Ophthalmic Suspension ... ⊙ 235
FML-S Liquifilm Sterile Ophthalmic Suspension ... ⊙ 238
Healon (Some cases) ... ⊙ 316
Healon 5 ... ⊙ 317
Healon GV ... ⊙ 320
HMS Sterile Ophthalmic Suspension ... ⊙ 240
Lotemax Sterile Ophthalmic Suspension 0.5% ... ⊙ 261
Meridia Capsules ... 481
Ocucoat (Some cases) ... ⊙ 330
Paxil (Rare) ... 1609
Permax Tablets (Infrequent) ... 1299
Poly-Pred Liquifilm Ophthalmic Suspension ... ⊙ 245
Pred Forte Ophthalmic Suspension ... ⊙ 246
Pred Mild Sterile Ophthalmic Suspension ... ⊙ 249
Pred-G Ophthalmic Suspension ... ⊙ 247
Prelone Syrup ... 2273
Rescula Ophthalmic Solution (Less than 1%) ... ⊙ 306
Salagen Tablets (Less than 1%) ... 2229
Sandostatin Injection (Less than 1%) ... 2394
Serzone Tablets (Rare) ... 1104
Solu-Medrol Sterile Powder ... 2855
TobraDex Ophthalmic Ointment ... 542
TobraDex Ophthalmic Suspension ... 541
Vancenase PocketHaler Nasal Inhaler (Rare) ... 3162
Vancenase AQ Nasal Spray 0.084% (Rare) ... 3163
Viagra Tablets ... 2732
▲ Vitravene for Injection (5% to 20%) ... ⊙ 310
▲ Voltaren Ophthalmic Sterile Ophthalmic Solution (5% to 15%) ... ⊙ 312

Iridocyclitis
(*see also under* Iritis)
Betagan (Rare) ... ⊙ 228
Cosopt Sterile Ophthalmic Solution (Less than 1%) ... 2065
Trusopt Sterile Ophthalmic Solution (Rare) ... 2196

Iris cysts
Humorsol Sterile Ophthalmic Solution ... 2102
Salagen Tablets (Rare) ... 2229

Iris pigmentation, increase in
Lumigan Ophthalmic Solution (1% to 3%) ... 553
Rescula Ophthalmic Solution (Less than 1%) ... ⊙ 306
Travatan Ophthalmic Solution (1% to 4%) ... 543

Iritis
(*see also under* Uveitis)
▲ Acular Ophthalmic Solution (1% to 10%) ... 544
▲ Acular PF Ophthalmic Solution (Approximately 1% to 10%) ... 544
Aredia for Injection (Rare) ... 2309
Arthrotec Tablets (Rare) ... 3195
Colazal Capsules ... 3069
Healon (Rare) ... ⊙ 316
Healon 5 (Rare) ... ⊙ 317
Lumigan Ophthalmic Solution (Less than 1%) ... 553
Neurontin Capsules (Rare) ... 2655
Neurontin Oral Solution (Rare) ... 2655
Neurontin Tablets (Rare) ... 2655
Norvir Capsules (Less than 2%) ... 487
Norvir Oral Solution (Less than 2%) ... 487
Ocucoat (Rare) ... ⊙ 330
Ophthetic Ophthalmic Solution (Sometimes) ... ⊙ 244
Prozac Pulvules, Liquid, and Weekly Capsules (Rare) ... 1238
Rescula Ophthalmic Solution (Less than 1%) ... ⊙ 306
Sarafem Pulvules (Rare) ... 1962
Tenex Tablets (3% or less) ... 2942
TheraCys Injection ... 823
Topamax Sprinkle Capsules (Rare) ... 2590
Topamax Tablets (Rare) ... 2590
Uniretic Tablets (Less than 1%) ... 3178
Viracept ... 532
Vistide Injection ... 1445
▲ Vitravene for Injection (5% to 20%) ... ⊙ 310
Voltaren Ophthalmic Sterile Ophthalmic Solution (Less than 5%) ... ⊙ 312
Xalatan Latanoprost Ophthalmic Solution ... ⊙ 320
Xalatan Sterile Ophthalmic Solution ... 2864
Zanaflex Tablets (Rare) ... 1305
Zonegran Capsules (Rare) ... 1307

Iritis, activation of latent
Humorsol Sterile Ophthalmic Solution ... 2102

Iron deficiency
Cuprimine Capsules ... 2075
Depen Titratable Tablets ... 3341
Epogen for Injection ... 582
Risperdal (Rare) ... 1796
Sandostatin Injection (Less than 1%) ... 2394
Syprine Capsules ... 2186

Irritability
▲ Acel-Imune (25%) ... 1851
▲ ActHIB Vaccine (10.1% to 77.9%) ... 798
▲ Aerobid/Aerobid-M (3% to 9%) ... 1363
Aquasol A Parenteral ... 593
Aricept Tablets (Frequent) ... 1270
Aricept Tablets (Frequent) ... 2665
Arthrotec Tablets (Rare) ... 3195
Attenuvax ... 2044
Benadryl Parenteral ... 2617
Bromfed Capsules (Extended-Release) ... 2269
Bromfed-PD Capsules (Extended-Release) ... 2269
Cafcit ... 1035
Cataflam Tablets (Less than 1%) ... 2315
Catapres-TTS (0.5% or less) ... 1038
Cedax Oral Suspension (0.1% to 1%) ... 1021
Ceftin for Oral Suspension (0.1% to 1%) ... 1898
Celontin Capsules ... 2618
Cipro I.V. (1% or less) ... 893
Cipro I.V. Pharmacy Bulk Package (Less than 1%) ... 897
Cipro (Less than 1%) ... 887
Claritin (At least one patient) ... 3100
Claritin-D 12 Hour Extended Release Tablets (Less frequent) ... 3102
Claritin-D 24 Hour Extended Release Tablets (Fewer than 2%) ... 3104
Clomid Tablets ... 735
Clozaril Tablets (Less than 1%) ... 2319
▲ Comvax (32.2% to 57.0%) ... 2056
Cylert Tablets ... 415
Cytovene ... 2959
Dipentum Capsules (Rare) ... 2803
Diphtheria & Tetanus Toxoids Adsorbed Purogenated for Pediatric Use ... 1857
Efudex ... 1733
Eldepryl Capsules ... 3266
Elspar for Injection ... 2092
Engerix-B Vaccine (Less than 1%) ... 1517
Extendryl ... 1361
Fortovase Capsules (Less than 2%) ... 2970
▲ Gabitril Tablets (10%) ... 1189
▲ Gamimune N, 5% Solvent/Detergent Treated (Among most common) ... 925
▲ Gamimune N, 10% Solvent/Detergent Treated (Among most common) ... 928
Gastrocrom Oral Concentrate (2 of 87 patients) ... 1162
Guaifed ... 2272
Halcion Tablets ... 2823
HibTITER (133 of 1,118 vaccinations) ... 1859
▲ Indapamide Tablets (Greater than or equal to 5%) ... 2286
▲ Infanrix Vaccine (28.8% to 36.3%) ... 1562
▲ Intron A for Injection (Up to 16%) ... 3120
Invirase Capsules (Less than 2%) ... 2979
Iopidine Sterile Ophthalmic Solution ... ⊙ 212
▲ IPOL Vaccine (6.7% to 64.5%) ... 809
▲ Lamictal (3.0%) ... 1567
Levoxyl Tablets ... 1819
Lexxel Tablets ... 608
Lufyllin Tablets ... 3347
Lufyllin-400 Tablets ... 3347
Lufyllin-GG Elixir ... 3348
Lufyllin-GG Tablets ... 3348
Maxalt Tablets (Infrequent) ... 2120
Maxalt-MLT Orally Disintegrating Tablets (Infrequent) ... 2120
Meruvax II ... 2130
M-M-R II ... 2118
Mumpsvax ... 2141
Narcan Injection ... 1322
▲ Nicotrol Nasal Spray (Over 5%) ... 2843
Novarel for Injection ... 1347
Liquid PedvaxHIB ... 2148
▲ PEG-Intron Powder for Injection (28%) ... 3140
Periactin Tablets ... 2155
Plaquenil Tablets ... 3082
Plendil Extended-Release Tablets (0.5% to 1.5%) ... 623
Pregnyl for Injection ... 2482
▲ Prevnar for Injection (68.9% to 72.8%) ... 1870
Prinivil Tablets (0.3% to 1.0%) ... 2164
Prinzide Tablets ... 2168
Proleukin for Injection ... 1199
▲ Prometrium Capsules (100 mg, 200 mg) (5% to 8%) ... 3261

Proventil Repetabs Tablets (Less than 1%)........ 3148
Pulmicort Respules (Less than 1%)........ 632
Pulmicort Turbuhaler Inhalation Powder (Rare)........ 636
▲ Rebetron Combination Therapy (23% to 32%)........ 3153
Recombivax HB (Greater than 1%).. 2178
Retrovir Capsules (1.6%)........ 1625
Retrovir IV Infusion (2%)........ 1629
Retrovir (1.6%)........ 1625
Rhinocort Nasal Inhaler (Rare)........ 640
▲ Roferon-A Injection (Less than 5% to 15%)........ 2996
Rynatan Tablets........ 3351
Serophene Tablets........ 3226
Singulair (Very rare)........ 2181
Skelaxin Tablets........ 1301
Soma Tablets........ 3353
Soma Compound Tablets (Infrequent or rare)........ 3354
Soma Compound w/Codeine Tablets (Infrequent or rare)........ 3355
Symmetrel (1% to 5%)........ 1328
Talacen Caplets (Rare)........ 3089
Talwin Nx Tablets........ 3090
Tasmar Tablets (1%)........ 3010
Tetanus & Diphtheria Toxoids Adsorbed for Adult Use........ 1880
Theo-Dur Extended-Release Tablets........ 1835
Tranxene........ 511
▲ Tripedia Vaccine (5% to 15%)........ 817
Twinrix Vaccine (Less than 1%)........ 1674
Uni-Dur Extended-Release Tablets... 1841
Uniphyl 400 mg and 600 mg Tablets........ 2903
Unithroid Tablets........ 3445
Varivax (Greater than or equal to 1%)........ 2202
Volmax Extended-Release Tablets (Less frequent)........ 2276
Voltaren Tablets (Less than 1%)........ 2315
Voltaren-XR Tablets (Less than 1%)........ 2315
Wellbutrin SR Sustained-Release Tablets (2% to 3%)........ 1684
▲ Xanax Tablets (33.1%)........ 2865
Zarontin Capsules........ 2659
Zarontin Syrup........ 2660
Zephrex Tablets........ 3091
Zephrex LA Tablets........ 3092
Zestoretic Tablets........ 695
Zestril Tablets (0.3% to 1.0%)........ 698
Zomig Tablets (Rare)........ 708
Zomig-ZMT Tablets (Rare)........ 708
▲ Zonegran Capsules (9%)........ 1307
Zyban Sustained-Release Tablets (Frequent)........ 1710

Irritation
Aclovate Cream (Approximately 2%)........ 1275
Analpram-HC........ 1338
Anusol-HC Cream 2.5% (Infrequent to frequent)........ 2237
Anusol-HC Suppositories........ 2238
Atrovent Inhalation Aerosol (1.6%).. 1030
Azelex Cream (Less than 1%)........ 547
Benoquin Cream 20%........ 1732
Bleph-10........ ⊙230
Capex Shampoo........ 1400
Cordran Lotion (Infrequent)........ 2438
Cordran Tape (Infrequent)........ 2439
Cormax Cream (0.5%)........ 2440
Cormax Ointment (0.5%)........ 2440
Cormax Scalp Application (Infrequent)........ 2441
Cutivate Cream (Infrequent)........ 1282
Cutivate Ointment (Less than 1%)........ 1284
DesOwen (Less than 2%)........ 1401
Diprolene Gel 0.05% (Less frequent)........ 3107
Dovonex Scalp Solution (1% to 5%)........ 1118
▲ Efudex (Among most frequent)........ 1733
Elocon Lotion 0.1% (Infrequent)........ 3111
Fluoroplex........ 552
▲ Lac-Hydrin Cream (Approximately 10% to 15%)........ 1118
Lac-Hydrin Lotion (Less frequent)... 1119
Lidex (Infrequent)........ 2020
Lindane Lotion USP 1% (Relatively infrequent)........ 559
Lindane Shampoo USP 1% (Relatively infrequent)........ 560
Locoid (Infrequent)........ 1341
Lotrimin AF Spray Powder, Spray Liquid, Spray Deodorant Powder, Shaker Powder and Jock Itch Spray Powder........ ▣742
Lotrisone........ 3129
Melanex Topical Solution........ 2300
▲ Nizoral 2% Cream (5%)........ 3620
Nizoral 2% Shampoo (Less than 1%)........ 2007
Olux Foam (Less than 2%)........ 1211
Pramosone........ 1343
Pred-G Ophthalmic Suspension........ ⊙247
Serevent Inhalation Aerosol (Rare).. 1633
Synalar (Infrequent)........ 2020
Temovate Cream........ 1301
▲ Temovate Gel (Among most frequent)........ 1303
Temovate Ointment (0.5%)........ 1301
Temovate Scalp Application (Infrequent)........ 1304
Temovate E Emollient (Less than 2%)........ 1302
Testoderm Transdermal Systems (2%)........ 574

Irritation, anal
Colyte with Flavor Packs for Oral Solution (Less frequent)........ 3170
Fleet Glycerin Laxatives........ 1359
GoLYTELY and Pineapple Flavor GoLYTELY for Oral Solution (Infrequent)........ 1068
NuLYTELY, Cherry Flavor, Lemon-Lime Flavor, and Orange Flavor NuLYTELY for Oral Solution (Less frequent)........ 1068
Zosyn (1.0% or less)........ 1890
Zosyn in Galaxy Containers (1.0% or less)........ 1894

Irritation, gastric
Accuretic Tablets........ 2614
Akineton........ 402
Aldoclor Tablets........ 2035
Aldoril Tablets........ 2039
Atacand HCT Tablets........ 597
Avalide Tablets........ 1070
Captopril Tablets (About 0.5% to 2%)........ 2281
Clorpres Tablets........ 1002
Combipres Tablets........ 1040
Corzide 40/5 Tablets........ 2247
Corzide 80/5 Tablets........ 2247
Dantrium Capsules (Rare)........ 2885
Diovan HCT Tablets........ 2338
Diucardin Tablets........ 3494
Diuril Oral........ 2087
Diuril Sodium Intravenous........ 2086
Furosemide Tablets........ 2284
HydroDIURIL Tablets........ 2108
Hyzaar........ 2109
Indapamide Tablets (Less than 5%)........ 2286
Inderide Tablets........ 3517
Inderide LA Long-Acting Capsules... 3519
Lotensin HCT Tablets........ 2367
Maxzide........ 1008
Micardis HCT Tablets........ 1051
Microzide Capsules........ 3414
Minizide Capsules........ 2700
Moduretic Tablets........ 2138
Monopril HCT........ 1094
Mylocel Tablets........ 2227
Norflex........ 1987
Prinzide Tablets........ 2168
Renese Tablets........ 2712
Timolide Tablets........ 2187
Uniretic Tablets........ 3178
Vaseretic Tablets........ 2204
Venastat Suppli-Cap Capsules (Rare)........ ▣833
Zestoretic Tablets........ 695
Ziac Tablets........ 1887

Irritation, gastrointestinal
Dibenzyline Capsules........ 3457
Fosamax Tablets........ 2095
Glucotrol XL Extended Release Tablets (Rare)........ 2693
▲ K-Lor Powder Packets (Among most common)........ 469
▲ Micro-K Extencaps (Among most common)........ 3311
Procardia XL Extended Release Tablets (Less than 1%)........ 2710
Tenoretic Tablets........ 690
Urocit-K Tablets (Some patients)........ 2232

Irritation, glossal
(*see under* Irritation, oral)

Irritation, local
Aldara Cream, 5% (More than 1%)........ 1978
Androderm Transdermal System CIII (Less than 1%)........ 3377
Astramorph/PF Injection, USP (Preservative-Free)........ 594
Auralgan Otic Solution........ 3485
Betasept Surgical Scrub........ 2895
Bleph-10........ ⊙230
Blephamide Ophthalmic Ointment... 547
Blephamide Ophthalmic Suspension........ 548
▲ Carac Cream (94.6%)........ 1222
▲ Cipro I.V. Pharmacy Bulk Package (Among most frequent)........ 897
Claforan Injection........ 732
▲ Cleocin Vaginal Cream (7%)........ 2788
▲ Climara Transdermal System (31%)........ 958
Cortisporin Ophthalmic Suspension........ ⊙297
Demerol........ 3079
Dermatop Emollient Cream........ 2517
Desenex........ ▣668
Desenex Jock Itch Spray Powder.. ▣668
Desferal Vials........ 2333
Duramorph Injection........ 1312
Edecrin (Occasional)........ 2091
Heparin Lock Flush Solution........ 3509
Heparin Sodium Injection........ 3511
HibTITER........ 1859
Infumorph 200 and Infumorph 500 Sterile Solutions........ 1314
Klaron Lotion 10%........ 1224
Locoid Lipocream Cream (Infrequent)........ 1342
Lovenox Injection........ 746
Mentax Cream (Less than 2%)........ 1009
Mepergan Injection........ 3539
Naftin Cream (2%)........ 2224
Nitro-Dur Transdermal Infusion System........ 1834
Nitro-Dur Transdermal Infusion System........ 3134
▲ Nizoral 2% Cream (5%)........ 3620
Novolin 70/30 Prefilled Disposable Insulin Delivery System........ 2425
Ovide Lotion........ 2023
Plexion (Rare)........ 2024
Polysporin Ophthalmic Ointment Sterile........ ⊙301
▲ Polytrim Ophthalmic Solution (Most frequent)........ 556
Proctocort Suppositories........ 2264
Psorcon E Cream........ 1227
Psorcon E Ointment........ 1228
Rifadin IV........ 765
Selsun Rx 2.5% Lotion, USP........ 3053
Sultrin Triple Sulfa Cream (Frequent)........ 2587
Topicort (Infrequent)........ 2025
Valstar Sterile Solution for Intravesical Instillation (Less than 1%)........ 1175
Vivelle Transdermal System........ 2412
Vivelle-Dot Transdermal System........ 2416
VōSoL HC Otic Solution (Very rare)........ 3356
Zebeta Tablets........ 1885

Irritation, nasal
Advair Diskus 100/50 (1% to 3%)........ 1448
Advair Diskus 250/50 (1% to 3%)... 1448
Advair Diskus 500/50 (1% to 3%)... 1448
Aerobid/Aerobid-M (1% to 3%)........ 1363
Atrovent Nasal Spray 0.03% (2.0%)........ 1032
▲ Beconase Inhalation Aerosol (11 in 100 patients)........ 1497
Beconase AQ Nasal Spray........ 1498
Claritin-D 12 Hour Extended Release Tablets (Less frequent)... 3102
Claritin-D 24 Hour Extended Release Tablets (Fewer than 2%)........ 3104
Efudex (Infrequent)........ 1733
Flonase Nasal Spray (1% to 3%)........ 1533
Maxalt Tablets (Infrequent)........ 2120
Maxalt-MLT Orally Disintegrating Tablets (Infrequent)........ 2120
▲ Miacalcin Nasal Spray (10.6%)........ 2375
Nasacort Nasal Inhaler (2.8%)........ 750
Nasalide Nasal Spray (5% or less).. 1295
Nasonex Nasal Spray........ 3131
Nicotrol Nasal Spray........ 2843
▲ Stadol NS Nasal Spray (3% to 9%).. 1108
▲ Synarel Nasal Solution for Endometriosis (10% of patients).. 3205
▲ Vancenase PocketHaler Nasal Inhaler (11 per 100 patients)........ 3162
Vancenase AQ Nasal Spray 0.084%........ 3163

Irritation, nasopharyngeal
▲ Beconase AQ Nasal Spray (24% of patients)........ 1498
Rhinocort Aqua Nasal Spray (2%)........ 642
▲ Rhinocort Nasal Inhaler (3% to 9%)........ 640

Irritation, oral
Aerobid/Aerobid-M (1% to 3%)........ 1363
Amerge Tablets (Rare)........ 1467
Axert Tablets (Rare)........ 2772
Flovent Rotadisk (1% to 3%)........ 1537
Furosemide Tablets........ 2284
Imitrex Nasal Spray........ 1554
▲ Nicotrol Inhaler (40%)........ 2840
Sandimmune (Rare)........ 2388

Irritation, oropharynx
Proventil Inhalation Aerosol........ 3142
Proventil Repetabs Tablets........ 3148
Proventil HFA Inhalation Aerosol........ 3150
Serevent Diskus........ 1637
Serevent Inhalation Aerosol (Rare).. 1633
Ventolin HFA Inhalation Aerosol........ 3618
Volmax Extended-Release Tablets... 2276

Irritation, perianal
(*see under* Irritation, anal)

Irritation, skin
(*see under* Irritation, local)

Irritation, vaginal
Ceftin for Oral Suspension (0.1% to 1%)........ 1898
Floxin I.V. (Less than 1%)........ 2526
Floxin Tablets (Less than 1%)........ 2529
Massengill Disposable Douches........ ▣752
Massengill Medicated Disposable Douche........ ▣753
▲ MetroGel-Vaginal Gel (9%)........ 1986
Nystatin Vaginal Tablets, USP (Rare)........ 2445
Sultrin Triple Sulfa Cream (Frequent)........ 2587
▲ Terazol 3 Vaginal Cream (5%)........ 2587
▲ Terazol 7 Vaginal Cream (3.1% of 521 patients)........ 2587

Irritation, vulvovaginal
(*see under* Irritation, vaginal)

Irritation at injection site
▲ Eulexin Capsules (3%)........ 3118
▲ Gammagard S/D (16%)........ 845
Humegon for Injection........ 2468
Nembutal Sodium Solution........ 485
Pepcid Injection Premixed (Infrequent)........ 2153
Pergonal for Injection........ 3223
Repronex for Intramuscular and Subcutaneous Injection........ 1347
Retrovir IV Infusion (Infrequent)........ 1629
Romazicon Injection........ 3000
Synercid I.V......... 775

Ischemia
▲ Lupron Injection (5% or more)........ 3279
▲ Prandin Tablets (0.5, 1, and 2 mg) (4%)........ 2432
Sandostatin Injection (Less than 1%)........ 2394
Sensorcaine........ 643
Sensorcaine-MPF Injection........ 643
▲ Vesanoid Capsules (3%)........ 3037

Ischemia, arteria basilaris
AK-Fluor Injection 10% and 25%........ ⊙202
Fluorescite Injection........ ⊙211

Ischemia, cerebral
Actiq (Less than 1%)........ 1184
Arimidex Tablets........ 659
Betagan........ ⊙228
Betaseron for SC Injection........ 988
Betimol Ophthalmic Solution........ ⊙324
Carteolol Hydrochloride Ophthalmic Solution USP, 1%........ ⊙258
Cosopt Sterile Ophthalmic Solution........ 2065
Effexor Tablets (Rare)........ 3495
Effexor XR Capsules (Rare)........ 3499
Enbrel for Injection (Infrequent)........ 1752
Enbrel for Injection (Infrequent)........ 3504
Gabitril Tablets (Infrequent)........ 1189
Imitrex Injection........ 1549
Imitrex Nasal Spray........ 1554
Imitrex Tablets (Rare)........ 1558
Nitrolingual Pumpspray (Occasional)........ 1355
Ocupress Ophthalmic Solution, 1% Sterile........ ⊙303
Paxil (Rare)........ 1609
Permax Tablets (Infrequent)........ 1299
Pletal Tablets (Less than 2%)........ 2605
Pletal Tablets (Less than 2%)........ 2848
Prozac Pulvules, Liquid, and Weekly Capsules (Rare)........ 1238
Quinaglute Dura-Tabs Tablets (2%).. 978
Remeron Tablets (Rare)........ 2483
Remeron SolTab Tablets (Rare)........ 2486
ReoPro Vials (0.3%)........ 1958
Rilutek Tablets (Rare)........ 772
Sarafem Pulvules (Rare)........ 1962
Seroquel Tablets (Infrequent)........ 684
Sonata Capsules (Rare)........ 3591
Sular Tablets (Less than or equal to 1%)........ 688
Tasmar Tablets (Infrequent)........ 3010
Thalomid Capsules........ 1154
Tikosyn Capsules (Less than or equal to 2%)........ 2717
Timolide Tablets........ 2187
Timolol GFS........ ⊙266
Timoptic in Ocudose........ 2192
Timoptic Sterile Ophthalmic Solution (Less frequent)........ 2190
Timoptic-XE Sterile Ophthalmic Gel Forming Solution........ 2194
Zoladex 3-month (1% to 5%)........ 706
Zomig Tablets (Rare)........ 708
Zomig-ZMT Tablets (Rare)........ 708

Ischemia, intestinal
Amerge Tablets........ 1467
Digitek Tablets (Rare)........ 1003
Imitrex Nasal Spray........ 1554
Lanoxicaps Capsules........ 1574
Lanoxin Injection........ 1581

Lanoxin Tablets 1587
Lanoxin Elixir Pediatric 1578
Lanoxin Injection Pediatric 1584

Ischemia, myocardial
Anzemet Injection (Rare) 719
Anzemet Tablets (Rare) 722
Arimidex Tablets 659
Brethine Ampuls 2314
Coreg Tablets (Less than or equal to 0.1%) 1508
Diprivan Injectable Emulsion (Less than 1%) 667
Enbrel for Injection (Infrequent) 1752
Enbrel for Injection (Infrequent) 3504
Ergamisol Tablets 1789
Femara Tablets (Less than or equal to 2%) 2351
Flolan for Injection (2%) 1528
Sterile FUDR (Remote possibility) 2974
Imitrex Injection (Extremely rare) 1549
Imitrex Nasal Spray 1554
Imitrex Tablets (Rare) 1558
Levlen 962
Levlite 21 Tablets 962
Levlite 28 Tablets 962
Maxalt Tablets (Very rare) 2120
Maxalt-MLT Orally Disintegrating Tablets (Very rare) 2120
Modicon 2563
Ortho-Novum 2563
Ortho-Novum 1/50□28 Tablets 2556
Ortho-Novum 2563
Ovcon 3364
Paxil (Rare) 1609
Pletal Tablets (Less than 2%) 2605
Pletal Tablets (Less than 2%) 2848
▲ Proleukin for Injection (3%) 1199
Protonix I.V. (Less than 1%) 3580
Protonix Tablets (Less than 1%) 3577
Rilutek Tablets (Infrequent) 772
Suprane Liquid for Inhalation (Less than 1%) 874
Tasmar Tablets (Infrequent) 3010
TNKase I.V. 1430
Trasylol Injection (1% to 2%) 909
Tri-Levlen 962
Ultracet Tablets 2597
Ultram Tablets (Infrequent) 2600
Uniretic Tablets (Less than 1%) 3178
Viagra Tablets (Less than 2%) 2732
Zomig Tablets 708
Zomig-ZMT Tablets 708

Ischemia, peripheral
Amicar Injection 3608
Amicar Syrup 3608
Amicar Tablets 3608
Anzemet Injection (Rare) 719
Anzemet Tablets (Rare) 722
Avonex 1013
Brevibloc Injection (Approximately 1%) 858
Cardura Tablets (0.3%) 2668
Coreg Tablets (0.1% to 1%) 1508
Cytovene 2959
Evoxac Capsules (Less than 1%) 1217
Exelon Capsules (Infrequent) 2342
Exelon Oral Solution (Infrequent) 2345
Felbatol 3343
Gengraf Capsules (1% to less than 3%) 457
Intron A for Injection (Less than 5%) 3120
Migranal Nasal Spray (Rare) 2376
Neoral Soft Gelatin Capsules (1% to less than 3%) 2380
Neoral Oral Solution (1% to less than 3%) 2380
Norvasc Tablets (More than 0.1% to 1%) 2704
Remicade for IV Injection (Less than 2%) 1178
▲ Requip Tablets (3%) 1621
Soriatane Capsules (Less than 1%) 3003
Teveten Tablets (Less than 1%) 3327
Trovan (Less than 1%) 2722
Ziac Tablets (0.4% to 0.7%) 1887
Zoloft (Infrequent) 2751

Ischemia, recurrent
Activase I.V. 1410
Retavase Vials 1182

Ischemia, transient
Imitrex Tablets 1558

Ischemia of digits
Zovirax for Injection (Less than 1%) 1708

Ischemic attacks, transient
Actimmune (Rare) 1772
Amerge Tablets 1467
Aricept Tablets (Infrequent) 1270
Aricept Tablets (Infrequent) 2665
Avalide Tablets 1070
Avapro Tablets (Less than 1%) 1074
Avapro Tablets (Less than 1%) 3076
Celexa (Rare) 1365
Clozaril Tablets (Several patients) 2319
Cognex Capsules (Infrequent) 1351
DynaCirc Capsules (0.5% to 1%) 2921
DynaCirc CR Tablets (0.5% to 1%) 2923
Epogen for Injection (0.4%) 582
Fareston Tablets (Less than 1% to 2%) 3237
Femara Tablets (Less than or equal to 2%) 2351
Fludara for Injection (Up to 1%) 995
Imitrex Injection 1549
Lupron Injection 3279
Meridia Capsules 481
Monopril Tablets (0.4% to 1.0%) 1091
Orthoclone OKT3 Sterile Solution (Less than 1%) 2498
PEG-Intron Powder for Injection (Less than or equal to 1%) 3140
Prinivil Tablets (0.3% to 1.0%) 2164
Prinzide Tablets 2168
Procrit for Injection (0.4%) 2502
Proleukin for Injection (Less than 1%) 1199
Roferon-A Injection (Infrequent) 2996
Tonocard Tablets 649
Viagra Tablets 2732
Vioxx (Less than 0.1%) 2213
Zestoretic Tablets 695
Zestril Tablets (0.3% to 1.0%) 698

Ischemic colitis
Imitrex Injection 1549
Imitrex Nasal Spray 1554
Imitrex Tablets 1558
Inderal 3513
Inderal LA Long-Acting Capsules 3516
Inderide Tablets 3517
Inderide LA Long-Acting Capsules 3519
Normodyne Tablets 3137
Sectral Capsules 3589
Timolide Tablets 2187
Timoptic in Ocudose 2192
Timoptic Sterile Ophthalmic Solution 2190

Ischemic disorders, life-threatening, aggravation of
Roferon-A Injection 2996

Itching
(*see under* Pruritus)

Itching, eyes
(*see under* Pruritus, ocular)

Itching, vulvovaginal
Ceftin Tablets (0.1% to 1%) 1898
Clozaril Tablets (Less than 1%) 2319
Hivid Tablets (Less than 1%) 2975
▲ MUSE Urethral Suppository (5.8%) 3335
Terazol 3 Vaginal Cream 2587
Terazol 7 Vaginal Cream (2.3% of 521 patients) 2587

IUD, difficult removal
ParaGard 2582

J

Jarisch-Herxheimer's reaction
(*see under* Herxheimer's reaction)

Jaundice (Less than 5%)
Abelcet Injection 1273
Accuretic Tablets 2614
Aceon Tablets (2 mg, 4 mg, 8 mg) 3249
Aciphex Tablets 1267
Aciphex Tablets 1783
Actiq (1% or greater) 1184
Aggrenox Capsules (Less than 1%) 1026
Aldoclor Tablets 2035
Aldomet Tablets 2037
Aldoril Tablets 2039
Aloprim for Injection (Less than 1%) 2292
Altace Capsules 2233
Amaryl Tablets (Isolated cases) 717
▲ Amphotec (5% or more) 1774
Anadrol-50 Tablets 3321
Anaprox Tablets (Rare; less than 1%) 2967
Anaprox DS Tablets (Rare; less than 1%) 2967
Ancobon Capsules 1730
Androderm Transdermal System CIII 3377
Android Capsules, 10 mg 1731
Antabuse Tablets 2444
Antabuse Tablets 3474
AquaMEPHYTON Injection 2042
Aquasol A Parenteral 593
Aricept Tablets (Infrequent) 1270
Aricept Tablets (Infrequent) 2665
Arthrotec Tablets (Rare) 3195
Asacol Delayed-Release Tablets (Rare) 2884
Atacand HCT Tablets 597
Avalide Tablets 1070
Avandia Tablets (Very rare) 1490
Avapro Tablets 1074
Avapro Tablets (Very rare) 3076
Axid Pulvules 1903
Axid Pulvules 2919
Azactam for Injection (Less than 1%) 1276
Azulfidine EN-tabs Tablets 2775
Biaxin/Biaxin XL (Infrequent) 403
Brevicon 28-Day Tablets 3380
Captopril Tablets 2281
Casodex Tablets (Rare) 662
Cataflam Tablets (Less than 1%) 2315
Cedax 1021
Ceftin 1898
Celebrex Capsules 2676
Celebrex Capsules 2780
Celexa (Rare) 1365
▲ CellCept Capsules (3% to 10%) 2951
▲ CellCept Intravenous (3% to 10%) 2951
▲ CellCept Oral Suspension (3% to 10%) 2951
▲ CellCept Tablets (3% to 10%) 2951
Chibroxin Sterile Ophthalmic Solution 2051
Cipro I.V. (1% or less) 893
Cipro I.V. Pharmacy Bulk Package (Less than 1%) 897
Cipro (Rare) 887
Claritin (Rare) 3100
Claritin-D 12 Hour Extended Release Tablets 3102
Cleocin HCl Capsules 2784
Cleocin Phosphate Sterile Solution 2785
Cleocin Vaginal Cream 2788
Cleocin Vaginal Ovules 2789
Clinoril Tablets (Less than 1%) 2053
Clorpres Tablets 1002
Clozaril Tablets 2319
Colazal Capsules 3069
Combipres Tablets 1040
Corzide 40/5 Tablets (Occasional) 2247
Corzide 80/5 Tablets (Occasional) 2247
Coumadin for Injection (Infrequent) 1243
Coumadin Tablets (Infrequent) 1243
Crixivan Capsules (Less than 2%) 2070
Cylert Tablets 415
Dantrium Capsules 2885
Dapsone Tablets USP 1780
Darvon-N/Darvocet-N (Rare) 1907
Darvon Pulvules 1909
Darvon Compound-65 Pulvules 1910
Darvon-N Tablets 1912
Depo-Provera Contraceptive Injection (Fewer than 1%) 2798
Diflucan Tablets, Injection, and Oral Suspension 2681
Diovan HCT Tablets 2338
Diucardin Tablets 3494
Dolobid Tablets (Less than 1 in 100) 2088
Doxil Injection (Less than 1%) 566
Dyazide Capsules 1515
Dyrenium Capsules (Rare) 3458
EC-Naprosyn Delayed-Release Tablets (Rare; less than 1%) 2967
Edecrin (Rare) 2091
Effexor Tablets (Rare) 3495
Effexor XR Capsules (Rare) 3499
Enalaprilat Injection 863
EryPed 446
Ery-Tab Tablets 448
Erythrocin Stearate Filmtab Tablets 452
Etrafon (Less frequent) 3115
Eulexin Capsules (Less than 1%) 3118
Felbatol 3343
Feldene Capsules (Occasional) 2685
Flexeril Tablets (Rare) 572
Flexeril Tablets (Rare) 2094
Floxin I.V. 2526
Floxin Tablets 2529
Fluothane Inhalation 3508
Fortaz 1541
Fortovase Capsules (Rare; less than 2%) 2970
Furosemide Tablets 2284
Geodon Capsules (Rare) 2688
Glucotrol Tablets (One case) 2692
Glucotrol XL Extended Release Tablets (One case) 2693
Halcion Tablets 2823
Haldol Decanoate 2535
Haldol Injection, Tablets and Concentrate 2533
Havrix Vaccine (Rare) 1544
Hivid Tablets (Less than 1%) 2975
HydroDIURIL Tablets 2108
Hyzaar 2109
Indapamide Tablets 2286
Inderide Tablets 3517
Inderide LA Long-Acting Capsules 3519
Indocin Capsules (Less than 1%) 2112
Indocin I.V. (Less than 1%) 2115
Indocin (Less than 1%) 2112
Intron A for Injection (Less than 5%) 3120
Invirase Capsules (Rare) 2979
Lamisil Tablets 2360
Leukeran Tablets 1591
Levaquin (Less than 0.3%) 2537
Levlen 962
Levlite 21 Tablets 962
Levlite 28 Tablets 962
Librium Capsules (Occasional) 1736
Librium for Injection (Occasional) 1737
Limbitrol (Rare) 1738
Lodine (Less than 1%) 3528
Lodine XL Extended-Release Tablets (Less than 1%) 3530
Lotensin HCT Tablets 2367
Loxitane Capsules (Rare) 3398
Luvox Tablets (25, 50, 100 mg) (Rare) 3256
Matulane Capsules 3246
Mavik Tablets (Rare) 478
Maxzide 1008
Mefoxin for Injection 2124
Mefoxin Premixed Intravenous Solution 2127
Merrem I.V. (0.1% to 1.0%) 673
Micardis HCT Tablets 1051
Microzide Capsules 3414
Midamor Tablets (Less than or equal to 1%) 2136
Mintezol 2137
Mobic Tablets (Less than 0.1%) 1054
Modicon 2563
Moduretic Tablets 2138
Monopril Tablets 1091
Monopril HCT 1094
Motrin Suspension, Oral Drops, Chewable Tablets, and Caplets (Rare; less than 1%) 2002
Mustargen for Injection (Infrequent) 2142
Mylotarg for Injection 3540
▲ Naprelan Tablets (3% to 9%) 1293
Naprosyn Suspension (Rare; less than 1%) 2967
Naprosyn Tablets (Rare; less than 1%) 2967
Nardil Tablets (Less frequent) 2653
Naropin Injection (Less than 1%) 612
Neurontin Capsules 2655
Neurontin Oral Solution 2655
Neurontin Tablets 2655
Niaspan Extended-Release Tablets 1846
Nilandron Tablets 753
Nimotop Capsules (Less than 1%) 904
Nizoral Tablets 1791
Norinyl 1 +35 28-Day Tablets 3380
Norinyl 1 + 50 28-Day Tablets 3380
Normodyne Injection 3135
Normodyne Tablets 3137
Noroxin Tablets 2145
Norpramin Tablets 755
Norvasc Tablets (Infrequent) 2704
Norvir Capsules 487
Norvir Oral Solution 487
▲ Novantrone for Injection (3% to 7%) 1760
Omnicef 493
Oncaspar (Greater than 1% but less than 5%) 756
Ortho-Cyclen/Ortho Tri-Cyclen 2573
Ortho-Novum 2563
Ortho-Novum 1/50□28 Tablets 2556
Ortho-Novum 2563
Ortho-Cyclen/Ortho Tri-Cyclen 2573
Orudis Capsules (Less than 1%) 3548
Oruvail Capsules (Less than 1%) 3548
Ovcon 3364
Oxandrin Tablets 1153
Paser Granules 1781
Paxil (Rare) 1609
Pediazole Suspension 3050
Pentasa Capsules 3239
Periactin Tablets 2155
Permax Tablets (Rare) 1299
Phenergan Injection 3553
Phenergan 3556
Photofrin for Injection (Less than 5%) 831
Ponstel Capsules (Occasional) 1356
Precose Tablets 906
PREVPAC (Infrequent) 3298
Priftin Tablets 758
Prilosec Delayed-Release Capsules (Rare) 628
Primaxin I.M. 2158
Primaxin I.V. (Less than 0.2%) 2160
Prinivil Tablets 2164
Prinzide Tablets 2168
▲ Prograf (3% to 15%) 1393
▲ Proleukin for Injection (11%) 1199
Protonix I.V. 3580
Protonix Tablets 3577
Reglan (Rare) 2935
Relafen Tablets (Less than 1%) 1617
Renese Tablets 2712
Rescriptor Tablets 526
Rifadin (Some patients) 765
Rifamate Capsules 767
Rifater Tablets 769
Rilutek Tablets (Infrequent) 772
Risperdal 1796
Robaxin Injectable 2938
Robaxin Tablets 2939

Rocephin Injectable Vials, ADD-Vantage, Galaxy, Bulk (Rare) 2993
Sandostatin Injection (Less than 1%) 2394
Sandostatin LAR Depot (1% to 4%) 2395
Septra Suspension 2265
Septra Tablets 2265
Septra DS Tablets 2265
Serentil 1057
Sinequan (Occasional) 2713
Skelaxin Tablets 1301
Soriatane Capsules (2 of 525 patients) 3003
Sporanox Capsules 1800
Sporanox Injection (1%) 1804
Sporanox Injection (1%) 2509
Stelazine 1640
Suprax 1877
Surmontil Capsules 3595
Tabloid Tablets (A few cases) 1642
Tambocor Tablets 1990
Tao Capsules 2716
Tapazole Tablets 1823
Tasmar Tablets 3010
Tenoretic Tablets 690
Testoderm Transdermal Systems 574
Thioridazine Hydrochloride Tablets 2289
Thorazine 1656
Tonocard Tablets (Less than 1%) 649
Trasylol Injection (1% to 2%) 909
Trecator-SC Tablets 3598
Trental Tablets (Rare) 784
Trilafon (Low incidence) 3160
Tri-Levlen 962
Tri-Norinyl-28 Tablets 3433
Trovan (Less than 1%) 2722
Twinrix Vaccine 1674
Uniretic Tablets (Less than 1%) 3178
Univasc Tablets 3181
Valium Injectable (Isolated reports) 3026
Valium Tablets (Isolated reports) 3047
Vaseretic Tablets 2204
Vasotec I.V. Injection 2207
Vasotec Tablets 2210
Vioxx 2213
Viracept 532
Viramune Oral Suspension 1060
Viramune Tablets 1060
Vistide Injection 1445
Vivactil Tablets 2217
Vivactil Tablets 2446
Voltaren Tablets (Less than 1%) 2315
Voltaren-XR Tablets (Less than 1%) 2315
Warfarin Sodium Tablets, USP 3302
Wellbutrin Tablets (Infrequent) 1680
Wellbutrin SR Sustained-Release Tablets (Infrequent) 1684
Xanax Tablets 2865
Zantac (Occasional) 1690
Zantac Injection 1688
Zantac Syrup (Occasional) 1690
Zestoretic Tablets 695
Ziac Tablets 1887
Zoloft (One or more patients) 2751
Zovirax 1706
Zyban Sustained-Release Tablets (Infrequent) 1710
Zyflo Filmtab Tablets (One patient) 524

Jaundice, cholestatic

Accupril Tablets (Rare) 2611
Accuretic Tablets 2614
Aceon Tablets (2 mg, 4 mg, 8 mg) (Rare) 3249
Activella Tablets 2764
Alesse-21 Tablets 3468
Alesse-28 Tablets 3473
Alora Transdermal System 3372
Altace Capsules (Rare) 2233
Amoxil Chewable Tablets 1471
Amoxil for Oral Suspension 1471
Amoxil 1471
Androderm Transdermal System CIII 3377
▲ Android Capsules, 10 mg (Among most common) 1731
Asacol Delayed-Release Tablets (Rare) 2884
Augmentin Chewable Tablets 1482
Augmentin Powder for Oral Suspension 1482
Augmentin Tablets 1485
Augmentin ES-600 Powder for Oral Suspension 1487
Avelox Tablets (0.05% to 1%) 879
Axid Pulvules (Rare) 1903
Axid Pulvules (Rare) 2919
Aygestin Tablets 1333
Azulfidine EN-tabs Tablets 2775
Bactrim 2949
Baycol Tablets 883
Brevicon 28-Day Tablets 3380
Captopril Tablets (Rare) 2281
Carbatrol Capsules 3234
Ceclor (Rare) 1905
Cefzil (Rare) 1076
▲ CellCept Capsules (11.9%) 2951
▲ CellCept Intravenous (11.9%) 2951
▲ CellCept Oral Suspension (11.9%) 2951
▲ CellCept Tablets (11.9%) 2951
Cenestin Tablets 1263
Chibroxin Sterile Ophthalmic Solution 2051
Cipro 887
Climara Transdermal System 958
Colazal Capsules 3069
Compazine 1505
Cyclessa Tablets 2450
Dapsone Tablets USP 1780
Darvon-N/Darvocet-N (Rare) 1907
Darvon Pulvules 1909
Darvon Compound-65 Pulvules 1910
Darvon-N Tablets (Rare) 1912
Delatestryl Injection 1151
Desogen Tablets 2458
DiaBeta Tablets (Rare) 741
Diabinese Tablets (Rare) 2680
Doxil Injection (Less than 1%) 566
Enalaprilat Injection (Rare) 863
Esclim Transdermal System 3460
Estinyl Tablets 3112
Estrace Vaginal Cream 3358
Estrace Tablets 3361
Estratest 3252
Estrostep 2627
Eulexin Capsules (Less than 1%) 3118
Famotidine Injection (Infrequent) 866
femhrt Tablets 2635
Floxin I.V. 2526
Floxin Tablets 2529
Geodon Capsules (Rare) 2688
Glucotrol Tablets (Rare) 2692
Keflex (Rare) 1237
Kefzol Vials, ADD-Vantage (Rare) 1951
Lescol Capsules 2361
Lescol Capsules 2925
Lescol XL Tablets 2361
Lescol XL Tablets 2925
Levlen 962
Levlite 21 Tablets 962
Levlite 28 Tablets 962
Levora Tablets 3389
Lexxel Tablets 608
Lipitor Tablets (Less than 2%) 2639
Lipitor Tablets (Less than 2%) 2696
Lodine (Less than 1%) 3528
Lodine XL Extended-Release Tablets (Less than 1%) 3530
Loestrin 21 Tablets 2642
Loestrin Fe Tablets 2642
Lo/Ovral Tablets 3532
Lo/Ovral-28 Tablets 3538
Lopid Tablets 2650
Lotrel Capsules (Rare) 2370
Low-Ogestrel-28 Tablets 3392
Lunelle Monthly Injection 2827
Macrobid Capsules (Rare) 2889
Macrodantin Capsules (Rare) 2891
Mandol Vials (Rare) 1953
Mavik Tablets (Rare) 478
Menest Tablets 2254
Merrem I.V. (0.1% to 1.0%) 673
Mevacor Tablets 2132
Microgestin Fe 1.5/30 Tablets 3407
Microgestin Fe 1/20 Tablets 3400
Mircette Tablets 2470
Modicon 2563
Monopril Tablets (Rare) 1091
Monurol Sachet 1375
Myleran Tablets (Rare) 1603
Necon 3415
Nordette-28 Tablets 2257
Norinyl 1 +35 28-Day Tablets 3380
Norinyl 1 + 50 28-Day Tablets 3380
Normodyne Injection 3135
Normodyne Tablets (Less common) 3137
Noroxin Tablets 2145
Ogen Tablets 2846
Ogestrel 0.5/50-28 Tablets 3428
Ortho Dienestrol Cream 2554
Ortho-Cept 21 Tablets 2546
Ortho-Cept 28 Tablets 2546
Ortho-Cyclen/Ortho Tri-Cyclen 2573
Ortho-Est Tablets 3464
Ortho-Novum 2563
Ortho-Novum 1/50□28 Tablets 2556
Ortho-Prefest Tablets 2570
Ortho-Cyclen/Ortho Tri-Cyclen 2573
Ovcon 3364
Ovral Tablets 3551
Ovral-28 Tablets 3552
Ovrette Tablets 3552
Oxandrin Tablets 1153
Pentasa Capsules 3239
Pepcid Injection (Infrequent) 2153
Pepcid for Oral Suspension (Infrequent) 2150
Pepcid RPD Orally Disintegrating Tablets (Infrequent) 2150
Pepcid Tablets (Infrequent) 2150
Phenergan 3556
Pravachol Tablets 1099
Premarin Intravenous 3563
Premarin Tablets 3566
Premarin Vaginal Cream 3570
Premphase Tablets 3572
Prempro Tablets 3572
Prilosec Delayed-Release Capsules (Rare) 628
Prinivil Tablets (0.3% to 1.0%) 2164
Prinzide Tablets (Rare) 2168
Procardia Capsules 2708
Procardia XL Extended Release Tablets 2710
▲ Prograf (3% to 15%) 1393
Prometrium Capsules (100 mg, 200 mg) 3261
Protonix I.V. (Less than 1%) 3580
Protonix Tablets (Less than 1%) 3577
Provera Tablets 2853
Prozac Pulvules, Liquid, and Weekly Capsules 1238
Relafen Tablets (1%) 1617
Robaxin Injectable 2938
Robaxin Tablets 2939
Sarafem Pulvules 1962
Septra Suspension 2265
Septra Tablets 2265
Septra DS Tablets 2265
Stelazine 1640
Tarka Tablets (Rare) 508
Tegretol/Tegretol-XR 2404
Testoderm Transdermal Systems 574
Testopel Pellets 3610
Testred Capsules, 10 mg 1746
Thalomid Capsules 1154
Ticlid Tablets (Rare) 3015
Timentin Injection- ADD-Vantage Vial (Rare) 1661
Timentin Injection-Galaxy Container (Rare) 1664
Timentin Injection-Pharmacy Bulk Package (Rare) 1666
Timentin for Intravenous Administration (Rare) 1658
Toradol 3018
Tri-Levlen 962
Tri-Norinyl-28 Tablets 3433
Triphasil-21 Tablets 3600
Triphasil-28 Tablets 3605
Trivora Tablets 3439
Uniretic Tablets (Rare) 3178
Univasc Tablets (Rare) 3181
Vaseretic Tablets (Rare) 2204
Vasotec I.V. Injection (Rare) 2207
Vasotec Tablets (0.5% to 1.0%) 2210
Vivelle Transdermal System 2412
Vivelle-Dot Transdermal System 2416
Yasmin 28 Tablets 980
Zestoretic Tablets (Rare) 695
Zestril Tablets (0.3% to 1.0%) 698
Zithromax Capsules, 250 mg (1% or less; rare) 2743
Zithromax for IV Infusion 2748
Zithromax for Oral Suspension, 1 g (1% or less; rare) 2743
Zithromax for Oral Suspension, 300 mg, 600 mg, 900 mg, 1200 mg (1% or less; rare) 2739
Zithromax Tablets, 250 mg (1% or less; rare) 2739
Zithromax Tablets, 600 mg (1% or less; rare) 2743
Zocor Tablets 2219
Zonegran Capsules (Rare) 1307
Zosyn 1890
Zosyn in Galaxy Containers 1894
Zovia 3449

Jaundice, fetal

Diuril Oral 2087
Diuril Sodium Intravenous 2086
HydroDIURIL Tablets 2108

Jaundice, hepatocellular

Aceon Tablets (2 mg, 4 mg, 8 mg) 3249
Augmentin Chewable Tablets 1482
Augmentin Powder for Oral Suspension 1482
Augmentin Tablets 1485
Augmentin ES-600 Powder for Oral Suspension 1487
Axid Pulvules (Rare) 1903
Axid Pulvules (Rare) 2919
Biaxin/Biaxin XL (Infrequent) 403
Carbatrol Capsules 3234
Enalaprilat Injection 863
Floxin I.V. 2526
Floxin Tablets 2529
Lexxel Tablets 608
Monopril Tablets 1091
PREVPAC (Infrequent) 3298
Prilosec Delayed-Release Capsules (Rare) 628
Prinivil Tablets (0.3% to 1.0%) 2164
Prinzide Tablets 2168
Tegretol/Tegretol-XR 2404
Ticlid Tablets (Rare) 3015
Vaseretic Tablets 2204
Vasotec I.V. Injection 2207
Vasotec Tablets (0.5% to 1.0%) 2210
Zantac (Occasional) 1690
Zestoretic Tablets 695
Zestril Tablets (0.3% to 1.0%) 698

Jaundice, intrahepatic

Minizide Capsules 2700

Jaundice, intrahepatic cholestatic

Accuretic Tablets 2614
Aldoclor Tablets 2035
Atacand HCT Tablets 597
Augmentin Chewable Tablets 1482
Augmentin Powder for Oral Suspension 1482
Augmentin Tablets 1485
Augmentin ES-600 Powder for Oral Suspension 1487
Avalide Tablets 1070
Clorpres Tablets 1002
Combipres Tablets 1040
Corzide 40/5 Tablets 2247
Corzide 80/5 Tablets 2247
Diovan HCT Tablets 2338
Diucardin Tablets 3494
Diuril Oral 2087
Diuril Sodium Intravenous 2086
Furosemide Tablets 2284
HydroDIURIL Tablets 2108
Hyzaar 2109
Indapamide Tablets 2286
Inderide Tablets 3517
Inderide LA Long-Acting Capsules 3519
Lotensin HCT Tablets 2367
Maxzide 1008
Micardis HCT Tablets 1051
Microzide Capsules 3414
Moduretic Tablets 2138
Monopril HCT 1094
Mykrox Tablets 1168
Prinzide Tablets 2168
Renese Tablets 2712
Tenoretic Tablets 690
Timolide Tablets 2187
Uniretic Tablets 3178
Vaseretic Tablets 2204
Zaroxolyn Tablets 1177
Zestoretic Tablets 695
Ziac Tablets 1887

Jaundice, neonatal

Aldoclor Tablets 2035
Aldoril Tablets 2039
AquaMEPHYTON Injection 2042
Compazine 1505
Diucardin Tablets 3494
Diuril Oral 2087
Diuril Sodium Intravenous 2086
Dyazide Capsules 1515
HydroDIURIL Tablets 2108
Inderide Tablets 3517
Inderide LA Long-Acting Capsules 3519
Levlen 962
Levlite 21 Tablets 962
Levlite 28 Tablets 962
Maxzide 1008
Mephyton Tablets 2129
Modicon 2563
Moduretic Tablets 2138
Mykrox Tablets 1168
▲ Naropin Injection (3.6%) 612
Ortho-Novum 2563
Ortho-Novum 1/50□28 Tablets 2556
Prinzide Tablets 2168
Stelazine 1640
Tenoretic Tablets 690
Thorazine 1656
Timolide Tablets 2187
Tri-Levlen 962
Vaseretic Tablets 2204
Zestoretic Tablets 695

Jaundice, obstructive

Thorazine 1656

Jaw tightness

Anectine Injection 1476
Imitrex Injection (Relatively common) 1549
Imitrex Tablets 1558
▲ Zomig Tablets (4% to 10%) 708
▲ Zomig-ZMT Tablets (4% to 10%) 708

Jerks

(*see under* Twitching)

Jitteriness

Compazine 1505
Etrafon 3115
Nardil Tablets (Less common) 2653
Procardia Capsules (2% or less) 2708
Reglan 2935
Stelazine 1640
Thorazine 1656

Joint cyst

Remicade (Less than 2%) 1178

Joint dislocation

Evoxac Capsules (Less than 1%) 1217

Joint disorder, unspecified

Actiq (1% or greater) 1184
▲ Actonel Tablets (6.8%) 2879
▲ Arava Tablets (4%) 724

Asacol Delayed-Release Tablets (2% or greater) 2884
Bicillin C-R 900/300 Injection 2240
Bicillin C-R Injection 2238
Bicillin L-A Injection 2242
▲ CellCept Capsules (3%) 2951
▲ CellCept Intravenous (3%) 2951
▲ CellCept Oral Suspension (3%) 2951
▲ CellCept Tablets (3%) 2951
Esclim Transdermal System 3460
▲ Humatrope Vials and Cartridges (2.3% to 5.8%) 1930
Hytrin Capsules (At least 1%) 464
Imitrex Nasal Spray (Infrequent) 1554
Keflex 1237
Lamictal (1.3%) 1567
▲ Lupron Depot 3.75 mg (7.8%) 3281
▲ Lupron Depot–3 Month 11.25 mg (7.8% to 8%) 3285
▲ Lupron Depot–3 Month 22.5 mg (11.7%) 3288
▲ Lupron Depot–4 Month 30 mg (4.2% to 16.3%) 3289
Meridia Capsules (1.1%) 481
Mirapex Tablets (Less than 1%) 2834
Myobloc Injectable Solution (2% or greater) 1291
Naprelan Tablets (Less than 3%) 1293
Norvir Capsules (Less than 2%) 487
Norvir Oral Solution (Less than 2%) 487
Oncaspar (Less than 1%) 756
Orgaran Injection (2.6%) 2480
▲ Prograf (3% to 15%) 1393
Protonix I.V. (Less than 1%) 3580
Protonix Tablets (Less than 1%) 3577
Provigil Tablets (1%) 1193
Sonata Capsules (Infrequent) 3591
Tasmar Tablets (Infrequent) 3010
Thalomid Capsules 1154
Tricor Capsules, Micronized 513
Vistide Injection 1445
Xenical Capsules (2.3%) 3043
Zoladex (1% or greater) 702
Zoladex 3-month 706

Joint effusion
Sandostatin Injection (Less than 1%) 2394
Sandostatin LAR Depot (Rare) 2395

Joint pain
(*see under* Arthralgia)

Joint stiffness
Amerge Tablets (Infrequent) 1467
Avalide Tablets 1070
Avapro Tablets (Less than 1%) 1074
Avapro Tablets (Less than 1%) 3076
Cipro I.V. (1% or less) 893
Cipro I.V. Pharmacy Bulk Package (Less than 1%) 897
Cipro (Less than 1%) 887
Imitrex Injection (Infrequent) 1549
Neurontin Capsules (Infrequent) 2655
Neurontin Oral Solution (Infrequent) 2655
Neurontin Tablets (Infrequent) 2655
Oncaspar 756
Procardia Capsules (2% or less) 2708
Xeloda Tablets (Less than 5%) 3039
Zyprexa Tablets 1973
Zyprexa ZYDIS Orally Disintegrating Tablets 1973

K

Kaposi's sarcoma
Fortovase Capsules (Less than 2%) 2970
▲ Serostim for Injection (1% to 10%) 3229

Kawasaki-like syndrome
Asacol Delayed-Release Tablets (One case) 2884
Azulfidine EN-tabs Tablets 2775
Pentasa Capsules (Less than 1%) 3239

Keratic precipitates, ocular
Vitravene for Injection (2% to 5%) ⊙ 310

Keratitis
Acular Ophthalmic Solution (Less than 5%) 544
▲ Acular PF Ophthalmic Solution (Approximately 1% to 10%) 544
Advair Diskus 100/50 (1% to 3%) 1448
Advair Diskus 250/50 (1% to 3%) 1448
Advair Diskus 500/50 (1% to 3%) 1448
Alomide Ophthalmic Solution (Less than 1%) ⊙ 204
Azopt Ophthalmic Suspension (1% to 5%) 536
Betagan ⊙ 228
Betimol Ophthalmic Solution (1% to 5%) ⊙ 324
Betoptic S Ophthalmic Suspension (Rare) 537
Botox Purified Neurotoxin Complex (Less than 1%) 549
Carteolol Hydrochloride Ophthalmic Solution USP, 1% ⊙ 258
Celexa (Rare) 1365
Ciloxan (Less than 1%) 538
Effexor Tablets (Rare) 3495
Effexor XR Capsules (Rare) 3499
Ellence Injection 2806
Emadine Ophthalmic Solution (Less than 5%) ⊙ 211
Engerix-B Vaccine 1517
Evoxac Capsules (Less than 1%) 1217
Flovent Diskus (1% to 3%) 3614
FML Ophthalmic Ointment (Occasional) ⊙ 237
FML Ophthalmic Suspension (Occasional) ⊙ 236
FML Forte Ophthalmic Suspension (Occasional) ⊙ 235
Geodon Capsules (Rare) 2688
Imitrex Injection 1549
Imitrex Nasal Spray 1554
Iopidine 0.5% Ophthalmic Solution (Less than 3%) ⊙ 213
Ocuflox Ophthalmic Solution 554
Ocupress Ophthalmic Solution, 1% Sterile ⊙ 303
Patanol Ophthalmic Solution (Less than 5%) 540
Pilopine HS Ophthalmic Gel ⊙ 217
Pred Forte Ophthalmic Suspension (Occasional) ⊙ 246
Pred Mild Sterile Ophthalmic Suspension (Occasional) ⊙ 249
Rescula Ophthalmic Solution (1% to 5%) ⊙ 306
Stromectol Tablets 2185
Symmetrel 1328
TheraCys Injection 823
Timolol GFS ⊙ 266
Timoptic Sterile Ophthalmic Solution (Less frequent) 2190
Timoptic-XE Sterile Ophthalmic Gel Forming Solution 2194
Travatan Ophthalmic Solution (1% to 4%) 543
Twinrix Vaccine 1674
Vexol 1% Ophthalmic Suspension (Less than 1%) ⊙ 222
Vistide Injection 1445
▲ Voltaren Ophthalmic Sterile Ophthalmic Solution (28%) ⊙ 312
Zaditor Ophthalmic Solution (Less than 5%) 2304
Zanaflex Tablets (Rare) 1305

Keratitis, bacterial
Chibroxin Sterile Ophthalmic Solution 2051
Decadron Phosphate Sterile Ophthalmic Ointment 2083
Decadron Phosphate Sterile Ophthalmic Solution 2084
Humorsol Sterile Ophthalmic Solution 2102
Trusopt Sterile Ophthalmic Solution 2196
Xalatan Latanoprost Ophthalmic Solution ⊙ 320
Xalatan Sterile Ophthalmic Solution 2864

Keratitis, epithelial
Ophthetic Ophthalmic Solution ⊙ 244

Keratitis, punctate
Albalon Ophthalmic Solution ⊙ 225
▲ Cosopt Sterile Ophthalmic Solution (5% to 30%) 2065
▲ Lumigan Ophthalmic Solution (3% to 10%) 553
Pred-G Ophthalmic Suspension (Occasional) ⊙ 247
Pred-G Sterile Ophthalmic Ointment ⊙ 248
▲ Rēv-Eyes Sterile Ophthalmic Eyedrops 0.5% (10% to 40%) ⊙ 265

Keratitis, superficial punctate
▲ Trusopt Sterile Ophthalmic Solution (10% to 15%) 2196
Viroptic Ophthalmic Solution Sterile ⊙ 301

Keratitis nigricans
Timoptic in Ocudose (Less frequent) 2192

Keratitis sicca
Viroptic Ophthalmic Solution Sterile ⊙ 301

Keratoconjunctivitis
Alrex Sterile Ophthalmic Suspension 0.2% (Less than 5%) ⊙ 256
Azopt Ophthalmic Suspension (Less than 1%) 536
Betaseron for SC Injection 988
Evoxac Capsules (Less than 1%) 1217
Gabitril Tablets (Infrequent) 1189
Geodon Capsules (Rare) 2688
Lotemax Sterile Ophthalmic Suspension 0.5% (Less than 5%) ⊙ 261
Naprelan Tablets (Less than 1%) 1293
Paxil (Rare) 1609
Remeron Tablets (Infrequent) 2483
Remeron SolTab Tablets (Infrequent) 2486
Serzone Tablets (Infrequent) 1104
Sular Tablets (Less than or equal to 1%) 688
Zyprexa Tablets (Rare) 1973
Zyprexa ZYDIS Orally Disintegrating Tablets (Rare) 1973

Keratopathy
Alomide Ophthalmic Solution (Less than 1%) ⊙ 204
Alphagan P Ophthalmic Solution (1% to 4%) 546
Ciloxan (Less than 1%) 538
Iopidine 0.5% Ophthalmic Solution (Less than 3%) ⊙ 213
Trilafon 3160
Vitrasert Implant (Less than 1%) ⊙ 254

Keratopathy, epithelial
Compazine 1505
Etrafon 3115
Stelazine 1640
Thorazine 1656
Viroptic Ophthalmic Solution Sterile ⊙ 301
▲ Xalatan Latanoprost Ophthalmic Solution (5% to 15%) ⊙ 320
▲ Xalatan Sterile Ophthalmic Solution (5% to 15%) 2864

Keratopathy, vortex
Mepron Suspension 1598

Keratosis
Gengraf Capsules (1% to less than 3%) 457
Neoral Soft Gelatin Capsules (1% to less than 3%) 2380
Neoral Oral Solution (1% to less than 3%) 2380

Keratosis pilaris
Azelex Cream (Rare) 547
Finevin Cream 962

Kernicterus, neonatal
AVC 1350
Azulfidine EN-tabs Tablets 2775
Bactrim 2949
Blephamide Ophthalmic Ointment 547
Pediazole Suspension 3050
Septra Suspension 2265
Septra Tablets 2265
Septra DS Tablets 2265
Silvadene Cream 1% 2267

Ketoniuria
Amerge Tablets (Rare) 1467

Ketosis
Betaseron for SC Injection 988
Cerebyx Injection (Infrequent) 2619
Clozaril Tablets (Sometimes) 2319
Doxil Injection (Less than 1%) 566
Geodon Capsules (Rare) 2688
Paxil (Rare) 1609
Sonata Capsules (Rare) 3591
Zyprexa Tablets (Infrequent) 1973
Zyprexa ZYDIS Orally Disintegrating Tablets (Infrequent) 1973

Kidney damage
Azulfidine EN-tabs Tablets 2775
Furosemide Tablets 2284
▲ Zenapax for Injection (2% to 5%) 3046

Kidney pain
(*see under* Pain, renal)

Kidney stones
(*see under* Nephrolithiasis)

L

Labia, fusion
Provera Tablets (Rare) 2853

Labor, slowing
Aggrenox Capsules 1026
Astramorph/PF Injection, USP (Preservative-Free) 594
Kadian Capsules (Less than 3%) 1335
Naropin Injection (Less than 1%) 612
Proventil Inhalation Solution 0.083% (Some reports) 3146
Proventil Repetabs Tablets (Some reports) 3148
Proventil Solution for Inhalation 0.5% (Some reports) 3144
Sensorcaine 643
Sensorcaine-MPF Injection 643

Laboratory abnormalities, unspecified
Betapace Tablets (1% to 4%) 950

Labyrinth disorder
Intron A for Injection (Less than 5%) 3120
Zoloft (Rare) 2751

Labyrinthitis
Amerge Tablets (Rare) 1467
Avonex 1013
Benadryl Parenteral 2617
Cognex Capsules (Rare) 1351
Effexor Tablets (Rare) 3495
Effexor XR Capsules (Rare) 3499
Neurontin Capsules (Rare) 2655
Neurontin Oral Solution (Rare) 2655
Neurontin Tablets (Rare) 2655
Nipent for Injection (Less than 3%) 3272
Periactin Tablets 2155
Rynatan Tablets 3351
Sonata Capsules (Rare) 3591

Laceration
Advair Diskus 100/50 (1% to 3%) 1448
Advair Diskus 250/50 (1% to 3%) 1448
Advair Diskus 500/50 (1% to 3%) 1448
Flovent Diskus (1% to 3%) 3614
Vioxx (Greater than 0.1% to 1.9%) 2213

Lacrimal duct, stenosis
Ergamisol Tablets 1789
Sterile FUDR (Remote possibility) 2974

Lacrimal gland, disorders
DDAVP Nasal Spray (Up to 2%) 738
DDAVP Rhinal Tube (Up to 2%) 738
Intron A for Injection (Less than 5%) 3120
Neurontin Capsules (Rare) 2655
Neurontin Oral Solution (Rare) 2655
Neurontin Tablets (Rare) 2655

Lacrimation
Adriamycin PFS/RDF Injection (Rare) 2767
Albalon Ophthalmic Solution ⊙ 225
Azopt Ophthalmic Suspension (Less than 1%) 536
▲ Botox Purified Neurotoxin Complex (10.0%) 549
Ciloxan (Less than 1%) 538
Claritin (At least one patient) 3100
Crolom Sterile Ophthalmic Solution USP 4% (Infrequent) ⊙ 259
Efudex 1733
Emadine Ophthalmic Solution (Less than 5%) ⊙ 211
Enalaprilat Injection 863
Sterile FUDR (Remote possibility) 2974
Heparin Lock Flush Solution 3509
Heparin Sodium Injection 3511
Hivid Tablets (Less than 1%) 2975
Humorsol Sterile Ophthalmic Solution 2102
Imitrex Injection (Infrequent) 1549
Imitrex Nasal Spray (Infrequent) 1554
Imitrex Tablets (Infrequent) 1558
Livostin (Approximately 1% to 3%) ⊙ 305
Maxalt Tablets (Infrequent) 2120
Maxalt-MLT Orally Disintegrating Tablets (Infrequent) 2120
Neurontin Capsules (Rare) 2655
Neurontin Oral Solution (Rare) 2655
Neurontin Tablets (Rare) 2655
Nipent for Injection (Less than 3%) 3272
Opticrom Ophthalmic Solution (Infrequent) 555
OptiPranolol Metipranolol Ophthalmic Solution 0.3% (A small number of patients) ⊙ 263
Pilopine HS Ophthalmic Gel ⊙ 217
▲ Salagen Tablets (6%) 2229
Tasmar Tablets (Infrequent) 3010
Tensilon Injectable 1745
Trusopt Sterile Ophthalmic Solution (Approximately 1% to 5%) 2196
Urecholine 2198
Urecholine Tablets 2445
Vanceril Double Strength Inhalation Aerosol (Fewer than 2%) 3167
Vaseretic Tablets 2204
Vasotec I.V. Injection 2207
Vasotec Tablets (0.5% to 1.0%) 2210
Vexol 1% Ophthalmic Suspension (Less than 1%) ⊙ 222
Zomig Tablets (Rare) 708
Zomig-ZMT Tablets (Rare) 708

Lacrimation, abnormal
Ambien Tablets (Rare) 3191
Arthrotec Tablets (Rare) 3195
Cardura Tablets (Less than 0.5%) 2668
Celexa (Infrequent) 1365
▲ CellCept Capsules (3% to 10%) 2951
▲ CellCept Intravenous (3% to 10%) 2951
▲ CellCept Oral Suspension (3% to 10%) 2951
▲ CellCept Tablets (3% to 10%) 2951

Claritin-D 12 Hour Extended Release Tablets (Less frequent) ... 3102
Claritin-D 24 Hour Extended Release Tablets (Fewer than 2%) ... 3104
Desmopressin Acetate Rhinal Tube (Up to 2%) ... 1345
Ergamisol Tablets (Up to 4%) ... 1789
Flumadine ... 1370
Lamictal (Rare) ... 1567
Miacalcin Nasal Spray (1% to 3%) ... 2375
Migranal Nasal Spray (Infrequent) ... 2376
Naprelan Tablets (Less than 1%) ... 1293
Nicotrol Nasal Spray (Common) ... 2843
Procardia XL Extended Release Tablets (1% or less) ... 2710
Remeron Tablets (Infrequent) ... 2483
Remeron SolTab Tablets (Infrequent) ... 2486
Requip Tablets (Infrequent) ... 1621
Risperdal (Rare) ... 1796
Rituxan for Infusion (1% to 5%) ... 1750
Rituxan I.V. (1% to 5%) ... 1428
Romazicon Injection (1% to 3%) ... 3000
Salagen Tablets (Less than 1%) ... 2229
Soriatane Capsules (Less than 1%) ... 3003
Topamax Sprinkle Capsules (Infrequent) ... 2590
Topamax Tablets (Infrequent) ... 2590
▲ Visudyne for Injection (1% to 10%) ... ⊙ 308
Voltaren Ophthalmic Sterile Ophthalmic Solution (Less than 5%) ... ⊙ 312
Zaditor Ophthalmic Solution (Less than 5%) ... 2304
Zebeta Tablets ... 1885
Ziac Tablets ... 1887
Zoloft (Rare) ... 2751

Lactation
Aldoclor Tablets ... 2035
Aldomet Tablets ... 2037
Aldoril Tablets ... 2039
Compazine ... 1505
Effexor Tablets (Rare) ... 3495
Etrafon ... 3115
Geodon Capsules (Infrequent) ... 2688
Haldol Decanoate ... 2535
Haldol Injection, Tablets and Concentrate ... 2533
Lamictal (Infrequent) ... 1567
▲ Lupron Depot 3.75 mg (Among most frequent) ... 3281
Lupron Depot–3 Month 11.25 mg (Less than 5%) ... 3285
Luvox Tablets (25, 50, 100 mg) (Infrequent) ... 3256
Navane Oral ... 2701
Navane Intramuscular ... 2703
Paxil (Rare) ... 1609
Permax Tablets (Infrequent) ... 1299
Prozac Pulvules, Liquid, and Weekly Capsules (Infrequent) ... 1238
Sarafem Pulvules (Infrequent) ... 1962
Serentil ... 1057
Stelazine ... 1640
Synarel Nasal Solution for Endometriosis (Less than 1%) ... 3205
Thioridazine Hydrochloride Tablets ... 2289
Thiothixene Capsules ... 2290
Thorazine ... 1656
Trilafon ... 3160
Zyprexa Tablets (Infrequent) ... 1973
Zyprexa ZYDIS Orally Disintegrating Tablets (Infrequent) ... 1973

Lactation, non-puerperal
Flumadine (Less than 0.3%) ... 1370
Risperdal (Infrequent) ... 1796
Sandostatin LAR Depot (Rare) ... 2395

Lactation, possible diminution
Alesse-21 Tablets ... 3468
Alesse-28 Tablets ... 3473
Brevicon 28-Day Tablets ... 3380
Desogen Tablets ... 2458
Estrostep ... 2627
Levlen ... 962
Levlite 21 Tablets ... 962
Levlite 28 Tablets ... 962
Levora Tablets ... 3389
Loestrin 21 Tablets ... 2642
Loestrin Fe Tablets ... 2642
Lo/Ovral Tablets ... 3532
Lo/Ovral-28 Tablets ... 3538
Low-Ogestrel-28 Tablets ... 3392
Lunelle Monthly Injection ... 2827
Microgestin Fe 1.5/30 Tablets ... 3407
Microgestin Fe 1/20 Tablets ... 3400
Mircette Tablets ... 2470
Modicon ... 2563
Necon ... 3415
Nordette-28 Tablets ... 2257
Norinyl 1 +35 28-Day Tablets ... 3380
Norinyl 1 + 50 28-Day Tablets ... 3380
Ogestrel 0.5/50-28 Tablets ... 3428
Ortho-Cept 21 Tablets ... 2546
Ortho-Cept 28 Tablets ... 2546
Ortho-Cyclen/Ortho Tri-Cyclen ... 2573
Ortho-Novum ... 2563
Ortho-Novum 1/50□28 Tablets ... 2556
Ortho-Novum ... 2563
Ortho-Cyclen/Ortho Tri-Cyclen ... 2573
Ovral Tablets ... 3551
Ovral-28 Tablets ... 3552
Ovrette Tablets ... 3552
Tri-Levlen ... 962
Tri-Norinyl-28 Tablets ... 3433
Triphasil-21 Tablets ... 3600
Triphasil-28 Tablets ... 3605
Trivora Tablets ... 3439
Zovia ... 3449

Lactation, suppression
Depo-Provera Contraceptive Injection (Fewer than 1%) ... 2798
Donnatal ... 2929
Donnatal Extentabs ... 2930
Donnatal Tablets ... 2929
Levsin/Levsinex/Levbid ... 3172
NuLev Orally Disintegrating Tablets ... 3176
Ovcon ... 3364
Robinul Forte Tablets ... 1358
Robinul Injectable ... 2940
Robinul Tablets ... 1358

Lactation abnormalities
Seroquel Tablets (Infrequent) ... 684
Thyrel TRH for Injection (Less frequent) ... 3630

Lactic acidosis
Aloprim for Injection (Less than 1%) ... 2292
Combivir Tablets ... 1502
Epivir ... 1520
Epivir-HBV ... 1524
Glucophage Tablets ... 1080
Glucophage XR Tablets ... 1080
Glucovance Tablets ... 1086
Hivid Tablets (Rare) ... 2975
Kaletra Capsules (Less than 2%) ... 471
Kaletra Oral Solution (Less than 2%) ... 471
Retrovir Capsules (Rare) ... 1625
Retrovir IV Infusion (Rare) ... 1629
Retrovir (Rare) ... 1625
Trizivir Tablets ... 1669
Videx ... 1138
Videx EC Capsules ... 1143
Zerit ... 1147

Lagophthalmos
Botox Purified Neurotoxin Complex ... 549

Language problems, unspecified
▲ Topamax Sprinkle Capsules (2.2% to 11.7%) ... 2590
▲ Topamax Tablets (2.2% to 11.7%) ... 2590

Laryngeal changes
Mexitil Capsules (About 1 in 1,000) ... 1047

Laryngeal stridor
Lotrel Capsules (About 0.5%) ... 2370
Monopril Tablets ... 1091

Laryngismus
Axert Tablets (Infrequent) ... 2772
▲ Copaxone for Injection (5%) ... 3306
Effexor Tablets (Infrequent) ... 3495
Effexor XR Capsules (Infrequent) ... 3499
Luvox Tablets (25, 50, 100 mg) ... 3256
Paxil ... 1609
Rescriptor Tablets (Less than 2%) ... 526
Roxicodone Tablets (Less than 3%) ... 3067
Salagen Tablets (Less than 1%) ... 2229
Topamax Sprinkle Capsules (Rare) ... 2590
Topamax Tablets (Rare) ... 2590
Trileptal Oral Suspension ... 2407
Trileptal Tablets ... 2407
Zoloft (Rare) ... 2751

Laryngitis
Aciphex Tablets ... 1267
Aciphex Tablets ... 1783
Aerobid/Aerobid-M (1% to 3%) ... 1363
Ambien Tablets (Rare) ... 3191
Astelin Nasal Spray (Infrequent) ... 3339
Avonex ... 1013
Axert Tablets (Rare) ... 2772
▲ Betaseron for SC Injection (6%) ... 988
Celebrex Capsules (0.1% to 1.9%) ... 2676
Celebrex Capsules (0.1% to 1.9%) ... 2780
Celexa (Rare) ... 1365
Claritin (At least one patient) ... 3100
Claritin-D 12 Hour Extended Release Tablets ... 3102
Claritin-D 24 Hour Extended Release Tablets ... 3104
Clozaril Tablets (Less than 1%) ... 2319
Copaxone for Injection (At least 2%) ... 3306
Doxil Injection (Less than 1%) ... 566
Effexor Tablets (Infrequent) ... 3495
Effexor XR Capsules (Infrequent) ... 3499
Evista Tablets (2.2%) ... 1915
Evoxac Capsules (Less than 1%) ... 1217
Exelon Capsules (Infrequent) ... 2342
Exelon Oral Solution (Infrequent) ... 2345
Flovent Diskus (1% to 3%) ... 3614
Flovent ... 1535
Flovent Rotadisk (1% to 3%) ... 1537
Fortovase Capsules (Less than 2%) ... 2970
Gabitril Tablets (Infrequent) ... 1189
Herceptin I.V. (At least one of the 958 patients) ... 1414
Invirase Capsules (Less than 2%) ... 2979
Lupron Depot–3 Month 11.25 mg ... 3285
Meridia Capsules (1.3%) ... 481
Monopril Tablets (0.2% to 1.0%) ... 1091
Monopril HCT ... 1094
Naprelan Tablets (Less than 1%) ... 1293
Neurontin Capsules (Rare) ... 2655
Neurontin Oral Solution (Rare) ... 2655
Neurontin Tablets (Rare) ... 2655
Permax Tablets (Infrequent) ... 1299
Prinivil Tablets (0.3% to 1.0%) ... 2164
Prinzide Tablets ... 2168
ProSom Tablets (Rare) ... 500
Prostin E2 Suppositories ... 2852
Protonix I.V. (Less than 1%) ... 3580
Protonix Tablets (Less than 1%) ... 3577
Protopic Ointment (Greater than or equal to 1%) ... 1397
▲ Pulmozyme Inhalation Solution (3% to 4%) ... 1426
Remeron Tablets (Rare) ... 2483
Remeron SolTab Tablets (Rare) ... 2486
Requip Tablets (Infrequent) ... 1621
Rilutek Tablets (Infrequent) ... 772
Salagen Tablets (Less than 1%) ... 2229
Serevent Inhalation Aerosol (1% to 3%) ... 1633
Serzone Tablets (Infrequent) ... 1104
Singulair (Greater than or equal to 2%) ... 2181
Sonata Capsules (Infrequent) ... 3591
Soriatane Capsules (Less than 1%) ... 3003
Sular Tablets (Less than or equal to 1%) ... 688
Tasmar Tablets (Infrequent) ... 3010
Trental Tablets (Less than 1%) ... 784
Tricor Capsules, Micronized ... 513
Uniretic Tablets (Less than 1%) ... 3178
Ventolin HFA Inhalation Aerosol (Less than 3%) ... 3618
Viagra Tablets (Less than 2%) ... 2732
Vioxx (Greater than 0.1% to 1.9%) ... 2213
Xeloda Tablets (Less than 5%) ... 3039
Zestoretic Tablets ... 695
Zestril Tablets (0.3% to 1.0%) ... 698
Zoloft (Rare) ... 2751
Zomig Tablets (Infrequent) ... 708
Zomig-ZMT Tablets (Infrequent) ... 708
Zyprexa Tablets (Rare) ... 1973
Zyprexa ZYDIS Orally Disintegrating Tablets (Rare) ... 1973

Laryngospasm
Advair Diskus 100/50 ... 1448
Advair Diskus 250/50 ... 1448
Advair Diskus 500/50 ... 1448
Atrovent Inhalation Aerosol ... 1030
Atrovent Nasal Spray 0.06% ... 1033
Blocadren Tablets ... 2046
Brevital Sodium for Injection, USP ... 1815
Carafate Suspension ... 731
Carafate Tablets ... 730
Combivent Inhalation Aerosol (Less than 2%) ... 1041
Corgard Tablets ... 2245
Corzide 40/5 Tablets ... 2247
Corzide 80/5 Tablets ... 2247
Cosopt Sterile Ophthalmic Solution ... 2065
Dilaudid Oral Liquid ... 445
Dilaudid Tablets - 8 mg ... 445
Dilaudid-HP (Less frequent) ... 443
Diprivan Injectable Emulsion (Less than 1%) ... 667
Dopram Injectable ... 2931
Haldol Decanoate ... 2535
Haldol Injection, Tablets and Concentrate ... 2533
Inderal ... 3513
Inderal LA Long-Acting Capsules ... 3516
Inderide Tablets ... 3517
Inderide LA Long-Acting Capsules ... 3519
MS Contin Tablets (Less frequent) ... 2896
MSIR (Less frequent) ... 2898
Nadolol Tablets ... 2288
Normodyne Tablets ... 3137
Numorphan ... 1324
Oramorph SR Tablets (Less frequent) ... 3062
Orthoclone OKT3 Sterile Solution (Less than 1%) ... 2498
Reglan ... 2935
Sectral Capsules ... 3589
Serevent Diskus (Rare) ... 1637
Serevent Inhalation Aerosol (Rare) ... 1633
▲ Suprane Liquid for Inhalation (3% to 50%) ... 874
Tenoretic Tablets ... 690
Tenormin ... 692
Tensilon Injectable ... 1745
Tessalon Capsules ... 1377
Timolide Tablets ... 2187
Timolol GFS ... ⊙ 266
Timoptic in Ocudose ... 2192
Timoptic Sterile Ophthalmic Solution ... 2190
Timoptic-XE Sterile Ophthalmic Gel Forming Solution ... 2194
Toprol-XL Tablets ... 651
Valium Injectable ... 3026
Versed Injection (Less than 1.0%) ... 3027
Versed Syrup (2%) ... 3033
Zebeta Tablets ... 1885
Ziac Tablets ... 1887
Zofran Injection ... 1698
Zofran ... 1703
Zofran ODT Orally Disintegrating Tablets ... 1703

Laryngotracheobronchitis
Prevnar for Injection ... 1870
Synagis Intramuscular (More than 1%) ... 2028

Lassitude
Azmacort Inhalation Aerosol ... 728
Beconase Inhalation Aerosol ... 1497
Beconase AQ Nasal Spray ... 1498
Bromfed Capsules (Extended-Release) ... 2269
Bromfed-PD Capsules (Extended-Release) ... 2269
Daranide Tablets ... 2077
Dexedrine ... 1512
Felbatol ... 3343
▲ Hytrin Capsules (7.4% to 11.3%) ... 464
Inderal ... 3513
Inderal LA Long-Acting Capsules ... 3516
Inderide Tablets ... 3517
Inderide LA Long-Acting Capsules ... 3519
▲ Mykrox Tablets (4.4%) ... 1168
Nasacort Nasal Inhaler ... 750
Neurontin Capsules (Rare) ... 2655
Neurontin Oral Solution (Rare) ... 2655
Neurontin Tablets (Rare) ... 2655
Pediazole Suspension ... 3050
Phenergan Injection ... 3553
Phenergan ... 3556
Plaquenil Tablets ... 3082
▲ Reglan (Approximately 10%) ... 2935
Risperdal ... 1796
Tonocard Tablets (0.8% to 1.6%) ... 649

Laughing, easy
▲ Marinol Capsules (8% to 24%) ... 3325

Laxative effect
Beelith Tablets ... 946
Ex•Lax Milk of Magnesia Liquid ... ▣ 670
Mag-Ox 400 Tablets ... 1024
Phillips' Chewable Tablets ... ▣ 615
Phillips' Milk of Magnesia Liquid (Original, Cherry, & Mint) ... ▣ 616
Uro-Mag Capsules ... 1024

LDH abnormalities
Ceftin Tablets (1.0%) ... 1898
▲ Emcyt Capsules (2% to 31%) ... 2810
Hivid Tablets (Less than 1%) ... 2975
Nimotop Capsules (0.4%; rare) ... 904
Sinemet Tablets ... 1253
Sinemet CR Tablets ... 1255
Vistide Injection ... 1445
Zithromax Capsules, 250 mg (Less than 1%) ... 2743
Zithromax for IV Infusion (1% to 3%) ... 2748
Zithromax for Oral Suspension, 1 g (Less than 1%) ... 2743
Zithromax for Oral Suspension, 300 mg, 600 mg, 900 mg, 1200 mg (Less than 1%) ... 2739
Zithromax Tablets, 250 mg (Less than 1%) ... 2739
Zithromax Tablets, 600 mg (Less than 1%) ... 2743

LDH increase
Abelcet Injection ... 1273
Accutane Capsules ... 2944
Adalat CC Tablets (Rare) ... 877
AmBisome for Injection (Less common) ... 1383
Amphotec (1% to 5%) ... 1774
Aricept Tablets (Infrequent) ... 1270
Aricept Tablets (Infrequent) ... 2665
Arthrotec Tablets (Rare) ... 3195
Asacol Delayed-Release Tablets ... 2884
Avelox Tablets (0.05% to 1%) ... 879
Azulfidine EN-tabs Tablets ... 2775
Biaxin/Biaxin XL (Less than 1%) ... 403
Cardizem Injectable ... 1018
Cardizem Lyo-Ject Syringe ... 1018
Cardizem Monovial ... 1018
Cardizem CD Capsules (Less than 1%) ... 1016
Ceclor ... 1905

Cefizox for Intramuscular or Intravenous Use ... 1390
Cefotan (1 in 700) ... 664
Cefzil ... 1076
▲ CellCept Capsules (3% to 23.2%) ... 2951
▲ CellCept Intravenous (3% to 23.2%) ... 2951
▲ CellCept Oral Suspension (3% to 23.2%) ... 2951
▲ CellCept Tablets (3% to 23.2%) ... 2951
Chibroxin Sterile Ophthalmic Solution ... 2051
▲ Cipro I.V. (Among most frequent) ... 893
▲ Cipro I.V. Pharmacy Bulk Package (Among most frequent) ... 897
Cipro (0.4%) ... 887
Claforan Injection (Less than 1%) ... 732
Colazal Capsules ... 3069
Corlopam Injection (0.5% to 5%) ... 412
Cuprimine Capsules (Few cases) ... 2075
Depacon Injection (Frequent) ... 416
Depakene (Frequent) ... 421
Depakote Sprinkle Capsules ... 426
Depakote Tablets (Frequent) ... 430
Depakote ER Tablets (Frequent) ... 436
Depen Titratable Tablets (Few reports) ... 3341
Doxil Injection (Less than 1%) ... 566
Duricef ... 1079
Effexor Tablets ... 3495
Effexor XR Capsules ... 3499
Evoxac Capsules ... 1217
Felbatol (Infrequent) ... 3343
Floxin I.V. ... 2526
Floxin Tablets ... 2529
▲ Fortaz (1 in 18) ... 1541
Foscavir Injection (Between 1% and 5%) ... 605
▲ Sterile FUDR (Among more common) ... 2974
Geodon Capsules (Infrequent) ... 2688
Glucotrol Tablets (Occasional) ... 2692
Glucotrol XL Extended Release Tablets (Occasional) ... 2693
Inderide Tablets ... 3517
Intron A for Injection (Less than 5%) ... 3120
Kefurox Vials, ADD-Vantage (1 in 75) ... 1948
Levaquin (Less than 0.3%) ... 2537
Lodosyn Tablets ... 1251
Lopid Tablets (Occasional) ... 2650
Lorabid Suspension and Pulvules ... 2251
▲ Lupron Depot 3.75 mg (Approximately 5% to 8%) ... 3281
Lupron Depot 7.5 mg (Greater than or equal to 5%) ... 3284
▲ Lupron Depot–4 Month 30 mg (Greater than or equal to 5%) ... 3289
Luvox Tablets (25, 50, 100 mg) (Rare) ... 3256
Mefoxin for Injection ... 2124
Mefoxin Premixed Intravenous Solution ... 2127
Megace Oral Suspension (1% to 3%) ... 1124
Meridia Capsules (1.6%) ... 481
Merrem I.V. (Greater than 0.2%) ... 673
Monopril Tablets ... 1091
Monopril HCT ... 1094
▲ Mylotarg for Injection (14% to 19%) ... 3540
Nebcin Vials, Hyporets & ADD-Vantage ... 1955
▲ Neupogen for Injection (27% to 58%) ... 587
Niaspan Extended-Release Tablets ... 1846
Noroxin Tablets (Less frequent) ... 2145
Omnicef (0.2%) ... 493
Paxil (Rare) ... 1609
Pentasa Capsules (Less than 1%) ... 3239
Pipracil (Less frequent) ... 1866
Prevacid Delayed-Release Capsules ... 3292
PREVPAC (Less than 1%) ... 3298
Priftin Tablets (Less than 1%) ... 758
Primaxin I.M. ... 2158
Primaxin I.V. ... 2160
Procardia Capsules (Rare) ... 2708
Procardia XL Extended Release Tablets (Rare) ... 2710
▲ Prograf (3% to 15%) ... 1393
▲ Rapamune Oral Solution and Tablets (3% to 20%) ... 3584
Requip Tablets (Infrequent) ... 1621
Rilutek Tablets (Rare) ... 772
Rituxan for Infusion (1% to 5%) ... 1750
Rituxan I.V. (1% to 5%) ... 1428
▲ Roferon-A Injection (Less than 1% to 10%) ... 2996
Sectral Capsules ... 3589
▲ Serostim for Injection (1% to 10%) ... 3229
Serzone Tablets (Infrequent) ... 1104
Sinemet Tablets ... 1253
Sinemet CR Tablets ... 1255
▲ Soriatane Capsules (Approximately 1 in 3 patients) ... 3003
Suprax ... 1877
Symmetrel ... 1328
Tarka Tablets ... 508
▲ Tazicef for Injection (1 in 18 patients) ... 1647
▲ Tazicef Galaxy Container (1 in 18 patients) ... 1650
▲ Tazicef Pharmacy Bulk Package (1 in 18 patients) ... 1653
▲ Tazidime Vials, Faspak & ADD-Vantage (1 in 18) ... 1966
Thalomid Capsules ... 1154
Tiazac Capsules (Less than 2%) ... 1378
Timentin Injection- ADD-Vantage Vial ... 1661
Timentin Injection-Galaxy Container ... 1664
Timentin Injection-Pharmacy Bulk Package ... 1666
Timentin for Intravenous Administration ... 1658
Toprol-XL Tablets ... 651
Unasyn for Injection ... 2728
Vantin Tablets and Oral Suspension ... 2860
Viracept ... 532
WinRho SDF ... 2297
Zinacef Injection (1 in 75 patients) ... 1696
Zinacef for Injection (1 in 75 patients) ... 1696
Zonegran Capsules (Rare) ... 1307
Zyvox (0.2% to 1.8%) ... 2871

LDL, increase
Anadrol-50 Tablets (Sometimes) ... 3321

LE cells test positive
(*see under* Lupus erythematosus)

Left ventricular dysfunction
Orthoclone OKT3 Sterile Solution (Less than 1%) ... 2498

Left ventricular ejection fraction, asymptomatic declines in
Idamycin PFS Injection ... 2825

Left ventricular ejection fraction, change
Novantrone for Injection ... 1760

Leg cramps, nocturnal
Prostin E2 Suppositories ... 2852

Legs, heaviness
Rum-K ... 1363
Uroqid-Acid No. 2 Tablets ... 947

Legs, restless
Ambien Tablets (Rare) ... 3191

Legs, stiffness
Colazal Capsules ... 3069
Gastrocrom Concentrate (Less common) ... 1162

Leiomyoma
femhrt Tablets ... 2635

LE-like reactions
(*see under* Lupus erythematosus)

Lens, pigmentation
Zyprexa Tablets (Rare) ... 1973
Zyprexa ZYDIS Orally Disintegrating Tablets (Rare) ... 1973

Lens changes, unspecified
Myleran Tablets ... 1603

Lens opacities, changes
Baycol Tablets ... 883
Cordarone Tablets ... 3487
Cosopt Sterile Ophthalmic Solution (1% to 5%) ... 2065
Etrafon ... 3115
Floxin I.V. ... 2526
Humorsol Sterile Ophthalmic Solution ... 2102
Isopto Carpine Ophthalmic Solution ... ⊙215
Lamisil Tablets ... 2360
Lescol Capsules ... 2361
Lescol Capsules ... 2925
Lescol XL Tablets ... 2361
Lescol XL Tablets ... 2925
Mevacor Tablets ... 2132
Pacerone Tablets ... 3331
Pilopine HS Ophthalmic Gel ... ⊙217
Pravachol Tablets ... 1099
Vitrasert Implant (Approximately 1% to 5%) ... ⊙254
Zocor Tablets ... 2219

Lens opacities, irregular
Floxin Tablets ... 2529
Serentil ... 1057
Thioridazine Hydrochloride Tablets ... 2289
Thorazine ... 1656

Lenticular deposits
Compazine ... 1505
Etrafon ... 3115
Stelazine ... 1640
Thioridazine Hydrochloride Tablets ... 2289
Thorazine ... 1656
Trilafon ... 3160

Lesions, anogenital
Declomycin Tablets ... 1855
Doryx Coated Pellet Filled Capsules ... 3357
Dynacin Capsules ... 2019
Minocin Intravenous ... 1862
Minocin Oral Suspension ... 1865
Minocin Pellet-Filled Capsules ... 1863
Monodox Capsules ... 2442
Periostat Tablets ... 1208
Vibramycin Calcium Oral Suspension Syrup ... 2735
Vibramycin Hyclate Capsules ... 2735
Vibramycin Monohydrate for Oral Suspension ... 2735
Vibra-Tabs Film Coated Tablets ... 2735

Lesions, bullous
Lodosyn Tablets ... 1251

Lesions, cerebrovascular
Imitrex Nasal Spray ... 1554

Lesions, corneal
Effexor Tablets (Infrequent) ... 3495
Effexor XR Capsules (Infrequent) ... 3499
Rescula Ophthalmic Solution (1% to 5%) ... ⊙306
Soriatane Capsules (1% to 5%) ... 3003
Vistide Injection ... 1445
Voltaren Ophthalmic Sterile Ophthalmic Solution (Less than 5%) ... ⊙312
Zyprexa Tablets (1%) ... 1973
Zyprexa ZYDIS Orally Disintegrating Tablets (1%) ... 1973

Lesions, cutaneous
Duranest Injections ... 600
Lupron Depot–3 Month 22.5 mg ... 3288
▲ Tonocard Tablets (0.4% to 12.2%) ... 649
Xylocaine Injections (Extremely rare) ... 653
Zestril Tablets (0.3% to 1.0%) ... 698

Lesions, erythema perstans-like
AquaMEPHYTON Injection ... 2042

Lesions, esophageal
Cataflam Tablets (Rare) ... 2315
Voltaren Tablets (Rare) ... 2315
Voltaren-XR Tablets (Rare) ... 2315

Lesions, follicular-pustular
Topicort Cream (0.8%) ... 2025

Lesions, gastrointestinal
K-Dur Microburst Release System ER Tablets ... 1832
Klor-Con M20/Klor-Con M10 Tablets ... 3329
K-Tab Filmtab Tablets ... 470
Micro-K ... 3311

Lesions, hepatic

Lesions, nerve root
LYMErix Vaccine (Greater than 1%) ... 1592

Lesions, neuro-ocular
Activella Tablets ... 2764
Modicon ... 2563
Ortho-Novum ... 2563
Ortho-Novum 1/50□28 Tablets ... 2556
Ortho-Novum ... 2563
Premphase Tablets ... 3572
Prempro Tablets ... 3572
Provera Tablets ... 2853

Lesions, oral
Avapro Tablets (Less than 1%) ... 1074
Avapro Tablets (Less than 1%) ... 3076
Vantin Tablets and Oral Suspension (Less than 1%) ... 2860
Vioxx (Greater than 0.1% to 1.9%) ... 2213
Viramune Oral Suspension ... 1060
Viramune Tablets ... 1060

Lesions, rectal mucosal
Testoderm Transdermal Systems (1%) ... 574

Lesions, retinal vascular
Activella Tablets ... 2764
Brevicon 28-Day Tablets ... 3380
Depo-Provera Contraceptive Injection ... 2798
Levlen ... 962
Levlite 21 Tablets ... 962
Levlite 28 Tablets ... 962
Modicon ... 2563
Norinyl 1 +35 28-Day Tablets ... 3380
Norinyl 1 + 50 28-Day Tablets ... 3380
Ortho-Cyclen/Ortho Tri-Cyclen ... 2573
Ortho-Novum ... 2563
Ortho-Novum 1/50□28 Tablets ... 2556
Ortho-Cyclen/Ortho Tri-Cyclen ... 2573
Premphase Tablets ... 3572
Prempro Tablets ... 3572
Provera Tablets ... 2853
Tri-Levlen ... 962
Tri-Norinyl-28 Tablets ... 3433

Lesions, scleroderma-like
AquaMEPHYTON Injection ... 2042

Lesions, spinal column, posterior
Azulfidine EN-tabs Tablets (Rare) ... 2775

Lesions, stenotic
Micro-K ... 3311

Lesions, upper motor neuron
Remicade for IV Injection (Less than 2%) ... 1178
Topamax Sprinkle Capsules (Infrequent) ... 2590
Topamax Tablets (Infrequent) ... 2590

Lethargy
Accutane Capsules ... 2944
ActHIB Vaccine ... 798
▲ Ambien Tablets (3%) ... 3191
Aquasol A Parenteral ... 593
Arimidex Tablets (1.2%) ... 659
Asacol Delayed-Release Tablets ... 2884
BeneFix for Injection ... 1432
Betagan (Rare) ... ⊙228
Betoptic S Ophthalmic Suspension (Rare) ... 537
Cataflam Tablets ... 2315
Catapres-TTS (3 of 101 patients) ... 1038
Celebrex Capsules ... 2676
Celebrex Capsules ... 2780
Cipro I.V. (1% or less) ... 893
Cipro I.V. Pharmacy Bulk Package (Less than 1%) ... 897
Cipro (Less than 1%) ... 887
Clozaril Tablets (1%) ... 2319
Cosmegen for Injection ... 2062
Coumadin for Injection (Infrequent) ... 1243
Coumadin Tablets (Infrequent) ... 1243
Demadex Tablets and Injection ... 2965
Depacon Injection ... 416
Depakote Sprinkle Capsules ... 426
Depakote Tablets ... 430
Dilaudid ... 441
Dilaudid Powder ... 441
Dilaudid Rectal Suppositories ... 441
Dilaudid Tablets ... 441
Diovan HCT Tablets ... 2338
Dipentum Capsules (1.8%) ... 2803
Diuril Sodium Intravenous ... 2086
Dyazide Capsules ... 1515
DynaCirc Capsules (0.5% to 1%) ... 2921
DynaCirc CR Tablets (0.5% to 1%) ... 2923
Ecotrin Enteric Coated Aspirin Low, Regular and Maximum Strength Tablets ... 1715
Eldepryl Capsules (1 of 49 patients) ... 3266
▲ Ellence Injection (1.1% to 45.8%) ... 2806
▲ Emcyt Capsules (4%) ... 2810
Ergamisol Tablets ... 1789
Eskalith ... 1527
Etrafon ... 3115
Fortovase Capsules (Less than 2%) ... 2970
Sterile FUDR ... 2974
Furosemide Tablets ... 2284
Gastrocrom Oral Concentrate (Less common) ... 1162
Gengraf Capsules (Rare) ... 457
Haldol Decanoate ... 2535
Haldol Injection, Tablets and Concentrate ... 2533
Hycodan ... 1316
Hycomine Compound Tablets ... 1317
Hycotuss Expectorant Syrup ... 1318
Inderal ... 3513
Inderal LA Long-Acting Capsules ... 3516
Inderide Tablets ... 3517
Invirase Capsules (Less than 2%) ... 2979
Kadian Capsules (Less than 3%) ... 1335
Levo-Dromoran ... 1734
▲ Levorphanol Tartrate Tablets (3% to 9%) ... 3059
Limbitrol ... 1738
Lithium Carbonate ... 3061
Lithium Citrate Syrup ... 3061
Lithobid Slow-Release Tablets ... 3255
Lortab ... 3319
Lortab Elixir ... 3317
Lupron Injection (Less than 5%) ... 3279
Matulane Capsules ... 3246
Maxidone Tablets CIII ... 3399
Maxzide ... 1008
Mithracin for Intravenous Use ... 903
Mononine Concentrate ... 794
▲ Mykrox Tablets (4.4%) ... 1168
Nebcin Vials, Hyporets & ADD-Vantage ... 1955
Neoral Soft Gelatin Capsules (Rare) ... 2380
Neoral Oral Solution (Rare) ... 2380
Norco 5/325 Tablets CIII ... 3424
Norco 7.5/325 Tablets CIII ... 3425

Norco 10/325 Tablets CIII 3425
Norco 10/325 Tablets CIII 3427
Orthoclone OKT3 Sterile Solution (Less than 1%) 2498
Prinzide Tablets 2168
Proleukin for Injection 1199
ReFacto Vials 1437
Rescriptor Tablets (Less than 2%) 526
RhoGAM Injection 2524
Roferon-A Injection (Less than 0.5% to 6%) 2996
Sandimmune (Rare) 2388
▲ Stadol NS Nasal Spray (3% to 9%) 1108
Tasmar Tablets (1% or more) 3010
Tenoretic Tablets (1% to 3%) 690
Tenormin (1% to 3%) 692
Thioridazine Hydrochloride Tablets (Extremely rare) 2289
Tonocard Tablets (0.8% to 1.6%) 649
Trilafon 3160
Trilisate (Less than 2%) 2901
Tussionex Pennkinetic Extended-Release Suspension 1174
Vaseretic Tablets 2204
▲ Verelan Capsules (3.2%) 3184
Versed Injection (Less than 1.0%) 3027
Vicodin Tablets 516
Vicodin ES Tablets 517
Vicodin HP Tablets 518
Vicodin Tuss Expectorant 519
Voltaren Tablets 2315
Voltaren-XR Tablets 2315
Warfarin Sodium Tablets, USP 3302
Zarontin Capsules 2659
Zarontin Syrup 2660
Zaroxolyn Tablets 1177
Zestoretic Tablets 695
Ziagen 1692
▲ Zoladex (5% to 8%) 702
Zoladex 3-month 706
Zovirax for Injection (Approximately 1%) 1708
Zydone Tablets 1330

Leukemia, acute
Herceptin I.V. (At least one of the 958 patients) 1414
Leukeran Tablets 1591
Nipent for Injection (Less than 3%) 3272

Leukemia, lymphoblastic
Permax Tablets (Rare) 1299

Leukemia, lymphocytic
Betaseron for SC Injection 988
Clomid Tablets 735
Mustargen for Injection 2142

Leukemia, myeloblastic, acute
Fortovase Capsules (Rare) 2970
Invirase Capsules (Rare) 2979

Leukemia, myelogenous
Ellence Injection 2806
Felbatol 3343
Thalomid Capsules 1154

Leukemia, unspecified
Depen Titratable Tablets 3341
Felbatol 3343
Genotropin Lyophilized Powder (A small number of children) 2818
Humatrope Vials and Cartridges 1930
Indocin (Rare) 2112
Norditropin Cartridges (A small number of children) 2420
Norditropin for Injection (A small number of children) 2419
Novantrone for Injection 1760
Nutropin AQ Injection (A small number of patients) 1420
Nutropin Depot for Injectable Suspension (A small number) 1423
Nutropin for Injection (A small number of patients) 1417
Plavix Tablets (Less than 1%) 1097
Plavix Tablets (Less than 1%) 3084
Saizen for Injection (Infrequent) 3225
Tasmar Tablets (Rare) 3010
Thalomid Capsules 1154
Ticlid Tablets (Rare) 3015
Trental Tablets (Rare) 784

Leukemia, polymorphocytic
Campath Ampules 992

Leukocytosis
Abelcet Injection 1273
Aceon Tablets (2 mg, 4 mg, 8 mg) 3249
Aciphex Tablets 1267
Aciphex Tablets 1783
▲ Adriamycin PFS/RDF Injection (High incidence) 2767
Amerge Tablets (Infrequent) 1467
Amphotec (1% to 5%) 1774
Arthrotec Tablets (Rare) 3195
Attenuvax 2044
Azactam for Injection (Less than 1%) 1276
Carbatrol Capsules 3234
Celexa (Infrequent) 1365
▲ CellCept Capsules (7.1% to 40.5%) 2951
▲ CellCept Intravenous (7.1% to 40.5%) 2951
▲ CellCept Oral Suspension (7.1% to 40.5%) 2951
▲ CellCept Tablets (7.1% to 40.5%) 2951
Cerebyx Injection (Infrequent) 2619
Chirocaine Injection (1.2%) 2909
Cipro I.V. (Rare) 893
Cipro I.V. Pharmacy Bulk Package (Rare) 897
Cipro (Less than 0.1%) 887
Clinoril Tablets (Less than 1 in 100) 2053
Clomid Tablets 735
Clozaril Tablets (Less than 1%) 2319
Colazal Capsules 3069
Corlopam Injection (0.5% to 5%) 412
Cuprimine Capsules 2075
Depen Titratable Tablets 3341
Diprivan Injectable Emulsion (Less than 1%) 667
Dynabac Tablets (0.1% to 1%) 2269
Effexor Tablets (Infrequent) 3495
Effexor XR Capsules (Infrequent) 3499
▲ Efudex (Among most frequent) 1733
Enalaprilat Injection 863
Eskalith 1527
Evoxac Capsules (Less than 1%) 1217
Exelon Capsules (Infrequent) 2342
Exelon Oral Solution (Infrequent) 2345
Felbatol (Infrequent) 3343
Ferrlecit Injection 3386
Floxin I.V. (More than or equal to 1%) 2526
Floxin Tablets (More than or equal to 1%) 2529
Geodon Capsules (Infrequent) 2688
Gliadel Wafer (1%) 1723
Haldol Decanoate 2535
Haldol Injection, Tablets and Concentrate 2533
INFeD Injection 3388
Lamictal (Infrequent) 1567
Lariam Tablets (Occasional) 2989
Levaquin (Less than 0.3%) 2537
Lexxel Tablets 608
Lithium Carbonate 3061
Lithium Citrate Syrup 3061
Lithobid Slow-Release Tablets 3255
Luvox Tablets (25, 50, 100 mg) (Infrequent) 3256
Meruvax II 2130
MetroGel-Vaginal Gel (1.7%) 1986
M-M-R II 2118
Moban 1320
Monopril Tablets 1091
Monopril HCT 1094
Mumpsvax 2141
Navane Oral (Occasional) 2701
Navane Intramuscular 2703
Nebcin Vials, Hyporets & ADD-Vantage 1955
Neupogen for Injection (Approximately 2%) 587
Nexium Delayed-Release Capsules (Less than 1%) 619
Orthoclone OKT3 Sterile Solution (Less than 1%) 2498
Ovidrel for Injection (Less than 2%) 3220
Panhematin for Injection 497
▲ Paser Granules (79% of 38 patients with drug-induced hepatitis) 1781
Paxil (Rare) 1609
Permax Tablets (Infrequent) 1299
Priftin Tablets (Less than 1%) 758
Prilosec Delayed-Release Capsules (Rare) 628
Primaxin I.V. 2160
Prinivil Tablets (0.3% to 1.0%) 2164
Prinzide Tablets 2168
▲ Prograf (3% to 32%) 1393
Prolastin 943
▲ Proleukin for Injection (9%) 1199
Protonix I.V. (Less than 1%) 3580
Protonix Tablets (Less than 1%) 3577
Protopic Ointment (Greater than or equal to 1%) 1397
Provigil Tablets (At least 1%) 1193
▲ Rapamune Oral Solution and Tablets (3% to 20%) 3584
ReoPro Vials (1.0%) 1958
Requip Tablets (Infrequent) 1621
Rilutek Tablets (Infrequent) 772
Risperdal (Rare) 1796
Rocephin Injectable Vials, ADD-Vantage, Galaxy, Bulk (Less than 0.1%) 2993
Serophene Tablets 3226
Seroquel Tablets (Infrequent) 684
Sonata Capsules (Rare) 3591
Suprane Liquid for Inhalation 874
Symmetrel 1328
Tao Capsules 2716
Tegretol/Tegretol-XR 2404
Thiothixene Capsules (Occasional) 2290
Trasylol Injection (1% to 2%) 909
▲ Trisenox Injection (50%) 1158
Vantin Tablets and Oral Suspension 2860
Vaseretic Tablets 2204
Vasotec I.V. Injection 2207
Vasotec Tablets (0.5% to 1.0%) 2210
▲ Vesanoid Capsules (About 40%) 3037
Vistide Injection 1445
Wellbutrin Tablets 1680
Wellbutrin SR Sustained-Release Tablets 1684
Zanaflex Tablets (Infrequent) 1305
Zestoretic Tablets 695
Zestril Tablets (0.3% to 1.0%) 698
Zovirax for Injection (Less than 1%) 1708
Zyban Sustained-Release Tablets 1710
Zyprexa Tablets (Infrequent) 1973
Zyprexa ZYDIS Orally Disintegrating Tablets (Infrequent) 1973

Leukocyturia
Primaxin I.M. 2158
Primaxin I.V. 2160
Sinemet CR Tablets (1% or greater) 1255

Leukoderma
Betaseron for SC Injection 988
Effexor Tablets (Rare) 3495
Effexor XR Capsules (Rare) 3499
Lamictal (Rare) 1567
Ultravate Cream (Less frequent) 1119
Ultravate Ointment (Less frequent) 1120

Leukoencephalopathy, multifocal progressive
Ergamisol Tablets 1789
Fortovase Capsules (Less than 2%) 2970
Invirase Capsules (Less than 2%) 2979

Leukoencephalopathy, unspecified
Taxol Injection (2%) 1129

Leukopenia
▲ Abelcet Injection (4%) 1273
Accuretic Tablets 2614
Accutane Capsules 2944
Aceon Tablets (2 mg, 4 mg, 8 mg) (0.1%) 3249
Aciphex Tablets 1267
Aciphex Tablets 1783
Actiq (Less than 1%) 1184
Adalat CC Tablets (Rare) 877
Adriamycin PFS/RDF Injection 2767
Aldoclor Tablets 2035
Aldomet Tablets 2037
Aldoril Tablets 2039
▲ Alferon N Injection (11%) 1770
Alkeran Tablets 1466
Aloprim for Injection (Less than 1%) 2292
Altace Capsules 2233
Amaryl Tablets 717
Ambien Tablets (Rare) 3191
Amicar Injection 3608
Amicar Syrup 3608
Amicar Tablets 3608
Amoxil Chewable Tablets 1471
Amoxil for Oral Suspension 1471
Amoxil 1471
Amphotec (1% to 5%) 1774
Anaprox Tablets (Less than 1%) 2967
Anaprox DS Tablets (Less than 1%) 2967
Ancef for Injection 1474
Ancef Injection 1474
Ancobon Capsules 1730
Aquasol A Parenteral 593
Arava Tablets (Rare) 724
Aredia for Injection (Up to 4%) 2309
Arimidex Tablets (2% to 5%) 659
Arthrotec Tablets (Rare) 3195
Asacol Delayed-Release Tablets 2884
Atacand Tablets (Very rare) 595
Atacand HCT Tablets 597
Atromid-S Capsules 3483
Augmentin Chewable Tablets 1482
Augmentin Powder for Oral Suspension 1482
Augmentin Tablets 1485
Augmentin ES-600 Powder for Oral Suspension 1487
Avalide Tablets 1070
Avelox Tablets (0.05% to 1%) 879
Bactrim 2949
Baycol Tablets 883
Betapace Tablets (Rare) 950
Betapace AF Tablets (Rare) 954
Bicillin C-R 900/300 Injection 2240
Bicillin C-R Injection 2238
Bicillin L-A Injection (Infrequent) 2242
Canasa Rectal Suppositories (One patient) 829
Carbatrol Capsules 3234
Cardizem Injectable 1018
Cardizem Lyo-Ject Syringe 1018
Cardizem Monovial 1018
Cardizem CD Capsules (Infrequent) 1016
Cardura Tablets 2668
▲ Casodex Tablets (2% to 5%) 662
Cataflam Tablets (Less than 1%) 2315
Ceclor CD Tablets 1279
Ceclor 1905
Cedax Capsules (0.1% to 1%) 1021
Cefizox for Intramuscular or Intravenous Use (Rare) 1390
Cefotan 664
Ceftin 1898
Cefzil (0.2%) 1076
Celexa (Infrequent) 1365
▲ CellCept Capsules (11.5% to 30.4%) 2951
▲ CellCept Intravenous (11.5% to 30.4%) 2951
▲ CellCept Oral Suspension (11.5% to 30.4%) 2951
▲ CellCept Tablets (11.5% to 45.8%) 2951
Celontin Capsules 2618
Ceptaz for Injection (Very rare) 1499
Cerebyx Injection (Infrequent) 2619
Chibroxin Sterile Ophthalmic Solution 2051
Cipro I.V. (Infrequent) 893
▲ Cipro I.V. Pharmacy Bulk Package (Among most frequent) 897
Cipro (0.4%) 887
Claforan Injection (Less than 1%) 732
Cleocin HCl Capsules 2784
Cleocin Phosphate Sterile Solution 2785
Cleocin Vaginal Cream 2788
Cleocin Vaginal Ovules 2789
Clinoril Tablets (Less than 1%) 2053
Clorpres Tablets 1002
▲ Clozaril Tablets (3%) 2319
Cognex Capsules (Rare) 1351
Colazal Capsules 3069
Combipres Tablets 1040
Compazine 1505
Concerta Extended-Release Tablets 1998
Concerta Tablets 561
Copaxone for Injection (Infrequent) 3306
Coreg Tablets (0.1% to 1%) 1508
Corzide 40/5 Tablets 2247
Corzide 80/5 Tablets 2247
Cosmegen for Injection 2062
Cuprimine Capsules (2%) 2075
▲ Cytovene (29%) 2959
Dantrium Capsules (Less frequent) 2885
Dantrium Intravenous 2886
Daranide Tablets 2077
Daraprim Tablets 1511
Depacon Injection 416
Depakene 421
Depakote Sprinkle Capsules 426
Depakote Tablets 430
Depakote ER Tablets (Greater than 1%) 436
▲ Depen Titratable Tablets (2%; up to 5%) 3341
DiaBeta Tablets 741
Diabinese Tablets 2680
Diamox ⊙269
Didronel Tablets (One report) 2888
Diflucan Tablets, Injection, and Oral Suspension 2681
Dilantin Infatabs (Occasional) 2624
Dilantin Kapseals (Occasional) 2622
Dilantin-125 Oral Suspension (Occasional) 2625
Diovan HCT Tablets 2338
Dipentum Capsules (Rare) 2803
Diucardin Tablets 3494
Diuril Oral 2087
Diuril Sodium Intravenous 2086
Dolobid Tablets (Less than 1 in 100) 2088
▲ Doxil Injection (About 42.2% to 60%) 566
Dyazide Capsules 1515
DynaCirc Capsules (0.5% to 1%) 2921
DynaCirc CR Tablets (0.5% to 1%) 2923
EC-Naprosyn Delayed-Release Tablets (Less than 1%) 2967
Effexor Tablets (Infrequent) 3495
Effexor XR Capsules (Infrequent) 3499
▲ Ellence Injection (1.5% to 80.3%) 2806
Elmiron Capsules (Less than or equal to 1%) 570
Elspar for Injection 2092
▲ Emcyt Capsules (4%) 2810
Enbrel for Injection 1752
Enbrel for Injection 3504
▲ Ergamisol Tablets (Less than 1% to 33%) 1789
Etrafon 3115
▲ Eulexin Capsules (3%) 3118
Evoxac Capsules (Less than 1%) 1217
Famotidine Injection (Rare) 866
Famvir Tablets (1.3%) 2348
Fareston Tablets 3237
▲ Felbatol (6.5%) 3343
Feldene Capsules (Occasional) 2685
Flexeril Tablets (Rare) 572

Flexeril Tablets (Rare) 2094
Floxin I.V. (More than or equal to 1%) 2526
Floxin Tablets (More than or equal to 1%) 2529
Fortaz (Very rare) 1541
▲ Foscavir Injection (5% or greater) 605
▲ Sterile FUDR (Among more common) 2974
Furosemide Tablets 2284
Gabitril Tablets (Infrequent) 1189
▲ Gemzar for Injection (15% to 71%) 1919
▲ Gengraf Capsules (1% to 6%) 457
Geocillin Tablets 2687
Geodon Capsules (Infrequent) 2688
Glucotrol Tablets 2692
Glucotrol XL Extended Release Tablets 2693
Grifulvin V Tablets Microsize and Oral Suspension Microsize (Rare) 2518
Gris-PEG Tablets (Rare) 2661
Haldol Decanoate 2535
Haldol Injection, Tablets and Concentrate 2533
▲ Herceptin I.V. (3%) 1414
▲ Hexalen Capsules (1% to 15%) 2226
▲ Hivid Tablets (Less than 1% to 13.1%) 2975
▲ Hycamtin for Injection (32% to 98%) 1546
HydroDIURIL Tablets 2108
Hyzaar 2109
▲ Ifex for Injection (Almost universal) 1123
Indapamide Tablets 2286
Inderide Tablets 3517
Inderide LA Long-Acting Capsules 3519
Indocin Capsules (Less than 1%) 2112
Indocin I.V. (Less than 1%) 2115
Indocin (Less than 1%) 2112
▲ Infergen (15% to 19%) 1777
▲ Intron A for Injection (Less than 5% to 68%) 3120
Kadian Capsules (Less than 3%) 1335
Kaletra Capsules (Less than 2%) 471
Kaletra Oral Solution (Less than 2%) 471
Kefurox Vials, ADD-Vantage (1 in 750) 1948
Kefzol Vials, ADD-Vantage 1951
Klonopin Tablets 2983
▲ Kytril Tablets (11%) 2988
Lamictal (Infrequent) 1567
▲ Lariam Tablets (Among most frequent) 2989
Lescol Capsules (Rare) 2361
Lescol Capsules (Rare) 2925
Lescol XL Tablets 2361
Lescol XL Tablets 2925
▲ Leukine (17%) 1755
Levaquin (Less than 0.3%) 2537
Lodine (Less than 1%) 3528
Lodine XL Extended-Release Tablets (Less than 1%) 3530
Lodosyn Tablets 1251
Lopid Tablets (Rare to occasional) 2650
Lorabid Suspension and Pulvules 2251
Lotensin HCT Tablets 2367
Loxitane Capsules (Rare) 3398
Lupron Depot 7.5 mg (Greater than or equal to 5%) 3284
▲ Lupron Depot–4 Month 30 mg (Greater than or equal to 5%) 3289
Luvox Tablets (25, 50, 100 mg) (Rare) 3256
Macrobid Capsules 2889
Macrodantin Capsules 2891
Matulane Capsules (Frequent) 3246
Mavik Tablets (Rare) 478
Maxzide 1008
Mefoxin for Injection 2124
Mefoxin Premixed Intravenous Solution 2127
Megace Oral Suspension (1% to 3%) 1124
Mepergan Injection (Very rare) 3539
▲ Mepron Suspension (4%) 1598
Meridia Capsules 481
Metadate CD Capsules 1164
Metadate ER Tablets 1167
Methylin Tablets 1995
Methylin ER Tablets 1995
MetroGel-Vaginal Gel (1.7%) 1986
Mevacor Tablets (Rare) 2132
Mexitil Capsules (About 1 in 1,000) 1047
Micardis HCT Tablets 1051
Microzide Capsules 3414
Miltown Tablets 3349
Minizide Capsules 2700
Mintezol 2137
▲ Mithracin for Intravenous Use (6%) 903
Moban 1320
Mobic Tablets (Less than 2%) 1054
Moduretic Tablets 2138
Monopril Tablets 1091
Monopril HCT 1094
▲ Mycobutin Capsules (17%) 2838
Mykrox Tablets 1168
Myleran Tablets 1603
Mylocel Tablets 2227
Naprelan Tablets (Less than 1%) 1293
Naprosyn Suspension (Less than 1%) 2967
Naprosyn Tablets (Less than 1%) 2967
Nardil Tablets (Less frequent) 2653
Navane Oral (Occasional) 2701
Navane Intramuscular (Occasional) 2703
▲ Navelbine Injection (12% to 81%) 1604
Nebcin Vials, Hyporets & ADD-Vantage 1955
▲ Neoral Soft Gelatin Capsules (1% to 6%) 2380
▲ Neoral Oral Solution (1% to 6%) 2380
Neptazane Tablets ⊙ 271
Neurontin Capsules (1.1%) 2655
Neurontin Oral Solution (1.1%) 2655
Neurontin Tablets (1.1%) 2655
Nexium Delayed-Release Capsules (Less than 1%) 619
▲ Nilandron Tablets (3%) 753
▲ Nipent for Injection (22% to 60%) 3272
Nizoral Tablets (Less than 1%) 1791
Nolvadex Tablets (0.4%) 678
Noroxin Tablets 2145
Norvasc Tablets (More than 0.1% to 1%) 2704
Norvir Capsules (Less than 2%) 487
Norvir Oral Solution (Less than 2%) 487
▲ Novantrone for Injection (9% to 19%) 1760
Omnicef 493
Oncaspar (Greater than 1% but less than 5%) 756
Orthoclone OKT3 Sterile Solution (Less than 1%) 2498
▲ Paraplatin for Injection (15% to 98%) 1126
Parnate Tablets 1607
Paser Granules 1781
Paxil (Infrequent) 1609
Pediazole Suspension 3050
Pentasa Capsules 3239
Pepcid Injection (Rare) 2153
Pepcid for Oral Suspension (Rare) 2150
Pepcid RPD Orally Disintegrating Tablets (Rare) 2150
Pepcid Tablets (Rare) 2150
Periactin Tablets 2155
Permapen Isoject 2706
Permax Tablets (Infrequent) 1299
Pfizerpen for Injection (Rare) 2707
Phenergan Injection 3553
Phenergan Suppositories 3556
Phenergan Syrup (Rare) 3554
Phenergan Tablets 3556
Phenergan with Codeine Syrup (Rare) 3557
Phenergan with Dextromethorphan Syrup (Rare) 3559
Phenergan VC Syrup (Rare) 3560
Phenergan VC with Codeine Syrup (Rare) 3561
Pipracil 1866
Plaquenil Tablets 3082
Plavix Tablets (Less than 1%) 1097
Plavix Tablets (Less than 1%) 3084
Podocon-25 Liquid 2608
Ponstel Capsules (Occasional) 1356
Prandin Tablets (0.5, 1, and 2 mg) (Less than 1%) 2432
Pravachol Tablets (Rare) 1099
Prevacid Delayed-Release Capsules (Less than 1%) 3292
PREVPAC 3298
Priftin Tablets (1.9%) 758
Primaxin I.M. 2158
Primaxin I.V. (Less than 0.2%) 2160
Prinzide Tablets 2168
Procardia Capsules (Less than 0.5%) 2708
▲ Prograf (3% to 15%) 1393
▲ Proleukin for Injection (16%) 1199
ProSom Tablets (Rare) 500
Protonix I.V. (Less than 1%) 3580
Protonix Tablets (Less than 1%) 3577
Protopic Ointment (Greater than or equal to 1%) 1397
Prozac Pulvules, Liquid, and Weekly Capsules (Rare) 1238
Purinethol Tablets (Frequent) 1615
▲ Rapamune Oral Solution and Tablets (9% to 13%) 3584
Reglan (A few cases) 2935
Relafen Tablets (Less than 1%) 1617
Remeron Tablets (Rare) 2483
Remeron SolTab Tablets (Rare) 2486
Remicade for IV Injection (Less than 2%) 1178
Renese Tablets 2712
Requip Tablets (Infrequent) 1621
Rescriptor Tablets 526
Rifamate Capsules 767
Rifater Tablets (Rare) 769
Rilutek Tablets (Infrequent) 772
Risperdal (Rare) 1796
Ritalin 2387
▲ Rituxan for Infusion (13%) 1750
▲ Rituxan I.V. (13%; Among most frequent) 1428
Robaxin Injectable 2938
Robaxin Tablets 2939
Rocephin Injectable Vials, ADD-Vantage, Galaxy, Bulk (2.1%) 2993
▲ Roferon-A Injection (1.5% to 49%) 2996
Roxicodone Tablets (Less than 3%) 3067
Rythmol Tablets – 150 mg, 225 mg, 300 mg (Less than 1%) 502
Salagen Tablets (Less than 1%) 2229
▲ Sandimmune (Up to 6%) 2388
Sarafem Pulvules (Rare) 1962
Septra Suspension 2265
Septra Tablets 2265
Septra DS Tablets 2265
Serentil 1057
Seroquel Tablets (Rare) 684
▲ Serostim for Injection (15.1%) 3229
Serzone Tablets (Infrequent) 1104
Silvadene Cream 1% (Several cases) 2267
▲ Simulect for Injection (3% to 10%) 2399
Sinemet Tablets 1253
Sinemet CR Tablets 1255
Sinequan (Occasional) 2713
Skelaxin Tablets 1301
Soma Tablets 3353
Soma Compound Tablets (Very rare) 3354
Soma Compound w/Codeine Tablets (Very rare) 3355
Stelazine 1640
Stromectol Tablets (One patient) 2185
Sular Tablets (Less than or equal to 1%) 688
Suprax (Less than 2%) 1877
Symmetrel (Less than 0.1%) 1328
Tabloid Tablets 1642
Tagamet (Approximately 1 per 100,000) 1644
Tambocor Tablets (Less than 1%) 1990
Tapazole Tablets 1823
Tarka Tablets (0.3% or more) 508
▲ Taxol Injection (17% to 90%) 1129
Taxotere for Injection Concentrate 778
Tazicef for Injection (Very rare) 1647
Tazicef Galaxy Container (Very rare) 1650
Tazicef Pharmacy Bulk Package (Very rare) 1653
Tazidime Vials, Faspak & ADD-Vantage (Very rare) 1966
Tegretol/Tegretol-XR 2404
Tenoretic Tablets 690
Teveten Tablets (0.3%) 3327
▲ Thalomid Capsules (16.7% to 25.5%) 1154
▲ TheraCys Injection (5%) 823
Thioplex for Injection 1765
Thioridazine Hydrochloride Tablets (Infrequent) 2289
Thiothixene Capsules (Occasional) 2290
Thorazine 1656
▲ Thymoglobulin for Injection (57.3%) 3071
Tiazac Capsules (Infrequent) 1378
Tice BCG, BCG Live (0.3%) 2489
Timentin Injection- ADD-Vantage Vial 1661
Timentin Injection-Galaxy Container 1664
Timentin Injection-Pharmacy Bulk Package 1666
Timentin for Intravenous Administration 1658
Timolide Tablets 2187
Tonocard Tablets (Less than 1%) 649
Topamax Sprinkle Capsules (1.6% to 2.7%) 2590
Topamax Tablets (1.6% to 2.7%) 2590
Toradol 3018
Trental Tablets (Less than 1%) 784
Tricor Capsules, Micronized 513
Trilafon 3160
Trileptal Oral Suspension 2407
Trileptal Tablets 2407
Trovan (Less than 1%) 2722
Unasyn for Injection 2728
Uniretic Tablets (Less than 1%) 3178
Urso Tablets 836
Valtrex Caplets (0.7% to 1.3%) 1676
Vantin Tablets and Oral Suspension 2860
Vascor Tablets (2 cases) 2602
Vaseretic Tablets 2204
Viagra Tablets (Less than 2%) 2732
▲ Videx (Less than 1% to 16%) 1138
Videx EC Capsules 1143
Vioxx 2213
Viracept 532
Vistide Injection 1445
Vivactil Tablets 2217
Vivactil Tablets 2446
Voltaren Tablets (Less than 1%) 2315
Voltaren-XR Tablets (Less than 1%) 2315
Wellbutrin Tablets 1680
Wellbutrin SR Sustained-Release Tablets 1684
Zanaflex Tablets (Infrequent) 1305
Zantac (A few patients) 1690
Zantac Injection (Few patients) 1688
Zantac Syrup (A few patients) 1690
Zarontin Capsules 2659
Zarontin Syrup 2660
Zaroxolyn Tablets 1177
Zestoretic Tablets (Rare) 695
Zestril Tablets (Rare) 698
Zinacef Injection (1 in 750 patients) 1696
Zinacef for Injection (1 in 750 patients) 1696
Zinecard for Injection 2869
Zithromax Capsules, 250 mg (Less than 1%) 2743
Zithromax for IV Infusion (Less than 1%) 2748
Zithromax for Oral Suspension, 1 g (Less than 1%) 2743
Zithromax for Oral Suspension, 300 mg, 600 mg, 900 mg, 1200 mg (Less than 1%) 2739
Zithromax Tablets, 250 mg (Less than 1%) 2739
Zithromax Tablets, 600 mg (Less than 1%) 2743
Zocor Tablets (Rare) 2219
Zoloft 2751
Zomig Tablets (Rare) 708
Zomig-ZMT Tablets (Rare) 708
Zonegran Capsules (Infrequent) 1307
Zosyn 1890
Zosyn in Galaxy Containers 1894
Zovirax Capsules 1706
Zovirax for Injection 1708
Zovirax 1706
Zyban Sustained-Release Tablets 1710
Zyflo Filmtab Tablets (1.0% of 1,678 patients) 524
Zyprexa Tablets (Frequent) 1973
Zyprexa ZYDIS Orally Disintegrating Tablets (Frequent) 1973

Leukopenia, transient

Maxipime for Injection 1285
Rifadin 765
Rifater Tablets 769

Leukoplakia, oral

Betaseron for SC Injection 988
Doxil Injection (Less than 1%) 566
Geodon Capsules (Rare) 2688
Intron A for Injection (Less than 5%) 3120
▲ Serostim for Injection (1% to 10%) 3229

Leukorrhea

Aciphex Tablets (Rare) 1267
Aciphex Tablets (Rare) 1783
Arimidex Tablets (1.8%) 659
Arthrotec Tablets (Rare) 3195
Avonex 1013
Betaseron for SC Injection 988
Ceclor CD Tablets (0.1% to 1%) 1279
▲ CombiPatch Transdermal System (8% to 10%) 2323
▲ Depo-Provera Contraceptive Injection (More than 5%) 2798
Doxil Injection (Less than 1%) 566
Effexor Tablets (Infrequent) 3495
Effexor XR Capsules (Infrequent) 3499
Esclim Transdermal System 3460
▲ Estring Vaginal Ring (7%) 2811
▲ Evista Tablets (3.3%) 1915
Evoxac Capsules (Less than 1%) 1217
Gengraf Capsules (1%) 457
Gonal-F for Injection (1.7%) 3216
Intron A for Injection (Less than 5%) 3120
Levaquin (0.1% to less than 0.5%) 2537
Lodine (Less than 1%) 3528
Lodine XL Extended-Release Tablets (Less than 1%) 3530
▲ Mirena Intrauterine System (5% or more) 974
Neoral Soft Gelatin Capsules (1%) 2380
Neoral Oral Solution (1%) 2380
Neurontin Capsules (Rare) 2655
Neurontin Oral Solution (Rare) 2655
Neurontin Tablets (Rare) 2655
▲ Norplant System (5% or greater) 3543
Omnicef (0.2%) 493
Ovidrel for Injection (Less than 2%) 3220
ParaGard T 380A Intrauterine Copper Contraceptive 2582
Paxil (Rare) 1609
Permax Tablets (Rare) 1299
▲ Prempro Tablets (5% to 6%) 3572
Prometrium Capsules (100 mg, 200 mg) (Less than 5%) 3261
Prozac Pulvules, Liquid, and Weekly Capsules (Infrequent) 1238
Remeron Tablets (Infrequent) 2483
Remeron SolTab Tablets (Infrequent) 2486
Risperdal (Infrequent) 1796
Seroquel Tablets (Infrequent) 684
Sonata Capsules (Rare) 3591

Soriatane Capsules (Less than 1%) 3003
Topamax Sprinkle Capsules (Frequent) 2590
Topamax Tablets (Frequent) 2590
Trileptal Oral Suspension 2407
Trileptal Tablets 2407
Trovan (Less than 1%) 2722
Uniretic Tablets (Less than 1%) 3178
Yasmin 28 Tablets (Greater than 1%) 980
Zoloft (Infrequent) 2751
Zosyn (1.0% or less) 1890
Zosyn in Galaxy Containers (1.0% or less) 1894
Zyrtec (Less than 2%) 2756
Zyrtec-D 12 Hour Extended Relief Tablets (Less than 2%) 2758

Lhermitte's sign

Copaxone for Injection (At least 2%) 3306

Libido, changes

Activella Tablets 2764
Adderall Tablets 3231
Adderall XR Capsules
Adipex-P 1406
Alesse-21 Tablets 3468
Alesse-28 Tablets 3473
Alora Transdermal System 3372
▲ Android Capsules, 10 mg (Among most common) 1731
Avalide Tablets 1070
Avapro Tablets (Less than 1%) 1074
Avapro Tablets (Less than 1%) 3076
Brevicon 28-Day Tablets 3380
Cenestin Tablets 1263
Climara Transdermal System 958
Cyclessa Tablets 2450
Desogen Tablets 2458
Desoxyn Tablets 440
Dexedrine 1512
DextroStat Tablets 3236
Esclim Transdermal System 3460
Estinyl Tablets 3112
Estrace Vaginal Cream 3358
Estrace Tablets 3361
Estratest 3252
Estrostep 2627
Etrafon 3115
femhrt Tablets 2635
Flexeril Tablets (Rare) 572
Flexeril Tablets (Rare) 2094
Fortovase Capsules (2.2%) 2970
Halcion Tablets 2823
Invirase Capsules (Less than 2%) 2979
Ionamin Capsules 1163
Levlen 962
Levlite 21 Tablets 962
Levlite 28 Tablets 962
Levora Tablets 3389
Librium Capsules (Isolated cases) 1736
Librium for Injection (Isolated cases) 1737
Limbitrol 1738
Loestrin 21 Tablets 2642
Loestrin Fe Tablets 2642
Lo/Ovral Tablets 3532
Lo/Ovral-28 Tablets 3538
Low-Ogestrel-28 Tablets 3392
Lunelle Monthly Injection 2827
Menest Tablets 2254
Microgestin Fe 1.5/30 Tablets 3407
Microgestin Fe 1/20 Tablets 3400
Mircette Tablets 2470
Modicon 2563
Monopril HCT (Less than 2%) 1094
Necon 3415
Neurontin Capsules (Infrequent) 2655
Neurontin Oral Solution (Infrequent) 2655
Neurontin Tablets (Infrequent) 2655
Nipent for Injection (Less than 3%) 3272
Nordette-28 Tablets 2257
Norinyl 1 +35 28-Day Tablets 3380
Norinyl 1 + 50 28-Day Tablets 3380
▲ Novantrone for Injection (4%) 1760
Ogen Tablets 2846
Ogestrel 0.5/50-28 Tablets 3428
Ortho Dienestrol Cream 2554
Ortho-Cept 21 Tablets 2546
Ortho-Cept 28 Tablets 2546
Ortho-Cyclen/Ortho Tri-Cyclen 2573
Ortho-Est Tablets 3464
Ortho-Novum 2563
Ortho-Novum 1/50□28 Tablets 2556
Ortho-Prefest Tablets 2570
Ortho-Cyclen/Ortho Tri-Cyclen 2573
Orudis Capsules (Rare) 3548
Oruvail Capsules (Rare) 3548
Ovcon 3364
Ovral Tablets 3551
Ovral-28 Tablets 3552
Ovrette Tablets 3552
Oxandrin Tablets 1153
Premarin Intravenous 3563
Premarin Tablets 3566
Premarin Vaginal Cream 3570
Premphase Tablets 3572
Prempro Tablets 3572
Provera Tablets 2853
Roferon-A Injection (Less than 4%) 2996
Serentil 1057
Sinequan 2713
Thioridazine Hydrochloride Tablets 2289
Trilafon 3160
Tri-Levlen 962
Tri-Norinyl-28 Tablets 3433
Triphasil-21 Tablets 3600
Triphasil-28 Tablets 3605
Trivora Tablets 3439
Valium Injectable 3026
Valium Tablets (Infrequent) 3047
Vivactil Tablets 2217
Vivactil Tablets 2446
Vivelle Transdermal System 2412
Vivelle-Dot Transdermal System 2416
▲ Xanax Tablets (7.1%) 2865
Yasmin 28 Tablets 980
Zovia 3449

Libido, loss

Baycol Tablets 883
Catapres Tablets (About 3 in 100 patients) 1037
Catapres-TTS (0.5% or less) 1038
Clorpres Tablets (About 3%) 1002
Combipres Tablets (About 3%) 1040
▲ Eulexin Capsules (36%) 3118
Klonopin Tablets (Infrequent) 2983
Lescol Capsules 2361
Lescol Capsules 2925
Lescol XL Tablets 2361
Lescol XL Tablets 2925
Mevacor Tablets (0.5% to 1.0%) 2132
Nolvadex Tablets 678
Orap Tablets 1407
Pravachol Tablets 1099
Roferon-A Injection (Infrequent) 2996
Vascor Tablets (0.5% to 2.0%) 2602
Zantac (Occasional) 1690
Ziac Tablets (0.4%) 1887
Zocor Tablets 2219

Libido decreased

Aciphex Tablets 1267
Aciphex Tablets 1783
Actiq (Less than 1%) 1184
Adalat CC Tablets (Less than 1.0%) 877
Aldoclor Tablets 2035
Aldomet Tablets 2037
Aldoril Tablets 2039
Ambien Tablets (Rare) 3191
Amerge Tablets (Rare) 1467
Anadrol-50 Tablets 3321
Androderm Transdermal System CIII (Less than 1%) 3377
AndroGel (Up to 3%) 3322
Aricept Tablets (Infrequent) 1270
Aricept Tablets (Infrequent) 2665
Asacol Delayed-Release Tablets 2884
Atromid-S Capsules 3483
Axid Pulvules 1903
Axid Pulvules 2919
Betaseron for SC Injection 988
Blocadren Tablets (0.6%) 2046
Bontril Slow-Release Capsules 576
Calcijex Injection 411
Cardura Tablets (0.8%) 2668
▲ Casodex Tablets (2% to 5%) 662
Celexa (2%) 1365
Claritin (At least one patient) 3100
Claritin-D 12 Hour Extended Release Tablets (Less frequent) 3102
Claritin-D 24 Hour Extended Release Tablets 3104
Clozaril Tablets (Less than 1%) 2319
Copaxone for Injection (Infrequent) 3306
Cordarone Tablets (1% to 3%) 3487
Coreg Tablets (0.1% to 1%) 1508
Corgard Tablets (1 to 5 per 1000 patients) 2245
Corzide 40/5 Tablets (1 to 5 of 1000 patients) 2247
Corzide 80/5 Tablets (1 to 5 of 1000 patients) 2247
Cosopt Sterile Ophthalmic Solution 2065
Cozaar Tablets (Less than 1%) 2067
▲ Crinone 8% Gel (10%) 3213
Cytotec Tablets (Infrequent) 3202
Delatestryl Injection 1151
Depo-Provera Contraceptive Injection (1% to 5%) 2798
Diovan HCT Tablets (Greater than 0.2%) 2338
Dolophine Hydrochloride Tablets 3056
▲ Duraclon Injection (3%) 3057
DynaCirc Capsules (0.5% to 1%) 2921
DynaCirc CR Tablets (0.5% to 1%) 2923
▲ Effexor Tablets (2% to 5.7%) 3495
▲ Effexor XR Capsules (3% to 6%) 3499
Estring Vaginal Ring (At least 1 report) 2811
Exelon Capsules (Infrequent) 2342
Exelon Oral Solution (Infrequent) 2345
Famotidine Injection (Infrequent) 866
Flomax Capsules (1.0% to 2.0%) 1044
Gabitril Tablets (Infrequent) 1189
Gengraf Capsules (1% to less than 3%) 457
Glucotrol XL Extended Release Tablets (Less than 1%) 2693
Hectorol Capsules 1064
Hectorol Injection 1066
Hytrin Capsules (0.6%) 464
Hyzaar 2109
Imdur Tablets (Less than or equal to 5%) 1826
Indapamide Tablets (Less than 5%) 2286
▲ Infergen (5%) 1777
Intron A for Injection (Up to 5%) 3120
Inversine Tablets 1850
Iopidine Sterile Ophthalmic Solution ⊙212
Kadian Capsules (Less than 3%) 1335
Kaletra Capsules (Less than 2%) 471
Kaletra Oral Solution (Less than 2%) 471
Klonopin Tablets (1%) 2983
Lamictal (Rare) 1567
Lexxel Tablets 608
Lipitor Tablets (Less than 2%) 2639
Lipitor Tablets (Less than 2%) 2696
Lopid Tablets 2650
Lotensin HCT Tablets (0.3% to 1%) 2367
Lotrel Capsules 2370
Lupron Depot 3.75 mg (Less than 5%) 3281
▲ Lupron Depot 7.5 mg (5.4%) 3284
▲ Lupron Depot–3 Month 11.25 mg (1.8% to 11%) 3285
Lupron Depot–3 Month 22.5 mg (Less than 5%) 3288
Lupron Depot–4 Month 30 mg (Less than 5%) 3289
Lupron Injection (Less than 5%) 3279
Luvox Tablets (25, 50, 100 mg) (2%) 3256
Mavik Tablets (0.3% to 1.0%) 478
Megace Oral Suspension (Up to 5%) 1124
Meridia Capsules 481
Mexitil Capsules (Less than 1% or about 4 in 1,000) 1047
Midamor Tablets (Less than or equal to 1%) 2136
Mirapex Tablets (1%) 2834
▲ Mirena Intrauterine System (5% or more) 974
Moduretic Tablets 2138
Monopril Tablets (0.2% to 1.0%) 1091
MS Contin Tablets (Less frequent) 2896
MSIR (Less frequent) 2898
Nadolol Tablets (1 to 5 of 1000 patients) 2288
Neoral Soft Gelatin Capsules (1% to less than 3%) 2380
Neoral Oral Solution (1% to less than 3%) 2380
▲ Nilandron Tablets (11%) 753
Norpramin Tablets 755
Norvir Capsules (Less than 2%) 487
Norvir Oral Solution (Less than 2%) 487
Oramorph SR Tablets (Less frequent) 3062
OxyContin Tablets 2912
Pacerone Tablets (1% to 3%) 3331
▲ Paxil (3% to 9%) 1609
Pepcid Injection (Infrequent) 2153
Pepcid for Oral Suspension (Infrequent) 2150
Pepcid RPD Orally Disintegrating Tablets (Infrequent) 2150
Pepcid Tablets (Infrequent) 2150
Permax Tablets (Infrequent) 1299
Plendil Extended-Release Tablets (0.5% to 1.5%) 623
Prevacid Delayed-Release Capsules (Less than 1%) 3292
PREVPAC (Less than 1%) 3298
Prinivil Tablets (0.4%) 2164
Prinzide Tablets (0.3% to 1%) 2168
Procardia XL Extended Release Tablets (1% or less) 2710
Propecia Tablets (1.8%) 2172
▲ Proscar Tablets (3.3%) 2175
ProSom Tablets (Rare) 500
Protonix I.V. (Less than 1%) 3580
Protonix Tablets (Less than 1%) 3577
Provigil Tablets (At least 1%) 1193
▲ Prozac Pulvules, Liquid, and Weekly Capsules (3% to 11%) 1238
Requip Tablets (Infrequent) 1621
Rescriptor Tablets (Less than 2%) 526
Rilutek Tablets (Infrequent) 772
Rocaltrol 2991
Roxanol 100 Concentrated Oral Solution 3066
Sandostatin Injection (Less than 1%) 2394
Sandostatin LAR Depot (Rare) 2395
▲ Sarafem Pulvules (4%) 1962
Seroquel Tablets (Rare) 684
Serzone Tablets (1%) 1104
Sonata Capsules (Infrequent) 3591
Soriatane Capsules (Less than 1%) 3003
Sporanox Capsules (0.2% to 1.2%) 1800
Sular Tablets (Less than or equal to 1%) 688
Surmontil Capsules 3595
Symmetrel (0.1% to 1%) 1328
▲ Synarel Nasal Solution for Endometriosis (22% of patients) 3205
Tambocor Tablets (Less than 1%) 1990
Tarka Tablets 508
Tasmar Tablets (Infrequent) 3010
Tenex Tablets (3% or less) 2942
Testoderm Transdermal Systems 574
Testopel Pellets 3610
Testred Capsules, 10 mg 1746
Thalomid Capsules 1154
Timolide Tablets (Less than 1%) 2187
Timolol GFS ⊙266
Timoptic in Ocudose 2192
Timoptic Sterile Ophthalmic Solution 2190
Timoptic-XE Sterile Ophthalmic Gel Forming Solution 2194
Topamax Sprinkle Capsules (Frequent) 2590
Topamax Tablets (Frequent) 2590
Toprol-XL Tablets 651
Tricor Capsules, Micronized (2%) 513
Trileptal Oral Suspension 2407
Trileptal Tablets 2407
Trovan (Less than 1%) 2722
Uniretic Tablets (Less than 1%) 3178
Vaseretic Tablets (0.5% to 2.0%) 2204
Vicoprofen Tablets (Less than 1%) 520
▲ Wellbutrin Tablets (3.1%) 1680
Wellbutrin SR Sustained-Release Tablets (Infrequent) 1684
▲ Xanax Tablets (14.4%) 2865
Zantac Injection 1688
Zebeta Tablets 1885
Zestoretic Tablets (0.3% to 1%) 695
Zestril Tablets (0.4%) 698
▲ Zoladex (61%) 702
▲ Zoloft (1% to 11%) 2751
Zonegran Capsules (Infrequent) 1307
Zyban Sustained-Release Tablets (Infrequent) 1710
Zyprexa Tablets (Infrequent) 1973
Zyprexa ZYDIS Orally Disintegrating Tablets (Infrequent) 1973
Zyrtec (Less than 2%) 2756
Zyrtec-D 12 Hour Extended Relief Tablets (Less than 2%) 2758

Libido increased

Anadrol-50 Tablets 3321
Androderm Transdermal System CIII 3377
AndroGel (One patient) 3322
Aricept Tablets (Frequent) 1270
Aricept Tablets (Frequent) 2665
Avonex 1013
Bontril Slow-Release Capsules 576
Celexa (Infrequent) 1365
Clozaril Tablets (Less than 1%) 2319
Cognex Capsules (Infrequent) 1351
Delatestryl Injection 1151
Depo-Provera Contraceptive Injection (Fewer than 1%) 2798
▲ Dostinex Tablets (Less than 10%) 2804
Effexor Tablets (Infrequent) 3495
Effexor XR Capsules (Infrequent) 3499
Exelon Capsules (Infrequent) 2342
Exelon Oral Solution (Infrequent) 2345
Gabitril Tablets (Infrequent) 1189
Gengraf Capsules (1% to less than 3%) 457
Haldol Decanoate 2535
Haldol Injection, Tablets and Concentrate 2533
Klonopin Tablets (Infrequent) 2983
Lamictal (Rare) 1567
Lodosyn Tablets 1251
Lotensin Tablets (Less than 1%) 2365
Lupron Injection 3279
Luvox Tablets (25, 50, 100 mg) (Infrequent) 3256
Meridia Capsules 481
Moban 1320
Neoral Soft Gelatin Capsules (1% to less than 3%) 2380
Neoral Oral Solution (1% to less than 3%) 2380
Neurontin Capsules (Rare) 2655
Neurontin Oral Solution (Rare) 2655
Neurontin Tablets (Rare) 2655
Norpramin Tablets 755
Paxil (Rare) 1609
Permax Tablets (Infrequent) 1299
Prozac Pulvules, Liquid, and Weekly Capsules (Infrequent) 1238
Remeron Tablets (Infrequent) 2483
Remeron SolTab Tablets (Infrequent) 2486
Reminyl Oral Solution (Infrequent) 1792
Reminyl Tablets (Infrequent) 1792
Requip Tablets (Infrequent) 1621
Rilutek Tablets (Infrequent) 772
Risperdal (Infrequent) 1796

Sarafem Pulvules (Infrequent) 1962
Seroquel Tablets (Infrequent) 684
Serzone Tablets (Infrequent) 1104
Sinemet Tablets 1253
Sinemet CR Tablets 1255
Surmontil Capsules 3595
Synarel Nasal Solution for Endometriosis (1% of patients) 3205
Tasmar Tablets (Infrequent) 3010
Testoderm Transdermal Systems (1%) 574
Testopel Pellets 3610
Testred Capsules, 10 mg 1746
Topamax Sprinkle Capsules (Rare) 2590
Topamax Tablets (Rare) 2590
Trileptal Oral Suspension 2407
Trileptal Tablets 2407
Vistide Injection 1445
Wellbutrin Tablets (Frequent) 1680
Wellbutrin SR Sustained-Release Tablets 1684
▲ Xanax Tablets (7.7%) 2865
Zarontin Capsules (Rare) 2659
Zarontin Syrup (Rare) 2660
▲ Zoladex (12%) 702
Zoloft (Rare) 2751
Zyban Sustained-Release Tablets 1710
Zyprexa Tablets 1973
Zyprexa ZYDIS Orally Disintegrating Tablets 1973

Lichen planus
Aralen Tablets 3075
Cuprimine Capsules 2075
Depen Titratable Tablets (Rare) 3341
Evoxac Capsules (Less than 1%) 1217
Felbatol 3343
Minipress Capsules (Less than 1%) 2699
Minizide Capsules (Rare) 2700
Pentasa Capsules (Less than 1%) 3239

Lichen planus, bullous
Normodyne Tablets 3137

Ligaments, calcification of
Accutane Capsules 2944

Light-headedness
Accupril Tablets 2611
Accuretic Tablets 2614
Adenocard Injection (2%) 1380
▲ Adenoscan (12%) 1381
Aldoclor Tablets 2035
Aldomet Tablets 2037
Alferon N Injection (One patient to 3%) 1770
Altace Capsules 2233
Ambien Tablets (2%) 3191
Anaprox Tablets (Less than 3%) 2967
Anaprox DS Tablets (Less than 3%) 2967
Beconase Inhalation Aerosol 1497
Beconase AQ Nasal Spray (Fewer than 5 per 100 patients) 1498
BeneFix for Injection (Two cases) 1432
▲ Betapace Tablets (4% to 12%) 950
Brevibloc Injection (Less than 1%) 858
Captopril Tablets 2281
▲ Cardura Tablets (Up to 23%) 2668
Chibroxin Sterile Ophthalmic Solution 2051
Cipro I.V. (1% or less) 893
Cipro I.V. Pharmacy Bulk Package (Less than 1%) 897
Cipro (Less than 1%) 887
Clomid Tablets (Fewer than 1%) 735
Colestid Tablets (Infrequent) 2791
Cutivate Ointment (Less than 1%) 1284
Dantrium Capsules (Less frequent) 2885
Dantrium Intravenous 2886
Darvon-N/Darvocet-N 1907
Darvon Pulvules 1909
Darvon Compound-65 Pulvules 1910
Darvon-N Tablets 1912
▲ Demerol (Among most frequent) 3079
Dilaudid Oral Liquid 445
Dilaudid Tablets - 8 mg 445
▲ Dilaudid-HP (Among most frequent) 443
Diovan HCT Tablets 2338
Dipentum Capsules 2803
Dolobid Tablets (Less than 1 in 100) 2088
▲ Dolophine Hydrochloride Tablets (Among most frequent) 3056
Duranest Injections 600
Dynacin Capsules 2019
EC-Naprosyn Delayed-Release Tablets (Less than 3%) 2967
ELA-Max Cream 1340
▲ Eldepryl Capsules (7 of 49 patients) 3266
Emla (Unlikely with cream) 602
Factrel (Rare) 3633
Floxin I.V. 2526
Floxin Tablets 2529
Fortovase Capsules (Less than 2%) 2970
▲ Gabitril Tablets (27%) 1189
Gammagard S/D (Occasional) 845
Gastrocrom Oral Concentrate (Less common) 1162
Glucophage Tablets (1% to 5%) 1080
▲ Halcion Tablets (4.9%) 2823
▲ Hytrin Capsules (28%) 464
Hyzaar 2109
Indapamide Tablets (Less than 5%) 2286
Inderal 3513
Inderal LA Long-Acting Capsules 3516
Inderide Tablets 3517
Inderide LA Long-Acting Capsules 3519
Indocin (Less than 1%) 2112
Inversine Tablets 1850
Invirase Capsules (Less than 2%) 2979
Ismo Tablets 3524
Isordil Sublingual Tablets 3525
Isordil Titradose Tablets 3526
Levaquin (0.1% to less than 1.0%) 2537
Lidoderm Patch 1319
▲ Lortab (Among most frequent) 3319
▲ Lortab Elixir (Among most frequent) 3317
Lotensin HCT Tablets 2367
Loxitane Capsules 3398
▲ Lupron Injection (5% or more) 3279
Mavik Tablets 478
▲ Maxidone Tablets CIII (Among most frequent) 3399
▲ Mepergan Injection (Among most frequent) 3539
▲ Mexitil Capsules (10.5% to 26.4%) 1047
Micardis HCT Tablets 1051
Minocin Intravenous 1862
Minocin Oral Suspension 1865
Minocin Pellet-Filled Capsules 1863
Monopril Tablets 1091
Monopril HCT 1094
Motofen Tablets (1 in 20) 577
▲ MS Contin Tablets (Among most frequent) 2896
▲ MSIR (Among most frequent) 2898
▲ Mykrox Tablets (10.2%) 1168
Naprelan Tablets (Less than 3%) 1293
Naprosyn Suspension (Less than 3%) 2967
Naprosyn Tablets (Less than 3%) 2967
Navane Oral 2701
Navane Intramuscular 2703
Nimotop Capsules (Less than 1%) 904
▲ Nitro-Dur Transdermal Infusion System (6%) 1834
▲ Nitro-Dur Transdermal Infusion System (6%) 3134
Nolvadex Tablets (Infrequent) 678
▲ Norco 5/325 Tablets CIII (Among most frequent) 3424
▲ Norco 7.5/325 Tablets CIII (Among most frequent) 3425
▲ Norco 10/325 Tablets CIII (Among most frequent) 3425
▲ Norco 10/325 Tablets CIII (Among most frequent) 3427
Norflex 1987
Noroxin Tablets 2145
Numorphan 1324
▲ Oramorph SR Tablets (Among most frequent) 3062
▲ OxyFast Oral Concentrate Solution (Among most frequent) 2916
▲ OxyIR Capsules (Among most frequent) 2916
Parafon Forte DSC Caplets (Occasional) 2582
▲ Percocet Tablets (Among most frequent) 1326
▲ Percodan Tablets (Among most frequent) 1327
▲ Percolone Tablets (Among most frequent) 1327
Phenergan with Codeine Syrup 3557
Phenergan VC with Codeine Syrup 3561
▲ Phrenilin (Among most frequent) 578
Prinivil Tablets 2164
Prinzide Tablets 2168
▲ Procardia Capsules (Approximately 10% to 27%) 2708
▲ Procardia XL Extended Release Tablets (1 in 8 patients) 2710
Prolastin (0.19%) 943
▲ Quinidex Extentabs (15%) 2933
Recombivax HB (Less than 1%) 2178
Robaxin Injectable 2938
Robaxin Tablets 2939
▲ Robaxisal Tablets (One in 20 to 25) 2939
▲ Roxanol (Among most frequent) 3066
▲ Roxicodone (Among most frequent) 3067
▲ Sedapap Tablets 50 mg/650 mg (Among the most frequent) 2225
Sensorcaine 643
Sensorcaine-MPF Injection 643
Serophene Tablets (Less than 1 in 100 patients) 3226
▲ Serzone Tablets (10%) 1104
▲ Symmetrel (5% to 10%) 1328
Talacen Caplets 3089
Talwin Nx Tablets 3090
Tambocor Tablets 1990
Tenoretic Tablets (1% to 3%) 690
Tenormin (1% to 3%) 692
Tequin Injection 1110
Tequin Tablets 1110
Thiothixene Capsules 2290
▲ Thrombate III (1 of 17) 944
Thyrel TRH for Injection 3630
Trilisate (Less than 2%) 2901
Trovan (1% to 2%) 2722
Tussi-Organidin NR Liquid 3350
Tussi-Organidin-S NR Liquid 3350
▲ Tylenol with Codeine (Among most frequent) 2595
▲ Tylox Capsules (Among most frequent) 2597
Uniretic Tablets (Less than 1%) 3178
Urecholine 2198
Vaseretic Tablets 2204
Vasotec Tablets 2210
Ventolin Inhalation Aerosol and Refill (Less than 1%) 1679
Versed Injection (Less than 1%) 3027
▲ Vicodin Tablets (Among most frequent) 516
▲ Vicodin ES Tablets (Among most frequent) 517
▲ Vicodin HP Tablets (Among most frequent) 518
▲ Xanax Tablets (20.8% to 29.8%) 2865
▲ Xylocaine Injections (Among most common) 653
Zaroxolyn Tablets 1177
▲ Zemplar Injection (5%) 522
Zestoretic Tablets 695
Zestril Tablets 698
Zovirax for Injection (Less than 1%) 1708
▲ Zydone Tablets (Among most frequent) 1330

Limb ischemia
Lovenox Injection 746

Limb reduction defects
Accupril Tablets 2611
Altace Capsules 2233
Captopril Tablets 2281
Cozaar Tablets 2067
Enalaprilat Injection 863
Hyzaar 2109
Lexxel Tablets 608
Lo/Ovral Tablets 3532
Lo/Ovral-28 Tablets 3538
Lotrel Capsules 2370
Low-Ogestrel-28 Tablets 3392
Monopril Tablets 1091
Nordette-28 Tablets 2257
Ogestrel 0.5/50-28 Tablets 3428
Ovral Tablets 3551
Ovral-28 Tablets 3552
Ovrette Tablets 3552
Prinivil Tablets 2164
Prinzide Tablets 2168
Proventil Inhalation Aerosol 3142
Proventil Inhalation Solution 0.083% 3146
Univasc Tablets 3181
Vaseretic Tablets 2204
Vasotec I.V. Injection 2207
Vasotec Tablets 2210
Ventolin Inhalation Aerosol and Refill 1679
Zestoretic Tablets 695
Zestril Tablets 698

Limbitis
▲ Stromectol Tablets (3.5% to 5.5%) 2185

Lipoatrophy
Imitrex Injection (Rare) 1549
▲ Nutropin Depot for Injectable Suspension (13%) 1423

Lipodystrophy
Genotropin Lyophilized Powder (Infrequent) 2818
Humalog 1926
Humalog Mix 75/25 Pen 1928
Humulin 50/50, 100 Units (Rare) 1934
Humulin 70/30, 100 Units (Rare) 1935
Humulin 70/30 Pen (Rare) 1936
Humulin L, 100 Units (Rare) 1937
Humulin R Regular (U-500) (Rare) 1943
Humulin N NPH Pen (Rare) 1940
Iletin II, Regular (Pork), 100 Units (Rare) 1947
Lantus Injection 742
NovoLog Injection 2427

Lipohypertrophy
Imitrex Injection (Rare) 1549

Lipoma
Avonex 1013
Cognex Capsules (Infrequent) 1351
Copaxone for Injection (Infrequent) 3306
Intron A for Injection (Less than 5%) 3120
Requip Tablets (Infrequent) 1621

Lipoprotein levels, changes
Accutane Capsules 2944
Carbatrol Capsules (Occasional) 3234
Humegon for Injection (Occasional) 2468
Levlen 962
Levlite 21 Tablets 962
Levlite 28 Tablets 962
▲ Soriatane Capsules (25% to 50%) 3003
Synarel Nasal Solution for Endometriosis 3205
Tegretol/Tegretol-XR (Occasional) 2404
Timolide Tablets 2187
Tri-Levlen 962
Triphasil-21 Tablets 3600
Vivelle Transdermal System 2412
Vivelle-Dot Transdermal System 2416
Zoladex 702
Zoladex 3-month 706

Lipoproteins, electrophoretic abnormalities
Sandimmune 2388

Lipotrophy
Humulin 50/50, 100 Units (Rare) 1934
Humulin 70/30, 100 Units (Rare) 1935
Humulin 70/30 Pen (Rare) 1936
Humulin L, 100 Units (Rare) 1937
Humulin R Regular (U-500) (Rare) 1943
Humulin N NPH Pen (Rare) 1940
Iletin II, Regular (Pork), 100 Units (Rare) 1947

Lips, enlargement
Dilantin Infatabs 2624
Dilantin Kapseals 2622
Dilantin-125 Oral Suspension 2625
Eskalith 1527

Lips, swelling
Altace Capsules 2233
Cataflam Tablets (Less than 1%) 2315
Levaquin 2537
Lithobid Slow-Release Tablets 3255
Propecia Tablets 2172
Proscar Tablets 2175
Tambocor Tablets (Less than 1%) 1990
Vaniqa Cream (Less than 1%) 1121
Voltaren Tablets (Less than 1%) 2315
Voltaren-XR Tablets (Less than 1%) 2315

Listlessness
Aricept Tablets (Infrequent) 1270
Aricept Tablets (Infrequent) 2665
Indocin (Greater than 1%) 2112
Rum-K 1363
Synvisc 3596

Livedo reticularis
Activase I.V. 1410
Felbatol 3343
Retavase Vials 1182
Streptase for Infusion 647
Symmetrel (1% to 5%) 1328

Liver, fatty
Aciphex Tablets (Rare) 1267
Aciphex Tablets (Rare) 1783
Effexor XR Capsules 3499
Geodon Capsules (Rare) 2688
Lescol Capsules 2361
Lescol Capsules 2925
Lescol XL Tablets 2361
Lescol XL Tablets 2925
Plavix Tablets (Less than 1%) 1097
Plavix Tablets (Less than 1%) 3084
Sandostatin LAR Depot (Rare) 2395
Sarafem Pulvules (Rare) 1962
Tricor Capsules, Micronized 513
Zyprexa Tablets (Rare) 1973
Zyprexa ZYDIS Orally Disintegrating Tablets (Rare) 1973

Liver abnormalities
Baycol Tablets 883
Catapres Tablets (About 1 in 100 patients) 1037
Clorpres Tablets 1002
Clozaril Tablets (1%) 2319
Combipres Tablets 1040
Compazine (A few observations) 1505
Effexor Tablets 3495
Famotidine Injection (Infrequent) 866
Nolvadex Tablets (Rare) 678
Oncaspar (Less than 1%) 756
Pepcid Injection (Infrequent) 2153
Pepcid for Oral Suspension (Infrequent) 2150
Pepcid RPD Orally Disintegrating Tablets (Infrequent) 2150
Pepcid Tablets (Infrequent) 2150
Pravachol Tablets 1099
Relafen Tablets (1%) 1617
Sectral Capsules 3589
▲ Tarka Tablets (3.2%) 508
Ziagen 1692
Zocor Tablets 2219

Liver damage

(*see under* Hepatotoxicity)

Liver disorders
Aldoclor Tablets 2035
Aldomet Tablets 2037
Aldoril Tablets 2039
Cosmegen for Injection 2062

Fortovase Capsules (Rare; less than 2%) 2970
Invirase Capsules (Rare) 2979
▲ Leukine (77%) 1755
Lo/Ovral Tablets 3532
Lo/Ovral-28 Tablets 3538
Low-Ogestrel-28 Tablets 3392
Ogestrel 0.5/50-28 Tablets 3428
Ovral Tablets 3551
Ovral-28 Tablets 3552
Ovrette Tablets 3552
Prozac Pulvules, Liquid, and Weekly Capsules (Rare) 1238
Pulmozyme Inhalation Solution 1426
Triphasil-21 Tablets 3600
Triphasil-28 Tablets 3605
▲ Vesanoid Capsules (3%) 3037

Liver dysfunction
(*see under* Hepatic dysfunction)

Liver function, changes
(*see under* Hepatic dysfunction)

Liver function, impaired
(*see under* Hepatic dysfunction)

Liver injury
Ancobon Capsules 1730
Cordarone Tablets (Common) 3487
Cylert Tablets 415
Eulexin Capsules 3118
Mexitil Capsules (Rare) 1047
Nilandron Tablets (Rare) 753
Pacerone Tablets (Common) 3331
Tasmar Tablets 3010
Trovan 2722
Vantin Tablets and Oral Suspension 2860

Liver pain
▲ Roferon-A Injection (3%) 2996

Liver tenderness
Actiq (Less than 1%) 1184

Liver transplant, need for
Antabuse Tablets 3474
Cylert Tablets 415
Felbatol 3343
Lamisil Tablets 2360
Serzone Tablets 1104
Trovan 2722

Liver tumors
(*see under* Hepatomas)

Loffler's syndrome
Paser Granules 1781

Loss of balance
(*see under* Balance, loss of)

Lower spinal segments deficit
Duranest Injections (Rare) 600

Lumbago
Klonopin Tablets (Infrequent) 2983
Prinivil Tablets (0.3% to 1.0%) 2164
Prinzide Tablets 2168
Zestoretic Tablets 695
Zestril Tablets (0.3% to 1.0%) 698

Lung consolidation
Survanta Intratracheal Suspension 3053

Lung development, hypoplastic
Accupril Tablets 2611
Altace Capsules 2233
Captopril Tablets 2281
Cozaar Tablets 2067
Enalaprilat Injection 863
Hyzaar 2109
Lexxel Tablets 608
Lotrel Capsules 2370
Monopril Tablets 1091
Monopril HCT 1094
Prinivil Tablets 2164
Prinzide Tablets 2168
Univasc Tablets 3181
Vaseretic Tablets 2204
Vasotec I.V. Injection 2207
Vasotec Tablets 2210
Zestoretic Tablets 695
Zestril Tablets 698

Lung disorders, unspecified
Accuretic Tablets 2614
Actiq (Less than 1%) 1184
▲ AmBisome for Injection (13.6% to 17.8%) 1383
▲ Amphotec (5% or more) 1774
Arava Tablets (1% to 3%) 724
▲ Casodex Tablets (2% to 5%) 662
Ceclor CD Tablets (0.1% to 1%) 1279
▲ CellCept Capsules (3% to 30.1%) 2951
▲ CellCept Intravenous (3% to 30.1%) 2951
▲ CellCept Oral Suspension (3% to 30.1%) 2951
▲ CellCept Tablets (3% to 30.1%) 2951
▲ DuoNeb Inhalation Solution (6.4%) 1233
▲ Leukine (20%) 1755
Lupron Depot–4 Month 30 mg (Less than 5%) 3289
Megace Oral Suspension (1% to 3%) 1124
Myobloc Injectable Solution (2% or greater) 1291
Naprelan Tablets (Less than 1%) 1293
▲ Nilandron Tablets (4%) 753
▲ Nipent for Injection (Up to 12%) 3272
Norvir Capsules (Less than 2%) 487
Norvir Oral Solution (Less than 2%) 487
▲ Prograf (3% to 15%) 1393
▲ Proleukin for Injection (24%) 1199
Protonix I.V. (Less than 1%) 3580
Protonix Tablets (Less than 1%) 3577
Protopic Ointment (Greater than or equal to 1%) 1397
▲ Provigil Tablets (4%) 1193
Pulmozyme Inhalation Solution 1426
Roxicodone Tablets (Less than 3%) 3067
Thalomid Capsules 1154
▲ Trasylol Injection (7%) 909
Ventolin HFA Inhalation Aerosol (Less than 3%) 3618
Vistide Injection 1445

Lung neoplasms, malignant
Prinzide Tablets 2168
Zestoretic Tablets 695
Zestril Tablets (0.3% to 1.0%) 698

Lupus erythematosus
Aldoclor Tablets 2035
Aldomet Tablets 2037
Aldoril Tablets 2039
Dapsone Tablets USP 1780
Depacon Injection 416
Depakene 421
Depakote Sprinkle Capsules 426
Depakote Tablets (1% to 5%) 430
Depakote ER Tablets (Greater than 1%) 436
Dilantin Infatabs 2624
Dilantin Kapseals 2622
Dilantin-125 Oral Suspension 2625
Gris-PEG Tablets 2661
Inderal (Rare) 3513
Inderal LA Long-Acting Capsules (Rare) 3516
Inderide LA Long-Acting Capsules (Rare) 3519
Rythmol Tablets – 150 mg, 225 mg, 300 mg (Less than 1%) 502
Tonocard Tablets (1.6%) 649
Zonegran Capsules (Rare) 1307

Lupus erythematosus, systemic
Atromid-S Capsules 3483
Bactrim 2949
Celontin Capsules 2618
Compazine 1505
Cosopt Sterile Ophthalmic Solution 2065
Declomycin Tablets 1855
Dilantin Infatabs 2624
Dilantin Kapseals 2622
Dilantin-125 Oral Suspension 2625
Etrafon 3115
Inderal (Extremely rare) 3513
Inderal LA Long-Acting Capsules (Extremely rare) 3516
Inderide Tablets (Extremely rare) 3517
Inderide LA Long-Acting Capsules (Extremely rare) 3519
Mexitil Capsules (About 4 in 10,000) 1047
Monodox Capsules 2442
Normodyne Tablets (Less common) 3137
Norplant System (Rare) 3543
Pediazole Suspension 3050
Procanbid Extended-Release Tablets (Fairly common) 2262
Quinaglute Dura-Tabs Tablets 978
Quinidex Extentabs 2933
Recombivax HB 2178
Sectral Capsules 3589
Septra Suspension 2265
Septra Tablets 2265
Septra DS Tablets 2265
Serentil 1057
Stelazine 1640
Syprine Capsules 2186
Thorazine 1656
Timolol GFS ⊙ 266
Timoptic in Ocudose (Less frequent) 2192
Timoptic Sterile Ophthalmic Solution (Less frequent) 2190
Timoptic-XE Sterile Ophthalmic Gel Forming Solution 2194
Trilafon 3160
Vibramycin Hyclate Intravenous 2737
Zarontin Capsules 2659
Zarontin Syrup 2660

Lupus erythematosus, systemic, exacerbation or activation of
Carbatrol Capsules 3234
Doryx Coated Pellet Filled Capsules 3357
Dyazide Capsules 1515
Dynacin Capsules 2019
Furosemide Tablets 2284
Maxzide 1008
Minocin Intravenous 1862
Minocin Oral Suspension 1865
Minocin Pellet-Filled Capsules 1863
Periostat Tablets 1208
Prinzide Tablets 2168
Tegretol/Tegretol-XR 2404
Tenoretic Tablets 690
Vaseretic Tablets 2204
Vibramycin Calcium Oral Suspension Syrup 2735
Vibramycin Hyclate Capsules 2735
Vibramycin Monohydrate for Oral Suspension 2735
Vibra-Tabs Film Coated Tablets 2735
Zaroxolyn Tablets 1177
Zestoretic Tablets 695

Lupus erythematosus syndrome
Azulfidine EN-tabs Tablets (Rare) 2775
Carbatrol Capsules (Isolated cases) 3234
Cuprimine Capsules 2075
Depen Titratable Tablets 3341
Evoxac Capsules (Less than 1%) 1217
Felbatol 3343
Mexitil Capsules (About 4 in 10,000) 1047
Motrin Suspension, Oral Drops, Chewable Tablets, and Caplets (Less than 1%) 2002
Naprelan Tablets (Less than 1%) 1293
Navane Oral 2701
Navane Intramuscular 2703
Permax Tablets (Rare) 1299
Remicade for IV Injection (Less than 2%) 1178
Rifamate Capsules 767
Roferon-A Injection (Rare) 2996
Tegretol/Tegretol-XR (Isolated cases) 2404
Thorazine 1656
Trileptal Oral Suspension 2407
Trileptal Tablets 2407

Lupus-like syndrome
Aldoclor Tablets 2035
Aldomet Tablets 2037
Aldoril Tablets 2039
Asacol Delayed-Release Tablets 2884
Baycol Tablets 883
Cuprimine Capsules 2075
Depen Titratable Tablets 3341
Dynacin Capsules 2019
Gastrocrom Oral Concentrate (Less common) 1162
Gris-PEG Tablets 2661
Lamictal 1567
Lescol Capsules (Rare) 2361
Lescol Capsules (Rare) 2925
Lescol XL Tablets 2361
Lescol XL Tablets 2925
Lopid Tablets 2650
Macrobid Capsules 2889
Macrodantin Capsules 2891
Mevacor Tablets (Rare) 2132
Minocin Intravenous 1862
Minocin Oral Suspension 1865
Minocin Pellet-Filled Capsules 1863
Nardil Tablets (Less frequent) 2653
PEG-Intron Powder for Injection (Less than or equal to 1%) 3140
Pravachol Tablets (Rare) 1099
Recombivax HB 2178
Rifater Tablets 769
Rituxan for Infusion (Less than 0.1%) 1750
Rituxan I.V. (Less than 0.1%) 1428
Sarafem Pulvules 1962
Tapazole Tablets 1823
Tegretol-XR Tablets (Isolated cases) 2404
Tenoretic Tablets 690
Tenormin 692
Tice BCG, BCG Live (Rare) 2489
Tonocard Tablets (1.6%) 649
Tricor Capsules, Micronized (Less than 1%) 513
Zocor Tablets (Rare) 2219
Zoloft 2751

Lyell's syndrome
Accutane Capsules 2944
Aldoclor Tablets 2035
Aldomet Tablets 2037
Aldoril Tablets 2039
Amoxil Chewable Tablets 1471
Amoxil for Oral Suspension 1471
Amoxil 1471
Anaprox Tablets (Less than 1%) 2967
Anaprox DS Tablets (Less than 1%) 2967
Ancobon Capsules 1730
Arava Tablets (Rare) 724
Arthrotec Tablets (Rare) 3195
Atacand HCT Tablets 597
Atromid-S Capsules 3483
Augmentin Chewable Tablets (Occasional) 1482
Augmentin Powder for Oral Suspension (Occasional) 1482
Augmentin Tablets (Occasional) 1485
Augmentin ES-600 Powder for Oral Suspension 1487
Avalide Tablets 1070
Azactam for Injection (Less than 1%) 1276
Azelex Cream (Less than 1%) 547
Azulfidine EN-tabs Tablets (Rare) 2775
Bactrim (Rare) 2949
Baycol Tablets (Rare) 883
Betoptic S Ophthalmic Suspension (Rare) 537
Biaxin/Biaxin XL 403
▲ Blephamide Ophthalmic Ointment (Among most often) 547
Blephamide Ophthalmic Suspension 548
Brevoxyl 3269
▲ Brevoxyl Cleansing (5 of 100 patients) 3269
Brevoxyl 3270
Carbatrol Capsules (Extremely rare) 3234
Ceclor CD Tablets (Rare) 1279
Ceclor (Rare) 1905
Cedax Capsules 1021
Cefizox for Intramuscular or Intravenous Use 1390
Cefotan 664
Ceftin 1898
Cefzil 1076
Celebrex Capsules (Less than 0.1%) 2676
Celebrex Capsules (Less than 0.1%) 2780
Celexa (3 cases) 1365
Ceptaz for Injection 1499
Chibroxin Sterile Ophthalmic Solution 2051
Cipro I.V. (1% or less) 893
Cipro I.V. Pharmacy Bulk Package (Less than 1%) 897
Cipro 887
Claritin-D 12 Hour Extended Release Tablets (Less frequent) 3102
▲ Cleocin T Topical (7% to 11%) 2790
Cleocin Vaginal Cream 2788
▲ Clindets Pledgets (Up to 11%) 3270
Clinoril Tablets (Less than 1%) 2053
Clorpres Tablets 1002
Combipres Tablets 1040
Condylox Topical Solution (Less than 5%) 2437
Cordarone Intravenous 3491
Cozaar Tablets (One subject) 2067
Cuprimine Capsules 2075
Daraprim Tablets 1511
Depacon Injection (Rare) 416
Depakene (Rare) 421
Depakote Sprinkle Capsules (Rare) 426
Depakote Tablets (Rare) 430
Depakote ER Tablets (Rare) 436
Depen Titratable Tablets (Rare) 3341
DesOwen (Less than 2%) 1401
Diamox Intravenous ⊙ 269
Diamox Sequels Sustained Release Capsules ⊙ 270
Diamox Tablets ⊙ 269
Diflucan Tablets, Injection, and Oral Suspension 2681
Dilantin Infatabs 2624
Dilantin Kapseals 2622
Dilantin-125 Oral Suspension 2625
Diovan HCT Tablets 2338
Diuril Oral 2087
Diuril Sodium Intravenous 2086
Dolobid Tablets (Less than 1 in 100) 2088
▲ Dovonex Ointment (1% to 10%) 1117
Duricef 1079
EC-Naprosyn Delayed-Release Tablets (Less than 1%) 2967
E.E.S. (Rare) 450
Effexor XR Capsules 3499
Emcyt Capsules (1%) 2810
Emgel 2% Topical Gel (Occasional) 1285
Enalaprilat Injection 863
EryPed (Rare) 446
Ethyol for Injection 2029
Eulexin Capsules 3118
Famotidine Injection (Very rare) 866
Felbatol 3343
Feldene Capsules (Rare) 2685
Floxin I.V. 2526
Floxin Tablets 2529
FML-S Liquifilm Sterile Ophthalmic Suspension ⊙ 238
Fortaz 1541

Foscavir Injection (Rare) 605
HydroDIURIL Tablets 2108
Hyzaar (One subject) 2109
Indocin Capsules (Less than 1%) 2112
Indocin I.V. (Less than 1%) 2115
Indocin (Less than 1%) 2112
Intron A for Injection (Less than 5%) 3120
Keflex (Rare) 1237
Kefurox Vials, ADD-Vantage 1948
Lac-Hydrin Lotion (1 in 60 patients) 1119
Lamictal (Rare) 1567
Lamisil Tablets (Isolated reports) 2360
Lescol Capsules (Rare) 2361
Lescol Capsules (Rare) 2925
Lescol XL Tablets 2361
Lescol XL Tablets 2925
Leukeran Tablets (Rare) 1591
Leustatin Injection (Isolated cases) 2495
Lexxel Tablets 608
Lipitor Tablets 2639
Lipitor Tablets 2696
Lodine (Less than 1%) 3528
Lodine XL Extended-Release Tablets (Less than 1%) 3530
Lorabid Suspension and Pulvules 2251
Lotrimin 3128
Lotrisone 3129
Luvox Tablets (25, 50, 100 mg) 3256
Maxalt Tablets 2120
Maxalt-MLT Orally Disintegrating Tablets 2120
Maxipime for Injection 1285
Mefoxin for Injection 2124
Mefoxin Premixed Intravenous Solution 2127
Merrem I.V. 673
Mevacor Tablets (Rare) 2132
Micardis HCT Tablets 1051
Microzide Capsules 3414
Mobic Tablets (Less than 0.1%) 1054
Moduretic Tablets 2138
Motrin Suspension, Oral Drops, Chewable Tablets, and Caplets (Less than 1%) 2002
▲ Naprelan Tablets (3% to 9%) 1293
Naprosyn Suspension (Less than 1%) 2967
Naprosyn Tablets (Less than 1%) 2967
Nebcin Vials, Hyporets & ADD-Vantage (Rare) 1955
Neptazane Tablets ⊙ 271
Noroxin Tablets 2145
Omnicef 493
Orudis Capsules (Less than 1%) 3548
Oruvail Capsules (Less than 1%) 3548
Pacerone Tablets 3331
Paxil 1609
PCE Dispertab Tablets (Rare) 498
Pediazole Suspension 3050
Pepcid Injection (Very rare) 2153
Pepcid for Oral Suspension (very rare) 2150
Pepcid RPD Orally Disintegrating Tablets (Very rare) 2150
Pepcid Tablets (Very rare) 2150
Phrenilin (Several cases) 578
Ponstel Capsules (Rare) 1356
Pravachol Tablets (Rare) 1099
Prilosec Delayed-Release Capsules (Very rare) 628
Primaxin I.M. 2158
Primaxin I.V. (Less than 0.2%) 2160
Prinivil Tablets (Rare) 2164
Prinzide Tablets (Rare) 2168
Procardia Capsules (Rare) 2708
Procardia XL Extended Release Tablets (Rare) 2710
Protonix I.V. 3580
Protonix Tablets 3577
Prozac Pulvules, Liquid, and Weekly Capsules 1238
Relafen Tablets (Less than 1%) 1617
▲ Renova 0.02% Cream (Almost all subjects) 2520
▲ Renova 0.05% Cream (Almost all subjects) 2519
Rifadin (Occasional) 765
Rifater Tablets 769
Rituxan for Infusion (Less than 0.1%) 1750
Rituxan I.V. (Less than 0.1%) 1428
Sarafem Pulvules 1962
Sedapap Tablets 50 mg/650 mg (Several cases) 2225
Septra Suspension 2265
Septra Tablets 2265
Septra DS Tablets 2265
▲ Soriatane Capsules (50% to 75%) 3003
Suprax 1877
Sustiva Capsules (Up to 3.5%) 1258
Tagamet (Very rare) 1644
Talacen Caplets (Rare) 3089
Talwin Nx Tablets 3090
Tamiflu Capsules 3008
Tamiflu Oral Suspension 3008
Tazicef for Injection 1647
Tazicef Galaxy Container 1650
Tazicef Pharmacy Bulk Package 1653
Tazidime Vials, Faspak & ADD-Vantage 1966
Tegretol/Tegretol-XR (Extremely rare) 2404
Tenoretic Tablets 690
Tiazac Capsules (Less than 2%) 1378
Timentin Injection- ADD-Vantage Vial 1661
Timentin Injection-Galaxy Container 1664
Timentin Injection-Pharmacy Bulk Package 1666
Timentin for Intravenous Administration 1658
Timolide Tablets 2187
Tolectin (Less than 1%) 2589
Toradol 3018
Trileptal Oral Suspension 2407
Trileptal Tablets 2407
Trovan 2722
Trusopt Sterile Ophthalmic Solution (Rare) 2196
Ultracet Tablets 2597
Ultram Tablets (Less than 1%) 2600
Vancocin HCl Capsules & Pulvules (Infrequent) 1972
Vancocin HCl Oral Solution (Infrequent) 1971
Vancocin HCl, Vials & ADD-Vantage (Infrequent) 1970
Vantin Tablets and Oral Suspension (Less than 1%) 2860
Vaseretic Tablets 2204
Vasotec I.V. Injection 2207
Vasotec Tablets (0.5% to 1.0%) 2210
Viramune Oral Suspension 1060
Viramune Tablets 1060
Xalatan Latanoprost Ophthalmic Solution ⊙ 320
Xalatan Sterile Ophthalmic Solution 2864
Zaroxolyn Tablets 1177
Zestoretic Tablets 695
Zestril Tablets (Rare) 698
Zinacef Injection (Rare) 1696
Zinacef for Injection (Rare) 1696
Zithromax Capsules, 250 mg (Rare) 2743
Zithromax for IV Infusion (Rare) 2748
Zithromax for Oral Suspension, 300 mg, 600 mg, 900 mg, 1200 mg (Rare) 2739
Zithromax Tablets, 250 mg (Rare) 2739
Zocor Tablets (Rare) 2219
Zovirax Capsules 1706
Zovirax for Injection 1708
Zovirax 1706

Lymph nodes, tender
ProSom Tablets (Rare) 500
Stromectol Tablets (1.9%) 2185

Lymphadenitis
Intron A for Injection (Less than or equal to 5%) 3120

Lymphadenopathy
AccuNeb Inhalation Solution (0.9% to 2.6%) 1230
Accutane Capsules 2944
Aciphex Tablets 1267
Aciphex Tablets 1783
Actiq (1% or greater) 1184
Adalat CC Tablets (Less than 1.0%) 877
Aerobid/Aerobid-M (1% to 3%) 1363
Alferon N Injection (1%) 1770
Ambien Tablets (Rare) 3191
Arthrotec Tablets (Rare) 3195
Asacol Delayed-Release Tablets 2884
Attenuvax (Less common) 2044
Avonex 1013
▲ Betaseron for SC Injection (14%) 988
Bicillin C-R 900/300 Injection 2240
Bicillin C-R Injection 2238
Bicillin L-A Injection 2242
Campath Ampules 992
Carbatrol Capsules 3234
Cardura Tablets (Less than 0.5%) 2668
Ceclor (Infrequent) 1905
Celexa (Infrequent) 1365
Cerebyx Injection (Infrequent) 2619
Cipro (0.3% to 1%) 887
Claritin-D 12 Hour Extended Release Tablets (Less frequent) 3102
Claritin-D 24 Hour Extended Release Tablets (Fewer than 2%) 3104
Cognex Capsules (Infrequent) 1351
Colazal Capsules 3069
Comvax 2056
▲ Copaxone for Injection (12%) 3306
Crixivan Capsules (Less than 2%) 2070
Cuprimine Capsules 2075
DaunoXome Injection (Less than or equal to 5%) 1442
Depen Titratable Tablets 3341
Dilantin Infatabs 2624
Dilantin Kapseals 2622
Dilantin-125 Oral Suspension 2625
Diphtheria & Tetanus Toxoids Adsorbed Purogenated for Pediatric Use 1857
Doxil Injection (Less than 1%) 566
Effexor Tablets (Infrequent) 3495
Effexor XR Capsules (Infrequent) 3499
Engerix-B Vaccine (Less than 1%) 1517
Epivir 1520
Epivir-HBV 1524
Evoxac Capsules (Less than 1%) 1217
Exelon Capsules (Infrequent) 2342
Exelon Oral Solution (Infrequent) 2345
Felbatol (Infrequent) 3343
Feldene Capsules (Rare) 2685
Ferrlecit Injection (Greater than 1%) 3386
FluShield Influenza Vaccine 3521
Fortovase Capsules (Less than 2%) 2970
Foscavir Injection (Between 1% and 5%) 605
Gabitril Tablets (Frequent) 1189
Gengraf Capsules (1% to less than 3%) 457
Geodon Capsules (Infrequent) 2688
Gonal-F for Injection 3216
Havrix Vaccine (Rare) 1544
Hivid Tablets (Less than 1% to 3%) 2975
Imitrex Nasal Spray (Rare) 1554
Imitrex Tablets (Rare) 1558
INFeD Injection 3388
▲ Infergen (4% to 6%) 1777
Intron A for Injection (Less than or equal to 5%) 3120
Invirase Capsules (Less than 2%) 2979
Kaletra Capsules (Less than 2%) 471
Kaletra Oral Solution (Less than 2%) 471
Klonopin Tablets 2983
Lamictal (Infrequent) 1567
Levaquin (Less than 0.3%) 2537
Lipitor Tablets (Less than 2%) 2639
Lipitor Tablets (Less than 2%) 2696
Lodine XL Extended-Release Tablets 3530
▲ Lupron Depot 3.75 mg (Among most frequent) 3281
Lupron Depot–3 Month 11.25 mg (Less than 5%) 3285
Lupron Depot–4 Month 30 mg (Less than 5%) 3289
Luvox Tablets (25, 50, 100 mg) (Infrequent) 3256
Meridia Capsules 481
Meruvax II 2130
Miacalcin Nasal Spray (1% to 3%) 2375
Mintezol 2137
M-M-R II 2118
Monopril Tablets (0.2% to 1.0%) 1091
Monopril HCT 1094
Monurol Sachet (Less than 1%) 1375
Mumpsvax 2141
Neoral Soft Gelatin Capsules (1% to less than 3%) 2380
Neoral Oral Solution (1% to less than 3%) 2380
Neurontin Capsules (Infrequent) 2655
Neurontin Oral Solution (Infrequent) 2655
Neurontin Tablets (Infrequent) 2655
Norvir Capsules (Less than 2%) 487
Norvir Oral Solution (Less than 2%) 487
Orthoclone OKT3 Sterile Solution (Less than 1%) 2498
OxyContin Tablets (Less than 1%) 2912
▲ Paser Granules (46% of 38 patients with drug-induced hepatitis) 1781
Paxil (Infrequent) 1609
Liquid PedvaxHIB 2148
Permax Tablets (Infrequent) 1299
Ponstel Capsules (Rare) 1356
Prometrium Capsules (100 mg, 200 mg) (Less than 5%) 3261
Protopic Ointment (1% to 3%) 1397
Quinaglute Dura-Tabs Tablets 978
Quinidex Extentabs 2933
▲ Rapamune Oral Solution and Tablets (3% to 20%) 3584
Recombivax HB (Less than 1%) 2178
Remeron Tablets (Rare) 2483
Remeron SolTab Tablets (Rare) 2486
Remicade for IV Injection 1178
Retrovir Capsules 1625
Retrovir IV Infusion 1629
Retrovir 1625
Rifamate Capsules 767
Rifater Tablets 769
Rilutek Tablets (Rare) 772
Risperdal (Rare) 1796
Salagen Tablets (Less than 1%) 2229
Seroquel Tablets (Infrequent) 684
▲ Serostim for Injection (14.1%) 3229
Serzone Tablets (Infrequent) 1104
Sonata Capsules (Infrequent) 3591
Tamiflu Capsules (1%) 3008
Tamiflu Oral Suspension (1%) 3008
Tapazole Tablets 1823
Tegretol/Tegretol-XR 2404
Tequin Injection (Less than 0.1%) 1110
Tequin Tablets (Less than 0.1%) 1110
Tetanus & Diphtheria Toxoids Adsorbed for Adult Use 1880
▲ Thalomid Capsules (5.6% to 12.5%) 1154
Tice BCG, BCG Live (Occasional) 2489
Tolectin (Less than 1%) 2589
Topamax Sprinkle Capsules (Infrequent) 2590
Topamax Tablets (Infrequent) 2590
Tricor Capsules, Micronized 513
Trileptal Oral Suspension (Up to 2%) 2407
Trileptal Tablets (Up to 2%) 2407
▲ Trisenox Injection (8%) 1158
Trizivir Tablets 1669
Twinrix Vaccine (Less than 1%) 1674
TYPHIM Vi Vaccine 825
Uniretic Tablets (Less than 1%) 3178
Vanceril Double Strength Inhalation Aerosol (Fewer than 2%) 3167
Varivax (Greater than or equal to 1%) 2202
Vistide Injection 1445
Wellbutrin Tablets (Rare) 1680
Wellbutrin SR Sustained-Release Tablets 1684
Xopenex Inhalation Solution 3207
Ziagen 1692
Zonegran Capsules (Infrequent) 1307
Zovirax Capsules 1706
Zovirax for Injection 1708
Zovirax 1706
Zyban Sustained-Release Tablets 1710
Zyflo Filmtab Tablets (Less common) 524
Zyprexa Tablets (Infrequent) 1973
Zyprexa ZYDIS Orally Disintegrating Tablets (Infrequent) 1973
Zyrtec (Less than 2%) 2756
Zyrtec-D 12 Hour Extended Relief Tablets (Less than 2%) 2758

Lymphadenopathy, cervical
Nexium Delayed-Release Capsules (Less than 1%) 619
Pulmicort Respules (1% to 3%) 632

Lymphadenopathy, post-cervical
Evoxac Capsules (Less than 1%) 1217

Lymphangitis, regional
Doxil Injection (Less than 1%) 566
Herceptin I.V. (At least one of the 958 patients) 1414

Lymphangitis, unspecified
Remicade for IV Injection (Less than 2%) 1178

Lymphedema
Actiq (1% or greater) 1184
Aromasin Tablets (Less frequent) 2769
Copaxone for Injection (Infrequent) 3306
Doxil Injection (Less than 1%) 566
Humatrope Vials and Cartridges 1930
Lupron Depot–3 Month 22.5 mg (Less than 5%) 3288
Paxil (Rare) 1609
Pima Syrup 1362
Prozac Pulvules, Liquid, and Weekly Capsules (Rare) 1238
Rabies Vaccine RabAvert (Uncommon) 1203
Requip Tablets (Infrequent) 1621
Sarafem Pulvules (Rare) 1962
Thalomid Capsules 1154
Xeloda Tablets (Less than 5%) 3039

Lymphedema, post-mastectomy
▲ Femara Tablets (7%) 2351

Lymphocele
▲ Rapamune Oral Solution and Tablets (3% to 20%) 3584
▲ Zenapax for Injection (Greater than 5%) 3046

Lymphocytes, decrease
(*see under* Lymphocytopenia)

Lymphocytes, increase
(*see under* Lymphocytosis)

Lymphocytopenia
▲ Betaseron for SC Injection (82%) 988
Ceclor CD Tablets (0.2%) 1279
Colazal Capsules 3069
Dipentum Capsules (Rare) 2803
Floxin I.V. (More than or equal to 1%) 2526
Floxin Tablets (More than or equal to 1%) 2529
Leukeran Tablets 1591
Levaquin (2.1% to 2.3%) 2537
Mavik Tablets (0.3% to 1.0%) 478
Mustargen for Injection 2142

Omnicef (0.8%) 493
Orthoclone OKT3 Sterile Solution (Less than 1%) 2498
Paxil (Rare) 1609
▲ Priftin Tablets (4.4%) 758
Requip Tablets (Infrequent) 1621
Rocephin Injectable Vials, ADD-Vantage, Galaxy, Bulk (Less than 1%) 2993
Stelazine Tablets 1640
Tarka Tablets 508
Topamax Sprinkle Capsules (Infrequent) 2590
Topamax Tablets (Infrequent) 2590
Trizivir Tablets 1669
Unasyn for Injection 2728
Vantin Tablets and Oral Suspension 2860
▲ Xanax Tablets (5.5% to 7.4%) 2865
▲ Xeloda Tablets (10% to 44%) 3039
Ziagen 1692

Lymphocytosis

Ceclor 1905
Celexa (Rare) 1365
Ceptaz for Injection (Very rare) 1499
Cipro I.V. (Infrequent) 893
▲ Cipro I.V. Pharmacy Bulk Package (Among most frequent) 897
Depacon Injection 416
Depakene 421
Depakote Sprinkle Capsules 426
Depakote Tablets 430
Depakote ER Tablets 436
Dynabac Tablets (0.1% to 1%) 2269
Effexor Tablets (Rare) 3495
Evoxac Capsules 1217
Floxin I.V. (More than or equal to 1%) 2526
Floxin Tablets (More than or equal to 1%) 2529
Fortaz (Very rare) 1541
Geodon Capsules (Rare) 2688
▲ Infergen (5% to 11%) 1777
Intron A for Injection (Less than 5%) 3120
Neurontin Capsules (Rare) 2655
Neurontin Oral Solution (Rare) 2655
Neurontin Tablets (Rare) 2655
Norvir Capsules (Less than 2%) 487
Norvir Oral Solution (Less than 2%) 487
Omnicef (0.2%) 493
Paxil (Rare) 1609
Permax Tablets (Rare) 1299
Primaxin I.M. 2158
Primaxin I.V. 2160
Prozac Pulvules, Liquid, and Weekly Capsules (Rare) 1238
Remeron Tablets (Rare) 2483
Remeron SolTab Tablets (Rare) 2486
Requip Tablets (Infrequent) 1621
Rocephin Injectable Vials, ADD-Vantage, Galaxy, Bulk (Less than 0.1%) 2993
Sarafem Pulvules (Rare) 1962
Sonata Capsules (Rare) 3591
Tazicef for Injection (Very rare) 1647
Tazicef Galaxy Container (Very rare) 1650
Tazicef Pharmacy Bulk Package (Very rare) 1653
Tazidime Vials, Faspak & ADD-Vantage (Very rare) 1966
Thalomid Capsules 1154
Topamax Sprinkle Capsules (Infrequent) 2590
Topamax Tablets (Infrequent) 2590
Unasyn for Injection 2728
Uniretic Tablets (Less than 1%) 3178
Vantin Tablets and Oral Suspension 2860

Lymphoma

Campath Ampules 992
CellCept Capsules (0.6% to 2.1%) 2951
CellCept Intravenous (0.6% to 2.1%) 2951
CellCept Oral Suspension (0.6% to 2.1%) 2951
CellCept Tablets (0.6% to 2.1%) 2951
Dilantin Infatabs 2624
Dilantin Kapseals 2622
Dilantin-125 Oral Suspension 2625
Felbatol 3343
▲ Gengraf Capsules (Less than 1% to 6%) 457
▲ Neoral Soft Gelatin Capsules (Less than 1% to 6%) 2380
▲ Neoral Oral Solution (Less than 1% to 6%) 2380
Orthoclone OKT3 Sterile Solution (Less than 1%) 2498
Prograf 1393
Rapamune Oral Solution and Tablets (0.4% to 1.4%) 3584
Remicade for IV Injection (Less than 2%) 1178
▲ Sandimmune (Less than 1% to 6%) 2388
Simulect for Injection (0.3%) 2399
Vioxx (Less than 0.1%) 2213
Vistide Injection 1445
Zenapax for Injection (Less than 1%) 3046

Lymphoma, lymphocytic

CellCept Capsules (0.6% to 1.0%) 2951
CellCept Intravenous (0.6% to 1.0%) 2951
CellCept Oral Suspension (0.6% to 1.0%) 2951
CellCept Tablets (0.6% to 1.0%) 2951
Dantrium Capsules (Less frequent) 2885
Dantrium Intravenous 2886

Lymphoma, non-Hodgkin's

Neurontin Capsules (Rare) 2655
Neurontin Oral Solution (Rare) 2655
Neurontin Tablets (Rare) 2655
Remicade for IV Injection 1178

Lymphoma-like disorder

Colazal Capsules 3069
Foscavir Injection (Between 1% and 5%) 605
Paser Granules 1781
Tegretol/Tegretol-XR 2404
Vitravene for Injection (2% to 5%) ⊙310

Lymphomonocytosis

Haldol Decanoate 2535
Haldol Injection, Tablets and Concentrate 2533

Lymphoproliferative disorder

Felbatol 3343
Orthoclone OKT3 Sterile Solution 2498
Rapamune Oral Solution and Tablets (0.4% to 1.4%) 3584
Remicade for IV Injection 1178
Simulect for Injection 2399

M

Maceration

Oxistat Cream (0.1%) 1298

Maceration, skin

DesOwen (Infrequent) 1401
Locoid Cream (Infrequent) 1341
Locoid Lipocream Cream (Infrequent) 1342
Locoid (Infrequent) 1341
Neurontin Capsules (Rare) 2655
Neurontin Oral Solution (Rare) 2655
Neurontin Tablets (Rare) 2655

Macrocytosis

Depacon Injection 416
Depakene 421
Depakote Sprinkle Capsules 426
Depakote Tablets (1% to 5%) 430
Depakote ER Tablets 436
Dilantin Kapseals 2622
Retrovir Capsules 1625
Retrovir IV Infusion 1629
Retrovir 1625

Maculae

Covera-HS Tablets (Less than 2%) 3199
Isoptin SR Tablets (1% or less) 467
Tarka Tablets 508
Verelan Capsules (1% or less) 3184
Verelan PM Capsules (2% or less) 3186

Macular degeneration

Cordarone Tablets 3487
Pacerone Tablets 3331

Macular hypopigmentation

Zyprexa Tablets (Rare) 1973
Zyprexa ZYDIS Orally Disintegrating Tablets (Rare) 1973

Maculopathy

Tolectin (Less than 1%) 2589

Malabsorption syndrome

Elspar for Injection 2092
Purinethol Tablets (Occasional) 1615
Sustiva Capsules 1258

Malaise

Abelcet Injection 1273
Accupril Tablets (0.5% to 1.0%) 2611
Accuretic Tablets (0.5% to 1%) 2614
Accutane Capsules 2944
Aceon Tablets (2 mg, 4 mg, 8 mg) (0.3% to 1%) 3249
Aciphex Tablets 1267
Aciphex Tablets 1783
Actiq (1% or greater) 1184
Aerobid/Aerobid-M (1% to 3%) 1363
Aggrenox Capsules (1.6%) 1026
▲ Agrylin Capsules (6.4%) 3232
▲ Alferon N Injection (9% to 65%) 1770
Altace Capsules (Less than 1%) 2233
Ambien Tablets (Infrequent) 3191
AmBisome for Injection (Less common) 1383
Amerge Tablets (2%) 1467
Amicar Injection 3608
Amicar Syrup 3608
Amicar Tablets 3608
Anaprox Tablets (Less than 1%) 2967
Anaprox DS Tablets (Less than 1%) 2967
Antabuse Tablets 3474
Apligraf (1.8%) 2305
Aquasol A Parenteral 593
Arava Tablets (1% to 3%) 724
Arimidex Tablets (2% to 5%) 659
Arthrotec Tablets (Rare) 3195
Asacol Delayed-Release Tablets (1% to 2%) 2884
Astelin Nasal Spray (Infrequent) 3339
Attenuvax 2044
Avelox Tablets (0.05% to 1%) 879
▲ Avonex (4%) 1013
Azactam for Injection (Less than 1%) 1276
Baycol Tablets (Rare) 883
▲ Betaseron for SC Injection (15%) 988
Biltricide Tablets 887
Buprenex Injectable (Infrequent) 2918
Calcium Disodium Versenate Injection 1980
▲ Campath Ampules (1% to 9%) 992
Captopril Tablets (0.5% to 2%) 2281
▲ Cardura Tablets (About 0.7% to 12%) 2668
Cataflam Tablets (Less than 1%) 2315
Catapres Tablets (About 1 in 100 patients) 1037
Catapres-TTS (0.5% or less) 1038
Ceclor CD Tablets (0.1% to 1%) 1279
Celestone Soluspan Injectable Suspension 3097
▲ CellCept Capsules (3%) 2951
▲ CellCept Intravenous (3%) 2951
▲ CellCept Oral Suspension (3%) 2951
▲ CellCept Tablets (3%) 2951
Cerebyx Injection (Infrequent) 2619
Cipro I.V. (1% or less) 893
Cipro I.V. Pharmacy Bulk Package (Less than 1%) 897
Cipro (Less than 1%) 887
Claritin (At least one patient to 2%) 3100
Claritin-D 12 Hour Extended Release Tablets (Less frequent) 3102
Claritin-D 24 Hour Extended Release Tablets (Fewer than 2%) 3104
Clinoril Tablets (Less than 1 in 100) 2053
Clorpres Tablets (About 1%) 1002
Clozaril Tablets (Less than 1%) 2319
Cognex Capsules (Frequent) 1351
Colazal Capsules 3069
Combipres Tablets (About 1%) 1040
▲ Combivir Tablets (27%) 1502
Copaxone for Injection (At least 2%) 3306
▲ Cordarone Tablets (4% to 9%) 3487
Coreg Tablets (1% to 2%) 1508
Cortone Acetate Injectable Suspension 2059
Cortone Acetate Tablets 2061
Cosmegen for Injection 2062
Coumadin for Injection (Infrequent) 1243
Coumadin Tablets (Infrequent) 1243
Crixivan Capsules (0.5%) 2070
Cylert Tablets 415
Cytovene (At least 3 subjects) 2959
▲ Dantrium Capsules (Among most frequent) 2885
▲ DaunoXome Injection (1% to 9%) 1442
Decadron Elixir 2078
Decadron Tablets 2079
Decadron Phosphate Injection 2081
Depacon Injection (1% to 5%) 416
Depakene (1% to 5%) 421
Depakote Sprinkle Capsules (1% to 5%) 426
Depakote Tablets (1% to 5%) 430
Depakote ER Tablets (Greater than 1%) 436
Diphtheria & Tetanus Toxoids Adsorbed Purogenated for Pediatric Use 1857
Dolobid Tablets (Less than 1 in 100) 2088
▲ Dostinex Tablets (1% to less than 10%) 2804
Doxil Injection (1% to 5%) 566
DTIC-Dome (Infrequent) 902
Duraclon Injection (1%) 3057
Dynabac Tablets (0.1% to 1%) 2269
EC-Naprosyn Delayed-Release Tablets (Less than 1%) 2967
Edecrin 2091
Effexor Tablets (Infrequent) 3495
Effexor XR Capsules (Infrequent) 3499
8-MOP Capsules 1727
Eldepryl Capsules 3266
Engerix-B Vaccine (Less than 1%) 1517
▲ Epivir (27%) 1520
▲ Epivir-HBV (24%) 1524
Ergamisol Tablets 1789
Etrafon 3115
Evoxac Capsules (Less than 1%) 1217
▲ Exelon Capsules (5%) 2342
▲ Exelon Oral Solution (5%) 2345
Felbatol (Frequent) 3343
Feldene Capsules (Occasional) 2685
Ferrlecit Injection (Greater than 1%) 3386
Flexeril Tablets (Less than 1%) 572
Flexeril Tablets (Less than 1%) 2094
▲ Flovent Diskus (1% to 16%) 3614
▲ Flovent (22% to 28%) 1535
Flovent Rotadisk 1537
Floxin I.V. (Less than 1%) 2526
Floxin Tablets (Less than 1%) 2529
▲ Fludara for Injection (6% to 8%) 995
FluShield Influenza Vaccine 3521
Fluzone Vaccine 802
Follistim for Injection 2465
Foradil Aerolizer 2354
Fortovase Capsules (Less than 2%) 2970
▲ Foscavir Injection (5% or greater) 605
Sterile FUDR 2974
Gabitril Tablets (Frequent) 1189
Gamimune N, 5% Solvent/Detergent Treated 925
Gamimune N, 10% Solvent/Detergent Treated 928
Gammar-P I.V. 787
Gastrocrom Oral Concentrate (1 report) 1162
Gemzar for Injection (Infrequent) 1919
Gengraf Capsules (1% to less than 3%) 457
Glucophage Tablets 1080
Glucophage XR Tablets 1080
Glucovance Tablets 1086
▲ Havrix Vaccine (1% to 10%) 1544
▲ Hectorol Capsules (27.9%) 1064
▲ Hectorol Injection (27.9%) 1066
Hivid Tablets (Less than 1%) 2975
Humegon for Injection 2468
Hycamtin for Injection (0.5% to 1.8%) 1546
Hydrocortone Tablets 2106
Hydrocortone Acetate Injectable Suspension 2103
Hydrocortone Phosphate Injection, Sterile 2105
Ifex for Injection (Less than 1%) 1123
Imdur Tablets (Less than or equal to 5%) 1826
Imitrex Injection (1.1%) 1549
Imitrex Tablets 1558
▲ Indapamide Tablets (Greater than or equal to 5%) 2286
Indocin (Greater than 1%) 2112
INFeD Injection 3388
▲ Infergen (2% to 11%) 1777
▲ Intron A for Injection (Up to 14%) 3120
Iopidine 0.5% Ophthalmic Solution (Less than 3%) ⊙213
Ismo Tablets (Fewer than 1%) 3524
Isoptin SR Tablets 467
Iveegam EN (0.3% to 0.8%) 849
▲ JE-VAX Vaccine (Approximately 10%) 811
Kadian Capsules (Less than 3%) 1335
Kaletra Capsules (Less than 2%) 471
Kaletra Oral Solution (Less than 2%) 471
Klonopin Tablets (Infrequent) 2983
Lamictal (2.3%) 1567
Lamisil Tablets 2360
Lescol Capsules (Rare) 2361
Lescol Capsules (Rare) 2925
▲ Lescol XL Tablets (3.8%) 2361
▲ Lescol XL Tablets (3.8%) 2925
▲ Leukine (57%) 1755
▲ Leustatin Injection (5% to 7%) 2495
Levaquin (0.1%) 2537
Lipitor Tablets (Less than 2%) 2639
Lipitor Tablets (Less than 2%) 2696
▲ Lodine (3% to 9%) 3528
▲ Lodine XL Extended-Release Tablets (3% to 9%) 3530
Lodosyn Tablets 1251
Luvox Tablets (25, 50, 100 mg) (Frequent) 3256
Macrobid Capsules (Less than 1%) 2889
Macrodantin Capsules (Common) 2891
Marinol Capsules (Less than 1%) 3325
Menomune-A/C/Y/W-135 Vaccine (2.5%) 813
Meruvax II 2130
Mevacor Tablets (Rare) 2132
Mexitil Capsules (Less than 1% or about 3 in 1,000) 1047
Micardis Tablets (More than 0.3%) 1049
Micardis HCT Tablets 1051
Minipress Capsules 2699
Mirapex Tablets (2% to 3%) 2834
Mithracin for Intravenous Use 903
M-M-R II 2118
Mobic Tablets (Less than 2%) 1054
Moduretic Tablets (Less than or equal to 1%) 2138
Motrin Suspension, Oral Drops, Chewable Tablets, and Caplets 2002
Myambutol Tablets 1290
▲ Mykrox Tablets (4.4%) 1168
Mylocel Tablets 2227
Myobloc Injectable Solution (2% or greater) 1291

▲ Nabi-HB (5%) 2295
Naprelan Tablets (Less than 1%) 1293
Naprosyn Suspension (Less than 1%) 2967
Naprosyn Tablets (Less than 1%) 2967
Nardil Tablets 2653
Naropin Injection (Less than 1%) 612
Neoral Soft Gelatin Capsules (1% to less than 3%) 2380
Neoral Oral Solution (1% to less than 3%) 2380
Neptazane Tablets ⊙271
Neurontin Capsules (Frequent) 2655
Neurontin Oral Solution (Frequent) 2655
Neurontin Tablets (Frequent) 2655
Nexium Delayed-Release Capsules (Less than 1%) 619
Nilandron Tablets (2%) 753
Norpramin Tablets 755
Norvasc Tablets (More than 0.1% to 1%) 2704
Norvir Capsules (0.7% to 1.7%) 487
Norvir Oral Solution (0.7% to 1.7%) 487
▲ Oncaspar (Greater than 5%) 756
Orthoclone OKT3 Sterile Solution (Less than 1%) 2498
Orudis Capsules (Greater than 1%) 3548
Oruvail Capsules (Greater than 1%) 3548
Ovidrel for Injection (Less than 2%) 3220
Oxsoralen-Ultra Capsules 1741
OxyContin Tablets (Less than 1%) 2912
▲ Pacerone Tablets (4% to 9%) 3331
Parafon Forte DSC Caplets (Occasional) 2582
Paraplatin for Injection 1126
Paxil (Frequent) 1609
▲ PEG-Intron Powder for Injection (7%) 3140
Pentasa Capsules (Less than 1%) 3239
Pergonal for Injection 3223
Permax Tablets (Infrequent) 1299
Persantine Tablets (Rare) 1057
Pletal Tablets (Less than 2%) 2605
Pletal Tablets (Less than 2%) 2848
Pneumovax 23 2156
Ponstel Capsules (Occasional) 1356
Pravachol Tablets (Rare) 1099
Prednisone 3064
Prevacid Delayed-Release Capsules (Less than 1%) 3292
PREVPAC (Less than 1%) 3298
Priftin Tablets 758
Prilosec Delayed-Release Capsules (Less than 1%) 628
Prinivil Tablets (0.3% to 1.0%) 2164
Prinzide Tablets 2168
Procanbid Extended-Release Tablets 2262
Procardia XL Extended Release Tablets (1% or less) 2710
▲ Proleukin for Injection (27%) 1199
▲ ProSom Tablets (5%) 500
Protonix I.V. (Less than 1%) 3580
Protonix Tablets (Less than 1%) 3577
Protopic Ointment (Greater than or equal to 1%) 1397
Proventil Inhalation Solution 0.083% (1.5%) 3146
Proventil Solution for Inhalation 0.5% (1.5%) 3144
Prozac Pulvules, Liquid, and Weekly Capsules (Infrequent) 1238
Pulmozyme Inhalation Solution 1426
Pyrazinamide Tablets 1876
▲ Rabies Vaccine RabAvert (15% to 20%) 1203
▲ Rapamune Oral Solution and Tablets (3% to 20%) 3584
Recombivax HB (Equal to or greater than 1%) 2178
Relafen Tablets (1%) 1617
Relenza Rotadisk (Less than 1.5%) 1619
Remeron Tablets (Frequent) 2483
Remeron SolTab Tablets (Frequent) 2486
Repronex for Intramuscular and Subcutaneous Injection 1347
▲ Requip Tablets (3%) 1621
Rescriptor Tablets (Less than 2%) 526
▲ Retrovir Capsules (8% to 53.2%) 1625
▲ Retrovir IV Infusion (8% to 53.2%) 1629
▲ Retrovir (8% to 53.2%) 1625
Rifadin 765
Rifamate Capsules 767
Rifater Tablets 769
Rilutek Tablets (0.4% to 1.2%) 772
Risperdal (Infrequent) 1796
Rituxan for Infusion (1% to 5%) 1750
Rituxan I.V. (1% to 5%) 1428
Roferon-A Injection (1%) 2996
Romazicon Injection (1% to 3%) 3000
▲ Rowasa Rectal Suspension Enema 4.0 grams/unit (60 mL) (3.44%) 3264
Sarafem Pulvules (Infrequent) 1962
Sectral Capsules 3589
Serevent Inhalation Aerosol (1% to 3%) 1633
Seroquel Tablets (Infrequent) 684
▲ Serostim for Injection (1% to 10%) 3229
Serzone Tablets (Infrequent) 1104
▲ Simulect for Injection (3% to 10%) 2399
Sinemet Tablets 1253
Sinemet CR Tablets 1255
Soriatane Capsules (Less than 1%) 3003
Sporanox Capsules (1% to 3%) 1800
Sular Tablets (Less than or equal to 1%) 688
Surmontil Capsules 3595
Sustiva Capsules (Less than 2%) 1258
Synvisc 3596
Tambocor Tablets (1% to 3%) 1990
Tarka Tablets (0.3% or more) 508
Tasmar Tablets (1%) 3010
Tenex Tablets (3% or less) 2942
Tetanus & Diphtheria Toxoids Adsorbed for Adult Use 1880
Tetanus and Diphtheria Toxoids Adsorbed For Adult Use (2%) 815
Tetanus Toxoid Adsorbed Purogenated 1882
Teveten Tablets (Less than 1%) 3327
▲ Thalomid Capsules (8.3%) 1154
▲ TheraCys Injection (40%) 823
▲ Thymoglobulin for Injection (13.4%) 3071
▲ Tice BCG, BCG Live (7.4%) 2489
▲ TOBI Solution for Inhalation (6.2%) 1206
Tonocard Tablets (Less than 1%) 649
Topamax Sprinkle Capsules (Frequent) 2590
Topamax Tablets (Frequent) 2590
Trental Tablets (Less than 1%) 784
Tricor Capsules, Micronized 513
Trileptal Oral Suspension 2407
Trileptal Tablets 2407
▲ Trizivir Tablets (44%) 1669
Trovan (Less than 1%) 2722
▲ TYPHIM Vi Vaccine (4.1% to 37%) 825
Ultram Tablets (1% to 5%) 2600
Unasyn for Injection (Less than 1%) 2728
Univasc Tablets (Less than 1%) 3181
Urecholine 2198
Urecholine Tablets 2445
▲ Valstar Sterile Solution for Intravesical Instillation (4%) 1175
Vantin Tablets and Oral Suspension (Less than 1%) 2860
Varivax (Greater than or equal to 1%) 2202
Venofer Injection (Greater than 1%) 580
Verelan Capsules 3184
Verelan PM Capsules 3186
▲ Vesanoid Capsules (66%) 3037
Viadur Implant (Less than 2%) 912
Viracept 532
Viramune Oral Suspension 1060
Viramune Tablets 1060
Vistide Injection 1445
Voltaren Tablets (Less than 1%) 2315
Voltaren-XR Tablets (Less than 1%) 2315
Warfarin Sodium Tablets, USP 3302
Wellbutrin SR Sustained-Release Tablets (Rare) 1684
Zanaflex Tablets (Infrequent) 1305
Zantac (Rare) 1690
Zantac Injection (Rare) 1688
Zantac Syrup (Rare) 1690
Zebeta Tablets 1885
Zestoretic Tablets 695
Zestril Tablets (0.3% to 1.0%) 698
Ziac Tablets 1887
▲ Ziagen (44%) 1692
▲ Zinecard for Injection (48% to 61%) 2869
Zithromax Capsules, 250 mg (1% or less) 2743
Zithromax for Oral Suspension, 300 mg, 600 mg, 900 mg, 1200 mg (1% or less) 2739
Zithromax Tablets, 250 mg (1% or less) 2739
Zocor Tablets (Rare) 2219
▲ Zofran Injection (5%) 1698
▲ Zofran (9% to 13%) 1703
▲ Zofran ODT Orally Disintegrating Tablets (9% to 13%) 1703
Zoladex (1% to 5%) 702
Zoladex 3-month 706
Zoloft (Frequent to 2%) 2751
Zomig Tablets (Infrequent) 708
Zomig-ZMT Tablets (Infrequent) 708
Zonegran Capsules (Infrequent) 1307
Zosyn (1.0% or less) 1890
Zosyn in Galaxy Containers (1.0% or less) 1894
▲ Zovirax (11.5%) 1706
Zyban Sustained-Release Tablets (Rare) 1710
Zyflo Filmtab Tablets (Less common) 524
Zyprexa Tablets (Infrequent) 1973
Zyprexa ZYDIS Orally Disintegrating Tablets (Infrequent) 1973
Zyrtec (Less than 2%) 2756
Zyrtec-D 12 Hour Extended Relief Tablets (Less than 2%) 2758

Malaria relapse
Aramine Injection 2043

Male pattern baldness
(*see under* Alopecia hereditaria)

Malignancies, secondary
Leukeran Tablets 1591

Malignancies, various types
Enbrel for Injection 1752
Enbrel for Injection 3504

Malignant hyperthermia
Anectine Injection 1476
Fluothane Inhalation 3508
Proleukin for Injection (Less than 1%) 1199
Robinul Injectable 2940
Sandostatin LAR Depot (Rare) 2395

Malignant hyperthermia, familial
Sensorcaine 643
Sensorcaine-MPF Injection 643

Malignant melanoma
Sinemet Tablets 1253
Sinemet CR Tablets 1255

Malignant neoplasms
CellCept Capsules (0.8% to 1.4%) 2951
CellCept Intravenous (0.8% to 1.4%) 2951
CellCept Oral Suspension (0.8% to 1.4%) 2951
CellCept Tablets (0.8% to 1.4%) 2951
Orthoclone OKT3 Sterile Solution (Less than 1%) 2498

Malodor, unspecified
Condylox Topical Solution (Less than 5%) 2437

Manic behavior
Ambien Tablets (Rare) 3191
Betaseron for SC Injection 988
Celexa 1365
Cipro I.V. (1% or less) 893
Cipro I.V. Pharmacy Bulk Package (Less than 1%) 897
Cipro (Less than 1%) 887
Copaxone for Injection (Infrequent) 3306
Effexor Tablets (0.5%) 3495
Effexor XR Capsules (0.5%) 3499
Evoxac Capsules (Less than 1%) 1217
Felbatol 3343
Floxin I.V. 2526
Floxin Tablets 2529
Halcion Tablets 2823
Herceptin I.V. (At least one of the 958 patients) 1414
Hivid Tablets (Less than 1%) 2975
Intron A for Injection (Less than 5%) 3120
Lamictal (Rare) 1567
Levaquin (Less than 0.3%) 2537
Levsin/Levsinex/Levbid 3172
Luvox Tablets (25, 50, 100 mg) (Approximately 1%) 3256
Nardil Tablets (Less frequent) 2653
Neurontin Capsules (Rare) 2655
Neurontin Oral Solution (Rare) 2655
Neurontin Tablets (Rare) 2655
Orthoclone OKT3 Sterile Solution (Less than 1%) 2498
Parnate Tablets 1607
Paxil (Infrequent) 1609
Permax Tablets (Infrequent) 1299
Protopam Chloride for Injection (Several cases) 3582
Prozac Pulvules, Liquid, and Weekly Capsules (0.1% to 0.8%) 1238
Remeron Tablets (Approximately 0.2%) 2483
Remeron SolTab Tablets (Approximately 0.2%) 2486
Requip Tablets (Infrequent) 1621
Rescriptor Tablets (Less than 2%) 526
Rilutek Tablets (Infrequent) 772
Risperdal 1796
Roferon-A Injection 2996
Rythmol Tablets – 150 mg, 225 mg, 300 mg (Less than 1%) 502
Seroquel Tablets (Infrequent) 684
Serzone Tablets (0.3% to 1.6%) 1104
Sustiva Capsules 1258
Symmetrel 1328
Tasmar Tablets (Infrequent) 3010
Tenex Tablets 2942
Topamax Sprinkle Capsules (Rare) 2590
Topamax Tablets (Rare) 2590
Trileptal Oral Suspension 2407
Trileptal Tablets 2407
Valtrex Caplets 1676
Wellbutrin Tablets (Frequent) 1680
Wellbutrin SR Sustained-Release Tablets 1684
Xanax Tablets 2865
Zoloft (0.4% to 2%) 2751
Zyban Sustained-Release Tablets 1710

Marrow aplasia
Aloprim for Injection (Less than 1%) 2292

Masculinization, female fetus
Oxandrin Tablets 1153

Mass, abdominal
(*see under* Abdominal mass)

Mastalgia
(*see under* Mastodynia)

Mastitis
Amerge Tablets (Rare) 1467
Aricept Tablets (Infrequent) 1270
Aricept Tablets (Infrequent) 2665
Doxil Injection (Less than 1%) 566
Effexor Tablets (Rare) 3495
Effexor XR Capsules (Rare) 3499
Humegon for Injection (Occasional) 2468
Intron A for Injection (Less than or equal to 5%) 3120
Paxil (Rare) 1609
Requip Tablets (Rare) 1621
Risperdal (Infrequent) 1796
Salagen Tablets (Less than 1%) 2229
Vistide Injection 1445
Zoloft (Rare) 2751
Zonegran Capsules (Rare) 1307

Mastodynia
Climara Transdermal System 958
Estrace Vaginal Cream 3358
Estrace Tablets 3361
Estratest 3252
Estring Vaginal Ring (Uncommon) 2811
Haldol Decanoate 2535
Menest Tablets 2254
Norplant System 3543
Ogen Tablets 2846
Ortho-Est Tablets 3464
Premarin Intravenous 3563
Premarin Tablets 3566
Premarin Vaginal Cream 3570
Premphase Tablets 3572
Prempro Tablets 3572

Mazzotti reactions, worsening of
Stromectol Tablets 2185

Medullary hypoplasia
Novantrone for Injection 1760

Megacolon, acquired
Felbatol 3343

Megacolon, toxic
Monurol Sachet 1375
Motofen Tablets 577
Numorphan 1324

Megaloblastic anemia
(*see under* Anemia, megaloblastic)

Megaloblastosis
Maxzide 1008

Melancholia
Celexa (Rare) 1365

Melanoma, skin
Clomid Tablets 735
Cognex Capsules (Rare) 1351
8-MOP Capsules 1727
Paxil 1609
Remicade for IV Injection (Less than 2%) 1178
Sinemet Tablets 1253
Sinemet CR Tablets 1255

Melanosis
Celexa (Rare) 1365
Copaxone for Injection (Infrequent) 3306
Intron A for Injection (Less than 5%) 3120
Lupron Depot–4 Month 30 mg (Less than 5%) 3289
Neurontin Capsules (Rare) 2655
Neurontin Oral Solution (Rare) 2655
Neurontin Tablets (Rare) 2655
Sonata Capsules (Rare) 3591

Melasma
(*see under* Chloasma)

Melasma, possibly persistent
Cyclessa Tablets 2450

Lunelle Monthly Injection 2827
Microgestin Fe 1.5/30 Tablets 3407
Microgestin Fe 1/20 Tablets 3400
Yasmin 28 Tablets 980

Melena (5%)

Abelcet Injection 1273
Aciphex Tablets 1267
Aciphex Tablets 1783
Aggrenox Capsules (1.9%) 1026
Agrylin Capsules (1% to 5%) 3232
Amphotec (1% to 5%) 1774
Anaprox Tablets (Less than 1%) 2967
Anaprox DS Tablets (Less than 1%) 2967
Arava Tablets (1% to 3%) 724
Aricept Tablets (Infrequent) 1270
Aricept Tablets (Infrequent) 2665
Arthrotec Tablets (Rare) 3195
Betaseron for SC Injection 988
Campath Ampules 992
▲ Carnitor Injection (2% to 6%) 3242
▲ Casodex Tablets (2% to 5%) 662
Cataflam Tablets (Less than 1%) 2315
Cedax 1021
Celebrex Capsules (0.1% to 1.9%) 2676
Celebrex Capsules (0.1% to 1.9%) 2780
▲ CellCept Capsules (3% to 10%) 2951
▲ CellCept Intravenous (3% to 10%) 2951
▲ CellCept Oral Suspension (3% to 10%) 2951
▲ CellCept Tablets (3% to 10%) 2951
Colazal Capsules 3069
Copaxone for Injection (Infrequent) 3306
Coreg Tablets (1% to 2%) 1508
DaunoXome Injection (Less than or equal to 5%) 1442
Diamox Intravenous (Occasional) .... ⊙ 269
Diamox Sequels Sustained Release Capsules .... ⊙ 270
Diamox Tablets (Occasional) .... ⊙ 269
Doxil Injection (Less than 1%) 566
EC-Naprosyn Delayed-Release Tablets (Less than 1%) 2967
Effexor Tablets (Infrequent) 3495
Effexor XR Capsules (Infrequent) 3499
Enalaprilat Injection 863
Evoxac Capsules (Less than 1%) 1217
Exelon Capsules (Infrequent) 2342
Exelon Oral Solution (Infrequent) 2345
Feldene Capsules (Occasional) 2685
Ferrlecit Injection (Greater than 1%) 3386
Fortovase Capsules (Less than 2%) 2970
Fosamax Tablets (1.3%) 2095
Foscavir Injection (Between 1% and 5%) 605
Gabitril Tablets (Infrequent) 1189
Geodon Capsules (Rare) 2688
Hivid Tablets (Less than 1%) 2975
Imdur Tablets (Less than or equal to 5%) 1826
Imitrex Injection 1549
Imitrex Nasal Spray (Rare) 1554
Imitrex Tablets (Rare) 1558
Innohep Injection 1248
Intron A for Injection (Less than 5%) 3120
Invirase Capsules (Less than 2%) 2979
Lamictal (Rare) 1567
[illegible] Tablets 608
Lipitor Tablets (Less than 2%) 2639
Lipitor Tablets (Less than 2%) 2696
Lodine (1% to 3%) 3528
Lodine XL Extended-Release Tablets (1% to 3%) 3530
Lotensin Tablets (Less than 1%) 2365
Lotensin HCT Tablets 2367
Luvox Tablets (25, 50, 100 mg) (Infrequent) 3256
Matulane Capsules 3246
Merrem I.V. (0.7%) 673
Mobic Tablets (Less than 2%) 1054
Motrin Suspension, Oral Drops, Chewable Tablets, and Caplets (Less than 1%) 2002
Naprelan Tablets (Less than 1%) 1293
Naprosyn Suspension (Less than 1%) 2967
Naprosyn Tablets (Less than 1%) 2967
Neptazane Tablets .... ⊙ 271
Nexium Delayed-Release Capsules (Less than 1%) 619
Nilandron Tablets (2%) 753
Omnicef 493
Orudis Capsules (Less than 1%) 3548
Oruvail Capsules (Less than 1%) 3548
▲ Pancrease Capsules (Among most frequent) 2580
Paxil (Rare) 1609
Pediazole Suspension 3050
Permax Tablets (Infrequent) 1299
▲ Photofrin for Injection (5%) 831
Pletal Tablets (Less than 2%) 2605
Pletal Tablets (Less than 2%) 2848
Ponstel Capsules (Occasional) 1356
Prevacid Delayed-Release Capsules (Less than 1%) 3292
PREVPAC (Less than 1%) 3298
Procardia XL Extended Release Tablets (1% or less) 2710
ProSom Tablets (Rare) 500
Protonix I.V. (Less than 1%) 3580
Protonix Tablets (Less than 1%) 3577
Prozac Pulvules, Liquid, and Weekly Capsules (Infrequent) 1238
Relafen Tablets (Less than 1%) 1617
Reminyl Oral Solution (Infrequent) 1792
Reminyl Tablets (Infrequent) 1792
Requip Tablets (Infrequent) 1621
Rilutek Tablets (Rare) 772
Risperdal (Infrequent) 1796
Salagen Tablets (Less than 1%) 2229
Sandostatin LAR Depot (1% to 4%) 2395
Sarafem Pulvules (Infrequent) 1962
Seroquel Tablets (Rare) 684
▲ Simulect for Injection (3% to 10%) 2399
Sonata Capsules (Infrequent) 3591
Soriatane Capsules (Less than 1%) 3003
Sular Tablets (Less than or equal to 1%) 688
Topamax Sprinkle Capsules (Infrequent) 2590
Topamax Tablets (Infrequent) 2590
Toradol 3018
Trovan (Less than 1%) 2722
Ultracet Tablets (Less than 1%) 2597
Uniretic Tablets (Less than 1%) 3178
Vaseretic Tablets 2204
Vasotec I.V. Injection 2207
Vasotec Tablets (0.5% to 1.0%) 2210
Vicoprofen Tablets (Less than 3%) 520
Vistide Injection 1445
Voltaren Tablets (Less than 1%) 2315
Voltaren-XR Tablets (Less than 1%) 2315
Zanaflex Tablets (Infrequent) 1305
Zithromax (1% or less) 2743
Zithromax for Oral Suspension, 300 mg, 600 mg, 900 mg, 1200 mg (1% or less) 2739
Zithromax Tablets, 250 mg (1% or less) 2739
Zithromax Tablets, 600 mg (1% or less) 2743
Zoloft (Rare) 2751
Zomig Tablets (Rare) 708
Zomig-ZMT Tablets (Rare) 708
Zonegran Capsules (Infrequent) 1307
Zosyn (1.0% or less) 1890
Zosyn in Galaxy Containers (1.0% or less) 1894
Zyprexa Tablets (Infrequent) 1973
Zyprexa ZYDIS Orally Disintegrating Tablets (Infrequent) 1973
Zyrtec (Less than 2%) 2756
Zyrtec-D 12 Hour Extended Relief Tablets (Less than 2%) 2758

Memory impairment

Cataflam Tablets (Less than 1%) 2315
Cogentin 2055
Copaxone for Injection (Infrequent) 3306
Cozaar Tablets (Less than 1%) 2067
Eldepryl Capsules 3266
Eskalith 1527
Halcion Tablets (0.5% to 0.9%) 2823
Hyzaar 2109
Imitrex Nasal Spray (Rare) 1554
Imitrex Tablets (Rare) 1558
▲ Klonopin Tablets (4%) 2983
Lamictal (2.4%) 1567
Lithobid Slow-Release Tablets 3255
Lodosyn Tablets 1251
▲ Lupron Depot 3.75 mg (Among most frequent) 3281
Lupron Depot–3 Month 11.25 mg (Less than 5%) 3285
Lupron Injection (Less than 5%) 3279
Maxalt Tablets (Infrequent) 2120
Maxalt-MLT Orally Disintegrating Tablets (Infrequent) 2120
Monopril Tablets (0.2% to 1.0%) 1091
Monopril HCT 1094
Prinivil Tablets (0.3% to 1.0%) 2164
Prinzide Tablets 2168
Rifamate Capsules (Uncommon) 767
Rifater Tablets (Uncommon) 769
Roferon-A Injection (Less than 4%) 2996
▲ Serzone Tablets (4%) 1104
Sinemet CR Tablets 1255
Timolide Tablets 2187
Tonocard Tablets (Less than 1%) 649
▲ Topamax Sprinkle Capsules (12.4% to 12.6%) 2590
▲ Topamax Tablets (12.4% to 12.6%) 2590
Transderm Scōp Transdermal Therapeutic System (Infrequent) 2302
▲ Vesanoid Capsules (3%) 3037
Voltaren Tablets (Less than 1%) 2315
Voltaren-XR Tablets (Less than 1%) 2315
Wellbutrin Tablets (Infrequent) 1680
Wellbutrin SR Sustained-Release Tablets (Up to 3%) 1684
▲ Xanax Tablets (33.1%) 2865
Zestoretic Tablets 695
Ziac Tablets 1887
▲ Zonegran Capsules (6%) 1307
Zyban Sustained-Release Tablets (Infrequent) 1710

Memory loss, short-term

Baycol Tablets 883
Blocadren Tablets 2046
Clozaril Tablets (Less than 1%) 2319
Corgard Tablets 2245
Corzide 40/5 Tablets 2247
Corzide 80/5 Tablets 2247
Cosopt Sterile Ophthalmic Solution 2065
Crinone (Less than 5%) 3213
Cytovene 2959
Ergamisol Tablets (10 out of 463 patients) 1789
Hivid Tablets (Less than 1%) 2975
Inderal 3513
Inderal LA Long-Acting Capsules 3516
Inderide Tablets 3517
Inderide LA Long-Acting Capsules 3519
Lescol Capsules 2361
Lescol Capsules 2925
Lescol XL Tablets 2361
Lescol XL Tablets 2925
Levsin/Levsinex/Levbid 3172
Meridia Capsules 481
Mevacor Tablets (0.5% to 1.0%) 2132
Mexitil Capsules (Less than 1% to about 9 in 1,000) 1047
Nadolol Tablets 2288
Normodyne Tablets 3137
Parnate Tablets 1607
Pravachol Tablets 1099
Rythmol Tablets – 150 mg, 225 mg, 300 mg (Less than 1%) 502
Sectral Capsules 3589
Tenoretic Tablets 690
Tenormin 692
Testoderm Transdermal Systems (1%) 574
Timolol GFS .... ⊙ 266
Timoptic in Ocudose 2192
Timoptic Sterile Ophthalmic Solution 2190
Timoptic-XE Sterile Ophthalmic Gel Forming Solution 2194
Toprol-XL Tablets 651
Zocor Tablets 2219

Meniere's syndrome

Imitrex Nasal Spray (Rare) 1554
Imitrex Tablets 1558

Meningism

Accuretic Tablets 2614
Albenza Tablets (Up to 1.0%) 1463
Neurontin Capsules (Rare) 2655
Neurontin Oral Solution (Rare) 2655
Neurontin Tablets (Rare) 2655
Nipent for Injection (Less than 3%) 3272
Sensorcaine 643
Sensorcaine-MPF Injection 643
▲ Serostim for Injection (1% to 10%) 3229

Meningismus

Naropin Injection 612

Meningitis

Arthrotec Tablets (Rare) 3195
Azulfidine EN-tabs Tablets (Rare) 2775
Betaseron for SC Injection 988
Campath Ampules 992
CellCept Capsules (Occasional) 2951
CellCept Intravenous (Occasional) 2951
CellCept Oral Suspension (Occasional) 2951
CellCept Tablets (Occasional) 2951
Cerebyx Injection (Infrequent) 2619
DaunoXome Injection (Less than or equal to 5%) 1442
Duraclon Injection 3057
Feldene Capsules (Rare) 2685
Foscavir Injection (Between 1% and 5%) 605
▲ Gliadel Wafer (4%) 1723
Lodine XL Extended-Release Tablets 3530
LYMErix Vaccine (Greater than 1%) 1592
Orthoclone OKT3 Sterile Solution (Less than 1%) 2498
Paxil (Rare) 1609
Permax Tablets (Infrequent) 1299
Proleukin for Injection (Less than 1%) 1199
Rabies Vaccine RabAvert (Ten cases) 1203
Tasmar Tablets (Rare) 3010

Meningitis, aseptic

Anaprox Tablets (Less than 1%) 2967
Anaprox DS Tablets (Less than 1%) 2967
Arthrotec Tablets (Rare) 3195
Bactrim 2949
Carbatrol Capsules (One case) 3234
Cataflam Tablets (Rare) 2315
EC-Naprosyn Delayed-Release Tablets (Less than 1%) 2967
Motrin Suspension, Oral Drops, Chewable Tablets, and Caplets (Rare; less than 1%) 2002
Mumpsvax 2141
▲ Naprelan Tablets (3% to 9%) 1293
Naprosyn Suspension (Less than 1%) 2967
Naprosyn Tablets (Less than 1%) 2967
Orudis Capsules (Less than 1%) 3548
Oruvail Capsules (Less than 1%) 3548
Sandoglobulin I.V. 2391
Septra Suspension 2265
Septra Tablets 2265
Septra DS Tablets 2265
Tegretol/Tegretol-XR (One case) 2404
Toradol 3018
Vicoprofen Tablets (Rare) 520
Vioxx (Less than 0.1%) 2213
Voltaren Tablets (Rare) 2315
Voltaren-XR Tablets (Rare) 2315

Meningitis, cryptococcal

Taxol Injection (2% to 3%) 1129

Meningitis, septic

Naropin Injection 612
Sensorcaine 643
Sensorcaine-MPF Injection 643

Menometrorrhagia

Orudis Capsules (Less than 1%) 3548
Oruvail Capsules (Less than 1%) 3548

Menopausal symptoms, unspecified

Vioxx (Greater than 0.1% to 1.9%) 2213

Menopause

Avonex 1013
Effexor Tablets (Rare) 3495
Effexor XR Capsules (Rare) 3499
Luvox Tablets (25, 50, 100 mg) (Infrequent) 3256
Permax Tablets (Infrequent) 1299
Sonata Capsules (Rare) 3591
Ultram Tablets (1% to 5%) 2600
Wellbutrin Tablets (Rare) 1680
Wellbutrin SR Sustained-Release Tablets 1684
Zyban Sustained-Release Tablets 1710

Menorrhagia

Aciphex Tablets (Rare) 1267
Aciphex Tablets (Rare) 1783
Arthrotec Tablets (Rare) 3195
Asacol Delayed-Release Tablets 2884
▲ Betaseron for SC Injection (6%) 988
Claritin (At least one patient) 3100
Claritin-D 12 Hour Extended Release Tablets 3102
Claritin-D 24 Hour Extended Release Tablets 3104
Clomid Tablets (1.3%) 735
CombiPatch Transdermal System (2% to 5%) 2323
Dipentum Capsules (Rare) 2803
Effexor Tablets (Infrequent) 3495
Effexor XR Capsules (Infrequent) 3499
Evoxac Capsules (Less than 1%) 1217
Floxin I.V. (Less than 1%) 2526
Floxin Tablets (Less than 1%) 2529
Gabitril Tablets (Infrequent) 1189
Geodon Capsules (Infrequent) 2688
Intron A for Injection (Less than 5%) 3120
Lamictal (Rare) 1567
Lunelle Monthly Injection 2827
Luvox Tablets (25, 50, 100 mg) (Infrequent) 3256
Motrin Suspension, Oral Drops, Chewable Tablets, and Caplets (Less than 1%) 2002
Naprelan Tablets (Less than 1%) 1293
Neurontin Capsules (Infrequent) 2655
Neurontin Oral Solution (Infrequent) 2655
Neurontin Tablets (Infrequent) 2655
▲ Novantrone for Injection (7%) 1760
Paxil (Infrequent) 1609
Pentasa Capsules (Less than 1%) 3239
Permax Tablets (Infrequent) 1299
Plavix Tablets (Less than 1%) 1097
Plavix Tablets (Less than 1%) 3084
Prozac Pulvules, Liquid, and Weekly Capsules (Infrequent) 1238
▲ Rapamune Oral Solution and Tablets (3% to 20%) 3584
Remeron Tablets (Rare) 2483
Remeron SolTab Tablets (Rare) 2486
Risperdal (Frequent) 1796
Salagen Tablets (Less than 1%) 2229
Seroquel Tablets (Infrequent) 684
Serzone Tablets (Infrequent) 1104
Sonata Capsules (Infrequent) 3591
Topamax Sprinkle Capsules (Frequent) 2590
Topamax Tablets (Frequent) 2590
Trileptal Oral Suspension 2407
Trileptal Tablets 2407

Vistide Injection 1445
Zanaflex Tablets (Infrequent) 1305
▲ Zoladex (4%) 702
Zoloft (Rare) 2751
Zonegran Capsules (Rare) 1307
Zyprexa Tablets (Infrequent) 1973
Zyprexa ZYDIS Orally Disintegrating Tablets (Infrequent) 1973
Zyrtec (Less than 2%) 2756
Zyrtec-D 12 Hour Extended Relief Tablets (Less than 2%) 2758

Menstrual disorders
Aceon Tablets (2 mg, 4 mg, 8 mg) (1.1%) 3249
▲ Aerobid/Aerobid-M (3% to 9%) 1363
Ambien Tablets (Infrequent) 3191
Anaprox Tablets (Less than 1%) 2967
Anaprox DS Tablets (Less than 1%) 2967
Arava Tablets (1% to 3%) 724
▲ Betaseron for SC Injection (17%) 988
Ceclor CD Tablets (0.1% to 1%) 1279
Celebrex Capsules (0.1% to 1.9%) 2676
Celebrex Capsules (0.1% to 1.9%) 2780
Cleocin Vaginal Ovules (Less than 1%) 2789
Colazal Capsules 3069
▲ CombiPatch Transdermal System (17% to 19%) 2323
Cortifoam Rectal Foam 3170
Cytotec Tablets (0.3%) 3202
Depakote ER Tablets (Greater than 1%) 436
EC-Naprosyn Delayed-Release Tablets (Less than 1%) 2967
Effexor Tablets (1%) 3495
Etrafon 3115
Evoxac Capsules (Less than 1%) 1217
Felbatol 3343
Gengraf Capsules (1%) 457
Gonal-F for Injection (2.5%) 3216
Lamictal (More than 1%) 1567
Lupron Depot 3.75 mg (Less than 5%) 3281
Lupron Depot–3 Month 11.25 mg (Less than 5%) 3285
Maxalt Tablets (Infrequent) 2120
Maxalt-MLT Orally Disintegrating Tablets (Infrequent) 2120
Meridia Capsules (Greater than or equal to 1%) 481
Monurol Sachet (Less than 1%) 1375
Mustargen for Injection 2142
▲ Naprelan Tablets (3% to 9%) 1293
Naprosyn Suspension (Less than 1%) 2967
Naprosyn Tablets (Less than 1%) 2967
Neoral Soft Gelatin Capsules (1%) 2380
Neoral Oral Solution (1%) 2380
Nexium Delayed-Release Capsules (Less than 1%) 619
▲ Nicotrol Nasal Spray (4%) 2843
▲ Nolvadex Tablets (5.7%) 678
▲ Novantrone for Injection (51% to 61%) 1760
ParaGard T 380A Intrauterine Copper Contraceptive 2582
▲ Periostat Tablets (4%) 1208
Provigil Tablets (At least 1%) 1193
Rifadin 765
Rifater Tablets 769
Sonata Capsules (Rare) 3591
Sporanox Capsules (Infrequent) 1800
Sporanox Injection (Rare) 1804
Sporanox Oral Solution 1808
Sporanox Oral Solution 2512
▲ Topamax Sprinkle Capsules (4.2%) 2590
▲ Topamax Tablets (4.2%) 2590
Trilafon 3160
Ultram Tablets (Less than 1%) 2600
Vaqta (1.1%) 2199
Vioxx (Greater than 0.1% to 1.9%) 2213
▲ Wellbutrin Tablets (4.7%) 1680
▲ Xanax Tablets (10.4%) 2865
Yasmin 28 Tablets (Greater than 1%) 980
Zoladex 702
Zoloft (Infrequent) 2751

Menstrual dysfunction
Luvox Tablets (25, 50, 100 mg) (Infrequent) 3256

Menstrual flow, changes
Alesse-21 Tablets 3468
Alesse-28 Tablets 3473
Aygestin Tablets 1333
Coumadin for Injection 1243
Coumadin Tablets 1243
Desogen Tablets 2458
Estinyl Tablets 3112
Estratest 3252
Estrostep 2627
Levlen 962
Levlite 21 Tablets 962
Levlite 28 Tablets 962
Levora Tablets 3389
Loestrin 21 Tablets 2642
Loestrin Fe Tablets 2642
Lo/Ovral Tablets 3532
Lo/Ovral-28 Tablets 3538
Low-Ogestrel-28 Tablets 3392
Menest Tablets 2254
Microgestin Fe 1.5/30 Tablets 3407
Microgestin Fe 1/20 Tablets 3400
Mircette Tablets 2470
Moban 1320
Modicon 2563
Necon 3415
Nordette-28 Tablets 2257
Ogestrel 0.5/50-28 Tablets 3428
Ortho Dienestrol Cream 2554
Ortho-Cept 21 Tablets 2546
Ortho-Cept 28 Tablets 2546
Ortho-Cyclen/Ortho Tri-Cyclen 2573
Ortho-Est Tablets 3464
Ortho-Novum 2563
Ortho-Novum 1/50□28 Tablets 2556
Ortho-Cyclen/Ortho Tri-Cyclen 2573
Ovcon 3364
Ovral Tablets 3551
Ovral-28 Tablets 3552
Ovrette Tablets 3552
ParaGard T 380A Intrauterine Copper Contraceptive 2582
Premarin Intravenous 3563
Premarin Vaginal Cream 3570
Provera Tablets 2853
Tarka Tablets 508
Tri-Levlen 962
Triphasil-21 Tablets 3600
Triphasil-28 Tablets 3605
Trivora Tablets 3439
Vivelle Transdermal System 2412
Vivelle-Dot Transdermal System 2416
Warfarin Sodium Tablets, USP 3302
Zovia 3449

Menstrual irregularities
Accutane Capsules 2944
Anadrol-50 Tablets 3321
▲ Android Capsules, 10 mg (Among most common) 1731
Arthrotec Tablets (Rare) 3195
Brevicon 28-Day Tablets 3380
Celestone Soluspan Injectable Suspension 3097
Celestone Syrup 3099
Claritin-D 12 Hour Extended Release Tablets (Less frequent) 3102
Compazine 1505
Cortone Acetate Injectable Suspension 2059
Cortone Acetate Tablets 2061
Covera-HS Tablets (Less than 2%) 3199
Decadron Elixir 2078
Decadron Tablets 2079
Decadron Phosphate Injection 2081
▲ Delatestryl Injection (Among most frequent) 1151
Depacon Injection 416
Depakene 421
Depakote Sprinkle Capsules 426
Depakote Tablets 430
Depakote ER Tablets 436
Depo-Medrol Injectable Suspension 2795
▲ Depo-Provera Contraceptive Injection (More than 5%) 2798
▲ Estratest (Among most common) 3252
Florinef Acetate Tablets 2250
Flovent Rotadisk (1% to 3%) 1537
Fortovase Capsules (Less than 2%) 2970
Halcion Tablets 2823
Haldol Decanoate 2535
Haldol Injection, Tablets and Concentrate 2533
Hydrocortone Tablets 2106
Hydrocortone Acetate Injectable Suspension 2103
Hydrocortone Phosphate Injection, Sterile 2105
Imitrex Nasal Spray 1554
▲ Infergen (2% to 6%) 1777
Intron A for Injection (Less than 5%) 3120
Isoptin SR Tablets (1% or less) 467
Klonopin Tablets (Infrequent) 2983
Levoxyl Tablets 1819
Librium Capsules (Isolated cases) 1736
Librium for Injection (Isolated cases) 1737
Limbitrol (Rare) 1738
Loxitane Capsules (Rare) 3398
▲ Micronor Tablets (Among most frequent) 2543
▲ Nolvadex Tablets (12.5% to 24.6%) 678
Norinyl 1 +35 28-Day Tablets 3380
Norinyl 1 + 50 28-Day Tablets 3380
▲ Nor-QD Tablets (Among most frequent) 3423
Oxandrin Tablets 1153
ParaGard T 380A Intrauterine Copper Contraceptive 2582
Pediapred Oral Solution 1170
Prednisone 3064
Prelone Syrup 2273
Prevacid Delayed-Release Capsules (Less than 1%) 3292
PREVPAC (Less than 1%) 3298
Prometrium Capsules (100 mg, 200 mg) 3261
Rifamate Capsules 767
Roferon-A Injection (2%) 2996
Sandostatin LAR Depot (1% to 4%) 2395
Serentil 1057
Solu-Medrol Sterile Powder 2855
Stelazine 1640
Testred Capsules, 10 mg 1746
Thioridazine Hydrochloride Tablets 2289
Tri-Norinyl-28 Tablets 3433
Trovan (Less than 1%) 2722
Unithroid Tablets 3445
Vantin Tablets and Oral Suspension (Less than 1%) 2860
Xanax Tablets 2865
▲ Xenical Capsules (9.8%) 3043
Zyprexa Tablets (Infrequent) 1973
Zyprexa ZYDIS Orally Disintegrating Tablets (Infrequent) 1973

Menstruation, early
Benadryl Parenteral 2617
Periactin Tablets 2155
Rynatan Tablets 3351

Menstruation, painful
ProSom Tablets (Infrequent) 500

Mental acuity, loss of
Crixivan Capsules (Less than 2%) 2070
Lodosyn Tablets 1251
Retrovir Capsules 1625
Retrovir IV Infusion 1629
Retrovir 1625
Sinemet Tablets 1253
Sinemet CR Tablets 1255
Tasmar Tablets (1%) 3010

Mental clouding
Compazine 1505
Dilaudid Ampules 441
Dilaudid Powder 441
Dilaudid Rectal Suppositories 441
Dilaudid Tablets 441
Halcion Tablets 2823
Hycodan 1316
Hycomine Compound Tablets 1317
Hycotuss Expectorant Syrup 1318
Lortab 3319
Lortab Elixir 3317
Maxidone Tablets CIII 3399
Norco 5/325 Tablets CIII 3424
Norco 7.5/325 Tablets CIII 3425
Norco 10/325 Tablets CIII 3425
Norco 10/325 Tablets CIII 3427
Numorphan 1324
Tussionex Pennkinetic Extended-Release Suspension 1174
Vicodin Tablets 516
Vicodin ES Tablets 517
Vicodin HP Tablets 518
Vicodin Tuss Expectorant 519
Vioxx (Greater than 0.1% to 1.9%) 2213
Zydone Tablets 1330

Mental confusion
(*see under* Confusion)

Mental depression
(*see under* Depression)

Mental perception, altered
Mykrox Tablets 1168

Mental performance, impairment
Aldoclor Tablets 2035
Aldomet Tablets 2037
Aldoril Tablets 2039
Alferon N Injection (1%) 1770
Ambien Tablets (Infrequent) 3191
Amerge Tablets (Infrequent) 1467
Anaprox Tablets (Less than 1%) 2967
Anaprox DS Tablets (Less than 1%) 2967
Arthrotec Tablets (Rare) 3195
Ativan Injection 3478
Cardura Tablets (Less than 0.5%) 2668
Celexa (Frequent) 1365
Claritin (At least one patient) 3100
Claritin-D 12 Hour Extended Release Tablets (Less frequent) 3102
Claritin-D 24 Hour Extended Release Tablets 3104
Clozaril Tablets 2319
Compazine 1505
Copaxone for Injection (Infrequent) 3306
Coreg Tablets (0.1% to 1%) 1508
Cosopt Sterile Ophthalmic Solution 2065
Demerol 3079
D.H.E. 45 Injection 2334
Dilaudid 441
Dilaudid Powder 441
Dilaudid Rectal Suppositories 441
Dilaudid Tablets 441
Dostinex Tablets (1%) 2804
EC-Naprosyn Delayed-Release Tablets (Less than 1%) 2967
Ergamisol Tablets (Less frequent) 1789
Eskalith 1527
Etrafon 3115
Exelon Capsules (Infrequent) 2342
Exelon Oral Solution (Infrequent) 2345
Felbatol 3343
Fludara for Injection (Up to 1%) 995
Flumadine (0.3% to 2.1%) 1370
Fortovase Capsules (Less than 2%) 2970
▲ Gabitril Tablets (6%) 1189
Gengraf Capsules (1% to less than 3%) 457
Grifulvin V Tablets Microsize and Oral Suspension Microsize 2518
Hivid Tablets (Less than 1%) 2975
Hycodan 1316
Hycomine Compound Tablets 1317
Hycotuss Expectorant Syrup 1318
Imdur Tablets (Less than or equal to 5%) 1826
Imitrex Injection (Rare) 1549
Imitrex Nasal Spray (Rare) 1554
Imitrex Tablets (Infrequent) 1558
▲ Intron A for Injection (Up to 14%) 3120
Inversine Tablets 1850
Invirase Capsules (Less than 2%) 2979
Kadian Capsules (Less than 3%) 1335
Klonopin Tablets (1% to 2%) 2983
Lamictal (1.7%) 1567
Levaquin (Less than 0.3%) 2537
Levsin/Levsinex/Levbid 3172
Limbitrol 1738
Lithobid Slow-Release Tablets 3255
Lortab 3319
Lortab Elixir 3317
Loxitane Capsules 3398
Maxalt Tablets (Frequent) 2120
Maxalt-MLT Orally Disintegrating Tablets (Infrequent) 2120
Maxidone Tablets CIII 3399
Meridia Capsules 481
Migranal Nasal Spray (Infrequent) 2376
Miltown Tablets 3349
MS Contin Tablets 2896
▲ Naprelan Tablets (3% to 9%) 1293
Naprosyn Suspension (Less than 1%) 2967
Naprosyn Tablets (less than 1%) 2967
Neoral Soft Gelatin Capsules (1% to less than 3%) 2380
Neoral Oral Solution (1% to less than 3%) 2380
▲ Nicotrol Nasal Spray (Over 5%) 2843
Norco 5/325 Tablets CIII 3424
Norco 7.5/325 Tablets CIII 3425
Norco 10/325 Tablets CIII 3425
Norco 10/325 Tablets CIII 3427
Norpramin Tablets 755
Orap Tablets 1407
Paxil (Frequent) 1609
Percocet Tablets 1326
Percodan Tablets 1327
Percolone Tablets 1327
Phenergan Injection 3553
Phenergan Suppositories 3556
Phenergan Syrup 3554
Phenergan Tablets 3556
Phenergan with Codeine Syrup 3557
Phenergan with Dextromethorphan Syrup 3559
Phenergan VC Syrup 3560
Phenergan VC with Codeine Syrup 3561
Prometrium Capsules (100 mg, 200 mg) (Less than 5%) 3261
ProSom Tablets 500
Prozac Pulvules, Liquid, and Weekly Capsules 1238
Rebetron Combination Therapy 3153
Remeron Tablets 2483
Remeron SolTab Tablets 2486
Requip Tablets (Infrequent) 1621
Rescriptor Tablets (Less than 2%) 526
Rifadin 765
Rifamate Capsules 767
Rifater Tablets 769
Risperdal (Infrequent) 1796
▲ Roferon-A Injection (4%) 2996
Ryna ▣ 768
Seroquel Tablets 684
▲ Serzone Tablets (3%) 1104
Sinemet Tablets 1253
Surmontil Capsules 3595
▲ Sustiva Capsules (1% to 9%) 1258
Tarka Tablets (Less frequent) 508
Timolide Tablets 2187
Timolol GFS ⊙ 266
Timoptic in Ocudose 2192
Timoptic Sterile Ophthalmic Solution 2190
Timoptic-XE Sterile Ophthalmic Gel Forming Solution 2194
▲ Topamax Sprinkle Capsules (6.7% to 15.4%) 2590
▲ Topamax Tablets (6.7% to 15.4%) 2590

Toradol (1% or less) 3018
Trovan (Less than 1%) 2722
Tussionex Pennkinetic Extended-Release Suspension 1174
Tylenol with Codeine 2595
Tylox Capsules 2597
Ultracet Tablets 2597
Ultram Tablets (Less than 1%) 2600
Vicodin Tablets 516
Vicodin ES Tablets 517
Vicodin HP Tablets 518
Vicodin Tuss Expectorant 519
Vistaril Intramuscular Solution (Seldom) 2738
Vivactil Tablets 2217
Vivactil Tablets 2446
Xanax Tablets 2865
Zarontin Capsules 2659
Zarontin Syrup 2660
Zebeta Tablets 1885
Zestril Tablets (0.3% to 1.0%) 698
Ziac Tablets 1887
Zoloft (1.3% to 2%) 2751
▲ Zonegran Capsules (6%) 1307
▲ Zyban Sustained-Release Tablets (9%) 1710
Zydone Tablets 1330
Zyrtec (Less than 2%) 2756
Zyrtec-D 12 Hour Extended Relief Tablets (Less than 2%) 2758

Mental slowness
Celontin Capsules 2618
Tonocard Tablets (Less than 1%) 649
▲ Topamax Sprinkle Capsules (8% to 15.4%) 2590
▲ Topamax Tablets (8% to 15.4%) 2590
▲ Zonegran Capsules (4%) 1307

Mental status, altered
Clozaril Tablets 2319
Cuprimine Capsules 2075
▲ Digitek Tablets (5%) 1003
Eldepryl Capsules 3266
Etrafon 3115
Haldol Decanoate 2535
▲ Idamycin PFS Injection (41%) 2825
Lanoxicaps Capsules 1574
Lanoxin Injection 1581
Lanoxin Tablets 1587
Lanoxin Elixir Pediatric 1578
Lanoxin Injection Pediatric 1584
Levaquin (Less than 0.3%) 2537
Moban 1320
Navane Oral 2701
Navane Intramuscular 2703
Oncaspar 756
Orap Tablets 1407
Orthoclone OKT3 Sterile Solution (Less than 1%) 2498
▲ Prograf (Approximately 55%) 1393
▲ Proleukin for Injection (73%) 1199
Risperdal 1796
▲ Roferon-A Injection (10% to 17%) 2996
Serentil 1057
Seroquel Tablets 684
Sinemet CR Tablets 1255
Stelazine 1640

Mesenteric arterial thrombosis
Blocadren Tablets 2046
Inderal 3513
Inderal LA Long-Acting Capsules 3516
Inderide Tablets 3517
Inderide LA Long-Acting Capsules 3519
Lo/Ovral Tablets 3532
Lo/Ovral-28 Tablets 3538
Low-Ogestrel-28 Tablets 3392
Nordette-28 Tablets 2257
Normodyne Tablets 3137
Ogestrel 0.5/50-28 Tablets 3428
Ovral Tablets 3551
Ovral-28 Tablets 3552
Ovrette Tablets 3552
Rilutek Tablets (Rare) 772
Sectral Capsules 3589
Tenoretic Tablets 690
Tenormin 692
Timolide Tablets 2187
Timoptic in Ocudose 2192
Timoptic Sterile Ophthalmic Solution 2190
Triphasil-21 Tablets 3600
Triphasil-28 Tablets 3605
Ziac Tablets 1887

Metabolic acidosis
(*see under* Acidosis, metabolic)

Metabolic changes
Clinoril Tablets (Rare) 2053
▲ Leukine (58%) 1755
▲ Neoral Soft Gelatin Capsules (9.3%) 2380
▲ Neoral Oral Solution (9.3%) 2380
Pravachol Tablets 1099

Methemoglobinemia
Americaine Anesthetic Lubricant (Rare) 1162
Americaine Otic Topical Anesthetic Ear Drops (Rare) 1162
Azulfidine EN-tabs Tablets (Rare) 2775
Bactrim 2949
Cipro I.V. 893
Cipro I.V. Pharmacy Bulk Package 897
Cipro 887
D.H.E. 45 Injection 2334
Eulexin Capsules 3118
Hurricaine Topical Anesthetic Gel, 1 oz. Fresh Mint, Wild Cherry, Pina Colada, Watermelon, 1/6 oz. Wild Cherry, Watermelon (Extremely rare) ▣618
Hurricaine Topical Anesthetic Liquid, 1 oz. Wild Cherry, Pina Colada, .25 ml Dry Handle Swab Wild Cherry, 1/6 oz. Wild Cherry (Extremely rare) ▣618
Hurricaine Topical Anesthetic Spray Extension Tubes (200) (Extremely rare) ▣618
Hurricaine Topical Anesthetic Spray Kit, 2 oz. Wild Cherry (Extremely rare) ▣618
Hurricaine Topical Anesthetic Spray, 2 oz. Wild Cherry (Extremely rare) ▣618
Ismo Tablets (Extremely rare) 3524
Isordil Sublingual Tablets (Extremely rare) 3525
Isordil Titradose Tablets (Extremely rare) 3526
Macrobid Capsules 2889
Macrodantin Capsules (Rare) 2891
Mepron Suspension 1598
Nitro-Dur Transdermal Infusion System (Very rare) 1834
Nitro-Dur Transdermal Infusion System (Very rare) 3134
Pediazole Suspension 3050
Reglan 2935
Septra Suspension 2265
Septra Tablets 2265
Septra DS Tablets 2265

Metrorrhagia
Aciphex Tablets 1267
Aciphex Tablets 1783
Aricept Tablets (Infrequent) 1270
Aricept Tablets (Infrequent) 2665
▲ Betaseron for SC Injection (15%) 988
▲ Cenestin Tablets (14%) 1263
Cleocin Vaginal Cream (Less than 1%) 2788
Copaxone for Injection (At least 2%) 3306
Depacon Injection (1% or more) 416
Depakene (1% or more) 421
Depakote Sprinkle Capsules 426
Depakote Tablets (1% to 5%) 430
Depakote ER Tablets (1% to 5%) 436
Floxin I.V. (Less than 1%) 2526
Floxin Tablets (Less than 1%) 2529
Gabitril Tablets (Frequent) 1189
Geodon Capsules (Infrequent) 2688
Lipitor Tablets (Less than 2%) 2639
Lipitor Tablets (Less than 2%) 2696
Lunelle Monthly Injection 2827
Luvox Tablets (25, 50, 100 mg) (Infrequent) 3256
Meridia Capsules (1%) 481
Naprelan Tablets (Less than 1%) 1293
Paxil (Rare) 1609
Pentasa Capsules (Less than 1%) 3239
Permax Tablets (Infrequent) 1299
Prozac Pulvules, Liquid, and Weekly Capsules (Infrequent) 1238
▲ Rapamune Oral Solution and Tablets (3% to 20%) 3584
Remeron Tablets (Rare) 2483
Remeron SolTab Tablets (Rare) 2486
Rescriptor Tablets (Less than 2%) 526
Rilutek Tablets (Infrequent) 772
Salagen Tablets (Less than 1%) 2229
Serzone Tablets (Infrequent) 1104
Sonata Capsules (Infrequent) 3591
Tequin Injection (Less than 0.1%) 1110
Tequin Tablets (Less than 0.1%) 1110
Thalomid Capsules 1154
Vantin Tablets and Oral Suspension (Less than 1%) 2860
Zanaflex Tablets (Rare) 1305
Zyprexa Tablets (Frequent) 1973
Zyprexa ZYDIS Orally Disintegrating Tablets (Frequent) 1973

Metyrapone test, altered results
Aygestin Tablets 1333
Estrace Vaginal Cream 3358
Estrace Tablets 3361
Estratest 3252
Provera Tablets 2853

Microangiopathy
Vitrasert Implant (Less than 1%) ⊙254

Microcephaly
Felbatol 3343

Microcephaly, fetal
Accutane Capsules 2944
Dilantin Infatabs 2624
Dilantin Kapseals 2622
Dilantin-125 Oral Suspension 2625

Microphthalmia, fetal
Accutane Capsules 2944

Microphthalmos
Thalomid Capsules 1154

Micropinna, fetal
Accutane Capsules 2944

Micturition, difficulty
Atrovent Inhalation Aerosol (Less than 1%) 1030
Benadryl Parenteral 2617
Blocadren Tablets 2046
▲ Casodex Tablets (2% to 5%) 662
Catapres Tablets (About 2 in 1,000 patients) 1037
Catapres-TTS (0.5% or less) 1038
Chemet Capsules (Up to 3.7%) 3078
Clorpres Tablets (About 2 in 1,000) 1002
Combipres Tablets (About 2 in 1,000) 1040
Combivent Inhalation Aerosol 1041
Cosopt Sterile Ophthalmic Solution 2065
Dantrium Capsules (Less frequent) 2885
Donnagel Liquid (Rare) ▣789
Duraclon Injection (About 0.2%) 3057
Effexor Tablets (2%) 3495
Effexor XR Capsules (Frequent) 3499
Flexeril Tablets (Rare) 572
Flexeril Tablets (Rare) 2094
Levo-Dromoran 1734
Levorphanol Tartrate Tablets (1% to 3%) 3059
Normodyne Tablets (Less common) 3137
Norpramin Tablets 755
OxyContin Tablets (Less than 1%) 2912
▲ Paxil (3%) 1609
Periactin Tablets 2155
ProAmatine Tablets (Rare) 3241
Proventil Repetabs Tablets (Less than 1%) 3148
Stadol NS Nasal Spray (Less than 1%) 1108
Timolide Tablets 2187
Timolol GFS ⊙266
Timoptic in Ocudose 2192
Timoptic Sterile Ophthalmic Solution 2190
Timoptic-XE Sterile Ophthalmic Gel Forming Solution 2194
Transderm Scōp Transdermal Therapeutic System (Infrequent) 2302
Urimax Tablets 1769
Urised Tablets 2876
Uroqid-Acid No. 2 Tablets (Occasional) 947
Vivactil Tablets 2217
Vivactil Tablets 2446
Volmax Extended-Release Tablets (Less frequent) 2276
▲ Xanax Tablets (12.2%) 2865
Zonegran Capsules (Infrequent) 1307
Zovirax for Injection (Less than 1%) 1708
Zyprexa Tablets (Infrequent) 1973
Zyprexa ZYDIS Orally Disintegrating Tablets (Infrequent) 1973

Micturition, painful
Uroqid-Acid No. 2 Tablets (Occasional) 947
Zoloft (Rare) 2751
Zovirax for Injection (Less than 1%) 1708

Micturition disturbances
Aceon Tablets (2 mg, 4 mg, 8 mg) (0.3% to 1%) 3249
Aciphex Tablets 1267
Aciphex Tablets 1783
Adalat CC Tablets (3% or less) 877
Ambien Tablets (Rare) 3191
Arava Tablets (1% to 3%) 724
Aricept Tablets (2%) 1270
Aricept Tablets (2%) 2665
Arthrotec Tablets (Rare) 3195
Astelin Nasal Spray (Infrequent) 3339
Avalide Tablets (2%) 1070
Benadryl Parenteral 2617
Bontril Slow-Release Capsules 576
Captopril Tablets (Approximately 1 to 2 of 1000 patients) 2281
Carbatrol Capsules 3234
Cardene I.V. (Rare) 3485
Cardura Tablets 2668
▲ Casodex Tablets (6%) 662
Cataflam Tablets (Less than 1%) 2315
Caverject Sterile Powder (Less than 1%) 2777
Celebrex Capsules (0.1% to 1.9%) 2676
Celebrex Capsules (0.1% to 1.9%) 2780
Celexa (At least 2%) 1365
▲ CellCept Capsules (3%) 2951
▲ CellCept Intravenous (3%) 2951
▲ CellCept Oral Suspension (3%) 2951
▲ CellCept Tablets (3%) 2951
Cipro I.V. (1% or less) 893
Cipro I.V. Pharmacy Bulk Package (Less than 1%) 897
Claritin (At least one patient) 3100
Claritin-D 12 Hour Extended Release Tablets (Less frequent) 3102
Claritin-D 24 Hour Extended Release Tablets (Fewer than 2%) 3104
Clomid Tablets (Fewer than 1%) 735
Clozaril Tablets (1%) 2319
▲ Cognex Capsules (3%) 1351
Colazal Capsules 3069
Copaxone for Injection (At least 2%) 3306
Coreg Tablets (0.1% to 1%) 1508
Covera-HS Tablets (Less than 2%) 3199
Cozaar Tablets (Less than 1%) 2067
Crinone (Less than 5%) 3213
Crixivan Capsules (Less than 2%) 2070
Cytovene (At least 3 subjects) 2959
Dantrium Capsules (Less frequent) 2885
Daranide Tablets 2077
▲ Demadex Tablets and Injection (6.7%) 2965
Depacon Injection (1% to 5%) 416
Depakene (1% to 5%) 421
Depakote Sprinkle Capsules (1% to 5%) 426
Depakote Tablets (1% to 5%) 430
Depakote ER Tablets (1% to 5%) 436
Detrol Tablets (1.7%) 3623
Diovan HCT Tablets (Greater than 0.2%) 2338
Dipentum Capsules (Rare) 2803
Dopram Injectable 2931
Duragesic Transdermal System (Less than 1%) 1786
Duramorph Injection 1312
Dynabac Tablets (0.1% to 1%) 2269
▲ Effexor Tablets (3%) 3495
Effexor XR Capsules (Frequent) 3499
Eldepryl Capsules 3266
Eskalith 1527
Estring Vaginal Ring (At least 1 report) 2811
Etrafon (Occasional) 3115
Evoxac Capsules (0.9%; less than 1%) 1217
Exelon Capsules (Infrequent) 2342
Exelon Oral Solution (Infrequent) 2345
Flexeril Tablets (Less than 1%) 572
Flexeril Tablets (Less than 1%) 2094
Floxin I.V. (Less than 1%) 2526
Floxin Tablets (Less than 1%) 2529
Flumadine 1370
Fortovase Capsules (Less than 2%) 2970
Gabitril Tablets (1% or more) 1189
Gastrocrom Oral Concentrate (Less common) 1162
Gengraf Capsules (1% to less than 3%) 457
Hivid Tablets (Less than 1%) 2975
Hytrin Capsules (At least 1%) 464
Hyzaar 2109
Ifex for Injection 1123
Imitrex Injection (Rare) 1549
Imitrex Nasal Spray (Infrequent) 1554
Imitrex Tablets (Infrequent) 1558
Indapamide Tablets (Less than 5%) 2286
Indocin (Rare) 2112
Intron A for Injection (Less than 5%) 3120
Invirase Capsules (Less than 2%) 2979
Ismo Tablets (Fewer than 1%) 3524
Isoptin SR Tablets (1% or less) 467
Klonopin Tablets (1%) 2983
Lamictal (Infrequent) 1567
Lexxel Tablets 608
Limbitrol 1738
Lipitor Tablets (Less than 2%) 2639
Lipitor Tablets (Less than 2%) 2696
Lodine (1% to 3%) 3528
Lodine XL Extended-Release Tablets (1% to 3%) 3530
Lodosyn Tablets 1251
Lotensin HCT Tablets (0.3% to 1%) 2367
Lupron Depot 7.5 mg (Less than 5%) 3284
▲ Lupron Injection (5% or more) 3279
▲ Luvox Tablets (25, 50, 100 mg) (3%) 3256
Matulane Capsules 3246
Maxalt Tablets (Infrequent) 2120
Maxalt-MLT Orally Disintegrating Tablets (Infrequent) 2120
Megace Oral Suspension (Up to 2%) 1124
Meridia Capsules 481
Micardis Tablets (More than 0.3%) 1049
Micardis HCT Tablets 1051
Midamor Tablets (Less than or equal to 1%) 2136

Migranal Nasal Spray (Infrequent)... 2376
Minipress Capsules (1% to 4%)...... 2699
Minizide Capsules (Rare)............ 2700
▲ Mirapex Tablets (6%) 2834
Mobic Tablets (0.1% to 2.4%)........ 1054
Moduretic Tablets.......................... 2138
Monopril Tablets (0.2% to 1.0%)..... 1091
Naprelan Tablets (Less than 1%).... 1293
Naropin Injection (Less than 1%)..... 612
Neoral Soft Gelatin Capsules (1% to less than 3%)....................... 2380
Neoral Oral Solution (1% to less than 3%)....................................... 2380
Neurontin Capsules (Infrequent)...... 2655
Neurontin Oral Solution (Infrequent)...................................... 2655
Neurontin Tablets (Infrequent)......... 2655
Nexium Delayed-Release Capsules (Less than 1%).............. 619
Norpramin Tablets......................... 755
Norvasc Tablets (More than 0.1% to 1%) 2704
Norvir Capsules (Less than 2%) 487
Norvir Oral Solution (Less than 2%) 487
Oncaspar (Less than 1%) 756
Orap Tablets 1407
Parnate Tablets 1607
▲ Paxil (3%) 1609
Pentasa Capsules (Less than 1%) ... 3239
Permax Tablets (2.7%) 1299
Plendil Extended-Release Tablets (0.5% to 1.5%) 623
Pletal Tablets (Less than 2%) 2605
Pletal Tablets (Less than 2%) 2848
Prilosec Delayed-Release Capsules (Less than 1%) 628
▲ ProAmatine Tablets (Among most frequent) 3241
▲ Prograf (3% to 15%) 1393
Proleukin for Injection (1%) 1199
Prosed/DS Tablets 3268
ProSom Tablets (Infrequent) 500
Prostigmin Injectable 1744
Prostigmin Tablets 1744
Protonix I.V. (Less than 1%) 3580
Protonix Tablets (Less than 1%) 3577
Prozac Pulvules, Liquid, and Weekly Capsules (Frequent) 1238
▲ Rapamune Oral Solution and Tablets (3% to 20%) 3584
Reglan 2935
Remeron Tablets (2%) 2483
Remeron SolTab Tablets (2%) 2486
Reminyl Oral Solution (Infrequent) ... 1792
Reminyl Tablets (Infrequent) 1792
ReoPro Vials (0.1%) 1958
Requip Tablets (Infrequent) 1621
Retrovir Capsules 1625
Retrovir IV Infusion 1629
Retrovir 1625
Risperdal 1796
Rynatan Tablets 3351
▲ Salagen Tablets (9% to 12%) 2229
Sarafem Pulvules (2%) 1962
▲ Sectral Capsules (3%) 3589
Serophene Tablets (Less than 1 in 100 patients) 3226
Seroquel Tablets (Infrequent) 684
Serzone Tablets (2%) 1104
▲ Simulect for Injection (3% to 10%) . 2399
Sinemet Tablets 1253
Sinemet CR Tablets (0.8%) 1255
Sonata Capsules (Infrequent) 3591
Surmontil Capsules 3595
Tarka Tablets 508
Tasmar Tablets (1% to 2%) 3010
Tegretol/Tegretol-XR 2404
Tenex Tablets (Less frequent) 2942
Tensilon Injectable 1745
Teveten Tablets (Less than 1%) 3327
▲ TheraCys Injection (40%) 823
▲ Tice BCG, BCG Live (40.4%) 2489
Topamax Sprinkle Capsules (Frequent) 2590
Topamax Tablets (Frequent) 2590
Toradol (1% or less) 3018
Tricor Capsules, Micronized 513
Trileptal Oral Suspension (1% to 2%) 2407
Trileptal Tablets (1% to 2%) 2407
Trovan (Less than 1%) 2722
Ultracet Tablets (Less than 1%) 2597
Ultram Tablets (1% to 5%) 2600
Uniretic Tablets (Less than 1%) 3178
Univasc Tablets (More than 1%) 3181
Urecholine 2198
Urecholine Tablets 2445
▲ Valstar Sterile Solution for Intravesical Instillation (30% to 61%) 1175
Verelan Capsules (1% or less) 3184
Verelan PM Capsules (2% or less) ... 3186
▲ Vesanoid Capsules (3%) 3037
▲ Viadur Implant (3.8%) 912
Viagra Tablets (Less than 2%) 2732
Vicoprofen Tablets (Less than 3%) .. 520
Vivactil Tablets 2217
Vivactil Tablets 2446
Voltaren Tablets (Less than 1%) 2315
Voltaren-XR Tablets (Less than 1%) 2315
Wellbutrin Tablets (2.5%)............... 1680
Wellbutrin SR Sustained-Release Tablets (2% to 5%)...................... 1684
▲ Zanaflex Tablets (3%) 1305
Zoladex (1% or greater).................. 702
Zoladex 3-month (1% to 5%)........... 706
Zoloft (Infrequent)........................... 2751
Zomig Tablets (Infrequent)............... 708
Zomig-ZMT Tablets (Infrequent)....... 708
Zyban Sustained-Release Tablets (Frequent)...................................... 1710
Zyprexa Tablets (Infrequent)............ 1973
Zyprexa ZYDIS Orally Disintegrating Tablets (Infrequent)...................................... 1973
Zyrtec (Less than 2%)...................... 2756
Zyrtec-D 12 Hour Extended Relief Tablets (Less than 2%)................ 2758

Migraine

AccuNeb Inhalation Solution (0.9% to 1.7%)............................. 1230
Aciphex Tablets 1267
Aciphex Tablets 1783
Actiq (1% or greater) 1184
Activella Tablets 2764
Agrylin Capsules (1% to 5%) 3232
Alesse-21 Tablets 3468
Alesse-28 Tablets 3473
Alora Transdermal System 3372
Ambien Tablets (Infrequent) 3191
Arava Tablets (1% to 3%) 724
Arthrotec Tablets (Rare) 3195
Asacol Delayed-Release Tablets (2% or greater) 2884
Aygestin Tablets 1333
▲ Betaseron for SC Injection (12%) ... 988
Brevicon 28-Day Tablets 3380
Cardura Tablets (Less than 0.5%) ... 2668
Celexa (Frequent) 1365
Cenestin Tablets 1263
Cerebyx Injection (Infrequent) 2619
Cipro HC Otic Suspension (One patient) 540
Claritin (At least one patient) 3100
Claritin-D 12 Hour Extended Release Tablets (Less frequent) ... 3102
Claritin-D 24 Hour Extended Release Tablets (Fewer than 2%) 3104
Climara Transdermal System 958
Clomid Tablets 735
Cognex Capsules (Infrequent) 1351
Colestid Tablets 2791
▲ Copaxone for Injection (5%) 3306
Coreg Tablets (Less than or equal to 0.1%) 1508
Cozaar Tablets (Less than 1%) 2067
Crinone (Less than 5%) 3213
Cyclessa Tablets 2450
Depo-Provera Contraceptive Injection 2798
Desogen Tablets 2458
Doxil Injection (Less than 1%) 566
Effexor Tablets (Frequent) 3495
Effexor XR Capsules (Frequent) 3499
Eldepryl Capsules 3266
Engerix-B Vaccine 1517
Esclim Transdermal System 3460
Estinyl Tablets 3112
Estrace Vaginal Cream 3358
Estrace Tablets 3361
Estratest 3252
Estring Vaginal Ring (1% to 3%) 2811
Estrostep 2627
Evista Tablets (2.4%) 1915
Evoxac Capsules (1% to 3%) 1217
Exelon Capsules (Infrequent) 2342
Exelon Oral Solution (Infrequent) 2345
Famvir Tablets (0.7% to 3.1%) 2348
Felbatol (Infrequent) 3343
femhrt Tablets 2635
Flovent Diskus (1% to 3%) 3614
Flovent Rotadisk (1% to 3%) 1537
Gabitril Tablets (Frequent) 1189
Gastrocrom Oral Concentrate (Less common) 1162
▲ Gengraf Capsules (3%) 457
Glucotrol XL Extended Release Tablets (Less than 1%) 2693
Hivid Tablets (Less than 1%) 2975
Hyzaar 2109
Imdur Tablets (Less than or equal to 5%) 1826
Imitrex Tablets 1558
Intron A for Injection (Less than 5%) 3120
Klonopin Tablets (Infrequent) 2983
Lamictal (Infrequent) 1567
Levlen 962
Levlite 21 Tablets 962
Levlite 28 Tablets 962
Levora Tablets 3389
Lipitor Tablets (Less than 2%) 2639
Lipitor Tablets (Less than 2%) 2696
Loestrin 21 Tablets 2642
Loestrin Fe Tablets 2642
Lo/Ovral Tablets 3532
Lo/Ovral-28 Tablets 3538
Low-Ogestrel-28 Tablets 3392
Lunelle Monthly Injection 2827
Luvox Tablets (25, 50, 100 mg)..... 3256
LYMErix Vaccine (Greater than 1%).. 1592
Maxair Autohaler............................ 1981
Maxair Inhaler (Less than 1%)......... 1984
Menest Tablets............................... 2254
Meridia Capsules (2.4%)................ 481
Miacalcin Nasal Spray (Less than 1%).. 2375
Micardis Tablets (More than 0.3%).. 1049
Micardis HCT Tablets..................... 1051
Microgestin Fe 1.5/30 Tablets....... 3407
Microgestin Fe 1/20 Tablets........... 3400
Mircette Tablets.............................. 2470
Modicon.. 2563
Monurol Sachet (Less than 1%)....... 1375
Myobloc Injectable Solution (2% or greater)...................................... 1291
Naprelan Tablets (Less than 1%)..... 1293
Necon... 3415
▲ Neoral Soft Gelatin Capsules (3%) .. 2380
▲ Neoral Oral Solution (3%) 2380
Neurontin Capsules (Infrequent)...... 2655
Neurontin Oral Solution (Infrequent)...................................... 2655
Neurontin Tablets (Infrequent)......... 2655
Nexium Delayed-Release Capsules (Less than 1%).............. 619
Niaspan Extended-Release Tablets... 1846
Nicotrol Nasal Spray (Less than 1%).. 2843
Nordette-28 Tablets....................... 2257
Norinyl 1 +35 28-Day Tablets......... 3380
Norinyl 1 + 50 28-Day Tablets........ 3380
Norplant System............................ 3543
Norvir Capsules (Less than 2%)...... 487
Norvir Oral Solution (Less than 2%).. 487
Ogen Tablets.................................. 2846
Ogestrel 0.5/50-28 Tablets........... 3428
Ortho Dienestrol Cream.................. 2554
Ortho-Cept 21 Tablets................... 2546
Ortho-Cept 28 Tablets.................... 2546
Ortho-Cyclen/Ortho Tri-Cyclen......... 2573
Ortho-Est Tablets............................ 3464
Ortho-Novum.................................. 2563
Ortho-Novum 1/50□28 Tablets......... 2556
Ortho-Prefest Tablets...................... 2570
Ortho-Cyclen/Ortho Tri-Cyclen......... 2573
Orudis Capsules (Less than 1%)...... 3548
Oruvail Capsules (Less than 1%)..... 3548
Ovcon... 3364
Ovral Tablets.................................. 3551
Ovral-28 Tablets............................. 3552
Ovrette Tablets............................... 3552
OxyContin Tablets (Less than 1%)... 2912
Paxil (Infrequent)............................. 1609
Permax Tablets (Rare)..................... 1299
Premarin Intravenous...................... 3563
Premarin Tablets............................. 3566
Premarin Vaginal Cream.................. 3570
Premphase Tablets......................... 3572
Prempro Tablets............................. 3572
Procardia XL Extended Release Tablets (1% or less)..................... 2710
Protonix I.V. (Greater than or equal to 1%)................................. 3580
Protonix Tablets (Greater than or equal to 1%)................................. 3577
Protopic Ointment (Greater than or equal to 1%)............................ 1397
Provera Tablets.............................. 2853
Provigil Tablets (At least 1%).......... 1193
Prozac Pulvules, Liquid, and Weekly Capsules (Infrequent)....... 1238
Pulmicort Turbuhaler Inhalation Powder (1% to 3%)...................... 636
Recombivax HB.............................. 2178
Remeron Tablets (Infrequent).......... 2483
Remeron SolTab Tablets (Infrequent)...................................... 2486
Requip Tablets (Infrequent)............. 1621
Rescriptor Tablets (Less than 2%)... 526
Rilutek Tablets (Infrequent).............. 772
Risperdal (Rare).............................. 1796
Roxicodone Tablets (Less than 3%)... 3067
Salagen Tablets (Less than 1%)....... 2229
Sandostatin LAR Depot (Rare)......... 2395
Sarafem Pulvules (Infrequent)......... 1962
Seroquel Tablets (Infrequent)........... 684
Serzone Tablets.............................. 1104
Soriatane Capsules (Less than 1%)... 3003
Sular Tablets (Less than or equal to 1%)... 688
Tasmar Tablets (Infrequent)............. 3010
Tequin Injection (Less than 0.1%).... 1110
Tequin Tablets (Less than 0.1%)...... 1110
Teveten Tablets (Less than 1%)....... 3327
Thalomid Capsules......................... 1154
Tikosyn Capsules (Less than or equal to 2%).................................. 2717
Topamax Sprinkle Capsules (Infrequent)...................................... 2590
Topamax Tablets (Infrequent).......... 2590
Tricor Capsules, Micronized (Less than 1%)... 513
Trileptal Oral Suspension................ 2407
Trileptal Tablets.............................. 2407
Tri-Levlen.. 962
Tri-Norinyl-28 Tablets..................... 3433
Triphasil-21 Tablets........................ 3600
Triphasil-28 Tablets........................ 3605
Trivora Tablets............................... 3439
Trovan (Less than 1%)..................... 2722
Ultracet Tablets (Less than 1%)....... 2597
Ultram Tablets (Infrequent).............. 2600
Uniretic Tablets (Less than 1%)........ 3178
Vanceril Double Strength Inhalation Aerosol (Fewer than 2%).. 3167
Vantin Tablets and Oral Suspension (Less than 1%)........... 2860
Viagra Tablets (Less than 2%)......... 2732
Vioxx (Greater than 0.1% to 1.9%).. 2213
Viracept... 532
Vistide Injection.............................. 1445
Vivelle Transdermal System............ 2412
Vivelle-Dot Transdermal System...... 2416
Xopenex Inhalation Solution (2.7%)... 3207
Yasmin 28 Tablets (Greater than 1%).. 980
Zanaflex Tablets (Infrequent) 1305
▲ Zoladex (1% to 7%) 702
Zoladex 3-month 706
Zoloft (Infrequent) 2751
Zovia 3449
Zyprexa Tablets (Infrequent) 1973
Zyprexa ZYDIS Orally Disintegrating Tablets (Infrequent) 1973
Zyrtec (Less than 2%) 2756
Zyrtec-D 12 Hour Extended Relief Tablets (Less than 2%) 2758

Migraine, aggravated

Migranal Nasal Spray (Rare) 2376
Nexium Delayed-Release Capsules (Less than 1%) 619

Miliaria

Aclovate (Infrequent) 1275
Analpram-HC 1338
Anusol-HC Cream 2.5% (Infrequent to frequent) 2237
Capex Shampoo 1400
Clobevate Gel 3271
▲ Cordran Lotion (More frequent) 2438
▲ Cordran Tape (More frequent) 2439
Cormax Cream (Infrequent) 2440
Cormax Ointment (Infrequent) 2440
Cormax Scalp Application (Infrequent) 2441
Cutivate Cream (Infrequent) 1282
Cutivate Ointment (Infrequent to more frequent) 1284
Dermatop Emollient Cream (Infrequent to frequent) 2517
DesOwen (Infrequent) 1401
Diprolene Gel 0.05% (Infrequent) 3107
Diprolene Lotion 0.05% (Infrequent) 3107
Diprolene Ointment 0.05% (Infrequent) 3108
Diprolene AF Cream 0.05% (Infrequent) 3106
Diprosone 3109
8-MOP Capsules 1727
Elocon Cream 0.1% (Infrequent) 3110
Elocon Lotion 0.1% (Infrequent) 3111
Elocon Ointment 0.1% (Infrequent) 3112
Lidex (Infrequent) 2020
Locoid Cream (Infrequent) 1341
Locoid Lipocream Cream (Infrequent) 1342
Locoid (Infrequent) 1341
Lotrisone 3129
Luxíq Foam 1210
Olux Foam 1211
Oxsoralen-Ultra Capsules 1741
Pramosone 1343
ProctoFoam-HC 3177
Psorcon E Cream 1227
Psorcon E Ointment 1228
Synalar (Infrequent) 2020
Temovate Cream 1301
Temovate Gel (Infrequent) 1303
Temovate Ointment 1301
Temovate Scalp Application (Infrequent) 1304
Temovate E Emollient (Infrequent) ... 1302
Topicort (Infrequent) 2025
Ultravate Cream 1119
Ultravate Ointment (Less Frequent) 1120

Miosis

Actiq (Less than 1%) 1184
▲ Buprenex Injectable (1% to 5%) 2918
Compazine 1505
Dibenzyline Capsules 3457
Dilaudid Oral Liquid (Less frequent) 445
Dilaudid Tablets - 8 mg (Less frequent) 445
Dilaudid-HP (Less frequent) 443
Duramorph Injection 1312
Effexor Tablets (Rare) 3495

Effexor XR Capsules (Rare) 3499
▲ Felbatol (6.5%) 3343
Kadian Capsules (Less than 3%) 1335
Mestinon 1740
MS Contin Tablets (Less frequent) 2896
MSIR (Less frequent) 2898
Navane Oral 2701
Navane Intramuscular 2703
Neurontin Capsules (Rare) 2655
Neurontin Oral Solution (Rare) 2655
Neurontin Tablets (Rare) 2655
Numorphan 1324
Ocufen Ophthalmic Solution ⊙242
Oramorph SR Tablets (Less frequent) 3062
Polocaine Injection, USP 625
Polocaine-MPF Injection, USP 625
Prostigmin Injectable 1744
Prostigmin Tablets 1744
Sensorcaine 643
Sensorcaine-MPF Injection 643
Serentil 1057
Soma Compound w/Codeine Tablets 3355
Stelazine 1640
Tensilon Injectable 1745
Thioridazine Hydrochloride Tablets 2289
Thiothixene Capsules 2290
Thorazine 1656
Tussi-Organidin NR Liquid 3350
Tussi-Organidin-S NR Liquid 3350
Urecholine 2198
Urecholine Tablets 2445
Versed Injection (Less than 1%) 3027
Vistide Injection 1445
Zyprexa Tablets (Rare) 1973
Zyprexa ZYDIS Orally Disintegrating Tablets (Rare) 1973

Miscarriage
Cytotec Tablets 3202
Efudex 1733
▲ Follistim for Injection (9.5% to 11%) 2465
Vantin Tablets and Oral Suspension 2860

Mitral insufficiency
Requip Tablets (Infrequent) 1621

Mitral regurgitation
Activase I.V. 1410
Retavase Vials 1182
TNKase I.V. 1430

Mitral valve disease
Effexor XR Capsules (Rare) 3499

Mitral valve prolapse
Effexor Tablets (Rare) 3495
Effexor XR Capsules (Rare) 3499

Moaning
Diprivan Injectable Emulsion (Less than 1%) 667

Mobility disorders, non-site specific
Amerge Tablets (Rare) 1467

Molluscum contagiosum
Fortovase Capsules (Less than 2%) 2970
Norvir Capsules (Less than 2%) 487
Norvir Oral Solution (Less than 2%) 487

Moniliasis
(*see under* Candidiasis)

Moniliasis, genital
(*see under* Candidiasis, genital)

Moniliasis, oral
(*see under* Candidiasis, oral)

Monocytosis
Celontin Capsules 2618
Cipro (Less than 0.1%) 887
Cuprimine Capsules 2075
Depen Titratable Tablets 3341
Dynabac Tablets (0.1% to 1%) 2269
Geodon Capsules (Rare) 2688
Paxil (Rare) 1609
Primaxin I.M. 2158
Primaxin I.V. 2160
Rocephin Injectable Vials, ADD-Vantage, Galaxy, Bulk (Rare) 2993
Unasyn for Injection 2728
Vantin Tablets and Oral Suspension 2860

Mononeuritis
Felbatol 3343

Mononeuropathy
Acel-Imune 1851

Monoplegia
Gliadel Wafer (2%) 1723
Imitrex Injection (Rare) 1549
Imitrex Nasal Spray (Rare) 1554
Imitrex Tablets (Infrequent) 1558

Mood changes
Adalat CC Tablets (Rare) 877
Aerobid/Aerobid-M (1% to 3%) 1363
Aygestin Tablets 1333
Betapace Tablets (Less than 1% to 3%) 950
Celestone Soluspan Injectable Suspension 3097
Clomid Tablets 735
Cortone Acetate Injectable Suspension 2059
Cortone Acetate Tablets 2061
Decadron Elixir 2078
Decadron Tablets 2079
Decadron Phosphate Injection 2081
Dilaudid 441
Dilaudid Oral Liquid (Less frequent) 445
Dilaudid Powder 441
Dilaudid Rectal Suppositories 441
Dilaudid Tablets 441
Dilaudid Tablets - 8 mg (Less frequent) 445
Dilaudid-HP (Less frequent) 443
Dipentum Capsules (Rare) 2803
Eldepryl Capsules 3266
Enbrel for Injection 1752
Enbrel for Injection 3504
Feldene Capsules (Rare) 2685
Florinef Acetate Tablets 2250
Hexalen Capsules 2226
Hivid Tablets (Less than 1%) 2975
Hycodan 1316
Hycomine Compound Tablets 1317
Hycotuss Expectorant Syrup 1318
Hydrocortone Tablets 2106
Hydrocortone Acetate Injectable Suspension 2103
Hydrocortone Phosphate Injection, Sterile 2105
Levlen 962
Levlite 21 Tablets 962
Levlite 28 Tablets 962
Levorphanol Tartrate Tablets 3059
Lortab 3319
Lortab Elixir 3317
Lupron Depot 3.75 mg 3281
Lupron Injection (Less than 5%) 3279
Marinol Capsules 3325
Maxidone Tablets CIII 3399
Meridia Capsules 481
Modicon 2563
Monopril Tablets (0.2% to 1.0%) 1091
Monopril HCT 1094
MS Contin Tablets (Less frequent) 2896
MSIR (Less frequent) 2898
Norco 5/325 Tablets CIII 3424
Norco 7.5/325 Tablets CIII 3425
Norco 10/325 Tablets CIII 3425
Norco 10/325 Tablets CIII 3427
Oncaspar 756
Oramorph SR Tablets (Less frequent) 3062
Orthoclone OKT3 Sterile Solution 2498
Ortho-Cyclen/Ortho Tri-Cyclen 2573
Ortho-Novum 2563
Ortho-Novum 1/50□28 Tablets 2556
Ortho-Cyclen/Ortho Tri-Cyclen 2573
Prednisone 3064
Prelone Syrup 2273
▲ Procardia Capsules (7%) 2708
▲ Procardia XL Extended Release Tablets (7%) 2710
Serophene Tablets 3226
Solu-Medrol Sterile Powder 2855
▲ Tonocard Tablets (1.5% to 11.0%) 649
▲ Topamax Sprinkle Capsules (3.5% to 10.1%) 2590
▲ Topamax Tablets (3.5% to 10.1%) 2590
Tri-Levlen 962
Tussionex Pennkinetic Extended-Release Suspension 1174
Univasc Tablets (Less than 1%) 3181
Versed Syrup (Less than 1%) 3033
Vicodin Tablets 516
Vicodin ES Tablets 517
Vicodin HP Tablets 518
Vicodin Tuss Expectorant 519
Vicoprofen Tablets (Less than 1%) 520
Wellbutrin Tablets (Infrequent) 1680
Zydone Tablets 1330

Moon face
Copaxone for Injection (Infrequent) 3306

Motion sickness
Aricept Tablets 1270
Aricept Tablets 2665
Evoxac Capsules (Less than 1%) 1217
Klonopin Tablets (Infrequent) 2983

Motor and phonic tics, exacerbations
Adderall Tablets 3231
Adderall XR Capsules
Dexedrine 1512
DextroStat Tablets 3236

Motor disturbances, reversible involuntary
Zantac (Rare) 1690
Zantac Injection (Rare) 1688
Zantac Syrup (Rare) 1690

Motor function, loss of
Neoral Soft Gelatin Capsules 2380
Neoral Oral Solution 2380
Sandimmune 2388

Motor restlessness
Compazine 1505
Etrafon 3115
Haldol Injection, Tablets and Concentrate 2533
Moban 1320
Navane Oral 2701
Navane Intramuscular 2703
Orap Tablets (Less frequent) 1407
Reglan 2935
Serentil 1057
Stelazine 1640
Thioridazine Hydrochloride Tablets 2289
Thorazine 1656

Motor skills, impairment
Ambien Tablets 3191
Amerge Tablets (Rare) 1467
Cogentin 2055
Compazine 1505
Dapsone Tablets USP 1780
Duranest Injections 600
Effexor Tablets 3495
Halcion Tablets 2823
Levsin/Levsinex/Levbid 3172
Moban 1320
Neurontin Capsules (Rare) 2655
Neurontin Oral Solution (Rare) 2655
Neurontin Tablets (Rare) 2655
Orap Tablets 1407
▲ Prograf (Approximately 55%) 1393
Proleukin for Injection (2%) 1199
Prozac Pulvules, Liquid, and Weekly Capsules 1238
Remeron Tablets 2483
Remeron SolTab Tablets 2486
Risperdal 1796
Robaxin Injectable 2938
Serzone Tablets 1104
Soma Compound Tablets 3354
Soma Compound w/Codeine Tablets 3355
Tonocard Tablets (Up to 1.2%) 649

Mouth, burning
Eldepryl Capsules 3266

Mouth, dry
(*see under* Xerostomia)

Mouth, fissuring in corner of
Parnate Tablets 1607

Mouth, puckering
Compazine 1505
Etrafon 3115
Haldol Decanoate 2535
Haldol Injection, Tablets and Concentrate 2533
Moban 1320
Navane Oral 2701
Navane Intramuscular 2703
Orap Tablets 1407
Serentil 1057
Stelazine 1640
Thorazine 1656
Trilafon 3160

Mouth, sore
Alferon N Injection (One patient) 1770
Flovent Diskus (1% to 3%) 3614
Gengraf Capsules (Rare) 457
▲ Imitrex Injection (4.9%) 1549
Neoral Soft Gelatin Capsules (Rare) 2380
Neoral Oral Solution (Rare) 2380
Oncaspar 756
Rifadin (Occasional) 765
Rifamate Capsules 767
Rifater Tablets (Occasional) 769

Movement, abnormal
Cognex Capsules (Infrequent) 1351
▲ Diprivan Injectable Emulsion (3% to 17%) 667
Gabitril Tablets (Infrequent) 1189
Hivid Tablets (Less than 1%) 2975
Lamictal (Rare) 1567
Neoral Soft Gelatin Capsules 2380
Neoral Oral Solution 2380
Oramorph SR Tablets (Less frequent) 3062
Orthoclone OKT3 Sterile Solution 2498
Prozac Pulvules, Liquid, and Weekly Capsules 1238
Sandimmune 2388
Sarafem Pulvules 1962
Zonegran Capsules (Infrequent) 1307
Zyprexa Tablets (1% to 5%) 1973
Zyprexa ZYDIS Orally Disintegrating Tablets (1% to 5%) 1973

Mucha-Habermann syndrome
Azulfidine EN-tabs Tablets (Rare) 2775

Mucocutaneous lymph node syndrome
(*see under* Kawasaki-like syndrome)

Mucormycosis
Desferal Vials (Rare) 2333

Mucosal pigmentation, changes
Aralen Tablets 3075
Intron A for Injection (Less than 5%) 3120
Minocin Oral Suspension 1865
Minocin Pellet-Filled Capsules 1863
Plaquenil Tablets 3082

Mucositis
Adriamycin PFS/RDF Injection 2767
Alferon N Injection (One patient) 1770
Aloprim for Injection (Less than 1%) 2292
AmBisome for Injection (Less common) 1383
Aphthasol Oral Paste (Infrequent) 1025
▲ Campath Ampules (1% to 14%) 992
Cerubidine for Injection 947
▲ Ellence Injection (8.9% to 58.5%) 2806
Evoxac Capsules (Less than 1%) 1217
Fludara for Injection (Up to 2%) 995
▲ Idamycin PFS Injection (50%) 2825
Intron A for Injection (Less than 5%) 3120
Myleran Tablets 1603
Mylocel Tablets 2227
▲ Mylotarg for Injection (35%) 3540
Navelbine Injection 1604
▲ Neumega for Injection (43%) 1434
▲ Neupogen for Injection (12%) 587
Neurontin Capsules (Rare) 2655
Neurontin Oral Solution (Rare) 2655
Neurontin Tablets (Rare) 2655
▲ Novantrone for Injection (18% to 29%) 1760
Oncaspar 756
▲ Paraplatin for Injection (1% to 10%) 1126
▲ Taxol Injection (18% to 45%) 1129
▲ Vesanoid Capsules (26%) 3037
Zithromax for IV Infusion (1% or less) 2748
▲ Zometa for Intravenous Infusion (5% to 10%) 3621

Mucous membrane, abnormalities
Aceon Tablets (2 mg, 4 mg, 8 mg) (0.3% to 1%) 3249
Actiq (Less than 1%) 1184
Baycol Tablets 883
Captopril Tablets (Approximately 1 in 1000 patients) 2281
Clinoril Tablets 2053
Dynacin Capsules 2019
Lescol Capsules 2361
Lescol Capsules 2925
Lescol XL Tablets 2361
Lescol XL Tablets 2925
▲ Leukine (75%) 1755
Mevacor Tablets 2132
Mexitil Capsules (About 1 in 1,000) 1047
Minocin Intravenous 1862
Minocin Oral Suspension 1865
Minocin Pellet-Filled Capsules 1863
Mintezol 2137
Monopril Tablets 1091
Naprelan Tablets (Less than 1%) 1293
Remeron Tablets 2483
Remeron SolTab Tablets 2486
Salagen Tablets (Less than 1%) 2229
Zocor Tablets 2219

Mucus, blood-tinted
Atrovent Nasal Spray 0.03% (2.0%) 1032
Flonase Nasal Spray (1% to 3%) 1533

Multiorgan system failure
Lamictal 1567
Levaquin 2537
Tasmar Tablets (One case) 3010

Muscle atrophy
Actiq (Less than 1%) 1184
Betaseron for SC Injection 988
Campath Ampules 992
Copaxone for Injection (Infrequent) 3306
Norcuron for Injection 2478
Permax Tablets (Rare) 1299

Virazole for Inhalation Solution ... 1747

Muscle cramp
(*see under* Cramping, muscular)

Muscle hypertonia
Trileptal Oral Suspension ... 2407
Trileptal Tablets ... 2407

Muscle hypotonia
Pipracil (Rare) ... 1866
▲ Xanax Tablets (6.3%) ... 2865

Muscle mass, loss
Celestone Soluspan Injectable Suspension ... 3097
Celestone Syrup ... 3099
Cortone Acetate Injectable Suspension ... 2059
Cortone Acetate Tablets ... 2061
Decadron Elixir ... 2078
Decadron Tablets ... 2079
Decadron Phosphate Injection ... 2081
Depo-Medrol Injectable Suspension ... 2795
Florinef Acetate Tablets ... 2250
Hydrocortone Tablets ... 2106
Hydrocortone Phosphate Injection, Sterile ... 2105
Pediapred Oral Solution ... 1170
Prednisone ... 3064
Prelone Syrup ... 2273
Solu-Medrol Sterile Powder ... 2855

Muscle movement, intraoperative
Dilaudid Oral Liquid (Less frequent) ... 445
Dilaudid Tablets - 8 mg (Less frequent) ... 445

Muscle rigidity
Advair Diskus 100/50 (1% to 3%) ... 1448
Advair Diskus 250/50 (1% to 3%) ... 1448
Advair Diskus 500/50 (1% to 3%) ... 1448
Amerge Tablets (Infrequent) ... 1467
Ceftin Tablets (0.1% to 1%) ... 1898
Clozaril Tablets ... 2319
Compazine ... 1505
Comtan Tablets ... 2328
Cozaar Tablets (Less than 1%) ... 2067
Cytotec Tablets (Infrequent) ... 3202
Dilaudid Oral Liquid (Less frequent) ... 445
Dilaudid Tablets - 8 mg (Less frequent) ... 445
Dilaudid-HP (Less frequent) ... 443
Etrafon ... 3115
Fortovase Capsules (Less than 2%) ... 2970
Haldol Decanoate ... 2535
Hivid Tablets (Less than 1%) ... 2975
Imitrex Injection (Rare) ... 1549
Imogam Rabies - HT (Uncommon) ... 805
Invirase Capsules (Less than 2%) ... 2979
Loxitane Capsules ... 3398
LYMErix Vaccine (0.95% to 2.47%) ... 1592
Miacalcin Nasal Spray (Less than 1%) ... 2375
Migranal Nasal Spray (1%; Rare) ... 2376
MS Contin Tablets (Less frequent) .. 2896
MSIR (Less frequent) ... 2898
Nardil Tablets (Less frequent) ... 2653
Navane Oral ... 2701
Navane Intramuscular ... 2703
Oramorph SR Tablets (Less frequent) ... 3062
▲ Orap Tablets (3 of 20 patients) ... 1407
Orthoclone OKT3 Sterile Solution ... 2498
Permax Tablets ... 1299
Phenergan ... 3556
ProSom Tablets (1%) ... 500
Reglan ... 2935
Risperdal ... 1796
Serentil ... 1057
Seroquel Tablets ... 684
Serzone Tablets (Infrequent) ... 1104
Stelazine ... 1640
Symmetrel (Uncommon) ... 1328
Tasmar Tablets (2%) ... 3010
Thioridazine Hydrochloride Tablets ... 2289
Thiothixene Capsules ... 2290
Thorazine ... 1656
Trilafon ... 3160
Versed Injection (0.3%) ... 3027
Wellbutrin Tablets ... 1680
Wellbutrin SR Sustained-Release Tablets ... 1684
Xanax Tablets (2.2%) ... 2865
Zyban Sustained-Release Tablets ... 1710

Muscle spasms
Advair Diskus 100/50 ... 1448
Advair Diskus 250/50 ... 1448
Advair Diskus 500/50 ... 1448
Aldoclor Tablets ... 2035
Aldoril Tablets ... 2039
Amerge Tablets (Infrequent) ... 1467
Aricept Tablets (Infrequent) ... 1270
Aricept Tablets (Infrequent) ... 2665
Atacand HCT Tablets ... 597
Avalide Tablets ... 1070
▲ Avonex (7%) ... 1013
Chirocaine Injection (Less than 1%) ... 2909
Clorpres Tablets ... 1002
Clozaril Tablets (1%) ... 2319
Combipres Tablets ... 1040
Corzide 40/5 Tablets ... 2247
Corzide 80/5 Tablets ... 2247
Diovan HCT Tablets ... 2338
Diucardin Tablets ... 3494
Diuril Oral ... 2087
Diuril Sodium Intravenous ... 2086
Dopram Injectable ... 2931
Etrafon ... 3115
Furosemide Tablets ... 2284
Halcion Tablets ... 2823
HydroDIURIL Tablets ... 2108
Hyzaar ... 2109
▲ Indapamide Tablets (Greater than or equal to 5%) ... 2286
Inderide Tablets ... 3517
Inderide LA Long-Acting Capsules ... 3519
Indocin I.V. (Less than 1%) ... 2115
Lamictal (1.0%) ... 1567
Lotensin HCT Tablets ... 2367
Loxitane Capsules ... 3398
Luvox Tablets (25, 50, 100 mg) (Infrequent) ... 3256
Maxalt Tablets (Infrequent) ... 2120
Maxalt-MLT Orally Disintegrating Tablets (Infrequent) ... 2120
Micardis HCT Tablets ... 1051
Microzide Capsules ... 3414
Migranal Nasal Spray (Rare) ... 2376
Minizide Capsules ... 2700
Moduretic Tablets (Less than or equal to 1%) ... 2138
Monopril HCT ... 1094
Parnate Tablets ... 1607
Prinzide Tablets ... 2168
Proleukin for Injection (1%) ... 1199
ProSom Tablets (Infrequent) ... 500
Prostigmin Injectable ... 1744
Prostigmin Tablets ... 1744
Renese Tablets ... 2712
Requip Tablets (1% or more) ... 1621
Retrovir Capsules ... 1625
Retrovir IV Infusion ... 1629
Retrovir ... 1625
Syprine Capsules ... 2186
Tenoretic Tablets ... 690
Timolide Tablets ... 2187
Tonocard Tablets (Less than 1%) ... 649
Uniretic Tablets ... 3178
Valium Injectable ... 3026
Valium Tablets ... 3047
Vancocin HCl Capsules & Pulvules ... 1972
Vancocin HCl Oral Solution ... 1971
Vancocin HCl, Vials & ADD-Vantage ... 1970
Vaseretic Tablets ... 2204
Vioxx (Greater than 0.1% to 1.9%) .. 2213
Wellbutrin Tablets (1.9%) ... 1680
Xanax Tablets (Rare) ... 2865
Zaroxolyn Tablets ... 1177
Zestoretic Tablets ... 695
Ziac Tablets ... 1887

Muscle twitching
(*see under* Fasciculations)

Muscle weakness
(*see under* Myasthenia)

Muscular disturbances
Copaxone for Injection (Infrequent) ... 3306
Felbatol ... 3343
▲ Foscavir Injection (5% or greater) .. 605
▲ Gengraf Capsules (12%) ... 457
Hivid Tablets (Less than 1%) ... 2975
Lescol Capsules ... 2361
Lescol Capsules ... 2925
Lescol XL Tablets ... 2361
Lescol XL Tablets ... 2925
▲ Neoral Soft Gelatin Capsules (12%) ... 2380
▲ Neoral Oral Solution (12%) ... 2380
Prometrium Capsules (100 mg, 200 mg) (Less than 5%) ... 3261
▲ Risperdal (17% to 34%) ... 1796
Roferon-A Injection (Less than 0.5%) ... 2996
Serevent Inhalation Aerosol (1% to 3%) ... 1633
Skelid Tablets (More than or equal to 1%) ... 3088
Vioxx (Greater than 0.1% to 1.9%) .. 2213
Zosyn (1.0% or less) ... 1890
Zosyn in Galaxy Containers (1.0% or less) ... 1894

Musculoskeletal contracture
Neurontin Capsules (Rare) ... 2655
Neurontin Oral Solution (Rare) ... 2655
Neurontin Tablets (Rare) ... 2655

Musculoskeletal symptoms, unspecified
Accutane Capsules ... 2944
Demadex Tablets and Injection ... 2965
▲ Epivir (12%) ... 1520
Flovent Diskus ... 3614
▲ Flovent (1% to 22%) ... 1535
Flovent Rotadisk (1% to 3%) ... 1537
Fortovase Capsules (0.6% to 2.0%) ... 2970
▲ Gengraf Capsules (13.2%) ... 457
Imdur Tablets (Less than or equal to 5%) ... 1826
▲ Infergen (4% to 7%) ... 1777
Invirase Capsules (0.6% to 2.0%) ... 2979
▲ Neoral Soft Gelatin Capsules (13.2%) ... 2380
▲ Neoral Oral Solution (13.2%) ... 2380
▲ Serostim for Injection (53.7%) ... 3229
Trasylol Injection (2%) ... 909

Musculoskeletal trauma
Apligraf (1.8%) ... 2305
Avalide Tablets ... 1070
Avapro Tablets (2%) ... 1074
Avapro Tablets (2%) ... 3076

Mutism
Lopid Tablets ... 2650
Luvox Tablets (25, 50, 100 mg) (Rare) ... 3256

Myalgia
Abelcet Injection ... 1273
Accolate Tablets (1.6%) ... 657
Accupril Tablets (1.5%) ... 2611
Accuretic Tablets (2.4%) ... 2614
Aceon Tablets (2 mg, 4 mg, 8 mg) (0.3% to 1.1%) ... 3249
Aciphex Tablets ... 1267
Aciphex Tablets ... 1783
▲ Actimmune (6%) ... 1772
Actiq (Less than 1%) ... 1184
Activella Tablets ... 2764
▲ Actonel Tablets (6.6%) ... 2879
▲ Actos Tablets (5.4%) ... 3275
Adalat CC Tablets (Less than 1.0%) ... 877
Aggrenox Capsules (1.2%) ... 1026
Agrylin Capsules (1% to 5%) ... 3232
Aldara Cream, 5% (1%) ... 1978
Aldoclor Tablets ... 2035
Aldomet Tablets ... 2037
Aldoril Tablets ... 2039
▲ Alferon N Injection (One patient to 45%) ... 1770
▲ Alphagan Ophthalmic Solution (Approximately 3% to 9%) ... 545
Altace Capsules (Less than 1%) ... 2233
▲ Ambien Tablets (1% to 7%) ... 3191
AmBisome for Injection (Less common) ... 1383
Amerge Tablets (Infrequent) ... 1467
Amicar Injection ... 3608
Amicar Syrup ... 3608
Amicar Tablets ... 3608
Amphotec (1% to 5%) ... 1774
Anaprox Tablets (Less than 1%) ... 2967
Anaprox DS Tablets (Less than 1%) ... 2967
Anectine Injection ... 1476
Anzemet Injection (Rare) ... 719
Anzemet Tablets (Rare) ... 722
Arava Tablets (1% to 3%) ... 724
▲ Aredia for Injection (26%) ... 2309
Arimidex Tablets (2% to 5%) ... 659
Arthrotec Tablets (Rare) ... 3195
▲ Asacol Delayed-Release Tablets (3%) ... 2884
Astelin Nasal Spray (1.5%) ... 3339
Atacand Tablets (0.5% or greater) .. 595
Atacand HCT Tablets (0.5% or greater) ... 597
Atromid-S Capsules (Less often) ... 3483
Augmentin Chewable Tablets ... 1482
Augmentin Powder for Oral Suspension ... 1482
Augmentin Tablets ... 1485
Augmentin ES-600 Powder for Oral Suspension ... 1487
Avalide Tablets ... 1070
Avapro Tablets (1% or greater) ... 1074
Avapro Tablets (1% or greater) ... 3076
Avelox Tablets (0.05% to 1%) ... 879
▲ Avonex (34%) ... 1013
Axert Tablets (Infrequent) ... 2772
Axid Pulvules (1.7%) ... 1903
Axid Pulvules (1.7%) ... 2919
Azactam for Injection (Less than 1%) ... 1276
Azmacort Inhalation Aerosol (1% to 3%) ... 728
Bactrim ... 2949
Baycol Tablets (2.5%) ... 883
Beconase Inhalation Aerosol ... 1497
Beconase AQ Nasal Spray ... 1498
Betapace Tablets (Rare) ... 950
Betapace AF Tablets (Rare) ... 954
▲ Betaseron for SC Injection (44%) ... 988
Calcijex Injection ... 411
Calcium Disodium Versenate Injection ... 1980
▲ Campath Ampules (11%) ... 992
Cancidas for Injection (Up to 3.1%) ... 2048
Captopril Tablets ... 2281
Carbatrol Capsules ... 3234
Cardura Tablets (1%) ... 2668
▲ Casodex Tablets (5%) ... 662
Catapres Tablets (About 6 in 1,000 patients) ... 1037
Catapres-TTS (0.5% or less) ... 1038
Ceclor CD Tablets (0.1% to 1%) ... 1279
Celebrex Capsules (0.1% to 1.9%) ... 2676
Celebrex Capsules (0.1% to 1.9%) ... 2780
Celexa (2%) ... 1365
▲ CellCept Capsules (3% to 12.5%) ... 2951
▲ CellCept Intravenous (3% to 12.5%) ... 2951
▲ CellCept Oral Suspension (3% to 12.5%) ... 2951
▲ CellCept Tablets (3% to 12.5%) ... 2951
▲ Cenestin Tablets (28%) ... 1263
Cerebyx Injection (Infrequent) ... 2619
Chibroxin Sterile Ophthalmic Solution ... 2051
Cipro I.V. ... 893
Cipro I.V. Pharmacy Bulk Package .. 897
Cipro ... 887
Claritin (At least one patient) ... 3100
Claritin-D 12 Hour Extended Release Tablets (Less frequent) ... 3102
Claritin-D 24 Hour Extended Release Tablets (Fewer than 2%) ... 3104
Clinoril Tablets (Less than 1 in 100) ... 2053
Clomid Tablets ... 735
Clorpres Tablets (About 6 in 1,000) ... 1002
Clozaril Tablets (1%) ... 2319
▲ Cognex Capsules (9%) ... 1351
Colazal Capsules (1%) ... 3069
Colestid Tablets ... 2791
Combipres Tablets (About 6 in 1,000) ... 1040
▲ Combivir Tablets (8%) ... 1502
Copaxone for Injection (At least 2%) ... 3306
▲ Coreg Tablets (3.4%) ... 1508
Cosmegen for Injection ... 2062
Coumadin for Injection ... 1243
Coumadin Tablets ... 1243
Cozaar Tablets (1.0%) ... 2067
▲ Crinone 4% Gel (8%) ... 3213
Crixivan Capsules (Less than 2%) ... 2070
Cytotec Tablets (Infrequent) ... 3202
Cytovene (At least 3 subjects) ... 2959
Dantrium Capsules (Less frequent) ... 2885
▲ DaunoXome Injection (Up to 7%) ... 1442
Demadex Tablets and Injection (1.6%) ... 2965
Depacon Injection (1% to 5%) ... 416
Depakene (1% to 5%) ... 421
Depakote Sprinkle Capsules (1% to 5%) ... 426
Depakote Tablets (1% to 5%) ... 430
Depakote ER Tablets (1% to 5%) ... 436
Desferal Vials ... 2333
D.H.E. 45 Injection ... 2334
DiaBeta Tablets ... 741
Diovan Capsules ... 2337
Diphtheria & Tetanus Toxoids Adsorbed Purogenated for Pediatric Use ... 1857
Diprivan Injectable Emulsion (Less than 1%) ... 667
Dolobid Tablets (Less than 1 in 100) ... 2088
Donnatal ... 2929
Donnatal Extentabs ... 2930
Donnatal Tablets ... 2929
Dostinex Tablets (2%) ... 2804
Doxil Injection (Less than 1% to 5%) ... 566
DTIC-Dome (Infrequent) ... 902
Duraclon Injection (About 0.6%) ... 3057
Dyazide Capsules ... 1515
Dynabac Tablets (0.1% to 1%) ... 2269
EC-Naprosyn Delayed-Release Tablets (Less than 1%) ... 2967
Effexor Tablets ... 3495
▲ Effexor XR Capsules (4%) ... 3499
Enalaprilat Injection ... 863
Engerix-B Vaccine (Less than 1%) ... 1517
▲ Epivir (8%) ... 1520
▲ Epivir-HBV (14%) ... 1524
Epogen for Injection (Rare) ... 582
Ergamisol Tablets (2% to 3%) ... 1789
▲ Evista Tablets (7.7%) ... 1915
Evoxac Capsules (1% to 3%) ... 1217
Exelon Capsules (Frequent) ... 2342
Exelon Oral Solution (Frequent) ... 2345
Famotidine Injection (Infrequent) ... 866
Felbatol (2.6%) ... 3343
▲ femhrt Tablets (7.8%) ... 2635
Ferrlecit Injection (Greater than 1%) ... 3386
Flexeril Tablets (Rare) ... 572
Flexeril Tablets (Rare) ... 2094
▲ Flolan for Injection (3% to 44%) ... 1528
▲ Flovent Diskus (1% to 12%) ... 3614
Flovent (1% to 3%) ... 1535
Flovent Rotadisk (1% to 3%) ... 1537

Floxin I.V. (Less than 1%)............... 2526
Floxin Tablets (Less than 1%).......... 2529
▲ Fludara for Injection (4% to 16%) 995
FluShield Influenza Vaccine............ 3521
Fluzone Vaccine.............................. 802
Fortovase Capsules (Less than 2%)..................................... 2970
▲ Fosamax Tablets (4.1% to approximately 6%)...................... 2095
Foscavir Injection (Between 1% and 5%)...................................... 605
Furosemide Tablets....................... 2284
Gabitril Tablets (1% to 5%)............ 1189
Gamimune N, 5% Solvent/Detergent Treated 925
Gamimune N, 10% Solvent/Detergent Treated.......... 928
Gammar-P I.V. 787
▲ Gastrocrom Oral Concentrate (3 of 87 patients)........................ 1162
Gemzar for Injection (Common)...... 1919
Gengraf Capsules (1% to less than 3%) 457
Genotropin Lyophilized Powder 2818
Geodon Capsules (1%) 2688
▲ Gleevec Capsules (7% to 18%) 2357
Glucophage Tablets (1% to 5%) 1080
Glucotrol XL Extended Release Tablets (Less than 3%) 2693
Glucovance Tablets 1086
Gonal-F for Injection 3216
Havrix Vaccine (Less than 1%) 1544
Hectorol Capsules 1064
Hectorol Injection 1066
Hivid Tablets (0.4%) 2975
▲ Humatrope Vials and Cartridges (9.1% to 13.5%)............................ 1930
Hytrin Capsules (At least 1%) 464
Hyzaar 2109
Imdur Tablets (Less than or equal to 5%).. 1826
Imitrex Injection (1.8%) 1549
Imitrex Nasal Spray (Infrequent) 1554
Imitrex Tablets (Frequent) 1558
▲ Imovax Rabies Vaccine (About 20%)... 807
INFeD Injection 3388
▲ Infergen (51% to 58%) 1777
▲ Intron A for Injection (3% to 75%) ... 3120
Invirase Capsules (0.3% to 1.0%) ... 2979
Iopidine 0.5% Ophthalmic Solution (0.2%) .... ⊙ 213
▲ JE-VAX Vaccine (Approximately 10%)... 811
Kaletra Capsules (Less than 2%) 471
Kaletra Oral Solution (Less than 2%) 471
Klonopin Tablets (1%) 2983
Lamictal (More than 1%) 1567
Lamisil Tablets 2360
▲ Lariam Tablets (Among most frequent) 2989
▲ Lescol Capsules (5.0%) 2361
▲ Lescol Capsules (5.0%) 2925
▲ Lescol XL Tablets (3.8%) 2361
▲ Lescol XL Tablets (3.8%) 2925
▲ Leukine (18%) 1755
▲ Leustatin Injection (7%) 2495
Levaquin (0.3% to less than 0.5%) .. 2537
Lexxel Tablets (Infrequent) 608
▲ Lipitor Tablets (Up to 5.6%) 2639
▲ Lipitor Tablets (Up to 5.6%) 2696
Lopid Tablets 2650
Lotensin Tablets (Less than 1%) 2365
Lotensin HCT Tablets (0.3% to 1%).. 2367
Lotrel Capsules 2370
Lupron Depot 3.75 mg (Less than 5%) 3281
Lupron Depot 7.5 mg (Less than 5%) 3284
Lupron Depot–3 Month 11.25 mg (0.6% to 1%) 3285
▲ Lupron Depot–4 Month 30 mg (Up to 8.2%) 3289
▲ Lupron Injection (5% or more) 3279
Luvox Tablets (25, 50, 100 mg) 3256
▲ LYMErix Vaccine (4.02% to 4.83%) 1592
Macrobid Capsules 2889
Macrodantin Capsules 2891
▲ Malarone (3% to 5%) 1596
Marinol Capsules (Less than 1%) 3325
Matulane Capsules 3246
▲ Mavik Tablets (4.7%) 478
Maxalt Tablets (Infrequent) 2120
Maxalt-MLT Orally Disintegrating Tablets (Infrequent) 2120
Maxzide 1008
Meridia Capsules (1.9%) 481
Meruvax II 2130
Mevacor Tablets (1.8% to 2.4%) 2132
Miacalcin Nasal Spray (1% to 3%) ... 2375
Micardis Tablets (1%) 1049
Micardis HCT Tablets 1051
Migranal Nasal Spray (Infrequent) ... 2376
M-M-R II 2118
Monopril Tablets (0.2% to 3.3%) 1091
Monopril HCT (Less than 2%) 1094
Monurol Sachet (Less than 1%) 1375
Mycobutin Capsules (2%) 2838
▲ Nabi-HB (5%) 2295
Naprelan Tablets (Less than 3%) 1293
Naprosyn Suspension (Less than 1%).. 2967
Naprosyn Tablets (Less than 1%)..... 2967
Naropin Injection (Less than 1%)..... 612
Nasacort Nasal Inhaler 750
Nascobal Gel................................. 3174
Nasonex Nasal Spray (Greater than or equal to 2%)................... 3131
Navelbine Injection (Less than 5%).. 1604
Neoral Soft Gelatin Capsules (1% to less than 3%)......................... 2380
Neoral Oral Solution (1% to less than 3%)...................................... 2380
▲ Neumega for Injection (Greater than or equal to 10%)................ 1434
Neupogen for Injection 587
Neurontin Capsules (2.0%)............. 2655
Neurontin Oral Solution (2.0%)....... 2655
Neurontin Tablets (2.0%)................ 2655
Niaspan Extended-Release Tablets 1846
▲ Nicotrol Nasal Spray (3%) 2843
Nimotop Capsules (Up to 1.4%) 904
▲ Nipent for Injection (11% to 19%) ... 3272
Nolvadex Tablets (2.8%) 678
Norditropin Cartridges 2420
Norditropin for Injection 2419
Noroxin Tablets 2145
▲ Norplant System (5% or greater) 3543
Norvasc Tablets (More than 0.1% to 1%) 2704
Norvir Capsules (1.7% to 2.2.%) 487
Norvir Oral Solution (1.7% to 2.2.%) 487
Oncaspar (Greater than 1% but less than 5%) 756
OptiPranolol Metipranolol Ophthalmic Solution 0.3% (A small number of patients) .... ⊙ 263
Orap Tablets (2.7%) 1407
Ortho Diaphragm Kits – All-Flex Arcing Spring; Ortho Coil Spring 2552
Orthoclone OKT3 Sterile Solution (Less than 1%) 2498
▲ Ortho-Prefest Tablets (5%) 2570
Orudis Capsules (Less than 1%) 3548
Oruvail Capsules (Less than 1%) 3548
Paxil (2%) 1609
Pentasa Capsules (Less than 1%) ... 3239
Pepcid Injection (Infrequent) 2153
Pepcid for Oral Suspension (Infrequent) 2150
Pepcid RPD Orally Disintegrating Tablets (Infrequent) 2150
Pepcid Tablets (Infrequent) 2150
Periostat Tablets (1%) 1208
Permax Tablets (1.1%) 1299
Persantine Tablets (Rare) 1057
Plendil Extended-Release Tablets (0.5% to 1.5%) 623
Pletal Tablets (2% to 3%) 2605
Pletal Tablets (2% to 3%) 2848
Pneumovax 23 2156
Pnu-Imune 23 (Occasional) 1868
Pravachol Tablets (0.6% to 2.7%) 1099
Prevacid Delayed-Release Capsules (Less than 1%) 3292
PREVPAC (Less than 1% to 3%) 3298
Prilosec Delayed-Release Capsules (Less than 1%) 628
Prinivil Tablets (0.3% to greater than 1%) 2164
Prinzide Tablets (0.3% to 1%) 2168
Procanbid Extended-Release Tablets (Fairly common) 2262
Procardia Capsules (Less than 0.5%) 2708
Procardia XL Extended Release Tablets (1% or less) 2710
Procrit for Injection (Rare) 2502
▲ Prograf (3% to 15%) 1393
▲ Proleukin for Injection (6%) 1199
Prometrium Capsules (100 mg, 200 mg) (Less than 5%) 3261
ProSom Tablets (Infrequent) 500
Prostin E2 Suppositories 2852
Protonix I.V. (Less than 1%) 3580
Protonix Tablets (Less than 1%) 3577
Protopic Ointment (Up to 3%) 1397
Provigil Tablets (At least 1%) 1193
Prozac Pulvules, Liquid, and Weekly Capsules (Less than 1%) 1238
Pulmicort Respules (1% to 3%) 632
Pulmicort Turbuhaler Inhalation Powder (1% to 3%) 636
Pyrazinamide Tablets (Frequent) 1876
Quinaglute Dura-Tabs Tablets 978
Quinidex Extentabs 2933
▲ Rapamune Oral Solution and Tablets (3% to 20%) 3584
▲ Rebetron Combination Therapy (61% to 64%) 3153
Recombivax HB (Less than 1%) 2178
ReFacto Vials 1437
Relenza Rotadisk (Less than 1.5%) 1619
Remeron Tablets (2%) 2483
Remeron SolTab Tablets (2%) 2486
Remicade for IV Injection (Less than 2%)...................................... 1178
ReoPro Vials (0.3%)....................... 1958
Requip Tablets (1% or more)........... 1621
Rescriptor Tablets (Less than 2%)... 526
▲ Retrovir Capsules (8%) 1625
▲ Retrovir IV Infusion (8%) 1629
▲ Retrovir (8%) 1625
Rhinocort Nasal Inhaler (Less than 1%).. 640
RhoGAM Injection 2524
Rifater Tablets (Frequent)................ 769
Risperdal (Infrequent)..................... 1796
▲ Rituxan for Infusion (7%) 1750
▲ Rituxan I.V. (7%) 1428
Rocaltrol 2991
▲ Roferon-A Injection (51% to 73%) ... 2996
Roxicodone Tablets (Less than 3%)... 3067
Salagen Tablets (1%)...................... 2229
Sandimmune (2% or less)............... 2388
Sandostatin Injection (Less than 1%) 2394
▲ Sandostatin LAR Depot (5% to 15%) 2395
Sectral Capsules (2%) 3589
Septra Suspension 2265
Septra Tablets 2265
Septra DS Tablets 2265
Serevent Inhalation Aerosol (1% to 3%) 1633
Serophene Tablets 3226
Serzone Tablets 1104
▲ Simulect for Injection (3% to 10%) . 2399
▲ Sonata Capsules (5% to 7%) 3591
▲ Soriatane Capsules (1% to 10%) 3003
Sporanox Capsules (1% to 3%) 1800
Sporanox Oral Solution (Less than 2%) 1808
Sporanox Oral Solution (Less than 2%) 2512
Streptase for Infusion 647
Stromectol Tablets (0.4%) 2185
Sular Tablets (Less than or equal to 1%) 688
Suprane Liquid for Inhalation (Less than 1%) 874
Sustiva Capsules (Less than 2%) 1258
▲ Synarel Nasal Solution for Endometriosis (10% of patients) .. 3205
Synercid I.V. (Less than 1%) 775
Synvisc 3596
Tagamet (Rare) 1644
Tambocor Tablets (Less than 1%) ... 1990
Tapazole Tablets 1823
Tarka Tablets (0.3% or more) 508
Tasmar Tablets (Frequent) 3010
▲ Taxol Injection (8% to 60%) 1129
Taxotere for Injection Concentrate .. 778
Tegretol/Tegretol-XR 2404
▲ Temodar Capsules (5%) 3157
Tenex Tablets (Less frequent) 2942
Tenoretic Tablets 690
Tequin Injection (Less than 0.1%) 1110
Tequin Tablets (Less than 0.1%) 1110
Testoderm Transdermal Systems (2%) 574
Tetanus & Diphtheria Toxoids Adsorbed for Adult Use 1880
Teveten Tablets (1% or greater) 3327
Thalomid Capsules 1154
▲ TheraCys Injection (7%) 823
Tiazac Capsules (2%) 1378
▲ Tice BCG, BCG Live (3%) 2489
Timentin Injection- ADD-Vantage Vial 1661
Timentin Injection-Galaxy Container 1664
Timentin Injection-Pharmacy Bulk Package 1666
Timentin for Intravenous Administration 1658
Timolide Tablets (Less than 1%) 2187
Tonocard Tablets (1.7%) 649
Topamax Sprinkle Capsules (1.2% to 1.8%) 2590
Topamax Tablets (1.2% to 1.8%) 2590
Toprol-XL Tablets 651
Toradol 3018
Tricor Capsules, Micronized (Less than 1%) 513
Tri-Nasal Spray (2.5% to 3.3%) 2274
▲ Trisenox Injection (25%) 1158
▲ Trizivir Tablets (8%) 1669
Trovan (Less than 1%) 2722
Twinrix Vaccine (Less than 1%) 1674
▲ TYPHIM Vi Vaccine (2% to 7.4%) 825
Uniretic Tablets (Less than 1%) 3178
Univasc Tablets (1.3%) 3181
Valstar Sterile Solution for Intravesical Instillation (1%) 1175
Vancenase AQ Nasal Spray 0.084% (2%) 3163
Vantin Tablets and Oral Suspension (Less than 1%) 2860
Vaqta (1.9%) 2199
Varivax (Greater than or equal to 1%) 2202
Vaseretic Tablets 2204
Vasotec I.V. Injection 2207
Vasotec Tablets (0.5% to 1.0%) 2210
Verelan Capsules (1.1%) 3184
▲ Vesanoid Capsules (14%) 3037
Viagra Tablets (Less than 2%)......... 2732
Vicoprofen Tablets (Less than 1%).. 520
Videx... 1138
Videx EC Capsules 1143
Vioxx (Greater than 0.1% to 1.9%).. 2213
Viracept 532
Viramune Oral Suspension.............. 1060
Viramune Tablets........................... 1060
Vistide Injection 1445
Warfarin Sodium Tablets, USP 3302
WelChol Tablets (2%)..................... 3073
Wellbutrin Tablets 1680
▲ Wellbutrin SR Sustained-Release Tablets (2% to 6%)..................... 1684
WinRho SDF 2297
Xalatan Latanoprost Ophthalmic Solution (1% to 2%)................. ⊙ 320
Xalatan Sterile Ophthalmic Solution (1% to 2%)................. 2864
Xeloda Tablets 3039
▲ Xenical Capsules (4.2%) 3043
Xopenex Inhalation Solution 3207
▲ YF-VAX Vaccine (2% to 5%) 827
Zantac (Rare)................................ 1690
Zantac Injection (Rare).................... 1688
Zantac Syrup (Rare)....................... 1690
Zebeta Tablets 1885
▲ Zenapax for Injection (2% to 5%) 3046
▲ Zerit (32%) 1147
Zestoretic Tablets (0.3% to 1%)...... 695
Zestril Tablets (0.3% to 1.0%)......... 698
Ziac Tablets (Up to 2.4%)............... 1887
Ziagen 1692
Zocor Tablets 2219
▲ Zofran Injection (10%) 1698
▲ Zoladex (3%) 702
Zoladex 3-month 706
Zoloft (Frequent)........................... 2751
Zometa for Intravenous Infusion...... 3621
Zomig Tablets (1% to 2%)............... 708
Zomig-ZMT Tablets (1% to 2%)........ 708
Zonegran Capsules (Infrequent)...... 1307
Zosyn (1.0% or less)...................... 1890
Zosyn in Galaxy Containers (1.0% or less)...................................... 1894
Zovirax Capsules 1706
Zovirax for Injection 1708
Zovirax 1706
Zyban Sustained-Release Tablets (2% to 4%).................................. 1710
▲ Zyflo Filmtab Tablets (3.2%) 524
Zyprexa Tablets 1973
Zyprexa ZYDIS Orally Disintegrating Tablets.................. 1973
Zyrtec (Less than 2%)..................... 2756
Zyrtec-D 12 Hour Extended Relief Tablets (Less than 2%)................ 2758

Myasthenia

Actiq (Less than 1%)...................... 1184
▲ Actonel Tablets (3.3%) 2879
Ambien Tablets (Rare)..................... 3191
Amicar Injection............................ 3608
Amicar Syrup 3608
Amicar Tablets 3608
Anaprox Tablets (Less than 1%)....... 2967
Anaprox DS Tablets (Less than 1%) 2967
Anectine Injection.......................... 1476
Aricept Tablets (Infrequent)............ 1270
Aricept Tablets (Infrequent)............ 2665
Atromid-S Capsules (Less often)..... 3483
Avalide Tablets 1070
Axert Tablets (Infrequent)............... 2772
Baycol Tablets 883
Betagan .... ⊙ 228
Campath Ampules 992
Cardura Tablets (1%)...................... 2668
Carnitor Tablets and Oral Solution.... 3245
Carteolol Hydrochloride Ophthalmic Solution USP, 1% ..... ⊙ 258
Celestone Soluspan Injectable Suspension 3097
Celestone Syrup 3099
Celexa (Infrequent) 1365
▲ CellCept Capsules (12.5%) 2951
▲ CellCept Intravenous (12.5%) 2951
▲ CellCept Oral Suspension (12.5%) . 2951
▲ CellCept Tablets (12.5%) 2951
Clozaril Tablets (1%)...................... 2319
Combivir Tablets............................ 1502
Compazine 1505
Copaxone for Injection (At least 2%) 3306
Cozaar Tablets (Less than 1%)........ 2067
Crixivan Capsules (Less than 2%).... 2070
Decadron Tablets 2079
Decadron Phosphate Injection......... 2081
Depakene (1% to 5%) 421
Depakote Tablets 430
Depakote ER Tablets (1% to 5%)..... 436
Depen Titratable Tablets................. 3341
Depo-Medrol Injectable Suspension 2795
Doxil Injection (Less than 1%)......... 566
EC-Naprosyn Delayed-Release Tablets (Less than 1%)................ 2967
Effexor XR Capsules (Infrequent)..... 3499
Epivir 1520
Ergamisol Tablets 1789
Eskalith 1527

Etrafon 3115
Evoxac Capsules (Less than 1%) 1217
Exelon Capsules (Infrequent) 2342
Exelon Oral Solution (Infrequent) 2345
Felbatol 3343
Florinef Acetate Tablets 2250
Foscavir Injection 605
Gabitril Tablets (1%) 1189
Hivid Tablets (Less than 1%) 2975
Humorsol Sterile Ophthalmic Solution (Infrequent) 2102
Hydrocortone Tablets 2106
Hydrocortone Acetate Injectable Suspension 2103
Hydrocortone Phosphate Injection, Sterile 2105
Hyzaar 2109
Imdur Tablets (Less than or equal to 5%) 1826
Intron A for Injection (Less than 5%) 3120
Klonopin Tablets 2983
Lescol Capsules 2361
Lescol Capsules 2925
Lescol XL Tablets 2361
Lescol XL Tablets 2925
Levaquin (Less than 0.3%) 2537
Levoxyl Tablets 1819
Lithium Carbonate 3061
Lithium Citrate Syrup 3061
Lithobid Slow-Release Tablets 3255
Lopid Tablets 2650
Lotensin HCT Tablets 2367
Maxzide 1008
Mestinon 1740
Mevacor Tablets 2132
Migranal Nasal Spray (Infrequent) 2376
Mirapex Tablets (1%) 2834
▲ Myobloc Injectable Solution (3% to 6%) 1291
▲ Naprelan Tablets (3% to 9%) 1293
Naprosyn Suspension (Less than 1%) 2967
Naprosyn Tablets (Less than 1%) 2967
▲ Navelbine Injection (Up to 15% to 20%) 1604
Norcuron for Injection 2478
Norvasc Tablets (Less than or equal to 0.1%) 2704
Norvir Capsules (Less than 2%) 487
Norvir Oral Solution (Less than 2%) 487
Ocupress Ophthalmic Solution, 1% Sterile .... ⊙ 303
Pediapred Oral Solution 1170
Plaquenil Tablets 3082
Pravachol Tablets 1099
Prednisone 3064
Prelone Syrup 2273
Prilosec Delayed-Release Capsules (Less than 1%) 628
Prostigmin Injectable 1744
Prostigmin Tablets 1744
Protopam Chloride for Injection 3582
Proventil Repetabs Tablets (2%) 3148
Recombivax HB 2178
ReFacto Vials 1437
Requip Tablets (Infrequent) 1621
Rescriptor Tablets (Less than 2%) 526
Retrovir Capsules 1625
Retrovir IV Infusion 1629
Retrovir 1625
Rifadin (Rare) 765
Rifamate Capsules 767
Rifater Tablets 769
Rythmol Tablets – 150 mg, 225 mg, 300 mg (Less than 1%) 502
Salagen Tablets (Less than 1%) 2229
Sarafem Pulvules (Rare) 1962
▲ Serostim for Injection (1% to 10%) 3229
Solu-Medrol Sterile Powder 2855
Sonata Capsules (Infrequent) 3591
Soriatane Capsules (Less than 1%) 3003
Stelazine 1640
Synercid I.V. (Less than 1%) 775
Tensilon Injectable 1745
Tequin Injection (Less than 0.1%) 1110
Tequin Tablets (Less than 0.1%) 1110
Thalomid Capsules 1154
Topamax Sprinkle Capsules (Frequent) 2590
Topamax Tablets (Frequent) 2590
Tricor Capsules, Micronized (Less than 1%) 513
Trilafon 3160
Trileptal Oral Suspension (1% to 2%) 2407
Trileptal Tablets (1% to 2%) 2407
Trizivir Tablets 1669
Trovan (Less than 1%) 2722
Unithroid Tablets 3445
Viagra Tablets (Less than 2%) 2732
Vioxx (Greater than 0.1% to 1.9%) 2213
Vistide Injection 1445
▲ Visudyne for Injection (1% to 10%) .... ⊙ 308
Wellbutrin Tablets 1680
Xanax Tablets 2865
Zocor Tablets 2219
Zoloft (Infrequent) 2751
Zomig Tablets (1% to 2%) 708
Zomig-ZMT Tablets (1% to 2%) 708
Zonegran Capsules (Infrequent) 1307
Zyrtec (Less than 2%) 2756
Zyrtec-D 12 Hour Extended Relief Tablets (Less than 2%) 2758

Myasthenia gravis
Abelcet Injection 1273
Avonex 1013
▲ Betaseron for SC Injection (13%) 988
Blocadren Tablets (Less than 1%) 2046
Captopril Tablets 2281
▲ Casodex Tablets (7%) 662
Cerebyx Injection (Frequent) 2619
Cuprimine Capsules 2075
Cytovene (At least 3 subjects) 2959
Depacon Injection (1% to 5%) 416
Depakote Sprinkle Capsules (1% to 5%) 426
Depakote Tablets (1% to 5%) 430
Depen Titratable Tablets 3341
Effexor Tablets (Infrequent) 3495
Eskalith (Rare) 1527
Lamictal (1.3%) 1567
Lipitor Tablets (Less than 2%) 2639
Lipitor Tablets (Less than 2%) 2696
Luvox Tablets (25, 50, 100 mg) (Infrequent) 3256
LYMErix Vaccine (Greater than 1%) 1592
Myleran Tablets (Rare) 1603
Naprelan Tablets (Less than 1%) 1293
Paxil (1%) 1609
▲ Prograf (3% to 15%) 1393
Prozac Pulvules, Liquid, and Weekly Capsules (Rare) 1238
Remeron Tablets (Frequent) 2483
Remeron SolTab Tablets (Frequent) 2486
Rilutek Tablets (Infrequent) 772
Sular Tablets (Less than or equal to 1%) 688
Syprine Capsules 2186
Timolide Tablets 2187
Tonocard Tablets (Less than 1%) 649
Viracept 532
Zanaflex Tablets (Frequent) 1305

Myasthenia gravis, exacerbation of
Betoptic S Ophthalmic Suspension 537
Chibroxin Sterile Ophthalmic Solution 2051
Cipro I.V. 893
Cipro I.V. Pharmacy Bulk Package (Less than 1%) 897
Cipro 887
Cosopt Sterile Ophthalmic Solution 2065
Floxin I.V. (Possible) 2526
Floxin Tablets (Possible) 2529
Mefoxin for Injection (A possibility) 2124
Mefoxin Premixed Intravenous Solution 2127
Mykrox Tablets (exacerbation of) 1168
Noroxin Tablets 2145
Timolol GFS .... ⊙ 266
Timoptic Sterile Ophthalmic Solution (Less frequent) 2190
Timoptic-XE Sterile Ophthalmic Gel Forming Solution 2194

Myasthenia gravis, increase
Betagan .... ⊙ 228
Betimol Ophthalmic Solution .... ⊙ 324
Timoptic in Ocudose (Less frequent) 2192

Myasthenia gravis-like syndrome
Clozaril Tablets 2319
Declomycin Tablets (Rare) 1855
Seroquel Tablets (Infrequent) 684

Mydriasis
Albalon Ophthalmic Solution .... ⊙ 225
Artane 1855
Betaseron for SC Injection 988
Blephamide Ophthalmic Ointment (Occasional) 547
Blephamide Ophthalmic Suspension 548
Caverject Sterile Powder (Less than 1%) 2777
Celexa (Rare) 1365
Cerebyx Injection (Infrequent) 2619
Claritin-D 12 Hour Extended Release Tablets (Less frequent) 3102
Claritin-D 24 Hour Extended Release Tablets (Fewer than 2%) 3104
Clear Eyes ACR Astringent/Lubricant Eye Redness Reliever .... ⊙ 322
Clear Eyes Lubricant Eye Redness Reliever .... ⊙ 322
Clozaril Tablets (Less than 1%) 2319
Cogentin 2055
Compazine 1505
Copaxone for Injection (Infrequent) 3306
Donnatal 2929
Donnatal Extentabs 2930
Donnatal Tablets 2929
Dopram Injectable 2931
Effexor Tablets (2%) 3495
Effexor XR Capsules (Frequent) 3499
Etrafon (Occasional) 3115
Evoxac Capsules (Less than 1%) 1217
Extendryl 1361
FML Ophthalmic Ointment (Occasional) .... ⊙ 237
FML Ophthalmic Suspension (Occasional) .... ⊙ 236
FML Forte Ophthalmic Suspension (Occasional) .... ⊙ 235
Healon GV .... ⊙ 320
Imitrex Nasal Spray 1554
Imitrex Tablets (Rare) 1558
Inversine Tablets 1850
Iopidine Sterile Ophthalmic Solution (Less than 2%) .... ⊙ 212
Levsin/Levsinex/Levbid 3172
Limbitrol 1738
Lodosyn Tablets 1251
Luvox Tablets (25, 50, 100 mg) (Infrequent) 3256
Meridia Capsules 481
Murine Tears Plus Lubricant Redness Reliever Eye Drops .... ⊙ 323
Navane Oral 2701
Navane Intramuscular 2703
Norflex 1987
Norpramin Tablets 755
NuLev Orally Disintegrating Tablets 3176
Ocufen Ophthalmic Solution .... ⊙ 242
Paxil (Infrequent) 1609
Pred Forte Ophthalmic Suspension (Occasional) .... ⊙ 246
Pred Mild Sterile Ophthalmic Suspension (Occasional) .... ⊙ 249
Propine Ophthalmic Solution .... ⊙ 250
Prozac Pulvules, Liquid, and Weekly Capsules (Infrequent) 1238
Quinaglute Dura-Tabs Tablets (Occasional) 978
Quinidex Extentabs (Occasional) 2933
Robinul Forte Tablets 1358
Robinul Injectable 2940
Robinul Tablets 1358
Rynatan Tablets 3351
Sarafem Pulvules (Infrequent) 1962
Serzone Tablets (Infrequent) 1104
Sinemet Tablets 1253
Sinemet CR Tablets 1255
Soma Tablets 3353
Soma Compound Tablets (Very rare) 3354
Soma Compound w/Codeine Tablets (Very rare) 3355
Stelazine 1640
Surmontil Capsules 3595
Symmetrel 1328
Testoderm Transdermal Systems (1%) 574
Thioridazine Hydrochloride Tablets 2289
Thiothixene Capsules 2290
Thorazine 1656
Topamax Sprinkle Capsules (Infrequent) 2590
Topamax Tablets (Infrequent) 2590
Transderm Scōp Transdermal Therapeutic System 2302
Trilafon (Occasional) 3160
Trileptal Oral Suspension 2407
Trileptal Tablets 2407
Viagra Tablets (Less than 2%) 2732
Vivactil Tablets 2217
Vivactil Tablets 2446
Wellbutrin Tablets (Infrequent) 1680
Wellbutrin SR Sustained-Release Tablets 1684
Zaditor Ophthalmic Solution (Less than 5%) 2304
Zoloft (Infrequent) 2751
Zyban Sustained-Release Tablets 1710
Zyprexa Tablets (Rare) 1973
Zyprexa ZYDIS Orally Disintegrating Tablets (Rare) 1973

Myelitis
Diphtheria & Tetanus Toxoids Adsorbed Purogenated for Pediatric Use 1857
Havrix Vaccine (Rare) 1544
Paxil (Rare) 1609
Permax Tablets (Rare) 1299
Rabies Vaccine RabAvert (One case) 1203
Recombivax HB 2178
Tetanus & Diphtheria Toxoids Adsorbed for Adult Use 1880
Twinrix Vaccine 1674
Zyrtec (Less than 2%) 2756
Zyrtec-D 12 Hour Extended Relief Tablets (Less than 2%) 2758

Myelitis, transverse
Asacol Delayed-Release Tablets (Rare) 2884
Azulfidine EN-tabs Tablets (Rare) 2775
Bicillin C-R 900/300 Injection 2240
Bicillin C-R Injection 2238
Bicillin L-A Injection 2242
Enbrel for Injection (Rare) 1752
Enbrel for Injection (Rare) 3504
Engerix-B Vaccine 1517
JE-VAX Vaccine (One case) 811
Recombivax HB 2178
Twinrix Vaccine 1674
Varivax 2202

Myelodysplastic syndrome
Azulfidine EN-tabs Tablets (Rare) 2775
Neupogen for Injection (Approximately 3%) 587

Myelofibrosis
Mexitil Capsules (About 2 in 10,000) 1047

Myelopathy
Cytovene 2959
Diphtheria & Tetanus Toxoids Adsorbed Purogenated for Pediatric Use 1857
Tetanus & Diphtheria Toxoids Adsorbed for Adult Use 1880

Myelopolyradiculoneuritis
Fortovase Capsules (Less than 2%) 2970
Invirase Capsules (Less than 2%) 2979

Myelosuppression
Adriamycin PFS/RDF Injection 2767
Alkeran for Injection 1465
▲ Cerubidine for Injection (All patients) 947
DaunoXome Injection 1442
Doxil Injection 566
▲ Fludara for Injection (Among most common) 995
Gemzar for Injection 1919
Hexalen Capsules 2226
Idamycin PFS Injection 2825
Ifex for Injection 1123
Leukeran Tablets 1591
Leustatin Injection (Frequent) 2495
▲ Myleran Tablets (Most frequent) 1603
Mylotarg for Injection 3540
▲ Navelbine Injection (53%) 1604
Novantrone for Injection 1760
Purinethol Tablets 1615
Roferon-A Injection 2996
▲ Tabloid Tablets (Most frequent) 1642
Temodar Capsules 3157
Zinecard for Injection 2869

Myelosuppression, persistent severe
Adriamycin PFS/RDF Injection 2767
Novantrone for Injection 1760

Myocardial hypertrophy
Prograf (Rare) 1393

Myocardial infarction
▲ Abelcet Injection (3%) 1273
Accupril Tablets (Rare) 2611
Accuretic Tablets (0.5% to 1%) 2614
Aceon Tablets (2 mg, 4 mg, 8 mg) (0.3% to 1%) 3249
Aciphex Tablets 1267
Aciphex Tablets 1783
Actimmune (Rare) 1772
Activella Tablets 2764
Adenoscan (Less than 1%) 1381
Agrylin Capsules 3232
Alesse-21 Tablets 3468
Alesse-28 Tablets 3473
Altace Capsules (Less than 1% to 1.7%) 2233
Ambien Tablets (Rare) 3191
Amerge Tablets 1467
Aricept Tablets (Infrequent) 1270
Aricept Tablets (Infrequent) 2665
Arimidex Tablets 659
Arthrotec Tablets (Rare) 3195
Atacand Tablets (Less frequently) 595
Atacand HCT Tablets (Less than 0.5%) 597
Avalide Tablets 1070
Avapro Tablets (Less than 1%) 1074
Avapro Tablets (Less than 1%) 3076
Betaseron for SC Injection 988
Brevicon 28-Day Tablets 3380
Campath Ampules 992
Captopril Tablets (2 to 3 of 1000 patients) 2281
Carbatrol Capsules 3234
Cardene I.V. 3485
Cardizem CD Capsules (Infrequent) 1016
Cardura Tablets (Less than 0.5%) 2668
Cataflam Tablets (Less than 1%) 2315
Celebrex Capsules (0.1% to 1.9%) 2676
Celebrex Capsules (0.1% to 1.9%) 2780

Celexa (Infrequent) 1365
Cipro I.V. (1% or less) 893
Cipro I.V. Pharmacy Bulk Package (Less than 1%) 897
Cipro (Less than 1%) 887
Climara Transdermal System 958
Clozaril Tablets (Several patients) 2319
Cognex Capsules (Infrequent) 1351
Corlopam Injection (0.5% to 5%) 412
Cosopt Sterile Ophthalmic Solution (Less than 1%) 2065
Covera-HS Tablets (Less than 2%) 3199
Cozaar Tablets (Less than 1%) 2067
Crixivan Capsules 2070
Cyclessa Tablets 2450
DDAVP Injection 4 mcg/mL (Rare) 737
Desmopressin Acetate Injection (Rare) 1344
Desogen Tablets 2458
D.H.E. 45 Injection (Extremely rare) 2334
Diprivan Injectable Emulsion (Less than 1%) 667
DynaCirc Capsules (0.5% to 1%) 2921
DynaCirc CR Tablets (0.5% to 1%) 2923
Effexor Tablets (Rare) 3495
Effexor XR Capsules (Infrequent) 3499
▲ Emcyt Capsules (3%) 2810
Enalaprilat Injection (0.5% to 1%) 863
Enbrel for Injection (Infrequent) 1752
Enbrel for Injection (Infrequent) 3504
Epogen for Injection (0.4%) 582
Estrace Vaginal Cream 3358
Estrace Tablets 3361
Estratest 3252
Estrostep 2627
Etrafon 3115
Evoxac Capsules (Less than 1%) 1217
Exelon Capsules (Frequent) 2342
Exelon Oral Solution (Frequent) 2345
Fareston Tablets (1%) 3237
Feiba VH 843
Feldene Capsules (Rare) 2685
Femara Tablets (Less than or equal to 2%) 2351
Ferrlecit Injection (Greater than 1%) 3386
Flexeril Tablets (Rare) 572
Flexeril Tablets (Rare) 2094
▲ Flolan for Injection (4%) 1528
Fludara for Injection (Up to 3%) 995
Gabitril Tablets (Infrequent) 1189
Gemzar for Injection (2%) 1919
Gengraf Capsules (1% to less than 3%) 457
Heparin Lock Flush Solution 3509
Heparin Sodium Injection 3511
Hyzaar 2109
Idamycin PFS Injection 2825
Imdur Tablets (Less than or equal to 5%) 1826
Imitrex Injection (Extremely rare) 1549
Imitrex Nasal Spray 1554
Imitrex Tablets (Rare) 1558
Innohep Injection 1248
Isoptin SR Tablets (1% or less) 467
Lamictal (Rare) 1567
Levaquin (0.3% to less than 0.5%) 2537
Levlen 962
Levlite 21 Tablets 962
Levlite 28 Tablets 962
Levora Tablets 3389
Levoxyl Tablets 1819
Lexxel Tablets 608
Limbitrol 1700
Lodine (Less than 1%) 3528
Lodine XL Extended-Release Tablets (Less than 1%) 3530
Lodosyn Tablets 1251
Loestrin 21 Tablets 2642
Loestrin Fe Tablets 2642
Lo/Ovral Tablets 3532
Lo/Ovral-28 Tablets 3538
Lotrel Capsules (Rare) 2370
Low-Ogestrel-28 Tablets 3392
Lunelle Monthly Injection 2827
Lupron Injection (Less than 5%) 3279
Luvox Tablets (25, 50, 100 mg) (Infrequent) 3256
Maxalt Tablets (Very rare) 2120
Maxalt-MLT Orally Disintegrating Tablets (Very rare) 2120
Menest Tablets 2254
Meridia Capsules 481
Merrem I.V. (0.1% to 1.0%) 673
Miacalcin Nasal Spray (Less than 1%) 2375
Microgestin Fe 1.5/30 Tablets 3407
Microgestin Fe 1/20 Tablets 3400
Mirapex Tablets (Less than 1%) 2834
Mircette Tablets 2470
Mobic Tablets (Less than 2%) 1054
Modicon 2563
Monopril Tablets (0.2% to 1.0%) 1091
Monopril HCT 1094
Naprelan Tablets (Less than 1%) 1293
Naropin Injection (Less than 1%) 612
Navelbine Injection (Rare) 1604
Necon 3415
Neoral Soft Gelatin Capsules (1% to less than 3%) 2380
Neoral Oral Solution (1% to less than 3%) 2380
▲ Neupogen for Injection (11 of 375 cancer patients) 587
Neurontin Capsules (Rare) 2655
Neurontin Oral Solution (Rare) 2655
Neurontin Tablets (Rare) 2655
Nordette-28 Tablets 2257
Norinyl 1 +35 28-Day Tablets 3380
Norinyl 1 + 50 28-Day Tablets 3380
Normodyne Injection 3135
Normodyne Tablets 3137
Noroxin Tablets (Less frequent) 2145
Norplant System 3543
Norpramin Tablets 755
Norvasc Tablets (Rare) 2704
Ogen Tablets 2846
Ogestrel 0.5/50-28 Tablets 3428
Omnicef 493
OptiPranolol Metipranolol Ophthalmic Solution 0.3% (A small number of patients) ⊙ 263
Ortho Dienestrol Cream 2554
Ortho-Cept 21 Tablets 2546
Ortho-Cept 28 Tablets 2546
Orthoclone OKT3 Sterile Solution (Less than 1%) 2498
Ortho-Cyclen/Ortho Tri-Cyclen 2573
Ortho-Est Tablets 3464
Ortho-Novum 2563
Ortho-Novum 1/50□28 Tablets 2556
Ortho-Cyclen/Ortho Tri-Cyclen 2573
Orudis Capsules (Rare) 3548
Oruvail Capsules (Rare) 3548
Ovcon 3364
Ovral Tablets 3551
Ovral-28 Tablets 3552
Ovrette Tablets 3552
Paxil (Rare) 1609
PEG-Intron Powder for Injection (Less than or equal to 1%) 3140
Permax Tablets (1.1%) 1299
Photofrin for Injection 831
Plendil Extended-Release Tablets (0.5% to 1.5%) 623
Pletal Tablets (Less than 2%) 2605
Pletal Tablets (Less than 2%) 2848
Ponstel Capsules (Rare) 1356
Prandin Tablets (0.5, 1, and 2 mg) (Less than or equal to 1%) 2432
Premarin Intravenous 3563
Premarin Tablets 3566
Premarin Vaginal Cream 3570
Premphase Tablets 3572
Prempro Tablets 3572
Prevacid Delayed-Release Capsules (Less than 1%) 3292
PREVPAC (Less than 1%) 3298
Prinivil Tablets (0.3% to 1.0%) 2164
Prinzide Tablets 2168
Procardia Capsules (Rare) 2708
▲ Procardia XL Extended Release Tablets (About 4%) 2710
Procrit for Injection (0.4%) 2502
Proleukin for Injection (2%) 1199
Prostin E2 Suppositories (Two cases) 2852
Prozac Pulvules, Liquid, and Weekly Capsules (Infrequent) 1238
Relafen Tablets (Less than 1%) 1617
Remeron Tablets (Infrequent) 2483
Remeron SolTab Tablets (Infrequent) 2486
Remicade for IV Injection (Less than 2%) 1178
Rilutek Tablets (Infrequent) 772
Risperdal (Infrequent) 1796
Rituxan I.V. 1428
Roferon-A Injection (Rare to infrequent) 2996
Salagen Tablets (One patient) 2229
Sandimmune (Rare) 2388
Sandostatin LAR Depot (Rare) 2395
Sarafem Pulvules (Infrequent) 1962
Sinemet Tablets 1253
Sinemet CR Tablets 1255
Streptase for Infusion 647
Sular Tablets (Less than or equal to 1%) 688
Suprane Liquid for Inhalation (Less than 1%) 874
Surmontil Capsules 3595
Tarka Tablets (Less frequent) 508
Tasmar Tablets (Infrequent) 3010
Taxol Injection (Rare) 1129
Tegretol/Tegretol-XR 2404
Tenex Tablets (Rare) 2942
Thalomid Capsules 1154
Thyrogen for Injection (One patient) 1441
Tiazac Capsules 1378
Tikosyn Capsules (Less than or equal to 2%) 2717
Tonocard Tablets (Less than 1%) 649
Toprol-XL Tablets (Greater than 1%) 651
▲ Trasylol Injection (6%) 909
Tricor Capsules, Micronized 513
Tri-Levlen 962
Tri-Norinyl-28 Tablets 3433
Triostat Injection (2%) 1825
Triphasil-21 Tablets 3600
Triphasil-28 Tablets 3605
Trivora Tablets 3439
Uniretic Tablets (Less than 1%) 3178
Unithroid Tablets 3445
Univasc Tablets (Less than 1%) 3181
Vascor Tablets (About 3% of patients) 2602
Vaseretic Tablets 2204
Vasotec I.V. Injection (0.5% to 1%) 2207
Vasotec Tablets (0.5% to 1.2%) 2210
Verelan Capsules (1% or less) 3184
Verelan PM Capsules (2% or less) 3186
▲ Vesanoid Capsules (3%) 3037
Viagra Tablets 2732
Vioxx (Less than 0.1%) 2213
Vivactil Tablets 2217
Vivactil Tablets 2446
Voltaren Tablets (Less than 1%) 2315
Voltaren-XR Tablets (Less than 1%) 2315
Wellbutrin Tablets (Rare) 1680
Wellbutrin SR Sustained-Release Tablets 1684
Yasmin 28 Tablets 980
Zanaflex Tablets (Rare) 1305
Zestoretic Tablets 695
Zestril Tablets (0.3% to 1.0%) 698
Zoladex (1% to 5%) 702
Zoladex 3-month 706
Zoloft (Rare) 2751
Zomig Tablets 708
Zomig-ZMT Tablets 708
Zosyn (1.0% or less) 1890
Zosyn in Galaxy Containers (1.0% or less) 1894
Zovia 3449
Zyban Sustained-Release Tablets 1710

Myocardial infarction, post-abrupt discontinuation

Inderal (Some cases) 3513
Inderal LA Long-Acting Capsules (Some cases) 3516
Tenoretic Tablets 690
Tenormin 692

Myocardial insufficiency

Idamycin PFS Injection 2825
Orthoclone OKT3 Sterile Solution 2498

Myocardial reinfarction

Activase I.V. 1410
TNKase I.V. 1430

Myocardial rupture

Activase I.V. 1410
Cortone Acetate Injectable Suspension 2059
Cortone Acetate Tablets 2061
Decadron Elixir 2078
Decadron Tablets 2079
Decadron Phosphate Injection 2081
Hydrocortone Tablets 2106
Hydrocortone Acetate Injectable Suspension 2103
Hydrocortone Phosphate Injection, Sterile 2105
Prednisone 3064
Retavase Vials 1182
TNKase I.V. 1430

Myocarditis

Aldoclor Tablets 2035
Aldomet Tablets 2037
Aldoril Tablets 2039
Asacol Delayed-Release Tablets (Rare) 2884
Cerubidine for Injection (Rare) 947
Clozaril Tablets 2319
Cytovene-IV (One report) 2959
Dipentum Capsules (One patient) 2803
Geodon Capsules (Rare) 2688
Pentasa Capsules (Infrequent) 3239
Proleukin for Injection (Less than 1% to 1%) 1199
Risperdal (Rare) 1796
▲ Vesanoid Capsules (3%) 3037

Myocarditis, allergic

Azulfidine EN-tabs Tablets (Rare) 2775
Bactrim 2949
Pediazole Suspension 3050
Septra Suspension 2265
Septra Tablets 2265
Septra DS Tablets 2265

Myocardium, depression

Naropin Injection 612
Nesacaine/Nesacaine MPF 617
Normodyne Tablets 3137
Sensorcaine 643
Sensorcaine-MPF Injection 643

Myoclonia

Aloprim for Injection (Less than 1%) 2292
Ativan Injection (Infrequent) 3478
Cerebyx Injection (Infrequent) 2619
Chibroxin Sterile Ophthalmic Solution 2051
Cipro I.V. 893
Cipro I.V. Pharmacy Bulk Package 897
Cipro 887
Clozaril Tablets (1%) 2319
Copaxone for Injection (Infrequent) 3306
Dilaudid 441
Dilaudid Oral Liquid 445
Dilaudid Powder 441
Dilaudid Tablets - 8 mg 445
Dilaudid-HP Injection 443
Diprivan Injectable Emulsion (Less than 1%) 667
Duramorph Injection 1312
Effexor Tablets (Infrequent) 3495
Effexor XR Capsules (Infrequent) 3499
Eldepryl Capsules 3266
Fortaz 1541
Gabitril Tablets (Frequent) 1189
Geodon Capsules (Rare) 2688
Imitrex Injection (Rare) 1549
Infumorph 200 and Infumorph 500 Sterile Solutions 1314
Kadian Capsules (Less than 3%) 1335
Lamictal (Infrequent) 1567
Leukeran Tablets (Rare) 1591
Luvox Tablets (25, 50, 100 mg) (Frequent) 3256
Mirapex Tablets (1%) 2834
Nardil Tablets (Common) 2653
Neurontin Capsules (Rare) 2655
Neurontin Oral Solution (Rare) 2655
Neurontin Tablets (Rare) 2655
Noroxin Tablets 2145
Orthoclone OKT3 Sterile Solution 2498
▲ Paxil (3%) 1609
Permax Tablets (Infrequent) 1299
Primaxin I.M. 2158
Primaxin I.V. (Less than 0.2%) 2160
▲ Prograf (3% to 15%) 1393
Prozac Pulvules, Liquid, and Weekly Capsules (Infrequent) 1238
Remeron Tablets (Rare) 2483
Remeron SolTab Tablets (Rare) 2486
Rilutek Tablets (Infrequent) 772
Sarafem Pulvules (Infrequent) 1962
Seroquel Tablets (Infrequent) 684
Serzone Tablets (Infrequent) 1104
Sonata Capsules (Rare) 3591
Tasmar Tablets (Infrequent) 3010
Vistide Injection 1445
Wellbutrin Tablets (Frequent) 1680
Zonegran Capsules (Rare) 1307
Zyprexa Tablets (1% to 5%) 1973
Zyprexa ZYDIS Orally Disintegrating Tablets (1% to 5%) 1973

Myoglobinemia

Anectine Injection 1476
Symmetrel (Uncommon) 1328

Myoglobinuria

Anectine Injection 1476
Baycol Tablets (Rare) 883
Bicillin C-R 900/300 Injection 2240
Bicillin C-R Injection 2238
Bicillin L-A Injection 2242
Fluothane Inhalation 3508
Haldol Decanoate 2535
Orap Tablets 1407
Risperdal 1796
Seroquel Tablets 684
Zocor Tablets (Rare) 2219

Myolysis

Ziagen 1692

Myopathy

Accuretic Tablets 2614
Actiq (Less than 1%) 1184
Amicar Injection 3608
Amicar Syrup 3608
Amicar Tablets 3608
Atromid-S Capsules 3483
Axert Tablets (Rare) 2772
Baycol Tablets 883
Betaseron for SC Injection 988
Cerebyx Injection (Infrequent) 2619
Cognex Capsules (Rare) 1351
Copaxone for Injection (Infrequent) 3306
Cordarone Tablets 3487
Cortone Acetate Tablets 2061
Darvon-N/Darvocet-N 1907
Darvon Pulvules 1909
Darvon Compound-65 Pulvules 1910
Darvon-N Tablets 1912
Effexor Tablets (Rare) 3495
Effexor XR Capsules (Rare) 3499
Foscavir Injection (Rare) 605
Geodon Capsules (Rare) 2688
Herceptin I.V. (At least one of the 958 patients) 1414
Hivid Tablets (Less than 1%) 2975
Lescol Capsules (Occasional) 2361
Lescol Capsules (Occasional) 2925
Lescol XL Tablets 2361
Lescol XL Tablets 2925
Lopid Tablets (Occasional) 2650
Luvox Tablets (25, 50, 100 mg) (Rare) 3256

Mevacor Tablets 2132
Normodyne Tablets (Less common) 3137
Paxil (2%) 1609
Pediapred Oral Solution 1170
Plaquenil Tablets 3082
Pravachol Tablets (Rare) 1099
Proleukin for Injection 1199
Prozac Pulvules, Liquid, and Weekly Capsules (Rare) 1238
ReoPro Vials (0.4%) 1958
Retrovir Capsules 1625
Retrovir IV Infusion 1629
Retrovir 1625
Rifadin (Rare) 765
Rifater Tablets (Rare) 769
Sarafem Pulvules (Rare) 1962
Sustiva Capsules 1258
Videx 1138
Videx EC Capsules 1143
Viracept 532
Zocor Tablets 2219
Zyprexa Tablets (Rare) 1973
Zyprexa ZYDIS Orally Disintegrating Tablets (Rare) 1973

Myopathy, steroid
Celestone Soluspan Injectable Suspension 3097
Celestone Syrup 3099
Cortone Acetate Injectable Suspension 2059
Decadron Elixir 2078
Decadron Tablets 2079
Decadron Phosphate Injection 2081
Depo-Medrol Injectable Suspension 2795
Florinef Acetate Tablets 2250
Hydrocortone Tablets 2106
Hydrocortone Acetate Injectable Suspension 2103
Hydrocortone Phosphate Injection, Sterile 2105
Prednisone 3064
Prelone Syrup 2273
Solu-Medrol Sterile Powder 2855

Myopia
Evoxac Capsules (Less than 1%) 1217
Humorsol Sterile Ophthalmic Solution 2102
Isopto Carpine Ophthalmic Solution ⊙215
Neptazane Tablets ⊙271
Pilopine HS Ophthalmic Gel ⊙217
Topamax Sprinkle Capsules (Infrequent) 2590
Topamax Tablets (Infrequent) 2590
Zarontin Capsules 2659
Zarontin Syrup 2660

Myopia, transient
Clorpres Tablets (Occasional) 1002
Combipres Tablets (Occasional) 1040
Cosopt Sterile Ophthalmic Solution 2065
Diamox Intravenous ⊙269
Diamox Sequels Sustained Release Capsules ⊙270
Diamox Tablets ⊙269
Trusopt Sterile Ophthalmic Solution 2196

Myosis
Doxil Injection (Less than 1%) 566
Etrafon (Occasional) 3115
Trilafon 3160

Myositis
Accuretic Tablets 2614
Advair Diskus 100/50 1448
Advair Diskus 250/50 1448
Advair Diskus 500/50 1448
Amicar Injection 3608
Amicar Syrup 3608
Amicar Tablets 3608
Atromid-S Capsules 3483
Baycol Tablets 883
Betaseron for SC Injection 988
Campath Ampules 992
Enalaprilat Injection 863
Foscavir Injection (Rare) 605
Hivid Tablets (Less than 1%) 2975
Imdur Tablets (Less than or equal to 5%) 1826
Lexxel Tablets 608
Lipitor Tablets (Less than 2%) 2639
Lipitor Tablets (Less than 2%) 2696
Lopid Tablets 2650
Mycobutin Capsules (Less than 1%; rare) 2838
Norvir Capsules (Less than 2%) 487
Norvir Oral Solution (Less than 2%) 487
Paxil (Rare) 1609
Permax Tablets (Infrequent) 1299
Proleukin for Injection 1199
Prozac Pulvules, Liquid, and Weekly Capsules (Rare) 1238
Remeron Tablets (Rare) 2483
Remeron SolTab Tablets (Rare) 2486
Retrovir Capsules 1625
Retrovir IV Infusion 1629
Retrovir 1625
Sarafem Pulvules (Rare) 1962
Serevent Inhalation Aerosol (1% to 3%) 1633
Sonata Capsules (Rare) 3591
Sular Tablets (Less than or equal to 1%) 688
Ticlid Tablets (Rare) 3015
Tricor Capsules, Micronized 513
Vaseretic Tablets 2204
Vasotec I.V. Injection 2207
Vasotec Tablets (0.5% to 1.0%) 2210
Vesanoid Capsules (Isolated cases) 3037

Myxedema
Eskalith 1527
Lithium Carbonate 3061
Lithium Citrate Syrup 3061
Lithobid Slow-Release Tablets 3255
Thalomid Capsules 1154

N

Nail discoloration
Evoxac Capsules (Less than 1%) 1217
Retrovir Capsules 1625
Retrovir IV Infusion 1629
Retrovir 1625

Nail disorders, unspecified
Celebrex Capsules (0.1% to 1.9%) 2676
Celebrex Capsules (0.1% to 1.9%) 2780
Evoxac Capsules (Less than 1%) 1217
Glucophage Tablets (1% to 5%) 1080
Kaletra Capsules (Less than 2%) 471
Kaletra Oral Solution (Less than 2%) 471
Penlac Nail Lacquer, Topical Solution (2%) 1225
Sustiva Capsules 1258
Tricor Capsules, Micronized 513
Vioxx (Greater than 0.1% to 1.9%) 2213
Vistide Injection 1445

Nails, changes of
Accutane Capsules 2944
Arava Tablets (1% to 3%) 724
Baycol Tablets 883
Copaxone for Injection (At least 2%) 3306
Effexor Tablets (Infrequent) 3495
Effexor XR Capsules (Infrequent) 3499
Ergamisol Tablets 1789
Fortovase Capsules (Less than 2%) 2970
Sterile FUDR (Remote possibility) 2974
Gengraf Capsules (1% to less than 3%) 457
Hivid Tablets (Less than 1%) 2975
Intron A for Injection (Less than 5%) 3120
Invirase Capsules (Less than 2%) 2979
Lescol Capsules 2361
Lescol Capsules 2925
Lescol XL Tablets 2361
Lescol XL Tablets 2925
Lupron Depot 3.75 mg (Less than 5%) 3281
Lupron Depot–3 Month 11.25 mg (Less than 5%) 3285
Mevacor Tablets 2132
Naprelan Tablets (Less than 1%) 1293
Neoral Soft Gelatin Capsules (1% to less than 3%) 2380
Neoral Oral Solution (1% to less than 3%) 2380
Oncaspar 756
Pentasa Capsules (Less than 1%) 3239
Pravachol Tablets 1099
Rescriptor Tablets (Less than 2%) 526
▲ Soriatane Capsules (25% to 50%) 3003
Taxol Injection (Uncommon) 1129
Taxotere for Injection Concentrate (2.6%) 778
▲ Thalomid Capsules (4.2%) 1154
Topamax Sprinkle Capsules (Infrequent) 2590
Topamax Tablets (Infrequent) 2590
Xeloda Tablets 3039
Zocor Tablets 2219

Nails, loss of
Sterile FUDR (Remote possibility) 2974

Nasal burning
▲ Astelin Nasal Spray (4.1%) 3339
Atrovent Nasal Spray 0.03% (2.0%) 1032
Atrovent Nasal Spray 0.06% (Less than 1%) 1033
▲ Beconase Inhalation Aerosol (11 in 100 patients) 1497
Flonase Nasal Spray (2.4% to 3.2%) 1533
Iopidine Sterile Ophthalmic Solution ⊙212
Nasacort Nasal Inhaler (Rare) 750
▲ Nasalide Nasal Spray (Approximately 45%) 1295
▲ Nasarel Nasal Solution 0.025% (13% to 44%) 1296
Nasonex Nasal Spray 3131
Neo-Synephrine ▣614
Neo-Synephrine 12 Hour ▣615
Nicotrol Nasal Spray (More common) 2843
Rhinocort Nasal Inhaler (Rare) 640
Tri-Nasal Spray (2%) 2274
▲ Vancenase PocketHaler Nasal Inhaler (11 per 100 patients) 3162
▲ Vancenase AQ Nasal Spray 0.084% (5%) 3163
Vicks Sinex Nasal Spray and Ultra Fine Mist ▣729

Nasal congestion
Adenoscan (Less than 1%) 1381
▲ Aerobid/Aerobid-M (15%) 1363
Alamast Ophthalmic Solution (Less than 5%) 3092
Aldoclor Tablets 2035
Aldomet Tablets 2037
Aldoril Tablets 2039
▲ Alocril Ophthalmic Solution (10% to 30%) 545
Amicar Injection 3608
Amicar Syrup 3608
Amicar Tablets 3608
Asacol Delayed-Release Tablets 2884
Astelin Nasal Spray 3339
▲ Atrovent Nasal Spray 0.03% (3.1%) 1032
Atrovent Nasal Spray 0.06% (1.1%) 1033
Azactam for Injection (Less than 1%) 1276
Betagan ⊙228
Betimol Ophthalmic Solution ⊙324
Brevibloc Injection (Less than 1%) 858
Calcium Disodium Versenate Injection 1980
Cardizem Injectable 1018
Cardizem Lyo-Ject Syringe 1018
Cardizem Monovial 1018
Cardizem CD Capsules (Less than 1%) 1016
Caverject Sterile Powder (1%) 2777
Cedax Capsules (0.1% to 1%) 1021
Chemet Capsules (0.7% to 3.7%) 3078
Claritin-D 12 Hour Extended Release Tablets (Less frequent) 3102
Claritin-D 24 Hour Extended Release Tablets (Fewer than 2%) 3104
Clozaril Tablets (1%) 2319
Combivent Inhalation Aerosol 1041
Compazine 1505
Corlopam Injection (2%) 412
Cosopt Sterile Ophthalmic Solution (1% to 5%) 2065
Cozaar Tablets (2.0%) 2067
DDAVP Nasal Spray (Occasional) 738
DDAVP Rhinal Tube (Occasional) 738
Demser Capsules (Infrequent) 2085
Desmopressin Acetate Rhinal Tube (Occasional) 1345
Dibenzyline Capsules 3457
DynaCirc CR Tablets (0.5% to 1%) 2923
Etrafon (Occasional) 3115
▲ Flovent Diskus (16%) 3614
▲ Flovent (8% to 22%) 1535
▲ Flovent Rotadisk (4% to 7%) 1537
▲ Hytrin Capsules (0.6% to 5.9%) 464
Hyzaar 2109
Imdur Tablets (Less than or equal to 5%) 1826
▲ Intron A for Injection (Up to 10%) 3120
Iveegam EN (0.91%) 849
Lexxel Tablets (Infrequent) 608
Limbitrol (Less common) 1738
Loxitane Capsules 3398
Maxalt Tablets (Infrequent) 2120
Maxalt-MLT Orally Disintegrating Tablets (Infrequent) 2120
Meridia Capsules 481
▲ Miacalcin Nasal Spray (10.6%) 2375
Midamor Tablets (Less than or equal to 1%) 2136
Minipress Capsules (1% to 4%) 2699
Minizide Capsules 2700
Moduretic Tablets (Less than or equal to 1%) 2138
Nasalide Nasal Spray (5% or less) 1295
Navane Oral 2701
Navane Intramuscular 2703
Orthoclone OKT3 Sterile Solution 2498
Periactin Tablets 2155
Phrenilin (Infrequent) 578
Prinivil Tablets (0.4%) 2164
Prinzide Tablets (0.3% to 1%) 2168
▲ Procardia Capsules (2% or less to 6%) 2708
▲ Procardia XL Extended Release Tablets (6%) 2710
Prometrium Capsules (100 mg, 200 mg) (Less than 5%) 3261
Proventil Inhalation Solution 0.083% (1%) 3146
Proventil Solution for Inhalation 0.5% (1%) 3144
Robaxin Injectable 2938
Robaxin Tablets 2939
Sedapap Tablets 50 mg/650 mg (Infrequent) 2225
▲ Serevent Diskus (9%) 1637
Serevent Inhalation Aerosol (1% to 3%) 1633
Singulair (1.6%) 2181
▲ Stadol NS Nasal Spray (13%) 1108
Stelazine 1640
Stimate Nasal Spray (Occasional) 796
Tessalon Capsules 1377
Thiothixene Capsules 2290
Thorazine 1656
Tiazac Capsules (Less than 2%) 1378
Timolol GFS ⊙266
Timoptic in Ocudose (Less frequent) 2192
Timoptic Sterile Ophthalmic Solution (Less frequent) 2190
Timoptic-XE Sterile Ophthalmic Gel Forming Solution 2194
Trental Tablets (Less than 1%) 784
Trilafon (Occasional) 3160
▲ Vanceril Double Strength Inhalation Aerosol (6%) 3167
Vaqta (1.1%) 2199
▲ Viagra Tablets (4%) 2732
Vioxx (Greater than 0.1% to 1.9%) 2213
▲ Xanax Tablets (7.3% to 17.4%) 2865
Zestoretic Tablets (0.3% to 1%) 695
Zestril Tablets (0.4%) 698

Nasal discharge, increase
Aredia for Injection (One patient) 2309
Flovent Diskus (1% to 3%) 3614
▲ Flovent (4% to 16%) 1535
Flovent Rotadisk (1% to 3%) 1537
Hivid Tablets (Less than 1%) 2975
Iopidine Sterile Ophthalmic Solution (Less than 2%) ⊙212
▲ Miacalcin Nasal Spray (10.6%) 2375
Neo-Synephrine ▣614
Neo-Synephrine 12 Hour ▣615
Vicks Sinex Nasal Spray and Ultra Fine Mist ▣729

Nasal drainage
Alferon N Injection (2%) 1770

Nasal drip, posterior
Aceon Tablets (2 mg, 4 mg, 8 mg) (0.3% to 1%) 3249
Advair Diskus 100/50 (1% to 3%) 1448
Advair Diskus 250/50 (1% to 3%) 1448
Advair Diskus 500/50 (1% to 3%) 1448
Aricept Tablets (Infrequent) 1270
Aricept Tablets (Infrequent) 2665
▲ Atrovent Nasal Spray 0.03% (3.1%) 1032
▲ Trisenox Injection (13%) 1158

Nasal itching
(*see under* Pruritus, rhinal)

Nasal mucosa, dryness
(*see under* Xeromycteria)

Nasal obstruction
Neurontin Oral Solution (Rare) 2655

Nasal septum, perforation
Beconase Inhalation Aerosol (Rare) 1497
Beconase AQ Nasal Spray (Rare) 1498
Flonase Nasal Spray (Rare) 1533
Nasacort Nasal Inhaler (Rare) 750
Nasacort AQ Nasal Spray (One patient) 752
Nasalide Nasal Spray (Rare) 1295
Nasarel Nasal Solution 0.025% (Rare) 1296
Nasonex Nasal Spray (Rare) 3131
Rhinocort Aqua Nasal Spray (Rare) 642
Rhinocort Nasal Inhaler (Less than 1%) 640
Vancenase PocketHaler Nasal Inhaler (Extremely rare) 3162
Vancenase AQ Nasal Spray 0.084% (Rare) 3163

Nasal stinging
Nasacort Nasal Inhaler (Rare) 750
NasalCrom Nasal Spray ▣719
▲ Nasarel Nasal Solution 0.025% (13% to 44%) 1296
Neo-Synephrine ▣614
Neo-Synephrine 12 Hour ▣615
Tri-Nasal Spray (2%) 2274
Vicks Sinex Nasal Spray and Ultra Fine Mist ▣729

Nasal stuffiness
Beconase AQ Nasal Spray (Fewer than 3 per 100 patients) 1498
Benadryl Parenteral 2617
Corgard Tablets (1 to 5 per 1000 patients) 2245
Corzide 40/5 Tablets (1 to 5 of 1000 patients) 2247
Corzide 80/5 Tablets (1 to 5 of 1000 patients) 2247

▲ Dostinex Tablets (Less than 10%) 2804
Loxitane Capsules 3398
Nadolol Tablets (1 to 5 of 1000 patients) 2288
▲ Normodyne Tablets (1% to 6%) 3137
Phenergan Injection 3553
Phenergan 3556
Rynatan Tablets 3351
Serentil 1057
Thioridazine Hydrochloride Tablets 2289

Nasal ulceration
Beconase Inhalation Aerosol (Rare) 1497
Beconase AQ Nasal Spray (Rare) 1498
Nasarel Nasal Solution 0.025% (1% or less) 1296
Nasonex Nasal Spray (Rare) 3131
Nicotrol Nasal Spray (More common) 2843
Vancenase PocketHaler Nasal Inhaler (Rare) 3162
Vancenase AQ Nasal Spray 0.084% (Rare) 3163

Nasolacrimal canals, obstruction
Humorsol Sterile Ophthalmic Solution 2102

Nasopharyngitis
Flovent Rotadisk (1% to 3%) 1537
▲ Gleevec Capsules (5% to 10%) 2357
Hivid Tablets (Less than 1%) 2975
▲ Serevent Inhalation Aerosol (14%) 1633
▲ Trisenox Injection (5%) 1158

Nausea (24%)
▲ Abelcet Injection (9%) 1273
▲ Accolate Tablets (3.1%) 657
AccuNeb Inhalation Solution (0.9% to 1.7%) 1230
Accupril Tablets (1.4% to 2.4%) 2611
Accuretic Tablets (1.8%) 2614
Accutane Capsules 2944
Aceon Tablets (2 mg, 4 mg, 8 mg) (2.3%) 3249
Aciphex Tablets 1267
Aciphex Tablets 1783
▲ Actimmune (10%) 1772
▲ Actiq (11% to 23%) 1184
Activase I.V. 1410
▲ Activella Tablets (3% to 10%) 2764
▲ Actonel Tablets (9.8% to 10.9%) 2879
Adalat CC Tablets (2%) 877
▲ Adderall XR Capsules (5%)
▲ Adenocard Injection (3%) 1380
Adriamycin PFS/RDF Injection (Frequent) 2767
▲ Advair Diskus 100/50 (4%) 1448
▲ Advair Diskus 250/50 (6%) 1448
▲ Advair Diskus 500/50 (4% to 6%) 1448
▲ Aerobid/Aerobid-M (25%) 1363
Aerolate 1361
▲ Agenerase Capsules (43% to 74%) 1454
▲ Agenerase Oral Solution (43% to 74%) 1459
Aggrastat (Less than 1%) 2031
▲ Aggrenox Capsules (16%) 1026
▲ Agrylin Capsules (17.1%) 3232
▲ AK-Fluor Injection 10% and 25% (Among most common) ⊙202
Albalon Ophthalmic Solution ⊙225
▲ Albenza Tablets (3.7% to 6.2%) 1463
Albumin (Human) 5% (Very rare) 838
Albumin (Human) 25% (Very rare) 839
Albuminar-5, U.S.P. 785
Albuminar-25, U.S.P. 786
Aldoclor Tablets 2035
Aldomet Tablets 2037
Aldoril Tablets 2039
Alesse-21 Tablets 3468
Alesse-28 Tablets 3473
▲ Alferon N Injection (4% to 48%) 1770
Alkeran for Injection 1465
Alkeran Tablets (Infrequent) 1466
Allegra (1.6%) 712
▲ Allegra-D Extended-Release Tablets (7.4%) 714
Alomide Ophthalmic Solution (Less than 1%) ⊙204
Aloprim for Injection (1.3%) 2292
▲ Alora Transdermal System (4.3% to 4.5%) 3372
Altace Capsules (Less than 1% to 2.2%) 2233
Alupent (1% to 4%) 1029
Amaryl Tablets (1.1%) 717
▲ Ambien Tablets (2% to 6%) 3191
▲ AmBisome for Injection (25.9% to 39.7%) 1383
▲ Amerge Tablets (4% to 5%) 1467
Amicar Injection 3608
Amicar Syrup 3608
Amicar Tablets 3608
Aminohippurate Sodium PAH Injection 2041
Amoxil Chewable Tablets 1471
Amoxil for Oral Suspension 1471
Amoxil 1471
▲ Amphotec (7% to 12%) 1774
Anadrol-50 Tablets 3321
▲ Anaprox Tablets (3% to 9%) 2967
▲ Anaprox DS Tablets (3% to 9%) 2967
Ancef for Injection (Rare) 1474
Ancef Injection (Rare) 1474
Ancobon Capsules 1730
Androderm Transdermal System CIII 3377
▲ Android Capsules, 10 mg (Among most common) 1731
Antabuse Tablets 3474
Antagon Injection (1.1%) 2447
Aphthasol Oral Paste (Infrequent) 1025
Aralen Tablets 3075
▲ Arava Tablets (9%) 724
▲ Aredia for Injection (53.5%) 2309
▲ Argatroban Injection (4.8%) 1478
▲ Aricept Tablets (11%) 1270
▲ Aricept Tablets (11%) 2665
▲ Arimidex Tablets (15.6% to 19.5%) 659
▲ Aromasin Tablets (18%) 2769
▲ Artane (30% to 50%) 1855
▲ Arthrotec Tablets (11%) 3195
▲ Asacol Delayed-Release Tablets (13%) 2884
Astelin Nasal Spray (2.8%) 3339
Astramorph/PF Injection, USP (Preservative-Free) (Frequent) 594
Atacand Tablets (More than 1%) 595
Atacand HCT Tablets (0.5% or greater) 597
Ativan Injection (Less than 1%) 3478
Ativan Tablets (Less frequent) 3482
▲ Atromid-S Capsules (Most common) 3483
Atrovent Inhalation Aerosol (2.8%) 1030
▲ Atrovent Inhalation Solution (4.1%) 1031
Atrovent Nasal Spray 0.03% (2.2%) 1032
▲ Augmentin Chewable Tablets (3%) 1482
▲ Augmentin Powder for Oral Suspension (3%) 1482
▲ Augmentin Tablets (3%) 1485
Augmentin ES-600 Powder for Oral Suspension 1487
▲ Avalide Tablets (3%) 1070
Avapro Tablets (1% or greater) 1074
Avapro Tablets (1% or greater) 3076
▲ Avelox Tablets (8%) 879
▲ Avonex (33%) 1013
Axert Tablets (1% to 2%) 2772
▲ Axid Pulvules (1.2% to 5.4%) 1903
▲ Axid Pulvules (1.2% to 5.4%) 2919
Aygestin Tablets 1333
Azactam for Injection (1 to 1.3%) 1276
Azopt Ophthalmic Suspension (Less than 1%) 536
▲ Azulfidine EN-tabs Tablets (19%) 2775
▲ Bactrim (Among most common) 2949
Bactroban Cream (1.1% to 4.9%) 1494
Bactroban Nasal (Less than 1%) 1495
Bactroban Ointment (Less than 1%) 1496
Baycol Tablets (2.4%) 883
▲ Genuine Bayer Professional Labeling (Aspirin Regimen Bayer) (7.6%) ▣608
Bebulin VH 840
Beconase AQ Nasal Spray (Fewer than 5 in 100 patients) 1498
Benadryl Parenteral 2617
BeneFix for Injection (16 cases) 1432
Betagan ⊙228
▲ Betapace Tablets (5% to 10%) 950
▲ Betapace AF Tablets (5.7% to 7.8%) 954
Betaseron for SC Injection 988
Betimol Ophthalmic Solution (1% to 5%) ⊙324
▲ Biaxin/Biaxin XL (3%) 403
Bicillin C-R 900/300 Injection 2240
Bicillin C-R Injection 2238
Bicillin L-A Injection 2242
Biltricide Tablets 887
Blocadren Tablets (0.6%) 2046
Bontril Slow-Release Capsules 576
Brethine Ampuls (1.3 to 3.9%) 2314
▲ Brethine Tablets (3%) 2313
▲ Brevibloc Injection (7%) 858
Brevicon 28-Day Tablets 3380
Brevital Sodium for Injection, USP 1815
Bromfed Capsules (Extended-Release) 2269
Bromfed-PD Capsules (Extended-Release) 2269
Buminate 5% Solution, USP (Occasional) 841
Buminate 25% Solution, USP (Occasional) 842
▲ Buprenex Injectable (5% to 10%) 2918
Calcijex Injection 411
Calcium Disodium Versenate Injection 1980
▲ Campath Ampules (2% to 54%) 992
▲ Cancidas for Injection (2.5% to 6%) 2048
Captopril Tablets (About 0.5% to 2%) 2281
Carafate Suspension (Less than 0.5%) 731
Carafate Tablets (Less than 0.5%) 730
▲ Carbatrol Capsules (Among most frequent) 3234
▲ Cardene I.V. (4.9%) 3485
Cardizem Injectable (Less than 1%) 1018
Cardizem Lyo-Ject Syringe (Less than 1%) 1018
Cardizem Monovial (Less than 1%) 1018
Cardizem CD Capsules (1.4%) 1016
Cardura Tablets (1.5% to 3%) 2668
▲ Carnitor Injection (5% to 12%) 3242
Carnitor Tablets and Oral Solution 3245
Carteolol Hydrochloride Ophthalmic Solution USP, 1% ⊙258
▲ Casodex Tablets (11%) 662
▲ Cataflam Tablets (3% to 9%) 2315
▲ Catapres Tablets (About 5 in 100 patients) 1037
Catapres-TTS (1 of 101 patients) 1038
Caverject Sterile Powder (Less than 1%) 2777
Ceclor CD Tablets (0.1% to 3.4%) 1279
Ceclor (Rare) 1905
▲ Cedax (4%) 1021
Cefizox for Intramuscular or Intravenous Use (Occasional) 1390
Cefobid Intravenous/Intramuscular (Rare) 2671
Cefobid Pharmacy Bulk Package - Not for Direct Infusion (Rare) 2673
Cefotan (1 in 700) 664
Ceftin (2.6%) 1898
▲ Cefzil (3.5%) 1076
▲ Celebrex Capsules (3.5%) 2676
▲ Celebrex Capsules (3.5%) 2780
▲ Celexa (8%) 1365
▲ CellCept Capsules (19.9% to 54%) 2951
▲ CellCept Intravenous (19.9% to 54%) 2951
▲ CellCept Oral Suspension (19.9% to 54%) 2951
▲ CellCept Tablets (19.9% to 54%) 2951
Celontin Capsules (Frequent) 2618
▲ Cenestin Tablets (18%) 1263
Ceptaz for Injection (One in 156 patients) 1499
▲ Cerebyx Injection (4.5% to 8.9%) 2619
▲ Cerezyme for Injection (5.4%) 1438
Cerubidine for Injection 947
Cervidil Vaginal Insert (Less than 1%) 1369
Cetrotide for Injection (1.3%) 3209
▲ Chemet Capsules (12.0% to 20.9%) 3078
▲ Chirocaine Injection (11.6%) 2909
New Formulation Chromagen OB Capsules 3094
Ciloxan (Less than 1%) 538
▲ Cipro I.V. (Among most frequent) 893
▲ Cipro I.V. Pharmacy Bulk Package (Among most frequent) 897
▲ Cipro (5.2%) 887
Claforan Injection (1.4%; rare) 732
Claritin (At least one patient) 3100
▲ Claritin-D 12 Hour Extended Release Tablets (3%) 3102
▲ Claritin-D 24 Hour Extended Release Tablets (3%) 3104
Cleocin HCl Capsules 2784
Cleocin Phosphate Sterile Solution 2785
Cleocin Vaginal Cream (Less than 1%) 2788
Cleocin Vaginal Ovules (Less than 1%) 2789
Climara Transdermal System 958
▲ Clinoril Tablets (3% to 9%) 2053
Clomid Tablets (2.2%) 735
▲ Clorpres Tablets (About 5%) 1002
▲ Clozaril Tablets (3% to 5% or more) 2319
Cogentin 2055
▲ Cognex Capsules (28%) 1351
Colace Capsules, Syrup, Liquid 3236
▲ Colazal Capsules (5%) 3069
Colestid Tablets (Less frequent) 2791
▲ Colyte with Flavor Packs for Oral Solution (Up to 50%) 3170
▲ CombiPatch Transdermal System (8% to 12%) 2323
▲ Combipres Tablets (About 5%) 1040
Combivent Inhalation Aerosol (2.0%) 1041
▲ Combivir Tablets (13% to 33%) 1502
Compazine 1505
▲ Comtan Tablets (14%) 2328
Concerta Extended-Release Tablets 1998
Concerta Tablets 561
▲ Copaxone for Injection (22%) 3306
▲ Cordarone Intravenous (3.9%) 3491
▲ Cordarone Tablets (10% to 33%) 3487
▲ Coreg Tablets (8.5%) 1508
Corgard Tablets (1 to 5 per 1000 patients) 2245
▲ Corlopam Injection (More than 5%) 412
Cortone Acetate Injectable Suspension 2059
Cortone Acetate Tablets 2061
Corvert Injection (1.9%) 2793
Corzide 40/5 Tablets (1 to 5 of 1000 patients) 2247
Corzide 80/5 Tablets (1 to 5 of 1000 patients) 2247
Cosmegen for Injection (Common) 2062
Cosopt Sterile Ophthalmic Solution (1% to 5%) 2065
Coumadin for Injection (Infrequent) 1243
Coumadin Tablets (Infrequent) 1243
Covera-HS Tablets (2.1% to 2.7%) 3199
Cozaar Tablets (1% or greater) 2067
▲ Creon 5 Capsules (Among most frequent) 3251
▲ Creon 10 Capsules (Among most frequent) 3251
▲ Creon 20 Capsules (Among most frequent) 3251
▲ Crinone (8%) 3213
▲ Crixivan Capsules (11.7%) 2070
Cuprimine Capsules (Greater than 1%) 2075
Cyclessa Tablets 2450
Cylert Tablets 415
CytoGam Intravenous (Less than 5.0%) 2026
▲ Cytotec Tablets (3.2%) 3202
Cytovene 2959
Dantrium Capsules (Rare) 2885
Dapsone Tablets USP 1780
▲ Daranide Tablets (Among the most common effects) 2077
▲ Darvon-N/Darvocet-N (Among most frequent) 1907
▲ Darvon Pulvules (Among most frequent) 1909
▲ Darvon Compound-65 Pulvules (Among most frequent) 1910
▲ Darvon-N Tablets (Among most frequent) 1912
▲ DaunoXome Injection (3% to 51%) 1442
DDAVP Injection 4 mcg/mL (Infrequent) 737
DDAVP Nasal Spray (Up to 2%) 738
DDAVP Rhinal Tube (Up to 2%) 738
DDAVP Tablets 739
Decadron Elixir 2078
Decadron Tablets 2079
Decadron Phosphate Injection 2081
Declomycin Tablets 1855
Delatestryl Injection 1151
Demadex Tablets and Injection (1.8%) 2965
▲ Demerol (Among most frequent) 3079
Demser Capsules (Infrequent) 2085
▲ Depacon Injection (3.2% to 48%) 416
▲ Depakene (34% to 48%) 421
▲ Depakote Sprinkle Capsules (26% to 48%) 426
▲ Depakote Tablets (22% to 48%) 430
▲ Depakote ER Tablets (15% to 48%) 436
▲ Depen Titratable Tablets (17%) 3341
▲ DepoCyt Injection (11%) 1197
▲ Depo-Provera Contraceptive Injection (More than 5%) 2798
Desferal Vials 2333
Desmopressin Acetate Injection (Infrequent) 1344
Desmopressin Acetate Rhinal Tube (Up to 2%) 1345
Desogen Tablets 2458
▲ Detrol Tablets (4.2%) 3623
D.H.E. 45 Injection 2334
DiaBeta Tablets (1.8%) 741
Diabinese Tablets (Less than 5%) 2680
Diamox Intravenous ⊙269
Diamox Sequels Sustained Release Capsules ⊙270
Diamox Tablets ⊙269
▲ Didronel Tablets (About 1 patient in 15; possibly 2 or 3 in 10) 2888
▲ Diflucan Tablets, Injection, and Oral Suspension (2% to 7%) 2681
▲ Digitek Tablets (4%) 1003
Dilantin Infatabs 2624
Dilantin Kapseals 2622
Dilantin-125 Oral Suspension 2625
Dilaudid (Infrequent) 441
Dilaudid Oral Liquid 445
Dilaudid Powder (Infrequent) 441
Dilaudid Rectal Suppositories (Infrequent) 441
Dilaudid Tablets (Infrequent) 441
Dilaudid Tablets - 8 mg 445
▲ Dilaudid-HP (Among most frequent) 443
Diovan Capsules (More than 1%) 2337
Diovan HCT Tablets (Greater than 0.2%) 2338
▲ Dipentum Capsules (5.0%) 2803
Diphtheria & Tetanus Toxoids Adsorbed Purogenated for Pediatric Use 1857
Diprivan Injectable Emulsion (Less than 1%) 667
▲ Ditropan XL Extended Release Tablets (8.9%) 564
Diucardin Tablets 3494
Diuril Oral 2087
Diuril Sodium Intravenous 2086
Dobutrex Solution Vials (1% to 3%) 1914
▲ Dolobid Tablets (3% to 9%) 2088

▲ Dolophine Hydrochloride Tablets (Among most frequent) ... 3056
Donnatal ... 2929
Donnatal Extentabs ... 2930
Donnatal Tablets ... 2929
Dopram Injectable ... 2931
Doryx Coated Pellet Filled Capsules ... 3357
▲ Dostinex Tablets (27% to 29%) ... 2804
▲ Doxil Injection (16.9% to 37.7%) ... 566
▲ DTIC-Dome (90% with the initial few doses) ... 902
DuoNeb Inhalation Solution (1.4%) .. 1233
▲ Duraclon Injection (7.9% to 13.2%) ... 3057
▲ Duragesic Transdermal System (10% or more) ... 1786
Duramorph Injection (Frequent) ... 1312
Duricef (Rare) ... 1079
Dyazide Capsules ... 1515
▲ Dynabac Tablets (5.9% to 8.3%) ... 2269
Dynacin Capsules ... 2019
DynaCirc Capsules (1% to 5.1%) ... 2921
DynaCirc CR Tablets ... 2923
Dyrenium Capsules (Rare) ... 3458
▲ EC-Naprosyn Delayed-Release Tablets (3% to 9%) ... 2967
Ecotrin Enteric Coated Aspirin Low, Regular and Maximum Strength Tablets ... 1715
Edecrin ... 2091
▲ E.E.S. (Among most frequent) ... 450
▲ Effexor Tablets (6% to 58.0%) ... 3495
▲ Effexor XR Capsules (31% to 43%) ... 3499
▲ 8-MOP Capsules (Most common; approximately 10%) ... 1727
▲ Eldepryl Capsules (10 of 49 patients) ... 3266
▲ Ellence Injection (22.1% to 92.4%) ... 2806
▲ Elmiron Capsules (4%) ... 570
Elspar for Injection ... 2092
▲ Emcyt Capsules (15%) ... 2810
Enalaprilat Injection (1.1%) ... 863
▲ Enbrel for Injection (15%) ... 1752
▲ Enbrel for Injection (15%) ... 3504
Engerix-B Vaccine (Less than 1%) ... 1517
EpiPen ... 1236
▲ Epivir (13% to 33%) ... 1520
▲ Epivir-HBV (15%) ... 1524
▲ Epogen for Injection (0.26% to 48%) ... 582
▲ Ergamisol Tablets (22% to 65%) ... 1789
▲ EryPed (Among most frequent) ... 446
▲ Ery-Tab Tablets (Among most frequent) ... 448
▲ Erythrocin Stearate Filmtab Tablets (Among most frequent) ... 452
▲ Erythromycin Base Filmtab Tablets (Among most frequent) ... 454
▲ Erythromycin Delayed-Release Capsules, USP (Among most frequent) ... 455
▲ Esclim Transdermal System (4.2% to 10.6%) ... 3460
Eskalith ... 1527
Estinyl Tablets ... 3112
Estrace Vaginal Cream ... 3358
Estrace Tablets ... 3361
Estratest ... 3252
▲ Estring Vaginal Ring (3%) ... 2811
Estrostep ... 2627
▲ Ethyol for Injection (8% to 19%) ... 2029
Etrafon (Occasional) ... 3115
▲ Eulexin Capsules (9% to 11%) ... 3118
▲ Evista Tablets (8.3% to 8.8%) ... 1915
▲ Evoxac Capsules (13.8%) ... 1217
▲ Exelon Capsules (47%) ... 2342
▲ Exelon Oral Solution (47%) ... 2345
Extendryl ... 1361
Factrel (Rare) ... 3633
Famotidine Injection (Infrequent) ... 866
▲ Famvir Tablets (7.2% to 12.5%) ... 2348
▲ Fareston Tablets (14%) ... 3237
▲ Felbatol (6.5% to 34.2%) ... 3343
▲ Feldene Capsules (1% to 10%) ... 2685
▲ Femara Tablets (13% to 17%) ... 2351
▲ femhrt Tablets (7.4%) ... 2635
Feosol Caplets ... 1717
Feosol Tablets (Occasional) ... 1717
Ferrlecit Injection (Greater than 1%) ... 3386
Flexeril Tablets (1% to 3%) ... 572
Flexeril Tablets (1% to 3%) ... 2094
▲ Flolan for Injection (32% to 67%) ... 1528
Flomax Capsules (2.0% to 3.9%) ... 1044
▲ Flonase Nasal Spray (2.6% to 4.8%) ... 1533
▲ Flovent Diskus (8% to 9%) ... 3614
▲ Flovent (1% to 22%) ... 1535
Flovent Rotadisk ... 1537
▲ Floxin I.V. (3% to 10%) ... 2526
Floxin Otic Solution (0.3%) ... 1219
▲ Floxin Tablets (3% to 10%) ... 2529
▲ Fludara for Injection (31% to 36%) ... 995
Flumadine (2.8%) ... 1370
Fluorescite Injection ... ⊙ 211
Fluothane Inhalation ... 3508
Follistim for Injection ... 2465
Foradil Aerolizer ... 2354
Fortaz (1 in 156 patients) ... 1541
▲ Fortovase Capsules (10.6% to 17.8%) ... 2970
Fosamax Tablets (0.6% to 3.6%) ... 2095
▲ Foscavir Injection (5% to 47%) ... 605
▲ Sterile FUDR (Among more common) ... 2974
Furosemide Tablets ... 2284
▲ Gabitril Tablets (11%) ... 1189
Gamimune N, 5% Solvent/Detergent Treated ... 925
Gamimune N, 10% Solvent/Detergent Treated ... 928
Gammagard S/D (Occasional) ... 845
Gammar-P I.V. ... 787
▲ Gastrocrom Oral Concentrate (3 of 87 patients) ... 1162
▲ Gemzar for Injection (58% to 71%) ... 1919
▲ Gengraf Capsules (2% to 18%) ... 457
Genotropin Lyophilized Powder (A small number of patients) ... 2818
Geocillin Tablets ... 2687
▲ Geodon Capsules (10%) ... 2688
Ginsana Sport Capsules ... ▣ 831
▲ Gleevec Capsules (55% to 68%) ... 2357
▲ Gliadel Wafer (4% to 9%) ... 1723
GlucaGen for Injection Diagnostic Kit (Occassional) ... 949
Glucagon for Injection Vials and Emergency Kit (Occasional) ... 1924
▲ Glucophage Tablets (25.5%) ... 1080
▲ Glucophage XR Tablets (6.5%) ... 1080
Glucotrol Tablets (1 in 70) ... 2692
Glucotrol XL Extended Release Tablets (Less than 3%) ... 2693
▲ Glucovance Tablets (7.6%) ... 1086
▲ GoLYTELY and Pineapple Flavor GoLYTELY for Oral Solution (Up to 50%) ... 1068
▲ Gonal-F for Injection (5.4% to 13.6%) ... 3216
Grifulvin V Tablets Microsize and Oral Suspension Microsize (Occasional) ... 2518
Gris-PEG Tablets (Occasional) ... 2661
Guaifed ... 2272
▲ Halcion Tablets (4.6%) ... 2823
Haldol Decanoate ... 2535
Haldol Injection, Tablets and Concentrate ... 2533
▲ Havrix Vaccine (1% to 10%) ... 1544
▲ Hectorol Capsules (21.3%) ... 1064
▲ Hectorol Injection (21.3%) ... 1066
Helixate Concentrate ... 788
Hemofil M (Extremely rare) ... 847
Heparin Lock Flush Solution ... 3509
Heparin Sodium Injection ... 3511
▲ Herceptin I.V. (8% to 33%) ... 1414
▲ Hexalen Capsules (1% to 33%) ... 2226
Hivid Tablets (Less than 1% to 3.4%) ... 2975
Humatrope Vials and Cartridges ... 1930
Humegon for Injection ... 2468
Humorsol Sterile Ophthalmic Solution (Rare) ... 2102
▲ Hycamtin for Injection (Less than 1% to 77%) ... 1546
Hycodan ... 1316
Hycomine Compound Tablets ... 1317
Hycotuss Expectorant Syrup ... 1318
Hydrocortone Tablets ... 2106
Hydrocortone Acetate Injectable Suspension ... 2103
Hydrocortone Phosphate Injection, Sterile ... 2105
HydroDIURIL Tablets ... 2108
▲ Hytrin Capsules (0.5% to 4.4%) ... 464
Hyzaar (1% or greater) ... 2109
▲ Idamycin PFS Injection (82%) ... 2825
▲ Ifex for Injection (58%) ... 1123
Imdur Tablets (Less than or equal to 5%) ... 1826
▲ Imitrex Injection (4%) ... 1549
▲ Imitrex Nasal Spray (11% to 13.5%) ... 1554
Imitrex Tablets ... 1558
▲ Imovax Rabies Vaccine (Up to 6%) ... 807
Indapamide Tablets (Less than 5%) ... 2286
Inderal ... 3513
Inderal LA Long-Acting Capsules ... 3516
Inderide Tablets ... 3517
Inderide LA Long-Acting Capsules ... 3519
▲ Indocin (3% to 9%) ... 2112
INFeD Injection ... 3388
▲ Infergen (30% to 40%) ... 1777
Infumorph 200 and Infumorph 500 Sterile Solutions ... 1314
Innohep Injection (1.7%) ... 1248
▲ Intron A for Injection (1% to 66%) ... 3120
Inversine Tablets ... 1850
Invirase Capsules (Up to 3.1%) ... 2979
Iopidine 0.5% Ophthalmic Solution (Less than 3%) ... ⊙ 213
Ismo Tablets (2% to 4%) ... 3524
Isoptin SR Tablets (2.7%) ... 467
Iveegam EN (0.3% to 0.8%) ... 849
▲ JE-VAX Vaccine (Approximately 10%) ... 811
▲ Kadian Capsules (Among most frequent) ... 1335
▲ Kaletra Capsules (2.2% to 15.5%) ... 471
▲ Kaletra Oral Solution (2.2% to 15.5%) ... 471
K-Dur Microburst Release System ER Tablets ... 1832
Keflex (Rare) ... 1237
Kefurox Vials, ADD-Vantage (1 in 440) ... 1948
Kefzol Vials, ADD-Vantage (Rare) ... 1951
Keppra Tablets (1% or more) ... 3314
Klonopin Tablets ... 2983
▲ Klor-Con M20/Klor-Con M10 Tablets (Among most common) ... 3329
▲ K-Lor Powder Packets (Among most common) ... 469
Koāte-DVI (0.7%) ... 931
Kogenate ... 934
Kogenate FS ... 936
K-Phos Neutral Tablets ... 946
K-Phos Original (Sodium Free) Tablets ... 947
Kristalose for Oral Solution ... 1007
▲ K-Tab Filmtab Tablets (Most common) ... 470
▲ Kytril Tablets (15% to 20%) ... 2988
▲ Lamictal (4% to 25%) ... 1567
Lamisil Tablets (2.6%) ... 2360
Lanoxicaps Capsules (Common) ... 1574
Lanoxin Injection ... 1581
Lanoxin Tablets (Common) ... 1587
Lanoxin Elixir Pediatric ... 1578
Lanoxin Injection Pediatric ... 1584
▲ Lariam Tablets (Among most frequent) ... 2989
▲ Lescol Capsules (3.2%) ... 2361
▲ Lescol Capsules (3.2%) ... 2925
Lescol XL Tablets (2.5%) ... 2361
Lescol XL Tablets (2.5%) ... 2925
Leukeran Tablets (Infrequent) ... 1591
▲ Leukine (58% to 90%) ... 1755
▲ Leustatin Injection (28%) ... 2495
▲ Levaquin (1.2% to 6.6%) ... 2537
Levbid Extended-Release Tablets ... 3172
Levlen ... 962
Levlite 21 Tablets ... 962
Levlite 28 Tablets ... 962
Levo-Dromoran ... 1734
Levora Tablets ... 3389
▲ Levorphanol Tartrate Tablets (3% to 9%) ... 3059
Levsin/Levsinex/Levbid ... 3172
Lexxel Tablets ... 608
Librium Capsules (Isolated cases) .. 1736
Librium for Injection (Isolated cases) ... 1737
Limbitrol ... 1738
Lipitor Tablets (Greater than or equal to 2%) ... 2639
Lipitor Tablets (Greater than or equal to 2%) ... 2696
Lithium Carbonate ... 3061
Lithium Citrate Syrup ... 3061
Lithobid Slow-Release Tablets ... 3255
Livostin (Approximately 1% to 3%) ... ⊙ 305
▲ Lodine (3% to 9%) ... 3528
▲ Lodine XL Extended-Release Tablets (3% to 9%) ... 3530
▲ Lodosyn Tablets (Among most common) ... 1251
Loestrin 21 Tablets ... 2642
Loestrin Fe Tablets ... 2642
▲ Lo/Ovral Tablets (10% or less) ... 3532
▲ Lo/Ovral-28 Tablets (10% or less) ... 3538
Lopid Tablets (2.5%) ... 2650
Lorabid Suspension and Pulvules (Up to 2.5%) ... 2251
▲ Lortab (Among most frequent) ... 3319
▲ Lortab Elixir (Among most frequent) ... 3317
Lotensin Tablets (1.5%) ... 2365
Lotensin HCT Tablets (1.4%) ... 2367
Lotrel Capsules ... 2370
▲ Lovenox Injection (3%) ... 746
▲ Low-Ogestrel-28 Tablets (10% or less) ... 3392
Loxitane Capsules ... 3398
Lufyllin Tablets ... 3347
Lufyllin-400 Tablets ... 3347
Lufyllin-GG Elixir ... 3348
Lufyllin-GG Tablets ... 3348
Lunelle Monthly Injection ... 2827
Lupron Depot 3.75 mg (Less than 5%) ... 3281
▲ Lupron Depot 7.5 mg (5.4%) ... 3284
▲ Lupron Depot–3 Month 11.25 mg (4.8% to 13%) ... 3285
Lupron Depot-PED 7.5 mg, 11.25 mg and 15 mg (Less than 2%) ... 3291
▲ Lupron Injection (5% or more) ... 3279
Lupron Injection Pediatric (Less than 2%) ... 3280
▲ Luvox Tablets (25, 50, 100 mg) (9% to 40%) ... 3256
LYMErix Vaccine (1.12%) ... 1592
▲ Macrobid Capsules (8%) ... 2889
▲ Macrodantin Capsules (Among most often) ... 2891
▲ Malarone (12%) ... 1596
Mandol Vials (Rare) ... 1953
▲ Marinol Capsules (3% to 10%) ... 3325
Massengill Disposable Douches ... ▣ 752
Massengill Medicated Disposable Douche ... ▣ 753
▲ Matulane Capsules (Among most frequent) ... 3246
Maxair Autohaler (1.3% to 1.7%) ... 1981
Maxair Inhaler (1.7%) ... 1984
▲ Maxalt Tablets (4% to 6%) ... 2120
▲ Maxalt-MLT Orally Disintegrating Tablets (4% to 6%) ... 2120
▲ Maxidone Tablets CIII (Among most frequent) ... 3399
Maxipime for Injection (0.1% to 2%) ... 1285
Maxzide ... 1008
Mefoxin for Injection (Rare) ... 2124
Mefoxin Premixed Intravenous Solution (Rare) ... 2127
▲ Megace Oral Suspension (Up to 5%) ... 1124
Menest Tablets ... 2254
▲ Mepergan Injection (Among most frequent) ... 3539
▲ Mepron Suspension (2.5% to 32%) ... 1598
▲ Meridia Capsules (5.9%) ... 481
▲ Merrem I.V. (3.8%) ... 673
Meruvax II ... 2130
Mestinon ... 1740
Metadate CD Capsules ... 1164
Metadate ER Tablets ... 1167
Methylin Tablets ... 1995
Methylin ER Tablets ... 1995
MetroCream ... 1404
MetroGel ... 1405
▲ MetroGel-Vaginal Gel (4%) ... 1986
MetroLotion ... 1405
Mevacor Tablets (1.9% to 4.7%) ... 2132
▲ Mexitil Capsules (39.3% to 39.6%) ... 1047
▲ Miacalcin Injection (About 10%) ... 2373
Miacalcin Nasal Spray (1% to 3%) ... 2375
Micardis Tablets (1%) ... 1049
Micardis HCT Tablets (2%) ... 1051
▲ Micro-K (Among most common) ... 3311
Microgestin Fe 1.5/30 Tablets ... 3407
Microgestin Fe 1/20 Tablets ... 3400
Micronor Tablets ... 2543
Microzide Capsules ... 3414
▲ Midamor Tablets (3% to 8%) ... 2136
▲ Migranal Nasal Spray (10%) ... 2376
Miltown Tablets ... 3349
▲ Minipress Capsules (4.9%) ... 2699
▲ Minizide Capsules (4.9%) ... 2700
Minocin Intravenous ... 1862
Minocin Oral Suspension ... 1865
Minocin Pellet-Filled Capsules ... 1863
Mintezol ... 2137
MiraLax Powder for Oral Solution ... 1069
▲ Mirapex Tablets (28%) ... 2834
Mircette Tablets ... 2470
▲ Mirena Intrauterine System (5% or more) ... 974
Mithracin for Intravenous Use ... 903
M-M-R II ... 2118
Moban (Occasional) ... 1320
Mobic Tablets (2.4% to 4.7%) ... 1054
Modicon ... 2563
▲ Moduretic Tablets (3% to 8%) ... 2138
Monoclate-P Concentrate ... 793
Monodox Capsules ... 2442
Mononine Concentrate ... 794
Monopril Tablets (1.2% to 2.2%) ... 1091
Monopril HCT (Less than 2%) ... 1094
▲ Monurol Sachet (4.1% to 5.2%) ... 1375
Motofen Tablets (1 in 15) ... 577
▲ Motrin Suspension, Oral Drops, Chewable Tablets, and Caplets (3% to 9%) ... 2002
▲ MS Contin Tablets (Among most frequent) ... 2896
▲ MSIR (Among most frequent) ... 2898
Mustargen for Injection ... 2142
Myambutol Tablets ... 1290
Mycelex Troche ... 573
▲ Mycobutin Capsules (6%) ... 2838
Mykrox Tablets (Less than 2%) ... 1168
Myleran Tablets ... 1603
Mylocel Tablets (Less frequently) ... 2227
▲ Mylotarg for Injection (38% to 51%) ... 3540
▲ Myobloc Injectable Solution (3% to 10%) ... 1291
▲ Nabi-HB (5%) ... 2295
Nadolol Tablets (1 to 5 of 1000 patients) ... 2288
▲ Naprelan Tablets (3% to 9%) ... 1293
▲ Naprosyn Suspension (3% to 9%) .. 2967
▲ Naprosyn Tablets (3% to 9%) ... 2967
Narcan Injection ... 1322
Nardil Tablets ... 2653
▲ Naropin Injection (More than 5% to 29.4%) ... 612
Nasalide Nasal Spray (5% or less) .. 1295
Nasarel Nasal Solution 0.025% (Greater than 1%) ... 1296
Nascobal Gel (One patient) ... 3174
Nasonex Nasal Spray (Greater than or equal to 2%) ... 3131
▲ Natrecor for Injection (4%) ... 3189
Navane Oral ... 2701
Navane Intramuscular ... 2703
▲ Navelbine Injection (Up to 34%) ... 1604
Nebcin Vials, Hyporets & ADD-Vantage ... 1955
Necon ... 3415
Nembutal Sodium Solution (Less than 1%) ... 485
▲ Neoral Soft Gelatin Capsules (2% to 18%) ... 2380
▲ Neoral Oral Solution (2% to 18%) ... 2380
Neptazane Tablets ... ⊙ 271

Nesacaine/Nesacaine MPF............ 617
▲ Neumega for Injection (77%) 1434
▲ Neupogen for Injection (10%; 57%)... 587
Neurontin Capsules.......................... 2655
▲ Neurontin Oral Solution (8.4%) 2655
Neurontin Tablets.............................. 2655
Nexium Delayed-Release Capsules (Greater than or equal to 1%).. 619
▲ Niaspan Extended-Release Tablets (2% to 8%)...................... 1846
Nicomide Tablets............................... 3247
▲ Nicotrol Inhaler (Greater than 3%) .. 2840
▲ Nicotrol Nasal Spray (5%) 2843
▲ Nilandron Tablets (23.9%) 753
Nimotop Capsules (Up to 1.4%)...... 904
▲ Nipent for Injection (53% to 63%) ... 3272
Nitrolingual Pumpspray (Uncommon)................................ 1355
Nitrostat Tablets............................... 2658
Nizoral Tablets (Approximately 3%)... 1791
▲ Nolvadex Tablets (2.1% to 25.7%) . 678
▲ Norco 5/325 Tablets CIII (Among most frequent)............................... 3424
▲ Norco 7.5/325 Tablets CIII (Among most frequent)................ 3425
▲ Norco 10/325 Tablets CIII (Among most frequent)................ 3425
▲ Norco 10/325 Tablets CIII (Among most frequent)................ 3427
▲ Nordette-28 Tablets (10% or less) .. 2257
Norditropin Cartridges (Small number of patients)..................... 2420
Norditropin for Injection (Small number of patients)..................... 2419
Norflex... 1987
Norinyl 1 +35 28-Day Tablets......... 3380
Norinyl 1 + 50 28-Day Tablets........ 3380
▲ Normodyne Injection (13%)............ 3135
▲ Normodyne Tablets (Less than 1% to 19%)................................... 3137
▲ Noroxin Tablets (2.6% to 4.2%) 2145
Norplant System............................... 3543
Norpramin Tablets............................ 755
Nor-QD Tablets................................. 3423
Norvasc Tablets (2.9%).................. 2704
▲ Norvir Capsules (23.1% to 26.2%)... 487
▲ Norvir Oral Solution (23.1% to 26.2%)... 487
▲ Novantrone for Injection (31% to 76%)... 1760
▲ Nubain Injection (6%) 1323
NuLev Orally Disintegrating Tablets... 3176
▲ NuLYTELY, Cherry Flavor, Lemon-Lime Flavor, and Orange Flavor NuLYTELY for Oral Solution (Among most common).................................... 1068
Numorphan....................................... 1324
Nutropin AQ Injection (A small number of patients).................... 1420
▲ Nutropin Depot for Injectable Suspension (8%).......................... 1423
Nutropin for Injection (A small number of patients).................... 1417
Ocuflox Ophthalmic Solution........ 554
Ocupress Ophthalmic Solution, 1% Sterile .... ⊙303
Ogen Tablets..................................... 2846
▲ Ogestrel 0.5/50-28 Tablets (10% or less).. 3428
▲ Omnicef (3%) 493
▲ Oncaspar (Greater than 5%) 756
OptiPranolol Metipranolol Ophthalmic Solution 0.3% (A small number of patients)........... ⊙263
▲ Oramorph SR Tablets (Among most frequent)............................. 3062
Orap Tablets...................................... 1407
▲ Organidin NR Liquid (Among most common)...................................... 3350
▲ Organidin NR Tablets (Among most common)............................. 3350
▲ Orgaran Injection (4.1% to 14.3%) . 2480
Ortho Dienestrol Cream.................. 2554
Ortho-Cept 21 Tablets..................... 2546
Ortho-Cept 28 Tablets..................... 2546
▲ Orthoclone OKT3 Sterile Solution (19%)... 2498
Ortho-Cyclen/Ortho Tri-Cyclen........ 2573
Ortho-Est Tablets............................. 3464
Ortho-Novum.................................... 2563
Ortho-Novum 1/50▫28 Tablets....... 2556
▲ Ortho-Prefest Tablets (6%) 2570
Ortho-Cyclen/Ortho Tri-Cyclen........ 2573
▲ Orudis Capsules (3% to 9%) 3548
▲ Oruvail Capsules (3% to 9%) 3548
Ovcon.. 3364
▲ Ovidrel for Injection (3.4%) 3220
▲ Ovral Tablets (10% or less) 3551
▲ Ovral-28 Tablets (10% or less) 3552
▲ Ovrette Tablets (10% or less) 3552
Oxandrin Tablets.............................. 1153
▲ Oxsoralen-Ultra Capsules (10%) 1741
▲ OxyContin Tablets (Less than 1% to 23%).. 2912
▲ OxyFast Oral Concentrate Solution (Among most frequent)... 2916
▲ OxyIR Capsules (Among most frequent)....................................... 2916

▲ Pacerone Tablets (10% to 33%) 3331
▲ Pancrease Capsules (Among most frequent)............................. 2580
▲ Paraplatin for Injection (75% to 96%)... 1126
Parnate Tablets................................ 1607
▲ Paser Granules (Among most common)...................................... 1781
Patanol Ophthalmic Solution (Less than 5%)........................... 540
▲ Paxil (1.9% to 36.3%) 1609
▲ PCE Dispertab Tablets (Among most frequent).............................. 498
▲ Pediazole Suspension (Among most frequent)............................. 3050
▲ PEG-Intron Powder for Injection (26%)... 3140
Pentasa Capsules (1.8% to 3.1%)... 3239
Pepcid Injection (Infrequent)........... 2153
Pepcid for Oral Suspension (Infrequent)................................... 2150
Pepcid RPD Orally Disintegrating Tablets (Infrequent) 2150
Pepcid Tablets (Infrequent) 2150
▲ Percocet Tablets (Among most frequent) 1326
▲ Percodan Tablets (Among most frequent) 1327
▲ Percolone Tablets (Among most frequent) 1327
Pergonal for Injection 3223
Periactin Tablets 2155
Peri-Colace Capsules and Syrup 3240
▲ Periostat Tablets (8%) 1208
▲ Permax Tablets (24.3%) 1299
Persantine Tablets (Rare) 1057
Phenergan Injection 3553
Phenergan Suppositories 3556
Phenergan Syrup 3554
Phenergan Tablets 3556
Phenergan with Codeine Syrup 3557
Phenergan with Dextromethorphan Syrup 3559
Phenergan VC Syrup 3560
Phenergan VC with Codeine Syrup .. 3561
PhosChol 579
PhosLo (Occasional) 1069
▲ Photofrin for Injection (24%) 831
▲ Phrenilin (Among most frequent) 578
Pima Syrup (Less frequent) 1362
Pipracil (Less frequent) 1866
Plaquenil Tablets 3082
Plasmanate (Occasional) 942
▲ Plavix Tablets (3.4%) 1097
▲ Plavix Tablets (3.4%) 3084
Plendil Extended-Release Tablets (1.0% to 1.7%) 623
▲ Pletal Tablets (6% to 7%) 2605
▲ Pletal Tablets (6% to 7%) 2848
Pneumovax 23 2156
Polocaine Injection, USP 625
Polocaine-MPF Injection, USP 625
▲ Ponstel Capsules (1% to 10%) 1356
Potaba (Infrequent) 1721
▲ Prandin Tablets (0.5, 1, and 2 mg) (3% to 5%) 2432
▲ Pravachol Tablets (2.9% to 7.3%) .. 1099
Prednisone 3064
Premarin Intravenous 3563
Premarin Tablets 3566
Premarin Vaginal Cream 3570
Premphase Tablets 3572
▲ Prempro Tablets (9% to 11%) 3572
Prevacid Delayed-Release Capsules (1.4%) 3292
PREVPAC (1.4% to 3%) 3298
Priftin Tablets (1.0%) 758
▲ Prilosec Delayed-Release Capsules (2.2% to 4.0%) 628
Primaxin I.M. (0.6%) 2158
Primaxin I.V. (2.0%) 2160
Prinivil Tablets (Greater than 1% to 2.0%) 2164
Prinzide Tablets (2.2%) 2168
ProAmatine Tablets (Rare) 3241
▲ Procanbid Extended-Release Tablets (3% to 4%) 2262
▲ Procardia Capsules (Approximately 10% to 11%) 2708
▲ Procardia XL Extended Release Tablets (3.3% to 11%) 2710
▲ Procrit for Injection (0.26% to 58%) 2502
▲ Prograf (32% to 46%) 1393
▲ Proleukin for Injection (35%) 1199
▲ Prometrium Capsules (100 mg, 200 mg) (8%) 3261
Prosed/DS Tablets 3268
▲ ProSom Tablets (4%) 500
Prostigmin Injectable 1744
Prostigmin Tablets 1744
▲ Prostin E2 Suppositories (Approximately one-third) 2852
Protonix I.V. (Greater than 1%) 3580
Protonix Tablets (Greater than or equal to 1%) 3577
Protopam Chloride for Injection 3582
Protopic Ointment (1% to 3%) 1397
▲ Proventil Inhalation Aerosol (Less than 15%) 3142
▲ Proventil Inhalation Solution 0.083% (3.1% to 4%) 3146
Proventil Repetabs Tablets (2% to 4%) 3148

▲ Proventil Solution for Inhalation 0.5% (3.1% to 4%).................... 3144
▲ Proventil HFA Inhalation Aerosol (10%).. 3150
Provera Tablets................................. 2853
▲ Provigil Tablets (13%) 1193
▲ Prozac Pulvules, Liquid, and Weekly Capsules (1% to 29%)...... 1238
▲ Pulmicort Turbuhaler Inhalation Powder (Up to 6%)...................... 636
Purinethol Tablets (Uncommon)...... 1615
Pyrazinamide Tablets...................... 1876
▲ Quinaglute Dura-Tabs Tablets (3%) . 978
▲ Quinidex Extentabs (Among most frequent)....................................... 2933
Qvar Inhalation Aerosol (Less than 1% to 2%)...................................... 1987
▲ Rapamune Oral Solution and Tablets (25% to 36%).................... 3584
▲ Rebetron Combination Therapy (38% to 47%).............................. 3153
Recombinate (Extremely rare) 853
Recombivax HB (Equal to or greater than 1%) 2178
ReFacto Vials 1437
Reglan 2935
▲ Relafen Tablets (3% to 9%) 1617
Relenza Rotadisk (Less than 3%) 1619
Remeron Tablets (1.5%) 2483
Remeron SolTab Tablets (1.5%) 2486
▲ Remicade for IV Injection (17%) 1178
▲ Reminyl Oral Solution (2% to 24%) . 1792
▲ Reminyl Tablets (2% to 24%) 1792
▲ Renagel Capsules (7%) 1439
▲ Renagel Tablets (7%) 1439
Renese Tablets 2712
▲ ReoPro Vials (18.4%) 1958
▲ Repronex for Intramuscular and Subcutaneous Injection (4% to 7.3%) 1347
▲ Requip Tablets (30% to 60%) 1621
▲ Rescriptor Tablets (4.9% to 10.8%) 526
Retavase Vials 1182
▲ Retrovir Capsules (0.8% to 61%) 1625
▲ Retrovir IV Infusion (1% to 61%) 1629
▲ Retrovir (0.8% to 61%) 1625
Rhinocort Nasal Inhaler (Less than 1%) 640
Rifadin (Some patients) 765
Rifamate Capsules (Some patients) 767
Rifater Tablets 769
▲ Rilutek Tablets (12.2% to 20.5%) ... 772
▲ Risperdal (4% to 6%) 1796
Ritalin 2387
▲ Rituxan for Infusion (18%) 1750
▲ Rituxan I.V. (18%) 1428
Robaxin Injectable 2938
Robaxin Tablets 2939
▲ Robaxisal Tablets (One in 20 to 25) 2939
Robinul Forte Tablets 1358
Robinul Injectable 2940
Robinul Tablets 1358
Rocaltrol 2991
Rocephin Injectable Vials, ADD-Vantage, Galaxy, Bulk (Less than 1%) 2993
▲ Roferon-A Injection (33% to 51%) ... 2996
▲ Romazicon Injection (11%) 3000
▲ Rowasa Rectal Suspension Enema 4.0 grams/unit (60 mL) (5.77%) 3264
▲ Roxanol (Among most frequent) 3066
▲ Roxicodone (Among most frequent) 3067
Rum-K 1363
Rynatan Tablets 3351
▲ Rythmol Tablets – 150 mg, 225 mg, 300 mg (2.8% to 10.7%) 502
Saizen for Injection (A small number of patients) 3225
▲ Salagen Tablets (6% to 15%) 2229
▲ Sandimmune (2% to 10%) 2388
Sandoglobulin I.V. 2391
▲ Sandostatin Injection (34% to 61%) 2394
▲ Sandostatin LAR Depot (10.3%) 2395
▲ Sarafem Pulvules (13% to 27%) 1962
▲ Sectral Capsules (4%) 3589
▲ Sedapap Tablets 50 mg/650 mg (Among the most frequent) 2225
Semprex-D Capsules (2%) 1172
Sensorcaine (Rare) 643
Sensorcaine-MPF Injection (Rare) 643
▲ Septra Suspension (Among most common) 2265
▲ Septra Tablets (Among most common) 2265
▲ Septra DS Tablets (Among most common) 2265
Serentil 1057
Serevent Diskus (1% to 3%) 1637
Serevent Inhalation Aerosol (1% to 3%) 1633
Serophene Tablets (Approximately 1 in 50 patients) .. 3226
▲ Serostim for Injection (25.9%) 3229
▲ Serzone Tablets (14% to 23%) 1104
▲ Simulect for Injection (Greater than or equal to 10%) 2399
▲ Sinemet Tablets (Among most common) 1253
▲ Sinemet CR Tablets (5.5%) 1255

Sinequan... 2713
Singulair (Greater than or equal to 2%).. 2181
Skelaxin Tablets 1301
▲ Skelid Tablets (9.3%) 3088
Solu-Medrol Sterile Powder............. 2855
Soma Tablets 3353
▲ Soma Compound Tablets (Among most common) 3354
Soma Compound w/Codeine Tablets 3355
▲ Sonata Capsules (7% to 8%) 3591
▲ Soriatane Capsules (1% to 10%) 3003
▲ Sporanox Capsules (3% to 10.6%) 1800
▲ Sporanox Injection (8%) 1804
▲ Sporanox Injection (8%) 2509
▲ Sporanox Oral Solution (10.3% to 11.1%) 1808
▲ Sporanox Oral Solution (10.3% to 11.1%) 2512
▲ Stadol NS Nasal Spray (13%) 1108
Starlix Tablets 2401
Stelazine 1640
Stimate Nasal Spray 796
Streptase for Infusion 647
Streptomycin Sulfate Injection 2714
Stromectol Tablets (1.8%) 2185
Sular Tablets (2%) 688
▲ Suprane Liquid for Inhalation (27%) 874
▲ Suprax (7%) 1877
Surmontil Capsules 3595
▲ Sustiva Capsules (2% to 16%) 1258
▲ Symmetrel (5% to 10%) 1328
▲ Synercid I.V. (4.6%) 775
Synvisc 3596
Tabloid Tablets (Less frequent) 1642
Talacen Caplets (Rare) 3089
Talwin Nx Tablets 3090
▲ Tambocor Tablets (8.9%) 1990
▲ Tamiflu Capsules (3.3% to 9.9%) 3008
▲ Tamiflu Oral Suspension (3.3% to 9.9%) 3008
Tao Capsules (Infrequent) 2716
Tapazole Tablets 1823
Tarka Tablets (0.3% to 1.5%) 508
▲ Tasmar Tablets (30% to 35%) 3010
▲ Taxol Injection (52% to 87%) 1129
Taxotere for Injection Concentrate .. 778
Tazicef for Injection (Less than 2%) 1647
Tazicef Galaxy Container (Less than 2%) 1650
Tazicef Pharmacy Bulk Package (Less than 2%) 1653
Tazidime Vials, Faspak & ADD-Vantage (1 in 156) 1966
▲ Tegretol/Tegretol-XR (Among most frequent) 2404
▲ Temodar Capsules (53%) 3157
Tenex Tablets (3% or less) 2942
▲ Tenoretic Tablets (3% to 4%) 690
▲ Tenormin (3% to 4%) 692
Tensilon Injectable 1745
▲ Tequin Injection (8%) 1110
▲ Tequin Tablets (8%) 1110
Tessalon Capsules 1377
Testoderm Transdermal Systems ... 574
Testopel Pellets 3610
Testred Capsules, 10 mg 1746
Tetanus & Diphtheria Toxoids Adsorbed for Adult Use 1880
Tetanus and Diphtheria Toxoids Adsorbed For Adult Use 815
Teveten Tablets (Less than 1%) 3327
▲ Thalomid Capsules (4.2%) 1154
Theo-Dur Extended-Release Tablets 1835
▲ TheraCys Injection (16%) 823
Thioplex for Injection 1765
Thioridazine Hydrochloride Tablets 2289
Thiothixene Capsules 2290
Thorazine 1656
▲ Thrombate III (3 of 17) 944
▲ Thymoglobulin for Injection (36.6%) 3071
Thyrel TRH for Injection 3630
▲ Thyrogen for Injection (10.5%) 1441
Tiazac Capsules (2%) 1378
▲ Tice BCG, BCG Live (3.0%) 2489
▲ Ticlid Tablets (7.0%) 3015
Timentin Injection- ADD-Vantage Vial 1661
Timentin Injection-Galaxy Container 1664
Timentin Injection-Pharmacy Bulk Package 1666
Timentin for Intravenous Administration 1658
Timolide Tablets (Less than 1%) 2187
Timolol GFS .... ⊙266
Timoptic in Ocudose (Less frequent) 2192
Timoptic Sterile Ophthalmic Solution (Less frequent) 2190
Timoptic-XE Sterile Ophthalmic Gel Forming Solution 2194
TNKase I.V. 1430
▲ TOBI Solution for Inhalation (11.2%) 1206
▲ Tolectin (11%) 2589

▲ Tonocard Tablets (14.5% to 24.6%)............ 649
▲ Topamax Sprinkle Capsules (11.5% to 13.8%)............ 2590
▲ Topamax Tablets (11.5% to 13.8%)............ 2590
Toprol-XL Tablets (About 1 of 100 patients)............ 651
▲ Toradol (12%)............ 3018
Transderm Scōp Transdermal Therapeutic System (Few patients)............ 2302
▲ Trasylol Injection (11%)............ 909
▲ Trecator-SC Tablets (Among most common)............ 3598
Trental Tablets (2.2%)............ 784
▲ Tricor Capsules, Micronized (4%)............ 513
Trilafon (Occasional)............ 3160
▲ Trileptal Oral Suspension (10% to 29%)............ 2407
▲ Trileptal Tablets (10% to 29%)............ 2407
Tri-Levlen............ 962
▲ Trilisate (Less than 20%)............ 2901
Tri-Nasal Spray (2% to 3%)............ 2274
Tri-Norinyl-28 Tablets............ 3433
▲ Triphasil-21 Tablets (10% or less)............ 3600
▲ Triphasil-28 Tablets (10% or less)............ 3605
▲ Trisenox Injection (75%)............ 1158
Trivora Tablets............ 3439
▲ Trizivir Tablets (12% to 60%)............ 1669
▲ Trovan (4% to 5%)............ 2722
Trusopt Sterile Ophthalmic Solution (Infrequent)............ 2196
Tussionex Pennkinetic Extended-Release Suspension............ 1174
Tussi-Organidin NR Liquid............ 3350
▲ Tussi-Organidin DM NR Liquid (Among most common)............ 3350
▲ Tussi-Organidin DM-S NR Liquid (Among most common)............ 3350
▲ Tussi-Organidin-S NR Liquid (Among most common)............ 3350
Twinrix Vaccine (2% to 4%)............ 1674
▲ Tylenol with Codeine (Among most frequent)............ 2595
▲ Tylox Capsules (Among most frequent)............ 2597
▲ TYPHIM Vi Vaccine (2% to 8.2%)............ 825
▲ Ultracet Tablets (3%)............ 2597
▲ Ultram Tablets (24% to 40%)............ 2600
Unasyn for Injection (Less than 1%)............ 2728
Uni-Dur Extended-Release Tablets............ 1841
Uniphyl 400 mg and 600 mg Tablets............ 2903
Uniretic Tablets (More than 1%)............ 3178
Univasc Tablets (More than 1%)............ 3181
Urecholine............ 2198
Urecholine Tablets............ 2445
Urimax Tablets............ 1769
Urobiotic-250 Capsules (Rare)............ 2731
Urocit-K Tablets (Some patients)............ 2232
Uroqid-Acid No. 2 Tablets............ 947
Urso Tablets............ 836
▲ Valcyte Tablets (8% to 30%)............ 3022
Valium Injectable............ 3026
Valium Tablets (Infrequent)............ 3047
▲ Valstar Sterile Solution for Intravesical Instillation (5%)............ 1175
▲ Valtrex Caplets (5% to 15%)............ 1676
Vanceril Double Strength Inhalation Aerosol (Fewer than 2%)............ 3167
Vancocin HCl Capsules & Pulvules (Infrequent)............ 1972
Vancocin HCl Oral Solution (Infrequent)............ 1971
Vancocin HCl, Vials & ADD-Vantage (Infrequent)............ 1970
Vaniqa Cream (0.7%)............ 1121
Vantin Tablets and Oral Suspension (1.4% to 3.8%)............ 2860
Vaqta (2.3%)............ 2199
Varivax (Greater than or equal to 1%)............ 2202
▲ Vascor Tablets (12.29% to 26.09%)............ 2602
Vaseretic Tablets (2.5%)............ 2204
Vasotec I.V. Injection (1.1%)............ 2207
Vasotec Tablets (1.3% to 1.4%)............ 2210
Venastat Suppli-Cap Capsules (Rare)............ ▣833
▲ Venofer Injection (Greater than 5%)............ 580
▲ Ventolin Inhalation Aerosol and Refill (Less than 6% to 15%)............ 1679
Verelan Capsules (2.7%)............ 3184
Verelan PM Capsules (1.7% to 2.7%)............ 3186
Versed Injection (2.8%)............ 3027
▲ Versed Syrup (4%)............ 3033
▲ Vesanoid Capsules (57%)............ 3037
Viadur Implant (Less than 2%)............ 912
Vibramycin Calcium Oral Suspension Syrup............ 2735
Vibramycin Hyclate Capsules............ 2735
Vibramycin Hyclate Intravenous............ 2737
Vibramycin Monohydrate for Oral Suspension............ 2735
Vibra-Tabs Film Coated Tablets............ 2735
▲ Vicodin Tablets (Among most frequent)............ 516
▲ Vicodin ES Tablets (Among most frequent)............ 517
▲ Vicodin HP Tablets (Among most frequent)............ 518
Vicodin Tuss Expectorant (More frequently in ambulatory than in recumbent patients)............ 519
▲ Vicoprofen Tablets (21%)............ 520
▲ Videx (7%)............ 1138
▲ Videx EC Capsules (21%)............ 1143
Vioxx (2.9%)............ 2213
▲ Viracept (2% to 7%)............ 532
▲ Viramune Oral Suspension (5%)............ 1060
▲ Viramune Tablets (5%)............ 1060
Visicol Tablets............ 1767
▲ Vistide Injection (7% to 69%)............ 1445
▲ Visudyne for Injection (1% to 10%)............ ⊙308
▲ Vitravene for Injection (5% to 20%)............ ⊙310
Vivactil Tablets............ 2217
Vivactil Tablets............ 2446
Vivelle Transdermal System............ 2412
Vivelle-Dot Transdermal System............ 2416
Vivotif Berna (Infrequent)............ 997
▲ Volmax Extended-Release Tablets (4.2%)............ 2276
Voltaren Ophthalmic Sterile Ophthalmic Solution (3% or less)............ ⊙312
▲ Voltaren Tablets (3% to 9%)............ 2315
▲ Voltaren-XR Tablets (3% to 9%)............ 2315
Warfarin Sodium Tablets, USP............ 3302
▲ WelChol Tablets (4%)............ 3073
▲ Wellbutrin Tablets (22.9%)............ 1680
▲ Wellbutrin SR Sustained-Release Tablets (0.8% to 18%)............ 1684
▲ Xanax Tablets (9.6% to 22.0%)............ 2865
▲ Xeloda Tablets (4%)............ 3039
▲ Xenical Capsules (3.6% to 8.1%)............ 3043
Xopenex Inhalation Solution............ 3207
X-Prep Liquid............ 2900
Xylocaine Injections (Less than 1%)............ 653
Yasmin 28 Tablets (Greater than 1%)............ 980
Yodoxin Tablets............ 1722
Zantac............ 1690
Zantac Injection............ 1688
Zantac Syrup............ 1690
Zarontin Capsules (Frequent)............ 2659
Zarontin Syrup (Frequent)............ 2660
Zaroxolyn Tablets............ 1177
Zebeta Tablets (1.5% to 2.2%)............ 1885
▲ Zemplar Injection (13%)............ 522
Zemuron Injection (Less than 1%)............ 2491
▲ Zenapax for Injection (Greater than 5%)............ 3046
Zephrex Tablets............ 3091
Zephrex LA Tablets............ 3092
▲ Zerit (38%)............ 1147
Zestoretic Tablets (2.2%)............ 695
Zestril Tablets (Greater than 1% to 2.0%)............ 698
Ziac Tablets (0.9% to 1.1%)............ 1887
▲ Ziagen (16% to 60%)............ 1692
Zinacef Injection (1 in 440 patients)............ 1696
Zinacef for Injection (1 in 440 patients)............ 1696
▲ Zinecard for Injection (51% to 77%)............ 2869
▲ Zithromax Capsules, 250 mg (1% to 18%)............ 2743
▲ Zithromax for IV Infusion (3.9% to 10.3%)............ 2748
▲ Zithromax for Oral Suspension, 1 g (3% to 5%)............ 2743
▲ Zithromax for Oral Suspension, 300 mg, 600 mg, 900 mg, 1200 mg (1% to 18%)............ 2739
▲ Zithromax Tablets, 250 mg (1% to 18%)............ 2739
▲ Zithromax Tablets, 600 mg (3% to 5%)............ 2743
Zocor Tablets (1.3%)............ 2219
▲ Zoladex (5% to 11%)............ 702
▲ Zoladex 3-month (9%)............ 706
▲ Zoloft (26% to 30%)............ 2751
▲ Zometa for Intravenous Infusion (29.1%)............ 3621
▲ Zomig Tablets (4% to 9%)............ 708
▲ Zomig-ZMT Tablets (4% to 9%)............ 708
▲ Zonegran Capsules (9%)............ 1307
▲ Zosyn (5.8% to 6.9%)............ 1890
▲ Zosyn in Galaxy Containers (5.8% to 6.9%)............ 1894
Zovia............ 3449
Zovirax Capsules (2.4% to 4.8%)............ 1706
▲ Zovirax for Injection (Approximately 7%)............ 1708
Zovirax (2.4% to 4.8%)............ 1706
▲ Zyban Sustained-Release Tablets (9%)............ 1710
▲ Zydone Tablets (Among most frequent)............ 1330
▲ Zyflo Filmtab Tablets (5.5%)............ 524
▲ Zyprexa Tablets (Up to 9%)............ 1973
▲ Zyprexa ZYDIS Orally Disintegrating Tablets (Up to 9%)............ 1973
Zyrtec (1.9% to 2.8%)............ 2756
Zyrtec-D 12 Hour Extended Relief Tablets............ 2758

Neck, redistribution/accumulation of body fat
Crixivan Capsules............ 2070

Neck, rigidity of
Aciphex Tablets............ 1267
Aciphex Tablets............ 1783
Amerge Tablets............ 1467
Axert Tablets (Infrequent)............ 2772
Depacon Injection (1% or more)............ 416
Depakene (1% or more)............ 421
Depakote Sprinkle Capsules............ 426
Depakote Tablets (1% to 5%)............ 430
Depakote ER Tablets (Greater than 1%)............ 436
Diprivan Injectable Emulsion (Less than 1%)............ 667
Effexor Tablets (Infrequent)............ 3495
Effexor XR Capsules (Infrequent)............ 3499
Eldepryl Capsules............ 3266
Hivid Tablets (Less than 1%)............ 2975
▲ Imitrex Injection (4.8%)............ 1549
Imitrex Nasal Spray............ 1554
Imitrex Tablets............ 1558
Ismo Tablets (Fewer than 1%)............ 3524
Lipitor Tablets (Less than 2%)............ 2639
Lipitor Tablets (Less than 2%)............ 2696
Luvox Tablets (25, 50, 100 mg) (Infrequent)............ 3256
Maxalt Tablets (Less than 2%)............ 2120
Maxalt-MLT Orally Disintegrating Tablets (Less than 2%)............ 2120
Naprelan Tablets (Less than 1%)............ 1293
Norvir Capsules (Less than 2%)............ 487
Norvir Oral Solution (Less than 2%)............ 487
Paxil (Rare)............ 1609
Pletal Tablets (Less than 2%)............ 2605
Pletal Tablets (Less than 2%)............ 2848
Prostin E2 Suppositories............ 2852
Protonix I.V. (Less than 1%)............ 3580
Protonix Tablets (Less than 1%)............ 3577
Remeron Tablets (Infrequent)............ 2483
Remeron SolTab Tablets (Infrequent)............ 2486
Rescriptor Tablets (Less than 2%)............ 526
Salagen Tablets (Less than 1%)............ 2229
Serzone Tablets (1%)............ 1104
▲ Thalomid Capsules (4.2%)............ 1154
Uniretic Tablets (Less than 1%)............ 3178
Varivax (Greater than or equal to 1%)............ 2202
Zonegran Capsules (Infrequent)............ 1307
Zyflo Filmtab Tablets (Less common)............ 524
Zyprexa Tablets (2% to 3%)............ 1973
Zyprexa ZYDIS Orally Disintegrating Tablets (2% to 3%)............ 1973

Neck tightness
Imitrex Injection (Relatively common)............ 1549

Necrolysis, digitus
Sustiva Capsules (Up to 3.5%)............ 1258

Necrolysis, epidermal
(*see under* Lyell's syndrome)

Necrosis
Aplisol Injection............ 2609
Benadryl Parenteral............ 2617
Betaseron for SC Injection (2%)............ 988
Bicillin C-R 900/300 Injection............ 2240
Bicillin C-R Injection............ 2238
Bicillin L-A Injection............ 2242
Captopril Tablets (Rare)............ 2281
Ceptaz for Injection............ 1499
Fortaz............ 1541
▲ Naprelan Tablets (3% to 9%)............ 1293
Sensorcaine............ 643
Sensorcaine-MPF Injection............ 643
Sustiva Capsules (Up to 3.5%)............ 1258
Taxol Injection (Rare)............ 1129
Tine Test, Tuberculin, Old............ 3631
Tubersol Diagnostic Antigen............ 3628

Necrosis, aseptic
Cortifoam Rectal Foam............ 3170
Cortone Acetate Tablets............ 2061

Necrosis, bone
Arava Tablets (1% to 3%)............ 724
Avonex............ 1013
Herceptin I.V. (At least one of the 958 patients)............ 1414
▲ Rapamune Oral Solution and Tablets (3% to 20%)............ 3584
Rilutek Tablets (Rare)............ 772
Vistide Injection............ 1445

Necrosis, bowel
Proleukin for Injection (Less than 1%)............ 1199

Necrosis, buccal
Orudis Capsules (Less than 1%)............ 3548
Oruvail Capsules (Less than 1%)............ 3548

Necrosis, cecal
Adriamycin PFS/RDF............ 2767

Necrosis, cutaneous
▲ Androderm Transdermal System CIII (12%)............ 3377
Aramine Injection............ 2043
Betaseron for SC Injection............ 988
Brevibloc Injection (Less than 1%)............ 858
Cognex Capsules (Rare)............ 1351
Coumadin for Injection (Less frequent)............ 1243
Coumadin Tablets (Less frequent)............ 1243
Dobutrex Solution Vials (Isolated cases)............ 1914
Doxil Injection (Less than 1%)............ 566
Effexor Tablets............ 3495
Ellence Injection............ 2806
Heparin Lock Flush Solution............ 3509
Heparin Sodium Injection............ 3511
Lovenox Injection............ 746
Naprelan Tablets (Less than 1%)............ 1293
Neurontin Capsules (Rare)............ 2655
Neurontin Oral Solution (Rare)............ 2655
Neurontin Tablets (Rare)............ 2655
Thalomid Capsules............ 1154
Vancocin HCl, Vials & ADD-Vantage............ 1970
Warfarin Sodium Tablets, USP............ 3302

Necrosis, femoral head avascular
Evoxac Capsules (Less than 1%)............ 1217
Pulmicort Respules (Less than 1%)............ 632

Necrosis, injection sites
Amicar Injection............ 3608
Amicar Syrup............ 3608
Amicar Tablets............ 3608

Necrosis, intestinal
Bicillin C-R 900/300 Injection............ 2240
Bicillin C-R Injection............ 2238
Bicillin L-A Injection............ 2242
Lanoxicaps Capsules (Very rare)............ 1574
Navelbine Injection............ 1604
Tabloid Tablets............ 1642

Necrosis, ischemic
Felbatol............ 3343
Plavix Tablets (Less than 1%)............ 1097
Plavix Tablets (Less than 1%)............ 3084

Necrosis, macular
Nebcin Vials, Hyporets & ADD-Vantage............ 1955

Necrosis, nasal
Rhinocort Nasal Inhaler (Rare)............ 640

Necrosis, papillary
Aggrenox Capsules............ 1026
Arthrotec Tablets (Rare)............ 3195
Cataflam Tablets (Rare)............ 2315
Ecotrin Enteric Coated Aspirin Low, Regular and Maximum Strength Tablets............ 1715
Voltaren Tablets (Rare)............ 2315
Voltaren-XR Tablets (Rare)............ 2315

Necrosis, renal papillary
Anaprox Tablets (Less than 1%)............ 2967
Anaprox DS Tablets (Less than 1%)............ 2967
Dapsone Tablets USP............ 1780
Darvon-N/Darvocet-N............ 1907
Darvon Pulvules............ 1909
Darvon Compound-65 Pulvules............ 1910
EC-Naprosyn Delayed-Release Tablets (Less than 1%)............ 2967
Lodine (Less than 1%)............ 3528
Lodine XL Extended-Release Tablets (Less than 1%)............ 3530
Motrin Suspension, Oral Drops, Chewable Tablets, and Caplets (Less than 1%)............ 2002
▲ Naprelan Tablets (3% to 9%)............ 1293
Naprosyn Suspension (Less than 1%)............ 2967
Naprosyn Tablets (Less than 1%)............ 2967
Relafen Tablets............ 1617
Vicoprofen Tablets............ 520

Necrosis, renal tubular
Calcium Disodium Versenate Injection............ 1980
▲ CellCept Capsules (6.3% to 10.0%)............ 2951
▲ CellCept Intravenous (6.3% to 10.0%)............ 2951
▲ CellCept Oral Suspension (6.3% to 10.0%)............ 2951
▲ CellCept Tablets (6.3% to 10.0%)............ 2951
Gamimune N, 5% Solvent/Detergent Treated............ 925
Gamimune N, 10% Solvent/Detergent Treated............ 928
Gammagard S/D............ 845
Gammar-P I.V.............. 787
Motrin Suspension, Oral Drops, Chewable Tablets, and Caplets (Less than 1%)............ 2002
▲ Prograf (3% to 15%)............ 1393
▲ Rapamune Oral Solution and Tablets (3% to 20%)............ 3584
Rifadin (Rare)............ 765

Sandoglobulin I.V. 2391
▲ Simulect for Injection (3% to 10%) 2399
Trasylol Injection (1% to 2%) 909
▲ Vesanoid Capsules (3%) 3037
▲ Zenapax for Injection (Greater than 5%) 3046

Necrosis, skin

Innohep Injection 1248

Necrosis, tissue

Adriamycin PFS/RDF Injection 2767
Cerubidine for Injection 947
Coumadin for Injection (Less frequent) 1243
Coumadin Tablets (Less frequent) 1243
DaunoXome Injection 1442
Ellence Injection 2806
Fragmin Injection (Rare) 2814
Idamycin PFS Injection 2825
Mepergan Injection 3539
Novantrone for Injection (Rare) 1760
Phenergan Injection 3553
Phenergan Tablets 3556
Silvadene Cream 1% (Infrequent) 2267
Warfarin Sodium Tablets, USP 3302

Necrotizing angiitis

Accuretic Tablets 2614
Aldoclor Tablets 2035
Aldoril Tablets 2039
Atacand HCT Tablets 597
Avalide Tablets 1070
Clorpres Tablets 1002
Combipres Tablets 1040
Cortifoam Rectal Foam 3170
Corzide 40/5 Tablets 2247
Corzide 80/5 Tablets 2247
Diovan HCT Tablets 2338
Diucardin Tablets 3494
Diuril Sodium Intravenous 2086
Dyazide Capsules 1515
Furosemide Tablets 2284
HydroDIURIL Tablets 2108
Hyzaar 2109
Indapamide Tablets 2286
Inderide Tablets 3517
Inderide LA Long-Acting Capsules 3519
Lodine (Less than 1%) 3528
Lodine XL Extended-Release Tablets (Less than 1%) 3530
Lotensin HCT Tablets 2367
Maxzide 1008
Micardis HCT Tablets 1051
Microzide Capsules 3414
Minizide Capsules 2700
Moduretic Tablets 2138
Mykrox Tablets 1168
Prinzide Tablets 2168
Renese Tablets 2712
Tenoretic Tablets 690
Uniretic Tablets 3178
Vaseretic Tablets 2204
Zaroxolyn Tablets 1177
Zestoretic Tablets 695
Ziac Tablets 1887

Necrotizing vasculitis

Concerta Extended-Release Tablets 1998
Concerta Tablets 561
Metadate CD Capsules 1164
Metadate ER Tablets 1167
Methylin Tablets 1995
Methylin ER Tablets 1995

Neonatal morbidity

Accuretic Tablets 2614
Aceon Tablets (2 mg, 4 mg, 8 mg) 3249
Altace Capsules 2233
Avalide Tablets 1070
Avapro Tablets 1074
Avapro Tablets 3076
Captopril Tablets 2281
Cozaar Tablets 2067
Enalaprilat Injection 863
Hyzaar 2109
Lexxel Tablets 608
Lotrel Capsules 2370
Mavik Tablets 478
Monopril Tablets 1091
Monopril HCT 1094
Prinivil Tablets 2164
Prinzide Tablets 2168
Uniretic Tablets (Several dozen cases) 3178
Univasc Tablets 3181
Vaseretic Tablets 2204
Vasotec I.V. Injection 2207
Vasotec Tablets 2210
Zestoretic Tablets 695
Zestril Tablets 698

Neonatal prematurity

Accupril Tablets 2611
Adderall Tablets 3231
Altace Capsules 2233
Captopril Tablets 2281
Cozaar Tablets 2067
Enalaprilat Injection 863
Hyzaar 2109
Monopril Tablets 1091
Prinivil Tablets 2164
Prinzide Tablets 2168
Univasc Tablets 3181
Vaseretic Tablets 2204
Vasotec I.V. Injection 2207
Vasotec Tablets 2210
Zestoretic Tablets 695
Zestril Tablets 698

Neoplasm
(*see under* Carcinoma, unspecified)

Neoplasm, brain, benign

Requip Tablets (Infrequent) 1621

Neoplasm, breast malignant

Evoxac Capsules (Less than 1%) 1217
Vioxx (Less than 0.1%) 2213

Neoplasm, laryngeal, malignant

Requip Tablets (Infrequent) 1621

Neoplasm, malignant

Alora Transdermal System 3372
Estratest 3252
Ortho Dienestrol Cream 2554
Orthoclone OKT3 Sterile Solution 2498
Pergonal for Injection 3223
Repronex for Intramuscular and Subcutaneous Injection (Infrequent) 1347

Neoplasm, prostatic malignant

Vioxx (Less than 0.1%) 2213

Neoplasms, hepatic

Androderm Transdermal System CIII (Rare) 3377
Android Capsules, 10 mg (Rare) 1731
Betaseron for SC Injection 988
Brevicon 28-Day Tablets 3380
Estratest (Rare) 3252
Norinyl 1 +35 28-Day Tablets 3380
Norinyl 1 + 50 28-Day Tablets 3380
Ortho-Cyclen/Ortho Tri-Cyclen 2573
Oxandrin Tablets 1153
Testoderm Transdermal Systems (Rare) 574
Testred Capsules, 10 mg (Rare) 1746
Tri-Norinyl-28 Tablets 3433

Nephritis

Aceon Tablets (2 mg, 4 mg, 8 mg) 3249
Azulfidine EN-tabs Tablets (Rare) 2775
Betaseron for SC Injection 988
Cipro (Less than 1%) 887
Lipitor Tablets (Less than 2%) 2639
Lipitor Tablets (Less than 2%) 2696
Paxil (Rare) 1609
Pediazole Suspension 3050
Rilutek Tablets (Rare) 772
Tapazole Tablets (Very rare) 1823
Timolide Tablets 2187
Toradol 3018
Zithromax (1% or less) 2743
Zithromax for Oral Suspension, 300 mg, 600 mg, 900 mg, 1200 mg (1% or less) 2739
Zithromax Tablets, 250 mg (1% or less) 2739
Zithromax Tablets, 600 mg (1% or less) 2743

Nephritis, interstitial

Accuretic Tablets 2614
Aggrenox Capsules 1026
Aldoclor Tablets 2035
Aldoril Tablets 2039
Anaprox Tablets (Less than 1%) 2967
Anaprox DS Tablets (Less than 1%) 2967
Arthrotec Tablets (Rare) 3195
Asacol Delayed-Release Tablets 2884
Atacand HCT Tablets 597
Augmentin Chewable Tablets (Rare) 1482
Augmentin Powder for Oral Suspension (Rare) 1482
Augmentin Tablets (Rare) 1485
Augmentin ES-600 Powder for Oral Suspension (Rare) 1487
Avalide Tablets 1070
Bactrim 2949
Captopril Tablets 2281
Cataflam Tablets (Rare) 2315
Ceclor CD Tablets 1279
Ceclor (Rare) 1905
Celebrex Capsules (Less than 0.1%) 2676
Celebrex Capsules (Less than 0.1%) 2780
Chibroxin Sterile Ophthalmic Solution 2051
Cipro I.V. (1% or less) 893
Cipro I.V. Pharmacy Bulk Package (Less than 1%) 897
Cipro (Less than 1%) 887
Claforan Injection (Occasional) 732
Clinoril Tablets (Less than 1 in 100) 2053
Clozaril Tablets 2319
Colazal Capsules 3069
Crixivan Capsules 2070
Diovan HCT Tablets 2338
Dipentum Capsules (Rare) 2803
Diuril Oral 2087
Diuril Sodium Intravenous 2086
Dolobid Tablets (Less than 1 in 100) 2088
Dyazide Capsules 1515
Dyrenium Capsules (Rare) 3458
EC-Naprosyn Delayed-Release Tablets (Less than 1%) 2967
Ecotrin Enteric Coated Aspirin Low, Regular and Maximum Strength Tablets 1715
Feldene Capsules (Occasional) 2685
Floxin I.V. 2526
Floxin Tablets 2529
Furosemide Tablets 2284
HydroDIURIL Tablets 2108
Hyzaar 2109
Indocin (Less than 1%) 2112
Keflex (Rare) 1237
Kefzol Vials, ADD-Vantage 1951
Lodine (Less than 1%) 3528
Lodine XL Extended-Release Tablets (Less than 1%) 3530
Maxzide 1008
Mefoxin for Injection 2124
Mefoxin Premixed Intravenous Solution 2127
Meridia Capsules (One patient) 481
Micardis HCT Tablets 1051
Microzide Capsules 3414
Mobic Tablets (Less than 0.1%) 1054
Moduretic Tablets 2138
Motrin Suspension, Oral Drops, Chewable Tablets, and Caplets 2002
▲ Naprelan Tablets (3% to 9%) 1293
Naprosyn Suspension (Less than 1%) 2967
Naprosyn Tablets (Less than 1%) 2967
Noroxin Tablets 2145
Orthoclone OKT3 Sterile Solution 2498
Orudis Capsules (Less than 1%) 3548
Oruvail Capsules (Less than 1%) 3548
PEG-Intron Powder for Injection (Less than or equal to 1%) 3140
Pentasa Capsules (Infrequent) 3239
Pipracil (Rare) 1866
Ponstel Capsules (Occasional) 1356
Prilosec Delayed-Release Capsules (Less than 1%) 628
Prinzide Tablets 2168
Proleukin for Injection (Less than 1%) 1199
Pyrazinamide Tablets (Rare) 1876
Relafen Tablets (Less than 1%) 1617
Rifadin (Rare) 765
Rifamate Capsules (Rare) 767
Rifater Tablets (Rare) 769
Septra Suspension 2265
Septra Tablets 2265
Septra DS Tablets 2265
Silvadene Cream 1% (Infrequent) 2267
Streptase for Infusion 647
Tagamet (Rare) 1644
Trovan (Less than 1%) 2722
Vancocin HCl Capsules & Pulvules (Rare) 1972
Vancocin HCl Oral Solution (Rare) 1971
Vancocin HCl, Vials & ADD-Vantage (Rare) 1970
Vaseretic Tablets 2204
Vioxx (Less than 0.1%) 2213
Voltaren Tablets (Rare) 2315
Voltaren-XR Tablets (Rare) 2315
Zestoretic Tablets 695
Ziac Tablets 1887
Zinacef Injection (Rare) 1696
Zinacef for Injection (Rare) 1696
Zithromax Capsules, 250 mg 2743
Zithromax for IV Infusion 2748
Zithromax for Oral Suspension, 300 mg, 600 mg, 900 mg, 1200 mg 2739
Zithromax Tablets, 250 mg 2739
Zosyn (Rare) 1890
Zosyn in Galaxy Containers (Rare) 1894

Nephritis, purpuric

Vantin Tablets and Oral Suspension 2860

Nephrocalcinosis

Rocaltrol 2991

Nephrolithiasis

Aceon Tablets (2 mg, 4 mg, 8 mg) (0.3% to 1%) 3249
Aciphex Tablets 1267
Aciphex Tablets 1783
Avonex 1013
Axid Pulvules 1903
Axid Pulvules 2919
Betaseron for SC Injection 988
Cardura Tablets (Less than 0.5%) 2668
Celebrex Capsules (0.1% to 1.9%) 2676
Celebrex Capsules (0.1% to 1.9%) 2780
Celexa (Rare) 1365
Cipro I.V. (1% or less) 893
Cipro I.V. Pharmacy Bulk Package (Less than 1%) 897
Cipro 887
Clinoril Tablets 2053
Cognex Capsules (Infrequent) 1351
Copaxone for Injection (Infrequent) 3306
▲ Crixivan Capsules (3.1%) 2070
Daranide Tablets 2077
Diamox ⊙269
Dyazide Capsules 1515
Dyrenium Capsules (Rare) 3458
Effexor Tablets (Infrequent) 3495
Effexor XR Capsules (Infrequent) 3499
Evoxac Capsules (Less than 1%) 1217
Exelon Capsules (Infrequent) 2342
Exelon Oral Solution (Infrequent) 2345
Floxin I.V. 2526
Floxin Tablets 2529
Fortovase Capsules (Rare) 2970
Foscavir Injection 605
Hivid Tablets (Less than 1%) 2975
Imdur Tablets (Less than or equal to 5%) 1826
Imitrex Injection (Rare) 1549
Imitrex Nasal Spray 1554
Imitrex Tablets 1558
Invirase Capsules (Rare) 2979
Kaletra Capsules (Less than 2%) 471
Kaletra Oral Solution (Less than 2%) 471
Lipitor Tablets (Less than 2%) 2639
Lipitor Tablets (Less than 2%) 2696
Lodine (Less than 1%) 3528
Lodine XL Extended-Release Tablets (Less than 1%) 3530
Luvox Tablets (25, 50, 100 mg) (Rare) 3256
Maxzide 1008
Miacalcin Nasal Spray (Less than 1%) 2375
Naprelan Tablets (Less than 1%) 1293
Neptazane Tablets ⊙271
Neurontin Capsules (Rare) 2655
Neurontin Oral Solution (Rare) 2655
Neurontin Tablets (Rare) 2655
Nipent for Injection (Less than 3%) 3272
Norvir Capsules (Less than 2%) 487
Norvir Oral Solution (Less than 2%) 487
Paxil (Rare) 1609
Permax Tablets (Infrequent) 1299
Prevacid Delayed-Release Capsules (Less than 1%) 3292
PREVPAC (Less than 1%) 3298
Protonix I.V. (Less than 1%) 3580
Protonix Tablets (Less than 1%) 3577
Relafen Tablets (Less than 1%) 1617
Remeron Tablets (Infrequent) 2483
Remeron SolTab Tablets (Infrequent) 2486
Reminyl Oral Solution (Infrequent) 1792
Reminyl Tablets (Infrequent) 1792
Requip Tablets (Infrequent) 1621
Rescriptor Tablets (Less than 2%) 526
Rilutek Tablets (Infrequent) 772
Rocephin Injectable Vials, ADD-Vantage, Galaxy, Bulk 2993
Sandostatin Injection (Less than 1%) 2394
▲ Sandostatin LAR Depot (5% to 15%) 2395
Serzone Tablets (Infrequent) 1104
Sonata Capsules (Infrequent) 3591
Sustiva Capsules (Up to 1%) 1258
Tasmar Tablets (Infrequent) 3010
Teveten Tablets (Less than 1%) 3327
Topamax Sprinkle Capsules (1.5%) 2590
Topamax Tablets (Frequent) 2590
Tricor Capsules, Micronized (Less than 1%) 513
Trileptal Oral Suspension 2407
Trileptal Tablets 2407
Uniretic Tablets (Less than 1%) 3178
Viracept 532
Vistide Injection 1445
Zanaflex Tablets (Infrequent) 1305
Zonegran Capsules (Rare) 1307

Nephropathy

AmBisome for Injection (Less common) 1383
Asacol Delayed-Release Tablets 2884
Bicillin C-R 900/300 Injection 2240
Bicillin C-R Injection 2238
Bicillin L-A Injection (Infrequent) 2242
Campath Ampules 992
Ceclor 1905
Cedax 1021
Cefizox for Intramuscular or Intravenous Use 1390
Cefotan 664
Ceftin 1898
Cefzil 1076
Ceptaz for Injection 1499
Duricef 1079
Fortaz 1541

Hivid Tablets (Less than 1%) 2975
Lorabid Suspension and Pulvules 2251
Maxipime for Injection 1285
Mefoxin for Injection 2124
Mefoxin Premixed Intravenous Solution 2127
Menomune-A/C/Y/W-135 Vaccine (Rare) 813
Nipent for Injection (Less than 3%) 3272
Omnicef 493
Permapen Isoject 2706
Pfizerpen for Injection (Rare) 2707
▲ Rapamune Oral Solution and Tablets (3% to 20%) 3584
Suprax 1877
Tazicef for Injection 1647
Tazicef Galaxy Container 1650
Tazicef Pharmacy Bulk Package 1653
Tazidime Vials, Faspak & ADD-Vantage 1966
Vantin Tablets and Oral Suspension 2860
Vistide Injection 1445
Zinacef Injection 1696
Zinacef for Injection 1696

Nephropathy, acute uric acid
Oncaspar 756

Nephropathy, proximal tubular
CytoGam Intravenous 2026
Gamimune N, 5% Solvent/Detergent Treated 925
Gamimune N, 10% Solvent/Detergent Treated 928
Gammagard S/D 845
Gammar-P I.V. 787
Sandoglobulin I.V. 2391

Nephrosclerosis, malignant
Naprelan Tablets (Less than 1%) 1293

Nephrosis, osmotic
CytoGam Intravenous 2026
Gamimune N, 5% Solvent/Detergent Treated 925
Gamimune N, 10% Solvent/Detergent Treated 928
Gammagard S/D 845
Gammar-P I.V. 787
Sandoglobulin I.V. 2391

Nephrosis, toxic
Accuretic Tablets 2614
Azulfidine EN-tabs Tablets (Rare) 2775
Bactrim 2949
Calcium Disodium Versenate Injection 1980
Evoxac Capsules (Less than 1%) 1217
Felbatol 3343
Neurontin Capsules (Rare) 2655
Neurontin Oral Solution (Rare) 2655
Neurontin Tablets (Rare) 2655
Pediazole Suspension 3050
Permax Tablets (Rare) 1299
Septra Suspension 2265
Septra Tablets 2265
Septra DS Tablets 2265
Silvadene Cream 1% 2267

Nephrotic syndrome
Anaprox Tablets (Occasional; less than 1%) 2967
Anaprox DS Tablets (Occasional; less than 1%) 2967
Arthrotec Tablets (Rare) 3195
Azulfidine EN-tabs Tablets (Rare) 2775
BayRab (Rare) 917
BayTet (Few isolated cases) 923
Captopril Tablets (Approximately 1 to 2 of 1000 patients) 2281
Cataflam Tablets (Rare) 2315
Clinoril Tablets (Less than 1 in 100) 2053
Cuprimine Capsules 2075
Dapsone Tablets USP 1780
Depen Titratable Tablets 3341
Dipentum Capsules (Rare) 2803
Dolobid Tablets (Rare) 2088
EC-Naprosyn Delayed-Release Tablets (Occasional; less than 1%) 2967
Feldene Capsules (Occasional) 2685
Indocin (Less than 1%) 2112
Motrin Suspension, Oral Drops, Chewable Tablets, and Caplets (Occasional) 2002
▲ Naprelan Tablets (3% to 9%) 1293
Naprosyn Suspension (Occasional; less than 1%) 2967
Naprosyn Tablets (Occasional; less than 1%) 2967
Orudis Capsules (Less than 1%) 3548
Oruvail Capsules (Less than 1%) 3548
Pentasa Capsules (Infrequent) 3239
Relafen Tablets (Less than 1%) 1617
Rythmol Tablets – 150 mg, 225 mg, 300 mg (Less than 1%) 502
Ticlid Tablets (Rare) 3015
Toradol 3018
Voltaren Tablets (Rare) 2315
Voltaren-XR Tablets (Rare) 2315

Nephrotoxicity
Anaprox Tablets 2967
Anaprox DS Tablets 2967
Canasa Rectal Suppositories 829
Cefotan (Rare) 664
Coly-Mycin M Parenteral 2243
Declomycin Tablets (No incidence, dose related) 1855
Depen Titratable Tablets 3341
EC-Naprosyn Delayed-Release Tablets 2967
Foscavir Injection 605
▲ Gengraf Capsules (25% to 38%) 457
▲ Ifex for Injection (6%) 1123
Leustatin Injection 2495
Minocin Intravenous 1862
Minocin Oral Suspension 1865
Minocin Pellet-Filled Capsules 1863
Naprosyn Suspension 2967
Naprosyn Tablets 2967
Nebcin Vials, Hyporets & ADD-Vantage 1955
▲ Neoral Soft Gelatin Capsules (25% to 38%) 2380
▲ Neoral Oral Solution (25% to 38%) 2380
Neosporin G.U. Irrigant Sterile 2256
Orudis Capsules 3548
Oruvail Capsules 3548
Paraplatin for Injection (Uncommon) 1126
▲ Prograf (36% to 52%) 1393
Relafen Tablets 1617
Roferon-A Injection (Unusual) 2996
Rowasa Rectal Suspension Enema 4.0 grams/unit (60 mL) 3264
▲ Sandimmune (25 to 38%) 2388
Streptomycin Sulfate Injection (Rare) 2714
▲ TheraCys Injection (10%) 823
TOBI Solution for Inhalation 1206
Vancocin HCl Capsules & Pulvules 1972
Vancocin HCl Oral Solution 1971
Vancocin HCl, Vials & ADD-Vantage 1970
Vicoprofen Tablets 520
▲ Vistide Injection (53%) 1445
Zinacef Injection 1696
Zinacef for Injection 1696

Nerve conduction, abnormal
Plaquenil Tablets 3082

Nerve deafness
M-M-R II 2118
Mumpsvax 2141
Plaquenil Tablets 3082

Nerve injury at injection site
Norplant System (Less than 1%) 3543

Nerve syndromes, compressed
Advair Diskus 100/50 (1% to 3%) 1448
Advair Diskus 250/50 (1% to 3%) 1448
Advair Diskus 500/50 (1% to 3%) 1448
Amerge Tablets (Rare) 1467

Nervousness
Accupril Tablets (0.5% to 1.0%) 2611
Accuretic Tablets (0.5% to 1%) 2614
Accutane Capsules 2944
Aceon Tablets (2 mg, 4 mg, 8 mg) (1.1%) 3249
Aciphex Tablets 1267
Aciphex Tablets 1783
Actifed Cold & Allergy Tablets ▣688
Actiq (1% to 2%) 1184
Activella Tablets 2764
Adalat CC Tablets (Rare) 877
▲ Adderall XR Capsules (6%)
Adenoscan (2%) 1381
Advil Cold and Sinus Caplets ▣771
Advil Cold and Sinus Tablets ▣771
▲ Aerobid/Aerobid-M (3% to 9%) 1363
Agrylin Capsules (1% to 5%) 3232
Albalon Ophthalmic Solution ⊙225
Alesse-21 Tablets 3468
Alesse-28 Tablets 3473
Alferon N Injection (1%) 1770
Allegra (Less than 1%) 712
Allegra-D Extended-Release Tablets (1.4%) 714
Altace Capsules (Less than 1%) 2233
▲ Alupent (6.8%) 1029
Ambien Tablets (1%) 3191
AmBisome for Injection (Less common) 1383
Amphotec (1% to 5%) 1774
AndroGel (Up to 3%) 3322
Aricept Tablets (Frequent) 1270
Aricept Tablets (Frequent) 2665
Arimidex Tablets (2% to 5%) 659
▲ Artane (30% to 50%) 1855
Arthrotec Tablets (Rare) 3195
Asacol Delayed-Release Tablets (2% or greater) 2884
Astelin Nasal Spray (Infrequent) 3339
▲ Atrovent Inhalation Aerosol (3.1%) 1030
Atrovent Inhalation Solution (0.5%) 1031
Avalide Tablets (1% or greater) 1070
Avapro Tablets (1% or greater) 1074
Avapro Tablets (1% or greater) 3076
Avelox Tablets (0.05% to 1%) 879
Axert Tablets (Rare) 2772
Axid Pulvules (1.1%) 1903
Axid Pulvules (1.1%) 2919
Bactrim 2949
Benadryl Allergy/Congestion Tablets ▣692
Benadryl Allergy & Sinus Liquid ▣693
Benadryl Allergy Sinus Headache Caplets & Gelcaps ▣693
Benadryl Parenteral 2617
Benylin Multi-Symptom Liquid ▣697
▲ Betaseron for SC Injection (8%) 988
Bicillin C-R 900/300 Injection 2240
Bicillin C-R Injection 2238
Bicillin L-A Injection 2242
Blocadren Tablets (Less than 1%) 2046
▲ Brethine Ampuls (16.9 to 38.0%) 2314
▲ Brethine Tablets (35%) 2313
Brevicon 28-Day Tablets 3380
Bromfed Capsules (Extended-Release) 2269
Bromfed-PD Capsules (Extended-Release) 2269
Campath Ampules 992
Captopril Tablets 2281
Cardizem Injectable 1018
Cardizem Lyo-Ject Syringe 1018
Cardizem Monovial 1018
Cardizem CD Capsules (Less than 1%) 1016
Cardura Tablets (2%) 2668
▲ Casodex Tablets (2% to 5%) 662
▲ Catapres Tablets (About 3 in 100 patients) 1037
Catapres-TTS (1 of 101 patients) 1038
Ceclor CD Tablets (0.1% to 1%) 1279
Ceclor (Rare) 1905
Cefzil (Less than 1%) 1076
Celebrex Capsules (0.1% to 1.9%) 2676
Celebrex Capsules (0.1% to 1.9%) 2780
▲ CellCept Capsules (11.4%) 2951
▲ CellCept Intravenous (11.4%) 2951
▲ CellCept Oral Suspension (11.4%) 2951
▲ CellCept Tablets (11.4%) 2951
Celontin Capsules 2618
▲ Cenestin Tablets (28%) 1263
Cerebyx Injection (Frequent) 2619
Cipro I.V. 893
Cipro I.V. Pharmacy Bulk Package 897
Cipro 887
▲ Claritin (4%) 3100
▲ Claritin-D 12 Hour Extended Release Tablets (5%) 3102
▲ Claritin-D 24 Hour Extended Release Tablets (3%) 3104
Clinoril Tablets (Greater than 1%) 2053
▲ Clorpres Tablets (About 3%) 1002
Cogentin 2055
Cognex Capsules (Frequent) 1351
Colazal Capsules 3069
▲ CombiPatch Transdermal System (5% to 6%) 2323
▲ Combipres Tablets (About 3%) 1040
Combivent Inhalation Aerosol (Less than 2%) 1041
Compazine 1505
▲ Concerta Extended-Release Tablets (Amongst most common) 1998
▲ Concerta Tablets (Amongst most common) 561
Contac Non-Drowsy 12 Hour Cold Caplets ▣745
Contac Non-Drowsy Timed Release 12 Hour Cold Caplets ▣746
Contac Severe Cold and Flu Caplets Maximum Strength ▣746
Contac Severe Cold and Flu Caplets Non-Drowsy ▣746
Copaxone for Injection (2%) 3306
Coreg Tablets (0.1% to 1%) 1508
Coricidin 'D' Cold, Flu & Sinus Tablets ▣737
Corlopam Injection (1% to 2%) 412
Cosopt Sterile Ophthalmic Solution 2065
Cozaar Tablets (Less than 1%) 2067
▲ Crinone 8% Gel (16%) 3213
Crixivan Capsules (Less than 2%) 2070
Cyclessa Tablets 2450
Dantrium Capsules (Less frequent) 2885
Daranide Tablets 2077
Demadex Tablets and Injection (1.1%) 2965
▲ Depacon Injection (0.9% to 11%) 416
▲ Depakene (11%) 421
▲ Depakote Sprinkle Capsules (7% to 11%) 426
▲ Depakote Tablets (1% to 11%) 430
Depakote ER Tablets (1% to 5%) 436
▲ Depo-Provera Contraceptive Injection (More than 5%) 2798
Desogen Tablets 2458
Detrol Tablets (1.1%) 3623
Dilantin Infatabs 2624
Dilantin Kapseals 2622
Dilantin-125 Oral Suspension 2625
Dilaudid Oral Liquid (Less frequent) 445
Dilaudid Tablets - 8 mg (Less frequent) 445
Dilaudid-HP 443
Ditropan XL Extended Release Tablets (2% to 5%) 564
Dolobid Tablets (Less than 1 in 100) 2088
Donnatal 2929
Donnatal Extentabs 2930
Donnatal Tablets 2929
▲ Dostinex Tablets (1% to less than 10%) 2804
Doxil Injection (Less than 1%) 566
Drixoral Allergy/Sinus Extended-Release Tablets ▣741
Drixoral Cold & Allergy Sustained-Action Tablets ▣740
Drixoral Cold & Flu Extended-Release Tablets ▣740
▲ Duraclon Injection (3%) 3057
▲ Duragesic Transdermal System (3% to 10%) 1786
Duranest Injections 600
Dynabac Tablets (0.1% to 1%) 2269
DynaCirc Capsules (0.5% to 1%) 2921
DynaCirc CR Tablets (0.5% to 1%) 2923
▲ Effexor Tablets (2% to 21.3%) 3495
▲ Effexor XR Capsules (10% to 12%) 3499
8-MOP Capsules 1727
ELA-Max Cream 1340
Eldepryl Capsules 3266
Emla (Unlikely with cream) 602
Enalaprilat Injection 863
EpiPen Jr. Auto-Injector 1236
Ergamisol Tablets (1% to 2%) 1789
Estring Vaginal Ring (At least 1 report) 2811
Estrostep 2627
Eulexin Capsules (1%) 3118
Exelon Capsules (2% or more) 2342
Exelon Oral Solution (2% or more) 2345
▲ Felbatol (7.0% to 16.1%) 3343
Feldene Capsules (Occasional) 2685
▲ femhrt Tablets (5.4%) 2635
Ferrlecit Injection (Two or more patients) 3386
Flexeril Tablets (1% to 3%) 572
Flexeril Tablets (1% to 3%) 2094
▲ Flolan for Injection (7% to 21%) 1528
Flovent Rotadisk (1% to 3%) 1537
Floxin I.V. (1% to 3%) 2526
Floxin Tablets (1% to 3%) 2529
Flumadine (1.3% to 2.1%) 1370
Foradil Aerolizer 2354
Foscavir Injection (Between 1% and 5%) 605
▲ Gabitril Tablets (10%) 1189
Gastrocrom Oral Concentrate (Less common) 1162
Gengraf Capsules (1% to less than 3%) 457
▲ Glucotrol XL Extended Release Tablets (3.6%) 2693
▲ Halcion Tablets (5.2%) 2823
Hivid Tablets (Less than 1%) 2975
Hytrin Capsules (2.3%) 464
Hyzaar 2109
Imdur Tablets (Less than or equal to 5%) 1826
Indapamide Tablets (Less than 5%) 2286
Indocin (Less than 1%) 2112
▲ Infergen (16% to 31%) 1777
Intron A for Injection (Up to 3%) 3120
Iopidine 0.5% Ophthalmic Solution (Less than 3%) ⊙213
Ismo Tablets (Fewer than 1%) 3524
Kaletra Capsules (Less than 2%) 471
Kaletra Oral Solution (Less than 2%) 471
▲ Keppra Tablets (4%) 3314
Klonopin Tablets (1% to 3%) 2983
Lamictal (Frequent) 1567
Levaquin (0.1% to less than 1.0%) 2537
Levbid Extended-Release Tablets 3172
Levlen 962
Levlite 21 Tablets 962
Levlite 28 Tablets 962
Levo-Dromoran 1734
Levora Tablets 3389
Levorphanol Tartrate Tablets (1% to 3%) 3059
Levoxyl Tablets 1819
Levsin/Levsinex/Levbid 3172
Lexxel Tablets 608
Lidoderm Patch 1319
Lodine (1% to 3%) 3528
Lodine XL Extended-Release Tablets (1% to 3%) 3530
Lodosyn Tablets 1251
Loestrin 21 Tablets 2642
Loestrin Fe Tablets 2642
Lo/Ovral Tablets 3532
Lo/Ovral-28 Tablets 3538
Lorabid Suspension and Pulvules 2251
Lotensin Tablets (Less than 1%) 2365

Lotensin HCT Tablets (0.3% to 1%) 2367
Lotrel Capsules 2370
Low-Ogestrel-28 Tablets 3392
Lunelle Monthly Injection 2827
Lupron Depot 3.75 mg (Less than 5%) 3281
▲ Lupron Depot–3 Month 11.25 mg (4.8% to 5%) 3285
Lupron Depot–3 Month 22.5 mg (Less than 5%) 3288
Lupron Depot-PED 7.5 mg, 11.25 mg and 15 mg (Less than 2%) 3291
Lupron Injection (Less than 5%) 3279
Lupron Injection Pediatric (Less than 2%) 3280
▲ Luvox Tablets (25, 50, 100 mg) (2% to 12%) 3256
Marinol Capsules (Greater than 1%) 3325
Matulane Capsules 3246
▲ Maxair Autohaler (4.5% to 6.9%) 1981
▲ Maxair Inhaler (4.5% to 6.9%) 1984
Maxalt Tablets (Infrequent) 2120
Maxalt-MLT Orally Disintegrating Tablets (Infrequent) 2120
▲ Meridia Capsules (5.2%) 481
Merrem I.V. (0.1% to 1.0%) 673
▲ Metadate CD Capsules (Among most common) 1164
▲ Metadate ER Tablets (Amongst most common) 1167
▲ Methylin Tablets (Among most common) 1995
▲ Methylin ER Tablets (Among most common) 1995
▲ Mexitil Capsules (5% to 11.3%) 1047
Micardis HCT Tablets 1051
Microgestin Fe 1.5/30 Tablets 3407
Microgestin Fe 1/20 Tablets 3400
Midamor Tablets (Less than or equal to 1%) 2136
Migranal Nasal Spray (Infrequent) 2376
Minipress Capsules (1% to 4%) 2699
Minizide Capsules 2700
Mirapex Tablets (1% or more) 2834
Mircette Tablets 2470
▲ Mirena Intrauterine System (5% or more) 974
Mobic Tablets (Less than 2%) 1054
Modicon 2563
Moduretic Tablets (Less than or equal to 1%) 2138
Monurol Sachet (Less than 1%) 1375
Motofen Tablets (1 in 200 to 1 in 600) 577
Motrin Suspension, Oral Drops, Chewable Tablets, and Caplets (1% to less than 3%) 2002
Motrin Sinus Headache Caplets 2005
MS Contin Tablets (Less frequent) 2896
MSIR (Less frequent) 2898
Mykrox Tablets (Less than 2%) 1168
Naprelan Tablets (Less than 1%) 1293
Narcan Injection 1322
Naropin Injection (Less than 1%) 612
Nascobal Gel 3174
Necon 3415
Nembutal Sodium Solution (Less than 1%) 485
Neoral Soft Gelatin Capsules (1% to less than 3%) 2380
Neoral Oral Solution (1% to less than 3%) 2380
▲ Neumega for Injection (Greater than or equal to 10%) 1434
Neurontin Capsules (2.4%) 2655
Neurontin Oral Solution (2.4%) 2655
Neurontin Tablets (2.4%) 2655
Nexium Delayed-Release Capsules (Less than 1%) 619
Nilandron Tablets (2%) 753
▲ Nipent for Injection (3% to 10%) 3272
Nordette-28 Tablets 2257
Norinyl 1 +35 28-Day Tablets 3380
Norinyl 1 + 50 28-Day Tablets 3380
Norplant System 3543
Norvasc Tablets (More than 0.1% to 1%) 2704
Norvir Capsules (Less than 2%) 487
Norvir Oral Solution (Less than 2%) 487
Nubain Injection (1% or less) 1323
NuLev Orally Disintegrating Tablets 3176
Numorphan 1324
Ogestrel 0.5/50-28 Tablets 3428
OptiPranolol Metipranolol Ophthalmic Solution 0.3% (A small number of patients) .... ⊙263
Oramorph SR Tablets (Less frequent) 3062
▲ Orap Tablets (8.3%) 1407
Ortho-Cept 21 Tablets 2546
Ortho-Cept 28 Tablets 2546
Ortho-Cyclen/Ortho Tri-Cyclen 2573
Ortho-Novum 2563
Ortho-Novum 1/50□28 Tablets 2556
Ortho-Cyclen/Ortho Tri-Cyclen 2573
▲ Orudis Capsules (3% to 9%) 3548
▲ Oruvail Capsules (3% to 9%) 3548
Ovcon 3364
Ovral Tablets 3551
Ovral-28 Tablets 3552
Ovrette Tablets 3552
Oxsoralen-Ultra Capsules 1741
OxyContin Tablets (Between 1% and 5%) 2912
▲ Paxil (4% to 9%) 1609
Periactin Tablets 2155
Permax Tablets (Frequent) 1299
Phenergan Injection 3553
Phenergan 3556
Phenergan VC Syrup 3560
Phenergan VC with Codeine Syrup .. 3561
Plaquenil Tablets 3082
Plendil Extended-Release Tablets (0.5% to 1.5%) 623
Ponstel Capsules (Occasional) 1356
Premphase Tablets 3572
Prempro Tablets 3572
Prevacid Delayed-Release Capsules (Less than 1%) 3292
PREVPAC (Less than 1%) 3298
Prilosec Delayed-Release Capsules (Less than 1%) 628
Primatene Tablets .... ▣780
Prinivil Tablets (0.3% to 1.0%) 2164
Prinzide Tablets 2168
ProAmatine Tablets (Less frequent) 3241
▲ Procardia Capsules (2% or less to 7%) 2708
▲ Procardia XL Extended Release Tablets (Less than 3% to 7%) 2710
▲ Prograf (3%) 1393
Prometrium Capsules (100 mg, 200 mg) 3261
▲ ProSom Tablets (8%) 500
Protonix I.V. (Less than 1%) 3580
Protonix Tablets (Less than 1%) 3577
▲ Proventil Inhalation Aerosol (Less than 10%) 3142
▲ Proventil Inhalation Solution 0.083% (4%) 3146
▲ Proventil Repetabs Tablets (2% to 20%) 3148
▲ Proventil Solution for Inhalation 0.5% (4%) 3144
▲ Proventil HFA Inhalation Aerosol (7%) 3150
Provera Tablets 2853
▲ Provigil Tablets (8%) 1193
▲ Prozac Pulvules, Liquid, and Weekly Capsules (11% to 16%) 1238
Quinidex Extentabs (2%) 2933
▲ Rebetron Combination Therapy (4% to 5%) 3153
Relafen Tablets (1% to 3%) 1617
Requip Tablets (1% or more) 1621
Rescriptor Tablets (Less than 2%) ... 526
Retrovir Capsules (1.6%) 1625
Retrovir IV Infusion (2%) 1629
Retrovir (1.6%) 1625
Rhinocort Nasal Inhaler (Less than 1%) 640
Risperdal (Frequent) 1796
▲ Ritalin (One of the two most common) 2387
Rituxan for Infusion (1% to 5%) 1750
Rituxan I.V. (1% to 5%) 1428
Robinul Forte Tablets 1358
Robinul Injectable 2940
Robinul Tablets 1358
Robitussin Maximum Strength Cough & Cold Liquid .... ▣785
Robitussin Pediatric Cough & Cold Formula Liquid .... ▣785
Robitussin-CF Liquid .... ▣783
Robitussin-DAC Syrup 2942
Robitussin-PE Liquid .... ▣782
Roferon-A Injection (Less than 3% to less than 5%) 2996
▲ Romazicon Injection (3% to 9%) 3000
Roxicodone Tablets (Less than 3%) 3067
Ryna .... ▣768
Rynatan Tablets 3351
Salagen Tablets (Less than 1%) 2229
Sandostatin LAR Depot (1% to 4%) 2395
▲ Sarafem Pulvules (7% to 14%) 1962
▲ Semprex-D Capsules (3%) 1172
Septra Suspension 2265
Septra Tablets 2265
Septra DS Tablets 2265
Serevent Inhalation Aerosol (1% to 3%) 1633
Serophene Tablets (Approximately 1 in 50 patients) 3226
▲ Serostim for Injection (1% to 10%) 3229
Sinemet Tablets 1253
Sinemet CR Tablets 1255
Sinutab Non-Drying Liquid Caps .... ▣706
Skelaxin Tablets 1301
Skelid Tablets (More than or equal to 1%) 3088
Sonata Capsules (Frequent) 3591
Stadol NS Nasal Spray (1% or greater) 1108
Sudafed 12 Hour Tablets .... ▣708
Sudafed 24 Hour Tablets .... ▣708
Children's Sudafed Cold & Cough Liquid .... ▣709
Sudafed Cold & Allergy Tablets .... ▣708
Sudafed Nasal Decongestant Tablets .... ▣710
Sudafed Sinus Headache Caplets .... ▣712
Sudafed Sinus Headache Tablets .. ▣712
Sular Tablets (Less than or equal to 1%) 688
Sustiva Capsules (1% to 2%) 1258
Symmetrel (1% to 5%) 1328
Synagis Intramuscular (More than 1%) 2028
Tasmar Tablets (Infrequent) 3010
Tenex Tablets (Less frequent) 2942
Tequin Injection (Less than 0.1%) 1110
Tequin Tablets (Less than 0.1%) 1110
Teveten Tablets (Less than 1%) 3327
▲ Thalomid Capsules (2.8% to 9.4%) 1154
TheraFlu Regular Strength Cold & Cough Night Time Hot Liquid .. ▣676
TheraFlu Regular Strength Cold & Sore Throat Night Time Hot Liquid .... ▣676
TheraFlu Maximum Strength Severe Cold & Congestion Night Time Caplets .... ▣678
Tiazac Capsules (Less than 2%) 1378
Timolide Tablets (Less than 1%) 2187
Timolol GFS .... ⊙266
Timoptic in Ocudose (Less frequent) 2192
Timoptic Sterile Ophthalmic Solution (Less frequent) 2190
Timoptic-XE Sterile Ophthalmic Gel Forming Solution 2194
▲ Tonocard Tablets (0.4% to 11.5%) . 649
▲ Topamax Sprinkle Capsules (13.3% to 20.6%) 2590
▲ Topamax Tablets (13.3% to 20.6%) 2590
Toradol (1% or less) 3018
Tranxene (Less common) 511
Trental Tablets 784
Triaminic Allergy Congestion Liquid .... ▣680
Triaminic Chest Congestion Liquid .... ▣680
Triaminic Cold & Allergy Liquid .... ▣681
Triaminic Cold & Allergy Softchews .... ▣683
Triaminic Cold & Cough Liquid .... ▣681
Triaminic Cold & Night Time Cough Liquid .... ▣681
Triaminic Cold, Cough & Fever Liquid .... ▣681
Triaminic Cough Liquid .... ▣682
Triaminic Cough & Congestion Liquid .... ▣682
Triaminic Cough & Sore Throat Liquid .... ▣682
Triaminic Cough & Sore Throat Softchews .... ▣684
Tricor Capsules, Micronized 513
Trileptal Oral Suspension (2% to 4%) 2407
Trileptal Tablets (2% to 4%) 2407
Tri-Levlen 962
Tri-Norinyl-28 Tablets 3433
Triphasil-21 Tablets 3600
Triphasil-28 Tablets 3605
Trivora Tablets 3439
Children's Tylenol Cold Suspension Liquid and Chewable Tablets 2015
Multi-Symptom Tylenol Cold Complete Formula Caplets 2010
Multi-Symptom Tylenol Cold Non-Drowsy Caplets and Gelcaps 2010
Maximum Strength Tylenol Flu NightTime Liquid 2011
Maximum Strength Tylenol Sinus NightTime Caplets 2012
Maximum Strength Tylenol Sinus Non-Drowsy Geltabs, Gelcaps, Caplets, and Tablets 2012
Ultracet Tablets (At least 1%) 2597
▲ Ultram Tablets (1% to 14%) 2600
Uniretic Tablets (Less than 1%) 3178
Unithroid Tablets 3445
Univasc Tablets (Less than 1%) 3181
Vantin Tablets and Oral Suspension (Less than 1%) 2860
Varivax (Greater than or equal to 1%) 2202
▲ Vascor Tablets (7.37% to 11.63%) 2602
Vaseretic Tablets (0.5% to 2.0%) 2204
Vasotec I.V. Injection 2207
Vasotec Tablets (0.5% to 1.0%) 2210
▲ Ventolin Inhalation Aerosol and Refill (1% to 10%) 1679
Versed Injection (Less than 1%) 3027
Vicks 44D Cough & Head Congestion Relief Liquid .... ▣724
Pediatric Vicks 44m Cough & Cold Relief .... ▣728
Vicks DayQuil LiquiCaps/Liquid Multi-Symptom Cold/Flu Relief .... ▣727
Children's Vicks NyQuil Cold/Cough Relief .... ▣726
▲ Vicoprofen Tablets (3% to 9%) 520
Vistide Injection 1445
▲ Volmax Extended-Release Tablets (8.5%) 2276
▲ Wellbutrin SR Sustained-Release Tablets (3% to 5%) 1684
▲ Xanax Tablets (4.1%) 2865
▲ Xopenex Inhalation Solution (2.8% to 9.6%) 3207
▲ Xylocaine Injections (Among most common) 653
Yasmin 28 Tablets (Greater than 1%) 980
▲ Zanaflex Tablets (3%) 1305
Zaroxolyn Tablets (Less than 2%) 1177
Zephrex Tablets 3091
Zephrex LA Tablets 3092
Zestoretic Tablets 695
Zestril Tablets (0.3% to 1.0%) 698
Zithromax Capsules, 250 mg (1% or less) 2743
Zithromax for IV Infusion (1% or less) 2748
Zithromax for Oral Suspension, 300 mg, 600 mg, 900 mg, 1200 mg (1% or less) 2739
Zithromax Tablets, 250 mg (1% or less) 2739
▲ Zoladex (3% to 5%) 702
Zoladex 3-month 706
▲ Zoloft (6%) 2751
Zonegran Capsules (2%) 1307
Zovia 3449
▲ Zyban Sustained-Release Tablets (4%) 1710
Zyflo Filmtab Tablets (Less common) 524
▲ Zyprexa Tablets (16%) 1973
▲ Zyprexa ZYDIS Orally Disintegrating Tablets (16%) 1973
Zyrtec (Less than 2%) 2756
Zyrtec-D 12 Hour Extended Relief Tablets (Less than 2%) 2758

Neural tube defects, unspecified

Clomid Tablets 735
Serophene Tablets 3226

Neuralgia

Aciphex Tablets 1267
Aciphex Tablets 1783
▲ Actonel Tablets (3.8%) 2879
Altace Capsules (Less than 1%) 2233
Ambien Tablets (Rare) 3191
Amerge Tablets (Rare) 1467
Arava Tablets (1% to 3%) 724
Aricept Tablets (Infrequent) 1270
Aricept Tablets (Infrequent) 2665
Arthrotec Tablets (Rare) 3195
Betaseron for SC Injection 988
Celebrex Capsules (0.1% to 1.9%) 2676
Celebrex Capsules (0.1% to 1.9%) 2780
Celexa (Infrequent) 1365
Coreg Tablets (Less than or equal to 0.1%) 1508
Crixivan Capsules (Less than 2%) 2070
Effexor Tablets (Infrequent) 3495
Effexor XR Capsules (Infrequent) 3499
Evoxac Capsules (Less than 1%) 1217
Exelon Capsules (Infrequent) 2342
Exelon Oral Solution (Infrequent) 2345
Hivid Tablets (Less than 1%) 2975
Imitrex Injection 1549
Imitrex Nasal Spray (Infrequent) 1554
Imitrex Tablets (Rare) 1558
Intron A for Injection (Less than 5%) 3120
Lamictal (Rare) 1567
Luvox Tablets (25, 50, 100 mg) (Infrequent) 3256
LYMErix Vaccine (Greater than 1%) 1592
Miacalcin Nasal Spray (Less than 1%) 2375
Naprelan Tablets (Less than 1%) 1293
Nipent for Injection (Less than 3%) 3272
Norvir Capsules (Less than 2%) 487
Norvir Oral Solution (Less than 2%) 487
Paxil (Rare) 1609
Permax Tablets (1.1%) 1299
Plavix Tablets (1% to 2.5%) 1097
Plavix Tablets (1% to 2.5%) 3084
Pletal Tablets (Less than 2%) 2605
Pletal Tablets (Less than 2%) 2848
Proleukin for Injection 1199
Protonix I.V. (Less than 1%) 3580
Protonix Tablets (Less than 1%) 3577
Prozac Pulvules, Liquid, and Weekly Capsules (Infrequent) 1238
Requip Tablets (Frequent) 1621
Roxicodone Tablets (Less than 3%) 3067
Sandostatin LAR Depot (1% to 4%) 2395

Sarafem Pulvules (Infrequent) 1962
Seroquel Tablets (Rare) 684
▲ Serostim for Injection (1% to 10%) 3229
Serzone Tablets (Infrequent) 1104
Sonata Capsules (Infrequent) 3591
Sustiva Capsules (Less than 2%) 1258
Tasmar Tablets (Infrequent) 3010
Thalomid Capsules 1154
Tricor Capsules, Micronized 513
Trileptal Oral Suspension 2407
Trileptal Tablets 2407
Uniretic Tablets (Less than 1%) 3178
Viagra Tablets (Less than 2%) 2732
Vicoprofen Tablets (Less than 1%) 520
Wellbutrin SR Sustained-Release Tablets 1684
Zanaflex Tablets (Infrequent) 1305
Zyban Sustained-Release Tablets 1710
Zyprexa Tablets (Rare) 1973
Zyprexa ZYDIS Orally Disintegrating Tablets (Rare) 1973

Neuralgia, occipital
Neurontin Capsules 2655
Neurontin Oral Solution 2655
Neurontin Tablets 2655

Neuralgia, trigeminal
LYMErix Vaccine (Greater than 1%) 1592

Neuritis
Ambien Tablets (Rare) 3191
Amerge Tablets (Rare) 1467
Arava Tablets (1% to 3%) 724
Benadryl Parenteral 2617
Clinoril Tablets (Rare) 2053
Cognex Capsules (Infrequent) 1351
Effexor Tablets (Rare) 3495
Effexor XR Capsules (Rare) 3499
Fluorescite Injection ⊙211
Gabitril Tablets (Infrequent) 1189
Hivid Tablets (Less than 1%) 2975
Imdur Tablets (Less than or equal to 5%) 1826
Intron A for Injection (Less than 5%) 3120
Lotrel Capsules (Infrequent) 2370
LYMErix Vaccine (Greater than 1%) 1592
Naprelan Tablets (Less than 1%) 1293
Nipent for Injection (Less than 3%) 3272
Periactin Tablets 2155
Permax Tablets (Rare) 1299
Proleukin for Injection 1199
ProSom Tablets (Rare) 500
Protonix I.V. (Less than 1%) 3580
Protonix Tablets (Less than 1%) 3577
Protopic Ointment (Greater than or equal to 1%) 1397
Prozac Pulvules, Liquid, and Weekly Capsules (Rare) 1238
Rynatan Tablets 3351
Sandostatin Injection (Less than 1%) 2394
Sarafem Pulvules (Rare) 1962
Soriatane Capsules (Less than 1%) 3003
Tapazole Tablets 1823
Teveten Tablets (Less than 1%) 3327
Thalomid Capsules 1154
Uniretic Tablets (Less than 1%) 3178

Neuritis, optic
Accutane Capsules 2944
Activella Tablets 2764
Alesse-21 Tablets 3468
Alesse-28 Tablets 3473
Antabuse Tablets 2444
Antabuse Tablets 3474
Attenuvax 2044
Aygestin Tablets 1333
Clomid Tablets 735
Copaxone for Injection (Infrequent) 3306
Cordarone Tablets 3487
Cuprimine Capsules 2075
Cyclessa Tablets 2450
Decadron Phosphate Sterile Ophthalmic Ointment 2083
Decadron Phosphate Sterile Ophthalmic Solution 2084
Depen Titratable Tablets 3341
Desferal Vials 2333
Doxil Injection (1% to 5%) 566
Elmiron Capsules (Less than or equal to 1%) 570
Enbrel for Injection 1752
Enbrel for Injection 3504
Engerix-B Vaccine 1517
Estratest 3252
Fluzone Vaccine 802
Levlen 962
Levlite 21 Tablets 962
Levlite 28 Tablets 962
Loestrin 21 Tablets 2642
Loestrin Fe Tablets 2642
Lo/Ovral Tablets 3532
Lo/Ovral-28 Tablets 3538
Low-Ogestrel-28 Tablets 3392
Macrobid Capsules (Rare) 2889
Macrodantin Capsules (Rare) 2891
Menest Tablets 2254
Meruvax II 2130
Microgestin Fe 1.5/30 Tablets 3407
Microgestin Fe 1/20 Tablets 3400
Mircette Tablets 2470
M-M-R II (Infrequent) 2118
Monurol Sachet (One patient) 1375
Motrin Suspension, Oral Drops, Chewable Tablets, and Caplets (Less than 1%) 2002
Mumpsvax 2141
Myambutol Tablets 1290
Necon 3415
Nordette-28 Tablets 2257
Ogestrel 0.5/50-28 Tablets 3428
Ortho Dienestrol Cream 2554
Ovral Tablets 3551
Ovral-28 Tablets 3552
Ovrette Tablets 3552
Pacerone Tablets 3331
Paser Granules 1781
Paxil 1609
Premarin Intravenous 3563
Premarin Vaginal Cream 3570
Premphase Tablets 3572
Prempro Tablets 3572
Proleukin for Injection (Less than 1%) 1199
Provera Tablets 2853
Prozac Pulvules, Liquid, and Weekly Capsules 1238
Quinaglute Dura-Tabs Tablets (Occasional) 978
Quinidex Extentabs (Occasional) 2933
Recombivax HB 2178
Rifamate Capsules (Uncommon) 767
Rifater Tablets (Uncommon) 769
Rituxan for Infusion (Less than 0.1%) 1750
Rituxan I.V. (Less than 0.1%) 1428
Sarafem Pulvules 1962
Serophene Tablets 3226
Trecator-SC Tablets (Rare) 3598
Tri-Levlen 962
Trivora Tablets 3439
Twinrix Vaccine 1674
Videx (Several patients) 1138
Videx EC Capsules 1143
Vitravene for Injection (2% to 5%) ⊙310
Yasmin 28 Tablets 980
Yodoxin Tablets 1722
Zanaflex Tablets (Infrequent) 1305
Zoloft 2751
Zovia 3449

Neuritis, peripheral
Antabuse Tablets 2444
Antabuse Tablets 3474
Bactrim 2949
Carbatrol Capsules 3234
Doxil Injection (Less than 1%) 566
Gabitril Tablets (Infrequent) 1189
Herceptin I.V. (2%) 1414
Kaletra Capsules (Less than 2%) 471
Kaletra Oral Solution (Less than 2%) 471
Lopid Tablets 2650
Myambutol Tablets 1290
Paxil (Rare) 1609
Pediazole Suspension 3050
Rilutek Tablets (Rare) 772
Septra Suspension 2265
Septra Tablets 2265
Septra DS Tablets 2265
Streptomycin Sulfate Injection 2714
Tegretol/Tegretol-XR 2404
Thalomid Capsules 1154
Trecator-SC Tablets (Rare) 3598
Zonegran Capsules (Infrequent) 1307

Neuritis, retrobulbar
Attenuvax 2044
Meruvax II 2130
M-M-R II 2118
Mumpsvax (Infrequent) 2141
Rabies Vaccine RabAvert (One case) 1203

Neurodermatitis
Aricept Tablets (Infrequent) 1270
Aricept Tablets (Infrequent) 2665

Neuroencephalopathy
Taxol Injection (Less than 1%) 1129

Neurofibromatosis
Serophene Tablets 3226

Neuroleptic malignant syndrome
Aricept Tablets 2665
Celexa (At least 3 patients) 1365
Clozaril Tablets (Several cases) 2319
Compazine 1505
Comtan Tablets 2328
Concerta Extended-Release Tablets (Very rare) 1998
Concerta Tablets (Very rare) 561
Effexor Tablets 3495
Effexor XR Capsules 3499
Etrafon 3115
Geodon Capsules 2688
Haldol Decanoate 2535
Haldol Injection, Tablets and Concentrate 2533
Lodosyn Tablets 1251
Loxitane Capsules 3398
Metadate CD Capsules (Very rare) 1164
Metadate ER Tablets (Very rare) 1167
Methylin Tablets (Very rare) 1995
Methylin ER Tablets (Very rare) 1995
Moban 1320
Navane Oral (Rare) 2701
Navane Intramuscular (Rare) 2703
Norpramin Tablets 755
Orap Tablets 1407
Paxil 1609
Permax Tablets 1299
Phenergan 3556
Prozac Pulvules, Liquid, and Weekly Capsules (Rare) 1238
Reglan (Rare) 2935
Risperdal 1796
Ritalin 2387
Sarafem Pulvules (Rare) 1962
Serentil 1057
Seroquel Tablets (0.1%) 684
Serzone Tablets (Rare) 1104
Sinemet Tablets (Sporadic cases) 1253
Sinemet CR Tablets (Sporadic cases) 1255
Stelazine 1640
Symmetrel 1328
Tegretol-XR Tablets (Isolated cases) 2404
Thioridazine Hydrochloride Tablets 2289
Thiothixene Capsules 2290
Thorazine 1656
Trilafon 3160
Zoloft 2751

Neurological disability, unspecified
Abelcet Injection 1273
Acel-Imune (Rare) 1851
Foscavir Injection (Less than 1%) 605
Hivid Tablets (Less than 1%) 2975
JE-VAX Vaccine (Two cases) 811
▲ Nipent for Injection (1% to 11%) 3272
Tice BCG, BCG Live (0.9%) 2489

Neuromuscular blockade
Coly-Mycin M Parenteral 2243
Nebcin Vials, Hyporets & ADD-Vantage 1955
Zemuron Injection 2491

Neuromuscular disorders, unspecified
Azulfidine EN-tabs Tablets 2775
Eulexin Capsules (2%) 3118
Lupron Depot 3.75 mg (Less than 5%) 3281
Lupron Depot 7.5 mg (Less than 5%) 3284
▲ Lupron Depot–3 Month 11.25 mg (1.8% to 7%) 3285
▲ Lupron Depot–3 Month 22.5 mg (9.6%) 3288
▲ Lupron Depot–4 Month 30 mg (4.2% to 6.1%) 3289

Neuromuscular excitability
Ceptaz for Injection 1499
Fortaz 1541
Tazidime Vials, Faspak & ADD-Vantage 1966
Zosyn 1890
Zosyn in Galaxy Containers 1894

Neuromyopathy
Aralen Tablets 3075
Plaquenil Tablets 3082

Neuro-ocular lesions
Triphasil-21 Tablets 3600
Triphasil-28 Tablets 3605

Neuropathic ulcer
▲ Apligraf (17%) 2305

Neuropathy
Accolate Tablets (Rare) 657
Aciphex Tablets 1267
Aciphex Tablets 1783
Actiq (Less than 1%) 1184
Altace Capsules (Less than 1%) 2233
Ambien Tablets (Rare) 3191
Axert Tablets (Rare) 2772
Betaseron for SC Injection 988
Bicillin C-R 900/300 Injection 2240
Bicillin C-R Injection 2238
Bicillin L-A Injection (Infrequent) 2242
▲ Casodex Tablets (2% to 5%) 662
Celebrex Capsules (0.1% to 1.9%) 2676
Celebrex Capsules (0.1% to 1.9%) 2780
▲ CellCept Capsules (3% to 10%) 2951
▲ CellCept Intravenous (3% to 10%) 2951
▲ CellCept Oral Suspension (3% to 10%) 2951
▲ CellCept Tablets (3% to 10%) 2951
▲ Chemet Capsules (1.0% to 12.7%) 3078
Cognex Capsules (Infrequent) 1351
▲ Combivir Tablets (12%) 1502
Cortifoam Rectal Foam 3170
Cuprimine Capsules 2075
Cytotec Tablets (Infrequent) 3202
▲ Cytovene (8%) 2959
▲ DaunoXome Injection (1% to 13%) 1442
Depen Titratable Tablets 3341
Diprivan Injectable Emulsion (Less than 1%) 667
Doxil Injection (Less than 1%) 566
Effexor Tablets (Infrequent) 3495
Effexor XR Capsules (Infrequent) 3499
Engerix-B Vaccine 1517
▲ Epivir (12%) 1520
Evoxac Capsules (Less than 1%) 1217
Flovent Diskus 3614
Flovent 1535
Flovent Rotadisk 1537
Fortovase Capsules (Less than 2%) 2970
▲ Foscavir Injection (5% or greater) 605
Gengraf Capsules (1% to less than 3%) 457
Geodon Capsules (Frequent) 2688
Havrix Vaccine (Rare) 1544
Herceptin I.V. (1%) 1414
Intron A for Injection (Less than 5%) 3120
Kaletra Capsules (Less than 2%) 471
Kaletra Oral Solution (Less than 2%) 471
Lupron Depot–4 Month 30 mg (Less than 5%) 3289
Luvox Tablets (25, 50, 100 mg) 3256
LYMErix Vaccine (Greater than 1%) 1592
Matulane Capsules 3246
Megace Oral Suspension (1% to 3%) 1124
Mykrox Tablets (Less than 2%) 1168
Naropin Injection (Less than 1%) 612
Neoral Soft Gelatin Capsules (1% to less than 3%) 2380
Neoral Oral Solution (1% to less than 3%) 2380
Nimotop Capsules (Less than 1%) 904
Nipent for Injection (Less than 3%) 3272
Norvir Capsules (Less than 2%) 487
Norvir Oral Solution (Less than 2%) 487
Paxil (Rare) 1609
Permapen Isoject 2706
Permax Tablets (Infrequent) 1299
Pfizerpen for Injection (Rare) 2707
Plaquenil Tablets 3082
▲ Prograf (3%) 1393
Proleukin for Injection 1199
Prozac Pulvules, Liquid, and Weekly Capsules (Infrequent) 1238
▲ Rapamune Oral Solution and Tablets (3% to 20%) 3584
ReFacto Vials 1437
Rescriptor Tablets (Less than 2%) 526
Roferon-A Injection (Less than 0.5%) 2996
Sandostatin LAR Depot (1% to 4%) 2395
Sarafem Pulvules (Infrequent) 1962
▲ Serostim for Injection (25.9%) 3229
▲ Simulect for Injection (3% to 10%) 2399
Singulair 2181
Sonata Capsules (Rare) 3591
Sporanox Capsules (Isolated cases) 1800
Sporanox Injection (Isolated cases) 1804
Sporanox Injection (Isolated cases) 2509
Sporanox Oral Solution (Isolated cases) 1808
Sporanox Oral Solution (Isolated cases) 2512
Sustiva Capsules 1258
Tambocor Tablets (Less than 1%) 1990
Tasmar Tablets (Infrequent) 3010
▲ Thalomid Capsules (8.3%) 1154
Topamax Sprinkle Capsules (Infrequent) 2590
Topamax Tablets (Infrequent) 2590
▲ Trizivir Tablets (12%) 1669
Twinrix Vaccine 1674
Urobiotic-250 Capsules 2731
Viagra Tablets (Less than 2%) 2732
▲ Videx (17% to 20%) 1138
▲ Videx EC Capsules (20%) 1143
Vistide Injection 1445
Vitravene for Injection (2% to 5%) ⊙310
Wellbutrin SR Sustained-Release Tablets 1684
Zanaflex Tablets (Rare) 1305
Zaroxolyn Tablets 1177
Zerit 1147
Zonegran Capsules (Infrequent) 1307
Zyban Sustained-Release Tablets 1710
Zyprexa Tablets (Rare) 1973
Zyprexa ZYDIS Orally Disintegrating Tablets (Rare) 1973

Neuropathy, autonomic
Taxol Injection (Rare) 1129

Neuropathy, median nerve
Vioxx (Greater than 0.1% to 1.9%) 2213

Neuropathy, optic
Cordarone Tablets 3487
Decadron Phosphate Injection 2081
Decadron Phosphate Sterile Ophthalmic Ointment 2083
Decadron Phosphate Sterile Ophthalmic Solution 2084
Healon GV ⊙320
Imitrex Injection 1549
Imitrex Nasal Spray 1554
Imitrex Tablets 1558
Pacerone Tablets 3331
Protonix I.V. 3580
Protonix Tablets 3577
Tolectin (Less than 1%) 2589

Neuropathy, peripheral
Abelcet Injection 1273
Ancobon Capsules 1730
Antabuse Tablets 2444
Antabuse Tablets 3474
Asacol Delayed-Release Tablets (Rare) 2884
Azulfidine EN-tabs Tablets (Rare) 2775
Baycol Tablets 883
Betapace Tablets (One case) 950
Chibroxin Sterile Ophthalmic Solution 2051
Cordarone Tablets (Common) 3487
Cozaar Tablets (Less than 1%) 2067
Crixivan Capsules (Less than 2%) 2070
Cuprimine Capsules 2075
Dapsone Tablets USP 1780
Depen Titratable Tablets 3341
Enalaprilat Injection 863
▲ Epivir (13%) 1520
Epivir-HBV 1524
Ergamisol Tablets 1789
Etrafon 3115
Exelon Capsules (Infrequent) 2342
Exelon Oral Solution (Infrequent) 2345
Flexeril Tablets (Rare) 572
Flexeril Tablets (Rare) 2094
Floxin I.V. 2526
Floxin Tablets 2529
Fludara for Injection 995
▲ Fortovase Capsules (1.0% to 11.3%) 2970
▲ Hexalen Capsules (9% to 31%) 2226
▲ Hivid Tablets (28% up to 1/3 of patients) 2975
Hyzaar 2109
▲ Idamycin PFS Injection (7%) 2825
Indocin Capsules (Less than 1%) 2112
Indocin I.V. (Less than 1%) 2115
Indocin (Less than 1%) 2112
▲ Invirase Capsules (1.0% to 11.3%) 2979
JE-VAX Vaccine (1 to 2.3 per million vaccines) 811
Lescol Capsules 2361
Lescol Capsules 2925
Lescol XL Tablets 2361
Lescol XL Tablets 2925
Leukeran Tablets 1591
Lexxel Tablets 608
Lipitor Tablets (Less than 2%) 2639
Lipitor Tablets (Less than 2%) 2696
Lodosyn Tablets 1251
Lupron Depot 3.75 mg 3281
Lupron Depot 7.5 mg 3284
Lupron Depot–3 Month 11.25 mg 3285
Lupron Depot–3 Month 22.5 mg 3288
Lupron Depot–4 Month 30 mg 3289
Lupron Depot-PED 7.5 mg, 11.25 mg and 15 mg 3291
Lupron Injection (Less than 5%) 3279
Macrobid Capsules 2889
Macrodantin Capsules 2891
Mevacor Tablets (0.5% to 1.0%) 2132
▲ Navelbine Injection (Up to 20%) 1604
Noroxin Tablets 2145
Norpramin Tablets 755
Norvasc Tablets (More than 0.1% to 1%) 2704
Norvir Capsules (Less than 2%) 487
Norvir Oral Solution (Less than 2%) 487
Pacerone Tablets (Common) 3331
▲ Paraplatin for Injection (4% to 16%) 1126
Pravachol Tablets 1099
Prinivil Tablets (0.3% to 1.0%) 2164
Prinzide Tablets 2168
Recombivax HB 2178
Requip Tablets (Infrequent) 1621
Rifamate Capsules 767
Rifater Tablets 769
Sinemet Tablets 1253
Sinemet CR Tablets 1255
Surmontil Capsules 3595
Sustiva Capsules (Less than 2%) 1258
▲ Taxol Injection (3% to 60%) 1129
Thalomid Capsules 1154
Ticlid Tablets (Rare) 3015
Tripedia Vaccine (A few cases) 817
▲ Valcyte Tablets (9%) 3022
Vaseretic Tablets 2204
Vasotec I.V. Injection 2207
Vasotec Tablets (0.5% to 1.0%) 2210
▲ Videx (34% to 51%) 1138
Videx EC Capsules 1143
Vivactil Tablets 2217
Vivactil Tablets 2446
Yodoxin Tablets 1722
▲ Zerit (4% to 24%) 1147
Zestoretic Tablets 695
Zestril Tablets (0.3% to 1.0%) 698
Zocor Tablets 2219

Neuropathy, peripheral sensory
Desferal Vials 2333
Norvir Capsules (Less than 2%) 487
Norvir Oral Solution (Less than 2%) 487

Neuropsychiatric disorders, life-threatening, aggravation of
Roferon-A Injection 2996

Neuropsychometrics performance, decrease
Blocadren Tablets 2046
Corgard Tablets 2245
Corzide 40/5 Tablets 2247
Corzide 80/5 Tablets 2247
Cosopt Sterile Ophthalmic Solution 2065
Inderal 3513
Inderal LA Long-Acting Capsules 3516
Inderide Tablets 3517
Inderide LA Long-Acting Capsules 3519
Nadolol Tablets 2288
Normodyne Tablets 3137
Sectral Capsules 3589
Tenoretic Tablets 690
Tenormin 692
Timolol GFS ⊙266
Timoptic in Ocudose 2192
Timoptic Sterile Ophthalmic Solution 2190
Timoptic-XE Sterile Ophthalmic Gel Forming Solution 2194
Toprol-XL Tablets 651

Neurosis, unspecified
Ambien Tablets (Rare) 3191
Avonex 1013
Betaseron for SC Injection 988
Cerebyx Injection (Infrequent) 2619
Cognex Capsules (Infrequent) 1351
Evoxac Capsules 1217
Exelon Capsules (Infrequent) 2342
Exelon Oral Solution (Infrequent) 2345
Gabitril Tablets (Infrequent) 1189
Intron A for Injection (Less than 5%) 3120
Lamictal (Rare) 1567
Neurontin Capsules (Rare) 2655
Neurontin Oral Solution (Rare) 2655
Neurontin Tablets (Rare) 2655
Nipent for Injection (Less than 3%) 3272
Paxil (Infrequent) 1609
Permax Tablets (Infrequent) 1299
Prozac Pulvules, Liquid, and Weekly Capsules (Infrequent) 1238
Remeron Tablets (Infrequent) 2483
Remeron SolTab Tablets (Infrequent) 2486
Requip Tablets (Infrequent) 1621
Sarafem Pulvules (Infrequent) 1962
Sustiva Capsules 1258
Topamax Sprinkle Capsules (Infrequent) 2590
Topamax Tablets (Infrequent) 2590
Uniretic Tablets (Less than 1%) 3178

Neurotoxicity
Hexalen Capsules 2226
Leustatin Injection (Rare) 2495
Nebcin Vials, Hyporets & ADD-Vantage 1955
▲ Paraplatin for Injection (5% to 28%) 1126
▲ Prograf (Approximately 55%) 1393
Streptomycin Sulfate Injection 2714
▲ Zinecard for Injection (10% to 17%) 2869

Neurotoxicity, peripheral
Navelbine Injection 1604

Neurovascular episodes
Bicillin C-R 900/300 Injection 2240
Bicillin C-R Injection 2238
ParaGard T 380A Intrauterine Copper Contraceptive 2582

Neutropenia
Accupril Tablets (Rare) 2611
Accuretic Tablets 2614
Accutane Capsules 2944
Aceon Tablets (2 mg, 4 mg, 8 mg) (0.1%) 3249
Aloprim for Injection (Less than 1%) 2292
Altace Capsules 2233
Ancef for Injection 1474
Ancef Injection 1474
Aredia for Injection (Up to 1%) 2309
Asacol Delayed-Release Tablets 2884
Atacand Tablets (Very rare) 595
▲ Azactam for Injection (Less than 1% to 11.3%) 1276
Bactrim 2949
▲ Betaseron for SC Injection (18%) 988
▲ Campath Ampules (64% to 85%) 992
Captopril Tablets 2281
Cardura Tablets 2668
Ceclor CD Tablets 1279
Ceclor (Rare) 1905
Cedax 1021
Cefizox for Intramuscular or Intravenous Use (Rare) 1390
Cefobid Intravenous/Intramuscular (1 in 50) 2671
Cefobid Pharmacy Bulk Package - Not for Direct Infusion (1 in 50) 2673
Cefotan 664
Ceftin 1898
Cefzil 1076
CellCept Capsules (Up to 2.0%) 2951
CellCept Intravenous (Up to 2.0%) 2951
CellCept Oral Suspension (Up to 2.0%) 2951
CellCept Tablets (Up to 2.0%) 2951
Ceptaz for Injection (Very rare) 1499
Chemet Capsules (0.5% to 1.5%) 3078
Chibroxin Sterile Ophthalmic Solution 2051
Claforan Injection (Less than 1%) 732
Cleocin HCl Capsules 2784
Cleocin Phosphate Sterile Solution 2785
Cleocin Vaginal Cream 2788
Cleocin Vaginal Ovules 2789
Clinoril Tablets (Less than 1 in 100) 2053
▲ Clozaril Tablets (3%) 2319
▲ Combivir Tablets (7.2%) 1502
Cordarone Intravenous 3491
Crixivan Capsules (1.1%) 2070
▲ Cytovene (6% to 22%) 2959
▲ DaunoXome Injection (15% to 36%) 1442
Declomycin Tablets 1855
▲ DepoCyt Injection (8% to 9%) 1197
Diflucan Tablets, Injection, and Oral Suspension 2681
Diovan Capsules (1.9%) 2337
Diovan HCT Tablets 2338
Dipentum Capsules (Rare) 2803
Doryx Coated Pellet Filled Capsules 3357
▲ Doxil Injection (44.2% to 51.7%) 566
Duricef 1079
Dynacin Capsules 2019
Edecrin 2091
▲ Ellence Injection (10.5% to 80.3%) 2806
Enalaprilat Injection (Several cases) 863
▲ Epivir (7.2% to 22%) 1520
Epivir-HBV 1524
Ergamisol Tablets (2 out of 463 patients) 1789
Famvir Tablets 2348
Floxin I.V. (More than or equal to 1%) 2526
Floxin Tablets (More than or equal to 1%) 2529
▲ Fludara for Injection (Among most common) 995
Fortaz (Very rare) 1541
Fortovase Capsules (1% to 2%) 2970
Gastrocrom Oral Concentrate (Less common) 1162
▲ Gemzar for Injection (18% to 63%) 1919
Geocillin Tablets 2687
▲ Gleevec Capsules (16% to 46%) 2357
Halcion Tablets (1.5%) 2823
▲ Hivid Tablets (16.9%) 2975
▲ Hycamtin for Injection (26% to 98%) 1546
▲ Intron A for Injection (Less than 5% to 92%) 3120
Invirase Capsules (1% to 2%) 2979
Iveegam EN (One case) 849
Keflex 1237
Kefurox Vials, ADD-Vantage (Less than 1 in 100) 1948
Kefzol Vials, ADD-Vantage 1951
Lamictal 1567
Lamisil Tablets (Isolated case) 2360
Leukeran Tablets 1591
▲ Leustatin Injection (70%) 2495
Lexxel Tablets (Several cases) 608
Lodine (Less than 1%) 3528
Lodine XL Extended-Release Tablets (Less than 1%) 3530
Lorabid Suspension and Pulvules 2251
Lotrel Capsules 2370
Mandol Vials 1953
Mavik Tablets (Rare) 478
Maxipime for Injection 1285
Mefoxin for Injection 2124
Mefoxin Premixed Intravenous Solution 2127
▲ Mepron Suspension (5%) 1598
Mexitil Capsules (About 1 in 1,000) 1047
Midamor Tablets (Rare) 2136
Minocin Intravenous 1862
Minocin Oral Suspension 1865
Minocin Pellet-Filled Capsules 1863
Moduretic Tablets 2138
Monodox Capsules 2442
Monopril Tablets 1091
Monopril HCT (Less than 2%) 1094
Motrin Suspension, Oral Drops, Chewable Tablets, and Caplets (Less than 1%) 2002
▲ Mycobutin Capsules (25%) 2838
▲ Mylotarg for Injection (98%) 3540
Nolvadex Tablets (Rare) 678
Noroxin Tablets (1.4%) 2145
Omnicef 493
Orthoclone OKT3 Sterile Solution (Less than 1%) 2498
Pacerone Tablets 3331
▲ Paraplatin for Injection (16% to 97%) 1126
▲ PEG-Intron Powder for Injection (6%) 3140
Periostat Tablets 1208
Pipracil 1866
Plavix Tablets (Less than 1%) 1097
Plavix Tablets (Less than 1%) 3084
Prevacid Delayed-Release Capsules (Less than 1%) 3292
PREVPAC 3298
▲ Priftin Tablets (5%) 758
Prilosec Delayed-Release Capsules (Rare) 628
Primaxin I.M. 2158
Primaxin I.V. (Less than 0.2%) 2160
Prinivil Tablets (Rare) 2164
Prinzide Tablets (Rare) 2168
Procanbid Extended-Release Tablets (Approximately 0.5%) 2262
Proleukin for Injection 1199
Reglan (A few cases) 2935
▲ Rescriptor Tablets (Less than 2% to 5.7%) 526
Retrovir Capsules 1625
Retrovir IV Infusion 1629
Retrovir 1625
Rilutek Tablets (Three cases) 772
▲ Rituxan for Infusion (1.9% to 7%) 1750
▲ Rituxan I.V. (1.9% to 7%) 1428
Rocephin Injectable Vials, ADD-Vantage, Galaxy, Bulk (Less than 1%) 2993
▲ Roferon-A Injection (Up to 68%) 2996
Septra Suspension 2265
Septra Tablets 2265
Septra DS Tablets 2265
Seroquel Tablets (Rare) 684
Sporanox Capsules (Rare) 1800
Sporanox Injection (Rare) 1804
Sporanox Injection (Rare) 2509
Sporanox Oral Solution (Rare) 1808
Sporanox Oral Solution (Rare) 2512
Suprax 1877
Symmetrel (Less than 0.1%) 1328
Tarka Tablets (Less frequent) 508
▲ Taxol Injection (52% to 90%) 1129
▲ Taxotere for Injection Concentrate (76%) 778
Tazicef for Injection (Very rare) 1647
Tazicef Galaxy Container (Very rare) 1650
Tazicef Pharmacy Bulk Package (Very rare) 1653
Tazidime Vials, Faspak & ADD-Vantage (Very rare) 1966
Temodar Capsules 3157
Tequin Injection (Less than 0.1%) 1110
Tequin Tablets (Less than 0.1%) 1110
Teveten Tablets (1.3%) 3327
Thalomid Capsules 1154
Ticlid Tablets (0.8% to 2.4%) 3015
Timentin Injection- ADD-Vantage Vial 1661
Timentin Injection-Galaxy Container 1664
Timentin Injection-Pharmacy Bulk Package 1666
Timentin for Intravenous Administration 1658
Tonocard Tablets (Less than 1%) 649
▲ Trisenox Injection (10%) 1158
▲ Trizivir Tablets (7.2%) 1669
Unasyn for Injection 2728
Uniretic Tablets (More than 1%) 3178
Univasc Tablets (More than 1%) 3181
▲ Valcyte Tablets (11% to 27%) 3022
Valium Injectable (Isolated reports) 3026
Valium Tablets (Isolated reports) 3047
Vancocin HCl Capsules & Pulvules (Several dozen cases) 1972
Vancocin HCl Oral Solution (Several dozen cases) 1971
Vancocin HCl, Vials & ADD-Vantage (Several dozen cases) 1970

Vantin Tablets and Oral Suspension 2860
Vascor Tablets (2 cases) 2602
Vaseretic Tablets (Rare) 2204
Vasotec I.V. Injection (Several cases) 2207
Vasotec Tablets (Rare) 2210
Vermox Chewable Tablets (Rare) 2017
Vibramycin Calcium Oral Suspension Syrup 2735
Vibramycin Hyclate Capsules 2735
Vibramycin Hyclate Intravenous 2737
Vibramycin Monohydrate for Oral Suspension 2735
Vibra-Tabs Film Coated Tablets 2735
▲ Viramune Oral Suspension (11.1%) 1060
▲ Viramune Tablets (11.1%) 1060
▲ Vistide Injection (20% to 43%) 1445
Vitravene for Injection (2% to 5%) ⊙310
Xanax Tablets (2.3% to 3.0%) 2865
Xeloda Tablets (2% to 3%) 3039
▲ Zerit (5%) 1147
Zestoretic Tablets (Rare) 695
Zestril Tablets (Rare) 698
Ziagen 1692
Zinacef Injection (Fewer than 1 in 100) 1696
Zinacef for Injection (Fewer than 1 in 100) 1696
Zithromax Capsules, 250 mg (Less than 1%) 2743
Zithromax for IV Infusion (Less than 1%) 2748
Zithromax for Oral Suspension, 1 g (Less than 1%) 2743
Zithromax for Oral Suspension, 300 mg, 600 mg, 900 mg, 1200 mg (Less than 1%) 2739
Zithromax Tablets, 250 mg (Less than 1%) 2739
Zithromax Tablets, 600 mg (Less than 1%) 2743
Zosyn 1890
Zosyn in Galaxy Containers 1894
Zovirax for Injection (Less than 1%) 1708

Neutropenia, congenital
Azulfidine EN-tabs Tablets (Rare) 2775

Neutropenia, febrile
▲ Trisenox Injection (8%) 1158

Neutrophilia
Dynabac Tablets (1.2%) 2269
Floxin I.V. (More than or equal to 1%) 2526
Floxin Tablets (More than or equal to 1%) 2529
Hivid Tablets (Less than 1%) 2975
Maxipime for Injection (0.1% to 1%) 1285
Priftin Tablets (Less than 1%) 758
Zovirax for Injection (Less than 1%) 1708

Neutrophils, decrease
(*see under* Neutropenia)

Nevi, pre-existing, increased growth of
Humatrope Vials and Cartridges (Rare) 1930
Nutropin AQ Injection (Rare) 1420
Nutropin for Injection (Rare) 1417

Night blindness
(*see under* Nyctalopia)

Night sweat
Aricept Tablets (Infrequent) 1270
Aricept Tablets (Infrequent) 2665
Crixivan Capsules (Less than 2%) 2070
Fortovase Capsules (Less than 2%) 2970
Gengraf Capsules (Rare) 457
▲ Gleevec Capsules (8% to 10%) 2357
Hivid Tablets (Less than 1%) 2975
Invirase Capsules (Less than 2%) 2979
Neoral Soft Gelatin Capsules (Rare) 2380
Neoral Oral Solution (Rare) 2380
Oncaspar (Greater than 1% but less than 5%) 756
▲ Prometrium Capsules (100 mg, 200 mg) (7%) 3261
▲ Rituxan for Infusion (Among most frequent) 1750
▲ Rituxan I.V. (Among most frequent) 1428
▲ Roferon-A Injection (8%) 2996
Sandimmune (Rare) 2388
▲ Trisenox Injection (8%) 1158
▲ Zenapax for Injection (2% to 5%) 3046

Night terrors
(*see under* Pavor nocturnus)

Nightmares
Aldoclor Tablets 2035
Aldomet Tablets 2037
Aldoril Tablets 2039
Axert Tablets (Rare) 2772
Biaxin/Biaxin XL 403
Blocadren Tablets 2046
Cataflam Tablets (Less than 1%) 2315
Catapres Tablets 1037
Catapres-TTS (0.5% or less) 1038
Cipro I.V. (1% or less) 893
Cipro I.V. Pharmacy Bulk Package (Less than 1%) 897
Cipro (Less than 1%) 887
Clorpres Tablets 1002
▲ Clozaril Tablets (4%) 2319
Combipres Tablets 1040
Cosopt Sterile Ophthalmic Solution 2065
Duraclon Injection (Rare) 3057
▲ Effexor XR Capsules (4% to 7%) 3499
Eldepryl Capsules 3266
Etrafon 3115
Floxin I.V. 2526
Floxin Tablets 2529
Halcion Tablets (Rare) 2823
Ismo Tablets (Fewer than 1%) 3524
Klonopin Tablets (Infrequent) 2983
Levaquin 2537
Lodosyn Tablets 1251
Marinol Capsules (Less than 1%) 3325
Matulane Capsules 3246
Meridia Capsules 481
Nardil Tablets (Infrequent) 2653
Naropin Injection (Less than 1%) 612
Nembutal Sodium Solution (Less than 1%) 485
Norpramin Tablets 755
Orudis Capsules (Rare) 3548
Oruvail Capsules (Rare) 3548
Plaquenil Tablets 3082
PREVPAC 3298
Relafen Tablets (Less than 1%) 1617
Rescriptor Tablets (Less than 2%) 526
Risperdal (Rare) 1796
Sinemet Tablets 1253
Sinemet CR Tablets 1255
Surmontil Capsules 3595
Tequin Injection 1110
Tequin Tablets 1110
Timolide Tablets 2187
Timolol GFS ⊙266
Timoptic in Ocudose 2192
Timoptic Sterile Ophthalmic Solution 2190
Timoptic-XE Sterile Ophthalmic Gel Forming Solution 2194
Toprol-XL Tablets 651
Trovan 2722
Vantin Tablets and Oral Suspension (Less than 1%) 2860
Ventolin Inhalation Aerosol and Refill (1%) 1679
Versed Injection (Less than 1%) 3027
Vivactil Tablets 2217
Vivactil Tablets 2446
Voltaren Tablets (Less than 1%) 2315
Voltaren-XR Tablets (Less than 1%) 2315

Nipple, supernumerary
Cetrotide for Injection 3209

Nitrogen balance, changes
(*see under* BUN levels, changes)

NMS
(*see under* Neuroleptic malignant syndrome)

Nocturia
Actiq (Less than 1%) 1184
Adalat CC Tablets (Less than 1.0%) 877
Ambien Tablets (Rare) 3191
Aricept Tablets (Frequent) 1270
Aricept Tablets (Frequent) 2665
Arthrotec Tablets (Rare) 3195
Avonex 1013
Betaseron for SC Injection 988
Calcijex Injection 411
Cardizem Injectable 1018
Cardizem Lyo-Ject Syringe 1018
Cardizem Monovial 1018
Cardizem CD Capsules (Less than 1%) 1016
Cardura Tablets 2668
▲ Casodex Tablets (9%) 662
Cataflam Tablets (Less than 1%) 2315
Catapres Tablets (About 1 in 100 patients) 1037
Ceclor CD Tablets (0.1% to 1%) 1279
Claritin-D 12 Hour Extended Release Tablets (Less frequent) 3102
Clorpres Tablets (About 1%) 1002
Cognex Capsules (Infrequent) 1351
Combipres Tablets (About 1%) 1040
Copaxone for Injection (Infrequent) 3306
Cozaar Tablets (Less than 1%) 2067
▲ Crinone 8% Gel (13%) 3213
Crixivan Capsules (Less than 2%) 2070
Dantrium Capsules (Less frequent) 2885
DaunoXome Injection (Less than or equal to 5%) 1442
Doxil Injection (Less than 1%) 566
Duraclon Injection (About 1%) 3057
DynaCirc Capsules (0.5% to 1%) 2921
DynaCirc CR Tablets (0.5% to 1%) 2923
Effexor Tablets (Infrequent) 3495
Effexor XR Capsules (Infrequent) 3499
Eldepryl Capsules 3266
Evoxac Capsules (Less than 1%) 1217
Exelon Capsules (Infrequent) 2342
Exelon Oral Solution (Infrequent) 2345
Fortovase Capsules (Less than 2%) 2970
Foscavir Injection (Between 1% and 5%) 605
Gabitril Tablets (Infrequent) 1189
Gengraf Capsules (1% to less than 3%) 457
Geodon Capsules (Rare) 2688
Hectorol Capsules 1064
Hectorol Injection 1066
Hivid Tablets (Less than 1%) 2975
Hyzaar 2109
Indapamide Tablets (Less than 5%) 2286
Intron A for Injection (Less than 5%) 3120
Klonopin Tablets 2983
Lipitor Tablets (Less than 2%) 2639
Lipitor Tablets (Less than 2%) 2696
Luvox Tablets (25, 50, 100 mg) (Infrequent) 3256
Matulane Capsules 3246
Miacalcin Injection 2373
Moduretic Tablets (Less than or equal to 1%) 2138
Mykrox Tablets (Less than 2%) 1168
Naprelan Tablets (Less than 1%) 1293
Neoral Soft Gelatin Capsules (1% to less than 3%) 2380
Neoral Oral Solution (1% to less than 3%) 2380
Neurontin Capsules (Rare) 2655
Neurontin Oral Solution (Rare) 2655
Neurontin Tablets (Rare) 2655
▲ Nilandron Tablets (6.7%) 753
Norpramin Tablets 755
Norvasc Tablets (More than 0.1% to 1%) 2704
Norvir Capsules (Less than 2%) 487
Norvir Oral Solution (Less than 2%) 487
Orap Tablets 1407
Paxil (Infrequent) 1609
Procardia Capsules (Less than 0.5%) 2708
Procardia XL Extended Release Tablets (1% or less) 2710
▲ Prograf (3% to 15%) 1393
ProSom Tablets (Rare) 500
Protonix I.V. (Less than 1%) 3580
Protonix Tablets (Less than 1%) 3577
Prozac Pulvules, Liquid, and Weekly Capsules (Infrequent) 1238
▲ Rapamune Oral Solution and Tablets (3% to 20%) 3584
Reminyl Oral Solution (Infrequent) 1792
Reminyl Tablets (Infrequent) 1792
Requip Tablets (Infrequent) 1621
Rescriptor Tablets (Less than 2%) 526
Rilutek Tablets (Rare) 772
Rocaltrol 2991
Sarafem Pulvules (Infrequent) 1962
Sectral Capsules (Up to 2%) 3589
Seroquel Tablets (Rare) 684
▲ Serostim for Injection (1% to 10%) 3229
Serzone Tablets (Infrequent) 1104
Sular Tablets (Less than or equal to 1%) 688
Tarka Tablets (Less frequent) 508
Tasmar Tablets (Infrequent) 3010
Tenex Tablets (Less frequent) 2942
Tiazac Capsules (Less than 2%) 1378
▲ Tice BCG, BCG Live (4.5%) 2489
Topamax Sprinkle Capsules (Infrequent) 2590
Topamax Tablets (Infrequent) 2590
Trilafon 3160
Uniretic Tablets (Less than 1%) 3178
▲ Valstar Sterile Solution for Intravesical Instillation (2% to 7%) 1175
Vantin Tablets and Oral Suspension (Less than 1%) 2860
▲ Viadur Implant (3.8%) 912
Viagra Tablets (Less than 2%) 2732
Vioxx (Greater than 0.1% to 1.9%) 2213
Vistide Injection 1445
Vivactil Tablets 2217
Vivactil Tablets 2446
Voltaren Tablets (Less than 1%) 2315
Voltaren-XR Tablets (Less than 1%) 2315
Wellbutrin Tablets (Frequent) 1680
Xeloda Tablets (Less than 5%) 3039
Zoloft (Infrequent) 2751
Zonegran Capsules (Infrequent) 1307

Nodal rhythm
Covera-HS Tablets 3199
Digitek Tablets 1003
Fluothane Inhalation 3508
Isoptin SR Tablets 467
Lanoxicaps Capsules (Common) 1574
Lanoxin Injection (Common) 1581
Lanoxin Tablets (Common) 1587
Lanoxin Elixir Pediatric (Common) 1578
Lanoxin Injection Pediatric (Common) 1584
Prostigmin Injectable 1744
Prostigmin Tablets 1744
Romazicon Injection (Less than 1%) 3000
Suprane Liquid for Inhalation (Greater than 1%) 874
Versed Injection (Less than 1%) 3027

Nodule, subcutaneous
Arava Tablets (1% to 3%) 724
Enbrel for Injection 1752
Enbrel for Injection 3504
Gabitril Tablets (Infrequent) 1189
Naprelan Tablets (Less than 1%) 1293
Neurontin Capsules (Rare) 2655
Neurontin Oral Solution (Rare) 2655
Neurontin Tablets (Rare) 2655
Permax Tablets (Rare) 1299
Uniretic Tablets (Less than 1%) 3178

Nodule at injection site
Genotropin Lyophilized Powder (Infrequent) 2818
Lovenox Injection 746
▲ Nutropin Depot for Injectable Suspension (61%) 1423

Noise intolerance
Neurontin Capsules (Rare) 2655
Neurontin Oral Solution (Rare) 2655
Neurontin Tablets (Rare) 2655

NPN elevation
Celebrex Capsules (0.1% to 1.9%) 2676
Celebrex Capsules (0.1% to 1.9%) 2780
▲ Coreg Tablets (5.8%) 1508
▲ Gengraf Capsules (18%) 457
Nebcin Vials, Hyporets & ADD-Vantage 1955
▲ Neoral Soft Gelatin Capsules (18%) 2380
▲ Neoral Oral Solution (18%) 2380
Sporanox Injection (2%) 1804
Sporanox Injection (2%) 2509

Nuchal rigidity
CytoGam Intravenous (Infrequent) 2026
Gamimune N, 5% Solvent/Detergent Treated (Infrequent) 925
Gamimune N, 10% Solvent/Detergent Treated (Infrequent) 928
Sandoglobulin I.V. 2391

Numbness
Acticin Cream 998
Adenocard Injection (1%) 1380
Aerobid/Aerobid-M (1% to 3%) 1363
Alferon N Injection (One patient to 3%) 1770
Aricept Tablets (Infrequent) 1270
Aricept Tablets (Infrequent) 2665
Avalide Tablets 1070
Avapro Tablets (Less than 1%) 1074
Avapro Tablets (Less than 1%) 3076
Botox Purified Neurotoxin Complex (Rare) 549
Calcium Disodium Versenate Injection 1980
Catapres-TTS (0.5% or less) 1038
Cefizox for Intramuscular or Intravenous Use (Rare) 1390
Clozaril Tablets (Less than 1%) 2319
DynaCirc Capsules (0.5% to 1%) 2921
DynaCirc CR Tablets (0.5% to 1%) 2923
ELA-Max Cream 1340
Elimite Cream (1 to 2% or less) 552
Emla (Unlikely with cream) 602
▲ Imitrex Injection (4.6%) 1549
Imitrex Nasal Spray (Infrequent) 1554
Imitrex Tablets (Frequent) 1558
INFeD Injection 3388
K-Phos Neutral Tablets 946
K-Phos Original (Sodium Free) Tablets (Less frequent) 947
Lidoderm Patch 1319
Limbitrol 1738
Lodosyn Tablets 1251
Loxitane Capsules 3398
Lupron Injection (Less than 5%) 3279
▲ Mexitil Capsules (2.4% to 3.8%) 1047
Mintezol 2137
Moduretic Tablets (Less than or equal to 1%) 2138
Monopril Tablets (0.4% to 1.0%) 1091
Monopril HCT (Less than 2%) 1094
Nebcin Vials, Hyporets & ADD-Vantage 1955
Nicotrol Nasal Spray (Less than 1%) 2843
Normodyne Injection (1%) 3135
Norplant System 3543
Norpramin Tablets 755

Nubain Injection (1% or less) 1323
Parnate Tablets 1607
Phrenilin (Infrequent) 578
Rifadin 765
Rifamate Capsules 767
Rifater Tablets 769
▲ Roferon-A Injection (3% to 12%) 2996
Rythmol Tablets – 150 mg, 225 mg, 300 mg (Less than 1%) 502
Saizen for Injection (Infrequent) 3225
Sedapap Tablets 50 mg/650 mg (Infrequent) 2225
Sinemet Tablets 1253
Sinemet CR Tablets 1255
Sinequan (Infrequent) 2713
Surmontil Capsules 3595
Tonocard Tablets (Less than 1%) 649
Vivactil Tablets 2217
Vivactil Tablets 2446
Xeloda Tablets 3039

Numbness, buccal mucosa

Azactam for Injection (Less than 1%) 1276
Clozaril Tablets (1%) 2319
Imitrex Injection 1549
Imitrex Nasal Spray (Infrequent) 1554
Nicotrol Nasal Spray (More common) 2843

Numbness, extremities

Bicillin C-R 900/300 Injection 2240
Bicillin C-R Injection 2238
Bicillin L-A Injection 2242
Cogentin 2055
Coly-Mycin M Parenteral 2243
Estrace Vaginal Cream 3358
Estrace Tablets 3361
Etrafon 3115
Fortovase Capsules (Less than 2%) 2970
Foscavir Injection 605
▲ Indapamide Tablets (Greater than or equal to 5%) 2286
Invirase Capsules (0.6% to 2.0%) 2979
Iopidine Sterile Ophthalmic Solution ⊙212
Levlen 962
Levlite 21 Tablets 962
Levlite 28 Tablets 962
Maxair Autohaler 1981
Maxair Inhaler (Less than 1%) 1984
MetroCream 1404
MetroLotion 1405
Modicon 2563
Myambutol Tablets 1290
Norpramin Tablets 755
Ortho-Cyclen/Ortho Tri-Cyclen 2573
Ortho-Est Tablets 3464
Ortho-Novum 2563
Ortho-Novum 1/50□28 Tablets 2556
Ortho-Cyclen/Ortho Tri-Cyclen 2573
Trilafon 3160
Tri-Levlen 962
Videx 1138
Videx EC Capsules 1143
Zerit 1147

Numbness, face

Fortovase Capsules (Less than 2%) 2970
Invirase Capsules (Less than 2%) 2979
Nicotrol Nasal Spray (More common) 2843

Numbness, feet

Uroqid-Acid No. 2 Tablets 947

Numbness, fingers

Alferon N Injection (One patient) 1770
Cormax Cream (Approximately 0.3%) 2440
Cormax Ointment (Approximately 0.3%) 2440
Cutivate Cream (1.0%) 1282
Hivid Tablets 2975
Olux Foam (Less than 2%) 1211
▲ Temovate Gel (Among most frequent) 1303
Temovate Ointment (Less frequent) 1301
Temovate E Emollient (Less than 2%) 1302

Numbness, hands

Alferon N Injection (One patient) 1770
Uroqid-Acid No. 2 Tablets 947

Numbness, lips

K-Phos Neutral Tablets 946
K-Phos Original (Sodium Free) Tablets (Less frequent) 947
Oncaspar 756
Sensorcaine 643
Sensorcaine-MPF Injection 643
Uroqid-Acid No. 2 Tablets 947

Numbness, mouth

(*see under* Numbness, buccal mucosa)

Numbness, nose

Nicotrol Nasal Spray (More common) 2843

Numbness, skin

Eskalith 1527
Lithium Carbonate 3061
Lithium Citrate Syrup 3061
Lithobid Slow-Release Tablets 3255
Vaniqa Cream (Less than 1%) 1121

Numbness, toes

Hivid Tablets 2975

Numbness/tingling, fingers and toes

D.H.E. 45 Injection 2334
Eldepryl Capsules 3266
MetroGel 1405

Nyctalopia

Accutane Capsules 2944
Aralen Tablets 3075
Arthrotec Tablets (Rare) 3195
Cataflam Tablets (Less than 1%) 2315
Desferal Vials 2333
▲ Nilandron Tablets (56.9%) 753
Paxil (Rare) 1609
Quinaglute Dura-Tabs Tablets (Occasional) 978
Quinidex Extentabs (Occasional) 2933
Serzone Tablets (Rare) 1104
▲ Soriatane Capsules (1% to 10%) 3003
Voltaren Tablets (Less than 1%) 2315
Voltaren-XR Tablets (Less than 1%) 2315

Nystagmus

Aricept Tablets (Infrequent) 1270
Aricept Tablets (Infrequent) 2665
Axert Tablets (Rare) 2772
Betaseron for SC Injection 988
Carbatrol Capsules 3234
▲ Cerebyx Injection (15.1% to 44.4%) 2619
Cipro I.V. (1% or less) 893
Cipro I.V. Pharmacy Bulk Package (Less than 1%) 897
Cipro 887
Clozaril Tablets (Less than 1%) 2319
Cylert Tablets 415
▲ Depacon Injection (1% to 8%) 416
▲ Depakene (7% to 8%) 421
▲ Depakote Sprinkle Capsules (1% to 8%) 426
▲ Depakote Tablets (7% to 8%) 430
Depakote ER Tablets (Greater than 1%) 436
▲ Dilantin Infatabs (Among most common) 2624
▲ Dilantin Kapseals (Among most common) 2622
▲ Dilantin-125 Oral Suspension (Among most common) 2625
Dilaudid Oral Liquid (Less frequent) 445
Dilaudid Tablets - 8 mg (Less frequent) 445
Dilaudid-HP (Less frequent) 443
Diprivan Injectable Emulsion (Less than 1%) 667
Effexor Tablets (Rare) 3495
Effexor XR Capsules (Rare) 3499
Ergamisol Tablets 1789
Eskalith 1527
Exelon Capsules (Infrequent) 2342
Exelon Oral Solution (Infrequent) 2345
Felbatol 3343
Floxin I.V. 2526
Floxin Tablets 2529
Sterile FUDR (Remote possibility) 2974
Gabitril Tablets (2%) 1189
Geodon Capsules (Rare) 2688
Kadian Capsules (Less than 3%) 1335
Klonopin Tablets 2983
Lamictal (1.0%) 1567
Lithium Carbonate 3061
Lithium Citrate Syrup 3061
Lithobid Slow-Release Tablets 3255
LYMErix Vaccine (Greater than 1%) 1592
Macrobid Capsules 2889
Macrodantin Capsules 2891
Matulane Capsules 3246
MS Contin Tablets (Less frequent) 2896
MSIR (Less frequent) 2898
Nardil Tablets (Less common) 2653
▲ Neurontin Capsules (8.3%) 2655
▲ Neurontin Oral Solution (8.3%) 2655
▲ Neurontin Tablets (8.3%) 2655
Noroxin Tablets 2145
Oramorph SR Tablets (Less frequent) 3062
Paxil (Rare) 1609
Plaquenil Tablets 3082
ProSom Tablets (Rare) 500
Remeron Tablets (Rare) 2483
Remeron SolTab Tablets (Rare) 2486
Rescriptor Tablets (Less than 2%) 526
Robaxin Injectable 2938
Robaxin Tablets 2939
▲ Serostim for Injection (1% to 10%) 3229
Sonata Capsules (Infrequent) 3591
Tambocor Tablets (Less than 1%) 1990
Tegretol/Tegretol-XR 2404
Thalomid Capsules 1154
Tonocard Tablets (Up to 1.1%) 649
▲ Topamax Sprinkle Capsules (15%) 2590
▲ Topamax Tablets (15%) 2590
▲ Trileptal Oral Suspension (5% to 26%) 2407
▲ Trileptal Tablets (5% to 26%) 2407
Valium Injectable 3026
Versed Injection (Less than 1% to 1.1%) 3027
Zoloft (Infrequent) 2751
▲ Zonegran Capsules (4%) 1307
Zyprexa Tablets (Rare) 1973
Zyprexa ZYDIS Orally Disintegrating Tablets (Rare) 1973

Nystagmus, horizontal

(*see under* Nystagmus)

O

Obesity

Celexa (Rare) 1365
Fortovase Capsules 2970
Kaletra Capsules (Less than 2%) 471
Kaletra Oral Solution (Less than 2%) 471

Obsessive compulsive symptoms

Zyprexa Tablets (Infrequent) 1973
Zyprexa ZYDIS Orally Disintegrating Tablets (Infrequent) 1973

Obstipation

Compazine 1505
Etrafon (Occasional) 3115
Serentil 1057
Stelazine 1640
Thioridazine Hydrochloride Tablets 2289
Thorazine 1656
Trilafon (Occasional) 3160

Obtundation

Orthoclone OKT3 Sterile Solution (Less than 1%) 2498
Roferon-A Injection (Rare) 2996
Zovirax for Injection (Approximately 1%) 1708

Occult bleeding

▲ Soma Compound Tablets (Among most common) 3354
Soma Compound w/Codeine Tablets 3355

Ocular, foreign body sensation

Alomide Ophthalmic Solution (1% to 5%) ⊙204
▲ Alphagan Ophthalmic Solution (Approximately 10% to 30%) 545
Azopt Ophthalmic Suspension (1% to 5%) 536
▲ Betimol Ophthalmic Solution (More than 5%) ⊙324
Betoptic S Ophthalmic Suspension (Small number of patients) 537
Cosopt Sterile Ophthalmic Solution (1% to 5%) 2065
Iopidine 0.5% Ophthalmic Solution (Less than 3%) ⊙213
Iopidine Sterile Ophthalmic Solution ⊙212
Ocuflox Ophthalmic Solution 554
Patanol Ophthalmic Solution (Less than 5%) 540
Quixin Ophthalmic Solution (1% to 3%) 3093
Timolol GFS (1% to 5%) ⊙266
Timoptic in Ocudose (Less frequent) 2192
Timoptic Sterile Ophthalmic Solution (Less frequent) 2190
Timoptic-XE Sterile Ophthalmic Gel Forming Solution (1% to 5%) 2194

Ocular allergy

Alomide Ophthalmic Solution (Less than 1%) ⊙204
▲ Alphagan Ophthalmic Solution (Approximately 10% to 30%) 545
▲ Trusopt Sterile Ophthalmic Solution (Approximately 10%) 2196
Voltaren Ophthalmic Sterile Ophthalmic Solution (Less than 5%) ⊙312

Ocular discomfort

Alamast Ophthalmic Solution (Less than 5%) 3092
▲ Alomide Ophthalmic Solution (Among most frequent) ⊙204
Amerge Tablets (Rare) 1467
Azopt Ophthalmic Suspension (1% to 5%) 536
▲ Betaxon Ophthalmic Suspension (11%) 537
▲ Betoptic S Ophthalmic Suspension (Most frequent) 537
Evoxac Capsules (1% to 3%) 1217
▲ Iopidine 0.5% Ophthalmic Solution (6%) ⊙213
▲ Ocuflox Ophthalmic Solution (Among most frequent) 554
Photofrin for Injection 831
Quixin Ophthalmic Solution (1% to 3%) 3093
Timolol GFS (1% to 5%) ⊙266
▲ Travatan Ophthalmic Solution (5% to 10%) 543
▲ Trusopt Sterile Ophthalmic Solution (Approximately one-third of patients) 2196
Vexol 1% Ophthalmic Suspension (1% to 5%) ⊙222

Ocular exudate

Alomide Ophthalmic Solution (1% to 5%) ⊙204
Betoptic S Ophthalmic Suspension (Small number of patients) 537
Cosopt Sterile Ophthalmic Solution (1% to 5%) 2065
Iopidine 0.5% Ophthalmic Solution (Less than 3%) ⊙213
Livostin (Approximately 1% to 3%) ⊙305
Timolol GFS (1% to 5%) ⊙266
Timoptic in Ocudose (Less frequent) 2192
Timoptic Sterile Ophthalmic Solution (Less frequent) 2190
Timoptic-XE Sterile Ophthalmic Gel Forming Solution (1% to 5%) 2194
Vexol 1% Ophthalmic Suspension (1% to 5%) ⊙222

Ocular hypotony

Iopidine Sterile Ophthalmic Solution ⊙212
▲ Vistide Injection (Five patients to more than 12%) 1445
Vitrasert Implant (Less than 1%) ⊙254
Vitravene for Injection (2% to 5%) ⊙310

Ocular infection

NeoDecadron Sterile Ophthalmic Solution 2144
Prelone Syrup 2273
Terra-Cortril Ophthalmic Suspension 2716
Trilafon 3160

Ocular lesions

Brevicon 28-Day Tablets 3380
Decadron Phosphate Sterile Ophthalmic Ointment 2083
Decadron Phosphate Sterile Ophthalmic Solution 2084
Norinyl 1 +35 28-Day Tablets 3380
Norinyl 1 + 50 28-Day Tablets 3380
Ovcon 3364
Tri-Norinyl-28 Tablets 3433

Ocular palsies

Attenuvax (Rare) 2044
M-M-R II (Rare) 2118
Mumpsvax 2141
Plaquenil Tablets 3082

Ocular perforation

Decadron Phosphate Sterile Ophthalmic Ointment 2083
Decadron Phosphate Sterile Ophthalmic Solution 2084

Ocular pressure

Zebeta Tablets 1885

Ocular tension, increase

Cortisporin Ophthalmic Suspension ⊙297
Decadron Phosphate Sterile Ophthalmic Ointment 2083
Decadron Phosphate Sterile Ophthalmic Solution 2084
Donnatal 2929
Donnatal Extentabs 2930
Donnatal Tablets 2929
Levsin/Levsinex/Levbid 3172
Norflex 1987
NuLev Orally Disintegrating Tablets 3176
Robinul Forte Tablets 1358
Robinul Injectable 2940
Robinul Tablets 1358
Ziac Tablets 1887

Ocular toxicity

Plaquenil Tablets 3082
TobraDex Ophthalmic Ointment (Less than 4%) 542
TobraDex Ophthalmic Suspension (Less than 4%) 541
Tobrex Ophthalmic Ointment (Less than 3 of 100 patients) ⊙220
Tobrex Ophthalmic Solution (Less than 3 of 100 patients) ⊙221

Oculogyric crises
Betaseron for SC Injection 988
Cognex Capsules (Rare) 1351
Compazine 1505
Cylert Tablets 415
Etrafon 3115
Geodon Capsules (Frequent) 2688
Haldol Decanoate (Frequent) 2535
Haldol Injection, Tablets and Concentrate 2533
Lodosyn Tablets 1251
Orap Tablets (Less frequent) 1407
Paxil 1609
Phenergan Injection 3553
Phenergan Suppositories 3556
Phenergan Syrup 3554
Phenergan Tablets 3556
Phenergan with Codeine Syrup 3557
Phenergan with Dextromethorphan Syrup 3559
Phenergan VC Syrup 3560
Phenergan VC with Codeine Syrup 3561
Reglan 2935
▲ Risperdal (17% to 34%) 1796
Serentil 1057
Sinemet Tablets 1253
Sinemet CR Tablets 1255
Stelazine 1640
Symmetrel (Less than 0.1%) 1328
Thioridazine Hydrochloride Tablets 2289
Thiothixene Capsules 2290
Thorazine 1656
Timolide Tablets 2187
Trilafon 3160
Trileptal Oral Suspension 2407
Trileptal Tablets 2407
Zofran Injection 1698
Zofran 1703
Zofran ODT Orally Disintegrating Tablets 1703
Zoloft 2751
Zonegran Capsules (Rare) 1307
Zyprexa Tablets (2% to 3%) 1973
Zyprexa ZYDIS Orally Disintegrating Tablets (2% to 3%) 1973

Oculomotor disturbances
Carbatrol Capsules 3234
Pravachol Tablets 1099
Tegretol/Tegretol-XR 2404

Oily evacuation
▲ Xenical Capsules (2.3% to 11.9%) 3043

Olfactory disorder, unspecified
Fortovase Capsules (Less than 2%) 2970

Oligohydramnios
Accupril Tablets 2611
Aceon Tablets (2 mg, 4 mg, 8 mg) 3249
Altace Capsules 2233
Avalide Tablets 1070
Avapro Tablets 1074
Avapro Tablets 3076
Captopril Tablets 2281
Cleocin Vaginal Cream (2%) 2788
Clinoril Tablets 2053
Cozaar Tablets 2067
Dolobid Tablets 2088
Enalaprilat Injection 863
Hyzaar 2109
Lexxel Tablets 608
Lotensin Tablets 2365
Lotrel Capsules 2370
Monopril Tablets 1091
Monopril HCT 1094
Prinivil Tablets 2164
Prinzide Tablets 2168
Uniretic Tablets 3178
Univasc Tablets 3181
Vaseretic Tablets 2204
Vasotec I.V. Injection 2207
Vasotec Tablets 2210
Zestoretic Tablets 695
Zestril Tablets 698

Oligomenorrhea
Brevicon 28-Day Tablets 3380
Levlen 962
Levlite 21 Tablets 962
Levlite 28 Tablets 962
Modicon 2563
Mustargen for Injection 2142
▲ Nolvadex Tablets (8.7%) 678
Norinyl 1 +35 28-Day Tablets 3380
Norinyl 1 + 50 28-Day Tablets 3380
Ortho-Cyclen/Ortho Tri-Cyclen 2573
Ortho-Novum 2563
Ortho-Novum 1/50□28 Tablets 2556
Ortho-Cyclen/Ortho Tri-Cyclen 2573
Sandostatin Injection (Less than 1%) 2394
Tri-Levlen 962
Tri-Norinyl-28 Tablets 3433

Oligospermia
Anadrol-50 Tablets 3321
Androderm Transdermal System CIII 3377
Android Capsules, 10 mg (At high dosages) 1731
▲ Azulfidine EN-tabs Tablets (Among most common) 2775
Nizoral Tablets 1791
Oxandrin Tablets 1153
Testoderm Transdermal Systems 574
Testopel Pellets 3610
Testred Capsules, 10 mg 1746

Oliguria
Abelcet Injection 1273
Actiq (Less than 1%) 1184
Aloprim for Injection (Less than 1%) 2292
Altace Capsules 2233
Amphotec (1% to 5%) 1774
Anzemet Injection (2.6%) 719
Anzemet Tablets (2.6%) 722
Arthrotec Tablets (Rare) 3195
Astramorph/PF Injection, USP (Preservative-Free) 594
Azulfidine EN-tabs Tablets (Rare) 2775
Bactrim 2949
Betaseron for SC Injection 988
Captopril Tablets (Approximately 1 to 2 of 1000 patients) 2281
Carbatrol Capsules 3234
Cataflam Tablets (Rare) 2315
Celexa (Rare) 1365
▲ CellCept Capsules (14.2%) 2951
▲ CellCept Intravenous (14.2%) 2951
▲ CellCept Oral Suspension (14.2%) 2951
▲ CellCept Tablets (14.2% to 17%) 2951
Cerebyx Injection (Infrequent) 2619
Claritin-D 24 Hour Extended Release Tablets (Fewer than 2%) 3104
Cleocin HCl Capsules (Rare) 2784
Cleocin Phosphate Sterile Solution (Rare) 2785
Cleocin Vaginal Cream (Rare) 2788
Cleocin Vaginal Ovules (Rare) 2789
Clomid Tablets 735
Corlopam Injection (0.5% to 5%) 412
CytoGam Intravenous 2026
Demadex Tablets and Injection 2965
Diovan HCT Tablets 2338
Diprivan Injectable Emulsion (Less than 1%) 667
Doxil Injection (Less than 1%) 566
Duragesic Transdermal System (Less than 1%) 1786
Duramorph Injection 1312
Dyazide Capsules 1515
Effexor Tablets (Rare) 3495
Enalaprilat Injection 863
Eskalith 1527
Evoxac Capsules 1217
Exelon Capsules (Infrequent) 2342
Exelon Oral Solution (Infrequent) 2345
Feldene Capsules (Occasional) 2685
Follistim for Injection 2465
Furosemide Tablets 2284
Gamimune N, 5% Solvent/Detergent Treated 925
Gamimune N, 10% Solvent/Detergent Treated 928
Gammagard S/D (Some patients) 845
Gammar-P I.V. 787
Geodon Capsules (Rare) 2688
Humegon for Injection 2468
Hyzaar 2109
Infumorph 200 and Infumorph 500 Sterile Solutions 1314
Lexxel Tablets 608
Lithium Carbonate 3061
Lithium Citrate Syrup 3061
Lithobid Slow-Release Tablets 3255
Lodine XL Extended-Release Tablets (Less than 1%) 3530
Lotrel Capsules 2370
Luvox Tablets (25, 50, 100 mg) (Rare) 3256
Maxzide 1008
Miltown Tablets (Rare) 3349
Monopril Tablets 1091
Monopril HCT 1094
Mykrox Tablets 1168
Naropin Injection (1% to 5%) 612
Nebcin Vials, Hyporets & ADD-Vantage 1955
Orthoclone OKT3 Sterile Solution (Less than 1%) 2498
Ovidrel for Injection (Less than 2%) 3220
Paxil (Rare) 1609
Pediazole Suspension 3050
Phenergan with Codeine Syrup 3557
Phenergan VC with Codeine Syrup 3561
Ponstel Capsules (Occasional) 1356
Primaxin I.M. 2158
Primaxin I.V. (2.2%) 2160
Prinivil Tablets (0.3% to 1.0%) 2164
Prinzide Tablets 2168
▲ Prograf (3% to 19%) 1393
▲ Proleukin for Injection (63%) 1199
ProSom Tablets (Rare) 500
Prozac Pulvules, Liquid, and Weekly Capsules (Rare) 1238
▲ Rapamune Oral Solution and Tablets (3% to 20%) 3584
Sandoglobulin I.V. 2391
Sarafem Pulvules (Rare) 1962
Septra Suspension 2265
Septra Tablets 2265
Septra DS Tablets 2265
Serophene Tablets 3226
Serzone Tablets (Rare) 1104
▲ Simulect for Injection (3% to 10%) 2399
Tasmar Tablets (Infrequent) 3010
Tegretol/Tegretol-XR 2404
Tenoretic Tablets 690
Thalomid Capsules 1154
Topamax Sprinkle Capsules (Infrequent) 2590
Topamax Tablets (Infrequent) 2590
Toradol (1% or less) 3018
Trasylol Injection (1% to 2%) 909
▲ Trisenox Injection (5%) 1158
Univasc Tablets (Less than 1%) 3181
Vaseretic Tablets 2204
Vasotec I.V. Injection 2207
Vasotec Tablets (0.5% to 1.0%) 2210
Voltaren Tablets (Rare) 2315
Voltaren-XR Tablets (Rare) 2315
Zaroxolyn Tablets 1177
▲ Zenapax for Injection (Greater than 5%) 3046
Zestoretic Tablets 695
Zestril Tablets (0.3% to 1.0%) 698
Zoloft (Rare) 2751
Zosyn (1.0% or less) 1890
Zosyn in Galaxy Containers (1.0% or less) 1894

Oliguria, neonatal
Altace Capsules 2233
Captopril Tablets 2281
Monopril Tablets 1091
Zestril Tablets 698

On-off phenomenon
Lodosyn Tablets 1251
Sinemet Tablets 1253
Sinemet CR Tablets (1.6%) 1255

Onychia
Evoxac Capsules (Less than 1%) 1217

Onycholysis
Adriamycin PFS/RDF Injection (A few cases) 2767
Feldene Capsules (Rare) 2685
Orudis Capsules (Less than 1%) 3548
Oruvail Capsules (Less than 1%) 3548
Taxotere for Injection Concentrate (0.8%) 778

Onychomycosis
Evoxac Capsules (Less than 1%) 1217

Opacity, punctate
Stromectol Tablets (1.4% to 1.8%) 2185

Ophthalmoplegia
Baycol Tablets 883
Betaseron for SC Injection 988
Lescol Capsules 2361
Lescol Capsules 2925
Lescol XL Tablets 2361
Lescol XL Tablets 2925
Mevacor Tablets 2132
Pravachol Tablets 1099
Zocor Tablets 2219

Opisthotonos
Compazine 1505
Diprivan Injectable Emulsion (Rare) 667
Etrafon 3115
Geodon Capsules (Rare) 2688
Haldol Decanoate (Frequent) 2535
Haldol Injection, Tablets and Concentrate 2533
Orap Tablets (Less frequent) 1407
Reglan 2935
Serentil 1057
Stelazine 1640
Thioridazine Hydrochloride Tablets 2289
Thorazine 1656
Trilafon 3160
Zyprexa Tablets (2% to 3%) 1973
Zyprexa ZYDIS Orally Disintegrating Tablets (2% to 3%) 1973

Optic atrophy
Aralen Tablets 3075
Eskalith 1527
Lithium Carbonate 3061
Lithium Citrate Syrup 3061
Plaquenil Tablets 3082
Rifater Tablets (Uncommon) 769
Yodoxin Tablets 1722
Zanaflex Tablets (Rare) 1305

Optic disorders
Effexor Tablets (Rare) 3495
Vitrasert Implant (Approximately 1% to 5%) ⊙254

Optic nerve, damage
Alrex Sterile Ophthalmic Suspension 0.2% ⊙256
Blephamide Ophthalmic Ointment (Infrequent) 547
Blephamide Ophthalmic Suspension (Infrequent) 548
Celestone Soluspan Injectable Suspension (Possible) 3097
Cortisporin Ophthalmic Suspension (Infrequent) ⊙297
Dapsone Tablets USP 1780
FML Ophthalmic Ointment (Infrequent) ⊙237
FML Ophthalmic Suspension (Infrequent) ⊙236
FML Forte Ophthalmic Suspension (Infrequent) ⊙235
FML-S Liquifilm Sterile Ophthalmic Suspension (Infrequent) ⊙238
HMS Sterile Ophthalmic Suspension (Rare) ⊙240
Lotemax Sterile Ophthalmic Suspension 0.5% ⊙261
NeoDecadron Sterile Ophthalmic Solution (Infrequent) 2144
Poly-Pred Liquifilm Ophthalmic Suspension (Infrequent) ⊙245
Pred Forte Ophthalmic Suspension (Infrequent) ⊙246
Pred Mild Sterile Ophthalmic Suspension (Infrequent) ⊙249
Pred-G Ophthalmic Suspension (Infrequent) ⊙247
Pred-G Sterile Ophthalmic Ointment ⊙248
Prelone Syrup 2273
Streptomycin Sulfate Injection 2714
Taxol Injection (Rare) 1129
Terra-Cortril Ophthalmic Suspension (Infrequent) 2716
TobraDex Ophthalmic Ointment (Infrequent) 542
TobraDex Ophthalmic Suspension (Infrequent) 541
Vexol 1% Ophthalmic Suspension ⊙222
Vitrasert Implant (Approximately 1% to 5%) ⊙254

Orchitis
Aciphex Tablets (Rare) 1267
Aciphex Tablets (Rare) 1783
M-M-R II 2118
Mumpsvax (Rare) 2141
Seroquel Tablets (Infrequent) 684
TheraCys Injection 823
Tice BCG, BCG Live (0.2%) 2489

Organic brain syndrome
Eskalith 1527
Lithium Carbonate 3061
Lithium Citrate Syrup 3061

Organomegaly
▲ Vesanoid Capsules (3%) 3037

Orgasmic dysfunction, female
▲ Effexor XR Capsules (4%) 3499
Prozac Pulvules, Liquid, and Weekly Capsules 1238
Sarafem Pulvules 1962

Oropharyngitis
▲ Roferon-A Injection (6% to 14%) 2996

Oropharynx, dry
▲ Atrovent Inhalation Aerosol (About 5 in 100) 1030
Proventil Inhalation Aerosol 3142
Proventil Repetabs Tablets 3148
Proventil HFA Inhalation Aerosol 3150
▲ Roferon-A Injection (6% to 14%) 2996
Tussionex Pennkinetic Extended-Release Suspension 1174
Ventolin HFA Inhalation Aerosol 3618
Volmax Extended-Release Tablets 2276

Orthopnea
Intron A for Injection (Less than or equal to 5%) 3120
Prinivil Tablets (0.3% to 1.0%) 2164
Prinzide Tablets 2168
Zestoretic Tablets 695
Zestril Tablets (0.3% to 1.0%) 698

Oscillopsia
Lamictal (Infrequent) 1567

Osteoarthritis
Remicade for IV Injection (Less than 2%) 1178
Vioxx (Greater than 0.1% to 1.9%) 2213

Osteoarticular pain
Cardizem Injectable 1018
Cardizem Lyo-Ject Syringe 1018
Cardizem Monovial 1018
Cardizem CD Capsules (Less than 1%) 1016
Tiazac Capsules (Less than 2%) 1378

Osteomalacia
Didronel Tablets 2888
Dilantin Kapseals 2622
Dilantin-125 Oral Suspension 2625

Osteomalacia, phosphate-induced
K-Phos Neutral Tablets 946
K-Phos Original (Sodium Free) Tablets 947
Uroqid-Acid No. 2 Tablets 947

Osteomalacia syndromes
Amphojel Suspension (Mint Flavor) ▣789
Maalox Antacid/Anti-Gas Oral Suspension ▣673
Maalox Max Maximum Strength Antacid/Anti-Gas Liquid 2300
Maalox Regular Strength Antacid/Antigas Liquid 2300
Mylanta 1813

Osteomyelitis
▲ Apligraf (2.7% to 8.9%) 2305
Campath Ampules 992
Copaxone for Injection (Infrequent) 3306
Enbrel for Injection 1752
Enbrel for Injection 3504
Evoxac Capsules (Less than 1%) 1217
Nipent for Injection (1%) 3272
Permax Tablets (Rare) 1299
Prozac Pulvules, Liquid, and Weekly Capsules (Rare) 1238
Regranex Gel 2586
Sarafem Pulvules (Rare) 1962
Tice BCG, BCG Live (Rare) 2489

Osteoporosis
Celestone Soluspan Injectable Suspension 3097
Celestone Syrup 3099
Celexa (Rare) 1365
▲ CellCept Capsules (3% to 10%) 2951
▲ CellCept Intravenous (3% to 10%) 2951
▲ CellCept Oral Suspension (3% to 10%) 2951
▲ CellCept Tablets (3% to 10%) 2951
Cognex Capsules (Infrequent) 1351
Cortifoam Rectal Foam 3170
Cortone Acetate Injectable Suspension 2059
Cortone Acetate Tablets 2061
Decadron Elixir 2078
Decadron Tablets 2079
Decadron Phosphate Injection 2081
Depo-Medrol Injectable Suspension 2795
Depo-Provera Contraceptive Injection (Fewer than 1%) 2798
Effexor Tablets (Rare) 3495
Effexor XR Capsules (Rare) 3499
Evoxac Capsules (Less than 1%) 1217
Florinef Acetate Tablets 2250
Flovent Diskus 3614
Fludara for Injection (Up to 2%) 995
Heparin Lock Flush Solution 3509
Heparin Sodium Injection 3511
Hydrocortone Tablets 2106
Hydrocortone Acetate Injectable Suspension 2103
Hydrocortone Phosphate Injection, Sterile 2105
Neupogen for Injection (Infrequent) 587
Neurontin Capsules (Rare) 2655
Neurontin Oral Solution (Rare) 2655
Neurontin Tablets (Rare) 2655
Paxil (Rare) 1609
Pediapred Oral Solution 1170
Permax Tablets (Rare) 1299
Prednisone 3064
Prelone Syrup 2273
▲ Prograf (3% to 15%) 1393
Prozac Pulvules, Liquid, and Weekly Capsules (Rare) 1238
Pulmicort Respules (Less than 1%) 632
▲ Rapamune Oral Solution and Tablets (3% to 20%) 3584
Remicade for IV Injection (Less than 2%) 1178
Requip Tablets (Infrequent) 1621
Rilutek Tablets (Rare) 772
Sarafem Pulvules (Rare) 1962
Solu-Medrol Sterile Powder 2855
Sonata Capsules (Rare) 3591
Topamax Sprinkle Capsules (Infrequent) 2590
Topamax Tablets (Infrequent) 2590
Zoladex 3-month (1% to 5%) 706
Zyprexa Tablets (Rare) 1973
Zyprexa ZYDIS Orally Disintegrating Tablets (Rare) 1973

Osteosclerosis
Effexor XR Capsules (Rare) 3499
femhrt Tablets 2635

Otitis externa
Ambien Tablets (Rare) 3191
Aricept Tablets (Infrequent) 1270
Aricept Tablets (Infrequent) 2665
Betaseron for SC Injection 988
Copaxone for Injection (Infrequent) 3306
Effexor Tablets (Rare) 3495
Effexor XR Capsules (Rare) 3499
Floxin Otic Solution (Single report) 1219
Gabitril Tablets (Infrequent) 1189
Imitrex Nasal Spray 1554
Infergen (1% to 2%) 1777
Meridia Capsules 481
Neurontin Capsules (Rare) 2655
Neurontin Oral Solution (Rare) 2655
Neurontin Tablets (Rare) 2655
Paxil (Rare) 1609
Protonix I.V. (Less than 1%) 3580
Protonix Tablets (Less than 1%) 3577
Singulair (Greater than or equal to 2%) 2181
Soriatane Capsules (Less than 1%) 3003
Teveten Tablets (Less than 1%) 3327
Trileptal Oral Suspension 2407
Trileptal Tablets 2407
Vistide Injection 1445

Otitis media
AccuNeb Inhalation Solution (0.9% to 4.3%) 1230
Aciphex Tablets 1267
Aciphex Tablets 1783
Actonel Tablets (2.5%) 2879
Allegra (2.4%) 712
Ambien Tablets (Rare) 3191
Aricept Tablets (Infrequent) 1270
Aricept Tablets (Infrequent) 2665
Attenuvax 2044
▲ Avonex (6%) 1013
Axert Tablets (Rare) 2772
Betaseron for SC Injection 988
Betaxon Ophthalmic Suspension (Less than 2%) 537
Campath Ampules 992
Ceclor CD Tablets (0.1% to 1%) 1279
Celebrex Capsules (0.1% to 1.9%) 2676
Celebrex Capsules (0.1% to 1.9%) 2780
Chemet Capsules (1.0% to 3.7%) 3078
Cognex Capsules (Infrequent) 1351
Comvax (0.5% to 2.7%) 2056
Depacon Injection (1% to 5%) 416
Depakene (1% to 5%) 421
Depakote Sprinkle Capsules (1% to 5%) 426
Depakote Tablets (1% to 5%) 430
Depakote ER Tablets (1% to 5%) 436
Doxil Injection (Less than 1%) 566
Effexor Tablets (Infrequent) 3495
Effexor XR Capsules (Infrequent) 3499
Estring Vaginal Ring (1% to 3%) 2811
Evoxac Capsules (1% to 3%) 1217
Exelon Capsules (Infrequent) 2342
Exelon Oral Solution (Infrequent) 2345
▲ Felbatol (3.4% to 9.7%) 3343
Flovent Diskus (1% to 3%) 3614
Flovent Rotadisk (1% to 3%) 1537
Fortovase Capsules (Less than 2%) 2970
Gabitril Tablets (Frequent) 1189
▲ Humatrope Vials and Cartridges (35.3%) 1930
Infergen (1% to 2%) 1777
Invirase Capsules (Less than 2%) 2979
Kaletra Capsules (Less than 2%) 471
Kaletra Oral Solution (Less than 2%) 471
Keppra Tablets (1% or more) 3314
Klonopin Tablets (Infrequent) 2983
Luvox Tablets (25, 50, 100 mg) (Infrequent) 3256
Meridia Capsules 481
Meruvax II 2130
Micardis Tablets (More than 0.3%) 1049
Micardis HCT Tablets 1051
M-M-R II 2118
Mumpsvax 2141
Myobloc Injectable Solution (2% or greater) 1291
Naprelan Tablets (Less than 1%) 1293
Nasacort AQ Nasal Spray 752
Nasonex Nasal Spray 3131
Neurontin Capsules (Infrequent) 2655
Neurontin Oral Solution (More than 2%) 2655
Neurontin Tablets (Infrequent) 2655
Nexium Delayed-Release Capsules (Less than 1%) 619
Orthoclone OKT3 Sterile Solution (Less than 1%) 2498
Paxil (Infrequent) 1609
▲ Liquid PedvaxHIB (Among most frequent) 2148
Permax Tablets (Infrequent) 1299
Prevacid Delayed-Release Capsules (Less than 1%) 3292
Prevnar for Injection 1870
PREVPAC (Less than 1%) 3298
▲ Prograf (3% to 15%) 1393
▲ Protopic Ointment (Up to 7%) 1397
▲ Pulmicort Respules (9% to 12%) 632
▲ Rapamune Oral Solution and Tablets (3% to 20%) 3584
Remeron Tablets (Rare) 2483
Remeron SolTab Tablets (Rare) 2486
Requip Tablets (Infrequent) 1621
Rescriptor Tablets 526
Sandostatin Injection (Less than 1%) 2394
▲ Sandostatin LAR Depot (5% to 15%) 2395
Singulair (Greater than or equal to 2%) 2181
Soriatane Capsules (Less than 1%) 3003
Sular Tablets (Less than or equal to 1%) 688
▲ Synagis Intramuscular (41.9%) 2028
▲ Tamiflu Capsules (8.9%) 3008
▲ Tamiflu Oral Suspension (8.9%) 3008
Tasmar Tablets (Infrequent) 3010
Teveten Tablets (Less than 1%) 3327
Tricor Capsules, Micronized 513
Uniretic Tablets (Less than 1%) 3178
Varivax (Greater than or equal to 1%) 2202
Vioxx (Greater than 0.1% to 1.9%) 2213
Vistide Injection 1445
▲ Xenical Capsules (2.9% to 4.3%) 3043
Zanaflex Tablets (Infrequent) 1305

Otitis media, serous
Helixate Concentrate 788
Kogenate FS 936

Otorrhea
Floxin Otic Solution (0.6%) 1219

Ototoxicity
Demadex Tablets and Injection 2965
Furosemide Tablets 2284
Nebcin Vials, Hyporets & ADD-Vantage 1955
Neosporin G.U. Irrigant Sterile 2256
▲ Paraplatin for Injection (1% to 13%) 1126
Streptomycin Sulfate Injection 2714
TOBI Solution for Inhalation 1206
Vancocin HCl Capsules & Pulvules 1972
Vancocin HCl Oral Solution 1971
Vancocin HCl, Vials & ADD-Vantage 1970
Zyrtec (Less than 2%) 2756
Zyrtec-D 12 Hour Extended Relief Tablets (Less than 2%) 2758

Ovarian cyst
Activella Tablets (0% to 7%) 2764
▲ Avonex (3%) 1013
Clomid Tablets 735
Copaxone for Injection (Infrequent) 3306
Effexor Tablets (Rare) 3495
Effexor XR Capsules (Rare) 3499
Evoxac Capsules (Less than 1%) 1217
Follistim for Injection (2.9%) 2465
▲ Gonal-F for Injection (15.3%) 3216
Humegon for Injection 2468
Nolvadex Tablets (2.8%) 678
▲ Ovidrel for Injection (3%) 3220
Pergonal for Injection 3223
Repronex for Intramuscular and Subcutaneous Injection 1347
Serophene Tablets 3226

Ovarian cysts, enlargement of existing
Synarel Nasal Solution for Central Precocious Puberty 3204
Synarel Nasal Solution for Endometriosis 3205

Ovarian disorder, unspecified
Evoxac Capsules (Less than 1%) 1217
Gonal-F for Injection (1.7%) 3216
▲ Repronex for Intramuscular and Subcutaneous Injection (3% to 8.3%) 1347
Salagen Tablets (Less than 1%) 2229
Wellbutrin Tablets (Rare) 1680

Ovarian enlargement
▲ Clomid Tablets (13.6%) 735
Follistim for Injection 2465
Gonal-F for Injection 3216
▲ Humegon for Injection (Approximately 20%) 2468
Ovidrel for Injection 3220
▲ Pergonal for Injection (Approximately 20%) 3223
▲ Repronex for Intramuscular and Subcutaneous Injection (Approximately 20%) 1347
▲ Serophene Tablets (Approximately 1 in 7 patients) 3226

Ovarian failure
Neurontin Capsules (Rare) 2655
Neurontin Oral Solution (Rare) 2655
Neurontin Tablets (Rare) 2655

Ovarian hyperstimulation syndrome
Antagon Injection (2.4%) 2447
▲ Cetrotide for Injection (3.5%) 3209
Clomid Tablets 735
▲ Follistim for Injection (5.2% to 7.6%) 2465
▲ Gonal-F for Injection (6.8%) 3216
Humegon for Injection (Approximately 0.4%) 2468
▲ Ovidrel for Injection (3%) 3220
Pergonal for Injection 3223
▲ Repronex for Intramuscular and Subcutaneous Injection (2% to 5.2%) 1347
Serophene Tablets 3226

Oversedation
Versed Injection (1.6%) 3027

Overstimulation
Adderall Tablets 3231
Adderall XR Capsules
Adipex-P 1406
Bontril Slow-Release Capsules 576
Desoxyn Tablets 440
Dexedrine 1512
DextroStat Tablets 3236
Eldepryl Capsules 3266
Halcion Tablets 2823
Ionamin Capsules 1163
Miltown Tablets 3349
Parafon Forte DSC Caplets (Occasional) 2582
Parnate Tablets 1607

Oxyhemoglobin desaturation
▲ Suprane Liquid for Inhalation (3% to 26%) 874

P

Pain (22%)
▲ Abelcet Injection (5%) 1273
Accolate Tablets (1.9%) 657
Aceon Tablets (2 mg, 4 mg, 8 mg) (0.3% to 1%) 3249
Actiq (1% or greater) 1184
▲ Actonel Tablets (13.6%) 2879
Adalat CC Tablets (Less than 1.0%) 877
Advair Diskus 100/50 (1% to 3%) 1448
Advair Diskus 250/50 (1% to 3%) 1448
Advair Diskus 500/50 (1% to 3%) 1448
▲ Aggrenox Capsules (6.4%) 1026
▲ Agrylin Capsules (15%) 3232
Aloprim for Injection (Less than 1%) 2292
▲ Alora Transdermal System (5.3% to 6.8%) 3372
Ambien Tablets (Rare) 3191
▲ AmBisome for Injection (14%) 1383
▲ Amphotec (5% or more) 1774
Androderm Transdermal System CIII (Less than 1%) 3377
Anzemet Injection (2.4%) 719
Aphthasol Oral Paste (1% to 2%) 1025
▲ Apligraf (1.8% to 7.1%) 2305
Arava Tablets (2%) 724
▲ Aredia for Injection (14.3%) 2309
▲ Argatroban Injection (4.6%) 1478
▲ Aricept Tablets (9%) 1270
▲ Aricept Tablets (9%) 2665
▲ Arimidex Tablets (10.7% to 15.4%) 659
▲ Aromasin Tablets (13%) 2769
▲ Asacol Delayed-Release Tablets (14%) 2884
Atacand HCT Tablets (0.5% or greater) 597
▲ Atrovent Inhalation Solution (4.1%) 1031
Avelox Tablets (0.05% to 1%) 879
▲ Avonex (24%) 1013
▲ Axid Pulvules (4.2%) 1903
▲ Axid Pulvules (4.2%) 2919
Azmacort Inhalation Aerosol (1% to 3%) 728
Bactroban Ointment (1.5%) 1496
Betapace Tablets (1% to 3%) 950
▲ Betaseron for SC Injection (52%) 988
Bicillin C-R 900/300 Injection 2240
Bicillin C-R Injection 2238
Bicillin L-A Injection 2242
▲ Campath Ampules (2% to 24%) 992
Cancidas for Injection (1.3% to 4.6%) 2048
Cardura Tablets (2%) 2668
▲ Carnitor Injection (21% to 35%) 3242
▲ Casodex Tablets (27%) 662
Ceclor CD Tablets (0.1% to 1%) 1279
Celebrex Capsules (0.1% to 1.9%) 2676
Celebrex Capsules (0.1% to 1.9%) 2780
▲ CellCept Capsules (3% to 75.8%) 2951
▲ CellCept Intravenous (3% to 75.8%) 2951
▲ CellCept Oral Suspension (3% to 75.8%) 2951
▲ CellCept Tablets (3% to 75.8%) 2951
▲ Cenestin Tablets (11%) 1263
▲ Chirocaine Injection (3.5%) 2909
Cipro I.V. Pharmacy Bulk Package (Less than 1%) 897
Colazal Capsules (2%) 3069
▲ CombiPatch Transdermal System (15% to 19%) 2323
Combivent Inhalation Aerosol (2.5%) 1041

▲ Combivir Tablets (12%) ... 1502
▲ Condylox Topical Solution (50% to 72%) ... 2437
▲ Copaxone for Injection (28%) ... 3306
▲ Coreg Tablets (8.6%) ... 1508
Coumadin for Injection (Infrequent) ... 1243
Coumadin Tablets (Infrequent) ... 1243
▲ Crinone 8% Gel (8%) ... 3213
Crixivan Capsules (Less than 2%) ... 2070
Cytotec Tablets (Infrequent) ... 3202
Cytovene (At least 3 subjects) ... 2959
Depacon Injection (1.3%) ... 416
▲ DepoCyt Injection (3% to 11%) ... 1197
Desferal Vials ... 2333
▲ Diphtheria & Tetanus Toxoids Adsorbed Purogenated for Pediatric Use (9.9%) ... 1857
▲ Ditropan XL Extended Release Tablets (6.8%) ... 564
▲ Doxil Injection (3.4% to 7.2%) ... 566
DuoNeb Inhalation Solution (1.3%) ... 1233
▲ Duraclon Injection (5%) ... 3057
Dynabac Tablets (2.2% to 2.9%) ... 2269
DynaCirc Capsules (0.5% to 1%) ... 2921
DynaCirc CR Tablets (0.5% to 1%) ... 2923
Effexor Tablets ... 3495
▲ Efudex (Among most frequent) ... 1733
Enbrel for Injection ... 1752
Enbrel for Injection ... 3504
▲ Evoxac Capsules (3.3%) ... 1217
Exelon Capsules (2% or more) ... 2342
Exelon Oral Solution (2% or more) ... 2345
Famvir Tablets (2.0% to 2.6%) ... 2348
▲ Felbatol (6.5%) ... 3343
▲ Femara Tablets (5%) ... 2351
▲ femhrt Tablets (3.9%) ... 2635
▲ Ferrlecit Injection (10%) ... 3386
Flonase Nasal Spray (1% to 3%) ... 1533
▲ Flovent Diskus (1% to 10%) ... 3614
Flovent (1% to 3%) ... 1535
Flovent Rotadisk (1% to 3%) ... 1537
Floxin I.V. (Less than 1%) ... 2526
Floxin Otic Solution (Single report) ... 1219
Floxin Tablets (Less than 1%) ... 2529
▲ Fludara for Injection (20% to 22%) ... 995
Fluorescite Injection ... ⊙ 211
Fluoroplex ... 552
FluShield Influenza Vaccine ... 3521
▲ Fortovase Capsules (3.3%) ... 2970
▲ Foscavir Injection (5% or greater) ... 605
▲ Gabitril Tablets (2% to 7%) ... 1189
Gammar-P I.V. ... 787
▲ Gemzar for Injection (7% to 48%) ... 1919
▲ Gengraf Capsules (6% to 13%) ... 457
▲ Gliadel Wafer (7%) ... 1723
Glucotrol XL Extended Release Tablets (Less than 3%) ... 2693
▲ Gonal-F for Injection (5.9%) ... 3216
Hectorol Injection ... 1066
▲ Herceptin I.V. (47%) ... 1414
Hivid Tablets (Less than 1%) ... 2975
▲ Humatrope Vials and Cartridges (6.25% to 13.6%) ... 1930
Humegon for Injection ... 2468
Hyalgan Solution ... 3080
Hycamtin for Injection (1.1% to 5.4%) ... 1546
▲ Indapamide Tablets (Greater than or equal to 5%) ... 2286
▲ Infergen (39% to 54%) ... 1777
Innohep Injection (1.5%) ... 1248
▲ Intron A for Injection (Up to 18%) ... 3120
Kadian Capsules (Less than 3%) ... 1335
Kaletra Capsules (0.3% to 2.4%) ... 471
Kaletra Oral Solution (0.3% to 2.4%) ... 471
▲ Keppra Tablets (7%) ... 3314
Klonopin Tablets (Infrequent) ... 2983
K-Phos Neutral Tablets ... 946
K-Phos Original (Sodium Free) Tablets (Less frequent) ... 947
Lamictal (Frequent) ... 1567
▲ Leukine (17%) ... 1755
Levaquin (1.4%) ... 2537
Levulan Kerastick (Up to 1%) ... 971
Librium for Injection ... 1737
Lovenox Injection ... 746
▲ Lupron Depot 3.75 mg (8.4%) ... 3281
▲ Lupron Depot 7.5 mg (23.2%) ... 3284
▲ Lupron Depot–3 Month 11.25 mg (8.4% to 19%) ... 3285
▲ Lupron Depot–3 Month 22.5 mg (26.6%) ... 3288
▲ Lupron Depot–4 Month 30 mg (4.2% to 32.7%) ... 3289
Lupron Depot-PED 7.5 mg, 11.25 mg and 15 mg (2%) ... 3291
▲ Lupron Injection (5% or more) ... 3279
Lupron Injection Pediatric ... 3280
Luvox Tablets (25, 50, 100 mg) ... 3256
Matulane Capsules ... 3246
▲ Megace Oral Suspension (Up to 6%) ... 1124
Menomune-A/C/Y/W-135 Vaccine (2% to 2.6%) ... 813
▲ Mepron Suspension (10%) ... 1598
Merrem I.V. (0.1% to 1.0%) ... 673
Micardis Tablets (1%) ... 1049
Micardis HCT Tablets (2% or greater) ... 1051
Minipress Capsules ... 2699
Mirapex Tablets (1% or more) ... 2834
Mobic Tablets (0.9% to 3.6%) ... 1054
Monopril Tablets (0.4% to 1.0%) ... 1091
Monurol Sachet (2.2%) ... 1375
▲ MUSE Urethral Suppository (3%) ... 3335
Mycobutin Capsules (1%) ... 2838
▲ Mylotarg for Injection (20% to 30%) ... 3540
▲ Myobloc Injectable Solution (6% to 13%) ... 1291
▲ Naprelan Tablets (3% to 9%) ... 1293
Naropin Injection (1% to 5%) ... 612
Nascobal Gel ... 3174
▲ Neoral Soft Gelatin Capsules (4.4% to 13%) ... 2380
▲ Neoral Oral Solution (4.4% to 13%) ... 2380
▲ Neumega for Injection (Greater than or equal to 10%) ... 1434
Neupogen for Injection (2%) ... 587
Nexium Delayed-Release Capsules (Less than 1%) ... 619
Niaspan Extended-Release Tablets (1% to 5%) ... 1846
▲ Nicotrol Inhaler (Greater than 3%) ... 2840
Nicotrol Nasal Spray (Less than 1%) ... 2843
▲ Nilandron Tablets (26.8%) ... 753
▲ Nipent for Injection (8% to 20%) ... 3272
Nolvadex Tablets (2.8%) ... 678
▲ Norplant System (3.7%) ... 3543
Norvasc Tablets (More than 0.1% to 1%) ... 2704
Norvir Capsules (Less than 2%) ... 487
Norvir Oral Solution (Less than 2%) ... 487
▲ Novantrone for Injection (8%) ... 1760
NovoSeven (1%) ... 2430
▲ Oncaspar (Greater than 5%) ... 756
▲ Orgaran Injection (8.7%) ... 2480
Orthoclone OKT3 Sterile Solution (Less than 1%) ... 2498
▲ Ortho-Prefest Tablets (6%) ... 2570
Orudis Capsules (Less than 1%) ... 3548
Oruvail Capsules (Less than 1%) ... 3548
Oxistat Lotion (0.4%) ... 1298
OxyContin Tablets (Less than 1%) ... 2912
Pancrease Capsules (Frequent) ... 2580
ParaGard T 380A Intrauterine Copper Contraceptive ... 2582
▲ Paraplatin for Injection (17% to 54%) ... 1126
Pergonal for Injection ... 3223
▲ Periostat Tablets (4%) ... 1208
▲ Permax Tablets (7.0%) ... 1299
▲ Photofrin for Injection (22%) ... 831
▲ Plavix Tablets (6.4%) ... 1097
▲ Plavix Tablets (6.4%) ... 3084
▲ Pravachol Tablets (1.4% to 10.0%) ... 1099
▲ Prempro Tablets (11% to 13%) ... 3572
Priftin Tablets (1.9%) ... 758
Prilosec Delayed-Release Capsules (Less than 1%) ... 628
Prinivil Tablets (0.3% to 1.0%) ... 2164
Prinzide Tablets ... 2168
▲ ProAmatine Tablets (4.9%) ... 3241
Procardia XL Extended Release Tablets (Less than 3%) ... 2710
▲ Prograf (24% to 63%) ... 1393
▲ Proleukin for Injection (12%) ... 1199
ProSom Tablets (2%) ... 500
Protonix I.V. (Greater than or equal to 1%) ... 3580
Protonix Tablets (Greater than or equal to 1%) ... 3577
Protopic Ointment (1% to 4%) ... 1397
Prozac Pulvules, Liquid, and Weekly Capsules (Less than 1%) ... 1238
▲ Pulmicort Turbuhaler Inhalation Powder (2% to 10%) ... 636
Qvar Inhalation Aerosol (1% to 5%) ... 1987
▲ Rapamune Oral Solution and Tablets (24% to 33%) ... 3584
ReFacto Vials ... 1437
Remicade for IV Injection (Less than 2%) ... 1178
▲ Renagel Capsules (13%) ... 1439
▲ Renagel Tablets (13%) ... 1439
▲ ReoPro Vials (3.4% to 5.4%) ... 1958
▲ Requip Tablets (8%) ... 1621
Rescriptor Tablets (Less than 2%) ... 526
Rescula Ophthalmic Solution (1% to 5%) ... ⊙ 306
Rituxan for Infusion (0.3%) ... 1750
Rituxan I.V. (0.3%) ... 1428
Robinul Injectable ... 2940
▲ Roferon-A Injection (24%) ... 2996
Roxicodone Tablets (Less than 3%) ... 3067
Rythmol Tablets – 150 mg, 225 mg, 300 mg (Less than 1%) ... 502
▲ Salagen Tablets (4%) ... 2229
▲ Sarafem Pulvules (9%) ... 1962
Serevent Diskus (1% to 3%) ... 1637
Serzone Tablets ... 1104
▲ Simulect for Injection (Greater than or equal to 10%) ... 2399
▲ Skelid Tablets (21.3%) ... 3088
▲ Soriatane Capsules (1% to 10%) ... 3003
Sporanox Capsules (2% to 3%) ... 1800
Sporanox Injection (1%) ... 1804
Sporanox Injection (1%) ... 2509
Sporanox Oral Solution (1.8% to 2.3%) ... 1808
Sporanox Oral Solution (1.8% to 2.3%) ... 2512
Stimate Nasal Spray ... 796
Sulfamylon Topical Solution ... 1011
Sustiva Capsules (Less than 2%) ... 1258
▲ Synagis Intramuscular (8.5%) ... 2028
Synercid I.V. (1.5% to 3.1%) ... 775
Tasmar Tablets (Infrequent) ... 3010
▲ Taxotere for Injection Concentrate (7 of 134 patients) ... 778
▲ Terazol 3 Vaginal Suppositories (3.9% of 284 patients) ... 2587
Terazol 7 Vaginal Cream (2.1% of 521 patients) ... 2587
Testoderm Transdermal Systems (2%) ... 574
▲ Tetanus & Diphtheria Toxoids Adsorbed for Adult Use (9.9%) ... 1880
Tetanus and Diphtheria Toxoids Adsorbed For Adult Use ... 815
Tetanus Toxoid Adsorbed Purogenated ... 1882
Teveten Tablets (Less than 1%) ... 3327
▲ Thalomid Capsules (8.3%) ... 1154
▲ Thymoglobulin for Injection (46.3%) ... 3071
Thyrogen for Injection (Four patients) ... 1441
▲ Tiazac Capsules (3% to 6%) ... 1378
Ticlid Tablets (0.5% to 1.0%) ... 3015
Tikosyn Capsules (Greater than 2%) ... 2717
Tine Test, Tuberculin, Old ... 3631
▲ TOBI Solution for Inhalation (8.1%) ... 1206
Topamax Sprinkle Capsules (More than 1%) ... 2590
Topamax Tablets (More than 1%) ... 2590
Travatan Ophthalmic Solution (1% to 5%) ... 543
▲ Tricor Capsules, Micronized (8%) ... 513
Tri-Nasal Spray (2%) ... 2274
▲ Trisenox Injection (15%) ... 1158
Trovan (Less than 1%) ... 2722
Uniretic Tablets (More than 1%) ... 3178
Univasc Tablets (More than 1%) ... 3181
▲ Vagifem Tablets (3% to 5%) ... 2857
▲ Vancenase AQ Nasal Spray 0.084% (4%) ... 3163
Vantin Tablets and Oral Suspension (Less than 1%) ... 2860
Vascor Tablets (0.5% to 2.0%) ... 2602
Venofer Injection (Greater than 1%) ... 580
Verelan PM Capsules (2.4%) ... 3186
▲ Vesanoid Capsules (37%) ... 3037
Viadur Implant (Less than 2%) ... 912
Viagra Tablets (Less than 2%) ... 2732
Vicoprofen Tablets (Less than 3%) ... 520
▲ Videx (6% to 7%) ... 1138
Videx EC Capsules ... 1143
Vioxx (Greater than 0.1% to 1.9%) ... 2213
Viracept ... 532
▲ Vistide Injection (25%) ... 1445
Vitravene for Injection (2% to 5%) ... ⊙ 310
Voltaren Ophthalmic Sterile Ophthalmic Solution (Less than 3%) ... ⊙ 312
Warfarin Sodium Tablets, USP ... 3302
▲ WelChol Tablets (5%) ... 3073
Wellbutrin Tablets (Infrequent) ... 1680
Wellbutrin SR Sustained-Release Tablets (2% to 3%) ... 1684
Xopenex Inhalation Solution (1.4% to 2.8%) ... 3207
▲ Zenapax for Injection (Greater than 5%) ... 3046
Zestoretic Tablets ... 695
Zestril Tablets (0.3% to 1.0%) ... 698
▲ Zoladex (8% to 17%) ... 702
▲ Zoladex 3-month (14%) ... 706
Zomig Tablets (2% to 3%) ... 708
Zomig-ZMT Tablets (2% to 3%) ... 708
Zosyn (1.7% to 3.2%) ... 1890
Zosyn in Galaxy Containers (1.7% to 3.2%) ... 1894
Zovirax Capsules ... 1706
Zovirax for Injection ... 1708
Zovirax Ointment ... 1707
Zovirax ... 1706
Zyban Sustained-Release Tablets (Infrequent) ... 1710
▲ Zyflo Filmtab Tablets (7.8%) ... 524
Zyrtec (Less than 2%) ... 2756
Zyrtec-D 12 Hour Extended Relief Tablets (Less than 2%) ... 2758

Pain, abdominal
(*see under* Abdominal pain/cramps)

Pain, arm
Cozaar Tablets (Less than 1%) ... 2067
Diovan HCT Tablets (Greater than 0.2%) ... 2338
▲ Femara Tablets (21% to 22%) ... 2351
Ferrlecit Injection (Greater than 1%) ... 3386
Hyzaar ... 2109
Lexxel Tablets ... 608
Norplant System ... 3543
Plendil Extended-Release Tablets (0.5% to 1.5%) ... 623
Prinzide Tablets ... 2168
Vaqta (1.3%) ... 2199
Vioxx (Greater than 0.1% to 1.9%) ... 2213
Zestoretic Tablets ... 695
Zestril Tablets (0.3% to 1.0%) ... 698

Pain, back
(*see under* Backache)

Pain, biliary
Campath Ampules ... 992
Lipitor Tablets (Less than 2%) ... 2639
Lipitor Tablets (Less than 2%) ... 2696
Luvox Tablets (25, 50, 100 mg) (Rare) ... 3256
Protonix I.V. (Less than 1%) ... 3580
Protonix Tablets (Less than 1%) ... 3577
Prozac Pulvules, Liquid, and Weekly Capsules (Rare) ... 1238
Remicade for IV Injection (Less than 2%) ... 1178
Requip Tablets (Rare) ... 1621
Rilutek Tablets (Rare) ... 772
Sarafem Pulvules (Rare) ... 1962
Sonata Capsules (Rare) ... 3591
Trileptal Oral Suspension ... 2407
Trileptal Tablets ... 2407

Pain, bone
Abelcet Injection ... 1273
Aciphex Tablets ... 1267
Aciphex Tablets ... 1783
Actiq (Less than 1%) ... 1184
▲ Actonel Tablets (4.6% to 4.9%) ... 2879
AmBisome for Injection (Less common) ... 1383
Amerge Tablets (Rare) ... 1467
Arava Tablets (1% to 3%) ... 724
▲ Aredia for Injection (At least 5% to 59.4%) ... 2309
▲ Arimidex Tablets (6.5% to 11.8%) ... 659
Avonex ... 1013
Calcijex Injection ... 411
▲ Casodex Tablets (4%) ... 662
Celexa (Infrequent) ... 1365
Copaxone for Injection (Infrequent) ... 3306
Crinone (Less than 5%) ... 3213
Depacon Injection ... 416
Depakene ... 421
Depakote Sprinkle Capsules ... 426
Depakote Tablets ... 430
Depakote ER Tablets ... 436
▲ Didronel Tablets (About 1 patient in 10 to about 2 in 10) ... 2888
Doxil Injection (Less than 1%) ... 566
Effexor Tablets (Infrequent) ... 3495
Effexor XR Capsules (Infrequent) ... 3499
Estring Vaginal Ring (2%) ... 2811
▲ Femara Tablets (20%) ... 2351
▲ Fosamax Tablets (4.1% to approximately 6%) ... 2095
Hectorol Capsules ... 1064
Hectorol Injection ... 1066
▲ Herceptin I.V. (7%) ... 1414
Hivid Tablets (Less than 1%) ... 2975
▲ Infergen (13% to 26%) ... 1777
Intron A for Injection (Less than 5%) ... 3120
Kadian Capsules (Less than 3%) ... 1335
K-Phos Neutral Tablets ... 946
K-Phos Original (Sodium Free) Tablets (Less frequent) ... 947
▲ Leukine (21%) ... 1755
Lupron Depot 7.5 mg (Less than 5%) ... 3284
▲ Lupron Injection (5% or more) ... 3279
Naprelan Tablets (Less than 1%) ... 1293
▲ Neumega for Injection (Greater than or equal to 10%) ... 1434
▲ Neupogen for Injection (22% to 33%) ... 587
▲ Nilandron Tablets (6.2%) ... 753
▲ Nolvadex Tablets (5.7%) ... 678
Oncaspar (Less than 1%) ... 756
Permax Tablets (Infrequent) ... 1299
Pletal Tablets (Less than 2%) ... 2605
Pletal Tablets (Less than 2%) ... 2848
Protonix I.V. (Less than 1%) ... 3580
Protonix Tablets (Less than 1%) ... 3577
Prozac Pulvules, Liquid, and Weekly Capsules (Infrequent) ... 1238
Remeron Tablets (Rare) ... 2483
Remeron SolTab Tablets (Rare) ... 2486
Rescriptor Tablets (Less than 2%) ... 526
Rifadin ... 765
Rifater Tablets ... 769
Risperdal (Rare) ... 1796
Rocaltrol ... 2991
▲ Roferon-A Injection (25% to 47%) ... 2996
Roxicodone Tablets (Less than 3%) ... 3067
Sarafem Pulvules (Infrequent) ... 1962
Seroquel Tablets (Infrequent) ... 684
▲ Soriatane Capsules (1% to 10%) ... 3003
Tasmar Tablets (1% or more) ... 3010
Tequin Injection (Less than 0.1%) ... 1110
Tequin Tablets (Less than 0.1%) ... 1110
▲ Trisenox Injection (23%) ... 1158
Uroqid-Acid No. 2 Tablets ... 947
▲ Vesanoid Capsules (77%) ... 3037
Viadur Implant (Less than 2%) ... 912

Viagra Tablets (Less than 2%)......... 2732
Vistide Injection......... 1445
Xeloda Tablets (Less than 5%)......... 3039
Zoladex (Small number of patients)......... 702
▲ Zoladex 3-month (6%)......... 706
▲ Zometa for Intravenous Infusion (11.6%)......... 3621
Zyprexa Tablets (Rare)......... 1973
Zyprexa ZYDIS Orally Disintegrating Tablets (Rare)......... 1973

Pain, cancer related
Tice BCG, BCG Live......... 2489
Zoladex (Occasional)......... 702
Zoladex 3-month......... 706

Pain, cervical
TYPHIM Vi Vaccine......... 825

Pain, dental
Advair Diskus 100/50 (1% to 3%)......... 1448
Advair Diskus 250/50 (1% to 3%)......... 1448
Advair Diskus 500/50 (1% to 3%)......... 1448
Azmacort Inhalation Aerosol (1% to 3%)......... 728
Claritin-D 12 Hour Extended Release Tablets (Less frequent)......... 3102
Cozaar Tablets (Less than 1%)......... 2067
Estring Vaginal Ring (1% to 3%)......... 2811
Evoxac Capsules (1% to 3%)......... 1217
Flovent Diskus (1% to 3%)......... 3614
Flovent (1% to 3%)......... 1535
Fortovase Capsules (Less than 2%)......... 2970
Hivid Tablets (Less than 1%)......... 2975
Hyzaar......... 2109
Imitrex Nasal Spray......... 1554
▲ Infergen (3% to 7%)......... 1777
Klonopin Tablets (Infrequent)......... 2983
Lexxel Tablets (Infrequent)......... 608
▲ Luvox Tablets (25, 50, 100 mg) (3%)......... 3256
Micardis Tablets (More than 0.3%)......... 1049
Micardis HCT Tablets......... 1051
▲ Periostat Tablets (7%)......... 1208
Requip Tablets (Infrequent)......... 1621
Risperdal (Up to 2%)......... 1796
Serevent Inhalation Aerosol (1% to 3%)......... 1633
Singulair (1.7%)......... 2181
Teveten Tablets (Less than 1%)......... 3327
▲ Thalomid Capsules (4.2%)......... 1154
Trileptal Oral Suspension (1% to 2%)......... 2407
Trileptal Tablets (1% to 2%)......... 2407
Vantin Tablets and Oral Suspension (Less than 1%)......... 2860
Vioxx (Greater than 0.1% to 1.9%)......... 2213
Wellbutrin Tablets (Infrequent)......... 1680
Zyprexa Tablets (Frequent)......... 1973
Zyprexa ZYDIS Orally Disintegrating Tablets (Frequent)......... 1973

Pain, ear
Aceon Tablets (2 mg, 4 mg, 8 mg) (0.3% to 1%)......... 3249
Actiq (Less than 1%)......... 1184
Adenoscan (Less than 1%)......... 1381
Advair Diskus 100/50......... 1448
Advair Diskus 250/50......... 1448
Advair Diskus 500/50......... 1448
Aricept Tablets (Infrequent)......... 1270
Aricept Tablets (Infrequent)......... 2665
Asacol Delayed-Release Tablets (2% or greater)......... 2884
Avalide Tablets......... 1070
Avapro Tablets (Less than 1%)......... 1074
Avapro Tablets (Less than 1%)......... 3076
Avonex......... 1013
Axert Tablets (Infrequent)......... 2772
Bactroban Nasal (Less than 1%)......... 1495
Betaseron for SC Injection......... 988
Betaxon Ophthalmic Suspension (Less than 2%)......... 537
Cardura Tablets (Less than 0.5%)......... 2668
Ceclor CD Tablets (0.1% to 1%)......... 1279
Celebrex Capsules (0.1% to 1.9%)......... 2676
Celebrex Capsules (0.1% to 1.9%)......... 2780
▲ CellCept Capsules (3% to 10%)......... 2951
▲ CellCept Intravenous (3% to 10%)......... 2951
▲ CellCept Oral Suspension (3% to 10%)......... 2951
▲ CellCept Tablets (3% to 10%)......... 2951
Cerebyx Injection (Infrequent)......... 2619
Claritin (At least one patient)......... 3100
Claritin-D 12 Hour Extended Release Tablets (Less frequent)......... 3102
Claritin-D 24 Hour Extended Release Tablets (Fewer than 2%)......... 3104
Cognex Capsules (Infrequent)......... 1351
Colazal Capsules......... 3069
DaunoXome Injection (Less than or equal to 5%)......... 1442
Depacon Injection......... 416
Depakene......... 421
Depakote Sprinkle Capsules......... 426
Depakote Tablets (1% to 5%)......... 430
Depakote ER Tablets......... 436
Diprivan Injectable Emulsion (Less than 1%)......... 667
Effexor Tablets (Frequent)......... 3495
Engerix-B Vaccine......... 1517
Evoxac Capsules (1% to 3%)......... 1217
Flovent Diskus (1% to 3%)......... 3614
Flovent Rotadisk (1% to 3%)......... 1537
Floxin Otic Solution (1%)......... 1219
Fortovase Capsules (Less than 2%)......... 2970
Gabitril Tablets (Frequent)......... 1189
Hivid Tablets (Less than 1%)......... 2975
Imdur Tablets (Less than or equal to 5%)......... 1826
Imitrex Nasal Spray (Rare)......... 1554
Imitrex Tablets (Infrequent)......... 1558
▲ Infergen (5%)......... 1777
Intron A for Injection (Less than or equal to 5%)......... 3120
Invirase Capsules (Less than 2%)......... 2979
Klonopin Tablets (Infrequent)......... 2983
Lamictal (1.8%)......... 1567
Lupron Depot–3 Month 11.25 mg......... 3285
Luvox Tablets (25, 50, 100 mg) (Infrequent)......... 3256
Maxalt Tablets (Infrequent)......... 2120
Maxalt-MLT Orally Disintegrating Tablets (Infrequent)......... 2120
Meridia Capsules (1.1%)......... 481
Miacalcin Nasal Spray (Less than 1%)......... 2375
Micardis Tablets (More than 0.3%)......... 1049
Micardis HCT Tablets......... 1051
Migranal Nasal Spray (Infrequent)......... 2376
Nasonex Nasal Spray (Greater than or equal to 2%)......... 3131
Neurontin Capsules (Infrequent)......... 2655
Neurontin Oral Solution (Infrequent)......... 2655
Neurontin Tablets (Infrequent)......... 2655
Nexium Delayed-Release Capsules (Less than 1%)......... 619
Nicotrol Nasal Spray (More common)......... 2843
Nipent for Injection (Less than 3%)......... 3272
Norvir Capsules (Less than 2%)......... 487
Norvir Oral Solution (Less than 2%)......... 487
Paxil (Infrequent)......... 1609
Permax Tablets (Infrequent)......... 1299
Phrenilin (Infrequent)......... 578
Pletal Tablets (Less than 2%)......... 2605
Pletal Tablets (Less than 2%)......... 2848
Prinzide Tablets (0.3% to 1%)......... 2168
▲ Prograf (3% to 15%)......... 1393
Prometrium Capsules (100 mg, 200 mg) (Less than 5%)......... 3261
ProSom Tablets (Infrequent)......... 500
Protonix I.V. (Less than 1%)......... 3580
Protonix Tablets (Less than 1%)......... 3577
Protopic Ointment (Greater than or equal to 1%)......... 1397
Provigil Tablets (At least 1%)......... 1193
Prozac Pulvules, Liquid, and Weekly Capsules (Frequent)......... 1238
Pulmicort Respules (1% to 3%)......... 632
Recombivax HB (Less than 1%)......... 2178
Remeron Tablets (Infrequent)......... 2483
Remeron SolTab Tablets (Infrequent)......... 2486
Requip Tablets (Infrequent)......... 1621
Rescriptor Tablets (Less than 2%)......... 526
[illegible]
Roferon-A Injection (Less than 1%)......... 2996
Salagen Tablets (Less than 1%)......... 2229
▲ Sandostatin LAR Depot (5% to 15%)......... 2395
Sarafem Pulvules (Frequent)......... 1962
Sedapap Tablets 50 mg/650 mg (Infrequent)......... 2225
Serevent Inhalation Aerosol (1% to 3%)......... 1633
Seroquel Tablets (1%)......... 684
▲ Serostim for Injection (1% to 10%)......... 3229
Serzone Tablets (Infrequent)......... 1104
Singulair (Greater than or equal to 2%)......... 2181
Sonata Capsules (Less than 1%)......... 3591
▲ Soriatane Capsules (1% to 10%)......... 3003
Stadol NS Nasal Spray (1% or greater)......... 1108
Sular Tablets (Less than or equal to 1%)......... 688
Tasmar Tablets (Infrequent)......... 3010
Tequin Injection (Less than 0.1%)......... 1110
Tequin Tablets (Less than 0.1%)......... 1110
Timolide Tablets......... 2187
▲ TOBI Solution for Inhalation (7.4%)......... 1206
Tonocard Tablets (Less than 1%)......... 649
Topamax Sprinkle Capsules (Rare)......... 2590
Topamax Tablets (Rare)......... 2590
Trental Tablets (Less than 1%)......... 784
Tricor Capsules, Micronized (1%)......... 513
Trileptal Oral Suspension (1% to 2%)......... 2407
Trileptal Tablets (1% to 2%)......... 2407
▲ Trisenox Injection (8%)......... 1158
Twinrix Vaccine......... 1674
Uniretic Tablets (Less than 1%)......... 3178
Vanceril Double Strength Inhalation Aerosol (Fewer than 2%)......... 3167
▲ Vesanoid Capsules (23%)......... 3037
Viagra Tablets (Less than 2%)......... 2732
Vioxx (Greater than 0.1% to 1.9%)......... 2213
Vistide Injection......... 1445
Zanaflex Tablets (Infrequent)......... 1305
Zebeta Tablets......... 1885
Zestoretic Tablets (0.3% to 1%)......... 695
Ziac Tablets......... 1887
Zoloft (Infrequent)......... 2751
Zomig Tablets (Infrequent)......... 708
Zomig-ZMT Tablets (Infrequent)......... 708
Zosyn (1.0% or less)......... 1890
Zosyn in Galaxy Containers (1.0% or less)......... 1894
Zyprexa Tablets (Infrequent)......... 1973
Zyprexa ZYDIS Orally Disintegrating Tablets (Infrequent)......... 1973
Zyrtec (Less than 2%)......... 2756
Zyrtec-D 12 Hour Extended Relief Tablets (Less than 2%)......... 2758

Pain, epigastric
(*see under* Distress, epigastric)

Pain, esophageal
Hivid Tablets (Less than 1%)......... 2975

Pain, extremities
Astelin Nasal Spray (Infrequent)......... 3339
▲ Betapace Tablets (2% to 7%)......... 950
Betimol Ophthalmic Solution (1% to 5%)......... ⊙ 324
Blocadren Tablets......... 2046
Cipro I.V. Pharmacy Bulk Package (Less than 1%)......... 897
Colestid Tablets (Infrequent)......... 2791
Cosopt Sterile Ophthalmic Solution......... 2065
Diprivan Injectable Emulsion (Less than 1%)......... 667
Flovent (1% to 3%)......... 1535
Floxin I.V. (Less than 1%)......... 2526
Floxin Tablets (Less than 1%)......... 2529
▲ Hytrin Capsules (3.5%)......... 464
Iopidine Sterile Ophthalmic Solution......... ⊙ 212
Levlen......... 962
Levlite 21 Tablets......... 962
Levlite 28 Tablets......... 962
Mavik Tablets (0.3% to 1.0%)......... 478
Oncaspar (Greater than 1% but less than 5%)......... 756
Rifadin......... 765
Rifater Tablets......... 769
Tarka Tablets (1.1%)......... 508
Timolol GFS......... ⊙ 266
Timoptic-XE Sterile Ophthalmic Gel Forming Solution......... 2194
Tri-Levlen......... 962
Uroqid-Acid No. 2 Tablets......... 947
▲ Viadur Implant (3.1%)......... 912
Videx......... 1138
Videx EC Capsules......... 1143
Zerit......... 1147
▲ Zyprexa Tablets (4%)......... 1973
▲ Zyprexa ZYDIS Orally Disintegrating Tablets (4%)......... 1973

Pain, eye
Aciphex Tablets......... 1267
Aciphex Tablets......... 1783
[illegible] (Less than 1%)......... ⊙ 204
▲ Alphagan Ophthalmic Solution (Approximately 3% to 9%)......... 545
Alphagan P Ophthalmic Solution (1% to 4%)......... 546
Alrex Sterile Ophthalmic Suspension 0.2% (Less than 5%)......... ⊙ 256
Ambien Tablets (Infrequent)......... 3191
Amerge Tablets (Rare)......... 1467
Asacol Delayed-Release Tablets......... 2884
Astelin Nasal Spray (Infrequent)......... 3339
Atrovent Inhalation Aerosol......... 1030
Atrovent Inhalation Solution (Less than 3%)......... 1031
Atrovent Nasal Spray 0.06%......... 1033
Avonex......... 1013
Axert Tablets (Rare)......... 2772
Azopt Ophthalmic Suspension (1% to 5%)......... 536
Betimol Ophthalmic Solution (1% to 5%)......... ⊙ 324
Betoptic S Ophthalmic Suspension (Small number of patients)......... 537
Cardura Tablets (1%)......... 2668
Celebrex Capsules (0.1% to 1.9%)......... 2676
Celebrex Capsules (0.1% to 1.9%)......... 2780
Celexa (Infrequent)......... 1365
Cerebyx Injection (Infrequent)......... 2619
Ciloxan (Less than 1%)......... 538
Cipro I.V. (1% or less)......... 893
Cipro I.V. Pharmacy Bulk Package (Less than 1%)......... 897
Cipro (Less than 1%)......... 887
Claritin (At least one patient)......... 3100
Claritin-D 12 Hour Extended Release Tablets (Less frequent)......... 3102
Claritin-D 24 Hour Extended Release Tablets (Fewer than 2%)......... 3104
Clomid Tablets......... 735
Cognex Capsules (Infrequent)......... 1351
Combivent Inhalation Aerosol......... 1041
▲ Copaxone for Injection (7%)......... 3306
Cosopt Sterile Ophthalmic Solution (1% to 5%)......... 2065
Crixivan Capsules (Less than 2%)......... 2070
DaunoXome Injection (Less than or equal to 5%)......... 1442
Depacon Injection (1% or more)......... 416
Depakene (1% or more)......... 421
Depakote Sprinkle Capsules......... 426
Depakote Tablets (1% to 5%)......... 430
Depakote ER Tablets (Greater than 1%)......... 436
Diprivan Injectable Emulsion (Less than 1%)......... 667
Doxil Injection (Less than 1%)......... 566
DuoNeb Inhalation Solution......... 1233
Effexor Tablets (Infrequent)......... 3495
Effexor XR Capsules (Infrequent)......... 3499
Eldepryl Capsules......... 3266
Epifrin Sterile Ophthalmic Solution......... ⊙ 235
Evoxac Capsules (1% to 3%)......... 1217
Exelon Capsules......... 2342
Exelon Oral Solution......... 2345
Flumadine......... 1370
Foscavir Injection (Between 1% and 5%)......... 605
Gabitril Tablets (Infrequent)......... 1189
Gengraf Capsules (1% to less than 3%)......... 457
Gliadel Wafer (1%)......... 1723
Glucotrol XL Extended Release Tablets (Less than 1%)......... 2693
Hivid Tablets (Less than 1%)......... 2975
Imitrex Nasal Spray......... 1554
▲ Infergen (4% to 5%)......... 1777
Intron A for Injection (Less than 5%)......... 3120
Iopidine 0.5% Ophthalmic Solution (Less than 1%)......... ⊙ 213
Livostin (Approximately 1% to 3%)......... ⊙ 305
Loprox Gel......... 2022
Lotemax Sterile Ophthalmic Suspension 0.5% (Less than 5%)......... ⊙ 261
▲ Lumigan Ophthalmic Solution (3% to 10%)......... 553
Luvox Tablets (25, 50, 100 mg) (Infrequent)......... 3256
Maxalt Tablets (Infrequent)......... 2120
Maxalt-MLT Orally Disintegrating Tablets (Infrequent)......... 2120
Meridia Capsules......... 481
Miacalcin Injection......... 2373
Migranal Nasal Spray (Rare)......... 2376
Minipress Capsules......... 2699
Naprelan Tablets (Less than 1%)......... 1293
Neoral Soft Gelatin Capsules (1% to less than 3%)......... 2380
Neoral Oral Solution (1% to less than 3%)......... 2380
Neurontin Capsules (Infrequent)......... 2655
Neurontin Oral Solution (Infrequent)......... 2655
Neurontin Tablets (Infrequent)......... 2655
Norvasc Tablets (More than 0.1% to 1%)......... 2704
Norvir Capsules (Less than 2%)......... 487
Norvir Oral Solution (Less than 2%)......... 487
Ocuflox Ophthalmic Solution......... 554
▲ Optivar Ophthalmic Solution (1% to 10%)......... 2273
Orudis Capsules (Less than 1%)......... 3548
Oruvail Capsules (Less than 1%)......... 3548
Paxil (Infrequent)......... 1609
Permax Tablets (Infrequent)......... 1299
Photofrin for Injection......... 831
Prevacid Delayed-Release Capsules (Less than 1%)......... 3292
PREVPAC (Less than 1%)......... 3298
ProSom Tablets (Infrequent)......... 500
Prostin E2 Suppositories......... 2852
Protopic Ointment (Greater than or equal to 1%)......... 1397
Provigil Tablets (At least 1%)......... 1193
Quixin Ophthalmic Solution (1% to 3%)......... 3093
Remeron Tablets (Infrequent)......... 2483
Remeron SolTab Tablets (Infrequent)......... 2486
Requip Tablets (Infrequent)......... 1621
Rescula Ophthalmic Solution (1% to 5%)......... ⊙ 306
Risperdal (Rare)......... 1796
Roferon-A Injection (Infrequent)......... 2996
Salagen Tablets (Less than 1%)......... 2229
Sectral Capsules (Up to 2%)......... 3589
Serophene Tablets......... 3226
Serzone Tablets (Frequent)......... 1104

Soma Tablets ... 3353
▲ Sonata Capsules (4%) ... 3591
▲ Soriatane Capsules (1% to 10%) ... 3003
Synarel Nasal Solution for Endometriosis (Less than 1%) ... 3205
Tambocor Tablets (Less than 1%) ... 1990
Tasmar Tablets (Infrequent) ... 3010
Tequin Injection (Less than 0.1%) ... 1110
Tequin Tablets (Less than 0.1%) ... 1110
Thalomid Capsules ... 1154
Timolol GFS (1% to 5%) ... ⊙266
Timoptic in Ocudose (Less frequent) ... 2192
Timoptic Sterile Ophthalmic Solution (Less frequent) ... 2190
Timoptic-XE Sterile Ophthalmic Gel Forming Solution (1% to 5%) .. 2194
Topamax Sprinkle Capsules (1.8% to 2%) ... 2590
Topamax Tablets (1.8% to 2%) ... 2590
▲ Travatan Ophthalmic Solution (5% to 10%) ... 543
Trovan (Less than 1%) ... 2722
Trusopt Sterile Ophthalmic Solution ... 2196
Vexol 1% Ophthalmic Suspension (1% to 5%) ... ⊙222
Viagra Tablets (Less than 2%) ... 2732
Vistide Injection ... 1445
▲ Vitravene for Injection (5% to 20%) ... ⊙310
Xalatan Latanoprost Ophthalmic Solution (1% to 4%) ... ⊙320
Xalatan Sterile Ophthalmic Solution (1% to 4%) ... 2864
Zaditor Ophthalmic Solution (Less than 5%) ... 2304
Zanaflex Tablets (Infrequent) ... 1305
Zebeta Tablets ... 1885
Ziac Tablets ... 1887
Zoloft (Infrequent) ... 2751
Zomig Tablets (Infrequent) ... 708
Zomig-ZMT Tablets (Infrequent) ... 708
Zyprexa Tablets (Infrequent) ... 1973
Zyprexa ZYDIS Orally Disintegrating Tablets (Infrequent) ... 1973
Zyrtec (Less than 2%) ... 2756
Zyrtec-D 12 Hour Extended Relief Tablets (Less than 2%) ... 2758

Pain, facial
▲ Carac Cream (43.6%) ... 1222
Fortovase Capsules (Less than 2%) ... 2970
Hivid Tablets (Less than 1%) ... 2975
Imitrex Injection (Infrequent) ... 1549
Imitrex Nasal Spray (Rare) ... 1554
Imitrex Tablets (Infrequent) ... 1558
Invirase Capsules (Less than 2%) ... 2979
Norvir Capsules (Less than 2%) ... 487
Norvir Oral Solution (Less than 2%) ... 487

Pain, female genitalia
Floxin Tablets (Less than 1%) ... 2529

Pain, flank
Aceon Tablets (2 mg, 4 mg, 8 mg) (0.3% to 1%) ... 3249
Actiq (Less than 1%) ... 1184
▲ Chemet Capsules (5.2% to 15.7%) ... 3078
Cleocin Vaginal Ovules (Less than 1%) ... 2789
Copaxone for Injection (Infrequent) ... 3306
Crixivan Capsules (Less than 2%) ... 2070
Enalaprilat Injection ... 863
Ferrlecit Injection ... 3386
Fludara for Injection ... 995
Geodon Capsules (Frequent) ... 2688
Hivid Tablets (Less than 1%) ... 2975
Lexxel Tablets ... 608
Neupogen for Injection (Infrequent) ... 587
Prinivil Tablets (0.3% to 1.0%) ... 2164
Prinzide Tablets ... 2168
Rescriptor Tablets (Less than 2%) ... 526
Tasmar Tablets (Frequent) ... 3010
TheraCys Injection (1%) ... 823
Toradol ... 3018
Vaseretic Tablets ... 2204
Vasotec I.V. Injection ... 2207
Vasotec Tablets (0.5% to 1.0%) ... 2210
▲ Vesanoid Capsules (9%) ... 3037
Zestoretic Tablets ... 695
Zestril Tablets (0.3% to 1.0%) ... 698
Zonegran Capsules (Infrequent) ... 1307

Pain, genital
▲ Condylox Topical Solution (50% to 72%) ... 2437
▲ TheraCys Injection (10%) ... 823

Pain, hand
Avelox Tablets (0.05% to 1%) ... 879

Pain, hip
Cozaar Tablets (Less than 1%) ... 2067
Gamimune N, 5% Solvent/Detergent Treated ... 925
Gamimune N, 10% Solvent/Detergent Treated ... 928
Hyzaar ... 2109
Lexxel Tablets ... 608
Plendil Extended-Release Tablets (0.5% to 1.5%) ... 623
Prinivil Tablets (0.3% to 1.0%) ... 2164
Prinzide Tablets ... 2168
Zestoretic Tablets ... 695
Zestril Tablets (0.3% to 1.0%) ... 698
Zyprexa Tablets (Infrequent) ... 1973
Zyprexa ZYDIS Orally Disintegrating Tablets (Infrequent) ... 1973

Pain, inguinal
Hivid Tablets (Less than 1%) ... 2975

Pain, jaw
Cipro I.V. (1% or less) ... 893
Cipro I.V. Pharmacy Bulk Package (Less than 1%) ... 897
▲ Flolan for Injection (54% to 75%) ... 1528
Fortovase Capsules (Less than 2%) ... 2970
Klonopin Tablets (Infrequent) ... 2983
Navelbine Injection (Less than 5%) .. 1604
▲ Nicotrol Inhaler (Over 3%) ... 2840
Permax Tablets (Infrequent) ... 1299
ProSom Tablets (Rare) ... 500

Pain, knee
Cozaar Tablets (Less than 1%) ... 2067
Hyzaar ... 2109
Klonopin Tablets (Infrequent) ... 2983
Lexxel Tablets (Infrequent) ... 608
Plendil Extended-Release Tablets (0.5% to 1.5%) ... 623
Prinivil Tablets (0.3% to 1.0%) ... 2164
Synvisc (2.2%) ... 3596
Zestril Tablets (0.3% to 1.0%) ... 698

Pain, limb
▲ Femara Tablets (8%) ... 2351
Meridia Capsules ... 481
▲ Trisenox Injection (13%) ... 1158

Pain, lower extremities
▲ Aceon Tablets (2 mg, 4 mg, 8 mg) (4.7%) ... 3249
Adalat CC Tablets (3% or less) ... 877
▲ Aggrastat (3%) ... 2031
Avelox Tablets (0.05% to 1%) ... 879
Baycol Tablets (2.2%) ... 883
Chemet Capsules (Up to 3.0%) ... 3078
Cipro (0.3% to 1%) ... 887
Clozaril Tablets (1%) ... 2319
Cozaar Tablets (1.0%) ... 2067
Crinone (Less than 5%) ... 3213
Crixivan Capsules (Less than 2%) ... 2070
Diovan HCT Tablets (Greater than 0.2%) ... 2338
DynaCirc Capsules (0.5% to 1%) ... 2921
DynaCirc CR Tablets (0.5% to 1%) .. 2923
Eldepryl Capsules (1 of 49 patients) ... 3266
Estrace Vaginal Cream ... 3358
Estrace Tablets ... 3361
Etrafon (Less frequent) ... 3115
▲ Femara Tablets (21% to 22%) ... 2351
Fortovase Capsules (Less than 2%) ... 2970
Hivid Tablets (Less than 1%) ... 2975
Hyzaar ... 2109
Klonopin Tablets (Infrequent) ... 2983
Lexxel Tablets (Infrequent) ... 608
Lopid Tablets ... 2650
Mevacor Tablets (0.5% to 1.0%) ... 2132
Micardis Tablets (More than 0.3%) .. 1049
Micardis HCT Tablets ... 1051
Midamor Tablets (Less than or equal to 1%) ... 2136
Moduretic Tablets ... 2138
▲ Nutropin Depot for Injectable Suspension (7%) ... 1423
Ortho-Est Tablets ... 3464
Phrenilin (Infrequent) ... 578
Plendil Extended-Release Tablets (0.5% to 1.5%) ... 623
Prilosec Delayed-Release Capsules (Less than 1%) ... 628
Prinivil Tablets (0.3% to 1.0%) ... 2164
Prinzide Tablets (0.3% to 1%) ... 2168
▲ ProSom Tablets (3%) ... 500
Rifamate Capsules ... 767
Rowasa Rectal Suspension Enema 4.0 grams/unit (60 mL) (2.09%) ... 3264
Sedapap Tablets 50 mg/650 mg (Infrequent) ... 2225
Seroquel Tablets (Infrequent) ... 684
▲ Simulect for Injection (3% to 10%) . 2399
Sinemet Tablets ... 1253
Sinemet CR Tablets ... 1255
Singulair (Greater than or equal to 2%) ... 2181
Tenex Tablets (Less frequent) ... 2942
Tenoretic Tablets (Up to 3%) ... 690
Tenormin (Up to 3%) ... 692
Timolide Tablets ... 2187
Timoptic in Ocudose ... 2192
Timoptic Sterile Ophthalmic Solution ... 2190
Topamax Sprinkle Capsules (2.4% to 3.5%) ... 2590
Topamax Tablets (2.4% to 3.5%) ... 2590
Vivelle Transdermal System ... 2412
Vivelle-Dot Transdermal System ... 2416
▲ Xenical Capsules (10.8%) ... 3043
Zestoretic Tablets (0.3% to 1%) ... 695
Zestril Tablets (0.3% to 1.0%) ... 698

Pain, medullary bone
▲ Neupogen for Injection (33%) ... 587

Pain, Mittelschmerz
Serophene Tablets ... 3226

Pain, muscle
(*see under* Myalgia)

Pain, musculoskeletal
▲ Advair Diskus 100/50 (4%) ... 1448
Advair Diskus 250/50 (2%) ... 1448
Advair Diskus 500/50 (2% to 4%) ... 1448
▲ Avalide Tablets (7%) ... 1070
Betapace AF Tablets (2.6% to 4.1%) ... 954
Cancidas for Injection (Up to 1.3%) ... 2048
Evoxac Capsules (2.8%) ... 1217
▲ Femara Tablets (21% to 22%) ... 2351
▲ Flovent Diskus (4%) ... 3614
Follistim for Injection ... 2465
▲ Fosamax Tablets (6%) ... 2095
▲ Gleevec Capsules (27% to 39%) ... 2357
Maxalt Tablets (Infrequent) ... 2120
Maxalt-MLT Orally Disintegrating Tablets (Infrequent) ... 2120
Monopril HCT (2%) ... 1094
Nasonex Nasal Spray (1% to 5%) ... 3131
▲ PEG-Intron Powder for Injection (56%) ... 3140
▲ Prometrium Capsules (100 mg, 200 mg) (12%) ... 3261
▲ Rebetron Combination Therapy (20% to 28%) ... 3153
▲ Trizivir Tablets (12%) ... 1669
Venofer Injection (Greater than 1%) ... 580
▲ Ventolin HFA Inhalation Aerosol (5%) ... 3618
Vioxx (Greater than 0.1% to 1.9%) .. 2213
▲ Zenapax for Injection (Greater than 5%) ... 3046

Pain, nasal
▲ Flovent (Up to 13%) ... 1535
Rhinocort Nasal Inhaler (Rare) ... 640

Pain, neck
(*see under* Torticollis)

Pain, nostril
DDAVP Nasal Spray (Up to 2%) ... 738
DDAVP Rhinal Tube (Up to 2%) ... 738
Desmopressin Acetate Rhinal Tube (Up to 2%) ... 1345

Pain, oral mucosa
Advair Diskus 100/50 (1% to 3%) ... 1448
Advair Diskus 250/50 (1% to 3%) ... 1448
Advair Diskus 500/50 (1% to 3%) ... 1448
Cipro (Less than 1%) ... 887
Flovent Diskus (1% to 3%) ... 3614
Floxin I.V. ... 2526
Floxin Tablets ... 2529

Pain, paranasal sinus
Advair Diskus 100/50 ... 1448
Advair Diskus 250/50 ... 1448
Advair Diskus 500/50 ... 1448

Pain, pelvic
Actiq (1% or greater) ... 1184
Adalat CC Tablets (Less than 1.0%) ... 877
▲ Aggrastat (6%) ... 2031
Alora Transdermal System (Up to 5.3%) ... 3372
Androderm Transdermal System CIII (Less than 1%) ... 3377
Arava Tablets (1% to 3%) ... 724
▲ Arimidex Tablets (4.5% to 6.9%) ... 659
Avelox Tablets (0.05% to 1%) ... 879
▲ Betaseron for SC Injection (6%) ... 988
▲ Casodex Tablets (13%) ... 662
Caverject Sterile Powder (Less than 1%) ... 2777
▲ CellCept Capsules (3%) ... 2951
▲ CellCept Intravenous (3%) ... 2951
▲ CellCept Oral Suspension (3%) ... 2951
▲ CellCept Tablets (3%) ... 2951
▲ Cerebyx Injection (4.4%) ... 2619
Clomid Tablets ... 735
▲ Depo-Provera Contraceptive Injection (More than 5%) ... 2798
Doxil Injection (Less than 1%) ... 566
Effexor Tablets (Infrequent) ... 3495
Effexor XR Capsules (Infrequent) ... 3499
Follistim for Injection ... 2465
Fortovase Capsules (Less than 2%) ... 2970
Gabitril Tablets (Infrequent) ... 1189
▲ Gonal-F for Injection (7.1%) ... 3216
▲ Gynazole-1 Vaginal Cream (5.7%) .. 3310
Hivid Tablets (Less than 1%) ... 2975
Humegon for Injection ... 2468
Intron A for Injection (Less than 5%) ... 3120
Invirase Capsules (Less than 2%) ... 2979
Klonopin Tablets (Infrequent) ... 2983
Luvox Tablets (25, 50, 100 mg) (Rare) ... 3256
Massengill Disposable Douches ... ▣752
Massengill Medicated Disposable Douche ... ▣753
MUSE Urethral Suppository (2%) ... 3335
Naprelan Tablets (Less than 1%) ... 1293
Nolvadex Tablets ... 678
Paxil (Rare) ... 1609
Permax Tablets (Infrequent) ... 1299
Pletal Tablets (Less than 2%) ... 2605
Pletal Tablets (Less than 2%) ... 2848
▲ Prempro Tablets (4% to 5%) ... 3572
Prinivil Tablets (0.3% to 1.0%) ... 2164
Prinzide Tablets ... 2168
Prozac Pulvules, Liquid, and Weekly Capsules (Infrequent) ... 1238
▲ Rapamune Oral Solution and Tablets (3% to 20%) ... 3584
▲ Repronex for Intramuscular and Subcutaneous Injection (1% to 3%) ... 1347
Sarafem Pulvules (Infrequent) ... 1962
Serophene Tablets ... 3226
Seroquel Tablets (Infrequent) ... 684
Serzone Tablets (Infrequent) ... 1104
Valstar Sterile Solution for Intravesical Instillation (1%) ... 1175
Vioxx (Greater than 0.1% to 1.9%) .. 2213
Zestoretic Tablets ... 695
Zestril Tablets (0.3% to 1.0%) ... 698
▲ Zoladex (9%) ... 702
▲ Zoladex 3-month (6%) ... 706
Zyprexa Tablets (Infrequent) ... 1973
Zyprexa ZYDIS Orally Disintegrating Tablets (Infrequent) ... 1973

Pain, penile
▲ Caverject Sterile Powder (2% to 37%) ... 2777
Hivid Tablets (Less than 1%) ... 2975
▲ MUSE Urethral Suppository (32%) .. 3335

Pain, perineal
Arthrotec Tablets (Rare) ... 3195
▲ Crinone 8% Gel (17%) ... 3213
Requip Tablets (Infrequent) ... 1621
Risperdal (Infrequent) ... 1796
Zosyn (1.0% or less) ... 1890
Zosyn in Galaxy Containers (1.0% or less) ... 1894

Pain, peripheral
Celebrex Capsules (0.1% to 1.9%) ... 2676
Celebrex Capsules (0.1% to 1.9%) ... 2780

Pain, pharynx
Prilosec Delayed-Release Capsules (Less than 1%) ... 628
Primaxin I.M. ... 2158
Primaxin I.V. (Less than 0.2%) ... 2160
Prinivil Tablets (0.3% to 1.0%) ... 2164
Prinzide Tablets (0.3% to 1%) ... 2168
Sinemet Tablets ... 1253
Sinemet CR Tablets ... 1255
Zestoretic Tablets (0.3% to 1%) ... 695
Zestril Tablets (0.3% to 1.0%) ... 698

Pain, pleural
Migranal Nasal Spray (Rare) ... 2376

Pain, postoperative
▲ Chirocaine Injection (7.3%) ... 2909
Evoxac Capsules (1% to 3%) ... 1217
▲ Ovidrel for Injection (4.7%) ... 3220
Vioxx (Greater than 0.1% to 1.9%) .. 2213

Pain, precordium
D.H.E. 45 Injection ... 2334
Imitrex Tablets ... 1558
Mykrox Tablets (2.7%) ... 1168
Phenergan VC with Codeine Syrup .. 3561
Trileptal Oral Suspension ... 2407
Trileptal Tablets ... 2407
Zoloft (Rare) ... 2751

Pain, prostate
Caverject Sterile Powder (2%) ... 2777
Lupron Depot 3.75 mg ... 3281
Lupron Depot 7.5 mg ... 3284
Lupron Depot–3 Month 11.25 mg ... 3285
Lupron Depot–3 Month 22.5 mg ... 3288
Lupron Depot–4 Month 30 mg ... 3289
Lupron Depot-PED 7.5 mg, 11.25 mg and 15 mg ... 3291
Lupron Injection ... 3279

Pain, rectum
Canasa Rectal Suppositories (1.8%) ... 829
Hivid Tablets (Less than 1%) ... 2975
Lexxel Tablets ... 608
Noroxin Tablets (0.3% to 1.0%) ... 2145
Remicade for IV Injection (Less than 2%) ... 1178

Rowasa Rectal Suspension Enema 4.0 grams/unit (60 mL) (1.23%) 3264
▲ Xenical Capsules (3.3% to 5.2%) 3043

Pain, renal
Actiq (Less than 1%) 1184
Ambien Tablets (Rare) 3191
Avonex 1013
Azopt Ophthalmic Suspension (Less than 1%) 536
Ceftin Tablets (0.1% to 1%) 1898
Celexa (Rare) 1365
Copaxone for Injection (Infrequent) 3306
Effexor Tablets (Infrequent) 3495
Effexor XR Capsules (Rare) 3499
Evoxac Capsules (Less than 1%) 1217
Lamictal (Rare) 1567
Monopril Tablets (0.4% to 1.0%) 1091
Naprelan Tablets (Less than 1%) 1293
Neurontin Capsules (Rare) 2655
Neurontin Oral Solution (Rare) 2655
Neurontin Tablets (Rare) 2655
Norvir Capsules (Less than 2%) 487
Norvir Oral Solution (Less than 2%) 487
Paxil (Rare) 1609
Protonix I.V. (Less than 1%) 3580
Protonix Tablets (Less than 1%) 3577
Prozac Pulvules, Liquid, and Weekly Capsules (Rare) 1238
▲ Rapamune Oral Solution and Tablets (3% to 20%) 3584
Rescriptor Tablets (Less than 2%) 526
Rilutek Tablets (Infrequent) 772
Sarafem Pulvules (Rare) 1962
Topamax Sprinkle Capsules (Infrequent) 2590
Topamax Tablets (Infrequent) 2590
Trileptal Oral Suspension 2407
Trileptal Tablets 2407
Zoloft (Rare) 2751

Pain, retrosternal
Fortovase Capsules (Less than 2%) 2970
Invirase Capsules (Less than 2%) 2979
Zofran Injection (2%) 1698

Pain, right hypochondrium
Trileptal Oral Suspension 2407
Trileptal Tablets 2407

Pain, right upper quadrant
Casodex Tablets 662
Fortovase Capsules (Rare) 2970
▲ Intron A for Injection (Less than 5% to 15%) 3120
Invirase Capsules (Rare) 2979
Isoptin SR Tablets 467
Lamisil Tablets 2360
Nilandron Tablets 753
▲ PEG-Intron Powder for Injection (8%) 3140
Procanbid Extended-Release Tablets 2262
Tarka Tablets (Several cases) 508

Pain, salivary gland
Evoxac Capsules (1% to 3%) 1217

Pain, shoulder
Brevibloc Injection (Less than 1%) 858
Cozaar Tablets (Less than 1%) 2067
Crixivan Capsules (Less than 2%) 2070
Engerix-B Vaccine (Less than 1%) 1517
Hytrin Capsules (At least 1%) 464
Hyzaar 2109
Klonopin Tablets (Infrequent) 2983
Lexxel Tablets (Infrequent) 608
Lodosyn Tablets 1251
Mevacor Tablets (0.5% to 1.0%) 2132
Moduretic Tablets 2138
Prinivil Tablets (0.3% to 1.0%) 2164
Prinzide Tablets (0.3% to 1%) 2168
Recombivax HB (Less than 1%) 2178
Serevent Inhalation Aerosol (1% to 3%) 1633
Sinemet Tablets 1253
Sinemet CR Tablets (1.0%) 1255
Tonocard Tablets (Less than 1%) 649
Zestoretic Tablets (0.3% to 1%) 695
Zestril Tablets (0.3% to 1.0%) 698
Zofran Injection (2%) 1698

Pain, skin
▲ Tazorac Gel (10% to 30%) 556

Pain, stomach
(*see under* Stomachache)

Pain, substernal
Aerolate 1361
Evoxac Capsules (Less than 1%) 1217
Levaquin Injection (Less than 0.5%) 2537
Sonata Capsules (Infrequent) 3591
Tenex Tablets (3% or less) 2942
Teveten Tablets (Less than 1%) 3327
Topamax Sprinkle Capsules (Rare) 2590
Topamax Tablets (Rare) 2590

Unasyn for Injection (Less than 1%) 2728

Pain, testicular
Caverject Sterile Powder (Less than 1%) 2777
Lupron Depot 7.5 mg (Less than 5%) 3284
Lupron Injection (Less than 5%) 3279
▲ MUSE Urethral Suppository (5%) 3335
Neurontin Capsules (Rare) 2655
Neurontin Oral Solution (Rare) 2655
Neurontin Tablets (Rare) 2655
Prilosec Delayed-Release Capsules (Less than 1%) 628
Propecia Tablets 2172
Proscar Tablets 2175
Rescriptor Tablets 526
▲ Viadur Implant (3.8%) 912

Pain, thoracic spine
▲ Chemet Capsules (5.2% to 15.7%) 3078
Primaxin I.M. 2158
Primaxin I.V. (Less than 0.2%) 2160

Pain, throat
DDAVP Nasal Spray 738
DDAVP Rhinal Tube 738
Desmopressin Acetate Rhinal Tube 1345

Pain, trunk
Diprivan Injectable Emulsion (Less than 1%) 667
▲ Epogen for Injection (3%) 582
Floxin I.V. (1% to 3%) 2526
Floxin Tablets (1% to 3%) 2529
▲ Leustatin Injection (6%) 2495
▲ Procrit for Injection (3%) 2502
Requip Tablets (Infrequent) 1621

Pain, tumor site
▲ Aromasin Tablets (8%) 2769
Herceptin I.V. 1414
Navelbine Injection 1604
Nolvadex Tablets 678

Pain, upper extremities
Aceon Tablets (2 mg, 4 mg, 8 mg) (0.2% to 2.8%) 3249
Cipro I.V. (1% or less) 893
Engerix-B Vaccine (Less than 1%) 1517
Hivid Tablets (Less than 1%) 2975
Lopid Tablets 2650
Midamor Tablets (Less than or equal to 1%) 2136
Moduretic Tablets 2138
Prinivil Tablets (0.3% to 1.0%) 2164
ProSom Tablets (Infrequent) 500
Rifamate Capsules 767
Thalomid Capsules 1154
Timolide Tablets 2187
Timoptic in Ocudose 2192
Timoptic Sterile Ophthalmic Solution 2190

Pain, urethral
Avonex 1013
Ceftin Tablets (0.1% to 1%) 1898
Cerebyx Injection (Infrequent) 2619
Mirapex Tablets (1% or more) 2834
Permax Tablets (Rare) 1299
Protonix I.V. (Less than 1%) 3580
Protonix Tablets (Less than 1%) 3577
Salagen Tablets (Less than 1%) 2229
▲ Valstar Sterile Solution for Intravesical Instillation (3%) 1175

Pain, urinary bladder
Duragesic Transdermal System (Less than 1%) 1786
Effexor Tablets (Infrequent) 3495
Effexor XR Capsules (Infrequent) 3499
Hivid Tablets (Less than 1%) 2975
▲ Rapamune Oral Solution and Tablets (3% to 20%) 3584
ReoPro Vials (0.1%) 1958
Sonata Capsules (Infrequent) 3591
▲ TheraCys Injection (7%) 823
Tice BCG, BCG Live 2489
▲ Valstar Sterile Solution for Intravesical Instillation (3%) 1175
Zonegran Capsules (Rare) 1307

Pain, urinary tract
Trileptal Oral Suspension 2407
Trileptal Tablets 2407

Pain, vaginal
Cleocin Vaginal Cream (Less than 1%) 2788
Cleocin Vaginal Ovules (1.9%) 2789
▲ Estring Vaginal Ring (5%) 2811
Floxin I.V. (Less than 1%) 2526
Hivid Tablets (Less than 1%) 2975
Neurontin Capsules (Rare) 2655
Neurontin Oral Solution (Rare) 2655
Neurontin Tablets (Rare) 2655
Prostin E2 Suppositories 2852
Vantin Tablets and Oral Suspension (Less than 1%) 2860

Pain, vulva
DDAVP Injection 4 mcg/mL (Infrequent) 737
Desmopressin Acetate Injection (Infrequent) 1344
Stimate Nasal Spray 796
▲ Terazol 3 Vaginal Suppositories (4.2% of 284 patients) 2587

Pain at application site
▲ Aldara Cream, 5% (Up to 12%) 1978
Cleocin Vaginal Ovules (Less than 1%) 2789
▲ Condylox Gel (11.5% to 23.7%) 2436
Loprox Gel 2022
Nystop Topical Powder USP (More common) 2608
▲ Sulfamylon Cream (One of two most frequent) 1011
Zovirax Ointment 1707

Pain at injection site
▲ ActHIB Vaccine (Among most common) 798
Actimmune 1772
Actiq (Less than 1%) 1184
Adagen Injection (Two patients) 1331
▲ Alferon N Injection (12%) 1770
Amicar Injection 3608
Amicar Syrup 3608
Amicar Tablets 3608
Amphotec (1% to 5%) 1774
Ancef for Injection (Infrequent) 1474
Ancef Injection (Infrequent) 1474
Anzemet Injection 719
AquaMEPHYTON Injection 2042
▲ Aredia for Injection (Up to 41%) 2309
▲ Ativan Injection (17%) 3478
Attenuvax 2044
Avonex 1013
▲ Azactam for Injection (1.5% to 12%) 1276
BayGam 914
BayHep B 915
Bicillin C-R 900/300 Injection 2240
Bicillin C-R Injection 2238
Bicillin L-A Injection 2242
▲ Botox Purified Neurotoxin Complex (2% to 10%) 549
Brethine Ampuls (0.5 to 2.6%) 2314
Brevital Sodium for Injection, USP 1815
Calcijex Injection (Occasional) 411
Calcium Disodium Versenate Injection 1980
Cardene I.V. (0.7%) 3485
Cefizox for Intramuscular or Intravenous Use (1% to 5%) 1390
Cefobid Intravenous/Intramuscular (Occasional) 2671
Cefobid Pharmacy Bulk Package - Not for Direct Infusion (Occasional) 2673
Ceptaz for Injection 1499
Cerebyx Injection (Frequent) 2619
Cipro I.V. (1% or less) 893
▲ Claforan Injection (4.3%) 732
Cleocin Phosphate Sterile Solution 2785
▲ Comvax (23.9% to 34.5%) 2056
▲ Copaxone for Injection (73%) 3306
Delatestryl Injection (Rare) 1151
Demerol 3079
Depacon Injection (2.6%) 416
Depo-Provera Contraceptive Injection (Fewer than 1%) 2798
Desferal Vials .... [illegible]
Dilaudid-HP (Rare) 443
▲ Diprivan Injectable Emulsion (10% to 17.6%) 667
Doxil Injection (Less than 1%) 566
Edecrin (Occasional) 2091
▲ Enbrel for Injection (37%) 1752
▲ Enbrel for Injection (37%) 3504
Engerix-B Vaccine (Less than 1%) 1517
Factrel (Occasional) 3633
▲ Flolan for Injection (13%) 1528
Fluorescite Injection .... ⊙211
FluShield Influenza Vaccine 3521
Follistim for Injection (1.7%) 2465
Fortaz 1541
Foscavir Injection (Between 1% and 5%) 605
Fragmin Injection (Up to 4.5%) 2814
▲ Gammagard S/D (16%) 845
Genotropin Lyophilized Powder (Infrequent) 2818
▲ Geref for Injection (Less than 6%) 3215
Gonal-F for Injection (2.5%) 3216
Humatrope Vials and Cartridges (Infrequent) 1930
Humegon for Injection 2468
▲ Hyalgan Solution (23%) 3080
Imitrex Injection 1549
▲ Imovax Rabies Vaccine (About 25%) 807
▲ Infanrix Vaccine (0.9% to 10.5%) 1562
INFeD Injection 3388
▲ Infergen (8% to 9%) 1777
Innohep Injection 1248
Intron A for Injection (Less than 5%) 3120
▲ IPOL Vaccine (13%) 809
Kefzol Vials, ADD-Vantage (Infrequent) 1951
Lantus Injection (2.7%) 742
▲ Leustatin Injection (9% to 19%) 2495
Levaquin Injection (2.7%) 2537
Lovenox Injection (2%) 746
▲ LYMErix Vaccine (21.87%) 1592
Mandol Vials (Infrequent) 1953
Maxipime for Injection (0.6%) 1285
Mepergan Injection 3539
Merrem I.V. (0.4%) 673
Meruvax II 2130
▲ Myobloc Injectable Solution (12% to 16%) 1291
▲ Nabi-HB (12%) 2295
Naropin Injection (Less than 1%) 612
Natrecor for Injection (At least 1%) 3189
▲ Navelbine Injection (Up to 13%) 1604
Nebcin Vials, Hyporets & ADD-Vantage 1955
Novantrone for Injection 1760
Novarel for Injection 1347
Nubain Injection 1323
▲ Nutropin Depot for Injectable Suspension (43% to 47%) 1423
Nutropin for Injection (Infrequent) 1417
Oncaspar (Greater than 1% but less than 5%) 756
▲ Orgaran Injection (7.6% to 13.7%) 2480
▲ Ovidrel for Injection (7.6% to 8.1%) 3220
Liquid PedvaxHIB 2148
Pergonal for Injection 3223
Pipracil (2%) 1866
▲ Pneumovax 23 (Common) 2156
▲ Pnu-Imune 23 (72%) 1868
Pregnyl for Injection 2482
Primaxin I.M. (1.2%) 2158
Primaxin I.V. (0.7%) 2160
Protonix I.V. (Greater than 1%) 3580
▲ Rabies Vaccine RabAvert (84%) 1203
Recombivax HB (Equal to or greater than 1%) 2178
ReoPro Vials (0.1%) 1958
Repronex for Intramuscular and Subcutaneous Injection 1347
Retrovir IV Infusion (Infrequent) 1629
Rituxan for Infusion (1% to 5%) 1750
Rituxan I.V. (1% to 5%) 1428
Robaxin Injectable 2938
Rocephin Injectable Vials, ADD-Vantage, Galaxy, Bulk (1%) 2993
Roferon-A Injection (Less than 1%) 2996
▲ Romazicon Injection (3% to 9%) 3000
Saizen for Injection (Infrequent) 3225
▲ Sandostatin Injection (7.7%) 2394
▲ Sandostatin LAR Depot (2% to 11%) 2395
▲ Serostim for Injection (1% to 10%) 3229
▲ Synercid I.V. (40% to 44.7%) 775
Synvisc 3596
Testopel Pellets 3610
Testred Capsules, 10 mg 1746
Thioplex for Injection 1765
Timentin Injection- ADD-Vantage Vial 1661
Timentin Injection-Galaxy Container 1664
Timentin Injection-Pharmacy Bulk Package 1666
Timentin for Intravenous Administration 1658
Toradol (2%) 3018
Tripedia Vaccine 817
▲ Trisenox Injection (20%) 1158
Tubersol Diagnostic Antigen 3628
▲ TYPHIM Vi Vaccine (Up to 56%) 825
▲ Unasyn for Injection (3% to 16%) 2728
Vancocin HCl, Vials & ADD-Vantage 1970
▲ Vaqta (1.2% to 51.1%) 2199
▲ Varivax (19.3% to 32.5%; less than 0.05%) 2202
▲ Versed Injection (3.7% to 5.0%) 3027
Zantac Injection 1688
▲ Zinecard for Injection (12% to 13%) 2869
▲ Zithromax for IV Infusion (6.5%) 2748
▲ Zofran Injection (4%) 1698
Zosyn (0.2%) 1890
Zosyn in Galaxy Containers (0.2%) 1894

Pain secondary to eczema
Bactroban Cream (One report) 1494

Pain with coitus
Condylox Topical Solution (Less than 5%) 2437

Pain, uterine

Palilalia
Nardil Tablets (Less common) 2653

Pallor
Advair Diskus 100/50 1448
Advair Diskus 250/50 1448
Advair Diskus 500/50 1448
Allegra-D Extended-Release Tablets 714
Ambien Tablets (Infrequent) 3191
Azulfidine EN-tabs Tablets 2775
Bicillin C-R 900/300 Injection 2240

Bicillin C-R Injection........ 2238
Bicillin L-A Injection........ 2242
Brevibloc Injection (Less than 1%)........ 858
Buprenex Injectable (Infrequent)........ 2918
Captopril Tablets (2 to 5 of 1000 patients)........ 2281
Cardura Tablets (Less than 0.5%)........ 2668
Catapres Tablets........ 1037
Catapres-TTS (0.5% or less)........ 1038
▲ CellCept Capsules (3% to 10%)........ 2951
▲ CellCept Intravenous (3% to 10%)........ 2951
▲ CellCept Oral Suspension (3% to 10%)........ 2951
▲ CellCept Tablets (3% to 10%)........ 2951
Claritin-D 12 Hour Extended Release Tablets........ 3102
Claritin-D 24 Hour Extended Release Tablets........ 3104
Clorpres Tablets........ 1002
Clozaril Tablets (Less than 1%)........ 2319
Combipres Tablets........ 1040
Cytotec Tablets (Infrequent)........ 3202
Dapsone Tablets USP........ 1780
Diphtheria & Tetanus Toxoids Adsorbed Purogenated for Pediatric Use........ 1857
Duraclon Injection........ 3057
Effexor Tablets (Rare)........ 3495
Effexor XR Capsules (Rare)........ 3499
▲ Emla (37%)........ 602
Enbrel for Injection........ 1752
Enbrel for Injection........ 3504
EpiPen........ 1236
Etrafon (Occasional)........ 3115
Evoxac Capsules (Less than 1%)........ 1217
▲ Flolan for Injection (21% to 32%)........ 1528
Flumadine (Less than 0.3%)........ 1370
Gabitril Tablets (Infrequent)........ 1189
Helixate Concentrate........ 788
Imitrex Injection (Rare)........ 1549
Imitrex Nasal Spray (Rare)........ 1554
Imitrex Tablets (Infrequent)........ 1558
Kadian Capsules (Less than 3%)........ 1335
Kogenate FS........ 936
Luvox Tablets (25, 50, 100 mg) (Infrequent)........ 3256
▲ Miacalcin Nasal Spray (10.6%)........ 2375
Nitrolingual Pumpspray........ 1355
Nitrostat Tablets........ 2658
Paxil (Rare)........ 1609
Prozac Pulvules, Liquid, and Weekly Capsules (Rare)........ 1238
ReoPro Vials (0.1%)........ 1958
Rescriptor Tablets (Less than 2%)........ 526
Risperdal (Rare)........ 1796
Rynatan Tablets........ 3351
Sarafem Pulvules (Rare)........ 1962
Septra Suspension........ 2265
Septra Tablets........ 2265
Septra DS Tablets........ 2265
▲ Serevent Diskus (9%)........ 1637
Serzone Tablets (Rare)........ 1104
Survanta Intratracheal Suspension (Less than 1%)........ 3053
Tetanus & Diphtheria Toxoids Adsorbed for Adult Use........ 1880
Thioridazine Hydrochloride Tablets........ 2289
Tonocard Tablets (Less than 1%)........ 649
Toradol (1% or less)........ 3018
Trilafon (Occasional)........ 3160
▲ Trisenox Injection (10%)........ 1158
▲ Vesanoid Capsules (6%)........ 3037
Vistide Injection........ 1445
Wellbutrin Tablets (Rare)........ 1680
WinRho SDF........ 2297
Zoloft (Rare)........ 2751
Zyprexa Tablets........ 1973
Zyprexa ZYDIS Orally Disintegrating Tablets........ 1973
Zyrtec (Less than 2%)........ 2756
Zyrtec-D 12 Hour Extended Relief Tablets (Less than 2%)........ 2758

Pallor, optic disc

Aralen Tablets........ 3075
Plaquenil Tablets........ 3082

Palmar-plantar erythrodysesthesia syndrome

▲ Doxil Injection (3.4% to 37.4%)........ 566
▲ Xeloda Tablets (11% to 13%)........ 3039

Palpebra superior, elevation

Iopidine Sterile Ophthalmic Solution (Less than 2%)........ ⊙ 212

Palpitations

Accupril Tablets (0.5% to 1.0%)........ 2611
Accuretic Tablets (0.5% to 1%)........ 2614
Accutane Capsules........ 2944
Aceon Tablets (2 mg, 4 mg, 8 mg) (0.9% to 1.1%)........ 3249
Aciphex Tablets........ 1267
Aciphex Tablets........ 1783
Actiq (1% or greater)........ 1184
Adalat CC Tablets (Less than 1.0%)........ 877
Adderall Tablets........ 3231
Adderall XR Capsules
Adenocard Injection (Less than 1%)........ 1380
Adenoscan (Less than 1%)........ 1381
Adipex-P........ 1406
Advair Diskus 100/50 (1% to 3%)........ 1448
Advair Diskus 250/50 (1% to 3%)........ 1448
Advair Diskus 500/50 (1% to 3%)........ 1448
▲ Aerobid/Aerobid-M (3% to 9%)........ 1363
Aerolate........ 1361
Aggrenox Capsules (Less than 1%)........ 1026
▲ Agrylin Capsules (26.1%)........ 3232
Allegra-D Extended-Release Tablets (1.9%)........ 714
Alphagan Ophthalmic Solution (Less than 3%)........ 545
Altace Capsules (Less than 1%)........ 2233
Alupent (1% to 4%)........ 1029
Ambien Tablets (2%)........ 3191
Amerge Tablets (Infrequent)........ 1467
Anaprox Tablets (Less than 3%)........ 2967
Anaprox DS Tablets (Less than 3%)........ 2967
Anzemet Injection (Rare)........ 719
Anzemet Tablets (Rare)........ 722
Arava Tablets (1% to 3%)........ 724
Arthrotec Tablets (Rare)........ 3195
Atacand Tablets (0.5% or greater)........ 595
Atacand HCT Tablets (0.5% or greater)........ 597
Atrovent Inhalation Aerosol (1.8%)........ 1030
Atrovent Inhalation Solution (Less than 3%)........ 1031
Atrovent Nasal Spray 0.06% (Less than 1%)........ 1033
Avelox Tablets (0.05% to 1%)........ 879
Avonex........ 1013
Axert Tablets (Infrequent)........ 2772
Benadryl Parenteral........ 2617
Betagan........ ⊙ 228
▲ Betapace Tablets (3% to 14%)........ 950
▲ Betaseron for SC Injection (8%)........ 988
Betimol Ophthalmic Solution........ ⊙ 324
Bicillin C-R 900/300 Injection........ 2240
Bicillin C-R Injection........ 2238
Bicillin L-A Injection........ 2242
Blocadren Tablets........ 2046
Bontril Slow-Release Capsules........ 576
▲ Brethine Ampuls (7.8% to 22.9%)........ 2314
▲ Brethine Tablets (5%)........ 2313
Bromfed Capsules (Extended-Release)........ 2269
Bromfed-PD Capsules (Extended-Release)........ 2269
Captopril Tablets (Approximately 1 of 100 patients)........ 2281
Cardizem Injectable........ 1018
Cardizem Lyo-Ject Syringe........ 1018
Cardizem Monovial........ 1018
Cardizem CD Capsules (Less than 1%)........ 1016
Cardura Tablets (1.2% to 2%)........ 2668
▲ Carnitor Injection (3% to 8%)........ 3242
Carteolol Hydrochloride Ophthalmic Solution USP, 1% (Occasional)........ ⊙ 258
Cataflam Tablets (Less than 1%)........ 2315
Catapres Tablets (About 5 in 1,000 patients)........ 1037
Catapres-TTS (0.5% or less)........ 1038
Ceclor CD Tablets (0.1% to 1%)........ 1279
Celebrex Capsules (0.1% to 1.9%)........ 2676
Celebrex Capsules (0.1% to 1.9%)........ 2780
Celexa (At least 2%)........ 1365
▲ CellCept Capsules (3%)........ 2951
▲ CellCept Intravenous (3%)........ 2951
▲ CellCept Oral Suspension (3%)........ 2951
▲ CellCept Tablets (3%)........ 2951
▲ Cenestin Tablets (21%)........ 1263
Cerebyx Injection (Infrequent)........ 2619
Cipro I.V. (1% or less)........ 893
Cipro I.V. Pharmacy Bulk Package (Less than 1%)........ 897
Cipro (Less than 1%)........ 887
Claritin (At least one patient)........ 3100
Claritin-D 12 Hour Extended Release Tablets (Less frequent)........ 3102
Claritin-D 24 Hour Extended Release Tablets (Fewer than 2%)........ 3104
Clinoril Tablets (Less than 1 in 100)........ 2053
Clomid Tablets........ 735
Clorpres Tablets (About 5 in 1,000)........ 1002
Clozaril Tablets (Less than 1%)........ 2319
Cognex Capsules (Infrequent)........ 1351
Colazal Capsules........ 3069
Combipres Tablets (About 5 in 1,000)........ 1040
Combivent Inhalation Aerosol (Less than 2%)........ 1041
Concerta Extended-Release Tablets........ 1998
Concerta Tablets........ 561
▲ Copaxone for Injection (17%)........ 3306
Coreg Tablets (More than 2%)........ 1508
Corlopam Injection (0.5% to 5%)........ 412
Corvert Injection (1.0%)........ 2793
Cosopt Sterile Ophthalmic Solution........ 2065
Covera-HS Tablets (Less than 2%)........ 3199
Cozaar Tablets (Less than 1%)........ 2067
Crixivan Capsules (Less than 2%)........ 2070
DaunoXome Injection (Less than or equal to 5%)........ 1442
Demerol........ 3079
Depacon Injection (1% to 5%)........ 416
Depakene (1% to 5%)........ 421
Depakote Sprinkle Capsules (1% to 5%)........ 426
Depakote Tablets (1% to 5%)........ 430
Depakote ER Tablets (Greater than 1%)........ 436
Desoxyn Tablets........ 440
Dexedrine........ 1512
DextroStat Tablets........ 3236
Digitek Tablets (1%)........ 1003
Dilaudid Oral Liquid........ 445
Dilaudid Tablets - 8 mg........ 445
Dilaudid-HP (Less frequent)........ 443
Diovan Capsules........ 2337
Diovan HCT Tablets (Greater than 0.2%)........ 2338
Dipentum Capsules (Rare)........ 2803
Ditropan XL Extended Release Tablets (2% to 5%)........ 564
Dobutrex Solution Vials (1% to 3%)........ 1914
Dolobid Tablets (Rare)........ 2088
Dolophine Hydrochloride Tablets........ 3056
Donnatal........ 2929
Donnatal Extentabs........ 2930
Donnatal Tablets........ 2929
▲ Dostinex Tablets (1% to less than 10%)........ 2804
Doxil Injection (Less than 1%)........ 566
DuoNeb Inhalation Solution........ 1233
Duraclon Injection (0.5%)........ 3057
Dynabac Tablets (0.1% to 1%)........ 2269
DynaCirc Capsules (1% to 5.1%)........ 2921
DynaCirc CR Tablets (1.2%)........ 2923
EC-Naprosyn Delayed-Release Tablets (Less than 3%)........ 2967
Effexor Tablets........ 3495
Eldepryl Capsules (1 of 49 patients)........ 3266
Enalaprilat Injection........ 863
Engerix-B Vaccine........ 1517
EpiPen........ 1236
Ery-Tab Tablets (Isolated reports)........ 448
Erythrocin Stearate Filmtab Tablets (Isolated reports)........ 452
Erythromycin Base Filmtab Tablets (Isolated reports)........ 454
Erythromycin Delayed-Release Capsules, USP (Isolated reports)........ 455
Etrafon........ 3115
Evoxac Capsules (1% to 3%)........ 1217
Exelon Capsules (Frequent)........ 2342
Exelon Oral Solution (Frequent)........ 2345
Extendryl........ 1361
Famotidine Injection (Infrequent)........ 866
Felbatol (Frequent)........ 3343
Feldene Capsules (Rare)........ 2685
Flexeril Tablets (Less than 1%)........ 572
Flexeril Tablets (Less than 1%)........ 2094
▲ Flolan for Injection (63%)........ 1528
Flomax Capsules (Infrequent)........ 1044
Flovent Diskus (1% to 3%)........ 3614
Floxin I.V. (Less than 1%)........ 2526
Floxin Tablets (Less than 1%)........ 2529
Flumadine (Less than 0.3%)........ 1370
Foradil Aerolizer........ 2354
Foscavir Injection (Between 1% and 5%)........ 605
Gabitril Tablets (Frequent)........ 1189
Gammar-P I.V........ 787
Gastrocrom Oral Concentrate (Less common)........ 1162
Glucophage Tablets (1% to 5%)........ 1080
Gonal-F for Injection........ 3216
Guaifed........ 2272
Hivid Tablets (Less than 1%)........ 2975
Hycomine Compound Tablets........ 1317
Hycotuss Expectorant Syrup........ 1318
▲ Hytrin Capsules (0.9% to 28%)........ 464
Hyzaar (1.4%)........ 2109
Imdur Tablets (Less than or equal to 5%)........ 1826
Imitrex Injection (Infrequent)........ 1549
Imitrex Nasal Spray (Infrequent)........ 1554
Imitrex Tablets (Up to 2%)........ 1558
Indapamide Tablets (Less than 5%)........ 2286
Indocin (Less than 1%)........ 2112
▲ Infergen (3% to 5%)........ 1777
Intron A for Injection (Less than 5%)........ 3120
Ionamin Capsules........ 1163
Iopidine Sterile Ophthalmic Solution........ ⊙ 212
Ismo Tablets (Fewer than 1%)........ 3524
Isoptin SR Tablets (1% or less)........ 467
Kadian Capsules (Less than 3%)........ 1335
Kaletra Capsules (Less than 2%)........ 471
Kaletra Oral Solution (Less than 2%)........ 471
Klonopin Tablets (Infrequent)........ 2983
Lamictal (1.0%)........ 1567
Lanoxicaps Capsules........ 1574
Lanoxin Injection........ 1581
Lanoxin Tablets........ 1587
Lanoxin Elixir Pediatric........ 1578
Lanoxin Injection Pediatric........ 1584
Levaquin........ 2537
Levbid Extended-Release Tablets........ 3172
Levo-Dromoran........ 1734
Levoxyl Tablets........ 1819
Levsin/Levsinex/Levbid........ 3172
Lexxel Tablets........ 608
Limbitrol........ 1738
Lipitor Tablets (Less than 2%)........ 2639
Lipitor Tablets (Less than 2%)........ 2696
Lodine (Less than 1%)........ 3528
Lodine XL Extended-Release Tablets (Less than 1%)........ 3530
Lodosyn Tablets........ 1251
Lotensin HCT Tablets (0.3% to 1%)........ 2367
Lotrel Capsules (0.5% to 0.3%)........ 2370
Lufyllin Tablets........ 3347
Lufyllin-400 Tablets........ 3347
Lufyllin-GG Elixir........ 3348
Lufyllin-GG Tablets........ 3348
▲ Lupron Depot 3.75 mg (Among most frequent)........ 3281
Lupron Depot–3 Month 11.25 mg (Less than 5%)........ 3285
▲ Luvox Tablets (25, 50, 100 mg) (3%)........ 3256
Marinol Capsules (Greater than 1%)........ 3325
Mavik Tablets (0.3% to 1.0%)........ 478
Maxair Autohaler (1.3% to 1.7%)........ 1981
Maxair Inhaler (1.3% to 1.7%)........ 1984
Maxalt Tablets (Frequent)........ 2120
Maxalt-MLT Orally Disintegrating Tablets (Frequent)........ 2120
Megace Oral Suspension (1% to 3%)........ 1124
Mepergan Injection........ 3539
Meridia Capsules (2%)........ 481
Metadate CD Capsules........ 1164
Metadate ER Tablets........ 1167
Methylin Tablets........ 1995
Methylin ER Tablets........ 1995
▲ Mexitil Capsules (4.3% to 7.5%)........ 1047
Miacalcin Nasal Spray (Less than 1%)........ 2375
Micardis Tablets (More than 0.3%)........ 1049
Micardis HCT Tablets........ 1051
Midamor Tablets (Less than or equal to 1%)........ 2136
Migranal Nasal Spray (Infrequent)........ 2376
Miltown Tablets........ 3349
▲ Minipress Capsules (5.3%)........ 2699
▲ Minizide Capsules (5.3%)........ 2700
Mirapex Tablets (Less than 1%)........ 2834
Mobic Tablets (Less than 2%)........ 1054
Moduretic Tablets........ 2138
Monopril Tablets (0.2% to 1.0%)........ 1091
Motrin Suspension, Oral Drops, Chewable Tablets, and Caplets (Less than 1%)........ 2002
MS Contin Tablets (Less frequent)........ 2896
MSIR (Less frequent)........ 2898
Mykrox Tablets (Less than 2%)........ 1168
Naprelan Tablets (Less than 3%)........ 1293
Naprosyn Suspension (Less than 3%)........ 2967
Naprosyn Tablets (Less than 3%)........ 2967
▲ Neumega for Injection (14%)........ 1434
Neurontin Capsules (Infrequent)........ 2655
Neurontin Oral Solution (Infrequent)........ 2655
Neurontin Tablets (Infrequent)........ 2655
Niaspan Extended-Release Tablets........ 1846
Nicotrol Inhaler (Occasional)........ 2840
▲ Nicotrol Nasal Spray (4%)........ 2843
Nicotrol Patch........ 2840
Nimotop Capsules (Less than 1%)........ 904
Nitrostat Tablets (Occasional)........ 2658
Norflex........ 1987
Noroxin Tablets (Less frequent)........ 2145
Norpramin Tablets........ 755
Norvasc Tablets (0.7% to 4.5%)........ 2704
Norvir Capsules (Less than 2%)........ 487
Norvir Oral Solution (Less than 2%)........ 487
NuLev Orally Disintegrating Tablets........ 3176
Numorphan........ 1324
Ocupress Ophthalmic Solution, 1% Sterile (Occasional)........ ⊙ 303
OptiPranolol Metipranolol Ophthalmic Solution 0.3% (A small number of patients)........ ⊙ 263
Oramorph SR Tablets (Less frequent)........ 3062
Orap Tablets........ 1407
Orudis Capsules (Less than 1%)........ 3548
Oruvail Capsules (Less than 1%)........ 3548
Parnate Tablets........ 1607
Paxil (2% to 3%)........ 1609
Pediazole Suspension........ 3050
Pentasa Capsules (Less than 1%)........ 3239
Pepcid Injection (Infrequent)........ 2153
Pepcid for Oral Suspension (Infrequent)........ 2150
Pepcid RPD Orally Disintegrating Tablets (Infrequent)........ 2150
Pepcid Tablets (Infrequent)........ 2150

Periactin Tablets 2155
Permax Tablets (2.1%) 1299
Persantine Tablets (Rare) 1057
Phenergan with Codeine Syrup 3557
Phenergan VC with Codeine Syrup 3561
Plavix Tablets (1% to 2.5%) 1097
Plavix Tablets (1% to 2.5%) 3084
Plendil Extended-Release Tablets (0.4% to 2.5%) 623
▲ Pletal Tablets (5% to 10%) 2605
▲ Pletal Tablets (5% to 10%) 2848
Ponstel Capsules (Rare) 1356
Prandin Tablets (0.5, 1, and 2 mg) (Less than or equal to 1%) 2432
Prevacid Delayed-Release Capsules (Less than 1%) 3292
PREVPAC (Less than 1%) 3298
Prilosec Delayed-Release Capsules (Less than 1%) 628
Primaxin I.M. 2158
Primaxin I.V. (Less than 0.2%) 2160
Prinivil Tablets (0.3% to 1.0%) 2164
Prinzide Tablets (0.3% to 1%) 2168
▲ Procardia Capsules (2% or less to 7%) 2708
▲ Procardia XL Extended Release Tablets (Less than 3% to 7%) 2710
Prometrium Capsules (100 mg, 200 mg) (Less than 5%) 3261
ProSom Tablets (Infrequent) 500
Protonix I.V. (Less than 1%) 3580
Protonix Tablets (Less than 1%) 3577
Protopic Ointment (Greater than or equal to 1%) 1397
▲ Proventil Inhalation Aerosol (Less than 10%) 3142
▲ Proventil Repetabs Tablets (5% to 8%) 3148
Proventil HFA Inhalation Aerosol (Less than 3%) 3150
Provigil Tablets (At least 1%) 1193
Prozac Pulvules, Liquid, and Weekly Capsules (2%) 1238
▲ Quinidex Extentabs (7%) 2933
▲ Rapamune Oral Solution and Tablets (3% to 20%) 3584
Recombivax HB (Less than 1%) 2178
ReFacto Vials 1437
Relafen Tablets (Less than 1%) 1617
Remicade for IV Injection (Less than 2%) 1178
Reminyl Oral Solution (Infrequent) 1792
Reminyl Tablets (Infrequent) 1792
ReoPro Vials (0.7%) 1958
▲ Requip Tablets (3%) 1621
Rescriptor Tablets (Less than 2%) 526
Rhinocort Aqua Nasal Spray (Rare) 642
Rifater Tablets 769
Rilutek Tablets (0.4% to 1.2%) 772
Risperdal (Infrequent) 1796
Ritalin 2387
Robinul Forte Tablets 1358
Robinul Injectable 2940
Robinul Tablets 1358
Rocephin Injectable Vials, ADD-Vantage, Galaxy, Bulk (Rare) 2993
Roferon-A Injection (Less than 3%) 2996
▲ Romazicon Injection (3% to 9%) 3000
Roxanol 3066
Roxicodone Tablets (Less than 3%) 3067
Rynatan Tablets 3351
Rythmol Tablets 150 mg, 225 mg, 300 mg (2% to 3.4%) 502
Salagen Tablets (Less than 1%) 2229
Sandostatin Injection (Less than 1%) 2394
▲ Sandostatin LAR Depot (5% to 15%) 2395
▲ Sarafem Pulvules (3%) 1962
Semprex-D Capsules 1172
Serentil 1057
Serevent Inhalation Aerosol (1% to 3%) 1633
Serophene Tablets 3226
Seroquel Tablets (Frequent) 684
Serzone Tablets 1104
Sinemet Tablets 1253
Sinemet CR Tablets 1255
Sonata Capsules (Infrequent) 3591
Stadol NS Nasal Spray (1% or greater) 1108
Stimate Nasal Spray 796
▲ Sular Tablets (3%) 688
Surmontil Capsules 3595
Sustiva Capsules (Less than 2%) 1258
Synarel Nasal Solution for Endometriosis (Less than 1%) 3205
Synercid I.V. (Less than 1%) 775
▲ Tambocor Tablets (6.1%) 1990
Tarka Tablets (0.3% or more) 508
Tasmar Tablets (Frequent) 3010
Tenex Tablets (3% or less) 2942
Tequin Injection (0.1% to 3%) 1110
Tequin Tablets (0.1% to 3%) 1110
Teveten Tablets (Less than 1%) 3327
Thalomid Capsules 1154
Theo-Dur Extended-Release Tablets 1835
Tiazac Capsules (Less than 2%) 1378
Tikosyn Capsules (Greater than 2%) 2717
Timolide Tablets 2187
Timolol GFS ⊙266
Timoptic in Ocudose (Less frequent) 2192
Timoptic Sterile Ophthalmic Solution (Less frequent) 2190
Timoptic-XE Sterile Ophthalmic Gel Forming Solution 2194
Tonocard Tablets (0.4% to 1.8%) 649
Topamax Sprinkle Capsules (Frequent) 2590
Topamax Tablets (Frequent) 2590
Toprol-XL Tablets (About 1 of 100 patients) 651
Toradol (1% or less) 3018
Trental Tablets 784
Tricor Capsules, Micronized (Less than 1%) 513
Trileptal Oral Suspension 2407
Trileptal Tablets 2407
▲ Trisenox Injection (10%) 1158
Trovan (Less than 1%) 2722
Twinrix Vaccine 1674
Ultracet Tablets (Less than 1%) 2597
Ultram Tablets (Infrequent) 2600
Uni-Dur Extended-Release Tablets 1841
Uniretic Tablets (Less than 1%) 3178
Unithroid Tablets 3445
Univasc Tablets (Less than 1%) 3181
Vantin Tablets and Oral Suspension (Less than 1%) 2860
▲ Vascor Tablets (2.27% to 6.52%) 2602
Vaseretic Tablets (0.5% to 2.0%) 2204
Vasotec I.V. Injection 2207
Vasotec Tablets (0.5% to 1.0%) 2210
Ventolin Inhalation Aerosol and Refill (Less than 1%) 1679
Ventolin HFA Inhalation Aerosol (Less than 3%) 3618
Verelan Capsules (1% or less) 3184
Verelan PM Capsules (2% or less) 3186
Viagra Tablets (Less than 2%) 2732
Vicodin Tuss Expectorant 519
Vicoprofen Tablets (Less than 3%) 520
Vioxx (Greater than 0.1% to 1.9%) 2213
Vivactil Tablets 2217
Vivactil Tablets 2446
Volmax Extended-Release Tablets (2.4%) 2276
Voltaren Tablets (Less than 1%) 2315
Voltaren-XR Tablets (Less than 1%) 2315
▲ Wellbutrin Tablets (3.7%) 1680
▲ Wellbutrin SR Sustained-Release Tablets (2% to 6%) 1684
▲ Xanax Tablets (7.7%) 2865
Zaroxolyn Tablets 1177
Zebeta Tablets 1885
▲ Zemplar Injection (3%) 522
Zephrex Tablets 3091
Zephrex LA Tablets 3092
Zestoretic Tablets (0.3% to 1%) 695
Zestril Tablets (0.3% to 1.0%) 698
Ziac Tablets 1887
Zithromax (1% or less) 2743
Zithromax for Oral Suspension, 300 mg, 600 mg, 900 mg, 1200 mg (1% or less) 2739
Zithromax Tablets, 250 mg (1% or less) 2739
Zithromax Tablets, 600 mg (1% or less) 2743
Zofran Injection 1698
Zoladex (1% or greater) 702
Zoladex 3-month 706
Zoloft (Frequent) 2751
Zomig Tablets (Less than 1% to 2%) 708
Zomig-ZMT Tablets (Less than 1% to 2%) 708
Zonegran Capsules (Infrequent) 1307
Zyban Sustained-Release Tablets (2%) 1710
Zyprexa Tablets (Infrequent) 1973
Zyprexa ZYDIS Orally Disintegrating Tablets (Infrequent) 1973
Zyrtec (Less than 2%) 2756
Zyrtec-D 12 Hour Extended Relief Tablets (Less than 2%) 2758

Palsies, skeletal muscles
Plaquenil Tablets 3082

Palsy, cranial nerve
Naropin Injection 612
Orthoclone OKT3 Sterile Solution (Less than 1%) 2498
Sensorcaine 643
Sensorcaine-MPF Injection 643

Palsy, extraocular
Protonix I.V. (Less than 1%) 3580
Protonix Tablets (Less than 1%) 3577

Palsy, nerve
Neurontin Capsules (Rare) 2655
Neurontin Oral Solution (Rare) 2655
Neurontin Tablets (Rare) 2655

Palsy, optic nerve
Symmetrel (0.1% to 1%) 1328

Palsy, peripheral nerve
Baycol Tablets 883
Lescol Capsules 2361
Lescol Capsules 2925
Lescol XL Tablets 2361
Lescol XL Tablets 2925
Mevacor Tablets 2132
Pravachol Tablets 1099
Zocor Tablets 2219

Pancolitis
Canasa Rectal Suppositories 829
Rowasa Rectal Suspension Enema 4.0 grams/unit (60 mL) 3264

Pancreatic disease, unspecified
Pulmozyme Inhalation Solution 1426

Pancreatic enzymes, increased
Norpramin Tablets 755

Pancreatic insufficiency
Remicade for IV Injection (Less than 2%) 1178

Pancreatitis
Accupril Tablets (Rare) 2611
Accuretic Tablets (0.5% to 1%) 2614
Accutane Capsules 2944
Aciphex Tablets 1267
Aciphex Tablets 1783
Actimmune (Rare) 1772
Activase I.V. 1410
Aggrenox Capsules 1026
Agrylin Capsules 3232
Aldoclor Tablets 2035
Aldomet Tablets 2037
Aldoril Tablets 2039
Altace Capsules (Less than 1%) 2233
Anaprox Tablets (Less than 1%) 2967
Anaprox DS Tablets (Less than 1%) 2967
Anzemet Injection (Rare) 719
Anzemet Tablets (Rare) 722
Aricept Tablets 1270
Aricept Tablets 2665
Arthrotec Tablets (Rare) 3195
Asacol Delayed-Release Tablets 2884
Atacand HCT Tablets 597
Atromid-S Capsules 3483
Avalide Tablets 1070
Azulfidine EN-tabs Tablets (Rare) 2775
Bactrim 2949
Baycol Tablets 883
Betaseron for SC Injection 988
Calcijex Injection 411
Campath Ampules 992
Canasa Rectal Suppositories 829
Captopril Tablets 2281
Carbatrol Capsules 3234
Cataflam Tablets (Less than 1%) 2315
Celebrex Capsules (Less than 0.1%) 2676
Celebrex Capsules (Less than 0.1%) 2780
Celestone Soluspan Injectable Suspension 3097
Celestone Syrup 3099
Celexa (At least 3 patients) 1365
CellCept Capsules 2951
CellCept Intravenous 2951
CellCept Oral Suspension 2951
CellCept Tablets 2951
Chibroxin Sterile Ophthalmic Solution 2051
Cipro I.V. (1% or less) 893
Cipro I.V. Pharmacy Bulk Package (Less than 1%) 897
Cipro 887
Clinoril Tablets (Less than 1 in 100) 2053
Clorpres Tablets 1002
Clozaril Tablets 2319
Cognex Capsules 1351
Colazal Capsules 3069
Combipres Tablets 1040
Combivir Tablets (Less than 0.5%) 1502
Copaxone for Injection (Infrequent) 3306
Cortifoam Rectal Foam 3170
Cortone Acetate Injectable Suspension 2059
Cortone Acetate Tablets 2061
Corzide 40/5 Tablets 2247
Corzide 80/5 Tablets 2247
Crixivan Capsules 2070
Cuprimine Capsules 2075
Cytovene 2959
Dapsone Tablets USP 1780
Decadron Elixir 2078
Decadron Tablets 2079
Decadron Phosphate Injection 2081
Declomycin Tablets 1855
Depacon Injection (1% to 5%) 416
Depakene 421
Depakote Sprinkle Capsules (1% to 5%) 426
Depakote Tablets (1% to 5%) 430
Depakote ER Tablets (1% to 5%) 436
Depen Titratable Tablets (Isolated cases) 3341
Depo-Medrol Injectable Suspension 2795
Diovan HCT Tablets 2338
Dipentum Capsules (Rare) 2803
Diprivan Injectable Emulsion (Very rare) 667
Diucardin Tablets 3494
Diuril Oral 2087
Diuril Sodium Intravenous 2086
Doxil Injection (Less than 1%) 566
Dyazide Capsules 1515
Dynacin Capsules 2019
EC-Naprosyn Delayed-Release Tablets (Less than 1%) 2967
Ecotrin Enteric Coated Aspirin Low, Regular and Maximum Strength Tablets 1715
Edecrin (Rare) 2091
Effexor Tablets 3495
Effexor XR Capsules 3499
Elspar for Injection 2092
Enalaprilat Injection 863
Enbrel for Injection (Infrequent) 1752
Enbrel for Injection (Infrequent) 3504
Epivir (Less than 0.5%) 1520
▲ Epivir-HBV (14% to 15%) 1524
Ergamisol Tablets (Less frequent) 1789
Estrace Vaginal Cream 3358
Estrace Tablets 3361
Exelon Capsules (Infrequent) 2342
Exelon Oral Solution (Infrequent) 2345
Felbatol 3343
Feldene Capsules (Rare) 2685
femhrt Tablets 2635
Florinef Acetate Tablets 2250
Fortovase Capsules (Less than 2%) 2970
Foscavir Injection (Between 1% and 5%) 605
Furosemide Tablets 2284
Gengraf Capsules (Rare) 457
Hectorol Capsules 1064
Hectorol Injection 1066
Herceptin I.V. (At least one of the 958 patients) 1414
Hivid Tablets (Rare) 2975
Humatrope Vials and Cartridges (Rare) 1930
Hydrocortone Tablets 2106
Hydrocortone Acetate Injectable Suspension 2103
Hydrocortone Phosphate Injection, Sterile 2105
HydroDIURIL Tablets 2108
Hyzaar 2109
Imitrex Injection 1549
Imitrex Nasal Spray (Rare) 1554
Imitrex Tablets 1558
Inderide Tablets 3517
Inderide LA Long-Acting Capsules 3519
Invirase Capsules (Rare) 2979
Kaletra Capsules (Less than 2%) 471
Kaletra Oral Solution (Less than 2%) 471
Lamictal 1567
Lescol Capsules 2361
Lescol Capsules 2925
Lescol XL Tablets 2361
Lescol XL Tablets 2925
Levaquin (Less than 0.3%) 2537
Lexxel Tablets 608
Lipitor Tablets (Less than 2%) 2639
Lipitor Tablets (Less than 2%) 2696
Lodine (Less than 1%) 3528
Lodine XL Extended-Release Tablets (Less than 1%) 3530
Lo/Ovral Tablets 3532
Lopid Tablets 2650
Lotensin Tablets (Less than 1%) 2365
Lotensin HCT Tablets (Rare) 2367
Lotrel Capsules (Rare) 2370
Luvox Tablets (25, 50, 100 mg) 3256
Macrobid Capsules 2889
Macrodantin Capsules 2891
Mavik Tablets (Rare) 478
Maxzide 1008
Mepron Suspension 1598
Mevacor Tablets 2132
Mexitil Capsules (Rare) 1047
Micardis HCT Tablets 1051
Microzide Capsules 3414
Minipress Capsules (Less than 1%) 2699
Minizide Capsules (Rare) 2700
Minocin Intravenous 1862
Minocin Oral Suspension 1865
Minocin Pellet-Filled Capsules 1863
M-M-R II 2118
Mobic Tablets (Less than 2%) 1054
Moduretic Tablets 2138
Monopril Tablets (0.2% to 1.0%) 1091
Monopril HCT 1094
Motofen Tablets 577
Motrin Suspension, Oral Drops, Chewable Tablets, and Caplets (Less than 1%) 2002
Mumpsvax 2141

Mykrox Tablets 1168
▲ Naprelan Tablets (3% to 9%) 1293
Naprosyn Suspension (Less than 1%) 2967
Naprosyn Tablets (Less than 1%) 2967
Navelbine Injection 1604
Neoral Soft Gelatin Capsules (Rare) 2380
Neoral Oral Solution (Rare) 2380
Neurontin Capsules (Rare) 2655
Neurontin Oral Solution (Rare) 2655
Neurontin Tablets (Rare) 2655
Nolvadex Tablets (Rare) 678
Noroxin Tablets (Rare) 2145
Norvasc Tablets (More than 0.1% to 1%) 2704
Norvir Capsules (Less than 2%) 487
Norvir Oral Solution (Less than 2%) 487
Nutropin AQ Injection (Rare) 1420
Nutropin Depot for Injectable Suspension (Rare) 1423
Nutropin for Injection (Rare) 1417
Ogen Tablets 2846
Oncaspar (1%) 756
Orudis Capsules (Rare) 3548
Oruvail Capsules (Rare) 3548
Pacerone Tablets 3331
Paxil 1609
Pediapred Oral Solution 1170
Pediazole Suspension 3050
Pentasa Capsules (Infrequent to less than 1%) 3239
Permax Tablets (Rare) 1299
Ponstel Capsules (Rare) 1356
Pravachol Tablets 1099
Prednisone 3064
Prelone Syrup 2273
Premarin Intravenous 3563
Premarin Tablets 3566
Premarin Vaginal Cream 3570
Premphase Tablets 3572
Prempro Tablets 3572
Priftin Tablets (Less than 1%) 758
Prilosec Delayed-Release Capsules (Less than 1%) 628
Prinivil Tablets (0.3% to 1.0%) 2164
Prinzide Tablets 2168
Proleukin for Injection (Less than 1%) 1199
Protonix I.V. 3580
Protonix Tablets 3577
Prozac Pulvules, Liquid, and Weekly Capsules (Rare) 1238
Purinethol Tablets 1615
Rapamune Oral Solution and Tablets (Less frequent) 3584
Relafen Tablets (Less than 1%) 1617
Remeron Tablets (Rare) 2483
Remeron SolTab Tablets (Rare) 2486
Remicade for IV Injection (Less than 2%) 1178
Renese Tablets 2712
Requip Tablets (Infrequent) 1621
Rescriptor Tablets (Less than 2%) 526
Retavase Vials 1182
Retrovir Capsules (Rare) 1625
Retrovir IV Infusion (Rare) 1629
Retrovir (Rare) 1625
Rilutek Tablets (Infrequent) 772
Risperdal 1796
Rocaltrol 2991
Roferon-A Injection (Infrequent) 2996
Rowasa Rectal Suspension Enema 4.0 grams/unit (60 mL) 3264
Salagen Tablets (Less than 1%) 2229
Sandimmune (Rare) 2388
Sandostatin Injection (Less than 1%) 2394
Sandostatin LAR Depot (Rare) 2395
Sarafem Pulvules (Rare) 1962
Septra Suspension 2265
Septra Tablets 2265
Septra DS Tablets 2265
Seroquel Tablets (Rare) 684
▲ Serostim for Injection (1% to 10%) 3229
Singulair (Very rare) 2181
Solu-Medrol Sterile Powder 2855
Soriatane Capsules 3003
Streptase for Infusion 647
Sustiva Capsules (Less than 2%) 1258
Synercid I.V. (Less than 1%) 775
Tagamet (Rare) 1644
Tarka Tablets 508
Taxol Injection (Rare) 1129
Tegretol/Tegretol-XR 2404
Tenoretic Tablets 690
Thalomid Capsules 1154
Timolide Tablets 2187
Tonocard Tablets (Less than 1%) 649
Topamax Sprinkle Capsules 2590
Topamax Tablets 2590
Toradol 3018
Tricor Capsules, Micronized (Less than 1%) 513
Triphasil-21 Tablets 3600
Trizivir Tablets (3 of 656 patients) 1669
Trovan 2722
Uniretic Tablets 3178
Univasc Tablets (Less than 1%) 3181
Urobiotic-250 Capsules 2731
Vaseretic Tablets 2204
Vasotec I.V. Injection 2207
Vasotec Tablets (0.5% to 1.0%) 2210
Vesanoid Capsules (Isolated cases) 3037
▲ Videx (3% to 27%) 1138
Videx EC Capsules (Less than 1%) 1143
Vioxx (Less than 0.1%) 2213
Viracept 532
Vistide Injection (Less than 1%) 1445
Vitravene for Injection (2% to 5%) ⊙ 310
Voltaren Tablets (Less than 1%) 2315
Voltaren-XR Tablets (Less than 1%) 2315
Zantac (Rare) 1690
Zantac Injection (Rare) 1688
Zantac Syrup (Rare) 1690
Zaroxolyn Tablets 1177
Zerit (Fewer than 1%) 1147
Zestoretic Tablets 695
Zestril Tablets (0.3% to 1.0%) 698
Ziac Tablets 1887
Ziagen 1692
Zocor Tablets 2219
Zoloft (Rare) 2751
Zomig Tablets (Rare) 708
Zomig-ZMT Tablets (Rare) 708
Zosyn (1.0% or less) 1890
Zosyn in Galaxy Containers (1.0% or less) 1894
Zyban Sustained-Release Tablets 1710

Pancreatitis, hemorrhagic

Hivid Tablets (Less than 1%) 2975

Pancytopenia

Aceon Tablets (2 mg, 4 mg, 8 mg) 3249
Actiq (1% or greater) 1184
Aggrenox Capsules 1026
Albenza Tablets (Rare) 1463
Aloprim for Injection (Less than 1%) 2292
Altace Capsules (Less than 1%) 2233
Amaryl Tablets 717
Ancobon Capsules 1730
Arthrotec Tablets (Rare) 3195
Asacol Delayed-Release Tablets 2884
Azactam for Injection (Less than 1%) 1276
▲ Campath Ampules (3% to 5%) 992
Captopril Tablets 2281
Carbatrol Capsules 3234
Ceclor 1905
Cedax 1021
Cefizox for Intramuscular or Intravenous Use 1390
Cefotan 664
Ceftin 1898
Cefzil 1076
Celontin Capsules 2618
Ceptaz for Injection 1499
Cipro I.V. (Rare) 893
Cipro I.V. Pharmacy Bulk Package (Rare) 897
Cipro (0.1%) 887
Cognex Capsules (Rare) 1351
Compazine 1505
Copaxone for Injection (Infrequent) 3306
Cordarone Intravenous 3491
Coreg Tablets (Less than or equal to 0.1%) 1508
Cosmegen for Injection 2062
Cytovene (At least 3 subjects) 2959
Daraprim Tablets 1511
Depacon Injection 416
Depakene 421
Depakote Sprinkle Capsules 426
Depakote Tablets 430
Depakote ER Tablets 436
DiaBeta Tablets (Occasional) 741
Diabinese Tablets 2680
Diamox ⊙ 269
Didronel Tablets (Rare) 2888
Dilantin Infatabs (Occasional) 2624
Dilantin Kapseals (Occasional) 2622
Dilantin-125 Oral Suspension (Occasional) 2625
Duricef 1079
Enbrel for Injection (Rare) 1752
Enbrel for Injection (Rare) 3504
Ergamisol Tablets 1789
Etrafon 3115
Famotidine Injection (Rare) 866
Felbatol 3343
Feldene Capsules (Rare) 2685
Flolan for Injection 1528
Floxin I.V. 2526
Floxin Tablets 2529
Fortaz 1541
Fortovase Capsules (Less than 2%) 2970
Foscavir Injection (Less than 1%) 605
Sterile FUDR (Remote possibility) 2974
Gastrocrom Oral Concentrate (Less common) 1162
Glucotrol Tablets 2692
Glucotrol XL Extended Release Tablets 2693
Herceptin I.V. (At least one of the 958 patients) 1414
Imitrex Injection 1549
Imitrex Nasal Spray 1554
Imitrex Tablets 1558
Invirase Capsules (Less than 2%) 2979
Kefurox Vials, ADD-Vantage 1948
Lamictal 1567
Leustatin Injection 2495
Lodine (Less than 1%) 3528
Lodine XL Extended-Release Tablets (Less than 1%) 3530
Lorabid Suspension and Pulvules 2251
Matulane Capsules 3246
Maxipime for Injection 1285
Mefoxin for Injection 2124
Mefoxin Premixed Intravenous Solution 2127
Monopril Tablets 1091
Monopril HCT 1094
Motrin Suspension, Oral Drops, Chewable Tablets, and Caplets (Less than 1%) 2002
Mustargen for Injection 2142
Myleran Tablets 1603
Navane Oral 2701
Navane Intramuscular 2703
Neptazane Tablets ⊙ 271
Nolvadex Tablets (Rare) 678
Omnicef 493
Oncaspar (Greater than 1% but less than 5%) 756
Orthoclone OKT3 Sterile Solution (Less than 1%) 2498
Pacerone Tablets 3331
Paxil 1609
Pentasa Capsules 3239
Pepcid Injection (Rare) 2153
Pepcid for Oral Suspension (Rare) 2150
Pepcid RPD Orally Disintegrating Tablets (Rare) 2150
Pepcid Tablets (Rare) 2150
Ponstel Capsules (Rare) 1356
Prevacid Delayed-Release Capsules (Less than 1%) 3292
PREVPAC 3298
Prilosec Delayed-Release Capsules (Rare) 628
Primaxin I.M. 2158
Primaxin I.V. 2160
Prozac Pulvules, Liquid, and Weekly Capsules 1238
Rapamune Oral Solution and Tablets (Rare) 3584
Remeron Tablets (Rare) 2483
Remeron SolTab Tablets (Rare) 2486
Rescriptor Tablets (Less than 2%) 526
Retrovir IV Infusion 1629
Rituxan for Infusion 1750
Rituxan I.V. 1428
Sandostatin LAR Depot (Rare) 2395
Sarafem Pulvules 1962
Serentil 1057
Soma Tablets 3353
Soma Compound Tablets (Very rare) 3354
Soma Compound w/Codeine Tablets (Very rare) 3355
Stelazine 1640
Suprax 1877
▲ Tabloid Tablets (Nearly all patients) 1642
Tagamet (Very rare) 1644
Tazicef for Injection 1647
Tazicef Galaxy Container 1650
Tazicef Pharmacy Bulk Package 1653
Tazidime Vials, Faspak & ADD-Vantage 1966
Tegretol/Tegretol-XR 2404
Thalomid Capsules 1154
Thioridazine Hydrochloride Tablets 2289
Thiothixene Capsules 2290
Thorazine 1656
Ticlid Tablets (Rare) 3015
Topamax Sprinkle Capsules (Rare) 2590
Topamax Tablets (Rare) 2590
Trental Tablets (Rare) 784
Trilafon 3160
Valcyte Tablets (Less than 5%) 3022
Vantin Tablets and Oral Suspension 2860
Vistide Injection 1445
Wellbutrin Tablets (Rare) 1680
Wellbutrin SR Sustained-Release Tablets 1684
Xeloda Tablets (Less than 5%) 3039
Zantac (Rare) 1690
Zantac Injection (Rare) 1688
Zantac Syrup (Rare) 1690
Zarontin Capsules 2659
Zarontin Syrup 2660
Zinacef Injection 1696
Zinacef for Injection 1696
Zoloft 2751
▲ Zometa for Intravenous Infusion (5% to 10%) 3621
Zyban Sustained-Release Tablets 1710

Panencephalitis, sclerosing, subacute

Attenuvax 2044
M-M-R II 2118

Panic

Ambien Tablets (Rare) 3191
Amerge Tablets (Rare) 1467
Celexa (Infrequent) 1365
Cozaar Tablets (Less than 1%) 2067
Effexor Tablets 3495
Effexor XR Capsules 3499
Hyzaar 2109
Imitrex Injection 1549
Imitrex Nasal Spray 1554
Imitrex Tablets 1558
Lamictal (Infrequent) 1567
Tasmar Tablets (1%) 3010
Trileptal Oral Suspension 2407
Trileptal Tablets 2407

Panniculitis

Attenuvax 2044
M-M-R II 2118

Papilledema

Accutane Capsules 2944
Aquasol A Parenteral 593
Betaseron for SC Injection 988
Brevicon 28-Day Tablets 3380
Celestone Soluspan Injectable Suspension 3097
Celestone Syrup 3099
Cordarone Tablets 3487
Cortone Acetate Injectable Suspension 2059
Cortone Acetate Tablets 2061
Decadron Elixir 2078
Decadron Tablets 2079
Decadron Phosphate Injection 2081
Depo-Medrol Injectable Suspension 2795
Depo-Provera Contraceptive Injection 2798
Effexor Tablets (Rare) 3495
Effexor XR Capsules (Rare) 3499
Eskalith 1527
Florinef Acetate Tablets 2250
Genotropin Lyophilized Powder (A small number of patients) 2818
Humatrope Vials and Cartridges 1930
Hydrocortone Tablets 2106
Hydrocortone Acetate Injectable Suspension 2103
Hydrocortone Phosphate Injection, Sterile 2105
Levlen 962
Levlite 21 Tablets 962
Levlite 28 Tablets 962
Lithium Carbonate 3061
Lithium Citrate Syrup 3061
Matulane Capsules 3246
Modicon 2563
Neumega for Injection (1.5%) 1434
Nizoral Tablets (Rare) 1791
Norinyl 1 +35 28-Day Tablets 3380
Norinyl 1 + 50 28-Day Tablets 3380
Norplant System 3543
Ortho-Cyclen/Ortho Tri-Cyclen 2573
Ortho-Novum 2563
Ortho-Novum 1/50▭28 Tablets 2556
Ortho-Cyclen/Ortho Tri-Cyclen 2573
Ovcon 3364
Pacerone Tablets 3331
Prednisone 3064
Premphase Tablets 3572
Prempro Tablets 3572
Provera Tablets 2853
Saizen for Injection (A small number of patients) 3225
Solu-Medrol Sterile Powder 2855
Soriatane Capsules (Less than 1%) 3003
Tri-Levlen 962
Tri-Norinyl-28 Tablets 3433

Papillitis

Attenuvax 2044
Meruvax II 2130
M-M-R II (Infrequent) 2118
Mumpsvax (Infrequent) 2141

Papilloma, scrotum

Testoderm Transdermal Systems (1%) 574

Papillomatosis

Fortovase Capsules (Less than 2%) 2970
Invirase Capsules (Less than 2%) 2979

Papules

Catapres-TTS (1 of 101 patients) 1038
Depen Titratable Tablets 3341
Duragesic Transdermal System (1% or greater) 1786
Oxistat Cream (0.1%) 1298
Yodoxin Tablets 1722

Papules, erythematous

(*see under* Erythema multiforme)

Paralysis

Accuretic Tablets 2614

Aloprim for Injection (Less than 1%) ... 2292
Baycol Tablets ... 883
Betapace Tablets (Rare) ... 950
Betapace AF Tablets (Rare) ... 954
Betaseron for SC Injection ... 988
Campath Ampules ... 992
Carbatrol Capsules ... 3234
Cerebyx Injection (Infrequent) ... 2619
Cognex Capsules (Infrequent) ... 1351
Coumadin for Injection ... 1243
Coumadin Tablets ... 1243
Depo-Provera Contraceptive Injection (Fewer than 1%) ... 2798
Evoxac Capsules ... 1217
Felbatol ... 3343
Gabitril Tablets (Infrequent) ... 1189
Hivid Tablets (Less than 1%) ... 2975
Imitrex Injection ... 1549
Imitrex Tablets (Rare) ... 1558
Lamictal (Rare) ... 1567
Levaquin (Less than 0.3%) ... 2537
Lovenox Injection (Rare) ... 746
Lupron Depot 7.5 mg ... 3284
Lupron Depot–3 Month 22.5 mg ... 3288
Lupron Depot–4 Month 30 mg (Less than 5%) ... 3289
Lupron Depot-PED 7.5 mg, 11.25 mg and 15 mg ... 3291
Lupron Injection ... 3279
Luvox Tablets (25, 50, 100 mg) (Infrequent) ... 3256
LYMErix Vaccine (Greater than 1%) ... 1592
Mirapex Tablets (1% or more) ... 2834
Naprelan Tablets (Less than 1%) ... 1293
Nipent for Injection (Less than 3%) ... 3272
Norvir Capsules (Less than 2%) ... 487
Norvir Oral Solution (Less than 2%) ... 487
Paxil (Infrequent) ... 1609
Permax Tablets (Infrequent) ... 1299
Prozac Pulvules, Liquid, and Weekly Capsules (Rare) ... 1238
Rabies Vaccine RabAvert (Seven cases) ... 1203
Remeron Tablets (Rare) ... 2483
Remeron SolTab Tablets (Rare) ... 2486
Requip Tablets (Infrequent) ... 1621
Rescriptor Tablets (Less than 2%) ... 526
Sarafem Pulvules (Rare) ... 1962
Sensorcaine ... 643
Sensorcaine-MPF Injection ... 643
Tegretol/Tegretol-XR ... 2404
Tikosyn Capsules (Less than or equal to 2%) ... 2717
Trileptal Oral Suspension ... 2407
Trileptal Tablets ... 2407
Warfarin Sodium Tablets, USP ... 3302
Zanaflex Tablets (Infrequent) ... 1305
Zyprexa Tablets (Rare) ... 1973
Zyprexa ZYDIS Orally Disintegrating Tablets (Rare) ... 1973
Zyrtec (Less than 2%) ... 2756
Zyrtec-D 12 Hour Extended Relief Tablets (Less than 2%) ... 2758

Paralysis, bladder
Etrafon (Occasional) ... 3115

Paralysis, extraocular muscles
Pravachol Tablets ... 1099

Paralysis, facial
Actiq (Less than 1%) ... 1184
Avonex ... 1013
Betaseron for SC Injection ... 988
Copaxone for Injection (Infrequent) ... 3306
Depo-Provera Contraceptive Injection (Fewer than 1%) ... 2798
Effexor Tablets (Rare) ... 3495
Effexor XR Capsules (Rare) ... 3499
Imitrex Tablets (Rare) ... 1558
Lescol Capsules ... 2361
Lescol Capsules ... 2925
Lescol XL Tablets ... 2361
Lescol XL Tablets ... 2925
Lipitor Tablets (Less than 2%) ... 2639
Lipitor Tablets (Less than 2%) ... 2696
Neurontin Capsules (Infrequent) ... 2655
Neurontin Oral Solution (Infrequent) ... 2655
Neurontin Tablets (Infrequent) ... 2655
Rilutek Tablets (Infrequent) ... 772
Sonata Capsules (Rare) ... 3591
Tikosyn Capsules (Less than or equal to 2%) ... 2717
Uniretic Tablets (Less than 1%) ... 3178
▲ Vesanoid Capsules (3%) ... 3037
Vistide Injection ... 1445
Zonegran Capsules (Rare) ... 1307
Zyprexa Tablets (Rare) ... 1973
Zyprexa ZYDIS Orally Disintegrating Tablets (Rare) ... 1973

Paralysis, flaccid
Diamox Intravenous (Occasional) ... ⊙269
Diamox Sequels Sustained Release Capsules ... ⊙270
Diamox Tablets (Occasional) ... ⊙269
Neptazane Tablets ... ⊙271
Rum-K ... 1363
Tikosyn Capsules (Less than or equal to 2%) ... 2717

Paralysis, legs
(*see under* Paralysis, lower extremities)

Paralysis, lower extremities
Naropin Injection ... 612
Polocaine Injection, USP ... 625
Polocaine-MPF Injection, USP ... 625
Sensorcaine ... 643
Sensorcaine-MPF Injection ... 643

Paralysis, oculomotor nerve
Cytovene ... 2959

Paralysis, radial nerve
Diphtheria & Tetanus Toxoids Adsorbed Purogenated for Pediatric Use ... 1857
Tetanus & Diphtheria Toxoids Adsorbed for Adult Use ... 1880
Tetanus and Diphtheria Toxoids Adsorbed For Adult Use ... 815
Tripedia Vaccine ... 817

Paralysis, respiratory
Polocaine Injection, USP ... 625
Polocaine-MPF Injection, USP ... 625
Sensorcaine ... 643
Sensorcaine-MPF Injection ... 643
Tensilon Injectable ... 1745

Paralysis, sensory motor
Demerol Tablets ... 3079

Paralysis, skeletal muscle
Anectine Injection ... 1476
Norcuron for Injection ... 2478

Paralysis, spinal cord
Lupron Depot 3.75 mg ... 3281
Lupron Depot–3 Month 11.25 mg ... 3285
Lupron Depot–4 Month 30 mg ... 3289

Paralysis, tongue
Maxalt Tablets (Rare) ... 2120
Maxalt-MLT Orally Disintegrating Tablets (Rare) ... 2120
Topamax Sprinkle Capsules (Rare) ... 2590
Topamax Tablets (Rare) ... 2590
Trovan (Less than 1%) ... 2722

Paralysis, vocal cord
Uniretic Tablets (Less than 1%) ... 3178

Paralysis agitans
(*see under* Parkinsonism)

Paranoia
Adalat CC Tablets (Rare) ... 877
Allegra-D Extended-Release Tablets (Less than 1%) ... 714
Aricept Tablets (Infrequent) ... 1270
Aricept Tablets (Infrequent) ... 2665
Artane (One case) ... 1855
Arthrotec Tablets (Rare) ... 3195
Betaseron for SC Injection ... 988
Celexa (Infrequent) ... 1365
Cipro I.V. (1% or less) ... 893
Cipro I.V. Pharmacy Bulk Package (Less than 1%) ... 897
Cipro ... 887
Clozaril Tablets (Less than 1%) ... 2319
Cognex Capsules (Infrequent) ... 1351
Copaxone for Injection (Infrequent) ... 3306
Duragesic Transdermal System (1% or greater) ... 1786
Effexor Tablets (Infrequent) ... 3495
Effexor XR Capsules (Infrequent) ... 3499
Etrafon ... 3115
Evoxac Capsules ... 1217
Exelon Capsules (2% or more) ... 2342
Exelon Oral Solution (2% or more) ... 2345
Felbatol ... 3343
Flexeril Tablets ... 572
Flexeril Tablets ... 2094
Floxin I.V. ... 2526
Floxin Tablets ... 2529
Gabitril Tablets (Frequent) ... 1189
Gliadel Wafer (1%) ... 1723
Hivid Tablets (Less than 1%) ... 2975
Lamictal (Infrequent) ... 1567
Levaquin (Less than 0.3%) ... 2537
Lodosyn Tablets ... 1251
Luvox Tablets (25, 50, 100 mg) (Infrequent) ... 3256
▲ Marinol Capsules (3% to 10%) ... 3325
Mirapex Tablets (Less than 1%) ... 2834
Neurontin Capsules (Infrequent) ... 2655
Neurontin Oral Solution (Infrequent) ... 2655
Neurontin Tablets (Infrequent) ... 2655
Orthoclone OKT3 Sterile Solution (Less than 1%) ... 2498
Paxil (Infrequent) ... 1609
Permax Tablets (Frequent) ... 1299
Procardia Capsules (Less than 0.5%) ... 2708
Prozac Pulvules, Liquid, and Weekly Capsules (Infrequent) ... 1238
Remeron Tablets (Infrequent) ... 2483
Remeron SolTab Tablets (Infrequent) ... 2486
Reminyl Oral Solution (Infrequent) ... 1792
Reminyl Tablets (Infrequent) ... 1792
Requip Tablets (Infrequent) ... 1621
Rescriptor Tablets (Less than 2%) ... 526
Rilutek Tablets (Infrequent) ... 772
Romazicon Injection (1% to 3%) ... 3000
Sandostatin Injection (Less than 1%) ... 2394
Sandostatin LAR Depot (Rare) ... 2395
Sarafem Pulvules (Infrequent) ... 1962
Seroquel Tablets (Infrequent) ... 684
Serzone Tablets (Infrequent) ... 1104
Sinemet Tablets ... 1253
Sinemet CR Tablets ... 1255
Sustiva Capsules ... 1258
Symmetrel ... 1328
Tasmar Tablets (Infrequent) ... 3010
Tequin Injection (Less than 0.1%) ... 1110
Tequin Tablets (Less than 0.1%) ... 1110
Topamax Sprinkle Capsules (Infrequent) ... 2590
Topamax Tablets (Infrequent) ... 2590
Trilafon ... 3160
Trileptal Oral Suspension ... 2407
Trileptal Tablets ... 2407
Trovan (Less than 1%) ... 2722
Ultracet Tablets (Less than 1%) ... 2597
Wellbutrin Tablets (Infrequent) ... 1680
Wellbutrin SR Sustained-Release Tablets ... 1684
Zoloft (Infrequent) ... 2751
Zyban Sustained-Release Tablets ... 1710
Zyprexa Tablets ... 1973
Zyprexa ZYDIS Orally Disintegrating Tablets ... 1973

Paraparesis
Leustatin Injection ... 2495
Orthoclone OKT3 Sterile Solution (Less than 1%) ... 2498

Paraplegia
Copaxone for Injection (Infrequent) ... 3306
Orthoclone OKT3 Sterile Solution ... 2498

Parapsoriasis varioliformis acuta
Azulfidine EN-tabs Tablets (Rare) ... 2775

Parathyroid disorder, unspecified
▲ Carnitor Injection (2% to 6%) ... 3242

Parathyroid hormone deficiency, fetal
Accutane Capsules ... 2944

Parathyroid neoplasm
Amerge Tablets (Rare) ... 1467

Parenchymatous organs, toxic damage
Tagamet (Highly unlikely) ... 1644

Paresis
Ambien Tablets (Rare) ... 3191
Cardura Tablets (Less than 0.5%) ... 2668
Cognex Capsules (Infrequent) ... 1351
Colazal Capsules ... 3005
Coreg Tablets (Less than or equal to 0.1%) ... 1508
Engerix-B Vaccine ... 1517
Exelon Capsules (Infrequent) ... 2342
Exelon Oral Solution (Infrequent) ... 2345
Fortovase Capsules (Less than 2%) ... 2970
Imdur Tablets (Less than or equal to 5%) ... 1826
Intron A for Injection (Less than 5%) ... 3120
Invirase Capsules (Less than 2%) ... 2979
Klonopin Tablets (Infrequent) ... 2983
Leukeran Tablets (Rare) ... 1591
Naropin Injection (Less than 1%) ... 612
Neurontin Capsules (Infrequent) ... 2655
Neurontin Oral Solution (Infrequent) ... 2655
Neurontin Tablets (Infrequent) ... 2655
▲ Requip Tablets (3%) ... 1621
Sandostatin LAR Depot (Rare) ... 2395
Tambocor Tablets (1% to 3%) ... 1990
Tasmar Tablets (1% or more) ... 3010
▲ Temodar Capsules (8%) ... 3157
Tenex Tablets (3% or less) ... 2942
Twinrix Vaccine ... 1674

Paresthesia
Accupril Tablets (0.5% to 1.0%) ... 2611
Accuretic Tablets (0.5% to 1%) ... 2614
Accutane Capsules ... 2944
Aceon Tablets (2 mg, 4 mg, 8 mg) (2.3%) ... 3249
Aciphex Tablets ... 1267
Aciphex Tablets ... 1783
Actiq (Less than 1%) ... 1184
Actonel Tablets (2.1%) ... 2879
Adalat CC Tablets (3% or less) ... 877
Adenoscan (2%) ... 1381
Advair Diskus 100/50 ... 1448
Advair Diskus 250/50 ... 1448
Advair Diskus 500/50 ... 1448
▲ Agenerase Capsules (26% to 31%) ... 1454
▲ Agenerase Oral Solution (26% to 31%) ... 1459
Aggrenox Capsules (Less than 1%) ... 1026
▲ Agrylin Capsules (5.9%) ... 3232
Aldoclor Tablets ... 2035
Aldomet Tablets ... 2037
Aldoril Tablets ... 2039
Altace Capsules (Less than 1%) ... 2233
Ambien Tablets (Infrequent) ... 3191
AmBisome for Injection (Less common) ... 1383
Amerge Tablets (1% to 2%) ... 1467
Amphotec (1% to 5%) ... 1774
Ancobon Capsules ... 1730
Androderm Transdermal System CIII (Less than 1%) ... 3377
AndroGel (Fewer than 1%) ... 3322
▲ Android Capsules, 10 mg (Among most common) ... 1731
Anzemet Injection (Infrequently) ... 719
Anzemet Tablets (Infrequently) ... 722
Arava Tablets (2%) ... 724
Aredia for Injection ... 2309
Aricept Tablets (Frequent) ... 1270
Aricept Tablets (Frequent) ... 2665
▲ Arimidex Tablets (4.6% to 6.1%) ... 659
Aromasin Tablets (Less frequent) ... 2769
Arthrotec Tablets (Rare) ... 3195
Asacol Delayed-Release Tablets (2% or greater) ... 2884
Astelin Nasal Spray ... 3339
Atacand Tablets (0.5% or greater) ... 595
Atacand HCT Tablets (0.5% or greater) ... 597
Atrovent Inhalation Aerosol (Less frequent) ... 1030
Avalide Tablets ... 1070
Avapro Tablets (Less than 1%) ... 1074
Avapro Tablets (Less than 1%) ... 3076
Avelox Tablets (0.05% to 1%) ... 879
Avonex ... 1013
Axert Tablets (1%) ... 2772
Azactam for Injection (Less than 1%) ... 1276
Baycol Tablets ... 883
Benadryl Parenteral ... 2617
Betagan ... ⊙228
Betapace Tablets (1% to 4%) ... 950
Betimol Ophthalmic Solution ... ⊙324
Blocadren Tablets (0.6%) ... 2046
Brethine Tablets (Less than 1%) ... 2313
Brevibloc Injection (Less than 1%) ... 858
Cancidas for Injection (1.3% to 3.1%) ... 2048
Captopril Tablets (About 0.5% to 2%) ... 2281
Carbatrol Capsules ... 3234
Cardene I.V. (0.7%) ... 3485
Cardizem Injectable (Less than 1%) ... 1018
Cardizem Lyo-Ject Syringe (Less than 1%) ... 1018
Cardizem Monovial (Less than 1%) ... 1018
Cardizem CD Capsules (Less than 1%) ... 1016
Cardura Tablets (1%) ... 2668
▲ Carnitor Injection (3% to 12%) ... 3242
▲ Casodex Tablets (6%) ... 662
Cataflam Tablets (Less than 1%) ... 2315
Ceclor CD Tablets ... 1279
Ceclor ... 1905
Cedax Capsules (0.1% to 1%) ... 1021
Cefizox for Intramuscular or Intravenous Use (1% to 5%) ... 1390
Celebrex Capsules (0.1% to 1.9%) ... 2676
Celebrex Capsules (0.1% to 1.9%) ... 2780
Celexa (Frequent) ... 1365
▲ CellCept Capsules (3% to 20.8%) ... 2951
▲ CellCept Intravenous (3% to 20.8%) ... 2951
▲ CellCept Oral Suspension (3% to 20.8%) ... 2951
▲ CellCept Tablets (3% to 20.8%) ... 2951
▲ Cenestin Tablets (33%) ... 1263
Ceptaz for Injection (Fewer than 1%) ... 1499
▲ Cerebyx Injection (7 of 16 volunteers; 3.9% to 4.4%) ... 2619
▲ Chemet Capsules (1.0% to 12.7%) ... 3078
Chibroxin Sterile Ophthalmic Solution ... 2051
Chirocaine Injection (1.8%) ... 2909
Cipro HC Otic Suspension (One patient) ... 540
Cipro I.V. (1% or less) ... 893
Cipro I.V. Pharmacy Bulk Package (Less than 1%) ... 897
Cipro (Less than 1%) ... 887
Claritin (At least one patient) ... 3100

Claritin-D 12 Hour Extended Release Tablets (Less frequent)... 3102
Claritin-D 24 Hour Extended Release Tablets (Fewer than 2%)... 3104
Clinoril Tablets (Less than 1%)... 2053
Clomid Tablets... 735
Clorpres Tablets... 1002
Clozaril Tablets... 2319
Cognex Capsules (Frequent)... 1351
Coly-Mycin M Parenteral... 2243
Combipres Tablets... 1040
Combivent Inhalation Aerosol (Less than 2%)... 1041
Copaxone for Injection (At least 2%)... 3306
▲ Cordarone Tablets (4% to 9%)... 3487
Coreg Tablets (2.0%)... 1508
Corgard Tablets (6 of 1000 patients)... 2245
Corzide 40/5 Tablets (6 of 100 patients)... 2247
Corzide 80/5 Tablets (6 of 100 patients)... 2247
Cosopt Sterile Ophthalmic Solution (1% to 5%)... 2065
Coumadin for Injection (Infrequent)... 1243
Coumadin Tablets (Infrequent)... 1243
Covera-HS Tablets (1%)... 3199
Cozaar Tablets (Less than 1%)... 2067
Crixivan Capsules (Less than 2%)... 2070
Cytovene... 2959
▲ Daranide Tablets (Among the most common effects)... 2077
Delatestryl Injection... 1151
Depacon Injection (0.9% to 5%)... 416
Depakene (1% to 5%)... 421
Depakote Sprinkle Capsules (1% to 5%)... 426
Depakote Tablets (1% to 5%)... 430
Depakote ER Tablets (1% to 5%)... 436
Depo-Provera Contraceptive Injection (Fewer than 1%)... 2798
Dermatop Emollient Cream (Less than 1%)... 2517
Detrol Tablets (1.1%)... 3623
D.H.E. 45 Injection (Occasional)... 2334
Diamox Sequels Sustained Release Capsules... ⊙270
Didronel Tablets... 2888
Dilaudid Oral Liquid (Less frequent)... 445
Dilaudid Tablets - 8 mg (Less frequent)... 445
Dilaudid-HP (Less frequent)... 443
Diovan Capsules... 2337
Diovan HCT Tablets (Greater than 0.2%)... 2338
Dipentum Capsules (Rare)... 2803
Diphtheria & Tetanus Toxoids Adsorbed Purogenated for Pediatric Use... 1857
Diprivan Injectable Emulsion (Less than 1%)... 667
Diucardin Tablets... 3494
Diuril Oral... 2087
Diuril Sodium Intravenous... 2086
Dolobid Tablets (Less than 1 in 100)... 2088
▲ Dostinex Tablets (1% to less than 10%)... 2804
Doxil Injection (Less than 1% to 7.8%)... 566
Duragesic Transdermal System (1% or greater)... 1786
Dyazide Capsules... 1515
Dynabac Tablets (0.1% to 1%)... 2269
DynaCirc Capsules (0.5% to 1%)... 2921
DynaCirc CR Tablets (0.5% to 1%)... 2923
▲ Effexor Tablets (3%)... 3495
▲ Effexor XR Capsules (3%)... 3499
Emla... 602
Enalaprilat Injection... 863
Enbrel for Injection... 1752
Enbrel for Injection... 3504
Engerix-B Vaccine... 1517
▲ Epivir (13%)... 1520
Epivir-HBV... 1524
▲ Epogen for Injection (11%)... 582
Ergamisol Tablets (2% to 3%)... 1789
Esclim Transdermal System... 3460
Estratest... 3252
Evoxac Capsules (Less than 1%)... 1217
Exelon Capsules (Frequent)... 2342
Exelon Oral Solution (Frequent)... 2345
Famotidine Injection (Infrequent)... 866
Famvir Tablets (0.9% to 2.6%)... 2348
▲ Felbatol (3.5%)... 3343
Feldene Capsules (Occasional)... 2685
▲ Ferrlecit Injection (6%)... 3386
Flexeril Tablets (Less than 1%)... 572
Flexeril Tablets (Less than 1%)... 2094
▲ Flolan for Injection (1% to 12%)... 1528
Floxin I.V. (Less than 1%)... 2526
Floxin Otic Solution (1%)... 1219
Floxin Tablets (Less than 1%)... 2529
▲ Fludara for Injection (4% to 12%)... 995
Fortaz (Less than 1%)... 1541
Fortovase Capsules (Less than 2%)... 2970
▲ Foscavir Injection (5% or greater)... 605
Furosemide Tablets... 2284
▲ Gabitril Tablets (3%)... 1189
Gastrocrom Oral Concentrate (Less common)... 1162
Gemzar for Injection (Less than 1%)... 1919
▲ Gengraf Capsules (1% to 11%)... 457
Geodon Capsules (Frequent)... 2688
Glucotrol XL Extended Release Tablets (Less than 3%)... 2693
Gonal-F for Injection... 3216
Halcion Tablets (Rare)... 2823
Havrix Vaccine (Rare)... 1544
▲ Herceptin I.V. (9%)... 1414
Humate-P Concentrate (2%)... 790
▲ Humatrope Vials and Cartridges (13.6% to 17.3%)... 1930
▲ Hycamtin for Injection (9%)... 1546
HydroDIURIL Tablets... 2108
Hytrin Capsules (0.8% to 1.9%)... 464
Hyzaar... 2109
Imdur Tablets (Less than or equal to 5%)... 1826
▲ Imitrex Injection (5%)... 1549
Imitrex Nasal Spray (Infrequent)... 1554
Imitrex Tablets (Frequent)... 1558
Indapamide Tablets... 2286
Inderide Tablets... 3517
Inderide LA Long-Acting Capsules... 3519
Indocin (Less than 1%)... 2112
INFeD Injection... 3388
▲ Infergen (9% to 13%)... 1777
▲ Intron A for Injection (1% to 21%)... 3120
Inversine Tablets... 1850
Invirase Capsules (0.3% to 3.1%)... 2979
Iopidine 0.5% Ophthalmic Solution (Less than 3%)... ⊙213
Iopidine Sterile Ophthalmic Solution... ⊙212
Isoptin SR Tablets (1% or less)... 467
Kadian Capsules (Less than 3%)... 1335
Kaletra Capsules (Less than 2%)... 471
Kaletra Oral Solution (Less than 2%)... 471
Keppra Tablets (2%)... 3314
Klonopin Tablets (Infrequent)... 2983
Lamictal (More than 1%)... 1567
Lescol Capsules... 2361
Lescol Capsules... 2925
Lescol XL Tablets... 2361
Lescol XL Tablets... 2925
▲ Leukine (11%)... 1755
Levaquin... 2537
Lexxel Tablets... 608
Lipitor Tablets (Less than 2%)... 2639
Lipitor Tablets (Less than 2%)... 2696
Lodine (Less than 1%)... 3528
Lodine XL Extended-Release Tablets (Less than 1%)... 3530
Lodosyn Tablets... 1251
Lopid Tablets (More common)... 2650
Lotensin Tablets (Less than 1%)... 2365
Lotensin HCT Tablets (0.3% to 1%)... 2367
Lotrisone (1.9%)... 3129
Loxitane Capsules... 3398
Lupron Depot 3.75 mg (Less than 5%)... 3281
Lupron Depot 7.5 mg (Less than 5%)... 3284
▲ Lupron Depot–3 Month 11.25 mg (1.2% to 7%)... 3285
Lupron Depot–3 Month 22.5 mg (Less than 5%)... 3288
▲ Lupron Depot–4 Month 30 mg (4.2% to 8.2%)... 3289
Lupron Injection (Less than 5%)... 3279
Luvox Tablets (25, 50, 100 mg)... 3256
Luxíq Foam (One patient)... 1210
▲ LYMErix Vaccine (3.6%)... 1592
Matulane Capsules... 3246
Mavik Tablets (0.3% to 1.0%)... 478
▲ Maxalt Tablets (3% to 4%)... 2120
▲ Maxalt-MLT Orally Disintegrating Tablets (3% to 4%)... 2120
Maxzide... 1008
Megace Oral Suspension (1% to 3%)... 1124
Meridia Capsules (2%)... 481
Merrem I.V. (0.1% to 1.0%)... 673
Meruvax II... 2130
Mevacor Tablets (0.5% to 1.0%)... 2132
Mexitil Capsules (2.4% to 3.8%)... 1047
Miacalcin Nasal Spray (1% to 3%)... 2375
Micardis Tablets (More than 0.3%)... 1049
Micardis HCT Tablets... 1051
Microzide Capsules... 3414
Midamor Tablets (Less than or equal to 1%)... 2136
Migranal Nasal Spray (2%)... 2376
Miltown Tablets... 3349
Minipress Capsules (Less than 1%)... 2699
Minizide Capsules (Rare)... 2700
Mirapex Tablets (1% or more)... 2834
M-M-R II... 2118
Mobic Tablets (Less than 2%)... 1054
Moduretic Tablets (Less than or equal to 1%)... 2138
Monopril Tablets (0.2% to 1.0%)... 1091
Monopril HCT (Less than 2%)... 1094
Monurol Sachet (Less than 1%)... 1375
Motrin Suspension, Oral Drops, Chewable Tablets, and Caplets (Less than 1%)... 2002
MS Contin Tablets (Less frequent)... 2896
MSIR (Less frequent)... 2898
Mycobutin Capsules (More than one patient)... 2838
Mykrox Tablets... 1168
Nadolol Tablets (6 of 1000 patients)... 2288
Naprelan Tablets (Less than 3%)... 1293
Narcan Injection (Infrequent)... 1322
Nardil Tablets (Less common)... 2653
▲ Naropin Injection (More than 5% to 6.9%)... 612
Nascobal Gel (One patient)... 3174
Natrecor for Injection (At least 1%)... 3189
▲ Navelbine Injection (Among most frequent)... 1604
▲ Neoral Soft Gelatin Capsules (1% to 11%)... 2380
▲ Neoral Oral Solution (1% to 11%)... 2380
Neptazane Tablets... ⊙271
Neumega for Injection... 1434
Neurontin Capsules (Frequent)... 2655
Neurontin Oral Solution (Frequent)... 2655
Neurontin Tablets (Frequent)... 2655
Nexium Delayed-Release Capsules (Less than 1%)... 619
▲ Nicotrol Inhaler (Greater than 3%)... 2840
Nicotrol Nasal Spray (Common)... 2843
▲ Nilandron Tablets (3%)... 753
▲ Nipent for Injection (3% to 10%)... 3272
Nizoral Tablets (Rare)... 1791
Normodyne Tablets (Up to 5%)... 3137
Noroxin Tablets... 2145
Norvasc Tablets (More than 0.1% to 1%)... 2704
Norvir Capsules (2.0% to 2.6%)... 487
Norvir Oral Solution (2.0% to 2.6%)... 487
Oncaspar (Greater than 1% but less than 5%)... 756
Oramorph SR Tablets (Less frequent)... 3062
Orudis Capsules (Less than 1%)... 3548
Oruvail Capsules (Less than 1%)... 3548
Ovidrel for Injection (Less than 2%)... 3220
OxyContin Tablets (Less than 1%)... 2912
▲ Pacerone Tablets (4% to 9%)... 3331
Paraplatin for Injection... 1126
Parnate Tablets... 1607
▲ Paxil (1.0% to 5.9%)... 1609
Pediazole Suspension... 3050
Pentasa Capsules (Less than 1%)... 3239
Pepcid Injection (Infrequent)... 2153
Pepcid for Oral Suspension (Infrequent)... 2150
Pepcid RPD Orally Disintegrating Tablets (Infrequent)... 2150
Pepcid Tablets (Infrequent)... 2150
Periactin Tablets... 2155
Permax Tablets (1.6%)... 1299
Persantine Tablets (Rare)... 1057
Plavix Tablets (1% to 2.5%)... 1097
Plavix Tablets (1% to 2.5%)... 3084
Plendil Extended-Release Tablets (1.2% to 1.6%)... 623
Pletal Tablets (2% or greater)... 2605
Pletal Tablets (2% or greater)... 2848
Pneumovax 23 (Rare)... 2156
Pnu-Imune 23... 1868
Podocon-25 Liquid... 2608
Polocaine Injection, USP... 625
Polocaine-MPF Injection, USP... 625
Ponstel Capsules (Occasional)... 1356
Prandin Tablets (0.5, 1, and 2 mg) (2% to 3%)... 2432
Pravachol Tablets... 1099
Prevacid Delayed-Release Capsules (Less than 1%)... 3292
PREVPAC (Less than 1%)... 3298
Prilosec Delayed-Release Capsules (Less than 1%)... 628
Primaxin I.M.... 2158
Primaxin I.V. (Less than 0.2%)... 2160
Prinivil Tablets (0.3% to 1.0%)... 2164
Prinzide Tablets (1.5%)... 2168
▲ ProAmatine Tablets (18.3%)... 3241
Procardia XL Extended Release Tablets (Less than 3%)... 2710
▲ Procrit for Injection (11%)... 2502
▲ Prograf (17% to 40%)... 1393
ProSom Tablets (Infrequent)... 500
Prostin E2 Suppositories... 2852
Protonix I.V. (Less than 1%)... 3580
Protonix Tablets (Less than 1%)... 3577
Protopic Ointment (Greater than or equal to 1%)... 1397
▲ Provigil Tablets (3%)... 1193
Prozac Pulvules, Liquid, and Weekly Capsules (Less than 1%)... 1238
Rabies Vaccine RabAvert (Rare)... 1203
▲ Rapamune Oral Solution and Tablets (3% to 20%)... 3584
Relafen Tablets (Less than 1%)... 1617
Remeron Tablets (Frequent)... 2483
Remeron SolTab Tablets (Frequent)... 2486
Reminyl Oral Solution (Infrequent)... 1792
Reminyl Tablets (Infrequent)... 1792
Renese Tablets... 2712
Requip Tablets (1% or more)... 1621
Rescriptor Tablets (Less than 2%)... 526
▲ Retrovir Capsules (6%)... 1625
▲ Retrovir IV Infusion (6%)... 1629
▲ Retrovir (6%)... 1625
Risperdal (Infrequent)... 1796
Rituxan for Infusion (1% to 5%)... 1750
Rituxan I.V. (1% to 5%)... 1428
▲ Roferon-A Injection (7% to 12%)... 2996
Romazicon Injection (1% to 3%)... 3000
Rynatan Tablets... 3351
Rythmol Tablets – 150 mg, 225 mg, 300 mg (Less than 1%)... 502
Salagen Tablets (Less than 1%)... 2229
Sandimmune (1% to 3%)... 2388
▲ Sandostatin LAR Depot (5% to 15%)... 2395
Sarafem Pulvules (Frequent)... 1962
Sensorcaine... 643
Sensorcaine-MPF Injection... 643
Serevent Diskus (1% to 3%)... 1637
Serophene Tablets... 3226
▲ Serzone Tablets (4%)... 1104
▲ Simulect for Injection (3% to 10%)... 2399
Sinemet Tablets... 1253
Sinemet CR Tablets (0.8%)... 1255
Sinequan (Infrequent)... 2713
▲ Skelid Tablets (4.0%)... 3088
▲ Sonata Capsules (3%)... 3591
▲ Soriatane Capsules (10% to 25%)... 3003
Stadol NS Nasal Spray (1% or greater)... 1108
Sular Tablets (Less than or equal to 1%)... 688
Sustiva Capsules (Less than 2%)... 1258
Symmetrel... 1328
Synarel Nasal Solution for Endometriosis (Less than 1%)... 3205
Synercid I.V. (Less than 1%)... 775
Synvisc... 3596
Talacen Caplets (Rare)... 3089
Talwin Nx Tablets... 3090
Tambocor Tablets (1% to 3%)... 1990
Tapazole Tablets... 1823
Tarka Tablets (Less frequent)... 508
Tasmar Tablets (1% to 3%)... 3010
▲ Taxotere for Injection Concentrate (7 of 134 patients)... 778
Tazicef for Injection (Less than 1%)... 1647
Tazicef Galaxy Container (Less than 1%)... 1650
Tazicef Pharmacy Bulk Package (Less than 1%)... 1653
Tazidime Vials, Faspak & ADD-Vantage (Less than 1%)... 1966
Tegretol/Tegretol-XR... 2404
▲ Temodar Capsules (9%)... 3157
Tenex Tablets (3% or less)... 2942
Tenoretic Tablets... 690
Tequin Injection (0.1% to 3%)... 1110
Tequin Tablets (0.1% to 3%)... 1110
Testoderm Transdermal Systems... 574
Testopel Pellets... 3610
Testred Capsules, 10 mg... 1746
Tetanus & Diphtheria Toxoids Adsorbed for Adult Use... 1880
Teveten Tablets (Less than 1%)... 3327
▲ Thalomid Capsules (5.6% to 15.6%)... 1154
Thyrogen for Injection (1.6%)... 1441
Tiazac Capsules (Less than 2%)... 1378
Tikosyn Capsules (Less than or equal to 2%)... 2717
Timolide Tablets... 2187
Timolol GFS... ⊙266
Timoptic in Ocudose (Less frequent)... 2192
Timoptic Sterile Ophthalmic Solution (Less frequent)... 2190
Timoptic-XE Sterile Ophthalmic Gel Forming Solution... 2194
▲ Tonocard Tablets (3.5% to 9.2%)... 649
▲ Topamax Sprinkle Capsules (14.6% to 15%)... 2590
▲ Topamax Tablets (14.6% to 15%)... 2590
Toradol (1% or less)... 3018
Tricor Capsules, Micronized (1%)... 513
▲ Trisenox Injection (33%)... 1158
Trovan (Less than 1%)... 2722
Trusopt Sterile Ophthalmic Solution... 2196
Twinrix Vaccine (Less than 1%)... 1674
Ultracet Tablets (Less than 1%)... 2597
Ultram Tablets (Less than 1%)... 2600
Ultravate Ointment (Less frequent)... 1120
Uniretic Tablets (Less than 1%)... 3178
▲ Valcyte Tablets (8%)... 3022
Vantin Tablets and Oral Suspension (Less than 1%)... 2860
Varivax... 2202
Vascor Tablets (2.46%)... 2602
Vaseretic Tablets (0.5% to 2.0%)... 2204
Vasotec I.V. Injection... 2207
Vasotec Tablets (0.5% to 1.0%)... 2210
Verelan Capsules (1% or less)... 3184
Verelan PM Capsules (2% or less)... 3186

Versed Injection (Less than 1%) 3027
▲ Vesanoid Capsules (17%) 3037
Viadur Implant (Less than 2%) 912
Viagra Tablets (Less than 2%) 2732
Vicoprofen Tablets (Less than 3%) 520
Vioxx (Greater than 0.1% to 1.9%) 2213
Viracept 532
Vistide Injection 1445
Voltaren Tablets (Less than 1%) 2315
Voltaren-XR Tablets (Less than 1%) 2315
Warfarin Sodium Tablets, USP 3302
Wellbutrin Tablets 1680
Wellbutrin SR Sustained-Release Tablets (1% to 2%) 1684
Xanax Tablets (2.4%) 2865
Xeloda Tablets (1%) 3039
Xopenex Inhalation Solution 3207
Zanaflex Tablets (Frequent) 1305
Zaroxolyn Tablets 1177
Zebeta Tablets 1885
▲ Zenapax for Injection (2% to 5%) 3046
Zestoretic Tablets (1.5%) 695
Zestril Tablets (0.3% to 1.0%) 698
Ziac Tablets 1887
Ziagen 1692
Zithromax Capsules, 250 mg 2743
Zithromax for IV Infusion 2748
Zithromax for Oral Suspension, 1 g 2743
Zithromax for Oral Suspension, 300 mg, 600 mg, 900 mg, 1200 mg 2739
Zithromax Tablets, 250 mg 2739
Zithromax Tablets, 600 mg 2743
Zocor Tablets 2219
Zofran Injection (2%) 1698
Zoladex (1% or greater) 702
Zoladex 3-month (1% to 5%) 706
▲ Zoloft (3%) 2751
▲ Zomig Tablets (5% to 9%) 708
▲ Zomig-ZMT Tablets (5% to 9%) 708
▲ Zonegran Capsules (4%) 1307
Zovirax 1706
Zyban Sustained-Release Tablets (Infrequent) 1710
Zyprexa Tablets 1973
Zyprexa ZYDIS Orally Disintegrating Tablets 1973
Zyrtec (Less than 2%) 2756
Zyrtec-D 12 Hour Extended Relief Tablets (Less than 2%) 2758

Paresthesia, circumoral
▲ Agenerase Capsules (26% to 31%) 1454
▲ Agenerase Oral Solution (26% to 31%) 1459
Cerebyx Injection (Infrequent) 2619
Coly-Mycin M Parenteral 2243
Copaxone for Injection (Infrequent) 3306
Effexor Tablets (Infrequent) 3495
Effexor XR Capsules (Infrequent) 3499
Gabitril Tablets (Infrequent) 1189
Geodon Capsules (Rare) 2688
▲ Norvir Capsules (2.6% to 5.9%) 487
▲ Norvir Oral Solution (2.6% to 5.9%) 487
Paxil (Rare) 1609
ProSom Tablets (Rare) 500
Prozac Pulvules, Liquid, and Weekly Capsules (Rare) 1238
Rilutek Tablets (1.3% to 3.3%) 772
Sarafem Pulvules (Rare) 1962
Sonata Capsules (Infrequent) 3591
Thalomid Capsules 1154
Zonegran Capsules (Rare) 1307
Zyprexa Tablets (Rare) 1973
Zyprexa ZYDIS Orally Disintegrating Tablets (Rare) 1973

Paresthesia, extremities
Diamox ⊙269
Etrafon 3115
Limbitrol 1738
Motofen Tablets 577
Norpramin Tablets 755
Rifater Tablets 769
Rum-K 1363
Surmontil Capsules 3595
Vivactil Tablets 2217
Vivactil Tablets 2446

Paresthesia, facial
DTIC-Dome 902
Nicotrol Nasal Spray (More common) 2843

Paresthesia, feet
Grifulvin V Tablets Microsize and Oral Suspension Microsize (Rare) 2518
Gris-PEG Tablets (Rare) 2661
Lupron Depot 7.5 mg 3284
Rifamate Capsules 767

Paresthesia, hands
Grifulvin V Tablets Microsize and Oral Suspension Microsize (Rare) 2518
Gris-PEG Tablets (Rare) 2661
Inderal 3513
Inderal LA Long-Acting Capsules 3516
Inderide Tablets 3517
Inderide LA Long-Acting Capsules 3519
Oncaspar 756
Rifamate Capsules 767

Paresthesia, oral
▲ Agenerase Capsules (26% to 31%) 1454
▲ Agenerase Oral Solution (26% to 31%) 1459
Crixivan Capsules 2070

Paresthesia, peripheral
▲ Agenerase Capsules (10% to 14%) 1454
▲ Agenerase Oral Solution (10% to 14%) 1459
▲ Norvir Capsules (5% to 6%) 487
▲ Norvir Oral Solution (5% to 6%) 487

Parkinsonism
Aldoclor Tablets 2035
Aldomet Tablets 2037
Aldoril Tablets 2039
Ancobon Capsules 1730
Clozaril Tablets (Less than 1%) 2319
Cognex Capsules (Infrequent) 1351
Compazine 1505
Demser Capsules 2085
Depakene 421
Depakote Tablets 430
Depakote ER Tablets 436
Etrafon 3115
Indocin (Less than 1%) 2112
Orap Tablets 1407
Risperdal (0.6% to 4.1%) 1796
Serentil 1057
Seroquel Tablets 684
Stelazine 1640
Trilafon 3160
▲ Zyprexa Tablets (8% to 20%) 1973
▲ Zyprexa ZYDIS Orally Disintegrating Tablets (8% to 20%) 1973

Parkinsonism, aggravation of
Cognex Capsules (Rare) 1351
Lamictal 1567
Reglan 2935
Requip Tablets (1% or more) 1621
Risperdal 1796

Parkinson-like symptoms
Actimmune (Rare) 1772
Compazine 1505
Elspar for Injection (Rare) 2092
Haldol Decanoate 2535
Haldol Injection, Tablets and Concentrate 2533
Moban 1320
Navane Oral 2701
Navane Intramuscular 2703
Oncaspar 756
Orap Tablets (Frequent) 1407
Reglan 2935

Paroniria
Allegra (Less than 1%) 712
Cardura Tablets (Less than 0.5%) 2668
Celexa (Infrequent) 1365
Claritin (At least one patient) 3100
Claritin-D 12 Hour Extended Release Tablets (Less frequent) 3102
Claritin-D 24 Hour Extended Release Tablets (Fewer than 2%) 3104
Coreg Tablets (0.1% to 1%) 1508
Evoxac Capsules (Less than 1%) 1217
Gengraf Capsules (1% to less than 3%) 457
Imdur Tablets (Less than or equal to 5%) 1826
Intron A for Injection (Less than 5%) 3120
Neoral Soft Gelatin Capsules (1% to less than 3%) 2380
Neoral Oral Solution (1% to less than 3%) 2380
Procardia XL Extended Release Tablets (1% or less) 2710
Reminyl Oral Solution (Infrequent) 1792
Reminyl Tablets (Infrequent) 1792
Zoloft (Infrequent) 2751
Zyrtec (Less than 2%) 2756
Zyrtec-D 12 Hour Extended Relief Tablets (Less than 2%) 2758

Paronychia
Accutane Capsules 2944
Crixivan Capsules 2070
Evoxac Capsules (Less than 1%) 1217
▲ Soriatane Capsules (10% to 25%) 3003

Parosmia
Ambien Tablets (Rare) 3191
Astelin Nasal Spray 3339
Axert Tablets (Rare) 2772
Betaseron for SC Injection 988
Cardura Tablets (Less than 0.5%) 2668
Cerebyx Injection (Infrequent) 2619
Colazal Capsules 3069
Doxil Injection (Less than 1%) 566
Effexor Tablets (Infrequent) 3495
Effexor XR Capsules (Infrequent) 3499
Evoxac Capsules (Less than 1%) 1217
Flumadine (Less than 0.3%) 1370
Gabitril Tablets (Infrequent) 1189
Hivid Tablets (Less than 1%) 2975
Intron A for Injection (Less than 5%) 3120
Iopidine 0.5% Ophthalmic Solution (0.2%) ⊙213
Lamictal (Rare) 1567
Levaquin Injection (Less than 0.5%) 2537
Lipitor Tablets (Less than 2%) 2639
Lipitor Tablets (Less than 2%) 2696
Luvox Tablets (25, 50, 100 mg) (Infrequent) 3256
Miacalcin Nasal Spray (Less than 1%) 2375
Nexium Delayed-Release Capsules (Less than 1%) 619
Norvasc Tablets (Less than or equal to 0.1%) 2704
Norvir Capsules (Less than 2%) 487
Norvir Oral Solution (Less than 2%) 487
Paxil (Rare) 1609
Prozac Pulvules, Liquid, and Weekly Capsules (Rare) 1238
Remeron Tablets (Rare) 2483
Remeron SolTab Tablets (Rare) 2486
Rescriptor Tablets 526
Sarafem Pulvules (Rare) 1962
Sonata Capsules (Less than 1% to 2%) 3591
Sustiva Capsules (Less than 2%) 1258
Tasmar Tablets (Infrequent) 3010
Tequin Injection (Less than 0.1%) 1110
Tequin Tablets (Less than 0.1%) 1110
Topamax Sprinkle Capsules (Infrequent) 2590
Topamax Tablets (Infrequent) 2590
Zomig Tablets (Infrequent) 708
Zomig-ZMT Tablets (Infrequent) 708
Zonegran Capsules (Infrequent) 1307
Zyrtec (Less than 2%) 2756
Zyrtec-D 12 Hour Extended Relief Tablets (Less than 2%) 2758

Parotid gland enlargement
Depacon Injection 416
Depakene 421
Depakote Sprinkle Capsules 426
Depakote Tablets 430
Depakote ER Tablets 436
Diprivan Injectable Emulsion (Less than 1%) 667
Etrafon (Rare) 3115
Limbitrol 1738
Norpramin Tablets 755
Salagen Tablets (Less than 1%) 2229
Surmontil Capsules 3595
Thalomid Capsules 1154
Thioridazine Hydrochloride Tablets (Rare) 2289
Trental Tablets (Less than 1%) 784
Videx 1138
Videx EC Capsules 1143

Parotid tenderness
Trilafon (Rare) 3160

Parotitis
Artane (Rare) 1855
Catapres Tablets (Rare) 1037
Clorpres Tablets (Rare) 1002
Combipres Tablets (Rare) 1040
Duraclon Injection (Rare) 3057
M-M-R II 2118
Mumpsvax (Very low) 2141
Vivactil Tablets 2217
Vivactil Tablets 2446

Patent ductus arteriosus
Accupril Tablets 2611
Altace Capsules 2233
Captopril Tablets 2281
Cozaar Tablets 2067
▲ Curosurf Intratracheal Suspension (60%) 1232
Enalaprilat Injection 863
Hyzaar 2109
▲ Infasurf Intratracheal Suspension (45% to 47%) 1372
Lotrel Capsules 2370
Monopril Tablets 1091
Prinivil Tablets 2164
Prinzide Tablets 2168
▲ Survanta Intratracheal Suspension (46.9%) 3053
Univasc Tablets 3181
Vaseretic Tablets 2204
Vasotec I.V. Injection 2207
Vasotec Tablets 2210
Zestoretic Tablets 695
Zestril Tablets 698

Pavor nocturnus
Zarontin Capsules 2659
Zarontin Syrup 2660

PBI decrease
Dyazide Capsules 1515
Estratest 3252
Maxzide 1008
Sinemet Tablets 1253

PBI increase
Aygestin Tablets 1333
Etrafon 3115
Provera Tablets 2853
Trilafon 3160

Pelger-Huet anomaly
Risperdal (Rare) 1796

Peliosis hepatis
Anadrol-50 Tablets 3321
Androderm Transdermal System CIII (Rare) 3377
Android Capsules, 10 mg (Rare) 1731
Delatestryl Injection 1151
Estratest 3252
Oxandrin Tablets 1153
Testoderm Transdermal Systems (Rare) 574
Testopel Pellets 3610
Testred Capsules, 10 mg (Rare) 1746

Pellagra
Rifamate Capsules 767
Rifater Tablets 769
Trecator-SC Tablets (Rare) 3598

Pelvic inflammatory disease
Avonex 1013
Flovent Rotadisk (1% to 3%) 1537
Massengill Disposable Douches ▣752
Massengill Medicated Disposable Douche ▣753
Migranal Nasal Spray (Rare) 2376
Mirena Intrauterine System 974
ParaGard T 380A Intrauterine Copper Contraceptive 2582

Pelvic inflammatory disease, exacerbation of
Ethiodol Injection (Infrequent) 3095

Pelvic pressure
▲ MetroGel-Vaginal Gel (3%) 1986
Nolvadex Tablets 678
▲ Zoladex (18%) 702

Pemphigoid-like lesion
Captopril Tablets 2281
Sinemet Tablets 1253
Sinemet CR Tablets 1255
Timolol GFS ⊙266
Timoptic in Ocudose 2192
Timoptic Sterile Ophthalmic Solution 2190
Timoptic-XE Sterile Ophthalmic Gel Forming Solution 2194

Pemphigus
Accupril Tablets (0.5% to 1.0%) 2611
Accuretic Tablets (0.5% to 1%) 2614
Arthrotec Tablets (Rare) 3195
Cuprimine Capsules 2075
Depen Titratable Tablets 3341
Enalaprilat Injection 863
Lexxel Tablets 608
Lotensin Tablets (Less than 1%) 2365
Lotensin HCT Tablets (Rare) 2367
Lotrel Capsules (Rare) 2370
Mavik Tablets (0.3% to 1.0%) 478
Prinivil Tablets (0.3% to 1.0%) 2164
Prinzide Tablets 2168
Rifadin (Occasional) 765
Rifamate Capsules (Occasional) 767
Rifater Tablets (Occasional) 769
Rituxan for Infusion (Less than 0.1%) 1750
Rituxan I.V. (Less than 0.1%) 1428
Uniretic Tablets (Less than 1%) 3178
Univasc Tablets (Less than 1%) 3181
Vaseretic Tablets 2204
Vasotec I.V. Injection 2207
Vasotec Tablets (0.5% to 1.0%) 2210
Zestril Tablets (0.3% to 1.0%) 698

Pemphigus, bullous
Aceon Tablets (2 mg, 4 mg, 8 mg) 3249
Captopril Tablets 2281
Efudex (Infrequent) 1733
Monopril Tablets 1091
Monopril HCT 1094
Nolvadex Tablets (Very rare) 678
Sinemet Tablets 1253
Sinemet CR Tablets 1255

Penile discharge, unspecified
Alferon N Injection (1%) 1770
ProSom Tablets (Rare) 500

Penile disorder, unspecified
AndroGel (Fewer than 1%) 3322
Avonex 1013
▲ Caverject Sterile Powder (3%) 2777
Fortovase Capsules (Less than 2%) 2970
Lupron Depot–3 Month 22.5 mg (Less than 5%) 3288
Norvir Capsules (Less than 2%) 487
Norvir Oral Solution (Less than 2%) 487

Requip Tablets (Infrequent) 1621
▲ Serostim for Injection (1% to 10%) 3229
Soriatane Capsules (Less than 1%) 3003

Penile erection, decrease
▲ Zoladex (18%) 702
▲ Zoladex 3-month (One of the two most common) 706

Penile erection, increase
(*see under* Priapism)

Penile erection, prolonged or inappropriate
Androderm Transdermal System CIII 3377
▲ Android Capsules, 10 mg (Among most common) 1731
Oxandrin Tablets 1153
Testoderm Transdermal Systems 574
Viagra Tablets 2732

Penile fibrosis
▲ Caverject (3%) 2777

Penis, decreased sensation
Eldepryl Capsules 3266

Penis, enlargement
Intron A for Injection (Less than or equal to 5%) 3120
Lupron Injection 3279
Oxandrin Tablets 1153

Penis, fibrotic plaques
(*see under* Peyronie's disease)

Penis, strange feeling of
▲ Caverject Sterile Powder (3%) 2777

Perforation, cervix (partial)
ParaGard 2582

Perianal sensation, loss of
Nesacaine/Nesacaine MPF 617
Polocaine Injection, USP 625
Polocaine-MPF Injection, USP 625
Sensorcaine 643
Sensorcaine-MPF Injection 643
Xylocaine Injections 653

Periarteritis
Tapazole Tablets 1823

Periarteritis nodosum
Bactrim 2949
Dilantin Infatabs 2624
Dilantin Kapseals 2622
Dilantin-125 Oral Suspension 2625
Pediazole Suspension 3050
Septra Suspension 2265
Septra Tablets 2265
Septra DS Tablets 2265

Pericardial effusion
Activase I.V. 1410
Betaseron for SC Injection 988
▲ CellCept Capsules (15.9%) 2951
▲ CellCept Intravenous (15.9%) 2951
▲ CellCept Oral Suspension (15.9%) 2951
▲ CellCept Tablets (15.9%) 2951
Clomid Tablets 735
Clozaril Tablets 2319
Doxil Injection (1% to 5%) 566
Fludara for Injection (One patient) 995
▲ Gleevec Capsules (2% to 16%) 2357
Herceptin I.V. (At least one of the 958 patients) 1414
▲ Leukine (25%) 1755
Neurontin Capsules (Rare) 2655
Neurontin Oral Solution (Rare) 2655
Neurontin Tablets (Rare) 2655
Nipent for Injection (Less than 3%) 3272
Permax Tablets (Rare) 1299
Proleukin for Injection (1%) 1199
Refludan for Injection 761
ReoPro Vials (0.4%) 1958
Retavase Vials 1182
Sonata Capsules (Rare) 3591
Tasmar Tablets 3010
Taxotere for Injection Concentrate (Less frequent) 778
TNKase I.V. 1430
Trasylol Injection (1% to 2%) 909
Vesanoid Capsules 3037

Pericardial rub
Neurontin Capsules (Rare) 2655
Neurontin Oral Solution (Rare) 2655
Neurontin Tablets (Rare) 2655

Pericardial tamponade
Azulfidine EN-tabs Tablets (Rare) 2775

Pericarditis
Activase I.V. 1410
Agrylin Capsules 3232
Aldoclor Tablets 2035
Aldomet Tablets 2037
Aldoril Tablets 2039
Asacol Delayed-Release Tablets (Rare) 2884
Avonex 1013
Azulfidine EN-tabs Tablets (Rare) 2775
Campath Ampules 992
Canasa Rectal Suppositories (Rare) 829
Cerubidine for Injection (Rare) 947
Clozaril Tablets 2319
Colazal Capsules 3069
Cytovene-IV (Two or more reports) 2959
Declomycin Tablets 1855
Dipentum Capsules (Rare) 2803
Doryx Coated Pellet Filled Capsules 3357
Dynacin Capsules 2019
Evoxac Capsules (Less than 1%) 1217
Luvox Tablets (25, 50, 100 mg) (Rare) 3256
Minocin Intravenous 1862
Minocin Oral Suspension 1865
Minocin Pellet-Filled Capsules 1863
Monodox Capsules 2442
Neurontin Capsules (Rare) 2655
Neurontin Oral Solution (Rare) 2655
Neurontin Tablets (Rare) 2655
Paser Granules 1781
Pentasa Capsules (Infrequent to less than 1%) 3239
Periostat Tablets 1208
Permax Tablets (Rare) 1299
Procanbid Extended-Release Tablets (Fairly common) 2262
Proleukin for Injection (Less than 1%) 1199
Retavase Vials 1182
Rilutek Tablets (Infrequent) 772
Rowasa Rectal Suspension Enema 4.0 grams/unit (60 mL) (Rare) 3264
Thalomid Capsules 1154
TNKase I.V. 1430
Tonocard Tablets (Less than 1%) 649
▲ Trasylol Injection (5%) 909
▲ Vesanoid Capsules (3%) 3037
Vibramycin Calcium Oral Suspension Syrup 2735
Vibramycin Hyclate Capsules 2735
Vibramycin Hyclate Intravenous 2737
Vibramycin Monohydrate for Oral Suspension 2735
Vibra-Tabs Film Coated Tablets 2735

Pericarditis, constrictive
Dostinex Tablets (One case) 2804

Perifollicular thickening
Thalomid Capsules 1154

Perinatal disorder, unspecified
Diprivan Injectable Emulsion (Less than 1%) 667

Periodontal destruction
Evoxac Capsules (Less than 1%) 1217

Periodontitis
Avonex 1013
Coreg Tablets (1% to 2%) 1508
Protonix I.V. (Less than 1%) 3580
Protonix Tablets (Less than 1%) 3577
Requip Tablets (Infrequent) 1621
Teveten Tablets (Less than 1%) 3327
Thalomid 1154

Periostitis
Bicillin C-R 900/300 Injection 2240
Bicillin C-R Injection 2238
Bicillin L-A Injection 2242

Peripheral nerve symptoms
Xylocaine Injections (Less than 1%) 653

Peripheral vascular collapse
Brevital Sodium for Injection, USP 1815

Peripheral vascular disorder, unspecified
Actiq (Less than 1%) 1184
Androderm Transdermal System CIII (Less than 1%) 3377
Aricept Tablets (Infrequent) 1270
Aricept Tablets (Infrequent) 2665
Avonex 1013
Betapace Tablets (1% to 3%) 950
▲ Betaseron for SC Injection (5%) 988
Caverject Sterile Powder (Less than 1%) 2777
▲ CellCept Capsules (3%) 2951
▲ CellCept Intravenous (3%) 2951
▲ CellCept Oral Suspension (3%) 2951
▲ CellCept Tablets (3%) 2951
Effexor Tablets (Infrequent) 3495
Effexor XR Capsules (Infrequent) 3499
▲ Flolan for Injection (96%) 1528
Gabitril Tablets (Infrequent) 1189
Lopid Tablets (More common) 2650
Lotensin HCT Tablets (0.3% or more) 2367
Nascobal Gel 3174
Neurontin Capsules (Infrequent) 2655
Neurontin Oral Solution (Infrequent) 2655
Neurontin Tablets (Infrequent) 2655
Norvir Capsules (Less than 2%) 487
Norvir Oral Solution (Less than 2%) 487
Orudis Capsules (Less than 1%) 3548
Oruvail Capsules (Less than 1%) 3548
Paxil (Infrequent) 1609
▲ Prograf (3% to 15%) 1393
Protopic Ointment (Greater than or equal to 1%) 1397
Prozac Pulvules, Liquid, and Weekly Capsules (Rare) 1238
▲ Rapamune Oral Solution and Tablets (3% to 20%) 3584
Rescriptor Tablets 526
Rilutek Tablets (Infrequent) 772
Sarafem Pulvules (Rare) 1962
Thalomid Capsules 1154
Tricor Capsules, Micronized 513
Uniretic Tablets (Less than 1%) 3178
▲ Visudyne for Injection (1% to 10%) ⊙308
Zoladex (1% to 5%) 702
Zoladex 3-month 706

Peripheral vascular insufficiency
Corzide 40/5 Tablets (2 of 100 patients) 2247
Corzide 80/5 Tablets (2 of 100 patients) 2247

Peripheral wasting
Crixivan Capsules 2070
Fortovase Capsules 2970

Peristalsis, increase
Mestinon 1740
Prostigmin Injectable 1744
Prostigmin Tablets 1744
Tensilon Injectable 1745

Peritonitis
Betaseron for SC Injection 988
Campath Ampules 992
▲ CellCept Capsules (10.1%) 2951
▲ CellCept Intravenous (10.1%) 2951
▲ CellCept Oral Suspension (10.1%) 2951
CellCept Tablets (10.1%) 2951
Epogen for Injection 582
Neupogen for Injection (2%) 587
ParaGard T 380A Intrauterine Copper Contraceptive 2582
Paxil (Rare) 1609
Photofrin for Injection (Less than 5%) 831
▲ Prograf (3% to 15%) 1393
▲ Rapamune Oral Solution and Tablets (3% to 20%) 3584
Remicade for IV Injection (Less than 2%) 1178
Rilutek Tablets (Infrequent) 772
▲ Taxol Injection (30%) 1129

Peritonitis, chemical
Vancocin HCl, Vials & ADD-Vantage 1970

Perleche
Neurontin Capsules (Rare) 2655
Neurontin Oral Solution (Rare) 2655
Neurontin Tablets (Rare) 2655

Personality changes
Ambien Tablets (Rare) 3191
Cardizem Injectable 1018
Cardizem Lyo-Ject Syringe 1018
Cardizem Monovial 1018
Cardizem CD Capsules (Less than 1%) 1016
Celestone Soluspan Injectable Suspension 3097
Cerebyx Injection (Infrequent) 2619
Cortone Acetate Injectable Suspension 2059
Cortone Acetate Tablets 2061
Decadron Elixir 2078
Decadron Tablets 2079
Depacon Injection (1% to 5%) 416
Depakene (1% to 5%) 421
Depakote Sprinkle Capsules (1% to 5%) 426
Depakote Tablets (1% to 5%) 430
Depakote ER Tablets (1% to 5%) 436
Eldepryl Capsules 3266
Enbrel for Injection 1752
Enbrel for Injection 3504
Evoxac Capsules 1217
Exelon Capsules (Infrequent) 2342
Exelon Oral Solution (Infrequent) 2345
Florinef Acetate Tablets 2250
Gabitril Tablets (Frequent) 1189
Hydrocortone Tablets 2106
Hydrocortone Acetate Injectable Suspension 2103
Hydrocortone Phosphate Injection, Sterile 2105
Imitrex Tablets (Rare) 1558
Intron A for Injection (Less than 5%) 3120
Lamictal (Infrequent) 1567
Levo-Dromoran 1734
▲ Lupron Depot 3.75 mg (Among most frequent) 3281
Lupron Depot–3 Month 11.25 mg (Less than 5%) 3285
Lupron Depot-PED 7.5 mg, 11.25 mg and 15 mg (Less than 2%) 3291
Lupron Injection Pediatric (Less than 2%) 3280
Neurontin Capsules (Rare) 2655
Neurontin Oral Solution (2.8%) 2655
Neurontin Tablets (Rare) 2655
Norvir Capsules (Less than 2%) 487
Norvir Oral Solution (Less than 2%) 487
Orudis Capsules (Rare) 3548
Oruvail Capsules (Rare) 3548
Permax Tablets (2.1%) 1299
Prednisone 3064
Prelone Syrup 2273
Prometrium Capsules (100 mg, 200 mg) (Less than 5%) 3261
Prozac Pulvules, Liquid, and Weekly Capsules (Infrequent) 1238
Requip Tablets (Infrequent) 1621
Rilutek Tablets (Infrequent) 772
Roxicodone Tablets (Less than 3%) 3067
Sarafem Pulvules (Infrequent) 1962
Solu-Medrol Sterile Powder 2855
Tiazac Capsules (Less than 2%) 1378
Topamax Sprinkle Capsules (Frequent) 2590
Topamax Tablets (Frequent) 2590
Trileptal Oral Suspension 2407
Trileptal Tablets 2407
Vistide Injection 1445
▲ Zyprexa Tablets (8%) 1973
▲ Zyprexa ZYDIS Orally Disintegrating Tablets (8%) 1973

Perspiration
(*see under* Diaphoresis)

Petechiae
Accuretic Tablets 2614
AmBisome for Injection (Less common) 1383
Amphotec (1% to 5%) 1774
Avonex 1013
Azactam for Injection (Less than 1%) 1276
Betaseron for SC Injection 988
Cardizem Injectable 1018
Cardizem Lyo-Ject Syringe 1018
Cardizem Monovial 1018
Cardizem CD Capsules (Less than 1%) 1016
Celestone Syrup 3099
▲ CellCept Capsules (3% to 10%) 2951
▲ CellCept Intravenous (3% to 10%) 2951
▲ CellCept Oral Suspension (3% to 10%) 2951
▲ CellCept Tablets (3% to 10%) 2951
Cerebyx Injection (Infrequent) 2619
Clozaril Tablets (Less than 1%) 2319
▲ Cognex Capsules (7%) 1351
Cortone Acetate Injectable Suspension 2059
Cortone Acetate Tablets 2061
Decadron Elixir 2078
Decadron Phosphate Injection 2081
Depacon Injection (1% to 5%) 416
Depakene (1% to 5%) 421
Depakote Sprinkle Capsules (1% to 5%) 426
Depakote Tablets (1% to 5%) 430
Depakote ER Tablets (Greater than 1%) 436
Depo-Medrol Injectable Suspension 2795
Doxil Injection (Less than 1%) 566
Emla 602
Engerix-B Vaccine (Less than 1%) 1517
Florinef Acetate Tablets 2250
Floxin I.V. 2526
Floxin Tablets 2529
Gabitril Tablets (Infrequent) 1189
▲ Gemzar for Injection (16%) 1919
▲ Gleevec Capsules (0.9% to 10%) 2357
Hydrocortone Tablets 2106
Hydrocortone Acetate Injectable Suspension 2103
Hydrocortone Phosphate Injection, Sterile 2105
Indocin Capsules (Less than 1%) 2112
Indocin I.V. (Less than 1%) 2115
Indocin (Less than 1%) 2112
Lac-Hydrin Lotion (Less frequent) 1119
Lamictal (Rare to infrequent) 1567
▲ Leukine (6%) 1755
▲ Leustatin Injection (8%) 2495
Lipitor Tablets (Less than 2%) 2639
Lipitor Tablets (Less than 2%) 2696
Matulane Capsules 3246
Meridia Capsules 481
Migranal Nasal Spray (Infrequent) 2376
Miltown Tablets 3349
Mustargen for Injection 2142
▲ Mylotarg for Injection (17% to 28%) 3540
▲ Neupogen for Injection (17%) 587

Nipent for Injection (Less than 3%) 3272
Norpramin Tablets 755
▲ Novantrone for Injection (7% to 11%) 1760
Oncaspar (Less than 1%) 756
Parafon Forte DSC Caplets (Rare) 2582
Permax Tablets (Infrequent) 1299
Prednisone 3064
Prilosec Delayed-Release Capsules 628
▲ Proleukin for Injection (4%) 1199
Prozac Pulvules, Liquid, and Weekly Capsules (Rare) 1238
Recombivax HB 2178
Remeron Tablets (Rare) 2483
Remeron SolTab Tablets (Rare) 2486
ReoPro Vials (0.3%) 1958
Rescriptor Tablets (Less than 2%) 526
Rilutek Tablets (Rare) 772
Roferon-A Injection (Rare) 2996
Sandostatin Injection (Less than 1%) 2394
Sandostatin LAR Depot (Rare) 2395
Sarafem Pulvules (Rare) 1962
Solu-Medrol Sterile Powder 2855
Sular Tablets (Less than or equal to 1%) 688
Surmontil Capsules 3595
Thalomid Capsules 1154
Tiazac Capsules (Less than 2%) 1378
▲ Trisenox Injection (8%) 1158
Twinrix Vaccine (Less than 1%) 1674
Uniretic Tablets (Less than 1%) 3178
Urobiotic-250 Capsules 2731
Vivactil Tablets 2217
Vivactil Tablets 2446
Zanaflex Tablets (Rare) 1305
Zonegran Capsules (Rare) 1307

Petechiae and ecchymosis
Celestone Soluspan Injectable Suspension (No incidence in labeling) 3097
Decadron Tablets 2079
Pediapred Oral Solution 1170
Prelone Syrup 2273

Petechial hemorrhage
Carbatrol Capsules 3234
Tegretol/Tegretol-XR 2404

Peyronie's disease
Avonex 1013
Blocadren Tablets 2046
Corgard Tablets 2245
Corzide 40/5 Tablets 2247
Corzide 80/5 Tablets 2247
Cosopt Sterile Ophthalmic Solution 2065
Dilantin Infatabs 2624
Dilantin Kapseals 2622
Dilantin-125 Oral Suspension 2625
Inderal (Rare) 3513
Inderal LA Long-Acting Capsules (Rare) 3516
Inderide Tablets (Rare) 3517
Inderide LA Long-Acting Capsules (Rare) 3519
Nadolol Tablets 2288
Normodyne Tablets (Less common) 3137
Requip Tablets (Rare) 1621
Sectral Capsules 3589
Tenoretic Tablets 690
Tenormin 692
Timolide Tablets 2187
Timolol GFS ⊙266
Timoptic in Ocudose 2192
Timoptic Sterile Ophthalmic Solution 2190
Timoptic-XE Sterile Ophthalmic Gel Forming Solution 2194
Toprol-XL Tablets (Fewer than 1 of 100,000 patients) 651
Zebeta Tablets 1885
Ziac Tablets (Very rare) 1887

Pharyngeal changes
Mexitil Capsules (About 1 in 1,000) 1047

Pharyngeal discomfort
Cozaar Tablets (Less than 1%) 2067
Hyzaar 2109
Lexxel Tablets 608
Nexium Delayed-Release Capsules (Less than 1%) 619
Prinzide Tablets (0.3% to 1.0%) 2168
Zestoretic Tablets (0.3% to 1.0%) 695

Pharyngeal secretion, increase
Iopidine Sterile Ophthalmic Solution ⊙212
Prostigmin Injectable 1744
Prostigmin Tablets 1744

Pharyngitis (11%)
Accupril Tablets (0.5% to 1.0%) 2611
Accuretic Tablets (1.1%) 2614
▲ Aceon Tablets (2 mg, 4 mg, 8 mg) (3.3%) 3249
Actiq (1% or greater) 1184
▲ Actonel Tablets (5.8%) 2879
▲ Actos Tablets (5.1%) 3275
Adalat CC Tablets (Less than 1.0%) 877
▲ Advair Diskus 100/50 (13%) 1448
▲ Advair Diskus 250/50 (10%) 1448
▲ Advair Diskus 500/50 (10% to 13%) 1448
Aerobid/Aerobid-M (1% to 3%) 1363
▲ Agrylin Capsules (6.8%) 3232
Alferon N Injection (1%) 1770
Aloprim for Injection (Less than 1%) 2292
Alphagan P Ophthalmic Solution (1% to 4%) 546
▲ Ambien Tablets (3%) 3191
AmBisome for Injection (Less common) 1383
Amphotec (1% to 5%) 1774
Apligraf (1.8% to 2.7%) 2305
▲ Arava Tablets (3%) 724
Aricept Tablets (Infrequent) 1270
Aricept Tablets (Infrequent) 2665
▲ Arimidex Tablets (6.1% to 9.3%) 659
▲ Aromasin Tablets (2% to 5%) 2769
▲ Asacol Delayed-Release Tablets (11%) 2884
▲ Astelin Nasal Spray (3.8%) 3339
Atacand Tablets (2%) 595
Atacand HCT Tablets (0.5% or greater) 597
▲ Atrovent Inhalation Solution (3.7%) 1031
▲ Atrovent Nasal Spray 0.03% (8.1%) 1032
Atrovent Nasal Spray 0.06% (Less than 1%) 1033
Avalide Tablets (1% or greater) 1070
Avapro Tablets (1% or greater) 1074
Avapro Tablets (1% or greater) 3076
Avelox Tablets (0.05% to 1%) 879
Axert Tablets (Infrequent) 2772
▲ Axid Pulvules (3.3%) 1903
▲ Axid Pulvules (3.3%) 2919
▲ Azmacort Inhalation Aerosol (7% to 25%) 728
Azopt Ophthalmic Suspension (Less than 1%) 536
Bactroban Nasal (0.5% to 4%) 1495
▲ Baycol Tablets (9.6%) 883
Betaxon Ophthalmic Suspension (Less than 2%) 537
▲ Campath Ampules (12%) 992
Cardura Tablets (Less than 0.5%) 2668
▲ Carnitor Injection (15% to 27%) 3242
▲ Casodex Tablets (8%) 662
Ceclor CD Tablets (1.4%) 1279
Celebrex Capsules (2.3%) 2676
Celebrex Capsules (2.3%) 2780
Celexa (At least 2%) 1365
▲ CellCept Capsules (9.5% to 18.3%) 2951
▲ CellCept Intravenous (9.5% to 18.3%) 2951
▲ CellCept Oral Suspension (9.5% to 18.3%) 2951
▲ CellCept Tablets (9.5% to 18.3%) 2951
▲ Cenestin Tablets (8%) 1263
Cerebyx Injection (Infrequent) 2619
Claritin (At least one patient) 3100
▲ Claritin-D 12 Hour Extended Release Tablets (3%) 3102
▲ Claritin-D 24 Hour Extended Release Tablets (5%) 3104
Cognex Capsules (Frequent) 1351
Colazal Capsules (2%) 3069
▲ CombiPatch Transdermal System (9%) 2323
Combivent Inhalation Aerosol (2.2%) 1041
▲ Concerta Extended-Release Tablets (4%) 1998
▲ Concerta Tablets (4%) 561
Copaxone for Injection (At least 2%) 3306
Coreg Tablets (1.5% to 3.1%) 1508
Cosmegen for Injection 2062
Cosopt Sterile Ophthalmic Solution (1% to 5%) 2065
Cozaar Tablets (1% or greater) 2067
Crinone (Less than 5%) 3213
Crixivan Capsules (Less than 2%) 2070
▲ Depacon Injection (0.6% to 8%) 416
▲ Depakene (8%) 421
▲ Depakote Sprinkle Capsules (2% to 8%) 426
▲ Depakote Tablets (At least 5% to 8%) 430
Depakote ER Tablets (1% to 5%) 436
Detrol Tablets (1.5%) 3623
Diovan Capsules (More than 1%) 2337
▲ Diovan HCT Tablets (3%) 2338
Diprivan Injectable Emulsion (Less than 1%) 667
Ditropan XL Extended Release Tablets (2% to 5%) 564
Doxil Injection (Less than 1% to 5.5%) 566
▲ DuoNeb Inhalation Solution (4.4%) 1233
Duragesic Transdermal System (1% or greater) 1786
Effexor Tablets 3495
▲ Effexor XR Capsules (7%) 3499
Elmiron Capsules (Less than or equal to 1%) 570
▲ Enbrel for Injection (7%) 1752
▲ Enbrel for Injection (7%) 3504
Epogen for Injection 582
Estring Vaginal Ring (1%) 2811
▲ Evista Tablets (5.3% to 7.6%) 1915
▲ Evoxac Capsules (5.2%) 1217
Exelon Capsules (2% or more) 2342
Exelon Oral Solution (2% or more) 2345
Famvir Tablets (2.6% to 2.7%) 2348
▲ Felbatol (2.6% to 9.7%) 3343
▲ Flolan for Injection (5%) 1528
▲ Flomax Capsules (5.1% to 5.8%) 1044
▲ Flonase Nasal Spray (6% to 7.8%) 1533
▲ Flovent (9% to 25%) 1535
▲ Flovent Rotadisk (6% to 13%) 1537
Floxin I.V. (1% to 3%) 2526
Floxin Otic Solution (Single report) 1219
Floxin Tablets (1% to 3%) 2529
▲ Fludara for Injection (Up to 9%) 995
FluShield Influenza Vaccine 3521
Fortovase Capsules (Less than 2%) 2970
Foscavir Injection (Between 1% and 5%) 605
Sterile FUDR 2974
▲ Gabitril Tablets (7%) 1189
Gastrocrom Oral Concentrate (Less common) 1162
▲ Gengraf Capsules (4%) 457
Glucotrol XL Extended Release Tablets (Less than 1%) 2693
Gonal-F for Injection (2.5%) 3216
Havrix Vaccine (Less than 1%) 1544
▲ Herceptin I.V. (12%) 1414
Hivid Tablets (Less than 1%) 2975
▲ Humatrope Vials and Cartridges (3.13% to 6.67%) 1930
Hytrin Capsules (At least 1%) 464
Hyzaar (1% or greater) 2109
Imdur Tablets (Less than or equal to 5%) 1826
Indapamide Tablets (Less than 5%) 2286
Inderal 3513
Inderal LA Long-Acting Capsules 3516
Inderide Tablets 3517
Inderide LA Long-Acting Capsules 3519
▲ Infergen (17% to 34%) 1777
▲ Intron A for Injection (1% to 31%) 3120
Invirase Capsules (Less than 2%) 2979
Iopidine 0.5% Ophthalmic Solution (Less than 3%) ⊙213
▲ Keppra Tablets (6%) 3314
Klonopin Tablets (2%) 2983
▲ Lamictal (9.8%) 1567
▲ Lescol Capsules (3.8%) 2361
▲ Lescol Capsules (3.8%) 2925
Lescol XL Tablets (2.4%) 2361
Lescol XL Tablets (2.4%) 2925
▲ Leukine (23%) 1755
Levaquin (0.5% to less than 1.0%) 2537
Lexxel Tablets (Infrequent) 608
Lipitor Tablets (Up to 2.5%) 2639
Lipitor Tablets (Up to 2.5%) 2696
Livostin (Approximately 1% to 3%) ⊙305
Lodine (Less than 1%) 3528
Lodine XL Extended-Release Tablets (Less than 1%) 3530
▲ Lotemax Sterile Ophthalmic Suspension 0.5% (Less than 15%) ⊙261
Lotrel Capsules 2370
Lupron Depot–3 Month 22.5 mg (Less than 5%) 3288
Luvox Tablets (25, 50, 100 mg) 3256
LYMErix Vaccine (2.19% to 2.52%) 1592
Maxalt Tablets (Infrequent) 2120
Maxalt-MLT Orally Disintegrating Tablets (Infrequent) 2120
Megace Oral Suspension (1% to 3%) 1124
▲ Meridia Capsules (10%) 481
Mexitil Capsules (Less than 1%) 1047
Miacalcin Nasal Spray (Less than 1%) 2375
Micardis Tablets (1%) 1049
Micardis HCT Tablets (Less than 2%) 1051
▲ Migranal Nasal Spray (3%) 2376
Mirapex Tablets (Less than 1%) 2834
Mobic Tablets (0.6% to 3.2%) 1054
Monopril Tablets (0.2% to 1.0%) 1091
Monopril HCT (Less than 2%) 1094
Monurol Sachet (2.5%) 1375
▲ Mylotarg for Injection (11% to 20%) 3540
▲ Naprelan Tablets (3% to 9%) 1293
▲ Nasacort AQ Nasal Spray (5.1%) 752
▲ Nasarel Nasal Solution 0.025% (3% to 9%) 1296
▲ Nasonex Nasal Spray (10 % to 12%) 3131
▲ Neoral Soft Gelatin Capsules (4%) 2380
▲ Neoral Oral Solution (4%) 2380
▲ Neumega for Injection (25%) 1434
Neurontin Capsules (2.8%) 2655
Neurontin Oral Solution 2655
Neurontin Tablets (2.8%) 2655
Nexium Delayed-Release Capsules (Less than 1%) 619
Nicotrol Nasal Spray (More common) 2843
▲ Nipent for Injection (8% to 10%) 3272
Norvir Capsules (0.4% to 2.6%) 487
Norvir Oral Solution (0.4% to 2.6%) 487
▲ Novantrone for Injection (19%) 1760
▲ Optivar Ophthalmic Solution (1% to 10%) 2273
▲ Ortho-Prefest Tablets (7%) 2570
Orudis Capsules (Less than 1%) 3548
Oruvail Capsules (Less than 1%) 3548
OxyContin Tablets (Less than 1%) 2912
Patanol Ophthalmic Solution (Less than 5%) 540
Paxil (2.1%) 1609
▲ PEG-Intron Powder for Injection (10%) 3140
Permax Tablets (Frequent) 1299
▲ Photofrin for Injection (11%) 831
Plendil Extended-Release Tablets (0.5% to 1.5%) 623
▲ Pletal Tablets (7% to 10%) 2605
▲ Pletal Tablets (7% to 10%) 2848
▲ Prempro Tablets (11%) 3572
Prevnar for Injection 1870
Prilosec Delayed-Release Capsules (1%) 628
Prinivil Tablets (0.3% to 1.0%) 2164
Prinzide Tablets 2168
▲ Prograf (3% to 15%) 1393
Prometrium Capsules (100 mg, 200 mg) (Less than 5%) 3261
ProSom Tablets (1%) 500
Prostin E2 Suppositories 2852
Protonix I.V. (Greater than or equal to 1%) 3580
Protonix Tablets (Greater than or equal to 1%) 3577
▲ Protopic Ointment (3% to 12%) 1397
Proventil Inhalation Solution 0.083% (Less than 1%) 3146
Proventil Solution for Inhalation 0.5% (Less than 1%) 3144
▲ Provigil Tablets (6%) 1193
▲ Prozac Pulvules, Liquid, and Weekly Capsules (3% to 11%) 1238
▲ Pulmicort Turbuhaler Inhalation Powder (5% to 10%) 636
▲ Pulmozyme Inhalation Solution (32% to 40%) 1426
Quixin Ophthalmic Solution (1% to 3%) 3093
▲ Qvar Inhalation Aerosol (8% to 27%) 1987
▲ Rapamune Oral Solution and Tablets (16% to 21%) 3584
Recombivax HB (Equal to or greater than 1%) 2178
ReFacto Vials 1437
▲ Remicade for IV Injection (8% to 26%) 1178
▲ Requip Tablets (6%) 1621
Rescula Ophthalmic Solution (1% to 5%) ⊙306
Retrovir Capsules 1625
Retrovir IV Infusion 1629
Retrovir 1625
▲ Rhinocort Aqua Nasal Spray (4%) 642
▲ Rhinocort Nasal Inhaler (3% to 9%) 640
Risperdal (2% to 3%) 1796
Roxicodone Tablets (Less than 3%) 3067
▲ Salagen Tablets (3%) 2229
▲ Sandostatin LAR Depot (5% to 15%) 2395
▲ Sarafem Pulvules (6% to 10%) 1962
Sectral Capsules (Up to 2%) 3589
▲ Semprex-D Capsules (3%) 1172
▲ Serevent Diskus (3% to 6%) 1637
Seroquel Tablets (Infrequent) 684
▲ Serostim for Injection (1% to 10%) 3229
▲ Serzone Tablets (6%) 1104
▲ Simulect for Injection (3% to 10%) 2399
Singulair (Greater than or equal to 2%) 2181
Skelid Tablets (2.7%) 3088
Soriatane Capsules (Less than 1%) 3003
Sporanox Oral Solution (Less than 2%) 1808
Sporanox Oral Solution (Less than 2%) 2512
▲ Stadol NS Nasal Spray (3% to 9%) 1108
Sular Tablets (Less than 1% to 5%) 688
▲ Suprane Liquid for Inhalation (3% to 10%) 874
Synagis Intramuscular (2.6%) 2028
Tasmar Tablets (Frequent) 3010
▲ Temodar Capsules (8%) 3157
Tequin Injection (0.1% to 3%) 1110
Tequin Tablets (0.1% to 3%) 1110
▲ Teveten Tablets (4%) 3327
▲ Thalomid Capsules (4.2%) 1154
▲ Tiazac Capsules (3%) 1378
▲ TOBI Solution for Inhalation (38.1%) 1206
▲ Topamax Sprinkle Capsules (2.8% to 7.1%) 2590
▲ Topamax Tablets (2.8% to 7.1%) 2590

Tricor Capsules, Micronized 513
Trileptal Oral Suspension (Up to 3%) 2407
Trileptal Tablets (Up to 3%) 2407
▲ Tri-Nasal Spray (10.3% to 13.7%) .. 2274
Trizivir Tablets 1669
Uniretic Tablets (More than 1%) 3178
Univasc Tablets (1.8%) 3181
▲ Vancenase AQ Nasal Spray 0.084% (12%) 3163
▲ Vanceril Double Strength Inhalation Aerosol (14%) 3167
Vaqta (Up to 2.7%) 2199
Varivax 2202
Vascor Tablets (0.5% to 2.0%) 2602
▲ Verelan PM Capsules (3%) 3186
Vexol 1% Ophthalmic Suspension (Less than 2%) .... ⊙ 222
Viagra Tablets (Less than 2%) 2732
Vicoprofen Tablets (Less than 3%) .. 520
Vioxx (Greater than 0.1% to 1.9%) .. 2213
Viracept 532
Vistide Injection 1445
▲ Visudyne for Injection (1% to 10%) .... ⊙ 308
▲ WelChol Tablets (3%) 3073
▲ Wellbutrin SR Sustained-Release Tablets (3% to 11%) 1684
Yasmin 28 Tablets (Greater than 1%) 980
Zaditor Ophthalmic Solution (Less than 5%) 2304
▲ Zanaflex Tablets (3%) 1305
Zebeta Tablets (2.2%) 1885
▲ Zenapax for Injection (2% to 5%) 3046
Zestoretic Tablets 695
Zestril Tablets (0.3% to 1.0%) 698
Ziac Tablets 1887
Ziagen 1692
▲ Zoladex (5% to 6%) 702
Zonegran Capsules (Frequent) 1307
Zosyn (1.0% or less) 1890
Zosyn in Galaxy Containers (1.0% or less) 1894
▲ Zyban Sustained-Release Tablets (3%) 1710
▲ Zyprexa Tablets (5%) 1973
▲ Zyprexa ZYDIS Orally Disintegrating Tablets (5%) 1973
▲ Zyrtec (2.0% to 6.2%) 2756
Zyrtec-D 12 Hour Extended Relief Tablets (2%) 2758

Pharyngoxerosis
Carbatrol Capsules 3234
Tegretol/Tegretol-XR 2404

Phenylketonuria

Phimosis
▲ Caverject Sterile Powder (3%) 2777

Phlebitis
Adalat CC Tablets (Less than 1.0%) 877
Ambien Tablets (Rare) 3191
Amphotec (1% to 5%) 1774
Ancef for Injection (Rare) 1474
Ancef Injection (Rare) 1474
Anzemet Injection (Rare) 719
Anzemet Tablets (Rare) 722
Arthrotec Tablets (Rare) 3195
Atromid-S Capsules 3483
Azactam for Injection (1.9% to 2.1%) 1276
BeneFix for Injection 1432
Campath Ampules 992
▲ Cancidas for Injection (11.3% to 15.7%) 2048
Cefizox for Intramuscular or Intravenous Use (1% to 5%) 1390
Cefobid Intravenous/Intramuscular (1 in 120) 2671
Cefobid Pharmacy Bulk Package - Not for Direct Infusion (1 in 120) 2673
Cefotan (1 in 300) 664
Celexa (Rare) 1365
Ceptaz for Injection (Fewer than 2%) 1499
Clomid Tablets 735
Clozaril Tablets (Less than 1%) 2319
Cognex Capsules (Infrequent) 1351
Cytotec Tablets (Infrequent) 3202
Cytovene (At least 3 subjects) 2959
Dantrium Capsules (Less frequent) 2885
Demerol 3079
Diphtheria & Tetanus Toxoids Adsorbed Purogenated for Pediatric Use 1857
Diprivan Injectable Emulsion (Rare) 667
Dobutrex Solution Vials (Occasional) 1914
Dopram Injectable 2931
Doxil Injection (Less than 1%) 566
Evoxac Capsules (Less than 1%) 1217
Floxin I.V. (Approximately 2%) 2526
Fludara for Injection (1% to 3%) 995
Fluorescite Injection .... ⊙ 211
Fortaz (1 in 69 patients) 1541
Gabitril Tablets (Infrequent) 1189
Geodon Capsules (Rare) 2688
Humate-P Concentrate (2%) 790
Ifex for Injection (2%) 1123
Imitrex Injection 1549
Imitrex Nasal Spray (Rare) 1554
Imitrex Tablets 1558
INFeD Injection 3388
Intron A for Injection (Less than or equal to 5%) 3120
Kefzol Vials, ADD-Vantage (Rare) 1951
Leustatin Injection (2%) 2495
Levaquin Injection (Less than 0.5%) 2537
Lipitor Tablets (Less than 2%) 2639
Lipitor Tablets (Less than 2%) 2696
Lodosyn Tablets 1251
▲ Lupron Injection (5% or more) 3279
Luvox Tablets (25, 50, 100 mg) (Rare) 3256
Maxipime for Injection (1.3%) 1285
Merrem I.V. (0.8%) 673
Mithracin for Intravenous Use 903
Naropin Injection (Less than 1%) 612
▲ Navelbine Injection (Up to 10%) 1604
Nipent for Injection (Less than 3%) 3272
Nolvadex Tablets (0.3%) 678
Norplant System (Less than 1%) 3543
Novantrone for Injection (Infrequent) 1760
Panhematin for Injection 497
Paxil (Rare) 1609
▲ Primaxin I.V. (3.1%) 2160
▲ Prograf (3% to 15%) 1393
▲ Proleukin for Injection (23%) 1199
Prozac Pulvules, Liquid, and Weekly Capsules (Rare) 1238
Remeron Tablets (Rare) 2483
Remeron SolTab Tablets (Rare) 2486
Requip Tablets (Infrequent) 1621
Retrovir Capsules (1.6%) 1625
Retrovir IV Infusion (2%) 1629
Retrovir (1.6%) 1625
Rifater Tablets 769
Rilutek Tablets (0.4% to 0.8%) 772
Risperdal (Rare) 1796
Rocephin Injectable Vials, ADD-Vantage, Galaxy, Bulk (Less than 1%) 2993
Sandostatin LAR Depot (1% to 4%) 2395
Sarafem Pulvules (Rare) 1962
Serophene Tablets (Rare) 3226
Sinemet Tablets 1253
Sinemet CR Tablets 1255
Synercid I.V. (Less than 1%) 775
Synvisc 3596
Taxol Injection (Rare) 1129
Taxotere for Injection Concentrate .. 778
Tazicef for Injection (Less than 2%) 1647
Tazicef Galaxy Container (Less than 2%) 1650
Tazicef Pharmacy Bulk Package (Less than 2%) 1653
Tazidime Vials, Faspak & ADD-Vantage (Less than 2%) 1966
Testoderm Transdermal Systems (1%) 574
Tetanus & Diphtheria Toxoids Adsorbed for Adult Use 1880
Topamax Sprinkle Capsules (Infrequent) 2590
Topamax Tablets (Infrequent) 2590
Trasylol Injection (1.0%) 909
Tricor Capsules, Micronized 513
Triostat Injection (1% or fewer) 1825
▲ Valium Injectable (Among most common) 3026
Vancocin HCl, Vials & ADD-Vantage 1970
Versed Injection (0.4%) 3027
▲ Vesanoid Capsules (11%) 3037
Vistide Injection 1445
Wellbutrin Tablets (Rare) 1680
Wellbutrin SR Sustained-Release Tablets 1684
Xeloda Tablets (Less than 5%) 3039
Zanaflex Tablets (Rare) 1305
▲ Zinecard for Injection (3% to 6%) ... 2869
Zosyn (1.3%) 1890
Zosyn in Galaxy Containers (1.3%) 1894
▲ Zovirax for Injection (Approximately 9%) 1708
Zyban Sustained-Release Tablets 1710

Phlebosclerosis
Adriamycin PFS/RDF Injection 2767

Phobia, unspecified
Imitrex Injection 1549

Phobic disorder
Cipro I.V. (1% or less) 893
Cipro I.V. Pharmacy Bulk Package (Less than 1%) 897
Cipro (Less than 1%) 887
Floxin I.V. 2526
Floxin Tablets 2529
Imitrex Tablets (Rare) 1558
Luvox Tablets (25, 50, 100 mg) (Infrequent) 3256
Zyprexa Tablets (Infrequent) 1973
Zyprexa ZYDIS Orally Disintegrating Tablets (Infrequent) 1973

Phocomelia
Thalomid Capsules 1154

Phonophobia
Imitrex Tablets (Frequent) 1558

Phosphaturia
Daranide Tablets 2077

Phosphenes
Clomid Tablets (1.5%) 735
Serophene Tablets 3226

Phospholipid concentration, increase
Estratest 3252
Triphasil-21 Tablets 3600
Triphasil-28 Tablets 3605

Phosphorus, decrease
Omnicef (0.3%) 493
Thalomid Capsules 1154

Photodermatosis
Advair Diskus 100/50 1448
Advair Diskus 250/50 1448
Advair Diskus 500/50 1448

Photodynamic reaction
Urobiotic-250 Capsules 2731

Photophobia
Accutane Capsules 2944
▲ Alocril Ophthalmic Solution (1% to 10%) 545
▲ Alphagan Ophthalmic Solution (Approximately 3% to 9%) 545
Alphagan P Ophthalmic Solution (1% to 4%) 546
▲ Alrex Sterile Ophthalmic Suspension 0.2% (5% to 15%) .... ⊙ 256
Amerge Tablets (Frequent) 1467
Betaseron for SC Injection 988
▲ Betimol Ophthalmic Solution (More than 5%) .... ⊙ 324
Betoptic S Ophthalmic Suspension (Small number of patients) 537
Botox Purified Neurotoxin Complex 549
Calcijex Injection 411
Cardura Tablets (Less than 0.5%) ... 2668
Carteolol Hydrochloride Ophthalmic Solution USP, 1% (Occasional) .... ⊙ 258
Celexa (Infrequent) 1365
Celontin Capsules 2618
Cerebyx Injection (Infrequent) 2619
Chibroxin Sterile Ophthalmic Solution 2051
Ciloxan (Less than 1%) 538
Claritin-D 12 Hour Extended Release Tablets (Less frequent) ... 3102
Clomid Tablets (1.5%) 735
Copaxone for Injection (Infrequent) 3306
▲ Cordarone Tablets (4% to 9%) 3487
Cosopt Sterile Ophthalmic Solution (Less than 1%) 2065
CytoGam Intravenous (Infrequent) ... 2026
Depakote ER Tablets (Greater than 1%) 436
Effexor Tablets (Infrequent) 3495
Effexor XR Capsules (Infrequent) 3499
Ergamisol Tablets 1789
Etrafon 3115
Floxin I.V. (Less than 1%) 2526
Floxin Tablets (Less than 1%) 2529
Sterile FUDR (Remote possibility) 2974
Gabitril Tablets (Infrequent) 1189
Gamimune N, 5% Solvent/Detergent Treated (Infrequent) 925
Gamimune N, 10% Solvent/Detergent Treated (Infrequent) 928
Geodon Capsules (Infrequent) 2688
Havrix Vaccine (Less than 1%) 1544
Hectorol Capsules 1064
Hectorol Injection 1066
Hivid Tablets (Less than 1%) 2975
Imdur Tablets (Less than or equal to 5%) 1826
Imitrex Injection (Infrequent) 1549
Imitrex Tablets (Frequent) 1558
Intron A for Injection (Less than 5%) 3120
Iopidine 0.5% Ophthalmic Solution (Less than 3%) .... ⊙ 213
Lacrisert Sterile Ophthalmic Insert 2117
Lamictal (Infrequent) 1567
Lodine (Less than 1%) 3528
Lodine XL Extended-Release Tablets (Less than 1%) 3530
▲ Lotemax Sterile Ophthalmic Suspension 0.5% (5% to 15%) .... ⊙ 261
Lumigan Ophthalmic Solution (1% to 3%) 553
Luvox Tablets (25, 50, 100 mg) (Infrequent) 3256
Matulane Capsules 3246
Maxalt Tablets (Rare) 2120
Maxalt-MLT Orally Disintegrating Tablets (Rare) 2120
Migranal Nasal Spray (Infrequent) ... 2376
Neurontin Capsules (Infrequent) 2655
Neurontin Oral Solution (Infrequent) 2655
Neurontin Tablets (Infrequent) 2655
Nilandron Tablets (2%) 753
Nipent for Injection (Less than 3%) 3272
Nizoral Tablets (Less than 1%) 1791
Norvir Capsules (Less than 2%) 487
Norvir Oral Solution (Less than 2%) 487
Ocuflox Ophthalmic Solution 554
Ocupress Ophthalmic Solution, 1% Sterile (Occasional) .... ⊙ 303
OptiPranolol Metipranolol Ophthalmic Solution 0.3% (A small number of patients) .... ⊙ 263
▲ Orthoclone OKT3 Sterile Solution (10%) 2498
▲ Pacerone Tablets (4% to 9%) 3331
Paxil (Rare) 1609
Permax Tablets (Infrequent) 1299
Photofrin for Injection 831
Plaquenil Tablets (Fairly common) 3082
Prinivil Tablets (0.3% to 1.0%) 2164
Prinzide Tablets 2168
ProSom Tablets (Infrequent) 500
Prozac Pulvules, Liquid, and Weekly Capsules (Infrequent) 1238
Quinaglute Dura-Tabs Tablets 978
Quinidex Extentabs 2933
Quixin Ophthalmic Solution (1% to 3%) 3093
Requip Tablets (Infrequent) 1621
Rescriptor Tablets (Less than 2%) ... 526
Rescula Ophthalmic Solution (1% to 5%) .... ⊙ 306
Retrovir Capsules 1625
Retrovir IV Infusion 1629
Retrovir 1625
▲ Rēv-Eyes Sterile Ophthalmic Eyedrops 0.5% (10% to 40%) .... ⊙ 265
Rilutek Tablets (Rare) 772
Risperdal (Rare) 1796
Rocaltrol 2991
Sandoglobulin I.V. 2391
Sarafem Pulvules (Infrequent) 1962
Serentil 1057
Serophene Tablets 3226
▲ Serostim for Injection (1% to 10%) . 3229
Serzone Tablets (Infrequent) 1104
Sonata Capsules (Infrequent) 3591
▲ Soriatane Capsules (1% to 10%) 3003
Tambocor Tablets (Less than 1%) 1990
Topamax Sprinkle Capsules (Infrequent) 2590
Topamax Tablets (Infrequent) 2590
Travatan Ophthalmic Solution (1% to 4%) 543
Trilafon 3160
Trileptal Oral Suspension 2407
Trileptal Tablets 2407
Trovan (Less than 1%) 2722
Trusopt Sterile Ophthalmic Solution (Approximately 1% to 5%) 2196
Twinrix Vaccine (Less than 1%) 1674
Vexol 1% Ophthalmic Suspension (Less than 1%) .... ⊙ 222
Viagra Tablets (Less than 2%) 2732
▲ Vitravene for Injection (5% to 20%) .... ⊙ 310
Xalatan Latanoprost Ophthalmic Solution (1% to 4%) .... ⊙ 320
Xalatan Sterile Ophthalmic Solution (1% to 4%) 2864
Zaditor Ophthalmic Solution (Less than 5%) 2304
Zestoretic Tablets 695
Zestril Tablets (0.3% to 1.0%) 698
Zoloft (Rare) 2751
Zonegran Capsules (Rare) 1307
Zosyn (1.0% or less) 1890
Zosyn in Galaxy Containers (1.0% or less) 1894

Photopsia
Ambien Tablets (Rare) 3191
Clomid Tablets 735
Evoxac Capsules (Less than 1%) 1217
Maxalt Tablets (Rare) 2120
Maxalt-MLT Orally Disintegrating Tablets (Rare) 2120
Risperdal (Rare) 1796
Serophene Tablets 3226
Vitravene for Injection (2% to 5%) .. ⊙ 310

Photosensitivity
Accupril Tablets (Rare) 2611
Accuretic Tablets (0.5% to 1%) 2614
Accutane Capsules 2944
Aciphex Tablets 1267
Aciphex Tablets 1783
Agrylin Capsules (1% to 5%) 3232
Aldoclor Tablets 2035

Aldoril Tablets 2039
Alferon N Injection (1%) 1770
Altace Capsules (Less than 1%) 2233
Amaryl Tablets (Less than 1%) 717
Ambien Tablets (Rare) 3191
Amerge Tablets (Rare) 1467
Anaprox Tablets (Less than 1%) 2967
Anaprox DS Tablets (Less than 1%) 2967
Ancobon Capsules 1730
Arthrotec Tablets (Rare) 3195
Atacand HCT Tablets 597
Avalide Tablets 1070
Avonex 1013
Axert Tablets (Rare) 2772
Azmacort Inhalation Aerosol (1% to 3%) 728
Azulfidine EN-tabs Tablets (Rare) 2775
Bactrim 2949
Baycol Tablets (Rare) 883
Benadryl Parenteral 2617
Betapace Tablets (Rare) 950
Betapace AF Tablets (Rare) 954
Betaseron for SC Injection 988
Captopril Tablets 2281
Carbatrol Capsules 3234
Cardizem Injectable 1018
Cardizem Lyo-Ject Syringe 1018
Cardizem Monovial 1018
Cardizem CD Capsules (Less than 1%) 1016
Cataflam Tablets (Less than 1%) 2315
Celebrex Capsules (0.1% to 1.9%) 2676
Celebrex Capsules (0.1% to 1.9%) 2780
Celexa (Infrequent) 1365
Cerebyx Injection (Infrequent) 2619
Chibroxin Sterile Ophthalmic Solution 2051
Cipro I.V. (1% or less) 893
Cipro I.V. Pharmacy Bulk Package (Less than 1%) 897
Cipro (Less than 1%) 887
Claritin (At least one patient) 3100
Claritin-D 12 Hour Extended Release Tablets 3102
Claritin-D 24 Hour Extended Release Tablets 3104
Clindagel 1401
Clinoril Tablets (Less than 1 in 100) 2053
Clorpres Tablets 1002
Clozaril Tablets 2319
Combipres Tablets 1040
Compazine 1505
Copaxone for Injection (Infrequent) 3306
▲ Cordarone Tablets (4% to 9%) 3487
Coreg Tablets (0.1% to 1%) 1508
Corzide 40/5 Tablets (Occasional) 2247
Corzide 80/5 Tablets (Occasional) 2247
Cozaar Tablets (Less than 1%) 2067
Dantrium Capsules 2885
Declomycin Tablets 1855
Depacon Injection 416
Depakene 421
Depakote Sprinkle Capsules 426
Depakote Tablets 430
Depakote ER Tablets 436
D.H.E. 45 Injection 2334
DiaBeta Tablets 741
Diabinese Tablets 2680
Diamox Intravenous (Occasional) ⊙269
Diamox Sequels Sustained Release Capsules ⊙270
Diamox Tablets (Occasional) ⊙269
Diovan HCT Tablets 2338
Dipentum Capsules (Rare) 2803
Diucardin Tablets 3494
Diuril Oral 2087
Diuril Sodium Intravenous 2086
Dolobid Tablets (Less than 1 in 100) 2088
Doryx Coated Pellet Filled Capsules 3357
Dyazide Capsules 1515
Dynacin Capsules (Rare) 2019
Dyrenium Capsules (Rare) 3458
EC-Naprosyn Delayed-Release Tablets (Less than 1%) 2967
Effexor Tablets (Infrequent) 3495
Effexor XR Capsules (Infrequent) 3499
▲ Efudex (Among most frequent) 1733
Eldepryl Capsules 3266
Elmiron Capsules (Less than or equal to 1%) 570
Enalaprilat Injection 863
Ergamisol Tablets 1789
Etrafon 3115
Eulexin Capsules 3118
Evoxac Capsules (Less than 1%) 1217
Felbatol (Rare) 3343
Feldene Capsules (Occasional) 2685
Flexeril Tablets (Rare) 572
Flexeril Tablets (Rare) 2094
Floxin I.V. 2526
Floxin Tablets 2529
Fortovase Capsules (Less than 2%) 2970
Fosamax Tablets (Occasional) 2095
Sterile FUDR (Remote possibility) 2974
Furosemide Tablets 2284
Gabitril Tablets (Infrequent) 1189
Gastrocrom Oral Concentrate (Less common) 1162
Geodon Capsules (Frequent) 2688
Glucotrol Tablets 2692
Grifulvin V Tablets Microsize and Oral Suspension Microsize 2518
Gris-PEG Tablets (Occasional) 2661
Haldol Decanoate (Isolated cases) 2535
Haldol Injection, Tablets and Concentrate (Isolated cases) 2533
Hivid Tablets (Less than 1%) 2975
HydroDIURIL Tablets 2108
Hyzaar 2109
Imitrex Injection 1549
Imitrex Nasal Spray 1554
Imitrex Tablets 1558
Indapamide Tablets 2286
Inderide Tablets 3517
Inderide LA Long-Acting Capsules 3519
Intron A for Injection (Less than 5%) 3120
Invirase Capsules (Less than 2%) 2979
Lamictal (Rare) 1567
Lescol Capsules (Rare) 2361
Lescol Capsules (Rare) 2925
Lescol XL Tablets 2361
Lescol XL Tablets 2925
Levulan Kerastick 971
Lexxel Tablets 608
Limbitrol 1738
Lipitor Tablets (Less than 2%) 2639
Lipitor Tablets (Less than 2%) 2696
Lodine (Less than 1%) 3528
Lodine XL Extended-Release Tablets (Less than 1%) 3530
Lopid Tablets 2650
Lotensin Tablets (Less than 1%) 2365
Lotensin HCT Tablets (0.3% or more) 2367
Lupron Depot 3.75 mg 3281
Lupron Depot 7.5 mg 3284
Lupron Depot–3 Month 11.25 mg 3285
Lupron Depot–3 Month 22.5 mg 3288
Lupron Depot–4 Month 30 mg 3289
Lupron Depot-PED 7.5 mg, 11.25 mg and 15 mg 3291
Luvox Tablets (25, 50, 100 mg) (Infrequent) 3256
Maxalt Tablets (Infrequent) 2120
Maxalt-MLT Orally Disintegrating Tablets (Infrequent) 2120
Maxzide 1008
Mepergan Injection (Extremely rare) 3539
Meridia Capsules 481
Mevacor Tablets (Rare) 2132
Micardis HCT Tablets 1051
Microzide Capsules 3414
Minizide Capsules 2700
Minocin Intravenous (Rare) 1862
Minocin Oral Suspension (Rare) 1865
Minocin Pellet-Filled Capsules (Rare) 1863
Mobic Tablets (Less than 2%) 1054
Moduretic Tablets 2138
Monodox Capsules 2442
Monopril Tablets (0.2% to 1.0%) 1091
Monopril HCT 1094
Motrin Suspension, Oral Drops, Chewable Tablets, and Caplets (Less than 1%) 2002
Mykrox Tablets 1168
▲ Naprelan Tablets (3% to 9%) 1293
Naprosyn Suspension (Less than 1%) 2967
Naprosyn Tablets (Less than 1%) 2967
Navane Oral 2701
Navane Intramuscular 2703
Neptazane Tablets ⊙271
Neurontin Capsules (Rare) 2655
Neurontin Oral Solution (Rare) 2655
Neurontin Tablets (Rare) 2655
Nipent for Injection (Less than 3%) 3272
Noroxin Tablets 2145
Norpramin Tablets 755
Norvir Capsules (Less than 2%) 487
Norvir Oral Solution (Less than 2%) 487
One-A-Day Tension & Mood Softgels ■808
Orudis Capsules (Less than 1%) 3548
Oruvail Capsules (Less than 1%) 3548
▲ Pacerone Tablets (4% to 9%) 3331
Paxil (Rare) 1609
Pediazole Suspension 3050
Pentasa Capsules (Less than 1%) 3239
Periactin Tablets 2155
Periostat Tablets 1208
Phenergan Injection 3553
Phenergan Suppositories 3556
Phenergan Syrup (Rare) 3554
Phenergan Tablets 3556
Phenergan with Codeine Syrup (Rare) 3557
Phenergan with Dextromethorphan Syrup (Rare) 3559
Phenergan VC Syrup (Rare) 3560
Phenergan VC with Codeine Syrup (Rare) 3561
▲ Photofrin for Injection (19% to 22%) 831
Plaquenil Tablets 3082
Polytrim Ophthalmic Solution 556
Ponstel Capsules (Occasional) 1356
Pravachol Tablets (Rare) 1099
Prinivil Tablets (0.3% to 1.0%) 2164
Prinzide Tablets 2168
Procardia Capsules (Rare) 2708
Procardia XL Extended Release Tablets (Rare) 2710
▲ Prograf (3% to 15%) 1393
ProSom Tablets (Rare) 500
Protopic Ointment (Greater than or equal to 1%) 1397
Prozac Pulvules, Liquid, and Weekly Capsules (Rare) 1238
Pyrazinamide Tablets (Rare) 1876
Quinaglute Dura-Tabs Tablets (Occasional) 978
Quinidex Extentabs (Occasional) 2933
Rapamune Oral Solution and Tablets 3584
Relafen Tablets (Less than 1%) 1617
Remeron Tablets (Infrequent) 2483
Remeron SolTab Tablets (Infrequent) 2486
Renese Tablets 2712
Requip Tablets (Infrequent) 1621
Rifater Tablets (Rare) 769
Rilutek Tablets (Infrequent) 772
Risperdal (Frequent) 1796
Roxicodone Tablets (Less than 3%) 3067
Rynatan Tablets 3351
Salagen Tablets (Less than 1%) 2229
Sarafem Pulvules (Rare) 1962
Septra Suspension 2265
Septra Tablets 2265
Septra DS Tablets 2265
Seroquel Tablets (Infrequent) 684
▲ Serostim for Injection (1% to 10%) 3229
Serzone Tablets (Infrequent) 1104
Sinequan (Occasional) 2713
Sonata Capsules (Less than 1%) 3591
Soriatane Capsules (Less than 1%) 3003
Stelazine (Occasional) 1640
Sular Tablets (One case) 688
Surmontil Capsules 3595
Tazorac Gel 556
Tegretol/Tegretol-XR 2404
Tenoretic Tablets 690
Thalomid Capsules 1154
Thioridazine Hydrochloride Tablets (Extremely rare) 2289
Thiothixene Capsules 2290
Thorazine (Occasional) 1656
Tiazac Capsules (Less than 2%) 1378
Timolide Tablets 2187
Topamax Sprinkle Capsules (Infrequent) 2590
Topamax Tablets (Infrequent) 2590
Trecator-SC Tablets (Rare) 3598
Tricor Capsules, Micronized (Less than 1%) 513
Trilafon 3160
Trileptal Oral Suspension 2407
Trileptal Tablets 2407
Trovan (Less than 1%) 2722
Uniretic Tablets (Less than 1%) 3178
Univasc Tablets (Less than 1%) 3181
Valtrex Caplets 1676
Vaseretic Tablets 2204
Vasotec I.V. Injection 2207
Vasotec Tablets (0.5% to 1.0%) 2210
Viagra Tablets (Less than 2%) 2732
Vibramycin Calcium Oral Suspension Syrup 2735
Vibramycin Hyclate Capsules 2735
Vibramycin Hyclate Intravenous 2737
Vibramycin Monohydrate for Oral Suspension 2735
Vibra-Tabs Film Coated Tablets 2735
Vistide Injection 1445
▲ Visudyne for Injection (1% to 10%) ⊙308
Vivactil Tablets 2217
Vivactil Tablets 2446
Voltaren Tablets (Less than 1%) 2315
Voltaren-XR Tablets (Less than 1%) 2315
Wellbutrin SR Sustained-Release Tablets (Infrequent) 1684
Xeloda Tablets (Less than 5%) 3039
Zaroxolyn Tablets 1177
Zestoretic Tablets 695
Zestril Tablets (0.3% to 1.0%) 698
Ziac Tablets 1887
Zithromax (1% or less) 2743
Zithromax for Oral Suspension, 300 mg, 600 mg, 900 mg, 1200 mg (1% or less) 2739
Zithromax Tablets, 250 mg (1% or less) 2739
Zithromax Tablets, 600 mg (1% or less) 2743
Zocor Tablets (Rare) 2219
Zoloft (Infrequent) 2751
Zomig Tablets (Infrequent) 708
Zomig-ZMT Tablets (Infrequent) 708
Zovirax Capsules 1706
Zovirax for Injection 1708
Zovirax 1706
Zyban Sustained-Release Tablets (Infrequent) 1710
Zyprexa Tablets (Infrequent) 1973
Zyprexa ZYDIS Orally Disintegrating Tablets (Infrequent) 1973
Zyrtec (Less than 2%) 2756
Zyrtec-D 12 Hour Extended Relief Tablets (Less than 2%) 2758

Phototoxicity

Cipro 887
Dapsone Tablets USP 1780
Floxin Tablets 2529
Levaquin (Less than 0.1%) 2537
Noroxin Tablets 2145
Zyrtec (Less than 2%) 2756
Zyrtec-D 12 Hour Extended Relief Tablets (Less than 2%) 2758

Phthisis bulbi

Vitrasert Implant (Less than 1%) ⊙254

Physical performance, impairment

Adipex-P 1406
Clozaril Tablets 2319
Compazine 1505
Demerol 3079
Dilaudid Ampules 441
Dilaudid Powder 441
Dilaudid Rectal Suppositories 441
Dilaudid Tablets 441
Etrafon 3115
Gris-PEG Tablets (Occasional) 2661
Hycodan 1316
Hycomine Compound Tablets 1317
Hycotuss Expectorant Syrup 1318
Kadian Capsules 1335
Lithobid Slow-Release Tablets 3255
Lortab 3319
Lortab Elixir 3317
Loxitane Capsules 3398
Maxidone Tablets CIII 3399
Miltown Tablets 3349
MS Contin Tablets 2896
Norco 5/325 Tablets CIII 3424
Norco 7.5/325 Tablets CIII 3425
Norco 10/325 Tablets CIII 3425
Norco 10/325 Tablets CIII 3427
Norpramin Tablets 755
Percocet Tablets 1326
Percodan Tablets 1327
Percolone Tablets 1327
Phenergan Injection 3553
Phenergan Suppositories 3556
Phenergan Syrup 3554
Phenergan Tablets 3556
Phenergan with Codeine Syrup 3557
Phenergan with Dextromethorphan Syrup 3559
Phenergan VC Syrup 3560
Phenergan VC with Codeine Syrup 3561
Soma Compound Tablets 3354
Surmontil Capsules 3595
Tussionex Pennkinetic Extended-Release Suspension 1174
Tylenol with Codeine 2595
Tylox Capsules 2597
Ultram Tablets 2600
Vicodin Tablets 516
Vicodin ES Tablets 517
Vicodin HP Tablets 518
Vicodin Tuss Expectorant 519
Vivactil Tablets 2217
Vivactil Tablets 2446
Zydone Tablets 1330

Pigmentation

Aquasol A Parenteral 593
Copaxone for Injection (Infrequent) 3306
Cortifoam Rectal Foam 3170
Cosmegen for Injection 2062
Cosopt Sterile Ophthalmic Solution 2065
Etrafon 3115
Genotropin Lyophilized Powder (Infrequent) 2818
Lupron Injection (Less than 5%) 3279
Minipress Capsules (Single report) 2699
Minizide Capsules (Single report) 2700
Plaquenil Tablets 3082
Risperdal (Frequent) 1796
Timolide Tablets (Less than 1%) 2187
Timolol GFS ⊙266
Timoptic in Ocudose 2192
Timoptic Sterile Ophthalmic Solution 2190

Timoptic-XE Sterile Ophthalmic Gel Forming Solution 2194
Trilafon 3160

Pigmentation disorders
Accutane Capsules 2944
Aralen Tablets 3075
Carbatrol Capsules 3234
Cordarone Tablets (Occasional) 3487
Declomycin Tablets 1855
Dynacin Capsules 2019
Sterile FUDR (Remote possibility) 2974
Gebauer's Ethyl Chloride 1409
Gengraf Capsules (1% to less than 3%) 457
Minocin Intravenous 1862
Minocin Oral Suspension 1865
Minocin Pellet-Filled Capsules 1863
Neoral Soft Gelatin Capsules (1% to less than 3%) 2380
Neoral Oral Solution (1% to less than 3%) 2380
Orudis Capsules (Less than 1%) 3548
Oruvail Capsules (Less than 1%) 3548
Pacerone Tablets (Occasional) 3331
Quinaglute Dura-Tabs Tablets 978
Quinidex Extentabs (Occasional) 2933
Retrovir Capsules 1625
Retrovir IV Infusion 1629
Retrovir 1625
▲ Serostim for Injection (1% to 10%) 3229
Tegretol/Tegretol-XR 2404
Thorazine 1656
▲ Xalatan Latanoprost Ophthalmic Solution (5% to 15%) ⊙320
▲ Xalatan Sterile Ophthalmic Solution (5% to 15%) 2864

Pill rolling motion
Compazine 1505
Stelazine 1640
Thioridazine Hydrochloride Tablets 2289
Thiothixene Capsules 2290
Thorazine 1656

Piloerection
Narcan Injection 1322
▲ ProAmatine Tablets (13.4%) 3241

Pilonidal cyst, infected
Gonal-F for Injection 3216

Pituitary apoplexy
Factrel 3633
Sandostatin Injection (Less than 1%) 2394
Thyrel TRH for Injection (Infrequent) 3630

Pituitary tumors
Clomid Tablets 735
Imitrex Nasal Spray (Rare) 1554

Pituitary unresponsiveness, secondary
Celestone Soluspan Injectable Suspension 3097
Celestone Syrup 3099
Cortone Acetate Injectable Suspension 2059
Cortone Acetate Tablets 2061
Decadron Elixir 2078
Decadron Tablets 2079
Decadron Phosphate Injection 2081
Depo-Medrol Injectable Suspension 2795
Florinef Acetate Tablets 2250
Hydrocortone Tablets 2106
Hydrocortone Acetate Injectable Suspension 2103
Hydrocortone Phosphate Injection, Sterile 2105
Pediapred Oral Solution 1170
Prednisone 3064
Prelone Syrup 2273
Solu-Medrol Sterile Powder 2855

Placental disorder, unspecified
Felbatol 3343

Plantar fasciitis
Evoxac Capsules (Less than 1%) 1217

Plaques, erythematous
AquaMEPHYTON 2042

Platelet, decrease
(*see under* Thrombocytopenia)

Platelet, increase
(*see under* Thrombocytosis)

Platelet disorder, unspecified
Felbatol (Rare) 3343
Foscavir Injection (Between 1% and 5%) 605
Hivid Tablets (Less than 1%) 2975
Levaquin (Less than 0.3%) 2537
Salagen Tablets (Less than 1%) 2229
Zoloft (Rare) 2751

Plethora
Talwin Nx Tablets 3090

Pleural effusion
Abelcet Injection 1273
Actiq (Less than 1%) 1184
Activase I.V. 1410
▲ AmBisome for Injection (12.5%) 1383
Amphotec (1% to 5%) 1774
▲ Aredia for Injection (10.7%) 2309
Betaseron for SC Injection 988
Campath Ampules 992
▲ CellCept Capsules (3% to 17%) 2951
▲ CellCept Intravenous (3% to 17%) 2951
▲ CellCept Oral Suspension (3% to 17%) 2951
▲ CellCept Tablets (3% to 34.3%) 2951
Cipro I.V. (1% or less) 893
Cipro I.V. Pharmacy Bulk Package (Less than 1%) 897
Clinoril Tablets (Less than 1 in 100) 2053
Clomid Tablets 735
Clozaril Tablets 2319
Dostinex Tablets (Rare) 2804
Doxil Injection (Less than 1%) 566
Ellence Injection 2806
Evoxac Capsules (Less than 1%) 1217
Felbatol 3343
Femara Tablets (Less frequent) 2351
▲ Flolan for Injection (4% to 7%) 1528
Follistim for Injection 2465
▲ Gleevec Capsules (2% to 16%) 2357
Herceptin I.V. 1414
Humegon for Injection 2468
Leukine 1755
Levaquin Injection (Less than 0.5%) 2537
Lupron Depot–3 Month 22.5 mg (Less than 5%) 3288
Macrobid Capsules 2889
Macrodantin Capsules 2891
Matulane Capsules 3246
▲ Neumega for Injection (10%) 1434
Permax Tablets (Rare to infrequent) 1299
▲ Photofrin for Injection (32%) 831
Prinivil Tablets (0.3% to 1.0%) 2164
Prinzide Tablets 2168
Procanbid Extended-Release Tablets (Fairly common) 2262
▲ Prograf (30% to 36%) 1393
▲ Proleukin for Injection (7%) 1199
▲ Rapamune Oral Solution and Tablets (3% to 20%) 3584
Remicade for IV Injection (Less than 2%) 1178
ReoPro Vials (1.3%) 1958
Rilutek Tablets (Infrequent) 772
Sandostatin LAR Depot (1% to 4%) 2395
Serophene Tablets 3226
Sonata Capsules (Rare) 3591
Sular Tablets (Less than or equal to 1%) 688
Synercid I.V. (Less than 1%) 775
Tasmar Tablets (Rare) 3010
▲ Taxotere for Injection Concentrate (6%) 778
▲ Trasylol Injection (7%) 909
▲ Trisenox Injection (20%) 1158
Vantin Tablets and Oral Suspension (Less than 1%) 2860
▲ Vesanoid Capsules (20%) 3037
▲ Zenapax for Injection (2% to 5%) 3046
Zestoretic Tablets 695
Zestril Tablets (0.3% to 1.0%) 698
▲ Zometa for Intravenous Infusion (5% to 10%) 3621
Zosyn (1.3%) 1890
Zosyn in Galaxy Containers (1.3%) 1894

Pleural effusion with pericarditis
Dantrium Capsules (Less frequent) 2885

Pleural friction rubs
Lupron Injection (Less than 5%) 3279

Pleuralgia
Intron A for Injection (Less than 5%) 3120
Monopril Tablets (0.4% to 1.0%) 1091
Procanbid Extended-Release Tablets (Fairly common) 2262

Pleurisy
Aerobid/Aerobid-M (1% to 3%) 1363
Aricept Tablets (Infrequent) 1270
Aricept Tablets (Infrequent) 2665
Campath Ampules 992
Claritin-D 24 Hour Extended Release Tablets (Fewer than 2%) 3104
Effexor Tablets (Rare) 3495
Effexor XR Capsules (Rare) 3499
Evoxac Capsules (Less than 1%) 1217
Klonopin Tablets (Infrequent) 2983
Remicade for IV Injection (Less than 2%) 1178
ReoPro Vials (1.3%) 1958
Requip Tablets (Infrequent) 1621
▲ Serostim for Injection (1% to 10%) 3229
Tonocard Tablets (Less than 1%) 649
Trileptal Oral Suspension 2407
Trileptal Tablets 2407

Pleuritis
Amerge Tablets (Rare) 1467
Asacol Delayed-Release Tablets 2884
Azulfidine EN-tabs Tablets (Rare) 2775
Pacerone Tablets 3331
Permax Tablets (Rare) 1299
Rituxan for Infusion (Less than 0.1%) 1750
Rituxan I.V. (Less than 0.1%) 1428

Pneumocystis carinii
Campath Ampules 992
CellCept Capsules (Up to 0.3%) 2951
CellCept Intravenous (Up to 0.3%) 2951
CellCept Oral Suspension (Up to 0.3%) 2951
CellCept Tablets (Up to 0.3%) 2951
▲ Serostim for Injection (1% to 10%) 3229
▲ Taxol Injection (14% to 21%) 1129

Pneumocystis carinii, susceptibility
▲ Doxil Injection (9.2%) 566
▲ Orthoclone OKT3 Sterile Solution (3.1%) 2498

Pneumonia
Accuretic Tablets 2614
Actiq (Less than 1%) 1184
▲ Actonel Tablets (3.1%) 2879
Advair Diskus 100/50 (1% to 3%) 1448
Advair Diskus 250/50 (1% to 3%) 1448
Advair Diskus 500/50 (1% to 3%) 1448
Aerobid/Aerobid-M (1% to 3%) 1363
Agrylin Capsules (1% to 5%) 3232
Ambien Tablets (Rare) 3191
AmBisome for Injection (Less common) 1383
Amerge Tablets (Infrequent) 1467
Arava Tablets (2%) 724
▲ Argatroban Injection (3.3%) 1478
Aricept Tablets (Infrequent) 1270
Aricept Tablets (Infrequent) 2665
Arthrotec Tablets (Rare) 3195
Avelox Tablets (0.05% to 1%) 879
Avonex 1013
Betaseron for SC Injection 988
Betaxon Ophthalmic Suspension (Less than 2%) 537
▲ Campath Ampules (10% to 16%) 992
Carbatrol Capsules 3234
▲ Casodex Tablets (4%) 662
Celebrex Capsules (0.1% to 1.9%) 2676
Celebrex Capsules (0.1% to 1.9%) 2780
Celexa (Infrequent) 1365
▲ CellCept Capsules (3.6% to 10.6%) 2951
▲ CellCept Intravenous (3.6% to 10.6%) 2951
▲ CellCept Oral Suspension (3.6% to 10.6%) 2951
▲ CellCept Tablets (3.6% to 13.7%) 2951
Cerebyx Injection (Frequent) 2619
Claritin-D 24 Hour Extended Release Tablets (Fewer than 2%) 3104
Clozaril Tablets (Less than 1%) 2319
Cognex Capsules (Frequent) 1351
Combivent Inhalation Aerosol (1.4%) 1041
Compazine 1505
Comvax 2056
Copaxone for Injection (Infrequent) 3306
Crixivan Capsules (Less than 2%) 2070
▲ Curosurf Intratracheal Suspension (17%) 1232
Cytotec Tablets (Infrequent) 3202
▲ Cytovene (13%) 2959
Depacon Injection (1% to 5%) 416
Depakene (1% to 5%) 421
Depakote Sprinkle Capsules (1% to 5%) 426
Depakote Tablets (1% to 5%) 430
Depakote ER Tablets (Greater than 1%) 436
Doxil Injection (1% to 5%) 566
DuoNeb Inhalation Solution 1233
Effexor Tablets (Infrequent) 3495
Effexor XR Capsules (Infrequent) 3499
Enalaprilat Injection 863
Enbrel for Injection 1752
Enbrel for Injection 3504
Evista Tablets (2.6%) 1915
Evoxac Capsules (1% to 3%) 1217
Felbatol 3343
Feldene Capsules (Rare) 2685
Ferrlecit Injection (Greater than 1%) 3386
▲ Flolan for Injection (5%) 1528
Flovent Diskus 3614
▲ Fludara for Injection (16% to 22%) 995
Fortovase Capsules (Less than 2%) 2970
Foscavir Injection (Between 1% and 5%) 605
Gabitril Tablets (Frequent) 1189
▲ Gengraf Capsules (1% to 6.2%) 457
Geodon Capsules (Infrequent) 2688
▲ Gleevec Capsules (1% to 10%) 2357
▲ Gliadel Wafer (4% to 9%) 1723
Hycamtin for Injection (2%) 1546
Imdur Tablets (Less than or equal to 5%) 1826
Innohep Injection (Greater than or equal to 1%) 1248
Intron A for Injection (Rare) 3120
Invirase Capsules (Less than 2%) 2979
Ismo Tablets (Fewer than 1%) 3524
Klonopin Tablets (Infrequent) 2983
Lamictal (Rare) 1567
▲ Leustatin Injection (6%) 2495
Lexxel Tablets 608
Lipitor Tablets (Less than 2%) 2639
Lipitor Tablets (Less than 2%) 2696
Lodine XL Extended-Release Tablets 3530
Lovenox Injection (0.82%) 746
Lupron Depot–3 Month 22.5 mg (Less than 5%) 3288
Lupron Injection (Less than 5%) 3279
Luvox Tablets (25, 50, 100 mg) (Rare) 3256
Megace Oral Suspension (Up to 2%) 1124
Miacalcin Nasal Spray (Less than 1%) 2375
Mirapex Tablets (Less than 1%) 2834
Myleran Tablets 1603
▲ Mylotarg for Injection (8% to 14%) 3540
Myobloc Injectable Solution (2% or greater) 1291
Naprelan Tablets (Less than 1%) 1293
Navelbine Injection 1604
▲ Neoral Soft Gelatin Capsules (1% to 6.2%) 2380
▲ Neoral Oral Solution (1% to 6.2%) 2380
Neurontin Capsules (Frequent) 2655
Neurontin Oral Solution (Frequent) 2655
Neurontin Tablets (Frequent) 2655
▲ Nilandron Tablets (5.3%) 753
▲ Nipent for Injection (5%) 3272
▲ Novantrone for Injection (9%) 1760
NovoSeven (1%) 2430
Omnicef 493
Orthoclone OKT3 Sterile Solution 2498
Paxil (Infrequent) 1609
Permax Tablets (Frequent) 1299
▲ Photofrin for Injection (18%) 831
Plavix Tablets (1% to 2.5%) 1097
Plavix Tablets (1% to 2.5%) 3084
Pletal Tablets (Less than 2%) 2605
Pletal Tablets (Less than 2%) 2848
Ponstel Capsules (Rare) 1356
Prevacid Delayed-Release Capsules (Less than 1%) 3292
Prevnar for Injection 1870
PREVPAC (Less than 1%) 3298
Prinivil Tablets (0.3% to 1.0%) 2164
Prinzide Tablets 2168
▲ Prograf (3% to 15%) 1393
Proleukin for Injection 1199
Protonix I.V. (Less than 1%) 3580
Protonix Tablets (Less than 1%) 3577
Protopic Ointment (1% to 2%) 1397
Provigil Tablets (At least 1%) 1193
Pulmozyme Inhalation Solution 1426
▲ Rapamune Oral Solution and Tablets (3% to 20%) 3584
Rebetron Combination Therapy 3153
▲ Refludan for Injection (4.4%) 761
Remeron Tablets (Infrequent) 2483
Remeron SolTab Tablets (Infrequent) 2486
▲ Remicade for IV Injection (Less than 2% to 26%) 1178
ReoPro Vials (1.0%) 1958
Rescriptor Tablets 526
Rilutek Tablets (More than 2%) 772
Risperdal (Infrequent) 1796
▲ Roferon-A Injection (Less than 3% to 11%) 2996
Salagen Tablets (Less than 1%) 2229
▲ Sandimmune (6.2% to 9.2%) 2388
Sandostatin Injection (Less than 1%) 2394
Sandostatin LAR Depot (1% to 4%) 2395
Serentil 1057
Serevent Inhalation Aerosol (1% to 3%) 1633
Seroquel Tablets (Infrequent) 684
▲ Serostim for Injection (1% to 10%) 3229
Serzone Tablets (Infrequent) 1104
▲ Simulect for Injection (3% to 10%) 2399
Sonata Capsules (Infrequent) 3591
Sporanox Oral Solution (1.5% to 2.0%) 1808
Sporanox Oral Solution (1.5% to 2.0%) 2512
Stelazine 1640
Synagis Intramuscular (More than 1%) 2028
Tamiflu Capsules (Less than 1.9%) 3008
Tamiflu Oral Suspension (Less than 1.9%) 3008
Tasmar Tablets (1% or more) 3010
▲ Taxol Injection (30%) 1129
Tegretol/Tegretol-XR 2404
Thalomid Capsules 1154
Tonocard Tablets (Less than 1%) 649

Toprol-XL Tablets (Greater than 1%) ... 651
▲ Trasylol Injection (4%) ... 909
Tricor Capsules, Micronized ... 513
Trileptal Oral Suspension (1% to 2%) ... 2407
Trileptal Tablets (1% to 2%) ... 2407
Uniretic Tablets (Less than 1%) ... 3178
Valstar Sterile Solution for Intravesical Instillation (1%) ... 1175
Vantin Tablets and Oral Suspension (Less than 1%) ... 2860
Vaseretic Tablets ... 2204
Vasotec I.V. Injection ... 2207
Vasotec Tablets (1.0%) ... 2210
Venofer Injection (Greater than 1%) ... 580
▲ Vesanoid Capsules (14%) ... 3037
Vicoprofen Tablets (Less than 1%) ... 520
Vioxx (Greater than 0.1% to 1.9%) ... 2213
Virazole for Inhalation Solution ... 1747
▲ Vistide Injection (9%) ... 1445
▲ Visudyne for Injection (1% to 10%) ... ⊙308
▲ Vitravene for Injection (5% to 20%) ... ⊙310
Wellbutrin Tablets (Rare) ... 1680
Wellbutrin SR Sustained-Release Tablets ... 1684
Xeloda Tablets (Less than 5%) ... 3039
Zanaflex Tablets (Infrequent) ... 1305
▲ Zemplar Injection (5%) ... 522
▲ Zerit Capsules (3% to 4%) ... 1147
Zestoretic Tablets ... 695
Zestril Tablets (0.3% to 1.0%) ... 698
Zoladex 3-month (1% to 5%) ... 706
Zyban Sustained-Release Tablets ... 1710
Zyprexa Tablets (Infrequent) ... 1973
Zyprexa ZYDIS Orally Disintegrating Tablets (Infrequent) ... 1973
Zyrtec (Less than 2%) ... 2756
Zyrtec-D 12 Hour Extended Relief Tablets (Less than 2%) ... 2758

Pneumonia, aspiration
Cerebyx Injection (Infrequent) ... 2619
Gliadel Wafer (1%) ... 1723
Neurontin Capsules (Rare) ... 2655
Neurontin Oral Solution (Rare) ... 2655
Neurontin Tablets (Rare) ... 2655
Zyprexa Tablets (Infrequent) ... 1973
Zyprexa ZYDIS Orally Disintegrating Tablets (Infrequent) ... 1973

Pneumonia, eosinophilic
▲ Asacol Delayed-Release Tablets (5% or greater) ... 2884
Omnicef ... 493
Prozac Pulvules, Liquid, and Weekly Capsules ... 1238
Relafen Tablets (Less than 1%) ... 1617
Sarafem Pulvules ... 1962

Pneumonia, interstitial
Aciphex Tablets ... 1267
Aciphex Tablets ... 1783
Betaseron for SC Injection ... 988
Leukeran Tablets ... 1591
Nilandron Tablets (2%) ... 753
Norvir Capsules (Less than 2%) ... 487
Norvir Oral Solution (Less than 2%) ... 487
Omnicef ... 493
Taxol Injection (Rare) ... 1130

Pneumonia, pneumocystis carinii
Thalomid Capsules ... 1154

Pneumonitis
Accuretic Tablets ... 2614
Aldoclor Tablets ... 2035
Aldoril Tablets ... 2039
Atacand HCT Tablets ... 597
Attenuvax ... 2044
Avalide Tablets ... 1070
Azulfidine EN-tabs Tablets (Rare) ... 2775
▲ Campath Ampules (13% to 21%) ... 992
Carbatrol Capsules ... 3234
Celexa (Rare) ... 1365
Clinoril Tablets (Less than 1 in 100) ... 2053
Corzide 40/5 Tablets (Occasional) ... 2247
Corzide 80/5 Tablets (Occasional) ... 2247
Cosmegen for Injection ... 2062
Diovan HCT Tablets ... 2338
Diucardin Tablets ... 3494
Diuril Oral ... 2087
Diuril Sodium Intravenous ... 2086
Felbatol ... 3343
Herceptin I.V. (Rare) ... 1414
HydroDIURIL Tablets ... 2108
Hyzaar ... 2109
Indapamide Tablets ... 2286
Inderide Tablets ... 3517
Inderide LA Long-Acting Capsules ... 3519
Intron A for Injection (Rare) ... 3120
Lotensin HCT Tablets ... 2367
Matulane Capsules ... 3246
Maxzide ... 1008
Micardis HCT Tablets ... 1051
Microzide Capsules ... 3414
M-M-R II ... 2118
Moduretic Tablets ... 2138
Monopril HCT ... 1094
Mykrox Tablets (Rare) ... 1168
Orthoclone OKT3 Sterile Solution ... 2498
Pediazole Suspension ... 3050
PEG-Intron Powder for Injection (Less than or equal to 1%) ... 3140
Photofrin for Injection ... 831
Prinzide Tablets ... 2168
Prometrium Capsules (100 mg, 200 mg) (Less than 5%) ... 3261
Quinaglute Dura-Tabs Tablets ... 978
Quinidex Extentabs ... 2933
Rapamune Oral Solution and Tablets ... 3584
Rebetron Combination Therapy ... 3153
Rituxan I.V. ... 1428
Roferon-A Injection (Infrequent) ... 2996
▲ Serostim for Injection (1% to 10%) ... 3229
Tegretol/Tegretol-XR ... 2404
Tice BCG, BCG Live (1.2%) ... 2489
Timolide Tablets ... 2187
Uniretic Tablets ... 3178
Varivax (Less than 1%) ... 2202
Vaseretic Tablets ... 2204
Zaroxolyn Tablets ... 1177
Zestoretic Tablets ... 695
Ziac Tablets ... 1887

Pneumonitis, allergic
Dyazide Capsules ... 1515
Floxin I.V. ... 2526
Floxin Tablets ... 2529
▲ Fludara for Injection (Up to 6%) ... 995
Levaquin ... 2537
Relafen Tablets (Less than 1%) ... 1617
Ticlid Tablets (Rare) ... 3015

Pneumonitis, eosinophilic
Accupril Tablets ... 2611
Aceon Tablets (2 mg, 4 mg, 8 mg) ... 3249
Anaprox Tablets (Less than 1%) ... 2967
Anaprox DS Tablets (Less than 1%) ... 2967
Captopril Tablets ... 2281
EC-Naprosyn Delayed-Release Tablets (Less than 1%) ... 2967
Enalaprilat Injection ... 863
Lexxel Tablets ... 608
Lotensin HCT Tablets ... 2367
Lotrel Capsules ... 2370
Monopril Tablets ... 1091
▲ Naprelan Tablets (3% to 9%) ... 1293
Naprosyn Suspension (Less than 1%) ... 2967
Naprosyn Tablets (Less than 1%) ... 2967
Prinivil Tablets ... 2164
Prinzide Tablets ... 2168
Uniretic Tablets ... 3178
Univasc Tablets ... 3181
Vaseretic Tablets ... 2204
Vasotec I.V. Injection ... 2207
Vasotec Tablets ... 2210
Zestoretic Tablets ... 695
Zestril Tablets (0.3% to 1.0%) ... 698

Pneumonitis, interstitial
Actimmune (Rare) ... 1772
Alkeran for Injection ... 1465
Alkeran Tablets ... 1466
Aredia for Injection (One case) ... 2309
Asacol Delayed-Release Tablets ... 2884
Casodex Tablets (Rare) ... 662
Cordarone Tablets ... 3487
Cuprimine Capsules (Rare) ... 2075
Depen Titratable Tablets ... 3341
Macrobid Capsules (Rare to common) ... 2889
Macrodantin Capsules (Rare) ... 2891
Novantrone for Injection ... 1760
Pacerone Tablets ... 3331
Relafen Tablets (Less than 1%) ... 1617
Tonocard Tablets (Less than 1%) ... 649

Pneumothorax
Actiq (Less than 1%) ... 1184
Betaseron for SC Injection ... 988
Campath Ampules ... 992
▲ CellCept Capsules (3% to 10%) ... 2951
▲ CellCept Intravenous (3% to 10%) ... 2951
▲ CellCept Oral Suspension (3% to 10%) ... 2951
▲ CellCept Tablets (3% to 10%) ... 2951
Cerebyx Injection (Infrequent) ... 2619
▲ Curosurf Intratracheal Suspension (21%) ... 1232
Doxil Injection (Less than 1%) ... 566
▲ Flolan for Injection (4%) ... 1528
Foscavir Injection (Between 1% and 5%) ... 605
Herceptin I.V. (At least one of the 958 patients) ... 1414
Intron A for Injection (Less than or equal to 5%) ... 3120
Permax Tablets (Rare) ... 1299
▲ Prograf (3% to 15%) ... 1393
Proleukin for Injection (1%) ... 1199
Prozac Pulvules, Liquid, and Weekly Capsules (Rare) ... 1238
Pulmozyme Inhalation Solution ... 1426
Remeron Tablets (Rare) ... 2483
Remeron SolTab Tablets (Rare) ... 2486
Remicade for IV Injection (Less than 2%) ... 1178
Rifater Tablets ... 769
Rilutek Tablets (Infrequent) ... 772
Sandostatin LAR Depot (Rare) ... 2395
Sarafem Pulvules (Rare) ... 1962
▲ Trasylol Injection (4%) ... 909
Virazole for Inhalation Solution ... 1747
Zosyn (1.3%) ... 1890
Zosyn in Galaxy Containers (1.3%) ... 1894

Poliomyelitis
Fortovase Capsules (Less than 2%) ... 2970
Invirase Capsules (Less than 2%) ... 2979

Pollakiuria
DynaCirc Capsules (1.5% to 3.4%) ... 2921
DynaCirc CR Tablets (0.5% to 1%) ... 2923

Polyarteritis nodosa
Azulfidine EN-tabs Tablets (Rare) ... 2775
Intron A for Injection (Less than 5%) ... 3120

Polyarthralgia
Declomycin Tablets ... 1855
Dynacin Capsules ... 2019
Eskalith ... 1527
Lithobid Slow-Release Tablets ... 3255
Minocin Intravenous ... 1862
Minocin Oral Suspension ... 1865
Minocin Pellet-Filled Capsules ... 1863
Primaxin I.M. ... 2158
Primaxin I.V. (Less than 0.2%) ... 2160

Polyarthralgia, migratory
Cuprimine Capsules (Some patients) ... 2075
Depen Titratable Tablets ... 3341

Polyarthritis
Cleocin HCl Capsules (Rare) ... 2784
Cleocin Phosphate Sterile Solution (Rare) ... 2785
Cleocin Vaginal Cream (Rare) ... 2788
Cleocin Vaginal Ovules (Rare) ... 2789
Fortovase Capsules (Rare) ... 2970
Invirase Capsules (Rare) ... 2979
▲ Roferon-A Injection (5%) ... 2996

Polycythemia
Androderm Transdermal System CIII ... 3377
▲ Android Capsules, 10 mg (Among most common) ... 1731
▲ CellCept Capsules (3% to 10%) ... 2951
▲ CellCept Intravenous (3% to 10%) ... 2951
▲ CellCept Oral Suspension (3% to 10%) ... 2951
▲ CellCept Tablets (3% to 10%) ... 2951
Delatestryl Injection ... 1151
Estratest ... 3252
Gastrocrom Oral Concentrate (Less common) ... 1162
Geodon Capsules (Rare) ... 2688
Oxandrin Tablets ... 1153
Permax Tablets (Rare) ... 1299
Pletal Tablets (Less than 2%) ... 2605
Pletal Tablets (Less than 2%) ... 2848
▲ Prograf (3% to 15%) ... 1393
▲ Rapamune Oral Solution and Tablets (3% to 20%) ... 3584
▲ Simulect for Injection (3% to 10%) ... 2399
Testoderm Transdermal Systems ... 574
Testopel Pellets ... 3610
Testred Capsules, 10 mg ... 1746
Topamax Sprinkle Capsules (Rare) ... 2590
Topamax Tablets (Rare) ... 2590

Polydipsia
Amerge Tablets (Infrequent) ... 1467
Aricept Tablets (Infrequent) ... 1270
Aricept Tablets (Infrequent) ... 2665
Calcijex Injection ... 411
Clozaril Tablets (Less than 1%) ... 2319
Eskalith ... 1527
Hectorol Capsules ... 1064
Hectorol Injection ... 1066
Imitrex Injection (Rare) ... 1549
Imitrex Nasal Spray ... 1554
Imitrex Tablets (Rare) ... 1558
Lithium Carbonate ... 3061
Lithium Citrate Syrup ... 3061
Lithobid Slow-Release Tablets (Occasional) ... 3255
Loxitane Capsules ... 3398
Navane Oral ... 2701
Navane Intramuscular ... 2703
Risperdal (Frequent) ... 1796
Rocaltrol ... 2991
Thiothixene Capsules ... 2290

Polymenorrhea
Sandostatin Injection (Less than 1%) ... 2394

Polymyalgia rheumatica
Baycol Tablets ... 883
Lescol Capsules (Rare) ... 2361
Lescol Capsules (Rare) ... 2925
Lescol XL Tablets ... 2361
Lescol XL Tablets ... 2925
LYMErix Vaccine ... 1592
Mevacor Tablets (Rare) ... 2132
Miacalcin Nasal Spray (Less than 1%) ... 2375
Nexium Delayed-Release Capsules (Less than 1%) ... 619
Pravachol Tablets (Rare) ... 1099
Requip Tablets (Infrequent) ... 1621
Zocor Tablets (Rare) ... 2219

Polymyositis
Campath Ampules ... 992
Cuprimine Capsules (Rare) ... 2075
Depen Titratable Tablets (Rare) ... 3341
Enbrel for Injection (Infrequent) ... 1752
Enbrel for Injection (Infrequent) ... 3504
Tagamet (Rare) ... 1644

Polyneuritis
Antabuse Tablets ... 2444
Antabuse Tablets ... 3474
Meruvax II ... 2130
M-M-R II ... 2118
Podocon-25 Liquid ... 2608

Polyneuropathy
Acel-Imune ... 1851
Dilantin Infatabs ... 2624
Dilantin Kapseals ... 2622
Dilantin-125 Oral Suspension ... 2625
Ifex for Injection (Less than 1%) ... 1123
Intron A for Injection (Less than 5%) ... 3120
Meruvax II (Isolated reports) ... 2130
M-M-R II ... 2118
Streptase for Infusion (Rare) ... 647

Polyneuropathy, peripheral
Leustatin Injection ... 2495

Polyphagia
Atromid-S Capsules ... 3483
Etrafon ... 3115
Trilafon ... 3160

Polyps, endometrial
Nolvadex Tablets ... 678

Polyps, gallbladder
Sandostatin Injection (Less than 1%) ... 2394
Sandostatin LAR Depot (Rare) ... 2395

Polyps, nasal
▲ Atrovent Nasal Spray 0.03% (3.1%) ... 1032
Pulmozyme Inhalation Solution ... 1426
Zyrtec (Less than 2%) ... 2756
Zyrtec-D 12 Hour Extended Relief Tablets (Less than 2%) ... 2758

Polyps, rectal
Lupron Injection (Less than 5%) ... 3279

Polyradiculoneuropathy
Depen Titratable Tablets ... 3341
Tripedia Vaccine ... 817

Polyuria
Aciphex Tablets ... 1267
Aciphex Tablets ... 1783
Ambien Tablets (Rare) ... 3191
Amerge Tablets (Infrequent) ... 1467
Anzemet Injection (Rare) ... 719
Anzemet Tablets (Rare) ... 722
Arthrotec Tablets (Rare) ... 3195
Avonex ... 1013
Betaseron for SC Injection ... 988
Calcijex Injection ... 411
Captopril Tablets (Approximately 1 to 2 of 1000 patients) ... 2281
Cardizem Injectable ... 1018
Cardizem Lyo-Ject Syringe ... 1018
Cardizem Monovial ... 1018
Cardizem CD Capsules (Less than 1%) ... 1016
Cardura Tablets (2%) ... 2668
Celexa (Frequent) ... 1365
Cerebyx Injection (Infrequent) ... 2619
Cipro I.V. (1% or less) ... 893
Cipro I.V. Pharmacy Bulk Package (Less than 1%) ... 897
Cipro (Less than 1%) ... 887
Claritin-D 12 Hour Extended Release Tablets (Less frequent) ... 3102
Clomid Tablets (Fewer than 1%) ... 735
Cognex Capsules (Infrequent) ... 1351
Colazal Capsules ... 3069
Cytotec Tablets (Infrequent) ... 3202
DaunoXome Injection (Less than or equal to 5%) ... 1442
Diamox Intravenous ... ⊙269
Diamox Sequels Sustained Release Capsules ... ⊙270

Diamox Tablets ⊙269
Effexor Tablets (Infrequent) 3495
Effexor XR Capsules (Infrequent) 3499
Elspar for Injection (Low) 2092
Eskalith 1527
Etrafon (Occasional) 3115
Evoxac Capsules (0.1%) 1217
Exelon Capsules (Infrequent) 2342
Exelon Oral Solution (Infrequent) 2345
Feldene Capsules (Occasional) 2685
Floxin I.V. 2526
Floxin Tablets 2529
Foscavir Injection (Between 1% and 5%) 605
Gabitril Tablets (Infrequent) 1189
Gengraf Capsules (1% to less than 3%) 457
Geodon Capsules (Infrequent) 2688
Glucotrol XL Extended Release Tablets (Less than 3%) 2693
Hectorol Capsules 1064
Hectorol Injection 1066
Hivid Tablets (Less than 1%) 2975
Imdur Tablets (Less than or equal to 5%) 1826
Indapamide Tablets (Less than 5%) 2286
Intron A for Injection (Less than 5%) 3120
Klonopin Tablets (Infrequent) 2983
Lamictal (Infrequent) 1567
Lexxel Tablets 608
Lithium Carbonate 3061
Lithium Citrate Syrup 3061
Lithobid Slow-Release Tablets (Occasional) 3255
Lodine XL Extended-Release Tablets (Less than 1%) 3530
Lotrel Capsules 2370
Luvox Tablets (25, 50, 100 mg) (Infrequent) 3256
Maxalt Tablets (Infrequent) 2120
Maxalt-MLT Orally Disintegrating Tablets (Infrequent) 2120
Midamor Tablets (Less than or equal to 1%) 2136
Moduretic Tablets 2138
Motrin Suspension, Oral Drops, Chewable Tablets, and Caplets (Less than 1%) 2002
Neoral Soft Gelatin Capsules (1% to less than 3%) 2380
Neoral Oral Solution (1% to less than 3%) 2380
Neptazane Tablets ⊙271
Nexium Delayed-Release Capsules (Less than 1%) 619
Norvasc Tablets (Less than or equal to 0.1%) 2704
Norvir Capsules (Less than 2%) 487
Norvir Oral Solution (Less than 2%) 487
OxyContin Tablets (Less than 1%) 2912
Paxil (Infrequent) 1609
Plendil Extended-Release Tablets (0.5% to 1.5%) 623
Ponstel Capsules (Occasional) 1356
Primaxin I.M. 2158
Primaxin I.V. (Less than 0.2%) 2160
Procardia Capsules (Less than 0.5%) 2708
Procardia XL Extended Release Tablets (Less than 3%) 2710
Prozac Pulvules, Liquid, and Weekly Capsules (Infrequent) 1238
▲ Rapamune Oral Solution and Tablets (3% to 20%) 3584
Remeron Tablets (Rare) 2483
Remeron SolTab Tablets (Rare) 2486
Requip Tablets (Infrequent) 1621
Rescriptor Tablets (Less than 2%) 526
Retrovir Capsules 1625
Retrovir IV Infusion 1629
Retrovir 1625
Risperdal (Frequent) 1796
Rocaltrol 2991
Sarafem Pulvules (Infrequent) 1962
Seroquel Tablets (Rare) 684
Serzone Tablets (Infrequent) 1104
Tambocor Tablets (Less than 1%) 1990
Tarka Tablets (Less frequent) 508
Tasmar Tablets (Infrequent) 3010
Teveten Tablets (Less than 1%) 3327
Tiazac Capsules (Less than 2%) 1378
Tonocard Tablets (Less than 1%) 649
Topamax Sprinkle Capsules (Infrequent) 2590
Topamax Tablets (Infrequent) 2590
Toradol (1% or less) 3018
Tricor Capsules, Micronized (1%) 513
Trilafon (Occasional) 3160
Trileptal Oral Suspension 2407
Trileptal Tablets 2407
Uniretic Tablets (Less than 1%) 3178
Vistide Injection 1445
Wellbutrin SR Sustained-Release Tablets (Infrequent) 1684
Ziac Tablets 1887
Zoloft (Infrequent) 2751
Zomig Tablets (Infrequent) 708
Zomig-ZMT Tablets (Infrequent) 708
Zonegran Capsules (Infrequent) 1307
Zyban Sustained-Release Tablets (Infrequent) 1710
Zyprexa Tablets (Infrequent) 1973
Zyprexa ZYDIS Orally Disintegrating Tablets (Infrequent) 1973
Zyrtec (Less than 2%) 2756
Zyrtec-D 12 Hour Extended Relief Tablets (Less than 2%) 2758

Porphyria
Alesse-21 Tablets 3468
Alesse-28 Tablets 3473
Arthrotec Tablets (Rare) 3195
Brevicon 28-Day Tablets 3380
Cenestin Tablets 1263
Cyclessa Tablets 2450
Desogen Tablets 2458
Esclim Transdermal System 3460
Estrostep 2627
Levlen 962
Levlite 21 Tablets 962
Levlite 28 Tablets 962
Levora Tablets 3389
Loestrin 21 Tablets 2642
Loestrin Fe Tablets 2642
Lo/Ovral Tablets 3532
Lo/Ovral-28 Tablets 3538
Low-Ogestrel-28 Tablets 3392
Lunelle Monthly Injection 2827
Luvox Tablets (25, 50, 100 mg) 3256
Microgestin Fe 1.5/30 Tablets 3407
Microgestin Fe 1/20 Tablets 3400
Mircette Tablets 2470
Modicon 2563
Necon 3415
Nordette-28 Tablets 2257
Norinyl 1 +35 28-Day Tablets 3380
Norinyl 1 + 50 28-Day Tablets 3380
Ogestrel 0.5/50-28 Tablets 3428
Ortho-Cept 21 Tablets 2546
Ortho-Cept 28 Tablets 2546
Ortho-Cyclen/Ortho Tri-Cyclen 2573
Ortho-Novum 2563
Ortho-Novum 1/50□28 Tablets 2556
Ortho-Cyclen/Ortho Tri-Cyclen 2573
Ovcon 3364
Ovral Tablets 3551
Ovral-28 Tablets 3552
Ovrette Tablets 3552
Paxil 1609
Plaquenil Tablets 3082
Pyrazinamide Tablets (Rare) 1876
Reglan 2935
Rifater Tablets (Rare) 769
Sulfamylon Cream (A single case) 1011
Sulfamylon Topical Solution 1011
Tri-Levlen 962
Tri-Norinyl-28 Tablets 3433
Triphasil-21 Tablets 3600
Triphasil-28 Tablets 3605
Trivora Tablets 3439
Yasmin 28 Tablets 980
Zovia 3449

Porphyria, aggravation of
Activella Tablets 2764
Alora Transdermal System 3372
Cataflam Tablets (One patient) 2315
Cerebyx Injection (Infrequent) 2619
Climara Transdermal System 958
Dilantin Infatabs 2624
Dilantin Kapseals (Isolated reports) 2622
Dilantin-125 Oral Suspension (Isolated reports) 2625
Epogen for Injection (Rare) 582
Estinyl Tablets 3112
Estrace Vaginal Cream 3358
Estrace Tablets 3361
Estratest 3252
femhrt Tablets 2635
Menest Tablets 2254
Miltown Tablets 3349
Ogen Tablets 2846
Ortho Dienestrol Cream 2554
Ortho-Est Tablets 3464
Ortho-Prefest Tablets 2570
Plaquenil Tablets 3082
Premarin Intravenous 3563
Premarin Tablets 3566
Premarin Vaginal Cream 3570
Premphase Tablets 3572
Prempro Tablets 3572
Procrit for Injection (Rare) 2502
Rifadin (Isolated reports) 765
Rifater Tablets (Isolated reports) 769
Vivelle Transdermal System 2412
Vivelle-Dot Transdermal System 2416
Voltaren Tablets (One patient) 2315
Voltaren-XR Tablets (One patient) 2315
Zantac (Rare) 1690
Zantac Injection (Rare) 1688
Zantac Syrup (Rare) 1690

Porphyria, cutaneous, drug-induced
Photofrin for Injection 831

Porphyria, hepatic cutaneous
Diabinese Tablets 2680
Glucotrol Tablets 2692
Glucotrol XL Extended Release Tablets 2693

Porphyria, intermittent, acute
Carbatrol Capsules 3234
Depacon Injection 416
Depakene 421
Depakote Sprinkle Capsules 426
Depakote Tablets 430
Depakote ER Tablets 436
Tegretol/Tegretol-XR 2404

Porphyria cutanea tarda
Amaryl Tablets (Less than 1%) 717
Anaprox Tablets (Less than 1%) 2967
Anaprox DS Tablets (Less than 1%) 2967
DiaBeta Tablets 741
Diabinese Tablets 2680
EC-Naprosyn Delayed-Release Tablets (Less than 1%) 2967
Glucotrol Tablets 2692
Myleran Tablets (Rare) 1603
▲ Naprelan Tablets (3% to 9%) 1293
Naprosyn Suspension (Less than 1%) 2967
Naprosyn Tablets (Less than 1%) 2967

Porphyria cutanea tarda, pseudo
Relafen Tablets (Less than 1%) 1617

Potassium loss
(*see under* Hypokalemia)

Potassium retention
(*see under* Hyperkalemia)

Potentia, decrease
Kadian Capsules (Less than 3%) 1335
Roxanol 100 Concentrated Oral Solution 3066

Pre syncope
Betapace Tablets (1% to 4%) 950

Precocious puberty
Novarel for Injection 1347
Pregnyl for Injection 2482

Pregnancy, accidental
Depo-Provera Contraceptive Injection (Fewer than 1%) 2798
Tricor Capsules, Micronized 513

Pregnancy, ectopic
Clomid Tablets 735
Depo-Provera Contraceptive Injection 2798
▲ Follistim for Injection (3%) 2465
Gonal-F for Injection 3216
Humegon for Injection 2468
Mirena Intrauterine System 974
Modicon 2563
Norplant System 3543
Ortho-Novum 2563
Ortho-Novum 1/50□28 Tablets 2556
Ovidrel for Injection (Less than 2%) 3220
ParaGard T 380A Intrauterine Copper Contraceptive 2582
Pergonal for Injection 3223
Repronex for Intramuscular and Subcutaneous Injection (1%) 1347
Serophene Tablets 3226

Pregnancy, multiple
Clomid Tablets (An increased chance) 735

Pregnancy, sensation of
Depo-Provera Contraceptive Injection (Fewer than 1%) 2798

Pregnancy tests, false positive
Compazine 1505
Etrafon 3115
Navane Oral 2701
Navane Intramuscular 2703
Phenergan Injection 3553
Serentil 1057
Stelazine 1640
Thioridazine Hydrochloride Tablets 2289
Thiothixene Capsules 2290
Thorazine 1656

Pregnancy tests, false results
Phenergan Injection 3553
Trilafon 3160

Pregnancy, prolonged
Aggrenox Capsules 1026

Premature ventricular contractions
Diprivan Injectable Emulsion (Less than 1%) 667
Imitrex Injection (Infrequent) 1549
Lexxel Tablets 608
Mexitil Capsules (1.0% to 1.9%) 1047
Prinivil Tablets (0.3% to 1.0%) 2164
Prinzide Tablets 2168
Rythmol Tablets – 150 mg, 225 mg, 300 mg (1.5%) 502
Tarka Tablets (0.3% or more) 508
Versed Injection (Less than 1%) 3027
Zestril Tablets (0.3% to 1.0%) 698

Premenstrual-like syndrome
Activella Tablets 2764
Alesse-21 Tablets 3468
Alesse-28 Tablets 3473
Brevicon 28-Day Tablets 3380
Crinone (Less than 5%) 3213
Crixivan Capsules (Less than 2%) 2070
Cyclessa Tablets 2450
Desogen Tablets 2458
Estinyl Tablets 3112
Estratest 3252
Estrostep 2627
femhrt Tablets 2635
Levlen 962
Levlite 21 Tablets 962
Levlite 28 Tablets 962
Levora Tablets 3389
Loestrin 21 Tablets 2642
Loestrin Fe Tablets 2642
Lo/Ovral Tablets 3532
Lo/Ovral-28 Tablets 3538
Low-Ogestrel-28 Tablets 3392
Lunelle Monthly Injection 2827
Luvox Tablets (25, 50, 100 mg) (Infrequent) 3256
Menest Tablets 2254
Microgestin Fe 1.5/30 Tablets 3407
Microgestin Fe 1/20 Tablets 3400
Mircette Tablets 2470
Modicon 2563
Necon 3415
Nordette-28 Tablets 2257
Norinyl 1 +35 28-Day Tablets 3380
Norinyl 1 + 50 28-Day Tablets 3380
Ogestrel 0.5/50-28 Tablets 3428
Ortho Dienestrol Cream 2554
Ortho-Cept 21 Tablets 2546
Ortho-Cept 28 Tablets 2546
Ortho-Cyclen/Ortho Tri-Cyclen 2573
Ortho-Novum 2563
Ortho-Novum 1/50□28 Tablets 2556
Ortho-Cyclen/Ortho Tri-Cyclen 2573
Ovcon 3364
Ovral Tablets 3551
Ovral-28 Tablets 3552
Ovrette Tablets 3552
Premarin Intravenous 3563
Premarin Vaginal Cream 3570
Premphase Tablets 3572
Prempro Tablets 3572
Provera Tablets 2853
Tri-Levlen 962
Tri-Norinyl-28 Tablets 3433
Triphasil-21 Tablets 3600
Triphasil-28 Tablets 3605
Trivora Tablets 3439
Yasmin 28 Tablets 980
Zovia 3449
Zyprexa Tablets (2%) 1973
Zyprexa ZYDIS Orally Disintegrating Tablets (2%) 1973

Preputium, irretraction of
Condylox Topical Solution (Less than 5%) 2437

Priapism
Anadrol-50 Tablets 3321
Androderm Transdermal System CIII 3377
Bicillin C-R 900/300 Injection 2240
Bicillin C-R Injection 2238
Bicillin L-A Injection 2242
Cardura Tablets 2668
▲ Caverject Sterile Powder (4%) 2777
Celexa (At least 3 patients) 1365
Clozaril Tablets 2319
Compazine 1505
Copaxone for Injection (Infrequent) 3306
Coumadin for Injection 1243
Coumadin Tablets 1243
Delatestryl Injection 1151
Effexor XR Capsules (Rare) 3499
Flomax Capsules (Rare) 1044
Haldol Decanoate 2535
Haldol Injection, Tablets and Concentrate 2533
Heparin Lock Flush Solution 3509
Heparin Sodium Injection 3511
Hytrin Capsules (Rare) 464
Innohep Injection 1248
Lodosyn Tablets 1251
Luvox Tablets (25, 50, 100 mg) (Several cases) 3256
Minipress Capsules (Less than 1%) 2699
Minizide Capsules (Rare) 2700
Moban 1320
MUSE Urethral Suppository (Less than 0.1%) 3335
Oxandrin Tablets 1153

Paxil ... 1609
Permax Tablets (Infrequent) ... 1299
Prozac Pulvules, Liquid, and Weekly Capsules (Rare) ... 1238
Rilutek Tablets (Infrequent) ... 772
Risperdal (Rare) ... 1796
Sarafem Pulvules ... 1962
Seroquel Tablets (One case) ... 684
Serzone Tablets (Rare) ... 1104
Sinemet Tablets ... 1253
Sinemet CR Tablets ... 1255
Stelazine ... 1640
Testoderm Transdermal Systems ... 574
Testopel Pellets ... 3610
Testred Capsules, 10 mg ... 1746
Thorazine ... 1656
Trileptal Oral Suspension ... 2407
Trileptal Tablets ... 2407
Viagra Tablets ... 2732
Warfarin Sodium Tablets, USP ... 3302
Zoloft (Rare) ... 2751
Zyprexa Tablets ... 1973
Zyprexa ZYDIS Orally Disintegrating Tablets ... 1973

Proarrhythmia
Betapace Tablets (Less than 1% to 5%) ... 950
Corvert Injection ... 2793
Procanbid Extended-Release Tablets ... 2262
Rythmol Tablets – 150 mg, 225 mg, 300 mg (1.2% to 4.7%) ... 502

Proctitis
Aciphex Tablets ... 1267
Aciphex Tablets ... 1783
Aloprim for Injection (Less than 1%) ... 2292
Avonex ... 1013
Betaseron for SC Injection ... 988
Cosmegen for Injection ... 2062
Doxil Injection (Less than 1%) ... 566
Effexor Tablets (Rare) ... 3495
Effexor XR Capsules (Rare) ... 3499
▲ Eulexin Capsules (8%) ... 3118
Indocin Capsules (Less than 1%) ... 2112
Indocin I.V. (Less than 1%) ... 2115
Indocin (Less than 1%) ... 2112
Miltown Tablets (Rare) ... 3349
Neurontin Capsules (Rare) ... 2655
Neurontin Oral Solution (Rare) ... 2655
Neurontin Tablets (Rare) ... 2655
Rilutek Tablets (Rare) ... 772
Urobiotic-250 Capsules (Rare) ... 2731
▲ Zoladex (8%) ... 702
▲ Zoladex 3-month (8%) ... 706
Zoloft (Rare) ... 2751

Proctitis, ulceration
Doxil Injection (Less than 1%) ... 566

Proctocolitis
Diabinese Tablets (Less than 1%) ... 2680

Prolactin levels, elevated
(*see under* Hyperprolactinemia)

Prolactinoma
Serophene Tablets ... 3226

Proptosis
Brevicon 28-Day Tablets ... 3380
Depo-Provera Contraceptive Injection ... 2798
femhrt Tablets ... 2635
Levlen ... 962
Levlite 21 Tablets ... 962
Levlite 28 Tablets ... 962
Modicon ... 2563
Norinyl 1 +35 28-Day Tablets ... 3380
Norinyl 1 + 50 28-Day Tablets ... 3380
Ortho-Cyclen/Ortho Tri-Cyclen ... 2573
Ortho-Novum ... 2563
Ortho-Novum 1/50□28 Tablets ... 2556
Ortho-Cyclen/Ortho Tri-Cyclen ... 2573
Ovcon ... 3364
Premphase Tablets ... 3572
Prempro Tablets ... 3572
Provera Tablets ... 2853
Tri-Levlen ... 962
Tri-Norinyl-28 Tablets ... 3433

Prostate disorders, unspecified
▲ Androderm Transdermal System CIII (5%) ... 3377
▲ AndroGel (3% to 5%) ... 3322
Arava Tablets (1% to 3%) ... 724
Atrovent Nasal Spray 0.03% ... 1032
Atrovent Nasal Spray 0.06% ... 1033
Avalide Tablets ... 1070
Avapro Tablets (Less than 1%) ... 1074
Avapro Tablets (Less than 1%) ... 3076
Avonex ... 1013
Caverject Sterile Powder (2%) ... 2777
Celebrex Capsules (0.1% to 1.9%) ... 2676
Celebrex Capsules (0.1% to 1.9%) ... 2780
Evoxac Capsules (Less than 1%) ... 1217
Lupron Depot–4 Month 30 mg (Less than 5%) ... 3289
Mirapex Tablets (Less than 1%) ... 2834
Naprelan Tablets (Less than 1%) ... 1293
Protonix I.V. (Less than 1%) ... 3580
Protonix Tablets (Less than 1%) ... 3577
Requip Tablets (Infrequent) ... 1621
Tasmar Tablets (Infrequent) ... 3010
Travatan Ophthalmic Solution (1% to 5%) ... 543
Tricor Capsules, Micronized ... 513
Ultracet Tablets (2%) ... 2597
Viadur Implant (Less than 2%) ... 912
Vistide Injection ... 1445
▲ Visudyne for Injection (1% to 10%) ... ⊙308
Wellbutrin SR Sustained-Release Tablets (Infrequent) ... 1684
Zyban Sustained-Release Tablets ... 1710

Prostate enlargement
AndroGel (Five patients) ... 3322
Caverject Sterile Powder (2%) ... 2777

Prostate specific antigen increase
Aciphex Tablets ... 1267
Aciphex Tablets ... 1783

Prostatic acid phosphatase, decreased
Lupron Depot (Greater than or equal to 5%) ... 3284

Prostatic cancer, transient worsening symptoms
Zoladex (A small percentage) ... 702
Zoladex 3-month (A small percentage) ... 706

Prostatic hypertrophy
Android Capsules, 10 mg ... 1731
Aricept Tablets (Infrequent) ... 1270
Aricept Tablets (Infrequent) ... 2665
Caverject Sterile Powder (2%) ... 2777
Eldepryl Capsules ... 3266
Fortovase Capsules (Less than 2%) ... 2970
Invirase Capsules (Less than 2%) ... 2979
Testoderm Transdermal Systems (1%) ... 574
▲ Vesanoid Capsules (3%) ... 3037

Prostatitis
Caverject Sterile Powder (2%) ... 2777
Effexor Tablets (Frequent) ... 3495
Effexor XR Capsules (Infrequent) ... 3499
ReoPro Vials (0.1%) ... 1958
▲ Testoderm Transdermal Systems (4%) ... 574
Tice BCG, BCG Live (0.3%) ... 2489

Prostration
Bicillin C-R 900/300 Injection ... 2240
Bicillin C-R Injection ... 2238
Bicillin L-A Injection ... 2242
Pfizerpen for Injection ... 2707

Protein bound iodine, lowered
(*see under* PBI decrease)

Protein catabolism
Celestone Soluspan Injectable Suspension ... 3097
Celestone Syrup ... 3099
Depo-Medrol Injectable Suspension ... [illegible]
Florinef Acetate Tablets ... 2250
Hydrocortone Tablets ... 2106
Hydrocortone Acetate Injectable Suspension ... 2103
Hydrocortone Phosphate Injection, Sterile ... 2105
Prednisone ... 3064
Solu-Medrol Sterile Powder ... 2855

Proteinuria
Accutane Capsules ... 2944
Aceon Tablets (2 mg, 4 mg, 8 mg) (1.0% to 1.5%) ... 3249
Aggrenox Capsules ... 1026
Altace Capsules ... 2233
Anaprox Tablets ... 2967
Anaprox DS Tablets ... 2967
Arthrotec Tablets (Rare) ... 3195
Atromid-S Capsules ... 3483
Azulfidine EN-tabs Tablets (Rare) ... 2775
▲ Betaseron for SC Injection (5%) ... 988
Bicillin C-R 900/300 Injection ... 2240
Bicillin C-R Injection ... 2238
Bicillin L-A Injection ... 2242
Calcium Disodium Versenate Injection ... 1980
Captopril Tablets (Approximately 1 of 100 patients) ... 2281
Cataflam Tablets (Less than 1%) ... 2315
Ceclor (Infrequent) ... 1905
Celontin Capsules ... 2618
Cleocin HCl Capsules (Rare) ... 2784
Cleocin Phosphate Sterile Solution (Rare) ... 2785
Cleocin Vaginal Cream (Rare) ... 2788
Cleocin Vaginal Ovules (Rare) ... 2789
Clinoril Tablets (Less than 1 in 100) ... 2053
Crixivan Capsules (Less than 2%) ... 2070
▲ Cuprimine Capsules (6%) ... 2075
▲ Depen Titratable Tablets (6%) ... 3341
Dipentum Capsules (Rare) ... 2803
Dolobid Tablets (Less than 1 in 100) ... 2088
EC-Naprosyn Delayed-Release Tablets ... 2967
Ecotrin Enteric Coated Aspirin Low, Regular and Maximum Strength Tablets ... 1715
Elspar for Injection (Infrequent) ... 2092
Feldene Capsules (Occasional) ... 2685
Floxin I.V. (More than or equal to 1%) ... 2526
Floxin Tablets (More than or equal to 1%) ... 2529
Fludara for Injection (Up to 1%) ... 995
▲ Gemzar for Injection (2% to 45%) ... 1919
Grifulvin V Tablets Microsize and Oral Suspension Microsize (Rare) ... 2518
Gris-PEG Tablets (Rare) ... 2661
Ifex for Injection (Rare) ... 1123
Indocin (Less than 1%) ... 2112
Intron A for Injection (Less than 5%) ... 3120
Lexxel Tablets (Infrequent) ... 608
Lodine XL Extended-Release Tablets (Less than 1%) ... 3530
Lotensin HCT Tablets ... 2367
Mithracin for Intravenous Use ... 903
Motrin Suspension, Oral Drops, Chewable Tablets, and Caplets ... 2002
Naprelan Tablets ... 1293
Naprosyn Suspension ... 2967
Naprosyn Tablets ... 2967
Nebcin Vials, Hyporets & ADD-Vantage ... 1955
Neupogen for Injection (Infrequent) ... 587
▲ Novantrone for Injection (6%) ... 1760
Ponstel Capsules (Occasional) ... 1356
▲ Priftin Tablets (4.7%) ... 758
Prilosec Delayed-Release Capsules (Less than 1%) ... 628
Primaxin I.M. ... 2158
Primaxin I.V. ... 2160
▲ Proleukin for Injection (12%) ... 1199
Rescriptor Tablets (Less than 2%) ... 526
Roferon-A Injection (Infrequent) ... 2996
Sinemet Tablets ... 1253
Sinemet CR Tablets ... 1255
Tarka Tablets (Less frequent) ... 508
Tolectin (Less than 1%) ... 2589
Toradol (1% or less) ... 3018
Ultram Tablets (Infrequent) ... 2600
Vantin Tablets and Oral Suspension (Less than 1%) ... 2860
Vaqta (Isolated reports) ... 2199
▲ Vistide Injection (48% to 88%) ... 1445
Voltaren Tablets (Less than 1%) ... 2315
Voltaren-XR Tablets (Less than 1%) ... 2315
Zosyn ... 1890
Zosyn in Galaxy Containers ... 1894

Proteinuria, increased
Chemet Capsules (Up to 3.7%) ... 3078
Noroxin Tablets (1.0%) ... 2145

Prothrombin, decrease
(*see under* Hypoprothrombinemia)

Prothrombin, increase
(*see under* Hyperprothrombinemia)

Prothrombin time, deviation
Avelox Tablets (0.05% to 1%) ... 879
Lupron Depot–3 Month 22.5 mg ... 3288
Rythmol Tablets – 150 mg, 225 mg, 300 mg (Less than 1%) ... 502
Thrombin-JMI ... 1824

Prothrombin time, elevation
Cancidas for Injection (1.3% to 1.5%) ... 2048
Ecotrin Enteric Coated Aspirin Low, Regular and Maximum Strength Tablets ... 1715

Prothrombin time, increase
(*see under* Prothrombin time prolongation)

Prothrombin time prolongation
Aggrenox Capsules ... 1026
▲ Amphotec (5% or more) ... 1774
Anadrol-50 Tablets ... 3321
Avelox Tablets (0.05% to 1%) ... 879
Azactam for Injection ... 1276
Biaxin/Biaxin XL (1%) ... 403
Cefizox for Intramuscular or Intravenous Use ... 1390
Cefotan ... 664
Ceftin ... 1898
Cefzil ... 1076
▲ CellCept Capsules (3% to 10%) ... 2951
▲ CellCept Intravenous (3% to 10%) ... 2951
▲ CellCept Oral Suspension (3% to 10%) ... 2951
▲ CellCept Tablets (3% to 10%) ... 2951
Ceptaz for Injection ... 1499
Cipro I.V. ... 893
Cipro I.V. Pharmacy Bulk Package (Less than 1%) ... 897
Cipro ... 887
Clinoril Tablets ... 2053
Colazal Capsules ... 3069
Duricef ... 1079
Elmiron Capsules (Less than or equal to 1%) ... 570
Felbatol ... 3343
Floxin I.V. ... 2526
Floxin Tablets ... 2529
Fortaz ... 1541
Sterile FUDR ... 2974
Infergen (1% to 3%) ... 1777
Kefurox Vials, ADD-Vantage ... 1948
Levaquin ... 2537
Lorabid Suspension and Pulvules (Rare) ... 2251
▲ Lupron Depot–4 Month 30 mg (Greater than or equal to 5%) ... 3289
Maxipime for Injection (1.6%) ... 1285
Mefoxin for Injection ... 2124
Mefoxin Premixed Intravenous Solution ... 2127
Merrem I.V. (Greater than 0.2%) ... 673
Niaspan Extended-Release Tablets ... 1846
Noroxin Tablets ... 2145
Oncaspar ... 756
Ortho-Cyclen/Ortho Tri-Cyclen ... 2573
Oxandrin Tablets ... 1153
Panhematin for Injection ... 497
PREVPAC (1%) ... 3298
Primaxin I.M. ... 2158
Primaxin I.V. ... 2160
Provera Tablets ... 2853
Rescriptor Tablets ... 526
Rocephin Injectable Vials, ADD-Vantage, Galaxy, Bulk (Less than 1%) ... 2993
Suprax (Rare) ... 1877
Tazicef for Injection ... 1647
Tazicef Galaxy Container ... 1650
Tazicef Pharmacy Bulk Package ... 1653
Tazidime Vials, Faspak & ADD-Vantage ... 1966
Timentin Injection- ADD-Vantage Vial ... 1661
Timentin Injection-Galaxy Container ... 1664
Timentin Injection-Pharmacy Bulk Package ... 1666
Timentin for Intravenous Administration ... 1658
Vantin Tablets and Oral Suspension ... 2860
Zinacef Injection ... 1696
Zinacef for Injection ... 1696
Zoloft ... 2751
Zosyn ... 1890
Zosyn in Galaxy Containers ... 1894

Pruritus
Abelcet Injection ... 1273
Accupril Tablets (0.5% to 1.0%) ... 2611
Accuretic Tablets (0.5% to 1%) ... 2614
Accutane Capsules ... 2944
Aceon Tablets (2 mg, 4 mg, 8 mg) (0.3% to 1%) ... 3249
Aciphex Tablets ... 1267
Aciphex Tablets ... 1783
Aclovate (Approximately 2%) ... 1275
▲ Acticin Cream (7%) ... 998
Actiq (Up to 5%) ... 1184
Activella Tablets ... 2764
▲ Actonel Tablets (3%) ... 2879
Adalat CC Tablets (Less than 1.0%) ... 877
▲ Aerobid/Aerobid-M (3% to 9%) ... 1363
Agenerase Capsules (1%) ... 1454
Agenerase Oral Solution (1%) ... 1459
Aggrenox Capsules (Less than 1%) ... 1026
▲ Agrylin Capsules (5.5%) ... 3232
AK-Fluor Injection 10% and 25% ... ⊙202
Albuminar-5, U.S.P. ... 785
Albuminar-25, U.S.P. ... 786
Alferon N Injection (2%) ... 1770
Alkeran for Injection ... 1465
Allegra (Rare) ... 712
Allegra-D Extended-Release Tablets (Rare) ... 714
Aloprim for Injection (Less than 1%) ... 2292
Altace Capsules (Less than 1%) ... 2233
Amaryl Tablets (Less than 1%) ... 717
Ambien Tablets (Infrequent) ... 3191
▲ AmBisome for Injection (10.8%) ... 1383
Amerge Tablets (Infrequent) ... 1467
Americaine Anesthetic Lubricant ... 1162
Americaine Otic Topical Anesthetic Ear Drops ... 1162
Amicar Injection ... 3608
Amicar Syrup ... 3608
Amicar Tablets ... 3608

▲ Amphotec (5% or more) 1774
Analpram-HC 1338
▲ Anaprox Tablets (3% to 9%) 2967
▲ Anaprox DS Tablets (3% to 9%) 2967
Ancef for Injection 1474
Ancef Injection 1474
Ancobon Capsules 1730
Anusol-HC Cream 2.5% (Infrequent to frequent) 2237
Anusol-HC Suppositories 2238
▲ Anzemet Injection (3.1%) 719
▲ Anzemet Tablets (3.1%) 722
▲ Apligraf (3.1%) 2305
Aralen Tablets 3075
▲ Arava Tablets (4%) 724
Aricept Tablets (Frequent) 1270
Aricept Tablets (Frequent) 2665
Arimidex Tablets (2% to 5%) 659
Aromasin Tablets (Less frequent) 2769
Arthrotec Tablets (Rare) 3195
▲ Asacol Delayed-Release Tablets (3%) 2884
Astelin Nasal Spray 3339
▲ Astramorph/PF Injection, USP (Preservative-Free) (High incidence) 594
Atacand HCT Tablets (0.5% or greater) 597
Atromid-S Capsules (Less often) 3483
Atrovent Inhalation Aerosol (Less frequent) 1030
Augmentin Chewable Tablets 1482
Augmentin Powder for Oral Suspension 1482
Augmentin Tablets 1485
Augmentin ES-600 Powder for Oral Suspension 1487
Avalide Tablets 1070
Avapro Tablets (Less than 1%) 1074
Avapro Tablets (Less than 1%) 3076
Avelox Tablets (0.05% to 1%) 879
Avonex 1013
Axert Tablets (Rare) 2772
Axid Pulvules (1.7%) 1903
Axid Pulvules (1.7%) 2919
Aygestin Tablets 1333
Azactam for Injection (Less than 1%) 1276
Azelex Cream (Approximately 1% to 5%) 547
▲ Azulfidine EN-tabs Tablets (Less frequent) 2775
Bactrim 2949
Bactroban Cream (Less than 1%) 1494
Bactroban Nasal (1%) 1495
Bactroban Ointment (1%) 1496
Baycol Tablets 883
Beano ⊡ 809
▲ Benzaclin Topical Gel (12%) 1220
Betagan (Rare) ⊙ 228
Betapace Tablets (Rare) 950
Betapace AF Tablets (Rare) 954
Bicillin C-R 900/300 Injection 2240
Bicillin C-R Injection 2238
Bicillin L-A Injection 2242
Blocadren Tablets (1.1%) 2046
Brevital Sodium for Injection, USP 1815
Buprenex Injectable (Less than 1%) 2918
Calcijex Injection 411
▲ Campath Ampules (1% to 24%) 992
Cancidas for Injection (Up to 2.5%) 2048
Capex Shampoo 1400
Captopril Tablets (About 2 of 100 patients) 2281
Carafate Suspension (Less than 0.5%) 731
Carafate Tablets (Less than 0.5%) 730
Cardizem Injectable (Less than 1%) 1018
Cardizem Lyo-Ject Syringe (Less than 1%) 1018
Cardizem Monovial (Less than 1%) 1018
Cardizem CD Capsules (Less than 1%) 1016
Cardura Tablets (1%) 2668
▲ Carnitor Injection (3% to 8%) 3242
Casodex Tablets (2% to 5%) 662
Cataflam Tablets (1% to 3%) 2315
Catapres Tablets (About 7 in 1,000 patients) 1037
▲ Catapres-TTS (51 of 101 patients) 1038
Caverject Sterile Powder (Less than 1%) 2777
Ceclor CD Tablets (1.4%) 1279
Ceclor (Less than 1 in 200) 1905
Cedax (0.1% to 1%) 1021
Cefizox for Intramuscular or Intravenous Use (1% to 5%) 1390
Cefotan (1 in 700) 664
Ceftin (0.1% to 1%) 1898
Celebrex Capsules (0.1% to 1.9%) 2676
Celebrex Capsules (0.1% to 1.9%) 2780
Celexa (Frequent) 1365
▲ CellCept Capsules (3%) 2951
▲ CellCept Intravenous (3%) 2951
▲ CellCept Oral Suspension (3%) 2951
▲ CellCept Tablets (3% to 14.1%) 2951
Ceptaz for Injection (2% of patients) 1499
▲ Cerebyx Injection (7 of 16 volunteers; 2.8% to 48.9%) 2619
▲ Cerezyme for Injection (Approximately 4%) 1438
Cerumenex Eardrops (1% of 2,700 patients) 2895
Cetrotide for Injection 3209
▲ Chemet Capsules (2.6% to 11.2%) 3078
▲ Chirocaine Injection (3.7%) 2909
Chloroptic Sterile Ophthalmic Ointment ⊙ 234
Cipro HC Otic Suspension (0.4%) 540
Cipro I.V. (1% or less) 893
Cipro I.V. Pharmacy Bulk Package (Less than 1%) 897
Cipro (Less than 1%) 887
Claforan Injection (2.4%) 732
Claritin (At least one patient) 3100
Claritin-D 12 Hour Extended Release Tablets (Less frequent) 3102
Claritin-D 24 Hour Extended Release Tablets (Fewer than 2%) 3104
Cleocin Phosphate Sterile Solution 2785
▲ Cleocin T Topical (7% to 11%) 2790
Cleocin Vaginal Cream (2%) 2788
Cleocin Vaginal Ovules (Less than 1%) 2789
Clindagel (1%) 1401
▲ Clindets Pledgets (7% to 11%) 3270
Clinoril Tablets (Greater than 1%) 2053
Clobevate Gel (Less than 2%) 3271
Clomid Tablets 735
Clorpres Tablets (About 7 in 1,000) 1002
Clozaril Tablets (Less than 1%) 2319
▲ Cognex Capsules (7%) 1351
Colazal Capsules 3069
Coly-Mycin M Parenteral 2243
Combipres Tablets (About 7 in 1,000) 1040
Combivent Inhalation Aerosol 1041
Compazine 1505
Comvax 2056
▲ Copaxone for Injection (18%) 3306
Cordran Lotion (Infrequent) 2438
Cordran Tape (Infrequent) 2439
Coreg Tablets (0.1% to 1%) 1508
Corgard Tablets (1 to 5 per 1000 patients) 2245
Cormax Cream (0.5%) 2440
Cormax Ointment (0.5%) 2440
Cormax Scalp Application (Infrequent) 2441
Cortisporin Ophthalmic Suspension ⊙ 297
Corzide 40/5 Tablets (1 to 5 of 1000 patients) 2247
Corzide 80/5 Tablets (1 to 5 of 1000 patients) 2247
Cosopt Sterile Ophthalmic Solution 2065
Coumadin for Injection (Infrequent) 1243
Coumadin Tablets (Infrequent) 1243
Cozaar Tablets (Less than 1%) 2067
Crinone 8% Gel (Less than 5%) 3213
Crixivan Capsules (Less than 2%) 2070
▲ Cuprimine Capsules (5%) 2075
Cutivate Cream (1.5% to 2.9%) 1282
Cutivate Ointment (Less than 1%) 1284
▲ Cytovene (6%) 2959
Dantrium Capsules (Less frequent) 2885
Daranide Tablets 2077
▲ DaunoXome Injection (Up to 7%) 1442
Demerol 3079
Depacon Injection (1% to 5%) 416
Depakene (1% to 5%) 421
Depakote Sprinkle Capsules (1% to 5%) 426
Depakote Tablets (1% to 5%) 430
Depakote ER Tablets (1% to 5%) 436
▲ Depen Titratable Tablets (5%) 3341
Dermatop Emollient Cream (Less than 1%) 2517
Desferal Vials 2333
DesOwen (Less than 2%) 1401
Detrol Tablets (1.3%) 3623
D.H.E. 45 Injection 2334
DiaBeta Tablets (1.5%) 741
Diabinese Tablets (Less than 3%) 2680
Didronel Tablets 2888
▲ Differin Cream (Less than 1% to 21%) 1402
▲ Differin Gel (10% to 40%) 1403
▲ Differin Solution/Pledgets (30% to 60%) 1404
Dilaudid Oral Liquid 445
Dilaudid Tablets - 8 mg 445
Dilaudid-HP (Less frequent) 443
Diovan Capsules 2337
Dipentum Capsules (1.3%) 2803
Diphtheria & Tetanus Toxoids Adsorbed Purogenated for Pediatric Use 1857
Diprivan Injectable Emulsion (2%) 667
Diprolene Gel 0.05% (2%) 3107
Diprolene Lotion 0.05% (Infrequent) 3107
Diprolene Ointment 0.05% (2 per 767 patients) 3108
Diprolene AF Cream 0.05% (Infrequent) 3106
Diprosone 3109
Dolobid Tablets (Less than 1 in 100) 2088
Dolophine Hydrochloride Tablets 3056
Dopram Injectable 2931
▲ Dostinex Tablets (1% to less than 10%) 2804
▲ Dovonex Cream (1% to 10%) 1116
▲ Dovonex Ointment (Approximately 10% to 15%) 1117
Doxil Injection (1% to 5%) 566
Drysol Solution 2663
DuoNeb Inhalation Solution (0.3%) 1233
Duraclon Injection (0.7%) 3057
▲ Duragesic Transdermal System (1% to 10%) 1786
▲ Duramorph Injection (High incidence; occasional) 1312
Dynabac Tablets (0.5% to 1.2%) 2269
DynaCirc Capsules (0.5% to 1%) 2921
DynaCirc CR Tablets (0.5% to 1%) 2923
▲ EC-Naprosyn Delayed-Release Tablets (3% to 9%) 2967
Effexor Tablets (1%) 3495
Effexor XR Capsules (Frequent) 3499
▲ Efudex (Among most frequent) 1733
▲ 8-MOP Capsules (Approximately 10%) 1727
▲ Elimite Cream (7%) 552
▲ Ellence Injection (0.3% to 8.9%) 2806
Elmiron Capsules (Less than or equal to 1%) 570
▲ Elocon Cream 0.1% (1.6% to approximately 7%) 3110
Elocon Lotion 0.1% (1 in 209 patients) 3111
▲ Elocon Ointment 0.1% (4.8% to approximately 7%) 3112
Emadine Ophthalmic Solution (Less than 5%) ⊙ 211
Emcyt Capsules (2%) 2810
Emgel 2% Topical Gel (Occasional) 1285
Emla (2%) 602
Enalaprilat Injection 863
Enbrel for Injection 1752
Enbrel for Injection 3504
Engerix-B Vaccine (Less than 1%) 1517
Epivir 1520
Epivir-HBV 1524
▲ Epogen for Injection (16%) 582
Ergamisol Tablets (1% to 2%) 1789
▲ Esclim Transdermal System (6.3% to 12.8%) 3460
Estring Vaginal Ring (At least 1 report) 2811
Etrafon 3115
Eulexin Capsules 3118
Evoxac Capsules (1% to 3%) 1217
Famotidine Injection (Infrequent) 866
Famvir Tablets (0.9% to 3.7%) 2348
Felbatol (Frequent) 3343
▲ Feldene Capsules (1% to 10%) 2685
Femara Tablets (1% to 2%) 2351
femhrt Tablets 2635
▲ Ferrlecit Injection (6%) 3386
Finevin Cream (1% to 5%) 962
Flexeril Tablets (Rare) 572
Flexeril Tablets (Rare) 2094
▲ Flolan for Injection (4%) 1528
Flomax Capsules 1044
Flonase Nasal Spray 1533
▲ Flovent Diskus (1% to 6%) 3614
Flovent 1535
Flovent Rotadisk 1537
Floxin I.V. (1% to 3%) 2526
Floxin Otic Solution (1% to 4%) 1219
Floxin Tablets (1% to 3%) 2529
Fludara for Injection (1% to 3%) 995
Fluorescite Injection ⊙ 211
Fluoroplex 552
FluShield Influenza Vaccine 3521
Fortaz (2%) 1541
Fortovase Capsules (Less than 2%) 2970
Foscavir Injection (Between 1% and 5%) 605
Fragmin Injection (Rare) 2814
Furosemide Tablets 2284
Gabitril Tablets (2%) 1189
Gamimune N, 5% Solvent/Detergent Treated 925
Gamimune N, 10% Solvent/Detergent Treated (A single incidence) 928
Gammar-P I.V. 787
▲ Gastrocrom Oral Concentrate (3 of 87 patients) 1162
▲ Gemzar for Injection (13%) 1919
Gengraf Capsules (1% to less than 3%) 457
Geocillin Tablets (Infrequent) 2687
▲ Gleevec Capsules (6% to 10%) 2357
Glucotrol Tablets (About 1 in 70) 2692
Glucotrol XL Extended Release Tablets (Less than 3%) 2693
Gonal-F for Injection 3216
Halcion Tablets 2823
Havrix Vaccine (Less than 1%) 1544
▲ Hectorol Capsules (8.2%) 1064
▲ Hectorol Injection (8.2%) 1066
Helixate Concentrate 788
Heparin Lock Flush Solution 3509
Heparin Sodium Injection 3511
Hexalen Capsules (Less than 1%) 2226
Hivid Tablets (Less than 1%) 2975
Humalog (Less common) 1926
Humalog Mix 75/25 Pen 1928
Humate-P Concentrate 790
▲ Hyalgan Solution (7%) 3080
Hycamtin for Injection (Rare) 1546
Hycodan 1316
Hytrin Capsules (At least 1%) 464
Hyzaar 2109
Imdur Tablets (Less than or equal to 5%) 1826
Imitrex Injection (Infrequent) 1549
Imitrex Nasal Spray (Infrequent) 1554
Imitrex Tablets (Infrequent) 1558
Indocin (Less than 1%) 2112
INFeD Injection 3388
▲ Infergen (11% to 14%) 1777
Infumorph 200 and Infumorph 500 Sterile Solutions (Occasional) 1314
Innohep Injection (Greater than or equal to 1%) 1248
▲ Intron A for Injection (Up to 11%) 3120
Invirase Capsules (Up to 0.6%) 2979
Iopidine Sterile Ophthalmic Solution ⊙ 212
Ismo Tablets (Fewer than 1%) 3524
Iveegam EN (1.6%) 849
JE-VAX Vaccine 811
Kadian Capsules (Less than 3%) 1335
Kaletra Capsules (Less than 2%) 471
Kaletra Oral Solution (Less than 2%) 471
Kefurox Vials, ADD-Vantage (Less than 1 in 250) 1948
Kefzol Vials, ADD-Vantage 1951
Klaron Lotion 10% (One of 105 patients) 1224
Klonopin Tablets (Infrequent) 2983
Kogenate FS 936
▲ Lac-Hydrin Cream (Approximately 5%) 1118
▲ Lamictal (3.1%) 1567
Lamisil Tablets (2.8%) 2360
Lantus Injection 742
Lariam Tablets (Less than 1%) 2989
Lescol Capsules 2361
Lescol Capsules 2925
Lescol XL Tablets 2361
Lescol XL Tablets 2925
▲ Leukine (23%) 1755
▲ Leustatin Injection (6%) 2495
Levaquin (0.5% to 1.6%) 2537
Levo-Dromoran 1734
▲ Levorphanol Tartrate Tablets (Greater than 10%) 3059
Levoxyl Tablets 1819
▲ Levulan Kerastick (1% to 25%) 971
Lexxel Tablets 608
Lidex (Infrequent) 2020
Limbitrol 1738
Lipitor Tablets (Less than 2%) 2639
Lipitor Tablets (Less than 2%) 2696
Lithium Carbonate 3061
Lithium Citrate Syrup 3061
Lithobid Slow-Release Tablets 3255
Locoid Cream (Infrequent) 1341
Locoid Lipocream Cream (Infrequent) 1342
Locoid (Infrequent) 1341
Lodine (1% to 3%) 3528
▲ Lodine XL Extended-Release Tablets (1% to 10%) 3530
Lodosyn Tablets 1251
Lopid Tablets 2650
Loprox Gel (1% to 5%) 2022
Loprox Lotion (2 patients) 2021
Lorabid Suspension and Pulvules 2251
Lortab 3319
Lortab Elixir 3317
Lotensin Tablets (Less than 1%) 2365
Lotensin HCT Tablets (0.3% or more) 2367
Lotrimin 3128
Lotrisone 3129
Lovenox Injection 746
Loxitane Capsules 3398
Lupron Injection (Less than 5%) 3279
Luvox Tablets (25, 50, 100 mg) 3256
▲ Luxiq Foam (2% to 44%) 1210
Macrobid Capsules (Less than 1%) 2889
Macrodantin Capsules 2891
▲ Malarone (6%) 1596
Mavik Tablets (0.3% to 1.0%) 478
Maxair Autohaler 1981
Maxair Inhaler (Less than 1%) 1984
Maxalt Tablets (Infrequent) 2120
Maxalt-MLT Orally Disintegrating Tablets (Infrequent) 2120
Maxidone Tablets CIII 3399
Maxipime for Injection (0.1% to 1%) 1285

Mefoxin for Injection ... 2124
Mefoxin Premixed Intravenous Solution ... 2127
Megace Oral Suspension (1% to 3%) ... 1124
▲ Mepron Suspension (5%) ... 1598
Meridia Capsules (Greater than or equal to 1%) ... 481
Merrem I.V. (1.6%) ... 673
MetroCream (Less than 3%) ... 1404
MetroGel-Vaginal Gel (Less than 1%) ... 1986
MetroLotion (1%) ... 1405
Mevacor Tablets (0.5% to 5.2%) ... 2132
Miacalcin Nasal Spray (Less than 1%) ... 2375
Micardis Tablets (More than 0.3%) ... 1049
Micardis HCT Tablets (Less than 2%) ... 1051
Midamor Tablets (Less than or equal to 1%) ... 2136
Migranal Nasal Spray (Infrequent) ... 2376
Minipress Capsules (Less than 1%) ... 2699
Minizide Capsules (Rare) ... 2700
Mintezol ... 2137
Mirapex Tablets (1% or more) ... 2834
Mobic Tablets (0.4% to 2.4%) ... 1054
Moduretic Tablets (Greater than 1%, less than 3%) ... 2138
Monopril Tablets (0.2% to 1.0%) ... 1091
Monopril HCT (Less than 2%) ... 1094
Monurol Sachet (Less than 1%) ... 1375
Motofen Tablets ... 577
Motrin Suspension, Oral Drops, Chewable Tablets, and Caplets (1% to less than 3%) ... 2002
MS Contin Tablets (Less frequent) ... 2896
MSIR (Less frequent) ... 2898
Myambutol Tablets ... 1290
Mycelex Troche ... 573
Mykrox Tablets (Less than 2%) ... 1168
Myobloc Injectable Solution (2% or greater) ... 1291
Nadolol Tablets (1 to 5 of 1000 patients) ... 2288
Naftin Cream (2%) ... 2224
Naftin Gel (1.0%) ... 2224
Naprelan Tablets (Less than 1%) ... 1293
▲ Naprosyn Suspension (3% to 9%) ... 2967
▲ Naprosyn Tablets (3% to 9%) ... 2967
Nardil Tablets (Less common) ... 2653
Naropin Injection (1% to 5%) ... 612
Natrecor for Injection (At least 1%) ... 3189
Navane Oral ... 2701
Navane Intramuscular ... 2703
Navelbine Injection ... 1604
Nebcin Vials, Hyporets & ADD-Vantage ... 1955
Neoral Soft Gelatin Capsules (1% to less than 3%) ... 2380
Neoral Oral Solution (1% to less than 3%) ... 2380
Nesacaine/Nesacaine MPF ... 617
Neurontin Capsules (1.3%) ... 2655
Neurontin Oral Solution (1.3%) ... 2655
Neurontin Tablets (1.3%) ... 2655
Niaspan Extended-Release Tablets (1% to 6%) ... 1846
Nicotrol Nasal Spray (2%) ... 2843
Nilandron Tablets (2%) ... 753
Nimotop Capsules (Less than 1%) ... 904
▲ Nipent for Injection (10% to 21%) ... 3272
▲ Nizoral 2% Cream (5%) ... 3620
Nizoral 2% Shampoo (One occurrence in 41 patients) ... 2007
Nizoral Tablets (1.5%) ... 1791
Norco 5/325 Tablets CIII ... 3424
Norco 7.5/325 Tablets CIII ... 3425
Norco 10/325 Tablets CIII ... 3425
Norco 10/325 Tablets CIII ... 3427
Norflex ... 1987
Normodyne Injection (1%) ... 3135
Normodyne Tablets (Rare) ... 3137
Noroxin Tablets (0.3% to 1.0%) ... 2145
Norplant System ... 3543
Norpramin Tablets ... 755
Norvasc Tablets (Less than 1% to 2%) ... 2704
Norvir Capsules (Less than 2%) ... 487
Norvir Oral Solution (Less than 2%) ... 487
NovoLog Injection ... 2427
NovoSeven (1%) ... 2430
Nubain Injection (1% or less) ... 1323
Numorphan ... 1324
▲ Nutropin Depot for Injectable Suspension (13%) ... 1423
Nystop Topical Powder USP (More common) ... 2608
Olux Foam (Less than 2%) ... 1211
Omnicef (0.2%) ... 493
Oncaspar (Less than 1%) ... 756
▲ Optivar Ophthalmic Solution (1% to 10%) ... 2273
Oramorph SR Tablets (Less frequent) ... 3062
▲ Orgaran Injection (3.9%) ... 2480
Orthoclone OKT3 Sterile Solution ... 2498
Orudis Capsules (Less than 1%) ... 3548
Oruvail Capsules (Less than 1%) ... 3548
Oxistat (1.6%) ... 1298
▲ Oxsoralen-Ultra Capsules (10%) ... 1741
▲ OxyContin Tablets (13%) ... 2912
OxyFast Oral Concentrate Solution ... 2916
OxyIR Capsules ... 2916
Paraplatin for Injection ... 1126
Patanol Ophthalmic Solution (Less than 5%) ... 540
Paxil (Frequent) ... 1609
Pediazole Suspension ... 3050
▲ PEG-Intron Powder for Injection (12%) ... 3140
Pentasa Capsules (Less than 1%) ... 3239
Pepcid Injection (Infrequent) ... 2153
Pepcid for Oral Suspension (Infrequent) ... 2150
Pepcid RPD Orally Disintegrating Tablets (Infrequent) ... 2150
Pepcid Tablets (Infrequent) ... 2150
Percocet Tablets ... 1326
Percodan Tablets ... 1327
Percolone Tablets ... 1327
Permax Tablets (Infrequent) ... 1299
Persantine Tablets ... 1057
Phenergan with Codeine Syrup (Infrequent) ... 3557
Phenergan VC with Codeine Syrup ... 3561
PhosLo (Isolated cases) ... 1069
Phrenilin (Infrequent) ... 578
Pipracil (Less frequent) ... 1866
Plaquenil Tablets ... 3082
▲ Plavix Tablets (3.3%) ... 1097
▲ Plavix Tablets (3.3%) ... 3084
Polocaine Injection, USP ... 625
Polocaine-MPF Injection, USP ... 625
▲ Ponstel Capsules (1% to 10%) ... 1356
Pramosone ... 1343
Pravachol Tablets ... 1099
Premphase Tablets ... 3572
▲ Prempro Tablets (8% to 10%) ... 3572
Prevacid Delayed-Release Capsules (Less than 1%) ... 3292
Prevnar for Injection ... 1870
PREVPAC (Less than 1%) ... 3298
Priftin Tablets (2.5%) ... 758
Prilosec Delayed-Release Capsules (Less than 1%) ... 628
Primaxin I.M. ... 2158
Primaxin I.V. (0.3%) ... 2160
Prinivil Tablets (Greater than 1%) ... 2164
Prinzide Tablets (0.3% to 1%) ... 2168
▲ ProAmatine Tablets (12.2%) ... 3241
Procanbid Extended-Release Tablets (Occasional) ... 2262
Procardia Capsules (2% or less) ... 2708
Procardia XL Extended Release Tablets (Less than 3%) ... 2710
▲ Procrit for Injection (14% to 22%) ... 2502
▲ Prograf (15% to 36%) ... 1393
▲ Proleukin for Injection (24%) ... 1199
Prometrium Capsules (100 mg, 200 mg) ... 3261
Proscar Tablets ... 2175
ProSom Tablets (1%) ... 500
▲ Protonix I.V. (4%) ... 3580
Protonix Tablets (Less than 1%) ... 3577
▲ Protopic Ointment (25% to 46%) ... 1397
Provera Tablets ... 2853
Provigil Tablets (At least 1%) ... 1193
Prozac Pulvules, Liquid, and Weekly Capsules (2.4% to 3%) ... 1238
Pulmicort Respules (1% to 3%) ... 632
Pyrazinamide Tablets ... 1876
Quinaglute Dura-Tabs Tablets ... 978
Quinidex Extentabs ... 2933
▲ Rapamune Oral Solution and Tablets (3% to 20%) ... 3584
▲ Rebetron Combination Therapy (13% to 21%) ... 3153
Recombivax HB (Less than 1%) ... 2178
ReFacto Vials ... 1437
Refludan for Injection (Uncommon) ... 761
▲ Relafen Tablets (3% to 9%) ... 1617
Remeron Tablets (Frequent) ... 2483
Remeron SolTab Tablets (Frequent) ... 2486
▲ Remicade for IV Injection (5% to 6%) ... 1178
▲ Renova 0.02% Cream (Almost all subjects) ... 2520
▲ Renova 0.05% Cream (Almost all subjects) ... 2519
ReoPro Vials (0.3%) ... 1958
Requip Tablets (Infrequent) ... 1621
Rescriptor Tablets (2.2% to 3.1%) ... 526
Retrovir Capsules ... 1625
Retrovir IV Infusion ... 1629
Retrovir ... 1625
▲ Rēv-Eyes Sterile Ophthalmic Eyedrops 0.5% (10% to 40%) ... ⊙265
Rhinocort Nasal Inhaler (Less than 1%) ... 640
Rifadin (Occasional) ... 765
Rifamate Capsules (Occasional) ... 767
Rifater Tablets (Occasional) ... 769
▲ Rilutek Tablets (2.5% to 3.8%) ... 772
Risperdal (Infrequent) ... 1796
▲ Rituxan for Infusion (10%) ... 1750
▲ Rituxan I.V. (10%) ... 1428
Robaxin Injectable ... 2938
Robaxin Tablets ... 2939
Robaxisal Tablets ... 2939
Robinul Injectable ... 2940
Rocaltrol ... 2991
Rocephin Injectable Vials, ADD-Vantage, Galaxy, Bulk (Less than 1%) ... 2993
▲ Roferon-A Injection (5% to 13%) ... 2996
Rogaine Extra Strength for Men Topical Solution ... ▣721
Rogaine for Women Topical Solution ... ▣721
Rowasa Rectal Suspension Enema 4.0 grams/unit (60 mL) (1.23%) ... 3264
Roxanol ... 3066
Roxicodone ... 3067
Rythmol Tablets – 150 mg, 225 mg, 300 mg (Less than 1%) ... 502
Salagen Tablets (1%) ... 2229
Sandimmune (Rare) ... 2388
Sandostatin Injection (1% to 4%) ... 2394
▲ Sandostatin LAR Depot (5% to 15%) ... 2395
Sectral Capsules (Up to 2%) ... 3589
Sedapap Tablets 50 mg/650 mg (Infrequent) ... 2225
Sensorcaine (Rare) ... 643
Sensorcaine-MPF Injection (Rare) ... 643
Septra Suspension ... 2265
Septra Tablets ... 2265
Septra DS Tablets ... 2265
Serentil ... 1057
Serophene Tablets ... 3226
Seroquel Tablets (Infrequent) ... 684
▲ Serostim for Injection (1% to 10%) ... 3229
Serzone Tablets (2%) ... 1104
▲ Simulect for Injection (3% to 10%) ... 2399
Sinemet Tablets ... 1253
Sinemet CR Tablets ... 1255
Sinequan (Occasional) ... 2713
Singulair ... 2181
Skelaxin Tablets ... 1301
Soma Tablets ... 3353
Soma Compound Tablets (Less common) ... 3354
Soma Compound w/Codeine Tablets (Rare) ... 3355
Sonata Capsules (Frequent) ... 3591
▲ Soriatane Capsules (25% to 50%) ... 3003
Sporanox Capsules (2.5% to 5%) ... 1800
Sporanox Injection (2.5% to 5%) ... 1804
Sporanox Injection (2.5% to 5%) ... 2509
Sporanox Oral Solution (Less than 2%) ... 1808
Sporanox Oral Solution (Less than 2%) ... 2512
Stadol NS Nasal Spray (1% or greater) ... 1108
Stelazine ... 1640
Streptase for Infusion ... 647
▲ Stromectol Tablets (2.8%; 27.5%) ... 2185
Sular Tablets (Less than or equal to 1%) ... 688
Sulfamylon Cream (2.8%) ... 1011
Sulfamylon Topical Solution (2.3%) ... 1011
Suprane Liquid for Inhalation (Less than 1%) ... 874
Suprax (Less than 2%) ... 1877
Surmontil Capsules ... 3595
Sustiva Capsules (1% to 2%) ... 1258
Symmetrel ... 1328
Synalar (Infrequent) ... 2020
Synarel Nasal Solution for Central Precocious Puberty (2.6%) ... 3204
Synercid I.V. (1.5%) ... 775
Synvisc ... 3596
Talwin Nx Tablets ... 3090
Tambocor Tablets (Less than 1%) ... 1990
Tapazole Tablets ... 1823
Tarka Tablets (Less frequent) ... 508
Tasmar Tablets (Infrequent) ... 3010
Taxotere for Injection Concentrate ... 778
Tazicef for Injection (2%) ... 1647
Tazicef Galaxy Container (2%) ... 1650
Tazicef Pharmacy Bulk Package (2%) ... 1653
Tazidime Vials, Faspak & ADD-Vantage (2%) ... 1966
▲ Tazorac Gel (10% to 30%) ... 556
▲ Temodar Capsules (8%) ... 3157
Temovate Cream (Less frequent) ... 1301
▲ Temovate Gel (Among most frequent) ... 1303
Temovate Ointment (0.5%) ... 1301
Temovate Scalp Application (1 of 294 patients; infrequent) ... 1304
Temovate E Emollient (Less than 2%) ... 1302
Tenex Tablets (3% or less) ... 2942
Tequin Injection (Less than 0.1%) ... 1110
Tequin Tablets (Less than 0.1%) ... 1110
Terazol 3 Vaginal Suppositories (1.8% of 284 patients) ... 2587
Tessalon Capsules ... 1377
▲ Testoderm Transdermal Systems (2% to 12%) ... 574
Tetanus & Diphtheria Toxoids Adsorbed for Adult Use ... 1880
Teveten Tablets (Less than 1%) ... 3327
▲ Thalomid Capsules (8.3%) ... 1154
Thiothixene Capsules ... 2290
Tiazac Capsules (Less than 2%) ... 1378
Ticlid Tablets (1.3%) ... 3015
Timentin Injection- ADD-Vantage Vial ... 1661
Timentin Injection-Galaxy Container ... 1664
Timentin Injection-Pharmacy Bulk Package ... 1666
Timentin for Intravenous Administration ... 1658
Timolide Tablets ... 2187
Timolol GFS ... ⊙266
Timoptic-XE Sterile Ophthalmic Gel Forming Solution ... 2194
Tine Test, Tuberculin, Old ... 3631
Tonocard Tablets (Less than 1%) ... 649
Topamax Sprinkle Capsules (1.8% to 3.2%) ... 2590
Topamax Tablets (1.8% to 3.2%) ... 2590
Topicort (Infrequent) ... 2025
▲ Toprol-XL Tablets (About 5 of 100 patients) ... 651
Toradol (Greater than 1%) ... 3018
Trasylol Injection ... 909
Trental Tablets (Less than 1%) ... 784
▲ Tricor Capsules, Micronized (3%) ... 513
Trilafon ... 3160
Trilisate (Less than 1%) ... 2901
▲ Trisenox Injection (33%) ... 1158
Trovan (2%) ... 2722
Trusopt Sterile Ophthalmic Solution ... 2196
Tussionex Pennkinetic Extended-Release Suspension ... 1174
Tussi-Organidin NR Liquid (Rare) ... 3350
Tussi-Organidin-S NR Liquid (Rare) ... 3350
Twinrix Vaccine (Less than 1%) ... 1674
Tylenol with Codeine ... 2595
Tylox Capsules ... 2597
Ultracet Tablets (2%) ... 2597
▲ Ultram Tablets (8% to 11%) ... 2600
Ultravate Cream ... 1119
Ultravate Ointment (1.6%) ... 1120
Unasyn for Injection (Less than 1%) ... 2728
Uniretic Tablets (Less than 1%) ... 3178
Unithroid Tablets ... 3445
Univasc Tablets (Less than 1%) ... 3181
Valstar Sterile Solution for Intravesical Instillation (Less than 1%) ... 1175
Vanceril Double Strength Inhalation Aerosol (2%) ... 3167
Vancocin HCl Capsules & Pulvules ... 1972
Vancocin HCl Oral Solution ... 1971
Vancocin HCl, Vials & ADD-Vantage ... 1970
▲ Vaniqa Cream (3.1%) ... 1121
Vaqta (Less than 1%) ... 2199
Varivax (Greater than or equal to 1%) ... 2202
Vaseretic Tablets (0.5% to 2.0%) ... 2204
Vasotec I.V. Injection ... 2207
Vasotec Tablets (0.5% to 1.0%) ... 2210
Venofer Injection (Greater than 1%) ... 580
Versed Injection (Less than 1%) ... 3027
▲ Vesanoid Capsules (20%) ... 3037
Vexol 1% Ophthalmic Suspension (1% to 5%) ... ⊙222
Viadur Implant (Less than 2%) ... 912
Viagra Tablets (Less than 2%) ... 2732
Vicodin Tablets ... 516
Vicodin ES Tablets ... 517
Vicodin HP Tablets ... 518
▲ Vicoprofen Tablets (3% to 9%) ... 520
▲ Videx (7% to 9%) ... 1138
Videx EC Capsules ... 1143
Vioxx (Greater than 0.1% to 1.9%) ... 2213
Viracept ... 532
Viramune Oral Suspension ... 1060
Viramune Tablets ... 1060
Vistide Injection ... 1445
Vivactil Tablets ... 2217
Vivactil Tablets ... 2446
Vivelle Transdermal System (One of the two most common) ... 2412
Vivelle-Dot Transdermal System (One of the two most common) ... 2416
Voltaren Tablets (1% to 3%) ... 2315
Voltaren-XR Tablets (1% to 3%) ... 2315
Warfarin Sodium Tablets, USP ... 3302
Wellbutrin Tablets (2.2%) ... 1680
Wellbutrin SR Sustained-Release Tablets (2% to 4%) ... 1684
WinRho SDF ... 2297
Xanax Tablets ... 2865
Xenical Capsules ... 3043
Xerac AC Solution ... 2663
Yasmin 28 Tablets ... 980
Yodoxin Tablets ... 1722
Zanaflex Tablets (Infrequent) ... 1305
Zantac Injection ... 1688
Zebeta Tablets ... 1885
Zemuron Injection (Less than 1%) ... 2491
▲ Zenapax for Injection (2% to 5%) ... 3046
Zestoretic Tablets (0.3% to 1%) ... 695
Zestril Tablets (Greater than 1%) ... 698
Ziac Tablets ... 1887

Zinacef Injection (Fewer than 1 in 250 patients) 1696
Zinacef for Injection (Fewer than 1 in 250 patients) 1696
Zithromax Capsules, 250 mg (1% or less) 2743
Zithromax for IV Infusion (1.9%) 2748
Zithromax for Oral Suspension, 300 mg, 600 mg, 900 mg, 1200 mg (1% or less) 2739
Zithromax Tablets, 250 mg (1% or less) 2739
Zocor Tablets 2219
Zofran Injection (2%) 1698
▲ Zofran (5%) 1703
▲ Zofran ODT Orally Disintegrating Tablets (5%) 1703
Zoladex (2%) 702
Zoladex 3-month (1% to 5%) 706
Zoloft (Infrequent) 2751
Zometa for Intravenous Infusion 3621
Zomig Tablets (Infrequent) 708
Zomig-ZMT Tablets (Infrequent) 708
Zonegran Capsules (Frequent) 1307
▲ Zosyn (3.1% to 3.2%) 1890
▲ Zosyn in Galaxy Containers (3.1% to 3.2%) 1894
Zovirax Capsules 1706
Zovirax for Injection (Approximately 2%) 1708
Zovirax Ointment 1707
Zovirax 1706
▲ Zyban Sustained-Release Tablets (3%) 1710
Zyflo Filmtab Tablets (Less common) 524
Zyprexa Tablets 1973
Zyprexa ZYDIS Orally Disintegrating Tablets 1973
Zyrtec (Less than 2%) 2756
Zyrtec-D 12 Hour Extended Relief Tablets (Less than 2%) 2758
Zyvox 2871

Pruritus, ear lobes
Miacalcin Injection 2373

Pruritus, exacerbation of
Cutivate Cream (0.8% to 3.0%) 1282

Pruritus, genital
Ancef for Injection 1474
Ancef Injection 1474
Avonex 1013
Ceclor CD Tablets 1279
Ceclor (Less than 1 in 100) 1905
Ceftin Tablets (0.1% to 1%) 1898
Cefzil (1.6%) 1076
Cipro I.V. (1%) 893
Cipro I.V. Pharmacy Bulk Package (1%) 897
Cipro (1%) 887
Cognex Capsules (Infrequent) 1351
▲ Condylox Topical Solution (50% to 65%) 2437
Crinone (2%) 3213
Duricef 1079
Estring Vaginal Ring (1% to 3%) 2811
Evoxac Capsules (Less than 1%) 1217
▲ Floxin I.V. (1% to 6%) 2526
▲ Floxin Tablets (1% to 6%) 2529
Gonal-F for Injection 3216
▲ Gynazole-1 Vaginal Cream (5.7%) 3310
Keflex 1237
Kefzol Vials, ADD-Vantage 1951
Levaquin (0.5% to less than 1.0%) 2537
Neurontin Capsules (Rare) 2655
Neurontin Oral Solution (Rare) 2655
Neurontin Tablets (Rare) 2655
Nolvadex Tablets (Infrequent) 678
Primaxin I.M. 2158
Primaxin I.V. (Less than 0.2%) 2160
ProSom Tablets (Infrequent) 500
Risperdal (Rare) 1796
Suprax (Les than 2%) 1877
▲ Terazol 3 Vaginal Cream (5%) 2587
Terazol 3 Vaginal Suppositories (1.8% of 284 patients) 2587
Terazol 7 Vaginal Cream (2.3% of 521 patients) 2587
Trileptal Oral Suspension 2407
Trileptal Tablets 2407
▲ Vagifem Tablets (6%) 2857
Vantin Tablets and Oral Suspension (Less than 1%) 2860
Zosyn (1.0% or less) 1890
Zosyn in Galaxy Containers (1.0% or less) 1894

Pruritus, injection site
▲ Alferon N Injection (12%) 1770
▲ Cardizem Injectable (3.9%) 1018
▲ Cardizem Lyo-Ject Syringe (3.9%) 1018
▲ Cardizem Monovial (3.9%) 1018
Cerezyme for Injection (Less than 1%) 1438
Cetrotide for Injection 3209
Cipro I.V. (1% or less) 893
▲ Copaxone for Injection (40%) 3306
Desferal Vials 2333
Diprivan Injectable Emulsion (Less than 1%) 667
▲ Enbrel for Injection (37%) 1752
▲ Enbrel for Injection (37%) 3504
Engerix-B Vaccine (Less than 1%) 1517
Factrel (Occasional) 3633
Gonal-F for Injection 3216
Humalog 1926
Humulin 50/50, 100 Units 1934
Humulin 70/30, 100 Units 1935
Humulin 70/30 Pen 1936
Humulin L, 100 Units 1937
Humulin R Regular (U-500) 1943
Humulin N NPH Pen 1940
Iletin II, Regular (Pork), 100 Units 1947
▲ Imovax Rabies Vaccine (About 25%) 807
Intron A for Injection (Less than 5%) 3120
Kogenate 934
Tubersol Diagnostic Antigen 3628
Vaqta (Less than 1%) 2199
▲ Varivax (19.3% to 32.5%) 2202
Velosulin BR Human Insulin 10 ml Vials 2435

Pruritus, localized
▲ Aldara Cream, 5% (22% to 32%) 1978
▲ Androderm Transdermal System CIII (37%) 3377
▲ Condylox Gel (7.8% to 32.2%) 2436
Eskalith 1527
Loprox Cream (1 out of 514 patients) 2021
Mentax Cream (Less than 2%) 1009
▲ Norplant System (3.7%) 3543
▲ Polytrim Ophthalmic Solution (Among most frequent) 556
Proctocort Suppositories 2264
ProctoFoam-HC 3177
Psorcon E Cream 1227
Psorcon E Ointment 1228

Pruritus, ocular
Alomide Ophthalmic Solution (1% to 5%) ⊙ 204
▲ Alphagan Ophthalmic Solution (Approximately 10% to 30%) 545
▲ Alphagan P Ophthalmic Solution (Approximately 10% to 20%) 546
▲ Alrex Sterile Ophthalmic Suspension 0.2% (5% to 15%) ⊙ 256
Aredia for Injection (One patient) 2309
Azopt Ophthalmic Suspension (1% to 5%) 536
▲ Betimol Ophthalmic Solution (More than 5%) ⊙ 324
Betoptic S Ophthalmic Suspension (Small number of patients) 537
▲ Carac Cream (5.4%) 1222
Chloroptic Sterile Ophthalmic Solution ⊙ 235
▲ Ciloxan (Less than 10%) 538
Clorpres Tablets 1002
Combipres Tablets 1040
▲ Cosopt Sterile Ophthalmic Solution (5% to 15%) 2065
Crolom Sterile Ophthalmic Solution USP 4% (Infrequent) ⊙ 259
Geocillin Tablets 2687
Imitrex Nasal Spray 1554
▲ Iopidine 0.5% Ophthalmic Solution (10%) ⊙ 213
▲ Lotemax Sterile Ophthalmic Suspension 0.5% (5% to 15%) ⊙ 261
▲ Lumigan Ophthalmic Solution (15% to 45%) 553
Maxalt Tablets (Infrequent) 2120
Maxalt-MLT Orally Disintegrating Tablets (Infrequent) 2120
Mykrox Tablets (Less than 2%) 1168
Neosporin Ophthalmic Ointment Sterile ⊙ 299
Neosporin Ophthalmic Solution Sterile ⊙ 300
Neurontin Capsules (Rare) 2655
Neurontin Oral Solution (Rare) 2655
Neurontin Tablets (Rare) 2655
Ocuflox Ophthalmic Solution 554
Opticrom Ophthalmic Solution (Infrequent) 555
▲ Polysporin Ophthalmic Ointment (Among those occurring most often) ⊙ 301
Quixin Ophthalmic Solution (Less than 1%) 3093
▲ Rescula Ophthalmic Solution (10% to 25%) ⊙ 306
Soriatane Capsules (1% to 5%) 3003
Stimate Nasal Spray 796
Sular Tablets (Less than or equal to 1%) 688
Timolol GFS (1% to 5%) ⊙ 266
Timoptic in Ocudose 2192
Timoptic Sterile Ophthalmic Solution 2190
Timoptic-XE Sterile Ophthalmic Gel Forming Solution 2194
TobraDex Ophthalmic Ointment (Less than 4%) 542
TobraDex Ophthalmic Suspension (Less than 4%) 541
Tobrex Ophthalmic Ointment (Less than 3 of 100 patients) ⊙ 220
Tobrex Ophthalmic Solution (Less than 3 of 100 patients) ⊙ 221
Transderm Scōp Transdermal Therapeutic System (Infrequent) 2302
▲ Travatan Ophthalmic Solution (5% to 10%) 543
Vantin Tablets and Oral Suspension (Less than 1%) 2860
Vaqta (Less than 1%) 2199
▲ Visudyne for Injection (1% to 10%) ⊙ 308
Voltaren Ophthalmic Sterile Ophthalmic Solution (Less than 5%) ⊙ 312
▲ Xalatan Latanoprost Ophthalmic Solution (5% to 15%) ⊙ 320
▲ Xalatan Sterile Ophthalmic Solution (5% to 15%) 2864
Zaditor Ophthalmic Solution (Less than 5%) 2304

Pruritus, oral
Imitrex Nasal Spray 1554

Pruritus, penile
▲ Caverject Sterile Powder (3%) 2777

Pruritus, rhinal
Atrovent Nasal Spray 0.03% (2.0%) 1032
▲ Miacalcin Nasal Spray (10.6%) 2375

Pruritus, vaginal
Cleocin Vaginal Ovules (Less than 1%) 2789

Pruritus ani
Ancef for Injection 1474
Ancef Injection 1474
Arthrotec Tablets (Rare) 3195
Celexa (Rare) 1365
Colazal Capsules 3069
Estring Vaginal Ring (At least 1 report) 2811
Fortovase Capsules (Less than 2%) 2970
Keflex 1237
Kefzol Vials, ADD-Vantage 1951
Nexium Delayed-Release Capsules (Less than 1%) 619
Noroxin Tablets (Less frequent) 2145
PREVPAC (Less than 3%) 3298
Trovan (Less than 1%) 2722
Yodoxin Tablets 1722

Pseudoaneurysm
ReoPro Vials (0.8%) 1958

Pseudofolliculitis barbae
▲ Vaniqa Cream (4.9%) 1121

Pseudolymphoma
Dilantin Infatabs 2624
Dilantin Kapseals 2622
Dilantin-125 Oral Suspension 2625

Pseudomembranous colitis
Amoxil Chewable Tablets 1471
Amoxil for Oral Suspension 1471
Amoxil 1471
Ancef for Injection 1474
Ancef Injection 1474
Augmentin Chewable Tablets 1482
Augmentin Powder for Oral Suspension 1482
Augmentin Tablets 1485
Augmentin ES-600 Powder for Oral Suspension 1487
Avelox Tablets 879
Azactam for Injection (Less than 1%) 1276
Benzaclin Topical Gel 1220
Biaxin/Biaxin XL 403
Bicillin C-R 900/300 Injection 2240
Bicillin C-R Injection 2238
Bicillin L-A Injection 2242
Campath Ampules 992
Ceclor CD Tablets 1279
Ceclor 1905
Cedax 1021
Cefizox for Intramuscular or Intravenous Use 1390
Cefobid Intravenous/Intramuscular 2671
Cefobid Pharmacy Bulk Package - Not for Direct Infusion 2673
▲ Cefotan (Most frequent) 664
Ceftin 1898
Cefzil (Rare) 1076
Ceptaz for Injection 1499
Chibroxin Sterile Ophthalmic Solution 2051
Cipro I.V. (1% or less) 893
Cipro I.V. Pharmacy Bulk Package (Less than 1%) 897
Cipro 887
Claforan Injection 732
Cleocin HCl Capsules 2784
Cleocin Phosphate Sterile Solution 2785
Cleocin T Topical (Rare) 2790
Cleocin Vaginal Cream 2788
Cleocin Vaginal Ovules 2789
Clindagel 1401
Duricef 1079
E.E.S. 450
EryPed 446
Ery-Tab Tablets (Rare) 448
Erythrocin Stearate Filmtab Tablets (Rare) 452
Erythromycin Base Filmtab Tablets (Rare) 454
Erythromycin Delayed-Release Capsules, USP (Rare) 455
Floxin I.V. 2526
Floxin Tablets 2529
Fortaz (Less frequent) 1541
Keflex 1237
Kefurox Vials, ADD-Vantage (1 in 440) 1948
Kefzol Vials, ADD-Vantage 1951
Levaquin (Less than 0.3%) 2537
Lorabid Suspension and Pulvules 2251
Macrobid Capsules 2889
Macrodantin Capsules 2891
Mandol Vials 1953
Maxipime for Injection (0.1% to 1%) 1285
Mefoxin for Injection 2124
Mefoxin Premixed Intravenous Solution 2127
Merrem I.V. 673
Noroxin Tablets 2145
Omnicef 493
PCE Dispertab Tablets 498
Pediazole Suspension (Rare) 3050
Pipracil (Rare) 1866
PREVPAC 3298
Priftin Tablets 758
Primaxin I.M. 2158
Primaxin I.V. (Less than 0.2%) 2160
Rifadin 765
Rifater Tablets 769
Rocephin Injectable Vials, ADD-Vantage, Galaxy, Bulk 2993
Septra Suspension 2265
Septra Tablets 2265
Septra DS Tablets 2265
Suprax (Several patients) 1877
Synercid I.V. 775
Tamiflu Capsules (Less than 1%) 3008
Tamiflu Oral Suspension (Less than 1%) 3008
Tazicef for Injection 1647
Tazicef Galaxy Container 1650
Tazicef Pharmacy Bulk Package 1653
Tazidime Vials, Faspak & ADD-Vantage 1966
Tequin Injection (Less than 0.1%) 1110
Tequin Tablets (Less than 0.1%) 1110
Timentin Injection- ADD-Vantage Vial 1661
Timentin Injection-Galaxy Container 1664
Timentin Injection-Pharmacy Bulk Package 1666
Timentin for Intravenous Administration 1658
Trovan (Less than 1%) 2722
Unasyn for Injection 2728
Vancocin HCl, Vials & ADD-Vantage 1970
Vantin Tablets and Oral Suspension (Less than 1%) 2860
Zinacef Injection 1696
Zinacef for Injection 1696
Zithromax Capsules, 250 mg 2743
Zithromax for IV Infusion 2748
Zithromax for Oral Suspension, 1 g 2743
Zithromax for Oral Suspension, 300 mg, 600 mg, 900 mg, 1200 mg 2739
Zithromax Tablets, 250 mg 2739
Zithromax Tablets, 600 mg 2743
Zosyn (One patient) 1890
Zosyn in Galaxy Containers (One patient) 1894
Zyvox 2871

Pseudomembranous enterocolitis
Bactrim 2949
Rilutek Tablets (Rare) 772
Septra Suspension 2265
Septra Tablets 2265
Septra DS Tablets 2265
Synercid I.V. (Less than 1%) 775

Pseudoparkinsonism
Compazine 1505
Navane Oral 2701
Navane Intramuscular 2703
Stelazine 1640
Thioridazine Hydrochloride Tablets (Infrequent) 2289
Thiothixene Capsules 2290
Thorazine 1656
Wellbutrin Tablets (1.5%) 1680

Pseudotumor cerebri
Accutane Capsules 2944
Celestone Soluspan Injectable Suspension 3097
Celestone Syrup 3099
Cordarone Tablets (Rare) 3487

Cortone Acetate Injectable Suspension 2059
Cortone Acetate Tablets 2061
Decadron Elixir 2078
Decadron Tablets 2079
Decadron Phosphate Injection 2081
Declomycin Tablets 1855
Depo-Medrol Injectable Suspension 2795
Dynacin Capsules 2019
Eskalith 1527
Hydrocortone Tablets 2106
Levoxyl Tablets 1819
Lithium Carbonate 3061
Lithium Citrate Syrup 3061
Lithobid Slow-Release Tablets 3255
Minocin Intravenous 1862
Minocin Oral Suspension 1865
Minocin Pellet-Filled Capsules 1863
Motrin Suspension, Oral Drops, Chewable Tablets, and Caplets (Less than 1%) 2002
Norplant System 3543
Pacerone Tablets (Rare) 3331
Pediapred Oral Solution 1170
Prednisone 3064
Soriatane Capsules (Less than 1%) 3003
Synthroid 505
Unithroid Tablets 3445
Vesanoid Capsules 3037

Psoriasis

Aciphex Tablets (Rare) 1267
Aciphex Tablets (Rare) 1783
Asacol Delayed-Release Tablets (Rare) 2884
Betaseron for SC Injection 988
Betaxon Ophthalmic Suspension (Less than 2%) 537
Celexa (Infrequent) 1365
Cognex Capsules (Infrequent) 1351
Colazal Capsules 3069
Copaxone for Injection (Infrequent) 3306
Doxil Injection (Less than 1%) 566
Effexor Tablets (Infrequent) 3495
Effexor XR Capsules (Infrequent) 3499
Eskalith 1527
Fortovase Capsules (Less than 2%) 2970
Gabitril Tablets (Infrequent) 1189
Intron A for Injection (Less than 5%) 3120
Lithobid Slow-Release Tablets 3255
Neurontin Capsules (Rare) 2655
Neurontin Oral Solution (Rare) 2655
Neurontin Tablets (Rare) 2655
Norvir Capsules (Less than 2%) 487
Norvir Oral Solution (Less than 2%) 487
Provigil Tablets (At least 1%) 1193
Prozac Pulvules, Liquid, and Weekly Capsules (Rare) 1238
Quinidex Extentabs 2933
Requip Tablets (Infrequent) 1621
Rilutek Tablets (Infrequent) 772
Roferon-A Injection (Less than 1%) 2996
Sarafem Pulvules (Rare) 1962
Seroquel Tablets (Rare) 684
Sonata Capsules (Rare) 3591
Thalomid Capsules 1154
Trileptal Oral Suspension 2407
Trileptal Tablets 2407
Uniretic Tablets (Less than 1%) 3178
Ziac Tablets 1887

Psoriasis, exacerbation of

Cormax Cream (Rare) 2440
Cormax Ointment (Rare) 2440
Cormax Scalp Application (Rare) 2441
Cosopt Sterile Ophthalmic Solution 2065
▲ Dovonex Cream (1% to 10%) 1116
▲ Dovonex Ointment (1% to 10%) 1117
Dovonex Scalp Solution (1% to 5%) 1118
Eskalith 1527
Intron A for Injection (Less than 5%) 3120
Lithium Carbonate 3061
Lithium Citrate Syrup 3061
Lithobid Slow-Release Tablets 3255
Neupogen for Injection (Infrequent) 587
Oxsoralen-Ultra Capsules 1741
PEG-Intron Powder for Injection (Less than or equal to 1%) 3140
Plaquenil Tablets 3082
Risperdal (Rare) 1796
Saizen for Injection (Infrequent) 3225
Soriatane Capsules (Less than 1%) 3003
Temovate Cream 1301
Temovate Scalp Application (Rare) 1304
Tenoretic Tablets 690
Tenormin 692
Timolol GFS ⊙266
Timoptic in Ocudose 2192
Timoptic Sterile Ophthalmic Solution 2190
Timoptic-XE Sterile Ophthalmic Gel Forming Solution 2194
Toprol-XL Tablets 651

Psoriasis, pustular

Cutivate Cream 1282
Cutivate Ointment 1284

Psoriasis, worsening of

▲ Tazorac Gel (10% to 30%) 556

Psychiatric disturbances

Accutane Capsules 2944
Aldoclor Tablets 2035
Aldomet Tablets 2037
Aldoril Tablets 2039
Aralen Tablets 3075
Artane (Rare) 1855
Arthrotec Tablets (Rare) 3195
Baycol Tablets 883
Chibroxin Sterile Ophthalmic Solution 2051
Clinoril Tablets (Less than 1 in 100) 2053
Cogentin 2055
Cortone Acetate Injectable Suspension 2059
Cortone Acetate Tablets 2061
Cosopt Sterile Ophthalmic Solution 2065
Cuprimine Capsules 2075
Decadron Elixir 2078
Decadron Tablets 2079
Decadron Phosphate Injection 2081
Didronel Tablets 2888
Famotidine Injection (Infrequent) 866
Florinef Acetate Tablets 2250
Fortovase Capsules (Less than 2%) 2970
▲ Gengraf Capsules (5.0%) 457
Hydrocortone Tablets 2106
Hydrocortone Acetate Injectable Suspension 2103
Hydrocortone Phosphate Injection, Sterile 2105
Indocin (Less than 1%) 2112
Infergen 1777
Invirase Capsules (Less than 2%) 2979
Lescol Capsules 2361
Lescol Capsules 2925
Lescol XL Tablets 2361
Lescol XL Tablets 2925
▲ Leukine (15%) 1755
Mintezol 2137
Nembutal Sodium Solution (Less than 1%) 485
Neoral Soft Gelatin Capsules 2380
Neoral Oral Solution 2380
Nizoral Tablets (Rare) 1791
Noroxin Tablets 2145
Pepcid Injection (Infrequent) 2153
Pepcid for Oral Suspension (Infrequent) 2150
Pepcid RPD Orally Disintegrating Tablets (Infrequent) 2150
Pepcid Tablets (Infrequent) 2150
Prednisone 3064
Prilosec Delayed-Release Capsules (Less than 1%) 628
Primaxin I.M. 2158
Primaxin I.V. (Less than 0.2%) 2160
Pulmicort Respules (Less than 1%) 632
Pulmicort Turbuhaler Inhalation Powder (Rare) 636
Sandimmune 2388
Solu-Medrol Sterile Powder 2855
Thioridazine Hydrochloride Tablets (Extremely rare) 2289
Timolol GFS ⊙266
Timoptic in Ocudose (Less frequent) 2192
Timoptic Sterile Ophthalmic Solution (Less frequent) 2190
Timoptic-XE Sterile Ophthalmic Gel Forming Solution 2194
Tonocard Tablets (Less than 1%) 649
Trecator-SC Tablets 3598
Zarontin Capsules 2659
Zarontin Syrup 2660

Psychic dependence

(*see under* Dependence, psychological)

Psychomotor retardation

Lithobid Slow-Release Tablets 3255
Serzone Tablets (2%) 1104
Sonata Capsules (Rare) 3591
▲ Topamax Sprinkle Capsules (16.8% to 25.1%) 2590
▲ Topamax Tablets (16.8% to 25.1%) 2590

Psychoses

Accutane Capsules 2944
Adderall Tablets (Rare) 3231
Adderall XR Capsules
Adipex-P 1406
Aldoclor Tablets 2035
Aldomet Tablets 2037
Aldoril Tablets 2039
Amphotec (1% to 5%) 1774
Ancobon Capsules 1730
Antabuse Tablets 2444
Antabuse Tablets 3474
Aralen Tablets (Rare) 3075
Aredia for Injection (Up to 4%) 2309
Avonex 1013
Betaseron for SC Injection 988
Biaxin/Biaxin XL 403
Bicillin L-A Injection 2242
Bontril Slow-Release Capsules (Rare) 576
Buprenex Injectable (Less than 1%) 2918
Cataflam Tablets (Rare) 2315
Cedax 1021
Celestone Soluspan Injectable Suspension 3097
Celexa (Infrequent) 1365
▲ CellCept Capsules (3% to 10%) 2951
▲ CellCept Intravenous (3% to 10%) 2951
▲ CellCept Oral Suspension (3% to 10%) 2951
▲ CellCept Tablets (3% to 10%) 2951
Celontin Capsules (Rare) 2618
Cerebyx Injection (Infrequent) 2619
Chibroxin Sterile Ophthalmic Solution 2051
Clinoril Tablets (Less than 1 in 100) 2053
Clomid Tablets 735
Cognex Capsules (Rare) 1351
Cortone Acetate Injectable Suspension 2059
Cortone Acetate Tablets 2061
Covera-HS Tablets (Less than 2%) 3199
Dapsone Tablets USP 1780
Decadron Elixir 2078
Decadron Tablets 2079
Decadron Phosphate Injection 2081
Depacon Injection 416
Depakene 421
Depakote Sprinkle Capsules 426
Depakote Tablets 430
Depakote ER Tablets (Greater than 1%) 436
Desoxyn Tablets (Rare) 440
Dexedrine (Rare at recommended doses) 1512
DextroStat Tablets (Rare) 3236
Effexor Tablets (Rare) 3495
Effexor XR Capsules (Infrequent) 3499
Exelon Capsules (Infrequent) 2342
Exelon Oral Solution (Infrequent) 2345
Felbatol 3343
Floxin I.V. 2526
Floxin Tablets 2529
Fortovase Capsules (Less than 2%) 2970
Gabitril Tablets (Infrequent) 1189
Gastrocrom Oral Concentrate (Less common) 1162
Hivid Tablets (Less than 1%) 2975
Hydrocortone Tablets 2106
Hydrocortone Acetate Injectable Suspension 2103
Hydrocortone Phosphate Injection, Sterile 2105
Indocin (Less than 1%) 2112
Invirase Capsules (Less than 2%) 2979
Ionamin Capsules (Rare) 1163
Isoptin SR Tablets (1% or less) 467
Klonopin Tablets 2983
Lamictal (Infrequent) 1567
Lanoxicaps Capsules 1574
Lanoxin Injection 1581
Lanoxin Elixir Pediatric 1578
Lanoxin Injection Pediatric 1584
Lariam Tablets 2989
Levsin/Levsinex/Levbid 3172
Luvox Tablets (25, 50, 100 mg) (Infrequent to frequent) 3256
Macrobid Capsules (Rare) 2889
Macrodantin Capsules (Rare) 2891
Mexitil Capsules (Less than 1% or about 2 in 1,000) 1047
Mirapex Tablets (1% or more) 2834
Nardil Tablets (Infrequent) 2653
Neurontin Capsules (Infrequent) 2655
Neurontin Oral Solution (Infrequent) 2655
Neurontin Tablets (Infrequent) 2655
Noroxin Tablets 2145
Orthoclone OKT3 Sterile Solution 2498
Paxil (Rare) 1609
Pediapred Oral Solution 1170
Pediazole Suspension 3050
Permax Tablets (2.1%; frequent) 1299
Plaquenil Tablets 3082
Prednisone 3064
Prelone Syrup 2273
PREVPAC 3298
Procanbid Extended-Release Tablets (Occasional) 2262
▲ Prograf (3% to 15%) 1393
Prozac Pulvules, Liquid, and Weekly Capsules (Infrequent) 1238
Pulmicort Respules (Less than 1%) 632
Pulmicort Turbuhaler Inhalation Powder (Rare) 636
Quinaglute Dura-Tabs Tablets 978
Quinidex Extentabs 2933
Rhinocort Nasal Inhaler (Rare) 640
Rifadin (Rare) 765
Rilutek Tablets (Rare) 772
Ritalin 2387
Rocaltrol (Rare) 2991
Roferon-A Injection 2996
Rythmol Tablets – 150 mg, 225 mg, 300 mg (Less than 1%) 502
Sarafem Pulvules (Infrequent) 1962
Serophene Tablets 3226
Sinemet Tablets 1253
Sinemet CR Tablets 1255
Solu-Medrol Sterile Powder 2855
Sustiva Capsules (Less than 2%) 1258
Symmetrel (0.1% to 1%) 1328
Tagamet 1644
Tarka Tablets 508
Tasmar Tablets (Infrequent) 3010
Tenoretic Tablets 690
Tenormin 692
Tequin Injection (Less than 0.1%) 1110
Tequin Tablets (Less than 0.1%) 1110
Thalomid Capsules 1154
Tonocard Tablets (Less than 1%) 649
Topamax Sprinkle Capsules (Frequent) 2590
Topamax Tablets (Frequent) 2590
Toradol 3018
Trilafon 3160
Valcyte Tablets (Less than 5%) 3022
Valtrex Caplets 1676
Verelan Capsules (1% or less) 3184
Verelan PM Capsules (2% or less) 3186
Voltaren Tablets (Rare) 2315
Voltaren-XR Tablets (Rare) 2315
Wellbutrin Tablets (Infrequent) 1680
Wellbutrin SR Sustained-Release Tablets 1684
Zarontin Capsules 2659
Zarontin Syrup 2660
Zoloft 2751
Zovirax Capsules 1706
Zovirax for Injection 1708
Zovirax 1706
Zyban Sustained-Release Tablets 1710

Psychoses, aggravation

Clozaril Tablets 2319
Cortone Acetate Injectable Suspension 2059
Cortone Acetate Tablets 2061
Decadron Elixir 2078
Decadron Tablets 2079
Decadron Phosphate Injection 2081
Etrafon 3115
Hydrocortone Tablets 2106
Hydrocortone Acetate Injectable Suspension 2103
Hydrocortone Phosphate Injection, Sterile 2105
Norpramin Tablets 755
Pediapred Oral Solution 1170
Prednisone 3064
Prelone Syrup 2273
Serentil 1057
Seroquel Tablets (Infrequent) 684
Solu-Medrol Sterile Powder 2855
Surmontil Capsules 3595
Thioridazine Hydrochloride Tablets 2289
Vivactil Tablets 2217
Vivactil Tablets 2446

Psychoses, toxic

Astramorph/PF Injection, USP (Preservative-Free) 594
Chibroxin Sterile Ophthalmic Solution 2051
Cipro I.V. (1% or less) 893
Cipro I.V. Pharmacy Bulk Package (Less than 1%) 897
Cipro 887
Concerta Extended-Release Tablets 1998
Concerta Tablets 561
Duramorph Injection 1312
Floxin I.V. 2526
Floxin Tablets 2529
Infumorph 200 and Infumorph 500 Sterile Solutions 1314
Levaquin 2537
Metadate CD Capsules 1164
Metadate ER Tablets 1167
Methylin Tablets 1995
Methylin ER Tablets 1995
Rifamate Capsules (Uncommon) 767
Rifater Tablets (Uncommon) 769
Ritalin 2387

Psychosis, activation

Carbatrol Capsules 3234
Compazine 1505
Stelazine 1640
Tegretol/Tegretol-XR 2404
Wellbutrin SR Sustained-Release Tablets 1684
Zyban Sustained-Release Tablets 1710

Psychosis, overt

Calcijex Injection (Rare) 411

Hectorol Capsules 1064
Hectorol Injection 1066
Pediapred Oral Solution 1170

Psychosis, paranoid
Zarontin Capsules (Rare) 2659
Zarontin Syrup (Rare) 2660

Psychotic episodes
(*see under* Psychoses)

Psychotic symptoms, paradoxical exacerbation
Haldol Decanoate 2535
Haldol Injection, Tablets and Concentrate 2533
Navane Oral (Infrequent) 2701
Navane Intramuscular (Infrequent) 2703
Thiothixene Capsules 2290

Ptosis, eyelids
Betagan ⊙228
Betaseron for SC Injection 988
Betimol Ophthalmic Solution ⊙324
Blephamide Ophthalmic Ointment (Occasional) 547
Blephamide Ophthalmic Suspension 548
Blocadren Tablets 2046
▲ Botox Purified Neurotoxin Complex (0.3% to 15.7%) 549
Carteolol Hydrochloride Ophthalmic Solution USP, 1% (Occasional) ⊙258
Celexa (Rare) 1365
Clozaril Tablets (Less than 1%) 2319
Cognex Capsules (Rare) 1351
Copaxone for Injection (Infrequent) 3306
Cosopt Sterile Ophthalmic Solution 2065
Depen Titratable Tablets 3341
FML Ophthalmic Ointment (Occasional) ⊙237
FML Ophthalmic Suspension (Occasional) ⊙236
FML Forte Ophthalmic Suspension (Occasional) ⊙235
Imdur Tablets (Less than or equal to 5%) 1826
Lamictal (Rare) 1567
Loxitane Capsules 3398
Lupron Depot–4 Month 30 mg (Less than 5%) 3289
Naprelan Tablets (Less than 1%) 1293
Naropin Injection (Less than 1%) 612
Neurontin Capsules (Infrequent) 2655
Neurontin Oral Solution (Infrequent) 2655
Neurontin Tablets (Infrequent) 2655
Ocupress Ophthalmic Solution, 1% Sterile (Occasional) ⊙303
Paxil (Rare) 1609
Pred Forte Ophthalmic Suspension (Occasional) ⊙246
Pred Mild Sterile Ophthalmic Suspension (Occasional) ⊙249
Rescula Ophthalmic Solution (Less than 1%) ⊙306
▲ Rēv-Eyes Sterile Ophthalmic Eyedrops 0.5% (10% to 40%) ⊙265
Serzone Tablets (Rare) 1104
Sonata Capsules (Rare) 3591
Tequin Injection (Less than 0.1%) 1110
Tequin Tablets (Less than 0.1%) 1110
Timolide Tablets 2187
Timolol GFS ⊙266
Timoptic in Ocudose (Less frequent) 2192
Timoptic Sterile Ophthalmic Solution (Less frequent) 2190
Timoptic-XE Sterile Ophthalmic Gel Forming Solution 2194
Topamax Sprinkle Capsules (Infrequent) 2590
Topamax Tablets (Infrequent) 2590
Trileptal Oral Suspension 2407
Trileptal Tablets 2407
Zoloft (Rare) 2751
Zyrtec (Less than 2%) 2756
Zyrtec-D 12 Hour Extended Relief Tablets (Less than 2%) 2758

Pubic hair, growth
▲ Synarel Nasal Solution for Central Precocious Puberty (5%) 3204

Pulmonary air leak
▲ Survanta Intratracheal Suspension (10.9%) 3053

Pulmonary allergy, unspecified
Idamycin PFS Injection (2%) 2825

Pulmonary apoplexy
Sandostatin LAR Depot (Rare) 2395

Pulmonary congestion
Aricept Tablets (Infrequent) 1270
Aricept Tablets (Infrequent) 2665
Avalide Tablets 1070
Avapro Tablets (Less than 1%) 1074
Avapro Tablets (Less than 1%) 3076
Evoxac Capsules (Less than 1%) 1217
Prinzide Tablets 2168
▲ Proleukin for Injection (54%) 1199
Vicoprofen Tablets (Less than 1%) 520
Vioxx (Greater than 0.1% to 1.9%) 2213
Zestoretic Tablets (0.3% to 1%) 695

Pulmonary disease, chronic interstitial obstructive
Dipentum Capsules (Rare) 2803

Pulmonary disease, chronic obstructive
Campath Ampules 992
Luvox Tablets (25, 50, 100 mg) (Rare) 3256
▲ Zoladex (5%) 702
Zoladex 3-month 706

Pulmonary distress
Betaxon Ophthalmic Suspension (Less than 2%) 537
Betoptic S Ophthalmic Suspension (Rare) 537
Follistim for Injection 2465
Humegon for Injection 2468
Serophene Tablets 3226

Pulmonary edema
(*see under* Edema, pulmonary)

Pulmonary embolism
(*see under* Embolism, pulmonary)

Pulmonary emphysema, interstitial
▲ Curosurf Intratracheal Suspension (21%) 1232
▲ Infasurf Intratracheal Suspension (7% to 10%) 1372
▲ Survanta Intratracheal Suspension (20.2%) 3053

Pulmonary fibrosis
Aceon Tablets (2 mg, 4 mg, 8 mg) (Less than 0.1%) 3249
Agrylin Capsules 3232
Alkeran for Injection 1465
Alkeran Tablets 1466
Campath Ampules 992
Casodex Tablets (Rare) 662
▲ CellCept Capsules (3% to 10%) 2951
▲ CellCept Intravenous (3% to 10%) 2951
▲ CellCept Oral Suspension (3% to 10%) 2951
▲ CellCept Tablets (3% to 10%) 2951
Cordarone Intravenous 3491
▲ Cordarone Tablets (4% to 9%) 3487
Cuprimine Capsules (Rare) 2075
Cytovene 2959
Depen Titratable Tablets 3341
Dostinex Tablets (Rare) 2804
Evoxac Capsules (Less than 1%) 1217
Herceptin I.V. (Rare) 1414
Leukeran Tablets 1591
Lupron Injection (Less than 5%) 3279
Macrobid Capsules (Rare to common) 2889
Macrodantin Capsules (Rare) 2891
Mexitil Capsules (Isolated reports) 1047
Myleran Tablets (Rare) 1603
Mylocel Tablets (Rare) 2227
Nilandron Tablets 753
▲ Pacerone Tablets (4% to 9%) 3331
Paxil (Rare) 1609
Pentasa Capsules (One case) 3239
Permax Tablets (Rare) 1299
Prozac Pulvules, Liquid, and Weekly Capsules (Rare) 1238
Tasmar Tablets (One case) 3010
Tonocard Tablets (Less than 1%) 649

Pulmonary function, changes
▲ Betapace Tablets (3% to 8%) 950
Diprivan Injectable Emulsion (Less than 1%) 667
Eulexin Capsules (Less than 1%) 3118
Follistim for Injection 2465
Humegon for Injection 2468
Ifex for Injection (Less than 1%) 1123
Intron A for Injection 3120
▲ Leukine (48%) 1755
Macrobid Capsules (Common) 2889
Macrodantin Capsules (Common) 2891
Mexitil Capsules (Isolated reports) 1047
Navelbine Injection (A few patients) 1604
▲ Novantrone for Injection (24% to 43%) 1760
Pergonal for Injection 3223
Repronex for Intramuscular and Subcutaneous Injection 1347
Virazole for Inhalation Solution 1747

Pulmonary function, decreased
Relenza Rotadisk 1619
▲ Rilutek Tablets (13.1% to 16%) 772

Pulmonary hemorrhage
(*see under* Hemorrhage, pulmonary)

Pulmonary hypersensitivity
Carbatrol Capsules 3234
Fludara for Injection 995
Tegretol/Tegretol-XR 2404

Pulmonary hypersensitivity, acute
Macrobid Capsules (Less than 1%) 2889
Macrodantin 2891

Pulmonary hypersensitivity, chronic
Timolide Tablets 2187

Pulmonary hypersensitivity, subacute
Macrodantin Capsules 2891

Pulmonary hypertension
Adipex-P (Rare) 1406
Agrylin Capsules 3232
Bicillin C-R 900/300 Injection 2240
Bicillin C-R Injection 2238
Bicillin L-A Injection 2242
▲ CellCept Capsules (3% to 10%) 2951
▲ CellCept Intravenous (3% to 10%) 2951
▲ CellCept Oral Suspension (3% to 10%) 2951
▲ CellCept Tablets (3% to 10%) 2951
Indocin I.V. (1% to 3%) 2115
Ionamin Capsules 1163
Paxil 1609
Permax Tablets (Rare) 1299
Prozac Pulvules, Liquid, and Weekly Capsules 1238
Sandostatin LAR Depot (Rare) 2395
Sarafem Pulvules 1962
Trasylol Injection (1% to 2%) 909
▲ Vesanoid Capsules (3%) 3037
Zoloft 2751

Pulmonary infarction
Enalaprilat Injection 863
Humegon for Injection 2468
Lexxel Tablets 608
Luvox Tablets (25, 50, 100 mg) (Rare) 3256
Prinivil Tablets (0.3% to 1.0%) 2164
Prinzide Tablets 2168
Vaseretic Tablets 2204
Vasotec I.V. Injection 2207
Vasotec Tablets (0.5% to 1.0%) 2210
Zestoretic Tablets 695
Zestril Tablets (0.3% to 1.0%) 698

Pulmonary infiltrates
Agrylin Capsules 3232
Bactrim 2949
Campath Ampules 992
DaunoXome Injection (Less than or equal to 5%) 1442
Declomycin Tablets 1855
Dynacin Capsules (Rare) 2019
Enalaprilat Injection 863
Fludara for Injection 995
Foscavir Injection (Between 1% and 5%) 605
Herceptin I.V. 1414
Imdur Tablets (Less than or equal to 5%) 1826
Intron A for Injection (Rare) 3120
Leustatin Injection 2495
Lexxel Tablets 608
Lodine 3528
Lodine XL Extended-Release Tablets 3530
Lupron Injection 3279
Macrobid Capsules 2889
Macrodantin Capsules 2891
Minocin Intravenous (Rare) 1862
Minocin Oral Suspension (Rare) 1865
Minocin Pellet-Filled Capsules (Rare) 1863
Myambutol Tablets 1290
Mylocel Tablets (Rare) 2227
Pediazole Suspension 3050
Pentasa Capsules (Less than 1%) 3239
Prinivil Tablets (0.3% to 1.0%) 2164
Prinzide Tablets 2168
Rebetron Combination Therapy 3153
Remicade for IV Injection (Less than 2%) 1178
Rituxan I.V. 1428
Septra Suspension (Rare) 2265
Septra Tablets (Rare) 2265
Septra DS Tablets (Rare) 2265
Vantin Tablets and Oral Suspension 2860
Vascor Tablets 2602
Vaseretic Tablets 2204
Vasotec I.V. Injection 2207
Vasotec Tablets (0.5% to 1.0%) 2210
▲ Vesanoid Capsules (6%) 3037
Zestoretic Tablets 695
Zestril Tablets (0.3% to 1.0%) 698

Pulmonary inflammation
Cordarone Tablets 3487
Pacerone Tablets 3331

Pulmonary insufficiency
Herceptin I.V. 1414

Pulmonary nodule
Sandostatin Injection (Less than 1%) 2394
Sandostatin LAR Depot (Rare) 2395

Pulmonary reembolism
Activase I.V. 1410

Pulmonary symptoms, worsening
Accolate Tablets (Rare) 657
Flovent Diskus 3614
Flovent 1535
Flovent Rotadisk 1537
Singulair 2181

Pulmonary toxicity, unspecified
Alkeran for Injection 1465
Alkeran Tablets 1466
▲ Cordarone Tablets (10% to 17%) 3487
▲ Idamycin PFS Injection (39%) 2825
▲ Pacerone Tablets (10% to 17%) 3331

Pulse, fast
Arco-Lase Plus Tablets 592
Caverject Sterile Powder (Less than 1%) 2777
Humalog (Less common) 1926
Humulin 50/50, 100 Units 1934
Humulin 70/30, 100 Units (Less common) 1935
Humulin 70/30 Pen (Less common) 1936
Humulin L, 100 Units (Less common) 1937
Humulin R Regular (U-500) 1943
Humulin N NPH Pen (Less common) 1940
Iletin II, Regular (Pork), 100 Units 1947
Levoxyl Tablets 1819
Children's Motrin Oral Suspension and Chewable Tablets 2006
Children's Motrin Oral Suspension ▣643
Infants' Motrin Concentrated Drops 2006
Junior Strength Motrin Caplets and Chewable Tablets 2006
Novolin 70/30 PenFill (Rare) 2423
Novolin 70/30 Prefilled Disposable Insulin Delivery System (Rare) 2425
Novolin N PenFill (Rare) 2423
Novolin R PenFill (Rare) 2423
Prosed/DS Tablets 3268
Unithroid Tablets 3445
Urimax Tablets 1769
Urised Tablets 2876
Velosulin BR Human Insulin 10 ml Vials 2435

Pulse changes
AquaMEPHYTON Injection 2042
Autoplex T 2294
Clozaril Tablets 2319
Compazine 1505
Concerta Extended-Release Tablets 1998
Concerta Tablets 561
Effexor Tablets 3495
Etrafon (Occasional) 3115
Haldol Decanoate 2535
Imitrex Injection (Rare) 1549
Imitrex Nasal Spray 1554
Loxitane Capsules 3398
Luvox Tablets (25, 50, 100 mg) (Infrequent) 3256
Mephyton Tablets (Rare) 2129
Metadate CD Capsules 1164
Metadate ER Tablets 1167
Methylin Tablets 1995
Methylin ER Tablets 1995
Moban 1320
Navane Oral 2701
Navane Intramuscular 2703
Norvasc Tablets (Less than or equal to 0.1%) 2704
Orap Tablets 1407
Plasbumin-5 (Rare) 939
Plasbumin-20 (Rare) 940
Plasbumin-25 (Rare) 941
Proplex T 851
Risperdal 1796
Ritalin 2387
Rituxan for Infusion (Two cases) 1750
Rituxan I.V. (Two cases) 1428
Serentil 1057
Seroquel Tablets (Infrequent) 684
Stelazine 1640
Trilafon (Occasional) 3160
▲ Versed Injection (Among most frequent) 3027

Pulse rate, depression
Acthrel for Injection (One patient) 3629

Lanoxicaps Capsules 1574
Lanoxin Injection 1581
ReoPro Vials (1.0%) 1958

Pulse, irregular
Phenergan 3556

Pupil enlargement

Pupillary atonia
Healon GV ⊙320

Pupils, unequal-sized
Hivid Tablets (Less than 1%) 2975

Purple toes syndrome
Activase I.V. 1410
Coumadin for Injection (Infrequent) 1243
Coumadin Tablets (Infrequent) 1243
Retavase Vials 1182
Streptase for Infusion 647
Warfarin Sodium Tablets, USP 3302

Purpura
Accuretic Tablets 2614
Aceon Tablets (2 mg, 4 mg, 8 mg) (0.1%) 3249
Adalat CC Tablets (Rare) 877
Aggrenox Capsules (1.4%) 1026
Aldoclor Tablets 2035
Aldoril Tablets 2039
Altace Capsules (Less than 1%) 2233
Ambien Tablets (Rare) 3191
AmBisome for Injection (Less common) 1383
Amerge Tablets (Rare) 1467
Anaprox Tablets (Less than 3%) 2967
Anaprox DS Tablets (Less than 3%) 2967
Anzemet Injection (Infrequently) 719
Anzemet Tablets (Infrequently) 722
Arthrotec Tablets (Rare) 3195
Attenuvax (Rare) 2044
Avalide Tablets 1070
Azactam for Injection (Less than 1%) 1276
Azulfidine EN-tabs Tablets (Rare) 2775
Bactrim 2949
Baycol Tablets 883
▲ Campath Ampules (8%) 992
Carbatrol Capsules 3234
Cardizem Injectable 1018
Cardizem Lyo-Ject Syringe 1018
Cardizem Monovial 1018
Cardizem CD Capsules (Infrequent) 1016
Cardura Tablets (Less than 0.5%) 2668
Cataflam Tablets (Less than 1%) 2315
Celexa (Infrequent) 1365
Chirocaine Injection (1.4%) 2909
Cipro I.V. (1% or less) 893
Cipro I.V. Pharmacy Bulk Package (Less than 1%) 897
Claritin (At least one patient) 3100
Claritin-D 12 Hour Extended Release Tablets 3102
Claritin-D 24 Hour Extended Release Tablets 3104
Clinoril Tablets (Less than 1 in 100) 2053
Clorpres Tablets (Few) 1002
Cognex Capsules (2%) 1351
Combipres Tablets (Few) 1040
Comtan Tablets (2%) 2328
Coreg Tablets (1% to 2%) 1508
Corzide 40/5 Tablets [illegible]
Corzide 80/5 Tablets 2247
Covera-HS Tablets (Less than 2%) 3199
Crinone (Less than 5%) 3213
Cytotec Tablets (Infrequent) 3202
Dapsone Tablets USP 1780
DiaBeta Tablets (Occasional) 741
Diovan HCT Tablets 2338
Diucardin Tablets 3494
Diuril Oral 2087
Diuril Sodium Intravenous 2086
Dyazide Capsules 1515
EC-Naprosyn Delayed-Release Tablets (Less than 3%) 2967
Emla 602
Engerix-B Vaccine 1517
Etrafon 3115
Evoxac Capsules (Less than 1%) 1217
Exelon Capsules (Infrequent) 2342
Exelon Oral Solution (Infrequent) 2345
▲ Felbatol (12.9%) 3343
Feldene Capsules (Occasional) 2685
Flexeril Tablets (Rare) 572
Flexeril Tablets (Rare) 2094
Florinef Acetate Tablets 2250
Floxin I.V. 2526
Floxin Tablets 2529
Furosemide Tablets 2284
Gastrocrom Oral Concentrate (Less common) 1162
Gengraf Capsules (2%) 457
Hivid Tablets (Less than 1%) 2975
HydroDIURIL Tablets 2108
Hyzaar 2109
Imdur Tablets (Less than or equal to 5%) 1826
Indapamide Tablets 2286
Inderide Tablets 3517
Inderide LA Long-Acting Capsules 3519
Indocin Capsules (Less than 1%) 2112
Indocin I.V. (Less than 1%) 2115
Indocin (Less than 1%) 2112
INFeD Injection 3388
Innohep Injection 1248
Intron A for Injection (Less than or equal to 5%) 3120
Isoptin SR Tablets (1% or less) 467
Lescol Capsules (Rare) 2361
Lescol Capsules (Rare) 2925
Lescol XL Tablets 2361
Lescol XL Tablets 2925
▲ Leustatin Injection (10%) 2495
Levaquin (0.3% to less than 0.5%) 2537
Limbitrol 1738
Lodine (Less than 1%) 3528
Lodine XL Extended-Release Tablets (Less than 1%) 3530
Lotensin HCT Tablets 2367
Lovenox Injection 746
Luvox Tablets (25, 50, 100 mg) (Rare) 3256
Matulane Capsules 3246
Maxzide 1008
Meruvax II 2130
Mevacor Tablets (Rare) 2132
Micardis HCT Tablets 1051
Microzide Capsules 3414
Minizide Capsules 2700
M-M-R II 2118
Mobic Tablets (Less than 2%) 1054
Moduretic Tablets 2138
Monopril HCT 1094
Motrin Suspension, Oral Drops, Chewable Tablets, and Caplets (Less than 1%) 2002
Mumpsvax (Extremely rare) 2141
Mykrox Tablets 1168
Naprelan Tablets (Less than 3%) 1293
Naprosyn Suspension (Less than 3%) 2967
Naprosyn Tablets (Less than 3%) 2967
Neoral Soft Gelatin Capsules (2%) 2380
Neoral Oral Solution (2%) 2380
Neurontin Capsules (Frequent) 2655
Neurontin Oral Solution (Frequent) 2655
Neurontin Tablets (Frequent) 2655
Nicotrol Nasal Spray (Less than 1%) 2843
Norpramin Tablets 755
Norvasc Tablets (More than 0.1% to 1%) 2704
NovoSeven (1%) 2430
Oncaspar (Less than 1%) 756
Orudis Capsules (Less than 1%) 3548
Oruvail Capsules (Less than 1%) 3548
Paxil (Infrequent) 1609
Pediazole Suspension 3050
Permax Tablets (Rare) 1299
▲ Plavix Tablets (5.3%) 1097
▲ Plavix Tablets (5.3%) 3084
Pletal Tablets (Less than 2%) 2605
Pletal Tablets (Less than 2%) 2848
Ponstel Capsules (Occasional) 1356
Pravachol Tablets (Rare) 1099
Priftin Tablets (Less than 1%) 758
Prilosec Delayed-Release Capsules 628
Prinzide Tablets 2168
Procardia Capsules (Less than 0.5%) 2708
Procardia XL Extended Release Tablets (1% or less) 2710
▲ Proleukin for Injection (4%) 11[illegible]
ProSom Tablets (Rare) 500
Prozac Pulvules, Liquid, and Weekly Capsules (Rare) 1238
Pulmicort Respules (1% to 3%) 632
Reminyl Oral Solution (Infrequent) 1792
Reminyl Tablets (Infrequent) 1792
Renese Tablets 2712
Requip Tablets (Infrequent) 1621
Rescriptor Tablets (Less than 2%) 526
Rifadin 765
Rifater Tablets 769
Rilutek Tablets (Rare) 772
Risperdal (Infrequent) 1796
Rythmol Tablets – 150 mg, 225 mg, 300 mg (Less than 1%) 502
Sarafem Pulvules (Rare) 1962
Septra Suspension 2265
Septra Tablets 2265
Septra DS Tablets 2265
▲ Serostim for Injection (1% to 10%) 3229
▲ Simulect for Injection (3% to 10%) 2399
Sinequan (Occasional) 2713
Sonata Capsules (Rare) 3591
▲ Soriatane Capsules (1% to 10%) 3003
Surmontil Capsules 3595
Tarka Tablets 508
Tegretol/Tegretol-XR 2404
Tenex Tablets (3% or less) 2942
Tenoretic Tablets 690
Tenormin 692
Teveten Tablets (Less than 1%) 3327
Thalomid Capsules 1154
Tiazac Capsules (Infrequent) 1378
Ticlid Tablets (2.2%) 3015
Timolide Tablets 2187
Tolectin (Less than 1%) 2589
Topamax Sprinkle Capsules (Infrequent) 2590
Topamax Tablets (Infrequent) 2590
Toradol (Greater than 1%) 3018
Trecator-SC Tablets 3598
Trental Tablets (Rare) 784
Trileptal Oral Suspension (Up to 2%) 2407
Trileptal Tablets (Up to 2%) 2407
Uniretic Tablets 3178
Urobiotic-250 Capsules 2731
Vaseretic Tablets 2204
Verelan Capsules (1% or less) 3184
Verelan PM Capsules (2% or less) 3186
Vivactil Tablets 2217
Vivactil Tablets 2446
Voltaren Tablets (Less than 1%) 2315
Voltaren-XR Tablets (Less than 1%) 2315
Zanaflex Tablets (Rare) 1305
Zaroxolyn Tablets 1177
Zebeta Tablets 1885
Zestoretic Tablets 695
Ziac Tablets 1887
Zocor Tablets (Rare) 2219
Zoloft (2%) 2751
Zosyn (1.0% or less) 1890
Zosyn in Galaxy Containers (1.0% or less) 1894
Zyrtec (Less than 2%) 2756
Zyrtec-D 12 Hour Extended Relief Tablets (Less than 2%) 2758

Purpura, allergic
Cataflam Tablets (Rare) 2315
Plavix Tablets (Less than 1%) 1097
Plavix Tablets (Less than 1%) 3084
Voltaren Tablets (Rare) 2315
Voltaren-XR Tablets (Rare) 2315

Purpura, anaphylactoid
Declomycin Tablets 1855
Doryx Coated Pellet Filled Capsules 3357
Dynacin Capsules 2019
Minocin Intravenous 1862
Minocin Oral Suspension 1865
Minocin Pellet-Filled Capsules 1863
Monodox Capsules 2442
Periostat Tablets 1208
Vibramycin Calcium Oral Suspension Syrup 2735
Vibramycin Hyclate Capsules 2735
Vibramycin Hyclate Intravenous 2737
Vibramycin Monohydrate for Oral Suspension 2735
Vibra-Tabs Film Coated Tablets 2735

Purpura, fulminous
Zovirax for Injection (Less than 1%) 1708

Purpura, nonthrombocytopenic
Blocadren Tablets 2046
Corgard Tablets 2245
Corzide 40/5 Tablets 2247
Corzide 80/5 Tablets 2247
Cosopt Sterile Ophthalmic Solution 2065
Edecrin (Rare) 2091
Inderal 3513
Inderal LA Long-Acting Capsules 3516
Inderide Tablets 3517
Inderide LA Long-Acting Capsules 3519
Miltown Tablets [illegible]
Nadolol Tablets 2288
Normodyne Tablets 3137
Sectral Capsules 3589
Timolide Tablets 2187
Timolol GFS ⊙266
Timoptic in Ocudose 2192
Timoptic Sterile Ophthalmic Solution 2190
Timoptic-XE Sterile Ophthalmic Gel Forming Solution 2194
Toprol-XL Tablets 651

Purpura, thrombocytopenic
Amoxil Chewable Tablets 1471
Amoxil for Oral Suspension 1471
Amoxil 1471
Atromid-S Capsules 3483
Augmentin Chewable Tablets 1482
Augmentin Powder for Oral Suspension 1482
Augmentin Tablets 1485
Augmentin ES-600 Powder for Oral Suspension 1487
Axid Pulvules (Rare) 1903
Axid Pulvules (Rare) 2919
Blocadren Tablets 2046
Compazine 1505
Concerta Extended-Release Tablets 1998
Concerta Tablets 561
Corgard Tablets 2245
Corzide 40/5 Tablets 2247
Corzide 80/5 Tablets 2247
Cosopt Sterile Ophthalmic Solution 2065
Cuprimine Capsules 2075
Diamox ⊙269
Etrafon 3115
Evoxac Capsules (Less than 1%) 1217
Genoptic Ophthalmic Ointment (Rare) ⊙239
Genoptic Sterile Ophthalmic Solution (Rare) ⊙239
Inderal 3513
Inderal LA Long-Acting Capsules 3516
Inderide Tablets 3517
Inderide LA Long-Acting Capsules 3519
Indocin Capsules (Less than 1%) 2112
Indocin I.V. (Less than 1%) 2115
Indocin (Less than 1%) 2112
Intron A for Injection (Less than 5%) 3120
Metadate CD Capsules 1164
Metadate ER Tablets 1167
Methylin Tablets 1995
Methylin ER Tablets 1995
Miltown Tablets (Rare) 3349
Nadolol Tablets 2288
Neptazane Tablets ⊙271
Normodyne Tablets 3137
Omnicef 493
Phenergan Injection 3553
Phenergan Tablets 3556
PREVPAC 3298
Prozac Pulvules, Liquid, and Weekly Capsules 1238
Quinaglute Dura-Tabs Tablets 978
Quinidex Extentabs 2933
Ritalin 2387
Sarafem Pulvules 1962
Sectral Capsules 3589
Stelazine 1640
Talacen Caplets (A few cases) 3089
Thorazine 1656
Timolide Tablets 2187
Timolol GFS ⊙266
Timoptic in Ocudose 2192
Timoptic Sterile Ophthalmic Solution 2190
Timoptic-XE Sterile Ophthalmic Gel Forming Solution 2194
Toprol-XL Tablets 651
Trilafon 3160
Vistide Injection 1445
Xeloda Tablets (Less than 5%) 3039
Zebeta Tablets 1885

Purpura, thrombocytopenic thrombotic
Cuprimine Capsules 2075
Depen Titratable Tablets 3341
Floxin I.V. 2526
Floxin Tablets 2529
Mycobutin Capsules (One patient) 2838
Norplant System 3543
Plavix Tablets (Rare) 1097
Plavix Tablets (Rare) 3084
Prevacid Delayed-Release Capsules (Less than 1%) 3292
▲ Rapamune Oral Solution and Tablets (3% to 20%) 3584
Risperdal (A single case) 1796
Ticlid Tablets (Rare) 3015
Valtrex Caplets 1676

Pustules, exanthematous
Plaquenil Tablets 3082

Pustules, scalp
Cormax Scalp Application (Approximately 1%) 2441
Nizoral 2% Shampoo (one occurrence in 41 patients) 2007
Temovate Scalp Application (3 of 294 patients) 1304

Pustules, unspecified
Duragesic Transdermal System (Less than 1%) 1786
Klonopin Tablets (Infrequent) 2983
Levulan Kerastick (Up to 4%) 971

Pustulosis, exanthematous
Augmentin ES-600 Powder for Oral Suspension 1487

Pustulosis, provocation
Cormax Cream (Rare) 2440
Cormax Ointment (Rare) 2440
Cormax Scalp Application (Rare) 2441
Temovate Scalp Application (Rare) 1304

Pyelitis
Amerge Tablets (Rare) 1467

Pyelonephritis
Actiq (Less than 1%) 1184
Ambien Tablets (Rare) 3191
Aricept Tablets (Infrequent) 1270
Aricept Tablets (Infrequent) 2665
Avonex 1013
Celexa (Rare) 1365
▲ CellCept Capsules (3%) 2951
▲ CellCept Intravenous (3%) 2951
▲ CellCept Oral Suspension (3%) 2951
▲ CellCept Tablets (3%) 2951
Cleocin Vaginal Cream (2%) 2788

Cleocin Vaginal Ovules (Less than 1%) 2789
Copaxone for Injection (Infrequent) 3306
Effexor Tablets (Rare) 3495
Effexor XR Capsules (Infrequent) 3499
Enbrel for Injection 1752
Enbrel for Injection 3504
Evoxac Capsules (Less than 1%) 1217
Gabitril Tablets (Infrequent) 1189
Gengraf Capsules (1% to less than 3%) 457
Herceptin I.V. (At least one of the 958 patients) 1414
Lupron Depot 3.75 mg 3281
Lupron Depot–3 Month 11.25 mg 3285
Miacalcin Nasal Spray (Less than 1%) 2375
Naprelan Tablets (Less than 1%) 1293
Neoral Soft Gelatin Capsules (1% to less than 3%) 2380
Neoral Oral Solution (1% to less than 3%) 2380
Norvir Capsules (Less than 2%) 487
Norvir Oral Solution (Less than 2%) 487
Permax Tablets (Rare) 1299
Prinivil Tablets (0.3% to 1.0%) 2164
Prinzide Tablets 2168
Protonix I.V. (Less than 1%) 3580
Protonix Tablets (Less than 1%) 3577
▲ Remicade for IV Injection (26%) 1178
Requip Tablets (Rare) 1621
Rilutek Tablets (Rare) 772
Uniretic Tablets (Less than 1%) 3178
Zanaflex Tablets (Infrequent) 1305
Zestril Tablets (0.3% to 1.0%) 698
Zoloft (Rare) 2751

Pyoderma gangrenosum
Asacol Delayed-Release Tablets (Rare) 2884

Pyogenic granuloma
Accutane Capsules 2944
▲ Soriatane Capsules (1% to 10%) 3003

Pyrexia
(see under Fever)

Pyridoxine deficiency
Macrodantin Capsules 2891
Rifamate Capsules 767
Rifater Tablets 769

Pyrosis
(see under Heartburn)

Pyuria
Accuretic Tablets 2614
Aricept Tablets (Infrequent) 1270
Aricept Tablets (Infrequent) 2665
Cognex Capsules (Infrequent) 1351
Colazal Capsules 3069
Effexor Tablets (Infrequent) 3495
Effexor XR Capsules (Infrequent) 3499
Evoxac Capsules (Less than 1%) 1217
Floxin I.V. (More than or equal to 1%) 2526
Floxin Tablets (More than or equal to 1%) 2529
Lexxel Tablets (Infrequent) 608
Naprelan Tablets (Less than 1%) 1293
Neurontin Capsules (Rare) 2655
Neurontin Oral Solution (Rare) 2655
Neurontin Tablets (Rare) 2655
Paxil (Rare) 1609
Permax Tablets (Infrequent) 1299
▲ Priftin Tablets (4.2%) 758
Prilosec Delayed-Release Capsules (Less than 1%) 628
▲ Prograf (3% to 15%) 1393
Provigil Tablets (At least 1%) 1193
▲ Rapamune Oral Solution and Tablets (3% to 20%) 3584
Requip Tablets (2%) 1621
Salagen Tablets (Less than 1%) 2229
Singulair (1%) 2181
Tice BCG, BCG Live (0.7%) 2489
Uniretic Tablets (More than 1%) 3178
Zosyn 1890
Zosyn in Galaxy Containers 1894
Zyprexa Tablets (Infrequent) 1973
Zyprexa ZYDIS Orally Disintegrating Tablets (Infrequent) 1973

Q

Quadriplegia
Orthoclone OKT3 Sterile Solution 2498
Soma Tablets 3353
Soma Compound Tablets (Very rare) 3354
Soma Compound w/Codeine Tablets (Very rare) 3355

Quncke's edema
(see also under Angioedema)
Protonix I.V. 3580
Protonix Tablets 3577

R

Radiation recall syndrome
Xeloda Tablets (Less than 5%) 3039

Radiculoneuropathy
Imitrex Injection 1549
Imitrex Tablets (Rare) 1558
Pneumovax 23 (Rare) 2156
Pnu-Imune 23 1868
Recombivax HB 2178

Rage
Librium Capsules 1736
Valium Tablets 3047
Xanax Tablets (Rare) 2865

Rales
Adalat CC Tablets (Less than 1.0%) 877
▲ Aredia for Injection (Up to 6%) 2309
Blocadren Tablets (0.6%) 2046
Brevibloc Injection (Less than 1%) 858
Cosopt Sterile Ophthalmic Solution 2065
Crixivan Capsules (Less than 2%) 2070
Hivid Tablets (Less than 1%) 2975
Imdur Tablets (Less than or equal to 5%) 1826
▲ Mylotarg for Injection (10% to 16%) 3540
ReoPro Vials (0.4%) 1958
Sular Tablets (Less than or equal to 1%) 688
Survanta Intratracheal Suspension 3053
Thalomid Capsules 1154
Timolide Tablets (Less than 1%) 2187
Timolol GFS ⊙ 266
Timoptic in Ocudose 2192
Timoptic Sterile Ophthalmic Solution 2190
Timoptic-XE Sterile Ophthalmic Gel Forming Solution 2194
▲ Trisenox Injection (10%) 1158
▲ Vesanoid Capsules (14%) 3037
▲ Zenapax for Injection (2% to 5%) 3046

Rash
▲ Abelcet Injection (4%) 1273
Accolate Tablets 657
Accupril Tablets (1.4%) 2611
Accutane Capsules 2944
Acel-Imune (1.2%) 1851
Aceon Tablets (2 mg, 4 mg, 8 mg) (2.3%) 3249
Aciphex Tablets 1267
Aciphex Tablets 1783
Acticin Cream 998
▲ Actimmune (17%) 1772
Actiq (1% to 2%) 1184
Activase I.V. (Very rare) 1410
Activella Tablets 2764
▲ Actonel Tablets (7.7% to 11.5%) 2879
Adalat CC Tablets (3% or less) 877
▲ Aerobid/Aerobid-M (3% to 9%) 1363
▲ Agenerase Capsules (20% to 27%) 1454
▲ Agenerase Oral Solution (20% to 27%) 1459
Aggrastat 2031
Aggrenox Capsules 1026
▲ Agrylin Capsules (8.3%) 3232
Albenza Tablets (Rare) 1463
Albumin (Human) 5% (Very rare) 838
Albumin (Human) 25% (Very rare) 839
Albuminar-5, U.S.P. 785
Albuminar-25, U.S.P. 786
Aldara Cream, 5% (More than 1%) 1978
Aldoclor Tablets 2035
Aldomet Tablets 2037
Aldoril Tablets 2039
Alkeran for Injection 1465
Alkeran Tablets 1466
Allegra (Rare) 712
Allegra-D Extended-Release Tablets (Rare) 714
Alomide Ophthalmic Solution (Less than 1%) ⊙ 204
Aloprim for Injection (1.5%) 2292
Alphagan P Ophthalmic Solution (1% to 4%) 546
Altace Capsules (Less than 1%) 2233
Ambien Tablets (2%) 3191
▲ AmBisome for Injection (22.2% to 24.8%) 1383
Amerge Tablets (Infrequent) 1467
Americaine Anesthetic Lubricant 1162
Americaine Otic Topical Anesthetic Ear Drops 1162
Amicar Injection 3608
Amicar Syrup 3608
Amicar Tablets 3608
Amoxil Chewable Tablets 1471
Amoxil for Oral Suspension 1471
Amoxil 1471
▲ Amphotec (5% or more) 1774
Anaprox Tablets (Less than 1%) 2967
Anaprox DS Tablets (Less than 1%) 2967
Ancef for Injection 1474
Ancef Injection 1474
Ancobon Capsules 1730
Androderm Transdermal System CIII (Less than 1% to 2%) 3377
Anectine Injection 1476
Anzemet Injection (Rare) 719
Anzemet Tablets (Rare) 722
▲ Apligraf (1.3% to 4.5%) 2305
▲ Arava Tablets (10%) 724
▲ Argatroban Injection (1% to 10%) 1478
Aricept Tablets 1270
Aricept Tablets 2665
▲ Arimidex Tablets (5.7% to 6.1%) 659
Aromasin Tablets (Less frequent) 2769
Artane (Rare) 1855
Arthrotec Tablets (Rare) 3195
▲ Asacol Delayed-Release Tablets (6%) 2884
Astelin Nasal Spray 3339
Atacand Tablets (0.5% or greater) 595
Atacand HCT Tablets (0.5% or greater) 597
Ativan Injection (Occasional) 3478
Atromid-S Capsules (Less often) 3483
Atrovent Inhalation Aerosol (1.2%) 1030
Atrovent Nasal Spray 0.03% (Infrequent) 1032
Atrovent Nasal Spray 0.06% (Rare) 1033
Attenuvax (Occasional) 2044
▲ Augmentin Chewable Tablets (3%) 1482
▲ Augmentin Powder for Oral Suspension (3%) 1482
▲ Augmentin Tablets (3%) 1485
Augmentin ES-600 Powder for Oral Suspension (1.1%) 1487
Avalide Tablets (1% or greater) 1070
Avapro Tablets (1% or greater) 1074
Avapro Tablets (1% or greater) 3076
Avelox Tablets (0.05% to 1%) 879
Avonex 1013
Axert Tablets (Rare) 2772
Axid Pulvules (1.9%) 1903
Axid Pulvules (1.9%) 2919
Azactam for Injection (1% to 4.3%) 1276
Azelex Cream (Less than 1%) 547
Azmacort Inhalation Aerosol (1% to 3%) 728
▲ Azulfidine EN-tabs Tablets (13%) 2775
▲ Bactrim (Among most common) 2949
Bactroban Cream (1.1%) 1494
Bactroban Nasal (Less than 1%) 1495
Bactroban Ointment (Less than 1%) 1496
▲ Baycol Tablets (3.3%) 883
BayRab (Rare) 917
Beano ▣ 809
Bebulin VH 840
Beconase Inhalation Aerosol (Rare) 1497
Beconase AQ Nasal Spray (Rare) 1498
BeneFix for Injection 1432
Betagan ⊙ 228
Betapace Tablets (2% to 5%) 950
▲ Betimol Ophthalmic Solution (More than 5%) ⊙ 324
▲ Biaxin/Biaxin XL (3%) 403
Bicillin C-R 900/300 Injection 2240
Bicillin C-R Injection 2238
Bicillin L-A Injection 2242
Blocadren Tablets (Less than 1%) 2046
Botox Purified Neurotoxin Complex (7 cases) 549
Brethine Tablets (Less than 1%) 2313
Brevicon 28-Day Tablets 3380
Buprenex Injectable (Infrequent) 2918
▲ Cafcit (8.7%) 1035
Calcium Disodium Versenate Injection 1980
▲ Campath Ampules (3% to 40%) 992
Canasa Rectal Suppositories (1.2%) 829
Cancidas for Injection (1.3% to 4.6%) 2048
▲ Captopril Tablets (About 4 to 7 of 100 patients) 2281
Carafate Suspension (Less than 0.5%) 731
Carafate Tablets (Less than 0.5%) 730
Carbatrol Capsules 3234
Cardizem Injectable 1018
Cardizem Lyo-Ject Syringe 1018
Cardizem Monovial 1018
Cardizem CD Capsules (1.2%) 1016
Cardura Tablets (1%) 2668
▲ Carnitor Injection (3% to 5%) 3242
Carteolol Hydrochloride Ophthalmic Solution USP, 1% ⊙ 258
▲ Casodex Tablets (6%) 662
Cataflam Tablets (1% to 3%) 2315
Catapres Tablets (About 1 in 100 patients) 1037
Catapres-TTS (0.5% or less) 1038
Caverject Sterile Powder (Less than 1%) 2777
Ceclor CD Tablets (0.1% to 1%) 1279
Ceclor 1905
Cedax (0.1% to 1%) 1021
Cefizox for Intramuscular or Intravenous Use (1% to 5%) 1390
Cefotan (1 in 150) 664
Ceftin (0.1% to 1%) 1898
Cefzil (0.9%) 1076
Celebrex Capsules 2676
Celebrex Capsules 2780
Celexa (Frequent) 1365
▲ CellCept Capsules (6.4% to 22.1%) 2951
▲ CellCept Intravenous (6.4% to 22.1%) 2951
▲ CellCept Oral Suspension (6.4% to 22.1%) 2951
▲ CellCept Tablets (6.4% to 22.1%) 2951
Ceptaz for Injection (2% of patients) 1499
Cerebyx Injection (Frequent) 2619
▲ Cerezyme for Injection (5.4%) 1438
Cerubidine for Injection (Rare) 947
Cerumenex Eardrops 2895
▲ Chemet Capsules (2.6% to 11.2%) 3078
Chibroxin Sterile Ophthalmic Solution 2051
Cipro HC Otic Suspension (One patient) 540
Cipro I.V. (Greater than 1%) 893
Cipro I.V. Pharmacy Bulk Package (Greater than 1%) 897
Cipro (1.1%) 887
Claforan Injection (2.4%) 732
Claritin (At least one patient) 3100
Claritin-D 12 Hour Extended Release Tablets (Less frequent) 3102
Claritin-D 24 Hour Extended Release Tablets 3104
Cleocin Vaginal Cream (Less than 1%) 2788
Cleocin Vaginal Ovules (Less than 1%) 2789
▲ Clinoril Tablets (3% to 9%) 2053
Clomid Tablets (Fewer than 1%) 735
Clorpres Tablets (1%) 1002
Clozaril Tablets (2%) 2319
Cogentin 2055
▲ Cognex Capsules (7%) 1351
Colace Capsules, Syrup, Liquid 3236
Colestid Tablets (Infrequent) 2791
Coly-Mycin M Parenteral 2243
▲ CombiPatch Transdermal System (5% to 6%) 2323
Combipres Tablets 1040
Combivent Inhalation Aerosol (Less than 2%; rare) 1041
▲ Combivir Tablets (9%) 1502
Compazine 1505
Comvax (0.8% to 0.9%) 2056
Concerta Extended-Release Tablets 1998
Concerta Tablets 561
Condylox Gel (Less common) 2436
▲ Copaxone for Injection (18%) 3306
Cordarone Tablets (Less than 1%) 3487
Coreg Tablets (More than 2%) 1508
Corgard Tablets 2245
Cortrosyn for Injection 2449
Corzide 40/5 Tablets (1 to 5 of 1000 patients) 2247
Corzide 80/5 Tablets (1 to 5 of 1000 patients) 2247
Cosopt Sterile Ophthalmic Solution (1% to 5%) 2065
Coumadin for Injection (Infrequent) 1243
Coumadin Tablets (Infrequent) 1243
Covera-HS Tablets (1.2% to 2%) 3199
Cozaar Tablets (Less than 1%) 2067
Crinone (Less than 5%) 3213
Crixivan Capsules 2070
Crolom Sterile Ophthalmic Solution USP 4% ⊙ 259
▲ Cuprimine Capsules (5%) 2075
Cylert Tablets 415
Cytotec Tablets (Infrequent) 3202
Cytovene 2959
Darvon-N/Darvocet-N 1907
Darvon Pulvules 1909
Darvon Compound-65 Pulvules 1910
Darvon-N Tablets (Less than 1%) 1912
DDAVP Nasal Spray 738
DDAVP Rhinal Tube 738
Demadex Tablets and Injection 2965
Demerol 3079
Depacon Injection (1% to 5%) 416
Depakene (1% to 5%) 421
Depakote Sprinkle Capsules (1% to 5%) 426
▲ Depakote Tablets (1% to 6%) 430
Depakote ER Tablets (1% to 5%) 436
▲ Depen Titratable Tablets (5%) 3341
▲ Depo-Provera Contraceptive Injection (More than 5%) 2798
Dermatop Emollient Cream (Less than 1%) 2517
Desferal Vials (Very rare) 2333
Desmopressin Acetate Rhinal Tube 1345
Detrol Tablets (1.9%) 3623
D.H.E. 45 Injection (Occasional) 2334
Differin Cream (Less than 1%) 1402
Diflucan Tablets, Injection, and Oral Suspension (1.8%) 2681
Digitek Tablets 1003
Dilantin Infatabs 2624
Dilantin Kapseals 2622
Dilantin-125 Oral Suspension 2625

Dilaudid Oral Liquid ... 445
Dilaudid Tablets - 8 mg ... 445
Dilaudid-HP (Less frequent) ... 443
Diovan Capsules ... 2337
Diovan HCT Tablets (Greater than 0.2%) ... 2338
Dipentum Capsules (2.3%) ... 2803
Diphtheria & Tetanus Toxoids Adsorbed Purogenated for Pediatric Use ... 1857
Diprivan Injectable Emulsion (Less than 1% to 5%) ... 667
Ditropan XL Extended Release Tablets (2% to 5%) ... 564
Diucardin Tablets ... 3494
Diuril Oral ... 2087
Diuril Sodium Intravenous ... 2086
Dobutrex Solution Vials (Occasional) ... 1914
▲ Dolobid Tablets (3% to 9%) ... 2088
Dolophine Hydrochloride Tablets ... 3056
▲ Donnazyme Tablets (Most frequent) ... 2931
▲ Dovonex Cream (1% to 10%) ... 1116
▲ Dovonex Ointment (1% to 10%) ... 1117
▲ Dovonex Scalp Solution (About 11%) ... 1118
▲ Doxil Injection (1% to 21.6%) ... 566
DuoNeb Inhalation Solution (0.3%) ... 1233
Duraclon Injection (1%) ... 3057
Duragesic Transdermal System (1% or greater) ... 1786
Duricef ... 1079
Dyazide Capsules ... 1515
Dynabac Tablets (1.4% to 1.6%) ... 2269
DynaCirc Capsules (1.5% to 2%) ... 2921
DynaCirc CR Tablets (1.3% to 2.6%) ... 2923
Dyrenium Capsules (Rare) ... 3458
EC-Naprosyn Delayed-Release Tablets (Less than 1%) ... 2967
Edecrin ... 2091
▲ Effexor Tablets (3%) ... 3495
Effexor XR Capsules (Frequent) ... 3499
▲ Efudex (Among most frequent) ... 1733
8-MOP Capsules ... 1727
Eldepryl Capsules ... 3266
Elimite Cream (1 to 2% or less) ... 552
▲ Ellence Injection (0.3% to 8.9%) ... 2806
▲ Elmiron Capsules (3%) ... 570
Elspar for Injection ... 2092
Emcyt Capsules (1%) ... 2810
Emla (Less than 1%) ... 602
Enalaprilat Injection (0.5% to 1%) ... 863
▲ Enbrel for Injection (14%) ... 1752
▲ Enbrel for Injection (14%) ... 3504
Engerix-B Vaccine (Less than 1%) ... 1517
▲ Epivir (9%) ... 1520
▲ Epivir-HBV (5%) ... 1524
Epogen for Injection (Rare) ... 582
Ergamisol Tablets (10 patients) ... 1789
Ery-Tab Tablets ... 448
Esclim Transdermal System (2.1% to 4.2%) ... 3460
Eskalith ... 1527
Ethyol for Injection (Rare) ... 2029
Etrafon ... 3115
▲ Eulexin Capsules (3% to 8%) ... 3118
▲ Evista Tablets (5.5%) ... 1915
▲ Evoxac Capsules (4.3%) ... 1217
Exelon Capsules (2% or more) ... 2342
Exelon Oral Solution (2% or more) ... 2345
Factrel ... 3633
Famotidine Injection (Infrequent) ... 866
Famvir Tablets (0.4% to 3.3%) ... 2348
Feiba VH ... 840
▲ Felbatol (3.4% to 9.7%) ... 3343
▲ Feldene Capsules (1% to 10%) ... 2685
▲ Femara Tablets (4% to 5%) ... 2351
femhrt Tablets ... 2635
Ferrlecit Injection (Greater than 1%) ... 3386
Finevin Cream (Less than 1%) ... 962
Flexeril Tablets (Less than 1%) ... 572
Flexeril Tablets (Less than 1%) ... 2094
▲ Flolan for Injection (10% to 25%) ... 1528
Flomax Capsules ... 1044
Flonase Nasal Spray ... 1533
Florinef Acetate Tablets ... 2250
▲ Flovent Diskus (8%) ... 3614
Flovent (1% to 3%) ... 1535
Floxin I.V. (1% to 3%) ... 2526
Floxin Otic Solution (1%) ... 1219
Floxin Tablets (1% to 3%) ... 2529
▲ Fludara for Injection (15%) ... 995
Flumadine (0.3% to 1%) ... 1370
Fluothane Inhalation (Rare) ... 3508
FluShield Influenza Vaccine ... 3521
Follistim for Injection ... 2465
Foradil Aerolizer (1.1%) ... 2354
Fortaz (2%) ... 1541
Fortovase Capsules (Up to 2.1%) ... 2970
Fosamax Tablets (Rare) ... 2095
▲ Foscavir Injection (5% or greater) ... 605
Fragmin Injection (Rare) ... 2814
Sterile FUDR ... 2974
Furosemide Tablets ... 2284
▲ Gabitril Tablets (5%) ... 1189
Gamimune N, 5% Solvent/Detergent Treated (Rare) ... 925
Gamimune N, 10% Solvent/Detergent Treated (A single incidence) ... 928
Gammar-P I.V. ... 787
Gastrocrom Oral Concentrate (2 of 87 patients) ... 1162
▲ Gemzar for Injection (28% to 30%) ... 1919
▲ Gengraf Capsules (1% to 8%) ... 457
Genotropin Lyophilized Powder (Infrequent) ... 2818
Geocillin Tablets (Infrequent) ... 2687
▲ Geodon Capsules (5%) ... 2688
▲ Gleevec Capsules (32% to 39%) ... 2357
▲ Gliadel Wafer (2% to 5%) ... 1723
GlucaGen for Injection Diagnostic Kit ... 949
Glucophage Tablets (1% to 5%) ... 1080
Glucotrol XL Extended Release Tablets (Less than 1%) ... 2693
▲ Glyset Tablets (4.3%) ... 2821
Grifulvin V Tablets Microsize and Oral Suspension Microsize ... 2518
Gris-PEG Tablets (Rare) ... 2661
Havrix Vaccine (Less than 1%) ... 1544
Helixate Concentrate (Two reports) ... 788
▲ Herceptin I.V. (18%) ... 1414
Hexalen Capsules (Less than 1%) ... 2226
HibTITER (1 of 1,118 vaccinations) ... 1859
▲ Hivid Tablets (3.4%) ... 2975
Humalog (Less common) ... 1926
Humalog Mix 75/25 Pen ... 1928
Humate-P Concentrate ... 790
Humegon for Injection ... 2468
Humulin 50/50, 100 Units ... 1934
Humulin 70/30, 100 Units (Less common) ... 1935
Humulin 70/30 Pen (Less common) ... 1936
Humulin L, 100 Units (Less common) ... 1937
Humulin R Regular (U-500) ... 1943
Humulin N NPH Pen (Less common) ... 1940
▲ Hyalgan Solution (14%) ... 3080
Hycamtin for Injection (Less than 1%) ... 1546
Hycodan ... 1316
HydroDIURIL Tablets ... 2108
Hytrin Capsules (At least 1%) ... 464
Hyzaar (1.4%) ... 2109
Idamycin PFS Injection ... 2825
Iletin II, Regular (Pork), 100 Units ... 1947
Imdur Tablets (Less than or equal to 2%) ... 1826
Imitrex Injection (Infrequent) ... 1549
Imitrex Nasal Spray (Infrequent) ... 1554
Imitrex Tablets (Rare to infrequent) ... 1558
IMUPlus Formula ... 3274
Inderide Tablets ... 3517
Inderide LA Long-Acting Capsules ... 3519
Indocin Capsules (Less than 1%) ... 2112
Indocin I.V. (Less than 1%) ... 2115
Indocin (Less than 1%) ... 2112
INFeD Injection ... 3388
▲ Infergen (13%) ... 1777
Innohep Injection (1.2%) ... 1248
▲ Intron A for Injection (Up to 25%) ... 3120
Invirase Capsules (Up to 2.1%) ... 2979
Ismo Tablets (Fewer than 1%) ... 3524
Isoptin SR Tablets (1.2% or less) ... 467
Iveegam EN (0.3% to 0.8%) ... 849
▲ JE-VAX Vaccine (5% to approximately 10%) ... 811
Kadian Capsules (Less than 3%) ... 1335
Kaletra Capsules (0.6% to 3.6%) ... 471
Kaletra Oral Solution (0.6% to 3.6%) ... 471
Keflex ... 1237
Kefurox Vials, ADD-Vantage (1 in 125) ... 1948
Kefzol Vials, ADD-Vantage ... 1951
Keppra Tablets (1% or more) ... 3314
Klonopin Tablets ... 2983
K-Lor Powder Packets (Rare) ... 469
Kogenate (Two reports) ... 934
Kogenate FS ... 936
K-Tab Filmtab Tablets (Rare) ... 470
Kytril Injection (Rare) ... 2986
▲ Lac-Hydrin Cream (Approximately 2% to 15%) ... 1118
▲ Lamictal (9% to 10%) ... 1567
▲ Lamisil Tablets (5.6%) ... 2360
Lantus Injection ... 742
▲ Lariam Tablets (Among most frequent) ... 2989
Lescol Capsules (2.3%) ... 2361
Lescol Capsules (2.3%) ... 2925
Lescol XL Tablets (1.6%) ... 2361
Lescol XL Tablets (1.6%) ... 2925
Leukeran Tablets (Rare) ... 1591
▲ Leukine (44% to 70%) ... 1755
▲ Leustatin Injection (10% to 27%) ... 2495
Levaquin (0.3% to 2.5%) ... 2537
Levo-Dromoran ... 1734
Levorphanol Tartrate Tablets (1% to 3%) ... 3059
Levoxyl Tablets ... 1819
Lexxel Tablets ... 608
Limbitrol ... 1738
Lipitor Tablets (1.1% to 3.9%) ... 2639
Lipitor Tablets (1.1% to 3.9%) ... 2696
Lithium Carbonate ... 3061
Lithium Citrate Syrup ... 3061
Livostin (Approximately 1% to 3%) ... ⊙305
Lodine (1% to 3%) ... 3528
Lodine XL Extended-Release Tablets (1% to 3%) ... 3530
Lodosyn Tablets ... 1251
Lo/Ovral Tablets ... 3532
Lo/Ovral-28 Tablets ... 3538
Lopid Tablets (1.7%) ... 2650
Loprox Gel (Less than 1%) ... 2022
Lorabid Suspension and Pulvules (0.7% to 2.9%) ... 2251
Lortab ... 3319
Lortab Elixir ... 3317
Lotensin Tablets (Less than 1%) ... 2365
Lotensin HCT Tablets (0.3% to 1%) ... 2367
Lotrel Capsules ... 2370
Lotrisone Cream (Less than 1%) ... 3129
Low-Ogestrel-28 Tablets ... 3392
Loxitane Capsules ... 3398
Lupron Depot 3.75 mg ... 3281
Lupron Depot 7.5 mg ... 3284
Lupron Depot–3 Month 11.25 mg ... 3285
Lupron Depot–3 Month 22.5 mg ... 3288
Lupron Depot–4 Month 30 mg ... 3289
Lupron Depot-PED 7.5 mg, 11.25 mg and 15 mg (2%) ... 3291
Luvox Tablets (25, 50, 100 mg) ... 3256
LYMErix Vaccine (1.35% to 3.07%) ... 1592
Matulane Capsules ... 3246
Mavik Tablets (0.3% to 1.0%) ... 478
Maxair Autohaler ... 1981
Maxair Inhaler (Less than 1%) ... 1984
Maxalt Tablets (Infrequent) ... 2120
Maxalt-MLT Orally Disintegrating Tablets (Infrequent) ... 2120
Maxidone Tablets CIII ... 3399
Maxipime for Injection (1.1% to 4%) ... 1285
Maxzide ... 1008
Mefoxin for Injection ... 2124
Mefoxin Premixed Intravenous Solution ... 2127
▲ Megace Oral Suspension (2% to 12%) ... 1124
Mepergan Injection ... 3539
▲ Mepron Suspension (6.3% to 46%) ... 1598
▲ Meridia Capsules (3.8%) ... 481
Merrem I.V. (1.4% to 3.5%) ... 673
Meruvax II ... 2130
Mestinon (Occasional) ... 1740
Metadate CD Capsules ... 1164
Metadate ER Tablets ... 1167
Methylin Tablets ... 1995
Methylin ER Tablets ... 1995
MetroGel-Vaginal Gel (Less than 1%) ... 1986
Mevacor Tablets (0.8% to 5.2%) ... 2132
▲ Mexitil Capsules (3.8% to 4.2%) ... 1047
Miacalcin Injection ... 2373
Micardis Tablets (More than 0.3%) ... 1049
Micardis HCT Tablets (2% or greater) ... 1051
Micro-K ... 3311
Microzide Capsules ... 3414
Midamor Tablets (Less than or equal to 1%) ... 2136
Midrin Capsules ... 3464
Migranal Nasal Spray (Infrequent) ... 2376
Minipress Capsules (1% to 4%) ... 2699
Minizide Capsules ... 2700
Mintezol ... 2137
Mirapex Tablets ... 2834
M-M-R II (Infrequent) ... 2118
Moban ... 1320
Mobic Tablets (0.3% to 3%) ... 1054
Modicon ... 2563
▲ Moduretic Tablets (3% to 8%) ... 2138
Monopril Tablets (0.2% to 1.0% or more) ... 1091
Monopril HCT (Less than 2%) ... 1094
Monurol Sachet (1.4%) ... 1375
▲ Motrin Suspension, Oral Drops, Chewable Tablets, and Caplets (3% to 9%) ... 2002
MS Contin Tablets (Less frequent) ... 2896
MSIR (Less frequent) ... 2898
▲ Mycobutin Capsules (11%) ... 2838
Mykrox Tablets (Less than 2%) ... 1168
▲ Mylotarg for Injection (22%) ... 3540
Nadolol Tablets (1 to 5 of 1000 patients) ... 2288
Naftin Gel (0.5%) ... 2224
▲ Naprelan Tablets (3% to 9%) ... 1293
Naprosyn Suspension (Less than 1%) ... 2967
Naprosyn Tablets (Less than 1%) ... 2967
Nardil Tablets (Less common) ... 2653
Naropin Injection (Less than 1%) ... 612
Natrecor for Injection (At least 1%) ... 3189
Navane Oral ... 2701
Navane Intramuscular ... 2703
Navelbine Injection (Less than 5%) ... 1604
Nebcin Vials, Hyporets & ADD-Vantage ... 1955
Nembutal Sodium Solution ... 485
▲ Neoral Soft Gelatin Capsules (1% to 8%) ... 2380
▲ Neoral Oral Solution (1% to 8%) ... 2380
Neptazane Tablets ... ⊙271
▲ Neumega for Injection (25%) ... 1434
▲ Neupogen for Injection (6%; 12%) ... 587
Neurontin Capsules ... 2655
Neurontin Oral Solution (More than 1%) ... 2655
Neurontin Tablets ... 2655
Nexium Delayed-Release Capsules (Less than 1%) ... 619
Niaspan Extended-Release Tablets (1% to 5%) ... 1846
Nicotrol Nasal Spray (Less than 1%) ... 2843
▲ Nilandron Tablets (5.3%) ... 753
Nimotop Capsules (Up to 2.4%) ... 904
▲ Nipent for Injection (26% to 43%) ... 3272
▲ Nolvadex Tablets (13%) ... 678
Norco 5/325 Tablets CIII ... 3424
Norco 7.5/325 Tablets CIII ... 3425
Norco 10/325 Tablets CIII ... 3425
Norco 10/325 Tablets CIII ... 3427
Nordette-28 Tablets ... 2257
Norinyl 1 +35 28-Day Tablets ... 3380
Norinyl 1 + 50 28-Day Tablets ... 3380
Normodyne Injection (Rare) ... 3135
Normodyne Tablets (1%) ... 3137
Noroxin Tablets (0.3% to 1.0%) ... 2145
Norplant System ... 3543
Norpramin Tablets ... 755
Norvasc Tablets (Less than 1% to 2%) ... 2704
Norvir Capsules (Up to 2.6%) ... 487
Norvir Oral Solution (Up to 2.6%) ... 487
Novantrone for Injection (Occasional) ... 1760
Novolin 70/30 PenFill (Rare) ... 2423
Novolin 70/30 Prefilled Disposable Insulin Delivery System (Rare) ... 2425
Novolin N PenFill (Rare) ... 2423
Novolin R PenFill (Rare) ... 2423
NovoLog Injection ... 2427
NovoSeven (1%) ... 2430
Numorphan ... 1324
Nystop Topical Powder USP ... 2608
Ocupress Ophthalmic Solution, 1% Sterile ... ⊙303
Ogestrel 0.5/50-28 Tablets ... 3428
Omnicef (0.9%) ... 493
▲ Oncaspar (Greater than 5%) ... 756
Opticrom Ophthalmic Solution (Rare) ... 555
OptiPranolol Metipranolol Ophthalmic Solution 0.3% (A small number of patients) ... ⊙263
Oramorph SR Tablets (Less frequent) ... 3062
▲ Orap Tablets (8.3%) ... 1407
Organidin NR Liquid (Rare) ... 3350
Organidin NR Tablets (Rare) ... 3350
Orgaran Injection (2.1% to 4.8%) ... 2480
Ortho Diaphragm Kits – All-Flex Arcing Spring; Ortho Coil Spring ... 2552
Orthoclone OKT3 Sterile Solution ... 2498
Ortho-Cyclen/Ortho Tri-Cyclen ... 2573
Ortho-Novum ... 2563
Ortho-Novum 1/50□28 Tablets ... 2556
Ortho-Cyclen/Ortho Tri-Cyclen ... 2573
Orudis Capsules (Greater than 1%) ... 3540
Oruvail Capsules (Greater than 1%) ... 3548
Ovidrel for Injection (Less than 2%) ... 3220
Ovral Tablets ... 3551
Ovrette Tablets ... 3552
Oxistat Cream (0.1%) ... 1298
Oxsoralen-Ultra Capsules ... 1741
OxyContin Tablets (Between 1% and 5%) ... 2912
OxyFast Oral Concentrate Solution ... 2916
OxyIR Capsules ... 2916
Pacerone Tablets (Less than 1%) ... 3331
Paraplatin for Injection ... 1126
Parnate Tablets (Rare) ... 1607
▲ Paser Granules (Among most common) ... 1781
Paxil (2% to 3%) ... 1609
Pediazole Suspension ... 3050
▲ PEG-Intron Powder for Injection (6%) ... 3140
Penlac Nail Lacquer, Topical Solution ... 1225
Pentasa Capsules (1.0% to 1.3%) ... 3239
Pepcid Injection (Infrequent) ... 2153
Pepcid for Oral Suspension (Infrequent) ... 2150
Pepcid RPD Orally Disintegrating Tablets (Infrequent) ... 2150
Pepcid Tablets (Infrequent) ... 2150
Percocet Tablets ... 1326
Percolone Tablets ... 1327
Pergonal for Injection ... 3223

Peri-Colace Capsules and Syrup ... 3240
▲ Periostat Tablets (4%) ... 1208
▲ Permax Tablets (3.2%) ... 1299
Persantine Tablets (2.3%) ... 1057
Pfizerpen for Injection ... 2707
Phenergan Suppositories ... 3556
Phenergan Syrup ... 3554
Phenergan with Codeine Syrup ... 3557
Phenergan with Dextromethorphan Syrup ... 3559
Phenergan VC Syrup ... 3560
Phenergan VC with Codeine Syrup .. 3561
Phrenilin (Infrequent) ... 578
Pipracil (1%) ... 1866
▲ Plavix Tablets (4.2%) ... 1097
▲ Plavix Tablets (4.2%) ... 3084
Plendil Extended-Release Tablets (0.2% to 2.0%) ... 623
Pletal Tablets (2% or greater) ... 2605
Pletal Tablets (2% or greater) ... 2848
Pneumovax 23 (Rare) ... 2156
Pnu-Imune 23 (Rare to infrequent) ... 1868
Polysporin Ophthalmic Ointment Sterile ... ⊙ 301
▲ Ponstel Capsules (1% to 10%) ... 1356
Potaba (Infrequent) ... 1721
Pravachol Tablets (1.3% to 4.0%) ... 1099
Precose Tablets (Rare) ... 906
Premarin Tablets ... 3566
Premphase Tablets ... 3572
▲ Prempro Tablets (4% to 6%) ... 3572
Prevacid Delayed-Release Capsules (Less than 1%) ... 3292
Prevnar for Injection (0.7% to 1.4%) ... 1870
PREVPAC (Less than 1%) ... 3298
▲ Priftin Tablets (3.6%) ... 758
Prilosec Delayed-Release Capsules (Less than 1% to 1.5%) ... 628
Primaxin I.M. (0.4%) ... 2158
Primaxin I.V. (1.5%) ... 2160
Prinivil Tablets (0.3% to 1.7%) ... 2164
Prinzide Tablets (1.2%) ... 2168
ProAmatine Tablets (2.4%; less frequent) ... 3241
Procardia XL Extended Release Tablets (Less than 3%) ... 2710
▲ Procrit for Injection (Rare to 16%) .. 2502
▲ Prograf (10% to 24%) ... 1393
Prolastin (Occasional) ... 943
Proleukin for Injection (1%) ... 1199
Propecia Tablets ... 2172
Proscar Tablets ... 2175
ProSom Tablets (Infrequent) ... 500
Prostigmin Injectable ... 1744
Prostigmin Tablets ... 1744
Prostin E2 Suppositories ... 2852
▲ Protonix I.V. (6%) ... 3580
Protonix Tablets (Less than 1% to 2%) ... 3577
▲ Protopic Ointment (2% to 5%) ... 1397
Proventil Inhalation Aerosol (Rare) ... 3142
Proventil Inhalation Solution 0.083% (Rare) ... 3146
Proventil Repetabs Tablets (2%) ... 3148
Proventil Solution for Inhalation 0.5% (Rare) ... 3144
Proventil HFA Inhalation Aerosol (Less than 3%) ... 3150
Provera Tablets ... 2853
Provigil Tablets (At least 1%) ... 1193
▲ Prozac Pulvules, Liquid, and Weekly Capsules (3% to 6%; 7% of 10,782 patients) ... 1238
Pulmicort Respules (Less than 1% to 4%) ... 632
Pulmicort Turbuhaler Inhalation Powder (Rare) ... 636
▲ Pulmozyme Inhalation Solution (3% to 12%) ... 1426
Purinethol Tablets ... 1615
Pyrazinamide Tablets ... 1876
▲ Quinaglute Dura-Tabs Tablets (6%) . 978
▲ Quinidex Extentabs (5%) ... 2933
Qvar Inhalation Aerosol (Rare) ... 1987
▲ Rapamune Oral Solution and Tablets (10% to 20%) ... 3584
▲ Rebetron Combination Therapy (20% to 28%) ... 3153
Recombivax HB (Less than 1%) ... 2178
ReFacto Vials ... 1437
Refludan for Injection (Uncommon) ... 761
Reglan (A few cases) ... 2935
▲ Relafen Tablets (3% to 9%) ... 1617
Remeron Tablets (Frequent) ... 2483
Remeron SolTab Tablets (Frequent) ... 2486
▲ Remicade for IV Injection (6% to 12%) ... 1178
Renese Tablets ... 2712
Repronex for Intramuscular and Subcutaneous Injection ... 1347
Requip Tablets (Infrequent) ... 1621
▲ Rescriptor Tablets (9.8% to 18%) ... 526
▲ Retrovir Capsules (17%) ... 1625
▲ Retrovir IV Infusion (17%) ... 1629
▲ Retrovir (17%) ... 1625
Rhinocort Nasal Inhaler (Rare) ... 640
Rifadin (Occasional) ... 765
Rifamate Capsules (Occasional) ... 767
Rifater Tablets (Occasional) ... 769
Risperdal (2% to 5%) ... 1796
Ritalin ... 2387
▲ Rituxan for Infusion (10%) ... 1750
▲ Rituxan I.V. (10%) ... 1428
Robaxin Injectable ... 2938
Robaxin Tablets ... 2939
Robaxisal Tablets ... 2939
Rocephin Injectable Vials, ADD-Vantage, Galaxy, Bulk (1.7%) ... 2993
▲ Roferon-A Injection (8% to 44%) ... 2996
Romazicon Injection (1% to 3%) ... 3000
Rowasa Rectal Suspension Enema 4.0 grams/unit (60 mL) (2.82%) ... 3264
Roxanol ... 3066
Roxicodone ... 3067
Rynatan Tablets ... 3351
Rythmol Tablets – 150 mg, 225 mg, 300 mg (2.6%) ... 502
Salagen Tablets (1% to 2%) ... 2229
Sandostatin Injection (Less than 1%) ... 2394
▲ Sandostatin LAR Depot (5% to 15%) ... 2395
▲ Sarafem Pulvules (5%) ... 1962
Sectral Capsules (2%) ... 3589
Sedapap Tablets 50 mg/650 mg ... 2225
▲ Septra Suspension (Among most common) ... 2265
▲ Septra Tablets (Among most common) ... 2265
▲ Septra DS Tablets (Among most common) ... 2265
Serentil ... 1057
▲ Serevent Diskus (4%) ... 1637
Serevent Inhalation Aerosol (Rare; 1% to 3%) ... 1633
▲ Seroquel Tablets (4%) ... 684
▲ Serostim for Injection (1% to 10%) . 3229
Serzone Tablets (2%) ... 1104
Silvadene Cream 1% (Infrequent) ... 2267
▲ Simulect for Injection (3% to 10%) . 2399
Sinemet Tablets ... 1253
Sinemet CR Tablets ... 1255
Sinequan (Occasional) ... 2713
Singulair (1.6% to 2% or greater) ... 2181
Skelaxin Tablets ... 1301
Skelid Tablets (2.7%) ... 3088
Soma Tablets ... 3353
Soma Compound Tablets (Less common) ... 3354
Soma Compound w/Codeine Tablets ... 3355
Sonata Capsules (Frequent) ... 3591
▲ Soriatane Capsules (1% to 10%) ... 3003
▲ Sporanox Capsules (3% to 8.6%) ... 1800
▲ Sporanox Injection (3%) ... 1804
▲ Sporanox Injection (3%) ... 2509
▲ Sporanox Oral Solution (4.0% to 4.8%) ... 1808
▲ Sporanox Oral Solution (4.0% to 4.8%) ... 2512
Stadol NS Nasal Spray (Less than 1%) ... 1108
Stelazine ... 1640
Stromectol Tablets (0.9%) ... 2185
Sular Tablets (Very rare) ... 688
▲ Sulfamylon Cream (4.6%) ... 1011
▲ Sulfamylon Topical Solution (4.6%) ... 1011
Suprax (Less than 2%) ... 1877
Surmontil Capsules ... 3595
▲ Sustiva Capsules (5% to 40%) ... 1258
Symmetrel (0.1% to 1%) ... 1328
▲ Synagis Intramuscular (25.6%) ... 2028
Synarel Nasal Solution for Central Precocious Puberty (2.6%) ... 3204
Synercid I.V. (2.5% to 3.1%) ... 775
Synthroid ... 505
Synvisc ... 3596
Tagamet ... 1644
Talacen Caplets (Infrequent) ... 3089
Talwin Nx Tablets (Infrequent) ... 3090
Tambocor Tablets (1% to 3%) ... 1990
Tamiflu Capsules ... 3008
Tamiflu Oral Suspension ... 3008
Tao Capsules ... 2716
Tapazole Tablets ... 1823
Tarka Tablets (0.3% or more) ... 508
Tasmar Tablets (Frequent) ... 3010
▲ Taxol Injection (12%) ... 1129
Taxotere for Injection Concentrate (0.9%) ... 778
Tazicef for Injection (2%) ... 1647
Tazicef Galaxy Container (2%) ... 1650
Tazicef Pharmacy Bulk Package (2%) ... 1653
Tazidime Vials, Faspak & ADD-Vantage (2%) ... 1966
▲ Tazorac Gel (1% to 10%) ... 556
Tegretol/Tegretol-XR ... 2404
▲ Temodar Capsules (8%) ... 3157
Tenex Tablets (Less frequent) ... 2942
Tenoretic Tablets ... 690
Tenormin ... 692
Tequin Injection (0.1% to 3%) ... 1110
Tequin Tablets (0.1% to 3%) ... 1110
Testoderm Transdermal Systems (1%) ... 574
Tetanus & Diphtheria Toxoids Adsorbed for Adult Use ... 1880
Tetanus and Diphtheria Toxoids Adsorbed For Adult Use ... 815
Teveten Tablets (Less than 1%) ... 3327
▲ Thalomid Capsules (20.8%) ... 1154
Theo-Dur Extended-Release Tablets ... 1835
TheraCys Injection (2%) ... 823
Thioplex for Injection ... 1765
Thiothixene Capsules ... 2290
Thyrogen for Injection (Greater than 1%) ... 1441
Tiazac Capsules (2%) ... 1378
Tice BCG, BCG Live (0.6%) ... 2489
▲ Ticlid Tablets (5.1%) ... 3015
▲ Tikosyn Capsules (3%) ... 2717
Timentin Injection- ADD-Vantage Vial ... 1661
Timentin Injection-Galaxy Container ... 1664
Timentin Injection-Pharmacy Bulk Package ... 1666
Timentin for Intravenous Administration ... 1658
Timolide Tablets (Less than 1%) ... 2187
Timolol GFS ... ⊙ 266
Timoptic in Ocudose (Less frequent) ... 2192
Timoptic Sterile Ophthalmic Solution (Less frequent) ... 2190
Timoptic-XE Sterile Ophthalmic Gel Forming Solution ... 2194
TNKase I.V. (Rare) ... 1430
▲ TOBI Solution for Inhalation (5.4%) . 1206
Tolectin ... 2589
▲ Tonocard Tablets (0.4% to 12.2%) . 649
▲ Topamax Sprinkle Capsules (3.2% to 4.4%) ... 2590
▲ Topamax Tablets (3.2% to 4.4%) ... 2590
▲ Toprol-XL Tablets (About 5 of 100 patients) ... 651
Toradol (Greater than 1%) ... 3018
Transderm Scōp Transdermal Therapeutic System (Infrequent) .. 2302
Tranxene ... 511
Trasylol Injection (2%) ... 909
Trecator-SC Tablets ... 3598
Trental Tablets (Less than 1%) ... 784
▲ Tricor Capsules, Micronized (6%) ... 513
Trileptal Oral Suspension (2% to 4%) ... 2407
Trileptal Tablets (2% to 4%) ... 2407
Trilisate (Less than 1%) ... 2901
Tri-Norinyl-28 Tablets ... 3433
Triphasil-21 Tablets ... 3600
Triphasil-28 Tablets ... 3605
▲ Trizivir Tablets (9%) ... 1669
Trovan (2%) ... 2722
Trusopt Sterile Ophthalmic Solution (Rare) ... 2196
Tussionex Pennkinetic Extended-Release Suspension ... 1174
Tussi-Organidin NR Liquid (Rare) ... 3350
Tussi-Organidin DM NR Liquid (Rare) ... 3350
Tussi-Organidin DM-S NR Liquid (Rare) ... 3350
Tussi-Organidin-S NR Liquid (Rare) ... 3350
Twinrix Vaccine (Less than 1%) ... 1674
Tylox Capsules ... 2597
Ultracet Tablets (At least 1%) ... 2597
Ultram Tablets (1% to 5%) ... 2600
Ultravate Cream (Less frequent) ... 1119
Ultravate Ointment (Less frequent) ... 1120
Unasyn for Injection (Less than 2%) ... 2728
Uni-Dur Extended-Release Tablets ... 1841
Uniretic Tablets (More than 1%) ... 3178
Unithroid Tablets ... 3445
Univasc Tablets (Less than 1% to 1.6%) ... 3181
Urised Tablets ... 2876
Urobiotic-250 Capsules ... 2731
Uroqid-Acid No. 2 Tablets (Occasional) ... 947
Urso Tablets ... 836
Valium Injectable ... 3026
Valium Tablets (Infrequent) ... 3047
▲ Valstar Sterile Solution for Intravesical Instillation (3%) ... 1175
Valtrex Caplets (0.4% to 1.1%) ... 1676
Vancenase PocketHaler Nasal Inhaler (Rare) ... 3162
Vanceril Inhalation Aerosol (Rare) ... 3165
Vanceril Double Strength Inhalation Aerosol (Rare) ... 3167
Vancocin HCl Capsules & Pulvules (Infrequent) ... 1972
Vancocin HCl Oral Solution (Infrequent) ... 1971
Vancocin HCl, Vials & ADD-Vantage (Infrequent) ... 1970
Vaniqa Cream (1.5%) ... 1121
Vantin Tablets and Oral Suspension (Less than 1% to 1.4%) ... 2860
Vaqta (Less than 1%) ... 2199
Varivax (Greater than or equal to 1%) ... 2202
Vascor Tablets (0.5% to 2.0%) ... 2602
Vaseretic Tablets (0.5% to 2.0%) ... 2204
Vasotec I.V. Injection (0.5% to 1.0%) ... 2207
Vasotec Tablets (0.5% to 1.4%) ... 2210
Velosulin BR Human Insulin 10 ml Vials ... 2435
Ventolin Inhalation Aerosol and Refill (Rare) ... 1679
Ventolin HFA Inhalation Aerosol ... 3618
Verelan Capsules (1% to 1.4%) ... 3184
Verelan PM Capsules (1.2% to 2%) ... 3186
Vermox Chewable Tablets (Rare) ... 2017
Versed Injection (Less than 1%) ... 3027
Versed Syrup (Less than 1%) ... 3033
▲ Vesanoid Capsules (54%) ... 3037
Viadur Implant (Less than 2%) ... 912
Viagra Tablets (2%) ... 2732
Vicodin Tablets ... 516
Vicodin ES Tablets ... 517
Vicodin HP Tablets ... 518
Vicoprofen Tablets (Less than 1%) .. 520
▲ Videx (7% to 9%) ... 1138
▲ Videx EC Capsules (10%) ... 1143
Vioxx (Greater than 0.1% to 1.9%) .. 2213
Viracept (Up to 4%) ... 532
▲ Viramune Oral Suspension (8% to 37%) ... 1060
▲ Viramune Tablets (8% to 37%) ... 1060
Virazole for Inhalation Solution ... 1747
▲ Vistide Injection (30%) ... 1445
▲ Visudyne for Injection (10% to 20%) ... ⊙ 308
▲ Vitravene for Injection (5% to 20%) ... ⊙ 310
Vivactil Tablets ... 2217
Vivactil Tablets ... 2446
Vivelle Transdermal System (Rare) ... 2412
Vivelle-Dot Transdermal System (Rare) ... 2416
Vivotif Berna ... 997
Volmax Extended-Release Tablets (Rare) ... 2276
Voltaren Tablets (1% to 3%) ... 2315
Voltaren-XR Tablets (1% to 3%) ... 2315
Warfarin Sodium Tablets, USP ... 3302
▲ Wellbutrin Tablets (8.0%) ... 1680
Wellbutrin SR Sustained-Release Tablets (0.9% to 5%) ... 1684
WinRho SDF ... 2297
Xalatan Latanoprost Ophthalmic Solution (1% to 2%) ... ⊙ 320
Xalatan Sterile Ophthalmic Solution (1% to 2%) ... 2864
▲ Xanax Tablets (10.8%) ... 2865
▲ Xenical Capsules (4.3%) ... 3043
Yasmin 28 Tablets ... 980
YF-VAX Vaccine (Uncommon) ... 827
Zaditor Ophthalmic Solution (Less than 5%) ... 2304
Zanaflex Tablets (Frequent) ... 1305
Zantac (Rare) ... 1690
Zantac Injection ... 1688
Zantac Syrup (Rare) ... 1690
Zaroxolyn Tablets ... 1177
Zebeta Tablets ... 1885
Zemuron Injection (Less than 1%) ... 2491
▲ Zenapax for Injection (2% to 5%) ... 3046
▲ Zerit (40%) ... 1147
Zestoretic Tablets (1.2%) ... 695
Zestril Tablets (0.01% to 1.7%) ... 698
Ziac Tablets ... 1887
▲ Ziagen (11%) ... 1692
Zinacef Injection (1 in 125 patients) ... 1696
Zinacef for Injection (1 in 125 patients) ... 1696
Zithromax Capsules, 250 mg (1% or less to 1.6%) ... 2743
Zithromax for IV Infusion (1.9%) ... 2748
Zithromax for Oral Suspension, 1 g (1% or less) ... 2743
Zithromax for Oral Suspension, 300 mg, 600 mg, 900 mg, 1200 mg (1% or less to 1.6%) ... 2739
Zithromax Tablets, 250 mg (1% or less to 1.6%) ... 2739
Zithromax Tablets, 600 mg (1% or less) ... 2743
Zofran Injection (Approximately 1%) ... 1698
Zofran (Approximately 1%) ... 1703
Zofran ODT Orally Disintegrating Tablets (Approximately 1%) ... 1703
▲ Zoladex (1% to 6%) ... 702
▲ Zoladex 3-month (8%) ... 706
▲ Zoloft (3%) ... 2751
Zometa for Intravenous Infusion ... 3621
Zomig Tablets (Infrequent) ... 708
Zomig-ZMT Tablets (Infrequent) ... 708
▲ Zonegran Capsules (3%) ... 1307
Zosyn (1.3% to 4.2%) ... 1890
Zosyn in Galaxy Containers (1.3% to 4.2%) ... 1894
Zovirax Capsules ... 1706
Zovirax for Injection (Approximately 2%) ... 1708
Zovirax Ointment ... 1707
Zovirax ... 1706
▲ Zyban Sustained-Release Tablets (3% to 4%) ... 1710
Zyflo Filmtab Tablets ... 524

Zyprexa Tablets 1973
Zyprexa ZYDIS Orally Disintegrating Tablets 1973
Zyrtec (Less than 2%) 2756
Zyrtec-D 12 Hour Extended Relief Tablets (Less than 2%) 2758
Zyvox (2%) 2871

Rash, allergic
Alesse-21 Tablets 3468
Alesse-28 Tablets 3473
Aygestin Tablets 1333
Brevicon 28-Day Tablets 3380
Cyclessa Tablets 2450
Desogen Tablets 2458
Estrostep 2627
Ginkoba Tablets (Very rare) ■□828
Levlen 962
Levlite 21 Tablets 962
Levlite 28 Tablets 962
Levora Tablets 3389
Loestrin 21 Tablets 2642
Loestrin Fe Tablets 2642
Lunelle Monthly Injection 2827
Microgestin Fe 1.5/30 Tablets 3407
Microgestin Fe 1/20 Tablets 3400
Mircette Tablets 2470
Modicon 2563
Necon 3415
Norinyl 1 +35 28-Day Tablets 3380
Norinyl 1 + 50 28-Day Tablets 3380
Ortho-Cept 21 Tablets 2546
Ortho-Cept 28 Tablets 2546
Ortho-Cyclen/Ortho Tri-Cyclen 2573
Ortho-Novum 2563
Ortho-Novum 1/50□28 Tablets 2556
Ortho-Cyclen/Ortho Tri-Cyclen 2573
Ovcon 3364
Parafon Forte DSC Caplets (Rare) 2582
Periactin Tablets 2155
Premphase Tablets 3572
Prempro Tablets 3572
Prometrium Capsules (100 mg, 200 mg) 3261
Tri-Levlen 962
Tri-Norinyl-28 Tablets 3433
Trivora Tablets 3439
Varivax (Greater than or equal to 1%) 2202
Zovia 3449

Rash, bullous
Exelon Capsules (Frequent) 2342
Exelon Oral Solution (Frequent) 2345
Lipitor Tablets 2639
Lipitor Tablets 2696
Orudis Capsules (Less than 1%) 3548
Oruvail Capsules (Less than 1%) 3548
▲ Zosyn (4.2%) 1890
▲ Zosyn in Galaxy Containers (4.2%) 1894

Rash, bullous erythrodermatous
Idamycin PFS Injection 2825

Rash, circumocular
Polytrim Ophthalmic Solution (Multiple reports) 556

Rash, diaper
▲ Augmentin ES-600 Powder for Oral Suspension (3.5%) 1487
Cedax Oral Suspension (0.1% to 1%) 1021
▲ Ceftin for Oral Suspension (3.4%) 1898
Cefzil (1.5%) 1076
Comvax (0.2% to 0.5%) 2056

Rash, drug
Benadryl Parenteral 2617
Nitrolingual Pumpspray 1355
Nitrostat Tablets 2658

Rash, eczematous
Exelon Capsules (Frequent) 2342
Exelon Oral Solution (Frequent) 2345
Thalomid Capsules 1154

Rash, erythematous (0.1%)
Blocadren Tablets 2046
▲ Campath Ampules (3% to 40%) 992
Carbatrol Capsules 3234
Celebrex Capsules (0.1% to 1.9%) 2676
Celebrex Capsules (0.1% to 1.9%) 2780
Celontin Capsules 2618
Clindagel 1401
▲ Cognex Capsules (7%) 1351
Colazal Capsules 3069
Coreg Tablets (0.1% to 1%) 1508
Cosopt Sterile Ophthalmic Solution 2065
Declomycin Tablets 1855
Denavir Cream (0.1%) 2332
Doryx Coated Pellet Filled Capsules 3357
DTIC-Dome (Infrequent) 902
Dynacin Capsules 2019
Evoxac Capsules (1% to 3%) 1217
Exelon Capsules (Frequent) 2342
Exelon Oral Solution (Frequent) 2345
▲ Femara Tablets (4% to 5%) 2351
Floxin Otic Solution (Single report) 1219
Foscavir Injection (Between 1% and 5%) 605
Hivid Tablets (Less than 1%) 2975
Hycamtin for Injection (Less than 1%) 1546
Inderal 3513
Inderal LA Long-Acting Capsules 3516
Inderide Tablets 3517
Inderide LA Long-Acting Capsules 3519
Innohep Injection (Greater than or equal to 1%) 1248
Intron A for Injection (Less than 5%) 3120
Miacalcin Nasal Spray (1% to 3%) 2375
Minocin Intravenous 1862
Minocin Oral Suspension 1865
Minocin Pellet-Filled Capsules 1863
Mobic Tablets (0.3% to 3%) 1054
Monodox Capsules 2442
Nexium Delayed-Release Capsules (Less than 1%) 619
Norvasc Tablets (More than 0.1% to 1%) 2704
Periostat Tablets 1208
Plavix Tablets (Less than 1%) 1097
Plavix Tablets (Less than 1%) 3084
Regranex Gel (2%) 2586
Sectral Capsules 3589
▲ Serostim for Injection (1% to 10%) 3229
▲ Soriatane Capsules (10% to 25%) 3003
Tegretol/Tegretol-XR 2404
Tenoretic Tablets 690
Tenormin 692
Thalomid Capsules 1154
Timolide Tablets 2187
Timolol GFS ⊙266
Timoptic in Ocudose 2192
Timoptic Sterile Ophthalmic Solution 2190
Timoptic-XE Sterile Ophthalmic Gel Forming Solution 2194
Topamax Sprinkle Capsules (Infrequent) 2590
Topamax Tablets (Infrequent) 2590
Trileptal Oral Suspension 2407
Trileptal Tablets 2407
Vibramycin Calcium Oral Suspension Syrup 2735
Vibramycin Hyclate Capsules 2735
Vibramycin Hyclate Intravenous 2737
Vibramycin Monohydrate for Oral Suspension 2735
Vibra-Tabs Film Coated Tablets 2735
Zarontin Capsules 2659
Zarontin Syrup 2660
Zoloft (Infrequent) 2751
▲ Zosyn (3.9%) 1890
▲ Zosyn in Galaxy Containers (3.9%) 1894
Zyrtec (Less than 2%) 2756
Zyrtec-D 12 Hour Extended Relief Tablets (Less than 2%) 2758

Rash, erythematous maculopapular
Amoxil Chewable Tablets 1471
Amoxil for Oral Suspension 1471
Amoxil 1471
Miltown Tablets 3349
Viramune Oral Suspension 1060
Viramune Tablets 1060

Rash, exfoliative
Exelon Capsules (Frequent) 2342
Exelon Oral Solution (Frequent) 2345
Quinaglute Dura-Tabs Tablets 978

Rash, facial
Venofer Injection (One patient) 580

Rash, female genitalia
Floxin I.V. (Less than 1%) 2526
Floxin Tablets (Less than 1%) 2529

Rash, follicular
Floxin Otic Solution (Single report) 1219
Hivid Tablets (Less than 1%) 2975
Zoloft (Rare) 2751

Rash, heat
Trileptal Oral Suspension 2407
Trileptal Tablets 2407

Rash, herpetic
(*see under* Eruptions, herpetic)

Rash, leg
DDAVP Nasal Spray 738
DDAVP Rhinal Tube 738
Desmopressin Acetate Rhinal Tube 1345

Rash, lichenoid
Normodyne Tablets (Less common) 3137
Permax Tablets (Rare) 1299

Rash, lupus erythematosus
Evoxac Capsules (Less than 1%) 1217

Rash, macular
Amerge Tablets (Rare) 1467

Rash, maculopapular
Abelcet Injection 1273
Accuretic Tablets 2614
Actiq (Less than 1%) 1184
Agenerase Capsules (1%) 1454
Agenerase Oral Solution (1%) 1459
▲ Amphotec (5% or more) 1774
Arava Tablets (1% to 3%) 724
Betaseron for SC Injection 988
▲ Campath Ampules (3% to 40%) 992
Captopril Tablets 2281
Catapres-TTS 1038
Ceclor CD Tablets (0.1% to 1%) 1279
Celebrex Capsules (0.1% to 1.9%) 2676
Celebrex Capsules (0.1% to 1.9%) 2780
Cerebyx Injection (Infrequent) 2619
Cleocin HCl Capsules 2784
Cleocin Phosphate Sterile Solution 2785
Cleocin Vaginal Cream 2788
Cleocin Vaginal Ovules 2789
▲ Cognex Capsules (7%) 1351
Copaxone for Injection (Infrequent) 3306
Coreg Tablets (0.1% to 1%) 1508
Declomycin Tablets 1855
Depacon Injection (1% or more) 416
Depakene (1% or more) 421
Depakote Sprinkle Capsules 426
Depakote Tablets (1% to 5%) 430
Depakote ER Tablets (Greater than 1%) 436
Didronel Tablets 2888
Digitek Tablets 1003
Doryx Coated Pellet Filled Capsules 3357
Doxil Injection (Less than 1% to 5%) 566
Dynacin Capsules 2019
Effexor Tablets (Infrequent) 3495
Effexor XR Capsules (Infrequent) 3499
Epivir 1520
Exelon Capsules (Frequent) 2342
Exelon Oral Solution (Frequent) 2345
▲ Femara Tablets (4% to 5%) 2351
Florinef Acetate Tablets 2250
Fortovase Capsules (Less than 2%) 2970
Foscavir Injection (Between 1% and 5%) 605
Sterile FUDR (Remote possibility) 2974
Gabitril Tablets (Infrequent) 1189
Geodon Capsules (Infrequent) 2688
Haldol Decanoate 2535
Haldol Injection, Tablets and Concentrate 2533
Hivid Tablets (Less than 1%) 2975
Hycamtin for Injection (Less than 1%) 1546
Intron A for Injection (Less than 5%) 3120
Invirase Capsules (Less than 2%) 2979
Kaletra Capsules (Less than 2%) 471
Kaletra Oral Solution (Less than 2%) 471
Lamictal (Infrequent) 1567
Lanoxicaps Capsules (Rare) 1574
Lanoxin Injection (Rare) 1581
Lanoxin Tablets (Rare) 1587
Lanoxin Elixir Pediatric (Rare) 1578
Lanoxin Injection Pediatric (Rare) 1584
Lodine (Less than 1%) 3528
Lodine XL Extended-Release Tablets (Less than 1%) 3530
Mandol Vials 1953
Minocin Intravenous 1862
Minocin Oral Suspension 1865
Minocin Pellet-Filled Capsules 1863
Mobic Tablets (0.3% to 3%) 1054
Monodox Capsules 2442
▲ Motrin Suspension, Oral Drops, Chewable Tablets, and Caplets (3% to 9%) 2002
Mylocel Tablets (Less frequently) 2227
Nexium Delayed-Release Capsules (Less than 1%) 619
Normodyne Tablets (Less common) 3137
Norvasc Tablets (More than 0.1% to 1%) 2704
Norvir Capsules (Less than 2%) 487
Norvir Oral Solution (Less than 2%) 487
Omnicef for Oral Suspension (0.2%) 493
Paxil (Rare) 1609
Periostat Tablets 1208
Plavix Tablets (Less than 1%) 1097
Plavix Tablets (Less than 1%) 3084
Priftin Tablets (1.1%) 758
Procanbid Extended-Release Tablets (Occasional) 2262
Protonix I.V. (Less than 1%) 3580
Protonix Tablets (Less than 1%) 3577
Protopic Ointment (2% to 4%) 1397
Prozac Pulvules, Liquid, and Weekly Capsules (Infrequent) 1238
Requip Tablets (Infrequent) 1621
▲ Rescriptor Tablets (4.5% to 6.6%) 526
Rifamate Capsules 767
Sarafem Pulvules (Infrequent) 1962
Seroquel Tablets (Infrequent) 684
Serzone Tablets (Infrequent) 1104
Sonata Capsules (Infrequent) 3591
Sular Tablets (Less than or equal to 1%) 688
▲ Sustiva Capsules (16.7% to 24.5%) 1258
Synarel Nasal Solution for Endometriosis (Less than 1%) 3205
Synercid I.V. (Less than 1%) 775
Tequin Injection (Less than 0.1%) 1110
Tequin Tablets (Less than 0.1%) 1110
Teveten Tablets (Less than 1%) 3327
▲ Thalomid Capsules (4.2%) 1154
Ticlid Tablets 3015
Toradol 3018
Tricor Capsules, Micronized 513
Trileptal Oral Suspension 2407
Trileptal Tablets 2407
Trizivir Tablets 1669
Uniretic Tablets (Less than 1%) 3178
Vantin Tablets and Oral Suspension (Less than 1%) 2860
Vibramycin Calcium Oral Suspension Syrup 2735
Vibramycin Hyclate Capsules 2735
Vibramycin Hyclate Intravenous 2737
Vibramycin Monohydrate for Oral Suspension 2735
Vibra-Tabs Film Coated Tablets 2735
Viracept 532
Wellbutrin SR Sustained-Release Tablets (Rare) 1684
Ziagen 1692
Zoloft (Infrequent) 2751
Zonegran Capsules (Infrequent) 1307
▲ Zosyn (4.2%) 1890
▲ Zosyn in Galaxy Containers (4.2%) 1894
Zyban Sustained-Release Tablets (Rare) 1710
Zyprexa Tablets (Rare) 1973
Zyprexa ZYDIS Orally Disintegrating Tablets (Rare) 1973
Zyrtec (Less than 2%) 2756
Zyrtec-D 12 Hour Extended Relief Tablets (Less than 2%) 2758

Rash, morbilliform
▲ Cleocin HCl Capsules (Among most frequent) 2784
▲ Cleocin Phosphate Sterile Solution (Among most frequent) 2785
▲ Cleocin Vaginal Cream (Most frequent) 2788
▲ Cleocin Vaginal Ovules (Among most frequent) 2789
▲ Dilantin Infatabs (Among most common) 2624
▲ Dilantin Kapseals (Among most common) 2622
▲ Dilantin-125 Oral Suspension (Among most common) 2625
Rifamate Capsules 767

Rash, oral
Advair Diskus 100/50 (1% to 3%) 1448
Advair Diskus 250/50 (1% to 3%) 1448
Advair Diskus 500/50 (1% to 3%) 1448

Rash, papular
Aclovate Cream (Approximately 2%) 1275
▲ Chemet Capsules (2.6% to 11.2%) 3078
Fortovase Capsules (Less than 2%) 2970
Migranal Nasal Spray (Rare) 2376
▲ Stromectol Tablets (22.7%) 2185

Rash, papular, neck
Alferon N Injection (1%) 1770

Rash, pemphigoid
Corgard Tablets 2245
Corzide 40/5 Tablets 2247
Corzide 80/5 Tablets 2247
Nadolol Tablets 2288

Rash, penile
Caverject Sterile Powder (1%) 2777

Rash, perianal
Mintezol 2137

Rash, petechial
Amphotec (1% to 5%) 1774
Feldene Capsules (Occasional) 2685
Sarafem Pulvules (Rare) 1962

Rash, pruritic
Amerge Tablets (Rare) 1467
▲ Captopril Tablets (About 4 to 7 of 100 patients) 2281
Carbatrol Capsules 3234
Fortovase Capsules (Less than 2%) 2970
Sterile FUDR (Remote possibility) 2974
Hivid Tablets (Less than 1%) 2975
Lithobid Slow-Release Tablets 3255
Miltown Tablets 3349
Premphase Tablets 3572
Prempro Tablets 3572
Skelaxin Tablets 1301
Tegretol/Tegretol-XR 2404

Rash, psoriaform
Coreg Tablets (0.1% to 1%) 1508
Cosopt Sterile Ophthalmic Solution 2065
Exelon Capsules (Frequent) 2342
Exelon Oral Solution (Frequent) 2345
▲ Femara Tablets (4% to 5%) 2351
Inderal (Rare) 3513
Inderal LA Long-Acting Capsules (Rare) 3516
Inderide Tablets (Rare) 3517
Inderide LA Long-Acting Capsules (Rare) 3519
Normodyne Tablets (Less common) 3137
Quinaglute Dura-Tabs Tablets 978
Requip Tablets (Infrequent) 1621
▲ Soriatane Capsules (1% to 10%) 3003
Tenoretic Tablets 690
Tenormin 692
Timolol GFS ⊙266
Timoptic in Ocudose 2192
Timoptic Sterile Ophthalmic Solution 2190
Timoptic-XE Sterile Ophthalmic Gel Forming Solution 2194

Rash, purpuric
Campath Ampules 992
Dilantin Infatabs 2624
Dilantin Kapseals 2622
Dilantin-125 Oral Suspension 2625
Orudis Capsules (Less than 1%) 3548
Oruvail Capsules (Less than 1%) 3548
Prozac Pulvules, Liquid, and Weekly Capsules (Rare) 1238
Rifamate Capsules 767
Sarafem Pulvules (Rare) 1962
Uniretic Tablets (Less than 1%) 3178

Rash, pustular
Cerebyx Injection (Infrequent) 2619
Copaxone for Injection (Frequent) 3306
Doxil Injection (Less than 1%) 566
Effexor Tablets (Rare) 3495
Effexor XR Capsules (Rare) 3499
Lamictal (Rare) 1567
▲ Protopic Ointment (3% to 8%) 1397
Prozac Pulvules, Liquid, and Weekly Capsules (Rare) 1238
Pulmicort Respules (1% to 3%) 632
Sarafem Pulvules (Rare) 1962
Sonata Capsules (Rare) 3591
▲ Stromectol Tablets (22.7%) 2185
Sular Tablets (Less than or equal to 1%) 688
Zoloft (Rare) 2751
Zonegran Capsules (Infrequent) 1307
Zyprexa Tablets (Rare) 1973
Zyprexa ZYDIS Orally Disintegrating Tablets (Rare) 1973

Rash, scarlatiniform
Dilantin Infatabs 2624
Dilantin Kapseals 2622
Dilantin-125 Oral Suspension 2625

Rash, urticarial
Captopril Tablets (Rare) 2281
DTIC-Dome (Infrequent) 902
Miltown Tablets 3349
Normodyne Tablets (Less common) 3137
▲ Stromectol Tablets (22.7%) 2185
Ticlid Tablets 3015
Trizivir Tablets 1669
Ziagen 1692
▲ Zosyn (4.2%) 1890
▲ Zosyn in Galaxy Containers (4.2%) 1894

Rash, varicella-like
Varivax (0.9% to 5.5%) 2202

Rash, vasculitic
Accolate Tablets (Rare) 657
Flovent Diskus 3614
Flovent 1535
Flovent Rotadisk 1537
Singulair 2181

Rash, vesiculobullous
Actiq (Less than 1%) 1184
AmBisome for Injection (Less common) 1383
Amphotec (1% to 5%) 1774
▲ Apligraf (8%) 2305
Betaseron for SC Injection 988
▲ CellCept Capsules (3% to 10%) 2951
CellCept Intravenous (3% to 10%) 2951
▲ CellCept Oral Suspension (3% to 10%) 2951
▲ CellCept Tablets (3% to 10%) 2951
Cleocin HCl Capsules 2784
▲ Cognex Capsules (7%) 1351
Copaxone for Injection (Infrequent) 3306
Depakote ER Tablets (Greater than 1%) 436
Doxil Injection (Less than 1% to 5%) 566
Effexor Tablets (Rare) 3495
Effexor XR Capsules (Rare) 3499
Foscavir Injection (Rare) 605
Gabitril Tablets (Infrequent) 1189
Geodon Capsules (Infrequent) 2688
Lamictal (Infrequent) 1567
Lodine (Less than 1%) 3528
Lodine XL Extended-Release Tablets (Less than 1%) 3530
Lovenox Injection 746
Megace Oral Suspension (1% to 3%) 1124
Norvir Capsules (Less than 2%) 487
Norvir Oral Solution (Less than 2%) 487
Paxil (Rare) 1609
Permax Tablets (Rare) 1299
Protopic Ointment (2% to 3%) 1397
Prozac Pulvules, Liquid, and Weekly Capsules (Infrequent) 1238
Rescriptor Tablets (Less than 2%) 526
Salagen Tablets (Less than 1%) 2229
Sarafem Pulvules (Infrequent) 1962
Serzone Tablets (Infrequent) 1104
Sonata Capsules (Infrequent) 3591
Tequin Injection (Less than 0.1%) 1110
Tequin Tablets (Less than 0.1%) 1110
Thalomid Capsules 1154
Vantin Tablets and Oral Suspension (Less than 1%) 2860
Zonegran Capsules (Infrequent) 1307
Zyprexa Tablets (2%) 1973
Zyprexa ZYDIS Orally Disintegrating Tablets (2%) 1973

Raynaud's phenomenon
Blocadren Tablets 2046
Captopril Tablets (2 to 3 of 1000 patients) 2281
Catapres Tablets (Rare) 1037
Catapres-TTS (0.5% or less) 1038
Clorpres Tablets (Rare) 1002
Combipres Tablets (Rare) 1040
Corgard Tablets (2 of 100 patients) 2245
Cosopt Sterile Ophthalmic Solution 2065
Duraclon Injection (Rare) 3057
Enalaprilat Injection 863
Imitrex Injection (Rare) 1549
Imitrex Nasal Spray 1554
Imitrex Tablets 1558
Inderal 3513
Inderal LA Long-Acting Capsules 3516
Inderide Tablets 3517
Inderide LA Long-Acting Capsules 3519
Lithobid Slow-Release Tablets 3255
Nadolol Tablets (2 of 100 patients) 2288
Roferon-A Injection (Infrequent) 2996
Sandostatin Injection (Less than 1%) 2394
Sandostatin LAR Depot (Rare) 2395
Tenoretic Tablets 690
Tenormin 692
Thalomid Capsules 1154
Timolide Tablets 2187
Timolol GFS ⊙266
Timoptic in Ocudose 2192
Timoptic Sterile Ophthalmic Solution 2190
Timoptic-XE Sterile Ophthalmic Gel Forming Solution 2194
Toprol-XL Tablets (About 1 of 100 patients) 651
Vaseretic Tablets 2204
Vasotec I.V. Injection 2207
Vasotec Tablets (0.5% to 1.0%) 2210

Rectal adenocarcinoma
Remicade for IV Injection (Less than 2%) 1178

Rectal bleeding
Accutane Capsules 2944
Aciphex Tablets 1267
Aciphex Tablets 1783
Actiq (1% or greater) 1184
Aggrenox Capsules (1.6%) 1026
Ambien Tablets (Rare) 3191
Arthrotec Tablets (Rare) 3195
Asacol Delayed-Release Tablets (2% or greater) 2884
Betaseron for SC Injection 988
▲ Casodex Tablets (2% to 5%) 662
Celexa (Rare) 1365
Clozaril Tablets (Less than 1%) 2319
Cognex Capsules (Infrequent) 1351
Colazal Capsules (2%) 3069
Copaxone for Injection (Infrequent) 3306
Demadex Tablets and Injection 2965
Depo-Provera Contraceptive Injection (Fewer than 1%) 2798
Dipentum Capsules (Rare) 2803
Effexor Tablets (Infrequent) 3495
Effexor XR Capsules (Infrequent) 3499
Eldepryl Capsules 3266
▲ Eulexin Capsules (14%) 3118
Evoxac Capsules (Less than 1%) 1217
Exelon Capsules (Infrequent) 2342
Exelon Oral Solution (Infrequent) 2345
Felbatol 3343
Feldene Capsules (Occasional) 2685
▲ Flolan for Injection (11%) 1528
Fortovase Capsules (Less than 2%) 2970
Foscavir Injection (Between 1% and 5%) 605
Gabitril Tablets (Infrequent) 1189
Gengraf Capsules (1%) 457
Geocillin Tablets 2687
Geodon Capsules (Infrequent) 2688
Hivid Tablets (Less than 1%) 2975
Imitrex Nasal Spray 1554
Indocin Capsules (Less than 1%) 2112
Indocin I.V. (Less than 1%) 2115
Indocin (Less than 1%) 2112
Innohep Injection 1248
Intron A for Injection (Less than 5%) 3120
Invirase Capsules (Less than 2%) 2979
Lipitor Tablets (Less than 2%) 2639
Lipitor Tablets (Less than 2%) 2696
Lodine XL Extended-Release Tablets (Less than 1%) 3530
Luvox Tablets (25, 50, 100 mg) (Infrequent) 3256
Naprelan Tablets (Less than 1%) 1293
Neoral Soft Gelatin Capsules (1%) 2380
Neoral Oral Solution (1%) 2380
Neurontin Capsules (Rare) 2655
Neurontin Oral Solution (Rare) 2655
Neurontin Tablets (Rare) 2655
Orudis Capsules (Less than 1%) 3548
Oruvail Capsules (Less than 1%) 3548
Paxil (Infrequent) 1609
Pentasa Capsules (Less than 1%) 3239
Pletal Tablets (Less than 2%) 2605
Pletal Tablets (Less than 2%) 2848
Ponstel Capsules (Occasional) 1356
Prevacid Delayed-Release Capsules (Less than 1%) 3292
PREVPAC (Less than 1%) 3298
Prometrium Capsules (100 mg, 200 mg) (Less than 5%) 3261
Protonix I.V. (Greater than or equal to 1%) 3580
Protonix Tablets (Less than 1%) 3577
Prozac Pulvules, Liquid, and Weekly Capsules (Rare) 1238
▲ Refludan for Injection (5.3%) 761
Relafen Tablets (Less than 1%) 1617
Reminyl Oral Solution (Infrequent) 1792
Reminyl Tablets (Infrequent) 1792
Requip Tablets (Infrequent) 1621
Retrovir Capsules 1625
Retrovir IV Infusion 1629
Retrovir 1625
Sandostatin LAR Depot (1% to 4%) 2395
Sarafem Pulvules (Rare) 1962
Seroquel Tablets (Infrequent) 684
Serzone Tablets (Infrequent) 1104
Sonata Capsules (Infrequent) 3591
Tequin Injection (Less than 0.1%) 1110
Tequin Tablets (Less than 0.1%) 1110
Toradol (1% or less) 3018
Tricor Capsules, Micronized 513
Trileptal Oral Suspension (Up to 2%) 2407
Trileptal Tablets (Up to 2%) 2407
Uniretic Tablets (Less than 1%) 3178
Vanceril Double Strength Inhalation Aerosol (Fewer than 2%) 3167
Vantin Tablets and Oral Suspension 2860
Viagra Tablets (Less than 2%) 2732
Xeloda Tablets (Less than 5%) 3039
▲ Zoladex (14%) 702
▲ Zoladex 3-month (14%) 706
Zoloft (Rare) 2751
Zonegran Capsules (Infrequent) 1307
Zyprexa Tablets (Infrequent) 1973
Zyprexa ZYDIS Orally Disintegrating Tablets (Infrequent) 1973
Zyrtec (Less than 2%) 2756
Zyrtec-D 12 Hour Extended Relief Tablets (Less than 2%) 2758

Rectal burning
Rowasa Rectal Suspension Enema 4.0 grams/unit (60 mL) (0.61%) 3264

Rectal discomfort
Fleet Glycerin Laxatives 1359
▲ Xenical Capsules (3.3% to 5.2%) 3043

Rectal disorders, unspecified
Actiq (1% or greater) 1184
Actonel Tablets (2.2%) 2879
Amphotec (1% to 5%) 1774
Asacol Delayed-Release Tablets (2% or greater) 2884
▲ CellCept Capsules (3%) 2951
▲ CellCept Intravenous (3%) 2951
▲ CellCept Oral Suspension (3%) 2951
▲ CellCept Tablets (3%) 2951
Cytotec Tablets (Infrequent) 3202
Dipentum Capsules (Rare) 2803
Evoxac Capsules (Less than 1%) 1217
Ferrlecit Injection (Greater than 1%) 3386
Meridia Capsules (1.2%) 481
Naprelan Tablets (Less than 1%) 1293
Nexium Delayed-Release Capsules (Less than 1%) 619
Norvir Capsules (Less than 2%) 487
Norvir Oral Solution (Less than 2%) 487
▲ Prograf (3% to 15%) 1393
Protonix I.V. (Greater than or equal to 1%) 3580
Protonix Tablets (Greater than or equal to 1%) 3577
Rescriptor Tablets (Less than 2%) 526
▲ Serostim for Injection (1% to 10%) 3229
Tasmar Tablets (Infrequent) 3010
Tricor Capsules, Micronized 513
Trovan (Less than 1%) 2722
Vantin Tablets and Oral Suspension (Less than 1%) 2860
Vistide Injection 1445
Wellbutrin Tablets (Rare) 1680

Rectal soreness
Rowasa Rectal Suspension Enema 4.0 grams/unit (60 mL) (0.61%) 3264

Rectal urgency
(*see under* Defecate, desire to)

Red blood cell, aplasia
Rituxan for Infusion (One case) 1750
Rituxan I.V. (One case) 1428

Red man syndrome
Vancocin HCl Capsules & Pulvules 1972
Vancocin HCl Oral Solution 1971
Vancocin HCl, Vials & ADD-Vantage 1970

Reflexes, abnormal
Neurontin Capsules (Frequent) 2655
Neurontin Oral Solution (Frequent) 2655
Neurontin Tablets (Frequent) 2655

Reflexes, increased
(*see under* Hyperreflexia)

Refraction disorder, unspecified
Tricor Capsules, Micronized 513
Vistide Injection 1445

Regurgitation
Amerge Tablets (Rare) 1467
Crixivan Capsules (2%) 2070
Fosamax Tablets (1.4% to 2.0%) 2095
Maxalt Tablets (Infrequent) 2120
Maxalt-MLT Orally Disintegrating Tablets (Infrequent) 2120
Mevacor Tablets (0.5% to 1.0%) 2132
Mylanta (Occasional) 1813
Plendil Extended-Release Tablets (0.5% to 1.5%) 623
Zyban Sustained-Release Tablets (Infrequent) 1710

Renal agenesis, unilateral, neonatal
Leukeran Tablets 1591

Renal calculi
(*see under* Nephrolithiasis)

Renal colic
Crixivan Capsules (Less than 2%) 2070
Daranide Tablets 2077
Noroxin Tablets (Less frequent) 2145
Timolide Tablets (Less than 1%) 2187
Zebeta Tablets 1885
Ziac Tablets 1887

Renal disease
Anaprox Tablets (Less than 1%) 2967
Anaprox DS Tablets (Less than 1%) 2967
EC-Naprosyn Delayed-Release Tablets (Less than 1%) 2967
▲ Naprelan Tablets (3% to 9%) 1293
Naprosyn Suspension (Less than 1%) 2967
Naprosyn Tablets (Less than 1%) 2967

Renal dysfunction
(*see under* Renal impairment)

Renal failure
▲ Abelcet Injection (5%) 1273
Accuretic Tablets 2614
ActHIB Vaccine 798
Actiq (1% or greater) 1184
Aggrenox Capsules (Less than 1%) 1026
Agrylin Capsules (6 of 551 patients) 3232
Aldoclor Tablets 2035
Aldoril Tablets 2039
Aloprim for Injection (1.2%) 2292

AmBisome for Injection (Less common) 1383
Amicar Injection 3608
Amicar Syrup 3608
Amicar Tablets 3608
Amphotec (1% to 5%) 1774
Anaprox Tablets (Less than 1%) 2967
Anaprox DS Tablets (Less than 1%) 2967
Ancobon Capsules 1730
Apligraf (1.3%) 2305
Aricept Tablets (Infrequent) 1270
Aricept Tablets (Infrequent) 2665
Arthrotec Tablets (Rare) 3195
Atacand HCT Tablets 597
Avalide Tablets 1070
Bactrim 2949
Betaseron for SC Injection 988
Bicillin C-R 900/300 Injection 2240
Bicillin C-R Injection 2238
Bicillin L-A Injection 2242
Cafcit (2.2%) 1035
Captopril Tablets (Approximately 1 to 2 of 1000 patients) 2281
Carbatrol Capsules 3234
▲ Carnitor Injection (6%) 3242
Cataflam Tablets 2315
▲ CellCept Capsules (3% to 10%) 2951
▲ CellCept Intravenous (3% to 10%) 2951
▲ CellCept Oral Suspension (3% to 10%) 2951
▲ CellCept Tablets (3% to 10%) 2951
Cerebyx Injection (Infrequent) 2619
Chibroxin Sterile Ophthalmic Solution 2051
Cipro I.V. (1% or less) 893
Cipro I.V. Pharmacy Bulk Package (Less than 1%) 897
Cipro (Less than 1%) 887
Clinoril Tablets (Less than 1 in 100) 2053
Clomid Tablets 735
Cognex Capsules (Rare) 1351
Corvert Injection (0.3%) 2793
Cytovene (At least 3 subjects) 2959
Diovan HCT Tablets 2338
Diprivan Injectable Emulsion (Less than 1%) 667
Diuril Oral 2087
Diuril Sodium Intravenous 2086
Dolobid Tablets (Less than 1 in 100) 2088
Dyrenium Capsules (One case) 3458
EC-Naprosyn Delayed-Release Tablets (Less than 1%) 2967
Ecotrin Enteric Coated Aspirin Low, Regular and Maximum Strength Tablets 1715
Effexor Tablets 3495
Effexor XR Capsules 3499
Enalaprilat Injection 863
Ergamisol Tablets (Less frequent) 1789
Feldene Capsules (Occasional) 2685
Floxin I.V. 2526
Fludara for Injection (Up to 1%) 995
Gabitril Tablets (Infrequent) 1189
Herceptin I.V. (At least one of the 958 patients) 1414
HydroDIURIL Tablets 2108
Hyzaar 2109
Ifex for Injection (1 episode) 1123
Indocin (Less than 1%) 2112
Lamictal (Rare) 1567
Levo-Dromoran 1734
Lexxel Tablets 608
Lodine (Less than 1%) 3528
Lodine XL Extended-Release Tablets (Less than 1%) 3530
Merrem I.V. (0.1% to 1.0%) 673
Micardis HCT Tablets 1051
Microzide Capsules 3414
Mobic Tablets (Less than 2%) 1054
Moduretic Tablets (Less than or equal to 1%) 2138
▲ Naprelan Tablets (Less than 1% to 9%) 1293
Naprosyn Suspension (Less than 1%) 2967
Naprosyn Tablets (Less than 1%) 2967
Nipent for Injection (Less than 3%) 3272
Noroxin Tablets 2145
Norvir Capsules (Less than 2%) 487
Norvir Oral Solution (Less than 2%) 487
▲ Novantrone for Injection (Up to 8%) 1760
Oncaspar 756
Orthoclone OKT3 Sterile Solution 2498
Orudis Capsules (Less than 1%) 3548
Oruvail Capsules (Less than 1%) 3548
Permax Tablets (Infrequent) 1299
Ponstel Capsules (Occasional) 1356
Prinzide Tablets 2168
▲ Prograf (3% to 15%) 1393
Prozac Pulvules, Liquid, and Weekly Capsules 1238
Relafen Tablets (Less than 1%) 1617
Remicade for IV Injection (Less than 2%) 1178
Rifadin 765
Rythmol Tablets – 150 mg, 225 mg, 300 mg (Less than 1%) 502
Sandostatin LAR Depot (Rare) 2395
Sarafem Pulvules 1962
Septra Suspension 2265
Septra Tablets 2265
Septra DS Tablets 2265
Tegretol/Tegretol-XR 2404
Tenormin (0.4%) 692
Ticlid Tablets (Rare) 3015
Timolide Tablets 2187
Tolectin (Less than 1%) 2589
Tonocard Tablets 649
Trasylol Injection (1% to 2%) 909
▲ Trisenox Injection (8%) 1158
Trizivir Tablets 1669
Valtrex Caplets 1676
Vancocin HCl Capsules & Pulvules (Rare) 1972
Vancocin HCl Oral Solution (Rare) 1971
Vancocin HCl, Vials & ADD-Vantage (Rare) 1970
Vaseretic Tablets 2204
Vasotec I.V. Injection 2207
Vasotec Tablets (0.5% to 1.0%) 2210
Vitravene for Injection (2% to 5%) ⊙ 310
Voltaren Tablets 2315
Voltaren-XR Tablets 2315
Zestoretic Tablets 695
Ziac Tablets 1887
Ziagen 1692
Zovirax Capsules 1706
Zovirax for Injection 1708
Zovirax 1706

Renal failure, acute

Abelcet Injection 1273
Accupril Tablets (Rare) 2611
Accuretic Tablets (0.5% to 1%) 2614
Aceon Tablets (2 mg, 4 mg, 8 mg) 3249
Activase I.V. 1410
Albenza Tablets 1463
Altace Capsules (Rare) 2233
Ambien Tablets (Rare) 3191
AmBisome for Injection (Less common) 1383
Amphotec (1% to 5%) 1774
Anectine Injection 1476
Anzemet Injection (Rare) 719
Anzemet Tablets (Rare) 722
Baycol Tablets (Rare) 883
Campath Ampules 992
Cataflam Tablets (Rare) 2315
Celebrex Capsules (Less than 0.1%) 2676
Celebrex Capsules (Less than 0.1%) 2780
▲ CellCept Capsules (3% to 10%) 2951
▲ CellCept Intravenous (3% to 10%) 2951
▲ CellCept Oral Suspension (3% to 10%) 2951
▲ CellCept Tablets (3% to 10%) 2951
Crixivan Capsules 2070
CytoGam Intravenous 2026
Declomycin Tablets (Rare) 1855
Dyazide Capsules 1515
Dyrenium Capsules 3458
Elspar for Injection 2092
Enalaprilat Injection (Rare) 863
Exelon Capsules (Infrequent) 2342
Exelon Oral Solution (Infrequent) 2345
Felbatol 3343
Floxin I.V. 2526
Floxin Tablets 2529
Fluothane Inhalation 3508
Foscavir Injection (Between 1% and 5%) 605
Gamimune N, 5% Solvent/Detergent Treated 925
Gamimune N, 10% Solvent/Detergent Treated 928
Gammagard S/D 845
Gammar-P I.V. 787
Haldol Decanoate 2535
Hivid Tablets (Less than 1%) 2975
Imitrex Injection 1549
Imitrex Nasal Spray 1554
Imitrex Tablets 1558
Indocin I.V. (Less than 1%) 2115
Lamictal (Rare) 1567
Levaquin (Less than 0.5%) 2537
Lipitor Tablets (Rare) 2639
Lipitor Tablets (Rare) 2696
Lotrel Capsules (Rare) 2370
Luvox Tablets (25, 50, 100 mg) 3256
Maxzide 1008
Mefoxin for Injection (Rare) 2124
Mefoxin Premixed Intravenous Solution (Rare) 2127
Mevacor Tablets 2132
Minocin Intravenous (Rare) 1862
Minocin Oral Suspension (Rare) 1865
Minocin Pellet-Filled Capsules (Rare) 1863
Monopril Tablets (Rare) 1091
Motrin Suspension, Oral Drops, Chewable Tablets, and Caplets (Less than 1%) 2002
Neurontin Capsules (Rare) 2655
Neurontin Oral Solution (Rare) 2655
Neurontin Tablets (Rare) 2655
Omnicef 493
Orap Tablets 1407
Paxil 1609
Pediazole Suspension 3050
Pravachol Tablets (Rare) 1099
Primaxin I.M. 2158
Primaxin I.V. (Less than 0.2%) 2160
Prinivil Tablets (0.3% to 1.3%) 2164
Prinzide Tablets 2168
Proleukin for Injection (Less than 1%) 1199
Requip Tablets (Rare) 1621
Rescriptor Tablets 526
Retavase Vials 1182
Rifadin (Rare) 765
Rifamate Capsules (Rare) 767
Rifater Tablets (Rare) 769
Risperdal 1796
Rituxan I.V. 1428
Sandoglobulin I.V. 2391
Seroquel Tablets (Rare) 684
Streptase for Infusion 647
Suprax 1877
Tenex Tablets (Rare) 2942
Thalomid Capsules 1154
Toradol 3018
Trasylol Injection (1% to 2%) 909
Trovan (Less than 1%) 2722
Vaseretic Tablets (Rare) 2204
Vasotec I.V. Injection (Rare) 2207
Vasotec Tablets (Rare) 2210
▲ Vesanoid Capsules (3%) 3037
Videx 1138
Videx EC Capsules 1143
Vioxx (Less than 0.1%) 2213
Voltaren Tablets (Rare) 2315
Voltaren-XR Tablets (Rare) 2315
Zestoretic Tablets (Rare) 695
Zestril Tablets (0.3% to 1.0%) 698
Zithromax Capsules, 250 mg 2743
Zithromax for IV Infusion 2748
Zithromax for Oral Suspension, 300 mg, 600 mg, 900 mg, 1200 mg 2739
Zithromax Tablets, 250 mg 2739
Zocor Tablets (Rare) 2219
Zoloft 2751

Renal failure, neonatal

Accupril Tablets 2611
Aceon Tablets (2 mg, 4 mg, 8 mg) 3249
Altace Capsules 2233
Captopril Tablets 2281
Cozaar Tablets 2067
Enalaprilat Injection 863
Hyzaar 2109
Lexxel Tablets 608
Lotrel Capsules 2370
Monopril Tablets 1091
Prinivil Tablets 2164
Prinzide Tablets 2168
Univasc Tablets 3181
Vaseretic Tablets 2204
Vasotec I.V. Injection 2207
Vasotec Tablets 2210
Zestoretic Tablets 695
Zestril Tablets 698

Renal failure, worsening of

Accupril Tablets (Rare) 2611
Vioxx (Less than 0.1%) 2213

Renal function impairment

(*see under* Renal impairment)

Renal impairment

Abelcet Injection 1273
Accuretic Tablets 2614
Agrylin Capsules (10 of 551 patients) 3232
Aldoclor Tablets 2035
Aldoril Tablets 2039
Alesse-21 Tablets 3468
Alesse-28 Tablets 3473
Aloprim for Injection (Less than 1%) 2292
Altace Capsules (Rare) 2233
Amphotec (1% to 5%) 1774
Argatroban Injection (2.8%) 1478
Asacol Delayed-Release Tablets 2884
Atacand HCT Tablets 597
Avalide Tablets 1070
Brevicon 28-Day Tablets 3380
Campath Ampules 992
Ceclor 1905
Cedax 1021
Cefotan 664
Ceftin 1898
Cefzil 1076
▲ CellCept Capsules (21.8%) 2951
▲ CellCept Intravenous (21.8%) 2951
▲ CellCept Oral Suspension (21.8%) 2951
▲ CellCept Tablets (21.8% to 25.6%) 2951
Ceptaz for Injection 1499
Cleocin HCl Capsules (Rare) 2784
Cleocin Phosphate Sterile Solution (Rare) 2785
Cleocin Vaginal Cream 2788
Cleocin Vaginal Ovules 2789
Clinoril Tablets (Less than 1 in 100) 2053
Coly-Mycin M Parenteral 2243
Cordarone Intravenous (Less than 2%) 3491
Coreg Tablets (1% to 2%) 1508
Cyclessa Tablets 2450
Cytovene (At least 3 subjects) 2959
Desferal Vials 2333
Desogen Tablets 2458
Diovan Capsules 2337
Diovan HCT Tablets 2338
Diuril Oral 2087
Diuril Sodium Intravenous 2086
Dolobid Tablets (Less than 1 in 100) 2088
Doxil Injection (Less than 1%) 566
DTIC-Dome (Few reports) 902
Duricef 1079
Effexor XR Capsules (Rare) 3499
Enalaprilat Injection 863
Estrace Vaginal Cream 3358
Estrace Tablets 3361
Estrostep 2627
Evoxac Capsules (Less than 1%) 1217
Felbatol 3343
▲ Feldene Capsules (1% to 10%) 2685
Fludara for Injection (Up to 1%) 995
Fortaz 1541
▲ Foscavir Injection (5% to 33%) 605
▲ Gengraf Capsules (25% to 38%) 457
Hivid Tablets (Less than 1%) 2975
HydroDIURIL Tablets 2108
Hyzaar 2109
Idamycin PFS Injection (No more than 1%) 2825
▲ Ifex for Injection (6%) 1123
▲ Indocin I.V. (41% of infants) 2115
Lescol Capsules 2361
Lescol Capsules 2925
Lescol XL Tablets 2361
Lescol XL Tablets 2925
▲ Leukine (8%) 1755
Levaquin (Less than 0.5%) 2537
Levlen 962
Levlite 21 Tablets 962
Levlite 28 Tablets 962
Levora Tablets 3389
Lexxel Tablets 608
Lithobid Slow-Release Tablets 3255
Loestrin 21 Tablets 2642
Loestrin Fe Tablets 2642
Lopid Tablets 2650
Lorabid Suspension and Pulvules 2251
Lunelle Monthly Injection 2827
Macrobid Capsules 2889
Macrodantin Capsules 2891
Maxipime for Injection 1285
Mefoxin for Injection 2124
Mefoxin Premixed Intravenous Solution 2127
Mepron Suspension 1598
Micardis HCT Tablets 1051
Microgestin Fe 1.5/30 Tablets 3407
Microgestin Fe 1/20 Tablets 3400
Microzide Capsules 3414
Mircette Tablets 2470
Modicon 2563
Moduretic Tablets (Less than or equal to 1%) 2138
Naprelan Tablets (Less than 1%) 1293
Nebcin Vials, Hyporets & ADD-Vantage 1955
Necon 3415
▲ Neoral Soft Gelatin Capsules (25% to 38%) 2380
▲ Neoral Oral Solution (25% to 38%) 2380
Nipent for Injection (Less than 3%) 3272
Nolvadex Tablets 678
Norinyl 1 +35 28-Day Tablets 3380
Norinyl 1 + 50 28-Day Tablets 3380
Nor-QD Tablets 3423
Omnicef 493
Oncaspar 756
Ortho-Cept 21 Tablets 2546
Ortho-Cept 28 Tablets 2546
Ortho-Cyclen/Ortho Tri-Cyclen 2573
Ortho-Novum 2563
Ortho-Novum 1/50▫28 Tablets 2556
Ortho-Cyclen/Ortho Tri-Cyclen 2573
Orudis Capsules (Greater than 1%) 3548
Oruvail Capsules (Greater than 1%) 3548
Ovcon 3364
Panhematin for Injection 497
Paxil (Rare) 1609
Plavix Tablets 1097
Plavix Tablets 3084
▲ Ponstel Capsules (1% to 10%) 1356
Prinivil Tablets (0.3% to 1.0%) 2164
Prinzide Tablets 2168
▲ Prograf (36% to 40%) 1393
Proleukin for Injection (2%) 1199
Refludan for Injection (1.8%) 761
ReoPro Vials (0.3%) 1958
▲ Sandimmune (25 to 38%) 2388
Sandoglobulin I.V. 2391
▲ Simulect for Injection (3% to 10%) 2399

Suprax 1877
Tazicef for Injection 1647
Tazicef Galaxy Container 1650
Tazicef Pharmacy Bulk Package 1653
Tazidime Vials, Faspak & ADD-Vantage 1966
Timolide Tablets 2187
Tonocard Tablets 649
Tranxene 511
▲ Trasylol Injection (5% to 30%) 909
Tricor Capsules, Micronized 513
Tri-Levlen 962
Tri-Norinyl-28 Tablets 3433
▲ Trisenox Injection (8%) 1158
Trivora Tablets 3439
Trovan (Less than 1%) 2722
Vantin Tablets and Oral Suspension 2860
Vaseretic Tablets 2204
Vasotec I.V. Injection 2207
Vasotec Tablets (0.5% to 1.0%) 2210
Viramune Oral Suspension 1060
Viramune Tablets 1060
Vistide Injection 1445
Yasmin 28 Tablets 980
Zestoretic Tablets 695
Zestril Tablets (0.3% to 1.0%) 698
Ziac Tablets 1887
Zovia 3449

Renal infarct
BeneFix for Injection (One patient) 1432

Renal insufficiency
Aggrenox Capsules (Less than 1%) 1026
Aloprim for Injection (1.2%) 2292
Captopril Tablets (Approximately 1 to 2 of 1000 patients) 2281
Crixivan Capsules (Some cases) 2070
Ecotrin Enteric Coated Aspirin Low, Regular and Maximum Strength Tablets 1715
Elspar for Injection 2092
Erythrocin Stearate Filmtab Tablets (Isolated reports) 452
Floxin I.V. 2526
Floxin Tablets 2529
Fortovase Capsules (Rare) 2970
Gamimune N, 5% Solvent/Detergent Treated (Isolated reports) 925
Gamimune N, 10% Solvent/Detergent Treated (Isolated reports) 928
Indocin Capsules (Less than 1%) 2112
Indocin I.V. (Less than 1%) 2115
Indocin (Less than 1%) 2112
Lodine (Less than 1%) 3528
Lodine XL Extended-Release Tablets (Less than 1%) 3530
Lopid Tablets 2650
Monopril Tablets (0.2% to 1.0%) 1091
Monopril HCT 1094
Neupogen for Injection (Two events) 587
Nipent for Injection (Less than 3%) 3272
Norvir Capsules 487
Norvir Oral Solution 487
Orthoclone OKT3 Sterile Solution 2498
Proleukin for Injection 1199
Rifadin (Rare) 765
Rifamate Capsules (Rare) 767
Rifater Tablets (Rare) 769
Risperdal (Rare) 1796
Sandostatin LAR Depot (Rare) 2395
Taxotere for Injection Concentrate 778
Univasc Tablets (Less than 1%) 3181
▲ Vesanoid Capsules (11%) 3037
▲ Zenapax for Injection (2% to 5%) 3046
Zoladex (1% to 5%) 702
Zoladex 3-month 706

Renal insufficiency, reversible
Actimmune (Rare) 1772

Renal precipitation
Rocephin Injectable Vials, ADD-Vantage, Galaxy, Bulk 2993

Renal rickets
Ifex for Injection 1123

Renal stones
(*see under* Nephrolithiasis)

Renal toxicity
(*see under* Nephrotoxicity)

Renal tubular damage
Betaseron for SC Injection 988
Cytovene 2959
Mylocel Tablets (Occasional) 2227
Vistide Injection 1445

Reproductive disorders, female
Amerge Tablets (Rare) 1467

Respiration, painful
Prinivil Tablets (0.3% to 1.0%) 2164
Prinzide Tablets 2168
Zestoretic Tablets 695
Zestril Tablets (0.3% to 1.0%) 698

Respiratory alkalosis
Aggrenox Capsules 1026
AmBisome for Injection (Less common) 1383
Campath Ampules 992
Coreg Tablets (Less than or equal to 0.1%) 1508
Ecotrin Enteric Coated Aspirin Low, Regular and Maximum Strength Tablets 1715
Geodon Capsules (Rare) 2688
Vistide Injection 1445

Respiratory arrest
Actiq 1184
Ancobon Capsules 1730
AquaMEPHYTON Injection 2042
Cipro I.V. (1% or less) 893
Cipro I.V. Pharmacy Bulk Package (Less than 1%) 897
Clozaril Tablets (Rare) 2319
Coly-Mycin M Parenteral 2243
Demerol 3079
Dilaudid Oral Liquid 445
Dilaudid Tablets - 8 mg 445
Dilaudid-HP 443
Duranest Injections 600
Emla (Unlikely with cream) 602
Floxin I.V. (Less than 1%) 2526
Floxin Tablets (Less than 1%) 2529
Fluothane Inhalation 3508
INFeD Injection 3388
Kadian Capsules 1335
Lidoderm Patch 1319
Mepergan Injection 3539
MS Contin Tablets 2896
MSIR 2898
Naropin Injection 612
Nesacaine/Nesacaine MPF 617
Nubain Injection (1% or less) 1323
Orthoclone OKT3 Sterile Solution 2498
OxyContin Tablets 2912
Proleukin for Injection (Less than 1%) 1199
Prostigmin Injectable 1744
Prostigmin Tablets 1744
Robinul Injectable 2940
Roxanol 3066
Roxicodone Tablets 3067
Sensorcaine 643
Sensorcaine-MPF Injection 643
Tonocard Tablets (Less than 1%) 649
Versed Syrup 3033
▲ Xylocaine Injections (Among most common) 653

Respiratory congestion, unspecified
Comvax (0.3% to 1.2%) 2056
Cozaar Tablets (Less than 1%) 2067
▲ Epogen for Injection (15%) 582
Hyzaar 2109
Lexxel Tablets 608
Maxalt Tablets (Infrequent) 2120
Maxalt-MLT Orally Disintegrating Tablets (Infrequent) 2120
▲ Procrit for Injection (15%) 2502
Versed Syrup (Less than 1%) 3033

Respiratory depression
Actiq 1184
Anectine Injection 1476
Arthrotec Tablets (Rare) 3195
Astramorph/PF Injection, USP (Preservative-Free) 594
Brevital Sodium for Injection, USP 1815
Campath Ampules 992
Dantrium Capsules (Less frequent) 2885
Demerol 3079
Dilaudid 441
Dilaudid Oral Liquid 445
Dilaudid Powder 441
Dilaudid Rectal Suppositories 441
Dilaudid Tablets 441
Dilaudid Tablets - 8 mg 445
Dilaudid-HP 443
Dolophine Hydrochloride Tablets 3056
Duramorph Injection 1312
Duranest Injections 600
Emla (Unlikely with cream) 602
Felbatol 3343
Feldene Capsules (Rare) 2685
Hycodan 1316
Hycomine Compound Tablets 1317
Hycotuss Expectorant Syrup 1318
Infumorph 200 and Infumorph 500 Sterile Solutions 1314
Kadian Capsules 1335
Klonopin Tablets 2983
Levo-Dromoran 1734
Lidoderm Patch 1319
Lodine XL Extended-Release Tablets 3530
Lortab 3319
Lortab Elixir 3317
Maxidone Tablets CIII 3399
Mepergan Injection 3539
MS Contin Tablets 2896
MSIR 2898
Nardil Tablets (Less frequent) 2653
Norco 5/325 Tablets CIII 3424
Norco 7.5/325 Tablets CIII 3425
Norco 10/325 Tablets CIII 3425
Norco 10/325 Tablets CIII 3427
Norcuron for Injection 2478
Numorphan 1324
Oramorph SR Tablets 3062
OxyContin Tablets 2912
OxyFast Oral Concentrate Solution 2916
OxyIR Capsules 2916
Percocet Tablets 1326
Phenergan 3556
Phenergan with Codeine Syrup 3557
Phenergan VC with Codeine Syrup 3561
ProSom Tablets 500
Prostigmin Injectable 1744
Prostigmin Tablets 1744
Roxanol 3066
Sensorcaine 643
Sensorcaine-MPF Injection 643
Streptase for Infusion 647
Survanta Intratracheal Suspension 3053
Talacen Caplets (Rare) 3089
Talwin Nx Tablets (Rare) 3090
Tussionex Pennkinetic Extended-Release Suspension 1174
Tussi-Organidin NR Liquid 3350
Tussi-Organidin-S NR Liquid 3350
Tylenol with Codeine 2595
Tylox Capsules 2597
Valium Injectable 3026
Versed Injection 3027
Versed Syrup (1%) 3033
Vicodin Tablets 516
Vicodin ES Tablets 517
Vicodin HP Tablets 518
Vicodin Tuss Expectorant 519
Vicoprofen Tablets 520
▲ Xylocaine Injections (Among most common) 653
Zydone Tablets 1330

Respiratory desaturation
Versed Syrup (Less than 1%) 3033

Respiratory difficulty
▲ Abelcet Injection (4%) 1273
▲ Acthrel for Injection (6%) 3629
Allegra-D Extended-Release Tablets 714
Ambien Tablets 3191
Carafate Suspension 731
Carafate Tablets 730
Cardene I.V. (Rare) 3485
Claritin-D 12 Hour Extended Release Tablets 3102
Claritin-D 24 Hour Extended Release Tablets 3104
EpiPen 1236
Felbatol 3343
Fortovase Capsules (Less than 2%) 2970
Haldol Decanoate 2535
Haldol Injection, Tablets and Concentrate 2533
Humorsol Sterile Ophthalmic Solution (Infrequent) 2102
INFeD Injection 3388
Invirase Capsules (Less than 2%) 2979
Kadian Capsules (Less than 3%) 1335
▲ Lupron Depot–4 Month 30 mg (4.2% to 8.2%) 3289
▲ Photofrin for Injection (10%) 831
Rilutek Tablets (More than 2%) 772
Rynatan Tablets 3351
Synvisc 3596
▲ Trasylol Injection (3%) 909
Versed Injection (Less than 1%) 3027
▲ Vesanoid Capsules (26%) 3037
Xylocaine Injections (Less than 1%) 653
Zyrtec-D 12 Hour Extended Relief Tablets 2758

Respiratory discharge, upper, unspecified
Emcyt Capsules (1%) 2810

Respiratory disorders, unspecified
Amphotec (1% to 5%) 1774
Ativan Injection (1.2%) 3478
▲ CellCept Capsules (3% to 10%) 2951
▲ CellCept Intravenous (3% to 10%) 2951
▲ CellCept Oral Suspension (3% to 10%) 2951
▲ CellCept Tablets (3% to 10%) 2951
▲ Colazal Capsules (4%) 3069
▲ CombiPatch Transdermal System (9% to 13%) 2323
Corlopam Injection (0.5% to 5%) 412
▲ Enbrel for Injection (5%) 1752
▲ Enbrel for Injection (5%) 3504
Evoxac Capsules (Less than 1%) 1217
▲ Flolan for Injection (7%) 1528
Fortovase Capsules (Less than 2%) 2970
Gabitril Tablets (Infrequent) 1189
▲ Geodon Capsules (8%) 2688
Innohep Injection (Greater than or equal to 1%) 1248
Intron A for Injection (Less than or equal to 5%) 3120
▲ Lupron Depot 7.5 mg (10.7%) 3284
Meridia Capsules 481
▲ Paxil (7%) 1609
Plasbumin-5 (Rare) 939
Plasbumin-20 (Rare) 940
Plasbumin-25 (Rare) 941
▲ Proleukin for Injection (11%) 1199
▲ Rituxan for Infusion (Among most frequent) 1750
▲ Rituxan I.V. (Among most frequent) 1428
▲ Simulect for Injection (3% to 10%) 2399
▲ TOBI Solution for Inhalation (31.4%) 1206
Trovan (Less than 1%) 2722
Zyrtec-D 12 Hour Extended Relief Tablets (Less than 2%) 2758

Respiratory distress
Accuretic Tablets 2614
Agrylin Capsules (1% to 5%) 3232
Aldoclor Tablets 2035
Aldoril Tablets 2039
Aloprim for Injection (Less than 1%) 2292
Americaine Otic Topical Anesthetic Ear Drops 1162
Aredia for Injection (One case) 2309
Atacand HCT Tablets 597
Atrovent Inhalation Solution (1.4%) 1031
Blocadren Tablets 2046
Cardura Tablets (1.1%) 2668
Ceclor CD Tablets (0.1% to 1%) 1279
Cerezyme for Injection 1438
Cipro I.V. (1% or less) 893
Cipro I.V. Pharmacy Bulk Package (Less than 1%) 897
Clomid Tablets 735
Coly-Mycin M Parenteral 2243
Combivent Inhalation Aerosol (2.5%) 1041
Comvax 2056
Cordarone Intravenous (2%) 3491
Corgard Tablets 2245
Corzide 40/5 Tablets 2247
Corzide 80/5 Tablets 2247
Cosopt Sterile Ophthalmic Solution 2065
Desferal Vials 2333
Diovan HCT Tablets 2338
Diucardin Tablets 3494
Diuril Oral 2087
Diuril Sodium Intravenous 2086
Duragesic Transdermal System (Less than 1%) 1786
Dyazide Capsules 1515
Elspar for Injection 2092
Floxin I.V. 2526
Floxin Tablets 2529
Follistim for Injection 2465
Foscavir Injection (Between 1% and 5%) 605
Glucagon for Injection Vials and Emergency Kit 1924
Glucovance Tablets 1086
Gonal-F for Injection 3216
Herceptin I.V. 1414
Hivid Tablets (Less than 1%) 2975
▲ Humatrope Vials and Cartridges (3.13% to 6.67%) 1930
Humegon for Injection 2468
HydroDIURIL Tablets 2108
Hyzaar 2109
Indapamide Tablets 2286
Inderal 3513
Inderal LA Long-Acting Capsules 3516
Inderide Tablets 3517
Inderide LA Long-Acting Capsules 3519
Indocin Capsules (Less than 1%) 2112
Indocin I.V. (Less than 1%) 2115
Indocin (Less than 1%) 2112
Lamictal (More than 1%) 1567
Leukine 1755
Lotensin HCT Tablets 2367
▲ Lupron Depot–3 Month 22.5 mg (6.4%) 3288
Maxzide 1008
▲ Mexitil Capsules (3.3% to 5.7%) 1047
Micardis HCT Tablets 1051
Microzide Capsules 3414
Moduretic Tablets 2138
Monopril HCT 1094
Mykrox Tablets (Rare) 1168
Nadolol Tablets 2288
Naprelan Tablets (Less than 1%) 1293
Normodyne Tablets 3137
Nubain Injection (1% or less) 1323
▲ Paraplatin for Injection (6% or less to 12%) 1126
Paxil 1609
Pergonal for Injection 3223
Phenergan VC Syrup 3560
Phenergan VC with Codeine Syrup 3561
Prinzide Tablets 2168
Procardia XL Extended Release Tablets (1% or less) 2710

▲ Prograf (3% to 15%) 1393
Remicade for IV Injection (Less than 2%) 1178
Repronex for Intramuscular and Subcutaneous Injection 1347
Rituxan I.V. 1428
Sandimmune 2388
Sectral Capsules 3589
Serevent Inhalation Aerosol 1633
Taxotere for Injection Concentrate 778
Tenoretic Tablets 690
Tenormin 692
Tice BCG, BCG Live (1.6%) 2489
Timolide Tablets 2187
Timolol GFS .... ⊙266
Timoptic in Ocudose 2192
Timoptic Sterile Ophthalmic Solution (Less frequent) 2190
Timoptic-XE Sterile Ophthalmic Gel Forming Solution 2194
Toprol-XL Tablets 651
Uniretic Tablets 3178
Vaseretic Tablets 2204
Virazole for Inhalation Solution 1747
Xeloda Tablets (Less than 5%) 3039
Zaroxolyn Tablets 1177
Zebeta Tablets 1885
Zestoretic Tablets 695
Ziac Tablets 1887

Respiratory distress, neonatal
Hycodan 1316
Hycotuss Expectorant Syrup 1318
Naropin Injection (1.5%) 612
Stadol NS Nasal Spray (Rare) 1108

Respiratory failure
▲ Abelcet Injection (8%) 1273
Actiq (Less than 1%) 1184
Aloprim for Injection (Less than 1%) 2292
AmBisome for Injection (Less common) 1383
Ativan Injection (2.4%) 3478
Betagan .... ⊙228
Betimol Ophthalmic Solution .... ⊙324
Betoptic S Ophthalmic Suspension (Rare) 537
Carteolol Hydrochloride Ophthalmic Solution USP, 1% .... ⊙258
Cosopt Sterile Ophthalmic Solution 2065
Crixivan Capsules (Less than 2%) 2070
Ocupress Ophthalmic Solution, 1% Sterile .... ⊙303
Omnicef 493
Orthoclone OKT3 Sterile Solution 2498
Photofrin for Injection 831
▲ Proleukin for Injection (Less than 1% to 9%) 1199
Pulmozyme Inhalation Solution 1426
Simulect for Injection 2399
Survanta Intratracheal Suspension 3053
Symmetrel 1328
Timolol GFS .... ⊙266
Timoptic in Ocudose (Less frequent) 2192
Timoptic Sterile Ophthalmic Solution (Less frequent) 2190
Timoptic-XE Sterile Ophthalmic Gel Forming Solution 2194

Respiratory insufficiency
Aloprim for Injection (Less than 1%) 2292
Campath Ampules 992
Chirocaine Injection (Less than 1%) 2909
Levaquin Injection (Less than 0.5%) 2537
Remicade for IV Injection 1178

Respiratory moniliasis
Rilutek Tablets (Infrequent) 772

Respiratory secretions, increased
▲ Suprane Liquid for Inhalation (3% to 21%) 874

Respiratory tract, hypersensitivity
Septra Suspension 2265
Septra Tablets 2265
Septra DS Tablets 2265

Restlessness
(*see under* Dysphoria)

Retardation, psychomotor
Eskalith 1527
Lithium Carbonate 3061
Lithium Citrate Syrup 3061
Roferon-A Injection (Infrequent) 2996

Retching
Bebulin VH 840
Imitrex Injection (Rare) 1549
Imitrex Nasal Spray 1554
Imitrex Tablets 1558
Rescriptor Tablets (Less than 2%) 526
Trileptal Oral Suspension 2407
Trileptal Tablets 2407
Versed Injection (Less than 1%) 3027

Reticulocytopenia
Cosmegen for Injection 2062

Reticulocytosis
▲ Dapsone Tablets USP (Almost all patients) 1780
Dipentum Capsules (Rare) 2803
Ticlid Tablets (Rare) 3015
Virazole for Inhalation Solution 1747

Retinal artery occlusion
Activase I.V. 1410
Imitrex Nasal Spray 1554
Imitrex Tablets 1558
Retavase Vials 1182
Streptase for Infusion 647

Retinal atrophy
Aralen Tablets 3075
Clinoril Tablets 2053
Plaquenil Tablets 3082

Retinal damage
Aralen Tablets 3075
Dapsone Tablets USP 1780
Neurontin Capsules (Rare) 2655
Neurontin Oral Solution (Rare) 2655
Neurontin Tablets (Rare) 2655
Plaquenil Tablets 3082
Vitrasert Implant (Less than 1%) .... ⊙254

Retinal degeneration
Aciphex Tablets 1267
Aciphex Tablets 1783
Uniretic Tablets (Less than 1%) 3178

Retinal detachment
▲ Cytovene (8%) 2959
Humorsol Sterile Ophthalmic Solution (Occasional) 2102
Isopto Carpine Ophthalmic Solution (Rare) .... ⊙215
Luvox Tablets (25, 50, 100 mg) (Rare) 3256
Permax Tablets (Rare) 1299
Pilopine HS Ophthalmic Gel .... ⊙217
Sonata Capsules (Rare) 3591
Sular Tablets (Less than or equal to 1%) 688
▲ Valcyte Tablets (15%) 3022
Vistide Injection 1445
▲ Vitrasert Implant (Approximately 10% to 20%) .... ⊙254
Xalatan Latanoprost Ophthalmic Solution (Extremely rare) .... ⊙320
Xalatan Sterile Ophthalmic Solution (Extremely rare) 2864

Retinal disorder, unspecified
Evoxac Capsules (Less than 1%) 1217
Lamisil Tablets 2360
Lotensin HCT Tablets (0.3% or more) 2367
Salagen Tablets (Less than 1%) 2229
Videx 1138
Vistide Injection 1445

Retinal ischemia
PEG-Intron Powder for Injection (Less than or equal to 1%) 3140

Retinal pigmentation disorders
Aralen Tablets 3075
Desferal Vials 2333
Plaquenil Tablets 3082
Videx (Several patients) 1138
Videx EC Capsules 1143
▲ Vitravene for Injection (5% to 20%) .... ⊙310

Retinal vascular disorder
Betimol Ophthalmic Solution .... ⊙324
Clomid Tablets 735
Intron A for Injection (Rare) 3120
Permax Tablets 1299
Protonix I.V. (Less than 1%) 3580
Protonix Tablets (Less than 1%) 3577
Serophene Tablets 3226
Viagra Tablets 2732
Virazole for Inhalation Solution 1747
Vitravene for Injection (2% to 5%) .... ⊙310

Retinitis
Attenuvax (Infrequent) 2044
Betaseron for SC Injection 988
Cytovene 2959
Doxil Injection (1% to 5%) 566
Indocin (Less than 1%) 2112
M-M-R II (Infrequent) 2118
▲ Serostim for Injection (1% to 10%) 3229

Retinitis, bilateral
TYPHIM Vi Vaccine 825

Retinitis, cytomegalovirus
Fortovase Capsules (Less than 2%) 2970

Retinoic-acid-APL syndrome
▲ Vesanoid Capsules (Up to 25%) 3037

Retinopathy
Aralen Tablets 3075
Cardizem Injectable 1018
Cardizem Lyo-Ject Syringe 1018
Cardizem Monovial 1018
Cardizem CD Capsules (Infrequent) 1016
Clinoril Tablets 2053
Desferal Vials 2333
Haldol Decanoate 2535
Haldol Injection, Tablets and Concentrate 2533
Minipress Capsules (Single report) 2699
Minizide Capsules (Single report) 2700
Neurontin Capsules (Rare) 2655
Neurontin Oral Solution (Rare) 2655
Neurontin Tablets (Rare) 2655
Nipent for Injection (Less than 3%) 3272
Nolvadex Tablets 678
Plaquenil Tablets (Rare) 3082
Roferon-A Injection (Rare) 2996
Tiazac Capsules (Infrequent) 1378
Tolectin (Less than 1%) 2589
Vitrasert Implant (Less than 1%) .... ⊙254

Retinopathy, pigmentary
Aralen Tablets 3075
Compazine 1505
Etrafon 3115
Stelazine 1640
Thioridazine Hydrochloride Tablets 2289
Thorazine 1656
Trilafon 3160

Retinopathy of prematurity
Cafcit (2.2%) 1035
Decadron Phosphate Injection 2081

Retrocollis
Etrafon 3115
Trilafon 3160

Retrolental fibroplasia
▲ Indocin I.V. (3% to 9%) 2115

Retroperitoneal fibrosis
Blocadren Tablets 2046
Cosopt Sterile Ophthalmic Solution 2065
D.H.E. 45 Injection (Occasional) 2334
Timolide Tablets 2187
Timolol GFS .... ⊙266
Timoptic in Ocudose (Less frequent) 2192
Timoptic Sterile Ophthalmic Solution (Less frequent) 2190
Timoptic-XE Sterile Ophthalmic Gel Forming Solution 2194

Retroperitoneum, redistribution/accumulation of body fat
Crixivan Capsules 2070

Retrosternal discomfort
Iopidine Sterile Ophthalmic Solution .... ⊙212

Reye's Syndrome, potential for development of
Aggrenox Capsules 1026
Alka-Seltzer .... ▣603
Alka-Seltzer Lemon Lime Antacid and Pain Reliever Effervescent Tablets .... ▣603
Alka-Seltzer Extra Strength Antacid and Pain Reliever Effervescent Tablets .... ▣603
Alka-Seltzer PM Effervescent Tablets .... ▣605
Genuine Bayer Tablets, Caplets and Gelcaps .... ▣606
Extra Strength Bayer Caplets and Gelcaps .... ▣610
Aspirin Regimen Bayer Children's Chewable Tablets (Orange or Cherry Flavored) .... ▣607
Aspirin Regimen Bayer Adult Low Strength 81 mg Tablets .... ▣606
Aspirin Regimen Bayer 81 mg Caplets with Calcium .... ▣607
Genuine Bayer Professional Labeling (Aspirin Regimen Bayer) .... ▣608
Extra Strength Bayer Arthritis Caplets .... ▣610
Extra Strength Bayer Plus Caplets .... ▣610
Extra Strength Bayer PM Caplets .... ▣611
BC Powder .... ▣619
BC Allergy Sinus Cold Powder .... ▣619
Arthritis Strength BC Powder .... ▣619
BC Sinus Cold Powder .... ▣619
Darvon Compound-65 Pulvules 1910
Ecotrin Enteric Coated Aspirin Low, Regular and Maximum Strength Tablets 1715
Excedrin Extra-Strength Tablets, Caplets, and Geltabs .... ▣629
Excedrin Migraine 1070
Goody's Body Pain Formula Powder .... ▣620
Goody's Extra Strength Headache Powder .... ▣620
Goody's Extra Strength Pain Relief Tablets .... ▣620
Momentum Backache Relief Extra Strength Caplets .... ▣666
Pepto-Bismol Maximum Strength Liquid (Rare) 2878
Pepto-Bismol Original Liquid, Original and Cherry Tablets and Easy-To-Swallow Caplets (Rare) 2878
Percodan Tablets 1327
Vanquish Caplets .... ▣617

Rhabdomyolysis
Aciphex Tablets 1267
Aciphex Tablets 1783
Activase I.V. 1410
Aggrenox Capsules 1026
Amicar Injection 3608
Amicar Syrup 3608
Amicar Tablets 3608
Anectine Injection (Rare) 1476
Atromid-S Capsules 3483
Azulfidine EN-tabs Tablets (Rare) 2775
Baycol Tablets (Rare) 883
Bicillin C-R 900/300 Injection 2240
Bicillin C-R Injection 2238
Bicillin L-A Injection 2242
Clozaril Tablets 2319
Combivir Tablets 1502
Comtan Tablets 2328
Cytovene 2959
Diprivan Injectable Emulsion (Very rare) 667
Ecotrin Enteric Coated Aspirin Low, Regular and Maximum Strength Tablets 1715
Epivir 1520
Epivir-HBV 1524
Felbatol 3343
Floxin I.V. 2526
Floxin Tablets 2529
Fluothane Inhalation 3508
Foscavir Injection (Rare) 605
Lamictal 1567
Lescol Capsules 2361
Lescol Capsules 2925
Lescol XL Tablets 2361
Lescol XL Tablets 2925
Levaquin (Less than 0.5%) 2537
Lipitor Tablets (Rare) 2639
Lipitor Tablets (Rare) 2696
Lopid Tablets 2650
Mevacor Tablets 2132
Mirapex Tablets (One case) 2834
Omnicef 493
Orap Tablets 1407
Pravachol Tablets (Rare) 1099
Proleukin for Injection 1199
Rescriptor Tablets 526
Retavase Vials 1182
Risperdal 1796
Seroquel Tablets 684
Streptase for Infusion 647
Tasmar Tablets 3010
Tricor Capsules, Micronized (Less than 1%) 513
Trizivir Tablets 1669
Videx (Rare) 1138
Videx EC Capsules 1143
Wellbutrin Tablets 1680
Wellbutrin SR Sustained-Release Tablets 1684
Zocor Tablets (Rare) 2219
Zyban Sustained-Release Tablets 1710

Rheumatic syndrome
Rifamate Capsules 767
Rifater Tablets 769

Rheumatism, articular
Advair Diskus 100/50 (1% to 3%) 1448
Advair Diskus 250/50 (1% to 3%) 1448
Advair Diskus 500/50 (1% to 3%) 1448
▲ Flovent Diskus (1% to 17%) 3614

Rheumatoid arthritis
Asacol Delayed-Release Tablets 2884
Atromid-S Capsules 3483
Effexor Tablets (Rare) 3495
Effexor XR Capsules (Rare) 3499
Evoxac Capsules (Less than 1%) 1217
LYMErix Vaccine 1592
Norplant System (Rare) 3543
PEG-Intron Powder for Injection (Less than or equal to 1%) 3140
Prozac Pulvules, Liquid, and Weekly Capsules (Rare) 1238
Rilutek Tablets (Rare) 772
Sarafem Pulvules (Rare) 1962
Zyprexa Tablets (Infrequent) 1973
Zyprexa ZYDIS Orally Disintegrating Tablets (Infrequent) 1973

Rheumatoid arthritis, worsening of
Remicade for IV Injection (Less than 2%) 1178

Rheumatoid factor, positive

Aldoclor Tablets 2035
Aldomet Tablets 2037
Aldoril Tablets 2039

Rheumatoid nodules

Remicade for IV Injection (Less than 2%) 1178

Rhinitis

Accuretic Tablets (2%) 2614
▲ Aceon Tablets (2 mg, 4 mg, 8 mg) (4.8%) 3249
Actiq (Less than 1%) 1184
▲ Actonel Tablets (5.7%) 2879
Adalat CC Tablets (3% or less) 877
Advair Diskus 100/50 (1% to 3%) 1448
Advair Diskus 250/50 (1% to 3%) 1448
Advair Diskus 500/50 (1% to 3%) 1448
▲ Aerobid/Aerobid-M (3% to 9%) 1363
Agrylin Capsules (1% to 5%) 3232
▲ Alamast Ophthalmic Solution (10% to 25%) 3092
▲ Alocril Ophthalmic Solution (1% to 10%) 545
Alphagan P Ophthalmic Solution (1% to 4%) 546
Ambien Tablets (1%) 3191
▲ AmBisome for Injection (11.1%) 1383
Amerge Tablets (Rare) 1467
▲ Amphotec (5% or more) 1774
Apligraf (1.8% to 2.5%) 2305
Arava Tablets (2%) 724
▲ Aredia for Injection (Up to 6%) 2309
Arimidex Tablets (2% to 5%) 659
▲ Aromasin Tablets (2% to 5%) 2769
▲ Asacol Delayed-Release Tablets (5% or greater) 2884
▲ Astelin Nasal Spray (5.6%) 3339
Atacand Tablets (2%) 595
Atacand HCT Tablets (0.5% or greater) 597
Atrovent Inhalation Solution (2.3%) 1031
Atrovent Nasal Spray 0.03% (2.0% to 5.1%) 1032
Attenuvax 2044
Avalide Tablets (1% or greater) 1070
Avapro Tablets (1% or greater) 1074
Avapro Tablets (1% or greater) 3076
Avelox Tablets (0.05% to 1%) 879
Axert Tablets (Infrequent) 2772
▲ Axid Pulvules (9.8%) 1903
▲ Axid Pulvules (9.8%) 2919
Azopt Ophthalmic Suspension (1% to 5%) 536
▲ Bactroban Nasal (1.0% to 6%) 1495
▲ Baycol Tablets (8.3%) 883
Betaxon Ophthalmic Suspension (Less than 2%) 537
Brevital Sodium for Injection, USP 1815
▲ Campath Ampules (7%) 992
Captopril Tablets 2281
Carafate Suspension 731
Carafate Tablets 730
▲ Cardura Tablets (3%) 2668
▲ Carnitor Injection (6% to 11%) 3242
▲ Casodex Tablets (4%) 662
▲ Ceclor CD Tablets (3.9%) 1279
Celebrex Capsules (2%) 2676
Celebrex Capsules (2%) 2780
▲ Celexa (5%) 1365
▲ CellCept Capsules (3% to 19%) 2951
▲ CellCept Intravenous (3% to 19%) 2951
▲ CellCept Oral Suspension (3% to 19%) 2951
▲ CellCept Tablets (3% to 19%) 2951
▲ Cenestin Tablets (8%) 1263
Cerebyx Injection (Infrequent) 2619
▲ Cognex Capsules (8%) 1351
Colazal Capsules (2%) 3069
▲ CombiPatch Transdermal System (19% to 22%) 2323
Combivent Inhalation Aerosol (1.1%) 1041
▲ Copaxone for Injection (14%) 3306
Coreg Tablets (More than 2%) 1508
Cozaar Tablets (Less than 1%) 2067
Crinone (Less than 5%) 3213
▲ DaunoXome Injection (Up to 12%) 1442
▲ DDAVP Nasal Spray (3% to 8%) 738
▲ DDAVP Rhinal Tube (3% to 8%) 738
Demadex Tablets and Injection (2.8%) 2965
▲ Depacon Injection (5%) 416
▲ Depakene (5%) 421
▲ Depakote Sprinkle Capsules (5%) 426
Depakote Tablets (1% to 5%) 430
Depakote ER Tablets (1% to 5%) 436
▲ Desmopressin Acetate Rhinal Tube (3% to 8%) 1345
Detrol Tablets (1.1%) 3623
Diovan Capsules (More than 1%) 2337
▲ Ditropan XL Extended Release Tablets (5.6%) 564
Dostinex Tablets (1%) 2804
Doxil Injection (Less than 1% to 5%) 566
Effexor Tablets 3495
▲ Effexor XR Capsules (8%) 3499
Elmiron Capsules (Less than or equal to 1%) 570
Emadine Ophthalmic Solution (Less than 5%) ⊙211
▲ Enbrel for Injection (16%) 1752
▲ Enbrel for Injection (16%) 3504
▲ Esclim Transdermal System (4.3% to 6.3%) 3460
▲ Evoxac Capsules (11.2%) 1217
▲ Exelon Capsules (4%) 2342
▲ Exelon Oral Solution (4%) 2345
▲ Felbatol (6.9%) 3343
▲ femhrt Tablets (15.1%) 2635
Ferrlecit Injection (Greater than 1%) 3386
▲ Flolan for Injection (21%) 1528
▲ Flomax Capsules (13.1% to 17.9%) 1044
▲ Flovent Diskus (4% to 13%) 3614
Flovent (1% to 3%) 1535
▲ Flovent Rotadisk (2% to 9%) 1537
Floxin Otic Solution (Single report) 1219
Fortovase Capsules (Less than 2%) 2970
Foscavir Injection (Between 1% and 5%) 605
Gabitril Tablets (1% or more) 1189
Gemzar for Injection (Infrequent) 1919
Gengraf Capsules (1% to 5.0%) 457
▲ Geodon Capsules (4%) 2688
Glucotrol XL Extended Release Tablets (Less than 3%) 2693
Gonal-F for Injection (0.8%) 3216
Helixate Concentrate 788
Heparin Lock Flush Solution 3509
Heparin Sodium Injection 3511
▲ Herceptin I.V. (14%) 1414
▲ Humatrope Vials and Cartridges (6.25% to 13.5%) 1930
Hytrin Capsules (At least 1% to 1.9%) 464
Hyzaar 2109
Imdur Tablets (Less than or equal to 5%) 1826
▲ Indapamide Tablets (Greater than or equal to 5%) 2286
▲ Infergen (7% to 13%) 1777
Intron A for Injection (Less than 5%) 3120
Invirase Capsules (Less than 2%) 2979
Iopidine 0.5% Ophthalmic Solution (Less than 3%) ⊙213
Kadian Capsules (Less than 3%) 1335
▲ Keppra Tablets (4%) 3314
Klonopin Tablets (2%) 2983
Kogenate FS 936
▲ Lamictal (13.6%) 1567
▲ Lescol Capsules (4.7%) 2361
▲ Lescol Capsules (4.7%) 2925
Lescol XL Tablets (1.5%) 2361
Lescol XL Tablets (1.5%) 2925
▲ Leukine (11%) 1755
Levaquin (0.5% to less than 1.0%) 2537
Lipitor Tablets (Greater than or equal to 2%) 2639
Lipitor Tablets (Greater than or equal to 2%) 2696
Lodine (Less than 1%) 3528
Lodine XL Extended-Release Tablets (Less than 1%) 3530
▲ Lorabid Suspension and Pulvules (1.6% to 6.3%) 2251
▲ Lotemax Sterile Ophthalmic Suspension 0.5% (Less than 15%) ⊙261
Lotensin HCT Tablets (More than 1%) 2367
Lupron Depot 3.75 mg (Less than 5%) 3281
Lupron Depot–3 Month 11.25 mg (Less than 5%) 3285
Luvox Tablets (25, 50, 100 mg) 3256
LYMErix Vaccine (1.41% to 2.41%) 1592
Marinol Capsules (Less than 1%) 3325
▲ Mepron Suspension (5% to 24%) 1598
▲ Meridia Capsules (10.2%) 481
Meruvax II 2130
▲ Miacalcin Nasal Spray (12%) 2375
Micardis Tablets (More than 0.3%) 1049
Micardis HCT Tablets 1051
▲ Migranal Nasal Spray (26%) 2376
Mirapex Tablets (1% or more) 2834
M-M-R II 2118
Monopril Tablets (0.2% to 1.0%) 1091
Monopril HCT (Less than 2%) 1094
▲ Monurol Sachet (4.5%) 1375
Motrin Suspension, Oral Drops, Chewable Tablets, and Caplets (Less than 1%) 2002
Mumpsvax 2141
MUSE Urethral Suppository (2%) 3335
▲ Mylotarg for Injection (8% to 14%) 3540
Myobloc Injectable Solution (1% to 5%) 1291
▲ Naprelan Tablets (3% to 9%) 1293
Nasacort AQ Nasal Spray (2% or greater) 752
Nascobal Gel (One patient) 3174
Nasonex Nasal Spray (Greater than or equal to 2%) 3131
Neoral Soft Gelatin Capsules (1% to 5.0%) 2380
Neoral Oral Solution (1% to 5.0%) 2380
▲ Neumega for Injection (42%) 1434
▲ Neurontin Capsules (4.1%) 2655
▲ Neurontin Oral Solution (4.1%) 2655
▲ Neurontin Tablets (4.1%) 2655
Nexium Delayed-Release Capsules (Less than 1%) 619
▲ Niaspan Extended-Release Tablets (2% to 5%) 1846
▲ Nicotrol Inhaler (23%) 2840
Nilandron Tablets (2%) 753
▲ Nipent for Injection (10% to 11%) 3272
Norvasc Tablets (Less than or equal to 0.1%) 2704
Norvir Capsules (Less than 2%) 487
Norvir Oral Solution (Less than 2%) 487
▲ Novantrone for Injection (10%) 1760
OptiPranolol Metipranolol Ophthalmic Solution 0.3% (A small number of patients) ⊙263
▲ Optivar Ophthalmic Solution (1% to 10%) 2273
Orudis Capsules (Less than 1%) 3548
Oruvail Capsules (Less than 1%) 3548
Patanol Ophthalmic Solution (Less than 5%) 540
Paxil (Frequent) 1609
▲ Permax Tablets (12.2%) 1299
▲ Plavix Tablets (4.2%) 1097
▲ Plavix Tablets (4.2%) 3084
▲ Pletal Tablets (7% to 12%) 2605
▲ Pletal Tablets (7% to 12%) 2848
▲ Prandin Tablets (0.5, 1, and 2 mg) (3% to 7%) 2432
Pravachol Tablets (0.1% to 4.0%) 1099
▲ Prempro Tablets (6% to 8%) 3572
Prilosec Delayed-Release Capsules (2%) 628
Prinivil Tablets (0.3% to 1.0%) 2164
Prinzide Tablets (0.3% to 1%) 2168
▲ Prograf (3% to 15%) 1393
▲ Proleukin for Injection (10%) 1199
ProSom Tablets (Infrequent) 500
Protonix I.V. (Greater than 1%) 3580
Protonix Tablets (Greater than or equal to 1%) 3577
▲ Protopic Ointment (3% to 5%) 1397
▲ Proventil HFA Inhalation Aerosol (16%) 3150
▲ Provigil Tablets (11%) 1193
Prozac Pulvules, Liquid, and Weekly Capsules (Less than 1%) 1238
▲ Pulmicort Respules (7% to 12%) 632
▲ Pulmicort Turbuhaler Inhalation Powder (2% to 6%) 636
▲ Pulmozyme Inhalation Solution (30%) 1426
▲ Qvar Inhalation Aerosol (3% to 8%) 1987
▲ Rapamune Oral Solution and Tablets (3% to 20%) 3584
Recombivax HB (Greater than 1%) 2178
ReFacto Vials 1437
▲ Remicade for IV Injection (6% to 9%) 1178
▲ Reminyl Oral Solution (4%) 1792
▲ Reminyl Tablets (4%) 1792
▲ Requip Tablets (4%) 1621
Rescriptor Tablets (Less than 2%) 526
Rescula Ophthalmic Solution (1% to 5%) ⊙306
Retrovir Capsules 1625
Retrovir IV Infusion 1629
Retrovir 1625
▲ Rilutek Tablets (7.8% to 8.9%) 772
▲ Risperdal (8% to 10%) 1796
▲ Rituxan for Infusion (0.3% to 8%) 1750
▲ Rituxan I.V. (0.3% to 8%) 1428
Roferon-A Injection (Less than 1% to 3%) 2996
Roxicodone Tablets (Less than 3%) 3067
▲ Salagen Tablets (5% to 14%) 2229
▲ Sandostatin LAR Depot (5% to 15%) 2395
▲ Sarafem Pulvules (23%) 1962
Sectral Capsules 3589
▲ Serevent Diskus (5%) 1637
Serevent Inhalation Aerosol (1% to 3%) 1633
▲ Seroquel Tablets (3%) 684
▲ Serostim for Injection (1% to 10%) 3229
Serzone Tablets 1104
▲ Simulect for Injection (3% to 10%) 2399
▲ Skelid Tablets (5.3%) 3088
▲ Soriatane Capsules (25% to 50%) 3003
▲ Sporanox Capsules (5% to 9%) 1800
Sporanox Oral Solution (Less than 2%) 1808
Sporanox Oral Solution (Less than 2%) 2512
▲ Stadol NS Nasal Spray (3% to 9%) 1108
Stimate Nasal Spray (Occasional) 796
Sular Tablets (Less than or equal to 1%) 688
▲ Synagis Intramuscular (28.7%) 2028
▲ Synarel Nasal Solution for Central Precocious Puberty (5%) 3204
Tasmar Tablets (Infrequent) 3010
Tenex Tablets (3% or less) 2942
▲ Teveten Tablets (4%) 3327
▲ Thalomid Capsules (4.2%) 1154
Tiazac Capsules (2%) 1378
▲ TOBI Solution for Inhalation (34.5%) 1206
Topamax Sprinkle Capsules (More than 1%) 2590
Topamax Tablets (More than 1%) 2590
Toradol (1% or less) 3018
▲ Tricor Capsules, Micronized (4%) 513
▲ Trileptal Oral Suspension (2% to 10%) 2407
▲ Trileptal Tablets (2% to 10%) 2407
Tri-Nasal Spray (2%) 2274
Trovan (Less than 1%) 2722
Uniretic Tablets (More than 1%) 3178
Univasc Tablets (More than 1%) 3181
Vantin Tablets and Oral Suspension (Less than 1%) 2860
Vascor Tablets (0.5% to 2.0%) 2602
Verelan PM Capsules (2.7%) 3186
Vexol 1% Ophthalmic Suspension (Less than 2%) ⊙222
Vicoprofen Tablets (Less than 3%) 520
Viracept 532
Vistide Injection 1445
Voltaren Ophthalmic Sterile Ophthalmic Solution (Less than 3%) ⊙312
▲ WelChol Tablets (3%) 3073
Wellbutrin SR Sustained-Release Tablets (At least 1%) 1684
▲ Xopenex Inhalation Solution (2.7% to 11.1%) 3207
▲ Zaditor Ophthalmic Solution (10% to 25%) 2304
▲ Zanaflex Tablets (3%) 1305
▲ Zebeta Tablets (2.9% to 4.0%) 1885
▲ Zenapax for Injection (2% to 5%) 3046
Zestoretic Tablets (0.3% to 1%) 695
Zestril Tablets (0.3% to 1.0%) 698
Ziac Tablets (0.7% to 0.9%) 1887
Zoladex (1% or greater) 702
Zoladex 3-month 706
Zoloft (Frequent) 2751
Zonegran Capsules (2%) 1307
Zosyn (1.2%) 1890
Zosyn in Galaxy Containers (1.2%) 1894
▲ Zyban Sustained-Release Tablets (12%) 1710
▲ Zyprexa Tablets (10%) 1973
▲ Zyprexa ZYDIS Orally Disintegrating Tablets (10%) 1973
Zyrtec (Less than 2%) 2756
Zyrtec-D 12 Hour Extended Relief Tablets (Less than 2%) 2758

Rhinitis, allergic

BeneFix for Injection 1432
Imitrex Injection 1549
Imitrex Nasal Spray 1554
Vioxx (Greater than 0.1% to 1.9%) 2213

Rhinitis, ulcerative

Atrovent Nasal Spray 0.03% (2.0%) 1032

Rhinorrhea

Aceon Tablets (2 mg, 4 mg, 8 mg) (0.3% to 1%) 3249
Advair Diskus 100/50 (1% to 3%) 1448
Advair Diskus 250/50 (1% to 3%) 1448
Advair Diskus 500/50 (1% to 3%) 1448
▲ Aerobid/Aerobid-M (3% to 9%) 1363
▲ Atrovent Nasal Spray 0.03% (3.1%) 1032
Beconase Inhalation Aerosol (1 per 100 patients) 1497
Beconase AQ Nasal Spray (Fewer than 3 per 100 patients) 1498
Calcijex Injection 411
Chemet Capsules (0.7% to 3.7%) 3078
Clozaril Tablets (Less than 1%) 2319
Colyte with Flavor Packs for Oral Solution (Isolated cases) 3170
Comvax (0.2% to 1.3%) 2056
Enalaprilat Injection 863
Flonase Nasal Spray (1% to 3%) 1533
Flovent Diskus (1% to 3%) 3614
Floxin I.V. (Less than 1%) 2526
Floxin Tablets (Less than 1%) 2529
GoLYTELY and Pineapple Flavor GoLYTELY for Oral Solution (Isolated cases) 1068
Hectorol Capsules 1064
Hectorol Injection 1066
Indapamide Tablets (Less than 5%) 2286
Intron A for Injection (Less than 5%) 3120
Klonopin Tablets 2983
Lexxel Tablets 608
Maxalt Tablets (Rare) 2120
Maxalt-MLT Orally Disintegrating Tablets (Rare) 2120
Nicotrol Nasal Spray (Common) 2843
NuLYTELY, Cherry Flavor, Lemon-Lime Flavor, and Orange Flavor NuLYTELY for Oral Solution (Isolated cases) 1068
Plendil Extended-Release Tablets (0.2% to 1.6%) 623
Prinivil Tablets (0.3% to 1.0%) 2164
Prinzide Tablets 2168
Rocaltrol 2991
▲ Roferon-A Injection (4% to 12%) 2996
Singulair (Greater than or equal to 2%) 2181
Soma Compound Tablets 3354

Soma Compound w/Codeine Tablets ... 3355
Vancenase PocketHaler Nasal Inhaler (1 per 100 patients) ... 3162
Vaseretic Tablets ... 2204
Vasotec I.V. Injection ... 2207
Vasotec Tablets (0.5% to 1.0%) ... 2210
Versed Syrup (0.25%) ... 3033
Zestoretic Tablets ... 695
Zestril Tablets (0.3% to 1.0%) ... 698

Rhonchi

Brevibloc Injection (Less than 1%) ... 858
Crixivan Capsules (Less than 2%) ... 2070
Hivid Tablets (Less than 1%) ... 2975
▲ Mylotarg for Injection (10% to 16%) ... 3540
ReoPro Vials (0.1%) ... 1958
Survanta Intratracheal Suspension ... 3053
▲ Trisenox Injection (8%) ... 1158
Versed Syrup (1%) ... 3033
Zemuron Injection (Less than 1%) ... 2491

Rigidity

Ambien Tablets (Rare) ... 3191
Brevibloc Injection (Less than 1%) ... 858
Cardura Tablets (Less than 0.5%) ... 2668
Cedax Oral Suspension (0.1% to 1%) ... 1021
Claritin (At least one patient) ... 3100
Claritin-D 12 Hour Extended Release Tablets (Less frequent) ... 3102
Claritin-D 24 Hour Extended Release Tablets (Fewer than 2%) ... 3104
▲ Clozaril Tablets (3%) ... 2319
Cytotec Tablets (Infrequent) ... 3202
▲ DaunoXome Injection (Up to 19%) ... 1442
Dipentum Capsules (Rare) ... 2803
Diprivan Injectable Emulsion (Less than 1%) ... 667
▲ Ergamisol Tablets (3% to 5%) ... 1789
Ethyol for Injection (Rare) ... 2029
Famvir Tablets (0.5% to 1.5%) ... 2348
Fareston Tablets ... 3237
Felbatol ... 3343
Flumadine ... 1370
▲ Foscavir Injection (5% or greater) ... 605
Gengraf Capsules (1% to less than 3%) ... 457
Hivid Tablets (Less than 1%) ... 2975
Hyzaar ... 2109
Imdur Tablets (Less than or equal to 5%) ... 1826
Imitrex Tablets (Rare) ... 1558
▲ Infergen (57% to 62%) ... 1777
▲ Intron A for Injection (Up to 42%) ... 3120
Ismo Tablets (Fewer than 1%) ... 3524
Moban ... 1320
Naropin Injection (1% to 5%) ... 612
Neoral Soft Gelatin Capsules (1% to less than 3%) ... 2380
Neoral Oral Solution (1% to less than 3%) ... 2380
Norvasc Tablets (More than 0.1% to 1%) ... 2704
▲ Orap Tablets (2 of 20 patients) ... 1407
▲ Orthoclone OKT3 Sterile Solution (8%) ... 2498
Pediazole Suspension ... 3050
Procardia XL Extended Release Tablets (1% or less) ... 2710
Proleukin for Injection ... 1199
Proventil HFA Inhalation Aerosol (Less than 3%) ... 3150
Risperdal (Infrequent) ... 1796
Romazicon Injection (Less than 1%) ... 3000
▲ Serostim for Injection (1% to 10%) ... 3229
▲ Soriatane Capsules (10% to 25%) ... 3003
Sporanox Oral Solution (Less than 2%) ... 1808
Sporanox Oral Solution (Less than 2%) ... 2512
Vanceril Double Strength Inhalation Aerosol (Fewer than 2%) ... 3167
▲ Xanax Tablets (4.2%) ... 2865
Zoloft (Infrequent) ... 2751
Zosyn (1.0% or less) ... 1890
Zosyn in Galaxy Containers (1.0% or less) ... 1894
Zovirax for Injection (Less than 1%) ... 1708
Zyrtec (Less than 2%) ... 2756
Zyrtec-D 12 Hour Extended Relief Tablets (Less than 2%) ... 2758

Rigors

AmBisome for Injection (Less common) ... 1383
Avonex ... 1013
▲ Campath Ampules (16% to 86%) ... 992
Celexa (Infrequent) ... 1365
Chirocaine Injection (2.9%) ... 2909
Evoxac Capsules (1.3%) ... 1217
Exelon Capsules (Frequent) ... 2342
Exelon Oral Solution (Frequent) ... 2345
Ferrlecit Injection (Greater than 1%) ... 3386
▲ Gengraf Capsules (3%) ... 457
Herceptin I.V. ... 1414
Levaquin Injection (Less than 0.5%) ... 2537
LYMErix Vaccine (1.74% to 2.78%) ... 1592
Migranal Nasal Spray (Infrequent) ... 2376
Nexium Delayed-Release Capsules (Less than 1%) ... 619
▲ PEG-Intron Powder for Injection (23%) ... 3140
▲ Rebetron Combination Therapy (32% to 42%) ... 3153
Requip Tablets (1% or more) ... 1621
Romazicon Injection (Less than 1%) ... 3000
▲ Sandostatin LAR Depot (5% to 15%) ... 2395
▲ Simulect for Injection (3% to 10%) ... 2399
Sporanox Injection (Less than 1%) ... 1804
Sporanox Injection (Less than 1%) ... 2509
Teveten Tablets (Less than 1%) ... 3327
▲ Tice BCG, BCG Live (3%) ... 2489
Topamax Sprinkle Capsules (0.4% to 1.8%) ... 2590
Topamax Tablets (0.4% to 1.8%) ... 2590
Trileptal Oral Suspension ... 2407
Trileptal Tablets ... 2407
▲ Trisenox Injection (38%) ... 1158
Ultracet Tablets (Less than 1%) ... 2597

Romberg test, positive

Neurontin Capsules (Infrequent) ... 2655
Neurontin Oral Solution (Infrequent) ... 2655
Neurontin Tablets (Infrequent) ... 2655

Rosacea

Elocon Cream 0.1% ... 3110
Elocon Ointment 0.1% ... 3112
Evoxac Capsules (Less than 1%) ... 1217
Vaniqa Cream (Less than 1%) ... 1121

Rosacea, worsening of

MetroCream (Less than 3%) ... 1404
MetroLotion (1%) ... 1405
Noritate Cream (One patient) ... 1224

Roseola

Prevnar for Injection ... 1870

S

S_3 gallop

(*see under* Ventricular gallop)

Saliva, discoloration

Lodosyn Tablets ... 1251
Mycobutin Capsules ... 2838
Rifadin ... 765
Sinemet Tablets ... 1253
Sinemet CR Tablets ... 1255

Salivary gland enlargement

Aciphex Tablets (Rare) ... 1267
Aciphex Tablets (Rare) ... 1783
Arava Tablets (1% to 3%) ... 724
Betaseron for SC Injection ... 988
Clozaril Tablets ... 2319
Copaxone for Injection (Frequent) ... 3306
Evoxac Capsules (1% to 3%) ... 1217
Gengraf Capsules (1% to less than 3%) ... 457
Hivid Tablets (Less than 1%) ... 2975
Imitrex Nasal Spray ... 1554
Lithobid Slow-Release Tablets ... 3255
Neoral Soft Gelatin Capsules (1% to less than 3%) ... 2380
Neoral Oral Solution (1% to less than 3%) ... 2380
Neurontin Capsules (Rare) ... 2655
Neurontin Oral Solution (Rare) ... 2655
Neurontin Tablets (Rare) ... 2655
Pediazole Suspension ... 3050
Permax Tablets (Infrequent) ... 1299
Prozac Pulvules, Liquid, and Weekly Capsules (Rare) ... 1238
Remeron Tablets (Rare) ... 2483
Remeron SolTab Tablets (Rare) ... 2486
Rilutek Tablets (Rare) ... 772
Salagen Tablets (Less than 1%) ... 2229
Sarafem Pulvules (Rare) ... 1962

Salivation

(*see under* Sialism)

Salivation, increase

(*see under* Sialism)

Salpingitis

Amerge Tablets (Rare) ... 1467
Betaseron for SC Injection ... 988
Effexor Tablets (Rare) ... 3495
Effexor XR Capsules (Rare) ... 3499
Gabitril Tablets (Infrequent) ... 1189
Permax Tablets (Infrequent) ... 1299
Salagen Tablets (Less than 1%) ... 2229
Wellbutrin SR Sustained-Release Tablets ... 1684
Zyban Sustained-Release Tablets ... 1710

Sarcoidosis

Risperdal (Rare) ... 1796

Sarcoma, bone

Permax Tablets (Infrequent) ... 1299

Sarcoma, multiple idiopathic hemorrhagic

(*see under* Kaposi's sarcoma)

Sarcoma, unspecified

Betaseron for SC Injection ... 988
Foscavir Injection (Between 1% and 5%) ... 605
Megace Oral Suspension (1% to 3%) ... 1124
Thalomid Capsules ... 1154
Vistide Injection ... 1445

Scabbing

▲ Aldara Cream, 5% (Up to 13%) ... 1978
Avita Cream ... 999
Condylox Gel (Less common) ... 2436
Levulan Kerastick (Up to 2%) ... 971

Scalp, dry

Nizoral 2% Shampoo ... 2007
Selsun Rx 2.5% Lotion, USP ... 3053

Scalp, oily

Nizoral 2% Shampoo ... 2007
Selsun Rx 2.5% Lotion, USP ... 3053

Scalp, tightness

Cormax Scalp Application (Approximately 0.3%) ... 2441
Temovate Scalp Application (1 of 294 patients) ... 1304

Scarring

Condylox Topical Solution (Less than 5%) ... 2437
▲ Efudex (Among most frequent) ... 1733
Fluoroplex (Occasional) ... 552
Tubersol Diagnostic Antigen ... 3628

Schizophrenia, precipitation

Nardil Tablets (Less frequent) ... 2653
Zyprexa Tablets ... 1973
Zyprexa ZYDIS Orally Disintegrating Tablets ... 1973

Sciatica

Ambien Tablets (Rare) ... 3191
Atacand HCT Tablets (0.5% or greater) ... 597
Vioxx (Greater than 0.1% to 1.9%) ... 2213
Wellbutrin Tablets (Rare) ... 1680

Sclera, discoloration

Hivid Tablets (Less than 1%) ... 2975
Minipress Capsules (1% to 4%) ... 2699
Minizide Capsules ... 2700
Serentil ... 1057
Ticlid Tablets ... 3015

Sclera, infection

Urobiotic-250 Capsules ... 2731

Scleral injection

Azulfidine EN-tabs Tablets (Rare) ... 2775
Bactrim ... 2949
Pediazole Suspension ... 3050
Prelone Syrup ... 2273
Septra Suspension ... 2265
Septra Tablets ... 2265
Septra DS Tablets ... 2265

Scleritis

Ambien Tablets (Infrequent) ... 3191
Aredia for Injection (Rare) ... 2309
Effexor Tablets (Rare) ... 3495
Effexor XR Capsules (Rare) ... 3499
Evoxac Capsules (Less than 1%) ... 1217
Prozac Pulvules, Liquid, and Weekly Capsules (Rare) ... 1238
Sarafem Pulvules (Rare) ... 1962

Scleroderma

Depo-Provera Contraceptive Injection (Fewer than 1%) ... 2798
Evoxac Capsules (Less than 1%) ... 1217
Soriatane Capsules (Less than 1%) ... 3003

Sclerosis

Vitrasert Implant (Less than 1%) ... ⊙254

Sclerosis, multiple

Enbrel for Injection ... 1752
Enbrel for Injection ... 3504
Engerix-B Vaccine (Less than 1%) ... 1517
Evoxac Capsules (Less than 1%) ... 1217
Havrix Vaccine (Rare) ... 1544
LYMErix Vaccine (Greater than 1%) ... 1592
Rabies Vaccine RabAvert (Two cases) ... 1203
Recombivax HB ... 2178
Twinrix Vaccine ... 1674

Sclerosis, skin

Norplant System (Rare) ... 3543
Parnate Tablets ... 1607

Scotomata

Adenoscan (Less than 1%) ... 1381
Amerge Tablets (Rare) ... 1467
Aralen Tablets ... 3075
Axert Tablets (Rare) ... 2772
Cataflam Tablets (Less than 1%) ... 2315
Cordarone Tablets ... 3487
Desferal Vials ... 2333
Eskalith ... 1527
Lithium Carbonate ... 3061
Lithium Citrate Syrup ... 3061
Lithobid Slow-Release Tablets ... 3255
Motrin Suspension, Oral Drops, Chewable Tablets, and Caplets (Less than 1%) ... 2002
Pacerone Tablets ... 3331
Plaquenil Tablets ... 3082
ProSom Tablets (Rare) ... 500
Quinaglute Dura-Tabs Tablets (Occasional) ... 978
Quinidex Extentabs (Occasional) ... 2933
Requip Tablets (Rare) ... 1621
Sandostatin LAR Depot (Rare) ... 2395
▲ Serzone Tablets (7%) ... 1104
Topamax Sprinkle Capsules (Infrequent) ... 2590
Topamax Tablets (Infrequent) ... 2590
Trental Tablets (Less than 1%) ... 784
Trileptal Oral Suspension ... 2407
Trileptal Tablets ... 2407
Trovan (Less than 1%) ... 2722
Voltaren Tablets (Less than 1%) ... 2315
Voltaren-XR Tablets (Less than 1%) ... 2315

Scotomata, scintillating

Clomid Tablets (1.5%) ... 735
Serophene Tablets ... 3226
Taxol Injection (Rare) ... 1129

Scrotal disorder, unspecified

Caverject Sterile Powder (Less than 1%) ... 2777

Seborrhea

Accutane Capsules ... 2944
Androderm Transdermal System CIII ... 3377
Avonex ... 1013
Betaseron for SC Injection ... 988
Cognex Capsules (Rare) ... 1351
Crinone (Less than 5%) ... 3213
Crixivan Capsules (Less than 2%) ... 2070
DaunoXome Injection (Less than or equal to 5%) ... 1442
Depacon Injection (1% or more) ... 416
Depakene (1% or more) ... 421
Depakote Sprinkle Capsules ... 426
Depakote Tablets (1% to 5%) ... 430
Depakote ER Tablets (Greater than 1%) ... 436
Effexor Tablets (Rare) ... 3495
Effexor XR Capsules (Rare) ... 3499
Evoxac Capsules (Less than 1%) ... 1217
Fludara for Injection (Up to 1%) ... 995
Fortovase Capsules (Less than 2%) ... 2970
Foscavir Injection (Between 1% and 5%) ... 605
Invirase Capsules (Less than 2%) ... 2979
Lamictal (Rare) ... 1567
Lipitor Tablets (Less than 2%) ... 2639
Lipitor Tablets (Less than 2%) ... 2696
Loxitane Capsules ... 3398
Lupron Depot-PED 7.5 mg, 11.25 mg and 15 mg (2%) ... 3291
Lupron Injection Pediatric ... 3280
Luvox Tablets (25, 50, 100 mg) (Infrequent) ... 3256
Neurontin Capsules (Infrequent) ... 2655
Neurontin Oral Solution (Infrequent) ... 2655
Neurontin Tablets (Infrequent) ... 2655
Norvir Capsules (Less than 2%) ... 487
Norvir Oral Solution (Less than 2%) ... 487
Paxil (Rare) ... 1609
Permax Tablets (Infrequent) ... 1299
Prozac Pulvules, Liquid, and Weekly Capsules (Rare) ... 1238
Remeron Tablets (Rare) ... 2483
Remeron SolTab Tablets (Rare) ... 2486
Requip Tablets (Infrequent) ... 1621
Rescriptor Tablets (Less than 2%) ... 526
Rilutek Tablets (Infrequent) ... 772
Risperdal (Up to 1%) ... 1796
Roferon-A Injection (Less than 1%) ... 2996
Salagen Tablets (Less than 1%) ... 2229
Sarafem Pulvules (Rare) ... 1962
Seroquel Tablets (Infrequent) ... 684
▲ Serostim for Injection (1% to 10%) ... 3229
▲ Soriatane Capsules (1% to 10%) ... 3003
Synagis Intramuscular (More than 1%) ... 2028
▲ Synarel Nasal Solution for Central Precocious Puberty (3%) ... 3204
▲ Synarel Nasal Solution for Endometriosis (8% of patients) ... 3205
Tasmar Tablets (Infrequent) ... 3010
Testoderm Transdermal Systems ... 574
Thalomid Capsules ... 1154
Topamax Sprinkle Capsules (Infrequent) ... 2590
Topamax Tablets (Infrequent) ... 2590
Trovan (Less than 1%) ... 2722
Vistide Injection ... 1445
▲ Zoladex (26%) ... 702

Zoladex 3-month 706
Zyprexa Tablets (Infrequent) 1973
Zyprexa ZYDIS Orally Disintegrating Tablets (Infrequent) 1973
Zyrtec (Less than 2%) 2756
Zyrtec-D 12 Hour Extended Relief Tablets (Less than 2%) 2758

Sedation

Aldoclor Tablets 2035
Aldomet Tablets 2037
Aldoril Tablets 2039
Amerge Tablets (Rare) 1467
Ancobon Capsules 1730
Ativan Injection 3478
▲ Ativan Tablets (15.9%) 3482
▲ Benadryl Parenteral (Among most frequent) 2617
▲ Buprenex Injectable (Most frequent) 2918
▲ Catapres Tablets (About 10 in 100 patients) 1037
Catapres-TTS (3 of 101 patients) 1038
▲ Clorpres Tablets (About 10%) 1002
▲ Clozaril Tablets (More than 5% to 39%) 2319
▲ Combipres Tablets (About 10%) 1040
Corgard Tablets (6 of 1000 patients) 2245
Corzide 40/5 Tablets (6 of 1000 patients) 2247
Corzide 80/5 Tablets (6 of 1000 patients) 2247
▲ Darvon-N/Darvocet-N (Among most frequent) 1907
▲ Darvon Pulvules (Among most frequent) 1909
▲ Darvon Compound-65 Pulvules (Among most frequent) 1910
▲ Darvon-N Tablets (Among most frequent) 1912
▲ Demerol (Among most frequent) 3079
▲ Demser Capsules (Almost all patients) 2085
Depacon Injection 416
Depakene 421
Depakote Tablets 430
Depakote ER Tablets 436
Dilaudid 441
Dilaudid Oral Liquid 445
Dilaudid Powder 441
Dilaudid Rectal Suppositories 441
Dilaudid Tablets 441
Dilaudid Tablets - 8 mg 445
▲ Dilaudid-HP (Among most frequent) 443
▲ Dolophine Hydrochloride Tablets (Among most frequent) 3056
Duraclon Injection 3057
Etrafon (Less frequent) 3115
Halcion Tablets 2823
Hycodan 1316
Hycomine Compound Tablets 1317
Hycotuss Expectorant Syrup 1318
Imitrex Injection (2.7%) 1549
Imitrex Nasal Spray (Infrequent) 1554
Imitrex Tablets 1558
Kadian Capsules (Less than 3%) 1335
▲ Lortab (Among most frequent) 3319
▲ Lortab Elixir (Among most frequent) 3317
▲ Maxidone Tablets CIII (Among most frequent) 3399
▲ Mepergan Injection (Among most frequent) 3539
Motofen Tablets 577
▲ MS Contin Tablets (Among most frequent) 2896
▲ MSIR (Among most frequent) 2898
Nadolol Tablets (6 of 1000 patients) 2288
Navane Oral 2701
Navane Intramuscular 2703
▲ Norco 5/325 Tablets CIII (Among most frequent) 3424
▲ Norco 7.5/325 Tablets CIII (Among most frequent) 3425
▲ Norco 10/325 Tablets CIII (Among most frequent) 3425
▲ Norco 10/325 Tablets CIII (Among most frequent) 3427
▲ Nubain Injection (36%) 1323
▲ Oramorph SR Tablets (Among most frequent) 3062
▲ Orap Tablets (14 of 20 patients) 1407
▲ OxyFast Oral Concentrate Solution (Among most frequent) 2916
▲ OxyIR Capsules (Among most frequent) 2916
▲ Percocet Tablets (Among most frequent) 1326
▲ Percodan Tablets (Among most frequent) 1327
▲ Percolone Tablets (Among most frequent) 1327
Periactin Tablets 2155
Phenergan Suppositories 3556
Phenergan Syrup 3554
Phenergan with Codeine Syrup 3557
Phenergan with Dextromethorphan Syrup 3559
Phenergan VC Syrup 3560
Phenergan VC with Codeine Syrup 3561
▲ Phrenilin (Among most frequent) 578
Roferon-A Injection (Infrequent) 2996
▲ Roxanol (Among most frequent) 3066
▲ Roxicodone (Among most frequent) 3067
▲ Ryna-12 S Suspension (Among most common) 3351
▲ Reformulated Rynatan Pediatric Suspension (Among most common) 3352
▲ Rynatan Tablets (Among most common) 3351
▲ Rynatuss Pediatric Suspension (Among most common) 3353
▲ Rynatuss Tablets (Among most common) 3353
▲ Sedapap Tablets 50 mg/650 mg (Among the most frequent) 2225
▲ Semprex-D Capsules (6% more common than with placebo) 1172
Soma Compound w/Codeine Tablets 3355
Talacen Caplets 3089
Talwin Nx Tablets 3090
▲ Tenex Tablets (5% to 39%) 2942
Tessalon Capsules 1377
Thiothixene Capsules 2290
▲ Tussi-12 S Suspension 3356
Tussi-12 Tablets 3356
Tussionex Pennkinetic Extended-Release Suspension 1174
▲ Tylenol with Codeine (Among most frequent) 2595
▲ Tylox Capsules (Among most frequent) 2597
Valcyte Tablets 3022
Versed Injection (1.6%) 3027
Versed Syrup (Less than 1%) 3033
▲ Vicodin Tablets (Among most frequent) 516
▲ Vicodin ES Tablets (Among most frequent) 517
▲ Vicodin HP Tablets (Among most frequent) 518
Vicodin Tuss Expectorant 519
▲ Wellbutrin Tablets (19.8%) 1680
Xanax Tablets 2865
▲ Zanaflex Tablets (48%) 1305
▲ Zofran Injection (8%) 1698
▲ Zofran (20%) 1703
▲ Zofran ODT Orally Disintegrating Tablets (20%) 1703
▲ Zydone Tablets (Among most frequent) 1330

Seizure control, loss of

Depakote Sprinkle Capsules 426

Seizures

(see also under Convulsions)

Accutane Capsules 2944
Acel-Imune (One child) 1851
Actimmune (Rare) 1772
Activase I.V. 1410
Agrylin Capsules 3232
Allegra-D Extended-Release Tablets 714
Aloprim for Injection (Less than 1%) 2292
▲ Aredia for Injection (3% to 4%) 2309
Attenuvax (Rare) 2044
▲ Avonex (3%) 1013
Azactam for Injection (Less than 1%) 1276
Bicillin C-R 900/300 Injection 2240
Bicillin C-R Injection 2238
Bicillin L-A Injection 2242
Brethine Ampuls (Rare) 2314
Brethine Tablets (Rare) 2313
Brevital Sodium for Injection, USP 1815
Carbatrol Capsules 3234
Carnitor Injection 3242
Carnitor Tablets and Oral Solution 3245
Ceclor 1905
Ceftin Tablets 1898
Cefzil 1076
Celexa (0.3%) 1365
Ceptaz for Injection (Fewer than 1%) 1499
Cipro I.V. Pharmacy Bulk Package (Less than 1%) 897
Claritin (Rare) 3100
Claritin-D 24 Hour Extended Release Tablets 3104
Clomid Tablets 735
▲ Clozaril Tablets (3% to approximately 5%) 2319
Combivir Tablets 1502
Dantrium Capsules (Less frequent) 2885
DDAVP Injection 4 mcg/mL (Rare) 737
DDAVP Nasal Spray (Rare) 738
DDAVP Rhinal Tube (Rare) 738
Desmopressin Acetate Injection (Rare) 1344
Diflucan Tablets, Injection, and Oral Suspension 2681
Dilaudid 441
Dilaudid Oral Liquid 445
Dilaudid Powder 441
Dilaudid Tablets - 8 mg 445
Dilaudid-HP Injection 443
Diprivan Injectable Emulsion (Less than 1%) 667
Duricef 1079
Ecotrin Enteric Coated Aspirin Low, Regular and Maximum Strength Tablets 1715
Effexor XR Capsules (Infrequent) 3499
Eldepryl Capsules 3266
Enbrel for Injection 1752
Enbrel for Injection 3504
Engerix-B Vaccine (Less than 1%) 1517
Epogen for Injection (1.1% to approximately 2.5%) 582
Ergamisol Tablets 1789
Ery-Tab Tablets (Isolated reports) 448
Erythrocin Stearate Filmtab Tablets (Isolated reports) 452
Erythromycin Base Filmtab Tablets (Isolated reports) 454
Erythromycin Delayed-Release Capsules, USP (Isolated reports) 455
Ethyol for Injection (Rare) 2029
Etrafon 3115
Floxin I.V. (Less than 1%) 2526
Floxin Tablets (Less than 1%) 2529
Fluothane Inhalation 3508
Fortaz 1541
Fortovase Capsules (Rare) 2970
▲ Foscavir Injection (5% to 10%) 605
Geodon Capsules (0.4%) 2688
Guaifed 2272
Hexalen Capsules (1%) 2226
HibTITER (One case) 1859
Hivid Tablets (Less than 1% to 1.3%) 2975
▲ Idamycin PFS Injection (4%) 2825
Ifex for Injection (Occasional) 1123
Imitrex Nasal Spray (Rare) 1554
Imitrex Tablets (Rare) 1558
INFeD Injection 3388
JE-VAX Vaccine (1 to 2.3 per million vaccines) 811
Kefzol Vials, ADD-Vantage 1951
K-Phos Neutral Tablets 946
Lariam Tablets 2989
Leukeran Tablets (Rare) 1591
Levoxyl Tablets (Rare) 1819
Lindane Lotion USP 1% (Exceedingly rare) 559
Lindane Shampoo USP 1% (Exceedingly rare) 560
Lorabid Suspension and Pulvules 2251
Loxitane Capsules 3398
Maxipime for Injection 1285
Mefoxin for Injection 2124
Mefoxin Premixed Intravenous Solution 2127
Meridia Capsules (0.1%) 481
Merrem I.V. (0.1% to 1.0%) 673
Mexitil Capsules (About 2 in 1,000) 1047
MS Contin Tablets (Less frequent) 2896
MSIR (Less frequent) 2898
Myleran Tablets 1603
Narcan Injection 1322
Navane Oral (Infrequent) 2701
Navane Intramuscular (Infrequent) 2703
Noroxin Tablets 2145
Norpramin Tablets 755
Norvir Capsules 487
Norvir Oral Solution 487
Novantrone for Injection (2% to 4%) 1760
Omnicef 493
Oramorph SR Tablets (Less frequent) 3062
Orap Tablets 1407
Orthoclone OKT3 Sterile Solution 2498
OxyContin Tablets (Less than 1%) 2912
Liquid PedvaxHIB (Infrequent) 2148
Primaxin I.M. 2158
Primaxin I.V. (0.4%) 2160
Prinzide Tablets 2168
▲ Procrit for Injection (1.1% to 10%) 2502
ProSom Tablets (Infrequent) 500
Prozac Pulvules, Liquid, and Weekly Capsules (0.1%) 1238
Remeron Tablets (One patient) 2483
Remeron SolTab Tablets (One patient) 2486
Retrovir Capsules (Rare; 0.8%) 1625
Retrovir IV Infusion (Rare; 1%) 1629
Retrovir (Rare; 0.8%) 1625
Risperdal (0.3%) 1796
Robinul Injectable 2940
Roferon-A Injection (Less than 1% to less than 4%) 2996
Romazicon Injection 3000
Rythmol Tablets – 150 mg, 225 mg, 300 mg (0.3%) 502
Saizen for Injection (Infrequent) 3225
Sandostatin Injection (Less than 1%) 2394
Serophene Tablets 3226
Seroquel Tablets (0.6%) 684
Serzone Tablets (One patient) 1104
Sinequan (Infrequent) 2713
Singulair (Very rare) 2181
Suprax 1877
Surmontil Capsules 3595
Tamiflu Capsules 3008
Tamiflu Oral Suspension 3008
Tazidime Vials, Faspak & ADD-Vantage 1966
Tegretol/Tegretol-XR 2404
Thiothixene Capsules 2290
Tonocard Tablets (Less than 1%) 649
Trizivir Tablets 1669
Ultracet Tablets 2597
Ultram Tablets (Less than 1%) 2600
Unithroid Tablets (Rare) 3445
Urecholine Tablets 2445
Uroqid-Acid No. 2 Tablets 947
Vaseretic Tablets 2204
Versed Injection (1.1%) 3027
Viagra Tablets 2732
Viracept 532
Vivactil Tablets 2217
Vivactil Tablets 2446
Wellbutrin Tablets (Frequent) 1680
Wellbutrin SR Sustained-Release Tablets (Approximately 0.1% to 0.4%) 1684
Xanax Tablets 2865
Zinacef Injection 1696
Zinacef for Injection 1696
Zovirax Capsules 1706
Zovirax for Injection (Approximately 1%) 1708
Zovirax 1706
Zyban Sustained-Release Tablets 1710
Zyprexa Tablets (0.9%) 1973
Zyprexa ZYDIS Orally Disintegrating Tablets (0.9%) 1973
Zyrtec-D 12 Hour Extended Relief Tablets 2758

Seizures, afebrile

Attenuvax 2044
M-M-R II 2118

Seizures, complex partial

Seizures, convulsive

Aralen Tablets 3075
Cipro I.V. (1% or less) 893
Cipro (Less than 1%) 887
Cylert Tablets 415
Etrafon 3115
Phenergan Injection 3553
Phenergan 3556
Reglan (Isolated reports) 2935
Robaxin Injectable 2938
Robaxin Tablets 2939
Serentil 1057
Thioridazine Hydrochloride Tablets (Infrequent) 2289
Thorazine 1656
Timentin Injection- ADD-Vantage Vial 1661
Timentin Injection-Galaxy Container 1664
Timentin Injection-Pharmacy Bulk Package 1666
Timentin for Intravenous Administration 1658
Trilafon 3160

Seizures, epileptiform

Eskalith 1527
Etrafon (A few instances) 3115
Lithium Carbonate 3061
Lithium Citrate Syrup 3061
Lithobid Slow-Release Tablets 3255

Seizures, exacerbation of

Enbrel for Injection (Rare) 1752
Enbrel for Injection (Rare) 3504
Lamictal (2.3%) 1567
Serzone Tablets (One patient) 1104
Topamax Sprinkle Capsules (More than 1%) 2590
Topamax Tablets (More than 1%) 2590

Seizures, febrile

Attenuvax 2044
M-M-R II 2118
Mumpsvax 2141
Prevnar for Injection 1870

Seizures, generalized

Chibroxin Sterile Ophthalmic Solution 2051
Leukeran Tablets (Rare) 1591
Noroxin Tablets 2145

Seizures, grand mal

Famotidine Injection (Infrequent) 866
▲ Foscavir Injection (5% or greater) 605
Haldol Decanoate 2535
Haldol Injection, Tablets and Concentrate 2533
Hivid Tablets (Less than 1%) 2975
Orap Tablets 1407
Pepcid Injection (Infrequent) 2153
Pepcid for Oral Suspension (Infrequent) 2150
Pepcid RPD Orally Disintegrating Tablets (Infrequent) 2150
Pepcid Tablets (Infrequent) 2150
Proleukin for Injection (1%) 1199
Serzone Tablets (Rare) 1104
Taxol Injection (Rare) 1129
Thorazine 1656

Topamax Sprinkle Capsules (Frequent) 2590
Topamax Tablets (Frequent) 2590
Zofran Injection (Rare) 1698
Zofran (Rare) 1703
Zofran ODT Orally Disintegrating Tablets (Rare) 1703

Seizures, neonatal
Captopril Tablets 2281
Versed Injection 3027

Seizures, non-febrile
Varivax 2202

Seminal volume, decrease in
Anadrol-50 Tablets 3321

Sensation, abnormal
(*see under* Paresthesia)

Sensation, disturbance of temperature
Amerge Tablets (Frequent) 1467
Dopram Injectable 2931
Duranest Injections 600
▲ Imitrex Injection (10.8%) 1549
Imitrex Nasal Spray (Infrequent) 1554
Imitrex Tablets (2% to 3%) 1558
Iopidine Sterile Ophthalmic Solution .... ⊙212
Lidoderm Patch 1319
Maxalt Tablets (Infrequent) 2120
Maxalt-MLT Orally Disintegrating Tablets (Infrequent) 2120
Tonocard Tablets (0.5% to 1.5%) 649
▲ Xylocaine Injections (Among most common) 653
▲ Zomig Tablets (5% to 7%) 708
▲ Zomig-ZMT Tablets (5% to 7%) 708

Sensation, heavy
Amerge Tablets (Frequent) 1467
▲ Imitrex Injection (7.3%) 1549
Imitrex Nasal Spray (Infrequent) 1554
Imitrex Tablets (Less than 1% to 2%) 1558
Nubain Injection (1% or less) 1323

Sensation, lightness
Imitrex Nasal Spray (Infrequent) 1554

Sensation of pressure/tightness
Amerge Tablets (Frequent) 1467
▲ Imitrex Injection (5.1 to 7.1%) 1549
Imitrex Nasal Spray (Infrequent) 1554
Imitrex Tablets (Less than 1% to 2%) 1558
Maxalt Tablets (Less than 2%) 2120
Maxalt-MLT Orally Disintegrating Tablets (Less than 2%) 2120
Zomig Tablets (2% to 4%) 708
Zomig-ZMT Tablets (2% to 4%) 708

Sensations, numbness
Duranest Injections 600
Lidoderm Patch 1319
▲ Xylocaine Injections (Among most common) 653

Sensations, pulsating
Imitrex Injection (Infrequent) 1549
Imitrex Nasal Spray 1554
Imitrex Tablets (Infrequent) 1558

Sensitivity, light
Cipro 887
▲ Nilandron Tablets (7.7%) 753
▲ Orap Tablets (1 of 20 patients) 1407
Symmetrel (0.1% to 1%) 1328

Sensitivity, sun
Avita Cream (Some individuals) 999
Avita Gel (Some individuals) 1000
Cipro 887
Dantrium Capsules 2885
Minocin Oral Suspension 1865
Renova 0.02% Cream 2520
Renova 0.05% Cream 2519
Retin-A Micro 0.1% 2522
Tegrin Dandruff Shampoo - Extra Conditioning .... ▣623
Tegrin Dandruff Shampoo - Fresh Herbal .... ▣624
Tegrin Skin Cream .... ▣624
Thorazine 1656

Sensitivity reactions
Aldara Cream, 5% (More than 1%) 1978
Auralgan Otic Solution 3485
AVC (Occasional) 1350
Bactroban Ointment 1496
BayRab (Occasional) 917
BayRho-D Full Dose (Extremely rare) 921
BayRho-D Mini-Dose (Extremely rare) 919
BayTet (Extremely rare) 923
Benoquin Cream 20% 1732
Betadine Skin Cleanser (Rare) 2895
Betasept Surgical Scrub 2895
Bleph-10 (Rare) .... ⊙230
Brevoxyl 3269
Brevoxyl 3270
Combivir Tablets 1502
Creon 10 Capsules 3251
Creon 20 Capsules 3251
FML-S Liquifilm Sterile Ophthalmic Suspension .... ⊙238
Gebauer's Ethyl Chloride (Extremely rare) 1409
Humegon for Injection 2468
Melanex Topical Solution 2300
Mykrox Tablets 1168
Nesacaine/Nesacaine MPF 617
Pergonal for Injection 3223
Polysporin Ophthalmic Ointment Sterile .... ⊙301
Polytrim Ophthalmic Solution (Rare) 556
Prinzide Tablets 2168
Provera Tablets 2853
Repronex for Intramuscular and Subcutaneous Injection 1347
Retrovir Capsules (Rare) 1625
Retrovir IV Infusion (Rare) 1629
Retrovir 1625
Sensorcaine 643
Sensorcaine-MPF Injection 643
Trusopt Sterile Ophthalmic Solution 2196
Tylenol, Children's (Rare) 2014
Junior Strength Tylenol Soft Chews Chewable Tablets (Rare) 2014
Maximum Strength Tylenol Allergy Sinus Caplets, Gelcaps, and Geltabs (Rare) 2010
Tylenol Severe Allergy Caplets (Rare) 2010
Maximum Strength Tylenol Flu NightTime Liquid (Rare) 2011
Vaseretic Tablets 2204
Zaroxolyn Tablets 1177
Zestoretic Tablets 695

Sensorium, clouded
Betapace Tablets (Rare) 950
Betapace AF Tablets (Rare) 954
Blocadren Tablets 2046
Corgard Tablets 2245
Corzide 40/5 Tablets 2247
Corzide 80/5 Tablets 2247
Cosopt Sterile Ophthalmic Solution 2065
Inderal 3513
Inderal LA Long-Acting Capsules 3516
Inderide Tablets 3517
Inderide LA Long-Acting Capsules 3519
Mexitil Capsules (1.9% to 2.6%) 1047
Nadolol Tablets 2288
Normodyne Tablets 3137
Sectral Capsules 3589
Tenoretic Tablets 690
Tenormin 692
Timolide Tablets 2187
Timolol GFS .... ⊙266
Timoptic in Ocudose 2192
Timoptic Sterile Ophthalmic Solution 2190
Timoptic-XE Sterile Ophthalmic Gel Forming Solution 2194
Toprol-XL Tablets 651
Xanax Tablets 2865
Zebeta Tablets 1885
Ziac Tablets 1887

Sensory deficit, persistent
Duranest Injections 600
Nesacaine/Nesacaine MPF 617

Sensory disturbances
Foscavir Injection (Between 1% and 5%) 605
▲ Leukine (6%) 1755
▲ Paraplatin for Injection (4% to 6%) 1126
Paxil 1609
▲ Prograf (Approximately 55%) 1393
▲ Proleukin for Injection (10%) 1199
▲ Wellbutrin Tablets (4.0%) 1680
Xanax Tablets 2865

Sepsis (Occasional)
▲ Abelcet Injection (7%) 1273
Actiq (1% or greater) 1184
Aloprim for Injection (Less than 1%) 2292
▲ AmBisome for Injection (7.4% to 14%) 1383
▲ Amphotec (5% or more) 1774
▲ Argatroban Injection (6%) 1478
Arthrotec Tablets (Rare) 3195
Avonex 1013
Betaseron for SC Injection 988
▲ Cafcit (4.3%) 1035
▲ Campath Ampules (10% to 15%) 992
▲ Casodex Tablets (2% to 5%) 662
Cathflo Activase 3611
▲ CellCept Capsules (17.6% to 19.7%) 2951
▲ CellCept Intravenous (17.6% to 19.7%) 2951
▲ CellCept Oral Suspension (17.6% to 19.7%) 2951
▲ CellCept Tablets (17.6% to 27.4%) 2951
Cerebyx Injection (Infrequent) 2619
Clozaril Tablets 2319
Cognex Capsules (Rare) 1351
▲ Cytovene (4%) 2959
Diprivan Injectable Emulsion (Less than 1%) 667
Doxil Injection (Less than 1% to 5%) 566
Enbrel for Injection 1752
Enbrel for Injection 3504
Ergamisol Tablets (2 out of 463 patients) 1789
Evoxac Capsules (Less than 1%) 1217
Felbatol 3343
Feldene Capsules (Occasional) 2685
Ferrlecit Injection (Greater than 1%) 3386
▲ Flolan for Injection (13% to 25%) 1528
▲ Foscavir Injection (5% or greater) 605
Gabitril Tablets (Infrequent) 1189
Gemzar for Injection (Less than 1%) 1919
Gliadel Wafer (1%) 1723
▲ Hycamtin for Injection (26%) 1546
▲ Infasurf Intratracheal Suspension (20% to 28%) 1372
Intron A for Injection (Less than 5%) 3120
Iveegam EN (One case) 849
▲ Leukine (11%) 1755
Lodine XL Extended-Release Tablets (Less than 1%) 3530
Merrem I.V. (0.1% to 1.0%) 673
Myleran Tablets 1603
▲ Mylotarg for Injection (19% to 36%) 3540
▲ Navelbine Injection (8%) 1604
▲ Nipent for Injection (3%) 3272
▲ Novantrone for Injection (31% to 34%) 1760
Oncaspar (Less than 1%) 756
Orthoclone OKT3 Sterile Solution 2498
Permax Tablets (Infrequent) 1299
Photofrin for Injection (Occasional) 831
Ponstel Capsules (Occasional) 1356
Pravachol Tablets 1099
Prevnar for Injection 1870
▲ Prograf (3% to 15%) 1393
▲ Proleukin for Injection (23%) 1199
Pulmozyme Inhalation Solution 1426
▲ Rapamune Oral Solution and Tablets (3% to 20%) 3584
▲ Refludan for Injection (3.5%) 761
▲ Remicade for IV Injection (26%) 1178
Requip Tablets (Infrequent) 1621
Rilutek Tablets (Infrequent) 772
Rituxan for Infusion 1750
Rituxan I.V. 1428
Roxicodone Tablets (Less than 3%) 3067
Rythmol Tablets – 150 mg, 225 mg, 300 mg (One case) 502
▲ Serostim for Injection (1% to 10%) 3229
▲ Simulect for Injection (3% to 10%) 2399
Survanta Intratracheal Suspension 3053
▲ Taxol Injection (30%) 1129
Thalomid Capsules 1154
TheraCys Injection 823
▲ Thymoglobulin for Injection (12.2%) 3071
Ticlid Tablets (Rare) 3015
Trasylol Injection (1% to 2%) 909
▲ Trisenox Injection (5%) 1158
Trovan (Less than 1%) 2722
Valcyte Tablets (Less than 5%) 3022
Vistide Injection 1445
▲ Vitravene for Injection (5% to 20%) .... ⊙310
Xeloda Tablets (Less than 5%) 3039
Zanaflex Tablets (Infrequent) 1305
▲ Zemplar Injection (5%) 522
▲ Zinecard for Injection (12% to 17%) 2869
Zoladex 3-month (1% to 5%) 706

Septic shock
Aloprim for Injection (Less than 1%) 2292
Enbrel for Injection 1752
Enbrel for Injection 3504
Oncaspar (Less than 1%) 756
Tonocard Tablets (Less than 1%) 649

Septicemia
▲ Curosurf Intratracheal Suspension (14%) 1232
▲ Gengraf Capsules (5.3%) 457
▲ Leustatin Injection (6%) 2495
▲ Neoral Soft Gelatin Capsules (5.3%) 2380
▲ Neoral Oral Solution (5.3%) 2380
Orudis Capsules (Rare) 3548
Oruvail Capsules (Rare) 3548
ParaGard T 380A Intrauterine Copper Contraceptive 2582
▲ Sandimmune (4.8% to 5.3%) 2388
Thioplex for Injection 1765
Tonocard Tablets (Less than 1%) 649
Vesanoid Capsules 3037
Zenapax for Injection 3046

Serositis
Aceon Tablets (2 mg, 4 mg, 8 mg) 3249
Enalaprilat Injection 863
Lexxel Tablets 608
Monopril Tablets 1091
Monopril HCT 1094
Vaseretic Tablets 2204
Vasotec I.V. Injection 2207
Vasotec Tablets (0.5% to 1.0%) 2210

Serotonin syndrome
Celexa (At least 3 patients) 1365
Effexor Tablets 3495
Effexor XR Capsules 3499
Imitrex Injection 1549
Imitrex Tablets 1558
Luvox Tablets (25, 50, 100 mg) 3256
Meridia Capsules 481
Paxil 1609
Prozac Pulvules, Liquid, and Weekly Capsules 1238
Zoloft 2751

Serum alkaline phosphatase, elevation
Abelcet Injection 1273
Accutane Capsules 2944
Aceon Tablets (2 mg, 4 mg, 8 mg) (0.3% to 1%) 3249
Adalat CC Tablets (Rare) 877
Ambien Tablets (Rare) 3191
▲ AmBisome for Injection (7.1% to 22.2%) 1383
▲ Amphotec (3% to 7%) 1774
Anadrol-50 Tablets 3321
Arimidex Tablets (2% to 5%) 659
Arthrotec Tablets (Rare) 3195
Asacol Delayed-Release Tablets 2884
Ativan Injection (Infrequent) 3478
Augmentin Chewable Tablets (Infrequent) 1482
Augmentin Powder for Oral Suspension (Infrequent) 1482
Augmentin Tablets (Infrequent) 1485
Augmentin ES-600 Powder for Oral Suspension (Infrequently) 1487
Axid Pulvules (Less common) 1903
Axid Pulvules (Less common) 2919
Azactam for Injection (Less than 1%) 1276
Azulfidine EN-tabs Tablets 2775
Baycol Tablets 883
Betaseron for SC Injection 988
Biaxin/Biaxin XL (Less than 1%) 403
Campath Ampules 992
▲ Cancidas for Injection (2.9% to 10.5%) 2048
Captopril Tablets 2281
Cardizem Injectable (Less than 1%) 1018
Cardizem Lyo-Ject Syringe (Less than 1%) 1018
Cardizem Monovial (Less than 1%) 1018
Cardizem CD Capsules (Less than 1%) 1016
▲ Casodex Tablets (2% to 5%) 662
Ceclor CD Tablets (0.3%) 1279
Ceclor (1 in 40) 1905
Cedax (0.1% to 1%) 1021
Cefizox for Intramuscular or Intravenous Use (1% to 5%) 1390
Cefotan (1 in 700) 664
Ceftin 1898
Cefzil (0.2%) 1076
Celebrex Capsules (0.1% to 1.9%) 2676
Celebrex Capsules (0.1% to 1.9%) 2780
Celexa (Infrequent) 1365
▲ CellCept Capsules (3%) 2951
▲ CellCept Intravenous (3%) 2951
▲ CellCept Oral Suspension (3%) 2951
▲ CellCept Tablets (3%) 2951
▲ Chemet Capsules (4.2% to 10.4%) 3078
Chibroxin Sterile Ophthalmic Solution 2051
▲ Cipro I.V. (Among most frequent) 893
▲ Cipro I.V. Pharmacy Bulk Package (Among most frequent) 897
Cipro (0.8%) 887
Claforan Injection (Less than 1%) 732
Colazal Capsules 3069
Colestid Tablets (One or more occasions) 2791
Coreg Tablets (1% to 2%) 1508
Covera-HS Tablets 3199
Cytotec Tablets (Infrequent) 3202
Depen Titratable Tablets (Few reports) 3341
Diflucan Tablets, Injection, and Oral Suspension 2681
▲ Doxil Injection (1.3% to 7.8%) 566
Duraclon Injection (Rare) 3057
Duricef 1079
Dynabac Tablets (0.1% to 1%) 2269
Effexor Tablets (Infrequent) 3495
Effexor XR Capsules (Infrequent) 3499
Elspar for Injection 2092
Ergamisol Tablets (Less frequent) 1789
Evoxac Capsules 1217
▲ Fareston Tablets (8% to 19%) 3237
Felbatol (Infrequent) 3343

Floxin I.V. (More than or equal to 1%) 2526
Floxin Tablets (More than or equal to 1%) 2529
▲ Fortaz (1 in 23) 1541
Fortovase Capsules (0.5%) 2970
Foscavir Injection (Between 1% and 5%) 605
▲ Sterile FUDR (Among more common) 2974
▲ Gemzar for Injection (55% to 77%) 1919
Geodon Capsules (Infrequent) 2688
Gleevec Capsules (0.2% to 4.6%) 2357
Glucotrol Tablets (Occasional) 2692
Glucotrol XL Extended Release Tablets (Occasional) 2693
▲ Hexalen Capsules (9%) 2226
Hivid Tablets (Less than 1%) 2975
Inderide Tablets 3517
▲ Intron A for Injection (Up to 13%) 3120
Isoptin SR Tablets 467
Kefzol Vials, ADD-Vantage 1951
Klonopin Tablets 2983
Lamictal (Infrequent) 1567
Lescol Capsules 2361
Lescol Capsules 2925
Lescol XL Tablets 2361
Lescol XL Tablets 2925
▲ Leukine (8%) 1755
Lopid Tablets (Occasional) 2650
Lorabid Suspension and Pulvules 2251
Mandol Vials 1953
Maxipime for Injection (0.1% to 1%) 1285
Mefoxin for Injection 2124
Mefoxin Premixed Intravenous Solution 2127
▲ Mepron Suspension (5% to 8%) 1598
Meridia Capsules (1.6%) 481
Merrem I.V. (Greater than 0.2%) 673
Mevacor Tablets 2132
Mithracin for Intravenous Use 903
Monopril Tablets 1091
Monopril HCT 1094
Monurol Sachet 1375
Mycobutin Capsules (Less than 1%) 2838
Navane Oral 2701
Navane Intramuscular 2703
▲ Neupogen for Injection (21% to 58%) 587
Nexium Delayed-Release Capsules (Less than 1%) 619
▲ Nilandron Tablets (3%) 753
Nimotop Capsules (0.2%; rare) 904
▲ Nolvadex Tablets (3.0%) 678
Noroxin Tablets (1.1%) 2145
Norpramin Tablets 755
Nutropin AQ Injection 1420
Nutropin for Injection 1417
Omnicef (0.2%) 493
Oxandrin Tablets 1153
▲ Paraplatin for Injection (24% to 37%) 1126
Paxil (Rare) 1609
Pentasa Capsules (Less than 1%) 3239
Pravachol Tablets 1099
Prevacid Delayed-Release Capsules 3292
PREVPAC (Less than 1%) 3298
Priftin Tablets (Less than 1%) 758
Prilosec Delayed-Release Capsules (Rare) 628
Primaxin I.M. 2158
Primaxin I.V. 2160
Procanbid Extended-Release Tablets 2262
Procardia Capsules (Rare) 2708
Procardia XL Extended Release Tablets (Rare) 2710
▲ Prograf (3% to 15%) 1393
▲ Proleukin for Injection (10%) 1199
Protonix I.V. (Less than 1%) 3580
Protonix Tablets (Less than 1%) 3577
Prozac Pulvules, Liquid, and Weekly Capsules (Rare) 1238
▲ Rapamune Oral Solution and Tablets (3% to 20%) 3584
Reminyl Oral Solution (Infrequent) 1792
Reminyl Tablets (Infrequent) 1792
Requip Tablets (Infrequent) 1621
Rescriptor Tablets (Less than 2%) 526
Rifadin 765
Rifamate Capsules 767
Rilutek Tablets (Infrequent) 772
Rocephin Injectable Vials, ADD-Vantage, Galaxy, Bulk (Less than 1%) 2993
▲ Roferon-A Injection (Up to 50%) 2996
Rythmol Tablets – 150 mg, 225 mg, 300 mg (0.2%) 502
Sarafem Pulvules (Rare) 1962
Sectral Capsules 3589
Seroquel Tablets (Infrequent) 684
▲ Serostim for Injection (1% to 10%) 3229
Sinemet Tablets 1253
Sinemet CR Tablets 1255
Solu-Medrol Sterile Powder 2855
Sporanox Injection (1%) 1804
Sporanox Injection (1%) 2509
Suprax (Less than 2%) 1877
Symmetrel 1328
Tambocor Tablets (Rare) 1990
Tarka Tablets (2.8%) 508
▲ Taxol Injection (22%) 1129
▲ Tazicef for Injection (1 in 23 patients) 1647
▲ Tazicef Galaxy Container (1 in 23 patients) 1650
▲ Tazicef Pharmacy Bulk Package (1 in 23 patients) 1653
▲ Tazidime Vials, Faspak & ADD-Vantage (1 in 23) 1966
Tequin Injection (Less than 0.1%) 1110
Tequin Tablets (Less than 0.1%) 1110
Teveten Tablets 3327
Thalomid Capsules 1154
Thiothixene Capsules 2290
Tiazac Capsules (Less than 2%) 1378
Timentin Injection- ADD-Vantage Vial 1661
Timentin Injection-Galaxy Container 1664
Timentin Injection-Pharmacy Bulk Package 1666
Timentin for Intravenous Administration 1658
Topamax Sprinkle Capsules (Infrequent) 2590
Topamax Tablets (Infrequent) 2590
Toprol-XL Tablets 651
Trovan (Greater than or equal to 1%) 2722
Unasyn for Injection 2728
Uniretic Tablets (Less than 1%) 3178
Vantin Tablets and Oral Suspension 2860
Verelan Capsules 3184
Verelan PM Capsules 3186
▲ Videx (1% to 9%) 1138
Videx EC Capsules 1143
Viracept 532
Vistide Injection 1445
Xanax Tablets (Less than 1% to 1.7%) 2865
Zinacef Injection (1 in 50 patients) 1696
Zinacef for Injection (1 in 50 patients) 1696
Zithromax Capsules, 250 mg (Less than 1%) 2743
Zithromax for IV Infusion (Less than 1%) 2748
Zithromax for Oral Suspension, 1 g (Less than 1%) 2743
Zithromax for Oral Suspension, 300 mg, 600 mg, 900 mg, 1200 mg (Less than 1%) 2739
Zithromax Tablets, 250 mg (Less than 1%) 2739
Zithromax Tablets, 600 mg (Less than 1%) 2743
Zocor Tablets 2219
Zomig Tablets (Rare) 708
Zomig-ZMT Tablets (Rare) 708
Zonegran Capsules 1307
Zosyn 1890
Zosyn in Galaxy Containers 1894
Zyprexa Tablets (Infrequent) 1973
Zyprexa ZYDIS Orally Disintegrating Tablets (Infrequent) 1973
Zyvox (0.2% to 3.5%) 2871

Serum amylase, elevation

Abelcet Injection 1273
AmBisome for Injection (Less common) 1383
Avelox Tablets (0.05% to 1%) 879
Cipro I.V. (Rare) 893
Cipro I.V. Pharmacy Bulk Package (Rare) 897
Cipro (Less than 0.1%) 887
Colazal Capsules 3069
Crixivan Capsules (1.0%) 2070
Cuprimine Capsules (Few cases) 2075
Cytotec Tablets (Infrequent) 3202
▲ Epivir (3% to 4.2%) 1520
Epivir-HBV (Less than 1%) 1524
Evoxac Capsules (1% to 3%) 1217
Fortovase Capsules (1% to 2%) 2970
Foscavir Injection (Less than 1%) 605
▲ Hivid Tablets (5.1%) 2975
Invirase Capsules (1% to 2%) 2979
Kadian Capsules 1335
▲ Mepron Suspension (1% to 8%) 1598
Niaspan Extended-Release Tablets 1846
Omnicef 493
Oncaspar (Less than 1%) 756
Pentasa Capsules (Less than 1%) 3239
Rescriptor Tablets (Up to 5.2%) 526
▲ Serostim for Injection (1% to 10%) 3229
▲ Sustiva Capsules (10%) 1258
Tequin Injection (Less than 0.1%) 1110
Tequin Tablets (Less than 0.1%) 1110
Uniretic Tablets (Less than 1%) 3178
▲ Videx (5% to 17%) 1138
Videx EC Capsules 1143
Viracept 532
▲ Zerit (14%) 1147

Serum bicarbonate content, variations

Cancidas for Injection (0.9%) 2048
Dynabac Tablets (1.4%) 2269
Hivid Tablets (Less than 1%) 2975
▲ Lupron Depot–4 Month 30 mg (Greater than or equal to 5%) 3289
▲ Prograf (3% to 15%) 1393
▲ Vistide Injection (Approximately 9%) 1445

Serum bilirubin, elevation
(*see under* Hyperbilirubinemia)

Serum bilirubin levels, abnormalities

Amerge Tablets (Rare) 1467
Cefzil (Less than 0.1%) 1076
Emcyt Capsules (1% to 2%) 2810
Kefurox Vials, ADD-Vantage (1 in 500) 1948
Sinemet Tablets 1253
Sinemet CR Tablets 1255
Xanax Tablets (Less than 1% to 1.6%) 2865

Serum calcium, depression
(*see under* Hypocalcemia)

Serum calcium decrease
(*see under* Hypocalcemia)

Serum cholesterol, increase
(*see under* Hypercholesterolemia)

Serum creatine phosphokinase, elevation

Aricept Tablets (Infrequent) 1270
Aricept Tablets (Infrequent) 2665
Arthrotec Tablets (Rare) 3195
Catapres Tablets (Rare) 1037
Ceclor CD Tablets (0.7%) 1279
▲ Cipro I.V. (Among most frequent) 893
▲ Cipro I.V. Pharmacy Bulk Package (Among most frequent) 897
Clorpres Tablets (Rare) 1002
Combipres Tablets (Rare) 1040
▲ Fortovase Capsules (Less than 2% to 12%) 2970
Foscavir Injection (Less than 1%) 605
Geodon Capsules (Infrequent) 2688
Haldol Decanoate 2535
Havrix Vaccine (Less than 1%) 1544
Hivid Tablets (0.8%) 2975
▲ Invirase Capsules (Less than 2% to 12%) 2979
Lipitor Tablets (Less than 2%) 2639
Lipitor Tablets (Less than 2%) 2696
Mirapex Tablets (1% or more) 2834
Norvir Capsules (0.9% to 3.4%) 487
Norvir Oral Solution (0.9% to 3.4%) 487
Prozac Pulvules, Liquid, and Weekly Capsules (Rare) 1238
Quinidex Extentabs 2933
Requip Tablets (Infrequent) 1621
Rescriptor Tablets (Less than 2%) 526
Risperdal (Infrequent) 1796
Sarafem Pulvules (Rare) 1962
Sular Tablets (Less than or equal to 1%) 688
Suprane Liquid for Inhalation (Less than 1%) 874
Symmetrel (Uncommon) 1328
Trasylol Injection (2%) 909
Videx 1138
Videx EC Capsules 1143
Viracept 532
Zithromax (1% to 2%) 2743
Zithromax for Oral Suspension, 300 mg, 600 mg, 900 mg, 1200 mg (1% to 2%) 2739
Zithromax Tablets, 250 mg (1% to 2%) 2739
Zithromax Tablets, 600 mg (1% to 2%) 2743
▲ Zocor Tablets (About 5% of patients) 2219

Serum creatinine, elevation

▲ Abelcet Injection (11%) 1273
Accupril Tablets (2%) 2611
▲ Accuretic Tablets (3%) 2614
Aceon Tablets (2 mg, 4 mg, 8 mg) (0.3% to 1%) 3249
Aloprim for Injection (Less than 1%) 2292
Altace Capsules (1.2% to 1.5%) 2233
▲ AmBisome for Injection (18.5% to 22.4%) 1383
▲ Amphotec (12% to 21%) 1774
Anadrol-50 Tablets 3321
Ancobon Capsules 1730
▲ AndroGel (3% to 6%) 3322
Asacol Delayed-Release Tablets 2884
Atacand Tablets (Infrequent) 595
Avalide Tablets (Less than 0.7%) 1070
Avapro Tablets (Less than 0.7%) 1074
Avapro Tablets (Less than 0.7%) 3076
▲ Azactam for Injection (5.8%) 1276
Bactrim 2949
Biaxin/Biaxin XL (Less than 1%) 403
Bicillin C-R 900/300 Injection 2240
Bicillin C-R Injection 2238
Bicillin L-A Injection 2242
Captopril Tablets 2281
▲ Casodex Tablets (2% to 5%) 662
Caverject Sterile Powder (Less than 1%) 2777
Ceclor CD Tablets (0.5%) 1279
Ceclor (Less than 1 in 500) 1905
Cedax (0.1% to 1%) 1021
Cefizox for Intramuscular or Intravenous Use (Occasional) 1390
Cefobid Intravenous/Intramuscular (1 in 48) 2671
Cefobid Pharmacy Bulk Package - Not for Direct Infusion (1 in 48) 2673
Cefotan 664
Ceftin 1898
Cefzil (0.1%) 1076
Celebrex Capsules (0.1% to 1.9%) 2676
Celebrex Capsules (0.1% to 1.9%) 2780
▲ CellCept Capsules (3% to 39.4%) 2951
▲ CellCept Intravenous (3% to 39.4%) 2951
▲ CellCept Oral Suspension (3% to 39.4%) 2951
▲ CellCept Tablets (3% to 39.4%) 2951
Ceptaz for Injection (Occasional) 1499
Chibroxin Sterile Ophthalmic Solution 2051
▲ Cipro I.V. (Among most frequent) 893
▲ Cipro I.V. Pharmacy Bulk Package (Among most frequent) 897
Cipro (1.1%) 887
Claforan Injection (Occasional) 732
Coly-Mycin M Parenteral 2243
Corlopam Injection (2%) 412
Cozaar Tablets (Less than 0.1%) 2067
CytoGam Intravenous 2026
▲ Cytovene (Up to 43%) 2959
Didronel Tablets 2888
Diovan Capsules (0.8%) 2337
Diovan HCT Tablets 2338
Diprivan Injectable Emulsion (Less than 1%) 667
Doxil Injection (Less than 1%) 566
Duricef 1079
Dyazide Capsules 1515
Dynabac Tablets (0.1% to 1%) 2269
Dyrenium Capsules (Rare) 3458
Effexor Tablets (Infrequent) 3495
Effexor XR Capsules (Infrequent) 3499
▲ Enalaprilat Injection (0.2% to 20%) 863
Ergamisol Tablets (Less frequent) 1789
Eulexin Capsules 3118
Famvir Tablets (0.2%) 2348
Floxin I.V. (More than or equal to 1%) 2526
Floxin Tablets (More than or equal to 1%) 2529
Fortaz (Occasional) 1541
▲ Foscavir Injection (5% to 27%) 605
Gamimune N, 5% Solvent/Detergent Treated 925
Gamimune N, 10% Solvent/Detergent Treated 928
Gammagard S/D 845
Gammar-P I.V. 787
▲ Gemzar for Injection (Up to 8%) 1919
▲ Gengraf Capsules (18% to 48%) 457
Geodon Capsules (Rare) 2688
Glucotrol Tablets (Occasional) 2692
Glucotrol XL Extended Release Tablets 2693
▲ Hexalen Capsules (7%) 2226
Hivid Tablets (Less than 1%) 2975
Hyzaar (0.8%) 2109
Ifex for Injection 1123
Indapamide Tablets (Less than 5%) 2286
Indocin I.V. 2115
Intron A for Injection (Up to 3%) 3120
Kefurox Vials, ADD-Vantage 1948
Lamictal (Rare) 1567
▲ Leukine (15%) 1755
Lexxel Tablets 608
Lodine (Less than 1%) 3528
Lodine XL Extended-Release Tablets (Less than 1%) 3530
Lodosyn Tablets 1251
Lorabid Suspension and Pulvules 2251
Lotensin Tablets (2%) 2365
Lotensin HCT Tablets 2367
Lotrel Capsules 2370
Lupron Depot 7.5 mg (Greater than or equal to 5%) 3284
Lupron Injection (Less than 5%) 3279
Macrobid Capsules 2889
Macrodantin Capsules 2891
Mandol Vials 1953
Mavik Tablets (1.1% to 4.7%) 478
Maxipime for Injection (0.1% to 1%) 1285
Maxzide 1008
Mefoxin for Injection 2124
Mefoxin Premixed Intravenous Solution 2127
Mepron Suspension (1%) 1598
Merrem I.V. (Greater than 0.2%) 673
Mithracin for Intravenous Use 903
Mobic Tablets (Less than 2%) 1054

Monopril Tablets 1091
Monopril HCT 1094
Motrin Suspension, Oral Drops, Chewable Tablets, and Caplets 2002
Mykrox Tablets 1168
Mylocel Tablets 2227
Naprelan Tablets (Less than 1%) 1293
Natrecor for Injection (At least 1%) 3189
Nebcin Vials, Hyporets & ADD-Vantage 1955
▲ Neoral Soft Gelatin Capsules (18% to 48%) 2380
▲ Neoral Oral Solution (18% to 48%) 2380
Nilandron Tablets (2%) 753
▲ Nipent for Injection (3% to 10%) 3272
Nolvadex Tablets (1.7%) 678
▲ Normodyne Injection (8%) 3135
Noroxin Tablets (Less frequent) 2145
Oncaspar 756
Oxandrin Tablets 1153
▲ Paraplatin for Injection (5% to 10%) 1126
Pediazole Suspension 3050
Pipracil 1866
Pletal Tablets (Less than 2%) 2605
Pletal Tablets (Less than 2%) 2848
Prevacid Delayed-Release Capsules 3292
PREVPAC (Less than 1%) 3298
Prilosec Delayed-Release Capsules (Less than 1%) 628
Primaxin I.M. 2158
Primaxin I.V. 2160
▲ Prinivil Tablets (About 2.0% to approximately 11.6%) 2164
Prinzide Tablets 2168
Procardia Capsules (Rare) 2708
Procardia XL Extended Release Tablets (Rare) 2710
▲ Prograf (24% to 39%) 1393
▲ Proleukin for Injection (33%) 1199
Protopic Ointment (Greater than or equal to 1%) 1397
▲ Rapamune Oral Solution and Tablets (35% to 40%) 3584
Rescriptor Tablets (Less than 2%) 526
▲ Rocaltrol (1 in 6) 2991
Rocephin Injectable Vials, ADD-Vantage, Galaxy, Bulk (Less than 1%) 2993
Sandimmune 2388
Sandoglobulin I.V. 2391
Sandostatin LAR Depot (Rare) 2395
Septra Suspension 2265
Septra Tablets 2265
Septra DS Tablets 2265
Sinemet Tablets 1253
Sinemet CR Tablets 1255
Sporanox Injection (2%) 1804
Sular Tablets (Less than or equal to 1%) 688
Suprax (Less than 2%) 1877
Symmetrel 1328
Tagamet 1644
Tazicef for Injection (Occasional) 1647
Tazicef Galaxy Container (Occasional) 1650
Tazicef Pharmacy Bulk Package (Occasional) 1653
Tazidime Vials, Faspak & ADD-Vantage (Occasional) 1966
Teveten Tablets (1.3%) 3327
Thalomid Capsules 1154
Timentin Injection- ADD-Vantage Vial 1661
Timentin Injection-Galaxy Container 1664
Timentin Injection-Pharmacy Bulk Package 1666
Timentin for Intravenous Administration 1658
Topamax Sprinkle Capsules (Infrequent) 2590
Topamax Tablets (Infrequent) 2590
Toradol 3018
▲ Trasylol Injection (18% to 21%) 909
Tricor Capsules, Micronized 513
Trilisate (Less than 1%) 2901
Trovan (Greater than or equal to 1%) 2722
Ultracet Tablets 2597
Ultram Tablets (Infrequent) 2600
Unasyn for Injection 2728
Uniretic Tablets (Less than 1%) 3178
Univasc Tablets (1% to 2%) 3181
Urso Tablets 836
Valtrex Caplets 1676
Vancocin HCl Capsules & Pulvules (Rare) 1972
Vancocin HCl Oral Solution (Rare) 1971
Vancocin HCl, Vials & ADD-Vantage (Rare) 1970
Vantin Tablets and Oral Suspension 2860
▲ Vaseretic Tablets (About 0.6% to 20%) 2204
▲ Vasotec I.V. Injection (0.2% to 20%) 2207
▲ Vasotec Tablets (About 0.2% to 20%) 2210
▲ Vistide Injection (8% to 53%) 1445
▲ Visudyne for Injection (1% to 10%) ⊙308
Xanax Tablets (1.9% to 2.2%) 2865
Zantac (Rare) 1690
Zantac Injection 1688
Zantac Syrup (Rare) 1690
Zaroxolyn Tablets 1177
Zebeta Tablets 1885
Zestoretic Tablets 695
Zestril Tablets (About 2.0%) 698
Ziagen 1692
Zinacef Injection 1696
Zinacef for Injection 1696
Zithromax Capsules, 250 mg (Less than 1%) 2743
▲ Zithromax for IV Infusion (4% to 6%) 2748
Zithromax for Oral Suspension, 1 g (Less than 1%) 2743
Zithromax for Oral Suspension, 300 mg, 600 mg, 900 mg, 1200 mg (Less than 1%) 2739
Zithromax Tablets, 250 mg (Less than 1%) 2739
Zithromax Tablets, 600 mg (Less than 1%) 2743
Zometa for Intravenous Infusion (2.3%) 3621
Zosyn 1890
Zosyn in Galaxy Containers 1894
Zovirax Capsules 1706
▲ Zovirax for Injection (5% to 10%) 1708
Zovirax 1706
Zyvox (0.2%) 2871

Serum electrolyte changes
(*see under* Electrolyte imbalance)

Serum fibrogen, decrease
Trental Tablets (Rare) 784

Serum folate, abnormal
Topamax Sprinkle Capsules (Rare) 2590
Topamax Tablets (Rare) 2590

Serum gastrin levels, increased
Nexium Delayed-Release Capsules (Less than 1%) 619

Serum lipase, elevation
▲ Epivir-HBV (10%) 1524
Hivid Tablets (Less than 1%) 2975
Oncaspar 756
Pentasa Capsules (Less than 1%) 3239
Rescriptor Tablets (Less than 2%) 526

Serum PBI levels, decrease
(*see under* PBI decrease)

Serum phosphorus, elevation
▲ Lupron Depot 3.75 mg (Approximately 5% to 8%) 3281
▲ Lupron Depot–4 Month 30 mg (Greater than or equal to 5%) 3289
Macrodantin Capsules 2891
Nutropin AQ Injection 1420
Nutropin for Injection 1417
Zebeta Tablets 1885

Serum phosphorus content, variations
Dynabac Tablets (0.1% to 1%) 2269
Macrobid Capsules (1% to 5%) 2889
Maxipime for Injection (Up to 2.8%) 1285

Serum potassium, reduction
(*see under* Hypokalemia)

Serum proteins, changes
Brevicon 28-Day Tablets 3380
Cancidas for Injection (Up to 3.1%) 2048
Dynabac Tablets (0.1% to 1%) 2269
Norinyl 1 +35 28-Day Tablets 3380
Norinyl 1 + 50 28-Day Tablets 3380
Tri-Norinyl-28 Tablets 3433

Serum sickness
Amoxil Chewable Tablets 1471
Amoxil for Oral Suspension 1471
Amoxil 1471
Antivenin (Black Widow Spider Antivenin) 2042
Augmentin Chewable Tablets 1482
Augmentin Powder for Oral Suspension 1482
Augmentin Tablets 1485
Augmentin ES-600 Powder for Oral Suspension 1487
Axid Pulvules (Rare) 1903
Axid Pulvules (Rare) 2919
Azulfidine EN-tabs Tablets (Rare) 2775
Bactrim 2949
Bicillin C-R 900/300 Injection 2240
Bicillin C-R Injection 2238
Bicillin L-A Injection 2242
Ceclor CD Tablets (One case) 1279
Ceclor (0.05% to 0.024%) 1905
Cedax 1021
Cefizox for Intramuscular or Intravenous Use 1390
Ceftin 1898
Cefzil (Rare) 1076
Copaxone for Injection (Infrequent) 3306
Doryx Coated Pellet Filled Capsules 3357
Duricef (Rare) 1079
Engerix-B Vaccine (Less than 1%) 1517
Feldene Capsules (Rare) 2685
Floxin I.V. 2526
Floxin Tablets 2529
Levoxyl Tablets 1819
Lorabid Suspension and Pulvules (Rare) 2251
Mefoxin for Injection 2124
Mefoxin Premixed Intravenous Solution 2127
Motrin Suspension, Oral Drops, Chewable Tablets, and Caplets (Less than 1%) 2002
Orthoclone OKT3 Sterile Solution 2498
Pediazole Suspension 3050
Periostat Tablets 1208
Permapen Isoject 2706
Pfizerpen for Injection 2707
Pneumovax 23 (Rare) 2156
PREVPAC 3298
Recombivax HB (Less than 1%) 2178
Rituxan for Infusion (Less than 0.1%) 1750
Rituxan I.V. (Less than 0.1%) 1428
Rocephin Injectable Vials, ADD-Vantage, Galaxy, Bulk (Rare) 2993
Septra Suspension 2265
Septra Tablets 2265
Septra DS Tablets 2265
Suprax (Less than 2%) 1877
Ticlid Tablets (Rare) 3015
Tolectin (Less than 1%) 2589
Twinrix Vaccine 1674
Unithroid Tablets 3445
Vantin Tablets and Oral Suspension 2860
Vibramycin Calcium Oral Suspension Syrup 2735
Vibramycin Hyclate Capsules 2735
Vibramycin Monohydrate for Oral Suspension 2735
Vibra-Tabs Film Coated Tablets 2735
Wellbutrin Tablets 1680
Wellbutrin SR Sustained-Release Tablets 1684
Zoloft 2751

Serum transaminase, elevation
Aricept Tablets (Infrequent) 1270
Aricept Tablets (Infrequent) 2665
Atromid-S Capsules 3483
Augmentin Chewable Tablets (Infrequent) 1482
Augmentin Powder for Oral Suspension (Infrequent) 1482
Augmentin Tablets (Infrequent) 1485
Augmentin ES-600 Powder for Oral Suspension (Infrequently) 1487
Bactrim 2949
Baycol Tablets 883
Captopril Tablets 2281
▲ Chemet Capsules (6% to 10% of patients) 3078
Clomid Tablets 735
▲ Cognex Capsules (29%) 1351
Concerta Extended Release Tablets 1998
Concerta Tablets 561
Cordarone Tablets 3487
Corlopam Injection (0.5% to 5%) 412
Covera-HS Tablets 3199
Depacon Injection (Frequent) 416
Depakene (Frequent) 421
Depakote Tablets (Frequent) 430
Depakote ER Tablets (Frequent) 436
DiaBeta Tablets (Isolated cases) 741
Diflucan Tablets, Injection, and Oral Suspension (Rare) 2681
Duricef 1079
Enbrel for Injection 1752
Enbrel for Injection 3504
Eulexin Capsules 3118
Fortovase Capsules (Isolated cases) 2970
▲ Sterile FUDR (Among more common) 2974
▲ Gemzar for Injection (Approximately two-thirds) 1919
Geodon Capsules (Infrequent) 2688
Gleevec Capsules (1.1% to 3.5%) 2357
Inderide Tablets 3517
Inderide LA Long-Acting Capsules 3519
Intron A for Injection (Less than 5%) 3120
Invirase Capsules (Isolated cases) 2979
Isoptin SR Tablets 467
Klonopin Tablets 2983
▲ Lariam Tablets (Among most frequent) 2989
Lescol Capsules 2361
Lescol Capsules 2925
Lescol XL Tablets 2361
Lescol XL Tablets 2925
Leustatin Injection 2495
Lopid Tablets 2650
▲ Lupron Depot–3 Month 11.25 mg (3%) 3285
Luvox Tablets (25, 50, 100 mg) (Frequent) 3256
Marinol Capsules (Less than 1%) 3325
Mavik Tablets (0.8% of patients) 478
Metadate CD Capsules 1164
Metadate ER Tablets 1167
Methylin Tablets 1995
Methylin ER Tablets 1995
Mevacor Tablets (1.9%) 2132
Mithracin for Intravenous Use 903
Monopril Tablets 1091
Monopril HCT 1094
Mylotarg for Injection (13 Patients) 3540
Nardil Tablets (Common) 2653
Navane Oral (Infrequent) 2701
Navane Intramuscular (Infrequent) 2703
Nebcin Vials, Hyporets & ADD-Vantage 1955
Niaspan Extended-Release Tablets 1846
▲ Normodyne Tablets (4%) 3137
Norvir Capsules 487
Norvir Oral Solution 487
Pacerone Tablets 3331
Paxil 1609
Plendil Extended-Release Tablets (Two episodes) 623
Pravachol Tablets 1099
Precose Tablets 906
Procanbid Extended-Release Tablets 2262
▲ Proleukin for Injection (56%) 1199
Prometrium Capsules (100 mg, 200 mg) 3261
Rifadin 765
▲ Rifamate Capsules (10% to 20%) 767
▲ Rifater Tablets (10% to 20% of patients) 769
Ritalin (Some instances) 2387
▲ Roferon-A Injection (Up to 50%) 2996
Rythmol Tablets – 150 mg, 225 mg, 300 mg (0.2%) 502
Septra Suspension 2265
Septra Tablets 2265
Septra DS Tablets 2265
Serophene Tablets 3226
Streptase for Infusion 647
Tagamet 1644
Tambocor Tablets (Rare) 1990
Thiothixene Capsules 2290
Ticlid Tablets (Rare) 3015
Toprol-XL Tablets 651
▲ Trasylol Injection (5%) 909
Tricor Capsules, Micronized 513
Trileptal Oral Suspension 2407
Trileptal Tablets 2407
Trilisate (Rare) 2901
Vaniqa Cream 1121
Vascor Tablets (Approximately 1%) 2602
Verelan Capsules 3184
Verelan PM Capsules 3186
Zocor Tablets (1%) 2219
Zofran 1703
Zofran ODT Orally Disintegrating Tablets 1703
Zovirax for Injection (1% to 2%) 1708
Zyflo Filmtab Tablets (Three patients) 524
Zyrtec (Occasional) 2756
Zyrtec-D 12 Hour Extended Relief Tablets (Occasional) 2758

Serum triglyceride, elevation
(*see under* Hypertriglyceridemia)

Sexual activity, decrease
▲ Catapres Tablets (About 3 in 100 patients) 1037
Catapres-TTS (0.5% or less) 1038
Clorpres Tablets (About 3%) 1002
Combipres Tablets (About 3%) 1040
▲ Duraclon Injection (3%) 3057
Risperdal (Frequent) 1796

Sexual dysfunction
Aceon Tablets (2 mg, 4 mg, 8 mg) (0.3% to 1.4%) 3249
Avalide Tablets 1070
Avapro Tablets (Less than 1%) 1074
Avapro Tablets (Less than 1%) 3076
Betapace Tablets (Less than 1% to 2%) 950
Cardizem Injectable 1018
Cardizem Lyo-Ject Syringe 1018
Cardizem Monovial 1018
Cardizem CD Capsules (Less than 1%) 1016
Cardura Tablets (2%) 2668
Catapres-TTS (2 of 101 patients) 1038
Celexa 1365
Copaxone for Injection (Infrequent) 3306
Duranest Injections 600
Effexor Tablets (2%) 3495
Effexor XR Capsules 3499

Eldepryl Capsules 3266
Eskalith 1527
Evoxac Capsules (Less than 1%) 1217
Geodon Capsules (Infrequent) 2688
Hivid Tablets (Less than 1%) 2975
Lithobid Slow-Release Tablets 3255
Luvox Tablets (25, 50, 100 mg) 3256
Maxzide 1008
Monopril Tablets (Less than 1.0% to 1.0%) 1091
Monopril HCT (Less than 2%) 1094
Nardil Tablets (Common) 2653
Naropin Injection 612
Nesacaine/Nesacaine MPF 617
Neurontin Capsules (Infrequent) 2655
Neurontin Oral Solution (Infrequent) 2655
Neurontin Tablets (Infrequent) 2655
Norvasc Tablets (Less than 1% to 2%) 2704
▲ Paxil (3.7% to 10.0%) 1609
Polocaine Injection, USP 625
Polocaine-MPF Injection, USP 625
Procardia Capsules (2% or less) 2708
Prozac Pulvules, Liquid, and Weekly Capsules 1238
Risperdal (Frequent) 1796
Roferon-A Injection (Infrequent) 2996
Sarafem Pulvules 1962
Sensorcaine 643
Tiazac Capsules (Less than 2%) 1378
Viracept 532
Wellbutrin Tablets (Frequent) 1680
▲ Xanax Tablets (7.4%) 2865
Xylocaine Injections 653
Ziac Tablets 1887
▲ Zoladex (21%) 702
▲ Zoladex 3-month (One of the two most common) 706
Zoloft (Frequent) 2751

Sexual maturity, accelerated
Lupron Depot-PED 7.5 mg, 11.25 mg and 15 mg (Less than 2%) 3291
Lupron Injection Pediatric (Less than 2%) 3280

SGOT changes
(*see under* Aspartate aminotransferase levels, changes in)

SGOT elevation
(*see under* Aspartate aminotransferase levels, elevation of)

SGPT changes
(*see under* Alanine aminotransferase levels, elevation of)

SGPT elevation
(*see under* Alanine aminotransferase levels, elevation of)

Shaking
(*see under* Tremors)

Shivering
(*see under* Tremors)

Shock
Abelcet Injection (Rare) 1273
Accuretic Tablets 2614
Acel-Imune (Rare) 1851
Actiq 1184
AK-Fluor Injection 10% and 25% ⊙202
Aleve Tablets, Caplets and Gelcaps ▣602
Amphotec (1% to 5%) 1774
AquaMEPHYTON Injection 2042
Betaseron for SC Injection 988
Bicillin L-A Injection 2242
Cerebyx Injection (Infrequent) 2619
Cordarone Intravenous (Less than 2%) 3491
Coumadin for Injection 1243
Coumadin Tablets 1243
Demerol 3079
Desferal Vials 2333
Dilaudid Oral Liquid 445
Dilaudid Tablets - 8 mg 445
Dilaudid-HP 443
Diphtheria & Tetanus Toxoids Adsorbed Purogenated for Pediatric Use (Rare) 1857
Doxil Injection (Less than 1%) 566
Effexor Tablets 3495
Effexor XR Capsules 3499
ELA-Max Cream 1340
ELA-Max 5 Cream 1340
Ellence Injection 2806
Emla 602
Etrafon (Occasional) 3115
▲ Flolan for Injection (5%) 1528
Floxin I.V. 2526
Floxin Tablets 2529
Fluorescite Injection ⊙211
Heparin Lock Flush Solution (Rare) 3509
Heparin Sodium Injection (Rare) 3511
Herceptin I.V. (At least one of the 958 patients) 1414
Humorsol Sterile Ophthalmic Solution (Infrequent) 2102
Hyalgan Solution (One case) 3080
Imitrex Injection 1549
Imitrex Nasal Spray 1554
Imitrex Tablets 1558
Indocin Capsules (Less than 1%) 2112
Indocin I.V. (Less than 1%) 2115
Indocin (Less than 1%) 2112
INFeD Injection 3388
Kadian Capsules 1335
Levo-Dromoran 1734
Lidoderm Patch (Rare) 1319
Mepergan Injection 3539
Merrem I.V. (0.1% to 1.0%) 673
Midamor Tablets 2136
Migranal Nasal Spray (Rare) 2376
Mobic Tablets (Less than 0.1%) 1054
Monopril Tablets (0.2%) 1091
Children's Motrin Oral Suspension and Chewable Tablets 2006
Children's Motrin Cold Oral Suspension 2007
Children's Motrin Oral Suspension ▣643
Infants' Motrin Concentrated Drops 2006
Junior Strength Motrin Caplets and Chewable Tablets 2006
Motrin IB Tablets, Caplets, and Gelcaps 2002
Motrin Sinus Headache Caplets 2005
MS Contin Tablets 2896
MSIR 2898
Nubain Injection (1% or less) 1323
Omnicef 493
Oramorph SR Tablets (Less frequent) 3062
Orthoclone OKT3 Sterile Solution (Less than 1%) 2498
Orudis Capsules (Rare) 3548
Oruvail Capsules (Rare) 3548
OxyContin Tablets 2912
Permax Tablets (Infrequent) 1299
Prevnar for Injection 1870
Proleukin for Injection (Less than 1%) 1199
Prozac Pulvules, Liquid, and Weekly Capsules (Rare) 1238
Rifadin (Rare) 765
Rifamate Capsules (Rare) 767
Rifater Tablets 769
Rilutek Tablets (Infrequent) 772
Roxanol 3066
Roxicodone Tablets 3067
Salagen Tablets (Rare) 2229
Sandoglobulin I.V. (Rare) 2391
Sarafem Pulvules (Rare) 1962
Tetanus & Diphtheria Toxoids Adsorbed for Adult Use (Rare) 1880
Thorazine 1656
Trasylol Injection (1% to 2%) 909
Trilafon 3160
Viagra Tablets (Less than 2%) 2732
Vistide Injection 1445
Warfarin Sodium Tablets, USP 3302
Zofran Injection (Rare) 1698
Zofran 1703
Zofran ODT Orally Disintegrating Tablets 1703

Shock, anaphylactic
(*see under* Anaphylactic shock)

Shock, hypovolemic
Prevacid Delayed-Release Capsules (Less than 1%) 3292
PREVPAC (Less than 1%) 3298

SIADH secretion syndrome
(*see under* ADH syndrome, inappropriate)

Sialadenitis
Accuretic Tablets 2614
Aldoclor Tablets 2035
Aldomet Tablets 2037
Aldoril Tablets 2039
Amerge Tablets (Rare) 1467
Atacand HCT Tablets 597
Avalide Tablets 1070
Corzide 40/5 Tablets (Occasional) 2247
Corzide 80/5 Tablets (Occasional) 2247
Diovan HCT Tablets 2338
Diucardin Tablets 3494
Diuril Oral 2087
Diuril Sodium Intravenous 2086
Dyazide Capsules 1515
Evoxac Capsules (1% to 3%) 1217
HydroDIURIL Tablets 2108
Hyzaar 2109
Indapamide Tablets 2286
Inderide Tablets 3517
Inderide LA Long-Acting Capsules 3519
Kaletra Capsules (Less than 2%) 471
Kaletra Oral Solution (Less than 2%) 471
Lotensin HCT Tablets 2367
Macrobid Capsules 2889
Macrodantin Capsules 2891
Maxzide 1008
Micardis HCT Tablets 1051
Microzide Capsules 3414
Moduretic Tablets 2138
Monopril HCT 1094
Mykrox Tablets (Rare) 1168
Permax Tablets (Rare) 1299
Prinzide Tablets 2168
Rescriptor Tablets (Less than 2%) 526
Timolide Tablets 2187
Trileptal Oral Suspension 2407
Trileptal Tablets 2407
Uniretic Tablets 3178
Vaseretic Tablets 2204
Videx 1138
Videx EC Capsules 1143
Zaroxolyn Tablets 1177
Zestoretic Tablets 695
Ziac Tablets 1887

Sialadenopathy
Tapazole Tablets 1823

Sialism
Albuminar-5, U.S.P. 785
Albuminar-25, U.S.P. 786
Alferon N Injection (1%) 1770
Altace Capsules (Less than 1%) 2233
Ambien Tablets (Rare) 3191
Anectine Injection 1476
Aricept Tablets (Infrequent) 1270
Aricept Tablets (Infrequent) 2665
Ativan Injection (Infrequent) 3478
Axert Tablets (Rare) 2772
Betaseron for SC Injection 988
Brevital Sodium for Injection, USP 1815
Ceftin for Oral Suspension (0.1% to 1%) 1898
Celexa (Frequent) 1365
Cerebyx Injection (Infrequent) 2619
Claritin (At least one patient) 3100
Claritin-D 24 Hour Extended Release Tablets 3104
▲ Clozaril Tablets (More than 5% to 31%) 2319
Cognex Capsules (Infrequent) 1351
Cordarone Tablets (1% to 3%) 3487
Diprivan Injectable Emulsion (Less than 1%) 667
Doxil Injection (Less than 1%) 566
Effexor Tablets (Rare) 3495
Effexor XR Capsules (Rare) 3499
Eskalith 1527
Etrafon (Occasional) 3115
Evoxac Capsules (2.2%) 1217
Exelon Capsules (Infrequent) 2342
Exelon Oral Solution (Infrequent) 2345
Gabitril Tablets (Infrequent) 1189
Geodon Capsules 2688
Haldol Decanoate 2535
Haldol Injection, Tablets and Concentrate 2533
Hivid Tablets (Less than 1%) 2975
Humorsol Sterile Ophthalmic Solution (Rare) 2102
Ifex for Injection (Less than 1%) 1123
Imitrex Injection 1549
Imitrex Nasal Spray 1554
Intron A for Injection (Less than 5%) 3120
Isopto Carbachol Ophthalmic Solution ⊙215
Klonopin Tablets 2983
Lamictal (Infrequent) 1567
Lithobid Slow-Release Tablets 3255
Lodosyn Tablets 1251
Loxitane Capsules 3398
Luvox Tablets (25, 50, 100 mg) (Infrequent) 3256
Megace Oral Suspension (1% to 3%) 1124
Meridia Capsules 481
Mestinon 1740
Mexitil Capsules (About 4 in 1,000) 1047
Mirapex Tablets (1% or more) 2834
Moban (Occasional) 1320
Navane Oral 2701
Navane Intramuscular 2703
Neurontin Capsules (Infrequent) 2655
Neurontin Oral Solution (Infrequent) 2655
Neurontin Tablets (Infrequent) 2655
▲ Orap Tablets (13.8%) 1407
Orudis Capsules (Less than 1%) 3548
Oruvail Capsules (Less than 1%) 3548
Pacerone Tablets (1% to 3%) 3331
Paxil (Infrequent) 1609
PhosChol 579
Prevacid Delayed-Release Capsules (Less than 1%) 3292
PREVPAC (Less than 1%) 3298
Primaxin I.M. 2158
Primaxin I.V. (Less than 0.2%) 2160
Prinivil Tablets (Greater than 1%) 2164
Prinzide Tablets 2168
▲ Prostigmin Injectable (Among most common) 1744
▲ Prostigmin Tablets (Among most common) 1744
Protonix I.V. 3580
Protonix Tablets 3577
Prozac Pulvules, Liquid, and Weekly Capsules (Infrequent) 1238
Remeron Tablets (Rare) 2483
Remeron SolTab Tablets (Rare) 2486
Reminyl Oral Solution (Infrequent) 1792
Reminyl Tablets (Infrequent) 1792
Requip Tablets (1% or more) 1621
Rescriptor Tablets (Less than 2%) 526
Risperdal (Up to 2%) 1796
Roferon-A Injection (Rare to infrequent) 2996
Sarafem Pulvules (Infrequent) 1962
Seroquel Tablets (Infrequent) 684
Serzone Tablets (Rare) 1104
Sinemet Tablets 1253
Sinemet CR Tablets 1255
Sonata Capsules (Rare) 3591
▲ Soriatane Capsules (1% to 10%) 3003
Suprane Liquid for Inhalation (Greater than 1%) 874
Tasmar Tablets (Infrequent) 3010
Tensilon Injectable 1745
Thiothixene Capsules (Infrequently) 2290
Topamax Sprinkle Capsules (Infrequent) 2590
Topamax Tablets (Infrequent) 2590
▲ Trecator-SC Tablets (Among most common) 3598
Trental Tablets (Less than 1%) 784
Trilafon 3160
Trovan (Less than 1%) 2722
Urecholine 2198
Urecholine Tablets 2445
Valium Injectable (Rare) 3026
Valium Tablets (Infrequent) 3047
Versed Injection (Less than 1%) 3027
Versed Syrup (Less than 1%) 3033
▲ Wellbutrin Tablets (3.4%) 1680
Wellbutrin SR Sustained-Release Tablets (Infrequent) 1684
▲ Xanax Tablets (4.2% to 5.6%) 2865
Zestril Tablets (Greater than 1%) 698
Zoloft (Infrequent) 2751
Zyban Sustained-Release Tablets 1710
Zyprexa Tablets (Frequent) 1973
Zyprexa ZYDIS Orally Disintegrating Tablets (Frequent) 1973
Zyrtec (Less than 2%) 2756
Zyrtec-D 12 Hour Extended Relief Tablets (Less than 2%) 2758

Sialorrhea
(*see under* Sialism)

Sialosis
(*see under* Sialism)

SICCA syndrome
(*see under* Sjögren's syndrome)

Sinoatrial block
Blocadren Tablets (Less than 1%) 2046
Flumadine (Less than 0.3%) 1370
Neurontin Capsules (Rare) 2655
Neurontin Oral Solution (Rare) 2655
Neurontin Tablets (Rare) 2655
Timolol GFS ⊙266
Timoptic in Ocudose (Less frequent) 2192
Timoptic-XE Sterile Ophthalmic Gel Forming Solution 2194

Sinoatrial node dysfunction
Cardene I.V. 3485
Cordarone Tablets 3487
Eskalith 1527
Lithobid Slow-Release Tablets 3255
Pacerone Tablets 3331

Sinus arrest
Catapres Tablets (Rare) 1037
Cordarone Tablets 3487
Nipent for Injection (Less than 3%) 3272
Pacerone Tablets 3331
Rythmol Tablets – 150 mg, 225 mg, 300 mg (Less than 1%) 502
Tambocor Tablets (1% to 3%) 1990
Tonocard Tablets (Less than 1%) 649

Sinus bradycardia
Aciphex Tablets 1267
Aciphex Tablets 1783
Activase I.V. 1410
Adenocard Injection 1380
Adenoscan 1381
Catapres Tablets (Rare) 1037
Catapres-TTS (0.5% or less) 1038
Cerebyx Injection (Infrequent) 2619
Clorpres Tablets (Rare) 1002
Combipres Tablets (Rare) 1040
Cordarone Intravenous (Less than 2%) 3491

Cordarone Tablets (2% to 5%)........ 3487
Corvert Injection (1.2%)........ 2793
Cozaar Tablets (Less than 1%)........ 2067
Digitek Tablets........ 1003
Duraclon Injection (Rare)........ 3057
Eldepryl Capsules........ 3266
Hyzaar........ 2109
Kytril Injection (Rare)........ 2986
Lanoxicaps Capsules........ 1574
Lanoxin Injection........ 1581
Lanoxin Tablets........ 1587
Lanoxin Elixir Pediatric........ 1578
Lanoxin Injection Pediatric........ 1584
Motrin Suspension, Oral Drops, Chewable Tablets, and Caplets (Less than 1%)........ 2002
Pacerone Tablets (2% to 5%)........ 3331
Retavase Vials........ 1182
▲ Sandostatin Injection (25%)........ 2394
Serzone Tablets (1.5%)........ 1104
Sonata Capsules (Rare)........ 3591
▲ Taxol Injection (23%)........ 1129
Uniretic Tablets (Less than 1%)........ 3178
Vascor Tablets (0.5% to 2.0%)........ 2602

Sinus congestion

▲ Aerobid/Aerobid-M (3% to 9%)........ 1363
Hivid Tablets (Less than 1%)........ 2975
▲ Lupron Injection (5% or more)........ 3279
Monopril HCT (Less than 2%)........ 1094
Mykrox Tablets (Less than 2%)........ 1168
Nasacort Nasal Inhaler (Fewer than 5%)........ 750
▲ Periostat Tablets (5%)........ 1208
▲ Serevent Diskus (9%)........ 1637
Serevent Inhalation Aerosol (1% to 3%)........ 1633
▲ Stadol NS Nasal Spray (3% to 9%)........ 1108
Tasmar Tablets (1% to 2%)........ 3010

Sinus discomfort

Aerobid/Aerobid-M (1% to 3%)........ 1363
Avalide Tablets........ 1070
Avapro Tablets (1% or greater)........ 1074
Avapro Tablets (1% or greater)........ 3076
Cozaar Tablets (1.5%)........ 2067
Hivid Tablets (Less than 1%)........ 2975
Imitrex Injection (2.2%)........ 1549
Imitrex Nasal Spray (0.8% to 2.4%)........ 1554
Maxalt Tablets (Infrequent)........ 2120
Maxalt-MLT Orally Disintegrating Tablets (Infrequent)........ 2120
Nicotrol Nasal Spray (More common)........ 2843

Sinus drainage

▲ Aerobid/Aerobid-M (3% to 9%)........ 1363
Alferon N Injection (2%)........ 1770

Sinus exit block

Adenoscan (Less than 1%)........ 1381

Sinus node dysfunction

Cardene I.V.........: 3485
Cardizem Injectable........ 1018
Cardizem Lyo-Ject Syringe........ 1018
Cardizem Monovial........ 1018
Eskalith........ 1527
Lithium Carbonate........ 3061
Lithium Citrate Syrup........ 3061

Sinus pause

Adenoscan (Less than 1%)........ 1381

Sinus syndrome, sick

Cardizem Injectable (Less than 1%)........ 1018
Cardizem Lyo-Ject Syringe (Less than 1%)........ 1018
Cardizem Monovial (Less than 1%)........ 1018
Exelon Capsules (Infrequent)........ 2342
Exelon Oral Solution (Infrequent)........ 2345
Photofrin for Injection........ 831
Rythmol Tablets – 150 mg, 225 mg, 300 mg (Less than 1%)........ 502
Tenoretic Tablets........ 690

Sinus tachycardia

Adenocard Injection........ 1380
Aramine Injection........ 2043
Corvert Injection (2.7%)........ 2793
Ellence Injection........ 2806
Etrafon........ 3115
Foscavir Injection (Between 1% and 5%)........ 605
Motrin Suspension, Oral Drops, Chewable Tablets, and Caplets (Less than 1%)........ 2002
▲ Proleukin for Injection (70%)........ 1199
▲ Taxol Injection (23%)........ 1129
Taxotere for Injection Concentrate (Rare)........ 778
Vascor Tablets (0.5% to 2.0%)........ 2602

Sinusitis

Accuretic Tablets (0.5% to 1%)........ 2614
Aceon Tablets (2 mg, 4 mg, 8 mg) (0.6% to 5.2%)........ 3249
Actiq (1% or greater)........ 1184
▲ Activella Tablets (7% to 11%)........ 2764
▲ Actonel Tablets (4.49%)........ 2879
▲ Actos Tablets (6.3%)........ 3275
▲ Advair Diskus 100/50 (4%)........ 1448
▲ Advair Diskus 250/50 (5%)........ 1448
▲ Advair Diskus 500/50 (4% to 5%)........ 1448
▲ Aerobid/Aerobid-M (3% to 9%)........ 1363
Agrylin Capsules (1% to 5%)........ 3232
Alamast Ophthalmic Solution (Less than 5%)........ 3092
Allegra (2.2%)........ 712
▲ Alora Transdermal System (6.8% to 10.6%)........ 3372
Alphagan P Ophthalmic Solution (1% to 4%)........ 546
▲ Ambien Tablets (4%)........ 3191
AmBisome for Injection (Less common)........ 1383
Amerge Tablets (Infrequent)........ 1467
Amphotec (1% to 5%)........ 1774
Arava Tablets (2%)........ 724
▲ Aredia for Injection (15.6%)........ 2309
Arimidex Tablets (2% to 5%)........ 659
Aromasin Tablets (Less frequent)........ 2769
Asacol Delayed-Release Tablets (2% or greater)........ 2884
▲ Astelin Nasal Spray (3.2%)........ 3339
Atacand Tablets (More than 1%)........ 595
Atacand HCT Tablets (0.5% or greater)........ 597
Atrovent Inhalation Solution (2.3%)........ 1031
▲ Avandia Tablets (3.2% to 5.3%)........ 1490
Avelox Tablets (0.05% to 1%)........ 879
▲ Avonex (18%)........ 1013
Axert Tablets (Infrequent)........ 2772
Axid Pulvules (2.4%)........ 1903
Axid Pulvules (2.4%)........ 2919
▲ Azmacort Inhalation Aerosol (2% to 9%)........ 728
▲ Baycol Tablets (4.7%)........ 883
▲ Betaseron for SC Injection (36%)........ 988
Betaxon Ophthalmic Suspension (Less than 2%)........ 537
Betimol Ophthalmic Solution (1% to 5%)........ ⊙ 324
Campath Ampules........ 992
Carac Cream (1.6%)........ 1222
Cardura Tablets (Less than 0.5%)........ 2668
Carnitor Injection (2% to 3%)........ 3242
Carteolol Hydrochloride Ophthalmic Solution USP, 1% (Occasional)........ ⊙ 258
▲ Casodex Tablets (2% to 5%)........ 662
Caverject Sterile Powder (2%)........ 2777
Ceclor CD Tablets (0.1% to 1%)........ 1279
Ceftin for Oral Suspension (0.1% to 1%)........ 1898
▲ Celebrex Capsules (5%)........ 2676
▲ Celebrex Capsules (5%)........ 2780
▲ Celexa (3%)........ 1365
▲ CellCept Capsules (3% to 26%)........ 2951
▲ CellCept Intravenous (3% to 26%)........ 2951
▲ CellCept Oral Suspension (3% to 26%)........ 2951
▲ CellCept Tablets (3% to 26%)........ 2951
Cerebyx Injection (Infrequent)........ 2619
Claritin (At least one patient)........ 3100
Claritin-D 12 Hour Extended Release Tablets (Less frequent)........ 3102
Claritin-D 24 Hour Extended Release Tablets (Fewer than 2%)........ 3104
Cognex Capsules (Frequent)........ 1351
Colazal Capsules (1%)........ 3069
▲ CombiPatch Transdermal System (10% to 12%)........ 2323
Combivent Inhalation Aerosol (2.3%)........ 1041
▲ Concerta Extended-Release Tablets (3%)........ 1998
▲ Concerta Tablets (3%)........ 561
Copaxone for Injection (At least 2%)........ 3306
▲ Coreg Tablets (5.4%)........ 1508
Cosopt Sterile Ophthalmic Solution (1% to 5%)........ 2065
Cozaar Tablets (1.0%)........ 2067
Crinone (Less than 5%)........ 3213
Crixivan Capsules (Less than 2%)........ 2070
▲ DaunoXome Injection (Up to 8%)........ 1442
Depacon Injection (1% to 5%)........ 416
Depakene (1% to 5%)........ 421
Depakote Sprinkle Capsules (1% to 5%)........ 426
Depakote Tablets (1% to 5%)........ 430
Depakote ER Tablets (1% to 5%)........ 436
Detrol Tablets (1.1%)........ 3623
Detrol LA Capsules (2%)........ 2801
Diovan Capsules (More than 1%)........ 2337
Diovan HCT Tablets (More than 2%)........ 2338
Ditropan XL Extended Release Tablets (2% to 5%)........ 564
Doxil Injection (Less than 1%)........ 566
DuoNeb Inhalation Solution........ 1233
Effexor XR Capsules (At least 2%)........ 3499
Emadine Ophthalmic Solution (Less than 5%)........ ⊙ 211
▲ Enbrel for Injection (5%)........ 1752
▲ Enbrel for Injection (5%)........ 3504
Esclim Transdermal System (2.1% to 4.2%)........ 3460
▲ Estring Vaginal Ring (4%)........ 2811
▲ Evista Tablets (7.9% to 10.3%)........ 1915
▲ Evoxac Capsules (12.3%)........ 1217
Famvir Tablets (1.3% to 2.6%)........ 2348
▲ Felbatol (3.5%)........ 3343
▲ femhrt Tablets (8.1%)........ 2635
▲ Flolan for Injection (4%)........ 1528
Flomax Capsules (2.2% to 3.7%)........ 1044
▲ Flovent Diskus (9% to 33%)........ 3614
▲ Flovent (3% to 22%)........ 1535
▲ Flovent Rotadisk (4% to 6%)........ 1537
Floxin Otic Solution (Single report)........ 1219
Fludara for Injection (Up to 5%)........ 995
Fortovase Capsules (Less than 2%)........ 2970
Foscavir Injection (Between 1% and 5%)........ 605
Gabitril Tablets (1% or more)........ 1189
Gengraf Capsules (Less than 1%)........ 457
▲ Gonal-F for Injection (5.1%)........ 3216
▲ Herceptin I.V. (9%)........ 1414
Hivid Tablets (Less than 1%)........ 2975
Hytrin Capsules (2.6%)........ 464
Hyzaar (1.2%)........ 2109
Imdur Tablets (Less than or equal to 5%)........ 1826
Imitrex Nasal Spray........ 1554
Indapamide Tablets (Less than 5%)........ 2286
▲ Infergen (12% to 17%)........ 1777
▲ Intron A for Injection (Up to 21%)........ 3120
Invirase Capsules (Less than 2%)........ 2979
Kaletra Capsules (Less than 2%)........ 471
Kaletra Oral Solution (Less than 2%)........ 471
Keppra Tablets (2%)........ 3314
▲ Klonopin Tablets (4%)........ 2983
Lescol Capsules (2.6%)........ 2361
Lescol Capsules (2.6%)........ 2925
▲ Lescol XL Tablets (3.5%)........ 2361
▲ Lescol XL Tablets (3.5%)........ 2925
Lexxel Tablets (Infrequent)........ 608
▲ Lipitor Tablets (Up to 6.4%)........ 2639
▲ Lipitor Tablets (Up to 6.4%)........ 2696
Lodine (Less than 1%)........ 3528
Lodine XL Extended-Release Tablets (Less than 1%)........ 3530
Lotensin Tablets (Less than 1%)........ 2365
Lotensin HCT Tablets (More than 1%)........ 2367
Lupron Depot–4 Month 30 mg (Less than 5%)........ 3289
Luvox Tablets (25, 50, 100 mg) (Frequent)........ 3256
▲ LYMErix Vaccine (3.07% to 3.16%)........ 1592
Marinol Capsules (Less than 1%)........ 3325
▲ Mepron Suspension (7%)........ 1598
▲ Meridia Capsules (5%)........ 481
Miacalcin Nasal Spray (1% to 3%)........ 2375
▲ Micardis Tablets (3%)........ 1049
▲ Micardis HCT Tablets (4%)........ 1051
Migranal Nasal Spray (1%)........ 2376
Mirapex Tablets (1% or more)........ 2834
▲ Mirena Intrauterine System (5% or more)........ 974
Monopril Tablets (0.2% to 1.0%)........ 1091
▲ Naprelan Tablets (3% to 9%)........ 1293
Nasacort AQ Nasal Spray........ 752
Nasarel Nasal Solution 0.025% (1% or less)........ 1296
▲ Nasonex Nasal Spray (4% to 5%)........ 3131
▲ Neoral Soft Gelatin Capsules (Less than 1% to 7%)........ 2380
Neoral Oral Solution (Less than 1%)........ 2380
Nexium Delayed-Release Capsules (Less than 1%)........ 619
▲ Nicotrol Inhaler (Over 3%)........ 2840
▲ Nipent for Injection (6%)........ 3272
▲ Novantrone for Injection (3% to 6%)........ 1760
Ocupress Ophthalmic Solution, 1% Sterile (Occasional)........ ⊙ 303
▲ Ortho-Prefest Tablets (8%)........ 2570
Patanol Ophthalmic Solution (Less than 5%)........ 540
Paxil (Infrequent to 4%)........ 1609
▲ PEG-Intron Powder for Injection (12%)........ 3140
▲ Periostat Tablets (3%)........ 1208
Permax Tablets (Infrequent)........ 1299
Plavix Tablets (1% to 2.5%)........ 1097
Plavix Tablets (1% to 2.5%)........ 3084
Plendil Extended-Release Tablets (0.5% to 1.5%)........ 623
Pletal Tablets (Less than 2%)........ 2605
Pletal Tablets (Less than 2%)........ 2848
▲ Prandin Tablets (0.5, 1, and 2 mg) (3% to 6%)........ 2432
▲ Prempro Tablets (7% to 8%)........ 3572
Prinivil Tablets (0.3% to 1.0%)........ 2164
Prinzide Tablets (0.3% to 1%)........ 2168
Procardia XL Extended Release Tablets (1% or less)........ 2710
▲ Prograf (3% to 15%)........ 1393
Prometrium Capsules (100 mg, 200 mg) (Less than 5%)........ 3261
ProSom Tablets (Infrequent)........ 500
Protonix I.V. (Greater than or equal to 1%)........ 3580
Protonix Tablets (Greater than or equal to 1%)........ 3577
▲ Protopic Ointment (2% to 7%)........ 1397
Provigil Tablets (At least 1%)........ 1193
▲ Prozac Pulvules, Liquid, and Weekly Capsules (Less than 1% to 6%)........ 1238
▲ Pulmicort Turbuhaler Inhalation Powder (2% to 16%)........ 636
Pulmozyme Inhalation Solution........ 1426
Qvar Inhalation Aerosol (Up to 3%)........ 1987
▲ Rapamune Oral Solution and Tablets (3% to 20%)........ 3584
▲ Rebetron Combination Therapy (9% to 12%)........ 3153
ReFacto Vials........ 1437
Relenza Rotadisk (2% to 3%)........ 1619
Remeron Tablets (Frequent)........ 2483
Remeron SolTab Tablets (Frequent)........ 2486
▲ Remicade for IV Injection (5% to 26%)........ 1178
▲ Requip Tablets (4%)........ 1621
Rescula Ophthalmic Solution (1% to 5%)........ ⊙ 306
Retrovir Capsules........ 1625
Retrovir IV Infusion........ 1629
Retrovir........ 1625
Rilutek Tablets (0.4% to 1.6%)........ 772
Risperdal (1% to 2%)........ 1796
Rituxan for Infusion (1% to 5%)........ 1750
Rituxan I.V. (1% to 5%)........ 1428
▲ Roferon-A Injection (Less than 1% to 11%)........ 2996
Roxicodone Tablets (Less than 3%)........ 3067
Salagen Tablets (1% to 4%)........ 2229
▲ Sandimmune (Less than 1% to 7%)........ 2388
▲ Sandostatin LAR Depot (5% to 15%)........ 2395
▲ Serevent Diskus (Greater than 3%)........ 1637
▲ Serostim for Injection (1% to 10%)........ 3229
Serzone Tablets........ 1104
▲ Simulect for Injection (3% to 10%)........ 2399
Singulair (Greater than or equal to 2%)........ 2181
▲ Skelid Tablets (5.3%)........ 3088
▲ Soriatane Capsules (1% to 10%)........ 3003
▲ Sporanox Capsules (3% to 7%)........ 1800
Sporanox Oral Solution (1.8% to 2.0%)........ 1808
Sporanox Oral Solution (1.8% to 2.0%)........ 2512
Stadol NS Nasal Spray (1% or greater)........ 1108
▲ Sular Tablets (3%)........ 688
Synagis Intramuscular (More than 1%)........ 2028
Tamiflu Capsules (1.7%)........ 3008
Tamiflu Oral Suspension (1.7%)........ 3008
Tasmar Tablets (1% or more)........ 3010
▲ Temodar Capsules (6%)........ 3157
Teveten Tablets (1% or greater)........ 3327
▲ Thalomid Capsules (4.2%)........ 1154
▲ TOBI Solution for Inhalation (8.1%)........ 1206
▲ Topamax Sprinkle Capsules (4% to 4.4%)........ 2590
▲ Topamax Tablets (4% to 4.4%)........ 2590
Travatan Ophthalmic Solution (1% to 5%)........ 543
Tricor Capsules, Micronized (1%)........ 513
Trileptal Oral Suspension (2% to 4%)........ 2407
Trileptal Tablets (2% to 4%)........ 2407
▲ Trisenox Injection (20%)........ 1158
Trovan (Less than 1%)........ 2722
Twinrix Vaccine........ 1674
Uniretic Tablets (More than 1%)........ 3178
Univasc Tablets (More than 1%)........ 3181
▲ Vagifem Tablets (3% to 5%)........ 2857
▲ Vanceril Double Strength Inhalation Aerosol (4%)........ 3167
Vantin Tablets and Oral Suspension (Less than 1%)........ 2860
▲ Verelan PM Capsules (3%)........ 3186
Viagra Tablets (Less than 2%)........ 2732
Vicoprofen Tablets (Less than 1%)........ 520
Vioxx (2.2%)........ 2213
Viracept........ 532
Vistide Injection........ 1445
▲ Vitravene for Injection (5% to 20%)........ ⊙ 310
WelChol Tablets (2%)........ 3073
Wellbutrin SR Sustained-Release Tablets (1% to 3%)........ 1684
Xopenex Inhalation Solution (1.4% to 4.2%)........ 3207
Yasmin 28 Tablets (Greater than 1%)........ 980
Zanaflex Tablets (Infrequent)........ 1305
Zebeta Tablets (2.2%)........ 1885
Zestoretic Tablets (0.3% to 1%)........ 695
Zestril Tablets (0.3% to 1.0%)........ 698
Ziac Tablets........ 1887
Zoladex (1% to 3%)........ 702
Zoladex 3-month........ 706
Zoloft (Infrequent)........ 2751
Zyban Sustained-Release Tablets (2%)........ 1710
Zyrtec (Less than 2%)........ 2756
Zyrtec-D 12 Hour Extended Relief Tablets (Less than 2%)........ 2758

Sjögren's syndrome

Mintezol........ 2137

Skin, anesthesia
(*see under* Numbness, skin)

Skin, bleeding
▲ Tazorac Gel (1% to 10%) ... 556
Vaniqa Cream (Less than 1%) ... 1121

Skin, burning of
▲ Cleocin T Topical (11%) ... 2790
Cleocin Vaginal Cream ... 2788
▲ Clindets Pledgets (10% to 11%) ... 3270
▲ Differin Cream (Less than 1% to 24%) ... 1402
▲ Differin Gel (10% to 40%) ... 1403
▲ Differin Solution/Pledgets (30% to 60%) ... 1404
Diprolene Lotion 0.05% (1%) ... 3107
Diprolene Ointment 0.05% (Infrequent) ... 3108
Diprolene AF Cream 0.05% (Infrequent) ... 3106
Diprosone ... 3109
▲ Dovonex Ointment (Approximately 10% to 15%) ... 1117
Drysol Solution ... 2663
8-MOP Capsules ... 1727
▲ Emgel 2% Topical Gel (Most common) ... 1285
Finevin Cream (1% to 5%) ... 962
Gastrocrom Oral Concentrate (Less common) ... 1162
Klonopin Tablets (Infrequent) ... 2983
Levulan Kerastick ... 971
▲ Loprox Gel (34%) ... 2022
Lotrisone Lotion (1.6%) ... 3129
▲ Luxíq Foam (2% to 44%) ... 1210
MetroCream (Less than 3%) ... 1404
MetroGel ... 1405
MetroLotion ... 1405
Nubain Injection (1% or less) ... 1323
Oxistat (1.7%) ... 1298
Oxsoralen Lotion 1% ... 1740
Oxsoralen-Ultra Capsules ... 1741
ProctoFoam-HC ... 3177
▲ Protopic Ointment (25% to 58%) ... 1397
Rogaine for Women Topical Solution ... ▣ 721
▲ Tazorac Gel (10% to 30%) ... 556
▲ Ultravate Cream (4.4%) ... 1119
Ultravate Ointment (1.6%) ... 1120
▲ Vaniqa Cream (3.5%) ... 1121

Skin, cracking
Aquasol A Parenteral ... 593
Clobevate Gel (Less than 2%) ... 3271
Cormax Cream (Approximately 0.3%) ... 2440
Cormax Ointment (Approximately 0.3%) ... 2440
Diprolene Gel 0.05% (Less frequent) ... 3107
Hivid Tablets (Less than 1%) ... 2975
Olux Foam (Less than 2%) ... 1211
Temovate Cream (Less frequent) ... 1301
▲ Temovate Gel (Among most frequent) ... 1303
Temovate Ointment (Less frequent) ... 1301
Temovate E Emollient (Less than 2%) ... 1302

Skin, dryness of
(*see under* Xerosis cutis)

Skin, eruptions of
▲ Anaprox Tablets (3% to 9%) ... 2967
▲ Anaprox DS Tablets (3% to 9%) ... 2967
Antabuse Tablets ... 2444
Antabuse Tablets (Occasional) ... 3474
Bactrim ... 2949
Biaxin/Biaxin XL ... 403
Cardizem CD Capsules (Infrequent) ... 1016
Cosmegen for Injection ... 2062
Daranide Tablets ... 2077
Depen Titratable Tablets (Rare) ... 3341
▲ EC-Naprosyn Delayed-Release Tablets (3% to 9%) ... 2967
E.E.S. ... 450
Ery-Tab Tablets ... 448
Erythrocin Stearate Filmtab Tablets ... 452
Flovent (1% to 3%) ... 1535
Floxin Tablets ... 2529
Imitrex Injection (Infrequent) ... 1549
Imitrex Nasal Spray (Infrequent) ... 1554
Levaquin (0.5% to less than 1.0%) .. 2537
Librium Capsules (Isolated cases) .. 1736
Librium for Injection (Isolated instances) ... 1737
▲ Naprelan Tablets (3% to 9%) ... 1293
▲ Naprosyn Suspension (3% to 9%) .. 2967
▲ Naprosyn Tablets (3% to 9%) ... 2967
Norvir Capsules ... 487
Norvir Oral Solution ... 487
Paser Granules ... 1781
PCE Dispertab Tablets (Rare) ... 498
Pediazole Suspension ... 3050
Pima Syrup ... 1362
Plaquenil Tablets ... 3082
PREVPAC ... 3298
Rifamate Capsules ... 767
Septra Suspension ... 2265
Septra Tablets ... 2265
Septra DS Tablets ... 2265
Serevent Inhalation Aerosol (1% to 3%) ... 1633
Tessalon Capsules ... 1377
Thioridazine Hydrochloride Tablets (Infrequent) ... 2289
Trasylol Injection ... 909
Yodoxin Tablets ... 1722

Skin, fluorescence
AK-Fluor Injection 10% and 25% ... ⊙ 202

Skin, fragile
Accutane Capsules ... 2944
Celestone Syrup ... 3099
Depo-Medrol Injectable Suspension ... 2795
Photofrin for Injection ... 831

Skin, fragility
Celestone Soluspan Injectable Suspension ... 3097
Cortone Acetate Injectable Suspension ... 2059
Cortone Acetate Tablets ... 2061
Cuprimine Capsules ... 2075
Decadron Elixir ... 2078
Decadron Tablets ... 2079
Decadron Phosphate Injection ... 2081
Depen Titratable Tablets ... 3341
Dermatop Emollient Cream (Two patients) ... 2517
Florinef Acetate Tablets ... 2250
Hydrocortone Tablets ... 2106
Hydrocortone Acetate Injectable Suspension ... 2103
Hydrocortone Phosphate Injection, Sterile ... 2105
Pediapred Oral Solution ... 1170
Prednisone ... 3064
Prelone Syrup ... 2273
Solu-Medrol Sterile Powder ... 2855

Skin, infection
Accutane Capsules ... 2944
Aceon Tablets (2 mg, 4 mg, 8 mg) (0.3% to 1%) ... 3249
Crixivan Capsules (Less than 2%) ... 2070
Cutivate Cream (0.8%) ... 1282
▲ Gengraf Capsules (7.0%) ... 457
▲ Neoral Soft Gelatin Capsules (7.0%) ... 2380
▲ Neoral Oral Solution (7.0%) ... 2380
Prinivil Tablets (0.3% to 1.0%) ... 2164
Prinzide Tablets ... 2168
▲ Sandimmune (7.0% to 10.1%) ... 2388
Zestoretic Tablets ... 695
Zestril Tablets (0.3% to 1.0%) ... 698

Skin, irritation of
Accuzyme Debriding Ointment (Occasional) ... 1725
Alora Transdermal System ... 3372
▲ Androderm Transdermal System CIII (5%) ... 3377
Betadine Solution ... 2895
Betadine Surgical Scrub (Rare) ... 2895
Blocadren Tablets ... 2046
Carac Cream (1.2%) ... 1222
Clobevate Gel (Less than 2%) ... 3271
Compazine ... 1505
Cosopt Sterile Ophthalmic Solution ... 2065
Cutivate Cream (0.8% to 4.5%) ... 1282
Differin Cream (1%) ... 1402
Differin Gel (Approximately 1% or less) ... 1403
Differin Solution/Pledgets (1% or less) ... 1404
Diprolene Lotion 0.05% (Less than 1%) ... 3107
Diprolene Ointment 0.05% (Infrequent) ... 3108
Diprolene AF Cream 0.05% (Infrequent) ... 3106
Diprosone ... 3109
▲ Dovonex Cream (Approximately 10% to 15%) ... 1116
▲ Dovonex Ointment (Approximately 10% to 15%) ... 1117
Elocon Cream 0.1% (Infrequent) ... 3110
Elocon Ointment 0.1% (Infrequent) ... 3112
Finevin Cream (Less than 1%) ... 962
Lotrimin ... 3128
Lotrisone ... 3129
Luxíq Foam ... 1210
MetroCream (Less than 3%) ... 1404
MetroGel ... 1405
MetroLotion ... 1405
Orap Tablets ... 1407
Oxistat Cream (0.4%) ... 1298
Panafil Ointment (Occasional) ... 1726
ProctoFoam-HC ... 3177
Rogaine Extra Strength for Men Topical Solution ... ▣ 721
Rogaine for Women Topical Solution ... ▣ 721
Selsun Rx 2.5% Lotion, USP ... 3053
Soriatane Capsules (Less than 1%) ... 3003
Stelazine ... 1640
▲ Tazorac Gel (10% to 30%) ... 556
Timolide Tablets ... 2187
Timolol GFS ... ⊙ 266
Timoptic in Ocudose ... 2192
Timoptic Sterile Ophthalmic Solution ... 2190
Timoptic-XE Sterile Ophthalmic Gel Forming Solution ... 2194
Tolectin (1% to 3%) ... 2589
Vaniqa Cream (1.8%) ... 1121
Vascor Tablets (0.5% to 2.0%) ... 2602
Xerac AC Solution ... 2663
Ziac Tablets ... 1887

Skin, lesions non-specific
Hivid Tablets (Less than 1%) ... 2975
Lupron Injection (Less than 5%) ... 3279
Prinivil Tablets (0.3% to 1.0%) ... 2164
Prinzide Tablets ... 2168
Procanbid Extended-Release Tablets (Fairly common) ... 2262
Roferon-A Injection (Infrequent) ... 2996
▲ Trisenox Injection (8%) ... 1158
Zestoretic Tablets ... 695

Skin, maceration
Analpram-HC ... 1338
Anusol-HC Cream 2.5% (Infrequent to frequent) ... 2237
Cordran Lotion (More frequent) ... 2438
Cordran Tape (More frequent) ... 2439
Cormax Cream (Infrequent) ... 2440
Cormax Ointment (Infrequent) ... 2440
Cormax Scalp Application (Infrequent) ... 2441
Diprolene Lotion 0.05% (Infrequent) ... 3107
Diprolene Ointment 0.05% (Infrequent) ... 3108
Diprolene AF Cream 0.05% (Infrequent) ... 3106
Diprosone ... 3109
Elocon Lotion 0.1% (Infrequent) ... 3111
Lidex (Infrequent) ... 2020
Lotrisone ... 3129
Pramosone ... 1343
ProctoFoam-HC ... 3177
Psorcon E Cream ... 1227
Psorcon E Ointment ... 1228
Sulfamylon Topical Solution ... 1011
Synalar (Infrequent) ... 2020
Temovate Scalp Application (Infrequent) ... 1304
Topicort (Infrequent) ... 2025
Ultravate Cream ... 1119
Ultravate Ointment ... 1120

Skin, oiliness
▲ Cleocin T Topical (1% to 18%) ... 2790
Cleocin Vaginal Cream ... 2788
▲ Clindets Pledgets (1% to 18%) ... 3270
Emgel 2% Topical Gel (Occasional) ... 1285

Skin, tenderness
Efudex ... 1733
Emgel 2% Topical Gel ... 1285
Imitrex Injection (Rare) ... 1549
Imitrex Nasal Spray ... 1554
Imitrex Tablets (Infrequent) ... 1558
Levulan Kerastick (Up to 2%) ... 971
Naftin Gel (0.5%) ... 2224

Skin, wrinkling
Amerge Tablets (Rare) ... 1467
Depen Titratable Tablets ... 3341
Imitrex Nasal Spray ... 1554
Imitrex Tablets (Rare) ... 1558
Photofrin for Injection ... 831

Skin atrophy
Aclovate (Infrequent) ... 1275
Analpram-HC ... 1338
Capex Shampoo ... 1400
Clobevate Gel (Less than 2%) ... 3271
Copaxone for Injection (Frequent) ... 3306
Cormax Cream (Approximately 0.3%) ... 2440
Cormax Ointment (Approximately 0.3%) ... 2440
Cormax Scalp Application (Infrequent) ... 2441
Cutivate Cream (Infrequent) ... 1282
Cutivate Ointment (Infrequent to more frequent) ... 1284
Dermatop Emollient Cream (1%) ... 2517
DesOwen (Infrequent) ... 1401
Diprolene Gel 0.05% (Less frequent) ... 3107
Diprolene Lotion 0.05% (Infrequent) ... 3107
Diprolene Ointment 0.05% (Infrequent) ... 3108
Diprolene AF Cream 0.05% (Infrequent) ... 3106
Diprosone ... 3109
Dovonex Ointment (Less than 1%) ... 1117
Dovonex Scalp Solution ... 1118
Effexor Tablets (Rare) ... 3495
Effexor XR Capsules (Rare) ... 3499
Elocon Cream 0.1% (1.6%) ... 3110
Elocon Lotion 0.1% (Infrequent) ... 3111
▲ Elocon Ointment 0.1% (4.8%) ... 3112
Lidex (Infrequent) ... 2020
Locoid Cream (Infrequent) ... 1341
Locoid Lipocream Cream (Infrequent) ... 1342
Locoid (Infrequent) ... 1341
Lotrisone ... 3129
Luxíq Foam ... 1210
Mylocel Tablets ... 2227
Olux Foam (Less than 2%) ... 1211
Pramosone ... 1343
ProctoFoam-HC ... 3177
Psorcon E Cream ... 1227
Psorcon E Ointment ... 1228
▲ Soriatane Capsules (10% to 25%) .. 3003
Synalar (Infrequent) ... 2020
Temovate Cream (Less frequent) ... 1301
▲ Temovate Gel (Among most frequent) ... 1303
Temovate Ointment (Less frequent) ... 1301
Temovate Scalp Application (Infrequent) ... 1304
Temovate E Emollient (Less than 2%) ... 1302
Topicort (Infrequent) ... 2025
Ultravate Cream (Less frequent) ... 1119
Ultravate Ointment (Less frequent) ... 1120

Skin discoloration
Aciphex Tablets (Rare) ... 1267
Aciphex Tablets (Rare) ... 1783
Actiq (Less than 1%) ... 1184
AK-Fluor Injection 10% and 25% ... ⊙ 202
AmBisome for Injection (Less common) ... 1383
Amphotec (1% to 5%) ... 1774
Android Capsules, 10 mg ... 1731
Aricept Tablets (Infrequent) ... 1270
Aricept Tablets (Infrequent) ... 2665
Avonex ... 1013
Azulfidine EN-tabs Tablets (Rare) ... 2775
Baycol Tablets ... 883
Brevibloc Injection (Less than 1%) ... 858
Carbatrol Capsules ... 3234
Celexa (Infrequent) ... 1365
Cerebyx Injection (Infrequent) ... 2619
Chirocaine Injection (Less than 1%) ... 2909
Compazine ... 1505
Condylox Gel (Less common) ... 2436
Cordarone Tablets (Less than 1%) .. 3487
Crinone (Less than 5%) ... 3213
Differin Cream (Less than 1%) ... 1402
Diphtheria & Tetanus Toxoids Adsorbed Purogenated for Pediatric Use ... 1857
Doxil Injection (Less than 1% to 5%) ... 566
Effexor Tablets (Rare) ... 3495
Effexor XR Capsules (Rare) ... 3499
Ergamisol Tablets (Up to 2%) ... 1789
Estrace Vaginal Cream ... 3358
Estrace Tablets ... 3361
Estratest ... 3252
Evoxac Capsules (Less than 1%) ... 1217
Fareston Tablets ... 3237
Fluorescite Injection ... ⊙ 211
FluShield Influenza Vaccine ... 3521
Fortovase Capsules (Less than 2%) ... 2970
Foscavir Injection (Between 1% and 5%) ... 605
Gabitril Tablets (Infrequent) ... 1189
INFeD Injection ... 3388
Intron A for Injection (Less than 5%) ... 3120
Invirase Capsules (Less than 2%) ... 2979
Kaletra Capsules (Less than 2%) ... 471
Kaletra Oral Solution (Less than 2%) ... 471
Lamictal (Rare) ... 1567
Lescol Capsules ... 2361
Lescol Capsules ... 2925
Lescol XL Tablets ... 2361
Lescol XL Tablets ... 2925
Luvox Tablets (25, 50, 100 mg) (Infrequent) ... 3256
Mevacor Tablets ... 2132
Minocin Oral Suspension ... 1865
Mycobutin Capsules (Less than 1%) ... 2838
Neumega for Injection ... 1434
Neurontin Capsules (Rare) ... 2655
Neurontin Oral Solution (Rare) ... 2655
Neurontin Tablets (Rare) ... 2655
Norvasc Tablets (Less than or equal to 0.1%) ... 2704
Novantrone for Injection ... 1760
Ortho-Est Tablets ... 3464
Orudis Capsules (Less than 1%) ... 3548
Oruvail Capsules (Less than 1%) ... 3548
Oxandrin Tablets ... 1153
Pacerone Tablets (Less than 1%) ... 3331
Paxil (Rare) ... 1609
Permax Tablets (Infrequent) ... 1299
Photofrin for Injection ... 831
Pravachol Tablets ... 1099

Priftin Tablets (Less than 1%) ... 758
▲ Prograf (3% to 15%) ... 1393
Prostin E2 Suppositories ... 2852
Protopic Ointment (Greater than or equal to 1%) ... 1397
Prozac Pulvules, Liquid, and Weekly Capsules (Infrequent) ... 1238
Psoriatec Cream ... 3247
Rescriptor Tablets ... 526
Retrovir IV Infusion ... 1629
Rifater Tablets ... 769
Sarafem Pulvules (Infrequent) ... 1962
Seroquel Tablets (Rare) ... 684
▲ Serostim for Injection (1% to 10%) ... 3229
Silvadene Cream 1% (Infrequent) ... 2267
Sonata Capsules (Rare) ... 3591
Stelazine ... 1640
Sular Tablets (Less than or equal to 1%) ... 688
Sustiva Capsules ... 1258
Tasmar Tablets (Infrequent) ... 3010
Taxol Injection ... 1129
▲ Tazorac Gel (1% to 10%) ... 556
Tegretol/Tegretol-XR ... 2404
Testoderm Transdermal Systems ... 574
Tetanus & Diphtheria Toxoids Adsorbed for Adult Use ... 1880
Thalomid Capsules ... 1154
Ticlid Tablets ... 3015
Topamax Sprinkle Capsules (Infrequent) ... 2590
Topamax Tablets (Infrequent) ... 2590
Trasylol Injection (1% to 2%) ... 909
Vanceril Double Strength Inhalation Aerosol (Fewer than 2%) ... 3167
Vistide Injection ... 1445
Zocor Tablets ... 2219
Zoladex (1% or greater) ... 702
Zoladex 3-month ... 706
Zoloft (Rare) ... 2751
Zyprexa Tablets (Rare) ... 1973
Zyprexa ZYDIS Orally Disintegrating Tablets (Rare) ... 1973

Skin disorder, unspecified
Agrylin Capsules (1% to 5%) ... 3232
AmBisome for Injection (Less common) ... 1383
Amphotec (1% to 5%) ... 1774
▲ Catapres-TTS (51 of 101 patients) ... 1038
Cefobid Intravenous/Intramuscular (1 in 45) ... 2671
Cefobid Pharmacy Bulk Package - Not for Direct Infusion (1 in 45) ... 2673
Compazine ... 1505
Crinone (Less than 5%) ... 3213
Crixivan Capsules (Less than 2%) ... 2070
Doxil Injection (1% to 5%) ... 566
▲ Epogen for Injection (7% to 10%) ... 582
EryPed ... 446
Evoxac Capsules (1% to 3%) ... 1217
Floxin Tablets ... 2529
Fortovase Capsules (Rare) ... 2970
Hivid Tablets (Less than 1%) ... 2975
Innohep Injection (Greater than or equal to 1%) ... 1248
Invirase Capsules (Rare) ... 2979
Klonopin Tablets (Infrequent) ... 2983
Lamisil Tablets (Isolated reports) ... 2360
Lanoxicaps Capsules (Rare) ... 1574
Lanoxin Injection (Rare) ... 1581
Lanoxin Elixir Pediatric (Rare) ... 1578
Lanoxin Injection Pediatric (Rare) ... 1584
▲ Leukine (77%) ... 1755
Levaquin Tablets (0.5% to less than 1.0%) ... 2537
▲ Levulan Kerastick (Up to 12%) ... 971
Lupron Depot 3.75 mg (Less than 5%) ... 3281
Lupron Depot 7.5 mg (Less than 5%) ... 3284
▲ Lupron Depot–3 Month 11.25 mg (3% to 10%) ... 3285
▲ Lupron Depot–3 Month 22.5 mg (8.5%) ... 3288
▲ Lupron Depot–4 Month 30 mg (Up to 12.2%) ... 3289
Lupron Injection (Less than 5%) ... 3279
Megace Oral Suspension (1% to 3%) ... 1124
▲ Mirena Intrauterine System (5% or more) ... 974
Monurol Sachet (Less than 1%) ... 1375
▲ Neoral Soft Gelatin Capsules (1% to 17.6%) ... 2380
▲ Neoral Oral Solution (1% to 17.6%) ... 2380
▲ Nipent for Injection (4% to 17%) ... 3272
▲ Nolvadex Tablets (18.7%) ... 678
ParaGard T 380A Intrauterine Copper Contraceptive ... 2582
Prilosec Delayed-Release Capsules (Very rare) ... 628
Primaxin I.M. ... 2158
Primaxin I.V. (Less than 0.2%) ... 2160
Prinivil Tablets (Rare) ... 2164
Prinzide Tablets (Rare) ... 2168
▲ Prograf (3% to 15%) ... 1393
Protonix I.V. (Less than 1%) ... 3580
Protonix Tablets (Less than 1%) ... 3577
Rescriptor Tablets (Less than 2%) ... 526
Rifadin ... 765
Rifater Tablets ... 769
Rilutek Tablets (Infrequent) ... 772
Romazicon Injection (1% to 3%) ... 3000
▲ Serostim for Injection (1% to 10%) ... 3229
Skelid Tablets (2.7%) ... 3088
Soriatane Capsules (Less than 1%) ... 3003
Sporanox Oral Solution (2.2% to 2.3%) ... 1808
Sporanox Oral Solution (2.2% to 2.3%) ... 2512
Streptomycin Sulfate Injection ... 2714
Taxol Injection ... 1129
Taxotere for Injection Concentrate ... 778
Tricor Capsules, Micronized ... 513
▲ Ultrase MT Capsules (Among most frequent) ... 835
▲ Vesanoid Capsules (14%) ... 3037
Xalatan Latanoprost Ophthalmic Solution (1% to 2%) ... ⊙320
Xalatan Sterile Ophthalmic Solution (1% to 2%) ... 2864
Zestoretic Tablets (Rare) ... 695
Zestril Tablets (Rare) ... 698
Zinecard for Injection (1%) ... 2869
Zithromax Capsules, 250 mg (Rare) ... 2743
Zithromax for IV Infusion (Rare) ... 2748
Zithromax for Oral Suspension, 300 mg, 600 mg, 900 mg, 1200 mg (Rare) ... 2739
Zithromax Tablets, 250 mg (Rare) ... 2739
Zoloft ... 2751
Zyrtec (Less than 2%) ... 2756
Zyrtec-D 12 Hour Extended Relief Tablets (Less than 2%) ... 2758

Skin eruptions
Permapen Isoject ... 2706

Skin eruptions, pleomorphic
Aralen Tablets ... 3075

Skin hypertrophy
Betaseron for SC Injection ... 988
▲ CellCept Capsules (3%) ... 2951
▲ CellCept Intravenous (3%) ... 2951
▲ CellCept Oral Suspension (3%) ... 2951
▲ CellCept Tablets (3%) ... 2951
Copaxone for Injection (Infrequent) ... 3306
Effexor Tablets (Infrequent) ... 3495
Effexor XR Capsules (Infrequent) ... 3499
Estring Vaginal Ring (1% to 3%) ... 2811
Evoxac Capsules (Less than 1%) ... 1217
Olux Foam (One case) ... 1211
Paxil (Rare) ... 1609
Pletal Tablets (Less than 2%) ... 2605
Pletal Tablets (Less than 2%) ... 2848
▲ Rapamune Oral Solution and Tablets (3% to 20%) ... 3584
Remeron Tablets (Rare) ... 2483
Remeron SolTab Tablets (Rare) ... 2486
Rescriptor Tablets ... 526
Sonata Capsules (Infrequent) ... 3591
Soriatane Capsules (Less than 1%) ... 3003
Vistide Injection ... 1445

Skin nodule
Amphotec (1% to 5%) ... 1774
Arava Tablets (1% to 3%) ... 724
Baycol Tablets ... 883
Celebrex Capsules (0.1% to 1.9%) ... 2676
Celebrex Capsules (0.1% to 1.9%) ... 2780
Cerebyx Injection (Infrequent) ... 2619
Copaxone for Injection (2%) ... 3306
Doxil Injection (Less than 1%) ... 566
Fortovase Capsules (Less than 2%) ... 2970
Gabitril Tablets (Infrequent) ... 1189
Imdur Tablets (Less than or equal to 5%) ... 1826
Imitrex Nasal Spray ... 1554
Imitrex Tablets (Rare) ... 1558
Invirase Capsules (Less than 2%) ... 2979
Lescol Capsules ... 2361
Lescol Capsules ... 2925
Lescol XL Tablets ... 2361
Lescol XL Tablets ... 2925
Lotrel Capsules ... 2370
Mevacor Tablets ... 2132
Neurontin Capsules (Rare) ... 2655
Neurontin Oral Solution (Rare) ... 2655
Neurontin Tablets (Rare) ... 2655
Permax Tablets (Rare) ... 1299
Photofrin for Injection ... 831
Pravachol Tablets ... 1099
Rescriptor Tablets (Less than 2%) ... 526
Rilutek Tablets (Rare) ... 772
Soriatane Capsules (Less than 1%) ... 3003
Zocor Tablets ... 2219
Zyrtec (Less than 2%) ... 2756
Zyrtec-D 12 Hour Extended Relief Tablets (Less than 2%) ... 2758

Skin odor, abnormal
▲ Soriatane Capsules (1% to 10%) ... 3003

Skin reactions
▲ Gengraf Capsules (1% to 17.6%) ... 457
Protopic Ointment (1% to 4%) ... 1397

Skin test reactions, suppression
Celestone Soluspan Injectable Suspension ... 3097
Cortone Acetate Injectable Suspension ... 2059
Cortone Acetate Tablets ... 2061
Decadron Elixir ... 2078
Decadron Tablets ... 2079
Decadron Phosphate Injection ... 2081
Florinef Acetate Tablets ... 2250
Hydrocortone Tablets ... 2106
Hydrocortone Acetate Injectable Suspension ... 2103
Hydrocortone Phosphate Injection, Sterile ... 2105
Pediapred Oral Solution ... 1170
Prednisone ... 3064
Prelone Syrup ... 2273
Solu-Medrol Sterile Powder ... 2855

Skull abnormalities, fetal
Accupril Tablets ... 2611
Accutane Capsules ... 2944
Aceon Tablets (2 mg, 4 mg, 8 mg) ... 3249
Altace Capsules ... 2233
Captopril Tablets ... 2281
Cozaar Tablets ... 2067
Enalaprilat Injection ... 863
Hyzaar ... 2109
Lexxel Tablets ... 608
Lotrel Capsules ... 2370
Monopril Tablets ... 1091
Prinivil Tablets ... 2164
Prinzide Tablets ... 2168
Univasc Tablets ... 3181
Vaseretic Tablets ... 2204
Vasotec I.V. Injection ... 2207
Vasotec Tablets ... 2210
Zestoretic Tablets ... 695
Zestril Tablets ... 698

Sleep disturbances
Aceon Tablets (2 mg, 4 mg, 8 mg) (2.5%) ... 3249
Adalat CC Tablets (Rare) ... 877
Advair Diskus 100/50 (1% to 3%) ... 1448
Advair Diskus 250/50 (1% to 3%) ... 1448
Advair Diskus 500/50 (1% to 3%) ... 1448
Allegra-D Extended-Release Tablets (Less than 1%) ... 714
Ambien Tablets (Infrequent) ... 3191
Amerge Tablets (Infrequent) ... 1467
Anzemet Injection (Infrequently) ... 719
Anzemet Tablets (Infrequently) ... 722
Arava Tablets (1% to 3%) ... 724
Astelin Nasal Spray (Infrequent) ... 3339
Ativan Tablets (Less frequent) ... 3482
Avalide Tablets ... 1070
Avapro Tablets (Less than 1%) ... 1074
Avapro Tablets (Less than 1%) ... 3076
▲ Avonex (19%) ... 1013
▲ Betapace Tablets (1% to 8%) ... 950
Celexa (At least 2%) ... 1365
▲ Clozaril Tablets (4%) ... 2319
▲ Combivir Tablets (11%) ... 1502
Copaxone for Injection (At least 2%) ... 3306
Cordarone Tablets (1% to 3%) ... 3487
Coreg Tablets (0.1% to 1%) ... 1508
Corgard Tablets ... 2245
Corzide 40/5 Tablets ... 2247
Corzide 80/5 Tablets ... 2247
Cozaar Tablets (Less than 1%) ... 2067
▲ Crinone (18%) ... 3213
Crixivan Capsules (Less than 2%) ... 2070
Depakote ER Tablets (Greater than 1%) ... 436
Effexor Tablets (Infrequent) ... 3495
Eldepryl Capsules ... 3266
▲ Epivir (11%) ... 1520
Flovent Diskus (1% to 3%) ... 3614
Floxin I.V. (1% to 3%) ... 2526
Floxin Tablets (1% to 3%) ... 2529
Fludara for Injection (1% to 3%) ... 995
Halcion Tablets ... 2823
▲ Hectorol Capsules (3.3%) ... 1064
▲ Hectorol Injection (3.3%) ... 1066
HibTITER ... 1859
Hyzaar ... 2109
Imitrex Injection (Rare) ... 1549
Imitrex Nasal Spray (Infrequent) ... 1554
Imitrex Tablets (Rare to infrequent) ... 1558
Klonopin Tablets (Infrequent) ... 2983
Lamictal (1.4%) ... 1567
Levaquin (0.1%) ... 2537
Lithium Carbonate ... 3061
Lithium Citrate Syrup ... 3061
Lupron Depot 7.5 mg (Less than 5%) ... 3284
Lupron Depot–3 Month 11.25 mg (Less than 5%) ... 3285
▲ Lupron Depot–3 Month 22.5 mg (8.5%) ... 3288
Lupron Depot–4 Month 30 mg (Less than 5%) ... 3289
▲ Lupron Injection (5% or more) ... 3279
Luvox Tablets (25, 50, 100 mg) (Infrequent) ... 3256
▲ Mexitil Capsules (7.1% to 7.5%) ... 1047
Mirapex Tablets (1%) ... 2834
Monopril Tablets (0.2% to 1.0%) ... 1091
Monopril HCT ... 1094
Nadolol Tablets ... 2288
Nardil Tablets (Common) ... 2653
Nexium Delayed-Release Capsules (Less than 1%) ... 619
Noroxin Tablets (Less frequent) ... 2145
Numorphan ... 1324
Pacerone Tablets (1% to 3%) ... 3331
▲ Prevnar for Injection (18.1% to 33.3%) ... 1870
Procardia Capsules (2% or less) ... 2708
ProSom Tablets (Infrequent) ... 500
Protonix I.V. (Less than 1%) ... 3580
Protonix Tablets (Less than 1%) ... 3577
Provigil Tablets (At least 1%) ... 1193
Prozac Pulvules, Liquid, and Weekly Capsules (Frequent) ... 1238
▲ Quinidex Extentabs (3%) ... 2933
Recombivax HB (Less than 1%) ... 2178
Rescriptor Tablets ... 526
Risperdal (Frequent) ... 1796
▲ Roferon-A Injection (5% to 11%) ... 2996
Sarafem Pulvules (Frequent) ... 1962
Serevent Diskus (1% to 3%) ... 1637
Sinemet CR Tablets ... 1255
Sonata Capsules (Rare) ... 3591
▲ Tasmar Tablets (24% to 25%) ... 3010
Tonocard Tablets (Less than 1%) ... 649
Tricor Capsules, Micronized (Less than 1%) ... 513
▲ Trizivir Tablets (7% to 11%) ... 1669
Ultram Tablets (1% to 5%) ... 2600
Univasc Tablets (Less than 1%) ... 3181
Valium Tablets ... 3047
Varivax (Greater than or equal to 1%) ... 2202
Verelan Capsules (1.4%) ... 3184
Versed Injection (Less than 1%) ... 3027
Viracept ... 532
▲ Visudyne for Injection (1% to 10%) ... ⊙308
▲ Wellbutrin Tablets (4.0%) ... 1680
Xanax Tablets (Rare) ... 2865
▲ Xenical Capsules (3.9%) ... 3043
Zarontin Capsules ... 2659
Zarontin Syrup ... 2660
Ziac Tablets ... 1887
▲ Ziagen (7%) ... 1692
Zyrtec (Less than 2%) ... 2756
Zyrtec-D 12 Hour Extended Relief Tablets (Less than 2%) ... 2758

Sleep talking
Sonata Capsules (Rare) ... 3591

Sleep walking
Neurontin Capsules ... 2655
Neurontin Oral Solution ... 2655
Neurontin Tablets ... 2655
Sonata Capsules (Rare) ... 3591

Sleepiness
(see under Drowsiness)

Sleeplessness
(see under Insomnia)

SLE-like syndrome
(see under Lupus erythematosus, systemic)

Sloughing
Aramine Injection ... 2043
Brevibloc Injection ... 858
Efudex ... 1733
Fluorescite Injection ... ⊙211
Gamimune N, 5% Solvent/Detergent Treated (One patient) ... 925
Gamimune N, 10% Solvent/Detergent Treated (One patient) ... 928
Iveegam EN (0.91%) ... 849
Navelbine Injection ... 1604
Norplant System ... 3543
Ophthetic Ophthalmic Solution ... ⊙244
Robaxin Injectable ... 2938

Sluggishness
Phrenilin (Infrequent) ... 578
Sedapap Tablets 50 mg/650 mg (Infrequent) ... 2225

Smell, loss of the sense
(see under Anosmia)

Smell disturbances
Amerge Tablets (Infrequent) ... 1467
Beconase Inhalation Aerosol (Rare) ... 1497
Beconase AQ Nasal Spray (Rare) ... 1498
Biaxin/Biaxin XL ... 403
Cordarone Tablets (1% to 3%) ... 3487
Ergamisol Tablets (1%) ... 1789
Flonase Nasal Spray ... 1533
Floxin I.V. ... 2526
Floxin Tablets ... 2529

Hivid Tablets (Less than 1%) 2975
Imitrex Injection (Rare) 1549
Imitrex Nasal Spray (Infrequent) 1554
Imitrex Tablets (Infrequent) 1558
Maxair Autohaler (0.6%) 1981
Maxair Inhaler (Less than 1%) 1984
Maxalt Tablets (Rare) 2120
Maxalt-MLT Orally Disintegrating Tablets (Rare) 2120
Migranal Nasal Spray (Infrequent) 2376
Nasalide Nasal Spray (5% or less) 1295
Nicotrol Nasal Spray (More common) 2843
Pacerone Tablets (1% to 3%) 3331
PREVPAC 3298
Rhinocort Nasal Inhaler (Less than 1%) 640
▲ Roferon-A Injection (3%) 2996
Rythmol Tablets – 150 mg, 225 mg, 300 mg (Less than 1%) 502
Timentin Injection- ADD-Vantage Vial 1661
Timentin Injection-Galaxy Container 1664
Timentin Injection-Pharmacy Bulk Package 1666
Timentin for Intravenous Administration 1658
Tonocard Tablets (Less than 1%) 649
Xanax Tablets 2865

Smoker's tongue
(*see under* Leukoplakia, oral)

Sneezing
Aceon Tablets (2 mg, 4 mg, 8 mg) (0.3% to 1%) 3249
Advair Diskus 100/50 (1% to 3%) 1448
Advair Diskus 250/50 (1% to 3%) 1448
Advair Diskus 500/50 (1% to 3%) 1448
▲ Aerobid/Aerobid-M (3% to 9%) 1363
Afrin Nasal Decongestant Children's Pump Mist ▣734
Afrin ▣733
Afrin No Drip Original Nasal Spray ▣735
Afrin No Drip Extra Moisturizing Nasal Spray ▣735
Afrin No Drip Severe Congestion Nasal Spray ▣735
Afrin No Drip Sinus Nasal Spray ▣735
Afrin Original Pump Mist ▣733
Alamast Ophthalmic Solution (Less than 5%) 3092
Alomide Ophthalmic Solution (Less than 1%) ⊙204
▲ Astelin Nasal Spray (3.1%) 3339
▲ Atrovent Nasal Spray 0.03% (3.1%) 1032
Axert Tablets (Rare) 2772
Azactam for Injection (Less than 1%) 1276
▲ Beconase Inhalation Aerosol (10 in 100 patients) 1497
▲ Beconase AQ Nasal Spray (4%) 1498
BeneFix for Injection (One case) 1432
Calcium Disodium Versenate Injection 1980
Claritin (At least one patient) 3100
Claritin-D 12 Hour Extended Release Tablets (Less frequent) 3102
Claritin-D 24 Hour Extended Release Tablets 3104
Clozaril Tablets (Less than 1%) 2319
Diprivan Injectable Emulsion (Less than 1%) 667
Ethyol for Injection 2029
Flovent Rotadisk (1% to 3%) 1537
Intron A for Injection (Less than or equal to 5%) 3120
Klonopin Tablets (Infrequent) 2983
Lexxel Tablets 608
Maxalt Tablets (Rare) 2120
Maxalt-MLT Orally Disintegrating Tablets (Rare) 2120
Naropin Injection 612
Nasacort Nasal Inhaler (Fewer than 5%) 750
Nasalide Nasal Spray (5% or less) 1295
Neo-Synephrine ▣614
Neo-Synephrine 12 Hour ▣615
Nesacaine/Nesacaine MPF 617
Nicotrol Nasal Spray (Common) 2843
Plendil Extended-Release Tablets (Up to 1.6%) 623
Polocaine Injection, USP 625
Polocaine-MPF Injection, USP 625
Rhinocort Nasal Inhaler (Less than 1%) 640
Sensorcaine (Rare) 643
Sensorcaine-MPF Injection (Rare) 643
Serevent Inhalation Aerosol (1% to 3%) 1633
Simulect for Injection 2399
Singulair (Greater than or equal to 2%) 2181
▲ Vancenase PocketHaler Nasal Inhaler (10 per 100 patients) 3162
▲ Vanceril Double Strength Inhalation Aerosol (3%) 3167
Versed Syrup (0.25%) 3033

Vicks Sinex Nasal Spray and Ultra Fine Mist ▣729

Snoring
Aricept Tablets (Infrequent) 1270
Aricept Tablets (Infrequent) 2665
Neurontin Capsules (Rare) 2655
Neurontin Oral Solution (Rare) 2655
Neurontin Tablets (Rare) 2655
Sonata Capsules (Infrequent) 3591

Social reaction, anti
(*see under* Sociopathy)

Sociopathy
DextroStat Tablets 3236
Neurontin Capsules (Rare) 2655
Neurontin Oral Solution (Rare) 2655
Neurontin Tablets (Rare) 2655
Paxil (Rare) 1609
Prozac Pulvules, Liquid, and Weekly Capsules (Rare) 1238
Sarafem Pulvules (Rare) 1962
Zyprexa Tablets (Infrequent) 1973
Zyprexa ZYDIS Orally Disintegrating Tablets (Infrequent) 1973

Sodium depletion
(*see under* Hyponatremia)

Sodium loss
(*see under* Hyponatremia)

Sodium retention
Celestone Soluspan Injectable Suspension 3097
Celestone Syrup 3099
Cortone Acetate Injectable Suspension 2059
Cortone Acetate Tablets 2061
Decadron Elixir 2078
Decadron Tablets 2079
Decadron Phosphate Injection 2081
Delatestryl Injection 1151
Depo-Medrol Injectable Suspension 2795
▲ Estratest (Among most common) 3252
Hydrocortone Tablets 2106
Hydrocortone Acetate Injectable Suspension 2103
Hydrocortone Phosphate Injection, Sterile 2105
Oxandrin Tablets 1153
Pediapred Oral Solution 1170
Prednisone 3064
Prelone Syrup 2273
Solu-Medrol Sterile Powder 2855
Testred Capsules, 10 mg 1746

Somatization
Zyprexa Tablets (Infrequent) 1973
Zyprexa ZYDIS Orally Disintegrating Tablets (Infrequent) 1973

Somnambulism
Ambien Tablets (Rare) 3191
Halcion Tablets 2823
Requip Tablets (Infrequent) 1621
Zoloft (Rare) 2751

Somnolence
(*see under* Drowsiness)

Sore throat
(*see under* Throat soreness)

Soreness, injection site
▲ Alferon N Injection (10%) 1770
BayRab 917
BayRho-D Full Dose 921
BayRho-D Mini-Dose 919
BayTet 923
▲ Comvax (23.9% to 34.5%) 2056
▲ Engerix-B Vaccine (22%) 1517
▲ FluShield Influenza Vaccine (Among most frequent) 3521
▲ Fluzone Vaccine (Most frequent) 802
▲ Havrix Vaccine (21% to 56%) 1544
Imogam Rabies - HT (Uncommon) 805
INFeD Injection 3388
▲ JE-VAX Vaccine (5.9% to 24.5%) 811
▲ LYMErix Vaccine (5% to 93.53%) 1592
▲ Pneumovax 23 (Common) 2156
▲ TYPHIM Vi Vaccine (13%) 825
▲ Varivax (19.3% to 32.5%) 2202

Soreness, vaginal
Condylox Gel (Less common) 2436
▲ Gynazole-1 Vaginal Cream (5.7%) 3310

Spasm, biliary tract
Demerol 3079
Dilaudid Oral Liquid 445
Dilaudid Tablets - 8 mg 445
Dilaudid-HP (Less frequent) 443
Dolophine Hydrochloride Tablets 3056
Levorphanol Tartrate Tablets 3059
MS Contin Tablets (Less frequent) 2896
MSIR (Less frequent) 2898
Numorphan 1324
Oramorph SR Tablets (Less frequent) 3062

Phenergan with Codeine Syrup 3557
Phenergan VC with Codeine Syrup 3561
Roxanol 3066
Trilafon 3160

Spasm, generalized
Colazal Capsules 3069
Fortovase Capsules (Less than 2%) 2970
Foscavir Injection (Between 1% and 5%) 605
Gabitril Tablets (Infrequent) 1189
Invirase Capsules (Less than 2%) 2979
Naprelan Tablets (Less than 1%) 1293
Paxil (Rare) 1609
Prinivil Tablets (0.3% to 1.0%) 2164
Prinzide Tablets 2168
▲ Prograf (3% to 15%) 1393
Zestoretic Tablets 695
Zestril Tablets (0.3% to 1.0%) 698
Zyprexa Tablets (2% to 3%) 1973
Zyprexa ZYDIS Orally Disintegrating Tablets (2% to 3%) 1973

Spasm, non-site specific
Amerge Tablets (Rare) 1467

Spasm, vesical sphincters
Hycomine Compound Tablets 1317
Hycotuss Expectorant Syrup 1318
Lortab 3319
Lortab Elixir 3317
Maxidone Tablets CIII 3399
Norco 5/325 Tablets CIII 3424
Norco 7.5/325 Tablets CIII 3425
Norco 10/325 Tablets CIII 3425
Norco 10/325 Tablets CIII 3427
Tussionex Pennkinetic Extended-Release Suspension 1174
Vicodin Tablets 516
Vicodin ES Tablets 517
Vicodin HP Tablets 518
Vicodin Tuss Expectorant 519
Zydone Tablets 1330

Spatial disorientation
Serophene Tablets 3226

Speech, bulbar type
Reglan 2935

Speech, compulsive

Speech, incoherent
Clozaril Tablets (Less than 1%) 2319
Sensorcaine 643
Sensorcaine-MPF Injection 643

Speech, slurring
Clozaril Tablets (1%) 2319
Coly-Mycin M Parenteral 2243
Corgard Tablets (1 to 5 per 1000 patients) 2245
Corzide 40/5 Tablets (1 to 5 of 1000 patients) 2247
Corzide 80/5 Tablets (1 to 5 of 1000 patients) 2247
▲ Dilantin Infatabs (Among most common) 2624
▲ Dilantin Kapseals (Among most common) 2622
▲ Dilantin-125 Oral Suspension (Among most common) 2625
Eskalith 1527
Etrafon 3115
Halcion Tablets 2823
Kadian Capsules (Less than 3%) 1335
Klonopin Tablets 2983
Lithium Carbonate 3061
Lithium Citrate Syrup 3061
Lithobid Slow-Release Tablets 3255
Loxitane Capsules 3398
Luvox Tablets (25, 50, 100 mg) (Rare) 3256
Matulane Capsules 3246
Miltown Tablets 3349
Nadolol Tablets (1 to 5 of 1000 patients) 2288
Serentil 1057
Sonata Capsules (Rare) 3591
Symmetrel (0.1% to 1%) 1328
Tonocard Tablets (Less than 1%) 649
Tranxene 511
Trilafon 3160
Valium Injectable 3026
Valium Tablets (Infrequent) 3047
Versed Injection (Less than 1%) 3027
Vicoprofen Tablets (Less than 1%) 520
Xanax Tablets 2865

Speech difficulties
Clozaril Tablets (Less than 1%) 2319
▲ Demser Capsules (10%) 2085
Marinol Capsules (Less than 1%) 3325
Mexitil Capsules (2.6%) 1047
Nubain Injection (1% or less) 1323
Stadol NS Nasal Spray (Less than 1%) 1108
Zyprexa Tablets (2%) 1973

Zyprexa ZYDIS Orally Disintegrating Tablets (2%) 1973

Speech disturbances
Accuretic Tablets 2614
Actiq (Less than 1%) 1184
Ambien Tablets (Infrequent) 3191
Amphotec (1% to 5%) 1774
▲ Avonex (3%) 1013
▲ Betaseron for SC Injection (3%) 988
Brevibloc Injection (Less than 1%) 858
Carbatrol Capsules 3234
Cerebyx Injection (Frequent) 2619
Copaxone for Injection (2%) 3306
Dantrium Capsules (Less frequent) 2885
Depakote Tablets (1% to 5%) 430
Depakote ER Tablets (1% to 5%) 436
Duragesic Transdermal System (1% or greater) 1786
Effexor Tablets (Infrequent) 3495
Effexor XR Capsules (Infrequent) 3499
Eldepryl Capsules 3266
Ergamisol Tablets 1789
Estrace Vaginal Cream 3358
Estrace Tablets 3361
Evoxac Capsules (Less than 1%) 1217
Fortovase Capsules (Less than 2%) 2970
▲ Gabitril Tablets (4%) 1189
Hivid Tablets (Less than 1%) 2975
Imitrex Injection 1549
Intron A for Injection (Less than 5%) 3120
Invirase Capsules (Less than 2%) 2979
Lamictal (2.5%) 1567
Levaquin (Less than 0.3%) 2537
Levbid Extended-Release Tablets 3172
Levlen 962
Levlite 21 Tablets 962
Levlite 28 Tablets 962
Levsin/Levsinex/Levbid 3172
Meridia Capsules 481
Migranal Nasal Spray (Rare) 2376
Mirapex Tablets (1% or more) 2834
Modicon 2563
NuLev Orally Disintegrating Tablets 3176
▲ Orap Tablets (2 of 20 patients) 1407
Ortho-Cyclen/Ortho Tri-Cyclen 2573
Ortho-Est Tablets 3464
Ortho-Novum 2563
Ortho-Novum 1/50□28 Tablets 2556
Ortho-Cyclen/Ortho Tri-Cyclen 2573
OxyContin Tablets (Less than 1%) 2912
Permax Tablets (1.1%) 1299
Prevacid Delayed-Release Capsules (Less than 1%) 3292
PREVPAC 3298
▲ Proleukin for Injection (7%) 1199
Prometrium Capsules (100 mg, 200 mg) (Less than 5%) 3261
Protonix I.V. 3580
Romazicon Injection (Less than 1%) 3000
Rythmol Tablets – 150 mg, 225 mg, 300 mg (Less than 1%) 502
Salagen Tablets (Less than 1%) 2229
Tambocor Tablets (Less than 1%) 1990
Tasmar Tablets (Frequent) 3010
Tegretol/Tegretol-XR 2404
Tonocard Tablets (Less than 1%) 649
▲ Topamax Sprinkle Capsules (13.8% to 16.8%) 2590
▲ Topamax Tablets (13.8% to 16.8%) 2590
Trileptal Oral Suspension (1% to 3%) 2407
Trileptal Tablets (1% to 3%) 2407
Tri-Levlen 962
Trovan (Less than 1%) 2722
Ultram Tablets (Infrequent) 2600
▲ Vesanoid Capsules (3%) 3037
Vistide Injection 1445
▲ Zanaflex Tablets (3%) 1305
▲ Zonegran Capsules (5%) 1307
Zyprexa Tablets (2%) 1973
Zyprexa ZYDIS Orally Disintegrating Tablets (2%) 1973

Spermatogenesis, changes
Cytovene-IV 2959
Thioplex for Injection 1765

Spermatogenesis, defective
Mustargen for Injection 2142

Spermatogenesis, inhibition
Cytovene-IV 2959

Spinal block
Duranest Injections 600
Naropin Injection 612
Nesacaine/Nesacaine MPF 617
Sensorcaine-MPF with Epinephrine Injection 643
Sensorcaine-MPF Injection 643
Xylocaine Injections 653

Spinal cord, compression
Zoladex 702
Zoladex 3-month (Isolated cases) 706

Spinal cord infarction
Activase I.V. ... 1410
Retavase Vials ... 1182
Streptase for Infusion ... 647

Spinal fracture
Lupron Depot 3.75 mg ... 3281
Lupron Depot 7.5 mg ... 3284
Lupron Depot–3 Month 11.25 mg ... 3285
Lupron Depot–3 Month 22.5 mg ... 3288
Lupron Depot–4 Month 30 mg ... 3289
Lupron Depot-PED 7.5 mg, 11.25 mg and 15 mg ... 3291
Lupron Injection ... 3279

Spinal stenosis
Remicade for IV Injection (Less than 2%) ... 1178

Spleen palpable
Thalomid Capsules ... 1154

Spleenomegaly
Flolan for Injection ... 1528

Splenic disorder, unspecified
Vistide Injection ... 1445

Splenic infarction
Campath Ampules ... 992
Remicade for IV Injection (Less than 2%) ... 1178

Splenomegaly
Aloprim for Injection (Less than 1%) ... 2292
Betaseron for SC Injection ... 988
Campath Ampules ... 992
Copaxone for Injection (Infrequent) ... 3306
DaunoXome Injection (Less than or equal to 5%) ... 1442
Epivir ... 1520
Epivir-HBV ... 1524
Fortovase Capsules (Less than 2%) ... 2970
Invirase Capsules (Less than 2%) ... 2979
Iveegam EN (One case) ... 849
▲ Neupogen for Injection (Approximately 30%) ... 587
Orthoclone OKT3 Sterile Solution ... 2498
Permax Tablets (Rare) ... 1299
Remicade for IV Injection (Less than 2%) ... 1178
RhoGAM Injection (One patient) ... 2524
Vistide Injection ... 1445

Spondylolisthesis
Remicade for IV Injection (Less than 2%) ... 1178

Spotting
Activella Tablets ... 2764
Alesse-21 Tablets ... 3468
Alesse-28 Tablets ... 3473
Alora Transdermal System ... 3372
Aygestin Tablets ... 1333
Brevicon 28-Day Tablets ... 3380
Cenestin Tablets ... 1263
Climara Transdermal System ... 958
Clomid Tablets (1.3%) ... 735
Cytotec Tablets (0.7%) ... 3202
Depo-Provera Contraceptive Injection ... 2798
Desogen Tablets ... 2458
Esclim Transdermal System ... 3460
Estinyl Tablets ... 3112
Estrace Vaginal Cream ... 3358
Estrace Tablets ... 3361
Estratest ... 3252
Estrostep ... 2627
femhrt Tablets ... 2635
Levlen (Sometimes) ... 962
Levlite 21 Tablets (Sometimes) ... 962
Levlite 28 Tablets (Sometimes) ... 962
Levora Tablets ... 3389
Loestrin 21 Tablets ... 2642
Loestrin Fe Tablets ... 2642
Lo/Ovral Tablets ... 3532
Lo/Ovral-28 Tablets ... 3538
Low-Ogestrel-28 Tablets ... 3392
Menest Tablets ... 2254
Microgestin Fe 1.5/30 Tablets ... 3407
Microgestin Fe 1/20 Tablets ... 3400
Mircette Tablets ... 2470
Modicon (Sometimes) ... 2563
Necon ... 3415
Nordette-28 Tablets ... 2257
Norinyl 1 +35 28-Day Tablets ... 3380
Norinyl 1 + 50 28-Day Tablets ... 3380
▲ Norplant System (17.1%) ... 3543
Ogen Tablets ... 2846
Ogestrel 0.5/50-28 Tablets ... 3428
Ortho-Cept 21 Tablets ... 2546
Ortho-Cept 28 Tablets ... 2546
Ortho-Cyclen/Ortho Tri-Cyclen ... 2573
Ortho-Est Tablets ... 3464
Ortho-Novum (Sometimes) ... 2563
Ortho-Novum 1/50□28 Tablets (Sometimes) ... 2556
Ortho-Prefest Tablets ... 2570
Ortho-Cyclen/Ortho Tri-Cyclen ... 2573
Ovcon (Sometimes) ... 3364
Ovral Tablets ... 3551
Ovral-28 Tablets ... 3552
Ovrette Tablets ... 3552
ParaGard T 380A Intrauterine Copper Contraceptive ... 2582
Premarin Intravenous ... 3563
Premarin Tablets ... 3566
Premarin Vaginal Cream ... 3570
Premphase Tablets ... 3572
Prempro Tablets ... 3572
Prometrium Capsules (100 mg, 200 mg) ... 3261
Provera Tablets ... 2853
Tri-Levlen (Sometimes) ... 962
Tri-Norinyl-28 Tablets (Sometimes) ... 3433
Triphasil-21 Tablets ... 3600
Triphasil-28 Tablets ... 3605
Trivora Tablets ... 3439
Verelan Capsules (1% or less) ... 3184
Verelan PM Capsules (2% or less) ... 3186
Vivelle Transdermal System ... 2412
Vivelle-Dot Transdermal System ... 2416
Zovia ... 3449

Spotting, oily
▲ Xenical Capsules (4.4% to 26.6%) ... 3043

Sputum, discoloration
Mycobutin Capsules ... 2838
Rifadin ... 765
Rifater Tablets ... 769
▲ TOBI Solution for Inhalation (21.3%) ... 1206

Sputum increased
Actiq (Less than 1%) ... 1184
▲ Aerobid/Aerobid-M (3% to 9%) ... 1363
Atrovent Inhalation Solution (1.4%) ... 1031
Celexa (Rare) ... 1365
▲ CellCept Capsules (3% to 10%) ... 2951
▲ CellCept Intravenous (3% to 10%) ... 2951
▲ CellCept Oral Suspension (3% to 10%) ... 2951
▲ CellCept Tablets (3% to 10%) ... 2951
Cerebyx Injection (Infrequent) ... 2619
Claritin-D 12 Hour Extended Release Tablets (Less frequent) ... 3102
Claritin-D 24 Hour Extended Release Tablets (Fewer than 2%) ... 3104
Combivent Inhalation Aerosol (Less than 2%) ... 1041
DaunoXome Injection (Less than or equal to 5%) ... 1442
Imdur Tablets (Less than or equal to 5%) ... 1826
Lupron Depot 7.5 mg (Less than 5%) ... 3284
Nicotrol Nasal Spray (Less than 1%) ... 2843
Paxil (Rare) ... 1609
Proventil Inhalation Solution 0.083% (1.5%) ... 3146
Proventil Solution for Inhalation 0.5% (1.5%) ... 3144
Pulmozyme Inhalation Solution ... 1426
Rilutek Tablets (More than 2%) ... 772
Risperdal (Rare) ... 1796
Salagen Tablets (Less than 1%) ... 2229
▲ Serostim for Injection (1% to 10%) ... 3229
Sonata Capsules (Rare) ... 3591
Soriatane Capsules (Less than 1%) ... 3003
Sporanox Oral Solution (2.0% to 2.6%) ... 1808
Sporanox Oral Solution (2.0% to 2.6%) ... 2512
▲ TOBI Solution for Inhalation (37.6%) ... 1206
Viagra Tablets (Less than 2%) ... 2732
Vistide Injection ... 1445
Zyrtec (Less than 2%) ... 2756
Zyrtec-D 12 Hour Extended Relief Tablets (Less than 2%) ... 2758

ST section changes
(*see under* EKG changes, ST section)

Status asthmaticus
Sandostatin Injection (Less than 1%) ... 2394
Sandostatin LAR Depot (Rare) ... 2395

Status epilepticus
Aloprim for Injection (Less than 1%) ... 2292
Carbatrol Capsules ... 3234
Clozaril Tablets ... 2319
Dilantin-125 Oral Suspension ... 2625
Felbatol ... 3343
Hivid Tablets (Less than 1%) ... 2975
Oncaspar ... 756
Paxil ... 1609
Tegretol/Tegretol-XR ... 2404
Xanax Tablets ... 2865

Steatorrhea
▲ Sandostatin LAR Depot (4% to 6%) ... 2395

Steatosis, hepatic
Combivir Tablets ... 1502
Epivir ... 1520
Epivir-HBV ... 1524
Ergamisol Tablets (Rare) ... 1789
Hivid Tablets (Rare) ... 2975
Retrovir Capsules ... 1625
Retrovir IV Infusion (Rare) ... 1629
Retrovir ... 1625
Trizivir Tablets ... 1669
Videx EC Capsules ... 1143
Zerit ... 1147

Steatosis, microvesicular
Orudis Capsules (Rare) ... 3548
Oruvail Capsules (Rare) ... 3548

Stenosis, aortic
Naprelan Tablets (Less than 1%) ... 1293
Tasmar Tablets (Infrequent) ... 3010

Stenosis, subglottic
Survanta Intratracheal Suspension ... 3053

Stevens-Johnson syndrome
Accuretic Tablets ... 2614
Agenerase Capsules (1%) ... 1454
Agenerase Oral Solution (1%) ... 1459
Aggrenox Capsules ... 1026
Aldoclor Tablets ... 2035
Aldoril Tablets ... 2039
Amoxil Chewable Tablets ... 1471
Amoxil for Oral Suspension ... 1471
Amoxil ... 1471
Anaprox Tablets (Less than 1%) ... 2967
Anaprox DS Tablets (Less than 1%) ... 2967
Ancef for Injection ... 1474
Ancef Injection ... 1474
Arava Tablets (Rare) ... 724
Arthrotec Tablets (Rare) ... 3195
Atacand HCT Tablets ... 597
Atromid-S Capsules ... 3483
Attenuvax ... 2044
Augmentin Chewable Tablets (Rare) ... 1482
Augmentin Powder for Oral Suspension (Rare) ... 1482
Augmentin Tablets (Rare) ... 1485
Augmentin ES-600 Powder for Oral Suspension ... 1487
Avalide Tablets ... 1070
Azulfidine EN-tabs Tablets (Rare) ... 2775
Bactrim (Rare) ... 2949
Baycol Tablets (Rare) ... 883
Betagan ... ⊙ 228
Biaxin/Biaxin XL (Rare) ... 403
Bleph-10 (Isolated incident) ... ⊙ 230
▲ Blephamide Ophthalmic Ointment (Among most often) ... 547
Blephamide Ophthalmic Suspension ... 548
Captopril Tablets ... 2281
Carbatrol Capsules (Extremely rare) ... 3234
Cataflam Tablets (Rare) ... 2315
Ceclor CD Tablets ... 1279
Ceclor (Rare) ... 1905
Cedax ... 1021
Cefizox for Intramuscular or Intravenous Use ... 1390
Cefotan ... 664
Ceftin ... 1000
Cefzil (Rare) ... 1076
Celebrex Capsules (Less than 0.1%) ... 2676
Celebrex Capsules (Less than 0.1%) ... 2780
Celontin Capsules ... 2618
Ceptaz for Injection ... 1499
Chibroxin Sterile Ophthalmic Solution ... 2051
Cipro I.V. (1% or less) ... 893
Cipro I.V. Pharmacy Bulk Package (Less than 1%) ... 897
Cipro ... 887
Cleocin HCl Capsules ... 2784
Cleocin Phosphate Sterile Solution ... 2785
Cleocin Vaginal Cream (Some cases) ... 2788
Cleocin Vaginal Ovules (Rare) ... 2789
Clinoril Tablets (Less than 1 in 100) ... 2053
Clozaril Tablets ... 2319
Combivir Tablets ... 1502
Comvax ... 2056
Cordarone Intravenous (Less than 2%) ... 3491
Covera-HS Tablets (Less than 2%) ... 3199
Crixivan Capsules ... 2070
Cytovene ... 2959
Daraprim Tablets ... 1511
Declomycin Tablets (Rare) ... 1855
Depacon Injection ... 416
Depakene ... 421
Depakote Sprinkle Capsules ... 426
Depakote Tablets ... 430
Depakote ER Tablets ... 436
Diamox Intravenous ... ⊙ 269
Diamox Sequels Sustained Release Capsules ... ⊙ 270
Diamox Tablets ... ⊙ 269
Didronel Tablets (A single case) ... 2888
Diflucan Tablets, Injection, and Oral Suspension ... 2681
Dilantin Infatabs ... 2624
Dilantin Kapseals ... 2622
Dilantin-125 Oral Suspension ... 2625
Diovan HCT Tablets ... 2338
Diuril Oral ... 2087
Diuril Sodium Intravenous ... 2086
Dolobid Tablets (Less than 1 in 100) ... 2088
Duricef (Rare) ... 1079
Dynacin Capsules (Rare) ... 2019
EC-Naprosyn Delayed-Release Tablets (Less than 1%) ... 2967
E.E.S. (Rare) ... 450
Effexor Tablets ... 3495
Effexor XR Capsules ... 3499
Enalaprilat Injection ... 863
Engerix-B Vaccine ... 1517
Ergamisol Tablets (Isolated cases) ... 1789
EryPed (Rare) ... 446
Ethyol for Injection (Rare) ... 2029
Exelon Capsules ... 2342
Exelon Oral Solution ... 2345
Felbatol (Rare) ... 3343
Feldene Capsules (Rare) ... 2685
Floxin I.V. ... 2526
Floxin Tablets ... 2529
FML-S Liquifilm Sterile Ophthalmic Suspension (Rare) ... ⊙ 238
Fortaz ... 1541
Fortovase Capsules (Rare) ... 2970
Foscavir Injection ... 605
HydroDIURIL Tablets ... 2108
Hyzaar ... 2109
Indapamide Tablets ... 2286
Indocin Capsules (Less than 1%) ... 2112
Indocin I.V. (Less than 1%) ... 2115
Indocin (Less than 1%) ... 2112
Invirase Capsules (Rare) ... 2979
Isoptin SR Tablets (1% or less) ... 467
Keflex (Rare) ... 1237
Kefurox Vials, ADD-Vantage ... 1948
Kefzol Vials, ADD-Vantage ... 1951
Lamictal (Rare) ... 1567
Lamisil Tablets (Isolated reports) ... 2360
Lariam Tablets ... 2989
Lescol Capsules (Rare) ... 2361
Lescol Capsules (Rare) ... 2925
Lescol XL Tablets ... 2361
Lescol XL Tablets ... 2925
Leukeran Tablets (Rare) ... 1591
Leustatin Injection (Isolated cases) ... 2495
Levaquin ... 2537
Lexxel Tablets ... 608
Lipitor Tablets ... 2639
Lipitor Tablets ... 2696
Lodine (Less than 1%) ... 3528
Lodine XL Extended-Release Tablets (Less than 1%) ... 3530
Lorabid Suspension and Pulvules ... 2251
Lotensin Tablets (Less than 1%) ... 2365
Lotensin HCT Tablets (Rare) ... 2367
Lotrel Capsules (Rare) ... 2370
Luvox Tablets (25, 50, 100 mg) ... 3256
Macrobid Capsules (Rare) ... 2889
Macrodantin Capsules (Rare) ... 2891
Maxipime for Injection ... 1285
Mefoxin for Injection ... 2124
Mefoxin Premixed Intravenous Solution ... 2127
Merrem I.V. ... 673
Meruvax II ... 2130
Mevacor Tablets (Rare) ... 2132
Mexitil Capsules (Rare) ... 1047
Micardis HCT Tablets ... 1051
Microzide Capsules ... 3414
Miltown Tablets (Rare) ... 3349
Minocin Intravenous (Rare) ... 1862
Minocin Oral Suspension (Rare) ... 1865
Minocin Pellet-Filled Capsules (Rare) ... 1863
Mintezol ... 2137
M-M-R II ... 2118
Mobic Tablets (Less than 0.1%) ... 1054
Moduretic Tablets ... 2138
Monopril HCT ... 1094
Motrin Suspension, Oral Drops, Chewable Tablets, and Caplets (Less than 1%) ... 2002
Mumpsvax ... 2141
▲ Naprelan Tablets (3% to 9%) ... 1293
Naprosyn Suspension (Less than 1%) ... 2967
Naprosyn Tablets (Less than 1%) ... 2967
Nebcin Vials, Hyporets & ADD-Vantage (Rare) ... 1955
Neptazane Tablets ... ⊙ 271
Neurontin Capsules ... 2655
Neurontin Oral Solution ... 2655
Neurontin Tablets ... 2655
Nolvadex Tablets (Very rare) ... 678
Noroxin Tablets ... 2145

Norvir Capsules (Rare) 487
Norvir Oral Solution (Rare) 487
Omnicef 493
Orthoclone OKT3 Sterile Solution 2498
Orudis Capsules (Less than 1%) 3548
Oruvail Capsules (Less than 1%) 3548
PCE Dispertab Tablets (Rare) 498
Pediazole Suspension 3050
Pipracil (Rare) 1866
Plaquenil Tablets 3082
Ponstel Capsules (Rare) 1356
Pravachol Tablets (Rare) 1099
PREVPAC (Rare) 3298
Prilosec Delayed-Release Capsules (Very rare) 628
Primaxin I.M. 2158
Primaxin I.V. 2160
Prinivil Tablets (Rare) 2164
Prinzide Tablets (Rare) 2168
Procardia Capsules (Rare) 2708
Procardia XL Extended Release Tablets (Rare) 2710
ProSom Tablets (Rare) 500
Protonix I.V. 3580
Protonix Tablets 3577
Prozac Pulvules, Liquid, and Weekly Capsules 1238
Recombivax HB 2178
Relafen Tablets (Less than 1%) 1617
Rescriptor Tablets (Less than 2%) 526
Rifadin (Occasional) 765
Sarafem Pulvules 1962
Septra Suspension 2265
Septra Tablets 2265
Septra DS Tablets 2265
Silvadene Cream 1% 2267
Skelid Tablets (Rare) 3088
Sporanox Capsules (Rare) 1800
Sporanox Injection (Rare) 1804
Sporanox Injection (Rare) 2509
Sporanox Oral Solution (Rare) 1808
Sporanox Oral Solution (Rare) 2512
Sultrin Triple Sulfa Cream (Frequent) 2587
Suprax (Less than 2%) 1877
Sustiva Capsules (Up to 3.5%) 1258
Tagamet (Very rare) 1644
Talacen Caplets 3089
Talwin Nx Tablets 3090
Tarka Tablets 508
Tazicef for Injection 1647
Tazicef Galaxy Container 1650
Tazicef Pharmacy Bulk Package 1653
Tazidime Vials, Faspak & ADD-Vantage 1966
Tegretol/Tegretol-XR (Extremely rare) 2404
Thalomid Capsules 1154
Tiazac Capsules (Less than 2%) 1378
Ticlid Tablets (Rare) 3015
Timentin Injection- ADD-Vantage Vial 1661
Timentin Injection-Galaxy Container 1664
Timentin Injection-Pharmacy Bulk Package 1666
Timentin for Intravenous Administration 1658
Timolide Tablets 2187
Tonocard Tablets (Less than 1%) 649
Toradol 3018
Trileptal Oral Suspension 2407
Trileptal Tablets 2407
Trizivir Tablets 1669
Trovan 2722
Trusopt Sterile Ophthalmic Solution (Rare) 2196
Twinrix Vaccine 1674
Ultracet Tablets 2597
Ultram Tablets (Less than 1%) 2600
Uniretic Tablets 3178
Vancocin HCl Capsules & Pulvules (Infrequent) 1972
Vancocin HCl Oral Solution (Infrequent) 1971
Vancocin HCl, Vials & ADD-Vantage (Infrequent) 1970
Vantin Tablets and Oral Suspension 2860
Varivax 2202
Vaseretic Tablets 2204
Vasotec I.V. Injection 2207
Vasotec Tablets (0.5% to 1.0%) 2210
Verelan Capsules (1% or less) 3184
Verelan PM Capsules (2% or less) 3186
Vioxx 2213
Viramune Oral Suspension 1060
Viramune Tablets 1060
Voltaren Tablets (Rare) 2315
Voltaren-XR Tablets (Rare) 2315
Wellbutrin Tablets (Rare) 1680
Wellbutrin SR Sustained-Release Tablets (Rare) 1684
Xanax Tablets 2865
Zarontin Capsules 2659
Zarontin Syrup 2660
Zaroxolyn Tablets 1177
Zestoretic Tablets 695
Zinacef Injection (Rare) 1696
Zinacef for Injection (Rare) 1696
Zithromax Capsules, 250 mg (Rare) 2743
Zithromax for IV Infusion (Rare) 2748
Zithromax for Oral Suspension, 300 mg, 600 mg, 900 mg, 1200 mg (Rare) 2739
Zithromax Tablets, 250 mg (Rare) 2739
Zocor Tablets (Rare) 2219
Zoloft 2751
Zosyn (Rare) 1890
Zosyn in Galaxy Containers (Rare) 1894
Zovirax Capsules 1706
Zovirax for Injection 1708
Zovirax 1706
Zyban Sustained-Release Tablets 1710

Stillbirths

Aggrenox Capsules 1026
Cetrotide for Injection (Two cases) 3209
Ecotrin Enteric Coated Aspirin Low, Regular and Maximum Strength Tablets 1715
Zyrtec-D 12 Hour Extended Relief Tablets (Rare) 2758

Stimulation

Sinemet Tablets 1253
Sinemet CR Tablets 1255
Sonata Capsules (Rare) 3591
Valium Injectable 3026
Valium Tablets 3047
Xanax Tablets (Rare) 2865

Stinging

Aci-Jel Therapeutic Vaginal Jelly (Occasional cases) 2525
Acticin Cream 998
▲ Acular Ophthalmic Solution (Up to 40%) 544
▲ Acular PF Ophthalmic Solution (Approximately 20%) 544
Adriamycin PFS/RDF Injection 2767
Afrin Nasal Decongestant Children's Pump Mist ▣ 734
Afrin ▣ 733
Afrin No Drip Original Nasal Spray ▣ 735
Afrin No Drip Extra Moisturizing Nasal Spray ▣ 735
Afrin No Drip Severe Congestion Nasal Spray ▣ 735
Afrin No Drip Sinus Nasal Spray ▣ 735
Afrin Original Pump Mist ▣ 733
Aldara Cream, 5% (More than 1%) 1978
▲ Alocril Ophthalmic Solution (10% to 30%) 545
▲ Alomide Ophthalmic Solution (Among most frequent) ⊙ 204
▲ Alphagan Ophthalmic Solution (Approximately 10% to 30%) 545
Americaine Anesthetic Lubricant 1162
Americaine Otic Topical Anesthetic Ear Drops 1162
Aphthasol Oral Paste (1% to 2%) 1025
Attenuvax 2044
Azelex Cream (Approximately 1% to 5%) 547
Bactroban Nasal (2%) 1495
Bactroban Ointment (1.5%) 1496
▲ Betagan (About 1 in 3 patients) ⊙ 228
▲ Betimol Ophthalmic Solution (1 in 8 patients) ⊙ 324
Bleph-10 ⊙ 230
Chloromycetin Ophthalmic Ointment, 1% (Occasional) ⊙ 296
Chloromycetin Ophthalmic Solution ⊙ 297
Chloroptic Sterile Ophthalmic Ointment ⊙ 234
Chloroptic Sterile Ophthalmic Solution ⊙ 235
Clobevate Gel (Less than 2%) 3271
▲ Condylox Gel (7%) 2436
Cormax Cream (Approximately 0.3%) 2440
Cormax Ointment (Approximately 0.3%) 2440
▲ Cormax Scalp Application (Approximately 10%) 2441
▲ Cosopt Sterile Ophthalmic Solution (Up to 30%) 2065
Cozaar Tablets (Less than 1%) 2067
Cutivate Cream (0.8%) 1282
▲ DesOwen (Approximately 3%) 1401
▲ Differin Cream (Less than 1% to 24%) 1402
Differin Gel (Approximately 1% or less) 1403
Differin Solution/Pledgets (1% or less) 1404
▲ Diprivan Injectable Emulsion (10% to 17.6%) 667
▲ Diprolene Gel 0.05% (6%) 3107
Diprolene AF Cream 0.05% (0.4%) 3106
▲ Dovonex Scalp Solution (Approximately 23%) 1118
Doxil Injection 566
Drysol Solution 2663
▲ Elimite Cream (10%) 552
▲ Elocon Cream 0.1% (Approximately 7%) 3110
▲ Elocon Ointment 0.1% (4.8% to approximately 7%) 3112
Emadine Ophthalmic Solution (Less than 5%) ⊙ 211
Finevin Cream (1% to 5%) 962
FML Ophthalmic Suspension ⊙ 236
FML Forte Ophthalmic Suspension ⊙ 235
HMS Sterile Ophthalmic Suspension (Occasional) ⊙ 240
Humorsol Sterile Ophthalmic Solution 2102
Hyzaar 2109
Idamycin PFS Injection 2825
Imitrex Injection (Infrequent) 1549
Isopto Carpine Ophthalmic Solution ⊙ 215
Klaron Lotion 10% 1224
▲ Lac-Hydrin Cream (Approximately 2% to 15%) 1118
▲ Lac-Hydrin Lotion (1 in 10 to 30 patients) 1119
Levulan Kerastick 971
▲ Livostin (29%) ⊙ 305
Lotrimin 3128
Lotrisone 3129
▲ Luxíq Foam (2% to 44%) 1210
Melanex Topical Solution 2300
Mentax Cream (Approximately 1%) 1009
Meruvax II 2130
MetroCream (Less than 3%) 1404
MetroLotion (1%) 1405
M-M-R II 2118
Monoclate-P Concentrate 793
Mumpsvax 2141
▲ Naftin Cream (6%) 2224
▲ Naftin Gel (5.0%) 2224
▲ Nasalide Nasal Spray (Approximately 45%) 1295
▲ Nizoral 2% Cream (5%) 3620
Ocufen Ophthalmic Solution ⊙ 242
Ocuflox Ophthalmic Solution 554
Olux Foam (Less than 2%) 1211
Ophthetic Ophthalmic Solution (Occasional) ⊙ 244
▲ Optivar Ophthalmic Solution (Approximately 30%) 2273
Oxistat (0.1%) 1298
Patanol Ophthalmic Solution (Less than 5%) 540
Polytrim Ophthalmic Solution 556
Pred Forte Ophthalmic Suspension ⊙ 246
Pred Mild Sterile Ophthalmic Suspension ⊙ 249
Pred-G Ophthalmic Suspension ⊙ 247
▲ Propine Ophthalmic Solution (6%) ⊙ 250
▲ Renova 0.02% Cream (Almost all subjects) 2520
▲ Renova 0.05% Cream (Almost all subjects) 2519
▲ Tazorac Gel (10% to 30%) 556
Temovate Cream (1%) 1301
▲ Temovate Gel (Among most frequent) 1303
Temovate Ointment (Less frequent) 1301
▲ Temovate Scalp Application (29 of 294 patients) 1304
▲ Temovate E Emollient (5%) 1302
▲ Timolol GFS (1 in 8 patients) ⊙ 266
▲ Timoptic in Ocudose (Approximately 1 in 8 patients) 2192
▲ Timoptic Sterile Ophthalmic Solution (Approximately 1 in 8 patients) 2190
▲ Timoptic-XE Sterile Ophthalmic Gel Forming Solution (1 in 8 patients) 2194
▲ Trusopt Sterile Ophthalmic Solution (Approximately one-third of patients) 2196
▲ Ultravate Cream (4.4%) 1119
Ultravate Ointment (1.6%) 1120
▲ Vaniqa Cream (4.1%) 1121
▲ Viroptic Ophthalmic Solution Sterile (4.6%) ⊙ 301
▲ Voltaren Ophthalmic Sterile Ophthalmic Solution (15%) ⊙ 312
VōSoL HC Otic Solution (Occasional) 3356
▲ Xalatan Latanoprost Ophthalmic Solution (5% to 15%) ⊙ 320
▲ Xalatan Sterile Ophthalmic Solution (5% to 15%) 2864
Xerac AC Solution 2663
▲ Zovirax Ointment (28.3%) 1707

Stomach, nervous

Clozaril Tablets (Less than 1%) 2319

Stomach atony

Tasmar Tablets (Rare) 3010

Stomach complaints

Stomachache

▲ Aerobid/Aerobid-M (10%) 1363
Aleve Tablets, Caplets and Gelcaps ▣ 602
Alomide Ophthalmic Solution (Less than 1%) ⊙ 204
▲ Genuine Bayer Professional Labeling (Aspirin Regimen Bayer) (14.5%) ▣ 608
Bontril Slow-Release Capsules 576
▲ Chemet Capsules (5.2% to 15.7%) 3078
Cylert Tablets 415
Ecotrin Enteric Coated Aspirin Low, Regular and Maximum Strength Tablets 1715
Fortovase Capsules (Less than 2%) 2970
Guaifed 2272
Invirase Capsules (Less than 2%) 2979
Klonopin Tablets (Infrequent) 2983
Koāte-DVI (0.7%) 931
K-Phos Neutral Tablets 946
K-Phos Original (Sodium Free) Tablets 947
Ortho-Cyclen/Ortho Tri-Cyclen 2573
PhosChol 579
Pima Syrup (Less frequent) 1362
▲ Serevent Inhalation Aerosol (4%) 1633
Stadol NS Nasal Spray (1% or greater) 1108
Uroqid-Acid No. 2 Tablets 947
▲ Ventolin Inhalation Aerosol and Refill (3%) 1679
Zofran Injection (2%) 1698

Stomatitis

Aciphex Tablets 1267
Aciphex Tablets 1783
Actiq (1% or greater) 1184
Adriamycin PFS/RDF Injection 2767
▲ Alferon N Injection (6%) 1770
AmBisome for Injection (Less common) 1383
▲ Amphotec (5% or more) 1774
Anaprox Tablets (Less than 3%) 2967
Anaprox DS Tablets (Less than 3%) 2967
Arava Tablets (1% to 3%) 724
Aredia for Injection (Up to 1%) 2309
Arthrotec Tablets (Rare) 3195
Asacol Delayed-Release Tablets 2884
Atromid-S Capsules 3483
Augmentin Chewable Tablets 1482
Augmentin Powder for Oral Suspension 1482
Augmentin Tablets 1485
Augmentin ES-600 Powder for Oral Suspension 1487
Avelox Tablets (0.05% to 1%) 879
Bactrim 2949
Biaxin/Biaxin XL 403
▲ Campath Ampules (1% to 14%) 992
Carbatrol Capsules 3234
Celebrex Capsules (0.1% to 1.9%) 2676
Celebrex Capsules (0.1% to 1.9%) 2780
Celexa (Infrequent) 1365
▲ CellCept Capsules (3% to 10%) 2951
▲ CellCept Intravenous (3% to 10%) 2951
▲ CellCept Oral Suspension (3% to 10%) 2951
▲ CellCept Tablets (3% to 10%) 2951
Claritin (At least one patient) 3100
Claritin-D 12 Hour Extended Release Tablets (Less frequent) 3102
Claritin-D 24 Hour Extended Release Tablets (Fewer than 2%) 3104
Clinoril Tablets (Less than 1 in 100) 2053
Cognex Capsules (Infrequent) 1351
Copaxone for Injection (Infrequent) 3306
▲ DaunoXome Injection (1% to 9%) 1442
Depacon Injection (1% or more) 416
Depakene (1% or more) 421
Depakote Sprinkle Capsules 426
Depakote Tablets (1% to 5%) 430
Depakote ER Tablets (1% to 5%) 436
Dipentum Capsules (1.0%) 2803
Dolobid Tablets (Less than 1 in 100) 2088
▲ Doxil Injection (5.2% to 37.4%) 566
EC-Naprosyn Delayed-Release Tablets (Less than 3%) 2967
Effexor Tablets (Infrequent) 3495
Effexor XR Capsules (Infrequent) 3499
Efudex 1733
Ellence Injection 2806
Enalaprilat Injection 863
Epivir 1520
Epivir-HBV 1524
▲ Ergamisol Tablets (3% to 39%) 1789
Estratest 3252
Etrafon 3115
Evoxac Capsules (Less than 1%) 1217
Feldene Capsules (Occasional) 2685
Flexeril Tablets (Rare) 572
Flexeril Tablets (Rare) 2094
▲ Fludara for Injection (Up to 9%) 995
Flumadine 1370
Fortovase Capsules (Less than 2%) 2970
▲ Sterile FUDR (Among more common) 2974
Gabitril Tablets (Frequent) 1189
Gastrocrom Oral Concentrate 1162
▲ Gemzar for Injection (10% to 15%) 1919
▲ Gengraf Capsules (6%) 457

Halcion Tablets 2823
Herceptin I.V. (At least one of the 958 patients) 1414
Hivid Tablets (Less than 1% to 3.0%) 2975
▲ Hycamtin for Injection (Less than 1% to 24%) 1546
Ifex for Injection (Less than 1%) 1123
Intron A for Injection (Less than 5%) 3120
Invirase Capsules (Less than 2%) 2979
Kaletra Capsules (Less than 2%) 471
Kaletra Oral Solution (Less than 2%) 471
Lamictal (Infrequent) 1567
▲ Leukine (24% to 62%) 1755
Lexxel Tablets 608
Limbitrol 1738
Lipitor Tablets (Less than 2%) 2639
Lipitor Tablets (Less than 2%) 2696
Luvox Tablets (25, 50, 100 mg) (Infrequent) 3256
Matulane Capsules 3246
Maxair Autohaler 1981
Maxair Inhaler (Less than 1%) 1984
Miltown Tablets (Rare) 3349
Mithracin for Intravenous Use 903
Mylocel Tablets (Less frequently) 2227
▲ Mylotarg for Injection (20% to 45%) 3540
Myobloc Injectable Solution (2% or greater) 1291
Naprelan Tablets (Less than 3%) 1293
Naprosyn Suspension (Less than 3%) 2967
Naprosyn Tablets (Less than 3%) 2967
▲ Navelbine Injection (Less than 20%) 1604
▲ Neoral Soft Gelatin Capsules (6%) 2380
▲ Neoral Oral Solution (6%) 2380
▲ Neupogen for Injection (5%) 587
Neurontin Capsules (Infrequent) 2655
Neurontin Oral Solution (Infrequent) 2655
Neurontin Tablets (Infrequent) 2655
Nicotrol Nasal Spray (Common) 2843
▲ Nipent for Injection (5% to 12%) 3272
Noroxin Tablets 2145
Norpramin Tablets 755
▲ Novantrone for Injection (15% to 29%) 1760
Omnicef 493
Orudis Capsules (Greater than 1%) 3548
Oruvail Capsules (Greater than 1%) 3548
OxyContin Tablets (Less than 1%) 2912
Paxil (Rare) 1609
Pediazole Suspension 3050
Ponstel Capsules (Occasional) 1356
Prevacid Delayed-Release Capsules (Less than 1%) 3292
PREVPAC (Less than 1% to 3%) 3298
▲ Prograf (3% to 15%) 1393
▲ Proleukin for Injection (22%) 1199
Protonix I.V. (Less than 1%) 3580
Protonix Tablets (Less than 1%) 3577
Prozac Pulvules, Liquid, and Weekly Capsules (Infrequent) 1238
▲ Rapamune Oral Solution and Tablets (3% to 20%) 3584
Relafen Tablets (1% to 3%) 1617
Remeron Tablets (Infrequent) 2483
Remeron SolTab Tablets (Infrequent) 2486
Requip Tablets (Infrequent) 1621
Rescriptor Tablets (Less than 2%) 526
Rilutek Tablets (0.8% to 1.2%) 772
Risperdal (Infrequent) 1796
Roferon-A Injection (Infrequent) 2996
Salagen Tablets (1% to 2%) 2229
Sandostatin LAR Depot (1% to 4%) 2395
Septra Suspension 2265
Septra Tablets 2265
Septra DS Tablets 2265
Seroquel Tablets (Infrequent) 684
Serzone Tablets (Infrequent) 1104
Sinequan 2713
Sonata Capsules (Infrequent) 3591
▲ Soriatane Capsules (1% to 10%) 3003
Surmontil Capsules 3595
Synercid I.V. (Less than 1%) 775
Tabloid Tablets (Less frequent) 1642
▲ Taxotere for Injection Concentrate (42.3%) 778
Tegretol/Tegretol-XR 2404
Tequin Injection (0.1% to 3%) 1110
Tequin Tablets (0.1% to 3%) 1110
Testred Capsules, 10 mg 1746
Thalomid Capsules 1154
Timentin Injection- ADD-Vantage Vial 1661
Timentin Injection-Galaxy Container 1664
Timentin Injection-Pharmacy Bulk Package 1666
Timentin for Intravenous Administration 1658
Tolectin (Less than 1%) 2589
Tonocard Tablets (Less than 1%) 649
Topamax Sprinkle Capsules (Infrequent) 2590
Topamax Tablets (Infrequent) 2590
Toradol (Greater than 1%) 3018
▲ Trecator-SC Tablets (Among most common) 3598
Trileptal Oral Suspension 2407
Trileptal Tablets 2407
Trovan (Less than 1%) 2722
Ultram Tablets (Infrequent) 2600
Unasyn for Injection 2728
Uniretic Tablets (Less than 1%) 3178
Urobiotic-250 Capsules (Rare) 2731
Vantin Tablets and Oral Suspension (Less than 1%) 2860
Vaseretic Tablets 2204
Vasotec I.V. Injection 2207
Vasotec Tablets (0.5% to 1.0%) 2210
Viagra Tablets (Less than 2%) 2732
Vioxx (Greater than 0.1% to 1.9%) 2213
Vistide Injection 1445
Vivactil Tablets 2217
Vivactil Tablets 2446
Wellbutrin Tablets (Frequent) 1680
Wellbutrin SR Sustained-Release Tablets (Infrequent) 1684
▲ Xeloda Tablets (4% to 7%) 3039
▲ Zinecard for Injection (26% to 34%) 2869
Zithromax for IV Infusion (1.9%) 2748
Zoloft (Rare) 2751
Zonegran Capsules (Infrequent) 1307
Zyban Sustained-Release Tablets (Infrequent) 1710
Zyprexa Tablets (Infrequent) 1973
Zyprexa ZYDIS Orally Disintegrating Tablets (Infrequent) 1973
Zyrtec (Less than 2%) 2756
Zyrtec-D 12 Hour Extended Relief Tablets (Less than 2%) 2758

Stomatitis, ulcerative

Agrylin Capsules (1% to 5%) 3232
AmBisome for Injection (Less common) 1383
Anaprox Tablets (Less than 1%) 2967
Anaprox DS Tablets (Less than 1%) 2967
Arthrotec Tablets (Rare) 3195
Astelin Nasal Spray (Infrequent) 3339
Bactroban Cream (Less than 1%) 1494
Betaseron for SC Injection 988
▲ Campath Ampules (1% to 14%) 992
Cataflam Tablets (Less than 1%) 2315
Colazal Capsules 3069
Copaxone for Injection (Frequent) 3306
Cosmegen for Injection 2062
Crixivan Capsules (Less than 2%) 2070
Cytovene (At least 3 subjects) 2959
Depen Titratable Tablets 3341
Doxil Injection (1% to 5%) 566
EC-Naprosyn Delayed-Release Tablets (Less than 1%) 2967
Evoxac Capsules (1% to 3%) 1217
Exelon Capsules (Infrequent) 2342
Exelon Oral Solution (Infrequent) 2345
Felbatol 3343
Foscavir Injection (Between 1% and 5%) 605
Gabitril Tablets (Infrequent) 1189
Indocin Capsules (Less than 1%) 2112
Indocin I.V. (Less than 1%) 2115
Indocin (Less than 1%) 2112
Intron A for Injection (Less than 5%) 3120
Kaletra Capsules (Less than 2%) 471
Kaletra Oral Solution (Less than 2%) 471
Lipitor Tablets (Less than 2%) 2639
Lipitor Tablets (Less than 2%) 2696
Lodine (Less than 1%) 3528
Lodine XL Extended-Release Tablets (Less than 1%) 3530
Mobic Tablets (Less than 2%) 1054
▲ Naprelan Tablets (Less than 1% to 9%) 1293
Naprosyn Suspension (Less than 1%) 2967
Naprosyn Tablets (Less than 1%) 2967
Neurontin Capsules (Rare) 2655
Neurontin Oral Solution (Rare) 2655
Neurontin Tablets (Rare) 2655
Nexium Delayed-Release Capsules (Less than 1%) 619
Paxil (Rare to infrequent) 1609
Permax Tablets (Rare) 1299
Protonix I.V. (Less than 1%) 3580
Protonix Tablets (Less than 1%) 3577
Prozac Pulvules, Liquid, and Weekly Capsules (Infrequent) 1238
Remeron Tablets (Rare) 2483
Remeron SolTab Tablets (Rare) 2486
Requip Tablets (Infrequent) 1621
Rescriptor Tablets (Less than 2%) 526
Sarafem Pulvules (Infrequent) 1962
▲ Serostim for Injection (1% to 10%) 3229
▲ Simulect for Injection (3% to 10%) 2399
Sonata Capsules (Rare) 3591
▲ Soriatane Capsules (1% to 10%) 3003
Sporanox Oral Solution (Less than 2%) 1808
Sporanox Oral Solution (Less than 2%) 2512
Trileptal Oral Suspension 2407
Trileptal Tablets 2407
Vistide Injection 1445
Voltaren Tablets (Less than 1%) 2315
Voltaren-XR Tablets (Less than 1%) 2315
Zoloft (Rare) 2751
Zonegran Capsules (Infrequent) 1307
Zosyn (1.0% or less) 1890
Zosyn in Galaxy Containers (1.0% or less) 1894
Zyprexa Tablets (Infrequent) 1973
Zyprexa ZYDIS Orally Disintegrating Tablets (Infrequent) 1973
Zyrtec (Less than 2%) 2756
Zyrtec-D 12 Hour Extended Relief Tablets (Less than 2%) 2758

Stool, bloody

(*see under* Hematochezia)

Stool, color changes

New Formulation Chromagen OB Capsules 3094
Coumadin for Injection 1243
Coumadin Tablets 1243
Fortovase Capsules (Less than 2%) 2970
Invirase Capsules (Less than 2%) 2979
Lamisil Tablets 2360
Levlen 962
Levlite 21 Tablets 962
Levlite 28 Tablets 962
Modicon 2563
Nizoral Tablets 1791
Ortho-Cyclen/Ortho Tri-Cyclen 2573
Ortho-Novum 2563
Ortho-Novum 1/50▫28 Tablets 2556
Ortho-Cyclen/Ortho Tri-Cyclen 2573
Pepto-Bismol Maximum Strength Liquid 2878
Pepto-Bismol Original Liquid, Original and Cherry Tablets and Easy-To-Swallow Caplets 2878
PREVPAC (Less than 3%) 3298
Prosed/DS Tablets 3268
▲ Sandostatin LAR Depot (4% to 6%) 2395
Sporanox Capsules 1800
Tasmar Tablets 3010
Ticlid Tablets 3015
Tri-Levlen 962
Warfarin Sodium Tablets, USP 3302

Stool, oily

▲ Xenical Capsules (5.5% to 20%) 3043

Stools, abnormal

Aciphex Tablets 1267
Aciphex Tablets 1783
Asacol Delayed-Release Tablets (2% or greater) 2884
Clozaril Tablets (Less than 1%) 2319
Colazal Capsules (1%) 3069
Dynabac Tablets (0.1% to 1%) 2269
Effexor Tablets (Rare) 3495
Effexor XR Capsules (Rare) 3499
Gabitril Tablets (Infrequent) 1189
Glucophage Tablets (1% to 5%) 1080
Hivid Tablets (Less than 1%) 2975
Kaletra Capsules (Up to 6%) 471
Kaletra Oral Solution (Up to 6%) 471
Monurol Sachet (Less than 1%) 1375
Nexium Delayed-Release Capsules (Less than 1%) 619
Norvir Capsules (Less than 2%) 487
Norvir Oral Solution (Less than 2%) 487
Omnicef (0.2%) 493
Pentasa Capsules (Less than 1%) 3239
▲ Pletal Tablets (12% to 15%) 2605
▲ Pletal Tablets (12% to 15%) 2848
Protonix I.V. (Less than 1%) 3580
Protonix Tablets (Less than 1%) 3577
▲ Relafen Tablets (3% to 9%) 1617
▲ Sandostatin Injection (Less than 10%) 2394
Tasmar Tablets (Infrequent) 3010
Ultrase MT Capsules (1.5%) 835
Vicoprofen Tablets (Less than 1%) 520
Zosyn (1.9% to 2.4%) 1890
Zosyn in Galaxy Containers (1.9% to 2.4%) 1894
Zyban Sustained-Release Tablets 1710

Stools, loose

▲ Agenerase Capsules (39% to 60%) 1454
▲ Agenerase Oral Solution (33% to 56%) 1459
Atromid-S Capsules (Less frequent) 3483
▲ Augmentin Chewable Tablets (9%) 1482
▲ Augmentin Powder for Oral Suspension (9%) 1482
▲ Augmentin Tablets (9%) 1485
Cedax (0.1% to 1%) 1021
▲ Cefobid Pharmacy Bulk Package - Not for Direct Infusion (1 in 30) 2673
▲ Ceftin (8.6%) 1898
▲ Chemet Capsules (12.0% to 20.9%) 3078
Claritin (At least one patient) 3100
Cognex Capsules 1351
Colestid Tablets (Less frequent) 2791
Dipentum Capsules 2803
Geocillin Tablets 2687
HeartBar 1212
Hivid Tablets (Less than 1%) 2975
Imdur Tablets (Less than or equal to 5%) 1826
▲ Intron A for Injection (Up to 10%) 3120
Magonate Natal Liquid 1362
Magonate Tablets and Liquid 1362
MetroGel-Vaginal Gel (1%) 1986
Noroxin Tablets (0.3% to 1.0%) 2145
Norvasc Tablets (Less than or equal to 0.1%) 2704
Pipracil (2%) 1866
▲ Sandostatin Injection (34% to 61%) 2394
▲ Suprax (6%) 1877
▲ Sustiva Capsules (39%) 1258
▲ Tonocard Tablets (Up to 6.8%) 649
▲ Trisenox Injection (10%) 1158
Trovan (Less than 1%) 2722
Urocit-K Tablets (Some patients) 2232
▲ Vantin Tablets and Oral Suspension (5.9% to 10.6%) 2860
▲ Zithromax Capsules, 250 mg (2% to 14%) 2743
▲ Zithromax for IV Infusion (4.3%) 2748
▲ Zithromax for Oral Suspension, 1 g (5% to 7%) 2743
▲ Zithromax for Oral Suspension, 300 mg, 600 mg, 900 mg, 1200 mg (2% to 14%) 2739
▲ Zithromax Tablets, 250 mg (2% to 14%) 2739
▲ Zithromax Tablets, 600 mg (5% to 7%) 2743
▲ Zoloft (20% to 24%) 2751

Strabismus

Aciphex Tablets 1267
Aciphex Tablets 1783
Lamictal (Rare) 1567
Neurontin Capsules (Rare) 2655
Neurontin Oral Solution (Rare) 2655
Neurontin Tablets (Rare) 2655
Prozac Pulvules, Liquid, and Weekly Capsules (Rare) 1238
Sarafem Pulvules (Rare) 1962
Topamax Sprinkle Capsules (Infrequent) 2590
Topamax Tablets (Infrequent) 2590
Versed Syrup (Less than 1%) 3033

Strabismus, bilateral

Cetrotide for Injection 3209

Strangury

Evoxac Capsules (Less than 1%) 1217

Striae

Aclovate (Infrequent) 1275
Analpram-HC 1338
Anusol-HC Cream 2.5% (Infrequent to frequent) 2237
Aricept Tablets (Infrequent) 1270
Aricept Tablets (Infrequent) 2665
Capex Shampoo 1400
Clobevate Gel 3271
Copaxone for Injection (Infrequent) 3306
Cordran Lotion (More frequent) 2438
Cordran Tape (More frequent) 2439
Cormax Cream (Infrequent) 2440
Cormax Ointment (Infrequent) 2440
Cormax Scalp Application (Infrequent) 2441
Cutivate Cream (Infrequent) 1282
Cutivate Ointment (Infrequent to more frequent) 1284
Dermatop Emollient Cream (Infrequent to frequent) 2517
DesOwen (Infrequent) 1401
Diprolene Gel 0.05% (Infrequent) 3107
Diprolene Lotion 0.05% (Infrequent) 3107
Diprolene Ointment 0.05% (Infrequent) 3108
Diprolene AF Cream 0.05% (Infrequent) 3106
Diprosone 3109
Effexor Tablets (Rare) 3495
Elocon Cream 0.1% (Infrequent) 3110
Elocon Lotion 0.1% (Infrequent) 3111
Elocon Ointment 0.1% (Infrequent) 3112
Florinef Acetate Tablets 2250
Lidex (Infrequent) 2020
Locoid Cream (Infrequent) 1341
Locoid Lipocream Cream (Infrequent) 1342
Locoid (Infrequent) 1341
Lotrisone 3129
Lupron Depot-PED 7.5 mg, 11.25 mg and 15 mg (Less than 2%) 3291

Lupron Injection Pediatric (Less than 2%) 3280
Luxíq Foam 1210
Olux Foam 1211
Pramosone 1343
ProctoFoam-HC 3177
Psorcon E Cream 1227
Psorcon E Ointment 1228
Synalar (Infrequent) 2020
Temovate Cream 1301
Temovate Gel (Infrequent) 1303
Temovate Ointment 1301
Temovate Scalp Application (Infrequent) 1304
Temovate E Emollient (Infrequent) 1302
Topicort (Infrequent) 2025
Ultravate Cream 1119
Ultravate Ointment 1120

Stridor

Advair Diskus 100/50 1448
Advair Diskus 250/50 1448
Advair Diskus 500/50 1448
Campath Ampules 992
Cedax Capsules 1021
Ceptaz for Injection 1499
Floxin I.V. 2526
Floxin Tablets 2529
Fortaz 1541
Foscavir Injection (Between 1% and 5%) 605
Nubain Injection (1% or less) 1323
Photofrin for Injection 831
Prozac Pulvules, Liquid, and Weekly Capsules (Rare) 1238
Pulmicort Respules (1% to 3%) 632
Refludan for Injection (Common) 761
Reglan (Rare) 2935
Rilutek Tablets (Infrequent) 772
Risperdal (Infrequent) 1796
Salagen Tablets (Less than 1%) 2229
Sarafem Pulvules (Rare) 1962
Serevent Diskus (Rare) 1637
Serevent Inhalation Aerosol (Rare) 1633
Trovan (Less than 1%) 2722
Versed Syrup (Less than 1%) 3033
Zofran Injection 1698
Zofran 1703
Zofran ODT Orally Disintegrating Tablets 1703
Zoloft (Rare) 2751
Zyprexa Tablets (Rare) 1973
Zyprexa ZYDIS Orally Disintegrating Tablets (Rare) 1973

Stroke

Accutane Capsules 2944
Activase I.V. (0.9%) 1410
Aloprim for Injection (Less than 1%) 2292
Amerge Tablets 1467
Amicar Injection 3608
Amicar Syrup 3608
Amicar Tablets 3608
Betapace Tablets (Less than 1% to 1%) 950
Brevicon 28-Day Tablets 3380
Clomid Tablets 735
Cytovene 2959
D.H.E. 45 Injection (Extremely rare) 2334
DynaCirc Capsules (0.5% to 1%) 2921
DynaCirc CR Tablets (0.5% to 1%) 2923
Enbrel for Injection 1752
Enbrel for Injection 3504
Estratest 3252
Etrafon 3115
Flexeril Tablets (Rare) 572
Flexeril Tablets (Rare) 2094
Fortovase Capsules (Less than 2%) 2970
Heparin Lock Flush Solution 3509
Heparin Sodium Injection 3511
Humegon for Injection 2468
Imitrex Injection 1549
Imitrex Tablets 1558
Integrilin Injection (0.5%) 1213
Integrilin Injection (0.5%) 1828
Intron A for Injection (Less than 5%) 3120
Limbitrol 1738
Lupron Injection 3279
▲ Mavik Tablets (3.3%) 478
Maxalt Tablets 2120
Maxalt-MLT Orally Disintegrating Tablets 2120
Menest Tablets 2254
Modicon 2563
Norinyl 1 +35 28-Day Tablets 3380
Norinyl 1 + 50 28-Day Tablets 3380
Norplant System 3543
Norpramin Tablets 755
Ortho Dienestrol Cream 2554
Ortho-Cyclen/Ortho Tri-Cyclen 2573
Ortho-Novum 2563
Ortho-Novum 1/50▭28 Tablets 2556
Ortho-Cyclen/Ortho Tri-Cyclen 2573
Ovcon 3364
Premarin Intravenous 3563
Premarin Vaginal Cream 3570
Prinivil Tablets (0.3% to 1.0%) 2164
Prinzide Tablets 2168
Proleukin for Injection (Less than 1%) 1199
Roferon-A Injection (Infrequent) 2996
Serophene Tablets 3226
Surmontil Capsules 3595
Testoderm Transdermal Systems (2%) 574
Tri-Norinyl-28 Tablets 3433
▲ Vesanoid Capsules (3%) 3037
Vivactil Tablets 2217
Vivactil Tablets 2446
Vivelle Transdermal System 2412
Vivelle-Dot Transdermal System 2416
Wellbutrin SR Sustained-Release Tablets (Infrequent) 1684
Zestoretic Tablets 695
Zestril Tablets (0.3% to 1.0%) 698
Zyban Sustained-Release Tablets (Infrequent) 1710

Stroke, hemorrhagic

Activase I.V. (0.7%) 1410
Femara Tablets (Less than or equal to 2%) 2351
Levlen 962
Levlite 21 Tablets 962
Levlite 28 Tablets 962
Modicon 2563
Ortho-Cyclen/Ortho Tri-Cyclen 2573
Ortho-Novum 2563
Ortho-Novum 1/50▭28 Tablets 2556
Ortho-Cyclen/Ortho Tri-Cyclen 2573
Tri-Levlen 962
Triphasil-21 Tablets 3600
Triphasil-28 Tablets 3605

Stroke, new ischemic

Activase I.V. 1410

Stroke, thrombotic

Levlen 962
Levlite 21 Tablets 962
Levlite 28 Tablets 962
Ortho-Cyclen/Ortho Tri-Cyclen 2573
Tri-Levlen 962
Triphasil-21 Tablets 3600
Triphasil-28 Tablets 3605

Strongyloidiasis hyperinfection

Tagamet (Extremely rare) 1644

Stuffiness, nasal

(*see under* Nasal congestion)

Stupor

Ambien Tablets (Infrequent) 3191
Amphotec (1% to 5%) 1774
Ativan Injection (1.2%) 3478
Betaseron for SC Injection 988
Celexa (Rare) 1365
▲ Cerebyx Injection (7.7%) 2619
Copaxone for Injection (Frequent) 3306
Duragesic Transdermal System (Less than 1%) 1786
Effexor Tablets (Infrequent) 3495
Effexor XR Capsules (Infrequent) 3499
Eskalith 1527
Felbatol (2.6%) 3343
Foscavir Injection (Between 1% and 5%) 605
Gabitril Tablets (Frequent) 1189
▲ Gliadel Wafer (6%) 1723
Hivid Tablets (Less than 1%) 2975
Lamictal (Infrequent) 1567
Levaquin (Less than 0.3%) 2537
Lithium Carbonate 3061
Lithium Citrate Syrup 3061
Lithobid Slow-Release Tablets 3255
Luvox Tablets (25, 50, 100 mg) (Infrequent) 3256
Migranal Nasal Spray (Rare) 2376
Moduretic Tablets (Less than or equal to 1%) 2138
Naropin Injection (Less than 1%) 612
Neurontin Capsules (Infrequent) 2655
Neurontin Oral Solution (Infrequent) 2655
Neurontin Tablets (Infrequent) 2655
Orthoclone OKT3 Sterile Solution 2498
OxyContin Tablets (Less than 1%) 2912
Paxil (Rare) 1609
Permax Tablets (Rare) 1299
PhosLo 1069
ProSom Tablets (Infrequent) 500
Prozac Pulvules, Liquid, and Weekly Capsules (Rare) 1238
Remeron Tablets (Rare) 2483
Remeron SolTab Tablets (Rare) 2486
Requip Tablets (Infrequent) 1621
Rilutek Tablets (Infrequent) 772
Risperdal (Infrequent) 1796
Romazicon Injection (Less than 1%) 3000
Sarafem Pulvules (Rare) 1962
Seroquel Tablets (Infrequent) 684
Sonata Capsules (Rare) 3591
Streptomycin Sulfate Injection 2714
Symmetrel 1328
Tambocor Tablets (Less than 1%) 1990
Topamax Sprinkle Capsules (Frequent) 2590
Topamax Tablets (Frequent) 2590
Toradol (1% or less) 3018
Trileptal Oral Suspension 2407
Trileptal Tablets 2407
Ultracet Tablets (Less than 1%) 2597
Zanaflex Tablets (Infrequent) 1305
Zyprexa Tablets (Infrequent) 1973
Zyprexa ZYDIS Orally Disintegrating Tablets (Infrequent) 1973

Stuttering

Seroquel Tablets (Rare) 684
Zyprexa Tablets (Infrequent) 1973
Zyprexa ZYDIS Orally Disintegrating Tablets (Infrequent) 1973

Stye

Cognex Capsules (Infrequent) 1351
Crolom Sterile Ophthalmic Solution USP 4% (Infrequent) ⊙259
Intron A for Injection (Less than 5%) 3120
Klonopin Tablets (Infrequent) 2983
Neurontin Capsules (Infrequent) 2655
Neurontin Oral Solution (Infrequent) 2655
Neurontin Tablets (Infrequent) 2655
Opticrom Ophthalmic Solution (Infrequent) 555

Sudden Infant Death Syndrome

Acel-Imune 1851
Felbatol 3343
Tripedia Vaccine 817

Suicidal ideation

Accutane Capsules 2944
Ambien Tablets 3191
Avelox Tablets 879
▲ Avonex (4%) 1013
Betaseron for SC Injection 988
Celontin Capsules (Rare) 2618
Cognex Capsules (Rare) 1351
Depakote Tablets 430
Effexor Tablets (Rare) 3495
Effexor XR Capsules (Rare) 3499
Exelon Capsules (Infrequent) 2342
Exelon Oral Solution (Infrequent) 2345
Floxin I.V. 2526
Floxin Tablets (Rare) 2529
Halcion Tablets 2823
Infergen 1777
Intron A for Injection (Rare) 3120
Klonopin Tablets (Infrequent) 2983
Lamictal (Rare) 1567
Levaquin (Rare) 2537
Lodosyn Tablets 1251
Lupron Depot 3.75 mg (Very rare) 3281
Lupron Depot–3 Month 11.25 mg (Very rare) 3285
Miltown Tablets 3349
Neurontin Capsules (Infrequent) 2655
Neurontin Oral Solution (Infrequent) 2655
Neurontin Tablets (Infrequent) 2655
Nizoral Tablets (Rare) 1791
PEG-Intron Powder for Injection (Less than or equal to 1%) 3140
Prozac Pulvules, Liquid, and Weekly Capsules (Less than 1%) 1238
Rebetron Combination Therapy (Less than 1%) 3153
Reglan (Less frequent) 2935
Remeron Tablets 2483
Remeron SolTab Tablets 2486
Roferon-A Injection 2996
Sarafem Pulvules 1962
Serzone Tablets (Infrequent) 1104
Sinemet Tablets 1253
Sinemet CR Tablets 1255
Symmetrel (Less than 0.1%) 1328
Trilafon 3160
Ultram Tablets (Infrequent) 2600
Viracept 532
Wellbutrin Tablets (Rare) 1680
Wellbutrin SR Sustained-Release Tablets (Infrequent) 1684
Xanax Tablets 2865
Zarontin Capsules (Rare) 2659
Zarontin Syrup (Rare) 2660
Zoloft (Rare) 2751
Zyban Sustained-Release Tablets (Infrequent) 1710

Suicide, attempt of

Accutane Capsules 2944
Ambien Tablets (Rare) 3191
Avonex (One patient) 1013
Betaseron for SC Injection 988
Celebrex Capsules 2780
Celexa (Frequent) 1365
Copaxone for Injection (Infrequent) 3306
D.H.E. 45 Injection 2334
Effexor Tablets (Infrequent) 3495
Effexor XR Capsules (Infrequent) 3499
Exelon Capsules (Infrequent) 2342
Exelon Oral Solution (Infrequent) 2345
Felbatol (Infrequent) 3343
Floxin I.V. (Rare) 2526
Floxin Tablets (Rare) 2529
Fortovase Capsules (Rare) 2970
Gabitril Tablets (Infrequent) 1189
Hivid Tablets (Less than 1%) 2975
Imitrex Tablets (Rare) 1558
Infergen 1777
Intron A for Injection (Rare; less than 5%) 3120
Invirase Capsules (Rare) 2979
Klonopin Tablets (Infrequent) 2983
Lamictal (Rare) 1567
Levaquin (Rare) 2537
Levo-Dromoran 1734
Lupron Depot 3.75 mg (Very rare) 3281
Lupron Depot–3 Month 11.25 mg (Very rare) 3285
Luvox Tablets (25, 50, 100 mg) (Infrequent) 3256
Mirapex Tablets (Less than 1%) 2834
Neurontin Capsules (Rare) 2655
Neurontin Oral Solution (Rare) 2655
Neurontin Tablets (Rare) 2655
Paxil 1609
PEG-Intron Powder for Injection (Less than or equal to 1%) 3140
Proleukin for Injection 1199
Prozac Pulvules, Liquid, and Weekly Capsules (Frequent) 1238
Rebetron Combination Therapy (Less than 1%) 3153
Remicade for IV Injection (Less than 2%) 1178
Requip Tablets (Rare) 1621
Rilutek Tablets (Infrequent) 772
Risperdal (1.2%) 1796
Roferon-A Injection 2996
Sandostatin LAR Depot (Rare) 2395
Sarafem Pulvules (Infrequent) 1962
Seroquel Tablets (Infrequent) 684
Serzone Tablets (Infrequent) 1104
Sustiva Capsules 1258
Symmetrel (Less than 0.1%) 1328
Thalomid Capsules 1154
Topamax Sprinkle Capsules (Frequent) 2590
Topamax Tablets (Frequent) 2590
Vivactil Tablets 2217
Vivactil Tablets 2446
Xanax Tablets 2865
Zanaflex Tablets (Rare) 1305
Zoloft 2751
Zyprexa Tablets (Frequent) 1973
Zyprexa ZYDIS Orally Disintegrating Tablets (Frequent) 1973

Sulfhemoglobinemia

Pediazole Suspension 3050

Sulfite, sensitivity to

Aramine Injection 2043
Compazine 1505
Decadron Phosphate Injection 2081
Dilaudid Oral Liquid 445
Dilaudid Tablets - 8 mg 445
Dobutrex Solution Vials 1914
Duranest Injections 600
Eldopaque Forte 4% Cream 1734
EpiPen 1236
Hydrocortone Phosphate Injection, Sterile 2105
Innohep Injection 1248
Lustra Cream 2023
Lustra-AF Cream 2023
Mepergan Injection 3539
Minocin Oral Suspension 1865
Moban 1320
Nebcin Vials, Hyporets & ADD-Vantage 1955
NeoDecadron Sterile Ophthalmic Solution 2144
Norflex Injection 1987
Orgaran Injection 2480
Phenergan Injection 3553
Pred Forte Ophthalmic Suspension ⊙246
Pred Mild Sterile Ophthalmic Suspension ⊙249
Sensorcaine 643
Sensorcaine-MPF Injection 643
Solaquin Forte 1734
Stelazine 1640
Streptomycin Sulfate Injection 2714
Tensilon Injectable 1745
Trilafon 3160
Tylenol with Codeine (Probably low) 2595
Tylox Capsules 2597
Vibramycin Calcium Oral Suspension Syrup 2735
Vibramycin Hyclate Capsules 2735
Vibramycin Monohydrate for Oral Suspension 2735
Vibra-Tabs Film Coated Tablets 2735
Xylocaine with Epinephrine Injection 653

Sunburn

Accutane Capsules 2944
Benzaclin Topical Gel (1%) 1220
Declomycin Tablets 1855
Differin Cream (2%) 1402

Differin Gel (Approximately 1% or less) 1403
Differin Solution/Pledgets (1% or less) 1404
Diovan HCT Tablets (Greater than 0.2%) 2338
Protopic Ointment (1% to 4%) 1397
▲ Soriatane Capsules (1% to 10%) 3003

Sunburn, exacerbation of
Imitrex Injection 1549
Imitrex Nasal Spray 1554
Imitrex Tablets 1558
Periostat Tablets 1208

Superinfection
Adriamycin PFS/RDF Injection 2767
Ancef for Injection 1474
Ancef Injection 1474
Augmentin Chewable Tablets 1482
Augmentin Powder for Oral Suspension 1482
Augmentin Tablets 1485
Ceclor 1905
Cefotan 664
Ceftin 1898
Cefzil (1.5%) 1076
Ceptaz for Injection 1499
Duricef 1079
Fortaz 1541
Keflex 1237
Kefzol Vials, ADD-Vantage 1951
Lorabid Suspension and Pulvules 2251
Macrobid Capsules 2889
Macrodantin Capsules 2891
Mefoxin for Injection 2124
Mefoxin Premixed Intravenous Solution 2127
Minocin Intravenous 1862
Minocin Oral Suspension 1865
Minocin Pellet-Filled Capsules 1863
Monodox Capsules 2442
Pipracil 1866
Primaxin I.M. 2158
Streptomycin Sulfate Injection 2714
Suprax 1877
Vancocin HCl, Vials & ADD-Vantage 1970
Vascor Tablets (0.5% to 2.0%) 2602
Zinacef Injection 1696
Zinacef for Injection 1696

Suppuration
Efudex 1733

Supraventricular contractions, premature
Paxil (Rare) 1609

Swallowing
Diprivan Injectable Emulsion (Less than 1%) 667

Swallowing, impairment
Captopril Tablets 2281
Compazine 1505
Coumadin for Injection 1243
Coumadin Tablets 1243
Dantrium Capsules (Rare) 2885
Dantrium Intravenous 2886
Gengraf Capsules (Rare) 457
Imitrex Injection 1549
Imitrex Nasal Spray 1554
Levaquin 2537
Mavik Tablets 478
Monopril Tablets 1091
Monopril HCT 1094
Neoral Soft Gelatin Capsules (Rare) 2380
Neoral Oral Solution (Rare) 2380
Orthoclone OKT3 Sterile Solution 2498
Phrenilin (Infrequent) 578
Prinivil Tablets 2164
Prinzide Tablets 2168
Sandimmune (Rare) 2388
Sedapap Tablets 50 mg/650 mg (Infrequent) 2225
Stelazine 1640
Thioridazine Hydrochloride Tablets 2289
Thorazine 1656
Vaseretic Tablets 2204
Vasotec Tablets 2210
Warfarin Sodium Tablets, USP 3302
Zestoretic Tablets 695
Zestril Tablets 698

Sweat discoloration
Mycobutin Capsules 2838
Priftin Tablets 758
Rifadin 765
Rifater Tablets 769
Sinemet Tablets 1253
Sinemet CR Tablets 1255

Sweat gland disorder
Soriatane Capsules (Less than 1%) 3003

Sweating
(*see under* Diaphoresis)

Sweating, decreased
(*see under* Hypohidrosis)

Sweet's syndrome
▲ Vesanoid Capsules (3%) 3037

Swelling, axillary
Depo-Provera Contraceptive Injection (Fewer than 1%) 2798

Swelling, edematous, ankles
Androderm Transdermal System CIII 3377
Android Capsules, 10 mg 1731
Eskalith 1527
Estratest 3252
Klonopin Tablets (Infrequent) 2983
Lithium Carbonate 3061
Lithium Citrate Syrup 3061
Lithobid Slow-Release Tablets 3255
Lo/Ovral Tablets 3532
Lo/Ovral-28 Tablets 3538
Low-Ogestrel-28 Tablets 3392
Modicon 2563
Ogestrel 0.5/50-28 Tablets 3428
Ortho-Cyclen/Ortho Tri-Cyclen 2573
Ortho-Novum 2563
Ortho-Novum 1/50▭28 Tablets 2556
Ortho-Cyclen/Ortho Tri-Cyclen 2573
Ovral Tablets 3551
Ovral-28 Tablets 3552
Ovrette Tablets 3552
Testoderm Transdermal Systems 574
Triphasil-21 Tablets 3600
Triphasil-28 Tablets 3605

Swelling, edematous, wrists
Eskalith 1527
Lithium Carbonate 3061
Lithium Citrate Syrup 3061
Lithobid Slow-Release Tablets 3255

Swelling, extremities
Avalide Tablets 1070
Avapro Tablets (Less than 1%) 1074
Avapro Tablets (Less than 1%) 3076
Colestid Tablets (Infrequent) 2791
Imitrex Injection (Rare) 1549
Imitrex Nasal Spray (Rare) 1554
Noroxin Tablets (Less frequent) 2145

Swelling, feet
K-Phos Neutral Tablets 946
Uroqid-Acid No. 2 Tablets 947

Swelling, joint
Ceftin for Oral Suspension (0.1% to 1%) 1898
Cozaar Tablets (Less than 1%) 2067
Hivid Tablets (Less than 1%) 2975
Hyzaar 2109
Imitrex Injection (Infrequent) 1549
Lexxel Tablets 608
Lithobid Slow-Release Tablets 3255
▲ Mykrox Tablets (3.1%) 1168
Neurontin Capsules (Infrequent) 2655
Neurontin Oral Solution (Infrequent) 2655
Neurontin Tablets (Infrequent) 2655
Priftin Tablets 758
Rifater Tablets 769

Swelling, legs
K-Phos Neutral Tablets 946
Uroqid-Acid No. 2 Tablets 947

Swelling, lower legs
(*see under* Swelling, legs)

Swelling, mouth
Acel-Imune (Rare) 1851
Felbatol (Rare) 3343
Tambocor Tablets (Less than 1%) 1990
Tripedia Vaccine (Rare) 817

Swelling, non-site specific
Amerge Tablets (Infrequent) 1467
Atromid-S Capsules 3483
Bactroban Ointment (Less than 1%) 1496
Cipro I.V. Pharmacy Bulk Package (Less than 1%) 897
Cortisporin Ophthalmic Suspension ⊙297
Coumadin for Injection 1243
Coumadin Tablets 1243
D.H.E. 45 Injection 2334
▲ Doxil Injection (3.4%) 566
Efudex 1733
Hyzaar (1.3%) 2109
▲ Lexxel Tablets (4.1%) 608
Oncaspar 756
Oxandrin Tablets 1153
Recombivax HB (Equal to or greater than 1%) 2178
Serevent Diskus 1637
Serevent Inhalation Aerosol (Rare) 1633
Sulfamylon Cream 1011
Sulfamylon Topical Solution 1011
TobraDex Ophthalmic Ointment (Less than 4%) 542
TobraDex Ophthalmic Suspension (Less than 4%) 541
Vaqta (Less than 1%) 2199
Viramune Oral Suspension 1060
Viramune Tablets 1060
Warfarin Sodium Tablets, USP 3302

Swelling, periorbital
Neosporin Ophthalmic Ointment Sterile ⊙299
Neosporin Ophthalmic Solution Sterile ⊙300
Ocuflox Ophthalmic Solution 554
Polysporin Ophthalmic Ointment Sterile ⊙301
Streptase for Infusion (Rare) 647

Swelling, salivary gland
Eskalith 1527
Flexeril Tablets (Rare) 572
Flexeril Tablets (Rare) 2094

Swelling at injection site
ActHIB Vaccine 798
▲ Aredia for Injection (Up to 41%) 2309
Attenuvax 2044
Avonex 1013
Azactam for Injection (2.4%) 1276
Cerebyx Injection (Infrequent) 2619
Cerezyme for Injection 1438
Cetrotide for Injection 3209
Cipro I.V. (1% or less) 893
▲ Comvax (27.2% to 27.6%) 2056
DDAVP Injection 4 mcg/mL (Occasional) 737
Desferal Vials 2333
Desmopressin Acetate Injection (Occasional) 1344
▲ Diphtheria & Tetanus Toxoids Adsorbed Purogenated for Pediatric Use (7.6%) 1857
▲ Enbrel for Injection (37%) 1752
▲ Enbrel for Injection (37%) 3504
▲ Engerix-B Vaccine (1% to 10%) 1517
Factrel 3633
Floxin I.V. (Approximately 2%) 2526
▲ Geref for Injection (1 patient in 6) 3215
Gonal-F for Injection 3216
▲ Havrix Vaccine (1% to 10%) 1544
HibTITER (Less than 1% to 1.7%) 1859
Humalog 1926
Humegon for Injection 2468
Humulin 50/50, 100 Units 1934
Humulin 70/30, 100 Units (Occasional) 1935
Humulin 70/30 Pen (Occasional) 1936
Humulin L, 100 Units (Occasional) 1937
Humulin R Regular (U-500) 1943
Humulin N NPH Pen (Occasional) 1940
Hyalgan Solution (Common) 3080
Iletin II, Regular (Pork), 100 Units 1947
Imitrex Injection 1549
▲ Imovax Rabies Vaccine (About 25%) 807
▲ Infanrix Vaccine (0.7% to 32.9%) 1562
INFeD Injection 3388
▲ IPOL Vaccine (Up to 11.4%) 809
▲ JE-VAX Vaccine (2.9% to approximately 20%) 811
▲ Leustatin Injection (9% to 19%) 2495
▲ Menomune-A/C/Y/W-135 Vaccine (92%) 813
Merrem I.V. (0.2%) 673
M-M-R II 2118
Novantrone for Injection 1760
Nubain Injection 1080
▲ Nutropin Depot for Injectable Suspension (8%) 1423
Liquid PedvaxHIB (0.9% to 2.5%) 2148
Pergonal for Injection 3223
Pneumovax 23 (Common) 2156
Pnu-Imune 23 (Rare) 1868
Repronex for Intramuscular and Subcutaneous Injection 1347
Saizen for Injection (Infrequent) 3225
▲ Synercid I.V. (17.3% to 18%) 775
▲ Synvisc (Among most common) 3596
Taxol Injection 1129
▲ Tetanus & Diphtheria Toxoids Adsorbed for Adult Use (7.6%) 1880
Timentin Injection- ADD-Vantage Vial 1661
Timentin Injection-Galaxy Container 1664
Timentin Injection-Pharmacy Bulk Package 1666
Timentin for Intravenous Administration 1658
Tripedia Vaccine 817
▲ Trisenox Injection (10%) 1158
▲ Vaqta (1.5% to 13.8%) 2199
▲ Varivax (19.3% to 32.5%) 2202
Velosulin BR Human Insulin 10 ml Vials 2435
Versed Injection (Less than 1%) 3027
Zemuron Injection (Less than 1%) 2491

Symphyseolysis
Remicade for IV Injection (Less than 2%) 1178

Syncope
Accupril Tablets (0.5% to 1.0%) 2611
Accuretic Tablets 2614
Accutane Capsules 2944
Aceon Tablets (2 mg, 4 mg, 8 mg) (0.3% to 1%) 3249
Aciphex Tablets 1267
Aciphex Tablets 1783
Actimmune (Rare) 1772
Adalat CC Tablets (Rare) 877
Aerobid/Aerobid-M (1% to 3%) 1363
Aggrenox Capsules (1%) 1026
Agrylin Capsules (1% to 5%) 3232
AK-Fluor Injection 10% and 25% ⊙202
Alphagan Ophthalmic Solution (Less than 3%) 545
Altace Capsules (Less than 1% to 2.1%) 2233
Ambien Tablets (Infrequent) 3191
Amerge Tablets (Infrequent) 1467
Amicar Injection 3608
Amicar Syrup 3608
Amicar Tablets 3608
Amphotec (1% to 5%) 1774
Antabuse Tablets 3474
Anzemet Injection (Rare) 719
Anzemet Tablets (Rare) 722
▲ Aredia for Injection (Up to 6%) 2309
Aricept Tablets (2%) 1270
Aricept Tablets (2%) 2665
Arthrotec Tablets (Rare) 3195
Attenuvax 2044
Avalide Tablets 1070
Avapro Tablets 1074
Avapro Tablets 3076
▲ Avonex (4%) 1013
Axert Tablets (Rare) 2772
Betagan ⊙228
Betapace Tablets (1% to 5%) 950
Betaseron for SC Injection 988
Betimol Ophthalmic Solution ⊙324
Bicillin C-R 900/300 Injection 2240
Bicillin C-R Injection 2238
Bicillin L-A Injection 2242
Blocadren Tablets (0.6%) 2046
Brevibloc Injection (Less than 1%) 858
Campath Ampules 992
Captopril Tablets 2281
Carbatrol Capsules 3234
Cardene I.V. (0.7%) 3485
Cardizem Injectable (Less than 1%) 1018
Cardizem Lyo-Ject Syringe (Less than 1%) 1018
Cardizem Monovial (Less than 1%) 1018
Cardizem CD Capsules (Less than 1%) 1016
▲ Cardura Tablets (0.5% to 23%) 2668
Carteolol Hydrochloride Ophthalmic Solution USP, 1% ⊙258
▲ Casodex Tablets (2% to 5%) 662
Catapres Tablets (Rare) 1037
Catapres-TTS (0.5% or less) 1038
Ceclor CD Tablets 1279
Ceclor 1905
Celebrex Capsules (Less than 0.1%) 2676
Celebrex Capsules (Less than 0.1%) 2780
Celexa (Infrequent) 1365
▲ CellCept Capsules (3% to 10%) 2951
▲ CellCept Intravenous (3% to 10%) 2951
▲ CellCept Oral Suspension (3% to 10%) 2951
▲ CellCept Tablets (3% to 10%) 2951
Cerebyx Injection (Infrequent) 2619
Chirocaine Injection (Less than 1%) 2909
Cipro I.V. (1% or less) 893
Cipro I.V. Pharmacy Bulk Package (Less than 1%) 897
Cipro (Less than 1%) 887
Claritin (At least one patient) 3100
Claritin-D 12 Hour Extended Release Tablets (Less frequent) 3102
Claritin-D 24 Hour Extended Release Tablets (Fewer than 2%) 3104
Clinoril Tablets (Less than 1%) 2053
Clomid Tablets 735
▲ Clozaril Tablets (More than 5% to 6%) 2319
Cognex Capsules (Frequent) 1351
Comtan Tablets 2328
Comvax 2056
▲ Copaxone for Injection (5 %) 3306
▲ Coreg Tablets (3.4%) 1508
Corvert Injection (0.3%) 2793
Cosopt Sterile Ophthalmic Solution 2065
Covera-HS Tablets (Less than 2%) 3199
Cozaar Tablets (Less than 1%) 2067
Crinone (Less than 5%) 3213
Crixivan Capsules (Less than 2%) 2070
Cytotec Tablets (Infrequent) 3202
DaunoXome Injection (Less than or equal to 5%) 1442
Demadex Tablets and Injection 2965
Demerol 3079

Depo-Provera Contraceptive Injection (Fewer than 1%) 2798
Dilaudid 441
Dilaudid Oral Liquid 445
Dilaudid Tablets - 8 mg 445
Dilaudid-HP (Less frequent) 443
Diovan Capsules (Less frequent) 2337
Diovan HCT Tablets (Greater than 0.2%) 2338
Diphtheria & Tetanus Toxoids Adsorbed Purogenated for Pediatric Use 1857
Diprivan Injectable Emulsion (Less than 1%) 667
Dolobid Tablets (Rare) 2088
Dolophine Hydrochloride Tablets 3056
▲ Dostinex Tablets (1% to less than 10%) 2804
Doxil Injection (Less than 1%) 566
Duraclon Injection (Rare) 3057
Duragesic Transdermal System (1% or greater) 1786
Dynabac Tablets (0.1% to 1%) 2269
DynaCirc Capsules (0.5% to 1%) 2921
DynaCirc CR Tablets (0.5% to 1%) 2923
Effexor Tablets (Infrequent) 3495
Effexor XR Capsules (Infrequent) 3499
▲ Eldepryl Capsules (7 of 49 patients) 3266
Enalaprilat Injection (0.5%) 863
Engerix-B Vaccine 1517
Eskalith 1527
Estrace Vaginal Cream 3358
Estrace Tablets 3361
Estring Vaginal Ring (1% to 3%) 2811
Etrafon 3115
Evoxac Capsules (Less than 1%) 1217
▲ Exelon Capsules (3%) 2342
▲ Exelon Oral Solution (3%) 2345
Feldene Capsules (Occasional) 2685
▲ Ferrlecit Injection (6%) 3386
Fleet Bisacodyl Laxatives 1359
Flexeril Tablets (Less than 1%) 572
Flexeril Tablets (Less than 1%) 2094
▲ Flolan for Injection (7%) 1528
Flomax Capsules (0.2% to 0.4%) 1044
Florinef Acetate Tablets 2250
Floxin I.V. (Less than 1%) 2526
Floxin Tablets (Less than 1%) 2529
Flumadine (Less than 0.3%) 1370
Fluorescite Injection ⊙211
Fortovase Capsules (Less than 2%) 2970
Gabitril Tablets (Frequent) 1189
Gamimune N, 5% Solvent/Detergent Treated 925
Gamimune N, 10% Solvent/Detergent Treated 928
Geodon Capsules (0.6%) 2688
Glucotrol XL Extended Release Tablets (Less than 3%) 2693
Halcion Tablets 2823
Havrix Vaccine (Rare) 1544
Herceptin I.V. (At least one of the 958 patients) 1414
Hivid Tablets (Less than 1%) 2975
▲ Hytrin Capsules (0.5% to 21%) 464
Hyzaar 2109
Imdur Tablets 1826
Imitrex Injection (Infrequent) 1549
Imitrex Nasal Spray (Infrequent) 1554
Imitrex Tablets (Rare to infrequent) 1558
Indocin (Less than 1%) 2112
INFeD Injection 3388
Intron A for Injection (Less than 5%) 3120
Inversine Tablets 1850
Invirase Capsules (Less than 2%) 2979
Ismo Tablets (Fewer than 1%) 3524
Isoptin SR Tablets (1% or less) 467
Isopto Carbachol Ophthalmic Solution ⊙215
Isordil Sublingual Tablets (Uncommon) 3525
Isordil Titradose Tablets (Uncommon) 3526
Kadian Capsules (Less than 3%) 1335
Kytril Tablets (Rare) 2988
Lamictal (Infrequent) 1567
Lariam Tablets (Less than 1%) 2989
Leukine 1755
Levaquin (Less than 0.3%) 2537
Levlen 962
Levlite 21 Tablets 962
Levlite 28 Tablets 962
Lexxel Tablets 608
Librium Capsules (Few instances) 1736
Librium for Injection (Isolated instances) 1737
Limbitrol 1738
Lipitor Tablets (Less than 2%) 2639
Lipitor Tablets (Less than 2%) 2696
Lithium Carbonate 3061
Lithium Citrate Syrup 3061
Lodine (Less than 1%) 3528
Lodine XL Extended-Release Tablets (Less than 1%) 3530
Lodosyn Tablets 1251
Lopid Tablets 2650
Lotensin Tablets (0.1%) 2365
Lotensin HCT Tablets (0.3% or more) 2367
Loxitane Capsules 3398
▲ Lupron Depot 3.75 mg (Among most frequent) 3281
Lupron Depot–3 Month 11.25 mg (Less than 5%) 3285
Lupron Depot-PED 7.5 mg, 11.25 mg and 15 mg (Less than 2%) 3291
Lupron Injection (Less than 5%) 3279
Lupron Injection Pediatric (Less than 2%) 3280
Luvox Tablets (25, 50, 100 mg) (Frequent) 3256
Matulane Capsules 3246
▲ Mavik Tablets (0.2% to 5.9%) 478
Maxair Autohaler 1981
Maxair Inhaler (Less than 1%) 1984
Maxalt Tablets (Rare) 2120
Maxalt-MLT Orally Disintegrating Tablets (Rare) 2120
Mepergan Injection 3539
Meridia Capsules 481
Merrem I.V. (0.1% to 1.0%) 673
Meruvax II 2130
Mexitil Capsules (Less than 1% or about 6 in 1,000) 1047
Miltown Tablets 3349
Minipress Capsules (1% to 4%) 2699
Minizide Capsules (Rare) 2700
Mirapex Tablets (1% or more) 2834
Mirena Intrauterine System 974
M-M-R II 2118
Mobic Tablets (Less than 2%) 1054
Modicon 2563
Moduretic Tablets (Less than or equal to 1%) 2138
Monopril Tablets (0.2% to 1.0%) 1091
Monopril HCT (Less than 2%) 1094
MS Contin Tablets (Less frequent) 2896
MSIR (Less frequent) 2898
Mumpsvax 2141
MUSE Urethral Suppository (0.4%) 3335
Mykrox Tablets 1168
Naprelan Tablets (Less than 1%) 1293
Naropin Injection (Less than 1%) 612
Navane Oral 2701
Navane Intramuscular 2703
Nembutal Sodium Solution (Less than 1%) 485
Nesacaine/Nesacaine MPF 617
▲ Neumega for Injection (13%) 1434
Neurontin Capsules (Infrequent) 2655
Neurontin Oral Solution (Infrequent) 2655
Neurontin Tablets (Infrequent) 2655
Niaspan Extended-Release Tablets 1846
Nilandron Tablets (2%) 753
Nipent for Injection (Less than 3%) 3272
▲ Nitro-Dur Transdermal Infusion System (4%) 1834
▲ Nitro-Dur Transdermal Infusion System (4%) 3134
Nitrostat Tablets 2658
Norflex 1987
Normodyne Injection (Rare) 3135
Normodyne Tablets (Rare) 3137
Norvasc Tablets (More than 0.1% to 1%) 2704
Norvir Capsules (Less than 2%) 487
Norvir Oral Solution (Less than 2%) 487
Nubain Injection (1% or less) 1323
Ocupress Ophthalmic Solution, 1% Sterile ⊙303
Oramorph SR Tablets (Less frequent) 3062
Orap Tablets 1407
Ortho Diaphragm Kits – All-Flex Arcing Spring; Ortho Coil Spring 2552
Ortho-Cyclen/Ortho Tri-Cyclen 2573
Ortho-Est Tablets 3464
Ortho-Novum 2563
Ortho-Novum 1/50□28 Tablets 2556
Ortho-Cyclen/Ortho Tri-Cyclen 2573
OxyContin Tablets (Less than 1%) 2912
ParaGard T 380A Intrauterine Copper Contraceptive 2582
Paxil (Frequent) 1609
Pediazole Suspension 3050
Periactin Tablets 2155
Permax Tablets (2.1%) 1299
Phenergan Injection 3553
Phenergan 3556
Phenergan with Codeine Syrup 3557
Phenergan VC with Codeine Syrup 3561
Phrenilin (Infrequent) 578
Plavix Tablets (1% to 2.5%) 1097
Plavix Tablets (1% to 2.5%) 3084
Plendil Extended-Release Tablets (0.5% to 1.5%) 623
Pletal Tablets (Less than 2%) 2605
Pletal Tablets (Less than 2%) 2848
Polocaine Injection, USP 625
Polocaine-MPF Injection, USP 625
Ponstel Capsules (Occasional) 1356
Prevacid Delayed-Release Capsules (Less than 1%) 3292
PREVPAC (Less than 1%) 3298
Prinivil Tablets (0.3% to 1.0%) 2164
Prinzide Tablets (0.8% to 0.1%) 2168
Procardia Capsules (Approximately 0.5%) 2708
Procardia XL Extended Release Tablets (1% or less) 2710
Proleukin for Injection (Less than 1%) 1199
Prometrium Capsules (100 mg, 200 mg) (Rare) 3261
ProSom Tablets (Rare) 500
Prostigmin Injectable 1744
Prostigmin Tablets 1744
Prostin E2 Suppositories 2852
Protonix I.V. (Less than 1%) 3580
Protonix Tablets (Less than 1%) 3577
Provigil Tablets (1%) 1193
Prozac Pulvules, Liquid, and Weekly Capsules (Infrequent) 1238
Pulmicort Turbuhaler Inhalation Powder (1% to 3%) 636
Quinaglute Dura-Tabs Tablets 978
Quinidex Extentabs (Many reports) 2933
▲ Rapamune Oral Solution and Tablets (3% to 20%) 3584
Recombivax HB 2178
Relafen Tablets (Less than 1%) 1617
Remeron Tablets (Infrequent) 2483
Remeron SolTab Tablets (Infrequent) 2486
Remicade for IV Injection (Less than 2%) 1178
Reminyl Oral Solution (Up to 2%) 1792
Reminyl Tablets (Up to 2%) 1792
▲ Requip Tablets (3% to 12%) 1621
Rescriptor Tablets (Less than 2%) 526
Retrovir Capsules 1625
Retrovir IV Infusion 1629
Retrovir 1625
Rilutek Tablets (Infrequent) 772
Risperdal (0.2%) 1796
Robaxin Tablets 2939
Roferon-A Injection (Less than 0.5% to less than 5%) 2996
Roxanol 3066
Rythmol Tablets – 150 mg, 225 mg, 300 mg (2.2%) 502
Salagen Tablets (Less than 1%) 2229
Sandostatin Injection (Less than 1%) 2394
Sandostatin LAR Depot (1% to 4%) 2395
Sarafem Pulvules (Infrequent) 1962
Sedapap Tablets 50 mg/650 mg (Infrequent) 2225
Sensorcaine 643
Sensorcaine-MPF Injection 643
Serentil 1057
Serophene Tablets 3226
Seroquel Tablets (1%) 684
Serzone Tablets (Infrequent) 1104
Sinemet Tablets 1253
Sinemet CR Tablets 1255
Skelid Tablets (More than or equal to 1%) 3088
Soma Tablets 3353
Soma Compound Tablets (Infrequent or rare) 3354
Soma Compound w/Codeine Tablets (Infrequent or rare) 3355
Sonata Capsules (Infrequent) 3591
Stadol NS Nasal Spray 1108
Sular Tablets (Less than or equal to 1%) 688
Sustiva Capsules (Less than 2%) 1258
Talacen Caplets (Infrequent) 3089
Talwin Nx Tablets 3090
Tambocor Tablets (1% to 3%) 1990
Tarka Tablets (0.1% to 0.3% or more) 508
▲ Tasmar Tablets (4% to 5%) 3010
Taxol Injection (Approximately 1%) 1129
Taxotere for Injection Concentrate 778
Tegretol/Tegretol-XR 2404
Tenex Tablets (Less frequent) 2942
Tenoretic Tablets 690
Tenormin 692
Tetanus & Diphtheria Toxoids Adsorbed for Adult Use 1880
Thalomid Capsules 1154
Thiothixene Capsules 2290
Thorazine 1656
Thyrel TRH for Injection (A small number of patients) 3630
Tiazac Capsules (Less than 2%) 1378
Tikosyn Capsules (Less than or equal to 2%) 2717
Timolide Tablets (Less than 1%) 2187
Timolol GFS ⊙266
Timoptic in Ocudose (Less frequent) 2192
Timoptic Sterile Ophthalmic Solution (Less frequent) 2190
Timoptic-XE Sterile Ophthalmic Gel Forming Solution 2194
Tonocard Tablets (Less than 1%) 649
Topamax Sprinkle Capsules (Infrequent) 2590
Topamax Tablets (Infrequent) 2590
Toprol-XL Tablets (Greater than 1%) 651
Toradol (1% or less) 3018
Trileptal Oral Suspension 2407
Trileptal Tablets 2407
Tri-Levlen 962
Trovan (Less than 1%) 2722
Twinrix Vaccine (Less than 1%) 1674
Ultram Tablets (Less than 1%) 2600
Uniretic Tablets (Less than 1%) 3178
Univasc Tablets (0.51%) 3181
Urecholine 2198
Valium Injectable 3026
Vantin Tablets and Oral Suspension (Less than 1%) 2860
Vascor Tablets (0.5% to 2.0%) 2602
Vaseretic Tablets (0.5% to 2.0%) 2204
Vasotec I.V. Injection (0.5%) 2207
Vasotec Tablets (0.5% to 2.2%) 2210
Verelan Capsules (1% or less) 3184
Verelan PM Capsules (2% or less) 3186
Versed Injection (Less than 1%) 3027
Viagra Tablets (Less than 2%) 2732
Vioxx (Greater than 0.1% to 1.9%) 2213
Vistide Injection 1445
Vivelle Transdermal System 2412
Vivelle-Dot Transdermal System 2416
Wellbutrin Tablets (1.2%) 1680
Wellbutrin SR Sustained-Release Tablets (Rare) 1684
▲ Xanax Tablets (3.1% to 3.8%) 2865
Xopenex Inhalation Solution 3207
Zanaflex Tablets (Infrequent) 1305
Zaroxolyn Tablets 1177
Zestoretic Tablets (0.1% to 0.8%) 695
Zestril Tablets (0.1% to 1.8%) 698
Ziac Tablets 1887
Zofran Injection (Rare) 1698
Zoloft (Infrequent) 2751
Zomig Tablets (Infrequent) 708
Zomig-ZMT Tablets (Infrequent) 708
Zonegran Capsules (Infrequent) 1307
Zosyn (1.0% or less) 1890
Zosyn in Galaxy Containers (1.0% or less) 1894
Zyban Sustained-Release Tablets (Rare) 1710
Zyprexa Tablets (0.6%) 1973
Zyprexa ZYDIS Orally Disintegrating Tablets (0.6%) 1973
Zyrtec (Less than 2%) 2756
Zyrtec-D 12 Hour Extended Relief Tablets (Less than 2%) 2758

Synechiae

Vitrasert Implant (Less than 1%) ⊙254

Synovitis

Actiq (Less than 1%) 1184
Arava Tablets (2%) 724
Avonex 1013
Celebrex Capsules (0.1% to 1.9%) 2676
Celebrex Capsules (0.1% to 1.9%) 2780
Cuprimine Capsules (Some patients) 2075
Depen Titratable Tablets 3341
Evoxac Capsules (Less than 1%) 1217
Levaquin Injection (Less than 0.5%) 2537
Lopid Tablets 2650
LYMErix Vaccine 1592
▲ Stromectol Tablets (9.3%) 2185
Viagra Tablets (Less than 2%) 2732

Systemic lupus erythematosus

(*see under* Lupus erythematosus, systemic)

T

T3, decrease

Aygestin Tablets 1333
Brevicon 28-Day Tablets 3380
Eskalith 1527
Estratest 3252
Lithium Carbonate 3061
Lithium Citrate Syrup 3061
Lithobid Slow-Release Tablets 3255
Norinyl 1 +35 28-Day Tablets 3380
Norinyl 1 + 50 28-Day Tablets 3380
Provera Tablets 2853
Tri-Norinyl-28 Tablets 3433

T4, decrease

Eskalith 1527
Lithium Carbonate 3061
Lithium Citrate Syrup 3061
Lithobid Slow-Release Tablets 3255

T4, increase

Brevicon 28-Day Tablets 3380
Estratest 3252
Nolvadex Tablets 678
Norinyl 1 +35 28-Day Tablets 3380
Norinyl 1 + 50 28-Day Tablets 3380
Ortho-Cyclen/Ortho Tri-Cyclen 2573

Tri-Norinyl-28 Tablets 3433

Tachyarrhythmia
Actimmune (Rare) 1772
Amerge Tablets (Infrequent) 1467
Ellence Injection 2806
Synvisc 3596

Tachyarrhythmias, supraventricular
Claritin (At least one patient) 3100
Claritin-D 12 Hour Extended Release Tablets 3102
Claritin-D 24 Hour Extended Release Tablets 3104
Digitek Tablets 1003
Lanoxicaps Capsules 1574
Lanoxin Injection 1581
Lanoxin Tablets 1587
Lanoxin Elixir Pediatric 1578
Lanoxin Injection Pediatric 1584

Tachycardia
AccuNeb Inhalation Solution 1230
Accupril Tablets (0.5% to 1.0%) 2611
Accuretic Tablets (0.5% to 1%) 2614
Accutane Capsules 2944
Aciphex Tablets 1267
Aciphex Tablets 1783
Acthrel for Injection 3629
Actiq (Less than 1%) 1184
Adalat CC Tablets (Less than 1.0%) 877
Adderall Tablets 3231
Adderall XR Capsules
Adipex-P 1406
Aerobid/Aerobid-M (1% to 3%) 1363
Aggrenox Capsules (Less than 1%) 1026
▲ Agrylin Capsules (7.5%) 3232
Albumin (Human) 5% (Very rare) 838
Albumin (Human) 25% (Very rare) 839
Alkeran for Injection (In some patients) 1465
Allegra-D Extended-Release Tablets 714
Alupent (Less than 1%) 1029
Ambien Tablets (Infrequent) 3191
▲ AmBisome for Injection (9.4% to 18.5%) 1383
▲ Amphotec (9% to 12%) 1774
Anectine Injection 1476
Anzemet Injection (2.2% to 3.3%) 719
Anzemet Tablets (2.2% to 3.3%) 722
Arava Tablets (1% to 3%) 724
▲ Aredia for Injection (Up to 6%) 2309
Artane 1855
Arthrotec Tablets (Rare) 3195
Astelin Nasal Spray (Infrequent) 3339
Atacand Tablets (0.5% or greater) 595
Atacand HCT Tablets (0.5% or greater) 597
Atrovent Inhalation Aerosol (Less frequent) 1030
Atrovent Inhalation Solution (Less than 3%) 1031
Atrovent Nasal Spray 0.03% 1032
Atrovent Nasal Spray 0.06% (Less than 1%) 1033
Avalide Tablets (1%) 1070
Avapro Tablets (1% or greater) 1074
Avapro Tablets (1% or greater) 3076
Avelox Tablets (0.05% to 1%) 879
Avonex 1013
Axert Tablets (Infrequent) 2772
Benadryl Parenteral 2617
▲ Betaseron for SC Injection (6%) 988
Betaxon Ophthalmic Suspension (Less than 2%) 537
Bicillin C-R 900/300 Injection 2240
Bicillin C-R Injection 2238
Bicillin L-A Injection 2242
Bontril Slow-Release Capsules 576
Brethine Ampuls (1.3% to 1.5%) 2314
▲ Brethine Tablets (3.5%) 2313
Brevital Sodium for Injection, USP 1815
Buprenex Injectable (Less than 1%) 2918
Cafcit 1035
Cancidas for Injection (Up to 1.3%) 2048
Captopril Tablets (Approximately 1 of 100 patients) 2281
▲ Cardene I.V. (3.5%) 3485
Cardizem Injectable 1018
Cardizem Lyo-Ject Syringe 1018
Cardizem Monovial 1018
Cardizem CD Capsules (Less than 1%) 1016
Cardura Tablets (0.3% to 0.9%) 2668
▲ Carnitor Injection (5% to 9%) 3242
Cataflam Tablets (Less than 1%) 2315
Catapres Tablets (About 5 in 1,000 patients) 1037
Catapres-TTS (0.5% or less) 1038
Ceftin Tablets (0.1% to 1%) 1898
Celebrex Capsules (0.1% to 1.9%) 2676
Celebrex Capsules (0.1% to 1.9%) 2780
Celexa (Frequent) 1365
▲ CellCept Capsules (3% to 20.1%) 2951
▲ CellCept Intravenous (3% to 20.1%) 2951
▲ CellCept Oral Suspension (3% to 20.1%) 2951
▲ CellCept Tablets (3% to 22%) 2951
Cerebyx Injection (2.2%) 2619
Chirocaine Injection (1.8%) 2909
Cipro I.V. (1% or less) 893
Cipro I.V. Pharmacy Bulk Package (Less than 1%) 897
Claritin (At least one patient) 3100
Claritin-D 12 Hour Extended Release Tablets (Less frequent) 3102
Claritin-D 24 Hour Extended Release Tablets (Fewer than 2%) 3104
Clinoril Tablets (Less than 1 in 100) 2053
Clomid Tablets 735
Clorpres Tablets (About 5 in 1,000) 1002
▲ Clozaril Tablets (More than 5% to 25%) 2319
Cogentin 2055
Cognex Capsules (Infrequent) 1351
Colestid Tablets (Infrequent) 2791
Combipres Tablets (About 5 in 1,000) 1040
Combivent Inhalation Aerosol (Less than 2%) 1041
Compazine 1505
Comvax 2056
Concerta Extended-Release Tablets 1998
Concerta Tablets 561
▲ Copaxone for Injection (5%) 3306
Coreg Tablets (0.1% to 1%) 1508
Corlopam Injection (2%) 412
Cortrosyn for Injection 2449
Corvert Injection (2.7%) 2793
Cozaar Tablets (Less than 1%) 2067
Dantrium Capsules (Less frequent) 2885
Dapsone Tablets USP 1780
DaunoXome Injection (Less than or equal to 5%) 1442
Demadex Tablets and Injection 2965
Demerol 3079
Depacon Injection (1% to 5%) 416
Depakene (1% to 5%) 421
Depakote Sprinkle Capsules (1% to 5%) 426
Depakote Tablets (1% to 5%) 430
Depakote ER Tablets (1% to 5%) 436
Depo-Provera Contraceptive Injection (Fewer than 1%) 2798
Desferal Vials 2333
Desoxyn Tablets 440
Detrol Tablets 3623
Detrol LA Capsules 2801
Dexedrine 1512
DextroStat Tablets 3236
D.H.E. 45 Injection 2334
Dibenzyline Capsules 3457
Digitek Tablets (2%) 1003
Dilaudid Oral Liquid 445
Dilaudid Tablets - 8 mg 445
Dilaudid-HP (Less frequent) 443
Diovan HCT Tablets (Greater than 0.2%) 2338
Dipentum Capsules (Rare) 2803
Diphtheria & Tetanus Toxoids Adsorbed Purogenated for Pediatric Use 1857
Diprivan Injectable Emulsion (Less than 1%) 667
Donnagel Liquid (Rare) ▣ 789
Donnatal 2929
Donnatal Extentabs 2930
Donnatal Tablets 2929
Doxil Injection (1% to 5%) 566
Duraclon Injection (0.5% to 2.6%) 3057
Duragesic Transdermal System 1786
Dyazide Capsules 1515
DynaCirc Capsules (1% to 3.4%) 2921
DynaCirc CR Tablets (0.5% to 1%) 2923
Ecotrin Enteric Coated Aspirin Low, Regular and Maximum Strength Tablets 1715
Effexor Tablets (2%) 3495
▲ Effexor XR Capsules (3%) 3499
Eldepryl Capsules 3266
Ellence Injection 2806
Engerix-B Vaccine 1517
EpiPen 1236
Epogen for Injection (0.31%) 582
Etrafon 3115
Evoxac Capsules (Less than 1%) 1217
Exelon Capsules (Infrequent) 2342
Exelon Oral Solution (Infrequent) 2345
Factrel (Rare) 3633
Felbatol (Frequent) 3343
Feldene Capsules (Occasional) 2685
▲ Ferrlecit Injection (5%) 3386
Flexeril Tablets (Less than 1%) 572
Flexeril Tablets (Less than 1%) 2094
▲ Flolan for Injection (1% to 43%) 1528
Floxin I.V. 2526
Floxin Otic Solution (Single report) 1219
Floxin Tablets 2529
Flumadine (Less than 0.3%) 1370
Fluothane Inhalation 3508
Foradil Aerolizer 2354
Furosemide Tablets 2284
Gabitril Tablets (Frequent) 1189
Gamimune N, 5% Solvent/Detergent Treated (One patient) 925
Gamimune N, 10% Solvent/Detergent Treated (One patient) 928
Gammar-P I.V. 787
Gastrocrom Oral Concentrate (Less common) 1162
Geodon Capsules (2%) 2688
GlucaGen for Injection Diagnostic Kit 949
Guaifed 2272
Halcion Tablets (0.5% to 0.9%) 2823
Haldol Decanoate 2535
Haldol Injection, Tablets and Concentrate 2533
▲ Herceptin I.V. (5%) 1414
Hivid Tablets (Less than 1%) 2975
Humegon for Injection 2468
Hycomine Compound Tablets 1317
Hytrin Capsules (0.6% to 1.9%) 464
Hyzaar 2109
Imdur Tablets (Less than or equal to 5%) 1826
Imitrex Injection (Infrequent) 1549
Imitrex Nasal Spray (Infrequent) 1554
Imitrex Tablets (Infrequent) 1558
Indocin Capsules (Less than 1%) 2112
Indocin I.V. (Less than 1%) 2115
Indocin (Less than 1%) 2112
INFeD Injection 3388
▲ Infergen (4%) 1777
Innohep Injection (Greater than or equal to 1%) 1248
Intron A for Injection (Less than 5%) 3120
Ionamin Capsules 1163
Kadian Capsules (Less than 3%) 1335
K-Phos Neutral Tablets 946
Kytril Injection (Rare) 2986
Lamictal (Infrequent) 1567
Lanoxicaps Capsules 1574
Lanoxin Injection 1581
Lanoxin Tablets 1587
Lanoxin Elixir Pediatric 1578
Lanoxin Injection Pediatric 1584
▲ Leukine (11%) 1755
▲ Leustatin Injection (6%) 2495
Levaquin (Less than 0.3%) 2537
Levbid Extended-Release Tablets 3172
Levo-Dromoran 1734
Levoxyl Tablets 1819
Levsin/Levsinex/Levbid 3172
Lexxel Tablets 608
Librium for Injection 1737
Limbitrol 1738
Lodine XL Extended-Release Tablets (Less than 1%) 3530
Lotensin HCT Tablets (0.3% or more) 2367
Loxitane Capsules 3398
Lufyllin Tablets 3347
Lufyllin-400 Tablets 3347
Lufyllin-GG Elixir 3348
Lufyllin-GG Tablets 3348
Lupron Depot 3.75 mg (Less than 5%) 3281
Lupron Depot-3 Month 11.25 mg (Less than 5%) 3285
Luvox Tablets (25, 50, 100 mg) (Frequent) 3256
Marinol Capsules (Greater than 1%) 3325
Matulane Capsules 3246
Maxair Autohaler (1.2% to 1.3%) 1981
Maxair Inhaler (1.2% to 1.3%) 1984
Maxalt Tablets (Infrequent) 2120
Maxalt-MLT Orally Disintegrating Tablets (Infrequent) 2120
Maxzide 1008
Mepergan Injection 3539
Meridia Capsules (2.6%) 481
Merrem I.V. (0.1% to 1.0%) 673
Metadate CD Capsules 1164
Metadate ER Tablets 1167
Methylin Tablets 1995
Methylin ER Tablets 1995
Miacalcin Nasal Spray (Less than 1%) 2375
Micardis Tablets (More than 0.3%) 1049
Micardis HCT Tablets (Less than 2%) 1051
Migranal Nasal Spray (Infrequent) 2376
Miltown Tablets 3349
Minipress Capsules (Less than 1%) 2699
Minizide Capsules (Rare) 2700
▲ Mirapex Tablets (17% to 27%) 2834
Moban 1320
Mobic Tablets (Less than 2%) 1054
Moduretic Tablets (Less than or equal to 1%) 2138
Monopril Tablets (0.4% to 1.0%) 1091
Motofen Tablets 577
MS Contin Tablets (Less frequent) 2896
MSIR (Less frequent) 2898
▲ Mylotarg for Injection (8% to 15%) 3540
Naprelan Tablets (Less than 1%) 1293
Narcan Injection 1322
Nardil Tablets (Less frequent) 2653
Naropin Injection (1% to 5%) 612
Natrecor for Injection (At least 1%) 3189
Navane Oral 2701
Navane Intramuscular 2703
Navelbine Injection 1604
Nesacaine/Nesacaine MPF 617
▲ Neumega for Injection (20%) 1434
Neupogen for Injection 587
Neurontin Capsules (Infrequent) 2655
Neurontin Oral Solution (Infrequent) 2655
Neurontin Tablets (Infrequent) 2655
Nexium Delayed-Release Capsules (Less than 1%) 619
Niaspan Extended-Release Tablets 1846
Nicotrol Inhaler (Occasional) 2840
Nicotrol Nasal Spray 2843
Nimotop Capsules (Up to 1.4%) 904
Nipent for Injection (Less than 3%) 3272
Norcuron for Injection (Rare) 2478
Norflex 1987
Normodyne Injection 3135
Normodyne Tablets 3137
Norpramin Tablets 755
Norvasc Tablets (More than 0.1% to 1%) 2704
Norvir Capsules (Less than 2%) 487
Norvir Oral Solution (Less than 2%) 487
Novantrone for Injection 1760
Nubain Injection (1% or less) 1323
NuLev Orally Disintegrating Tablets 3176
Numorphan 1324
Oncaspar (Greater than 1% but less than 5%) 756
Oramorph SR Tablets (Less frequent) 3062
Orap Tablets 1407
▲ Orthoclone OKT3 Sterile Solution (10%) 2498
Orudis Capsules (Less than 1%) 3548
Oruvail Capsules (Less than 1%) 3548
Parnate Tablets 1607
Paxil (Frequent) 1609
Pediazole Suspension 3050
Pergonal for Injection 3223
Periactin Tablets 2155
Permax Tablets (Infrequent) 1299
Persantine Tablets (Rare) 1057
Phenergan Injection 3553
Phenergan 3556
Phenergan with Codeine Syrup 3557
Phenergan VC with Codeine Syrup 3561
▲ Photofrin for Injection (6%) 831
Phrenilin (Infrequent) 578
Plendil Extended-Release Tablets (0.5% to 1.5%) 623
▲ Pletal Tablets (4%) 2605
▲ Pletal Tablets (4%) 2848
Polocaine Injection, USP 625
Polocaine-MPF Injection, USP 625
Ponstel Capsules (Occasional) 1356
Prilosec Delayed-Release Capsules (Less than 1%) 628
Primaxin I.M. 2158
Primaxin I.V. (1.5%) 2160
Prinzide Tablets 2168
Procardia XL Extended Release Tablets (1% or less) 2710
Procrit for Injection (0.31%) 2502
▲ Prograf (3% to 15%) 1393
Prolastin (Occasional) 943
▲ Proleukin for Injection (23%) 1199
Propine Ophthalmic Solution ⊙ 250
Prostigmin Injectable 1744
Prostigmin Tablets 1744
Protonix I.V. (Less than 1%) 3580
Protonix Tablets (Less than 1%) 3577
Protopam Chloride for Injection 3582
▲ Proventil Inhalation Aerosol (10%) 3142
Proventil Inhalation Solution 0.083% (1%) 3146
▲ Proventil Repetabs Tablets (5% to 8%) 3148
Proventil Solution for Inhalation 0.5% (1%) 3144
▲ Proventil HFA Inhalation Aerosol (7%) 3150
Provigil Tablets (At least 1%) 1193
Prozac Pulvules, Liquid, and Weekly Capsules (Infrequent) 1238
▲ Rapamune Oral Solution and Tablets (3% to 20%) 3584
Recombivax HB 2178
ReFacto Vials 1437
Remicade for IV Injection (Less than 2%) 1178
Repronex for Intramuscular and Subcutaneous Injection 1347
Requip Tablets (2%) 1621
Rescriptor Tablets (Less than 2%) 526
Rilutek Tablets (1.3% to 2.0%) 772
▲ Risperdal (3% to 5%) 1796
Ritalin 2387

▲ Rituxan for Infusion (Among most frequent) 1750
▲ Rituxan I.V. (Among most frequent) 1428
Robinul Forte Tablets 1358
Robinul Injectable 2940
Robinul Tablets 1358
Romazicon Injection (Less than 1%) 3000
Roxicodone Tablets (Less than 3%) 3067
Rynatan Tablets 3351
Salagen Tablets (2%) 2229
Sandimmune 2388
Sandostatin Injection (Less than 1%) 2394
Sandostatin LAR Depot (1% to 4%) 2395
Sarafem Pulvules (Infrequent) 1962
Sedapap Tablets 50 mg/650 mg (Infrequent) 2225
Semprex-D Capsules 1172
Sensorcaine (Rare) 643
Sensorcaine-MPF Injection (Rare) 643
Serentil 1057
Serevent Inhalation Aerosol (1% to 3%) 1633
Serophene Tablets 3226
▲ Seroquel Tablets (7%) 684
▲ Serostim for Injection (11.2%) 3229
Serzone Tablets (Infrequent) 1104
▲ Simulect for Injection (3% to 10%) 2399
Sinequan (Occasional) 2713
Soma Tablets 3353
Soma Compound Tablets 3354
Soma Compound w/Codeine Tablets 3355
Sonata Capsules (Infrequent) 3591
Stadol NS Nasal Spray (Infrequent) 1108
Stelazine 1640
Stimate Nasal Spray 796
Streptase for Infusion (Occasional) 647
▲ Stromectol Tablets (3.5%) 2185
Sular Tablets (Very rare) 688
Suprane Liquid for Inhalation (Greater than 1%) 874
Surmontil Capsules 3595
Survanta Intratracheal Suspension 3053
Sustiva Capsules (Less than 2%) 1258
Symmetrel 1328
Tagamet (Rare) 1644
Talacen Caplets (Infrequent) 3089
Talwin Nx Tablets 3090
Tambocor Tablets (1% to 3%) 1990
Tarka Tablets (0.3% or more) 508
Tasmar Tablets (Infrequent) 3010
Taxol Injection (2%) 1129
Taxotere for Injection Concentrate 778
Tenex Tablets (Less frequent) 2942
Tenoretic Tablets 690
Tenormin 692
Tequin Injection (Less than 0.1%) 1110
Tequin Tablets (Less than 0.1%) 1110
Tetanus & Diphtheria Toxoids Adsorbed for Adult Use 1880
Teveten Tablets (Less than 1%) 3327
Thalomid Capsules 1154
Thiothixene Capsules 2290
Thorazine 1656
▲ Thymoglobulin for Injection (26.8%) 3071
Tiazac Capsules (Less than 2%) 1378
▲ Tonocard Tablets (3.2%) 649
Trasylol Injection (2%) 909
Trental Tablets (Rare) 784
Tricor Capsules, Micronized (Less than 1%) 513
Trilafon 3160
Trileptal Oral Suspension 2407
Trileptal Tablets 2407
▲ Triostat Injection (3%) 1825
▲ Trisenox Injection (55%) 1158
Trovan (Less than 1%) 2722
Twinrix Vaccine 1674
Ultracet Tablets (Less than 1%) 2597
Ultram Tablets (Less than 1%) 2600
Uniretic Tablets (Less than 1%) 3178
Unithroid Tablets 3445
Uroqid-Acid No. 2 Tablets 947
Valtrex Caplets 1676
Vanceril Double Strength Inhalation Aerosol (Fewer than 2%) 3167
Vaseretic Tablets (0.5% to 2.0%) 2204
▲ Ventolin Inhalation Aerosol and Refill (10%) 1679
Ventolin HFA Inhalation Aerosol (Less than 3%) 3618
Versed Injection (Less than 1%) 3027
Viagra Tablets (Less than 2%) 2732
Vicoprofen Tablets (Less than 1%) 520
Vioxx (Greater than 0.1% to 1.9%) 2213
Virazole for Inhalation Solution (Infrequent) 1747
Vistide Injection 1445
Vivactil Tablets 2217
Vivactil Tablets 2446
Volmax Extended-Release Tablets (2.7%) 2276
Voltaren Tablets (Less than 1%) 2315
Voltaren-XR Tablets (Less than 1%) 2315
▲ Wellbutrin Tablets (10.8%) 1680
Wellbutrin SR Sustained-Release Tablets (Infrequent) 1684
▲ Xanax Tablets (7.7% to 15.4%) 2865
Xopenex Inhalation Solution (2.7%) 3207
Zantac (Rare) 1690
Zantac Injection (Rare) 1688
Zantac Syrup (Rare) 1690
Zaroxolyn Tablets 1177
Zemuron Injection (Less than 1%) 2491
▲ Zenapax for Injection (Greater than 5%) 3046
Zephrex Tablets 3091
Zephrex LA Tablets 3092
Zestoretic Tablets 695
Zofran Injection (Rare) 1698
Zofran (Rare) 1703
Zofran ODT Orally Disintegrating Tablets (Rare) 1703
Zoladex (1% or greater) 702
Zoladex 3-month 706
Zoloft (Infrequent) 2751
Zomig Tablets (Rare) 708
Zomig-ZMT Tablets (Rare) 708
Zonegran Capsules (Infrequent) 1307
Zosyn (1.0% or less) 1890
Zosyn in Galaxy Containers (1.0% or less) 1894
Zyban Sustained-Release Tablets (Infrequent) 1710
▲ Zyprexa Tablets (4%) 1973
▲ Zyprexa ZYDIS Orally Disintegrating Tablets (4%) 1973
Zyrtec (Less than 2%) 2756
Zyrtec-D 12 Hour Extended Relief Tablets (Less than 2%) 2758

Tachycardia, junctional

Digitek Tablets 1003
▲ Lanoxicaps Capsules (Among most common) 1574
Lanoxin Injection 1581
Lanoxin Tablets 1587
Lanoxin Elixir Pediatric 1578
▲ Lanoxin Injection Pediatric (Among most common) 1584
Romazicon Injection (1 of 446 patients) 3000

Tachycardia, nodal

Diprivan Injectable Emulsion (1.6%) 667

Tachycardia, reflex

Urecholine 2198
Urecholine Tablets 2445

Tachycardia, supraventricular

Aciphex Tablets (Rare) 1267
Aciphex Tablets (Rare) 1783
Advair Diskus 100/50 1448
Advair Diskus 250/50 1448
Advair Diskus 500/50 1448
Aggrenox Capsules (Less than 1%) 1026
Amphotec (1% to 5%) 1774
Aricept Tablets (Infrequent) 1270
Aricept Tablets (Infrequent) 2665
▲ Campath Ampules (3% to 11%) 992
Cardene I.V. (0.7%) 3485
▲ CellCept Capsules (3% to 10%) 2951
▲ CellCept Intravenous (3% to 10%) 2951
▲ CellCept Oral Suspension (3% to 10%) 2951
▲ CellCept Tablets (3% to 10%) 2951
Corvert Injection (2.7%) 2793
Diprivan Injectable Emulsion (Less than 1%) 667
Effexor Tablets 3495
Effexor XR Capsules 3499
Evoxac Capsules (Less than 1%) 1217
Exelon Capsules (Infrequent) 2342
Exelon Oral Solution (Infrequent) 2345
Felbatol (Rare) 3343
▲ Flolan for Injection (8%) 1528
Fludara for Injection (Up to 3%) 995
Hytrin Capsules (Occasional) 464
Ismo Tablets (Fewer than 1%) 3524
Levaquin Injection (Less than 0.5%) 2537
Meridia Capsules 481
Photofrin for Injection 831
Pletal Tablets (Less than 2%) 2605
Pletal Tablets (Less than 2%) 2848
▲ Proleukin for Injection (12%) 1199
Proventil Repetabs Tablets 3148
Reglan 2935
Reminyl Oral Solution (Infrequent) 1792
Reminyl Tablets (Infrequent) 1792
ReoPro Vials (1.0%) 1958
Requip Tablets (Infrequent) 1621
Retavase Vials 1182
Rilutek Tablets (Rare) 772
Rituxan for Infusion 1750
Rituxan I.V. 1428
Rythmol Tablets – 150 mg, 225 mg, 300 mg (Less than 1%) 502
Serevent Diskus 1637
Serevent Inhalation Aerosol 1633
Sular Tablets (Less than or equal to 1%) 688
Taxol Injection (Rare) 1129
▲ Tenormin (11.5%) 692
Tikosyn Capsules (Greater than 2%) 2717
▲ Trasylol Injection (4%) 909
Ventolin Inhalation Aerosol and Refill 1679
Ventolin HFA Inhalation Aerosol 3618
Zofran Injection 1698
Zosyn (1.0% or less to 1.3%) 1890
Zosyn in Galaxy Containers (1.0% or less to 1.3%) 1894

Tachycardia, ventricular

Aciphex Tablets (Rare) 1267
Aciphex Tablets (Rare) 1783
Activase I.V. 1410
Adenocard Injection 1380
Adenoscan 1381
Advair Diskus 100/50 1448
Advair Diskus 250/50 1448
Advair Diskus 500/50 1448
Ambien Tablets (Rare) 3191
Aramine Injection 2043
▲ Argatroban Injection (4.8%) 1478
Axid Pulvules (2 individuals) 1903
Axid Pulvules (2 individuals) 2919
Betapace Tablets 950
Betapace AF Tablets 954
Biaxin/Biaxin XL (Rare) 403
Campath Ampules 992
Cardene I.V. (0.7%) 3485
Cardizem Injectable (Less than 1%) 1018
Cardizem Lyo-Ject Syringe (Less than 1%) 1018
Cardizem Monovial (Less than 1%) 1018
▲ CellCept Capsules (3% to 10%) 2951
▲ CellCept Intravenous (3% to 10%) 2951
▲ CellCept Oral Suspension (3% to 10%) 2951
▲ CellCept Tablets (3% to 10%) 2951
Cordarone Intravenous (2.4%) 3491
Corvert Injection (0.2% to 4.9%) 2793
Cozaar Tablets (Less than 1%) 2067
Cytovene 2959
Demadex Tablets and Injection 2965
D.H.E. 45 Injection 2334
Digitek Tablets 1003
Diprivan Injectable Emulsion (Less than 1%) 667
Dobutrex Solution Vials (Rare) 1914
Dopram Injectable 2931
Dynabac Tablets (Rare) 2269
E.E.S. (Rare) 450
Effexor Tablets 3495
Effexor XR Capsules 3499
Ellence Injection 2806
EryPed (Rare) 446
Ery-Tab Tablets (Occasional reports) 448
Erythrocin Stearate Filmtab Tablets (Occasional reports) 452
Erythromycin Base Filmtab Tablets (Occasional reports) 454
Erythromycin Delayed-Release Capsules, USP (Occasional reports) 455
Hyzaar 2109
Imdur Tablets (Less than or equal to 5%) 1826
Imitrex Injection (Extremely rare) 1549
Imitrex Tablets (Rare) 1558
Lanoxicaps Capsules 1574
Lanoxin Injection 1581
Lanoxin Tablets 1587
Lanoxin Elixir Pediatric 1578
Lanoxin Injection Pediatric 1584
Luvox Tablets (25, 50, 100 mg) 3256
Meridia Capsules 481
Narcan Injection (Several instances) 1322
Naropin Injection 612
▲ Natrecor for Injection (3%) 3189
Norpramin Tablets 755
Norvasc Tablets (More than 0.1% to 1%) 2704
Paxil 1609
PCE Dispertab Tablets (Rare) 498
Pediazole Suspension (Rare) 3050
Permax Tablets (Infrequent) 1299
Pletal Tablets (Less than 2%) 2605
Pletal Tablets (Less than 2%) 2848
PREVPAC (Rare) 3298
Primacor Injection (1% to 2.8%) 3086
Prinivil Tablets (0.3% to 1.0%) 2164
Prinzide Tablets 2168
Prozac Pulvules, Liquid, and Weekly Capsules 1238
Quinaglute Dura-Tabs Tablets 978
Quinidex Extentabs 2933
Reminyl Oral Solution (Infrequent) 1792
Reminyl Tablets (Infrequent) 1792
ReoPro Vials (1.4%) 1958
Requip Tablets (Rare) 1621
Retavase Vials 1182
Rilutek Tablets (Rare) 772
Risperdal (Rare) 1796
Rituxan for Infusion 1750
Rituxan I.V. 1428
Robinul Injectable 2940
Romazicon Injection (1 of 446 patients) 3000
▲ Rythmol Tablets – 150 mg, 225 mg, 300 mg (3.4%) 502
Sarafem Pulvules 1962
Sensorcaine 643
Sensorcaine-MPF Injection 643
Serentil 1057
Serevent Inhalation Aerosol (3 patients) 1633
Sonata Capsules (Rare) 3591
Survanta Intratracheal Suspension 3053
Tambocor Tablets (0.4%) 1990
Taxol Injection (Approximately 1%) 1129
▲ Tenormin (16%) 692
▲ Tikosyn Capsules (2.6% to 13.2%) 2717
Toprol-XL Tablets (Greater than 1%) 651
Trasylol Injection (1% to 2%) 909
Vascor Tablets (0.5% to 2.0%) 2602
Zanaflex Tablets (Rare) 1305
Zestril Tablets (0.3% to 1.0%) 698
Zithromax Capsules, 250 mg 2743
Zithromax for IV Infusion 2748
Zithromax for Oral Suspension, 300 mg, 600 mg, 900 mg, 1200 mg 2739
Zithromax Tablets, 250 mg 2739
Zofran Injection 1698
Zoloft 2751
Zomig Tablets 708
Zomig-ZMT Tablets 708
Zosyn (1.0% or less) 1890
Zosyn in Galaxy Containers (1.0% or less) 1894

Tachypnea

Abelcet Injection 1273
Actimmune (Rare) 1772
Aggrenox Capsules 1026
Cancidas for Injection (Up to 1.3%) 2048
Diprivan Injectable Emulsion (Less than 1%) 667
Dopram Injectable 2931
Follistim for Injection 2465
Humegon for Injection 2468
Lufyllin Tablets 3347
Lufyllin-400 Tablets 3347
Lufyllin-GG Elixir 3348
Lufyllin-GG Tablets 3348
Maxalt Tablets (Rare) 2120
Maxalt-MLT Orally Disintegrating Tablets (Rare) 2120
Nardil Tablets (Less frequent) 2653
Orthoclone OKT3 Sterile Solution 2498
Pergonal for Injection 3223
▲ Proleukin for Injection (8%) 1199
Repronex for Intramuscular and Subcutaneous Injection 1347
Retrovir Capsules 1625
Retrovir IV Infusion 1629
Retrovir 1625
Roferon-A Injection (Rare to infrequent) 2996
Sensorcaine 643
Sensorcaine-MPF Injection 643
Sulfamylon Cream 1011
Sulfamylon Topical Solution 1011
Survanta Intratracheal Suspension 3053
Symmetrel 1328
Theo-Dur Extended-Release Tablets 1835
▲ Trisenox Injection (8%) 1158
Uni-Dur Extended-Release Tablets 1841
Versed Injection (Less than 1%) 3027

Talkativeness

Carbatrol Capsules 3234
Tegretol/Tegretol-XR 2404
Xanax Tablets (2.2%) 2865

Tardive dyskinesia

Clozaril Tablets 2319
Cognex Capsules (Rare) 1351
Compazine 1505
Depacon Injection (1% or more) 416
Depakene (1% or more) 421
Depakote Sprinkle Capsules 426
Depakote Tablets (1% to 5%) 430
Depakote ER Tablets (Greater than 1%) 436
Effexor Tablets 3495
Effexor XR Capsules 3499
Eldepryl Capsules 3266
Etrafon 3115
Geodon Capsules 2688
Haldol Decanoate 2535
Haldol Injection, Tablets and Concentrate 2533
Loxitane Capsules 3398
Luvox Tablets (25, 50, 100 mg) (Rare) 3256
Moban 1320
Navane Oral 2701
Navane Intramuscular 2703

Orap Tablets ... 1407
Reglan ... 2935
Risperdal ... 1796
Serentil ... 1057
Seroquel Tablets ... 684
Sinequan (Infrequent) ... 2713
Stelazine ... 1640
Thioridazine Hydrochloride Tablets ... 2289
Thiothixene Capsules ... 2290
Thorazine ... 1656
Trilafon ... 3160
Wellbutrin Tablets ... 1680
Wellbutrin SR Sustained-Release Tablets ... 1684
Zyban Sustained-Release Tablets ... 1710
Zyprexa Tablets (Up to 2%) ... 1973
Zyprexa ZYDIS Orally Disintegrating Tablets (Up to 2%) ... 1973

Tardive dyskinesia, unmasking of
Wellbutrin Tablets ... 1680

Tardive dystonia
(*see under* Dystonia, tardive)

Taste, altered (0.2%)
Actiq (Less than 1%) ... 1184
Adalat CC Tablets (Rare) ... 877
Advair Diskus 100/50 (1% to 3%) ... 1448
Advair Diskus 250/50 (1% to 3%) ... 1448
Advair Diskus 500/50 (1% to 3%) ... 1448
▲ Agenerase Capsules (2% to 10%) ... 1454
▲ Agenerase Oral Solution (2% to 10%) ... 1459
Alferon N Injection (1%) ... 1770
Alphagan Ophthalmic Solution (Less than 3%) ... 545
Alphagan P Ophthalmic Solution (Less than 1%) ... 546
Altace Capsules (Less than 1%) ... 2233
Ambien Tablets (Infrequent) ... 3191
Amerge Tablets (Rare) ... 1467
Antabuse Tablets ... 2444
Anzemet Injection (Infrequently) ... 719
Anzemet Tablets (Infrequently) ... 722
AquaMEPHYTON Injection ... 2042
Arava Tablets (1% to 3%) ... 724
Arthrotec Tablets (Rare) ... 3195
Asacol Delayed-Release Tablets ... 2884
Atrovent Nasal Spray 0.03% (Less than 2%) ... 1032
Atrovent Nasal Spray 0.06% (Less than 1%) ... 1033
Axert Tablets (Infrequent) ... 2772
Azactam for Injection (Less than 1%) ... 1276
Bactroban Nasal (0.8% to 3%) ... 1495
Baycol Tablets ... 883
BeneFix for Injection (10 cases) ... 1432
Betaseron for SC Injection ... 988
Betaxon Ophthalmic Suspension (Less than 2%) ... 537
▲ Biaxin/Biaxin XL (3%) ... 403
Bicillin C-R 900/300 Injection ... 2240
Bicillin C-R Injection ... 2238
Bicillin L-A Injection ... 2242
Brevibloc Injection ... 858
Captopril Tablets (Approximately 2 to 4 of 100 patients) ... 2281
Cardura Tablets (Less than 0.5%) ... 2668
▲ Carnitor Injection (2% to 9%) ... 3242
Carteolol Hydrochloride Ophthalmic Solution USP, 1% (Occasional) ... ⊙258
Cataflam Tablets (Less than 1%) ... 2315
Catapres-TTS (1 of 101 patients) ... 1038
Cedax Capsules (0.1% to 1%) ... 1021
Celebrex Capsules (0.1% to 1.9%) ... 2676
Celebrex Capsules (0.1% to 1.9%) ... 2780
Celexa (Frequent) ... 1365
▲ Cerebyx Injection (3.3%; frequent) ... 2619
Claritin (At least one patient) ... 3100
Claritin-D 12 Hour Extended Release Tablets (Less frequent) ... 3102
Claritin-D 24 Hour Extended Release Tablets (Fewer than 2%) ... 3104
Cognex Capsules (Infrequent) ... 1351
Colazal Capsules ... 3069
Combivent Inhalation Aerosol (Less than 2%) ... 1041
Comtan Tablets (1%) ... 2328
Copaxone for Injection (At least 2%) ... 3306
Cordarone Tablets (1% to 3%) ... 3487
▲ Cosopt Sterile Ophthalmic Solution (Up to 30%) ... 2065
Coumadin for Injection (Infrequent) ... 1243
Coumadin Tablets (Infrequent) ... 1243
Cozaar Tablets (Less than 1%) ... 2067
Crixivan Capsules (2.6%) ... 2070
▲ Cuprimine Capsules (12%) ... 2075
Cytotec Tablets (Infrequent) ... 3202
Cytovene (At least 3 subjects) ... 2959
Dantrium Capsules (Less frequent) ... 2885
DaunoXome Injection (Less than or equal to 5%) ... 1442
Denavir Cream (0.2%) ... 2332
Depacon Injection (1% to 5%) ... 416
Depakene (1% to 5%) ... 421
Depakote Sprinkle Capsules (1% to 5%) ... 426
Depakote Tablets (1% to 5%) ... 430
Depakote ER Tablets (Greater than 1%) ... 436
Diamox Intravenous ... ⊙269
Diamox Sequels Sustained Release Capsules ... ⊙270
Diamox Tablets ... ⊙269
Diflucan Tablets, Injection, and Oral Suspension (1%) ... 2681
Dilaudid Oral Liquid ... 445
Dilaudid Tablets - 8 mg ... 445
Dilaudid-HP (Less frequent) ... 443
Diprivan Injectable Emulsion (Less than 1%) ... 667
Doxil Injection (Less than 1% to 5%) ... 566
DuoNeb Inhalation Solution ... 1233
Dynabac Tablets (0.1% to 1%) ... 2269
Effexor Tablets (2%) ... 3495
Effexor XR Capsules (Frequent) ... 3499
Eldepryl Capsules ... 3266
Enalaprilat Injection ... 863
Enbrel for Injection ... 1752
Enbrel for Injection ... 3504
▲ Ergamisol Tablets (8%) ... 1789
Eskalith ... 1527
Evoxac Capsules (Less than 1%) ... 1217
Exelon Capsules (Infrequent) ... 2342
Exelon Oral Solution (Infrequent) ... 2345
Famotidine Injection (Infrequent) ... 866
▲ Felbatol (6.1%) ... 3343
Flonase Nasal Spray ... 1533
Floxin I.V. ... 2526
▲ Floxin Otic Solution (7%) ... 1219
Floxin Tablets ... 2529
Flumadine (Less than 0.3%) ... 1370
FML Ophthalmic Suspension ... ⊙236
FML Forte Ophthalmic Suspension ... ⊙235
▲ Fortovase Capsules (4.4%) ... 2970
Fosamax Tablets (0.5%) ... 2095
Foscavir Injection (Between 1% and 5%) ... 605
Gabitril Tablets (Infrequent) ... 1189
Gastrocrom Oral Concentrate (Less common) ... 1162
Gengraf Capsules (1% to less than 3%) ... 457
Glucophage Tablets (1% to 5%) ... 1080
Glucophage XR Tablets (1% to 5%) ... 1080
Halcion Tablets (Rare) ... 2823
Helixate Concentrate ... 788
Hivid Tablets (Less than 1%) ... 2975
Hyzaar ... 2109
Imitrex Injection (Infrequent) ... 1549
▲ Imitrex Nasal Spray (13.5% to 24.5%) ... 1554
Imitrex Tablets ... 1558
INFeD Injection ... 3388
▲ Infergen (3%) ... 1777
▲ Intron A for Injection (Up to 24%) ... 3120
Invirase Capsules (Less than 2%) ... 2979
Iopidine 0.5% Ophthalmic Solution (Less than 3%) ... ⊙213
Iopidine Sterile Ophthalmic Solution ... ⊙212
Kaletra Capsules (Less than 2%) ... 471
Kaletra Oral Solution (Less than 2%) ... 471
Kogenate ... 934
Kogenate FS ... 936
Kytril Injection (2%) ... 2986
Lamictal (Infrequent) ... 1567
Lamisil Tablets (2.8%) ... 2360
Lescol Capsules ... 2361
Lescol Capsules ... 2925
Lescol XL Tablets ... 2361
Lescol XL Tablets ... 2925
Levaquin (0.2% to less than 1.0%) ... 2537
Lexxel Tablets ... 608
Limbitrol ... 1738
Lipitor Tablets (Less than 2%) ... 2639
Lipitor Tablets (Less than 2%) ... 2696
Lithobid Slow-Release Tablets ... 3255
Lodine (Less than 1%) ... 3528
Lodine XL Extended-Release Tablets (Less than 1%) ... 3530
Lodosyn Tablets ... 1251
Lopid Tablets (More common) ... 2650
Lotensin HCT Tablets (0.3% to 1%) ... 2367
Lupron Depot 3.75 mg (Less than 5%) ... 3281
Lupron Depot–3 Month 11.25 mg (Less than 5%) ... 3285
Lupron Injection (Less than 5%) ... 3279
▲ Luvox Tablets (25, 50, 100 mg) (3%) ... 3256
Maxair Autohaler (0.6%) ... 1981
Maxair Inhaler (Less than 1%) ... 1984
Maxzide ... 1008
▲ Mepron Suspension (3%) ... 1598
Meridia Capsules (2.2%) ... 481
MetroGel-Vaginal Gel (2%) ... 1986
Mevacor Tablets ... 2132
Mexitil Capsules (About 5 in 1,000) ... 1047
Miacalcin Nasal Spray (Less than 1%) ... 2375
▲ Migranal Nasal Spray (8%) ... 2376
Mirapex Tablets (2% to 3%) ... 2834
Mobic Tablets (Less than 2%) ... 1054
Monopril Tablets (0.2% to 1.0%) ... 1091
Monopril HCT ... 1094
MS Contin Tablets (Less frequent) ... 2896
MSIR (Less frequent) ... 2898
▲ Mycobutin Capsules (3%) ... 2838
Myobloc Injectable Solution (2% or greater) ... 1291
Neoral Soft Gelatin Capsules (1% to less than 3%) ... 2380
Neoral Oral Solution (1% to less than 3%) ... 2380
Neptazane Tablets ... ⊙271
Neurontin Capsules (Infrequent) ... 2655
Neurontin Oral Solution (Infrequent) ... 2655
Neurontin Tablets (Infrequent) ... 2655
Nexium Delayed-Release Capsules (Less than 1% to 6.6%) ... 619
▲ Nicotrol Inhaler (Over 3%) ... 2840
Nicotrol Nasal Spray (More common) ... 2843
Nipent for Injection (Less than 3%) ... 3272
Normodyne Injection (1%) ... 3135
Normodyne Tablets (1%) ... 3137
Norvasc Tablets (Less than or equal to 0.1%) ... 2704
▲ Norvir Capsules (5.4% to 10.3%) ... 487
▲ Norvir Oral Solution (5.4% to 10.3%) ... 487
Ocupress Ophthalmic Solution, 1% Sterile (Occasional) ... ⊙303
Oramorph SR Tablets (Less frequent) ... 3062
▲ Orap Tablets (1 of 20 patients) ... 1407
Orudis Capsules (Less than 1%) ... 3548
Oruvail Capsules (Less than 1%) ... 3548
OxyContin Tablets (Less than 1%) ... 2912
Pacerone Tablets (1% to 3%) ... 3331
Paraplatin for Injection (1%) ... 1126
Patanol Ophthalmic Solution (Less than 5%) ... 540
Paxil (2%) ... 1609
Pepcid Injection (Infrequent) ... 2153
Pepcid for Oral Suspension (Infrequent) ... 2150
Pepcid RPD Orally Disintegrating Tablets (Infrequent) ... 2150
Pepcid Tablets (Infrequent) ... 2150
Permax Tablets (1.6%) ... 1299
Pravachol Tablets ... 1099
Prevacid Delayed-Release Capsules (Less than 1%) ... 3292
▲ PREVPAC (3% to 5%) ... 3298
▲ Prilosec Delayed-Release Capsules (Less than 1% to 15%) ... 628
Primaxin I.M. ... 2158
Primaxin I.V. (Less than 0.2%) ... 2160
Prinivil Tablets ... 2164
Prinzide Tablets ... 2168
Procardia XL Extended Release Tablets (1% or less) ... 2710
▲ Proleukin for Injection (7%) ... 1199
ProSom Tablets (Infrequent) ... 500
Protonix I.V. (Less than 1%) ... 3580
Protonix Tablets (Less than 1%) ... 3577
Protopic Ointment (Greater than or equal to 1%) ... 1397
Proventil Inhalation Aerosol ... 3142
Proventil Repetabs Tablets ... 3148
▲ Proventil HFA Inhalation Aerosol (4%) ... 3150
Provigil Tablets (At least 1%) ... 1193
Prozac Pulvules, Liquid, and Weekly Capsules (Frequent) ... 1238
Pulmicort Turbuhaler Inhalation Powder (1% to 3%) ... 636
▲ Rebetron Combination Therapy (6% to 8%) ... 3153
ReFacto Vials ... 1437
Relafen Tablets (Less than 1%) ... 1617
Rescriptor Tablets (Less than 2%) ... 526
▲ Retrovir Capsules (5%) ... 1625
▲ Retrovir IV Infusion (5%) ... 1629
▲ Retrovir (5%) ... 1625
Rituxan for Infusion (1% to 5%) ... 1750
Rituxan I.V. (1% to 5%) ... 1428
▲ Roferon-A Injection (Less than 4% to 25%) ... 2996
▲ Rythmol Tablets – 150 mg, 225 mg, 300 mg (3% to 22.6%) ... 502
Salagen Tablets (1%) ... 2229
Sandostatin LAR Depot (1% to 4%) ... 2395
Sarafem Pulvules (Frequent) ... 1962
Seroquel Tablets (Infrequent) ... 684
Serzone Tablets (2%) ... 1104
Sinemet Tablets ... 1253
Sinemet CR Tablets ... 1255
Sinequan ... 2713
▲ Soriatane Capsules (1% to 10%) ... 3003
Sporanox Oral Solution (Less than 2%) ... 1808
Sporanox Oral Solution (Less than 2%) ... 2512
Sular Tablets (Less than or equal to 1%) ... 688
Surmontil Capsules ... 3595
Sustiva Capsules (Less than 2%) ... 1258
Tambocor Tablets (Less than 1%) ... 1990
Tasmar Tablets (1% or more) ... 3010
Tenex Tablets (3% or less) ... 2942
Tequin Injection (0.1% to 3%) ... 1110
Tequin Tablets (0.1% to 3%) ... 1110
Timentin Injection- ADD-Vantage Vial ... 1661
Timentin Injection-Galaxy Container ... 1664
Timentin Injection-Pharmacy Bulk Package ... 1666
Timentin for Intravenous Administration ... 1658
▲ TOBI Solution for Inhalation (6.6%) ... 1206
Tonocard Tablets (Less than 1%) ... 649
Topamax Sprinkle Capsules (Infrequent) ... 2590
Topamax Tablets (Infrequent) ... 2590
Toradol (1% or less) ... 3018
Trileptal Oral Suspension ... 2407
Trileptal Tablets ... 2407
▲ Tri-Nasal Spray (5% to 7.8%) ... 2274
Trovan (Less than 1%) ... 2722
Univasc Tablets (Less than 1%) ... 3181
Vanceril Double Strength Inhalation Aerosol (Fewer than 2%) ... 3167
Vantin Tablets and Oral Suspension (Less than 1%) ... 2860
Vascor Tablets (0.5% to 2.0%) ... 2602
Vaseretic Tablets ... 2204
Vasotec I.V. Injection ... 2207
Vasotec Tablets (0.5% to 1.0%) ... 2210
Ventolin Inhalation Aerosol and Refill ... 1679
Vexol 1% Ophthalmic Suspension (Less than 2%) ... ⊙222
Vistide Injection ... 1445
Volmax Extended-Release Tablets ... 2276
Voltaren Tablets (Less than 1%) ... 2315
Voltaren-XR Tablets (Less than 1%) ... 2315
Warfarin Sodium Tablets, USP ... 3302
Wellbutrin SR Sustained-Release Tablets (2% to 4%) ... 1684
Xanax Tablets ... 2865
Zebeta Tablets ... 1885
Zestoretic Tablets ... 695
Zestril Tablets (0.3% to 1.0%) ... 698
Ziac Tablets ... 1887
Zithromax Capsules, 250 mg (Rare) ... 2743
Zithromax for IV Infusion (Rare) ... 2748
Zithromax for Oral Suspension, 300 mg, 600 mg, 900 mg, 1200 mg (Rare) ... 2739
Zithromax Tablets, 250 mg (Rare) ... 2739
Zocor Tablets ... 2219
Zonegran Capsules (2%) ... 1307
Zosyn (1.0% or less) ... 1890
Zosyn in Galaxy Containers (1.0% or less) ... 1894
Zyban Sustained-Release Tablets (2% to 3%) ... 1710
Zyprexa Tablets (Infrequent) ... 1973
Zyprexa ZYDIS Orally Disintegrating Tablets (Infrequent) ... 1973
Zyrtec (Less than 2%) ... 2756
Zyrtec-D 12 Hour Extended Relief Tablets (Less than 2%) ... 2758
Zyvox (0.9% to 1.8%) ... 2871

Taste, bad
Alupent Inhalation Solution (Less frequent) ... 1029
Aricept Tablets (Infrequent) ... 1270
Aricept Tablets (Infrequent) ... 2665
▲ Ciloxan (Less than 10%) ... 538
Cipro I.V. (1% or less) ... 893
Cipro I.V. Pharmacy Bulk Package (Less than 1%) ... 897
Cipro (Less than 1%) ... 887
Cleocin Phosphate Sterile Solution (Occasional) ... 2785
Emadine Ophthalmic Solution (Less than 5%) ... ⊙211
Fluorescite Injection ... ⊙211
Imitrex Injection ... 1549
▲ Imitrex Nasal Spray (13.5% to 24.5%) ... 1554
Imitrex Tablets ... 1558
Moduretic Tablets (Less than or equal to 1%) ... 2138
Rhinocort Nasal Inhaler (Less than 1%) ... 640
▲ Thrombate III (3 of 17) ... 944
Thyrel TRH for Injection ... 3630
Trental Tablets (Less than 1%) ... 784
Vicoprofen Tablets (Less than 1%) ... 520

Taste, bitter
▲ Astelin Nasal Spray (19.4%) ... 3339

▲ Azopt Ophthalmic Suspension (5% to 10%) ⊙ 536
Ceftin Tablets 1898
Chibroxin Sterile Ophthalmic Solution 2051
Clinoril Tablets (Less than 1 in 100) 2053
Clozaril Tablets (Less than 1%) 2319
Colace Capsules, Syrup, Liquid 3236
▲ Cosopt Sterile Ophthalmic Solution (Up to 30%) 2065
Mykrox Tablets (Less than 2%) 1168
Noroxin Tablets (Less frequent) 2145
Nubain Injection (1% or less) 1323
▲ Optivar Ophthalmic Solution (Approximately 10%) 2273
▲ Procanbid Extended-Release Tablets (3% to 4%) 2262
Risperdal (Rare) 1796
▲ Trusopt Sterile Ophthalmic Solution (Approximately one-quarter of patients) 2196
Versed Injection (Less than 1%) 3027
Zaroxolyn Tablets 1177

Taste, changes
(*see under* Taste, altered)

Taste, loss
(*see under* Ageusia)

Taste, metallic
Adenocard Injection (Less than 1%) 1380
Adenoscan (Less than 1%) 1381
Antabuse Tablets 2444
Antabuse Tablets (Small number of patients) 3474
Calcijex Injection 411
▲ Chemet Capsules (12.0% to 20.9%) 3078
Cleocin Phosphate Sterile Solution (Occasional) 2785
Clinoril Tablets (Less than 1 in 100) 2053
Eskalith 1527
Hectorol Capsules 1064
Hectorol Injection 1066
Lithium Carbonate 3061
Lithium Citrate Syrup 3061
Lithobid Slow-Release Tablets 3255
MetroCream 1404
MetroGel 1405
MetroLotion 1405
Pima Syrup 1362
Robaxin Injectable 2938
Robaxin Tablets 2939
Rocaltrol 2991
Sensorcaine 643
Sensorcaine-MPF Injection 643
▲ Trecator-SC Tablets (Among most common) 3598

Taste, salty
Lithobid Slow-Release Tablets 3255
Miacalcin Injection 2373

Taste, unpleasant
Adderall Tablets 3231
Adderall XR Capsules
Adipex-P 1406
▲ Aerobid/Aerobid-M (10%) 1363
▲ Alocril Ophthalmic Solution (10% to 30%) ⊙ 545
Avelox Tablets (1%) 879
▲ Azopt Ophthalmic Suspension (5% to 10%) ⊙ 536
Beconase Inhalation Aerosol 1497
Beconase AQ Nasal Spray 1498
▲ Ceftin for Oral Suspension (5.0%) 1898
Desoxyn Tablets 440
Dexedrine 1512
DextroStat Tablets 3236
Efudex 1733
Etrafon 3115
Flexeril Tablets (1% to 3%) 572
Flexeril Tablets (1% to 3%) 2094
Flonase Nasal Spray (Less than 1%) 1533
Fortovase Capsules (Less than 2%) 2970
Ionamin Capsules 1163
Mephyton Tablets 2129
Mycelex Troche 573
Norpramin Tablets 755
Rimso-50 Solution 1267
▲ Stadol NS Nasal Spray (3% to 9%) 1108
Vivactil Tablets 2217
Vivactil Tablets 2446

Tears, discoloration
Mycobutin Capsules 2838
Priftin Tablets 758
Rifadin 765
Rifater Tablets 769

Teeth, discoloration
Declomycin Tablets 1855
Doryx Coated Pellet Filled Capsules 3357
Dynacin Capsules (In children less than 8 years of age; rare in adults) 2019
Minocin Intravenous (Rare) 1862
Minocin Oral Suspension (Rare) 1865
Minocin Pellet-Filled Capsules (Rare) 1863
Monodox Capsules 2442
Neurontin Capsules (Rare) 2655
Neurontin Oral Solution (Rare) 2655
Neurontin Tablets (Rare) 2655
Periostat Tablets 1208
Primaxin I.M. 2158
Primaxin I.V. (Less than 0.2%) 2160
Urobiotic-250 Capsules 2731
Ventolin Inhalation Aerosol and Refill 1679
Vibramycin Calcium Oral Suspension Syrup 2735
Vibramycin Hyclate Capsules 2735
Vibramycin Hyclate Intravenous 2737
Vibramycin Monohydrate for Oral Suspension 2735
Vibra-Tabs Film Coated Tablets (May occur in infants and children under eight) 2735

Teeth, mottling of enamel
(*see under* Teeth, discoloration)

Teeth grinding
Celexa (Infrequent) 1365
Zoloft (Infrequent) 2751

Telangiectasia
Avonex 1013
Clobevate Gel (Less than 2%) 3271
Cormax Cream (Approximately 0.3%) 2440
Cormax Ointment (Approximately 0.3%) 2440
Dermatop Emollient Cream (Three patients) 2517
Diprolene Gel 0.05% (Less frequent) 3107
Efudex 1733
Fluoroplex 552
Olux Foam (Less than 2%) 1211
▲ Temovate Gel (Among most frequent) 1303
Temovate Ointment (Less frequent) 1301
Temovate E Emollient (Less than 2%) 1302
Tricor Capsules, Micronized (Less than 1%) 513
Ultravate Ointment (Less frequent) 1120

Telogen effluvium
Lariam Tablets 2989

Temperature disturbances, cutaneous
▲ Emla (7%) 602
Wellbutrin Tablets (1.9%) 1680

Temperature elevation
(*see under* Hyperthermia)

Temporal bone, swelling
Lupron Injection (Less than 5%) 3279

Tenderness
Aldara Cream, 5% (More than 1%) 1978
Americaine Anesthetic Lubricant 1162
Americaine Otic Topical Anesthetic Ear Drops 1162
Bactroban Ointment (Less than 1%) 1496
Condylox Gel (Less common) 2436
Condylox Topical Solution (Less than 5%) 2437
Cormax Scalp Application (Approximately 0.3%) 2441
Efudex (Infrequent) 1733
HibTITER (0.3% to 3.7%) 1859
▲ Menomune-A/C/Y/W-135 Vaccine (9% to 64%) 813
Mevacor Tablets 2132
▲ Miacalcin Nasal Spray (10.6%) 2375
M-M-R II 2118
Oncaspar 756
▲ Prevnar for Injection (25.2% to 36.5%) 1870
Recombivax HB (Equal to or greater than 1%) 2178
Tabloid Tablets 1642
Temovate Scalp Application (1 of 294 patients) 1304
Tetanus Toxoid Adsorbed Purogenated 1882
Vivelle Transdermal System 2412
Vivelle-Dot Transdermal System 2416
Zocor Tablets 2219

Tenderness, elbow
Temovate E Emollient (Less than 2%) 1302

Tenderness, right upper quadrant
Cataflam Tablets 2315
Celebrex Capsules 2676
Celebrex Capsules 2780
Eulexin Capsules 3118
Normodyne Injection 3135
Tasmar Tablets 3010
Voltaren Tablets 2315
Voltaren-XR Tablets 2315

Tenderness at injection site
▲ Acel-Imune (26% to 38%) 1851
▲ ActHIB Vaccine (1.1% to 66.9%) 798
▲ Actimmune (14%) 1772
BayGam 914
BayHep B 915
Cefizox for Intramuscular or Intravenous Use (1% to 5%) 1390
▲ Claforan Injection (4.3%) 732
▲ Diphtheria & Tetanus Toxoids Adsorbed Purogenated for Pediatric Use (19%) 1857
FluShield Influenza Vaccine 3521
Imogam Rabies - HT (Uncommon) 805
▲ Infanrix Vaccine (4.0% to 5.2%) 1562
▲ IPOL Vaccine (Up to 29.4%) 809
▲ JE-VAX Vaccine (Approximately 20%) 811
Rocephin Injectable Vials, ADD-Vantage, Galaxy, Bulk (1%) 2993
Taxol Injection 1129
▲ Tetanus & Diphtheria Toxoids Adsorbed for Adult Use (19%) 1880
▲ Tetanus and Diphtheria Toxoids Adsorbed For Adult Use (19%) 815
▲ Tripedia Vaccine (2% to 35%) 817
▲ TYPHIM Vi Vaccine (Up to 98%) 825
Vancocin HCl, Vials & ADD-Vantage 1970
▲ Vaqta (1.7% to 52.7%) 2199
▲ Versed Injection (5.6%) 3027

Tendinitis
Ambien Tablets (Rare) 3191
Celebrex Capsules (0.1% to 1.9%) 2676
Celebrex Capsules (0.1% to 1.9%) 2780
Cipro I.V. 893
Cipro I.V. Pharmacy Bulk Package 897
Cipro 887
Claritin-D 24 Hour Extended Release Tablets (Fewer than 2%) 3104
Cognex Capsules (Infrequent) 1351
Evoxac Capsules (Less than 1%) 1217
Floxin I.V. 2526
Floxin Tablets 2529
Intron A for Injection (Less than 5%) 3120
Klonopin Tablets (Infrequent) 2983
Levaquin (Less than 0.3%) 2537
Lexxel Tablets (Infrequent) 608
LYMErix Vaccine (1.92%) 1592
Neurontin Capsules 2655
Neurontin Oral Solution (Infrequent) 2655
Neurontin Tablets 2655
Noroxin Tablets 2145
Requip Tablets (Infrequent) 1621
Teveten Tablets (Less than 1%) 3327
Trovan (Less than 1%) 2722
Vioxx (Greater than 0.1% to 1.9%) 2213

Tendinous contracture
Gabitril Tablets (Infrequent) 1189
Lamictal (Rare) 1567
Lipitor Tablets (Less than 2%) 2639
Lipitor Tablets (Less than 2%) 2696
Luvox Tablets (25, 50, 100 mg) (Infrequent) 3256
Serzone Tablets (Rare) 1104

Tendon disorder, unspecified
Actiq (Less than 1%) 1184
▲ Actonel Tablets (3%) 2879
Cipro I.V. 893
Gengraf Capsules (1% to less than 3%) 457
Imdur Tablets (Less than or equal to 5%) 1826
Naprelan Tablets (Less than 3%) 1293
Neoral Soft Gelatin Capsules (1% to less than 3%) 2380
Neoral Oral Solution (1% to less than 3%) 2380
Remicade for IV Injection (Less than 2%) 1178
Rescriptor Tablets (Less than 2%) 526
Salagen Tablets (Less than 1%) 2229

Tendon reflexes, depression of
Plaquenil Tablets 3082

Tendon rupture
Arava Tablets (1% to 3%) 724
Chibroxin Sterile Ophthalmic Solution 2051
Cipro I.V. 893
Cipro I.V. Pharmacy Bulk Package 897
Cipro 887
Cortone Acetate Injectable Suspension 2059
Cortone Acetate Tablets 2061
Decadron Elixir 2078
Decadron Tablets 2079
Decadron Phosphate Injection 2081
Effexor Tablets (Rare) 3495
Effexor XR Capsules (Rare) 3499
Floxin I.V. 2526
Floxin Tablets 2529
Hydrocortone Tablets 2106
Hydrocortone Acetate Injectable Suspension 2103
Hydrocortone Phosphate Injection, Sterile 2105
Levaquin 2537
Noroxin Tablets 2145
Prednisone 3064
Remeron Tablets (Rare) 2483
Remeron SolTab Tablets (Rare) 2486
Solu-Medrol Sterile Powder 2855
Trovan 2722
Viagra Tablets (Less than 2%) 2732

Tendonitis
Betaxon Ophthalmic Suspension (Less than 2%) ⊙ 537
Chibroxin Sterile Ophthalmic Solution 2051
Soriatane Capsules (Less than 1%) 3003
Xenical Capsules (2%) 3043

Tendons, calcification of
Accutane Capsules 2944

Tenesmus
Ambien Tablets (Rare) 3191
Arthrotec Tablets (Rare) 3195
Asacol Delayed-Release Tablets (2% or greater) 2884
Betaseron for SC Injection 988
Celebrex Capsules (0.1% to 1.9%) 2676
Celebrex Capsules (0.1% to 1.9%) 2780
Cerebyx Injection (Infrequent) 2619
Colazal Capsules 3069
Copaxone for Injection (Infrequent) 3306
DaunoXome Injection (1% to 4%) 1442
Doxil Injection (Less than 1%) 566
Evoxac Capsules (Less than 1%) 1217
Exelon Capsules (Infrequent) 2342
Exelon Oral Solution (Infrequent) 2345
Ismo Tablets (Fewer than 1%) 3524
Lipitor Tablets (Less than 2%) 2639
Lipitor Tablets (Less than 2%) 2696
Naropin Injection (Less than 1%) 612
Norvir Capsules (Less than 2%) 487
Norvir Oral Solution (Less than 2%) 487
Prevacid Delayed-Release Capsules (Less than 1%) 3292
PREVPAC (Less than 1%) 3298
Rilutek Tablets (Infrequent) 772
▲ Sandostatin LAR Depot (4% to 6%) 2395
Soriatane Capsules (Less than 1%) 3003
Valstar Sterile Solution for Intravesical Instillation (Less than 1%) 1175
Zoloft (Rare) 2751

Tenosynovitis
▲ Arava Tablets (3%) 724
Azmacort Inhalation Aerosol (1% to 3%) 728
Betaseron for SC Injection 988
Copaxone for Injection (Infrequent) 3306
Effexor Tablets (Infrequent) 3495
Effexor XR Capsules (Infrequent) 3499
Evoxac Capsules (Less than 1%) 1217
Geodon Capsules (Infrequent) 2688
Lipitor Tablets (Less than 2%) 2639
Lipitor Tablets (Less than 2%) 2696
Lupron Depot 3.75 mg 3281
Lupron Depot 7.5 mg 3284
Lupron Depot–3 Month 11.25 mg 3285
Lupron Depot–3 Month 22.5 mg 3288
Lupron Depot–4 Month 30 mg 3289
Lupron Depot-PED 7.5 mg, 11.25 mg and 15 mg 3291
Luvox Tablets (25, 50, 100 mg) (Infrequent) 3256
Meridia Capsules (1.2%) 481
Paxil (Rare) 1609
Permax Tablets (Infrequent) 1299
Protonix I.V. (Less than 1%) 3580
Protonix Tablets (Less than 1%) 3577
Prozac Pulvules, Liquid, and Weekly Capsules (Infrequent) 1238
Remeron Tablets (Infrequent) 2483
Remeron SolTab Tablets (Infrequent) 2486
Rescriptor Tablets (Less than 2%) 526
Salagen Tablets (Less than 1%) 2229
Sarafem Pulvules (Infrequent) 1962
Serzone Tablets (Infrequent) 1104
Sonata Capsules (Infrequent) 3591
Sular Tablets (Less than or equal to 1%) 688
Tasmar Tablets (Infrequent) 3010
Tricor Capsules, Micronized 513
Uniretic Tablets (Less than 1%) 3178
Viagra Tablets (Less than 2%) 2732
Zomig Tablets (Infrequent) 708
Zomig-ZMT Tablets (Infrequent) 708

Tenseness
Allegra-D Extended-Release Tablets ... 714
Claritin-D 12 Hour Extended Release Tablets ... 3102
Claritin-D 24 Hour Extended Release Tablets ... 3104
Clomid Tablets (Fewer than 1%) ... 735
▲ Indapamide Tablets (Greater than or equal to 5%) ... 2286
Loxitane Capsules ... 3398
Prostin E2 Suppositories ... 2852
Zyrtec-D 12 Hour Extended Relief Tablets ... 2758

Testes, size decrease
▲ Lupron Depot 7.5 mg (5.4%) ... 3284
▲ Lupron Injection (5% or more) ... 3279

Testicular atrophy
Anadrol-50 Tablets ... 3321
▲ Lupron Depot 7.5 mg (5.4%) ... 3284
▲ Lupron Depot–3 Month 22.5 mg (20.2%) ... 3288
Lupron Depot–4 Month 30 mg (Less than 5%) ... 3289
▲ Nilandron Tablets (16.3%) ... 753
Oxandrin Tablets ... 1153
▲ Viadur Implant (3.8%) ... 912

Testicular disorder, unspecified
Androderm Transdermal System CIII (Less than 1%) ... 3377
AndroGel (Up to 3%) ... 3322
Avonex ... 1013
Caverject Sterile Powder (Less than 1%) ... 2777
Lupron Depot–3 Month 22.5 mg (Less than 5%) ... 3288
▲ Rapamune Oral Solution and Tablets (3% to 20%) ... 3584
Tenex Tablets (3% or less) ... 2942
Vivelle Transdermal System ... 2412
Vivelle-Dot Transdermal System ... 2416

Testicular function, inhibited
Alkeran for Injection ... 1465
Anadrol-50 Tablets ... 3321
Oxandrin Tablets ... 1153

Testicular hypotrophy
Cytovene ... 2959

Testicular swelling
Etrafon ... 3115
Flexeril Tablets (Rare) ... 572
Flexeril Tablets (Rare) ... 2094
Hivid Tablets (Less than 1%) ... 2975
Limbitrol ... 1738
Neurontin Capsules (Rare) ... 2655
Neurontin Oral Solution (Rare) ... 2655
Neurontin Tablets (Rare) ... 2655
Norpramin Tablets ... 755
Sinequan ... 2713
Surmontil Capsules ... 3595
Vivactil Tablets ... 2217
Vivactil Tablets ... 2446
Wellbutrin Tablets (Infrequent) ... 1680

Testosterone, decreased physiologic effects
Lupron Injection ... 3279
Zoladex ... 702

Testosterone serum levels, transient increase
Zoladex 3-month ... 706

Tetany
Ambien Tablets (Rare) ... 3191
Aredia for Injection (Rare) ... 2309
Furosemide Tablets ... 2284
Imitrex Injection ... 1549
Imitrex Nasal Spray (Rare) ... 1554
Imitrex Tablets (Rare) ... 1558
Paxil (Rare) ... 1609
▲ Rapamune Oral Solution and Tablets (3% to 20%) ... 3584
Rescriptor Tablets (Less than 2%) ... 526
Rilutek Tablets (Rare) ... 772
Trileptal Oral Suspension ... 2407
Trileptal Tablets ... 2407
Zomig Tablets (Rare) ... 708
Zomig-ZMT Tablets (Rare) ... 708

Thermoregulatory mechanisms, interference
Astramorph/PF Injection, USP (Preservative-Free) ... 594
Compazine ... 1505
Duramorph Injection ... 1312
Infumorph 200 and Infumorph 500 Sterile Solutions ... 1314

Thinking abnormality
Actiq (1% to 2%) ... 1184
Ambien Tablets (Rare) ... 3191
AmBisome for Injection (Less common) ... 1383
▲ Amphotec (5% or more) ... 1774
Androderm Transdermal System CIII (Less than 1%) ... 3377
Astelin Nasal Spray (Infrequent) ... 3339
Ativan Injection (Less than 1%) ... 3478
Brevibloc Injection (Less than 1%) ... 858
Campath Ampules ... 992
Cardura Tablets (Less than 0.5%) ... 2668
▲ CellCept Capsules (3% to 10%) ... 2951
▲ CellCept Intravenous (3% to 10%) ... 2951
▲ CellCept Oral Suspension (3% to 10%) ... 2951
▲ CellCept Tablets (3% to 10%) ... 2951
Cerebyx Injection (Frequent) ... 2619
▲ Cognex Capsules (3%) ... 1351
Coreg Tablets (0.1% to 1%) ... 1508
Cytovene (At least 3 subjects) ... 2959
DaunoXome Injection (Less than or equal to 5%) ... 1442
DDAVP Tablets ... 739
▲ Depacon Injection (6%) ... 416
▲ Depakene (6%) ... 421
▲ Depakote Sprinkle Capsules (6%) ... 426
▲ Depakote Tablets (1% to 6%) ... 430
Depakote ER Tablets (1% to 5%) ... 436
Diprivan Injectable Emulsion (Less than 1%) ... 667
Doxil Injection (Less than 1%) ... 566
Duragesic Transdermal System (1% or greater) ... 1786
Effexor Tablets (2%) ... 3495
Effexor XR Capsules ... 3499
Evoxac Capsules (Less than 1%) ... 1217
▲ Felbatol (6.5%) ... 3343
Flexeril Tablets (Less than 1%) ... 572
Flexeril Tablets (Less than 1%) ... 2094
▲ Gabitril Tablets (6%) ... 1189
Gliadel Wafer (2%) ... 1723
Halcion Tablets ... 2823
Hivid Tablets (Less than 1%) ... 2975
▲ Infergen (8% to 10%) ... 1777
Intron A for Injection (Less than 5%) ... 3120
Kadian Capsules (Less than 3%) ... 1335
Kaletra Capsules (Less than 2%) ... 471
Kaletra Oral Solution (Less than 2%) ... 471
Keppra Tablets (1% or more) ... 3314
Lamictal (Frequent) ... 1567
Levo-Dromoran ... 1734
Levorphanol Tartrate Tablets (1% to 3%) ... 3059
Lithobid Slow-Release Tablets ... 3255
Lupron Depot–4 Month 30 mg (Less than 5%) ... 3289
Luvox Tablets (25, 50, 100 mg) ... 3256
▲ Marinol Capsules (3% to 10%) ... 3325
Megace Oral Suspension (1% to 3%) ... 1124
Meridia Capsules (Greater than or equal to 1%) ... 481
Mirapex Tablets (2% to 3%) ... 2834
Nembutal Sodium Solution (Less than 1%) ... 485
Neurontin Capsules (1.7%) ... 2655
Neurontin Oral Solution (1.7%) ... 2655
Neurontin Tablets (1.7%) ... 2655
Nipent for Injection (Less than 3%) ... 3272
Norvir Capsules (Up to 0.7%) ... 487
Norvir Oral Solution (Up to 0.7%) ... 487
OxyContin Tablets (Between 1% and 5%) ... 2912
Paxil (Infrequent) ... 1609
Permax Tablets (Frequent) ... 1299
Prevacid Delayed-Release Capsules (Less than 1%) ... 3292
PREVPAC (Less than 1%) ... 3298
ProAmatine Tablets (Less frequent) ... 3241
▲ Prograf (3% to 15%) ... 1393
ProSom Tablets (2%) ... 500
Protonix I.V. (Less than 1%) ... 3580
Protonix Tablets (Less than 1%) ... 3577
Provigil Tablets (At least 1%) ... 1193
Prozac Pulvules, Liquid, and Weekly Capsules (Less than 1%) ... 1238
▲ Remeron Tablets (3%) ... 2483
▲ Remeron SolTab Tablets (3%) ... 2486
ReoPro Vials (2.1%) ... 1958
Rilutek Tablets (Infrequent) ... 772
Salagen Tablets (Less than 1%) ... 2229
▲ Sarafem Pulvules (3% to 6%) ... 1962
Seroquel Tablets (Infrequent) ... 684
▲ Serostim for Injection (1% to 10%) ... 3229
Serzone Tablets (Infrequent) ... 1104
Sonata Capsules (Frequent) ... 3591
Sular Tablets (Less than or equal to 1%) ... 688
Symmetrel (0.1% to 1%) ... 1328
Tasmar Tablets (Infrequent) ... 3010
Tequin Injection (Less than 0.1%) ... 1110
Tequin Tablets (Less than 0.1%) ... 1110
Thalomid Capsules ... 1154
Toradol (1% or less) ... 3018
Trileptal Oral Suspension (2%) ... 2407
Trileptal Tablets (2%) ... 2407
Trovan (Less than 1%) ... 2722
Ultracet Tablets (Less than 1%) ... 2597
Vicoprofen Tablets (Less than 3%) ... 520
Wellbutrin Tablets (Infrequent) ... 1680
Wellbutrin SR Sustained-Release Tablets ... 1684
Zanaflex Tablets (Infrequent) ... 1305
Zoladex (1% or greater) ... 702
Zoladex 3-month ... 706
Zoloft (2%) ... 2751
Zyban Sustained-Release Tablets (1%) ... 1710
Zyprexa Tablets ... 1973
Zyprexa ZYDIS Orally Disintegrating Tablets ... 1973
Zyrtec (Less than 2%) ... 2756
Zyrtec-D 12 Hour Extended Relief Tablets (Less than 2%) ... 2758

Thirst
(*see under* Dipsesis)

Thrashing
Diprivan Injectable Emulsion (Less than 1%) ... 667

Throat, aching
Zebeta Tablets ... 1885

Throat, burning
Astelin Nasal Spray (Infrequent) ... 3339
Diprivan Injectable Emulsion (Less than 1%) ... 667
Eldepryl Capsules ... 3266
Emcyt Capsules (1%) ... 2810
Rhinocort Aqua Nasal Spray (Rare) ... 642

Throat, dryness of
Accupril Tablets (0.5% to 1.0%) ... 2611
Accuretic Tablets (0.5% to 1%) ... 2614
Aerobid/Aerobid-M (1% to 3%) ... 1363
Atrovent Nasal Spray 0.03% (Less than 2%) ... 1032
Atrovent Nasal Spray 0.06% (1.4%) ... 1033
Azmacort Inhalation Aerosol ... 728
Beconase Inhalation Aerosol ... 1497
Beconase AQ Nasal Spray ... 1498
Benadryl Parenteral ... 2617
Catapres-TTS (2 of 101 patients) ... 1038
Claritin-D 12 Hour Extended Release Tablets (Less frequent) ... 3102
Clozaril Tablets (Less than 1%) ... 2319
Cognex Capsules (Infrequent) ... 1351
Flonase Nasal Spray ... 1533
Lexxel Tablets ... 608
Maxalt Tablets (Infrequent) ... 2120
Maxalt-MLT Orally Disintegrating Tablets (Infrequent) ... 2120
Neurontin Capsules (1.7%) ... 2655
Neurontin Oral Solution (1.7%) ... 2655
Neurontin Tablets (1.7%) ... 2655
Periactin Tablets ... 2155
Robinul Forte Tablets ... 1358
Robinul Injectable ... 2940
Robinul Tablets ... 1358
Rynatan Tablets ... 3351
Vantin Tablets and Oral Suspension (Less than 1%) ... 2860
Vioxx (Greater than 0.1% to 1.9%) ... 2213
Xopenex Inhalation Solution ... 3207

Throat, presence of hard nodule
Lupron Depot 7.5 mg (Less than 5%) ... 3284
Lupron Injection ... 3279

Throat, swelling of
Floxin I.V. ... 2526
Floxin Tablets ... 2529
Miacalcin Injection (A few cases) ... 2373
Miacalcin Nasal Spray (Few reports) ... 2375
Rhinocort Aqua Nasal Spray (Rare) ... 642

Throat, tightness
Adenocard Injection (Less than 1%) ... 1380
Alferon N Injection (1%) ... 1770
Benadryl Parenteral ... 2617
Campath Ampules ... 992
▲ Doxil Injection (Approximately 6.8%) ... 566
Etrafon ... 3115
Levaquin ... 2537
Maxalt Tablets (Less than 2%) ... 2120
Maxalt-MLT Orally Disintegrating Tablets (Less than 2%) ... 2120
Paxil (2%) ... 1609
Thyrel TRH for Injection (Less frequent) ... 3630
Trilafon ... 3160
Unasyn for Injection (Less than 1%) ... 2728

Throat irritation
Advair Diskus 100/50 ... 1448
Advair Diskus 250/50 ... 1448
Advair Diskus 500/50 ... 1448
Aerobid/Aerobid-M (1% to 3%) ... 1363
Allegra (Greater than 1%) ... 712
Allegra-D Extended-Release Tablets (2.3%) ... 714
Alupent (1% to 4%) ... 1029
Aredia for Injection (One patient) ... 2309
Azmacort Inhalation Aerosol ... 728
Beconase Inhalation Aerosol ... 1497
Clozaril Tablets (1%) ... 2319
Colace Capsules, Syrup, Liquid ... 3236
Cosopt Sterile Ophthalmic Solution ... 2065
Dostinex Tablets (1%) ... 2804
▲ Epivir-HBV (13%) ... 1524
Flonase Nasal Spray ... 1533
▲ Flovent Diskus (10% to 13%) ... 3614
Flovent ... 1535
Flovent Rotadisk ... 1537
Nasacort Nasal Inhaler (Fewer than 5%) ... 750
▲ Nicotrol Inhaler (40%) ... 2840
Nicotrol Nasal Spray (Common) ... 2843
Norvir Capsules (1.7% to 2.6%) ... 487
Norvir Oral Solution (1.7% to 2.6%) ... 487
Paxil (2%) ... 1609
Rhinocort Aqua Nasal Spray (Rare) ... 642
▲ Rituxan for Infusion (6%) ... 1750
▲ Rituxan I.V. (6%) ... 1428
▲ Roferon-A Injection (21%) ... 2996
Trusopt Sterile Ophthalmic Solution ... 2196
▲ Ventolin Inhalation Aerosol and Refill (6%) ... 1679
▲ Ventolin HFA Inhalation Aerosol (10%) ... 3618

Throat soreness
Aceon Tablets (2 mg, 4 mg, 8 mg) ... 3249
▲ Adenoscan (15%) ... 1381
Advair Diskus 100/50 ... 1448
Advair Diskus 250/50 ... 1448
Advair Diskus 500/50 ... 1448
▲ Aerobid/Aerobid-M (20%) ... 1363
Altace Capsules ... 2233
Aricept Tablets (Frequent) ... 1270
Aricept Tablets (Frequent) ... 2665
Azulfidine EN-tabs Tablets ... 2775
Blocadren Tablets ... 2046
Captopril Tablets ... 2281
Carbatrol Capsules ... 3234
Chemet Capsules (0.7% to 3.7%) ... 3078
Clozaril Tablets ... 2319
Compazine ... 1505
Corgard Tablets ... 2245
Corzide 40/5 Tablets ... 2247
Corzide 80/5 Tablets ... 2247
Cosopt Sterile Ophthalmic Solution ... 2065
Dapsone Tablets USP ... 1780
Demadex Tablets and Injection (1.6%) ... 2965
Depen Titratable Tablets ... 3341
DuoNeb Inhalation Solution ... 1233
Enalaprilat Injection ... 863
Etrafon ... 3115
Flovent Diskus ... 3614
Flovent ... 1535
Flovent Rotadisk ... 1537
Hivid Tablets (Less than 1%) ... 2975
▲ Imitrex Injection (3.3%) ... 1549
Inderal ... 3513
Inderal LA Long-Acting Capsules ... 3516
Inderide Tablets ... 3517
Inderide LA Long-Acting Capsules ... 3519
Kogenate ... 934
Lexxel Tablets ... 608
Mavik Tablets (0.3% to 1.0%) ... 478
Maxair Autohaler ... 1981
Maxair Inhaler (Less than 1%) ... 1984
Meruvax II ... 2130
M-M-R II ... 2118
Monopril Tablets ... 1091
Mykrox Tablets (Less than 2%) ... 1168
Nadolol Tablets ... 2288
Nasalide Nasal Spray (5% or less) ... 1295
Nascobal Gel (Three patients) ... 3174
▲ Neupogen for Injection (4%) ... 587
Normodyne Tablets ... 3137
Ortho Diaphragm Kits – All-Flex Arcing Spring; Ortho Coil Spring ... 2552
▲ Periostat Tablets (5%) ... 1208
Prinivil Tablets ... 2164
Prinzide Tablets ... 2168
▲ Procardia Capsules (6%) ... 2708
▲ Procardia XL Extended Release Tablets (6%) ... 2710
Remeron Tablets ... 2483
Remeron SolTab Tablets ... 2486
Remicade for IV Injection ... 1178
Rowasa Rectal Suspension Enema 4.0 grams/unit (60 mL) (2.33%) ... 3264
Rythmol Tablets – 150 mg, 225 mg, 300 mg ... 502
Sectral Capsules ... 3589
Septra Suspension ... 2265
Septra Tablets ... 2265
Septra DS Tablets ... 2265
▲ Serevent Inhalation Aerosol (8%) ... 1633
Stelazine ... 1640
Stimate Nasal Spray ... 796
Taxol Injection ... 1129
Tegretol/Tegretol-XR ... 2404
Tenoretic Tablets ... 690
Tenormin ... 692
Ticlid Tablets ... 3015

Timolol GFS ⊙266
Timoptic in Ocudose 2192
Timoptic Sterile Ophthalmic Solution 2190
Timoptic-XE Sterile Ophthalmic Gel Forming Solution 2194
Tonocard Tablets 649
Toprol-XL Tablets 651
Trental Tablets (Less than 1%) 784
▲ Trisenox Injection (40%) 1158
Univasc Tablets 3181
Valium Injectable 3026
Vaseretic Tablets 2204
Vasotec I.V. Injection 2207
Vasotec Tablets (0.5% to 1.0%) 2210
Zebeta Tablets 1885
Zestoretic Tablets 695
Zestril Tablets 698
Ziac Tablets 1887

Throbbing, localized

Catapres-TTS (1 of 101 patients) 1038

Thrombocythemia

(*see under* Thrombocytosis)

Thrombocytopenia

▲ Abelcet Injection (5%) 1273
Accupril Tablets (Rare) 2611
Accuretic Tablets (0.5% to 1%) 2614
Accutane Capsules 2944
Aceon Tablets (2 mg, 4 mg, 8 mg) 3249
Aciphex Tablets 1267
Aciphex Tablets 1783
Actiq (1% or greater) 1184
Adalat CC Tablets (Rare) 877
Aggrastat 2031
Aggrenox Capsules 1026
Agrylin Capsules (1% to 5%) 3232
Albenza Tablets (Rare) 1463
Aldoclor Tablets 2035
Aldomet Tablets 2037
Aldoril Tablets 2039
Alkeran Tablets 1466
Aloprim for Injection (Less than 1%) 2292
Altace Capsules (Less than 1%) 2233
Amaryl Tablets 717
AmBisome for Injection (Less common) 1383
Amerge Tablets (Rare) 1467
Amicar Injection 3608
Amicar Syrup 3608
Amicar Tablets 3608
Amoxil Chewable Tablets 1471
Amoxil for Oral Suspension 1471
Amoxil 1471
▲ Amphotec (1% to 7%) 1774
Anaprox Tablets (Less than 1%) 2967
Anaprox DS Tablets (Less than 1%) 2967
Ancef for Injection 1474
Ancef Injection 1474
Ancobon Capsules 1730
Anzemet Injection (Infrequently) 719
Anzemet Tablets (Infrequently) 722
Aquasol A Parenteral 593
Arava Tablets (Rare) 724
▲ Aredia for Injection (14%) 2309
Aricept Tablets (Infrequent) 1270
Aricept Tablets (Infrequent) 2665
Arthrotec Tablets (Rare) 3195
Asacol Delayed-Release Tablets 2884
Atacand Tablets 595
Atacand HCT Tablets 597
Attenuvax (Rare) 2044
Augmentin Chewable Tablets 1482
Augmentin Powder for Oral Suspension 1482
Augmentin Tablets 1485
Augmentin ES-600 Powder for Oral Suspension 1487
Avalide Tablets 1070
Avelox Tablets (0.05% to 1%) 879
Axid Pulvules (One patient) 1903
Axid Pulvules (One patient) 2919
Azactam for Injection (Less than 1%) 1276
Bactrim 2949
Baycol Tablets 883
Benadryl Parenteral 2617
Betapace Tablets (Rare) 950
Betapace AF Tablets (Rare) 954
Betaseron for SC Injection 988
Bicillin C-R 900/300 Injection 2240
Bicillin C-R Injection 2238
Bicillin L-A Injection (Infrequent) 2242
▲ Campath Ampules (50% to 72%) 992
Canasa Rectal Suppositories (One patient) 829
Captopril Tablets 2281
Carbatrol Capsules 3234
Cardene I.V. (Rare) 3485
Cardizem Injectable 1018
Cardizem Lyo-Ject Syringe 1018
Cardizem Monovial 1018
Cardizem CD Capsules (Infrequent) 1016
Cardura Tablets 2668
Cataflam Tablets (Less than 1%) 2315
Catapres Tablets (Rare) 1037
Cathflo Activase 3611
Ceclor CD Tablets 1279
Ceclor (Rare) 1905
Cedax (0.1% to 1%) 1021
Cefizox for Intramuscular or Intravenous Use (Rare) 1390
Cefotan 664
Ceftin 1898
Cefzil (Rare) 1076
Celebrex Capsules (0.1% to 1.9%) 2676
Celebrex Capsules (0.1% to 1.9%) 2780
Celexa (At least 3 patients) 1365
▲ CellCept Capsules (8.2% to 23.5%) 2951
▲ CellCept Intravenous (8.2% to 23.5%) 2951
▲ CellCept Oral Suspension (8.2% to 23.5%) 2951
▲ CellCept Tablets (8.2% to 38.3%) 2951
Ceptaz for Injection (Very rare) 1499
Cerebyx Injection (Infrequent) 2619
Chibroxin Sterile Ophthalmic Solution 2051
▲ Cipro I.V. (Among most frequent) 893
▲ Cipro I.V. Pharmacy Bulk Package (Among most frequent) 897
Cipro (0.1%) 887
Claforan Injection (Less than 1%) 732
Claritin (At least one patient) 3100
Cleocin HCl Capsules 2784
Cleocin Phosphate Sterile Solution 2785
Cleocin Vaginal Cream 2788
Cleocin Vaginal Ovules 2789
Clinoril Tablets (Less than 1 in 100) 2053
Clorpres Tablets 1002
Clozaril Tablets 2319
Cognex Capsules (Rare) 1351
Combipres Tablets 1040
Combivir Tablets (0.4%) 1502
Comvax 2056
Cordarone Intravenous (Less than 2%) 3491
Cordarone Tablets 3487
Coreg Tablets (1.1% to 2.0%) 1508
Corzide 40/5 Tablets 2247
Corzide 80/5 Tablets 2247
Cosmegen for Injection 2062
Crixivan Capsules (0.5%) 2070
▲ Cuprimine Capsules (4%) 2075
Cytotec Tablets (Infrequent) 3202
▲ Cytovene (5%) 2959
Dantrium Capsules (Less frequent) 2885
Daranide Tablets 2077
Daraprim Tablets 1511
Declomycin Tablets 1855
Demser Capsules (Rare) 2085
▲ Depacon Injection (1% to 24%) 416
▲ Depakene (24%) 421
▲ Depakote Sprinkle Capsules (1% to 24%) 426
▲ Depakote Tablets (24%) 430
▲ Depakote ER Tablets (24%) 436
▲ Depen Titratable Tablets (4%; up to 5%) 3341
▲ DepoCyt Injection (5% to 8%) 1197
DiaBeta Tablets 741
Diabinese Tablets 2680
Diflucan Tablets, Injection, and Oral Suspension 2681
Digitek Tablets 1003
Dilantin Infatabs (Occasional) 2624
Dilantin Kapseals (Occasional) 2622
Dilantin-125 Oral Suspension (Occasional) 2625
Diovan HCT Tablets 2338
Dipentum Capsules (Rare) 2803
Diucardin Tablets 3494
Diuril Oral 2087
Diuril Sodium Intravenous 2086
Dobutrex Solution Vials (Isolated cases) 1914
Dolobid Tablets (Less than 1 in 100) 2088
Dolophine Hydrochloride Tablets 3056
Doryx Coated Pellet Filled Capsules 3357
▲ Doxil Injection (6.5% to 24.2%) 566
Duraclon Injection (Rare) 3057
Duricef 1079
Dyazide Capsules 1515
Dynabac Tablets (0.1% to 1%) 2269
Dynacin Capsules 2019
Dyrenium Capsules (Rare) 3458
EC-Naprosyn Delayed-Release Tablets (Less than 1%) 2967
Ecotrin Enteric Coated Aspirin Low, Regular and Maximum Strength Tablets 1715
Edecrin (Rare) 2091
Effexor Tablets (Infrequent) 3495
Efudex 1733
▲ Ellence Injection (4.6% to 48.8%) 2806
Elmiron Capsules (Less than or equal to 1%) 570
Emcyt Capsules (1%) 2810
Enalaprilat Injection (Rare) 863
Enbrel for Injection 1752
Enbrel for Injection 3504
Engerix-B Vaccine 1517
Epivir (Up to 0.4%) 1520
▲ Epivir-HBV (4%) 1524
▲ Ergamisol Tablets (Up to 10%) 1789
Etrafon 3115
Eulexin Capsules (1%) 3118
Evoxac Capsules (Less than 1%) 1217
Exelon Capsules (Infrequent) 2342
Exelon Oral Solution (Infrequent) 2345
Famotidine Injection (Rare) 866
Fareston Tablets 3237
Felbatol (Infrequent) 3343
Feldene Capsules (Occasional) 2685
Flexeril Tablets (Rare) 572
Flexeril Tablets (Rare) 2094
▲ Flolan for Injection (4%) 1528
Floxin I.V. (More than or equal to 1%) 2526
Floxin Tablets (More than or equal to 1%) 2529
▲ Fludara for Injection (Among most common) 995
Fortaz (Very rare) 1541
Fortovase Capsules (Rare) 2970
Foscavir Injection (Between 1% and 5%) 605
Fragmin Injection (Less than 1%) 2814
▲ Sterile FUDR (Among more common) 2974
Furosemide Tablets 2284
Gabitril Tablets (Infrequent) 1189
▲ Gemzar for Injection (15% to 47%) 1919
Gengraf Capsules (2% or less) 457
Geocillin Tablets 2687
Geodon Capsules (Rare) 2688
▲ Gleevec Capsules (Less than 1% to 31%) 2357
Gliadel Wafer (1%) 1723
Glucotrol Tablets 2692
Glucotrol XL Extended Release Tablets 2693
▲ Heparin Lock Flush Solution (0 to 30%) 3509
▲ Heparin Sodium Injection (0 to 30%) 3511
▲ Hexalen Capsules (3% to 10%) 2226
Hivid Tablets (Less than 1% to 1.3%) 2975
▲ Hycamtin for Injection (26% to 63%) 1546
HydroDIURIL Tablets 2108
Hytrin Capsules 464
Hyzaar 2109
▲ Ifex for Injection (About 20%) 1123
Imdur Tablets (Less than or equal to 5%) 1826
Imitrex Injection 1549
Imitrex Nasal Spray 1554
Imitrex Tablets 1558
Indapamide Tablets 2286
Inderide Tablets 3517
Inderide LA Long-Acting Capsules 3519
Indocin I.V. (1% to 3%) 2115
▲ Infergen (18% to 19%) 1777
Innohep Injection (1%) 1248
Integrilin Injection 1213
Integrilin Injection 1828
▲ Intron A for Injection (Less than 5% to 15%) 3120
Invirase Capsules (Rare) 2979
Kadian Capsules (Less than 3%) 1335
Keflex 1237
Kefurox Vials, ADD-Vantage (Rare) 1948
Kefzol Vials, ADD-Vantage 1951
Klonopin Tablets 2983
▲ Kytril Tablets (3%) 2988
Lamictal (Rare) 1567
Lamisil Tablets (Rare) 2360
Lariam Tablets (Occasional) 2989
Lescol Capsules (Rare) 2361
Lescol Capsules (Rare) 2925
Lescol XL Tablets 2361
Lescol XL Tablets 2925
▲ Leukine (19%) 1755
▲ Leustatin Injection (12%) 2495
Levaquin (Less than 0.5%) 2537
Lexxel Tablets (Rare) 608
Limbitrol 1738
Lipitor Tablets (Less than 2%) 2639
Lipitor Tablets (Less than 2%) 2696
Lodine (Less than 1%) 3528
Lodine XL Extended-Release Tablets (Less than 1%) 3530
Lodosyn Tablets 1251
Lopid Tablets (Rare) 2650
Lorabid Suspension and Pulvules 2251
Lortab 3319
Lortab Elixir 3317
Lotensin Tablets (Less than 1%) 2365
Lotensin HCT Tablets (Rare) 2367
Lotrel Capsules (Rare) 2370
Lovenox Injection (1.8%) 746
Loxitane Capsules (Rare) 3398
▲ Lupron Depot–3 Month 22.5 mg (More than or equal to 5%) 3288
▲ Lupron Depot–4 Month 30 mg (Greater than or equal to 5%) 3289
Luvox Tablets (25, 50, 100 mg) (Infrequent) 3256
Macrobid Capsules 2889
Macrodantin Capsules 2891
Mandol Vials (Rare) 1953
Matulane Capsules (Frequent) 3246
Mavik Tablets (0.3% to 1.0%) 478
Maxidone Tablets CIII 3399
Maxipime for Injection 1285
Maxzide 1008
Mefoxin for Injection 2124
Mefoxin Premixed Intravenous Solution 2127
Mepron Suspension 1598
Meridia Capsules 481
Merrem I.V. (Greater than 0.2%) 673
Meruvax II 2130
Mevacor Tablets (Rare) 2132
Mexitil Capsules (About 2 in 1,000) 1047
Micardis HCT Tablets 1051
Microzide Capsules 3414
Minizide Capsules 2700
Minocin Intravenous 1862
Minocin Oral Suspension 1865
Minocin Pellet-Filled Capsules 1863
Mithracin for Intravenous Use 903
M-M-R II 2118
Mobic Tablets (Less than 2%) 1054
Moduretic Tablets 2138
Monodox Capsules 2442
Monopril Tablets 1091
Monopril HCT 1094
Monurol Sachet 1375
Motrin Suspension, Oral Drops, Chewable Tablets, and Caplets (Less than 1%) 2002
Mumpsvax 2141
Mustargen for Injection 2142
▲ Mycobutin Capsules (5%; rare) 2838
Mykrox Tablets (Rare) 1168
Myleran Tablets 1603
Mylocel Tablets 2227
▲ Mylotarg for Injection (99%) 3540
Naprelan Tablets (Less than 1%) 1293
Naprosyn Suspension (Less than 1%) 2967
Naprosyn Tablets (Less than 1%) 2967
Navane Oral 2701
Navane Intramuscular 2703
Navelbine Injection (1% to 4%) 1604
Nebcin Vials, Hyporets & ADD-Vantage 1955
Neoral Soft Gelatin Capsules (2% or less) 2380
Neoral Oral Solution (2% or less) 2380
▲ Neupogen for Injection (Fewer than 6% to 12%) 587
Neurontin Capsules (Infrequent) 2655
Neurontin Oral Solution (Infrequent) 2655
Neurontin Tablets (Infrequent) 2655
Nexium Delayed-Release Capsules (Less than 1%) 619
Niaspan Extended-Release Tablets 1846
Nimotop Capsules (0.3%; rare) 904
▲ Nipent for Injection (6% to 32%) 3272
Nizoral Tablets (Less than 1%) 1791
Nolvadex Tablets (1.5%) 678
Norco 5/325 Tablets CIII 3424
Norco 7.5/325 Tablets CIII 3425
Norco 10/325 Tablets CIII 3425
Norco 10/325 Tablets CIII 3427
Noroxin Tablets (1.0%) 2145
Norpramin Tablets 755
Norvasc Tablets (More than 0.1% to 1%) 2704
Norvir Capsules (Less than 2%) 487
Norvir Oral Solution (Less than 2%) 487
Omnicef 493
▲ Oncaspar (Greater than 1% but less than 5%) 756
Orthoclone OKT3 Sterile Solution 2498
Orudis Capsules (Less than 1%) 3548
Oruvail Capsules (Less than 1%) 3548
Pacerone Tablets 3331
Panhematin for Injection 497
▲ Paraplatin for Injection (22% to 70%) 1126
Parnate Tablets 1607
Paser Granules 1781
Paxil 1609
Pediazole Suspension 3050
Liquid PedvaxHIB (One child) 2148
▲ PEG-Intron Powder for Injection (7%) 3140
Pentasa Capsules (Less than 1%) 3239
Pepcid Injection (Rare) 2153
Pepcid for Oral Suspension (Rare) 2150
Pepcid RPD Orally Disintegrating Tablets (Rare) 2150
Pepcid Tablets (Rare) 2150
Periactin Tablets 2155
Periostat Tablets 1208
Permapen Isoject 2706
Permax Tablets (Infrequent) 1299
Pfizerpen for Injection (Rare) 2707
Phenergan Suppositories 3556
Phenergan Syrup 3554
Phenergan with Codeine Syrup (Rare) 3557

Phenergan with Dextromethorphan Syrup (Rare)... 3559
Phenergan VC Syrup... 3560
Phenergan VC with Codeine Syrup.. 3561
Phrenilin (Infrequent)... 578
Pipracil... 1866
Plaquenil Tablets... 3082
Plavix Tablets (1% to 2.5%)... 1097
Plavix Tablets (1% to 2.5%)... 3084
Pneumovax 23... 2156
Pnu-Imune 23 (Rare)... 1868
Podocon-25 Liquid... 2608
Ponstel Capsules (Occasional)... 1356
Prandin Tablets (0.5, 1, and 2 mg) (Less than 1%)... 2432
Pravachol Tablets (Rare)... 1099
Prevacid Delayed-Release Capsules (Less than 1%)... 3292
PREVPAC... 3298
Priftin Tablets (Less than 1%)... 758
Prilosec Delayed-Release Capsules (Rare)... 628
Primacor Injection (0.4%)... 3086
Primaxin I.M. ... 2158
Primaxin I.V. (Less than 0.2%)... 2160
Prinivil Tablets (Rare)... 2164
Prinzide Tablets (Rare)... 2168
Procanbid Extended-Release Tablets (Approximately 0.5%)... 2262
Procardia Capsules (Less than 0.5%)... 2708
Procardia XL Extended Release Tablets (Some patients)... 2710
▲ Prograf (3% to 24%)... 1393
▲ Proleukin for Injection (37%)... 1199
Protonix I.V. (Less than 1%)... 3580
Protonix Tablets (Less than 1%)... 3577
Prozac Pulvules, Liquid, and Weekly Capsules (Rare)... 1238
Purinethol Tablets (Frequent)... 1615
Pyrazinamide Tablets (Rare)... 1876
▲ Rapamune Oral Solution and Tablets (13% to 30%)... 3584
Recombivax HB... 2178
Relafen Tablets (Less than 1%)... 1617
Remeron Tablets (Rare)... 2483
Remeron SolTab Tablets (Rare)... 2486
Remicade for IV Injection (Less than 2%)... 1178
Reminyl Oral Solution (Infrequent)... 1792
Reminyl Tablets (Infrequent)... 1792
Renese Tablets... 2712
ReoPro Vials (0.7% to 5.2%)... 1958
Requip Tablets (Infrequent)... 1621
Rescriptor Tablets (Up to 1.5%)... 526
▲ Retrovir Capsules (12%)... 1625
▲ Retrovir IV Infusion (12%)... 1629
▲ Retrovir (12%)... 1625
Rifadin (Rare)... 765
Rifamate Capsules... 767
Rifater Tablets (Rare)... 769
Risperdal (Rare)... 1796
▲ Rituxan for Infusion (1.3% to 8%)... 1750
▲ Rituxan I.V. (1.3% to 8%)... 1428
Rocephin Injectable Vials, ADD-Vantage, Galaxy, Bulk (Less than 1%)... 2993
▲ Roferon-A Injection (4.5% to 62%).. 2996
Rynatan Tablets... 3351
Rythmol Tablets – 150 mg, 225 mg, 300 mg (Less than 1%)... 502
Sandimmune (2% or less; occasional)... 2388
Sandostatin LAR Depot (Rare)... 2395
Sarafem Pulvules (Rare)... 1962
Sedapap Tablets 50 mg/650 mg... 2225
Septra Suspension... 2265
Septra Tablets... 2265
Septra DS Tablets... 2265
Serentil... 1057
Seroquel Tablets (Rare)... 684
▲ Serostim for Injection (1% to 10%)... 3229
Silvadene Cream 1%... 2267
▲ Simulect for Injection (3% to 10%)... 2399
Sinemet Tablets... 1253
Sinemet CR Tablets... 1255
Sinequan (Occasional)... 2713
Stelazine... 1640
Suprax (Less than 2%)... 1877
Surmontil Capsules... 3595
Synvisc (Rare)... 3596
Tabloid Tablets... 1642
Tagamet (Approximately 3 per 1,000,000)... 1644
Tambocor Tablets (Less than 1%)... 1990
Tapazole Tablets... 1823
Tarka Tablets... 508
Tasmar Tablets (Rare)... 3010
Taxol Injection (Uncommon)... 1129
▲ Taxotere for Injection Concentrate (7.5%)... 778
Tazicef for Injection (Very rare)... 1647
Tazicef Galaxy Container (Very rare)... 1650
Tazicef Pharmacy Bulk Package (Very rare)... 1653
Tazidime Vials, Faspak & ADD-Vantage (Very rare)... 1966
Tegretol/Tegretol-XR... 2404
Temodar Capsules... 3157
Tenoretic Tablets... 690
Tenormin... 692
Teveten Tablets (0.3%)... 3327
Thalomid Capsules... 1154
TheraCys Injection (1%)... 823
Thioplex for Injection... 1765
Thioridazine Hydrochloride Tablets... 2289
Thiothixene Capsules... 2290
▲ Thymoglobulin for Injection (36.6%)... 3071
Tiazac Capsules (Infrequent)... 1378
Tice BCG, BCG Live (0.3%)... 2489
Ticlid Tablets (Rare)... 3015
Timentin Injection- ADD-Vantage Vial... 1661
Timentin Injection-Galaxy Container... 1664
Timentin Injection-Pharmacy Bulk Package... 1666
Timentin for Intravenous Administration... 1658
Timolide Tablets... 2187
Tolectin (Less than 1%)... 2589
Tonocard Tablets (Less than 1%)... 649
Topamax Sprinkle Capsules (Infrequent)... 2590
Topamax Tablets (Infrequent)... 2590
Toradol... 3018
Trasylol Injection (2%)... 909
Trecator-SC Tablets... 3598
Trental Tablets (Rare)... 784
Tricor Capsules, Micronized... 513
Trileptal Oral Suspension... 2407
Trileptal Tablets... 2407
▲ Trisenox Injection (13%)... 1158
Trizivir Tablets (0.4%)... 1669
Trovan (Less than 1%)... 2722
Twinrix Vaccine... 1674
Unasyn for Injection... 2728
Uniretic Tablets... 3178
Urso Tablets... 836
▲ Valcyte Tablets (6%)... 3022
Valtrex Caplets (0.1% to 1.2%)... 1676
Vancocin HCl Capsules & Pulvules (Rare)... 1972
Vancocin HCl Oral Solution (Rare)... 1971
Vancocin HCl, Vials & ADD-Vantage (Rare)... 1970
Vantin Tablets and Oral Suspension... 2860
Varivax... 2202
Vaseretic Tablets (Rare)... 2204
Vasotec I.V. Injection (Rare)... 2207
Vasotec Tablets (Rare)... 2210
Vibramycin Calcium Oral Suspension Syrup... 2735
Vibramycin Hyclate Capsules... 2735
Vibramycin Hyclate Intravenous... 2737
Vibramycin Monohydrate for Oral Suspension... 2735
Vibra-Tabs Film Coated Tablets... 2735
Vicodin Tablets... 516
Vicodin ES Tablets... 517
Vicodin HP Tablets... 518
▲ Videx (2% to 7%)... 1138
Videx EC Capsules... 1143
Vioxx... 2213
Viracept... 532
Viramune Oral Suspension (0.8%)... 1060
Viramune Tablets (0.8%)... 1060
Vistide Injection... 1445
Vitravene for Injection (2% to 5%).. ⊙ 310
Vivactil Tablets... 2217
Vivactil Tablets... 2446
Voltaren Tablets (Less than 1%)... 2315
Voltaren-XR Tablets (Less than 1%)... 2315
Wellbutrin Tablets... 1680
Xeloda Tablets (1% to 3%)... 3039
Zanaflex Tablets (Rare)... 1305
Zantac (A few patients)... 1690
Zantac Injection (Few patients)... 1688
Zantac Syrup (A few patients)... 1690
Zaroxolyn Tablets... 1177
Zebeta Tablets... 1885
▲ Zerit (3%)... 1147
Zestoretic Tablets (Rare)... 695
Zestril Tablets (Rare)... 698
Ziac Tablets... 1887
Zinacef Injection (Rare)... 1696
Zinacef for Injection (Rare)... 1696
Zinecard for Injection... 2869
Zithromax Capsules, 250 mg (Less than 1%)... 2743
Zithromax for IV Infusion (Less than 1%)... 2748
Zithromax for Oral Suspension, 1 g (Less than 1%)... 2743
Zithromax for Oral Suspension, 300 mg, 600 mg, 900 mg, 1200 mg (Less than 1%)... 2739
Zithromax Tablets, 250 mg (Less than 1%)... 2739
Zithromax Tablets, 600 mg (Less than 1%)... 2743
Zocor Tablets (Rare)... 2219
Zoloft... 2751
▲ Zometa for Intravenous Infusion (5% to 10%)... 3621
Zomig Tablets (Rare)... 708
Zomig-ZMT Tablets (Rare)... 708
Zonegran Capsules (Rare)... 1307
Zosyn... 1890
Zosyn in Galaxy Containers... 1894
Zovirax Capsules... 1706
Zovirax for Injection (Less than 1%)... 1708
Zovirax... 1706
Zyrtec (Rare)... 2756
Zyrtec-D 12 Hour Extended Relief Tablets (Rare)... 2758
Zyvox (2.4%)... 2871

Thrombocytopenia, autoimmune idiopathic

Campath Ampules... 992

Thrombocytopenia, immune

PEG-Intron Powder for Injection (Less than or equal to 1%)... 3140
Ticlid Tablets (Rare)... 3015

Thrombocytopenia, neonatal

Dyazide Capsules (Rare)... 1515
HydroDIURIL Tablets... 2108
Prinzide Tablets... 2168
Zestoretic Tablets... 695

Thrombocytopenic purpura

(*see under* Purpura, thrombocytopenic)

Thrombocytosis

Accutane Capsules... 2944
Aggrenox Capsules... 1026
Ancef for Injection... 1474
Ancef Injection... 1474
Aricept Tablets (Infrequent)... 1270
Aricept Tablets (Infrequent)... 2665
Arthrotec Tablets (Rare)... 3195
Augmentin Chewable Tablets (Less than 1%)... 1482
Augmentin Powder for Oral Suspension (Less than 1%)... 1482
Augmentin Tablets (Less than 1%)... 1485
Avelox Tablets (0.05% to 1%)... 879
Azactam for Injection (Less than 1% to 3.6%)... 1276
Campath Ampules... 992
Cedax (0.1% to 1%)... 1021
Cefizox for Intramuscular or Intravenous Use (1% to 5%)... 1390
Cefotan (1 in 300)... 664
Celebrex Capsules (0.1% to 1.9%)... 2676
Celebrex Capsules (0.1% to 1.9%)... 2780
Ceptaz for Injection (One in 45)... 1499
Chemet Capsules (0.5% to 1.5%)... 3078
▲ Cipro I.V. (Among most frequent)... 893
▲ Cipro I.V. Pharmacy Bulk Package (Among most frequent)... 897
Cipro (0.1%)... 887
Clozaril Tablets... 2319
Colazal Capsules... 3069
Cuprimine Capsules... 2075
Demser Capsules (Rare)... 2085
Depen Titratable Tablets... 3341
▲ Dynabac Tablets (3.8%)... 2269
Effexor Tablets (Infrequent)... 3495
Estratest... 3252
Evoxac Capsules (Less than 1%)... 1217
Floxin I.V. (More than or equal to 1%)... 2526
Floxin Tablets (More than or equal to 1%)... 2529
Fortaz (1 in 45)... 1541
Geodon Capsules (Rare)... 2688
Kefzol Vials, ADD-Vantage... 1951
Lovenox Injection... 746
Maxipime for Injection (0.1% to 1%)... 1285
Merrem I.V. (Greater than 0.2%)... 673
Monurol Sachet... 1375
Motrin Suspension, Oral Drops, Chewable Tablets, and Caplets... 2002
Neumega for Injection... 1434
Paxil (Rare)... 1609
Pentasa Capsules (Less than 1%)... 3239
Permax Tablets (Rare)... 1299
Prevacid Delayed-Release Capsules... 3292
PREVPAC... 3298
Priftin Tablets (1.1%)... 758
Primaxin I.M.... 2158
Primaxin I.V.... 2160
Prozac Pulvules, Liquid, and Weekly Capsules (Rare)... 1238
▲ Rocephin Injectable Vials, ADD-Vantage, Galaxy, Bulk (5.1%)... 2993
Salagen Tablets (Less than 1%)... 2229
Sarafem Pulvules (Rare)... 1962
Tazicef for Injection (1 in 45 patients)... 1647
Tazicef Galaxy Container (1 in 45 patients)... 1650
Tazicef Pharmacy Bulk Package (1 in 45 patients)... 1653
Tazidime Vials, Faspak & ADD-Vantage (1 in 45)... 1966
Ticlid Tablets... 3015
Topamax Sprinkle Capsules (Infrequent)... 2590
Topamax Tablets (Infrequent)... 2590
Trovan (Less than 1%)... 2722
Unasyn for Injection... 2728
Vantin Tablets and Oral Suspension... 2860
Zanaflex Tablets (Rare)... 1305
Zosyn... 1890
Zosyn in Galaxy Containers... 1894
Zovirax for Injection (Less than 1%)... 1708
Zyprexa Tablets (Infrequent)... 1973
Zyprexa ZYDIS Orally Disintegrating Tablets (Infrequent)... 1973

Thromboembolic complications

Activella Tablets... 2764
Arimidex Tablets (1.6% to 3.4%)... 659
Atromid-S Capsules... 3483
Brevicon 28-Day Tablets... 3380
Estratest... 3252
Femara Tablets (Less than or equal to 2%)... 2351
Heparin Lock Flush Solution... 3509
Heparin Sodium Injection... 3511
Humegon for Injection... 2468
Levlen... 962
Levlite 21 Tablets... 962
Levlite 28 Tablets... 962
Megace Oral Suspension (1% to 3%)... 1124
Menest Tablets... 2254
Modicon... 2563
Mononine Concentrate... 794
Nordette-28 Tablets... 2257
Norinyl 1 +35 28-Day Tablets... 3380
Norinyl 1 + 50 28-Day Tablets... 3380
Norplant System... 3543
Ortho Dienestrol Cream... 2554
Ortho-Cyclen/Ortho Tri-Cyclen... 2573
Ortho-Est Tablets... 3464
Ortho-Novum... 2563
Ortho-Novum 1/50□28 Tablets... 2556
Ortho-Cyclen/Ortho Tri-Cyclen... 2573
Ovcon... 3364
Premarin Intravenous... 3563
Premarin Vaginal Cream... 3570
Premphase Tablets... 3572
Prempro Tablets... 3572
Provera Tablets... 2853
Serophene Tablets (Rare)... 3226
Ticlid Tablets... 3015
Tri-Levlen... 962
Tri-Norinyl-28 Tablets... 3433
Triphasil-21 Tablets... 3600
Triphasil-28 Tablets... 3605

Thromboembolic disease

(*see under* Thromboembolic complications)

Thromboembolism

Activase I.V.... 1410
Brevicon 28-Day Tablets... 3380
CombiPatch Transdermal System... 2323
Cortone Acetate Injectable Suspension... 2059
Cortone Acetate Tablets... 2061
Decadron Elixir... 2078
Decadron Tablets... 2079
Decadron Phosphate Injection... 2081
Estrace Vaginal Cream... 3358
Estrace Tablets... 3361
Estratest... 3252
Hydrocortone Tablets... 2106
Hydrocortone Acetate Injectable Suspension... 2103
Hydrocortone Phosphate Injection, Sterile... 2105
Innohep Injection... 1248
Lo/Ovral Tablets... 3532
Lo/Ovral-28 Tablets... 3538
Low-Ogestrel-28 Tablets... 3392
Modicon... 2563
Nordette-28 Tablets... 2257
Norinyl 1 +35 28-Day Tablets... 3380
Norinyl 1 + 50 28-Day Tablets... 3380
Ogestrel 0.5/50-28 Tablets... 3428
Ortho Dienestrol Cream... 2554
Ortho-Cyclen/Ortho Tri-Cyclen... 2573
Ortho-Est Tablets... 3464
Ortho-Novum... 2563
Ortho-Novum 1/50□28 Tablets... 2556
Ortho-Cyclen/Ortho Tri-Cyclen... 2573
Ovcon... 3364
Ovral Tablets... 3551
Ovral-28 Tablets... 3552
Ovrette Tablets... 3552
Prednisone... 3064
Premarin Tablets... 3566
Premarin Vaginal Cream... 3570
Tegretol-XR Tablets... 2404
Tri-Norinyl-28 Tablets... 3433
Triphasil-21 Tablets... 3600
Triphasil-28 Tablets... 3605

Thromboembolism, arterial
Alesse-21 Tablets 3468
Alesse-28 Tablets 3473
Brevicon 28-Day Tablets 3380
Cyclessa Tablets 2450
Desogen Tablets 2458
Estrostep 2627
Levlen 962
Levlite 21 Tablets 962
Levlite 28 Tablets 962
Levora Tablets 3389
Loestrin 21 Tablets 2642
Loestrin Fe Tablets 2642
Lunelle Monthly Injection 2827
Microgestin Fe 1.5/30 Tablets 3407
Microgestin Fe 1/20 Tablets 3400
Mircette Tablets 2470
Modicon 2563
Necon 3415
Norinyl 1 +35 28-Day Tablets 3380
Norinyl 1 + 50 28-Day Tablets 3380
Ortho-Cept 21 Tablets 2546
Ortho-Cept 28 Tablets 2546
Ortho-Cyclen/Ortho Tri-Cyclen 2573
Ortho-Novum 2563
Ortho-Novum 1/50□28 Tablets 2556
Ortho-Cyclen/Ortho Tri-Cyclen 2573
Ovcon 3364
Pergonal for Injection 3223
Repronex for Intramuscular and Subcutaneous Injection 1347
Tri-Levlen 962
Tri-Norinyl-28 Tablets 3433
Trivora Tablets 3439
Yasmin 28 Tablets 980
Zovia 3449

Thromboembolism, venous
femhrt Tablets 2635
Ortho-Prefest Tablets 2570
Premarin Intravenous 3563
Premarin Tablets 3566

Thrombopenia
(*see under* Thrombocytopenia)

Thrombophlebitis
Abelcet Injection 1273
Aciphex Tablets (Rare) 1267
Aciphex Tablets (Rare) 1783
Actiq (Less than 1%) 1184
Activella Tablets 2764
AK-Fluor Injection 10% and 25% ⊙202
Alesse-21 Tablets 3468
Alesse-28 Tablets 3473
Aloprim for Injection (Less than 1%) 2292
Anzemet Injection (Rare) 719
Anzemet Tablets (Rare) 722
Arimidex Tablets (2% to 5%) 659
Azactam for Injection (1.9%) 1276
Betaseron for SC Injection 988
Brevibloc Injection (Less than 1%) 858
Brevicon 28-Day Tablets 3380
Brevital Sodium for Injection, USP 1815
Campath Ampules 992
▲ Cancidas for Injection (11.3% to 15.7%) 2048
Carbatrol Capsules 3234
Celebrex Capsules (Less than 0.1%) 2676
Celebrex Capsules (Less than 0.1%) 2780
Cerebyx Injection (Infrequent) 2619
Cipro I.V. (1% or less) 893
Cipro I.V. Pharmacy Bulk Package (Less than 1%) 897
Cleocin Phosphate Sterile Solution 2785
Climara Transdermal System 958
Clomid Tablets 735
Clozaril Tablets (Less than 1%) 2319
Cortifoam Rectal Foam 3170
Cuprimine Capsules (Rare) 2075
Cyclessa Tablets 2450
Dantrium Intravenous 2886
Depen Titratable Tablets (Rare) 3341
Depo-Provera Contraceptive Injection (Fewer than 1%) 2798
Desogen Tablets 2458
Doxil Injection (Less than 1%) 566
Effexor Tablets (Infrequent) 3495
Effexor XR Capsules (Infrequent) 3499
▲ Emcyt Capsules (3%) 2810
Enbrel for Injection (Infrequent) 1752
Enbrel for Injection (Infrequent) 3504
Epogen for Injection (Rare) 582
Ergamisol Tablets 1789
Estrace Vaginal Cream 3358
Estrace Tablets 3361
Estratest 3252
Estring Vaginal Ring (At least 1 report) 2811
Estrostep 2627
Fareston Tablets (Less than 1% to 2%) 3237
Felbatol 3343
Femara Tablets (Less than or equal to 2%) 2351
Florinef Acetate Tablets 2250
Fluorescite Injection ⊙211
Fortovase Capsules (Rare; up to 1%) 2970
Sterile FUDR 2974
Furosemide Tablets 2284
Gabitril Tablets (Infrequent) 1189
Geodon Capsules (Rare) 2688
Imitrex Nasal Spray 1554
Imitrex Tablets 1558
Indocin Capsules (Rare) 2112
Indocin I.V. 2115
Indocin (Rare) 2112
Invirase Capsules (Rare; up to 1%) 2979
Kaletra Capsules (Less than 2%) 471
Kaletra Oral Solution (Less than 2%) 471
Kefurox Vials, ADD-Vantage (1 in 60) 1948
Klonopin Tablets (Infrequent) 2983
Levlen 962
Levlite 21 Tablets 962
Levlite 28 Tablets 962
Levora Tablets 3389
Loestrin 21 Tablets 2642
Loestrin Fe Tablets 2642
Lo/Ovral Tablets 3532
Lo/Ovral-28 Tablets 3538
Low-Ogestrel-28 Tablets 3392
Lunelle Monthly Injection 2827
Mandol Vials (Rare) 1953
Mefoxin for Injection 2124
Mefoxin Premixed Intravenous Solution 2127
Megace Oral Suspension 1124
Menest Tablets 2254
Merrem I.V. (0.8%) 673
Miacalcin Nasal Spray (Less than 1%) 2375
Microgestin Fe 1.5/30 Tablets 3407
Microgestin Fe 1/20 Tablets 3400
Mircette Tablets 2470
Modicon 2563
Mustargen for Injection 2142
Necon 3415
Neurontin Capsules (Rare) 2655
Neurontin Oral Solution (Rare) 2655
Neurontin Tablets (Rare) 2655
Nordette-28 Tablets 2257
Norinyl 1 +35 28-Day Tablets 3380
Norinyl 1 + 50 28-Day Tablets 3380
Norplant System 3543
Ogen Tablets 2846
Ogestrel 0.5/50-28 Tablets 3428
Ortho Dienestrol Cream 2554
Ortho-Cept 21 Tablets 2546
Ortho-Cept 28 Tablets 2546
Ortho-Cyclen/Ortho Tri-Cyclen 2573
Ortho-Est Tablets 3464
Ortho-Novum 2563
Ortho-Novum 1/50□28 Tablets 2556
Ortho-Cyclen/Ortho Tri-Cyclen 2573
Ovcon 3364
Ovral Tablets 3551
Ovral-28 Tablets 3552
Ovrette Tablets 3552
Paxil (Rare) 1609
Permax Tablets (Infrequent) 1299
▲ Pipracil (4%) 1866
Premarin Intravenous 3563
Premarin Tablets 3566
Premarin Vaginal Cream 3570
Premphase Tablets 3572
Prempro Tablets 3572
▲ Primaxin I.V. (3.1%) 2160
Procrit for Injection (Rare) 2502
Protonix I.V. (Less than 1%) 3580
Protonix Tablets (Less than 1%) 3577
Provera Tablets 2853
Prozac Pulvules, Liquid, and Weekly Capsules (Rare) 1238
▲ Rapamune Oral Solution and Tablets (3% to 20%) 3584
ReFacto Vials 1437
Relafen Tablets (Less than 1%) 1617
Remicade for IV Injection (Less than 2%) 1178
ReoPro Vials (0.1%) 1958
Risperdal (Rare) 1796
Robaxin Injectable 2938
Roferon-A Injection (Rare) 2996
Romazicon Injection (1% to 3%) 3000
Roxicodone Tablets (Less than 3%) 3067
Sandostatin Injection (Less than 1%) 2394
Sarafem Pulvules (Rare) 1962
Serophene Tablets 3226
Seroquel Tablets (Infrequent) 684
Sonata Capsules (Rare) 3591
Sustiva Capsules (Less than 2%) 1258
Synercid I.V. (1.7% to 2.4%) 775
Taxotere for Injection Concentrate 778
Tegretol/Tegretol-XR 2404
Thalomid Capsules 1154
Timentin Injection- ADD-Vantage Vial 1661
Timentin Injection-Galaxy Container 1664
Timentin Injection-Pharmacy Bulk Package 1666
Timentin for Intravenous Administration 1658
Trasylol Injection (1% to 2%) 909
Tri-Levlen 962
Tri-Norinyl-28 Tablets 3433
Triphasil-21 Tablets 3600
Triphasil-28 Tablets 3605
Trivora Tablets 3439
Trovan (Less than 1%) 2722
▲ Unasyn for Injection (3%) 2728
Vancocin HCl, Vials & ADD-Vantage 1970
Yasmin 28 Tablets 980
Zinacef Injection (1 in 60 patients) 1696
Zinacef for Injection (1 in 60 patients) 1696
Zomig Tablets (Rare) 708
Zomig-ZMT Tablets (Rare) 708
Zonegran Capsules (Infrequent) 1307
Zosyn (0.2% to 1.3%) 1890
Zosyn in Galaxy Containers (0.2% to 1.3%) 1894
Zovia 3449

Thrombophlebitis, deep-vein
Cardene I.V. (Rare) 3485
Effexor Tablets 3495
Effexor XR Capsules 3499
Evoxac Capsules (Less than 1%) 1217
Exelon Capsules (Infrequent) 2342
Exelon Oral Solution (Infrequent) 2345
▲ Gliadel Wafer (4% to 9%) 1723
Humegon for Injection 2468
Innohep Injection (Greater than or equal to 1%) 1248
Lamictal (Rare) 1567
Lupron Depot–4 Month 30 mg (Less than 5%) 3289
Naprelan Tablets (Less than 1%) 1293
Nipent for Injection (Less than 3%) 3272
▲ Prograf (3% to 15%) 1393
Requip Tablets (Rare) 1621

Thrombophlebitis, leg
Innohep Injection (Greater than or equal to 1%) 1248
Requip Tablets (Rare) 1621

Thromboplastin decrease
Amphotec (1% to 5%) 1774

Thromboplastin time, increase
Azactam for Injection 1276
▲ CellCept Capsules (3% to 10%) 2951
▲ CellCept Intravenous (3% to 10%) 2951
▲ CellCept Oral Suspension (3% to 10%) 2951
▲ CellCept Tablets (3% to 10%) 2951
Elmiron Capsules (Less than or equal to 1%) 570
Merrem I.V. (Greater than 0.2%) 673
Oncaspar (Greater than 1% but less than 5%) 756
Panhematin for Injection 497
Viramune Oral Suspension 1060
Viramune Tablets 1060
Zosyn 1890
Zosyn in Galaxy Containers 1894

Thrombosis
Accuretic Tablets 2614
Ambien Tablets (Rare) 3191
Amicar Injection 3608
Amicar Syrup 3608
Amicar Tablets 3608
Betaseron for SC Injection 988
▲ CellCept Capsules (3%) 2951
▲ CellCept Intravenous (3%) 2951
▲ CellCept Oral Suspension (3%) 2951
▲ CellCept Tablets (3%) 2951
Colazal Capsules 3069
Demadex Tablets and Injection 2965
Diprivan Injectable Emulsion (Rare) 667
Doxil Injection (Less than 1%) 566
Emcyt Capsules 2810
Estratest 3252
Exelon Capsules (Infrequent) 2342
Exelon Oral Solution (Infrequent) 2345
Fareston Tablets (Less than 1%) 3237
Foscavir Injection (Between 1% and 5%) 605
Herceptin I.V. (At least one of the 958 patients) 1414
Hivid Tablets (Less than 1%) 2975
Humegon for Injection 2468
Imitrex Nasal Spray 1554
Imitrex Tablets (Rare) 1558
Konÿne 80 937
Leukine 1755
Leustatin Injection (2%) 2495
Lovenox Injection (Rare) 746
▲ Lupron Injection (5% or more) 3279
Mustargen for Injection 2142
NovoSeven (Two patients) 2430
Oncaspar (Greater than 1% but less than 5%) 756
Ovcon 3364
Paxil (Rare) 1609
Pipracil 1866
Premarin Intravenous 3563
Premarin Vaginal Cream 3570
Proleukin for Injection (1%) 1199
Proplex T 851
Protonix I.V. (Less than 1%) 3580
Protonix Tablets (Less than 1%) 3577
Prozac Pulvules, Liquid, and Weekly Capsules (Rare) 1238
▲ Rapamune Oral Solution and Tablets (3% to 20%) 3584
▲ Renagel Capsules (10%) 1439
▲ Renagel Tablets (10%) 1439
Requip Tablets (Rare) 1621
Rilutek Tablets (Rare) 772
Salagen Tablets (Less than 1%) 2229
Sarafem Pulvules (Rare) 1962
▲ Simulect for Injection (3% to 10%) 2399
Tasmar Tablets (Rare) 3010
Thalomid Capsules 1154
Thrombin-JMI 1824
TNKase I.V. 1430
Trasylol Injection (1% to 2%) 909
▲ Valium Injectable (Among most common) 3026
▲ Zenapax for Injection (Greater than 5%) 3046

Thrombosis, arterial
Orthoclone OKT3 Sterile Solution 2498
Sandostatin LAR Depot (Rare) 2395
Trasylol Injection (1% to 2%) 909

Thrombosis, cerebral
(*see under* Cerebral thrombosis)

Thrombosis, coronary
(*see under* Coronary thrombosis)

Thrombosis, glomerular capillary
Gengraf Capsules 457
Neoral Soft Gelatin Capsules 2380
Neoral Oral Solution 2380
Sandimmune 2388

Thrombosis, mesenteric
Alesse-21 Tablets 3468
Alesse-28 Tablets 3473
Brevicon 28-Day Tablets 3380
Cyclessa Tablets 2450
Estratest 3252
Estrostep 2627
Levlen 962
Levlite 21 Tablets 962
Levlite 28 Tablets 962
Levora Tablets 3389
Loestrin 21 Tablets 2642
Loestrin Fe Tablets 2642
Lunelle Monthly Injection 2827
Menest Tablets 2254
Microgestin Fe 1.5/30 Tablets 3407
Microgestin Fe 1/20 Tablets 3400
Mircette Tablets 2470
Necon 3415
Norinyl 1 +35 28-Day Tablets 3380
Norinyl 1 + 50 28-Day Tablets 3380
Ortho Dienestrol Cream 2554
Ovcon 3364
Premarin Intravenous 3563
Premarin Vaginal Cream 3570
Tri-Levlen 962
Tri-Norinyl-28 Tablets 3433
Trivora Tablets 3439
Yasmin 28 Tablets 980
Zovia 3449

Thrombosis, mesenteric arterial
Corgard Tablets 2245
Corzide 40/5 Tablets 2247
Corzide 80/5 Tablets 2247
Cosopt Sterile Ophthalmic Solution 2065
Nadolol Tablets 2288
Timolol GFS ⊙266
Timoptic-XE Sterile Ophthalmic Gel Forming Solution 2194
Zebeta Tablets 1885

Thrombosis, portal vein
Femara Tablets (Less than or equal to 2%) 2351

Thrombosis, pulmonary
Neurontin Capsules (Rare) 2655
Neurontin Oral Solution (Rare) 2655
Neurontin Tablets (Rare) 2655
Trasylol Injection (1% to 2%) 909

Thrombosis, renal artery
Epogen for Injection (Rare) 582
Procrit for Injection (Rare) 2502

Thrombosis, retinal vascular
Activella Tablets 2764
Alesse-21 Tablets 3468
Alesse-28 Tablets 3473
Aygestin Tablets 1333
Brevicon 28-Day Tablets 3380
Clomid Tablets 735
Cyclessa Tablets 2450
Depo-Provera Contraceptive Injection 2798
Epogen for Injection (Rare) 582

Estratest 3252
Estrostep 2627
Imitrex Tablets 1558
Levlen 962
Levlite 21 Tablets 962
Levlite 28 Tablets 962
Levora Tablets 3389
Loestrin 21 Tablets 2642
Loestrin Fe Tablets 2642
Lo/Ovral Tablets 3532
Lo/Ovral-28 Tablets 3538
Low-Ogestrel-28 Tablets 3392
Lunelle Monthly Injection 2827
Menest Tablets 2254
Microgestin Fe 1.5/30 Tablets 3407
Microgestin Fe 1/20 Tablets 3400
Mircette Tablets 2470
Modicon 2563
Necon 3415
Nordette-28 Tablets 2257
Norinyl 1 +35 28-Day Tablets 3380
Norinyl 1 + 50 28-Day Tablets 3380
Ogestrel 0.5/50-28 Tablets 3428
Ortho Dienestrol Cream 2554
Ortho-Cyclen/Ortho Tri-Cyclen 2573
Ortho-Novum 2563
Ortho-Novum 1/50□28 Tablets 2556
Ortho-Cyclen/Ortho Tri-Cyclen 2573
Ovcon 3364
Ovral Tablets 3551
Ovral-28 Tablets 3552
Ovrette Tablets 3552
PEG-Intron Powder for Injection (Less than or equal to 1%) 3140
Premarin Intravenous 3563
Premarin Vaginal Cream 3570
Premphase Tablets 3572
Prempro Tablets 3572
Procrit for Injection (Rare) 2502
Provera Tablets (Occasional) 2853
Sandostatin LAR Depot (Rare) 2395
Serophene Tablets 3226
Tri-Levlen 962
Tri-Norinyl-28 Tablets 3433
Triphasil-21 Tablets 3600
Triphasil-28 Tablets 3605
Trivora Tablets 3439
Yasmin 28 Tablets 980
Zovia 3449

Thrombosis, sagittal sinus
Oncaspar 756

Thrombosis, venous
Actimmune (Rare) 1772
Activase I.V. 1410
Aricept Tablets (Infrequent) 1270
Aricept Tablets (Infrequent) 2665
Campath Ampules 992
Cathflo Activase 3611
Clomid Tablets 735
Clozaril Tablets 2319
Cyclessa Tablets 2450
Depo-Provera Contraceptive Injection (Fewer than 1%) 2798
Desogen Tablets 2458
Enbrel for Injection (Infrequent) 1752
Enbrel for Injection (Infrequent) 3504
Epogen for Injection (Rare) 582
Femara Tablets (Less than or equal to 2%) 2351
femhrt Tablets 2635
Fludara for Injection (1% to 3%) 995
Kaletra Capsules (Less than 2%) 471
Kaletra Oral Solution (Less than 2%) 471
Loestrin 21 Tablets 2642
Loestrin Fe Tablets 2642
Mepergan Injection 3539
Microgestin Fe 1.5/30 Tablets 3407
Microgestin Fe 1/20 Tablets 3400
Mircette Tablets 2470
Modicon 2563
Mykrox Tablets 1168
Naropin Injection (Less than 1%) 612
Navelbine Injection 1604
Necon 3415
Nimotop Capsules (Less than 1%) 904
Nolvadex Tablets (0.8%) 678
Norplant System 3543
Oncaspar 756
Ortho-Cept 21 Tablets 2546
Ortho-Cept 28 Tablets 2546
Orthoclone OKT3 Sterile Solution 2498
Ortho-Cyclen/Ortho Tri-Cyclen 2573
Ortho-Novum 2563
Ortho-Novum 1/50□28 Tablets 2556
Ortho-Cyclen/Ortho Tri-Cyclen 2573
Phenergan Injection 3553
Pipracil (Less frequent) 1866
▲ Procrit for Injection (Up to 10%) 2502
Retavase Vials 1182
Taxol Injection (Approximately 1%) 1129
Taxotere for Injection Concentrate 778
Topamax Sprinkle Capsules (Infrequent) 2590
Topamax Tablets (Infrequent) 2590
Trivora Tablets 3439
Vioxx (Less than 0.1%) 2213
Xeloda Tablets (Less than 5%) 3039
Yasmin 28 Tablets 980
Zaroxolyn Tablets 1177
Zovia 3449

Thrombosis of vascular access
Epogen for Injection (0.25%) 582
Furosemide Tablets 2284
Procrit for Injection 2502

Thrombotic events, unspecified
Aygestin Tablets 1333
DDAVP Injection 4 mcg/mL (Rare) 737
Desmopressin Acetate Injection (Rare) 1344
Neumega for Injection 1434
Procrit for Injection 2502

Thrombotic vascular disease
Accutane Capsules 2944
Ortho Dienestrol Cream 2554
Ortho-Cyclen/Ortho Tri-Cyclen 2573

Thrush, oral
(*see under* Candidiasis, oral)

Thymol turbidity test, positive
Atromid-S Capsules 3483
Cuprimine Capsules 2075
Depen Titratable Tablets (Few reports) 3341

Thymus gland abnormalities, fetal
Accutane Capsules 2944

Thyroid adenoma
Permax Tablets (Rare) 1299

Thyroid binding globulin, increase
(*see under* T4, increase)

Thyroid disease, exacerbation
Proleukin for Injection 1199

Thyroid disorders
(*see under* T3, decrease; T4, decrease; T4, increase)

Thyroid function test, abnormal
Baycol Tablets 883
Depacon Injection 416
Depakene 421
Depakote Sprinkle Capsules 426
Depakote Tablets 430
Depakote ER Tablets 436
Dynacin Capsules (Very rare) 2019
▲ Infergen (4% to 9%) 1777
Lescol Capsules 2361
Lescol Capsules 2925
Lescol XL Tablets 2361
Lescol XL Tablets 2925
Mevacor Tablets 2132
Minocin Intravenous (Very rare) 1862
Minocin Oral Suspension (Very rare) 1865
Minocin Pellet-Filled Capsules (Very rare) 1863
Pravachol Tablets 1099
Proleukin for Injection 1199
Provera Tablets 2853
Roferon-A Injection (Infrequent) 2996
Zocor Tablets 2219

Thyroid gland discoloration
Declomycin Tablets 1855
Doryx Coated Pellet Filled Capsules 3357
Dynacin Capsules 2019
Minocin Intravenous 1862
Minocin Oral Suspension 1865
Minocin Pellet-Filled Capsules 1863
Monodox Capsules 2442
Vibramycin Calcium Oral Suspension Syrup 2735
Vibramycin Hyclate Capsules 2735
Vibramycin Hyclate Intravenous 2737
Vibramycin Monohydrate for Oral Suspension 2735
Vibra-Tabs Film Coated Tablets 2735

Thyroid gland enlargement
Lupron Injection (Less than 5%) 3279

Thyroid hormone, changes
(*see under* T3, decrease; T4, decrease; T4, increase)

Thyroid nodule
Effexor Tablets (Rare) 3495
Effexor XR Capsules (Rare) 3499
ProSom Tablets (Rare) 500

Thyroid stimulating hormone elevation
Aciphex Tablets 1267
Aciphex Tablets 1783

Thyroiditis
Cuprimine Capsules 2075
Depen Titratable Tablets (Extremely rare) 3341
Effexor Tablets (Rare) 3495
Effexor XR Capsules (Rare) 3499
Paxil (Rare) 1609
Sular Tablets (Less than or equal to 1%) 688

Thyrotoxicosis
Synthroid 505

Tics
Lamictal 1567

Tingling
Acticin Cream 998
Azelex Cream (Approximately 1% to 5%) 547
Calcium Disodium Versenate Injection 1980
Cipro I.V. 893
Cipro 887
Condylox Gel (Less common) 2436
Condylox Topical Solution (Less than 5%) 2437
Decadron Phosphate Injection 2081
DynaCirc Capsules (0.5% to 1%) 2921
DynaCirc CR Tablets (0.5% to 1%) 2923
Elimite Cream (1 to 2% or less) 552
▲ Elocon Ointment 0.1% (4.8%) 3112
Engerix-B Vaccine (Less than 1%) 1517
Finevin Cream (1% to 5%) 962
Floxin I.V. 2526
Floxin Tablets 2529
Gengraf Capsules (Rare) 457
▲ Imitrex Injection (13.5%) 1549
Imitrex Nasal Spray (Infrequent) 1554
▲ Imitrex Tablets (4% to 8%) 1558
Konȳne 80 937
K-Phos Neutral Tablets 946
K-Phos Original (Sodium Free) Tablets (Less frequent) 947
Neoral Soft Gelatin Capsules (Rare) 2380
Neoral Oral Solution (Rare) 2380
▲ Niaspan Extended-Release Tablets (Among most common) 1846
Noroxin Tablets 2145
Norplant System 3543
Norpramin Tablets 755
Nubain Injection (1% or less) 1323
Oxistat Lotion (0.4%) 1298
Phrenilin (Infrequent) 578
▲ Protopic Ointment (1% to 8%) 1397
Rescriptor Tablets (Less than 2%) 526
Sandimmune (Rare) 2388
Sedapap Tablets 50 mg/650 mg (Infrequent) 2225
Taxol Injection 1129
Thyrel TRH for Injection (Less frequent) 3630
Trovan 2722
Twinrix Vaccine (Less than 1%) 1674

Tingling, ears
Koāte-DVI (0.7%) 931

Tingling, extremities
Coly-Mycin M Parenteral 2243
Diamox Sequels Sustained Release Capsules ⊙270
Etrafon 3115
Hivid Tablets 2975
Hydrocortone Phosphate Injection, Sterile 2105
Indapamide Tablets (Less than 5%) 2286
Limbitrol 1738
MetroCream 1404
MetroLotion 1405
Myambutol Tablets 1290
Neptazane Tablets ⊙271
Nicotrol Nasal Spray (Common) 2843
Norpramin Tablets 755
Surmontil Capsules 3595
Videx 1138
Videx EC Capsules 1143
Vivactil Tablets 2217
Vivactil Tablets 2446
Zerit 1147

Tingling, feet
Alferon N Injection (1%) 1770
Uroqid-Acid No. 2 Tablets 947

Tingling, fingers
Noroxin Tablets (0.3% to 1.0%) 2145

Tingling, hands
Adenocard Injection (1%) 1380
Koāte-DVI (0.7%) 931
Uroqid-Acid No. 2 Tablets 947

Tingling, legs
Alferon N Injection (1%) 1770

Tingling, lips
K-Phos Neutral Tablets 946
K-Phos Original (Sodium Free) Tablets (Less frequent) 947
Sensorcaine 643
Sensorcaine-MPF Injection 643
Uroqid-Acid No. 2 Tablets 947

Tingling, mouth
Coly-Mycin M Parenteral 2243
Foscavir Injection 605
Sensorcaine 643
Sensorcaine-MPF Injection 643

Tingling, scalp
Cormax Scalp Application (Approximately 0.6%) 2441
▲ Dovonex Scalp Solution (Approximately 23%) 1118
▲ Normodyne Injection (7%) 3135
Normodyne Tablets (Less common) 3137
Temovate Scalp Application (2 of 294 patients) 1304

Tingling, skin
Nebcin Vials, Hyporets & ADD-Vantage 1955
▲ Normodyne Injection (7%) 3135
Vaniqa Cream (2.2%) 1121

Tinnitus
Abelcet Injection 1273
Accutane Capsules 2944
Aceon Tablets (2 mg, 4 mg, 8 mg) (1.5%) 3249
Aciphex Tablets 1267
Aciphex Tablets 1783
Actiq (1% or greater) 1184
▲ Actonel Tablets (3.3%) 2879
Adalat CC Tablets (Less than 1.0%) 877
Aggrenox Capsules (Less than 1%) 1026
Agrylin Capsules (1% to 5%) 3232
Alferon N Injection (One patient) 1770
Alka-Seltzer ▣603
Alka-Seltzer Lemon Lime Antacid and Pain Reliever Effervescent Tablets ▣603
Alka-Seltzer Extra Strength Antacid and Pain Reliever Effervescent Tablets ▣603
Alka-Seltzer PM Effervescent Tablets ▣605
Altace Capsules (Less than 1%) 2233
Ambien Tablets (Infrequent) 3191
Amerge Tablets (Infrequent) 1467
Amicar Injection 3608
Amicar Syrup 3608
Amicar Tablets 3608
Amphotec (1% to 5%) 1774
▲ Anaprox Tablets (3% to 9%) 2967
▲ Anaprox DS Tablets (3% to 9%) 2967
Anzemet Injection (Infrequently) 719
Anzemet Tablets (Infrequently) 722
Aralen Tablets (1 patient) 3075
Aricept Tablets (Infrequent) 1270
Aricept Tablets (Infrequent) 2665
Arthrotec Tablets (Rare) 3195
Asacol Delayed-Release Tablets 2884
Atacand HCT Tablets (0.5% or greater) 597
Atrovent Nasal Spray 0.06% (Less than 1%) 1033
Avelox Tablets (0.05% to 1%) 879
Axert Tablets (Rare) 2772
Azactam for Injection (Less than 1%) 1276
Azulfidine EN-tabs Tablets (Rare) 2775
Bactrim 2949
Genuine Bayer Tablets, Caplets and Gelcaps ▣606
Extra Strength Bayer Caplets and Gelcaps ▣610
Aspirin Regimen Bayer Children's Chewable Tablets (Orange or Cherry Flavored) ▣607
Aspirin Regimen Bayer 81 mg Caplets with Calcium ▣607
Aspirin Regimen Bayer Regular Strength 325 mg Caplets ▣606
Genuine Bayer Professional Labeling (Aspirin Regimen Bayer) ▣608
Extra Strength Bayer Arthritis Caplets ▣610
Extra Strength Bayer PM Caplets ▣611
BC Powder ▣619
Arthritis Strength BC Powder ▣619
Benadryl Parenteral 2617
Betaxon Ophthalmic Suspension (Less than 2%) 537
Biaxin/Biaxin XL 403
Bicillin L-A Injection 2242
Blocadren Tablets (Less than 1%) 2046
Buprenex Injectable (Less than 1%) 2918
Carbatrol Capsules 3234
Cardene I.V. (Rare) 3485
Cardizem Injectable 1018
Cardizem Lyo-Ject Syringe 1018
Cardizem Monovial 1018
Cardizem CD Capsules (Less than 1%) 1016
Cardura Tablets (1%) 2668
Cataflam Tablets (1% to 3%) 2315

Celebrex Capsules (0.1% to 1.9%) 2676
Celebrex Capsules (0.1% to 1.9%) 2780
Celexa (Infrequent) 1365
▲ CellCept Capsules (3% to 10%) 2951
▲ CellCept Intravenous (3% to 10%) 2951
▲ CellCept Oral Suspension (3% to 10%) 2951
▲ CellCept Tablets (3% to 10%) 2951
▲ Cerebyx Injection (8.9%) 2619
Chibroxin Sterile Ophthalmic Solution 2051
Cipro I.V. (1% or less) 893
Cipro I.V. Pharmacy Bulk Package (Less than 1%) 897
Cipro (Less than 1%) 887
Claritin (At least one patient) 3100
Claritin-D 12 Hour Extended Release Tablets (Less frequent) 3102
Claritin-D 24 Hour Extended Release Tablets (Fewer than 2%) 3104
Clinoril Tablets (Greater than 1%) 2053
Clomid Tablets 735
Cognex Capsules (Infrequent) 1351
Colazal Capsules 3069
Copaxone for Injection (At least 2%) 3306
Coreg Tablets (0.1% to 1%) 1508
Corgard Tablets (1 to 5 per 1000 patients) 2245
Corzide 40/5 Tablets (1 to 5 of 1000 patients) 2247
Corzide 80/5 Tablets (1 to 5 of 1000 patients) 2247
Cosopt Sterile Ophthalmic Solution 2065
Covera-HS Tablets (Less than 2%) 3199
Cozaar Tablets (Less than 1%) 2067
Cuprimine Capsules (Greater than 1%) 2075
Cytotec Tablets (Infrequent) 3202
Cytovene (At least 3 subjects) 2959
Dapsone Tablets USP 1780
Daranide Tablets 2077
DaunoXome Injection (Less than or equal to 5%) 1442
Declomycin Tablets 1855
Demadex Tablets and Injection 2965
▲ Depacon Injection (1% to 7%) 416
▲ Depakene (7%) 421
▲ Depakote Sprinkle Capsules (1% to 7%) 426
▲ Depakote Tablets (1% to 7%) 430
Depakote ER Tablets (1% to 5%) 436
Depen Titratable Tablets 3341
Desferal Vials 2333
Diamox Intravenous ⊙ 269
Diamox Sequels Sustained Release Capsules ⊙ 270
Diamox Tablets ⊙ 269
Diovan HCT Tablets (Greater than 0.2%) 2338
Dipentum Capsules (Rare) 2803
Diprivan Injectable Emulsion (Less than 1%) 667
Dolobid Tablets (Greater than 1 in 100) 2088
Doxil Injection (Less than 1%) 566
▲ Duraclon Injection (5.3%) 3057
Duranest Injections 600
Dynabac Tablets (0.1% to 1%) 2269
▲ EC-Naprosyn Delayed-Release Tablets (3% to 9%) 2967
Ecotrin Enteric Coated Aspirin Low, Regular and Maximum Strength Tablets 1715
Edecrin 2091
Effexor Tablets (2%) 3495
Effexor XR Capsules (Frequent) 3499
ELA-Max Cream 1340
Eldepryl Capsules 3266
Elmiron Capsules (Less than or equal to 1%) 570
Emla (Unlikely with cream) 602
Enalaprilat Injection 863
Engerix-B Vaccine 1517
Eskalith 1527
Etrafon 3115
Evoxac Capsules (Less than 1%) 1217
Excedrin Extra-Strength Tablets, Caplets, and Geltabs ▣ 629
Exelon Capsules (Frequent) 2342
Exelon Oral Solution (Frequent) 2345
Famotidine Injection (Infrequent) 866
▲ Feldene Capsules (1% to 10%) 2685
Flexeril Tablets (Less than 1%) 572
Flexeril Tablets (Less than 1%) 2094
Floxin I.V. (Less than 1%) 2526
Floxin Otic Solution (0.3%) 1219
Floxin Tablets (Less than 1%) 2529
Flumadine (0.3% to 1%) 1370
Fortovase Capsules (Less than 2%) 2970
Furosemide Tablets 2284
Gabitril Tablets (Frequent) 1189
Gastrocrom Oral Concentrate (Less common) 1162
Gengraf Capsules (1% to less than 3%) 457
Geodon Capsules (Infrequent) 2688
Halcion Tablets (Rare) 2823
Hivid Tablets (Less than 1%) 2975
Hytrin Capsules (At least 1%) 464
Hyzaar 2109
Imdur Tablets (Less than or equal to 5%) 1826
Imitrex Nasal Spray 1554
Indocin (Greater than 1%) 2112
▲ Infergen (4% to 6%) 1777
Intron A for Injection (Less than 5%) 3120
Invirase Capsules (Less than 2%) 2979
Isoptin SR Tablets (1% or less) 467
Kaletra Capsules (Less than 2%) 471
Kaletra Oral Solution (Less than 2%) 471
Lamictal (1.1%) 1567
▲ Lariam Tablets (Among most frequent) 2989
Levaquin (0.3% to less than 0.5%) 2537
Lexxel Tablets 608
Lidoderm Patch 1319
Lipitor Tablets (Less than 2%) 2639
Lipitor Tablets (Less than 2%) 2696
Lithium Carbonate 3061
Lithium Citrate Syrup 3061
Lithobid Slow-Release Tablets 3255
Lodine (1% to 3%) 3528
Lodine XL Extended-Release Tablets (1% to 3%) 3530
Lotensin HCT Tablets (0.3% to 1%) 2367
Lotrel Capsules (Infrequent) 2370
Lupron Depot–3 Month 22.5 mg (Less than 5%) 3288
Luvox Tablets (25, 50, 100 mg) 3256
Marinol Capsules (Less than 1%) 3325
Maxalt Tablets (Infrequent) 2120
Maxalt-MLT Orally Disintegrating Tablets (Infrequent) 2120
Meridia Capsules 481
Mexitil Capsules (1.9% to 2.4%) 1047
Miacalcin Nasal Spray (Less than 1%) 2375
Micardis Tablets (More than 0.3%) 1049
Micardis HCT Tablets 1051
Midamor Tablets (Less than or equal to 1%) 2136
Migranal Nasal Spray (Infrequent) 2376
Minipress Capsules (Less than 1%) 2699
Minizide Capsules (Rare) 2700
Mintezol 2137
Mirapex Tablets (2%) 2834
Mobic Tablets (Less than 2%) 1054
Moduretic Tablets 2138
Momentum Backache Relief Extra Strength Caplets ▣ 666
Monopril Tablets (0.2% to 1.0%) 1091
Monopril HCT (Less than 2%) 1094
Motrin Suspension, Oral Drops, Chewable Tablets, and Caplets (1% to less than 3%) 2002
Mustargen for Injection (Infrequent) 2142
Mykrox Tablets (Less than 2%) 1168
Myobloc Injectable Solution (2% or greater) 1291
Nadolol Tablets (1 to 5 of 1000 patients) 2288
▲ Naprelan Tablets (3% to 9%) 1293
▲ Naprosyn Suspension (3% to 9%) 2967
▲ Naprosyn Tablets (3% to 9%) 2967
Naropin Injection (Less than 1%) 612
Nebcin Vials, Hyporets & ADD-Vantage 1955
Neoral Soft Gelatin Capsules (1% to less than 3%) 2380
Neoral Oral Solution (1% to less than 3%) 2380
Neptazane Tablets ⊙ 271
Nesacaine/Nesacaine MPF 617
Neurontin Capsules (Infrequent) 2655
Neurontin Oral Solution (Infrequent) 2655
Neurontin Tablets (Infrequent) 2655
Nexium Delayed-Release Capsules (Less than 1%) 619
Nipent for Injection (Less than 3%) 3272
Noroxin Tablets 2145
Norpramin Tablets 755
Norvasc Tablets (More than 0.1% to 1%) 2704
Norvir Capsules (Less than 2%) 487
Norvir Oral Solution (Less than 2%) 487
Orthoclone OKT3 Sterile Solution 2498
Orudis Capsules (Greater than 1%) 3548
Oruvail Capsules (Greater than 1%) 3548
OxyContin Tablets (Less than 1%) 2912
Parnate Tablets 1607
Paxil (Frequent) 1609
Pediazole Suspension 3050
Pepcid Injection (Infrequent) 2153
Pepcid for Oral Suspension (Infrequent) 2150
Pepcid RPD Orally Disintegrating Tablets (Infrequent) 2150
Pepcid Tablets (Infrequent) 2150
Pepto-Bismol Maximum Strength Liquid 2878
Pepto-Bismol Original Liquid, Original and Cherry Tablets and Easy-To-Swallow Caplets 2878
Periactin Tablets 2155
Permax Tablets (Infrequent) 1299
Phenergan Injection 3553
Phenergan 3556
Phrenilin (Infrequent) 578
Plaquenil Tablets 3082
Pletal Tablets (Less than 2%) 2605
Pletal Tablets (Less than 2%) 2848
Polocaine Injection, USP 625
Polocaine-MPF Injection, USP 625
▲ Ponstel Capsules (1% to 10%) 1356
Prevacid Delayed-Release Capsules (Less than 1%) 3292
PREVPAC (Less than 1%) 3298
Prilosec Delayed-Release Capsules (Less than 1%) 628
Primaxin I.M. 2158
Primaxin I.V. (Less than 0.2%) 2160
Prinivil Tablets (0.3% to 1.0%) 2164
Prinzide Tablets (0.3% to 1%) 2168
Procardia Capsules (Less than 0.5%) 2708
Procardia XL Extended Release Tablets (1% or less) 2710
▲ Prograf (3% to 15%) 1393
ProSom Tablets (Infrequent) 500
Protonix I.V. (Less than 1%) 3580
Protonix Tablets (Less than 1%) 3577
Proventil Repetabs Tablets (2%) 3148
Proventil HFA Inhalation Aerosol (Less than 3%) 3150
Prozac Pulvules, Liquid, and Weekly Capsules (Frequent) 1238
Quinaglute Dura-Tabs Tablets 978
Quinidex Extentabs 2933
▲ Rapamune Oral Solution and Tablets (3% to 20%) 3584
Recombivax HB (Less than 1%) 2178
▲ Relafen Tablets (3% to 9%) 1617
Requip Tablets (Infrequent) 1621
Rescriptor Tablets (Less than 2%) 526
Rifater Tablets 769
Risperdal (Rare) 1796
Romazicon Injection (Less than 1%) 3000
Rynatan Tablets 3351
Rythmol Tablets – 150 mg, 225 mg, 300 mg (Less than 1% to 1.9%) 502
Salagen Tablets (1% to 2%) 2229
Sandimmune (2% or less) 2388
Sandostatin LAR Depot (1% to 4%) 2395
Sarafem Pulvules (Frequent) 1962
Sedapap Tablets 50 mg/650 mg (Infrequent) 2225
Sensorcaine 643
Sensorcaine-MPF Injection 643
Septra Suspension 2265
Septra Tablets 2265
Septra DS Tablets 2265
Serophene Tablets 3226
Seroquel Tablets (Infrequent) 684
Serzone Tablets (Up to 3%) 1104
Sinequan (Occasional) 2713
Soma Compound Tablets 3354
Soma Compound w/Codeine Tablets 3355
Sonata Capsules (Infrequent) 3591
▲ Soriatane Capsules (Less than 1% to 10%) 3003
Sporanox Capsules (Infrequent) 1800
Sporanox Oral Solution (Less than 2%) 1808
Sporanox Oral Solution (Less than 2%) 2512
▲ Stadol NS Nasal Spray (3% to 9%) 1108
Streptomycin Sulfate Injection 2714
Sular Tablets (Less than or equal to 1%) 688
Surmontil Capsules 3595
Sustiva Capsules (Less than 2%) 1258
Talacen Caplets (Rare) 3089
Talwin Nx Tablets 3090
Tambocor Tablets (1% to 3%) 1990
Tarka Tablets (Less frequent) 508
Tasmar Tablets (Frequent) 3010
Tegretol/Tegretol-XR 2404
Tenex Tablets (3% or less) 2942
Tequin Injection (0.1% to 3%) 1110
Tequin Tablets (0.1% to 3%) 1110
Teveten Tablets (Less than 1%) 3327
Thalomid Capsules 1154
Tiazac Capsules (Less than 2%) 1378
Ticlid Tablets (0.5% to 1.0%) 3015
Timolide Tablets 2187
Timolol GFS ⊙ 266
Timoptic in Ocudose 2192
Timoptic Sterile Ophthalmic Solution 2190
Timoptic-XE Sterile Ophthalmic Gel Forming Solution 2194
▲ TOBI Solution for Inhalation (3%) 1206
Tolectin (1% to 3%) 2589
Tonocard Tablets (0.4% to 1.5%) 649
Topamax Sprinkle Capsules (Frequent) 2590
Topamax Tablets (Frequent) 2590
Toprol-XL Tablets 651
Toradol (1% or less) 3018
Tricor Capsules, Micronized (Less than 1%) 513
Trileptal Oral Suspension 2407
Trileptal Tablets 2407
▲ Trilisate (Less than 20%) 2901
▲ Trisenox Injection (5%) 1158
Trovan (Less than 1%) 2722
Twinrix Vaccine 1674
Ultracet Tablets (Less than 1%) 2597
Ultram Tablets (Infrequent) 2600
Uniretic Tablets (Less than 1%) 3178
Univasc Tablets (Less than 1%) 3181
Vancenase AQ Nasal Spray 0.084% (2%) 3163
Vancocin HCl Capsules & Pulvules (Rare) 1972
Vancocin HCl Oral Solution (Rare) 1971
Vancocin HCl, Vials & ADD-Vantage (Rare) 1970
Vantin Tablets and Oral Suspension (Less than 1%) 2860
▲ Vascor Tablets (Up to 6.52%) 2602
Vaseretic Tablets (0.5% to 2.0%) 2204
Vasotec I.V. Injection 2207
Vasotec Tablets (0.5% to 1.0%) 2210
Verelan Capsules 3184
Verelan PM Capsules (2% or less) 3186
Viagra Tablets (Less than 2%) 2732
Vicoprofen Tablets (Less than 3%) 520
Vioxx (Greater than 0.1% to 1.9%) 2213
Vistide Injection 1445
Vivactil Tablets 2217
Vivactil Tablets 2446
Voltaren Tablets (1% to 3%) 2315
Voltaren-XR Tablets (1% to 3%) 2315
Wellbutrin Tablets 1680
▲ Wellbutrin SR Sustained-Release Tablets (6%) 1684
▲ Xanax Tablets (6.6%) 2865
▲ Xylocaine Injections (Among most common) 653
Zanaflex Tablets (Infrequent) 1305
Zebeta Tablets 1885
Zestoretic Tablets (0.3% to 1%) 695
Zestril Tablets (0.3% to 1.0%) 698
Ziac Tablets 1887
Zithromax Capsules, 250 mg 2743
Zithromax for IV Infusion (Rare) 2748
Zithromax for Oral Suspension, 300 mg, 600 mg, 900 mg, 1200 mg 2739
Zithromax Tablets, 250 mg 2739
Zoloft (Frequent) 2751
Zomig Tablets (Infrequent) 708
Zomig-ZMT Tablets (Infrequent) 708
Zonegran Capsules (Frequent) 1307
Zosyn (1.0% or less) 1890
Zosyn in Galaxy Containers (1.0% or less) 1894
Zyban Sustained-Release Tablets (1%) 1710
Zyprexa Tablets (Infrequent) 1973
Zyprexa ZYDIS Orally Disintegrating Tablets (Infrequent) 1973
Zyrtec (Less than 2%) 2756
Zyrtec-D 12 Hour Extended Relief Tablets (Less than 2%) 2758

Tiredness

(*see under* Fatigue)

Tissue turgor, increased

▲ Serostim for Injection (27.3%) 3229

Tobacco misuse

Zyprexa Tablets (Infrequent) 1973
Zyprexa ZYDIS Orally Disintegrating Tablets (Infrequent) 1973

Toenails, ingrown

Crixivan Capsules 2070

Toes, discoloration

Eskalith (A few reports) 1527
Lithium Carbonate (A single report) 3061
Lithium Citrate Syrup 3061
Lithobid Slow-Release Tablets (A few reports) 3255

Tolerance

Adipex-P 1406
Astelin Nasal Spray 3339
Astramorph/PF Injection, USP (Preservative-Free) 594
Carnitor Tablets and Oral Solution 3245
DextroStat Tablets 3236
Dilaudid Oral Liquid 445
Dilaudid Tablets - 8 mg 445
Duragesic Transdermal System 1786
Duramorph Injection 1312
Hycodan 1316
Hycomine Compound Tablets 1317
Hycotuss Expectorant Syrup 1318

Infumorph 200 and Infumorph 500 Sterile Solutions 1314
Isordil Sublingual Tablets 3525
Isordil Titradose Tablets 3526
Kadian Capsules (Less than 3%) 1335
Lortab 3319
Lortab Elixir 3317
MS Contin Tablets 2896
Nembutal Sodium Solution 485
Nitrostat Tablets 2658
Oramorph SR Tablets 3062
Percocet Tablets 1326
Percodan Tablets 1327
Percolone Tablets 1327
Phrenilin 578
Ritalin 2387
Roxanol 3066
Sedapap Tablets 50 mg/650 mg (Infrequent) 2225
Tylenol with Codeine 2595
Vicodin Tablets 516
Vicodin HP Tablets 518
Vicodin Tuss Expectorant 519
Vicoprofen Tablets 520
Zemuron Injection (Rare) 2491

Tolerance, diminished
Duranest Injections 600
Sensorcaine 643
Sensorcaine-MPF Injection 643
Timolide Tablets 2187
Xylocaine Injections 653

Tongue, black hairy
(*see under* Glossotrichia)

Tongue, burning
Halcion Tablets 2823
Imitrex Injection 1549
Imitrex Nasal Spray (Infrequent) 1554
Imitrex Tablets 1558
Lodosyn Tablets 1251
Sinemet Tablets 1253
Sinemet CR Tablets 1255

Tongue, fine vermicular movements
Compazine 1505
Eskalith 1527
Etrafon 3115
Haldol Decanoate 2535
Haldol Injection, Tablets and Concentrate 2533
Lithobid Slow-Release Tablets 3255
Moban 1320
Navane Oral 2701
Navane Intramuscular 2703
Orap Tablets 1407
Reglan 2935
Stelazine 1640
Thioridazine Hydrochloride Tablets 2289
Thiothixene Capsules 2290
Thorazine 1656

Tongue, furry
Geocillin Tablets 2687

Tongue, geographic
Evoxac Capsules (Less than 1%) 1217

Tongue, mucosal atrophy
Prilosec Delayed-Release Capsules (Less than 1%) 628

Tongue, protrusion
Compazine 1505
Etrafon 3115
Haldol Decanoate 2535
Haldol Injection, Tablets and Concentrate 2533
Loxitane Capsules 3398
Moban 1320
Navane Oral 2701
Navane Intramuscular 2703
Orap Tablets 1407
Phenergan Suppositories 3556
Phenergan Syrup 3554
Phenergan with Codeine Syrup 3557
Phenergan with Dextromethorphan Syrup 3559
Phenergan VC Syrup 3560
Phenergan VC with Codeine Syrup 3561
Prozac Pulvules, Liquid, and Weekly Capsules (One case) 1238
Reglan 2935
Sarafem Pulvules (One case) 1962
Serentil 1057
Stelazine 1640
Thioridazine Hydrochloride Tablets 2289
Thiothixene Capsules 2290
Thorazine 1656
Trilafon 3160

Tongue, rounding
Etrafon 3115
Trilafon 3160

Tongue, sore
(*see under* Glossodynia)

Tongue, swelling
(*see under* Glossoncus)

Tongue discoloration
Aldomet Tablets 2037
Biaxin/Biaxin XL 403
Claritin-D 12 Hour Extended Release Tablets (Less frequent) 3102
Colazal Capsules 3069
Copaxone for Injection (Infrequent) 3306
Effexor Tablets (Rare) 3495
Effexor XR Capsules (Rare) 3499
Etrafon 3115
Evoxac Capsules (Less than 1%) 1217
Paxil (Rare) 1609
Pepto-Bismol Maximum Strength Liquid 2878
Pepto-Bismol Original Liquid, Original and Cherry Tablets and Easy-To-Swallow Caplets 2878
PREVPAC (Less than 3%) 3298
Prilosec Delayed-Release Capsules (2%) 628
Primaxin I.M. 2158
Primaxin I.V. (Less than 0.2%) 2160
Protonix I.V. (Less than 1%) 3580
Protonix Tablets (Less than 1%) 3577
Remeron Tablets (Rare) 2483
Remeron SolTab Tablets (Rare) 2486
Rilutek Tablets (Rare) 772
Risperdal (Rare) 1796
Sonata Capsules (Rare) 3591
Thalomid Capsules 1154
Trilafon 3160
Uniretic Tablets (Less than 1%) 3178
Vistide Injection 1445
Zyprexa Tablets (Rare) 1973
Zyprexa ZYDIS Orally Disintegrating Tablets (Rare) 1973
Zyrtec (Less than 2%) 2756
Zyrtec-D 12 Hour Extended Relief Tablets (Less than 2%) 2758
Zyvox (0.2% to 1.1%) 2871

Tongue disorder, unspecified
Avonex 1013
▲ Cerebyx Injection (4.4%) 2619
Evoxac Capsules (Less than 1%) 1217
Flovent Diskus (1% to 3%) 3614
Gengraf Capsules (1% to less than 3%) 457
Hivid Tablets (Less than 1%) 2975
Neoral Soft Gelatin Capsules (1% to less than 3%) 2380
Neoral Oral Solution (1% to less than 3%) 2380
Nexium Delayed-Release Capsules (Less than 1%) 619
PREVPAC (Less than 3%) 3298
Salagen Tablets (Less than 1%) 2229
▲ Soriatane Capsules (1% to 10%) 3003
Tasmar Tablets (Infrequent) 3010

Tongue numbness
(*see under* Numbness, buccal mucosa)

Tonsillitis
Flovent Diskus (1% to 3%) 3614
Flovent Rotadisk (1% to 3%) 1537
Foradil Aerolizer (1.2%) 2354
Gengraf Capsules (1% to less than 3%) 457
Neoral Soft Gelatin Capsules (1% to less than 3%) 2380
Neoral Oral Solution (1% to less than 3%) 2380
Synvisc 3596
Vioxx (Greater than 0.1% to 1.9%) 2213

Tooth development, impaired
Urobiotic-250 Capsules 2731
Vibramycin Hyclate Intravenous 2737

Tooth discoloration
Augmentin ES-600 Powder for Oral Suspension (Very rare) 1487
Biaxin/Biaxin XL 403
PREVPAC 3298
Urobiotic-250 Capsules (Contraindicated in pregnancy) 2731

Tooth disorder
Actiq (Less than 1%) 1184
Actonel Tablets (2.1%) 2879
▲ Actos Tablets (5.3%) 3275
Arava Tablets (1% to 3%) 724
Aricept Tablets (Frequent) 1270
Aricept Tablets (Frequent) 2665
Avonex 1013
Axid Pulvules (1.0%) 1903
Axid Pulvules (1.0%) 2919
Celebrex Capsules (0.1% to 1.9%) 2676
Celebrex Capsules (0.1% to 1.9%) 2780
Claritin-D 24 Hour Extended Release Tablets (Fewer than 2%) 3104
▲ CombiPatch Transdermal System (4% to 6%) 2323
Crinone (Less than 5%) 3213
Depakote ER Tablets (1% to 5%) 436
Dostinex Tablets (1%) 2804
Estring Vaginal Ring (1% to 3%) 2811
Evoxac Capsules (1% to 3%) 1217
Flomax Capsules (1.2% to 2.0%) 1044
Flovent Diskus (1% to 3%) 3614
Flovent (1% to 3%) 1535
Fortovase Capsules (Less than 2%) 2970
Gengraf Capsules (1% to less than 3%) 457
Gonal-F for Injection 3216
Invirase Capsules (Less than 2%) 2979
Ismo Tablets (Fewer than 1%) 3524
Klonopin Tablets (Infrequent) 2983
▲ Lamictal (3.2%) 1567
Lescol Capsules (2.1%) 2361
Lescol Capsules (2.1%) 2925
Lescol XL Tablets (1.4%) 2361
Lescol XL Tablets (1.4%) 2925
Lotensin HCT Tablets (0.3% or more) 2367
▲ Luvox Tablets (25, 50, 100 mg) (3%) 3256
Meridia Capsules (Greater than or equal to 1%) 481
Mirapex Tablets (1% or more) 2834
Myobloc Injectable Solution (2% or greater) 1291
Naprelan Tablets (Less than 1%) 1293
Neoral Soft Gelatin Capsules (1% to less than 3%) 2380
Neoral Oral Solution (1% to less than 3%) 2380
Neurontin Oral Solution (1.5%) 2655
▲ Nicotrol Inhaler (Over 3%) 2840
▲ Nicotrol Nasal Spray (4%) 2843
▲ Nipent for Injection (3% to 10%) 3272
▲ Ortho-Prefest Tablets (5%) 2570
Paxil (Rare) 1609
▲ Periostat Tablets (6%) 1208
Prandin Tablets (0.5, 1, and 2 mg) (Less than 1% to 2%) 2432
Prometrium Capsules (100 mg, 200 mg) 3261
Protopic Ointment (Greater than or equal to 1%) 1397
Provigil Tablets (At least 1%) 1193
Rilutek Tablets (Up to 1.2%) 772
Roferon-A Injection (Infrequent) 2996
Salagen Tablets (Less than 1%) 2229
Serzone Tablets 1104
Skelid Tablets (2.7%) 3088
Tasmar Tablets (Frequent) 3010
Thalomid Capsules 1154
Tricor Capsules, Micronized 513
Trovan (Less than 1%) 2722
Vantin Tablets and Oral Suspension (Less than 1%) 2860
Versed Injection (Less than 1%) 3027
Wellbutrin SR Sustained-Release Tablets (At least 1%) 1684
▲ Xenical Capsules (2.9% to 4.3%) 3043
Zyprexa Tablets 1973
Zyprexa ZYDIS Orally Disintegrating Tablets 1973
Zyrtec (Less than 2%) 2756
Zyrtec-D 12 Hour Extended Relief Tablets (Less than 2%) 2758

Torsade de pointes
Betapace Tablets (Up to 5.8%) 950
Betapace AF Tablets 954
Biaxin/Biaxin XL (Rare) 403
Celexa (At least 3 patients) 1365
Cordarone Intravenous 3491
Corvert Injection 2793
Cytovene 2959
Dynabac Tablets (Rare) 2269
E.E.S. (Rare) 450
EryPed (Rare) 446
Erythrocin Stearate Filmtab Tablets (Rare) 452
Erythromycin Base Filmtab Tablets (Rare) 454
Felbatol 3343
Haldol Decanoate 2535
Haldol Injection, Tablets and Concentrate 2533
Levaquin 2537
Luvox Tablets (25, 50, 100 mg) 3256
Meridia Capsules 481
Paxil 1609
PCE Dispertab Tablets (Rare) 498
Pediazole Suspension (Rare) 3050
PREVPAC (Rare) 3298
Prozac Pulvules, Liquid, and Weekly Capsules 1238
Quinidex Extentabs 2933
Remeron Tablets (Four cases) 2483
Remeron SolTab Tablets (Four cases) 2486
Sarafem Pulvules 1962
Tambocor Tablets (Rare) 1990
▲ Tikosyn Capsules (Up to 10.5%) 2717
Vascor Tablets 2602
Zithromax 2743
Zoloft 2751

Torticollis
Aceon Tablets (2 mg, 4 mg, 8 mg) (1.4%) 3249
Actiq (1% or greater) 1184
▲ Actonel Tablets (5.3%) 2879
Adalat CC Tablets (Less than 1.0%) 877
Adenocard Injection (Less than 1%) 1380
▲ Adenoscan (15%) 1381
Agrylin Capsules (1% to 5%) 3232
AmBisome for Injection (Less common) 1383
Amphotec (1% to 5%) 1774
Arava Tablets (1% to 3%) 724
Arimidex Tablets (2% to 5%) 659
Asacol Delayed-Release Tablets 2884
Axert Tablets (Infrequent) 2772
Betaseron for SC Injection 988
▲ Botox Purified Neurotoxin Complex (11%) 549
Cardene I.V. (Rare) 3485
▲ Casodex Tablets (2% to 5%) 662
Ceclor CD Tablets (0.1% to 1%) 1279
Cipro I.V. (1% or less) 893
Cipro I.V. Pharmacy Bulk Package (Less than 1%) 897
Cipro (Less than 1%) 887
Claritin-D 12 Hour Extended Release Tablets (Less frequent) 3102
Clozaril Tablets (1%) 2319
Compazine 1505
▲ Copaxone for Injection (8%) 3306
Depacon Injection (1% or more) 416
Depakene (1% or more) 421
Depakote Sprinkle Capsules 426
Depakote Tablets (1% to 5%) 430
Depakote ER Tablets (1% or more) 436
Diprivan Injectable Emulsion (Less than 1%) 667
Doxil Injection (Less than 1%) 566
Dynabac Tablets (0.1% to 1%) 2269
DynaCirc CR Tablets (0.5% to 1%) 2923
Effexor Tablets (Frequent) 3495
▲ Effexor XR Capsules (3%) 3499
Engerix-B Vaccine (Less than 1%) 1517
Etrafon 3115
▲ Flolan for Injection (84%) 1528
Gabitril Tablets (Frequent) 1189
Geodon Capsules (Rare) 2688
Gliadel Wafer (2%) 1723
Hivid Tablets (Less than 1%) 2975
Hytrin Capsules (At least 1%) 464
Imdur Tablets (Less than or equal to 5%) 1826
▲ Imitrex Injection (4.8%) 1549
▲ Infergen (8% to 14%) 1777
Klonopin Tablets (Infrequent) 2983
Lamictal (2.4%) 1567
Lexxel Tablets 608
Lipitor Tablets (Less than 2%) 2639
Lipitor Tablets (Less than 2%) 2696
Lotensin HCT Tablets (0.3% or more) 2367
Lupron Depot–4 Month 30 mg (Less than 5%) 3289
Luvox Tablets (25, 50, 100 mg) (Rare to infrequent) 3256
Meridia Capsules (1.6%) 481
Mirapex Tablets (1.6%) 2834
Moduretic Tablets 2138
▲ Myobloc Injectable Solution (Up to 17%) 1291
Naprelan Tablets (Less than 1%) 1293
▲ Nicotrol Inhaler (Over 3%) 2840
Norvir Capsules (Less than 2%) 487
Norvir Oral Solution (Less than 2%) 487
Orap Tablets (2.7%) 1407
▲ Orthoclone OKT3 Sterile Solution (14%) 2498
OxyContin Tablets (Less than 1%) 2912
Paxil (Infrequent) 1609
Permax Tablets (2.7%) 1299
Phenergan Suppositories 3556
Phenergan Syrup 3554
Phenergan with Codeine Syrup 3557
Phenergan with Dextromethorphan Syrup 3559
Phenergan VC Syrup 3560
Phenergan VC with Codeine Syrup 3561
Prinivil Tablets (0.3% to 1.0%) 2164
Prinzide Tablets 2168
ProSom Tablets (Infrequent) 500
Protonix I.V. (Greater than or equal to 1%) 3580
Protonix Tablets (Greater than or equal to 1%) 3577
Protopic Ointment (Greater than or equal to 1%) 1397
Provigil Tablets (2%) 1193
Pulmicort Turbuhaler Inhalation Powder (1% to 3%) 636
Recombivax HB (Less than 1%) 2178
Reglan 2935
Remeron Tablets (Infrequent) 2483
Remeron SolTab Tablets (Infrequent) 2486

Requip Tablets (Infrequent) 1621
Risperdal (Rare) 1796
Roxicodone Tablets (Less than 3%) 3067
Salagen Tablets (Less than 1%) 2229
Serentil 1057
Serevent Inhalation Aerosol (1% to 3%) 1633
Seroquel Tablets (Infrequent) 684
Serzone Tablets 1104
Sonata Capsules (Infrequent) 3591
Stelazine 1640
Tasmar Tablets (2%) 3010
Tequin Injection (Less than 0.1%) 1110
Tequin Tablets (Less than 0.1%) 1110
▲ Thalomid Capsules (4.2%) 1154
Thioridazine Hydrochloride Tablets 2289
Thorazine 1656
Tiazac Capsules (1%) 1378
Tonocard Tablets (Less than 1%) 649
Trilafon 3160
▲ Trisenox Injection (13%) 1158
Uniretic Tablets (Less than 1%) 3178
Vistide Injection 1445
Wellbutrin SR Sustained-Release Tablets (At least 1%) 1684
Zanaflex Tablets (Infrequent) 1305
Zebeta Tablets 1885
Zestoretic Tablets 695
Zestril Tablets (0.3% to 1.0%) 698
Ziac Tablets 1887
Zyban Sustained-Release Tablets (2%) 1710
Zyflo Filmtab Tablets (Less common) 524
Zyprexa Tablets (2% to 3%) 1973
Zyprexa ZYDIS Orally Disintegrating Tablets (2% to 3%) 1973

Total proteins, decrease
(*see under* Hypoproteinemia)

Tourette's syndrome
Adderall Tablets 3231
Adderall XR Capsules
Concerta Extended-Release Tablets (Rare) 1998
Concerta Tablets (Rare) 561
Cylert Tablets 415
Desoxyn Tablets 440
Dexedrine 1512
DextroStat Tablets 3236
Meridia Capsules 481
Metadate CD Capsules (Rare) 1164
Metadate ER Tablets (Rare) 1167
Methylin Tablets 1995
Methylin ER Tablets 1995
Ritalin (Rare) 2387

Toxic granulation
Efudex 1733

Toxic shock syndrome
Ortho Diaphragm Kits – All-Flex Arcing Spring; Ortho Coil Spring 2552

Toxicity, hepatic
Cordarone Tablets 3487
Declomycin Tablets (Rare) 1855
Hexalen Capsules (Less than 1%) 2226
Pacerone Tablets 3331
Parafon Forte DSC Caplets (Rare) 2582
Urobiotic-250 Capsules 2731

Toxoplasmosis
Doxil Injection 566

Tracheitis
Advair Diskus 100/50 1448
Advair Diskus 250/50 1448
Advair Diskus 500/50 1448
Amerge Tablets (Rare) 1467
Liquid PedvaxHIB (One case) 2148
▲ Serevent Diskus (7%) 1637
Serevent Inhalation Aerosol (1% to 3%) 1633

Tracheobronchitis
Avalide Tablets 1070
Avapro Tablets (Less than 1%) 1074
Avapro Tablets (Less than 1%) 3076
Betapace AF Tablets (0.7% to 3.3%) 954
Monopril Tablets (0.4% to 1.0%) 1091

Transaminase, elevation
(*see under* Serum transaminase, elevation)

Trauma
Caverject Sterile Powder (2%) 2777
Exelon Capsules (Frequent) 2342
Exelon Oral Solution (Frequent) 2345
Fortovase Capsules (Less than 2%) 2970
▲ Gengraf Capsules (4%) 457
▲ Neoral Soft Gelatin Capsules (4%) 2380
▲ Neoral Oral Solution (4%) 2380
▲ Simulect for Injection (3% to 10%) 2399
Singulair (1%) 2181
Starlix Tablets (2.9%) 2401
Vioxx (Greater than 0.1% to 1.9%) 2213

Trauma, unspecified
Ambien Tablets (Infrequent) 3191
Decadron Phosphate Sterile Ophthalmic Ointment 2083
Decadron Phosphate Sterile Ophthalmic Solution 2084
Effexor Tablets (2%) 3495
Fortovase Capsules (Less than 2%) 2970
Humorsol Sterile Ophthalmic Solution 2102
Invirase Capsules (Less than 2%) 2979
▲ Lescol Capsules (5.1%) 2361
▲ Lescol Capsules (5.1%) 2925
▲ Lescol XL Tablets (4.2%) 2361
▲ Lescol XL Tablets (4.2%) 2925
Neurontin Capsules (Frequent) 2655
Neurontin Oral Solution (Frequent) 2655
Neurontin Tablets (Frequent) 2655
Paxil (1.4%) 1609
Pravachol Tablets 1099
Prinzide Tablets (0.3% to 1%) 2168
Rescriptor Tablets (Less than 2%) 526
Zestoretic Tablets (0.3% to 1%) 695

Trembling
(*see under* Tremors)

Tremor, fine hand
Eskalith 1527
Lithium Carbonate 3061
Lithium Citrate Syrup 3061
Lithobid Slow-Release Tablets 3255
▲ Vascor Tablets (3.02% to 9.30%) 2602

Tremors
Aciphex Tablets 1267
Aciphex Tablets 1783
Adalat CC Tablets (Rare) 877
Adderall Tablets 3231
Adderall XR Capsules
Adenoscan (Less than 1%) 1381
Adipex-P 1406
Advair Diskus 100/50 (1% to 3%) 1448
Advair Diskus 250/50 (1% to 3%) 1448
Advair Diskus 500/50 (1% to 3%) 1448
▲ Aerobid/Aerobid-M (3% to 9%) 1363
Alferon N Injection (One patient) 1770
Aloprim for Injection (Less than 1%) 2292
Altace Capsules (Less than 1%) 2233
Alupent (1% to 4%) 1029
Ambien Tablets (Infrequent) 3191
AmBisome for Injection (Less common) 1383
Amerge Tablets (Infrequent) 1467
▲ Amphotec (5% or more) 1774
Anzemet Injection (Infrequently) 719
Anzemet Tablets (Infrequently) 722
Aricept Tablets (Frequent) 1270
Aricept Tablets (Frequent) 2665
Arthrotec Tablets (Rare) 3195
Asacol Delayed-Release Tablets 2884
Atarax Tablets & Syrup (Rare) 2667
Ativan Injection (Infrequent) 3478
Atromid-S Capsules 3483
Atrovent Inhalation Aerosol (Less frequent) 1030
Atrovent Inhalation Solution (0.9%) 1031
Avalide Tablets 1070
Avapro Tablets (Less than 1%) 1074
Avapro Tablets (Less than 1%) 3076
Avelox Tablets (0.05% to 1%) 879
Axert Tablets (Infrequent) 2772
Baycol Tablets 883
Benadryl Parenteral 2617
Betaseron for SC Injection 988
Biaxin/Biaxin XL 403
Bicillin C-R 900/300 Injection 2240
Bicillin C-R Injection 2238
Bicillin L-A Injection 2242
Bontril Slow-Release Capsules 576
▲ Brethine Ampuls (7.8 to 38.0%) 2314
▲ Brethine Tablets (15%) 2313
Buprenex Injectable (Infrequent) 2918
Calcium Disodium Versenate Injection 1980
▲ Campath Ampules (7%) 992
Cardizem Injectable 1018
Cardizem Lyo-Ject Syringe 1018
Cardizem Monovial 1018
Cardizem CD Capsules (Less than 1%) 1016
Cardura Tablets (Less than 0.5%) 2668
Cataflam Tablets (Less than 1%) 2315
Ceclor CD Tablets (0.1% to 1%) 1279
▲ Celexa (8%) 1365
▲ CellCept Capsules (11.0% to 24.2%) 2951
▲ CellCept Intravenous (11.0% to 24.2%) 2951
▲ CellCept Oral Suspension (11.0% to 24.2%) 2951
▲ CellCept Tablets (11.0% to 33.9%) 2951
▲ Cerebyx Injection (3.3% to 9.5%) 2619
Chibroxin Sterile Ophthalmic Solution 2051
Chirocaine Injection (Less than 1%) 2909
Cipro I.V. (1% or less) 893
Cipro I.V. Pharmacy Bulk Package (Less than 1%) 897
Cipro (Less than 1%) 887
Claritin (At least one patient) 3100
Claritin-D 12 Hour Extended Release Tablets (Less frequent) 3102
Claritin-D 24 Hour Extended Release Tablets (Fewer than 2%) 3104
▲ Clozaril Tablets (More than 5% to 6%) 2319
Cognex Capsules (2%) 1351
Colazal Capsules 3069
Combivent Inhalation Aerosol (Less than 2%) 1041
Compazine 1505
▲ Copaxone for Injection (7%) 3306
▲ Cordarone Tablets (4% to 9%) 3487
Covera-HS Tablets (Less than 2%) 3199
Cozaar Tablets (Less than 1%) 2067
Crinone (Less than 5%) 3213
Crixivan Capsules (Less than 2%) 2070
Cytovene (At least 3 subjects) 2959
Daranide Tablets 2077
DaunoXome Injection (Less than or equal to 5%) 1442
Demerol 3079
▲ Demser Capsules (10%) 2085
▲ Depacon Injection (0.6% to 57%) 416
▲ Depakene (25% to 57%) 421
▲ Depakote Sprinkle Capsules (19% to 57%) 426
▲ Depakote Tablets (9% to 57%) 430
Depakote ER Tablets (1% to 5%) 436
Desoxyn Tablets 440
Dexedrine 1512
DextroStat Tablets 3236
Dilantin Infatabs (Rare) 2624
Dilantin Kapseals (Rare) 2622
Dilantin-125 Oral Suspension (Rare) 2625
Dilaudid Oral Liquid (Less frequent) 445
Dilaudid Tablets - 8 mg (Less frequent) 445
Dilaudid-HP (Less frequent) 443
Dipentum Capsules (Rare) 2803
Diprivan Injectable Emulsion (Less than 1%) 667
Duraclon Injection 3057
Duragesic Transdermal System (1% or greater) 1786
Duranest Injections 600
Dyazide Capsules 1515
Dynabac Tablets (0.1% to 1%) 2269
▲ Effexor Tablets (5% to 10.2%) 3495
▲ Effexor XR Capsules (5%) 3499
ELA-Max Cream 1340
Eldepryl Capsules 3266
Elspar for Injection 2092
Emla (Unlikely with cream) 602
EpiPen 1236
Eskalith 1527
Etrafon 3115
Evoxac Capsules (1% to 3%) 1217
▲ Exelon Capsules (4%) 2342
▲ Exelon Oral Solution (4%) 2345
▲ Felbatol (6.1%) 3343
Feldene Capsules (Occasional) 2685
Flexeril Tablets (Less than 1%) 572
Flexeril Tablets (Less than 1%) 2094
▲ Flolan for Injection (7% to 21%) 1528
Floxin I.V. (Less than 1%) 2526
Floxin Tablets (Less than 1%) 2529
Flumadine (Less than 0.3%) 1370
Fluothane Inhalation 3508
Foradil Aerolizer (1.9%) 2354
Fortovase Capsules (Less than 2%) 2970
Foscavir Injection (Between 1% and 5%) 605
▲ Gabitril Tablets (9%) 1189
Gammar-P I.V. 787
▲ Gengraf Capsules (13%) 457
Geodon Capsules (Frequent) 2688
▲ Glucotrol XL Extended Release Tablets (3.6%) 2693
Hivid Tablets (Less than 1%) 2975
Hyzaar 2109
Imdur Tablets (Less than or equal to 5%) 1826
Imitrex Injection (Infrequent) 1549
Imitrex Nasal Spray (Infrequent) 1554
Imitrex Tablets (Rare to infrequent) 1558
INFeD Injection 3388
Intron A for Injection (Less than 5%) 3120
Inversine Tablets 1850
Invirase Capsules (Less than 2%) 2979
Ionamin Capsules 1163
Isoptin SR Tablets (1% or less) 467
Kadian Capsules (Less than 3%) 1335
Kaletra Capsules (Less than 2%) 471
Kaletra Oral Solution (Less than 2%) 471
Keppra Tablets (1% or more) 3314
Klonopin Tablets (Infrequent) 2983
▲ Lamictal (3% to 4.4%) 1567
Lescol Capsules 2361
Lescol Capsules 2925
Lescol XL Tablets 2361
Lescol XL Tablets 2925
Leukeran Tablets (Rare) 1591
Levaquin (0.1% to less than 0.5%) 2537
Levoxyl Tablets 1819
Lexxel Tablets 608
Lidoderm Patch 1319
Limbitrol (Less common) 1738
Lithium Carbonate 3061
Lithium Citrate Syrup 3061
Lithobid Slow-Release Tablets 3255
Lodine XL Extended-Release Tablets (Less than 1%) 3530
Lodosyn Tablets 1251
Lotrel Capsules 2370
Loxitane Capsules 3398
▲ Luvox Tablets (25, 50, 100 mg) (5%) 3256
LYMErix Vaccine (Greater than 1%) 1592
Matulane Capsules 3246
▲ Maxair Autohaler (1.3% to 6.0%) 1981
▲ Maxair Inhaler (1.3% to 6.0%) 1984
Maxalt Tablets (Frequent) 2120
Maxalt-MLT Orally Disintegrating Tablets (Frequent) 2120
Mepergan Injection 3539
Meridia Capsules 481
Mevacor Tablets (0.5% to 1.0%) 2132
▲ Mexitil Capsules (12.6% to 13.2%) 1047
Midamor Tablets (Less than or equal to 1%) 2136
Migranal Nasal Spray (Infrequent) 2376
Mirapex Tablets (1% or more) 2834
Moban 1320
Mobic Tablets (Less than 2%) 1054
Moduretic Tablets 2138
Monopril Tablets (0.2% to 1.0%) 1091
Monopril HCT 1094
MS Contin Tablets (Less frequent) 2896
MSIR (Less frequent) 2898
Myobloc Injectable Solution (2% or greater) 1291
Narcan Injection 1322
Nardil Tablets (Common) 2653
Naropin Injection (Less than 1%) 612
Natrecor for Injection (At least 1%) 3189
▲ Neoral Soft Gelatin Capsules (12% to 55%) 2380
▲ Neoral Oral Solution (12% to 55%) 2380
Nesacaine/Nesacaine MPF 617
▲ Neurontin Capsules (6.8%) 2655
▲ Neurontin Oral Solution (6.8%) 2655
▲ Neurontin Tablets (6.8%) 2655
Nexium Delayed-Release Capsules (Less than 1%) 619
Nicotrol Nasal Spray (Under 5%) 2843
Norflex 1987
Noroxin Tablets 2145
Norpramin Tablets 755
Norvasc Tablets (More than 0.1% to 1%) 2704
Norvir Capsules (Less than 2%) 487
Norvir Oral Solution (Less than 2%) 487
Nubain Injection (1% or less) 1323
Oramorph SR Tablets (Less frequent) 3062
Orap Tablets (2.7%) 1407
▲ Orthoclone OKT3 Sterile Solution (13%) 2498
OxyContin Tablets (Less than 1%) 2912
▲ Pacerone Tablets (4% to 9%) 3331
Parnate Tablets 1607
▲ Paxil (5% to 14.7%) 1609
Periactin Tablets 2155
▲ Permax Tablets (4.2%) 1299
Phenergan Injection 3553
Phenergan 3556
Phenergan VC Syrup 3560
Phenergan VC with Codeine Syrup 3561
Polocaine Injection, USP 625
Polocaine-MPF Injection, USP 625
Ponstel Capsules (Occasional) 1356
Pravachol Tablets 1099
Prilosec Delayed-Release Capsules (Less than 1%) 628
Primacor Injection (0.4%) 3086
Primaxin I.M. 2158
Primaxin I.V. (Less than 0.2%) 2160
Prinivil Tablets (0.3% to 1.0%) 2164
Prinzide Tablets 2168
▲ Procardia Capsules (2% or less to 8%) 2708
▲ Procardia XL Extended Release Tablets (1% or less to 8%) 2710
▲ Prograf (48% to 56%) 1393
ProSom Tablets (Rare) 500
Prostin E2 Suppositories 2852
Protonix I.V. (Less than 1%) 3580
Protonix Tablets (Less than 1%) 3577
▲ Proventil Inhalation Aerosol (Less than 15%) 3142
▲ Proventil Inhalation Solution 0.083% (10.7% to 20%) 3146
▲ Proventil Repetabs Tablets (6% to 20%) 3148

▲ Proventil Solution for Inhalation 0.5% (10.7% to 20%) 3144
▲ Proventil HFA Inhalation Aerosol (7%) 3150
Provigil Tablets (1%) 1193
▲ Prozac Pulvules, Liquid, and Weekly Capsules (10% to 13%) 1238
Quinidex Extentabs (2%) 2933
▲ Rapamune Oral Solution and Tablets (21% to 31%) 3584
Reglan 2935
Relafen Tablets (Less than 1%) 1617
Remeron Tablets (2%) 2483
Remeron SolTab Tablets (2%) 2486
▲ Reminyl Oral Solution (3%) 1792
▲ Reminyl Tablets (3%) 1792
Requip Tablets (1% or more) 1621
Rescriptor Tablets (Less than 2%) 526
Retrovir Capsules 1625
Retrovir IV Infusion 1629
Retrovir 1625
Rilutek Tablets (Frequent) 772
▲ Risperdal (17% to 34%) 1796
Roferon-A Injection (Less than 0.5% to less than 3%) 2996
▲ Romazicon Injection (3% to 9%) 3000
Roxicodone Tablets (Less than 3%) 3067
Rynatan Tablets 3351
Rythmol Tablets – 150 mg, 225 mg, 300 mg (2%) 502
Salagen Tablets (2%) 2229
▲ Sandimmune (12 to 55%) 2388
Sandostatin Injection (Less than 1%) 2394
Sandostatin LAR Depot (1% to 4%) 2395
▲ Sarafem Pulvules (12%) 1962
Sedapap Tablets 50 mg/650 mg (Infrequent) 2225
Sensorcaine 643
Sensorcaine-MPF Injection 643
Serentil 1057
▲ Serevent Inhalation Aerosol (4%) 1633
▲ Serostim for Injection (1% to 10%) 3229
Serzone Tablets (2%) 1104
▲ Simulect for Injection (Greater than or equal to 10%) 2399
Sinemet Tablets 1253
Sinemet CR Tablets 1255
Sinequan (Infrequent) 2713
Soma Tablets 3353
Soma Compound Tablets (Infrequent or rare) 3354
Soma Compound w/Codeine Tablets (Infrequent or rare) 3355
Sonata Capsules (2%) 3591
Sporanox Capsules (2%) 1800
Stadol NS Nasal Spray (1% or greater) 1108
Stelazine 1640
Streptase for Infusion (1% to 4%) 647
Stromectol Tablets (0.9%) 2185
Sular Tablets (Less than or equal to 1%) 688
Surmontil Capsules 3595
Sustiva Capsules (Less than 2%) 1258
Symmetrel 1328
Synvisc 3596
Talacen Caplets (Rare) 3089
Talwin Nx Tablets (Rare) 3090
▲ Tambocor Tablets (4.7%) 1990
Tarka Tablets 508
Tasmar Tablets (Frequent) 3010
Tenex Tablets (Less frequent) 2942
Tequin Injection (0.1% to 3%) 1110
Tequin Tablets (0.1% to 3%) 1110
Teveten Tablets (Less than 1%) 3327
▲ Thalomid Capsules (4.2%) 1154
Theo-Dur Extended-Release Tablets 1835
Thioridazine Hydrochloride Tablets 2289
Thorazine 1656
Tiazac Capsules (Less than 2%) 1378
▲ Tonocard Tablets (2.9% to 21.6%) 649
▲ Topamax Sprinkle Capsules (8.8% to 13.8%) 2590
▲ Topamax Tablets (8.8% to 13.8%) 2590
Toradol (1% or less) 3018
Tranxene 511
Trental Tablets (0.3%) 784
▲ Trileptal Oral Suspension (3% to 16%) 2407
▲ Trileptal Tablets (3% to 16%) 2407
▲ Trisenox Injection (13%) 1158
Trovan (Less than 1%) 2722
TYPHIM Vi Vaccine 825
Ultracet Tablets (At least 1%) 2597
▲ Ultram Tablets (Less than 1% to 14%) 2600
Unithroid Tablets 3445
Valium Injectable 3026
Valium Tablets (Infrequent) 3047
Vantin Tablets and Oral Suspension (Less than 1%) 2860
▲ Vascor Tablets (0.5% to 6.98%) 2602
▲ Ventolin Inhalation Aerosol and Refill (Less than 1% to 15%) 1679
Verelan Capsules (1% or less) 3184
Verelan PM Capsules (2% or less) 3186
▲ Vesanoid Capsules (3%) 3037
Viagra Tablets (Less than 2%) 2732
Vicoprofen Tablets (Less than 1%) 520
Vistaril Capsules (Rare) 2738
Vistaril Intramuscular Solution (Rare) 2738
Vistaril Oral Suspension (Rare) 2738
Vistide Injection 1445
Vivactil Tablets 2217
Vivactil Tablets 2446
▲ Volmax Extended-Release Tablets (24.2%) 2276
Voltaren Tablets (Less than 1%) 2315
Voltaren-XR Tablets (Less than 1%) 2315
▲ Wellbutrin Tablets (21.1%) 1680
▲ Wellbutrin SR Sustained-Release Tablets (3% to 6%) 1684
▲ Xanax Tablets (4.0%) 2865
▲ Xopenex Inhalation Solution (6.8%) 3207
▲ Xylocaine Injections (Among most common) 653
Zanaflex Tablets (Infrequent) 1305
Zebeta Tablets 1885
▲ Zenapax for Injection (Greater than 5%) 3046
Zestoretic Tablets 695
Zestril Tablets (0.3% to 1.0%) 698
Ziac Tablets 1887
Zocor Tablets 2219
▲ Zofran Injection (7%) 1698
▲ Zofran (5%) 1703
▲ Zofran ODT Orally Disintegrating Tablets (5%) 1703
▲ Zoloft (5% to 11%) 2751
Zonegran Capsules (Frequent) 1307
Zosyn (1.0% or less) 1890
Zosyn in Galaxy Containers (1.0% or less) 1894
Zovirax Capsules 1706
Zovirax for Injection (Approximately 1%) 1708
Zovirax 1706
Zyban Sustained-Release Tablets (1% to 2%) 1710
▲ Zyprexa Tablets (Up to 20%) 1973
▲ Zyprexa ZYDIS Orally Disintegrating Tablets (Up to 20%) 1973
Zyrtec (Less than 2%) 2756
Zyrtec-D 12 Hour Extended Relief Tablets (Less than 2%) 2758

Tremulousness
(*see under* Tremors)

Trigeminal neuralgia
(*see under* Neuralgia, trigeminal)

Trigeminy
Digitek Tablets 1003
Lanoxicaps Capsules 1574
Lanoxin Injection 1581
Lanoxin Tablets 1587
Lanoxin Elixir Pediatric 1578
Lanoxin Injection Pediatric 1584
Rituxan for Infusion (One case) 1750
Rituxan I.V. (One case) 1428

Triglycerides, increase
(*see under* Hypertriglyceridemia)

Trismus
Ceftin Tablets (0.1% to 1%) 1898
Compazine 1505
Demser Capsules 2085
Duranest Injections (Rare) 600
Effexor Tablets (Frequent) 3495
Effexor XR Capsules (2%) 3499
Etrafon 3115
Geodon Capsules (Rare) 2688
Lodosyn Tablets 1251
Luvox Tablets (25, 50, 100 mg) (Rare) 3256
Paxil (Rare) 1609
Reglan 2935
Rilutek Tablets (Rare) 772
Serentil 1057
Sinemet Tablets 1253
Sinemet CR Tablets 1255
Sonata Capsules (Rare) 3591
Stelazine 1640
Thioridazine Hydrochloride Tablets 2289
Thorazine 1656
Trilafon 3160

Tubal damage
ParaGard T 380A Intrauterine Copper Contraceptive 2582

Tuberculosis
Campath Ampules 992
CellCept Capsules 2951
CellCept Intravenous 2951
CellCept Oral Suspension 2951
CellCept Tablets 2951
Enbrel for Injection 1752
Enbrel for Injection 3504

Tuberculosis, disseminated
Remicade for IV Injection (One patient) 1178

Tubulopathy
Orudis Capsules (Rare) 3548
Oruvail Capsules (Rare) 3548

Tumor flare
▲ Arimidex Tablets (3%) 659
Fareston Tablets 3237
Fortovase Capsules (Less than 2%) 2970
Gengraf Capsules (1% to less than 3%) 457
Invirase Capsules (Less than 2%) 2979
Neoral Soft Gelatin Capsules (1% to less than 3%) 2380
Neoral Oral Solution (1% to less than 3%) 2380
▲ Zoladex (23%) 702

Tumor lysis syndrome
Aloprim for Injection (Less than 1%) 2292
Ellence Injection 2806
Fludara for Injection (Up to 1%) 995
Leustatin Injection (Rare) 2495
Mylotarg for Injection 3540
Rituxan I.V. 1428

Tumors, malignant

T-wave flattening
(*see under* EKG changes, T-wave)

Twitching
Aciphex Tablets (Rare) 1267
Aciphex Tablets (Rare) 1783
Aloprim for Injection (Less than 1%) 2292
Anzemet Injection (Rare) 719
Anzemet Tablets (Rare) 722
Brevital Sodium for Injection, USP 1815
Cardura Tablets (Less than 0.5%) 2668
Cataflam Tablets (Less than 1%) 2315
Cerebyx Injection (Infrequent) 2619
Clozaril Tablets (Less than 1%) 2319
Cognex Capsules (Infrequent) 1351
Compazine 1505
Depacon Injection (1% to 5%) 416
Depakene (1% to 5%) 421
Depakote Tablets (1% to 5%) 430
Depakote ER Tablets (Greater than 1%) 436
Desoxyn Tablets 440
Dilantin Infatabs 2624
Dilantin Kapseals 2622
Dilantin-125 Oral Suspension 2625
Diprivan Injectable Emulsion (Less than 1%) 667
Duranest Injections 600
Effexor Tablets (1%) 3495
Effexor XR Capsules (2%) 3499
ELA-Max Cream 1340
Emla (Unlikely with cream) 602
Eskalith 1527
Gabitril Tablets (1% or more) 1189
Hivid Tablets (Less than 1%) 2975
Imitrex Tablets (Rare) 1558
Klonopin Tablets (Infrequent) 2983
Lamictal (Infrequent) 1567
Lidoderm Patch 1319
Lithium Carbonate 3061
Lithium Citrate Syrup 3061
Lithobid Slow-Release Tablets 3255
Luvox Tablets (25, 50, 100 mg) (Infrequent) 3256
Meridia Capsules 481
Mirapex Tablets (2%) 2834
Nardil Tablets (Common) 2653
Neurontin Capsules (1.3%) 2655
Neurontin Oral Solution (1.3%) 2655
Neurontin Tablets (1.3%) 2655
Nipent for Injection (Less than 3%) 3272
Norvasc Tablets (Less than or equal to 0.1%) 2704
Norvir Capsules (Less than 2%) 487
Norvir Oral Solution (Less than 2%) 487
OxyContin Tablets (Between 1% and 5%) 2912
Permax Tablets (1.1%) 1299
ProSom Tablets (Infrequent) 500
Remeron Tablets (Frequent) 2483
Remeron SolTab Tablets (Frequent) 2486
Retrovir Capsules 1625
Retrovir IV Infusion 1629
Retrovir 1625
Salagen Tablets (Less than 1%) 2229
Sensorcaine 643
Sensorcaine-MPF Injection 643
Seroquel Tablets (Infrequent) 684
Serzone Tablets (Infrequent) 1104
Stelazine 1640
Tambocor Tablets (Less than 1%) 1990
Tasmar Tablets (Infrequent) 3010
Trilafon 3160
Triostat Injection (1% or fewer) 1825
Vistide Injection 1445
Voltaren Tablets (Less than 1%) 2315
Voltaren-XR Tablets (Less than 1%) 2315
Wellbutrin SR Sustained-Release Tablets (1% to 2%) 1684
▲ Xylocaine Injections (Among most common) 653
Zebeta Tablets 1885
Ziac Tablets 1887
Zoloft (Infrequent to 2%) 2751
Zomig Tablets (Rare) 708
Zomig-ZMT Tablets (Rare) 708
Zonegran Capsules (Infrequent) 1307
Zyban Sustained-Release Tablets (Infrequent) 1710
Zyprexa Tablets (1% to 5%) 1973
Zyprexa ZYDIS Orally Disintegrating Tablets (1% to 5%) 1973
Zyrtec (Less than 2%) 2756
Zyrtec-D 12 Hour Extended Relief Tablets (Less than 2%) 2758

Twitching, lid muscle
Humorsol Sterile Ophthalmic Solution 2102
Neurontin Capsules (Infrequent) 2655
Neurontin Oral Solution (Infrequent) 2655
Neurontin Tablets (Infrequent) 2655
Salagen Tablets (Rare) 2229

Tympanic membrane perforation
Imdur Tablets (Less than or equal to 5%) 1826

Typhlitis
Adriamycin PFS/RDF Injection 2767
Taxol Injection (Rare) 1129

U

Ulceration
Adriamycin PFS/RDF Injection 2767
Aldara Cream, 5% (Up to 5%) 1978
Aplisol Injection 2609
Cerumenex Eardrops 2895
Condylox Gel (Less common) 2436
Condylox Topical Solution (Less than 5%) 2437
▲ Efudex (Among most frequent) 1733
Eulexin Capsules 3118
Heparin Lock Flush Solution 3509
Heparin Sodium Injection 3511
K-Tab Filmtab Tablets 470
Micro-K 3311
Norplant System 3543
Tine Test, Tuberculin, Old 3631
Tubersol Diagnostic Antigen 3628

Ulceration, tongue
Claritin-D 24 Hour Extended Release Tablets (Fewer than 2%) 3104
Evoxac Capsules (Less than 1%) 1217
Fortovase Capsules (Up to 3.8%) 2970
Hivid Tablets (Less than 1%) 2975
Invirase Capsules (Up to 3.8%) 2979
Rescriptor Tablets (Less than 2%) 526
▲ Serostim for Injection (1% to 10%) 3229
Soriatane Capsules (Less than 1%) 3003
Zoloft (Rare) 2751

Ulcers
Paxil (Rare) 1609
Remeron Tablets (Infrequent) 2483
Remeron SolTab Tablets (Infrequent) 2486
▲ Vesanoid Capsules (3%) 3037
Zoladex (1% to 5%) 702
Zoladex 3-month 706

Ulcers, anal
Hivid Tablets (Less than 1%) 2975

Ulcers, aphthous
Captopril Tablets (About 0.5% to 2%) 2281

Ulcers, corneal
Acular PF Ophthalmic Solution 544
Copaxone for Injection (Infrequent) 3306
FML Ophthalmic Ointment (Occasional) ⊙237
FML Ophthalmic Suspension (Occasional) ⊙236
FML Forte Ophthalmic Suspension (Occasional) ⊙235
Genoptic Ophthalmic Ointment ⊙239
Genoptic Sterile Ophthalmic Solution ⊙239
Luvox Tablets (25, 50, 100 mg) (Rare) 3256
Poly-Pred Liquifilm Ophthalmic Suspension ⊙245

Ulcers, cutaneous
Actiq (1% or greater) 1184
AmBisome for Injection (Less common) 1383
Amphotec (1% to 5%) 1774
Arava Tablets (1% to 3%) 724
Aricept Tablets (Infrequent) 1270
Aricept Tablets (Infrequent) 2665
Arthrotec Tablets (Rare) 3195

Avonex 1013
Betaseron for SC Injection 988
Bicillin C-R 900/300 Injection 2240
Bicillin C-R Injection 2238
Bicillin L-A Injection 2242
▲ CellCept Capsules (3%) 2951
▲ CellCept Intravenous (3%) 2951
▲ CellCept Oral Suspension (3%) 2951
▲ CellCept Tablets (3%) 2951
Cognex Capsules (Rare) 1351
Colazal Capsules 3069
Doxil Injection (Less than 1%) 566
▲ Duraclon Injection (5%) 3057
Enbrel for Injection 1752
Enbrel for Injection 3504
Eskalith 1527
Evoxac Capsules (Less than 1%) 1217
Exelon Capsules (Infrequent) 2342
Exelon Oral Solution (Infrequent) 2345
▲ Flolan for Injection (39%) 1528
Fortovase Capsules (Less than 2%) 2970
Foscavir Injection (Between 1% and 5%) 605
Gabitril Tablets (Infrequent) 1189
Gengraf Capsules 457
Herceptin I.V. (At least one of the 958 patients) 1414
Hivid Tablets (Less than 1%) 2975
Invirase Capsules (Less than 2%) 2979
Levaquin Injection (Less than 0.5%) 2537
Lipitor Tablets (Less than 2%) 2639
Lipitor Tablets (Less than 2%) 2696
Lithium Carbonate 3061
Lithium Citrate Syrup 3061
Lithobid Slow-Release Tablets 3255
Miacalcin Nasal Spray (Less than 1%) 2375
Mylocel Tablets (Less frequently) 2227
Naprelan Tablets (Less than 1%) 1293
Neoral Soft Gelatin Capsules 2380
Neoral Oral Solution 2380
Paxil (Rare) 1609
Permax Tablets (Infrequent) 1299
Plavix Tablets (1% to 2.5%) 1097
Plavix Tablets (1% to 2.5%) 3084
▲ Prograf (3% to 15%) 1393
Protonix I.V. (Less than 1%) 3580
Protonix Tablets (Less than 1%) 3577
Prozac Pulvules, Liquid, and Weekly Capsules (Infrequent) 1238
▲ Rapamune Oral Solution and Tablets (3% to 20%) 3584
Remeron Tablets (Rare) 2483
Remeron SolTab Tablets (Rare) 2486
Requip Tablets (Infrequent) 1621
Rilutek Tablets (Infrequent) 772
Risperdal (Rare) 1796
Salagen Tablets (Less than 1%) 2229
Sarafem Pulvules (Infrequent) 1962
▲ Serostim for Injection (1% to 10%) 3229
▲ Simulect for Injection (3% to 10%) 2399
▲ Soriatane Capsules (1% to 10%) 3003
Sular Tablets (Less than or equal to 1%) 688
Tricor Capsules, Micronized 513
Trovan (Less than 1%) 2722
Viagra Tablets (Less than 2%) 2732
Zanaflex Tablets (Frequent) 1305
Zyprexa Tablets (Infrequent) 1973
Zyprexa ZYDIS Orally Disintegrating Tablets (Infrequent) 1973

Ulcers, duodenal
Agrylin Capsules 3232
Ancobon Capsules 1730
Aricept Tablets (Infrequent) 1270
Aricept Tablets (Infrequent) 2665
Baycol Tablets 883
Betaseron for SC Injection 988
Campath Ampules 992
Celexa (Rare) 1365
Cognex Capsules (Rare) 1351
Copaxone for Injection (Infrequent) 3306
Dostinex Tablets (Rare) 2804
Exelon Capsules (Infrequent) 2342
Exelon Oral Solution (Infrequent) 2345
▲ Feldene Capsules (1% to 10%) 2685
Fosamax Tablets (Rare) 2095
Sterile FUDR 2974
Indocin Capsules (Less than 1%) 2112
Indocin I.V. (Less than 1%) 2115
Indocin (Less than 1%) 2112
Lipitor Tablets (Less than 2%) 2639
Lipitor Tablets (Less than 2%) 2696
Lodosyn Tablets 1251
Lupron Depot–3 Month 22.5 mg (Less than 5%) 3288
Meridia Capsules 481
Mobic Tablets (Less than 2%) 1054
Motrin Suspension, Oral Drops, Chewable Tablets, and Caplets (Less than 1%) 2002
Pentasa Capsules (Less than 1%) 3239
Pletal Tablets (Less than 2%) 2605
Pletal Tablets (Less than 2%) 2848
Proleukin for Injection (Less than 1%) 1199
Prozac Pulvules, Liquid, and Weekly Capsules (Rare) 1238
Relafen Tablets (Less than 1%) 1617
Sarafem Pulvules (Rare) 1962
Sinemet Tablets 1253
Sinemet CR Tablets 1255
Sonata Capsules (Rare) 3591
Tasmar Tablets (Rare) 3010
Taxotere for Injection Concentrate 778
Tricor Capsules, Micronized 513
Trileptal Oral Suspension 2407
Trileptal Tablets 2407
Trilisate (Rare) 2901
Vioxx (Less than 0.1%) 2213
Zonegran Capsules (Infrequent) 1307
Zosyn (1.3%) 1890
Zosyn in Galaxy Containers (1.3%) 1894

Ulcers, duodenal, hemorrhagic
Mobic Tablets (Less than 2%) 1054

Ulcers, esophageal
Actonel Tablets 2879
Copaxone for Injection (Infrequent) 3306
Declomycin Tablets 1855
Doxil Injection (Less than 1%) 566
Effexor Tablets (Rare) 3495
Fortovase Capsules (Less than 2%) 2970
Fosamax Tablets (1.5%) 2095
Herceptin I.V. (At least one of the 958 patients) 1414
Hivid Tablets (Less than 1%) 2975
Naprelan Tablets (Less than 1%) 1293
Nexium Delayed-Release Capsules (Less than 1%) 619
Pentasa Capsules (Less than 1%) 3239
Periostat Tablets 1208
Permax Tablets (Rare) 1299
Prozac Pulvules, Liquid, and Weekly Capsules (Rare) 1238
Sarafem Pulvules (Rare) 1962
Skelid Tablets 3088
Urobiotic-250 Capsules (Rare) 2731
Vioxx (Less than 0.1%) 2213
Zyprexa Tablets (Rare) 1973
Zyprexa ZYDIS Orally Disintegrating Tablets (Rare) 1973

Ulcers, gastric
Actonel Tablets 2879
Agrylin Capsules 3232
Amerge Tablets (Rare) 1467
Celexa (Rare) 1365
Evoxac Capsules (Less than 1%) 1217
Exelon Capsules (Infrequent) 2342
Exelon Oral Solution (Infrequent) 2345
Gengraf Capsules (1% to less than 3%) 457
Meridia Capsules 481
Mobic Tablets (Less than 2%) 1054
Neoral Soft Gelatin Capsules (1% to less than 3%) 2380
Neoral Oral Solution (1% to less than 3%) 2380
Nexium Delayed-Release Capsules (Less than 1%) 619
Plavix Tablets (Less than 1%) 1097
Plavix Tablets (Less than 1%) 3084
Pletal Tablets (Less than 2%) 2605
Pletal Tablets (Less than 2%) 2848
Remicade for IV Injection (Less than 2%) 1178
Requip Tablets (Infrequent) 1621
Sandostatin Injection (Less than 1%) 2394
Sandostatin LAR Depot (Rare) 2395
Skelid Tablets 3088
Thalomid Capsules 1154
Trileptal Oral Suspension 2407
Trileptal Tablets 2407
Vioxx (Less than 0.1%) 2213
Zonegran Capsules (Infrequent) 1307

Ulcers, gastrointestinal (Less than 5%)
Adriamycin PFS/RDF Injection 2767
Aggrenox Capsules (Less than 1%) 1026
Anaprox Tablets (Less than 1% to 4%) 2967
Anaprox DS Tablets (Less than 1% to 4%) 2967
Arthrotec Tablets 3195
Cataflam Tablets 2315
Clinoril Tablets 2053
Clozaril Tablets (Less than 1%) 2319
Cosmegen for Injection 2062
Dolobid Tablets 2088
Dostinex Tablets (Rare) 2804
EC-Naprosyn Delayed-Release Tablets (Less than 1% to 4%) 2967
Ecotrin Enteric Coated Aspirin Low, Regular and Maximum Strength Tablets 1715
Effexor Tablets (Infrequent) 3495
Effexor XR Capsules (Infrequent) 3499
Ergamisol Tablets 1789
Felbatol 3343
Fortovase Capsules (Less than 2%) 2970
Sterile FUDR 2974
Indocin Capsules (Less than 1%) 2112
Indocin I.V. (Less than 1%) 2115
Indocin (Less than 1%) 2112
Intron A for Injection (Less than 5%) 3120
K-Dur Microburst Release System ER Tablets 1832
Klor-Con M20/Klor-Con M10 Tablets 3329
K-Tab Filmtab Tablets 470
Lodine 3528
▲ Lodine XL Extended-Release Tablets (1% to 10%) 3530
Luvox Tablets (25, 50, 100 mg) (Infrequent) 3256
Micro-K 3311
Motrin Suspension, Oral Drops, Chewable Tablets, and Caplets (Less than 1% to 4%) 2002
▲ Naprelan Tablets (3% to 9%) 1293
Naprosyn Suspension (Less than 1% to 4%) 2967
Naprosyn Tablets (Less than 1% to 4%) 2967
Orudis Capsules (Less than 1%) 3548
Oruvail Capsules (Less than 1%) 3548
Paxil (Rare) 1609
Photofrin for Injection (Less than 5%) 831
Plavix Tablets (Less than 1%) 1097
Plavix Tablets (Less than 1%) 3084
▲ Ponstel Capsules (1% to 10%) 1356
Purinethol Tablets 1615
Relafen Tablets (1%) 1617
Rilutek Tablets (Infrequent) 772
Sandostatin Injection (Less than 1%) 2394
Sandostatin LAR Depot (Rare) 2395
Tolectin (Less than 1%) 2589
Toradol 3018
Trilisate (Less than 1%) 2901
Voltaren Tablets 2315
Voltaren-XR Tablets 2315
Wellbutrin Tablets (Rare) 1680
Zomig Tablets (Rare) 708
Zomig-ZMT Tablets (Rare) 708

Ulcers, intestinal
Cytovene 2959
Lodine (Less than 1%) 3528
Lodine XL Extended-Release Tablets (Less than 1%) 3530
Orudis Capsules (Less than 1%) 3548
Oruvail Capsules (Less than 1%) 3548

Ulcers, leg
Colazal Capsules 3069
Enbrel for Injection 1752
Enbrel for Injection 3504
Imdur Tablets (Less than or equal to 5%) 1826
Neurontin Capsules (Rare) 2655
Neurontin Oral Solution (Rare) 2655
Neurontin Tablets (Rare) 2655

Ulcers, oral mucosal
Aciphex Tablets 1267
Aciphex Tablets 1783
Actiq (Less than 1%) 1184
Advair Diskus 100/50 (1% to 3%) 1448
Advair Diskus 250/50 (1% to 3%) 1448
Advair Diskus 500/50 (1% to 3%) 1448
Alkeran for Injection (Infrequent) 1465
Alkeran Tablets (Infrequent) 1466
Amphotec (1% to 5%) 1774
▲ Arava Tablets (3%) 724
Asacol Delayed-Release Tablets 2884
Atrovent Inhalation Aerosol (Less frequent) 1030
Azactam for Injection (Less than 1%) 1276
Carbatrol Capsules 3234
Ceftin Tablets (0.1% to 1%) 1898
▲ CellCept Capsules (3%) 2951
▲ CellCept Intravenous (3%) 2951
▲ CellCept Oral Suspension (3%) 2951
▲ CellCept Tablets (3%) 2951
Cipro I.V. (1% or less) 893
Cipro I.V. Pharmacy Bulk Package (Less than 1%) 897
Clozaril Tablets 2319
Combivent Inhalation Aerosol 1041
Copaxone for Injection (Infrequent) 3306
Cuprimine Capsules (Some patients) 2075
Depakote ER Tablets (Greater than 1%) 436
Depen Titratable Tablets (Some patients) 3341
Doxil Injection (1% to 5%) 566
Dynabac Tablets (0.1% to 1%) 2269
Effexor Tablets (Infrequent) 3495
Effexor XR Capsules (Infrequent) 3499
Elmiron Capsules (Less than or equal to 1%) 570
▲ Enbrel for Injection (6%) 1752
▲ Enbrel for Injection (6%) 3504
Flovent Diskus (1% to 3%) 3614
Gabitril Tablets (1%) 1189
Hivid Tablets (Less than 1% up to 3.0%) 2975
Intron A for Injection (Less than 5%) 3120
Lamictal (Infrequent) 1567
Leukeran Tablets (Infrequent) 1591
Lipitor Tablets (Less than 2%) 2639
Lipitor Tablets (Less than 2%) 2696
Meridia Capsules 481
Naprelan Tablets (Less than 1%) 1293
Noroxin Tablets (Less frequent) 2145
Norvir Capsules (Less than 2%) 487
Norvir Oral Solution (Less than 2%) 487
Paxil (Infrequent) 1609
Pentasa Capsules (Less than 1%) 3239
ProAmatine Tablets (Rare) 3241
ProSom Tablets (Rare) 500
Protonix I.V. (Less than 1%) 3580
Protonix Tablets (Less than 1%) 3577
Provigil Tablets (1%) 1193
Prozac Pulvules, Liquid, and Weekly Capsules (Infrequent) 1238
▲ Rapamune Oral Solution and Tablets (3% to 20%) 3584
Rescriptor Tablets (Less than 2%) 526
Retrovir Capsules 1625
Retrovir IV Infusion 1629
Retrovir 1625
Sarafem Pulvules (Infrequent) 1962
Seroquel Tablets (Infrequent) 684
Serzone Tablets (Infrequent) 1104
Sonata Capsules (Infrequent) 3591
Sular Tablets (Less than or equal to 1%) 688
Tasmar Tablets (Infrequent) 3010
Tegretol/Tegretol-XR 2404
Tequin Injection (0.1% to 3%) 1110
Tequin Tablets (0.1% to 3%) 1110
Trizivir Tablets 1669
Vantin Tablets and Oral Suspension (Less than 1%) 2860
Vicoprofen Tablets (Less than 3%) 520
Vioxx (Greater than 0.1% to 1.9%) 2213
Viracept 532
Vistide Injection 1445
Wellbutrin SR Sustained-Release Tablets (Infrequent) 1684
Ziagen 1692
Zonegran Capsules (Rare) 1307
Zyban Sustained-Release Tablets (2%) 1710
Zyprexa Tablets (Infrequent) 1973
Zyprexa ZYDIS Orally Disintegrating Tablets (Infrequent) 1973

Ulcers, oropharyngeal
Fosamax Tablets 2095

Ulcers, peptic
Aricept Tablets (Infrequent) 1270
Aricept Tablets (Infrequent) 2665
Arthrotec Tablets (Rare) 3195
Atromid-S Capsules 3483
Betaseron for SC Injection 988
Campath Ampules 992
Captopril Tablets (About 0.5% to 2%) 2281
Cataflam Tablets (0.6% to 4%) 2315
▲ CellCept Capsules (3% to 10%) 2951
▲ CellCept Intravenous (3% to 10%) 2951
▲ CellCept Oral Suspension (3% to 10%) 2951
▲ CellCept Tablets (3% to 10%) 2951
Clinoril Tablets (Less than 1 in 100) 2053
Cognex Capsules (Infrequent) 1351
Colestid Tablets (Rare) 2791
Cortifoam Rectal Foam 3170
Cuprimine Capsules (Less than 1%) 2075
Dolobid Tablets (Less than 1 in 100) 2088
Effexor Tablets (Infrequent) 3495
Effexor XR Capsules 3499
Evoxac Capsules (Less than 1%) 1217
▲ Feldene Capsules (1% to 10%) 2685
Florinef Acetate Tablets 2250
Fosamax Tablets (Rare) 2095
Gengraf Capsules (1% to less than 3%) 457
Hydrocortone Tablets 2106
Hydrocortone Acetate Injectable Suspension 2103
Hydrocortone Phosphate Injection, Sterile 2105
Imdur Tablets (Less than or equal to 5%) 1826
Imitrex Injection (Rare) 1549
Imitrex Nasal Spray 1554
Imitrex Tablets (Rare) 1558
Indocin Capsules (Less than 1%) 2112
Indocin I.V. (Less than 1%) 2115
Indocin (Less than 1%) 2112
Lamictal (Rare) 1567
Lipitor Tablets (Less than 2%) 2639
Lipitor Tablets (Less than 2%) 2696
Lupron Depot 7.5 mg (Less than 5%) 3284
Lupron Injection (Less than 5%) 3279

Mexitil Capsules (About 8 in 10,000) 1047
Midamor Tablets (Rare) 2136
Moduretic Tablets 2138
Naprelan Tablets (Less than 1%) 1293
Neoral Soft Gelatin Capsules (1% to less than 3%) 2380
Neoral Oral Solution (1% to less than 3%) 2380
Neurontin Capsules (Rare) 2655
Neurontin Oral Solution (Rare) 2655
Neurontin Tablets (Rare) 2655
Niaspan Extended-Release Tablets 1846
Omnicef 493
Orudis Capsules (Less than 1%) 3548
Oruvail Capsules (Less than 1%) 3548
Paxil (Rare) 1609
Permax Tablets (Rare to infrequent) 1299
Pletal Tablets (Less than 2%) 2605
Pletal Tablets (Less than 2%) 2848
Prednisone 3064
Protonix I.V. (Less than 1%) 3580
Protonix Tablets (Less than 1%) 3577
Prozac Pulvules, Liquid, and Weekly Capsules (Infrequent) 1238
Relafen Tablets (0.3%) 1617
Requip Tablets (Infrequent) 1621
Sandimmune (2% or less) 2388
Sandostatin Injection (Less than 1%) 2394
Sandostatin LAR Depot (Rare) 2395
Sarafem Pulvules (Infrequent) 1962
Serzone Tablets (Infrequent) 1104
Solu-Medrol Sterile Powder 2855
Sonata Capsules (Rare) 3591
Ticlid Tablets (Rare) 3015
Tolectin (1% to 3%) 2589
Toradol 3018
Tricor Capsules, Micronized 513
Urso Tablets 836
Voltaren Tablets (0.6% to 4%) 2315
Voltaren-XR Tablets (0.6% to 4%) 2315
Wellbutrin SR Sustained-Release Tablets 1684
Ziac Tablets 1887
Zosyn (1.0% or less) 1890
Zosyn in Galaxy Containers (1.0% or less) 1894
Zyban Sustained-Release Tablets 1710

Ulcers, peptic, aggravation of
Eldepryl Capsules 3266
Niaspan Extended-Release Tablets 1846

Ulcers, peptic, hemorrhagic
Imdur Tablets (Less than or equal to 5%) 1826
Mobic Tablets (Less than 2%) 1054
Prozac Pulvules, Liquid, and Weekly Capsules (Rare) 1238
Sarafem Pulvules (Rare) 1962
Zoloft (Rare) 2751

Ulcers, peptic, reactivation of
Depen Titratable Tablets (Isolated cases) 3341
Didronel Tablets (A few patients) 2888

Ulcers, peptic with or without perforation
Asacol Delayed-Release Tablets (Rare) 2884
Cataflam Tablets (Approximately 1% to 4%) 2315
Cognex Capsules 1351
Didronel Tablets (One report) 2888
Lodine (Less than 1%) 3528
Lodine XL Extended-Release Tablets (Less than 1%) 3530
Voltaren Tablets (Approximately 1% to 4%) 2315
Voltaren-XR Tablets (Approximately 1% to 4%) 2315

Ulcers, peptic with perforation and hemorrhage
Anaprox Tablets (Approximately 1% to 4%) 2967
Anaprox DS Tablets (Approximately 1% to 4%) 2967
Cataflam Tablets (Approximately 1% to 4%) 2315
Celestone Soluspan Injectable Suspension 3097
Celestone Syrup 3099
Cortone Acetate Injectable Suspension 2059
Cortone Acetate Tablets 2061
Decadron Elixir 2078
Decadron Tablets 2079
Decadron Phosphate Injection 2081
Depo-Medrol Injectable Suspension 2795
EC-Naprosyn Delayed-Release Tablets (Approximately 1% to 4%) 2967
Hydrocortone Tablets 2106
Lodine (Less than 1%) 3528
Lodine XL Extended-Release Tablets (Less than 1%) 3530
Mobic Tablets (Less than 2%) 1054
Motrin Suspension, Oral Drops, Chewable Tablets, and Caplets (Less than 1%) 2002
Naprosyn Suspension (Approximately 1% to 4%) 2967
Naprosyn Tablets (Approximately 1% to 4%) 2967
Pediapred Oral Solution 1170
Prednisone 3064
Prelone Syrup 2273
Solu-Medrol Sterile Powder 2855
Voltaren Tablets (Approximately 1% to 4%) 2315
Voltaren-XR Tablets (Approximately 1% to 4%) 2315

Ulcers, vulvovaginal
Foscavir Injection (One case) 605
Hivid Tablets (Less than 1%) 2975

Unconsciousness
(*see under* Consciousness, loss of)

Underventilation
(*see under* Hypoventilation)

Unsteadiness
Ativan Injection 3478
▲ Ativan Tablets (3.4%) 3482
▲ Carbatrol Capsules (Among most frequent) 3234
Kadian Capsules 1335
Matulane Capsules 3246
Tambocor Tablets 1990
▲ Tegretol/Tegretol-XR (Among most frequent) 2404
Tonocard Tablets (Up to 1.2%) 649

Upper respiratory symptoms
▲ Alphagan Ophthalmic Solution (Approximately 3% to 9%) 545
▲ Bactroban Nasal (5%) 1495
Betapace Tablets (1% to 5%) 950
Engerix-B Vaccine (Less than 1%) 1517
▲ Neoral Soft Gelatin Capsules (13%) 2380
▲ Neoral Oral Solution (13%) 2380
Tarka Tablets (2.4%) 508
Varivax (Greater than or equal to 1%) 2202
▲ Vesanoid Capsules (63%) 3037
▲ Wellbutrin Tablets (5.0%) 1680

Uremia
(*see under* Azotemia)

Ureteral obstruction
Remicade for IV Injection (Less than 2%) 1178
Zoladex 702
Zoladex 3-month (Isolated cases) 706

Ureteral spasm
Dilaudid 441
Dilaudid Powder 441
Dilaudid Rectal Suppositories 441
Dilaudid Tablets 441
Hycodan 1316
Hycomine Compound Tablets 1317
Hycotuss Expectorant Syrup 1318
Lortab 3319
Lortab Elixir 3317
Maxidone Tablets CIII 3399
Norco 5/325 Tablets CIII 3424
Norco 7.5/325 Tablets CIII 3425
Norco 10/325 Tablets CIII 3425
Norco 10/325 Tablets CIII 3427
Tussionex Pennkinetic Extended-Release Suspension 1174
Vicodin Tablets 516
Vicodin ES Tablets 517
Vicodin HP Tablets 518
Vicodin Tuss Expectorant 519
Zydone Tablets 1330

Urethral disorder
Estring Vaginal Ring (At least 1 report) 2811
Evoxac Capsules (Less than 1%) 1217
Foscavir Injection (Between 1% and 5%) 605

Urethritis
Betaseron for SC Injection 988
Copaxone for Injection (Infrequent) 3306
Gabitril Tablets (Infrequent) 1189
Imitrex Injection 1549
Imitrex Nasal Spray 1554
Norvir Capsules (Less than 2%) 487
Norvir Oral Solution (Less than 2%) 487
Paxil (Rare to infrequent) 1609
Protonix I.V. (Less than 1%) 3580
Protonix Tablets (Less than 1%) 3577
Remeron Tablets (Rare) 2483
Remeron SolTab Tablets (Rare) 2486
Sonata Capsules (Rare) 3591
Tice BCG, BCG Live (1.2%) 2489
Valstar Sterile Solution for Intravesical Instillation (Less than 1%) 1175
Vistide Injection 1445

Uric acid level, increase
(*see under* Hyperuricemia)

Uricaciduria
▲ Lupron Depot–4 Month 30 mg (Greater than or equal to 5%) 3289
Permax Tablets (Rare) 1299

Urinary bladder, inflammation of
Amerge Tablets (Infrequent) 1467

Urinary bladder, irritability
Neosporin G.U. Irrigant Sterile 2256

Urinary bladder malignancies
Permax Tablets (Rare) 1299

Urinary calculi
Adalat CC Tablets (Less than 1.0%) 877

Urinary casts
▲ Priftin Tablets (3.9%) 758
Primaxin I.M. 2158
Primaxin I.V. 2160
Rocephin Injectable Vials, ADD-Vantage, Galaxy, Bulk (Less than 1%) 2993
Unasyn for Injection 2728
Uniretic Tablets (Less than 1%) 3178
Vistide Injection 1445

Urinary cytology, abnormal
Orthoclone OKT3 Sterile Solution 2498

Urinary difficulty
(*see under* Micturition, difficulty)

Urinary disturbances
Avapro Tablets (Less than 1%) 1074
Avapro Tablets (Less than 1%) 3076
Eldepryl Capsules 3266
▲ Lupron Depot 7.5 mg (12.5%) 3284
Lupron Depot–3 Month 11.25 mg 3285
▲ Lupron Depot–3 Month 22.5 mg (14.9%) 3288
▲ Lupron Depot–4 Month 30 mg (10.2% to 16.7%) 3289
▲ Neoral Soft Gelatin Capsules (24.2%) 2380
▲ Neoral Oral Solution (24.2%) 2380
TheraCys Injection 823
Trilafon (Occasional) 3160

Urinary findings, abnormal
Ceclor (Less than 1 in 200) 1905
Clozaril Tablets (2%) 2319

Urinary frequency
(*see under* Micturition disturbances)

Urinary glucose, false-positive
Augmentin Chewable Tablets 1482
Augmentin Powder for Oral Suspension 1482
Augmentin Tablets 1485
Ceclor 1905
Cedax 1021
Ceftin 1898
Ceptaz for Injection 1499
Fortaz 1541
Keflex 1237
Mefoxin for Injection 2124
Mefoxin Premixed Intravenous Solution 2127
Tazicef for Injection 1647
Tazicef Galaxy Container 1650
Tazicef Pharmacy Bulk Package 1653
Tazidime Vials, Faspak & ADD-Vantage 1966

Urinary hesitancy
Artane 1855
Dilaudid Oral Liquid 445
Dilaudid Tablets - 8 mg 445
Dilaudid-HP (Less frequent) 443
Ditropan XL Extended Release Tablets (2% to 5%) 564
Dolophine Hydrochloride Tablets 3056
Donnatal 2929
Donnatal Extentabs 2930
Donnatal Tablets 2929
Eldepryl Capsules 3266
Fludara for Injection (Up to 3%) 995
Kadian Capsules (Less than 3%) 1335
Levsin/Levsinex/Levbid 3172
Mexitil Capsules (Less than 1% or about 2 in 1,000) 1047
MS Contin Tablets (Less frequent) 2896
MSIR (Less frequent) 2898
Norflex 1987
NuLev Orally Disintegrating Tablets 3176
Numorphan 1324
Oramorph SR Tablets (Less frequent) 3062
▲ Paxil (3%) 1609
ProSom Tablets (Infrequent) 500
Retrovir Capsules 1625
Retrovir IV Infusion 1629
Retrovir 1625
Robinul Forte Tablets 1358
Robinul Injectable 2940
Robinul Tablets 1358
Roxanol 100 Concentrated Oral Solution 3066
Valium Injectable 3026
Valium Tablets (Infrequent) 3047

Urinary incontinence
Aciphex Tablets (Rare) 1267
Aciphex Tablets (Rare) 1783
Actiq (Less than 1%) 1184
Ambien Tablets (Infrequent) 3191
AmBisome for Injection (Less common) 1383
Amerge Tablets (Rare) 1467
Amphotec (1% to 5%) 1774
Androderm Transdermal System CIII (Less than 1%) 3377
Aricept Tablets (Frequent) 1270
Aricept Tablets (Frequent) 2665
Avonex 1013
Betaseron for SC Injection 988
Cardura Tablets (1%) 2668
Casodex Tablets (2%) 662
Celebrex Capsules (0.1% to 1.9%) 2676
Celebrex Capsules (0.1% to 1.9%) 2780
Celexa (Infrequent) 1365
▲ CellCept Capsules (3% to 10%) 2951
▲ CellCept Intravenous (3% to 10%) 2951
▲ CellCept Oral Suspension (3% to 10%) 2951
▲ CellCept Tablets (3% to 10%) 2951
Cerebyx Injection (Infrequent) 2619
Chirocaine Injection (1.2%) 2909
Claritin (At least one patient) 3100
Clozaril Tablets (1%) 2319
▲ Cognex Capsules (3%) 1351
Copaxone for Injection (At least 2%) 3306
Dantrium Capsules (Less frequent) 2885
Depacon Injection (1% to 5%) 416
Depakene (1% to 5%) 421
Depakote Sprinkle Capsules (1% to 5%) 426
Depakote Tablets (1% to 5%) 430
Depakote ER Tablets (Greater than 1%) 436
DepoCyt Injection (Less than 3%) 1197
D.H.E. 45 Injection 2334
Effexor Tablets (Infrequent) 3495
Effexor XR Capsules (Infrequent) 3499
Eskalith 1527
Estring Vaginal Ring (1% to 3%) 2811
Etrafon (Occasional) 3115
Evoxac Capsules (Less than 1%) 1217
Exelon Capsules (2% or more) 2342
Exelon Oral Solution (2% or more) 2345
▲ Felbatol (6.5%) 3343
Gabitril Tablets (Frequent) 1189
Gengraf Capsules (1% to less than 3%) 457
Gliadel Wafer (2%) 1723
Humorsol Sterile Ophthalmic Solution (Rare) 2102
Hytrin Capsules (At least 1%) 464
Intron A for Injection (Less than 5%) 3120
Klonopin Tablets (Infrequent) 2983
Lamictal (Infrequent) 1567
Lipitor Tablets (Less than 2%) 2639
Lipitor Tablets (Less than 2%) 2696
Lithium Carbonate 3061
Lithium Citrate Syrup 3061
Lithobid Slow-Release Tablets 3255
Lodosyn Tablets 1251
Lupron Depot–4 Month 30 mg (Less than 5%) 3289
Lupron Depot-PED 7.5 mg, 11.25 mg and 15 mg (Less than 2%) 3291
Lupron Injection (Less than 5%) 3279
Lupron Injection Pediatric (Less than 2%) 3280
Luvox Tablets (25, 50, 100 mg) (Infrequent) 3256
Megace Oral Suspension (1% to 3%) 1124
Mirapex Tablets (2.1%) 2834
Naprelan Tablets (Less than 1%) 1293
Naropin Injection (Less than 1%) 612
Neoral Soft Gelatin Capsules (1% to less than 3%) 2380
Neoral Oral Solution (1% to less than 3%) 2380
Neurontin Capsules (Infrequent) 2655
Neurontin Oral Solution (Infrequent) 2655
Neurontin Tablets (Infrequent) 2655
Ovidrel for Injection (Less than 2%) 3220
Parnate Tablets 1607
Paxil (Infrequent) 1609
Permax Tablets (Frequent) 1299

Polocaine Injection, USP ... 625
Polocaine-MPF Injection, USP ... 625
▲ Prograf (3% to 15%) ... 1393
ProSom Tablets (Rare) ... 500
Prozac Pulvules, Liquid, and Weekly Capsules (Infrequent) ... 1238
▲ Rapamune Oral Solution and Tablets (3% to 20%) ... 3584
Reglan ... 2935
Remeron Tablets (Infrequent) ... 2483
Remeron SolTab Tablets (Infrequent) ... 2486
Reminyl Oral Solution (Greater than or equal to 2%) ... 1792
Reminyl Tablets (Greater than or equal to 2%) ... 1792
ReoPro Vials (0.1%) ... 1958
Requip Tablets (2%) ... 1621
Rilutek Tablets (Infrequent) ... 772
Risperdal (Infrequent) ... 1796
Salagen Tablets (1% to 2%) ... 2229
Sarafem Pulvules (Infrequent) ... 1962
Sensorcaine ... 643
Sensorcaine-MPF Injection ... 643
Serentil ... 1057
Seroquel Tablets (Infrequent) ... 684
Serzone Tablets (Infrequent) ... 1104
Sinemet Tablets ... 1253
Sinemet CR Tablets ... 1255
Sonata Capsules (Infrequent) ... 3591
Tasmar Tablets (Frequent) ... 3010
▲ Temodar Capsules (8%) ... 3157
Tenex Tablets (3% or less) ... 2942
Tensilon Injectable ... 1745
Teveten Tablets (Less than 1%) ... 3327
▲ TheraCys Injection (6%) ... 823
Thioridazine Hydrochloride Tablets ... 2289
Tice BCG, BCG Live (2.4%) ... 2489
Topamax Sprinkle Capsules (Frequent) ... 2590
Topamax Tablets (Frequent) ... 2590
Travatan Ophthalmic Solution (1% to 5%) ... 543
▲ Trisenox Injection (5%) ... 1158
Trovan (Less than 1%) ... 2722
▲ Valstar Sterile Solution for Intravesical Instillation (7% to 22%) ... 1175
Viagra Tablets (Less than 2%) ... 2732
Vicoprofen Tablets (Less than 1%) ... 520
Vistide Injection ... 1445
Wellbutrin Tablets (Rare) ... 1680
Wellbutrin SR Sustained-Release Tablets ... 1684
Zoladex 3-month (1% to 5%) ... 706
Zoloft (Infrequent) ... 2751
Zonegran Capsules (Infrequent) ... 1307
Zosyn (1.0% or less) ... 1890
Zosyn in Galaxy Containers (1.0% or less) ... 1894
Zyban Sustained-Release Tablets ... 1710
Zyprexa Tablets (Frequent) ... 1973
Zyprexa ZYDIS Orally Disintegrating Tablets (Frequent) ... 1973
Zyrtec (Less than 2%) ... 2756
Zyrtec-D 12 Hour Extended Relief Tablets (Less than 2%) ... 2758

Urinary obstruction

Campath Ampules ... 992
Luvox Tablets (25, 50, 100 mg) (Infrequent) ... 3256
Salagen Tablets (Less than 1%) ... 2229
Tice BCG, BCG Live (0.3%) ... 2489

Urinary retention

Aceon Tablets (2 mg, 4 mg, 8 mg) (0.3% to 1%) ... 3249
Actiq (Less than 1%) ... 1184
Akineton ... 402
Ambien Tablets (Rare) ... 3191
Amphotec (1% to 5%) ... 1774
Anzemet Injection (2%) ... 719
Artane ... 1855
Astelin Nasal Spray ... 3339
▲ Astramorph/PF Injection, USP (Preservative-Free) (Approximately 90% of males; somewhat less in females) ... 594
Atrovent Inhalation Solution (Less than 3%) ... 1031
Atrovent Nasal Spray 0.03% ... 1032
Atrovent Nasal Spray 0.06% ... 1033
Avonex ... 1013
Benadryl Parenteral ... 2617
Betaseron for SC Injection ... 988
Brevibloc Injection (Less than 1%) ... 858
Buprenex Injectable (Less than 1%) ... 2918
Campath Ampules ... 992
Carbatrol Capsules ... 3234
▲ Casodex Tablets (2% to 5%) ... 662
Catapres Tablets (About 1 in 1,000 patients) ... 1037
Celexa (Infrequent) ... 1365
Cerebyx Injection (Infrequent) ... 2619
Cipro I.V. (1% or less) ... 893
Cipro I.V. Pharmacy Bulk Package (Less than 1%) ... 897
Cipro (Less than 1%) ... 887
Claritin (At least one patient) ... 3100
Claritin-D 12 Hour Extended Release Tablets (Less frequent) ... 3102
Claritin-D 24 Hour Extended Release Tablets (Fewer than 2%) ... 3104
Clorpres Tablets (About 1 in 1,000) ... 1002
Clozaril Tablets (1%) ... 2319
Cogentin ... 2055
Cognex Capsules (Infrequent) ... 1351
Combipres Tablets (About 1 in 1,000) ... 1040
Compazine ... 1505
Copaxone for Injection (At least 2%) ... 3306
Dantrium Capsules (Less frequent) ... 2885
Demerol ... 3079
Detrol Tablets (1.7%) ... 3623
Detrol LA Capsules ... 2801
Dilaudid ... 441
Dilaudid Oral Liquid ... 445
Dilaudid Powder ... 441
Dilaudid Rectal Suppositories ... 441
Dilaudid Tablets ... 441
Dilaudid Tablets - 8 mg ... 445
Dilaudid-HP (Less frequent) ... 443
Diprivan Injectable Emulsion (Less than 1%) ... 667
Ditropan XL Extended Release Tablets (2% to 5%) ... 564
Dolophine Hydrochloride Tablets ... 3056
Donnatal ... 2929
Donnatal Extentabs ... 2930
Donnatal Tablets ... 2929
Dopram Injectable ... 2931
Duraclon Injection (About 0.1%) ... 3057
▲ Duragesic Transdermal System (3% to 10%) ... 1786
Duramorph Injection (Frequent in males; less frequent in females) ... 1312
Effexor Tablets (1%) ... 3495
Effexor XR Capsules (Frequent) ... 3499
Eldepryl Capsules (1 of 49 patients) ... 3266
Etrafon (Occasional) ... 3115
Evoxac Capsules ... 1217
Exelon Capsules (Infrequent) ... 2342
Exelon Oral Solution (Infrequent) ... 2345
Extendryl ... 1361
Felbatol ... 3343
Flexeril Tablets (Less than 1%) ... 572
Flexeril Tablets (Less than 1%) ... 2094
Floxin I.V. (Less than 1%) ... 2526
Floxin Tablets (Less than 1%) ... 2529
Foscavir Injection (Between 1% and 5%) ... 605
Gabitril Tablets (Infrequent) ... 1189
Geodon Capsules (Infrequent) ... 2688
Halcion Tablets ... 2823
Haldol Decanoate ... 2535
Haldol Injection, Tablets and Concentrate ... 2533
Hivid Tablets (Less than 1%) ... 2975
Hycodan ... 1316
Hycomine Compound Tablets ... 1317
Hycotuss Expectorant Syrup ... 1318
Infumorph 200 and Infumorph 500 Sterile Solutions (Frequent) ... 1314
Innohep Injection (Greater than or equal to 1%) ... 1248
Inversine Tablets ... 1850
Kadian Capsules (Less than 3%) ... 1335
Klonopin Tablets (Infrequent) ... 2983
Lamictal (Infrequent) ... 1567
Levbid Extended-Release Tablets ... 3172
Levo-Dromoran ... 1734
Levsin/Levsinex/Levbid ... 3172
Limbitrol ... 1738
Lodosyn Tablets ... 1251
Lortab ... 3319
Lortab Elixir ... 3317
Loxitane Capsules ... 3398
Luvox Tablets (25, 50, 100 mg) (1%) ... 3256
Maxidone Tablets CIII ... 3399
Mepergan Injection ... 3539
Mexitil Capsules (Less than 1% or about 2 in 1,000) ... 1047
Mirapex Tablets (1% or more) ... 2834
Moban ... 1320
Motofen Tablets ... 577
MS Contin Tablets (Less frequent) ... 2896
MSIR (Less frequent) ... 2898
Naprelan Tablets (Less than 1%) ... 1293
Nardil Tablets (Less common) ... 2653
Naropin Injection (1% to 5%) ... 612
Neurontin Capsules (Infrequent) ... 2655
Neurontin Oral Solution (Infrequent) ... 2655
Neurontin Tablets (Infrequent) ... 2655
Norco 5/325 Tablets CIII ... 3424
Norco 7.5/325 Tablets CIII ... 3425
Norco 10/325 Tablets CIII ... 3425
Norco 10/325 Tablets CIII ... 3427
Norflex ... 1987
Normodyne Tablets (Less common) ... 3137
Norpramin Tablets ... 755
Norvir Capsules (Less than 2%) ... 487
Norvir Oral Solution (Less than 2%) ... 487
NuLev Orally Disintegrating Tablets ... 3176
Numorphan ... 1324
Oramorph SR Tablets (Less frequent) ... 3062
Organan Injection (2.0%) ... 2480
OxyContin Tablets (Less than 1%) ... 2912
Parnate Tablets ... 1607
Paxil (Infrequent) ... 1609
Pediazole Suspension ... 3050
Periactin Tablets ... 2155
Permax Tablets (Infrequent) ... 1299
Phenergan with Codeine Syrup ... 3557
Phenergan VC with Codeine Syrup ... 3561
Polocaine Injection, USP ... 625
Polocaine-MPF Injection, USP ... 625
Prevacid Delayed-Release Capsules (Less than 1%) ... 3292
PREVPAC ... 3298
▲ ProAmatine Tablets (Among most frequent) ... 3241
Proleukin for Injection (1%) ... 1199
Prosed/DS Tablets ... 3268
Prostin E2 Suppositories ... 2852
Provigil Tablets (1%) ... 1193
Prozac Pulvules, Liquid, and Weekly Capsules (Infrequent) ... 1238
▲ Rapamune Oral Solution and Tablets (3% to 20%) ... 3584
Remeron Tablets (Infrequent) ... 2483
Remeron SolTab Tablets (Infrequent) ... 2486
Reminyl Oral Solution (Infrequent) ... 1792
Reminyl Tablets (Infrequent) ... 1792
ReoPro Vials (0.4%) ... 1958
Rilutek Tablets (Infrequent) ... 772
Risperdal (Rare) ... 1796
Robinul Forte Tablets ... 1358
Robinul Injectable ... 2940
Robinul Tablets ... 1358
Roxanol 100 Concentrated Oral Solution ... 3066
Rynatan Tablets ... 3351
Sarafem Pulvules (Infrequent) ... 1962
Sensorcaine ... 643
Sensorcaine-MPF Injection ... 643
Serentil ... 1057
Seroquel Tablets (Infrequent) ... 684
Serzone Tablets (2%) ... 1104
▲ Simulect for Injection (3% to 10%) ... 2399
Sinemet Tablets ... 1253
Sinemet CR Tablets ... 1255
Sinequan ... 2713
Sonata Capsules (Rare) ... 3591
Stelazine ... 1640
Surmontil Capsules ... 3595
Symmetrel (0.1% to 1%) ... 1328
Tagamet (Rare) ... 1644
Talacen Caplets (Rare) ... 3089
Talwin Nx Tablets ... 3090
Tambocor Tablets (Less than 1%) ... 1990
Tasmar Tablets (Infrequent) ... 3010
Tegretol/Tegretol-XR ... 2404
Thioplex for Injection ... 1765
Thioridazine Hydrochloride Tablets ... 2289
Thorazine ... 1656
Tonocard Tablets (Less than 1%) ... 649
Topamax Sprinkle Capsules (Infrequent) ... 2590
Topamax Tablets (Infrequent) ... 2590
Toradol (1% or less) ... 3018
▲ Trasylol Injection (3%) ... 909
Tussionex Pennkinetic Extended-Release Suspension ... 1174
Ultracet Tablets (Less than 1%) ... 2597
Ultram Tablets (1% to 5%) ... 2600
Unasyn for Injection (Less than 1%) ... 2728
Uniretic Tablets (Less than 1%) ... 3178
Urimax Tablets ... 1769
Urised Tablets ... 2876
▲ Valstar Sterile Solution for Intravesical Instillation (4%) ... 1175
Viadur Implant (Less than 2%) ... 912
Vicodin Tablets ... 516
Vicodin ES Tablets ... 517
Vicodin HP Tablets ... 518
Vicodin Tuss Expectorant ... 519
Vicoprofen Tablets (Less than 1%) ... 520
Vioxx (Greater than 0.1% to 1.9%) ... 2213
Vistide Injection ... 1445
Vivactil Tablets ... 2217
Vivactil Tablets ... 2446
Wellbutrin Tablets (1.9%) ... 1680
Wellbutrin SR Sustained-Release Tablets ... 1684
Xanax Tablets ... 2865
Zanaflex Tablets (Infrequent) ... 1305
▲ Zenapax for Injection (2% to 5%) ... 3046
▲ Zofran Injection (3%) ... 1698
▲ Zofran (5%) ... 1703
▲ Zofran ODT Orally Disintegrating Tablets (5%) ... 1703
Zoladex 3-month (1% to 5%) ... 706
Zoloft (Infrequent) ... 2751
Zonegran Capsules (Infrequent) ... 1307
Zosyn (1.0% or less) ... 1890
Zosyn in Galaxy Containers (1.0% or less) ... 1894
Zyban Sustained-Release Tablets ... 1710
Zydone Tablets ... 1330
Zyprexa Tablets (Infrequent) ... 1973
Zyprexa ZYDIS Orally Disintegrating Tablets (Infrequent) ... 1973
Zyrtec (Less than 2%) ... 2756
Zyrtec-D 12 Hour Extended Relief Tablets (Less than 2%) ... 2758

Urinary sediment, abnormalities

Crixivan Capsules (Less than 2%) ... 2070
Dyazide Capsules ... 1515
Roferon-A Injection (Infrequent) ... 2996

Urinary tract, burning of

Rowasa Rectal Suspension Enema 4.0 grams/unit (60 mL) (0.61%) ... 3264

Urinary tract, obstruction

Cognex Capsules (Rare) ... 1351
Lupron Injection (Less than 5%) ... 3279
Zoladex (1% to 5%) ... 702
Zoladex 3-month (1% to 5%) ... 706

Urinary tract dilatation

Etrafon ... 3115
Limbitrol ... 1738
Norpramin Tablets ... 755
Surmontil Capsules ... 3595

Urinary tract disorder, unspecified

Amphotec (1% to 5%) ... 1774
▲ Casodex Tablets (2% to 5%) ... 662
▲ CellCept Capsules (3% to 10.6%) ... 2951
▲ CellCept Intravenous (3% to 10.6%) ... 2951
▲ CellCept Oral Suspension (3% to 10.6%) ... 2951
▲ CellCept Tablets (3% to 10.6%) ... 2951
▲ Cleocin Vaginal Cream (11%) ... 2788
▲ Leukine (14%) ... 1755
Lupron Depot 3.75 mg ... 3281
▲ Nilandron Tablets (7.2%) ... 753
Pravachol Tablets (0.7% to 2.4%) ... 1099
Protonix I.V. (Less than 1%) ... 3580
Protonix Tablets (Less than 1%) ... 3577
Tasmar Tablets (Infrequent) ... 3010
▲ Zenapax for Injection (2% to 5%) ... 3046
▲ Zoladex (13%) ... 702
Zoladex 3-month (1% to 5%) ... 706
Zyban Sustained-Release Tablets ... 1710

Urinary tract irritation

Orudis Capsules (Greater than 1%) ... 3548
Oruvail Capsules (Greater than 1%) ... 3548

Urinary urgency

Actiq (1% or greater) ... 1184
Adenoscan (Less than 1%) ... 1381
Amerge Tablets (Rare) ... 1467
Aricept Tablets (Infrequent) ... 1270
Aricept Tablets (Infrequent) ... 2665
Asacol Delayed-Release Tablets ... 2884
Avonex ... 1013
▲ Betaseron for SC Injection (4%) ... 988
▲ Casodex Tablets (2% to 5%) ... 662
Caverject Sterile Powder (Less than 1%) ... 2777
Clozaril Tablets (1%) ... 2319
Cognex Capsules (Infrequent) ... 1351
▲ Copaxone for Injection (10%) ... 3306
Effexor Tablets (Infrequent) ... 3495
Effexor XR Capsules (Infrequent) ... 3499
Gabitril Tablets (Infrequent) ... 1189
Isopto Carbachol Ophthalmic Solution (Frequent) ... ⊙215
Lexxel Tablets ... 608
Lipitor Tablets (Less than 2%) ... 2639
Lipitor Tablets (Less than 2%) ... 2696
Lupron Depot 7.5 mg (Less than 5%) ... 3284
▲ Lupron Injection (5% or more) ... 3279
Luvox Tablets (25, 50, 100 mg) (Infrequent) ... 3256
Neurontin Capsules (Rare) ... 2655
Neurontin Oral Solution (Infrequent) ... 2655
Neurontin Tablets (Rare) ... 2655
Nubain Injection (1% or less) ... 1323
Paxil (Infrequent) ... 1609
Plendil Extended-Release Tablets (0.5% to 1.5%) ... 623
▲ ProAmatine Tablets (Among most frequent) ... 3241
ProSom Tablets (Infrequent) ... 500
Prozac Pulvules, Liquid, and Weekly Capsules (Infrequent) ... 1238
Remeron Tablets (Rare) ... 2483
Remeron SolTab Tablets (Rare) ... 2486
Rilutek Tablets (Infrequent) ... 772
Salagen Tablets (Less than 1%) ... 2229
Sarafem Pulvules (Infrequent) ... 1962
Serzone Tablets (Infrequent) ... 1104
Sonata Capsules (Infrequent) ... 3591
▲ TheraCys Injection (18%) ... 823
Thyrel TRH for Injection ... 3630
▲ Tice BCG, BCG Live (5.8%) ... 2489

▲ Valstar Sterile Solution for Intravesical Instillation (27% to 57%) ... 1175
Viadur Implant (Less than 2%) ... 912
Wellbutrin SR Sustained-Release Tablets (Up to 2%) ... 1684
Zanaflex Tablets (Infrequent) ... 1305
Zomig Tablets (Infrequent) ... 708
Zomig-ZMT Tablets (Infrequent) ... 708
Zyban Sustained-Release Tablets (Infrequent) ... 1710

Urination, difficult
(*see under* Micturition, difficulty)

Urination, impaired
Actiq (1% or greater) ... 1184
AndroGel (Fewer than 1%) ... 3322

Urination, painful
(*see under* Micturition, painful)

Urine, abnormal
Aciphex Tablets ... 1267
Aciphex Tablets ... 1783
Ceclor CD Tablets ... 1279
Chirocaine Injection (1.8%) ... 2909
Crixivan Capsules (Less than 2%) ... 2070
Diprivan Injectable Emulsion (Less than 1%) ... 667
Evoxac Capsules (Less than 1%) ... 1217
Gengraf Capsules (1% to less than 3%) ... 457
Kaletra Capsules (Less than 2%) ... 471
Kaletra Oral Solution (Less than 2%) ... 471
Lamictal (Rare) ... 1567
Lithobid Slow-Release Tablets ... 3255
Naprelan Tablets (Less than 1%) ... 1293
Neoral Soft Gelatin Capsules (1% to less than 3%) ... 2380
Neoral Oral Solution (1% to less than 3%) ... 2380
▲ Novantrone for Injection (5% to 11%) ... 1760
Provigil Tablets (1%) ... 1193
Rilutek Tablets (Infrequent) ... 772
Soriatane Capsules (Less than 1%) ... 3003
Viracept ... 532

Urine, cells in
Accutane Capsules ... 2944
Merrem I.V. (Greater than 0.2%) ... 673
Sinemet Tablets ... 1253
TheraCys Injection (1%) ... 823
Zovirax for Injection (Less than 1%) ... 1708

Urine, color change
Adriamycin PFS/RDF Injection ... 2767
AK-Fluor Injection 10% and 25% ... ⊙ 202
Antabuse Tablets ... 3474
Azulfidine EN-tabs Tablets (Rare) ... 2775
Casodex Tablets ... 662
Cerubidine for Injection ... 947
Claritin (At least one patient) ... 3100
Claritin-D 12 Hour Extended Release Tablets ... 3102
Claritin-D 24 Hour Extended Release Tablets ... 3104
Clinoril Tablets (Less than 1%) ... 2053
▲ Comtan Tablets (10%) ... 2328
Coumadin for Injection ... 1243
Coumadin Tablets ... 1243
Desferal Vials ... 2333
Diprivan Injectable Emulsion (Less than 1%) ... 667
Eulexin Capsules ... 3118
Fluorescite Injection ... ⊙ 211
Klonopin Tablets (Infrequent) ... 2983
Lamisil Tablets ... 2360
Levlen ... 962
Levlite 21 Tablets ... 962
Levlite 28 Tablets ... 962
Lodosyn Tablets ... 1251
Maxzide ... 1008
MetroGel-Vaginal Gel (Less than 1%) ... 1986
Modicon ... 2563
▲ Mycobutin Capsules (30%) ... 2838
Nilandron Tablets ... 753
Nizoral Tablets ... 1791
Normodyne Injection ... 3135
Novantrone for Injection ... 1760
Ortho-Cyclen/Ortho Tri-Cyclen ... 2573
Ortho-Novum ... 2563
Ortho-Novum 1/50□28 Tablets ... 2556
Ortho-Novum ... 2563
Ortho-Cyclen/Ortho Tri-Cyclen ... 2573
Parafon Forte DSC Caplets (Rare) ... 2582
Priftin Tablets ... 758
Primaxin I.M. ... 2158
Primaxin I.V. (Less than 0.2%) ... 2160
Prosed/DS Tablets ... 3268
Pyrazinamide Tablets ... 1876
Rifadin ... 765
Rifater Tablets ... 769
Sectral Capsules ... 3589
Sinemet Tablets ... 1253
Sinemet CR Tablets ... 1255
Sporanox Capsules ... 1800
▲ Tasmar Tablets (2% to 7%) ... 3010
Ticlid Tablets ... 3015
Tri-Levlen ... 962
Urimax Tablets ... 1769
Urised Tablets ... 2876
Warfarin Sodium Tablets, USP ... 3302

Urine, fluorescence
AK-Fluor Injection 10% and 25% ... ⊙ 202

Urine, microscopic deposits
Carbatrol Capsules ... 3234
Tegretol/Tegretol-XR ... 2404

Urine, output low
(*see under* Hypouresis)

Urine, presence of RBC's
(*see under* Hematuria)

Urine, presence of urobilinogen
Primaxin I.M. ... 2158
Primaxin I.V. ... 2160

Urine flow decreased
Chirocaine Injection (1%) ... 2909
Evoxac Capsules (Less than 1%) ... 1217

Urolithiasis
Cosopt Sterile Ophthalmic Solution (Less than 1%) ... 2065
Crixivan Capsules (Less than 2%) ... 2070
Effexor Tablets (Rare) ... 3495
Effexor XR Capsules (Rare) ... 3499
Kytril Injection (Rare) ... 2986
Paxil (Rare) ... 1609
Permax Tablets (Infrequent) ... 1299
Tricor Capsules, Micronized ... 513
Trusopt Sterile Ophthalmic Solution (Rare) ... 2196
Vioxx (Less than 0.1%) ... 2213

Urticaria
Accolate Tablets ... 657
AccuNeb Inhalation Solution (0.9% to 1.7%) ... 1230
Accuretic Tablets ... 2614
Accutane Capsules ... 2944
Acel-Imune ... 1851
Aciphex Tablets ... 1267
Aciphex Tablets ... 1783
ActHIB Vaccine ... 798
Actiq (Less than 1%) ... 1184
Activase I.V. (Very rare) ... 1410
Adalat CC Tablets (Rare) ... 877
Adderall Tablets ... 3231
Adderall XR Capsules
Adipex-P ... 1406
Adriamycin PFS/RDF Injection (Occasional) ... 2767
Advair Diskus 100/50 (1% to 3%) ... 1448
Advair Diskus 250/50 (1% to 3%) ... 1448
Advair Diskus 500/50 (1% to 3%) ... 1448
Aerobid/Aerobid-M (1% to 3%) ... 1363
Aggrastat ... 2031
Aggrenox Capsules (Less than 1%) ... 1026
▲ Agrylin Capsules (8.3%) ... 3232
AK-Fluor Injection 10% and 25% ... ⊙ 202
Albenza Tablets (Rare) ... 1463
Albuminar-5, U.S.P. ... 785
Albuminar-25, U.S.P. ... 786
Aldoclor Tablets ... 2035
Aldoril Tablets ... 2039
Aleve Tablets, Caplets and Gelcaps ... ◙ 002
Alferon N Injection ... 1770
Alkeran for Injection ... 1465
Allegra (Rare) ... 712
Allegra-D Extended-Release Tablets (Rare) ... 714
Aloprim for Injection (Less than 1%) ... 2292
Altace Capsules (Less than 1%) ... 2233
Amaryl Tablets (Less than 1%) ... 717
Ambien Tablets (Rare) ... 3191
AmBisome for Injection (Less common) ... 1383
Amerge Tablets (Infrequent) ... 1467
Americaine Anesthetic Lubricant ... 1162
Americaine Otic Topical Anesthetic Ear Drops ... 1162
Amoxil Chewable Tablets ... 1471
Amoxil for Oral Suspension ... 1471
Amoxil ... 1471
Amphotec (1% to 5%) ... 1774
Anaprox Tablets (Less than 1%) ... 2967
Anaprox DS Tablets (Less than 1%) ... 2967
Ancobon Capsules ... 1730
Anzemet Injection (Rare) ... 719
Anzemet Tablets (Rare) ... 722
Arava Tablets (Rare) ... 724
Aricept Tablets (Frequent) ... 1270
Aricept Tablets (Frequent) ... 2665
Arthrotec Tablets (Rare) ... 3195
Asacol Delayed-Release Tablets ... 2884
Astramorph/PF Injection, USP (Preservative-Free) ... 594
Atacand HCT Tablets ... 597
Atromid-S Capsules (Less often) ... 3483
Atrovent Inhalation Aerosol ... 1030
Atrovent Inhalation Solution (Less than 3%) ... 1031
Atrovent Nasal Spray 0.06% (Rare) ... 1033
Attenuvax (Rare) ... 2044
▲ Augmentin Chewable Tablets (3%) ... 1482
▲ Augmentin Powder for Oral Suspension (3%) ... 1482
▲ Augmentin Tablets (3%) ... 1485
Augmentin ES-600 Powder for Oral Suspension ... 1487
Avalide Tablets (Rare) ... 1070
Avapro Tablets (Rare) ... 1074
Avapro Tablets (Less than 1%) ... 3076
Avelox Tablets (0.05% to 1%) ... 879
▲ Avonex (5%) ... 1013
Axid Pulvules (More frequent) ... 1903
Axid Pulvules (More frequent) ... 2919
Aygestin Tablets ... 1333
Azactam for Injection (Less than 1%) ... 1276
Azmacort Inhalation Aerosol (Rare) ... 728
Azopt Ophthalmic Suspension (Less than 1%) ... 536
▲ Azulfidine EN-tabs Tablets (Less frequent) ... 2775
▲ Bactrim (Among most common) ... 2949
Bactroban Cream (One report) ... 1494
Baycol Tablets (Rare) ... 883
BayGam ... 914
BayHep B ... 915
Bebulin VH ... 840
Beconase Inhalation Aerosol (Rare) ... 1497
Beconase AQ Nasal Spray (Rare) ... 1498
Benadryl Parenteral ... 2617
BeneFix for Injection (One case) ... 1432
Betagan (Rare) ... ⊙ 228
Betaseron for SC Injection ... 988
Betimol Ophthalmic Solution ... ⊙ 324
Betoptic S Ophthalmic Suspension (Rare) ... 537
Biaxin/Biaxin XL ... 403
Bicillin C-R 900/300 Injection ... 2240
Bicillin C-R Injection ... 2238
Bicillin L-A Injection ... 2242
Biltricide Tablets (Rare) ... 887
Brevital Sodium for Injection, USP ... 1815
Buminate 5% Solution, USP (Occasional) ... 841
Buminate 25% Solution, USP (Occasional) ... 842
Buprenex Injectable (Rare) ... 2918
▲ Campath Ampules (5% to 30%) ... 992
Carafate Suspension ... 731
Carafate Tablets ... 730
Carbatrol Capsules ... 3234
Cardizem Injectable ... 1018
Cardizem Lyo-Ject Syringe ... 1018
Cardizem Monovial ... 1018
Cardizem CD Capsules (Less than 1%) ... 1016
Cataflam Tablets (Less than 1%) ... 2315
Catapres Tablets (About 5 in 1,000 patients) ... 1037
Catapres-TTS (2 cases of 3,539 patients) ... 1038
Ceclor CD Tablets (0.1% to 1%) ... 1279
Ceclor (Less than 1 in 200) ... 1905
Cedax (0.1% to 1%) ... 1021
Cefotan ... 664
Ceftin (0.1% to 1%) ... 1898
Cefzil (0.1%) ... 1076
Celebrex Capsules (0.1% to 1.9%) ... 2676
Celebrex Capsules (0.1% to 1.9%) ... 2780
Celexa (Infrequent) ... 1365
Ceptaz for Injection ... 1499
Cerebyx Injection (Infrequent) ... 2619
▲ Cerezyme for Injection (Approximately 4%) ... 1438
Chibroxin Sterile Ophthalmic Solution ... 2051
Chloroptic Sterile Ophthalmic Ointment ... ⊙ 234
Chloroptic Sterile Ophthalmic Solution ... ⊙ 235
Cipro HC Otic Suspension (One patient) ... 540
Cipro I.V. (1% or less) ... 893
Cipro I.V. Pharmacy Bulk Package (Less than 1%) ... 897
Cipro (Less than 1%) ... 887
Claforan Injection (Less frequent) ... 732
Claritin (At least one patient) ... 3100
Claritin-D 12 Hour Extended Release Tablets (Less frequent) ... 3102
Claritin-D 24 Hour Extended Release Tablets (Fewer than 2%) ... 3104
Cleocin HCl Capsules ... 2784
Cleocin Phosphate Sterile Solution ... 2785
Cleocin Vaginal Cream (Less than 1%) ... 2788
Cleocin Vaginal Ovules ... 2789
Clorpres Tablets (About 5 in 1,000) ... 1002
Clozaril Tablets (Less than 1%) ... 2319
▲ Cognex Capsules (7%) ... 1351
Colestid Tablets (Rare) ... 2791
Coly-Mycin M Parenteral ... 2243
Colyte with Flavor Packs for Oral Solution (Isolated cases) ... 3170
Combipres Tablets (About 5 in 1,000) ... 1040
Combivent Inhalation Aerosol (Less than 2%; rare) ... 1041
Combivir Tablets ... 1502
Compazine ... 1505
Comvax ... 2056
Concerta Extended-Release Tablets ... 1998
Concerta Tablets ... 561
▲ Copaxone for Injection (5%) ... 3306
Cortone Acetate Injectable Suspension ... 2059
Cortone Acetate Tablets ... 2061
Corzide 40/5 Tablets ... 2247
Corzide 80/5 Tablets ... 2247
Cosopt Sterile Ophthalmic Solution ... 2065
Coumadin for Injection (Infrequent) ... 1243
Coumadin Tablets (Infrequent) ... 1243
Covera-HS Tablets (Less than 2%) ... 3199
Cozaar Tablets (Less than 1%) ... 2067
Crinone (Less than 5%) ... 3213
Crixivan Capsules (Less than 2%) ... 2070
Cuprimine Capsules ... 2075
Cutivate Ointment (Less than 1%) ... 1284
Dantrium Capsules (Less frequent) ... 2885
Dantrium Intravenous (Rare) ... 2886
Decadron Elixir ... 2078
Decadron Tablets ... 2079
Decadron Phosphate Injection ... 2081
Declomycin Tablets ... 1855
Demerol ... 3079
Demser Capsules (Rare) ... 2085
Depen Titratable Tablets ... 3341
Dermatop Emollient Cream (Less than 1%) ... 2517
Desferal Vials ... 2333
Desoxyn Tablets ... 440
Dexedrine ... 1512
DextroStat Tablets ... 3236
D.H.E. 45 Injection ... 2334
DiaBeta Tablets (1.5%) ... 741
Diabinese Tablets (Approximately 1% or less) ... 2680
Diamox Intravenous (Occasional) ... ⊙ 269
Diamox Sequels Sustained Release Capsules ... ⊙ 270
Diamox Tablets (Occasional) ... ⊙ 269
Didronel Tablets ... 2888
Dilaudid Oral Liquid ... 445
Dilaudid Tablets - 8 mg ... 445
Dilaudid-HP (Less frequent) ... 443
Diovan HCT Tablets ... 2338
Diphtheria & Tetanus Toxoids Adsorbed Purogenated for Pediatric Use ... 1857
Diprivan Injectable Emulsion (Less than 1%) ... 667
Diucardin Tablets ... 3494
Diuril Oral ... 2087
Diuril Sodium Intravenous ... 2086
Dolobid Tablets (Less than 1 in 100) ... 2088
Dolophine Hydrochloride Tablets ... 3056
Donnatal ... 2929
Donnatal Extentabs ... 2930
Donnatal Tablets ... 2929
Doryx Coated Pellet Filled Capsules ... 3357
Doxil Injection (1% to 5%) ... 566
DuoNeb Inhalation Solution (0.3%) ... 1233
Duraclon Injection (0.5%) ... 3057
Duramorph Injection ... 1312
Duranest Injections ... 600
Duricef ... 1079
Dyazide Capsules ... 1515
Dynabac Tablets (0.5% to 1.2%) ... 2269
Dynacin Capsules ... 2019
DynaCirc Capsules (0.5% to 1%) ... 2921
DynaCirc CR Tablets (0.5% to 1%) ... 2923
EC-Naprosyn Delayed-Release Tablets (Less than 1%) ... 2967
Ecotrin Enteric Coated Aspirin Low, Regular and Maximum Strength Tablets ... 1715
E.E.S. ... 450
Effexor Tablets (Infrequent) ... 3495
Effexor XR Capsules ... 3499
Efudex ... 1733
8-MOP Capsules ... 1727
ELA-Max Cream ... 1340
ELA-Max 5 Cream ... 1340
Ellence Injection ... 2806
Elmiron Capsules (Less than or equal to 1%) ... 570
Elspar for Injection ... 2092
Emla ... 602
Enalaprilat Injection ... 863
Enbrel for Injection ... 1752
Enbrel for Injection ... 3504
Engerix-B Vaccine (Less than 1%) ... 1517
Epivir ... 1520
Epivir-HBV ... 1524

Epogen for Injection (Rare) 582
Ergamisol Tablets (Less than 1%) 1789
EryPed 446
Ery-Tab Tablets 448
Erythrocin Stearate Filmtab Tablets 452
Erythromycin Base Filmtab Tablets 454
Erythromycin Delayed-Release Capsules, USP 455
Ethyol for Injection 2029
Etrafon 3115
Evoxac Capsules (Less than 1%) 1217
Exelon Capsules (Infrequent) 2342
Exelon Oral Solution (Infrequent) 2345
Factrel (Rare) 3633
Famotidine Injection (Infrequent) 866
Famvir Tablets (Infrequent) 2348
Feiba VH 843
Felbatol (Infrequent) 3343
Feldene Capsules (Rare) 2685
Flexeril Tablets (Less than 1%) 572
Flexeril Tablets (Less than 1%) 2094
▲ Flolan for Injection (25%) 1528
Flomax Capsules 1044
Flonase Nasal Spray (Less than 1%) 1533
Florinef Acetate Tablets 2250
Flovent Diskus 3614
Flovent (Rare) 1535
Flovent Rotadisk (1% to 3%) 1537
Floxin I.V. (Less than 1%) 2526
Floxin Otic Solution (Single report) 1219
Floxin Tablets (Less than 1%) 2529
Fluorescite Injection (Very rare) ⊙ 211
FluShield Influenza Vaccine (Rare) 3521
Fluzone Vaccine (Rare) 802
Follistim for Injection 2465
Fortaz 1541
Fortovase Capsules (Less than 2%) 2970
Fosamax Tablets 2095
Furosemide Tablets 2284
Gabitril Tablets (Infrequent) 1189
Gamimune N, 10% Solvent/Detergent Treated (A single incidence) 928
Gammagard S/D (Occasional) 845
Gastrocrom Oral Concentrate (Less common) 1162
Gengraf Capsules (1% to less than 3%) 457
Geocillin Tablets (Infrequent) 2687
Geodon Capsules (Infrequent) 2688
▲ Geref for Injection (1 patient in 6) 3215
Glucagon for Injection Vials and Emergency Kit 1924
Glucotrol Tablets (About 1 in 70) 2692
Glucotrol XL Extended Release Tablets (Less than 1%) 2693
GoLYTELY and Pineapple Flavor GoLYTELY for Oral Solution (Isolated cases) 1068
Grifulvin V Tablets Microsize and Oral Suspension Microsize (Occasional) 2518
Gris-PEG Tablets 2661
Havrix Vaccine (Less than 1%) 1544
Hemofil M (Extremely rare) 847
Heparin Lock Flush Solution 3509
Heparin Sodium Injection 3511
HibTITER 1859
Hivid Tablets (Less than 1% to 3.4%) 2975
Humate-P Concentrate 790
Hycamtin for Injection (Less than 1%) 1546
Hydrocortone Tablets 2106
Hydrocortone Acetate Injectable Suspension 2103
Hydrocortone Phosphate Injection, Sterile 2105
HydroDIURIL Tablets 2108
Hyzaar 2109
IC-Green ⊙ 203
Idamycin PFS Injection 2825
Imitrex Injection 1549
Imitrex Nasal Spray 1554
Imitrex Tablets 1558
Imogam Rabies - HT 805
IMUPlus Formula 3274
Inderide Tablets 3517
Inderide LA Long-Acting Capsules 3519
Indocin Capsules (Less than 1%) 2112
Indocin I.V. (Less than 1%) 2115
Indocin (Less than 1%) 2112
INFeD Injection 3388
Infumorph 200 and Infumorph 500 Sterile Solutions 1314
Intron A for Injection (Rare; Less than 5%) 3120
Invirase Capsules (Less than 2%) 2979
Ionamin Capsules 1163
Isoptin SR Tablets (1% or less) 467
JE-VAX Vaccine 811
Keflex 1237
Kefurox Vials, ADD-Vantage (Less than 1 in 250) 1948
Kytril Tablets (Rare) 2988
Lamictal (Infrequent) 1567
Lamisil Tablets (1.1%) 2360
Lescol Capsules (Rare) 2361
Lescol Capsules (Rare) 2925
Lescol XL Tablets 2361
Lescol XL Tablets 2925
Leukeran Tablets 1591
Leustatin Injection 2495
Levaquin (0.1% to less than 0.5%) 2537
Levbid Extended-Release Tablets 3172
Levo-Dromoran 1734
▲ Levorphanol Tartrate Tablets (3% to 9%) 3059
Levoxyl Tablets 1819
Levsin/Levsinex/Levbid 3172
Lexxel Tablets 608
Lidoderm Patch (Rare) 1319
Limbitrol 1738
Lipitor Tablets (Less than 2%) 2639
Lipitor Tablets (Less than 2%) 2696
Lodine (Less than 1%) 3528
Lodine XL Extended-Release Tablets (Less than 1%) 3530
Lodosyn Tablets 1251
Lopid Tablets 2650
Lorabid Suspension and Pulvules 2251
Lotensin HCT Tablets 2367
Lotrimin 3128
Lotrisone 3129
Lovenox Injection 746
Lupron Depot 3.75 mg 3281
Lupron Depot 7.5 mg 3284
Lupron Depot–3 Month 11.25 mg 3285
Lupron Depot–3 Month 22.5 mg 3288
Lupron Depot–4 Month 30 mg 3289
Lupron Depot-PED 7.5 mg, 11.25 mg and 15 mg 3291
Luvox Tablets (25, 50, 100 mg) (Infrequent) 3256
LYMErix Vaccine (Very rare) 1592
Macrobid Capsules (Less than 1%) 2889
Macrodantin Capsules 2891
Mandol Vials 1953
Matulane Capsules 3246
Maxalt Tablets (Infrequent) 2120
Maxalt-MLT Orally Disintegrating Tablets (Infrequent) 2120
Maxipime for Injection (0.1% to 1%) 1285
Maxzide 1008
Mefoxin for Injection 2124
Mefoxin Premixed Intravenous Solution 2127
Mepergan Injection 3539
Meridia Capsules 481
Merrem I.V. (0.1% to 1.0%) 673
Meruvax II 2130
Metadate CD Capsules 1164
Metadate ER Tablets 1167
Methylin Tablets 1995
Methylin ER Tablets 1995
Mevacor Tablets (Rare) 2132
Micardis HCT Tablets 1051
Microzide Capsules 3414
Migranal Nasal Spray (Rare) 2376
Minipress Capsules 2699
Minizide Capsules 2700
Minocin Intravenous 1862
Minocin Oral Suspension 1865
Minocin Pellet-Filled Capsules 1863
MiraLax Powder for Oral Solution (Occasional) 1069
M-M-R II 2118
Mobic Tablets (Less than 2%) 1054
Moduretic Tablets 2138
Monodox Capsules 2442
Mononine Concentrate 794
Monopril Tablets (0.2% to 1.0%) 1091
Monopril HCT 1094
Motofen Tablets 577
Children's Motrin Oral Suspension and Chewable Tablets 2006
Children's Motrin Cold Oral Suspension 2007
Children's Motrin Oral Suspension ▣ 643
Motrin Suspension, Oral Drops, Chewable Tablets, and Caplets (Less than 1%) 2002
Infants' Motrin Concentrated Drops 2006
Junior Strength Motrin Caplets and Chewable Tablets 2006
Motrin IB Tablets, Caplets, and Gelcaps 2002
Motrin Sinus Headache Caplets 2005
MS Contin Tablets (Less frequent) 2896
MSIR (Less frequent) 2898
Mumpsvax (Extremely rare) 2141
Mykrox Tablets 1168
Myleran Tablets 1603
Naprelan Tablets (Less than 1%) 1293
Naprosyn Suspension (Less than 1%) 2967
Naprosyn Tablets (Less than 1%) 2967
Naropin Injection (Less than 1%) 612
Navane Oral 2701
Navane Intramuscular 2703
Navelbine Injection 1604
Nebcin Vials, Hyporets & ADD-Vantage 1955
Neoral Soft Gelatin Capsules (1% to less than 3%) 2380
Neoral Oral Solution (1% to less than 3%) 2380
Neptazane Tablets ⊙ 271
Nesacaine/Nesacaine MPF 617
Neupogen for Injection 587
Neurontin Capsules (Infrequent) 2655
Neurontin Oral Solution (Infrequent) 2655
Neurontin Tablets (Infrequent) 2655
Nexium Delayed-Release Capsules (Less than 1%) 619
Niaspan Extended-Release Tablets 1846
▲ Nipent for Injection (3% to 10%) 3272
Nizoral Tablets (Several cases) 1791
Norflex (Rare) 1987
Normodyne Injection (Rare) 3135
Normodyne Tablets (Rare) 3137
Noroxin Tablets (Less frequent) 2145
Norplant System 3543
Norpramin Tablets 755
Norvasc Tablets (Less than or equal to 0.1%) 2704
Norvir Capsules (Less than 2%) 487
Norvir Oral Solution (Less than 2%) 487
Novantrone for Injection (Occasional) 1760
Nubain Injection (1% or less) 1323
NuLev Orally Disintegrating Tablets 3176
NuLYTELY, Cherry Flavor, Lemon-Lime Flavor, and Orange Flavor NuLYTELY for Oral Solution (Isolated cases) 1068
Numorphan 1324
▲ Oncaspar (Greater than 5%) 756
Oramorph SR Tablets (Less frequent) 3062
Organidin NR Liquid (Rare) 3350
Organidin NR Tablets (Rare) 3350
Orthoclone OKT3 Sterile Solution 2498
Orudis Capsules (Less than 1%) 3548
Oruvail Capsules (Less than 1%) 3548
Oxsoralen-Ultra Capsules 1741
ParaGard T 380A Intrauterine Copper Contraceptive 2582
Paraplatin for Injection 1126
Parnate Tablets 1607
Paxil (Infrequent) 1609
PCE Dispertab Tablets 498
Pediazole Suspension 3050
Liquid PedvaxHIB (Two children) 2148
PEG-Intron Powder for Injection (Less than or equal to 1%) 3140
Pentasa Capsules (Less than 1%) 3239
Pepcid Injection (Infrequent) 2153
Pepcid for Oral Suspension (Infrequent) 2150
Pepcid RPD Orally Disintegrating Tablets (Infrequent) 2150
Pepcid Tablets (Infrequent) 2150
Pergonal for Injection 3223
Periactin Tablets 2155
Periostat Tablets 1208
Permapen Isoject 2706
Pfizerpen for Injection 2707
Phenergan Injection 3553
Phenergan 3556
Phenergan with Codeine Syrup 3557
Phenergan VC with Codeine Syrup 3561
Pima Syrup 1362
Plaquenil Tablets 3082
Plasbumin-5 (Rare) 939
Plasbumin-20 (Rare) 940
Plasbumin-25 (Rare) 941
Plasmanate (Occasional) 942
Plavix Tablets (Less than 1%) 1097
Plavix Tablets (Less than 1%) 3084
Plendil Extended-Release Tablets (0.5% to 1.5%) 623
Pletal Tablets (Less than 2%) 2605
Pletal Tablets (Less than 2%) 2848
Pneumovax 23 (Rare) 2156
Pnu-Imune 23 (Rare) 1868
Polocaine Injection, USP 625
Polocaine-MPF Injection, USP 625
Ponstel Capsules (Rare) 1356
Pravachol Tablets (Rare) 1099
Prednisone 3064
Premphase Tablets 3572
Prempro Tablets 3572
Prevacid Delayed-Release Capsules (Less than 1%) 3292
Prevnar for Injection (0.7% to 1.4%) 1870
PREVPAC (Less than 1%) 3298
Priftin Tablets (Less than 1%) 758
Prilosec Delayed-Release Capsules (Less than 1%) 628
Primaxin I.M. 2158
Primaxin I.V. (0.2%) 2160
Prinivil Tablets (0.3% to 1.0%) 2164
Prinzide Tablets 2168
Procanbid Extended-Release Tablets (Occasional) 2262
Procardia Capsules (2% or less) 2708
Procardia XL Extended Release Tablets (1% or less) 2710
Procrit for Injection (Rare) 2502
Proleukin for Injection (2%) 1199
Propecia Tablets 2172
Proscar Tablets 2175
ProSom Tablets (Infrequent) 500
Prostigmin Injectable 1744
Prostigmin Tablets 1744
Protonix I.V. (Less than 1%) 3580
Protonix Tablets (Less than 1%) 3577
▲ Protopic Ointment (3% to 5%) 1397
Proventil Inhalation Aerosol (Rare) 3142
Proventil Inhalation Solution 0.083% (Rare) 3146
Proventil Repetabs Tablets 3148
Proventil Solution for Inhalation 0.5% (Rare) 3144
Proventil HFA Inhalation Aerosol (Rare) 3150
Provera Tablets 2853
Prozac Pulvules, Liquid, and Weekly Capsules (Infrequent) 1238
Pulmicort Turbuhaler Inhalation Powder (Rare) 636
Pulmozyme Inhalation Solution 1426
Pyrazinamide Tablets 1876
Quinaglute Dura-Tabs Tablets 978
Quinidex Extentabs 2933
Qvar Inhalation Aerosol (Rare) 1987
Rebetron Combination Therapy 3153
Recombinate (Extremely rare) 853
Recombivax HB (Less than 1%) 2178
ReFacto Vials 1437
Refludan for Injection (Uncommon) 761
Reglan (A few cases) 2935
Relafen Tablets (1%) 1617
Relenza Rotadisk (Less than 1.5%) 1619
Remeron Tablets (Rare) 2483
Remeron SolTab Tablets (Rare) 2486
Remicade for IV Injection 1178
Renese Tablets 2712
Repronex for Intramuscular and Subcutaneous Injection 1347
Requip Tablets (Infrequent) 1621
Rescriptor Tablets (Less than 2%) 526
Retrovir Capsules 1625
Retrovir IV Infusion 1629
Retrovir 1625
Rhinocort Nasal Inhaler (Rare) 640
Rifadin (Occasional) 765
Rifamate Capsules (Occasional) 767
Rifater Tablets (Occasional) 769
Rilutek Tablets (Infrequent) 772
Risperdal (Rare) 1796
Ritalin 2387
▲ Rituxan for Infusion (1% to 8%) 1750
▲ Rituxan I.V. (1% to 8%) 1428
Robaxin Injectable 2938
Robaxin Tablets 2939
Robaxisal Tablets 2939
Robinul Forte Tablets 1358
Robinul Injectable 2940
Robinul Tablets 1358
Rocaltrol (One case) 2991
Roferon-A Injection (Less than 3%; rare) 2996
Roxanol 3066
Roxicodone Tablets (Less than 3%) 3067
Rynatan Tablets 3351
Sandostatin Injection (Less than 1%) 2394
Sandostatin LAR Depot (1% to 4%) 2395
Sensorcaine (Rare) 643
Sensorcaine-MPF Injection (Rare) 643
▲ Septra Suspension (Among most common) 2265
▲ Septra Tablets (Among most common) 2265
▲ Septra DS Tablets (Among most common) 2265
▲ Serevent Diskus (3%) 1637
Serevent Inhalation Aerosol (Rare; 1% to 3%) 1633
Serophene Tablets (Less than 1 in 100 patients) 3226
Serzone Tablets (Infrequent) 1104
Singulair (Greater than or equal to 2%) 2181
Solu-Medrol Sterile Powder 2855
Soma Compound Tablets (Less common) 3354
Soma Compound w/Codeine Tablets 3355
Sonata Capsules (Infrequent) 3591
Soriatane Capsules (Less than 1%) 3003
Sporanox Capsules 1800
Sporanox Injection 1804
Sporanox Injection 2509
Sporanox Oral Solution 1808
Sporanox Oral Solution 2512
Stadol NS Nasal Spray (Less than 1%) 1108
Stelazine 1640
Streptase for Infusion 647
Stromectol Tablets (0.9%) 2185
Sular Tablets (Less than or equal to 1%) 688

Sulfamylon Cream.......................... 1011
Sulfamylon Topical Solution........... 1011
Suprax (Less than 2%).................... 1877
Surmontil Capsules........................ 3595
Sustiva Capsules (Less than 2%).... 1258
Synarel Nasal Solution for Central Precocious Puberty (2.6%).......... 3204
Synarel Nasal Solution for Endometriosis (Less than 1%)...... 3205
Synercid I.V. (Less than 1%)........... 775
Synthroid... 505
Synvisc 3596
Talacen Caplets (Rare)................... 3089
Talwin Nx Tablets (Rare)................ 3090
Tambocor Tablets (Less than 1%)... 1990
Tao Capsules (Infrequent).............. 2716
Tapazole Tablets............................ 1823
Tarka Tablets.................................. 508
Tasmar Tablets (Infrequent)........... 3010
Taxol Injection (2%)........................ 1129
Tazicef for Injection........................ 1647
Tazicef Galaxy Container 1650
Tazicef Pharmacy Bulk Package 1653
Tazidime Vials, Faspak & ADD-Vantage 1966
Tegretol/Tegretol-XR 2404
Tenoretic Tablets 690
Tetanus & Diphtheria Toxoids Adsorbed for Adult Use 1880
Tetanus and Diphtheria Toxoids Adsorbed For Adult Use 815
Thalomid Capsules 1154
Thioplex for Injection 1765
Thioridazine Hydrochloride Tablets (Infrequent).................... 2289
Thiothixene Capsules 2290
Thorazine (Occasional)................... 1656
▲ Thrombate III (1 of 17) 944
Thyrogen for Injection (Greater than 1%)................................. 1441
Ticlid Tablets (0.5% to 1.0%) 3015
Timentin Injection- ADD-Vantage Vial 1661
Timentin Injection-Galaxy Container 1664
Timentin Injection-Pharmacy Bulk Package 1666
Timentin for Intravenous Administration 1658
Timolide Tablets 2187
Timolol GFS .... ⊙266
Timoptic in Ocudose (Less frequent) 2192
Timoptic Sterile Ophthalmic Solution (Less frequent)................ 2190
Timoptic-XE Sterile Ophthalmic Gel Forming Solution 2194
TNKase I.V. (Rare) 1430
Tolectin (Less than 1%) 2589
Tonocard Tablets (Less than 1%) 649
Topamax Sprinkle Capsules (Infrequent) 2590
Topamax Tablets (Infrequent) 2590
Toradol (1% or less) 3018
Trental Tablets (Less than 1%) 784
Tricor Capsules, Micronized 513
Trilafon 3160
Trilisate (Rare) 2901
Tripedia Vaccine (Rare) 817
▲ Trisenox Injection (8%) 1158
Trizivir Tablets 1669
Trovan (Less than 1%) 2722
Trusopt Sterile Ophthalmic Solution 2196
Tussi Organidin NR Liquid (Rare) 3350
Tussi-Organidin DM NR Liquid (Rare) 3350
Tussi-Organidin DM-S NR Liquid (Rare) 3350
Tussi-Organidin-S NR Liquid (Rare) .. 3350
Twinrix Vaccine (Less than 1%) 1674
TYPHIM Vi Vaccine 825
Ultracet Tablets 2597
Ultram Tablets (Less than 1%) 2600
Ultravate Ointment (Less frequent) 1120
Unasyn for Injection 2728
Uniretic Tablets (Less than 1%) 3178
Unithroid Tablets 3445
Univasc Tablets (Less than 1%) 3181
Valium Injectable 3026
Valtrex Caplets 1676
Vancenase PocketHaler Nasal Inhaler (Rare) 3162
Vanceril Inhalation Aerosol (Rare) 3165
Vanceril Double Strength Inhalation Aerosol (Rare) 3167
Vancocin HCl Capsules & Pulvules .. 1972
Vancocin HCl Oral Solution 1971
Vancocin HCl, Vials & ADD-Vantage 1970
Vantin Tablets and Oral Suspension (Less than 1%) 2860
Vaqta (Less than 1%) 2199
Varivax (Greater than or equal to 1%) 2202
Vaseretic Tablets 2204
Vasotec I.V. Injection 2207
Vasotec Tablets (0.5% to 1.0%) 2210
Velosulin BR Human Insulin 10 ml Vials 2435
Ventolin Inhalation Aerosol and Refill (Rare)................................. 1679
Ventolin HFA Inhalation Aerosol....... 3618
Verelan Capsules (1% or less)......... 3184
Verelan PM Capsules (2% or less).... 3186
Vermox Chewable Tablets (Rare)..... 2017
Versed Injection (Less than 1%)...... 3027
Viagra Tablets (Less than 2%)......... 2732
Vibramycin Calcium Oral Suspension Syrup 2735
Vibramycin Hyclate Capsules........... 2735
Vibramycin Hyclate Intravenous....... 2737
Vibramycin Monohydrate for Oral Suspension 2735
Vibra-Tabs Film Coated Tablets....... 2735
Vicoprofen Tablets (Less than 1%).. 520
Vioxx (Greater than 0.1% to 1.9%).. 2213
Viracept... 532
Viramune Oral Suspension............... 1060
Viramune Tablets............................. 1060
Vistide Injection............................... 1445
Vivactil Tablets 2217
Vivactil Tablets 2446
Vivotif Berna (Infrequent) 997
Volmax Extended-Release Tablets (Rare)... 2276
Voltaren Tablets (Less than 1%) 2315
Voltaren-XR Tablets (Less than 1%)... 2315
Warfarin Sodium Tablets, USP 3302
Wellbutrin Tablets 1680
Wellbutrin SR Sustained-Release Tablets (1% to 2%) 1684
Xenical Capsules 3043
Xylocaine Injections (Extremely rare) 653
YF-VAX Vaccine (Uncommon) 827
Yodoxin Tablets 1722
Zanaflex Tablets (Infrequent) 1305
Zarontin Capsules 2659
Zarontin Syrup 2660
Zaroxolyn Tablets 1177
Zestoretic Tablets 695
Zestril Tablets (0.3% to 1.0%) 698
Ziac Tablets 1887
Zinacef Injection (Fewer than 1 in 250 patients) 1696
Zinacef for Injection (Fewer than 1 in 250 patients) 1696
Zinecard for Injection (2%) 2869
Zithromax Capsules, 250 mg (1% or less) 2743
Zithromax for IV Infusion 2748
Zithromax for Oral Suspension, 300 mg, 600 mg, 900 mg, 1200 mg (1% or less) 2739
Zithromax Tablets, 250 mg (1% or less) 2739
Zocor Tablets (Rare) 2219
Zofran Injection (Rare) 1698
Zofran 1703
Zofran ODT Orally Disintegrating Tablets 1703
Zoladex (Rare) 702
Zoladex 3-month (Rare) 706
Zoloft (Infrequent) 2751
Zomig Tablets (Infrequent) 708
Zomig-ZMT Tablets (Infrequent) 708
Zonegran Capsules (Infrequent) 1307
Zovirax Capsules 1706
Zovirax for Injection 1708
Zovirax 1706
Zyban Sustained-Release Tablets (1% to 2%) 1710
Zyflo Filmtab Tablets 504
Zyprexa Tablets (Infrequent) 1973
Zyprexa ZYDIS Orally Disintegrating Tablets (Infrequent) 1973
Zyrtec (Less than 2%) 2756
Zyrtec-D 12 Hour Extended Relief Tablets (Less than 2%) 2758

Urticaria, hemorrhagic

Dolophine Hydrochloride Tablets (Rare) 3056
Roxanol (Rare) 3066

Urticaria pigmentosa

Rabies Vaccine RabAvert (One case) 1203

Urticarial reaction, generalized

Celontin Capsules 2618
Emgel 2% Topical Gel 1285

Uterine contractions, abnormal

Cervidil Vaginal Insert (2.0% to 4.7%) 1369
▲ Prepidil Gel (6.6%) 2851

Uterine contractions, altered

Astramorph/PF Injection, USP (Preservative-Free) 594
Proventil Inhalation Solution 0.083% 3146
Proventil Solution for Inhalation 0.5% 3144

Uterine contractions, production of

Cytotec Tablets 3202

Uterine fibroids

Activella (0% to 5%)........................ 2764

Uterine fibromyomata, increase in size

Alora Transdermal System 3372
Betaseron for SC Injection.............. 988
Cenestin Tablets.............................. 1263
Climara Transdermal System........... 958
Esclim Transdermal System 3460
Estinyl Tablets 3112
Estrace Vaginal Cream.................... 3358
Estrace Tablets 3361
Estratest.. 3252
femhrt Tablets................................. 2635
Menest Tablets................................ 2254
Nolvadex Tablets (A few reports)..... 678
Ogen Tablets 2846
Ortho Dienestrol Cream.................. 2554
Ortho-Est Tablets............................ 3464
Ortho-Prefest Tablets...................... 2570
Premarin Intravenous 3563
Premarin Tablets 3566
Premarin Vaginal Cream 3570
Premphase Tablets 3572
Prempro Tablets 3572
Prozac Pulvules, Liquid, and Weekly Capsules (Rare) 1238
Sarafem Pulvules (Rare) 1962
Serzone Tablets (Rare) 1104
Vivelle Transdermal System 2412
Vivelle-Dot Transdermal System 2416
Zanaflex Tablets (Infrequent) 1305
Zyprexa Tablets (Infrequent) 1973
Zyprexa ZYDIS Orally Disintegrating Tablets (Infrequent) 1973

Uterine inertia

Tasmar Tablets (Infrequent) 3010

Uterine rupture

Cervidil Vaginal Insert 1369
Cytotec Tablets 3202
Prepidil Gel 2851
Prostin E2 Suppositories 2852

Uterine spasm

Effexor Tablets (Rare) 3495
Effexor XR Capsules (Rare) 3499
Paxil (Rare) 1609

Uterotonic effect

D.H.E. 45 Injection 2334

Uveitis

Alrex Sterile Ophthalmic Suspension 0.2% (Less than 5%) .... ⊙256
Aredia for Injection (Rare) 2309
Betaseron for SC Injection 988
Blephamide Ophthalmic Ointment ... 547
Blephamide Ophthalmic Suspension 548
Effexor Tablets (Rare) 3495
Effexor XR Capsules (Rare) 3499
FML Ophthalmic Ointment .... ⊙237
FML Ophthalmic Suspension .... ⊙236
FML Forte Ophthalmic Suspension .... ⊙235
Fosamax Tablets (Rare) 2095
Healon GV (Rare) .... ⊙320
Humorsol Sterile Ophthalmic Solution 2102
Lamictal (Rare) 1567
Lotemax Sterile Ophthalmic Suspension 0.5% (Less than 5%) .... ⊙261
Mycobutin Capsules (Rare) 2838
Nipent for Injection (Less than 3%) 3272
Norvir Capsules (Less than 2%) 487
Norvir Oral Solution (Less than 2%) 487
OptiPranolol Metipranolol Ophthalmic Solution 0.3% .... ⊙263
Pred Forte Ophthalmic Suspension .... ⊙246
Pred Mild Sterile Ophthalmic Suspension .... ⊙249
Quinaglute Dura-Tabs Tablets 978
Quinidex Extentabs 2933
Rituxan for Infusion (Less than 0.1%) 1750
Rituxan I.V. (Less than 0.1%) 1428
Stromectol Tablets 2185
TheraCys Injection 823
Vistide Injection 1445
Vitrasert Implant (Approximately 1% to 5%) .... ⊙254
▲ Vitravene for Injection (5% to 20%) .... ⊙310
Xalatan Latanoprost Ophthalmic Solution .... ⊙320
Xalatan Sterile Ophthalmic Solution 2864

V

Vagina, dryness

Arimidex Tablets (1.2% to 1.9%) 659
Clomid Tablets (Fewer than 1%) 735
Crinone (Less than 5%)................... 3213
Intron A for Injection (Less than 5%)... 3120
Massengill Disposable Douches.... ▣752
Massengill Medicated Disposable Douche .... ▣753
Nolvadex Tablets (Infrequent).......... 678
Prometrium Capsules (100 mg, 200 mg) (Less than 6%) 3261
Risperdal (Frequent) 1796
▲ Synarel Nasal Solution for Endometriosis (19% of patients).. 3205

Vagina, warm feeling in

Prepidil Gel (1.5%).......................... 2851

Vaginal adenosis

Estrace Vaginal Cream.................... 3358
Estrace Tablets................................ 3361
Ortho-Est Tablets............................ 3464
Premarin Tablets............................. 3566
Vivelle Transdermal System............ 2412
Vivelle-Dot Transdermal System...... 2416

Vaginal burning

Floxin I.V. (Less than 1%)............... 2526
Floxin Tablets (Less than 1%).......... 2529
▲ Gynazole-1 Vaginal Cream (5.7%) .. 3310
▲ MUSE Urethral Suppository (5.8%).. 3335
▲ Terazol 3 Vaginal Cream (5%) 2587
▲ Terazol 3 Vaginal Suppositories (15.2% of 284 patients).............. 2587
▲ Terazol 7 Vaginal Cream (5.2% of 521 patients) 2587

Vaginal candidiasis

Activella Tablets 2764
Alesse-21 Tablets............................ 3468
Alesse-28 Tablets............................ 3473
Alora Transdermal System 3372
Arava Tablets (1% to 3%)................ 724
Avelox Tablets (0.05% to 1%).......... 879
Azactam for Injection (Less than 1%)... 1276
Brevicon 28-Day Tablets................. 3380
Cefotan... 664
Ceftin (Less frequent)...................... 1898
Cenestin Tablets............................. 1263
Cipro I.V. 893
Cipro I.V. Pharmacy Bulk Package .. 897
Cipro... 887
Cleocin Vaginal Ovules (1.5%)......... 2789
Climara Transdermal System.......... 958
Clozaril Tablets (Less than 1%)....... 2319
▲ Copaxone for Injection (8%) 3306
Cyclessa Tablets............................. 2450
Desogen Tablets 2458
Doxil Injection (Less than 1%).......... 566
▲ Esclim Transdermal System (4.2% to 8.5%)............................. 3460
Estinyl Tablets 3112
Estrace Vaginal Cream.................... 3358
Estrace Tablets 3361
Estratest.. 3252
Estrostep 2627
femhrt Tablets................................. 2635
Flovent Rotadisk (1% to 3%)........... 1537
Floxin I.V... 2526
Floxin Tablets 2529
Lamictal (Infrequent)....................... 1567
Levlen 962
Levlite 21 Tablets............................ 962
Levlite 28 Tablets............................ 962
Levora Tablets................................ 3389
Loestrin 21 Tablets 2642
Loestrin Fe Tablets.......................... 2642
Lo/Ovral Tablets.............................. 3532
Lo/Ovral-28 Tablets......................... 3538
Low-Ogestrel-28 Tablets................. 3392
Lunelle Monthly Injection................. 2827
Menest Tablets................................ 2254
Meridia Capsules (1.2%).................. 481
▲ MetroGel-Vaginal Gel (10%) 1986
Microgestin Fe 1.5/30 Tablets 3407
Microgestin Fe 1/20 Tablets 3400
Mircette Tablets.............................. 2470
Modicon.. 2563
Myobloc Injectable Solution (2% or greater).................................... 1291
Necon 3415
Nordette-28 Tablets......................... 2257
Norinyl 1 +35 28-Day Tablets.......... 3380
Norinyl 1 + 50 28-Day Tablets......... 3380
Noroxin Tablets............................... 2145
Ogen Tablets 2846
Ogestrel 0.5/50-28 Tablets............... 3428
▲ Omnicef (5%) 493
Ortho Dienestrol Cream................... 2554
Ortho-Cept 21 Tablets 2546
Ortho-Cept 28 Tablets 2546
Ortho-Cyclen/Ortho Tri-Cyclen......... 2573
Ortho-Est Tablets............................. 3464
Ortho-Novum 2563
Ortho-Novum 1/50□28 Tablets......... 2556
Ortho-Prefest Tablets....................... 2570
Ortho-Cyclen/Ortho Tri-Cyclen......... 2573
Ovcon 3364
Ovral Tablets................................... 3551
Ovral-28 Tablets.............................. 3552
Ovrette Tablets................................ 3552
Periostat Tablets 1208

Premarin Tablets 3566
Premarin Vaginal Cream 3570
Premphase Tablets 3572
Prempro Tablets 3572
Prometrium Capsules (100 mg, 200 mg) (Less than 5%) 3261
Protopic Ointment (Greater than or equal to 1%) 1397
Salagen Tablets (Less than 1%) 2229
Seroquel Tablets (Infrequent) 684
Tricor Capsules, Micronized 513
Tri-Levlen 962
Tri-Norinyl-28 Tablets 3433
Triphasil-21 Tablets 3600
Triphasil-28 Tablets 3605
Trivora Tablets 3439
▲ Vantin Tablets and Oral Suspension (3.1%) 2860
Vivelle Transdermal System 2412
Vivelle-Dot Transdermal System 2416
Yasmin 28 Tablets (Greater than 1%) 980
Zinacef Injection 1696
Zinacef for Injection 1696
Zovia 3449
Zyvox (1% to 1.6%) 2871

Vaginal discharge

▲ Alora Transdermal System (4.5% to 5.3%) 3372
Ceftin Tablets (0.1% to 1%) 1898
Cleocin Vaginal Ovules (Less than 1%) 2789
▲ Crinone (11%) 3213
▲ Fareston Tablets (13%) 3237
Floxin I.V. (1% to 3%) 2526
Floxin Tablets (1% to 3%) 2529
Fortovase Capsules (Less than 2%) 2970
Hivid Tablets (Less than 1%) 2975
Invirase Capsules (Less than 2%) 2979
Keflex 1237
Lupron Depot-PED 7.5 mg, 11.25 mg and 15 mg (2%) 3291
Lupron Injection Pediatric 3280
Massengill Disposable Douches ▣ 752
▲ MetroGel-Vaginal Gel (12%) 1986
▲ Nolvadex Tablets (29.6%) 678
ParaGard T 380A Intrauterine Copper Contraceptive 2582
▲ Prometrium Capsules (100 mg, 200 mg) (10%) 3261
ProSom Tablets (Infrequent) 500
▲ Synarel Nasal Solution for Central Precocious Puberty (3%) 3204

Vaginal pressure

Adenoscan (Less than 1%) 1381

Vaginismus

Prostin E2 Suppositories 2852

Vaginitis

Aceon Tablets (2 mg, 4 mg, 8 mg) (0.3% to 1%) 3249
Actiq (1% or greater) 1184
Alesse-21 Tablets 3468
Alesse-28 Tablets 3473
▲ Alora Transdermal System (3.2% to 3.4%) 3372
Ambien Tablets (Infrequent) 3191
Amerge Tablets (Rare) 1467
Ancef for Injection 1474
Ancef Injection 1474
Aricept Tablets (Infrequent) 1270
Aricept Tablets (Infrequent) 2665
Augmentin Chewable Tablets (1%) 1482
Augmentin Powder for Oral Suspension (1%) 1482
Augmentin Tablets (1%) 1485
Avelox Tablets (0.05% to 1%) 879
▲ Avonex (4%) 1013
Azactam for Injection (Less than 1%) 1276
Brevicon 28-Day Tablets 3380
Ceclor CD Tablets (2.4%) 1279
Ceclor (Less than 1 in 100) 1905
Cedax Capsules (0.1% to 1%) 1021
Cefizox for Intramuscular or Intravenous Use (Rare) 1390
Cefotan 664
▲ Ceftin Tablets (0.1% to 5.4%) 1898
Cefzil (1.6%) 1076
Celebrex Capsules (0.1% to 1.9%) 2676
Celebrex Capsules (0.1% to 1.9%) 2780
Ceptaz for Injection (Fewer than 1%) 1499
Cerebyx Injection (Infrequent) 2619
Cipro I.V. (1% or less) 893
Cipro I.V. Pharmacy Bulk Package (Less than 1%) 897
Cipro (Less than 1% to 2%) 887
Claforan Injection (Less than 1%) 732
Claritin (At least one patient) 3100
Claritin-D 12 Hour Extended Release Tablets (Less frequent) 3102
Claritin-D 24 Hour Extended Release Tablets (Fewer than 2%) 3104
Cleocin Phosphate Sterile Solution 2785
▲ Cleocin Vaginal Cream (16% to 33%) 2788
Cleocin Vaginal Ovules (Less than 1%) 2789
▲ CombiPatch Transdermal System (9% to 13%) 2323
Copaxone for Injection (At least 2%) 3306
Cyclessa Tablets 2450
Depacon Injection (1% to 5%) 416
Depakene (1% to 5%) 421
Depakote Sprinkle Capsules (1% to 5%) 426
Depakote Tablets (1% to 5%) 430
Depakote ER Tablets (Greater than 1%) 436
▲ Depo-Provera Contraceptive Injection (More than 5%) 2798
Desogen Tablets 2458
Doxil Injection (Less than 1%) 566
Duricef 1079
Dynabac Tablets (0.4% to 1.2%) 2269
Effexor Tablets (Frequent) 3495
Effexor XR Capsules (Frequent) 3499
▲ Estring Vaginal Ring (5%) 2811
Estrostep 2627
▲ Evista Tablets (4.3%) 1915
Evoxac Capsules (1% to 3%) 1217
▲ femhrt Tablets (5.4%) 2635
Flovent Rotadisk (1% to 3%) 1537
Floxin I.V. (1% to 5%) 2526
Floxin Tablets (1% to 5%) 2529
Fortaz (Less than 1%) 1541
Gabitril Tablets (Frequent) 1189
Geocillin Tablets 2687
▲ Infergen (5% to 8%) 1777
Keflex 1237
Kefzol Vials, ADD-Vantage 1951
Klonopin Tablets (1%) 2983
▲ Lamictal (4.1%) 1567
Levaquin (0.8% to 1.8%) 2537
Levlen 962
Levlite 21 Tablets 962
Levlite 28 Tablets 962
Levora Tablets 3389
Loestrin 21 Tablets 2642
Loestrin Fe Tablets 2642
Lo/Ovral Tablets 3532
Lo/Ovral-28 Tablets 3538
Lorabid Suspension and Pulvules (1.3%) 2251
Low-Ogestrel-28 Tablets 3392
Lunelle Monthly Injection 2827
▲ Lupron Depot 3.75 mg (11.4%) 3281
▲ Lupron Depot–3 Month 11.25 mg (11.4% to 28%) 3285
Lupron Depot-PED 7.5 mg, 11.25 mg and 15 mg (2%) 3291
Lupron Injection Pediatric 3280
Luvox Tablets (25, 50, 100 mg) (Infrequent) 3256
Maxipime for Injection (0.1% to 1%) 1285
Mefoxin for Injection 2124
Mefoxin Premixed Intravenous Solution 2127
Microgestin Fe 1.5/30 Tablets 3407
Microgestin Fe 1/20 Tablets 3400
Migranal Nasal Spray (Rare) 2376
Mircette Tablets 2470
▲ Mirena Intrauterine System (5% or more) 974
Modicon 2563
▲ Monurol Sachet (5.5% to 7.6%) 1375
Naprelan Tablets (Less than 1%) 1293
Necon 3415
Nexium Delayed-Release Capsules (Less than 1%) 619
Nordette-28 Tablets 2257
Norinyl 1 +35 28-Day Tablets 3380
Norinyl 1 + 50 28-Day Tablets 3380
▲ Norplant System (5% or greater) 3543
Ogestrel 0.5/50-28 Tablets 3428
Omnicef (1%) 493
Ortho-Cept 21 Tablets 2546
Ortho-Cept 28 Tablets 2546
Ortho-Cyclen/Ortho Tri-Cyclen 2573
Ortho-Novum 2563
Ortho-Novum 1/50□28 Tablets 2556
▲ Ortho-Prefest Tablets (7%) 2570
Ortho-Cyclen/Ortho Tri-Cyclen 2573
Ovcon 3364
Ovidrel for Injection (Less than 2%) 3220
Ovral Tablets 3551
Ovral-28 Tablets 3552
Ovrette Tablets 3552
ParaGard T 380A Intrauterine Copper Contraceptive 2582
Paxil (Infrequent) 1609
Permax Tablets (Infrequent) 1299
Pletal Tablets (Less than 2%) 2605
Pletal Tablets (Less than 2%) 2848
▲ Prempro Tablets (7%) 3572
PREVPAC (Less than 3%) 3298
▲ Prograf (3% to 15%) 1393
Prometrium Capsules (100 mg, 200 mg) (Less than 5%) 3261
Prostin E2 Suppositories 2852
Protonix I.V. (Less than 1%) 3580
Protonix Tablets (Less than 1%) 3577
Remeron Tablets (Infrequent) 2483
Remeron SolTab Tablets (Infrequent) 2486
Rocephin Injectable Vials, ADD-Vantage, Galaxy, Bulk (Occasional) 2993
Salagen Tablets (1% to 2%) 2229
Sandostatin Injection (Less than 1%) 2394
Seroquel Tablets (Infrequent) 684
Serzone Tablets (2%) 1104
Sonata Capsules (Infrequent) 3591
Sular Tablets (Less than or equal to 1%) 688
Suprax (Less than 2%) 1877
Synercid I.V. (Less than 1%) 775
Tasmar Tablets (Infrequent) 3010
Tazicef for Injection (Less than 1%) 1647
Tazicef Galaxy Container (Less than 1%) 1650
Tazicef Pharmacy Bulk Package (Less than 1%) 1653
Tazidime Vials, Faspak & ADD-Vantage (Less than 1%) 1966
▲ Tequin Injection (6%) 1110
▲ Tequin Tablets (6%) 1110
Topamax Sprinkle Capsules (Frequent) 2590
Topamax Tablets (Frequent) 2590
Tricor Capsules, Micronized (1%) 513
Trileptal Oral Suspension (Up to 2%) 2407
Trileptal Tablets (Up to 2%) 2407
Tri-Levlen 962
Tri-Norinyl-28 Tablets 3433
Triphasil-21 Tablets 3600
Triphasil-28 Tablets 3605
Trivora Tablets 3439
Trovan (Less than 1%) 2722
Uniretic Tablets (Less than 1%) 3178
Urobiotic-250 Capsules (Rare) 2731
▲ Vagifem Tablets (3% to 5%) 2857
Vantin Tablets and Oral Suspension (Less than 1%) 2860
Vioxx (Greater than 0.1% to 1.9%) 2213
Wellbutrin Tablets (Infrequent) 1680
Wellbutrin SR Sustained-Release Tablets 1684
Xenical Capsules (2.6% to 3.8%) 3043
Yasmin 28 Tablets (Greater than 1%) 980
Zanaflex Tablets (Infrequent) 1305
Zinacef Injection 1696
Zinacef for Injection 1696
Zithromax Capsules, 250 mg (1% or less to 2%) 2743
Zithromax for IV Infusion (2.8%) 2748
Zithromax for Oral Suspension, 1 g (1% or less to 1%) 2743
Zithromax for Oral Suspension, 300 mg, 600 mg, 900 mg, 1200 mg (1% or less to 2%) 2739
Zithromax Tablets, 250 mg (1% or less to 2%) 2739
Zithromax Tablets, 600 mg (1% or less to 1%) 2743
▲ Zoladex (1% to 75%) 702
Zosyn (1.0% or less) 1890
Zosyn in Galaxy Containers (1.0% or less) 1894
Zovia 3449
Zyban Sustained-Release Tablets 1710
Zyflo Filmtab Tablets (Less common) 524
Zyprexa Tablets 1973
Zyprexa ZYDIS Orally Disintegrating Tablets 1973
Zyrtec (Less than 2%) 2756
Zyrtec-D 12 Hour Extended Relief Tablets (Less than 2%) 2758

Vaginitis, atrophic

Evoxac Capsules (Less than 1%) 1217
Exelon Capsules (Infrequent) 2342
Exelon Oral Solution (Infrequent) 2345
Imdur Tablets (Less than or equal to 5%) 1826
Soriatane Capsules (Less than 1%) 3003
Zoloft (Rare) 2751

Varices, esophageal

Myleran Tablets 1603
Nexium Delayed-Release Capsules (Less than 1%) 619
Tabloid Tablets 1642

Varicocele

Gonal-F for Injection 3216

Vascular access, clotting

▲ Epogen for Injection (0.25 to 7%) 582
▲ Procrit for Injection (0.25 to 7%) 2502

Vascular complications, unspecified

Avonex 1013
Betaxon Ophthalmic Suspension (Less than 2%) 537
▲ Carnitor Injection (2% to 6%) 3242
▲ Flolan for Injection (95%) 1528
Follistim for Injection 2465
Gonal-F for Injection 3216
Ortho-Cyclen/Ortho Tri-Cyclen 2573
Pergonal for Injection 3223
ReoPro Vials (1.8%) 1958
Repronex for Intramuscular and Subcutaneous Injection 1347
Sandostatin LAR Depot (1% to 4%) 2395
Tricor Capsules, Micronized 513
Vistide Injection 1445
Zofran (Rare) 1703
Zofran ODT Orally Disintegrating Tablets (Rare) 1703

Vascular insufficiency

Corgard Tablets (2 of 100 patients) 2245
Zonegran Capsules (Infrequent) 1307

Vasculitis

Accuretic Tablets 2614
Accutane Capsules 2944
Aceon Tablets (2 mg, 4 mg, 8 mg) 3249
Advair Diskus 100/50 1448
Advair Diskus 250/50 1448
Advair Diskus 500/50 1448
Aldoclor Tablets 2035
Aldomet Tablets 2037
Aldoril Tablets 2039
Alkeran for Injection 1465
Alkeran Tablets 1466
Altace Capsules (Less than 1%) 2233
Anaprox Tablets (Less than 1%) 2967
Anaprox DS Tablets (Less than 1%) 2967
Arava Tablets (1% to 3%) 724
Arthrotec Tablets (Rare) 3195
Atacand HCT Tablets 597
Attenuvax 2044
Avalide Tablets 1070
Axid Pulvules (Rare) 1903
Axid Pulvules (Rare) 2919
Azulfidine EN-tabs Tablets (Rare) 2775
Baycol Tablets 883
Captopril Tablets 2281
Celebrex Capsules (Less than 0.1%) 2676
Celebrex Capsules (Less than 0.1%) 2780
Chibroxin Sterile Ophthalmic Solution 2051
Cipro I.V. (1% or less) 893
Cipro I.V. Pharmacy Bulk Package (Less than 1%) 897
Cipro 887
Clorpres Tablets 1002
Clozaril Tablets 2319
Combipres Tablets 1040
Combivir Tablets 1502
Cordarone Tablets (Rare) 3487
Corzide 40/5 Tablets 2247
Corzide 80/5 Tablets 2247
Coumadin for Injection (Infrequent) 1243
Coumadin Tablets (Infrequent) 1243
Covera-HS Tablets (Less than 2%) 3199
Cytovene Capsules 2959
Depen Titratable Tablets (Rare) 3341
DiaBeta Tablets 741
Diovan HCT Tablets 2338
Diucardin Tablets 3494
Diuril Oral 2087
Diuril Sodium Intravenous 2086
Dyazide Capsules 1515
EC-Naprosyn Delayed-Release Tablets (Less than 1%) 2967
Enalaprilat Injection 863
Evoxac Capsules (Less than 1%) 1217
Felbatol 3343
Feldene Capsules (Rare) 2685
Floxin I.V. (Less than 1%) 2526
Floxin Tablets (Less than 1%) 2529
FluShield Influenza Vaccine 3521
Furosemide Tablets 2284
HydroDIURIL Tablets 2108
Hyzaar 2109
Inderide Tablets 3517
Inderide LA Long-Acting Capsules 3519
Isoptin SR Tablets (1% or less) 467
Kaletra Capsules (Less than 2%) 471
Kaletra Oral Solution (Less than 2%) 471
Lamictal 1567
Lescol Capsules (Rare) 2361
Lescol Capsules (Rare) 2925
Lescol XL Tablets 2361
Lescol XL Tablets 2925
Lexxel Tablets 608
Lodine (Less than 1%) 3528
Lodine XL Extended-Release Tablets (Less than 1%) 3530
Lopid Tablets 2650
Luvox Tablets (25, 50, 100 mg) 3256
Maxzide 1008
Meruvax II 2130
Mevacor Tablets (Rare) 2132
Micardis HCT Tablets 1051
Minipress Capsules 2699
Minizide Capsules 2700
M-M-R II 2118

Mobic Tablets (Less than 2%) 1054
Moduretic Tablets 2138
Monopril Tablets 1091
Monopril HCT 1094
Mumpsvax (Rare) 2141
▲ Naprelan Tablets (3% to 9%) 1293
Naprosyn Suspension (Less than 1%) 2967
Naprosyn Tablets (Less than 1%) 2967
Nipent for Injection (Less than 3%) 3272
Noroxin Tablets 2145
Norvasc Tablets (More than 0.1% to 1%) 2704
Orthoclone OKT3 Sterile Solution 2498
Pacerone Tablets (Rare) 3331
Paser Granules 1781
Pediazole Suspension 3050
Permax Tablets (Rare) 1299
Ponstel Capsules (Rare) 1356
Pravachol Tablets (Rare) 1099
Prinivil Tablets (0.3% to 1.0%) 2164
Prinzide Tablets 2168
Quinaglute Dura-Tabs Tablets 978
Quinidex Extentabs 2933
Recombivax HB 2178
Relafen Tablets (Less than 1%) 1617
Renese Tablets 2712
Retrovir Capsules (Rare) 1625
Retrovir IV Infusion (Rare) 1629
Retrovir (Rare) 1625
Rifadin (Occasional) 765
Rifamate Capsules 767
Rifater Tablets 769
Ritalin 2387
Rituxan for Infusion (Less than 0.1%) 1750
Rituxan I.V. (Less than 0.1%) 1428
Roferon-A Injection (Rare) 2996
Sporanox Capsules (1%) 1800
Tarka Tablets 508
Tegretol/Tegretol-XR 2404
Tenoretic Tablets 690
Ticlid Tablets (Rare) 3015
Timolide Tablets 2187
Tonocard Tablets (Less than 1%) 649
Trizivir Tablets 1669
Vancocin HCl Capsules & Pulvules (Rare) 1972
Vancocin HCl Oral Solution (Rare) 1971
Vancocin HCl, Vials & ADD-Vantage (Rare) 1970
Vaseretic Tablets 2204
Vasotec I.V. Injection 2207
Vasotec Tablets (0.5% to 1.0%) 2210
Verelan Capsules (1% or less) 3184
Verelan PM Capsules (2% or less) 3186
Warfarin Sodium Tablets, USP 3302
Zantac 1690
Zantac Injection 1688
Zantac Syrup 1690
Zestoretic Tablets 695
Zestril Tablets (0.3% to 1.0%) 698
Ziac Tablets 1887
Zocor Tablets (Rare) 2219
Zoloft 2751

Vasculitis, allergic

Aggrenox Capsules 1026
Amaryl Tablets (Rare) 717
Amoxil Chewable Tablets 1471
Amoxil for Oral Suspension 1471
Amoxil 1471
Bicillin C-R 900/300 Injection 2240
Bicillin C-R Injection 2238
Bicillin L-A Injection 2242
Imitrex Nasal Spray 1554
Imitrex Tablets 1558
Lodine (Less than 1%) 3528
Lodine XL Extended-Release Tablets (Less than 1%) 3530
Omnicef 493
Vioxx 2213

Vasculitis, central nervous system

Imitrex Nasal Spray 1554
Imitrex Tablets 1558

Vasculitis, cutaneous

Atacand HCT Tablets 597
Avalide Tablets 1070
Clorpres Tablets 1002
Combipres Tablets 1040
Corzide 40/5 Tablets 2247
Corzide 80/5 Tablets 2247
Depacon Injection 416
Depakene 421
Depakote Sprinkle Capsules 426
Depakote Tablets 430
Depakote ER Tablets 436
Diovan HCT Tablets 2338
Diucardin Tablets 3494
Diuril Oral 2087
Diuril Sodium Intravenous 2086
Enbrel for Injection 1752
Enbrel for Injection 3504
HydroDIURIL Tablets 2108
Hyzaar 2109
Inderide Tablets 3517
Inderide LA Long-Acting Capsules 3519
Lodine (Rare) 3528
Lodine XL Extended-Release Tablets (Less than 1%) 3530
Maxzide 1008
Micardis HCT Tablets 1051
Minizide Capsules 2700
Moduretic Tablets 2138
Mykrox Tablets 1168
Neupogen for Injection (Infrequent) 587
Prinzide Tablets 2168
Renese Tablets 2712
Tenoretic Tablets 690
Timolide Tablets 2187
Vaseretic Tablets 2204
Zaroxolyn Tablets 1177
Zebeta Tablets 1885
Zestoretic Tablets 695
Ziac Tablets 1887

Vasculitis, eosinophilic

Accolate Tablets (Rare) 657

Vasculitis, leukocytoclastic

Cardizem Injectable 1018
Cardizem Lyo-Ject Syringe 1018
Cardizem Monovial 1018
Cardizem CD Capsules (A number of cases) 1016
Lexxel Tablets 608
Rescriptor Tablets (Less than 2%) 526
Tiazac Capsules 1378

Vasculitis, renal

Cuprimine Capsules (Rare) 2075
Depen Titratable Tablets 3341

Vasoconstriction

Fortovase Capsules (Rare) 2970
Invirase Capsules (Rare) 2979
Survanta Intratracheal Suspension (Less than 1%) 3053

Vasodilation

Accupril Tablets (0.5% to 1.0%) 2611
Accuretic Tablets (1%) 2614
Aceon Tablets (2 mg, 4 mg, 8 mg) (0.3% to 1%) 3249
Aciphex Tablets (Rare) 1267
Aciphex Tablets (Rare) 1783
Actiq (Up to 2%) 1184
Agrylin Capsules (1% to 5%) 3232
AmBisome for Injection (Less common) 1383
Amphotec (1% to 5%) 1774
AndroGel (Fewer than 1%) 3322
Arava Tablets (1% to less than 3%) 724
▲ Argatroban Injection (1% to 10%) 1478
Aricept Tablets (Frequent) 1270
Aricept Tablets (Frequent) 2665
▲ Arimidex Tablets (25.3%) 659
Asacol Delayed-Release Tablets (2% or greater) 2884
Avelox Tablets (0.05% to 1%) 879
▲ Avonex (4%) 1013
Axert Tablets (Infrequent) 2772
Betapace Tablets (1% to 3%) 950
Bicillin C-R 900/300 Injection 2240
Bicillin C-R Injection 2238
Bicillin L-A Injection 2242
Brethine Tablets (1%) 2313
Cardene I.V. (0.7%) 3485
Cardizem Injectable (1.7%) 1018
Cardizem Lyo-Ject Syringe (1.7%) 1018
Cardizem Monovial (1.7%) 1018
Caverject Sterile Powder (Less than 1%) 2777
Ceclor CD Tablets 1279
Ceclor 1905
▲ CellCept Capsules (3%) 2951
▲ CellCept Intravenous (3%) 2951
▲ CellCept Oral Suspension (3%) 2951
▲ CellCept Tablets (3%) 2951
▲ Cerebyx Injection (5.6%) 2619
▲ Copaxone for Injection (27%) 3306
Cosopt Sterile Ophthalmic Solution 2065
Cytovene (At least 3 subjects) 2959
DDAVP Nasal Spray 738
DDAVP Rhinal Tube 738
Depacon Injection (0.9%) 416
Depakene (1% or more) 421
Depakote Sprinkle Capsules 426
Depakote Tablets (1% to 5%) 430
Depakote ER Tablets (1% to 5%) 436
Desmopressin Acetate Rhinal Tube 1345
Ditropan XL Extended Release Tablets (2% to 5%) 564
Dynabac Tablets (0.1% to 1%) 2269
▲ Effexor Tablets (2.3% to 5.6%) 3495
▲ Effexor XR Capsules (4% to 6%) 3499
Enbrel for Injection 1752
Enbrel for Injection 3504
Ferrlecit Injection 3386
Flexeril Tablets (Less than 1%) 572
Flexeril Tablets (Less than 1%) 2094
▲ Flolan for Injection (Most common) 1528
Floxin I.V. (Less than 1%) 2526
Floxin Tablets (Less than 1%) 2529
Gabitril Tablets (2%) 1189
Humate-P Concentrate (2%) 790
Hytrin Capsules (At least 1%) 464
Imitrex Injection (Rare) 1549
Imitrex Nasal Spray 1554
Imitrex Tablets (Rare) 1558
Kadian Capsules (Less than 3%) 1335
Lamictal (Infrequent) 1567
Levaquin 2537
Lipitor Tablets (Less than 2%) 2639
Lipitor Tablets (Less than 2%) 2696
Lorabid Suspension and Pulvules 2251
Lotrel Capsules 2370
Lupron Depot-PED 7.5 mg, 11.25 mg and 15 mg (Less than 2%) 3291
Lupron Injection Pediatric (Less than 2%) 3280
▲ Luvox Tablets (25, 50, 100 mg) (3%) 3256
Marinol Capsules (Greater than 1%) 3325
Meridia Capsules (2.4%) 481
Mirapex Tablets (1% or more) 2834
Myobloc Injectable Solution (2% or greater) 1291
Naprelan Tablets (Less than 1%) 1293
Navelbine Injection 1604
▲ Neumega for Injection (19%) 1434
Neurontin Capsules (1.1%) 2655
Neurontin Oral Solution (1.1%) 2655
Neurontin Tablets (1.1%) 2655
Nitrostat Tablets 2658
Norvir Capsules (1.3% to 1.7%) 487
Norvir Oral Solution (1.3% to 1.7%) 487
Orudis Capsules (Less than 1%) 3548
Oruvail Capsules (Less than 1%) 3548
OxyContin Tablets (Less than 1%) 2912
▲ Paxil (3% to 4%) 1609
Pentasa Capsules (Less than 1%) 3239
▲ Permax Tablets (3.2%) 1299
Pletal Tablets (Less than 2%) 2605
Pletal Tablets (Less than 2%) 2848
Prevacid Delayed-Release Capsules (Less than 1%) 3292
PREVPAC (Less than 1%) 3298
ProAmatine Tablets (Less frequent) 3241
▲ Proleukin for Injection (13%) 1199
Protonix I.V. (Less than 1%) 3580
Protonix Tablets (Less than 1%) 3577
Protopic Ointment (Greater than or equal to 1%) 1397
Provigil Tablets (1%) 1193
Prozac Pulvules, Liquid, and Weekly Capsules (2% to 3%) 1238
▲ Rapamune Oral Solution and Tablets (3% to 20%) 3584
ReFacto Vials 1437
Remeron Tablets (Frequent) 2483
Remeron SolTab Tablets (Frequent) 2486
Rescriptor Tablets (Less than 2%) 526
Retrovir Capsules 1625
Retrovir IV Infusion 1629
Retrovir 1625
Roxicodone Tablets (Less than 3%) 3067
▲ Sarafem Pulvules (3%) 1962
Seroquel Tablets (Infrequent) 684
▲ Serzone Tablets (4%) 1104
Sonata Capsules (Infrequent) 3591
▲ Stadol NS Nasal Spray (3% to 9%) 1108
Stimate Nasal Spray 796
▲ Sular Tablets (4%) 688
Suprane Liquid for Inhalation (Less than 1%) 874
Synercid I.V. (Less than 1%) 775
Tasmar Tablets (Infrequent) 3010
Tequin Injection (0.1% to 3%) 1110
Tequin Tablets (0.1% to 3%) 1110
Thalomid Capsules 1154
▲ Tiazac Capsules (4%) 1378
Timolide Tablets 2187
Timolol GFS ⊙ 266
Timoptic in Ocudose 2192
Timoptic Sterile Ophthalmic Solution 2190
Timoptic-XE Sterile Ophthalmic Gel Forming Solution 2194
Tricor Capsules, Micronized 513
Ultracet Tablets 2597
Ultram Tablets (1% to 5%) 2600
Valstar Sterile Solution for Intravesical Instillation (2%) 1175
Vantin Tablets and Oral Suspension (Less than 1%) 2860
Vascor Tablets (0.5% to 2.0%) 2602
▲ Viadur Implant (67.9%) 912
Vicoprofen Tablets (Less than 3%) 520
Vistide Injection 1445
Wellbutrin SR Sustained-Release Tablets (Infrequent) 1684
WinRho SDF 2297
Zanaflex Tablets (Infrequent) 1305
▲ Zoladex (57%) 702
Zoloft (Rare) 2751
Zyban Sustained-Release Tablets (Infrequent) 1710
Zyprexa Tablets (Infrequent) 1973
Zyprexa ZYDIS Orally Disintegrating Tablets (Infrequent) 1973

Vasodilation, peripheral

Aggrenox Capsules 1026
Persantine Tablets 1057

Vasomotor disturbances

Aminohippurate Sodium PAH Injection 2041
Urecholine Tablets 2445
Xanax Tablets (2.0%) 2865

Vasomotor flushes

▲ Clomid Tablets (10.4%) 735
▲ Serophene Tablets (Approximately 1 in 10 patients) 3226

Vasospasm, coronary artery

Amerge Tablets 1467
Imitrex Tablets 1558
Migranal Nasal Spray 2376
Zomig Tablets 708
Zomig-ZMT Tablets 708

Vasospasm, rebound

Nimotop Capsules (Less than 1%) 904

Vasospasm, unspecified

Betaseron for SC Injection 988
Bicillin C-R 900/300 Injection 2240
Bicillin C-R Injection 2238
Bicillin L-A Injection 2242
▲ CellCept Capsules (3% to 10%) 2951
▲ CellCept Intravenous (3% to 10%) 2951
▲ CellCept Oral Suspension (3% to 10%) 2951
▲ CellCept Tablets (3% to 10%) 2951
D.H.E. 45 Injection (Occasional) 2334
Prozac Pulvules, Liquid, and Weekly Capsules (Rare) 1238
Sarafem Pulvules (Rare) 1962
Topamax Sprinkle Capsules (Rare) 2590
Topamax Tablets (Rare) 2590

Vasovagal episode

Aggrastat (2%) 2031
Alferon N Injection (2%) 1770
Bicillin C-R 900/300 Injection 2240
Bicillin C-R Injection 2238
Bicillin L-A Injection 2242
Caverject Sterile Powder (Less than 1%) 2777
Iopidine Sterile Ophthalmic Solution ⊙ 212
Naropin Injection (Less than 1%) 612
Tonocard Tablets (Less than 1%) 649
Versed Injection (Less than 1%) 3027

Veins, varicosis

Ambien Tablets (Rare) 3191
Amerge Tablets (Rare) 1467
Arava Tablets (1% to 3%) 724
Betaseron for SC Injection 988
Copaxone for Injection (Infrequent) 3306
Depo-Provera Contraceptive Injection (Fewer than 1%) 2798
Imdur Tablets (Less than or equal to 5%) 1826
Lupron Depot–3 Month 22.5 mg (Less than 5%) 3288
Paxil (Rare) 1609
Permax Tablets (Infrequent) 1299
Pletal Tablets (Less than 2%) 2605
Pletal Tablets (Less than 2%) 2848
Requip Tablets (Infrequent) 1621
Serzone Tablets (Rare) 1104
Tricor Capsules, Micronized 513
▲ Visudyne for Injection (1% to 10%) ⊙ 308
Zoladex 3-month (1% to 5%) 706

Venous infection at injection site

Primaxin I.V. (0.1%) 2160

Venous insufficiency

Vioxx (Greater than 0.1% to 1.9%) 2213

Venous leak

▲ Caverject Sterile Powder (3%) 2777

Venous thrombophlebitis

Xeloda Tablets (Less than 5%) 3039

Ventilator dependence

Virazole for Inhalation Solution 1747

Ventricular arrhythmias

Adenoscan (Less than 1%) 1381
Anectine Injection (Rare) 1476
▲ Betapace Tablets (4.3% of 3,257 patients) 950
Betapace AF Tablets 954
Biaxin/Biaxin XL 403
Campath Ampules 992
Cardizem Injectable (Less than 1%) 1018
Cardizem Lyo-Ject Syringe (Less than 1%) 1018
Cardizem Monovial (Less than 1%) 1018
Celexa (At least 3 patients) 1365
Corvert Injection 2793

Digitek Tablets 1003
Doxil Injection (Less than 1%) 566
Dynabac Tablets (Rare) 2269
E.E.S. (Rare) 450
EryPed (Rare) 446
Erythrocin Stearate Filmtab Tablets (Rare) 452
Erythromycin Base Filmtab Tablets (Rare) 454
Foscavir Injection 605
Lanoxicaps Capsules (Less common) 1574
Lanoxin Injection 1581
Lanoxin Tablets (Less common) 1587
Lanoxin Elixir Pediatric (Less common) 1578
Lanoxin Injection Pediatric (Less common) 1584
Lufyllin Tablets 3347
Lufyllin-400 Tablets 3347
Lufyllin-GG Elixir 3348
Lufyllin-GG Tablets 3348
Mexitil Capsules (1.0% to 1.9%) 1047
Naropin Injection 612
Nesacaine/Nesacaine MPF 617
Normodyne Injection (1%) 3135
PCE Dispertab Tablets (Rare) 498
Pediazole Suspension (Rare) 3050
PREVPAC (Rare) 3298
▲ Primacor Injection (12.1%) 3086
Procardia Capsules (Fewer than 0.5%) 2708
Procardia XL Extended Release Tablets (Fewer than 0.5%) 2710
▲ Proleukin for Injection (3%) 1199
Prozac Pulvules, Liquid, and Weekly Capsules (Rare) 1238
Remeron Tablets (Four cases) 2483
Remeron SolTab Tablets (Four cases) 2486
ReoPro Vials (0.3%) 1958
Rituxan for Infusion (Four patients) 1750
Rituxan I.V. (Four patients) 1428
Sarafem Pulvules (Rare) 1962
Sensorcaine 643
Sensorcaine-MPF Injection 643
Serentil 1057
▲ Tambocor Tablets (7% to 13%) 1990
Theo-Dur Extended-Release Tablets 1835
▲ Tikosyn Capsules (2.6% to 15.8%) 2717
▲ Tonocard Tablets (10.9%) 649
Trasylol Injection (1% to 2%) 909
Uni-Dur Extended-Release Tablets 1841
Viagra Tablets 2732

Ventricular arrhythmias, post-abrupt discontinuation
Tenormin 692

Ventricular bigeminy
Azactam for Injection (Less than 1%) 1276

Ventricular contractions, premature
Adenocard Injection 1380
Amerge Tablets (Infrequent) 1467
Arthrotec Tablets (Rare) 3195
Azactam for Injection (Less than 1%) 1276
Cataflam Tablets (Less than 1%) 2315
Clozaril Tablets (Less than 1%) 2319
Diprivan Injectable Emulsion (Less than 1%) 667
▲ Dobutrex Solution Vials (Approximately 5%) 1914
Ellence Injection 2806
Gastrocrom Oral Concentrate (Less common) 1162
Indapamide Tablets (Less than 5%) 2286
Ismo Tablets (Fewer than 1%) 3524
Lanoxin Injection (Less common) 1581
Lanoxin Injection Pediatric (Less common) 1584
Norpramin Tablets 755
▲ Proleukin for Injection (5%) 1199
▲ Tonocard Tablets (10.9%) 649
Vascor Tablets (0.5% to 2.0%) 2602
Vioxx (Greater than 0.1% to 1.9%) 2213
Voltaren Tablets (Less than 1%) 2315
Voltaren-XR Tablets (Less than 1%) 2315
Zantac (Rare) 1690
Zantac Injection (Rare) 1688
Zantac Syrup (Rare) 1690
Zofran Injection 1698

Ventricular contractions, premature, multifocal
Digitek Tablets 1003
Lanoxicaps Capsules (Common) 1574
Lanoxin Injection 1581
▲ Lanoxin Tablets (Among most common) 1587
Lanoxin Elixir Pediatric (Less common) 1578
Lanoxin Injection Pediatric (Less common) 1584

Ventricular contractions, premature, unifocal
Digitek Tablets 1003
Lanoxicaps Capsules (Common) 1574
Lanoxin Injection 1581
▲ Lanoxin Tablets (Among most common) 1587
Lanoxin Elixir Pediatric (Less common) 1578
Lanoxin Injection Pediatric (Less common) 1584

Ventricular dilation, left-side
Retrovir Capsules (0.8%) 1625
Retrovir IV Infusion (1%) 1629
Retrovir (0.8%) 1625

Ventricular dysfunction
Herceptin I.V. 1414
Prograf (Rare) 1393
Taxotere for Injection Concentrate 778

Ventricular ectopic beats
Cipro (Less than 1%) 887
Digibind Powder 1514
Dobutrex Solution Vials 1914
Hivid Tablets (Less than 1%) 2975
Imitrex Tablets 1558
Kytril Injection (Rare) 2986
▲ Primacor Injection (8.5%) 3086
Quinaglute Dura-Tabs Tablets 978

Ventricular extrasystoles
Aceon Tablets (2 mg, 4 mg, 8 mg) (0.3% to 1%) 3249
Amphotec (1% to 5%) 1774
Betaseron for SC Injection 988
Brethine Tablets (1.5%) 2313
Cardene I.V. (1.4%) 3485
Cardizem Injectable 1018
Cardizem Lyo-Ject Syringe 1018
Cardizem Monovial 1018
Cardizem CD Capsules (Less than 1%) 1016
▲ CellCept Capsules (3% to 10%) 2951
▲ CellCept Intravenous (3% to 10%) 2951
▲ CellCept Oral Suspension (3% to 10%) 2951
▲ CellCept Tablets (3% to 10%) 2951
Cerebyx Injection (Infrequent) 2619
Claritin-D 12 Hour Extended Release Tablets (Less frequent) 3102
▲ Corvert Injection (5.1%) 2793
Digitek Tablets (1%) 1003
Effexor Tablets 3495
Effexor XR Capsules 3499
Fluothane Inhalation 3508
Lanoxicaps Capsules 1574
Lanoxin Injection 1581
Lanoxin Tablets 1587
Lanoxin Elixir Pediatric 1578
Lanoxin Injection Pediatric 1584
Lotrel Capsules (Infrequent) 2370
▲ Natrecor for Injection (3%) 3189
Neurontin Capsules (Rare) 2655
Neurontin Oral Solution (Rare) 2655
Neurontin Tablets (Rare) 2655
Nipent for Injection (Less than 3%) 3272
Paxil (Rare) 1609
Permax Tablets (Infrequent) 1299
Pletal Tablets (Less than 2%) 2605
Pletal Tablets (Less than 2%) 2848
Proleukin for Injection (Less than 1%) 1199
Provigil Tablets (At least 1%) 1193
Prozac Pulvules, Liquid, and Weekly Capsules (Rare) 1238
Remeron Tablets (Infrequent) 2483
Remeron SolTab Tablets (Infrequent) 2486
Rilutek Tablets (Infrequent) 772
Risperdal (Rare) 1796
Romazicon Injection (Less than 1%) 3000
Sarafem Pulvules (Rare) 1962
Serzone Tablets (Infrequent) 1104
Sonata Capsules (Infrequent) 3591
Sular Tablets (Less than or equal to 1%) 688
Tiazac Capsules (Less than 2%) 1378
▲ Trasylol Injection (6%) 909
Tricor Capsules, Micronized 513
Uniretic Tablets (Less than 1%) 3178
Zanaflex Tablets (Rare) 1305
Zonegran Capsules (Rare) 1307
Zyprexa Tablets (Infrequent) 1973
Zyprexa ZYDIS Orally Disintegrating Tablets (Infrequent) 1973

Ventricular failure
Flolan for Injection 1528
Tonocard Tablets (Up to 1.4%) 649

Ventricular fibrillations
Abelcet Injection 1273
Adenocard Injection (Rare) 1380
Aloprim for Injection (Less than 1%) 2292
Betapace Tablets 950
Betaseron for SC Injection 988
Cardizem Injectable (Less than 1%) 1018
Cardizem Lyo-Ject Syringe (Less than 1%) 1018
Cardizem Monovial (Less than 1%) 1018
Celebrex Capsules (Less than 0.1%) 2676
Celebrex Capsules (Less than 0.1%) 2780
Clozaril Tablets 2319
Cordarone Intravenous (Less than 2%) 3491
Covera-HS Tablets 3199
D.H.E. 45 Injection 2334
Digitek Tablets 1003
Diprivan Injectable Emulsion (Less than 1%) 667
Dopram Injectable 2931
DynaCirc Capsules (0.5% to 1%) 2921
DynaCirc CR Tablets (0.5% to 1%) 2923
Hyzaar 2109
Imitrex Injection (Rare) 1549
Imitrex Tablets (Rare) 1558
Isoptin SR Tablets 467
Lanoxicaps Capsules 1574
Lanoxin Injection 1581
Lanoxin Tablets 1587
Lanoxin Elixir Pediatric 1578
Lanoxin Injection Pediatric 1584
Levaquin Injection (Less than 0.5%) 2537
Meridia Capsules 481
Narcan Injection (Several instances) 1322
Naropin Injection 612
Norpramin Tablets 755
Paxil 1609
Primacor Injection (0.2%) 3086
Procanbid Extended-Release Tablets 2262
Prozac Pulvules, Liquid, and Weekly Capsules (Rare) 1238
Quinaglute Dura-Tabs Tablets 978
Quinidex Extentabs 2933
Refludan for Injection 761
Retavase Vials 1182
Rilutek Tablets (Rare) 772
Rituxan I.V. 1428
Robinul Injectable 2940
Sarafem Pulvules (Rare) 1962
Sensorcaine 643
Sensorcaine-MPF Injection 643
▲ Tikosyn Capsules (Up to 4.6%) 2717
Tonocard Tablets (Less than 1%) 649
Trasylol Injection (2%) 909
Uniretic Tablets (Less than 1%) 3178
Zomig Tablets 708
Zomig-ZMT Tablets 708
Zosyn (1.0% or less) 1890
Zosyn in Galaxy Containers (1.0% or less) 1894

Ventricular flutter
Quinidex Extentabs 2933

Ventricular gallop
Herceptin I.V. 1414
Retrovir Capsules (0.8%) 1625
Retrovir IV Infusion (1%) 1629
Retrovir (0.8%) 1625

Ventricular irregularities
Ancobon Capsules 1730
Cerubidine for Injection 947
Verelan Capsules (1% or less) 3184

Ventricular irritation
Tenoretic Tablets 690
Timolide Tablets 2187
Vaseretic Tablets 2204
Zestoretic Tablets 695

Ventricular response, rapid
Verelan Capsules 3184
Verelan PM Capsules 3186

Venus sequelae
Diprivan Injectable Emulsion (Rare) 667

Verruca
Copaxone for Injection (Frequent) 3306
Evoxac Capsules (Less than 1%) 1217
Fortovase Capsules (2.2%) 2970
Invirase Capsules (Less than 2%) 2979
Prometrium Capsules (100 mg, 200 mg) (Less than 5%) 3261
Risperdal (Rare) 1796
▲ Serostim for Injection (1% to 10%) 3229
Soriatane Capsules (Less than 1%) 3003

Vertebral compression fractures
Celestone Syrup 3099
Cortone Acetate Injectable Suspension 2059
Cortone Acetate Tablets 2061
Decadron Elixir 2078
Decadron Phosphate Injection 2081
Depo-Medrol Injectable Suspension 2795
Pediapred Oral Solution 1170

Vertical deviation
▲ Botox Purified Neurotoxin Complex (2.1% to 16.9%) 549

Vertigo
Abelcet Injection 1273
Accupril Tablets (0.5% to 1.0%) 2611
Accuretic Tablets (1%) 2614
Aceon Tablets (2 mg, 4 mg, 8 mg) (0.3% to 1%) 3249
Aciphex Tablets 1267
Aciphex Tablets 1783
Actiq (Up to 1%) 1184
▲ Actonel Tablets (3.3%) 2879
Adalat CC Tablets (3% or less) 877
Aerobid/Aerobid-M (1% to 3%) 1363
Albenza Tablets (Less than 1.0% to 1.2%) 1463
Aldoclor Tablets 2035
Aldoril Tablets 2039
Altace Capsules (Less than 1% to 1.5%) 2233
Ambien Tablets (Frequent) 3191
Amerge Tablets (Frequent) 1467
Anaprox Tablets (Less than 3%) 2967
Anaprox DS Tablets (Less than 3%) 2967
Ancobon Capsules 1730
Androderm Transdermal System CIII (Less than 1%) 3377
Anzemet Injection (Infrequently) 719
Anzemet Tablets (Infrequently) 722
Arava Tablets (1% to 3%) 724
Aricept Tablets (Frequent) 1270
Aricept Tablets (Frequent) 2665
Arthrotec Tablets (Rare) 3195
Asacol Delayed-Release Tablets 2884
Astelin Nasal Spray (Infrequent) 3339
Atacand Tablets (0.5% or greater) 595
Atacand HCT Tablets (0.5% or greater) 597
Avalide Tablets 1070
Avapro Tablets 1074
Avapro Tablets 3076
Avelox Tablets (0.05% to 1%) 879
Axert Tablets (Infrequent) 2772
Azactam for Injection (Less than 1%) 1276
Azulfidine EN-tabs Tablets (Rare) 2775
Bactrim 2949
Baycol Tablets 883
Benadryl Parenteral 2617
Betapace Tablets (Rare) 950
Betapace AF Tablets (Rare) 954
Betaxon Ophthalmic Suspension (Less than 2%) 537
Betoptic S Ophthalmic Suspension (Rare) 537
Biaxin/Biaxin XL 403
Blocadren Tablets (0.6%) 2046
▲ Buprenex Injectable (5% to 10%) 2918
Carafate Suspension (Less than 0.5%) 731
Carafate Tablets (Less than 0.5%) 730
▲ Cardura Tablets (2% to 23%) 2668
▲ Carnitor Injection (2% to 6%) 3242
Ceclor CD Tablets 1279
Celebrex Capsules (0.1% to 1.9%) 2676
Celebrex Capsules (0.1% to 1.9%) 2780
Celestone Soluspan Injectable Suspension 3097
Celestone Syrup 3099
Celexa (Infrequent) 1365
▲ CellCept Capsules (3% to 10%) 2951
▲ CellCept Intravenous (3% to 10%) 2951
▲ CellCept Oral Suspension (3% to 10%) 2951
▲ CellCept Tablets (3% to 10%) 2951
▲ Cenestin Tablets (17%) 1263
Cerebyx Injection (2.2%) 2619
Claritin (At least one patient) 3100
Claritin-D 12 Hour Extended Release Tablets (Less frequent) 3102
Claritin-D 24 Hour Extended Release Tablets (Fewer than 2%) 3104
Cleocin Vaginal Cream (Less than 1%) 2788
Clinoril Tablets (Less than 1 in 100) 2053
Clomid Tablets (Fewer than 1%) 735
Clorpres Tablets 1002
▲ Clozaril Tablets (More than 5% to 19%) 2319
Cognex Capsules (Frequent) 1351
Coly-Mycin M Parenteral 2243
Combipres Tablets 1040
▲ Copaxone for Injection (6%) 3306
Coreg Tablets (1% to 2%) 1508
Cortone Acetate Injectable Suspension 2059
Cortone Acetate Tablets 2061
Corzide 40/5 Tablets 2247
Corzide 80/5 Tablets 2247
Cosopt Sterile Ophthalmic Solution 2065
Cozaar Tablets (Less than 1%) 2067

Crixivan Capsules (Less than 2%).... 2070
Dapsone Tablets USP.... 1780
Decadron Elixir.... 2078
Decadron Tablets.... 2079
Decadron Phosphate Injection.... 2081
Depacon Injection (1% or more).... 416
Depakene (1% or more).... 421
Depakote Sprinkle Capsules.... 426
Depakote Tablets (1% to 5%).... 430
Depakote ER Tablets (1% to 5%).... 436
Depo-Medrol Injectable Suspension.... 2795
▲ Detrol Tablets (8.6%).... 3623
Diovan Capsules.... 2337
Diovan HCT Tablets (Greater than 0.2%).... 2338
Dipentum Capsules (1.0%).... 2803
Diucardin Tablets.... 3494
Diuril Oral.... 2087
Diuril Sodium Intravenous.... 2086
Dolobid Tablets (Less than 1 in 100).... 2088
Dostinex Tablets (1% to 4%).... 2804
Doxil Injection (Less than 1%).... 566
Duragesic Transdermal System (Less than 1%).... 1786
Dyazide Capsules.... 1515
Dynabac Tablets (2.1% to 2.3%).... 2269
Dynacin Capsules.... 2019
EC-Naprosyn Delayed-Release Tablets (Less than 3%).... 2967
Edecrin.... 2091
Effexor Tablets (Frequent).... 3495
Effexor XR Capsules (Frequent).... 3499
Eldepryl Capsules.... 3266
Enalaprilat Injection.... 863
Engerix-B Vaccine.... 1517
Ery-Tab Tablets (Isolated reports).... 448
Erythrocin Stearate Filmtab Tablets (Isolated reports).... 452
Erythromycin Base Filmtab Tablets (Isolated reports).... 454
Erythromycin Delayed-Release Capsules, USP (Isolated reports).... 455
Eskalith.... 1527
Evoxac Capsules (1% to 3%).... 1217
Exelon Capsules (2% or more).... 2342
Exelon Oral Solution (2% or more).... 2345
Fareston Tablets.... 3237
Feldene Capsules (Occasional).... 2685
Femara Tablets (Less frequent).... 2351
Flexeril Tablets (Less than 1%).... 572
Flexeril Tablets (Less than 1%).... 2094
Flomax Capsules (0.6% to 1.0%).... 1044
Florinef Acetate Tablets.... 2250
Floxin I.V. (Less than 1%).... 2526
Floxin Otic Solution (0.5% to 1%).... 1219
Floxin Tablets (Less than 1%).... 2529
Furosemide Tablets.... 2284
Gabitril Tablets (Frequent).... 1189
Gengraf Capsules (1% to less than 3%).... 457
Geodon Capsules (Frequent).... 2688
Glucotrol XL Extended Release Tablets (Less than 1%).... 2693
Haldol Decanoate.... 2535
Haldol Injection, Tablets and Concentrate.... 2533
Havrix Vaccine (Less than 1%).... 1544
Hexalen Capsules.... 2226
Hivid Tablets (Less than 1%).... 2975
Hydrocortone Tablets.... 2106
Hydrocortone Acetate Injectable Suspension.... 2103
Hydrocortone Phosphate Injection, Sterile.... 2105
HydroDIURIL Tablets.... 2108
▲ Hytrin Capsules (0.5% to 21%).... 464
Hyzaar.... 2109
Imdur Tablets (Less than or equal to 5%).... 1826
▲ Imitrex Injection (11.9%).... 1549
Imitrex Nasal Spray (1% to 1.7%).... 1554
Imitrex Tablets.... 1558
Indapamide Tablets (Less than 5%).... 2286
Inderide Tablets.... 3517
Inderide LA Long-Acting Capsules.... 3519
Indocin (Greater than 1%).... 2112
▲ Intron A for Injection (Less than 5% to 23%).... 3120
Kadian Capsules (Less than 3%).... 1335
▲ Keppra Tablets (3%).... 3314
Klonopin Tablets (Infrequent).... 2983
Lamictal (1.1%).... 1567
Lariam Tablets.... 2989
Lescol Capsules.... 2361
Lescol Capsules.... 2925
Lescol XL Tablets.... 2361
Lescol XL Tablets.... 2925
Levaquin (Less than 0.5%).... 2537
Lexxel Tablets.... 608
Lithium Carbonate.... 3061
Lithium Citrate Syrup.... 3061
Lithobid Slow-Release Tablets.... 3255
Lodine XL Extended-Release Tablets (Less than 1%).... 3530
Lopid Tablets (1.5%).... 2650
Lotensin HCT Tablets (1.5%).... 2367
▲ Lupron Depot–3 Month 22.5 mg (6.4%).... 3288
▲ Lupron Depot–4 Month 30 mg (6.1% to 8.3%).... 3289
Luvox Tablets (25, 50, 100 mg) (Infrequent).... 3256
Macrobid Capsules.... 2889
Macrodantin Capsules.... 2891
Mavik Tablets (0.3% to 1.0%).... 478
Maxalt Tablets (Infrequent).... 2120
Maxalt-MLT Orally Disintegrating Tablets (Infrequent).... 2120
Maxzide.... 1008
Meridia Capsules.... 481
Mevacor Tablets (0.5% to 1.0%).... 2132
Miacalcin Nasal Spray (Less than 1%).... 2375
Micardis Tablets (More than 0.3%).. 1049
Micardis HCT Tablets.... 1051
Microzide Capsules.... 3414
Midamor Tablets (Less than or equal to 1%).... 2136
Migranal Nasal Spray (Infrequent) ... 2376
Miltown Tablets.... 3349
Minipress Capsules (1% to 4%).... 2699
Minizide Capsules.... 2700
Minocin Intravenous.... 1862
Minocin Oral Suspension.... 1865
Minocin Pellet-Filled Capsules.... 1863
Mirapex Tablets (1% or more).... 2834
Mobic Tablets (Less than 2%).... 1054
Moduretic Tablets (Less than or equal to 1%).... 2138
Monopril Tablets (0.2% to 1.0%).... 1091
Monopril HCT.... 1094
Mustargen for Injection (Infrequent).... 2142
Myobloc Injectable Solution (2% or greater).... 1291
Naprelan Tablets (Less than 1%).... 1293
Naprosyn Suspension (Less than 3%).... 2967
Naprosyn Tablets (Less than 3%).... 2967
Naropin Injection (Less than 1%).... 612
Nebcin Vials, Hyporets & ADD-Vantage.... 1955
Neoral Soft Gelatin Capsules (1% to less than 3%).... 2380
Neoral Oral Solution (1% to less than 3%).... 2380
Neurontin Capsules (Frequent).... 2655
Neurontin Oral Solution (Frequent) .. 2655
Neurontin Tablets (Frequent).... 2655
Nexium Delayed-Release Capsules (Less than 1%).... 619
Nipent for Injection (Less than 3%).... 3272
Nitrostat Tablets (Occasional).... 2658
Normodyne Injection (1%).... 3135
Normodyne Tablets (2%).... 3137
Norvasc Tablets (More than 0.1% to 1%).... 2704
Norvir Capsules (Less than 2%).... 487
Norvir Oral Solution (Less than 2%).... 487
▲ Nubain Injection (5%).... 1323
Orthoclone OKT3 Sterile Solution.... 2498
Orudis Capsules (Less than 1%).... 3548
Oruvail Capsules (Less than 1%).... 3548
OxyContin Tablets (Less than 1%).... 2912
Paxil (Frequent).... 1609
Pediapred Oral Solution.... 1170
Pediazole Suspension.... 3050
Periactin Tablets.... 2155
Permax Tablets (Infrequent).... 1299
Plaquenil Tablets.... 3082
Plavix Tablets (1% to 2.5%).... 1097
Plavix Tablets (1% to 2.5%).... 3084
Pletal Tablets (1% to 3%).... 2605
Pletal Tablets (1% to 3%).... 2848
Ponstel Capsules (Occasional).... 1356
Pravachol Tablets.... 1099
Prednisone.... 3064
Prelone Syrup.... 2273
PREVPAC.... 3298
Prilosec Delayed-Release Capsules (Less than 1%).... 628
Primaxin I.M..... 2158
Primaxin I.V. (Less than 0.2%).... 2160
Prinivil Tablets (0.2%).... 2164
Prinzide Tablets (0.3% to 1%).... 2168
Procardia XL Extended Release Tablets (1% or less).... 2710
Protonix I.V. (Less than 1%).... 3580
Protonix Tablets (Less than 1%).... 3577
Protopic Ointment (Greater than or equal to 1%).... 1397
Proventil Inhalation Aerosol.... 3142
Proventil Repetabs Tablets.... 3148
Proventil HFA Inhalation Aerosol.... 3150
Prozac Pulvules, Liquid, and Weekly Capsules (Infrequent).... 1238
Quinaglute Dura-Tabs Tablets.... 978
Quinidex Extentabs.... 2933
Relafen Tablets (Less than 1%).... 1617
Remeron Tablets (Frequent).... 2483
Remeron SolTab Tablets (Frequent).... 2486
Reminyl Oral Solution (Infrequent) ... 1792
Reminyl Tablets (Infrequent).... 1792
Renese Tablets.... 2712
Requip Tablets (2%).... 1621
Rescriptor Tablets (Less than 2%).... 526
Retrovir Capsules.... 1625
Retrovir IV Infusion.... 1629
Retrovir.... 1625
Rifater Tablets.... 769
▲ Rilutek Tablets (2.5% to 4.5%).... 772
Risperdal (Infrequent).... 1796
Robaxin Injectable.... 2938
Robaxin Tablets.... 2939
Roferon-A Injection (Less than 3% to less than 5%).... 2996
▲ Romazicon Injection (10%).... 3000
Rynatan Tablets.... 3351
Rythmol Tablets – 150 mg, 225 mg, 300 mg (Less than 1%).... 502
Sandostatin LAR Depot (1% to 4%).... 2395
Sarafem Pulvules (Infrequent).... 1962
Septra Suspension.... 2265
Septra Tablets.... 2265
Septra DS Tablets.... 2265
Seroquel Tablets (Infrequent).... 684
Serzone Tablets (Infrequent).... 1104
Skelid Tablets (More than or equal to 1%).... 3088
Solu-Medrol Sterile Powder.... 2855
Soma Tablets.... 3353
Soma Compound Tablets (Less frequent).... 3354
Soma Compound w/Codeine Tablets.... 3355
Sonata Capsules (Less than 1%).... 3591
Sporanox Capsules (1%).... 1800
Stadol NS Nasal Spray (Less than 1%).... 1108
Stromectol Tablets (0.9%).... 2185
Sular Tablets (Less than or equal to 1%).... 688
Sustiva Capsules (Less than 2%).... 1258
Tambocor Tablets (1% to 3%).... 1990
Tamiflu Capsules (0.3% to 1%).... 3008
Tamiflu Oral Suspension (0.3% to 1%).... 3008
Tapazole Tablets.... 1823
Tarka Tablets (Less frequent).... 508
Tasmar Tablets (Frequent).... 3010
Tenex Tablets (Less frequent).... 2942
Tenoretic Tablets (2%).... 690
Tenormin (2%).... 692
Tequin Injection (0.1% to 3%).... 1110
Tequin Tablets (0.1% to 3%).... 1110
Teveten Tablets (Less than 1%).... 3327
▲ Thalomid Capsules (8.3%).... 1154
Timolide Tablets.... 2187
Timolol GFS.... ⊙ 266
Timoptic in Ocudose.... 2192
Timoptic Sterile Ophthalmic Solution.... 2190
Timoptic-XE Sterile Ophthalmic Gel Forming Solution.... 2194
▲ Tonocard Tablets (8.0% to 25.3%) . 649
Topamax Sprinkle Capsules (Frequent).... 2590
Topamax Tablets (Frequent).... 2590
Toprol-XL Tablets (1.8%).... 651
Toradol (1% or less).... 3018
Tricor Capsules, Micronized (Less than 1%).... 513
▲ Trileptal Oral Suspension (2% to 15%).... 2407
▲ Trileptal Tablets (2% to 15%).... 2407
Trovan (Less than 1%).... 2722
Twinrix Vaccine (Less than 1%).... 1674
Ultracet Tablets (Less than 1%).... 2597
▲ Ultram Tablets (26% to 33%).... 2600
Uniretic Tablets (More than 1%).... 3178
Valium Injectable.... 3026
Valium Tablets (Infrequent).... 3047
Vancocin HCl Capsules & Pulvules (Rare).... 1972
Vancocin HCl Oral Solution (Rare) ... 1971
Vancocin HCl, Vials & ADD-Vantage (Rare).... 1970
Vaniqa Cream (0.1%).... 1121
Vantin Tablets and Oral Suspension (Less than 1%).... 2860
Vascor Tablets (0.5% to 2.0%).... 2602
Vaseretic Tablets (0.5% to 2.0%).... 2204
Vasotec I.V. Injection.... 2207
Vasotec Tablets (1.6%).... 2210
Versed Syrup (Less than 1%).... 3033
Viagra Tablets (Less than 2%).... 2732
Vicoprofen Tablets (Less than 1%).. 520
Vioxx (Greater than 0.1% to 1.9%).. 2213
Vistide Injection.... 1445
▲ Visudyne for Injection (1% to 10%).... ⊙ 308
Volmax Extended-Release Tablets.... 2276
Wellbutrin Tablets (Infrequent).... 1680
Wellbutrin SR Sustained-Release Tablets (Infrequent).... 1684
Yodoxin Tablets.... 1722
Zanaflex Tablets (Infrequent).... 1305
Zantac (Rare).... 1690
Zantac Injection.... 1688
Zantac Syrup (Rare).... 1690
Zaroxolyn Tablets.... 1177
Zebeta Tablets.... 1885
Zestoretic Tablets (0.3% to 1%).... 695
Zestril Tablets (0.2%).... 698
Ziac Tablets.... 1887
Zithromax (1% or less).... 2743
Zithromax for Oral Suspension, 300 mg, 600 mg, 900 mg, 1200 mg (1% or less).... 2739
Zithromax Tablets, 250 mg (1% or less).... 2739
Zithromax Tablets, 600 mg (1% or less).... 2743
Zocor Tablets.... 2219
Zoloft (Infrequent).... 2751
Zomig Tablets (2%).... 708
Zomig-ZMT Tablets (2%).... 708
Zonegran Capsules (Infrequent).... 1307
Zosyn (1.0% or less).... 1890
Zosyn in Galaxy Containers (1.0% or less).... 1894
Zyban Sustained-Release Tablets (Infrequent).... 1710
Zyprexa Tablets (Infrequent).... 1973
Zyprexa ZYDIS Orally Disintegrating Tablets (Infrequent).... 1973
Zyrtec (Less than 2%).... 2756
Zyrtec-D 12 Hour Extended Relief Tablets (Less than 2%).... 2758

Vesical spasm

Dilaudid.... 441
Dilaudid Powder.... 441
Dilaudid Rectal Suppositories.... 441
Dilaudid Tablets.... 441
Hycodan.... 1316

Vesiculation

Adriamycin PFS/RDF Injection.... 2767
Aldara Cream, 5% (Up to 3%).... 1978
Aplisol Injection.... 2609
Attenuvax.... 2044
▲ Catapres-TTS (7 of 101 patients).... 1038
Cipro I.V. (1% or less).... 893
Condylox Topical Solution (Less than 5%).... 2437
Diprolene Ointment 0.05% (1 per 767 patients).... 3108
8-MOP Capsules.... 1727
Levulan Kerastick (Up to 4%).... 971
M-M-R II.... 2118
Oxsoralen-Ultra Capsules.... 1741
Tine Test, Tuberculin, Old.... 3631
Topicort LP Cream (0.8%).... 2025
Tubersol Diagnostic Antigen.... 3628
Ultram Tablets (Less than 1%).... 2600

Vesiculobullous reaction

Feldene Capsules (Rare).... 2685
Floxin I.V..... 2526
Floxin Tablets.... 2529
Motrin Suspension, Oral Drops, Chewable Tablets, and Caplets (Less than 1%).... 2002

Vestibular disturbances

Navelbine Injection.... 1604

Vestibular dysfunction

Cipro I.V. Pharmacy Bulk Package (Less than 1%).... 897
Gengraf Capsules (1% to less than 3%).... 457
Neoral Soft Gelatin Capsules (1% to less than 3%).... 2380
Neoral Oral Solution (1% to less than 3%).... 2380
Rilutek Tablets (Rare).... 772
Streptomycin Sulfate Injection.... 2714

Virilization

Anadrol-50 Tablets.... 3321
Androderm Transdermal System CIII.... 3377
▲ Android Capsules, 10 mg (Among most common).... 1731
▲ Delatestryl Injection (Among most frequent).... 1151
▲ Estratest (Among most common).... 3252
Intron A for Injection (Less than 5%).... 3120
Oxandrin Tablets.... 1153
Testoderm Transdermal Systems.... 574
Testred Capsules, 10 mg.... 1746

Virilization, female fetus

▲ Android Capsules, 10 mg (Among most common).... 1731
Delatestryl Injection.... 1151
Testred Capsules, 10 mg.... 1746

Vision, blurred

Accuretic Tablets.... 2614
Aciphex Tablets.... 1267
Aciphex Tablets.... 1783
Acular Ophthalmic Solution (Rare).... 544
Acular PF Ophthalmic Solution.... 544
Adenocard Injection (Less than 1%).... 1380
Adenoscan (Less than 1%).... 1381
Aerobid/Aerobid-M (1% to 3%).... 1363
Akineton.... 402
Albalon Ophthalmic Solution.... ⊙ 225
Aldoclor Tablets.... 2035
Aldoril Tablets.... 2039
▲ Alferon N Injection (3% to 6%).... 1770

▲ Alomide Ophthalmic Solution (1% to 5%) ⊙204
▲ Alphagan Ophthalmic Solution (Approximately 10% to 30%) 545
▲ Alrex Sterile Ophthalmic Suspension 0.2% (5% to 15%) ⊙256
Amaryl Tablets (0.4%) 717
Amerge Tablets (Infrequent) 1467
Antivert, Antivert/25, & Antivert/50 Tablets (Rare) 2664
Aralen Tablets 3075
Arava Tablets (1% to 3%) 724
Arco-Lase Plus Tablets 592
Aricept Tablets (Frequent) 1270
Aricept Tablets (Frequent) 2665
▲ Artane (30% to 50%) 1855
Arthrotec Tablets (Rare) 3195
Asacol Delayed-Release Tablets 2884
Atacand HCT Tablets 597
Ativan Injection (Occasional) 3478
Atromid-S Capsules 3483
Atrovent Inhalation Aerosol (1.2%) 1030
Atrovent Nasal Spray 0.03% (Less than 2%) 1032
Atrovent Nasal Spray 0.06% (Less than 1%) 1033
Avalide Tablets 1070
▲ Azopt Ophthalmic Suspension (5% to 10%) 536
Baycol Tablets 883
Benadryl Parenteral 2617
Betaxon Ophthalmic Suspension (2%) 537
Betimol Ophthalmic Solution (1% to 5%) ⊙324
Betoptic S Ophthalmic Suspension (Small number of patients) 537
Bicillin C-R 900/300 Injection 2240
Bicillin C-R Injection 2238
Bicillin L-A Injection 2242
Bontril Slow-Release Capsules 576
Bromfed Capsules (Extended-Release) 2269
Bromfed-PD Capsules (Extended-Release) 2269
Captopril Tablets 2281
Carbatrol Capsules 3234
Carteolol Hydrochloride Ophthalmic Solution USP, 1% (Occasional) ⊙258
Cataflam Tablets (Less than 1%) 2315
Catapres Tablets 1037
Catapres-TTS (0.5% or less) 1038
Celebrex Capsules (0.1% to 1.9%) 2676
Celebrex Capsules (0.1% to 1.9%) 2780
Celontin Capsules 2618
Ciloxan (Less than 1%) 538
Cipro I.V. (1% or less) 893
Cipro I.V. Pharmacy Bulk Package (Less than 1%) 897
Cipro (Less than 1%) 887
Claritin (At least one patient) 3100
Claritin-D 12 Hour Extended Release Tablets (Less frequent) 3102
Clinoril Tablets (Less than 1 in 100) 2053
Clomid Tablets (1.5%) 735
Clorpres Tablets 1002
Cogentin 2055
Combipres Tablets 1040
Combivent Inhalation Aerosol 1041
Compazine 1505
Concerta Extended-Release Tablets 1998
Concerta Tablets 561
Corgard Tablets (1 to 5 per 1000 patients) 2245
Corzide 40/5 Tablets (1 to 5 of 1000 patients) 2247
Corzide 80/5 Tablets (1 to 5 of 1000 patients) 2247
▲ Cosopt Sterile Ophthalmic Solution (5% to 15%) 2065
Covera-HS Tablets (Less than 2%) 3199
Cozaar Tablets (Less than 1%) 2067
Crixivan Capsules (Less than 2%) 2070
Dapsone Tablets USP 1780
Decadron Phosphate Sterile Ophthalmic Ointment 2083
Decadron Phosphate Sterile Ophthalmic Solution 2084
Declomycin Tablets 1855
▲ Depacon Injection (8% to 12%) 416
▲ Depakene (8% to 12%) 421
▲ Depakote Sprinkle Capsules (4% to 12%) 426
▲ Depakote Tablets (8% to 12%) 430
▲ Depakote ER Tablets (8% to 12%) 436
Desferal Vials 2333
Detrol Tablets 3623
Detrol LA Capsules 2801
DiaBeta Tablets 741
Digitek Tablets 1003
Dilaudid Oral Liquid (Less frequent) 445
Dilaudid Tablets - 8 mg (Less frequent) 445
Dilaudid-HP (Less frequent) 443
Diovan HCT Tablets 2338
Dipentum Capsules (Rare) 2803
▲ Ditropan XL Extended Release Tablets (7.7%) 564
Diucardin Tablets 3494
Diuril Oral 2087
Diuril Sodium Intravenous 2086
Dolobid Tablets (Less than 1 in 100) 2088
Donnagel Liquid (Rare) ▣789
Donnatal 2929
Donnatal Extentabs 2930
Donnatal Tablets 2929
DuoNeb Inhalation Solution 1233
Duraclon Injection (Rare) 3057
Duragesic Transdermal System 1786
Duranest Injections 600
Dyazide Capsules 1515
Edecrin 2091
▲ Effexor Tablets (6%) 3495
▲ Effexor XR Capsules (4% to 8%) 3499
ELA-Max Cream 1340
Eldepryl Capsules 3266
Emadine Ophthalmic Solution (Less than 5%) ⊙211
Emla (Unlikely with cream) 602
Enalaprilat Injection 863
Ergamisol Tablets (1% to 2%) 1789
Eskalith 1527
Etrafon (Occasional) 3115
Extendryl 1361
Fareston Tablets 3237
Feldene Capsules (Occasional) 2685
Flexeril Tablets (1% to 3%) 572
Flexeril Tablets (1% to 3%) 2094
Flonase Nasal Spray 1533
Floxin I.V. 2526
Floxin Tablets 2529
FML Ophthalmic Suspension ⊙236
FML Forte Ophthalmic Suspension ⊙235
Furosemide Tablets 2284
Glucotrol XL Extended Release Tablets (Less than 3%) 2693
Haldol Decanoate 2535
Haldol Injection, Tablets and Concentrate 2533
Hivid Tablets (Less than 1%) 2975
Humorsol Sterile Ophthalmic Solution 2102
Hycomine Compound Tablets 1317
Hycotuss Expectorant Syrup 1318
HydroDIURIL Tablets 2108
Hytrin Capsules (0.6% to 1.6%) 464
Hyzaar 2109
Inderide Tablets 3517
Inderide LA Long-Acting Capsules 3519
Indocin (Less than 1%) 2112
Intron A for Injection (Less than 5%) 3120
Inversine Tablets 1850
Iopidine 0.5% Ophthalmic Solution (Less than 3%) ⊙213
Iopidine Sterile Ophthalmic Solution ⊙212
Ismo Tablets (Fewer than 1%) 3524
Isoptin SR Tablets (1% or less) 467
Kadian Capsules (Less than 3%) 1335
Klonopin Tablets (1%) 2983
Koāte-DVI (0.7%) 931
Lacrisert Sterile Ophthalmic Insert 2117
▲ Lamictal (11% to 25%) 1567
Lanoxicaps Capsules 1574
Lanoxin Injection 1581
Lanoxin Tablets 1587
Lanoxin Elixir Pediatric 1578
Lanoxin Injection Pediatric 1584
Levsin/Levsinex/Levbid 3172
Lexxel Tablets 608
Librium for Injection (Isolated instances) 1737
Lidoderm Patch 1319
▲ Limbitrol (Among most frequent) 1738
Lithium Carbonate 3061
Lithium Citrate Syrup 3061
Lithobid Slow-Release Tablets 3255
Lodine (1% to 3%) 3528
Lodine XL Extended-Release Tablets (1% to 3%) 3530
Lodosyn Tablets 1251
Lopid Tablets 2650
▲ Lotemax Sterile Ophthalmic Suspension 0.5% (5% to 15%) ⊙261
Lotensin HCT Tablets 2367
Loxitane Capsules 3398
Lupron Injection (Less than 5%) 3279
▲ Luvox Tablets (25, 50, 100 mg) (3%) 3256
Maxalt Tablets (Infrequent) 2120
Maxalt-MLT Orally Disintegrating Tablets (Infrequent) 2120
Maxzide 1008
Mepergan Injection (Occasional) 3539
Meridia Capsules 481
Metadate CD Capsules 1164
Metadate ER Tablets 1167
Methylin Tablets 1995
Methylin ER Tablets 1995
Mevacor Tablets (0.9% to 1.5%) 2132
▲ Mexitil Capsules (5.7% to 7.5%) 1047
Miacalcin Nasal Spray (Less than 1%) 2375
Micardis HCT Tablets 1051
Microzide Capsules 3414
Minipress Capsules (1% to 4%) 2699
Minizide Capsules 2700
Minocin Intravenous 1862
Minocin Oral Suspension 1865
Minocin Pellet-Filled Capsules 1863
Mintezol 2137
Moban (Occasional) 1320
Moduretic Tablets 2138
Monopril HCT 1094
Motofen Tablets (Less frequent) 577
Motrin Suspension, Oral Drops, Chewable Tablets, and Caplets (Less than 1%) 2002
MS Contin Tablets (Less frequent) 2896
MSIR (Less frequent) 2898
Mykrox Tablets 1168
Nadolol Tablets (1 to 5 of 1000 patients) 2288
Nardil Tablets (Less common) 2653
Naropin Injection 612
Navane Oral 2701
Navane Intramuscular 2703
Nesacaine/Nesacaine MPF 617
Neumega for Injection 1434
Norflex 1987
Noroxin Tablets (Less frequent) 2145
Norpramin Tablets 755
Norvir Capsules (Less than 2%) 487
Norvir Oral Solution (Less than 2%) 487
▲ Novantrone for Injection (3%) 1760
Nubain Injection (1% or less) 1323
NuLev Orally Disintegrating Tablets 3176
Ocuflox Ophthalmic Solution 554
Ocupress Ophthalmic Solution, 1% Sterile (Occasional) ⊙303
OptiPranolol Metipranolol Ophthalmic Solution 0.3% (A small number of patients) ⊙263
▲ Optivar Ophthalmic Solution (1% to 10%) 2273
Oramorph SR Tablets (Less frequent) 3062
Orap Tablets 1407
Orthoclone OKT3 Sterile Solution 2498
Parnate Tablets 1607
Patanol Ophthalmic Solution (Less than 5%) 540
▲ Paxil (2.0% to 7.8%) 1609
Periactin Tablets 2155
Phenergan Injection 3553
Phenergan Suppositories 3556
Phenergan Syrup (Occasional) 3554
Phenergan Tablets 3556
Phenergan with Codeine Syrup (Occasional) 3557
Phenergan with Dextromethorphan Syrup (Occasional) 3559
Phenergan VC Syrup (Occasional) 3560
Phenergan VC with Codeine Syrup (Occasional) 3561
Plaquenil Tablets (Fairly common) 3082
Polocaine Injection, USP 625
Polocaine-MPF Injection, USP 625
Ponstel Capsules (Occasional) 1356
Pred Forte Ophthalmic Suspension ⊙246
Prinivil Tablets (0.3% to 1.0%) 2164
Prinzide Tablets (0.3% to 1%) 2168
Procardia Capsules (2% or less) 2708
Propine Ophthalmic Solution ⊙250
Prosed/DS Tablets 3268
Prostin E2 Suppositories 2852
Protonix I.V. 3580
Protopam Chloride for Injection 3582
Quinaglute Dura-Tabs Tablets 978
Quinidex Extentabs 2933
Rescriptor Tablets 526
Rēv-Eyes Sterile Ophthalmic Eyedrops 0.5% (Less frequently) ⊙265
Ritalin 2387
Robaxin Injectable 2938
Robaxin Tablets 2939
Robaxisal Tablets 2939
Robinul Forte Tablets 1358
Robinul Injectable 2940
Robinul Tablets 1358
▲ Romazicon Injection (1% to 9%) 3000
Rynatan Tablets 3351
▲ Rythmol Tablets – 150 mg, 225 mg, 300 mg (2.0% to 5.7%) 502
Salagen Tablets (1% to 2%) 2229
Sandostatin Injection (1% to 4%) 2394
Sensorcaine 643
Sensorcaine-MPF Injection 643
Serentil 1057
Serophene Tablets (Occasionally) 3226
▲ Serzone Tablets (3% to 9%) 1104
Sinemet Tablets 1253
Sinemet CR Tablets 1255
Sinequan 2713
▲ Soriatane Capsules (1% to 10%) 3003
Stadol NS Nasal Spray (1% or greater) 1108
Stelazine 1640
Surmontil Capsules 3595
Talacen Caplets (Infrequent) 3089
Talwin Nx Tablets 3090
Tambocor Tablets 1990
Tarka Tablets (Less frequent) 508
Tasmar Tablets (1% or more) 3010
Tegretol/Tegretol-XR 2404
▲ Temodar Capsules (5%) 3157
Tenex Tablets (Less frequent) 2942
Thioplex for Injection 1765
Thioridazine Hydrochloride Tablets 2289
Thiothixene Capsules (Infrequently) 2290
Timolide Tablets 2187
▲ Timolol GFS (1 in 3 patients) ⊙266
Timoptic-XE Sterile Ophthalmic Gel Forming Solution 2194
▲ Tonocard Tablets (1.3% to 10.0%) 649
Toprol-XL Tablets 651
Toradol (1% or less) 3018
Transderm Scōp Transdermal Therapeutic System 2302
Tranxene (Less common) 511
Travatan Ophthalmic Solution (1% to 4%) 543
Trecator-SC Tablets 3598
Trental Tablets (Less than 1%) 784
Tricor Capsules, Micronized (1%) 513
Trilafon (Occasional) 3160
▲ Trisenox Injection (10%) 1158
Trusopt Sterile Ophthalmic Solution (Approximately 1% to 5%) 2196
Uniretic Tablets 3178
Urimax Tablets 1769
Urised Tablets 2876
Valium Injectable 3026
Valium Tablets (Infrequent) 3047
Vascor Tablets (0.5% to 2.0%) 2602
Vaseretic Tablets 2204
Vasotec I.V. Injection 2207
Vasotec Tablets (0.5% to 1.0%) 2210
Verelan Capsules (1% or less) 3184
Verelan PM Capsules (2% or less) 3186
Versed Injection (Less than 1%) 3027
Versed Syrup (Less than 1%) 3033
▲ Vexol 1% Ophthalmic Suspension (1% to 5%) ⊙222
▲ Viagra Tablets (3%) 2732
Vicodin Tuss Expectorant 519
Vioxx (Greater than 0.1% to 1.9%) 2213
▲ Visudyne for Injection (10% to 20%) ⊙308
▲ Vitravene for Injection (5% to 20%) ⊙310
Vivactil Tablets 2217
Vivactil Tablets 2446
Voltaren Ophthalmic Sterile Ophthalmic Solution (Less than 5%) ⊙312
Voltaren Tablets (Less than 1%) 2315
Voltaren-XR Tablets (Less than 1%) 2315
▲ Wellbutrin Tablets (14.6%) 1680
▲ Xalatan Latanoprost Ophthalmic Solution (5% to 15%) ⊙320
▲ Xalatan Sterile Ophthalmic Solution (5% to 15%) 2864
▲ Xanax Tablets (6.2% to 21.0%) 2865
▲ Xylocaine Injections (Among most common) 653
Zantac (Rare) 1690
Zantac Injection (Rare) 1688
Zantac Syrup (Rare) 1690
Zaroxolyn Tablets 1177
▲ Zenapax for Injection (2% to 5%) 3046
Zestoretic Tablets (0.3% to 1%) 695
Zestril Tablets (0.3% to 1.0%) 698
Ziac Tablets 1887
Zofran Injection 1698

Vision, changes

(*see under* Visual disturbances)

Vision, color tinge to

▲ Viagra Tablets (3%) 2732

Vision, complete loss

Brevicon 28-Day Tablets 3380
Depo-Provera Contraceptive Injection 2798
Levlen 962
Levlite 21 Tablets 962
Levlite 28 Tablets 962
Modicon 2563
Norinyl 1 +35 28-Day Tablets 3380
Norinyl 1 + 50 28-Day Tablets 3380
Ortho-Cyclen/Ortho Tri-Cyclen 2573
Ortho-Novum 2563
Ortho-Novum 1/50▫28 Tablets 2556
Ortho-Cyclen/Ortho Tri-Cyclen 2573
Ovcon 3364
Plaquenil Tablets (One case) 3082
Premphase Tablets 3572
Prempro Tablets 3572
Provera Tablets 2853
Tri-Levlen 962
Tri-Norinyl-28 Tablets 3433

Vision, double
(*see under* Diplopia)

Vision, loss of
- Cognex Capsules (Rare) 1351
- Cordarone Tablets 3487
- Desferal Vials 2333
- femhrt Tablets 2635
- Imitrex Injection 1549
- Imitrex Nasal Spray 1554
- Imitrex Tablets 1558
- Nipent for Injection (Less than 3%) 3272
- Pacerone Tablets 3331
- Paraplatin for Injection 1126
- Prinivil Tablets (0.3% to 1.0%) 2164
- Prinzide Tablets 2168
- Procardia Capsules 2708
- Serophene Tablets 3226
- ▲ Visudyne for Injection (1% to 10%) ⊙308
- Zestoretic Tablets 695
- Zestril Tablets (0.3% to 1.0%) 698

Vision, loss of color
- Cipro I.V. (1% or less) 893
- Cipro (Less than 1%) 887
- Motrin Suspension, Oral Drops, Chewable Tablets, and Caplets 2002

Vision, obscured by enlarged iris cysts
- Humorsol Sterile Ophthalmic Solution 2102

Vision, partial loss
- Brevicon 28-Day Tablets 3380
- Depo-Provera Contraceptive Injection 2798
- Levlen 962
- Levlite 21 Tablets 962
- Levlite 28 Tablets 962
- Mintezol 2137
- Modicon 2563
- Motrin Suspension, Oral Drops, Chewable Tablets, and Caplets (Less than 1%) 2002
- Norinyl 1 +35 28-Day Tablets 3380
- Norinyl 1 + 50 28-Day Tablets 3380
- Ortho-Cyclen/Ortho Tri-Cyclen 2573
- Ortho-Novum 2563
- Ortho-Novum 1/50□28 Tablets 2556
- Ortho-Cyclen/Ortho Tri-Cyclen 2573
- Ovcon 3364
- Premphase Tablets 3572
- Prempro Tablets 3572
- Provera Tablets 2853
- Tri-Levlen 962
- Tri-Norinyl-28 Tablets 3433

Vision, peripheral, decreased
- Vitravene for Injection (2% to 5%) ⊙310

Vision, temporary loss of
- Clomid Tablets 735
- Soma Tablets 3353
- Soma Compound Tablets (Very rare) 3354
- Soma Compound w/Codeine Tablets 3355
- Sular Tablets (Less than or equal to 1%) 688
- Viagra Tablets 2732

Vision, tunnel
- Serophene Tablets 3226

Vision abnormalities
(*see under* Visual disturbances)

Visual acuity, defects
- Alphagan P Ophthalmic Solution (1% to 4%) 546
- Alrex Sterile Ophthalmic Suspension 0.2% ⊙256
- Betoptic S Ophthalmic Suspension (Small number of patients) 537
- Blephamide Ophthalmic Ointment 547
- Blephamide Ophthalmic Suspension 548
- Cipro I.V. (1% or less) 893
- Cipro I.V. Pharmacy Bulk Package (Less than 1%) 897
- Cipro (Less than 1%) 887
- Cortisporin Ophthalmic Suspension ⊙297
- Cozaar Tablets (Less than 1%) 2067
- Desferal Vials 2333
- FML Ophthalmic Ointment ⊙237
- FML Ophthalmic Suspension ⊙236
- FML Forte Ophthalmic Suspension ⊙235
- FML-S Liquifilm Sterile Ophthalmic Suspension ⊙238
- HMS Sterile Ophthalmic Suspension ⊙240
- Hyzaar 2109
- Intron A for Injection 3120
- Isopto Carbachol Ophthalmic Solution ⊙215
- Isopto Carpine Ophthalmic Solution (Frequent) ⊙215
- Lotemax Sterile Ophthalmic Suspension 0.5% ⊙261
- Myambutol Tablets 1290
- Pilopine HS Ophthalmic Gel ⊙217
- Plaquenil Tablets 3082
- Pred Forte Ophthalmic Suspension ⊙246
- Pred Mild Sterile Ophthalmic Suspension ⊙249
- Pred-G Ophthalmic Suspension ⊙247
- Pred-G Sterile Ophthalmic Ointment ⊙248
- Rescula Ophthalmic Solution (Less than 1%) ⊙306
- Roferon-A Injection (Less than 1%) 2996
- Serophene Tablets 3226
- Symmetrel (0.1% to 1%) 1328
- TobraDex Ophthalmic Ointment 542
- TobraDex Ophthalmic Suspension 541
- ▲ Travatan Ophthalmic Solution (5% to 10%) 543
- ▲ Vesanoid Capsules (6%) 3037
- Vexol 1% Ophthalmic Suspension ⊙222
- ▲ Visudyne for Injection (10% to 20%) ⊙308
- ▲ Vitrasert Implant (Approximately 10% to 20%) ⊙254
- ▲ Vitravene for Injection (5% to 20%) ⊙310

Visual disturbances
- Accuretic Tablets 2614
- Accutane Capsules 2944
- Aciphex Tablets 1267
- Aciphex Tablets 1783
- Actiq (1% to 2%) 1184
- Activella Tablets 2764
- Acular Ophthalmic Solution (Rare) 544
- Acular PF Ophthalmic Solution 544
- Adalat CC Tablets (Less than 1.0%) 877
- Agrylin Capsules (1% to 5%) 3232
- Alferon N Injection (1%) 1770
- ▲ Alphagan Ophthalmic Solution (Approximately 3% to 9%) 545
- ▲ Alphagan P Ophthalmic Solution (Approximately 5% to 9%) 546
- ▲ Alrex Sterile Ophthalmic Suspension 0.2% (5% to 15%) ⊙256
- Altace Capsules (Less than 1%) 2233
- Ambien Tablets (Frequent) 3191
- Anaprox Tablets (Less than 3%) 2967
- Anaprox DS Tablets (Less than 3%) 2967
- Anzemet Injection (Infrequently) 719
- Anzemet Tablets (Infrequently) 722
- Aralen Tablets 3075
- Arthrotec Tablets (Rare) 3195
- Asacol Delayed-Release Tablets (2% or greater) 2884
- Astelin Nasal Spray 3339
- Avalide Tablets 1070
- Avapro Tablets (Less than 1%) 1074
- Avapro Tablets (Less than 1%) 3076
- Avonex 1013
- Baycol Tablets 883
- Betagan ⊙228
- Betapace Tablets (1% to 5%) 950
- Betapace AF Tablets (0.8% to 2.6%) 954
- ▲ Betaseron for SC Injection (7%) 988
- ▲ Betimol Ophthalmic Solution (More than 5%) ⊙324
- Blephamide Ophthalmic Suspension 548
- Blocadren Tablets 2046
- Brevibloc Injection (Less than 1%) 858
- Brevicon 28-Day Tablets 3380
- Buprenex Injectable (Less than 1%) 2918
- Cardura Tablets (1.4% to 2%) 2668
- Carteolol Hydrochloride Ophthalmic Solution USP, 1% (Occasional) ⊙258
- Celexa (At least 2%) 1365
- Cipro I.V. (1% or less) 893
- Cipro I.V. Pharmacy Bulk Package (Less than 1%) 897
- Cipro (Less than 1%) 887
- Claritin-D 24 Hour Extended Release Tablets (Fewer than 2%) 3104
- Clinoril Tablets (Less than 1 in 100) 2053
- Clomid Tablets (1.5%) 735
- ▲ Clozaril Tablets (5% or more) 2319
- Colazal Capsules 3069
- Comvax 2056
- Concerta Extended-Release Tablets 1998
- Concerta Tablets 561
- Copaxone for Injection (At least 2%) 3306
- ▲ Cordarone Tablets (4% to 9%) 3487
- ▲ Coreg Tablets (5.0%) 1508
- Corgard Tablets 2245
- Corzide 40/5 Tablets 2247
- Corzide 80/5 Tablets 2247
- Cosopt Sterile Ophthalmic Solution 2065
- Cuprimine Capsules 2075
- Cytotec Tablets (Infrequent) 3202
- Cytovene (At least 3 subjects) 2959
- Dantrium Capsules (Less frequent) 2885
- Darvon-N/Darvocet-N 1907
- Darvon Pulvules 1909
- Darvon Compound-65 Pulvules 1910
- Darvon-N Tablets 1912
- ▲ DaunoXome Injection (3%) 1442
- Declomycin Tablets 1855
- Demerol 3079
- Depacon Injection (1% to 5%) 416
- Depakene (1% to 5%) 421
- Depakote Sprinkle Capsules (1% to 5%) 426
- Depakote Tablets (1% to 5%) 430
- Depakote ER Tablets (1% to 5%) 436
- Desferal Vials 2333
- ▲ Detrol Tablets (4.7%) 3623
- Detrol LA Capsules (1%) 2801
- Digitek Tablets 1003
- Dilaudid Oral Liquid (Less frequent) 445
- Dilaudid Tablets - 8 mg (Less frequent) 445
- Dilaudid-HP (Less frequent) 443
- Diovan HCT Tablets (Greater than 0.2%) 2338
- Diprivan Injectable Emulsion (Less than 1%) 667
- Dolobid Tablets (Less than 1 in 100) 2088
- Dolophine Hydrochloride Tablets 3056
- ▲ Dostinex Tablets (1% to less than 10%) 2804
- Doxil Injection (Less than 1%) 566
- DynaCirc Capsules (0.5% to 1%) 2921
- DynaCirc CR Tablets (0.5% to 1%) 2923
- EC-Naprosyn Delayed-Release Tablets (Less than 3%) 2967
- Effexor Tablets (Frequent) 3495
- ▲ Effexor XR Capsules (4% to 8%) 3499
- Engerix-B Vaccine 1517
- Estrace Vaginal Cream 3358
- Estrace Tablets 3361
- Estring Vaginal Ring (At least 1 report) 2811
- Evoxac Capsules (1% to 3%) 1217
- Fareston Tablets 3237
- ▲ Felbatol (5.3%) 3343
- femhrt Tablets 2635
- Ferrlecit Injection (Greater than 1%) 3386
- ▲ Flolan for Injection (4%) 1528
- Floxin I.V. (1% to 3%) 2526
- Floxin Tablets (1% to 3%) 2529
- ▲ Fludara for Injection (3% to 15%) 995
- FML Ophthalmic Suspension ⊙236
- FML Forte Ophthalmic Suspension ⊙235
- FML-S Liquifilm Sterile Ophthalmic Suspension ⊙238
- Fortovase Capsules (Less than 2%) 2970
- ▲ Foscavir Injection (5% or greater) 605
- Sterile FUDR (Remote possibility) 2974
- Gabitril Tablets (Frequent) 1189
- Gengraf Capsules (1% to less than 3%) 457
- Genotropin Lyophilized Powder (A small number of patients) 2818
- ▲ Geodon Capsules (3%) 2688
- Halcion Tablets (0.5% to 0.9%) 2823
- Haldol Decanoate 2535
- Haldol Injection, Tablets and Concentrate 2533
- Hivid Tablets (Less than 1%) 2975
- Humatrope Vials and Cartridges 1930
- Hytrin Capsules (At least 1%) 464
- Imdur Tablets (Less than or equal to 5%) 1826
- Imitrex Injection (1.1%) 1549
- Imitrex Nasal Spray (Infrequent) 1554
- Imitrex Tablets (Up to 3%) 1558
- Inderal 3513
- Inderal LA Long-Acting Capsules 3516
- Inderide Tablets 3517
- Inderide LA Long-Acting Capsules 3519
- ▲ Infergen (3% to 5%) 1777
- Intron A for Injection (Less than 5%) 3120
- Invirase Capsules (Less than 2%) 2979
- Iopidine 0.5% Ophthalmic Solution (Less than 1%) ⊙213
- Iopidine Sterile Ophthalmic Solution ⊙212
- Kaletra Capsules (Less than 2%) 471
- Kaletra Oral Solution (Less than 2%) 471
- Klonopin Tablets (Infrequent) 2983
- ▲ Lamictal (3.4%) 1567
- Lamisil Tablets (1.1%) 2360
- Lanoxicaps Capsules 1574
- Lanoxin Injection 1581
- Lanoxin Tablets 1587
- Lanoxin Elixir Pediatric 1578
- Lanoxin Injection Pediatric 1584
- Lariam Tablets 2989
- Levaquin (Less than 0.5%) 2537
- Levlen 962
- Levlite 21 Tablets 962
- Levlite 28 Tablets 962
- Levo-Dromoran 1734
- Levorphanol Tartrate Tablets (1% to 3%) 3059
- Lexxel Tablets 608
- Livostin (Approximately 1% to 3%) ⊙305
- Lodine (Less than 1%) 3528
- Lodine XL Extended-Release Tablets (Less than 1%) 3530
- ▲ Lotemax Sterile Ophthalmic Suspension 0.5% (5% to 15%) ⊙261
- Lotensin HCT Tablets (0.3% or more) 2367
- ▲ Lumigan Ophthalmic Solution (3% to 10%) 553
- Lupron Depot–3 Month 22.5 mg (Less than 5%) 3288
- Marinol Capsules (Less than 1%) 3325
- Mepergan Injection 3539
- Meridia Capsules 481
- Metadate CD Capsules 1164
- Metadate ER Tablets 1167
- Methylin Tablets 1995
- Methylin ER Tablets 1995
- ▲ Mexitil Capsules (5.7% to 7.5%) 1047
- Micardis Tablets (More than 0.3%) 1049
- Micardis HCT Tablets 1051
- Midamor Tablets (Less than or equal to 1%) 2136
- Migranal Nasal Spray (Infrequent) 2376
- Miltown Tablets 3349
- Mirapex Tablets (1% or more) 2834
- Mobic Tablets (Less than 2%) 1054
- Modicon (Rare) 2563
- Moduretic Tablets (Less than or equal to 1%) 2138
- Monopril Tablets (0.2% to 1.0%) 1091
- Monopril HCT 1094
- MS Contin Tablets (Less frequent) 2896
- MSIR (Less frequent) 2898
- Myambutol Tablets 1290
- Myobloc Injectable Solution (2% or greater) 1291
- Nadolol Tablets 2288
- Naprelan Tablets (Less than 3%) 1293
- Naprosyn Suspension (Less than 3%) 2967
- Naprosyn Tablets (Less than 3%) 2967
- Naropin Injection (Less than 1%) 612
- Neoral Soft Gelatin Capsules (1% to less than 3%) 2380
- Neoral Oral Solution (1% to less than 3%) 2380
- Neurontin Capsules (Frequent) 2655
- Neurontin Oral Solution (Frequent) 2655
- Neurontin Tablets (Frequent) 2655
- Nexium Delayed-Release Capsules (Less than 1%) 619
- Nicotrol Nasal Spray (Less than 1%) 2843
- ▲ Nilandron Tablets (6.2%) 753
- Nipent for Injection (Less than 3%) 3272
- Nolvadex Tablets 678
- Norditropin Cartridges (Small number of patients) 2420
- Norditropin for Injection (Small number of patients) 2419
- Norinyl 1 +35 28-Day Tablets 3380
- Norinyl 1 + 50 28-Day Tablets 3380
- Normodyne Tablets (1%) 3137
- Noroxin Tablets 2145
- Norplant System 3543
- Norvasc Tablets (More than 0.1% to 1%) 2704
- Norvir Capsules (Less than 2%) 487
- Norvir Oral Solution (Less than 2%) 487
- Nutropin AQ Injection (A small number of patients) 1420
- Nutropin Depot for Injectable Suspension 1423
- Nutropin for Injection (A small number of patients) 1417
- Ocupress Ophthalmic Solution, 1% Sterile (Occasional) ⊙303
- OptiPranolol Metipranolol Ophthalmic Solution 0.3% (A small number of patients) ⊙263
- Oramorph SR Tablets (Less frequent) 3062
- ▲ Orap Tablets (5.5%) 1407
- Ortho-Cyclen/Ortho Tri-Cyclen 2573
- Ortho-Est Tablets 3464
- Ortho-Novum (Rare) 2563
- Ortho-Novum 1/50□28 Tablets (Rare) 2556
- Ortho-Cyclen/Ortho Tri-Cyclen 2573
- Orudis Capsules (Greater than 1%) 3548
- Oruvail Capsules (Greater than 1%) 3548
- OxyContin Tablets (Less than 1%) 2912
- ▲ Pacerone Tablets (4% to 9%) 3331
- Paraplatin for Injection (1%) 1126
- Paxil (2% to 4%) 1609
- ▲ Permax Tablets (5.8%) 1299
- Phenergan with Codeine Syrup 3557
- Phenergan VC with Codeine Syrup 3561

Photofrin for Injection 831
Plaquenil Tablets 3082
Plendil Extended-Release Tablets (0.5% to 1.5%) 623
Pred Forte Ophthalmic Suspension .... ⊙ 246
Premphase Tablets 3572
Prempro Tablets 3572
Procardia XL Extended Release Tablets (1% or less) 2710
▲ Prograf (3% to 15%) 1393
▲ Proleukin for Injection (7%) 1199
Prometrium Capsules (100 mg, 200 mg) (Less than 5%) 3261
ProSom Tablets (Infrequent) 500
Prostigmin Injectable 1744
Prostigmin Tablets 1744
Protonix I.V. (Less than 1%) 3580
Protonix Tablets (Less than 1%) 3577
Provigil Tablets (2%) 1193
▲ Prozac Pulvules, Liquid, and Weekly Capsules (3%) 1238
▲ Quinidex Extentabs (3%) 2933
Quixin Ophthalmic Solution (1% to 3%) 3093
▲ Rapamune Oral Solution and Tablets (3% to 20%) 3584
Recombivax HB (Less than 1%) 2178
Reglan 2935
Relafen Tablets (Less than 1%) 1617
ReoPro Vials (0.7%) 1958
▲ Requip Tablets (6%) 1621
▲ Rescula Ophthalmic Solution (5% to 10%) .... ⊙ 306
Rifadin 765
Rifamate Capsules 767
Rifater Tablets 769
Risperdal (1% to 2%) 1796
Ritalin (Rare) 2387
▲ Roferon-A Injection (5% to 6%) 2996
▲ Romazicon Injection (1% to 9%) 3000
Roxanol 3066
Rythmol Tablets – 150 mg, 225 mg, 300 mg (Less than 1% to 1.9%) 502
Saizen for Injection (A small number of patients) 3225
Salagen Tablets (1%) 2229
Sandimmune (Rare) 2388
Sandostatin Injection (1% to 4%) 2394
Sandostatin LAR Depot (1% to 4%) 2395
▲ Sarafem Pulvules (3%) 1962
Sectral Capsules (2%) 3589
Serophene Tablets (Approximately 1 in 50 patients) 3226
Seroquel Tablets (Infrequent) 684
▲ Serostim for Injection (1% to 10%) 3229
▲ Serzone Tablets (Up to 10%) 1104
▲ Simulect for Injection (3% to 10%) 2399
Sonata Capsules (Less than 1% to 2%) 3591
▲ Soriatane Capsules (1% to 10%) 3003
Sporanox Oral Solution (Less than 2%) 1808
Sporanox Oral Solution (Less than 2%) 2512
Sular Tablets (Less than or equal to 1%) 688
Sustiva Capsules 1258
Symmetrel (0.1% to 1%) 1328
Talacen Caplets (Infrequent) 3089
Talwin Nx Tablets 3090
▲ Tambocor Tablets (15.9%) 1990
Taxol Injection (Rare) 1129
▲ Temodar Capsules (5%) 3157
Tenex Tablets (3% or less) 2942
Tenoretic Tablets 690
Tenormin 692
Tequin Injection (0.1% to 3%) 1110
Tequin Tablets (0.1% to 3%) 1110
Terra-Cortril Ophthalmic Suspension 2716
Teveten Tablets (Less than 1%) 3327
Thorazine 1656
Timolide Tablets 2187
Timolol GFS .... ⊙ 266
Timoptic in Ocudose (Less frequent) 2192
Timoptic Sterile Ophthalmic Solution (Less frequent) 2190
Timoptic-XE Sterile Ophthalmic Gel Forming Solution 2194
Tolectin (1% to 3%) 2589
▲ Tonocard Tablets (1.3% to 10.0%) 649
▲ Topamax Sprinkle Capsules (10.5% to 14.2%) 2590
▲ Topamax Tablets (10.5% to 14.2%) 2590
Toradol (1% or less) 3018
Travatan Ophthalmic Solution (1% to 4%) 543
Tricor Capsules, Micronized 513
▲ Trileptal Oral Suspension (2% to 14%) 2407
▲ Trileptal Tablets (2% to 14%) 2407
Tri-Levlen 962
Tri-Norinyl-28 Tablets 3433
Trovan (Less than 1%) 2722
Twinrix Vaccine 1674
Ultracet Tablets (Less than 1%) 2597
Ultram Tablets (1% to 5%) 2600
Uniretic Tablets (Less than 1%) 3178
Valtrex Caplets 1676
Versed Injection (Less than 1%) 3027
▲ Vesanoid Capsules (17%) 3037
▲ Viagra Tablets (3%) 2732
Vicoprofen Tablets (Less than 1%) 520
Vistide Injection 1445
▲ Visudyne for Injection (10% to 20%) .... ⊙ 308
▲ Vitravene for Injection (5% to 20%) .... ⊙ 310
Vivelle Transdermal System 2412
Vivelle-Dot Transdermal System 2416
Voltaren Ophthalmic Sterile Ophthalmic Solution (Less than 5%) .... ⊙ 312
Wellbutrin Tablets (Infrequent) 1680
Zebeta Tablets 1885
Ziac Tablets 1887
▲ Zoloft (4%) 2751
Zovirax Capsules 1706
Zovirax for Injection 1708
Zovirax 1706

Visual disturbances, flashing lights

Clomid Tablets (1.5%) 735

Visual field defect

Agrylin Capsules (1% to 5%) 3232
Alphagan P Ophthalmic Solution (1% to 4%) 546
Alrex Sterile Ophthalmic Suspension 0.2% .... ⊙ 256
Betaseron for SC Injection 988
Blephamide Ophthalmic Ointment 547
Blephamide Ophthalmic Suspension 548
Cerebyx Injection (Infrequent) 2619
Cognex Capsules (Infrequent) 1351
Cortisporin Ophthalmic Suspension .... ⊙ 297
Cosopt Sterile Ophthalmic Solution (1% to 5%) 2065
Doxil Injection (Less than 1%) 566
Effexor Tablets (Infrequent) 3495
Effexor XR Capsules (Infrequent) 3499
Eskalith 1527
▲ Fareston Tablets (4%) 3237
FML Ophthalmic Ointment .... ⊙ 237
FML Ophthalmic Suspension .... ⊙ 236
FML Forte Ophthalmic Suspension .... ⊙ 235
FML-S Liquifilm Sterile Ophthalmic Suspension .... ⊙ 238
Gabitril Tablets (Infrequent) 1189
Geodon Capsules (Rare) 2688
Gliadel Wafer (2%) 1723
HMS Sterile Ophthalmic Suspension .... ⊙ 240
Intron A for Injection 3120
Klonopin Tablets (Infrequent) 2983
Lotemax Sterile Ophthalmic Suspension 0.5% .... ⊙ 261
Luvox Tablets (25, 50, 100 mg) (Infrequent) 3256
Neurontin Capsules (Infrequent) 2655
Neurontin Oral Solution (Infrequent) 2655
Neurontin Tablets (Infrequent) 2655
Nexium Delayed-Release Capsules (Less than 1%) 619
Norvir Capsules (Less than 2%) 487
Norvir Oral Solution (Less than 2%) 487
Paxil (Infrequent) 1609
Permax Tablets (Infrequent) 1299
Pred Forte Ophthalmic Suspension .... ⊙ 246
Pred Mild Sterile Ophthalmic Suspension .... ⊙ 249
Pred-G Ophthalmic Suspension .... ⊙ 247
Prevacid Delayed-Release Capsules (Less than 1%) 3292
PREVPAC (Less than 1%) 3298
ProAmatine Tablets (Rare) 3241
Prozac Pulvules, Liquid, and Weekly Capsules (Rare) 1238
Quinaglute Dura-Tabs Tablets 978
Quinidex Extentabs 2933
Romazicon Injection (1% to 3%) 3000
Sandostatin LAR Depot (Rare) 2395
Sarafem Pulvules (Rare) 1962
Serzone Tablets (2%) 1104
Sonata Capsules (Rare) 3591
TobraDex Ophthalmic Ointment 542
TobraDex Ophthalmic Suspension 541
Topamax Sprinkle Capsules (Infrequent) 2590
Topamax Tablets (Infrequent) 2590
Trovan (Less than 1%) 2722
▲ Vesanoid Capsules (3%) 3037
Vexol 1% Ophthalmic Suspension .... ⊙ 222
Vistide Injection 1445
▲ Visudyne for Injection (10% to 20%) .... ⊙ 308
Vitravene for Injection (2% to 5%) .... ⊙ 310
Zanaflex Tablets (Infrequent) 1305
Zoloft (Rare) 2751
Zonegran Capsules (Infrequent) 1307
Zyrtec (Less than 2%) 2756
Zyrtec-D 12 Hour Extended Relief Tablets (Less than 2%) 2758

Visual impairment

Abelcet Injection 1273
Ciloxan (Less than 1%) 538
Cordarone Tablets 3487
Levlen (Rare) 962
Levlite 21 Tablets (Rare) 962
Levlite 28 Tablets (Rare) 962
Ortho-Cyclen/Ortho Tri-Cyclen (Rare) 2573
Pacerone Tablets 3331
Tri-Levlen (Rare) 962

Visual trails

▲ Serzone Tablets (7%) 1104

Vitamin B_{12} deficiency

Nexium Delayed-Release Capsules (Less than 1%) 619

Vitamin D, increased requirement

Skelid Tablets (2.7%) 3088

Vitiligo

Azelex Cream (Rare) 547
Finevin Cream (Rare) 962
Intron A for Injection (Less than 5%) 3120
Proleukin for Injection 1199
Trileptal Oral Suspension 2407
Trileptal Tablets 2407

Vitreous detachment

Cosopt Sterile Ophthalmic Solution (1% to 5%) 2065
Evoxac Capsules (Less than 1%) 1217
Serophene Tablets 3226
Viagra Tablets 2732

Vitreous disorder, unspecified

Betaxon Ophthalmic Suspension (Less than 2%) 537
Clomid Tablets 735
Cytovene (At least 3 subjects) 2959
Rescula Ophthalmic Solution (1% to 5%) .... ⊙ 306

Vitreous floaters

Alphagan P Ophthalmic Solution (1% to 4%) 546
Avonex 1013
Cataflam Tablets (Less than 1%) 2315
Miacalcin Nasal Spray (Less than 1%) 2375
Sular Tablets (Less than or equal to 1%) 688
Voltaren Tablets (Less than 1%) 2315
Voltaren-XR Tablets (Less than 1%) 2315

Vitreous opacity

Vitravene (2% to 5%) .... ⊙ 310

Voice, deepening of

Anadrol-50 Tablets 3321
▲ Android Capsules, 10 mg (Among most common) 1731
▲ Delatestryl Injection (Among most frequent) 1151
Estratest 3252
Oxandrin Tablets 1153
Testred Capsules, 10 mg 1746

Voice, hoarseness

Estratest 3252

Voice, loss of

(*see under* Aphonia)

Voice alteration

Accutane Capsules 2944
Actiq (Less than 1%) 1184
Azmacort Inhalation Aerosol (1% to 3%) 728
▲ CellCept Capsules (3% to 10%) 2951
▲ CellCept Intravenous (3% to 10%) 2951
▲ CellCept Oral Suspension (3% to 10%) 2951
▲ CellCept Tablets (3% to 10%) 2951
Copaxone for Injection (Infrequent) 3306
Doxil Injection (Less than 1%) 566
DuoNeb Inhalation Solution (More than 1%) 1233
Effexor Tablets (Infrequent) 3495
Effexor XR Capsules (Infrequent) 3499
Flonase Nasal Spray 1533
Gabitril Tablets (Infrequent) 1189
Imitrex Injection 1549
Imitrex Nasal Spray (Rare) 1554
Imitrex Tablets (Rare) 1558
Kadian Capsules (Less than 3%) 1335
Lotensin HCT Tablets 2367
Lupron Depot–4 Month 30 mg (Less than 5%) 3289
▲ Mirapex Tablets (3%) 2834
Monopril Tablets (0.4% to 1.0%) 1091
OxyContin Tablets (Less than 1%) 2912
Paxil (Infrequent) 1609
Permax Tablets (Infrequent) 1299
▲ Prograf (3% to 15%) 1393
Protonix I.V. (Less than 1%) 3580
Protonix Tablets (Less than 1%) 3577
▲ Pulmicort Turbuhaler Inhalation Powder (1% to 6%) 636
▲ Pulmozyme Inhalation Solution (12% to 18%) 1426
Salagen Tablets (2%) 2229
Serzone Tablets (Infrequent) 1104
Sonata Capsules (Infrequent) 3591
Thalomid Capsules 1154
▲ TOBI Solution for Inhalation (13%) 1206
Uniretic Tablets (Less than 1%) 3178
▲ Zoladex (3%) 702
Zoladex 3-month 706
Zomig Tablets (Rare) 708
Zomig-ZMT Tablets (Rare) 708
Zyprexa Tablets (Infrequent) 1973
Zyprexa ZYDIS Orally Disintegrating Tablets (Infrequent) 1973

Vomiting

▲ Abelcet Injection (3% to 8%) 1273
Accolate Tablets (1.5%) 657
Accupril Tablets (1.4% to 2.4%) 2611
Accuretic Tablets (1.8%) 2614
Accutane Capsules 2944
Acel-Imune (2% to 3%) 1851
Aceon Tablets (2 mg, 4 mg, 8 mg) (1.5%) 3249
Aciphex Tablets 1267
Aciphex Tablets 1783
▲ ActHIB Vaccine (1.5% to 5.4%) 798
▲ Actimmune (13%) 1772
▲ Actiq (6% to 15%) 1184
Activase I.V. 1410
Activella Tablets 2764
Adalat CC Tablets (Less than 1.0%) 877
▲ Adderall XR Capsules (7%)
Adriamycin PFS/RDF Injection (Frequent) 2767
▲ Advair Diskus 100/50 (4%) 1448
▲ Advair Diskus 250/50 (6%) 1448
▲ Advair Diskus 500/50 (4% to 6%) 1448
▲ Aerobid/Aerobid-M (25%) 1363
Aerolate 1361
▲ Agenerase Capsules (24% to 34%) 1454
▲ Agenerase Oral Solution (24% to 34%) 1459
▲ Aggrenox Capsules (8.4%) 1026
▲ Agrylin Capsules (9.7%) 3232
AK-Fluor Injection 10% and 25% .... ⊙ 202
▲ Albenza Tablets (3.7% to 6.2%) 1463
Albuminar-5, U.S.P. 785
Albuminar-25, U.S.P. 786
Aldoclor Tablets 2035
Aldomet Tablets 2037
Aldoril Tablets 2039
Alesse-21 Tablets 3468
Alesse-28 Tablets 3473
▲ Alferon N Injection (3% to 29%) 1770
Alkeran for Injection 1465
Alkeran Tablets (Infrequent) 1466
Aloprim for Injection (1.2%) 2292
Alora Transdermal System 3372
Altace Capsules (Less than 1% to 2%) 2233
Alupent (1% to 4%) 1029
Amaryl Tablets (Less than 1%) 717
Ambien Tablets (1%) 3191
▲ AmBisome for Injection (22.4% to 31.8%) 1383
Amerge Tablets (Frequent) 1467
Amicar Injection 3608
Amicar Syrup 3608
Amicar Tablets 3608
Aminohippurate Sodium PAH Injection 2041
Amoxil Chewable Tablets 1471
Amoxil for Oral Suspension 1471
Amoxil 1471
▲ Amphotec (6% to 11%) 1774
Anadrol-50 Tablets 3321
Anaprox Tablets (Less than 1%) 2967
Anaprox DS Tablets (Less than 1%) 2967
Ancef for Injection (Rare) 1474
Ancef Injection (Rare) 1474
Ancobon Capsules 1730
Androderm Transdermal System CIII 3377
Antabuse Tablets 3474
Aquasol A Parenteral 593
Aralen Tablets 3075
▲ Arava Tablets (3%) 724
▲ Aredia for Injection (35.7%) 2309
▲ Argatroban Injection (4.2%) 1478
▲ Aricept Tablets (5%) 1270
▲ Aricept Tablets (5%) 2665
▲ Arimidex Tablets (7.5% to 10.6%) 659
▲ Aromasin Tablets (7%) 2769
Artane 1855
Arthrotec Tablets (Rare) 3195
▲ Asacol Delayed-Release Tablets (5%) 2884
Astelin Nasal Spray (Infrequent) 3339
Astramorph/PF Injection, USP (Preservative-Free) (Frequent) 594
Atacand Tablets (More than 1%) 595
Atacand HCT Tablets (0.5% or greater) 597
Ativan Injection (Less than 1%) 3478
Atromid-S Capsules (Less frequent) 3483

Atrovent Inhalation Aerosol............ 1030
Augmentin Chewable Tablets (1%).. 1482
Augmentin Powder for Oral Suspension (1%)........................ 1482
Augmentin Tablets (1%)................... 1485
Augmentin ES-600 Powder for Oral Suspension (2.2%).................. 1487
▲ Avalide Tablets (3%) 1070
Avapro Tablets (1% or greater)....... 1074
Avapro Tablets (1% or greater)....... 3076
Avelox Tablets (2%)........................ 879
Avonex.. 1013
Axert Tablets (Infrequent)................ 2772
Axid Pulvules (1.2% to 3.6%)........... 1903
Axid Pulvules (1.2% to 3.6%)........... 2919
Azactam for Injection (1% to 1.3%)... 1276
Azmacort Inhalation Aerosol (1% to 3%)... 728
▲ Azulfidine EN-tabs Tablets (Among most common)........................... 2775
▲ Bactrim (Among most common) 2949
Baycol Tablets (Rare)..................... 883
Genuine Bayer Professional Labeling (Aspirin Regimen Bayer) (2.1%).......................... ▣ 608
Benadryl Parenteral........................ 2617
BeneFix for Injection....................... 1432
▲ Betapace Tablets (5% to 10%) 950
▲ Betapace AF Tablets (5.7% to 7.8%)... 954
▲ Betaseron for SC Injection (21%) ... 988
▲ Biaxin/Biaxin XL (6%) 403
Bicillin C-R 900/300 Injection......... 2240
Bicillin C-R Injection........................ 2238
Bicillin L-A Injection........................ 2242
Blocadren Tablets (Less than 1%)... 2046
Brethine Ampuls (1.3% to 3.9%)..... 2314
Brethine Tablets (Less than 1%)...... 2313
Brevibloc Injection (About 1%)........ 858
Brevicon 28-Day Tablets................. 3380
Brevital Sodium for Injection, USP... 1815
Buprenex Injectable (1% to 5%)....... 2918
Calcijex Injection............................ 411
Calcium Disodium Versenate Injection... 1980
▲ Campath Ampules (4% to 41%) 992
Cancidas for Injection (1.2% to 3.1%)... 2048
Captopril Tablets (About 0.5% to 2%).. 2281
Carafate Suspension (Less than 0.5%)... 731
Carafate Tablets (Less than 0.5%).. 730
▲ Carbatrol Capsules (Among most frequent)...................................... 3234
▲ Cardene I.V. (4.9%) 3485
Cardizem Injectable (Less than 1%).. 1018
Cardizem Lyo-Ject Syringe (Less than 1%)....................................... 1018
Cardizem Monovial (Less than 1%).. 1018
Cardizem CD Capsules (Less than 1%).. 1016
Cardura Tablets.............................. 2668
▲ Carnitor Injection (9% to 12%) 3242
Carnitor Tablets and Oral Solution... 3245
▲ Casodex Tablets (5%) 662
Cataflam Tablets (Less than 1%)..... 2315
▲ Catapres Tablets (About 5 in 100 patients)....................................... 1037
Catapres-TTS (0.5% or less)........... 1038
Ceclor CD Tablets (0.1% to 1%)....... 1279
Ceclor (Rare).................................... 1905
Cedax (Greater than or equal to 1%).. 1021
Cefizox for Intramuscular or Intravenous Use (Occasional)....... 1390
Cefobid Intravenous/Intramuscular (Rare)... 2671
Cefobid Pharmacy Bulk Package - Not for Direct Infusion (Rare)........ 2673
Cefotan.. 664
Ceftin (2.6%)................................... 1898
Cefzil (1%)....................................... 1076
Celebrex Capsules (0.1% to 1.9%)... 2676
Celebrex Capsules (0.1% to 1.9%)... 2780
▲ Celexa (4%) 1365
▲ CellCept Capsules (12.5% to 33.9%)... 2951
▲ CellCept Intravenous (12.5% to 33.9%)... 2951
▲ CellCept Oral Suspension (12.5% to 33.9%)..................................... 2951
▲ CellCept Tablets (12.5% to 33.9%)... 2951
Celontin Capsules (Frequent).......... 2618
▲ Cenestin Tablets (7%) 1263
Ceptaz for Injection (One in 500 patients)....................................... 1499
Cerebyx Injection (2.2% to 2.8%).... 2619
Cerezyme for Injection.................... 1438
Cerubidine for Injection................... 947
Cervidil Vaginal Insert (Less than 1%).. 1369
▲ Chemet Capsules (12.0% to 20.9%)... 3078
▲ Chirocaine Injection (8.3%) 2909
New Formulation Chromagen OB Capsules.................................... 3094
Cipro I.V. (1% or less)..................... 893
Cipro I.V. Pharmacy Bulk Package (Less than 1%)............................ 897
Cipro (2.0%).................................... 887
Claforan Injection (1.4%; rare)......... 732
Claritin (At least one patient).......... 3100
Claritin-D 12 Hour Extended Release Tablets (Less frequent)... 3102
Claritin-D 24 Hour Extended Release Tablets (Fewer than 2%).. 3104
Cleocin HCl Capsules...................... 2784
Cleocin Phosphate Sterile Solution.. 2785
Cleocin Vaginal Cream (Less than 1%).. 2788
Cleocin Vaginal Ovules (Less than 1%).. 2789
Climara Transdermal System.......... 958
Clinoril Tablets (Greater than 1%).... 2053
Clomid Tablets (2.2%)..................... 735
▲ Clorpres Tablets (About 5%) 1002
▲ Clozaril Tablets (3%) 2319
Cogentin.. 2055
▲ Cognex Capsules (28%) 1351
▲ Colazal Capsules (4%) 3069
Colestid Tablets (Less frequent)...... 2791
Colyte with Flavor Packs for Oral Solution (Less frequent)............... 3170
▲ Combipres Tablets (About 5%) 1040
Combivent Inhalation Aerosol (Less than 2%)............................ 1041
▲ Combivir Tablets (13%) 1502
Compazine...................................... 1505
▲ Comtan Tablets (4%) 2328
Comvax (1.0% to 2.5%)................... 2056
▲ Concerta Extended-Release Tablets (4%).................................. 1998
▲ Concerta Tablets (4%) 561
Condylox Topical Solution (Less than 5%)....................................... 2437
▲ Copaxone for Injection (6%) 3306
Cordarone Intravenous (Less than 2%).. 3491
▲ Cordarone Tablets (10% to 33%) 3487
▲ Coreg Tablets (6.3%) 1508
Corgard Tablets (1 to 5 per 1000 patients)....................................... 2245
Corlopam Injection (1% to 2%)......... 412
Corzide 40/5 Tablets (1 to 5 of 1000 patients)............................ 2247
Corzide 80/5 Tablets (1 to 5 of 1000 patients)............................ 2247
Cosmegen for Injection (Common)....................................... 2062
Cosopt Sterile Ophthalmic Solution (1% to 5%)...................... 2065
Coumadin for Injection (Infrequent)................................... 1243
Coumadin Tablets (Infrequent)......... 1243
Cozaar Tablets (Less than 1%)......... 2067
▲ Creon 5 Capsules (Among most frequent)...................................... 3251
▲ Creon 10 Capsules (Among most frequent)...................................... 3251
▲ Creon 20 Capsules (Among most frequent)...................................... 3251
▲ Crinone 8% Gel (5%) 3213
▲ Crixivan Capsules (4.1%) 2070
Cuprimine Capsules (Greater than 1%).. 2075
Cyclessa Tablets 2450
CytoGam Intravenous (Less than 5.0%)... 2026
Cytotec Tablets (1.3%)..................... 3202
▲ Cytovene (13%) 2959
Dantrium Capsules (Rare)................ 2885
Dapsone Tablets USP...................... 1780
▲ Daranide Tablets (Among the most common effects).................. 2077
Daraprim Tablets............................. 1511
▲ Darvon-N/Darvocet-N (Among most frequent)............................ 1907
▲ Darvon Pulvules (Among most frequent)...................................... 1909
▲ Darvon Compound-65 Pulvules (Among most frequent)................ 1910
▲ Darvon-N Tablets (Among most frequent)...................................... 1912
▲ DaunoXome Injection (3% to 20%) . 1442
Declomycin Tablets......................... 1855
Demadex Tablets and Injection........ 2965
▲ Demerol (Among most frequent) 3079
Demser Capsules (Infrequent).......... 2085
▲ Depacon Injection (1.3% to 27%) 416
▲ Depakene (23% to 27%) 421
▲ Depakote Sprinkle Capsules (15% to 27%).. 426
▲ Depakote Tablets (11% to 27%) 430
▲ Depakote ER Tablets (7% to 27%) .. 436
▲ Depen Titratable Tablets (17%) 3341
▲ DepoCyt Injection (3% to 12%) 1197
Desferal Vials.................................. 2333
Desogen Tablets 2458
▲ Detrol Tablets (4.2%) 3623
D.H.E. 45 Injection.......................... 2334
Diabinese Tablets (Less than 2%).... 2680
Diamox Intravenous......................... ⊙ 269
Diamox Sequels Sustained Release Capsules......................... ⊙ 270
Diamox Tablets .... ⊙ 269
▲ Diflucan Tablets, Injection, and Oral Suspension (1.7% to 5.4%).. 2681
Digitek Tablets (2%)........................ 1003
Dilantin Infatabs............................. 2624
Dilantin Kapseals............................ 2622
Dilantin-125 Oral Suspension.......... 2625
Dilaudid (Infrequent)........................ 441
Dilaudid Oral Liquid......................... 445
Dilaudid Powder (Infrequent)........... 441
Dilaudid Rectal Suppositories (Infrequent)................................. 441
Dilaudid Tablets (Infrequent)............ 441
Dilaudid Tablets - 8 mg 445
▲ Dilaudid-HP (Among most frequent)...................................... 443
Diovan Capsules (Less frequent)...... 2337
Diovan HCT Tablets (Greater than 0.2%)... 2338
Dipentum Capsules (1.0%).............. 2803
Diphtheria & Tetanus Toxoids Adsorbed Purogenated for Pediatric Use (2.6%)................... 1857
Diprivan Injectable Emulsion (Less than 1%) 667
Diucardin Tablets 3494
Diuril Oral 2087
Diuril Sodium Intravenous 2086
Dolobid Tablets (Greater than 1 in 100) 2088
▲ Dolophine Hydrochloride Tablets (Among most frequent) 3056
Donnatal 2929
Donnatal Extentabs 2930
Donnatal Tablets 2929
Dopram Injectable 2931
Doryx Coated Pellet Filled Capsules 3357
Dostinex Tablets (2% to 4%) 2804
▲ Doxil Injection (7.8% to 22.4%) 566
▲ DTIC-Dome (90% with the initial few doses) 902
▲ Duraclon Injection (5% to 10.5%) 3057
▲ Duragesic Transdermal System (10% or more) 1786
Duramorph Injection (Frequent) 1312
Duranest Injections 600
Duricef (Rare) 1079
Dyazide Capsules 1515
Dynabac Tablets (1.1% to 3%) 2269
Dynacin Capsules 2019
DynaCirc Capsules 2921
DynaCirc CR Tablets (0.5% to 1%) .. 2923
Dyrenium Capsules (Rare) 3458
EC-Naprosyn Delayed-Release Tablets (Less than 1%) 2967
Ecotrin Enteric Coated Aspirin Low, Regular and Maximum Strength Tablets 1715
Edecrin 2091
▲ E.E.S. (Among most frequent) 450
▲ Effexor Tablets (6% to 7.9%) 3495
▲ Effexor XR Capsules (4% to 6%) 3499
ELA-Max Cream 1340
Eldepryl Capsules 3266
▲ Ellence Injection (22.1% to 92.4%) 2806
Elmiron Capsules (Less than or equal to 1%) 570
Elspar for Injection 2092
Emcyt Capsules (1%) 2810
Emla (Unlikely with cream) 602
Enalaprilat Injection 863
▲ Enbrel for Injection (5%) 1752
▲ Enbrel for Injection (5%) 3504
Engerix-B Vaccine (Less than 1%) ... 1517
EpiPen 1236
▲ Epivir (13%) 1520
▲ Epivir-HBV (15%) 1524
▲ Epogen for Injection (0.26% to 22%) 582
▲ Ergamisol Tablets (6% to 20%) 1789
▲ EryPed (Among most frequent) 446
▲ Ery-Tab Tablets (Among most frequent) 448
▲ Erythrocin Stearate Filmtab Tablets (Among most frequent) 452
▲ Erythromycin Base Filmtab Tablets (Among most frequent) 454
▲ Erythromycin Delayed-Release Capsules, USP (Among most frequent) 455
Esclim Transdermal System 3460
Eskalith 1527
Estinyl Tablets 3112
Estrace Vaginal Cream 3358
Estrace Tablets 3361
Estratest 3252
Estring Vaginal Ring (At least 1 report) 2811
Estrostep 2627
▲ Ethyol for Injection (8% to 19%) 2029
Etrafon (Occasional) 3115
▲ Eulexin Capsules (11%) 3118
▲ Evista Tablets (3.4% to 4.8%) 1915
▲ Evoxac Capsules (4.6%) 1217
▲ Exelon Capsules (31%) 2342
▲ Exelon Oral Solution (31%) 2345
Famotidine Injection (Infrequent) 866
Famvir Tablets (1.3% to 4.8%) 2348
▲ Fareston Tablets (4%) 3237
▲ Felbatol (8.6% to 38.7%) 3343
▲ Feldene Capsules (1% to 10%) 2685
▲ Femara Tablets (4%) 2351
▲ femhrt Tablets (7.4%) 2635
Flexeril Tablets (Less than 1%)........ 572
Flexeril Tablets (Less than 1%)........ 2094
▲ Flolan for Injection (32% to 67%) ... 1528
Flomax Capsules (Infrequent).......... 1044
▲ Flonase Nasal Spray (2.6% to 4.8%)... 1533
▲ Flovent Diskus (8% to 9%) 3614
▲ Flovent (1% to 22%) 1535
Flovent Rotadisk............................... 1537
Floxin I.V. (1% to 4%)...................... 2526
Floxin Otic Solution (0.3%).............. 1219
Floxin Tablets (1% to 4%)................ 2529
▲ Fludara for Injection (31% to 36%) . 995
Flumadine (1.7%)............................. 1370
Fluorescite Injection .... ⊙ 211
Fluothane Inhalation........................ 3508
FluShield Influenza Vaccine............. 3521
Follistim for Injection 2465
Fortaz (1 in 500 patients)................. 1541
▲ Fortovase Capsules (2.9% to 4.4%)... 2970
Fosamax Tablets (1.0%).................. 2095
▲ Foscavir Injection (5% to 26%) 605
Sterile FUDR (Among more common) 2974
Furosemide Tablets 2284
▲ Gabitril Tablets (7%) 1189
Gamimune N, 5% Solvent/Detergent Treated 925
Gamimune N, 10% Solvent/Detergent Treated 928
Gammagard S/D (Occasional) 845
Gammar-P I.V. 787
Gastrocrom Oral Concentrate 1162
▲ Gemzar for Injection (58% to 71%) 1919
▲ Gengraf Capsules (2% to 10%) 457
Genotropin Lyophilized Powder (A small number of patients) 2818
Geocillin Tablets 2687
Geodon Capsules (Frequent) 2688
▲ Gleevec Capsules (28% to 54%) 2357
▲ Gliadel Wafer (8%) 1723
GlucaGen for Injection Diagnostic Kit (Occassional) 949
Glucagon for Injection Vials and Emergency Kit (Occasional) 1924
▲ Glucophage Tablets (25.5%) 1080
▲ Glucophage XR Tablets (6.5%) 1080
Glucotrol XL Extended Release Tablets (Less than 3%) 2693
▲ Glucovance Tablets (7.6%) 1086
GoLYTELY and Pineapple Flavor GoLYTELY for Oral Solution (Infrequent) 1068
Gonal-F for Injection (2.5%) 3216
Grifulvin V Tablets Microsize and Oral Suspension Microsize (Occasional) 2518
Gris-PEG Tablets (Occasional) 2661
▲ Halcion Tablets (4.6%) 2823
Haldol Decanoate 2535
Haldol Injection, Tablets and Concentrate 2533
Havrix Vaccine (Less than 1%) 1544
▲ Hectorol Capsules (21.3%) 1064
▲ Hectorol Injection (21.3%) 1066
Heparin Lock Flush Solution 3509
Heparin Sodium Injection 3511
▲ Herceptin I.V. (8% to 23%) 1414
▲ Hexalen Capsules (1% to 33%) 2226
HibTITER (9 of 1,118 vaccinations) 1859
Hivid Tablets (Less than 1%) 2975
Humatrope Vials and Cartridges 1930
Humegon for Injection 2468
Humorsol Sterile Ophthalmic Solution (Rare) 2102
▲ Hycamtin for Injection (Less than 1% to 58%) 1546
Hycodan 1316
Hycomine Compound Tablets 1317
Hycotuss Expectorant Syrup 1318
HydroDIURIL Tablets 2108
Hytrin Capsules (At least 1%) 464
Hyzaar 2109
▲ Idamycin PFS Injection (82%) 2825
▲ Ifex for Injection (58%) 1123
Imdur Tablets (Less than or equal to 5%) 1826
▲ Imitrex Injection (4%) 1549
▲ Imitrex Nasal Spray (11% to 13.5%) 1554
Imitrex Tablets 1558
Indapamide Tablets (Less than 5%) 2286
Inderal 3513
Inderal LA Long-Acting Capsules 3516
Inderide Tablets 3517
Inderide LA Long-Acting Capsules 3519
Indocin I.V. (1% to 3%) 2115
▲ Infanrix Vaccine (3.3% to 6.6.%) 1562
INFeD Injection 3388
▲ Infergen (12% to 13%) 1777
Infumorph 200 and Infumorph 500 Sterile Solutions 1314
Innohep Injection (1%) 1248
▲ Intron A for Injection (1% to 66%) .. 3120
Inversine Tablets 1850
Invirase Capsules (Less than 2%) 2979
Iopidine Sterile Ophthalmic Solution .... ⊙ 212
IPOL Vaccine (Up to 2.8%) 809

(▣ Described in PDR For Nonprescription Drugs) Incidence data in parenthesis; ▲ 3% or more (⊙ Described in PDR For Ophthalmic Medicines™)

Ismo Tablets (Fewer than 1% to 4%) 3524
Isopto Carbachol Ophthalmic Solution ⊙215
Iveegam EN (0.3% to 0.8%) 849
▲ JE-VAX Vaccine (Approximately 10%) 811
Kadian Capsules (Less than 3%) 1335
Kaletra Capsules (1.6% to 4.8%) 471
Kaletra Oral Solution (1.6% to 4.8%) 471
K-Dur Microburst Release System ER Tablets 1832
Keflex (Rare) 1237
Kefurox Vials, ADD-Vantage 1948
Kefzol Vials, ADD-Vantage (Rare) 1951
Keppra Tablets (1% or more) 3314
▲ Klor-Con M20/Klor-Con M10 Tablets (Among most common) 3329
▲ K-Lor Powder Packets (Among most common) 469
Kogenate (Three reports) 934
K-Phos Neutral Tablets 946
K-Phos Original (Sodium Free) Tablets 947
Kristalose for Oral Solution 1007
▲ K-Tab Filmtab Tablets (Most common) 470
▲ Kytril Tablets (9% to 12%) 2988
▲ Lamictal (9% to 18%) 1567
Lamisil Tablets 2360
Lanoxicaps Capsules (Common) 1574
Lanoxin Injection (Common) 1581
Lanoxin Tablets (Common) 1587
Lanoxin Elixir Pediatric 1578
Lanoxin Injection Pediatric 1584
▲ Lariam Tablets (Among most frequent) 2989
Lescol Capsules 2361
Lescol Capsules 2925
Lescol XL Tablets 2361
Lescol XL Tablets 2925
Leukeran Tablets (Infrequent) 1591
▲ Leukine (46% to 85%) 1755
▲ Leustatin Injection (13%) 2495
Levaquin (0.2% to 2.1%) 2537
Levbid Extended-Release Tablets 3172
Levlen 962
Levlite 21 Tablets 962
Levlite 28 Tablets 962
Levo-Dromoran 1734
Levora Tablets 3389
▲ Levorphanol Tartrate Tablets (3% to 9%) 3059
Levoxyl Tablets 1819
Levsin/Levsinex/Levbid 3172
Lexxel Tablets 608
Lidoderm Patch 1319
Limbitrol 1738
Lipitor Tablets (Less than 2%) 2639
Lipitor Tablets (Less than 2%) 2696
Lithium Carbonate 3061
Lithium Citrate Syrup 3061
Lithobid Slow-Release Tablets 3255
Lodine (1% to 3%) 3528
Lodine XL Extended-Release Tablets (1% to 3%) 3530
Loestrin 21 Tablets 2642
Loestrin Fe Tablets 2642
▲ Lo/Ovral Tablets (10% or less) 3532
▲ Lo/Ovral-28 Tablets (10% or less) 3538
Lopid Tablets (2.5%) 2650
Lorabid Suspension and Pulvules (0.5% to 3.3%) 2251
▲ Lortab (Among most frequent) 3319
▲ Lortab Elixir (Among most frequent) 3317
Lotensin Tablets (Less than 1%) 2365
Lotensin HCT Tablets (0.3% to 1%) 2367
▲ Low-Ogestrel-28 Tablets (10% or less) 3392
Loxitane Capsules 3398
Lufyllin Tablets 3347
Lufyllin-400 Tablets 3347
Lufyllin-GG Elixir 3348
Lufyllin-GG Tablets 3348
Lunelle Monthly Injection 2827
Lupron Depot 3.75 mg (Less than 5%) 3281
▲ Lupron Depot 7.5 mg (5.4%) 3284
▲ Lupron Depot–3 Month 11.25 mg (4.8% to 13%) 3285
Lupron Depot-PED 7.5 mg, 11.25 mg and 15 mg (Less than 2%) 3291
▲ Lupron Injection (5% or more) 3279
Lupron Injection Pediatric (Less than 2%) 3280
Luvox Tablets (25, 50, 100 mg) (2% to 5%) 3256
Macrobid Capsules (Less than 1%) 2889
▲ Macrodantin Capsules (Among most often) 2891
▲ Malarone (Less than 1% to 7%) 1596
Mandol Vials (Rare) 1953
▲ Marinol Capsules (3% to 10%) 3325
▲ Matulane Capsules (Among most frequent) 3246
Mavik Tablets (0.3% to 1.0%) 478
Maxair Autohaler 1981
Maxair Inhaler (Less than 1%) 1984
Maxalt Tablets (Frequent) 2120
Maxalt-MLT Orally Disintegrating Tablets (Frequent) 2120
▲ Maxidone Tablets CIII (Among most frequent) 3399
Maxipime for Injection (0.1% to 1%) 1285
Maxzide 1008
Mefoxin for Injection (Rare) 2124
Mefoxin Premixed Intravenous Solution (Rarely) 2127
▲ Megace Oral Suspension (Up to 6%) 1124
Menest Tablets 2254
▲ Mepergan Injection (Among most frequent) 3539
▲ Mepron Suspension (1.3% to 22%) 1598
Meridia Capsules (1.5%) 481
Merrem I.V. (1.0% to 3.9%) 673
Meruvax II 2130
Mestinon 1740
▲ MetroGel-Vaginal Gel (4%) 1986
Mevacor Tablets (0.5% to 1.0%) 2132
▲ Mexitil Capsules (39.3% to 39.6%) 1047
▲ Miacalcin Injection (About 10%) 2373
Miacalcin Nasal Spray (Less than 1% to 1.8%) 2375
Micardis Tablets (More than 0.3%) 1049
Micardis HCT Tablets (Less than 2%) 1051
▲ Micro-K (Among most common) 3311
Microgestin Fe 1.5/30 Tablets 3407
Microgestin Fe 1/20 Tablets 3400
Microzide Capsules 3414
▲ Midamor Tablets (3% to 8%) 2136
▲ Migranal Nasal Spray (4%) 2376
Miltown Tablets 3349
Minipress Capsules (1% to 4%) 2699
Minizide Capsules (Rare) 2700
Minocin Intravenous 1862
Minocin Oral Suspension 1865
Minocin Pellet-Filled Capsules 1863
Mintezol 2137
Mirapex Tablets (1% or more) 2834
Mircette Tablets 2470
Mithracin for Intravenous Use 903
M-M-R II 2118
Mobic Tablets (0.6% to 1.8%) 1054
Modicon 2563
Moduretic Tablets (Less than or equal to 1%) 2138
Monodox Capsules 2442
Mononine Concentrate 794
Monopril Tablets (1.2% to 2.2%) 1091
Monopril HCT (Less than 2%) 1094
Monurol Sachet (Less than 1%) 1375
Motofen Tablets (1 in 30) 577
Motrin Suspension, Oral Drops, Chewable Tablets, and Caplets (1% to less than 3%) 2002
▲ MS Contin Tablets (Among most frequent) 2896
▲ MSIR (Among most frequent) 2898
Mustargen for Injection 2142
Myambutol Tablets 1290
Mycelex Troche 573
Mycobutin Capsules (1%) 2838
Mykrox Tablets (Less than 2%) 1168
Myleran Tablets 1603
Mylocel Tablets (Less frequently) 2227
▲ Mylotarg for Injection (32% to 44%) 3540
Myobloc Injectable Solution (2% or greater) 1291
Nadolol Tablets (1 to 5 of 1000 patients) 2288
Naprelan Tablets (Less than 3%) 1293
Naprosyn Suspension (Less than 1%) 2967
Naprosyn Tablets (Less than 1%) 2967
Narcan Injection 1322
Nardil Tablets 2653
▲ Naropin Injection (More than 5% to 14.6%) 612
Nasacort AQ Nasal Spray 752
Nasalide Nasal Spray (5% or less) 1295
Nascobal Gel 3174
Nasonex Nasal Spray (1% to 5%) 3131
Natrecor for Injection (1%) 3189
Navane Oral 2701
Navane Intramuscular 2703
▲ Navelbine Injection (Up to 15% but less than 20%) 1604
Nebcin Vials, Hyporets & ADD-Vantage 1955
Necon 3415
Nembutal Sodium Solution (Less than 1%) 485
▲ Neoral Soft Gelatin Capsules (2% to 10%) 2380
▲ Neoral Oral Solution (2% to 10%) 2380
Neptazane Tablets ⊙271
Nesacaine Injection 617
▲ Neumega for Injection (77%) 1434
▲ Neupogen for Injection (7% to 57%) 587
Neurontin Capsules (More than 1%) 2655
▲ Neurontin Oral Solution (8.4%) 2655
Neurontin Tablets (More than 1%) 2655
Nexium Delayed-Release Capsules (Less than 1%) 619
Nicomide Tablets 3247
▲ Nilandron Tablets (5.7%) 753
Nimotop Capsules (Less than 1%) 904
▲ Nipent for Injection (53% to 63%) 3272
Nitrolingual Pumpspray (Uncommon) 1355
Nitrostat Tablets 2658
Nizoral Tablets (Approximately 3%) 1791
▲ Nolvadex Tablets (2.1% to 25%) 678
▲ Norco 5/325 Tablets CIII (Among most frequent) 3424
▲ Norco 7.5/325 Tablets CIII (Among most frequent) 3425
▲ Norco 10/325 Tablets CIII (Among most frequent) 3425
▲ Norco 10/325 Tablets CIII (Among most frequent) 3427
▲ Nordette-28 Tablets (10% or less) 2257
Norditropin Cartridges (Small number of patients) 2420
Norditropin for Injection (Small number of patients) 2419
Norflex 1987
Norinyl 1 +35 28-Day Tablets 3380
Norinyl 1 + 50 28-Day Tablets 3380
▲ Normodyne Injection (4%) 3135
Normodyne Tablets (Up to 3%) 3137
Noroxin Tablets (0.3 to 1.0%) 2145
Norplant System 3543
Norpramin Tablets 755
Norvasc Tablets (More than 0.1% to 1%) 2704
▲ Norvir Capsules (12.8% to 15.2%) 487
▲ Norvir Oral Solution (12.8% to 15.2%) 487
▲ Novantrone for Injection (31% to 72%) 1760
NovoSeven (1%) 2430
▲ Nubain Injection (6%) 1323
NuLev Orally Disintegrating Tablets 3176
NuLYTELY, Cherry Flavor, Lemon-Lime Flavor, and Orange Flavor NuLYTELY for Oral Solution (Less frequent) 1068
Numorphan 1324
Nutropin AQ Injection (A small number of patients) 1420
▲ Nutropin Depot for Injectable Suspension (5%) 1423
Nutropin for Injection (A small number of patients) 1417
Ogen Tablets 2846
▲ Ogestrel 0.5/50-28 Tablets (10% or less) 3428
Omnicef (0.6%) 493
▲ Oncaspar (Greater than 5%) 756
▲ Oramorph SR Tablets (Among most frequent) 3062
Orap Tablets 1407
▲ Organidin NR Liquid (Among most common) 3350
▲ Organidin NR Tablets (Among most common) 3350
Orgaran Injection (2.9%) 2480
Ortho Diaphragm Kits – All-Flex Arcing Spring; Ortho Coil Spring 2552
Ortho Dienestrol Cream 2554
Ortho-Cept 21 Tablets 2546
Ortho-Cept 28 Tablets 2546
▲ Orthoclone OKT3 Sterile Solution (19%) 2498
Ortho-Cyclen/Ortho Tri-Cyclen 2573
Ortho-Est Tablets 3464
Ortho-Novum 2563
Ortho-Novum 1/50□28 Tablets 2556
Ortho-Prefest Tablets 2570
Ortho-Cyclen/Ortho Tri-Cyclen 2573
Orudis Capsules (Greater than 1%) 3548
Oruvail Capsules (Greater than 1%) 3548
Ovcon 3364
Ovidrel for Injection (2.5%) 3220
▲ Ovral Tablets (10% or less) 3551
▲ Ovral-28 Tablets (10% or less) 3552
▲ Ovrette Tablets (10% or less) 3552
Oxandrin Tablets 1153
▲ OxyContin Tablets (Less than 1% to 12%) 2912
▲ OxyFast Oral Concentrate Solution (Among most frequent) 2916
▲ OxyIR Capsules (Among most frequent) 2916
▲ Pacerone Tablets (10% to 33%) 3331
▲ Pancrease Capsules (Among most frequent) 2580
▲ Pancrease MT Capsules (Among most frequent) 2581
▲ Paraplatin for Injection (65% to 93%) 1126
▲ Paser Granules (Among most common) 1781
Paxil (1% to 3%) 1609
▲ PCE Dispertab Tablets (Among most frequent) 498
▲ Pediazole Suspension (Among most frequent) 3050
▲ PEG-Intron Powder for Injection (7%) 3140
Pentasa Capsules (1.5%) 3239
Pepcid Injection (Infrequent) 2153
Pepcid for Oral Suspension (Infrequent) 2150
Pepcid RPD Orally Disintegrating Tablets (Infrequent) 2150
Pepcid Tablets (Infrequent) 2150
▲ Percocet Tablets (Among most frequent) 1326
▲ Percodan Tablets (Among most frequent) 1327
▲ Percolone Tablets (Among most frequent) 1327
Pergonal for Injection 3223
Periactin Tablets 2155
Periostat Tablets 1208
Permax Tablets (2.7%; frequent) 1299
Persantine Tablets 1057
Phenergan Injection 3553
Phenergan Suppositories 3556
Phenergan Syrup 3554
Phenergan Tablets 3556
Phenergan with Codeine Syrup 3557
Phenergan with Dextromethorphan Syrup 3559
Phenergan VC Syrup 3560
Phenergan VC with Codeine Syrup 3561
PhosLo 1069
▲ Photofrin for Injection (17%) 831
▲ Phrenilin (Among most frequent) 578
Pima Syrup (Less frequent) 1362
Pipracil (Less than 2%) 1866
Plaquenil Tablets (Rare) 3082
Plavix Tablets (1% to 2.5%) 1097
Plavix Tablets (1% to 2.5%) 3084
Plendil Extended-Release Tablets (0.5% to 1.5%) 623
Pletal Tablets (2% or greater) 2605
Pletal Tablets (2% or greater) 2848
Pneumovax 23 2156
Polocaine Injection, USP 625
Polocaine-MPF Injection, USP 625
▲ Ponstel Capsules (1% to 10%) 1356
Prandin Tablets (0.5, 1, and 2 mg) (2% to 3%) 2432
▲ Pravachol Tablets (2.9% to 7.3%) 1099
Premarin Intravenous 3563
Premarin Tablets 3566
Premarin Vaginal Cream 3570
Premphase Tablets 3572
Prempro Tablets 3572
Prevacid Delayed-Release Capsules (Less than 1%) 3292
▲ Prevnar for Injection (9.6% to 17.9%) 1870
▲ PREVPAC (3% to 6%) 3298
Priftin Tablets (1.4%) 758
Prilosec Delayed-Release Capsules (1.5% to 3.2%) 628
Primaxin I.M. (0.3%) 2158
Primaxin I.V. (Up to 1.5%) 2160
Prinivil Tablets (0.3% to 1.0%) 2164
Prinzide Tablets (1.4%) 2168
▲ Procanbid Extended-Release Tablets (3% to 4%) 2262
Procardia XL Extended Release Tablets (1% or less) 2710
▲ Procrit for Injection (0.26% to 29%) 2502
▲ Prograf (14% to 29%) 1393
▲ Proleukin for Injection (50%) 1199
▲ Prometrium Capsules (100 mg, 200 mg) (Less than 5% to 8%) 3261
Prosed/DS Tablets 3268
ProSom Tablets (Infrequent) 500
Prostigmin Injectable 1744
Prostigmin Tablets 1744
▲ Prostin E2 Suppositories (Approximately two-thirds) 2852
Protonix I.V. (Greater than 1%) 3580
Protonix Tablets (Greater than or equal to 1%) 3577
Protopic Ointment (1% to 5%) 1397
Proventil Inhalation Aerosol 3142
Proventil Repetabs Tablets (1% to 4%) 3148
▲ Proventil HFA Inhalation Aerosol (7%) 3150
Provigil Tablets (1%) 1193
▲ Prozac Pulvules, Liquid, and Weekly Capsules (3%) 1238
Pulmicort Respules (2% to 4%) 632
Pulmicort Turbuhaler Inhalation Powder (1% to 3%) 636
Purinethol Tablets (Uncommon) 1615
Pyrazinamide Tablets 1876
▲ Quinaglute Dura-Tabs Tablets (3%) 978
▲ Quinidex Extentabs (Among most frequent) 2933
▲ Rapamune Oral Solution and Tablets (19% to 25%) 3584
▲ Rebetron Combination Therapy (9% to 12%) 3153
Recombivax HB (Less to greater than 1%) 2178
ReFacto Vials 1437
Relafen Tablets (1% to 3%) 1617
Relenza Rotadisk (1% to 2%) 1619
Remeron Tablets (Frequent) 2483
Remeron SolTab Tablets (Frequent) 2486

▲ Remicade for IV Injection (7% to 9%) 1178
▲ Reminyl Oral Solution (1% to 13%) 1792
▲ Reminyl Tablets (1% to 13%) 1792
▲ Renagel Capsules (12%) 1439
▲ Renagel Tablets (12%) 1439
Renese Tablets 2712
▲ ReoPro Vials (11.4%) 1958
Repronex for Intramuscular and Subcutaneous Injection 1347
▲ Requip Tablets (7% to 12%) 1621
Rescriptor Tablets (2.4% to 2.8%) 526
Retavase Vials 1182
▲ Retrovir Capsules (4.8% to 25%) 1625
▲ Retrovir IV Infusion (6% to 25%) 1629
▲ Retrovir (4.8% to 25%) 1625
Rifadin (Some patients) 765
Rifamate Capsules (Some patients) 767
Rifater Tablets 769
▲ Rilutek Tablets (4.2% to 4.5%) 772
▲ Risperdal (5% to 7%) 1796
▲ Rituxan for Infusion (7%) 1750
▲ Rituxan I.V. (7%) 1428
Robaxin Injectable 2938
Robaxin Tablets 2939
Robaxisal Tablets 2939
Robinul Forte Tablets 1358
Robinul Injectable 2940
Robinul Tablets 1358
Rocaltrol 2991
Rocephin Injectable Vials, ADD-Vantage, Galaxy, Bulk (Less than 1%) 2993
▲ Roferon-A Injection (17% to 39%) 2996
▲ Romazicon Injection (11%) 3000
▲ Roxanol (Among most frequent) 3066
▲ Roxicodone (Among most frequent) 3067
Rum-K 1363
Rynatan Tablets 3351
▲ Rythmol Tablets – 150 mg, 225 mg, 300 mg (2.8% to 11%) 502
Saizen for Injection (A small number of patients) 3225
▲ Salagen Tablets (4%) 2229
▲ Sandimmune (2 to 10%) 2388
Sandoglobulin I.V. 2391
▲ Sandostatin Injection (Less than 10%) 2394
▲ Sandostatin LAR Depot (6.5%) 2395
▲ Sarafem Pulvules (3%) 1962
Sectral Capsules (Up to 2%) 3589
▲ Sedapap Tablets 50 mg/650 mg (Among the most frequent) 2225
Sensorcaine (Rare) 643
Sensorcaine-MPF Injection (Rare) 643
▲ Septra Suspension (Among most common) 2265
▲ Septra Tablets (Among most common) 2265
▲ Septra DS Tablets (Among most common) 2265
Serentil 1057
Serevent Inhalation Aerosol (1% to 3%) 1633
Serophene Tablets (Approximately 1 in 50 patients) 3226
▲ Serostim for Injection (11.7%) 3229
Serzone Tablets (Up to 2%) 1104
▲ Simulect for Injection (Greater than or equal to 10%) 2399
Sinemet Tablets 1253
Sinemet CR Tablets (1.8%) 1255
Sinequan 2713
Singulair 2181
Skelaxin Tablets 1301
▲ Skelid Tablets (4.0%) 3088
Solu-Medrol Sterile Powder 2855
Soma Tablets 3353
▲ Soma Compound Tablets (Among most common) 3354
Soma Compound w/Codeine Tablets 3355
Soriatane Capsules 3003
▲ Sporanox Capsules (5.1%) 1800
▲ Sporanox Injection (4%) 1804
▲ Sporanox Injection (4%) 2509
▲ Sporanox Oral Solution (5.5% to 7.1%) 1808
▲ Sporanox Oral Solution (5.5% to 7.1%) 2512
▲ Stadol NS Nasal Spray (13%) 1108
Stelazine 1640
Stimate Nasal Spray 796
Streptomycin Sulfate Injection 2714
Stromectol Tablets (0.9%) 2185
▲ Suprane Liquid for Inhalation (16%) 874
Suprax (Less than 2%) 1877
Surmontil Capsules 3595
▲ Sustiva Capsules (3% to 16%) 1258
Symmetrel (0.1% to 1%) 1328
Synagis Intramuscular (More than 1%) 2028
Synercid I.V. (2.7% to 3.7%) 775
Tabloid Tablets (Less frequent) 1642
Talacen Caplets (Occasional) 3089
Talwin Nx Tablets 3090
Tambocor Tablets (1% to 3%) 1990
▲ Tamiflu Capsules (2.1% to 15%) 3008
▲ Tamiflu Oral Suspension (2.1% to 15%) 3008
Tao Capsules (Infrequent) 2716
Tapazole Tablets 1823
▲ Tasmar Tablets (8% to 10%) 3010
▲ Taxol Injection (52% to 87%) 1129
Taxotere for Injection Concentrate 778
Tazicef for Injection (Less than 2%) 1647
Tazicef Galaxy Container (Less than 2%) 1650
Tazicef Pharmacy Bulk Package (Less than 2%) 1653
Tazidime Vials, Faspak & ADD-Vantage (1 in 500) 1966
▲ Tegretol/Tegretol-XR (Among most frequent) 2404
▲ Temodar Capsules (42%) 3157
Tenoretic Tablets 690
Tensilon Injectable 1745
Tequin Injection (0.1% to 3%) 1110
Tequin Tablets (0.1% to 3%) 1110
Testoderm Transdermal Systems 574
Tetanus & Diphtheria Toxoids Adsorbed for Adult Use (2.6%) 1880
Teveten Tablets (Less than 1%) 3327
Thalomid Capsules 1154
Theo-Dur Extended-Release Tablets 1835
▲ TheraCys Injection (16%) 823
Thioplex for Injection 1765
Thioridazine Hydrochloride Tablets 2289
Thiothixene Capsules 2290
Thyrogen for Injection (2.1%) 1441
Tiazac Capsules (Less than 2%) 1378
▲ Tice BCG, BCG Live (3.0%) 2489
Ticlid Tablets (1.9%) 3015
Timentin Injection- ADD-Vantage Vial 1661
Timentin Injection-Galaxy Container 1664
Timentin Injection-Pharmacy Bulk Package 1666
Timentin for Intravenous Administration 1658
Timolide Tablets 2187
Timolol GFS ⊙ 266
Timoptic in Ocudose 2192
Timoptic Sterile Ophthalmic Solution 2190
Timoptic-XE Sterile Ophthalmic Gel Forming Solution 2194
TNKase I.V. 1430
▲ TOBI Solution for Inhalation (14%) 1206
▲ Tolectin (3% to 9%) 2589
▲ Tonocard Tablets (4.6% to 9.0%) 649
Topamax Sprinkle Capsules (Frequent) 2590
Topamax Tablets (Frequent) 2590
Toradol (Greater than 1%) 3018
Transderm Scōp Transdermal Therapeutic System (Few patients) 2302
▲ Trasylol Injection (3%) 909
▲ Trecator-SC Tablets (Among most common) 3598
Trental Tablets (1.2%) 784
▲ Tricor Capsules, Micronized (4%) 513
Trilafon (Occasional) 3160
▲ Trileptal Oral Suspension (5% to 36%) 2407
▲ Trileptal Tablets (5% to 36%) 2407
Tri-Levlen 962
▲ Trilisate (Less than 20%) 2901
Tri-Nasal Spray (1.5% to 2.7%) 2274
Tri-Norinyl-28 Tablets 3433
Tripedia Vaccine (Up to 2%) 817
▲ Triphasil-21 Tablets (10% or less) 3600
▲ Triphasil-28 Tablets (10% or less) 3605
▲ Trisenox Injection (58%) 1158
Trivora Tablets 3439
▲ Trizivir Tablets (12% to 30%) 1669
▲ Trovan (1% to 3%) 2722
Tussionex Pennkinetic Extended-Release Suspension 1174
Tussi-Organidin NR Liquid 3350
▲ Tussi-Organidin DM NR Liquid (Among most common) 3350
▲ Tussi-Organidin DM-S NR Liquid (Among most common) 3350
▲ Tussi-Organidin-S NR Liquid (Among most common) 3350
Twinrix Vaccine (Up to 1%) 1674
▲ Tylenol with Codeine (Among most frequent) 2595
▲ Tylox Capsules (Among most frequent) 2597
TYPHIM Vi Vaccine (Up to 1.9%) 825
Ultracet Tablets (At least 1%) 2597
▲ Ultram Tablets (9% to 17%) 2600
Unasyn for Injection (Less than 1%) 2728
Uni-Dur Extended-Release Tablets 1841
Uniphyl 400 mg and 600 mg Tablets 2903
Uniretic Tablets (Less than 1%) 3178
Unithroid Tablets 3445
Univasc Tablets (less than 1%) 3181
Urecholine 2198
Urimax Tablets 1769
Urobiotic-250 Capsules 2731
Urocit-K Tablets (Some patients) 2232
Uroqid-Acid No. 2 Tablets 947
Urso Tablets 836
▲ Valcyte Tablets (21%) 3022
Valstar Sterile Solution for Intravesical Instillation (2%) 1175
Valtrex Caplets (Less than 1% to 6%) 1676
Vantin Tablets and Oral Suspension (1%) 2860
Vaqta (1.0%) 2199
Varivax (Greater than or equal to 1%) 2202
Vaseretic Tablets (0.5% to 2.0%) 2204
Vasotec I.V. Injection 2207
Vasotec Tablets (1.3%) 2210
▲ Venofer Injection (Greater than 5%) 580
▲ Ventolin Inhalation Aerosol and Refill (6%) 1679
Versed Injection (2.6%) 3027
▲ Versed Syrup (8%) 3033
▲ Vesanoid Capsules (57%) 3037
Viagra Tablets (Less than 2%) 2732
Vibramycin Calcium Oral Suspension Syrup 2735
Vibramycin Hyclate Capsules 2735
Vibramycin Hyclate Intravenous 2737
Vibramycin Monohydrate for Oral Suspension 2735
Vibra-Tabs Film Coated Tablets 2735
▲ Vicodin Tablets (Among most frequent) 516
▲ Vicodin ES Tablets (Among most frequent) 517
▲ Vicodin HP Tablets (Among most frequent) 518
Vicodin Tuss Expectorant (More frequently in ambulatory than in recumbent patients) 519
▲ Vicoprofen Tablets (3% to 9%) 520
▲ Videx (7%) 1138
▲ Videx EC Capsules (13%) 1143
Vioxx (Greater than 0.1% to 1.9%) 2213
Viracept 532
▲ Viramune Oral Suspension (2% to 15%) 1060
▲ Viramune Tablets (2% to 15%) 1060
Visicol Tablets 1767
▲ Vistide Injection (8% to 69%) 1445
▲ Vitravene for Injection (5% to 20%) ⊙ 310
Vivactil Tablets 2217
Vivactil Tablets 2446
Vivelle Transdermal System 2412
Vivelle-Dot Transdermal System 2416
Vivotif Berna (Infrequent) 997
▲ Volmax Extended-Release Tablets (4.2%) 2276
Voltaren Ophthalmic Sterile Ophthalmic Solution (3% or less) ⊙ 312
Voltaren Tablets (Less than 1%) 2315
Voltaren-XR Tablets (Less than 1%) 2315
Warfarin Sodium Tablets, USP 3302
▲ Wellbutrin Tablets (22.9%) 1680
Wellbutrin SR Sustained-Release Tablets (2% to 4%) 1684
▲ Xanax Tablets (9.6% to 22.0%) 2865
▲ Xeloda Tablets (3% to 4%) 3039
▲ Xenical Capsules (3.8%) 3043
Xopenex Inhalation Solution 3207
X-Prep Liquid (Rare) 2900
▲ Xylocaine Injections (Among most common) 653
Yasmin 28 Tablets (Greater than 1%) 980
Yodoxin Tablets 1722
▲ Zanaflex Tablets (3%) 1305
Zantac 1690
Zantac Injection 1688
Zantac Syrup 1690
Zarontin Capsules (Frequent) 2659
Zarontin Syrup (Frequent) 2660
Zaroxolyn Tablets 1177
Zebeta Tablets (1.1% to 1.5%) 1885
▲ Zemplar Injection (8%) 522
Zemuron Injection (Less than 1%) 2491
▲ Zenapax for Injection (Greater than 5%) 3046
▲ Zerit (38%) 1147
Zestoretic Tablets (1.4%) 695
Zestril Tablets (0.3% to 1.0%) 698
Ziac Tablets 1887
▲ Ziagen (16% to 30%) 1692
Zinacef Injection 1696
Zinacef for Injection 1696
▲ Zinecard for Injection (42% to 59%) 2869
▲ Zithromax Capsules, 250 mg (1% or less to 7%) 2743
Zithromax for IV Infusion (1.4% to 2.8%) 2748
Zithromax for Oral Suspension, 1 g (1% or less to 2%) 2743
▲ Zithromax for Oral Suspension, 300 mg, 600 mg, 900 mg, 1200 mg (1% or less to 7%) 2739
▲ Zithromax Tablets, 250 mg (1% or less to 7%) 2739
Zithromax Tablets, 600 mg (1% or less to 2%) 2743
Zocor Tablets 2219
Zoladex (1% to 5%) 702
Zoladex 3-month 706
▲ Zoloft (4%) 2751
▲ Zometa for Intravenous Infusion (14%) 3621
Zonegran Capsules (Frequent) 1307
Zosyn (2.6% to 3.3%) 1890
Zosyn in Galaxy Containers (2.6% to 3.3%) 1894
Zovia 3449
Zovirax Capsules (2.7%) 1706
▲ Zovirax for Injection (Approximately 7%) 1708
Zovirax (2.7%) 1706
Zyban Sustained-Release Tablets (Frequent) 1710
▲ Zydone Tablets (Among most frequent) 1330
Zyflo Filmtab Tablets (Less common) 524
Zyprexa Tablets (Frequent) 1973
Zyprexa ZYDIS Orally Disintegrating Tablets (Frequent) 1973
Zyrtec (2.3% to 2.5%) 2756
Zyrtec-D 12 Hour Extended Relief Tablets 2758
Zyvox (0.9% to 3.7%) 2871

Vulva, dryness
(*see under* Vagina, dryness)

Vulvar disorder
▲ Cleocin Vaginal Cream (6%) 2788
▲ Cleocin Vaginal Ovules (3.4%) 2789
Estring Vaginal Ring (At least 1 report) 2811
Hivid Tablets (Less than 1% to 3.4%) 2975

Vulvitis
Prostin E2 Suppositories 2852
Zovirax Ointment (0.3%) 1707

Vulvovaginal disorder, unspecified
Lunelle Monthly Injection 2827

Vulvovaginitis
Flovent Rotadisk (1% to 3%) 1537
Seroquel Tablets (Infrequent) 684
▲ Zoladex (5%) 702

W

Walking disorders
Imitrex Nasal Spray (Rare) 1554
Tonocard Tablets (Up to 1.2%) 649

Warmth
Aceon Tablets (2 mg, 4 mg, 8 mg) (0.3% to 1%) 3249
▲ Adalat CC Tablets (4%) 877
Alomide Ophthalmic Solution (Less than 1%) ⊙ 204
Bicillin C-R 900/300 Injection 2240
Bicillin C-R Injection 2238
Buprenex Injectable (Less than 1%) 2918
Cancidas for Injection (Up to 1.5%) 2048
Dopram Injectable 2931
Emla (Unlikely with cream) 602
Ethyol for Injection 2029
▲ Imitrex Injection (10.8%) 1549
Imitrex Nasal Spray (Infrequent) 1554
▲ Luvox Tablets (25, 50, 100 mg) (3%) 3256
Miacalcin Injection 2373
▲ Niaspan Extended-Release Tablets (Among most common) 1846
Nubain Injection (1% or less) 1323
Plendil Extended-Release Tablets (Up to 1.5%) 623
▲ Procardia Capsules (25%) 2708
▲ Procardia XL Extended Release Tablets (25%) 2710
Recombivax HB (Less than 1%) 2178
Sarapin 1727
Stadol NS Nasal Spray (1% or greater) 1108
Tripedia Vaccine 817
Urecholine Tablets 2445
Xanax Tablets (1.3%) 2865

Warmth at injection site
Bicillin L-A Injection 2242
Diphtheria & Tetanus Toxoids Adsorbed Purogenated for Pediatric Use 1857
HibTITER (Less than 1% to 1.8%) 1859
Hyalgan Solution 3080
Nubain Injection 1323
Pneumovax 23 (Common) 2156
Rocephin Injectable Vials, ADD-Vantage, Galaxy, Bulk 2993
Tetanus & Diphtheria Toxoids Adsorbed for Adult Use 1880
Tetanus and Diphtheria Toxoids Adsorbed For Adult Use 815
▲ Vaqta (0.6% to 17.4%) 2199
Versed Injection (Less than 1%) 3027

Warts
(*see under* Verruca)

Wasting syndrome
Fortovase Capsules (Less than 2%) ... 2970
Invirase Capsules (Less than 2%) ... 2979

Water intoxication
Aloprim for Injection (Less than 1%) ... 2292
Carbatrol Capsules ... 3234
DDAVP Injection 4 mcg/mL ... 737
DDAVP Nasal Spray ... 738
DDAVP Rhinal Tube ... 738
DDAVP Tablets ... 739
Desmopressin Acetate Injection ... 1344
Seroquel Tablets (Infrequent) ... 684
Stimate Nasal Spray ... 796
Tegretol/Tegretol-XR ... 2404
Zyprexa Tablets (Infrequent) ... 1973
Zyprexa ZYDIS Orally Disintegrating Tablets (Infrequent) ... 1973

Water retention
(*see also under* Edema)
Testred Capsules, 10 mg ... 1746

WBC, immature
▲ Betaseron for SC Injection (16%) ... 988
Cipro I.V. (Infrequent) ... 893
▲ Cipro I.V. Pharmacy Bulk Package (Among most frequent) ... 897
▲ Clozaril Tablets (3%) ... 2319
Lupron Depot 3.75 mg ... 3281
Lupron Depot 7.5 mg ... 3284
Lupron Depot–3 Month 11.25 mg ... 3285
Lupron Depot–4 Month 30 mg ... 3289
Lupron Depot-PED 7.5 mg, 11.25 mg and 15 mg ... 3291
Merrem I.V. (Greater than 0.2%) ... 673
Naprelan Tablets (Less than 1%) ... 1293
Neurontin Capsules (1.1%) ... 2655
Neurontin Oral Solution (Rare) ... 2655
Neurontin Tablets (1.1%) ... 2655
Zebeta Tablets ... 1885

WBC counts, fluctuation
Aciphex Tablets ... 1267
Aciphex Tablets ... 1783
Cytotec Tablets (Infrequent) ... 3202
Dopram Injectable ... 2931
Effexor Tablets (Infrequent) ... 3495
Foscavir Injection (Between 1% and 5%) ... 605
Sterile FUDR ... 2974
Halcion Tablets (1.7 to 2.1%) ... 2823
Hivid Tablets (Less than 1%) ... 2975
Levaquin (Less than 0.5%) ... 2537
Lopid Tablets ... 2650
▲ Lupron Depot 3.75 mg (Approximately 5% to 8%) ... 3281
▲ Lupron Depot–3 Month 22.5 mg (More than or equal to 5%) ... 3288
Maxipime for Injection (0.1% to 1%) ... 1285
Monurol Sachet ... 1375
Neurontin Capsules (Rare) ... 2655
Neurontin Oral Solution (1.1%) ... 2655
Neurontin Tablets (Rare) ... 2655
Noroxin Tablets (1.3% to 1.4%) ... 2145
Prevacid Delayed-Release Capsules ... 3292
PREVPAC ... 3298
Primaxin I.M. ... 2158
▲ Synarel Nasal Solution for Endometriosis (10% to 15%) ... 3205
Uniretic Tablets (Less than 1%) ... 3178
▲ Visudyne for Injection (1% to 10%) ... ⊙ 308
Xanax Tablets (1.4% to 2.3%) ... 2865

Weakness
(*see under* Asthenia)

Weakness, feet
K-Phos Neutral Tablets ... 946
K-Phos Original (Sodium Free) Tablets (Less frequent) ... 947
Monopril Tablets (0.4% to 1.0%) ... 1091
Roferon-A Injection (Infrequent) ... 2996
Uroqid-Acid No. 2 Tablets ... 947

Weakness, hands
K-Phos Neutral Tablets ... 946
K-Phos Original (Sodium Free) Tablets (Less frequent) ... 947
Monopril Tablets (0.4% to 1.0%) ... 1091
Roferon-A Injection (Infrequent) ... 2996
Uroqid-Acid No. 2 Tablets ... 947

Weakness, legs
Dantrium Intravenous ... 2886
D.H.E. 45 Injection ... 2334
K-Phos Neutral Tablets ... 946
K-Phos Original (Sodium Free) Tablets (Less frequent) ... 947
Lupron Injection (A few cases) ... 3279
Uroqid-Acid No. 2 Tablets ... 947
▲ Vesanoid Capsules (3%) ... 3037

Weakness, local
Cosopt Sterile Ophthalmic Solution ... 2065
Timolol GFS ... ⊙ 266
Timoptic in Ocudose (Less frequent) ... 2192
Timoptic Sterile Ophthalmic Solution ... 2190
Timoptic-XE Sterile Ophthalmic Gel Forming Solution ... 2194

Weight change, unspecified
Arthrotec Tablets (Rare) ... 3195
Aygestin Tablets ... 1333
Betapace Tablets (1% to 2%) ... 950
Cytotec Tablets (Infrequent) ... 3202
▲ Depo-Provera Contraceptive Injection (More than 5%) ... 2798
Feldene Capsules (Occasional) ... 2685
Flexeril Tablets (Rare) ... 572
Flexeril Tablets (Rare) ... 2094
Lodine (Less than 1%) ... 3528
Lodine XL Extended-Release Tablets (Less than 1%) ... 3530
Lo/Ovral Tablets ... 3532
Lo/Ovral-28 Tablets ... 3538
Low-Ogestrel-28 Tablets ... 3392
Loxitane Capsules ... 3398
Lupron Depot 3.75 mg (Less than 5%) ... 3281
Monopril Tablets (0.2% to 1.0% or more) ... 1091
Monopril HCT ... 1094
Nordette-28 Tablets ... 2257
Norpramin Tablets ... 755
Ogestrel 0.5/50-28 Tablets ... 3428
Ovral Tablets ... 3551
Ovral-28 Tablets ... 3552
Ovrette Tablets ... 3552
Ponstel Capsules (Occasional) ... 1356
Trental Tablets (Less than 1%) ... 784
Triphasil-21 Tablets ... 3600
Triphasil-28 Tablets ... 3605
Univasc Tablets (Less than 1%) ... 3181
Vivactil Tablets ... 2217
Vivactil Tablets ... 2446

Weight changes, increase or decrease
Activella Tablets ... 2764
Alesse-21 Tablets ... 3468
Alesse-28 Tablets ... 3473
Climara Transdermal System ... 958
Cyclessa Tablets ... 2450
Desogen Tablets ... 2458
Esclim Transdermal System ... 3460
Estinyl Tablets ... 3112
Estratest ... 3252
Estring Vaginal Ring (At least 1 report) ... 2811
Estrostep ... 2627
femhrt Tablets ... 2635
Klonopin Tablets (Infrequent) ... 2983
Levlen ... 962
Levlite 21 Tablets ... 962
Levlite 28 Tablets ... 962
Levora Tablets ... 3389
Menest Tablets ... 2254
Moban ... 1320
Ogen Tablets ... 2846
Ortho-Cept 21 Tablets ... 2546
Ortho-Cept 28 Tablets ... 2546
Ortho-Cyclen/Ortho Tri-Cyclen ... 2573
Ortho-Est Tablets ... 3464
Ortho-Prefest Tablets ... 2570
Ortho-Cyclen/Ortho Tri-Cyclen ... 2573
Ovcon ... 3364
Premphase Tablets ... 3572
Prempro Tablets ... 3572
Prometrium Capsules (100 mg, 200 mg) ... 3261
Provera Tablets ... 2853
Rescriptor Tablets (Less than 2%) ... 526
Tri-Levlen ... 962
Yasmin 28 Tablets ... 980

Weight decrease
(*see under* Weight loss)

Weight gain
Aciphex Tablets ... 1267
Aciphex Tablets ... 1783
Activella Tablets (0% to 9%) ... 2764
Advair Diskus 100/50 ... 1448
Advair Diskus 250/50 ... 1448
Advair Diskus 500/50 ... 1448
Aerobid/Aerobid-M (1% to 3%) ... 1363
Aldoclor Tablets ... 2035
Aldomet Tablets ... 2037
Aldoril Tablets ... 2039
Alora Transdermal System ... 3372
Altace Capsules (Less than 1%) ... 2233
▲ Amphotec (5% or more) ... 1774
Aricept Tablets (Infrequent) ... 1270
Aricept Tablets (Infrequent) ... 2665
Arimidex Tablets (1.5% to 4.1%) ... 659
Astelin Nasal Spray (2.0%) ... 3339
Atromid-S Capsules ... 3483
Avandia Tablets ... 1490
Azmacort Inhalation Aerosol (1% to 3%) ... 728
▲ Betaseron for SC Injection (4%) ... 988
Brevicon 28-Day Tablets ... 3380
Cardizem Injectable ... 1018
Cardizem Lyo-Ject Syringe ... 1018
Cardizem Monovial ... 1018
Cardizem CD Capsules (Less than 1%) ... 1016
Cardura Tablets (0.5% to 1%) ... 2668
▲ Carnitor Injection (2% to 6%) ... 3242
▲ Casodex Tablets (2% to 5%) ... 662
Catapres Tablets (About 1 in 100 patients) ... 1037
Catapres-TTS (0.5% or less) ... 1038
Celebrex Capsules (0.1% to 1.9%) ... 2676
Celebrex Capsules (0.1% to 1.9%) ... 2780
Celexa (Frequent) ... 1365
▲ CellCept Capsules (3% to 15.6%) ... 2951
▲ CellCept Intravenous (3% to 15.6%) ... 2951
▲ CellCept Oral Suspension (3% to 15.6%) ... 2951
▲ CellCept Tablets (3% to 15.6%) ... 2951
Claritin (At least one patient) ... 3100
Claritin-D 12 Hour Extended Release Tablets (Less frequent) ... 3102
Claritin-D 24 Hour Extended Release Tablets (Fewer than 2%) ... 3104
Clomid Tablets (Fewer than 1%) ... 735
Clorpres Tablets (About 1%) ... 1002
▲ Clozaril Tablets (4%) ... 2319
Cognex Capsules (Infrequent) ... 1351
Colazal Capsules ... 3069
Combipres Tablets (About 1%) ... 1040
Compazine ... 1505
▲ Copaxone for Injection (3%) ... 3306
▲ Coreg Tablets (9.7%) ... 1508
Corgard Tablets (1 to 5 per 1000 patients) ... 2245
Cortifoam Rectal Foam ... 3170
Cortone Acetate Injectable Suspension ... 2059
Cortone Acetate Tablets ... 2061
DDAVP Tablets ... 739
Decadron Elixir ... 2078
Decadron Tablets ... 2079
Decadron Phosphate Injection ... 2081
▲ Depacon Injection (4% to 9%) ... 416
▲ Depakene (9%) ... 421
▲ Depakote Sprinkle Capsules (4% to 9%) ... 426
▲ Depakote Tablets (8% to 9%) ... 430
Depakote ER Tablets (1% to 5%) ... 436
Detrol Tablets (1.5%) ... 3623
▲ Dostinex Tablets (Less than 10%) ... 2804
Doxil Injection (Less than 1%) ... 566
Duraclon Injection (0.1%) ... 3057
DynaCirc Capsules ... 2921
DynaCirc CR Tablets (0.5% to 1%) ... 2923
Effexor Tablets (Frequent) ... 3495
Effexor XR Capsules (Frequent) ... 3499
Enbrel for Injection ... 1752
Enbrel for Injection ... 3504
Eskalith ... 1527
Estrace Vaginal Cream ... 3358
Estrace Tablets ... 3361
Etrafon ... 3115
▲ Evista Tablets (8.8%) ... 1915
Evoxac Capsules (Less than 1%) ... 1217
Felbatol (Frequent) ... 3343
Femara Tablets (2%) ... 2351
▲ Flolan for Injection (6%) ... 1528
Florinef Acetate Tablets ... 2250
Flovent Diskus ... 3614
Flovent ... 1535
Flovent Rotadisk ... 1537
Follistim for Injection ... 2465
Fortovase Capsules (Less than 2%) ... 2970
Gabitril Tablets (Frequent) ... 1189
Gengraf Capsules (1% to less than 3%) ... 457
▲ Geodon Capsules (10%) ... 2688
▲ Gleevec Capsules (4% to 14%) ... 2357
▲ Gonal-F for Injection (3.6%) ... 3216
▲ Hectorol Capsules (4.9%) ... 1064
▲ Hectorol Injection (4.9%) ... 1066
Humegon for Injection ... 2468
Hydrocortone Tablets ... 2106
Hydrocortone Acetate Injectable Suspension ... 2103
Hydrocortone Phosphate Injection, Sterile ... 2105
Hytrin Capsules (0.5%) ... 464
Imitrex Injection ... 1549
Imitrex Nasal Spray ... 1554
Imitrex Tablets (Rare) ... 1558
Indocin Capsules (Less than 1%) ... 2112
Indocin I.V. (Less than 1%) ... 2115
Indocin (Less than 1%) ... 2112
Intron A for Injection (Less than or equal to 5%) ... 3120
Invirase Capsules (Less than 2%) ... 2979
Keppra Tablets (1% or more) ... 3314
K-Phos Neutral Tablets ... 946
Lamictal (Frequent) ... 1567
▲ Leukine (8%) ... 1755
Limbitrol ... 1738
Lipitor Tablets (Less than 2%) ... 2639
Lipitor Tablets (Less than 2%) ... 2696
Lithium Carbonate ... 3061
Lithium Citrate Syrup ... 3061
Lithobid Slow-Release Tablets ... 3255
Lodosyn Tablets ... 1251
Lunelle Monthly Injection ... 2827
Lupron Depot 7.5 mg (Less than 5%) ... 3284
▲ Lupron Depot–3 Month 11.25 mg (3% to 13%) ... 3285
Lupron Depot-PED 7.5 mg, 11.25 mg and 15 mg (Less than 2%) ... 3291
Lupron Injection ... 3279
Lupron Injection Pediatric (Less than 2%) ... 3280
Luvox Tablets (25, 50, 100 mg) (Frequent) ... 3256
Maxair Autohaler ... 1981
Maxair Inhaler (Less than 1%) ... 1984
Miacalcin Nasal Spray (Less than 1%) ... 2375
Micronor Tablets (Rare) ... 2543
Mirapex Tablets (1% or more) ... 2834
▲ Mirena Intrauterine System (5% or more) ... 974
Mobic Tablets (Less than 2%) ... 1054
Modicon ... 2563
Motrin Suspension, Oral Drops, Chewable Tablets, and Caplets ... 2002
Nadolol Tablets (1 to 5 of 1000 patients) ... 2288
Nardil Tablets (Common) ... 2653
Navane Oral ... 2701
Navane Intramuscular ... 2703
Neoral Soft Gelatin Capsules (1% to less than 3%) ... 2380
Neoral Oral Solution (1% to less than 3%) ... 2380
Neurontin Capsules (2.9%) ... 2655
Neurontin Oral Solution (2.9% to 3.4%) ... 2655
Neurontin Tablets (2.9%) ... 2655
Nexium Delayed-Release Capsules (Less than 1%) ... 619
▲ Nicotrol Nasal Spray (Over 5%) ... 2843
▲ Nolvadex Tablets (38.1%) ... 678
Norinyl 1 +35 28-Day Tablets ... 3380
Norinyl 1 + 50 28-Day Tablets ... 3380
Norplant System ... 3543
Nor-QD Tablets (Rare) ... 3423
Norvasc Tablets (More than 0.1% to 1%) ... 2704
▲ Novantrone for Injection (14%) ... 1760
Orap Tablets ... 1407
Ortho Dienestrol Cream ... 2554
Ortho-Novum ... 2563
Ortho-Novum 1/50◻28 Tablets ... 2556
Orudis Capsules (Less than 1%) ... 3548
Oruvail Capsules (Less than 1%) ... 3548
Ovidrel for Injection (Less than 2%) ... 3220
Paxil (Frequent) ... 1609
Periactin Tablets ... 2155
Permax Tablets (1.6%; frequent) ... 1299
Prednisone ... 3064
Premarin Intravenous ... 3563
Premarin Tablets ... 3566
Premarin Vaginal Cream ... 3570
Prevacid Delayed-Release Capsules (Less than 1%) ... 3292
PREVPAC (Less than 1%) ... 3298
Prilosec Delayed-Release Capsules (Less than 1%) ... 628
Prinivil Tablets (0.3% to 1.0%) ... 2164
Prinzide Tablets ... 2168
Procardia XL Extended Release Tablets (1% or less) ... 2710
▲ Prograf (3% to 15%) ... 1393
▲ Proleukin for Injection (16%) ... 1199
ProSom Tablets (Rare) ... 500
Protonix I.V. (Less than 1%) ... 3580
Protonix Tablets (Less than 1%) ... 3577
Provigil Tablets (At least 1%) ... 1193
Prozac Pulvules, Liquid, and Weekly Capsules (Frequent) ... 1238
Pulmicort Turbuhaler Inhalation Powder (1% to 3%) ... 636
▲ Rapamune Oral Solution and Tablets (8% to 21%) ... 3584
Relafen Tablets (Less than 1%) ... 1617
▲ Remeron Tablets (7.5% to 12%) ... 2483
▲ Remeron SolTab Tablets (7.5% to 12%) ... 2486
Requip Tablets (Infrequent) ... 1621
Rilutek Tablets (Infrequent) ... 772
▲ Risperdal (18%) ... 1796
Sarafem Pulvules (Frequent) ... 1962
Serentil ... 1057
Serophene Tablets (Less than 1 in 100 patients) ... 3226
Seroquel Tablets (2%) ... 684
Serzone Tablets ... 1104
▲ Simulect for Injection (3% to 10%) ... 2399
Sinemet Tablets ... 1253
Sinemet CR Tablets ... 1255
Sinequan (Occasional) ... 2713
Sonata Capsules (Infrequent) ... 3591
Soriatane Capsules (Less than 1%) ... 3003
Stelazine (Occasional) ... 1640
Sular Tablets (Less than or equal to 1%) ... 688

Surmontil Capsules 3595
▲ Synarel Nasal Solution for Endometriosis (8% of patients) 3205
Taxotere for Injection Concentrate 778
▲ Temodar Capsules (5%) 3157
Thalomid Capsules 1154
Thioridazine Hydrochloride Tablets 2289
Thiothixene Capsules 2290
Tiazac Capsules (Less than 2%) 1378
▲ Tolectin (3% to 9%) 2589
Topamax Sprinkle Capsules (Frequent) 2590
Topamax Tablets (Frequent) 2590
Toradol (1% or less) 3018
Tricor Capsules, Micronized 513
Trilafon 3160
Trileptal Oral Suspension (1% to 2%) 2407
Trileptal Tablets (1% to 2%) 2407
Trilisate (Less than 1%) 2901
Tri-Norinyl-28 Tablets 3433
▲ Trisenox Injection (13%) 1158
Trovan (Less than 1%) 2722
Uniretic Tablets (Less than 1%) 3178
Uroqid-Acid No. 2 Tablets 947
Vantin Tablets and Oral Suspension (Less than 1%) 2860
▲ Vesanoid Capsules (23%) 3037
Viadur Implant (2.3%) 912
Vioxx (Greater than 0.1% to 1.9%) 2213
Vistide Injection 1445
Vivelle Transdermal System 2412
Vivelle-Dot Transdermal System 2416
▲ Wellbutrin Tablets (9.4% to 13.6%) 1680
Wellbutrin SR Sustained-Release Tablets (2% to 3%) 1684
▲ Xanax Tablets (2.7% to 27.2%) 2865
Zebeta Tablets 1885
Zestoretic Tablets 695
Zestril Tablets (0.3% to 1.0%) 698
Ziac Tablets 1887
Zoladex (1% to 5%) 702
Zoladex 3-month 706
Zoloft (Frequent) 2751
Zonegran Capsules (Infrequent) 1307
Zyban Sustained-Release Tablets (Infrequent) 1710
▲ Zyprexa Tablets (5.6% to 6%) 1973
▲ Zyprexa ZYDIS Orally Disintegrating Tablets (5.6% to 6%) 1973
Zyrtec (Less than 2%) 2756
Zyrtec-D 12 Hour Extended Relief Tablets (Less than 2%) 2758

Weight loss

Abelcet Injection 1273
Accuretic Tablets 2614
Accutane Capsules 2944
Aciphex Tablets 1267
Aciphex Tablets 1783
▲ Actimmune (6%) 1772
Actiq (Less than 1%) 1184
Adalat CC Tablets (Less than 1.0%) 877
Adderall Tablets 3231
Adderall XR Capsules (1.2% to 4%)
Alferon N Injection (1%) 1770
Alkeran for Injection 1465
Alkeran Tablets 1466
Alora Transdermal System 3372
Ambien Tablets (Rare) 3191
Amphotec (1% to 5%) 1774
▲ Arava Tablets (4%) 724
▲ Aricept Tablets (3%) 1270
▲ Aricept Tablets (3%) 2665
Arimidex Tablets (2% to 5%) 659
▲ Betaseron for SC Injection (4%) 988
Blocadren Tablets 2046
Brevicon 28-Day Tablets 3380
Calcijex Injection 411
Captopril Tablets 2281
Cardura Tablets (Less than 0.5%) 2668
▲ Carnitor Injection (3% to 8%) 3242
▲ Casodex Tablets (4%) 662
Cataflam Tablets (Rare) 2315
Celexa (Frequent) 1365
▲ CellCept Capsules (3% to 10%) 2951
▲ CellCept Intravenous (3% to 10%) 2951
▲ CellCept Oral Suspension (3% to 10%) 2951
▲ CellCept Tablets (3% to 10%) 2951
Celontin Capsules 2618
Clomid Tablets (Fewer than 1%) 735
Clozaril Tablets 2319
Cogentin 2055
▲ Cognex Capsules (3%) 1351
Colazal Capsules 3069
Concerta Extended-Release Tablets 1998
Concerta Tablets 561
Copaxone for Injection (Infrequent) 3306
Cosopt Sterile Ophthalmic Solution 2065
Cylert Tablets 415
Cytovene (At least 3 subjects) 2959
Daranide Tablets 2077
▲ Depacon Injection (6%) 416
▲ Depakene (6%) 421
▲ Depakote Sprinkle Capsules (6%) 426
▲ Depakote Tablets (6%) 430
Depakote ER Tablets (Greater than 1%) 436
Dexedrine 1512
DextroStat Tablets 3236
▲ Dostinex Tablets (Less than 10%) 2804
Doxil Injection (1% to 5%) 566
Duragesic Transdermal System 1786
Effexor Tablets (1%) 3495
▲ Effexor XR Capsules (3%) 3499
Eldepryl Capsules (1 of 49 patients) 3266
Elspar for Injection 2092
Eskalith 1527
Estrace Vaginal Cream 3358
Estrace Tablets 3361
Etrafon 3115
Evoxac Capsules (Less than 1%) 1217
▲ Exelon Capsules (3%) 2342
▲ Exelon Oral Solution (3%) 2345
▲ Felbatol (3.4% to 6.5%) 3343
▲ Femara Tablets (6%) 2351
▲ Flolan for Injection (27% to 45%) 1528
Floxin I.V. (Less than 1%) 2526
Floxin Tablets (Less than 1%) 2529
Fortovase Capsules (Less than 2%) 2970
Foscavir Injection (Between 1% and 5%) 605
Gabitril Tablets (Frequent) 1189
Gengraf Capsules (1% to less than 3%) 457
Hectorol Capsules 1064
Hectorol Injection 1066
Herceptin I.V. (At least one of the 958 patients) 1414
Hivid Tablets (Less than 1%) 2975
Imitrex Injection 1549
Imitrex Nasal Spray (Rare) 1554
Imitrex Tablets (Rare) 1558
Indapamide Tablets (Less than 5%) 2286
▲ Infergen (5%) 1777
▲ Intron A for Injection (Less than 1% to 10%) 3120
Invirase Capsules (Less than 2%) 2979
Kaletra Capsules (Less than 2%) 471
Kaletra Oral Solution (Less than 2%) 471
Lamictal (Infrequent) 1567
Lamisil Tablets 2360
▲ Leukine (37%) 1755
Levaquin (Less than 0.5%) 2537
Levoxyl Tablets 1819
Limbitrol 1738
Lithium Carbonate 3061
Lithium Citrate Syrup 3061
Lithobid Slow-Release Tablets 3255
Lodosyn Tablets 1251
Lopid Tablets 2650
Lunelle Monthly Injection 2827
▲ Lupron Depot–3 Month 11.25 mg (3% to 13%) 3285
Lupron Depot–4 Month 30 mg (Less than 5%) 3289
Luvox Tablets (25, 50, 100 mg) (Frequent) 3256
Metadate CD Capsules 1164
Metadate ER Tablets 1167
Methylin Tablets 1995
Methylin ER Tablets 1995
Mirapex Tablets (2%) 2834
Mobic Tablets (Less than 2%) 1054
Modicon 2563
Myleran Tablets 1603
Naprelan Tablets (Less than 1%) 1293
Neoral Soft Gelatin Capsules (1% to less than 3%) 2380
Neoral Oral Solution (1% to less than 3%) 2380
Neurontin Capsules (Infrequent) 2655
Neurontin Oral Solution (Infrequent) 2655
Neurontin Tablets (Infrequent) 2655
Nexium Delayed-Release Capsules (Less than 1%) 619
Nilandron Tablets (2%) 753
▲ Nolvadex Tablets (22.6%) 678
Norinyl 1 +35 28-Day Tablets 3380
Norinyl 1 + 50 28-Day Tablets 3380
Norvir Capsules (Less than 2%) 487
Norvir Oral Solution (Less than 2%) 487
▲ Novantrone for Injection (17%) 1760
Oncaspar (Less than 1%) 756
Orap Tablets 1407
Ortho Dienestrol Cream 2554
Ortho-Novum 2563
Ortho-Novum 1/50□28 Tablets 2556
Orudis Capsules (Less than 1%) 3548
Oruvail Capsules (Less than 1%) 3548
Pancrease Capsules (Frequent) 2580
Paxil (Frequent) 1609
▲ PEG-Intron Powder for Injection (11%) 3140
Permax Tablets (Frequent) 1299
▲ Photofrin for Injection (9%) 831
Plaquenil Tablets 3082
Premarin Intravenous 3563
Premarin Tablets 3566
Premarin Vaginal Cream 3570
Prevacid Delayed-Release Capsules (Less than 1%) 3292
PREVPAC (Less than 1%) 3298
Prinivil Tablets (0.3% to 1.0%) 2164
Prinzide Tablets 2168
▲ Proleukin for Injection (5%) 1199
ProSom Tablets (Rare) 500
Protonix I.V. (Less than 1%) 3580
Protonix Tablets (Less than 1%) 3577
Prozac Pulvules, Liquid, and Weekly Capsules (1% to 4%) 1238
Pulmozyme Inhalation Solution 1426
▲ Rapamune Oral Solution and Tablets (3% to 20%) 3584
Relafen Tablets (Less than 1%) 1617
Remeron Tablets (Infrequent) 2483
Remeron SolTab Tablets (Infrequent) 2486
Remicade for IV Injection (Less than 2%) 1178
▲ Reminyl Oral Solution (5% to 7%) 1792
▲ Reminyl Tablets (5% to 7%) 1792
Requip Tablets (1% or more) 1621
Retrovir Capsules (0.8%) 1625
Retrovir IV Infusion (1%) 1629
Retrovir (0.8%) 1625
▲ Rilutek Tablets (3.7% to 4.6%) 772
Risperdal (Infrequent) 1796
Ritalin 2387
Rocaltrol 2991
▲ Roferon-A Injection (25% to 33%) 2996
Sandimmune (Rare) 2388
Sandostatin Injection (Less than 1%) 2394
▲ Sandostatin LAR Depot (5% to 15%) 2395
▲ Sarafem Pulvules (3%) 1962
Seroquel Tablets (Infrequent) 684
Serzone Tablets (Infrequent) 1104
Sinemet Tablets 1253
Sinemet CR Tablets 1255
Sonata Capsules (Rare) 3591
Sporanox Oral Solution (Less than 2%) 1808
Sporanox Oral Solution (Less than 2%) 2512
Sular Tablets (Less than or equal to 1%) 688
Surmontil Capsules 3595
Synarel Nasal Solution for Endometriosis (1% of patients) 3205
Tice BCG, BCG Live (2.2%) 2489
Timolide Tablets 2187
Timolol GFS ⊙266
Timoptic in Ocudose 2192
Timoptic Sterile Ophthalmic Solution 2190
Timoptic-XE Sterile Ophthalmic Gel Forming Solution 2194
▲ TOBI Solution for Inhalation (10.1%) 1206
▲ Tolectin (3% to 9%) 2589
▲ Topamax Sprinkle Capsules (4.4% to 12.6%) 2590
▲ Topamax Tablets (4.4% to 12.6%) 2590
▲ Trecator-SC Tablets (Among most common) 3598
Tricor Capsules, Micronized (Less than 1%) 513
Trileptal Oral Suspension 2407
Trileptal Tablets 2407
Tri-Norinyl-28 Tablets 3433
▲ Trisenox Injection (8%) 1158
Trovan (Less than 1%) 2722
Ultracet Tablets (Less than 1%) 2607
Ultram Tablets (Less than 1%) 2600
Unithroid Tablets 3445
▲ Vesanoid Capsules (17%) 3037
Vicoprofen Tablets (Less than 1%) 520
Vistide Injection 1445
Vitravene for Injection (2% to 5%) ⊙310
Vivelle Transdermal System 2412
Vivelle-Dot Transdermal System 2416
Voltaren Tablets (Rare) 2315
Voltaren-XR Tablets (Rare) 2315
▲ Wellbutrin Tablets (23.2% to 28%) 1680
▲ Wellbutrin SR Sustained-Release Tablets (14% to 19%) 1684
▲ Xanax Tablets (2.3% to 22.6%) 2865
Zanaflex Tablets (Infrequent) 1305
Zarontin Capsules (Frequent) 2659
Zarontin Syrup (Frequent) 2660
Zestoretic Tablets 695
Zestril Tablets (0.3% to 1.0%) 698
Zoloft (2%) 2751
▲ Zonegran Capsules (3%) 1307
Zyprexa Tablets (Frequent) 1973
Zyprexa ZYDIS Orally Disintegrating Tablets (Frequent) 1973

Wenckebach block

Buprenex Injectable (Less than 1%) 2918
Digitek Tablets 1003
Lanoxin Injection 1581
Lanoxin Tablets 1587
Lanoxin Elixir Pediatric 1578
Lanoxin Injection Pediatric 1584

Wenckebach's period

(*see under* A-V conduction, prolongation)

Wheals

Astramorph/PF Injection, USP (Preservative-Free) 594
Attenuvax (Rare) 2044
Cortrosyn for Injection (Single instance) 2449
Demerol 3079
Desferal Vials 2333
Dilaudid-HP (Less frequent) 443
Duramorph Injection 1312
Infumorph 200 and Infumorph 500 Sterile Solutions 1314
Levulan Kerastick (1% to 7%) 971
Mepergan Injection 3539
Meruvax II 2130
M-M-R II 2118
Mumpsvax (Extremely rare) 2141

Wheezing

Abelcet Injection 1273
Advair Diskus 100/50 (1% to 3%) 1448
Advair Diskus 250/50 (1% to 3%) 1448
Advair Diskus 500/50 (1% to 3%) 1448
▲ Aerobid/Aerobid-M (3% to 9%) 1363
Aleve Tablets, Caplets and Gelcaps ▣602
Alferon N Injection 1770
Aricept Tablets (Infrequent) 1270
Aricept Tablets (Infrequent) 2665
Avalide Tablets 1070
Avapro Tablets (Less than 1%) 1074
Avapro Tablets (Less than 1%) 3076
Azactam for Injection (Less than 1%) 1276
Azmacort Inhalation Aerosol 728
Beconase Inhalation Aerosol (Rare) 1497
Beconase AQ Nasal Spray (Rare) 1498
Benadryl Parenteral 2617
Brevibloc Injection (Less than 1%) 858
▲ Claritin (4%) 3100
Claritin-D 12 Hour Extended Release Tablets (Less frequent) 3102
Claritin-D 24 Hour Extended Release Tablets (Fewer than 2%) 3104
Clozaril Tablets (Less than 1%) 2319
Combivent Inhalation Aerosol 1041
CytoGam Intravenous (Less than 5.0%) 2026
Depen Titratable Tablets 3341
Diprivan Injectable Emulsion (Less than 1%) 667
DuoNeb Inhalation Solution 1233
Epivir 1520
Epivir-HBV 1524
Flonase Nasal Spray 1533
Flovent Diskus 3614
Flovent 1535
Flovent Rotadisk 1537
Gamimune N, 5% Solvent/Detergent Treated 925
Gamimune N, 10% Solvent/Detergent Treated 928
Gammar-P I.V. 787
Hivid Tablets (Less than 1%) 2975
Humalog (Less common) 1926
Humalog Mix 75/25 Pen (Less common) 1928
Humulin 50/50, 100 Units 1934
Humulin 70/30, 100 Units (Less common) 1935
Humulin 70/30 Pen (Less common) 1936
Humulin L, 100 Units (Less common) 1937
Humulin R Regular (U-500) 1943
Humulin N NPH Pen (Less common) 1940
Iletin II, Regular (Pork), 100 Units 1947
Imitrex Tablets 1558
INFeD Injection 3388
Intron A for Injection (Less than or equal to 5%) 3120
JE-VAX Vaccine 811
Levoxyl Tablets 1819
Maxair Autohaler 1981
Maxair Inhaler (Less than 1%) 1984
Maxalt Tablets 2120
Maxalt-MLT Orally Disintegrating Tablets 2120
Children's Motrin Cold Oral Suspension 2007
Motrin IB Tablets, Caplets, and Gelcaps 2002
Motrin Sinus Headache Caplets 2005
Nasonex Nasal Spray 3131
Neupogen for Injection 587
Nimotop Capsules (Less than 1%) 904
Normodyne Injection (1%) 3135
NovoLog Injection 2427
Nubain Injection (1% or less) 1323
▲ Orthoclone OKT3 Sterile Solution (13%) 2498
Periactin Tablets 2155
Prevnar for Injection 1870
Prinivil Tablets (0.3% to 1.0%) 2164

Prinzide Tablets 2168
▲ Procardia Capsules (6%) 2708
▲ Procardia XL Extended Release Tablets (6%) 2710
▲ Proleukin for Injection (6%) 1199
Prostin E2 Suppositories 2852
Proventil Inhalation Solution 0.083% (1% to 1.5%) 3146
Proventil Solution for Inhalation 0.5% (1% to 1.5%) 3144
Pulmozyme Inhalation Solution 1426
Rhinocort Aqua Nasal Spray (Rare) 642
Rhinocort Nasal Inhaler (Less than 1%) 640
Rifadin 765
Rifater Tablets 769
Rynatan Tablets 3351
Sandimmune 2388
Sectral Capsules (Up to 2%) 3589
Serevent Inhalation Aerosol (1% to 3%) 1633
Simulect for Injection 2399
Sular Tablets (Less than or equal to 1%) 688
Survanta Intratracheal Suspension 3053
Synagis Intramuscular (More than 1%) 2028
Tenoretic Tablets (Up to 3%) 690
Tenormin (Up to 3%) 692
Thioplex for Injection 1765
Tonocard Tablets 649
Toprol-XL Tablets (About 1 of 100 patients) 651
▲ Trisenox Injection (13%) 1158
Unithroid Tablets 3445
Vancenase AQ Nasal Spray 0.084% (Rare) 3163
Vancocin HCl Capsules & Pulvules 1972
Vancocin HCl Oral Solution 1971
Vancocin HCl, Vials & ADD-Vantage 1970
Vantin Tablets and Oral Suspension (Less than 1%) 2860
Vaqta (Less than 1%) 2199
Versed Injection (Less than 1%) 3027
▲ Vesanoid Capsules (14%) 3037
Xopenex Inhalation Solution 3207
Zemuron Injection (Less than 1%) 2491
Zestoretic Tablets 695
Zestril Tablets (0.3% to 1.0%) 698

White-clot syndrome
Heparin Lock Flush Solution 3509
Heparin Sodium Injection 3511

Withdrawal reactions
Ambien Tablets (Rare) 3191
Aricept Tablets (Infrequent) 1270
Aricept Tablets (Infrequent) 2665
Astramorph/PF Injection, USP (Preservative-Free) 594
Betapace Tablets 950
Catapres Tablets 1037
Catapres-TTS (0.5% or less) 1038
Celexa (At least 3 patients) 1365
Darvon-N/Darvocet-N 1907
Dexedrine 1512
Dilaudid 441
Dilaudid Powder 441
Dilaudid Rectal Suppositories 441
Dilaudid Tablets 441
Duraclon Injection (1%) 3057
Effexor Tablets (Rare) 3495
Effexor XR Capsules (Rare) 3499
Halcion Tablets 2823
Infumorph 200 and Infumorph 500 Sterile Solutions 1314
Kadian Capsules (Less than 3%) 1335
Klonopin Tablets 2983
Levo-Dromoran 1734
Levorphanol Tartrate Tablets 3059
Librium Capsules 1736
Librium for Injection 1737
Lortab 3319
Lortab Elixir 3317
Luvox Tablets (25, 50, 100 mg) (Rare) 3256
MS Contin Tablets 2896
MSIR 2898
Nembutal Sodium Solution 485
OxyContin Tablets (Less than 1%) 2912
Paxil (Rare) 1609
ProSom Tablets 500
Remeron Tablets (Rare) 2483
Remeron SolTab Tablets (Rare) 2486
Risperdal (Rare) 1796
Stadol NS Nasal Spray (2 patients) 1108
Tranxene 511
Ultracet Tablets (Less than 1%) 2597
Valium Injectable 3026
Valium Tablets 3047
Xanax Tablets 2865
Zoloft (Rare) 2751
Zyprexa Tablets (Infrequent) 1973
Zyprexa ZYDIS Orally Disintegrating Tablets (Infrequent) 1973

Wound healing, impaired
Blephamide Ophthalmic Ointment (Infrequent) 547
Blephamide Ophthalmic Suspension 548
Celestone Soluspan Injectable Suspension 3097
Celestone Syrup 3099
Cortifoam Rectal Foam 3170
Cortisporin Ophthalmic Suspension ⊙297
Cortone Acetate Injectable Suspension 2059
Cortone Acetate Tablets 2061
Decadron Elixir 2078
Decadron Tablets 2079
Decadron Phosphate Injection 2081
Depo-Medrol Injectable Suspension 2795
Florinef Acetate Tablets 2250
FML Ophthalmic Ointment (Infrequent) ⊙237
FML Ophthalmic Suspension ⊙236
FML Forte Ophthalmic Suspension (Infrequent) ⊙235
FML-S Liquifilm Sterile Ophthalmic Suspension ⊙238
Hydrocortone Tablets 2106
Hydrocortone Acetate Injectable Suspension 2103
Hydrocortone Phosphate Injection, Sterile 2105
NeoDecadron Sterile Ophthalmic Solution 2144
Ocufen Ophthalmic Solution ⊙242
Pediapred Oral Solution 1170
Poly-Pred Liquifilm Ophthalmic Suspension ⊙245
Pred Forte Ophthalmic Suspension ⊙246
Pred Mild Sterile Ophthalmic Suspension (Infrequent) ⊙249
Pred-G Ophthalmic Suspension ⊙247
Pred-G Sterile Ophthalmic Ointment ⊙248
Prednisone 3064
Prelone Syrup 2273
Rhinocort Nasal Inhaler 640
Solu-Medrol Sterile Powder 2855
Terra-Cortril Ophthalmic Suspension 2716
TobraDex Ophthalmic Ointment 542
TobraDex Ophthalmic Suspension 541
▲ Zenapax for Injection (Greater than 5%) 3046
▲ Zofran (28%) 1703
▲ Zofran ODT Orally Disintegrating Tablets (28%) 1703

Wound infection
Enbrel for Injection 1752
Enbrel for Injection 3504
▲ Gengraf Capsules (7%) 457
▲ Neoral Soft Gelatin Capsules (7.0%) 2380
▲ Neoral Oral Solution (7.0%) 2380
▲ Sandimmune (7.0% to 10.1%) 2388

Wrist fracture
Vioxx (Greater than 0.1% to 1.9%) 2213

Wrist-drop
Fludara for Injection (One case) 995
Rilutek Tablets (Rare) 772

X

Xanthomas, eruptive
Accutane Capsules 2944

Xanthopsia
Accuretic Tablets 2614
Aldoclor Tablets 2035
Aldoril Tablets 2039
Atacand HCT Tablets 597
Avalide Tablets 1070
Clorpres Tablets 1002
Combipres Tablets 1040
Corzide 40/5 Tablets (Occasional) 2247
Corzide 80/5 Tablets (Occasional) 2247
Digitek Tablets 1003
Diovan HCT Tablets 2338
Diucardin Tablets 3494
Diuril Oral 2087
Diuril Sodium Intravenous 2086
Dyazide Capsules 1515
Furosemide Tablets 2284
HydroDIURIL Tablets 2108
Hyzaar (One subject) 2109
Indapamide Tablets 2286
Inderide Tablets 3517
Inderide LA Long-Acting Capsules 3519
Lanoxicaps Capsules 1574
Lanoxin Injection 1581
Lanoxin Tablets 1587
Lanoxin Elixir Pediatric 1578
Lanoxin Injection Pediatric 1584
Lotensin HCT Tablets 2367
Maxzide 1008
Micardis HCT Tablets 1051
Microzide Capsules 3414
Minizide Capsules 2700
Mintezol 2137
Moduretic Tablets 2138
Monopril HCT 1094
Mykrox Tablets (Rare) 1168
Normodyne Tablets (Less common) 3137
Prinzide Tablets 2168
Renese Tablets 2712
Tenoretic Tablets 690
Timolide Tablets 2187
Uniretic Tablets 3178
Vaseretic Tablets 2204
Zaroxolyn Tablets 1177
Zestoretic Tablets 695
Ziac Tablets 1887

Xeroderma
(*see under* Xerosis cutis)

Xeromycteria
Accutane Capsules 2944
Alomide Ophthalmic Solution (Less than 1%) ⊙204
Alphagan Ophthalmic Solution (Less than 3%) 545
Alphagan P Ophthalmic Solution (Less than 1%) 546
AmBisome for Injection (Less common) 1383
▲ Atrovent Nasal Spray 0.03% (5.1%) 1032
▲ Atrovent Nasal Spray 0.06% (4.8%) 1033
Beconase Inhalation Aerosol 1497
Beconase AQ Nasal Spray 1498
Benadryl Parenteral 2617
Catapres Tablets 1037
Claritin (At least one patient) 3100
Claritin-D 12 Hour Extended Release Tablets 3102
Claritin-D 24 Hour Extended Release Tablets 3104
Clorpres Tablets 1002
Combipres Tablets 1040
Ditropan XL Extended Release Tablets (2% to 5%) 564
Duraclon Injection (Rare) 3057
Flonase Nasal Spray (Less than 1%) 1533
Hivid Tablets (Less than 1%) 2975
Iopidine 0.5% Ophthalmic Solution (2%) ⊙213
Iopidine Sterile Ophthalmic Solution ⊙212
Maxalt Tablets (Infrequent) 2120
Maxalt-MLT Orally Disintegrating Tablets (Infrequent) 2120
▲ Miacalcin Nasal Spray (10.6%) 2375
▲ Nasarel Nasal Solution 0.025% (3% to 9%) 1296
Periactin Tablets 2155
Rynatan Tablets 3351
Symmetrel (1% to 5%) 1328

Xerophthalmia
Accutane Capsules 2944
Aciphex Tablets 1267
Aciphex Tablets 1783
▲ Actonel Tablets (3.3%) 2879
Acular Ophthalmic Solution (Rare) 544
Acular PF Ophthalmic Solution 544
Alamast Ophthalmic Solution (Less than 5%) 3092
Alomide Ophthalmic Solution (1% to 5%) ⊙204
▲ Alphagan Ophthalmic Solution (Approximately 3% to 9%) 545
Alphagan P Ophthalmic Solution (1% to 4%) 546
▲ Alrex Sterile Ophthalmic Suspension 0.2% (5% to 15%) ⊙256
AmBisome for Injection (Less common) 1383
Amerge Tablets (Rare) 1467
Aricept Tablets (Infrequent) 1270
Aricept Tablets (Infrequent) 2665
Astelin Nasal Spray 3339
Axert Tablets (Rare) 2772
Azopt Ophthalmic Suspension (1% to 5%) 536
Betaseron for SC Injection 988
▲ Betimol Ophthalmic Solution (More than 5%) ⊙324
Betoptic S Ophthalmic Suspension (Small number of patients) 537
Blocadren Tablets 2046
Botox Purified Neurotoxin Complex 549
Catapres Tablets 1037
Catapres-TTS (0.5% or less) 1038
Celexa (Infrequent) 1365
Ciloxan (Less than 1%) 538
Clorpres Tablets 1002
Cognex Capsules (Infrequent) 1351
Combipres Tablets 1040
Copaxone for Injection (Infrequent) 3306
Cordarone Tablets 3487
Corgard Tablets (1 to 5 per 1000 patients) 2245
Corzide 40/5 Tablets (1 to 5 of 1000 patients) 2247
Corzide 80/5 Tablets (1 to 5 of 1000 patients) 2247
Cosopt Sterile Ophthalmic Solution (1% to 5%) 2065
Crinone (Less than 5%) 3213
Cytovene 2959
Depacon Injection (1% or more) 416
Depakene (1% or more) 421
Depakote Sprinkle Capsules 426
Depakote Tablets (1% to 5%) 430
Depakote ER Tablets (Greater than 1%) 436
▲ Detrol Tablets (3.8%) 3623
▲ Detrol LA Capsules (3%) 2801
Dipentum Capsules (Rare) 2803
▲ Ditropan XL Extended Release Tablets (6.1%) 564
Duraclon Injection (Rare) 3057
Effexor Tablets (Infrequent) 3495
Effexor XR Capsules (Infrequent) 3499
Enalaprilat Injection 863
Enbrel for Injection 1752
Enbrel for Injection 3504
Evoxac Capsules (1% to 3%) 1217
▲ Fareston Tablets (9%) 3237
Flonase Nasal Spray 1533
Fortovase Capsules (Less than 2%) 2970
Geodon Capsules (Infrequent) 2688
Hivid Tablets (Less than 1%) 2975
Inderal (Rare) 3513
Inderal LA Long-Acting Capsules (Rare) 3516
Inderide Tablets (Rare) 3517
Inderide LA Long-Acting Capsules 3519
Intron A for Injection (Less than 5%) 3120
Invirase Capsules (Less than 2%) 2979
Iopidine 0.5% Ophthalmic Solution (Less than 3%) ⊙213
Iopidine Sterile Ophthalmic Solution ⊙212
Klonopin Tablets (Infrequent) 2983
Lamictal (Rare) 1567
Lexxel Tablets 608
Lipitor Tablets (Less than 2%) 2639
Lipitor Tablets (Less than 2%) 2696
Livostin (Approximately 1% to 3%) ⊙305
▲ Lotemax Sterile Ophthalmic Suspension 0.5% (5% to 15%) ⊙261
▲ Lumigan Ophthalmic Solution (3% to 10%) 553
Lupron Depot–3 Month 22.5 mg (Less than 5%) 3288
Luvox Tablets (25, 50, 100 mg) (Infrequent) 3256
Maxalt Tablets (Infrequent) 2120
Maxalt-MLT Orally Disintegrating Tablets (Infrequent) 2120
Meridia Capsules 481
Mintezol 2137
Motrin Suspension, Oral Drops, Chewable Tablets, and Caplets (Less than 1%) 2002
Nadolol Tablets (1 to 5 of 1000 patients) 2288
Neurontin Capsules (Infrequent) 2655
Neurontin Oral Solution (Infrequent) 2655
Neurontin Tablets (Infrequent) 2655
Nipent for Injection (Less than 3%) 3272
Normodyne Tablets 3137
Norvasc Tablets (Less than or equal to 0.1%) 2704
Ocuflox Ophthalmic Solution 554
Pacerone Tablets 3331
Patanol Ophthalmic Solution (Less than 5%) 540
Prozac Pulvules, Liquid, and Weekly Capsules (Infrequent) 1238
Quixin Ophthalmic Solution (Less than 1%) 3093
Requip Tablets (2%) 1621
Rescriptor Tablets (Less than 2%) 526
▲ Rescula Ophthalmic Solution (10% to 25%) ⊙306
Rēv-Eyes Sterile Ophthalmic Eyedrops 0.5% (Less frequently) ⊙265
Risperdal (Infrequent) 1796
Salagen Tablets (Less than 1%) 2229
Sarafem Pulvules (Infrequent) 1962
Sectral Capsules (Up to 2%) 3589
Seroquel Tablets (Infrequent) 684
Serzone Tablets (Infrequent) 1104
Sonata Capsules (Infrequent) 3591
▲ Soriatane Capsules (10% to 25%) 3003
Tenoretic Tablets 690
Tenormin 692
Teveten Tablets (Less than 1%) 3327
Timolide Tablets 2187
Timolol GFS ⊙266
Timoptic in Ocudose 2192
Timoptic Sterile Ophthalmic Solution 2190
Timoptic-XE Sterile Ophthalmic Gel Forming Solution 2194

- Topamax Sprinkle Capsules (Infrequent) 2590
- Topamax Tablets (Infrequent) 2590
- Toprol-XL Tablets (Rare) 651
- Transderm Scōp Transdermal Therapeutic System (Infrequent) 2302
- Travatan Ophthalmic Solution (1% to 4%) 543
- Trileptal Oral Suspension 2407
- Trileptal Tablets 2407
- ▲ Trisenox Injection (8%) 1158
- Trovan (Less than 1%) 2722
- Trusopt Sterile Ophthalmic Solution (Approximately 1% to 5%) 2196
- Vaseretic Tablets 2204
- Vasotec I.V. Injection 2207
- Vasotec Tablets (0.5% to 1.0%) 2210
- Vexol 1% Ophthalmic Suspension (Less than 1%) ⊙222
- Viagra Tablets (Less than 2%) 2732
- Vicoprofen Tablets (Less than 1%) 520
- Videx 1138
- Videx EC Capsules 1143
- Vistide Injection 1445
- ▲ Visudyne for Injection (1% to 10%) ⊙308
- Wellbutrin SR Sustained-Release Tablets (Infrequent) 1684
- Xalatan Latanoprost Ophthalmic Solution (1% to 4%) ⊙320
- Xalatan Sterile Ophthalmic Solution (1% to 4%) 2864
- Zoladex (1% or greater) 702
- Zoladex 3-month 706
- Zoloft (Rare) 2751
- Zomig Tablets (Infrequent) 708
- Zomig-ZMT Tablets (Infrequent) 708
- Zyban Sustained-Release Tablets (Infrequent) 1710
- Zyprexa Tablets (Infrequent) 1973
- Zyprexa ZYDIS Orally Disintegrating Tablets (Infrequent) 1973
- Zyrtec (Less than 2%) 2756
- Zyrtec-D 12 Hour Extended Relief Tablets (Less than 2%) 2758

Xerosis cutis

- Accutane Capsules 2944
- Aceon Tablets (2 mg, 4 mg, 8 mg) (0.3% to 1%) 3249
- Aciphex Tablets (Rare) 1267
- Aciphex Tablets (Rare) 1783
- AmBisome for Injection (Less common) 1383
- Amerge Tablets (Rare) 1467
- AndroGel (Fewer than 1%) 3322
- ▲ Apligraf (3.6%) 2305
- Aquasol A Parenteral 593
- Arava Tablets (2%) 724
- Asacol Delayed-Release Tablets 2884
- Atromid-S Capsules 3483
- Avelox Tablets (0.05% to 1%) 879
- Bactroban Cream (One report) 1494
- Bactroban Ointment (Less than 1%) 1496
- Baycol Tablets 883
- ▲ Benzaclin Topical Gel (3%) 1220
- Cafcit (2.2%) 1035
- ▲ Carac Cream (83.4%) 1222
- Cardura Tablets (Less than 0.5%) 2668
- ▲ Casodex Tablets (2% to 5%) 662
- Celebrex Capsules (0.1% to 1.9%) 2676
- Celebrex Capsules (0.1% to 1.9%) 2780
- Celexa (Infrequent) 1365
- Claritin (At least one patient) 3100
- Claritin-D 12 Hour Extended Release Tablets (Less frequent) 3102
- Claritin-D 24 Hour Extended Release Tablets 3104
- ▲ Cleocin T Topical (18% to 23%) 2790
- Clinac BPO Gel USP 1339
- Clindagel 1401
- ▲ Clindets Pledgets (18% to 23%) 3270
- Clobevate Gel 3271
- Cognex Capsules (Infrequent) 1351
- Copaxone for Injection (Infrequent) 3306
- Corgard Tablets (1 to 5 per 1000 patients) 2245
- Cortifoam Rectal Foam 3170
- Corzide 40/5 Tablets (1 to 5 of 1000 patients) 2247
- Corzide 80/5 Tablets (1 to 5 of 1000 patients) 2247
- Cozaar Tablets (Less than 1%) 2067
- Crixivan Capsules (Less than 2%) 2070
- Cutivate Cream (0.8%) 1282
- Cytovene (At least 3 subjects) 2959
- DaunoXome Injection (Less than or equal to 5%) 1442
- Depacon Injection (1% to 5%) 416
- Depakene (1% to 5%) 421
- Depakote Sprinkle Capsules (1% to 5%) 426
- Depakote Tablets (1% to 5%) 430
- Depakote ER Tablets (Greater than 1%) 436
- Depo-Provera Contraceptive Injection (Fewer than 1%) 2798
- DesOwen (Less than 2%) 1401
- Detrol Tablets (1.7%) 3623
- ▲ Differin Cream (Less than 1% to 38%) 1402
- ▲ Differin Gel (10% to 40%) 1403
- ▲ Differin Solution/Pledgets (30% to 60%) 1404
- ▲ Diprolene Gel 0.05% (4%) 3107
- Diprolene Lotion 0.05% (Infrequent) 3107
- Diprolene Ointment 0.05% (Infrequent) 3108
- Diprolene AF Cream 0.05% (Infrequent) 3106
- Diprosone 3109
- Ditropan XL Extended Release Tablets (2% to 5%) 564
- Donnagel Liquid (Rare) ▣789
- ▲ Dovonex Ointment (1% to 10%) 1117
- Dovonex Scalp Solution (1% to 5%) 1118
- ▲ Doxil Injection (5.5%) 566
- Effexor Tablets (Infrequent) 3495
- Effexor XR Capsules (Infrequent) 3499
- Elocon Cream 0.1% (Infrequent) 3110
- Elocon Ointment 0.1% (Infrequent) 3112
- Emcyt Capsules (2%) 2810
- Emgel 2% Topical Gel (Occasional) 1285
- Ergamisol Tablets 1789
- Eskalith 1527
- Evoxac Capsules (Less than 1%) 1217
- Famotidine Injection (Infrequent) 866
- Finevin Cream (Less than 1%) 962
- Follistim for Injection 2465
- Fortovase Capsules (Less than 2%) 2970
- Sterile FUDR (Remote possibility) 2974
- Gabitril Tablets (Frequent) 1189
- Gengraf Capsules (1% to less than 3%) 457
- Hivid Tablets (Less than 1%) 2975
- Hyzaar 2109
- Imitrex Injection 1549
- Imitrex Nasal Spray 1554
- Imitrex Tablets (Rare) 1558
- ▲ Infergen (2% to 6%) 1777
- ▲ Intron A for Injection (Up to 10%) 3120
- Invirase Capsules (Less than 2%) 2979
- Kaletra Capsules (Less than 2%) 471
- Kaletra Oral Solution (Less than 2%) 471
- Klonopin Tablets (Infrequent) 2983
- Lac-Hydrin Cream (Approximately 2%) 1118
- Lac-Hydrin Lotion (Less frequent) 1119
- Lamictal (Infrequent) 1567
- Lescol Capsules 2361
- Lescol Capsules 2925
- Lescol XL Tablets 2361
- Lescol XL Tablets 2925
- Lexxel Tablets 608
- Lipitor Tablets (Less than 2%) 2639
- Lipitor Tablets (Less than 2%) 2696
- Lithium Carbonate 3061
- Lithium Citrate Syrup 3061
- Lithobid Slow-Release Tablets 3255
- Loprox Gel 2022
- Lotrisone 3129
- Lupron Injection (Less than 5%) 3279
- Luvox Tablets (25, 50, 100 mg) (Infrequent) 3256
- Luxiq Foam 1210
- MetroCream 1404
- MetroGel 1405
- MetroLotion (1%) 1405
- Mevacor Tablets 2132
- Mexitil Capsules (About 1 in 1,000) 1047
- Mirapex Tablets (Less than 1%) 2834
- Motofen Tablets 577
- Mykrox Tablets (Less than 2%) 1168
- Myleran Tablets (Rare) 1603
- Naprelan Tablets (Less than 1%) 1293
- Neoral Soft Gelatin Capsules (1% to less than 3%) 2380
- Neoral Oral Solution (1% to less than 3%) 2380
- Neurontin Capsules (Infrequent) 2655
- Neurontin Oral Solution (Infrequent) 2655
- Neurontin Tablets (Infrequent) 2655
- Niaspan Extended-Release Tablets 1846
- ▲ Nilandron Tablets (5.3%) 753
- ▲ Nipent for Injection (3% to 10%) 3272
- Nizoral 2% Shampoo (One occurrence in 41 patients) 2007
- Norvasc Tablets (Less than or equal to 0.1%) 2704
- Norvir Capsules (Less than 2%) 487
- Norvir Oral Solution (Less than 2%) 487
- Olux Foam (One case) 1211
- OxyContin Tablets (Less than 1%) 2912
- Paxil (Infrequent) 1609
- ▲ PEG-Intron Powder for Injection (11%) 3140
- Pentasa Capsules (Less than 1%) 3239
- Pepcid Injection (Infrequent) 2153
- Pepcid for Oral Suspension (Infrequent) 2150
- Pepcid RPD Orally Disintegrating Tablets (Infrequent) 2150
- Pepcid Tablets (Infrequent) 2150
- Permax Tablets (Infrequent) 1299
- Pletal Tablets (Less than 2%) 2605
- Pletal Tablets (Less than 2%) 2848
- Pravachol Tablets 1099
- Prilosec Delayed-Release Capsules (Less than 1%) 628
- ProAmatine Tablets (Rare) 3241
- ProctoFoam-HC 3177
- ▲ Proleukin for Injection (15%) 1199
- ProSom Tablets (Rare) 500
- Protonix Tablets (Less than 1%) 3577
- Protopic Ointment (Up to 3%) 1397
- Provigil Tablets (1%) 1193
- Psorcon E Cream 1227
- Psorcon E Ointment 1228
- Remeron Tablets (Infrequent) 2483
- Remeron SolTab Tablets (Infrequent) 2486
- ▲ Renova 0.02% Cream (Almost all subjects) 2520
- ▲ Renova 0.05% Cream (Almost all subjects) 2519
- Rescriptor Tablets (Less than 2%) 526
- Risperdal (2% to 4%) 1796
- ▲ Roferon-A Injection (5% to 17%) 2996
- Salagen Tablets (Less than 1%) 2229
- Serzone Tablets (Infrequent) 1104
- Sonata Capsules (Infrequent) 3591
- ▲ Soriatane Capsules (25% to 50%) 3003
- Sular Tablets (Less than or equal to 1%) 688
- Taxotere for Injection Concentrate 778
- ▲ Tazorac Gel (1% to 10%) 556
- Tequin Injection (Less than 0.1%) 1110
- Tequin Tablets (Less than 0.1%) 1110
- Thalomid Capsules 1154
- Topamax Sprinkle Capsules (Infrequent) 2590
- Topamax Tablets (Infrequent) 2590
- ▲ Trisenox Injection (15%) 1158
- Ultravate Cream (Less frequent) 1119
- Ultravate Ointment (Less frequent) 1120
- Uniretic Tablets (Less than 1%) 3178
- ▲ Vaniqa Cream (3.3%) 1121
- Varivax (Greater than or equal to 1%) 2202
- ▲ Vesanoid Capsules (77%) 3037
- Vioxx (Greater than 0.1% to 1.9%) 2213
- Vistide Injection 1445
- Wellbutrin Tablets (Infrequent) 1680
- Xenical Capsules (2.1%) 3043
- Zanaflex Tablets (Infrequent) 1305
- Zocor Tablets 2219
- Zoladex (1% or greater) 702
- Zoladex 3-month 706
- Zoloft (Infrequent) 2751
- Zonegran Capsules (Infrequent) 1307
- Zosyn (1.0% or less) 1890
- Zosyn in Galaxy Containers (1.0% or less) 1894
- Zyban Sustained-Release Tablets (2%) 1710
- Zyprexa Tablets (Infrequent) 1973
- Zyprexa ZYDIS Orally Disintegrating Tablets (Infrequent) 1973
- Zyrtec (Less than 2%) 2756
- Zyrtec-D 12 Hour Extended Relief Tablets (Less than 2%) 2758

Xerostomia

- Accupril Tablets (0.5% to 1.0%) 2611
- Accuretic Tablets (0.5% to 1%) 2614
- Accutane Capsules 2944
- Aceon Tablets (2 mg, 4 mg, 8 mg) (0.3% to 1%) 3249
- Aciphex Tablets 1267
- Aciphex Tablets 1783
- Actiq (1% to 2%) 1184
- Adalat CC Tablets (Less than 1.0%) 877
- Adderall Tablets 3231
- Adderall XR Capsules
- Adenoscan (Less than 1%) 1381
- Adipex-P 1406
- Advair Diskus 100/50 1448
- Advair Diskus 250/50 1448
- Advair Diskus 500/50 1448
- Akineton 402
- Aldoclor Tablets 2035
- Aldomet Tablets 2037
- Aldoril Tablets 2039
- Alferon N Injection (One patient) 1770
- Allegra-D Extended-Release Tablets (2.8%) 714
- ▲ Alphagan Ophthalmic Solution (Approximately 10% to 30%) 545
- ▲ Alphagan P Ophthalmic Solution (Approximately 5% to 9%) 546
- Altace Capsules (Less than 1%) 2233
- ▲ Ambien Tablets (3%) 3191
- AmBisome for Injection (Less common) 1383
- ▲ Amphotec (5% or more) 1774
- Ancobon Capsules 1730
- Antivert, Antivert/25, & Antivert/50 Tablets 2664
- Arava Tablets (1% to 3%) 724
- Arco-Lase Plus Tablets 592
- Aricept Tablets (Infrequent) 1270
- Aricept Tablets (Infrequent) 2665
- ▲ Arimidex Tablets (4.5% to 5.7%) 659
- ▲ Artane (30% to 50%) 1855
- Arthrotec Tablets (Rare) 3195
- Asacol Delayed-Release Tablets 2884
- Astelin Nasal Spray (2.8%) 3339
- Atarax Tablets & Syrup 2667
- Atrovent Inhalation Aerosol (2.4%) 1030
- ▲ Atrovent Inhalation Solution (3.2%) 1031
- Atrovent Nasal Spray 0.03% (Less than 2%) 1032
- Atrovent Nasal Spray 0.06% (1.4%) 1033
- Avalide Tablets 1070
- Avelox Tablets (0.05% to 1%) 879
- Avonex 1013
- Axert Tablets (1%) 2772
- Axid Pulvules (1.4%) 1903
- Axid Pulvules (1.4%) 2919
- Azmacort Inhalation Aerosol (1% to 3%) 728
- Azopt Ophthalmic Suspension (Less than 1%) 536
- Bactroban Nasal (Less than 1%) 1495
- Benadryl Parenteral 2617
- Betaseron for SC Injection 988
- ▲ Betimol Ophthalmic Solution (More than 5%) ⊙324
- Bontril Slow-Release Capsules 576
- Brethine Ampuls (Less than 0.5%) 2314
- Brethine Tablets (1.5%) 2313
- Brevibloc Injection (Less than 1%) 858
- Bromfed Capsules (Extended-Release) 2269
- Bromfed-PD Capsules (Extended-Release) 2269
- Calcijex Injection 411
- Captopril Tablets (About 0.5% to 2%) 2281
- Carafate Suspension (Less than 0.5%) 731
- Carafate Tablets (Less than 0.5%) 730
- Carbatrol Capsules 3234
- Cardizem Injectable (Less than 1%) 1018
- Cardizem Lyo-Ject Syringe (Less than 1%) 1018
- Cardizem Monovial (Less than 1%) 1018
- Cardizem CD Capsules (Less than 1%) 1016
- Cardura Tablets (1.4% to 2%) 2668
- ▲ Casodex Tablets (2% to 5%) 662
- Cataflam Tablets (Less than 1%) 2315
- ▲ Catapres Tablets (40 of 100 patients) 1037
- ▲ Catapres-TTS (25 of 101 patients) 1038
- Caverject Sterile Powder (Less than 1%) 2777
- Cedax Capsules (0.1% to 1%) 1021
- Celebrex Capsules (0.1% to 1.9%) 2676
- Celebrex Capsules (0.1% to 1.9%) 2780
- ▲ Celexa (20%) 1365
- ▲ CellCept Capsules (3% to 10%) 2951
- ▲ CellCept Intravenous (3% to 10%) 2951
- ▲ CellCept Oral Suspension (3% to 10%) 2951
- ▲ CellCept Tablets (3% to 10%) 2951
- ▲ Cerebyx Injection (4.4%) 2619
- Cipro I.V. (1% or less) 893
- Cipro I.V. Pharmacy Bulk Package (Less than 1%) 897
- ▲ Claritin (3%) 3100
- ▲ Claritin-D 12 Hour Extended Release Tablets (14%) 3102
- ▲ Claritin-D 24 Hour Extended Release Tablets (8%) 3104
- Clinoril Tablets (Less than 1%) 2053
- ▲ Clorpres Tablets (40%) 1002
- ▲ Clozaril Tablets (More than 5% to 6%) 2319
- Cogentin 2055
- Cognex Capsules (Infrequent) 1351
- Colazal Capsules (1%) 3069
- ▲ Combipres Tablets (40%) 1040
- Combivent Inhalation Aerosol (Less than 2%) 1041
- Compazine 1505
- ▲ Comtan Tablets (3%) 2328
- Copaxone for Injection (At least 2%) 3306
- Coreg Tablets (0.1% to 1%) 1508
- Corgard Tablets (1 to 5 per 1000 patients) 2245
- Corzide 40/5 Tablets (1 to 5 of 1000 patients) 2247
- Corzide 80/5 Tablets (1 to 5 of 1000 patients) 2247
- Cosopt Sterile Ophthalmic Solution (Less than 1%) 2065
- Covera-HS Tablets (Less than 2%) 3199
- Cozaar Tablets (Less than 1%) 2067
- Crinone (Less than 5%) 3213
- Crixivan Capsules (0.5%) 2070

(▣ Described in PDR For Nonprescription Drugs) Incidence data in parenthesis; ▲ 3% or more (⊙ Described in PDR For Ophthalmic Medicines™)

Cytovene (At least 3 subjects) 2959
DaunoXome Injection (Less than or equal to 5%) 1442
Demadex Tablets and Injection 2965
Demerol 3079
Demser Capsules (Infrequent) 2085
Depacon Injection (1% or more) 416
Depakene (1% or more) 421
Depakote Sprinkle Capsules 426
Depakote Tablets (1% to 5%) 430
Depakote ER Tablets (1% to 5%) 436
Desoxyn Tablets 440
▲ Detrol Tablets (39.5%) 3623
▲ Detrol LA Capsules (23.4%) 2801
Dexedrine 1512
DextroStat Tablets 3236
Dilaudid Oral Liquid 445
Dilaudid Tablets - 8 mg 445
Dilaudid-HP (Less frequent) 443
Diovan Capsules 2337
Diovan HCT Tablets (Greater than 0.2%) 2338
Dipentum Capsules (Rare) 2803
Diprivan Injectable Emulsion (Less than 1%) 667
▲ Ditropan XL Extended Release Tablets (60.8%) 564
Diuril Sodium Intravenous 2086
Dolophine Hydrochloride Tablets 3056
Donnagel Liquid (Rare) .... ▣789
Donnatal 2929
Donnatal Extentabs 2930
Donnatal Tablets 2929
▲ Dostinex Tablets (2% to less than 10%) 2804
▲ Duraclon Injection (13.2%) 3057
▲ Duragesic Transdermal System (10% or more) 1786
Dyazide Capsules 1515
Dynabac Tablets (0.1% to 1%) 2269
DynaCirc Capsules 2921
DynaCirc CR Tablets (0.5% to 1%) 2923
Dyrenium Capsules (Rare) 3458
▲ Effexor Tablets (2% to 22%) 3495
▲ Effexor XR Capsules (12% to 23%) 3499
▲ Eldepryl Capsules (3 of 49 patients) 3266
Emadine Ophthalmic Solution (Less than 5%) .... ⊙211
Enalaprilat Injection 863
Enbrel for Injection 1752
Enbrel for Injection 3504
Eskalith 1527
Etrafon (Occasional) 3115
Evoxac Capsules (1% to 3%) 1217
Exelon Capsules (Infrequent) 2342
Exelon Oral Solution (Infrequent) 2345
Extendryl 1361
Famotidine Injection (Infrequent) 866
Felbatol (2.6%) 3343
Feldene Capsules (Occasional) 2685
Ferrlecit Injection (Two or more patients) 3386
▲ Flexeril Tablets (7% to 27%) 572
▲ Flexeril Tablets (7% to 27%) 2094
Floxin I.V. (1% to 3%) 2526
Floxin Otic Solution (0.5%) 1219
Floxin Tablets (1% to 3%) 2529
Flumadine (1.5%) 1370
Foradil Aerolizer 2354
Fortovase Capsules (Less than 2%) 2970
Foscavir Injection (Between 1% and 5%) 605
Furosemide Tablets 2284
Gabitril Tablets (1% or more) 1189
Gengraf Capsules (1% to less than 3%) 457
Geocillin Tablets 2687
▲ Geodon Capsules (4%) 2688
Halcion Tablets (Rare) 2823
Haldol Decanoate 2535
Haldol Injection, Tablets and Concentrate 2533
Hectorol Capsules 1064
Hectorol Injection 1066
Hivid Tablets (Less than 1%) 2975
HydroDIURIL Tablets 2108
Hytrin Capsules (At least 1%) 464
Hyzaar 2109
Imdur Tablets (Less than or equal to 5%) 1826
Imitrex Injection 1549
Imitrex Nasal Spray (Infrequent) 1554
Imitrex Tablets 1558
▲ Infergen (4% to 6%) 1777
▲ Intron A for Injection (Up to 28%) 3120
Inversine Tablets 1850
Invirase Capsules (Less than 2%) 2979
Ionamin Capsules 1163
▲ Iopidine 0.5% Ophthalmic Solution (10%) .... ⊙213
Iopidine Sterile Ophthalmic Solution .... ⊙212
Isoptin SR Tablets (1% or less) 467
Kadian Capsules (Less than 3%) 1335
Kaletra Capsules (Less than 2%) 471
Kaletra Oral Solution (Less than 2%) 471
Klonopin Tablets 2983
Lamictal (1.0%) 1567
Levaquin (0.5% to less than 1.0%) 2537
Levbid Extended-Release Tablets 3172
Levo-Dromoran 1734
Levorphanol Tartrate Tablets (1% to 3%) 3059
Levsin/Levsinex/Levbid 3172
Lexxel Tablets 608
▲ Limbitrol (Among most frequent) 1738
Lipitor Tablets (Less than 2%) 2639
Lipitor Tablets (Less than 2%) 2696
Lithium Carbonate 3061
Lithium Citrate Syrup 3061
Lithobid Slow-Release Tablets 3255
Livostin (Approximately 1% to 3%) .... ⊙305
Lodine (Less than 1%) 3528
Lodine XL Extended-Release Tablets (Less than 1%) 3530
Lodosyn Tablets 1251
Lotensin HCT Tablets (0.3% to 1%) 2367
Lotrel Capsules 2370
Loxitane Capsules 3398
Lupron Depot 3.75 mg (Less than 5%) 3281
Lupron Depot–3 Month 11.25 mg (Less than 5%) 3285
Lupron Depot–3 Month 22.5 mg (Less than 5%) 3288
▲ Luvox Tablets (25, 50, 100 mg) (1% to 14%) 3256
Matulane Capsules 3246
Maxair Autohaler (1.3%) 1981
Maxair Inhaler (Less than 1% to 1.3%) 1984
▲ Maxalt Tablets (3%) 2120
▲ Maxalt-MLT Orally Disintegrating Tablets (3%) 2120
Maxzide 1008
Megace Oral Suspension (1% to 3%) 1124
Mepergan Injection 3539
▲ Meridia Capsules (17.2%) 481
MetroGel-Vaginal Gel (Less than 1%) 1986
Mevacor Tablets (0.5% to 1.0%) 2132
Mexitil Capsules (2.8%) 1047
Miacalcin Nasal Spray (Less than 1%) 2375
Micardis Tablets (More than 0.3%) 1049
Micardis HCT Tablets 1051
Midamor Tablets (Less than or equal to 1%) 2136
Migranal Nasal Spray (1%) 2376
Minipress Capsules (1% to 4%) 2699
Minizide Capsules (Rare) 2700
Mintezol 2137
▲ Mirapex Tablets (1% to 7%) 2834
Moban (Occasional) 1320
Mobic Tablets (Less than 2%) 1054
Moduretic Tablets 2138
Monopril Tablets (0.2% to 1.0%) 1091
Monopril HCT 1094
Monurol Sachet (Less than 1%) 1375
Motofen Tablets (1 in 30) 577
Motrin Suspension, Oral Drops, Chewable Tablets, and Caplets (Less than 1%) 2002
MS Contin Tablets (Less frequent) 2896
MSIR (Less frequent) 2898
Mykrox Tablets (Less than 2%) 1168
▲ Myobloc Injectable Solution (3% to 34%) 1291
Nadolol Tablets (1 to 5 of 1000 patients) 2288
Nardil Tablets (Common) 2653
Navane Oral 2701
Navane Intramuscular 2703
Neoral Soft Gelatin Capsules (1% to less than 3%) 2380
Neoral Oral Solution (1% to less than 3%) 2380
Neurontin Capsules (1.7%) 2655
Neurontin Oral Solution (1.7%) 2655
Neurontin Tablets (1.7%) 2655
Nexium Delayed-Release Capsules (Greater than or equal to 1%) 619
Niaspan Extended-Release Tablets 1846
Nicotrol Nasal Spray (Less than 1%) 2843
Nilandron Tablets (2%) 753
Norflex 1987
Noroxin Tablets (0.3 to 1.0%) 2145
Norpramin Tablets 755
Norvasc Tablets (More than 0.1% to 1%) 2704
Norvir Capsules (Less than 2%) 487
Norvir Oral Solution (Less than 2%) 487
▲ Nubain Injection (4%) 1323
NuLev Orally Disintegrating Tablets 3176
Numorphan 1324
Oramorph SR Tablets (Less frequent) 3062
▲ Orap Tablets (5 of 20 patients) 1407
Orudis Capsules (Less than 1%) 3548
Oruvail Capsules (Less than 1%) 3548
▲ OxyContin Tablets (6%) 2912
Parnate Tablets 1607
▲ Paxil (1.0% to 20.6%) 1609
Pepcid Injection (Infrequent) 2153
Pepcid for Oral Suspension (Infrequent) 2150
Pepcid RPD Orally Disintegrating Tablets (Infrequent) 2150
Pepcid Tablets (Infrequent) 2150
Periactin Tablets 2155
▲ Permax Tablets (3.7%; frequent) 1299
Phenergan Injection 3553
Phenergan Suppositories 3556
Phenergan Syrup 3554
Phenergan Tablets 3556
Phenergan with Codeine Syrup 3557
Phenergan with Dextromethorphan Syrup 3559
Phenergan VC Syrup 3560
Phenergan VC with Codeine Syrup 3561
Phrenilin (Infrequent) 578
Plendil Extended-Release Tablets (0.5% to 1.5%) 623
Ponstel Capsules (Occasional) 1356
Prevacid Delayed-Release Capsules (Less than 1%) 3292
PREVPAC (Less than 1% to 3%) 3298
Prilosec Delayed-Release Capsules (Less than 1%) 628
Prinivil Tablets (0.3% to 1.0%) 2164
Prinzide Tablets (0.3% to 1%) 2168
ProAmatine Tablets (Less frequent) 3241
Procardia XL Extended Release Tablets (Less than 3%) 2710
Prometrium Capsules (100 mg, 200 mg) (Less than 5%) 3261
Prosed/DS Tablets 3268
ProSom Tablets (Frequent) 500
Protonix I.V. (Less than 1%) 3580
Protonix Tablets (Less than 1%) 3577
Proventil HFA Inhalation Aerosol (Less than 3%) 3150
▲ Provigil Tablets (5%) 1193
▲ Prozac Pulvules, Liquid, and Weekly Capsules (9% to 12%) 1238
Pulmicort Turbuhaler Inhalation Powder (1% to 3%) 636
Relafen Tablets (1% to 3%) 1617
▲ Remeron Tablets (25%) 2483
▲ Remeron SolTab Tablets (25%) 2486
Reminyl Oral Solution (Infrequent) 1792
Reminyl Tablets (Infrequent) 1792
Renese Tablets 2712
ReoPro Vials (0.1%) 1958
▲ Requip Tablets (5%) 1621
Rescriptor Tablets (Less than 2%) 526
Rhinocort Nasal Inhaler (1% to 3%) 640
Rilutek Tablets (2.0% to 3.0%) 772
Robinul Forte Tablets 1358
Robinul Injectable 2940
Robinul Tablets 1358
Rocaltrol 2991
▲ Romazicon Injection (3% to 9%) 3000
Roxanol 3066
Roxicodone Tablets (Less than 3%) 3067
Rynatan Tablets 3351
▲ Rythmol Tablets – 150 mg, 225 mg, 300 mg (2.0% to 5.7%) 502
Salagen Tablets (Less than 1%) 2229
Sandostatin LAR Depot (1% to 4%) 2395
▲ Sarafem Pulvules (11%) 1962
Sedapap Tablets 50 mg/650 mg (Infrequent) 2225
▲ Semprex-D Capsules (7%) 1172
Serentil 1057
Serevent Inhalation Aerosol (1% to 3%) 1633
▲ Seroquel Tablets (7%) 684
▲ Serostim for Injection (1% to 10%) 3229
▲ Serzone Tablets (25%) 1104
Sinemet Tablets 1253
Sinemet CR Tablets (1.4%) 1255
Sinequan 2713
Skelid Tablets (More than or equal to 1%) 3088
Sonata Capsules (Frequent) 3591
▲ Stadol NS Nasal Spray (3% to 9%) 1108
Stelazine 1640
Sular Tablets (Less than or equal to 1%) 688
Surmontil Capsules (Rare) 3595
Symmetrel (1% to 5%) 1328
Tambocor Tablets (Less than 1%) 1990
Tarka Tablets (0.3% or more) 508
▲ Tasmar Tablets (5% to 6%) 3010
Tegretol/Tegretol-XR 2404
▲ Tenex Tablets (5% to 54%) 2942
Tenoretic Tablets 690
Tenormin 692
Teveten Tablets (Less than 1%) 3327
▲ Thalomid Capsules (8.3% to 9.4%) 1154
Thioridazine Hydrochloride Tablets 2289
Thiothixene Capsules 2290
Thorazine (Occasional) 1656
Thyrel TRH for Injection 3630
Tiazac Capsules (Less than 2%) 1378
Timolol GFS .... ⊙266
Timoptic in Ocudose (Less frequent) 2192
Timoptic Sterile Ophthalmic Solution (Less frequent) 2190
Timoptic-XE Sterile Ophthalmic Gel Forming Solution 2194
Tonocard Tablets (Less than 1%) 649
Topamax Sprinkle Capsules (2.7% to 3.2%) 2590
Topamax Tablets (2.7% to 3.2%) 2590
Toprol-XL Tablets (About 1 of 100 patients) 651
Toradol (1% or less) 3018
▲ Transderm Scōp Transdermal Therapeutic System (About two-thirds) 2302
Tranxene (Less common) 511
Trental Tablets (Less than 1%) 784
Tricor Capsules, Micronized (Less than 1%) 513
Trilafon 3160
Trileptal Oral Suspension (Up to 3%) 2407
Trileptal Tablets (Up to 3%) 2407
▲ Trisenox Injection (8%) 1158
Trovan (Less than 1%) 2722
Trusopt Sterile Ophthalmic Solution 2196
Ultracet Tablets (2%) 2597
▲ Ultram Tablets (5% to 10%) 2600
Uniretic Tablets (Less than 1%) 3178
Univasc Tablets (Less than 1%) 3181
Urimax Tablets 1769
Urised Tablets 2876
Vanceril Inhalation Aerosol (Few patients) 3165
Vanceril Double Strength Inhalation Aerosol (Some patients) 3167
Vantin Tablets and Oral Suspension (Less than 1%) 2860
Vascor Tablets (0.5% to 3.40%) 2602
Vaseretic Tablets (0.5% to 2.0%) 2204
Vasotec I.V. Injection 2207
Vasotec Tablets (0.5% to 1.0%) 2210
Verelan Capsules (1% or less) 3184
Verelan PM Capsules (2% or less) 3186
Viadur Implant (Less than 2%) 912
Viagra Tablets (Less than 2%) 2732
▲ Vicoprofen Tablets (3% to 9%) 520
Videx 1138
Videx EC Capsules 1143
Vioxx (Greater than 0.1% to 1.9%) 2213
Vistaril Capsules 2738
Vistaril Intramuscular Solution 2738
Vistaril Oral Suspension 2738
Vistide Injection 1445
Vivactil Tablets 2217
Vivactil Tablets 2446
Voltaren Tablets (Less than 1%) 2315
Voltaren-XR Tablets (Less than 1%) 2315
▲ Wellbutrin Tablets (27.6%) 1680
▲ Wellbutrin SR Sustained-Release Tablets (17% to 24%) 1684
▲ Xanax Tablets (14.7%) 2865
Xopenex Inhalation Solution 3207
Zaditor Ophthalmic Solution (Less than 5%) 2304
▲ Zanaflex Tablets (49% to 88%) 1305
Zaroxolyn Tablets 1177
Zebeta Tablets (0.7% to 1.3%) 1885
▲ Zemplar Injection (3%) 522
Zestoretic Tablets (0.3% to 1%) 695
Zestril Tablets (0.3% to 1.0%) 698
Ziac Tablets 1887
Zofran (1% to 2%) 1703
Zofran ODT Orally Disintegrating Tablets (1% to 2%) 1703
Zoladex (1% or greater) 702
Zoladex 3-month 706
▲ Zoloft (15%) 2751
▲ Zomig Tablets (3% to 5%) 708
▲ Zomig-ZMT Tablets (3% to 5%) 708
Zonegran Capsules (2%) 1307
▲ Zyban Sustained-Release Tablets (10% to 11%) 1710
▲ Zyprexa Tablets (3% to 22%) 1973
▲ Zyprexa ZYDIS Orally Disintegrating Tablets (3% to 22%) 1973
Zyrtec (Less than 2% to 5%) 2756
Zyrtec-D 12 Hour Extended Relief Tablets (5%) 2758

Y

Yawning

Ambien Tablets (Rare) 3191
Celexa (2%) 1365
▲ Effexor Tablets (3% to 8%) 3495
▲ Effexor XR Capsules (3% to 6%) 3499
Evoxac Capsules 1217
Imitrex Injection (Rare) 1549
Imitrex Nasal Spray 1554
Imitrex Tablets 1558
Klonopin Tablets (Infrequent) 2983

Luvox Tablets (25, 50, 100 mg) (2%) ... 3256
Maxalt Tablets (Infrequent) ... 2120
Maxalt-MLT Orally Disintegrating Tablets (Infrequent) ... 2120
Meridia Capsules ... 481
Migranal Nasal Spray (Rare) ... 2376
Narcan Injection ... 1322
▲ Normodyne Injection (3%) ... 3135
▲ Paxil (4%) ... 1609
▲ Prozac Pulvules, Liquid, and Weekly Capsules (3% to 11%) ... 1238
▲ Requip Tablets (3%) ... 1621
Rilutek Tablets (Infrequent) ... 772
Risperdal (Rare) ... 1796
Salagen Tablets (Less than 1%) ... 2229
▲ Sarafem Pulvules (5%) ... 1962
Serzone Tablets (Rare) ... 1104
Tonocard Tablets (Less than 1%) ... 649
Versed Injection (Less than 1%) ... 3027
Zoloft (Frequent) ... 2751
Zomig Tablets (Infrequent) ... 708
Zomig-ZMT Tablets (Infrequent) ... 708

Z

Zinc deficiency

Calcium Disodium Versenate Injection ... 1980

SECTION 4

INDICATIONS INDEX

This section lists in alphabetical order every indication cited in *PDR®* and its companion volumes, with cross-references to each product entry in which the indication is found. For easy comparison, each listing includes the product's brand name, generic ingredients, and manufacturer. Page numbers refer to the 2002 editions of *PDR®* and *PDR for Ophthalmic Medicines™* and the 2001 edition of *PDR for Nonprescription Drugs and Dietary Supplements™*, which is published later each year. A key to the symbols denoting the companion volumes appears in the bottom margin.

Because *PDR®* publishes only official product labeling, only approved indications are cited here. No unapproved uses are listed.

This index is intended to assist you in identifying the extent and nature of your prescribing alternatives as quickly and easily as possible. However, it is by its nature only an extract of the official labeling as it appears in *PDR®*. For more definitive information, always consult the underlying *PDR®* text.

A

Abdominal cramps
(*see under* Cramps, abdominal, symptomatic relief of)

Abdominal distress, symptomatic relief of
- Levsin/Levsinex/Levbid (Hyoscyamine Sulfate) Schwarz ... 3172
- NuLev Orally Disintegrating Tablets (Hyoscyamine Sulfate) Schwarz ... 3176

Abrasions, pain associated with
(*see under* Pain, topical relief of)

Abrasions, skin
(*see under* Infections, skin, bacterial, minor)

Abscess, cutaneous
(*see also under* Infections, skin and skin structure)
- Levaquin (Levofloxacin) Ortho-McNeil ... 2537
- Zosyn (Piperacillin Sodium, Tazobactam Sodium) Lederle ... 1890
- Zosyn in Galaxy Containers (Piperacillin Sodium, Tazobactam Sodium) Lederle ... 1894

Abscess, hepatic
(*see under* Infections, intra-abdominal)

Abscess, intra-abdominal
(*see also under* Infections, intra-abdominal)
- Cleocin HCl Capsules (Clindamycin Hydrochloride) Pharmacia & Upjohn ... 2784
- Cleocin Phosphate Sterile Solution (Clindamycin Phosphate) Pharmacia & Upjohn ... 2785
- Mefoxin for Injection (Cefoxitin Sodium) Merck ... 2124
- Mefoxin Premixed Intravenous Solution (Cefoxitin Sodium) Merck ... 2127

Abscess, lung
(*see also under* Infections, lower respiratory tract)
- Cleocin HCl Capsules (Clindamycin Hydrochloride) Pharmacia & Upjohn ... 2784
- Cleocin Phosphate Sterile Solution (Clindamycin Phosphate) Pharmacia & Upjohn ... 2785
- Mefoxin for Injection (Cefoxitin Sodium) Merck ... 2124
- Mefoxin Premixed Intravenous Solution (Cefoxitin Sodium) Merck ... 2127

Abscess, tubo-ovarian
(*see under* Infections, gynecologic)

Aches
(*see under* Pain, general)

Aches, muscular
(*see under* Pain, muscular, temporary relief of)

Aches due to common cold
(*see under* Pain associated with upper respiratory infection)

Acid indigestion
(*see under* Hyperacidity, gastric, symptomatic relief of)

Acinetobacter calcoaceticus infections
- Minocin Oral Suspension (Minocycline Hydrochloride) Lederle ... 1865
- Primaxin I.M. (Cilastatin Sodium, Imipenem) Merck ... 2158
- Rocephin Injectable Vials, ADD-Vantage, Galaxy, Bulk (Ceftriaxone Sodium) Roche Laboratories ... 2993
- Unasyn for Injection (Ampicillin Sodium, Sulbactam Sodium) Pfizer ... 2728

Acinetobacter calcoaceticus infections, ocular
- Chibroxin Sterile Ophthalmic Solution (Norfloxacin) Merck ... 2051
- Quixin Ophthalmic Solution (Levofloxacin) Santen ... 3093
- TobraDex Ophthalmic Ointment (Dexamethasone, Tobramycin) Alcon ... 542
- TobraDex Ophthalmic Suspension (Dexamethasone, Tobramycin) Alcon ... 541

Acinetobacter calcoaceticus skin and skin structure infections
- Primaxin I.M. (Cilastatin Sodium, Imipenem) Merck ... 2158
- Unasyn for Injection (Ampicillin Sodium, Sulbactam Sodium) Pfizer ... 2728

Acinetobacter species infections
- Claforan Injection (Cefotaxime Sodium) Aventis ... 732
- Declomycin Tablets (Demeclocycline Hydrochloride) Lederle ... 1855
- Doryx Coated Pellet Filled Capsules (Doxycycline Hyclate) Warner Chilcott ... 3357
- Dynacin Capsules (Minocycline Hydrochloride) Medicis ... 2019
- Minocin Intravenous (Minocycline Hydrochloride) Lederle ... 1862
- Minocin Oral Suspension (Minocycline Hydrochloride) Lederle ... 1865
- Minocin Pellet-Filled Capsules (Minocycline Hydrochloride) Lederle ... 1863
- Monodox Capsules (Doxycycline Monohydrate) Oclassen ... 2442
- Primaxin I.M. (Cilastatin Sodium, Imipenem) Merck ... 2158
- Primaxin I.V. (Cilastatin Sodium, Imipenem) Merck ... 2160
- Vibramycin Calcium Oral Suspension Syrup (Doxycycline Calcium) Pfizer ... 2735
- Vibramycin Hyclate Capsules (Doxycycline Hyclate) Pfizer ... 2735
- Vibramycin Hyclate Intravenous (Doxycycline Hyclate) Pfizer ... 2737
- Vibramycin Monohydrate for Oral Suspension (Doxycycline Monohydrate) Pfizer ... 2735
- Vibra-Tabs Film Coated Tablets (Doxycycline Hyclate) Pfizer ... 2735

Acinetobacter species lower respiratory tract infections
- Primaxin I.V. (Cilastatin Sodium, Imipenem) Merck ... 2160

Acinetobacter species skin and skin structure infections
- Claforan Injection (Cefotaxime Sodium) Aventis ... 732
- Primaxin I.M. (Cilastatin Sodium, Imipenem) Merck ... 2158
- Primaxin I.V. (Cilastatin Sodium, Imipenem) Merck ... 2160
- Rocephin Injectable Vials, ADD-Vantage, Galaxy, Bulk (Ceftriaxone Sodium) Roche Laboratories ... 2993

Acne, cystic, severe recalcitrant
- Accutane Capsules (Isotretinoin) Roche Laboratories ... 2944

Acne rosacea
- Nicomide Tablets (Folic Acid, Nicotinamide, Zinc Oxide) Sirius Laboratories, Inc. ... 3247
- Plexion (Sodium Sulfacetamide, Sulfur) Medicis ... 2024

Acne rosacea, ocular
- Decadron Phosphate Sterile Ophthalmic Ointment (Dexamethasone Sodium Phosphate) Merck ... 2083
- Decadron Phosphate Sterile Ophthalmic Solution (Dexamethasone Sodium Phosphate) Merck ... 2084

Acne vulgaris
- Avita Cream (Tretinoin) Bertek ... 999
- Avita Gel (Tretinoin) Bertek ... 1000
- Azelex Cream (Azelaic Acid) Allergan ... 547
- Benzaclin Topical Gel (Benzoyl Peroxide, Clindamycin Phosphate) Dermik ... 1220
- Brevoxyl (Benzoyl Peroxide) Stiefel ... 3269
- Brevoxyl Cleansing (Benzoyl Peroxide) Stiefel ... 3269

Brevoxyl (Benzoyl Peroxide) Stiefel . 3270
Cleocin T Topical (Clindamycin Phosphate) Pharmacia & Upjohn .. 2790
Clinac BPO Gel USP (Benzoyl Peroxide) Ferndale 1339
Clindagel (Clindamycin Phosphate) Galderma 1401
Clindets Pledgets (Clindamycin Phosphate) Stiefel 3270
Declomycin Tablets (Demeclocycline Hydrochloride) Lederle 1855
Differin Cream (Adapalene) Galderma 1402
Differin Gel (Adapalene) Galderma... 1403
Differin Solution/Pledgets (Adapalene) Galderma 1404
Doryx Coated Pellet Filled Capsules (Doxycycline Hyclate) Warner Chilcott 3357
Emgel 2% Topical Gel (Erythromycin) Elan 1285
Finevin Cream (Azelaic Acid) Berlex 962
Klaron Lotion 10% (Sulfacetamide Sodium) Dermik 1224
Monodox Capsules (Doxycycline Monohydrate) Oclassen 2442
Nicomide Tablets (Folic Acid, Nicotinamide, Zinc Oxide) Sirius Laboratories, Inc. 3247
Ortho-Cyclen/Ortho Tri-Cyclen (Ethinyl Estradiol, Norgestimate) Ortho-McNeil 2573
Plexion (Sodium Sulfacetamide, Sulfur) Medicis 2024
Retin-A Micro 0.1% (Tretinoin) Ortho Dermatological 2522
Tazorac Gel (Tazarotene) Allergan ... 556
Triaz Cleanser (Benzoyl Peroxide) Medicis 2026
Triaz Gel (Benzoyl Peroxide) Medicis 2026
Vibramycin Calcium Oral Suspension Syrup (Doxycycline Calcium) Pfizer 2735
Vibramycin Hyclate Capsules (Doxycycline Hyclate) Pfizer 2735
Vibramycin Monohydrate for Oral Suspension (Doxycycline Monohydrate) Pfizer 2735
Vibra-Tabs Film Coated Tablets (Doxycycline Hyclate) Pfizer 2735

Acneiform eruptions, severe, adjunct in
Dynacin Capsules (Minocycline Hydrochloride) Medicis 2019
Minocin Oral Suspension (Minocycline Hydrochloride) Lederle 1865
Minocin Pellet-Filled Capsules (Minocycline Hydrochloride) Lederle 1863

Acquired immunodeficiency syndrome
(*see under* Infections, human immunodeficiency virus)

Acromegaly
Sandostatin Injection Novartis 2394
Sandostatin LAR Depot (Octreotide Acetate) Novartis 2395

Actinomyces species infection
(*see under* Actinomycosis)

Actinomycosis
Declomycin Tablets (Demeclocycline Hydrochloride) Lederle 1855
Doryx Coated Pellet Filled Capsules (Doxycycline Hyclate) Warner Chilcott 3357
Dynacin Capsules (Minocycline Hydrochloride) Medicis 2019
Minocin Intravenous (Minocycline Hydrochloride) Lederle 1862
Minocin Oral Suspension (Minocycline Hydrochloride) Lederle 1865
Minocin Pellet-Filled Capsules (Minocycline Hydrochloride) Lederle 1863
Monodox Capsules (Doxycycline Monohydrate) Oclassen 2442
Pfizerpen for Injection (Penicillin G Potassium) Pfizer 2707
Vibramycin Calcium Oral Suspension Syrup (Doxycycline Calcium) Pfizer 2735
Vibramycin Hyclate Capsules (Doxycycline Hyclate) Pfizer 2735
Vibramycin Hyclate Intravenous (Doxycycline Hyclate) Pfizer 2737
Vibramycin Monohydrate for Oral Suspension (Doxycycline Monohydrate) Pfizer 2735
Vibra-Tabs Film Coated Tablets (Doxycycline Hyclate) Pfizer 2735

Addison's disease
(*see under* Adrenocortical insufficiency)

Adenocarcinoma, gastrointestinal, palliative management of
(*see under* Carcinoma, gastrointestinal, palliative management of)

Adenomatous polyposis, familial
Celebrex Capsules (Celecoxib) Pfizer 2676
Celebrex Capsules (Celecoxib) Pharmacia & Upjohn 2780

Adenosine deaminase, enzyme replacement therapy for
Adagen Injection (Pegademase Bovine) Enzon 1331

Adrenal hyperplasia, congenital
Celestone Soluspan Injectable Suspension (Betamethasone Acetate, Betamethasone Sodium Phosphate) Schering 3097
Celestone Syrup (Betamethasone) Schering 3099
Cortone Acetate Injectable Suspension (Cortisone Acetate) Merck 2059
Cortone Acetate Tablets (Cortisone Acetate) Merck 2061
Decadron Elixir (Dexamethasone) Merck 2078
Decadron Tablets (Dexamethasone) Merck 2079
Decadron Phosphate Injection (Dexamethasone Sodium Phosphate) Merck 2081
Depo-Medrol Injectable Suspension (Methylprednisolone Acetate) Pharmacia & Upjohn 2795
Hydrocortone Tablets (Hydrocortisone) Merck 2106
Hydrocortone Phosphate Injection, Sterile (Hydrocortisone Sodium Phosphate) Merck 2105
Pediapred Oral Solution (Prednisolone Sodium Phosphate) Celltech 1170
Prednisone (Prednisone) Roxane 3064
Prelone Syrup (Prednisolone) Muro . 2273
Solu-Medrol Sterile Powder (Methylprednisolone Sodium Succinate) Pharmacia & Upjohn 2855

Adrenocortical hyperfunction, diagnostic testing of
Decadron Elixir (Dexamethasone) Merck 2078
Decadron Tablets (Dexamethasone) Merck 2079
Decadron Phosphate Injection (Dexamethasone Sodium Phosphate) Merck 2081

Adrenocortical insufficiency
Celestone Soluspan Injectable Suspension (Betamethasone Acetate, Betamethasone Sodium Phosphate) Schering 3097
Celestone Syrup (Betamethasone) Schering 3099
Cortone Acetate Injectable Suspension (Cortisone Acetate) Merck 2059
Cortone Acetate Tablets (Cortisone Acetate) Merck 2061
Decadron Elixir (Dexamethasone) Merck 2078
Decadron Tablets (Dexamethasone) Merck 2079
Decadron Phosphate Injection (Dexamethasone Sodium Phosphate) Merck 2081
Depo-Medrol Injectable Suspension (Methylprednisolone Acetate) Pharmacia & Upjohn 2795
Florinef Acetate Tablets (Fludrocortisone Acetate) Monarch 2250
Hydrocortone Tablets (Hydrocortisone) Merck 2106
Hydrocortone Phosphate Injection, Sterile (Hydrocortisone Sodium Phosphate) Merck 2105
Pediapred Oral Solution (Prednisolone Sodium Phosphate) Celltech 1170
Prednisone (Prednisone) Roxane 3064
Prelone Syrup (Prednisolone) Muro . 2273
Solu-Medrol Sterile Powder (Methylprednisolone Sodium Succinate) Pharmacia & Upjohn 2855

Adrenocortical insufficiency, diagnosis of
Cortrosyn for Injection (Cosyntropin) Organon 2449

Aerobacter aerogenes infections
(*see under* Enterobacter aerogenes infections)

Aeromonas hydrophila infections, ocular
Chibroxin Sterile Ophthalmic Solution (Norfloxacin) Merck 2051

Agammaglobulinemias, congenital
Gamimune N, 5% Solvent/Detergent Treated (Globulin, Immune (Human)) Bayer Biological 925
Gamimune N, 10% Solvent/Detergent Treated (Globulin, Immune (Human)) Bayer Biological 928
Gammagard S/D (Globulin, Immune (Human)) Baxter Healthcare 845
Iveegam EN (Globulin, Immune (Human)) Baxter Healthcare 849

AIDS
(*see under* Infections, human immunodeficiency virus)

AIDS related complex
(*see under* Infections, acquired immunodeficiency syndrome-related complex)

Airway obstruction disorders
(*see under* Bronchial asthma; Emphysema)

Albinism
(*see under* Hypopigmentation, skin)

Alcohol withdrawal, acute, symptomatic relief of
Librium Capsules (Chlordiazepoxide Hydrochloride) ICN 1736
Librium for Injection (Chlordiazepoxide Hydrochloride) ICN 1737
Tranxene (Clorazepate Dipotassium) Abbott 511
Valium Injectable (Diazepam) Roche Laboratories 3026
Valium Tablets (Diazepam) Roche Products 3047
Vistaril Intramuscular (Hydroxyzine Hydrochloride) Pfizer 2738

Alcoholism, chronic, an aid in the management of
Antabuse Tablets (Disulfiram) Odyssey 2444
Antabuse Tablets (Disulfiram) Wyeth-Ayerst 3474
Vistaril Intramuscular Solution (Hydroxyzine Hydrochloride) Pfizer 2738

Allergic reactions, drug-induced
(*see under* Hypersensitivity reactions, drug-induced)

Allergic reactions, general
Celestone Soluspan Injectable Suspension (Betamethasone Acetate, Betamethasone Sodium Phosphate) Schering 3097
Celestone Syrup (Betamethasone) Schering 3099
Cortone Acetate Injectable Suspension (Cortisone Acetate) Merck 2059
Cortone Acetate Tablets (Cortisone Acetate) Merck 2061
Decadron Elixir (Dexamethasone) Merck 2078
Decadron Tablets (Dexamethasone) Merck 2079
Decadron Phosphate Injection (Dexamethasone Sodium Phosphate) Merck 2081
Depo-Medrol Injectable Suspension (Methylprednisolone Acetate) Pharmacia & Upjohn 2795
EpiPen (Epinephrine) Dey 1236
Hydrocortone Tablets (Hydrocortisone) Merck 2106
Hydrocortone Phosphate Injection, Sterile (Hydrocortisone Sodium Phosphate) Merck 2105
Pediapred Oral Solution (Prednisolone Sodium Phosphate) Celltech 1170
Phenergan Injection (Promethazine Hydrochloride) Wyeth-Ayerst 3553
Prednisone (Prednisone) Roxane 3064
Prelone Syrup (Prednisolone) Muro . 2273
Solu-Medrol Sterile Powder (Methylprednisolone Sodium Succinate) Pharmacia & Upjohn 2855
Vistaril Intramuscular Solution (Hydroxyzine Hydrochloride) Pfizer 2738

Allergic reactions associated with blood or plasma
Benadryl Parenteral (Diphenhydramine Hydrochloride) Parke-Davis 2617
Periactin Tablets (Cyproheptadine Hydrochloride) Merck 2155
Phenergan Injection (Promethazine Hydrochloride) Wyeth-Ayerst 3553
Phenergan Suppositories (Promethazine Hydrochloride) Wyeth-Ayerst 3556
Phenergan Syrup (Promethazine Hydrochloride) Wyeth-Ayerst 3554
Phenergan Tablets (Promethazine Hydrochloride) Wyeth-Ayerst 3556

Allergic rhinitis
(*see under* Rhinitis, allergic)

Alopecia, androgenetic
Propecia Tablets (Finasteride) Merck 2172

Alopecia areata
Celestone Soluspan Injectable Suspension (Betamethasone Acetate, Betamethasone Sodium Phosphate) Schering 3097
Decadron Phosphate Injection (Dexamethasone Sodium Phosphate) Merck 2081
Hydrocortone Acetate Injectable Suspension (Hydrocortisone Acetate) Merck 2103

Alzheimer's disease
(*see under* Dementia, Alzheimer's type)

Amebiasis, acute intestinal
E.E.S. (Erythromycin Ethylsuccinate) Abbott 450
EryPed (Erythromycin Ethylsuccinate) Abbott 446
Ery-Tab Tablets (Erythromycin) Abbott 448
Erythrocin Stearate Filmtab Tablets (Erythromycin Stearate) Abbott 452
Erythromycin Base Filmtab Tablets (Erythromycin) Abbott 454
Erythromycin Delayed-Release Capsules, USP (Erythromycin) Abbott 455
PCE Dispertab Tablets (Erythromycin) Abbott 498
Yodoxin Tablets (Iodoquinol) Glenwood 1722

Amebiasis, acute intestinal, adjunct in
Declomycin Tablets (Demeclocycline Hydrochloride) Lederle 1855
Doryx Coated Pellet Filled Capsules (Doxycycline Hyclate) Warner Chilcott 3357
Dynacin Capsules (Minocycline Hydrochloride) Medicis 2019
Minocin Intravenous (Minocycline Hydrochloride) Lederle 1862
Minocin Oral Suspension (Minocycline Hydrochloride) Lederle 1865
Minocin Pellet-Filled Capsules (Minocycline Hydrochloride) Lederle 1863
Monodox Capsules (Doxycycline Monohydrate) Oclassen 2442
Vibramycin Calcium Oral Suspension Syrup (Doxycycline Calcium) Pfizer 2735
Vibramycin Hyclate Capsules (Doxycycline Hyclate) Pfizer 2735
Vibramycin Hyclate Intravenous (Doxycycline Hyclate) Pfizer 2737
Vibramycin Monohydrate for Oral Suspension (Doxycycline Monohydrate) Pfizer 2735
Vibra-Tabs Film Coated Tablets (Doxycycline Hyclate) Pfizer 2735

Amebiasis, extraintestinal
Aralen Tablets (Chloroquine Phosphate) Sanofi-Synthelabo 3075

Amenorrhea, secondary
Aygestin Tablets (Norethindrone Acetate) ESI Lederle 1333
Crinone (Progesterone) Serono 3213
Prometrium Capsules (100 mg, 200 mg) (Progesterone) Solvay ... 3261

Provera Tablets (Medroxyprogesterone Acetate) Pharmacia & Upjohn 2853

Amyotrophic lateral sclerosis
(*see under* Sclerosis, amyotrophic lateral)

Analgesia
(*see under* Pain, general)

Anaphylactic reactions, adjunctive therapy in
Benadryl Parenteral (Diphenhydramine Hydrochloride) Parke-Davis 2617
Periactin Tablets (Cyproheptadine Hydrochloride) Merck 2155
Phenergan Injection (Promethazine Hydrochloride) Wyeth-Ayerst 3553
Phenergan Suppositories (Promethazine Hydrochloride) Wyeth-Ayerst 3556
Phenergan Syrup (Promethazine Hydrochloride) Wyeth-Ayerst 3554
Phenergan Tablets (Promethazine Hydrochloride) Wyeth-Ayerst 3556

Anaphylactoid reactions
EpiPen (Epinephrine) Dey 1236

Ancylostoma duodenale infections
Mintezol (Thiabendazole) Merck 2137
Vermox Chewable Tablets (Mebendazole) McNeil Consumer 2017

Androgen, absence or deficiency of
Androderm Transdermal System CIII (Testosterone) Watson 3377
AndroGel (Testosterone) Unimed 3322
Android Capsules, 10 mg (Methyltestosterone) ICN 1731

Anemia, aplastic, acquired
Anadrol-50 (Oxymetholone) Unimed 3321

Anemia, AZT-treated HIV-infected patients, treatment of
Epogen for Injection (Epoetin Alfa) Amgen 582
Procrit for Injection (Epoetin Alfa) Ortho Biotech 2502

Anemia, chemotherapy-induced in cancer patients
Epogen for Injection (Epoetin Alfa) Amgen 582
Procrit for Injection (Epoetin Alfa) Ortho Biotech 2502

Anemia, hemolytic, acquired
Celestone Soluspan Injectable Suspension (Betamethasone Acetate, Betamethasone Sodium Phosphate) Schering 3097
Celestone Syrup (Betamethasone) Schering 3099
Cortone Acetate Injectable Suspension (Cortisone Acetate) Merck 2059
Cortone Acetate Tablets (Cortisone Acetate) Merck 2061
Decadron Elixir (Dexamethasone) Merck 2078
Decadron Tablets (Dexamethasone) Merck 2079
Decadron Phosphate Injection (Dexamethasone Sodium Phosphate) Merck 2081
Depo-Medrol Injectable Suspension (Methylprednisolone Acetate) Pharmacia & Upjohn 2795
Hydrocortone Tablets (Hydrocortisone) Merck 2106
Hydrocortone Phosphate Injection, Sterile (Hydrocortisone Sodium Phosphate) Merck 2105
Pediapred Oral Solution (Prednisolone Sodium Phosphate) Celltech 1170
Prednisone (Prednisone) Roxane 3064
Prelone Syrup (Prednisolone) Muro 2273
Solu-Medrol Sterile Powder (Methylprednisolone Sodium Succinate) Pharmacia & Upjohn 2855

Anemia, hypoplastic
Anadrol-50 Tablets (Oxymetholone) Unimed 3321

Anemia, hypoplastic, congenital
Celestone Soluspan Injectable Suspension (Betamethasone Acetate, Betamethasone Sodium Phosphate) Schering 3097
Celestone Syrup (Betamethasone) Schering 3099
Cortone Acetate Injectable Suspension (Cortisone Acetate) Merck 2059
Cortone Acetate Tablets (Cortisone Acetate) Merck 2061
Decadron Elixir (Dexamethasone) Merck 2078
Decadron Tablets (Dexamethasone) Merck 2079
Decadron Phosphate Injection (Dexamethasone Sodium Phosphate) Merck 2081
Depo-Medrol Injectable Suspension (Methylprednisolone Acetate) Pharmacia & Upjohn 2795
Hydrocortone Tablets (Hydrocortisone) Merck 2106
Hydrocortone Phosphate Injection, Sterile (Hydrocortisone Sodium Phosphate) Merck 2105
Pediapred Oral Solution (Prednisolone Sodium Phosphate) Celltech 1170
Prednisone (Prednisone) Roxane 3064
Prelone Syrup (Prednisolone) Muro 2273
Solu-Medrol Sterile Powder (Methylprednisolone Sodium Succinate) Pharmacia & Upjohn 2855

Anemia, iron deficiency
Feosol Caplets (Iron Carbonyl) GlaxoSmithKline Consumer 1717
Feosol Tablets (Ferrous Sulfate) GlaxoSmithKline Consumer 1717
May-Vita Elixir (Vitamins with Minerals) Merz 2224
Niferex (Polysaccharide-Iron Complex) Schwarz 3176
Niferex-150 Capsules (Polysaccharide-Iron Complex) Schwarz 3176
Nu-Iron 150 Capsules (Polysaccharide-Iron Complex) Merz 2224
Slow Fe Tablets (Ferrous Sulfate) Novartis Consumer .... ■ 827
Slow Fe with Folic Acid Tablets (Ferrous Sulfate, Folic Acid) Novartis Consumer .... ■ 828
Venofer Injection (Iron Sucrose) American Regent 580

Anemia, myelofibrosis
Anadrol-50 Tablets (Oxymetholone) Unimed 3321

Anemia, pernicious
Nascobal Gel (Vitamin B_{12}) Schwarz 3174

Anemia, RBC
(*see under* Erythroblastopenia)

Anemia, surgical procedure-induced, to reduce the need for allogeneic blood transfusions
Epogen for Injection (Epoetin Alfa) Amgen 582
Procrit for Injection (Epoetin Alfa) Ortho Biotech 2502

Anemia, uterine leiomyomata-induced, preoperative adjunct
Lupron Depot 3.75 mg (Leuprolide Acetate) TAP 3281
Lupron Depot–3 Month 11.25 mg (Leuprolide Acetate) TAP 3285

Anemia associated with chronic renal failure
Epogen for Injection (Epoetin Alfa) Amgen 582
Procrit for Injection (Epoetin Alfa) Ortho Biotech 2502

Anemias, deficient red cell production
Anadrol-50 Tablets (Oxymetholone) Unimed 3321

Anesthesia, general
Brevital Sodium for Injection, USP (Methohexital Sodium) Jones 1815
Diprivan Injectable Emulsion (Propofol) AstraZeneca 667
Fluothane Inhalation (Halothane) Wyeth-Ayerst 3508
Suprane Liquid for Inhalation (Desflurane) Baxter Anesthesia 874
Versed Injection (Midazolam Hydrochloride) Roche Laboratories 3027

Anesthesia, general, adjunct in
Anectine Injection (Succinylcholine Chloride) GlaxoSmithKline 1476
Atarax Tablets & Syrup (Hydroxyzine Hydrochloride) Pfizer 2667
Ativan Injection (Lorazepam) Wyeth-Ayerst 3478
Brevital Sodium for Injection, USP (Methohexital Sodium) Jones 1815
Levsin Injection (Hyoscyamine Sulfate) Schwarz 3172
Mepergan Injection (Meperidine Hydrochloride, Promethazine Hydrochloride) Wyeth-Ayerst 3539
Nembutal Sodium Solution (Pentobarbital Sodium) Abbott 485
Norcuron for Injection (Vecuronium Bromide) Organon 2478
Nubain Injection (Nalbuphine Hydrochloride) Endo Labs 1323
Numorphan Injection (Oxymorphone Hydrochloride) Endo Labs 1324
Phenergan Injection (Promethazine Hydrochloride) Wyeth-Ayerst 3553
Phenergan Suppositories (Promethazine Hydrochloride) Wyeth-Ayerst 3556
Phenergan Syrup (Promethazine Hydrochloride) Wyeth-Ayerst 3554
Phenergan Tablets (Promethazine Hydrochloride) Wyeth-Ayerst 3556
Robinul Injectable (Glycopyrrolate) Robins 2940
Thorazine (Chlorpromazine Hydrochloride) GlaxoSmithKline 1656
Versed Injection (Midazolam Hydrochloride) Roche Laboratories 3027
Versed Syrup (Midazolam Hydrochloride) Roche Laboratories 3033
Zemuron Injection (Rocuronium Bromide) Organon 2491

Anesthesia, general, supplement to
(*see under* Anesthesia, general, adjunct in)

Anesthesia, local
Americaine Anesthetic Lubricant (Benzocaine) Celltech 1162
Chirocaine Injection (Levobupivacaine Hydrochloride) Purdue Pharma 2909
Duranest Injections (Etidocaine Hydrochloride) AstraZeneca LP 600
Emla (Lidocaine, Prilocaine) AstraZeneca LP 602
Hurricaine Topical Anesthetic Gel, 1 oz. Fresh Mint, Wild Cherry, Pina Colada, Watermelon, 1/6 oz. Wild Cherry, Watermelon (Benzocaine) Beutlich .... ■ 618
Hurricaine Topical Anesthetic Liquid, 1 oz. Wild Cherry, Pina Colada, .25 ml Dry Handle Swab Wild Cherry, 1/6 oz. Wild Cherry (Benzocaine) Beutlich .... ■ 618
Hurricaine Topical Anesthetic Spray Extension Tubes (200) (Benzocaine) Beutlich .... ■ 618
Hurricaine Topical Anesthetic Spray Kit, 2 oz. Wild Cherry (Benzocaine) Beutlich .... ■ 618
Hurricaine Topical Anesthetic Spray, 2 oz. Wild Cherry (Benzocaine) Beutlich .... ■ 618
Naropin Injection (Ropivacaine Hydrochloride) AstraZeneca LP 612
Nesacaine/Nesacaine MPF (Chloroprocaine Hydrochloride) AstraZeneca LP 617
Polocaine Injection, USP (Mepivacaine Hydrochloride) AstraZeneca LP 625
Polocaine-MPF Injection, USP (Mepivacaine Hydrochloride) AstraZeneca LP 625
Sensorcaine (Bupivacaine Hydrochloride) AstraZeneca LP 643
Sensorcaine-MPF Injection (Bupivacaine Hydrochloride) AstraZeneca LP 643
Xylocaine Injections (Lidocaine Hydrochloride) AstraZeneca LP 653

Anesthesia, local, adjunct in
Diprivan Injectable Emulsion (Propofol) AstraZeneca 667
Levsin Injection (Hyoscyamine Sulfate) Schwarz 3172
Mepergan Injection (Meperidine Hydrochloride, Promethazine Hydrochloride) Wyeth-Ayerst 3539
Phenergan Injection (Promethazine Hydrochloride) Wyeth-Ayerst 3553

Anesthesia, local, diagnostic procedures
Sensorcaine (Bupivacaine Hydrochloride) AstraZeneca LP 643
Sensorcaine-MPF Injection (Bupivacaine Hydrochloride) AstraZeneca LP 643

Anesthesia, local, genital mucous membrane
Emla (Lidocaine, Prilocaine) AstraZeneca LP 602

Anesthesia, local, obstetrical procedures
Americaine Anesthetic Lubricant (Benzocaine) Celltech 1162
Chirocaine Injection (Levobupivacaine Hydrochloride) Purdue Pharma 2909
Naropin Injection (Ropivacaine Hydrochloride) AstraZeneca LP 612
Sensorcaine (Bupivacaine Hydrochloride) AstraZeneca LP 643
Sensorcaine-MPF Injection (Bupivacaine Hydrochloride) AstraZeneca LP 643

Anesthesia, local, ocular
Ophthetic Ophthalmic Solution (Proparacaine Hydrochloride) Allergan .... ⊙ 244

Anesthesia, local, oral cavity
Hurricaine Topical Anesthetic Gel, 1 oz. Fresh Mint, Wild Cherry, Pina Colada, Watermelon, 1/6 oz. Wild Cherry, Watermelon (Benzocaine) Beutlich .... ■ 618
Hurricaine Topical Anesthetic Liquid, 1 oz. Wild Cherry, Pina Colada, .25 ml Dry Handle Swab Wild Cherry, 1/6 oz. Wild Cherry (Benzocaine) Beutlich .... ■ 618
Hurricaine Topical Anesthetic Spray Extension Tubes (200) (Benzocaine) Beutlich .... ■ 618
Hurricaine Topical Anesthetic Spray Kit, 2 oz. Wild Cherry (Benzocaine) Beutlich .... ■ 618
Hurricaine Topical Anesthetic Spray, 2 oz. Wild Cherry (Benzocaine) Beutlich .... ■ 618

Anesthesia, local, oral surgical procedures
Sensorcaine (Bupivacaine Hydrochloride) AstraZeneca LP 643
Sensorcaine-MPF Injection (Bupivacaine Hydrochloride) AstraZeneca LP 643

Anesthesia, local, pharyngeal
Americaine Anesthetic Lubricant (Benzocaine) Celltech 1162
Hurricaine Topical Anesthetic Gel, 1 oz. Fresh Mint, Wild Cherry, Pina Colada, Watermelon, 1/6 oz. Wild Cherry, Watermelon (Benzocaine) Beutlich .... ■ 618
Hurricaine Topical Anesthetic Liquid, 1 oz. Wild Cherry, Pina Colada, .25 ml Dry Handle Swab Wild Cherry, 1/6 oz. Wild Cherry (Benzocaine) Beutlich .... ■ 618
Hurricaine Topical Anesthetic Spray Extension Tubes (200) (Benzocaine) Beutlich .... ■ 618
Hurricaine Topical Anesthetic Spray Kit, 2 oz. Wild Cherry (Benzocaine) Beutlich .... ■ 618
Hurricaine Topical Anesthetic Spray, 2 oz. Wild Cherry (Benzocaine) Beutlich .... ■ 618

Anesthesia, local, spinal
Sensorcaine (Bupivacaine Hydrochloride) AstraZeneca LP 643
Sensorcaine-MPF Injection (Bupivacaine Hydrochloride) AstraZeneca LP 643

Anesthesia, local, surgical procedures
Naropin Injection (Ropivacaine Hydrochloride) AstraZeneca LP 612
Sensorcaine (Bupivacaine Hydrochloride) AstraZeneca LP 643
Sensorcaine-MPF Injection (Bupivacaine Hydrochloride) AstraZeneca LP 643

Anesthesia, local, therapeutic procedures
Sensorcaine (Bupivacaine Hydrochloride) AstraZeneca LP 643
Sensorcaine-MPF Injection (Bupivacaine Hydrochloride) AstraZeneca LP 643

Anesthesia, regional
Chirocaine Injection (Levobupivacaine Hydrochloride) Purdue Pharma 2909
Naropin Injection (Ropivacaine Hydrochloride) AstraZeneca LP 612
Polocaine Injection, USP (Mepivacaine Hydrochloride) AstraZeneca LP 625
Polocaine-MPF Injection, USP (Mepivacaine Hydrochloride) AstraZeneca LP 625
Sensorcaine (Bupivacaine Hydrochloride, Epinephrine Bitartrate) AstraZeneca LP 643
Sensorcaine-MPF Injection (Bupivacaine Hydrochloride) AstraZeneca LP 643
Xylocaine Injections (Lidocaine Hydrochloride) AstraZeneca LP 653

Anesthesia, regional, adjunct in
Diprivan Injectable Emulsion (Propofol) AstraZeneca 667

Anesthesia care sedation, monitored
Diprivan Injectable Emulsion (Propofol) AstraZeneca 667

Angina
(*see under* Angina pectoris)

Angina, chronic stable
Cardizem CD Capsules (Diltiazem Hydrochloride) Biovail 1016
Ecotrin Enteric Coated Aspirin Low, Regular and Maximum Strength Tablets (Aspirin) GlaxoSmithKline Consumer 1715
Inderal Tablets (Propranolol Hydrochloride) Wyeth-Ayerst 3513
Norvasc Tablets (Amlodipine Besylate) Pfizer 2704
Procardia Capsules (Nifedipine) Pfizer 2708
Procardia XL Extended Release Tablets (Nifedipine) Pfizer 2710
Tiazac Capsules (Diltiazem Hydrochloride) Forest 1378
Vascor Tablets (Bepridil Hydrochloride) Ortho-McNeil 2602

Angina, classic effort-associated
(*see under* Angina, chronic stable)

Angina, crescendo
(*see under* Angina, unstable)

Angina, pre-infarction
(*see under* Angina, unstable)

Angina, Prinzmetal's
Norvasc Tablets (Amlodipine Besylate) Pfizer 2704
Procardia Capsules (Nifedipine) Pfizer 2708
Procardia XL Extended Release Tablets (Nifedipine) Pfizer 2710

Angina, unstable
Genuine Bayer Professional Labeling (Aspirin Regimen Bayer) (Aspirin) Bayer Consumer .... ◘608
Ecotrin Enteric Coated Aspirin Low, Regular and Maximum Strength Tablets (Aspirin) GlaxoSmithKline Consumer 1715
Fragmin Injection (Dalteparin Sodium) Pharmacia & Upjohn 2814

Angina, variant
(*see under* Angina, Prinzmetal's)

Angina, vasospastic
(*see under* Angina, Prinzmetal's)

Angina pectoris
Corgard Tablets (Nadolol) Monarch 2245
Covera-HS Tablets (Verapamil Hydrochloride) Searle 3199
Imdur Tablets (Isosorbide Mononitrate) Key 1826
Inderal (Propranolol Hydrochloride) Wyeth-Ayerst 3513
Inderal LA Long-Acting Capsules (Propranolol Hydrochloride) Wyeth-Ayerst 3516
Ismo Tablets (Isosorbide Mononitrate) Wyeth-Ayerst 3524
Isordil Titradose Tablets (Isosorbide Dinitrate) Wyeth-Ayerst 3526
Nitro-Dur Transdermal Infusion System (Nitroglycerin) Key 1834
Nitro-Dur Transdermal Infusion System (Nitroglycerin) Schering 3134
Nitrolingual Pumpspray (Nitroglycerin) First Horizon 1355
Procardia Capsules (Nifedipine) Pfizer 2708
Tenormin (Atenolol) AstraZeneca 692
Toprol-XL Tablets (Metoprolol Succinate) AstraZeneca LP 651

Angina pectoris, acute, prophylaxis
Isordil Sublingual Tablets (Isosorbide Dinitrate) Wyeth-Ayerst 3525
Nitrolingual Pumpspray (Nitroglycerin) First Horizon 1355
Nitrostat Tablets (Nitroglycerin) Parke-Davis 2658

Angioedema, adjunctive therapy in
Extendryl (Chlorpheniramine Maleate, Methscopolamine Nitrate, Phenylephrine Hydrochloride) Fleming 1361
Periactin Tablets (Cyproheptadine Hydrochloride) Merck 2155
Phenergan Suppositories (Promethazine Hydrochloride) Wyeth-Ayerst 3556
Phenergan Syrup (Promethazine Hydrochloride) Wyeth-Ayerst 3554
Phenergan Tablets (Promethazine Hydrochloride) Wyeth-Ayerst 3556

Angiography, fluorescein, fundus
AK-Fluor Injection 10% and 25% (Fluorescein Sodium) Akorn .... ⊙202
Fluorescite Injection (Fluorescein Sodium) Alcon .... ⊙211

Angiography, fluorescein, iris vasculature
AK-Fluor Injection 10% and 25% (Fluorescein Sodium) Akorn .... ⊙202
Fluorescite Injection (Fluorescein Sodium) Alcon .... ⊙211

Ankylosing spondylitis
Anaprox Tablets (Naproxen Sodium) Roche Laboratories 2967
Anaprox DS Tablets (Naproxen Sodium) Roche Laboratories 2967
Genuine Bayer Professional Labeling (Aspirin Regimen Bayer) (Aspirin) Bayer Consumer .... ◘608
Extra Strength Bayer Arthritis Caplets (Aspirin) Bayer Consumer .... ◘610
Cataflam Tablets (Diclofenac Potassium) Novartis 2315
Celestone Soluspan Injectable Suspension (Betamethasone Acetate, Betamethasone Sodium Phosphate) Schering 3097
Celestone Syrup (Betamethasone) Schering 3099
Clinoril Tablets (Sulindac) Merck 2053
Cortone Acetate Injectable Suspension (Cortisone Acetate) Merck 2059
Cortone Acetate Tablets (Cortisone Acetate) Merck 2061
Decadron Elixir (Dexamethasone) Merck 2078
Decadron Tablets (Dexamethasone) Merck 2070
Decadron Phosphate Injection (Dexamethasone Sodium Phosphate) Merck 2081
Depo-Medrol Injectable Suspension (Methylprednisolone Acetate) Pharmacia & Upjohn 2795
EC-Naprosyn Delayed-Release Tablets (Naproxen) Roche Laboratories 2967
Ecotrin Enteric Coated Aspirin Low, Regular and Maximum Strength Tablets (Aspirin) GlaxoSmithKline Consumer 1715
Hydrocortone Tablets (Hydrocortisone) Merck 2106
Hydrocortone Phosphate Injection, Sterile (Hydrocortisone Sodium Phosphate) Merck 2105
Indocin (Indomethacin) Merck 2112
Naprelan Tablets (Naproxen Sodium) Elan 1293
Naprosyn Suspension (Naproxen) Roche Laboratories 2967
Naprosyn Tablets (Naproxen) Roche Laboratories 2967
Pediapred Oral Solution (Prednisolone Sodium Phosphate) Celltech 1170
Prednisone (Prednisone) Roxane 3064
Prelone Syrup (Prednisolone) Muro 2273
Solu-Medrol Sterile Powder (Methylprednisolone Sodium Succinate) Pharmacia & Upjohn 2855
Traumeel Injection Solution (Homeopathic Formulations) Heel 1726
Voltaren Tablets (Diclofenac Sodium) Novartis 2315

Anorexia associated with weight loss, AIDS-induced
Marinol Capsules (Dronabinol) Unimed 3325
Megace Oral Suspension (Megestrol Acetate) Bristol-Myers Squibb Oncology/Immunology 1124

Anterior segment inflammation
(*see under* Inflammation, anterior segment)

Anthrax
(*see under* B. anthracis infections)

Anticholinesterase drugs, overdosage, treatment of
Levsin/Levsinex/Levbid (Hyoscyamine Sulfate) Schwarz 3172
NuLev Orally Disintegrating Tablets (Hyoscyamine Sulfate) Schwarz 3176
Protopam Chloride for Injection (Pralidoxime Chloride) Wyeth-Ayerst 3582

Antithrombin III deficiency, hereditary
Thrombate III (Antithrombin III) Bayer Biological 944

Anxiety, generalized non-psychotic, short-term treatment of
Compazine (Prochlorperazine) GlaxoSmithKline 1505
Stelazine (Trifluoperazine Hydrochloride) GlaxoSmithKline 1640

Anxiety, mental depression-induced
Ativan Tablets (Lorazepam) Wyeth-Ayerst 3482
Etrafon (Amitriptyline Hydrochloride, Perphenazine) Schering 3115
Limbitrol (Amitriptyline Hydrochloride, Chlordiazepoxide) ICN 1738
Sinequan (Doxepin Hydrochloride) Pfizer 2713
Vistaril Intramuscular Solution (Hydroxyzine Hydrochloride) Pfizer 2738
Xanax Tablets (Alprazolam) Pharmacia & Upjohn 2865

Anxiety, preoperative
Ativan Injection (Lorazepam) Wyeth-Ayerst 3478
Librium Capsules (Chlordiazepoxide Hydrochloride) ICN 1736
Librium for Injection (Chlordiazepoxide Hydrochloride) ICN 1737
Thorazine (Chlorpromazine Hydrochloride) GlaxoSmithKline 1656
Valium Injectable (Diazepam) Roche Laboratories 3026
Vistaril Capsules (Hydroxyzine Pamoate) Pfizer 2738
Vistaril Intramuscular Solution (Hydroxyzine Hydrochloride) Pfizer 2738
Vistaril Oral Suspension (Hydroxyzine Pamoate) Pfizer 2738

Anxiety, short-term symptomatic relief of
Atarax Tablets & Syrup (Hydroxyzine Hydrochloride) Pfizer 2667
Ativan Tablets (Lorazepam) Wyeth-Ayerst 3482
Effexor XR Capsules (Venlafaxine Hydrochloride) Wyeth-Ayerst 3499
Hyland's Nerve Tonic Tablets and Caplets (Homeopathic Formulations) Standard Homeopathic .... ◘766
Librium Capsules (Chlordiazepoxide Hydrochloride) ICN 1736
Librium for Injection (Chlordiazepoxide Hydrochloride) ICN 1737
Miltown Tablets (Meprobamate) Wallace 3349
Paxil (Paroxetine Hydrochloride) GlaxoSmithKline 1609
Tranxene (Clorazepate Dipotassium) Abbott 511
Valium Injectable (Diazepam) Roche Laboratories 3026
Valium Tablets (Diazepam) Roche Products 3047
Vistaril Capsules (Hydroxyzine Pamoate) Pfizer 2738
Vistaril Intramuscular Solution (Hydroxyzine Hydrochloride) Pfizer 2738
Vistaril Oral Suspension (Hydroxyzine Pamoate) Pfizer 2738
Xanax Tablets (Alprazolam) Pharmacia & Upjohn 2865

Anxiety disorder, social
Paxil (Paroxetine Hydrochloride) GlaxoSmithKline 1609

Anxiety disorders, management of
Ativan Tablets (Lorazepam) Wyeth-Ayerst 3482
Etrafon (Amitriptyline Hydrochloride, Perphenazine) Schering 3115
Librium Capsules (Chlordiazepoxide Hydrochloride) ICN 1736
Librium for Injection (Chlordiazepoxide Hydrochloride) ICN 1737
Miltown Tablets (Meprobamate) Wallace 3349
Phenergan Injection (Promethazine Hydrochloride) Wyeth-Ayerst 3553
Phenergan Suppositories (Promethazine Hydrochloride) Wyeth-Ayerst 3556
Phenergan Syrup (Promethazine Hydrochloride) Wyeth-Ayerst 3554
Phenergan Tablets (Promethazine Hydrochloride) Wyeth-Ayerst 3556
Tranxene (Clorazepate Dipotassium) Abbott 511
Valium Injectable (Diazepam) Roche Laboratories 3026
Valium Tablets (Diazepam) Roche Products 3047
Vistaril Intramuscular Solution (Hydroxyzine Hydrochloride) Pfizer 2738
Xanax Tablets (Alprazolam) Pharmacia & Upjohn 2865

Aphthous ulcers
(*see also under* Stomatitis, recurrent aphthous, symptomatic relief of)
Aphthasol Oral Paste (Amlexanox) Block 1025

Apnea of prematurity
Cafcit (Caffeine Citrate) Boehringer Ingelheim 1035

Appendicitis, gangrenous
Primaxin I.M. (Cilastatin Sodium, Imipenem) Merck 2158

Appendicitis with peritonitis
Merrem I.V. (Meropenem) AstraZeneca 673
Primaxin I.M. (Cilastatin Sodium, Imipenem) Merck 2158
Zosyn (Piperacillin Sodium, Tazobactam Sodium) Lederle 1890
Zosyn in Galaxy Containers (Piperacillin Sodium, Tazobactam Sodium) Lederle 1894

Appetite, suppression of
(*see under* Obesity, exogenous)

Apprehension
(*see under* Anxiety disorders, management of)

ARC
(*see under* Infections, acquired immunodeficiency syndrome-related complex)

Arrhythmias
Inderal (Propranolol Hydrochloride) Wyeth-Ayerst 3513
Quinidex Extentabs (Quinidine Sulfate) Robins 2933
Tonocard Tablets (Tocainide Hydrochloride) AstraZeneca LP 649

Arrhythmias, supraventricular
Inderal (Propranolol Hydrochloride) Wyeth-Ayerst 3513

Arrhythmias, ventricular
Betapace Tablets (Sotalol Hydrochloride) Berlex 950
Cordarone Intravenous (Amiodarone Hydrochloride) Wyeth-Ayerst 3491
Procanbid Extended-Release Tablets (Procainamide Hydrochloride) Monarch 2262
Quinaglute Dura-Tabs Tablets (Quinidine Gluconate) Berlex 978
Quinidex Extentabs (Quinidine Sulfate) Robins 2933
Rythmol Tablets – 150 mg, 225 mg, 300 mg (Propafenone Hydrochloride) Abbott 502
Sectral Capsules (Acebutolol Hydrochloride) Wyeth-Ayerst 3589
Tambocor Tablets (Flecainide Acetate) 3M 1990

Arrhythmias, ventricular, life-threatening
Cordarone Tablets (Amiodarone Hydrochloride) Wyeth-Ayerst 3487
Mexitil Capsules (Mexiletine Hydrochloride) Boehringer Ingelheim..... 1047
Pacerone Tablets (Amiodarone Hydrochloride) Upsher-Smith........ 3331
Procanbid Extended-Release Tablets (Procainamide Hydrochloride) Monarch........................ 2262
Tambocor Tablets (Flecainide Acetate) 3M 1990
Tonocard Tablets (Tocainide Hydrochloride) AstraZeneca LP.... 649

Arrhythmias due to thyrotoxicosis, adjunct to
Inderal (Propranolol Hydrochloride) Wyeth-Ayerst 3513

Arteriovenous cannulae, occlusion of
Streptase for Infusion (Streptokinase) AstraZeneca LP 647

Arthralgia, topical relief of
(*see under* Pain, topical relief of)

Arthritis
(*see also under* Osteoarthritis; Rheumatoid arthritis)
Goody's Body Pain Formula Powder (Acetaminophen, Aspirin, Acetaminophen, Aspirin) Block ....◘620
Trilisate (Choline Magnesium Trisalicylate) Purdue Frederick 2901

Arthritis, acute, gouty
Celestone Soluspan Injectable Suspension (Betamethasone Acetate, Betamethasone Sodium Phosphate) Schering 3097
Celestone Syrup (Betamethasone) Schering 3099
Clinoril Tablets (Sulindac) Merck 2053
Cortone Acetate Injectable Suspension (Cortisone Acetate) Merck 2059
Cortone Acetate Tablets (Cortisone Acetate) Merck 2061
Decadron Elixir (Dexamethasone) Merck 2078
Decadron Tablets (Dexamethasone) Merck 2079
Decadron Phosphate Injection (Dexamethasone Sodium Phosphate) Merck 2081
Depo-Medrol Injectable Suspension (Methylprednisolone Acetate) Pharmacia & Upjohn 2795
Hydrocortone Tablets (Hydrocortisone) Merck 2106
Hydrocortone Acetate Injectable Suspension (Hydrocortisone Acetate) Merck 2103
Hydrocortone Phosphate Injection, Sterile (Hydrocortisone Sodium Phosphate) Merck 2105
Indocin (Indomethacin) Merck 2112
Pediapred Oral Solution (Prednisolone Sodium Phosphate) Celltech 1170
Prednisone (Prednisone) Roxane 3064
Prelone Syrup (Prednisolone) Muro .2273
Solu-Medrol Sterile Powder (Methylprednisolone Sodium Succinate) Pharmacia & Upjohn 2855

Arthritis, gonorrheal
Pfizerpen for Injection (Penicillin G Potassium) Pfizer 2707

Arthritis, juvenile
Anaprox Tablets (Naproxen Sodium) Roche Laboratories 2967
Anaprox DS Tablets (Naproxen Sodium) Roche Laboratories 2967
Azulfidine EN-tabs Tablets (Sulfasalazine) Pharmacia & Upjohn ...2775
EC-Naprosyn Delayed-Release Tablets (Naproxen) Roche Laboratories 2967
Motrin Suspension, Oral Drops, Chewable Tablets, and Caplets (Ibuprofen) McNeil Consumer 2002
Naprosyn Suspension (Naproxen) Roche Laboratories 2967
Naprosyn Tablets (Naproxen) Roche Laboratories 2967
Trilisate (Choline Magnesium Trisalicylate) Purdue Frederick 2901

Arthritis, osteo-
(*see under* Osteoarthritis)

Arthritis, psoriatic
Genuine Bayer Professional Labeling (Aspirin Regimen Bayer) (Aspirin) Bayer Consumer ....◘608
Extra Strength Bayer Arthritis Caplets (Aspirin) Bayer Consumer ....◘610
Celestone Soluspan Injectable Suspension (Betamethasone Acetate, Betamethasone Sodium Phosphate) Schering............. 3097
Celestone Syrup (Betamethasone) Schering 3099
Cortone Acetate Injectable Suspension (Cortisone Acetate) Merck... 2059
Cortone Acetate Tablets (Cortisone Acetate) Merck 2061
Decadron Elixir (Dexamethasone) Merck.. 2078
Decadron Tablets (Dexamethasone) Merck 2079
Decadron Phosphate Injection (Dexamethasone Sodium Phosphate) Merck 2081
Depo-Medrol Injectable Suspension (Methylprednisolone Acetate) Pharmacia & Upjohn 2795
Ecotrin Enteric Coated Aspirin Low, Regular and Maximum Strength Tablets (Aspirin) GlaxoSmithKline Consumer 1715
Hydrocortone Tablets (Hydrocortisone) Merck 2106
Hydrocortone Phosphate Injection, Sterile (Hydrocortisone Sodium Phosphate) Merck 2105
Pediapred Oral Solution (Prednisolone Sodium Phosphate) Celltech 1170
Prednisone (Prednisone) Roxane 3064
Prelone Syrup (Prednisolone) Muro .2273
Solu-Medrol Sterile Powder (Methylprednisolone Sodium Succinate) Pharmacia & Upjohn 2855

Arthritis, rheumatoid
(*see under* Rheumatoid arthritis)

Arthritis, topical adjunct to
BenGay External Analgesic Products (Menthol, Methyl Salicylate) Pfizer Inc., Warner-Lambert Healthcare ....◘696
Thera-Gesic Creme (Menthol, Methyl Salicylate) Mission 2233

Ascariasis, as secondary therapy in
Mintezol (Thiabendazole) Merck 2137

Ascaris lumbricoides infections
Vermox Chewable Tablets (Mebendazole) McNeil Consumer 2017

Aspergillosis
Abelcet Injection (Amphotericin B) Elan 1273
AmBisome for Injection (Amphotericin B) Fujisawa 1383
Amphotec (Amphotericin B, Cholesteryl Sulfate Complex) InterMune 1774
Cancidas for Injection (Caspofungin acetate) Merck 2048
Sporanox Capsules (Itraconazole) Janssen 1800
Sporanox Injection (Itraconazole) Janssen 1804
Sporanox Injection (Itraconazole) Ortho Biotech 2509

Aspergillus fumigatus infections
(*see under* Aspergillosis)

Asthma, bronchial
(*see under* Bronchial asthma)

Asthmatic attack, acute, in children age 6 years and older, treatment of
Alupent Inhalation Aerosol (Metaproterenol Sulfate) Boehringer Ingelheim 1029

Astrocytoma, anaplastic
Temodar Capsules (Temozolomide) Schering 3157

Athetosis, adjunctive therapy in
Valium Injectable (Diazepam) Roche Laboratories 3026
Valium Tablets (Diazepam) Roche Products 3047

Athlete's foot
(*see under* Tinea pedis infections)

Atrial extrasystoles
Inderal (Propranolol Hydrochloride) Wyeth-Ayerst 3513

Atrial fibrillation
Betapace AF Tablets (Sotalol Hydrochloride) Berlex 954
Brevibloc Injection (Esmolol Hydrochloride) Baxter Anesthesia 858
Cardizem Injectable (Diltiazem Hydrochloride) Biovail 1018
Cardizem Lyo-Ject Syringe (Diltiazem Hydrochloride) Biovail 1018
Cardizem Monovial (Diltiazem Hydrochloride) Biovail 1018
Corvert Injection (Ibutilide Fumarate) Pharmacia & Upjohn 2793
Digitek Tablets (Digoxin) Bertek 1003
Lanoxicaps Capsules (Digoxin) GlaxoSmithKline.......................... 1574
Lanoxin Injection (Digoxin) GlaxoSmithKline.......................... 1581
Lanoxin Tablets (Digoxin) GlaxoSmithKline 1587
Lanoxin Elixir Pediatric (Digoxin) GlaxoSmithKline 1578
Lanoxin Injection Pediatric (Digoxin) GlaxoSmithKline 1584
Quinaglute Dura-Tabs Tablets (Quinidine Gluconate) Berlex 978
Quinidex Extentabs (Quinidine Sulfate) Robins 2933
Tikosyn Capsules (Dofetilide) Pfizer 2717

Atrial fibrillation, paroxysmal
Rythmol Tablets – 150 mg, 225 mg, 300 mg (Propafenone Hydrochloride) Abbott 502
Tambocor Tablets (Flecainide Acetate) 3M 1990

Atrial fibrillation with embolism
Coumadin for Injection (Warfarin Sodium) DuPont 1243
Coumadin Tablets (Warfarin Sodium) DuPont 1243
Warfarin Sodium Tablets, USP (Warfarin Sodium) Taro 3302

Atrial flutter
Betapace AF Tablets (Sotalol Hydrochloride) Berlex 954
Brevibloc Injection (Esmolol Hydrochloride) Baxter Anesthesia 858
Cardizem Injectable (Diltiazem Hydrochloride) Biovail 1018
Cardizem Lyo-Ject Syringe (Diltiazem Hydrochloride) Biovail 1018
Cardizem Monovial (Diltiazem Hydrochloride) Biovail 1018
Corvert Injection (Ibutilide Fumarate) Pharmacia & Upjohn 2793
Inderal (Propranolol Hydrochloride) Wyeth-Ayerst 3513
Quinaglute Dura-Tabs Tablets (Quinidine Gluconate) Berlex 978
Quinidex Extentabs (Quinidine Sulfate) Robins 2933
Rythmol Tablets – 150 mg, 225 mg, 300 mg (Propafenone Hydrochloride) Abbott 502
Tikosyn Capsules (Dofetilide) Pfizer 2717

Attention deficit disorders with hyperactivity
Adderall Tablets (Amphetamine Aspartate, Amphetamine Sulfate, Dextroamphetamine Saccharate, Dextroamphetamine Sulfate) Shire US 3231
Adderall XR Capsules (Amphetamine Aspartate, Amphetamine Sulfate, Dextroamphetamine Saccharate, Dextroamphetamine Sulfate) Shire US ....
Concerta Extended-Release Tablets (Methylphenidate Hydrochloride) McNeil Consumer 1998
Concerta Tablets (Methylphenidate Hydrochloride) Alza 561
Cylert Tablets (Pemoline) Abbott 415
Desoxyn Tablets (Methamphetamine Hydrochloride) Abbott 440
Dexedrine (Dextroamphetamine Sulfate) GlaxoSmithKline 1512
DextroStat Tablets (Dextroamphetamine Sulfate) Shire US 3236
Metadate CD Capsules (Methylphenidate Hydrochloride) Celltech 1164
Metadate ER Tablets (Methylphenidate Hydrochloride) Celltech 1167
Methylin Tablets (Methylphenidate Hydrochloride) Mallinckrodt 1995
Methylin ER Tablets (Methylphenidate Hydrochloride) Mallinckrodt ..1995
Ritalin (Methylphenidate Hydrochloride) Novartis 2387

B

B. anthracis infections
Cipro (Ciprofloxacin) Bayer............. 887
Declomycin Tablets (Demeclocycline Hydrochloride) Lederle 1855
Doryx Coated Pellet Filled Capsules (Doxycycline Hyclate) Warner Chilcott.............................. 3357
Dynacin Capsules (Minocycline Hydrochloride) Medicis 2019
Minocin Intravenous (Minocycline Hydrochloride) Lederle................. 1862
Minocin Oral Suspension (Minocycline Hydrochloride) Lederle 1865
Minocin Pellet-Filled Capsules (Minocycline Hydrochloride) Lederle.. 1863
Monodox Capsules (Doxycycline Monohydrate) Oclassen 2442
Pfizerpen for Injection (Penicillin G Potassium) Pfizer 2707
Vibramycin Calcium Oral Suspension Syrup (Doxycycline Calcium) Pfizer 2735
Vibramycin Hyclate Capsules (Doxycycline Hyclate) Pfizer 2735
Vibramycin Hyclate Intravenous (Doxycycline Hyclate) Pfizer 2737
Vibramycin Monohydrate for Oral Suspension (Doxycycline Monohydrate) Pfizer 2735
Vibra-Tabs Film Coated Tablets (Doxycycline Hyclate) Pfizer 2735

B. distasonis infections
Mefoxin for Injection (Cefoxitin Sodium) Merck 2124
Mefoxin Premixed Intravenous Solution (Cefoxitin Sodium) Merck 2127
Primaxin I.M. (Cilastatin Sodium, Imipenem) Merck 2158

B. distasonis intra-abdominal infections
Mefoxin for Injection (Cefoxitin Sodium) Merck 2124
Mefoxin Premixed Intravenous Solution (Cefoxitin Sodium) Merck 2127
Primaxin I.M. (Cilastatin Sodium, Imipenem) Merck 2158

B. distasonis peritonitis
Mefoxin for Injection (Cefoxitin Sodium) Merck 2124
Mefoxin Premixed Intravenous Solution (Cefoxitin Sodium) Merck 2127

B. fragilis gynecologic infections
Cefobid Intravenous/Intramuscular (Cefoperazone) Pfizer 2671
Cefobid Pharmacy Bulk Package - Not for Direct Infusion (Cefoperazone Sodium) Pfizer 2673
Cefotan (Cefotetan) AstraZeneca 664
Claforan Injection (Cefotaxime Sodium) Aventis 732
Mefoxin for Injection (Cefoxitin Sodium) Merck 2124
Mefoxin Premixed Intravenous Solution (Cefoxitin Sodium) Merck 2127
Pipracil (Piperacillin Sodium) Lederle 1866
Primaxin I.V. (Cilastatin Sodium, Imipenem) Merck 2160
Unasyn for Injection (Ampicillin Sodium, Sulbactam Sodium) Pfizer 2728

B. fragilis infections
Cefizox for Intramuscular or Intravenous Use (Ceftizoxime Sodium) Fujisawa 1390
Cefobid Intravenous/Intramuscular (Cefoperazone) Pfizer 2671
Cefobid Pharmacy Bulk Package - Not for Direct Infusion (Cefoperazone Sodium) Pfizer 2673
Cefotan (Cefotetan) AstraZeneca 664
Cipro I.V. (Ciprofloxacin) Bayer 893
Cipro I.V. Pharmacy Bulk Package (Ciprofloxacin) Bayer 897
Cipro (Ciprofloxacin) Bayer 887
Claforan Injection (Cefotaxime Sodium) Aventis 732
Mefoxin for Injection (Cefoxitin Sodium) Merck 2124
Mefoxin Premixed Intravenous Solution (Cefoxitin Sodium) Merck 2127
Merrem I.V. (Meropenem) AstraZeneca 673
Pipracil (Piperacillin Sodium) Lederle 1866

Primaxin I.M. (Cilastatin Sodium, Imipenem) Merck ... 2158
Primaxin I.V. (Cilastatin Sodium, Imipenem) Merck ... 2160
Rocephin Injectable Vials, ADD-Vantage, Galaxy, Bulk (Ceftriaxone Sodium) Roche Laboratories ... 2993
Tazicef for Injection (Ceftazidime) GlaxoSmithKline ... 1647
Tazicef Galaxy Container (Ceftazidime Sodium) GlaxoSmithKline ... 1650
Tazicef Pharmacy Bulk Package (Ceftazidime) GlaxoSmithKline ... 1653
Tazidime Vials, Faspak & ADD-Vantage (Ceftazidime) Lilly ... 1966
Timentin Injection- ADD-Vantage Vial (Clavulanate Potassium, Ticarcillin Disodium) GlaxoSmithKline ... 1661
Timentin Injection-Galaxy Container (Clavulanate Potassium, Ticarcillin Disodium) GlaxoSmithKline ... 1664
Timentin Injection-Pharmacy Bulk Package (Clavulanate Potassium, Ticarcillin Disodium) GlaxoSmithKline ... 1666
Timentin for Intravenous Administration (Clavulanate Potassium, Ticarcillin Disodium) GlaxoSmithKline ... 1658
Trovan (Alatrofloxacin Mesylate) Pfizer ... 2722
Unasyn for Injection (Ampicillin Sodium, Sulbactam Sodium) Pfizer ... 2728
Zosyn (Piperacillin Sodium, Tazobactam Sodium) Lederle ... 1890
Zosyn in Galaxy Containers (Piperacillin Sodium, Tazobactam Sodium) Lederle ... 1894

B. fragilis intra-abdominal infections
Cefizox for Intramuscular or Intravenous Use (Ceftizoxime Sodium) Fujisawa ... 1390
Cefobid Intravenous/Intramuscular (Cefoperazone) Pfizer ... 2671
Cefobid Pharmacy Bulk Package - Not for Direct Infusion (Cefoperazone Sodium) Pfizer ... 2673
Cipro I.V. (Ciprofloxacin) Bayer ... 893
Cipro I.V. Pharmacy Bulk Package (Ciprofloxacin) Bayer ... 897
Cipro (Ciprofloxacin) Bayer ... 887
Fortaz (Ceftazidime Sodium) GlaxoSmithKline ... 1541
Maxipime for Injection (Cefepime Hydrochloride) Elan ... 1285
Mefoxin for Injection (Cefoxitin Sodium) Merck ... 2124
Mefoxin Premixed Intravenous Solution (Cefoxitin Sodium) Merck ... 2127
Merrem I.V. (Meropenem) AstraZeneca ... 673
Pipracil (Piperacillin Sodium) Lederle ... 1866
Primaxin I.M. (Cilastatin Sodium, Imipenem) Merck ... 2158
Primaxin I.V. (Cilastatin Sodium, Imipenem) Merck ... 2160
Rocephin Injectable Vials, ADD-Vantage, Galaxy, Bulk (Ceftriaxone Sodium) Roche Laboratories ... 2993
Tazicef for Injection (Ceftazidime) GlaxoSmithKline ... 1647
Tazicef Galaxy Container (Ceftazidime Sodium) GlaxoSmithKline ... 1650
Tazicef Pharmacy Bulk Package (Ceftazidime) GlaxoSmithKline ... 1653
Tazidime Vials, Faspak & ADD-Vantage (Ceftazidime) Lilly ... 1966
Timentin Injection- ADD-Vantage Vial (Clavulanate Potassium, Ticarcillin Disodium) GlaxoSmithKline ... 1661
Timentin Injection-Galaxy Container (Clavulanate Potassium, Ticarcillin Disodium) GlaxoSmithKline ... 1664
Timentin Injection-Pharmacy Bulk Package (Clavulanate Potassium, Ticarcillin Disodium) GlaxoSmithKline ... 1666
Timentin for Intravenous Administration (Clavulanate Potassium, Ticarcillin Disodium) GlaxoSmithKline ... 1658
Trovan (Alatrofloxacin Mesylate) Pfizer ... 2722
Unasyn for Injection (Ampicillin Sodium, Sulbactam Sodium) Pfizer ... 2728

B. fragilis peritonitis
Cefobid Intravenous/Intramuscular (Cefoperazone) Pfizer ... 2671
Cefobid Pharmacy Bulk Package - Not for Direct Infusion (Cefoperazone Sodium) Pfizer ... 2673
Mefoxin for Injection (Cefoxitin Sodium) Merck ... 2124
Mefoxin Premixed Intravenous Solution (Cefoxitin Sodium) Merck ... 2127
Merrem I.V. (Meropenem) AstraZeneca ... 673
Timentin Injection- ADD-Vantage Vial (Clavulanate Potassium, Ticarcillin Disodium) GlaxoSmithKline ... 1661
Timentin Injection-Galaxy Container (Clavulanate Potassium, Ticarcillin Disodium) GlaxoSmithKline ... 1664
Timentin Injection-Pharmacy Bulk Package (Clavulanate Potassium, Ticarcillin Disodium) GlaxoSmithKline ... 1666
Timentin for Intravenous Administration (Clavulanate Potassium, Ticarcillin Disodium) GlaxoSmithKline ... 1658
Zosyn (Piperacillin Sodium, Tazobactam Sodium) Lederle ... 1890
Zosyn in Galaxy Containers (Piperacillin Sodium, Tazobactam Sodium) Lederle ... 1894

B. fragilis septicemia
Cefizox for Intramuscular or Intravenous Use (Ceftizoxime Sodium) Fujisawa ... 1390
Mefoxin for Injection (Cefoxitin Sodium) Merck ... 2124
Mefoxin Premixed Intravenous Solution (Cefoxitin Sodium) Merck ... 2127
Primaxin I.V. (Cilastatin Sodium, Imipenem) Merck ... 2160

B. fragilis skin and skin structure infections
Cefizox for Intramuscular or Intravenous Use (Ceftizoxime Sodium) Fujisawa ... 1390
Mefoxin for Injection (Cefoxitin Sodium) Merck ... 2124
Mefoxin Premixed Intravenous Solution (Cefoxitin Sodium) Merck ... 2127
Pipracil (Piperacillin Sodium) Lederle ... 1866
Primaxin I.M. (Cilastatin Sodium, Imipenem) Merck ... 2158
Primaxin I.V. (Cilastatin Sodium, Imipenem) Merck ... 2160
Rocephin Injectable Vials, ADD-Vantage, Galaxy, Bulk (Ceftriaxone Sodium) Roche Laboratories ... 2993
Unasyn for Injection (Ampicillin Sodium, Sulbactam Sodium) Pfizer ... 2728

B. intermedius infections
Primaxin I.M. (Cilastatin Sodium, Imipenem) Merck ... 2158

B. melaninogenicus endometritis
Timentin Injection- ADD-Vantage Vial (Clavulanate Potassium, Ticarcillin Disodium) GlaxoSmithKline ... 1661
Timentin Injection-Galaxy Container (Clavulanate Potassium, Ticarcillin Disodium) GlaxoSmithKline ... 1664
Timentin Injection-Pharmacy Bulk Package (Clavulanate Potassium, Ticarcillin Disodium) GlaxoSmithKline ... 1666
Timentin for Intravenous Administration (Clavulanate Potassium, Ticarcillin Disodium) GlaxoSmithKline ... 1658

B. melaninogenicus infections
Timentin Injection- ADD-Vantage Vial (Clavulanate Potassium, Ticarcillin Disodium) GlaxoSmithKline ... 1661
Timentin Injection-Galaxy Container (Clavulanate Potassium, Ticarcillin Disodium) GlaxoSmithKline ... 1664
Timentin Injection-Pharmacy Bulk Package (Clavulanate Potassium, Ticarcillin Disodium) GlaxoSmithKline ... 1666
Timentin for Intravenous Administration (Clavulanate Potassium, Ticarcillin Disodium) GlaxoSmithKline ... 1658

B. ovatus infections
Mefoxin for Injection (Cefoxitin Sodium) Merck ... 2124
Mefoxin Premixed Intravenous Solution (Cefoxitin Sodium) Merck ... 2127
Zosyn (Piperacillin Sodium, Tazobactam Sodium) Lederle ... 1890
Zosyn in Galaxy Containers (Piperacillin Sodium, Tazobactam Sodium) Lederle ... 1894

B. ovatus intra-abdominal infections
Mefoxin for Injection (Cefoxitin Sodium) Merck ... 2124
Mefoxin Premixed Intravenous Solution (Cefoxitin Sodium) Merck ... 2127

B. ovatus peritonitis
Mefoxin for Injection (Cefoxitin Sodium) Merck ... 2124
Mefoxin Premixed Intravenous Solution (Cefoxitin Sodium) Merck ... 2127
Zosyn (Piperacillin Sodium, Tazobactam Sodium) Lederle ... 1890
Zosyn in Galaxy Containers (Piperacillin Sodium, Tazobactam Sodium) Lederle ... 1894

B. pertussis infections
E.E.S. (Erythromycin Ethylsuccinate) Abbott ... 450
EryPed (Erythromycin Ethylsuccinate) Abbott ... 446
Ery-Tab Tablets (Erythromycin) Abbott ... 448
Erythrocin Stearate Filmtab Tablets (Erythromycin Stearate) Abbott ... 452
Erythromycin Base Filmtab Tablets (Erythromycin) Abbott ... 454
Erythromycin Delayed-Release Capsules, USP (Erythromycin) Abbott ... 455
PCE Dispertab Tablets (Erythromycin) Abbott ... 498

B. pertussis respiratory tract infections
E.E.S. (Erythromycin Ethylsuccinate) Abbott ... 450
EryPed (Erythromycin Ethylsuccinate) Abbott ... 446
Ery-Tab Tablets (Erythromycin) Abbott ... 448
Erythrocin Stearate Filmtab Tablets (Erythromycin Stearate) Abbott ... 452
Erythromycin Base Filmtab Tablets (Erythromycin) Abbott ... 454
Erythromycin Delayed-Release Capsules, USP (Erythromycin) Abbott ... 455
PCE Dispertab Tablets (Erythromycin) Abbott ... 498

B. thetaiotaomicron infections
Mefoxin for Injection (Cefoxitin Sodium) Merck ... 2124
Mefoxin Premixed Intravenous Solution (Cefoxitin Sodium) Merck ... 2127
Merrem I.V. (Meropenem) AstraZeneca ... 673
Primaxin I.M. (Cilastatin Sodium, Imipenem) Merck ... 2158
Zosyn (Piperacillin Sodium, Tazobactam Sodium) Lederle ... 1890
Zosyn in Galaxy Containers (Piperacillin Sodium, Tazobactam Sodium) Lederle ... 1894

B. thetaiotaomicron intra-abdominal infections
Mefoxin for Injection (Cefoxitin Sodium) Merck ... 2124
Mefoxin Premixed Intravenous Solution (Cefoxitin Sodium) Merck ... 2127
Merrem I.V. (Meropenem) AstraZeneca ... 673
Primaxin I.M. (Cilastatin Sodium, Imipenem) Merck ... 2158

B. thetaiotaomicron peritonitis
Mefoxin for Injection (Cefoxitin Sodium) Merck ... 2124
Mefoxin Premixed Intravenous Solution (Cefoxitin Sodium) Merck ... 2127
Merrem I.V. (Meropenem) AstraZeneca ... 673
Zosyn (Piperacillin Sodium, Tazobactam Sodium) Lederle ... 1890
Zosyn in Galaxy Containers (Piperacillin Sodium, Tazobactam Sodium) Lederle ... 1894

B. vulgatus infections
Cefotan (Cefotetan) AstraZeneca ... 664
Zosyn (Piperacillin Sodium, Tazobactam Sodium) Lederle ... 1890
Zosyn in Galaxy Containers (Piperacillin Sodium, Tazobactam Sodium) Lederle ... 1894

B. vulgatus intra-abdominal infections
Cefotan (Cefotetan) AstraZeneca ... 664

B. vulgatus peritonitis
Zosyn (Piperacillin Sodium, Tazobactam Sodium) Lederle ... 1890
Zosyn in Galaxy Containers (Piperacillin Sodium, Tazobactam Sodium) Lederle ... 1894

Backache, systemic, symptomatic relief of
Advil (Ibuprofen) Whitehall-Robins ... ▣771
Aleve Tablets, Caplets and Gelcaps (Naproxen Sodium) Bayer Consumer ... ▣602
Goody's Extra Strength Headache Powder (Acetaminophen, Aspirin, Caffeine) Block ... ▣620
Goody's Extra Strength Pain Relief Tablets (Acetaminophen, Aspirin, Caffeine) Block ... ▣620
Momentum Backache Relief Extra Strength Caplets (Magnesium Salicylate) Medtech ... ▣666
Motrin IB Tablets, Caplets, and Gelcaps (Ibuprofen) McNeil Consumer ... 2002
Orudis KT Tablets (Ketoprofen) Whitehall-Robins ... ▣778
Traumeel Injection Solution (Homeopathic Formulations) Heel ... 1726
Tylenol (Acetaminophen) McNeil Consumer ... 2009

Backache, temporary relief of
(*see under* Pain, topical relief of)

Bacteremia
(*see under* Septicemia, bacterial)

Bacteriuria, asymptomatic
Geocillin Tablets (Carbenicillin Indanyl Sodium) Pfizer ... 2687

Bacteriuria associated with cystitis, elimination or suppression of
(*see also under* Infections, urinary tract)
Uroqid-Acid No. 2 Tablets (Methenamine Mandelate, Sodium Acid Phosphate) Beach ... 947

Bacteriuria associated with polynephritis, elimination or suppression of
(*see under* Infections, urinary tract)

Bacteroides distasonis infections
(*see under* B. distasonis infections)

Bacteroides fragilis infections
(*see under* B. fragilis infections)

Bacteroides ovatus infections
(*see under* B. ovatus infections)

Bacteroides species bone and joint infections
Cefizox for Intramuscular or Intravenous Use (Ceftizoxime Sodium) Fujisawa ... 1390

Bacteroides species gynecologic infections
Cefobid Intravenous/Intramuscular (Cefoperazone) Pfizer ... 2671
Cefobid Pharmacy Bulk Package - Not for Direct Infusion (Cefoperazone Sodium) Pfizer ... 2673
Cefotan (Cefotetan) AstraZeneca ... 664
Claforan Injection (Cefotaxime Sodium) Aventis ... 732
Mefoxin for Injection (Cefoxitin Sodium) Merck ... 2124
Mefoxin Premixed Intravenous Solution (Cefoxitin Sodium) Merck ... 2127
Primaxin I.M. (Cilastatin Sodium, Imipenem) Merck ... 2158
Primaxin I.V. (Cilastatin Sodium, Imipenem) Merck ... 2160
Unasyn for Injection (Ampicillin Sodium, Sulbactam Sodium) Pfizer ... 2728

Bacteroides species infections
(*see also under* B. distasonis infections; B. fragilis infections; B. ovatus infections; B. thetaiotaomicron infections; B. vulgatus infections)

Cefizox for Intramuscular or Intravenous Use (Ceftizoxime Sodium) Fujisawa 1390
Cefobid Intravenous/Intramuscular (Cefoperazone) Pfizer 2671
Cefobid Pharmacy Bulk Package - Not for Direct Infusion (Cefoperazone Sodium) Pfizer 2673
Cefotan (Cefotetan) AstraZeneca 664
Ceptaz for Injection (Ceftazidime) GlaxoSmithKline 1499
Claforan Injection (Cefotaxime Sodium) Aventis 732
Declomycin Tablets (Demeclocycline Hydrochloride) Lederle 1855
Fortaz (Ceftazidime Sodium) GlaxoSmithKline 1541
Mefoxin for Injection (Cefoxitin Sodium) Merck 2124
Mefoxin Premixed Intravenous Solution (Cefoxitin Sodium) Merck 2127
Minocin Intravenous (Minocycline Hydrochloride) Lederle 1862
Pipracil (Piperacillin Sodium) Lederle 1866
Primaxin I.M. (Cilastatin Sodium, Imipenem) Merck 2158
Primaxin I.V. (Cilastatin Sodium, Imipenem) Merck 2160
Tazicef for Injection (Ceftazidime) GlaxoSmithKline 1647
Tazicef Galaxy Container (Ceftazidime Sodium) GlaxoSmithKline 1650
Tazicef Pharmacy Bulk Package (Ceftazidime) GlaxoSmithKline 1653
Tazidime Vials, Faspak & ADD-Vantage (Ceftazidime) Lilly 1966
Unasyn for Injection (Ampicillin Sodium, Sulbactam Sodium) Pfizer 2728
Vibramycin Hyclate Intravenous (Doxycycline Hyclate) Pfizer 2737

Bacteroides species intra-abdominal infections
Cefizox for Intramuscular or Intravenous Use (Ceftizoxime Sodium) Fujisawa 1390
Cefobid Intravenous/Intramuscular (Cefoperazone) Pfizer 2671
Cefobid Pharmacy Bulk Package - Not for Direct Infusion (Cefoperazone Sodium) Pfizer 2673
Cefotan (Cefotetan) AstraZeneca 664
Ceptaz for Injection (Ceftazidime) GlaxoSmithKline 1499
Claforan Injection (Cefotaxime Sodium) Aventis 732
Fortaz (Ceftazidime Sodium) GlaxoSmithKline 1541
Mefoxin for Injection (Cefoxitin Sodium) Merck 2124
Mefoxin Premixed Intravenous Solution (Cefoxitin Sodium) Merck 2127
Pipracil (Piperacillin Sodium) Lederle 1866
Primaxin I.M. (Cilastatin Sodium, Imipenem) Merck 2158
Primaxin I.V. (Cilastatin Sodium, Imipenem) Merck 2160
Tazicef for Injection (Ceftazidime) GlaxoSmithKline 1647
Tazicef Galaxy Container (Ceftazidime Sodium) GlaxoSmithKline 1650
Tazicef Pharmacy Bulk Package (Ceftazidime) GlaxoSmithKline 1653
Tazidime Vials, Faspak & ADD-Vantage (Ceftazidime) Lilly 1966
Unasyn for Injection (Ampicillin Sodium, Sulbactam Sodium) Pfizer 2728

Bacteroides species lower respiratory tract infections
Cefizox for Intramuscular or Intravenous Use (Ceftizoxime Sodium) Fujisawa 1390
Mefoxin for Injection (Cefoxitin Sodium) Merck 2124
Mefoxin Premixed Intravenous Solution (Cefoxitin Sodium) Merck 2127

Bacteroides species lung abscess
Mefoxin for Injection (Cefoxitin Sodium) Merck 2124
Mefoxin Premixed Intravenous Solution (Cefoxitin Sodium) Merck 2127

Bacteroides species peritonitis
Mefoxin for Injection (Cefoxitin Sodium) Merck 2124
Mefoxin Premixed Intravenous Solution (Cefoxitin Sodium) Merck 2127
Primaxin I.M. (Cilastatin Sodium, Imipenem) Merck 2158

Bacteroides species pneumonia
Mefoxin for Injection (Cefoxitin Sodium) Merck 2124
Mefoxin Premixed Intravenous Solution (Cefoxitin Sodium) Merck 2127

Bacteroides species septicemia
Cefizox for Intramuscular or Intravenous Use (Ceftizoxime Sodium) Fujisawa 1390
Mefoxin for Injection (Cefoxitin Sodium) Merck 2124
Mefoxin Premixed Intravenous Solution (Cefoxitin Sodium) Merck 2127
Pipracil (Piperacillin Sodium) Lederle 1866
Primaxin I.V. (Cilastatin Sodium, Imipenem) Merck 2160

Bacteroides species skin and skin structure infections
Cefizox for Intramuscular or Intravenous Use (Ceftizoxime Sodium) Fujisawa 1390
Claforan Injection (Cefotaxime Sodium) Aventis 732
Mefoxin for Injection (Cefoxitin Sodium) Merck 2124
Mefoxin Premixed Intravenous Solution (Cefoxitin Sodium) Merck 2127
Primaxin I.M. (Cilastatin Sodium, Imipenem) Merck 2158
Primaxin I.V. (Cilastatin Sodium, Imipenem) Merck 2160

Bacteroides thetaiotaomicron infections
(*see under* B. thetaiotaomicron infections)

Bacteroides vulgatus infections
(*see under* B. vulgatus infections)

Baldness, male pattern of vertex of scalp
Propecia Tablets (Finasteride) Merck 2172
Rogaine Extra Strength for Men Topical Solution (Minoxidil) Pharmacia Consumer .... ▣ 721

Barber's itch
(*see under* Folliculitis barbae)

Bartonella bacilliformis infections
Declomycin Tablets (Demeclocycline Hydrochloride) Lederle 1855
Doryx Coated Pellet Filled Capsules (Doxycycline Hyclate) Warner Chilcott 3357
Dynacin Capsules (Minocycline Hydrochloride) Medicis 2019
Minocin Intravenous (Minocycline Hydrochloride) Lederle 1862
Minocin Oral Suspension (Minocycline Hydrochloride) Lederle 1865
Minocin Pellet-Filled Capsules (Minocycline Hydrochloride) Lederle 1863
Monodox Capsules (Doxycycline Monohydrate) Oclassen 2442
Vibramycin Calcium Oral Suspension Syrup (Doxycycline Calcium) Pfizer 2735
Vibramycin Hyclate Capsules (Doxycycline Hyclate) Pfizer 2735
Vibramycin Hyclate Intravenous (Doxycycline Hyclate) Pfizer 2737
Vibramycin Monohydrate for Oral Suspension (Doxycycline Monohydrate) Pfizer 2735
Vibra-Tabs Film Coated Tablets (Doxycycline Hyclate) Pfizer 2735

Bartonellosis
Dynacin Capsules (Minocycline Hydrochloride) Medicis 2019
Minocin Oral Suspension (Minocycline Hydrochloride) Lederle 1865
Minocin Pellet-Filled Capsules (Minocycline Hydrochloride) Lederle 1863
Monodox Capsules (Doxycycline Monohydrate) Oclassen 2442

Bedsores
(*see under* Ulcers, decubitus, adjunctive therapy in)

Behavioral problems, severe, in children
Haldol Injection, Tablets and Concentrate (Haloperidol) Ortho-McNeil 2533
Thorazine (Chlorpromazine Hydrochloride) GlaxoSmithKline 1656

Bejel
Bicillin L-A Injection (Penicillin G Benzathine) Monarch 2242
Permapen Isoject (Penicillin G Benzathine) Pfizer 2706

Benzodiazepine overdose, management of
Romazicon Injection (Flumazenil) Roche Laboratories 3000

Berylliosis
Celestone Soluspan Injectable Suspension (Betamethasone Acetate, Betamethasone Sodium Phosphate) Schering 3097
Celestone Syrup (Betamethasone) Schering 3099
Cortone Acetate Injectable Suspension (Cortisone Acetate) Merck 2059
Cortone Acetate Tablets (Cortisone Acetate) Merck 2061
Decadron Elixir (Dexamethasone) Merck 2078
Decadron Tablets (Dexamethasone) Merck 2079
Decadron Phosphate Injection (Dexamethasone Sodium Phosphate) Merck 2081
Depo-Medrol Injectable Suspension (Methylprednisolone Acetate) Pharmacia & Upjohn 2795
Hydrocortone Tablets (Hydrocortisone) Merck 2106
Hydrocortone Phosphate Injection, Sterile (Hydrocortisone Sodium Phosphate) Merck 2105
Pediapred Oral Solution (Prednisolone Sodium Phosphate) Celltech 1170
Prednisone (Prednisone) Roxane 3064
Prelone Syrup (Prednisolone) Muro 2273
Solu-Medrol Sterile Powder (Methylprednisolone Sodium Succinate) Pharmacia & Upjohn 2855

Bifidobacterium species gynecologic infections
Primaxin I.V. (Cilastatin Sodium, Imipenem) Merck 2160

Biotin, deficiency of
Biotin Capsules (Biotin) Mericon 2223

Bipolar disorder
(*see under* Mania, bipolar)

Bites, black widow spider
Antivenin (Black Widow Spider Antivenin) (Black Widow Spider Antivenin (Equine)) Merck 2042

Bites, crotalidae
(*see under* Envenomation, pit viper)

Bites, insect
Benadryl Itch Stopping Cream Original Strength (Diphenhydramine Hydrochloride, Zinc Acetate) Pfizer Inc., Warner-Lambert Healthcare .... ▣ 695
Benadryl Gel (Diphenhydramine Hydrochloride) Pfizer Inc., Warner-Lambert Healthcare .... ▣ 695
Benadryl Spray (Diphenhydramine Hydrochloride, Zinc Acetate) Pfizer Inc., Warner-Lambert Healthcare .... ▣ 696
Cortaid (Hydrocortisone) Pharmacia Consumer .... ▣ 717
Cortizone•5 (Hydrocortisone) Pfizer Inc., Warner-Lambert Healthcare .... ▣ 699
Cortizone•10 (Hydrocortisone) Pfizer Inc., Warner-Lambert Healthcare .... ▣ 699
Cortizone•10 Plus Creme (Hydrocortisone) Pfizer Inc., Warner-Lambert Healthcare .... ▣ 700
Cortizone•10 Quick Shot Spray (Hydrocortisone) Pfizer Inc., Warner-Lambert Healthcare .... ▣ 699
Cortizone for Kids Creme (Hydrocortisone) Pfizer Inc., Warner-Lambert Healthcare .... ▣ 699
EpiPen (Epinephrine) Dey 1236

Bites, pit vipers
(*see under* Envenomation, pit viper)

Bladder carcinoma, transitional cell
(*see under* Carcinoma, bladder, transitional cell)

Blastomycosis
Nizoral Tablets (Ketoconazole) Janssen 1791
Sporanox Capsules (Itraconazole) Janssen 1800
Sporanox Injection (Itraconazole) Janssen 1804
Sporanox Injection (Itraconazole) Ortho Biotech 2509

Blastomycosis, North American
(*see under* Blastomycosis)

Bleeding, control of in patients with Factor VIII inhibitors
Autoplex T (Anti-Inhibitor Coagulant Complex) Nabi 2294

Bleeding, fibrinolytic
Amicar Injection (Aminocaproic Acid) Xanodyne 3608
Amicar Syrup (Aminocaproic Acid) Xanodyne 3608
Amicar Tablets (Aminocaproic Acid) Xanodyne 3608

Bleeding, upper gastrointestinal, in critically ill
Tagamet (Cimetidine Hydrochloride) GlaxoSmithKline 1644

Bleeding associated with hemophilia A
Autoplex T (Anti-Inhibitor Coagulant Complex) Nabi 2294
Bebulin VH (Factor IX Complex) Baxter Healthcare 840
Feiba VH (Anti-Inhibitor Coagulant Complex) Baxter Healthcare 843
Konyne 80 (Factor IX Complex) Bayer Biological 937
NovoSeven (Antihemophilic Factor (Recombinant)) Novo Nordisk 2430
Proplex T (Factor IX Complex) Baxter Healthcare 851

Blepharitis
Genoptic Ophthalmic Ointment (Gentamicin Sulfate) Allergan .... ⊙ 239
Genoptic Sterile Ophthalmic Solution (Gentamicin Sulfate) Allergan .... ⊙ 239
Neosporin Ophthalmic Ointment Sterile (Bacitracin Zinc, Neomycin Sulfate, Polymyxin B Sulfate) Monarch .... ⊙ 299
Neosporin Ophthalmic Solution Sterile (Gramicidin, Neomycin Sulfate, Polymyxin B Sulfate) Monarch .... ⊙ 300
Polysporin Ophthalmic Ointment Sterile (Bacitracin Zinc, Polymyxin B Sulfate, Bacitracin Zinc, Polymyxin B Sulfate) Monarch .... ⊙ 301
Pred Mild Sterile Ophthalmic Suspension (Prednisolone Acetate) Allergan .... ⊙ 249

Blepharitis, fungal
Natacyn Antifungal Ophthalmic Suspension (Natamycin) Alcon .... ⊙ 216

Blepharoconjunctivitis
Genoptic Ophthalmic Ointment (Gentamicin Sulfate) Allergan .... ⊙ 239
Genoptic Sterile Ophthalmic Solution (Gentamicin Sulfate) Allergan .... ⊙ 239
Neosporin Ophthalmic Ointment Sterile (Bacitracin Zinc, Neomycin Sulfate, Polymyxin B Sulfate) Monarch .... ⊙ 299
Neosporin Ophthalmic Solution Sterile (Gramicidin, Neomycin Sulfate, Polymyxin B Sulfate) Monarch .... ⊙ 300
Polysporin Ophthalmic Ointment Sterile (Bacitracin Zinc, Polymyxin B Sulfate, Bacitracin Zinc, Polymyxin B Sulfate) Monarch .... ⊙ 301
Polytrim Ophthalmic Solution (Polymyxin B Sulfate, Trimethoprim Sulfate) Allergan 556

Blepharospasm
Botox Purified Neurotoxin Complex (Botulinum Toxin Type A) Allergan 549

Blood clotting, prevention of in arterial surgery
Heparin Sodium Injection (Heparin Sodium) Wyeth-Ayerst 3511

Blood clotting, prevention of in blood transfusion
Heparin Lock Flush Solution (Heparin Sodium) Wyeth-Ayerst 3509

Blood clotting, prevention of in cardiac surgery
Heparin Sodium Injection (Heparin Sodium) Wyeth-Ayerst 3511

Blood clotting, prevention of in dialysis procedures
Heparin Lock Flush (Heparin Sodium) Wyeth-Ayerst 3509

Blood loss, perioperative, reduction of
Trasylol Injection (Aprotinin) Bayer 909

Body aches
(*see under* Pain, general)

Boils, symptomatic relief of
(*see under* Furunculosis, symptomatic relief of)

Bone disease, metabolic, with chronic renal failure
(*see under* Osteodystrophy, renal)

Bone marrow transplantation, allogeneic or autologous, delayed or failed
Leukine (Sargramostim) Immunex 1755

Bone marrow transplantation, to decrease the risk of septicemia
Gamimune N, 5% Solvent/Detergent Treated (Globulin, Immune (Human)) Bayer Biological 925
Gamimune N, 10% Solvent/Detergent Treated (Globulin, Immune (Human)) Bayer Biological 928

Bone mass, loss of
(*see under* Osteoporosis)

Bordetella pertussis
(*see under* B. pertussis infections)

Borrelia burgdorferi infection
Ceftin Tablets (Cefuroxime Axetil) Lifecycle Ventures 1898

Borrelia recurrentis infection
Declomycin Tablets (Demeclocycline Hydrochloride) Lederle 1855
Doryx Coated Pellet Filled Capsules (Doxycycline Hyclate) Warner Chilcott 3357
Dynacin Capsules (Minocycline Hydrochloride) Medicis 2019
Minocin Intravenous (Minocycline Hydrochloride) Lederle 1862
Minocin Oral Suspension (Minocycline Hydrochloride) Lederle 1865
Minocin Pellet-Filled Capsules (Minocycline Hydrochloride) Lederle 1863
Monodox Capsules (Doxycycline Monohydrate) Oclassen 2442
Vibramycin Calcium Oral Suspension Syrup (Doxycycline Calcium) Pfizer 2735
Vibramycin Hyclate Capsules (Doxycycline Hyclate) Pfizer 2735
Vibramycin Hyclate Intravenous (Doxycycline Hyclate) Pfizer 2737
Vibramycin Monohydrate for Oral Suspension (Doxycycline Monohydrate) Pfizer 2735
Vibra-Tabs Film Coated Tablets (Doxycycline Hyclate) Pfizer 2735

Bowel, evacuation of
Colyte with Flavor Packs for Oral Solution (Polyethylene Glycol, Potassium Chloride, Sodium Bicarbonate, Sodium Chloride, Sodium Sulfate) Schwarz 3170
Fleet Bisacodyl Laxatives (Bisacodyl) Fleet 1359
Fleet Enema (Sodium Phosphate) Fleet 1359
Fleet Mineral Oil Enema (Mineral Oil) Fleet 1360
Fleet Phospho-soda (Sodium Phosphate) Fleet 1360
Fleet Prep Kits (Sodium Phosphate) Fleet 1361
GoLYTELY and Pineapple Flavor GoLYTELY for Oral Solution (Polyethylene Glycol, Potassium Chloride, Sodium Bicarbonate, Sodium Chloride, Sodium Sulfate) Braintree 1068
NuLYTELY, Cherry Flavor, Lemon-Lime Flavor, and Orange Flavor NuLYTELY for Oral Solution (Polyethylene Glycol, Potassium Chloride, Sodium Bicarbonate, Sodium Chloride) Braintree 1068
Purge Liquid (Castor Oil) Fleming .... ▣633
Visicol Tablets (Sodium Phosphate) Inkine 1767
X-Prep Liquid (Senna) Purdue Frederick 2900

Bowel, irritable, syndrome
Citrucel Caplets (Methylcellulose) SmithKline Beecham Consumer .... ▣745
Citrucel Orange Flavor Powder (Methylcellulose) SmithKline Beecham Consumer .... ▣744
Citrucel Sugar Free Orange Flavor Powder (Methylcellulose) SmithKline Beecham Consumer .... ▣745
Levsin/Levsinex/Levbid (Hyoscyamine Sulfate) Schwarz 3172
Metamucil (Psyllium Preparations) Procter & Gamble 2877
Mitrolan Chewable Tablets (Calcium Polycarbophil) Wyeth-Ayerst .... ▣789
NuLev Orally Disintegrating Tablets (Hyoscyamine Sulfate) Schwarz 3176

Bowel, irritable, syndrome, possibly effective in, adjunctive therapy
Donnatal (Atropine Sulfate, Hyoscyamine Sulfate, Phenobarbital, Scopolamine Hydrobromide) Robins 2929
Donnatal Extentabs (Atropine Sulfate, Hyoscyamine Sulfate, Phenobarbital, Scopolamine Hydrobromide) Robins 2930
Donnatal Tablets (Atropine Sulfate, Hyoscyamine Sulfate, Phenobarbital, Scopolamine Hydrobromide) Robins 2929

Branhamella catarrhalis
(*see under* M. catarrhalis infections)

Breast cancer
(*see under* Carcinoma, breast)

Breast carcinoma
(*see under* Carcinoma, breast)

Bromhidrosis, topical relief of
(*see under* Hyperhidrosis, topical relief of)

Bronchial asthma
Accolate Tablets (Zafirlukast) AstraZeneca 657
AccuNeb Inhalation Solution (Albuterol Sulfate) Dey 1230
Advair Diskus 100/50 (Fluticasone Propionate, Salmeterol Xinafoate) GlaxoSmithKline 1448
Advair Diskus 250/50 (Fluticasone Propionate, Salmeterol Xinafoate) GlaxoSmithKline 1448
Advair Diskus 500/50 (Fluticasone Propionate, Salmeterol Xinafoate) GlaxoSmithKline 1448
Aerobid/Aerobid-M (Flunisolide) Forest 1363
Aerolate (Theophylline) Fleming 1361
Alupent (Metaproterenol Sulfate) Boehringer Ingelheim 1029
Atrovent Inhalation Aerosol (Ipratropium Bromide) Boehringer Ingelheim 1030
Azmacort Inhalation Aerosol (Triamcinolone Acetonide) Aventis 728
Brethine Ampuls (Terbutaline Sulfate) Novartis 2314
Brethine Tablets (Terbutaline Sulfate) Novartis 2313
Celestone Soluspan Injectable Suspension (Betamethasone Acetate, Betamethasone Sodium Phosphate) Schering 3097
Celestone Syrup (Betamethasone) Schering 3099
Combivent Inhalation Aerosol (Albuterol Sulfate, Ipratropium Bromide) Boehringer Ingelheim 1041
Cortone Acetate Injectable Suspension (Cortisone Acetate) Merck 2059
Cortone Acetate Tablets (Cortisone Acetate) Merck 2061
Decadron Elixir (Dexamethasone) Merck 2078
Decadron Tablets (Dexamethasone) Merck 2079
Decadron Phosphate Injection (Dexamethasone Sodium Phosphate) Merck 2081
Depo-Medrol Injectable Suspension (Methylprednisolone Acetate) Pharmacia & Upjohn 2795
DuoNeb Inhalation Solution (Albuterol Sulfate, Ipratropium Bromide) Dey 1233
Flovent Diskus (Fluticasone Propionate) GlaxoSmithKline 3614
Flovent (Fluticasone Propionate) GlaxoSmithKline 1535
Flovent Rotadisk (Fluticasone Propionate) GlaxoSmithKline 1537
Foradil Aerolizer (Formoterol Fumarate) Novartis 2354
Hydrocortone Tablets (Hydrocortisone) Merck 2106
Hydrocortone Phosphate Injection, Sterile (Hydrocortisone Sodium Phosphate) Merck 2105
Lufyllin Tablets (Dyphylline) Wallace 3347
Lufyllin-400 Tablets (Dyphylline) Wallace 3347
Lufyllin-GG Elixir (Dyphylline, Guaifenesin) Wallace 3348
Lufyllin-GG Tablets (Dyphylline, Guaifenesin) Wallace 3348
Maxair Autohaler (Pirbuterol Acetate) 3M 1981
Maxair Inhaler (Pirbuterol Acetate) 3M 1984
Pediapred Oral Solution (Prednisolone Sodium Phosphate) Celltech 1170
Pima Syrup (Potassium Iodide) Fleming 1362
Prednisone (Prednisone) Roxane 3064
Prelone Syrup (Prednisolone) Muro 2273
Primatene Mist (Epinephrine) Whitehall-Robins .... ▣779
Primatene Tablets (Ephedrine Hydrochloride, Guaifenesin) Whitehall-Robins .... ▣780
Proventil Inhalation Aerosol (Albuterol) Schering 3142
Proventil Inhalation Solution 0.083% (Albuterol Sulfate) Schering 3146
Proventil Repetabs Tablets (Albuterol Sulfate) Schering 3148
Proventil Solution for Inhalation 0.5% (Albuterol Sulfate) Schering 3144
Proventil HFA Inhalation Aerosol (Albuterol Sulfate) Schering 3150
Pulmicort Respules (Budesonide) AstraZeneca LP 632
Pulmicort Turbuhaler Inhalation Powder (Budesonide) AstraZeneca LP 636
Qvar Inhalation Aerosol (Beclomethasone Dipropionate) 3M 1987
Serevent Diskus (Salmeterol Xinafoate) GlaxoSmithKline 1637
Serevent Inhalation Aerosol (Salmeterol Xinafoate) GlaxoSmithKline 1633
Singulair (Montelukast Sodium) Merck 2181
Solu-Medrol Sterile Powder (Methylprednisolone Sodium Succinate) Pharmacia & Upjohn 2855
Theo-Dur Extended-Release Tablets (Theophylline) Key 1835
Uni-Dur Extended-Release Tablets (Theophylline) Key 1841
Uniphyl 400 mg and 600 mg Tablets (Theophylline) Purdue Frederick 2903
Vanceril Inhalation Aerosol (Beclomethasone Dipropionate) Schering 3165
Vanceril Double Strength Inhalation Aerosol (Beclomethasone Dipropionate) Schering 3167
Ventolin Inhalation Aerosol and Refill (Albuterol) GlaxoSmithKline 1679
Ventolin HFA Inhalation Aerosol (Albuterol Sulfate) GlaxoSmithKline 3618
Volmax Extended-Release Tablets (Albuterol Sulfate) Muro 2276
Xopenex Inhalation Solution (Levalbuterol Hydrochloride) Sepracor 3207
Zyflo Filmtab Tablets (Zileuton) Abbott 524

Bronchial congestion
Comtrex Deep Chest Cold & Congestion Relief Softgels (Acetaminophen, Dextromethorphan Hydrobromide, Guaifenesin, Pseudoephedrine Hydrochloride) Bristol-Myers .... ▣627
Guaifed (Guaifenesin, Pseudoephedrine Hydrochloride) Muro 2272
Organidin NR Liquid (Guaifenesin) Wallace 3350
Organidin NR Tablets (Guaifenesin) Wallace 3350
Robitussin Liquid (Guaifenesin) Whitehall-Robins .... ▣782
Robitussin A-C Syrup (Codeine Phosphate, Guaifenesin) Robins 2942
Robitussin Cold Softgels Severe Congestion (Guaifenesin, Pseudoephedrine Hydrochloride) Whitehall-Robins .... ▣782
Robitussin-DAC Syrup (Codeine Phosphate, Guaifenesin, Pseudoephedrine Hydrochloride) Robins 2942
Robitussin DM Infant Drops (Dextromethorphan Hydrobromide, Guaifenesin) Whitehall-Robins .... ▣783
Robitussin-DM Liquid (Dextromethorphan Hydrobromide, Guaifenesin) Whitehall-Robins .... ▣783
Robitussin-PE Liquid (Guaifenesin, Pseudoephedrine Hydrochloride) Whitehall-Robins .... ▣782
Sudafed Non-Drying Sinus Liquid Caps (Guaifenesin, Pseudoephedrine Hydrochloride) Pfizer Inc., Warner-Lambert Healthcare .... ▣712
Triaminic Chest Congestion Liquid (Guaifenesin, Pseudoephedrine Hydrochloride) Novartis Consumer .... ▣680
Vicks 44E Cough & Chest Congestion Relief Liquid (Dextromethorphan Hydrobromide, Guaifenesin) Procter & Gamble .... ▣725
Pediatric Vicks 44e Cough & Chest Congestion Relief Liquid (Dextromethorphan Hydrobromide, Guaifenesin) Procter & Gamble .... ▣728

Bronchitis, acute
Azactam for Injection (Aztreonam) Elan 1276
Cefzil (Cefprozil) Bristol-Myers Squibb 1076
Dynabac Tablets (Dirithromycin) Muro 2269
Lorabid Suspension and Pulvules (Loracarbef) Monarch 2251
Omnicef (Cefdinir) Abbott 493
Suprax (Cefixime) Lederle 1877

Bronchitis, chronic
Atrovent Inhalation Aerosol (Ipratropium Bromide) Boehringer Ingelheim 1030
Brethine Ampuls (Terbutaline Sulfate) Novartis 2314
Brethine Tablets (Terbutaline Sulfate) Novartis 2313
Pima Syrup (Potassium Iodide) Fleming 1362
Theo-Dur Extended-Release Tablets (Theophylline) Key 1835
Uniphyl 400 mg and 600 mg Tablets (Theophylline) Purdue Frederick 2903

Bronchitis, chronic, acute exacerbation of
Avelox Tablets (Moxifloxacin Hydrochloride) Bayer 879
Bactrim (Sulfamethoxazole, Trimethoprim) Roche Laboratories 2949
Biaxin/Biaxin XL (Clarithromycin) Abbott 403
Ceclor CD Tablets (Cefaclor) Elan 1279
Cedax (Ceftibuten Dihydrate) Biovail 1021
Ceftin Tablets (Cefuroxime Axetil) Lifecycle Ventures 1898
Cefzil (Cefprozil) Bristol-Myers Squibb 1076
Cipro (Ciprofloxacin) Bayer 887
Floxin I.V. (Ofloxacin) Ortho-McNeil 2526
Floxin Tablets (Ofloxacin) Ortho-McNeil 2529
Levaquin (Levofloxacin) Ortho-McNeil 2537
Lorabid Suspension and Pulvules (Loracarbef) Monarch 2251
Omnicef (Cefdinir) Abbott 493
Primaxin I.M. (Cilastatin Sodium, Imipenem) Merck 2158
Septra Suspension (Sulfamethoxazole, Trimethoprim) Monarch 2265
Septra Tablets (Sulfamethoxazole, Trimethoprim) Monarch 2265
Septra DS Tablets (Sulfamethoxazole, Trimethoprim) Monarch 2265
Suprax (Cefixime) Lederle 1877
Tequin Injection (Gatifloxacin) Bristol-Myers Squibb 1110
Tequin Tablets (Gatifloxacin) Bristol-Myers Squibb 1110
Vantin Tablets and Oral Suspension (Cefpodoxime Proxetil) Pharmacia & Upjohn 2860

Bronchospasm, exercise-induced
Foradil Aerolizer (Formoterol Fumarate) Novartis 2354
Proventil Inhalation Aerosol (Albuterol) Schering 3142
Proventil HFA Inhalation Aerosol (Albuterol Sulfate) Schering 3150
Serevent Diskus (Salmeterol Xinafoate) GlaxoSmithKline 1637

Serevent Inhalation Aerosol (Salmeterol Xinafoate) GlaxoSmithKline 1633
Ventolin Inhalation Aerosol and Refill (Albuterol) GlaxoSmithKline .. 1679

Bronchospasm, prevention and relief of
Serevent Diskus (Salmeterol Xinafoate) GlaxoSmithKline 1637
Uni-Dur Extended-Release Tablets (Theophylline) Key 1841
Ventolin Inhalation Aerosol and Refill (Albuterol) GlaxoSmithKline .. 1679
Xopenex Inhalation Solution (Levalbuterol Hydrochloride) Sepracor .. 3207

Bronchospasm, reversible
(*see also under* Bronchial asthma)
AccuNeb Inhalation Solution (Albuterol Sulfate) Dey 1230
Alupent (Metaproterenol Sulfate) Boehringer Ingelheim 1029
Atrovent Inhalation Aerosol (Ipratropium Bromide) Boehringer Ingelheim 1030
Atrovent Inhalation Solution (Ipratropium Bromide) Boehringer Ingelheim 1031
Brethine Ampuls (Terbutaline Sulfate) Novartis 2314
Brethine Tablets (Terbutaline Sulfate) Novartis 2313
Lufyllin Tablets (Dyphylline) Wallace 3347
Lufyllin-400 Tablets (Dyphylline) Wallace 3347
Lufyllin-GG Elixir (Dyphylline, Guaifenesin) Wallace 3348
Lufyllin-GG Tablets (Dyphylline, Guaifenesin) Wallace 3348
Maxair Inhaler (Pirbuterol Acetate) 3M 1984
Proventil Inhalation Aerosol (Albuterol) Schering 3142
Proventil Inhalation Solution 0.083% (Albuterol Sulfate) Schering 3146
Proventil Repetabs Tablets (Albuterol Sulfate) Schering 3148
Proventil Solution for Inhalation 0.5% (Albuterol Sulfate) Schering 3144
Proventil HFA Inhalation Aerosol (Albuterol Sulfate) Schering 3150
Serevent Inhalation Aerosol (Salmeterol Xinafoate) GlaxoSmithKline 1633
Theo-Dur Extended-Release Tablets (Theophylline) Key 1835
Uniphyl 400 mg and 600 mg Tablets (Theophylline) Purdue Frederick 2903
Ventolin Inhalation Aerosol and Refill (Albuterol) GlaxoSmithKline .. 1679
Ventolin HFA Inhalation Aerosol (Albuterol Sulfate) GlaxoSmithKline 3618
Volmax Extended-Release Tablets (Albuterol Sulfate) Muro 2276
Xopenex Inhalation Solution (Levalbuterol Hydrochloride) Sepracor .. 3207

Bronchospasm associated with chronic obstructive pulmonary disease
Alupent (Metaproterenol Sulfate) Boehringer Ingelheim 1029
Atrovent Inhalation Aerosol (Ipratropium Bromide) Boehringer Ingelheim 1030
Atrovent Inhalation Solution (Ipratropium Bromide) Boehringer Ingelheim 1031
Brethine Ampuls (Terbutaline Sulfate) Novartis 2314
Brethine Tablets (Terbutaline Sulfate) Novartis 2313
Lufyllin Tablets (Dyphylline) Wallace 3347
Lufyllin-400 Tablets (Dyphylline) Wallace 3347
Lufyllin-GG Elixir (Dyphylline, Guaifenesin) Wallace 3348
Lufyllin-GG Tablets (Dyphylline, Guaifenesin) Wallace 3348
Maxair Autohaler (Pirbuterol Acetate) 3M 1981
Serevent Inhalation Aerosol (Salmeterol Xinafoate) GlaxoSmithKline 1633
Uni-Dur Extended-Release Tablets (Theophylline) Key 1841
Uniphyl 400 mg and 600 mg Tablets (Theophylline) Purdue Frederick 2903

Brucella species infections
Streptomycin Sulfate Injection (Streptomycin Sulfate) Pfizer 2714

Brucella species infections, adjunct in
Declomycin Tablets (Demeclocycline Hydrochloride) Lederle 1855
Doryx Coated Pellet Filled Capsules (Doxycycline Hyclate) Warner Chilcott 3357
Dynacin Capsules (Minocycline Hydrochloride) Medicis 2019
Minocin Intravenous (Minocycline Hydrochloride) Lederle 1862
Minocin Oral Suspension (Minocycline Hydrochloride) Lederle 1865
Minocin Pellet-Filled Capsules (Minocycline Hydrochloride) Lederle 1863
Monodox Capsules (Doxycycline Monohydrate) Oclassen 2442
Vibramycin Calcium Oral Suspension Syrup (Doxycycline Calcium) Pfizer 2735
Vibramycin Hyclate Capsules (Doxycycline Hyclate) Pfizer 2735
Vibramycin Hyclate Intravenous (Doxycycline Hyclate) Pfizer 2737
Vibramycin Monohydrate for Oral Suspension (Doxycycline Monohydrate) Pfizer 2735
Vibra-Tabs Film Coated Tablets (Doxycycline Hyclate) Pfizer 2735

Brucellosis
Dynacin Capsules (Minocycline Hydrochloride) Medicis 2019
Minocin Oral Suspension (Minocycline Hydrochloride) Lederle 1865
Minocin Pellet-Filled Capsules (Minocycline Hydrochloride) Lederle 1863
Monodox Capsules (Doxycycline Monohydrate) Oclassen 2442

Bruises, topical relief of
(*see under* Pain, topical relief of)

Bubble boy disease
(*see under* Adenosine deaminase, enzyme replacement therapy for)

Bulbar conjunctiva inflammation
Blephamide Ophthalmic Suspension (Prednisolone Acetate, Sulfacetamide Sodium) Allergan 548
Cortisporin Ophthalmic Suspension (Hydrocortisone, Neomycin Sulfate, Polymyxin B Sulfate, Hydrocortisone, Neomycin Sulfate, Polymyxin B Sulfate) Monarch .... ⊙297
FML Ophthalmic Ointment (Fluorometholone) Allergan .... ⊙237
FML Ophthalmic Suspension (Fluorometholone) Allergan .... ⊙236
FML Forte Ophthalmic Suspension (Fluorometholone) Allergan .... ⊙235
FML-S Liquifilm Sterile Ophthalmic Suspension (Fluorometholone, Sulfacetamide Sodium) Allergan .. ⊙238
Lotemax Sterile Ophthalmic Suspension 0.5% (Loteprednol Etabonate) Bausch & Lomb .... ⊙261
Poly-Pred Liquifilm Ophthalmic Suspension (Neomycin Sulfate, Polymyxin B Sulfate, Prednisolone Acetate) Allergan .... ⊙245
Pred Forte Ophthalmic Suspension (Prednisolone Acetate) Allergan .... ⊙246
Pred-G Ophthalmic Suspension (Gentamicin Sulfate, Prednisolone Acetate) Allergan .... ⊙247
Pred-G Sterile Ophthalmic Ointment (Gentamicin Sulfate, Prednisolone Acetate) Allergan ... ⊙248
TobraDex Ophthalmic Ointment (Dexamethasone, Tobramycin) Alcon 542
TobraDex Ophthalmic Suspension (Dexamethasone, Tobramycin) Alcon 541

Bulimia nervosa
Prozac Pulvules, Liquid, and Weekly Capsules (Fluoxetine Hydrochloride) Dista 1238

Burn wound infections
(*see under* Infections, burn wound)

Burns, maintenance of electrolyte balance
Albumin (Human) 5% (Albumin (human)) Baxter Healthcare 838
Albumin (Human) 25% (Albumin (human)) Baxter Healthcare 839
Albuminar-5, U.S.P. (Albumin (human)) Aventis Behring 785
Albuminar-25, U.S.P. (Albumin (human)) Aventis Behring 786
Buminate 5% Solution, USP (Albumin (human)) Baxter Healthcare ... 841
Buminate 25% Solution, USP (Albumin (human)) Baxter Healthcare 842
Plasbumin-5 (Albumin (human)) Bayer Biological 939
Plasbumin-20 (Albumin (human)) Bayer Biological 940
Plasbumin-25 (Albumin (human)) Bayer Biological 941

Burns, minor
A + D Original Ointment (Lanolin, Petrolatum) Schering-Plough .... ▣733
Bactine First Aid Liquid (Benzalkonium Chloride, Lidocaine Hydrochloride) Bayer Consumer .... ▣611
Betadine Brand Plus First Aid Antibiotics & Pain Reliever Ointment (Bacitracin Zinc, Polymyxin B Sulfate, Pramoxine Hydrochloride) Purdue Frederick .. 2894
Betadine Ointment (Povidone Iodine) Purdue Frederick 2894
Betadine Solution (Povidone Iodine) Purdue Frederick 2895
Desitin Ointment (Cod Liver Oil, Zinc Oxide) Pfizer Inc., Warner-Lambert Healthcare .... ▣700
ELA-Max Cream (Lidocaine) Ferndale 1340
Polysporin Ointment (Bacitracin Zinc, Polymyxin B Sulfate) Pfizer Inc., Warner-Lambert Healthcare .... ▣706
Polysporin Powder (Bacitracin Zinc, Polymyxin B Sulfate) Pfizer Inc., Warner-Lambert Healthcare .... ▣706

Burns, pain associated with
(*see under* Pain, topical relief of)

Burns, second- and third-degree, adjunctive therapy in
Silvadene Cream 1% (Silver Sulfadiazine) Monarch 2267
Sulfamylon Topical Solution (Mafenide Acetate) Bertek 1011

Burns, to prevent hemoconcentration
Albumin (Human) 5% (Albumin (human)) Baxter Healthcare 838
Albumin (Human) 25% (Albumin (human)) Baxter Healthcare 839
Albuminar-5, U.S.P. (Albumin (human)) Aventis Behring 785
Albuminar-25, U.S.P. (Albumin (human)) Aventis Behring 786
Plasbumin-5 (Albumin (human)) Bayer Biological 939
Plasbumin-20 (Albumin (human)) Bayer Biological 940
Plasbumin-25 (Albumin (human)) Bayer Biological 941

Bursitis
Anaprox Tablets (Naproxen Sodium) Roche Laboratories 2967
Anaprox DS Tablets (Naproxen Sodium) Roche Laboratories 2967
Celestone Soluspan Injectable Suspension (Betamethasone Acetate, Betamethasone Sodium Phosphate) Schering 3097
Celestone Syrup (Betamethasone) Schering 3099
Cortone Acetate Injectable Suspension (Cortisone Acetate) Merck 2059
Cortone Acetate Tablets (Cortisone Acetate) Merck 2061
Decadron Elixir (Dexamethasone) Merck 2078
Decadron Tablets (Dexamethasone) Merck 2079
Decadron Phosphate Injection (Dexamethasone Sodium Phosphate) Merck 2081
Depo-Medrol Injectable Suspension (Methylprednisolone Acetate) Pharmacia & Upjohn 2795
Hydrocortone Tablets (Hydrocortisone) Merck 2106
Hydrocortone Acetate Injectable Suspension (Hydrocortisone Acetate) Merck 2103
Hydrocortone Phosphate Injection, Sterile (Hydrocortisone Sodium Phosphate) Merck 2105
Indocin (Indomethacin) Merck 2112
Naprelan Tablets (Naproxen Sodium) Elan 1293
Naprosyn Suspension (Naproxen) Roche Laboratories 2967
Naprosyn Tablets (Naproxen) Roche Laboratories 2967
Pediapred Oral Solution (Prednisolone Sodium Phosphate) Celltech 1170
Prednisone (Prednisone) Roxane 3064
Prelone Syrup (Prednisolone) Muro . 2273
Solu-Medrol Sterile Powder (Methylprednisolone Sodium Succinate) Pharmacia & Upjohn 2855
Traumeel Injection Solution (Homeopathic Formulations) Heel 1726

Bursitis, subacromial, acute, symptomatic relief of
Clinoril Tablets (Sulindac) Merck 2053
Indocin (Indomethacin) Merck 2112
Trilisate (Choline Magnesium Trisalicylate) Purdue Frederick 2901

C

C. difficile infection
(*see under* Colitis, pseudomembranous, antibiotic-associated)

C. diphtheriae infections
E.E.S. (Erythromycin Ethylsuccinate) Abbott 450
EryPed (Erythromycin Ethylsuccinate) Abbott 446
Ery-Tab Tablets (Erythromycin) Abbott 448
Erythrocin Stearate Filmtab Tablets (Erythromycin Stearate) Abbott 452
Erythromycin Base Filmtab Tablets (Erythromycin) Abbott 454
Erythromycin Delayed-Release Capsules, USP (Erythromycin) Abbott 455
PCE Dispertab Tablets (Erythromycin) Abbott 498
Pfizerpen for Injection (Penicillin G Potassium) Pfizer 2707

C. minutissimum infections
E.E.S. (Erythromycin Ethylsuccinate) Abbott 450
EryPed (Erythromycin Ethylsuccinate) Abbott 446
Ery-Tab Tablets (Erythromycin) Abbott 448
Erythrocin Stearate Filmtab Tablets (Erythromycin Stearate) Abbott 452
Erythromycin Base Filmtab Tablets (Erythromycin) Abbott 454
Erythromycin Delayed-Release Capsules, USP (Erythromycin) Abbott 455
PCE Dispertab Tablets (Erythromycin) Abbott 498

Cachexia associated with weight loss, AIDS-induced
Megace Oral Suspension (Megestrol Acetate) Bristol-Myers Squibb Oncology/Immunology 1124
Serostim for Injection (Somatropin) Serono 3229

Calcium deficiency
(*see under* Hypocalcemia)

Calluses
(*see under* Hyperkeratosis skin disorders)

Campylobacter fetus infections
Declomycin Tablets (Demeclocycline Hydrochloride) Lederle 1855
Doryx Coated Pellet Filled Capsules (Doxycycline Hyclate) Warner Chilcott 3357
Dynacin Capsules (Minocycline Hydrochloride) Medicis 2019
Minocin Intravenous (Minocycline Hydrochloride) Lederle 1862
Minocin Oral Suspension (Minocycline Hydrochloride) Lederle 1865
Minocin Pellet-Filled Capsules (Minocycline Hydrochloride) Lederle 1863
Monodox Capsules (Doxycycline Monohydrate) Oclassen 2442
Vibramycin Calcium Oral Suspension Syrup (Doxycycline Calcium) Pfizer 2735
Vibramycin Hyclate Capsules (Doxycycline Hyclate) Pfizer 2735
Vibramycin Hyclate Intravenous (Doxycycline Hyclate) Pfizer 2737
Vibramycin Monohydrate for Oral Suspension (Doxycycline Monohydrate) Pfizer 2735

Vibra-Tabs Film Coated Tablets (Doxycycline Hyclate) Pfizer 2735

Campylobacter jejuni infectious diarrhea
Cipro (Ciprofloxacin) Bayer............ 887

Cancer, prostatic
(*see under* Carcinoma, prostate, palliative treatment of)

Cancerous conditions, unspecified, adjunctive therapy in
Iscar Mali Injection (Homeopathic Formulations) Weleda 3456
Iscar Mali Special Injection (Homeopathic Formulations) Weleda 3456
Iscar Pini Injection (Homeopathic Formulations) Weleda 3456
Iscar Quercus Injection (Homeopathic Formulations) Weleda 3456
Iscar Quercus Special Injection (Homeopathic Formulations) Weleda 3456

Candida albicans infections
AVC (Sulfanilamide) Fielding 1350
Betadine Medicated Douche (Povidone Iodine) Purdue Frederick 2894
Gynazole-1 Vaginal Cream (Butoconazole Nitrate) Ther-Rx 3310
Loprox Cream (Ciclopirox Olamine) Medicis 2021
Loprox Gel (Ciclopirox) Medicis 2022
Loprox Lotion (Ciclopirox Olamine) Medicis 2021
Lotrimin (Clotrimazole) Schering 3128
Mycelex-7 Combination-Pack Vaginal Inserts & External Vulvar Cream (Clotrimazole) Bayer Consumer ....▣614
Mycelex-7 Vaginal Cream (Clotrimazole) Bayer Consumer ....▣614
Nystop Topical Powder USP (Nystatin) Paddock 2608

Candida infections, serious
Ancobon (Flucytosine) ICN 1730

Candidemia
Diflucan (Fluconazole) Pfizer 2681

Candidiasis, cutaneous
Loprox Cream (Ciclopirox Olamine) Medicis 2021
Loprox Gel (Ciclopirox) Medicis 2022
Loprox Lotion (Ciclopirox Olamine) Medicis 2021
Lotrimin (Clotrimazole) Schering 3128
Nizoral 2% Cream (Ketoconazole) Janssen 3620
Nystop Topical Powder USP (Nystatin) Paddock 2608

Candidiasis, disseminated
Diflucan (Fluconazole) Pfizer 2681

Candidiasis, esophageal
Sporanox Oral Solution (Itraconazole) Janssen 1808
Sporanox Oral Solution (Itraconazole) Ortho Biotech 2512

Candidiasis, mucocutaneous, chronic
Nizoral Tablets (Ketoconazole) Janssen 1791

Candidiasis, oropharyngeal
Diflucan Tablets, Injection, and Oral Suspension (Fluconazole) Pfizer 2681
Mycelex Troche (Clotrimazole) Alza 573
Nizoral Tablets (Ketoconazole) Janssen 1791
Sporanox Oral Solution (Itraconazole) Janssen 1808
Sporanox Oral Solution (Itraconazole) Ortho Biotech 2512

Candidiasis, systemic
Abelcet Injection (Amphotericin B) Elan 1273
AmBisome for Injection (Amphotericin B) Fujisawa 1383

Candidiasis, unspecified
Nizoral Tablets (Ketoconazole) Janssen 1791

Candidiasis, vaginal
Diflucan Tablets, Injection, and Oral Suspension (Fluconazole) Pfizer 2681
Gynazole-1 Vaginal Cream (Butoconazole Nitrate) Ther-Rx 3310
Gyne-Lotrimin 3, 3-Day Cream (Clotrimazole) Schering-Plough ...▣741
Mycelex-3 Vaginal Cream with 3 Disposable Applicators (Butoconazole Nitrate) Bayer Consumer.................................▣613
Mycelex-3 Vaginal Cream in 3 Pre-filled Applicators (Butoconazole Nitrate) Bayer Consumer ....▣613
Mycelex-7 Combination-Pack Vaginal Inserts & External Vulvar Cream (Clotrimazole) Bayer Consumer ....▣614
Mycelex-7 Vaginal Cream with 7 Disposable Applicators (Clotrimazole) Bayer Consumer ....▣614
Nystatin Vaginal Tablets, USP (Nystatin) Odyssey......................2445
Terazol 3 Vaginal Cream (Terconazole) Ortho-McNeil 2587
Terazol 3 Vaginal Suppositories (Terconazole) Ortho-McNeil 2587
Terazol 7 Vaginal Cream (Terconazole) Ortho-McNeil 2587

Candiduria
Nizoral Tablets (Ketoconazole) Janssen 1791

Canker sores
(*see under* Stomatitis, recurrent aphthous, symptomatic relief of)

Carbuncles
(*see under* Furunculosis, symptomatic relief of)

Carcinoma, bladder, transitional cell
Adriamycin PFS/RDF Injection (Doxorubicin Hydrochloride) Pharmacia & Upjohn 2767

Carcinoma, breast
Adriamycin PFS/RDF Injection (Doxorubicin Hydrochloride) Pharmacia & Upjohn 2767
Arimidex Tablets (Anastrozole) AstraZeneca 659
Aromasin Tablets (Exemestane) Pharmacia & Upjohn 2769
Ellence Injection (Epirubicin Hydrochloride) Pharmacia & Upjohn 2806
Fareston Tablets (Toremifene Citrate) Shire US 3237
Femara Tablets (Letrozole) Novartis 2351
Herceptin I.V. (Trastuzumab) Genentech 1414
Nolvadex Tablets (Tamoxifen Citrate) AstraZeneca 678
Taxol Injection (Paclitaxel) Bristol-Myers Squibb Oncology/Immunology 1129
Thioplex for Injection (Thiotepa) Immunex 1765
Xeloda Tablets (Capecitabine) Roche Laboratories 3039

Carcinoma, breast, metastatic, treatment of
Android Capsules, 10 mg (Methyltestosterone) ICN 1731
Delatestryl Injection (Testosterone Enanthate) BTG 1151
Fareston Tablets (Toremifene Citrate) Shire US 3237
Herceptin I.V. (Trastuzumab) Genentech 1414
Nolvadex Tablets (Tamoxifen Citrate) AstraZeneca 678
Taxol Injection (Paclitaxel) Bristol-Myers Squibb Oncology/Immunology 1129
Taxotere for Injection Concentrate (Docetaxel) Aventis 778
Xeloda Tablets (Capecitabine) Roche Laboratories 3039

Carcinoma, breast, osteolytic bone metastases of
Aredia for Injection (Pamidronate Disodium) Novartis 2309

Carcinoma, breast, palliative therapy in
Estinyl Tablets (Ethinyl Estradiol) Schering 3112
Estrace Tablets (Estradiol) Warner Chilcott 3361
Menest Tablets (Estrogens, Esterified) Monarch 2254
Premarin Tablets (Estrogens, Conjugated) Wyeth-Ayerst 3566
Testred Capsules, 10 mg (Methyltestosterone) ICN 1746
Zoladex (Goserelin Acetate) AstraZeneca 702

Carcinoma, breast, to reduce the incidence of
Nolvadex Tablets (Tamoxifen Citrate) AstraZeneca 678

Carcinoma, bronchogenic
Adriamycin PFS/RDF Injection (Doxorubicin Hydrochloride) Pharmacia & Upjohn 2767
Mustargen for Injection (Mechlorethamine Hydrochloride) Merck....2142

Carcinoma, colon, Dukes' stage C, adjunctive treatment in
Ergamisol Tablets (Levamisole Hydrochloride) Janssen...............1789

Carcinoma, esophageal, obstructing, palliative treatment of
Photofrin for Injection (Porfimer Sodium) Axcan Scandipharm 831

Carcinoma, gastric
Adriamycin PFS/RDF Injection (Doxorubicin Hydrochloride) Pharmacia & Upjohn 2767

Carcinoma, gastrointestinal, palliative management of
Sterile FUDR (Floxuridine) Roche Laboratories 2974

Carcinoma, lung, non-small cell
Gemzar for Injection (Gemcitabine Hydrochloride) Lilly 1919
Navelbine Injection (Vinorelbine Tartrate) GlaxoSmithKline 1604
Photofrin for Injection (Porfimer Sodium) Axcan Scandipharm 831
Taxol Injection (Paclitaxel) Bristol-Myers Squibb Oncology/Immunology 1129
Taxotere for Injection Concentrate (Docetaxel) Aventis 778

Carcinoma, lung, small cell
Hycamtin for Injection (Topotecan Hydrochloride) GlaxoSmithKline 1546

Carcinoma, metastatic, palliative treatment of
Mustargen for Injection (Mechlorethamine Hydrochloride) Merck 2142

Carcinoma, ovary
Adriamycin PFS/RDF Injection (Doxorubicin Hydrochloride) Pharmacia & Upjohn 2767
Alkeran Tablets (Melphalan) GlaxoSmithKline 1466
Doxil Injection (Doxorubicin Hydrochloride) Alza 566
Hexalen Capsules (Altretamine) MGI 2226
Hycamtin for Injection (Topotecan Hydrochloride) GlaxoSmithKline ...1546
Mylocel Tablets (Hydroxyurea) MGI ..2227
Paraplatin for Injection (Carboplatin) Bristol-Myers Squibb Oncology/Immunology 1126
Taxol Injection (Paclitaxel) Bristol-Myers Squibb Oncology/Immunology 1129
Thioplex for Injection (Thiotepa) Immunex 1765

Carcinoma, pancreas
Gemzar for Injection (Gemcitabine Hydrochloride) Lilly 1919

Carcinoma, prostate
Eulexin Capsules (Flutamide) Schering 3118

Carcinoma, prostate, adjunctive therapy in
Casodex Tablets (Bicalutamide) AstraZeneca 662
Eulexin Capsules (Flutamide) Schering 3118
Nilandron Tablets (Nilutamide) Aventis 753
Novantrone for Injection (Mitoxantrone Hydrochloride) Immunex ..1760
Zoladex (Goserelin Acetate) AstraZeneca 702
Zoladex 3-month (Goserelin Acetate) AstraZeneca 706

Carcinoma, prostate, palliative treatment of
Emcyt Capsules (Estramustine Phosphate Sodium) Pharmacia & Upjohn 2810
Estinyl Tablets (Ethinyl Estradiol) Schering 3112
Estrace Tablets (Estradiol) Warner Chilcott 3361
Lupron Depot 7.5 mg (Leuprolide Acetate) TAP 3284
Lupron Depot–3 Month 22.5 mg (Leuprolide Acetate) TAP 3288
Lupron Depot–4 Month 30 mg (Leuprolide Acetate) TAP............. 3289
Lupron Injection (Leuprolide Acetate) TAP 3279
Menest Tablets (Estrogens, Esterified) Monarch 2254
Premarin Tablets (Estrogens, Conjugated) Wyeth-Ayerst 3566
Viadur Implant (Leuprolide Acetate) Bayer 912
Zoladex (Goserelin Acetate) AstraZeneca 702
Zoladex 3-month (Goserelin Acetate) AstraZeneca 706

Carcinoma, renal cell, metastatic, in adults
Proleukin for Injection (Aldesleukin) Chiron 1199

Carcinoma, superficial basal cell
Efudex (Fluorouracil) ICN................ 1733

Carcinoma, testicular, germ cell
Ifex for Injection (Ifosfamide) Bristol-Myers Squibb Oncology/Immunology 1123

Carcinoma, testis, advanced
Cosmegen for Injection (Dactinomycin) Merck 2062
Mithracin for Intravenous Use (Plicamycin) Bayer 903

Carcinoma, thyroid
Adriamycin PFS/RDF Injection (Doxorubicin Hydrochloride) Pharmacia & Upjohn 2767
Cytomel Tablets (Liothyronine Sodium) Jones 1817
Levothroid Tablets (Levothyroxine Sodium) Forest 1373
Levoxyl Tablets (Levothyroxine Sodium) Jones 1819
Synthroid (Levothyroxine Sodium) Abbott 505
Unithroid Tablets (Levothyroxine Sodium) Watson 3445

Carcinoma, thyroid, adjunctive diagnostic tool for serum thyroglobulin testing
Thyrogen for Injection (Thyrotropin alfa) Genzyme 1441

Carcinoma, urinary bladder, *in-situ*
TheraCys Injection (BCG, Live (Intravesical)) Aventis Pasteur 823
Tice BCG, BCG Live (BCG Vaccine) Organon 2489
Valstar Sterile Solution for Intravesical Instillation (Valrubicin) Celltech 1175

Carcinoma, urinary bladder, superficial papillary
Thioplex for Injection (Thiotepa) Immunex 1765

Cardiac arrhythmias
(*see under* Arrhythmias)

Cardiac decompensation
Dobutrex Solution Vials (Dobutamine Hydrochloride) Lilly 1914

Cardiac failure
(*see under* Congestive heart failure, adjunct in)

Cardiac ischemic complications, acute, prevention of, adjunct to PTCA
ReoPro Vials (Abciximab) Lilly 1958

Cardiomyopathy, doxorubicin-induced, to reduce the incidence and severity of
Zinecard for Injection (Dexrazoxane) Pharmacia & Upjohn 2869

Cardiopulmonary bypass surgery, adjunct in
Albumin (Human) 25% (Albumin (human)) Baxter Healthcare 839
Buminate 5% Solution, USP (Albumin (human)) Baxter Healthcare ... 841
Buminate 25% Solution, USP (Albumin (human)) Baxter Healthcare 842
Plasbumin-5 (Albumin (human)) Bayer Biological 939
Plasbumin-20 (Albumin (human)) Bayer Biological 940
Plasbumin-25 (Albumin (human)) Bayer Biological 941

Carnitine, deficiency of
Carnitor Injection (Levocarnitine) Sigma-Tau ... 3242
Carnitor Tablets and Oral Solution (Levocarnitine) Sigma-Tau ... 3245

Catabolic or tissue depleting processes, adjunctive therapy
Oxandrin Tablets (Oxandrolone) BTG ... 1153

Cataract extraction, surgical aid in
Amvisc Plus (Sodium Hyaluronate) Bausch & Lomb Surgical ... ⊙ 329
Healon (Sodium Hyaluronate) Pharmacia & Upjohn ... ⊙ 316
Healon GV (Sodium Hyaluronate) Pharmacia & Upjohn ... ⊙ 320
Ocucoat (Hydroxypropyl Methylcellulose) Bausch & Lomb Surgical ... ⊙ 330

Cellulitis, pelvic
(*see under* Pelvic cellulitis)

Central cranial diabetes insipidus
(*see under* Diabetes insipidus)

Central nervous system depression, drug-induced
Dopram Injectable (Doxapram Hydrochloride) Robins ... 2931

Cephalalgia, histaminic
Imitrex Injection (Sumatriptan Succinate) GlaxoSmithKline ... 1549

Cerebral edema
(*see under* Edema, cerebral)

Cerumen, removal of
Auralgan Otic Solution (Antipyrine, Benzocaine, Glycerin) Wyeth-Ayerst ... 3485
Cerumenex Eardrops (Triethanolamine Polypeptide Oleate-Condensate) Purdue Frederick ... 2895
Debrox Drops (Carbamide Peroxide) SmithKline Beecham Consumer ... ▣ 747

Cervicitis
Zithromax (Azithromycin Dihydrate) Pfizer ... 2743
Zithromax for Oral Suspension, 300 mg, 600 mg, 900 mg, 1200 mg (Azithromycin Dihydrate) Pfizer ... 2739
Zithromax Tablets, 250 mg (Azithromycin Dihydrate) Pfizer ... 2739
Zithromax Tablets, 600 mg (Azithromycin Dihydrate) Pfizer ... 2743

Cervicitis, mild, adjunct
Amino-Cerv (L-Cystine, Inositol, Methionine, Sodium Propionate, Urea) Milex ... 2231

Cervix, ripening of, in pregnant women at or near term
Cervidil Vaginal Insert (Dinoprostone) Forest ... 1369
Prepidil Gel (Dinoprostone) Pharmacia & Upjohn ... 2851

Chancroid
Declomycin Tablets (Demeclocycline Hydrochloride) Lederle ... 1855
Doryx Coated Pellet Filled Capsules (Doxycycline Hyclate) Warner Chilcott ... 3357
Dynacin Capsules (Minocycline Hydrochloride) Medicis ... 2019
Minocin Intravenous (Minocycline Hydrochloride) Lederle ... 1862
Minocin Oral Suspension (Minocycline Hydrochloride) Lederle ... 1865
Minocin Pellet-Filled Capsules (Minocycline Hydrochloride) Lederle ... 1863
Monodox Capsules (Doxycycline Monohydrate) Oclassen ... 2442
Vibramycin Calcium Oral Suspension Syrup (Doxycycline Calcium) Pfizer ... 2735
Vibramycin Hyclate Capsules (Doxycycline Hyclate) Pfizer ... 2735
Vibramycin Hyclate Intravenous (Doxycycline Hyclate) Pfizer ... 2737
Vibramycin Monohydrate for Oral Suspension (Doxycycline Monohydrate) Pfizer ... 2735
Vibra-Tabs Film Coated Tablets (Doxycycline Hyclate) Pfizer ... 2735
Zithromax Capsules, 250 mg (Azithromycin Dihydrate) Pfizer ... 2743
Zithromax for Oral Suspension, 300 mg, 600 mg, 900 mg, 1200 mg (Azithromycin Dihydrate) Pfizer ... 2739
Zithromax Tablets, 250 mg (Azithromycin Dihydrate) Pfizer ... 2739

Chickenpox
(*see under* Varicella, acute, treatment of)

Chlamydia pneumoniae infections
Avelox Tablets (Moxifloxacin Hydrochloride) Bayer ... 879
Biaxin/Biaxin XL (Clarithromycin) Abbott ... 403
Levaquin (Levofloxacin) Ortho-McNeil ... 2537
Tequin Injection (Gatifloxacin) Bristol-Myers Squibb ... 1110
Tequin Tablets (Gatifloxacin) Bristol-Myers Squibb ... 1110
Trovan (Alatrofloxacin Mesylate) Pfizer ... 2722
Zithromax Capsules, 250 mg (Azithromycin Dihydrate) Pfizer ... 2743
Zithromax for IV Infusion (Azithromycin Dihydrate) Pfizer ... 2748
Zithromax for Oral Suspension, 300 mg, 600 mg, 900 mg, 1200 mg (Azithromycin Dihydrate) Pfizer ... 2739
Zithromax Tablets, 250 mg (Azithromycin Dihydrate) Pfizer ... 2739

Chlamydia pneumoniae lower respiratory tract infections
Avelox Tablets (Moxifloxacin Hydrochloride) Bayer ... 879
Biaxin/Biaxin XL (Clarithromycin) Abbott ... 403
Levaquin (Levofloxacin) Ortho-McNeil ... 2537
Tequin Injection (Gatifloxacin) Bristol-Myers Squibb ... 1110
Tequin Tablets (Gatifloxacin) Bristol-Myers Squibb ... 1110
Trovan (Alatrofloxacin Mesylate) Pfizer ... 2722
Zithromax Capsules, 250 mg (Azithromycin Dihydrate) Pfizer ... 2743
Zithromax for IV Infusion (Azithromycin Dihydrate) Pfizer ... 2748
Zithromax for Oral Suspension, 300 mg, 600 mg, 900 mg, 1200 mg (Azithromycin Dihydrate) Pfizer ... 2739
Zithromax Tablets, 250 mg (Azithromycin Dihydrate) Pfizer ... 2739

Chlamydia psittaci infection
Declomycin Tablets (Demeclocycline Hydrochloride) Lederle ... 1855
Doryx Coated Pellet Filled Capsules (Doxycycline Hyclate) Warner Chilcott ... 3357
Dynacin Capsules (Minocycline Hydrochloride) Medicis ... 2019
Minocin Intravenous (Minocycline Hydrochloride) Lederle ... 1862
Minocin Oral Suspension (Minocycline Hydrochloride) Lederle ... 1865
Minocin Pellet-Filled Capsules (Minocycline Hydrochloride) Lederle ... 1863
Monodox Capsules (Doxycycline Monohydrate) Oclassen ... 2442
Vibramycin Calcium Oral Suspension Syrup (Doxycycline Calcium) Pfizer ... 2735
Vibramycin Hyclate Capsules (Doxycycline Hyclate) Pfizer ... 2735
Vibramycin Hyclate Intravenous (Doxycycline Hyclate) Pfizer ... 2737
Vibramycin Monohydrate for Oral Suspension (Doxycycline Monohydrate) Pfizer ... 2735
Vibra-Tabs Film Coated Tablets (Doxycycline Hyclate) Pfizer ... 2735

Chlamydia trachomatis conjunctivitis of the newborn
E.E.S. (Erythromycin Ethylsuccinate) Abbott ... 450
EryPed (Erythromycin Ethylsuccinate) Abbott ... 446
Ery-Tab Tablets (Erythromycin) Abbott ... 448
Erythrocin Stearate Filmtab Tablets (Erythromycin Stearate) Abbott ... 452
Erythromycin Base Filmtab Tablets (Erythromycin) Abbott ... 454
Erythromycin Delayed-Release Capsules, USP (Erythromycin) Abbott ... 455
Monodox Capsules (Doxycycline Monohydrate) Oclassen ... 2442
PCE Dispertab Tablets (Erythromycin) Abbott ... 498

Chlamydia trachomatis endocervical infections
Doryx Coated Pellet Filled Capsules (Doxycycline Hyclate) Warner Chilcott ... 3357
E.E.S. (Erythromycin Ethylsuccinate) Abbott ... 450
EryPed (Erythromycin Ethylsuccinate) Abbott ... 446
Ery-Tab Tablets (Erythromycin) Abbott ... 448
Erythrocin Stearate Filmtab Tablets (Erythromycin Stearate) Abbott ... 452
Erythromycin Base Filmtab Tablets (Erythromycin) Abbott ... 454
Erythromycin Delayed-Release Capsules, USP (Erythromycin) Abbott ... 455
Minocin Oral Suspension (Minocycline Hydrochloride) Lederle ... 1865
Monodox Capsules (Doxycycline Monohydrate) Oclassen ... 2442
PCE Dispertab Tablets (Erythromycin) Abbott ... 498
Vibramycin Calcium Oral Suspension Syrup (Doxycycline Calcium) Pfizer ... 2735
Vibramycin Hyclate Capsules (Doxycycline Hyclate) Pfizer ... 2735
Vibramycin Monohydrate for Oral Suspension (Doxycycline Monohydrate) Pfizer ... 2735
Vibra-Tabs Film Coated Tablets (Doxycycline Hyclate) Pfizer ... 2735

Chlamydia trachomatis gynecologic infections
Floxin I.V. (Ofloxacin) Ortho-McNeil ... 2526
Floxin Tablets (Ofloxacin) Ortho-McNeil ... 2529

Chlamydia trachomatis infections
Doryx Coated Pellet Filled Capsules (Doxycycline Hyclate) Warner Chilcott ... 3357
Dynacin Capsules (Minocycline Hydrochloride) Medicis ... 2019
E.E.S. (Erythromycin Ethylsuccinate) Abbott ... 450
EryPed (Erythromycin Ethylsuccinate) Abbott ... 446
Ery-Tab Tablets (Erythromycin) Abbott ... 448
Erythrocin Stearate Filmtab Tablets (Erythromycin Stearate) Abbott ... 452
Erythromycin Base Filmtab Tablets (Erythromycin) Abbott ... 454
Erythromycin Delayed-Release Capsules, USP (Erythromycin) Abbott ... 455
Floxin I.V. (Ofloxacin) Ortho-McNeil ... 2526
Floxin Tablets (Ofloxacin) Ortho-McNeil ... 2529
Minocin Oral Suspension (Minocycline Hydrochloride) Lederle ... 1865
Minocin Pellet-Filled Capsules (Minocycline Hydrochloride) Lederle ... 1863
Monodox Capsules (Doxycycline Monohydrate) Oclassen ... 2442
PCE Dispertab Tablets (Erythromycin) Abbott ... 498
Vibramycin Calcium Oral Suspension Syrup (Doxycycline Calcium) Pfizer ... 2735
Vibramycin Hyclate Capsules (Doxycycline Hyclate) Pfizer ... 2735
Vibramycin Monohydrate for Oral Suspension (Doxycycline Monohydrate) Pfizer ... 2735
Vibra-Tabs Film Coated Tablets (Doxycycline Hyclate) Pfizer ... 2735
Zithromax Capsules, 250 mg (Azithromycin Dihydrate) Pfizer ... 2743
Zithromax for IV Infusion (Azithromycin Dihydrate) Pfizer ... 2748
Zithromax for Oral Suspension, 1 g (Azithromycin Dihydrate) Pfizer ... 2743
Zithromax for Oral Suspension, 300 mg, 600 mg, 900 mg, 1200 mg (Azithromycin Dihydrate) Pfizer ... 2739
Zithromax Tablets, 250 mg (Azithromycin Dihydrate) Pfizer ... 2739
Zithromax Tablets, 600 mg (Azithromycin Dihydrate) Pfizer ... 2743

Chlamydia trachomatis infections, ocular
(*see under* Trachoma)

Chlamydia trachomatis nongonococcal cervicitis
Floxin I.V. (Ofloxacin) Ortho-McNeil ... 2526
Floxin Tablets (Ofloxacin) Ortho-McNeil ... 2529
Zithromax (Azithromycin Dihydrate) Pfizer ... 2743
Zithromax for Oral Suspension, 300 mg, 600 mg, 900 mg, 1200 mg (Azithromycin Dihydrate) Pfizer ... 2739
Zithromax Tablets, 250 mg (Azithromycin Dihydrate) Pfizer ... 2739
Zithromax Tablets, 600 mg (Azithromycin Dihydrate) Pfizer ... 2743

Chlamydia trachomatis nongonococcal urethritis
Dynacin Capsules (Minocycline Hydrochloride) Medicis ... 2019
Floxin I.V. (Ofloxacin) Ortho-McNeil ... 2526
Floxin Tablets (Ofloxacin) Ortho-McNeil ... 2529
Minocin Oral Suspension (Minocycline Hydrochloride) Lederle ... 1865
Minocin Pellet-Filled Capsules (Minocycline Hydrochloride) Lederle ... 1863
Zithromax (Azithromycin Dihydrate) Pfizer ... 2743
Zithromax for Oral Suspension, 300 mg, 600 mg, 900 mg, 1200 mg (Azithromycin Dihydrate) Pfizer ... 2739
Zithromax Tablets, 250 mg (Azithromycin Dihydrate) Pfizer ... 2739
Zithromax Tablets, 600 mg (Azithromycin Dihydrate) Pfizer ... 2743

Chlamydia trachomatis pneumonia of infancy
E.E.S. (Erythromycin Ethylsuccinate) Abbott ... 450
EryPed (Erythromycin Ethylsuccinate) Abbott ... 446
Ery-Tab Tablets (Erythromycin) Abbott ... 448
Erythrocin Stearate Filmtab Tablets (Erythromycin Stearate) Abbott ... 452
Erythromycin Base Filmtab Tablets (Erythromycin) Abbott ... 454
Erythromycin Delayed-Release Capsules, USP (Erythromycin) Abbott ... 455
PCE Dispertab Tablets (Erythromycin) Abbott ... 498

Chlamydia trachomatis rectal infections
Doryx Coated Pellet Filled Capsules (Doxycycline Hyclate) Warner Chilcott ... 3357
E.E.S. (Erythromycin Ethylsuccinate) Abbott ... 450
EryPed (Erythromycin Ethylsuccinate) Abbott ... 446
Ery-Tab Tablets (Erythromycin) Abbott ... 448
Erythrocin Stearate Filmtab Tablets (Erythromycin Stearate) Abbott ... 452
Erythromycin Base Filmtab Tablets (Erythromycin) Abbott ... 454
Erythromycin Delayed-Release Capsules, USP (Erythromycin) Abbott ... 455
Minocin Oral Suspension (Minocycline Hydrochloride) Lederle ... 1865
Monodox Capsules (Doxycycline Monohydrate) Oclassen ... 2442
PCE Dispertab Tablets (Erythromycin) Abbott ... 498
Vibramycin Calcium Oral Suspension Syrup (Doxycycline Calcium) Pfizer ... 2735
Vibramycin Hyclate Capsules (Doxycycline Hyclate) Pfizer ... 2735
Vibramycin Monohydrate for Oral Suspension (Doxycycline Monohydrate) Pfizer ... 2735
Vibra-Tabs Film Coated Tablets (Doxycycline Hyclate) Pfizer ... 2735

Chlamydia trachomatis urethral infections
Doryx Coated Pellet Filled Capsules (Doxycycline Hyclate) Warner Chilcott ... 3357
E.E.S. (Erythromycin Ethylsuccinate) Abbott ... 450
EryPed (Erythromycin Ethylsuccinate) Abbott ... 446
Ery-Tab Tablets (Erythromycin) Abbott ... 448
Erythrocin Stearate Filmtab Tablets (Erythromycin Stearate) Abbott ... 452
Erythromycin Base Filmtab Tablets (Erythromycin) Abbott ... 454
Erythromycin Delayed-Release Capsules, USP (Erythromycin) Abbott ... 455

Monodox Capsules (Doxycycline Monohydrate) Oclassen ... 2442
PCE Dispertab Tablets (Erythromycin) Abbott ... 498
Vibramycin Calcium Oral Suspension Syrup (Doxycycline Calcium) Pfizer ... 2735
Vibramycin Hyclate Capsules (Doxycycline Hyclate) Pfizer ... 2735
Vibramycin Monohydrate for Oral Suspension (Doxycycline Monohydrate) Pfizer ... 2735
Vibra-Tabs Film Coated Tablets (Doxycycline Hyclate) Pfizer ... 2735

Chlamydia trachomatis urogenital infections during pregnancy
E.E.S. (Erythromycin Ethylsuccinate) Abbott ... 450
EryPed (Erythromycin Ethylsuccinate) Abbott ... 446
Ery-Tab Tablets (Erythromycin) Abbott ... 448
Erythrocin Stearate Filmtab Tablets (Erythromycin Stearate) Abbott ... 452
Erythromycin Base Filmtab Tablets (Erythromycin) Abbott ... 454
Erythromycin Delayed-Release Capsules, USP (Erythromycin) Abbott ... 455
PCE Dispertab Tablets (Erythromycin) Abbott ... 498

Chloasma
(*see under* Hyperpigmentation, skin, bleaching of)

Cholangitis
(*see under* Infections, intra-abdominal)

Cholecystitis, acute
(*see under* Infections, intra-abdominal)

Cholera
Doryx Coated Pellet Filled Capsules (Doxycycline Hyclate) Warner Chilcott ... 3357
Dynacin Capsules (Minocycline Hydrochloride) Medicis ... 2019
Minocin Oral Suspension (Minocycline Hydrochloride) Lederle ... 1865
Minocin Pellet-Filled Capsules (Minocycline Hydrochloride) Lederle ... 1863
Monodox Capsules (Doxycycline Monohydrate) Oclassen ... 2442
Vibramycin Hyclate Capsules (Doxycycline Hyclate) Pfizer ... 2735

Cholesterol levels, elevated
(*see under* Hypercholesterolemia, primary, adjunct to diet)

Chorea, prophylaxis of
Bicillin L-A Injection (Penicillin G Benzathine) Monarch ... 2242
Permapen Isoject (Penicillin G Benzathine) Pfizer ... 2706

Chorioretinitis
Celestone Soluspan Injectable Suspension (Betamethasone Acetate, Betamethasone Sodium Phosphate) Schering ... 3097
Celestone Syrup (Betamethasone) Schering ... 3099
Cortone Acetate Injectable Suspension (Cortisone Acetate) Merck ... 2059
Cortone Acetate Tablets (Cortisone Acetate) Merck ... 2061
Decadron Elixir (Dexamethasone) Merck ... 2078
Decadron Tablets (Dexamethasone) Merck ... 2079
Decadron Phosphate Injection (Dexamethasone Sodium Phosphate) Merck ... 2081
Depo-Medrol Injectable Suspension (Methylprednisolone Acetate) Pharmacia & Upjohn ... 2795
Hydrocortone Tablets (Hydrocortisone) Merck ... 2106
Hydrocortone Phosphate Injection, Sterile (Hydrocortisone Sodium Phosphate) Merck ... 2105
Pediapred Oral Solution (Prednisolone Sodium Phosphate) Celltech ... 1170
Prednisone (Prednisone) Roxane ... 3064
Prelone Syrup (Prednisolone) Muro ... 2273
Solu-Medrol Sterile Powder (Methylprednisolone Sodium Succinate) Pharmacia & Upjohn ... 2855

Choroiditis
Celestone Soluspan Injectable Suspension (Betamethasone Acetate, Betamethasone Sodium Phosphate) Schering ... 3097
Celestone Syrup (Betamethasone) Schering ... 3099
Cortone Acetate Injectable Suspension (Cortisone Acetate) Merck ... 2059
Cortone Acetate Tablets (Cortisone Acetate) Merck ... 2061
Decadron Elixir (Dexamethasone) Merck ... 2078
Decadron Tablets (Dexamethasone) Merck ... 2079
Decadron Phosphate Injection (Dexamethasone Sodium Phosphate) Merck ... 2081
Depo-Medrol Injectable Suspension (Methylprednisolone Acetate) Pharmacia & Upjohn ... 2795
Hydrocortone Tablets (Hydrocortisone) Merck ... 2106
Hydrocortone Phosphate Injection, Sterile (Hydrocortisone Sodium Phosphate) Merck ... 2105
Pediapred Oral Solution (Prednisolone Sodium Phosphate) Celltech ... 1170
Prednisone (Prednisone) Roxane ... 3064
Prelone Syrup (Prednisolone) Muro ... 2273
Solu-Medrol Sterile Powder (Methylprednisolone Sodium Succinate) Pharmacia & Upjohn ... 2855

Christmas disease
(*see under* Hemophilia B)

Chromomycosis
Nizoral Tablets (Ketoconazole) Janssen ... 1791

Cirrhosis, biliary
Urso Tablets (Ursodiol) Axcan Scandipharm ... 836

Citrobacter diversus infections
Cipro I.V. (Ciprofloxacin) Bayer ... 893
Cipro I.V. Pharmacy Bulk Package (Ciprofloxacin) Bayer ... 897
Cipro (Ciprofloxacin) Bayer ... 887
Floxin I.V. (Ofloxacin) Ortho-McNeil ... 2526
Floxin Tablets (Ofloxacin) Ortho-McNeil ... 2529

Citrobacter diversus urinary tract infections
Cipro I.V. (Ciprofloxacin) Bayer ... 893
Cipro I.V. Pharmacy Bulk Package (Ciprofloxacin) Bayer ... 897
Cipro (Ciprofloxacin) Bayer ... 887
Floxin I.V. (Ofloxacin) Ortho-McNeil ... 2526
Floxin Tablets (Ofloxacin) Ortho-McNeil ... 2529

Citrobacter freundii infections
Azactam for Injection (Aztreonam) Elan ... 1276
Cipro I.V. (Ciprofloxacin) Bayer ... 893
Cipro I.V. Pharmacy Bulk Package (Ciprofloxacin) Bayer ... 897
Cipro (Ciprofloxacin) Bayer ... 887
Claforan Injection (Cefotaxime Sodium) Aventis ... 732
Noroxin Tablets (Norfloxacin) Merck ... 2145

Citrobacter freundii intra-abdominal infections
Azactam for Injection (Aztreonam) Elan ... 1276

Citrobacter freundii skin and skin structure infections
Cipro I.V. (Ciprofloxacin) Bayer ... 893
Cipro I.V. Pharmacy Bulk Package (Ciprofloxacin) Bayer ... 897
Cipro (Ciprofloxacin) Bayer ... 887
Claforan Injection (Cefotaxime Sodium) Aventis ... 732

Citrobacter freundii urinary tract infections
Cipro I.V. (Ciprofloxacin) Bayer ... 893
Cipro I.V. Pharmacy Bulk Package (Ciprofloxacin) Bayer ... 897
Cipro (Ciprofloxacin) Bayer ... 887
Noroxin Tablets (Norfloxacin) Merck ... 2145

Citrobacter species infections
Azactam for Injection (Aztreonam) Elan ... 1276
Ceptaz for Injection (Ceftazidime) GlaxoSmithKline ... 1499
Claforan Injection (Cefotaxime Sodium) Aventis ... 732
Fortaz (Ceftazidime Sodium) GlaxoSmithKline ... 1541
Nebcin Vials, Hyporets & ADD-Vantage (Tobramycin Sulfate) Lilly ... 1955
Primaxin I.M. (Cilastatin Sodium, Imipenem) Merck ... 2158
Primaxin I.V. (Cilastatin Sodium, Imipenem) Merck ... 2160
Tazicef for Injection (Ceftazidime) GlaxoSmithKline ... 1647
Tazicef Galaxy Container (Ceftazidime Sodium) GlaxoSmithKline ... 1650
Tazicef Pharmacy Bulk Package (Ceftazidime) GlaxoSmithKline ... 1653
Tazidime Vials, Faspak & ADD-Vantage (Ceftazidime) Lilly ... 1966
Timentin Injection- ADD-Vantage Vial (Clavulanate Potassium, Ticarcillin Disodium) GlaxoSmithKline ... 1661
Timentin Injection-Galaxy Container (Clavulanate Potassium, Ticarcillin Disodium) GlaxoSmithKline ... 1664
Timentin Injection-Pharmacy Bulk Package (Clavulanate Potassium, Ticarcillin Disodium) GlaxoSmithKline ... 1666
Timentin for Intravenous Administration (Clavulanate Potassium, Ticarcillin Disodium) GlaxoSmithKline ... 1658

Citrobacter species intra-abdominal infections
Azactam for Injection (Aztreonam) Elan ... 1276
Primaxin I.V. (Cilastatin Sodium, Imipenem) Merck ... 2160

Citrobacter species lower respiratory tract infections
Ceptaz for Injection (Ceftazidime) GlaxoSmithKline ... 1499
Fortaz (Ceftazidime Sodium) GlaxoSmithKline ... 1541
Tazicef for Injection (Ceftazidime) GlaxoSmithKline ... 1647
Tazicef Galaxy Container (Ceftazidime Sodium) GlaxoSmithKline ... 1650
Tazicef Pharmacy Bulk Package (Ceftazidime) GlaxoSmithKline ... 1653
Tazidime Vials, Faspak & ADD-Vantage (Ceftazidime) Lilly ... 1966

Citrobacter species skin and skin structure infections
Azactam for Injection (Aztreonam) Elan ... 1276
Claforan Injection (Cefotaxime Sodium) Aventis ... 732
Primaxin I.M. (Cilastatin Sodium, Imipenem) Merck ... 2158
Primaxin I.V. (Cilastatin Sodium, Imipenem) Merck ... 2160

Citrobacter species urinary tract infections
Azactam for Injection (Aztreonam) Elan ... 1276
Claforan Injection (Cefotaxime Sodium) Aventis ... 732
Nebcin Vials, Hyporets & ADD-Vantage (Tobramycin Sulfate) Lilly ... 1955
Timentin Injection- ADD-Vantage Vial (Clavulanate Potassium, Ticarcillin Disodium) GlaxoSmithKline ... 1661
Timentin Injection-Galaxy Container (Clavulanate Potassium, Ticarcillin Disodium) GlaxoSmithKline ... 1664
Timentin Injection-Pharmacy Bulk Package (Clavulanate Potassium, Ticarcillin Disodium) GlaxoSmithKline ... 1666
Timentin for Intravenous Administration (Clavulanate Potassium, Ticarcillin Disodium) GlaxoSmithKline ... 1658

Claudication, intermittent
Pletal Tablets (Cilostazol) Otsuka America ... 2605
Pletal Tablets (Cilostazol) Pharmacia & Upjohn ... 2848
Trental Tablets (Pentoxifylline) Aventis ... 784

Clonorchiasis
Biltricide (Praziquantel) Bayer ... 887

Clostridium species gynecologic infections
Cefobid Intravenous/Intramuscular (Cefoperazone) Pfizer ... 2671
Cefobid Pharmacy Bulk Package - Not for Direct Infusion (Cefoperazone Sodium) Pfizer ... 2673
Claforan Injection (Cefotaxime Sodium) Aventis ... 732
Mefoxin for Injection (Cefoxitin Sodium) Merck ... 2124
Mefoxin Premixed Intravenous Solution (Cefoxitin Sodium) Merck ... 2127

Clostridium species infections
Cefobid Intravenous/Intramuscular (Cefoperazone) Pfizer ... 2671
Cefobid Pharmacy Bulk Package - Not for Direct Infusion (Cefoperazone Sodium) Pfizer ... 2673
Cefotan (Cefotetan) AstraZeneca ... 664
Claforan Injection (Cefotaxime Sodium) Aventis ... 732
Declomycin Tablets (Demeclocycline Hydrochloride) Lederle ... 1855
Doryx Coated Pellet Filled Capsules (Doxycycline Hyclate) Warner Chilcott ... 3357
Dynacin Capsules (Minocycline Hydrochloride) Medicis ... 2019
Mefoxin for Injection (Cefoxitin Sodium) Merck ... 2124
Mefoxin Premixed Intravenous Solution (Cefoxitin Sodium) Merck ... 2127
Minocin Intravenous (Minocycline Hydrochloride) Lederle ... 1862
Minocin Oral Suspension (Minocycline Hydrochloride) Lederle ... 1865
Minocin Pellet-Filled Capsules (Minocycline Hydrochloride) Lederle ... 1863
Monodox Capsules (Doxycycline Monohydrate) Oclassen ... 2442
Pfizerpen for Injection (Penicillin G Potassium) Pfizer ... 2707
Pipracil (Piperacillin Sodium) Lederle ... 1866
Primaxin I.V. (Cilastatin Sodium, Imipenem) Merck ... 2160
Rocephin Injectable Vials, ADD-Vantage, Galaxy, Bulk (Ceftriaxone Sodium) Roche Laboratories ... 2993
Vibramycin Calcium Oral Suspension Syrup (Doxycycline Calcium) Pfizer ... 2735
Vibramycin Hyclate Capsules (Doxycycline Hyclate) Pfizer ... 2735
Vibramycin Hyclate Intravenous (Doxycycline Hyclate) Pfizer ... 2737
Vibramycin Monohydrate for Oral Suspension (Doxycycline Monohydrate) Pfizer ... 2735
Vibra-Tabs Film Coated Tablets (Doxycycline Hyclate) Pfizer ... 2735

Clostridium species intra-abdominal infections
Cefotan (Cefotetan) AstraZeneca ... 664
Claforan Injection (Cefotaxime Sodium) Aventis ... 732
Mefoxin for Injection (Cefoxitin Sodium) Merck ... 2124
Mefoxin Premixed Intravenous Solution (Cefoxitin Sodium) Merck ... 2127
Primaxin I.V. (Cilastatin Sodium, Imipenem) Merck ... 2160
Rocephin Injectable Vials, ADD-Vantage, Galaxy, Bulk (Ceftriaxone Sodium) Roche Laboratories ... 2993

Clostridium species peritonitis
Mefoxin for Injection (Cefoxitin Sodium) Merck ... 2124
Mefoxin Premixed Intravenous Solution (Cefoxitin Sodium) Merck ... 2127

Clostridium species septicemia
Cefobid Intravenous/Intramuscular (Cefoperazone) Pfizer ... 2671
Cefobid Pharmacy Bulk Package - Not for Direct Infusion (Cefoperazone Sodium) Pfizer ... 2673

Clostridium species skin and skin structure infections
Mefoxin for Injection (Cefoxitin Sodium) Merck ... 2124
Mefoxin Premixed Intravenous Solution (Cefoxitin Sodium) Merck ... 2127

CNS depression
(*see under* Central nervous system depression, drug-induced)

Coagulation, disseminated intravascular
(*see under* Coagulopathies, consumptive)

Coagulopathies, consumptive
Heparin Sodium Injection (Heparin Sodium) Wyeth-Ayerst 3511

Coccidioidomycosis
Nizoral Tablets (Ketoconazole) Janssen 1791

Coitus, adjunct in
Natural Arousal Cream (L-Arginine) Strategic Science .... ▣840
Natural Sensation Cream (L-Arginine) Strategic Science .... ▣841
Vitara Cream (Dehydroepiandrosterone (DHEA), N-Methylnicotinate) Products on Demand .... ▣731

Cold, common, symptomatic relief of
(*see also under* Influenza syndrome, symptomatic relief of)
Actifed Cold & Allergy Tablets (Pseudoephedrine Hydrochloride, Triprolidine Hydrochloride) Pfizer Inc., Warner-Lambert Healthcare .... ▣688
Actifed Cold & Sinus Caplets and Tablets (Acetaminophen, Chlorpheniramine Maleate, Pseudoephedrine Hydrochloride) Pfizer Inc., Warner-Lambert Healthcare .... ▣688
Afrin Nasal Decongestant Children's Pump Mist (Phenylephrine Hydrochloride) Schering-Plough .... ▣734
Afrin (Oxymetazoline Hydrochloride) Schering-Plough .... ▣733
Afrin No Drip Original Nasal Spray (Oxymetazoline Hydrochloride) Schering-Plough .... ▣735
Afrin No Drip Extra Moisturizing Nasal Spray (Oxymetazoline Hydrochloride) Schering-Plough .... ▣735
Afrin No Drip Severe Congestion Nasal Spray (Oxymetazoline Hydrochloride) Schering-Plough .... ▣735
Afrin No Drip Sinus Nasal Spray (Oxymetazoline Hydrochloride) Schering-Plough .... ▣735
Afrin Original Pump Mist (Oxymetazoline Hydrochloride) Schering-Plough .... ▣733
Afrin Saline Aromatic Mist (Menthol, Sodium Chloride) Schering-Plough .... ▣734
Alka-Seltzer Plus Cold & Sinus Medicine Liqui-Gels (Acetaminophen, Pseudoephedrine Hydrochloride) Bayer Consumer .... ▣604
BC Cold Powder (Aspirin, Chlorpheniramine Maleate, Pseudoephedrine Hydrochloride) Block .... ▣619
Benadryl Allergy Chewables (Diphenhydramine Hydrochloride) Pfizer Inc., Warner-Lambert Healthcare .... ▣689
Benadryl Allergy Liquid (Diphenhydramine Hydrochloride) Pfizer Inc., Warner-Lambert Healthcare .... ▣690
Benadryl Allergy/Cold Tablets (Acetaminophen, Diphenhydramine Hydrochloride, Pseudoephedrine Hydrochloride) Pfizer Inc., Warner-Lambert Healthcare .... ▣691
Benadryl Allergy/Congestion Tablets (Diphenhydramine Hydrochloride, Pseudoephedrine Hydrochloride) Pfizer Inc., Warner-Lambert Healthcare .... ▣692
Benadryl Allergy & Sinus Liquid (Diphenhydramine Hydrochloride, Pseudoephedrine Hydrochloride) Pfizer Inc., Warner-Lambert Healthcare .... ▣693
Benadryl Allergy & Sinus Fastmelt Tablets (Diphenhydramine Citrate, Pseudoephedrine Hydrochloride) Pfizer Inc., Warner-Lambert Healthcare .... ▣693
Benadryl Allergy Sinus Headache Caplets & Gelcaps (Acetaminophen, Diphenhydramine Hydrochloride, Pseudoephedrine Hydrochloride) Pfizer Inc., Warner-Lambert Healthcare .... ▣693
Benadryl Children's Allergy/Cold Fastmelt Tablets (Diphenhydramine Citrate, Pseudoephedrine Hydrochloride) Pfizer Inc., Warner-Lambert Healthcare .... ▣692
Benadryl Dye-Free Allergy Liqui-Gels Softgels (Diphenhydramine Hydrochloride) Pfizer Inc., Warner-Lambert Healthcare .... ▣690
Biomune OSF Express Spray (Homeopathic Formulations) Matol .... ▣640
Chlor-Trimeton Allergy/Decongestant Tablets (Chlorpheniramine Maleate, Pseudoephedrine Sulfate) Schering-Plough .... ▣736
Comtrex Acute Head Cold & Sinus Pressure Relief Tablets (Acetaminophen, Brompheniramine Maleate, Pseudoephedrine Hydrochloride) Bristol-Myers .... ▣627
Contac Non-Drowsy 12 Hour Cold Caplets (Pseudoephedrine Hydrochloride) SmithKline Beecham Consumer .... ▣745
Contac Non-Drowsy Timed Release 12 Hour Cold Caplets (Pseudoephedrine Hydrochloride) SmithKline Beecham Consumer .... ▣746
Coricidin 'D' Cold, Flu & Sinus Tablets (Acetaminophen, Chlorpheniramine Maleate, Pseudoephedrine Sulfate) Schering-Plough .... ▣737
Coricidin/Coricidin D (Acetaminophen, Chlorpheniramine Maleate) Schering-Plough .... ▣738
Dimetapp Elixir (Brompheniramine Maleate, Pseudoephedrine Hydrochloride) Whitehall-Robins .... ▣777
Dimetapp Cold and Fever Suspension (Acetaminophen, Brompheniramine Maleate, Pseudoephedrine Hydrochloride) Whitehall-Robins .... ▣775
Drixoral Allergy/Sinus Extended-Release Tablets (Acetaminophen, Dexbrompheniramine Maleate, Pseudoephedrine Sulfate) Schering-Plough .... ▣741
Drixoral Cold & Allergy Sustained-Action Tablets (Dexbrompheniramine Maleate, Pseudoephedrine Sulfate) Schering-Plough .... ▣740
Drixoral Cold & Flu Extended-Release Tablets (Acetaminophen, Dexbrompheniramine Maleate, Pseudoephedrine Sulfate) Schering-Plough .... ▣740
Hyland's Cold Tablets with Zinc (Homeopathic Formulations) Standard Homeopathic .... ▣765
Natru-Vent Nasal Spray, Adult Strength (Xylometazoline Hydrochloride) Boehringer Ingelheim .... ▣624
Natru-Vent Nasal Spray, Pediatric Strength (Xylometazoline Hydrochloride) Boehringer Ingelheim .... ▣625
Neo-Synephrine (Phenylephrine Hydrochloride) Bayer Consumer .... ▣614
Neo-Synephrine 12 Hour Nasal Spray (Oxymetazoline Hydrochloride) Bayer Consumer .... ▣615
PediaCare Cough-Cold Liquid (Chlorpheniramine Maleate, Dextromethorphan Hydrobromide, Pseudoephedrine Hydrochloride) Pharmacia Consumer .... ▣719
Robitussin-PE Liquid (Guaifenesin, Pseudoephedrine Hydrochloride) Whitehall-Robins .... ▣782
Ryna-12 S Suspension (Phenylephrine Tannate, Pyrilamine Tannate) Wallace 3351
Reformulated Rynatan Pediatric Suspension (Chlorpheniramine Tannate, Phenylephrine Tannate) Wallace 3352
Rynatan Tablets (Azatadine Maleate, Pseudoephedrine Sulfate) Wallace 3351
Sinutab Sinus Allergy Medication, Maximum Strength Formula, Tablets & Caplets (Acetaminophen, Chlorpheniramine Maleate, Pseudoephedrine Hydrochloride) Pfizer Inc., Warner-Lambert Healthcare .... ▣707
Children's Sudafed Nasal Decongestant Chewables (Pseudoephedrine Hydrochloride) Pfizer Inc., Warner-Lambert Healthcare .... ▣711
Children's Sudafed Nasal Decongestant Liquid Medication (Pseudoephedrine Hydrochloride) Pfizer Inc., Warner-Lambert Healthcare .... ▣711
Sudafed Cold & Allergy Tablets (Chlorpheniramine Maleate, Pseudoephedrine Hydrochloride) Pfizer Inc., Warner-Lambert Healthcare .... ▣708
Sudafed Cold & Sinus Liquid Caps (Acetaminophen, Pseudoephedrine Hydrochloride) Pfizer Inc., Warner-Lambert Healthcare .... ▣710
Sudafed Nasal Decongestant Tablets (Pseudoephedrine Hydrochloride) Pfizer Inc., Warner-Lambert Healthcare .... ▣710
Triaminic Allergy Congestion Liquid (Pseudoephedrine Hydrochloride) Novartis Consumer .... ▣680
Triaminic Cold & Allergy Liquid (Chlorpheniramine Maleate, Pseudoephedrine Hydrochloride) Novartis Consumer .... ▣681
Triaminic Cold & Allergy Softchews (Chlorpheniramine Maleate, Pseudoephedrine Hydrochloride) Novartis Consumer .... ▣683
Children's Tylenol Cold Suspension Liquid and Chewable Tablets (Acetaminophen, Chlorpheniramine Maleate, Pseudoephedrine Hydrochloride) McNeil Consumer 2015
Vicks Sinex Nasal Spray and Ultra Fine Mist (Phenylephrine Hydrochloride) Procter & Gamble .... ▣729
Vicks Sinex 12-Hour Nasal Spray and Ultra Fine Mist (Oxymetazoline Hydrochloride) Procter & Gamble .... ▣729
Vicks Vapor Inhaler (Levmetamfetamine) Procter & Gamble .... ▣730
Zephrex Tablets (Guaifenesin, Pseudoephedrine Hydrochloride) Sanofi-Synthelabo 3091
Zephrex LA Tablets (Guaifenesin, Pseudoephedrine Hydrochloride) Sanofi-Synthelabo 3092

Cold sores
(*see under* Herpetic manifestations, oral, symptomatic relief of)

Colic, biliary, symptomatic relief of
Levsin/Levsinex/Levbid (Hyoscyamine Sulfate) Schwarz 3172
NuLev Orally Disintegrating Tablets (Hyoscyamine Sulfate) Schwarz 3176

Colic, renal, symptomatic relief of
Levsin/Levsinex/Levbid (Hyoscyamine Sulfate) Schwarz 3172
NuLev Orally Disintegrating Tablets (Hyoscyamine Sulfate) Schwarz 3176

Colic, symptomatic relief of
Hyland's Colic Tablets (Dioscorea, Homeopathic Formulations) Standard Homeopathic .... ▣765
Levsin/Levsinex/Levbid (Hyoscyamine Sulfate) Schwarz 3172
NuLev Orally Disintegrating Tablets (Hyoscyamine Sulfate) Schwarz 3176

Colitis, mucous
(*see under* Bowel, irritable, syndrome)

Colitis, pseudomembranous, antibiotic-associated
Vancocin HCl Capsules & Pulvules (Vancomycin Hydrochloride) Lilly 1972
Vancocin HCl Oral Solution (Vancomycin Hydrochloride) Lilly 1971
Vancocin HCl, Vials & ADD-Vantage (Vancomycin Hydrochloride) Lilly 1970

Colitis, ulcerative
Anusol-HC Suppositories (Hydrocortisone Acetate) Monarch 2238
Asacol Delayed-Release Tablets (Mesalamine) Procter & Gamble Pharmaceuticals 2884
Azulfidine EN-tabs Tablets (Sulfasalazine) Pharmacia & Upjohn 2775
Celestone Soluspan Injectable Suspension (Betamethasone Acetate, Betamethasone Sodium Phosphate) Schering 3097
Celestone Syrup (Betamethasone) Schering 3099
Colazal Capsules (Balsalazide Disodium) Salix 3069
Cortone Acetate Injectable Suspension (Cortisone Acetate) Merck 2059
Cortone Acetate Tablets (Cortisone Acetate) Merck 2061
Decadron Elixir (Dexamethasone) Merck 2078
Decadron Tablets (Dexamethasone) Merck 2079
Decadron Phosphate Injection (Dexamethasone Sodium Phosphate) Merck 2081
Depo-Medrol Injectable Suspension (Methylprednisolone Acetate) Pharmacia & Upjohn 2795
Dipentum Capsules (Olsalazine Sodium) Pharmacia & Upjohn 2803
Hydrocortone Tablets (Hydrocortisone) Merck 2106
Hydrocortone Phosphate Injection, Sterile (Hydrocortisone Sodium Phosphate) Merck 2105
Pediapred Oral Solution (Prednisolone Sodium Phosphate) Celltech 1170
Pentasa Capsules (Mesalamine) Shire US 3239
Prednisone (Prednisone) Roxane 3064
Prelone Syrup (Prednisolone) Muro 2273
Rowasa Rectal Suspension Enema 4.0 grams/unit (60 mL) (Mesalamine) Solvay 3264
Solu-Medrol Sterile Powder (Methylprednisolone Sodium Succinate) Pharmacia & Upjohn 2855

Collagen disease
Celestone Soluspan Injectable Suspension (Betamethasone Acetate, Betamethasone Sodium Phosphate) Schering 3097
Celestone Syrup (Betamethasone) Schering 3099
Cortone Acetate Injectable Suspension (Cortisone Acetate) Merck 2059
Cortone Acetate Tablets (Cortisone Acetate) Merck 2061
Decadron Elixir (Dexamethasone) Merck 2078
Decadron Tablets (Dexamethasone) Merck 2079
Decadron Phosphate Injection (Dexamethasone Sodium Phosphate) Merck 2081
Depo-Medrol Injectable Suspension (Methylprednisolone Acetate) Pharmacia & Upjohn 2795
Hydrocortone Tablets (Hydrocortisone) Merck 2106
Hydrocortone Phosphate Injection, Sterile (Hydrocortisone Sodium Phosphate) Merck 2105
Pediapred Oral Solution (Prednisolone Sodium Phosphate) Celltech 1170
Prednisone (Prednisone) Roxane 3064
Prelone Syrup (Prednisolone) Muro 2273
Solu-Medrol Sterile Powder (Methylprednisolone Sodium Succinate) Pharmacia & Upjohn 2855

Colon, irritable
(*see under* Bowel, irritable, syndrome)

Colon, spastic
(*see under* Bowel, irritable, syndrome)

Colorectal polyps, adenomatous
Celebrex Capsules (Celecoxib) Pfizer 2676
Celebrex Capsules (Celecoxib) Pharmacia & Upjohn 2780

Colostomies, reduction in odor, adjunct to
Devrom Chewable Tablets (Bismuth Subgallate) Parthenon .... ▣685

Condylomata acuminata
Aldara Cream, 5% (Imiquimod) 3M 1978
Alferon N Injection (Interferon alfa-N3 (Human Leukocyte Derived)) Interferon 1770
Condylox Topical Solution (Podofilox) Oclassen 2437
Intron A for Injection (Interferon alfa-2B, Recombinant) Schering 3120
Podocon-25 Liquid (Podophyllin) Paddock 2608

Condylomata acuminata, topical treatment of
Condylox Gel (Podofilox) Oclassen 2436

Congestive heart failure, adjunct in (*see also under* Edema, adjunctive therapy in)

Accupril Tablets (Quinapril Hydrochloride) Parke-Davis 2611
Altace Capsules (Ramipril) Monarch 2233
Captopril Tablets (Captopril) Mylan .. 2281
Coreg Tablets (Carvedilol) GlaxoSmithKline 1508
Demadex Tablets and Injection (Torsemide) Roche Laboratories .. 2965
Diamox (Acetazolamide Sodium) Lederle .... ⊙ 269
Diucardin Tablets (Hydroflumethiazide) Wyeth-Ayerst 3494
Diuril Oral (Chlorothiazide) Merck 2087
Diuril Sodium Intravenous (Chlorothiazide Sodium) Merck 2086
Dyrenium Capsules (Triamterene) WellSpring 3458
Edecrin (Ethacrynic Acid) Merck 2091
Furosemide Tablets (Furosemide) Mylan 2284
HydroDIURIL Tablets (Hydrochlorothiazide) Merck 2108
Indapamide Tablets (Indapamide) Mylan 2286
Lanoxicaps Capsules (Digoxin) GlaxoSmithKline 1574
Lanoxin Injection (Digoxin) GlaxoSmithKline 1581
Lanoxin Tablets (Digoxin) GlaxoSmithKline 1587
Lanoxin Elixir Pediatric (Digoxin) GlaxoSmithKline 1578
Lanoxin Injection Pediatric (Digoxin) GlaxoSmithKline 1584
Mavik Tablets (Trandolapril) Abbott .. 478
Microzide Capsules (Hydrochlorothiazide) Watson 3414
Midamor Tablets (Amiloride Hydrochloride) Merck 2136
Moduretic Tablets (Amiloride Hydrochloride, Hydrochlorothiazide) Merck 2138
Monopril Tablets (Fosinopril Sodium) Bristol-Myers Squibb 1091
Natrecor for Injection (Nesiritide) Scios Inc. 3189
Primacor Injection (Milrinone Lactate) Sanofi-Synthelabo 3086
Prinivil Tablets (Lisinopril) Merck 2164
Renese Tablets (Polythiazide) Pfizer 2712
Toprol-XL Tablets (Metoprolol Succinate) AstraZeneca LP 651
Vasotec Tablets (Enalapril Maleate) Merck 2210
Zaroxolyn Tablets (Metolazone) Celltech 1177
Zestril Tablets (Lisinopril) AstraZeneca 698

Conjunctival hyperemia, reduction of signs and symptoms (*see under* Ocular redness)

Conjunctival inflammation, bulbar, steroid-responsive

Blephamide Ophthalmic Ointment (Prednisolone Acetate, Sulfacetamide Sodium) Allergan 547
Decadron Phosphate Sterile Ophthalmic Ointment (Dexamethasone Sodium Phosphate) Merck 2083
Decadron Phosphate Sterile Ophthalmic Solution (Dexamethasone Sodium Phosphate) Merck 2084
NeoDecadron Sterile Ophthalmic Solution (Dexamethasone Sodium Phosphate, Neomycin Sulfate) Merck 2144
Terra-Cortril Ophthalmic Suspension (Hydrocortisone Acetate, Oxytetracycline Hydrochloride) Pfizer 2716

Conjunctival inflammation, palpebral, steroid-responsive

Blephamide Ophthalmic Ointment (Prednisolone Acetate, Sulfacetamide Sodium) Allergan 547
Decadron Phosphate Sterile Ophthalmic Ointment (Dexamethasone Sodium Phosphate) Merck 2083
Decadron Phosphate Sterile Ophthalmic Solution (Dexamethasone Sodium Phosphate) Merck 2084
NeoDecadron Sterile Ophthalmic Solution (Dexamethasone Sodium Phosphate, Neomycin Sulfate) Merck 2144
Terra-Cortril Ophthalmic Suspension (Hydrocortisone Acetate, Oxytetracycline Hydrochloride) Pfizer 2716

Conjunctivitis, allergic

Alamast Ophthalmic Solution (Pemirolast Potassium) Santen 3092
Alocril Ophthalmic Solution (Nedocromil Sodium) Allergan 545
Alrex Sterile Ophthalmic Suspension 0.2% (Loteprednol Etabonate) Bausch & Lomb .... ⊙ 256
Celestone Soluspan Injectable Suspension (Betamethasone Acetate, Betamethasone Sodium Phosphate) Schering 3097
Celestone Syrup (Betamethasone) Schering 3099
Cortone Acetate Injectable Suspension (Cortisone Acetate) Merck 2059
Cortone Acetate Tablets (Cortisone Acetate) Merck 2061
Decadron Elixir (Dexamethasone) Merck 2078
Decadron Tablets (Dexamethasone) Merck 2079
Decadron Phosphate Injection (Dexamethasone Sodium Phosphate) Merck 2081
Decadron Phosphate Sterile Ophthalmic Ointment (Dexamethasone Sodium Phosphate) Merck 2083
Decadron Phosphate Sterile Ophthalmic Solution (Dexamethasone Sodium Phosphate) Merck 2084
Depo-Medrol Injectable Suspension (Methylprednisolone Acetate) Pharmacia & Upjohn 2795
Emadine Ophthalmic Solution (Emedastine Difumarate) Alcon .... ⊙ 211
HMS Sterile Ophthalmic Suspension (Medrysone) Allergan .... ⊙ 240
Hydrocortone Tablets (Hydrocortisone) Merck 2106
Hydrocortone Phosphate Injection, Sterile (Hydrocortisone Sodium Phosphate) Merck 2105
Livostin (Levocabastine Hydrochloride) Novartis Ophthalmics .... ⊙ 305
Optivar Ophthalmic Solution (Azelastine Hydrochloride) Muro 2273
Patanol Ophthalmic Solution (Olopatadine Hydrochloride) Alcon 540
Pediapred Oral Solution (Prednisolone Sodium Phosphate) Celltech 1170
Periactin Tablets (Cyproheptadine Hydrochloride) Merck 2155
Phenergan Suppositories (Promethazine Hydrochloride) Wyeth-Ayerst 3556
Phenergan Syrup (Promethazine Hydrochloride) Wyeth-Ayerst 3554
Phenergan Tablets (Promethazine Hydrochloride) Wyeth-Ayerst 3556
Prednisone (Prednisone) Roxane 3064
Prelone Syrup (Prednisolone) Muro 2273
Solu-Medrol Sterile Powder (Methylprednisolone Sodium Succinate) Pharmacia & Upjohn 2855
Zaditor Ophthalmic Solution (Ketotifen Fumarate) Novartis Ophthalmics 2304

Conjunctivitis, bacterial

Chibroxin Sterile Ophthalmic Solution (Norfloxacin) Merck 2051
Ciloxan (Ciprofloxacin Hydrochloride) Alcon 538
Neosporin Ophthalmic Ointment Sterile (Bacitracin Zinc, Neomycin Sulfate, Polymyxin B Sulfate) Monarch .... ⊙ 299
Neosporin Ophthalmic Solution Sterile (Gramicidin, Neomycin Sulfate, Polymyxin B Sulfate) Monarch .... ⊙ 300
Ocuflox Ophthalmic Solution (Ofloxacin) Allergan 554
Polysporin Ophthalmic Ointment (Bacitracin Zinc, Polymyxin B Sulfate, Bacitracin Zinc, Polymyxin B Sulfate) Monarch .... ⊙ 301
Polytrim Ophthalmic Solution (Polymyxin B Sulfate, Trimethoprim Sulfate) Allergan 556
Quixin Ophthalmic Solution (Levofloxacin) Santen 3093

Conjunctivitis, fungal

Natacyn Antifungal Ophthalmic Suspension (Natamycin) Alcon .... ⊙ 216

Conjunctivitis, granular (*see under* Trachoma)

Conjunctivitis, inclusion

Declomycin Tablets (Demeclocycline Hydrochloride) Lederle 1855
Doryx Coated Pellet Filled Capsules (Doxycycline Hyclate) Warner Chilcott 3357
Dynacin Capsules (Minocycline Hydrochloride) Medicis 2019
Minocin Intravenous (Minocycline Hydrochloride) Lederle 1862
Minocin Oral Suspension (Minocycline Hydrochloride) Lederle 1865
Minocin Pellet-Filled Capsules (Minocycline Hydrochloride) Lederle 1863
Monodox Capsules (Doxycycline Monohydrate) Oclassen 2442
Vibramycin Calcium Oral Suspension Syrup (Doxycycline Calcium) Pfizer 2735
Vibramycin Hyclate Capsules (Doxycycline Hyclate) Pfizer 2735
Vibramycin Monohydrate for Oral Suspension (Doxycycline Monohydrate) Pfizer 2735
Vibra-Tabs Film Coated Tablets (Doxycycline Hyclate) Pfizer 2735

Conjunctivitis, infective

Blephamide Ophthalmic Ointment (Prednisolone Acetate, Sulfacetamide Sodium) Allergan 547
Blephamide Ophthalmic Suspension (Prednisolone Acetate, Sulfacetamide Sodium) Allergan 548
Decadron Phosphate Sterile Ophthalmic Ointment (Dexamethasone Sodium Phosphate) Merck 2083
Decadron Phosphate Sterile Ophthalmic Solution (Dexamethasone Sodium Phosphate) Merck 2084
FML-S Liquifilm Sterile Ophthalmic Suspension (Fluorometholone, Sulfacetamide Sodium) Allergan .. ⊙ 238
NeoDecadron Sterile Ophthalmic Solution (Dexamethasone Sodium Phosphate, Neomycin Sulfate) Merck 2144
Poly-Pred Liquifilm Ophthalmic Suspension (Neomycin Sulfate, Polymyxin B Sulfate, Prednisolone Acetate) Allergan .... ⊙ 245
Pred-G Ophthalmic Suspension (Gentamicin Sulfate, Prednisolone Acetate) Allergan .... ⊙ 247
Pred-G Sterile Ophthalmic Ointment (Gentamicin Sulfate, Prednisolone Acetate) Allergan .. ⊙ 248
Terra-Cortril Ophthalmic Suspension (Hydrocortisone Acetate, Oxytetracycline Hydrochloride) Pfizer 2716
TobraDex Ophthalmic Ointment (Dexamethasone, Tobramycin) Alcon 542
TobraDex Ophthalmic Suspension (Dexamethasone, Tobramycin) Alcon 541

Conjunctivitis, neonatal

Ery-Tab Tablets (Erythromycin) Abbott 448
Erythrocin Stearate Filmtab Tablets (Erythromycin Stearate) Abbott 452
Erythromycin Base Filmtab Tablets (Erythromycin) Abbott 454
Erythromycin Delayed-Release Capsules, USP (Erythromycin) Abbott 455
PCE Dispertab Tablets (Erythromycin) Abbott 498

Conjunctivitis, unspecified

Bleph-10 (Sulfacetamide Sodium) Allergan .... ⊙ 230
Genoptic Ophthalmic Ointment (Gentamicin Sulfate) Allergan .... ⊙ 239
Genoptic Sterile Ophthalmic Solution (Gentamicin Sulfate) Allergan .... ⊙ 239
Pred Mild Sterile Ophthalmic Suspension (Prednisolone Acetate) Allergan .... ⊙ 249

Conjunctivitis, vernal

Alomide Ophthalmic Solution (Lodoxamide Tromethamine) Alcon .... ⊙ 204
Crolom Sterile Ophthalmic Solution USP 4% (Cromolyn Sodium) Bausch & Lomb .... ⊙ 259
HMS Sterile Ophthalmic Suspension (Medrysone) Allergan .... ⊙ 240
Opticrom Ophthalmic Solution (Cromolyn Sodium) Allergan 555

Constipation, chronic

Kristalose for Oral Solution (Lactulose) Bertek 1007
Metamucil (Psyllium Preparations) Procter & Gamble 2877
Perdiem Fiber Therapy (Psyllium Preparations) Novartis Consumer 2301
Peri-Colace Capsules and Syrup (Casanthranol, Docusate Sodium) Shire US 3240
Senokot Granules (Senna) Purdue Frederick 2901
Senokot Syrup (Senna) Purdue Frederick .... ▣ 732
Senokot Tablets (Senna) Purdue Frederick 2901
Senokot-S Tablets (Docusate Sodium, Senna) Purdue Frederick 2901
SenokotXTRA Tablets (Senna) Purdue Frederick 2901

Constipation, temporary

Ceo-Two Evacuant Suppository (Potassium Bitartrate, Sodium Bicarbonate) Beutlich .... ▣ 618
Citrucel Caplets (Methylcellulose) SmithKline Beecham Consumer .... ▣ 745
Citrucel Orange Flavor Powder (Methylcellulose) SmithKline Beecham Consumer .... ▣ 744
Citrucel Sugar Free Orange Flavor Powder (Methylcellulose) SmithKline Beecham Consumer .... ▣ 745
Colace Capsules, Syrup, Liquid (Docusate Sodium) Shire US 3236
Correctol Laxative Tablets and Caplets (Bisacodyl) Schering-Plough .... ▣ 739
Dulcolax Suppositories (Bisacodyl) Novartis Consumer .... ▣ 668
Dulcolax Tablets (Bisacodyl) Novartis Consumer .... ▣ 668
Ex•Lax Gentle Strength Caplets (Sennosides, Docusate Sodium) Novartis Consumer .... ▣ 670
Ex•Lax Regular Strength Pills (Sennosides) Novartis Consumer .... ▣ 670
Ex•Lax Regular Strength Chocolated Pieces (Sennosides) Novartis Consumer .... ▣ 669
Ex•Lax Maximum Strength Pills (Sennosides) Novartis Consumer .... ▣ 670
Ex•Lax Milk of Magnesia Liquid (Magnesium Hydroxide) Novartis Consumer .... ▣ 670
Ex•Lax Stool Softener Caplets (Docusate Sodium) Novartis Consumer .... ▣ 671
FiberCon Caplets (Calcium Polycarbophil) Lederle Consumer .... ▣ 639
Fleet Bisacodyl Laxatives (Bisacodyl) Fleet 1359
Fleet Enema (Sodium Phosphate) Fleet 1359
Fleet Glycerin Laxatives (Glycerin) Fleet 1359
Fleet Mineral Oil Enema (Mineral Oil) Fleet 1360
Fleet Phospho-soda (Sodium Phosphate) Fleet 1360
Iscar Mali Injection (Homeopathic Formulations) Weleda 3456
Iscar Mali Special Injection (Homeopathic Formulations) Weleda 3456
Iscar Pini Injection (Homeopathic Formulations) Weleda 3456
Iscar Quercus Injection (Homeopathic Formulations) Weleda 3456
Iscar Quercus Special Injection (Homeopathic Formulations) Weleda 3456
Maltsupex Powder, Liquid, Tablets (Malt Soup Extract) Wallace .... ▣ 767
MiraLax Powder for Oral Solution (Polyethylene Glycol) Braintree 1069
Mitrolan Chewable Tablets (Calcium Polycarbophil) Wyeth-Ayerst .... ▣ 789
Nature's Remedy Tablets (Sennosides) Block .... ▣ 621
Perdiem Overnight Relief (Psyllium Preparations, Senna) Novartis Consumer 2301
Peri-Colace Capsules and Syrup (Casanthranol, Docusate Sodium) Shire US 3240
Phillips' Chewable Tablets (Magnesium Hydroxide) Bayer Consumer .... ▣ 615
Phillips' FiberCaps Caplets (Calcium Polycarbophil) Bayer Consumer .... ▣ 615
Phillips' Liqui-Gels (Docusate Sodium) Bayer Consumer .... ▣ 616
Phillips' Milk of Magnesia Liquid (Original, Cherry, & Mint) (Magnesium Hydroxide) Bayer Consumer .... ▣ 616

Purge Liquid (Castor Oil) Fleming .. ▣633
Senokot Granules (Senna) Purdue Frederick 2901
Senokot Syrup (Senna) Purdue Frederick .... ▣732
Senokot Children's Syrup (Senna) Purdue Frederick 2900
Senokot Tablets (Senna) Purdue Frederick 2901
Senokot-S Tablets (Docusate Sodium, Senna) Purdue Frederick 2901
SenokotXTRA Tablets (Senna) Purdue Frederick 2901
Surfak Liqui-Gels (Docusate Calcium) Pharmacia Consumer .... ▣721

Contact lenses, fitting of, adjunct in

Fluor-I-Strip A.T. Ophthalmic Strips 1 mg (Fluorescein Sodium) Bausch & Lomb .... ⊙260
Fluor-I-Strip Ophthalmic Strips 9 mg (Fluorescein Sodium) Bausch & Lomb .... ⊙260

Contraception

(*see under* Pregnancy, prevention of)

Convulsive disorders, adjunctive therapy in

Valium Tablets (Diazepam) Roche Products 3047

Convulsive episodes, control of

Nembutal Sodium Solution (Pentobarbital Sodium) Abbott 485

Corneal edema

(*see under* Edema, corneal, temporary relief of)

Corneal erosions, recurrent

Lacrisert Sterile Ophthalmic Insert (Hydroxypropyl Cellulose) Merck 2117

Corneal inflammation, steroid-responsive

Blephamide Ophthalmic Ointment (Prednisolone Acetate, Sulfacetamide Sodium) Allergan 547
Blephamide Ophthalmic Suspension (Prednisolone Acetate, Sulfacetamide Sodium) Allergan 548
Cortisporin Ophthalmic Suspension (Hydrocortisone, Neomycin Sulfate, Polymyxin B Sulfate, Hydrocortisone, Neomycin Sulfate, Polymyxin B Sulfate) Monarch .... ⊙297
Decadron Phosphate Sterile Ophthalmic Ointment (Dexamethasone Sodium Phosphate) Merck 2083
Decadron Phosphate Sterile Ophthalmic Solution (Dexamethasone Sodium Phosphate) Merck 2084
FML Ophthalmic Ointment (Fluorometholone) Allergan .... ⊙237
FML Ophthalmic Suspension (Fluorometholone) Allergan .... ⊙236
FML Forte Ophthalmic Suspension (Fluorometholone) Allergan .... ⊙235
FML-S Liquifilm Sterile Ophthalmic Suspension (Fluorometholone, Sulfacetamide Sodium) Allergan .. ⊙238
Lotemax Sterile Ophthalmic Suspension 0.5% (Loteprednol Etabonate) Bausch & Lomb .... ⊙261
NeoDecadron Sterile Ophthalmic Solution (Dexamethasone Sodium Phosphate, Neomycin Sulfate) Merck 2144
Poly-Pred Liquifilm Ophthalmic Suspension (Neomycin Sulfate, Polymyxin B Sulfate, Prednisolone Acetate) Allergan .... ⊙245
Pred Forte Ophthalmic Suspension (Prednisolone Acetate) Allergan .... ⊙246
Pred-G Ophthalmic Suspension (Gentamicin Sulfate, Prednisolone Acetate) Allergan .... ⊙247
Pred-G Sterile Ophthalmic Ointment (Gentamicin Sulfate, Prednisolone Acetate) Allergan ... ⊙248
Terra-Cortril Ophthalmic Suspension (Hydrocortisone Acetate, Oxytetracycline Hydrochloride) Pfizer 2716
TobraDex Ophthalmic Ointment (Dexamethasone, Tobramycin) Alcon 542
TobraDex Ophthalmic Suspension (Dexamethasone, Tobramycin) Alcon 541

Corneal injury, chemical

Blephamide Ophthalmic Ointment (Prednisolone Acetate, Sulfacetamide Sodium) Allergan 547
Blephamide Ophthalmic Suspension (Prednisolone Acetate, Sulfacetamide Sodium) Allergan 548
Cortisporin Ophthalmic Suspension (Hydrocortisone, Neomycin Sulfate, Polymyxin B Sulfate, Hydrocortisone, Neomycin Sulfate, Polymyxin B Sulfate) Monarch .... ⊙297
Decadron Phosphate Sterile Ophthalmic Ointment (Dexamethasone Sodium Phosphate) Merck 2083
Decadron Phosphate Sterile Ophthalmic Solution (Dexamethasone Sodium Phosphate) Merck 2084
FML-S Liquifilm Sterile Ophthalmic Suspension (Fluorometholone, Sulfacetamide Sodium) Allergan .. ⊙238
NeoDecadron Sterile Ophthalmic Solution (Dexamethasone Sodium Phosphate, Neomycin Sulfate) Merck 2144
Poly-Pred Liquifilm Ophthalmic Suspension (Neomycin Sulfate, Polymyxin B Sulfate, Prednisolone Acetate) Allergan .... ⊙245
Pred Mild Sterile Ophthalmic Suspension (Prednisolone Acetate) Allergan .... ⊙249
Pred-G Ophthalmic Suspension (Gentamicin Sulfate, Prednisolone Acetate) Allergan .... ⊙247
Pred-G Sterile Ophthalmic Ointment (Gentamicin Sulfate, Prednisolone Acetate) Allergan ... ⊙248
Terra-Cortril Ophthalmic Suspension (Hydrocortisone Acetate, Oxytetracycline Hydrochloride) Pfizer 2716
TobraDex Ophthalmic Ointment (Dexamethasone, Tobramycin) Alcon 542
TobraDex Ophthalmic Suspension (Dexamethasone, Tobramycin) Alcon 541

Corneal injury, foreign bodies

Blephamide Ophthalmic Ointment (Prednisolone Acetate, Sulfacetamide Sodium) Allergan 547
Blephamide Ophthalmic Suspension (Prednisolone Acetate, Sulfacetamide Sodium) Allergan 548
Cortisporin Ophthalmic Suspension (Hydrocortisone, Neomycin Sulfate, Polymyxin B Sulfate, Hydrocortisone, Neomycin Sulfate, Polymyxin B Sulfate) Monarch .... ⊙297
Decadron Phosphate Sterile Ophthalmic Ointment (Dexamethasone Sodium Phosphate) Merck 2083
Decadron Phosphate Sterile Ophthalmic Solution (Dexamethasone Sodium Phosphate) Merck 2084
FML-S Liquifilm Sterile Ophthalmic Suspension (Fluorometholone, Sulfacetamide Sodium) Allergan .. ⊙238
NeoDecadron Sterile Ophthalmic Solution (Dexamethasone Sodium Phosphate, Neomycin Sulfate) Merck 2144
Poly-Pred Liquifilm Ophthalmic Suspension (Neomycin Sulfate, Polymyxin B Sulfate, Prednisolone Acetate) Allergan .... ⊙245
Pred-G Ophthalmic Suspension (Gentamicin Sulfate, Prednisolone Acetate) Allergan .... ⊙247
Pred-G Sterile Ophthalmic Ointment (Gentamicin Sulfate, Prednisolone Acetate) Allergan ... ⊙248
Terra-Cortril Ophthalmic Suspension (Hydrocortisone Acetate, Oxytetracycline Hydrochloride) Pfizer 2716
TobraDex Ophthalmic Ointment (Dexamethasone, Tobramycin) Alcon 542
TobraDex Ophthalmic Suspension (Dexamethasone, Tobramycin) Alcon 541

Corneal injury, radiation

Blephamide Ophthalmic Ointment (Prednisolone Acetate, Sulfacetamide Sodium) Allergan 547
Blephamide Ophthalmic Suspension (Prednisolone Acetate, Sulfacetamide Sodium) Allergan 548
Cortisporin Ophthalmic Suspension (Hydrocortisone, Neomycin Sulfate, Polymyxin B Sulfate, Hydrocortisone, Neomycin Sulfate, Polymyxin B Sulfate) Monarch .... ⊙297
FML-S Liquifilm Sterile Ophthalmic Suspension (Fluorometholone, Sulfacetamide Sodium) Allergan .. ⊙238
NeoDecadron Sterile Ophthalmic Solution (Dexamethasone Sodium Phosphate, Neomycin Sulfate) Merck 2144
Poly-Pred Liquifilm Ophthalmic Suspension (Neomycin Sulfate, Polymyxin B Sulfate, Prednisolone Acetate) Allergan .... ⊙245
Pred-G Ophthalmic Suspension (Gentamicin Sulfate, Prednisolone Acetate) Allergan .... ⊙247
Pred-G Sterile Ophthalmic Ointment (Gentamicin Sulfate, Prednisolone Acetate) Allergan ... ⊙248
Terra-Cortril Ophthalmic Suspension (Hydrocortisone Acetate, Oxytetracycline Hydrochloride) Pfizer 2716
TobraDex Ophthalmic Ointment (Dexamethasone, Tobramycin) Alcon 542
TobraDex Ophthalmic Suspension (Dexamethasone, Tobramycin) Alcon 541

Corneal injury, thermal burns

Blephamide Ophthalmic Ointment (Prednisolone Acetate, Sulfacetamide Sodium) Allergan 547
Blephamide Ophthalmic Suspension (Prednisolone Acetate, Sulfacetamide Sodium) Allergan 548
Cortisporin Ophthalmic Suspension (Hydrocortisone, Neomycin Sulfate, Polymyxin B Sulfate, Hydrocortisone, Neomycin Sulfate, Polymyxin B Sulfate) Monarch .... ⊙297
Decadron Phosphate Sterile Ophthalmic Ointment (Dexamethasone Sodium Phosphate) Merck 2083
Decadron Phosphate Sterile Ophthalmic Solution (Dexamethasone Sodium Phosphate) Merck 2084
FML-S Liquifilm Sterile Ophthalmic Suspension (Fluorometholone, Sulfacetamide Sodium) Allergan .. ⊙238
NeoDecadron Sterile Ophthalmic Solution (Dexamethasone Sodium Phosphate, Neomycin Sulfate) Merck 2144
Poly-Pred Liquifilm Ophthalmic Suspension (Neomycin Sulfate, Polymyxin B Sulfate, Prednisolone Acetate) Allergan .... ⊙245
Pred Mild Sterile Ophthalmic Suspension (Prednisolone Acetate) Allergan .... ⊙249
Pred-G Ophthalmic Suspension (Gentamicin Sulfate, Prednisolone Acetate) Allergan .... ⊙247
Pred-G Sterile Ophthalmic Ointment (Gentamicin Sulfate, Prednisolone Acetate) Allergan ... ⊙248
Terra-Cortril Ophthalmic Suspension (Hydrocortisone Acetate, Oxytetracycline Hydrochloride) Pfizer 2716
TobraDex Ophthalmic Ointment (Dexamethasone, Tobramycin) Alcon 542
TobraDex Ophthalmic Suspension (Dexamethasone, Tobramycin) Alcon 541

Corneal marginal ulcers, allergic

Celestone Syrup (Betamethasone) Schering 3099
Cortone Acetate Injectable Suspension (Cortisone Acetate) Merck 2059
Cortone Acetate Tablets (Cortisone Acetate) Merck 2061
Decadron Elixir (Dexamethasone) Merck 2078
Decadron Tablets (Dexamethasone) Merck 2079
Decadron Phosphate Injection (Dexamethasone Sodium Phosphate) Merck 2081
Depo-Medrol Injectable Suspension (Methylprednisolone Acetate) Pharmacia & Upjohn 2795
Hydrocortone Tablets (Hydrocortisone) Merck 2106
Hydrocortone Phosphate Injection, Sterile (Hydrocortisone Sodium Phosphate) Merck 2105
Pediapred Oral Solution (Prednisolone Sodium Phosphate) Celltech 1170
Prednisone (Prednisone) Roxane 3064
Prelone Syrup (Prednisolone) Muro . 2273
Solu-Medrol Sterile Powder (Methylprednisolone Sodium Succinate) Pharmacia & Upjohn 2855

Corneal sensitivity, decreased

Lacrisert Sterile Ophthalmic Insert (Hydroxypropyl Cellulose) Merck 2117

Corneal transplant, surgical aid in

Healon (Sodium Hyaluronate) Pharmacia & Upjohn .... ⊙316
Healon GV (Sodium Hyaluronate) Pharmacia & Upjohn .... ⊙320

Corneal ulcers

Bleph-10 (Sulfacetamide Sodium) Allergan .... ⊙230
Celestone Soluspan Injectable Suspension (Betamethasone Acetate, Betamethasone Sodium Phosphate) Schering 3097
Ciloxan Ophthalmic Solution (Ciprofloxacin Hydrochloride) Alcon 538
Genoptic Ophthalmic Ointment (Gentamicin Sulfate) Allergan .... ⊙239
Genoptic Sterile Ophthalmic Solution (Gentamicin Sulfate) Allergan .... ⊙239

Corns

(*see under* Hyperkeratosis skin disorders)

Coronary angioplasty or atherectomy, percutaneous transluminal, adjunct in

ReoPro Vials (Abciximab) Lilly 1958

Coronary artery disease, reducing the risk of

Lopid Tablets (Gemfibrozil) Parke-Davis 2650
Metamucil Dietary Fiber Supplement (Psyllium Preparations) Procter & Gamble .... ▣834
Mevacor Tablets (Lovastatin) Merck 2132
Zocor Tablets (Simvastatin) Merck .. 2219

Coronary atherosclerosis, to slow the progression of

(*see also under* Coronary artery disease, reducing the risk of)

Lescol Capsules (Fluvastatin Sodium) Novartis 2361
Lescol Capsules (Fluvastatin Sodium) Reliant 2925
Lescol XL Tablets (Fluvastatin Sodium) Novartis 2361
Lescol XL Tablets (Fluvastatin Sodium) Reliant 2925
Mevacor Tablets (Lovastatin) Merck 2132
Niaspan Extended-Release Tablets (Niacin) Kos 1846
Pravachol (Pravastatin Sodium) Bristol-Myers Squibb 1099

Coronary syndrome, acute

(*see also under* Coronary angioplasty or atherectomy, percutaneous transluminal, adjunct in; Cardiac ischemic complications, acute, prevention of, adjunct to PTCA)

Aggrastat (Tirofiban Hydrochloride) Merck 2031
Ecotrin Enteric Coated Aspirin Low, Regular and Maximum Strength Tablets (Aspirin) GlaxoSmithKline Consumer 1715
Fragmin Injection (Dalteparin Sodium) Pharmacia & Upjohn 2814
Integrilin Injection (Eptifibatide) COR 1213
Integrilin Injection (Eptifibatide) Key 1828
Lovenox Injection (Enoxaparin) Aventis 746

Corynebacterium diphtheriae

(*see under* C. diphtheriae infections)

Corynebacterium minutissimum

(*see under* C. minutissimum infections)

Corynebacterium vaginitis

MetroGel-Vaginal Gel (Metronidazole) 3M 1986

(▣ Described in PDR For Nonprescription Drugs) (⊙ Described in PDR For Ophthalmic Medicines™)

Coryza, acute
(*see under* Cold, common, symptomatic relief of)

Cough, symptomatic relief of

Benadryl Allergy Liquid (Diphenhydramine Hydrochloride) Pfizer Inc., Warner-Lambert Healthcare ▣ 690
Benylin Adult Formula Cough Suppressant Liquid (Dextromethorphan Hydrobromide) Pfizer Inc., Warner-Lambert Healthcare ▣ 696
Benylin Cough Suppressant/Expectorant Liquid (Dextromethorphan Hydrobromide, Guaifenesin) Pfizer Inc., Warner-Lambert Healthcare ▣ 697
Benylin Pediatric Cough Suppressant Liquid (Dextromethorphan Hydrobromide) Pfizer Inc., Warner-Lambert Healthcare ▣ 698
Coricidin HBP Cough & Cold Tablets (Chlorpheniramine Maleate, Dextromethorphan Hydrobromide) Schering-Plough ▣ 738
Coricidin HBP Maximum Strength Flu Tablets (Acetaminophen, Chlorpheniramine Maleate, Dextromethorphan Hydrobromide) Schering-Plough ▣ 738
Delsym Extended-Release Suspension (Dextromethorphan Polistirex) Medeva ▣ 664
Halls Mentho-Lyptus Drops (Menthol) Pfizer Inc., Warner-Lambert Group ▣ 686
Halls Sugar Free (Menthol) Pfizer Inc., Warner-Lambert Group ▣ 686
Halls Plus Cough Drops (Menthol, Pectin) Pfizer Inc., Warner-Lambert Group ▣ 686
Hycodan (Homatropine Methylbromide, Hydrocodone Bitartrate) Endo Labs 1316
Hycotuss Expectorant Syrup (Guaifenesin, Hydrocodone Bitartrate) Endo Labs 1318
Robitussin A-C Syrup (Codeine Phosphate, Guaifenesin) Robins 2942
Robitussin Cough Drops (Menthol) Whitehall-Robins ▣ 781
Robitussin Honey Cough Drops (Menthol) Whitehall-Robins ▣ 784
Robitussin Honey Cough Liquid Whitehall-Robins ▣ 784
Robitussin Pediatric Cough & Cold Formula Liquid (Dextromethorphan Hydrobromide, Pseudoephedrine Hydrochloride) Whitehall-Robins ▣ 785
Robitussin Maximum Strength Cough Suppressant Liquid (Dextromethorphan Hydrobromide) Whitehall-Robins ▣ 784
Robitussin Pediatric Cough Suppressant Liquid (Dextromethorphan Hydrobromide) Whitehall-Robins ▣ 784
Robitussin Honey Calmers Throat Drops (Menthol) Whitehall-Robins ▣ 783
Robitussin Sugar Free Throat Drops (Menthol) Whitehall-Robins ▣ 786
Robitussin DM Infant Drops (Dextromethorphan Hydrobromide, Guaifenesin) Whitehall-Robins ▣ 783
Robitussin-DM Liquid (Dextromethorphan Hydrobromide, Guaifenesin) Whitehall-Robins ▣ 783
Tessalon Capsules (Benzonatate) Forest 1377
TheraFlu Maximum Strength Severe Cold & Congestion Night Time Caplets (Acetaminophen, Chlorpheniramine Maleate, Dextromethorphan Hydrobromide, Pseudoephedrine Hydrochloride) Novartis Consumer ▣ 678
TheraFlu Maximum Strength Severe Cold & Congestion Night Time Hot Liquid (Acetaminophen, Chlorpheniramine Maleate, Dextromethorphan Hydrobromide, Pseudoephedrine Hydrochloride) Novartis Consumer ▣ 678
Triaminic Cough Liquid (Dextromethorphan Hydrobromide, Pseudoephedrine Hydrochloride) Novartis Consumer ▣ 682
Triaminic Cough Softchews (Dextromethorphan Hydrobromide) Novartis Consumer ▣ 684
Triaminic Cough & Congestion Liquid (Dextromethorphan Hydrobromide, Pseudoephedrine Hydrochloride) Novartis Consumer ▣ 682
Triaminic Cough & Sore Throat Liquid (Acetaminophen, Dextromethorphan Hydrobromide, Pseudoephedrine Hydrochloride) Novartis Consumer ▣ 682
Triaminic Cough & Sore Throat Softchews (Acetaminophen, Dextromethorphan Hydrobromide, Pseudoephedrine Hydrochloride) Novartis Consumer ▣ 684
Tussi-12 S Suspension (Carbetapentane Tannate, Chlorpheniramine Tannate) Wallace 3356
Tussi-12 Tablets (Carbetapentane Tannate, Chlorpheniramine Tannate) Wallace 3356
Tussionex Pennkinetic Extended-Release Suspension (Chlorpheniramine Polistirex, Hydrocodone Polistirex) Celltech 1174
Tussi-Organidin NR Liquid (Codeine Phosphate, Guaifenesin) Wallace 3350
Tussi-Organidin DM NR Liquid (Dextromethorphan Hydrobromide, Guaifenesin) Wallace 3350
Tussi-Organidin DM-S NR Liquid (Dextromethorphan Hydrobromide, Guaifenesin) Wallace 3350
Tussi-Organidin-S NR Liquid (Codeine Phosphate, Guaifenesin) Wallace 3350
Vicks 44 Cough Relief Liquid (Dextromethorphan Hydrobromide) Procter & Gamble ▣ 724
Vicks 44E Cough & Chest Congestion Relief Liquid (Dextromethorphan Hydrobromide, Guaifenesin) Procter & Gamble ▣ 725
Pediatric Vicks 44e Cough & Chest Congestion Relief Liquid (Dextromethorphan Hydrobromide, Guaifenesin) Procter & Gamble ▣ 728
Vicks Cough Drops, Menthol and Cherry Flavors (Menthol) Procter & Gamble ▣ 726
Vicodin Tuss Expectorant (Guaifenesin, Hydrocodone Bitartrate) Abbott 519

Cough, whooping
(*see under* Pertussis)

Cough and nasal congestion, symptomatic relief of

Benadryl Children's Allergy/Cold Fastmelt Tablets (Diphenhydramine Citrate, Pseudoephedrine Hydrochloride) Pfizer Inc., Warner-Lambert Healthcare ▣ 692
Benylin Multi-Symptom Liquid (Dextromethorphan Hydrobromide, Guaifenesin, Pseudoephedrine Hydrochloride) Pfizer Inc., Warner-Lambert Healthcare ▣ 697
Comtrex Flu Therapy & Fever Relief Nighttime Tablets (Acetaminophen, Chlorpheniramine Maleate, Pseudoephedrine Hydrochloride) Bristol-Myers ▣ 628
Comtrex Maximum Strength Multi-Symptom Cold & Cough Relief Tablets and Caplets (Acetaminophen, Chlorpheniramine Maleate, Dextromethorphan Hydrobromide, Pseudoephedrine Hydrochloride) Bristol-Myers ▣ 626
Contac Severe Cold and Flu Caplets Maximum Strength (Acetaminophen, Chlorpheniramine Maleate, Dextromethorphan Hydrobromide, Pseudoephedrine Hydrochloride) SmithKline Beecham Consumer ▣ 746
Contac Severe Cold and Flu Caplets Non-Drowsy (Acetaminophen, Dextromethorphan Hydrobromide, Pseudoephedrine Hydrochloride) SmithKline Beecham Consumer ▣ 746
Dimetapp DM Cold & Cough Elixir (Brompheniramine Maleate, Dextromethorphan Hydrobromide, Pseudoephedrine Hydrochloride) Whitehall-Robins ▣ 775
Dimetapp Nighttime Flu Liquid (Acetaminophen, Brompheniramine Maleate, Dextromethorphan Hydrobromide, Pseudoephedrine Hydrochloride) Whitehall-Robins ▣ 776
Dimetapp Non-Drowsy Flu Syrup (Acetaminophen, Dextromethorphan Hydrobromide, Pseudoephedrine Hydrochloride) Whitehall-Robins ▣ 777
Dimetapp Infant Drops Decongestant Plus Cough (Dextromethorphan Hydrobromide, Pseudoephedrine Hydrochloride) Whitehall-Robins ▣ 776
Guaifed (Guaifenesin, Pseudoephedrine Hydrochloride) Muro 2272
Hycomine Compound Tablets (Acetaminophen, Caffeine, Chlorpheniramine Maleate, Hydrocodone Bitartrate, Phenylephrine Hydrochloride) Endo Labs 1317
PediaCare Cough-Cold Liquid (Chlorpheniramine Maleate, Dextromethorphan Hydrobromide, Pseudoephedrine Hydrochloride) Pharmacia Consumer ▣ 719
PediaCare Infants' Drops Decongestant Plus Cough (Dextromethorphan Hydrobromide, Pseudoephedrine Hydrochloride) Pharmacia Consumer ▣ 719
PediaCare NightRest Cough-Cold Liquid (Chlorpheniramine Maleate, Dextromethorphan Hydrobromide, Pseudoephedrine Hydrochloride) Pharmacia Consumer ▣ 719
Phenergan with Codeine Syrup (Codeine Phosphate, Promethazine Hydrochloride) Wyeth-Ayerst 3557
Phenergan with Dextromethorphan Syrup (Dextromethorphan Hydrobromide, Promethazine Hydrochloride) Wyeth-Ayerst 3559
Phenergan VC Syrup (Phenylephrine Hydrochloride, Promethazine Hydrochloride) Wyeth-Ayerst 3560
Phenergan VC with Codeine Syrup (Codeine Phosphate, Phenylephrine Hydrochloride, Promethazine Hydrochloride) Wyeth-Ayerst 3561
Relief Nasal & Throat Spray (Homeopathic Formulations) Body Wise ▣ 811
Robitussin Cold Caplets Cold & Congestion (Dextromethorphan Hydrobromide, Guaifenesin, Pseudoephedrine Hydrochloride) Whitehall-Robins ▣ 780
Robitussin Cold Softgels Cold & Congestion (Dextromethorphan Hydrobromide, Guaifenesin, Pseudoephedrine Hydrochloride) Whitehall-Robins ▣ 780
Robitussin Cold Caplets Multi-Symptom Cold & Flu (Acetaminophen, Dextromethorphan Hydrobromide, Guaifenesin, Pseudoephedrine Hydrochloride) Whitehall-Robins ▣ 781
Robitussin Cold Softgels Multi-Symptom Cold & Flu (Acetaminophen, Dextromethorphan Hydrobromide, Guaifenesin, Pseudoephedrine Hydrochloride) Whitehall-Robins ▣ 781
Robitussin Cough & Cold Infant Drops (Dextromethorphan Hydrobromide, Guaifenesin, Pseudoephedrine Hydrochloride) Whitehall-Robins ▣ 782
Robitussin Maximum Strength Cough & Cold Liquid (Dextromethorphan Hydrobromide, Pseudoephedrine Hydrochloride) Whitehall-Robins ▣ 785
Robitussin Multi Symptom Honey Flu Liquid (Acetaminophen, Dextromethorphan Hydrobromide, Pseudoephedrine Hydrochloride) Whitehall-Robins ▣ 785
Robitussin Nighttime Honey Flu Liquid (Acetaminophen, Chlorpheniramine Maleate, Dextromethorphan Hydrobromide, Pseudoephedrine Hydrochloride) Whitehall-Robins ▣ 786
Robitussin-CF Liquid (Dextromethorphan Hydrobromide, Guaifenesin, Pseudoephedrine Hydrochloride) Whitehall-Robins ▣ 783
Robitussin-DAC Syrup (Codeine Phosphate, Guaifenesin, Pseudoephedrine Hydrochloride) Robins 2942
Ryna-C Liquid (Chlorpheniramine Maleate, Codeine Phosphate, Pseudoephedrine Hydrochloride) Wallace ▣ 768
Rynatuss Pediatric Suspension (Carbetapentane Tannate, Chlorpheniramine Tannate, Ephedrine Tannate, Phenylephrine Tannate) Wallace 3353
Rynatuss Tablets (Carbetapentane Tannate, Chlorpheniramine Tannate, Ephedrine Tannate, Phenylephrine Tannate) Wallace 3353
Children's Sudafed Cold & Cough Liquid (Dextromethorphan Hydrobromide, Pseudoephedrine Hydrochloride) Pfizer Inc., Warner-Lambert Healthcare ▣ 709
Sudafed Cold & Cough Liquid Caps (Acetaminophen, Dextromethorphan Hydrobromide, Guaifenesin, Pseudoephedrine Hydrochloride) Pfizer Inc., Warner-Lambert Healthcare ▣ 709
TheraFlu Regular Strength Cold & Cough Night Time Hot Liquid (Acetaminophen, Chlorpheniramine Maleate, Dextromethorphan Hydrobromide, Pseudoephedrine Hydrochloride) Novartis Consumer ▣ 676
TheraFlu Regular Strength Cold & Sore Throat Night Time Hot Liquid (Acetaminophen, Chlorpheniramine Maleate, Pseudoephedrine Hydrochloride) Novartis Consumer ▣ 676
TheraFlu Maximum Strength Flu & Congestion Non-Drowsy Hot Liquid (Acetaminophen, Dextromethorphan Hydrobromide, Guaifenesin, Pseudoephedrine Hydrochloride) Novartis Consumer ▣ 677
TheraFlu Maximum Strength Flu & Cough Night Time Hot Liquid (Acetaminophen, Chlorpheniramine Maleate, Dextromethorphan Hydrobromide, Pseudoephedrine Hydrochloride) Novartis Consumer ▣ 678
TheraFlu Maximum Strength Severe Cold & Congestion Non-Drowsy Caplets (Acetaminophen, Dextromethorphan Hydrobromide, Pseudoephedrine Hydrochloride) Novartis Consumer ▣ 679
Triaminic Cold & Cough Liquid (Chlorpheniramine Maleate, Dextromethorphan Hydrobromide, Pseudoephedrine Hydrochloride) Novartis Consumer ▣ 681
Triaminic Cold & Cough Softchews (Chlorpheniramine Maleate, Dextromethorphan Hydrobromide, Pseudoephedrine Hydrochloride) Novartis Consumer ▣ 683
Triaminic Cold & Night Time Cough Liquid (Chlorpheniramine Maleate, Dextromethorphan Hydrobromide, Pseudoephedrine Hydrochloride) Novartis Consumer ▣ 681
Triaminic Cold, Cough & Fever Liquid (Acetaminophen, Chlorpheniramine Maleate, Dextromethorphan Hydrobromide, Pseudoephedrine Hydrochloride) Novartis Consumer ▣ 681
Triaminic Cough Liquid (Dextromethorphan Hydrobromide, Pseudoephedrine Hydrochloride) Novartis Consumer ▣ 682
Triaminic Cough & Congestion Liquid (Dextromethorphan Hydrobromide, Pseudoephedrine Hydrochloride) Novartis Consumer ▣ 682
Triaminic Cough & Sore Throat Liquid (Acetaminophen, Dextromethorphan Hydrobromide, Pseudoephedrine Hydrochloride) Novartis Consumer ▣ 682
Triaminic Cough & Sore Throat Softchews (Acetaminophen, Dextromethorphan Hydrobromide, Pseudoephedrine Hydrochloride) Novartis Consumer ▣ 684
Triaminic Vapor Patch-Cherry Scent (Camphor, Menthol) Novartis Consumer ▣ 684
Triaminic Vapor Patch-Menthol Scent (Camphor, Menthol) Novartis Consumer ▣ 684
Children's Tylenol Cold Plus Cough Suspension Liquid and Chewable Tablets (Acetaminophen, Chlorpheniramine Maleate, Dextromethorphan Hydrobromide, Pseudoephedrine Hydrochloride) McNeil Consumer 2015

Children's Tylenol Flu Suspension Liquid (Acetaminophen, Chlorpheniramine Maleate, Dextromethorphan Hydrobromide, Pseudoephedrine Hydrochloride) McNeil Consumer 2015
Infants' Tylenol Cold Decongestant and Fever Reducer Concentrated Drops Plus Cough (Acetaminophen, Dextromethorphan Hydrobromide, Pseudoephedrine Hydrochloride) McNeil Consumer 2015
Multi-Symptom Tylenol Cold Complete Formula Caplets (Acetaminophen, Chlorpheniramine Maleate, Dextromethorphan Hydrobromide, Pseudoephedrine Hydrochloride) McNeil Consumer 2010
Multi-Symptom Tylenol Cold Non-Drowsy Caplets and Gelcaps (Acetaminophen, Dextromethorphan Hydrobromide, Pseudoephedrine Hydrochloride) McNeil Consumer 2010
Multi-Symptom Tylenol Cold Severe Congestion Non-Drowsy Caplets (Acetaminophen, Dextromethorphan Hydrobromide, Guaifenesin, Pseudoephedrine Hydrochloride) McNeil Consumer 2011
Maximum Strength Tylenol Flu NightTime Liquid (Acetaminophen, Dextromethorphan Hydrobromide, Doxylamine Succinate, Pseudoephedrine Hydrochloride) McNeil Consumer 2011
Maximum Strength Tylenol Flu Non-Drowsy Gelcaps (Acetaminophen, Dextromethorphan Hydrobromide, Pseudoephedrine Hydrochloride) McNeil Consumer 2011
Vicks 44D Cough & Head Congestion Relief Liquid (Dextromethorphan Hydrobromide, Pseudoephedrine Hydrochloride) Procter & Gamble .... ▣ 724
Vicks 44M Cough, Cold & Flu Relief Liquid (Acetaminophen, Chlorpheniramine Maleate, Dextromethorphan Hydrobromide, Pseudoephedrine Hydrochloride) Procter & Gamble .... ▣ 725
Vicks DayQuil LiquiCaps/Liquid Multi-Symptom Cold/Flu Relief (Acetaminophen, Dextromethorphan Hydrobromide, Pseudoephedrine Hydrochloride) Procter & Gamble .... ▣ 727
Children's Vicks NyQuil Cold/Cough Relief (Chlorpheniramine Maleate, Dextromethorphan Hydrobromide, Pseudoephedrine Hydrochloride) Procter & Gamble .... ▣ 726
Vicks NyQuil LiquiCaps/Liquid Multi-Symptom Cold/Flu Relief, Original and Cherry Flavors (Acetaminophen, Dextromethorphan Hydrobromide, Doxylamine Succinate, Pseudoephedrine Hydrochloride) Procter & Gamble .... ▣ 727
Vicks VapoRub (Camphor, Menthol) Procter & Gamble .... ▣ 730
Vicks VapoSteam (Camphor) Procter & Gamble .... ▣ 730

Cradle cap
(*see under* Dermatitis, seborrheic)

Cramps, abdominal, symptomatic relief of
Donnagel Liquid (Attapulgite) Wyeth-Ayerst .... ▣ 789
Levsin/Levsinex/Levbid (Hyoscyamine Sulfate) Schwarz 3172
NuLev Orally Disintegrating Tablets (Hyoscyamine Sulfate) Schwarz 3176

Cramps, leg
(*see under* Leg muscle cramps)

Creeping eruptions
(*see under* Larva migrans, cutaneous)

Cretinism
(*see under* Hypothyroidism, replacement or supplemental therapy in)

Crohn's disease
Remicade for IV Injection (Infliximab) Centocor 1178

Cryptitis, temporary relief of
Anusol-HC Suppositories (Hydrocortisone Acetate) Monarch 2238
Proctocort Suppositories (Hydrocortisone Acetate) Monarch 2264

Cryptococcosis
Abelcet Injection (Amphotericin B) Elan 1273
AmBisome for Injection (Amphotericin B) Fujisawa 1383
Ancobon (Flucytosine) ICN 1730

Cryptococcus meningitis
Diflucan Tablets, Injection, and Oral Suspension (Fluconazole) Pfizer 2681

Cryptococcus strains pulmonary infections
Ancobon (Flucytosine) ICN 1730

Cryptorchidism, prepubertal
Novarel for Injection (Chorionic Gonadotropin) Ferring 1347
Pregnyl for Injection (Chorionic Gonadotropin) Organon 2482

Cushing's syndrome, ACTH-dependent, differential diagnosis of
Acthrel for Injection (Corticorelin Ovine Triflutate) Ferring 3629

Cushing's syndrome, diagnosis of
(*see under* Adrenocortical hyperfunction, diagnostic testing of)

Cuts, minor, infection from
(*see under* Infections, skin, bacterial, minor)

Cuts, minor, pain associated with
(*see under* Pain, topical relief of)

Cyclitis
Decadron Phosphate Sterile Ophthalmic Ointment (Dexamethasone Sodium Phosphate) Merck 2083
Decadron Phosphate Sterile Ophthalmic Solution (Dexamethasone Sodium Phosphate) Merck 2084

Cystic fibrosis, adjunctive therapy in
Pulmozyme Inhalation Solution (Dornase Alfa) Genentech 1426
TOBI Solution for Inhalation (Tobramycin) Chiron 1206

Cystic tumors
Celestone Soluspan Injectable Suspension (Betamethasone Acetate, Betamethasone Sodium Phosphate) Schering 3097

Cystinuria
Cuprimine Capsules (Penicillamine) Merck 2075
Depen Titratable Tablets (Penicillamine) Wallace 3341

Cystitis
Azactam for Injection (Aztreonam) Elan 1276
Ceclor (Cefaclor) Lilly 1905
Cipro (Ciprofloxacin) Bayer 887
Floxin I.V. (Ofloxacin) Ortho-McNeil 2526
Floxin Tablets (Ofloxacin) Ortho-McNeil 2529
Lorabid Suspension and Pulvules (Loracarbef) Monarch 2251
Macrobid Capsules (Nitrofurantoin Monohydrate) Procter & Gamble Pharmaceuticals 2889
Monurol Sachet (Fosfomycin Tromethamine) Forest 1375
Noroxin Tablets (Norfloxacin) Merck 2145
Tequin Injection (Gatifloxacin) Bristol-Myers Squibb 1110
Tequin Tablets (Gatifloxacin) Bristol-Myers Squibb 1110
Urised Tablets (Atropine Sulfate, Benzoic Acid, Hyoscyamine, Methenamine, Methylene Blue, Phenyl Salicylate) PolyMedica 2876
Uroqid-Acid No. 2 Tablets (Methenamine Mandelate, Sodium Acid Phosphate) Beach 947
Vantin Tablets and Oral Suspension (Cefpodoxime Proxetil) Pharmacia & Upjohn 2860

Cystitis, interstitial, symptomatic relief of
Elmiron Capsules (Pentosan Polysulfate Sodium) Alza 570
Rimso-50 Solution (Dimethyl Sulfoxide) Edwards 1267

Cystitis, lacking substantial evidence of effectiveness in
Urobiotic-250 Capsules (Oxytetracycline Hydrochloride, Phenazopyridine Hydrochloride, Sulfamethizole) Pfizer 2731

Cytomegalovirus disease associated with renal transplantation, prophylaxis of
CytoGam Intravenous (Cytomegalovirus Immune Globulin) MedImmune 2026

Cytomegalovirus disease associated with transplant patients
Cytovene (Ganciclovir) Roche Laboratories 2959

D

Dacryocystitis
Genoptic Ophthalmic Ointment (Gentamicin Sulfate) Allergan .... ⊙ 239
Genoptic Sterile Ophthalmic Solution (Gentamicin Sulfate) Allergan .... ⊙ 239

Dandruff
(*see also under* Dermatitis, seborrheic)
Head & Shoulders Dandruff Shampoo (Pyrithione Zinc) Procter & Gamble 2876
Head & Shoulders Dandruff Shampoo Dry Scalp (Pyrithione Zinc) Procter & Gamble 2876
Head & Shoulders Intensive Treatment Dandruff and Seborrheic Dermatitis Shampoo (Selenium Sulfide) Procter & Gamble 2877
Nizoral A-D Shampoo (Ketoconazole) McNeil Consumer 2008
Selsun Rx 2.5% Lotion, USP (Selenium Sulfide) Ross 3053
Tegrin Dandruff Shampoo - Extra Conditioning (Coal Tar) Block .... ▣ 623
Tegrin Dandruff Shampoo - Fresh Herbal (Coal Tar) Block .... ▣ 624

Dehydration, prevention of
Pedialyte Oral Electrolyte Maintenance Solution (Electrolyte Supplement) Ross 3049
Rehydralyte Oral Electrolyte Rehydration Solution (Electrolyte Supplement) Ross 3052

Dementia, Alzheimer's type
Aricept Tablets (Donepezil Hydrochloride) Eisai 1270
Aricept Tablets (Donepezil Hydrochloride) Pfizer 2665
Cognex Capsules (Tacrine Hydrochloride) First Horizon 1351
Exelon Capsules (Rivastigmine Tartrate) Novartis 2342
Exelon Oral Solution (Rivastigmine Tartrate) Novartis 2345
Reminyl Oral Solution (Galantamine Hydrobromide) Janssen 1792
Reminyl Tablets (Galantamine Hydrobromide) Janssen 1792

Dental caries, prophylaxis
Listermint Alcohol-Free Mouthrinse (Sodium Fluoride) Pfizer Inc., Warner-Lambert Healthcare .... ▣ 703

Dental plaque, prevention of
Listerine Mouthrinse (Eucalyptol, Menthol, Methyl Salicylate) Pfizer Inc., Warner-Lambert Healthcare .... ▣ 702
Tartar Control Listerine Mouthrinse (Eucalyptol, Menthol, Methyl Salicylate) Pfizer Inc., Warner-Lambert Healthcare .... ▣ 702

Depression, atypical
(*see under* Depression, mental, nonendogenous)

Depression, bipolar
(*see under* Depression, manic-depressive)

Depression, major, without melancholia
Parnate Tablets (Tranylcypromine Sulfate) GlaxoSmithKline 1607

Depression, manic-depressive
(*see also under* Mania, bipolar)
Depakote Tablets (Divalproex Sodium) Abbott 430
Eskalith (Lithium Carbonate) GlaxoSmithKline 1527
Lithium Carbonate (Lithium Carbonate) Roxane 3061
Lithium Citrate Syrup (Lithium Citrate) Roxane 3061
Lithobid Slow-Release Tablets (Lithium Carbonate) Solvay 3255
Sinequan (Doxepin Hydrochloride) Pfizer 2713
Thorazine (Chlorpromazine Hydrochloride) GlaxoSmithKline 1656
Zyprexa Tablets (Olanzapine) Lilly 1973
Zyprexa ZYDIS Orally Disintegrating Tablets (Olanzapine) Lilly 1973

Depression, mental, nonendogenous
Nardil Tablets (Phenelzine Sulfate) Parke-Davis 2653

Depression, neurotic
(*see under* Depression, mental, nonendogenous)

Depression, relief of symptoms
Celexa (Citalopram Hydrobromide) Forest 1365
Effexor Tablets (Venlafaxine Hydrochloride) Wyeth-Ayerst 3495
Effexor XR Capsules (Venlafaxine Hydrochloride) Wyeth-Ayerst 3499
Etrafon (Amitriptyline Hydrochloride, Perphenazine) Schering 3115
Limbitrol (Amitriptyline Hydrochloride, Chlordiazepoxide) ICN 1738
Norpramin Tablets (Desipramine Hydrochloride) Aventis 755
Paxil (Paroxetine Hydrochloride) GlaxoSmithKline 1609
Prozac Pulvules, Liquid, and Weekly Capsules (Fluoxetine Hydrochloride) Dista 1238
Remeron Tablets (Mirtazapine) Organon 2483
Remeron SolTab Tablets (Mirtazapine) Organon 2486
Serzone Tablets (Nefazodone Hydrochloride) Bristol-Myers Squibb 1104
Sinequan (Doxepin Hydrochloride) Pfizer 2713
Sonata Capsules (Zaleplon) Wyeth-Ayerst 3591
Surmontil Capsules (Trimipramine Maleate) Wyeth-Ayerst 3595
Vivactil Tablets (Protriptyline Hydrochloride) Merck 2217
Vivactil Tablets (Protriptyline Hydrochloride) Odyssey 2446
Wellbutrin Tablets (Bupropion Hydrochloride) GlaxoSmithKline 1680
Wellbutrin SR Sustained-Release Tablets (Bupropion Hydrochloride) GlaxoSmithKline 1684
Zoloft (Sertraline Hydrochloride) Pfizer 2751

Dermatitis, atopic
Celestone Soluspan Injectable Suspension (Betamethasone Acetate, Betamethasone Sodium Phosphate) Schering 3097
Celestone Syrup (Betamethasone) Schering 3099
Cortizone•5 (Hydrocortisone) Pfizer Inc., Warner-Lambert Healthcare .... ▣ 699
Cortizone•10 (Hydrocortisone) Pfizer Inc., Warner-Lambert Healthcare .... ▣ 699
Cortizone•10 Plus Creme (Hydrocortisone) Pfizer Inc., Warner-Lambert Healthcare .... ▣ 700
Cortizone•10 Quick Shot Spray (Hydrocortisone) Pfizer Inc., Warner-Lambert Healthcare .... ▣ 699
Cortone Acetate Injectable Suspension (Cortisone Acetate) Merck 2059
Cortone Acetate Tablets (Cortisone Acetate) Merck 2061
Decadron Elixir (Dexamethasone) Merck 2078
Decadron Tablets (Dexamethasone) Merck 2079
Decadron Phosphate Injection (Dexamethasone Sodium Phosphate) Merck 2081
Depo-Medrol Injectable Suspension (Methylprednisolone Acetate) Pharmacia & Upjohn 2795
Hydrocortone Tablets (Hydrocortisone) Merck 2106

Hydrocortone Phosphate Injection, Sterile (Hydrocortisone Sodium Phosphate) Merck 2105
Pediapred Oral Solution (Prednisolone Sodium Phosphate) Celltech 1170
Prednisone (Prednisone) Roxane 3064
Prelone Syrup (Prednisolone) Muro . 2273
Protopic Ointment (Tacrolimus) Fujisawa 1397
Solu-Medrol Sterile Powder (Methylprednisolone Sodium Succinate) Pharmacia & Upjohn 2855

Dermatitis, contact
(*see also under* Dermatoses, corticosteroid-responsive)
Benadryl Itch Relief Stick Extra Strength (Diphenhydramine Hydrochloride, Zinc Acetate) Pfizer Inc., Warner-Lambert Healthcare .... ▣695
Benadryl Cream (Diphenhydramine Hydrochloride, Zinc Acetate) Pfizer Inc., Warner-Lambert Healthcare .... ▣695
Benadryl Gel (Diphenhydramine Hydrochloride) Pfizer Inc., Warner-Lambert Healthcare .... ▣695
Benadryl Spray (Diphenhydramine Hydrochloride, Zinc Acetate) Pfizer Inc., Warner-Lambert Healthcare .... ▣696
Caladryl (Pramoxine Hydrochloride, Zinc Acetate) Pfizer Inc., Warner-Lambert Healthcare .... ▣698
Celestone Soluspan Injectable Suspension (Betamethasone Acetate, Betamethasone Sodium Phosphate) Schering 3097
Celestone Syrup (Betamethasone) Schering 3099
Cortaid Sensitive Skin Cream (Hydrocortisone Acetate) Pharmacia Consumer .... ▣717
Cortizone•5 (Hydrocortisone) Pfizer Inc., Warner-Lambert Healthcare .... ▣699
Cortizone•10 (Hydrocortisone) Pfizer Inc., Warner-Lambert Healthcare .... ▣699
Cortizone•10 Plus Creme (Hydrocortisone) Pfizer Inc., Warner-Lambert Healthcare .... ▣700
Cortizone•10 Quick Shot Spray (Hydrocortisone) Pfizer Inc., Warner-Lambert Healthcare .... ▣699
Cortizone for Kids Creme (Hydrocortisone) Pfizer Inc., Warner-Lambert Healthcare .... ▣699
Cortone Acetate Injectable Suspension (Cortisone Acetate) Merck 2059
Cortone Acetate Tablets (Cortisone Acetate) Merck 2061
Decadron Elixir (Dexamethasone) Merck 2078
Decadron Tablets (Dexamethasone) Merck 2079
Decadron Phosphate Injection (Dexamethasone Sodium Phosphate) Merck 2081
Depo-Medrol Injectable Suspension (Methylprednisolone Acetate) Pharmacia & Upjohn 2795
Hydrocortone Tablets (Hydrocortisone) Merck 2106
Hydrocortone Phosphate Injection, Sterile (Hydrocortisone Sodium Phosphate) Merck 2105
Pediapred Oral Solution (Prednisolone Sodium Phosphate) Celltech 1170
Prednisone (Prednisone) Roxane 3064
Solu-Medrol Sterile Powder (Methylprednisolone Sodium Succinate) Pharmacia & Upjohn 2855
Vistaril (Hydroxyzine Pamoate) Pfizer 2738
Zanfel Urushiol Wash Zanfel .... ▣790

Dermatitis, corticosteroid-responsive, anal region
Analpram-HC (Hydrocortisone Acetate, Pramoxine Hydrochloride) Ferndale 1338

Dermatitis, exfoliative
Celestone Soluspan Injectable Suspension (Betamethasone Acetate, Betamethasone Sodium Phosphate) Schering 3097
Celestone Syrup (Betamethasone) Schering 3099
Cortone Acetate Injectable Suspension (Cortisone Acetate) Merck 2059
Cortone Acetate Tablets (Cortisone Acetate) Merck 2061
Decadron Elixir (Dexamethasone) Merck 2078
Decadron Tablets (Dexamethasone) Merck 2079
Decadron Phosphate Injection (Dexamethasone Sodium Phosphate) Merck 2081
Depo-Medrol Injectable Suspension (Methylprednisolone Acetate) Pharmacia & Upjohn 2795
Hydrocortone Tablets (Hydrocortisone) Merck 2106
Hydrocortone Phosphate Injection, Sterile (Hydrocortisone Sodium Phosphate) Merck 2105
Pediapred Oral Solution (Prednisolone Sodium Phosphate) Celltech 1170
Prednisone (Prednisone) Roxane 3064
Prelone Syrup (Prednisolone) Muro . 2273
Solu-Medrol Sterile Powder (Methylprednisolone Sodium Succinate) Pharmacia & Upjohn 2855

Dermatitis, herpetiformis
Dapsone Tablets USP (Dapsone) Jacobus 1780

Dermatitis, herpetiformis bullous
Celestone Soluspan Injectable Suspension (Betamethasone Acetate, Betamethasone Sodium Phosphate) Schering 3097
Celestone Syrup (Betamethasone) Schering 3099
Cortone Acetate Injectable Suspension (Cortisone Acetate) Merck 2059
Cortone Acetate Tablets (Cortisone Acetate) Merck 2061
Decadron Elixir (Dexamethasone) Merck 2078
Decadron Tablets (Dexamethasone) Merck 2079
Decadron Phosphate Injection (Dexamethasone Sodium Phosphate) Merck 2081
Depo-Medrol Injectable Suspension (Methylprednisolone Acetate) Pharmacia & Upjohn 2795
Hydrocortone Tablets (Hydrocortisone) Merck 2106
Hydrocortone Phosphate Injection, Sterile (Hydrocortisone Sodium Phosphate) Merck 2105
Pediapred Oral Solution (Prednisolone Sodium Phosphate) Celltech 1170
Prednisone (Prednisone) Roxane 3064
Prelone Syrup (Prednisolone) Muro . 2273
Solu-Medrol Sterile Powder (Methylprednisolone Sodium Succinate) Pharmacia & Upjohn 2855

Dermatitis, seborrheic
Capex Shampoo (Fluocinolone Acetonide) Galderma 1400
Cortaid Intensive Therapy Cream (Hydrocortisone) Pharmacia Consumer .... ▣717
Cortizone•10 (Hydrocortisone) Pfizer Inc., Warner-Lambert Healthcare .... ▣699
Cortizone•10 Plus Creme (Hydrocortisone) Pfizer Inc., Warner-Lambert Healthcare .... ▣700
Cortizone•10 Quick Shot Spray (Hydrocortisone) Pfizer Inc., Warner-Lambert Healthcare .... ▣699
Cortizone for Kids Creme (Hydrocortisone) Pfizer Inc., Warner-Lambert Healthcare .... ▣699
Head & Shoulders Intensive Treatment Dandruff and Seborrheic Dermatitis Shampoo (Selenium Sulfide) Procter & Gamble 2877
Nizoral 2% Cream (Ketoconazole) Janssen 3620
Plexion (Sodium Sulfacetamide, Sulfur) Medicis 2024
Selsun Rx 2.5% Lotion, USP (Selenium Sulfide) Ross 3053
Tegrin Dandruff Shampoo - Extra Conditioning (Coal Tar) Block .... ▣623
Tegrin Dandruff Shampoo - Fresh Herbal (Coal Tar) Block .... ▣624
Tegrin Skin Cream (Coal Tar) Block .... ▣624

Dermatitis, seborrheic, severe
Celestone Soluspan Injectable Suspension (Betamethasone Acetate, Betamethasone Sodium Phosphate) Schering 3097
Celestone Syrup (Betamethasone) Schering 3099
Cortone Acetate Injectable Suspension (Cortisone Acetate) Merck 2059
Cortone Acetate Tablets (Cortisone Acetate) Merck 2061
Decadron Elixir (Dexamethasone) Merck 2078
Decadron Tablets (Dexamethasone) Merck 2079
Decadron Phosphate Injection (Dexamethasone Sodium Phosphate) Merck 2081
Depo-Medrol Injectable Suspension (Methylprednisolone Acetate) Pharmacia & Upjohn 2795
Hydrocortone Tablets (Hydrocortisone) Merck 2106
Hydrocortone Phosphate Injection, Sterile (Hydrocortisone Sodium Phosphate) Merck 2105
Pediapred Oral Solution (Prednisolone Sodium Phosphate) Celltech 1170
Prednisone (Prednisone) Roxane 3064
Prelone Syrup (Prednisolone) Muro . 2273
Solu-Medrol Sterile Powder (Methylprednisolone Sodium Succinate) Pharmacia & Upjohn 2855

Dermatomyositis, possibly effective in
Potaba (Aminobenzoate Potassium) Glenwood 1721

Dermatomyositis, systemic
Celestone Syrup (Betamethasone) Schering 3099
Cortone Acetate Injectable Suspension (Cortisone Acetate) Merck 2059
Cortone Acetate Tablets (Cortisone Acetate) Merck 2061
Depo-Medrol Injectable Suspension (Methylprednisolone Acetate) Pharmacia & Upjohn 2795
Hydrocortone Tablets (Hydrocortisone) Merck 2106
Hydrocortone Phosphate Injection, Sterile (Hydrocortisone Sodium Phosphate) Merck 2105
Pediapred Oral Solution (Prednisolone Sodium Phosphate) Celltech 1170
Prednisone (Prednisone) Roxane 3064
Prelone Syrup (Prednisolone) Muro . 2273
Solu-Medrol Sterile Powder (Methylprednisolone Sodium Succinate) Pharmacia & Upjohn 2855

Dermatoses, corticosteroid-responsive
(*see also under* Skin, inflammatory conditions)
Aclovate (Alclometasone Dipropionate) Elan 1275
Clobevate Gel (Clobetasol Propionate) Stiefel 3271
Cordran Lotion (Flurandrenolide) Oclassen 2438
Cordran Tape (Flurandrenolide) Oclassen 2439
Cormax Cream (Clobetasol Propionate) Oclassen 2440
Cormax Ointment (Clobetasol Propionate) Oclassen 2440
Cormax Scalp Application (Clobetasol Propionate) Oclassen 2441
Cutivate Cream (Fluticasone Propionate) Elan 1282
Cutivate Ointment (Fluticasone Propionate) Elan 1284
Dermatop Emollient Cream (Prednicarbate) Ortho Dermatological .. 2517
DesOwen (Desonide) Galderma 1401
Diprolene Gel 0.05% (Betamethasone Dipropionate) Schering 3107
Diprolene Ointment 0.05% (Betamethasone Dipropionate) Schering 3108
Diprolene AF Cream 0.05% (Betamethasone Dipropionate) Schering 3106
Diprosone (Betamethasone Dipropionate) Schering 3109
Elocon Cream 0.1% (Mometasone Furoate) Schering 3110
Elocon Lotion 0.1% (Mometasone Furoate) Schering 3111
Elocon Ointment 0.1% (Mometasone Furoate) Schering 3112
Lidex (Fluocinonide) Medicis 2020
Locoid Cream (Hydrocortisone Butyrate) Ferndale 1341
Locoid Lipocream Cream (Hydrocortisone Butyrate) Ferndale 1342
Locoid (Hydrocortisone Butyrate) Ferndale 1341
Luxíq Foam (Betamethasone Valerate) Connetics 1210
Olux Foam (Clobetasol Propionate) Connetics 1211
Pramosone (Hydrocortisone Acetate, Pramoxine Hydrochloride) Ferndale 1343
Prelone Syrup (Prednisolone) Muro . 2273
ProctoFoam-HC (Hydrocortisone Acetate, Pramoxine Hydrochloride) Schwarz 3177
Psorcon E Cream (Diflorasone Diacetate) Dermik 1227
Psorcon E Ointment (Diflorasone Diacetate) Dermik 1228
Synalar (Fluocinolone Acetonide) Medicis 2020
Temovate Cream (Clobetasol Propionate) Elan 1301
Temovate Gel (Clobetasol Propionate) Elan 1303
Temovate Ointment (Clobetasol Propionate) Elan 1301
Temovate Scalp Application (Clobetasol Propionate) Elan 1304
Temovate E Emollient (Clobetasol Propionate) Elan 1302
Topicort (Desoximetasone) Medicis 2025
Ultravate Cream Bristol-Myers Squibb Dermatology 1119
Ultravate Ointment Bristol-Myers Squibb Dermatology 1120

Dermatoses, steroid-responsive, with secondary infection
Anusol-HC Cream 2.5% (Hydrocortisone) Monarch 2237

Dermographism
Periactin Tablets (Cyproheptadine Hydrochloride) Merck 2155
Phenergan Suppositories (Promethazine Hydrochloride) Wyeth-Ayerst 3556
Phenergan Syrup (Promethazine Hydrochloride) Wyeth-Ayerst 3554
Phenergan Tablets (Promethazine Hydrochloride) Wyeth-Ayerst 3556

Diabetes insipidus
DDAVP Injection 4 mcg/mL (Desmopressin Acetate) Aventis 737
DDAVP Nasal Spray (Desmopressin Acetate) Aventis 738
DDAVP Rhinal Tube (Desmopressin Acetate) Aventis 738
DDAVP Tablets (Desmopressin Acetate) Aventis 739
Desmopressin Acetate Injection (Desmopressin Acetate) Ferring ... 1344
Desmopressin Acetate Rhinal Tube (Desmopressin Acetate) Ferring 1345

Diabetes mellitus
(*see under* Hyperglycemia, control of, adjunct to diet)

Diabetes mellitus, insulin-dependent
Humalog (Insulin Lispro, Human) Lilly 1926
Humalog Mix 75/25 Pen (Insulin Lispro, Human, Insulin Lispro Protamine, Human) Lilly 1928
Humulin 50/50, 100 Units (Insulin, Human Regular and Human NPH Mixture) Lilly 1934
Humulin 70/30, 100 Units (Insulin, Human Regular and Human NPH Mixture) Lilly 1935
Humulin 70/30 Pen (Insulin, Human Regular and Human NPH Mixture) Lilly 1936
Humulin L, 100 Units (Insulin, Human, Zinc Suspension) Lilly 1937
Humulin N, 100 Units (Insulin, Human NPH) Lilly 1939
Humulin R Regular (U-500) (Insulin, Human Regular) Lilly 1943
Humulin R, 100 Units (Insulin, Human Regular) Lilly 1941
Humulin U, 100 Units (Insulin, Human, Zinc Suspension) Lilly 1943
Humulin N NPH Pen (Insulin, Human NPH) Lilly 1940
Iletin II, Lente (Pork), 100 Units (Insulin, Zinc Suspension) Lilly 1945
Iletin II, NPH (Pork), 100 Units (Insulin, NPH) Lilly 1946
Iletin II, Regular (Pork), 100 Units (Insulin, Regular) Lilly 1947
Lantus Injection (Insulin glargine) Aventis 742
Novolin 70/30 Human Insulin 10 ml Vials (Insulin, Human Regular and Human NPH Mixture) Novo Nordisk 2421
Novolin 70/30 PenFill (Insulin, Human Regular and Human NPH Mixture) Novo Nordisk 2423

Novolin 70/30 Prefilled Disposable Insulin Delivery System (Insulin, Human Regular and Human NPH Mixture) Novo Nordisk 2425
Novolin L Human Insulin 10 ml Vials (Insulin, Human, Zinc Suspension) Novo Nordisk.......... 2422
Novolin N Human Insulin 10 ml Vials (Insulin, Human NPH) Novo Nordisk 2422
Novolin N PenFill (Insulin, Human NPH) Novo Nordisk.......... 2423
Novolin N Prefilled Syringe Disposable Insulin Delivery System (Insulin, Human NPH) Novo Nordisk 2425
Novolin R Human Insulin 10 ml Vials (Insulin, Human Regular) Novo Nordisk 2423
Novolin R PenFill (Insulin, Human Regular) Novo Nordisk.......... 2423
Novolin R Prefilled Syringe Disposable Insulin Delivery System (Insulin, Human Regular) Novo Nordisk 2425
NovoLog Injection Novo Nordisk 2427
Velosulin BR Human Insulin 10 ml Vials (Insulin, Human Regular) Novo Nordisk 2435

Diabetes mellitus, non-insulin-dependent
Actos Tablets (Pioglitazone Hydrochloride) Takeda 3275
Amaryl Tablets (Glimepiride) Aventis 717
Avandia Tablets (Rosiglitazone Maleate) GlaxoSmithKline 1490
DiaBeta Tablets (Glyburide) Aventis . 741
Diabinese Tablets (Chlorpropamide) Pfizer 2680
Glucophage Tablets (Metformin Hydrochloride) Bristol-Myers Squibb 1080
Glucophage XR Tablets (Metformin Hydrochloride) Bristol-Myers Squibb 1080
Glucotrol Tablets (Glipizide) Pfizer 2692
Glucotrol XL Extended Release Tablets (Glipizide) Pfizer 2693
Glucovance Tablets (Glyburide, Metformin Hydrochloride) Bristol-Myers Squibb 1086
Glyset Tablets (Miglitol) Pharmacia & Upjohn 2821
Prandin Tablets (0.5, 1, and 2 mg) (Repaglinide) Novo Nordisk 2432
Precose Tablets (Acarbose) Bayer .. 906
Starlix Tablets (Nateglinide) Novartis 2401

Diabetic nephropathy
(*see under* Nephropathy, diabetic)

Diaper rash
(*see under* Rash, diaper)

Diarrhea, adjunctive therapy in
Imodium A-D Liquid and Caplets (Loperamide Hydrochloride) McNeil Consumer 2001
Imodium Advanced Caplets and Chewable Tablets (Loperamide Hydrochloride, Simethicone) McNeil Consumer 2001
Pedialyte Oral Electrolyte Maintenance Solution (Electrolyte Supplement) Ross 3049
Rehydralyte Oral Electrolyte Rehydration Solution (Electrolyte Supplement) Ross 3052

Diarrhea, bacterial
(*see under* Diarrhea, infectious)

Diarrhea, E. coli-induced
Bactrim (Sulfamethoxazole, Trimethoprim) Roche Laboratories 2949
Cipro (Ciprofloxacin) Bayer 887
Septra Suspension (Sulfamethoxazole, Trimethoprim) Monarch 2265
Septra Tablets (Sulfamethoxazole, Trimethoprim) Monarch 2265
Septra DS Tablets (Sulfamethoxazole, Trimethoprim) Monarch 2265

Diarrhea, infectious
Cipro (Ciprofloxacin) Bayer 887

Diarrhea, protozoal
(*see under* Diarrhea, infectious)

Diarrhea, symptomatic relief of
Donnagel Liquid (Attapulgite) Wyeth-Ayerst .... ▣789
Imodium A-D Liquid and Caplets (Loperamide Hydrochloride) McNeil Consumer 2001
Imodium Advanced Caplets and Chewable Tablets (Loperamide Hydrochloride, Simethicone) McNeil Consumer 2001
Motofen Tablets (Atropine Sulfate, Difenoxin Hydrochloride) Amarin... 577
Pepto-Bismol Maximum Strength Liquid (Bismuth Subsalicylate) Procter & Gamble.......... 2878
Pepto-Bismol Original Liquid, Original and Cherry Tablets and Easy-To-Swallow Caplets (Bismuth Subsalicylate) Procter & Gamble 2878

Diarrhea, traveler's
Bactrim (Sulfamethoxazole, Trimethoprim) Roche Laboratories.......... 2949
Imodium A-D Liquid and Caplets (Loperamide Hydrochloride) McNeil Consumer 2001
Septra Suspension (Sulfamethoxazole, Trimethoprim) Monarch.......... 2265
Septra Tablets (Sulfamethoxazole, Trimethoprim) Monarch.......... 2265
Septra DS Tablets (Sulfamethoxazole, Trimethoprim) Monarch.......... 2265

Diarrhea associated with vasoactive intestinal peptide tumors
Sandostatin Injection Novartis.......... 2394
Sandostatin LAR Depot (Octreotide Acetate) Novartis.......... 2395

Diet, supplementation of
Active Calcium Tablets (Calcium Citrate, Vitamin D) USANA 3335
ActoTherm Caplets (Herbals with Vitamins & Minerals) AdvoCare... ▣794
Advantin Capsules (Herbals, Multiple) AdvoCare .... ▣794
Aflexa Tablets (Glucosamine) McNeil Consumer 1997
Ag-Immune Capsules Body Wise.... ▣810
All-Basic Capsules (Amino Acid Preparations) Montiff 2268
Alluna Sleep Tablets (Valeriana officinalis) SmithKline Beecham Consumer.......... ▣837
Ambrotose Capsules Mannatech ... ▣819
Ambrotose Powder (Glucosamine Hydrochloride) Mannatech.......... ▣819
Ambrotose with Lecithin Capsules (Lecithin) Mannatech ... ▣819
Antioxidant Booster Caplets (Herbals with Vitamins & Minerals) AdvoCare .... ▣794
Beano (Alpha Galactosidase Enzyme) Block .... ▣809
Beta-C Tablets (Bioflavonoids, Allium sativum, Hesperidin Complex, Vitamin A, Vitamin C) Body Wise .... ▣811
Bevitamel Tablets (Folic Acid, Melatonin, Vitamin B_{12}) Westlake 3459
BioChoice Immune[26] Powder and Capsules (Egg Product) Legacy for Life .... ▣818
BioChoice Immune Support Powder (Vitamins with Minerals, Egg Product) Legacy for Life.......... ▣818
BioLean Capsules and Tablets (Amino Acid Preparations, Herbals, Multiple, Ephedra) Wellness International.......... ▣842
BioLean Accelerator Tablets (Amino Acid Preparations, Herbals, Multiple) Wellness International... ▣842
BioLean Free Tablets (Amino Acid Preparations, Ginkgo biloba, Ginseng) Wellness International .. ▣843
BioLean LipoTrim Capsules (Herbals with Minerals) Wellness International.......... ▣843
Biomune OSF Plus Capsules (Astragalus, Whey, Colostrum) Matol .... ▣820
Bios Life 2 Drink Mix (Fiber, Vitamins with Minerals) Unicity.......... 3321
BodyLean Powder (Amino Acid Preparations, Vitamins with Minerals) AdvoCare .... ▣795
Brite-Life Caplets (Hypericum, Vitamin B_6) AdvoCare.......... ▣795
Caltrate 600 Tablets (Calcium Carbonate) Lederle Consumer.... ▣814
Caltrate 600 PLUS (Calcium Carbonate, Vitamin D, Vitamins with Minerals) Lederle Consumer.......... ▣815
Caltrate 600 + D Tablets (Calcium Carbonate, Vitamin D) Lederle Consumer .... ▣814
Caltrate 600 + Soy Tablets (Calcium Carbonate) Lederle Consumer.......... ▣814
Cardio Essentials Capsules (Coenzyme Q-10) Unicity 3321
CardiOptima Drink Mix Packets (Amino Acid Preparations, Herbals with Vitamins & Minerals) AdvoCare .... ▣795
Catalyst Capsules (Amino Acid Preparations) AdvoCare .... ▣796
Centrum Echinacea Softgels (Echinacea angustifolia) Whitehall-Robins .... ▣852
Centrum Focused Formulas Bone Health Tablets (Minerals, Multiple, Vitamin D) Lederle Consumer.......... ▣815
Centrum Focused Formulas Energy Tablets (Ginseng, Vitamin B Complex) Lederle Consumer.......... ▣816
Centrum Focused Formulas Heart Tablets (Coenzyme Q-10, Allium sativum, Vitamins with Minerals) Lederle Consumer ...... ▣816
Centrum Focused Formulas Mental Clarity Tablets (Ginkgo biloba, Vitamins with Minerals) Lederle Consumer.......... ▣816
Centrum Focused Formulas Prostate Softgels (Serenoa repens, Vitamin A) Lederle Consumer .... ▣816
Centrum Ginkgo Biloba Softgels (Ginkgo biloba) Whitehall-Robins .... ▣852
Centrum Ginseng Softgels (Ginseng) Whitehall-Robins .... ▣853
Centrum Kids Complete Children's Chewables (Vitamins with Minerals) Lederle Consumer .... ▣817
Centrum Performance Multivitamin-Multimineral Tablets (Vitamins with Minerals) Lederle Consumer .... ▣817
Centrum Saw Palmetto Softgels (Serenoa repens) Whitehall-Robins .... ▣853
Centrum St. John's Wort Softgels (Hypericum) Whitehall-Robins .... ▣853
Centrum Tablets (Vitamins with Minerals) Lederle Consumer .... ▣815
Centrum Silver Tablets (Vitamins with Minerals) Lederle Consumer .... ▣818
C-Grams Caplets (Vitamin C) AdvoCare .... ▣795
Chelated Mineral Tablets (Minerals, Multiple) USANA 3335
Coffeccino Beverage Mix AdvoCare .... ▣796
Cold Season Nutrition Booster Capsules (Astragalus, Herbals, Multiple, Echinacea) AdvoCare ... ▣796
CoQuinone Capsules (Coenzyme Q-10, Lipoic Acid) USANA 3335
CorePlex Capsules (Allium sativum, Ginkgo biloba, Herbals with Vitamins & Minerals) AdvoCare .... ▣796
D-Cal Chewable Caplets (Calcium Carbonate, Vitamin D) A & Z Pharm .... ▣794
DHEA Plus Capsules (Dehydroepiandrosterone (DHEA), Ginkgo biloba) Wellness International ...... ▣844
Fat Metabolizer + Capsules (Herbals with Minerals) Youngevity .... ▣854
FemEssence Capsules AdvoCare .. ▣796
Fiber 10 Packets (Carboxymethylcellulose Sodium, Lactobacillus Acidophilus, Psyllium Preparations, Herbals, Multiple) AdvoCare .... ▣797
Food for Thought Drink Mix (Amino Acid Preparations, Vitamins with Minerals) Wellness International .... ▣844
Ginkoba Tablets (Ginkgo biloba) Pharmaton .... ▣828
Ginkoba M/E Suppli-Cap Capsules (Ginkgo biloba, Ginseng) Pharmaton .... ▣829
Ginsana Sport Capsules Pharmaton .... ▣831
Gluca-Balance Capsules (Amino Acid Preparations) Montiff 2269
HGH-Turn Back the Hands of Time Capsules (Amino Acid Preparations, Minerals, Multiple) Youngevity .... ▣854
Immunocal Powder Sachets (Whey Protein Isolate) Immunotec 1766
IMUPlus Formula (Whey Protein Isolate) Swiss Bioceutical 3274
Intelectol Tablets (Vinpocetine) Covex .... ▣813
IntelleQ Capsules (Amino Acid Preparations, Ginkgo biloba, Herbals with Vitamins) AdvoCare .... ▣797
Lipoflavonoid Caplets (Bioflavonoids, Vitamins, Multiple) Numark .... ▣828
LipoTrol Caplets AdvoCare .... ▣797
Macro-Mineral Complex Caplets (Herbals with Vitamins & Minerals) AdvoCare .... ▣797
Mass Appeal Tablets (Amino Acid Preparations) Wellness International.......... ▣845
Mega Antioxidant Tablets (Vitamins, Multiple) USANA 3335
Metabolic Nutrition System (Herbals with Vitamins & Minerals, Hypericum, Ginseng, Ephedra) AdvoCare.......... ▣798
MetaBoost Caplets AdvoCare.......... ▣798
Metamucil Dietary Fiber Supplement (Psyllium Preparations) Procter & Gamble.......... ▣834
Meyenberg Goat Milk (Goat Milk) Meyenberg.......... ▣823
Movana Tablets (Hypericum) Pharmaton .... ▣832
One-A-Day Bedtime & Rest Tablets (Calcium Carbonate, Valeriana officinalis, Herbals with Minerals, Kava-Kava) Bayer Consumer .... ▣805
One-A-Day Cholesterol Health Tablets (Allium sativum, Herbals with Vitamins, Vitamin E) Bayer Consumer .... ▣805
One-A-Day Energy Formula Tablets (Chromium Picolinate, Ginseng, Vitamin B Complex) Bayer Consumer .... ▣806
One-A-Day Joint Health Tablets (Glucosamine Sulfate, Herbals with Vitamins) Bayer Consumer .. ▣806
One-A-Day Memory & Concentration Tablets (Choline, Ginkgo biloba, Vitamin B_6, Vitamin B_{12}) Bayer Consumer .... ▣807
One-A-Day Menopause Health Tablets (Black Cohosh, Lecithin, Vitamin E) Bayer Consumer .... ▣808
One-A-Day Prostate Health Softgels (Serenoa repens, Zinc, Pumpkin) Bayer Consumer .... ▣808
One-A-Day Tension & Mood Softgels (Hypericum, Vitamin B Complex With Vitamin C, Kava-Kava) Bayer Consumer .... ▣808
Perfect Meal (Amino Acid Preparations, Lactobacillus Acidophilus, Vitamins with Minerals) AdvoCare .... ▣798
Performance Gold Caplets (Golden Root, Ginseng, Whey) AdvoCare .... ▣798
Performance Optimizer System (Amino Acid Preparations, Herbals with Vitamins & Minerals, Serenoa repens, Ginseng, Herbals, Multiple) AdvoCare .... ▣798
Peridin-C Tablets (Bioflavonoids, Hesperidin Complex, Hesperidin Methyl Chalcone, Vitamin C) Beutlich .... ▣618
PhytAloe Capsules (Aloe vera, Herbals, Multiple) Mannatech .... ▣819
PhytAloe Powder (Aloe vera, Herbals, Multiple) Mannatech .... ▣819
Phyto-Vite Tablets (Bioflavonoids, Ginkgo biloba, Herbals with Vitamins & Minerals) Wellness International .... ▣849
Probiotica Tablets (Lactobacillus Reuteri) McNeil Consumer 2008
Proflavanol Tablets (Dietary Supplement) USANA 3335
ProForm Bars AdvoCare .... ▣799
ProMotion Capsules (Glucosamine Hydrochloride) AdvoCare .... ▣800
Prostatonin Softgel Capsules (Herbals, Multiple) Pharmaton .... ▣832
Proxeed Powder (Acetyl-L-Carnitine Hydrochloride, Levocarnitine Fumarate, Citric Acid) Sigma-Tau .... ▣835
Pro-Xtreme Drink Mix (Amino Acid Preparations) Wellness International .... ▣845
Remifemin Menopause Tablets (Black Cohosh) SmithKline Beecham Consumer .... ▣839
ReSource Wellness AllerPro Capsules (Herbals, Multiple) Novartis Consumer .... ▣824
ReSource Wellness CalciWise Soft Chews (Calcium Carbonate, Vitamins with Minerals) Novartis Consumer .... ▣824
ReSource Wellness EnVigor Caplets (Ginkgo biloba, Herbals with Vitamins & Minerals, Ginseng) Novartis Consumer .... ▣824

ReSource Wellness FlexTend Caplets (Glucosamine Sulfate, Vitamins with Minerals) Novartis Consumer ▣825
ReSource Wellness ForSight Caplets (Dicalcium Phosphate, Vitamins with Minerals) Novartis Consumer ▣825
ReSource Wellness MemorAble Softgels (Ginkgo biloba, Lecithin, Herbals with Vitamins) Novartis Consumer ▣825
ReSource Wellness ResistEx Capsules (Ginseng, Echinacea) Novartis Consumer ▣826
ReSource Wellness 2nd Wind Capsules (Ginseng) Novartis Consumer ▣826
ReSource Wellness StayCalm Caplets (Valeriana officinalis, Herbals with Vitamins & Minerals, Hypericum) Novartis Consumer ▣826
ReSource Wellness VeinTain Caplets (Herbals with Vitamins & Minerals) Novartis Consumer ▣827
ProBiotic Restore Capsules (Lactobacillus Acidophilus) AdvoCare ▣799
Right Choice A.M. Multi Formula Caplets (Herbals with Vitamins) Body Wise ▣811
Right Choice P.M. Multi Formula Caplets (Minerals, Multiple) Body Wise ▣812
Satiete Tablets (Amino Acid Preparations, Ginkgo biloba, Herbals with Vitamins & Minerals, Hypericum) Wellness International ▣846
Second Look Capsules AdvoCare ▣800
Slow-Mag Tablets (Calcium Carbonate, Magnesium Chloride) Shire ▣835
Spark! Beverage Mix (Amino Acid Preparations, Vitamins with Minerals) AdvoCare ▣800
StePHan Clarity Capsules (Amino Acid Preparations, Ginkgo biloba, Herbals with Vitamins) Wellness International ▣844
StePHan Elasticity Capsules (Amino Acid Preparations, Herbals with Vitamins & Minerals) Wellness International ▣847
StePHan Elixir Capsules (Amino Acid Preparations, Ginkgo biloba, Herbals with Vitamins & Minerals) Wellness International ▣848
StePHan Essential Capsules (Amino Acid Preparations, Vitamins with Minerals) Wellness International ▣848
StePHan Feminine Capsules (Amino Acid Preparations, Vitamin E) Wellness International ▣848
StePHan Flexibility Capsules (Amino Acid Preparations, Vitamins with Minerals) Wellness International ▣848
StePHan Lovpil Capsules (Amino Acid Preparations, Herbals with Vitamins & Minerals) Wellness International ▣849
StePHan Masculine Capsules (Amino Acid Preparations, Herbals with Minerals) Wellness International ▣849
StePHan Protector Capsules (Amino Acid Preparations, Astragalus) Wellness International ▣850
StePHan Relief Capsules (Amino Acid Preparations, Psyllium Preparations, Herbals with Vitamins) Wellness International ▣850
StePHan Tranquility Capsules (Amino Acid Preparations, Valeriana officinalis, Herbals with Vitamins & Minerals) Wellness International ▣851
Super Anti-Oxidant Cell Protector Capsules (Herbals, Multiple) Youngevity ▣854
Super Food Soy Shake (Amino Acid Preparations, Herbals with Vitamins & Minerals, Lactobacillus Acidophilus) Youngevity ▣854
SuperEPA 2000 Softgels (Docosahexaenoic Acid (DHA), EPA (Eicosapentaenoic Acid)) Advanced Nutritional 526
Sure2Endure Tablets (Herbals with Vitamins & Minerals, Glucosamine Hydrochloride) Wellness International ▣851
System 3-4-3 Capsules (Allium sativum, Herbals with Vitamins & Minerals, Lactobacillus Acidophilus, Psyllium Preparations, Senna, Herbals, Multiple, Echinacea) AdvoCare ▣800
Thermo-E Caplets (Herbals with Vitamins & Minerals, Ephedra) AdvoCare ▣801
Thermo-G Caplets AdvoCare ▣801
Transfer Factor Capsules (Colostrum) 4Life ▣814
Ultra Zn Tablets (Herbals, Multiple) Advanced Nutritional 526
Venastat Suppli-Cap Capsules (Horse Chestnut Seed Extract) Pharmaton ▣833
Vitamist Intra-Oral Spray (Vitamins with Minerals) Mayor ▣821
Winrgy Drink Mix (Amino Acid Preparations, Vitamins with Minerals) Wellness International ▣852
Wobenzym Tablets Marlyn 1997
ZZZ Spray Liquid (5-hydroxytryptophan, Herbals with Vitamins & Minerals, Melatonin) AdvoCare ▣801

Digestive disorders, symptomatic relief of
Arco-Lase Tablets (Amylase, Cellulase, Lipase, Protease) Arco 592
Arco-Lase Plus Tablets (Amylase, Cellulase, Hyoscyamine Sulfate, Lipase, Phenobarbital, Protease) Arco 592
DDS-Acidophilus Capsules, Tablets, and Powder (Lactobacillus Acidophilus) UAS Labs ▣767

Digestive insufficiencies, symptomatic relief of
Arco-Lase Tablets (Amylase, Cellulase, Lipase, Protease) Arco 592
Arco-Lase Plus Tablets (Amylase, Cellulase, Hyoscyamine Sulfate, Lipase, Phenobarbital, Protease) Arco 592

Digoxin intoxication, life-threatening
Digibind Powder (Digoxin Immune Fab (Ovine)) GlaxoSmithKline 1514

Diphtheria
(*see under* C. diphtheriae infections)

Diphtheroid endocarditis
Vancocin HCl, Vials & ADD-Vantage (Vancomycin Hydrochloride) Lilly 1970

Diplococcus pneumoniae infections
(*see under* S. pneumoniae infections)

Diuresis, induction of in edema due to lupus erythematosus
Celestone Syrup (Betamethasone) Schering 3099
Cortone Acetate Injectable Suspension (Cortisone Acetate) Merck 2059
Cortone Acetate Tablets (Cortisone Acetate) Merck 2061
Decadron Elixir (Dexamethasone) Merck 2078
Decadron Tablets (Dexamethasone) Merck 2079
Decadron Phosphate Injection (Dexamethasone Sodium Phosphate) Merck 2081
Depo-Medrol Injectable Suspension (Methylprednisolone Acetate) Pharmacia & Upjohn 2795
Hydrocortone Tablets (Hydrocortisone) Merck 2106
Hydrocortone Phosphate Injection, Sterile (Hydrocortisone Sodium Phosphate) Merck 2105
Pediapred Oral Solution (Prednisolone Sodium Phosphate) Celltech 1170
Prednisone (Prednisone) Roxane 3064
Prelone Syrup (Prednisolone) Muro 2273
Solu-Medrol Sterile Powder (Methylprednisolone Sodium Succinate) Pharmacia & Upjohn 2855

Diuresis, induction of in nephrotic syndrome
Celestone Syrup (Betamethasone) Schering 3099
Cortone Acetate Injectable Suspension (Cortisone Acetate) Merck 2059
Cortone Acetate Tablets (Cortisone Acetate) Merck 2061
Decadron Elixir (Dexamethasone) Merck 2078
Decadron Tablets (Dexamethasone) Merck 2079
Decadron Phosphate Injection (Dexamethasone Sodium Phosphate) Merck 2081
Depo-Medrol Injectable Suspension (Methylprednisolone Acetate) Pharmacia & Upjohn 2795
Hydrocortone Tablets (Hydrocortisone) Merck 2106
Hydrocortone Phosphate Injection, Sterile (Hydrocortisone Sodium Phosphate) Merck 2105
Pediapred Oral Solution (Prednisolone Sodium Phosphate) Celltech 1170
Prednisone (Prednisone) Roxane 3064
Prelone Syrup (Prednisolone) Muro 2273
Solu-Medrol Sterile Powder (Methylprednisolone Sodium Succinate) Pharmacia & Upjohn 2855

Donovania granulomatis infection
(*see under* Granuloma inguinale)

Drowsiness, symptomatic relief of
Vivarin (Caffeine) SmithKline Beecham Consumer ▣763

Ductus arteriosus, patent, palliative maintenance
Indocin I.V. (Indomethacin Sodium Trihydrate) Merck 2115

Dukes' stage C colon cancer
(*see under* Carcinoma, colon, Dukes' stage C, adjunctive treatment in)

Duodenal ulcers, active, short-term treatment of
Aciphex Tablets (Rabeprazole Sodium) Eisai 1267
Aciphex Tablets (Rabeprazole Sodium) Janssen 1783
Axid Pulvules (Nizatidine) Lilly 1903
Axid Pulvules (Nizatidine) Reliant 2919
Carafate Suspension (Sucralfate) Aventis 731
Carafate Tablets (Sucralfate) Aventis 730
Famotidine Injection (Famotidine) Baxter Anesthesia 866
Pepcid Injection (Famotidine) Merck 2153
Pepcid for Oral Suspension (Famotidine) Merck 2150
Pepcid RPD Orally Disintegrating Tablets (Famotidine) Merck 2150
Pepcid Tablets (Famotidine) Merck 2150
Prevacid Delayed-Release Capsules (Lansoprazole) TAP 3292
Prilosec Delayed-Release Capsules (Omeprazole) AstraZeneca LP 628
Tagamet (Cimetidine Hydrochloride) GlaxoSmithKline 1644
Zantac (Ranitidine Hydrochloride) GlaxoSmithKline 1690
Zantac Injection (Ranitidine Hydrochloride) GlaxoSmithKline 1688
Zantac Syrup (Ranitidine Hydrochloride) GlaxoSmithKline 1690

Duodenal ulcers, adjunctive therapy for
Donnatal (Atropine Sulfate, Hyoscyamine Sulfate, Phenobarbital, Scopolamine Hydrobromide) Robins 2929
Donnatal Extentabs (Atropine Sulfate, Hyoscyamine Sulfate, Phenobarbital, Scopolamine Hydrobromide) Robins 2930
Donnatal Tablets (Atropine Sulfate, Hyoscyamine Sulfate, Phenobarbital, Scopolamine Hydrobromide) Robins 2929

Duodenal ulcers, maintenance therapy for
Axid Pulvules (Nizatidine) Lilly 1903
Axid Pulvules (Nizatidine) Reliant 2919
Carafate Tablets (Sucralfate) Aventis 730
Famotidine Injection (Famotidine) Baxter Anesthesia 866
Pepcid Injection (Famotidine) Merck 2153
Pepcid for Oral Suspension (Famotidine) Merck 2150
Pepcid RPD Orally Disintegrating Tablets (Famotidine) Merck 2150
Pepcid Tablets (Famotidine) Merck 2150
Prevacid Delayed-Release Capsules (Lansoprazole) TAP 3292
Tagamet (Cimetidine Hydrochloride) GlaxoSmithKline 1644
Zantac (Ranitidine Hydrochloride) GlaxoSmithKline 1690

Duodenal ulcers, to reduce the risk of recurrence
Prilosec Delayed-Release Capsules (Omeprazole) AstraZeneca LP 628

Dysbetalipoproteinemia
Atromid-S Capsules (Clofibrate) Wyeth-Ayerst 3483
Lipitor Tablets (Atorvastatin Calcium) Parke-Davis 2639
Lipitor Tablets (Atorvastatin Calcium) Pfizer 2696

Dysentery, amoebic
(*see under* Amebiasis, acute intestinal)

Dysmenorrhea, primary
Anaprox Tablets (Naproxen Sodium) Roche Laboratories 2967
Anaprox DS Tablets (Naproxen Sodium) Roche Laboratories 2967
Cataflam Tablets (Diclofenac Potassium) Novartis 2315
EC-Naprosyn Delayed-Release Tablets (Naproxen) Roche Laboratories 2967
Motrin Suspension, Oral Drops, Chewable Tablets, and Caplets (Ibuprofen) McNeil Consumer 2002
Naprelan Tablets (Naproxen Sodium) Elan 1293
Naprosyn Suspension (Naproxen) Roche Laboratories 2967
Naprosyn Tablets (Naproxen) Roche Laboratories 2967
Orudis Capsules (Ketoprofen) Wyeth-Ayerst 3548
Ponstel Capsules (Mefenamic Acid) First Horizon 1356
Vioxx (Rofecoxib) Merck 2213

Dyspepsia
(*see under* Digestive disorders, symptomatic relief of)

Dysphoric disorder, premenstrual
Sarafem Pulvules (Fluoxetine Hydrochloride) Lilly 1962

Dystonia, cervical
Botox Purified Neurotoxin Complex (Botulinum Toxin Type A) Allergan 549
Myobloc Injectable Solution (Botulinum Toxin Type B) Elan 1291

E

E. cloacae gynecologic infections
Azactam for Injection (Aztreonam) Elan 1276
Timentin Injection- ADD-Vantage Vial (Clavulanate Potassium, Ticarcillin Disodium) GlaxoSmithKline 1661
Timentin Injection-Galaxy Container (Clavulanate Potassium, Ticarcillin Disodium) GlaxoSmithKline 1664
Timentin Injection-Pharmacy Bulk Package (Clavulanate Potassium, Ticarcillin Disodium) GlaxoSmithKline 1666
Timentin for Intravenous Administration (Clavulanate Potassium, Ticarcillin Disodium) GlaxoSmithKline 1658

E. coli biliary tract infections
Ancef for Injection (Cefazolin Sodium) GlaxoSmithKline 1474
Ancef Injection (Cefazolin Sodium) GlaxoSmithKline 1474
Kefzol Vials, ADD-Vantage (Cefazolin Sodium) Lilly 1951

E. coli bone and joint infections
Nebcin Vials, Hyporets & ADD-Vantage (Tobramycin Sulfate) Lilly 1955
Rocephin Injectable Vials, ADD-Vantage, Galaxy, Bulk (Ceftriaxone Sodium) Roche Laboratories 2993

E. coli central nervous system infections
Claforan Injection (Cefotaxime Sodium) Aventis 732

E. coli genital infections
Ancef for Injection (Cefazolin Sodium) GlaxoSmithKline 1474
Ancef Injection (Cefazolin Sodium) GlaxoSmithKline 1474

E. coli gynecological infections
Azactam for Injection (Aztreonam) Elan ... 1276
Cefizox for Intramuscular or Intravenous Use (Ceftizoxime Sodium) Fujisawa ... 1390
Cefobid Intravenous/Intramuscular (Cefoperazone) Pfizer ... 2671
Cefobid Pharmacy Bulk Package - Not for Direct Infusion (Cefoperazone Sodium) Pfizer ... 2673
Cefotan (Cefotetan) AstraZeneca ... 664
Ceptaz for Injection (Ceftazidime) GlaxoSmithKline ... 1499
Claforan Injection (Cefotaxime Sodium) Aventis ... 732
Fortaz (Ceftazidime Sodium) GlaxoSmithKline ... 1541
Mefoxin for Injection (Cefoxitin Sodium) Merck ... 2124
Mefoxin Premixed Intravenous Solution (Cefoxitin Sodium) Merck ... 2127
Primaxin I.M. (Cilastatin Sodium, Imipenem) Merck ... 2158
Primaxin I.V. (Cilastatin Sodium, Imipenem) Merck ... 2160
Tazicef for Injection (Ceftazidime) GlaxoSmithKline ... 1647
Tazicef Galaxy Container (Ceftazidime Sodium) GlaxoSmithKline ... 1650
Tazicef Pharmacy Bulk Package (Ceftazidime) GlaxoSmithKline ... 1653
Tazidime Vials, Faspak & ADD-Vantage (Ceftazidime) Lilly ... 1966
Timentin Injection- ADD-Vantage Vial (Clavulanate Potassium, Ticarcillin Disodium) GlaxoSmithKline ... 1661
Timentin Injection-Galaxy Container (Clavulanate Potassium, Ticarcillin Disodium) GlaxoSmithKline ... 1664
Timentin Injection-Pharmacy Bulk Package (Clavulanate Potassium, Ticarcillin Disodium) GlaxoSmithKline ... 1666
Timentin for Intravenous Administration (Clavulanate Potassium, Ticarcillin Disodium) GlaxoSmithKline ... 1658
Unasyn for Injection (Ampicillin Sodium, Sulbactam Sodium) Pfizer ... 2728
Zosyn (Piperacillin Sodium, Tazobactam Sodium) Lederle ... 1890
Zosyn in Galaxy Containers (Piperacillin Sodium, Tazobactam Sodium) Lederle ... 1894

E. coli infections
Amoxil Chewable Tablets (Amoxicillin) GlaxoSmithKline ... 1471
Amoxil for Oral Suspension (Amoxicillin) GlaxoSmithKline ... 1471
Amoxil (Amoxicillin) GlaxoSmithKline ... 1471
Ancef for Injection (Cefazolin Sodium) GlaxoSmithKline ... 1474
Ancef Injection (Cefazolin Sodium) GlaxoSmithKline ... 1474
Augmentin Chewable Tablets (Amoxicillin, Clavulanate Potassium) GlaxoSmithKline ... 1482
Augmentin Powder for Oral Suspension (Amoxicillin, Clavulanate Potassium) GlaxoSmithKline ... 1482
Augmentin Tablets (Amoxicillin, Clavulanate Potassium) GlaxoSmithKline ... 1485
Azactam for Injection (Aztreonam) Elan ... 1276
Bactrim (Sulfamethoxazole, Trimethoprim) Roche Laboratories ... 2949
Ceclor (Cefaclor) Lilly ... 1905
Cefizox for Intramuscular or Intravenous Use (Ceftizoxime Sodium) Fujisawa ... 1390
Cefobid Intravenous/Intramuscular (Cefoperazone) Pfizer ... 2671
Cefobid Pharmacy Bulk Package - Not for Direct Infusion (Cefoperazone Sodium) Pfizer ... 2673
Cefotan (Cefotetan) AstraZeneca ... 664
Ceftin Tablets (Cefuroxime Axetil) Lifecycle Ventures ... 1898
Ceptaz for Injection (Ceftazidime) GlaxoSmithKline ... 1499
Cipro I.V. (Ciprofloxacin) Bayer ... 893
Cipro I.V. Pharmacy Bulk Package (Ciprofloxacin) Bayer ... 897
Cipro (Ciprofloxacin) Bayer ... 887
Claforan Injection (Cefotaxime Sodium) Aventis ... 732
Declomycin Tablets (Demeclocycline Hydrochloride) Lederle ... 1855
Doryx Coated Pellet Filled Capsules (Doxycycline Hyclate) Warner Chilcott ... 3357
Duricef (Cefadroxil) Bristol-Myers Squibb ... 1079
Dynacin Capsules (Minocycline Hydrochloride) Medicis ... 2019
Floxin I.V. (Ofloxacin) Ortho-McNeil ... 2526
Floxin Tablets (Ofloxacin) Ortho-McNeil ... 2529
Fortaz (Ceftazidime Sodium) GlaxoSmithKline ... 1541
Geocillin Tablets (Carbenicillin Indanyl Sodium) Pfizer ... 2687
Keflex (Cephalexin) Dista ... 1237
Kefurox Vials, ADD-Vantage (Cefuroxime Sodium) Lilly ... 1948
Kefzol Vials, ADD-Vantage (Cefazolin Sodium) Lilly ... 1951
Levaquin (Levofloxacin) Ortho-McNeil ... 2537
Lorabid Suspension and Pulvules (Loracarbef) Monarch ... 2251
Macrobid Capsules (Nitrofurantoin Monohydrate) Procter & Gamble Pharmaceuticals ... 2889
Macrodantin Capsules (Nitrofurantoin) Procter & Gamble Pharmaceuticals ... 2891
Mandol Vials (Cefamandole Nafate) Lilly ... 1953
Maxipime for Injection (Cefepime Hydrochloride) Elan ... 1285
Mefoxin for Injection (Cefoxitin Sodium) Merck ... 2124
Mefoxin Premixed Intravenous Solution (Cefoxitin Sodium) Merck ... 2127
Merrem I.V. (Meropenem) AstraZeneca ... 673
Minocin Intravenous (Minocycline Hydrochloride) Lederle ... 1862
Minocin Oral Suspension (Minocycline Hydrochloride) Lederle ... 1865
Minocin Pellet-Filled Capsules (Minocycline Hydrochloride) Lederle ... 1863
Monodox Capsules (Doxycycline Monohydrate) Oclassen ... 2442
Monurol Sachet (Fosfomycin Tromethamine) Forest ... 1375
Nebcin Vials, Hyporets & ADD-Vantage (Tobramycin Sulfate) Lilly ... 1955
Noroxin Tablets (Norfloxacin) Merck ... 2145
Pfizerpen for Injection (Penicillin G Potassium) Pfizer ... 2707
Pipracil (Piperacillin Sodium) Lederle ... 1866
Primaxin I.M. (Cilastatin Sodium, Imipenem) Merck ... 2158
Primaxin I.V. (Cilastatin Sodium, Imipenem) Merck ... 2160
Rocephin Injectable Vials, ADD-Vantage, Galaxy, Bulk (Ceftriaxone Sodium) Roche Laboratories ... 2993
Septra Suspension (Sulfamethoxazole, Trimethoprim) Monarch ... 2265
Septra Tablets (Sulfamethoxazole, Trimethoprim) Monarch ... 2265
Septra DS Tablets (Sulfamethoxazole, Trimethoprim) Monarch ... 2265
Suprax (Cefixime) Lederle ... 1877
Tazicef for Injection (Ceftazidime) GlaxoSmithKline ... 1647
Tazicef Galaxy Container (Ceftazidime Sodium) GlaxoSmithKline ... 1650
Tazicef Pharmacy Bulk Package (Ceftazidime) GlaxoSmithKline ... 1653
Tazidime Vials, Faspak & ADD-Vantage (Ceftazidime) Lilly ... 1966
Timentin Injection- ADD-Vantage Vial (Clavulanate Potassium, Ticarcillin Disodium) GlaxoSmithKline ... 1661
Timentin Injection-Galaxy Container (Clavulanate Potassium, Ticarcillin Disodium) GlaxoSmithKline ... 1664
Timentin Injection-Pharmacy Bulk Package (Clavulanate Potassium, Ticarcillin Disodium) GlaxoSmithKline ... 1666
Timentin for Intravenous Administration (Clavulanate Potassium, Ticarcillin Disodium) GlaxoSmithKline ... 1658
Trovan (Alatrofloxacin Mesylate) Pfizer ... 2722
Unasyn for Injection (Ampicillin Sodium, Sulbactam Sodium) Pfizer ... 2728
Vantin Tablets and Oral Suspension (Cefpodoxime Proxetil) Pharmacia & Upjohn ... 2860
Vibramycin Calcium Oral Suspension Syrup (Doxycycline Calcium) Pfizer ... 2735
Vibramycin Hyclate Capsules (Doxycycline Hyclate) Pfizer ... 2735
Vibramycin Hyclate Intravenous (Doxycycline Hyclate) Pfizer ... 2737
Vibramycin Monohydrate for Oral Suspension (Doxycycline Monohydrate) Pfizer ... 2735
Vibra-Tabs Film Coated Tablets (Doxycycline Hyclate) Pfizer ... 2735
Zinacef Injection (Cefuroxime) GlaxoSmithKline ... 1696
Zinacef for Injection (Cefuroxime) GlaxoSmithKline ... 1696
Zosyn (Piperacillin Sodium, Tazobactam Sodium) Lederle ... 1890
Zosyn in Galaxy Containers (Piperacillin Sodium, Tazobactam Sodium) Lederle ... 1894

E. coli infections, ocular
Blephamide Ophthalmic Ointment (Prednisolone Acetate, Sulfacetamide Sodium) Allergan ... 547
Blephamide Ophthalmic Suspension (Prednisolone Acetate, Sulfacetamide Sodium) Allergan ... 548
Chloromycetin Ophthalmic Ointment, 1% (Chloramphenicol) Monarch ... ⊙296
Chloromycetin Ophthalmic Solution (Chloramphenicol) Monarch ... ⊙297
Chloroptic Sterile Ophthalmic Ointment (Chloramphenicol) Allergan ... ⊙234
Cortisporin Ophthalmic Suspension (Hydrocortisone, Neomycin Sulfate, Polymyxin B Sulfate, Hydrocortisone, Neomycin Sulfate, Polymyxin B Sulfate) Monarch ... ⊙297
FML-S Liquifilm Sterile Ophthalmic Suspension (Fluorometholone, Sulfacetamide Sodium) Allergan ... ⊙238
Genoptic Ophthalmic Ointment (Gentamicin Sulfate) Allergan ... ⊙239
Genoptic Sterile Ophthalmic Solution (Gentamicin Sulfate) Allergan ... ⊙239
NeoDecadron Sterile Ophthalmic Solution (Dexamethasone Sodium Phosphate, Neomycin Sulfate) Merck ... 2144
Poly-Pred Liquifilm Ophthalmic Suspension (Neomycin Sulfate, Polymyxin B Sulfate, Prednisolone Acetate) Allergan ... ⊙245
Pred-G Ophthalmic Suspension (Gentamicin Sulfate, Prednisolone Acetate) Allergan ... ⊙247
Pred-G Sterile Ophthalmic Ointment (Gentamicin Sulfate, Prednisolone Acetate) Allergan ... ⊙248
Terra-Cortril Ophthalmic Suspension (Hydrocortisone Acetate, Oxytetracycline Hydrochloride) Pfizer ... 2716
TobraDex Ophthalmic Ointment (Dexamethasone, Tobramycin) Alcon ... 542
TobraDex Ophthalmic Suspension (Dexamethasone, Tobramycin) Alcon ... 541

E. coli intra-abdominal infections
Azactam for Injection (Aztreonam) Elan ... 1276
Cefizox for Intramuscular or Intravenous Use (Ceftizoxime Sodium) Fujisawa ... 1390
Cefobid Intravenous/Intramuscular (Cefoperazone) Pfizer ... 2671
Cefobid Pharmacy Bulk Package - Not for Direct Infusion (Cefoperazone Sodium) Pfizer ... 2673
Cefotan (Cefotetan) AstraZeneca ... 664
Ceptaz for Injection (Ceftazidime) GlaxoSmithKline ... 1499
Cipro I.V. (Ciprofloxacin) Bayer ... 893
Cipro I.V. Pharmacy Bulk Package (Ciprofloxacin) Bayer ... 897
Cipro (Ciprofloxacin) Bayer ... 887
Claforan Injection (Cefotaxime Sodium) Aventis ... 732
Fortaz (Ceftazidime Sodium) GlaxoSmithKline ... 1541
Maxipime for Injection (Cefepime Hydrochloride) Elan ... 1285
Mefoxin for Injection (Cefoxitin Sodium) Merck ... 2124
Mefoxin Premixed Intravenous Solution (Cefoxitin Sodium) Merck ... 2127
Merrem I.V. (Meropenem) AstraZeneca ... 673
Nebcin Vials, Hyporets & ADD-Vantage (Tobramycin Sulfate) Lilly ... 1955
Pipracil (Piperacillin Sodium) Lederle ... 1866
Primaxin I.M. (Cilastatin Sodium, Imipenem) Merck ... 2158
Primaxin I.V. (Cilastatin Sodium, Imipenem) Merck ... 2160
Rocephin Injectable Vials, ADD-Vantage, Galaxy, Bulk (Ceftriaxone Sodium) Roche Laboratories ... 2993
Tazicef for Injection (Ceftazidime) GlaxoSmithKline ... 1647
Tazicef Galaxy Container (Ceftazidime Sodium) GlaxoSmithKline ... 1650
Tazicef Pharmacy Bulk Package (Ceftazidime) GlaxoSmithKline ... 1653
Tazidime Vials, Faspak & ADD-Vantage (Ceftazidime) Lilly ... 1966
Timentin Injection- ADD-Vantage Vial (Clavulanate Potassium, Ticarcillin Disodium) GlaxoSmithKline ... 1661
Timentin Injection-Galaxy Container (Clavulanate Potassium, Ticarcillin Disodium) GlaxoSmithKline ... 1664
Timentin Injection-Pharmacy Bulk Package (Clavulanate Potassium, Ticarcillin Disodium) GlaxoSmithKline ... 1666
Timentin for Intravenous Administration (Clavulanate Potassium, Ticarcillin Disodium) GlaxoSmithKline ... 1658
Trovan (Alatrofloxacin Mesylate) Pfizer ... 2722
Unasyn for Injection (Ampicillin Sodium, Sulbactam Sodium) Pfizer ... 2728

E. coli lower respiratory tract infections
Azactam for Injection (Aztreonam) Elan ... 1276
Cefizox for Intramuscular or Intravenous Use (Ceftizoxime Sodium) Fujisawa ... 1390
Cefotan (Cefotetan) AstraZeneca ... 664
Ceptaz for Injection (Ceftazidime) GlaxoSmithKline ... 1499
Cipro I.V. (Ciprofloxacin) Bayer ... 893
Cipro I.V. Pharmacy Bulk Package (Ciprofloxacin) Bayer ... 897
Cipro (Ciprofloxacin) Bayer ... 887
Claforan Injection (Cefotaxime Sodium) Aventis ... 732
Fortaz (Ceftazidime Sodium) GlaxoSmithKline ... 1541
Kefurox Vials, ADD-Vantage (Cefuroxime Sodium) Lilly ... 1948
Mefoxin for Injection (Cefoxitin Sodium) Merck ... 2124
Mefoxin Premixed Intravenous Solution (Cefoxitin Sodium) Merck ... 2127
Nebcin Vials, Hyporets & ADD-Vantage (Tobramycin Sulfate) Lilly ... 1955
Pipracil (Piperacillin Sodium) Lederle ... 1866
Primaxin I.V. (Cilastatin Sodium, Imipenem) Merck ... 2160
Rocephin Injectable Vials, ADD-Vantage, Galaxy, Bulk (Ceftriaxone Sodium) Roche Laboratories ... 2993
Tazicef for Injection (Ceftazidime) GlaxoSmithKline ... 1647
Tazicef Galaxy Container (Ceftazidime Sodium) GlaxoSmithKline ... 1650
Tazicef Pharmacy Bulk Package (Ceftazidime) GlaxoSmithKline ... 1653
Tazidime Vials, Faspak & ADD-Vantage (Ceftazidime) Lilly ... 1966
Trovan (Alatrofloxacin Mesylate) Pfizer ... 2722
Zinacef Injection (Cefuroxime) GlaxoSmithKline ... 1696
Zinacef for Injection (Cefuroxime) GlaxoSmithKline ... 1696

E. coli meningitis
Rocephin Injectable Vials, ADD-Vantage, Galaxy, Bulk (Ceftriaxone Sodium) Roche Laboratories ... 2993

E. coli peritonitis
Cefobid Intravenous/Intramuscular (Cefoperazone) Pfizer ... 2671
Cefobid Pharmacy Bulk Package - Not for Direct Infusion (Cefoperazone Sodium) Pfizer ... 2673
Ceptaz for Injection (Ceftazidime) GlaxoSmithKline ... 1499
Fortaz (Ceftazidime Sodium) GlaxoSmithKline ... 1541
Mandol Vials (Cefamandole Nafate) Lilly ... 1953
Mefoxin for Injection (Cefoxitin Sodium) Merck ... 2124
Mefoxin Premixed Intravenous Solution (Cefoxitin Sodium) Merck ... 2127
Merrem I.V. (Meropenem) AstraZeneca ... 673

Nebcin Vials, Hyporets & ADD-Vantage (Tobramycin Sulfate) Lilly 1955
Tazidime Vials, Faspak & ADD-Vantage (Ceftazidime) Lilly 1966
Timentin Injection- ADD-Vantage Vial (Clavulanate Potassium, Ticarcillin Disodium) GlaxoSmithKline 1661
Timentin Injection-Galaxy Container (Clavulanate Potassium, Ticarcillin Disodium) GlaxoSmithKline 1664
Timentin Injection-Pharmacy Bulk Package (Clavulanate Potassium, Ticarcillin Disodium) GlaxoSmithKline 1666
Timentin for Intravenous Administration (Clavulanate Potassium, Ticarcillin Disodium) GlaxoSmithKline 1658
Zosyn (Piperacillin Sodium, Tazobactam Sodium) Lederle 1890
Zosyn in Galaxy Containers (Piperacillin Sodium, Tazobactam Sodium) Lederle 1894

E. coli prostatitis
Ancef for Injection (Cefazolin Sodium) GlaxoSmithKline 1474
Ancef Injection (Cefazolin Sodium) GlaxoSmithKline 1474
Cipro I.V. (Ciprofloxacin) Bayer 893
Cipro I.V. Pharmacy Bulk Package (Ciprofloxacin) Bayer 897
Cipro (Ciprofloxacin) Bayer 887
Floxin I.V. (Ofloxacin) Ortho-McNeil 2526
Floxin Tablets (Ofloxacin) Ortho-McNeil 2529
Geocillin Tablets (Carbenicillin Indanyl Sodium) Pfizer 2687
Keflex (Cephalexin) Dista 1237
Noroxin Tablets (Norfloxacin) Merck 2145

E. coli respiratory tract infections
Cefobid Intravenous/Intramuscular (Cefoperazone) Pfizer 2671
Cefobid Pharmacy Bulk Package - Not for Direct Infusion (Cefoperazone Sodium) Pfizer 2673

E. coli septicemia
Ancef for Injection (Cefazolin Sodium) GlaxoSmithKline 1474
Ancef Injection (Cefazolin Sodium) GlaxoSmithKline 1474
Azactam for Injection (Aztreonam) Elan 1276
Cefizox for Intramuscular or Intravenous Use (Ceftizoxime Sodium) Fujisawa 1390
Cefobid Intravenous/Intramuscular (Cefoperazone) Pfizer 2671
Cefobid Pharmacy Bulk Package - Not for Direct Infusion (Cefoperazone Sodium) Pfizer 2673
Ceptaz for Injection (Ceftazidime) GlaxoSmithKline 1499
Cipro I.V. (Ciprofloxacin) Bayer 893
Claforan Injection (Cefotaxime Sodium) Aventis 732
Fortaz (Ceftazidime Sodium) GlaxoSmithKline 1541
Kefurox Vials, ADD-Vantage (Cefuroxime Sodium) Lilly 1948
Kefzol Vials, ADD-Vantage (Cefazolin Sodium) Lilly 1951
Mefoxin for Injection (Cefoxitin Sodium) Merck 2124
Mefoxin Premixed Intravenous Solution (Cefoxitin Sodium) Merck 2127
Nebcin Vials, Hyporets & ADD-Vantage (Tobramycin Sulfate) Lilly 1955
Pfizerpen for Injection (Penicillin G Potassium) Pfizer 2707
Primaxin I.V. (Cilastatin Sodium, Imipenem) Merck 2160
Rocephin Injectable Vials, ADD-Vantage, Galaxy, Bulk (Ceftriaxone Sodium) Roche Laboratories 2993
Tazicef for Injection (Ceftazidime) GlaxoSmithKline 1647
Tazicef Galaxy Container (Ceftazidime Sodium) GlaxoSmithKline 1650
Tazicef Pharmacy Bulk Package (Ceftazidime) GlaxoSmithKline 1653
Tazidime Vials, Faspak & ADD-Vantage (Ceftazidime) Lilly 1966
Timentin Injection- ADD-Vantage Vial (Clavulanate Potassium, Ticarcillin Disodium) GlaxoSmithKline 1661
Timentin Injection-Galaxy Container (Clavulanate Potassium, Ticarcillin Disodium) GlaxoSmithKline 1664
Timentin Injection-Pharmacy Bulk Package (Clavulanate Potassium, Ticarcillin Disodium) GlaxoSmithKline 1666
Timentin for Intravenous Administration (Clavulanate Potassium, Ticarcillin Disodium) GlaxoSmithKline 1658
Zinacef Injection (Cefuroxime) GlaxoSmithKline 1696
Zinacef for Injection (Cefuroxime) GlaxoSmithKline 1696

E. coli skin and skin structure infections
Amoxil Chewable Tablets (Amoxicillin) GlaxoSmithKline 1471
Amoxil for Oral Suspension (Amoxicillin) GlaxoSmithKline 1471
Amoxil (Amoxicillin) GlaxoSmithKline 1471
Augmentin Chewable Tablets (Amoxicillin, Clavulanate Potassium) GlaxoSmithKline 1482
Augmentin Powder for Oral Suspension (Amoxicillin, Clavulanate Potassium) GlaxoSmithKline 1482
Augmentin Tablets (Amoxicillin, Clavulanate Potassium) GlaxoSmithKline 1485
Azactam for Injection (Aztreonam) Elan 1276
Cefizox for Intramuscular or Intravenous Use (Ceftizoxime Sodium) Fujisawa 1390
Cefotan (Cefotetan) AstraZeneca 664
Ceptaz for Injection (Ceftazidime) GlaxoSmithKline 1499
Cipro I.V. (Ciprofloxacin) Bayer 893
Cipro I.V. Pharmacy Bulk Package (Ciprofloxacin) Bayer 897
Cipro (Ciprofloxacin) Bayer 887
Claforan Injection (Cefotaxime Sodium) Aventis 732
Fortaz (Ceftazidime Sodium) GlaxoSmithKline 1541
Kefurox Vials, ADD-Vantage (Cefuroxime Sodium) Lilly 1948
Mandol Vials (Cefamandole Nafate) Lilly 1953
Mefoxin for Injection (Cefoxitin Sodium) Merck 2124
Mefoxin Premixed Intravenous Solution (Cefoxitin Sodium) Merck 2127
Nebcin Vials, Hyporets & ADD-Vantage (Tobramycin Sulfate) Lilly 1955
Pipracil (Piperacillin Sodium) Lederle 1866
Primaxin I.M. (Cilastatin Sodium, Imipenem) Merck 2158
Primaxin I.V. (Cilastatin Sodium, Imipenem) Merck 2160
Rocephin Injectable Vials, ADD-Vantage, Galaxy, Bulk (Ceftriaxone Sodium) Roche Laboratories 2993
Tazicef for Injection (Ceftazidime) GlaxoSmithKline 1647
Tazicef Galaxy Container (Ceftazidime Sodium) GlaxoSmithKline 1650
Tazicef Pharmacy Bulk Package (Ceftazidime) GlaxoSmithKline 1653
Tazidime Vials, Faspak & ADD-Vantage (Ceftazidime) Lilly 1966
Timentin Injection- ADD-Vantage Vial (Clavulanate Potassium, Ticarcillin Disodium) GlaxoSmithKline 1661
Timentin Injection-Galaxy Container (Clavulanate Potassium, Ticarcillin Disodium) GlaxoSmithKline 1664
Timentin Injection-Pharmacy Bulk Package (Clavulanate Potassium, Ticarcillin Disodium) GlaxoSmithKline 1666
Timentin for Intravenous Administration (Clavulanate Potassium, Ticarcillin Disodium) GlaxoSmithKline 1658
Trovan (Alatrofloxacin Mesylate) Pfizer 2722
Unasyn for Injection (Ampicillin Sodium, Sulbactam Sodium) Pfizer 2728
Zinacef Injection (Cefuroxime) GlaxoSmithKline 1696
Zinacef for Injection (Cefuroxime) GlaxoSmithKline 1696

E. coli urinary tract infections
Ancef for Injection (Cefazolin Sodium) GlaxoSmithKline 1474
Ancef Injection (Cefazolin Sodium) GlaxoSmithKline 1474
Augmentin Chewable Tablets (Amoxicillin, Clavulanate Potassium) GlaxoSmithKline 1482
Augmentin Powder for Oral Suspension (Amoxicillin, Clavulanate Potassium) GlaxoSmithKline 1482
Augmentin Tablets (Amoxicillin, Clavulanate Potassium) GlaxoSmithKline 1485
Azactam for Injection (Aztreonam) Elan 1276
Bactrim (Sulfamethoxazole, Trimethoprim) Roche Laboratories 2949
Ceclor (Cefaclor) Lilly 1905
Cefizox for Intramuscular or Intravenous Use (Ceftizoxime Sodium) Fujisawa 1390
Cefobid Intravenous/Intramuscular (Cefoperazone) Pfizer 2671
Cefobid Pharmacy Bulk Package - Not for Direct Infusion (Cefoperazone Sodium) Pfizer 2673
Cefotan (Cefotetan) AstraZeneca 664
Ceftin Tablets (Cefuroxime Axetil) Lifecycle Ventures 1898
Ceptaz for Injection (Ceftazidime) GlaxoSmithKline 1499
Cipro I.V. (Ciprofloxacin) Bayer 893
Cipro I.V. Pharmacy Bulk Package (Ciprofloxacin) Bayer 897
Cipro (Ciprofloxacin) Bayer 887
Claforan Injection (Cefotaxime Sodium) Aventis 732
Duricef (Cefadroxil) Bristol-Myers Squibb 1079
Floxin I.V. (Ofloxacin) Ortho-McNeil 2526
Floxin Tablets (Ofloxacin) Ortho-McNeil 2529
Fortaz (Ceftazidime Sodium) GlaxoSmithKline 1541
Geocillin Tablets (Carbenicillin Indanyl Sodium) Pfizer 2687
Keflex (Cephalexin) Dista 1237
Kefurox Vials, ADD-Vantage (Cefuroxime Sodium) Lilly 1948
Kefzol Vials, ADD-Vantage (Cefazolin Sodium) Lilly 1951
Levaquin (Levofloxacin) Ortho-McNeil 2537
Lorabid Suspension and Pulvules (Loracarbef) Monarch 2251
Macrobid Capsules (Nitrofurantoin Monohydrate) Procter & Gamble Pharmaceuticals 2889
Macrodantin Capsules (Nitrofurantoin) Procter & Gamble Pharmaceuticals 2891
Mandol Vials (Cefamandole Nafate) Lilly 1953
Maxipime for Injection (Cefepime Hydrochloride) Elan 1285
Mefoxin for Injection (Cefoxitin Sodium) Merck 2124
Mefoxin Premixed Intravenous Solution (Cefoxitin Sodium) Merck 2127
Monurol Sachet (Fosfomycin Tromethamine) Forest 1375
Nebcin Vials, Hyporets & ADD-Vantage (Tobramycin Sulfate) Lilly 1955
Noroxin Tablets (Norfloxacin) Merck 2145
Pipracil (Piperacillin Sodium) Lederle 1866
Primaxin I.V. (Cilastatin Sodium, Imipenem) Merck 2160
Rocephin Injectable Vials, ADD-Vantage, Galaxy, Bulk (Ceftriaxone Sodium) Roche Laboratories 2993
Septra Suspension (Sulfamethoxazole, Trimethoprim) Monarch 2265
Septra Tablets (Sulfamethoxazole, Trimethoprim) Monarch 2265
Septra DS Tablets (Sulfamethoxazole, Trimethoprim) Monarch 2265
Streptomycin Sulfate Injection (Streptomycin Sulfate) Pfizer 2714
Suprax (Cefixime) Lederle 1877
Tazicef for Injection (Ceftazidime) GlaxoSmithKline 1647
Tazicef Galaxy Container (Ceftazidime Sodium) GlaxoSmithKline 1650
Tazicef Pharmacy Bulk Package (Ceftazidime) GlaxoSmithKline 1653
Tazidime Vials, Faspak & ADD-Vantage (Ceftazidime) Lilly 1966
Tequin Injection (Gatifloxacin) Bristol-Myers Squibb 1110
Tequin Tablets (Gatifloxacin) Bristol-Myers Squibb 1110
Timentin Injection- ADD-Vantage Vial (Clavulanate Potassium, Ticarcillin Disodium) GlaxoSmithKline 1661
Timentin Injection-Galaxy Container (Clavulanate Potassium, Ticarcillin Disodium) GlaxoSmithKline 1664
Timentin Injection-Pharmacy Bulk Package (Clavulanate Potassium, Ticarcillin Disodium) GlaxoSmithKline 1666
Timentin for Intravenous Administration (Clavulanate Potassium, Ticarcillin Disodium) GlaxoSmithKline 1658
Vantin Tablets and Oral Suspension (Cefpodoxime Proxetil) Pharmacia & Upjohn 2860
Zinacef Injection (Cefuroxime) GlaxoSmithKline 1696
Zinacef for Injection (Cefuroxime) GlaxoSmithKline 1696

E. coli-induced diarrhea
(*see under* Diarrhea, E. coli-induced)

Ear, infection
(*see under* Otitis externa; Otitis media, acute)

Ear wax removal
(*see under* Cerumen, removal of)

Echinococcus granulosus infections
Albenza Tablets (Albendazole) GlaxoSmithKline 1463

Eczema, unspecified
(*see under* Skin, inflammatory conditions)

Edema, adjunctive therapy in
Demadex Tablets and Injection (Torsemide) Roche Laboratories 2965
Diamox (Acetazolamide Sodium) Lederle .... ⊙269
Diucardin Tablets (Hydroflumethiazide) Wyeth-Ayerst 3494
Diuril Oral (Chlorothiazide) Merck 2087
Diuril Sodium Intravenous (Chlorothiazide Sodium) Merck 2086
Dyazide Capsules (Hydrochlorothiazide, Triamterene) GlaxoSmithKline 1515
Dyrenium Capsules (Triamterene) WellSpring 3458
Edecrin (Ethacrynic Acid) Merck 2091
Furosemide Tablets (Furosemide) Mylan 2284
HydroDIURIL Tablets (Hydrochlorothiazide) Merck 2108
Indapamide Tablets (Indapamide) Mylan 2286
Maxzide (Hydrochlorothiazide, Triamterene) Bertek 1008
Microzide Capsules (Hydrochlorothiazide) Watson 3414
Renese Tablets (Polythiazide) Pfizer 2712
Zaroxolyn Tablets (Metolazone) Celltech 1177

Edema, cerebral
Decadron Tablets (Dexamethasone) Merck 2079
Decadron Phosphate Injection (Dexamethasone Sodium Phosphate) Merck 2081

Edema, corneal, temporary relief of
Muro 128 Sterile Ophthalmic Ointment (Sodium Chloride) Bausch & Lomb .... ⊙262
Muro 128 Sterile Ophthalmic Solution 2% and 5% (Sodium Chloride) Bausch & Lomb .... ⊙262

Electrolytes, depletion of
Pedialyte Oral Electrolyte Maintenance Solution (Electrolyte Supplement) Ross 3049
Rehydralyte Oral Electrolyte Rehydration Solution (Electrolyte Supplement) Ross 3052

Embolism, atrial fibrillation with
(*see under* Atrial fibrillation with embolism)

Embolism, peripheral arterial
Heparin Sodium Injection (Heparin Sodium) Wyeth-Ayerst 3511

Embolism, pulmonary
Activase I.V. (Alteplase, Recombinant) Genentech 1410
Coumadin for Injection (Warfarin Sodium) DuPont 1243
Coumadin Tablets (Warfarin Sodium) DuPont 1243
Heparin Sodium Injection (Heparin Sodium) Wyeth-Ayerst 3511
Lovenox Injection (Enoxaparin) Aventis 746
Warfarin Sodium Tablets, USP (Warfarin Sodium) Taro 3302

Embolism, pulmonary, acute, lysis of
Activase I.V. (Alteplase, Recombinant) Genentech ... 1410
Streptase for Infusion (Streptokinase) AstraZeneca LP ... 647

Embolism, pulmonary, prophylaxis of
Coumadin for Injection (Warfarin Sodium) DuPont ... 1243
Coumadin Tablets (Warfarin Sodium) DuPont ... 1243
Warfarin Sodium Tablets, USP (Warfarin Sodium) Taro ... 3302

Embolism, systemic, post-myocardial infarction, prophylaxis
Coumadin for Injection (Warfarin Sodium) DuPont ... 1243
Coumadin Tablets (Warfarin Sodium) DuPont ... 1243
Warfarin Sodium Tablets, USP (Warfarin Sodium) Taro ... 3302

Emphysema
Atrovent Inhalation Aerosol (Ipratropium Bromide) Boehringer Ingelheim ... 1030
Brethine Ampuls (Terbutaline Sulfate) Novartis ... 2314
Brethine Tablets (Terbutaline Sulfate) Novartis ... 2313
Pima Syrup (Potassium Iodide) Fleming ... 1362
Uniphyl 400 mg and 600 mg Tablets (Theophylline) Purdue Frederick ... 2903

Emphysema, panacinar, due to congenital Alpha1-antitrypsin deficiency
Prolastin (Alpha[1] -Proteinase Inhibitor (Human)) Bayer Biological ... 943

Empyema
Cleocin HCl Capsules (Clindamycin Hydrochloride) Pharmacia & Upjohn ... 2784
Cleocin Phosphate Sterile Solution (Clindamycin Phosphate) Pharmacia & Upjohn ... 2785
Pfizerpen for Injection (Penicillin G Potassium) Pfizer ... 2707

Endocarditis, bacterial
Ancef for Injection (Cefazolin Sodium) GlaxoSmithKline ... 1474
Ancef Injection (Cefazolin Sodium) GlaxoSmithKline ... 1474
Kefzol Vials, ADD-Vantage (Cefazolin Sodium) Lilly ... 1951
Pfizerpen for Injection (Penicillin G Potassium) Pfizer ... 2707
Primaxin I.V. (Cilastatin Sodium, Imipenem) Merck ... 2160
Vancocin HCl, Vials & ADD-Vantage (Vancomycin Hydrochloride) Lilly ... 1970

Endocarditis, bacterial, prophylaxis
Erythrocin Stearate Filmtab Tablets (Erythromycin Stearate) Abbott ... 452
Erythromycin Base Filmtab Tablets (Erythromycin) Abbott ... 454
Erythromycin Delayed-Release Capsules, USP (Erythromycin) Abbott ... 455
Pfizerpen for Injection (Penicillin G Potassium) Pfizer ... 2707
Vancocin HCl, Vials & ADD-Vantage (Vancomycin Hydrochloride) Lilly ... 1970

Endocarditis, erysipeloid
Pfizerpen for Injection (Penicillin G Potassium) Pfizer ... 2707

Endocarditis, fungal
Ancobon Capsules (Flucytosine) ICN ... 1730

Endocarditis, gonorrheal
Pfizerpen for Injection (Penicillin G Potassium) Pfizer ... 2707

Endocrine adenomas, multiple (*see also under* Hypersecretory conditions, pathological)
Famotidine Injection (Famotidine) Baxter Anesthesia ... 866
Pepcid Injection (Famotidine) Merck ... 2153
Pepcid for Oral Suspension (Famotidine) Merck ... 2150
Pepcid RPD Orally Disintegrating Tablets (Famotidine) Merck ... 2150
Pepcid Tablets (Famotidine) Merck ... 2150
Prilosec Delayed-Release Capsules (Omeprazole) AstraZeneca LP ... 628
Tagamet (Cimetidine Hydrochloride) GlaxoSmithKline ... 1644

Endocrine disorders
Celestone Soluspan Injectable Suspension (Betamethasone Acetate, Betamethasone Sodium Phosphate) Schering ... 3097
Celestone Syrup (Betamethasone) Schering ... 3099
Cortone Acetate Injectable Suspension (Cortisone Acetate) Merck ... 2059
Cortone Acetate Tablets (Cortisone Acetate) Merck ... 2061
Decadron Elixir (Dexamethasone) Merck ... 2078
Decadron Tablets (Dexamethasone) Merck ... 2079
Decadron Phosphate Injection (Dexamethasone Sodium Phosphate) Merck ... 2081
Depo-Medrol Injectable Suspension (Methylprednisolone Acetate) Pharmacia & Upjohn ... 2795
Hydrocortone Tablets (Hydrocortisone) Merck ... 2106
Hydrocortone Phosphate Injection, Sterile (Hydrocortisone Sodium Phosphate) Merck ... 2105
Pediapred Oral Solution (Prednisolone Sodium Phosphate) Celltech ... 1170
Prednisone (Prednisone) Roxane ... 3064
Prelone Syrup (Prednisolone) Muro ... 2273
Solu-Medrol Sterile Powder (Methylprednisolone Sodium Succinate) Pharmacia & Upjohn ... 2855

Endometrial hyperplasia
Provera Tablets (Medroxyprogesterone Acetate) Pharmacia & Upjohn ... 2853

Endometrial hyperplasia, prevention of
Prometrium Capsules (100 mg, 200 mg) (Progesterone) Solvay ... 3261

Endometrial thinning, prior to endometrial ablation
Zoladex (Goserelin Acetate) AstraZeneca ... 702

Endometriosis
Aygestin Tablets (Norethindrone Acetate) ESI Lederle ... 1333
Lupron Depot 3.75 mg (Leuprolide Acetate) TAP ... 3281
Lupron Depot–3 Month 11.25 mg (Leuprolide Acetate) TAP ... 3285
Synarel Nasal Solution for Endometriosis (Nafarelin Acetate) Searle ... 3205
Timentin Injection-Galaxy Container (Clavulanate Potassium, Ticarcillin Disodium) GlaxoSmithKline ... 1664
Zoladex (Goserelin Acetate) AstraZeneca ... 702

Endometritis (*see also under* Infections, gynecologic)
Azactam for Injection (Aztreonam) Elan ... 1276
Cefobid Intravenous/Intramuscular (Cefoperazone) Pfizer ... 2671
Cefobid Pharmacy Bulk Package - Not for Direct Infusion (Cefoperazone Sodium) Pfizer ... 2673
Ceptaz for Injection (Ceftazidime) GlaxoSmithKline ... 1499
Claforan Injection (Cefotaxime Sodium) Aventis ... 732
Cleocin HCl Capsules (Clindamycin Hydrochloride) Pharmacia & Upjohn ... 2784
Cleocin Phosphate Sterile Solution (Clindamycin Phosphate) Pharmacia & Upjohn ... 2785
Fortaz (Ceftazidime Sodium) GlaxoSmithKline ... 1541
Mefoxin for Injection (Cefoxitin Sodium) Merck ... 2124
Mefoxin Premixed Intravenous Solution (Cefoxitin Sodium) Merck ... 2127
Pipracil (Piperacillin Sodium) Lederle ... 1866
Tazicef for Injection (Ceftazidime) GlaxoSmithKline ... 1647
Tazicef Galaxy Container (Ceftazidime Sodium) GlaxoSmithKline ... 1650
Tazicef Pharmacy Bulk Package (Ceftazidime) GlaxoSmithKline ... 1653
Tazidime Vials, Faspak & ADD-Vantage (Ceftazidime) Lilly ... 1966
Timentin Injection- ADD-Vantage Vial (Clavulanate Potassium, Ticarcillin Disodium) GlaxoSmithKline ... 1661
Timentin Injection-Pharmacy Bulk Package (Clavulanate Potassium, Ticarcillin Disodium) GlaxoSmithKline ... 1666
Timentin for Intravenous Administration (Clavulanate Potassium, Ticarcillin Disodium) GlaxoSmithKline ... 1658

Endomyometritis
Primaxin I.M. (Cilastatin Sodium, Imipenem) Merck ... 2158
Trovan (Alatrofloxacin Mesylate) Pfizer ... 2722

Entamoeba histolytica (*see under* Amebiasis, acute intestinal)

Enteritis
Septra Suspension (Sulfamethoxazole, Trimethoprim) Monarch ... 2265
Septra Tablets (Sulfamethoxazole, Trimethoprim) Monarch ... 2265
Septra DS Tablets (Sulfamethoxazole, Trimethoprim) Monarch ... 2265

Enteritis, regional, systemic therapy for
Celestone Soluspan Injectable Suspension (Betamethasone Acetate, Betamethasone Sodium Phosphate) Schering ... 3097
Celestone Syrup (Betamethasone) Schering ... 3099
Cortone Acetate Injectable Suspension (Cortisone Acetate) Merck ... 2059
Cortone Acetate Tablets (Cortisone Acetate) Merck ... 2061
Decadron Elixir (Dexamethasone) Merck ... 2078
Decadron Tablets (Dexamethasone) Merck ... 2079
Decadron Phosphate Injection (Dexamethasone Sodium Phosphate) Merck ... 2081
Depo-Medrol Injectable Suspension (Methylprednisolone Acetate) Pharmacia & Upjohn ... 2795
Hydrocortone Tablets (Hydrocortisone) Merck ... 2106
Hydrocortone Phosphate Injection, Sterile (Hydrocortisone Sodium Phosphate) Merck ... 2105
Pediapred Oral Solution (Prednisolone Sodium Phosphate) Celltech ... 1170
Prednisone (Prednisone) Roxane ... 3064
Prelone Syrup (Prednisolone) Muro ... 2273
Solu-Medrol Sterile Powder (Methylprednisolone Sodium Succinate) Pharmacia & Upjohn ... 2855

Enterobacter aerogenes infections
Declomycin Tablets (Demeclocycline Hydrochloride) Lederle ... 1855
Doryx Coated Pellet Filled Capsules (Doxycycline Hyclate) Warner Chilcott ... 3357
Dynacin Capsules (Minocycline Hydrochloride) Medicis ... 2019
Floxin I.V. (Ofloxacin) Ortho-McNeil ... 2526
Floxin Tablets (Ofloxacin) Ortho-McNeil ... 2529
Minocin Intravenous (Minocycline Hydrochloride) Lederle ... 1862
Minocin Oral Suspension (Minocycline Hydrochloride) Lederle ... 1865
Minocin Pellet-Filled Capsules (Minocycline Hydrochloride) Lederle ... 1863
Monodox Capsules (Doxycycline Monohydrate) Oclassen ... 2442
Noroxin Tablets (Norfloxacin) Merck ... 2145
Pfizerpen for Injection (Penicillin G Potassium) Pfizer ... 2707
Rocephin Injectable Vials, ADD-Vantage, Galaxy, Bulk (Ceftriaxone Sodium) Roche Laboratories ... 2993
Vibramycin Calcium Oral Suspension Syrup (Doxycycline Calcium) Pfizer ... 2735
Vibramycin Hyclate Capsules (Doxycycline Hyclate) Pfizer ... 2735
Vibramycin Hyclate Intravenous (Doxycycline Hyclate) Pfizer ... 2737
Vibramycin Monohydrate for Oral Suspension (Doxycycline Monohydrate) Pfizer ... 2735
Vibra-Tabs Film Coated Tablets (Doxycycline Hyclate) Pfizer ... 2735

Enterobacter aerogenes infections, ocular
Genoptic Ophthalmic Ointment (Gentamicin Sulfate) Allergan ... ⊙239
Genoptic Sterile Ophthalmic Solution (Gentamicin Sulfate) Allergan ... ⊙239
Pred-G Ophthalmic Suspension (Gentamicin Sulfate, Prednisolone Acetate) Allergan ... ⊙247
Pred-G Sterile Ophthalmic Ointment (Gentamicin Sulfate, Prednisolone Acetate) Allergan ... ⊙248
TobraDex Ophthalmic Ointment (Dexamethasone, Tobramycin) Alcon ... 542
TobraDex Ophthalmic Suspension (Dexamethasone, Tobramycin) Alcon ... 541

Enterobacter aerogenes lower respiratory tract infections
Rocephin Injectable Vials, ADD-Vantage, Galaxy, Bulk (Ceftriaxone Sodium) Roche Laboratories ... 2993

Enterobacter aerogenes urinary tract infections
Floxin I.V. (Ofloxacin) Ortho-McNeil ... 2526
Floxin Tablets (Ofloxacin) Ortho-McNeil ... 2529
Noroxin Tablets (Norfloxacin) Merck ... 2145

Enterobacter cloacae bone and joint infections
Cipro I.V. (Ciprofloxacin) Bayer ... 893
Cipro I.V. Pharmacy Bulk Package (Ciprofloxacin) Bayer ... 897
Cipro (Ciprofloxacin) Bayer ... 887

Enterobacter cloacae infections
Azactam for Injection (Aztreonam) Elan ... 1276
Cipro I.V. (Ciprofloxacin) Bayer ... 893
Cipro I.V. Pharmacy Bulk Package (Ciprofloxacin) Bayer ... 897
Cipro (Ciprofloxacin) Bayer ... 887
Levaquin (Levofloxacin) Ortho-McNeil ... 2537
Noroxin Tablets (Norfloxacin) Merck ... 2145
Primaxin I.M. (Cilastatin Sodium, Imipenem) Merck ... 2158
Rocephin Injectable Vials, ADD-Vantage, Galaxy, Bulk (Ceftriaxone Sodium) Roche Laboratories ... 2993
Timentin Injection- ADD-Vantage Vial (Clavulanate Potassium, Ticarcillin Disodium) GlaxoSmithKline ... 1661
Timentin Injection-Galaxy Container (Clavulanate Potassium, Ticarcillin Disodium) GlaxoSmithKline ... 1664
Timentin Injection-Pharmacy Bulk Package (Clavulanate Potassium, Ticarcillin Disodium) GlaxoSmithKline ... 1666
Timentin for Intravenous Administration (Clavulanate Potassium, Ticarcillin Disodium) GlaxoSmithKline ... 1658

Enterobacter cloacae infections, ocular
Ocuflox Ophthalmic Solution (Ofloxacin) Allergan ... 554

Enterobacter cloacae lower respiratory tract infections
Cipro I.V. (Ciprofloxacin) Bayer ... 893
Cipro I.V. Pharmacy Bulk Package (Ciprofloxacin) Bayer ... 897
Cipro (Ciprofloxacin) Bayer ... 887

Enterobacter cloacae skin and skin structure infections
Cipro I.V. (Ciprofloxacin) Bayer ... 893
Cipro I.V. Pharmacy Bulk Package (Ciprofloxacin) Bayer ... 897
Cipro (Ciprofloxacin) Bayer ... 887
Primaxin I.M. (Cilastatin Sodium, Imipenem) Merck ... 2158
Rocephin Injectable Vials, ADD-Vantage, Galaxy, Bulk (Ceftriaxone Sodium) Roche Laboratories ... 2993

Enterobacter cloacae urinary tract infections
Azactam for Injection (Aztreonam) Elan ... 1276
Cipro I.V. (Ciprofloxacin) Bayer ... 893
Cipro I.V. Pharmacy Bulk Package (Ciprofloxacin) Bayer ... 897
Cipro (Ciprofloxacin) Bayer ... 887

Levaquin (Levofloxacin) Ortho-McNeil ... 2537
Noroxin Tablets (Norfloxacin) Merck ... 2145
Timentin Injection- ADD-Vantage Vial (Clavulanate Potassium, Ticarcillin Disodium) GlaxoSmithKline ... 1661
Timentin Injection-Galaxy Container (Clavulanate Potassium, Ticarcillin Disodium) GlaxoSmithKline ... 1664
Timentin Injection-Pharmacy Bulk Package (Clavulanate Potassium, Ticarcillin Disodium) GlaxoSmithKline ... 1666
Timentin for Intravenous Administration (Clavulanate Potassium, Ticarcillin Disodium) GlaxoSmithKline ... 1658

Enterobacter species bone and joint infections
Ceptaz for Injection (Ceftazidime) GlaxoSmithKline ... 1499
Fortaz (Ceftazidime Sodium) GlaxoSmithKline ... 1541
Nebcin Vials, Hyporets & ADD-Vantage (Tobramycin Sulfate) Lilly ... 1955
Primaxin I.V. (Cilastatin Sodium, Imipenem) Merck ... 2160
Rocephin Injectable Vials, ADD-Vantage, Galaxy, Bulk (Ceftriaxone Sodium) Roche Laboratories ... 2993
Tazicef for Injection (Ceftazidime) GlaxoSmithKline ... 1647
Tazicef Galaxy Container (Ceftazidime Sodium) GlaxoSmithKline ... 1650
Tazicef Pharmacy Bulk Package (Ceftazidime) GlaxoSmithKline ... 1653
Tazidime Vials, Faspak & ADD-Vantage (Ceftazidime) Lilly ... 1966

Enterobacter species gynecologic infections
Azactam for Injection (Aztreonam) Elan ... 1276
Claforan Injection (Cefotaxime Sodium) Aventis ... 732
Primaxin I.V. (Cilastatin Sodium, Imipenem) Merck ... 2160
Timentin Injection- ADD-Vantage Vial (Clavulanate Potassium, Ticarcillin Disodium) GlaxoSmithKline ... 1661
Timentin Injection-Galaxy Container (Clavulanate Potassium, Ticarcillin Disodium) GlaxoSmithKline ... 1664
Timentin Injection-Pharmacy Bulk Package (Clavulanate Potassium, Ticarcillin Disodium) GlaxoSmithKline ... 1666
Timentin for Intravenous Administration (Clavulanate Potassium, Ticarcillin Disodium) GlaxoSmithKline ... 1658

Enterobacter species infections
Ancef for Injection (Cefazolin Sodium) GlaxoSmithKline ... 1474
Ancef Injection (Cefazolin Sodium) GlaxoSmithKline ... 1474
Augmentin Chewable Tablets (Amoxicillin, Clavulanate Potassium) GlaxoSmithKline ... 1482
Augmentin Powder for Oral Suspension (Amoxicillin, Clavulanate Potassium) GlaxoSmithKline ... 1482
Augmentin Tablets (Amoxicillin, Clavulanate Potassium) GlaxoSmithKline ... 1485
Azactam for Injection (Aztreonam) Elan ... 1276
Bactrim (Sulfamethoxazole, Trimethoprim) Roche Laboratories ... 2949
Cefizox for Intramuscular or Intravenous Use (Ceftizoxime Sodium) Fujisawa ... 1390
Cefobid Intravenous/Intramuscular (Cefoperazone) Pfizer ... 2671
Cefobid Pharmacy Bulk Package - Not for Direct Infusion (Cefoperazone Sodium) Pfizer ... 2673
Ceptaz for Injection (Ceftazidime) GlaxoSmithKline ... 1499
Claforan Injection (Cefotaxime Sodium) Aventis ... 732
Fortaz (Ceftazidime Sodium) GlaxoSmithKline ... 1541
Geocillin Tablets (Carbenicillin Indanyl Sodium) Pfizer ... 2687
Kefurox Vials, ADD-Vantage (Cefuroxime Sodium) Lilly ... 1948
Kefzol Vials, ADD-Vantage (Cefazolin Sodium) Lilly ... 1951
Macrodantin Capsules (Nitrofurantoin) Procter & Gamble Pharmaceuticals ... 2891
Maxipime for Injection (Cefepime Hydrochloride) Elan ... 1285
Nebcin Vials, Hyporets & ADD-Vantage (Tobramycin Sulfate) Lilly ... 1955
Pipracil (Piperacillin Sodium) Lederle ... 1866
Primaxin I.V. (Cilastatin Sodium, Imipenem) Merck ... 2160
Rocephin Injectable Vials, ADD-Vantage, Galaxy, Bulk (Ceftriaxone Sodium) Roche Laboratories ... 2993
Septra Suspension (Sulfamethoxazole, Trimethoprim) Monarch ... 2265
Septra Tablets (Sulfamethoxazole, Trimethoprim) Monarch ... 2265
Septra DS Tablets (Sulfamethoxazole, Trimethoprim) Monarch ... 2265
Tazicef for Injection (Ceftazidime) GlaxoSmithKline ... 1647
Tazicef Galaxy Container (Ceftazidime Sodium) GlaxoSmithKline ... 1650
Tazicef Pharmacy Bulk Package (Ceftazidime) GlaxoSmithKline ... 1653
Tazidime Vials, Faspak & ADD-Vantage (Ceftazidime) Lilly ... 1966
Timentin Injection- ADD-Vantage Vial (Clavulanate Potassium, Ticarcillin Disodium) GlaxoSmithKline ... 1661
Timentin Injection-Galaxy Container (Clavulanate Potassium, Ticarcillin Disodium) GlaxoSmithKline ... 1664
Timentin Injection-Pharmacy Bulk Package (Clavulanate Potassium, Ticarcillin Disodium) GlaxoSmithKline ... 1666
Timentin for Intravenous Administration (Clavulanate Potassium, Ticarcillin Disodium) GlaxoSmithKline ... 1658
Unasyn for Injection (Ampicillin Sodium, Sulbactam Sodium) Pfizer ... 2728
Zinacef Injection (Cefuroxime) GlaxoSmithKline ... 1696
Zinacef for Injection (Cefuroxime) GlaxoSmithKline ... 1696

Enterobacter species infections, ocular
Pred-G Sterile Ophthalmic Ointment (Gentamicin Sulfate, Prednisolone Acetate) Allergan ... ⊙248

Enterobacter species intra-abdominal infections
Azactam for Injection (Aztreonam) Elan ... 1276
Cefizox for Intramuscular or Intravenous Use (Ceftizoxime Sodium) Fujisawa ... 1390
Mandol Vials (Cefamandole Nafate) Lilly ... 1953
Maxipime for Injection (Cefepime Hydrochloride) Elan ... 1285
Nebcin Vials, Hyporets & ADD-Vantage (Tobramycin Sulfate) Lilly ... 1955
Primaxin I.V. (Cilastatin Sodium, Imipenem) Merck ... 2160
Unasyn for Injection (Ampicillin Sodium, Sulbactam Sodium) Pfizer ... 2728

Enterobacter species lower respiratory tract infections
Azactam for Injection (Aztreonam) Elan ... 1276
Cefizox for Intramuscular or Intravenous Use (Ceftizoxime Sodium) Fujisawa ... 1390
Ceptaz for Injection (Ceftazidime) GlaxoSmithKline ... 1499
Claforan Injection (Cefotaxime Sodium) Aventis ... 732
Fortaz (Ceftazidime Sodium) GlaxoSmithKline ... 1541
Maxipime for Injection (Cefepime Hydrochloride) Elan ... 1285
Nebcin Vials, Hyporets & ADD-Vantage (Tobramycin Sulfate) Lilly ... 1955
Primaxin I.V. (Cilastatin Sodium, Imipenem) Merck ... 2160
Tazicef for Injection (Ceftazidime) GlaxoSmithKline ... 1647
Tazicef Galaxy Container (Ceftazidime Sodium) GlaxoSmithKline ... 1650
Tazicef Pharmacy Bulk Package (Ceftazidime) GlaxoSmithKline ... 1653
Tazidime Vials, Faspak & ADD-Vantage (Ceftazidime) Lilly ... 1966

Enterobacter species prostatitis
Geocillin Tablets (Carbenicillin Indanyl Sodium) Pfizer ... 2687

Enterobacter species respiratory tract infections
Cefobid Intravenous/Intramuscular (Cefoperazone) Pfizer ... 2671
Cefobid Pharmacy Bulk Package - Not for Direct Infusion (Cefoperazone Sodium) Pfizer ... 2673
Ceptaz for Injection (Ceftazidime) GlaxoSmithKline ... 1499

Enterobacter species septicemia
Azactam for Injection (Aztreonam) Elan ... 1276
Pipracil (Piperacillin Sodium) Lederle ... 1866
Primaxin I.V. (Cilastatin Sodium, Imipenem) Merck ... 2160

Enterobacter species skin and skin structure infections
Azactam for Injection (Aztreonam) Elan ... 1276
Cefizox for Intramuscular or Intravenous Use (Ceftizoxime Sodium) Fujisawa ... 1390
Ceptaz for Injection (Ceftazidime) GlaxoSmithKline ... 1499
Claforan Injection (Cefotaxime Sodium) Aventis ... 732
Fortaz (Ceftazidime Sodium) GlaxoSmithKline ... 1541
Kefurox Vials, ADD-Vantage (Cefuroxime Sodium) Lilly ... 1948
Mandol Vials (Cefamandole Nafate) Lilly ... 1953
Nebcin Vials, Hyporets & ADD-Vantage (Tobramycin Sulfate) Lilly ... 1955
Primaxin I.V. (Cilastatin Sodium, Imipenem) Merck ... 2160
Tazicef for Injection (Ceftazidime) GlaxoSmithKline ... 1647
Tazicef Galaxy Container (Ceftazidime Sodium) GlaxoSmithKline ... 1650
Tazicef Pharmacy Bulk Package (Ceftazidime) GlaxoSmithKline ... 1653
Tazidime Vials, Faspak & ADD-Vantage (Ceftazidime) Lilly ... 1966
Unasyn for Injection (Ampicillin Sodium, Sulbactam Sodium) Pfizer ... 2728
Zinacef Injection (Cefuroxime) GlaxoSmithKline ... 1696
Zinacef for Injection (Cefuroxime) GlaxoSmithKline ... 1696

Enterobacter species urinary tract infections
Ancef for Injection (Cefazolin Sodium) GlaxoSmithKline ... 1474
Ancef Injection (Cefazolin Sodium) GlaxoSmithKline ... 1474
Augmentin Chewable Tablets (Amoxicillin, Clavulanate Potassium) GlaxoSmithKline ... 1482
Augmentin Powder for Oral Suspension (Amoxicillin, Clavulanate Potassium) GlaxoSmithKline ... 1482
Augmentin Tablets (Amoxicillin, Clavulanate Potassium) GlaxoSmithKline ... 1485
Azactam for Injection (Aztreonam) Elan ... 1276
Bactrim (Sulfamethoxazole, Trimethoprim) Roche Laboratories ... 2949
Ceptaz for Injection (Ceftazidime) GlaxoSmithKline ... 1499
Claforan Injection (Cefotaxime Sodium) Aventis ... 732
Fortaz (Ceftazidime Sodium) GlaxoSmithKline ... 1541
Geocillin Tablets (Carbenicillin Indanyl Sodium) Pfizer ... 2687
Kefzol Vials, ADD-Vantage (Cefazolin Sodium) Lilly ... 1951
Macrodantin Capsules (Nitrofurantoin) Procter & Gamble Pharmaceuticals ... 2891
Mandol Vials (Cefamandole Nafate) Lilly ... 1953
Nebcin Vials, Hyporets & ADD-Vantage (Tobramycin Sulfate) Lilly ... 1955
Primaxin I.V. (Cilastatin Sodium, Imipenem) Merck ... 2160
Septra Suspension (Sulfamethoxazole, Trimethoprim) Monarch ... 2265
Septra Tablets (Sulfamethoxazole, Trimethoprim) Monarch ... 2265
Septra DS Tablets (Sulfamethoxazole, Trimethoprim) Monarch ... 2265
Tazicef for Injection (Ceftazidime) GlaxoSmithKline ... 1647
Tazicef Galaxy Container (Ceftazidime Sodium) GlaxoSmithKline ... 1650
Tazicef Pharmacy Bulk Package (Ceftazidime) GlaxoSmithKline ... 1653
Tazidime Vials, Faspak & ADD-Vantage (Ceftazidime) Lilly ... 1966

Enterobiasis
Pin-X Pinworm Treatment (Pyrantel Pamoate) Effcon ... ▣632
Vermox Chewable Tablets (Mebendazole) McNeil Consumer ... 2017

Enterobius vermicularis infestation
(*see under* Enterobiasis)

Enterococci infections
(*see under* Streptococci group D infections)

Enterococci species genital infections
Ancef for Injection (Cefazolin Sodium) GlaxoSmithKline ... 1474
Ancef Injection (Cefazolin Sodium) GlaxoSmithKline ... 1474

Enterococci species gynecologic infections
Claforan (Cefotaxime Sodium) Aventis ... 732

Enterococci species urinary tract infections
Ancef for Injection (Cefazolin Sodium) GlaxoSmithKline ... 1474
Ancef Injection (Cefazolin Sodium) GlaxoSmithKline ... 1474
Claforan Injection (Cefotaxime Sodium) Aventis ... 732
Geocillin Tablets (Carbenicillin Indanyl Sodium) Pfizer ... 2687
Macrodantin Capsules (Nitrofurantoin) Procter & Gamble Pharmaceuticals ... 2891

Enterococcus faecium, vancomycin-resistant bacteremia
Synercid I.V. (Dalfopristin, Quinupristin) Aventis ... 775
Zyvox (Linezolid) Pharmacia & Upjohn ... 2871

Enterococcus faecium, vancomycin-resistant infections
Synercid I.V. (Dalfopristin, Quinupristin) Aventis ... 775
Zyvox (Linezolid) Pharmacia & Upjohn ... 2871

Enterocolitis, acute, possibly effective in, adjunctive therapy
Donnatal (Atropine Sulfate, Hyoscyamine Sulfate, Phenobarbital, Scopolamine Hydrobromide) Robins ... 2929
Donnatal Extentabs (Atropine Sulfate, Hyoscyamine Sulfate, Phenobarbital, Scopolamine Hydrobromide) Robins ... 2930
Donnatal Tablets (Atropine Sulfate, Hyoscyamine Sulfate, Phenobarbital, Scopolamine Hydrobromide) Robins ... 2929

Enterocolitis, staphylococcal
Vancocin HCl Capsules & Pulvules (Vancomycin Hydrochloride) Lilly ... 1972
Vancocin HCl Oral Solution (Vancomycin Hydrochloride) Lilly ... 1971
Vancocin HCl, Vials & ADD-Vantage (Vancomycin Hydrochloride) Lilly ... 1970

Enuresis, nocturnal, primary
DDAVP Nasal Spray (Desmopressin Acetate) Aventis ... 738
DDAVP Rhinal Tube (Desmopressin Acetate) Aventis ... 738
DDAVP Tablets (Desmopressin Acetate) Aventis ... 739
Desmopressin Acetate Rhinal Tube (Desmopressin Acetate) Ferring ... 1345

Envenomation, Micrurus fulvius
Antivenin (Micrurus fulvius) (Antivenin (Micrurus Fulvius)) Wyeth-Ayerst ... 3477

Envenomation, pit viper
Antivenin Polyvalent (Antivenin (Crotalidae) Polyvalent) Wyeth-Ayerst ... 3475

Epicondylitis
Celestone Soluspan Injectable Suspension (Betamethasone Acetate, Betamethasone Sodium Phosphate) Schering ... 3097

Celestone Syrup (Betamethasone) Schering 3099
Cortone Acetate Injectable Suspension (Cortisone Acetate) Merck 2059
Cortone Acetate Tablets (Cortisone Acetate) Merck 2061
Decadron Elixir (Dexamethasone) Merck 2078
Decadron Tablets (Dexamethasone) Merck 2079
Decadron Phosphate Injection (Dexamethasone Sodium Phosphate) Merck 2081
Depo-Medrol Injectable Suspension (Methylprednisolone Acetate) Pharmacia & Upjohn 2795
Hydrocortone Tablets (Hydrocortisone) Merck 2106
Hydrocortone Acetate Injectable Suspension (Hydrocortisone Acetate) Merck 2103
Hydrocortone Phosphate Injection, Sterile (Hydrocortisone Sodium Phosphate) Merck 2105
Pediapred Oral Solution (Prednisolone Sodium Phosphate) Celltech 1170
Prednisone (Prednisone) Roxane 3064
Prelone Syrup (Prednisolone) Muro 2273
Solu-Medrol Sterile Powder (Methylprednisolone Sodium Succinate) Pharmacia & Upjohn 2855
Traumeel Injection Solution (Homeopathic Formulations) Heel 1726

Epidermophyton floccosum infections
Grifulvin V Tablets Microsize and Oral Suspension Microsize (Griseofulvin) Ortho Dermatological 2518
Gris-PEG Tablets (Griseofulvin) Pedinol 2661
Loprox Cream (Ciclopirox Olamine) Medicis 2021
Loprox Gel (Ciclopirox) Medicis 2022
Loprox Lotion (Ciclopirox Olamine) Medicis 2021
Lotrimin (Clotrimazole) Schering 3128
Lotrisone (Betamethasone Dipropionate, Clotrimazole) Schering 3129
Mentax Cream (Butenafine Hydrochloride) Bertek 1009
Naftin Cream (Naftifine Hydrochloride) Merz 2224
Naftin Gel (Naftifine Hydrochloride) Merz 2224
Nizoral 2% Cream (Ketoconazole) Janssen 3620
Oxistat (Oxiconazole Nitrate) Elan 1298

Epididymitis
Ancef for Injection (Cefazolin Sodium) GlaxoSmithKline 1474
Ancef Injection (Cefazolin Sodium) GlaxoSmithKline 1474

Epilepsy, centrencephalic
(*see under* Seizures, centrencephalic)

Epilepsy, generalized
(*see under* Seizures, generalized, tonic-clonic)

Epilepsy, grand mal
(*see under* Seizures, generalized, tonic-clonic)

Epilepsy, petit mal
(*see under* Seizures, generalized, absence)

Epilepticus, status
Ativan Injection (Lorazepam) Wyeth-Ayerst 3478
Cerebyx Injection (Fosphenytoin Sodium) Parke-Davis 2619
Nembutal Sodium Solution (Pentobarbital Sodium) Abbott 485
Valium Injectable (Diazepam) Roche Laboratories 3026

Epinephrine sensitivity, ocular, treatment of
HMS (Medrysone) Allergan .... ⊙240

Episiotomy, topical debriding in
(*see under* Wounds, debridement of)

Erectile dysfunction
Caverject Sterile Powder (Alprostadil) Pharmacia & Upjohn 2777
MUSE Urethral Suppository (Alprostadil) Vivus 3335
Viagra Tablets (Sildenafil Citrate) Pfizer 2732

Erectile dysfunction, diagnosis of
Caverject Sterile Powder (Alprostadil) Pharmacia & Upjohn 2777

Erysipelas
Bicillin C-R 900/300 Injection (Penicillin G Benzathine, Penicillin G Procaine) Monarch 2240
Bicillin C-R Injection (Penicillin G Benzathine, Penicillin G Procaine) Monarch 2238
Duricef (Cefadroxil) Bristol-Myers Squibb 1079

Erysipeloid
Pfizerpen (Penicillin G Potassium) Pfizer 2707

Erythema multiforme, severe
(*see under* Stevens-Johnson syndrome)

Erythema nodosum leprosum
Thalomid Capsules (Thalidomide) Celgene 1154

Erythrasma
E.E.S. (Erythromycin Ethylsuccinate) Abbott 450
EryPed (Erythromycin Ethylsuccinate) Abbott 446
Ery-Tab Tablets (Erythromycin) Abbott 448
Erythrocin Stearate Filmtab Tablets (Erythromycin Stearate) Abbott 452
Erythromycin Base Filmtab Tablets (Erythromycin) Abbott 454
Erythromycin Delayed-Release Capsules, USP (Erythromycin) Abbott 455
PCE Dispertab Tablets (Erythromycin) Abbott 498

Erythroblastopenia
Celestone Soluspan Injectable Suspension (Betamethasone Acetate, Betamethasone Sodium Phosphate) Schering 3097
Celestone Syrup (Betamethasone) Schering 3099
Cortone Acetate Injectable Suspension (Cortisone Acetate) Merck 2059
Cortone Acetate Tablets (Cortisone Acetate) Merck 2061
Decadron Elixir (Dexamethasone) Merck 2078
Decadron Tablets (Dexamethasone) Merck 2079
Decadron Phosphate Injection (Dexamethasone Sodium Phosphate) Merck 2081
Depo-Medrol Injectable Suspension (Methylprednisolone Acetate) Pharmacia & Upjohn 2795
Hydrocortone Tablets (Hydrocortisone) Merck 2106
Hydrocortone Phosphate Injection, Sterile (Hydrocortisone Sodium Phosphate) Merck 2105
Pediapred Oral Solution (Prednisolone Sodium Phosphate) Celltech 1170
Prednisone (Prednisone) Roxane 3064
Prelone Syrup (Prednisolone) Muro 2273
Solu-Medrol Sterile Powder (Methylprednisolone Sodium Succinate) Pharmacia & Upjohn 2855

Erythroblastosis fetalis, prevention of
BayRho-D Full Dose (Rh_0 (D) Immune Globulin (Human)) Bayer Biological 921

Escherichia coli
(*see under* E. coli infections)

Esophagitis, erosive
(*see also under* Gastroesophageal reflux disease)
Axid Pulvules (Nizatidine) Lilly 1903
Axid Pulvules (Nizatidine) Reliant 2919
Nexium Delayed-Release Capsules (Esomeprazole Magnesium) AstraZeneca LP 619
Prevacid Delayed-Release Capsules (Lansoprazole) TAP 3292
Prilosec Delayed-Release Capsules (Omeprazole) AstraZeneca LP 628
Protonix Tablets (Pantoprazole Sodium) Wyeth-Ayerst 3577
Tagamet (Cimetidine Hydrochloride) GlaxoSmithKline 1644
Zantac (Ranitidine Hydrochloride) GlaxoSmithKline 1690

Esotropia, accommodative
Humorsol Sterile Ophthalmic Solution (Demecarium Bromide) Merck 2102

Estrogen, deficiency
(*see under* Hypoestrogenism)

Eubacterium species infections
Primaxin I.V. (Cilastatin Sodium, Imipenem) Merck 2160

Ewing's sarcoma, palliative treatment of
Cosmegen for Injection (Dactinomycin) Merck 2062

Extrapyramidal reactions, drug-induced
Akineton (Biperiden Hydrochloride) Abbott 402
Artane (Trihexyphenidyl Hydrochloride) Lederle 1855
Cogentin (Benztropine Mesylate) Merck 2055
Symmetrel (Amantadine Hydrochloride) Endo Labs 1328

Eye, anterior segment inflammation
(*see under* Inflammation, anterior segment)

Eye and its adnexa, external infections of
Genoptic Ophthalmic Ointment (Gentamicin Sulfate) Allergan .... ⊙239
Genoptic Sterile Ophthalmic Solution (Gentamicin Sulfate) Allergan .... ⊙239
Polysporin Ophthalmic Ointment Sterile (Bacitracin Zinc, Polymyxin B Sulfate, Bacitracin Zinc, Polymyxin B Sulfate) Monarch .... ⊙301
Tobrex Ophthalmic Ointment (Tobramycin) Alcon .... ⊙220
Tobrex Ophthalmic Solution (Tobramycin) Alcon .... ⊙221

Eyes, anterior segment, staining of
Fluor-I-Strip A.T. Ophthalmic Strips 1 mg (Fluorescein Sodium) Bausch & Lomb .... ⊙260
Fluor-I-Strip Ophthalmic Strips 9 mg (Fluorescein Sodium) Bausch & Lomb .... ⊙260

Eyes, burning, reduction of
Refresh Tears Lubricant Eye Drops (Carboxymethylcellulose Sodium) Allergan .... ⊙251
Tears Naturale Forte Lubricant Eye Drops (Dextran 70, Hydroxypropyl Methylcellulose) Alcon 541
Tears Naturale Free Lubricant Eye Drops (Dextran 70, Hydroxypropyl Methylcellulose) Alcon 541

Eyes, cleansing of
Collyrium Eye Wash (Boric Acid, Sodium Borate) Bausch & Lomb, Inc .... ⊙252
Eye Wash Solution (Boric Acid, Sodium Borate, Sodium Chloride) Bausch & Lomb, Inc .... ⊙252
Eye•Scrub Pads (PEG-200 Glyceryl Tallowate) Novartis Ophthalmics .... ⊙304

Eyes, diagnostic procedures, adjunct in
Fluor-I-Strip A.T. Ophthalmic Strips 1 mg (Fluorescein Sodium) Bausch & Lomb .... ⊙260
Fluor-I-Strip Ophthalmic Strips 9 mg (Fluorescein Sodium) Bausch & Lomb .... ⊙260

Eyes, dry
(*see under* Keratoconjunctivitis sicca)

Eyes, external infections of
Genoptic Ophthalmic Ointment (Gentamicin Sulfate) Allergan .... ⊙239
Genoptic Sterile Ophthalmic Solution (Gentamicin Sulfate) Allergan .... ⊙239

Eyes, inflammation
(*see under* Ocular inflammation)

Eyes, irrigation of
(*see also under* Eyes, cleansing of)
Eye Wash Solution (Boric Acid, Sodium Borate, Sodium Chloride) Bausch & Lomb, Inc .... ⊙252

Eyes, irritation, symptomatic relief of
All Clear Eye Drops (Naphazoline Hydrochloride, Polyethylene Glycol) Bausch & Lomb, Inc .... ⊙252
All Clear AR Eye Drops (Hydroxypropyl Methylcellulose, Naphazoline Hydrochloride) Bausch & Lomb, Inc .... ⊙252
Clear Eyes CLR Soothing Drops (Glycerin, Hydroxypropyl Methylcellulose, Sodium Chloride) Ross .... ⊙322
GenTeal Eye Drops (Hydroxypropyl Methylcellulose) Novartis Ophthalmics .... ⊙304
GenTeal Gel (Hydroxypropyl Methylcellulose) Novartis Ophthalmics .... ⊙304
GenTeal Mild Eye Drops (Polyethylene Glycol, Polyvinyl Alcohol) Novartis Ophthalmics .... ⊙304
Murine Tears Lubricant Eye Drops (Polyvinyl Alcohol, Povidone) Ross .... ⊙323
Murine Tears Plus Lubricant Redness Reliever Eye Drops (Polyvinyl Alcohol, Povidone, Tetrahydrozoline Hydrochloride) Ross .... ⊙323
Refresh Tears Lubricant Eye Drops (Carboxymethylcellulose Sodium) Allergan .... ⊙251
Tears Naturale Forte Lubricant Eye Drops (Dextran 70, Hydroxypropyl Methylcellulose) Alcon 541
Tears Naturale Free Lubricant Eye Drops (Dextran 70, Hydroxypropyl Methylcellulose) Alcon 541
Advanced Relief Visine Eye Drops (Dextran 70, Polyethylene Glycol, Povidone, Tetrahydrozoline Hydrochloride) Pfizer Consumer .... ⊙313
Visine Original Eye Drops (Tetrahydrozoline Hydrochloride) Pfizer Consumer .... ⊙315
Visine A.C. Seasonal Relief From Pollen & Dust Eye Drops (Tetrahydrozoline Hydrochloride, Zinc Sulfate) Pfizer Consumer .... ⊙314
Visine For Contacts Rewetting Drops (Glycerin, Hydroxypropyl Methylcellulose) Pfizer Consumer .... ⊙314
Visine L.R. Long Lasting Eye Drops (Oxymetazoline Hydrochloride) Pfizer Consumer .... ⊙315
Visine Tears Eye Drops (Glycerin, Hydroxypropyl Methylcellulose, Polyethylene Glycol) Pfizer Consumer .... ⊙315
Visine Tears Preservative Free Eye Drops (Glycerin, Hydroxypropyl Methylcellulose, Polyethylene Glycol) Pfizer Consumer .... ⊙315

Eyes, itching, reduction of
Ryna Liquid (Chlorpheniramine Maleate, Pseudoephedrine Hydrochloride) Wallace .... ■768
Triaminic Cold & Allergy Softchews (Chlorpheniramine Maleate, Pseudoephedrine Hydrochloride) Novartis Consumer .... ■683
Tylenol Severe Allergy Caplets (Acetaminophen, Diphenhydramine Hydrochloride) McNeil Consumer 2010
Vasocon-A Eye Drops (Antazoline Phosphate, Naphazoline Hydrochloride) Novartis Ophthalmics .... ⊙307

Eyes, lubrication of
(*see also under* Keratoconjunctivitis sicca)
Computer Eye Drops (Glycerin) Bausch & Lomb, Inc .... ⊙252

Eyes, red
(*see under* Ocular redness)

Eyes, surgery, adjunct to
Acular PF Ophthalmic Solution (Ketorolac Tromethamine) Allergan 544
Amvisc Plus (Sodium Hyaluronate) Bausch & Lomb Surgical .. ⊙329
Healon (Sodium Hyaluronate) Pharmacia & Upjohn .... ⊙316
Healon 5 (Sodium Hyaluronate) Pharmacia & Upjohn .... ⊙317
Miochol-E System Pak (Acetylcholine Chloride) Novartis Ophthalmics .... ⊙305
Miochol-E with Steri-Tags (Acetylcholine Chloride) Novartis Ophthalmics .... ⊙305

Ocucoat (Hydroxypropyl Methylcellulose) Bausch & Lomb Surgical .... ⊙330

Eyes, surgical procedures, irrigation of
(*see under* Eyes, cleansing of)

Eyes, watery
(*see under* Lacrimation, symptomatic relief of)

F

Factor IX, deficiency of
Bebulin VH (Factor IX Complex) Baxter Healthcare 840
Konÿne 80 (Factor IX Complex) Bayer Biological 937
Proplex T (Factor IX Complex) Baxter Healthcare 851

Fatigue, symptomatic relief of
Vivarin (Caffeine) SmithKline Beecham Consumer .... ▣763

Female castration
(*see under* Ovaries, castration of)

Fever, reduction of
Advil (Ibuprofen) Whitehall-Robins .... ▣771
Children's Advil Oral Suspension (Ibuprofen) Whitehall-Robins .... ▣773
Children's Advil Chewable Tablets (Ibuprofen) Whitehall-Robins .... ▣773
Infants' Advil Drops (Ibuprofen) Whitehall-Robins .... ▣773
Junior Strength Advil Tablets (Ibuprofen) Whitehall-Robins .... ▣773
Junior Strength Advil Chewable Tablets (Ibuprofen) Whitehall-Robins .... ▣773
Aleve Tablets, Caplets and Gelcaps (Naproxen Sodium) Bayer Consumer .... ▣602
Genuine Bayer Tablets, Caplets and Gelcaps (Aspirin) Bayer Consumer .... ▣606
Extra Strength Bayer Caplets and Gelcaps (Aspirin) Bayer Consumer .... ▣610
Aspirin Regimen Bayer Children's Chewable Tablets (Orange or Cherry Flavored) (Aspirin) Bayer Consumer .... ▣607
Extra Strength Bayer Plus Caplets (Aspirin, Calcium Carbonate) Bayer Consumer .... ▣610
BC Powder (Aspirin, Caffeine, Salicylamide) Block .... ▣619
Goody's Extra Strength Headache Powder (Acetaminophen, Aspirin, Caffeine) Block .... ▣620
Goody's Extra Strength Pain Relief Tablets (Acetaminophen, Aspirin, Caffeine) Block .... ▣620
Children's Motrin Oral Suspension and Chewable Tablets (Ibuprofen) McNeil Consumer 2006
Children's Motrin Oral Suspension (Ibuprofen) McNeil Consumer .... ▣643
Motrin Suspension, Oral Drops, Chewable Tablets, and Caplets (Ibuprofen) McNeil Consumer 2002
Infants' Motrin Concentrated Drops (Ibuprofen) McNeil Consumer 2006
Junior Strength Motrin Caplets and Chewable Tablets (Ibuprofen) McNeil Consumer 2006
Motrin IB Tablets, Caplets, and Gelcaps (Ibuprofen) McNeil Consumer 2002
Orudis KT Tablets (Ketoprofen) Whitehall-Robins .... ▣778
Trilisate (Choline Magnesium Trisalicylate) Purdue Frederick 2901
Tylenol, Children's (Acetaminophen) McNeil Consumer 2014
Junior Strength Tylenol Soft Chews Chewable Tablets (Acetaminophen) McNeil Consumer 2014
Tylenol (Acetaminophen) McNeil Consumer 2009
Maximum Strength Tylenol Sore Throat Adult Liquid (Acetaminophen) McNeil Consumer 2013
Vanquish Caplets (Acetaminophen, Aluminum Hydroxide, Aspirin, Caffeine, Magnesium Hydroxide) Bayer Consumer .... ▣617

Fever, San Joaquin
(*see under* Coccidioidomycosis)

Fever, unspecified
Percogesic Aspirin-Free Coated Tablets (Acetaminophen, Phenyltoloxamine Citrate) Medtech .... ▣667
Extra Strength Percogesic Aspirin-Free Coated Caplets (Acetaminophen, Diphenhydramine Hydrochloride) Medtech .... ▣665

Fever, valley
(*see under* Coccidioidomycosis)

Fever associated with common cold
Advil Cold and Sinus Caplets (Ibuprofen, Pseudoephedrine Hydrochloride) Whitehall-Robins .... ▣771
Advil Cold and Sinus Tablets (Ibuprofen, Pseudoephedrine Hydrochloride) Whitehall-Robins .... ▣771
Advil Flu & Body Ache Caplets (Ibuprofen, Pseudoephedrine Hydrochloride) Whitehall-Robins .... ▣772
Aleve Cold & Sinus Caplets (Naproxen Sodium, Pseudoephedrine Hydrochloride) Bayer Consumer .... ▣603
BC Cold Powder (Aspirin, Chlorpheniramine Maleate, Pseudoephedrine Hydrochloride) Block .... ▣619
Benadryl Severe Allergy & Sinus Headache Caplets (Acetaminophen, Diphenhydramine Hydrochloride, Pseudoephedrine Hydrochloride) Pfizer Inc., Warner-Lambert Healthcare .... ▣694
Comtrex Flu Therapy & Fever Relief Daytime Caplets (Acetaminophen, Pseudoephedrine Hydrochloride) Bristol-Myers .... ▣628
Contac Severe Cold and Flu Caplets Maximum Strength (Acetaminophen, Chlorpheniramine Maleate, Dextromethorphan Hydrobromide, Pseudoephedrine Hydrochloride) SmithKline Beecham Consumer .... ▣746
Contac Severe Cold and Flu Caplets Non-Drowsy (Acetaminophen, Dextromethorphan Hydrobromide, Pseudoephedrine Hydrochloride) SmithKline Beecham Consumer .... ▣746
Coricidin HBP Maximum Strength Flu Tablets (Acetaminophen, Chlorpheniramine Maleate, Dextromethorphan Hydrobromide) Schering-Plough .... ▣738
Children's Motrin Cold Oral Suspension (Ibuprofen, Pseudoephedrine Hydrochloride) McNeil Consumer 2007
Motrin Sinus Headache Caplets (Ibuprofen, Pseudoephedrine Hydrochloride) McNeil Consumer 2005
TheraFlu Regular Strength Cold & Sore Throat Night Time Hot Liquid (Acetaminophen, Chlorpheniramine Maleate, Pseudoephedrine Hydrochloride) Novartis Consumer .... ▣676
Children's Tylenol Cold Suspension Liquid and Chewable Tablets (Acetaminophen, Chlorpheniramine Maleate, Pseudoephedrine Hydrochloride) McNeil Consumer 2015
Infants' Tylenol Cold Decongestant and Fever Reducer Concentrated Drops Plus Cough (Acetaminophen, Dextromethorphan Hydrobromide, Pseudoephedrine Hydrochloride) McNeil Consumer 2015
Multi-Symptom Tylenol Cold Complete Formula Caplets (Acetaminophen, Chlorpheniramine Maleate, Dextromethorphan Hydrobromide, Pseudoephedrine Hydrochloride) McNeil Consumer 2010
Multi-Symptom Tylenol Cold Non-Drowsy Caplets and Gelcaps (Acetaminophen, Dextromethorphan Hydrobromide, Pseudoephedrine Hydrochloride) McNeil Consumer 2010

Fever blisters
(*see under* Herpetic manifestations, oral, symptomatic relief of)

Fiber, deficiency of
Metamucil Dietary Fiber Supplement (Psyllium Preparations) Procter & Gamble .... ▣834

Flatulence, relief of
Arco-Lase Tablets (Amylase, Cellulase, Lipase, Protease) Arco 592
Beano (Alpha Galactosidase Enzyme) Block .... ▣809
Maximum Strength Gas Aid Softgels (Simethicone) McNeil Consumer 2001
Gas-X Chewable Tablets (Simethicone) Novartis Consumer .... ▣671
Extra Strength Gas-X Liquid (Simethicone) Novartis Consumer .... ▣671
Gas-X (Simethicone) Novartis Consumer .... ▣671
Maximum Strength Gas-X Softgels (Simethicone) Novartis Consumer .... ▣671
Hyland's Colic Tablets (Dioscorea, Homeopathic Formulations) Standard Homeopathic .... ▣765
Maalox Max Maximum Strength Antacid/Anti-Gas Liquid (Aluminum Hydroxide, Magnesium Hydroxide, Simethicone) Novartis Consumer 2300
Fast-Acting Mylanta Liquid Antacid (Aluminum Hydroxide, Magnesium Hydroxide, Simethicone) J&J • Merck 1813
Mylanta Gas Relief (Simethicone) J&J • Merck 1814
Mylicon Infants' Drops (Simethicone) J&J • Merck 1813
Phazyme-125 mg Quick Dissolve Chewable Tablets (Simethicone) Block .... ▣622
Phazyme-180 mg Ultra Strength Softgels (Simethicone) Block .... ▣622

Flu symptoms
(*see under* Influenza syndrome, symptomatic relief of)

Fluoride and calcium, deficiency of
Florical Capsules and Tablets (Calcium Carbonate, Sodium Fluoride) Mericon 2223
Monocal Tablets (Calcium Carbonate, Sodium Monofluorophosphate) Mericon 2223

Folic acid deficiency, prevention of
Slow Fe with Folic Acid Tablets (Ferrous Sulfate, Folic Acid) Novartis Consumer .... ▣828

Folliculitis barbae
Grifulvin V Tablets Microsize and Oral Suspension Microsize (Griseofulvin) Ortho Dermatological 2518
Gris-PEG Tablets (Griseofulvin) Pedinol 2661

Francisella tularensis infections
Declomycin Tablets (Demeclocycline Hydrochloride) Lederle 1855
Doryx Coated Pellet Filled Capsules (Doxycycline Hyclate) Warner Chilcott 3357
Dynacin Capsules (Minocycline Hydrochloride) Medicis 2019
Minocin Intravenous (Minocycline Hydrochloride) Lederle 1862
Minocin Oral Suspension (Minocycline Hydrochloride) Lederle 1865
Minocin Pellet-Filled Capsules (Minocycline Hydrochloride) Lederle 1863
Monodox Capsules (Doxycycline Monohydrate) Oclassen 2442
Streptomycin Sulfate Injection (Streptomycin Sulfate) Pfizer 2714
Vibramycin Calcium Oral Suspension Syrup (Doxycycline Calcium) Pfizer 2735
Vibramycin Hyclate Capsules (Doxycycline Hyclate) Pfizer 2735
Vibramycin Hyclate Intravenous (Doxycycline Hyclate) Pfizer 2737
Vibramycin Monohydrate for Oral Suspension (Doxycycline Monohydrate) Pfizer 2735
Vibra-Tabs Film Coated Tablets (Doxycycline Hyclate) Pfizer 2735

Fungal infections, skin
(*see under* Infections, mycotic, cutaneous)

Furunculosis
Levaquin (Levofloxacin) Ortho-McNeil 2537

Furunculosis, symptomatic relief of
Panafil Ointment (Chlorophyllin Copper Complex Sodium, Papain, Urea) Healthpoint 1726

Fusobacterium fusiformisans spirochete infections
Pfizerpen for Injection (Penicillin G Potassium) Pfizer 2707

Fusobacterium nucleatum gynecologic infections
Claforan (Cefotaxime Sodium) Aventis 732

Fusobacterium species gynecologic infections
Cefotan (Cefotetan) AstraZeneca 664
Claforan Injection (Cefotaxime Sodium) Aventis 732

Fusobacterium species infections
Cefotan (Cefotetan) AstraZeneca 664
Claforan Injection (Cefotaxime Sodium) Aventis 732
Primaxin I.M. (Cilastatin Sodium, Imipenem) Merck 2158
Primaxin I.V. (Cilastatin Sodium, Imipenem) Merck 2160

Fusobacterium species intra-abdominal infections
Primaxin I.M. (Cilastatin Sodium, Imipenem) Merck 2158
Primaxin I.V. (Cilastatin Sodium, Imipenem) Merck 2160

Fusospirochetosis
Declomycin Tablets (Demeclocycline Hydrochloride) Lederle 1855
Doryx Coated Pellet Filled Capsules (Doxycycline Hyclate) Warner Chilcott 3357
Dynacin Capsules (Minocycline Hydrochloride) Medicis 2019
Minocin Intravenous (Minocycline Hydrochloride) Lederle 1862
Minocin Oral Suspension (Minocycline Hydrochloride) Lederle 1865
Minocin Pellet-Filled Capsules (Minocycline Hydrochloride) Lederle 1863
Monodox Capsules (Doxycycline Monohydrate) Oclassen 2442
Pfizerpen for Injection (Penicillin G Potassium) Pfizer 2707
Vibramycin Calcium Oral Suspension Syrup (Doxycycline Calcium) Pfizer 2735
Vibramycin Hyclate Capsules (Doxycycline Hyclate) Pfizer 2735
Vibramycin Hyclate Intravenous (Doxycycline Hyclate) Pfizer 2737
Vibramycin Monohydrate for Oral Suspension (Doxycycline Monohydrate) Pfizer 2735
Vibra-Tabs Film Coated Tablets (Doxycycline Hyclate) Pfizer 2735

G

Gag reflex, suppression
Cetacaine Topical Anesthetic (Benzocaine, Butyl Aminobenzoate, Tetracaine Hydrochloride) Cetylite 1196
Hurricaine Topical Anesthetic Gel, 1 oz. Fresh Mint, Wild Cherry, Pina Colada, Watermelon, 1/6 oz. Wild Cherry, Watermelon (Benzocaine) Beutlich .... ▣618
Hurricaine Topical Anesthetic Liquid, 1 oz. Wild Cherry, Pina Colada, .25 ml Dry Handle Swab Wild Cherry, 1/6 oz. Wild Cherry (Benzocaine) Beutlich .... ▣618
Hurricaine Topical Anesthetic Spray Extension Tubes (200) (Benzocaine) Beutlich .... ▣618
Hurricaine Topical Anesthetic Spray Kit, 2 oz. Wild Cherry (Benzocaine) Beutlich .... ▣618
Hurricaine Topical Anesthetic Spray, 2 oz. Wild Cherry (Benzocaine) Beutlich .... ▣618

Gardnerella vaginalis infections
MetroGel-Vaginal Gel (Metronidazole) 3M 1986
Primaxin I.V. (Cilastatin Sodium, Imipenem) Merck 2160

Gardnerella vaginalis vaginitis
(*see under* H. vaginalis vaginitis)

Gastric emptying, delayed
Reglan (Metoclopramide Hydrochloride) Robins ... 2935

Gastric ulcer, nonsteroidal anti-inflammatory drug induced
Prevacid Delayed-Release Capsules (Lansoprazole) TAP ... 3292

Gastric ulcers, active, benign, short-term treatment of
Axid Pulvules (Nizatidine) Lilly ... 1903
Axid Pulvules (Nizatidine) Reliant ... 2919
Famotidine Injection (Famotidine) Baxter Anesthesia ... 866
Pepcid Injection (Famotidine) Merck ... 2153
Pepcid for Oral Suspension (Famotidine) Merck ... 2150
Pepcid RPD Orally Disintegrating Tablets (Famotidine) Merck ... 2150
Pepcid Tablets (Famotidine) Merck ... 2150
Prevacid Delayed-Release Capsules (Lansoprazole) TAP ... 3292
Prilosec Delayed-Release Capsules (Omeprazole) AstraZeneca LP ... 628
Tagamet (Cimetidine Hydrochloride) GlaxoSmithKline ... 1644
Zantac (Ranitidine Hydrochloride) GlaxoSmithKline ... 1690

Gastric ulcers, nonsteroidal anti-inflammatory drug-induced, prevention of
Cytotec Tablets (Misoprostol) Searle ... 3202

Gastroesophageal reflux, symptomatic
Reglan (Metoclopramide Hydrochloride) Robins ... 2935

Gastroesophageal reflux disease
Aciphex Tablets (Rabeprazole Sodium) Eisai ... 1267
Aciphex Tablets (Rabeprazole Sodium) Janssen ... 1783
Axid Pulvules (Nizatidine) Lilly ... 1903
Axid Pulvules (Nizatidine) Reliant ... 2919
Famotidine Injection (Famotidine) Baxter Anesthesia ... 866
Nexium Delayed-Release Capsules (Esomeprazole Magnesium) AstraZeneca LP ... 619
Pepcid Injection (Famotidine) Merck ... 2153
Pepcid for Oral Suspension (Famotidine) Merck ... 2150
Pepcid RPD Orally Disintegrating Tablets (Famotidine) Merck ... 2150
Pepcid Tablets (Famotidine) Merck ... 2150
Prevacid Delayed-Release Capsules (Lansoprazole) TAP ... 3292
Prilosec Delayed-Release Capsules (Omeprazole) AstraZeneca LP ... 628
Protonix I.V. (Pantoprazole Sodium) Wyeth-Ayerst ... 3580
Protonix Tablets (Pantoprazole Sodium) Wyeth-Ayerst ... 3577
Tagamet (Cimetidine Hydrochloride) GlaxoSmithKline ... 1644
Zantac (Ranitidine Hydrochloride) GlaxoSmithKline ... 1690

Gastrointestinal hypermotility, symptomatic relief of
Arco-Lase Plus Tablets (Amylase, Cellulase, Hyoscyamine Sulfate, Lipase, Phenobarbital, Protease) Arco ... 592
Levsin/Levsinex/Levbid (Hyoscyamine Sulfate) Schwarz ... 3172
NuLev Orally Disintegrating Tablets (Hyoscyamine Sulfate) Schwarz ... 3176

Gastroparesis, diabetic
(*see also under* Gastric emptying, delayed)
Reglan (Metoclopramide Hydrochloride) Robins ... 2935

Gaucher disease, Type 1
Cerezyme for Injection (Imiglucerase) Genzyme ... 1438

Gelineau's syndrome
(*see under* Narcolepsy)

Genital warts
(*see under* Condylomata acuminata)

GERD
(*see under* Gastroesophageal reflux disease)

German measles
(*see under* Rubella, prophylaxis)

Gestational trophoblastic disease, non-metastatic
Prostin E2 Suppositories (Dinoprostone) Pharmacia & Upjohn ... 2852

Gestational trophoblastic neoplasia
Cosmegen for Injection (Dactinomycin) Merck ... 2062

Gibraltar fever
(*see under* Brucellosis)

Gilchrist's disease
(*see under* Blastomycosis)

Gingivitis
Listerine Mouthrinse (Eucalyptol, Menthol, Methyl Salicylate) Pfizer Inc., Warner-Lambert Healthcare ... ▣702
Cool Mint Listerine Mouthrinse (Eucalyptol, Menthol, Methyl Salicylate, Thymol) Pfizer Inc., Warner-Lambert Healthcare ... ▣702
FreshBurst Listerine Mouthrinse (Eucalyptol, Menthol, Methyl Salicylate, Thymol) Pfizer Inc., Warner-Lambert Healthcare ... ▣702
Tartar Control Listerine Mouthrinse (Eucalyptol, Menthol, Methyl Salicylate) Pfizer Inc., Warner-Lambert Healthcare ... ▣702

Gingivitis, necrotizing ulcerative
(*see under* Fusospirochetosis)

Glaucoma, angle-closure, acute
Daranide Tablets (Dichlorphenamide) Merck ... 2077
Diamox Intravenous (Acetazolamide Sodium) Lederle ... ⊙269
Diamox Sequels Sustained Release Capsules (Acetazolamide) Lederle ... ⊙270
Diamox Tablets (Acetazolamide) Lederle ... ⊙269
Neptazane Tablets (Methazolamide) Lederle ... ⊙271

Glaucoma, angle-closure, acute, preoperative
Diamox (Acetazolamide Sodium) Lederle ... ⊙269

Glaucoma, chronic open-angle
Betagan (Levobunolol Hydrochloride) Allergan ... ⊙228
Betaxon Ophthalmic Suspension (Levobetaxolol Hydrochloride) Alcon ... 537
Betoptic S Ophthalmic Suspension (Betaxolol Hydrochloride) Alcon ... 537
Carteolol Hydrochloride Ophthalmic Solution USP, 1% (Carteolol Hydrochloride) Bausch & Lomb ... ⊙258
Daranide Tablets (Dichlorphenamide) Merck ... 2077
Diamox Intravenous (Acetazolamide Sodium) Lederle ... ⊙269
Diamox Sequels Sustained Release Capsules (Acetazolamide) Lederle ... ⊙270
Diamox Tablets (Acetazolamide) Lederle ... ⊙269
Epifrin Sterile Ophthalmic Solution (Epinephrine) Allergan ... ⊙235
Neptazane Tablets (Methazolamide) Lederle ... ⊙271
Ocupress Ophthalmic Solution, 1% Sterile (Carteolol Hydrochloride) Novartis Ophthalmics ... ⊙303
OptiPranolol Metipranolol Ophthalmic Solution 0.3% (Metipranolol) Bausch & Lomb ... ⊙263
Propine Ophthalmic Solution (Dipivefrin Hydrochloride) Allergan ... ⊙250
Timolol GFS (Timolol Maleate) Falcon ... ⊙266
Timoptic in Ocudose (Timolol Maleate) Merck ... 2192
Timoptic Sterile Ophthalmic Solution (Timolol Maleate) Merck ... 2190
Timoptic-XE Sterile Ophthalmic Gel Forming Solution (Timolol Maleate) Merck ... 2194

Glaucoma, open-angle
Alphagan Ophthalmic Solution (Brimonidine Tartrate) Allergan ... 545
Alphagan P Ophthalmic Solution (Brimonidine Tartrate) Allergan ... 546
Azopt Ophthalmic Suspension (Brinzolamide) Alcon ... 536
Cosopt Sterile Ophthalmic Solution (Dorzolamide Hydrochloride, Timolol Maleate) Merck ... 2065
Humorsol Sterile Ophthalmic Solution (Demecarium Bromide) Merck ... 2102
Lumigan Ophthalmic Solution (Bimatoprost) Allergan ... 553
Rescula Ophthalmic Solution (Unoprostone isopropyl) Novartis Ophthalmics ... ⊙306
Travatan Ophthalmic Solution (Travoprost) Alcon ... 543
Trusopt Sterile Ophthalmic Solution (Dorzolamide Hydrochloride) Merck ... 2196
Xalatan Latanoprost Ophthalmic Solution (Latanoprost) Pharmacia & Upjohn ... ⊙320
Xalatan Sterile Ophthalmic Solution (Latanoprost) Pharmacia & Upjohn ... 2864

Glaucoma, secondary
Daranide Tablets (Dichlorphenamide) Merck ... 2077
Diamox Intravenous (Acetazolamide Sodium) Lederle ... ⊙269
Diamox Sequels Sustained Release Capsules (Acetazolamide) Lederle ... ⊙270
Diamox Tablets (Acetazolamide) Lederle ... ⊙269
Neptazane Tablets (Methazolamide) Lederle ... ⊙271

Glaucoma, unspecified
Isopto Carbachol Ophthalmic Solution (Carbachol) Alcon ... ⊙215

Glaucoma filtration, surgical aid in
Healon (Sodium Hyaluronate) Pharmacia & Upjohn ... ⊙316
Healon GV (Sodium Hyaluronate) Pharmacia & Upjohn ... ⊙320

Glioblastoma multiforme, recurrent, adjunctive therapy in
Gliadel Wafer (Carmustine (BCNU)) Guilford ... 1723

Glomerulonephritis, acute, prophylaxis
Bicillin L-A Injection (Penicillin G Benzathine) Monarch ... 2242

Goiter, euthyroid, treatment or prevention of
Synthroid (Levothyroxine Sodium) Abbott ... 505

Goiter, suppression of pituitary TSH in
Cytomel Tablets (Liothyronine Sodium) Jones ... 1817
Levothroid Tablets (Levothyroxine Sodium) Forest ... 1373
Levoxyl Tablets (Levothyroxine Sodium) Jones ... 1819
Synthroid (Levothyroxine Sodium) Abbott ... 505
Unithroid Tablets (Levothyroxine Sodium) Watson ... 3445

Gonococcal infections, uncomplicated
Doryx Coated Pellet Filled Capsules (Doxycycline Hyclate) Warner Chilcott ... 3357
Pipracil (Piperacillin Sodium) Lederle ... 1866
Rocephin Injectable Vials, ADD-Vantage, Galaxy, Bulk (Ceftriaxone Sodium) Roche Laboratories ... 2993
Vantin Tablets and Oral Suspension (Cefpodoxime Proxetil) Pharmacia & Upjohn ... 2860
Vibramycin Calcium Oral Suspension Syrup (Doxycycline Calcium) Pfizer ... 2735
Vibramycin Hyclate Capsules (Doxycycline Hyclate) Pfizer ... 2735
Vibramycin Monohydrate for Oral Suspension (Doxycycline Monohydrate) Pfizer ... 2735
Vibra-Tabs Film Coated Tablets (Doxycycline Hyclate) Pfizer ... 2735
Zinacef Injection (Cefuroxime) GlaxoSmithKline ... 1696
Zinacef for Injection (Cefuroxime) GlaxoSmithKline ... 1696

Gonorrhea
(*see also under* N. gonorrhoeae infections)
Amoxil Chewable Tablets (Amoxicillin) GlaxoSmithKline ... 1471
Amoxil for Oral Suspension (Amoxicillin) GlaxoSmithKline ... 1471
Amoxil (Amoxicillin) GlaxoSmithKline ... 1471
Cefizox for Intramuscular or Intravenous Use (Ceftizoxime Sodium) Fujisawa ... 1390
Claforan Injection (Cefotaxime Sodium) Aventis ... 732
Kefurox Vials, ADD-Vantage (Cefuroxime Sodium) Lilly ... 1948
Rocephin Injectable Vials, ADD-Vantage, Galaxy, Bulk (Ceftriaxone Sodium) Roche Laboratories ... 2993
Zinacef Injection (Cefuroxime) GlaxoSmithKline ... 1696
Zinacef for Injection (Cefuroxime) GlaxoSmithKline ... 1696

Gonorrhea, cervical/urethral
Cefizox for Intramuscular or Intravenous Use (Ceftizoxime Sodium) Fujisawa ... 1390
Cipro (Ciprofloxacin) Bayer ... 887
Floxin I.V. (Ofloxacin) Ortho-McNeil ... 2526
Floxin Tablets (Ofloxacin) Ortho-McNeil ... 2529
Noroxin Tablets (Norfloxacin) Merck ... 2145
Rocephin Injectable Vials, ADD-Vantage, Galaxy, Bulk (Ceftriaxone Sodium) Roche Laboratories ... 2993
Vantin Tablets and Oral Suspension (Cefpodoxime Proxetil) Pharmacia & Upjohn ... 2860

Gonorrhea, pharyngeal
Rocephin (Ceftriaxone Sodium) Roche Laboratories ... 2993

Gonorrhea, uncomplicated
Cefizox for Intramuscular or Intravenous Use (Ceftizoxime Sodium) Fujisawa ... 1390
Ceftin Tablets (Cefuroxime Axetil) Lifecycle Ventures ... 1898
Cipro (Ciprofloxacin) Bayer ... 887
Monodox Capsules (Doxycycline Monohydrate) Oclassen ... 2442
Noroxin Tablets (Norfloxacin) Merck ... 2145
Rocephin Injectable Vials, ADD-Vantage, Galaxy, Bulk (Ceftriaxone Sodium) Roche Laboratories ... 2993
Suprax Tablets (Cefixime) Lederle ... 1877

Gout, acute
Anaprox Tablets (Naproxen Sodium) Roche Laboratories ... 2967
Anaprox DS Tablets (Naproxen Sodium) Roche Laboratories ... 2967
Naprelan Tablets (Naproxen Sodium) Elan ... 1293
Naprosyn Suspension (Naproxen) Roche Laboratories ... 2967
Naprosyn Tablets (Naproxen) Roche Laboratories ... 2967

Grand mal epilepsy
(*see under* Seizures, generalized, tonic-clonic)

Granuloma annulare, infiltrated inflammatory lesions of
Celestone Soluspan Injectable Suspension (Betamethasone Acetate, Betamethasone Sodium Phosphate) Schering ... 3097
Decadron Phosphate Injection (Dexamethasone Sodium Phosphate) Merck ... 2081
Hydrocortone Acetate Injectable Suspension (Hydrocortisone Acetate) Merck ... 2103

Granuloma inguinale
Declomycin Tablets (Demeclocycline Hydrochloride) Lederle ... 1855
Doryx Coated Pellet Filled Capsules (Doxycycline Hyclate) Warner Chilcott ... 3357
Dynacin Capsules (Minocycline Hydrochloride) Medicis ... 2019
Minocin Intravenous (Minocycline Hydrochloride) Lederle ... 1862
Minocin Oral Suspension (Minocycline Hydrochloride) Lederle ... 1865
Minocin Pellet-Filled Capsules (Minocycline Hydrochloride) Lederle ... 1863
Monodox Capsules (Doxycycline Monohydrate) Oclassen ... 2442
Streptomycin Sulfate Injection (Streptomycin Sulfate) Pfizer ... 2714
Vibramycin Calcium Oral Suspension Syrup (Doxycycline Calcium) Pfizer ... 2735

Vibramycin Hyclate Capsules (Doxycycline Hyclate) Pfizer 2735
Vibramycin Hyclate Intravenous (Doxycycline Hyclate) Pfizer 2737
Vibramycin Monohydrate for Oral Suspension (Doxycycline Monohydrate) Pfizer 2735
Vibra-Tabs Film Coated Tablets (Doxycycline Hyclate) Pfizer 2735

Granulomatous disease, chronic
Actimmune (Interferon Gamma-1B) InterMune 1772

Growth failure, chronic renal insufficiency-induced in children
Nutropin AQ Injection (Somatropin) Genentech 1420
Nutropin for Injection (Somatropin) Genentech 1417

Growth hormone secretion, inadequate
Genotropin Lyophilized Powder (Somatropin) Pharmacia & Upjohn 2818
Geref for Injection (Sermorelin Acetate) Serono 3215
Humatrope Vials and Cartridges (Somatropin) Lilly 1930
Norditropin Cartridges (Somatropin) Novo Nordisk 2420
Norditropin for Injection (Somatropin) Novo Nordisk 2419
Nutropin AQ Injection (Somatropin) Genentech 1420
Nutropin Depot for Injectable Suspension (Somatropin) Genentech 1423
Nutropin for Injection (Somatropin) Genentech 1417
Saizen for Injection (Somatropin) Serono 3225

Gums, sore
(*see under* Pain, dental)

H

H. aegypticus infections, ocular
TobraDex Ophthalmic Ointment (Dexamethasone, Tobramycin) Alcon 542
TobraDex Ophthalmic Suspension (Dexamethasone, Tobramycin) Alcon 541

H. ducreyi infections
Declomycin Tablets (Demeclocycline Hydrochloride) Lederle 1855
Doryx Coated Pellet Filled Capsules (Doxycycline Hyclate) Warner Chilcott 3357
Dynacin Capsules (Minocycline Hydrochloride) Medicis 2019
Minocin Intravenous (Minocycline Hydrochloride) Lederle 1862
Minocin Oral Suspension (Minocycline Hydrochloride) Lederle 1865
Minocin Pellet-Filled Capsules (Minocycline Hydrochloride) Lederle 1863
Monodox Capsules (Doxycycline Monohydrate) Oclassen 2442
Streptomycin Sulfate Injection (Streptomycin Sulfate) Pfizer 2714
Vibramycin Calcium Oral Suspension Syrup (Doxycycline Calcium) Pfizer 2735
Vibramycin Hyclate Capsules (Doxycycline Hyclate) Pfizer 2735
Vibramycin Hyclate Intravenous (Doxycycline Hyclate) Pfizer 2737
Vibramycin Monohydrate for Oral Suspension (Doxycycline Monohydrate) Pfizer 2735
Vibra-Tabs Film Coated Tablets (Doxycycline Hyclate) Pfizer 2735
Zithromax Capsules, 250 mg (Azithromycin Dihydrate) Pfizer 2743
Zithromax for IV Infusion (Azithromycin Dihydrate) Pfizer 2748
Zithromax for Oral Suspension, 300 mg, 600 mg, 900 mg, 1200 mg (Azithromycin Dihydrate) Pfizer 2739
Zithromax Tablets, 250 mg (Azithromycin Dihydrate) Pfizer 2739

H. influenzae, central nervous system infections
Ceptaz for Injection (Ceftazidime) GlaxoSmithKline 1499
Claforan Injection (Cefotaxime Sodium) Aventis 732
Fortaz (Ceftazidime Sodium) GlaxoSmithKline 1541
Tazicef for Injection (Ceftazidime) GlaxoSmithKline 1647
Tazicef Galaxy Container (Ceftazidime Sodium) GlaxoSmithKline 1650
Tazicef Pharmacy Bulk Package (Ceftazidime) GlaxoSmithKline 1653
Tazidime Vials, Faspak & ADD-Vantage (Ceftazidime) Lilly 1966

H. influenzae, skin and skin structure infections
Mandol Vials (Cefamandole Nafate) Lilly 1953

H. influenzae bacteremia
Ceptaz for Injection (Ceftazidime) GlaxoSmithKline 1499

H. influenzae bronchitis
Avelox Tablets (Moxifloxacin Hydrochloride) Bayer 879
Bactrim (Sulfamethoxazole, Trimethoprim) Roche Laboratories 2949
Biaxin/Biaxin XL (Clarithromycin) Abbott 403
Ceclor CD Tablets (Cefaclor) Elan 1279
Cedax (Ceftibuten Dihydrate) Biovail 1021
Ceftin Tablets (Cefuroxime Axetil) Lifecycle Ventures 1898
Cefzil (Cefprozil) Bristol-Myers Squibb 1076
Floxin I.V. (Ofloxacin) Ortho-McNeil 2526
Floxin Tablets (Ofloxacin) Ortho-McNeil 2529
Levaquin (Levofloxacin) Ortho-McNeil 2537
Lorabid Suspension and Pulvules (Loracarbef) Monarch 2251
Omnicef (Cefdinir) Abbott 493
Septra Suspension (Sulfamethoxazole, Trimethoprim) Monarch 2265
Septra Tablets (Sulfamethoxazole, Trimethoprim) Monarch 2265
Septra DS Tablets (Sulfamethoxazole, Trimethoprim) Monarch 2265
Suprax Tablets (Cefixime) Lederle 1877
Tequin Injection (Gatifloxacin) Bristol-Myers Squibb 1110
Tequin Tablets (Gatifloxacin) Bristol-Myers Squibb 1110
Vantin Tablets and Oral Suspension (Cefpodoxime Proxetil) Pharmacia & Upjohn 2860

H. influenzae infections
Amoxil Chewable Tablets (Amoxicillin) GlaxoSmithKline 1471
Amoxil for Oral Suspension (Amoxicillin) GlaxoSmithKline 1471
Amoxil (Amoxicillin) GlaxoSmithKline 1471
Ancef for Injection (Cefazolin Sodium) GlaxoSmithKline 1474
Ancef Injection (Cefazolin Sodium) GlaxoSmithKline 1474
Augmentin Chewable Tablets (Amoxicillin, Clavulanate Potassium) GlaxoSmithKline 1482
Augmentin Powder for Oral Suspension (Amoxicillin, Clavulanate Potassium) GlaxoSmithKline 1482
Augmentin Tablets (Amoxicillin, Clavulanate Potassium) GlaxoSmithKline 1485
Augmentin ES-600 Powder for Oral Suspension (Amoxicillin, Clavulanate Potassium) GlaxoSmithKline 1487
Avelox Tablets (Moxifloxacin Hydrochloride) Bayer 879
Azactam for Injection (Aztreonam) Elan 1276
Bactrim (Sulfamethoxazole, Trimethoprim) Roche Laboratories 2949
Biaxin/Biaxin XL (Clarithromycin) Abbott 403
Ceclor CD Tablets (Cefaclor) Elan 1279
Ceclor (Cefaclor) Lilly 1905
Cedax (Ceftibuten Dihydrate) Biovail 1021
Cefizox for Intramuscular or Intravenous Use (Ceftizoxime Sodium) Fujisawa 1390
Cefotan (Cefotetan) AstraZeneca 664
Ceftin (Cefuroxime Axetil) Lifecycle Ventures 1898
Cefzil (Cefprozil) Bristol-Myers Squibb 1076
Ceptaz for Injection (Ceftazidime) GlaxoSmithKline 1499
Cipro I.V. (Ciprofloxacin) Bayer 893
Cipro (Ciprofloxacin) Bayer 887
Claforan Injection (Cefotaxime Sodium) Aventis 732
Declomycin Tablets (Demeclocycline Hydrochloride) Lederle 1855
Dynacin Capsules (Minocycline Hydrochloride) Medicis 2019
E.E.S. (Erythromycin Ethylsuccinate) Abbott 450
EryPed (Erythromycin Ethylsuccinate) Abbott 446
Ery-Tab Tablets (Erythromycin) Abbott 448
Erythrocin Stearate Filmtab Tablets (Erythromycin Stearate) Abbott 452
Erythromycin Base Filmtab Tablets (Erythromycin) Abbott 454
Erythromycin Delayed-Release Capsules, USP (Erythromycin) Abbott 455
Floxin I.V. (Ofloxacin) Ortho-McNeil 2526
Floxin Tablets (Ofloxacin) Ortho-McNeil 2529
Fortaz (Ceftazidime Sodium) GlaxoSmithKline 1541
Keflex (Cephalexin) Dista 1237
Kefurox Vials, ADD-Vantage (Cefuroxime Sodium) Lilly 1948
Kefzol Vials, ADD-Vantage (Cefazolin Sodium) Lilly 1951
Levaquin (Levofloxacin) Ortho-McNeil 2537
Lorabid Suspension and Pulvules (Loracarbef) Monarch 2251
Mefoxin for Injection (Cefoxitin Sodium) Merck 2124
Mefoxin Premixed Intravenous Solution (Cefoxitin Sodium) Merck 2127
Merrem I.V. (Meropenem) AstraZeneca 673
Minocin Intravenous (Minocycline Hydrochloride) Lederle 1862
Minocin Oral Suspension (Minocycline Hydrochloride) Lederle 1865
Minocin Pellet-Filled Capsules (Minocycline Hydrochloride) Lederle 1863
Monodox Capsules (Doxycycline Monohydrate) Oclassen 2442
Omnicef (Cefdinir) Abbott 493
PCE Dispertab Tablets (Erythromycin) Abbott 498
Pipracil (Piperacillin Sodium) Lederle 1866
Primaxin I.M. (Cilastatin Sodium, Imipenem) Merck 2158
Primaxin I.V. (Cilastatin Sodium, Imipenem) Merck 2160
Rocephin Injectable Vials, ADD-Vantage, Galaxy, Bulk (Ceftriaxone Sodium) Roche Laboratories 2993
Septra Suspension (Sulfamethoxazole, Trimethoprim) Monarch 2265
Septra Tablets (Sulfamethoxazole, Trimethoprim) Monarch 2265
Septra DS Tablets (Sulfamethoxazole, Trimethoprim) Monarch 2265
Suprax (Cefixime) Lederle 1877
Tazicef for Injection (Ceftazidime) GlaxoSmithKline 1647
Tazicef Galaxy Container (Ceftazidime Sodium) GlaxoSmithKline 1650
Tazicef Pharmacy Bulk Package (Ceftazidime) GlaxoSmithKline 1653
Tazidime Vials, Faspak & ADD-Vantage (Ceftazidime) Lilly 1966
Tequin Injection (Gatifloxacin) Bristol-Myers Squibb 1110
Tequin Tablets (Gatifloxacin) Bristol-Myers Squibb 1110
Timentin Injection- ADD-Vantage Vial (Clavulanate Potassium, Ticarcillin Disodium) GlaxoSmithKline 1661
Timentin Injection-Galaxy Container (Clavulanate Potassium, Ticarcillin Disodium) GlaxoSmithKline 1664
Timentin Injection-Pharmacy Bulk Package (Clavulanate Potassium, Ticarcillin Disodium) GlaxoSmithKline 1666
Timentin for Intravenous Administration (Clavulanate Potassium, Ticarcillin Disodium) GlaxoSmithKline 1658
Trovan (Alatrofloxacin Mesylate) Pfizer 2722
Vantin Tablets and Oral Suspension (Cefpodoxime Proxetil) Pharmacia & Upjohn 2860
Zinacef Injection (Cefuroxime) GlaxoSmithKline 1696
Zinacef for Injection (Cefuroxime) GlaxoSmithKline 1696
Zithromax Capsules, 250 mg (Azithromycin Dihydrate) Pfizer 2743
Zithromax for IV Infusion (Azithromycin Dihydrate) Pfizer 2748
Zithromax for Oral Suspension, 1 g (Azithromycin Dihydrate) Pfizer 2743
Zithromax for Oral Suspension, 300 mg, 600 mg, 900 mg, 1200 mg (Azithromycin Dihydrate) Pfizer 2739
Zithromax Tablets, 250 mg (Azithromycin Dihydrate) Pfizer 2739
Zithromax Tablets, 600 mg (Azithromycin Dihydrate) Pfizer 2743
Zosyn (Piperacillin Sodium, Tazobactam Sodium) Lederle 1890
Zosyn in Galaxy Containers (Piperacillin Sodium, Tazobactam Sodium) Lederle 1894

H. influenzae infections, ocular
Blephamide Ophthalmic Ointment (Prednisolone Acetate, Sulfacetamide Sodium) Allergan 547
Blephamide Ophthalmic Suspension (Prednisolone Acetate, Sulfacetamide Sodium) Allergan 548
Chibroxin Sterile Ophthalmic Solution (Norfloxacin) Merck 2051
Chloromycetin Ophthalmic Ointment, 1% (Chloramphenicol) Monarch .... ⊙296
Chloromycetin Ophthalmic Solution (Chloramphenicol) Monarch .... ⊙297
Chloroptic Sterile Ophthalmic Ointment (Chloramphenicol) Allergan .... ⊙234
Ciloxan (Ciprofloxacin Hydrochloride) Alcon 538
Cortisporin Ophthalmic Suspension (Hydrocortisone, Neomycin Sulfate, Polymyxin B Sulfate, Hydrocortisone, Neomycin Sulfate, Polymyxin B Sulfate) Monarch .... ⊙297
FML-S Liquifilm Sterile Ophthalmic Suspension (Fluorometholone, Sulfacetamide Sodium) Allergan .... ⊙238
Genoptic Ophthalmic Ointment (Gentamicin Sulfate) Allergan .... ⊙239
Genoptic Sterile Ophthalmic Solution (Gentamicin Sulfate) Allergan .... ⊙239
NeoDecadron Sterile Ophthalmic Solution (Dexamethasone Sodium Phosphate, Neomycin Sulfate) Merck 2144
Ocuflox Ophthalmic Solution (Ofloxacin) Allergan 554
Poly-Pred Liquifilm Ophthalmic Suspension (Neomycin Sulfate, Polymyxin B Sulfate, Prednisolone Acetate) Allergan .... ⊙245
Polytrim Ophthalmic Solution (Polymyxin B Sulfate, Trimethoprim Sulfate) Allergan 556
Pred-G Ophthalmic Suspension (Gentamicin Sulfate, Prednisolone Acetate) Allergan .... ⊙247
Pred-G Sterile Ophthalmic Ointment (Gentamicin Sulfate, Prednisolone Acetate) Allergan .... ⊙248
Quixin Ophthalmic Solution (Levofloxacin) Santen 3093
TobraDex Ophthalmic Ointment (Dexamethasone, Tobramycin) Alcon 542
TobraDex Ophthalmic Suspension (Dexamethasone, Tobramycin) Alcon 541

H. influenzae infections, treatment adjunct
Streptomycin Sulfate Injection (Streptomycin Sulfate) Pfizer 2714

H. influenzae lower respiratory tract infections
Amoxil Chewable Tablets (Amoxicillin) GlaxoSmithKline 1471
Amoxil for Oral Suspension (Amoxicillin) GlaxoSmithKline 1471
Amoxil (Amoxicillin) GlaxoSmithKline 1471
Augmentin Chewable Tablets (Amoxicillin, Clavulanate Potassium) GlaxoSmithKline 1482
Augmentin Powder for Oral Suspension (Amoxicillin, Clavulanate Potassium) GlaxoSmithKline 1482
Augmentin Tablets (Amoxicillin, Clavulanate Potassium) GlaxoSmithKline 1485
Azactam for Injection (Aztreonam) Elan 1276
Biaxin/Biaxin XL (Clarithromycin) Abbott 403
Ceclor (Cefaclor) Lilly 1905
Cefizox for Intramuscular or Intravenous Use (Ceftizoxime Sodium) Fujisawa 1390
Cefobid Intravenous/Intramuscular (Cefoperazone) Pfizer 2671
Cefobid Pharmacy Bulk Package - Not for Direct Infusion (Cefoperazone Sodium) Pfizer 2673
Cefotan (Cefotetan) AstraZeneca 664

Cefzil (Cefprozil) Bristol-Myers Squibb ... 1076
Ceptaz for Injection (Ceftazidime) GlaxoSmithKline ... 1499
Cipro I.V. (Ciprofloxacin) Bayer ... 893
Cipro I.V. Pharmacy Bulk Package (Ciprofloxacin) Bayer ... 897
Cipro (Ciprofloxacin) Bayer ... 887
Claforan Injection (Cefotaxime Sodium) Aventis ... 732
Floxin I.V. (Ofloxacin) Ortho-McNeil ... 2526
Floxin Tablets (Ofloxacin) Ortho-McNeil ... 2529
Fortaz (Ceftazidime Sodium) GlaxoSmithKline ... 1541
Kefurox Vials, ADD-Vantage (Cefuroxime Sodium) Lilly ... 1948
Levaquin (Levofloxacin) Ortho-McNeil ... 2537
Lorabid Suspension and Pulvules (Loracarbef) Monarch ... 2251
Mandol Vials (Cefamandole Nafate) Lilly ... 1953
Mefoxin for Injection (Cefoxitin Sodium) Merck ... 2124
Mefoxin Premixed Intravenous Solution (Cefoxitin Sodium) Merck ... 2127
Pipracil (Piperacillin Sodium) Lederle ... 1866
Primaxin I.M. (Cilastatin Sodium, Imipenem) Merck ... 2158
Primaxin I.V. (Cilastatin Sodium, Imipenem) Merck ... 2160
Rocephin Injectable Vials, ADD-Vantage, Galaxy, Bulk (Ceftriaxone Sodium) Roche Laboratories ... 2993
Tazicef for Injection (Ceftazidime) GlaxoSmithKline ... 1647
Tazicef Galaxy Container (Ceftazidime Sodium) GlaxoSmithKline ... 1650
Tazicef Pharmacy Bulk Package (Ceftazidime) GlaxoSmithKline ... 1653
Tazidime Vials, Faspak & ADD-Vantage (Ceftazidime) Lilly ... 1966
Tequin Injection (Gatifloxacin) Bristol-Myers Squibb ... 1110
Tequin Tablets (Gatifloxacin) Bristol-Myers Squibb ... 1110
Timentin Injection- ADD-Vantage Vial (Clavulanate Potassium, Ticarcillin Disodium) GlaxoSmithKline ... 1661
Timentin Injection-Galaxy Container (Clavulanate Potassium, Ticarcillin Disodium) GlaxoSmithKline ... 1664
Timentin Injection-Pharmacy Bulk Package (Clavulanate Potassium, Ticarcillin Disodium) GlaxoSmithKline ... 1666
Timentin for Intravenous Administration (Clavulanate Potassium, Ticarcillin Disodium) GlaxoSmithKline ... 1658
Trovan (Alatrofloxacin Mesylate) Pfizer ... 2722
Vantin Tablets and Oral Suspension (Cefpodoxime Proxetil) Pharmacia & Upjohn ... 2860
Zinacef Injection (Cefuroxime) GlaxoSmithKline ... 1696
Zinacef for Injection (Cefuroxime) GlaxoSmithKline ... 1696
Zithromax Capsules, 250 mg (Azithromycin Dihydrate) Pfizer ... 2743
Zithromax for IV Infusion (Azithromycin Dihydrate) Pfizer ... 2748
Zithromax for Oral Suspension, 1 g (Azithromycin Dihydrate) Pfizer ... 2743
Zithromax for Oral Suspension, 300 mg, 600 mg, 900 mg, 1200 mg (Azithromycin Dihydrate) Pfizer ... 2739
Zithromax Tablets, 250 mg (Azithromycin Dihydrate) Pfizer ... 2739
Zithromax Tablets, 600 mg (Azithromycin Dihydrate) Pfizer ... 2743
Zosyn (Piperacillin Sodium, Tazobactam Sodium) Lederle ... 1890
Zosyn in Galaxy Containers (Piperacillin Sodium, Tazobactam Sodium) Lederle ... 1894

H. influenzae meningitis
Cefizox for Intramuscular or Intravenous Use (Ceftizoxime Sodium) Fujisawa ... 1390
Fortaz (Ceftazidime Sodium) GlaxoSmithKline ... 1541
Merrem I.V. (Meropenem) AstraZeneca ... 673
Rocephin Injectable Vials, ADD-Vantage, Galaxy, Bulk (Ceftriaxone Sodium) Roche Laboratories ... 2993
Tazicef for Injection (Ceftazidime) GlaxoSmithKline ... 1647
Tazicef Galaxy Container (Ceftazidime Sodium) GlaxoSmithKline ... 1650
Tazicef Pharmacy Bulk Package (Ceftazidime) GlaxoSmithKline ... 1653
Tazidime Vials, Faspak & ADD-Vantage (Ceftazidime) Lilly ... 1966
Zinacef Injection (Cefuroxime) GlaxoSmithKline ... 1696
Zinacef for Injection (Cefuroxime) GlaxoSmithKline ... 1696

H. influenzae otitis media
Augmentin Chewable Tablets (Amoxicillin, Clavulanate Potassium) GlaxoSmithKline ... 1482
Augmentin Powder for Oral Suspension (Amoxicillin, Clavulanate Potassium) GlaxoSmithKline ... 1482
Augmentin Tablets (Amoxicillin, Clavulanate Potassium) GlaxoSmithKline ... 1485
Augmentin ES-600 Powder for Oral Suspension (Amoxicillin, Clavulanate Potassium) GlaxoSmithKline ... 1487
Bactrim (Sulfamethoxazole, Trimethoprim) Roche Laboratories ... 2949
Biaxin/Biaxin XL (Clarithromycin) Abbott ... 403
Ceclor (Cefaclor) Lilly ... 1905
Cedax (Ceftibuten Dihydrate) Biovail ... 1021
Ceftin (Cefuroxime Axetil) Lifecycle Ventures ... 1898
Cefzil (Cefprozil) Bristol-Myers Squibb ... 1076
Keflex (Cephalexin) Dista ... 1237
Lorabid Suspension and Pulvules (Loracarbef) Monarch ... 2251
Omnicef (Cefdinir) Abbott ... 493
Pediazole Suspension (Erythromycin Ethylsuccinate, Sulfisoxazole Acetyl) Ross ... 3050
Rocephin Injectable Vials, ADD-Vantage, Galaxy, Bulk (Ceftriaxone Sodium) Roche Laboratories ... 2993
Septra Suspension (Sulfamethoxazole, Trimethoprim) Monarch ... 2265
Septra Tablets (Sulfamethoxazole, Trimethoprim) Monarch ... 2265
Septra DS Tablets (Sulfamethoxazole, Trimethoprim) Monarch ... 2265
Suprax (Cefixime) Lederle ... 1877
Vantin Tablets and Oral Suspension (Cefpodoxime Proxetil) Pharmacia & Upjohn ... 2860
Zithromax Capsules, 250 mg (Azithromycin Dihydrate) Pfizer ... 2743
Zithromax for Oral Suspension, 300 mg, 600 mg, 900 mg, 1200 mg (Azithromycin Dihydrate) Pfizer ... 2739
Zithromax Tablets, 250 mg (Azithromycin Dihydrate) Pfizer ... 2739

H. influenzae pneumonia
Avelox Tablets (Moxifloxacin Hydrochloride) Bayer ... 879
Biaxin/Biaxin XL (Clarithromycin) Abbott ... 403
Omnicef (Cefdinir) Abbott ... 493
Tequin Injection (Gatifloxacin) Bristol-Myers Squibb ... 1110
Tequin Tablets (Gatifloxacin) Bristol-Myers Squibb ... 1110

H. influenzae respiratory tract infections
Ancef for Injection (Cefazolin Sodium) GlaxoSmithKline ... 1474
Ancef Injection (Cefazolin Sodium) GlaxoSmithKline ... 1474
Cefobid Intravenous/Intramuscular (Cefoperazone) Pfizer ... 2671
Cefobid Pharmacy Bulk Package - Not for Direct Infusion (Cefoperazone Sodium) Pfizer ... 2673
Declomycin Tablets (Demeclocycline Hydrochloride) Lederle ... 1855
Doryx Coated Pellet Filled Capsules (Doxycycline Hyclate) Warner Chilcott ... 3357
Dynacin Capsules (Minocycline Hydrochloride) Medicis ... 2019
Kefzol Vials, ADD-Vantage (Cefazolin Sodium) Lilly ... 1951
Minocin Intravenous (Minocycline Hydrochloride) Lederle ... 1862
Minocin Oral Suspension (Minocycline Hydrochloride) Lederle ... 1865
Minocin Pellet-Filled Capsules (Minocycline Hydrochloride) Lederle ... 1863
Monodox Capsules (Doxycycline Monohydrate) Oclassen ... 2442
Streptomycin Sulfate Injection (Streptomycin Sulfate) Pfizer ... 2714
Vibramycin Calcium Oral Suspension Syrup (Doxycycline Calcium) Pfizer ... 2735
Vibramycin Hyclate Capsules (Doxycycline Hyclate) Pfizer ... 2735
Vibramycin Hyclate Intravenous (Doxycycline Hyclate) Pfizer ... 2737
Vibramycin Monohydrate for Oral Suspension (Doxycycline Monohydrate) Pfizer ... 2735
Vibra-Tabs Film Coated Tablets (Doxycycline Hyclate) Pfizer ... 2735

H. influenzae septicemia
Ceptaz for Injection (Ceftazidime) GlaxoSmithKline ... 1499
Fortaz (Ceftazidime Sodium) GlaxoSmithKline ... 1541
Kefurox Vials, ADD-Vantage (Cefuroxime Sodium) Lilly ... 1948
Rocephin Injectable Vials, ADD-Vantage, Galaxy, Bulk (Ceftriaxone Sodium) Roche Laboratories ... 2993
Tazicef for Injection (Ceftazidime) GlaxoSmithKline ... 1647
Tazicef Galaxy Container (Ceftazidime Sodium) GlaxoSmithKline ... 1650
Tazicef Pharmacy Bulk Package (Ceftazidime) GlaxoSmithKline ... 1653
Tazidime Vials, Faspak & ADD-Vantage (Ceftazidime) Lilly ... 1966
Zinacef Injection (Cefuroxime) GlaxoSmithKline ... 1696
Zinacef for Injection (Cefuroxime) GlaxoSmithKline ... 1696

H. influenzae sinusitis
Augmentin Chewable Tablets (Amoxicillin, Clavulanate Potassium) GlaxoSmithKline ... 1482
Augmentin Powder for Oral Suspension (Amoxicillin, Clavulanate Potassium) GlaxoSmithKline ... 1482
Augmentin Tablets (Amoxicillin, Clavulanate Potassium) GlaxoSmithKline ... 1485
Avelox Tablets (Moxifloxacin Hydrochloride) Bayer ... 879
Biaxin/Biaxin XL (Clarithromycin) Abbott ... 403
Ceftin Tablets (Cefuroxime Axetil) Lifecycle Ventures ... 1898
Cefzil (Cefprozil) Bristol-Myers Squibb ... 1076
Cipro I.V. (Ciprofloxacin) Bayer ... 893
Cipro I.V. Pharmacy Bulk Package (Ciprofloxacin) Bayer ... 897
Cipro (Ciprofloxacin) Bayer ... 887
Levaquin (Levofloxacin) Ortho-McNeil ... 2537
Lorabid Suspension and Pulvules (Loracarbef) Monarch ... 2251
Omnicef (Cefdinir) Abbott ... 493
Tequin Injection (Gatifloxacin) Bristol-Myers Squibb ... 1110
Tequin Tablets (Gatifloxacin) Bristol-Myers Squibb ... 1110
Vantin Tablets and Oral Suspension (Cefpodoxime Proxetil) Pharmacia & Upjohn ... 2860

H. influenzae upper respiratory tract infections
Cefobid Intravenous/Intramuscular (Cefoperazone) Pfizer ... 2671
Cefobid Pharmacy Bulk Package - Not for Direct Infusion (Cefoperazone Sodium) Pfizer ... 2673
E.E.S. (Erythromycin Ethylsuccinate) Abbott ... 450
EryPed (Erythromycin Ethylsuccinate) Abbott ... 446
Ery-Tab Tablets (Erythromycin) Abbott ... 448
Erythrocin Stearate Filmtab Tablets (Erythromycin Stearate) Abbott ... 452
Erythromycin Base Filmtab Tablets (Erythromycin) Abbott ... 454
Erythromycin Delayed-Release Capsules, USP (Erythromycin) Abbott ... 455
PCE Dispertab Tablets (Erythromycin) Abbott ... 498
Septra Suspension (Sulfamethoxazole, Trimethoprim) Monarch ... 2265
Septra Tablets (Sulfamethoxazole, Trimethoprim) Monarch ... 2265
Septra DS Tablets (Sulfamethoxazole, Trimethoprim) Monarch ... 2265

H. parainfluenzae bronchitis
Avelox Tablets (Moxifloxacin Hydrochloride) Bayer ... 879
Ceftin Tablets (Cefuroxime Axetil) Lifecycle Ventures ... 1898
Levaquin (Levofloxacin) Ortho-McNeil ... 2537
Tequin Injection (Gatifloxacin) Bristol-Myers Squibb ... 1110
Tequin Tablets (Gatifloxacin) Bristol-Myers Squibb ... 1110

H. parainfluenzae infections
Avelox Tablets (Moxifloxacin Hydrochloride) Bayer ... 879
Ceftin Tablets (Cefuroxime Axetil) Lifecycle Ventures ... 1898
Cipro I.V. Pharmacy Bulk Package (Ciprofloxacin) Bayer ... 897
Cipro (Ciprofloxacin) Bayer ... 887
Claforan Injection (Cefotaxime Sodium) Aventis ... 732
Levaquin (Levofloxacin) Ortho-McNeil ... 2537
Primaxin I.V. (Cilastatin Sodium, Imipenem) Merck ... 2160
Rocephin Injectable Vials, ADD-Vantage, Galaxy, Bulk (Ceftriaxone Sodium) Roche Laboratories ... 2993
Tequin Injection (Gatifloxacin) Bristol-Myers Squibb ... 1110
Tequin Tablets (Gatifloxacin) Bristol-Myers Squibb ... 1110

H. parainfluenzae lower respiratory tract infections
Cipro I.V. (Ciprofloxacin) Bayer ... 893
Cipro I.V. Pharmacy Bulk Package (Ciprofloxacin) Bayer ... 897
Cipro (Ciprofloxacin) Bayer ... 887
Claforan Injection (Cefotaxime Sodium) Aventis ... 732
Levaquin (Levofloxacin) Ortho-McNeil ... 2537
Primaxin I.V. (Cilastatin Sodium, Imipenem) Merck ... 2160
Rocephin Injectable Vials, ADD-Vantage, Galaxy, Bulk (Ceftriaxone Sodium) Roche Laboratories ... 2993
Suprax for Oral Suspension (Cefixime) Lederle ... 1877
Tequin Injection (Gatifloxacin) Bristol-Myers Squibb ... 1110
Tequin Tablets (Gatifloxacin) Bristol-Myers Squibb ... 1110

H. parainfluenzae pneumonia
Omnicef (Cefdinir) Abbott ... 493
Tequin Injection (Gatifloxacin) Bristol-Myers Squibb ... 1110
Tequin Tablets (Gatifloxacin) Bristol-Myers Squibb ... 1110

H. pylori infection and duodenal ulcer, adjunct in
Amoxil Chewable Tablets (Amoxicillin) GlaxoSmithKline ... 1471
Amoxil for Oral Suspension (Amoxicillin) GlaxoSmithKline ... 1471
Amoxil (Amoxicillin) GlaxoSmithKline ... 1471
Biaxin/Biaxin XL (Clarithromycin) Abbott ... 403
Nexium Delayed-Release Capsules (Esomeprazole Magnesium) AstraZeneca LP ... 619
Prevacid Delayed-Release Capsules (Lansoprazole) TAP ... 3292
PREVPAC (Amoxicillin, Clarithromycin, Lansoprazole) TAP ... 3298
Prilosec Delayed-Release Capsules (Omeprazole) AstraZeneca LP ... 628

H. vaginalis vaginitis
MetroGel-Vaginal Gel (Metronidazole) 3M ... 1986
Sultrin Triple Sulfa Cream (Sulfabenzamide, Sulfacetamide, Sulfathiazole) Ortho-McNeil ... 2587

Haemophilus influenzae
(*see under* H. influenzae infections)

Hair, cleansing of
Bio-Complex 5000 Revitalizing Conditioner (Octyl Methoxycinnamate) Wellness International ... 769
Bio-Complex 5000 Revitalizing Shampoo (Octyl Methoxycinnamate) Wellness International ... 770

Hair, facial, reduction of
Vaniqa Cream (Eflornithine Hydrochloride) Bristol-Myers Squibb Dermatology ... 1121

Hair loss or thinning of the frontoparietal areas, females
Rogaine for Women Topical Solution (Minoxidil) Pharmacia Consumer ... 721

Hairy cell leukemias
(*see under* Leukemia, hairy cell)

Halitosis, adjunctive therapy in
Cēpacol Antiseptic Mouthwash/Gargle, Original (Cetylpyridinium Chloride) Williams .... ▣786
Cēpacoll Antiseptic Mouthwash/Gargle, Mint (Cetylpyridinium Chloride) Williams ...... ▣786
Certs Cool Mint Drops (Breath Freshener) Pfizer Inc., Warner-Lambert Group .... ▣685
Certs Powerful Mints (Breath Freshener) Pfizer Inc., Warner-Lambert Group .... ▣686
Listerine Mouthrinse (Eucalyptol, Menthol, Methyl Salicylate) Pfizer Inc., Warner-Lambert Healthcare .... ▣702
FreshBurst Listerine Mouthrinse (Eucalyptol, Menthol, Methyl Salicylate, Thymol) Pfizer Inc., Warner-Lambert Healthcare .... ▣702
Tartar Control Listerine Mouthrinse (Eucalyptol, Menthol, Methyl Salicylate) Pfizer Inc., Warner-Lambert Healthcare .... ▣702
Listermint Alcohol-Free Mouthrinse (Sodium Fluoride) Pfizer Inc., Warner-Lambert Healthcare .... ▣703
Trident Advantage Mints (Breath Freshener) Pfizer Inc., Warner-Lambert Group .... ▣687
Trident Advantage Sugarless Gum (Breath Freshener) Pfizer Inc., Warner-Lambert Group .... ▣687

Hansen's disease
(*see under* Leprosy)

Hashimoto's thyroiditis
Synthroid (Levothyroxine Sodium) Abbott 505

Hay fever
(*see under* Pollinosis)

Headache
Children's Advil Oral Suspension (Ibuprofen) Whitehall-Robins .... ▣773
Children's Advil Chewable Tablets (Ibuprofen) Whitehall-Robins .... ▣773
Infants' Advil Drops (Ibuprofen) Whitehall-Robins .... ▣773
Junior Strength Advil Tablets (Ibuprofen) Whitehall-Robins .... ▣773
Junior Strength Advil Chewable Tablets (Ibuprofen) Whitehall-Robins .... ▣773
Alka-Seltzer (Aspirin, Citric Acid, Sodium Bicarbonate) Bayer Consumer .... ▣603
Alka-Seltzer Lemon Lime Antacid and Pain Reliever Effervescent Tablets (Aspirin, Citric Acid, Sodium Bicarbonate) Bayer Consumer .... ▣603
Alka-Seltzer Extra Strength Antacid and Pain Reliever Effervescent Tablets (Aspirin, Citric Acid, Sodium Bicarbonate) Bayer Consumer .... ▣603
Genuine Bayer Tablets, Caplets and Gelcaps (Aspirin) Bayer Consumer .... ▣606
Extra Strength Bayer Caplets and Gelcaps (Aspirin) Bayer Consumer .... ▣610
Aspirin Regimen Bayer Children's Chewable Tablets (Orange or Cherry Flavored) (Aspirin) Bayer Consumer .... ▣607
Extra Strength Bayer Plus Caplets (Aspirin, Calcium Carbonate) Bayer Consumer .... ▣610
BC Powder (Aspirin, Caffeine, Salicylamide) Block .... ▣619
Ecotrin Enteric Coated Aspirin Low, Regular and Maximum Strength Tablets (Aspirin) GlaxoSmithKline Consumer 1715
Aspirin Free Excedrin Caplets and Geltabs (Acetaminophen, Caffeine) Bristol-Myers .... ▣628
Excedrin Extra-Strength Tablets, Caplets, and Geltabs (Acetaminophen, Aspirin, Caffeine) Bristol-Myers .... ▣629
Excedrin PM Tablets, Caplets, and Geltabs (Acetaminophen, Diphenhydramine Citrate) Bristol-Myers .... ▣631
Goody's Body Pain Formula Powder (Acetaminophen, Aspirin, Acetaminophen, Aspirin) Block .... ▣620
Goody's Extra Strength Headache Powder (Acetaminophen, Aspirin, Caffeine) Block .... ▣620
Goody's Extra Strength Pain Relief Tablets (Acetaminophen, Aspirin, Caffeine) Block .... ▣620
Goody's PM Powder (Acetaminophen, Diphenhydramine Citrate) Block .... ▣621
Maximum Strength Midol Teen Caplets (Acetaminophen, Pamabrom) Bayer Consumer .... ▣612
Children's Motrin Oral Suspension and Chewable Tablets (Ibuprofen) McNeil Consumer 2006
Children's Motrin Oral Suspension (Ibuprofen) McNeil Consumer .... ▣643
Infants' Motrin Concentrated Drops (Ibuprofen) McNeil Consumer 2006
Junior Strength Motrin Caplets and Chewable Tablets (Ibuprofen) McNeil Consumer 2006
Motrin IB Tablets, Caplets, and Gelcaps (Ibuprofen) McNeil Consumer 2002
Orudis KT Tablets (Ketoprofen) Whitehall-Robins .... ▣778
Sui-Shen-An Liquid (Herbals, Multiple) Headache Relief 1725
Junior Strength Tylenol Soft Chews Chewable Tablets (Acetaminophen) McNeil Consumer 2014
Tylenol (Acetaminophen) McNeil Consumer 2009
Maximum Strength Tylenol Sore Throat Adult Liquid (Acetaminophen) McNeil Consumer 2013
Vanquish Caplets (Acetaminophen, Aluminum Hydroxide, Aspirin, Caffeine, Magnesium Hydroxide) Bayer Consumer .... ▣617

Headache, cluster
(*see under* Cephalalgia, histaminic)

Headache, migraine
Advil Migraine Liquigels (Ibuprofen) Whitehall-Robins .... ▣772
Amerge Tablets (Naratriptan Hydrochloride) GlaxoSmithKline ... 1467
Axert Tablets (Almotriptan Malate) Pharmacia & Upjohn 2772
D.H.E. 45 Injection (Dihydroergotamine Mesylate) Novartis 2334
Excedrin Migraine (Acetaminophen, Aspirin, Caffeine) Bristol-Myers 1070
Imitrex Injection (Sumatriptan Succinate) GlaxoSmithKline 1549
Imitrex Nasal Spray (Sumatriptan) GlaxoSmithKline 1554
Imitrex Tablets (Sumatriptan Succinate) GlaxoSmithKline 1558
Maxalt Tablets (Rizatriptan Benzoate) Merck 2120
Maxalt-MLT Orally Disintegrating Tablets (Rizatriptan Benzoate) Merck 2120
Migranal Nasal Spray (Dihydroergotamine Mesylate) Novartis 2376
Motrin Migraine Pain Caplets (Ibuprofen) McNeil Consumer 2005
Zomig Tablets (Zolmitriptan) AstraZeneca 708
Zomig-ZMT Tablets (Zolmitriptan) AstraZeneca 708

Headache, migraine, possibly effective in
Midrin Capsules (Acetaminophen, Dichloralphenazone, Isometheptene Mucate) Women First 3464

Headache, migraine, prophylaxis of
Blocadren Tablets (Timolol Maleate) Merck 2046
Depakote Tablets (Divalproex Sodium) Abbott 430
Depakote ER Tablets (Divalproex Sodium) Abbott 436
Inderal (Propranolol Hydrochloride) Wyeth-Ayerst 3513
Inderal LA Long-Acting Capsules (Propranolol Hydrochloride) Wyeth-Ayerst 3516

Headache, sinus, symptomatic relief of
(*see under* Sinus headache)

Headache, tension
(*see also under* Pain, unspecified)
Phrenilin (Acetaminophen, Butalbital) Amarin 578
Sedapap Tablets 50 mg/650 mg (Acetaminophen, Butalbital) Merz 2225

Headache, vascular
(*see under* Headache, migraine)

Headache accompanied by insomnia
Alka-Seltzer PM Effervescent Tablets (Aspirin, Diphenhydramine Citrate) Bayer Consumer .... ▣605
Extra Strength Bayer PM Caplets (Aspirin, Diphenhydramine Hydrochloride) Bayer Consumer .... ▣611
Excedrin PM Tablets, Caplets, and Geltabs (Acetaminophen, Diphenhydramine Citrate) Bristol-Myers .... ▣631
Goody's PM Powder (Acetaminophen, Diphenhydramine Citrate) Block .... ▣621
Percogesic Aspirin-Free Coated Tablets (Acetaminophen, Phenyltoloxamine Citrate) Medtech .... ▣667
Extra Strength Percogesic Aspirin-Free Coated Caplets (Acetaminophen, Diphenhydramine Hydrochloride) Medtech ..... ▣665
Extra Strength Tylenol PM Caplets, Geltabs, and Gelcaps (Acetaminophen, Diphenhydramine Hydrochloride) McNeil Consumer 2012

Headache associated with common cold
(*see also under* Sinus headache)
Advil Cold and Sinus Caplets (Ibuprofen, Pseudoephedrine Hydrochloride) Whitehall-Robins .... ▣771
Advil Cold and Sinus Tablets (Ibuprofen, Pseudoephedrine Hydrochloride) Whitehall-Robins .. ▣771
Advil Flu & Body Ache Caplets (Ibuprofen, Pseudoephedrine Hydrochloride) Whitehall-Robins .. ▣772
Aleve Cold & Sinus Caplets (Naproxen Sodium, Pseudoephedrine Hydrochloride) Bayer Consumer .... ▣603
Benadryl Severe Allergy & Sinus Headache Caplets (Acetaminophen, Diphenhydramine Hydrochloride, Pseudoephedrine Hydrochloride) Pfizer Inc., Warner-Lambert Healthcare .... ▣694
Comtrex Flu Therapy & Fever Relief Daytime Caplets (Acetaminophen, Pseudoephedrine Hydrochloride) Bristol-Myers .... ▣628
Coricidin HBP Maximum Strength Flu Tablets (Acetaminophen, Chlorpheniramine Maleate, Dextromethorphan Hydrobromide) Schering-Plough .... ▣738
Children's Motrin Cold Oral Suspension (Ibuprofen, Pseudoephedrine Hydrochloride) McNeil Consumer 2007
Motrin Sinus Headache Caplets (Ibuprofen, Pseudoephedrine Hydrochloride) McNeil Consumer 2005
Children's Tylenol Cold Suspension Liquid and Chewable Tablets (Acetaminophen, Chlorpheniramine Maleate, Pseudoephedrine Hydrochloride) McNeil Consumer 2015

Headache with gastric hyperacidity
Alka-Seltzer (Aspirin, Citric Acid, Sodium Bicarbonate) Bayer Consumer .... ▣603
Alka-Seltzer Lemon Lime Antacid and Pain Reliever Effervescent Tablets (Aspirin, Citric Acid, Sodium Bicarbonate) Bayer Consumer .... ▣603
Alka-Seltzer Extra Strength Antacid and Pain Reliever Effervescent Tablets (Aspirin, Citric Acid, Sodium Bicarbonate) Bayer Consumer .... ▣603

Headache with upset stomach
Alka-Seltzer (Aspirin, Citric Acid, Sodium Bicarbonate) Bayer Consumer .... ▣603
Alka-Seltzer Lemon Lime Antacid and Pain Reliever Effervescent Tablets (Aspirin, Citric Acid, Sodium Bicarbonate) Bayer Consumer .... ▣603
Alka-Seltzer Extra Strength Antacid and Pain Reliever Effervescent Tablets (Aspirin, Citric Acid, Sodium Bicarbonate) Bayer Consumer .... ▣603

Heart, allogeneic transplants, prophylaxis of organ rejection in
CellCept Capsules (Mycophenolate Mofetil) Roche Laboratories 2951
CellCept Intravenous (Mycophenolate Mofetil Hydrochloride) Roche Laboratories 2951
CellCept Oral Suspension (Mycophenolate Mofetil) Roche Laboratories 2951
CellCept Tablets (Mycophenolate Mofetil) Roche Laboratories 2951
Gengraf Capsules (Cyclosporine) Abbott 457
Neoral Soft Gelatin Capsules (Cyclosporine) Novartis 2380
Neoral Oral Solution (Cyclosporine) Novartis 2380
Orthoclone OKT3 Sterile Solution (Muromonab-CD3) Ortho Biotech .. 2498
Sandimmune (Cyclosporine) Novartis 2388

Heart failure
(*see under* Congestive heart failure, adjunct in)

Heart failure, congestive
(*see under* Congestive heart failure, adjunct in)

Heartburn
(*see under* Hyperacidity, gastric, symptomatic relief of)

Hematopoietic progenitor cells, mobilization of
Neupogen for Injection (Filgrastim) Amgen 587

Hemolytic disease, newborn
Buminate 25% Solution, USP (Albumin (human)) Baxter Healthcare 842

Hemolytic disease, Rh, prevention of
(*see under* Erythroblastosis fetalis, prevention of)

Hemolytic disease, unspecified
Albumin (Human) 25% (Albumin (human)) Baxter Healthcare 839
Plasbumin-20 (Albumin (human)) Bayer Biological 940
Plasbumin-25 (Albumin (human)) Bayer Biological 941

Hemophilia, congenital with antibodies to Factor VIII:C
Kogenate (Antihemophilic Factor (Recombinant)) Bayer Biological 934

Hemophilia A
DDAVP Injection 4 mcg/mL (Desmopressin Acetate) Aventis 737
Desmopressin Acetate Injection (Desmopressin Acetate) Ferring ... 1344
Helixate Concentrate (Antihemophilic Factor (Recombinant)) Aventis Behring 788
Hemofil M (Antihemophilic Factor (Human)) Baxter Healthcare 847
Humate-P Concentrate (Antihemophilic Factor (Human)) Aventis Behring 790
Koāte-DVI (Antihemophilic Factor (Human)) Bayer Biological 931
Koāte-HP (Antihemophilic Factor (Human)) Bayer Biological 932
Kogenate (Antihemophilic Factor (Recombinant)) Bayer Biological ... 934
Kogenate FS (Antihemophilic Factor (Recombinant)) Bayer Biological 936
Monoclate-P Concentrate (Antihemophilic Factor (Human)) Aventis Behring 793
Recombinate (Antihemophilic Factor (Recombinant)) Baxter Healthcare 853
ReFacto Vials (Antihemophilic Factor (Recombinant)) Genetics 1437
Stimate Nasal Spray (Desmopressin Acetate) Aventis Behring . 796

Hemophilia B
Bebulin VH (Factor IX Complex) Baxter Healthcare 840
BeneFix for Injection (Antihemophilic Factor (Recombinant)) Genetics 1432
Konȳne 80 (Factor IX Complex) Bayer Biological 937
Mononine Concentrate (Factor IX (Human)) Aventis Behring 794

NovoSeven (Antihemophilic Factor (Recombinant)) Novo Nordisk....... 2430
Proplex T (Factor IX Complex) Baxter Healthcare....................... 851

Hemorrhage, coumarin anticoagulant-induced, reversal of
Konÿne 80 (Factor IX Complex) Bayer Biological 937

Hemorrhage, postpartum, control of
AquaMEPHYTON Injection (Vitamin K_1) Merck 2042

Hemorrhage, subarachnoid, resulting in neurological deficits
Nimotop Capsules (Nimodipine) Bayer 904

Hemorrhoidal pain
(*see under* Pain, anorectal)

Hemorrhoids
Anusol Ointment (Mineral Oil, Pramoxine Hydrochloride, Zinc Oxide) Pfizer Inc., Warner-Lambert Healthcare ....▣688
Anusol Suppositories (Starch) Pfizer Inc., Warner-Lambert Healthcare ....▣689
Anusol-HC Suppositories (Hydrocortisone Acetate) Monarch 2238
Preparation H Cream (Glycerin, Petrolatum, Phenylephrine Hydrochloride, Shark Liver Oil) Whitehall-Robins ....▣778
Preparation H Cooling Gel (Phenylephrine Hydrochloride) Whitehall-Robins ....▣778
Preparation H (Mineral Oil, Petrolatum, Phenylephrine Hydrochloride, Shark Liver Oil) Whitehall-Robins ....▣778
Preparation H Medicated Wipes (Witch Hazel) Whitehall-Robins .....▣779
Proctocort Suppositories (Hydrocortisone Acetate) Monarch 2264
Tucks Pre-moistened Pads (Witch Hazel) Pfizer Inc., Warner-Lambert Healthcare ....▣713

Hemostasis, an aid in
Amicar Injection (Aminocaproic Acid) Xanodyne 3608
Amicar Syrup (Aminocaproic Acid) Xanodyne 3608
Amicar Tablets (Aminocaproic Acid) Xanodyne 3608
DDAVP Injection 4 mcg/mL (Desmopressin Acetate) Aventis 737
Desmopressin Acetate Injection (Desmopressin Acetate) Ferring ...1344
Thrombin-JMI (Thrombin) Jones 1824
Tisseel VH (Fibrin Sealant) Baxter Healthcare 854
Trasylol Injection (Aprotinin) Bayer ... 909

Hepatitis A, prophylaxis
BayGam (Globulin, Immune (Human)) Bayer Biological 914

Hepatitis B, chronic
Epivir-HBV (Lamivudine) GlaxoSmithKline..............................1524
Intron A for Injection (Interferon alfa-2B, Recombinant) Schering ...3120

Hepatitis B virus, postexposure prophylaxis
BayHep B (Hepatitis B Immune Globulin (Human)) Bayer Biological 915
Nabi-HB (Hepatitis B Immune Globulin (Human)) Nabi 2295

Hepatitis C, chronic
Infergen (Interferon Alfacon-1) InterMune 1777
Intron A for Injection (Interferon alfa-2B, Recombinant) Schering ...3120
PEG-Intron Powder for Injection (Peginterferon Alfa-2B) Schering ..3140
Rebetron Combination Therapy (Interferon alfa-2B, Recombinant, Ribavirin) Schering 3153
Roferon-A Injection (Interferon alfa-2A, Recombinant) Roche Laboratories 2996

Herellea vaginicola
(*see under* Acinetobacter calcoaceticus infections, ocular)

Herpes, genital, initial and recurrent episodes
Famvir Tablets (Famciclovir) Novartis 2348
Zovirax Capsules (Acyclovir) GlaxoSmithKline.......................... 1706
Zovirax for Injection (Acyclovir Sodium) GlaxoSmithKline 1708
Zovirax (Acyclovir) GlaxoSmithKline.......................... 1706

Herpes genitalis
Valtrex Caplets (Valacyclovir Hydrochloride) GlaxoSmithKline.... 1676
Zovirax Capsules (Acyclovir) GlaxoSmithKline.......................... 1706
Zovirax for Injection (Acyclovir Sodium) GlaxoSmithKline 1708
Zovirax Ointment (Acyclovir) GlaxoSmithKline.......................... 1707
Zovirax (Acyclovir) GlaxoSmithKline.......................... 1706

Herpes simplex infections, ocular
Viroptic (Trifluridine) Monarch......... ⊙301

Herpes simplex virus encephalitis
Zovirax for Injection (Acyclovir Sodium) GlaxoSmithKline 1708

Herpes simplex virus infections
Denavir Cream (Penciclovir) Novartis 2332
Famvir Tablets (Famciclovir) Novartis 2348
Zovirax for Injection (Acyclovir Sodium) GlaxoSmithKline 1708
Zovirax Ointment (Acyclovir) GlaxoSmithKline 1707

Herpes simplex virus mucocutaneous infection
Famvir Tablets (Famciclovir) Novartis 2348
Foscavir Injection (Foscarnet Sodium) AstraZeneca LP 605
Zovirax for Injection (Acyclovir Sodium) GlaxoSmithKline 1708
Zovirax Ointment (Acyclovir) GlaxoSmithKline 1707

Herpes zoster infections
Famvir Tablets (Famciclovir) Novartis 2348
Valtrex Caplets (Valacyclovir Hydrochloride) GlaxoSmithKline ...1676
Zovirax (Acyclovir) GlaxoSmithKline..........................1706

Herpes zoster ophthalmicus
Celestone Soluspan Injectable Suspension (Betamethasone Acetate, Betamethasone Sodium Phosphate) Schering 3097
Celestone Syrup (Betamethasone) Schering 3099
Cortone Acetate Injectable Suspension (Cortisone Acetate) Merck 2059
Cortone Acetate Tablets (Cortisone Acetate) Merck 2061
Decadron Elixir (Dexamethasone) Merck 2078
Decadron Tablets (Dexamethasone) Merck 2079
Decadron Phosphate Injection (Dexamethasone Sodium Phosphate) Merck 2081
Depo-Medrol Injectable Suspension (Methylprednisolone Acetate) Pharmacia & Upjohn 2795
Hydrocortone Tablets (Hydrocortisone) Merck 2106
Hydrocortone Phosphate Injection, Sterile (Hydrocortisone Sodium Phosphate) Merck 2105
Pediapred Oral Solution (Prednisolone Sodium Phosphate) Celltech 1170
Prednisone (Prednisone) Roxane 3064
Prelone Syrup (Prednisolone) Muro .2273
Solu-Medrol Sterile Powder (Methylprednisolone Sodium Succinate) Pharmacia & Upjohn 2855

Herpetic manifestations, oral, symptomatic relief of
(*see also under* Herpes simplex virus infections)
Abreva Cream (Docosanol) SmithKline Beecham Consumer ....▣744
Cēpacol Viractin (Tetracaine) Williams ....▣788
Denavir Cream (Penciclovir) Novartis 2332
Zilactin/Dermaflex (Benzyl Alcohol) Zila Consumer ....▣790

Hiccup
Thorazine (Chlorpromazine Hydrochloride) GlaxoSmithKline ...1656

Histoplasmosis
Nizoral Tablets (Ketoconazole) Janssen.. 1791
Sporanox Capsules (Itraconazole) Janssen.. 1800
Sporanox Injection (Itraconazole) Janssen.. 1804
Sporanox Injection (Itraconazole) Ortho Biotech............................ 2509

HIV Infection
(*see under* Infections, human immunodeficiency virus)

Hodgkin's disease
Adriamycin PFS/RDF Injection (Doxorubicin Hydrochloride) Pharmacia & Upjohn.................. 2767
Leukeran Tablets (Chlorambucil) GlaxoSmithKline.......................... 1591
Thioplex for Injection (Thiotepa) Immunex 1765

Hodgkin's disease, adjunctive therapy in
Leukine (Sargramostim) Immunex 1755

Hodgkin's disease, secondary line therapy in
DTIC-Dome (Dacarbazine) Bayer 902

Hodgkin's disease, stages III and IV, palliative treatment of
Matulane Capsules (Procarbazine Hydrochloride) Sigma-Tau 3246
Mustargen for Injection (Mechlorethamine Hydrochloride) Merck 2142

Hookworm, American
(*see under* Necator americanus infections)

Hookworm infections
(*see under* Ancylostoma duodenale infections)

Horton's headache
(*see under* Cephalalgia, histaminic)

Hydatid disease, cystic
Albenza Tablets (Albendazole) GlaxoSmithKline 1463

Hyperacidity, gastric, symptomatic relief of
Alka-Seltzer Heartburn Relief Tablets (Citric Acid, Sodium Bicarbonate) Bayer Consumer ....▣604
Amphojel Suspension (Mint Flavor) (Aluminum Hydroxide) Wyeth-Ayerst ....▣789
Ex•Lax Milk of Magnesia Liquid (Magnesium Hydroxide) Novartis Consumer ....▣670
Gaviscon Extra Strength Liquid (Aluminum Hydroxide, Magnesium Carbonate) SmithKline Beecham Consumer ....▣751
Gaviscon Extra Strength Tablets (Aluminum Hydroxide, Magnesium Carbonate) SmithKline Beecham Consumer ....▣751
Gaviscon Regular Strength Liquid (Aluminum Hydroxide, Magnesium Carbonate) SmithKline Beecham Consumer ....▣751
Gaviscon Regular Strength Tablets (Aluminum Hydroxide, Magnesium Trisilicate) SmithKline Beecham Consumer .▣750
Maalox Antacid/Anti-Gas Oral Suspension (Aluminum Hydroxide, Magnesium Hydroxide, Simethicone) Novartis Consumer ....▣673
Maalox Max Maximum Strength Antacid/Anti-Gas Liquid (Aluminum Hydroxide, Magnesium Hydroxide, Simethicone) Novartis Consumer 2300
Maalox Regular Strength Antacid/Antigas Liquid (Aluminum Hydroxide, Magnesium Hydroxide) Novartis Consumer 2300
Quick Dissolve Maalox Max Maximum Strength Antacid/Antigas Tablets (Calcium Carbonate) Novartis Consumer 2301
Quick Dissolve Maalox Regular Strength Antacid Tablets (Calcium Carbonate) Novartis Consumer 2301
Mag-Ox 400 Tablets (Magnesium Oxide) Blaine 1024
Marblen Suspension (Calcium Carbonate, Magnesium Carbonate) Fleming ....▣633
Children's Mylanta J&J • Merck .....▣634
Fast-Acting Mylanta Antacid Gelcaps (Calcium Carbonate, Magnesium Hydroxide) J&J • Merck.. 1813
Mylanta (Aluminum Hydroxide, Magnesium Hydroxide, Simethicone) J&J • Merck........................ 1813
Fast-Acting Mylanta Ultra Tabs (Calcium Carbonate, Magnesium Hydroxide) J&J • Merck............. 1813
Mylanta Supreme Liquid J&J • Merck..▣636
Extra Strength Mylanta Calci Tabs Tablets (Calcium Carbonate) J&J • Merck...........................▣636
Nexium Delayed-Release Capsules (Esomeprazole Magnesium) AstraZeneca LP 619
Pepcid AC (Famotidine) J&J • Merck... 1814
Pepcid Complete Chewable Tablets (Calcium Carbonate, Famotidine, Magnesium Hydroxide) J&J • Merck 1815
Phillips' Chewable Tablets (Magnesium Hydroxide) Bayer Consumer ....▣615
Phillips' Milk of Magnesia Liquid (Original, Cherry, & Mint) (Magnesium Hydroxide) Bayer Consumer ....▣616
Prelief Tablets and Granulate (Calcium Glycerophosphate) AK Pharma ....▣801
Prilosec Delayed-Release Capsules (Omeprazole) AstraZeneca LP 628
Rolaids Tablets (Calcium Carbonate, Magnesium Hydroxide) Pfizer Inc., Warner-Lambert Healthcare ....▣706
Extra Strength Rolaids Tablets (Calcium Carbonate, Magnesium Hydroxide) Pfizer Inc., Warner-Lambert Healthcare ....▣706
Tagamet HB 200 Suspension (Cimetidine) SmithKline Beecham Consumer ....▣762
Tagamet HB 200 Tablets (Cimetidine) SmithKline Beecham Consumer ....▣761
Titralac (Calcium Carbonate) 3M ....▣640
3M Titralac Plus Antacid Tablets (Calcium Carbonate, Simethicone) 3M ....▣640
Tums (Calcium Carbonate) SmithKline Beecham Consumer .▣763
Uro-Mag Capsules (Magnesium Oxide) Blaine 1024
Zantac 75 Tablets (Ranitidine Hydrochloride) Pfizer Inc., Warner-Lambert Healthcare ....▣717

Hyperbetalipoproteinemia
(*see under* Hyperlipoproteinemia, types IIa and IIb, adjunct to diet)

Hypercalcemia associated with cancer
Aredia for Injection (Pamidronate Disodium) Novartis 2309
Celestone Soluspan Injectable Suspension (Betamethasone Acetate, Betamethasone Sodium Phosphate) Schering 3097
Celestone Syrup (Betamethasone) Schering 3099
Cortone Acetate Injectable Suspension (Cortisone Acetate) Merck 2059
Cortone Acetate Tablets (Cortisone Acetate) Merck 2061
Decadron Elixir (Dexamethasone) Merck 2078
Decadron Tablets (Dexamethasone) Merck 2079
Decadron Phosphate Injection (Dexamethasone Sodium Phosphate) Merck 2081
Depo-Medrol Injectable Suspension (Methylprednisolone Acetate) Pharmacia & Upjohn 2795
Hydrocortone Tablets (Hydrocortisone) Merck 2106
Hydrocortone Phosphate Injection, Sterile (Hydrocortisone Sodium Phosphate) Merck 2105
Mithracin for Intravenous Use (Plicamycin) Bayer 903
Pediapred Oral Solution (Prednisolone Sodium Phosphate) Celltech 1170
Prednisone (Prednisone) Roxane 3064
Prelone Syrup (Prednisolone) Muro .2273
Solu-Medrol Sterile Powder (Methylprednisolone Sodium Succinate) Pharmacia & Upjohn 2855
Zometa for Intravenous Infusion (Zoledronic acid) Novartis 3621

Hypercalcemic emergencies, adjunct in
Miacalcin Injection (Calcitonin-Salmon) Novartis ... 2373

Hypercalciuria associated with cancer
Mithracin for Intravenous Use (Plicamycin) Bayer ... 903

Hypercapnia, acute, with COPD
(*see under* Respiratory insufficiency, acute, with chronic obstructive pulmonary disease)

Hypercholesterolemia, primary, adjunct to diet
Baycol Tablets (Cerivastatin Sodium) Bayer ... 883
Colestid Tablets (Colestipol Hydrochloride) Pharmacia & Upjohn ... 2791
Lescol Capsules (Fluvastatin Sodium) Novartis ... 2361
Lescol Capsules (Fluvastatin Sodium) Reliant ... 2925
Lescol XL Tablets (Fluvastatin Sodium) Novartis ... 2361
Lescol XL Tablets (Fluvastatin Sodium) Reliant ... 2925
Lipitor Tablets (Atorvastatin Calcium) Parke-Davis ... 2639
Lipitor Tablets (Atorvastatin Calcium) Pfizer ... 2696
Mevacor Tablets (Lovastatin) Merck ... 2132
Niaspan Extended-Release Tablets (Niacin) Kos ... 1846
Pravachol Tablets (Pravastatin Sodium) Bristol-Myers Squibb ... 1099
Tricor Capsules, Micronized (Fenofibrate) Abbott ... 513
WelChol Tablets (Colesevelam Hydrochloride) Sankyo ... 3073
Zocor Tablets (Simvastatin) Merck ... 2219

Hyperglycemia, control of, adjunct to diet
(*see also under* Diabetes mellitus, insulin-dependent; Diabetes mellitus, non-insulin-dependent)
Actos Tablets (Pioglitazone Hydrochloride) Takeda ... 3275
Amaryl Tablets (Glimepiride) Aventis ... 717
Avandia Tablets (Rosiglitazone Maleate) GlaxoSmithKline ... 1490
DiaBeta Tablets (Glyburide) Aventis ... 741
Diabinese Tablets (Chlorpropamide) Pfizer ... 2680
Glucophage Tablets (Metformin Hydrochloride) Bristol-Myers Squibb ... 1080
Glucophage XR Tablets (Metformin Hydrochloride) Bristol-Myers Squibb ... 1080
Glucotrol Tablets (Glipizide) Pfizer ... 2692
Glucotrol XL Extended Release Tablets (Glipizide) Pfizer ... 2693
Glucovance Tablets (Glyburide, Metformin Hydrochloride) Bristol-Myers Squibb ... 1086
Glyset Tablets (Miglitol) Pharmacia & Upjohn ... 2821
Prandin Tablets (0.5, 1, and 2 mg) (Repaglinide) Novo Nordisk ... 2432
Precose Tablets (Acarbose) Bayer ... 906
Starlix Tablets (Nateglinide) Novartis ... 2401

Hyperhidrosis, topical relief of
Drysol Solution (Aluminum Chloride) Persōn & Covey ... 2663
Xerac AC Solution (Aluminum Chloride) Persōn & Covey ... 2663

Hyperhidrosis associated with Parkinsonism
Levsin/Levsinex/Levbid (Hyoscyamine Sulfate) Schwarz ... 3172
NuLev Orally Disintegrating Tablets (Hyoscyamine Sulfate) Schwarz ... 3176

Hyperkeratosis skin disorders
Lac-Hydrin Lotion (Ammonium Lactate) Bristol-Myers Squibb Dermatology ... 1119

Hyperlipoproteinemia, type III, adjunct to diet
Atromid-S Capsules (Clofibrate) Wyeth-Ayerst ... 3483

Hyperlipoproteinemia, types IIa and IIb, adjunct to diet
Baycol Tablets (Cerivastatin Sodium) Bayer ... 883
Lescol Capsules (Fluvastatin Sodium) Novartis ... 2361
Lescol Capsules (Fluvastatin Sodium) Reliant ... 2925
Lescol XL Tablets (Fluvastatin Sodium) Novartis ... 2361
Lescol XL Tablets (Fluvastatin Sodium) Reliant ... 2925
Lipitor Tablets (Atorvastatin Calcium) Parke-Davis ... 2639
Lipitor Tablets (Atorvastatin Calcium) Pfizer ... 2696
Mevacor Tablets (Lovastatin) Merck ... 2132
Niaspan Extended-Release Tablets (Niacin) Kos ... 1846
Pravachol Tablets (Pravastatin Sodium) Bristol-Myers Squibb ... 1099
Zocor Tablets (Simvastatin) Merck ... 2219

Hyperlipoproteinemia, types IV and V, adjunct to diet
Atromid-S Capsules (Clofibrate) Wyeth-Ayerst ... 3483
Lopid Tablets (Gemfibrozil) Parke-Davis ... 2650
Niaspan Extended-Release Tablets (Niacin) Kos ... 1846
Tricor Capsules, Micronized (Fenofibrate) Abbott ... 513
Zocor Tablets (Simvastatin) Merck ... 2219

Hyperparathyroidism, secondary
Hectorol Capsules (Doxercalciferol) Bone Care ... 1064
Hectorol Injection Bone Care ... 1066
Rocaltrol (Calcitriol) Roche Laboratories ... 2991
Zemplar Injection (Paricalcitol) Abbott ... 522

Hyperphosphatemia
PhosLo (Calcium Acetate) Braintree ... 1069
Renagel Capsules (Sevelamer Hydrochloride) Genzyme ... 1439
Renagel Tablets (Sevelamer Hydrochloride) Genzyme ... 1439

Hyperpigmentation, mottled, adjunct in
Renova 0.02% Cream (Tretinoin) Ortho Dermatological ... 2520
Renova 0.05% Cream (Tretinoin) Ortho Dermatological ... 2519

Hyperpigmentation, skin, bleaching of
Alustra Cream (Hydroquinone) Medicis ... 2018
Eldopaque Forte 4% Cream (Hydroquinone) ICN ... 1734
Eldoquin Forte 4% Cream (Hydroquinone) ICN ... 1734
Lustra Cream (Hydroquinone) Medicis ... 2023
Lustra-AF Cream (Hydroquinone) Medicis ... 2023
Melanex Topical Solution (Hydroquinone) Neutrogena ... 2300
Solaquin Forte (Dioxybenzone, Hydroquinone, Oxybenzone, Padimate O (Octyl Dimethyl Paba)) ICN ... 1734

Hyperprolactinemia-associated dysfunctions
Dostinex Tablets (Cabergoline) Pharmacia & Upjohn ... 2804

Hypersecretory conditions, pathological
Aciphex Tablets (Rabeprazole Sodium) Eisai ... 1267
Aciphex Tablets (Rabeprazole Sodium) Janssen ... 1783
Famotidine Injection (Famotidine) Baxter Anesthesia ... 866
Pepcid Injection (Famotidine) Merck ... 2153
Pepcid for Oral Suspension (Famotidine) Merck ... 2150
Pepcid RPD Orally Disintegrating Tablets (Famotidine) Merck ... 2150
Pepcid Tablets (Famotidine) Merck ... 2150
Prevacid Delayed-Release Capsules (Lansoprazole) TAP ... 3292
Prilosec Delayed-Release Capsules (Omeprazole) AstraZeneca LP ... 628
Tagamet (Cimetidine Hydrochloride) GlaxoSmithKline ... 1644
Zantac (Ranitidine Hydrochloride) GlaxoSmithKline ... 1690
Zantac Injection (Ranitidine Hydrochloride) GlaxoSmithKline ... 1688
Zantac Syrup (Ranitidine Hydrochloride) GlaxoSmithKline ... 1690

Hypersecretory conditions, pre-operative, symptomatic relief of
Levsin/Levsinex/Levbid (Hyoscyamine Sulfate) Schwarz ... 3172
NuLev Orally Disintegrating Tablets (Hyoscyamine Sulfate) Schwarz ... 3176
Robinul Injectable (Glycopyrrolate) Robins ... 2940

Hypersensitivity reactions, drug-induced
Celestone Soluspan Injectable Suspension (Betamethasone Acetate, Betamethasone Sodium Phosphate) Schering ... 3097
Celestone Syrup (Betamethasone) Schering ... 3099
Cortone Acetate Injectable Suspension (Cortisone Acetate) Merck ... 2059
Cortone Acetate Tablets (Cortisone Acetate) Merck ... 2061
Decadron Elixir (Dexamethasone) Merck ... 2078
Decadron Tablets (Dexamethasone) Merck ... 2079
Decadron Phosphate Injection (Dexamethasone Sodium Phosphate) Merck ... 2081
Depo-Medrol Injectable Suspension (Methylprednisolone Acetate) Pharmacia & Upjohn ... 2795
EpiPen (Epinephrine) Dey ... 1236
Hydrocortone Tablets (Hydrocortisone) Merck ... 2106
Hydrocortone Phosphate Injection, Sterile (Hydrocortisone Sodium Phosphate) Merck ... 2105
Pediapred Oral Solution (Prednisolone Sodium Phosphate) Celltech ... 1170
Prednisone (Prednisone) Roxane ... 3064
Prelone Syrup (Prednisolone) Muro ... 2273
Solu-Medrol Sterile Powder (Methylprednisolone Sodium Succinate) Pharmacia & Upjohn ... 2855

Hypertension
Accupril Tablets (Quinapril Hydrochloride) Parke-Davis ... 2611
Accuretic Tablets (Hydrochlorothiazide, Quinapril Hydrochloride) Parke-Davis ... 2614
Aceon Tablets (2 mg, 4 mg, 8 mg) (Perindopril Erbumine) Solvay ... 3249
Adalat CC Tablets (Nifedipine) Bayer ... 877
Aldoclor Tablets (Chlorothiazide, Methyldopa) Merck ... 2035
Aldomet Tablets (Methyldopa) Merck ... 2037
Aldoril Tablets (Hydrochlorothiazide, Methyldopa) Merck ... 2039
Altace Capsules (Ramipril) Monarch ... 2233
Atacand Tablets (Candesartan Cilexetil) AstraZeneca LP ... 595
Atacand HCT Tablets (Hydrochlorothiazide, Candesartan Cilexetil) AstraZeneca LP ... 597
Avalide Tablets (Irbesartan, Hydrochlorothiazide) Bristol-Myers Squibb ... 1070
Avapro Tablets (Irbesartan) Bristol-Myers Squibb ... 1074
Avapro Tablets (Irbesartan) Sanofi-Synthelabo ... 3076
Blocadren Tablets (Timolol Maleate) Merck ... 2046
Captopril Tablets (Captopril) Mylan ... 2281
Cardene I.V. (Nicardipine Hydrochloride) Wyeth-Ayerst ... 3485
Cardizem CD Capsules (Diltiazem Hydrochloride) Biovail ... 1016
Cardura Tablets (Doxazosin Mesylate) Pfizer ... 2668
Catapres Tablets (Clonidine Hydrochloride) Boehringer Ingelheim ... 1037
Catapres-TTS (Clonidine) Boehringer Ingelheim ... 1038
Clorpres Tablets (Chlorthalidone, Clonidine Hydrochloride) Bertek ... 1002
Combipres Tablets (Chlorthalidone, Clonidine Hydrochloride) Boehringer Ingelheim ... 1040
Coreg Tablets (Carvedilol) GlaxoSmithKline ... 1508
Corgard Tablets (Nadolol) Monarch ... 2245
Corlopam Injection (Fenoldopam Mesylate) Abbott ... 412
Corzide 40/5 Tablets (Bendroflumethiazide, Nadolol) Monarch ... 2247
Corzide 80/5 Tablets (Bendroflumethiazide, Nadolol) Monarch ... 2247
Covera-HS Tablets (Verapamil Hydrochloride) Searle ... 3199
Cozaar Tablets (Losartan Potassium) Merck ... 2067
Demadex Tablets and Injection (Torsemide) Roche Laboratories ... 2965
Diovan Capsules (Valsartan) Novartis ... 2337
Diovan HCT Tablets (Hydrochlorothiazide, Valsartan) Novartis ... 2338
Diucardin Tablets (Hydroflumethiazide) Wyeth-Ayerst ... 3494
Diuril Oral (Chlorothiazide) Merck ... 2087
Dyazide Capsules (Hydrochlorothiazide, Triamterene) GlaxoSmithKline ... 1515
DynaCirc Capsules (Isradipine) Reliant ... 2921
DynaCirc CR Tablets (Isradipine) Reliant ... 2923
Enalaprilat Injection (Enalaprilat) Baxter Anesthesia ... 863
Furosemide Tablets (Furosemide) Mylan ... 2284
HydroDIURIL Tablets (Hydrochlorothiazide) Merck ... 2108
Hytrin Capsules (Terazosin Hydrochloride) Abbott ... 464
Hyzaar (Hydrochlorothiazide, Losartan Potassium) Merck ... 2109
Indapamide Tablets (Indapamide) Mylan ... 2286
Inderal (Propranolol Hydrochloride) Wyeth-Ayerst ... 3513
Inderal LA Long-Acting Capsules (Propranolol Hydrochloride) Wyeth-Ayerst ... 3516
Inderide Tablets (Hydrochlorothiazide, Propranolol Hydrochloride) Wyeth-Ayerst ... 3517
Inderide LA Long-Acting Capsules (Hydrochlorothiazide, Propranolol Hydrochloride) Wyeth-Ayerst ... 3519
Inversine Tablets (Mecamylamine Hydrochloride) Layton ... 1850
Isoptin SR Tablets (Verapamil Hydrochloride) Abbott ... 467
Lexxel Tablets (Enalapril Maleate, Felodipine) AstraZeneca LP ... 608
Lotensin Tablets (Benazepril Hydrochloride) Novartis ... 2365
Lotensin HCT Tablets (Benazepril Hydrochloride, Hydrochlorothiazide) Novartis ... 2367
Lotrel Capsules (Amlodipine Besylate, Benazepril Hydrochloride) Novartis ... 2370
Mavik Tablets (Trandolapril) Abbott ... 478
Maxzide (Hydrochlorothiazide, Triamterene) Bertek ... 1008
Micardis Tablets (Telmisartan) Boehringer Ingelheim ... 1049
Micardis HCT Tablets (Hydrochlorothiazide, Telmisartan) Boehringer Ingelheim ... 1051
Microzide Capsules (Hydrochlorothiazide) Watson ... 3414
Midamor Tablets (Amiloride Hydrochloride) Merck ... 2136
Minipress Capsules (Prazosin Hydrochloride) Pfizer ... 2699
Minizide Capsules (Polythiazide, Prazosin Hydrochloride) Pfizer ... 2700
Moduretic Tablets (Amiloride Hydrochloride, Hydrochlorothiazide) Merck ... 2138
Monopril Tablets (Fosinopril Sodium) Bristol-Myers Squibb ... 1091
Monopril HCT (Fosinopril Sodium, Hydrochlorothiazide) Bristol-Myers Squibb ... 1094
Mykrox Tablets (Metolazone) Celltech ... 1168
Nadolol Tablets (Nadolol) Mylan ... 2288
Normodyne Injection (Labetalol Hydrochloride) Schering ... 3135
Normodyne Tablets (Labetalol Hydrochloride) Schering ... 3137
Norvasc Tablets (Amlodipine Besylate) Pfizer ... 2704
Plendil Extended-Release Tablets (Felodipine) AstraZeneca LP ... 623
Prinivil Tablets (Lisinopril) Merck ... 2164
Prinzide Tablets (Hydrochlorothiazide, Lisinopril) Merck ... 2168
Procardia XL Extended Release Tablets (Nifedipine) Pfizer ... 2710
Renese Tablets (Polythiazide) Pfizer ... 2712
Sectral Capsules (Acebutolol Hydrochloride) Wyeth-Ayerst ... 3589
Sular Tablets (Nisoldipine) AstraZeneca ... 688
Tarka Tablets (Trandolapril, Verapamil Hydrochloride) Abbott ... 508
Tenex Tablets (Guanfacine Hydrochloride) Robins ... 2942
Tenoretic Tablets (Atenolol, Chlorthalidone) AstraZeneca ... 690
Tenormin (Atenolol) AstraZeneca ... 692
Teveten Tablets (Eprosartan Mesylate) Unimed ... 3327

Tiazac Capsules (Diltiazem Hydrochloride) Forest ... 1378
Timolide Tablets (Hydrochlorothiazide, Timolol Maleate) Merck ... 2187
Toprol-XL Tablets (Metoprolol Succinate) AstraZeneca LP ... 651
Uniretic Tablets (Hydrochlorothiazide, Moexipril Hydrochloride) Schwarz ... 3178
Univasc Tablets (Moexipril Hydrochloride) Schwarz ... 3181
Vaseretic Tablets (Enalapril Maleate, Hydrochlorothiazide) Merck ... 2204
Vasotec I.V. Injection (Enalaprilat) Merck ... 2207
Vasotec Tablets (Enalapril Maleate) Merck ... 2210
Verelan Capsules (Verapamil Hydrochloride) Schwarz ... 3184
Verelan PM Capsules (Verapamil Hydrochloride) Schwarz ... 3186
Zaroxolyn Tablets (Metolazone) Celltech ... 1177
Zebeta Tablets (Bisoprolol Fumarate) Lederle ... 1885
Zestoretic Tablets (Hydrochlorothiazide, Lisinopril) AstraZeneca ... 695
Zestril Tablets (Lisinopril) AstraZeneca ... 698
Ziac Tablets (Bisoprolol Fumarate, Hydrochlorothiazide) Lederle ... 1887

Hypertension, adjunctive treatment
Resperate Device (Device) InterCure ... 1770

Hypertension, essential
(*see under* Hypertension)

Hypertension, malignant
Corlopam Injection (Fenoldopam Mesylate) Abbott ... 412
Inversine Tablets (Mecamylamine Hydrochloride) Layton ... 1850

Hypertension, ocular
(*see also under* Glaucoma, chronic open-angle; Glaucoma, secondary)
Alphagan Ophthalmic Solution (Brimonidine Tartrate) Allergan ... 545
Alphagan P Ophthalmic Solution (Brimonidine Tartrate) Allergan ... 546
Azopt Ophthalmic Suspension (Brinzolamide) Alcon ... 536
Betagan (Levobunolol Hydrochloride) Allergan ... ⊙228
Betaxon Ophthalmic Suspension (Levobetaxolol Hydrochloride) Alcon ... 537
Betimol Ophthalmic Solution (Timolol Hemihydrate) Santen ... ⊙324
Betoptic S Ophthalmic Suspension (Betaxolol Hydrochloride) Alcon ... 537
Carteolol Hydrochloride Ophthalmic Solution USP, 1% (Carteolol Hydrochloride) Bausch & Lomb ... ⊙258
Cosopt Sterile Ophthalmic Solution (Dorzolamide Hydrochloride, Timolol Maleate) Merck ... 2065
Isopto Carbachol Ophthalmic Solution (Carbachol) Alcon ... ⊙215
Isopto Carpine Ophthalmic Solution (Pilocarpine Hydrochloride) Alcon ... ⊙215
Lumigan Ophthalmic Solution (Bimatoprost) Allergan ... 553
Ocupress Ophthalmic Solution, 1% Sterile (Carteolol Hydrochloride) Novartis Ophthalmics ... ⊙303
OptiPranolol Metipranolol Ophthalmic Solution 0.3% (Metipranolol) Bausch & Lomb ... ⊙263
Pilopine HS Ophthalmic Gel (Pilocarpine Hydrochloride) Alcon ... ⊙217
Rescula Ophthalmic Solution (Unoprostone isopropyl) Novartis Ophthalmics ... ⊙306
Timolol GFS (Timolol Maleate) Falcon ... ⊙266
Timoptic in Ocudose (Timolol Maleate) Merck ... 2192
Timoptic Sterile Ophthalmic Solution (Timolol Maleate) Merck ... 2190
Timoptic-XE Sterile Ophthalmic Gel Forming Solution (Timolol Maleate) Merck ... 2194
Travatan Ophthalmic Solution (Travoprost) Alcon ... 543
Trusopt Sterile Ophthalmic Solution (Dorzolamide Hydrochloride) Merck ... 2196
Xalatan Latanoprost Ophthalmic Solution (Latanoprost) Pharmacia & Upjohn ... ⊙320
Xalatan Sterile Ophthalmic Solution (Latanoprost) Pharmacia & Upjohn ... 2864

Hypertension, ocular, post-surgical
Iopidine Sterile Ophthalmic Solution (Apraclonidine Hydrochloride) Alcon ... ⊙212

Hypertension, ocular, short-term reduction of
Iopidine 0.5% Ophthalmic Solution (Apraclonidine Hydrochloride) Alcon ... ⊙213

Hypertension, pulmonary
Flolan for Injection (Epoprostenol Sodium) GlaxoSmithKline ... 1528

Hypertension, severe
Corlopam Injection (Fenoldopam Mesylate) Abbott ... 412

Hypertension associated with anesthesia
Brevibloc (Esmolol Hydrochloride) Baxter Anesthesia ... 858

Hypertensive crises
(*see under* Hypertension)

Hypertensive episodes, control of, in pheochromocytoma
(*see also under* Pheochromocytoma, adjunctive therapy)
Dibenzyline Capsules (Phenoxybenzamine Hydrochloride) WellSpring ... 3457

Hyperthermia, malignant, prophylaxis
Dantrium Capsules (Dantrolene Sodium) Procter & Gamble Pharmaceuticals ... 2885
Dantrium Intravenous (Dantrolene Sodium) Procter & Gamble Pharmaceuticals ... 2886

Hyperthyroidism
Tapazole Tablets Jones ... 1823

Hypertriglyceridemia, adjunct to diet
(*see also under* Dysbetalipoproteinemia)
Atromid-S Capsules (Clofibrate) Wyeth-Ayerst ... 3483
Lescol Capsules (Fluvastatin Sodium) Novartis ... 2361
Lescol Capsules (Fluvastatin Sodium) Reliant ... 2925
Lescol XL Tablets (Fluvastatin Sodium) Novartis ... 2361
Lescol XL Tablets (Fluvastatin Sodium) Reliant ... 2925
Lipitor Tablets (Atorvastatin Calcium) Parke-Davis ... 2639
Lipitor Tablets (Atorvastatin Calcium) Pfizer ... 2696
Pravachol Tablets (Pravastatin Sodium) Bristol-Myers Squibb ... 1099
Tricor Capsules, Micronized (Fenofibrate) Abbott ... 513
Zocor Tablets (Simvastatin) Merck ... 2219

Hypnotic
(*see under* Sleep, induction of)

Hypoalbuminemia
Buminate 5% Solution, USP (Albumin (human)) Baxter Healthcare ... 841
Buminate 25% Solution, USP (Albumin (human)) Baxter Healthcare ... 842

Hypocalcemia
Caltrate 600 Tablets (Calcium Carbonate) Lederle Consumer ... ▣814
Caltrate 600 + Soy Tablets (Calcium Carbonate) Lederle Consumer ... ▣814
Citracal Liquitab Tablets (Calcium Citrate) Mission ... ▣823
Citracal Tablets (Calcium Citrate) Mission ... 2231
Citracal Caplets + D (Calcium Citrate, Vitamin D) Mission ... ▣823
Extra Strength Mylanta Calci Tabs Tablets (Calcium Carbonate) J&J • Merck ... ▣636
One-A-Day Calcium Plus Chewable Tablets (Calcium Carbonate, Magnesium Carbonate, Vitamin D) Bayer Consumer ... ▣805
Os-Cal Chewable Tablets (Calcium Carbonate) SmithKline Beecham Consumer ... ▣838
Os-Cal 500 Tablets (Calcium) SmithKline Beecham Consumer ... ▣839
Rocaltrol (Calcitriol) Roche Laboratories ... 2991

Hypocalcemia associated with chronic renal failure
Calcijex Injection (Calcitriol) Abbott ... 411
Rocaltrol (Calcitriol) Roche Laboratories ... 2991

Hypocalcemia with vitamin D, deficiency of
Caltrate 600 PLUS (Calcium Carbonate, Vitamin D, Vitamins with Minerals) Lederle Consumer ... ▣815
Caltrate 600 + D Tablets (Calcium Carbonate, Vitamin D) Lederle Consumer ... ▣814
D-Cal Chewable Caplets (Calcium Carbonate, Vitamin D) A & Z Pharm ... ▣794
Os-Cal 250 + D Tablets (Calcium, Vitamin D) SmithKline Beecham Consumer ... ▣838
Os-Cal 500 + D Tablets (Calcium, Vitamin D) SmithKline Beecham Consumer ... ▣839

Hypoestrogenism
Alora Transdermal System (Estradiol) Watson ... 3372
Climara Transdermal System (Estradiol) Berlex ... 958
CombiPatch Transdermal System (Estradiol, Norethindrone Acetate) Novartis ... 2323
Esclim Transdermal System (Estradiol) Women First ... 3460
Estinyl Tablets (Ethinyl Estradiol) Schering ... 3112
Estrace Tablets (Estradiol) Warner Chilcott ... 3361
Ogen Tablets (Estropipate) Pharmacia & Upjohn ... 2846
Ortho-Est Tablets (Estropipate) Women First ... 3464
Premarin Tablets (Estrogens, Conjugated) Wyeth-Ayerst ... 3566
Vivelle Transdermal System (Estradiol) Novartis ... 2412
Vivelle-Dot Transdermal System (Estradiol) Novartis ... 2416

Hypogammaglobulinemia, prevention of bacterial infections
Gammar-P I.V. (Immune Globulin (Human)) Aventis Behring ... 787

Hypoglycemia
GlucaGen for Injection Diagnostic Kit (Glucagon) Bedford ... 949
Glucagon for Injection Vials and Emergency Kit (Glucagon) Lilly ... 1924

Hypogonadism, female
Menest Tablets (Estrogens, Esterified) Monarch ... 2254
Ogen Tablets (Estropipate) Pharmacia & Upjohn ... 2846
Ortho-Est Tablets (Estropipate) Women First ... 3464

Hypogonadism, hypogonadotropic, in males
Androderm Transdermal System CIII (Testosterone) Watson ... 3377
AndroGel (Testosterone) Unimed ... 3322
Android Capsules, 10 mg (Methyltestosterone) ICN ... 1731
Delatestryl Injection (Testosterone Enanthate) BTG ... 1151
Humegon for Injection (Menotropins) Organon ... 2468
Novarel for Injection (Chorionic Gonadotropin) Ferring ... 1347
Pergonal for Injection (Menotropins) Serono ... 3223
Pregnyl for Injection (Chorionic Gonadotropin) Organon ... 2482
Repronex for Intramuscular and Subcutaneous Injection (Menotropins) Ferring ... 1347
Testoderm Transdermal Systems (Testosterone) Alza ... 574
Testopel Pellets (Testosterone) Bartor ... 3610
Testred Capsules, 10 mg (Methyltestosterone) ICN ... 1746

Hypogonadism, hypogonadotropic, secondary, adjunctive therapy in
Humegon for Injection (Menotropins) Organon ... 2468
Pergonal for Injection (Menotropins) Serono ... 3223
Repronex for Intramuscular and Subcutaneous Injection (Menotropins) Ferring ... 1347

Hypogonadism, male, primary
Androderm Transdermal System CIII (Testosterone) Watson ... 3377
AndroGel (Testosterone) Unimed ... 3322
Android Capsules, 10 mg (Methyltestosterone) ICN ... 1731
Delatestryl Injection (Testosterone Enanthate) BTG ... 1151
Testoderm Transdermal Systems (Testosterone) Alza ... 574
Testopel Pellets (Testosterone) Bartor ... 3610

Hypokalemia
K-Dur Microburst Release System ER Tablets (Potassium Chloride) Key ... 1832
Klor-Con M20/Klor-Con M10 Tablets (Potassium Chloride) Upsher-Smith ... 3329
K-Lor Powder Packets (Potassium Chloride) Abbott ... 469
K-Tab Filmtab Tablets (Potassium Chloride) Abbott ... 470
Micro-K (Potassium Chloride) Ther-Rx ... 3311
Rum-K (Potassium Chloride) Fleming ... 1363

Hypomagnesemia
Magonate Natal Liquid (Magnesium Gluconate) Fleming ... 1362
Magonate Tablets and Liquid (Magnesium Gluconate) Fleming ... 1362
Mag-Ox 400 Tablets (Magnesium Oxide) Blaine ... 1024
Slow-Mag Tablets (Calcium Carbonate, Magnesium Chloride) Shire ... ▣835
Uro-Mag Capsules (Magnesium Oxide) Blaine ... 1024

Hypophosphatemia
K-Phos Neutral Tablets (Potassium Phosphate, Sodium Phosphate) Beach ... 946

Hypopigmentation, skin
Benoquin Cream 20% (Monobenzone) ICN ... 1732
8-MOP Capsules (Methoxsalen) ICN ... 1727
Oxsoralen Lotion 1% (Methoxsalen) ICN ... 1740

Hypoproteinemia
Albumin (Human) 25% (Albumin (human)) Baxter Healthcare ... 839
Albuminar-5, U.S.P. (Albumin (human)) Aventis Behring ... 785
Albuminar-25, U.S.P. (Albumin (human)) Aventis Behring ... 786
Buminate 5% Solution, USP (Albumin (human)) Baxter Healthcare ... 841
Buminate 25% Solution, USP (Albumin (human)) Baxter Healthcare ... 842
Plasbumin-20 (Albumin (human)) Bayer Biological ... 940
Plasbumin-25 (Albumin (human)) Bayer Biological ... 941

Hypoprothrombinemia, drug-induced
AquaMEPHYTON Injection (Vitamin K_1) Merck ... 2042
Mephyton Tablets (Vitamin K_1) Merck ... 2129

Hypoprothrombinemia, salicylate-induced
AquaMEPHYTON Injection (Vitamin K_1) Merck ... 2042
Mephyton Tablets (Vitamin K_1) Merck ... 2129

Hypoprothrombinemia, secondary factors-induced
AquaMEPHYTON Injection (Vitamin K_1) Merck ... 2042
Mephyton Tablets (Vitamin K_1) Merck ... 2129

Hypoprothrombinemia due to antibacterial therapy
AquaMEPHYTON Injection (Vitamin K_1) Merck ... 2042

Hypotension, orthostatic
ProAmatine Tablets (Midodrine Hydrochloride) Shire US ... 3241

Hypotension, shock associated with brain damage due to trauma, adjunct to
Aramine (Metaraminol Bitartrate) Merck ... 2043

(▣ Described in PDR For Nonprescription Drugs)   (⊙ Described in PDR For Ophthalmic Medicines™)

Hypothalamic-pituitary gonadotropic function, diagnostic evaluation of
Factrel (Gonadorelin Hydrochloride) Wyeth-Ayerst 3633

Hypothyroidism, ordinary
(*see under* Hypothyroidism, replacement or supplemental therapy in)

Hypothyroidism, primary
(*see under* Hypothyroidism, replacement or supplemental therapy in)

Hypothyroidism, replacement or supplemental therapy in
Cytomel Tablets (Liothyronine Sodium) Jones........ 1817
Levothroid Tablets (Levothyroxine Sodium) Forest........ 1373
Levoxyl Tablets (Levothyroxine Sodium) Jones........ 1819
Synthroid (Levothyroxine Sodium) Abbott........ 505
Triostat Injection (Liothyronine Sodium) Jones........ 1825
Unithroid Tablets (Levothyroxine Sodium) Watson........ 3445

Hypothyroidism, secondary
(*see under* Hypothyroidism, replacement or supplemental therapy in)

Hypothyroidism, tertiary
(*see under* Hypothyroidism, replacement or supplemental therapy in)

Hypovolemia
Albumin (Human) 25% (Albumin (human)) Baxter Healthcare........ 839
Buminate 5% Solution, USP (Albumin (human)) Baxter Healthcare ... 841
Buminate 25% Solution, USP (Albumin (human)) Baxter Healthcare........ 842
Plasbumin-5 (Albumin (human)) Bayer Biological........ 939

Hysteria, acute
Vistaril Intramuscular Solution (Hydroxyzine Hydrochloride) Pfizer........ 2738

Hysterosalpingography, diagnostic aid in
Ethiodol Injection (Ethiodized Oil) Savage........ 3095

I

Ichthyosis vulgaris
Lac-Hydrin Cream (Ammonium Lactate) Bristol-Myers Squibb Dermatology........ 1118
Lac-Hydrin Lotion (Ammonium Lactate) Bristol-Myers Squibb Dermatology........ 1119

Idiopathic thrombocytopenic purpura
(*see under* Purpura, idiopathic thrombocytopenic)

Ileostomies, reduction in odor, adjunct to
Devrom Chewable Tablets (Bismuth Subgallate) Parthenon .... ▣685

Immunization, diphtheria, tetanus, pertussis, and haemophilus influenzae type B
ActHIB Vaccine (Haemophilus B Conjugate Vaccine) Aventis Pasteur........ 798

Immunization, diphtheria, tetanus and pertussis
Acel-Imune (Diphtheria & Tetanus Toxoids and Acellular Pertussis Vaccine Adsorbed) Lederle........ 1851
Infanrix Vaccine (Diphtheria & Tetanus Toxoids and Acellular Pertussis Vaccine Adsorbed) GlaxoSmithKline........ 1562
Tripedia Vaccine (Diphtheria & Tetanus Toxoids and Acellular Pertussis Vaccine Adsorbed) Aventis Pasteur........ 817

Immunization, diphtheria and tetanus
Diphtheria & Tetanus Toxoids Adsorbed Purogenated for Pediatric Use (Diphtheria & Tetanus Toxoids Adsorbed, (For Pediatric Use)) Lederle........ 1857
Tetanus & Diphtheria Toxoids Adsorbed for Adult Use (Tetanus & Diphtheria Toxoids Adsorbed) Lederle........ 1880
Tetanus and Diphtheria Toxoids Adsorbed For Adult Use (Tetanus & Diphtheria Toxoids Adsorbed) Aventis Pasteur........ 815

Immunization, haemophilus influenzae type B
ActHIB Vaccine (Haemophilus B Conjugate Vaccine) Aventis Pasteur........ 798
HibTITER (Haemophilus B Conjugate Vaccine) Lederle........ 1859
Liquid PedvaxHIB (Haemophilus B Conjugate Vaccine) Merck........ 2148

Immunization, haemophilus influenzae type B and hepatitis B virus
Comvax (Haemophilus B Conjugate Vaccine, Hepatitis B Vaccine, Recombinant) Merck........ 2056

Immunization, hepatitis A and B virus
Twinrix Vaccine (Hepatitis A Vaccine, Inactivated, Hepatitis B Vaccine, Recombinant) GlaxoSmithKline........ 1674

Immunization, hepatitis A virus
Havrix Vaccine (Hepatitis A Vaccine, Inactivated) GlaxoSmithKline........ 1544
Vaqta (Hepatitis A Vaccine, Inactivated) Merck........ 2199

Immunization, hepatitis B virus
Engerix-B Vaccine (Hepatitis B Vaccine, Recombinant) GlaxoSmithKline........ 1517
Recombivax HB (Hepatitis B Vaccine, Recombinant) Merck........ 2178

Immunization, influenza virus, types A and B
FluShield Influenza Vaccine (Influenza Virus Vaccine) Wyeth-Ayerst........ 3521
Fluzone Vaccine (Influenza Virus Vaccine) Aventis Pasteur........ 802

Immunization, Japanese encephalitis
JE-VAX Vaccine (Japanese Encephalitis Vaccine Inactivated) Aventis Pasteur........ 811

Immunization, Lyme disease
LYMErix Vaccine (Lyme Disease Vaccine (Recombinant OspA)) GlaxoSmithKline........ 1592

Immunization, meningococcal
Menomune-A/C/Y/W-135 Vaccine (Meningococcal Polysaccharide Vaccine) Aventis Pasteur........ 813

Immunization, poliovirus 1, 2, and 3
IPOL Vaccine (Poliovirus Vaccine Inactivated, Trivalent Types 1,2,3) Aventis Pasteur........ 809

Immunization, rabies
Imovax Rabies Vaccine (Rabies Vaccine) Aventis Pasteur........ 807
Rabies Vaccine RabAvert (Rabies Vaccine) Chiron........ 1203

Immunization, tetanus
BayTet (Tetanus Immune Globulin (Human)) Bayer Biological........ 923
Tetanus Toxoid Adsorbed Purogenated (Tetanus Toxoid, Adsorbed) Lederle........ 1882

Immunization, typhoid fever
TYPHIM Vi Vaccine (Typhoid Vi Polysaccharide Vaccine) Aventis Pasteur........ 825
Vivotif Berna (Typhoid Vaccine Live Oral TY21a) Berna........ 997

Immunization, varicella
Varivax (Varicella Virus Vaccine Live) Merck........ 2202

Immunization, yellow fever
YF-VAX Vaccine (Yellow Fever Vaccine) Aventis Pasteur........ 827

Immunodeficiencies
BayGam (Globulin, Immune (Human)) Bayer Biological........ 914
Gamimune N, 5% Solvent/Detergent Treated (Globulin, Immune (Human)) Bayer Biological........ 925
Gamimune N, 10% Solvent/Detergent Treated (Globulin, Immune (Human)) Bayer Biological........ 928
Gammagard S/D (Globulin, Immune (Human)) Baxter Healthcare........ 845
Iveegam EN (Globulin, Immune (Human)) Baxter Healthcare........ 849
Sandoglobulin I.V. (Globulin, Immune (Human)) Novartis........ 2391

Immunodeficiency disease, severe combined
(*see under* Adenosine deaminase, enzyme replacement therapy for)

Impetigo contagiosa
Bactroban Ointment (Mupirocin) GlaxoSmithKline........ 1496
Ceftin for Oral Suspension (Cefuroxime Axetil) Lifecycle Ventures........ 1898
Levaquin (Levofloxacin) Ortho-McNeil........ 2537

Impotence, male
(*see under* Erectile dysfunction)

Indigestion
(*see under* Digestive disorders, symptomatic relief of)

Infections, acquired immunodeficiency syndrome-related complex
AmBisome for Injection (Amphotericin B) Fujisawa........ 1383
Bactrim (Sulfamethoxazole, Trimethoprim) Roche Laboratories........ 2949
Biaxin/Biaxin XL (Clarithromycin) Abbott........ 403
Cytovene (Ganciclovir) Roche Laboratories........ 2959
DaunoXome Injection (Daunorubicin Citrate) Gilead........ 1442
Doxil Injection (Doxorubicin Hydrochloride) Alza........ 566
Famvir Tablets (Famciclovir) Novartis........ 2348
Foscavir Injection (Foscarnet Sodium) AstraZeneca LP........ 605
Gamimune N, 5% Solvent/Detergent Treated (Globulin, Immune (Human)) Bayer Biological........ 925
Gamimune N, 10% Solvent/Detergent Treated (Globulin, Immune (Human)) Bayer Biological........ 928
Intron A for Injection (Interferon alfa-2B, Recombinant) Schering ... 3120
Marinol Capsules (Dronabinol) Unimed........ 3325
Mycobutin Capsules (Rifabutin) Pharmacia & Upjohn........ 2838
Retrovir IV Infusion (Zidovudine) GlaxoSmithKline........ 1629
Roferon-A Injection (Interferon alfa-2A, Recombinant) Roche Laboratories........ 2996
Septra Suspension (Sulfamethoxazole, Trimethoprim) Monarch........ 2265
Septra Tablets (Sulfamethoxazole, Trimethoprim) Monarch........ 2265
Septra DS Tablets (Sulfamethoxazole, Trimethoprim) Monarch........ 2265
Serostim for Injection (Somatropin) Serono........ 3229
Sporanox Capsules (Itraconazole) Janssen........ 1800
Sporanox Injection (Itraconazole) Janssen........ 1804
Sporanox Injection (Itraconazole) Ortho Biotech........ 2509
Taxol Injection (Paclitaxel) Bristol-Myers Squibb Oncology/Immunology........ 1129
Valcyte Tablets (Valganciclovir Hydrochloride) Roche Laboratories........ 3022
Vistide Injection (Cidofovir) Gilead ... 1445
Vitrasert Implant (Ganciclovir) Bausch & Lomb Surgical .... ⊙254
WinRho SDF (Rh_0 (D) Immune Globulin (Human)) Nabi........ 2297

Infections, aerobic organisms
Cefizox for Intramuscular or Intravenous Use (Ceftizoxime Sodium) Fujisawa........ 1390
Ceptaz for Injection (Ceftazidime) GlaxoSmithKline........ 1499
Fortaz (Ceftazidime Sodium) GlaxoSmithKline........ 1541
Mefoxin for Injection (Cefoxitin Sodium) Merck........ 2124
Mefoxin Premixed Intravenous Solution (Cefoxitin Sodium) Merck........ 2127
Tazicef for Injection (Ceftazidime) GlaxoSmithKline........ 1647
Tazicef Galaxy Container (Ceftazidime Sodium) GlaxoSmithKline........ 1650
Tazicef Pharmacy Bulk Package (Ceftazidime) GlaxoSmithKline........ 1653
Tazidime Vials, Faspak & ADD-Vantage (Ceftazidime) Lilly........ 1966

Infections, anaerobic cocci
Cefizox for Intramuscular or Intravenous Use (Ceftizoxime Sodium) Fujisawa........ 1390
Claforan Injection (Cefotaxime Sodium) Aventis........ 732
Pipracil (Piperacillin Sodium) Lederle........ 1866

Infections, anaerobic organisms
Cefobid Intravenous/Intramuscular (Cefoperazone) Pfizer........ 2671
Cefobid Pharmacy Bulk Package - Not for Direct Infusion (Cefoperazone Sodium) Pfizer........ 2673
Ceptaz for Injection (Ceftazidime) GlaxoSmithKline........ 1499
Cleocin HCl Capsules (Clindamycin Hydrochloride) Pharmacia & Upjohn........ 2784
Cleocin Phosphate Sterile Solution (Clindamycin Phosphate) Pharmacia & Upjohn........ 2785
Fortaz (Ceftazidime Sodium) GlaxoSmithKline........ 1541
Mefoxin for Injection (Cefoxitin Sodium) Merck........ 2124
Mefoxin Premixed Intravenous Solution (Cefoxitin Sodium) Merck........ 2127
Pipracil (Piperacillin Sodium) Lederle........ 1866
Primaxin I.V. (Cilastatin Sodium, Imipenem) Merck........ 2160
Tazicef for Injection (Ceftazidime) GlaxoSmithKline........ 1647
Tazicef Galaxy Container (Ceftazidime Sodium) GlaxoSmithKline........ 1650
Tazicef Pharmacy Bulk Package (Ceftazidime) GlaxoSmithKline........ 1653
Tazidime Vials, Faspak & ADD-Vantage (Ceftazidime) Lilly........ 1966

Infections, beta-lactamase producing organisms
Augmentin Chewable Tablets (Amoxicillin, Clavulanate Potassium) GlaxoSmithKline........ 1482
Augmentin Powder for Oral Suspension (Amoxicillin, Clavulanate Potassium) GlaxoSmithKline........ 1482
Augmentin Tablets (Amoxicillin, Clavulanate Potassium) GlaxoSmithKline........ 1485
Ceclor CD Tablets (Cefaclor) Elan........ 1279
Ceftin (Cefuroxime Axetil) Lifecycle Ventures........ 1898
Cefzil (Cefprozil) Bristol-Myers Squibb........ 1076
Lorabid Suspension and Pulvules (Loracarbef) Monarch........ 2251
Merrem I.V. (Meropenem) AstraZeneca........ 673
Unasyn for Injection (Ampicillin Sodium, Sulbactam Sodium) Pfizer........ 2728
Vantin Tablets and Oral Suspension (Cefpodoxime Proxetil) Pharmacia & Upjohn........ 2860
Zosyn (Piperacillin Sodium, Tazobactam Sodium) Lederle........ 1890
Zosyn in Galaxy Containers (Piperacillin Sodium, Tazobactam Sodium) Lederle........ 1894

Infections, biliary tract
Ancef for Injection (Cefazolin Sodium) GlaxoSmithKline........ 1474
Ancef Injection (Cefazolin Sodium) GlaxoSmithKline........ 1474
Kefzol Vials, ADD-Vantage (Cefazolin Sodium) Lilly........ 1951
Pipracil (Piperacillin Sodium) Lederle........ 1866

Infections, bone and joint
Ancef for Injection (Cefazolin Sodium) GlaxoSmithKline........ 1474
Ancef Injection (Cefazolin Sodium) GlaxoSmithKline........ 1474

Cefizox for Intramuscular or Intravenous Use (Ceftizoxime Sodium) Fujisawa ... 1390
Cefotan (Cefotetan) AstraZeneca ... 664
Ceptaz for Injection (Ceftazidime) GlaxoSmithKline ... 1499
Cipro I.V. (Ciprofloxacin) Bayer ... 893
Cipro I.V. Pharmacy Bulk Package (Ciprofloxacin) Bayer ... 897
Cipro (Ciprofloxacin) Bayer ... 887
Claforan Injection (Cefotaxime Sodium) Aventis ... 732
Cleocin Phosphate Sterile Solution (Clindamycin Phosphate) Pharmacia & Upjohn ... 2785
Fortaz (Ceftazidime Sodium) GlaxoSmithKline ... 1541
Keflex (Cephalexin) Dista ... 1237
Kefurox Vials, ADD-Vantage (Cefuroxime Sodium) Lilly ... 1948
Kefzol Vials, ADD-Vantage (Cefazolin Sodium) Lilly ... 1951
Mandol Vials (Cefamandole Nafate) Lilly ... 1953
Mefoxin for Injection (Cefoxitin Sodium) Merck ... 2124
Mefoxin Premixed Intravenous Solution (Cefoxitin Sodium) Merck ... 2127
Nebcin Vials, Hyporets & ADD-Vantage (Tobramycin Sulfate) Lilly ... 1955
Pipracil (Piperacillin Sodium) Lederle ... 1866
Primaxin I.V. (Cilastatin Sodium, Imipenem) Merck ... 2160
Rocephin Injectable Vials, ADD-Vantage, Galaxy, Bulk (Ceftriaxone Sodium) Roche Laboratories ... 2993
Tazicef for Injection (Ceftazidime) GlaxoSmithKline ... 1647
Tazicef Galaxy Container (Ceftazidime Sodium) GlaxoSmithKline ... 1650
Tazicef Pharmacy Bulk Package (Ceftazidime) GlaxoSmithKline ... 1653
Tazidime Vials, Faspak & ADD-Vantage (Ceftazidime) Lilly ... 1966
Timentin Injection- ADD-Vantage Vial (Clavulanate Potassium, Ticarcillin Disodium) GlaxoSmithKline ... 1661
Timentin Injection-Galaxy Container (Clavulanate Potassium, Ticarcillin Disodium) GlaxoSmithKline ... 1664
Timentin Injection-Pharmacy Bulk Package (Clavulanate Potassium, Ticarcillin Disodium) GlaxoSmithKline ... 1666
Timentin for Intravenous Administration (Clavulanate Potassium, Ticarcillin Disodium) GlaxoSmithKline ... 1658
Zinacef Injection (Cefuroxime) GlaxoSmithKline ... 1696
Zinacef Injection (Cefuroxime) GlaxoSmithKline ... 1696

Infections, burn wound
(*see also under* Infections, skin, bacterial, minor)
Azactam for Injection (Aztreonam) Elan ... 1276
Sulfamylon Cream (Mafenide Acetate) Bertek ... 1011

Infections, central nervous system
Ceptaz for Injection (Ceftazidime) GlaxoSmithKline ... 1499
Claforan Injection (Cefotaxime Sodium) Aventis ... 732
Fortaz (Ceftazidime Sodium) GlaxoSmithKline ... 1541
Nebcin Vials, Hyporets & ADD-Vantage (Tobramycin Sulfate) Lilly ... 1955
Tazicef for Injection (Ceftazidime) GlaxoSmithKline ... 1647
Tazicef Galaxy Container (Ceftazidime Sodium) GlaxoSmithKline ... 1650
Tazicef Pharmacy Bulk Package (Ceftazidime) GlaxoSmithKline ... 1653
Tazidime Vials, Faspak & ADD-Vantage (Ceftazidime) Lilly ... 1966

Infections, cutaneous dermatophyte, severe recalcitrant
Nizoral Tablets (Ketoconazole) Janssen ... 1791

Infections, fenestration cavities
Cortisporin-TC Otic Suspension (Colistin Sulfate, Hydrocortisone Acetate, Neomycin Sulfate, Thonzonium Bromide) Monarch ... 2246

Infections, fungal, systemic
Abelcet Injection (Amphotericin B) Elan ... 1273
Diflucan Tablets, Injection, and Oral Suspension (Fluconazole) Pfizer ... 2681

Infections, genitourinary tract
Ancef for Injection (Cefazolin Sodium) GlaxoSmithKline ... 1474
Ancef Injection (Cefazolin Sodium) GlaxoSmithKline ... 1474
Claforan Injection (Cefotaxime Sodium) Aventis ... 732
Keflex (Cephalexin) Dista ... 1237
Kefzol Vials, ADD-Vantage (Cefazolin Sodium) Lilly ... 1951
Pfizerpen for Injection (Penicillin G Potassium) Pfizer ... 2707

Infections, genitourinary tract, lacking substantial evidence of effectiveness in
Urobiotic-250 Capsules (Oxytetracycline Hydrochloride, Phenazopyridine Hydrochloride, Sulfamethizole) Pfizer ... 2731

Infections, gram-negative bacteria
Amoxil Chewable Tablets (Amoxicillin) GlaxoSmithKline ... 1471
Amoxil for Oral Suspension (Amoxicillin) GlaxoSmithKline ... 1471
Amoxil (Amoxicillin) GlaxoSmithKline ... 1471
Cefizox for Intramuscular or Intravenous Use (Ceftizoxime Sodium) Fujisawa ... 1390
Cefobid Intravenous/Intramuscular (Cefoperazone) Pfizer ... 2671
Cefobid Pharmacy Bulk Package - Not for Direct Infusion (Cefoperazone Sodium) Pfizer ... 2673
Coly-Mycin M Parenteral (Colistimethate Sodium) Monarch ... 2243
Mefoxin for Injection (Cefoxitin Sodium) Merck ... 2124
Mefoxin Premixed Intravenous Solution (Cefoxitin Sodium) Merck ... 2127
Minocin Oral Suspension (Minocycline Hydrochloride) Lederle ... 1865
Monodox Capsules (Doxycycline Monohydrate) Oclassen ... 2442
Ocuflox Ophthalmic Solution (Ofloxacin) Allergan ... 554
Primaxin I.V. (Cilastatin Sodium, Imipenem) Merck ... 2160

Infections, gram-positive anaerobic cocci
Cefobid Intravenous/Intramuscular (Cefoperazone) Pfizer ... 2671
Cefobid Pharmacy Bulk Package - Not for Direct Infusion (Cefoperazone Sodium) Pfizer ... 2673
Cefotan (Cefotetan) AstraZeneca ... 664
Mefoxin for Injection (Cefoxitin Sodium) Merck ... 2124
Mefoxin Premixed Intravenous Solution (Cefoxitin Sodium) Merck ... 2127

Infections, gram-positive bacteria
Amoxil Chewable Tablets (Amoxicillin) GlaxoSmithKline ... 1471
Amoxil for Oral Suspension (Amoxicillin) GlaxoSmithKline ... 1471
Amoxil (Amoxicillin) GlaxoSmithKline ... 1471
Minocin Oral Suspension (Minocycline Hydrochloride) Lederle ... 1865
Monodox Capsules (Doxycycline Monohydrate) Oclassen ... 2442
Ocuflox Ophthalmic Solution (Ofloxacin) Allergan ... 554
Primaxin I.V. (Cilastatin Sodium, Imipenem) Merck ... 2160

Infections, gynecologic
Azactam for Injection (Aztreonam) Elan ... 1276
Cefobid Intravenous/Intramuscular (Cefoperazone) Pfizer ... 2671
Cefobid Pharmacy Bulk Package - Not for Direct Infusion (Cefoperazone Sodium) Pfizer ... 2673
Cefotan (Cefotetan) AstraZeneca ... 664
Ceptaz for Injection (Ceftazidime) GlaxoSmithKline ... 1499
Claforan Injection (Cefotaxime Sodium) Aventis ... 732
Cleocin HCl Capsules (Clindamycin Hydrochloride) Pharmacia & Upjohn ... 2784
Cleocin Phosphate Sterile Solution (Clindamycin Phosphate) Pharmacia & Upjohn ... 2785
Ery-Tab Tablets (Erythromycin) Abbott ... 448
Erythrocin Stearate Filmtab Tablets (Erythromycin Stearate) Abbott ... 452
Erythromycin Base Filmtab Tablets (Erythromycin) Abbott ... 454
Erythromycin Delayed-Release Capsules, USP (Erythromycin) Abbott ... 455
Fortaz (Ceftazidime Sodium) GlaxoSmithKline ... 1541
Mefoxin for Injection (Cefoxitin Sodium) Merck ... 2124
Mefoxin Premixed Intravenous Solution (Cefoxitin Sodium) Merck ... 2127
PCE Dispertab Tablets (Erythromycin) Abbott ... 498
Pipracil (Piperacillin Sodium) Lederle ... 1866
Primaxin I.M. (Cilastatin Sodium, Imipenem) Merck ... 2158
Primaxin I.V. (Cilastatin Sodium, Imipenem) Merck ... 2160
Tazicef for Injection (Ceftazidime) GlaxoSmithKline ... 1647
Tazicef Galaxy Container (Ceftazidime Sodium) GlaxoSmithKline ... 1650
Tazicef Pharmacy Bulk Package (Ceftazidime) GlaxoSmithKline ... 1653
Tazidime Vials, Faspak & ADD-Vantage (Ceftazidime) Lilly ... 1966
Timentin Injection- ADD-Vantage Vial (Clavulanate Potassium, Ticarcillin Disodium) GlaxoSmithKline ... 1661
Timentin Injection-Galaxy Container (Clavulanate Potassium, Ticarcillin Disodium) GlaxoSmithKline ... 1664
Timentin Injection-Pharmacy Bulk Package (Clavulanate Potassium, Ticarcillin Disodium) GlaxoSmithKline ... 1666
Timentin for Intravenous Administration (Clavulanate Potassium, Ticarcillin Disodium) GlaxoSmithKline ... 1658
Unasyn for Injection (Ampicillin Sodium, Sulbactam Sodium) Pfizer ... 2728
Vantin Tablets and Oral Suspension (Cefpodoxime Proxetil) Pharmacia & Upjohn ... 2860
Zosyn (Piperacillin Sodium, Tazobactam Sodium) Lederle ... 1890
Zosyn in Galaxy Containers (Piperacillin Sodium, Tazobactam Sodium) Lederle ... 1894

Infections, human immunodeficiency virus
Agenerase Capsules (Amprenavir) GlaxoSmithKline ... 1454
Agenerase Oral Solution (Amprenavir) GlaxoSmithKline ... 1459
Combivir Tablets (Lamivudine, Zidovudine) GlaxoSmithKline ... 1502
Crixivan Capsules (Indinavir Sulfate) Merck ... 2070
Epivir (Lamivudine) GlaxoSmithKline ... 1520
Fortovase Capsules (Saquinavir) Roche Laboratories ... 2970
Hivid Tablets (Zalcitabine) Roche Laboratories ... 2975
Invirase Capsules (Saquinavir Mesylate) Roche Laboratories ... 2979
Kaletra Capsules (Lopinavir, Ritonavir) Abbott ... 471
Kaletra Oral Solution (Lopinavir, Ritonavir) Abbott ... 471
Norvir Capsules (Ritonavir) Abbott ... 487
Norvir Oral Solution (Ritonavir) Abbott ... 487
Rescriptor Tablets (Delavirdine Mesylate) Agouron ... 526
Retrovir Capsules (Zidovudine) GlaxoSmithKline ... 1625
Retrovir IV Infusion (Zidovudine) GlaxoSmithKline ... 1629
Retrovir (Zidovudine) GlaxoSmithKline ... 1625
Sustiva Capsules (Efavirenz) DuPont ... 1258
Trizivir Tablets (Lamivudine, Abacavir Sulfate, Zidovudine) GlaxoSmithKline ... 1669
Videx (Didanosine) Bristol-Myers Squibb Oncology/Immunology ... 1138
Videx EC Capsules (Didanosine) Bristol-Myers Squibb Oncology/Immunology ... 1143
Viracept (Nelfinavir Mesylate) Agouron ... 532
Viramune Oral Suspension (Nevirapine) Boehringer Ingelheim ... 1060
Viramune Tablets (Nevirapine) Boehringer Ingelheim ... 1060
Zerit (Stavudine) Bristol-Myers Squibb Oncology/Immunology ... 1147
Ziagen (Abacavir Sulfate) GlaxoSmithKline ... 1692

Infections, intra-abdominal
Azactam for Injection (Aztreonam) Elan ... 1276
Cefizox for Intramuscular or Intravenous Use (Ceftizoxime Sodium) Fujisawa ... 1390
Cefobid Intravenous/Intramuscular (Cefoperazone) Pfizer ... 2671
Cefobid Pharmacy Bulk Package - Not for Direct Infusion (Cefoperazone Sodium) Pfizer ... 2673
Cefotan (Cefotetan) AstraZeneca ... 664
Ceptaz for Injection (Ceftazidime) GlaxoSmithKline ... 1499
Cipro I.V. (Ciprofloxacin) Bayer ... 893
Cipro I.V. Pharmacy Bulk Package (Ciprofloxacin) Bayer ... 897
Cipro (Ciprofloxacin) Bayer ... 887
Claforan Injection (Cefotaxime Sodium) Aventis ... 732
Cleocin HCl Capsules (Clindamycin Hydrochloride) Pharmacia & Upjohn ... 2784
Cleocin Phosphate Sterile Solution (Clindamycin Phosphate) Pharmacia & Upjohn ... 2785
Fortaz (Ceftazidime Sodium) GlaxoSmithKline ... 1541
Maxipime for Injection (Cefepime Hydrochloride) Elan ... 1285
Mefoxin for Injection (Cefoxitin Sodium) Merck ... 2124
Mefoxin Premixed Intravenous Solution (Cefoxitin Sodium) Merck ... 2127
Merrem I.V. (Meropenem) AstraZeneca ... 673
Nebcin Vials, Hyporets & ADD-Vantage (Tobramycin Sulfate) Lilly ... 1955
Pipracil (Piperacillin Sodium) Lederle ... 1866
Primaxin I.M. (Cilastatin Sodium, Imipenem) Merck ... 2158
Primaxin I.V. (Cilastatin Sodium, Imipenem) Merck ... 2160
Rocephin Injectable Vials, ADD-Vantage, Galaxy, Bulk (Ceftriaxone Sodium) Roche Laboratories ... 2993
Tazicef for Injection (Ceftazidime) GlaxoSmithKline ... 1647
Tazicef Galaxy Container (Ceftazidime Sodium) GlaxoSmithKline ... 1650
Tazicef Pharmacy Bulk Package (Ceftazidime) GlaxoSmithKline ... 1653
Tazidime Vials, Faspak & ADD-Vantage (Ceftazidime) Lilly ... 1966
Timentin Injection- ADD-Vantage Vial (Clavulanate Potassium, Ticarcillin Disodium) GlaxoSmithKline ... 1661
Timentin Injection-Galaxy Container (Clavulanate Potassium, Ticarcillin Disodium) GlaxoSmithKline ... 1664
Timentin Injection-Pharmacy Bulk Package (Clavulanate Potassium, Ticarcillin Disodium) GlaxoSmithKline ... 1666
Timentin for Intravenous Administration (Clavulanate Potassium, Ticarcillin Disodium) GlaxoSmithKline ... 1658
Trovan (Alatrofloxacin Mesylate) Pfizer ... 2722
Unasyn for Injection (Ampicillin Sodium, Sulbactam Sodium) Pfizer ... 2728

Infections, lacrimal sac
(*see under* Dacryocystitis)

Infections, liver flukes
(*see under* Clonorchiasis)

Infections, lower respiratory tract
Amoxil Chewable Tablets (Amoxicillin) GlaxoSmithKline ... 1471
Amoxil for Oral Suspension (Amoxicillin) GlaxoSmithKline ... 1471
Amoxil (Amoxicillin) GlaxoSmithKline ... 1471
Augmentin Chewable Tablets (Amoxicillin, Clavulanate Potassium) GlaxoSmithKline ... 1482
Augmentin Powder for Oral Suspension (Amoxicillin, Clavulanate Potassium) GlaxoSmithKline ... 1482
Augmentin Tablets (Amoxicillin, Clavulanate Potassium) GlaxoSmithKline ... 1485
Avelox Tablets (Moxifloxacin Hydrochloride) Bayer ... 879
Azactam for Injection (Aztreonam) Elan ... 1276

Biaxin/Biaxin XL (Clarithromycin) Abbott ... 403
Ceclor (Cefaclor) Lilly ... 1905
Cedax (Ceftibuten Dihydrate) Biovail ... 1021
Cefizox for Intramuscular or Intravenous Use (Ceftizoxime Sodium) Fujisawa ... 1390
Cefotan (Cefotetan) AstraZeneca ... 664
Cefzil (Cefprozil) Bristol-Myers Squibb ... 1076
Ceptaz for Injection (Ceftazidime) GlaxoSmithKline ... 1499
Cipro I.V. (Ciprofloxacin) Bayer ... 893
Cipro I.V. Pharmacy Bulk Package (Ciprofloxacin) Bayer ... 897
Cipro (Ciprofloxacin) Bayer ... 887
Claforan Injection (Cefotaxime Sodium) Aventis ... 732
Cleocin HCl Capsules (Clindamycin Hydrochloride) Pharmacia & Upjohn ... 2784
Cleocin Phosphate Sterile Solution (Clindamycin Phosphate) Pharmacia & Upjohn ... 2785
E.E.S. (Erythromycin Ethylsuccinate) Abbott ... 450
EryPed (Erythromycin Ethylsuccinate) Abbott ... 446
Ery-Tab Tablets (Erythromycin) Abbott ... 448
Erythrocin Stearate Filmtab Tablets (Erythromycin Stearate) Abbott ... 452
Erythromycin Base Filmtab Tablets (Erythromycin) Abbott ... 454
Erythromycin Delayed-Release Capsules, USP (Erythromycin) Abbott ... 455
Floxin I.V. (Ofloxacin) Ortho-McNeil ... 2526
Floxin Tablets (Ofloxacin) Ortho-McNeil ... 2529
Fortaz (Ceftazidime Sodium) GlaxoSmithKline ... 1541
Kefurox Vials, ADD-Vantage (Cefuroxime Sodium) Lilly ... 1948
Lorabid Suspension and Pulvules (Loracarbef) Monarch ... 2251
Mandol Vials (Cefamandole Nafate) Lilly ... 1953
Mefoxin for Injection (Cefoxitin Sodium) Merck ... 2124
Mefoxin Premixed Intravenous Solution (Cefoxitin Sodium) Merck ... 2127
Nebcin Vials, Hyporets & ADD-Vantage (Tobramycin Sulfate) Lilly ... 1955
Omnicef (Cefdinir) Abbott ... 493
PCE Dispertab Tablets (Erythromycin) Abbott ... 498
Pfizerpen for Injection (Penicillin G Potassium) Pfizer ... 2707
Pipracil (Piperacillin Sodium) Lederle ... 1866
Primaxin I.M. (Cilastatin Sodium, Imipenem) Merck ... 2158
Primaxin I.V. (Cilastatin Sodium, Imipenem) Merck ... 2160
Rocephin Injectable Vials, ADD-Vantage, Galaxy, Bulk (Ceftriaxone Sodium) Roche Laboratories ... 2993
Tazicef for Injection (Ceftazidime) GlaxoSmithKline ... 1647
Tazicef Galaxy Container (Ceftazidime Sodium) GlaxoSmithKline ... 1650
Tazicef Pharmacy Bulk Package (Ceftazidime) GlaxoSmithKline ... 1653
Tazidime Vials, Faspak & ADD-Vantage (Ceftazidime) Lilly ... 1966
Tequin Injection (Gatifloxacin) Bristol-Myers Squibb ... 1110
Tequin Tablets (Gatifloxacin) Bristol-Myers Squibb ... 1110
Timentin Injection- ADD-Vantage Vial (Clavulanate Potassium, Ticarcillin Disodium) GlaxoSmithKline ... 1661
Timentin Injection-Galaxy Container (Clavulanate Potassium, Ticarcillin Disodium) GlaxoSmithKline ... 1664
Timentin Injection-Pharmacy Bulk Package (Clavulanate Potassium, Ticarcillin Disodium) GlaxoSmithKline ... 1666
Timentin for Intravenous Administration (Clavulanate Potassium, Ticarcillin Disodium) GlaxoSmithKline ... 1658
Trovan (Alatrofloxacin Mesylate) Pfizer ... 2722
Vantin Tablets and Oral Suspension (Cefpodoxime Proxetil) Pharmacia & Upjohn ... 2860
Zinacef Injection (Cefuroxime) GlaxoSmithKline ... 1696
Zinacef for Injection (Cefuroxime) GlaxoSmithKline ... 1696
Zithromax Capsules, 250 mg (Azithromycin Dihydrate) Pfizer ... 2743
Zithromax for IV Infusion (Azithromycin Dihydrate) Pfizer ... 2748
Zithromax for Oral Suspension, 1 g (Azithromycin Dihydrate) Pfizer ... 2743
Zithromax for Oral Suspension, 300 mg, 600 mg, 900 mg, 1200 mg (Azithromycin Dihydrate) Pfizer ... 2739
Zithromax Tablets, 250 mg (Azithromycin Dihydrate) Pfizer ... 2739
Zithromax Tablets, 600 mg (Azithromycin Dihydrate) Pfizer ... 2743
Zosyn (Piperacillin Sodium, Tazobactam Sodium) Lederle ... 1890
Zosyn in Galaxy Containers (Piperacillin Sodium, Tazobactam Sodium) Lederle ... 1894

Infections, lower respiratory tract, RSV-induced

Virazole for Inhalation Solution (Ribavirin) ICN ... 1747

Infections, lower respiratory tract, RSV-induced, prevention of

Synagis Intramuscular (Palivizumab) MedImmune ... 2028

Infections, mastoidectomy

Cortisporin-TC Otic Suspension (Colistin Sulfate, Hydrocortisone Acetate, Neomycin Sulfate, Thonzonium Bromide) Monarch ... 2246

Infections, mycotic, cutaneous

Nystop (Nystatin) Paddock ... 2608

Infections, ocular, bacterial

Bleph-10 (Sulfacetamide Sodium) Allergan ... ⊙ 230
Chloromycetin Ophthalmic Ointment, 1% (Chloramphenicol) Monarch ... ⊙ 296
Chloromycetin Ophthalmic Solution (Chloramphenicol) Monarch ... ⊙ 297
Chloroptic Sterile Ophthalmic Ointment (Chloramphenicol) Allergan ... ⊙ 234
Chloroptic Sterile Ophthalmic Solution (Chloramphenicol) Allergan ... ⊙ 235
Cortisporin Ophthalmic Suspension (Hydrocortisone, Neomycin Sulfate, Polymyxin B Sulfate, Hydrocortisone, Neomycin Sulfate, Polymyxin B Sulfate) Monarch ... ⊙ 297
NeoDecadron Sterile Ophthalmic Solution (Dexamethasone Sodium Phosphate, Neomycin Sulfate) Merck ... 2144
Neosporin Ophthalmic Ointment Sterile (Bacitracin Zinc, Neomycin Sulfate, Polymyxin B Sulfate) Monarch ... ⊙ 299
Neosporin Ophthalmic Solution Sterile (Gramicidin, Neomycin Sulfate, Polymyxin B Sulfate) Monarch ... ⊙ 300
Ocuflox Ophthalmic Solution (Ofloxacin) Allergan ... 554
Polysporin Ophthalmic Ointment (Bacitracin Zinc, Polymyxin B Sulfate, Bacitracin Zinc, Polymyxin B Sulfate) Monarch ... ⊙ 301
Polytrim Ophthalmic Solution (Polymyxin B Sulfate, Trimethoprim Sulfate) Allergan ... 556
Quixin Ophthalmic Solution (Levofloxacin) Santen ... 3093
Terra-Cortril Ophthalmic Suspension (Hydrocortisone Acetate, Oxytetracycline Hydrochloride) Pfizer ... 2716

Infections, perioperative, reduction of the incidence of

Ancef for Injection (Cefazolin Sodium) GlaxoSmithKline ... 1474
Ancef Injection (Cefazolin Sodium) GlaxoSmithKline ... 1474
Cefotan (Cefotetan) AstraZeneca ... 664
Claforan Injection (Cefotaxime Sodium) Aventis ... 732
Kefurox Vials, ADD-Vantage (Cefuroxime Sodium) Lilly ... 1948
Kefzol Vials, ADD-Vantage (Cefazolin Sodium) Lilly ... 1951
Mandol Vials (Cefamandole Nafate) Lilly ... 1953
Mefoxin for Injection (Cefoxitin Sodium) Merck ... 2124
Mefoxin Premixed Intravenous Solution (Cefoxitin Sodium) Merck ... 2127
Pipracil (Piperacillin Sodium) Lederle ... 1866
Rocephin Injectable Vials, ADD-Vantage, Galaxy, Bulk (Ceftriaxone Sodium) Roche Laboratories ... 2993
Zinacef Injection (Cefuroxime) GlaxoSmithKline ... 1696
Zinacef for Injection (Cefuroxime) GlaxoSmithKline ... 1696

Infections, polymicrobic

Ceptaz for Injection (Ceftazidime) GlaxoSmithKline ... 1499
Fortaz (Ceftazidime Sodium) GlaxoSmithKline ... 1541
Primaxin I.V. (Cilastatin Sodium, Imipenem) Merck ... 2160
Tazicef for Injection (Ceftazidime) GlaxoSmithKline ... 1647
Tazicef Galaxy Container (Ceftazidime Sodium) GlaxoSmithKline ... 1650
Tazicef Pharmacy Bulk Package (Ceftazidime) GlaxoSmithKline ... 1653
Tazidime Vials, Faspak & ADD-Vantage (Ceftazidime) Lilly ... 1966

Infections, respiratory tract, unspecified

Ancef for Injection (Cefazolin Sodium) GlaxoSmithKline ... 1474
Ancef Injection (Cefazolin Sodium) GlaxoSmithKline ... 1474
Cefobid Intravenous/Intramuscular (Cefoperazone) Pfizer ... 2671
Cefobid Pharmacy Bulk Package - Not for Direct Infusion (Cefoperazone Sodium) Pfizer ... 2673
Doryx Coated Pellet Filled Capsules (Doxycycline Hyclate) Warner Chilcott ... 3357
Dynacin Capsules (Minocycline Hydrochloride) Medicis ... 2019
E.E.S. (Erythromycin Ethylsuccinate) Abbott ... 450
EryPed (Erythromycin Ethylsuccinate) Abbott ... 446
Erythrocin Stearate Filmtab Tablets (Erythromycin Stearate) Abbott ... 452
Erythromycin Base Filmtab Tablets (Erythromycin) Abbott ... 454
Erythromycin Delayed-Release Capsules, USP (Erythromycin) Abbott ... 455
Keflex (Cephalexin) Dista ... 1237
Kefzol Vials, ADD-Vantage (Cefazolin Sodium) Lilly ... 1951
Minocin Oral Suspension (Minocycline Hydrochloride) Lederle ... 1865
Monodox Capsules (Doxycycline Monohydrate) Oclassen ... 2442
Omnicef (Cefdinir) Abbott ... 493
PCE Dispertab Tablets (Erythromycin) Abbott ... 498
Pfizerpen for Injection (Penicillin G Potassium) Pfizer ... 2707
Vibramycin Hyclate Capsules (Doxycycline Hyclate) Pfizer ... 2735

Infections, skin, bacterial, minor

Bactine First Aid Liquid (Benzalkonium Chloride, Lidocaine Hydrochloride) Bayer Consumer ... ▣ 611
Bactroban Ointment (Mupirocin) GlaxoSmithKline ... 1496
Betadine Brand First Aid Antibiotics & Moisturizer Ointment (Bacitracin Zinc, Polymyxin B Sulfate) Purdue Frederick ... 2894
Betadine Brand Plus First Aid Antibiotics & Pain Reliever Ointment (Bacitracin Zinc, Polymyxin B Sulfate, Pramoxine Hydrochloride) Purdue Frederick ... 2894
Betadine Ointment (Povidone Iodine) Purdue Frederick ... 2894
Betadine PrepStick Applicator (Povidone Iodine) Purdue Frederick ... 2894
Betadine Solution (Povidone Iodine) Purdue Frederick ... 2895
Clorpactin WCS-90 (Sodium Oxychlorosene) Guardian ... 1723
Neosporin Ointment (Bacitracin Zinc, Neomycin, Polymyxin B Sulfate) Pfizer Inc., Warner-Lambert Healthcare ... ▣ 704
Neosporin + Pain Relief Maximum Strength Cream (Neomycin, Polymyxin B Sulfate, Pramoxine Hydrochloride) Pfizer Inc., Warner-Lambert Healthcare ... ▣ 704
Neosporin + Pain Relief Maximum Strength Ointment (Bacitracin Zinc, Neomycin, Polymyxin B Sulfate, Pramoxine Hydrochloride) Pfizer Inc., Warner-Lambert Healthcare ... ▣ 704
Polysporin Ointment (Bacitracin Zinc, Polymyxin B Sulfate) Pfizer Inc., Warner-Lambert Healthcare ... ▣ 706
Polysporin Powder (Bacitracin Zinc, Polymyxin B Sulfate) Pfizer Inc., Warner-Lambert Healthcare ... ▣ 706

Infections, skin and skin structure

Amoxil Chewable Tablets (Amoxicillin) GlaxoSmithKline ... 1471
Amoxil for Oral Suspension (Amoxicillin) GlaxoSmithKline ... 1471
Amoxil (Amoxicillin) GlaxoSmithKline ... 1471
Ancef for Injection (Cefazolin Sodium) GlaxoSmithKline ... 1474
Ancef Injection (Cefazolin Sodium) GlaxoSmithKline ... 1474
Augmentin Chewable Tablets (Amoxicillin, Clavulanate Potassium) GlaxoSmithKline ... 1482
Augmentin Powder for Oral Suspension (Amoxicillin, Clavulanate Potassium) GlaxoSmithKline ... 1482
Augmentin Tablets (Amoxicillin, Clavulanate Potassium) GlaxoSmithKline ... 1485
Avelox Tablets (Moxifloxacin Hydrochloride) Bayer ... 879
Azactam for Injection (Aztreonam) Elan ... 1276
Bactroban Cream (Mupirocin Calcium) GlaxoSmithKline ... 1494
Biaxin/Biaxin XL (Clarithromycin) Abbott ... 403
Bicillin C-R 900/300 Injection (Penicillin G Benzathine, Penicillin G Procaine) Monarch ... 2240
Bicillin C-R Injection (Penicillin G Benzathine, Penicillin G Procaine) Monarch ... 2238
Ceclor (Cefaclor) Lilly ... 1905
Cefizox for Intramuscular or Intravenous Use (Ceftizoxime Sodium) Fujisawa ... 1390
Cefobid Intravenous/Intramuscular (Cefoperazone) Pfizer ... 2671
Cefobid Pharmacy Bulk Package - Not for Direct Infusion (Cefoperazone Sodium) Pfizer ... 2673
Cefotan (Cefotetan) AstraZeneca ... 664
Ceftin Tablets (Cefuroxime Axetil) Lifecycle Ventures ... 1898
Cefzil (Cefprozil) Bristol-Myers Squibb ... 1076
Ceptaz for Injection (Ceftazidime) GlaxoSmithKline ... 1499
Cipro I.V. (Ciprofloxacin) Bayer ... 893
Cipro I.V. Pharmacy Bulk Package (Ciprofloxacin) Bayer ... 897
Cipro (Ciprofloxacin) Bayer ... 887
Claforan Injection (Cefotaxime Sodium) Aventis ... 732
Cleocin HCl Capsules (Clindamycin Hydrochloride) Pharmacia & Upjohn ... 2784
Cleocin Phosphate Sterile Solution (Clindamycin Phosphate) Pharmacia & Upjohn ... 2785
Duricef (Cefadroxil) Bristol-Myers Squibb ... 1079
Dynabac Tablets (Dirithromycin) Muro ... 2269
Dynacin Capsules (Minocycline Hydrochloride) Medicis ... 2019
E.E.S. (Erythromycin Ethylsuccinate) Abbott ... 450
EryPed (Erythromycin Ethylsuccinate) Abbott ... 446
Ery-Tab Tablets (Erythromycin) Abbott ... 448
Erythrocin Stearate Filmtab Tablets (Erythromycin Stearate) Abbott ... 452
Erythromycin Base Filmtab Tablets (Erythromycin) Abbott ... 454
Erythromycin Delayed-Release Capsules, USP (Erythromycin) Abbott ... 455
Floxin I.V. (Ofloxacin) Ortho-McNeil ... 2526
Floxin Tablets (Ofloxacin) Ortho-McNeil ... 2529
Fortaz (Ceftazidime Sodium) GlaxoSmithKline ... 1541
Keflex (Cephalexin) Dista ... 1237
Kefurox Vials, ADD-Vantage (Cefuroxime Sodium) Lilly ... 1948
Kefzol Vials, ADD-Vantage (Cefazolin Sodium) Lilly ... 1951
Levaquin (Levofloxacin) Ortho-McNeil ... 2537
Lorabid Suspension and Pulvules (Loracarbef) Monarch ... 2251
Mandol Vials (Cefamandole Nafate) Lilly ... 1953
Maxipime for Injection (Cefepime Hydrochloride) Elan ... 1285

Mefoxin for Injection (Cefoxitin Sodium) Merck ... 2124
Mefoxin Premixed Intravenous Solution (Cefoxitin Sodium) Merck ... 2127
Minocin Oral Suspension (Minocycline Hydrochloride) Lederle ... 1865
Monodox Capsules (Doxycycline Monohydrate) Oclassen ... 2442
Nebcin Vials, Hyporets & ADD-Vantage (Tobramycin Sulfate) Lilly ... 1955
Omnicef (Cefdinir) Abbott ... 493
PCE Dispertab Tablets (Erythromycin) Abbott ... 498
Pipracil (Piperacillin Sodium) Lederle ... 1866
Primaxin I.M. (Cilastatin Sodium, Imipenem) Merck ... 2158
Primaxin I.V. (Cilastatin Sodium, Imipenem) Merck ... 2160
Rocephin Injectable Vials, ADD-Vantage, Galaxy, Bulk (Ceftriaxone Sodium) Roche Laboratories ... 2993
Synercid I.V. (Dalfopristin, Quinupristin) Aventis ... 775
Tazicef for Injection (Ceftazidime) GlaxoSmithKline ... 1647
Tazicef Galaxy Container (Ceftazidime Sodium) GlaxoSmithKline ... 1650
Tazicef Pharmacy Bulk Package (Ceftazidime) GlaxoSmithKline ... 1653
Tazidime Vials, Faspak & ADD-Vantage (Ceftazidime) Lilly ... 1966
Timentin Injection- ADD-Vantage Vial (Clavulanate Potassium, Ticarcillin Disodium) GlaxoSmithKline ... 1661
Timentin Injection-Galaxy Container (Clavulanate Potassium, Ticarcillin Disodium) GlaxoSmithKline ... 1664
Timentin Injection-Pharmacy Bulk Package (Clavulanate Potassium, Ticarcillin Disodium) GlaxoSmithKline ... 1666
Timentin for Intravenous Administration (Clavulanate Potassium, Ticarcillin Disodium) GlaxoSmithKline ... 1658
Trovan (Alatrofloxacin Mesylate) Pfizer ... 2722
Unasyn for Injection (Ampicillin Sodium, Sulbactam Sodium) Pfizer ... 2728
Vantin Tablets and Oral Suspension (Cefpodoxime Proxetil) Pharmacia & Upjohn ... 2860
Zinacef Injection (Cefuroxime) GlaxoSmithKline ... 1696
Zinacef for Injection (Cefuroxime) GlaxoSmithKline ... 1696
Zithromax (Azithromycin Dihydrate) Pfizer ... 2743
Zithromax for Oral Suspension, 300 mg, 600 mg, 900 mg, 1200 mg (Azithromycin Dihydrate) Pfizer ... 2739
Zithromax Tablets, 250 mg (Azithromycin Dihydrate) Pfizer ... 2739
Zithromax Tablets, 600 mg (Azithromycin Dihydrate) Pfizer ... 2743
Zosyn (Piperacillin Sodium, Tazobactam Sodium) Lederle ... 1890
Zosyn in Galaxy Containers (Piperacillin Sodium, Tazobactam Sodium) Lederle ... 1894
Zyvox (Linezolid) Pharmacia & Upjohn ... 2871

Infections, soft tissues
(*see under* Infections, skin and skin structure)

Infections, superficial, external auditory canal
(*see under* Otitis externa)

Infections, tapeworm
Albenza Tablets (Albendazole) GlaxoSmithKline ... 1463

Infections, upper respiratory tract
Amoxil Chewable Tablets (Amoxicillin) GlaxoSmithKline ... 1471
Amoxil for Oral Suspension (Amoxicillin) GlaxoSmithKline ... 1471
Amoxil (Amoxicillin) GlaxoSmithKline ... 1471
Avelox Tablets (Moxifloxacin Hydrochloride) Bayer ... 879
Bactrim (Sulfamethoxazole, Trimethoprim) Roche Laboratories ... 2949
Biaxin/Biaxin XL (Clarithromycin) Abbott ... 403
Bicillin C-R 900/300 Injection (Penicillin G Benzathine, Penicillin G Procaine) Monarch ... 2240
Bicillin C-R Injection (Penicillin G Benzathine, Penicillin G Procaine) Monarch ... 2238
Bicillin L-A Injection (Penicillin G Benzathine) Monarch ... 2242
Ceclor (Cefaclor) Lilly ... 1905
Cedax (Ceftibuten Dihydrate) Biovail ... 1021
Cefzil (Cefprozil) Bristol-Myers Squibb ... 1076
Doryx Coated Pellet Filled Capsules (Doxycycline Hyclate) Warner Chilcott ... 3357
Duricef (Cefadroxil) Bristol-Myers Squibb ... 1079
Dynacin Capsules (Minocycline Hydrochloride) Medicis ... 2019
E.E.S. (Erythromycin Ethylsuccinate) Abbott ... 450
EryPed (Erythromycin Ethylsuccinate) Abbott ... 446
Ery-Tab Tablets (Erythromycin) Abbott ... 448
Erythrocin Stearate Filmtab Tablets (Erythromycin Stearate) Abbott ... 452
Erythromycin Base Filmtab Tablets (Erythromycin) Abbott ... 454
Erythromycin Delayed-Release Capsules, USP (Erythromycin) Abbott ... 455
Lorabid Suspension and Pulvules (Loracarbef) Monarch ... 2251
Minocin Oral Suspension (Minocycline Hydrochloride) Lederle ... 1865
Monodox Capsules (Doxycycline Monohydrate) Oclassen ... 2442
Omnicef (Cefdinir) Abbott ... 493
PCE Dispertab Tablets (Erythromycin) Abbott ... 498
Permapen Isoject (Penicillin G Benzathine) Pfizer ... 2706
Septra Suspension (Sulfamethoxazole, Trimethoprim) Monarch ... 2265
Septra Tablets (Sulfamethoxazole, Trimethoprim) Monarch ... 2265
Septra DS Tablets (Sulfamethoxazole, Trimethoprim) Monarch ... 2265
Suprax (Cefixime) Lederle ... 1877
Tequin Injection (Gatifloxacin) Bristol-Myers Squibb ... 1110
Tequin Tablets (Gatifloxacin) Bristol-Myers Squibb ... 1110
Vantin Tablets and Oral Suspension (Cefpodoxime Proxetil) Pharmacia & Upjohn ... 2860
Vibramycin Hyclate Capsules (Doxycycline Hyclate) Pfizer ... 2735
Zithromax (Azithromycin Dihydrate) Pfizer ... 2743
Zithromax for Oral Suspension, 300 mg, 600 mg, 900 mg, 1200 mg (Azithromycin Dihydrate) Pfizer ... 2739
Zithromax Tablets, 250 mg (Azithromycin Dihydrate) Pfizer ... 2739
Zithromax Tablets, 600 mg (Azithromycin Dihydrate) Pfizer ... 2743

Infections, urinary bladder, prophylaxis of
Neosporin G.U. Irrigant Sterile (Neomycin Sulfate, Polymyxin B Sulfate) Monarch ... 2256

Infections, urinary tract
Amoxil Chewable Tablets (Amoxicillin) GlaxoSmithKline ... 1471
Amoxil for Oral Suspension (Amoxicillin) GlaxoSmithKline ... 1471
Amoxil (Amoxicillin) GlaxoSmithKline ... 1471
Ancef for Injection (Cefazolin Sodium) GlaxoSmithKline ... 1474
Ancef Injection (Cefazolin Sodium) GlaxoSmithKline ... 1474
Augmentin Chewable Tablets (Amoxicillin, Clavulanate Potassium) GlaxoSmithKline ... 1482
Augmentin Powder for Oral Suspension (Amoxicillin, Clavulanate Potassium) GlaxoSmithKline ... 1482
Augmentin Tablets (Amoxicillin, Clavulanate Potassium) GlaxoSmithKline ... 1485
Azactam for Injection (Aztreonam) Elan ... 1276
Bactrim (Sulfamethoxazole, Trimethoprim) Roche Laboratories ... 2949
Ceclor (Cefaclor) Lilly ... 1905
Cefizox for Intramuscular or Intravenous Use (Ceftizoxime Sodium) Fujisawa ... 1390
Cefobid Intravenous/Intramuscular (Cefoperazone) Pfizer ... 2671
Cefobid Pharmacy Bulk Package - Not for Direct Infusion (Cefoperazone Sodium) Pfizer ... 2673
Cefotan (Cefotetan) AstraZeneca ... 664
Ceftin Tablets (Cefuroxime Axetil) Lifecycle Ventures ... 1898
Ceptaz for Injection (Ceftazidime) GlaxoSmithKline ... 1499
Cipro I.V. (Ciprofloxacin) Bayer ... 893
Cipro I.V. Pharmacy Bulk Package (Ciprofloxacin) Bayer ... 897
Cipro (Ciprofloxacin) Bayer ... 887
Duricef (Cefadroxil) Bristol-Myers Squibb ... 1079
Dynacin Capsules (Minocycline Hydrochloride) Medicis ... 2019
Floxin I.V. (Ofloxacin) Ortho-McNeil ... 2526
Floxin Tablets (Ofloxacin) Ortho-McNeil ... 2529
Fortaz (Ceftazidime Sodium) GlaxoSmithKline ... 1541
Geocillin Tablets (Carbenicillin Indanyl Sodium) Pfizer ... 2687
Kefurox Vials, ADD-Vantage (Cefuroxime Sodium) Lilly ... 1948
Kefzol Vials, ADD-Vantage (Cefazolin Sodium) Lilly ... 1951
Levaquin (Levofloxacin) Ortho-McNeil ... 2537
Lorabid Suspension and Pulvules (Loracarbef) Monarch ... 2251
Macrobid Capsules (Nitrofurantoin Monohydrate) Procter & Gamble Pharmaceuticals ... 2889
Macrodantin Capsules (Nitrofurantoin) Procter & Gamble Pharmaceuticals ... 2891
Mandol Vials (Cefamandole Nafate) Lilly ... 1953
Maxipime for Injection (Cefepime Hydrochloride) Elan ... 1285
Mefoxin for Injection (Cefoxitin Sodium) Merck ... 2124
Mefoxin Premixed Intravenous Solution (Cefoxitin Sodium) Merck ... 2127
Minocin Oral Suspension (Minocycline Hydrochloride) Lederle ... 1865
Monodox Capsules (Doxycycline Monohydrate) Oclassen ... 2442
Monurol Sachet (Fosfomycin Tromethamine) Forest ... 1375
Nebcin Vials, Hyporets & ADD-Vantage (Tobramycin Sulfate) Lilly ... 1955
Noroxin Tablets (Norfloxacin) Merck ... 2145
Pipracil (Piperacillin Sodium) Lederle ... 1866
Primaxin I.V. (Cilastatin Sodium, Imipenem) Merck ... 2160
Rocephin Injectable Vials, ADD-Vantage, Galaxy, Bulk (Ceftriaxone Sodium) Roche Laboratories ... 2993
Septra Suspension (Sulfamethoxazole, Trimethoprim) Monarch ... 2265
Septra Tablets (Sulfamethoxazole, Trimethoprim) Monarch ... 2265
Septra DS Tablets (Sulfamethoxazole, Trimethoprim) Monarch ... 2265
Suprax (Cefixime) Lederle ... 1877
Tazicef for Injection (Ceftazidime) GlaxoSmithKline ... 1647
Tazicef Galaxy Container (Ceftazidime Sodium) GlaxoSmithKline ... 1650
Tazicef Pharmacy Bulk Package (Ceftazidime) GlaxoSmithKline ... 1653
Tazidime Vials, Faspak & ADD-Vantage (Ceftazidime) Lilly ... 1966
Tequin Injection (Gatifloxacin) Bristol-Myers Squibb ... 1110
Tequin Tablets (Gatifloxacin) Bristol-Myers Squibb ... 1110
Timentin Injection- ADD-Vantage Vial (Clavulanate Potassium, Ticarcillin Disodium) GlaxoSmithKline ... 1661
Timentin Injection-Galaxy Container (Clavulanate Potassium, Ticarcillin Disodium) GlaxoSmithKline ... 1664
Timentin Injection-Pharmacy Bulk Package (Clavulanate Potassium, Ticarcillin Disodium) GlaxoSmithKline ... 1666
Timentin for Intravenous Administration (Clavulanate Potassium, Ticarcillin Disodium) GlaxoSmithKline ... 1658
Urimax Tablets (Belladonna Alkaloids, Hyoscyamine Sulfate, Methenamine, Methylene Blue, Phenyl Salicylate, Sodium Biphosphate) Integrity Pharmaceutical ... 1769
Urised Tablets (Atropine Sulfate, Benzoic Acid, Hyoscyamine, Methenamine, Methylene Blue, Phenyl Salicylate) PolyMedica ... 2876
Uroqid-Acid No. 2 Tablets (Methenamine Mandelate, Sodium Acid Phosphate) Beach ... 947
Vantin Tablets and Oral Suspension (Cefpodoxime Proxetil) Pharmacia & Upjohn ... 2860
Zinacef Injection (Cefuroxime) GlaxoSmithKline ... 1696
Zinacef for Injection (Cefuroxime) GlaxoSmithKline ... 1696

Infections, urinary tract, systemic candidal
Diflucan Tablets, Injection, and Oral Suspension (Fluconazole) Pfizer ... 2681

Infections, vaginal cuff, post-surgical
Cleocin HCl Capsules (Clindamycin Hydrochloride) Pharmacia & Upjohn ... 2784
Cleocin Phosphate Sterile Solution (Clindamycin Phosphate) Pharmacia & Upjohn ... 2785

Infections, venereal
(*see also under* Bejel; Gonorrhea; Pinta; Yaws)
Bicillin L-A Injection (Penicillin G Benzathine) Monarch ... 2242

Infections, vulvovaginal mycotic, Candida species
AVC (Sulfanilamide) Fielding ... 1350

Infectious diarrhea
(*see under* Diarrhea, infectious)

Infertility, progesterone deficiency-induced
Crinone (Progesterone) Serono ... 3213

Inflammation, anorectal
Analpram-HC (Hydrocortisone Acetate, Pramoxine Hydrochloride) Ferndale ... 1338
Anusol-HC Suppositories (Hydrocortisone Acetate) Monarch ... 2238
Cortizone•5 (Hydrocortisone) Pfizer Inc., Warner-Lambert Healthcare ... ▣699
Cortizone•10 (Hydrocortisone) Pfizer Inc., Warner-Lambert Healthcare ... ▣699
Cortizone•10 Plus Creme (Hydrocortisone) Pfizer Inc., Warner-Lambert Healthcare ... ▣700
Proctocort Suppositories (Hydrocortisone Acetate) Monarch ... 2264
ProctoFoam-HC (Hydrocortisone Acetate, Pramoxine Hydrochloride) Schwarz ... 3177

Inflammation, anterior segment
Blephamide Ophthalmic Ointment (Prednisolone Acetate, Sulfacetamide Sodium) Allergan ... 547
Blephamide Ophthalmic Suspension (Prednisolone Acetate, Sulfacetamide Sodium) Allergan ... 548
Celestone Soluspan Injectable Suspension (Betamethasone Acetate, Betamethasone Sodium Phosphate) Schering ... 3097
Celestone Syrup (Betamethasone) Schering ... 3099
Cortisporin Ophthalmic Suspension (Hydrocortisone, Neomycin Sulfate, Polymyxin B Sulfate, Hydrocortisone, Neomycin Sulfate, Polymyxin B Sulfate) Monarch ... ⊙297
Cortone Acetate Injectable Suspension (Cortisone Acetate) Merck ... 2059
Cortone Acetate Tablets (Cortisone Acetate) Merck ... 2061
Decadron Elixir (Dexamethasone) Merck ... 2078
Decadron Tablets (Dexamethasone) Merck ... 2079
Decadron Phosphate Injection (Dexamethasone Sodium Phosphate) Merck ... 2081
Decadron Phosphate Sterile Ophthalmic Ointment (Dexamethasone Sodium Phosphate) Merck ... 2083
Decadron Phosphate Sterile Ophthalmic Solution (Dexamethasone Sodium Phosphate) Merck ... 2084
Depo-Medrol Injectable Suspension (Methylprednisolone Acetate) Pharmacia & Upjohn ... 2795
FML Ophthalmic Ointment (Fluorometholone) Allergan ... ⊙237
FML Ophthalmic Suspension (Fluorometholone) Allergan ... ⊙236
FML Forte Ophthalmic Suspension (Fluorometholone) Allergan ... ⊙235

FML-S Liquifilm Sterile Ophthalmic Suspension (Fluorometholone, Sulfacetamide Sodium) Allergan.. ⊙ 238
Hydrocortone Tablets (Hydrocortisone) Merck 2106
Hydrocortone Phosphate Injection, Sterile (Hydrocortisone Sodium Phosphate) Merck.......... 2105
Lotemax Sterile Ophthalmic Suspension 0.5% (Loteprednol Etabonate) Bausch & Lomb .... ⊙ 261
NeoDecadron Sterile Ophthalmic Solution (Dexamethasone Sodium Phosphate, Neomycin Sulfate) Merck.......... 2144
Pediapred Oral Solution (Prednisolone Sodium Phosphate) Celltech.......... 1170
Poly-Pred Liquifilm Ophthalmic Suspension (Neomycin Sulfate, Polymyxin B Sulfate, Prednisolone Acetate) Allergan.......... ⊙ 245
Pred Forte Ophthalmic Suspension (Prednisolone Acetate) Allergan .... ⊙ 246
Pred-G Ophthalmic Suspension (Gentamicin Sulfate, Prednisolone Acetate) Allergan .... ⊙ 247
Pred-G Sterile Ophthalmic Ointment (Gentamicin Sulfate, Prednisolone Acetate) Allergan ..... ⊙ 248
Prednisone (Prednisone) Roxane 3064
Prelone Syrup (Prednisolone) Muro . 2273
Solu-Medrol Sterile Powder (Methylprednisolone Sodium Succinate) Pharmacia & Upjohn 2855
Terra-Cortril Ophthalmic Suspension (Hydrocortisone Acetate, Oxytetracycline Hydrochloride) Pfizer 2716
TobraDex Ophthalmic Ointment (Dexamethasone, Tobramycin) Alcon 542
TobraDex Ophthalmic Suspension (Dexamethasone, Tobramycin) Alcon 541

Influenza A virus, acute illness, treatment of
Relenza Rotadisk (Zanamivir) GlaxoSmithKline 1619
Tamiflu Capsules (Oseltamivir Phosphate) Roche Laboratories ... 3008
Tamiflu Oral Suspension (Oseltamivir Phosphate) Roche Laboratories 3008

Influenza A virus, respiratory tract illness, chemoprophylaxis of
Flumadine (Rimantadine Hydrochloride) Forest 1370
Symmetrel (Amantadine Hydrochloride) Endo Labs 1328
Tamiflu Capsules (Oseltamivir Phosphate) Roche Laboratories ... 3008
Tamiflu Oral Suspension (Oseltamivir Phosphate) Roche Laboratories 3008

Influenza A virus, respiratory tract illness, treatment of
Flumadine (Rimantadine Hydrochloride) Forest 1370
Symmetrel (Amantadine Hydrochloride) Endo Labs 1328

Influenza syndrome, symptomatic relief of
Advil Cold and Sinus Caplets (Ibuprofen, Pseudoephedrine Hydrochloride) Whitehall-Robins .... ▣ 771
Advil Cold and Sinus Tablets (Ibuprofen, Pseudoephedrine Hydrochloride) Whitehall-Robins .. ▣ 771
Advil Flu & Body Ache Caplets (Ibuprofen, Pseudoephedrine Hydrochloride) Whitehall-Robins .. ▣ 772
Aleve Cold & Sinus Caplets (Naproxen Sodium, Pseudoephedrine Hydrochloride) Bayer Consumer .... ▣ 603
Alka-Seltzer Plus Liqui-Gels (Acetaminophen, Chlorpheniramine Maleate, Pseudoephedrine Hydrochloride) Bayer Consumer .... ▣ 604
Alka-Seltzer Plus Cold & Flu Medicine Liqui-Gels (Acetaminophen, Dextromethorphan Hydrobromide, Pseudoephedrine Hydrochloride) Bayer Consumer .... ▣ 604
Benadryl Allergy (Diphenhydramine Hydrochloride) Pfizer Inc., Warner-Lambert Healthcare .... ▣ 691
Benadryl Severe Allergy & Sinus Headache Caplets (Acetaminophen, Diphenhydramine Hydrochloride, Pseudoephedrine Hydrochloride) Pfizer Inc., Warner-Lambert Healthcare .... ▣ 694
Benadryl Dye-Free Allergy Liquid (Diphenhydramine Hydrochloride) Pfizer Inc., Warner-Lambert Healthcare .... ▣ 690
Benylin Multi-Symptom Liquid (Dextromethorphan Hydrobromide, Guaifenesin, Pseudoephedrine Hydrochloride) Pfizer Inc., Warner-Lambert Healthcare .... ▣ 697
Biomune OSF Express Spray (Homeopathic Formulations) Matol .... ▣ 640
Children's Cēpacol Sore Throat (Acetaminophen, Pseudoephedrine Hydrochloride) Williams .... ▣ 788
Comtrex Deep Chest Cold & Congestion Relief Softgels (Acetaminophen, Dextromethorphan Hydrobromide, Guaifenesin, Pseudoephedrine Hydrochloride) Bristol-Myers .... ▣ 627
Comtrex Flu Therapy & Fever Relief Daytime Caplets (Acetaminophen, Pseudoephedrine Hydrochloride) Bristol-Myers .... ▣ 628
Comtrex Flu Therapy & Fever Relief Nighttime Tablets (Acetaminophen, Chlorpheniramine Maleate, Pseudoephedrine Hydrochloride) Bristol-Myers .... ▣ 628
Contac Severe Cold and Flu Caplets Maximum Strength (Acetaminophen, Chlorpheniramine Maleate, Dextromethorphan Hydrobromide, Pseudoephedrine Hydrochloride) SmithKline Beecham Consumer . ▣ 746
Contac Severe Cold and Flu Caplets Non-Drowsy (Acetaminophen, Dextromethorphan Hydrobromide, Pseudoephedrine Hydrochloride) SmithKline Beecham Consumer .... ▣ 746
Coricidin HBP Maximum Strength Flu Tablets (Acetaminophen, Chlorpheniramine Maleate, Dextromethorphan Hydrobromide) Schering-Plough .... ▣ 738
Dimetapp Nighttime Flu Liquid (Acetaminophen, Brompheniramine Maleate, Dextromethorphan Hydrobromide, Pseudoephedrine Hydrochloride) Whitehall-Robins .... ▣ 776
Dimetapp Non-Drowsy Flu Syrup (Acetaminophen, Dextromethorphan Hydrobromide, Pseudoephedrine Hydrochloride) Whitehall-Robins .... ▣ 777
Drixoral Cold & Flu Extended-Release Tablets (Acetaminophen, Dexbrompheniramine Maleate, Pseudoephedrine Sulfate) Schering-Plough .... ▣ 740
Excedrin Extra-Strength Tablets, Caplets, and Geltabs (Acetaminophen, Aspirin, Caffeine) Bristol-Myers .... ▣ 629
Extendryl (Chlorpheniramine Maleate, Methscopolamine Nitrate, Phenylephrine Hydrochloride) Fleming 1361
Kronofed-A (Chlorpheniramine Maleate, Pseudoephedrine Hydrochloride) Ferndale 1341
Children's Motrin Cold Oral Suspension (Ibuprofen, Pseudoephedrine Hydrochloride) McNeil Consumer 2007
Motrin Sinus Headache Caplets (Ibuprofen, Pseudoephedrine Hydrochloride) McNeil Consumer 2005
Oscillococcinum Pellets (Anas Barbariae Hepatis et Cordis Extractum) Boiron .... ▣ 625
PediaCare NightRest Cough-Cold Liquid (Chlorpheniramine Maleate, Dextromethorphan Hydrobromide, Pseudoephedrine Hydrochloride) Pharmacia Consumer .... ▣ 719
Phenergan with Codeine Syrup (Codeine Phosphate, Promethazine Hydrochloride) Wyeth-Ayerst 3557
Phenergan with Dextromethorphan Syrup (Dextromethorphan Hydrobromide, Promethazine Hydrochloride) Wyeth-Ayerst 3559
Phenergan VC Syrup (Phenylephrine Hydrochloride, Promethazine Hydrochloride) Wyeth-Ayerst 3560
Phenergan VC with Codeine Syrup (Codeine Phosphate, Phenylephrine Hydrochloride, Promethazine Hydrochloride) Wyeth-Ayerst 3561
Robitussin Cold Caplets Multi-Symptom Cold & Flu (Acetaminophen, Dextromethorphan Hydrobromide, Guaifenesin, Pseudoephedrine Hydrochloride) Whitehall-Robins .... ▣ 781
Robitussin Cold Softgels Multi-Symptom Cold & Flu (Acetaminophen, Dextromethorphan Hydrobromide, Guaifenesin, Pseudoephedrine Hydrochloride) Whitehall-Robins .... ▣ 781
Robitussin Multi Symptom Honey Flu Liquid (Acetaminophen, Dextromethorphan Hydrobromide, Pseudoephedrine Hydrochloride) Whitehall-Robins .... ▣ 785
Robitussin Nighttime Honey Flu Liquid (Acetaminophen, Chlorpheniramine Maleate, Dextromethorphan Hydrobromide, Pseudoephedrine Hydrochloride) Whitehall-Robins .... ▣ 786
Ryna (Chlorpheniramine Maleate, Pseudoephedrine Hydrochloride) Wallace .... ▣ 768
Reformulated Rynatan Pediatric Suspension (Chlorpheniramine Tannate, Phenylephrine Tannate) Wallace 3352
Sudafed Cold & Cough Liquid Caps (Acetaminophen, Dextromethorphan Hydrobromide, Guaifenesin, Pseudoephedrine Hydrochloride) Pfizer Inc., Warner-Lambert Healthcare .... ▣ 709
Sudafed Severe Cold (Acetaminophen, Dextromethorphan Hydrobromide, Pseudoephedrine Hydrochloride) Pfizer Inc., Warner-Lambert Healthcare .... ▣ 711
TheraFlu Regular Strength Cold & Sore Throat Night Time Hot Liquid (Acetaminophen, Chlorpheniramine Maleate, Pseudoephedrine Hydrochloride) Novartis Consumer .... ▣ 676
TheraFlu Maximum Strength Flu & Congestion Non-Drowsy Hot Liquid (Acetaminophen, Dextromethorphan Hydrobromide, Guaifenesin, Pseudoephedrine Hydrochloride) Novartis Consumer .... ▣ 677
TheraFlu Maximum Strength Flu & Cough Night Time Hot Liquid (Acetaminophen, Chlorpheniramine Maleate, Dextromethorphan Hydrobromide, Pseudoephedrine Hydrochloride) Novartis Consumer .... ▣ 678
TheraFlu Maximum Strength Flu & Sore Throat Night Time Hot Liquid (Acetaminophen, Chlorpheniramine Maleate, Pseudoephedrine Hydrochloride) Novartis Consumer .... ▣ 677
TheraFlu Maximum Strength Severe Cold & Congestion Night Time Caplets (Acetaminophen, Chlorpheniramine Maleate, Dextromethorphan Hydrobromide, Pseudoephedrine Hydrochloride) Novartis Consumer .... ▣ 678
TheraFlu Maximum Strength Severe Cold & Congestion Night Time Hot Liquid (Acetaminophen, Chlorpheniramine Maleate, Dextromethorphan Hydrobromide, Pseudoephedrine Hydrochloride) Novartis Consumer .... ▣ 678
TheraFlu Maximum Strength Severe Cold & Congestion Non-Drowsy (Acetaminophen, Dextromethorphan Hydrobromide, Pseudoephedrine Hydrochloride) Novartis Consumer .... ▣ 679
Triaminic Cold & Cough Liquid (Chlorpheniramine Maleate, Dextromethorphan Hydrobromide, Pseudoephedrine Hydrochloride) Novartis Consumer .... ▣ 681
Triaminic Cold & Night Time Cough Liquid (Chlorpheniramine Maleate, Dextromethorphan Hydrobromide, Pseudoephedrine Hydrochloride) Novartis Consumer .... ▣ 681
Triaminic Cold, Cough & Fever Liquid (Acetaminophen, Chlorpheniramine Maleate, Dextromethorphan Hydrobromide, Pseudoephedrine Hydrochloride) Novartis Consumer .... ▣ 681
Triaminic Cough & Sore Throat Liquid (Acetaminophen, Dextromethorphan Hydrobromide, Pseudoephedrine Hydrochloride) Novartis Consumer .... ▣ 682
Triaminic Cough & Sore Throat Softchews (Acetaminophen, Dextromethorphan Hydrobromide, Pseudoephedrine Hydrochloride) Novartis Consumer ...... ▣ 684
Tussionex Pennkinetic Extended-Release Suspension (Chlorpheniramine Polistirex, Hydrocodone Polistirex) Celltech.. 1174
Children's Tylenol Suspension Liquid and Soft Chews Chewable Tablets (Acetaminophen) McNeil Consumer.......... 2014
Maximum Strength Tylenol Allergy Sinus NightTime Caplets (Acetaminophen, Diphenhydramine Hydrochloride, Pseudoephedrine Hydrochloride) McNeil Consumer 2010
Multi-Symptom Tylenol Cold Complete Formula Caplets (Acetaminophen, Chlorpheniramine Maleate, Dextromethorphan Hydrobromide, Pseudoephedrine Hydrochloride) McNeil Consumer 2010
Multi-Symptom Tylenol Cold Non-Drowsy Caplets and Gelcaps (Acetaminophen, Dextromethorphan Hydrobromide, Pseudoephedrine Hydrochloride) McNeil Consumer 2010
Maximum Strength Tylenol Flu NightTime Gelcaps (Acetaminophen, Diphenhydramine Hydrochloride, Pseudoephedrine Hydrochloride) McNeil Consumer 2011
Maximum Strength Tylenol Flu NightTime Liquid (Acetaminophen, Dextromethorphan Hydrobromide, Doxylamine Succinate, Pseudoephedrine Hydrochloride) McNeil Consumer 2011
Maximum Strength Tylenol Flu Non-Drowsy Gelcaps (Acetaminophen, Dextromethorphan Hydrobromide, Pseudoephedrine Hydrochloride) McNeil Consumer 2011
Vicks 44M Cough, Cold & Flu Relief Liquid (Acetaminophen, Chlorpheniramine Maleate, Dextromethorphan Hydrobromide, Pseudoephedrine Hydrochloride) Procter & Gamble .... ▣ 725
Pediatric Vicks 44m Cough & Cold Relief (Chlorpheniramine Maleate, Dextromethorphan Hydrobromide, Pseudoephedrine Hydrochloride) Procter & Gamble .... ▣ 728
Vicks DayQuil LiquiCaps/Liquid Multi-Symptom Cold/Flu Relief (Acetaminophen, Dextromethorphan Hydrobromide, Pseudoephedrine Hydrochloride) Procter & Gamble .... ▣ 727
Children's Vicks NyQuil Cold/Cough Relief (Chlorpheniramine Maleate, Dextromethorphan Hydrobromide, Pseudoephedrine Hydrochloride) Procter & Gamble .... ▣ 726
Vicks NyQuil LiquiCaps/Liquid Multi-Symptom Cold/Flu Relief, Original and Cherry Flavors (Acetaminophen, Dextromethorphan Hydrobromide, Doxylamine Succinate, Pseudoephedrine Hydrochloride) Procter & Gamble .... ▣ 727

Insect bites, pain due to
(*see under* Pain, topical relief of)

Insomnia
(*see under* Sleep, induction of)

Intermittent claudication
(*see under* Claudication, intermittent)

Intertrigo
(*see under* Skin, inflammatory conditions)

Intraocular pressure, elevation
(*see under* Hypertension, ocular)

Intravascular device, maintenance of patency
Cathflo Activase (Alteplase, Recombinant) Genentech 3611
Heparin Lock Flush Solution (Heparin Sodium) Wyeth-Ayerst 3509

Intubation, endotracheal
Anectine Injection (Succinylcholine Chloride) GlaxoSmithKline 1476
Norcuron for Injection (Vecuronium Bromide) Organon 2478
Zemuron Injection (Rocuronium Bromide) Organon 2491

Intubation, small bowel
Reglan (Metoclopramide Hydrochloride) Robins........ 2935

Iridectomy, post-, adjunct
Humorsol Sterile Ophthalmic Solution (Demecarium Bromide) Merck 2102

Iridocyclitis
Celestone Soluspan Injectable Suspension (Betamethasone Acetate, Betamethasone Sodium Phosphate) Schering........ 3097
Celestone Syrup (Betamethasone) Schering 3099
Cortone Acetate Injectable Suspension (Cortisone Acetate) Merck 2059
Cortone Acetate Tablets (Cortisone Acetate) Merck 2061
Decadron Elixir (Dexamethasone) Merck 2078
Decadron Tablets (Dexamethasone) Merck 2079
Decadron Phosphate Injection (Dexamethasone Sodium Phosphate) Merck 2081
Depo-Medrol Injectable Suspension (Methylprednisolone Acetate) Pharmacia & Upjohn 2795
Hydrocortone Tablets (Hydrocortisone) Merck 2106
Hydrocortone Phosphate Injection, Sterile (Hydrocortisone Sodium Phosphate) Merck 2105
Pediapred Oral Solution (Prednisolone Sodium Phosphate) Celltech 1170
Prednisone (Prednisone) Roxane 3064
Prelone Syrup (Prednisolone) Muro 2273
Solu-Medrol Sterile Powder (Methylprednisolone Sodium Succinate) Pharmacia & Upjohn 2855

Iritis
Celestone Soluspan Injectable Suspension (Betamethasone Acetate, Betamethasone Sodium Phosphate) Schering 3097
Celestone Syrup (Betamethasone) Schering 3099
Cortone Acetate Injectable Suspension (Cortisone Acetate) Merck 2059
Cortone Acetate Tablets (Cortisone Acetate) Merck 2061
Decadron Elixir (Dexamethasone) Merck 2078
Decadron Tablets (Dexamethasone) Merck 2079
Decadron Phosphate Injection (Dexamethasone Sodium Phosphate) Merck 2081
Decadron Phosphate Sterile Ophthalmic Ointment (Dexamethasone Sodium Phosphate) Merck 2083
Decadron Phosphate Sterile Ophthalmic Solution (Dexamethasone Sodium Phosphate) Merck 2084
Depo-Medrol Injectable Suspension (Methylprednisolone Acetate) Pharmacia & Upjohn 2795
Hydrocortone Tablets (Hydrocortisone) Merck 2106
Hydrocortone Phosphate Injection, Sterile (Hydrocortisone Sodium Phosphate) Merck 2105
Pediapred Oral Solution (Prednisolone Sodium Phosphate) Celltech 1170
Prednisone (Prednisone) Roxane 3064
Prelone Syrup (Prednisolone) Muro 2273
Solu-Medrol Sterile Powder (Methylprednisolone Sodium Succinate) Pharmacia & Upjohn 2855

Iron deficiency
Feosol Caplets (Iron Carbonyl) GlaxoSmithKline Consumer 1717
Feosol Tablets (Ferrous Sulfate) GlaxoSmithKline Consumer 1717
Fergon Iron Tablets (Ferrous Gluconate) Bayer Consumer .... ▣802
Ferrlecit Injection (Sodium Ferric Gluconate) Watson 3386
INFeD Injection (Iron Dextran) Watson 3388
Slow Fe Tablets (Ferrous Sulfate) Novartis Consumer .... ▣827

Iron intoxication, acute
Desferal (Deferoxamine Mesylate) Novartis 2333

Irritable bowel syndrome
(*see under* Bowel, irritable, syndrome)

Ischemic attacks, transient
Genuine Bayer Professional Labeling (Aspirin Regimen Bayer) (Aspirin) Bayer Consumer .... ▣608
Ecotrin Enteric Coated Aspirin Low, Regular and Maximum Strength Tablets (Aspirin) GlaxoSmithKline Consumer 1715
Pravachol Tablets (Pravastatin Sodium) Bristol-Myers Squibb 1099
Zocor Tablets (Simvastatin) Merck 2219

Isoimmunization, prevention of in Rho(D) negative individuals
BayRho-D Full Dose (Rh_o (D) Immune Globulin (Human)) Bayer Biological 921

Isoimmunization, prevention of in Rho(D) negative women
BayRho-D Mini-Dose (Rh_o (D) Immune Globulin (Human)) Bayer Biological 919
MICRhoGAM Injection (Rh_o (D) Immune Globulin (Human)) Ortho-Clinical 2524
RhoGAM Injection (Rh_o (D) Immune Globulin (Human)) Ortho-Clinical 2524

Itching, skin
(*see under* Pruritus, topical relief of)

Itching, sunburn
(*see under* Pruritus, topical relief of)

J

Jock itch
(*see under* Tinea cruris infections)

Joint pain
(*see under* Pain, arthritic, minor)

K

K. pneumoniae bacteremia
Rocephin (Ceftriaxone Sodium) Roche Laboratories 2993

K. pneumoniae central nervous system infections
Claforan Injection (Cefotaxime Sodium) Aventis 732

K. pneumoniae genitourinary tract infections
Keflex (Cephalexin) Dista 1237

K. pneumoniae gynecologic infections
Azactam for Injection (Aztreonam) Elan 1276
Primaxin I.M. (Cilastatin Sodium, Imipenem) Merck 2158
Timentin Injection- ADD-Vantage Vial (Clavulanate Potassium, Ticarcillin Disodium) GlaxoSmithKline 1661
Timentin Injection-Galaxy Container (Clavulanate Potassium, Ticarcillin Disodium) GlaxoSmithKline 1664
Timentin Injection-Pharmacy Bulk Package (Clavulanate Potassium, Ticarcillin Disodium) GlaxoSmithKline 1666
Timentin for Intravenous Administration (Clavulanate Potassium, Ticarcillin Disodium) GlaxoSmithKline 1658

K. pneumoniae infections
Avelox Tablets (Moxifloxacin Hydrochloride) Bayer 879
Azactam for Injection (Aztreonam) Elan 1276
Cefobid Intravenous/Intramuscular (Cefoperazone) Pfizer 2671
Cefobid Pharmacy Bulk Package - Not for Direct Infusion (Cefoperazone Sodium) Pfizer 2673
Cefotan (Cefotetan) AstraZeneca 664
Ceftin Tablets (Cefuroxime Axetil) Lifecycle Ventures 1898
Cipro I.V. (Ciprofloxacin) Bayer 893
Cipro I.V. Pharmacy Bulk Package (Ciprofloxacin) Bayer 897
Cipro (Ciprofloxacin) Bayer 887
Claforan Injection (Cefotaxime Sodium) Aventis 732
Floxin I.V. (Ofloxacin) Ortho-McNeil 2526
Floxin Tablets (Ofloxacin) Ortho-McNeil 2529
Keflex (Cephalexin) Dista 1237
Levaquin (Levofloxacin) Ortho-McNeil 2537
Maxipime for Injection (Cefepime Hydrochloride) Elan 1285
Merrem I.V. (Meropenem) AstraZeneca 673
Noroxin Tablets (Norfloxacin) Merck........ 2145
Primaxin I.M. (Cilastatin Sodium, Imipenem) Merck........ 2158
Rocephin Injectable Vials, ADD-Vantage, Galaxy, Bulk (Ceftriaxone Sodium) Roche Laboratories........ 2993
Suprax for Oral Suspension (Cefixime) Lederle........ 1877
Tequin Injection (Gatifloxacin) Bristol-Myers Squibb........ 1110
Tequin Tablets (Gatifloxacin) Bristol-Myers Squibb 1110
Timentin Injection- ADD-Vantage Vial (Clavulanate Potassium, Ticarcillin Disodium) GlaxoSmithKline 1661
Timentin Injection-Galaxy Container (Clavulanate Potassium, Ticarcillin Disodium) GlaxoSmithKline 1664
Timentin Injection-Pharmacy Bulk Package (Clavulanate Potassium, Ticarcillin Disodium) GlaxoSmithKline 1666
Timentin for Intravenous Administration (Clavulanate Potassium, Ticarcillin Disodium) GlaxoSmithKline 1658
Trovan (Alatrofloxacin Mesylate) Pfizer 2722
Unasyn for Injection (Ampicillin Sodium, Sulbactam Sodium) Pfizer 2728
Vantin Tablets and Oral Suspension (Cefpodoxime Proxetil) Pharmacia & Upjohn 2860

K. pneumoniae infections, ocular
Genoptic Ophthalmic Ointment (Gentamicin Sulfate) Allergan .... ⊙239
Genoptic Sterile Ophthalmic Solution (Gentamicin Sulfate) Allergan .... ⊙239
Pred-G Sterile Ophthalmic Ointment (Gentamicin Sulfate, Prednisolone Acetate) Allergan .... ⊙248

K. pneumoniae intra-abdominal infections
Azactam for Injection (Aztreonam) Elan 1276
Cefotan (Cefotetan) AstraZeneca 664
Cipro I.V. (Ciprofloxacin) Bayer 893
Cipro I.V. Pharmacy Bulk Package (Ciprofloxacin) Bayer 897
Cipro (Ciprofloxacin) Bayer 887
Maxipime for Injection (Cefepime Hydrochloride) Elan 1285
Merrem I.V. (Meropenem) AstraZeneca 673
Primaxin I.M. (Cilastatin Sodium, Imipenem) Merck 2158
Rocephin Injectable Vials, ADD-Vantage, Galaxy, Bulk (Ceftriaxone Sodium) Roche Laboratories 2993
Timentin Injection- ADD-Vantage Vial (Clavulanate Potassium, Ticarcillin Disodium) GlaxoSmithKline 1661
Timentin Injection-Galaxy Container (Clavulanate Potassium, Ticarcillin Disodium) GlaxoSmithKline 1664
Timentin Injection-Pharmacy Bulk Package (Clavulanate Potassium, Ticarcillin Disodium) GlaxoSmithKline 1666
Timentin for Intravenous Administration (Clavulanate Potassium, Ticarcillin Disodium) GlaxoSmithKline 1658
Trovan (Alatrofloxacin Mesylate) Pfizer 2722
Unasyn for Injection (Ampicillin Sodium, Sulbactam Sodium) Pfizer 2728

K. pneumoniae lower respiratory tract infections
Azactam for Injection (Aztreonam) Elan 1276
Cefotan (Cefotetan) AstraZeneca 664
Cipro I.V. (Ciprofloxacin) Bayer 893
Cipro I.V. Pharmacy Bulk Package (Ciprofloxacin) Bayer 897
Cipro (Ciprofloxacin) Bayer 887
Levaquin (Levofloxacin) Ortho-McNeil 2537
Maxipime for Injection (Cefepime Hydrochloride) Elan 1285
Rocephin Injectable Vials, ADD-Vantage, Galaxy, Bulk (Ceftriaxone Sodium) Roche Laboratories 2993
Trovan (Alatrofloxacin Mesylate) Pfizer 2722

K. pneumoniae pneumonia, treatment, adjunct
Streptomycin Sulfate Injection (Streptomycin Sulfate) Pfizer 2714

K. pneumoniae prostatitis
Keflex (Cephalexin) Dista 1237

K. pneumoniae respiratory tract infections
Avelox Tablets (Moxifloxacin Hydrochloride) Bayer 879
Cefobid Intravenous/Intramuscular (Cefoperazone) Pfizer 2671
Cefobid Pharmacy Bulk Package - Not for Direct Infusion (Cefoperazone Sodium) Pfizer 2673

K. pneumoniae septicemia
Azactam for Injection (Aztreonam) Elan 1276
Cefobid Intravenous/Intramuscular (Cefoperazone) Pfizer 2671
Cefobid Pharmacy Bulk Package - Not for Direct Infusion (Cefoperazone Sodium) Pfizer 2673
Rocephin Injectable Vials, ADD-Vantage, Galaxy, Bulk (Ceftriaxone Sodium) Roche Laboratories 2993

K. pneumoniae skin and skin structure infections
Azactam for Injection (Aztreonam) Elan 1276
Cefotan (Cefotetan) AstraZeneca 664
Cipro I.V. (Ciprofloxacin) Bayer 893
Cipro I.V. Pharmacy Bulk Package (Ciprofloxacin) Bayer 897
Cipro (Ciprofloxacin) Bayer 887
Primaxin I.M. (Cilastatin Sodium, Imipenem) Merck 2158
Rocephin Injectable Vials, ADD-Vantage, Galaxy, Bulk (Ceftriaxone Sodium) Roche Laboratories 2993
Unasyn for Injection (Ampicillin Sodium, Sulbactam Sodium) Pfizer 2728

K. pneumoniae urinary tract infections
Azactam for Injection (Aztreonam) Elan 1276
Cefotan (Cefotetan) AstraZeneca 664
Ceftin Tablets (Cefuroxime Axetil) Lifecycle Ventures 1898
Cipro I.V. (Ciprofloxacin) Bayer 893
Cipro I.V. Pharmacy Bulk Package (Ciprofloxacin) Bayer 897
Cipro (Ciprofloxacin) Bayer 887
Floxin I.V. (Ofloxacin) Ortho-McNeil 2526
Floxin Tablets (Ofloxacin) Ortho-McNeil 2529
Levaquin (Levofloxacin) Ortho-McNeil 2537
Maxipime for Injection (Cefepime Hydrochloride) Elan 1285
Noroxin Tablets (Norfloxacin) Merck 2145
Rocephin Injectable Vials, ADD-Vantage, Galaxy, Bulk (Ceftriaxone Sodium) Roche Laboratories 2993
Streptomycin Sulfate Injection (Streptomycin Sulfate) Pfizer 2714
Tequin Injection (Gatifloxacin) Bristol-Myers Squibb 1110
Tequin Tablets (Gatifloxacin) Bristol-Myers Squibb 1110
Vantin Tablets and Oral Suspension (Cefpodoxime Proxetil) Pharmacia & Upjohn 2860

Kaposi's sarcoma, AIDS-related
DaunoXome Injection (Daunorubicin Citrate) Gilead 1442
Doxil Injection (Doxorubicin Hydrochloride) Alza 566
Intron A for Injection (Interferon alfa-2B, Recombinant) Schering 3120
Roferon-A Injection (Interferon alfa-2A, Recombinant) Roche Laboratories 2996
Taxol Injection (Paclitaxel) Bristol-Myers Squibb Oncology/Immunology 1129

Kawasaki syndrome
Gammagard S/D (Globulin, Immune (Human)) Baxter Healthcare 845

Iveegam EN (Globulin, Immune (Human)) Baxter Healthcare ... 849

Keloids
Celestone Soluspan Injectable Suspension (Betamethasone Acetate, Betamethasone Sodium Phosphate) Schering ... 3097
Decadron Phosphate Injection (Dexamethasone Sodium Phosphate) Merck ... 2081
Hydrocortone Acetate Injectable Suspension (Hydrocortisone Acetate) Merck ... 2103

Keratitis
Celestone Soluspan Injectable Suspension (Betamethasone Acetate, Betamethasone Sodium Phosphate) Schering ... 3097
Celestone Syrup (Betamethasone) Schering ... 3099
Cortone Acetate Injectable Suspension (Cortisone Acetate) Merck ... 2059
Cortone Acetate Tablets (Cortisone Acetate) Merck ... 2061
Decadron Elixir (Dexamethasone) Merck ... 2078
Decadron Tablets (Dexamethasone) Merck ... 2079
Decadron Phosphate Injection (Dexamethasone Sodium Phosphate) Merck ... 2081
Depo-Medrol Injectable Suspension (Methylprednisolone Acetate) Pharmacia & Upjohn ... 2795
Genoptic Ophthalmic Ointment (Gentamicin Sulfate) Allergan ... ⊙239
Genoptic Sterile Ophthalmic Solution (Gentamicin Sulfate) Allergan ... ⊙239
Hydrocortone Tablets (Hydrocortisone) Merck ... 2106
Hydrocortone Phosphate Injection, Sterile (Hydrocortisone Sodium Phosphate) Merck ... 2105
Neosporin Ophthalmic Ointment Sterile (Bacitracin Zinc, Neomycin Sulfate, Polymyxin B Sulfate) Monarch ... ⊙299
Neosporin Ophthalmic Solution Sterile (Gramicidin, Neomycin Sulfate, Polymyxin B Sulfate) Monarch ... ⊙300
Pediapred Oral Solution (Prednisolone Sodium Phosphate) Celltech ... 1170
Polysporin Ophthalmic Ointment Sterile (Bacitracin Zinc, Polymyxin B Sulfate, Bacitracin Zinc, Polymyxin B Sulfate) Monarch ... ⊙301
Prednisone (Prednisone) Roxane ... 3064
Prelone Syrup (Prednisolone) Muro ... 2273
Solu-Medrol Sterile Powder (Methylprednisolone Sodium Succinate) Pharmacia & Upjohn ... 2855

Keratitis, dendritic
Viroptic (Trifluridine) Monarch ... ⊙301

Keratitis, exposure
Lacrisert Sterile Ophthalmic Insert (Hydroxypropyl Cellulose) Merck ... 2117

Keratitis, fungal
Natacyn (Natamycin) Alcon ... ⊙216

Keratitis, herpes zoster
Decadron Phosphate Sterile Ophthalmic Ointment (Dexamethasone Sodium Phosphate) Merck ... 2083
Decadron Phosphate Sterile Ophthalmic Solution (Dexamethasone Sodium Phosphate) Merck ... 2084

Keratitis, punctate, superficial
Decadron Phosphate Sterile Ophthalmic Ointment (Dexamethasone Sodium Phosphate) Merck ... 2083
Decadron Phosphate Sterile Ophthalmic Solution (Dexamethasone Sodium Phosphate) Merck ... 2084

Keratitis, recurrent epithelial
(*see under* Keratitis, dendritic)

Keratitis, vernal
Alomide Ophthalmic Solution (Lodoxamide Tromethamine) Alcon ... ⊙204
Crolom Sterile Ophthalmic Solution USP 4% (Cromolyn Sodium) Bausch & Lomb ... ⊙259
Opticrom Ophthalmic Solution (Cromolyn Sodium) Allergan ... 555

Keratitis sicca
(*see under* Keratoconjunctivitis sicca)

Keratoconjunctivitis, acute
Viroptic (Trifluridine) Monarch ... ⊙301

Keratoconjunctivitis, unspecified
Genoptic Ophthalmic Ointment (Gentamicin Sulfate) Allergan ... ⊙239
Genoptic Sterile Ophthalmic Solution (Gentamicin Sulfate) Allergan ... ⊙239
Neosporin Ophthalmic Ointment Sterile (Bacitracin Zinc, Neomycin Sulfate, Polymyxin B Sulfate) Monarch ... ⊙299
Neosporin Ophthalmic Solution Sterile (Gramicidin, Neomycin Sulfate, Polymyxin B Sulfate) Monarch ... ⊙300
Polysporin Ophthalmic Ointment Sterile (Bacitracin Zinc, Polymyxin B Sulfate, Bacitracin Zinc, Polymyxin B Sulfate) Monarch ... ⊙301

Keratoconjunctivitis, vernal
Alomide Ophthalmic Solution (Lodoxamide Tromethamine) Alcon ... ⊙204
Crolom Sterile Ophthalmic Solution USP 4% (Cromolyn Sodium) Bausch & Lomb ... ⊙259
Opticrom Ophthalmic Solution (Cromolyn Sodium) Allergan ... 555

Keratoconjunctivitis sicca
Bion Tears Lubricant Eye Drops (Dextran 70, Hydroxypropyl Methylcellulose) Alcon ... 538
Celluvisc Lubricant Eye Drops (Carboxymethylcellulose Sodium) Allergan ... ⊙234
Clear Eyes ACR Astringent/Lubricant Eye Redness Reliever (Glycerin, Naphazoline Hydrochloride, Zinc Sulfate) Ross ... ⊙322
Computer Eye Drops (Glycerin) Bausch & Lomb, Inc ... ⊙252
GenTeal Eye Drops (Hydroxypropyl Methylcellulose) Novartis Ophthalmics ... ⊙304
GenTeal Gel (Hydroxypropyl Methylcellulose) Novartis Ophthalmics ... ⊙304
GenTeal Mild Eye Drops (Polyethylene Glycol, Polyvinyl Alcohol) Novartis Ophthalmics ... ⊙304
Lacrisert Sterile Ophthalmic Insert (Hydroxypropyl Cellulose) Merck ... 2117
Moisture Eyes Eye Drops (Glycerin, Propylene Glycol) Bausch & Lomb, Inc ... ⊙252
Moisture Eyes Preservative Free Eye Drops (Propylene Glycol) Bausch & Lomb, Inc ... ⊙253
Moisture Eyes PM Preservative Free Eye Ointment (Mineral Oil, Petrolatum, White) Bausch & Lomb, Inc ... ⊙253
Moisture Eyes Protect and Preservative-Free Moisture Eyes Protect (Dextran 70, Hydroxypropyl Methylcellulose) Bausch & Lomb, Inc ... ⊙253
Refresh P.M. Lubricant Eye Ointment (Mineral Oil, Petrolatum, White) Allergan ... ⊙251
Refresh Plus Lubricant Eye Drops (Carboxymethylcellulose Sodium) Allergan ... ⊙251
Refresh Tears Lubricant Eye Drops (Carboxymethylcellulose Sodium) Allergan ... ⊙251
Tears Naturale Forte Lubricant Eye Drops (Dextran 70, Hydroxypropyl Methylcellulose) Alcon ... 541
Tears Naturale Free Lubricant Eye Drops (Dextran 70, Hydroxypropyl Methylcellulose) Alcon ... 541

Keratosis, actinic
Carac Cream (Fluorouracil) Dermik ... 1222
Efudex (Fluorouracil) ICN ... 1733
Fluoroplex (Fluorouracil) Allergan ... 552
Levulan Kerastick (Aminolevulinic Acid Hydrochloride) Berlex ... 971

Keratosis, solar
Carac Cream (Fluorouracil) Dermik ... 1222
Efudex (Fluorouracil) ICN ... 1733

Keratosis palmaris
(*see under* Hyperkeratosis skin disorders)

Keratosis pilaris
(*see under* Hyperkeratosis skin disorders)

Keratosis plantaris
(*see under* Hyperkeratosis skin disorders)

Klebsiella oxytoca infections
Azactam for Injection (Aztreonam) Elan ... 1276
Rocephin (Ceftriaxone Sodium) Roche Laboratories ... 2993

Klebsiella pneumoniae infections
(*see under* K. pneumoniae infections)

Klebsiella species bacteremia
Ceptaz for Injection (Ceftazidime) GlaxoSmithKline ... 1499

Klebsiella species biliary tract infections
Ancef for Injection (Cefazolin Sodium) GlaxoSmithKline ... 1474
Ancef Injection (Cefazolin Sodium) GlaxoSmithKline ... 1474
Kefzol Vials, ADD-Vantage (Cefazolin Sodium) Lilly ... 1951

Klebsiella species bone and joint infections
Ceptaz for Injection (Ceftazidime) GlaxoSmithKline ... 1499
Fortaz (Ceftazidime Sodium) GlaxoSmithKline ... 1541
Nebcin Vials, Hyporets & ADD-Vantage (Tobramycin Sulfate) Lilly ... 1955
Tazicef for Injection (Ceftazidime) GlaxoSmithKline ... 1647
Tazicef Galaxy Container (Ceftazidime Sodium) GlaxoSmithKline ... 1650
Tazicef Pharmacy Bulk Package (Ceftazidime) GlaxoSmithKline ... 1653
Tazidime Vials, Faspak & ADD-Vantage (Ceftazidime) Lilly ... 1966

Klebsiella species genital tract infections
Ancef for Injection (Cefazolin Sodium) GlaxoSmithKline ... 1474
Ancef Injection (Cefazolin Sodium) GlaxoSmithKline ... 1474

Klebsiella species gynecologic infections
Claforan Injection (Cefotaxime Sodium) Aventis ... 732
Primaxin I.V. (Cilastatin Sodium, Imipenem) Merck ... 2160

Klebsiella species infections
Ancef for Injection (Cefazolin Sodium) GlaxoSmithKline ... 1474
Ancef Injection (Cefazolin Sodium) GlaxoSmithKline ... 1474
Augmentin Chewable Tablets (Amoxicillin, Clavulanate Potassium) GlaxoSmithKline ... 1482
Augmentin Powder for Oral Suspension (Amoxicillin, Clavulanate Potassium) GlaxoSmithKline ... 1482
Augmentin Tablets (Amoxicillin, Clavulanate Potassium) GlaxoSmithKline ... 1485
Bactrim (Sulfamethoxazole, Trimethoprim) Roche Laboratories ... 2949
Ceclor (Cefaclor) Lilly ... 1905
Cefizox for Intramuscular or Intravenous Use (Ceftizoxime Sodium) Fujisawa ... 1390
Cefobid Intravenous/Intramuscular (Cefoperazone) Pfizer ... 2671
Cefobid Pharmacy Bulk Package - Not for Direct Infusion (Cefoperazone Sodium) Pfizer ... 2673
Cefotan (Cefotetan) AstraZeneca ... 664
Ceptaz for Injection (Ceftazidime) GlaxoSmithKline ... 1499
Claforan Injection (Cefotaxime Sodium) Aventis ... 732
Declomycin Tablets (Demeclocycline Hydrochloride) Lederle ... 1855
Doryx Coated Pellet Filled Capsules (Doxycycline Hyclate) Warner Chilcott ... 3357
Duricef (Cefadroxil) Bristol-Myers Squibb ... 1079
Dynacin Capsules (Minocycline Hydrochloride) Medicis ... 2019
Fortaz (Ceftazidime Sodium) GlaxoSmithKline ... 1541
Kefurox Vials, ADD-Vantage (Cefuroxime Sodium) Lilly ... 1948
Kefzol Vials, ADD-Vantage (Cefazolin Sodium) Lilly ... 1951
Macrodantin Capsules (Nitrofurantoin) Procter & Gamble Pharmaceuticals ... 2891
Mefoxin for Injection (Cefoxitin Sodium) Merck ... 2124
Mefoxin Premixed Intravenous Solution (Cefoxitin Sodium) Merck ... 2127
Minocin Intravenous (Minocycline Hydrochloride) Lederle ... 1862
Minocin Oral Suspension (Minocycline Hydrochloride) Lederle ... 1865
Minocin Pellet-Filled Capsules (Minocycline Hydrochloride) Lederle ... 1863
Monodox Capsules (Doxycycline Monohydrate) Oclassen ... 2442
Nebcin Vials, Hyporets & ADD-Vantage (Tobramycin Sulfate) Lilly ... 1955
Pipracil (Piperacillin Sodium) Lederle ... 1866
Primaxin I.V. (Cilastatin Sodium, Imipenem) Merck ... 2160
Septra Suspension (Sulfamethoxazole, Trimethoprim) Monarch ... 2265
Septra Tablets (Sulfamethoxazole, Trimethoprim) Monarch ... 2265
Septra DS Tablets (Sulfamethoxazole, Trimethoprim) Monarch ... 2265
Tazicef for Injection (Ceftazidime) GlaxoSmithKline ... 1647
Tazicef Galaxy Container (Ceftazidime Sodium) GlaxoSmithKline ... 1650
Tazicef Pharmacy Bulk Package (Ceftazidime) GlaxoSmithKline ... 1653
Tazidime Vials, Faspak & ADD-Vantage (Ceftazidime) Lilly ... 1966
Timentin Injection- ADD-Vantage Vial (Clavulanate Potassium, Ticarcillin Disodium) GlaxoSmithKline ... 1661
Timentin Injection-Galaxy Container (Clavulanate Potassium, Ticarcillin Disodium) GlaxoSmithKline ... 1664
Timentin Injection-Pharmacy Bulk Package (Clavulanate Potassium, Ticarcillin Disodium) GlaxoSmithKline ... 1666
Timentin for Intravenous Administration (Clavulanate Potassium, Ticarcillin Disodium) GlaxoSmithKline ... 1658
Unasyn for Injection (Ampicillin Sodium, Sulbactam Sodium) Pfizer ... 2728
Vibramycin Calcium Oral Suspension Syrup (Doxycycline Calcium) Pfizer ... 2735
Vibramycin Hyclate Capsules (Doxycycline Hyclate) Pfizer ... 2735
Vibramycin Hyclate Intravenous (Doxycycline Hyclate) Pfizer ... 2737
Vibramycin Monohydrate for Oral Suspension (Doxycycline Monohydrate) Pfizer ... 2735
Vibra-Tabs Film Coated Tablets (Doxycycline Hyclate) Pfizer ... 2735
Zinacef Injection (Cefuroxime) GlaxoSmithKline ... 1696
Zinacef for Injection (Cefuroxime) GlaxoSmithKline ... 1696

Klebsiella species intra-abdominal infections
Azactam for Injection (Aztreonam) Elan ... 1276
Cefizox for Intramuscular or Intravenous Use (Ceftizoxime Sodium) Fujisawa ... 1390
Cefotan (Cefotetan) AstraZeneca ... 664
Ceptaz for Injection (Ceftazidime) GlaxoSmithKline ... 1499
Claforan Injection (Cefotaxime Sodium) Aventis ... 732
Fortaz (Ceftazidime Sodium) GlaxoSmithKline ... 1541
Mefoxin for Injection (Cefoxitin Sodium) Merck ... 2124
Mefoxin Premixed Intravenous Solution (Cefoxitin Sodium) Merck ... 2127
Nebcin Vials, Hyporets & ADD-Vantage (Tobramycin Sulfate) Lilly ... 1955
Primaxin I.V. (Cilastatin Sodium, Imipenem) Merck ... 2160
Tazicef for Injection (Ceftazidime) GlaxoSmithKline ... 1647
Tazicef Galaxy Container (Ceftazidime Sodium) GlaxoSmithKline ... 1650
Tazicef Pharmacy Bulk Package (Ceftazidime) GlaxoSmithKline ... 1653
Tazidime Vials, Faspak & ADD-Vantage (Ceftazidime) Lilly ... 1966
Unasyn for Injection (Ampicillin Sodium, Sulbactam Sodium) Pfizer ... 2728

Klebsiella species lower respiratory tract infections
Cefizox for Intramuscular or Intravenous Use (Ceftizoxime Sodium) Fujisawa ... 1390
Cefotan (Cefotetan) AstraZeneca ... 664
Ceptaz for Injection (Ceftazidime) GlaxoSmithKline ... 1499
Claforan Injection (Cefotaxime Sodium) Aventis ... 732
Fortaz (Ceftazidime Sodium) GlaxoSmithKline ... 1541
Mandol Vials (Cefamandole Nafate) Lilly ... 1953
Mefoxin for Injection (Cefoxitin Sodium) Merck ... 2124
Mefoxin Premixed Intravenous Solution (Cefoxitin Sodium) Merck ... 2127
Nebcin Vials, Hyporets & ADD-Vantage (Tobramycin Sulfate) Lilly ... 1955
Pipracil (Piperacillin Sodium) Lederle ... 1866
Primaxin I.V. (Cilastatin Sodium, Imipenem) Merck ... 2160
Tazicef for Injection (Ceftazidime) GlaxoSmithKline ... 1647
Tazicef Galaxy Container (Ceftazidime Sodium) GlaxoSmithKline ... 1650
Tazicef Pharmacy Bulk Package (Ceftazidime) GlaxoSmithKline ... 1653
Tazidime Vials, Faspak & ADD-Vantage (Ceftazidime) Lilly ... 1966
Timentin Injection- ADD-Vantage Vial (Clavulanate Potassium, Ticarcillin Disodium) GlaxoSmithKline ... 1661
Timentin Injection-Galaxy Container (Clavulanate Potassium, Ticarcillin Disodium) GlaxoSmithKline ... 1664
Timentin Injection-Pharmacy Bulk Package (Clavulanate Potassium, Ticarcillin Disodium) GlaxoSmithKline ... 1666
Timentin for Intravenous Administration (Clavulanate Potassium, Ticarcillin Disodium) GlaxoSmithKline ... 1658
Zinacef Injection (Cefuroxime) GlaxoSmithKline ... 1696
Zinacef for Injection (Cefuroxime) GlaxoSmithKline ... 1696

Klebsiella species prostatitis
Ancef for Injection (Cefazolin Sodium) GlaxoSmithKline ... 1474
Ancef Injection (Cefazolin Sodium) GlaxoSmithKline ... 1474

Klebsiella species respiratory tract infections
Ancef for Injection (Cefazolin Sodium) GlaxoSmithKline ... 1474
Ancef Injection (Cefazolin Sodium) GlaxoSmithKline ... 1474
Ceptaz for Injection (Ceftazidime) GlaxoSmithKline ... 1499
Doryx Coated Pellet Filled Capsules (Doxycycline Hyclate) Warner Chilcott ... 3357
Dynacin Capsules (Minocycline Hydrochloride) Medicis ... 2019
Kefzol Vials, ADD-Vantage (Cefazolin Sodium) Lilly ... 1951
Minocin Intravenous (Minocycline Hydrochloride) Lederle ... 1862
Minocin Oral Suspension (Minocycline Hydrochloride) Lederle ... 1865
Minocin Pellet-Filled Capsules (Minocycline Hydrochloride) Lederle ... 1863
Monodox Capsules (Doxycycline Monohydrate) Oclassen ... 2442
Vibramycin Calcium Oral Suspension Syrup (Doxycycline Calcium) Pfizer ... 2735
Vibramycin Hyclate Capsules (Doxycycline Hyclate) Pfizer ... 2735
Vibramycin Hyclate Intravenous (Doxycycline Hyclate) Pfizer ... 2737
Vibramycin Monohydrate for Oral Suspension (Doxycycline Monohydrate) Pfizer ... 2735
Vibra-Tabs Film Coated Tablets (Doxycycline Hyclate) Pfizer ... 2735

Klebsiella species septicemia
Ancef for Injection (Cefazolin Sodium) GlaxoSmithKline ... 1474
Ancef Injection (Cefazolin Sodium) GlaxoSmithKline ... 1474
Cefizox for Intramuscular or Intravenous Use (Ceftizoxime Sodium) Fujisawa ... 1390
Ceptaz for Injection (Ceftazidime) GlaxoSmithKline ... 1499
Claforan Injection (Cefotaxime Sodium) Aventis ... 732
Fortaz (Ceftazidime Sodium) GlaxoSmithKline ... 1541
Kefurox Vials, ADD-Vantage (Cefuroxime Sodium) Lilly ... 1948
Kefzol Vials, ADD-Vantage (Cefazolin Sodium) Lilly ... 1951
Mefoxin for Injection (Cefoxitin Sodium) Merck ... 2124
Mefoxin Premixed Intravenous Solution (Cefoxitin Sodium) Merck ... 2127
Nebcin Vials, Hyporets & ADD-Vantage (Tobramycin Sulfate) Lilly ... 1955
Pipracil (Piperacillin Sodium) Lederle ... 1866
Primaxin I.V. (Cilastatin Sodium, Imipenem) Merck ... 2160
Tazicef for Injection (Ceftazidime) GlaxoSmithKline ... 1647
Tazicef Galaxy Container (Ceftazidime Sodium) GlaxoSmithKline ... 1650
Tazicef Pharmacy Bulk Package (Ceftazidime) GlaxoSmithKline ... 1653
Tazidime Vials, Faspak & ADD-Vantage (Ceftazidime) Lilly ... 1966
Timentin Injection- ADD-Vantage Vial (Clavulanate Potassium, Ticarcillin Disodium) GlaxoSmithKline ... 1661
Timentin Injection-Galaxy Container (Clavulanate Potassium, Ticarcillin Disodium) GlaxoSmithKline ... 1664
Timentin Injection-Pharmacy Bulk Package (Clavulanate Potassium, Ticarcillin Disodium) GlaxoSmithKline ... 1666
Timentin for Intravenous Administration (Clavulanate Potassium, Ticarcillin Disodium) GlaxoSmithKline ... 1658
Zinacef Injection (Cefuroxime) GlaxoSmithKline ... 1696
Zinacef for Injection (Cefuroxime) GlaxoSmithKline ... 1696

Klebsiella species skin and skin structure infections
Augmentin Chewable Tablets (Amoxicillin, Clavulanate Potassium) GlaxoSmithKline ... 1482
Augmentin Powder for Oral Suspension (Amoxicillin, Clavulanate Potassium) GlaxoSmithKline ... 1482
Augmentin Tablets (Amoxicillin, Clavulanate Potassium) GlaxoSmithKline ... 1485
Cefizox for Intramuscular or Intravenous Use (Ceftizoxime Sodium) Fujisawa ... 1390
Ceptaz for Injection (Ceftazidime) GlaxoSmithKline ... 1499
Claforan Injection (Cefotaxime Sodium) Aventis ... 732
Fortaz (Ceftazidime Sodium) GlaxoSmithKline ... 1541
Kefurox Vials, ADD-Vantage (Cefuroxime Sodium) Lilly ... 1948
Mefoxin for Injection (Cefoxitin Sodium) Merck ... 2124
Mefoxin Premixed Intravenous Solution (Cefoxitin Sodium) Merck ... 2127
Nebcin Vials, Hyporets & ADD-Vantage (Tobramycin Sulfate) Lilly ... 1955
Pipracil (Piperacillin Sodium) Lederle ... 1866
Primaxin I.V. (Cilastatin Sodium, Imipenem) Merck ... 2160
Tazicef for Injection (Ceftazidime) GlaxoSmithKline ... 1647
Tazicef Galaxy Container (Ceftazidime Sodium) GlaxoSmithKline ... 1650
Tazicef Pharmacy Bulk Package (Ceftazidime) GlaxoSmithKline ... 1653
Tazidime Vials, Faspak & ADD-Vantage (Ceftazidime) Lilly ... 1966
Timentin Injection- ADD-Vantage Vial (Clavulanate Potassium, Ticarcillin Disodium) GlaxoSmithKline ... 1661
Timentin Injection-Galaxy Container (Clavulanate Potassium, Ticarcillin Disodium) GlaxoSmithKline ... 1664
Timentin Injection-Pharmacy Bulk Package (Clavulanate Potassium, Ticarcillin Disodium) GlaxoSmithKline ... 1666
Timentin for Intravenous Administration (Clavulanate Potassium, Ticarcillin Disodium) GlaxoSmithKline ... 1658
Unasyn for Injection (Ampicillin Sodium, Sulbactam Sodium) Pfizer ... 2728
Zinacef Injection (Cefuroxime) GlaxoSmithKline ... 1696
Zinacef for Injection (Cefuroxime) GlaxoSmithKline ... 1696

Klebsiella species urinary tract infections
Ancef for Injection (Cefazolin Sodium) GlaxoSmithKline ... 1474
Ancef Injection (Cefazolin Sodium) GlaxoSmithKline ... 1474
Augmentin Chewable Tablets (Amoxicillin, Clavulanate Potassium) GlaxoSmithKline ... 1482
Augmentin Powder for Oral Suspension (Amoxicillin, Clavulanate Potassium) GlaxoSmithKline ... 1482
Augmentin Tablets (Amoxicillin, Clavulanate Potassium) GlaxoSmithKline ... 1485
Bactrim (Sulfamethoxazole, Trimethoprim) Roche Laboratories ... 2949
Ceclor (Cefaclor) Lilly ... 1905
Cefizox for Intramuscular or Intravenous Use (Ceftizoxime Sodium) Fujisawa ... 1390
Cefotan (Cefotetan) AstraZeneca ... 664
Ceptaz for Injection (Ceftazidime) GlaxoSmithKline ... 1499
Claforan Injection (Cefotaxime Sodium) Aventis ... 732
Declomycin Tablets (Demeclocycline Hydrochloride) Lederle ... 1855
Doryx Coated Pellet Filled Capsules (Doxycycline Hyclate) Warner Chilcott ... 3357
Duricef (Cefadroxil) Bristol-Myers Squibb ... 1079
Dynacin Capsules (Minocycline Hydrochloride) Medicis ... 2019
Fortaz (Ceftazidime Sodium) GlaxoSmithKline ... 1541
Kefurox Vials, ADD-Vantage (Cefuroxime Sodium) Lilly ... 1948
Kefzol Vials, ADD-Vantage (Cefazolin Sodium) Lilly ... 1951
Macrodantin Capsules (Nitrofurantoin) Procter & Gamble Pharmaceuticals ... 2891
Mandol Vials (Cefamandole Nafate) Lilly ... 1953
Mefoxin for Injection (Cefoxitin Sodium) Merck ... 2124
Mefoxin Premixed Intravenous Solution (Cefoxitin Sodium) Merck ... 2127
Minocin Intravenous (Minocycline Hydrochloride) Lederle ... 1862
Minocin Oral Suspension (Minocycline Hydrochloride) Lederle ... 1865
Minocin Pellet-Filled Capsules (Minocycline Hydrochloride) Lederle ... 1863
Monodox Capsules (Doxycycline Monohydrate) Oclassen ... 2442
Nebcin Vials, Hyporets & ADD-Vantage (Tobramycin Sulfate) Lilly ... 1955
Primaxin I.V. (Cilastatin Sodium, Imipenem) Merck ... 2160
Septra Suspension (Sulfamethoxazole, Trimethoprim) Monarch ... 2265
Septra Tablets (Sulfamethoxazole, Trimethoprim) Monarch ... 2265
Septra DS Tablets (Sulfamethoxazole, Trimethoprim) Monarch ... 2265
Tazicef for Injection (Ceftazidime) GlaxoSmithKline ... 1647
Tazicef Galaxy Container (Ceftazidime Sodium) GlaxoSmithKline ... 1650
Tazicef Pharmacy Bulk Package (Ceftazidime) GlaxoSmithKline ... 1653
Tazidime Vials, Faspak & ADD-Vantage (Ceftazidime) Lilly ... 1966
Timentin Injection- ADD-Vantage Vial (Clavulanate Potassium, Ticarcillin Disodium) GlaxoSmithKline ... 1661
Timentin Injection-Galaxy Container (Clavulanate Potassium, Ticarcillin Disodium) GlaxoSmithKline ... 1664
Timentin Injection-Pharmacy Bulk Package (Clavulanate Potassium, Ticarcillin Disodium) GlaxoSmithKline ... 1666
Timentin for Intravenous Administration (Clavulanate Potassium, Ticarcillin Disodium) GlaxoSmithKline ... 1658
Vibramycin Calcium Oral Suspension Syrup (Doxycycline Calcium) Pfizer ... 2735
Vibramycin Hyclate Capsules (Doxycycline Hyclate) Pfizer ... 2735
Vibramycin Hyclate Intravenous (Doxycycline Hyclate) Pfizer ... 2737
Vibramycin Monohydrate for Oral Suspension (Doxycycline Monohydrate) Pfizer ... 2735
Vibra-Tabs Film Coated Tablets (Doxycycline Hyclate) Pfizer ... 2735
Zinacef Injection (Cefuroxime) GlaxoSmithKline ... 1696
Zinacef for Injection (Cefuroxime) GlaxoSmithKline ... 1696

Klebsiella-Enterobacter species infections, ocular
Blephamide Ophthalmic Ointment (Prednisolone Acetate, Sulfacetamide Sodium) Allergan ... 547
Blephamide Ophthalmic Suspension (Prednisolone Acetate, Sulfacetamide Sodium) Allergan ... 548
Chloromycetin Ophthalmic Ointment, 1% (Chloramphenicol) Monarch ... ⊙296
Chloromycetin Ophthalmic Solution (Chloramphenicol) Monarch ... ⊙297
Chloroptic Sterile Ophthalmic Ointment (Chloramphenicol) Allergan ... ⊙234
Cortisporin Ophthalmic Suspension (Hydrocortisone, Neomycin Sulfate, Polymyxin B Sulfate, Hydrocortisone, Neomycin Sulfate, Polymyxin B Sulfate) Monarch ... ⊙297
FML-S Liquifilm Sterile Ophthalmic Suspension (Fluorometholone, Sulfacetamide Sodium) Allergan ... ⊙238
NeoDecadron Sterile Ophthalmic Solution (Dexamethasone Sodium Phosphate, Neomycin Sulfate) Merck ... 2144
Poly-Pred Liquifilm Ophthalmic Suspension (Neomycin Sulfate, Polymyxin B Sulfate, Prednisolone Acetate) Allergan ... ⊙245
Pred-G Ophthalmic Suspension (Gentamicin Sulfate, Prednisolone Acetate) Allergan ... ⊙247
TobraDex Ophthalmic Ointment (Dexamethasone, Tobramycin) Alcon ... 542
TobraDex Ophthalmic Suspension (Dexamethasone, Tobramycin) Alcon ... 541

Koch-Weeks bacillus infections, ocular
(*see under* H. aegypticus infections, ocular)

L

Lacrimation, symptomatic relief of
Benadryl Allergy Kapseal Capsules (Diphenhydramine Hydrochloride) Pfizer Inc., Warner-Lambert Healthcare ... ▣691
Benadryl Allergy Liquid (Diphenhydramine Hydrochloride) Pfizer Inc., Warner-Lambert Healthcare ... ▣690
Benadryl Allergy Ultratab Tablets (Diphenhydramine Hydrochloride) Pfizer Inc., Warner-Lambert Healthcare ... ▣691
Benadryl Allergy Sinus Headache Caplets & Gelcaps (Acetaminophen, Diphenhydramine Hydrochloride, Pseudoephedrine Hydrochloride) Pfizer Inc., Warner-Lambert Healthcare ... ▣693
Chlor-Trimeton Allergy Tablets (Chlorpheniramine Maleate) Schering-Plough ... ▣735
Dimetapp Elixir (Brompheniramine Maleate, Pseudoephedrine Hydrochloride) Whitehall-Robins ... ▣777
Ryna Liquid (Chlorpheniramine Maleate, Pseudoephedrine Hydrochloride) Wallace ... ▣768
Tylenol Severe Allergy Caplets (Acetaminophen, Diphenhydramine Hydrochloride) McNeil Consumer ... 2010

Lactobacillus acidophilus, deficiency of
DDS-Acidophilus Capsules, Tablets, and Powder (Lactobacillus Acidophilus) UAS Labs ... ▣767

Lactose intolerance
Lactaid (Lactase (beta-d-Galactosidase)) McNeil Consumer ... 2002
Lactaid Ultra Caplets and Chewable Tablets (Lactase (beta-d-Galactosidase)) McNeil Consumer ... 2002
Lactaid Drops McNeil Consumer ... ▣822

Larva migrans, cutaneous
Mintezol (Thiabendazole) Merck ... 2137

Laryngeal edema, acute noninfectious, adjunctive therapy in
Celestone Soluspan Injectable Suspension (Betamethasone Acetate, Betamethasone Sodium Phosphate) Schering 3097
Cortone Acetate Injectable Suspension (Cortisone Acetate) Merck 2059
Decadron Phosphate Injection (Dexamethasone Sodium Phosphate) Merck 2081
Hydrocortone Phosphate Injection, Sterile (Hydrocortisone Sodium Phosphate) Merck 2105
Solu-Medrol Sterile Powder (Methylprednisolone Sodium Succinate) Pharmacia & Upjohn 2855

LDL cholesterol, elevation
(*see under* Hyperlipoproteinemia, types IIa and IIb, adjunct to diet)

Lead encephalopathy
Calcium Disodium Versenate (Calcium Disodium Edetate) 3M 1980

Lead poisoning
Chemet Capsules (Succimer) Sanofi-Synthelabo 3078

Leg muscle cramps
Hyland's Leg Cramps with Quinine Tablets (Homeopathic Formulations) Standard Homeopathic .... ■765

Legionella pneumophila infections
(*see under* Legionnaires' disease)

Legionnaires' disease
Dynabac Tablets (Dirithromycin) Muro 2269
E.E.S. (Erythromycin Ethylsuccinate) Abbott 450
EryPed (Erythromycin Ethylsuccinate) Abbott 446
Ery-Tab Tablets (Erythromycin) Abbott 448
Erythrocin Stearate Filmtab Tablets (Erythromycin Stearate) Abbott 452
Erythromycin Base Filmtab Tablets (Erythromycin) Abbott 454
Erythromycin Delayed-Release Capsules, USP (Erythromycin) Abbott 455
Levaquin (Levofloxacin) Ortho-McNeil 2537
PCE Dispertab Tablets (Erythromycin) Abbott 498
Tequin Injection (Gatifloxacin) Bristol-Myers Squibb 1110
Tequin Tablets (Gatifloxacin) Bristol-Myers Squibb 1110
Trovan (Alatrofloxacin Mesylate) Pfizer 2722
Zithromax for IV Infusion (Azithromycin Dihydrate) Pfizer 2748

Lennox-Gastaut syndrome
Felbatol (Felbamate) Wallace 3343
Klonopin Tablets (Clonazepam) Roche Laboratories 2983
Lamictal (Lamotrigine) GlaxoSmithKline 1567

Lens, intraocular, implantation of, surgical aid in
Healon (Sodium Hyaluronate) Pharmacia & Upjohn .... ⊙316
Ocucoat (Hydroxypropyl Methylcellulose) Bausch & Lomb Surgical .... ⊙330

Leprosy
Dapsone Tablets USP (Dapsone) Jacobus 1780

Leukemia, acute, palliative management of in childhood
Cortone Acetate Injectable Suspension (Cortisone Acetate) Merck 2059
Cortone Acetate Tablets (Cortisone Acetate) Merck 2061
Decadron Elixir (Dexamethasone) Merck 2078
Decadron Tablets (Dexamethasone) Merck 2079
Decadron Phosphate Injection (Dexamethasone Sodium Phosphate) Merck 2081
Hydrocortone Tablets (Hydrocortisone) Merck 2106
Hydrocortone Phosphate Injection, Sterile (Hydrocortisone Sodium Phosphate) Merck 2105
Pediapred Oral Solution (Prednisolone Sodium Phosphate) Celltech 1170
Prednisone (Prednisone) Roxane 3064
Prelone Syrup (Prednisolone) Muro 2273
Solu-Medrol Sterile Powder (Methylprednisolone Sodium Succinate) Pharmacia & Upjohn 2855

Leukemia, acute, promyelocytic
Trisenox Injection (Arsenic Trioxide) Cell Therapeutics 1158
Vesanoid Capsules (Tretinoin) Roche Laboratories 3037

Leukemia, acute erythroid
Cerubidine for Injection (Daunorubicin Hydrochloride) Bedford 947

Leukemia, acute lymphoblastic
Adriamycin PFS/RDF Injection (Doxorubicin Hydrochloride) Pharmacia & Upjohn 2767
Oncaspar (Pegaspargase) Aventis 756
Purinethol Tablets (Mercaptopurine) GlaxoSmithKline 1615

Leukemia, acute lymphocytic
Cerubidine for Injection (Daunorubicin Hydrochloride) Bedford 947
Elspar for Injection (Asparaginase) Merck 2092
Purinethol Tablets (Mercaptopurine) GlaxoSmithKline 1615

Leukemia, acute monocytic
Cerubidine for Injection (Daunorubicin Hydrochloride) Bedford 947

Leukemia, acute myeloblastic
Adriamycin PFS/RDF Injection (Doxorubicin Hydrochloride) Pharmacia & Upjohn 2767

Leukemia, acute myelogenous
Cerubidine for Injection (Daunorubicin Hydrochloride) Bedford 947
Idamycin PFS Injection (Idarubicin Hydrochloride) Pharmacia & Upjohn 2825
Leukine (Sargramostim) Immunex 1755

Leukemia, acute myeloid, adjunctive therapy in
Neupogen for Injection (Filgrastim) Amgen 587

Leukemia, acute myeloid, CD33 positive
Mylotarg for Injection (Gemtuzumab ozogamicin) Wyeth-Ayerst 3540

Leukemia, acute nonlymphocytic
Cerubidine for Injection (Daunorubicin Hydrochloride) Bedford 947
Novantrone for Injection (Mitoxantrone Hydrochloride) Immunex 1760
Tabloid Tablets (Thioguanine) GlaxoSmithKline 1642

Leukemia, adjunctive therapy in
Aloprim for Injection (Allopurinol Sodium) Nabi 2292

Leukemia, chronic lymphocytic
Leukeran Tablets (Chlorambucil) GlaxoSmithKline 1591
Mustargen for Injection (Mechlorethamine Hydrochloride) Merck 2142

Leukemia, chronic lymphocytic, B-cell
Campath Ampules (Alemtuzumab) Berlex 992
Fludara for Injection (Fludarabine Phosphate) Berlex 995

Leukemia, chronic lymphocytic, B-cell, prevention of bacterial infection in
Gammagard S/D (Globulin, Immune (Human)) Baxter Healthcare 845

Leukemia, chronic myeloid
Gleevec Capsules (Imatinib mesylate) Novartis 2357
Mustargen for Injection (Mechlorethamine Hydrochloride) Merck 2142
Myleran Tablets (Busulfan) GlaxoSmithKline 1603
Mylocel Tablets (Hydroxyurea) MGI 2227
Roferon-A Injection (Interferon alfa-2A, Recombinant) Roche Laboratories 2996

Leukemia, hairy cell
Intron A for Injection (Interferon alfa-2B, Recombinant) Schering 3120
Leustatin Injection (Cladribine) Ortho Biotech 2495
Roferon-A Injection (Interferon alfa-2A, Recombinant) Roche Laboratories 2996

Leukemia, hairy cell, alpha-interferon-refractory
Nipent for Injection (Pentostatin) SuperGen 3272

Leukemia, lymphoblastic, adjunctive therapy in
Leukine (Sargramostim) Immunex 1755

Leukemias, palliative management of
Celestone Soluspan Injectable Suspension (Betamethasone Acetate, Betamethasone Sodium Phosphate) Schering 3097
Celestone Syrup (Betamethasone) Schering 3099
Cortone Acetate Injectable Suspension (Cortisone Acetate) Merck 2059
Cortone Acetate Tablets (Cortisone Acetate) Merck 2061
Decadron Elixir (Dexamethasone) Merck 2078
Decadron Tablets (Dexamethasone) Merck 2079
Decadron Phosphate Injection (Dexamethasone Sodium Phosphate) Merck 2081
Depo-Medrol Injectable Suspension (Methylprednisolone Acetate) Pharmacia & Upjohn 2795
Hydrocortone Tablets (Hydrocortisone) Merck 2106
Hydrocortone Phosphate Injection, Sterile (Hydrocortisone Sodium Phosphate) Merck 2105
Pediapred Oral Solution (Prednisolone Sodium Phosphate) Celltech 1170
Prednisone (Prednisone) Roxane 3064
Prelone Syrup (Prednisolone) Muro 2273
Solu-Medrol Sterile Powder (Methylprednisolone Sodium Succinate) Pharmacia & Upjohn 2855

Lice, body
(*see under* Pediculosis, human)

Lice, head
(*see under* Pediculosis, human)

Lice, pubic
(*see under* Pediculosis, human)

Lichen planus
Celestone Soluspan Injectable Suspension (Betamethasone Acetate, Betamethasone Sodium Phosphate) Schering 3097
Decadron Phosphate Injection (Dexamethasone Sodium Phosphate) Merck 2081
Hydrocortone Acetate Injectable Suspension (Hydrocortisone Acetate) Merck 2103

Lichen simplex chronicus
Celestone Soluspan Injectable Suspension (Betamethasone Acetate, Betamethasone Sodium Phosphate) Schering 3097
Decadron Phosphate Injection (Dexamethasone Sodium Phosphate) Merck 2081
Hydrocortone Acetate Injectable Suspension (Hydrocortisone Acetate) Merck 2103

Listeria monocytogenes infections
Declomycin Tablets (Demeclocycline Hydrochloride) Lederle 1855
Doryx Coated Pellet Filled Capsules (Doxycycline Hyclate) Warner Chilcott 3357
Dynacin Capsules (Minocycline Hydrochloride) Medicis 2019
E.E.S. (Erythromycin Ethylsuccinate) Abbott 450
EryPed (Erythromycin Ethylsuccinate) Abbott 446
Ery-Tab Tablets (Erythromycin) Abbott 448
Erythrocin Stearate Filmtab Tablets (Erythromycin Stearate) Abbott 452
Erythromycin Base Filmtab Tablets (Erythromycin) Abbott 454
Erythromycin Delayed-Release Capsules, USP (Erythromycin) Abbott 455
Minocin Intravenous (Minocycline Hydrochloride) Lederle 1862
Minocin Oral Suspension (Minocycline Hydrochloride) Lederle 1865
Minocin Pellet-Filled Capsules (Minocycline Hydrochloride) Lederle 1863
Monodox Capsules (Doxycycline Monohydrate) Oclassen 2442
PCE Dispertab Tablets (Erythromycin) Abbott 498
Pfizerpen for Injection (Penicillin G Potassium) Pfizer 2707
Vibramycin Calcium Oral Suspension Syrup (Doxycycline Calcium) Pfizer 2735
Vibramycin Hyclate Capsules (Doxycycline Hyclate) Pfizer 2735
Vibramycin Hyclate Intravenous (Doxycycline Hyclate) Pfizer 2737
Vibramycin Monohydrate for Oral Suspension (Doxycycline Monohydrate) Pfizer 2735
Vibra-Tabs Film Coated Tablets (Doxycycline Hyclate) Pfizer 2735

Listeriosis
Dynacin Capsules (Minocycline Hydrochloride) Medicis 2019
E.E.S. (Erythromycin Ethylsuccinate) Abbott 450
EryPed (Erythromycin Ethylsuccinate) Abbott 446
Minocin Oral Suspension (Minocycline Hydrochloride) Lederle 1865
Minocin Pellet-Filled Capsules (Minocycline Hydrochloride) Lederle 1863
Monodox Capsules (Doxycycline Monohydrate) Oclassen 2442
PCE Dispertab Tablets (Erythromycin) Abbott 498

Liver, allogeneic transplants, prophylaxis of organ rejection in
CellCept Capsules (Mycophenolate Mofetil) Roche Laboratories 2951
CellCept Intravenous (Mycophenolate Mofetil Hydrochloride) Roche Laboratories 2951
CellCept Oral Suspension (Mycophenolate Mofetil) Roche Laboratories 2951
CellCept Tablets (Mycophenolate Mofetil) Roche Laboratories 2951
Gengraf Capsules (Cyclosporine) Abbott 457
Neoral Soft Gelatin Capsules (Cyclosporine) Novartis 2380
Neoral Oral Solution (Cyclosporine) Novartis 2380
Orthoclone OKT3 Sterile Solution (Muromonab-CD3) Ortho Biotech 2498
Prograf (Tacrolimus) Fujisawa 1393
Sandimmune (Cyclosporine) Novartis 2388

Liver failure, acute
Albumin (Human) 25% (Albumin (human)) Baxter Healthcare 839
Plasbumin-5 (Albumin (human)) Bayer Biological 939
Plasbumin-20 (Albumin (human)) Bayer Biological 940
Plasbumin-25 (Albumin (human)) Bayer Biological 941

Locoregional solid malignancies
Cosmegen for Injection (Dactinomycin) Merck 2062

Loeffler's syndrome
Celestone Soluspan Injectable Suspension (Betamethasone Acetate, Betamethasone Sodium Phosphate) Schering 3097
Celestone Syrup (Betamethasone) Schering 3099
Cortone Acetate Injectable Suspension (Cortisone Acetate) Merck 2059
Cortone Acetate Tablets (Cortisone Acetate) Merck 2061
Decadron Elixir (Dexamethasone) Merck 2078
Decadron Tablets (Dexamethasone) Merck 2079
Decadron Phosphate Injection (Dexamethasone Sodium Phosphate) Merck 2081
Depo-Medrol Injectable Suspension (Methylprednisolone Acetate) Pharmacia & Upjohn 2795
Hydrocortone Tablets (Hydrocortisone) Merck 2106

(■ Described in PDR For Nonprescription Drugs) (⊙ Described in PDR For Ophthalmic Medicines™)

Hydrocortone Phosphate Injection, Sterile (Hydrocortisone Sodium Phosphate) Merck 2105
Pediapred Oral Solution (Prednisolone Sodium Phosphate) Celltech 1170
Prednisone (Prednisone) Roxane 3064
Prelone Syrup (Prednisolone) Muro . 2273
Solu-Medrol Sterile Powder (Methylprednisolone Sodium Succinate) Pharmacia & Upjohn 2855

Lou Gehrig's disease
(*see under* Sclerosis, amyotrophic lateral)

Lubrication, sexual
(*see under* Coitus, adjunct in)

Lung abscess
(*see under* Abscess, lung)

Lupus erythematosus, systemic
Extra Strength Bayer Arthritis Caplets (Aspirin) Bayer Consumer .... ▣610
Celestone Soluspan Injectable Suspension (Betamethasone Acetate, Betamethasone Sodium Phosphate) Schering 3097
Celestone Syrup (Betamethasone) Schering 3099
Cortone Acetate Injectable Suspension (Cortisone Acetate) Merck 2059
Cortone Acetate Tablets (Cortisone Acetate) Merck 2061
Decadron Elixir (Dexamethasone) Merck 2078
Decadron Tablets (Dexamethasone) Merck 2079
Decadron Phosphate Injection (Dexamethasone Sodium Phosphate) Merck 2081
Depo-Medrol Injectable Suspension (Methylprednisolone Acetate) Pharmacia & Upjohn 2795
Ecotrin Enteric Coated Aspirin Low, Regular and Maximum Strength Tablets (Aspirin) GlaxoSmithKline Consumer 1715
Hydrocortone Tablets (Hydrocortisone) Merck 2106
Hydrocortone Phosphate Injection, Sterile (Hydrocortisone Sodium Phosphate) Merck 2105
Pediapred Oral Solution (Prednisolone Sodium Phosphate) Celltech 1170
Plaquenil Tablets (Hydroxychloroquine Sulfate) Sanofi-Synthelabo .. 3082
Prednisone (Prednisone) Roxane 3064
Prelone Syrup (Prednisolone) Muro . 2273
Solu-Medrol Sterile Powder (Methylprednisolone Sodium Succinate) Pharmacia & Upjohn 2855

Lupus erythematosus discoides
Celestone Soluspan Injectable Suspension (Betamethasone Acetate, Betamethasone Sodium Phosphate) Schering 3097
Decadron Phosphate Injection (Dexamethasone Sodium Phosphate) Merck 2081
Hydrocortone Acetate Injectable Suspension (Hydrocortisone Acetate) Merck 2103
Plaquenil Tablets (Hydroxychloroquine Sulfate) Sanofi-Synthelabo .. 3082

Luteinizing hormone surge, premature, inhibition of
Antagon Injection (Ganirelix acetate) Organon 2447
Cetrotide for Injection (Cetrorelix Acetate) Serono 3209

Lyme disease
(*see under* Borrelia burgdorferi infection)

Lymphogranuloma venereum
Declomycin Tablets (Demeclocycline Hydrochloride) Lederle 1855
Doryx Coated Pellet Filled Capsules (Doxycycline Hyclate) Warner Chilcott 3357
Dynacin Capsules (Minocycline Hydrochloride) Medicis 2019
Minocin Intravenous (Minocycline Hydrochloride) Lederle 1862
Minocin Oral Suspension (Minocycline Hydrochloride) Lederle 1865
Minocin Pellet-Filled Capsules (Minocycline Hydrochloride) Lederle 1863
Monodox Capsules (Doxycycline Monohydrate) Oclassen 2442
Vibramycin Calcium Oral Suspension Syrup (Doxycycline Calcium) Pfizer 2735
Vibramycin Hyclate Capsules (Doxycycline Hyclate) Pfizer 2735
Vibramycin Hyclate Intravenous (Doxycycline Hyclate) Pfizer 2737
Vibramycin Monohydrate for Oral Suspension (Doxycycline Monohydrate) Pfizer 2735
Vibra-Tabs Film Coated Tablets (Doxycycline Hyclate) Pfizer 2735

Lymphography, diagnostic aid in
Ethiodol Injection (Ethiodized Oil) Savage 3095

Lymphoma, cutaneous T-cell
8-MOP Capsules (Methoxsalen) ICN 1727

Lymphoma, non-Hodgkin's, follicular
Intron A for Injection (Interferon alfa-2B, Recombinant) Schering 3120

Lymphoma, unspecified, adjunctive therapy in
Aloprim for Injection (Allopurinol Sodium) Nabi 2292

Lymphomas, giant follicular
Leukeran Tablets (Chlorambucil) GlaxoSmithKline 1591

Lymphomas, Hodgkin's
(*see under* Hodgkin's disease)

Lymphomas, malignant
Adriamycin PFS/RDF Injection (Doxorubicin Hydrochloride) Pharmacia & Upjohn 2767
Leukeran (Chlorambucil) GlaxoSmithKline 1591

Lymphomas, non-Hodgkin's
Mustargen for Injection (Mechlorethamine Hydrochloride) Merck 2142
Rituxan for Infusion (Rituximab) IDEC 1750
Rituxan I.V. (Rituximab) Genentech .. 1428
Thioplex for Injection (Thiotepa) Immunex 1765

Lymphomas, non-Hodgkin's, adjunctive therapy in
Leukine (Sargramostim) Immunex 1755

Lymphomas, palliative management of in adults
Celestone Soluspan Injectable Suspension (Betamethasone Acetate, Betamethasone Sodium Phosphate) Schering 3097
Celestone Syrup (Betamethasone) Schering 3099
Cortone Acetate Injectable Suspension (Cortisone Acetate) Merck 2059
Cortone Acetate Tablets (Cortisone Acetate) Merck 2061
Decadron Elixir (Dexamethasone) Merck 2078
Decadron Tablets (Dexamethasone) Merck 2079
Decadron Phosphate Injection (Dexamethasone Sodium Phosphate) Merck 2081
Depo-Medrol Injectable Suspension (Methylprednisolone Acetate) Pharmacia & Upjohn 2795
Hydrocortone Tablets (Hydrocortisone) Merck 2106
Hydrocortone Phosphate Injection, Sterile (Hydrocortisone Sodium Phosphate) Merck 2105
Pediapred Oral Solution (Prednisolone Sodium Phosphate) Celltech 1170
Prednisone (Prednisone) Roxane 3064
Prelone Syrup (Prednisolone) Muro . 2273
Solu-Medrol Sterile Powder (Methylprednisolone Sodium Succinate) Pharmacia & Upjohn 2855

Lymphomatous meningitis
DepoCyt Injection (Cytarabine Liposome) Chiron 1197

Lymphosarcoma
(*see under* Lymphomas, non-Hodgkin's)

M

M. catarrhalis, otitis media
Augmentin Chewable Tablets (Amoxicillin, Clavulanate Potassium) GlaxoSmithKline 1482
Augmentin Powder for Oral Suspension (Amoxicillin, Clavulanate Potassium) GlaxoSmithKline 1482
Augmentin Tablets (Amoxicillin, Clavulanate Potassium) GlaxoSmithKline 1485
Augmentin ES-600 Powder for Oral Suspension (Amoxicillin, Clavulanate Potassium) GlaxoSmithKline 1487
Biaxin/Biaxin XL (Clarithromycin) Abbott 403
Cedax (Ceftibuten Dihydrate) Biovail 1021
Ceftin (Cefuroxime Axetil) Lifecycle Ventures 1898
Cefzil (Cefprozil) Bristol-Myers Squibb 1076
Keflex (Cephalexin) Dista 1237
Lorabid Suspension and Pulvules (Loracarbef) Monarch 2251
Omnicef (Cefdinir) Abbott 493
Rocephin Injectable Vials, ADD-Vantage, Galaxy, Bulk (Ceftriaxone Sodium) Roche Laboratories 2993
Suprax (Cefixime) Lederle 1877
Vantin Tablets and Oral Suspension (Cefpodoxime Proxetil) Pharmacia & Upjohn 2860
Zithromax Capsules, 250 mg (Azithromycin Dihydrate) Pfizer 2743
Zithromax for Oral Suspension, 300 mg, 600 mg, 900 mg, 1200 mg (Azithromycin Dihydrate) Pfizer 2739
Zithromax Tablets, 250 mg (Azithromycin Dihydrate) Pfizer 2739

M. catarrhalis infections
Augmentin Chewable Tablets (Amoxicillin, Clavulanate Potassium) GlaxoSmithKline 1482
Augmentin Powder for Oral Suspension (Amoxicillin, Clavulanate Potassium) GlaxoSmithKline 1482
Augmentin Tablets (Amoxicillin, Clavulanate Potassium) GlaxoSmithKline 1485
Avelox Tablets (Moxifloxacin Hydrochloride) Bayer 879
Biaxin/Biaxin XL (Clarithromycin) Abbott 403
Ceclor CD Tablets (Cefaclor) Elan ... 1279
Cedax (Ceftibuten Dihydrate) Biovail 1021
Ceftin (Cefuroxime Axetil) Lifecycle Ventures 1898
Cefzil (Cefprozil) Bristol-Myers Squibb 1076
Cipro (Ciprofloxacin) Bayer 887
Dynabac Tablets (Dirithromycin) Muro 2269
Keflex (Cephalexin) Dista 1237
Levaquin (Levofloxacin) Ortho-McNeil 2537
Lorabid Suspension and Pulvules (Loracarbef) Monarch 2251
Omnicef (Cefdinir) Abbott 493
Suprax (Cefixime) Lederle 1877
Tequin Injection (Gatifloxacin) Bristol-Myers Squibb 1110
Tequin Tablets (Gatifloxacin) Bristol-Myers Squibb 1110
Trovan (Alatrofloxacin Mesylate) Pfizer 2722
Vantin Tablets and Oral Suspension (Cefpodoxime Proxetil) Pharmacia & Upjohn 2860
Zithromax Capsules, 250 mg (Azithromycin Dihydrate) Pfizer 2743
Zithromax for IV Infusion (Azithromycin Dihydrate) Pfizer 2748
Zithromax for Oral Suspension, 1 g (Azithromycin Dihydrate) Pfizer . 2743
Zithromax for Oral Suspension, 300 mg, 600 mg, 900 mg, 1200 mg (Azithromycin Dihydrate) Pfizer 2739
Zithromax Tablets, 250 mg (Azithromycin Dihydrate) Pfizer 2739
Zithromax Tablets, 600 mg (Azithromycin Dihydrate) Pfizer 2743

M. catarrhalis lower respiratory tract infections
Augmentin Chewable Tablets (Amoxicillin, Clavulanate Potassium) GlaxoSmithKline 1482
Augmentin Powder for Oral Suspension (Amoxicillin, Clavulanate Potassium) GlaxoSmithKline 1482
Augmentin Tablets (Amoxicillin, Clavulanate Potassium) GlaxoSmithKline 1485
Avelox Tablets (Moxifloxacin Hydrochloride) Bayer 879
Biaxin/Biaxin XL (Clarithromycin) Abbott 403
Ceclor CD Tablets (Cefaclor) Elan ... 1279
Cedax (Ceftibuten Dihydrate) Biovail 1021
Cefzil (Cefprozil) Bristol-Myers Squibb 1076
Cipro (Ciprofloxacin) Bayer 887
Dynabac Tablets (Dirithromycin) Muro 2269
Levaquin (Levofloxacin) Ortho-McNeil 2537
Lorabid Suspension and Pulvules (Loracarbef) Monarch 2251
Omnicef (Cefdinir) Abbott 493
Tequin Injection (Gatifloxacin) Bristol-Myers Squibb 1110
Tequin Tablets (Gatifloxacin) Bristol-Myers Squibb 1110
Trovan (Alatrofloxacin Mesylate) Pfizer 2722
Vantin Tablets and Oral Suspension (Cefpodoxime Proxetil) Pharmacia & Upjohn 2860
Zithromax Capsules, 250 mg (Azithromycin Dihydrate) Pfizer 2743
Zithromax for IV Infusion (Azithromycin Dihydrate) Pfizer 2748
Zithromax for Oral Suspension, 1 g (Azithromycin Dihydrate) Pfizer . 2743
Zithromax for Oral Suspension, 300 mg, 600 mg, 900 mg, 1200 mg (Azithromycin Dihydrate) Pfizer 2739
Zithromax Tablets, 250 mg (Azithromycin Dihydrate) Pfizer 2739
Zithromax Tablets, 600 mg (Azithromycin Dihydrate) Pfizer 2743

M. catarrhalis pneumonia
Avelox Tablets (Moxifloxacin Hydrochloride) Bayer 879
Omnicef (Cefdinir) Abbott 493
Tequin Injection (Gatifloxacin) Bristol-Myers Squibb 1110
Tequin Tablets (Gatifloxacin) Bristol-Myers Squibb 1110

M. catarrhalis sinusitis
Augmentin Chewable Tablets (Amoxicillin, Clavulanate Potassium) GlaxoSmithKline 1482
Augmentin Powder for Oral Suspension (Amoxicillin, Clavulanate Potassium) GlaxoSmithKline 1482
Augmentin Tablets (Amoxicillin, Clavulanate Potassium) GlaxoSmithKline 1485
Avelox Tablets (Moxifloxacin Hydrochloride) Bayer 879
Biaxin/Biaxin XL (Clarithromycin) Abbott 403
Cefzil (Cefprozil) Bristol-Myers Squibb 1076
Cipro I.V. (Ciprofloxacin) Bayer 893
Cipro I.V. Pharmacy Bulk Package (Ciprofloxacin) Bayer 897
Cipro (Ciprofloxacin) Bayer 887
Levaquin (Levofloxacin) Ortho-McNeil 2537
Lorabid Suspension and Pulvules (Loracarbef) Monarch 2251
Vantin Tablets and Oral Suspension (Cefpodoxime Proxetil) Pharmacia & Upjohn 2860

Macular degeneration
Visudyne for Injection (Verteporfin) Novartis Ophthalmics .... ⊙308

Magnesium deficiency
(*see under* Hypomagnesemia)

Malaria
(*see under* P. falciparum infections; P. malariae infections; P. ovale infections; P. vivax infections)

Malaria, prophylaxis of
Daraprim Tablets (Pyrimethamine) GlaxoSmithKline 1511
Doryx Coated Pellet Filled Capsules (Doxycycline Hyclate) Warner Chilcott 3357
Lariam Tablets (Mefloquine Hydrochloride) Roche Laboratories 2989
Vibramycin Hyclate Capsules (Doxycycline Hyclate) Pfizer 2735

Malassezia furfur
(*see under* Pityrosporon orbiculare infections)

Malignant effusion, serosal cavities
Thioplex for Injection (Thiotepa) Immunex 1765

Mania, bipolar
Zyprexa Tablets (Olanzapine) Lilly.... 1973
Zyprexa ZYDIS Orally Disintegrating Tablets (Olanzapine) Lilly.................................... 1973

Manic episodes associated with bipolar disorder
Depakote Tablets (Divalproex Sodium) Abbott 430
Eskalith (Lithium Carbonate) GlaxoSmithKline.......................... 1527
Lithobid Slow-Release Tablets (Lithium Carbonate) Solvay 3255

Mastocytosis, systemic
Gastrocrom Oral Concentrate (Cromolyn Sodium) Celltech......... 1162
Prilosec Delayed-Release Capsules (Omeprazole) AstraZeneca LP 628
Tagamet (Cimetidine Hydrochloride) GlaxoSmithKline 1644
Zantac (Ranitidine Hydrochloride) GlaxoSmithKline 1690

Measles, prevention or modification of
BayGam (Globulin, Immune (Human)) Bayer Biological 914

Measles, prophylaxis
Attenuvax (Measles Virus Vaccine Live) Merck 2044
M-M-R II (Measles, Mumps & Rubella Virus Vaccine, Live) Merck 2118

Meibomianitis, acute
Genoptic Ophthalmic Ointment (Gentamicin Sulfate) Allergan ......⊙239
Genoptic Sterile Ophthalmic Solution (Gentamicin Sulfate) Allergan ....⊙239

Melanin hyperpigmentation
(*see under* Hyperpigmentation, skin, bleaching of)

Melanoma
DTIC-Dome (Dacarbazine) Bayer 902
Intron A for Injection (Interferon alfa-2B, Recombinant) Schering ...3120
Mylocel Tablets (Hydroxyurea) MGI ..2227
Proleukin for Injection (Aldesleukin) Chiron 1199

Melasma
(*see under* Hyperpigmentation, skin, bleaching of)

Meningitis
Cefizox for Intramuscular or Intravenous Use (Ceftizoxime Sodium) Fujisawa 1390
Ceptaz for Injection (Ceftazidime) GlaxoSmithKline 1499
Claforan Injection (Cefotaxime Sodium) Aventis 732
Fortaz (Ceftazidime Sodium) GlaxoSmithKline 1541
Kefurox Vials, ADD-Vantage (Cefuroxime Sodium) Lilly 1948
Merrem I.V. (Meropenem) AstraZeneca 673
Nebcin Vials, Hyporets & ADD-Vantage (Tobramycin Sulfate) Lilly 1955
Pfizerpen for Injection (Penicillin G Potassium) Pfizer 2707
Rocephin Injectable Vials, ADD-Vantage, Galaxy, Bulk (Ceftriaxone Sodium) Roche Laboratories 2993
Tazicef for Injection (Ceftazidime) GlaxoSmithKline 1647
Tazicef Galaxy Container (Ceftazidime Sodium) GlaxoSmithKline 1650
Tazicef Pharmacy Bulk Package (Ceftazidime) GlaxoSmithKline 1653
Tazidime Vials, Faspak & ADD-Vantage (Ceftazidime) Lilly 1966
Zinacef Injection (Cefuroxime) GlaxoSmithKline 1696
Zinacef for Injection (Cefuroxime) GlaxoSmithKline 1696

Meningitis, meningococcal, treatment of
Pfizerpen for Injection (Penicillin G Potassium) Pfizer 2707

Meningitis, tuberculous
Celestone Soluspan Injectable Suspension (Betamethasone Acetate, Betamethasone Sodium Phosphate) Schering............. 3097
Celestone Syrup (Betamethasone) Schering 3099
Cortone Acetate Injectable Suspension (Cortisone Acetate) Merck.. 2059
Cortone Acetate Tablets (Cortisone Acetate) Merck 2061
Decadron Elixir (Dexamethasone) Merck.. 2078
Decadron Tablets (Dexamethasone) Merck 2079
Decadron Phosphate Injection (Dexamethasone Sodium Phosphate) Merck 2081
Depo-Medrol Injectable Suspension (Methylprednisolone Acetate) Pharmacia & Upjohn 2795
Hydrocortone Tablets (Hydrocortisone) Merck 2106
Hydrocortone Phosphate Injection, Sterile (Hydrocortisone Sodium Phosphate) Merck 2105
Pediapred Oral Solution (Prednisolone Sodium Phosphate) Celltech 1170
Prednisone (Prednisone) Roxane 3064
Prelone Syrup (Prednisolone) Muro .2273
Solu-Medrol Sterile Powder (Methylprednisolone Sodium Succinate) Pharmacia & Upjohn 2855

Menopause, vasomotor symptoms of
Activella Tablets (Estradiol, Norethindrone Acetate) Pharmacia & Upjohn 2764
Alora Transdermal System (Estradiol) Watson 3372
Cenestin Tablets (Estrogens, Conjugated, Synthetic A) Duramed 1263
Climara Transdermal System (Estradiol) Berlex 958
CombiPatch Transdermal System (Estradiol, Norethindrone Acetate) Novartis 2323
Esclim Transdermal System (Estradiol) Women First 3460
Estinyl Tablets (Ethinyl Estradiol) Schering 3112
Estrace Tablets (Estradiol) Warner Chilcott 3361
Estratest (Estrogens, Esterified, Methyltestosterone) Solvay 3252
Estring Vaginal Ring (Estradiol) Pharmacia & Upjohn 2811
femhrt Tablets (Ethinyl Estradiol, Norethindrone Acetate) Parke-Davis 2635
Hyland's MenoCalm Tablets (Homeopathic Formulations) Standard Homeopathic ....▣765
Menest Tablets (Estrogens, Esterified) Monarch 2254
Ogen Tablets (Estropipate) Pharmacia & Upjohn 2846
Ortho-Est Tablets (Estropipate) Women First 3464
Ortho-Prefest Tablets (Estradiol, Norgestimate) Ortho-McNeil 2570
Premarin Tablets (Estrogens, Conjugated) Wyeth-Ayerst 3566
Premphase Tablets (Estrogens, Conjugated, Medroxyprogesterone Acetate) Wyeth-Ayerst 3572
Prempro Tablets (Estrogens, Conjugated, Medroxyprogesterone Acetate) Wyeth-Ayerst 3572
Vivelle Transdermal System (Estradiol) Novartis 2412
Vivelle-Dot Transdermal System (Estradiol) Novartis 2416

Menstrual cramps
(*see under* Pain, menstrual)

Menstrual syndrome, pre-, management of
(*see also under* Dysphoric disorder, premenstrual)
Maximum Strength Midol Menstrual Caplets and Gelcaps (Acetaminophen, Caffeine, Pyrilamine Maleate) Bayer Consumer ....▣612
Maximum Strength Midol PMS Caplets and Gelcaps (Acetaminophen, Pamabrom, Pyrilamine Maleate) Bayer Consumer ....▣613
Women's Tylenol Menstrual Relief Caplets (Acetaminophen, Pamabrom) McNeil Consumer 2013

Microsporum audouinii infections
Grifulvin V Tablets Microsize and Oral Suspension Microsize (Griseofulvin) Ortho Dermatological 2518
Gris-PEG Tablets (Griseofulvin) Pedinol.. 2661

Microsporum canis infections
Grifulvin V Tablets Microsize and Oral Suspension Microsize (Griseofulvin) Ortho Dermatological............................... 2518
Gris-PEG Tablets (Griseofulvin) Pedinol.. 2661
Loprox Cream (Ciclopirox Olamine) Medicis 2021
Loprox Gel (Ciclopirox) Medicis....... 2022
Loprox Lotion (Ciclopirox Olamine) Medicis 2021
Lotrimin (Clotrimazole) Schering 3128
Lotrisone (Betamethasone Dipropionate, Clotrimazole) Schering...... 3129

Microsporum gypseum infections
Grifulvin V Tablets Microsize and Oral Suspension Microsize (Griseofulvin) Ortho Dermatological...................................2518
Gris-PEG Tablets (Griseofulvin) Pedinol 2661

Migraine headache
(*see under* Headache, migraine)

Mima-Herellea species infections
(*see under* Acinetobacter species infections)

Miosis, intraoperative, inhibition of
Ocufen Ophthalmic Solution (Flurbiprofen Sodium) Allergan ....⊙242

Miosis, production of
Humorsol Sterile Ophthalmic Solution (Demecarium Bromide) Merck 2102
Isopto Carpine Ophthalmic Solution (Pilocarpine Hydrochloride) Alcon ....⊙215
Miochol-E System Pak (Acetylcholine Chloride) Novartis Ophthalmics ....⊙305
Miochol-E with Steri-Tags (Acetylcholine Chloride) Novartis Ophthalmics ....⊙305
Pilopine HS Ophthalmic Gel (Pilocarpine Hydrochloride) Alcon ......⊙217
Rēv-Eyes Sterile Ophthalmic Eyedrops 0.5% (Dapiprazole Hydrochloride) Bausch & Lomb ..⊙265

Moraxella catarrhalis
(*see under* M. catarrhalis infections)

Moraxella lacunata infections, ocular
Chloromycetin Ophthalmic Ointment, 1% (Chloramphenicol) Monarch ....⊙296
Chloromycetin Ophthalmic Solution (Chloramphenicol) Monarch ....⊙297
Chloroptic Sterile Ophthalmic Ointment (Chloramphenicol) Allergan ....⊙234
TobraDex Ophthalmic Ointment (Dexamethasone, Tobramycin) Alcon 542
TobraDex Ophthalmic Suspension (Dexamethasone, Tobramycin) Alcon 541

Morganella morganii infections
Bactrim (Sulfamethoxazole, Trimethoprim) Roche Laboratories 2949
Cefizox for Intramuscular or Intravenous Use (Ceftizoxime Sodium) Fujisawa 1390
Cefotan (Cefotetan) AstraZeneca 664
Ceptaz for Injection (Ceftazidime) GlaxoSmithKline 1499
Cipro I.V. (Ciprofloxacin) Bayer 893
Cipro I.V. Pharmacy Bulk Package (Ciprofloxacin) Bayer 897
Cipro (Ciprofloxacin) Bayer 887
Claforan Injection (Cefotaxime Sodium) Aventis 732
Fortaz (Ceftazidime Sodium) GlaxoSmithKline 1541
Geocillin Tablets (Carbenicillin Indanyl Sodium) Pfizer 2687
Mefoxin for Injection (Cefoxitin Sodium) Merck 2124
Mefoxin Premixed Intravenous Solution (Cefoxitin Sodium) Merck 2127
Nebcin Vials, Hyporets & ADD-Vantage (Tobramycin Sulfate) Lilly 1955
Primaxin I.V. (Cilastatin Sodium, Imipenem) Merck.............................. 2160
Rocephin Injectable Vials, ADD-Vantage, Galaxy, Bulk (Ceftriaxone Sodium) Roche Laboratories.............................. 2993
Septra Suspension (Sulfamethoxazole, Trimethoprim) Monarch...... 2265
Septra Tablets (Sulfamethoxazole, Trimethoprim) Monarch.................. 2265
Septra DS Tablets (Sulfamethoxazole, Trimethoprim) Monarch...... 2265
Tazicef for Injection (Ceftazidime) GlaxoSmithKline.............................. 1647
Tazicef Galaxy Container (Ceftazidime Sodium) GlaxoSmithKline..... 1650
Tazicef Pharmacy Bulk Package (Ceftazidime) GlaxoSmithKline...... 1653

Morganella morganii infections, ocular
TobraDex Ophthalmic Ointment (Dexamethasone, Tobramycin) Alcon 542
TobraDex Ophthalmic Suspension (Dexamethasone, Tobramycin) Alcon 541

Morganella morganii skin and skin structure infections
Cipro I.V. (Ciprofloxacin) Bayer 893
Cipro I.V. Pharmacy Bulk Package (Ciprofloxacin) Bayer 897
Cipro (Ciprofloxacin) Bayer 887
Claforan Injection (Cefotaxime Sodium) Aventis 732
Primaxin I.V. (Cilastatin Sodium, Imipenem) Merck 2160
Rocephin Injectable Vials, ADD-Vantage, Galaxy, Bulk (Ceftriaxone Sodium) Roche Laboratories 2993
Tazicef for Injection (Ceftazidime) GlaxoSmithKline 1647
Tazicef Galaxy Container (Ceftazidime Sodium) GlaxoSmithKline 1650
Tazicef Pharmacy Bulk Package (Ceftazidime) GlaxoSmithKline 1653
Tazidime Vials, Faspak & ADD-Vantage (Ceftazidime) Lilly 1966

Morganella morganii urinary tract infections
Bactrim (Sulfamethoxazole, Trimethoprim) Roche Laboratories 2949
Cefizox for Intramuscular or Intravenous Use (Ceftizoxime Sodium) Fujisawa 1390
Cefotan (Cefotetan) AstraZeneca 664
Ceptaz for Injection (Ceftazidime) GlaxoSmithKline 1499
Cipro I.V. (Ciprofloxacin) Bayer 893
Cipro I.V. Pharmacy Bulk Package (Ciprofloxacin) Bayer 897
Cipro (Ciprofloxacin) Bayer 887
Claforan Injection (Cefotaxime Sodium) Aventis 732
Geocillin Tablets (Carbenicillin Indanyl Sodium) Pfizer 2687
Mefoxin for Injection (Cefoxitin Sodium) Merck 2124
Mefoxin Premixed Intravenous Solution (Cefoxitin Sodium) Merck 2127
Primaxin I.V. (Cilastatin Sodium, Imipenem) Merck 2160
Rocephin Injectable Vials, ADD-Vantage, Galaxy, Bulk (Ceftriaxone Sodium) Roche Laboratories 2993
Septra Suspension (Sulfamethoxazole, Trimethoprim) Monarch 2265
Septra Tablets (Sulfamethoxazole, Trimethoprim) Monarch 2265
Septra DS Tablets (Sulfamethoxazole, Trimethoprim) Monarch 2265
Tazicef for Injection (Ceftazidime) GlaxoSmithKline 1647
Tazicef Galaxy Container (Ceftazidime Sodium) GlaxoSmithKline 1650
Tazicef Pharmacy Bulk Package (Ceftazidime) GlaxoSmithKline 1653
Tazidime Vials, Faspak & ADD-Vantage (Ceftazidime) Lilly 1966

Morphea, possibly effective in
Potaba (Aminobenzoate Potassium) Glenwood 1721

Motion sickness
Antivert, Antivert/25, & Antivert/50 Tablets (Meclizine Hydrochloride) Pfizer 2664
Benadryl Parenteral (Diphenhydramine Hydrochloride) Parke-Davis ..2617
Dramamine (Dimenhydrinate) Pharmacia Consumer ....▣718

Dramamine Less Drowsy Tablets (Meclizine Hydrochloride) Pharmacia Consumer .... ▣ 718
Phenergan Injection (Promethazine Hydrochloride) Wyeth-Ayerst 3553
Phenergan Suppositories (Promethazine Hydrochloride) Wyeth-Ayerst 3556
Phenergan Syrup (Promethazine Hydrochloride) Wyeth-Ayerst 3554
Phenergan Tablets (Promethazine Hydrochloride) Wyeth-Ayerst 3556
Transderm Scōp Transdermal Therapeutic System (Scopolamine) Novartis Consumer 2302

Mountain sickness, acute
Diamox Intravenous (Acetazolamide Sodium) Lederle .... ⊙ 269
Diamox Sequels Sustained Release Capsules (Acetazolamide) Lederle .... ⊙ 270
Diamox Tablets (Acetazolamide) Lederle .... ⊙ 269

Mucormycosis
(*see under* Zygomycosis)

Multiple follicles, development of in an ART program
Follistim for Injection (Follitropin Beta) Organon 2465

Multiple sclerosis, acute exacerbations of
(*see under* Sclerosis, multiple, acute exacerbations of)

Mumps, prophylaxis
M-M-R II (Measles, Mumps & Rubella Virus Vaccine, Live) Merck 2118
Mumpsvax (Mumps Virus Vaccine, Live) Merck 2141

Muscle spasm
(*see under* Spasticity, muscle, symptomatic alleviation of)

Muscles, skeletal, relaxation, preoperative
Anectine Injection (Succinylcholine Chloride) GlaxoSmithKline 1476
Norcuron for Injection (Vecuronium Bromide) Organon 2478
Zemuron Injection (Rocuronium Bromide) Organon 2491

Musculo-skeletal discomfort, adjunct in
Flexeril Tablets (Cyclobenzaprine Hydrochloride) Alza 572
Flexeril Tablets (Cyclobenzaprine Hydrochloride) Merck 2094
Norflex (Orphenadrine Citrate) 3M ... 1987
Parafon Forte DSC Caplets (Chlorzoxazone) Ortho-McNeil 2582
Robaxin Injectable (Methocarbamol) Robins 2938
Robaxin Tablets (Methocarbamol) Robins 2939
Robaxisal Tablets (Aspirin, Methocarbamol) Robins 2939
Skelaxin Tablets (Metaxalone) Elan .. 1301
Soma Compound Tablets (Aspirin, Carisoprodol) Wallace 3354
Soma Compound w/Codeine Tablets (Aspirin, Carisoprodol, Codeine Phosphate) Wallace 3355

Myalgia
(*see under* Pain, muscular, temporary relief of)

Myalgia, topical relief of
(*see under* Pain, topical relief of)

Myasthenia gravis, differential diagnosis of
Tensilon Injectable (Edrophonium Chloride) ICN 1745

Myasthenia gravis, treatment of
Mestinon (Pyridostigmine Bromide) ICN 1740
Prostigmin Injectable (Neostigmine Methylsulfate) ICN 1744
Prostigmin Tablets (Neostigmine Bromide) ICN 1744
Tensilon Injectable (Edrophonium Chloride) ICN 1745

Mycobacterium avium complex (MAC) disease, disseminated
Biaxin/Biaxin XL (Clarithromycin) Abbott 403
Mycobutin Capsules (Rifabutin) Pharmacia & Upjohn 2838

Mycobacterium avium complex (MAC) disease, disseminated, prophylaxis of
Biaxin/Biaxin XL (Clarithromycin) Abbott 403
Zithromax (Azithromycin Dihydrate) Pfizer 2743

Mycobacterium intracellulare infections
Biaxin/Biaxin XL (Clarithromycin) Abbott 403

Mycobacterium leprae infections
(*see under* Leprosy)

Mycobacterium marinum infections
Dynacin Capsules (Minocycline Hydrochloride) Medicis 2019
Minocin Oral Suspension (Minocycline Hydrochloride) Lederle 1865
Minocin Pellet-Filled Capsules (Minocycline Hydrochloride) Lederle 1863

Mycobacterium tuberculosis, aid in the detection of
Aplisol Injection (Tuberculin, Purified Protein Derivative, Diluted) Parkedale 2609

Mycobacterium tuberculosis infection
Streptomycin Sulfate Injection (Streptomycin Sulfate) Pfizer 2714
Trecator-SC Tablets (Ethionamide) Wyeth-Ayerst 3598

Mycoplasma hominis pelvic inflammatory disease
Zithromax for IV Infusion (Azithromycin Dihydrate) Pfizer 2748

Mycoplasma pneumoniae infection
Avelox Tablets (Moxifloxacin Hydrochloride) Bayer 879
Biaxin/Biaxin XL (Clarithromycin) Abbott 403
Declomycin Tablets (Demeclocycline Hydrochloride) Lederle 1855
Doryx Coated Pellet Filled Capsules (Doxycycline Hyclate) Warner Chilcott 3357
Dynabac Tablets (Dirithromycin) Muro 2269
Dynacin Capsules (Minocycline Hydrochloride) Medicis 2019
E.E.S. (Erythromycin Ethylsuccinate) Abbott 450
EryPed (Erythromycin Ethylsuccinate) Abbott 446
Ery-Tab Tablets (Erythromycin) Abbott 448
Erythrocin Stearate Filmtab Tablets (Erythromycin Stearate) Abbott 452
Erythromycin Base Filmtab Tablets (Erythromycin) Abbott 454
Erythromycin Delayed-Release Capsules, USP (Erythromycin) Abbott 455
Levaquin (Levofloxacin) Ortho-McNeil 2537
Minocin Intravenous (Minocycline Hydrochloride) Lederle 1862
Minocin Oral Suspension (Minocycline Hydrochloride) Lederle 1865
Minocin Pellet-Filled Capsules (Minocycline Hydrochloride) Lederle 1863
Monodox Capsules (Doxycycline Monohydrate) Oclassen 2442
PCE Dispertab Tablets (Erythromycin) Abbott 498
Tequin Injection (Gatifloxacin) Bristol-Myers Squibb 1110
Tequin Tablets (Gatifloxacin) Bristol-Myers Squibb 1110
Vibramycin Calcium Oral Suspension Syrup (Doxycycline Calcium) Pfizer 2735
Vibramycin Hyclate Capsules (Doxycycline Hyclate) Pfizer 2735
Vibramycin Hyclate Intravenous (Doxycycline Hyclate) Pfizer 2737
Vibramycin Monohydrate for Oral Suspension (Doxycycline Monohydrate) Pfizer 2735
Vibra-Tabs Film Coated Tablets (Doxycycline Hyclate) Pfizer 2735
Zithromax Capsules, 250 mg (Azithromycin Dihydrate) Pfizer 2743
Zithromax for IV Infusion (Azithromycin Dihydrate) Pfizer 2748
Zithromax for Oral Suspension, 300 mg, 600 mg, 900 mg, 1200 mg (Azithromycin Dihydrate) Pfizer 2739
Zithromax Tablets, 250 mg (Azithromycin Dihydrate) Pfizer 2739

Mycoplasma pneumoniae respiratory tract infections
Biaxin/Biaxin XL (Clarithromycin) Abbott 403
Dynabac Tablets (Dirithromycin) Muro 2269
Dynacin Capsules (Minocycline Hydrochloride) Medicis 2019
E.E.S. (Erythromycin Ethylsuccinate) Abbott 450
EryPed (Erythromycin Ethylsuccinate) Abbott 446
Ery-Tab Tablets (Erythromycin) Abbott 448
Erythrocin Stearate Filmtab Tablets (Erythromycin Stearate) Abbott 452
Erythromycin Base Filmtab Tablets (Erythromycin) Abbott 454
Erythromycin Delayed-Release Capsules, USP (Erythromycin) Abbott 455
Levaquin (Levofloxacin) Ortho-McNeil 2537
Monodox Capsules (Doxycycline Monohydrate) Oclassen 2442
PCE Dispertab Tablets (Erythromycin) Abbott 498
Zithromax Capsules, 250 mg (Azithromycin Dihydrate) Pfizer 2743
Zithromax for IV Infusion (Azithromycin Dihydrate) Pfizer 2748
Zithromax for Oral Suspension, 300 mg, 600 mg, 900 mg, 1200 mg (Azithromycin Dihydrate) Pfizer 2739
Zithromax Tablets, 250 mg (Azithromycin Dihydrate) Pfizer 2739

Mycosis fungoides
Celestone Soluspan Injectable Suspension (Betamethasone Acetate, Betamethasone Sodium Phosphate) Schering 3097
Celestone Syrup (Betamethasone) Schering 3099
Cortone Acetate Injectable Suspension (Cortisone Acetate) Merck 2059
Cortone Acetate Tablets (Cortisone Acetate) Merck 2061
Decadron Elixir (Dexamethasone) Merck 2078
Decadron Tablets (Dexamethasone) Merck 2079
Decadron Phosphate Injection (Dexamethasone Sodium Phosphate) Merck 2081
Depo-Medrol Injectable Suspension (Methylprednisolone Acetate) Pharmacia & Upjohn 2795
Hydrocortone Tablets (Hydrocortisone) Merck 2106
Hydrocortone Phosphate Injection, Sterile (Hydrocortisone Sodium Phosphate) Merck 2105
Mustargen for Injection (Mechlorethamine Hydrochloride) Merck 2142
Pediapred Oral Solution (Prednisolone Sodium Phosphate) Celltech 1170
Prednisone (Prednisone) Roxane 3064
Prelone Syrup (Prednisolone) Muro . 2273
Solu-Medrol Sterile Powder (Methylprednisolone Sodium Succinate) Pharmacia & Upjohn 2855

Mydriasis, reversal of
Isopto Carpine Ophthalmic Solution (Pilocarpine Hydrochloride) Alcon .... ⊙ 215

Myeloid recovery, acceleration of
Leukine (Sargramostim) Immunex 1755

Myeloma, multiple
Alkeran Tablets (Melphalan) GlaxoSmithKline 1466

Myeloma, multiple, adjunct in
Alkeran for Injection (Melphalan Hydrochloride) GlaxoSmithKline ... 1465
Aredia for Injection (Pamidronate Disodium) Novartis 2309

Myocardial infarction, acute
Activase I.V. (Alteplase, Recombinant) Genentech 1410
Genuine Bayer Professional Labeling (Aspirin Regimen Bayer) (Aspirin) Bayer Consumer .... ▣ 608
Ecotrin Enteric Coated Aspirin Low, Regular and Maximum Strength Tablets (Aspirin) GlaxoSmithKline Consumer 1715
Integrilin Injection (Eptifibatide) COR 1213
Integrilin Injection (Eptifibatide) Key 1828
Plavix Tablets (Clopidogrel Bisulfate) Bristol-Myers Squibb 1097
Plavix Tablets (Clopidogrel Bisulfate) Sanofi-Synthelabo 3084
Retavase Vials (Reteplase) Centocor 1182
Streptase for Infusion (Streptokinase) AstraZeneca LP..................... 647
TNKase I.V. (Tenecteplase) Genentech.. 1430

Myocardial infarction, non-Q-wave
Aggrastat (Tirofiban Hydrochloride) Merck.. 2031
Fragmin Injection (Dalteparin Sodium) Pharmacia & Upjohn 2814
Integrilin Injection (Eptifibatide) COR 1213
Integrilin Injection (Eptifibatide) Key 1828
Lovenox Injection (Enoxaparin) Aventis 746
ReoPro Vials (Abciximab) Lilly 1958

Myocardial infarction, post, left ventricular dysfunction
Captopril Tablets (Captopril) Mylan 2281
Mavik Tablets (Trandolapril) Abbott .. 478

Myocardial infarction, prophylaxis, adjunct in
Mevacor Tablets (Lovastatin) Merck 2132

Myocardial infarction, to reduce the risk of
Altace Capsules (Ramipril) Monarch 2233
Niaspan Extended-Release Tablets (Niacin) Kos 1846
Pravachol Tablets (Pravastatin Sodium) Bristol-Myers Squibb 1099
Zocor Tablets (Simvastatin) Merck .. 2219

Myocardial infarction, treatment adjunct
Altace Capsules (Ramipril) Monarch 2233
Mavik Tablets (Trandolapril) Abbott .. 478
Prinivil Tablets (Lisinopril) Merck 2164
Zestril Tablets (Lisinopril) AstraZeneca 698

Myocardial perfusion imaging, thallium, adjunct in
Adenoscan (Adenosine) Fujisawa 1381

Myocardial reinfarction, prophylaxis
Genuine Bayer Professional Labeling (Aspirin Regimen Bayer) (Aspirin) Bayer Consumer .... ▣ 608
Blocadren Tablets (Timolol Maleate) Merck 2046
Coumadin for Injection (Warfarin Sodium) DuPont 1243
Coumadin Tablets (Warfarin Sodium) DuPont 1243
Ecotrin Enteric Coated Aspirin Low, Regular and Maximum Strength Tablets (Aspirin) GlaxoSmithKline Consumer 1715
Inderal (Propranolol Hydrochloride) Wyeth-Ayerst 3513
Plavix Tablets (Clopidogrel Bisulfate) Bristol-Myers Squibb 1097
Plavix Tablets (Clopidogrel Bisulfate) Sanofi-Synthelabo 3084
Tenormin (Atenolol) AstraZeneca 692
Warfarin Sodium Tablets, USP (Warfarin Sodium) Taro 3302

Myocardial revascularization procedures, to reduce the risk of
Pravachol Tablets (Pravastatin Sodium) Bristol-Myers Squibb 1099
Zocor Tablets (Simvastatin) Merck .. 2219

Myxedema
(*see under* Hypothyroidism, replacement or supplemental therapy in)

Myxedema coma/precoma
(*see also under* Hypothyroidism, replacement or supplemental therapy in)
Triostat Injection (Liothyronine Sodium) Jones 1825

N

N. gonorrhoeae endocervical infections
Cefizox for Intramuscular or Intravenous Use (Ceftizoxime Sodium) Fujisawa 1390
Ceftin Tablets (Cefuroxime Axetil) Lifecycle Ventures 1898
Cipro (Ciprofloxacin) Bayer 887
Noroxin Tablets (Norfloxacin) Merck 2145
Rocephin Injectable Vials, ADD-Vantage, Galaxy, Bulk (Ceftriaxone Sodium) Roche Laboratories 2993
Vantin Tablets and Oral Suspension (Cefpodoxime Proxetil) Pharmacia & Upjohn 2860
Zithromax Capsules, 250 mg (Azithromycin Dihydrate) Pfizer 2743
Zithromax for Oral Suspension, 300 mg, 600 mg, 900 mg, 1200 mg (Azithromycin Dihydrate) Pfizer 2739
Zithromax Tablets, 250 mg (Azithromycin Dihydrate) Pfizer 2739

N. gonorrhoeae epididymo-orchitis, acute
Monodox Capsules (Doxycycline Monohydrate) Oclassen 2442

N. gonorrhoeae gynecologic infections
Cefobid Intravenous/Intramuscular (Cefoperazone) Pfizer 2671
Cefobid Pharmacy Bulk Package - Not for Direct Infusion (Cefoperazone Sodium) Pfizer 2673
Cefotan (Cefotetan) AstraZeneca 664
Dynacin Capsules (Minocycline Hydrochloride) Medicis 2019
Erythrocin Stearate Filmtab Tablets (Erythromycin Stearate) Abbott 452
Erythromycin Base Filmtab Tablets (Erythromycin) Abbott 454
Erythromycin Delayed-Release Capsules, USP (Erythromycin) Abbott 455
Floxin I.V. (Ofloxacin) Ortho-McNeil 2526
Floxin Tablets (Ofloxacin) Ortho-McNeil 2529
Mefoxin for Injection (Cefoxitin Sodium) Merck 2124
Mefoxin Premixed Intravenous Solution (Cefoxitin Sodium) Merck 2127
Minocin Pellet-Filled Capsules (Minocycline Hydrochloride) Lederle 1863
Noroxin Tablets (Norfloxacin) Merck 2145
PCE Dispertab Tablets (Erythromycin) Abbott 498

N. gonorrhoeae infections
Amoxil Chewable Tablets (Amoxicillin) GlaxoSmithKline 1471
Amoxil for Oral Suspension (Amoxicillin) GlaxoSmithKline 1471
Amoxil (Amoxicillin) GlaxoSmithKline 1471
Cefizox for Intramuscular or Intravenous Use (Ceftizoxime Sodium) Fujisawa 1390
Cefobid Intravenous/Intramuscular (Cefoperazone) Pfizer 2671
Cefobid Pharmacy Bulk Package - Not for Direct Infusion (Cefoperazone Sodium) Pfizer 2673
Cefotan (Cefotetan) AstraZeneca 664
Ceftin Tablets (Cefuroxime Axetil) Lifecycle Ventures 1898
Ceptaz for Injection (Ceftazidime) GlaxoSmithKline 1499
Cipro (Ciprofloxacin) Bayer 887
Claforan Injection (Cefotaxime Sodium) Aventis 732
Declomycin Tablets (Demeclocycline Hydrochloride) Lederle 1855
Doryx Coated Pellet Filled Capsules (Doxycycline Hyclate) Warner Chilcott 3357
Dynacin Capsules (Minocycline Hydrochloride) Medicis 2019
E.E.S. (Erythromycin Ethylsuccinate) Abbott 450
EryPed (Erythromycin Ethylsuccinate) Abbott 446
Ery-Tab Tablets (Erythromycin) Abbott 448
Erythrocin Stearate Filmtab Tablets (Erythromycin Stearate) Abbott 452
Erythromycin Base Filmtab Tablets (Erythromycin) Abbott 454
Erythromycin Delayed-Release Capsules, USP (Erythromycin) Abbott 455
Floxin I.V. (Ofloxacin) Ortho-McNeil 2526
Floxin Tablets (Ofloxacin) Ortho-McNeil 2529
Fortaz (Ceftazidime Sodium) GlaxoSmithKline 1541
Kefurox Vials, ADD-Vantage (Cefuroxime Sodium) Lilly 1948
Mefoxin for Injection (Cefoxitin Sodium) Merck 2124
Mefoxin Premixed Intravenous Solution (Cefoxitin Sodium) Merck 2127
Minocin Intravenous (Minocycline Hydrochloride) Lederle 1862
Minocin Oral Suspension (Minocycline Hydrochloride) Lederle 1865
Minocin Pellet-Filled Capsules (Minocycline Hydrochloride) Lederle 1863
Monodox Capsules (Doxycycline Monohydrate) Oclassen 2442
Noroxin Tablets (Norfloxacin) Merck 2145
PCE Dispertab Tablets (Erythromycin) Abbott 498
Pfizerpen for Injection (Penicillin G Potassium) Pfizer 2707
Pipracil (Piperacillin Sodium) Lederle 1866
Rocephin Injectable Vials, ADD-Vantage, Galaxy, Bulk (Ceftriaxone Sodium) Roche Laboratories 2993
Suprax Tablets (Cefixime) Lederle 1877
Tazicef for Injection (Ceftazidime) GlaxoSmithKline 1647
Tazicef Galaxy Container (Ceftazidime Sodium) GlaxoSmithKline 1650
Tazicef Pharmacy Bulk Package (Ceftazidime) GlaxoSmithKline 1653
Tazidime Vials, Faspak & ADD-Vantage (Ceftazidime) Lilly 1966
Tequin Injection (Gatifloxacin) Bristol-Myers Squibb 1110
Tequin Tablets (Gatifloxacin) Bristol-Myers Squibb 1110
Vantin Tablets and Oral Suspension (Cefpodoxime Proxetil) Pharmacia & Upjohn 2860
Vibramycin Calcium Oral Suspension Syrup (Doxycycline Calcium) Pfizer 2735
Vibramycin Hyclate Capsules (Doxycycline Hyclate) Pfizer 2735
Vibramycin Hyclate Intravenous (Doxycycline Hyclate) Pfizer 2737
Vibramycin Monohydrate for Oral Suspension (Doxycycline Monohydrate) Pfizer 2735
Vibra-Tabs Film Coated Tablets (Doxycycline Hyclate) Pfizer 2735
Zinacef Injection (Cefuroxime) GlaxoSmithKline 1696
Zinacef for Injection (Cefuroxime) GlaxoSmithKline 1696
Zithromax Capsules, 250 mg (Azithromycin Dihydrate) Pfizer 2743
Zithromax for IV Infusion (Azithromycin Dihydrate) Pfizer 2748
Zithromax for Oral Suspension, 300 mg, 600 mg, 900 mg, 1200 mg (Azithromycin Dihydrate) Pfizer 2739
Zithromax Tablets, 250 mg (Azithromycin Dihydrate) Pfizer 2739

N. gonorrhoeae infections, ocular
Genoptic Ophthalmic Ointment (Gentamicin Sulfate) Allergan ⊙239
Genoptic Sterile Ophthalmic Solution (Gentamicin Sulfate) Allergan ⊙239
Pred-G Ophthalmic Suspension (Gentamicin Sulfate, Prednisolone Acetate) Allergan ⊙247
Pred-G Sterile Ophthalmic Ointment (Gentamicin Sulfate, Prednisolone Acetate) Allergan ⊙248

N. gonorrhoeae pelvic inflammatory disease
Cefizox for Intramuscular or Intravenous Use (Ceftizoxime Sodium) Fujisawa 1390
Cefobid Intravenous/Intramuscular (Cefoperazone) Pfizer 2671
Cefobid Pharmacy Bulk Package - Not for Direct Infusion (Cefoperazone Sodium) Pfizer 2673
E.E.S. (Erythromycin Ethylsuccinate) Abbott 450
EryPed (Erythromycin Ethylsuccinate) Abbott 446
Ery-Tab Tablets (Erythromycin) Abbott 448
Mefoxin for Injection (Cefoxitin Sodium) Merck 2124
Mefoxin Premixed Intravenous Solution (Cefoxitin Sodium) Merck 2127
Rocephin Injectable Vials, ADD-Vantage, Galaxy, Bulk (Ceftriaxone Sodium) Roche Laboratories 2993
Zithromax for IV Infusion (Azithromycin Dihydrate) Pfizer 2748

N. gonorrhoeae pharyngeal infections
Rocephin Injectable Vials, ADD-Vantage, Galaxy, Bulk (Ceftriaxone Sodium) Roche Laboratories 2993

N. gonorrhoeae rectal infections
Ceftin Tablets (Cefuroxime Axetil) Lifecycle Ventures 1898
Rocephin Injectable Vials, ADD-Vantage, Galaxy, Bulk (Ceftriaxone Sodium) Roche Laboratories 2993
Vantin Tablets and Oral Suspension (Cefpodoxime Proxetil) Pharmacia & Upjohn 2860

N. gonorrhoeae urethral infections
Ceftin Tablets (Cefuroxime Axetil) Lifecycle Ventures 1898
Cipro (Ciprofloxacin) Bayer 887
Dynacin Capsules (Minocycline Hydrochloride) Medicis 2019
Floxin I.V. (Ofloxacin) Ortho-McNeil 2526
Minocin Oral Suspension (Minocycline Hydrochloride) Lederle 1865
Noroxin Tablets (Norfloxacin) Merck 2145
Rocephin Injectable Vials, ADD-Vantage, Galaxy, Bulk (Ceftriaxone Sodium) Roche Laboratories 2993
Tequin Injection (Gatifloxacin) Bristol-Myers Squibb 1110
Tequin Tablets (Gatifloxacin) Bristol-Myers Squibb 1110
Vantin Tablets and Oral Suspension (Cefpodoxime Proxetil) Pharmacia & Upjohn 2860
Zithromax Capsules, 250 mg (Azithromycin Dihydrate) Pfizer 2743
Zithromax for Oral Suspension, 300 mg, 600 mg, 900 mg, 1200 mg (Azithromycin Dihydrate) Pfizer 2739
Zithromax Tablets, 250 mg (Azithromycin Dihydrate) Pfizer 2739

N. gonorrhoeae urinary tract infections
Claforan Injection (Cefotaxime Sodium) Aventis 732
Kefurox Vials, ADD-Vantage (Cefuroxime Sodium) Lilly 1948

N. meningitidis, asymptomatic carriers of
Minocin Oral Suspension (Minocycline Hydrochloride) Lederle 1865
Rifadin (Rifampin) Aventis 765

N. meningitidis central nervous system infections
Claforan Injection (Cefotaxime Sodium) Aventis 732
Tazicef for Injection (Ceftazidime) GlaxoSmithKline 1647
Tazicef Galaxy Container (Ceftazidime Sodium) GlaxoSmithKline 1650
Tazicef Pharmacy Bulk Package (Ceftazidime) GlaxoSmithKline 1653

N. meningitidis infections
Ceptaz for Injection (Ceftazidime) GlaxoSmithKline 1499
Claforan Injection (Cefotaxime Sodium) Aventis 732
Fortaz (Ceftazidime Sodium) GlaxoSmithKline 1541
Merrem I.V. (Meropenem) AstraZeneca 673
Minocin Intravenous (Minocycline Hydrochloride) Lederle 1862
Minocin Oral Suspension (Minocycline Hydrochloride) Lederle 1865
Minocin Pellet-Filled Capsules (Minocycline Hydrochloride) Lederle 1863
Rocephin Injectable Vials, ADD-Vantage, Galaxy, Bulk (Ceftriaxone Sodium) Roche Laboratories 2993
Tazicef for Injection (Ceftazidime) GlaxoSmithKline 1647
Tazicef Galaxy Container (Ceftazidime Sodium) GlaxoSmithKline 1650
Tazicef Pharmacy Bulk Package (Ceftazidime) GlaxoSmithKline 1653
Tazidime Vials, Faspak & ADD-Vantage (Ceftazidime) Lilly 1966
Vibramycin Hyclate Intravenous (Doxycycline Hyclate) Pfizer 2737
Zinacef Injection (Cefuroxime) GlaxoSmithKline 1696
Zinacef for Injection (Cefuroxime) GlaxoSmithKline 1696

N. meningitidis meningitis
Ceptaz for Injection (Ceftazidime) GlaxoSmithKline 1499
Fortaz (Ceftazidime Sodium) GlaxoSmithKline 1541
Kefurox Vials, ADD-Vantage (Cefuroxime Sodium) Lilly 1948
Merrem I.V. (Meropenem) AstraZeneca 673
Rocephin Injectable Vials, ADD-Vantage, Galaxy, Bulk (Ceftriaxone Sodium) Roche Laboratories 2993
Tazicef for Injection (Ceftazidime) GlaxoSmithKline 1647
Tazicef Galaxy Container (Ceftazidime Sodium) GlaxoSmithKline 1650
Tazicef Pharmacy Bulk Package (Ceftazidime) GlaxoSmithKline 1653
Tazidime Vials, Faspak & ADD-Vantage (Ceftazidime) Lilly 1966
Zinacef Injection (Cefuroxime) GlaxoSmithKline 1696
Zinacef for Injection (Cefuroxime) GlaxoSmithKline 1696

Narcolepsy
Adderall Tablets (Amphetamine Aspartate, Amphetamine Sulfate, Dextroamphetamine Saccharate, Dextroamphetamine Sulfate) Shire US 3231
Dexedrine (Dextroamphetamine Sulfate) GlaxoSmithKline 1512
DextroStat Tablets (Dextroamphetamine Sulfate) Shire US 3236
Metadate ER Tablets (Methylphenidate Hydrochloride) Celltech 1167
Methylin Tablets (Methylphenidate Hydrochloride) Mallinckrodt 1995
Methylin ER Tablets (Methylphenidate Hydrochloride) Mallinckrodt 1995
Provigil Tablets (Modafinil) Cephalon 1193
Ritalin (Methylphenidate Hydrochloride) Novartis 2387

Narcotic addiction, detoxification treatment of
Dolophine (Methadone Hydrochloride) Roxane 3056

Nasal congestion, symptomatic relief of
Actifed Cold & Allergy Tablets (Pseudoephedrine Hydrochloride, Triprolidine Hydrochloride) Pfizer Inc., Warner-Lambert Healthcare ▣688
Actifed Cold & Sinus Caplets and Tablets (Acetaminophen, Chlorpheniramine Maleate, Pseudoephedrine Hydrochloride) Pfizer Inc., Warner-Lambert Healthcare ▣688
Afrin Nasal Decongestant Children's Pump Mist (Phenylephrine Hydrochloride) Schering-Plough ▣734
Afrin (Oxymetazoline Hydrochloride) Schering-Plough ▣733
Afrin No Drip Original Nasal Spray (Oxymetazoline Hydrochloride) Schering-Plough ▣735
Afrin No Drip Extra Moisturizing Nasal Spray (Oxymetazoline Hydrochloride) Schering-Plough ▣735
Afrin No Drip Severe Congestion Nasal Spray (Oxymetazoline Hydrochloride) Schering-Plough ▣735
Afrin No Drip Sinus Nasal Spray (Oxymetazoline Hydrochloride) Schering-Plough ▣735
Afrin Original Pump Mist (Oxymetazoline Hydrochloride) Schering-Plough ▣733
Alka-Seltzer Plus Cold & Sinus Medicine Liqui-Gels (Acetaminophen, Pseudoephedrine Hydrochloride) Bayer Consumer ▣604
Allegra-D Extended-Release Tablets (Fexofenadine Hydrochloride, Pseudoephedrine Hydrochloride) Aventis 714
BC Cold Powder (Aspirin, Chlorpheniramine Maleate, Pseudoephedrine Hydrochloride) Block ▣619

Benadryl Allergy/Cold Tablets (Acetaminophen, Diphenhydramine Hydrochloride, Pseudoephedrine Hydrochloride) Pfizer Inc., Warner-Lambert Healthcare ▣691
Benadryl Allergy/Congestion Tablets (Diphenhydramine Hydrochloride, Pseudoephedrine Hydrochloride) Pfizer Inc., Warner-Lambert Healthcare ▣692
Benadryl Allergy & Sinus Liquid (Diphenhydramine Hydrochloride, Pseudoephedrine Hydrochloride) Pfizer Inc., Warner-Lambert Healthcare ▣693
Benadryl Allergy Sinus Headache Caplets & Gelcaps (Acetaminophen, Diphenhydramine Hydrochloride, Pseudoephedrine Hydrochloride) Pfizer Inc., Warner-Lambert Healthcare ▣693
Bromfed Capsules (Extended-Release) (Brompheniramine Maleate, Pseudoephedrine Hydrochloride) Muro 2269
Bromfed-PD Capsules (Extended-Release) (Brompheniramine Maleate, Pseudoephedrine Hydrochloride) Muro 2269
Chlor-Trimeton Allergy/Decongestant Tablets (Chlorpheniramine Maleate, Pseudoephedrine Sulfate) Schering-Plough ▣736
Comtrex Acute Head Cold & Sinus Pressure Relief Tablets (Acetaminophen, Brompheniramine Maleate, Pseudoephedrine Hydrochloride) Bristol-Myers ▣627
Contac Non-Drowsy 12 Hour Cold Caplets (Pseudoephedrine Hydrochloride) SmithKline Beecham Consumer ▣745
Contac Non-Drowsy Timed Release 12 Hour Cold Caplets (Pseudoephedrine Hydrochloride) SmithKline Beecham Consumer ▣746
Coricidin 'D' Cold, Flu & Sinus Tablets (Acetaminophen, Chlorpheniramine Maleate, Pseudoephedrine Sulfate) Schering-Plough ▣737
Dimetapp Elixir (Brompheniramine Maleate, Pseudoephedrine Hydrochloride) Whitehall-Robins ▣777
Dimetapp Cold and Fever Suspension (Acetaminophen, Brompheniramine Maleate, Pseudoephedrine Hydrochloride) Whitehall-Robins ▣775
Dimetapp Infant Drops Decongestant (Pseudoephedrine Hydrochloride) Whitehall-Robins ▣775
Drixoral Allergy/Sinus Extended-Release Tablets (Acetaminophen, Dexbrompheniramine Maleate, Pseudoephedrine Sulfate) Schering-Plough ▣741
Drixoral Cold & Allergy Sustained-Action Tablets (Dexbrompheniramine Maleate, Pseudoephedrine Sulfate) Schering-Plough ▣740
Drixoral Cold & Flu Extended-Release Tablets (Acetaminophen, Dexbrompheniramine Maleate, Pseudoephedrine Sulfate) Schering-Plough ▣740
Drixoral Nasal Decongestant Long-Acting Non-Drowsy Tablets (Pseudoephedrine Sulfate) Schering-Plough ▣740
Kronofed-A (Chlorpheniramine Maleate, Pseudoephedrine Hydrochloride) Ferndale 1341
Natru-Vent Nasal Spray, Adult Strength (Xylometazoline Hydrochloride) Boehringer Ingelheim ▣624
Natru-Vent Nasal Spray, Pediatric Strength (Xylometazoline Hydrochloride) Boehringer Ingelheim ▣625
Neo-Synephrine (Phenylephrine Hydrochloride) Bayer Consumer ▣614
Neo-Synephrine 12 Hour (Oxymetazoline Hydrochloride) Bayer Consumer ▣615
PediaCare Infants' Drops Decongestant (Pseudoephedrine Hydrochloride) Pharmacia Consumer ▣719
Robitussin Cold Softgels Severe Congestion (Guaifenesin, Pseudoephedrine Hydrochloride) Whitehall-Robins ▣782
Robitussin Pediatric Cough & Cold Formula Liquid (Dextromethorphan Hydrobromide, Pseudoephedrine Hydrochloride) Whitehall-Robins ▣785
Robitussin-PE Liquid (Guaifenesin, Pseudoephedrine Hydrochloride) Whitehall-Robins ▣782
Ryna Liquid (Chlorpheniramine Maleate, Pseudoephedrine Hydrochloride) Wallace ▣768
Ryna-12 S Suspension (Phenylephrine Tannate, Pyrilamine Tannate) Wallace 3351
Reformulated Rynatan Pediatric Suspension (Chlorpheniramine Tannate, Phenylephrine Tannate) Wallace 3352
Rynatan Tablets (Azatadine Maleate, Pseudoephedrine Sulfate) Wallace 3351
Semprex-D Capsules (Acrivastine, Pseudoephedrine Hydrochloride) Celltech 1172
Singlet Caplets (Acetaminophen, Chlorpheniramine Maleate, Pseudoephedrine Hydrochloride) SmithKline Beecham Consumer ▣761
Sinutab Sinus Allergy Medication, Maximum Strength Formula, Tablets & Caplets (Acetaminophen, Chlorpheniramine Maleate, Pseudoephedrine Hydrochloride) Pfizer Inc., Warner-Lambert Healthcare ▣707
Sinutab Sinus Medication, Maximum Strength Without Drowsiness Formula, Tablets & Caplets (Acetaminophen, Pseudoephedrine Hydrochloride) Pfizer Inc., Warner-Lambert Healthcare ▣707
Sudafed 12 Hour Tablets (Pseudoephedrine Hydrochloride) Pfizer Inc., Warner-Lambert Healthcare ▣708
Sudafed 24 Hour Tablets (Pseudoephedrine Hydrochloride) Pfizer Inc., Warner-Lambert Healthcare ▣708
Children's Sudafed Nasal Decongestant Chewables (Pseudoephedrine Hydrochloride) Pfizer Inc., Warner-Lambert Healthcare ▣711
Children's Sudafed Nasal Decongestant Liquid Medication (Pseudoephedrine Hydrochloride) Pfizer Inc., Warner-Lambert Healthcare ▣711
Sudafed Cold & Sinus Liquid Caps (Acetaminophen, Pseudoephedrine Hydrochloride) Pfizer Inc., Warner-Lambert Healthcare ▣710
Sudafed Nasal Decongestant Tablets (Pseudoephedrine Hydrochloride) Pfizer Inc., Warner-Lambert Healthcare ▣710
Sudafed Non-Drying Sinus Liquid Caps (Guaifenesin, Pseudoephedrine Hydrochloride) Pfizer Inc., Warner-Lambert Healthcare ▣712
Sudafed Sinus Headache Caplets (Acetaminophen, Pseudoephedrine Hydrochloride) Pfizer Inc., Warner-Lambert Healthcare ▣712
Sudafed Sinus Headache Tablets (Acetaminophen, Pseudoephedrine Hydrochloride) Pfizer Inc., Warner-Lambert Healthcare ▣712
Tavist Sinus Non-Drowsy Coated Caplets (Acetaminophen, Pseudoephedrine Hydrochloride) Novartis Consumer ▣676
Triaminic Allergy Congestion Liquid (Pseudoephedrine Hydrochloride) Novartis Consumer ▣680
Triaminic Chest Congestion Liquid (Guaifenesin, Pseudoephedrine Hydrochloride) Novartis Consumer ▣680
Children's Tylenol Allergy-D Liquid (Acetaminophen, Diphenhydramine Hydrochloride, Pseudoephedrine Hydrochloride) McNeil Consumer 2014
Children's Tylenol Flu Suspension Liquid (Acetaminophen, Chlorpheniramine Maleate, Dextromethorphan Hydrobromide, Pseudoephedrine Hydrochloride) McNeil Consumer 2015
Infants' Tylenol Cold Decongestant and Fever Reducer Concentrated Drops (Acetaminophen, Pseudoephedrine Hydrochloride) McNeil Consumer 2015
Maximum Strength Tylenol Allergy Sinus Caplets, Gelcaps, and Geltabs (Acetaminophen, Chlorpheniramine Maleate, Pseudoephedrine Hydrochloride) McNeil Consumer 2010
Maximum Strength Tylenol Sinus NightTime Caplets (Acetaminophen, Doxylamine Succinate, Pseudoephedrine Hydrochloride) McNeil Consumer 2012
Vicks Sinex Nasal Spray and Ultra Fine Mist (Phenylephrine Hydrochloride) Procter & Gamble ▣729
Vicks Sinex 12-Hour Nasal Spray and Ultra Fine Mist (Oxymetazoline Hydrochloride) Procter & Gamble ▣729
Zephrex Tablets (Guaifenesin, Pseudoephedrine Hydrochloride) Sanofi-Synthelabo 3091
Zephrex LA Tablets (Guaifenesin, Pseudoephedrine Hydrochloride) Sanofi-Synthelabo 3092

Nasal irritation, symptomatic relief of
Afrin Extra Moisturizing Saline Mist (Sodium Chloride) Schering-Plough ▣734

Nausea
(*see also under* Motion sickness)
Emetrol Oral Solution (Lemon-Mint & Cherry Flavors) (Dextrose, Levulose, Phosphoric Acid) Pharmacia Consumer ▣718
Vistaril Intramuscular Solution (Hydroxyzine Hydrochloride) Pfizer 2738

Nausea, emetogenic, cancer chemotherapy-induced
Anzemet Injection (Dolasetron Mesylate) Aventis 719
Anzemet Tablets (Dolasetron Mesylate) Aventis 722
Kytril Injection (Granisetron Hydrochloride) Roche Laboratories 2986
Kytril Tablets (Granisetron Hydrochloride) Roche Laboratories 2988
Marinol Capsules (Dronabinol) Unimed 3325
Reglan (Metoclopramide Hydrochloride) Robins 2935
Zofran Injection (Ondansetron Hydrochloride) GlaxoSmithKline 1698
Zofran (Ondansetron Hydrochloride) GlaxoSmithKline 1703
Zofran ODT Orally Disintegrating Tablets (Ondansetron) GlaxoSmithKline 1703

Nausea, emetogenic, radiation therapy-induced
Kytril Tablets (Granisetron Hydrochloride) Roche Laboratories 2988
Zofran (Ondansetron Hydrochloride) GlaxoSmithKline 1703
Zofran ODT Orally Disintegrating Tablets (Ondansetron) GlaxoSmithKline 1703

Nausea, postoperative
Anzemet Injection (Dolasetron Mesylate) Aventis 719
Anzemet Tablets (Dolasetron Mesylate) Aventis 722
Phenergan Injection (Promethazine Hydrochloride) Wyeth-Ayerst 3553
Phenergan Suppositories (Promethazine Hydrochloride) Wyeth-Ayerst 3556
Phenergan Syrup (Promethazine Hydrochloride) Wyeth-Ayerst 3554
Phenergan Tablets (Promethazine Hydrochloride) Wyeth-Ayerst 3556
Reglan (Metoclopramide Hydrochloride) Robins 2935
Zofran Injection (Ondansetron Hydrochloride) GlaxoSmithKline 1698
Zofran (Ondansetron Hydrochloride) GlaxoSmithKline 1703
Zofran ODT Orally Disintegrating Tablets (Ondansetron) GlaxoSmithKline 1703

Nausea, severe, control of
Compazine (Prochlorperazine) GlaxoSmithKline 1505
Thorazine (Chlorpromazine Hydrochloride) GlaxoSmithKline 1656
Trilafon (Perphenazine) Schering 3160

Necator americanus infections
Mintezol (Thiabendazole) Merck 2137
Vermox Chewable Tablets (Mebendazole) McNeil Consumer 2017

Necrobiosis lipoidica diabeticorum
Celestone Soluspan Injectable Suspension (Betamethasone Acetate, Betamethasone Sodium Phosphate) Schering 3097
Decadron Phosphate Injection (Dexamethasone Sodium Phosphate) Merck 2081
Hydrocortone Acetate Injectable Suspension (Hydrocortisone Acetate) Merck 2103

Neisseria gonorrhoeae
(*see under* N. gonorrhoeae infections)

Neisseria meningitidis
(*see under* N. gonorrhoeae infections)

Neisseria species infections, ocular
Chloromycetin Ophthalmic Ointment, 1% (Chloramphenicol) Monarch ⊙296
Chloromycetin Ophthalmic Solution (Chloramphenicol) Monarch ⊙297
Chloroptic Sterile Ophthalmic Ointment (Chloramphenicol) Allergan ⊙234
Cortisporin Ophthalmic Suspension (Hydrocortisone, Neomycin Sulfate, Polymyxin B Sulfate, Hydrocortisone, Neomycin Sulfate, Polymyxin B Sulfate) Monarch ⊙297
NeoDecadron Sterile Ophthalmic Solution (Dexamethasone Sodium Phosphate, Neomycin Sulfate) Merck 2144
Poly-Pred Liquifilm Ophthalmic Suspension (Neomycin Sulfate, Polymyxin B Sulfate, Prednisolone Acetate) Allergan ⊙245
Pred-G Ophthalmic Suspension (Gentamicin Sulfate, Prednisolone Acetate) Allergan ⊙247
Terra-Cortril Ophthalmic Suspension (Hydrocortisone Acetate, Oxytetracycline Hydrochloride) Pfizer 2716
TobraDex Ophthalmic Ointment (Dexamethasone, Tobramycin) Alcon 542
TobraDex Ophthalmic Suspension (Dexamethasone, Tobramycin) Alcon 541

Nephroblastoma
(*see under* Wilms' tumor)

Nephrolithiasis, calcium
Urocit-K Tablets (Potassium Citrate) Mission 2232

Nephropathy, diabetic
Captopril Tablets (Captopril) Mylan 2281

Nephrosis, acute, adjunctive therapy
Albumin (Human) 25% (Albumin (human)) Baxter Healthcare 839
Buminate 25% Solution, USP (Albumin (human)) Baxter Healthcare 842
Plasbumin-20 (Albumin (human)) Bayer Biological 940
Plasbumin-25 (Albumin (human)) Bayer Biological 941

Neuralgia
(*see under* Pain, neurogenic)

Neuralgia, glossopharyngeal
Carbatrol Capsules (Carbamazepine) Shire US 3234
Tegretol/Tegretol-XR (Carbamazepine) Novartis 2404

Neuralgia, postherpetic
Lidoderm Patch (Lidocaine) Endo Labs 1319

Neuralgia, trigeminal
Carbatrol Capsules (Carbamazepine) Shire US 3234
Sarapin (Sarraceniaceae) High Chemical 1727
Tegretol/Tegretol-XR (Carbamazepine) Novartis 2404

Neuritis, peripheral, acute
(*see under* Pain, neurogenic)

Neuroblastoma
Adriamycin PFS/RDF Injection (Doxorubicin Hydrochloride) Pharmacia & Upjohn ... 2767

Neurocysticercosis
Albenza Tablets (Albendazole) GlaxoSmithKline ... 1463

Neurodermatitis
(*see under* Lichen simplex chronicus)

Neurological deficits, post-SAH, improvement of
Nimotop Capsules (Nimodipine) Bayer ... 904

Neuromuscular blockade, nondepolarizing, reversal of
Prostigmin Injectable (Neostigmine Methylsulfate) ICN ... 1744
Tensilon Injectable (Edrophonium Chloride) ICN ... 1745

Neutropenia, chemotherapy-induced
Neupogen for Injection (Filgrastim) Amgen ... 587

Neutropenia, febrile, to decrease the incidence of infection
AmBisome for Injection (Amphotericin B) Fujisawa ... 1383
Cipro I.V. (Ciprofloxacin) Bayer ... 893
Cipro I.V. Pharmacy Bulk Package (Ciprofloxacin) Bayer ... 897
Maxipime for Injection (Cefepime Hydrochloride) Elan ... 1285
Neupogen (Filgrastim) Amgen ... 587

Neutropenia-related clinical sequelae, post-bone marrow transplant
Neupogen for Injection (Filgrastim) Amgen ... 587

Niacin, deficiency of
Nicotinex Elixir (Niacin) Fleming ... ▣633

Nicolas-Favre disease
(*see under* Lymphogranuloma venereum)

Nose, itchy
(*see under* Pruritus, rhinopharyngeal, symptomatic relief of)

Nose, runny
(*see under* Rhinorrhea)

Nutrients, deficiency of
Beelith Tablets (Magnesium Oxide, Vitamin B_6) Beach ... 946
EleCare Powder (Amino Acid Preparations, Vitamins with Minerals) Ross ... 3049
Ginsana (Ginseng) Pharmaton ... ▣830
HeartBar (Amino Acid Preparations, Vitamins, Multiple) Cooke ... 1212
Marlyn Formula 50 Capsules (Amino Acid Preparations, Vitamin B_6) Marlyn ... 1997
One-A-Day Garlic Softgels (Garlic Oil) Bayer Consumer ... ▣806
One-A-Day Men's Tablets (Vitamins with Minerals) Bayer Consumer ... ▣808
PediaSure Enteral Formula (Enteral Nutrition) Ross ... 3052
PediaSure Formula (Entereal Nutrition) Ross ... 3052
PhosChol (Phosphatidylcholine) American Lecithin ... 579

Nutrients, deficiency of, stress-induced
(*see under* Nutrients, deficiency of)

Nutrients, deficiency of, surgery-induced
(*see under* Nutrients, deficiency of)

O

Obesity, exogenous
Adipex-P (Phentermine Hydrochloride) Gate ... 1406
Bontril Slow-Release Capsules (Phendimetrazine Tartrate) Amarin ... 576
Desoxyn Tablets (Methamphetamine Hydrochloride) Abbott ... 440
Ionamin Capsules (Phentermine Resin) Celltech ... 1163
Meridia Capsules (Sibutramine Hydrochloride Monohydrate) Abbott ... 481
Xenical Capsules (Orlistat) Roche Laboratories ... 3043

Obsessive compulsive disorder
Luvox Tablets (25, 50, 100 mg) (Fluvoxamine Maleate) Solvay ... 3256
Paxil (Paroxetine Hydrochloride) GlaxoSmithKline ... 1609
Prozac Pulvules, Liquid, and Weekly Capsules (Fluoxetine Hydrochloride) Dista ... 1238
Zoloft (Sertraline Hydrochloride) Pfizer ... 2751

Ocular congestion, symptomatic relief of
Albalon Ophthalmic Solution (Naphazoline Hydrochloride) Allergan ... ⊙225

Ocular inflammation
Poly-Pred Liquifilm Ophthalmic Suspension (Neomycin Sulfate, Polymyxin B Sulfate, Prednisolone Acetate) Allergan ... ⊙245
Pred Mild Sterile Ophthalmic Suspension (Prednisolone Acetate) Allergan ... ⊙249

Ocular inflammation, postoperative
Acular Ophthalmic Solution (Ketorolac Tromethamine) Allergan ... 544
Vexol 1% Ophthalmic Suspension (Rimexolone) Alcon ... ⊙222
Voltaren Ophthalmic Sterile Ophthalmic Solution (Diclofenac Sodium) Novartis Ophthalmics ... ⊙312

Ocular inflammation, steroid-responsive
Decadron Phosphate Sterile Ophthalmic Ointment (Dexamethasone Sodium Phosphate) Merck ... 2083
Decadron Phosphate Sterile Ophthalmic Solution (Dexamethasone Sodium Phosphate) Merck ... 2084
FML Ophthalmic Suspension (Fluorometholone) Allergan ... ⊙236
Lotemax Sterile Ophthalmic Suspension 0.5% (Loteprednol Etabonate) Bausch & Lomb ... ⊙261
Pred Forte Ophthalmic Suspension (Prednisolone Acetate) Allergan ... ⊙246

Ocular inflammation with bacterial infection, steroid-responsive
Blephamide Ophthalmic Ointment (Prednisolone Acetate, Sulfacetamide Sodium) Allergan ... 547
Blephamide Ophthalmic Suspension (Prednisolone Acetate, Sulfacetamide Sodium) Allergan ... 548
Cortisporin Ophthalmic Suspension (Hydrocortisone, Neomycin Sulfate, Polymyxin B Sulfate, Hydrocortisone, Neomycin Sulfate, Polymyxin B Sulfate) Monarch ... ⊙297
FML-S Liquifilm Sterile Ophthalmic Suspension (Fluorometholone, Sulfacetamide Sodium) Allergan ... ⊙238
NeoDecadron Sterile Ophthalmic Solution (Dexamethasone Sodium Phosphate, Neomycin Sulfate) Merck ... 2144
Poly-Pred Liquifilm Ophthalmic Suspension (Neomycin Sulfate, Polymyxin B Sulfate, Prednisolone Acetate) Allergan ... ⊙245
Pred-G Ophthalmic Suspension (Gentamicin Sulfate, Prednisolone Acetate) Allergan ... ⊙247
Pred-G Sterile Ophthalmic Ointment (Gentamicin Sulfate, Prednisolone Acetate) Allergan ... ⊙248
Terra-Cortril Ophthalmic Suspension (Hydrocortisone Acetate, Oxytetracycline Hydrochloride) Pfizer ... 2716
TobraDex Ophthalmic Ointment (Dexamethasone, Tobramycin) Alcon ... 542
TobraDex Ophthalmic Suspension (Dexamethasone, Tobramycin) Alcon ... 541

Ocular redness
All Clear Eye Drops (Naphazoline Hydrochloride, Polyethylene Glycol) Bausch & Lomb, Inc ... ⊙252
All Clear AR Eye Drops (Hydroxypropyl Methylcellulose, Naphazoline Hydrochloride) Bausch & Lomb, Inc ... ⊙252
Clear Eyes ACR Astringent/Lubricant Eye Redness Reliever (Glycerin, Naphazoline Hydrochloride, Zinc Sulfate) Ross ... ⊙322
Clear Eyes Lubricant Eye Redness Reliever (Glycerin, Naphazoline Hydrochloride) Ross ... ⊙322
Murine Tears Plus Lubricant Redness Reliever Eye Drops (Polyvinyl Alcohol, Povidone, Tetrahydrozoline Hydrochloride) Ross ... ⊙323
Naphcon-A Ophthalmic Solution (Naphazoline Hydrochloride, Pheniramine Maleate) Alcon ... 540
Opcon-A Eye Drops (Naphazoline Hydrochloride, Pheniramine Maleate) Bausch & Lomb, Inc ... ⊙253
Vasocon-A Eye Drops (Antazoline Phosphate, Naphazoline Hydrochloride) Novartis Ophthalmics ... ⊙307
Visine Original Eye Drops (Tetrahydrozoline Hydrochloride) Pfizer Consumer ... ⊙315
Visine A.C. Seasonal Relief From Pollen & Dust Eye Drops (Tetrahydrozoline Hydrochloride, Zinc Sulfate) Pfizer Consumer ... ⊙314
Advanced Relief Visine Eye Drops (Dextran 70, Polyethylene Glycol, Povidone, Tetrahydrozoline Hydrochloride) Pfizer Consumer ... ⊙313
Visine L.R. Long Lasting Eye Drops (Oxymetazoline Hydrochloride) Pfizer Consumer ... ⊙315
Visine-A Eye Allergy Relief Eye Drops (Naphazoline Hydrochloride, Pheniramine Maleate) Pfizer Consumer ... ⊙314
Visine-A Eye Drops (Naphazoline Hydrochloride, Pheniramine Maleate) Pfizer Inc., Warner-Lambert Healthcare ... ▣714

Onchocerciasis
Stromectol Tablets (Ivermectin) Merck ... 2185

Onychomycosis
(*see under* Tinea unguium infections)

Ophthalmia, Egyptian
(*see under* Trachoma)

Ophthalmia, sympathetic
Celestone Soluspan Injectable Suspension (Betamethasone Acetate, Betamethasone Sodium Phosphate) Schering ... 3097
Celestone Syrup (Betamethasone) Schering ... 3099
Cortone Acetate Injectable Suspension (Cortisone Acetate) Merck ... 2059
Cortone Acetate Tablets (Cortisone Acetate) Merck ... 2061
Decadron Elixir (Dexamethasone) Merck ... 2078
Decadron Tablets (Dexamethasone) Merck ... 2079
Decadron Phosphate Injection (Dexamethasone Sodium Phosphate) Merck ... 2081
Depo-Medrol Injectable Suspension (Methylprednisolone Acetate) Pharmacia & Upjohn ... 2795
Hydrocortone Tablets (Hydrocortisone) Merck ... 2106
Hydrocortone Phosphate Injection, Sterile (Hydrocortisone Sodium Phosphate) Merck ... 2105
Pediapred Oral Solution (Prednisolone Sodium Phosphate) Celltech ... 1170
Prednisone (Prednisone) Roxane ... 3064
Prelone Syrup (Prednisolone) Muro ... 2273
Solu-Medrol Sterile Powder (Methylprednisolone Sodium Succinate) Pharmacia & Upjohn ... 2855

Ophthalmic angiography, adjunct in
IC-Green Akorn ... ⊙203

Opioids, acute overdosage, diagnosis of
Narcan Injection (Naloxone Hydrochloride) Endo Labs ... 1322

Optic neuritis
Celestone Soluspan Injectable Suspension (Betamethasone Acetate, Betamethasone Sodium Phosphate) Schering ... 3097
Celestone Syrup (Betamethasone) Schering ... 3099
Cortone Acetate Injectable Suspension (Cortisone Acetate) Merck ... 2059
Cortone Acetate Tablets (Cortisone Acetate) Merck ... 2061
Decadron Elixir (Dexamethasone) Merck ... 2078
Decadron Tablets (Dexamethasone) Merck ... 2079
Decadron Phosphate Injection (Dexamethasone Sodium Phosphate) Merck ... 2081
Depo-Medrol Injectable Suspension (Methylprednisolone Acetate) Pharmacia & Upjohn ... 2795
Hydrocortone Tablets (Hydrocortisone) Merck ... 2106
Hydrocortone Phosphate Injection, Sterile (Hydrocortisone Sodium Phosphate) Merck ... 2105
Pediapred Oral Solution (Prednisolone Sodium Phosphate) Celltech ... 1170
Prednisone (Prednisone) Roxane ... 3064
Prelone Syrup (Prednisolone) Muro ... 2273
Solu-Medrol Sterile Powder (Methylprednisolone Sodium Succinate) Pharmacia & Upjohn ... 2855

Ornithosis
(*see under* Chlamydia psittaci infection)

Ossification, heterotopic
Didronel Tablets (Etidronate Disodium) Procter & Gamble Pharmaceuticals ... 2888

Osteitis deformans
(*see under* Paget's disease of bone)

Osteitis fibrosa
(*see under* Osteodystrophy)

Osteoarthritis
Anaprox Tablets (Naproxen Sodium) Roche Laboratories ... 2967
Anaprox DS Tablets (Naproxen Sodium) Roche Laboratories ... 2967
Arthrotec Tablets (Diclofenac Sodium, Misoprostol) Searle ... 3195
Genuine Bayer Professional Labeling (Aspirin Regimen Bayer) (Aspirin) Bayer Consumer ... ▣608
Extra Strength Bayer Arthritis Caplets (Aspirin) Bayer Consumer ... ▣610
Cataflam Tablets (Diclofenac Potassium) Novartis ... 2315
Celebrex Capsules (Celecoxib) Pfizer ... 2676
Celebrex Capsules (Celecoxib) Pharmacia & Upjohn ... 2780
Clinoril Tablets (Sulindac) Merck ... 2053
Dolobid Tablets (Diflunisal) Merck ... 2088
EC-Naprosyn Delayed-Release Tablets (Naproxen) Roche Laboratories ... 2967
Ecotrin Enteric Coated Aspirin Low, Regular and Maximum Strength Tablets (Aspirin) GlaxoSmithKline Consumer ... 1715
Feldene Capsules (Piroxicam) Pfizer ... 2685
Hyalgan Solution (Sodium Hyaluronate) Sanofi-Synthelabo ... 3080
Indocin (Indomethacin) Merck ... 2112
Lodine (Etodolac) Wyeth-Ayerst ... 3528
Lodine XL Extended-Release Tablets (Etodolac) Wyeth-Ayerst ... 3530
Mobic Tablets (Meloxicam) Boehringer Ingelheim ... 1054
Motrin Suspension, Oral Drops, Chewable Tablets, and Caplets (Ibuprofen) McNeil Consumer ... 2002
Naprelan Tablets (Naproxen Sodium) Elan ... 1293
Naprosyn Suspension (Naproxen) Roche Laboratories ... 2967
Naprosyn Tablets (Naproxen) Roche Laboratories ... 2967
Orudis Capsules (Ketoprofen) Wyeth-Ayerst ... 3548
Oruvail Capsules (Ketoprofen) Wyeth-Ayerst ... 3548
Relafen Tablets (Nabumetone) GlaxoSmithKline ... 1617
Synvisc (Hylan G-F 20) Wyeth-Ayerst ... 3596
Tolectin (Tolmetin Sodium) Ortho-McNeil ... 2589
Traumeel Injection Solution (Homeopathic Formulations) Heel ... 1726

Trilisate (Choline Magnesium Trisalicylate) Purdue Frederick 2901
Tylenol (Acetaminophen) McNeil Consumer 2009
Vioxx (Rofecoxib) Merck 2213
Voltaren Tablets (Diclofenac Sodium) Novartis 2315
Voltaren-XR Tablets (Diclofenac Sodium) Novartis 2315

Osteoarthritis, post-traumatic
Celestone Soluspan Injectable Suspension (Betamethasone Acetate, Betamethasone Sodium Phosphate) Schering 3097
Celestone Syrup (Betamethasone) Schering 3099
Cortone Acetate Injectable Suspension (Cortisone Acetate) Merck 2059
Cortone Acetate Tablets (Cortisone Acetate) Merck 2061
Decadron Elixir (Dexamethasone) Merck 2078
Decadron Tablets (Dexamethasone) Merck 2079
Decadron Phosphate Injection (Dexamethasone Sodium Phosphate) Merck 2081
Depo-Medrol Injectable Suspension (Methylprednisolone Acetate) Pharmacia & Upjohn 2795
Hydrocortone Tablets (Hydrocortisone) Merck 2106
Hydrocortone Acetate Injectable Suspension (Hydrocortisone Acetate) Merck 2103
Hydrocortone Phosphate Injection, Sterile (Hydrocortisone Sodium Phosphate) Merck 2105
Pediapred Oral Solution (Prednisolone Sodium Phosphate) Celltech 1170
Prednisone (Prednisone) Roxane 3064
Prelone Syrup (Prednisolone) Muro 2273
Solu-Medrol Sterile Powder (Methylprednisolone Sodium Succinate) Pharmacia & Upjohn 2855

Osteoarthritis, synovitis of
Celestone Soluspan Injectable Suspension (Betamethasone Acetate, Betamethasone Sodium Phosphate) Schering 3097
Celestone Syrup (Betamethasone) Schering 3099
Cortone Acetate Injectable Suspension (Cortisone Acetate) Merck 2059
Cortone Acetate Tablets (Cortisone Acetate) Merck 2061
Decadron Elixir (Dexamethasone) Merck 2078
Decadron Tablets (Dexamethasone) Merck 2079
Decadron Phosphate Injection (Dexamethasone Sodium Phosphate) Merck 2081
Depo-Medrol Injectable Suspension (Methylprednisolone Acetate) Pharmacia & Upjohn 2795
Hydrocortone Tablets (Hydrocortisone) Merck 2106
Hydrocortone Acetate Injectable Suspension (Hydrocortisone Acetate) Merck 2103
Hydrocortone Phosphate Injection, Sterile (Hydrocortisone Sodium Phosphate) Merck 2105
Pediapred Oral Solution (Prednisolone Sodium Phosphate) Celltech 1170
Prednisone (Prednisone) Roxane 3064
Prelone Syrup (Prednisolone) Muro 2273
Solu-Medrol Sterile Powder (Methylprednisolone Sodium Succinate) Pharmacia & Upjohn 2855

Osteodystrophy
Rocaltrol (Calcitriol) Roche Laboratories 2991

Osteodystrophy, renal
Calcijex Injection (Calcitriol) Abbott 411

Osteolytic bone lesions, multiple myeloma-induced
Aredia for Injection (Pamidronate Disodium) Novartis 2309

Osteomalacia
(*see under* Osteodystrophy)

Osteomyelitis, acute hematogenous
Cleocin Phosphate Sterile Solution (Clindamycin Phosphate) Pharmacia & Upjohn 2785

Osteoporosis
Activella Tablets (Estradiol, Norethindrone Acetate) Pharmacia & Upjohn 2764
Actonel Tablets (Risedronate Sodium) Procter & Gamble Pharmaceuticals 2879
Climara Transdermal System (Estradiol) Berlex 958
Estrace Tablets (Estradiol) Warner Chilcott 3361
Evista Tablets (Raloxifene Hydrochloride) Lilly 1915
femhrt Tablets (Ethinyl Estradiol, Norethindrone Acetate) Parke-Davis 2635
Fosamax Tablets (Alendronate Sodium) Merck 2095
Ogen Tablets (Estropipate) Pharmacia & Upjohn 2846
Ortho-Est Tablets (Estropipate) Women First 3464
Ortho-Prefest Tablets (Estradiol, Norgestimate) Ortho-McNeil 2570
Premarin Tablets (Estrogens, Conjugated) Wyeth-Ayerst 3566
Premphase Tablets (Estrogens, Conjugated, Medroxyprogesterone Acetate) Wyeth-Ayerst 3572
Prempro Tablets (Estrogens, Conjugated, Medroxyprogesterone Acetate) Wyeth-Ayerst 3572
Vivelle Transdermal System (Estradiol) Novartis 2412

Osteoporosis, corticosteroid-induced
Actonel Tablets (Risedronate Sodium) Procter & Gamble Pharmaceuticals 2879
Fosamax Tablets (Alendronate Sodium) Merck 2095

Osteoporosis, postmenopausal, treatment adjunct
Miacalcin Injection (Calcitonin-Salmon) Novartis 2373
Miacalcin Nasal Spray (Calcitonin-Salmon) Novartis 2375

Otitis externa
Cipro HC Otic Suspension (Ciprofloxacin Hydrochloride, Hydrocortisone) Alcon 540
Cortisporin-TC Otic Suspension (Colistin Sulfate, Hydrocortisone Acetate, Neomycin Sulfate, Thonzonium Bromide) Monarch 2246
Floxin Otic Solution (Ofloxacin) Daiichi 1219
VōSoL HC Otic Solution (Acetic Acid, Hydrocortisone) Wallace 3356

Otitis externa, symptomatic relief of
Americaine Otic Topical Anesthetic Ear Drops (Benzocaine) Celltech 1162

Otitis externa with inflammation
Decadron Phosphate Sterile Ophthalmic Solution (Dexamethasone Sodium Phosphate) Merck 2084
VōSoL HC Otic Solution (Acetic Acid, Hydrocortisone) Wallace 3356

Otitis media, acute
Amoxil Chewable Tablets (Amoxicillin) GlaxoSmithKline 1471
Amoxil for Oral Suspension (Amoxicillin) GlaxoSmithKline 1471
Amoxil (Amoxicillin) GlaxoSmithKline 1471
Augmentin Chewable Tablets (Amoxicillin, Clavulanate Potassium) GlaxoSmithKline 1482
Augmentin Powder for Oral Suspension (Amoxicillin, Clavulanate Potassium) GlaxoSmithKline 1482
Augmentin Tablets (Amoxicillin, Clavulanate Potassium) GlaxoSmithKline 1485
Augmentin ES-600 Powder for Oral Suspension (Amoxicillin, Clavulanate Potassium) GlaxoSmithKline 1487
Bactrim (Sulfamethoxazole, Trimethoprim) Roche Laboratories 2949
Biaxin/Biaxin XL (Clarithromycin) Abbott 403
Bicillin C-R 900/300 Injection (Penicillin G Benzathine, Penicillin G Procaine) Monarch 2240
Bicillin C-R Injection (Penicillin G Benzathine, Penicillin G Procaine) Monarch 2238
Ceclor (Cefaclor) Lilly 1905
Cedax (Ceftibuten Dihydrate) Biovail 1021
Ceftin (Cefuroxime Axetil) Lifecycle Ventures 1898
Cefzil (Cefprozil) Bristol-Myers Squibb 1076
Ery-Tab Tablets (Erythromycin) Abbott 448
Erythrocin Stearate Filmtab Tablets (Erythromycin Stearate) Abbott 452
Erythromycin Base Filmtab Tablets (Erythromycin) Abbott 454
Floxin Otic Solution (Ofloxacin) Daiichi 1219
Keflex (Cephalexin) Dista 1237
Lorabid Suspension and Pulvules (Loracarbef) Monarch 2251
Omnicef (Cefdinir) Abbott 493
Pediazole Suspension (Erythromycin Ethylsuccinate, Sulfisoxazole Acetyl) Ross 3050
Rocephin Injectable Vials, ADD-Vantage, Galaxy, Bulk (Ceftriaxone Sodium) Roche Laboratories 2993
Septra Suspension (Sulfamethoxazole, Trimethoprim) Monarch 2265
Septra Tablets (Sulfamethoxazole, Trimethoprim) Monarch 2265
Septra DS Tablets (Sulfamethoxazole, Trimethoprim) Monarch 2265
Suprax (Cefixime) Lederle 1877
Vantin Tablets and Oral Suspension (Cefpodoxime Proxetil) Pharmacia & Upjohn 2860
Zithromax Capsules, 250 mg (Azithromycin Dihydrate) Pfizer 2743
Zithromax for Oral Suspension, 300 mg, 600 mg, 900 mg, 1200 mg (Azithromycin Dihydrate) Pfizer 2739
Zithromax Tablets, 250 mg (Azithromycin Dihydrate) Pfizer 2739

Otitis media, acute, adjuvant therapy
Americaine Otic Topical Anesthetic Ear Drops (Benzocaine) Celltech 1162
Auralgan Otic Solution (Antipyrine, Benzocaine, Glycerin) Wyeth-Ayerst 3485
Biomune OSF Express Spray (Homeopathic Formulations) Matol ..... ▣640
Children's Tylenol Sinus Suspension Liquid (Acetaminophen, Pseudoephedrine Hydrochloride) McNeil Consumer 2017
Zephrex Tablets (Guaifenesin, Pseudoephedrine Hydrochloride) Sanofi-Synthelabo 3091
Zephrex LA Tablets (Guaifenesin, Pseudoephedrine Hydrochloride) Sanofi-Synthelabo 3092

Otitis media, adjunctive therapy
Hyland's Earache Tablets (Homeopathic Formulations) Standard Homeopathic ..... ▣765

Otitis media, chronic suppurative
Floxin Otic Solution (Ofloxacin) Daiichi 1219

Otitis media, H. influenzae-induced
(*see under* H. influenzae otitis media)

Otitis media, S. pneumoniae-induced
(*see under* S. pneumoniae otitis media)

Otitis media, S. pyogenes-induced
(*see under* S. pyogenes otitis media)

Otitis media, Staphylococci-induced
(*see under* Staphylococci otitis media)

Ovarian failure, primary
Alora Transdermal System (Estradiol) Watson 3372
CombiPatch Transdermal System (Estradiol, Norethindrone Acetate) Novartis 2323
Esclim Transdermal System (Estradiol) Women First 3460
Estrace Tablets (Estradiol) Warner Chilcott 3361
Menest Tablets (Estrogens, Esterified) Monarch 2254
Ogen Tablets (Estropipate) Pharmacia & Upjohn 2846
Ortho-Est Tablets (Estropipate) Women First 3464
Premarin Tablets (Estrogens, Conjugated) Wyeth-Ayerst 3566
Vivelle Transdermal System (Estradiol) Novartis 2412
Vivelle-Dot Transdermal System (Estradiol) Novartis 2416

Ovaries, castration of
Alora Transdermal System (Estradiol) Watson 3372
CombiPatch Transdermal System (Estradiol, Norethindrone Acetate) Novartis 2323
Estrace Tablets (Estradiol) Warner Chilcott 3361
Menest Tablets (Estrogens, Esterified) Monarch 2254
Ogen Tablets (Estropipate) Pharmacia & Upjohn 2846
Ortho-Est Tablets (Estropipate) Women First 3464
Premarin Tablets (Estrogens, Conjugated) Wyeth-Ayerst 3566
Vivelle Transdermal System (Estradiol) Novartis 2412
Vivelle-Dot Transdermal System (Estradiol) Novartis 2416

Ovary, adenocarcinoma
(*see under* Carcinoma, ovary)

Ovulation, induction of
Clomid Tablets (Clomiphene Citrate) Aventis 735
Follistim for Injection (Follitropin Beta) Organon 2465
Gonal-F for Injection (Follitropin Alfa) Serono 3216
Humegon for Injection (Menotropins) Organon 2468
Novarel for Injection (Chorionic Gonadotropin) Ferring 1347
Ovidrel for Injection (Choriogonadotropin Alfa) Serono 3220
Pergonal for Injection (Menotropins) Serono 3223
Pregnyl for Injection (Chorionic Gonadotropin) Organon 2482
Repronex for Intramuscular and Subcutaneous Injection (Menotropins) Ferring 1347
Serophene Tablets (Clomiphene Citrate) Serono 3226

Oxyuriasis
(*see under* Enterobiasis)

P

P. aeruginosa bacteremia
Ceptaz (Ceftazidime) GlaxoSmithKline 1499

P. aeruginosa bone and joint infections
Cipro I.V. (Ciprofloxacin) Bayer 893
Cipro I.V. Pharmacy Bulk Package (Ciprofloxacin) Bayer 897
Cipro (Ciprofloxacin) Bayer 887
Claforan Injection (Cefotaxime Sodium) Aventis 732
Fortaz (Ceftazidime Sodium) GlaxoSmithKline 1541
Nebcin Vials, Hyporets & ADD-Vantage (Tobramycin Sulfate) Lilly 1955
Pipracil (Piperacillin Sodium) Lederle 1866
Primaxin I.V. (Cilastatin Sodium, Imipenem) Merck 2160
Tazicef for Injection (Ceftazidime) GlaxoSmithKline 1647
Tazicef Galaxy Container (Ceftazidime Sodium) GlaxoSmithKline 1650
Tazicef Pharmacy Bulk Package (Ceftazidime) GlaxoSmithKline 1653
Tazidime Vials, Faspak & ADD-Vantage (Ceftazidime) Lilly 1966

P. aeruginosa infection, cystic fibrosis
TOBI Solution for Inhalation (Tobramycin) Chiron 1206

P. aeruginosa infections
Azactam for Injection (Aztreonam) Elan 1276
Cefizox for Intramuscular or Intravenous Use (Ceftizoxime Sodium) Fujisawa 1390
Cefobid Intravenous/Intramuscular (Cefoperazone) Pfizer 2671
Cefobid Pharmacy Bulk Package - Not for Direct Infusion (Cefoperazone Sodium) Pfizer 2673
Ceptaz (Ceftazidime) GlaxoSmithKline 1499
Cipro I.V. (Ciprofloxacin) Bayer 893

Cipro I.V. Pharmacy Bulk Package (Ciprofloxacin) Bayer.................. 897
Cipro (Ciprofloxacin) Bayer............. 887
Claforan Injection (Cefotaxime Sodium) Aventis.............................. 732
Coly-Mycin M Parenteral (Colistimethate Sodium) Monarch........... 2243
Cortisporin Ophthalmic Suspension (Hydrocortisone, Neomycin Sulfate, Polymyxin B Sulfate, Hydrocortisone, Neomycin Sulfate, Polymyxin B Sulfate) Monarch............................ ⊙297
Floxin I.V. (Ofloxacin) Ortho-McNeil .. 2526
Floxin Tablets (Ofloxacin) Ortho-McNeil 2529
Fortaz (Ceftazidime Sodium) GlaxoSmithKline........................... 1541
Levaquin (Levofloxacin) Ortho-McNeil 2537
Maxipime for Injection (Cefepime Hydrochloride) Elan 1285
Merrem I.V. (Meropenem) AstraZeneca 673
Nebcin Vials, Hyporets & ADD-Vantage (Tobramycin Sulfate) Lilly 1955
Noroxin Tablets (Norfloxacin) Merck 2145
Pipracil (Piperacillin Sodium) Lederle 1866
Primaxin I.M. (Cilastatin Sodium, Imipenem) Merck 2158
Primaxin I.V. (Cilastatin Sodium, Imipenem) Merck 2160
Rocephin Injectable Vials, ADD-Vantage, Galaxy, Bulk (Ceftriaxone Sodium) Roche Laboratories 2993
Tazicef for Injection (Ceftazidime) GlaxoSmithKline 1647
Tazicef Galaxy Container (Ceftazidime Sodium) GlaxoSmithKline 1650
Tazicef Pharmacy Bulk Package (Ceftazidime) GlaxoSmithKline 1653
Tazidime Vials, Faspak & ADD-Vantage (Ceftazidime) Lilly 1966
Timentin Injection- ADD-Vantage Vial (Clavulanate Potassium, Ticarcillin Disodium) GlaxoSmithKline 1661
Timentin Injection-Galaxy Container (Clavulanate Potassium, Ticarcillin Disodium) GlaxoSmithKline 1664
Timentin Injection-Pharmacy Bulk Package (Clavulanate Potassium, Ticarcillin Disodium) GlaxoSmithKline 1666
Timentin for Intravenous Administration (Clavulanate Potassium, Ticarcillin Disodium) GlaxoSmithKline 1658
TOBI Solution for Inhalation (Tobramycin) Chiron 1206
Trovan (Alatrofloxacin Mesylate) Pfizer 2722

P. aeruginosa infections, ocular

Ciloxan (Ciprofloxacin Hydrochloride) Alcon 538
Genoptic Ophthalmic Ointment (Gentamicin Sulfate) Allergan ......⊙239
Genoptic Sterile Ophthalmic Solution (Gentamicin Sulfate) Allergan ....⊙239
Ocuflox Ophthalmic Solution (Ofloxacin) Allergan 554
Poly-Pred Liquifilm Ophthalmic Suspension (Neomycin Sulfate, Polymyxin B Sulfate, Prednisolone Acetate) Allergan ....⊙245
Polytrim Ophthalmic Solution (Polymyxin B Sulfate, Trimethoprim Sulfate) Allergan 556
Pred-G Ophthalmic Suspension (Gentamicin Sulfate, Prednisolone Acetate) Allergan ....⊙247
Pred-G Sterile Ophthalmic Ointment (Gentamicin Sulfate, Prednisolone Acetate) Allergan ...⊙248
TobraDex Ophthalmic Ointment (Dexamethasone, Tobramycin) Alcon 542
TobraDex Ophthalmic Suspension (Dexamethasone, Tobramycin) Alcon 541

P. aeruginosa intra-abdominal infections

Azactam for Injection (Aztreonam) Elan 1276
Cefobid Intravenous/Intramuscular (Cefoperazone) Pfizer 2671
Cefobid Pharmacy Bulk Package - Not for Direct Infusion (Cefoperazone Sodium) Pfizer 2673
Cipro I.V. (Ciprofloxacin) Bayer 893
Cipro I.V. Pharmacy Bulk Package (Ciprofloxacin) Bayer 897
Cipro (Ciprofloxacin) Bayer 887
Maxipime for Injection (Cefepime Hydrochloride) Elan 1285
Merrem I.V. (Meropenem) AstraZeneca 673
Pipracil (Piperacillin Sodium) Lederle.................................... 1866
Primaxin I.M. (Cilastatin Sodium, Imipenem) Merck.......................... 2158
Primaxin I.V. (Cilastatin Sodium, Imipenem) Merck.......................... 2160

P. aeruginosa lower respiratory tract infections

Azactam for Injection (Aztreonam) Elan 1276
Ceptaz for Injection (Ceftazidime) GlaxoSmithKline........................... 1499
Cipro I.V. (Ciprofloxacin) Bayer........ 893
Cipro I.V. Pharmacy Bulk Package (Ciprofloxacin) Bayer..................... 897
Cipro (Ciprofloxacin) Bayer............. 887
Claforan Injection (Cefotaxime Sodium) Aventis 732
Fortaz (Ceftazidime Sodium) GlaxoSmithKline 1541
Maxipime for Injection (Cefepime Hydrochloride) Elan 1285
Nebcin Vials, Hyporets & ADD-Vantage (Tobramycin Sulfate) Lilly 1955
Pipracil (Piperacillin Sodium) Lederle 1866
Tazicef for Injection (Ceftazidime) GlaxoSmithKline 1647
Tazicef Galaxy Container (Ceftazidime Sodium) GlaxoSmithKline 1650
Tazicef Pharmacy Bulk Package (Ceftazidime) GlaxoSmithKline 1653
Tazidime Vials, Faspak & ADD-Vantage (Ceftazidime) Lilly 1966
Trovan (Alatrofloxacin Mesylate) Pfizer 2722

P. aeruginosa meningitis

Ceptaz for Injection (Ceftazidime) GlaxoSmithKline 1499
Fortaz (Ceftazidime Sodium) GlaxoSmithKline 1541
Tazicef for Injection (Ceftazidime) GlaxoSmithKline 1647
Tazicef Galaxy Container (Ceftazidime Sodium) GlaxoSmithKline 1650
Tazicef Pharmacy Bulk Package (Ceftazidime) GlaxoSmithKline 1653
Tazidime Vials, Faspak & ADD-Vantage (Ceftazidime) Lilly 1966

P. aeruginosa otitis externa

Cipro HC Otic Suspension (Ciprofloxacin Hydrochloride, Hydrocortisone) Alcon 540
Floxin Otic Solution (Ofloxacin) Daiichi 1219

P. aeruginosa respiratory tract infections

Cefobid Intravenous/Intramuscular (Cefoperazone) Pfizer 2671
Cefobid Pharmacy Bulk Package - Not for Direct Infusion (Cefoperazone Sodium) Pfizer 2673

P. aeruginosa septicemia

Azactam for Injection (Aztreonam) Elan 1276
Cefobid Intravenous/Intramuscular (Cefoperazone) Pfizer 2671
Cefobid Pharmacy Bulk Package - Not for Direct Infusion (Cefoperazone Sodium) Pfizer 2673
Ceptaz for Injection (Ceftazidime) GlaxoSmithKline 1499
Fortaz (Ceftazidime Sodium) GlaxoSmithKline 1541
Nebcin Vials, Hyporets & ADD-Vantage (Tobramycin Sulfate) Lilly 1955
Pipracil (Piperacillin Sodium) Lederle 1866
Primaxin I.V. (Cilastatin Sodium, Imipenem) Merck 2160
Tazicef for Injection (Ceftazidime) GlaxoSmithKline 1647
Tazicef Galaxy Container (Ceftazidime Sodium) GlaxoSmithKline 1650
Tazicef Pharmacy Bulk Package (Ceftazidime) GlaxoSmithKline 1653
Tazidime Vials, Faspak & ADD-Vantage (Ceftazidime) Lilly 1966
Timentin Injection- ADD-Vantage Vial (Clavulanate Potassium, Ticarcillin Disodium) GlaxoSmithKline 1661
Timentin Injection-Galaxy Container (Clavulanate Potassium, Ticarcillin Disodium) GlaxoSmithKline 1664
Timentin Injection-Pharmacy Bulk Package (Clavulanate Potassium, Ticarcillin Disodium) GlaxoSmithKline 1666
Timentin for Intravenous Administration (Clavulanate Potassium, Ticarcillin Disodium) GlaxoSmithKline........................... 1658

P. aeruginosa skin and skin structure infections

Azactam for Injection (Aztreonam) Elan 1276
Cefobid Intravenous/Intramuscular (Cefoperazone) Pfizer 2671
Cefobid Pharmacy Bulk Package - Not for Direct Infusion (Cefoperazone Sodium) Pfizer.............. 2673
Ceptaz for Injection (Ceftazidime) GlaxoSmithKline............................ 1499
Cipro I.V. (Ciprofloxacin) Bayer........ 893
Cipro I.V. Pharmacy Bulk Package (Ciprofloxacin) Bayer..................... 897
Cipro (Ciprofloxacin) Bayer............. 887
Fortaz (Ceftazidime Sodium) GlaxoSmithKline............................ 1541
Nebcin Vials, Hyporets & ADD-Vantage (Tobramycin Sulfate) Lilly 1955
Pipracil (Piperacillin Sodium) Lederle 1866
Primaxin I.M. (Cilastatin Sodium, Imipenem) Merck 2158
Primaxin I.V. (Cilastatin Sodium, Imipenem) Merck 2160
Rocephin Injectable Vials, ADD-Vantage, Galaxy, Bulk (Ceftriaxone Sodium) Roche Laboratories 2993
Tazicef for Injection (Ceftazidime) GlaxoSmithKline 1647
Tazicef Galaxy Container (Ceftazidime Sodium) GlaxoSmithKline 1650
Tazicef Pharmacy Bulk Package (Ceftazidime) GlaxoSmithKline 1653
Tazidime Vials, Faspak & ADD-Vantage (Ceftazidime) Lilly 1966
Trovan (Alatrofloxacin Mesylate) Pfizer 2722

P. aeruginosa urinary tract infections

Azactam for Injection (Aztreonam) Elan 1276
Cefizox for Intramuscular or Intravenous Use (Ceftizoxime Sodium) Fujisawa 1390
Cefobid Intravenous/Intramuscular (Cefoperazone) Pfizer 2671
Cefobid Pharmacy Bulk Package - Not for Direct Infusion (Cefoperazone Sodium) Pfizer 2673
Ceptaz for Injection (Ceftazidime) GlaxoSmithKline 1499
Cipro I.V. (Ciprofloxacin) Bayer 893
Cipro I.V. Pharmacy Bulk Package (Ciprofloxacin) Bayer 897
Cipro (Ciprofloxacin) Bayer 887
Claforan Injection (Cefotaxime Sodium) Aventis 732
Floxin I.V. (Ofloxacin) Ortho-McNeil ..2526
Floxin Tablets (Ofloxacin) Ortho-McNeil 2529
Fortaz (Ceftazidime Sodium) GlaxoSmithKline 1541
Levaquin (Levofloxacin) Ortho-McNeil 2537
Nebcin Vials, Hyporets & ADD-Vantage (Tobramycin Sulfate) Lilly 1955
Noroxin Tablets (Norfloxacin) Merck 2145
Primaxin I.V. (Cilastatin Sodium, Imipenem) Merck 2160
Tazicef for Injection (Ceftazidime) GlaxoSmithKline 1647
Tazicef Galaxy Container (Ceftazidime Sodium) GlaxoSmithKline 1650
Tazicef Pharmacy Bulk Package (Ceftazidime) GlaxoSmithKline 1653
Tazidime Vials, Faspak & ADD-Vantage (Ceftazidime) Lilly 1966
Timentin Injection- ADD-Vantage Vial (Clavulanate Potassium, Ticarcillin Disodium) GlaxoSmithKline 1661
Timentin Injection-Galaxy Container (Clavulanate Potassium, Ticarcillin Disodium) GlaxoSmithKline 1664
Timentin Injection-Pharmacy Bulk Package (Clavulanate Potassium, Ticarcillin Disodium) GlaxoSmithKline 1666
Timentin for Intravenous Administration (Clavulanate Potassium, Ticarcillin Disodium) GlaxoSmithKline 1658

P. falciparum infections

Aralen Tablets (Chloroquine Phosphate) Sanofi-Synthelabo 3075
Daraprim Tablets (Pyrimethamine) GlaxoSmithKline 1511
Doryx Coated Pellet Filled Capsules (Doxycycline Hyclate) Warner Chilcott.............................. 3357
Lariam Tablets (Mefloquine Hydrochloride) Roche Laboratories 2989
Malarone (Atovaquone, Proguanil Hydrochloride) GlaxoSmithKline.... 1596
Plaquenil Tablets (Hydroxychloroquine Sulfate) Sanofi-Synthelabo .. 3082
Vibramycin Hyclate Capsules (Doxycycline Hyclate) Pfizer 2735

P. inconstans group B urinary tract infections

Claforan Injection (Cefotaxime Sodium) Aventis.............................. 732

P. malariae infections

Aralen Tablets (Chloroquine Phosphate) Sanofi-Synthelabo 3075
Daraprim Tablets (Pyrimethamine) GlaxoSmithKline.......................... 1511
Plaquenil Tablets (Hydroxychloroquine Sulfate) Sanofi-Synthelabo .. 3082

P. mirabilis biliary tract infections

Ancef for Injection (Cefazolin Sodium) GlaxoSmithKline 1474
Ancef Injection (Cefazolin Sodium) GlaxoSmithKline 1474
Kefzol Vials, ADD-Vantage (Cefazolin Sodium) Lilly 1951

P. mirabilis bone and joint infections

Cefizox for Intramuscular or Intravenous Use (Ceftizoxime Sodium) Fujisawa 1390
Claforan Injection (Cefotaxime Sodium) Aventis 732
Keflex (Cephalexin) Dista 1237
Rocephin Injectable Vials, ADD-Vantage, Galaxy, Bulk (Ceftriaxone Sodium) Roche Laboratories 2993

P. mirabilis genitourinary tract infections

Ancef for Injection (Cefazolin Sodium) GlaxoSmithKline 1474
Ancef Injection (Cefazolin Sodium) GlaxoSmithKline 1474
Azactam for Injection (Aztreonam) Elan 1276
Keflex (Cephalexin) Dista 1237

P. mirabilis gynecologic infections

Cefotan (Cefotetan) AstraZeneca 664
Claforan Injection (Cefotaxime Sodium) Aventis 732

P. mirabilis infections

Amoxil Chewable Tablets (Amoxicillin) GlaxoSmithKline 1471
Amoxil for Oral Suspension (Amoxicillin) GlaxoSmithKline 1471
Amoxil (Amoxicillin) GlaxoSmithKline 1471
Ancef for Injection (Cefazolin Sodium) GlaxoSmithKline 1474
Ancef Injection (Cefazolin Sodium) GlaxoSmithKline 1474
Azactam for Injection (Aztreonam) Elan 1276
Bactrim (Sulfamethoxazole, Trimethoprim) Roche Laboratories 2949
Ceclor (Cefaclor) Lilly 1905
Cefizox for Intramuscular or Intravenous Use (Ceftizoxime Sodium) Fujisawa 1390
Cefobid Intravenous/Intramuscular (Cefoperazone) Pfizer 2671
Cefobid Pharmacy Bulk Package - Not for Direct Infusion (Cefoperazone Sodium) Pfizer 2673
Cefotan (Cefotetan) AstraZeneca 664
Ceptaz for Injection (Ceftazidime) GlaxoSmithKline 1499
Cipro I.V. (Ciprofloxacin) Bayer 893
Cipro I.V. Pharmacy Bulk Package (Ciprofloxacin) Bayer 897
Cipro (Ciprofloxacin) Bayer 887
Claforan Injection (Cefotaxime Sodium) Aventis 732
Duricef (Cefadroxil) Bristol-Myers Squibb 1079
Floxin I.V. (Ofloxacin) Ortho-McNeil ..2526
Floxin Tablets (Ofloxacin) Ortho-McNeil 2529
Fortaz (Ceftazidime Sodium) GlaxoSmithKline 1541
Geocillin Tablets (Carbenicillin Indanyl Sodium) Pfizer 2687
Keflex (Cephalexin) Dista 1237
Kefzol Vials, ADD-Vantage (Cefazolin Sodium) Lilly 1951
Levaquin (Levofloxacin) Ortho-McNeil 2537

Maxipime for Injection (Cefepime Hydrochloride) Elan ... 1285
Mefoxin for Injection (Cefoxitin Sodium) Merck ... 2124
Mefoxin Premixed Intravenous Solution (Cefoxitin Sodium) Merck ... 2127
Noroxin Tablets (Norfloxacin) Merck ... 2145
Pfizerpen for Injection (Penicillin G Potassium) Pfizer ... 2707
Pipracil (Piperacillin Sodium) Lederle ... 1866
Rocephin Injectable Vials, ADD-Vantage, Galaxy, Bulk (Ceftriaxone Sodium) Roche Laboratories ... 2993
Septra Suspension (Sulfamethoxazole, Trimethoprim) Monarch ... 2265
Septra Tablets (Sulfamethoxazole, Trimethoprim) Monarch ... 2265
Septra DS Tablets (Sulfamethoxazole, Trimethoprim) Monarch ... 2265
Suprax (Cefixime) Lederle ... 1877
Tazicef for Injection (Ceftazidime) GlaxoSmithKline ... 1647
Tazicef Galaxy Container (Ceftazidime Sodium) GlaxoSmithKline ... 1650
Tazicef Pharmacy Bulk Package (Ceftazidime) GlaxoSmithKline ... 1653
Tazidime Vials, Faspak & ADD-Vantage (Ceftazidime) Lilly ... 1966
Tequin Injection (Gatifloxacin) Bristol-Myers Squibb ... 1110
Tequin Tablets (Gatifloxacin) Bristol-Myers Squibb ... 1110
Trovan (Alatrofloxacin Mesylate) Pfizer ... 2722
Unasyn for Injection (Ampicillin Sodium, Sulbactam Sodium) Pfizer ... 2728
Vantin Tablets and Oral Suspension (Cefpodoxime Proxetil) Pharmacia & Upjohn ... 2860

P. mirabilis infections, ocular
Chibroxin Sterile Ophthalmic Solution (Norfloxacin) Merck ... 2051
Ocuflox Ophthalmic Solution (Ofloxacin) Allergan ... 554
TobraDex Ophthalmic Ointment (Dexamethasone, Tobramycin) Alcon ... 542
TobraDex Ophthalmic Suspension (Dexamethasone, Tobramycin) Alcon ... 541

P. mirabilis intra-abdominal infections
Cipro I.V. (Ciprofloxacin) Bayer ... 893
Cipro I.V. Pharmacy Bulk Package (Ciprofloxacin) Bayer ... 897
Cipro (Ciprofloxacin) Bayer ... 887
Claforan Injection (Cefotaxime Sodium) Aventis ... 732

P. mirabilis lower respiratory tract infections
Azactam for Injection (Aztreonam) Elan ... 1276
Cefizox for Intramuscular or Intravenous Use (Ceftizoxime Sodium) Fujisawa ... 1390
Cefotan (Cefotetan) AstraZeneca ... 664
Ceptaz for Injection (Ceftazidime) GlaxoSmithKline ... 1499
Cipro I.V. (Ciprofloxacin) Bayer ... 893
Cipro I.V. Pharmacy Bulk Package (Ciprofloxacin) Bayer ... 897
Cipro (Ciprofloxacin) Bayer ... 887
Claforan Injection (Cefotaxime Sodium) Aventis ... 732
Fortaz (Ceftazidime Sodium) GlaxoSmithKline ... 1541
Mandol Vials (Cefamandole Nafate) Lilly ... 1953
Rocephin Injectable Vials, ADD-Vantage, Galaxy, Bulk (Ceftriaxone Sodium) Roche Laboratories ... 2993
Tazicef for Injection (Ceftazidime) GlaxoSmithKline ... 1647
Tazicef Galaxy Container (Ceftazidime Sodium) GlaxoSmithKline ... 1650
Tazicef Pharmacy Bulk Package (Ceftazidime) GlaxoSmithKline ... 1653
Tazidime Vials, Faspak & ADD-Vantage (Ceftazidime) Lilly ... 1966

P. mirabilis otitis externa
Cipro HC Otic Suspension (Ciprofloxacin Hydrochloride, Hydrocortisone) Alcon ... 540

P. mirabilis otitis media
Floxin Otic Solution (Ofloxacin) Daiichi ... 1219

P. mirabilis prostatitis
Ancef for Injection (Cefazolin Sodium) GlaxoSmithKline ... 1474
Ancef Injection (Cefazolin Sodium) GlaxoSmithKline ... 1474
Cipro I.V. (Ciprofloxacin) Bayer ... 893
Cipro I.V. Pharmacy Bulk Package (Ciprofloxacin) Bayer ... 897
Cipro (Ciprofloxacin) Bayer ... 887
Geocillin Tablets (Carbenicillin Indanyl Sodium) Pfizer ... 2687
Keflex (Cephalexin) Dista ... 1237

P. mirabilis respiratory tract infections
Cefobid Intravenous/Intramuscular (Cefoperazone) Pfizer ... 2671
Cefobid Pharmacy Bulk Package - Not for Direct Infusion (Cefoperazone Sodium) Pfizer ... 2673

P. mirabilis septicemia
Ancef for Injection (Cefazolin Sodium) GlaxoSmithKline ... 1474
Ancef Injection (Cefazolin Sodium) GlaxoSmithKline ... 1474
Azactam for Injection (Aztreonam) Elan ... 1276
Kefzol Vials, ADD-Vantage (Cefazolin Sodium) Lilly ... 1951
Pipracil (Piperacillin Sodium) Lederle ... 1866

P. mirabilis skin and skin structure infections
Azactam for Injection (Aztreonam) Elan ... 1276
Cefizox for Intramuscular or Intravenous Use (Ceftizoxime Sodium) Fujisawa ... 1390
Ceptaz for Injection (Ceftazidime) GlaxoSmithKline ... 1499
Cipro I.V. (Ciprofloxacin) Bayer ... 893
Cipro I.V. Pharmacy Bulk Package (Ciprofloxacin) Bayer ... 897
Cipro (Ciprofloxacin) Bayer ... 887
Claforan Injection (Cefotaxime Sodium) Aventis ... 732
Floxin I.V. (Ofloxacin) Ortho-McNeil ... 2526
Floxin Tablets (Ofloxacin) Ortho-McNeil ... 2529
Fortaz (Ceftazidime Sodium) GlaxoSmithKline ... 1541
Mandol Vials (Cefamandole Nafate) Lilly ... 1953
Mefoxin for Injection (Cefoxitin Sodium) Merck ... 2124
Mefoxin Premixed Intravenous Solution (Cefoxitin Sodium) Merck ... 2127
Pipracil (Piperacillin Sodium) Lederle ... 1866
Rocephin Injectable Vials, ADD-Vantage, Galaxy, Bulk (Ceftriaxone Sodium) Roche Laboratories ... 2993
Tazicef for Injection (Ceftazidime) GlaxoSmithKline ... 1647
Tazicef Galaxy Container (Ceftazidime Sodium) GlaxoSmithKline ... 1650
Tazicef Pharmacy Bulk Package (Ceftazidime) GlaxoSmithKline ... 1653
Tazidime Vials, Faspak & ADD-Vantage (Ceftazidime) Lilly ... 1966
Trovan (Alatrofloxacin Mesylate) Pfizer ... 2722
Unasyn for Injection (Ampicillin Sodium, Sulbactam Sodium) Pfizer ... 2728

P. mirabilis urinary tract infections
Ancef for Injection (Cefazolin Sodium) GlaxoSmithKline ... 1474
Ancef Injection (Cefazolin Sodium) GlaxoSmithKline ... 1474
Azactam for Injection (Aztreonam) Elan ... 1276
Bactrim (Sulfamethoxazole, Trimethoprim) Roche Laboratories ... 2949
Ceclor (Cefaclor) Lilly ... 1905
Cefizox for Intramuscular or Intravenous Use (Ceftizoxime Sodium) Fujisawa ... 1390
Cefotan (Cefotetan) AstraZeneca ... 664
Ceptaz for Injection (Ceftazidime) GlaxoSmithKline ... 1499
Cipro I.V. (Ciprofloxacin) Bayer ... 893
Cipro I.V. Pharmacy Bulk Package (Ciprofloxacin) Bayer ... 897
Cipro (Ciprofloxacin) Bayer ... 887
Claforan Injection (Cefotaxime Sodium) Aventis ... 732
Duricef (Cefadroxil) Bristol-Myers Squibb ... 1079
Floxin I.V. (Ofloxacin) Ortho-McNeil ... 2526
Floxin Tablets (Ofloxacin) Ortho-McNeil ... 2529
Fortaz (Ceftazidime Sodium) GlaxoSmithKline ... 1541
Geocillin Tablets (Carbenicillin Indanyl Sodium) Pfizer ... 2687
Keflex (Cephalexin) Dista ... 1237
Kefzol Vials, ADD-Vantage (Cefazolin Sodium) Lilly ... 1951
Levaquin (Levofloxacin) Ortho-McNeil ... 2537
Maxipime for Injection (Cefepime Hydrochloride) Elan ... 1285
Mefoxin for Injection (Cefoxitin Sodium) Merck ... 2124
Mefoxin Premixed Intravenous Solution (Cefoxitin Sodium) Merck ... 2127
Noroxin Tablets (Norfloxacin) Merck ... 2145
Rocephin Injectable Vials, ADD-Vantage, Galaxy, Bulk (Ceftriaxone Sodium) Roche Laboratories ... 2993
Septra Suspension (Sulfamethoxazole, Trimethoprim) Monarch ... 2265
Septra Tablets (Sulfamethoxazole, Trimethoprim) Monarch ... 2265
Septra DS Tablets (Sulfamethoxazole, Trimethoprim) Monarch ... 2265
Suprax (Cefixime) Lederle ... 1877
Tazicef for Injection (Ceftazidime) GlaxoSmithKline ... 1647
Tazicef Galaxy Container (Ceftazidime Sodium) GlaxoSmithKline ... 1650
Tazicef Pharmacy Bulk Package (Ceftazidime) GlaxoSmithKline ... 1653
Tazidime Vials, Faspak & ADD-Vantage (Ceftazidime) Lilly ... 1966
Tequin Injection (Gatifloxacin) Bristol-Myers Squibb ... 1110
Tequin Tablets (Gatifloxacin) Bristol-Myers Squibb ... 1110
Vantin Tablets and Oral Suspension (Cefpodoxime Proxetil) Pharmacia & Upjohn ... 2860

P. ovale infections
Aralen Tablets (Chloroquine Phosphate) Sanofi-Synthelabo ... 3075
Daraprim Tablets (Pyrimethamine) GlaxoSmithKline ... 1511
Plaquenil Tablets (Hydroxychloroquine Sulfate) Sanofi-Synthelabo ... 3082

P. vivax infections
Aralen Tablets (Chloroquine Phosphate) Sanofi-Synthelabo ... 3075
Daraprim Tablets (Pyrimethamine) GlaxoSmithKline ... 1511
Lariam Tablets (Mefloquine Hydrochloride) Roche Laboratories ... 2989
Plaquenil Tablets (Hydroxychloroquine Sulfate) Sanofi-Synthelabo ... 3082

P. vulgaris infections
Bactrim (Sulfamethoxazole, Trimethoprim) Roche Laboratories ... 2949
Cefizox for Intramuscular or Intravenous Use (Ceftizoxime Sodium) Fujisawa ... 1390
Cefotan (Cefotetan) AstraZeneca ... 664
Cipro I.V. (Ciprofloxacin) Bayer ... 893
Cipro I.V. Pharmacy Bulk Package (Ciprofloxacin) Bayer ... 897
Cipro (Ciprofloxacin) Bayer ... 887
Claforan Injection (Cefotaxime Sodium) Aventis ... 732
Geocillin Tablets (Carbenicillin Indanyl Sodium) Pfizer ... 2687
Mefoxin for Injection (Cefoxitin Sodium) Merck ... 2124
Mefoxin Premixed Intravenous Solution (Cefoxitin Sodium) Merck ... 2127
Noroxin Tablets (Norfloxacin) Merck ... 2145
Primaxin I.V. (Cilastatin Sodium, Imipenem) Merck ... 2160
Rocephin Injectable Vials, ADD-Vantage, Galaxy, Bulk (Ceftriaxone Sodium) Roche Laboratories ... 2993
Septra Suspension (Sulfamethoxazole, Trimethoprim) Monarch ... 2265
Septra Tablets (Sulfamethoxazole, Trimethoprim) Monarch ... 2265
Septra DS Tablets (Sulfamethoxazole, Trimethoprim) Monarch ... 2265

P. vulgaris infections, ocular
TobraDex Ophthalmic Ointment (Dexamethasone, Tobramycin) Alcon ... 542
TobraDex Ophthalmic Suspension (Dexamethasone, Tobramycin) Alcon ... 541

P. vulgaris skin and skin structure infections
Cipro I.V. (Ciprofloxacin) Bayer ... 893
Cipro I.V. Pharmacy Bulk Package (Ciprofloxacin) Bayer ... 897
Cipro (Ciprofloxacin) Bayer ... 887
Claforan Injection (Cefotaxime Sodium) Aventis ... 732
Primaxin I.V. (Cilastatin Sodium, Imipenem) Merck ... 2160

P. vulgaris urinary tract infections
Bactrim (Sulfamethoxazole, Trimethoprim) Roche Laboratories ... 2949
Cefizox for Intramuscular or Intravenous Use (Ceftizoxime Sodium) Fujisawa ... 1390
Cefotan (Cefotetan) AstraZeneca ... 664
Claforan Injection (Cefotaxime Sodium) Aventis ... 732
Geocillin Tablets (Carbenicillin Indanyl Sodium) Pfizer ... 2687
Mefoxin for Injection (Cefoxitin Sodium) Merck ... 2124
Mefoxin Premixed Intravenous Solution (Cefoxitin Sodium) Merck ... 2127
Noroxin Tablets (Norfloxacin) Merck ... 2145
Primaxin I.V. (Cilastatin Sodium, Imipenem) Merck ... 2160
Rocephin Injectable Vials, ADD-Vantage, Galaxy, Bulk (Ceftriaxone Sodium) Roche Laboratories ... 2993
Septra Suspension (Sulfamethoxazole, Trimethoprim) Monarch ... 2265
Septra Tablets (Sulfamethoxazole, Trimethoprim) Monarch ... 2265
Septra DS Tablets (Sulfamethoxazole, Trimethoprim) Monarch ... 2265

Paget's disease of bone
Actonel Tablets (Risedronate Sodium) Procter & Gamble Pharmaceuticals ... 2879
Aredia for Injection (Pamidronate Disodium) Novartis ... 2309
Didronel Tablets (Etidronate Disodium) Procter & Gamble Pharmaceuticals ... 2888
Fosamax Tablets (Alendronate Sodium) Merck ... 2095
Miacalcin Injection (Calcitonin-Salmon) Novartis ... 2373
Skelid Tablets (Tiludronate Disodium) Sanofi-Synthelabo ... 3088

Pain, abdominal
(*see under* Cramps, abdominal, symptomatic relief of)

Pain, anal
(*see under* Pain, anorectal)

Pain, anogenital
Preparation H Cream (Glycerin, Petrolatum, Phenylephrine Hydrochloride, Shark Liver Oil) Whitehall-Robins ... ▣ 778
Preparation H Cooling Gel (Phenylephrine Hydrochloride) Whitehall-Robins ... ▣ 778
Preparation H (Mineral Oil, Petrolatum, Phenylephrine Hydrochloride, Shark Liver Oil) Whitehall-Robins ... ▣ 778

Pain, anorectal
ELA-Max 5 Cream (Lidocaine) Ferndale ... 1340

Pain, arthritic, minor
Advil (Ibuprofen) Whitehall-Robins ... ▣ 771
Aleve Tablets, Caplets and Gelcaps (Naproxen Sodium) Bayer Consumer ... ▣ 602
Genuine Bayer Tablets, Caplets and Gelcaps (Aspirin) Bayer Consumer ... ▣ 606
Extra Strength Bayer Caplets and Gelcaps (Aspirin) Bayer Consumer ... ▣ 610
Bayer, Aspirin Regimen (Aspirin) Bayer Consumer ... ▣ 606
Extra Strength Bayer Arthritis Caplets (Aspirin) Bayer Consumer ... ▣ 610
Extra Strength Bayer Plus Caplets (Aspirin, Calcium Carbonate) Bayer Consumer ... ▣ 610
BC Powder (Aspirin, Caffeine, Salicylamide) Block ... ▣ 619
Arthritis Strength BC Powder (Aspirin, Caffeine, Salicylamide) Block ... ▣ 619
Ecotrin Enteric Coated Aspirin Low, Regular and Maximum Strength Tablets (Aspirin) GlaxoSmithKline Consumer ... 1715
Aspirin Free Excedrin Caplets and Geltabs (Acetaminophen, Caffeine) Bristol-Myers ... ▣ 628

Excedrin Extra-Strength Tablets, Caplets, and Geltabs (Acetaminophen, Aspirin, Caffeine) Bristol-Myers ▣629
Goody's Extra Strength Headache Powder (Acetaminophen, Aspirin, Caffeine) Block ▣620
Goody's Extra Strength Pain Relief Tablets (Acetaminophen, Aspirin, Caffeine) Block ▣620
Motrin IB Tablets, Caplets, and Gelcaps (Ibuprofen) McNeil Consumer 2002
Orudis KT Tablets (Ketoprofen) Whitehall-Robins ▣778
Percogesic Aspirin-Free Coated Tablets (Acetaminophen, Phenyltoloxamine Citrate) Medtech ▣667
Extra Strength Percogesic Aspirin-Free Coated Caplets (Acetaminophen, Diphenhydramine Hydrochloride) Medtech ▣665
Traumeel Injection Solution (Homeopathic Formulations) Heel 1726
Tylenol (Acetaminophen) McNeil Consumer 2009
Vanquish Caplets (Acetaminophen, Aluminum Hydroxide, Aspirin, Caffeine, Magnesium Hydroxide) Bayer Consumer ▣617

Pain, dental
Advil (Ibuprofen) Whitehall-Robins ▣771
Children's Advil Oral Suspension (Ibuprofen) Whitehall-Robins ▣773
Children's Advil Chewable Tablets (Ibuprofen) Whitehall-Robins ▣773
Infants' Advil Drops (Ibuprofen) Whitehall-Robins ▣773
Junior Strength Advil Tablets (Ibuprofen) Whitehall-Robins ▣773
Junior Strength Advil Chewable Tablets (Ibuprofen) Whitehall-Robins ▣773
Aleve Tablets, Caplets and Gelcaps (Naproxen Sodium) Bayer Consumer ▣602
Baby Anbesol Gel (Benzocaine) Whitehall-Robins ▣774
Junior Anbesol Gel (Benzocaine) Whitehall-Robins ▣774
Anbesol (Benzocaine) Whitehall-Robins ▣774
Genuine Bayer Tablets, Caplets and Gelcaps (Aspirin) Bayer Consumer ▣606
Extra Strength Bayer Caplets and Gelcaps (Aspirin) Bayer Consumer ▣610
Aspirin Regimen Bayer Children's Chewable Tablets (Orange or Cherry Flavored) (Aspirin) Bayer Consumer ▣607
Extra Strength Bayer Plus Caplets (Aspirin, Calcium Carbonate) Bayer Consumer ▣610
BC Powder (Aspirin, Caffeine, Salicylamide) Block ▣619
Arthritis Strength BC Powder (Aspirin, Caffeine, Salicylamide) Block ▣619
Aspirin Free Excedrin Caplets and Geltabs (Acetaminophen, Caffeine) Bristol-Myers ▣628
Excedrin Extra-Strength Tablets, Caplets, and Geltabs (Acetaminophen, Aspirin, Caffeine) Bristol-Myers ▣629
Goody's Extra Strength Headache Powder (Acetaminophen, Aspirin, Caffeine) Block ▣620
Goody's Extra Strength Pain Relief Tablets (Acetaminophen, Aspirin, Caffeine) Block ▣620
Hyland's Teething Gel (Homeopathic Formulations) Standard Homeopathic ▣766
Hyland's Teething Tablets (Belladonna Alkaloids, Homeopathic Formulations) Standard Homeopathic ▣766
Children's Motrin Oral Suspension and Chewable Tablets (Ibuprofen) McNeil Consumer 2006
Children's Motrin Oral Suspension (Ibuprofen) McNeil Consumer ▣643
Infants' Motrin Concentrated Drops (Ibuprofen) McNeil Consumer 2006
Junior Strength Motrin Caplets and Chewable Tablets (Ibuprofen) McNeil Consumer 2006
Motrin IB Tablets, Caplets, and Gelcaps (Ibuprofen) McNeil Consumer 2002
Orudis KT Tablets (Ketoprofen) Whitehall-Robins ▣778
Percogesic Aspirin-Free Coated Tablets (Acetaminophen, Phenyltoloxamine Citrate) Medtech ▣667
Extra Strength Percogesic Aspirin-Free Coated Caplets (Acetaminophen, Diphenhydramine Hydrochloride) Medtech ▣665
Tylenol, Children's (Acetaminophen) McNeil Consumer 2014
Tylenol (Acetaminophen) McNeil Consumer 2009
Vanquish Caplets (Acetaminophen, Aluminum Hydroxide, Aspirin, Caffeine, Magnesium Hydroxide) Bayer Consumer ▣617
Vioxx (Rofecoxib) Merck 2213
Zilactin Baby Gel (Benzocaine) Zila Consumer ▣791

Pain, ear
Americaine Otic Topical Anesthetic Ear Drops (Benzocaine) Celltech 1162

Pain, general
Advil (Ibuprofen) Whitehall-Robins ▣771
Aleve Tablets, Caplets and Gelcaps (Naproxen Sodium) Bayer Consumer ▣602
Alka-Seltzer (Aspirin, Citric Acid, Sodium Bicarbonate) Bayer Consumer ▣603
Alka-Seltzer Lemon Lime Antacid and Pain Reliever Effervescent Tablets (Aspirin, Citric Acid, Sodium Bicarbonate) Bayer Consumer ▣603
Alka-Seltzer Extra Strength Antacid and Pain Reliever Effervescent Tablets (Aspirin, Citric Acid, Sodium Bicarbonate) Bayer Consumer ▣603
Alka-Seltzer PM Effervescent Tablets (Aspirin, Diphenhydramine Citrate) Bayer Consumer ▣605
Genuine Bayer Tablets, Caplets and Gelcaps (Aspirin) Bayer Consumer ▣606
Extra Strength Bayer Caplets and Gelcaps (Aspirin) Bayer Consumer ▣610
Aspirin Regimen Bayer Children's Chewable Tablets (Orange or Cherry Flavored) (Aspirin) Bayer Consumer ▣607
Bayer, Aspirin Regimen (Aspirin) Bayer Consumer ▣606
Genuine Bayer Professional Labeling (Aspirin Regimen Bayer) (Aspirin) Bayer Consumer ▣608
Extra Strength Bayer PM Caplets (Aspirin, Diphenhydramine Hydrochloride) Bayer Consumer ▣611
Aspirin Free Excedrin Caplets and Geltabs (Acetaminophen, Caffeine) Bristol-Myers ▣628
Goody's Body Pain Formula Powder (Acetaminophen, Aspirin, Acetaminophen, Aspirin) Block ▣620
Momentum Backache Relief Extra Strength Caplets (Magnesium Salicylate) Medtech ▣666
Children's Motrin Oral Suspension and Chewable Tablets (Ibuprofen) McNeil Consumer 2006
Children's Motrin Oral Suspension (Ibuprofen) McNeil Consumer ▣643
Infants' Motrin Concentrated Drops (Ibuprofen) McNeil Consumer 2006
Motrin IB Tablets, Caplets, and Gelcaps (Ibuprofen) McNeil Consumer 2002
Percogesic Aspirin-Free Coated Tablets (Acetaminophen, Phenyltoloxamine Citrate) Medtech ▣667
Extra Strength Percogesic Aspirin-Free Coated Caplets (Acetaminophen, Diphenhydramine Hydrochloride) Medtech ▣665
Traumeel Injection Solution (Homeopathic Formulations) Heel 1726
Trilisate (Choline Magnesium Trisalicylate) Purdue Frederick 2901
Tylenol, Children's (Acetaminophen) McNeil Consumer 2014
Junior Strength Tylenol Soft Chews Chewable Tablets (Acetaminophen) McNeil Consumer 2014
Tylenol (Acetaminophen) McNeil Consumer 2009
Extra Strength Tylenol PM Caplets, Geltabs, and Gelcaps (Acetaminophen, Diphenhydramine Hydrochloride) McNeil Consumer 2012
Maximum Strength Tylenol Sore Throat Adult Liquid (Acetaminophen) McNeil Consumer 2013
Vanquish Caplets (Acetaminophen, Aluminum Hydroxide, Aspirin, Caffeine, Magnesium Hydroxide) Bayer Consumer ▣617

Pain, hemorrhoidal
(*see under* Pain, anorectal)

Pain, intractable chronic
(*see also under* Pain, severe)
Infumorph 200 and Infumorph 500 Sterile Solutions (Morphine Sulfate) Elkins-Sinn 1314

Pain, menstrual
Advil (Ibuprofen) Whitehall-Robins ▣771
Aleve Tablets, Caplets and Gelcaps (Naproxen Sodium) Bayer Consumer ▣602
Genuine Bayer Tablets, Caplets and Gelcaps (Aspirin) Bayer Consumer ▣606
Extra Strength Bayer Caplets and Gelcaps (Aspirin) Bayer Consumer ▣610
Extra Strength Bayer Plus Caplets (Aspirin, Calcium Carbonate) Bayer Consumer ▣610
BC Powder (Aspirin, Caffeine, Salicylamide) Block ▣619
Aspirin Free Excedrin Caplets and Geltabs (Acetaminophen, Caffeine) Bristol-Myers ▣628
Excedrin Extra-Strength Tablets, Caplets, and Geltabs (Acetaminophen, Aspirin, Caffeine) Bristol-Myers ▣629
Goody's Extra Strength Headache Powder (Acetaminophen, Aspirin, Caffeine) Block ▣620
Goody's Extra Strength Pain Relief Tablets (Acetaminophen, Aspirin, Caffeine) Block ▣620
Maximum Strength Midol Menstrual Caplets and Gelcaps (Acetaminophen, Caffeine, Pyrilamine Maleate) Bayer Consumer ▣612
Maximum Strength Midol PMS Caplets and Gelcaps (Acetaminophen, Pamabrom, Pyrilamine Maleate) Bayer Consumer ▣613
Motrin IB Tablets, Caplets, and Gelcaps (Ibuprofen) McNeil Consumer 2002
Orudis KT Tablets (Ketoprofen) Whitehall-Robins ▣778
Percogesic Aspirin-Free Coated Tablets (Acetaminophen, Phenyltoloxamine Citrate) Medtech ▣667
Extra Strength Percogesic Aspirin-Free Coated Caplets (Acetaminophen, Diphenhydramine Hydrochloride) Medtech ▣665
Tylenol (Acetaminophen) McNeil Consumer 2009
Women's Tylenol Menstrual Relief Caplets (Acetaminophen, Pamabrom) McNeil Consumer 2013
Vanquish Caplets (Acetaminophen, Aluminum Hydroxide, Aspirin, Caffeine, Magnesium Hydroxide) Bayer Consumer ▣617

Pain, mild
Advil (Ibuprofen) Whitehall-Robins ▣771
Children's Advil Oral Suspension (Ibuprofen) Whitehall-Robins ▣773
Children's Advil Chewable Tablets (Ibuprofen) Whitehall-Robins ▣773
Infants' Advil Drops (Ibuprofen) Whitehall-Robins ▣773
Junior Strength Advil Tablets (Ibuprofen) Whitehall-Robins ▣773
Junior Strength Advil Chewable Tablets (Ibuprofen) Whitehall-Robins ▣773
Aleve Tablets, Caplets and Gelcaps (Naproxen Sodium) Bayer Consumer ▣602
Aspirin Regimen Bayer 81 mg Caplets with Calcium (Aspirin, Calcium Carbonate) Bayer Consumer ▣607
Ecotrin Enteric Coated Aspirin Low, Regular and Maximum Strength Tablets (Aspirin) GlaxoSmithKline Consumer 1715
Excedrin Extra-Strength Tablets, Caplets, and Geltabs (Acetaminophen, Aspirin, Caffeine) Bristol-Myers ▣629
Goody's Body Pain Formula Powder (Acetaminophen, Aspirin, Acetaminophen, Aspirin) Block ▣620
Goody's Extra Strength Headache Powder (Acetaminophen, Aspirin, Caffeine) Block ▣620
Goody's Extra Strength Pain Relief Tablets (Acetaminophen, Aspirin, Caffeine) Block ▣620
Junior Strength Motrin Caplets and Chewable Tablets (Ibuprofen) McNeil Consumer 2006
Motrin IB Tablets, Caplets, and Gelcaps (Ibuprofen) McNeil Consumer 2002
Orudis KT Tablets (Ketoprofen) Whitehall-Robins ▣778
Junior Strength Tylenol Soft Chews Chewable Tablets (Acetaminophen) McNeil Consumer 2014
Tylenol (Acetaminophen) McNeil Consumer 2009

Pain, mild to moderate
Anaprox Tablets (Naproxen Sodium) Roche Laboratories 2967
Anaprox DS Tablets (Naproxen Sodium) Roche Laboratories 2967
Darvon-N/Darvocet-N (Acetaminophen, Propoxyphene Napsylate) Lilly 1907
Darvon Pulvules (Propoxyphene Hydrochloride) Lilly 1909
Darvon Compound-65 Pulvules (Aspirin, Caffeine, Propoxyphene Hydrochloride) Lilly 1910
Darvon-N Tablets (Propoxyphene Napsylate) Lilly 1912
Dolobid Tablets (Diflunisal) Merck 2088
Motrin Suspension, Oral Drops, Chewable Tablets, and Caplets (Ibuprofen) McNeil Consumer 2002
Naprelan Tablets (Naproxen Sodium) Elan 1293
Naprosyn Suspension (Naproxen) Roche Laboratories 2967
Naprosyn Tablets (Naproxen) Roche Laboratories 2967
Orudis Capsules (Ketoprofen) Wyeth-Ayerst 3548
Ponstel Capsules (Mefenamic Acid) First Horizon 1356
Talacen Caplets (Pentazocine Hydrochloride) Sanofi-Synthelabo 3089
Trilisate (Choline Magnesium Trisalicylate) Purdue Frederick 2901
Tylenol with Codeine Elixir (Acetaminophen, Codeine Phosphate) Ortho-McNeil 2595

Pain, mild to moderate, acute musculo-skeletal
Parafon Forte DSC Caplets (Chlorzoxazone) Ortho-McNeil 2582
Soma Tablets (Carisoprodol) Wallace 3353
Soma Compound Tablets (Aspirin, Carisoprodol) Wallace 3354
Soma Compound w/Codeine Tablets (Aspirin, Carisoprodol, Codeine Phosphate) Wallace 3355

Pain, moderate to moderately severe
Lortab (Acetaminophen, Hydrocodone Bitartrate) UCB 3319
Lortab Elixir (Acetaminophen, Hydrocodone Bitartrate) UCB 3317
Maxidone Tablets CIII (Acetaminophen, Hydrocodone Bitartrate) Watson 3399
Norco 5/325 Tablets CIII (Acetaminophen, Hydrocodone Bitartrate) Watson 3424
Norco 7.5/325 Tablets CIII (Acetaminophen, Hydrocodone Bitartrate) Watson 3425
Norco 10/325 Tablets CIII (Acetaminophen, Hydrocodone Bitartrate) Watson 3425
Norco 10/325 Tablets CIII (Acetaminophen, Hydrocodone Bitartrate) Watson 3427
OxyFast Oral Concentrate Solution (Oxycodone Hydrochloride) Purdue Pharma 2916
OxyIR Capsules (Oxycodone Hydrochloride) Purdue Pharma 2916
Percocet Tablets (Acetaminophen, Oxycodone Hydrochloride) Endo Labs 1326
Percodan Tablets (Aspirin, Oxycodone Hydrochloride, Oxycodone Terephthalate) Endo Labs 1327
Percolone Tablets (Oxycodone Hydrochloride) Endo Labs 1327
Roxicodone (Oxycodone Hydrochloride) Roxane 3067
Toradol (Ketorolac Tromethamine) Roche Laboratories 3018
Tylenol with Codeine Tablets (Acetaminophen, Codeine Phosphate) Ortho-McNeil 2595

Tylox Capsules (Acetaminophen, Oxycodone Hydrochloride) Ortho-McNeil ... 2597
Ultram Tablets (Tramadol Hydrochloride) Ortho-McNeil ... 2600
Vicodin Tablets (Acetaminophen, Hydrocodone Bitartrate) Abbott ... 516
Vicodin ES Tablets (Acetaminophen, Hydrocodone Bitartrate) Abbott ... 517
Vicodin HP Tablets (Acetaminophen, Hydrocodone Bitartrate) Abbott ... 518
Zydone Tablets (Acetaminophen, Hydrocodone Bitartrate) Endo Labs ... 1330

Pain, moderate to severe
Astramorph/PF Injection, USP (Preservative-Free) (Morphine Sulfate) AstraZeneca LP ... 594
Buprenex Injectable (Buprenorphine Hydrochloride) Reckitt Benckiser ... 2918
Demerol (Meperidine Hydrochloride) Sanofi-Synthelabo ... 3079
Dilaudid (Hydromorphone Hydrochloride) Abbott ... 441
Dilaudid Oral Liquid (Hydromorphone Hydrochloride) Abbott ... 445
Dilaudid Powder (Hydromorphone Hydrochloride) Abbott ... 441
Dilaudid Rectal Suppositories (Hydromorphone Hydrochloride) Abbott ... 441
Dilaudid Tablets (Hydromorphone Hydrochloride) Abbott ... 441
Dilaudid Tablets - 8 mg (Hydromorphone Hydrochloride) Abbott.. 445
Dilaudid-HP (Hydromorphone Hydrochloride) Abbott ... 443
Duragesic Transdermal System (Fentanyl) Janssen ... 1786
Duramorph Injection (Morphine Sulfate) Elkins-Sinn ... 1312
Kadian Capsules (Morphine Sulfate) Faulding ... 1335
Levo-Dromoran (Levorphanol Tartrate) ICN ... 1734
MS Contin Tablets (Morphine Sulfate) Purdue Frederick ... 2896
MSIR (Morphine Sulfate) Purdue Frederick ... 2898
Nubain Injection (Nalbuphine Hydrochloride) Endo Labs ... 1323
Numorphan (Oxymorphone Hydrochloride) Endo Labs ... 1324
OxyContin Tablets (Oxycodone Hydrochloride) Purdue Pharma ... 2912
Stadol NS Nasal Spray (Butorphanol Tartrate) Bristol-Myers Squibb ... 1108
Talwin Nx Tablets (Naloxone Hydrochloride, Pentazocine Hydrochloride) Sanofi-Synthelabo ... 3090
Vicoprofen Tablets (Hydrocodone Bitartrate, Ibuprofen) Abbott ... 520
Vioxx (Rofecoxib) Merck ... 2213

Pain, muscular, temporary relief of
Aleve Tablets, Caplets and Gelcaps (Naproxen Sodium) Bayer Consumer ... ▣602
Alka-Seltzer (Aspirin, Citric Acid, Sodium Bicarbonate) Bayer Consumer ... ▣603
Alka-Seltzer Lemon Lime Antacid and Pain Reliever Effervescent Tablets (Aspirin, Citric Acid, Sodium Bicarbonate) Bayer Consumer ... ▣603
Alka-Seltzer Extra Strength Antacid and Pain Reliever Effervescent Tablets (Aspirin, Citric Acid, Sodium Bicarbonate) Bayer Consumer ... ▣603
Extra Strength Bayer Caplets and Gelcaps (Aspirin) Bayer Consumer ... ▣610
Bayer, Aspirin Regimen (Aspirin) Bayer Consumer ... ▣606
Extra Strength Bayer Plus Caplets (Aspirin, Calcium Carbonate) Bayer Consumer ... ▣610
Aspirin Free Excedrin Caplets and Geltabs (Acetaminophen, Caffeine) Bristol-Myers ... ▣628
Excedrin Extra-Strength Tablets, Caplets, and Geltabs (Acetaminophen, Aspirin, Caffeine) Bristol-Myers ... ▣629
Goody's Body Pain Formula Powder (Acetaminophen, Aspirin, Acetaminophen, Aspirin) Block ... ▣620
Hyland's Arnisport Tablets (Homeopathic Formulations) Standard Homeopathic ... ▣764

Maximum Strength Midol Teen Caplets (Acetaminophen, Pamabrom) Bayer Consumer ... ▣612
Momentum Backache Relief Extra Strength Caplets (Magnesium Salicylate) Medtech ... ▣666
Traumeel Injection Solution (Homeopathic Formulations) Heel ... 1726
Junior Strength Tylenol Soft Chews Chewable Tablets (Acetaminophen) McNeil Consumer ... 2014
Tylenol (Acetaminophen) McNeil Consumer ... 2009
Vanquish Caplets (Acetaminophen, Aluminum Hydroxide, Aspirin, Caffeine, Magnesium Hydroxide) Bayer Consumer ... ▣617

Pain, neurogenic
BC Powder (Aspirin, Caffeine, Salicylamide) Block ... ▣619
Arthritis Strength BC Powder (Aspirin, Caffeine, Salicylamide) Block ... ▣619
Sarapin (Sarraceniaceae) High Chemical ... 1727
Tegretol/Tegretol-XR (Carbamazepine) Novartis ... 2404
Vanquish Caplets (Acetaminophen, Aluminum Hydroxide, Aspirin, Caffeine, Magnesium Hydroxide) Bayer Consumer ... ▣617

Pain, obstetrical
Nubain Injection (Nalbuphine Hydrochloride) Endo Labs ... 1323

Pain, ocular
Acular PF Ophthalmic Solution (Ketorolac Tromethamine) Allergan ... 544
Voltaren Ophthalmic Sterile Ophthalmic Solution (Diclofenac Sodium) Novartis Ophthalmics ... ⊙312

Pain, oral mucosal and gingival
Cēpacol Maximum Spray (Dyclonine Hydrochloride) Williams ... ▣787
Cēpacol Maximum Strength Sore Throat Spray, Honey Lemon Flavor Williams ... ▣787
Cetacaine Topical Anesthetic (Benzocaine, Butyl Aminobenzoate, Tetracaine Hydrochloride) Cetylite ... 1196

Pain, postoperative, relief of
Chirocaine Injection (Levobupivacaine Hydrochloride) Purdue Pharma ... 2909
Naropin Injection (Ropivacaine Hydrochloride) AstraZeneca LP ... 612
Vioxx (Rofecoxib) Merck ... 2213

Pain, pre- and postoperative, adjunct to
Phenergan Injection (Promethazine Hydrochloride) Wyeth-Ayerst ... 3553

Pain, pre- and postoperative, relief of
Gebauer's Ethyl Chloride (Ethyl Chloride) Gebauer ... 1409
Levo-Dromoran (Levorphanol Tartrate) ICN ... 1734
Mepergan Injection (Meperidine Hydrochloride, Promethazine Hydrochloride) Wyeth-Ayerst ... 3539
Nubain Injection (Nalbuphine Hydrochloride) Endo Labs ... 1323
Toradol (Ketorolac Tromethamine) Roche Laboratories ... 3018

Pain, prepartum
(*see under* Pain, obstetrical)

Pain, severe
Actiq (Fentanyl Citrate) Cephalon ... 1184
Astramorph/PF Injection, USP (Preservative-Free) (Morphine Sulfate) AstraZeneca LP ... 594
Dolophine Hydrochloride Tablets (Methadone Hydrochloride) Roxane ... 3056
Duraclon Injection (Clonidine Hydrochloride) Roxane ... 3057
Duramorph Injection (Morphine Sulfate) Elkins-Sinn ... 1312
Kadian Capsules (Morphine Sulfate) Faulding ... 1335
Levorphanol Tartrate Tablets (Levorphanol Tartrate) Roxane ... 3059
Oramorph SR Tablets (Morphine Sulfate) Roxane ... 3062
Roxanol (Morphine Sulfate) Roxane ... 3066

Pain, short-term management of
Toradol (Ketorolac Tromethamine) Roche Laboratories ... 3018
Ultracet Tablets (Acetaminophen, Tramadol Hydrochloride) Ortho-McNeil ... 2597

Pain, teething
(*see under* Pain, dental)

Pain, topical relief of
Benadryl Cream (Diphenhydramine Hydrochloride, Zinc Acetate) Pfizer Inc., Warner-Lambert Healthcare ... ▣695
Benadryl Gel (Diphenhydramine Hydrochloride) Pfizer Inc., Warner-Lambert Healthcare ... ▣695
Benadryl Spray (Diphenhydramine Hydrochloride, Zinc Acetate) Pfizer Inc., Warner-Lambert Healthcare ... ▣696
BenGay External Analgesic Products (Menthol, Methyl Salicylate) Pfizer Inc., Warner-Lambert Healthcare ... ▣696
Dermoplast Hospital Strength Spray (Benzocaine, Menthol) Medtech ... ▣666
ELA-Max Cream (Lidocaine) Ferndale ... 1340
Emla (Lidocaine, Prilocaine) AstraZeneca LP ... 602
Gebauer's Ethyl Chloride (Ethyl Chloride) Gebauer ... 1409
Lidoderm Patch (Lidocaine) Endo Labs ... 1319
Nature's Own Pain Expeller Cream (L-Arginine, Capsaicin) Strategic Science ... ▣841
Smile's Prid Salve (Homeopathic Formulations) Standard Homeopathic ... ▣766
Thera-Gesic Creme (Menthol, Methyl Salicylate) Mission ... 2233
Vicks VapoRub (Camphor, Menthol) Procter & Gamble ... ▣730
Zilactin-B Gel (Benzocaine) Zila Consumer ... ▣790

Pain, unspecified
Extra Strength Bayer Plus Caplets (Aspirin, Calcium Carbonate) Bayer Consumer ... ▣610
Cataflam Tablets (Diclofenac Potassium) Novartis ... 2315
Ecotrin Enteric Coated Aspirin Low, Regular and Maximum Strength Tablets (Aspirin) GlaxoSmithKline Consumer ... 1715
Lodine (Etodolac) Wyeth-Ayerst ... 3528

Pain, urinary tract
Urimax Tablets (Belladonna Alkaloids, Hyoscyamine Sulfate, Methenamine, Methylene Blue, Phenyl Salicylate, Sodium Biphosphate) Integrity Pharmaceutical ... 1769

Pain associated with arthritis, topical
(*see under* Pain, topical relief of)

Pain associated with sports injuries
(*see under* Pain, topical relief of)

Pain associated with upper respiratory infection
Actifed Cold & Sinus Caplets and Tablets (Acetaminophen, Chlorpheniramine Maleate, Pseudoephedrine Hydrochloride) Pfizer Inc., Warner-Lambert Healthcare ... ▣688
Children's Advil Oral Suspension (Ibuprofen) Whitehall-Robins ... ▣773
Children's Advil Chewable Tablets (Ibuprofen) Whitehall-Robins ... ▣773
Advil Cold and Sinus Caplets (Ibuprofen, Pseudoephedrine Hydrochloride) Whitehall-Robins .. ▣771
Advil Cold and Sinus Tablets (Ibuprofen, Pseudoephedrine Hydrochloride) Whitehall-Robins .. ▣771
Advil Flu & Body Ache Caplets (Ibuprofen, Pseudoephedrine Hydrochloride) Whitehall-Robins .. ▣772
Infants' Advil Drops (Ibuprofen) Whitehall-Robins ... ▣773
Junior Strength Advil Tablets (Ibuprofen) Whitehall-Robins ... ▣773
Junior Strength Advil Chewable Tablets (Ibuprofen) Whitehall-Robins ... ▣773
Aleve Cold & Sinus Caplets (Naproxen Sodium, Pseudoephedrine Hydrochloride) Bayer Consumer ... ▣603

BC Cold Powder (Aspirin, Chlorpheniramine Maleate, Pseudoephedrine Hydrochloride) Block ... ▣619
Benadryl Severe Allergy & Sinus Headache Caplets (Acetaminophen, Diphenhydramine Hydrochloride, Pseudoephedrine Hydrochloride) Pfizer Inc., Warner-Lambert Healthcare ... ▣694
Children's Cēpacol Sore Throat (Acetaminophen, Pseudoephedrine Hydrochloride) Williams ... ▣788
Comtrex Flu Therapy & Fever Relief Daytime Caplets (Acetaminophen, Pseudoephedrine Hydrochloride) Bristol-Myers ... ▣628
Contac Severe Cold and Flu Caplets Maximum Strength (Acetaminophen, Chlorpheniramine Maleate, Dextromethorphan Hydrobromide, Pseudoephedrine Hydrochloride) SmithKline Beecham Consumer .. ▣746
Contac Severe Cold and Flu Caplets Non-Drowsy (Acetaminophen, Dextromethorphan Hydrobromide, Pseudoephedrine Hydrochloride) SmithKline Beecham Consumer ... ▣746
Coricidin 'D' Cold, Flu & Sinus Tablets (Acetaminophen, Chlorpheniramine Maleate, Pseudoephedrine Sulfate) Schering-Plough ... ▣737
Coricidin HBP Cold & Flu Tablets (Acetaminophen, Chlorpheniramine Maleate) Schering-Plough ... ▣738
Coricidin HBP Maximum Strength Flu Tablets (Acetaminophen, Chlorpheniramine Maleate, Dextromethorphan Hydrobromide) Schering-Plough ... ▣738
Coricidin HBP Night-Time Cold & Flu Tablets (Acetaminophen, Diphenhydramine Hydrochloride) Schering-Plough ... ▣738
Drixoral Cold & Flu Extended-Release Tablets (Acetaminophen, Dexbrompheniramine Maleate, Pseudoephedrine Sulfate) Schering-Plough ... ▣740
Children's Motrin Oral Suspension and Chewable Tablets (Ibuprofen) McNeil Consumer ... 2006
Children's Motrin Cold Oral Suspension (Ibuprofen, Pseudoephedrine Hydrochloride) McNeil Consumer ... 2007
Children's Motrin Oral Suspension (Ibuprofen) McNeil Consumer ... ▣643
Children's Motrin Cold Oral Suspension (Ibuprofen, Pseudoephedrine Hydrochloride) McNeil Consumer ... ▣645
Infants' Motrin Concentrated Drops (Ibuprofen) McNeil Consumer ... 2006
Junior Strength Motrin Caplets and Chewable Tablets (Ibuprofen) McNeil Consumer ... 2006
Motrin Sinus Headache Caplets (Ibuprofen, Pseudoephedrine Hydrochloride) McNeil Consumer ... 2005
Sinutab Sinus Allergy Medication, Maximum Strength Formula, Tablets & Caplets (Acetaminophen, Chlorpheniramine Maleate, Pseudoephedrine Hydrochloride) Pfizer Inc., Warner-Lambert Healthcare ... ▣707
Sinutab Sinus Medication, Maximum Strength Without Drowsiness Formula, Tablets & Caplets (Acetaminophen, Pseudoephedrine Hydrochloride) Pfizer Inc., Warner-Lambert Healthcare ... ▣707
Tavist Sinus Non-Drowsy Coated Caplets (Acetaminophen, Pseudoephedrine Hydrochloride) Novartis Consumer ... ▣676
TheraFlu Regular Strength Cold & Sore Throat Night Time Hot Liquid (Acetaminophen, Chlorpheniramine Maleate, Pseudoephedrine Hydrochloride) Novartis Consumer ... ▣676
Children's Tylenol Cold Suspension Liquid and Chewable Tablets (Acetaminophen, Chlorpheniramine Maleate, Pseudoephedrine Hydrochloride) McNeil Consumer ... 2015
Infants' Tylenol Cold Decongestant and Fever Reducer Concentrated Drops (Acetaminophen, Pseudoephedrine Hydrochloride) McNeil Consumer ... 2015

Multi-Symptom Tylenol Cold Complete Formula Caplets (Acetaminophen, Chlorpheniramine Maleate, Dextromethorphan Hydrobromide, Pseudoephedrine Hydrochloride) McNeil Consumer ... 2010
Multi-Symptom Tylenol Cold Non-Drowsy Caplets and Gelcaps (Acetaminophen, Dextromethorphan Hydrobromide, Pseudoephedrine Hydrochloride) McNeil Consumer ... 2010

Pain due to common cold
(*see under* Pain associated with upper respiratory infection)

Pain with gastric hyperacidity
Alka-Seltzer (Aspirin, Citric Acid, Sodium Bicarbonate) Bayer Consumer ... ▣603
Alka-Seltzer Lemon Lime Antacid and Pain Reliever Effervescent Tablets (Aspirin, Citric Acid, Sodium Bicarbonate) Bayer Consumer ... ▣603
Alka-Seltzer Extra Strength Antacid and Pain Reliever Effervescent Tablets (Aspirin, Citric Acid, Sodium Bicarbonate) Bayer Consumer ... ▣603

Palpebral conjunctiva inflammation
Blephamide Ophthalmic Suspension (Prednisolone Acetate, Sulfacetamide Sodium) Allergan ... 548
Cortisporin Ophthalmic Suspension (Hydrocortisone, Neomycin Sulfate, Polymyxin B Sulfate, Hydrocortisone, Neomycin Sulfate, Polymyxin B Sulfate) Monarch ... ⊙297
FML Ophthalmic Ointment (Fluorometholone) Allergan ... ⊙237
FML Ophthalmic Suspension (Fluorometholone) Allergan ... ⊙236
FML Forte Ophthalmic Suspension (Fluorometholone) Allergan ... ⊙235
FML-S Liquifilm Sterile Ophthalmic Suspension (Fluorometholone, Sulfacetamide Sodium) Allergan ... ⊙238
Lotemax Sterile Ophthalmic Suspension 0.5% (Loteprednol Etabonate) Bausch & Lomb ... ⊙261
Poly-Pred Liquifilm Ophthalmic Suspension (Neomycin Sulfate, Polymyxin B Sulfate, Prednisolone Acetate) Allergan ... ⊙245
Pred Forte Ophthalmic Suspension (Prednisolone Acetate) Allergan ... ⊙246
Pred-G Ophthalmic Suspension (Gentamicin Sulfate, Prednisolone Acetate) Allergan ... ⊙247
Pred-G Sterile Ophthalmic Ointment (Gentamicin Sulfate, Prednisolone Acetate) Allergan ... ⊙248
TobraDex Ophthalmic Ointment (Dexamethasone, Tobramycin) Alcon ... 542
TobraDex Ophthalmic Suspension (Dexamethasone, Tobramycin) Alcon ... 541

Pancreas, disseminated adenocarcinoma
(*see under* Carcinoma, pancreas)

Pancreatic cystic fibrosis
Creon 10 Capsules (Pancrelipase) Solvay ... 3251
Creon 20 Capsules (Pancrelipase) Solvay ... 3251
Pancrease Capsules (Pancrelipase) Ortho-McNeil ... 2580
Pancrease MT Capsules (Pancrelipase) Ortho-McNeil ... 2581
Viokase (Pancrelipase) Axcan Scandipharm ... 837

Pancreatic insufficiency
Creon 5 Capsules (Pancrelipase) Solvay ... 3251
Creon 10 Capsules (Pancrelipase) Solvay ... 3251
Creon 20 Capsules (Pancrelipase) Solvay ... 3251
Donnazyme Tablets (Pancreatin) Robins ... 2931
Pancrease Capsules (Pancrelipase) Ortho-McNeil ... 2580
Pancrease MT Capsules (Pancrelipase) Ortho-McNeil ... 2581
Ultrase Capsules (Pancrelipase) Axcan Scandipharm ... 835
Ultrase MT Capsules (Pancrelipase) Axcan Scandipharm ... 835
Viokase (Pancrelipase) Axcan Scandipharm ... 837

Pancreatitis, adjunctive therapy
Albumin (Human) 5% (Albumin (human)) Baxter Healthcare ... 838
Albumin (Human) 25% (Albumin (human)) Baxter Healthcare ... 839
Plasbumin-5 (Albumin (human)) Bayer Biological ... 939
Plasbumin-20 (Albumin (human)) Bayer Biological ... 940
Plasbumin-25 (Albumin (human)) Bayer Biological ... 941

Panic disorder
Klonopin Tablets (Clonazepam) Roche Laboratories ... 2983
Paxil (Paroxetine Hydrochloride) GlaxoSmithKline ... 1609
Xanax Tablets (Alprazolam) Pharmacia & Upjohn ... 2865
Zoloft (Sertraline Hydrochloride) Pfizer ... 2751

Papillitis
(*see under* Optic neuritis)

Paracoccidioidomycosis
Nizoral Tablets (Ketoconazole) Janssen ... 1791

Paralysis agitans
(*see under* Parkinson's disease)

Parkinson's disease
Akineton (Biperiden Hydrochloride) Abbott ... 402
Artane (Trihexyphenidyl Hydrochloride) Lederle ... 1855
Benadryl Parenteral (Diphenhydramine Hydrochloride) Parke-Davis ... 2617
Cogentin (Benztropine Mesylate) Merck ... 2055
Comtan Tablets (Entacapone) Novartis ... 2328
Eldepryl Capsules (Selegiline Hydrochloride) Somerset ... 3266
Levsin/Levsinex/Levbid (Hyoscyamine Sulfate) Schwarz ... 3172
Lodosyn Tablets (Carbidopa) DuPont ... 1251
Mirapex Tablets (Pramipexole Dihydrochloride) Pharmacia & Upjohn ... 2834
NuLev Orally Disintegrating Tablets (Hyoscyamine Sulfate) Schwarz ... 3176
Permax Tablets (Pergolide Mesylate) Elan ... 1299
Requip Tablets (Ropinirole Hydrochloride) GlaxoSmithKline ... 1621
Sinemet Tablets (Carbidopa, Levodopa) DuPont ... 1253
Sinemet CR Tablets (Carbidopa, Levodopa) DuPont ... 1255
Symmetrel (Amantadine Hydrochloride) Endo Labs ... 1328
Tasmar Tablets (Tolcapone) Roche Laboratories ... 3010

Pasteurella pestis
(*see under* Yersinia pestis infections)

Pasteurella tularensis
(*see under* Francisella tularensis infections)

PCP
(*see under* Pneumocystis carinii pneumonia)

Pediculosis, human
Ovide Lotion (Malathion) Medicis ... 2023
Maximum Strength Rid Mousse (Piperonyl Butoxide, Pyrethrins) Bayer Consumer ... ▣617
Maximum Strength Rid Shampoo (Piperonyl Butoxide, Pyrethrum Extract) Bayer Consumer ... ▣616

Pediculosis capitis infestation
Lindane Shampoo USP 1% (Lindane) Alpharma ... 560
Nix Creme Rinse (Permethrin) Pfizer Inc., Warner-Lambert Healthcare ... ▣704
Ovide Lotion (Malathion) Medicis ... 2023
Permethrin Lotion (Permethrin) Alpharma ... ▣602

Pediculosis pubis infestation
Lindane Shampoo USP 1% (Lindane) Alpharma ... 560

Pelvic cellulitis
(*see also under* Infections, gynecologic)
Azactam for Injection (Aztreonam) Elan ... 1276
Ceptaz for Injection (Ceftazidime) GlaxoSmithKline ... 1499
Claforan Injection (Cefotaxime Sodium) Aventis ... 732
Cleocin HCl Capsules (Clindamycin Hydrochloride) Pharmacia & Upjohn ... 2784
Cleocin Phosphate Sterile Solution (Clindamycin Phosphate) Pharmacia & Upjohn ... 2785
Fortaz (Ceftazidime Sodium) GlaxoSmithKline ... 1541
Mefoxin for Injection (Cefoxitin Sodium) Merck ... 2124
Mefoxin Premixed Intravenous Solution (Cefoxitin Sodium) Merck ... 2127
Pipracil (Piperacillin Sodium) Lederle ... 1866
Tazicef for Injection (Ceftazidime) GlaxoSmithKline ... 1647
Tazicef Galaxy Container (Ceftazidime Sodium) GlaxoSmithKline ... 1650
Tazicef Pharmacy Bulk Package (Ceftazidime) GlaxoSmithKline ... 1653
Tazidime Vials, Faspak & ADD-Vantage (Ceftazidime) Lilly ... 1966

Pelvic inflammatory disease
(*see also under* Infections, gynecologic)
Cefizox for Intramuscular or Intravenous Use (Ceftizoxime Sodium) Fujisawa ... 1390
Cefobid Intravenous/Intramuscular (Cefoperazone) Pfizer ... 2671
Cefobid Pharmacy Bulk Package - Not for Direct Infusion (Cefoperazone Sodium) Pfizer ... 2673
Claforan Injection (Cefotaxime Sodium) Aventis ... 732
E.E.S. (Erythromycin Ethylsuccinate) Abbott ... 450
EryPed (Erythromycin Ethylsuccinate) Abbott ... 446
Floxin I.V. (Ofloxacin) Ortho-McNeil ... 2526
Floxin Tablets (Ofloxacin) Ortho-McNeil ... 2529
Mefoxin for Injection (Cefoxitin Sodium) Merck ... 2124
Mefoxin Premixed Intravenous Solution (Cefoxitin Sodium) Merck ... 2127
PCE Dispertab Tablets (Erythromycin) Abbott ... 498
Pipracil (Piperacillin Sodium) Lederle ... 1866
Rocephin Injectable Vials, ADD-Vantage, Galaxy, Bulk (Ceftriaxone Sodium) Roche Laboratories ... 2993
Zithromax for IV Infusion (Azithromycin Dihydrate) Pfizer ... 2748

Pemphigus
Celestone Soluspan Injectable Suspension (Betamethasone Acetate, Betamethasone Sodium Phosphate) Schering ... 3097
Celestone Syrup (Betamethasone) Schering ... 3099
Cortone Acetate Injectable Suspension (Cortisone Acetate) Merck ... 2059
Cortone Acetate Tablets (Cortisone Acetate) Merck ... 2061
Decadron Elixir (Dexamethasone) Merck ... 2078
Decadron Tablets (Dexamethasone) Merck ... 2079
Decadron Phosphate Injection (Dexamethasone Sodium Phosphate) Merck ... 2081
Depo-Medrol Injectable Suspension (Methylprednisolone Acetate) Pharmacia & Upjohn ... 2795
Hydrocortone Tablets (Hydrocortisone) Merck ... 2106
Hydrocortone Phosphate Injection, Sterile (Hydrocortisone Sodium Phosphate) Merck ... 2105
Pediapred Oral Solution (Prednisolone Sodium Phosphate) Celltech ... 1170
Prednisone (Prednisone) Roxane ... 3064
Prelone Syrup (Prednisolone) Muro ... 2273
Solu-Medrol Sterile Powder (Methylprednisolone Sodium Succinate) Pharmacia & Upjohn ... 2855

Pemphigus, possibly effective in
Potaba (Aminobenzoate Potassium) Glenwood ... 1721

Penicillin therapy, an adjuvant to
E.E.S. (Erythromycin Ethylsuccinate) Abbott ... 450
EryPed (Erythromycin Ethylsuccinate) Abbott ... 446
PCE Dispertab Tablets (Erythromycin) Abbott ... 498

Peptic ulcer, adjunctive therapy in
Levsin Drops (Hyoscyamine Sulfate) Schwarz ... 3172
Robinul Forte Tablets (Glycopyrrolate) First Horizon ... 1358
Robinul Injectable (Glycopyrrolate) Robins ... 2940
Robinul Tablets (Glycopyrrolate) First Horizon ... 1358

Peptococcus niger gynecologic infections
Cefotan (Cefotetan) AstraZeneca ... 664
Mefoxin Premixed Intravenous Solution (Cefoxitin Sodium) Merck ... 2127

Peptococcus niger infections
Cefotan (Cefotetan) AstraZeneca ... 664
Mefoxin Premixed Intravenous Solution (Cefoxitin Sodium) Merck ... 2127

Peptococcus niger skin and skin structure infections
Cefotan (Cefotetan) AstraZeneca ... 664
Mefoxin Premixed Intravenous Solution (Cefoxitin Sodium) Merck ... 2127

Peptococcus species bone and joint infections
Cefizox for Intramuscular or Intravenous Use (Ceftizoxime Sodium) Fujisawa ... 1390

Peptococcus species gynecologic infections
Claforan Injection (Cefotaxime Sodium) Aventis ... 732
Primaxin I.V. (Cilastatin Sodium, Imipenem) Merck ... 2160

Peptococcus species infections
Cefizox for Intramuscular or Intravenous Use (Ceftizoxime Sodium) Fujisawa ... 1390
Claforan Injection (Cefotaxime Sodium) Aventis ... 732
Primaxin I.V. (Cilastatin Sodium, Imipenem) Merck ... 2160

Peptococcus species intra-abdominal infections
Cefizox for Intramuscular or Intravenous Use (Ceftizoxime Sodium) Fujisawa ... 1390
Claforan Injection (Cefotaxime Sodium) Aventis ... 732
Primaxin I.M. (Cilastatin Sodium, Imipenem) Merck ... 2158
Primaxin I.V. (Cilastatin Sodium, Imipenem) Merck ... 2160

Peptococcus species skin and skin structure infections
Cefizox for Intramuscular or Intravenous Use (Ceftizoxime Sodium) Fujisawa ... 1390
Claforan Injection (Cefotaxime Sodium) Aventis ... 732
Primaxin I.V. (Cilastatin Sodium, Imipenem) Merck ... 2160

Peptostreptococcus species bone and joint infections
Cefizox for Intramuscular or Intravenous Use (Ceftizoxime Sodium) Fujisawa ... 1390

Peptostreptococcus species endometritis
Mefoxin for Injection (Cefoxitin Sodium) Merck ... 2124
Mefoxin Premixed Intravenous Solution (Cefoxitin Sodium) Merck ... 2127

Peptostreptococcus species gynecologic infections
Cefotan (Cefotetan) AstraZeneca ... 664
Claforan Injection (Cefotaxime Sodium) Aventis ... 732
Mefoxin for Injection (Cefoxitin Sodium) Merck ... 2124
Mefoxin Premixed Intravenous Solution (Cefoxitin Sodium) Merck ... 2127
Primaxin I.M. (Cilastatin Sodium, Imipenem) Merck ... 2158
Primaxin I.V. (Cilastatin Sodium, Imipenem) Merck ... 2160

Peptostreptococcus species infections

Cefizox for Intramuscular or Intravenous Use (Ceftizoxime Sodium) Fujisawa 1390
Cefotan (Cefotetan) AstraZeneca 664
Claforan Injection (Cefotaxime Sodium) Aventis 732
Mefoxin for Injection (Cefoxitin Sodium) Merck 2124
Mefoxin Premixed Intravenous Solution (Cefoxitin Sodium) Merck 2127
Merrem I.V. (Meropenem) AstraZeneca 673
Primaxin I.M. (Cilastatin Sodium, Imipenem) Merck 2158
Primaxin I.V. (Cilastatin Sodium, Imipenem) Merck 2160
Rocephin Injectable Vials, ADD-Vantage, Galaxy, Bulk (Ceftriaxone Sodium) Roche Laboratories 2993
Trovan (Alatrofloxacin Mesylate) Pfizer 2722

Peptostreptococcus species intra-abdominal infections

Cefizox for Intramuscular or Intravenous Use (Ceftizoxime Sodium) Fujisawa 1390
Claforan Injection (Cefotaxime Sodium) Aventis 732
Merrem I.V. (Meropenem) AstraZeneca 673
Primaxin I.M. (Cilastatin Sodium, Imipenem) Merck 2158
Primaxin I.V. (Cilastatin Sodium, Imipenem) Merck 2160
Rocephin Injectable Vials, ADD-Vantage, Galaxy, Bulk (Ceftriaxone Sodium) Roche Laboratories 2993
Trovan (Alatrofloxacin Mesylate) Pfizer 2722

Peptostreptococcus species peritonitis

Merrem I.V. (Meropenem) AstraZeneca 673

Peptostreptococcus species skin and skin structure infections

Cefizox for Intramuscular or Intravenous Use (Ceftizoxime Sodium) Fujisawa 1390
Cefotan (Cefotetan) AstraZeneca 664
Claforan Injection (Cefotaxime Sodium) Aventis 732
Mefoxin for Injection (Cefoxitin Sodium) Merck 2124
Mefoxin Premixed Intravenous Solution (Cefoxitin Sodium) Merck 2127
Primaxin I.V. (Cilastatin Sodium, Imipenem) Merck 2160
Rocephin Injectable Vials, ADD-Vantage, Galaxy, Bulk (Ceftriaxone Sodium) Roche Laboratories 2993

Periodontitis, adjunct to scaling and planing

Periostat Tablets (Doxycycline Hyclate) CollaGenex 1208

Peripheral blood progenitor cell transplantation
(*see under* Hematopoietic progenitor cells, mobilization of)

Peritonitis
(*see also under* Infections, intra-abdominal)

Azactam for Injection (Aztreonam) Elan 1276
Cefobid Intravenous/Intramuscular (Cefoperazone) Pfizer 2671
Cefobid Pharmacy Bulk Package - Not for Direct Infusion (Cefoperazone Sodium) Pfizer 2673
Ceptaz for Injection (Ceftazidime) GlaxoSmithKline 1499
Claforan Injection (Cefotaxime Sodium) Aventis 732
Cleocin HCl Capsules (Clindamycin Hydrochloride) Pharmacia & Upjohn 2784
Cleocin Phosphate Sterile Solution (Clindamycin Phosphate) Pharmacia & Upjohn 2785
Diflucan Tablets, Injection, and Oral Suspension (Fluconazole) Pfizer 2681
Fortaz (Ceftazidime Sodium) GlaxoSmithKline 1541
Mandol Vials (Cefamandole Nafate) Lilly 1953
Mefoxin for Injection (Cefoxitin Sodium) Merck 2124
Mefoxin Premixed Intravenous Solution (Cefoxitin Sodium) Merck 2127
Nebcin Vials, Hyporets & ADD-Vantage (Tobramycin Sulfate) Lilly 1955
Tazicef for Injection (Ceftazidime) GlaxoSmithKline 1647
Tazicef Galaxy Container (Ceftazidime Sodium) GlaxoSmithKline 1650
Tazicef Pharmacy Bulk Package (Ceftazidime) GlaxoSmithKline 1653
Tazidime Vials, Faspak & ADD-Vantage (Ceftazidime) Lilly 1966
Timentin Injection- ADD-Vantage Vial (Clavulanate Potassium, Ticarcillin Disodium) GlaxoSmithKline 1661
Timentin Injection-Galaxy Container (Clavulanate Potassium, Ticarcillin Disodium) GlaxoSmithKline 1664
Timentin Injection-Pharmacy Bulk Package (Clavulanate Potassium, Ticarcillin Disodium) GlaxoSmithKline 1666
Timentin for Intravenous Administration (Clavulanate Potassium, Ticarcillin Disodium) GlaxoSmithKline 1658

Peritonitis, adjunctive therapy

Albumin (Human) 5% (Albumin (human)) Baxter Healthcare 838
Albumin (Human) 25% (Albumin (human)) Baxter Healthcare 839
Plasbumin-5 (Albumin (human)) Bayer Biological 939
Plasbumin-20 (Albumin (human)) Bayer Biological 940
Plasbumin-25 (Albumin (human)) Bayer Biological 941

Peritonitis, candidal

Diflucan Tablets, Injection, and Oral Suspension (Fluconazole) Pfizer 2681

Pertussis

E.E.S. (Erythromycin Ethylsuccinate) Abbott 450
EryPed (Erythromycin Ethylsuccinate) Abbott 446
Ery-Tab Tablets (Erythromycin) Abbott 448
Erythrocin Stearate Filmtab Tablets (Erythromycin Stearate) Abbott 452
Erythromycin Base Filmtab Tablets (Erythromycin) Abbott 454
Erythromycin Delayed-Release Capsules, USP (Erythromycin) Abbott 455
PCE Dispertab Tablets (Erythromycin) Abbott 498

Petit mal epilepsy
(*see under* Seizures, generalized, absence)

Peyronie's disease, possibly effective in

Potaba (Aminobenzoate Potassium) Glenwood 1721

Pharyngitis, symptomatic relief of

Children's Advil Oral Suspension (Ibuprofen) Whitehall-Robins .... ▣773
Children's Advil Chewable Tablets (Ibuprofen) Whitehall-Robins .... ▣773
Infants' Advil Drops (Ibuprofen) Whitehall-Robins .... ▣773
Junior Strength Advil Tablets (Ibuprofen) Whitehall-Robins .... ▣773
Junior Strength Advil Chewable Tablets (Ibuprofen) Whitehall-Robins .... ▣773
Aspirin Regimen Bayer Children's Chewable Tablets (Orange or Cherry Flavored) (Aspirin) Bayer Consumer .... ▣607
Benadryl Allergy/Cold Tablets (Acetaminophen, Diphenhydramine Hydrochloride, Pseudoephedrine Hydrochloride) Pfizer Inc., Warner-Lambert Healthcare .... ▣691
Celestial Seasonings Soothers Throat Drops (Menthol, Pectin) Pfizer Inc., Warner-Lambert Group .... ▣685
Children's Cēpacol Sore Throat (Acetaminophen, Pseudoephedrine Hydrochloride) Williams .... ▣788
Cēpacol Maximum Strength Sugar Free Sore Throat Lozenges, Cherry Flavor (Benzocaine, Menthol) Williams .... ▣787
Cēpacol Maximum Strength Sugar Free Sore Throat Lozenges, Cool Mint Flavor (Benzocaine, Menthol) Williams... ▣787
Cēpacol Maximum Strength Sore Throat Lozenges, Cherry Flavor (Benzocaine, Menthol) Williams .... ▣787
Cēpacol Maximum Strength Sore Throat Lozenges, Mint Flavor (Benzocaine, Menthol) Williams... ▣787
Cēpacol Regular Strength Sore Throat Lozenges, Cherry Flavor (Menthol) Williams .... ▣787
Cēpacol Regular Strength Sore Throat Lozenges, Original Mint Flavor (Menthol) Williams .... ▣787
Cēpacol Maximum Spray (Dyclonine Hydrochloride) Williams .... ▣787
Cēpacol Maximum Strength Sore Throat Spray, Honey Lemon Flavor Williams .... ▣787
Junior Strength Motrin Caplets and Chewable Tablets (Ibuprofen) McNeil Consumer 2006
Relief Nasal & Throat Spray (Homeopathic Formulations) Body Wise .... ▣811
TheraFlu Regular Strength Cold & Sore Throat Night Time Hot Liquid (Acetaminophen, Chlorpheniramine Maleate, Pseudoephedrine Hydrochloride) Novartis Consumer .... ▣676
TheraFlu Maximum Strength Flu & Cough Night Time Hot Liquid (Acetaminophen, Chlorpheniramine Maleate, Dextromethorphan Hydrobromide, Pseudoephedrine Hydrochloride) Novartis Consumer .... ▣678
TheraFlu Maximum Strength Flu & Sore Throat Night Time Hot Liquid (Acetaminophen, Chlorpheniramine Maleate, Pseudoephedrine Hydrochloride) Novartis Consumer .... ▣677
Children's Tylenol Allergy-D Liquid (Acetaminophen, Diphenhydramine Hydrochloride, Pseudoephedrine Hydrochloride) McNeil Consumer 2014
Children's Tylenol Cold Plus Cough Suspension Liquid and Chewable Tablets (Acetaminophen, Chlorpheniramine Maleate, Dextromethorphan Hydrobromide, Pseudoephedrine Hydrochloride) McNeil Consumer 2015
Infants' Tylenol Cold Decongestant and Fever Reducer Concentrated Drops Plus Cough (Acetaminophen, Dextromethorphan Hydrobromide, Pseudoephedrine Hydrochloride) McNeil Consumer 2015
Tylenol Severe Allergy Caplets (Acetaminophen, Diphenhydramine Hydrochloride) McNeil Consumer 2010
Multi-Symptom Tylenol Cold Complete Formula Caplets (Acetaminophen, Chlorpheniramine Maleate, Dextromethorphan Hydrobromide, Pseudoephedrine Hydrochloride) McNeil Consumer 2010
Multi-Symptom Tylenol Cold Non-Drowsy Caplets and Gelcaps (Acetaminophen, Dextromethorphan Hydrobromide, Pseudoephedrine Hydrochloride) McNeil Consumer 2010
Multi-Symptom Tylenol Cold Severe Congestion Non-Drowsy Caplets (Acetaminophen, Dextromethorphan Hydrobromide, Guaifenesin, Pseudoephedrine Hydrochloride) McNeil Consumer 2011
Maximum Strength Tylenol Sore Throat Adult Liquid (Acetaminophen) McNeil Consumer 2013

Pharyngitis, treatment of

Biaxin/Biaxin XL (Clarithromycin) Abbott 403
Ceclor CD Tablets (Cefaclor) Elan ... 1279
Ceclor (Cefaclor) Lilly 1905
Cedax (Ceftibuten Dihydrate) Biovail 1021
Ceftin (Cefuroxime Axetil) Lifecycle Ventures 1898
Cefzil (Cefprozil) Bristol-Myers Squibb 1076
Duricef (Cefadroxil) Bristol-Myers Squibb 1079
Dynabac Tablets (Dirithromycin) Muro 2269
E.E.S. (Erythromycin Ethylsuccinate) Abbott 450
EryPed (Erythromycin Ethylsuccinate) Abbott 446
Ery-Tab Tablets (Erythromycin) Abbott 448
Erythrocin Stearate Filmtab Tablets (Erythromycin Stearate) Abbott 452
Erythromycin Base Filmtab Tablets (Erythromycin) Abbott 454
Lorabid Suspension and Pulvules (Loracarbef) Monarch 2251
Omnicef (Cefdinir) Abbott 493
PCE Dispertab Tablets (Erythromycin) Abbott 498
Permapen Isoject (Penicillin G Benzathine) Pfizer 2706
Suprax (Cefixime) Lederle 1877
Vantin Tablets and Oral Suspension (Cefpodoxime Proxetil) Pharmacia & Upjohn 2860
Zithromax (Azithromycin Dihydrate) Pfizer 2743
Zithromax for Oral Suspension, 300 mg, 600 mg, 900 mg, 1200 mg (Azithromycin Dihydrate) Pfizer 2739
Zithromax Tablets, 250 mg (Azithromycin Dihydrate) Pfizer 2739
Zithromax Tablets, 600 mg (Azithromycin Dihydrate) Pfizer 2743

Pheochromocytoma

Demser Capsules (Metyrosine) Merck 2085
Dibenzyline Capsules (Phenoxybenzamine Hydrochloride) WellSpring 3457

Pheochromocytoma, adjunctive therapy

Demser Capsules (Metyrosine) Merck 2085
Inderal (Propranolol Hydrochloride) Wyeth-Ayerst 3513

Phosphorus deficiency
(*see under* Hypophosphatemia)

Photophobia

Acular PF Ophthalmic Solution (Ketorolac Tromethamine) Allergan 544
Voltaren Ophthalmic Sterile Ophthalmic Solution (Diclofenac Sodium) Novartis Ophthalmics .... ⊙312

Phycomycosis
(*see under* Zygomycosis)

Piles
(*see under* Hemorrhoids)

Pinta

Bicillin L-A Injection (Penicillin G Benzathine) Monarch 2242
Permapen Isoject (Penicillin G Benzathine) Pfizer 2706

Pinworm infestation
(*see under* Enterobiasis)

Pityrosporon orbiculare infections

Loprox Cream (Ciclopirox Olamine) Medicis 2021
Loprox Gel (Ciclopirox) Medicis 2022
Loprox Lotion (Ciclopirox Olamine) Medicis 2021
Lotrimin (Clotrimazole) Schering 3128
Nizoral 2% Cream (Ketoconazole) Janssen 3620
Nizoral 2% Shampoo (Ketoconazole) McNeil Consumer 2007
Oxistat (Oxiconazole Nitrate) Elan ... 1298
Selsun Rx 2.5% Lotion, USP (Selenium Sulfide) Ross 3053

Plague

Dynacin Capsules (Minocycline Hydrochloride) Medicis 2019
Minocin Oral Suspension (Minocycline Hydrochloride) Lederle 1865
Minocin Pellet-Filled Capsules (Minocycline Hydrochloride) Lederle 1863
Monodox Capsules (Doxycycline Monohydrate) Oclassen 2442

Plasmodium infection
(*see under* P. falciparum infections; P. malariae infections; P. ovale infections; P. vivax infections)

Platelet transfusions, reduction of the need for

Neumega for Injection (Oprelvekin) Genetics 1434

PMDD
(*see under* Dysphoric disorder, premenstrual)

PMS
(*see under* Menstrual syndrome, pre-, management of)

Pneumococcal disease, immunization against
Pneumovax 23 (Pneumococcal Vaccine, Polyvalent) Merck 2156
Pnu-Imune 23 (Pneumococcal Vaccine, Polyvalent) Lederle 1868
Prevnar for Injection (Pneumococcal vaccine, diphtheria conjugate) Lederle 1870

Pneumocystis carinii pneumonia
Bactrim (Sulfamethoxazole, Trimethoprim) Roche Laboratories 2949
Mepron Suspension (Atovaquone) GlaxoSmithKline 1598
Septra Suspension (Sulfamethoxazole, Trimethoprim) Monarch 2265
Septra Tablets (Sulfamethoxazole, Trimethoprim) Monarch 2265
Septra DS Tablets (Sulfamethoxazole, Trimethoprim) Monarch 2265

Pneumonia
(*see also under* Infections, lower respiratory tract)
Avelox Tablets (Moxifloxacin Hydrochloride) Bayer 879
Azactam for Injection (Aztreonam) Elan 1276
Biaxin/Biaxin XL (Clarithromycin) Abbott 403
Bicillin C-R 900/300 Injection (Penicillin G Benzathine, Penicillin G Procaine) Monarch 2240
Bicillin C-R Injection (Penicillin G Benzathine, Penicillin G Procaine) Monarch 2238
Ceclor (Cefaclor) Lilly 1905
Ceptaz for Injection (Ceftazidime) GlaxoSmithKline 1499
Claforan Injection (Cefotaxime Sodium) Aventis 732
Cleocin HCl Capsules (Clindamycin Hydrochloride) Pharmacia & Upjohn 2784
Cleocin Phosphate Sterile Solution (Clindamycin Phosphate) Pharmacia & Upjohn 2785
Dynabac Tablets (Dirithromycin) Muro 2269
Ery-Tab Tablets (Erythromycin) Abbott 448
Erythrocin Stearate Filmtab Tablets (Erythromycin Stearate) Abbott 452
Erythromycin Base Filmtab Tablets (Erythromycin) Abbott 454
Floxin I.V. (Ofloxacin) Ortho-McNeil .. 2526
Floxin Tablets (Ofloxacin) Ortho-McNeil 2529
Fortaz (Ceftazidime Sodium) GlaxoSmithKline 1541
Kefurox Vials, ADD-Vantage (Cefuroxime Sodium) Lilly 1948
Levaquin (Levofloxacin) Ortho-McNeil 2537
Lorabid Suspension and Pulvules (Loracarbef) Monarch 2251
Mandol Vials (Cefamandole Nafate) Lilly 1953
Maxipime for Injection (Cefepime Hydrochloride) Elan 1285
Mefoxin for Injection (Cefoxitin Sodium) Merck 2124
Mefoxin Premixed Intravenous Solution (Cefoxitin Sodium) Merck 2127
Omnicef (Cefdinir) Abbott 493
Pfizerpen for Injection (Penicillin G Potassium) Pfizer 2707
Tao Capsules (Troleandomycin) Pfizer 2716
Tazicef for Injection (Ceftazidime) GlaxoSmithKline 1647
Tazicef Galaxy Container (Ceftazidime Sodium) GlaxoSmithKline 1650
Tazicef Pharmacy Bulk Package (Ceftazidime) GlaxoSmithKline 1653
Tazidime Vials, Faspak & ADD-Vantage (Ceftazidime) Lilly 1966
Tequin Injection (Gatifloxacin) Bristol-Myers Squibb 1110
Tequin Tablets (Gatifloxacin) Bristol-Myers Squibb 1110
Trovan (Alatrofloxacin Mesylate) Pfizer 2722
Vantin Tablets and Oral Suspension (Cefpodoxime Proxetil) Pharmacia & Upjohn 2860
Vibramycin Hyclate Intravenous (Doxycycline Hyclate) Pfizer 2737
Zinacef Injection (Cefuroxime) GlaxoSmithKline 1696
Zinacef for Injection (Cefuroxime) GlaxoSmithKline 1696
Zithromax Capsules, 250 mg (Azithromycin Dihydrate) Pfizer..... 2743
Zithromax for IV Infusion (Azithromycin Dihydrate) Pfizer 2748
Zithromax for Oral Suspension, 1 g (Azithromycin Dihydrate) Pfizer . 2743
Zithromax for Oral Suspension, 300 mg, 600 mg, 900 mg, 1200 mg (Azithromycin Dihydrate) Pfizer 2739
Zithromax Tablets, 250 mg (Azithromycin Dihydrate) Pfizer..... 2739
Zithromax Tablets, 600 mg (Azithromycin Dihydrate) Pfizer..... 2743
Zyvox (Linezolid) Pharmacia & Upjohn 2871

Pneumonia, candidal
Diflucan Tablets, Injection, and Oral Suspension (Fluconazole) Pfizer 2681

Pneumonia, nosocomial
(*see also under* Infections, lower respiratory tract)
Cipro I.V. (Ciprofloxacin) Bayer 893
Cipro I.V. Pharmacy Bulk Package (Ciprofloxacin) Bayer 897
Trovan (Alatrofloxacin Mesylate) Pfizer 2722
Zosyn (Piperacillin Sodium, Tazobactam Sodium) Lederle 1890
Zosyn in Galaxy Containers (Piperacillin Sodium, Tazobactam Sodium) Lederle 1894
Zyvox (Linezolid) Pharmacia & Upjohn 2871

Pneumonia, pneumocystis carinii
(*see under* Pneumocystis carinii pneumonia)

Pneumonitis, aspiration
Celestone Soluspan Injectable Suspension (Betamethasone Acetate, Betamethasone Sodium Phosphate) Schering 3097
Celestone Syrup (Betamethasone) Schering 3099
Cortone Acetate Injectable Suspension (Cortisone Acetate) Merck 2059
Cortone Acetate Tablets (Cortisone Acetate) Merck 2061
Decadron Elixir (Dexamethasone) Merck 2078
Decadron Tablets (Dexamethasone) Merck 2079
Decadron Phosphate Injection (Dexamethasone Sodium Phosphate) Merck 2081
Depo-Medrol Injectable Suspension (Methylprednisolone Acetate) Pharmacia & Upjohn 2795
Hydrocortone Tablets (Hydrocortisone) Merck 2106
Hydrocortone Phosphate Injection, Sterile (Hydrocortisone Sodium Phosphate) Merck 2105
Pediapred Oral Solution (Prednisolone Sodium Phosphate) Celltech 1170
Prednisone (Prednisone) Roxane 3064
Prelone Syrup (Prednisolone) Muro . 2273
Solu-Medrol Sterile Powder (Methylprednisolone Sodium Succinate) Pharmacia & Upjohn 2855

Poison ivy
(*see under* Dermatitis, contact)

Poison oak
(*see under* Dermatitis, contact)

Poison sumac
(*see under* Dermatitis, contact)

Poisoning, pesticides and chemicals of organophosphate class
Protopam Chloride for Injection (Pralidoxime Chloride) Wyeth-Ayerst 3582

Poliomyelitis, prevention of
(*see under* Immunization, poliovirus 1, 2, and 3)

Pollinosis
(*see also under* Rhinitis, seasonal allergic)
Actifed Cold & Allergy Tablets (Pseudoephedrine Hydrochloride, Triprolidine Hydrochloride) Pfizer Inc., Warner-Lambert Healthcare .... ■688
Afrin Nasal Decongestant Children's Pump Mist (Phenylephrine Hydrochloride) Schering-Plough .... ■734
Afrin (Oxymetazoline Hydrochloride) Schering-Plough .... ■733
Afrin No Drip Original Nasal Spray (Oxymetazoline Hydrochloride) Schering-Plough .... ■735
Afrin No Drip Extra Moisturizing Nasal Spray (Oxymetazoline Hydrochloride) Schering-Plough .. ■735
Afrin No Drip Severe Congestion Nasal Spray (Oxymetazoline Hydrochloride) Schering-Plough .. ■735
Afrin No Drip Sinus Nasal Spray (Oxymetazoline Hydrochloride) Schering-Plough .... ■735
Afrin Original Pump Mist (Oxymetazoline Hydrochloride) Schering-Plough .... ■733
Benadryl Allergy Chewables (Diphenhydramine Hydrochloride) Pfizer Inc., Warner-Lambert Healthcare .... ■689
Benadryl Allergy Liquid (Diphenhydramine Hydrochloride) Pfizer Inc., Warner-Lambert Healthcare .... ■690
Benadryl Allergy/Congestion Tablets (Diphenhydramine Hydrochloride, Pseudoephedrine Hydrochloride) Pfizer Inc., Warner-Lambert Healthcare .... ■692
Benadryl Allergy Sinus Headache Caplets & Gelcaps (Acetaminophen, Diphenhydramine Hydrochloride, Pseudoephedrine Hydrochloride) Pfizer Inc., Warner-Lambert Healthcare .... ■693
Benadryl Dye-Free Allergy Liquid (Diphenhydramine Hydrochloride) Pfizer Inc., Warner-Lambert Healthcare .... ■690
Benadryl Dye-Free Allergy Liqui-Gels Softgels (Diphenhydramine Hydrochloride) Pfizer Inc., Warner-Lambert Healthcare .... ■690
Chlor-Trimeton Allergy Tablets (Chlorpheniramine Maleate) Schering-Plough .... ■735
Chlor-Trimeton Allergy/Decongestant Tablets (Chlorpheniramine Maleate, Pseudoephedrine Sulfate) Schering-Plough .... ■736
Dimetapp Elixir (Brompheniramine Maleate, Pseudoephedrine Hydrochloride) Whitehall-Robins .... ■777
Drixoral Cold & Allergy Sustained-Action Tablets (Dexbrompheniramine Maleate, Pseudoephedrine Sulfate) Schering-Plough .... ■740
Kronofed-A (Chlorpheniramine Maleate, Pseudoephedrine Hydrochloride) Ferndale 1341
Natru-Vent Nasal Spray, Adult Strength (Xylometazoline Hydrochloride) Boehringer Ingelheim .... ■624
Natru-Vent Nasal Spray, Pediatric Strength (Xylometazoline Hydrochloride) Boehringer Ingelheim .... ■625
Neo-Synephrine (Phenylephrine Hydrochloride) Bayer Consumer .... ■614
Neo-Synephrine 12 Hour Nasal Spray (Oxymetazoline Hydrochloride) Bayer Consumer .... ■615
PediaCare Cough-Cold Liquid (Chlorpheniramine Maleate, Dextromethorphan Hydrobromide, Pseudoephedrine Hydrochloride) Pharmacia Consumer .... ■719
Sudafed Cold & Allergy Tablets (Chlorpheniramine Maleate, Pseudoephedrine Hydrochloride) Pfizer Inc., Warner-Lambert Healthcare .... ■708
Tavist 12 Hour Allergy Tablets (Clemastine Fumarate) Novartis Consumer .... ■676
Triaminic Cold & Allergy Liquid (Chlorpheniramine Maleate, Pseudoephedrine Hydrochloride) Novartis Consumer .... ■681
Children's Tylenol Allergy-D Liquid (Acetaminophen, Diphenhydramine Hydrochloride, Pseudoephedrine Hydrochloride) McNeil Consumer 2014
Tylenol Severe Allergy Caplets (Acetaminophen, Diphenhydramine Hydrochloride) McNeil Consumer 2010
Vicks Sinex Nasal Spray and Ultra Fine Mist (Phenylephrine Hydrochloride) Procter & Gamble .... ■729
Vicks Sinex 12-Hour Nasal Spray and Ultra Fine Mist (Oxymetazoline Hydrochloride) Procter & Gamble .... ■729

Polycythemia vera
Mustargen for Injection (Mechlorethamine Hydrochloride) Merck 2142

Polydipsia, temporary, management of
DDAVP Nasal Spray (Desmopressin Acetate) Aventis 738
DDAVP Rhinal Tube (Desmopressin Acetate) Aventis 738
Desmopressin Acetate Rhinal Tube (Desmopressin Acetate) Ferring 1345

Polymyositis
(*see under* Dermatomyositis, systemic)

Polyps, nasal, prevention of recurrence
Beconase Inhalation Aerosol (Beclomethasone Dipropionate) GlaxoSmithKline 1497
Beconase AQ Nasal Spray (Beclomethasone Dipropionate Monohydrate) GlaxoSmithKline 1498
Vancenase PocketHaler Nasal Inhaler (Beclomethasone Dipropionate) Schering 3162
Vancenase AQ Nasal Spray 0.084% (Beclomethasone Dipropionate) Schering 3163

Polyuria, temporary, management of
DDAVP Nasal Spray (Desmopressin Acetate) Aventis 738
DDAVP Rhinal Tube (Desmopressin Acetate) Aventis 738
Desmopressin Acetate Rhinal Tube (Desmopressin Acetate) Ferring 1345

Porphyria, acute intermittent, adjunctive therapy in
Thorazine (Chlorpromazine Hydrochloride) GlaxoSmithKline ... 1656

Porphyria, acute intermittent, amelioration of recurrent attacks of
Panhematin (Hemin) Abbott 497

Postnasal drip
(*see under* Cold, common, symptomatic relief of)

Prader-Willi syndrome
Genotropin Lyophilized Powder (Somatropin) Pharmacia & Upjohn 2818

Pregnancy, diagnosis of
e.p.t. Pregnancy Test (HCG Monoclonal Antibody) Pfizer Inc., Warner-Lambert Healthcare .... ■701

Pregnancy, prevention of
Alesse-21 Tablets (Ethinyl Estradiol, Levonorgestrel) Wyeth-Ayerst 3468
Alesse-28 Tablets (Ethinyl Estradiol, Levonorgestrel) Wyeth-Ayerst .. 3473
Brevicon 28-Day Tablets (Ethinyl Estradiol, Norethindrone) Watson 3380
Cyclessa Tablets (Desogestrel, Ethinyl Estradiol) Organon 2450
Depo-Provera Contraceptive Injection (Medroxyprogesterone Acetate) Pharmacia & Upjohn 2798
Desogen Tablets (Desogestrel, Ethinyl Estradiol) Organon 2458
Estrostep (Ethinyl Estradiol, Norethindrone Acetate) Parke-Davis .. 2627
Levlen (Ethinyl Estradiol, Levonorgestrel) Berlex 962
Levlite 21 Tablets (Ethinyl Estradiol, Levonorgestrel) Berlex 962
Levlite 28 Tablets (Ethinyl Estradiol, Levonorgestrel) Berlex 962
Levora Tablets (Ethinyl Estradiol, Levonorgestrel) Watson 3389
Loestrin 21 Tablets (Ethinyl Estradiol, Norethindrone Acetate) Parke-Davis 2642

Loestrin Fe Tablets (Ethinyl Estradiol, Ferrous Fumarate, Norethindrone Acetate) Parke-Davis ... 2642
Lo/Ovral Tablets (Ethinyl Estradiol, Norgestrel) Wyeth-Ayerst ... 3532
Lo/Ovral-28 Tablets (Ethinyl Estradiol, Norgestrel) Wyeth-Ayerst ... 3538
Low-Ogestrel-28 Tablets (Ethinyl Estradiol, Norgestrel) Watson ... 3392
Lunelle Monthly Injection (Estradiol Cypionate, Medroxyprogesterone Acetate) Pharmacia & Upjohn ... 2827
Microgestin Fe 1.5/30 Tablets (Ethinyl Estradiol, Norethindrone Acetate) Watson ... 3407
Microgestin Fe 1/20 Tablets (Ethinyl Estradiol, Norethindrone Acetate) Watson ... 3400
Micronor Tablets (Norethindrone) Ortho-McNeil ... 2543
Mircette Tablets (Desogestrel, Ethinyl Estradiol) Organon ... 2470
Mirena Intrauterine System (Levonorgestrel) Berlex ... 974
Modicon (Ethinyl Estradiol, Norethindrone) Ortho-McNeil ... 2563
Necon (Ethinyl Estradiol, Norethindrone) Watson ... 3415
Nordette-28 Tablets (Ethinyl Estradiol, Levonorgestrel) Monarch ... 2257
Norinyl 1 +35 28-Day Tablets (Ethinyl Estradiol, Norethindrone) Watson ... 3380
Norinyl 1 + 50 28-Day Tablets (Mestranol, Norethindrone) Watson ... 3380
Norplant System (Levonorgestrel) Wyeth-Ayerst ... 3543
Nor-QD Tablets (Norethindrone) Watson ... 3423
Ogestrel 0.5/50-28 Tablets (Ethinyl Estradiol, Norgestrel) Watson ... 3428
Ortho Diaphragm Kits – All-Flex Arcing Spring; Ortho Coil Spring (Diaphragm) Ortho-McNeil ... 2552
Ortho-Cept 21 Tablets (Desogestrel, Ethinyl Estradiol) Ortho-McNeil ... 2546
Ortho-Cept 28 Tablets (Desogestrel, Ethinyl Estradiol) Ortho-McNeil ... 2546
Ortho-Cyclen/Ortho Tri-Cyclen (Ethinyl Estradiol, Norgestimate) Ortho-McNeil ... 2573
Ortho-Novum (Ethinyl Estradiol, Norethindrone) Ortho-McNeil ... 2563
Ortho-Novum 1/50◻28 Tablets (Mestranol, Norethindrone) Ortho-McNeil ... 2556
Ovcon (Ethinyl Estradiol, Norethindrone) Warner Chilcott ... 3364
Ovral Tablets (Ethinyl Estradiol, Norgestrel) Wyeth-Ayerst ... 3551
Ovral-28 Tablets (Ethinyl Estradiol, Norgestrel) Wyeth-Ayerst ... 3552
Ovrette Tablets (Norgestrel) Wyeth-Ayerst ... 3552
ParaGard T 380A Intrauterine Copper Contraceptive (Copper, Intrauterine) Ortho-McNeil ... 2582
Tri-Levlen (Ethinyl Estradiol, Levonorgestrel) Berlex ... 962
Tri-Norinyl-28 Tablets (Ethinyl Estradiol, Norethindrone) Watson ... 3433
Triphasil-21 Tablets (Ethinyl Estradiol, Levonorgestrel) Wyeth-Ayerst ... 3600
Triphasil-28 Tablets (Ethinyl Estradiol, Levonorgestrel) Wyeth-Ayerst ... 3605
Trivora Tablets (Ethinyl Estradiol, Levonorgestrel) Watson ... 3439
Yasmin 28 Tablets (Ethinyl Estradiol, Drospirenone) Berlex ... 980
Zovia (Ethinyl Estradiol, Ethynodiol Diacetate) Watson ... 3449

Pregnancy, termination of, from 12th through the 20th gestational week
Prostin E2 Suppositories (Dinoprostone) Pharmacia & Upjohn ... 2852

Pregnancy, vitamin supplement for
(*see under* Vitamin deficiency, postpartum; Vitamin deficiency, prenatal)

Premenstrual dysphoric disorder
(*see under* Dysphoric disorder, premenstrual)

Premenstrual syndrome
(*see under* Menstrual syndrome, pre-, management of)

Prinzmetal's angina
(*see under* Angina, Prinzmetal's)

Proctitis, temporary relief of
Anusol-HC Suppositories (Hydrocortisone Acetate) Monarch ... 2238

Proctitis, ulcerative
Canasa Rectal Suppositories (Mesalamine) Axcan Scandipharm ... 829
Cortifoam Rectal Foam (Hydrocortisone Acetate) Schwarz ... 3170
Proctocort Suppositories (Hydrocortisone Acetate) Monarch ... 2264
Rowasa Rectal Suspension Enema 4.0 grams/unit (60 mL) (Mesalamine) Solvay ... 3264

Proctosigmoiditis, ulcerative
Rowasa Rectal Suspension Enema 4.0 grams/unit (60 mL) (Mesalamine) Solvay ... 3264

Propionibacterium species gynecologic infections
Primaxin I.V. (Cilastatin Sodium, Imipenem) Merck ... 2160

Prostatic cancer
(*see under* Carcinoma, prostate)

Prostatic cancer, palliative treatment of
(*see under* Carcinoma, prostate, palliative treatment of)

Prostatic hyperplasia, benign, symptomatic treatment
Cardura Tablets (Doxazosin Mesylate) Pfizer ... 2668
Flomax Capsules (Tamsulosin Hydrochloride) Boehringer Ingelheim ... 1044
Hytrin Capsules (Terazosin Hydrochloride) Abbott ... 464
Proscar Tablets (Finasteride) Merck ... 2175

Prostatitis
Ancef for Injection (Cefazolin Sodium) GlaxoSmithKline ... 1474
Ancef Injection (Cefazolin Sodium) GlaxoSmithKline ... 1474
Cipro I.V. (Ciprofloxacin) Bayer ... 893
Cipro I.V. Pharmacy Bulk Package (Ciprofloxacin) Bayer ... 897
Cipro (Ciprofloxacin) Bayer ... 887
Floxin I.V. (Ofloxacin) Ortho-McNeil ... 2526
Floxin Tablets (Ofloxacin) Ortho-McNeil ... 2529
Geocillin Tablets (Carbenicillin Indanyl Sodium) Pfizer ... 2687
Keflex (Cephalexin) Dista ... 1237
Noroxin Tablets (Norfloxacin) Merck ... 2145

Prostatitis, lacking substantial evidence of effectiveness in
Urobiotic-250 Capsules (Oxytetracycline Hydrochloride, Phenazopyridine Hydrochloride, Sulfamethizole) Pfizer ... 2731

Proteinuria, remission of in nephrotic syndrome
Celestone Soluspan Injectable Suspension (Betamethasone Acetate, Betamethasone Sodium Phosphate) Schering ... 3097
Celestone Syrup (Betamethasone) Schering ... 3099
Cortone Acetate Injectable Suspension (Cortisone Acetate) Merck ... 2059
Cortone Acetate Tablets (Cortisone Acetate) Merck ... 2061
Decadron Elixir (Dexamethasone) Merck ... 2078
Decadron Tablets (Dexamethasone) Merck ... 2079
Decadron Phosphate Injection (Dexamethasone Sodium Phosphate) Merck ... 2081
Depo-Medrol Injectable Suspension (Methylprednisolone Acetate) Pharmacia & Upjohn ... 2795
Hydrocortone Tablets (Hydrocortisone) Merck ... 2106
Hydrocortone Phosphate Injection, Sterile (Hydrocortisone Sodium Phosphate) Merck ... 2105
Pediapred Oral Solution (Prednisolone Sodium Phosphate) Celltech ... 1170
Prednisone (Prednisone) Roxane ... 3064
Prelone Syrup (Prednisolone) Muro ... 2273
Solu-Medrol Sterile Powder (Methylprednisolone Sodium Succinate) Pharmacia & Upjohn ... 2855

Proteus, indole-positive, infections
(*see under* Morganella morganii infections)

Proteus mirabilis
(*see under* P. mirabilis infections)

Proteus species bone and joint infections
Nebcin Vials, Hyporets & ADD-Vantage (Tobramycin Sulfate) Lilly ... 1955

Proteus species gynecologic infections
Primaxin I.V. (Cilastatin Sodium, Imipenem) Merck ... 2160

Proteus species infections
Cefobid Intravenous/Intramuscular (Cefoperazone) Pfizer ... 2671
Cefobid Pharmacy Bulk Package - Not for Direct Infusion (Cefoperazone Sodium) Pfizer ... 2673
Cefotan (Cefotetan) AstraZeneca ... 664
Ceptaz for Injection (Ceftazidime) GlaxoSmithKline ... 1499
Fortaz (Ceftazidime Sodium) GlaxoSmithKline ... 1541
Nebcin Vials, Hyporets & ADD-Vantage (Tobramycin Sulfate) Lilly ... 1955
Pipracil (Piperacillin Sodium) Lederle ... 1866
Primaxin I.V. (Cilastatin Sodium, Imipenem) Merck ... 2160
Tazicef for Injection (Ceftazidime) GlaxoSmithKline ... 1647
Tazicef Galaxy Container (Ceftazidime Sodium) GlaxoSmithKline ... 1650
Tazicef Pharmacy Bulk Package (Ceftazidime) GlaxoSmithKline ... 1653
Tazidime Vials, Faspak & ADD-Vantage (Ceftazidime) Lilly ... 1966

Proteus species infections, ocular, indole-negative
Pred-G Ophthalmic Suspension (Gentamicin Sulfate, Prednisolone Acetate) Allergan ... ⊙247

Proteus species intra-abdominal infections
Primaxin I.V. (Cilastatin Sodium, Imipenem) Merck ... 2160

Proteus species septicemia
Cefobid Intravenous/Intramuscular (Cefoperazone) Pfizer ... 2671
Cefobid Pharmacy Bulk Package - Not for Direct Infusion (Cefoperazone Sodium) Pfizer ... 2673

Proteus species skin and skin structure infections
Ceptaz for Injection (Ceftazidime) GlaxoSmithKline ... 1499
Fortaz (Ceftazidime Sodium) GlaxoSmithKline ... 1541
Nebcin Vials, Hyporets & ADD-Vantage (Tobramycin Sulfate) Lilly ... 1955
Tazicef for Injection (Ceftazidime) GlaxoSmithKline ... 1647
Tazicef Galaxy Container (Ceftazidime Sodium) GlaxoSmithKline ... 1650
Tazicef Pharmacy Bulk Package (Ceftazidime) GlaxoSmithKline ... 1653
Tazidime Vials, Faspak & ADD-Vantage (Ceftazidime) Lilly ... 1966

Proteus species urinary tract infections
Cefotan (Cefotetan) AstraZeneca ... 664
Ceptaz for Injection (Ceftazidime) GlaxoSmithKline ... 1499
Fortaz (Ceftazidime Sodium) GlaxoSmithKline ... 1541
Mandol Vials (Cefamandole Nafate) Lilly ... 1953
Nebcin Vials, Hyporets & ADD-Vantage (Tobramycin Sulfate) Lilly ... 1955
Streptomycin Sulfate Injection (Streptomycin Sulfate) Pfizer ... 2714
Tazicef for Injection (Ceftazidime) GlaxoSmithKline ... 1647
Tazicef Galaxy Container (Ceftazidime Sodium) GlaxoSmithKline ... 1650
Tazicef Pharmacy Bulk Package (Ceftazidime) GlaxoSmithKline ... 1653
Tazidime Vials, Faspak & ADD-Vantage (Ceftazidime) Lilly ... 1966

Proteus vulgaris
(*see under* P. vulgaris infections)

Prothrombin deficiency, anticoagulant-induced
AquaMEPHYTON Injection (Vitamin K_1) Merck ... 2042
Mephyton Tablets (Vitamin K_1) Merck ... 2129

Providencia rettgeri infections
Cefizox for Intramuscular or Intravenous Use (Ceftizoxime Sodium) Fujisawa ... 1390
Cefotan (Cefotetan) AstraZeneca ... 664
Cipro I.V. (Ciprofloxacin) Bayer ... 893
Cipro I.V. Pharmacy Bulk Package (Ciprofloxacin) Bayer ... 897
Cipro (Ciprofloxacin) Bayer ... 887
Claforan Injection (Cefotaxime Sodium) Aventis ... 732
Geocillin Tablets (Carbenicillin Indanyl Sodium) Pfizer ... 2687
Mefoxin for Injection (Cefoxitin Sodium) Merck ... 2124
Mefoxin Premixed Intravenous Solution (Cefoxitin Sodium) Merck ... 2127
Primaxin I.V. (Cilastatin Sodium, Imipenem) Merck ... 2160

Providencia rettgeri skin and skin structure infections
Claforan Injection (Cefotaxime Sodium) Aventis ... 732
Primaxin I.V. (Cilastatin Sodium, Imipenem) Merck ... 2160

Providencia rettgeri urinary tract infections
Cefizox for Intramuscular or Intravenous Use (Ceftizoxime Sodium) Fujisawa ... 1390
Cefotan (Cefotetan) AstraZeneca ... 664
Cipro I.V. (Ciprofloxacin) Bayer ... 893
Cipro I.V. Pharmacy Bulk Package (Ciprofloxacin) Bayer ... 897
Cipro (Ciprofloxacin) Bayer ... 887
Claforan Injection (Cefotaxime Sodium) Aventis ... 732
Geocillin Tablets (Carbenicillin Indanyl Sodium) Pfizer ... 2687
Mefoxin for Injection (Cefoxitin Sodium) Merck ... 2124
Mefoxin Premixed Intravenous Solution (Cefoxitin Sodium) Merck ... 2127
Primaxin I.V. (Cilastatin Sodium, Imipenem) Merck ... 2160

Providencia species infections
Mefoxin for Injection (Cefoxitin Sodium) Merck ... 2124
Mefoxin Premixed Intravenous Solution (Cefoxitin Sodium) Merck ... 2127
Nebcin Vials, Hyporets & ADD-Vantage (Tobramycin Sulfate) Lilly ... 1955

Providencia species urinary tract infections
Mefoxin for Injection (Cefoxitin Sodium) Merck ... 2124
Nebcin Vials, Hyporets & ADD-Vantage (Tobramycin Sulfate) Lilly ... 1955

Providencia stuartii infections
Cipro I.V. (Ciprofloxacin) Bayer ... 893
Cipro I.V. Pharmacy Bulk Package (Ciprofloxacin) Bayer ... 897
Cipro (Ciprofloxacin) Bayer ... 887

Providencia stuartii skin and skin structure infections
Cipro I.V. (Ciprofloxacin) Bayer ... 893
Cipro I.V. Pharmacy Bulk Package (Ciprofloxacin) Bayer ... 897
Cipro (Ciprofloxacin) Bayer ... 887

Pruritus
Drysol Solution (Aluminum Chloride) Person & Covey ... 2663

Pruritus, anogenital
Analpram-HC (Hydrocortisone Acetate, Pramoxine Hydrochloride) Ferndale ... 1338
Cortaid (Hydrocortisone) Pharmacia Consumer ... ▣717
Cortizone•5 (Hydrocortisone) Pfizer Inc., Warner-Lambert Healthcare ... ▣699
Cortizone•10 (Hydrocortisone) Pfizer Inc., Warner-Lambert Healthcare ... ▣699
Cortizone•10 Plus Creme (Hydrocortisone) Pfizer Inc., Warner-Lambert Healthcare ... ▣700

Cortizone for Kids Creme (Hydrocortisone) Pfizer Inc., Warner-Lambert Healthcare .... ▣699
Preparation H Cream (Glycerin, Petrolatum, Phenylephrine Hydrochloride, Shark Liver Oil) Whitehall-Robins .... ▣778
Preparation H Cooling Gel (Phenylephrine Hydrochloride) Whitehall-Robins .... ▣778
Preparation H (Mineral Oil, Petrolatum, Phenylephrine Hydrochloride, Shark Liver Oil) Whitehall-Robins .... ▣778
Preparation H Medicated Wipes (Witch Hazel) Whitehall-Robins .... ▣779
ProctoFoam-HC (Hydrocortisone Acetate, Pramoxine Hydrochloride) Schwarz 3177
Tucks Pre-moistened Pads (Witch Hazel) Pfizer Inc., Warner-Lambert Healthcare .... ▣713

Pruritus, ocular
Acular Ophthalmic Solution (Ketorolac Tromethamine) Allergan 544
Naphcon-A Ophthalmic Solution (Naphazoline Hydrochloride, Pheniramine Maleate) Alcon 540
Opcon-A Eye Drops (Naphazoline Hydrochloride, Pheniramine Maleate) Bausch & Lomb, Inc ..... ⊙253
Visine-A Eye Allergy Relief Eye Drops (Naphazoline Hydrochloride, Pheniramine Maleate) Pfizer Consumer .... ⊙314
Visine-A Eye Drops (Naphazoline Hydrochloride, Pheniramine Maleate) Pfizer Inc., Warner-Lambert Healthcare .... ▣714

Pruritus, rhinopharyngeal, symptomatic relief of
Benadryl Allergy Kapseal Capsules (Diphenhydramine Hydrochloride) Pfizer Inc., Warner-Lambert Healthcare .... ▣691
Benadryl Allergy Liquid (Diphenhydramine Hydrochloride) Pfizer Inc., Warner-Lambert Healthcare .... ▣690
Benadryl Allergy Ultratab Tablets (Diphenhydramine Hydrochloride) Pfizer Inc., Warner-Lambert Healthcare .... ▣691
Benadryl Allergy/Congestion Tablets (Diphenhydramine Hydrochloride, Pseudoephedrine Hydrochloride) Pfizer Inc., Warner-Lambert Healthcare .... ▣692
Benadryl Allergy Sinus Headache Caplets & Gelcaps (Acetaminophen, Diphenhydramine Hydrochloride, Pseudoephedrine Hydrochloride) Pfizer Inc., Warner-Lambert Healthcare .... ▣693
Triaminic Cold & Allergy Softchews (Chlorpheniramine Maleate, Pseudoephedrine Hydrochloride) Novartis Consumer .... ▣683
Tylenol Severe Allergy Caplets (Acetaminophen, Diphenhydramine Hydrochloride) McNeil Consumer 2010

Pruritus, systemic relief of
Atarax Tablets & Syrup (Hydroxyzine Hydrochloride) Pfizer 2667
Vistaril Capsules (Hydroxyzine Pamoate) Pfizer 2738
Vistaril Intramuscular Solution (Hydroxyzine Hydrochloride) Pfizer 2738
Vistaril Oral Suspension (Hydroxyzine Pamoate) Pfizer 2738

Pruritus, topical relief of
(*see also under* Pruritus, systemic relief of)
Aclovate (Alclometasone Dipropionate) Elan 1275
Anusol HC-1 Hydrocortisone Anti-Itch Cream (Hydrocortisone Acetate) Pfizer Inc., Warner-Lambert Healthcare .... ▣689
Anusol-HC Cream 2.5% (Hydrocortisone) Monarch 2237
Benadryl Itch Relief Stick Extra Strength (Diphenhydramine Hydrochloride, Zinc Acetate) Pfizer Inc., Warner-Lambert Healthcare .... ▣695
Benadryl Cream (Diphenhydramine Hydrochloride, Zinc Acetate) Pfizer Inc., Warner-Lambert Healthcare .... ▣695
Benadryl Gel (Diphenhydramine Hydrochloride) Pfizer Inc., Warner-Lambert Healthcare .... ▣695
Benadryl Spray (Diphenhydramine Hydrochloride, Zinc Acetate) Pfizer Inc., Warner-Lambert Healthcare .... ▣696
Clobevate Gel (Clobetasol Propionate) Stiefel 3271
Cordran Lotion (Flurandrenolide) Oclassen 2438
Cordran Tape (Flurandrenolide) Oclassen 2439
Cortizone•5 (Hydrocortisone) Pfizer Inc., Warner-Lambert Healthcare .... ▣699
Cortizone•10 (Hydrocortisone) Pfizer Inc., Warner-Lambert Healthcare .... ▣699
Cortizone•10 Plus Creme (Hydrocortisone) Pfizer Inc., Warner-Lambert Healthcare .... ▣700
Cortizone•10 Quick Shot Spray (Hydrocortisone) Pfizer Inc., Warner-Lambert Healthcare .... ▣699
Cutivate Cream (Fluticasone Propionate) Elan 1282
Cutivate Ointment (Fluticasone Propionate) Elan 1284
Dermatop Emollient Cream (Prednicarbate) Ortho Dermatological .. 2517
Dermoplast Hospital Strength Spray (Benzocaine, Menthol) Medtech .... ▣666
DesOwen (Desonide) Galderma 1401
Diprolene Lotion 0.05% (Betamethasone Dipropionate) Schering 3107
Diprolene Ointment 0.05% (Betamethasone Dipropionate) Schering 3108
Diprolene AF Cream 0.05% (Betamethasone Dipropionate) Schering 3106
Diprosone (Betamethasone Dipropionate) Schering 3109
Elocon Cream 0.1% (Mometasone Furoate) Schering 3110
Elocon Lotion 0.1% (Mometasone Furoate) Schering 3111
Elocon Ointment 0.1% (Mometasone Furoate) Schering 3112
Lac-Hydrin Lotion (Ammonium Lactate) Bristol-Myers Squibb Dermatology 1119
Lidex (Fluocinonide) Medicis 2020
Locoid Cream (Hydrocortisone Butyrate) Ferndale 1341
Locoid Lipocream Cream (Hydrocortisone Butyrate) Ferndale 1342
Locoid (Hydrocortisone Butyrate) Ferndale 1341
Luxíq Foam (Betamethasone Valerate) Connetics 1210
Massengill Medicated Soft Cloth Towelette (Hydrocortisone) SmithKline Beecham Consumer.. ▣753
Olux Foam (Clobetasol Propionate) Connetics 1211
Pramosone (Hydrocortisone Acetate, Pramoxine Hydrochloride) Ferndale 1343
Psorcon E Cream (Diflorasone Diacetate) Dermik 1227
Psorcon E Ointment (Diflorasone Diacetate) Dermik 1228
Synalar (Fluocinolone Acetonide) Medicis 2020
Temovate Gel (Clobetasol Propionate) Elan 1303
Temovate Scalp Application (Clobetasol Propionate) Elan 1304
Topicort (Desoximetasone) Medicis 2025
Ultravate Cream (Halobetasol Propionate) Bristol-Myers Squibb Dermatology 1119
Ultravate Ointment (Halobetasol Propionate) Bristol-Myers Squibb Dermatology 1120

Pruritus, vaginal
Betadine Medicated Douche (Povidone Iodine) Purdue Frederick 2894
Cortaid (Hydrocortisone Acetate) Pharmacia Consumer .... ▣717

Pruritus ani
(*see also under* Pruritus, anogenital)
Anusol-HC Suppositories (Hydrocortisone Acetate) Monarch 2238
ELA-Max 5 Cream (Lidocaine) Ferndale 1340
Proctocort Suppositories (Hydrocortisone Acetate) Monarch 2264

Pseudomonas aeruginosa infections
(*see under* P. aeruginosa infections)

Pseudomonas species bone and joint infections
Claforan Injection (Cefotaxime Sodium) Aventis 732

Pseudomonas species infections
Cefizox for Intramuscular or Intravenous Use (Ceftizoxime Sodium) Fujisawa 1390
Ceptaz for Injection (Ceftazidime) GlaxoSmithKline 1499
Claforan Injection (Cefotaxime Sodium) Aventis 732
Fortaz (Ceftazidime Sodium) GlaxoSmithKline 1541
Geocillin Tablets (Carbenicillin Indanyl Sodium) Pfizer 2687
Pipracil (Piperacillin Sodium) Lederle 1866
Tazicef for Injection (Ceftazidime) GlaxoSmithKline 1647
Tazicef Galaxy Container (Ceftazidime Sodium) GlaxoSmithKline 1650
Tazicef Pharmacy Bulk Package (Ceftazidime) GlaxoSmithKline 1653
Tazidime Vials, Faspak & ADD-Vantage (Ceftazidime) Lilly 1966

Pseudomonas species infections, ocular
Blephamide Ophthalmic Suspension (Prednisolone Acetate, Sulfacetamide Sodium) Allergan 548
Chibroxin Sterile Ophthalmic Solution (Norfloxacin) Merck 2051

Pseudomonas species lower respiratory tract infections
Claforan Injection (Cefotaxime Sodium) Aventis 732
Tazicef for Injection (Ceftazidime) GlaxoSmithKline 1647
Tazicef Galaxy Container (Ceftazidime Sodium) GlaxoSmithKline 1650
Tazicef Pharmacy Bulk Package (Ceftazidime) GlaxoSmithKline 1653
Tazidime Vials, Faspak & ADD-Vantage (Ceftazidime) Lilly 1966

Pseudomonas species septicemia
Timentin Injection- ADD-Vantage Vial (Clavulanate Potassium, Ticarcillin Disodium) GlaxoSmithKline 1661
Timentin Injection-Galaxy Container (Clavulanate Potassium, Ticarcillin Disodium) GlaxoSmithKline 1664
Timentin Injection-Pharmacy Bulk Package (Clavulanate Potassium, Ticarcillin Disodium) GlaxoSmithKline 1666
Timentin for Intravenous Administration (Clavulanate Potassium, Ticarcillin Disodium) GlaxoSmithKline 1658

Pseudomonas species skin and skin structure infections
Claforan Injection (Cefotaxime Sodium) Aventis 732

Pseudomonas species urinary tract infections
Cefizox for Intramuscular or Intravenous Use (Ceftizoxime Sodium) Fujisawa 1390
Claforan Injection (Cefotaxime Sodium) Aventis 732
Geocillin Tablets (Carbenicillin Indanyl Sodium) Pfizer 2687
Timentin Injection- ADD-Vantage Vial (Clavulanate Potassium, Ticarcillin Disodium) GlaxoSmithKline 1661
Timentin Injection-Galaxy Container (Clavulanate Potassium, Ticarcillin Disodium) GlaxoSmithKline 1664
Timentin Injection-Pharmacy Bulk Package (Clavulanate Potassium, Ticarcillin Disodium) GlaxoSmithKline 1666
Timentin for Intravenous Administration (Clavulanate Potassium, Ticarcillin Disodium) GlaxoSmithKline 1658

Psittacosis
(*see under* Chlamydia psittaci infection)

Psoriasis
Cortaid Intensive Therapy Cream (Hydrocortisone) Pharmacia Consumer .... ▣717
Cortizone•5 (Hydrocortisone) Pfizer Inc., Warner-Lambert Healthcare .... ▣699
Cortizone for Kids Creme (Hydrocortisone) Pfizer Inc., Warner-Lambert Healthcare .... ▣699
Dovonex Cream (Calcipotriene) Bristol-Myers Squibb Dermatology 1116
Dovonex Ointment (Calcipotriene) Bristol-Myers Squibb Dermatology 1117
Dovonex Scalp Solution (Calcipotriene) Bristol-Myers Squibb Dermatology 1118
Oxsoralen-Ultra Capsules (Methoxsalen) ICN 1741
Psoriatec Cream (Anthralin) Sirius Laboratories, Inc. 3247
Tegrin Dandruff Shampoo - Extra Conditioning (Coal Tar) Block...... ▣623
Tegrin Dandruff Shampoo - Fresh Herbal (Coal Tar) Block .... ▣624
Tegrin Skin Cream (Coal Tar) Block .... ▣624

Psoriasis, erythrodermic
Soriatane (Acitretin) Roche Laboratories 3003

Psoriasis, severe
Celestone Soluspan Injectable Suspension (Betamethasone Acetate, Betamethasone Sodium Phosphate) Schering 3097
Celestone Syrup (Betamethasone) Schering 3099
Cortone Acetate Injectable Suspension (Cortisone Acetate) Merck 2059
Cortone Acetate Tablets (Cortisone Acetate) Merck 2061
Decadron Elixir (Dexamethasone) Merck 2078
Decadron Tablets (Dexamethasone) Merck 2079
Decadron Phosphate Injection (Dexamethasone Sodium Phosphate) Merck 2081
Depo-Medrol Injectable Suspension (Methylprednisolone Acetate) Pharmacia & Upjohn 2795
Hydrocortone Tablets (Hydrocortisone) Merck 2106
Hydrocortone Phosphate Injection, Sterile (Hydrocortisone Sodium Phosphate) Merck 2105
Pediapred Oral Solution (Prednisolone Sodium Phosphate) Celltech 1170
Prednisone (Prednisone) Roxane 3064
Prelone Syrup (Prednisolone) Muro . 2273
Solu-Medrol Sterile Powder (Methylprednisolone Sodium Succinate) Pharmacia & Upjohn 2855

Psoriasis, severe recalcitrant
8-MOP Capsules (Methoxsalen) ICN 1727
Gengraf Capsules (Cyclosporine) Abbott 457
Neoral Soft Gelatin Capsules (Cyclosporine) Novartis 2380
Neoral Oral Solution (Cyclosporine) Novartis 2380

Psoriatic arthritis
(*see under* Arthritis, psoriatic)

Psoriatic plaques
Celestone Soluspan Injectable Suspension (Betamethasone Acetate, Betamethasone Sodium Phosphate) Schering 3097
Decadron Phosphate Injection (Dexamethasone Sodium Phosphate) Merck 2081
Dovonex Cream (Calcipotriene) Bristol-Myers Squibb Dermatology 1116
Dovonex Ointment (Calcipotriene) Bristol-Myers Squibb Dermatology 1117
Gengraf Capsules (Cyclosporine) Abbott 457
Hydrocortone Acetate Injectable Suspension (Hydrocortisone Acetate) Merck 2103
Neoral Soft Gelatin Capsules (Cyclosporine) Novartis 2380
Neoral Oral Solution (Cyclosporine) Novartis 2380

Psoriatic plaques, stable
Tazorac Gel (Tazarotene) Allergan 556

Psychotic disorders, management of the manifestations in severely ill
Clozaril Tablets (Clozapine) Novartis 2319

Psychotic disorders, management of the manifestations of
(*see also under* Psychotic disorders,

management of the manifestations in severely ill)
- Compazine (Prochlorperazine) GlaxoSmithKline 1505
- Geodon Capsules (Ziprasidone Hydrochloride) Pfizer 2688
- Haldol Decanoate (Haloperidol Decanoate) Ortho-McNeil 2535
- Haldol Injection, Tablets and Concentrate (Haloperidol) Ortho-McNeil 2533
- Loxitane Capsules (Loxapine Succinate) Watson 3398
- Moban (Molindone Hydrochloride) Endo Labs 1320
- Navane Oral (Thiothixene) Pfizer 2701
- Navane Intramuscular (Thiothixene Hydrochloride) Pfizer 2703
- Risperdal (Risperidone) Janssen 1796
- Serentil (Mesoridazine Besylate) Boehringer Ingelheim 1057
- Seroquel Tablets (Quetiapine Fumarate) AstraZeneca 684
- Stelazine (Trifluoperazine Hydrochloride) GlaxoSmithKline 1640
- Thioridazine Hydrochloride Tablets (Thioridazine Hydrochloride) Mylan 2289
- Thiothixene Capsules (Thiothixene) Mylan 2290
- Thorazine (Chlorpromazine Hydrochloride) GlaxoSmithKline 1656
- Trilafon (Perphenazine) Schering 3160
- Zyprexa Tablets (Olanzapine) Lilly 1973
- Zyprexa ZYDIS Orally Disintegrating Tablets (Olanzapine) Lilly 1973

Psychotic disorders with depressive symptoms
- Etrafon (Amitriptyline Hydrochloride, Perphenazine) Schering 3115

Puberty, central precocious
- Lupron Depot-PED 7.5 mg, 11.25 mg and 15 mg (Leuprolide Acetate) TAP 3291
- Lupron Injection Pediatric (Leuprolide Acetate) TAP 3280
- Synarel Nasal Solution for Central Precocious Puberty (Nafarelin Acetate) Searle 3204

Puberty, delayed, in male
- Android Capsules, 10 mg (Methyltestosterone) ICN 1731
- Delatestryl Injection (Testosterone Enanthate) BTG 1151
- Testopel Pellets (Testosterone) Bartor 3610
- Testred Capsules, 10 mg (Methyltestosterone) ICN 1746

Pulmonary disease, obstruction, exacerbation of
- Zithromax (Azithromycin Dihydrate) Pfizer 2743
- Zithromax for Oral Suspension, 300 mg, 900 mg, 600 mg, 1200 mg (Azithromycin Dihydrate) Pfizer 2739
- Zithromax Tablets, 250 mg (Azithromycin Dihydrate) Pfizer 2739
- Zithromax Tablets, 600 mg (Azithromycin Dihydrate) Pfizer 2743

Pulmonary emphysema
(*see under* Emphysema)

Purpura, idiopathic thrombocytopenic
- Celestone Syrup (Betamethasone) Schering 3099
- Cortone Acetate Tablets (Cortisone Acetate) Merck 2061
- Decadron Elixir (Dexamethasone) Merck 2078
- Decadron Tablets (Dexamethasone) Merck 2079
- Decadron Phosphate Injection (Dexamethasone Sodium Phosphate) Merck 2081
- Depo-Medrol Injectable Suspension (Methylprednisolone Acetate) Pharmacia & Upjohn 2795
- Gamimune N, 5% Solvent/Detergent Treated (Globulin, Immune (Human)) Bayer Biological 925
- Gamimune N, 10% Solvent/Detergent Treated (Globulin, Immune (Human)) Bayer Biological 928
- Gammagard S/D (Globulin, Immune (Human)) Baxter Healthcare 845
- Hydrocortone Tablets (Hydrocortisone) Merck 2106
- Hydrocortone Phosphate Injection, Sterile (Hydrocortisone Sodium Phosphate) Merck 2105
- Pediapred Oral Solution (Prednisolone Sodium Phosphate) Celltech 1170
- Prednisone (Prednisone) Roxane 3064
- Prelone Syrup (Prednisolone) Muro 2273
- Sandoglobulin I.V. (Globulin, Immune (Human)) Novartis 2391
- Solu-Medrol Sterile Powder (Methylprednisolone Sodium Succinate) Pharmacia & Upjohn 2855
- WinRho SDF (Rh_0 (D) Immune Globulin (Human)) Nabi 2297

Pyelitis
- Uroqid-Acid No. 2 Tablets (Methenamine Mandelate, Sodium Acid Phosphate) Beach 947

Pyelitis, lacking substantial evidence of effectiveness in
- Urobiotic-250 Capsules (Oxytetracycline Hydrochloride, Phenazopyridine Hydrochloride, Sulfamethizole) Pfizer 2731

Pyelonephritis
- Azactam for Injection (Aztreonam) Elan 1276
- Ceclor (Cefaclor) Lilly 1905
- Levaquin (Levofloxacin) Ortho-McNeil 2537
- Lorabid Suspension and Pulvules (Loracarbef) Monarch 2251
- Maxipime for Injection (Cefepime Hydrochloride) Elan 1285
- Tequin Injection (Gatifloxacin) Bristol-Myers Squibb 1110
- Tequin Tablets (Gatifloxacin) Bristol-Myers Squibb 1110
- Uroqid-Acid No. 2 Tablets (Methenamine Mandelate, Sodium Acid Phosphate) Beach 947

Pyelonephritis, lacking substantial evidence of effectiveness in
- Urobiotic-250 Capsules (Oxytetracycline Hydrochloride, Phenazopyridine Hydrochloride, Sulfamethizole) Pfizer 2731

Pyoderma gangrenosum
- Levaquin (Levofloxacin) Ortho-McNeil 2537

Q

Q fever
- Declomycin Tablets (Demeclocycline Hydrochloride) Lederle 1855
- Doryx Coated Pellet Filled Capsules (Doxycycline Hyclate) Warner Chilcott 3357
- Dynacin Capsules (Minocycline Hydrochloride) Medicis 2019
- Minocin Intravenous (Minocycline Hydrochloride) Lederle 1862
- Minocin Oral Suspension (Minocycline Hydrochloride) Lederle 1865
- Minocin Pellet-Filled Capsules (Minocycline Hydrochloride) Lederle 1863
- Monodox Capsules (Doxycycline Monohydrate) Oclassen 2442
- Vibramycin Calcium Oral Suspension Syrup (Doxycycline Calcium) Pfizer 2735
- Vibramycin Hyclate Capsules (Doxycycline Hyclate) Pfizer 2735
- Vibramycin Hyclate Intravenous (Doxycycline Hyclate) Pfizer 2737
- Vibramycin Monohydrate for Oral Suspension (Doxycycline Monohydrate) Pfizer 2735
- Vibra-Tabs Film Coated Tablets (Doxycycline Hyclate) Pfizer 2735

R

Rabies, postexposure prophylaxis
- BayRab (Rabies Immune Globulin (Human)) Bayer Biological 917
- Imogam Rabies - HT (Rabies Immune Globulin (Human)) Aventis Pasteur 805
- Imovax Rabies Vaccine (Rabies Vaccine) Aventis Pasteur 807

Radiography, gastrointestinal tract, adjunct in
- GlucaGen for Injection Diagnostic Kit (Glucagon) Bedford 949
- Glucagon for Injection Vials and Emergency Kit (Glucagon) Lilly 1924
- Reglan (Metoclopramide Hydrochloride) Robins 2935

Rash, diaper
- A + D Original Ointment (Lanolin, Petrolatum) Schering-Plough .... ▣733
- A + D Ointment with Zinc Oxide (Dimethicone, Zinc Oxide) Schering-Plough .... ▣733
- Balmex Diaper Rash Ointment (Zinc Oxide) Block .... ▣619
- Balmex Medicated Plus Baby Powder (Corn Starch, Zinc Oxide) Block .... ▣619
- Desitin Baby Powder (Corn Starch, Zinc Oxide) Pfizer Inc., Warner-Lambert Healthcare .... ▣700
- Desitin Creamy Ointment (Zinc Oxide) Pfizer Inc., Warner-Lambert Healthcare .... ▣700
- Desitin Ointment (Cod Liver Oil, Zinc Oxide) Pfizer Inc., Warner-Lambert Healthcare .... ▣700

Rash, drug
(*see under* Hypersensitivity reactions, drug-induced)

Rash, unspecified
(*see under* Skin, inflammatory conditions)

Rat-bite fever
(*see under* Spirillum minus infections)

RDS
(*see under* Respiratory distress syndrome)

Reiter's syndrome
- Genuine Bayer Professional Labeling (Aspirin Regimen Bayer) (Aspirin) Bayer Consumer .... ▣608
- Extra Strength Bayer Arthritis Caplets (Aspirin) Bayer Consumer .... ▣610
- Ecotrin Enteric Coated Aspirin Low, Regular and Maximum Strength Tablets (Aspirin) GlaxoSmithKline Consumer 1715

Relapsing fever
(*see under* Borrelia recurrentis infection)

Renal allogeneic transplants, prophylaxis of organ rejection in
- CellCept Capsules (Mycophenolate Mofetil) Roche Laboratories 2951
- CellCept Intravenous (Mycophenolate Mofetil Hydrochloride) Roche Laboratories 2951
- CellCept Oral Suspension (Mycophenolate Mofetil) Roche Laboratories 2951
- CellCept Tablets (Mycophenolate Mofetil) Roche Laboratories 2951
- Zenapax for Injection (Daclizumab) Roche Laboratories 3046

Renal dialysis, adjunctive therapy
- Albumin (Human) 25% (Albumin (human)) Baxter Healthcare 839
- Plasbumin-20 (Albumin (human)) Bayer Biological 940
- Plasbumin-25 (Albumin (human)) Bayer Biological 941

Renal plasma flow, estimation of
- Aminohippurate Sodium PAH Injection (Aminohippurate Sodium) Merck 2041

Renal toxicity, cumulative, cisplatin-induced
- Ethyol for Injection (Amifostine) MedImmune Oncology 2029

Renal transplantation, prevention of rejection in
- CellCept Capsules (Mycophenolate Mofetil) Roche Laboratories 2951
- CellCept Intravenous (Mycophenolate Mofetil Hydrochloride) Roche Laboratories 2951
- CellCept Oral Suspension (Mycophenolate Mofetil) Roche Laboratories 2951
- CellCept Tablets (Mycophenolate Mofetil) Roche Laboratories 2951
- Gengraf Capsules (Cyclosporine) Abbott 457
- Neoral Soft Gelatin Capsules (Cyclosporine) Novartis 2380
- Neoral Oral Solution (Cyclosporine) Novartis 2380
- Orthoclone OKT3 Sterile Solution (Muromonab-CD3) Ortho Biotech 2498
- Prograf (Tacrolimus) Fujisawa 1393
- Rapamune Oral Solution and Tablets (Sirolimus) Wyeth-Ayerst 3584
- Sandimmune (Cyclosporine) Novartis 2388
- Simulect for Injection (Basiliximab) Novartis 2399
- Thymoglobulin for Injection (Antithymocyte Globulin) SangStat 3071

Renal tubular acidosis, management of
- Urocit-K Tablets (Potassium Citrate) Mission 2232

Renal tubular secretory mechanism, measurement of the functional capacity of
- Aminohippurate Sodium PAH Injection (Aminohippurate Sodium) Merck 2041

Respiratory depression, post-anesthesia
- Dopram Injectable (Doxapram Hydrochloride) Robins 2931
- Tensilon Injectable (Edrophonium Chloride) ICN 1745

Respiratory distress syndrome
- Albumin (Human) 25% (Albumin (human)) Baxter Healthcare 839
- Buminate 25% Solution, USP (Albumin (human)) Baxter Healthcare 842
- Curosurf Intratracheal Suspension (Poractant alfa) Dey 1232
- Infasurf Intratracheal Suspension (Calfactant) Forest 1372
- Plasbumin-20 (Albumin (human)) Bayer Biological 940
- Plasbumin-25 (Albumin (human)) Bayer Biological 941
- Survanta Intratracheal Suspension (Beractant) Ross 3053

Respiratory insufficiency, acute, with chronic obstructive pulmonary disease
- Dopram Injectable (Doxapram Hydrochloride) Robins 2931

Respiratory symptoms, upper, relief of
(*see under* Influenza syndrome, symptomatic relief of)

Respiratory syncytial virus (RSV) infections
(*see under* Infections, lower respiratory tract, RSV-induced)

Retinal attachment, surgical aid in
- Healon (Sodium Hyaluronate) Pharmacia & Upjohn .... ⊙316

Retinitis, cytomegalovirus
- Cytovene (Ganciclovir) Roche Laboratories 2959
- Foscavir Injection (Foscarnet Sodium) AstraZeneca LP 605
- Valcyte Tablets (Valganciclovir Hydrochloride) Roche Laboratories 3022
- Vistide Injection (Cidofovir) Gilead 1445
- Vitrasert Implant (Ganciclovir) Bausch & Lomb Surgical .... ⊙254
- Vitravene for Injection (Fomivirsen Sodium) Novartis Ophthalmics .... ⊙310

Rhabdomyosarcoma
- Cosmegen for Injection (Dactinomycin) Merck 2062

Rheumatic carditis, acute
- Celestone Soluspan Injectable Suspension (Betamethasone Acetate, Betamethasone Sodium Phosphate) Schering 3097
- Celestone Syrup (Betamethasone) Schering 3099
- Cortone Acetate Injectable Suspension (Cortisone Acetate) Merck 2059
- Cortone Acetate Tablets (Cortisone Acetate) Merck 2061
- Decadron Elixir (Dexamethasone) Merck 2078
- Decadron Tablets (Dexamethasone) Merck 2079
- Decadron Phosphate Injection (Dexamethasone Sodium Phosphate) Merck 2081

Depo-Medrol Injectable Suspension (Methylprednisolone Acetate) Pharmacia & Upjohn 2795
Hydrocortone Tablets (Hydrocortisone) Merck 2106
Hydrocortone Phosphate Injection, Sterile (Hydrocortisone Sodium Phosphate) Merck 2105
Pediapred Oral Solution (Prednisolone Sodium Phosphate) Celltech 1170
Prednisone (Prednisone) Roxane 3064
Prelone Syrup (Prednisolone) Muro . 2273
Solu-Medrol Sterile Powder (Methylprednisolone Sodium Succinate) Pharmacia & Upjohn 2855

Rheumatic fever, prophylaxis of

Bicillin L-A Injection (Penicillin G Benzathine) Monarch 2242
E.E.S. (Erythromycin Ethylsuccinate) Abbott 450
EryPed (Erythromycin Ethylsuccinate) Abbott 446
Erythromycin Base Filmtab Tablets (Erythromycin) Abbott 454
Erythromycin Delayed-Release Capsules, USP (Erythromycin) Abbott 455
PCE Dispertab Tablets (Erythromycin) Abbott 498
Permapen Isoject (Penicillin G Benzathine) Pfizer 2706

Rheumatoid arthritis

Anaprox Tablets (Naproxen Sodium) Roche Laboratories 2967
Anaprox DS Tablets (Naproxen Sodium) Roche Laboratories 2967
Arava Tablets (Leflunomide) Aventis 724
Arthrotec Tablets (Diclofenac Sodium, Misoprostol) Searle 3195
Azulfidine EN-tabs Tablets (Sulfasalazine) Pharmacia & Upjohn ... 2775
Genuine Bayer Professional Labeling (Aspirin Regimen Bayer) (Aspirin) Bayer Consumer ...... ▣608
Extra Strength Bayer Arthritis Caplets (Aspirin) Bayer Consumer ...... ▣610
Cataflam Tablets (Diclofenac Potassium) Novartis 2315
Celebrex Capsules (Celecoxib) Pfizer 2676
Celebrex Capsules (Celecoxib) Pharmacia & Upjohn 2780
Celestone Soluspan Injectable Suspension (Betamethasone Acetate, Betamethasone Sodium Phosphate) Schering 3097
Celestone Syrup (Betamethasone) Schering 3099
Clinoril Tablets (Sulindac) Merck 2053
Cortone Acetate Injectable Suspension (Cortisone Acetate) Merck 2059
Cortone Acetate Tablets (Cortisone Acetate) Merck 2061
Cuprimine Capsules (Penicillamine) Merck 2075
Decadron Elixir (Dexamethasone) Merck 2078
Decadron Tablets (Dexamethasone) Merck 2079
Decadron Phosphate Injection (Dexamethasone Sodium Phosphate) Merck 2081
Depen Titratable Tablets (Penicillamine) Wallace 3341
Depo-Medrol Injectable Suspension (Methylprednisolone Acetate) Pharmacia & Upjohn 2795
Dolobid Tablets (Diflunisal) Merck 2088
EC-Naprosyn Delayed-Release Tablets (Naproxen) Roche Laboratories 2967
Ecotrin Enteric Coated Aspirin Low, Regular and Maximum Strength Tablets (Aspirin) GlaxoSmithKline Consumer 1715
Enbrel for Injection (Etanercept) Immunex 1752
Enbrel for Injection (Etanercept) Wyeth-Ayerst 3504
Feldene Capsules (Piroxicam) Pfizer 2685
Gengraf Capsules (Cyclosporine) Abbott 457
Hydrocortone Tablets (Hydrocortisone) Merck 2106
Hydrocortone Acetate Injectable Suspension (Hydrocortisone Acetate) Merck 2103
Hydrocortone Phosphate Injection, Sterile (Hydrocortisone Sodium Phosphate) Merck 2105
Indocin (Indomethacin) Merck 2112
Lodine (Etodolac) Wyeth-Ayerst 3528
Lodine XL Extended-Release Tablets (Etodolac) Wyeth-Ayerst ... 3530
Motrin Suspension, Oral Drops, Chewable Tablets, and Caplets (Ibuprofen) McNeil Consumer 2002
Naprelan Tablets (Naproxen Sodium) Elan 1293
Naprosyn Suspension (Naproxen) Roche Laboratories 2967
Naprosyn Tablets (Naproxen) Roche Laboratories 2967
Neoral Soft Gelatin Capsules (Cyclosporine) Novartis 2380
Neoral Oral Solution (Cyclosporine) Novartis 2380
Orudis Capsules (Ketoprofen) Wyeth-Ayerst 3548
Oruvail Capsules (Ketoprofen) Wyeth-Ayerst 3548
Pediapred Oral Solution (Prednisolone Sodium Phosphate) Celltech 1170
Plaquenil Tablets (Hydroxychloroquine Sulfate) Sanofi-Synthelabo ... 3082
Prednisone (Prednisone) Roxane 3064
Prelone Syrup (Prednisolone) Muro . 2273
Relafen Tablets (Nabumetone) GlaxoSmithKline 1617
Remicade for IV Injection (Infliximab) Centocor 1178
Solu-Medrol Sterile Powder (Methylprednisolone Sodium Succinate) Pharmacia & Upjohn 2855
Tolectin (Tolmetin Sodium) Ortho-McNeil 2589
Trilisate (Choline Magnesium Trisalicylate) Purdue Frederick 2901
Voltaren Tablets (Diclofenac Sodium) Novartis 2315
Voltaren-XR Tablets (Diclofenac Sodium) Novartis 2315

Rheumatoid arthritis, juvenile

Genuine Bayer Professional Labeling (Aspirin Regimen Bayer) (Aspirin) Bayer Consumer ...... ▣608
Extra Strength Bayer Arthritis Caplets (Aspirin) Bayer Consumer ...... ▣610
Celestone Soluspan Injectable Suspension (Betamethasone Acetate, Betamethasone Sodium Phosphate) Schering 3097
Celestone Syrup (Betamethasone) Schering 3099
Cortone Acetate Injectable Suspension (Cortisone Acetate) Merck 2059
Cortone Acetate Tablets (Cortisone Acetate) Merck 2061
Decadron Elixir (Dexamethasone) Merck 2078
Decadron Tablets (Dexamethasone) Merck 2079
Decadron Phosphate Injection (Dexamethasone Sodium Phosphate) Merck 2081
Depo-Medrol Injectable Suspension (Methylprednisolone Acetate) Pharmacia & Upjohn 2795
Ecotrin Enteric Coated Aspirin Low, Regular and Maximum Strength Tablets (Aspirin) GlaxoSmithKline Consumer 1715
Enbrel for Injection (Etanercept) Immunex 1752
Enbrel for Injection (Etanercept) Wyeth-Ayerst 3504
Hydrocortone Tablets (Hydrocortisone) Merck 2106
Hydrocortone Phosphate Injection, Sterile (Hydrocortisone Sodium Phosphate) Merck 2105
Pediapred Oral Solution (Prednisolone Sodium Phosphate) Celltech 1170
Prednisone (Prednisone) Roxane 3064
Prelone Syrup (Prednisolone) Muro . 2273
Solu-Medrol Sterile Powder (Methylprednisolone Sodium Succinate) Pharmacia & Upjohn 2855
Tolectin (Tolmetin Sodium) Ortho-McNeil 2589
Trilisate (Choline Magnesium Trisalicylate) Purdue Frederick 2901

Rhinitis, acute, drying agent in

Levsin/Levsinex/Levbid (Hyoscyamine Sulfate) Schwarz 3172
NuLev Orally Disintegrating Tablets (Hyoscyamine Sulfate) Schwarz 3176

Rhinitis, allergic

Actifed Cold & Allergy Tablets (Pseudoephedrine Hydrochloride, Triprolidine Hydrochloride) Pfizer Inc., Warner-Lambert Healthcare ...... ▣688
Atrovent Nasal Spray 0.03% (Ipratropium Bromide) Boehringer Ingelheim 1032
Dimetapp Elixir (Brompheniramine Maleate, Pseudoephedrine Hydrochloride) Whitehall-Robins ...... ▣777
Extendryl (Chlorpheniramine Maleate, Methscopolamine Nitrate, Phenylephrine Hydrochloride) Fleming 1361
NasalCrom Nasal Spray (Cromolyn Sodium) Pharmacia Consumer ...... ▣719
Natru-Vent Saline Nasal Spray (Sodium Chloride) Boehringer Ingelheim ...... ▣625
Ocean Nasal Mist (Sodium Chloride) Fleming ...... ▣633
Phenergan Suppositories (Promethazine Hydrochloride) Wyeth-Ayerst 3556
Phenergan Syrup (Promethazine Hydrochloride) Wyeth-Ayerst 3554
Phenergan Tablets (Promethazine Hydrochloride) Wyeth-Ayerst 3556
Ryna Liquid (Chlorpheniramine Maleate, Pseudoephedrine Hydrochloride) Wallace ...... ▣768
Ryna-12 S Suspension (Phenylephrine Tannate, Pyrilamine Tannate) Wallace 3351
Reformulated Rynatan Pediatric Suspension (Chlorpheniramine Tannate, Phenylephrine Tannate) Wallace 3352
Rynatan Tablets (Azatadine Maleate, Pseudoephedrine Sulfate) Wallace 3351
Semprex-D Capsules (Acrivastine, Pseudoephedrine Hydrochloride) Celltech 1172
Vancenase AQ Nasal Spray 0.084% (Beclomethasone Dipropionate) Schering 3163

Rhinitis, perennial allergic

Atrovent Nasal Spray 0.03% (Ipratropium Bromide) Boehringer Ingelheim 1032
Beconase Inhalation Aerosol (Beclomethasone Dipropionate) GlaxoSmithKline 1497
Beconase AQ Nasal Spray (Beclomethasone Dipropionate Monohydrate) GlaxoSmithKline 1498
Bromfed Capsules (Extended-Release) (Brompheniramine Maleate, Pseudoephedrine Hydrochloride) Muro 2269
Bromfed-PD Capsules (Extended-Release) (Brompheniramine Maleate, Pseudoephedrine Hydrochloride) Muro 2269
Celestone Soluspan Injectable Suspension (Betamethasone Acetate, Betamethasone Sodium Phosphate) Schering 3097
Celestone Syrup (Betamethasone) Schering 3099
Cortone Acetate Injectable Suspension (Cortisone Acetate) Merck 2059
Cortone Acetate Tablets (Cortisone Acetate) Merck 2061
Decadron Elixir (Dexamethasone) Merck 2078
Decadron Tablets (Dexamethasone) Merck 2079
Decadron Phosphate Injection (Dexamethasone Sodium Phosphate) Merck 2081
Depo-Medrol Injectable Suspension (Methylprednisolone Acetate) Pharmacia & Upjohn 2795
Flonase Nasal Spray (Fluticasone Propionate) GlaxoSmithKline 1533
Hydrocortone Tablets (Hydrocortisone) Merck 2106
Hydrocortone Phosphate Injection, Sterile (Hydrocortisone Sodium Phosphate) Merck 2105
Nasacort Nasal Inhaler (Triamcinolone Acetonide) Aventis 750
Nasacort AQ Nasal Spray (Triamcinolone Acetonide) Aventis 752
NasalCrom Nasal Spray (Cromolyn Sodium) Pharmacia Consumer ...... ▣719
Nasalide Nasal Spray (Flunisolide) Elan 1295
Nasarel Nasal Solution 0.025% (Flunisolide) Elan 1296
Nasonex Nasal Spray (Mometasone Furoate Monohydrate) Schering 3131
Pediapred Oral Solution (Prednisolone Sodium Phosphate) Celltech 1170
Periactin Tablets (Cyproheptadine Hydrochloride) Merck 2155
Prednisone (Prednisone) Roxane 3064
Prelone Syrup (Prednisolone) Muro . 2273
Rhinocort Aqua Nasal Spray (Budesonide) AstraZeneca LP 642
Rhinocort Nasal Inhaler (Budesonide) AstraZeneca LP 640
Solu-Medrol Sterile Powder (Methylprednisolone Sodium Succinate) Pharmacia & Upjohn 2855
Tri-Nasal Spray (Triamcinolone Acetonide) Muro 2274
Vancenase PocketHaler Nasal Inhaler (Beclomethasone Dipropionate) Schering 3162
Zyrtec (Cetirizine Hydrochloride) Pfizer 2756
Zyrtec-D 12 Hour Extended Relief Tablets (Cetirizine Hydrochloride, Pseudoephedrine Hydrochloride) Pfizer 2758

Rhinitis, seasonal allergic

Actifed Cold & Sinus Caplets and Tablets (Acetaminophen, Chlorpheniramine Maleate, Pseudoephedrine Hydrochloride) Pfizer Inc., Warner-Lambert Healthcare ...... ▣688
Allegra (Fexofenadine Hydrochloride) Aventis 712
Allegra-D Extended-Release Tablets (Fexofenadine Hydrochloride, Pseudoephedrine Hydrochloride) Aventis 714
Astelin Nasal Spray (Azelastine Hydrochloride) Wallace 3339
Beconase Inhalation Aerosol (Beclomethasone Dipropionate) GlaxoSmithKline 1497
Beconase AQ Nasal Spray (Beclomethasone Dipropionate Monohydrate) GlaxoSmithKline 1498
Benadryl Allergy Liquid (Diphenhydramine Hydrochloride) Pfizer Inc., Warner-Lambert Healthcare ...... ▣690
Benadryl Allergy/Congestion Tablets (Diphenhydramine Hydrochloride, Pseudoephedrine Hydrochloride) Pfizer Inc., Warner-Lambert Healthcare ...... ▣692
Benadryl Allergy & Sinus Liquid (Diphenhydramine Hydrochloride, Pseudoephedrine Hydrochloride) Pfizer Inc., Warner-Lambert Healthcare ...... ▣693
Benadryl Allergy Sinus Headache Caplets & Gelcaps (Acetaminophen, Diphenhydramine Hydrochloride, Pseudoephedrine Hydrochloride) Pfizer Inc., Warner-Lambert Healthcare ...... ▣693
Bromfed Capsules (Extended-Release) (Brompheniramine Maleate, Pseudoephedrine Hydrochloride) Muro 2269
Bromfed-PD Capsules (Extended-Release) (Brompheniramine Maleate, Pseudoephedrine Hydrochloride) Muro 2269
Celestone Soluspan Injectable Suspension (Betamethasone Acetate, Betamethasone Sodium Phosphate) Schering 3097
Celestone Syrup (Betamethasone) Schering 3099
Claritin (Loratadine) Schering 3100
Claritin-D 12 Hour Extended Release Tablets (Loratadine, Pseudoephedrine Sulfate) Schering 3102
Claritin-D 24 Hour Extended Release Tablets (Loratadine, Pseudoephedrine Sulfate) Schering 3104
Cortone Acetate Injectable Suspension (Cortisone Acetate) Merck 2059
Cortone Acetate Tablets (Cortisone Acetate) Merck 2061
Decadron Elixir (Dexamethasone) Merck 2078
Decadron Tablets (Dexamethasone) Merck 2079
Decadron Phosphate Injection (Dexamethasone Sodium Phosphate) Merck 2081
Depo-Medrol Injectable Suspension (Methylprednisolone Acetate) Pharmacia & Upjohn 2795
Flonase Nasal Spray (Fluticasone Propionate) GlaxoSmithKline 1533
Hydrocortone Tablets (Hydrocortisone) Merck 2106
Hydrocortone Phosphate Injection, Sterile (Hydrocortisone Sodium Phosphate) Merck 2105
Nasacort Nasal Inhaler (Triamcinolone Acetonide) Aventis 750
Nasacort AQ Nasal Spray (Triamcinolone Acetonide) Aventis 752

NasalCrom Nasal Spray (Cromolyn Sodium) Pharmacia Consumer .... ▣719
Nasalide Nasal Spray (Flunisolide) Elan 1295
Nasarel Nasal Solution 0.025% (Flunisolide) Elan 1296
Nasonex Nasal Spray (Mometasone Furoate Monohydrate) Schering 3131
Pediapred Oral Solution (Prednisolone Sodium Phosphate) Celltech 1170
Periactin Tablets (Cyproheptadine Hydrochloride) Merck 2155
Prednisone (Prednisone) Roxane 3064
Prelone Syrup (Prednisolone) Muro . 2273
Rhinocort Aqua Nasal Spray (Budesonide) AstraZeneca LP 642
Rhinocort Nasal Inhaler (Budesonide) AstraZeneca LP 640
Sinutab Sinus Allergy Medication, Maximum Strength Formula, Tablets & Caplets (Acetaminophen, Chlorpheniramine Maleate, Pseudoephedrine Hydrochloride) Pfizer Inc., Warner-Lambert Healthcare .... ▣707
Sinutab Sinus Medication, Maximum Strength Without Drowsiness Formula, Tablets & Caplets (Acetaminophen, Pseudoephedrine Hydrochloride) Pfizer Inc., Warner-Lambert Healthcare .... ▣707
Solu-Medrol Sterile Powder (Methylprednisolone Sodium Succinate) Pharmacia & Upjohn 2855
Tri-Nasal Spray (Triamcinolone Acetonide) Muro 2274
Vancenase PocketHaler Nasal Inhaler (Beclomethasone Dipropionate) Schering 3162
Zyrtec (Cetirizine Hydrochloride) Pfizer 2756
Zyrtec-D 12 Hour Extended Relief Tablets (Cetirizine Hydrochloride, Pseudoephedrine Hydrochloride) Pfizer 2758

Rhinitis, vasomotor
Astelin Nasal Spray (Azelastine Hydrochloride) Wallace 3339
Beconase AQ Nasal Spray (Beclomethasone Dipropionate Monohydrate) GlaxoSmithKline 1498
Bromfed Capsules (Extended-Release) (Brompheniramine Maleate, Pseudoephedrine Hydrochloride) Muro 2269
Bromfed-PD Capsules (Extended-Release) (Brompheniramine Maleate, Pseudoephedrine Hydrochloride) Muro 2269
Periactin Tablets (Cyproheptadine Hydrochloride) Merck 2155
Phenergan Suppositories (Promethazine Hydrochloride) Wyeth-Ayerst 3556
Phenergan Syrup (Promethazine Hydrochloride) Wyeth-Ayerst 3554
Phenergan Tablets (Promethazine Hydrochloride) Wyeth-Ayerst 3556
Vancenase AQ Nasal Spray 0.084% (Beclomethasone Dipropionate) Schering 3163

Rhinitis sicca
Afrin Extra Moisturizing Saline Mist (Sodium Chloride) Schering-Plough .... ▣734

Rhinorrhea
Allegra-D Extended-Release Tablets (Fexofenadine Hydrochloride, Pseudoephedrine Hydrochloride) Aventis 714
Atrovent Nasal Spray 0.03% (Ipratropium Bromide) Boehringer Ingelheim 1032
Atrovent Nasal Spray 0.06% (Ipratropium Bromide) Boehringer Ingelheim 1033
Benadryl Allergy Chewables (Diphenhydramine Hydrochloride) Pfizer Inc., Warner-Lambert Healthcare .... ▣689
Benadryl Allergy Kapseal Capsules (Diphenhydramine Hydrochloride) Pfizer Inc., Warner-Lambert Healthcare .... ▣691
Benadryl Allergy Liquid (Diphenhydramine Hydrochloride) Pfizer Inc., Warner-Lambert Healthcare .... ▣690
Benadryl Allergy Ultratab Tablets (Diphenhydramine Hydrochloride) Pfizer Inc., Warner-Lambert Healthcare .... ▣691
Benadryl Allergy/Congestion Tablets (Diphenhydramine Hydrochloride, Pseudoephedrine Hydrochloride) Pfizer Inc., Warner-Lambert Healthcare .... ▣692
Benadryl Allergy Sinus Headache Caplets & Gelcaps (Acetaminophen, Diphenhydramine Hydrochloride, Pseudoephedrine Hydrochloride) Pfizer Inc., Warner-Lambert Healthcare .... ▣693
Benadryl Dye-Free Allergy Liquid (Diphenhydramine Hydrochloride) Pfizer Inc., Warner-Lambert Healthcare .... ▣690
Benadryl Dye-Free Allergy Liqui-Gels Softgels (Diphenhydramine Hydrochloride) Pfizer Inc., Warner-Lambert Healthcare .... ▣690
Chlor-Trimeton Allergy Tablets (Chlorpheniramine Maleate) Schering-Plough .... ▣735
Chlor-Trimeton Allergy/Decongestant Tablets (Chlorpheniramine Maleate, Pseudoephedrine Sulfate) Schering-Plough .... ▣736
Comtrex Acute Head Cold & Sinus Pressure Relief Tablets (Acetaminophen, Brompheniramine Maleate, Pseudoephedrine Hydrochloride) Bristol-Myers .... ▣627
Dimetapp Elixir (Brompheniramine Maleate, Pseudoephedrine Hydrochloride) Whitehall-Robins .... ▣777
Dimetapp Cold and Fever Suspension (Acetaminophen, Brompheniramine Maleate, Pseudoephedrine Hydrochloride) Whitehall-Robins .... ▣775
PediaCare Cough-Cold Liquid (Chlorpheniramine Maleate, Dextromethorphan Hydrobromide, Pseudoephedrine Hydrochloride) Pharmacia Consumer .... ▣719
Ryna (Chlorpheniramine Maleate, Pseudoephedrine Hydrochloride) Wallace .... ▣768
Tavist 12 Hour Allergy Tablets (Clemastine Fumarate) Novartis Consumer .... ▣676
Triaminic Cold & Allergy Softchews (Chlorpheniramine Maleate, Pseudoephedrine Hydrochloride) Novartis Consumer .... ▣683
Maximum Strength Tylenol Allergy Sinus Caplets, Gelcaps, and Geltabs (Acetaminophen, Chlorpheniramine Maleate, Pseudoephedrine Hydrochloride) McNeil Consumer 2010
Tylenol Severe Allergy Caplets (Acetaminophen, Diphenhydramine Hydrochloride) McNeil Consumer 2010

Rickets
Rocaltrol (Calcitriol) Roche Laboratories 2991

Rickettsiae
Declomycin Tablets (Demeclocycline Hydrochloride) Lederle 1855
Doryx Coated Pellet Filled Capsules (Doxycycline Hyclate) Warner Chilcott 3357
Dynacin Capsules (Minocycline Hydrochloride) Medicis 2019
Minocin Intravenous (Minocycline Hydrochloride) Lederle 1862
Minocin Oral Suspension (Minocycline Hydrochloride) Lederle 1865
Minocin Pellet-Filled Capsules (Minocycline Hydrochloride) Lederle 1863
Monodox Capsules (Doxycycline Monohydrate) Oclassen 2442
Vibramycin Calcium Oral Suspension Syrup (Doxycycline Calcium) Pfizer 2735
Vibramycin Hyclate Capsules (Doxycycline Hyclate) Pfizer 2735
Vibramycin Hyclate Intravenous (Doxycycline Hyclate) Pfizer 2737
Vibramycin Monohydrate for Oral Suspension (Doxycycline Monohydrate) Pfizer 2735
Vibra-Tabs Film Coated Tablets (Doxycycline Hyclate) Pfizer 2735

Rickettsialpox
Declomycin Tablets (Demeclocycline Hydrochloride) Lederle 1855
Doryx Coated Pellet Filled Capsules (Doxycycline Hyclate) Warner Chilcott 3357
Dynacin Capsules (Minocycline Hydrochloride) Medicis 2019
Minocin Intravenous (Minocycline Hydrochloride) Lederle 1862
Minocin Oral Suspension (Minocycline Hydrochloride) Lederle 1865
Minocin Pellet-Filled Capsules (Minocycline Hydrochloride) Lederle 1863
Monodox Capsules (Doxycycline Monohydrate) Oclassen 2442
Vibramycin Calcium Oral Suspension Syrup (Doxycycline Calcium) Pfizer 2735
Vibramycin Hyclate Capsules (Doxycycline Hyclate) Pfizer 2735
Vibramycin Hyclate Intravenous (Doxycycline Hyclate) Pfizer 2737
Vibramycin Monohydrate for Oral Suspension (Doxycycline Monohydrate) Pfizer 2735
Vibra-Tabs Film Coated Tablets (Doxycycline Hyclate) Pfizer 2735

Ringworm infections of the body
(*see under* Tinea corporis infections)

Ringworm infections of the feet
(*see under* Tinea pedis infections)

Ringworm infections of the groin
(*see under* Tinea cruris infections)

Ringworm infections of the nails
(*see under* Tinea unguium infections)

Ringworm infections of the scalp
(*see under* Tinea capitis infections)

Rocky Mountain spotted fever
Declomycin Tablets (Demeclocycline Hydrochloride) Lederle 1855
Doryx Coated Pellet Filled Capsules (Doxycycline Hyclate) Warner Chilcott 3357
Dynacin Capsules (Minocycline Hydrochloride) Medicis 2019
Minocin Intravenous (Minocycline Hydrochloride) Lederle 1862
Minocin Oral Suspension (Minocycline Hydrochloride) Lederle 1865
Minocin Pellet-Filled Capsules (Minocycline Hydrochloride) Lederle 1863
Monodox Capsules (Doxycycline Monohydrate) Oclassen 2442
Vibramycin Calcium Oral Suspension Syrup (Doxycycline Calcium) Pfizer 2735
Vibramycin Hyclate Capsules (Doxycycline Hyclate) Pfizer 2735
Vibramycin Hyclate Intravenous (Doxycycline Hyclate) Pfizer 2737
Vibramycin Monohydrate for Oral Suspension (Doxycycline Monohydrate) Pfizer 2735
Vibra-Tabs Film Coated Tablets (Doxycycline Hyclate) Pfizer 2735

Rosacea
MetroCream (Metronidazole) Galderma 1404
MetroGel (Metronidazole) Galderma 1405
MetroLotion (Metronidazole) Galderma 1405
Noritate Cream (Metronidazole) Dermik 1224

Roundworm, common
(*see under* Ascaris lumbricoides infections)

Rubella, prophylaxis
Meruvax II (Rubella Virus Vaccine Live) Merck 2130
M-M-R II (Measles, Mumps & Rubella Virus Vaccine, Live) Merck 2118

S

S. agalactiae gynecologic infections
Cefobid Intravenous/Intramuscular (Cefoperazone) Pfizer 2671
Cefobid Pharmacy Bulk Package - Not for Direct Infusion (Cefoperazone Sodium) Pfizer 2673
Cefotan (Cefotetan) AstraZeneca 664

S. agalactiae infections
Cefizox for Intramuscular or Intravenous Use (Ceftizoxime Sodium) Fujisawa 1390
Cefobid Intravenous/Intramuscular (Cefoperazone) Pfizer 2671
Cefobid Pharmacy Bulk Package - Not for Direct Infusion (Cefoperazone Sodium) Pfizer 2673
Cefotan (Cefotetan) AstraZeneca 664
Noroxin Tablets (Norfloxacin) Merck 2145
Zithromax (Azithromycin Dihydrate) Pfizer 2743
Zithromax for Oral Suspension, 300 mg, 600 mg, 900 mg, 1200 mg (Azithromycin Dihydrate) Pfizer 2739
Zithromax Tablets, 250 mg (Azithromycin Dihydrate) Pfizer 2739
Zithromax Tablets, 600 mg (Azithromycin Dihydrate) Pfizer 2743
Zyvox (Linezolid) Pharmacia & Upjohn 2871

S. agalactiae pelvic inflammatory disease
Cefizox for Intramuscular or Intravenous Use (Ceftizoxime Sodium) Fujisawa 1390
Cefobid Intravenous/Intramuscular (Cefoperazone) Pfizer 2671
Cefobid Pharmacy Bulk Package - Not for Direct Infusion (Cefoperazone Sodium) Pfizer 2673

S. agalactiae septicemia
Cefobid Intravenous/Intramuscular (Cefoperazone) Pfizer 2671
Cefobid Pharmacy Bulk Package - Not for Direct Infusion (Cefoperazone Sodium) Pfizer 2673

S. agalactiae skin and skin structure infections
Trovan (Alatrofloxacin Mesylate) Pfizer 2722
Zithromax (Azithromycin Dihydrate) Pfizer 2743
Zithromax for Oral Suspension, 300 mg, 600 mg, 900 mg, 1200 mg (Azithromycin Dihydrate) Pfizer 2739
Zithromax Tablets, 250 mg (Azithromycin Dihydrate) Pfizer 2739
Zithromax Tablets, 600 mg (Azithromycin Dihydrate) Pfizer 2743
Zyvox (Linezolid) Pharmacia & Upjohn 2871

S. agalactiae urinary tract infections
Noroxin Tablets (Norfloxacin) Merck 2145

S. aureus (non-penicillinase producing) infections
Cefotan (Cefotetan) AstraZeneca 664
Claforan Injection (Cefotaxime Sodium) Aventis 732
Mefoxin for Injection (Cefoxitin Sodium) Merck 2124
Mefoxin Premixed Intravenous Solution (Cefoxitin Sodium) Merck 2127
Primaxin I.V. (Cilastatin Sodium, Imipenem) Merck 2160

S. aureus (penicillinase and non-penicillinase producing strains) skin and skin structure infections
Mandol Vials (Cefamandole Nafate) Lilly 1953
Mefoxin for Injection (Cefoxitin Sodium) Merck 2124
Mefoxin Premixed Intravenous Solution (Cefoxitin Sodium) Merck 2127
Nebcin Vials, Hyporets & ADD-Vantage (Tobramycin Sulfate) Lilly 1955
Zinacef Injection (Cefuroxime) GlaxoSmithKline 1696
Zinacef for Injection (Cefuroxime) GlaxoSmithKline 1696

S. aureus (penicillinase producing) infections
Cefotan (Cefotetan) AstraZeneca 664
Cefzil (Cefprozil) Bristol-Myers Squibb 1076
Claforan Injection (Cefotaxime Sodium) Aventis 732
Kefzol Vials, ADD-Vantage (Cefazolin Sodium) Lilly 1951
Lorabid Suspension and Pulvules (Loracarbef) Monarch 2251
Mefoxin for Injection (Cefoxitin Sodium) Merck 2124
Mefoxin Premixed Intravenous Solution (Cefoxitin Sodium) Merck 2127
Primaxin I.M. (Cilastatin Sodium, Imipenem) Merck 2158
Primaxin I.V. (Cilastatin Sodium, Imipenem) Merck 2160

S. aureus biliary tract infections
Ancef for Injection (Cefazolin Sodium) GlaxoSmithKline 1474
Ancef Injection (Cefazolin Sodium) GlaxoSmithKline 1474
Kefzol Vials, ADD-Vantage (Cefazolin Sodium) Lilly 1951

S. aureus bone and joint infections
Ancef for Injection (Cefazolin Sodium) GlaxoSmithKline 1474
Ancef Injection (Cefazolin Sodium) GlaxoSmithKline 1474
Cefizox for Intramuscular or Intravenous Use (Ceftizoxime Sodium) Fujisawa 1390
Cefotan (Cefotetan) AstraZeneca 664
Ceptaz for Injection (Ceftazidime) GlaxoSmithKline 1499
Claforan Injection (Cefotaxime Sodium) Aventis 732
Cleocin Phosphate Sterile Solution (Clindamycin Phosphate) Pharmacia & Upjohn 2785
Fortaz (Ceftazidime Sodium) GlaxoSmithKline 1541
Kefurox Vials, ADD-Vantage (Cefuroxime Sodium) Lilly 1948
Kefzol Vials, ADD-Vantage (Cefazolin Sodium) Lilly 1951
Mandol Vials (Cefamandole Nafate) Lilly 1953
Mefoxin for Injection (Cefoxitin Sodium) Merck 2124
Mefoxin Premixed Intravenous Solution (Cefoxitin Sodium) Merck 2127
Nebcin Vials, Hyporets & ADD-Vantage (Tobramycin Sulfate) Lilly 1955
Primaxin I.V. (Cilastatin Sodium, Imipenem) Merck 2160
Rocephin Injectable Vials, ADD-Vantage, Galaxy, Bulk (Ceftriaxone Sodium) Roche Laboratories 2993
Tazicef for Injection (Ceftazidime) GlaxoSmithKline 1647
Tazicef Galaxy Container (Ceftazidime Sodium) GlaxoSmithKline 1650
Tazicef Pharmacy Bulk Package (Ceftazidime) GlaxoSmithKline 1653
Tazidime Vials, Faspak & ADD-Vantage (Ceftazidime) Lilly 1966
Timentin Injection- ADD-Vantage Vial (Clavulanate Potassium, Ticarcillin Disodium) GlaxoSmithKline 1661
Timentin Injection-Galaxy Container (Clavulanate Potassium, Ticarcillin Disodium) GlaxoSmithKline 1664
Timentin Injection-Pharmacy Bulk Package (Clavulanate Potassium, Ticarcillin Disodium) GlaxoSmithKline 1666
Timentin for Intravenous Administration (Clavulanate Potassium, Ticarcillin Disodium) GlaxoSmithKline 1658
Zinacef Injection (Cefuroxime) GlaxoSmithKline 1696
Zinacef for Injection (Cefuroxime) GlaxoSmithKline 1696

S. aureus endocarditis
Ancef for Injection (Cefazolin Sodium) GlaxoSmithKline 1474
Ancef Injection (Cefazolin Sodium) GlaxoSmithKline 1474
Kefzol Vials, ADD-Vantage (Cefazolin Sodium) Lilly 1951
Primaxin I.V. (Cilastatin Sodium, Imipenem) Merck 2160

S. aureus gynecologic infections
Cefotan (Cefotetan) AstraZeneca 664
Primaxin I.V. (Cilastatin Sodium, Imipenem) Merck 2160
Timentin Injection- ADD-Vantage Vial (Clavulanate Potassium, Ticarcillin Disodium) GlaxoSmithKline 1661
Timentin Injection-Galaxy Container (Clavulanate Potassium, Ticarcillin Disodium) GlaxoSmithKline 1664
Timentin Injection-Pharmacy Bulk Package (Clavulanate Potassium, Ticarcillin Disodium) GlaxoSmithKline 1666
Timentin for Intravenous Administration (Clavulanate Potassium, Ticarcillin Disodium) GlaxoSmithKline 1658

S. aureus infection, eradication of nasal colonization of
Bactroban Nasal (Mupirocin Calcium) GlaxoSmithKline 1495

S. aureus infections
Ancef for Injection (Cefazolin Sodium) GlaxoSmithKline 1474
Ancef Injection (Cefazolin Sodium) GlaxoSmithKline 1474
Augmentin Chewable Tablets (Amoxicillin, Clavulanate Potassium) GlaxoSmithKline 1482
Augmentin Powder for Oral Suspension (Amoxicillin, Clavulanate Potassium) GlaxoSmithKline 1482
Augmentin Tablets (Amoxicillin, Clavulanate Potassium) GlaxoSmithKline 1485
Avelox Tablets (Moxifloxacin Hydrochloride) Bayer 879
Bactroban Ointment (Mupirocin) GlaxoSmithKline 1496
Biaxin/Biaxin XL (Clarithromycin) Abbott 403
Ceclor (Cefaclor) Lilly 1905
Cefizox for Intramuscular or Intravenous Use (Ceftizoxime Sodium) Fujisawa 1390
Cefobid Intravenous/Intramuscular (Cefoperazone) Pfizer 2671
Cefobid Pharmacy Bulk Package - Not for Direct Infusion (Cefoperazone Sodium) Pfizer 2673
Cefotan (Cefotetan) AstraZeneca 664
Ceftin (Cefuroxime Axetil) Lifecycle Ventures 1898
Cefzil (Cefprozil) Bristol-Myers Squibb 1076
Ceptaz for Injection (Ceftazidime) GlaxoSmithKline 1499
Cipro I.V. (Ciprofloxacin) Bayer 893
Cipro (Ciprofloxacin) Bayer 887
Claforan Injection (Cefotaxime Sodium) Aventis 732
Cleocin HCl Capsules (Clindamycin Hydrochloride) Pharmacia & Upjohn 2784
Cleocin Phosphate Sterile Solution (Clindamycin Phosphate) Pharmacia & Upjohn 2785
Declomycin Tablets (Demeclocycline Hydrochloride) Lederle 1855
Dynabac Tablets (Dirithromycin) Muro 2269
Dynacin Capsules (Minocycline Hydrochloride) Medicis 2019
E.E.S. (Erythromycin Ethylsuccinate) Abbott 450
EryPed (Erythromycin Ethylsuccinate) Abbott 446
Ery-Tab Tablets (Erythromycin) Abbott 448
Erythrocin Stearate Filmtab Tablets (Erythromycin Stearate) Abbott 452
Erythromycin Base Filmtab Tablets (Erythromycin) Abbott 454
Erythromycin Delayed-Release Capsules, USP (Erythromycin) Abbott 455
Floxin I.V. (Ofloxacin) Ortho-McNeil 2526
Floxin Tablets (Ofloxacin) Ortho-McNeil 2529
Fortaz (Ceftazidime Sodium) GlaxoSmithKline 1541
Kefurox Vials, ADD-Vantage (Cefuroxime Sodium) Lilly 1948
Kefzol Vials, ADD-Vantage (Cefazolin Sodium) Lilly 1951
Levaquin (Levofloxacin) Ortho-McNeil 2537
Lorabid Suspension and Pulvules (Loracarbef) Monarch 2251
Macrodantin Capsules (Nitrofurantoin) Procter & Gamble Pharmaceuticals 2891
Mandol Vials (Cefamandole Nafate) Lilly 1953
Maxipime for Injection (Cefepime Hydrochloride) Elan 1285
Mefoxin for Injection (Cefoxitin Sodium) Merck 2124
Mefoxin Premixed Intravenous Solution (Cefoxitin Sodium) Merck 2127
Minocin Intravenous (Minocycline Hydrochloride) Lederle 1862
Minocin Oral Suspension (Minocycline Hydrochloride) Lederle 1865
Minocin Pellet-Filled Capsules (Minocycline Hydrochloride) Lederle 1863
Monodox Capsules (Doxycycline Monohydrate) Oclassen 2442
Nebcin Vials, Hyporets & ADD-Vantage (Tobramycin Sulfate) Lilly 1955
Noroxin Tablets (Norfloxacin) Merck 2145
PCE Dispertab Tablets (Erythromycin) Abbott 498
Primaxin I.M. (Cilastatin Sodium, Imipenem) Merck 2158
Primaxin I.V. (Cilastatin Sodium, Imipenem) Merck 2160
Rocephin Injectable Vials, ADD-Vantage, Galaxy, Bulk (Ceftriaxone Sodium) Roche Laboratories 2993
Tazicef for Injection (Ceftazidime) GlaxoSmithKline 1647
Tazicef Galaxy Container (Ceftazidime Sodium) GlaxoSmithKline 1650
Tazicef Pharmacy Bulk Package (Ceftazidime) GlaxoSmithKline 1653
Tazidime Vials, Faspak & ADD-Vantage (Ceftazidime) Lilly 1966
Tequin Injection (Gatifloxacin) Bristol-Myers Squibb 1110
Tequin Tablets (Gatifloxacin) Bristol-Myers Squibb 1110
Timentin Injection- ADD-Vantage Vial (Clavulanate Potassium, Ticarcillin Disodium) GlaxoSmithKline 1661
Timentin Injection-Galaxy Container (Clavulanate Potassium, Ticarcillin Disodium) GlaxoSmithKline 1664
Timentin Injection-Pharmacy Bulk Package (Clavulanate Potassium, Ticarcillin Disodium) GlaxoSmithKline 1666
Timentin for Intravenous Administration (Clavulanate Potassium, Ticarcillin Disodium) GlaxoSmithKline 1658
Trovan (Alatrofloxacin Mesylate) Pfizer 2722
Unasyn for Injection (Ampicillin Sodium, Sulbactam Sodium) Pfizer 2728
Vantin Tablets and Oral Suspension (Cefpodoxime Proxetil) Pharmacia & Upjohn 2860
Zinacef Injection (Cefuroxime) GlaxoSmithKline 1696
Zinacef for Injection (Cefuroxime) GlaxoSmithKline 1696
Zithromax Capsules, 250 mg (Azithromycin Dihydrate) Pfizer 2743
Zithromax for IV Infusion (Azithromycin Dihydrate) Pfizer 2748
Zithromax for Oral Suspension, 1 g (Azithromycin Dihydrate) Pfizer 2743
Zithromax for Oral Suspension, 300 mg, 600 mg, 900 mg, 1200 mg (Azithromycin Dihydrate) Pfizer 2739
Zithromax Tablets, 250 mg (Azithromycin Dihydrate) Pfizer 2739
Zithromax Tablets, 600 mg (Azithromycin Dihydrate) Pfizer 2743
Zosyn (Piperacillin Sodium, Tazobactam Sodium) Lederle 1890
Zosyn in Galaxy Containers (Piperacillin Sodium, Tazobactam Sodium) Lederle 1894
Zyvox (Linezolid) Pharmacia & Upjohn 2871

S. aureus infections, ocular
Blephamide Ophthalmic Ointment (Prednisolone Acetate, Sulfacetamide Sodium) Allergan 547
Blephamide Ophthalmic Suspension (Prednisolone Acetate, Sulfacetamide Sodium) Allergan 548
Chibroxin Sterile Ophthalmic Solution (Norfloxacin) Merck 2051
Chloromycetin Ophthalmic Ointment, 1% (Chloramphenicol) Monarch .... ⊙296
Chloromycetin Ophthalmic Solution (Chloramphenicol) Monarch .... ⊙297
Chloroptic Sterile Ophthalmic Ointment (Chloramphenicol) Allergan .... ⊙234
Ciloxan (Ciprofloxacin Hydrochloride) Alcon 538
Cortisporin Ophthalmic Suspension (Hydrocortisone, Neomycin Sulfate, Polymyxin B Sulfate, Hydrocortisone, Neomycin Sulfate, Polymyxin B Sulfate) Monarch .... ⊙297
FML-S Liquifilm Sterile Ophthalmic Suspension (Fluorometholone, Sulfacetamide Sodium) Allergan .... ⊙238
Genoptic Ophthalmic Ointment (Gentamicin Sulfate) Allergan .... ⊙239
Genoptic Sterile Ophthalmic Solution (Gentamicin Sulfate) Allergan .... ⊙239
NeoDecadron Sterile Ophthalmic Solution (Dexamethasone Sodium Phosphate, Neomycin Sulfate) Merck 2144
Ocuflox Ophthalmic Solution (Ofloxacin) Allergan 554
Poly-Pred Liquifilm Ophthalmic Suspension (Neomycin Sulfate, Polymyxin B Sulfate, Prednisolone Acetate) Allergan .... ⊙245
Polytrim Ophthalmic Solution (Polymyxin B Sulfate, Trimethoprim Sulfate) Allergan 556
Pred-G Ophthalmic Suspension (Gentamicin Sulfate, Prednisolone Acetate) Allergan .... ⊙247
Pred-G Sterile Ophthalmic Ointment (Gentamicin Sulfate, Prednisolone Acetate) Allergan .... ⊙248
Quixin Ophthalmic Solution (Levofloxacin) Santen 3093
Terra-Cortril Ophthalmic Suspension (Hydrocortisone Acetate, Oxytetracycline Hydrochloride) Pfizer 2716
TobraDex Ophthalmic Ointment (Dexamethasone, Tobramycin) Alcon 542
TobraDex Ophthalmic Suspension (Dexamethasone, Tobramycin) Alcon 541

S. aureus intra-abdominal infections
Ceptaz for Injection (Ceftazidime) GlaxoSmithKline 1499
Fortaz (Ceftazidime Sodium) GlaxoSmithKline 1541
Primaxin I.V. (Cilastatin Sodium, Imipenem) Merck 2160
Tazicef for Injection (Ceftazidime) GlaxoSmithKline 1647
Tazicef Galaxy Container (Ceftazidime Sodium) GlaxoSmithKline 1650
Tazicef Pharmacy Bulk Package (Ceftazidime) GlaxoSmithKline 1653
Tazidime Vials, Faspak & ADD-Vantage (Ceftazidime) Lilly 1966

S. aureus lower respiratory tract infections
Cefizox for Intramuscular or Intravenous Use (Ceftizoxime Sodium) Fujisawa 1390
Cefotan (Cefotetan) AstraZeneca 664
Ceptaz for Injection (Ceftazidime) GlaxoSmithKline 1499
Claforan Injection (Cefotaxime Sodium) Aventis 732
Cleocin HCl Capsules (Clindamycin Hydrochloride) Pharmacia & Upjohn 2784
Cleocin Phosphate Sterile Solution (Clindamycin Phosphate) Pharmacia & Upjohn 2785
Fortaz (Ceftazidime Sodium) GlaxoSmithKline 1541
Levaquin (Levofloxacin) Ortho-McNeil 2537
Mefoxin for Injection (Cefoxitin Sodium) Merck 2124
Nebcin Vials, Hyporets & ADD-Vantage (Tobramycin Sulfate) Lilly 1955
Primaxin I.V. (Cilastatin Sodium, Imipenem) Merck 2160
Rocephin Injectable Vials, ADD-Vantage, Galaxy, Bulk (Ceftriaxone Sodium) Roche Laboratories 2993
Tazicef for Injection (Ceftazidime) GlaxoSmithKline 1647
Tazicef Galaxy Container (Ceftazidime Sodium) GlaxoSmithKline 1650
Tazicef Pharmacy Bulk Package (Ceftazidime) GlaxoSmithKline 1653
Tazidime Vials, Faspak & ADD-Vantage (Ceftazidime) Lilly 1966
Tequin Injection (Gatifloxacin) Bristol-Myers Squibb 1110
Tequin Tablets (Gatifloxacin) Bristol-Myers Squibb 1110
Timentin Injection- ADD-Vantage Vial (Clavulanate Potassium, Ticarcillin Disodium) GlaxoSmithKline 1661
Timentin Injection-Galaxy Container (Clavulanate Potassium, Ticarcillin Disodium) GlaxoSmithKline 1664
Timentin Injection-Pharmacy Bulk Package (Clavulanate Potassium, Ticarcillin Disodium) GlaxoSmithKline 1666
Timentin for Intravenous Administration (Clavulanate Potassium, Ticarcillin Disodium) GlaxoSmithKline 1658
Trovan (Alatrofloxacin Mesylate) Pfizer 2722
Zinacef Injection (Cefuroxime) GlaxoSmithKline 1696

Zinacef for Injection (Cefuroxime) GlaxoSmithKline 1696
Zithromax for IV Infusion (Azithromycin Dihydrate) Pfizer 2748
Zosyn (Piperacillin Sodium, Tazobactam Sodium) Lederle 1890
Zosyn in Galaxy Containers (Piperacillin Sodium, Tazobactam Sodium) Lederle 1894
Zyvox (Linezolid) Pharmacia & Upjohn 2871

S. aureus meningitis
Kefurox Vials, ADD-Vantage (Cefuroxime Sodium) Lilly 1948
Zinacef Injection (Cefuroxime) GlaxoSmithKline 1696
Zinacef for Injection (Cefuroxime) GlaxoSmithKline 1696

S. aureus otitis externa
Cipro HC Otic Suspension (Ciprofloxacin Hydrochloride, Hydrocortisone) Alcon 540
Floxin Otic Solution (Ofloxacin) Daiichi 1219

S. aureus respiratory tract infections
Ancef for Injection (Cefazolin Sodium) GlaxoSmithKline 1474
Ancef Injection (Cefazolin Sodium) GlaxoSmithKline 1474
Avelox Tablets (Moxifloxacin Hydrochloride) Bayer 879
Cefobid Intravenous/Intramuscular (Cefoperazone) Pfizer 2671
Cefobid Pharmacy Bulk Package - Not for Direct Infusion (Cefoperazone Sodium) Pfizer 2673
Kefzol Vials, ADD-Vantage (Cefazolin Sodium) Lilly 1951

S. aureus septicemia
Ancef for Injection (Cefazolin Sodium) GlaxoSmithKline 1474
Ancef Injection (Cefazolin Sodium) GlaxoSmithKline 1474
Cefizox for Intramuscular or Intravenous Use (Ceftizoxime Sodium) Fujisawa 1390
Cefobid Intravenous/Intramuscular (Cefoperazone) Pfizer 2671
Cefobid Pharmacy Bulk Package - Not for Direct Infusion (Cefoperazone Sodium) Pfizer 2673
Ceptaz for Injection (Ceftazidime) GlaxoSmithKline 1499
Claforan Injection (Cefotaxime Sodium) Aventis 732
Cleocin Phosphate Sterile Solution (Clindamycin Phosphate) Pharmacia & Upjohn 2785
Fortaz (Ceftazidime Sodium) GlaxoSmithKline 1541
Kefurox Vials, ADD-Vantage (Cefuroxime Sodium) Lilly 1948
Kefzol Vials, ADD-Vantage (Cefazolin Sodium) Lilly 1951
Mefoxin for Injection (Cefoxitin Sodium) Merck 2124
Mefoxin Premixed Intravenous Solution (Cefoxitin Sodium) Merck 2127
Primaxin I.V. (Cilastatin Sodium, Imipenem) Merck 2160
Rocephin Injectable Vials, ADD-Vantage, Galaxy, Bulk (Ceftriaxone Sodium) Roche Laboratories 2993
Tazicef for Injection (Ceftazidime) GlaxoSmithKline 1647
Tazicef Galaxy Container (Ceftazidime Sodium) GlaxoSmithKline 1650
Tazicef Pharmacy Bulk Package (Ceftazidime) GlaxoSmithKline 1653
Tazidime Vials, Faspak & ADD-Vantage (Ceftazidime) Lilly 1966
Timentin Injection- ADD-Vantage Vial (Clavulanate Potassium, Ticarcillin Disodium) GlaxoSmithKline 1661
Timentin Injection-Galaxy Container (Clavulanate Potassium, Ticarcillin Disodium) GlaxoSmithKline 1664
Timentin Injection-Pharmacy Bulk Package (Clavulanate Potassium, Ticarcillin Disodium) GlaxoSmithKline 1666
Timentin for Intravenous Administration (Clavulanate Potassium, Ticarcillin Disodium) GlaxoSmithKline 1658
Zinacef Injection (Cefuroxime) GlaxoSmithKline 1696
Zinacef for Injection (Cefuroxime) GlaxoSmithKline 1696

S. aureus skin and skin structure infections
Ancef for Injection (Cefazolin Sodium) GlaxoSmithKline 1474
Ancef Injection (Cefazolin Sodium) GlaxoSmithKline 1474
Augmentin Chewable Tablets (Amoxicillin, Clavulanate Potassium) GlaxoSmithKline 1482
Augmentin Powder for Oral Suspension (Amoxicillin, Clavulanate Potassium) GlaxoSmithKline 1482
Augmentin Tablets (Amoxicillin, Clavulanate Potassium) GlaxoSmithKline 1485
Avelox Tablets (Moxifloxacin Hydrochloride) Bayer 879
Bactroban Cream (Mupirocin Calcium) GlaxoSmithKline 1494
Bactroban Ointment (Mupirocin) GlaxoSmithKline 1496
Biaxin/Biaxin XL (Clarithromycin) Abbott 403
Ceclor (Cefaclor) Lilly 1905
Cefizox for Intramuscular or Intravenous Use (Ceftizoxime Sodium) Fujisawa 1390
Cefobid Intravenous/Intramuscular (Cefoperazone) Pfizer 2671
Cefobid Pharmacy Bulk Package - Not for Direct Infusion (Cefoperazone Sodium) Pfizer 2673
Cefotan (Cefotetan) AstraZeneca 664
Ceftin Tablets (Cefuroxime Axetil) Lifecycle Ventures 1898
Cefzil (Cefprozil) Bristol-Myers Squibb 1076
Ceptaz for Injection (Ceftazidime) GlaxoSmithKline 1499
Cipro I.V. (Ciprofloxacin) Bayer 893
Cipro I.V. Pharmacy Bulk Package (Ciprofloxacin) Bayer 897
Cipro (Ciprofloxacin) Bayer 887
Claforan Injection (Cefotaxime Sodium) Aventis 732
Cleocin HCl Capsules (Clindamycin Hydrochloride) Pharmacia & Upjohn 2784
Cleocin Phosphate Sterile Solution (Clindamycin Phosphate) Pharmacia & Upjohn 2785
Dynabac Tablets (Dirithromycin) Muro 2269
Dynacin Capsules (Minocycline Hydrochloride) Medicis 2019
E.E.S. (Erythromycin Ethylsuccinate) Abbott 450
EryPed (Erythromycin Ethylsuccinate) Abbott 446
Ery-Tab Tablets (Erythromycin) Abbott 448
Erythrocin Stearate Filmtab Tablets (Erythromycin Stearate) Abbott 452
Erythromycin Base Filmtab Tablets (Erythromycin) Abbott 454
Erythromycin Delayed-Release Capsules, USP (Erythromycin) Abbott 455
Floxin I.V. (Ofloxacin) Ortho-McNeil 2526
Floxin Tablets (Ofloxacin) Ortho-McNeil 2529
Fortaz (Ceftazidime Sodium) GlaxoSmithKline 1541
Kefurox Vials, ADD-Vantage (Cefuroxime Sodium) Lilly 1948
Kefzol Vials, ADD-Vantage (Cefazolin Sodium) Lilly 1951
Levaquin (Levofloxacin) Ortho-McNeil 2537
Lorabid Suspension and Pulvules (Loracarbef) Monarch 2251
Mandol Vials (Cefamandole Nafate) Lilly 1953
Maxipime for Injection (Cefepime Hydrochloride) Elan 1285
Mefoxin for Injection (Cefoxitin Sodium) Merck 2124
Mefoxin Premixed Intravenous Solution (Cefoxitin Sodium) Merck 2127
Minocin Intravenous (Minocycline Hydrochloride) Lederle 1862
Minocin Oral Suspension (Minocycline Hydrochloride) Lederle 1865
Minocin Pellet-Filled Capsules (Minocycline Hydrochloride) Lederle 1863
Monodox Capsules (Doxycycline Monohydrate) Oclassen 2442
Nebcin Vials, Hyporets & ADD-Vantage (Tobramycin Sulfate) Lilly 1955
Omnicef (Cefdinir) Abbott 493
PCE Dispertab Tablets (Erythromycin) Abbott 498
Primaxin I.M. (Cilastatin Sodium, Imipenem) Merck 2158
Primaxin I.V. (Cilastatin Sodium, Imipenem) Merck 2160
Rocephin Injectable Vials, ADD-Vantage, Galaxy, Bulk (Ceftriaxone Sodium) Roche Laboratories 2993
Synercid I.V. (Dalfopristin, Quinupristin) Aventis 775
Tazicef for Injection (Ceftazidime) GlaxoSmithKline 1647
Tazicef Galaxy Container (Ceftazidime Sodium) GlaxoSmithKline 1650
Tazicef Pharmacy Bulk Package (Ceftazidime) GlaxoSmithKline 1653
Tazidime Vials, Faspak & ADD-Vantage (Ceftazidime) Lilly 1966
Timentin Injection- ADD-Vantage Vial (Clavulanate Potassium, Ticarcillin Disodium) GlaxoSmithKline 1661
Timentin Injection-Galaxy Container (Clavulanate Potassium, Ticarcillin Disodium) GlaxoSmithKline 1664
Timentin Injection-Pharmacy Bulk Package (Clavulanate Potassium, Ticarcillin Disodium) GlaxoSmithKline 1666
Timentin for Intravenous Administration (Clavulanate Potassium, Ticarcillin Disodium) GlaxoSmithKline 1658
Trovan (Alatrofloxacin Mesylate) Pfizer 2722
Unasyn for Injection (Ampicillin Sodium, Sulbactam Sodium) Pfizer 2728
Vantin Tablets and Oral Suspension (Cefpodoxime Proxetil) Pharmacia & Upjohn 2860
Zinacef Injection (Cefuroxime) GlaxoSmithKline 1696
Zinacef for Injection (Cefuroxime) GlaxoSmithKline 1696
Zithromax (Azithromycin Dihydrate) Pfizer 2743
Zithromax for Oral Suspension, 300 mg, 600 mg, 900 mg, 1200 mg (Azithromycin Dihydrate) Pfizer 2739
Zithromax Tablets, 250 mg (Azithromycin Dihydrate) Pfizer 2739
Zithromax Tablets, 600 mg (Azithromycin Dihydrate) Pfizer 2743
Zosyn (Piperacillin Sodium, Tazobactam Sodium) Lederle 1890
Zosyn in Galaxy Containers (Piperacillin Sodium, Tazobactam Sodium) Lederle 1894
Zyvox (Linezolid) Pharmacia & Upjohn 2871

S. aureus urinary tract infections
Cefizox for Intramuscular or Intravenous Use (Ceftizoxime Sodium) Fujisawa 1390
Claforan Injection (Cefotaxime Sodium) Aventis 732
Macrodantin Capsules (Nitrofurantoin) Procter & Gamble Pharmaceuticals 2891
Nebcin Vials, Hyporets & ADD-Vantage (Tobramycin Sulfate) Lilly 1955
Noroxin Tablets (Norfloxacin) Merck 2145
Primaxin I.V. (Cilastatin Sodium, Imipenem) Merck 2160
Timentin Injection- ADD-Vantage Vial (Clavulanate Potassium, Ticarcillin Disodium) GlaxoSmithKline 1661
Timentin Injection-Galaxy Container (Clavulanate Potassium, Ticarcillin Disodium) GlaxoSmithKline 1664
Timentin Injection-Pharmacy Bulk Package (Clavulanate Potassium, Ticarcillin Disodium) GlaxoSmithKline 1666
Timentin for Intravenous Administration (Clavulanate Potassium, Ticarcillin Disodium) GlaxoSmithKline 1658

S. bovis endocarditis
Vancocin HCl, Vials & ADD-Vantage (Vancomycin Hydrochloride) Lilly 1970

S. epidermis bone and joint infections
Primaxin I.V. (Cilastatin Sodium, Imipenem) Merck 2160

S. epidermis endocarditis, early-onset prosthetic valve
Vancocin HCl, Vials & ADD-Vantage (Vancomycin Hydrochloride) Lilly 1970

S. epidermis gynecologic infections
Cefobid Intravenous/Intramuscular (Cefoperazone) Pfizer 2671
Cefobid Pharmacy Bulk Package - Not for Direct Infusion (Cefoperazone Sodium) Pfizer 2673
Cefotan (Cefotetan) AstraZeneca 664
Claforan Injection (Cefotaxime Sodium) Aventis 732
Primaxin I.V. (Cilastatin Sodium, Imipenem) Merck 2160
Timentin Injection- ADD-Vantage Vial (Clavulanate Potassium, Ticarcillin Disodium) GlaxoSmithKline 1661
Timentin Injection-Galaxy Container (Clavulanate Potassium, Ticarcillin Disodium) GlaxoSmithKline 1664
Timentin Injection-Pharmacy Bulk Package (Clavulanate Potassium, Ticarcillin Disodium) GlaxoSmithKline 1666
Timentin for Intravenous Administration (Clavulanate Potassium, Ticarcillin Disodium) GlaxoSmithKline 1658

S. epidermis infections
Cefizox for Intramuscular or Intravenous Use (Ceftizoxime Sodium) Fujisawa 1390
Cefobid Intravenous/Intramuscular (Cefoperazone) Pfizer 2671
Cefobid Pharmacy Bulk Package - Not for Direct Infusion (Cefoperazone Sodium) Pfizer 2673
Cefotan (Cefotetan) AstraZeneca 664
Cipro I.V. (Ciprofloxacin) Bayer 893
Cipro I.V. Pharmacy Bulk Package (Ciprofloxacin) Bayer 897
Cipro (Ciprofloxacin) Bayer 887
Claforan Injection (Cefotaxime Sodium) Aventis 732
Mefoxin for Injection (Cefoxitin Sodium) Merck 2124
Mefoxin Premixed Intravenous Solution (Cefoxitin Sodium) Merck 2127
Noroxin Tablets (Norfloxacin) Merck 2145
Primaxin I.V. (Cilastatin Sodium, Imipenem) Merck 2160
Rocephin Injectable Vials, ADD-Vantage, Galaxy, Bulk (Ceftriaxone Sodium) Roche Laboratories 2993
Timentin Injection- ADD-Vantage Vial (Clavulanate Potassium, Ticarcillin Disodium) GlaxoSmithKline 1661
Timentin Injection-Galaxy Container (Clavulanate Potassium, Ticarcillin Disodium) GlaxoSmithKline 1664
Timentin Injection-Pharmacy Bulk Package (Clavulanate Potassium, Ticarcillin Disodium) GlaxoSmithKline 1666
Timentin for Intravenous Administration (Clavulanate Potassium, Ticarcillin Disodium) GlaxoSmithKline 1658
Vancocin HCl, Vials & ADD-Vantage (Vancomycin Hydrochloride) Lilly 1970

S. epidermis infections, ocular
Chibroxin Sterile Ophthalmic Solution (Norfloxacin) Merck 2051
Ciloxan (Ciprofloxacin Hydrochloride) Alcon 538
Genoptic Ophthalmic Ointment (Gentamicin Sulfate) Allergan .... ⊙ 239
Genoptic Sterile Ophthalmic Solution (Gentamicin Sulfate) Allergan .... ⊙ 239
Ocuflox Ophthalmic Solution (Ofloxacin) Allergan 554
Polytrim Ophthalmic Solution (Polymyxin B Sulfate, Trimethoprim Sulfate) Allergan 556
Quixin Ophthalmic Solution (Levofloxacin) Santen 3093
TobraDex Ophthalmic Ointment (Dexamethasone, Tobramycin) Alcon 542
TobraDex Ophthalmic Suspension (Dexamethasone, Tobramycin) Alcon 541

S. epidermis intra-abdominal infections
Cefizox for Intramuscular or Intravenous Use (Ceftizoxime Sodium) Fujisawa 1390
Primaxin I.V. (Cilastatin Sodium, Imipenem) Merck 2160

S. epidermis meningitis
Rocephin Injectable Vials, ADD-Vantage, Galaxy, Bulk (Ceftriaxone Sodium) Roche Laboratories ... 2993

S. epidermis pelvic inflammatory disease
Cefobid Intravenous/Intramuscular (Cefoperazone) Pfizer ... 2671
Cefobid Pharmacy Bulk Package - Not for Direct Infusion (Cefoperazone Sodium) Pfizer ... 2673

S. epidermis skin and skin structure infections
Cefizox for Intramuscular or Intravenous Use (Ceftizoxime Sodium) Fujisawa ... 1390
Cefotan (Cefotetan) AstraZeneca ... 664
Cipro I.V. (Ciprofloxacin) Bayer ... 893
Cipro I.V. Pharmacy Bulk Package (Ciprofloxacin) Bayer ... 897
Cipro (Ciprofloxacin) Bayer ... 887
Claforan Injection (Cefotaxime Sodium) Aventis ... 732
Mefoxin for Injection (Cefoxitin Sodium) Merck ... 2124
Mefoxin Premixed Intravenous Solution (Cefoxitin Sodium) Merck ... 2127
Primaxin I.V. (Cilastatin Sodium, Imipenem) Merck ... 2160
Rocephin Injectable Vials, ADD-Vantage, Galaxy, Bulk (Ceftriaxone Sodium) Roche Laboratories ... 2993

S. epidermis urinary tract infections
Cipro I.V. (Ciprofloxacin) Bayer ... 893
Cipro I.V. Pharmacy Bulk Package (Ciprofloxacin) Bayer ... 897
Cipro (Ciprofloxacin) Bayer ... 887
Claforan Injection (Cefotaxime Sodium) Aventis ... 732
Mandol Vials (Cefamandole Nafate) Lilly ... 1953
Noroxin Tablets (Norfloxacin) Merck ... 2145

S. faecalis, endocardial infections, treatment adjunct
Vancocin HCl, Vials & ADD-Vantage (Vancomycin Hydrochloride) Lilly ... 1970

S. faecalis gynecologic infections
Pipracil (Piperacillin Sodium) Lederle ... 1866

S. faecalis infections
Amoxil Chewable Tablets (Amoxicillin) GlaxoSmithKline ... 1471
Amoxil for Oral Suspension (Amoxicillin) GlaxoSmithKline ... 1471
Amoxil (Amoxicillin) GlaxoSmithKline ... 1471
Cipro I.V. (Ciprofloxacin) Bayer ... 893
Cipro (Ciprofloxacin) Bayer ... 887
Geocillin Tablets (Carbenicillin Indanyl Sodium) Pfizer ... 2687
Levaquin (Levofloxacin) Ortho-McNeil ... 2537
Monurol Sachet (Fosfomycin Tromethamine) Forest ... 1375
Noroxin Tablets (Norfloxacin) Merck ... 2145
Pipracil (Piperacillin Sodium) Lederle ... 1866

S. faecalis urinary tract infections
Cipro I.V. (Ciprofloxacin) Bayer ... 893
Cipro (Ciprofloxacin) Bayer ... 887
Levaquin (Levofloxacin) Ortho-McNeil ... 2537
Monurol Sachet (Fosfomycin Tromethamine) Forest ... 1375
Noroxin Tablets (Norfloxacin) Merck ... 2145

S. pneumoniae bone and joint infections
Rocephin Injectable Vials, ADD-Vantage, Galaxy, Bulk (Ceftriaxone Sodium) Roche Laboratories ... 2993

S. pneumoniae bronchitis
Avelox Tablets (Moxifloxacin Hydrochloride) Bayer ... 879
Bactrim (Sulfamethoxazole, Trimethoprim) Roche Laboratories ... 2949
Biaxin/Biaxin XL (Clarithromycin) Abbott ... 403
Ceclor CD Tablets (Cefaclor) Elan ... 1279
Cedax (Ceftibuten Dihydrate) Biovail ... 1021
Ceftin Tablets (Cefuroxime Axetil) Lifecycle Ventures ... 1898
Cefzil (Cefprozil) Bristol-Myers Squibb ... 1076
Dynabac Tablets (Dirithromycin) Muro ... 2269
Floxin I.V. (Ofloxacin) Ortho-McNeil ... 2526
Floxin Tablets (Ofloxacin) Ortho-McNeil ... 2529
Levaquin (Levofloxacin) Ortho-McNeil ... 2537
Lorabid Suspension and Pulvules (Loracarbef) Monarch ... 2251
Omnicef (Cefdinir) Abbott ... 493
Septra Suspension (Sulfamethoxazole, Trimethoprim) Monarch ... 2265
Septra Tablets (Sulfamethoxazole, Trimethoprim) Monarch ... 2265
Septra DS Tablets (Sulfamethoxazole, Trimethoprim) Monarch ... 2265
Suprax (Cefixime) Lederle ... 1877
Tequin Injection (Gatifloxacin) Bristol-Myers Squibb ... 1110
Tequin Tablets (Gatifloxacin) Bristol-Myers Squibb ... 1110
Vantin Tablets and Oral Suspension (Cefpodoxime Proxetil) Pharmacia & Upjohn ... 2860

S. pneumoniae central nervous system infections
Claforan Injection (Cefotaxime Sodium) Aventis ... 732
Fortaz (Ceftazidime Sodium) GlaxoSmithKline ... 1541
Tazicef for Injection (Ceftazidime) GlaxoSmithKline ... 1647
Tazicef Galaxy Container (Ceftazidime Sodium) GlaxoSmithKline ... 1650
Tazicef Pharmacy Bulk Package (Ceftazidime) GlaxoSmithKline ... 1653
Tazidime Vials, Faspak & ADD-Vantage (Ceftazidime) Lilly ... 1966

S. pneumoniae infections
Amoxil Chewable Tablets (Amoxicillin) GlaxoSmithKline ... 1471
Amoxil for Oral Suspension (Amoxicillin) GlaxoSmithKline ... 1471
Amoxil (Amoxicillin) GlaxoSmithKline ... 1471
Ancef for Injection (Cefazolin Sodium) GlaxoSmithKline ... 1474
Ancef Injection (Cefazolin Sodium) GlaxoSmithKline ... 1474
Augmentin Tablets (Amoxicillin, Clavulanate Potassium) GlaxoSmithKline ... 1485
Augmentin ES-600 Powder for Oral Suspension (Amoxicillin, Clavulanate Potassium) GlaxoSmithKline ... 1487
Avelox Tablets (Moxifloxacin Hydrochloride) Bayer ... 879
Bactrim (Sulfamethoxazole, Trimethoprim) Roche Laboratories ... 2949
Biaxin/Biaxin XL (Clarithromycin) Abbott ... 403
Bicillin C-R 900/300 Injection (Penicillin G Benzathine, Penicillin G Procaine) Monarch ... 2240
Bicillin C-R Injection (Penicillin G Benzathine, Penicillin G Procaine) Monarch ... 2238
Ceclor CD Tablets (Cefaclor) Elan ... 1279
Ceclor (Cefaclor) Lilly ... 1905
Cedax (Ceftibuten Dihydrate) Biovail ... 1021
Cefizox for Intramuscular or Intravenous Use (Ceftizoxime Sodium) Fujisawa ... 1390
Cefobid Intravenous/Intramuscular (Cefoperazone) Pfizer ... 2671
Cefobid Pharmacy Bulk Package - Not for Direct Infusion (Cefoperazone Sodium) Pfizer ... 2673
Cefotan (Cefotetan) AstraZeneca ... 664
Ceftin (Cefuroxime Axetil) Lifecycle Ventures ... 1898
Cefzil (Cefprozil) Bristol-Myers Squibb ... 1076
Ceptaz for Injection (Ceftazidime) GlaxoSmithKline ... 1499
Cipro I.V. (Ciprofloxacin) Bayer ... 893
Cipro I.V. Pharmacy Bulk Package (Ciprofloxacin) Bayer ... 897
Cipro (Ciprofloxacin) Bayer ... 887
Claforan Injection (Cefotaxime Sodium) Aventis ... 732
Cleocin HCl Capsules (Clindamycin Hydrochloride) Pharmacia & Upjohn ... 2784
Cleocin Phosphate Sterile Solution (Clindamycin Phosphate) Pharmacia & Upjohn ... 2785
Declomycin Tablets (Demeclocycline Hydrochloride) Lederle ... 1855
Doryx Coated Pellet Filled Capsules (Doxycycline Hyclate) Warner Chilcott ... 3357
Dynabac Tablets (Dirithromycin) Muro ... 2269
Dynacin Capsules (Minocycline Hydrochloride) Medicis ... 2019
E.E.S. (Erythromycin Ethylsuccinate) Abbott ... 450
EryPed (Erythromycin Ethylsuccinate) Abbott ... 446
Ery-Tab Tablets (Erythromycin) Abbott ... 448
Erythrocin Stearate Filmtab Tablets (Erythromycin Stearate) Abbott ... 452
Erythromycin Base Filmtab Tablets (Erythromycin) Abbott ... 454
Erythromycin Delayed-Release Capsules, USP (Erythromycin) Abbott ... 455
Floxin I.V. (Ofloxacin) Ortho-McNeil ... 2526
Floxin Tablets (Ofloxacin) Ortho-McNeil ... 2529
Fortaz (Ceftazidime Sodium) GlaxoSmithKline ... 1541
Keflex (Cephalexin) Dista ... 1237
Kefurox Vials, ADD-Vantage (Cefuroxime Sodium) Lilly ... 1948
Kefzol Vials, ADD-Vantage (Cefazolin Sodium) Lilly ... 1951
Levaquin (Levofloxacin) Ortho-McNeil ... 2537
Lorabid Suspension and Pulvules (Loracarbef) Monarch ... 2251
Maxipime for Injection (Cefepime Hydrochloride) Elan ... 1285
Mefoxin for Injection (Cefoxitin Sodium) Merck ... 2124
Mefoxin Premixed Intravenous Solution (Cefoxitin Sodium) Merck ... 2127
Merrem I.V. (Meropenem) AstraZeneca ... 673
Minocin Intravenous (Minocycline Hydrochloride) Lederle ... 1862
Minocin Oral Suspension (Minocycline Hydrochloride) Lederle ... 1865
Minocin Pellet-Filled Capsules (Minocycline Hydrochloride) Lederle ... 1863
Monodox Capsules (Doxycycline Monohydrate) Oclassen ... 2442
Omnicef (Cefdinir) Abbott ... 493
PCE Dispertab Tablets (Erythromycin) Abbott ... 498
Pfizerpen for Injection (Penicillin G Potassium) Pfizer ... 2707
Pipracil (Piperacillin Sodium) Lederle ... 1866
Primaxin I.M. (Cilastatin Sodium, Imipenem) Merck ... 2158
Primaxin I.V. (Cilastatin Sodium, Imipenem) Merck ... 2160
Rocephin Injectable Vials, ADD-Vantage, Galaxy, Bulk (Ceftriaxone Sodium) Roche Laboratories ... 2993
Suprax (Cefixime) Lederle ... 1877
Tao Capsules (Troleandomycin) Pfizer ... 2716
Tazicef for Injection (Ceftazidime) GlaxoSmithKline ... 1647
Tazicef Galaxy Container (Ceftazidime Sodium) GlaxoSmithKline ... 1650
Tazicef Pharmacy Bulk Package (Ceftazidime) GlaxoSmithKline ... 1653
Tazidime Vials, Faspak & ADD-Vantage (Ceftazidime) Lilly ... 1966
Tequin Injection (Gatifloxacin) Bristol-Myers Squibb ... 1110
Tequin Tablets (Gatifloxacin) Bristol-Myers Squibb ... 1110
Trovan (Alatrofloxacin Mesylate) Pfizer ... 2722
Vantin Tablets and Oral Suspension (Cefpodoxime Proxetil) Pharmacia & Upjohn ... 2860
Vibramycin Hyclate Capsules (Doxycycline Hyclate) Pfizer ... 2735
Vibramycin Hyclate Intravenous (Doxycycline Hyclate) Pfizer ... 2737
Zinacef Injection (Cefuroxime) GlaxoSmithKline ... 1696
Zinacef for Injection (Cefuroxime) GlaxoSmithKline ... 1696
Zithromax Capsules, 250 mg (Azithromycin Dihydrate) Pfizer ... 2743
Zithromax for IV Infusion (Azithromycin Dihydrate) Pfizer ... 2748
Zithromax for Oral Suspension, 1 g (Azithromycin Dihydrate) Pfizer ... 2743
Zithromax for Oral Suspension, 300 mg, 600 mg, 900 mg, 1200 mg (Azithromycin Dihydrate) Pfizer ... 2739
Zithromax Tablets, 250 mg (Azithromycin Dihydrate) Pfizer ... 2739
Zithromax Tablets, 600 mg (Azithromycin Dihydrate) Pfizer ... 2743
Zyvox (Linezolid) Pharmacia & Upjohn ... 2871

S. pneumoniae infections, ocular
Blephamide Ophthalmic Ointment (Prednisolone Acetate, Sulfacetamide Sodium) Allergan ... 547
Blephamide Ophthalmic Suspension (Prednisolone Acetate, Sulfacetamide Sodium) Allergan ... 548
Chibroxin Sterile Ophthalmic Solution (Norfloxacin) Merck ... 2051
Chloromycetin Ophthalmic Ointment, 1% (Chloramphenicol) Monarch ... ⊙296
Chloromycetin Ophthalmic Solution (Chloramphenicol) Monarch ... ⊙297
Chloroptic Sterile Ophthalmic Ointment (Chloramphenicol) Allergan ... ⊙234
Ciloxan (Ciprofloxacin Hydrochloride) Alcon ... 538
FML-S Liquifilm Sterile Ophthalmic Suspension (Fluorometholone, Sulfacetamide Sodium) Allergan ... ⊙238
Genoptic Ophthalmic Ointment (Gentamicin Sulfate) Allergan ... ⊙239
Genoptic Sterile Ophthalmic Solution (Gentamicin Sulfate) Allergan ... ⊙239
Ocuflox Ophthalmic Solution (Ofloxacin) Allergan ... 554
Polytrim Ophthalmic Solution (Polymyxin B Sulfate, Trimethoprim Sulfate) Allergan ... 556
Pred-G Ophthalmic Suspension (Gentamicin Sulfate, Prednisolone Acetate) Allergan ... ⊙247
Pred-G Sterile Ophthalmic Ointment (Gentamicin Sulfate, Prednisolone Acetate) Allergan ... ⊙248
Quixin Ophthalmic Solution (Levofloxacin) Santen ... 3093
Terra-Cortril Ophthalmic Suspension (Hydrocortisone Acetate, Oxytetracycline Hydrochloride) Pfizer ... 2716
TobraDex Ophthalmic Ointment (Dexamethasone, Tobramycin) Alcon ... 542
TobraDex Ophthalmic Suspension (Dexamethasone, Tobramycin) Alcon ... 541

S. pneumoniae lower respiratory tract infections
Biaxin/Biaxin XL (Clarithromycin) Abbott ... 403
Ceclor (Cefaclor) Lilly ... 1905
Cefizox for Intramuscular or Intravenous Use (Ceftizoxime Sodium) Fujisawa ... 1390
Cefotan (Cefotetan) AstraZeneca ... 664
Cefzil (Cefprozil) Bristol-Myers Squibb ... 1076
Ceptaz for Injection (Ceftazidime) GlaxoSmithKline ... 1499
Cipro I.V. (Ciprofloxacin) Bayer ... 893
Cipro I.V. Pharmacy Bulk Package (Ciprofloxacin) Bayer ... 897
Cipro (Ciprofloxacin) Bayer ... 887
Claforan Injection (Cefotaxime Sodium) Aventis ... 732
Cleocin HCl Capsules (Clindamycin Hydrochloride) Pharmacia & Upjohn ... 2784
Cleocin Phosphate Sterile Solution (Clindamycin Phosphate) Pharmacia & Upjohn ... 2785
E.E.S. (Erythromycin Ethylsuccinate) Abbott ... 450
EryPed (Erythromycin Ethylsuccinate) Abbott ... 446
Ery-Tab Tablets (Erythromycin) Abbott ... 448
Erythrocin Stearate Filmtab Tablets (Erythromycin Stearate) Abbott ... 452
Erythromycin Base Filmtab Tablets (Erythromycin) Abbott ... 454
Erythromycin Delayed-Release Capsules, USP (Erythromycin) Abbott ... 455
Floxin I.V. (Ofloxacin) Ortho-McNeil ... 2526
Floxin Tablets (Ofloxacin) Ortho-McNeil ... 2529
Fortaz (Ceftazidime Sodium) GlaxoSmithKline ... 1541
Kefurox Vials, ADD-Vantage (Cefuroxime Sodium) Lilly ... 1948
Levaquin (Levofloxacin) Ortho-McNeil ... 2537
Lorabid Suspension and Pulvules (Loracarbef) Monarch ... 2251
Mandol Vials (Cefamandole Nafate) Lilly ... 1953
Maxipime for Injection (Cefepime Hydrochloride) Elan ... 1285
Mefoxin for Injection (Cefoxitin Sodium) Merck ... 2124

Mefoxin Premixed Intravenous Solution (Cefoxitin Sodium) Merck 2127
Omnicef (Cefdinir) Abbott 493
PCE Dispertab Tablets (Erythromycin) Abbott 498
Primaxin I.M. (Cilastatin Sodium, Imipenem) Merck 2158
Rocephin Injectable Vials, ADD-Vantage, Galaxy, Bulk (Ceftriaxone Sodium) Roche Laboratories 2993
Tao Capsules (Troleandomycin) Pfizer 2716
Tazicef for Injection (Ceftazidime) GlaxoSmithKline 1647
Tazicef Galaxy Container (Ceftazidime Sodium) GlaxoSmithKline 1650
Tazicef Pharmacy Bulk Package (Ceftazidime) GlaxoSmithKline 1653
Tazidime Vials, Faspak & ADD-Vantage (Ceftazidime) Lilly 1966
Trovan (Alatrofloxacin Mesylate) Pfizer 2722
Vantin Tablets and Oral Suspension (Cefpodoxime Proxetil) Pharmacia & Upjohn 2860
Zinacef Injection (Cefuroxime) GlaxoSmithKline 1696
Zinacef for Injection (Cefuroxime) GlaxoSmithKline 1696
Zithromax Capsules, 250 mg (Azithromycin Dihydrate) Pfizer 2743
Zithromax for IV Infusion (Azithromycin Dihydrate) Pfizer 2748
Zithromax for Oral Suspension, 1 g (Azithromycin Dihydrate) Pfizer 2743
Zithromax for Oral Suspension, 300 mg, 600 mg, 900 mg, 1200 mg (Azithromycin Dihydrate) Pfizer 2739
Zithromax Tablets, 250 mg (Azithromycin Dihydrate) Pfizer 2739
Zithromax Tablets, 600 mg (Azithromycin Dihydrate) Pfizer 2743
Zyvox (Linezolid) Pharmacia & Upjohn 2871

S. pneumoniae meningitis

Cefizox for Intramuscular or Intravenous Use (Ceftizoxime Sodium) Fujisawa 1390
Ceptaz for Injection (Ceftazidime) GlaxoSmithKline 1499
Fortaz (Ceftazidime Sodium) GlaxoSmithKline 1541
Kefurox Vials, ADD-Vantage (Cefuroxime Sodium) Lilly 1948
Merrem I.V. (Meropenem) AstraZeneca 673
Rocephin Injectable Vials, ADD-Vantage, Galaxy, Bulk (Ceftriaxone Sodium) Roche Laboratories 2993
Tazicef for Injection (Ceftazidime) GlaxoSmithKline 1647
Tazicef Galaxy Container (Ceftazidime Sodium) GlaxoSmithKline 1650
Tazicef Pharmacy Bulk Package (Ceftazidime) GlaxoSmithKline 1653
Tazidime Vials, Faspak & ADD-Vantage (Ceftazidime) Lilly 1966
Zinacef Injection (Cefuroxime) GlaxoSmithKline 1696
Zinacef for Injection (Cefuroxime) GlaxoSmithKline 1696

S. pneumoniae otitis media

Augmentin Tablets (Amoxicillin, Clavulanate Potassium) GlaxoSmithKline 1485
Augmentin ES-600 Powder for Oral Suspension (Amoxicillin, Clavulanate Potassium) GlaxoSmithKline 1487
Bactrim (Sulfamethoxazole, Trimethoprim) Roche Laboratories 2949
Biaxin/Biaxin XL (Clarithromycin) Abbott 403
Bicillin C-R 900/300 Injection (Penicillin G Benzathine, Penicillin G Procaine) Monarch 2240
Bicillin C-R Injection (Penicillin G Benzathine, Penicillin G Procaine) Monarch 2238
Ceclor (Cefaclor) Lilly 1905
Ceftin (Cefuroxime Axetil) Lifecycle Ventures 1898
Cefzil (Cefprozil) Bristol-Myers Squibb 1076
Ery-Tab Tablets (Erythromycin) Abbott 448
Erythrocin Stearate Filmtab Tablets (Erythromycin Stearate) Abbott 452
Erythromycin Base Filmtab Tablets (Erythromycin) Abbott 454
Keflex (Cephalexin) Dista 1237
Lorabid Suspension and Pulvules (Loracarbef) Monarch 2251
Omnicef (Cefdinir) Abbott 493
Rocephin Injectable Vials, ADD-Vantage, Galaxy, Bulk (Ceftriaxone Sodium) Roche Laboratories 2993
Septra Suspension (Sulfamethoxazole, Trimethoprim) Monarch 2265
Septra Tablets (Sulfamethoxazole, Trimethoprim) Monarch 2265
Septra DS Tablets (Sulfamethoxazole, Trimethoprim) Monarch 2265
Suprax (Cefixime) Lederle 1877
Vantin Tablets and Oral Suspension (Cefpodoxime Proxetil) Pharmacia & Upjohn 2860
Zithromax Capsules, 250 mg (Azithromycin Dihydrate) Pfizer 2743
Zithromax for Oral Suspension, 300 mg, 600 mg, 900 mg, 1200 mg (Azithromycin Dihydrate) Pfizer 2739
Zithromax Tablets, 250 mg (Azithromycin Dihydrate) Pfizer 2739

S. pneumoniae pharyngitis

EryPed (Erythromycin Ethylsuccinate) Abbott 446
Ery-Tab Tablets (Erythromycin) Abbott 448
Erythrocin Stearate Filmtab Tablets (Erythromycin Stearate) Abbott 452
Erythromycin Base Filmtab Tablets (Erythromycin) Abbott 454
Erythromycin Delayed-Release Capsules, USP (Erythromycin) Abbott 455
PCE Dispertab Tablets (Erythromycin) Abbott 498

S. pneumoniae respiratory tract infections

Ancef for Injection (Cefazolin Sodium) GlaxoSmithKline 1474
Ancef Injection (Cefazolin Sodium) GlaxoSmithKline 1474
Cefobid Intravenous/Intramuscular (Cefoperazone) Pfizer 2671
Cefobid Pharmacy Bulk Package - Not for Direct Infusion (Cefoperazone Sodium) Pfizer 2673
Dynabac Tablets (Dirithromycin) Muro 2269
Keflex (Cephalexin) Dista 1237
Kefzol Vials, ADD-Vantage (Cefazolin Sodium) Lilly 1951

S. pneumoniae septicemia

Ancef for Injection (Cefazolin Sodium) GlaxoSmithKline 1474
Ancef Injection (Cefazolin Sodium) GlaxoSmithKline 1474
Cefizox for Intramuscular or Intravenous Use (Ceftizoxime Sodium) Fujisawa 1390
Cefobid Intravenous/Intramuscular (Cefoperazone) Pfizer 2671
Cefobid Pharmacy Bulk Package - Not for Direct Infusion (Cefoperazone Sodium) Pfizer 2673
Ceptaz for Injection (Ceftazidime) GlaxoSmithKline 1499
Claforan Injection (Cefotaxime Sodium) Aventis 732
Fortaz (Ceftazidime Sodium) GlaxoSmithKline 1541
Kefurox Vials, ADD-Vantage (Cefuroxime Sodium) Lilly 1948
Kefzol Vials, ADD-Vantage (Cefazolin Sodium) Lilly 1951
Mefoxin for Injection (Cefoxitin Sodium) Merck 2124
Mefoxin Premixed Intravenous Solution (Cefoxitin Sodium) Merck 2127
Pipracil (Piperacillin Sodium) Lederle 1866
Rocephin Injectable Vials, ADD-Vantage, Galaxy, Bulk (Ceftriaxone Sodium) Roche Laboratories 2993
Tazicef for Injection (Ceftazidime) GlaxoSmithKline 1647
Tazicef Galaxy Container (Ceftazidime Sodium) GlaxoSmithKline 1650
Tazicef Pharmacy Bulk Package (Ceftazidime) GlaxoSmithKline 1653
Tazidime Vials, Faspak & ADD-Vantage (Ceftazidime) Lilly 1966
Zinacef Injection (Cefuroxime) GlaxoSmithKline 1696
Zinacef for Injection (Cefuroxime) GlaxoSmithKline 1696

S. pneumoniae sinusitis

Avelox Tablets (Moxifloxacin Hydrochloride) Bayer 879
Biaxin/Biaxin XL (Clarithromycin) Abbott 403
Ceftin Tablets (Cefuroxime Axetil) Lifecycle Ventures 1898
Cefzil (Cefprozil) Bristol-Myers Squibb 1076
Cipro I.V. (Ciprofloxacin) Bayer 893
Cipro I.V. Pharmacy Bulk Package (Ciprofloxacin) Bayer 897
Cipro (Ciprofloxacin) Bayer 887
Levaquin (Levofloxacin) Ortho-McNeil 2537
Tequin Injection (Gatifloxacin) Bristol-Myers Squibb 1110
Tequin Tablets (Gatifloxacin) Bristol-Myers Squibb 1110
Vantin Tablets and Oral Suspension (Cefpodoxime Proxetil) Pharmacia & Upjohn 2860

S. pneumoniae upper respiratory tract infections

Biaxin/Biaxin XL (Clarithromycin) Abbott 403
Doryx Coated Pellet Filled Capsules (Doxycycline Hyclate) Warner Chilcott 3357
Dynacin Capsules (Minocycline Hydrochloride) Medicis 2019
E.E.S. (Erythromycin Ethylsuccinate) Abbott 450
EryPed (Erythromycin Ethylsuccinate) Abbott 446
Ery-Tab Tablets (Erythromycin) Abbott 448
Erythrocin Stearate Filmtab Tablets (Erythromycin Stearate) Abbott 452
Erythromycin Base Filmtab Tablets (Erythromycin) Abbott 454
Erythromycin Delayed-Release Capsules, USP (Erythromycin) Abbott 455
Minocin Oral Suspension (Minocycline Hydrochloride) Lederle 1865
Minocin Pellet-Filled Capsules (Minocycline Hydrochloride) Lederle 1863
Monodox Capsules (Doxycycline Monohydrate) Oclassen 2442
PCE Dispertab Tablets (Erythromycin) Abbott 498
Vibramycin Hyclate Capsules (Doxycycline Hyclate) Pfizer 2735

S. pyogenes bone and joint infections

Claforan Injection (Cefotaxime Sodium) Aventis 732

S. pyogenes infections

Bactroban Ointment (Mupirocin) GlaxoSmithKline 1496
Biaxin/Biaxin XL (Clarithromycin) Abbott 403
Ceclor CD Tablets (Cefaclor) Elan 1279
Ceclor (Cefaclor) Lilly 1905
Cedax (Ceftibuten Dihydrate) Biovail 1021
Cefizox for Intramuscular or Intravenous Use (Ceftizoxime Sodium) Fujisawa 1390
Cefobid Intravenous/Intramuscular (Cefoperazone) Pfizer 2671
Cefobid Pharmacy Bulk Package - Not for Direct Infusion (Cefoperazone Sodium) Pfizer 2673
Cefotan (Cefotetan) AstraZeneca 664
Ceftin (Cefuroxime Axetil) Lifecycle Ventures 1898
Cefzil (Cefprozil) Bristol-Myers Squibb 1076
Ceptaz for Injection (Ceftazidime) GlaxoSmithKline 1499
Cipro I.V. (Ciprofloxacin) Bayer 893
Cipro I.V. Pharmacy Bulk Package (Ciprofloxacin) Bayer 897
Cipro (Ciprofloxacin) Bayer 887
Claforan Injection (Cefotaxime Sodium) Aventis 732
Cleocin HCl Capsules (Clindamycin Hydrochloride) Pharmacia & Upjohn 2784
Cleocin Phosphate Sterile Solution (Clindamycin Phosphate) Pharmacia & Upjohn 2785
Dynabac Tablets (Dirithromycin) Muro 2269
E.E.S. (Erythromycin Ethylsuccinate) Abbott 450
EryPed (Erythromycin Ethylsuccinate) Abbott 446
Ery-Tab Tablets (Erythromycin) Abbott 448
Erythrocin Stearate Filmtab Tablets (Erythromycin Stearate) Abbott 452
Erythromycin Base Filmtab Tablets (Erythromycin) Abbott 454
Erythromycin Delayed-Release Capsules, USP (Erythromycin) Abbott 455
Floxin I.V. (Ofloxacin) Ortho-McNeil 2526
Floxin Tablets (Ofloxacin) Ortho-McNeil 2529
Fortaz (Ceftazidime Sodium) GlaxoSmithKline 1541
Keflex (Cephalexin) Dista 1237
Kefurox Vials, ADD-Vantage (Cefuroxime Sodium) Lilly 1948
Levaquin (Levofloxacin) Ortho-McNeil 2537
Lorabid Suspension and Pulvules (Loracarbef) Monarch 2251
Maxipime for Injection (Cefepime Hydrochloride) Elan 1285
Omnicef (Cefdinir) Abbott 493
PCE Dispertab Tablets (Erythromycin) Abbott 498
Primaxin I.M. (Cilastatin Sodium, Imipenem) Merck 2158
Primaxin I.V. (Cilastatin Sodium, Imipenem) Merck 2160
Rocephin Injectable Vials, ADD-Vantage, Galaxy, Bulk (Ceftriaxone Sodium) Roche Laboratories 2993
Suprax (Cefixime) Lederle 1877
Tao Capsules (Troleandomycin) Pfizer 2716
Tazicef for Injection (Ceftazidime) GlaxoSmithKline 1647
Tazicef Galaxy Container (Ceftazidime Sodium) GlaxoSmithKline 1650
Tazicef Pharmacy Bulk Package (Ceftazidime) GlaxoSmithKline 1653
Tazidime Vials, Faspak & ADD-Vantage (Ceftazidime) Lilly 1966
Trovan I.V. (Alatrofloxacin Mesylate) Pfizer 2722
Vantin Tablets and Oral Suspension (Cefpodoxime Proxetil) Pharmacia & Upjohn 2860
Zinacef Injection (Cefuroxime) GlaxoSmithKline 1696
Zinacef for Injection (Cefuroxime) GlaxoSmithKline 1696
Zithromax (Azithromycin Dihydrate) Pfizer 2743
Zithromax for Oral Suspension, 300 mg, 600 mg, 900 mg, 1200 mg (Azithromycin Dihydrate) Pfizer 2739
Zithromax Tablets, 250 mg (Azithromycin Dihydrate) Pfizer 2739
Zithromax Tablets, 600 mg (Azithromycin Dihydrate) Pfizer 2743
Zyvox (Linezolid) Pharmacia & Upjohn 2871

S. pyogenes infections, ocular

Genoptic Ophthalmic Ointment (Gentamicin Sulfate) Allergan ⊙239
Genoptic Sterile Ophthalmic Solution (Gentamicin Sulfate) Allergan ⊙239
Pred-G Sterile Ophthalmic Ointment (Gentamicin Sulfate, Prednisolone Acetate) Allergan ⊙248

S. pyogenes lower respiratory tract infections

Ceclor (Cefaclor) Lilly 1905
Claforan Injection (Cefotaxime Sodium) Aventis 732
E.E.S. (Erythromycin Ethylsuccinate) Abbott 450
EryPed (Erythromycin Ethylsuccinate) Abbott 446
Ery-Tab Tablets (Erythromycin) Abbott 448
Erythrocin Stearate Filmtab Tablets (Erythromycin Stearate) Abbott 452
Erythromycin Base Filmtab Tablets (Erythromycin) Abbott 454
Erythromycin Delayed-Release Capsules, USP (Erythromycin) Abbott 455
Kefurox Vials, ADD-Vantage (Cefuroxime Sodium) Lilly 1948
PCE Dispertab Tablets (Erythromycin) Abbott 498
Zinacef Injection (Cefuroxime) GlaxoSmithKline 1696
Zinacef for Injection (Cefuroxime) GlaxoSmithKline 1696

S. pyogenes otitis media

Ceclor (Cefaclor) Lilly 1905
Cedax (Ceftibuten Dihydrate) Biovail 1021
Ceftin (Cefuroxime Axetil) Lifecycle Ventures 1898
Lorabid Suspension and Pulvules (Loracarbef) Monarch 2251
Suprax (Cefixime) Lederle 1877

S. pyogenes pharyngitis

Biaxin/Biaxin XL (Clarithromycin) Abbott 403
Ceclor CD Tablets (Cefaclor) Elan 1279
Ceclor (Cefaclor) Lilly 1905
Cedax (Ceftibuten Dihydrate) Biovail 1021

(▣ Described in PDR For Nonprescription Drugs)   (⊙ Described in PDR For Ophthalmic Medicines™)

Ceftin (Cefuroxime Axetil) Lifecycle Ventures 1898
Cefzil (Cefprozil) Bristol-Myers Squibb 1076
Dynabac Tablets (Dirithromycin) Muro 2269
Lorabid Suspension and Pulvules (Loracarbef) Monarch 2251
Omnicef (Cefdinir) Abbott 493
Suprax (Cefixime) Lederle 1877
Vantin Tablets and Oral Suspension (Cefpodoxime Proxetil) Pharmacia & Upjohn 2860
Zithromax (Azithromycin Dihydrate) Pfizer 2743
Zithromax for Oral Suspension, 300 mg, 600 mg, 900 mg, 1200 mg (Azithromycin Dihydrate) Pfizer 2739
Zithromax Tablets, 250 mg (Azithromycin Dihydrate) Pfizer 2739
Zithromax Tablets, 600 mg (Azithromycin Dihydrate) Pfizer 2743

S. pyogenes respiratory tract infections
Cefobid Intravenous/Intramuscular (Cefoperazone) Pfizer 2671
Cefobid Pharmacy Bulk Package - Not for Direct Infusion (Cefoperazone Sodium) Pfizer 2673
Keflex (Cephalexin) Dista 1237

S. pyogenes skin and skin structure infections
Avelox Tablets (Moxifloxacin Hydrochloride) Bayer 879
Bactroban Cream (Mupirocin Calcium) GlaxoSmithKline 1494
Biaxin/Biaxin XL (Clarithromycin) Abbott 403
Ceclor (Cefaclor) Lilly 1905
Cefizox for Intramuscular or Intravenous Use (Ceftizoxime Sodium) Fujisawa 1390
Cefobid Intravenous/Intramuscular (Cefoperazone) Pfizer 2671
Cefobid Pharmacy Bulk Package - Not for Direct Infusion (Cefoperazone Sodium) Pfizer 2673
Cefotan (Cefotetan) AstraZeneca 664
Ceftin Tablets (Cefuroxime Axetil) Lifecycle Ventures 1898
Cefzil (Cefprozil) Bristol-Myers Squibb 1076
Ceptaz for Injection (Ceftazidime) GlaxoSmithKline 1499
Cipro I.V. (Ciprofloxacin) Bayer 893
Cipro I.V. Pharmacy Bulk Package (Ciprofloxacin) Bayer 897
Cipro (Ciprofloxacin) Bayer 887
Claforan Injection (Cefotaxime Sodium) Aventis 732
Cleocin HCl Capsules (Clindamycin Hydrochloride) Pharmacia & Upjohn 2784
Cleocin Phosphate Sterile Solution (Clindamycin Phosphate) Pharmacia & Upjohn 2785
E.E.S. (Erythromycin Ethylsuccinate) Abbott 450
EryPed (Erythromycin Ethylsuccinate) Abbott 446
Ery-Tab Tablets (Erythromycin) Abbott 448
Erythrocin Stearate Filmtab Tablets (Erythromycin Stearate) Abbott 452
Erythromycin Base Filmtab Tablets (Erythromycin) Abbott 454
Erythromycin Delayed-Release Capsules, USP (Erythromycin) Abbott 455
Floxin I.V. (Ofloxacin) Ortho-McNeil 2526
Floxin Tablets (Ofloxacin) Ortho-McNeil 2529
Fortaz (Ceftazidime Sodium) GlaxoSmithKline 1541
Levaquin (Levofloxacin) Ortho-McNeil 2537
Lorabid Suspension and Pulvules (Loracarbef) Monarch 2251
Mandol Vials (Cefamandole Nafate) Lilly 1953
Maxipime for Injection (Cefepime Hydrochloride) Elan 1285
Omnicef (Cefdinir) Abbott 493
PCE Dispertab Tablets (Erythromycin) Abbott 498
Primaxin I.M. (Cilastatin Sodium, Imipenem) Merck 2158
Primaxin I.V. (Cilastatin Sodium, Imipenem) Merck 2160
Rocephin Injectable Vials, ADD-Vantage, Galaxy, Bulk (Ceftriaxone Sodium) Roche Laboratories 2993
Synercid I.V. (Dalfopristin, Quinupristin) Aventis 775
Tazicef for Injection (Ceftazidime) GlaxoSmithKline 1647
Tazicef Galaxy Container (Ceftazidime Sodium) GlaxoSmithKline 1650
Tazicef Pharmacy Bulk Package (Ceftazidime) GlaxoSmithKline 1653
Tazidime Vials, Faspak & ADD-Vantage (Ceftazidime) Lilly 1966
Trovan I.V. (Alatrofloxacin Mesylate) Pfizer 2722
Vantin Tablets and Oral Suspension (Cefpodoxime Proxetil) Pharmacia & Upjohn 2860
Zinacef Injection (Cefuroxime) GlaxoSmithKline 1696
Zinacef for Injection (Cefuroxime) GlaxoSmithKline 1696
Zithromax (Azithromycin Dihydrate) Pfizer 2743
Zithromax for Oral Suspension, 300 mg, 600 mg, 900 mg, 1200 mg (Azithromycin Dihydrate) Pfizer 2739
Zithromax Tablets, 250 mg (Azithromycin Dihydrate) Pfizer 2739
Zithromax Tablets, 600 mg (Azithromycin Dihydrate) Pfizer 2743
Zyvox (Linezolid) Pharmacia & Upjohn 2871

S. pyogenes tonsillitis
Biaxin/Biaxin XL (Clarithromycin) Abbott 403
Ceclor CD Tablets (Cefaclor) Elan 1279
Ceclor (Cefaclor) Lilly 1905
Cedax (Ceftibuten Dihydrate) Biovail 1021
Ceftin (Cefuroxime Axetil) Lifecycle Ventures 1898
Cefzil (Cefprozil) Bristol-Myers Squibb 1076
Dynabac Tablets (Dirithromycin) Muro 2269
Lorabid Suspension and Pulvules (Loracarbef) Monarch 2251
Omnicef (Cefdinir) Abbott 493
Suprax (Cefixime) Lederle 1877
Vantin Tablets and Oral Suspension (Cefpodoxime Proxetil) Pharmacia & Upjohn 2860
Zithromax (Azithromycin Dihydrate) Pfizer 2743
Zithromax for Oral Suspension, 300 mg, 600 mg, 900 mg, 1200 mg (Azithromycin Dihydrate) Pfizer 2739
Zithromax Tablets, 250 mg (Azithromycin Dihydrate) Pfizer 2739
Zithromax Tablets, 600 mg (Azithromycin Dihydrate) Pfizer 2743

S. pyogenes upper respiratory tract infections
Biaxin/Biaxin XL (Clarithromycin) Abbott 403
Ceclor (Cefaclor) Lilly 1905
E.E.S. (Erythromycin Ethylsuccinate) Abbott 450
EryPed (Erythromycin Ethylsuccinate) Abbott 446
Ery-Tab Tablets (Erythromycin) Abbott 448
Erythrocin Stearate Filmtab Tablets (Erythromycin Stearate) Abbott 452
Erythromycin Base Filmtab Tablets (Erythromycin) Abbott 454
Erythromycin Delayed-Release Capsules, USP (Erythromycin) Abbott 455
Omnicef (Cefdinir) Abbott 493
PCE Dispertab Tablets (Erythromycin) Abbott 498
Suprax (Cefixime) Lederle 1877
Tao Capsules (Troleandomycin) Pfizer 2716
Zithromax (Azithromycin Dihydrate) Pfizer 2743
Zithromax for Oral Suspension, 300 mg, 600 mg, 900 mg, 1200 mg (Azithromycin Dihydrate) Pfizer 2739
Zithromax Tablets, 250 mg (Azithromycin Dihydrate) Pfizer 2739
Zithromax Tablets, 600 mg (Azithromycin Dihydrate) Pfizer 2743

S. saprophyticus urinary tract infections
Cipro I.V. Pharmacy Bulk Package (Ciprofloxacin) Bayer 897
Cipro (Ciprofloxacin) Bayer 887
Lorabid Suspension and Pulvules (Loracarbef) Monarch 2251
Macrobid Capsules (Nitrofurantoin Monohydrate) Procter & Gamble Pharmaceuticals 2889
Noroxin Tablets (Norfloxacin) Merck 2145
Vantin Tablets and Oral Suspension (Cefpodoxime Proxetil) Pharmacia & Upjohn 2860

S. viridans endocarditis
Erythrocin Stearate Filmtab Tablets (Erythromycin Stearate) Abbott 452
Erythromycin Base Filmtab Tablets (Erythromycin) Abbott 454
Vancocin HCl, Vials & ADD-Vantage (Vancomycin Hydrochloride) Lilly 1970

S. warnerii infections, ocular
Chibroxin Sterile Ophthalmic Solution (Norfloxacin) Merck 2051

SAH
(*see under* Hemorrhage, subarachnoid, resulting in neurological deficits)

Salmonella species infections
Pfizerpen (Penicillin G Potassium) Pfizer 2707

Salmonella typhi infections
Cipro (Ciprofloxacin) Bayer 887

Salt, substitute for
Chlor-3 (Potassium Chloride) Fleming 1361

Sarcoidosis, symptomatic
Celestone Soluspan Injectable Suspension (Betamethasone Acetate, Betamethasone Sodium Phosphate) Schering 3097
Celestone Syrup (Betamethasone) Schering 3099
Cortone Acetate Injectable Suspension (Cortisone Acetate) Merck 2059
Cortone Acetate Tablets (Cortisone Acetate) Merck 2061
Decadron Elixir (Dexamethasone) Merck 2078
Decadron Tablets (Dexamethasone) Merck 2079
Decadron Phosphate Injection (Dexamethasone Sodium Phosphate) Merck 2081
Depo-Medrol Injectable Suspension (Methylprednisolone Acetate) Pharmacia & Upjohn 2795
Hydrocortone Tablets (Hydrocortisone) Merck 2106
Hydrocortone Phosphate Injection, Sterile (Hydrocortisone Sodium Phosphate) Merck 2105
Pediapred Oral Solution (Prednisolone Sodium Phosphate) Celltech 1170
Prednisone (Prednisone) Roxane 3064
Prelone Syrup (Prednisolone) Muro 2273
Solu-Medrol Sterile Powder (Methylprednisolone Sodium Succinate) Pharmacia & Upjohn 2855

Sarcoma botryoides
Cosmegen for Injection (Dactinomycin) Merck 2062

Sarcomas, soft tissue and bone
Adriamycin PFS/RDF Injection (Doxorubicin Hydrochloride) Pharmacia & Upjohn 2767

Sarcoptes scabiei infestations
Acticin Cream (Permethrin) Bertek 998
Elimite Cream (Permethrin) Allergan 552
Lindane Lotion USP 1% (Lindane) Alpharma 559

Scabies
(*see under* Sarcoptes scabiei infestations)

Scarlatina
Bicillin C-R 900/300 Injection (Penicillin G Benzathine, Penicillin G Procaine) Monarch 2240
Bicillin C-R Injection (Penicillin G Benzathine, Penicillin G Procaine) Monarch 2238

Scarlet fever
(*see under* Scarlatina)

Schistosoma haematobium infections
Biltricide (Praziquantel) Bayer 887

Schizophrenia
(*see under* Psychotic disorders, management of the manifestations of)

Schizophrenia with depression
(*see under* Psychotic disorders with depressive symptoms)

Sciatica, temporary relief of
BC Powder (Aspirin, Caffeine, Salicylamide) Block 619
Arthritis Strength BC Powder (Aspirin, Caffeine, Salicylamide) Block 619
Sarapin (Sarraceniaceae) High Chemical 1727

Scleroderma, linear, possibly effective in
Potaba (Aminobenzoate Potassium) Glenwood 1721

Sclerosis, amyotrophic lateral
Rilutek Tablets (Riluzole) Aventis 772

Sclerosis, multiple, acute exacerbations of
Pediapred Oral Solution (Prednisolone Sodium Phosphate) Celltech 1170
Solu-Medrol Sterile Powder (Methylprednisolone Sodium Succinate) Pharmacia & Upjohn 2855

Sclerosis, multiple, relapsing-remitting
Avonex (Interferon Beta-1a) Biogen 1013
Betaseron for SC Injection (Interferon Beta-1b) Berlex 988
Copaxone for Injection (Glatiramer Acetate) Teva Neuroscience 3306
Novantrone for Injection (Mitoxantrone Hydrochloride) Immunex 1760

Seborrhea
(*see under* Dandruff)

Sedation
(*see also under* Sleep, induction of)
Nembutal Sodium Solution (Pentobarbital Sodium) Abbott 485
Phenergan Injection (Promethazine Hydrochloride) Wyeth-Ayerst 3553
Phenergan Suppositories (Promethazine Hydrochloride) Wyeth-Ayerst 3556
Phenergan Syrup (Promethazine Hydrochloride) Wyeth-Ayerst 3554
Phenergan Tablets (Promethazine Hydrochloride) Wyeth-Ayerst 3556

Sedation, benzodiazepine-induced, complete or partial reversal of
Romazicon Injection (Flumazenil) Roche Laboratories 3000

Sedation, conscious, prediagnostic procedures
Versed (Midazolam Hydrochloride) Roche Laboratories 3027

Sedation, conscious, pre-endoscopic or therapeutic procedures
Versed Syrup (Midazolam Hydrochloride) Roche Laboratories 3033

Sedation, obstetric
Phenergan Injection (Promethazine Hydrochloride) Wyeth-Ayerst 3553
Phenergan Suppositories (Promethazine Hydrochloride) Wyeth-Ayerst 3556
Phenergan Syrup (Promethazine Hydrochloride) Wyeth-Ayerst 3554
Phenergan Tablets (Promethazine Hydrochloride) Wyeth-Ayerst 3556

Sedation, postoperative
Vistaril (Hydroxyzine Pamoate) Pfizer 2738

Sedation, preoperative
Atarax Tablets & Syrup (Hydroxyzine Hydrochloride) Pfizer 2667
Ativan Injection (Lorazepam) Wyeth-Ayerst 3478
Mepergan Injection (Meperidine Hydrochloride, Promethazine Hydrochloride) Wyeth-Ayerst 3539
Versed Injection (Midazolam Hydrochloride) Roche Laboratories 3027
Versed Syrup (Midazolam Hydrochloride) Roche Laboratories 3033
Vistaril (Hydroxyzine Pamoate) Pfizer 2738

Seizures, absence, adjunctive therapy in
Depacon Injection (Valproate Sodium) Abbott 416

Depakene (Valproic Acid) Abbott 421
Depakote Sprinkle Capsules (Divalproex Sodium) Abbott 426
Depakote Tablets (Divalproex Sodium) Abbott 430

Seizures, akinetic
Klonopin Tablets (Clonazepam) Roche Laboratories 2983

Seizures, centrencephalic
(*see also under* Seizures, generalized, absence; Seizures, generalized, tonic-clonic)
Diamox (Acetazolamide Sodium) Lederle ..... ⊙269

Seizures, convulsive, severe recurrent, adjunct in
Valium Injectable (Diazepam) Roche Laboratories 3026

Seizures, focal
Carbatrol Capsules (Carbamazepine) Shire US 3234
Depakote Sprinkle Capsules (Divalproex Sodium) Abbott 426
Depakote Tablets (Divalproex Sodium) Abbott 430
Felbatol (Felbamate) Wallace 3343
Keppra Tablets (Levetiracetam) UCB 3314
Lamictal (Lamotrigine) GlaxoSmithKline 1567
Tegretol/Tegretol-XR (Carbamazepine) Novartis 2404
Tranxene T-TAB Tablets (Clorazepate Dipotassium) Abbott 511
Trileptal Oral Suspension (Oxcarbazepine) Novartis 2407
Trileptal Tablets (Oxcarbazepine) Novartis 2407

Seizures, focal, adjunctive therapy in
Depakote Sprinkle Capsules (Divalproex Sodium) Abbott 426
Felbatol (Felbamate) Wallace 3343
Neurontin Capsules (Gabapentin) Parke-Davis 2655
Neurontin Oral Solution (Gabapentin) Parke-Davis 2655
Neurontin Tablets (Gabapentin) Parke-Davis 2655
Topamax Sprinkle Capsules (Topiramate) Ortho-McNeil 2590
Topamax Tablets (Topiramate) Ortho-McNeil 2590
Tranxene (Clorazepate Dipotassium) Abbott 511
Trileptal Oral Suspension (Oxcarbazepine) Novartis 2407
Trileptal Tablets (Oxcarbazepine) Novartis 2407

Seizures, generalized, absence
Celontin Capsules (Methsuximide) Parke-Davis 2618
Depacon Injection (Valproate Sodium) Abbott 416
Depakene (Valproic Acid) Abbott 421
Depakote Sprinkle Capsules (Divalproex Sodium) Abbott 426
Depakote Tablets (Divalproex Sodium) Abbott 430
Diamox (Acetazolamide Sodium) Lederle ..... ⊙269
Klonopin Tablets (Clonazepam) Roche Laboratories 2983
Zarontin Capsules (Ethosuximide) Parke-Davis 2659
Zarontin Syrup (Ethosuximide) Parke-Davis 2660

Seizures, generalized, tonic-clonic
Carbatrol Capsules (Carbamazepine) Shire US 3234
Diamox (Acetazolamide Sodium) Lederle ..... ⊙269
Dilantin Infatabs (Phenytoin) Parke-Davis 2624
Dilantin Kapseals (Phenytoin Sodium) Parke-Davis 2622
Dilantin-125 Oral Suspension (Phenytoin) Parke-Davis 2625
Tegretol/Tegretol-XR (Carbamazepine) Novartis 2404
Topamax Sprinkle Capsules (Topiramate) Ortho-McNeil 2590
Topamax Tablets (Topiramate) Ortho-McNeil 2590

Seizures, multiple, adjunctive therapy in
Depacon Injection (Valproate Sodium) Abbott 416
Depakene (Valproic Acid) Abbott 421
Depakote Tablets (Divalproex Sodium) Abbott 430

Seizures, myoclonic
Klonopin Tablets (Clonazepam) Roche Laboratories 2983

Seizures, neurosurgery-induced
Cerebyx Injection (Fosphenytoin Sodium) Parke-Davis 2619
Dilantin Infatabs (Phenytoin) Parke-Davis 2624
Dilantin Kapseals (Phenytoin Sodium) Parke-Davis 2622

Seizures, neurosurgery-induced, prophylaxis of
Cerebyx Injection (Fosphenytoin Sodium) Parke-Davis 2619
Dilantin Infatabs (Phenytoin) Parke-Davis 2624
Dilantin Kapseals (Phenytoin Sodium) Parke-Davis 2622

Seizures, partial
(*see under* Seizures, focal)

Seizures, partial, adjunctive therapy in
Gabitril Tablets (Tiagabine Hydrochloride) Cephalon 1189
Zonegran Capsules (Zonisamide) Elan 1307

Seizures, psychomotor
Carbatrol Capsules (Carbamazepine) Shire US 3234
Dilantin Infatabs (Phenytoin) Parke-Davis 2624
Dilantin Kapseals (Phenytoin Sodium) Parke-Davis 2622
Dilantin-125 Oral Suspension (Phenytoin) Parke-Davis 2625
Tegretol-XR Tablets (Carbamazepine) Novartis 2404

Senile lentigines
(*see under* Hyperpigmentation, skin, bleaching of)

Sepsis, burn wound
Silvadene Cream 1% (Silver Sulfadiazine) Monarch 2267

Septic shock, treatment adjunct
Narcan Injection (Naloxone Hydrochloride) Endo Labs 1322

Septicemia, anaerobic bacterial
Cefobid Intravenous/Intramuscular (Cefoperazone) Pfizer 2671
Cefobid Pharmacy Bulk Package - Not for Direct Infusion (Cefoperazone Sodium) Pfizer 2673

Septicemia, bacterial
Ancef for Injection (Cefazolin Sodium) GlaxoSmithKline 1474
Ancef Injection (Cefazolin Sodium) GlaxoSmithKline 1474
Azactam for Injection (Aztreonam) Elan 1276
Cefizox for Intramuscular or Intravenous Use (Ceftizoxime Sodium) Fujisawa 1390
Cefobid Intravenous/Intramuscular (Cefoperazone) Pfizer 2671
Cefobid Pharmacy Bulk Package - Not for Direct Infusion (Cefoperazone Sodium) Pfizer 2673
Ceptaz for Injection (Ceftazidime) GlaxoSmithKline 1499
Cipro I.V. (Ciprofloxacin) Bayer 893
Claforan Injection (Cefotaxime Sodium) Aventis 732
Cleocin HCl Capsules (Clindamycin Hydrochloride) Pharmacia & Upjohn 2784
Cleocin Phosphate Sterile Solution (Clindamycin Phosphate) Pharmacia & Upjohn 2785
Fortaz (Ceftazidime Sodium) GlaxoSmithKline 1541
Kefurox Vials, ADD-Vantage (Cefuroxime Sodium) Lilly 1948
Kefzol Vials, ADD-Vantage (Cefazolin Sodium) Lilly 1951
Mandol Vials (Cefamandole Nafate) Lilly 1953
Maxipime for Injection (Cefepime Hydrochloride) Elan 1285
Mefoxin for Injection (Cefoxitin Sodium) Merck 2124
Mefoxin Premixed Intravenous Solution (Cefoxitin Sodium) Merck 2127
Merrem I.V. (Meropenem) AstraZeneca 673
Nebcin Vials, Hyporets & ADD-Vantage (Tobramycin Sulfate) Lilly 1955
Pfizerpen for Injection (Penicillin G Potassium) Pfizer 2707
Pipracil (Piperacillin Sodium) Lederle 1866
Primaxin I.V. (Cilastatin Sodium, Imipenem) Merck 2160
Rocephin Injectable Vials, ADD-Vantage, Galaxy, Bulk (Ceftriaxone Sodium) Roche Laboratories 2993
Synercid I.V. (Dalfopristin, Quinupristin) Aventis 775
Tazicef for Injection (Ceftazidime) GlaxoSmithKline 1647
Tazicef Galaxy Container (Ceftazidime Sodium) GlaxoSmithKline 1650
Tazicef Pharmacy Bulk Package (Ceftazidime) GlaxoSmithKline 1653
Tazidime Vials, Faspak & ADD-Vantage (Ceftazidime) Lilly 1966
Timentin Injection- ADD-Vantage Vial (Clavulanate Potassium, Ticarcillin Disodium) GlaxoSmithKline 1661
Timentin Injection-Galaxy Container (Clavulanate Potassium, Ticarcillin Disodium) GlaxoSmithKline 1664
Timentin Injection-Pharmacy Bulk Package (Clavulanate Potassium, Ticarcillin Disodium) GlaxoSmithKline 1666
Timentin for Intravenous Administration (Clavulanate Potassium, Ticarcillin Disodium) GlaxoSmithKline 1658
Vancocin HCl, Vials & ADD-Vantage (Vancomycin Hydrochloride) Lilly 1970
Zinacef Injection (Cefuroxime) GlaxoSmithKline 1696
Zinacef for Injection (Cefuroxime) GlaxoSmithKline 1696
Zyvox (Linezolid) Pharmacia & Upjohn 2871

Septicemia, candida
Ancobon (Flucytosine) ICN 1730

Septicemia, gram-negative bacillary, treatment adjunct
Streptomycin Sulfate Injection (Streptomycin Sulfate) Pfizer 2714

Serratia marcescens bone and joint infections
Cipro I.V. (Ciprofloxacin) Bayer 893
Cipro I.V. Pharmacy Bulk Package (Ciprofloxacin) Bayer 897
Cipro (Ciprofloxacin) Bayer 887

Serratia marcescens infections
Azactam for Injection (Aztreonam) Elan 1276
Cefizox for Intramuscular or Intravenous Use (Ceftizoxime Sodium) Fujisawa 1390
Cefotan (Cefotetan) AstraZeneca 664
Cipro I.V. (Ciprofloxacin) Bayer 893
Cipro I.V. Pharmacy Bulk Package (Ciprofloxacin) Bayer 897
Cipro (Ciprofloxacin) Bayer 887
Claforan Injection (Cefotaxime Sodium) Aventis 732
Noroxin Tablets (Norfloxacin) Merck 2145
Primaxin I.V. (Cilastatin Sodium, Imipenem) Merck 2160
Rocephin Injectable Vials, ADD-Vantage, Galaxy, Bulk (Ceftriaxone Sodium) Roche Laboratories 2993
Timentin Injection- ADD-Vantage Vial (Clavulanate Potassium, Ticarcillin Disodium) GlaxoSmithKline 1661
Timentin Injection-Galaxy Container (Clavulanate Potassium, Ticarcillin Disodium) GlaxoSmithKline 1664
Timentin Injection-Pharmacy Bulk Package (Clavulanate Potassium, Ticarcillin Disodium) GlaxoSmithKline 1666
Timentin for Intravenous Administration (Clavulanate Potassium, Ticarcillin Disodium) GlaxoSmithKline 1658

Serratia marcescens infections, ocular
Chibroxin Sterile Ophthalmic Solution (Norfloxacin) Merck 2051
Ciloxan Ophthalmic Solution (Ciprofloxacin Hydrochloride) Alcon 538
Genoptic Ophthalmic Ointment (Gentamicin Sulfate) Allergan ..... ⊙239
Genoptic Sterile Ophthalmic Solution (Gentamicin Sulfate) Allergan ..... ⊙239
Ocuflox Ophthalmic Solution (Ofloxacin) Allergan 554
Pred-G Ophthalmic Suspension (Gentamicin Sulfate, Prednisolone Acetate) Allergan ..... ⊙247
Pred-G Sterile Ophthalmic Ointment (Gentamicin Sulfate, Prednisolone Acetate) Allergan ..... ⊙248
Quixin Ophthalmic Solution (Levofloxacin) Santen 3093

Serratia marcescens lower respiratory tract infections
Azactam for Injection (Aztreonam) Elan 1276
Cefotan (Cefotetan) AstraZeneca 664
Claforan Injection (Cefotaxime Sodium) Aventis 732
Primaxin I.V. (Cilastatin Sodium, Imipenem) Merck 2160
Rocephin Injectable Vials, ADD-Vantage, Galaxy, Bulk (Ceftriaxone Sodium) Roche Laboratories 2993

Serratia marcescens skin and skin structure infections
Azactam for Injection (Aztreonam) Elan 1276
Claforan Injection (Cefotaxime Sodium) Aventis 732
Rocephin Injectable Vials, ADD-Vantage, Galaxy, Bulk (Ceftriaxone Sodium) Roche Laboratories 2993

Serratia marcescens urinary tract infections
Azactam for Injection (Aztreonam) Elan 1276
Cefizox for Intramuscular or Intravenous Use (Ceftizoxime Sodium) Fujisawa 1390
Cipro I.V. (Ciprofloxacin) Bayer 893
Cipro (Ciprofloxacin) Bayer 887
Claforan Injection (Cefotaxime Sodium) Aventis 732
Noroxin Tablets (Norfloxacin) Merck 2145
Timentin Injection- ADD-Vantage Vial (Clavulanate Potassium, Ticarcillin Disodium) GlaxoSmithKline 1661
Timentin Injection-Galaxy Container (Clavulanate Potassium, Ticarcillin Disodium) GlaxoSmithKline 1664
Timentin Injection-Pharmacy Bulk Package (Clavulanate Potassium, Ticarcillin Disodium) GlaxoSmithKline 1666
Timentin for Intravenous Administration (Clavulanate Potassium, Ticarcillin Disodium) GlaxoSmithKline 1658

Serratia species infections
Azactam for Injection (Aztreonam) Elan 1276
Cefizox for Intramuscular or Intravenous Use (Ceftizoxime Sodium) Fujisawa 1390
Ceptaz for Injection (Ceftazidime) GlaxoSmithKline 1499
Fortaz (Ceftazidime Sodium) GlaxoSmithKline 1541
Nebcin Vials, Hyporets & ADD-Vantage (Tobramycin Sulfate) Lilly 1955
Pipracil (Piperacillin Sodium) Lederle 1866
Primaxin I.V. (Cilastatin Sodium, Imipenem) Merck 2160
Tazicef for Injection (Ceftazidime) GlaxoSmithKline 1647
Tazicef Galaxy Container (Ceftazidime Sodium) GlaxoSmithKline 1650
Tazicef Pharmacy Bulk Package (Ceftazidime) GlaxoSmithKline 1653
Tazidime Vials, Faspak & ADD-Vantage (Ceftazidime) Lilly 1966

Serratia species lower respiratory tract infections
Cefizox for Intramuscular or Intravenous Use (Ceftizoxime Sodium) Fujisawa 1390
Ceptaz for Injection (Ceftazidime) GlaxoSmithKline 1499
Fortaz (Ceftazidime Sodium) GlaxoSmithKline 1541
Nebcin Vials, Hyporets & ADD-Vantage (Tobramycin Sulfate) Lilly 1955
Tazicef for Injection (Ceftazidime) GlaxoSmithKline 1647
Tazicef Galaxy Container (Ceftazidime Sodium) GlaxoSmithKline 1650

Tazicef Pharmacy Bulk Package (Ceftazidime) GlaxoSmithKline...... 1653
Tazidime Vials, Faspak & ADD-Vantage (Ceftazidime) Lilly.... 1966

Serratia species septicemia
Azactam for Injection (Aztreonam) Elan.................................. 1276
Cefizox for Intramuscular or Intravenous Use (Ceftizoxime Sodium) Fujisawa.......................... 1390
Ceptaz for Injection (Ceftazidime) GlaxoSmithKline........................... 1499
Claforan Injection (Cefotaxime Sodium) Aventis........................ 732
Fortaz (Ceftazidime Sodium) GlaxoSmithKline........................... 1541
Pipracil (Piperacillin Sodium) Lederle.. 1866
Primaxin I.V. (Cilastatin Sodium, Imipenem) Merck........................ 2160
Tazicef for Injection (Ceftazidime) GlaxoSmithKline........................... 1647
Tazicef Galaxy Container (Ceftazidime Sodium) GlaxoSmithKline 1650
Tazicef Pharmacy Bulk Package (Ceftazidime) GlaxoSmithKline 1653
Tazidime Vials, Faspak & ADD-Vantage (Ceftazidime) Lilly 1966

Serratia species skin and skin structure infections
Cefizox for Intramuscular or Intravenous Use (Ceftizoxime Sodium) Fujisawa 1390
Ceptaz for Injection (Ceftazidime) GlaxoSmithKline 1499
Fortaz (Ceftazidime Sodium) GlaxoSmithKline 1541
Pipracil (Piperacillin Sodium) Lederle 1866
Primaxin I.V. (Cilastatin Sodium, Imipenem) Merck 2160
Tazicef for Injection (Ceftazidime) GlaxoSmithKline 1647
Tazicef Galaxy Container (Ceftazidime Sodium) GlaxoSmithKline 1650
Tazicef Pharmacy Bulk Package (Ceftazidime) GlaxoSmithKline 1653
Tazidime Vials, Faspak & ADD-Vantage (Ceftazidime) Lilly 1966

Serratia species urinary tract infections
Cefizox for Intramuscular or Intravenous Use (Ceftizoxime Sodium) Fujisawa 1390
Cipro I.V. Pharmacy Bulk Package (Ciprofloxacin) Bayer 897
Nebcin Vials, Hyporets & ADD-Vantage (Tobramycin Sulfate) Lilly 1955

Serum sickness
Celestone Soluspan Injectable Suspension (Betamethasone Acetate, Betamethasone Sodium Phosphate) Schering 3097
Celestone Syrup (Betamethasone) Schering 3099
Cortone Acetate Injectable Suspension (Cortisone Acetate) Merck 2059
Cortone Acetate Tablets (Cortisone Acetate) Merck 2061
Decadron Elixir (Dexamethasone) Merck 2078
Decadron Tablets (Dexamethasone) Merck 2079
Decadron Phosphate Injection (Dexamethasone Sodium Phosphate) Merck 2081
Depo-Medrol Injectable Suspension (Methylprednisolone Acetate) Pharmacia & Upjohn 2795
Hydrocortone Tablets (Hydrocortisone) Merck 2106
Hydrocortone Phosphate Injection, Sterile (Hydrocortisone Sodium Phosphate) Merck 2105
Pediapred Oral Solution (Prednisolone Sodium Phosphate) Celltech 1170
Prednisone (Prednisone) Roxane 3064
Prelone Syrup (Prednisolone) Muro ..2273
Solu-Medrol Sterile Powder (Methylprednisolone Sodium Succinate) Pharmacia & Upjohn 2855

Shigella flexneri enteritis
Bactrim (Sulfamethoxazole, Trimethoprim) Roche Laboratories 2949
Septra Suspension (Sulfamethoxazole, Trimethoprim) Monarch 2265
Septra Tablets (Sulfamethoxazole, Trimethoprim) Monarch 2265
Septra DS Tablets (Sulfamethoxazole, Trimethoprim) Monarch 2265

Shigella flexneri infectious diarrhea
Cipro (Ciprofloxacin) Bayer............. 887

Shigella sonnei enteritis
Bactrim (Sulfamethoxazole, Trimethoprim) Roche Laboratories............................... 2949
Septra Suspension (Sulfamethoxazole, Trimethoprim) Monarch...... 2265
Septra Tablets (Sulfamethoxazole, Trimethoprim) Monarch.................. 2265
Septra DS Tablets (Sulfamethoxazole, Trimethoprim) Monarch...... 2265

Shigella sonnei infectious diarrhea
Cipro (Ciprofloxacin) Bayer............. 887

Shigella species infections
Declomycin Tablets (Demeclocycline Hydrochloride) Lederle 1855
Doryx Coated Pellet Filled Capsules (Doxycycline Hyclate) Warner Chilcott.............................. 3357
Dynacin Capsules (Minocycline Hydrochloride) Medicis 2019
Minocin Intravenous (Minocycline Hydrochloride) Lederle 1862
Minocin Oral Suspension (Minocycline Hydrochloride) Lederle 1865
Minocin Pellet-Filled Capsules (Minocycline Hydrochloride) Lederle 1863
Monodox Capsules (Doxycycline Monohydrate) Oclassen 2442
Pfizerpen for Injection (Penicillin G Potassium) Pfizer 2707
Vibramycin Calcium Oral Suspension Syrup (Doxycycline Calcium) Pfizer 2735
Vibramycin Hyclate Capsules (Doxycycline Hyclate) Pfizer 2735
Vibramycin Hyclate Intravenous (Doxycycline Hyclate) Pfizer 2737
Vibramycin Monohydrate for Oral Suspension (Doxycycline Monohydrate) Pfizer 2735
Vibra-Tabs Film Coated Tablets (Doxycycline Hyclate) Pfizer 2735

Shigellosis
Bactrim (Sulfamethoxazole, Trimethoprim) Roche Laboratories 2949
Septra Suspension (Sulfamethoxazole, Trimethoprim) Monarch 2265
Septra Tablets (Sulfamethoxazole, Trimethoprim) Monarch 2265
Septra DS Tablets (Sulfamethoxazole, Trimethoprim) Monarch 2265

Shingles
(*see under* Herpes zoster infections)

Shock, emergency treatment of
Albumin (Human) 5% (Albumin (human)) Baxter Healthcare 838
Albumin (Human) 25% (Albumin (human)) Baxter Healthcare 839
Albuminar-5, U.S.P. (Albumin (human)) Aventis Behring 785
Albuminar-25, U.S.P. (Albumin (human)) Aventis Behring 786
Plasbumin-5 (Albumin (human)) Bayer Biological 939
Plasbumin-20 (Albumin (human)) Bayer Biological 940
Plasbumin-25 (Albumin (human)) Bayer Biological 941
Plasmanate (Plasma Protein Fraction (Human)) Bayer Biological 942

Shock, suspected adrenocortical insufficiency
Celestone Soluspan Injectable Suspension (Betamethasone Acetate, Betamethasone Sodium Phosphate) Schering 3097
Cortone Acetate Injectable Suspension (Cortisone Acetate) Merck 2059
Decadron Phosphate Injection (Dexamethasone Sodium Phosphate) Merck 2081
Hydrocortone Phosphate Injection, Sterile (Hydrocortisone Sodium Phosphate) Merck 2105
Solu-Medrol Sterile Powder (Methylprednisolone Sodium Succinate) Pharmacia & Upjohn 2855

Shoulder, acute painful
(*see under* Bursitis, subacromial, acute, symptomatic relief of)

Sialorrhea associated with Parkinsonism
Levsin/Levsinex/Levbid (Hyoscyamine Sulfate) Schwarz 3172
NuLev Orally Disintegrating Tablets (Hyoscyamine Sulfate) Schwarz 3176

Sinus congestion, symptomatic relief of
Actifed Cold & Sinus Caplets and Tablets (Acetaminophen, Chlorpheniramine Maleate, Pseudoephedrine Hydrochloride) Pfizer Inc., Warner-Lambert Healthcare .... ■688
Afrin (Oxymetazoline Hydrochloride) Schering-Plough .... ■733
Afrin No Drip Original Nasal Spray (Oxymetazoline Hydrochloride) Schering-Plough .... ■735
Afrin No Drip Extra Moisturizing Nasal Spray (Oxymetazoline Hydrochloride) Schering-Plough .. ■735
Afrin No Drip Severe Congestion Nasal Spray (Oxymetazoline Hydrochloride) Schering-Plough .. ■735
Afrin No Drip Sinus Nasal Spray (Oxymetazoline Hydrochloride) Schering-Plough .... ■735
Afrin Original Pump Mist (Oxymetazoline Hydrochloride) Schering-Plough .... ■733
Benadryl Allergy & Sinus Fastmelt Tablets (Diphenhydramine Citrate, Pseudoephedrine Hydrochloride) Pfizer Inc., Warner-Lambert Healthcare .... ■693
Children's Cēpacol Sore Throat (Acetaminophen, Pseudoephedrine Hydrochloride) Williams .... ■788
Chlor-Trimeton Allergy/Decongestant Tablets (Chlorpheniramine Maleate, Pseudoephedrine Sulfate) Schering-Plough .... ■736
Coricidin 'D' Cold, Flu & Sinus Tablets (Acetaminophen, Chlorpheniramine Maleate, Pseudoephedrine Sulfate) Schering-Plough .... ■737
Dimetapp Elixir (Brompheniramine Maleate, Pseudoephedrine Hydrochloride) Whitehall-Robins .... ■777
Drixoral Allergy/Sinus Extended-Release Tablets (Acetaminophen, Dexbrompheniramine Maleate, Pseudoephedrine Sulfate) Schering-Plough ..... ■741
Sinutab Non-Drying Liquid Caps (Guaifenesin, Pseudoephedrine Hydrochloride) Pfizer Inc., Warner-Lambert Healthcare .... ■706
Sinutab Sinus Allergy Medication, Maximum Strength Formula, Tablets & Caplets (Acetaminophen, Chlorpheniramine Maleate, Pseudoephedrine Hydrochloride) Pfizer Inc., Warner-Lambert Healthcare .... ■707
Sinutab Sinus Medication, Maximum Strength Without Drowsiness Formula, Tablets & Caplets (Acetaminophen, Pseudoephedrine Hydrochloride) Pfizer Inc., Warner-Lambert Healthcare .... ■707
Tavist Sinus Non-Drowsy Coated Caplets (Acetaminophen, Pseudoephedrine Hydrochloride) Novartis Consumer .... ■676
Triaminic Cold & Allergy Liquid (Chlorpheniramine Maleate, Pseudoephedrine Hydrochloride) Novartis Consumer .... ■681
Triaminic Cold & Cough Liquid (Chlorpheniramine Maleate, Dextromethorphan Hydrobromide, Pseudoephedrine Hydrochloride) Novartis Consumer ...... ■681
Triaminic Cold & Night Time Cough Liquid (Chlorpheniramine Maleate, Dextromethorphan Hydrobromide, Pseudoephedrine Hydrochloride) Novartis Consumer .... ■681
Triaminic Cold, Cough & Fever Liquid (Acetaminophen, Chlorpheniramine Maleate, Dextromethorphan Hydrobromide, Pseudoephedrine Hydrochloride) Novartis Consumer .... ■681
Children's Tylenol Sinus Suspension Liquid (Acetaminophen, Pseudoephedrine Hydrochloride) McNeil Consumer 2017
Tylenol Allergy Sinus (Acetaminophen, Chlorpheniramine Maleate, Pseudoephedrine Hydrochloride) McNeil Consumer 2010
Maximum Strength Tylenol Sinus NightTime Caplets (Acetaminophen, Doxylamine Succinate, Pseudoephedrine Hydrochloride) McNeil Consumer 2012
Maximum Strength Tylenol Sinus Non-Drowsy Geltabs, Gelcaps, Caplets, and Tablets (Acetaminophen, Pseudoephedrine Hydrochloride) McNeil Consumer 2012
Vicks Sinex Nasal Spray and Ultra Fine Mist (Phenylephrine Hydrochloride) Procter & Gamble......................... ■729
Vicks Sinex 12-Hour Nasal Spray and Ultra Fine Mist (Oxymetazoline Hydrochloride) Procter & Gamble......................... ■729

Sinus headache
Actifed Cold & Sinus Caplets and Tablets (Acetaminophen, Chlorpheniramine Maleate, Pseudoephedrine Hydrochloride) Pfizer Inc., Warner-Lambert Healthcare .... ■688
Alka-Seltzer Plus Cold & Sinus Medicine Liqui-Gels (Acetaminophen, Pseudoephedrine Hydrochloride) Bayer Consumer .... ■604
Benadryl Severe Allergy & Sinus Headache Caplets (Acetaminophen, Diphenhydramine Hydrochloride, Pseudoephedrine Hydrochloride) Pfizer Inc., Warner-Lambert Healthcare .... ■694
Comtrex Flu Therapy & Fever Relief Daytime Caplets (Acetaminophen, Pseudoephedrine Hydrochloride) Bristol-Myers ...... ■628
Coricidin 'D' Cold, Flu & Sinus Tablets (Acetaminophen, Chlorpheniramine Maleate, Pseudoephedrine Sulfate) Schering-Plough .... ■737
Drixoral Allergy/Sinus Extended-Release Tablets (Acetaminophen, Dexbrompheniramine Maleate, Pseudoephedrine Sulfate) Schering-Plough ..... ■741
Singlet Caplets (Acetaminophen, Chlorpheniramine Maleate, Pseudoephedrine Hydrochloride) SmithKline Beecham Consumer .... ■761
Sinutab Sinus Allergy Medication, Maximum Strength Formula, Tablets & Caplets (Acetaminophen, Chlorpheniramine Maleate, Pseudoephedrine Hydrochloride) Pfizer Inc., Warner-Lambert Healthcare .... ■707
Sinutab Sinus Medication, Maximum Strength Without Drowsiness Formula, Tablets & Caplets (Acetaminophen, Pseudoephedrine Hydrochloride) Pfizer Inc., Warner-Lambert Healthcare .... ■707
Sudafed Cold & Sinus Liquid Caps (Acetaminophen, Pseudoephedrine Hydrochloride) Pfizer Inc., Warner-Lambert Healthcare .... ■710
Sudafed Sinus Headache Caplets (Acetaminophen, Pseudoephedrine Hydrochloride) Pfizer Inc., Warner-Lambert Healthcare .... ■712
Sudafed Sinus Headache Tablets (Acetaminophen, Pseudoephedrine Hydrochloride) Pfizer Inc., Warner-Lambert Healthcare .... ■712
Tavist Sinus Non-Drowsy Coated Caplets (Acetaminophen, Pseudoephedrine Hydrochloride) Novartis Consumer .... ■676
Children's Tylenol Sinus Suspension Liquid (Acetaminophen, Pseudoephedrine Hydrochloride) McNeil Consumer 2017
Tylenol Allergy Sinus (Acetaminophen, Chlorpheniramine Maleate, Pseudoephedrine Hydrochloride) McNeil Consumer 2010
Maximum Strength Tylenol Sinus NightTime Caplets (Acetaminophen, Doxylamine Succinate, Pseudoephedrine Hydrochloride) McNeil Consumer 2012
Maximum Strength Tylenol Sinus Non-Drowsy Geltabs, Gelcaps, Caplets, and Tablets (Acetaminophen, Pseudoephedrine Hydrochloride) McNeil Consumer 2012

Sinusitis, adjunctive therapy
Actifed Cold & Sinus Caplets and Tablets (Acetaminophen, Chlorpheniramine Maleate, Pseudoephedrine Hydrochloride) Pfizer Inc., Warner-Lambert Healthcare .... ▣688
Advil Cold and Sinus Caplets (Ibuprofen, Pseudoephedrine Hydrochloride) Whitehall-Robins .. ▣771
Advil Cold and Sinus Tablets (Ibuprofen, Pseudoephedrine Hydrochloride) Whitehall-Robins .. ▣771
Advil Flu & Body Ache Caplets (Ibuprofen, Pseudoephedrine Hydrochloride) Whitehall-Robins .. ▣772
Afrin (Oxymetazoline Hydrochloride) Schering-Plough .... ▣733
Afrin No Drip Original Nasal Spray (Oxymetazoline Hydrochloride) Schering-Plough .... ▣735
Afrin No Drip Extra Moisturizing Nasal Spray (Oxymetazoline Hydrochloride) Schering-Plough .. ▣735
Afrin No Drip Severe Congestion Nasal Spray (Oxymetazoline Hydrochloride) Schering-Plough .. ▣735
Afrin No Drip Sinus Nasal Spray (Oxymetazoline Hydrochloride) Schering-Plough .... ▣735
Afrin Original Pump Mist (Oxymetazoline Hydrochloride) Schering-Plough .... ▣733
Aleve Cold & Sinus Caplets (Naproxen Sodium, Pseudoephedrine Hydrochloride) Bayer Consumer .... ▣603
Alka-Seltzer Plus Cold & Sinus Medicine Liqui-Gels (Acetaminophen, Pseudoephedrine Hydrochloride) Bayer Consumer .... ▣604
Benadryl Severe Allergy & Sinus Headache Caplets (Acetaminophen, Diphenhydramine Hydrochloride, Pseudoephedrine Hydrochloride) Pfizer Inc., Warner-Lambert Healthcare .... ▣694
Comtrex Acute Head Cold & Sinus Pressure Relief Tablets (Acetaminophen, Brompheniramine Maleate, Pseudoephedrine Hydrochloride) Bristol-Myers .... ▣627
Comtrex Flu Therapy & Fever Relief Daytime Caplets (Acetaminophen, Pseudoephedrine Hydrochloride) Bristol-Myers .... ▣628
Contac Non-Drowsy 12 Hour Cold Caplets (Pseudoephedrine Hydrochloride) SmithKline Beecham Consumer .... ▣745
Contac Non-Drowsy Timed Release 12 Hour Cold Caplets (Pseudoephedrine Hydrochloride) SmithKline Beecham Consumer .... ▣746
Dimetapp Cold and Fever Suspension (Acetaminophen, Brompheniramine Maleate, Pseudoephedrine Hydrochloride) Whitehall-Robins .... ▣775
Drixoral Cold & Flu Extended-Release Tablets (Acetaminophen, Dexbrompheniramine Maleate, Pseudoephedrine Sulfate) Schering-Plough ...... ▣740
Excedrin Extra-Strength Tablets, Caplets, and Geltabs (Acetaminophen, Aspirin, Caffeine) Bristol-Myers .... ▣629
Kronofed-A (Chlorpheniramine Maleate, Pseudoephedrine Hydrochloride) Ferndale 1341
Children's Motrin Cold Oral Suspension (Ibuprofen, Pseudoephedrine Hydrochloride) McNeil Consumer 2007
Motrin Sinus Headache Caplets (Ibuprofen, Pseudoephedrine Hydrochloride) McNeil Consumer 2005
Natru-Vent Nasal Spray, Adult Strength (Xylometazoline Hydrochloride) Boehringer Ingelheim .... ▣624
Natru-Vent Nasal Spray, Pediatric Strength (Xylometazoline Hydrochloride) Boehringer Ingelheim .... ▣625
Neo-Synephrine (Phenylephrine Hydrochloride) Bayer Consumer .... ▣614
Neo-Synephrine 12 Hour Nasal Spray (Oxymetazoline Hydrochloride) Bayer Consumer .... ▣615
Ryna-12 S Suspension (Phenylephrine Tannate, Pyrilamine Tannate) Wallace 3351
Reformulated Rynatan Pediatric Suspension (Chlorpheniramine Tannate, Phenylephrine Tannate) Wallace 3352
Rynatan Tablets (Azatadine Maleate, Pseudoephedrine Sulfate) Wallace 3351
Sinutab Sinus Allergy Medication, Maximum Strength Formula, Tablets & Caplets (Acetaminophen, Chlorpheniramine Maleate, Pseudoephedrine Hydrochloride) Pfizer Inc., Warner-Lambert Healthcare .... ▣707
Sinutab Sinus Medication, Maximum Strength Without Drowsiness Formula, Tablets & Caplets (Acetaminophen, Pseudoephedrine Hydrochloride) Pfizer Inc., Warner-Lambert Healthcare .... ▣707
Children's Sudafed Nasal Decongestant Chewables (Pseudoephedrine Hydrochloride) Pfizer Inc., Warner-Lambert Healthcare .... ▣711
Sudafed Cold & Sinus Liquid Caps (Acetaminophen, Pseudoephedrine Hydrochloride) Pfizer Inc., Warner-Lambert Healthcare .... ▣710
Sudafed Non-Drying Sinus Liquid Caps (Guaifenesin, Pseudoephedrine Hydrochloride) Pfizer Inc., Warner-Lambert Healthcare .... ▣712
Sudafed Sinus Headache Caplets (Acetaminophen, Pseudoephedrine Hydrochloride) Pfizer Inc., Warner-Lambert Healthcare .... ▣712
Sudafed Sinus Headache Tablets (Acetaminophen, Pseudoephedrine Hydrochloride) Pfizer Inc., Warner-Lambert Healthcare .... ▣712
Tavist Sinus Non-Drowsy Coated Caplets (Acetaminophen, Pseudoephedrine Hydrochloride) Novartis Consumer .... ▣676
Triaminic Allergy Congestion Liquid (Pseudoephedrine Hydrochloride) Novartis Consumer ...... ▣680
Triaminic Chest Congestion Liquid (Guaifenesin, Pseudoephedrine Hydrochloride) Novartis Consumer .... ▣680
Maximum Strength Tylenol Allergy Sinus Caplets, Gelcaps, and Geltabs (Acetaminophen, Chlorpheniramine Maleate, Pseudoephedrine Hydrochloride) McNeil Consumer 2010
Zephrex Tablets (Guaifenesin, Pseudoephedrine Hydrochloride) Sanofi-Synthelabo 3091
Zephrex LA Tablets (Guaifenesin, Pseudoephedrine Hydrochloride) Sanofi-Synthelabo 3092

Sinusitis, treatment of
Augmentin Chewable Tablets (Amoxicillin, Clavulanate Potassium) GlaxoSmithKline 1482
Augmentin Powder for Oral Suspension (Amoxicillin, Clavulanate Potassium) GlaxoSmithKline 1482
Augmentin Tablets (Amoxicillin, Clavulanate Potassium) GlaxoSmithKline 1485
Avelox Tablets (Moxifloxacin Hydrochloride) Bayer 879
Biaxin/Biaxin XL (Clarithromycin) Abbott 403
Ceftin Tablets (Cefuroxime Axetil) Lifecycle Ventures 1898
Cefzil (Cefprozil) Bristol-Myers Squibb 1076
Cipro I.V. (Ciprofloxacin) Bayer 893
Cipro I.V. Pharmacy Bulk Package (Ciprofloxacin) Bayer 897
Cipro (Ciprofloxacin) Bayer 887
Levaquin (Levofloxacin) Ortho-McNeil 2537
Lorabid Suspension and Pulvules (Loracarbef) Monarch 2251
Omnicef (Cefdinir) Abbott 493
Tequin Injection (Gatifloxacin) Bristol-Myers Squibb 1110
Tequin Tablets (Gatifloxacin) Bristol-Myers Squibb 1110
Vantin Tablets and Oral Suspension (Cefpodoxime Proxetil) Pharmacia & Upjohn 2860

Sjögren's syndrome
Evoxac Capsules (Cevimeline Hydrochloride) Daiichi 1217
Salagen Tablets (Pilocarpine Hydrochloride) MGI 2229

Skin, bactericidal/virucidal cleansing of
Betadine PrepStick Plus Applicator (Povidone Iodine) Purdue Frederick 2894
Betadine Skin Cleanser (Povidone Iodine) Purdue Frederick 2895
Betadine Surgical Scrub (Povidone Iodine) Purdue Frederick 2895

Skin, bacteriostatic cleansing of
Betadine PrepStick Plus Applicator (Povidone Iodine) Purdue Frederick 2894
Betasept Surgical Scrub (Chlorhexidine Gluconate) Purdue Frederick 2895
Clinical Care Antimicrobial Wound Cleanser (Benzethonium Chloride) Care-Tech................................ ▣632
Techni-Care Surgical Scrub, Prep and Wound Decontaminant (Chloroxylenol, Cocamidopropyl PG-Dimonium Chloride Phosphate) Care-Tech .... ▣632

Skin, dry, moisturization of
Doctor Ginsberg's Psoria Rid Cream Strategic Science .... ▣840
Lac-Hydrin Lotion (Ammonium Lactate) Bristol-Myers Squibb Dermatology 1119
Lubriderm Advanced Therapy Creamy Lotion (Cetyl Alcohol, Glycerin, Mineral Oil) Pfizer Inc., Warner-Lambert Healthcare .... ▣703
Lubriderm Seriously Sensitive Lotion (Glycerin, Mineral Oil, Petrolatum) Pfizer Inc., Warner-Lambert Healthcare .... ▣703
Lubriderm Skin Therapy Moisturizing Lotion (Lanolin, Mineral Oil, Petrolatum) Pfizer Inc., Warner-Lambert Healthcare .... ▣703
StePHan Bio-Nutritional Daytime Hydrating Creme (Vitamin E) Wellness International .... ▣770
StePHan Bio-Nutritional Eye-Firming Concentrate (Moisturizing Formula) Wellness International .... ▣770
StePHan Bio-Nutritional Nighttime Moisture Creme (Moisturizing Formula) Wellness International .. ▣770
StePHan Bio-Nutritional Ultra Hydrating Fluid (Moisturizing Formula) Wellness International .. ▣770

Skin, emollient cleansing of
Bio-Complex 5000 Gentle Foaming Cleanser (Aloe vera) Wellness International .... ▣769
StePHan Bio-Nutritional Refreshing Moisture Gel (Moisturizing Formula) Wellness International .... ▣770

Skin, facial, tactile roughness of, adjunct in
Renova 0.02% Cream (Tretinoin) Ortho Dermatological 2520
Renova 0.05% Cream (Tretinoin) Ortho Dermatological 2519

Skin, fine wrinkles, mitigation of
Renova 0.02% Cream (Tretinoin) Ortho Dermatological 2520
Renova 0.05% Cream (Tretinoin) Ortho Dermatological 2519

Skin, hyperpigmentation
(*see under* Hyperpigmentation, skin, bleaching of)

Skin, inflammatory conditions
(*see also under* Dermatitis, contact; Dermatoses, corticosteroid-responsive; Rash, diaper)
Cortaid Intensive Therapy Cream (Hydrocortisone) Pharmacia Consumer .... ▣717
Cortizone•5 (Hydrocortisone) Pfizer Inc., Warner-Lambert Healthcare .... ▣699
Cortizone for Kids Creme (Hydrocortisone) Pfizer Inc., Warner-Lambert Healthcare .... ▣699
Cutivate Cream (Fluticasone Propionate) Elan 1282
Cutivate Ointment (Fluticasone Propionate) Elan 1284
Dermatop Emollient Cream (Prednicarbate) Ortho Dermatological ...2517
Diprolene Gel 0.05% (Betamethasone Dipropionate) Schering 3107
Diprolene Lotion 0.05% (Betamethasone Dipropionate) Schering 3107

Skin, irritation, minor, pain associated with
(*see under* Pain, topical relief of)

Skin, irritation, minor, temporary relief of
Caladryl Clear Lotion (Pramoxine Hydrochloride, Zinc Acetate) Pfizer Inc., Warner-Lambert Healthcare........ ▣698
Desitin Baby Powder (Corn Starch, Zinc Oxide) Pfizer Inc., Warner-Lambert Healthcare........ ▣700
Domeboro (Aluminum Sulfate) Bayer Consumer .... ▣611
Smile's Prid Salve (Homeopathic Formulations) Standard Homeopathic .... ▣766

Skin abscesses
(*see under* Infections, skin and skin structure)

Skin care
Warm Cream (L-Arginine) Strategic Science .... ▣841

Skin infections, bacterial, minor
(*see under* Infections, skin, bacterial, minor)

Skin lacerations, infected
(*see under* Infections, skin and skin structure)

Skin ulcers, venous insufficiency-induced, non-infected
Apligraf (Graftskin) Novartis 2305

Sleep, induction of
(*see also under* Sedation)
Ambien Tablets (Zolpidem Tartrate) Searle 3191
Halcion Tablets (Triazolam) Pharmacia & Upjohn 2823
Hyland's Calms Forté Tablets and Caplets (Homeopathic Formulations) Standard Homeopathic ..... ▣764
Nembutal Sodium Solution (Pentobarbital Sodium) Abbott 485
Nytol Natural Tablets (Aconite, Ignatius Beans) Block .... ▣622
Nytol QuickCaps Caplets (Diphenhydramine Hydrochloride) Block .... ▣622
Maximum Strength Nytol QuickGels Softgels (Diphenhydramine Hydrochloride) Block ..... ▣621
ProSom Tablets (Estazolam) Abbott 500
Simply Sleep Caplets (Diphenhydramine Hydrochloride) McNeil Consumer 2008
Sleep-Tite Caplets (Herbals, Multiple) Wellness International .... ▣850
Sominex Original Formula Tablets (Diphenhydramine Hydrochloride) SmithKline Beecham Consumer .... ▣761
Sonata Capsules (Zaleplon) Wyeth-Ayerst 3591
Unisom SleepTabs (Doxylamine Succinate) Pfizer Inc., Warner-Lambert Healthcare .... ▣713
Unisom Maximum Strength SleepGels (Diphenhydramine Hydrochloride) Pfizer Inc., Warner-Lambert Healthcare .... ▣713
Versed Injection (Midazolam Hydrochloride) Roche Laboratories 3027

Smoking cessation, temporary aid to
Nicoderm CQ Patch (Nicotine) GlaxoSmithKline Consumer 1717
Nicorette Gum (Nicotine Polacrilex) GlaxoSmithKline Consumer ..1720
Nicotrol Inhaler (Nicotine) Pharmacia & Upjohn 2840
Nicotrol Nasal Spray (Nicotine) Pharmacia & Upjohn 2843
Nicotrol Patch (Nicotine) Pharmacia & Upjohn 2840
Zyban Sustained-Release Tablets (Bupropion Hydrochloride) GlaxoSmithKline 1710

Sneezing
Benadryl Allergy Kapseal Capsules (Diphenhydramine Hydrochloride) Pfizer Inc., Warner-Lambert Healthcare .... ▣691

Benadryl Allergy Liquid (Diphenhydramine Hydrochloride) Pfizer Inc., Warner-Lambert Healthcare ⊡690
Benadryl Allergy Ultratab Tablets (Diphenhydramine Hydrochloride) Pfizer Inc., Warner-Lambert Healthcare ⊡691
Benadryl Allergy/Congestion Tablets (Diphenhydramine Hydrochloride, Pseudoephedrine Hydrochloride) Pfizer Inc., Warner-Lambert Healthcare ⊡692
Benadryl Allergy Sinus Headache Caplets & Gelcaps (Acetaminophen, Diphenhydramine Hydrochloride, Pseudoephedrine Hydrochloride) Pfizer Inc., Warner-Lambert Healthcare ⊡693
Benadryl Dye-Free Allergy Liquid (Diphenhydramine Hydrochloride) Pfizer Inc., Warner-Lambert Healthcare ⊡690
Benadryl Dye-Free Allergy Liqui-Gels Softgels (Diphenhydramine Hydrochloride) Pfizer Inc., Warner-Lambert Healthcare ⊡690
Chlor-Trimeton Allergy Tablets (Chlorpheniramine Maleate) Schering-Plough ⊡735
Dimetapp Elixir (Brompheniramine Maleate, Pseudoephedrine Hydrochloride) Whitehall-Robins ⊡777
Ryna (Chlorpheniramine Maleate, Pseudoephedrine Hydrochloride) Wallace ⊡768
Tylenol Severe Allergy Caplets (Acetaminophen, Diphenhydramine Hydrochloride) McNeil Consumer 2010

Social phobia
(*see under* Anxiety disorder, social)

Somatotropin deficiency syndrome
Humatrope Vials and Cartridges (Somatropin) Lilly 1930

Sour stomach
(*see under* Hyperacidity, gastric, symptomatic relief of)

Spasm, skeletal muscle
Flexeril Tablets (Cyclobenzaprine Hydrochloride) Alza 572
Flexeril Tablets (Cyclobenzaprine Hydrochloride) Merck 2094
Valium Injectable (Diazepam) Roche Laboratories 3026
Valium Tablets (Diazepam) Roche Products 3047

Spasticity, cerebral palsy-induced
(*see under* Spasticity, upper motor neuron disorder-induced)

Spasticity, multiple sclerosis-induced
(*see under* Spasticity, upper motor neuron disorder-induced)

Spasticity, muscle, symptomatic alleviation of
Flexeril Tablets (Cyclobenzaprine Hydrochloride) Alza 572
Flexeril Tablets (Cyclobenzaprine Hydrochloride) Merck 2094
Zanaflex Tablets (Tizanidine Hydrochloride) Elan 1305

Spasticity, spinal cord injury-induced
(*see under* Spasticity, upper motor neuron disorder-induced)

Spasticity, stroke-induced
(*see under* Spasticity, upper motor neuron disorder-induced)

Spasticity, upper motor neuron disorder-induced
Dantrium Capsules (Dantrolene Sodium) Procter & Gamble Pharmaceuticals 2885
Valium Injectable (Diazepam) Roche Laboratories 3026
Valium Tablets (Diazepam) Roche Products 3047
Zanaflex Tablets (Tizanidine Hydrochloride) Elan 1305

Spermatogenesis, stimulation of, adjunctive therapy in
Gonal-F for Injection (Follitropin Alfa) Serono 3216
Humegon for Injection (Menotropins) Organon 2468

Spirillum minus infections
Pfizerpen for Injection (Penicillin G Potassium) Pfizer 2707

Spirochetes species infections
(*see also under* Borrelia recurrentis infection)
Minocin Intravenous (Minocycline Hydrochloride) Lederle 1862
Minocin Oral Suspension (Minocycline Hydrochloride) Lederle 1865
Minocin Pellet-Filled Capsules (Minocycline Hydrochloride) Lederle 1863
Vibramycin Hyclate Intravenous (Doxycycline Hyclate) Pfizer 2737

Sprains, topical relief of
(*see under* Pain, topical relief of)

Staphylococcal enterocolitis
(*see under* Enterocolitis, staphylococcal)

Staphylococci, coagulase-negative, infections, ocular
Pred-G Ophthalmic Suspension (Gentamicin Sulfate, Prednisolone Acetate) Allergan ⊙247
TobraDex Ophthalmic Ointment (Dexamethasone, Tobramycin) Alcon 542
TobraDex Ophthalmic Suspension (Dexamethasone, Tobramycin) Alcon 541

Staphylococci, coagulase-positive, infections, ocular
Pred-G Ophthalmic Suspension (Gentamicin Sulfate, Prednisolone Acetate) Allergan ⊙247
TobraDex Ophthalmic Ointment (Dexamethasone, Tobramycin) Alcon 542
TobraDex Ophthalmic Suspension (Dexamethasone, Tobramycin) Alcon 541

Staphylococci, nonpenicillinase-producing, infections
Amoxil Chewable Tablets (Amoxicillin) GlaxoSmithKline 1471
Amoxil for Oral Suspension (Amoxicillin) GlaxoSmithKline 1471
Amoxil (Amoxicillin) GlaxoSmithKline 1471

Staphylococci, penicillinase-producing, infections
Mefoxin for Injection (Cefoxitin Sodium) Merck 2124
Mefoxin Premixed Intravenous Solution (Cefoxitin Sodium) Merck 2127

Staphylococci bone and joint infections
Keflex (Cephalexin) Dista 1237
Vancocin HCl Injection (Vancomycin Hydrochloride) Lilly 1970

Staphylococci otitis media
Ceclor (Cefaclor) Lilly 1905
Keflex (Cephalexin) Dista 1237

Staphylococci septicemia
Vancocin HCl, Vials & ADD-Vantage (Vancomycin Hydrochloride) Lilly 1970

Staphylococci skin and skin structure infections
Duricef (Cefadroxil) Bristol-Myers Squibb 1079
Keflex (Cephalexin) Dista 1237
Vancocin HCl, Vials & ADD-Vantage (Vancomycin Hydrochloride) Lilly 1970

Staphylococcus aureus
(*see under* S. aureus infections)

Staphylococcus epidermidis
(*see under* S. epidermis infections)

Staphylococcus species, coagulase-negative, infections
Ceclor (Cefaclor) Lilly 1905

Staphylococcus species infections
Duricef (Cefadroxil) Bristol-Myers Squibb 1079
Keflex (Cephalexin) Dista 1237
Nebcin Vials, Hyporets & ADD-Vantage (Tobramycin Sulfate) Lilly 1955
Pfizerpen for Injection (Penicillin G Potassium) Pfizer 2707
Vancocin HCl, Vials & ADD-Vantage (Vancomycin Hydrochloride) Lilly 1970

Status epilepticus
(*see under* Epilepticus, status)

Steatorrhea, adjunctive therapy in
Ultrase MT Capsules (Pancrelipase) Axcan Scandipharm 835

Stenosis, hypertrophic subaortic
Inderal (Propranolol Hydrochloride) Wyeth-Ayerst 3513
Inderal LA Long-Acting Capsules (Propranolol Hydrochloride) Wyeth-Ayerst 3516

Stevens-Johnson syndrome
Celestone Soluspan Injectable Suspension (Betamethasone Acetate, Betamethasone Sodium Phosphate) Schering 3097
Celestone Syrup (Betamethasone) Schering 3099
Cortone Acetate Injectable Suspension (Cortisone Acetate) Merck 2059
Cortone Acetate Tablets (Cortisone Acetate) Merck 2061
Decadron Elixir (Dexamethasone) Merck 2078
Decadron Tablets (Dexamethasone) Merck 2079
Decadron Phosphate Injection (Dexamethasone Sodium Phosphate) Merck 2081
Depo-Medrol Injectable Suspension (Methylprednisolone Acetate) Pharmacia & Upjohn 2795
Hydrocortone Tablets (Hydrocortisone) Merck 2106
Hydrocortone Phosphate Injection, Sterile (Hydrocortisone Sodium Phosphate) Merck 2105
Pediapred Oral Solution (Prednisolone Sodium Phosphate) Celltech 1170
Prednisone (Prednisone) Roxane 3064
Prelone Syrup (Prednisolone) Muro 2273
Solu-Medrol Sterile Powder (Methylprednisolone Sodium Succinate) Pharmacia & Upjohn 2855

Stiff-man syndrome, adjunctive therapy in
Valium Injectable (Diazepam) Roche Laboratories 3026
Valium Tablets (Diazepam) Roche Products 3047

Stomach, sour
(*see under* Hyperacidity, gastric, symptomatic relief of)

Stomach, upset
(*see under* Digestive disorders, symptomatic relief of)

Stomatitis, recurrent aphthous, symptomatic relief of
Gly-Oxide Liquid (Carbamide Peroxide) SmithKline Beecham Consumer ⊡751
Zilactin Gel (Benzyl Alcohol) Zila Consumer ⊡790
Zilactin-B Gel (Benzocaine) Zila Consumer ⊡790

Strabismus
Botox Purified Neurotoxin Complex (Botulinum Toxin Type A) Allergan 549

Strabismus, accommodative convergent
(*see under* Esotropia, accommodative)

Strep throat
(*see under* Streptococci species upper respiratory tract infections)

Streptococcal pharyngitis
Duricef (Cefadroxil) Bristol-Myers Squibb 1079
E.E.S. (Erythromycin Ethylsuccinate) Abbott 450
Omnicef (Cefdinir) Abbott 493
Suprax (Cefixime) Lederle 1877

Streptococci biliary tract infections
Kefzol Vials, ADD-Vantage (Cefazolin Sodium) Lilly 1951

Streptococci group A beta-hemolytic endocarditis
Ancef for Injection (Cefazolin Sodium) GlaxoSmithKline 1474
Ancef Injection (Cefazolin Sodium) GlaxoSmithKline 1474

Streptococci group A beta-hemolytic infections
(*see also under* Erysipelas)
Ancef for Injection (Cefazolin Sodium) GlaxoSmithKline 1474
Ancef Injection (Cefazolin Sodium) GlaxoSmithKline 1474
Ceclor (Cefaclor) Lilly 1905
Kefzol Vials, ADD-Vantage (Cefazolin Sodium) Lilly 1951
Mandol Vials (Cefamandole Nafate) Lilly 1953
Primaxin I.V. (Cilastatin Sodium, Imipenem) Merck 2160

Streptococci group A beta-hemolytic otitis media
Ceclor (Cefaclor) Lilly 1905

Streptococci group A beta-hemolytic skin and skin structure infections
Ceptaz for Injection (Ceftazidime) GlaxoSmithKline 1499
Fortaz (Ceftazidime Sodium) GlaxoSmithKline 1541
Kefzol Vials, ADD-Vantage (Cefazolin Sodium) Lilly 1951
Mandol Vials (Cefamandole Nafate) Lilly 1953
Primaxin I.V. (Cilastatin Sodium, Imipenem) Merck 2160
Tazicef for Injection (Ceftazidime) GlaxoSmithKline 1647
Tazicef Galaxy Container (Ceftazidime Sodium) GlaxoSmithKline 1650
Tazicef Pharmacy Bulk Package (Ceftazidime) GlaxoSmithKline 1653
Tazidime Vials, Faspak & ADD-Vantage (Ceftazidime) Lilly 1966

Streptococci group A beta-hemolytic species infections, ocular
Pred-G Ophthalmic Suspension (Gentamicin Sulfate, Prednisolone Acetate) Allergan ⊙247
Pred-G Sterile Ophthalmic Ointment (Gentamicin Sulfate, Prednisolone Acetate) Allergan ⊙248
TobraDex Ophthalmic Ointment (Dexamethasone, Tobramycin) Alcon 542
TobraDex Ophthalmic Suspension (Dexamethasone, Tobramycin) Alcon 541

Streptococci group A beta-hemolytic upper respiratory tract infections
Ceclor (Cefaclor) Lilly 1905
Duricef (Cefadroxil) Bristol-Myers Squibb 1079
PCE Dispertab Tablets (Erythromycin) Abbott 498
Tao Capsules (Troleandomycin) Pfizer 2716

Streptococci group B infections
Mefoxin for Injection (Cefoxitin Sodium) Merck 2124
Mefoxin Premixed Intravenous Solution (Cefoxitin Sodium) Merck 2127
Primaxin I.V. (Cilastatin Sodium, Imipenem) Merck 2160

Streptococci group D bone and joint infections
Primaxin I.V. (Cilastatin Sodium, Imipenem) Merck 2160

Streptococci group D gynecologic infections
Primaxin I.M. (Cilastatin Sodium, Imipenem) Merck 2158

Streptococci group D infections
Ancef for Injection (Cefazolin Sodium) GlaxoSmithKline 1474
Ancef Injection (Cefazolin Sodium) GlaxoSmithKline 1474
Claforan Injection (Cefotaxime Sodium) Aventis 732

Mandol Vials (Cefamandole Nafate) Lilly ... 1953
Pipracil (Piperacillin Sodium) Lederle ... 1866
Primaxin I.V. (Cilastatin Sodium, Imipenem) Merck ... 2160

Streptococci group D intra-abdominal infections
Pipracil (Piperacillin Sodium) Lederle ... 1866
Primaxin I.M. (Cilastatin Sodium, Imipenem) Merck ... 2158
Primaxin I.V. (Cilastatin Sodium, Imipenem) Merck ... 2160

Streptococci group D skin and skin structure infections
Primaxin I.M. (Cilastatin Sodium, Imipenem) Merck ... 2158
Primaxin I.V. (Cilastatin Sodium, Imipenem) Merck ... 2160

Streptococci group D urinary tract infections
Mandol Vials (Cefamandole Nafate) Lilly ... 1953

Streptococci infections, ocular
Chloromycetin Ophthalmic Ointment, 1% (Chloramphenicol) Monarch ... ⊙296
Chloromycetin Ophthalmic Solution (Chloramphenicol) Monarch ... ⊙297
Quixin Ophthalmic Solution (Levofloxacin) Santen ... 3093
Terra-Cortril Ophthalmic Suspension (Hydrocortisone Acetate, Oxytetracycline Hydrochloride) Pfizer ... 2716
TobraDex Ophthalmic Ointment (Dexamethasone, Tobramycin) Alcon ... 542
TobraDex Ophthalmic Suspension (Dexamethasone, Tobramycin) Alcon ... 541

Streptococci non-hemolytic species infections, ocular
Pred-G Ophthalmic Suspension (Gentamicin Sulfate, Prednisolone Acetate) Allergan ... ⊙247
TobraDex Ophthalmic Ointment (Dexamethasone, Tobramycin) Alcon ... 542
TobraDex Ophthalmic Suspension (Dexamethasone, Tobramycin) Alcon ... 541

Streptococci skin and skin structure infections
Cefizox for Intramuscular or Intravenous Use (Ceftizoxime Sodium) Fujisawa ... 1390
Cefotan (Cefotetan) AstraZeneca ... 664
Duricef (Cefadroxil) Bristol-Myers Squibb ... 1079
Keflex (Cephalexin) Dista ... 1237
Kefzol Vials, ADD-Vantage (Cefazolin Sodium) Lilly ... 1951
Mefoxin for Injection (Cefoxitin Sodium) Merck ... 2124
Mefoxin Premixed Intravenous Solution (Cefoxitin Sodium) Merck ... 2127

Streptococci species otitis media
Keflex (Cephalexin) Dista ... 1237

Streptococci species upper respiratory tract infections
Bicillin C-R 900/300 Injection (Penicillin G Benzathine, Penicillin G Procaine) Monarch ... 2240
Bicillin C-R Injection (Penicillin G Benzathine, Penicillin G Procaine) Monarch ... 2238
Bicillin L-A Injection (Penicillin G Benzathine) Monarch ... 2242
Ceftin (Cefuroxime Axetil) Lifecycle Ventures ... 1898
Omnicef (Cefdinir) Abbott ... 493
Permapen Isoject (Penicillin G Benzathine) Pfizer ... 2706
Suprax (Cefixime) Lederle ... 1877

Streptococci (viridans group) infections, ocular
Blephamide Ophthalmic Suspension (Prednisolone Acetate, Sulfacetamide Sodium) Allergan ... 548
Ciloxan (Ciprofloxacin Hydrochloride) Alcon ... 538
FML-S Liquifilm Sterile Ophthalmic Suspension (Fluorometholone, Sulfacetamide Sodium) Allergan ... ⊙238
Polytrim Ophthalmic Solution (Polymyxin B Sulfate, Trimethoprim Sulfate) Allergan ... 556
Quixin Ophthalmic Solution (Levofloxacin) Santen ... 3093

Streptococcus agalactiae infections
(*see under* S. agalactiae infections)

Streptococcus faecalis
(*see under* S. faecalis infections)

Streptococcus pneumoniae
(*see under* S. pneumoniae infections)

Streptococcus pyogenes
(*see under* S. pyogenes infections)

Streptococcus species bone and joint infections
Cefizox for Intramuscular or Intravenous Use (Ceftizoxime Sodium) Fujisawa ... 1390
Claforan Injection (Cefotaxime Sodium) Aventis ... 732

Streptococcus species gynecologic infections
Cefotan (Cefotetan) AstraZeneca ... 664
Claforan Injection (Cefotaxime Sodium) Aventis ... 732

Streptococcus species infections
Amoxil Chewable Tablets (Amoxicillin) GlaxoSmithKline ... 1471
Amoxil for Oral Suspension (Amoxicillin) GlaxoSmithKline ... 1471
Amoxil (Amoxicillin) GlaxoSmithKline ... 1471
Bactroban Ointment (Mupirocin) GlaxoSmithKline ... 1496
Cefizox for Intramuscular or Intravenous Use (Ceftizoxime Sodium) Fujisawa ... 1390
Cefotan (Cefotetan) AstraZeneca ... 664
Claforan Injection (Cefotaxime Sodium) Aventis ... 732
Cleocin HCl Capsules (Clindamycin Hydrochloride) Pharmacia & Upjohn ... 2784
Cleocin Phosphate Sterile Solution (Clindamycin Phosphate) Pharmacia & Upjohn ... 2785
Declomycin Tablets (Demeclocycline Hydrochloride) Lederle ... 1855
Duricef (Cefadroxil) Bristol-Myers Squibb ... 1079
Kefzol Vials, ADD-Vantage (Cefazolin Sodium) Lilly ... 1951
Minocin Intravenous (Minocycline Hydrochloride) Lederle ... 1862
Omnicef (Cefdinir) Abbott ... 493
Pfizerpen for Injection (Penicillin G Potassium) Pfizer ... 2707
Suprax (Cefixime) Lederle ... 1877
Vibramycin Hyclate Intravenous (Doxycycline Hyclate) Pfizer ... 2737

Streptococcus species intra-abdominal infections
Cefizox for Intramuscular or Intravenous Use (Ceftizoxime Sodium) Fujisawa ... 1390
Cefotan (Cefotetan) AstraZeneca ... 664
Claforan Injection (Cefotaxime Sodium) Aventis ... 732

Streptococcus species lower respiratory tract infections
Cefizox for Intramuscular or Intravenous Use (Ceftizoxime Sodium) Fujisawa ... 1390

Streptococcus species respiratory tract infections
Cleocin HCl Capsules (Clindamycin Hydrochloride) Pharmacia & Upjohn ... 2784
Cleocin Phosphate Sterile Solution (Clindamycin Phosphate) Pharmacia & Upjohn ... 2785

Streptococcus species septicemia
Cefizox for Intramuscular or Intravenous Use (Ceftizoxime Sodium) Fujisawa ... 1390
Claforan Injection (Cefotaxime Sodium) Aventis ... 732
Cleocin Phosphate Sterile Solution (Clindamycin Phosphate) Pharmacia & Upjohn ... 2785

Streptococcus tonsillitis
(*see under* Streptococci species upper respiratory tract infections)

Streptococcus viridans group infections
Blephamide Ophthalmic Ointment (Prednisolone Acetate, Sulfacetamide Sodium) Allergan ... 547
Merrem I.V. (Meropenem) AstraZeneca ... 673
Primaxin I.M. (Cilastatin Sodium, Imipenem) Merck ... 2158
Rocephin Injectable Vials, ADD-Vantage, Galaxy, Bulk (Ceftriaxone Sodium) Roche Laboratories ... 2993
Streptomycin Sulfate Injection (Streptomycin Sulfate) Pfizer ... 2714

Stress disorder, post-traumatic
Zoloft (Sertraline Hydrochloride) Pfizer ... 2751

Stroke, ischemic
Activase I.V. (Alteplase, Recombinant) Genentech ... 1410

Stroke, to reduce the risk of
Aggrenox Capsules (Aspirin, Dipyridamole) Boehringer Ingelheim ... 1026
Altace Capsules (Ramipril) Monarch ... 2233
Coumadin for Injection (Warfarin Sodium) DuPont ... 1243
Coumadin Tablets (Warfarin Sodium) DuPont ... 1243
Plavix Tablets (Clopidogrel Bisulfate) Bristol-Myers Squibb ... 1097
Plavix Tablets (Clopidogrel Bisulfate) Sanofi-Synthelabo ... 3084
Pravachol Tablets (Pravastatin Sodium) Bristol-Myers Squibb ... 1099
Ticlid Tablets (Ticlopidine Hydrochloride) Roche Laboratories ... 3015
Warfarin Sodium Tablets, USP (Warfarin Sodium) Taro ... 3302
Zocor Tablets (Simvastatin) Merck ... 2219

Strongyloidiasis
Mintezol (Thiabendazole) Merck ... 2137
Stromectol Tablets (Ivermectin) Merck ... 2185

Sunburn, acute, prophylaxis
Lubriderm Daily UV Lotion (Octyl Methoxycinnamate, Octyl Salicylate, Oxybenzone) Pfizer Inc., Warner-Lambert Healthcare ... ▣703

Sunburn, pain associated with
(*see under* Pain, topical relief of)

Sympathetic ophthalmia
(*see under* Ophthalmia, sympathetic)

Synechial formation
Humorsol Sterile Ophthalmic Solution (Demecarium Bromide) Merck ... 2102

Syphilis
(*see under* T. pallidum infections)

T

T. pallidum infections
Bicillin L-A Injection (Penicillin G Benzathine) Monarch ... 2242
Declomycin Tablets (Demeclocycline Hydrochloride) Lederle ... 1855
Doryx Coated Pellet Filled Capsules (Doxycycline Hyclate) Warner Chilcott ... 3357
Dynacin Capsules (Minocycline Hydrochloride) Medicis ... 2019
E.E.S. (Erythromycin Ethylsuccinate) Abbott ... 450
EryPed (Erythromycin Ethylsuccinate) Abbott ... 446
Ery-Tab Tablets (Erythromycin) Abbott ... 448
Erythrocin Stearate Filmtab Tablets (Erythromycin Stearate) Abbott ... 452
Erythromycin Base Filmtab Tablets (Erythromycin) Abbott ... 454
Erythromycin Delayed-Release Capsules, USP (Erythromycin) Abbott ... 455
Minocin Intravenous (Minocycline Hydrochloride) Lederle ... 1862
Minocin Oral Suspension (Minocycline Hydrochloride) Lederle ... 1865
Minocin Pellet-Filled Capsules (Minocycline Hydrochloride) Lederle ... 1863
Monodox Capsules (Doxycycline Monohydrate) Oclassen ... 2442
PCE Dispertab Tablets (Erythromycin) Abbott ... 498
Permapen Isoject (Penicillin G Benzathine) Pfizer ... 2706
Pfizerpen for Injection (Penicillin G Potassium) Pfizer ... 2707
Vibramycin Calcium Oral Suspension Syrup (Doxycycline Calcium) Pfizer ... 2735
Vibramycin Hyclate Capsules (Doxycycline Hyclate) Pfizer ... 2735
Vibramycin Hyclate Intravenous (Doxycycline Hyclate) Pfizer ... 2737
Vibramycin Monohydrate for Oral Suspension (Doxycycline Monohydrate) Pfizer ... 2735
Vibra-Tabs Film Coated Tablets (Doxycycline Hyclate) Pfizer ... 2735

T. vaginalis infections
Betadine Medicated Douche (Povidone Iodine) Purdue Frederick ... 2894

Tachyarrhythmias, catecholamine-induced, during anesthesia
Inderal (Propranolol Hydrochloride) Wyeth-Ayerst ... 3513

Tachycardia, noncompensatory sinus
Brevibloc Injection (Esmolol Hydrochloride) Baxter Anesthesia ... 858

Tachycardia, paroxysmal supraventricular
Adenocard Injection (Adenosine) Fujisawa ... 1380
Cardizem Injectable (Diltiazem Hydrochloride) Biovail ... 1018
Cardizem Lyo-Ject Syringe (Diltiazem Hydrochloride) Biovail ... 1018
Cardizem Monovial (Diltiazem Hydrochloride) Biovail ... 1018
Inderal (Propranolol Hydrochloride) Wyeth-Ayerst ... 3513
Rythmol Tablets – 150 mg, 225 mg, 300 mg (Propafenone Hydrochloride) Abbott ... 502
Tambocor Tablets (Flecainide Acetate) 3M ... 1990

Tachycardia, paroxysmal supraventricular associated with Wolff-Parkinson-White syndrome
(*see under* Wolff-Parkinson-White syndrome)

Tachycardia, supraventricular
Brevibloc Injection (Esmolol Hydrochloride) Baxter Anesthesia ... 858
Tambocor Tablets (Flecainide Acetate) 3M ... 1990

Tachycardia, ventricular
Betapace Tablets (Sotalol Hydrochloride) Berlex ... 950
Inderal (Propranolol Hydrochloride) Wyeth-Ayerst ... 3513
Quinaglute Dura-Tabs Tablets (Quinidine Gluconate) Berlex ... 978
Tambocor Tablets (Flecainide Acetate) 3M ... 1990
Tonocard Tablets (Tocainide Hydrochloride) AstraZeneca LP ... 649

Tachycardia, ventricular, recurrent hemodynamically unstable
Cordarone Intravenous (Amiodarone Hydrochloride) Wyeth-Ayerst ... 3491
Cordarone Tablets (Amiodarone Hydrochloride) Wyeth-Ayerst ... 3487
Pacerone Tablets (Amiodarone Hydrochloride) Upsher-Smith ... 3331

Tachycardia, ventricular, sustained
Mexitil Capsules (Mexiletine Hydrochloride) Boehringer Ingelheim ... 1047
Procanbid Extended-Release Tablets (Procainamide Hydrochloride) Monarch ... 2262
Quinidex Extentabs (Quinidine Sulfate) Robins ... 2933
Rythmol Tablets – 150 mg, 225 mg, 300 mg (Propafenone Hydrochloride) Abbott ... 502
Tambocor Tablets (Flecainide Acetate) 3M ... 1990

Tachycardias, paroxysmal atrial
(*see under* Tachycardia, paroxysmal supraventricular)

Tachycardias, sinus, persistent
Inderal (Propranolol Hydrochloride) Wyeth-Ayerst ... 3513

Taenia solium infections
Albenza Tablets (Albendazole) GlaxoSmithKline 1463

Tapeworm infections
(*see under* Infections, tapeworm)

Tendinitis
Anaprox Tablets (Naproxen Sodium) Roche Laboratories 2967
Anaprox DS Tablets (Naproxen Sodium) Roche Laboratories 2967
Clinoril Tablets (Sulindac) Merck 2053
Indocin (Indomethacin) Merck 2112
Naprelan Tablets (Naproxen Sodium) Elan 1293
Naprosyn Suspension (Naproxen) Roche Laboratories 2967
Naprosyn Tablets (Naproxen) Roche Laboratories 2967
Traumeel Injection Solution (Homeopathic Formulations) Heel 1726

Tenosynovitis, acute nonspecific
Celestone Soluspan Injectable Suspension (Betamethasone Acetate, Betamethasone Sodium Phosphate) Schering 3097
Celestone Syrup (Betamethasone) Schering 3099
Cortone Acetate Injectable Suspension (Cortisone Acetate) Merck 2059
Cortone Acetate Tablets (Cortisone Acetate) Merck 2061
Decadron Elixir (Dexamethasone) Merck 2078
Decadron Tablets (Dexamethasone) Merck 2079
Decadron Phosphate Injection (Dexamethasone Sodium Phosphate) Merck 2081
Depo-Medrol Injectable Suspension (Methylprednisolone Acetate) Pharmacia & Upjohn 2795
Hydrocortone Tablets (Hydrocortisone) Merck 2106
Hydrocortone Acetate Injectable Suspension (Hydrocortisone Acetate) Merck 2103
Hydrocortone Phosphate Injection, Sterile (Hydrocortisone Sodium Phosphate) Merck 2105
Pediapred Oral Solution (Prednisolone Sodium Phosphate) Celltech 1170
Prednisone (Prednisone) Roxane 3064
Prelone Syrup (Prednisolone) Muro 2273
Solu-Medrol Sterile Powder (Methylprednisolone Sodium Succinate) Pharmacia & Upjohn 2855

Testis, advanced carcinoma of
(*see under* Carcinoma, testis, advanced)

Testosterone, deficiency of
(*see under* Androgen, absence or deficiency of)

Tetanus
BayTet (Tetanus Immune Globulin (Human)) Bayer Biological 923
Pfizerpen for Injection (Penicillin G Potassium) Pfizer 2707

Tetanus, treatment adjunct
Thorazine (Chlorpromazine Hydrochloride) GlaxoSmithKline 1656
Valium Injectable (Diazepam) Roche Laboratories 3026

Threadworm infestations
(*see under* Strongyloidiasis)

Throat, itchy
(*see under* Pruritus, rhinopharyngeal, symptomatic relief of)

Throat, sore
(*see under* Pharyngitis, symptomatic relief of)

Thrombocythemia
Agrylin Capsules (Anagrelide Hydrochloride) Shire US 3232

Thrombocytopenia, heparin-induced
Argatroban Injection (Argatroban) GlaxoSmithKline 1478
Refludan for Injection (Lepirudin) Aventis 761

Thrombocytopenia, prevention of
Neumega for Injection (Oprelvekin) Genetics 1434

Thrombocytopenia, secondary
Celestone Soluspan Injectable Suspension (Betamethasone Acetate, Betamethasone Sodium Phosphate) Schering 3097
Celestone Syrup (Betamethasone) Schering 3099
Cortone Acetate Tablets (Cortisone Acetate) Merck 2061
Decadron Elixir (Dexamethasone) Merck 2078
Decadron Tablets (Dexamethasone) Merck 2079
Decadron Phosphate Injection (Dexamethasone Sodium Phosphate) Merck 2081
Depo-Medrol Injectable Suspension (Methylprednisolone Acetate) Pharmacia & Upjohn 2795
Hydrocortone Tablets (Hydrocortisone) Merck 2106
Hydrocortone Phosphate Injection, Sterile (Hydrocortisone Sodium Phosphate) Merck 2105
Pediapred Oral Solution (Prednisolone Sodium Phosphate) Celltech 1170
Prednisone (Prednisone) Roxane 3064
Prelone Syrup (Prednisolone) Muro 2273
Solu-Medrol Sterile Powder (Methylprednisolone Sodium Succinate) Pharmacia & Upjohn 2855

Thromboembolic complications
Coumadin for Injection (Warfarin Sodium) DuPont 1243
Coumadin Tablets (Warfarin Sodium) DuPont 1243
Refludan for Injection (Lepirudin) Aventis 761
Warfarin Sodium Tablets, USP (Warfarin Sodium) Taro 3302

Thromboembolism, postoperative, adjunct in
Persantine Tablets (Dipyridamole) Boehringer Ingelheim 1057

Thrombosis, coronary artery, acute, lysis of
Streptase for Infusion (Streptokinase) AstraZeneca LP 647

Thrombosis, venous
Coumadin for Injection (Warfarin Sodium) DuPont 1243
Coumadin Tablets (Warfarin Sodium) DuPont 1243
Heparin Sodium Injection (Heparin Sodium) Wyeth-Ayerst 3511
Innohep Injection (Tinzaparin sodium) DuPont 1248
Streptase for Infusion (Streptokinase) AstraZeneca LP 647
Warfarin Sodium Tablets, USP (Warfarin Sodium) Taro 3302

Thrombosis, venous, prophylaxis of
Coumadin for Injection (Warfarin Sodium) DuPont 1243
Coumadin Tablets (Warfarin Sodium) DuPont 1243
Fragmin Injection (Dalteparin Sodium) Pharmacia & Upjohn 2814
Lovenox Injection (Enoxaparin) Aventis 746
Orgaran Injection (Danaparoid Sodium) Organon 2480
Warfarin Sodium Tablets, USP (Warfarin Sodium) Taro 3302

Thrush
(*see under* Candidiasis, oropharyngeal)

Thyroid function, aid in the diagnosis of
Cytomel Tablets (Liothyronine Sodium) Jones 1817
Levothroid Tablets (Levothyroxine Sodium) Forest 1373
Levoxyl Tablets (Levothyroxine Sodium) Jones 1819
Synthroid (Levothyroxine Sodium) Abbott 505
Thyrel TRH for Injection (Protirelin) Ferring 3630
Unithroid Tablets (Levothyroxine Sodium) Watson 3445

Thyroiditis, chronic lymphocytic
(*see under* Hashimoto's thyroiditis)

Thyroiditis, nonsuppurative
Celestone Soluspan Injectable Suspension (Betamethasone Acetate, Betamethasone Sodium Phosphate) Schering 3097
Celestone Syrup (Betamethasone) Schering 3099
Cortone Acetate Injectable Suspension (Cortisone Acetate) Merck 2059
Cortone Acetate Tablets (Cortisone Acetate) Merck 2061
Decadron Elixir (Dexamethasone) Merck 2078
Decadron Tablets (Dexamethasone) Merck 2079
Decadron Phosphate Injection (Dexamethasone Sodium Phosphate) Merck 2081
Depo-Medrol Injectable Suspension (Methylprednisolone Acetate) Pharmacia & Upjohn 2795
Hydrocortone Tablets (Hydrocortisone) Merck 2106
Hydrocortone Phosphate Injection, Sterile (Hydrocortisone Sodium Phosphate) Merck 2105
Pediapred Oral Solution (Prednisolone Sodium Phosphate) Celltech 1170
Prednisone (Prednisone) Roxane 3064
Prelone Syrup (Prednisolone) Muro 2273
Solu-Medrol Sterile Powder (Methylprednisolone Sodium Succinate) Pharmacia & Upjohn 2855

Tick fevers
Declomycin Tablets (Demeclocycline Hydrochloride) Lederle 1855
Doryx Coated Pellet Filled Capsules (Doxycycline Hyclate) Warner Chilcott 3357
Dynacin Capsules (Minocycline Hydrochloride) Medicis 2019
Minocin Intravenous (Minocycline Hydrochloride) Lederle 1862
Minocin Oral Suspension (Minocycline Hydrochloride) Lederle 1865
Minocin Pellet-Filled Capsules (Minocycline Hydrochloride) Lederle 1863
Monodox Capsules (Doxycycline Monohydrate) Oclassen 2442
Vibramycin Calcium Oral Suspension Syrup (Doxycycline Calcium) Pfizer 2735
Vibramycin Hyclate Capsules (Doxycycline Hyclate) Pfizer 2735
Vibramycin Hyclate Intravenous (Doxycycline Hyclate) Pfizer 2737
Vibramycin Monohydrate for Oral Suspension (Doxycycline Monohydrate) Pfizer 2735
Vibra-Tabs Film Coated Tablets (Doxycycline Hyclate) Pfizer 2735

Tinea barbae
(*see under* Folliculitis barbae)

Tinea capitis infections
Grifulvin V Tablets Microsize and Oral Suspension Microsize (Griseofulvin) Ortho Dermatological 2518
Gris-PEG Tablets (Griseofulvin) Pedinol 2661
Lamisil AT Cream (Terbinafine Hydrochloride) Novartis Consumer .... ▣672
Lamisil AT Solution (Terbinafine Hydrochloride) Novartis Consumer .... ▣672

Tinea corporis infections
Desenex Spray Powder (Miconazole Nitrate) Novartis Consumer .... ▣668
Desenex Jock Itch Spray Powder (Miconazole Nitrate) Novartis Consumer .... ▣668
Grifulvin V Tablets Microsize and Oral Suspension Microsize (Griseofulvin) Ortho Dermatological 2518
Gris-PEG Tablets (Griseofulvin) Pedinol 2661
Loprox Cream (Ciclopirox Olamine) Medicis 2021
Loprox Gel (Ciclopirox) Medicis 2022
Loprox Lotion (Ciclopirox Olamine) Medicis 2021
Lotrimin AF Cream, Lotion, Solution, and Jock Itch Cream (Clotrimazole) Schering-Plough .... ▣742
Lotrimin AF Spray Powder, Spray Liquid, Spray Deodorant Powder, Shaker Powder and Jock Itch Spray Powder (Miconazole Nitrate) Schering-Plough .... ▣742
Lotrimin (Clotrimazole) Schering 3128
Lotrisone (Betamethasone Dipropionate, Clotrimazole) Schering 3129
Mentax Cream (Butenafine Hydrochloride) Bertek 1009
Naftin Cream (Naftifine Hydrochloride) Merz 2224
Naftin Gel (Naftifine Hydrochloride) Merz 2224
Nizoral 2% Cream (Ketoconazole) Janssen 3620
Oxistat (Oxiconazole Nitrate) Elan 1298

Tinea cruris infections
Desenex Liquid Spray (Miconazole Nitrate) Novartis Consumer .... ▣668
Grifulvin V Tablets Microsize and Oral Suspension Microsize (Griseofulvin) Ortho Dermatological 2518
Gris-PEG Tablets (Griseofulvin) Pedinol 2661
Loprox Cream (Ciclopirox Olamine) Medicis 2021
Loprox Gel (Ciclopirox) Medicis 2022
Loprox Lotion (Ciclopirox Olamine) Medicis 2021
Lotrimin AF Cream, Lotion, Solution, and Jock Itch Cream (Clotrimazole) Schering-Plough .... ▣742
Lotrimin AF Spray Powder, Spray Liquid, Spray Deodorant Powder, Shaker Powder and Jock Itch Spray Powder (Miconazole Nitrate) Schering-Plough .... ▣742
Lotrimin (Clotrimazole) Schering 3128
Lotrisone (Betamethasone Dipropionate, Clotrimazole) Schering 3129
Mentax Cream (Butenafine Hydrochloride) Bertek 1009
Naftin Cream (Naftifine Hydrochloride) Merz 2224
Naftin Gel (Naftifine Hydrochloride) Merz 2224
Nizoral 2% Cream (Ketoconazole) Janssen 3620
Oxistat (Oxiconazole Nitrate) Elan 1298

Tinea pedis infections
Desenex (Miconazole Nitrate) Novartis Consumer .... ▣668
Desenex Jock Itch Spray Powder (Miconazole Nitrate) Novartis Consumer .... ▣668
Gordochom Solution (Chloroxylenol, Undecylenic Acid) Gordon 1722
Grifulvin V Tablets Microsize and Oral Suspension Microsize (Griseofulvin) Ortho Dermatological 2518
Gris-PEG Tablets (Griseofulvin) Pedinol 2661
Lamisil AT Cream (Terbinafine Hydrochloride) Novartis Consumer .... ▣672
Lamisil AT Solution (Terbinafine Hydrochloride) Novartis Consumer .... ▣672
Loprox Cream (Ciclopirox Olamine) Medicis 2021
Loprox Gel (Ciclopirox) Medicis 2022
Loprox Lotion (Ciclopirox Olamine) Medicis 2021
Lotrimin AF Cream, Lotion, Solution, and Jock Itch Cream (Clotrimazole) Schering-Plough .... ▣742
Lotrimin AF Spray Powder, Spray Liquid, Spray Deodorant Powder, Shaker Powder and Jock Itch Spray Powder (Miconazole Nitrate) Schering-Plough .... ▣742
Lotrimin (Clotrimazole) Schering 3128
Lotrisone (Betamethasone Dipropionate, Clotrimazole) Schering 3129
Mentax Cream (Butenafine Hydrochloride) Bertek 1009
Naftin Cream (Naftifine Hydrochloride) Merz 2224
Naftin Gel (Naftifine Hydrochloride) Merz 2224
Oxistat (Oxiconazole Nitrate) Elan 1298

Tinea unguium infections
Grifulvin V Tablets Microsize and Oral Suspension Microsize (Griseofulvin) Ortho Dermatological 2518
Gris-PEG Tablets (Griseofulvin) Pedinol 2661
Lamisil Tablets (Terbinafine Hydrochloride) Novartis 2360
Penlac Nail Lacquer, Topical Solution (Ciclopirox) Dermik 1225
Sporanox Capsules (Itraconazole) Janssen 1800

Tinea versicolor infections
(*see under* Pityrosporon orbiculare infections)

Tonsillitis
Biaxin/Biaxin XL (Clarithromycin) Abbott 403
Ceclor CD Tablets (Cefaclor) Elan 1279
Ceclor (Cefaclor) Lilly 1905
Cedax (Ceftibuten Dihydrate) Biovail 1021
Ceftin (Cefuroxime Axetil) Lifecycle Ventures 1898
Cefzil (Cefprozil) Bristol-Myers Squibb 1076

Duricef (Cefadroxil) Bristol-Myers Squibb 1079
Dynabac Tablets (Dirithromycin) Muro 2269
E.E.S. (Erythromycin Ethylsuccinate) Abbott 450
EryPed (Erythromycin Ethylsuccinate) Abbott 446
Lorabid Suspension and Pulvules (Loracarbef) Monarch 2251
Omnicef (Cefdinir) Abbott 493
PCE Dispertab Tablets (Erythromycin) Abbott 498
Suprax (Cefixime) Lederle 1877
Vantin Tablets and Oral Suspension (Cefpodoxime Proxetil) Pharmacia & Upjohn 2860
Zithromax (Azithromycin Dihydrate) Pfizer 2743
Zithromax for Oral Suspension, 300 mg, 600 mg, 900 mg, 1200 mg (Azithromycin Dihydrate) Pfizer 2739
Zithromax Tablets, 250 mg (Azithromycin Dihydrate) Pfizer 2739
Zithromax Tablets, 600 mg (Azithromycin Dihydrate) Pfizer 2743

Tooth, hypersensitivity of
Sensodyne Original Flavor (Potassium Nitrate, Sodium Fluoride) Block .... ■623
Sensodyne Cool Gel (Potassium Nitrate, Sodium Fluoride) Block .... ■623
Sensodyne Extra Whitening (Potassium Nitrate, Sodium Monofluorophosphate) Block .... ■623
Sensodyne Fresh Mint (Potassium Nitrate, Sodium Fluoride) Block .... ■623
Sensodyne Tartar Control (Potassium Nitrate, Sodium Fluoride) Block .... ■623
Sensodyne Tartar Control Plus Whitening (Potassium Nitrate, Sodium Fluoride) Block .... ■623
Sensodyne with Baking Soda (Potassium Nitrate, Sodium Fluoride) Block .... ■623

Torulosis
(*see under* Cryptococcosis)

Tourette, Gilles de la, syndrome
Haldol Injection, Tablets and Concentrate (Haloperidol) Ortho-McNeil 2533
Orap Tablets (Pimozide) Gate 1407

Toxicity, drug, unspecified
Liqui-Char Activated Charcoal Jones 1823

Toxoplasmosis, adjunctive therapy in
Daraprim Tablets (Pyrimethamine) GlaxoSmithKline 1511

Trachoma
Declomycin Tablets (Demeclocycline Hydrochloride) Lederle 1855
Doryx Coated Pellet Filled Capsules (Doxycycline Hyclate) Warner Chilcott 3357
Dynacin Capsules (Minocycline Hydrochloride) Medicis 2019
Minocin Intravenous (Minocycline Hydrochloride) Lederle 1862
Minocin Oral Suspension (Minocycline Hydrochloride) Lederle 1865
Minocin Pellet-Filled Capsules (Minocycline Hydrochloride) Lederle 1863
Monodox Capsules (Doxycycline Monohydrate) Oclassen 2442
Vibramycin Calcium Oral Suspension Syrup (Doxycycline Calcium) Pfizer 2735
Vibramycin Hyclate Capsules (Doxycycline Hyclate) Pfizer 2735
Vibramycin Hyclate Intravenous (Doxycycline Hyclate) Pfizer 2737
Vibramycin Monohydrate for Oral Suspension (Doxycycline Monohydrate) Pfizer 2735
Vibra-Tabs Film Coated Tablets (Doxycycline Hyclate) Pfizer 2735

Trachoma, adjunct in
Bleph-10 (Sulfacetamide Sodium) Allergan .... ⊙230

Tremor, essential
Inderal (Propranolol Hydrochloride) Wyeth-Ayerst 3513

Treponema pallidum
(*see under* T. pallidum infections)

Treponema pertenue infections
(*see under* Yaws)

Trichinosis
Mintezol (Thiabendazole) Merck 2137

Trichinosis with myocardial involvement
Celestone Soluspan Injectable Suspension (Betamethasone Acetate, Betamethasone Sodium Phosphate) Schering 3097
Celestone Syrup (Betamethasone) Schering 3099
Cortone Acetate Injectable Suspension (Cortisone Acetate) Merck 2059
Cortone Acetate Tablets (Cortisone Acetate) Merck 2061
Decadron Elixir (Dexamethasone) Merck 2078
Decadron Tablets (Dexamethasone) Merck 2079
Decadron Phosphate Injection (Dexamethasone Sodium Phosphate) Merck 2081
Depo-Medrol Injectable Suspension (Methylprednisolone Acetate) Pharmacia & Upjohn 2795
Hydrocortone Tablets (Hydrocortisone) Merck 2106
Hydrocortone Phosphate Injection, Sterile (Hydrocortisone Sodium Phosphate) Merck 2105
Pediapred Oral Solution (Prednisolone Sodium Phosphate) Celltech 1170
Prednisone (Prednisone) Roxane 3064
Prelone Syrup (Prednisolone) Muro 2273
Solu-Medrol Sterile Powder (Methylprednisolone Sodium Succinate) Pharmacia & Upjohn 2855

Trichinosis with neurologic involvement
Celestone Soluspan Injectable Suspension (Betamethasone Acetate, Betamethasone Sodium Phosphate) Schering 3097
Celestone Syrup (Betamethasone) Schering 3099
Cortone Acetate Injectable Suspension (Cortisone Acetate) Merck 2059
Cortone Acetate Tablets (Cortisone Acetate) Merck 2061
Decadron Elixir (Dexamethasone) Merck 2078
Decadron Tablets (Dexamethasone) Merck 2079
Decadron Phosphate Injection (Dexamethasone Sodium Phosphate) Merck 2081
Depo-Medrol Injectable Suspension (Methylprednisolone Acetate) Pharmacia & Upjohn 2795
Hydrocortone Tablets (Hydrocortisone) Merck 2106
Hydrocortone Phosphate Injection, Sterile (Hydrocortisone Sodium Phosphate) Merck 2105
Pediapred Oral Solution (Prednisolone Sodium Phosphate) Celltech 1170
Prednisone (Prednisone) Roxane 3064
Prelone Syrup (Prednisolone) Muro 2273
Solu-Medrol Sterile Powder (Methylprednisolone Sodium Succinate) Pharmacia & Upjohn 2855

Trichophyton crateriform infections
Grifulvin V Tablets Microsize and Oral Suspension Microsize (Griseofulvin) Ortho Dermatological 2518
Gris-PEG Tablets (Griseofulvin) Pedinol 2661

Trichophyton gallinae infections
Grifulvin V Tablets Microsize and Oral Suspension Microsize (Griseofulvin) Ortho Dermatological 2518
Gris-PEG Tablets (Griseofulvin) Pedinol 2661

Trichophyton interdigitalis infections
Grifulvin V Tablets Microsize and Oral Suspension Microsize (Griseofulvin) Ortho Dermatological 2518
Gris-PEG Tablets (Griseofulvin) Pedinol 2661

Trichophyton megnini infections
Grifulvin V Tablets Microsize and Oral Suspension Microsize (Griseofulvin) Ortho Dermatological 2518
Gris-PEG Tablets (Griseofulvin) Pedinol 2661

Trichophyton mentagrophytes infections
Grifulvin V Tablets Microsize and Oral Suspension Microsize (Griseofulvin) Ortho Dermatological 2518
Gris-PEG Tablets (Griseofulvin) Pedinol 2661
Loprox Cream (Ciclopirox Olamine) Medicis 2021
Loprox Gel (Ciclopirox) Medicis 2022
Loprox Lotion (Ciclopirox Olamine) Medicis 2021
Lotrimin (Clotrimazole) Schering 3128
Lotrisone (Betamethasone Dipropionate, Clotrimazole) Schering 3129
Mentax Cream (Butenafine Hydrochloride) Bertek 1009
Naftin Cream (Naftifine Hydrochloride) Merz 2224
Naftin Gel (Naftifine Hydrochloride) Merz 2224
Nizoral 2% Cream (Ketoconazole) Janssen 3620
Oxistat (Oxiconazole Nitrate) Elan 1298

Trichophyton rubrum infections
Grifulvin V Tablets Microsize and Oral Suspension Microsize (Griseofulvin) Ortho Dermatological 2518
Gris-PEG Tablets (Griseofulvin) Pedinol 2661
Loprox Cream (Ciclopirox Olamine) Medicis 2021
Loprox Gel (Ciclopirox) Medicis 2022
Loprox Lotion (Ciclopirox Olamine) Medicis 2021
Lotrimin (Clotrimazole) Schering 3128
Lotrisone (Betamethasone Dipropionate, Clotrimazole) Schering 3129
Mentax Cream (Butenafine Hydrochloride) Bertek 1009
Naftin Cream (Naftifine Hydrochloride) Merz 2224
Naftin Gel (Naftifine Hydrochloride) Merz 2224
Nizoral 2% Cream (Ketoconazole) Janssen 3620
Oxistat (Oxiconazole Nitrate) Elan 1298
Penlac Nail Lacquer, Topical Solution (Ciclopirox) Dermik 1225

Trichophyton schoenleini infections
Grifulvin V Tablets Microsize and Oral Suspension Microsize (Griseofulvin) Ortho Dermatological 2518
Gris-PEG Tablets (Griseofulvin) Pedinol 2661

Trichophyton sulfureum infections
Grifulvin V Tablets Microsize and Oral Suspension Microsize (Griseofulvin) Ortho Dermatological 2518
Gris-PEG Tablets (Griseofulvin) Pedinol 2661

Trichophyton tonsurans infections
Grifulvin V Tablets Microsize and Oral Suspension Microsize (Griseofulvin) Ortho Dermatological 2518
Gris-PEG Tablets (Griseofulvin) Pedinol 2661
Mentax Cream (Butenafine Hydrochloride) Bertek 1009
Naftin Gel (Naftifine Hydrochloride) Merz 2224

Trichophyton verrucosum infections
Grifulvin V Tablets Microsize and Oral Suspension Microsize (Griseofulvin) Ortho Dermatological 2518
Gris-PEG Tablets (Griseofulvin) Pedinol 2661

Trichuriasis, as secondary therapy
Mintezol (Thiabendazole) Merck 2137

Trichuris trichiura infections
Vermox Chewable Tablets (Mebendazole) McNeil Consumer 2017

Triglyceride levels, elevated
(*see under* Hypertriglyceridemia, adjunct to diet)

Trigonitis
Urised Tablets (Atropine Sulfate, Benzoic Acid, Hyoscyamine, Methenamine, Methylene Blue, Phenyl Salicylate) PolyMedica 2876

Tuberculin-sensitivity, detection of
Tine Test, Tuberculin, Old (Tuberculin, Old) Lederle 3631

Tuberculosis, diagnostic aid in
Tubersol Diagnostic Antigen (Tuberculin, Purified Protein Derivative For Mantoux Test) Aventis Pasteur 3628

Tuberculosis, pulmonary
Myambutol Tablets (Ethambutol Hydrochloride) Elan 1290
Priftin Tablets (Rifapentine) Aventis 758
Rifadin (Rifampin) Aventis 765
Rifamate Capsules (Isoniazid, Rifampin) Aventis 767
Rifater Tablets (Isoniazid, Pyrazinamide, Rifampin) Aventis 769
Streptomycin Sulfate Injection (Streptomycin Sulfate) Pfizer 2714

Tuberculosis, pulmonary, disseminated
Celestone Soluspan Injectable Suspension (Betamethasone Acetate, Betamethasone Sodium Phosphate) Schering 3097
Celestone Syrup (Betamethasone) Schering 3099
Cortone Acetate Injectable Suspension (Cortisone Acetate) Merck 2059
Cortone Acetate Tablets (Cortisone Acetate) Merck 2061
Decadron Elixir (Dexamethasone) Merck 2078
Decadron Tablets (Dexamethasone) Merck 2079
Decadron Phosphate Injection (Dexamethasone Sodium Phosphate) Merck 2081
Depo-Medrol Injectable Suspension (Methylprednisolone Acetate) Pharmacia & Upjohn 2795
Hydrocortone Tablets (Hydrocortisone) Merck 2106
Hydrocortone Phosphate Injection, Sterile (Hydrocortisone Sodium Phosphate) Merck 2105
Pediapred Oral Solution (Prednisolone Sodium Phosphate) Celltech 1170
Prednisone (Prednisone) Roxane 3064
Prelone Syrup (Prednisolone) Muro 2273
Solu-Medrol Sterile Powder (Methylprednisolone Sodium Succinate) Pharmacia & Upjohn 2855

Tuberculosis, pulmonary, fulminating
Celestone Soluspan Injectable Suspension (Betamethasone Acetate, Betamethasone Sodium Phosphate) Schering 3097
Celestone Syrup (Betamethasone) Schering 3099
Cortone Acetate Injectable Suspension (Cortisone Acetate) Merck 2059
Cortone Acetate Tablets (Cortisone Acetate) Merck 2061
Decadron Elixir (Dexamethasone) Merck 2078
Decadron Tablets (Dexamethasone) Merck 2079
Decadron Phosphate Injection (Dexamethasone Sodium Phosphate) Merck 2081
Depo-Medrol Injectable Suspension (Methylprednisolone Acetate) Pharmacia & Upjohn 2795
Hydrocortone Tablets (Hydrocortisone) Merck 2106
Hydrocortone Phosphate Injection, Sterile (Hydrocortisone Sodium Phosphate) Merck 2105
Pediapred Oral Solution (Prednisolone Sodium Phosphate) Celltech 1170
Prednisone (Prednisone) Roxane 3064
Prelone Syrup (Prednisolone) Muro 2273
Solu-Medrol Sterile Powder (Methylprednisolone Sodium Succinate) Pharmacia & Upjohn 2855

Tuberculosis, pulmonary, prophylaxis of
Tice BCG, BCG Live (BCG Vaccine) Organon 2489

Tuberculosis, treatment
Myambutol Tablets (Ethambutol Hydrochloride) Elan 1290

Priftin Tablets (Rifapentine) Aventis .. 758
Pyrazinamide Tablets (Pyrazinamide) Lederle 1876
Rifadin (Rifampin) Aventis 765
Rifamate Capsules (Isoniazid, Rifampin) Aventis 767
Streptomycin Sulfate Injection (Streptomycin Sulfate) Pfizer 2714
Trecator-SC Tablets (Ethionamide) Wyeth-Ayerst 3598

Tuberculosis, treatment adjunct
Paser Granules (Aminosalicylic Acid) Jacobus 1781
Pyrazinamide Tablets (Pyrazinamide) Lederle 1876

Tuberculosis meningitis, adjunctive therapy in
(*see under* Meningitis, tuberculous)

Tularemia
Doryx Coated Pellet Filled Capsules (Doxycycline Hyclate) Warner Chilcott 3357
Dynacin Capsules (Minocycline Hydrochloride) Medicis 2019
Minocin Oral Suspension (Minocycline Hydrochloride) Lederle 1865
Minocin Pellet-Filled Capsules (Minocycline Hydrochloride) Lederle 1863
Monodox Capsules (Doxycycline Monohydrate) Oclassen 2442
Vibramycin Hyclate Capsules (Doxycycline Hyclate) Pfizer 2735

Tumors, benign epithelial
(*see under* Warts, common, removal of; Warts, plantar, removal of)

Tumors, carcinoid, symptomatic relief of
Sandostatin Injection Novartis 2394
Sandostatin LAR Depot (Octreotide Acetate) Novartis 2395

Turner's syndrome
Humatrope Vials and Cartridges (Somatropin) Lilly 1930
Nutropin AQ Injection (Somatropin) Genentech 1420
Nutropin for Injection (Somatropin) Genentech 1417

Typhoid fever
Cipro (Ciprofloxacin) Bayer 887

Typhus fever
Declomycin Tablets (Demeclocycline Hydrochloride) Lederle 1855
Doryx Coated Pellet Filled Capsules (Doxycycline Hyclate) Warner Chilcott 3357
Dynacin Capsules (Minocycline Hydrochloride) Medicis 2019
Minocin Intravenous (Minocycline Hydrochloride) Lederle 1862
Minocin Oral Suspension (Minocycline Hydrochloride) Lederle 1865
Minocin Pellet-Filled Capsules (Minocycline Hydrochloride) Lederle 1863
Monodox Capsules (Doxycycline Monohydrate) Oclassen 2442
Vibramycin Calcium Oral Suspension Syrup (Doxycycline Calcium) Pfizer 2735
Vibramycin Hyclate Capsules (Doxycycline Hyclate) Pfizer 2735
Vibramycin Hyclate Intravenous (Doxycycline Hyclate) Pfizer 2737
Vibramycin Monohydrate for Oral Suspension (Doxycycline Monohydrate) Pfizer 2735
Vibra-Tabs Film Coated Tablets (Doxycycline Hyclate) Pfizer 2735

Typhus group infection
Declomycin Tablets (Demeclocycline Hydrochloride) Lederle 1855
Doryx Coated Pellet Filled Capsules (Doxycycline Hyclate) Warner Chilcott 3357
Dynacin Capsules (Minocycline Hydrochloride) Medicis 2019
Minocin Intravenous (Minocycline Hydrochloride) Lederle 1862
Minocin Oral Suspension (Minocycline Hydrochloride) Lederle 1865
Minocin Pellet-Filled Capsules (Minocycline Hydrochloride) Lederle 1863
Monodox Capsules (Doxycycline Monohydrate) Oclassen 2442
Vibramycin Hyclate Capsules (Doxycycline Hyclate) Pfizer 2735
Vibramycin Hyclate Intravenous (Doxycycline Hyclate) Pfizer 2737

U

Ulcerative colitis
(*see under* Colitis, ulcerative)

Ulcers, decubitus, adjunctive therapy in
Granulex Aerosol (Balsam Peru, Castor Oil, Trypsin) Bertek 1007
Panafil Ointment (Chlorophyllin Copper Complex Sodium, Papain, Urea) Healthpoint 1726

Ulcers, decubitus, reduction of possible occurrence of
Betadine Solution (Povidone Iodine) Purdue Frederick 2895

Ulcers, dermal
Primaxin I.M. (Cilastatin Sodium, Imipenem) Merck 2158

Ulcers, diabetic, adjunctive therapy in
Accuzyme Debriding Ointment (Papain, Urea) Healthpoint 1725
Panafil Ointment (Chlorophyllin Copper Complex Sodium, Papain, Urea) Healthpoint 1726

Ulcers, diabetic neuropathic
Apligraf (Graftskin) Novartis 2305
Regranex Gel (Becaplermin) Ortho-McNeil 2586

Ulcers, varicose, adjunctive therapy in
Accuzyme Debriding Ointment (Papain, Urea) Healthpoint 1725
Panafil Ointment (Chlorophyllin Copper Complex Sodium, Papain, Urea) Healthpoint 1726

Uncinariasis, as secondary therapy
Mintezol (Thiabendazole) Merck 2137

Ureaplasma urealyticum urethritis
E.E.S. Granules (Erythromycin Ethylsuccinate) Abbott 450
Minocin Oral Suspension (Minocycline Hydrochloride) Lederle 1865

Ureaplasma urealyticum urethritis, nongonococcal
Doryx Coated Pellet Filled Capsules (Doxycycline Hyclate) Warner Chilcott 3357
Dynacin Capsules (Minocycline Hydrochloride) Medicis 2019
E.E.S. (Erythromycin Ethylsuccinate) Abbott 450
EryPed (Erythromycin Ethylsuccinate) Abbott 446
Minocin Oral Suspension (Minocycline Hydrochloride) Lederle 1865
Minocin Pellet-Filled Capsules (Minocycline Hydrochloride) Lederle 1863
Monodox Capsules (Doxycycline Monohydrate) Oclassen 2442
PCE Dispertab Tablets (Erythromycin) Abbott 498
Vibramycin Calcium Oral Suspension Syrup (Doxycycline Calcium) Pfizer 2735
Vibramycin Hyclate Capsules (Doxycycline Hyclate) Pfizer 2735
Vibramycin Monohydrate for Oral Suspension (Doxycycline Monohydrate) Pfizer 2735
Vibra-Tabs Film Coated Tablets (Doxycycline Hyclate) Pfizer 2735

Urethritis
E.E.S. Granules (Erythromycin Ethylsuccinate) Abbott 450
Urised Tablets (Atropine Sulfate, Benzoic Acid, Hyoscyamine, Methenamine, Methylene Blue, Phenyl Salicylate) PolyMedica 2876
Zithromax (Azithromycin Dihydrate) Pfizer 2743
Zithromax for Oral Suspension, 300 mg, 600 mg, 900 mg, 1200 mg (Azithromycin Dihydrate) Pfizer 2739
Zithromax Tablets, 250 mg (Azithromycin Dihydrate) Pfizer 2739
Zithromax Tablets, 600 mg (Azithromycin Dihydrate) Pfizer 2743

Urethritis, atrophic
Estrace Tablets (Estradiol) Warner Chilcott 3361
Premarin Tablets (Estrogens, Conjugated) Wyeth-Ayerst 3566

Urethritis, Chlamydia trachomatis, nongonococcal
Doryx Coated Pellet Filled Capsules (Doxycycline Hyclate) Warner Chilcott 3357
Floxin I.V. (Ofloxacin) Ortho-McNeil .. 2526
Monodox Capsules (Doxycycline Monohydrate) Oclassen 2442
Vibramycin Calcium Oral Suspension Syrup (Doxycycline Calcium) Pfizer 2735
Vibramycin Hyclate Capsules (Doxycycline Hyclate) Pfizer 2735
Vibramycin Monohydrate for Oral Suspension (Doxycycline Monohydrate) Pfizer 2735
Vibra-Tabs Film Coated Tablets (Doxycycline Hyclate) Pfizer 2735
Zithromax (Azithromycin Dihydrate) Pfizer 2743

Urethritis, lacking substantial evidence of effectiveness in
Urobiotic-250 Capsules (Oxytetracycline Hydrochloride, Phenazopyridine Hydrochloride, Sulfamethizole) Pfizer 2731

Urethritis, nongonococcal
E.E.S. (Erythromycin Ethylsuccinate) Abbott 450
EryPed (Erythromycin Ethylsuccinate) Abbott 446
PCE Dispertab Tablets (Erythromycin) Abbott 498

Urethritis, uncomplicated gonococcal
Dynacin Capsules (Minocycline Hydrochloride) Medicis 2019
Minocin Oral Suspension (Minocycline Hydrochloride) Lederle 1865
Minocin Pellet-Filled Capsules (Minocycline Hydrochloride) Lederle 1863
Pipracil (Piperacillin Sodium) Lederle 1866

Uric acid lithiasis
(*see under* Urolithiasis, management of)

Urinary bladder, overactive
Detrol Tablets (Tolterodine Tartrate) Pharmacia & Upjohn ....
Detrol LA Capsules (Tolterodine Tartrate) Pharmacia & Upjohn 2801
Ditropan XL Extended Release Tablets (Oxybutynin Chloride) Alza 564

Urinary bladder with retention, neurogenic atony of
Urecholine (Bethanechol Chloride) Merck 2198
Urecholine Tablets (Bethanechol Chloride) Odyssey 2445

Urinary retention, acute postoperative
Prostigmin Injectable (Neostigmine Methylsulfate) ICN 1744
Urecholine (Bethanechol Chloride) Merck 2198
Urecholine Tablets (Bethanechol Chloride) Odyssey 2445

Urinary retention, postpartum nonobstructive
Urecholine (Bethanechol Chloride) Merck 2198
Urecholine Tablets (Bethanechol Chloride) Odyssey 2445

Urinary tract, hypermotility, control of symptoms
Levsin/Levsinex/Levbid (Hyoscyamine Sulfate) Schwarz 3172
NuLev Orally Disintegrating Tablets (Hyoscyamine Sulfate) Schwarz 3176
Prosed/DS (Atropine Sulfate, Benzoic Acid, Hyoscyamine Sulfate, Methenamine, Methylene Blue, Phenyl Salicylate) Star 3268

Urinary tract, lower, hypermotility disorders
Urimax Tablets (Belladonna Alkaloids, Hyoscyamine Sulfate, Methenamine, Methylene Blue, Phenyl Salicylate, Sodium Biphosphate) Integrity Pharmaceutical 1769
Urised Tablets (Atropine Sulfate, Benzoic Acid, Hyoscyamine, Methenamine, Methylene Blue, Phenyl Salicylate) PolyMedica 2876

Urinary tract pain, relief of
(*see under* Pain, urinary tract)

Urine, acidification of
K-Phos Original (Sodium Free) Tablets (Potassium Acid Phosphate) Beach 947

Urolithiasis, management of
Urocit-K Tablets (Potassium Citrate) Mission 2232

Urticaria, chronic
(*see also under* Urticarial manifestations, relief of)
Allegra (Fexofenadine Hydrochloride) Aventis 712
Atarax Tablets & Syrup (Hydroxyzine Hydrochloride) Pfizer 2667
Claritin (Loratadine) Schering 3100
Vistaril (Hydroxyzine Pamoate) Pfizer 2738
Zyrtec (Cetirizine Hydrochloride) Pfizer 2756

Urticaria, cold
Periactin Tablets (Cyproheptadine Hydrochloride) Merck 2155

Urticarial manifestations, relief of
(*see also under* Urticaria, chronic)
Extendryl (Chlorpheniramine Maleate, Methscopolamine Nitrate, Phenylephrine Hydrochloride) Fleming 1361
Periactin Tablets (Cyproheptadine Hydrochloride) Merck 2155
Phenergan Suppositories (Promethazine Hydrochloride) Wyeth-Ayerst 3556
Phenergan Syrup (Promethazine Hydrochloride) Wyeth-Ayerst 3554
Phenergan Tablets (Promethazine Hydrochloride) Wyeth-Ayerst 3556
Vistaril Intramuscular Solution (Hydroxyzine Hydrochloride) Pfizer 2738

Urticarial transfusion reactions
Celestone Soluspan Injectable Suspension (Betamethasone Acetate, Betamethasone Sodium Phosphate) Schering 3097
Cortone Acetate Injectable Suspension (Cortisone Acetate) Merck 2059
Decadron Phosphate Injection (Dexamethasone Sodium Phosphate) Merck 2081
Hydrocortone Phosphate Injection, Sterile (Hydrocortisone Sodium Phosphate) Merck 2105
Solu-Medrol Sterile Powder (Methylprednisolone Sodium Succinate) Pharmacia & Upjohn 2855

Uterine bleeding, abnormal
Aygestin Tablets (Norethindrone Acetate) ESI Lederle 1333
Climara Transdermal System (Estradiol) Berlex 958
Premarin Intravenous (Estrogens, Conjugated) Wyeth-Ayerst 3563
Provera Tablets (Medroxyprogesterone Acetate) Pharmacia & Upjohn 2853

Uterine contents, evacuation of
Prostin E2 Suppositories (Dinoprostone) Pharmacia & Upjohn 2852

Uveitis, chronic anterior, steroid-responsive
Blephamide Ophthalmic Ointment (Prednisolone Acetate, Sulfacetamide Sodium) Allergan 547
Blephamide Ophthalmic Suspension (Prednisolone Acetate, Sulfacetamide Sodium) Allergan 548
Cortisporin Ophthalmic Suspension (Hydrocortisone, Neomycin Sulfate, Polymyxin B Sulfate, Hydrocortisone, Neomycin Sulfate, Polymyxin B Sulfate) Monarch .... ⊙ 297
FML-S Liquifilm Sterile Ophthalmic Suspension (Fluorometholone, Sulfacetamide Sodium) Allergan .. ⊙ 238
NeoDecadron Sterile Ophthalmic Solution (Dexamethasone Sodium Phosphate, Neomycin Sulfate) Merck 2144
Poly-Pred Liquifilm Ophthalmic Suspension (Neomycin Sulfate, Polymyxin B Sulfate, Prednisolone Acetate) Allergan .... ⊙ 245
Pred-G Ophthalmic Suspension (Gentamicin Sulfate, Prednisolone Acetate) Allergan .... ⊙ 247

Pred-G Sterile Ophthalmic Ointment (Gentamicin Sulfate, Prednisolone Acetate) Allergan.... ⊙248
Terra-Cortril Ophthalmic Suspension (Hydrocortisone Acetate, Oxytetracycline Hydrochloride) Pfizer 2716
TobraDex Ophthalmic Ointment (Dexamethasone, Tobramycin) Alcon.......... 542
TobraDex Ophthalmic Suspension (Dexamethasone, Tobramycin) Alcon.......... 541
Vexol 1% Ophthalmic Suspension (Rimexolone) Alcon .... ⊙222

Uveitis, diffuse posterior
Celestone Soluspan Injectable Suspension (Betamethasone Acetate, Betamethasone Sodium Phosphate) Schering.......... 3097
Celestone Syrup (Betamethasone) Schering 3099
Cortone Acetate Injectable Suspension (Cortisone Acetate) Merck 2059
Cortone Acetate Tablets (Cortisone Acetate) Merck 2061
Decadron Elixir (Dexamethasone) Merck 2078
Decadron Tablets (Dexamethasone) Merck 2079
Decadron Phosphate Injection (Dexamethasone Sodium Phosphate) Merck 2081
Depo-Medrol Injectable Suspension (Methylprednisolone Acetate) Pharmacia & Upjohn 2795
Hydrocortone Tablets (Hydrocortisone) Merck 2106
Hydrocortone Phosphate Injection, Sterile (Hydrocortisone Sodium Phosphate) Merck 2105
Pediapred Oral Solution (Prednisolone Sodium Phosphate) Celltech 1170
Prednisone (Prednisone) Roxane 3064
Prelone Syrup (Prednisolone) Muro 2273
Solu-Medrol Sterile Powder (Methylprednisolone Sodium Succinate) Pharmacia & Upjohn 2855

V

Vagina, cleansing of
Massengill Feminine Cleansing Wash (Cleanser) SmithKline Beecham Consumer .... ▣753
Massengill Disposable Douches (Vinegar) SmithKline Beecham Consumer .... ▣752

Vaginal acidity, restoration of, adjunctive therapy for
Aci-Jel Therapeutic Vaginal Jelly (Acetic Acid, Oxyquinoline Sulfate) Ortho-McNeil 2525

Vaginal and anogenital areas, external, cleansing of
Betadine Medicated Douche (Povidone Iodine) Purdue Frederick 2894
Betadine Solution (Povidone Iodine) Purdue Frederick 2895
Massengill Baby Powder Scent Soft Cloth Towelette (Lactic Acid, Potassium Sorbate, Sodium Lactate) SmithKline Beecham Consumer .... ▣753
Preparation H Medicated Wipes (Witch Hazel) Whitehall-Robins .... ▣779
Tucks Pre-moistened Pads (Witch Hazel) Pfizer Inc., Warner-Lambert Healthcare .... ▣713

Vaginal atrophy
Activella Tablets (Estradiol, Norethindrone Acetate) Pharmacia & Upjohn 2764
Alora Transdermal System (Estradiol) Watson 3372
Esclim Transdermal System (Estradiol) Women First 3460
Ortho-Prefest Tablets (Estradiol, Norgestimate) Ortho-McNeil 2570
Premphase Tablets (Estrogens, Conjugated, Medroxyprogesterone Acetate) Wyeth-Ayerst 3572
Prempro Tablets (Estrogens, Conjugated, Medroxyprogesterone Acetate) Wyeth-Ayerst 3572
Vivelle Transdermal System (Estradiol) Novartis 2412
Vivelle-Dot Transdermal System (Estradiol) Novartis 2416

Vaginitis
(*see under* Vaginosis, bacterial)

Vaginitis, atrophic
Climara Transdermal System (Estradiol) Berlex 958
CombiPatch Transdermal System (Estradiol, Norethindrone Acetate) Novartis 2323
Estrace Vaginal Cream (Estradiol) Warner Chilcott 3358
Estrace Tablets (Estradiol) Warner Chilcott 3361
Estring Vaginal Ring (Estradiol) Pharmacia & Upjohn 2811
Menest Tablets (Estrogens, Esterified) Monarch 2254
Ogen Tablets (Estropipate) Pharmacia & Upjohn 2846
Ortho Dienestrol Cream (Dienestrol) Ortho-McNeil 2554
Ortho-Est Tablets (Estropipate) Women First 3464
Premarin Tablets (Estrogens, Conjugated) Wyeth-Ayerst 3566
Premarin Vaginal Cream (Estrogens, Conjugated) Wyeth-Ayerst 3570
Vagifem Tablets (Estradiol) Pharmacia & Upjohn 2857

Vaginitis, symptomatic relief of irritation and itching
Betadine Medicated Douche (Povidone Iodine) Purdue Frederick 2894
Massengill Medicated Disposable Douche (Povidone Iodine) SmithKline Beecham Consumer .... ▣753
Massengill Medicated Soft Cloth Towelette (Hydrocortisone) SmithKline Beecham Consumer .... ▣753

Vaginosis, bacterial
Cleocin Vaginal Cream (Clindamycin Phosphate) Pharmacia & Upjohn 2788
Cleocin Vaginal Ovules (Clindamycin Phosphate) Pharmacia & Upjohn 2789
MetroGel-Vaginal Gel (Metronidazole) 3M 1986
Sultrin Triple Sulfa Cream (Sulfabenzamide, Sulfacetamide, Sulfathiazole) Ortho-McNeil 2587

Varicella, acute, treatment of
Zovirax (Acyclovir) GlaxoSmithKline 1706

Varicella, prevention or modification of
BayGam (Globulin, Immune (Human)) Bayer Biological 914

Vasopressin-sensitive diabetes insipidus
(*see under* Diabetes insipidus)

Ventilation, mechanical, facilitation of
Anectine Injection (Succinylcholine Chloride) GlaxoSmithKline 1476
Norcuron for Injection (Vecuronium Bromide) Organon 2478
Zemuron Injection (Rocuronium Bromide) Organon 2491

Ventricular arrhythmias
(*see under* Arrhythmias, ventricular)

Ventricular dysfunction, left, asymptomatic
(*see also under* Myocardial infarction, post, left ventricular dysfunction)
Vasotec Tablets (Enalapril Maleate) Merck 2210

Ventricular extrasystoles, premature
Inderal (Propranolol Hydrochloride) Wyeth-Ayerst 3513

Ventricular fibrillation
Cordarone Intravenous (Amiodarone Hydrochloride) Wyeth-Ayerst 3491
Cordarone Tablets (Amiodarone Hydrochloride) Wyeth-Ayerst 3487
Pacerone Tablets (Amiodarone Hydrochloride) Upsher-Smith 3331

Ventricular tachycardia, sustained
(*see under* Tachycardia, ventricular, sustained)

Ventriculitis
(*see also under* Infections, central nervous system)
Claforan Injection (Cefotaxime Sodium) Aventis 732

Verrucae plantaris
(*see under* Warts, plantar, removal of)

Verrucae vulgaris infection
(*see under* Warts, common, removal of)

Vertigo, possibly effective in
Antivert, Antivert/25, & Antivert/50 Tablets (Meclizine Hydrochloride) Pfizer 2664

Vibrio cholerae infections
Declomycin Tablets (Demeclocycline Hydrochloride) Lederle 1855
Doryx Coated Pellet Filled Capsules (Doxycycline Hyclate) Warner Chilcott.......... 3357
Dynacin Capsules (Minocycline Hydrochloride) Medicis 2019
Minocin Intravenous (Minocycline Hydrochloride) Lederle.......... 1862
Minocin Oral Suspension (Minocycline Hydrochloride) Lederle 1865
Minocin Pellet-Filled Capsules (Minocycline Hydrochloride) Lederle 1863
Monodox Capsules (Doxycycline Monohydrate) Oclassen 2442
Vibramycin Calcium Oral Suspension Syrup (Doxycycline Calcium) Pfizer 2735
Vibramycin Hyclate Capsules (Doxycycline Hyclate) Pfizer 2735
Vibramycin Hyclate Intravenous (Doxycycline Hyclate) Pfizer 2737
Vibramycin Monohydrate for Oral Suspension (Doxycycline Monohydrate) Pfizer 2735
Vibra-Tabs Film Coated Tablets (Doxycycline Hyclate) Pfizer 2735

Vibrio comma
(*see under* Vibrio cholerae infections)

Vibrio fetus infections
(*see under* Campylobacter fetus infections)

Vincent's gingivitis
(*see under* Fusospirochetosis)

Vincent's infection
(*see under* Fusospirochetosis)

Vincent's pharyngitis
(*see under* Fusospirochetosis)

VIPomas diarrhea
(*see under* Diarrhea associated with vasoactive intestinal peptide tumors)

Vitamin, multiple, deficiency of
Hep-Forte Capsules (Vitamins with Minerals) Marlyn 1997
Mega Antioxidant Tablets (Vitamins, Multiple) USANA 3335

Vitamin A, deficiency of
Aquasol A Parenteral (Vitamin A) AstraZeneca LP 593

Vitamin and mineral, multiple, deficiency of
Bugs Bunny Children's Multivitamin Plus Extra C Chewable Tablets (Sugar Free) (Vitamins with Minerals) Bayer Consumer .... ▣804
Bugs Bunny Children's Multivitamin Plus Iron Chewable Tablets (Vitamins with Iron) Bayer Consumer .... ▣802
Bugs Bunny Complete Children's Multivitamin/Multimineral Chewable Tablets (Sugar Free) (Vitamins with Minerals) Bayer Consumer .... ▣803
Centrum Kids Complete Children's Chewables (Vitamins with Minerals) Lederle Consumer .... ▣817
Centrum Performance Multivitamin-Multimineral Tablets (Vitamins with Minerals) Lederle Consumer .... ▣817
Centrum Tablets (Vitamins with Minerals) Lederle Consumer .... ▣815
Centrum Silver Tablets (Vitamins with Minerals) Lederle Consumer .... ▣818
Flintstones Original Children's Multivitamin Chewable Tablets (Vitamins, Multiple) Bayer Consumer .... ▣802
Flintstones Children's Multivitamin Plus Calcium Chewable Tablets (Vitamins with Minerals) Bayer Consumer .... ▣804
Flintstones Children's Multivitamin Plus Extra C Chewable Tablets (Vitamins, Multiple) Bayer Consumer .... ▣804
Flintstones Children's Multivitamin Plus Iron Chewable Tablets (Vitamins with Iron) Bayer Consumer .... ▣802
Flintstones Complete Children's Mutivitamin/Multimineral Chewable Tablets (Vitamins with Minerals) Bayer Consumer .... ▣803
May-Vita Elixir (Vitamins with Minerals) Merz 2224
MDR Fitness Tabs for Men and Women (Vitamins with Minerals) MDR 2018
Megadose Tablets (Vitamins with Minerals) Arco 593
Ocuvite Lutein Vitamin and Mineral Supplement (Vitamins with Minerals) Bausch & Lomb .... ⊙263
Ocuvite Vitamin and Mineral Supplement (Vitamins with Minerals) Bausch & Lomb .... ⊙263
Ocuvite Extra Vitamin and Mineral Supplement (Vitamins with Minerals) Bausch & Lomb .... ⊙263
One-A-Day Essential Tablets (Vitamins with Minerals) Bayer Consumer .... ▣806
One-A-Day 50 Plus Tablets (Vitamins with Minerals) Bayer Consumer .... ▣804
One-A-Day Kids Complete Tablets (Vitamins with Minerals) Bayer Consumer .... ▣806
One-A-Day Maximum Tablets (Vitamins with Minerals) Bayer Consumer .... ▣807
One-A-Day Women's Tablets (Vitamins with Minerals) Bayer Consumer .... ▣809
Vitasana Gelcaps (Herbals with Vitamins & Minerals, Ginseng) Pharmaton .... ▣834

Vitamin B complex, deficiency of
Eldertonic (Vitamins with Minerals) Merz 2223
Mega-B Tablets (Vitamin B Complex) Arco 592

Vitamin B complex and C, deficiency of
Nephrocaps (Vitamins, Multiple) Fleming 1362

Vitamin B12, deficiency of
Nascobal Gel (Vitamin B[12]) Schwarz 3174

Vitamin C, deficiency of
Halls Defense Drops (Vitamin C) Pfizer Inc., Warner-Lambert Group .... ▣687

Vitamin deficiency, postpartum
New Formulation Chromagen OB Capsules (Ferrous Fumarate, Vitamins with Minerals, Vitamins, Prenatal) Savage 3094
Citracal Prenatal Rx Tablets (Vitamins, Prenatal) Mission 2231
Materna Tablets (Vitamins with Minerals, Vitamins, Prenatal) Lederle 1862
NataChew Tablets (Ferrous Fumarate, Vitamins with Iron, Vitamins, Prenatal) Warner Chilcott 3364
Nestabs RX Tablets (Vitamins with Minerals, Vitamins, Prenatal) Fielding 1351
Obegyn Prenatal Supplement (Vitamins, Prenatal) Fleming 1362
PreCare Chewable Tablets (Vitamins, Prenatal) Ther-Rx 3312
PreCare Conceive Tablets (Vitamins, Prenatal) Ther-Rx 3312
PreCare Prenatal Caplets (Vitamins, Prenatal) Ther-Rx 3313
StrongStart Caplets (Vitamins with Minerals, Vitamins, Prenatal) Savage 3096
StrongStart Chewable (Vitamins with Minerals, Vitamins, Prenatal) Savage 3097
StuartNatal Plus 3 Tablets (Vitamins, Prenatal) Integrity Pharmaceutical 1769

Vitamin deficiency, prenatal
New Formulation Chromagen OB Capsules (Ferrous Fumarate, Vitamins with Minerals, Vitamins, Prenatal) Savage 3094

Citracal Prenatal Rx Tablets (Vitamins, Prenatal) Mission 2231
Materna Tablets (Vitamins with Minerals, Vitamins, Prenatal) Lederle 1862
NataChew Tablets (Ferrous Fumarate, Vitamins with Iron, Vitamins, Prenatal) Warner Chilcott 3364
Nestabs RX Tablets (Vitamins with Minerals, Vitamins, Prenatal) Fielding 1351
Obegyn Prenatal Supplement (Vitamins, Prenatal) Fleming 1362
PreCare Chewable Tablets (Vitamins, Prenatal) Ther-Rx 3312
PreCare Conceive Tablets (Vitamins, Prenatal) Ther-Rx 3312
PreCare Prenatal Caplets (Vitamins, Prenatal) Ther-Rx 3313
PremesisRx Tablets (Vitamin B_6, Vitamins, Prenatal) Ther-Rx 3313
StrongStart Caplets (Vitamins with Minerals, Vitamins, Prenatal) Savage 3096
StrongStart Chewable (Vitamins with Minerals, Vitamins, Prenatal) Savage 3097
StuartNatal Plus 3 Tablets (Vitamins, Prenatal) Integrity Pharmaceutical 1769

Vitamin E, deficiency of
Nutr-E-Sol Liquid (Vitamin E) Advanced Nutritional 526
Unique E Vitamin E Capsules (Vitamin E) Grace 1723

Vitamins A, C and E and zinc deficiency
One-A-Day Antioxidant Softgels (Vitamins with Minerals) Bayer Consumer .... ■805

Vitiligo
(*see under* Hypopigmentation, skin)

Vomiting
(*see also under* Motion sickness)
Vistaril Intramuscular Solution (Hydroxyzine Hydrochloride) Pfizer 2738

Vomiting, emetogenic, cancer chemotherapy-induced
Anzemet Injection (Dolasetron Mesylate) Aventis 719
Anzemet Tablets (Dolasetron Mesylate) Aventis 722
Kytril Injection (Granisetron Hydrochloride) Roche Laboratories 2986
Kytril Tablets (Granisetron Hydrochloride) Roche Laboratories 2988
Marinol Capsules (Dronabinol) Unimed 3325
Reglan (Metoclopramide Hydrochloride) Robins 2935
Zofran Injection (Ondansetron Hydrochloride) GlaxoSmithKline 1698
Zofran (Ondansetron Hydrochloride) GlaxoSmithKline 1703
Zofran ODT Orally Disintegrating Tablets (Ondansetron) GlaxoSmithKline 1703

Vomiting, emetogenic, radiation therapy-induced
Kytril Tablets (Granisetron Hydrochloride) Roche Laboratories 2988
Zofran (Ondansetron Hydrochloride) GlaxoSmithKline 1703
Zofran ODT Orally Disintegrating Tablets (Ondansetron) GlaxoSmithKline 1703

Vomiting, postoperative
Anzemet Injection (Dolasetron Mesylate) Aventis 719
Anzemet Tablets (Dolasetron Mesylate) Aventis 722
Phenergan Injection (Promethazine Hydrochloride) Wyeth-Ayerst 3553
Phenergan Suppositories (Promethazine Hydrochloride) Wyeth-Ayerst 3556
Phenergan Syrup (Promethazine Hydrochloride) Wyeth-Ayerst 3554
Phenergan Tablets (Promethazine Hydrochloride) Wyeth-Ayerst 3556
Reglan (Metoclopramide Hydrochloride) Robins 2935
Vistaril Intramuscular Solution (Hydroxyzine Hydrochloride) Pfizer 2738
Zofran Injection (Ondansetron Hydrochloride) GlaxoSmithKline 1698
Zofran (Ondansetron Hydrochloride) GlaxoSmithKline 1703
Zofran ODT Orally Disintegrating Tablets (Ondansetron) GlaxoSmithKline 1703

Vomiting, postpartum, adjunctive therapy in
Vistaril Intramuscular Solution (Hydroxyzine Hydrochloride) Pfizer 2738

Vomiting, severe, control of
Compazine (Prochlorperazine) GlaxoSmithKline 1505
Thorazine (Chlorpromazine Hydrochloride) GlaxoSmithKline 1656
Trilafon (Perphenazine) Schering 3160

von Willebrand's disease, type 1
DDAVP Injection 4 mcg/mL (Desmopressin Acetate) Aventis 737
Desmopressin Acetate Injection (Desmopressin Acetate) Ferring ... 1344
Stimate Nasal Spray (Desmopressin Acetate) Aventis Behring .. 796

Vulvae, kraurosis
Climara Transdermal System (Estradiol) Berlex 958
Estrace Vaginal Cream (Estradiol) Warner Chilcott 3358
Estring Vaginal Ring (Estradiol) Pharmacia & Upjohn 2811
Menest Tablets (Estrogens, Esterified) Monarch 2254
Ogen Tablets (Estropipate) Pharmacia & Upjohn 2846
Ortho Dienestrol Cream (Dienestrol) Ortho-McNeil 2554
Ortho-Est Tablets (Estropipate) Women First 3464
Premarin Vaginal Cream (Estrogens, Conjugated) Wyeth-Ayerst .. 3570

Vulvar atrophy
Activella Tablets (Estradiol, Norethindrone Acetate) Pharmacia & Upjohn 2764
Alora Transdermal System (Estradiol) Watson 3372
CombiPatch Transdermal System (Estradiol, Norethindrone Acetate) Novartis 2323
Esclim Transdermal System (Estradiol) Women First 3460
Ortho-Prefest Tablets (Estradiol, Norgestimate) Ortho-McNeil 2570
Premphase Tablets (Estrogens, Conjugated, Medroxyprogesterone Acetate) Wyeth-Ayerst 3572
Prempro Tablets (Estrogens, Conjugated, Medroxyprogesterone Acetate) Wyeth-Ayerst 3572
Vivelle Transdermal System (Estradiol) Novartis 2412
Vivelle-Dot Transdermal System (Estradiol) Novartis 2416

Vulvovaginal candidiasis
(*see under* Candidiasis, vaginal)

Vulvovaginitis
AVC (Sulfanilamide) Fielding 1350

W

Warts, common, removal of
Clear Away Gel with Aloe Wart Remover System (Salicylic Acid) Schering-Plough .... ■736
Clear Away Liquid Wart Remover System (Salicylic Acid) Schering-Plough .... ■736
Clear Away One Step Wart Remover (Salicylic Acid) Schering-Plough .... ■737
Clear Away One Step Wart Remover for Kids (Salicylic Acid) Schering-Plough .... ■737
Clear Away One Step Plantar Wart Remover (Salicylic Acid) Schering-Plough .... ■737
Compound W One Step Pads for Kids (Salicylic Acid) Medtech ...... ■664
Compound W One Step Plantar Pads (Salicylic Acid) Medtech ..... ■664
Compound W One Step Wart Remover Pads (Salicylic Acid) Medtech .... ■664
Compound W Wart Remover Gel (Salicylic Acid) Medtech .... ■665
Compound W Wart Remover Liquid (Salicylic Acid) Medtech ... ■665
Wart-Off Liquid (Salicylic Acid) Pfizer Inc., Warner-Lambert Healthcare .... ■716

Warts, genital
(*see under* Condylomata acuminata)

Warts, plantar, removal of
Clear Away Gel with Aloe Wart Remover System (Salicylic Acid) Schering-Plough .... ■736
Clear Away Liquid Wart Remover System (Salicylic Acid) Schering-Plough .... ■736
Clear Away One Step Wart Remover (Salicylic Acid) Schering-Plough .... ■737
Clear Away One Step Wart Remover for Kids (Salicylic Acid) Schering-Plough .... ■737
Clear Away One Step Plantar Wart Remover (Salicylic Acid) Schering-Plough .... ■737
Compound W One Step Pads for Kids (Salicylic Acid) Medtech ...... ■664
Compound W One Step Plantar Pads (Salicylic Acid) Medtech ..... ■664
Compound W One Step Wart Remover Pads (Salicylic Acid) Medtech .... ■664
Compound W Wart Remover Gel (Salicylic Acid) Medtech .... ■665
Compound W Wart Remover Liquid (Salicylic Acid) Medtech ... ■665
Wart-Off Liquid (Salicylic Acid) Pfizer Inc., Warner-Lambert Healthcare .... ■716

Water, body, depletion of
(*see under* Dehydration, prevention of)

Weight, body, management of
Oxandrin Tablets (Oxandrolone) BTG 1153

Wheezing, symptomatic relief of
(*see also under* Bronchial asthma)
Primatene Mist (Epinephrine) Whitehall-Robins .... ■779

Whipworm infection
(*see under* Trichuris trichiura infections)

Whooping cough
(*see under* Pertussis)

Wilms' tumor
Adriamycin PFS/RDF Injection (Doxorubicin Hydrochloride) Pharmacia & Upjohn 2767
Cosmegen for Injection (Dactinomycin) Merck 2062

Wilson's disease
Cuprimine Capsules (Penicillamine) Merck 2075
Depen Titratable Tablets (Penicillamine) Wallace 3341
Syprine Capsules (Trientine Hydrochloride) Merck 2186

Wiskott-Aldrich syndrome
Gamimune N, 5% Solvent/Detergent Treated (Globulin, Immune (Human)) Bayer Biological 925
Gamimune N, 10% Solvent/Detergent Treated (Globulin, Immune (Human)) Bayer Biological 928
Gammagard S/D (Globulin, Immune (Human)) Baxter Healthcare 845
Iveegam EN (Globulin, Immune (Human)) Baxter Healthcare 849

Wolff-Parkinson-White syndrome
Adenocard Injection (Adenosine) Fujisawa 1380

Wound care, adjunctive therapy in
Betasept Surgical Scrub (Chlorhexidine Gluconate) Purdue Frederick 2895
Desitin Ointment (Cod Liver Oil, Zinc Oxide) Pfizer Inc., Warner-Lambert Healthcare .... ■700
Granulex Aerosol (Balsam Peru, Castor Oil, Trypsin) Bertek 1007
Humatrix Microclysmic Burn/Wound Healing Gel (Collagen, Chondroitin Sulfate) Care-Tech .... ■632
Panafil Ointment (Chlorophyllin Copper Complex Sodium, Papain, Urea) Healthpoint 1726
Preparation H Medicated Wipes (Witch Hazel) Whitehall-Robins .... ■779
Tucks Pre-moistened Pads (Witch Hazel) Pfizer Inc., Warner-Lambert Healthcare .... ■713

Wounds, debridement of
Accuzyme Debriding Ointment (Papain, Urea) Healthpoint 1725
Collagenase Santyl Ointment (Collagenase) Smith & Nephew 3248
Granulex Aerosol (Balsam Peru, Castor Oil, Trypsin) Bertek 1007
Panafil Ointment (Chlorophyllin Copper Complex Sodium, Papain, Urea) Healthpoint 1726

Wounds, removal of exudates, aids in
Panafil Ointment (Chlorophyllin Copper Complex Sodium, Papain, Urea) Healthpoint 1726

Wrinkles, fine
(*see under* Skin, fine wrinkles, mitigation of)

X

Xerosis
Lac-Hydrin Cream (Ammonium Lactate) Bristol-Myers Squibb Dermatology 1118
Lac-Hydrin Lotion (Ammonium Lactate) Bristol-Myers Squibb Dermatology 1119

Xerostomia, radiotherapy-induced
Ethyol for Injection (Amifostine) MedImmune Oncology 2029
Salagen Tablets (Pilocarpine Hydrochloride) MGI 2229

XO syndrome
(*see under* Turner's syndrome)

Y

Yaws
Bicillin L-A Injection (Penicillin G Benzathine) Monarch 2242
Declomycin Tablets (Demeclocycline Hydrochloride) Lederle 1855
Doryx Coated Pellet Filled Capsules (Doxycycline Hyclate) Warner Chilcott 3357
Dynacin Capsules (Minocycline Hydrochloride) Medicis 2019
Minocin Intravenous (Minocycline Hydrochloride) Lederle 1862
Minocin Oral Suspension (Minocycline Hydrochloride) Lederle 1865
Minocin Pellet-Filled Capsules (Minocycline Hydrochloride) Lederle 1863
Monodox Capsules (Doxycycline Monohydrate) Oclassen 2442
Vibramycin Calcium Oral Suspension Syrup (Doxycycline Calcium) Pfizer 2735
Vibramycin Hyclate Capsules (Doxycycline Hyclate) Pfizer 2735
Vibramycin Hyclate Intravenous (Doxycycline Hyclate) Pfizer 2737
Vibramycin Monohydrate for Oral Suspension (Doxycycline Monohydrate) Pfizer 2735
Vibra-Tabs Film Coated Tablets (Doxycycline Hyclate) Pfizer 2735

Yersinia pestis infections
Declomycin Tablets (Demeclocycline Hydrochloride) Lederle 1855
Doryx Coated Pellet Filled Capsules (Doxycycline Hyclate) Warner Chilcott 3357
Dynacin Capsules (Minocycline Hydrochloride) Medicis 2019
Minocin Intravenous (Minocycline Hydrochloride) Lederle 1862
Minocin Oral Suspension (Minocycline Hydrochloride) Lederle 1865
Minocin Pellet-Filled Capsules (Minocycline Hydrochloride) Lederle 1863
Monodox Capsules (Doxycycline Monohydrate) Oclassen 2442
Streptomycin Sulfate Injection (Streptomycin Sulfate) Pfizer 2714
Vibramycin Calcium Oral Suspension Syrup (Doxycycline Calcium) Pfizer 2735
Vibramycin Hyclate Capsules (Doxycycline Hyclate) Pfizer 2735
Vibramycin Hyclate Intravenous (Doxycycline Hyclate) Pfizer 2737
Vibramycin Monohydrate for Oral Suspension (Doxycycline Monohydrate) Pfizer 2735

Vibra-Tabs Film Coated Tablets (Doxycycline Hyclate) Pfizer 2735

Z

Zollinger-Ellison syndrome

Aciphex Tablets (Rabeprazole Sodium) Eisai 1267
Aciphex Tablets (Rabeprazole Sodium) Janssen 1783
Famotidine Injection (Famotidine) Baxter Anesthesia........................ 866
Pepcid Injection (Famotidine) Merck.. 2153
Pepcid for Oral Suspension (Famotidine) Merck 2150
Pepcid RPD Orally Disintegrating Tablets (Famotidine) Merck 2150
Pepcid Tablets (Famotidine) Merck.. 2150
Prevacid Delayed-Release Capsules (Lansoprazole) TAP....... 3292
Prilosec Delayed-Release Capsules (Omeprazole) AstraZeneca LP........................... 628
Tagamet (Cimetidine Hydrochloride) GlaxoSmithKline.................. 1644
Zantac (Ranitidine Hydrochloride) GlaxoSmithKline.......................... 1690

Zygomycosis

Abelcet Injection (Amphotericin B) Elan 1273

SECTION 5

OFF-LABEL TREATMENT GUIDE

This section identifies medications routinely used—but never officially approved—for nearly 1,000 indications. The entries include only those off-label uses well documented in the peer-reviewed literature. The information is drawn from knowledge bases maintained by MICROMEDEX, Inc., an affiliate of *PDR*® and the world leader in evaluative clinical drug information. Medications are listed by generic name and include all drugs described in *PDR*® and its companion volumes, as well as other currently available products. All listings are alphabetical.

Acetaminophen overdose, management of
Cimetidine

Acetylator status, determination of
Procainamide Hydrochloride

Acinetobacter calcoaceticus infections
Gentamicin Sulfate, Injectable

Acinetobacter species infections
Tobramycin Sulfate, Injectable

Acne, cystic, adjunctive treatment for
Isotretinoin

Acne, unspecified
Chloramphenicol
Cimetidine

Acrodermatitis enteropathica
Zinc

Adenoma, islet cell, insulin-secreting
Dextrose

Adenoma, islet cell, insulin-secreting, diagnosis of
Calcium

Adrenal hyperplasia, congenital
Flutamide

Aeromonas hydrophila infections
Ciprofloxacin, Systemic
Gentamicin Sulfate, Injectable
Ofloxacin, Systemic

Agitation, dementia related
Carbamazepine

Agoraphobia
Imipramine

Airway obstruction, post-extubation
Dexamethasone, Injectable
Dexamethasone, Oral

Akathisia
Clonidine

Akathisia, neuroleptic-induced
Propranolol Hydrochloride

Alcohol intoxication, management of
Lorazepam

Alcohol withdrawal, acute, symptomatic relief of
Clonidine

Alcoholism, associated with related depression
Fluoxetine Hydrochloride

Alkalosis, metabolic
Hydrochloric Acid

Alopecia, androgenetic
Cimetidine

Amenorrhea
Levothyroxine Sodium
Liothyronine Sodium

Amniotic fluid volume determination
Aminohippurate Sodium

Anaphylaxis, treatment of
Cimetidine

Ancylostoma duodenale infections
Albendazole

Anemia, sickle cell
Deferoxamine Mesylate

Anemia, surgical procedure or trauma-induced
Erythropoietins

Anesthesia, general, adjunct in
Calcium
Diazepam

Anesthesia, local
Diphenhydramine Hydrochloride

Anesthesia, local, obstetrical procedures
Isoproterenol

Anesthesia, post, shivering
Nalbuphine Hydrochloride

Anesthesia, spinal
Dibucaine

Anesthesia, surgical, prolongation of
Clonidine
Esmolol Hydrochloride

Angina pectoris
Acebutolol Hydrochloride
Bisoprolol Fumarate
Carteolol Hydrochloride, Oral
Esmolol Hydrochloride
Labetalol Hydrochloride
Levocarnitine
Penbutolol Sulfate
Pindolol
Sotalol Hydrochloride
Timolol Maleate, Oral

Angina, unstable
Acetylcysteine
Diltiazem
Nifedipine

Angiography, penile vasculature
Alprostadil

Angiomatosis, bacillary
Doxycycline
Minocycline Hydrochloride
Tetracycline Hydrochloride, Oral

Angioplasty, aid to
Papaverine Hydrochloride

Ankylosing spondylitis
Flurbiprofen, Oral
Piroxicam

Anorectal conditions
Phenolphthalein

Anorexia nervosa
Cisapride
Cyproheptadine Hydrochloride

Anorexia, non-AIDS related
Megestrol Acetate

Antidiuretic hormone secretion, inappropriate, syndrome of
Demeclocycline Hydrochloride
Urea, Injectable

Antisepsis, catheter
Chlorhexidine Gluconate

Antiseptic, surgical
Benzalkonium Chloride
Iodine

Anxiety disorders, management of
Chlorpromazine
Propranolol Hydrochloride

Aorta insufficiency, severe
Propranolol Hydrochloride

Aortic insufficiency
Hydralazine Hydrochloride

Aortic regurgitation
Enalapril
Quinapril Hydrochloride

Aortic stenosis
Sodium Nitroprusside

Apnea, neonatal
Caffeine

Appendicitis with peritonitis
Netilmicin Sulfate

Appendicitis, perforated
Netilmicin Sulfate

Appetite, stimulation of
Cyproheptadine Hydrochloride

Arachnoiditis
Hyaluronidase

Arrhythmias
Magnesium
Metoprolol
Nadolol
Phentolamine Mesylate
Potassium Chloride, Oral
Timolol Maleate, Oral

Arrhythmias, supraventricular
Sotalol Hydrochloride

Arrhythmias, supraventricular, diagnosis of
Adenosine

Arrhythmias, ventricular
Bepridil Hydrochloride
Flecainide Acetate

Arteriography, to improve visualization of
Tolazoline Hydrochloride

Ascariasis
Albendazole
Piperazine

Ascites
Albumin, Normal Serum, Human

Asthma, diagnosis of
Carbachol
Histamine Phosphate

Asthma, nocturnal
Theophylline

Ataxia, hereditary
Acetazolamide

Atherosclerosis
Colestipol Hydrochloride

Atrial fibrillation
Procainamide Hydrochloride

Atrial flutter
Procainamide Hydrochloride

Attention deficit disorders with hyperactivity
Desipramine Hydrochloride

Autonomic dysreflexia
Nifedipine

Bacillus cereus, subtilis
Vancomycin Hydrochloride

Balantidiasis
Tetracycline Hydrochloride, Oral

Barotrauma
Pseudoephedrine Hydrochloride

Barrett's esophagus
Cimetidine
Methylene Blue
Omeprazole

Bartter's syndrome
Captopril

Behavior, aggressive
Lithium Carbonate
Propranolol Hydrochloride

Biliary tract disorders
Nitroglycerin

Bite wounds
Amoxicillin with Clavulanate Potassium
Oxacillin Sodium
Tetracycline Hydrochloride, Oral

Bites, insect, prevention of
Permethrin

Bites, poisonous
Prazosin Hydrochloride

Bladder disease, neurogenic
Verapamil Hydrochloride

Bladder instability
Dantrolene Sodium

Bladder irrigation
Mannitol, Injectable
Polymyxin B Sulfate

Bleeding, gastrointestinal
Isosorbide Dinitrate
Isosorbide Mononitrate
Nadolol
Nitroglycerin
Propranolol Hydrochloride

Bleeding, gastrointestinal, drug-induced
Dinoprostone

Blepharitis
Polymyxin B Sulfate

Bone marrow transplantation, allogeneic or autologous, adjunctive therapy in
Busulfan

Borrelia burgdorferi infection
Amoxicillin
Ceftriaxone Sodium
Clarithromycin
Doxycycline
Penicillin G Sodium
Penicillin V Potassium

Bowel syndrome, short
Cimetidine

Bowel, evacuation of
Mannitol, Injectable

Bowel, irritable, syndrome
Amitriptyline Hydrochloride

Bronchial asthma
Astemizole
Atropine Sulfate, Injectable
Azelastine Hydrochloride
Cetirizine Hydrochloride
Ipratropium Bromide
Loratadine
Methotrexate
Olopatadine Hydrochloride
Salmeterol/Fluticasone
Troleandomycin

Bronchopulmonary dysplasia, chronic
Furosemide
Hydrochlorothiazide
Spironolactone

Brucellosis
Gentamicin Sulfate, Injectable

Bulimia nervosa
Flutamide
Isocarboxazid
Phenelzine Sulfate

Burns, adjunctive therapy in
Cimetidine

Burns, alkali
Acetic Acid, Topical

Burns, recovery phase, weight gain, aid in the management of
Oxandrolone

Cachexia associated with weight loss, AIDS-induced
Oxandrolone

Calcinosis
Diltiazem

Calymmatobacterium granulomatis
Gentamicin Sulfate, Injectable
Tetracycline Hydrochloride, Oral

Campylobacter jejuni infectious diarrhea
Erythromycin, Injectable
Erythromycin, Oral

Candidiasis, systemic
Miconazole

Candidiasis, unspecified
Amphotericin B, Topical

Candidiasis, vaginal
Natamycin

Cannulation, radial artery
Aspirin

Carcinoma, adrenal cortex
Aminoglutethimide

Carcinoma, basal cell
Porfimer Sodium

Carcinoma, bladder
Ifosfamide
Methotrexate
Mitomycin
Vinblastine Sulfate

Carcinoma, brain
Hydroxyurea
Methotrexate

Carcinoma, breast
Aminoglutethimide
Gemcitabine Hydrochloride
Idarubicin Hydrochloride
Ifosfamide
Medroxyprogesterone Acetate, Oral
Prednisolone, Systemic
Trimetrexate Glucuronate
Vinorelbine Tartrate

Carcinoma, cervix
Cisplatin
Fluorouracil, Systemic
Fluorouracil, Topical
Ifosfamide
Vinorelbine Tartrate

Carcinoma, colorectal, adjunctive therapy in
Floxuridine
Leucovorin Calcium
Trimetrexate Glucuronate

Carcinoma, endometrial
Doxorubicin Hydrochloride

Carcinoma, esophageal
Bleomycin Sulfate
Fluorouracil, Systemic
Fluorouracil, Topical

Carcinoma, gastrointestinal
Hydroxyurea

Carcinoma, head and neck
Carboplatin
Fluorouracil, Systemic
Fluorouracil, Topical
Trimetrexate Glucuronate

Carcinoma, islet cell
Doxorubicin Hydrochloride
Fluorouracil, Systemic
Fluorouracil, Topical

Carcinoma, liver
Floxuridine
Fluorouracil, Systemic
Fluorouracil, Topical
Ifosfamide
Vincristine Sulfate

Carcinoma, lung, non-small cell
Carboplatin
Ifosfamide
Irinotecan Hydrochloride
Paclitaxel
Trimetrexate Glucuronate

Carcinoma, lung, small cell
Ifosfamide
Vincristine Sulfate

Carcinoma, ovary
Busulfan
Dactinomycin
Ifosfamide
Megestrol Acetate
Tamoxifen Citrate

Carcinoma, prostate
Aminoglutethimide
Megestrol Acetate
Vitamin E

Carcinoma, renal
Cimetidine
Interferon Alfa-2A
Interferon Alfa-2B

Carcinoma, renal cell
Megestrol Acetate

Carcinoma, testicular
Vincristine Sulfate

Carcinoma, thyroid
Levothyroxine Sodium
Liothyronine Sodium

Carcinoma, verrucous (wart)
Bleomycin Sulfate

Cardiomyopathy, hypertrophic
Diltiazem
Ethanol
Nifedipine
Verapamil Hydrochloride

Cardioplegia solutions
Dextrose

Cardiopulmonary resuscitation
Isoproterenol

Cardiovascular bypass surgery, treatment adjunct
Dipyridamole, Oral
Ticlopidine Hydrochloride

Cardiovascular disorders, diagnosis of
Papaverine Hydrochloride

Cardiovascular surgery, aid in
Droperidol and Fentanyl Citrate
Milrinone Lactate

Caroli's syndrome
Ursodiol

Cataract extraction, surgical aid in
Carbachol

Catatonia
Amobarbital Sodium

Catheter occlusion
Ethanol
Hydrochloric Acid
Streptokinase

Catheter patency, arterial
Papaverine Hydrochloride

Cephalalgia, histaminic
Lithium Carbonate
Verapamil Hydrochloride

Cerebral palsy
Botulinum Toxin Type A

Cerebrovascular insufficiency
Cyclandelate

Cerebrovascular reserve, determination of
Acetazolamide

Cerumen, removal of
Hydrogen Peroxide

Cervix, ripening of, in pregnant women at or near term
Dinoprostone, Cervical
Dinoprostone, Vaginal
Misoprostol

Chancroid
Amoxicillin with Clavulanate Potassium
Ceftriaxone Sodium
Ciprofloxacin, Systemic
Enoxacin
Erythromycin, Injectable
Erythromycin, Oral
Ofloxacin, Systemic

Chest syndrome, acute
Dexamethasone, Injectable
Dexamethasone, Oral

Chlamydia infections, unspecified
Oxytetracycline Hydrochloride

Chlamydia pneumoniae infections
Clarithromycin

Chlamydia psittaci infection
Chloramphenicol

Chlamydia trachomatis conjunctivitis of the newborn
Silver Nitrate

Chlamydia trachomatis infections
Sparfloxacin

Chlamydia trachomatis, ophthalmia neonatorum, prophylaxis of
Silver Nitrate

Cholera
Ciprofloxacin, Systemic
Enoxacin
Lomefloxacin Hydrochloride
Norfloxacin, Oral
Ofloxacin, Systemic

Choriocarcinoma
Dactinomycin
Methotrexate

Cirrhosis, biliary
Nalmefene Hydrochloride

Coccidioidomycosis
Miconazole

Colic, ureteral, symptomatic relief of
Butorphanol Tartrate

Colitis, pseudomembranous, antibiotic-associated
Ciprofloxacin, Systemic
Metronidazole, Systemic

Colitis, pseudomembranous, unspecified
Bacitracin

Colitis, ulcerative
Folic Acid
Sucralfate

Colitis, ulcerative, maintenance therapy for
Mesalamine

Colonic surgery, prophylaxis
Doxycycline

Condylomata acuminata
Fluorouracil, Systemic
Fluorouracil, Topical

Conjunctivitis, unspecified
Lomefloxacin Hydrochloride

Constipation
Cisapride

Coronary artery bypass graft, myocardial protection
Diltiazem
Nifedipine

Coronary artery disease, diagnostic aid in
Dobutamine Hydrochloride

Corynebacterium JK
Erythromycin, Injectable
Erythromycin, Oral
Gentamicin Sulfate, Injectable

Corynebacterium infections, unspecified
Vancomycin Hydrochloride

Crohn's disease
Mesalamine
Omeprazole

Croup
Dexamethasone, Injectable
Dexamethasone, Oral
Epinephrine, Systemic

Cryptococcosis
Fluconazole

Cushing's disease, management of clinical features
Cyproheptadine Hydrochloride
Metyrapone

Cushing's syndrome
Mitotane

Cystic fibrosis
Amikacin Sulfate
Aztreonam
Ceftazidime
Ciprofloxacin, Systemic
Cisapride
Imipenem/Cilastatin
Minocycline Hydrochloride
Netilmicin Sulfate
Pancreatin

Cystinuria
Captopril

Cysts, Mucoid
Sodium Tetradecyl Sulfate

Decontamination, alimentary tract
Ciprofloxacin, Systemic

Dehydration, treatment of, oral therapy
Dextrose

Dementia, Alzheimer's type
Propranolol Hydrochloride
Vitamin E

Dental hygiene, adjunct to
Zinc

Dental procedures, adjunct to
Novobiocin Sodium
Propantheline Bromide

Dental stains, treatment adjunct
Carbamide Peroxide

Depression, mental, endogenous
Nortriptyline Hydrochloride

Depression, relief of symptoms
Buspirone Hydrochloride
Clomipramine Hydrochloride
Imipramine
Nortriptyline Hydrochloride
Pindolol

Dermatitis, actinic
Azathioprine

Dermatitis, atopic
Tacrolimus
Urea, Topical

Dermatitis, unspecified
Tacrolimus

Dermatomycosis, systemic
Itraconazole

Dermatomyositis, systemic
Tioconazole

Dermatosis, bullous
Colchicine

Dermographism
Cimetidine

Diabetes insipidus
Chlorpropamide

Diabetes mellitus, diagnosis of
Dextrose

Dialysis, unspecified
Deferoxamine Mesylate

Diarrhea
Ampicillin
Clonidine
Octreotide Acetate
Sucralfate

Diarrhea, acquired immune deficiency syndrome-induced
Octreotide Acetate

Diarrhea, infantile, adjunct in
Cholestyramine

Diarrhea, infectious
Levofloxacin
Ofloxacin, Systemic

Diarrhea, radiation-induced
Sucralfate

Diarrhea, traveler's
Doxycycline
Loperamide Hydrochloride

Diarrhea, traveler's, prevention of
Norfloxacin, Oral

Diet, supplementation of
Ergocalciferol

Digestive disorders, symptomatic relief of
Bismuth Subsalicylate
Cisapride
Omeprazole
Ranitidine Hydrochloride

Diphtheria, prevention or treatment of
Diphtheria Toxoid, Adsorbed

Disinfection, topical
Hydrogen Peroxide

Dracunculus infections
Metronidazole, Systemic

Drug overdose, unspecified
Propranolol Hydrochloride

Duodenal ulcers, adjunctive therapy for
Misoprostol

Duodenal ulcers, maintenance therapy for
Omeprazole

Duodenitis
Cimetidine

Dyskinesia, tardive
Diltiazem
Metoclopramide Hydrochloride
Verapamil Hydrochloride

Dysmenorrhea, unspecified, symptomatic relief of
Nifedipine
Piroxicam

Dyspepsia, non-ulcer
Cimetidine

Dysphoric disorder, premenstrual
Sertraline Hydrochloride

Dysthymia
Sertraline Hydrochloride

Dystonia
Botulinum Toxin Type A

Dystrophy, sympathetic reflex
Bretylium Tosylate

E. coli infections
Ceftriaxone Sodium

Ear, infection, unspecified
Piperacillin Sodium

Ear, middle, surgical procedures
Labetalol Hydrochloride

Echocardiography stress test
Adenosine
Atropine Sulfate, Injectable
Dobutamine Hydrochloride

Eclampsia
Phenytoin

Edema, cerebral
Glycerin

Edema, drug-related
Bumetanide

Edema, pulmonary, adjunctive treatment of
Nifedipine
Nitroglycerin

Eikenella corradens infections
Erythromycin, Injectable
Erythromycin, Oral

Electroconvulsive therapy
Caffeine
Esmolol Hydrochloride

Empyema
Vancomycin Hydrochloride

Endocarditis, bacterial, prophylaxis
Amoxicillin
Clindamycin, Systemic

Endocarditis, prosthetic valve
Warfarin Sodium

Endocarditis, streptococcal
Ceftriaxone Sodium

Endocarditis, unspecified
Amoxicillin
Ciprofloxacin, Systemic
Kanamycin Sulfate

Endocarditis, unspecified, prophylaxis
Ampicillin
Cefazolin Sodium
Clarithromycin
Gentamicin Sulfate, Injectable

Endometrial thinning
Goserelin Acetate

Endometriosis
Megestrol Acetate

Endothelial dysfunction
Vitamin C

Entamoeba polecki
Metronidazole, Systemic

Enteritis
Levofloxacin

Enteritis, campylobacter
Chloramphenicol

Enterocolitis, necrotizing
Kanamycin Sulfate

Epididymitis
Ceftriaxone Sodium
Doxycycline
Ofloxacin, Systemic

Epidural, post, backache prophylaxis
Dexamethasone, Injectable
Dexamethasone, Oral

Epilepsy
Allopurinol
Medium Chain Triglycerides
Midazolam Hydrochloride

Epilepsy, intractable
Lamotrigine

Epilepticus, status
Phenobarbital

Erectile dysfunction
Isosorbide Dinitrate
Papaverine Hydrochloride
Phentolamine Mesylate

Erythrocytosis, treatment of
Captopril
Enalapril
Lisinopril
Losartan Potassium

Erythroderma
Coal Tar

Erythromelalgia
Sodium Nitroprusside

Esophageal disorders, unspecified
Botulinum Toxin Type A

Esophageal varices, hemorrhage from
Octreotide Acetate
Sodium Nitroprusside
Sodium Tetradecyl Sulfate

Esophagitis, reflux
Cisapride
Sucralfate

Esophagitis, refractory
Omeprazole

Esophagitis, unspecified, maintenance therapy of
Famotidine

Ewing's sarcoma, palliative treatment of
Ifosfamide

Extrapyramidal reactions, drug-induced
Diphenhydramine Hydrochloride

Extravasation, cytotoxic drugs
Sodium Thiosulfate

Eyes, infections of
Oxacillin Sodium
Piperacillin Sodium
Ticarcillin Disodium
Vancomycin Hydrochloride

Eyes, laser surgery, adjunct to
Pilocarpine, Ophthalmic

Fertilization, in vitro, adjunct in
Clomiphene Citrate
Nafarelin Acetate
Progesterone

Fetal maturation
Levothyroxine Sodium

Fever, familial mediterranean
Colchicine

Fever, unspecified
Diclofenac, Oral

Fissure, anal
Isosorbide Dinitrate
Nitroglycerin

Fistula, gastrointestinal
Octreotide Acetate

Fluorosis
Vitamin C

Fluorosis, pediatric
Calcium

Flushing, niacin-induced
Aspirin

Folic acid antagonists, overdosage of
Folic Acid

Francisella tularensis infections
Tetracycline Hydrochloride, Oral

Frostbite, possibly effective in
Tetanus Immune Globulin

Fusobacterium species infections
Penicillin G Sodium

Gangrene
Pentoxifylline

Gastric emptying, delayed
Omeprazole

Gastric ulcers, maintenance therapy for
Lansoprazole
Sucralfate

Gastritis
Sucralfate

Gastritis, drug-induced
Famotidine
Ranitidine Hydrochloride

Gastritis, hemorrhagic
Ethanolamine Oleate
Omeprazole

Gastrointestinal imaging
Metrizamide

Gastrointestinal ulcers, unspecified, nsaid-induced
Omeprazole

Gastrointestinal, stress ulcer prophylaxis
Ranitidine Hydrochloride
Sucralfate

Gestational trophoblastic disease, unspecified
Ifosfamide

Gestational trophoblastic neoplasm
Vincristine Sulfate

Giardiasis
Tinidazole

Gingivitis
Chlorhexidine Gluconate
Minocycline Hydrochloride

Gland, salivary, dysfunction of
Pilocarpine Hydrochloride, Oral

Glaucoma, unspecified
Clonidine
Diltiazem
Fluorouracil, Systemic
Fluorouracil, Topical
Guanethidine Monosulfate
Nifedipine
Verapamil Hydrochloride

Glomerular filtration rate, measurement of
Cimetidine
Mannitol, Injectable

Gnathostomiasis
Albendazole

Gonococcal infections, disseminated
Ceftriaxone Sodium

Gout, management of signs and symptoms
Piroxicam

Graft-versus-host disease (GVHD)
Cyclosporine
Methotrexate
Methylprednisolone

Growth hormone secretion, inadequate
Oxandrolone

Growth, stimulation of
Fluoxymesterone
Oxandrolone

Guillain-Barre syndrome
Immune Globulin

Gustatory sweating
Glycopyrrolate

Gynecologic surgery
Etidocaine Hydrochloride

H. influenzae bronchitis
Cotrimoxazole

H. influenzae infections
Ceftriaxone Sodium
Tetracycline Hydrochloride, Oral

H. influenzae upper respiratory tract infections
Cotrimoxazole

Headache
Butorphanol Tartrate
Diclofenac, Oral
Prochlorperazine

Headache, migraine
Cyproheptadine Hydrochloride
Diltiazem
Metoprolol
Nadolol
Verapamil Hydrochloride

Heart surgery, open, treatment adjunct
Amrinone Lactate

Heart transplant, to reduce the incidence of rejection, adjunct in
Dobutamine Hydrochloride
Rabbit Antithymocyte Globulin

Heart transplantation, postoperative
Dobutamine Hydrochloride

Heart transplantation, preoperative
Milrinone Lactate

Heart-lung transplant, to reduce the incidence of rejection, adjunct in
Rabbit Antithymocyte Globulin

Helicobacter pylori-induced peptic ulceration/gastritis
Ciprofloxacin, Systemic
Clarithromycin
Lansoprazole
Nizatidine
Ranitidine Hydrochloride
Tetracycline Hydrochloride, Oral
Tinidazole

Hemangioma
Bleomycin Sulfate

Hemarthrosis
Factor IX (Human)

Hemodialysis, adjunct in
Levocarnitine
Mannitol, Injectable

Hemophilia, unspecified
Danazol

Hemorrhage, gastrointestinal, unspecified
Cimetidine
Epinephrine, Systemic
Famotidine
Ranitidine Hydrochloride
Tranexamic Acid

Hemorrhage, intraventricular
Vitamin E

Hemorrhage, upper gastrointestinal
Thrombin

Hepatic dysfunction
Factor IX (Human)

Hepatic porphyria
Hemin

Hepatitis, alcoholic
Prednisolone, Systemic

Hepatitis, unspecified
Ursodiol

Hernia, diaphragmatic, congenital
Tolazoline Hydrochloride

Herpes simplex virus infections
Cimetidine
Zinc

Herpes zoster infections
Cimetidine

Hirsutism
Cimetidine
Finasteride
Flutamide
Spironolactone

Hodgkin's disease
Ifosfamide
Mitoxantrone Hydrochloride

Homocysteinemia
Folic Acid

Horner's syndrome, diagnosis of
Cocaine Hydrochloride

Hyperaldosteronism, unspecified
Captopril
Enalapril

Hypercalcemia, unspecified
Alendronate Sodium

Hypercalciuria, unspecified
Hydrochlorothiazide
Indapamide
Potassium Chloride, Oral

Hypercholesterolemia
Lovastatin
Magnesium
Neomycin Sulfate

Hyperemesis gravidarum
Diphenhydramine Hydrochloride
Droperidol
Ondansetron Hydrochloride

Hypereosinophilic syndrome
Hydroxyurea

Hyperhidrosis
Methenamine Mandelate

Hyperimmunoglobulinemia E
Cimetidine

Hyperkalemia
Albuterol

Hyperlipidemia
Orlistat
Oxandrolone
Terazosin Hydrochloride

Hyperlipoproteinemia, type III, adjunct to diet
Fenofibrate

Hyperlipoproteinemia, types IIa and IIb, adjunct to diet
Fenofibrate

Hyperlipoproteinemia, unspecified
Levocarnitine

Hyperparathyroidism
Calcitriol
Cimetidine

Hyperparathyroidism, primary
Calcium

Hyperphosphatemia
Sucralfate

Hyperprolactinemia
Pergolide Mesylate

Hypersensitivity reactions, radiocontrast media-induced
Cimetidine
Diphenhydramine Hydrochloride

Hypertension
Ethacrynic Acid
Levobunolol Hydrochloride, Ophthalmic
Magnesium
Metipranolol
Sotalol Hydrochloride

Hypertension associated with surgical procedures
Clonidine
Esmolol Hydrochloride
Guanabenz Acetate
Isradipine
Magnesium
Nifedipine

Hypertension, intracranial
Dihydroergotamine Mesylate

Hypertension, malignant
Captopril
Clonidine
Minoxidil, Oral
Nifedipine

Hypertension, portal
Clonidine

Hypertension, pregnancy
Diazoxide
Isradipine
Methyldopa
Nifedipine
Nisoldipine

Hypertension, preoperative
Droperidol and Fentanyl Citrate

Hypertension, pulmonary
Adenosine
Alprostadil
Amlodipine Besylate
Nifedipine

Hypertension, renal
Captopril
Enalapril
Lisinopril
Nifedipine
Ramipril

Hypertension, renal, associated with renography
Captopril
Enalapril

Hypertensive emergency
Labetalol Hydrochloride

Hyperthyroidism
Diltiazem
Nadolol
Potassium Perchlorate
Propranolol Hydrochloride

Hypogammaglobulinemia
Cimetidine

Hypogonadism, hypogonadotrophic, unspecified
Urofollitropin

Hypokalemia
Magnesium

Hyponatremia
Fludrocortisone Acetate

Hypotension
Midodrine Hydrochloride
Propranolol Hydrochloride

Hypotension, orthostatic
Fludrocortisone Acetate

Ileus, meconium
Acetylcysteine

Ileus, paralytic
Metoclopramide Hydrochloride

Ileus, postoperative
Cisapride

Immunodeficiencies
Vitamin E

Immunomodulator, for cancer patients
Cimetidine

Infection, tendency to
Norfloxacin, Oral
Vitamin A

Infections, anaerobic organisms
Penicillin G Sodium

Infections, bacterial, various types
Cefpirome
Ceftriaxone Sodium
Ticarcillin/Clavulanic Acid

Infections, balnei
Minocycline Hydrochloride

Infections, biliary tract
Cefoperazone Sodium
Cefoperazone/Sulbactam
Ofloxacin, Systemic

Infections, bone and joint
Aztreonam
Cefadroxil Monohydrate
Ofloxacin, Systemic

Infections, catheter exit-site
Mupirocin

Infections, contaminated surgery of ruptured viscus, prophylaxis of
Clindamycin, Systemic

Infections, dientamobea
Tetracycline Hydrochloride, Oral

Infections, ear, nose and throat
Enoxacin
Ofloxacin, Systemic
Oxacillin Sodium
Ticarcillin/Clavulanic Acid

Infections, ehrlichia chaffeensis
Doxycycline
Tetracycline Hydrochloride, Oral

Infections, genitourinary tract
Doxycycline

Infections, gram-negative bacteria
Aztreonam
Kanamycin Sulfate

Infections, gynecologic
Cefoperazone/Sulbactam
Levofloxacin

Infections, gynecologic, prophylaxis of
Ampicillin Sodium and Sulbactam Sodium

Infections, head and neck surgery, prophylaxis of
Clindamycin, Systemic

Infections, intra-abdominal
Cefoperazone/Sulbactam
Ciprofloxacin, Systemic
Clindamycin, Systemic
Tobramycin Sulfate, Injectable

Infections, lower respiratory tract
Cloxacillin Sodium
Nafcillin Sodium
Oxacillin Sodium

Infections, lower respiratory tract, RSV-induced
Prednisolone, Systemic

Infections, neurological, unspecified
Nafcillin Sodium

Infections, ocular, neonatal prophylaxis
Penicillin G Sodium

Infections, ocular, unspecified
Tetracycline Hydrochloride, Oral

Infections, perinatal, prevention of
Ceftazidime

Infections, post-urologic surgery, prophylaxis in
Enoxacin

Infections, prevention of
Ofloxacin, Systemic

Infections, respiratory tract, unspecified
Acetylcysteine
Cefadroxil Monohydrate
Enoxacin
Gramicidin

Infections, sinus
Piperacillin Sodium

Infections, skeletal
Cloxacillin Sodium
Nafcillin Sodium
Oxacillin Sodium

Infections, skin and skin structure
Enoxacin
Gramicidin

Infections, surgical, appendectomy, prevention of
Ampicillin Sodium and Sulbactam Sodium
Tinidazole

Infections, surgical, cardiac, prevention of
Cefuroxime Sodium

Infections, surgical, colorectal, prevention of
Ampicillin Sodium and Sulbactam Sodium
Tinidazole

Infections, surgical, genitourinary, prevention of
Ampicillin Sodium and Sulbactam Sodium

Infections, surgical, gynecologic, prevention of
Ampicillin Sodium and Sulbactam Sodium
Metronidazole, Systemic

Infections, surgical, head and neck, prevention of
Gentamicin Sulfate, Injectable

Infections, surgical, non-colorectal, prevention of
Tinidazole

Infections, surgical, ophthalmic, prevention of
Gentamicin Sulfate, Injectable
Tobramycin Sulfate, Injectable

Infections, surgical, ruptured viscus, prevention of
Gentamicin Sulfate, Injectable

Infections, surgical, thoracic, prevention of
Cefuroxime Sodium

Infections, surgical, unspecified
Cefoperazone Sodium
Kanamycin Sulfate

Infections, surgical, unspecified, prevention of
Aztreonam
Cloxacillin Sodium
Minocycline Hydrochloride
Nafcillin Sodium
Oxacillin Sodium
Penicillin G Sodium
Ticarcillin Disodium

Infections, urinary tract
Ceftibuten
Kanamycin Sulfate
Sparfloxacin

Infections, urinary tract, post-prostatectomy, prophylaxis of
Cephalexin

Infections, urinary tract, prevention of
Cotrimoxazole

Infections, uterine, peripartum
Gentamicin Sulfate, Injectable

Infections, xanthomonas
Cotrimoxazole
Enoxacin
Lomefloxacin Hydrochloride
Ofloxacin, Systemic

Infertility
Doxycycline
Gonadotropin, Chorionic
Progesterone
Urofollitropin

Infertility, female
Gonadorelin Hydrochloride

Inflammatory bowel disease
Azathioprine
Sulfasalazine
Vancomycin Hydrochloride

Inflammatory conditions, unspecified
Diclofenac Sodium and Misoprostol

Intoxication, bromide
Ethacrynic Acid

Intracarotid procedure
Amobarbital Sodium

Intraocular pressure, postcycloplegic
Apraclonidine Hydrochloride

Intubation, endotracheal
Etidocaine Hydrochloride
Propofol
Tubocurarine Chloride

Iris cyst formation
Phenylephrine Hydrochloride

Irrigation, antibacterial
Hydrogen Peroxide

Ischemia, mesenteric
Papaverine Hydrochloride

Ischemia, myocardial
Metoprolol
Nitroglycerin

Ischemia, myocardial, silent
Isosorbide Dinitrate
Isosorbide Mononitrate

Ischemic tissue damage, prevention of
Allopurinol

Isovaleric acidemia
Glycine

Jaundice, neonatal, evaluation of
Phenobarbital

Kaposi's sarcoma
Gonadotropin, Chorionic
Paclitaxel
Vincristine Sulfate

Kaposi's sarcoma, AIDS-related
Bleomycin Sulfate

Keratinization disorders
Acitretin

Labial adhesions
Dienestrol

Labor, induction of
Castor Oil

Labor, preterm, management of
Albuterol
Amlodipine Besylate
Amoxicillin
Ampicillin
Diltiazem
Erythromycin, Injectable
Erythromycin, Oral
Indomethacin
Isoxsuprine Hydrochloride
Isradipine
Nicardipine Hydrochloride
Nifedipine
Nisoldipine
Terbutaline Sulfate
Verapamil Hydrochloride

Lactation, inhibition of
Cabergoline

Lactation, stimulation of
Metoclopramide Hydrochloride

Larva migrans, cutaneous
Ethyl Chloride

Laser vaporization
Cocaine Hydrochloride

Lavage, unspecified
Povidone-Iodine

Legionnaires' disease
Clarithromycin

Leishmaniasis, cutaneous
Sodium Chloride, Irrigation

Leishmaniasis, unspecified, prophylaxis of
Allopurinol
Pentamidine Isethionate
Permethrin

Leprosy
Minocycline Hydrochloride
Ofloxacin, Systemic

Leptospirosis
Doxycycline
Penicillin G Sodium

Leptotrichia buccalis infections
Erythromycin, Injectable
Erythromycin, Oral
Penicillin G Sodium

Lesch-Nyhan syndrome
Allopurinol

Leukemia, acute
Fludarabine Phosphate

Leukemia, acute lymphoblastic
Mitoxantrone Hydrochloride

Leukemia, acute myelogenous
Methotrexate

Leukemia, acute, promyelocytic
Arsenic Trioxide

Leukemia, chronic
Vincristine Sulfate

Leukemia, chronic lymphocytic
Doxorubicin Hydrochloride

Leukemia, chronic myeloid
Asparaginase
Methotrexate

Leukemia, unspecified
Topotecan Hydrochloride

Lichen planus
Acitretin

Lipid peroxidation
Zinc

Listeriosis
Ampicillin
Gentamicin Sulfate, Injectable

Liver transplantation
Alprostadil

Lung transplant
Muromonab-CD3

Lupus anticoagulant
Dicumarol

Lupus erythematosus, systemic
Quinacrine

Lymphoma, cutaneous T-cell
Isotretinoin

Lymphoma, follicular
Fludarabine Phosphate

Lymphoma, unspecified
Fludarabine Phosphate

Lymphomas, non-Hodgkin's
Idarubicin Hydrochloride
Ifosfamide
Leucovorin Calcium
Procarbazine Hydrochloride
Teniposide

M. catarrhalis infections
Cotrimoxazole
Erythromycin, Injectable
Erythromycin, Oral

Magnetic resonance imaging
Barium Sulfate

Malaria, prophylaxis of
Permethrin

Measles
Vitamin A

Meckel's diverticulitis
Cimetidine

Mediterranean spotted fever
Ciprofloxacin, Systemic

Melanoma
BCG
Dactinomycin
Megestrol Acetate

Menetrier's disease
Cimetidine

Meniere's disease
Hydrochlorothiazide
Streptomycin Sulfate

Meningitis
Ampicillin Sodium and Sulbactam Sodium
Aztreonam
Dexamethasone, Injectable
Dexamethasone, Oral

Meningitis, Mollaret's
Colchicine

Meningitis, meningococcal, treatment of
Trovafloxacin Mesylate

Meningoencephalitis, viral
Glycerin

Menopause, male
Gonadotropin, Chorionic

Menopause, management of the manifestations of
Estrogens, Conjugated
Megestrol Acetate

Menopause, vasomotor symptoms of
Clonidine
Methyldopa

Menorrhagia
Naproxen
Tranexamic Acid

Mental capacity, idiopathic, decline in
Prochlorperazine

Metagonimus yokogawai infection
Praziquantel

Mitral insufficiency
Hydralazine Hydrochloride

Mitral regurgitation
Ramipril

Mitral valve prolapse
Magnesium
Propranolol Hydrochloride

Molluscum contagiosum
Cantharidin
Cimetidine

Morganella morganii infections
Enoxacin

Mountain sickness
Dexamethasone, Injectable
Dexamethasone, Oral
Methazolamide

Mucositis
Povidone-Iodine

Mucositis, radiation-induced
Sucralfate

Multiple sclerosis
Cladribine
Pemoline
Prednisolone, Systemic

Myasthenia gravis, treatment of
Atracurium Besylate

Mycobacterium avium complex (MAC) infections
Ciprofloxacin, Systemic
Clofazimine

Mycobacterium infections, unspecified
Amikacin Sulfate
Capreomycin Sulfate
Clarithromycin
Doxycycline

Mycobacterium tuberculosis infection
Ciprofloxacin, Systemic

Mycobacterium, atypical, infections
Vancomycin Hydrochloride

Mycoplasma infections, unspecified
Tetracycline Hydrochloride, Oral

Mycoplasma pneumoniae infection
Doxycycline

Mycoplasmas, genital
Erythromycin, Injectable
Erythromycin, Oral

Mycosis fungoides
Carmustine
Cimetidine
Fludarabine Phosphate
Methoxsalen

Mydriasis, diagnosis of
Pilocarpine, Ophthalmic

Myeloma, multiple
Dexamethasone, Injectable
Dexamethasone, Oral
Doxorubicin Hydrochloride
Ifosfamide
Topotecan Hydrochloride
Vincristine Sulfate

Myocardial imaging, technetium-99m
Adenosine

Myocardial infarction, post, unspecified
Acebutolol Hydrochloride
Esmolol Hydrochloride
Labetalol Hydrochloride

Myocardial infarction, treatment adjunct
Alprostadil
Benazepril Hydrochloride
Diltiazem
Dipyridamole, Oral
Dobutamine Hydrochloride
Enalapril
Fosinopril Sodium
Insulin
Isosorbide Dinitrate
Isosorbide Mononitrate
Levocarnitine
Moexipril Hydrochloride
Nalbuphine Hydrochloride
Nisoldipine
Nitroglycerin
Phentolamine Mesylate
Potassium Chloride, Oral
Quinapril Hydrochloride
Quinidine Sulfate
Sodium Nitroprusside
Trandolapril
Verapamil Hydrochloride

Myoclonus, palatal
Botulinum Toxin Type A

N. meningitidis, carriers of
Ceftriaxone Sodium
Ciprofloxacin, Systemic

Nail psoriasis
Calcipotriene

Narcolepsy
Pemoline

Narcotic addiction, detoxification treatment of
Propoxyphene Hydrochloride

Narcotic effects, postoperative
Naloxone Hydrochloride

Nausea, emetogenic, cancer chemotherapy-induced
Droperidol

Nausea, postoperative
Dexamethasone, Injectable
Dexamethasone, Oral
Dimenhydrinate, Injectable
Granisetron Hydrochloride

Nephropathy
Benazepril Hydrochloride
Captopril
Enalapril
Fosinopril Sodium
Lisinopril
Moexipril Hydrochloride
Quinapril Hydrochloride
Ramipril
Trandolapril

Nephropathy, diabetic
Enalapril
Insulin

Nephrotoxicity, cisplatin-induced
Cimetidine

Nephrotoxicity, unspecified
Clonidine

Nerve damage
Thrombin

Nerve damage, nerve agent induced, prophylaxis of
Pyridostigmine Bromide

Neuralgia, postherpetic
Gabapentin

Neuralgia, trigeminal
Glycerin
Lamotrigine

Neuromuscular blockade
Clonidine

Neuropathy, diabetic
Desipramine Hydrochloride
Insulin

Neutropenia, febrile, to decrease the incidence of infection
Amikacin Sulfate
Cefoperazone/Sulbactam
Ceftazidime
Floxacillin
Gentamicin Sulfate, Injectable
Netilmicin Sulfate
Piperacillin Sodium
Ticarcillin Disodium
Tobramycin Sulfate, Injectable
Vancomycin Hydrochloride

Neutropenia, to decrease the incidence of infection
Nalidixic Acid

Nitrate tolerance, treatment of
Acetylcysteine

Nocardia infections, unspecified
Amikacin Sulfate
Cotrimoxazole

Nutrients, deficiency of
Levocarnitine

Obesity, unspecified
Diazoxide

Obsessive compulsive disorder
Clonidine

Obstetrics, use in
Clonidine
Methylene Blue
Streptokinase

Ocular inflammation
Indomethacin

Ophthalmia neonatorum
Povidone-Iodine

Ophthalmic disorders, diagnosis of
Proparacaine Hydrochloride

Ophthalmology, use in
Glycerin

Oral lesions, unspecified
Clobetasol Propionate

Ossification, heterotopic, prevention of
Indomethacin

Osteoarthritis
Chondroitin Sulfate
Mefenamic Acid
Vitamin E

Osteoporosis
Alendronate Sodium
Calcium

Osteoporosis, biliary cirrhosis associated
Calcitriol

Osteosarcoma
Bleomycin Sulfate
Ifosfamide

Otitis media
Ciprofloxacin, Systemic
Penicillin V Potassium
Prednisolone, Systemic
Xylometazoline

Otomycosis
Gentian Violet

Ovarian syndrome, polycystic
Follitropin Alpha

Ovulation, induction of
Leuprolide Acetate

P. falciparum infections
Atovaquone/Proguanil

P. malariae infections
Deferoxamine Mesylate
Doxycycline
Minocycline Hydrochloride

P. mallei infections
Doxycycline
Streptomycin Sulfate
Tetracycline Hydrochloride, Oral

P. maltophilia infections
Ciprofloxacin, Systemic
Ofloxacin, Systemic

Paget's disease of bone
Plicamycin

Pain, cancer
Fentanyl

Pain, dental
Celecoxib
Diclofenac Sodium and Misoprostol
Flurbiprofen, Oral
Rofecoxib

Pain, episiotomy
Meclofenamate Sodium

Pain, general
Clonidine
Guanethidine Monosulfate
Indomethacin
Metoclopramide Hydrochloride
Nifedipine
Suprofen

Pain, gynecologic
Flurbiprofen, Oral

Pain, intrapleural
Bupivacaine, Bupivacaine with Epinephrine, and Bupivacaine Spinal in Dextrose

Pain, neuropathic
Oxycodone Hydrochloride

Pain, obstetrical
Butorphanol Tartrate
Epinephrine, Systemic
Fentanyl
Isoflurane

Pain, postoperative, relief of
Bupivacaine, Bupivacaine with Epinephrine, and Bupivacaine Spinal in Dextrose
Clonidine
Glycopyrrolate

Pain, soft tissue
Diclofenac, Oral
Piroxicam

Pain, unspecified
Phentolamine Mesylate

Palsy, sixth nerve
Botulinum Toxin Type A

Pancreas transplantation, to reduce the incidence of rejection, adjunct in
Muromonab-CD3

Pancreatic insufficiency
Cimetidine

Panic disorder
Clomipramine Hydrochloride
Clonidine
Imipramine

Panic disorder, diagnosis of
Sodium Lactate

Paralysis, fetal
Pancuronium Bromide

Parkinson's disease
Apomorphine
Cabergoline
Selegiline Hydrochloride

Pelvic congestion
Dihydroergotamine Mesylate

Pemphigus
Tetracycline Hydrochloride, Oral

Peptic ulcer, adjunctive therapy in
Doxepin Hydrochloride
Furazolidone
Metoclopramide Hydrochloride
Omeprazole
Oxytetracycline Hydrochloride

Peptic ulcer, drug-induced
Cimetidine

Periodontitis
Tetracycline Hydrochloride, Oral

Peripheral vascular disease
Alprostadil

Pertechnetate administration for imaging, to decrease the accumulation of
Potassium Perchlorate

Pharyngitis, treatment of
Amoxicillin

Pheochromocytoma
Doxazosin Mesylate
Esmolol Hydrochloride

Pheochromocytoma, diagnosis of
Clonidine

Pheochromocytoma, malignant
Vincristine Sulfate

Pityrosporon orbiculare infections
Sulfur

Pleural effusion, malignant
Doxycycline

Pleural effusion, unspecified
Mitoxantrone Hydrochloride
Quinacrine

Pneumocystis carinii pneumonia
Dexamethasone, Injectable
Dexamethasone, Oral
Hydrocortisone, Systemic
Methylprednisolone
Prednisolone, Systemic
Pyrimethamine and Sulfadoxine
Triamcinolone

Pneumocystis carinii pneumonia, prophylaxis
Cotrimoxazole

Pneumonia, aspiration, prophylaxis
Cisapride

Pneumonitis, aspiration, prophylaxis
Cimetidine
Metoclopramide Hydrochloride
Ranitidine Hydrochloride

Pneumothorax
Quinacrine
Talc

Poisoning, ethylene glycol
Ethanol

Polycythemia vera
Hydroxyurea

Polyneuropathy
Amitriptyline Hydrochloride

Polyneuropathy, chronic inflammatory demyelinating
Immune Globulin

Pre-eclampsia
Nitroglycerin
Phenytoin

Pregnancy, ectopic
Dextrose
Methotrexate

Pregnancy, prevention of
Megestrol Acetate
Nafarelin Acetate

Pregnancy, termination of
Mannitol, Injectable
Methotrexate
Misoprostol
Urea, Injectable

Pregnancy, toxemia of
Aspirin

Priapism
Epinephrine, Systemic
Phenylephrine Hydrochloride

Proctalgia fugax
Diltiazem

Proctitis
Doxycycline
Sucralfate

Proctosigmoiditis, radiation-induced
Sucralfate

Prostatic hyperplasia, benign, symptomatic treatment
Finasteride
Flutamide
Megestrol Acetate

Prostatitis
Minocycline Hydrochloride

Protein C, deficiency of
Warfarin Sodium

Protein S, deficiency of
Warfarin Sodium

Providencia species infections
Enoxacin
Ofloxacin, Systemic

Providencia stuartii infections
Ceftazidime
Ceftriaxone Sodium
Ciprofloxacin, Systemic
Norfloxacin, Oral

Pruritus
Cyproheptadine Hydrochloride
Nalbuphine Hydrochloride
Propofol

Pruritus, drug-induced
Cimetidine

Pseudomonas species infections
Chloramphenicol

Psoriasis
Calcitriol
Capsaicin
Cimetidine
Nalidixic Acid
Propylthiouracil
Sulfasalazine
Tacrolimus

Psoriasis, vulgaris
Muromonab-CD3

Psychiatric disorders, aid in the evaluation of
Amobarbital Sodium

Psychological changes, postmenopausal
Estrogens, Conjugated

Psychosis, unspecified
Midazolam Hydrochloride

Ptosis
Phenylephrine Hydrochloride

Puberty, delayed
Oxandrolone

Pulmonary disease, chronic, obstructive
Albuterol

Purpura, idiopathic thrombocytopenic
Vincristine Sulfate

Purpura, thrombotic, thrombocytopenic
Aspirin
Dipyridamole, Oral

Pustulosis palmaris et plantaris
Methoxsalen

Q fever
Ofloxacin, Systemic

Radial keratotomy, post, relieving symptoms of
Diclofenac, Oral

Radioiodine therapy, protection against
Amifostine

Raynaud's disease
Alprostadil
Amlodipine Besylate
Nifedipine
Phenoxybenzamine Hydrochloride
Prazosin Hydrochloride
Verapamil Hydrochloride

Raynaud's phenomenon
Diltiazem
Losartan Potassium
Nicardipine Hydrochloride
Nisoldipine

Rectal ulcers
Sucralfate

Regurgitation, in infants
Cisapride

Renal allograft transplants, prophylaxis of organ rejection
Muromonab-CD3

Renal calculi
Nifedipine

Renal transplants, unspecified, prophylaxis of organ rejection
Rabbit Antithymocyte Globulin

Respiratory depression, CNS depressant overdosage-induced, treatment adjunct
Nalbuphine Hydrochloride

Respiratory distress syndrome
Betamethasone
Dexamethasone, Injectable
Dexamethasone, Oral
Methylprednisolone

Restenosis, prevention of
Vitamin C

Restless leg syndrome
Levodopa

Retinoblastoma
Teniposide

Retinopathy, diabetic
Insulin
Lisinopril

Reye's syndrome
Mannitol, Injectable

Rhabdomyosarcoma
Cyclophosphamide

Rheumatic fever, prophylaxis of
Penicillin G Sodium

Rheumatoid arthritis
Minocycline Hydrochloride
Rimexolone

Rhinitis, perennial allergic
Astemizole

Rhinitis, seasonal allergic
Hydroxyzine

Rickets
Calcitriol

Rickettsiae
Ciprofloxacin, Systemic

S. pyogenes infections
Penicillin V Potassium

Salmonella infection, carrier of
Ciprofloxacin, Systemic

Salmonella species infections
Ceftriaxone Sodium
Ciprofloxacin, Systemic
Norfloxacin, Oral
Ofloxacin, Systemic

Sarcoidosis
Pentoxifylline

Sarcoma, soft tissue
Ifosfamide

Scleroderma, esophageal
Ranitidine Hydrochloride

Sclerosis, systemic
Methoxsalen

Sclerotherapy
Dextrose
Doxycycline
Povidone-Iodine

Sedation, pediatric, during procedures
Chlorpromazine

Sedation, preoperative
Clonidine
Zolpidem Tartrate

Sedative addiction
Phenobarbital

Seizures, febrile
Phenobarbital

Seizures, focal
Gabapentin

Seizures, generalized, unspecified
Gabapentin
Topiramate

Seizures, malarial
Phenobarbital

Seizures, neurosurgery-induced, prophylaxis of
Phenobarbital

Seizures, posttraumatic
Phenytoin

Seizures, unspecified, adjunctive therapy in
Lorazepam
Paramethadione

Sepsis, biliary
Ciprofloxacin, Systemic

Sepsis, surgical
Netilmicin Sulfate

Septic shock, treatment adjunct
Dobutamine Hydrochloride
Epinephrine, Systemic
Milrinone Lactate

Septicemia, nonspecific
Ethanol

Serratia species infections
Ceftriaxone Sodium
Enoxacin

Sexual dysfunction
Cyproheptadine Hydrochloride
Paroxetine Hydrochloride

Sexually transmitted diseases, prevention of
Doxycycline

Sexually transmitted diseases, treatment of
Levofloxacin

Shigella species infections
Ofloxacin, Systemic

Shivering
Dexamethasone, Injectable
Dexamethasone, Oral

Shivering, postanesthetic
Methylphenidate Hydrochloride

Shivering, postoperative
Clonidine

Shock, septic
Norepinephrine Bitartrate

Sialorrhea
Benztropine Mesylate
Clonidine

Sickle cell crisis
Nalbuphine Hydrochloride

Sinusitis
Amoxicillin
Cephalexin
Dexbrompheniramine Maleate
Erythromycin Ethylsuccinate with Sulfisoxazole Acetyl
Flunisolide

Skin conditions, premalignant
Etretinate

Skin disorders
Acrivastine

Skin ulcers
Pentoxifylline

Skin, dry, moisturization of
Urea, Topical

Sleep, induction of, long term treatment
Zolpidem Tartrate

Spasm, arterial
Sodium Nitroprusside

Spasm, hemifacial
Botulinum Toxin Type A

Spasms, infantile
Cosyntropin

Spasticity, unspecified
Botulinum Toxin Type A
Clonidine

Speech disorders
Botulinum Toxin Type A

Sperm motility, improvement of
Pentoxifylline

Spinal cord injury
Terazosin Hydrochloride

Spinal cord protection, intraoperative
Papaverine Hydrochloride

Spirillum minus infections
Streptomycin Sulfate

Staphylococci, penicillinase-producing, infections
Floxacillin

Staphylococcus species infections
Enoxacin
Penicillin V Potassium

Steatorrhea, adjunctive therapy in
Cimetidine

Sterilization, female
Quinacrine

Stomatitis
Sucralfate

Stomatitis, recurrent aphthous, symptomatic relief of
Mesalamine

Streptobacillus moniliformis infections
Streptomycin Sulfate

Streptococcal infections, neonatal, prophylaxis of
Ampicillin

Streptococci group B infections
Clindamycin, Systemic

Streptococci group B infections, prophylaxis of
Penicillin G Sodium

Streptococci group D infections
Ciprofloxacin, Systemic
Gentamicin Sulfate, Injectable
Norfloxacin, Oral
Ofloxacin, Systemic

Streptococci species infections
Vancomycin Hydrochloride

Stress disorder, post-traumatic
Propranolol Hydrochloride

Stroke, to reduce the risk of
Lovastatin

Stroke, unspecified
Streptokinase

Superior vena cava syndrome
Streptokinase

Surgery, adjunct in
Dextrose
Gentian Violet
Oxymetazoline
Phentolamine Mesylate

Surgery, ophthalmic, adjunct to
Botulinum Toxin Type A

Surgical procedures, ear, nose and throat
Cocaine Hydrochloride

Syncope
Metoprolol
Midodrine Hydrochloride

Syncope, diagnosis of
Adenosine

Syndrome X
Doxazosin Mesylate

T-cell function, improvement of
Arginine Hydrochloride

T. pallidum infections
Cephradine

Tachyarrhythmias, supraventricular, intrauterine
Digoxin

Teeth, bleaching of
Hydrogen Peroxide

Telangiectasias
Estropipate

Tetanus
Amobarbital Sodium
Pancuronium Bromide

Thalassemia major
Deferoxamine Mesylate

Thrombocythemia
Aspirin
Hydroxyurea

Thrombocytopenia, antenatal and neonatal
Immune Globulin

Thrombocytopenia, unspecified
Immune Globulin

Thromboembolic complications
Dipyridamole, Oral

Thromboembolic complications, prosthetic heart valve related, prevention of
Aspirin

Thrombosis, atrial, acute, lysis of
Streptokinase

Thrombosis, deep venous, prophylaxis of
Enoxaparin Sodium

Thrombosis, deep venous, treatment of
Enoxaparin Sodium

Thrombosis, lysis of, during coronary artery bypass graft
Urokinase

Thrombosis, prosthetic heart valve
Streptokinase

Thrombosis, renal vein
Streptokinase

Thrombosis, unspecified
Stanozolol
Urokinase

Thrombosis, ventricular, lysis of
Streptokinase

Thyroid stimulating hormone, hypersecretion of
Octreotide Acetate

Thyroid storm
Esmolol Hydrochloride

Tinea pedis infections
Salicylic Acid

Tinea unguium infections
Tioconazole

Tissue preservation
Papaverine Hydrochloride

Tomography, computed, single photon emisson (SPECT), stress test
Dipyridamole, Oral
Dobutamine Hydrochloride

Tomography, computerized, for hepatic imaging
Ethiodized Oil

Tomography, positron emission (PET), stress test
Dobutamine Hydrochloride

Tooth, hypersensitivity of
Magnesium
Sodium Fluoride

Torsade de Pointes
Mexiletine Hydrochloride

Torticollis
Pancuronium Bromide

Tourette, Gilles de la, syndrome
Clonidine

Toxicity, drug, unspecified
Esmolol Hydrochloride

Toxicity, ergotamine
Sodium Nitroprusside

Toxicity, inhalation, unspecified
Acetylcysteine

Toxicity, nitrous oxide
Leucovorin Calcium

Transplantation complications, unspecified
Diltiazem
Lisinopril

Transurethral prostatic resection, adjunct in
Ciprofloxacin, Systemic
Enoxacin

Transurethral surgical procedures, adjunct in
Bupivacaine, Bupivacaine with Epinephrine, and Bupivacaine Spinal in Dextrose

Trauma, treatment adjunct
Bendroflumethiazide

Tremor, unspecified
Botulinum Toxin Type A
Propranolol Hydrochloride

Tuberculosis, treatment
Kanamycin Sulfate
Ofloxacin, Systemic

Tularemia
Streptomycin Sulfate

Tumors, brain, metastatic, palliative therapy in
Thioguanine

Tumors, brain, palliative therapy in
Procarbazine Hydrochloride
Teniposide
Vincristine Sulfate

Tumors, carcinoid, symptomatic relief of
Streptozocin

Tumors, germ cell
Vinblastine Sulfate

Tumors, gynecological
Ferumoxsil

Tumors, sinus
Dactinomycin

Turner's syndrome
Oxandrolone

Typhus group infection
Doxycycline

Ulcers, decubitus, adjunctive therapy in
Silver Sulfadiazine

Ulcers, gastric
Misoprostol
Sucralfate

Ulcers, unspecified
Glycine

Ureaplasma urealyticum infections
Clarithromycin
Erythromycin, Injectable
Erythromycin, Oral

Urethritis
Lomefloxacin Hydrochloride
Oxytetracycline Hydrochloride
Penicillin G Procaine
Sparfloxacin

Urethritis, non-gonococcal
Tetracycline Hydrochloride, Oral

Urine, alkalinization of
Sodium Lactate

Urolithiasis, management of
Bendroflumethiazide
Pentosan Polysulfate Sodium

Uterine bleeding
Estrogens, Esterified

Uterine contractions, drug-induced, inhibition of
Ritodrine Hydrochloride

Uterine contractions, inhibition of
Nitroglycerin

Vaginal disinfection, obstetrical
Chlorhexidine Gluconate

Vaginitis, trichomonas
Tinidazole

Vaginosis, bacterial
Boric Acid
Tinidazole

Vaginosis, bacterial, oral
Clindamycin, Systemic

Vascular prosthesis
Aspirin

Vasculitis
Aspirin
Colchicine
Prednisolone, Systemic

Venous vasodilation, induction of, for IV access
Nitroglycerin

Ventriculography, diagnostic aid in
Dobutamine Hydrochloride

Vertigo
Astemizole

Vibrio vulnificus
Doxycycline

Voice disorders
Botulinum Toxin Type A

Vomiting, emetogenic, cancer chemotherapy-induced
Dexamethasone, Injectable
Dexamethasone, Oral
Droperidol

Vomiting, emetogenic, radiation therapy-induced
Granisetron Hydrochloride

Vomiting, postoperative
Dexamethasone, Injectable
Dexamethasone, Oral
Dimenhydrinate, Injectable
Granisetron Hydrochloride

Vomiting, pregnancy induced
Meclizine Hydrochloride

Vulvovaginitis
Boric Acid

Warts
Bleomycin Sulfate
Cantharidin
Cimetidine
Podophyllum

Water, intoxication of
Mannitol, Injectable

Water, purification of
Iodine

Wheezing, in infants, symptomatic relief of
Epinephrine, Systemic

Whipple's disease
Streptomycin Sulfate

Withdrawal, glutethimide
Phenobarbital

Withdrawal, narcotic, adjunctive therapy in
Clonidine
Opium
Phenobarbital

Withdrawal, nicotine, treatment adjunct
Clonidine

Wolff-Parkinson-White syndrome
Flecainide Acetate
Procainamide Hydrochloride

Wound care, adjunctive therapy in
Benzalkonium Chloride
Magnesium
Oxacillin Sodium

Wounds, disinfection of
Iodine

Yaws
Penicillin G Sodium

Yersinia enterocolitica infections
Amikacin Sulfate
Ciprofloxacin, Systemic
Gentamicin Sulfate, Injectable
Tobramycin Sulfate, Injectable

Yersinia infections, unspecified
Ofloxacin, Systemic

Zollinger-Ellison syndrome
Cimetidine

SECTION 6

CONTRAINDICATIONS INDEX

This section lists in alphabetical order every medical condition cited as a contraindication in *PDR*® and its companion volumes, with cross-references to all product entries in which the contraindication is found. Page numbers refer to the 2002 editions of *PDR*® and *PDR For Ophthalmic Medicines™* and the 2001 edition of *PDR For Nonprescription Drugs and Dietary Supplements™*, which is published later in the year. A key to the symbols denoting the companion volumes appears in the bottom margin.

These listings will enable you to quickly identify drugs that generally threaten to be inappropriate in the presence of a given complication. However, a drug's suitability is sometimes affected by the severity of the complicating condition, the age or gender of the patient, and the drug's route of administration. In ambiguous situations, a quick review of the underlying *PDR*® text may therefore prove helpful.

Note, too, that the index does not list other drugs and dietary items whose use would present a contraindication. Contraindicated combinations can be found in the Interactions Index and the Food Interactions Cross-Reference. Hypersensitivity to the product's ingredients—an almost universal contraindication—also has not been indexed here. If the clinical picture includes the risk of allergic reaction, be sure to check individual product labeling for additional information.

A

Abortion, infected
Mirena Intrauterine System 974
ParaGard T 380A Intrauterine Copper Contraceptive 2582

Abortion, missed
Aygestin Tablets 1333
Crinone 3213
Premphase Tablets........................ 3572
Prometrium Capsules (100 mg, 200 mg) 3261
Provera Tablets 2853

Abortion, threatened
Coumadin for Injection 1243
Coumadin Tablets.......................... 1243
Warfarin Sodium Tablets, USP 3302

Abscess, intestinal
Cortifoam Rectal Foam................... 3170

Achalasia, esophageal
Fosamax Tablets 2095

Achalasia, unspecified
Donnatal 2929
Donnatal Extentabs 2930
Donnatal Tablets 2929
Levsin/Levsinex/Levbid................... 3172
NuLev Orally Disintegrating Tablets 3176
Robinul Forte Tablets 1358
Robinul Injectable.......................... 2940
Robinul Tablets.............................. 1358

Acid base imbalance, uncorrected
(*see under* Acidosis, hyperchloremic; Acidosis, metabolic, unspecified; Ketoacidosis, diabetic)

Acidosis, hyperchloremic
Daranide Tablets 2077

Acidosis, metabolic, unspecified
(*see also under* Ketoacidosis, diabetic)
Glucophage Tablets 1080
Glucophage XR Tablets 1080
Glucovance Tablets 1086

Acquired immune deficiency syndrome
(*see also under* Human immunodeficiency virus)
Attenuvax 2044
Meruvax II 2130
M-M-R II.. 2118
Mumpsvax..................................... 2141
ParaGard T 380A Intrauterine Copper Contraceptive 2582
Tice BCG, BCG Live 2489
Varivax.. 2202
YF-VAX Vaccine 827

Actinomycosis, genital
Mirena Intrauterine System 974
ParaGard T 380A Intrauterine Copper Contraceptive 2582

Adams-Stokes syndrome
Cerebyx Injection........................... 2619

Addison's disease, untreated
Rum-K 1363

Adenoma, hepatic
Alesse-21 Tablets.......................... 3468
Alesse-28 Tablets.......................... 3473
Brevicon 28-Day Tablets 3380
Cyclessa Tablets 2450
Desogen Tablets............................ 2458
Estrostep 2627
Levlen 962
Levlite 21 Tablets........................... 962
Levlite 28 Tablets........................... 962
Levora Tablets............................... 3389
Loestrin 21 Tablets 2642
Loestrin Fe Tablets........................ 2642
Lo/Ovral Tablets............................ 3532
Lo/Ovral-28 Tablets 3538
Low-Ogestrel-28 Tablets 3392
Lunelle Monthly Injection................ 2827
Microgestin Fe 1.5/30 Tablets 3407
Microgestin Fe 1/20 Tablets 3400
Mircette Tablets 2470
Modicon 2563
Necon 3415
Nordette-28 Tablets....................... 2257
Norinyl 1 +35 28-Day Tablets 3380
Norinyl 1 + 50 28-Day Tablets 3380
Ogestrel 0.5/50-28 Tablets............ 3428
Ortho-Cept 21 Tablets.................... 2546
Ortho-Cept 28 Tablets.................... 2546
Ortho-Cyclen/Ortho Tri-Cyclen......... 2573
Ortho-Novum 2563
Ortho-Novum 1/50□28 Tablets....... 2556
Ortho-Novum 2563
Ortho-Cyclen/Ortho Tri-Cyclen......... 2573
Ovcon.. 3364
Ovral Tablets 3551
Ovral-28 Tablets 3552
Ovrette Tablets 3552
Tri-Levlen 962
Tri-Norinyl-28 Tablets 3433
Triphasil-21 Tablets 3600
Triphasil-28 Tablets 3605
Trivora Tablets 3439
Yasmin 28 Tablets........................... 980
Zovia 3449

Adrenal cortical insufficiency
(*see under* Addison's disease, untreated; Adrenal insufficiency, uncorrected; Adrenal insufficiency, unspecified)

Adrenal dysfunction, uncontrolled
Ovidrel for Injection 3220

Adrenal dysfunction, uncorrected
(*see also under* Adrenal insufficiency, uncorrected)
Clomid Tablets 735
Follistim for Injection..................... 2465
Gonal-F for Injection 3216
Humegon for Injection 2468
Pergonal for Injection 3223
Repronex for Intramuscular and Subcutaneous Injection 1347
Serophene Tablets 3226

Adrenal gland failure
(*see under* Adrenal insufficiency, unspecified)

Adrenal insufficiency, uncorrected
(*see also under* Addison's disease, untreated; Adrenal dysfunction, uncorrected)
Cytomel Tablets............................. 1817
Levothroid Tablets 1373
Levoxyl Tablets 1819
Synthroid... 505
Unithroid Tablets 3445

Adrenal insufficiency, unspecified
Daranide Tablets 2077
Triostat Injection........................... 1825
Urocit-K Tablets 2232
Yasmin 28 Tablets........................... 980

Adrenocortical insufficiency
(*see under* Adrenal insufficiency, uncorrected; Adrenal insufficiency, unspecified)

Agitated states
(*see under* Agitation)

Agitation
Adderall Tablets............................ 3231
Adipex-P 1406
Bontril Slow-Release Capsules 576
Concerta Extended-Release Tablets 1998
Concerta Tablets 561
Desoxyn Tablets 440
Dexedrine...................................... 1512
DextroStat Tablets......................... 3236
Ionamin Capsules 1163
Metadate CD Capsules 1164
Metadate ER Tablets 1167
Methylin Tablets 1995
Methylin ER Tablets....................... 1995
Ritalin 2387

Agranulocytosis, history of
Clozaril Tablets.............................. 2319
Cuprimine Capsules 2075
Depen Titratable Tablets................. 3341

AIDS
(*see under* Acquired immune deficiency syndrome)

Albinism
8-MOP Capsules............................. 1727
Oxsoralen-Ultra Capsules 1741

Alcoholism
Roxanol 3066

Alcoholism, unsupervised
Coumadin for Injection 1243
Coumadin Tablets 1243
Warfarin Sodium Tablets, USP 3302

Allograft
(*see under* Bone marrow transplantation; Organ allograft)

Amino acid metabolism disorders
(*see under* Electrolyte imbalance, uncorrected)

Amniocentesis, genetic
MICRhoGAM Injection 2524

Anastomosis, unspecified
(*see also under* Ileocolostomy)
Cortifoam Rectal Foam 3170
Roxanol 3066
Urecholine 2198
Urecholine Tablets 2445

Anemia, aplastic, history of
Cuprimine Capsules 2075
Depen Titratable Tablets 3341
Ticlid Tablets 3015

Anemia, hemolytic, history of
Cefotan 664
Skelaxin Tablets 1301

Anemia, megaloblastic, unspecified
(*see also under* Anemia, pernicious)
Bactrim 2949
Daraprim Tablets 1511
Septra Suspension 2265
Septra Tablets 2265
Septra DS Tablets 2265

Anemia, non-iron deficiency, unspecified
Ferrlecit Injection 3386
INFeD Injection 3388
Venofer Injection 580

Anemia, sickle cell
Caverject Sterile Powder 2777
MUSE Urethral Suppository 3335

Anemia, unspecified
Albumin (Human) 5% 838
Albumin (Human) 25% 839
Albuminar-5, U.S.P. 785
Albuminar-25, U.S.P. 786
Buminate 5% Solution, USP 841
Buminate 25% Solution, USP 842
Mylocel Tablets 2227
Nitrostat Tablets 2658
Plasbumin-5 939
Plasbumin-20 940
Plasbumin-25 941
Plasmanate 942

Anemia, unspecified, history of
Skelaxin Tablets 1301

Anesthesia, general
Nardil Tablets 2653
Parnate Tablets 1607

Anesthesia, local
(*see also under* Anesthesia, major regional lumbar block; Anesthesia, obstetrical, paracervical block; Denervation, skeletal muscle)
Nardil Tablets 2653
Parnate Tablets 1607

Anesthesia, major regional lumbar block
Coumadin for Injection 1243
Coumadin Tablets 1243
Warfarin Sodium Tablets, USP 3302

Anesthesia, obstetrical, paracervical block
Sensorcaine 643
Sensorcaine-MPF Injection 643

Anesthesia, obstetrical, unspecified
Fluothane Inhalation 3508

Aneurysm
(*see also under* Cerebrovascular accident)
Activase I.V. 1410
Aggrastat 2031
Coumadin for Injection 1243
Coumadin Tablets 1243
ReoPro Vials 1958
Retavase Vials 1182
TNKase I.V. 1430
Warfarin Sodium Tablets, USP 3302

Angina pectoris
Amerge Tablets 1467
Axert Tablets 2772
D.H.E. 45 Injection 2334
Imitrex Injection 1549
Imitrex Nasal Spray 1554
Imitrex Tablets 1558
Maxalt Tablets 2120
Maxalt-MLT Orally Disintegrating Tablets 2120
Migranal Nasal Spray 2376
Zomig Tablets 708
Zomig-ZMT Tablets 708

Angina, Prinzmetal's
Amerge Tablets 1467
Axert Tablets 2772
D.H.E. 45 Injection 2334
Imitrex Injection 1549
Imitrex Nasal Spray 1554
Imitrex Tablets 1558
Maxalt Tablets 2120
Maxalt-MLT Orally Disintegrating Tablets 2120
Migranal Nasal Spray 2376
Zomig Tablets 708
Zomig-ZMT Tablets 708

Angina, unspecified, history of
Proleukin for Injection 1199

Angina, unstable
Visicol Tablets 1767

Angioedema, hereditary
Prinivil Tablets 2164
Prinzide Tablets 2168
Vaseretic Tablets 2204
Vasotec I.V. Injection 2207
Vasotec Tablets 2210

Angioedema, idiopathic
Prinivil Tablets 2164
Prinzide Tablets 2168
Vaseretic Tablets 2204
Vasotec I.V. Injection 2207
Vasotec Tablets 2210

Angulation, penile
Caverject Sterile Powder 2777
MUSE Urethral Suppository 3335

Anorexia nervosa
Meridia Capsules 481
Wellbutrin Tablets 1680
Wellbutrin SR Sustained-Release Tablets 1684
Zyban Sustained-Release Tablets 1710

Antepartum prophylaxis
MICRhoGAM Injection 2524

Anuria
Accuretic Tablets 2614
Aldoclor Tablets 2035
Aldoril Tablets 2039
Avalide Tablets 1070
Calcium Disodium Versenate Injection 1980
Clorpres Tablets 1002
Combipres Tablets 1040
Corzide 40/5 Tablets 2247
Corzide 80/5 Tablets 2247
Demadex Tablets and Injection 2905
Desferal Vials 2333
Diovan HCT Tablets 2338
Diucardin Tablets 3494
Diuril Oral 2087
Diuril Sodium Intravenous 2086
Dyazide Capsules 1515
Dyrenium Capsules 3458
Edecrin 2091
Furosemide Tablets 2284
HydroDIURIL Tablets 2108
Hyzaar 2109
Indapamide Tablets 2286
Inderide Tablets 3517
Inderide LA Long-Acting Capsules 3519
Lotensin HCT Tablets 2367
Macrobid Capsules 2889
Macrodantin Capsules 2891
Maxzide 1008
Micardis HCT Tablets 1051
Microzide Capsules 3414
Midamor Tablets 2136
Minizide Capsules 2700
Moduretic Tablets 2138
Monopril HCT 1094
Mykrox Tablets 1168
Prinzide Tablets 2168
Renese Tablets 2712
Tenoretic Tablets 690
Timolide Tablets 2187
Uniretic Tablets 3178
Vaseretic Tablets 2204
Zaroxolyn Tablets 1177
Zestoretic Tablets 695
Ziac Tablets 1887

Anxiety
Concerta Extended-Release Tablets 1998
Concerta Tablets 561
Metadate CD Capsules 1164
Metadate ER Tablets 1167
Methylin Tablets 1995
Methylin ER Tablets 1995
Ritalin 2387

Aortic coarctation
(*see under* Stenosis, aortic)

Aortic dissection
Aggrastat 2031

Aortic stenosis
(*see under* Stenosis, aortic)

Aphakia
8-MOP Capsules 1727
Oxsoralen-Ultra Capsules 1741

Apoplexy, cerebral
(*see under* Cerebrovascular accident)

Appendicitis
Dulcolax Suppositories ▣668
Dulcolax Tablets ▣668

Arrhythmia, cardiac, history of
Proleukin for Injection 1199
Serentil 1057

Arrhythmia, cardiac, unspecified
(*see also under* Arrhythmia, ventricular, unspecified; Bradycardia, sinus; Bradycardia, unspecified; Fibrillation, atrial; Fibrillation, ventricular; Flutter, atrial; Heart block, first degree; Heart block, greater than first degree; Heart block, sinoatrial; Heart block, unspecified; Lown-Ganong-Levine syndrome; PR Syndrome, short; Q-T interval prolongation; Sick sinus syndrome; Sinus node dysfunction, unspecified; Tachycardia, unspecified; Tachycardia, ventricular; Tachycardia, ventricular, history of; Torsade de pointes; Wolff-Parkinson-White syndrome)
Flexeril Tablets 572
Flexeril Tablets 2094
Quinidex Extentabs 2933
Roxanol 3066
Rythmol Tablets – 150 mg, 225 mg, 300 mg 502
Urimax Tablets 1769

Arrhythmia, ventricular, unspecified
(*see also under* Fibrillation, ventricular; Tachycardia, ventricular; Tachycardia, ventricular, history of; Ventricular dysfunction, left)
Quinidex Extentabs 2933

Arterial disease, unspecified
(*see under* Angina pectoris; Angina, Prinzmetal's; Angina, unstable; Arteriosclerosis, unspecified; Arteriovenous malformation; Coronary artery disease; Coronary artery vasospasm; Stenosis, aortic; Stenosis, subaortic)

Arteriosclerosis, unspecified
(*see also under* Coronary artery disease; Stenosis, aortic; Stenosis, subaortic)
Adderall Tablets 3231
Adipex-P 1406
Bontril Slow-Release Capsules 576
Desoxyn Tablets 440
Dexedrine 1512
DextroStat Tablets 3236
Ionamin Capsules 1163

Arteriovenous malformation
Activase I.V. 1410
Aggrastat 2031
ReoPro Vials 1958
Retavase Vials 1182
TNKase I.V. 1430

Ascites
Visicol Tablets 1767

Asthma, acute
(*see also under* Status asthmaticus)
Advair Diskus 100/50 1448
Advair Diskus 250/50 1448
Advair Diskus 500/50 1448
Astramorph/PF Injection, USP (Preservative-Free) 594
Azmacort Inhalation Aerosol 728
Bromfed Capsules (Extended-Release) 2269
Bromfed-PD Capsules (Extended-Release) 2269
Dopram Injectable 2931
Duramorph Injection 1312
Flovent Diskus 3614
Flovent Rotadisk 1537
Kadian Capsules 1335
MS Contin Tablets 2896
MSIR 2898
Oramorph SR Tablets 3062
OxyContin Tablets 2912
OxyFast Oral Concentrate Solution 2916
OxyIR Capsules 2916
Pulmicort Respules 632
Pulmicort Turbuhaler Inhalation Powder 636
Qvar Inhalation Aerosol 1987
Roxanol 3066
Roxicodone Tablets 3067
Urecholine 2198
Urecholine Tablets 2445
Vanceril Inhalation Aerosol 3165
Vanceril Double Strength Inhalation Aerosol 3167

Asthma, history of
Betagan ⊙228
Betimol Ophthalmic Solution ⊙324
Blocadren Tablets 2046
Carteolol Hydrochloride Ophthalmic Solution USP, 1% ⊙258
Cosopt Sterile Ophthalmic Solution 2065
Ocupress Ophthalmic Solution, 1% Sterile ⊙303
OptiPranolol Metipranolol Ophthalmic Solution 0.3% ⊙263
Timolide Tablets 2187
Timolol GFS ⊙266
Timoptic in Ocudose 2192
Timoptic Sterile Ophthalmic Solution 2190
Timoptic-XE Sterile Ophthalmic Gel Forming Solution 2194

Asthma, unspecified
Adenoscan 1381
Betagan ⊙228
Betapace Tablets 950
Betapace AF Tablets 954
Betimol Ophthalmic Solution ⊙324
Blocadren Tablets 2046
Carteolol Hydrochloride Ophthalmic Solution USP, 1% ⊙258
Coreg Tablets 1508
Corgard Tablets 2245
Corzide 40/5 Tablets 2247
Corzide 80/5 Tablets 2247
Cosopt Sterile Ophthalmic Solution 2065
Inderal 3513
Inderal LA Long-Acting Capsules 3516
Inderide Tablets 3517
Inderide LA Long-Acting Capsules 3519
Kadian Capsules 1335
Mestinon Syrup 1740
MS Contin Tablets 2896
MSIR 2898
Nadolol Tablets 2288
Normodyne Injection 3135
Normodyne Tablets 3137
Ocupress Ophthalmic Solution, 1% Sterile ⊙303
OptiPranolol Metipranolol Ophthalmic Solution 0.3% ⊙263
Oramorph SR Tablets 3062
OxyContin Tablets 2912
OxyFast Oral Concentrate Solution 2916
OxyIR Capsules 2916
Phenergan Suppositories 3556
Phenergan Syrup 3554
Phenergan Tablets 3556
Phenergan with Codeine Syrup 3557
Phenergan with Dextromethorphan Syrup 3559
Phenergan VC Syrup 3560
Phenergan VC with Codeine Syrup 3561
Roxicodone Tablets 3067
Rynatan Tablets 3351
Salagen Tablets 2229
Timolide Tablets 2187
Timolol GFS ⊙266

Timoptic in Ocudose 2192
Timoptic Sterile Ophthalmic Solution 2190
Timoptic-XE Sterile Ophthalmic Gel Forming Solution 2194
Urecholine 2198
Urecholine Tablets 2445

Asthmatic attack
(*see under* Asthma, acute)

Atony, intestinal
Donnatal 2929
Donnatal Extentabs 2930
Donnatal Tablets 2929
Levsin/Levsinex/Levbid 3172
NuLev Orally Disintegrating Tablets 3176
Robinul Forte Tablets 1358
Robinul Injectable 2940
Robinul Tablets 1358

Atresia, pulmonary
Indocin I.V. 2115

Atrial fibrillation
(*see under* Fibrillation, atrial)

Atrial flutter
(*see under* Flutter, atrial)

Atrioventricular block
(*see under* Heart block, first degree; Heart block, greater than first degree; Heart block, unspecified)

AV block
(*see under* Heart block, first degree; Heart block, greater than first degree; Heart block, unspecified)

Azotemia
(*see also under* Uremia)
Edecrin 2091

B

Bacterial endocarditis
(*see under* Endocarditis, bacterial)

Balanitis
MUSE Urethral Suppository 3335

Bedridden
(*see under* Debilitation)

Bilirubinemia
Cognex Capsules 1351

Birthmarks
Podocon-25 Liquid 2608

Bladder neck obstruction
(*see under* Obstruction, bladder neck)

Bleeding disorders, unspecified
(*see also under* Bleeding tendencies; Hemophilia; Thrombocytopathy, unspecified; Thrombocytopenia, unspecified; Thrombocytopenic purpura, history of)
Indocin I.V. 2115
Mithracin for Intravenous Use 903
Soma Compound Tablets 3354
Soma Compound w/Codeine Tablets 3355
Ticlid Tablets 3015

Bleeding tendencies
Activase I.V. 1410
Aggrastat 2031
Astramorph/PF Injection, USP (Preservative-Free) 594
Coumadin for Injection 1243
Coumadin Tablets 1243
Mithracin for Intravenous Use 903
Orgaran Injection 2480
ReoPro Vials 1958
Retavase Vials 1182
TNKase I.V. 1430
Toradol 3018
Warfarin Sodium Tablets, USP 3302

Bleeding, abnormal, unspecified
(*see also under* Hematuria)
Indocin I.V. 2115
Orgaran Injection 2480
Pergonal for Injection 3223
Repronex for Intramuscular and Subcutaneous Injection 1347

Bleeding, arterial
Niaspan Extended-Release Tablets 1846

Bleeding, cerebrovascular
(*see under* Bleeding, intracranial; Cerebrovascular accident)

Bleeding, gastrointestinal
Indocin I.V. 2115
Plavix Tablets 1097
Plavix Tablets 3084
Reglan 2935
ReoPro Vials 1958
Ticlid Tablets 3015
Toradol 3018

Bleeding, gastrointestinal, history of
Proleukin for Injection 1199
Toradol 3018

Bleeding, genital, abnormal
(*see also under* Bleeding, genitourinary)
Activella Tablets 2764
Alesse-21 Tablets 3468
Alesse-28 Tablets 3473
Alora Transdermal System 3372
Aygestin Tablets 1333
Brevicon 28-Day Tablets 3380
Cenestin Tablets 1263
Cervidil Vaginal Insert 1369
Climara Transdermal System 958
Clomid Tablets 735
CombiPatch Transdermal System 2323
Crinone 3213
Cyclessa Tablets 2450
Depo-Provera Contraceptive Injection 2798
Desogen Tablets 2458
Esclim Transdermal System 3460
Estinyl Tablets 3112
Estrace Tablets 3361
Estratest 3252
Estring Vaginal Ring 2811
Estrostep 2627
femhrt Tablets 2635
Follistim for Injection 2465
Gonal-F for Injection 3216
Humegon for Injection 2468
Levlen 962
Levlite 21 Tablets 962
Levlite 28 Tablets 962
Levora Tablets 3389
Loestrin 21 Tablets 2642
Loestrin Fe Tablets 2642
Lo/Ovral Tablets 3532
Lo/Ovral-28 Tablets 3538
Low-Ogestrel-28 Tablets 3392
Lunelle Monthly Injection 2827
Lupron Depot 3.75 mg 3281
Lupron Depot–3 Month 11.25 mg 3285
Menest Tablets 2254
Microgestin Fe 1.5/30 Tablets 3407
Microgestin Fe 1/20 Tablets 3400
Micronor Tablets 2543
Mircette Tablets 2470
Mirena Intrauterine System 974
Modicon 2563
Necon 3415
Nordette-28 Tablets 2257
Norinyl 1 +35 28-Day Tablets 3380
Norinyl 1 + 50 28-Day Tablets 3380
Norplant System 3543
Nor-QD Tablets 3423
Ogen Tablets 2846
Ogestrel 0.5/50-28 Tablets 3428
Ortho Dienestrol Cream 2554
Ortho-Cept 21 Tablets 2546
Ortho-Cept 28 Tablets 2546
Ortho-Cyclen/Ortho Tri-Cyclen 2573
Ortho-Est Tablets 3464
Ortho-Novum 2563
Ortho-Novum 1/50□28 Tablets 2556
Ortho-Novum 2563
Ortho-Prefest Tablets 2570
Ortho-Cyclen/Ortho Tri-Cyclen 2573
Ovcon 3364
Ovidrel for Injection 3220
Ovral Tablets 3551
Ovral-28 Tablets 3552
Ovrette Tablets 3552
ParaGard T 380A Intrauterine Copper Contraceptive 2582
Pergonal for Injection 3223
Premarin Intravenous 3563
Premarin Tablets 3566
Premarin Vaginal Cream 3570
Premphase Tablets 3572
Prempro Tablets 3572
Prepidil Gel 2851
Prometrium Capsules (100 mg, 200 mg) 3261
Provera Tablets 2853
Repronex for Intramuscular and Subcutaneous Injection 1347
Serophene Tablets 3226
Synarel Nasal Solution for Central Precocious Puberty 3204
Synarel Nasal Solution for Endometriosis 3205
Tri-Levlen 962
Tri-Norinyl-28 Tablets 3433
Triphasil-21 Tablets 3600
Triphasil-28 Tablets 3605
Trivora Tablets 3439
Vagifem Tablets 2857
Vivelle Transdermal System 2412
Vivelle-Dot Transdermal System 2416
Yasmin 28 Tablets 980
Zovia 3449

Bleeding, genitourinary
(*see also under* Bleeding, genital, abnormal)
ReoPro Vials 1958

Bleeding, history of
Aggrastat 2031
Duraclon Injection 3057
Integrilin Injection 1213
Integrilin Injection 1828
Oncaspar 756

Bleeding, internal, unspecified
(*see also under* Hematuria)
Activase I.V. 1410
ReoPro Vials 1958
Retavase Vials 1182
Streptase for Infusion 647
TNKase I.V. 1430

Bleeding, intracranial
(*see also under* Cerebrovascular accident)
Aggrastat 2031
Coumadin for Injection 1243
Coumadin Tablets 1243
Indocin I.V. 2115
Plavix Tablets 1097
Plavix Tablets 3084
Ticlid Tablets 3015
Toradol 3018
Trental Tablets 784
Warfarin Sodium Tablets, USP 3302

Bleeding, rectal
Dulcolax Suppositories ◘668
Dulcolax Tablets ◘668
Indocin Suppositories 2112

Bleeding, retinal
Trental Tablets 784

Bleeding, unspecified
(*see also under* Bleeding, internal, unspecified; Hematuria; Hemostasis, incomplete)
Argatroban Injection 1478
Coumadin for Injection 1243
Coumadin Tablets 1243
Fragmin Injection 2814
Heparin Lock Flush Solution 3509
Heparin Sodium Injection 3511
Humegon for Injection 2468
Innohep Injection 1248
Lovenox Injection 746
Nicotinex Elixir ◘633
Paraplatin for Injection 1126
Ticlid Tablets 3015
Warfarin Sodium Tablets, USP 3302

Bleeding, uterine
(*see under* Bleeding, genital, abnormal)

Bleeding, vaginal, abnormal
(*see under* Bleeding, genital, abnormal)

Blood circulation, poor
Podocon-25 Liquid 2608

Blood dyscrasias, history of
Felbatol 3343

Blood dyscrasias, unspecified
(*see also under* Agranulocytosis, history of; Anemia, aplastic, history of; Anemia, hemolytic, history of; Anemia, megaloblastic, unspecified; Anemia, non-iron deficiency, unspecified; Anemia, pernicious; Anemia, sickle cell; Anemia, unspecified; Anemia, unspecified, history of; Bleeding disorders, unspecified; Granulocytopenia, history of; Hemophilia; Leukopenia; Neutropenia; Thrombocytopathy, unspecified; Thrombocytopenia, unspecified; Thrombocytopenic purpura, history of)
Attenuvax 2044
Coumadin for Injection 1243
Coumadin Tablets 1243
Etrafon 3115
Meruvax II 2130
M-M-R II 2118
Mumpsvax 2141
Navane Oral 2701
Navane Intramuscular 2703
Stelazine 1640
Thiothixene Capsules 2290
Ticlid Tablets 3015
Trilafon 3160
Varivax 2202
Warfarin Sodium Tablets, USP 3302

Blood vessel, major, tumors eroding into
Photofrin for Injection 831

Bone marrow aplasia
(*see under* Bone marrow depression)

Bone marrow damage
(*see under* Bone marrow depression)

Bone marrow depression
Adriamycin PFS/RDF Injection 2767
Etrafon 3115
Sterile FUDR 2974
Hexalen Capsules 2226
Hycamtin for Injection 1546
Ifex for Injection 1123
Mithracin for Intravenous Use 903
Mylocel Tablets 2227
Paraplatin for Injection 1126
Stelazine 1640
Thioplex for Injection 1765
Trilafon 3160

Bone marrow depression, history of
Carbatrol Capsules 3234
Tegretol/Tegretol-XR 2404

Bone marrow function impairment
(*see under* Bone marrow depression)

Bone marrow hypoplasia
(*see under* Bone marrow depression)

Bone marrow reserve, inadequate
Matulane Capsules 3246

Bone marrow transplantation
Adagen Injection 1331

Bowel disease, inflammatory
(*see under* Inflammation, gastrointestinal tract)

Bowel ischemia, history of
Amerge Tablets 1467
Imitrex Nasal Spray 1554
Imitrex Tablets 1558
Proleukin for Injection 1199

Bowel obstruction
(*see under* Bowel ischemia, history of; Obstruction, gastrointestinal tract)

Bowel perforation
(*see under* Perforation, gastrointestinal tract)

Bowel perforation, history of
(*see under* Perforation, gastrointestinal tract, history of)

Bradycardia, sinus
Adenoscan 1381
Betagan ⊙228
Betapace Tablets 950
Betapace AF Tablets 954
Betaxon Ophthalmic Suspension 537
Betimol Ophthalmic Solution ⊙324
Betoptic S Ophthalmic Suspension 537
Blocadren Tablets 2046
Brevibloc Injection 858
Cerebyx Injection 2619
Cordarone Intravenous 3491
Cordarone Tablets 3487
Corgard Tablets 2245
Corzide 40/5 Tablets 2247
Corzide 80/5 Tablets 2247
Inderal 3513
Inderal LA Long-Acting Capsules 3516
Inderide Tablets 3517
Inderide LA Long-Acting Capsules 3519
Nadolol Tablets 2288

Ocupress Ophthalmic Solution, 1% Sterile ⊙ 303
OptiPranolol Metipranolol Ophthalmic Solution 0.3% ⊙ 263
Pacerone Tablets 3331
Tenoretic Tablets 690
Tenormin 692
Timolide Tablets 2187
Timolol GFS ⊙ 266
Timoptic in Ocudose 2192
Timoptic Sterile Ophthalmic Solution 2190
Timoptic-XE Sterile Ophthalmic Gel Forming Solution 2194
Toprol-XL Tablets 651
Zebeta Tablets 1885
Ziac Tablets 1887

Bradycardia, unspecified
Cordarone Tablets 3487
Coreg Tablets 1508
Normodyne Injection 3135
Normodyne Tablets 3137
Pacerone Tablets 3331
Rythmol Tablets – 150 mg, 225 mg, 300 mg 502
Sectral Capsules 3589
Urecholine 2198
Urecholine Tablets 2445

Brain damage
(*see also under* Hypothalamic damage; Motor neuron injury)
Etrafon 3115
Trilafon 3160

Brain tumor
(*see under* Tumor, pituitary, unspecified)

Breast cancer
(*see under* Carcinoma, breast, male; Carcinoma, breast, unspecified)

Breastfeeding
Atromid-S Capsules 3483
Bactrim 2949
Baycol Tablets 883
Benadryl Parenteral 2617
Cetrotide for Injection 3209
Cuprimine Capsules 2075
Depen Titratable Tablets 3341
D.H.E. 45 Injection 2334
Doxil Injection 566
Estratest 3252
Evista Tablets 1915
Guaifed 2272
Hycamtin for Injection 1546
Lescol Capsules 2361
Lescol Capsules 2925
Lescol XL Tablets 2361
Lescol XL Tablets 2925
Lipitor Tablets 2639
Lipitor Tablets 2696
Lupron Depot 3.75 mg 3281
Lupron Depot–3 Month 11.25 mg 3285
Mevacor Tablets 2132
Migranal Nasal Spray 2376
Orthoclone OKT3 Sterile Solution 2498
Pediazole Suspension 3050
Periactin Tablets 2155
Pravachol Tablets 1099
Ryna-12 S Suspension 3351
Reformulated Rynatan Pediatric Suspension 3352
Rynatuss Pediatric Suspension 3353
Septra Suspension 2265
Septra Tablets 2265
Septra DS Tablets 2265
Sultrin Triple Sulfa Cream 2587
Synarel Nasal Solution for Central Precocious Puberty 3204
Synarel Nasal Solution for Endometriosis 3205
Tapazole Tablets 1823
Tice BCG, BCG Live 2489
Toradol 3018
Zephrex LA Tablets 3092
Zocor Tablets 2219
Zoladex 702

Breathing problems, unspecified
(*see under* Pulmonary disorders, unspecified; Respiratory illness, febrile; Respiratory illness, unspecified)

Bronchial asthma
(*see under* Asthma, acute; Asthma, history of; Asthma, unspecified)

Bronchoesophageal, fistula, existence of
Photofrin for Injection 831

Bronchography
Ethiodol Injection 3095

Bronchospastic disorders, unspecified
(*see also under* Asthma, acute; Asthma, history of; Asthma, unspecified; Emphysema)
Coreg Tablets 1508
Rythmol Tablets – 150 mg, 225 mg, 300 mg 502

Bulimia
Wellbutrin Tablets 1680
Wellbutrin SR Sustained-Release Tablets 1684
Zyban Sustained-Release Tablets 1710

Bundle branch block
(*see under* Heart block, unspecified)

Burns
Anectine Injection 1476

C

CAD
(*see under* Coronary artery disease)

Cancer
(*see under* Carcinoma, breast, male; Carcinoma, breast, unspecified; Carcinoma, cervical; Carcinoma, endometrium; Carcinoma, female reproductive organs; Carcinoma, genital, unspecified; Carcinoma, hepatic; Carcinoma, prostate; Carcinoma, skin, unspecified; Carcinoma, uterine; Neoplasm, bone marrow system, malignant; Neoplasm, lymphatic system, malignant)

Cancer, prevention of
TheraCys Injection 823

Carcinoma, breast, male
(*see also under* Carcinoma, breast, unspecified)
Anadrol-50 Tablets 3321
Androderm Transdermal System CIII 3377
AndroGel 3322
Android Capsules, 10 mg 1731
Delatestryl Injection 1151
Oxandrin Tablets 1153
Testoderm Transdermal Systems 574

Carcinoma, breast, unspecified
(*see also under* Carcinoma, breast, male; Neoplasm, estrogen dependent)
Activella Tablets 2764
Alesse-21 Tablets 3468
Alesse-28 Tablets 3473
Alora Transdermal System 3372
Anadrol-50 Tablets 3321
Aygestin Tablets 1333
Brevicon 28-Day Tablets 3380
Cenestin Tablets 1263
Climara Transdermal System 958
CombiPatch Transdermal System 2323
Crinone 3213
Cyclessa Tablets 2450
Depo-Provera Contraceptive Injection 2798
Desogen Tablets 2458
Esclim Transdermal System 3460
Estinyl Tablets 3112
Estrace Tablets 3361
Estratest 3252
Estring Vaginal Ring 2811
Estrostep 2627
femhrt Tablets 2635
Follistim for Injection 2465
Levlen 962
Levlite 21 Tablets 962
Levlite 28 Tablets 962
Levora Tablets 3389
Loestrin 21 Tablets 2642
Loestrin Fe Tablets 2642
Lo/Ovral Tablets 3532
Lo/Ovral-28 Tablets 3538
Low-Ogestrel-28 Tablets 3392
Lunelle Monthly Injection 2827
Menest Tablets 2254
Microgestin Fe 1.5/30 Tablets 3407
Microgestin Fe 1/20 Tablets 3400
Micronor Tablets 2543
Mircette Tablets 2470
Mirena Intrauterine System 974
Modicon 2563
Necon 3415
Nordette-28 Tablets 2257
Norinyl 1 +35 28-Day Tablets 3380
Norinyl 1 + 50 28-Day Tablets 3380
Norplant System 3543
Nor-QD Tablets 3423
Ogen Tablets 2846
Ogestrel 0.5/50-28 Tablets 3428
Ortho Dienestrol Cream 2554
Ortho-Cept 21 Tablets 2546
Ortho-Cept 28 Tablets 2546
Ortho-Cyclen/Ortho Tri-Cyclen 2573
Ortho-Est Tablets 3464
Ortho-Novum 2563
Ortho-Novum 1/50□28 Tablets 2556
Ortho-Novum 2563
Ortho-Prefest Tablets 2570
Ortho-Cyclen/Ortho Tri-Cyclen 2573
Ovcon 3364
Ovral Tablets 3551
Ovral-28 Tablets 3552
Ovrette Tablets 3552
Oxandrin Tablets 1153
Premarin Intravenous 3563
Premarin Tablets 3566
Premarin Vaginal Cream 3570
Premphase Tablets 3572
Prempro Tablets 3572
Prometrium Capsules (100 mg, 200 mg) 3261
Provera Tablets 2853
Tri-Levlen 962
Tri-Norinyl-28 Tablets 3433
Triphasil-21 Tablets 3600
Triphasil-28 Tablets 3605
Trivora Tablets 3439
Vagifem Tablets 2857
Vivelle Transdermal System 2412
Vivelle-Dot Transdermal System 2416
Yasmin 28 Tablets 980
Zovia 3449

Carcinoma, cervical
(*see also under* Carcinoma, female reproductive organs; Carcinoma, genital, unspecified)
Mirena Intrauterine System 974
ParaGard T 380A Intrauterine Copper Contraceptive 2582

Carcinoma, endometrium
(*see also under* Carcinoma, female reproductive organs; Carcinoma, uterine)
Alesse-21 Tablets 3468
Alesse-28 Tablets 3473
Brevicon 28-Day Tablets 3380
Cyclessa Tablets 2450
Desogen Tablets 2458
Estrostep 2627
Levlen 962
Levlite 21 Tablets 962
Levlite 28 Tablets 962
Levora Tablets 3389
Loestrin 21 Tablets 2642
Loestrin Fe Tablets 2642
Lo/Ovral Tablets 3532
Lo/Ovral-28 Tablets 3538
Low-Ogestrel-28 Tablets 3392
Lunelle Monthly Injection 2827
Microgestin Fe 1.5/30 Tablets 3407
Microgestin Fe 1/20 Tablets 3400
Mircette Tablets 2470
Modicon 2563
Necon 3415
Nordette-28 Tablets 2257
Norinyl 1 +35 28-Day Tablets 3380
Norinyl 1 + 50 28-Day Tablets 3380
Ogestrel 0.5/50-28 Tablets 3428
Ortho-Cept 21 Tablets 2546
Ortho-Cept 28 Tablets 2546
Ortho-Cyclen/Ortho Tri-Cyclen 2573
Ortho-Novum 2563
Ortho-Novum 1/50□28 Tablets 2556
Ortho-Novum 2563
Ortho-Cyclen/Ortho Tri-Cyclen 2573
Ovcon 3364
Ovral Tablets 3551
Ovral-28 Tablets 3552
Ovrette Tablets 3552
Tri-Levlen 962
Tri-Norinyl-28 Tablets 3433
Triphasil-21 Tablets 3600
Triphasil-28 Tablets 3605
Trivora Tablets 3439
Yasmin 28 Tablets 980
Zovia 3449

Carcinoma, female reproductive organs
(*see also under* Carcinoma, cervical; Carcinoma, endometrium; Carcinoma, genital, unspecified; Carcinoma, uterine)
Follistim for Injection 2465
Gonal-F for Injection 3216

Carcinoma, genital, unspecified
(*see also under* Carcinoma, cervical; Carcinoma, female reproductive organs; Carcinoma, prostate)
Crinone 3213
Prometrium Capsules (100 mg, 200 mg) 3261
Provera Tablets 2853

Carcinoma, hepatic
Alesse-21 Tablets 3468
Alesse-28 Tablets 3473
Brevicon 28-Day Tablets 3380
Cyclessa Tablets 2450
Desogen Tablets 2458
Estrostep 2627
Levlen 962
Levlite 21 Tablets 962
Levlite 28 Tablets 962
Levora Tablets 3389
Loestrin 21 Tablets 2642
Loestrin Fe Tablets 2642
Lo/Ovral Tablets 3532
Lo/Ovral-28 Tablets 3538
Low-Ogestrel-28 Tablets 3392
Lunelle Monthly Injection 2827
Microgestin Fe 1.5/30 Tablets 3407
Microgestin Fe 1/20 Tablets 3400
Micronor Tablets 2543
Mircette Tablets 2470
Mirena Intrauterine System 974
Modicon 2563
Necon 3415
Nordette-28 Tablets 2257
Norinyl 1 +35 28-Day Tablets 3380
Norinyl 1 + 50 28-Day Tablets 3380
Norplant System 3543
Ogestrel 0.5/50-28 Tablets 3428
Ortho-Cept 21 Tablets 2546
Ortho-Cept 28 Tablets 2546
Ortho-Cyclen/Ortho Tri-Cyclen 2573
Ortho-Novum 2563
Ortho-Novum 1/50□28 Tablets 2556
Ortho-Novum 2563
Ortho-Cyclen/Ortho Tri-Cyclen 2573
Ovcon 3364
Ovral Tablets 3551
Ovral-28 Tablets 3552
Ovrette Tablets 3552
Tri-Levlen 962
Tri-Norinyl-28 Tablets 3433
Triphasil-21 Tablets 3600
Triphasil-28 Tablets 3605
Trivora Tablets 3439
Yasmin 28 Tablets 980
Zovia 3449

Carcinoma, ovarian
(*see under* Carcinoma, female reproductive organs)

Carcinoma, prostate
(*see also under* Carcinoma, genital, unspecified; Neoplasm, androgen dependent)
Anadrol-50 Tablets 3321
Androderm Transdermal System CIII 3377
AndroGel 3322
Android Capsules, 10 mg 1731
Delatestryl Injection 1151
Novarel for Injection 1347
Oxandrin Tablets 1153
Pregnyl for Injection 2482
Testoderm Transdermal Systems 574

Carcinoma, skin, unspecified
(*see also under* Melanoma, history of)
Oxsoralen Lotion 1% 1740

Carcinoma, squamous cell, unspecified
8-MOP Capsules 1727
Oxsoralen-Ultra Capsules 1741

Carcinoma, uterine
(*see also under* Carcinoma, endometrium; Carcinoma, female reproductive organs)
Mirena Intrauterine System 974
ParaGard T 380A Intrauterine Copper Contraceptive 2582

Cardiac arrhythmia
(*see under* Arrhythmia, cardiac, unspecified)

Cardiac decompensation
(*see under* Heart failure, unspecified)

Cardiac dilation
Daranide Tablets 2077

Cardiac disease
(*see under* Cardiovascular disorders, unspecified)

Cardiac dysfunction
(*see under* Cardiovascular disorders, unspecified)

Cardiac failure
(*see under* Heart failure, unspecified)

Cardiac failure, NYHA class IV decompensated
Coreg Tablets 1508
Toprol-XL Tablets 651

Cardiac insufficiency
(*see under* Cardiovascular disorders, unspecified)

Cardiac rhythm disturbances, unspecified
(*see under* Arrhythmia, cardiac, unspecified)

Cardiogenic shock
Betagan ⊙ 228
Betapace Tablets 950
Betapace AF Tablets 954
Betaxon Ophthalmic Suspension 537
Betimol Ophthalmic Solution ⊙ 324
Betoptic S Ophthalmic Suspension 537
Blocadren Tablets 2046
Brevibloc Injection 858
Cardizem Injectable 1018
Cardizem Lyo-Ject Syringe 1018
Cardizem Monovial 1018
Carteolol Hydrochloride Ophthalmic Solution USP, 1% ⊙ 258
Cordarone Intravenous 3491
Coreg Tablets 1508
Corgard Tablets 2245
Corzide 40/5 Tablets 2247
Corzide 80/5 Tablets 2247
Cosopt Sterile Ophthalmic Solution 2065
Covera-HS Tablets 3199
Inderal 3513
Inderal LA Long-Acting Capsules 3516
Inderide Tablets 3517
Inderide LA Long-Acting Capsules 3519
Isoptin SR Tablets 467
Mexitil Capsules 1047
Nadolol Tablets 2288
Natrecor for Injection 3189
Normodyne Injection 3135
Normodyne Tablets 3137
Ocupress Ophthalmic Solution, 1% Sterile ⊙ 303
OptiPranolol Metipranolol Ophthalmic Solution 0.3% ⊙ 263
Rythmol Tablets – 150 mg, 225 mg, 300 mg 502
Sectral Capsules 3589
Tambocor Tablets 1990
Tarka Tablets 508
Tenoretic Tablets 690
Tenormin 692
Timolide Tablets 2187
Timolol GFS ⊙ 266
Timoptic in Ocudose 2192
Timoptic Sterile Ophthalmic Solution 2190
Timoptic-XE Sterile Ophthalmic Gel Forming Solution 2194
Toprol-XL Tablets 651
Zebeta Tablets 1885
Ziac Tablets 1887

Cardiopulmonary bypass
Plasmanate 942

Cardiospasm
Norflex 1987
Prosed/DS Tablets 3268
Urised Tablets 2876

Cardiovascular collapse
(*see under* Shock, unspecified)

Cardiovascular disorders, unspecified
(*see also under* Adams-Stokes syndrome; Angina pectoris; Angina, Prinzmetal's; Angina, unstable; Arrhythmia, cardiac, unspecified; Cardiogenic shock; Cardiospasm; Congestive heart failure, uncontrolled; Congestive heart failure, unspecified; Cor pulmonale; Coronary artery disease; Coronary occlusion; ECG changes, history of; Endocarditis, bacterial; Heart disease, ischemic; Heart failure, unspecified; Hypertension, unspecified; Myocardial infarction; Myocardial infarction, history of; Pericardial effusion)
Adderall Tablets 3231
Adipex-P 1406
Antabuse Tablets 2444
Antabuse Tablets 3474
Bontril Slow-Release Capsules 576
Cortifoam Rectal Foam 3170
Desoxyn Tablets 440
Dexedrine 1512
DextroStat Tablets 3236
Dopram Injectable 2931
Extendryl 1361
Hycomine Compound Tablets 1317
Imitrex Injection 1549
Indocin I.V. 2115
Ionamin Capsules 1163
Kronofed-A 1341
Lithium Carbonate 3061
Lithium Citrate Syrup 3061
Lunelle Monthly Injection 2827
Midrin Capsules 3464
Parnate Tablets 1607
Prostin E2 Suppositories 2852

Cardiovascular status, unstable in acute hemorrhage
Donnatal 2929
Donnatal Extentabs 2930
Donnatal Tablets 2929
Levsin/Levsinex/Levbid 3172
NuLev Orally Disintegrating Tablets 3176
Robinul Forte Tablets 1358
Robinul Injectable 2940
Robinul Tablets 1358

Cavernosal fibrosis
(*see under* Fibrosis, cavernosal)

Cellular immune deficiency
(*see under* Immunodeficiency, unspecified)

Central nervous system depression
Clozaril Tablets 2319
Compazine 1505
Etrafon 3115
Haldol Decanoate 2535
Haldol Injection, Tablets and Concentrate 2533
Loxitane Capsules 3398
Moban 1320
Navane Oral 2701
Navane Intramuscular 2703
Orap Tablets 1407
Phenergan Injection 3553
Roxanol 3066
Serentil 1057
Stelazine 1640
Thioridazine Hydrochloride Tablets 2289
Thiothixene Capsules 2290
Thorazine 1656
Trilafon 3160

Cephalopelvic disproportion
Cervidil Vaginal Insert 1369
Prepidil Gel 2851

Cerebral apoplexy
(*see under* Cerebrovascular accident)

Cerebral vascular accident
(*see under* Cerebrovascular accident)

Cerebral vascular disease
(*see also under* Bleeding, intracranial; Cerebrovascular accident)
Alesse-21 Tablets 3468
Alesse-28 Tablets 3473
Brevicon 28-Day Tablets 3380
Cyclessa Tablets 2450
Depo-Provera Contraceptive Injection 2798
Desogen Tablets 2458
Estrostep 2627
Levlen 962
Levlite 21 Tablets 962
Levlite 28 Tablets 962
Levora Tablets 3389
Loestrin 21 Tablets 2642
Loestrin Fe Tablets 2642
Lo/Ovral Tablets 3532
Lo/Ovral-28 Tablets 3538
Low-Ogestrel-28 Tablets 3392
Lunelle Monthly Injection 2827
Microgestin Fe 1.5/30 Tablets 3407
Microgestin Fe 1/20 Tablets 3400
Mircette Tablets 2470
Modicon 2563
Necon 3415
Nordette-28 Tablets 2257
Norinyl 1 +35 28-Day Tablets 3380
Norinyl 1 + 50 28-Day Tablets 3380
Ogestrel 0.5/50-28 Tablets 3428
Ortho-Cept 21 Tablets 2546
Ortho-Cept 28 Tablets 2546
Ortho-Cyclen/Ortho Tri-Cyclen 2573
Ortho-Novum 2563
Ortho-Novum 1/50□28 Tablets 2556
Ortho-Novum 2563
Ortho-Cyclen/Ortho Tri-Cyclen 2573
Ovcon 3364
Ovral Tablets 3551
Ovral-28 Tablets 3552
Ovrette Tablets 3552
Parnate Tablets 1607
Tri-Levlen 962
Tri-Norinyl-28 Tablets 3433
Triphasil-21 Tablets 3600
Triphasil-28 Tablets 3605
Trivora Tablets 3439
Yasmin 28 Tablets 980
Zovia 3449

Cerebral vascular disease, history of
(*see under* Cerebrovascular accident, history of)

Cerebrospinal pressure, increased
Roxanol 3066

Cerebrovascular accident
(*see also under* Bleeding, intracranial)
Amerge Tablets 1467
Aygestin Tablets 1333
CombiPatch Transdermal System 2323
Dopram Injectable 2931
Imitrex Injection 1549
Imitrex Nasal Spray 1554
Imitrex Tablets 1558
Premphase Tablets 3572
Prempro Tablets 3572
Prometrium Capsules (100 mg, 200 mg) 3261
Provera Tablets 2853
ReoPro Vials 1958
Streptase for Infusion 647

Cerebrovascular accident, history of
Activase I.V. 1410
Aggrastat 2031
Aygestin Tablets 1333
Integrilin Injection 1213
Integrilin Injection 1828
Premphase Tablets 3572
Prempro Tablets 3572
Provera Tablets 2853
ReoPro Vials 1958
Retavase Vials 1182
TNKase I.V. 1430

Cerebrovascular defects
(*see under* Cerebral vascular disease)

Cerebrovascular disorders, unspecified
(*see under* Cerebral vascular disease; Neurological disorders, unspecified)

Cerebrovascular hemorrhage
(*see under* Bleeding, intracranial; Cerebrovascular accident)

Cerebrovascular syndrome
Amerge Tablets 1467
Imitrex Nasal Spray 1554
Imitrex Tablets 1558

Cervicitis, untreated
Mirena Intrauterine System 974
ParaGard T 380A Intrauterine Copper Contraceptive 2582

Cesarean section, history of
Cervidil Vaginal Insert 1369
Prepidil Gel 2851

Chest pain, unspecified, history of
(*see also under* Angina, unspecified, history of)
Proleukin for Injection 1199

CHF
(*see under* Congestive heart failure, uncontrolled; Congestive heart failure, unspecified)

Chicken pox
(*see under* Varicella)

Children below the age of 4 years
Agenerase Oral Solution 1459

Cholestasis
Xenical Capsules 3043

Chronic obstructive pulmonary disease
(*see also under* Asthma, history of; Asthma, unspecified; Emphysema)
Betagan ⊙ 228
Betimol Ophthalmic Solution ⊙ 324
Blocadren Tablets 2046
Carteolol Hydrochloride Ophthalmic Solution USP, 1% ⊙ 258
Cosopt Sterile Ophthalmic Solution 2065
Dilaudid 441
Dilaudid Powder 441
Dilaudid Rectal Suppositories 441
Dilaudid Tablets 441
Ocupress Ophthalmic Solution, 1% Sterile ⊙ 303
OptiPranolol Metipranolol Ophthalmic Solution 0.3% ⊙ 263
Timolide Tablets 2187
Timolol GFS ⊙ 266
Timoptic in Ocudose 2192
Timoptic Sterile Ophthalmic Solution 2190
Timoptic-XE Sterile Ophthalmic Gel Forming Solution 2194

Circulatory collapse
(*see under* Shock, unspecified)

Cirrhosis, primary biliary
Atromid-S Capsules 3483
Lopid Tablets 2650
Tricor Capsules, Micronized 513

Cirrhosis, unspecified
Aldoclor Tablets 2035
Aldomet Tablets 2037
Aldoril Tablets 2039
Dantrium Capsules 2885
Glyset Tablets 2821
Precose Tablets 906

Coagulation disorders
(*see under* Bleeding disorders, unspecified; Hemophilia)

Coagulation, intravascular, active
Amicar Injection 3608
Amicar Syrup 3608
Amicar Tablets 3608

Coagulation, intravascular, disseminated
Autoplex T 2294

Colitis, toxic
Colyte with Flavor Packs for Oral Solution 3170
GoLYTELY and Pineapple Flavor GoLYTELY for Oral Solution 1068
NuLYTELY, Cherry Flavor, Lemon-Lime Flavor, and Orange Flavor NuLYTELY for Oral Solution 1068
Tri-Levlen 28 Tablets 962

Colitis, ulcerative
Donnatal 2929
Donnatal Extentabs 2930
Donnatal Tablets 2929
Glyset Tablets 2821
Levsin/Levsinex/Levbid 3172
NuLev Orally Disintegrating Tablets 3176

Precose Tablets........ 906
Robinul Forte Tablets........ 1358
Robinul Injectable........ 2940
Robinul Tablets........ 1358

Colitis, ulcerative, history of
Benzaclin Topical Gel........ 1220
Cleocin T Topical........ 2790
Cleocin Vaginal Cream........ 2788
Cleocin Vaginal Ovules........ 2789
Clindagel........ 1401
Clindets Pledgets........ 3270

Colitis, unspecified
(*see also under* Colitis, ulcerative; Enterocolitis, necrotizing)
Visicol Tablets........ 1767

Colitis, unspecified, history of
Benzaclin Topical Gel........ 1220
Cleocin T Topical........ 2790
Cleocin Vaginal Cream........ 2788
Cleocin Vaginal Ovules........ 2789
Clindagel........ 1401

Collagen diseases, unspecified
(*see under* Lupus erythematosus)

Colonic ulceration
(*see under* Colitis, ulcerative)

Coma, diabetic
Amaryl Tablets........ 717
DiaBeta Tablets........ 741
Diabinese Tablets........ 2680
Glucophage Tablets........ 1080
Glucophage XR Tablets........ 1080
Glucotrol Tablets........ 2692
Glucotrol XL Extended Release Tablets........ 2693

Coma, hepatic
(*see also under* Precoma, hepatic)
Mykrox Tablets........ 1168
Zaroxolyn Tablets........ 1177

Coma, unspecified
Clozaril Tablets........ 2319
Compazine........ 1505
Etrafon........ 3115
Haldol Decanoate........ 2535
Haldol Injection, Tablets and Concentrate........ 2533
Loxitane Capsules........ 3398
Moban........ 1320
Navane Oral........ 2701
Navane Intramuscular........ 2703
Orap Tablets........ 1407
Phenergan Injection........ 3553
Phenergan........ 3556
Serentil........ 1057
Stelazine........ 1640
Thioridazine Hydrochloride Tablets... 2289
Thiothixene Capsules........ 2290
Thorazine........ 1656
Trilafon........ 3160

Coma, unspecified, history of
Proleukin for Injection........ 1199

Comatose states
(*see under* Coma, diabetic; Coma, hepatic; Coma, unspecified)

Conduction disorders, cardiac
(*see under* Arrhythmia, cardiac, unspecified)

Conduction disturbances
(*see under* Arrhythmia, cardiac, unspecified)

Confusion, drug-induced
Tasmar Tablets........ 3010

Congestive heart failure, uncontrolled
Betapace Tablets........ 950
Betapace AF Tablets........ 954
Rythmol Tablets – 150 mg, 225 mg, 300 mg........ 502

Congestive heart failure, unspecified
Flexeril Tablets........ 572
Flexeril Tablets........ 2094
Flolan for Injection........ 1528
Glucophage Tablets........ 1080
Glucophage XR Tablets........ 1080
Glucovance Tablets........ 1086
Inderal........ 3513
Inderal LA Long-Acting Capsules........ 3516
Inderide Tablets........ 3517
Inderide LA Long-Acting Capsules........ 3519
Nardil Tablets........ 2653
Plasbumin-5........ 939
Plasbumin-20........ 940
Plasbumin-25........ 941
Plasmanate........ 942
Pletal Tablets........ 2605
Pletal Tablets........ 2848
Sporanox Capsules........ 1800
Urimax Tablets........ 1769
Visicol Tablets........ 1767

Constipation, severe chronic
Visicol Tablets........ 1767

Convulsions, history of
(*see under* Convulsive disorders, history of; Seizure disorders, history of)

Convulsive disorders
(*see also under* Adams-Stokes syndrome; Seizure disorders, unspecified)
Dopram Injectable........ 2931
Roxanol........ 3066

Convulsive disorders, history of
(*see also under* Seizure disorders, history of)
Acel-Imune........ 1851

COPD
(*see under* Chronic obstructive pulmonary disease)

Cor pulmonale
Dilaudid........ 441
Dilaudid Powder........ 441
Dilaudid Rectal Suppositories........ 441
Dilaudid Tablets........ 441

Corneal foreign body removal
Blephamide Ophthalmic Suspension........ 548
Poly-Pred Liquifilm Ophthalmic Suspension........ ⊙ 245
Pred-G Sterile Ophthalmic Ointment........ ⊙ 248
Terra-Cortril Ophthalmic Suspension........ 2716
TobraDex Ophthalmic Ointment........ 542
TobraDex Ophthalmic Suspension... 541

Coronary artery disease
(*see also under* Coronary artery vasospasm; Stenosis, aortic; Stenosis, subaortic)
Alesse-21 Tablets........ 3468
Alesse-28 Tablets........ 3473
Allegra-D Extended-Release Tablets........ 714
Brevicon 28-Day Tablets........ 3380
Bromfed Capsules (Extended-Release)........ 2269
Bromfed-PD Capsules (Extended-Release)........ 2269
Claritin-D 12 Hour Extended Release Tablets........ 3102
Claritin-D 24 Hour Extended Release Tablets........ 3104
Cortifoam Rectal Foam........ 3170
Cyclessa Tablets........ 2450
Desogen Tablets........ 2458
D.H.E. 45 Injection........ 2334
Estrostep........ 2627
Guaifed........ 2272
[illegible]
Levlite 21 Tablets........ 962
Levlite 28 Tablets........ 962
Levora Tablets........ 3389
Loestrin 21 Tablets........ 2642
Loestrin Fe Tablets........ 2642
Lo/Ovral Tablets........ 3532
Lo/Ovral-28 Tablets........ 3538
Low-Ogestrel-28 Tablets........ 3392
Lunelle Monthly Injection........ 2827
Microgestin Fe 1.5/30 Tablets........ 3407
Microgestin Fe 1/20 Tablets........ 3400
Mircette Tablets........ 2470
Modicon........ 2563
Necon........ 3415
Nordette-28 Tablets........ 2257
Norinyl 1 +35 28-Day Tablets........ 3380
Norinyl 1 + 50 28-Day Tablets........ 3380
Ogestrel 0.5/50-28 Tablets........ 3428
Ortho-Cept 21 Tablets........ 2546
Ortho-Cept 28 Tablets........ 2546
Ortho-Cyclen/Ortho Tri-Cyclen........ 2573
Ortho-Novum........ 2563
Ortho-Novum 1/50□28 Tablets........ 2556
Ortho-Novum........ 2563
Ortho-Cyclen/Ortho Tri-Cyclen........ 2573
Ovcon........ 3364
Ovral Tablets........ 3551
Ovral-28 Tablets........ 3552
Ovrette Tablets........ 3552
Rynatan Tablets........ 3351
Semprex-D Capsules........ 1172
Tri-Levlen........ 962
Tri-Norinyl-28 Tablets........ 3433
Triphasil-21 Tablets........ 3600
Triphasil-28 Tablets........ 3605
Trivora Tablets........ 3439
Urecholine........ 2198
Urecholine Tablets........ 2445
Urimax Tablets........ 1769
Yasmin 28 Tablets........ 980
Zephrex Tablets........ 3091
Zephrex LA Tablets........ 3092
Zovia........ 3449
Zyrtec-D 12 Hour Extended Relief Tablets........ 2758

Coronary artery vasospasm
(*see also under* Angina pectoris; Angina, Prinzmetal's; Angina, unstable)
Axert Tablets........ 2772
D.H.E. 45 Injection........ 2334
Imitrex Injection........ 1549
Maxalt Tablets........ 2120
Maxalt-MLT Orally Disintegrating Tablets........ 2120
Migranal Nasal Spray........ 2376
Zomig Tablets........ 708
Zomig-ZMT Tablets........ 708

Coronary heart disease
(*see under* Cardiovascular disorders, unspecified)

Coronary insufficiency
(*see under* Cardiovascular disorders, unspecified)

Coronary occlusion
(*see also under* Myocardial infarction)
Antabuse Tablets........ 2444
Antabuse Tablets........ 3474

Cramps, heat
(*see under* Heat cramps)

Creatinine clearance, abnormal
(*see under* Renal dysfunction)

Critical illness, acute
Genotropin Lyophilized Powder........ 2818
Norditropin Cartridges........ 2420
Norditropin for Injection........ 2419
Nutropin AQ Injection........ 1420
Nutropin Depot for Injectable Suspension........ 1423
Nutropin for Injection........ 1417
Saizen for Injection........ 3225
Serostim for Injection........ 3229

Cysticercosis, ocular
Biltricide Tablets........ 887

Cysts, ovarian
Clomid Tablets........ 735
Follistim for Injection........ 2465
Gonal-F for Injection........ 3216
Humegon for Injection........ 2468
Ovidrel for Injection........ 3220
Pergonal for Injection........ 3223
Repronex for Intramuscular and Subcutaneous Injection........ 1347
Serophene Tablets........ 3226

D

Debilitation
Lithium Carbonate........ 3061
Lithium Citrate Syrup........ 3061
Periactin Tablets........ 2155
Robinul Forte Tablets........ 1358
Robinul Tablets........ 1358

Deep vein thrombophlebitis, history of
(*see under* Thrombophlebitis, history of)

Dehydration, unspecified
Lithium Carbonate........ 3061
Lithium Citrate Syrup........ 3061
Rum-K........ 1363
Urocit-K Tablets........ 2232
Uroqid-Acid No. 2 Tablets........ 947

Delirium tremens
Roxanol........ 3066

Delivery, traumatic, history of
Prepidil Gel........ 2851

Delivery, unspecified
Dilaudid Oral Liquid........ 445
Dilaudid Tablets - 8 mg........ 445
Dilaudid-HP........ 443
Macrobid Capsules........ 2889
Macrodantin Capsules........ 2891
Toradol........ 3018

Delivery, vaginal
Prepidil Gel........ 2851

Dendritic keratitis
(*see under* Herpes simplex keratitis)

Denervation, skeletal muscle
Anectine Injection........ 1476

Dermatitis
(*see under* Inflammation, local; Intertrigo; Rash)

Diabetes mellitus
Urocit-K Tablets........ 2232

Diabetes mellitus, type 1, sole therapy
Prandin Tablets (0.5, 1, and 2 mg)........ 2432
Starlix Tablets........ 2401

Diabetes with vascular involvement
Lunelle Monthly Injection........ 2827

Diabetes, unspecified
Cortifoam Rectal Foam........ 3170
Hycomine Compound Tablets........ 1317
Podocon-25 Liquid........ 2608

Diabetic gastroparesis
(*see under* Gastroparesis, diabetic)

Diabetic ketoacidosis
(*see under* Ketoacidosis, diabetic)

Diabetic nephropathy
(*see under* Nephropathy, diabetic)

Diarrhea, infectious
Motofen Tablets........ 577

Diarrhea, severe
Edecrin........ 2091

Diet, sodium restricted
Fleet Phospho-soda........ 1360

Discharge, otic
Americaine Otic Topical Anesthetic Ear Drops........ 1162

Disease, infectious, unspecified
Mustargen for Injection........ 2142

Dissecting aorta
Coumadin for Injection........ 1243
Coumadin Tablets........ 1243
Warfarin Sodium Tablets, USP........ 3302

Diverticulitis
Cortifoam Rectal Foam........ 3170

Drug abuse, history of
Adderall Tablets........ 3231
Adipex-P........ 1406
Bontril Slow-Release Capsules........ 576
Desoxyn Tablets........ 440
Dexedrine........ 1512
DextroStat Tablets........ 3236
Ionamin Capsules........ 1163

Drug abuse, unspecified
ParaGard T 380A Intrauterine Copper Contraceptive........ 2582

Dysgammaglobulinemia
Attenuvax........ 2044
Meruvax II........ 2130
M-M-R II........ 2118
Mumpsvax........ 2141
Varivax........ 2202

E

Ear infection, fungal
(*see under* Infection, otic, fungal)

Eardrum perforation
(*see under* Tympanic membrane perforation)

ECG, QT syndrome, long
Serentil........ 1057
Tikosyn Capsules........ 2717

ECG changes, history of
Proleukin for Injection........ 1199

Eclampsia
Coumadin for Injection........ 1243
Coumadin Tablets........ 1243
Warfarin Sodium Tablets, USP........ 3302

Edema, pulmonary
Albumin (Human) 5%........ 838
Albumin (Human) 25%........ 839

Effusion, pericardial
(*see under* Pericardial effusion)

Electrocardiogram changes
(*see under* ECG changes, history of)

Electrolyte depletion
(*see under* Electrolyte imbalance, uncorrected)

Electrolyte disturbances
(*see under* Electrolyte imbalance, uncorrected)

Electrolyte imbalance, uncorrected
(*see also under* Hypercalcemia; Hyperkalemia; Hyperphosphatemia; Hypocalcemia; Hypokalemia; Hyponatremia)
Edecrin ... 2091
Rythmol Tablets – 150 mg, 225 mg, 300 mg ... 502

Emergency, obstetric
Prepidil Gel ... 2851

Emphysema
Dilaudid ... 441
Dilaudid Powder ... 441
Dilaudid Rectal Suppositories ... 441
Dilaudid Tablets ... 441

Encephalopathy, history of
Acel-Imune ... 1851

Endocarditis, bacterial
Coumadin for Injection ... 1243
Coumadin Tablets ... 1243
Warfarin Sodium Tablets, USP ... 3302

Endometrial cancer
(*see under* Carcinoma, endometrium)

Endometritis, postpartum
Mirena Intrauterine System ... 974
ParaGard T 380A Intrauterine Copper Contraceptive ... 2582

Enteritis, history of
Benzaclin Topical Gel ... 1220
Cleocin T Topical ... 2790
Cleocin Vaginal Cream ... 2788
Cleocin Vaginal Ovules ... 2789
Clindagel ... 1401
Clindets Pledgets ... 3270

Enterobiasis, prophylactic treatment for
Mintezol ... 2137

Enterocolitis, necrotizing
Indocin I.V. ... 2115

Epilepsy
Dopram Injectable ... 2931
Reglan ... 2935
Urecholine ... 2198
Urecholine Tablets ... 2445

Epilepsy, uncontrolled
(*see also under* Status epilepticus)
Clozaril Tablets ... 2319

Epiphyses, closed
Genotropin Lyophilized Powder ... 2818
Humatrope Vials and Cartridges ... 1930
Norditropin Cartridges ... 2420
Norditropin for Injection ... 2419
Nutropin AQ Injection ... 1420
Nutropin Depot for Injectable Suspension ... 1423
Nutropin for Injection ... 1417

Epiphyses, fused
(*see under* Epiphyses, closed)

Epithelial herpes simplex keratitis
(*see under* Herpes simplex keratitis)

Esophageal abnormalities, unspecified
(*see also under* Achalasia, esophageal; Esophageal compression; Esophagitis, reflux; Stricture, esophageal)
Fosamax Tablets ... 2095

Esophageal achalasia
(*see under* Achalasia, esophageal)

Esophageal compression
K-Dur Microburst Release System ER Tablets ... 1832
Klor-Con M20/Klor-Con M10 Tablets ... 3329
Micro-K ... 3311

Esophageal stricture
(*see under* Stricture, esophageal)

Esophagitis, reflux
Donnatal ... 2929
Donnatal Extentabs ... 2930
Donnatal Tablets ... 2929

Exanthematous conditions
(*see under* Rash)

Exercise, strenuous physical
Urocit-K Tablets ... 2232

Eye infection
(*see under* Cysticercosis, ocular; Infection, ophthalmic, fungal; Infection, ophthalmic, mycobacterial; Infection, ophthalmic, viral; Iritis, acute)

Eye surgery
(*see under* Surgery, ophthalmic)

F

Fallot's tetralogy
(*see under* Tetralogy of Fallot)

Febrile illness
(*see under* Fever; Infection, febrile; Respiratory illness, febrile)

Fecal impaction
Citrucel Orange Flavor Powder ... ▣ 744
Citrucel Sugar Free Orange Flavor Powder ... ▣ 745
Metamucil Dietary Fiber Supplement ... ▣ 834
Metamucil ... 2877

Fetal distress, non-imminent delivery
Cervidil Vaginal Insert ... 1369
Prepidil Gel ... 2851

Fever
(*see also under* Infection, febrile; Respiratory illness, febrile)
Acel-Imune ... 1851
Diphtheria & Tetanus Toxoids Adsorbed Purogenated for Pediatric Use ... 1857
FluShield Influenza Vaccine ... 3521
Imovax Rabies Vaccine ... 807
Infanrix Vaccine ... 1562
IPOL Vaccine ... 809
Pnu-Imune 23 ... 1868
Tasmar Tablets ... 3010
Tetanus & Diphtheria Toxoids Adsorbed for Adult Use ... 1880
Tetanus Toxoid Adsorbed Purogenated ... 1882
TheraCys Injection ... 823
Tice BCG, BCG Live ... 2489
Tripedia Vaccine ... 817

Fibrillation, atrial
Cardizem Injectable ... 1018
Cardizem Lyo-Ject Syringe ... 1018
Cardizem Monovial ... 1018
Covera-HS Tablets ... 3199
Isoptin SR Tablets ... 467
Verelan Capsules ... 3184
Verelan PM Capsules ... 3186

Fibrillation, ventricular
Digitek Tablets ... 1003
Lanoxicaps Capsules ... 1574
Lanoxin Injection ... 1581
Lanoxin Tablets ... 1587
Lanoxin Elixir Pediatric ... 1578
Lanoxin Injection Pediatric ... 1584

Fibrinolysis
Autoplex T ... 2294

Fibrosis, cavernosal
Caverject Sterile Powder ... 2777
MUSE Urethral Suppository ... 3335

Fibrosis, pulmonary
(*see under* Pulmonary fibrosis)

Fibrosis, unspecified
(*see under* Fibrosis, cavernosal; Pulmonary fibrosis)

Fibrotic processes
(*see under* Fibrosis, cavernosal; Pulmonary fibrosis)

Fistula
Cortifoam Rectal Foam ... 3170

Flail chest
Dopram Injectable ... 2931

Fluid overload
Orthoclone OKT3 Sterile Solution ... 2498

Flutter, atrial
Cardizem Injectable ... 1018
Cardizem Lyo-Ject Syringe ... 1018
Cardizem Monovial ... 1018
Covera-HS Tablets ... 3199
Isoptin SR Tablets ... 467
Verelan Capsules ... 3184
Verelan PM Capsules ... 3186

Fungal infections
(*see under* Actinomycosis, genital; Infection, fungal, unspecified; Infection, ophthalmic, fungal; Infection, otic, fungal; Infection, systemic, fungal; Lesions, skin, fungal)

G

Gallbladder disease, unspecified
Lopid Tablets ... 2650
Tricor Capsules, Micronized ... 513

Gastric retention
Colyte with Flavor Packs for Oral Solution ... 3170
Detrol Tablets ... 3623
Detrol LA Capsules ... 2801
Ditropan XL Extended Release Tablets ... 564
GoLYTELY and Pineapple Flavor GoLYTELY for Oral Solution ... 1068
NuLYTELY, Cherry Flavor, Lemon-Lime Flavor, and Orange Flavor NuLYTELY for Oral Solution ... 1068
Tri-Levlen 28 Tablets ... 962
Visicol Tablets ... 1767

Gastroenteritis
Dulcolax Suppositories ... ▣ 668
Dulcolax Tablets ... ▣ 668

Gastrointestinal disorders
(*see under* Bleeding, gastrointestinal; Esophageal abnormalities, unspecified; Gastric retention; Gastroparesis, diabetic; Hernia, hiatal; Inflammation, gastrointestinal tract; Intestinal disorders, unspecified; Obstruction, gastrointestinal tract; Perforation, gastrointestinal tract; Spasms, gastrointestinal; Ulcer, gastrointestinal)

Gastrointestinal obstruction
(*see under* Obstruction, gastrointestinal tract)

Gastrointestinal perforation
(*see under* Perforation, gastrointestinal tract)

Gastroparesis, diabetic
K-Dur Microburst Release System ER Tablets ... 1832
Klor-Con M20/Klor-Con M10 Tablets ... 3329
K-Tab Filmtab Tablets ... 470
Micro-K ... 3311

General anesthesia
(*see under* Anesthesia, general)

Genital bleeding
(*see under* Bleeding, genital, abnormal)

Glaucoma, angle closure
Akineton ... 402
Albalon Ophthalmic Solution ... ⊙ 225
Allegra-D Extended-Release Tablets ... 714
Ativan Injection ... 3478
Ativan Tablets ... 3482
Bromfed Capsules (Extended-Release) ... 2269
Bromfed-PD Capsules (Extended-Release) ... 2269
Claritin-D 12 Hour Extended Release Tablets ... 3102
Claritin-D 24 Hour Extended Release Tablets ... 3104
Detrol Tablets ... 3623
Detrol LA Capsules ... 2801
Ditropan XL Extended Release Tablets ... 564
Epifrin Sterile Ophthalmic Solution ... ⊙ 235
Evoxac Capsules ... 1217
Klonopin Tablets ... 2983
Lodosyn Tablets ... 1251
Periactin Tablets ... 2155
Rynatan Tablets ... 3351
Salagen Tablets ... 2229
Sinemet Tablets ... 1253
Sinemet CR Tablets ... 1255
Transderm Scōp Transdermal Therapeutic System ... 2302
Tranxene ... 511
Valium Injectable ... 3026
Valium Tablets ... 3047
Versed Injection ... 3027
Versed Syrup ... 3033
Xanax Tablets ... 2865
Zyrtec-D 12 Hour Extended Relief Tablets ... 2758

Glaucoma, narrow angle
(*see under* Glaucoma, angle closure)

Glaucoma, open angle, untreated
Klonopin Tablets ... 2983
Valium Injectable ... 3026
Valium Tablets ... 3047
Versed Injection ... 3027
Versed Syrup ... 3033
Xanax Tablets ... 2865

Glaucoma, pupillary block
Isopto Carpine Ophthalmic Solution ... ⊙ 215

Glaucoma, unspecified
Adderall Tablets ... 3231
Adipex-P ... 1406
Arco-Lase Plus Tablets ... 592
Bontril Slow-Release Capsules ... 576
Concerta Extended-Release Tablets ... 1998
Concerta Tablets ... 561
Desoxyn Tablets ... 440
Dexedrine ... 1512
DextroStat Tablets ... 3236
Donnatal ... 2929
Donnatal Extentabs ... 2930
Donnatal Tablets ... 2929
Extendryl ... 1361
Inversine Tablets ... 1850
Ionamin Capsules ... 1163
Levsin/Levsinex/Levbid ... 3172
Metadate CD Capsules ... 1164
Metadate ER Tablets ... 1167
Methylin Tablets ... 1995
Methylin ER Tablets ... 1995
Midrin Capsules ... 3464
Norflex ... 1987
NuLev Orally Disintegrating Tablets ... 3176
Prosed/DS Tablets ... 3268
Ritalin ... 2387
Robinul Forte Tablets ... 1358
Robinul Injectable ... 2940
Robinul Tablets ... 1358
Sinequan ... 2713
Urimax Tablets ... 1769
Urised Tablets ... 2876

Glomerulonephritis
Cortifoam Rectal Foam ... 3170

Gout, acute
Pyrazinamide Tablets ... 1876
Rifater Tablets ... 769

Granulocytopenia, history of
Clozaril Tablets ... 2319

Guillain-Barre syndrome, history of
FluShield Influenza Vaccine ... 3521

H

Head injury
(*see also under* Trauma, intracranial)
Dopram Injectable ... 2931
Roxanol ... 3066

Headache
(*see under* Headache, history of; Migraine, basilar; Migraine, hemiplegic)

Headache, history of
Parnate Tablets 1607

Headaches with focal neurological symptoms
Lunelle Monthly Injection 2827

Heart attack
(*see under* Myocardial infarction)

Heart block, greater than first degree
Adenocard Injection 1380
Adenoscan 1381
Betagan ⊙ 228
Betapace Tablets 950
Betapace AF Tablets 954
Betaxon Ophthalmic Suspension 537
Betimol Ophthalmic Solution ⊙ 324
Betoptic S Ophthalmic Suspension 537
Blocadren Tablets 2046
Brevibloc Injection 858
Cardizem Injectable 1018
Cardizem Lyo-Ject Syringe 1018
Cardizem Monovial 1018
Cardizem CD Capsules 1016
Carteolol Hydrochloride Ophthalmic Solution USP, 1% ⊙ 258
Cerebyx Injection 2619
Cordarone Intravenous 3491
Cordarone Tablets 3487
Coreg Tablets 1508
Corgard Tablets 2245
Corzide 40/5 Tablets 2247
Corzide 80/5 Tablets 2247
Covera-HS Tablets 3199
Inderal 3513
Inderal LA Long-Acting Capsules 3516
Inderide Tablets 3517
Inderide LA Long-Acting Capsules 3519
Isoptin SR Tablets 467
Mexitil Capsules 1047
Nadolol Tablets 2288
Normodyne Injection 3135
Normodyne Tablets 3137
Ocupress Ophthalmic Solution, 1% Sterile ⊙ 303
OptiPranolol Metipranolol Ophthalmic Solution 0.3% ⊙ 263
Pacerone Tablets 3331
Sectral Capsules 3589
Tambocor Tablets 1990
Tarka Tablets 508
Tenoretic Tablets 690
Tenormin 692
Tiazac Capsules 1378
Timolide Tablets 2187
Timolol GFS ⊙ 266
Timoptic in Ocudose 2192
Timoptic Sterile Ophthalmic Solution 2190
Timoptic-XE Sterile Ophthalmic Gel Forming Solution 2194
Tonocard Tablets 649
Toprol-XL Tablets 651
Verelan Capsules 3184
Verelan PM Capsules 3186
Zebeta Tablets 1885
Ziac Tablets 1887

Heart block, sinoatrial
Cerebyx Injection 2619
Rythmol Tablets – 150 mg, 225 mg, 300 mg 502

Heart block, unspecified
Cerebyx Injection 2619
Flexeril Tablets 572
Flexeril Tablets 2094
Primaxin I.M. 2158
Procanbid Extended-Release Tablets 2262
Quinaglute Dura-Tabs Tablets 978
Quinidex Extentabs 2933
Rythmol Tablets – 150 mg, 225 mg, 300 mg 502
Tambocor Tablets 1990

Heart damage
(*see under* Cardiovascular disorders, unspecified)

Heart disease, ischemic
(*see also under* Angina pectoris; Ischemia, silent; Myocardial infarction)
Amerge Tablets 1467
Axert Tablets 2772
D.H.E. 45 Injection 2334
Imitrex Injection 1549
Imitrex Nasal Spray 1554
Imitrex Tablets 1558
Maxalt Tablets 2120
Maxalt-MLT Orally Disintegrating Tablets 2120
Migranal Nasal Spray 2376
Zomig Tablets 708
Zomig-ZMT Tablets 708

Heart disease, severe organic
ProAmatine Tablets 3241

Heart disease, unspecified
(*see under* Cardiovascular disorders, unspecified)

Heart failure, unspecified
(*see also under* Congestive heart failure, unspecified)
Albumin (Human) 5% 838
Albumin (Human) 25% 839
Albuminar-5, U.S.P. 785
Albuminar-25, U.S.P. 786
Betagan ⊙ 228
Betaxon Ophthalmic Suspension 537
Betimol Ophthalmic Solution ⊙ 324
Betoptic S Ophthalmic Suspension 537
Blocadren Tablets 2046
Brevibloc Injection 858
Buminate 5% Solution, USP 841
Buminate 25% Solution, USP 842
Carteolol Hydrochloride Ophthalmic Solution USP, 1% ⊙ 258
Corgard Tablets 2245
Corzide 40/5 Tablets 2247
Corzide 80/5 Tablets 2247
Cosopt Sterile Ophthalmic Solution 2065
Geodon Capsules 2688
Inversine Tablets 1850
Nadolol Tablets 2288
Normodyne Injection 3135
Normodyne Tablets 3137
Ocupress Ophthalmic Solution, 1% Sterile ⊙ 303
OptiPranolol Metipranolol Ophthalmic Solution 0.3% ⊙ 263
Orthoclone OKT3 Sterile Solution 2498
Roxanol 3066
Sectral Capsules 3589
Tenoretic Tablets 690
Tenormin 692
Timolide Tablets 2187
Timolol GFS ⊙ 266
Timoptic in Ocudose 2192
Timoptic Sterile Ophthalmic Solution 2190
Timoptic-XE Sterile Ophthalmic Gel Forming Solution 2194
Toprol-XL Tablets 651
Zebeta Tablets 1885
Ziac Tablets 1887

Heat cramps
Rum-K 1363

Hematologic disorders
(*see under* Bleeding disorders, unspecified; Blood dyscrasias, unspecified)

Hematopoietic disorders
(*see under* Blood dyscrasias, unspecified; Bone marrow depression)

Hematuria
Tice BCG, BCG Live 2489

Hemochromatosis
New Formulation Chromagen OB Capsules 3094

Hemophilia
Orgaran Injection 2480

Hemorrhage
(*see under* Bleeding disorders, unspecified; Bleeding tendencies; Bleeding, abnormal, unspecified; Bleeding, gastrointestinal; Bleeding, gastrointestinal, history of; Bleeding, genital, abnormal; Bleeding, genitourinary; Bleeding, history of; Bleeding, internal, unspecified; Bleeding, intracranial; Bleeding, rectal; Bleeding, retinal; Bleeding, unspecified; Cardiovascular status, unstable in acute hemorrhage)

Hemorrhagic diathesis
(*see under* Bleeding tendencies)

Hemorrhagic stroke
Aggrastat 2031
Orgaran Injection 2480

Hemosiderosis
New Formulation Chromagen OB Capsules 3094

Hemostasis, incomplete
Toradol 3018

Hemostatic disorders
(*see under* Bleeding disorders, unspecified)

Hepatic adenoma
(*see under* Adenoma, hepatic)

Hepatic cancer
(*see under* Carcinoma, hepatic)

Hepatic coma
(*see under* Coma, hepatic)

Hepatic damage
(*see under* Liver dysfunction)

Hepatic disease
(*see under* Liver disease, unspecified)

Hepatic dysfunction
(*see under* Liver dysfunction)

Hepatic failure
(*see under* Liver failure)

Hepatic impairment
(*see under* Liver dysfunction)

Hepatic injury
(*see under* Liver dysfunction)

Hepatic insufficiency
(*see under* Liver dysfunction)

Hepatic precoma
(*see under* Precoma, hepatic)

Hepatitis
Aldoclor Tablets 2035
Aldomet Tablets 2037
Aldoril Tablets 2039
Calcium Disodium Versenate Injection 1980
Dantrium Capsules 2885

Hepatitis, autoimmune
PEG-Intron Powder for Injection 3140
Rebetron Combination Therapy 3153

Hepatitis, history of
Rifamate Capsules 767

Hepatocellular failure
(*see under* Liver failure)

Hernia, hiatal
Donnatal 2929
Donnatal Extentabs 2930
Donnatal Tablets 2929

Herpes genitalia
Prepidil Gel 2851

Herpes simplex, otic
Cipro HC Otic Suspension 540

Herpes simplex keratitis
Alrex Sterile Ophthalmic Suspension 0.2% ⊙ 256
Blephamide Ophthalmic Ointment 547
Blephamide Ophthalmic Suspension 548
Cortifoam Rectal Foam 3170
Cortisporin Ophthalmic Suspension Sterile ⊙ 297
Decadron Phosphate Sterile Ophthalmic Ointment 2083
Decadron Phosphate Sterile Ophthalmic Solution 2084
FML Ophthalmic Ointment ⊙ 237
FML Ophthalmic Suspension ⊙ 236
FML Forte Ophthalmic Suspension ⊙ 235
FML-S Liquifilm Sterile Ophthalmic Suspension ⊙ 238
HMS Sterile Ophthalmic Suspension ⊙ 240
Lotemax Sterile Ophthalmic Suspension 0.5% ⊙ 261
NeoDecadron Sterile Ophthalmic Solution 2144
Poly-Pred Liquifilm Ophthalmic Suspension ⊙ 245
Pred Forte Ophthalmic Suspension ⊙ 246
Pred Mild Sterile Ophthalmic Suspension ⊙ 249
Pred-G Ophthalmic Suspension ⊙ 247
Pred-G Sterile Ophthalmic Ointment ⊙ 248
Terra-Cortril Ophthalmic Suspension 2716
TobraDex Ophthalmic Ointment 542
TobraDex Ophthalmic Suspension 541
Vexol 1% Ophthalmic Suspension ⊙ 222

Herpes simplex, unspecified
Cortisporin-TC Otic Suspension 2246
VōSoL HC Otic Solution 3356

Herpes zoster
Cosmegen for Injection 2062

Hiatal hernia
(*see under* Hernia, hiatal)

HIV
(*see under* Human immunodeficiency virus)

Human immunodeficiency virus
(*see also under* Acquired immune deficiency syndrome)
Attenuvax 2044
Mumpsvax 2141
Tice BCG, BCG Live 2489
Varivax 2202

Hypercalcemia
Calcijex Injection 411
Dovonex Cream 1116
Dovonex Ointment 1117
Dovonex Scalp Solution 1118
Hectorol Capsules 1064
Hectorol Injection 1066
Oxandrin Tablets 1153
PhosLo 1069
Rocaltrol 2991

Hypercarbia
OxyContin Tablets 2912
OxyFast Oral Concentrate Solution 2916
OxyIR Capsules 2916
Roxicodone Tablets 3067

Hyperkalemia
Dyazide Capsules 1515
Dyrenium Capsules 3458
K-Dur Microburst Release System ER Tablets 1832
Klor-Con M20/Klor-Con M10 Tablets 3329
K-Lor Powder Packets 469
K-Phos Original (Sodium Free) Tablets 947
K-Tab Filmtab Tablets 470
Maxzide 1008
Micro-K 3311
Midamor Tablets 2136
Moduretic Tablets 2138
Rum-K 1363
Urocit-K Tablets 2232

Hyperphosphatemia
K-Phos Neutral Tablets 946
K-Phos Original (Sodium Free) Tablets 947
Uroqid-Acid No. 2 Tablets 947

Hypersensitivity associated with ALT elevations
Cognex Capsules 1351

Hypertension, excessive supine
ProAmatine Tablets 3241

Hypertension, intracranial, history of
Norplant System 3543

Hypertension, malignant
Coumadin for Injection 1243
Coumadin Tablets 1243
Warfarin Sodium Tablets, USP 3302

Hypertension, uncontrolled
Activase I.V. 1410
Aggrastat 2031
Amerge Tablets 1467
Axert Tablets 2772
D.H.E. 45 Injection 2334
Dostinex Tablets 2804
Epogen for Injection 582
Gengraf Capsules 457
Imitrex Nasal Spray 1554
Imitrex Tablets 1558
Integrilin Injection 1213
Integrilin Injection 1828
Maxalt Tablets 2120
Maxalt-MLT Orally Disintegrating Tablets 2120
Migranal Nasal Spray 2376
Neoral Soft Gelatin Capsules 2380
Neoral Oral Solution 2380
Procrit for Injection 2502
ReoPro Vials 1958
Retavase Vials 1182
Streptase for Infusion 647
TNKase I.V. 1430

Zomig Tablets ... 708
Zomig-ZMT Tablets ... 708

Hypertension, unspecified
Adderall Tablets ... 3231
Adipex-P ... 1406
Allegra-D Extended-Release Tablets ... 714
Bontril Slow-Release Capsules ... 576
Bromfed Capsules (Extended-Release) ... 2269
Bromfed-PD Capsules (Extended-Release) ... 2269
Claritin-D 12 Hour Extended Release Tablets ... 3102
Claritin-D 24 Hour Extended Release Tablets ... 3104
Cortifoam Rectal Foam ... 3170
Desoxyn Tablets ... 440
Dexedrine ... 1512
DextroStat Tablets ... 3236
Dopram Injectable ... 2931
Extendryl ... 1361
Guaifed ... 2272
Hycomine Compound Tablets ... 1317
Imitrex Injection ... 1549
Inversine Tablets ... 1850
Ionamin Capsules ... 1163
Kronofed-A ... 1341
Lunelle Monthly Injection ... 2827
Midrin Capsules ... 3464
Parnate Tablets ... 1607
Phenergan VC Syrup ... 3560
Phenergan VC with Codeine Syrup ... 3561
Rynatan Tablets ... 3351
Semprex-D Capsules ... 1172
Zephrex Tablets ... 3091
Zephrex LA Tablets ... 3092
Zyrtec-D 12 Hour Extended Relief Tablets ... 2758

Hyperthermia, malignant, history of
Anectine Injection ... 1476
Suprane Liquid for Inhalation ... 874

Hyperthyroidism
(*see also under* Thyrotoxicosis; Thyrotoxicosis, untreated)
Adderall Tablets ... 3231
Adipex-P ... 1406
Bontril Slow-Release Capsules ... 576
Cortifoam Rectal Foam ... 3170
Desoxyn Tablets ... 440
Dexedrine ... 1512
DextroStat Tablets ... 3236
Extendryl ... 1361
Flexeril Tablets ... 572
Flexeril Tablets ... 2094
Hycomine Compound Tablets ... 1317
Ionamin Capsules ... 1163
Iscar Mali Injection ... 3456
Iscar Mali Special Injection ... 3456
Iscar Pini Injection ... 3456
Iscar Quercus Injection ... 3456
Iscar Quercus Special Injection ... 3456
Pima Syrup ... 1362
Rynatan Tablets ... 3351
Urecholine ... 2198
Urecholine Tablets ... 2445

Hyperviscosity syndrome
MUSE Urethral Suppository ... 3335

Hypervitaminosis A
Aquasol A Parenteral ... 593

Hypervitaminosis D
(*see under* Toxicity, vitamin D)

Hypervolemia
Plasmanate ... 942

Hypocalcemia
Actonel Tablets ... 2879
Fosamax Tablets ... 2095

Hypogammaglobulinemia
(*see also under* Immunodeficiency, unspecified)
Attenuvax ... 2044
Meruvax II ... 2130
M-M-R II ... 2118
Mumpsvax ... 2141
Varivax ... 2202

Hypoglycemia, unspecified
Humalog ... 1926
Humulin R Regular (U-500) ... 1943
NovoLog Injection ... 2427

Hypokalemia
Betapace AF Tablets ... 954
Daranide Tablets ... 2077

Hypomotility syndrome
Visicol Tablets ... 1767

Hyponatremia
Daranide Tablets ... 2077
Lithium Carbonate ... 3061
Lithium Citrate Syrup ... 3061

Hypophosphatemia
Renagel Capsules ... 1439
Renagel Tablets ... 1439

Hypospadias, severe
MUSE Urethral Suppository ... 3335

Hypotension, unspecified
Cardizem Injectable ... 1018
Cardizem Lyo-Ject Syringe ... 1018
Cardizem Monovial ... 1018
Cardizem CD Capsules ... 1016
Covera-HS Tablets ... 3199
Isoptin SR Tablets ... 467
Natrecor for Injection ... 3189
Nicotinex Elixir ... ▣633
Normodyne Injection ... 3135
Normodyne Tablets ... 3137
Rythmol Tablets – 150 mg, 225 mg, 300 mg ... 502
Tarka Tablets ... 508
Tiazac Capsules ... 1378
Urecholine ... 2198
Urecholine Tablets ... 2445
Verelan Capsules ... 3184
Verelan PM Capsules ... 3186

Hypothalamic damage
Etrafon ... 3115
Trilafon ... 3160

Hypovolemia
(*see under* Shock, unspecified)

I

IgA deficiencies, selective
(*see under* Immunoglobulin A deficiency)

Ileocolostomy
Activase I.V. ... 1410

Ileus, paralytic
Donnatal ... 2929
Donnatal Extentabs ... 2930
Donnatal Tablets ... 2929
Kadian Capsules ... 1335
Levsin/Levsinex/Levbid ... 3172
MS Contin Tablets ... 2896
MSIR ... 2898
NuLev Orally Disintegrating Tablets ... 3176
Oramorph SR Tablets ... 3062
OxyContin Tablets ... 2912
OxyFast Oral Concentrate Solution ... 2916
OxyIR Capsules ... 2916
Robinul Forte Tablets ... 1358
Robinul Injectable ... 2940
Robinul Tablets ... 1358
Roxicodone Tablets ... 3067

Ileus, unspecified
(*see also under* Ileus, paralytic)
Colyte with Flavor Packs for Oral Solution ... 3170
GoLYTELY and Pineapple Flavor GoLYTELY for Oral Solution ... 1068
Tri-Levlen 28 Tablets ... 962
Visicol Tablets ... 1767

Illness, unspecified
Tetanus and Diphtheria Toxoids Adsorbed For Adult Use ... 815

Immunodeficiency, family history of
Meruvax II ... 2130
M-M-R II ... 2118
Mumpsvax ... 2141

Immunodeficiency, history of
Attenuvax ... 2044
Varivax ... 2202

Immunodeficiency, unspecified
(*see also under* Acquired immune deficiency syndrome; Dysgammaglobulinemia; Human immunodeficiency virus; Hypogammaglobulinemia; Immunodeficiency, family history of; Immunodeficiency, history of; Immunoglobulin A deficiency; Immunosuppression)
Attenuvax ... 2044
Meruvax II ... 2130
M-M-R II ... 2118
Mumpsvax ... 2141
TheraCys Injection ... 823
Tice BCG, BCG Live ... 2489
Varivax ... 2202
Vivotif Berna ... 997

Immunodeficient state
(*see under* Immunodeficiency, unspecified)

Immunoglobulin A deficiency
BayGam ... 914
CytoGam Intravenous ... 2026
Gamimune N, 5% Solvent/Detergent Treated ... 925
Gamimune N, 10% Solvent/Detergent Treated ... 928
Gammar-P I.V. ... 787
Sandoglobulin I.V. ... 2391

Immunosuppression
Attenuvax ... 2044
Meruvax II ... 2130
M-M-R II ... 2118
Mumpsvax ... 2141
TheraCys Injection ... 823
Tice BCG, BCG Live ... 2489
Varivax ... 2202
Vivotif Berna ... 997

Impulse generation disorders
(*see under* Arrhythmia, cardiac, unspecified)

Increased intracranial pressure
(*see under* Intracranial pressure, increased)

Infants
Agenerase Oral Solution ... 1459
Bactrim ... 2949
Benadryl Parenteral ... 2617
Cardizem Injectable ... 1018
Cardizem Lyo-Ject Syringe ... 1018
Cardizem Monovial ... 1018
Caverject Sterile Powder ... 2777
Dopram Injectable ... 2931
Lindane Shampoo USP 1% ... 560
Macrobid Capsules ... 2889
Macrodantin Capsules ... 2891
Ovide Lotion ... 2023
Pediazole Suspension ... 3050
Periactin Tablets ... 2155
Robinul Injectable ... 2940
Ryna-12 S Suspension ... 3351
Reformulated Rynatan Pediatric Suspension ... 3352
Rynatuss Pediatric Suspension ... 3353
Septra Suspension ... 2265
Septra Tablets ... 2265
Septra DS Tablets ... 2265

Infants, premature
Benadryl Parenteral ... 2617
Lindane Lotion USP 1% ... 559
Periactin Tablets ... 2155

Infection, external ear canal, viral
Cipro HC Otic Suspension ... 540

Infection, bacterial, unspecified
(*see under* Endocarditis, bacterial)

Infection, febrile
Attenuvax ... 2044
Infanrix Vaccine ... 1562
Meruvax II ... 2130
M-M-R II ... 2118
Mumpsvax ... 2141
TheraCys Injection ... 823
Varivax ... 2202

Infection, fungal
(*see under* Actinomycosis, genital; Infection, fungal, unspecified; Infection, ophthalmic, fungal; Infection, otic, fungal; Infection, systemic, fungal; Lesions, skin, fungal)

Infection, fungal, unspecified
(*see also under* Actinomycosis, genital)
Cortifoam Rectal Foam ... 3170

Infection, injection site
Botox Purified Neurotoxin Complex ... 549
Duraclon Injection ... 3057
Hyalgan Solution ... 3080
Synvisc ... 3596

Infection, mycobacterial
(*see under* Infection, ophthalmic, mycobacterial; Tuberculosis, unspecified)

Infection, nasal, untreated
Nasarel Nasal Solution 0.025% ... 1296

Infection, ophthalmic, cysticercosis
(*see under* Cysticercosis, ocular)

Infection, ophthalmic, fungal
Alrex Sterile Ophthalmic Suspension 0.2% ... ⊙256
Blephamide Ophthalmic Ointment ... 547
Blephamide Ophthalmic Suspension ... 548
Cortisporin Ophthalmic Suspension Sterile ... ⊙297
Decadron Phosphate Sterile Ophthalmic Ointment ... 2083
Decadron Phosphate Sterile Ophthalmic Solution ... 2084
FML Ophthalmic Ointment ... ⊙237
FML Ophthalmic Suspension ... ⊙236
FML Forte Ophthalmic Suspension ... ⊙235
FML-S Liquifilm Sterile Ophthalmic Suspension ... ⊙238
HMS Sterile Ophthalmic Suspension ... ⊙240
Lotemax Sterile Ophthalmic Suspension 0.5% ... ⊙261
NeoDecadron Sterile Ophthalmic Solution ... 2144
Poly-Pred Liquifilm Ophthalmic Suspension ... ⊙245
Pred Forte Ophthalmic Suspension ... ⊙246
Pred Mild Sterile Ophthalmic Suspension ... ⊙249
Pred-G Ophthalmic Suspension ... ⊙247
Pred-G Sterile Ophthalmic Ointment ... ⊙248
Terra-Cortril Ophthalmic Suspension ... 2716
TobraDex Ophthalmic Ointment ... 542
TobraDex Ophthalmic Suspension ... 541
Vexol 1% Ophthalmic Suspension ... ⊙222

Infection, ophthalmic, mycobacterial
(*see also under* Tuberculosis, unspecified)
Alrex Sterile Ophthalmic Suspension 0.2% ... ⊙256
Blephamide Ophthalmic Ointment ... 547
Blephamide Ophthalmic Suspension ... 548
Cortisporin Ophthalmic Suspension Sterile ... ⊙297
Decadron Phosphate Sterile Ophthalmic Ointment ... 2083
Decadron Phosphate Sterile Ophthalmic Solution ... 2084
FML Ophthalmic Ointment ... ⊙237
FML Ophthalmic Suspension ... ⊙236
FML Forte Ophthalmic Suspension ... ⊙235
FML-S Liquifilm Sterile Ophthalmic Suspension ... ⊙238
HMS Sterile Ophthalmic Suspension ... ⊙240
Lotemax Sterile Ophthalmic Suspension 0.5% ... ⊙261
NeoDecadron Sterile Ophthalmic Solution ... 2144
Poly-Pred Liquifilm Ophthalmic Suspension ... ⊙245
Pred Forte Ophthalmic Suspension ... ⊙246
Pred Mild Sterile Ophthalmic Suspension ... ⊙249
Pred-G Ophthalmic Suspension ... ⊙247
Pred-G Sterile Ophthalmic Ointment ... ⊙248
Terra-Cortril Ophthalmic Suspension ... 2716
TobraDex Ophthalmic Ointment ... 542
TobraDex Ophthalmic Suspension ... 541
Vexol 1% Ophthalmic Suspension ... ⊙222

Infection, ophthalmic, unspecified
(*see under* Cysticercosis, ocular; Iritis, acute)

Infection, ophthalmic, untreated
Pred Forte Ophthalmic Suspension ... ⊙246
Pred Mild Sterile Ophthalmic Suspension ... ⊙249

Infection, ophthalmic, viral
(*see also under* Herpes simplex keratitis)
Blephamide Ophthalmic Ointment ... 547
Blephamide Ophthalmic Suspension ... 548
Cortisporin Ophthalmic Suspension Sterile ... ⊙297

- Decadron Phosphate Sterile Ophthalmic Ointment ... 2083
- Decadron Phosphate Sterile Ophthalmic Solution ... 2084
- FML Ophthalmic Ointment ... ⊙ 237
- FML Ophthalmic Suspension ... ⊙ 236
- FML Forte Ophthalmic Suspension ... ⊙ 235
- HMS Sterile Ophthalmic Suspension ... ⊙ 240
- Lotemax Sterile Ophthalmic Suspension 0.5% ... ⊙ 261
- NeoDecadron Sterile Ophthalmic Solution ... 2144
- Poly-Pred Liquifilm Ophthalmic Suspension ... ⊙ 245
- Pred Forte Ophthalmic Suspension ... ⊙ 246
- Pred Mild Sterile Ophthalmic Suspension ... ⊙ 249
- Pred-G Ophthalmic Suspension ... ⊙ 247
- Pred-G Sterile Ophthalmic Ointment ... ⊙ 248
- Terra-Cortril Ophthalmic Suspension ... 2716
- TobraDex Ophthalmic Ointment ... 542
- TobraDex Ophthalmic Suspension ... 541
- Vexol 1% Ophthalmic Suspension ... ⊙ 222

Infection, otic
(*see under* Infection, otic, fungal; Otitis media)

Infection, otic, fungal
- Decadron Phosphate Sterile Ophthalmic Solution ... 2084

Infection, respiratory
(*see also under* Respiratory illness, febrile; Respiratory illness, unspecified; Tuberculosis, unspecified)
- Fluzone Vaccine ... 802

Infection, scalp
- Cormax Scalp Application ... 2441
- Temovate Scalp Application ... 1304

Infection, skin, fungal
(*see under* Lesions, skin, fungal)

Infection, systemic, fungal
- Celestone Soluspan Injectable Suspension ... 3097
- Cortifoam Rectal Foam ... 3170
- Cortone Acetate Injectable Suspension ... 2059
- Cortone Acetate Tablets ... 2061
- Decadron Elixir ... 2078
- Decadron Tablets ... 2079
- Decadron Phosphate Injection ... 2081
- Depo-Medrol Injectable Suspension ... 2795
- Florinef Acetate Tablets ... 2250
- Hydrocortone Tablets ... 2106
- Hydrocortone Acetate Injectable Suspension ... 2103
- Hydrocortone Phosphate Injection, Sterile ... 2105
- Pediapred Oral Solution ... 1170
- Prednisone ... 3064
- Prelone Syrup ... 2273
- Solu-Medrol Sterile Powder ... 2855

Infection, unspecified
- Astramorph/PF Injection, USP (Preservative-Free) ... 594
- Cortifoam Rectal Foam ... 3170
- Diphtheria & Tetanus Toxoids Adsorbed Purogenated for Pediatric Use ... 1857
- Sterile FUDR ... 2974
- Tetanus & Diphtheria Toxoids Adsorbed for Adult Use ... 1880
- Tetanus Toxoid Adsorbed Purogenated ... 1882
- Tripedia Vaccine ... 817

Infection, untreated
(*see also under* Infection, nasal, untreated; Infection, ophthalmic, untreated)
- Indocin I.V. ... 2115
- Vexol 1% Ophthalmic Suspension ... ⊙ 222

Infection, urinary tract
(*see also under* Glomerulonephritis; Nephritis)
- TheraCys Injection ... 823
- Tice BCG, BCG Live ... 2489
- Valstar Sterile Solution for Intravesical Instillation ... 1175

Infection, vaginal
(*see under* Cervicitis, untreated; Vaginitis, untreated; Vaginosis, bacterial, untreated)

Infection, viral
(*see under* Herpes genitalia; Herpes simplex keratitis; Herpes simplex, unspecified; Herpes zoster; Human immunodeficiency virus; Infection, ophthalmic, viral; Lesions, skin, viral; Varicella)

Infertility, non-anovulatory
- Humegon for Injection ... 2468
- Pergonal for Injection ... 3223
- Repronex for Intramuscular and Subcutaneous Injection ... 1347

Infertility, non-hypogonadotropic
- Humegon for Injection ... 2468
- Pergonal for Injection ... 3223
- Repronex for Intramuscular and Subcutaneous Injection ... 1347

Infertility, treatment of
- Synthroid ... 505

Inflammation, gastrointestinal tract
(*see also under* Abscess, intestinal; Colitis, toxic; Colitis, ulcerative; Colitis, ulcerative, history of; Colitis, unspecified; Colitis, unspecified, history of; Diverticulitis; Enteritis, history of; Enterocolitis, necrotizing; Esophagitis, reflux; Gastroenteritis; Ulcer, gastrointestinal)
- Glyset Tablets ... 2821
- Ponstel Capsules ... 1356
- Precose Tablets ... 906

Inflammation, local
- Sarapin ... 1727

Inflammation, uveal
(*see under* Uveitis)

Inflammatory bowel disease
(*see under* Inflammation, gastrointestinal tract)

Intertriginous areas
(*see under* Intertrigo)

Intertrigo
- Cordran Tape ... 2439

Intestinal atony
(*see under* Atony, intestinal)

Intestinal disorders, unspecified
(*see also under* Atony, intestinal; Bowel ischemia, history of; Inflammation, gastrointestinal tract; Megacolon, toxic; Megacolon, unspecified; Obstruction, gastrointestinal tract; Perforation, gastrointestinal tract)
- Glyset Tablets ... 2821
- Precose Tablets ... 906

Intestinal obstruction
(*see under* Obstruction, gastrointestinal tract)

Intoxication, acute
- Ultracet Tablets ... 2597

Intoxication, unspecified
- Ultram Tablets ... 2600

Intracranial pressure, increased
- Dilaudid ... 441
- Dilaudid Powder ... 441
- Dilaudid Rectal Suppositories ... 441
- Dilaudid Tablets ... 441
- Hycomine Compound Tablets ... 1317
- Hycotuss Expectorant Syrup ... 1318
- Nitrostat Tablets ... 2658
- Romazicon Injection ... 3000
- Roxanol ... 3066
- Vicodin Tuss Expectorant ... 519

Intracranial trauma
(*see under* Trauma, intracranial)

Intraocular injection
- Vistide Injection ... 1445

Intravascular clotting process, active
(*see under* Coagulation, intravascular, active)

Intubation, history of
- Proleukin for Injection ... 1199

Iridocyclitis
(*see also under* Uveitis)
- Humorsol Sterile Ophthalmic Solution ... 2102

Iritis, acute
(*see also under* Iridocyclitis; Uveitis)
- Evoxac Capsules ... 1217
- Isopto Carbachol Ophthalmic Solution ... ⊙ 215
- Isopto Carpine Ophthalmic Solution ... ⊙ 215
- Pilopine HS Ophthalmic Gel ... ⊙ 217
- Rēv-Eyes Sterile Ophthalmic Eyedrops 0.5% ... ⊙ 265
- Salagen Tablets ... 2229

Iron overload, evidence of
- Ferrlecit Injection ... 3386

Ischemia, silent
- Amerge Tablets ... 1467
- Axert Tablets ... 2772
- D.H.E. 45 Injection ... 2334
- Imitrex Injection ... 1549
- Imitrex Nasal Spray ... 1554
- Imitrex Tablets ... 1558
- Maxalt Tablets ... 2120
- Maxalt-MLT Orally Disintegrating Tablets ... 2120
- Migranal Nasal Spray ... 2376
- Zomig Tablets ... 708
- Zomig-ZMT Tablets ... 708

Ischemia, unspecified
- Imitrex Injection ... 1549

Ischemic attacks, transient
- Amerge Tablets ... 1467
- Imitrex Injection ... 1549
- Imitrex Nasal Spray ... 1554
- Imitrex Tablets ... 1558

Ischemic heart disease
(*see under* Heart disease, ischemic)

Ischemic myocardial disease
(*see under* Heart disease, ischemic)

J

Jaundice, cholestatic of pregnancy, history of
- Alesse-21 Tablets ... 3468
- Alesse-28 Tablets ... 3473
- Brevicon 28-Day Tablets ... 3380
- Cyclessa Tablets ... 2450
- Desogen Tablets ... 2458
- Estrostep ... 2627
- Levlen ... 962
- Levlite 21 Tablets ... 962
- Levlite 28 Tablets ... 962
- Levora Tablets ... 3389
- Loestrin 21 Tablets ... 2642
- Loestrin Fe Tablets ... 2642
- Lo/Ovral Tablets ... 3532
- Lo/Ovral-28 Tablets ... 3538
- Low-Ogestrel-28 Tablets ... 3392
- Lunelle Monthly Injection ... 2827
- Microgestin Fe 1.5/30 Tablets ... 3407
- Microgestin Fe 1/20 Tablets ... 3400
- Mircette Tablets ... 2470
- Modicon ... 2563
- Necon ... 3415
- Nordette-28 Tablets ... 2257
- Norinyl 1 +35 28-Day Tablets ... 3380
- Norinyl 1 + 50 28-Day Tablets ... 3380
- Ogestrel 0.5/50-28 Tablets ... 3428
- Ortho-Cept 21 Tablets ... 2546
- Ortho-Cept 28 Tablets ... 2546
- Ortho-Cyclen/Ortho Tri-Cyclen ... 2573
- Ortho-Novum ... 2563
- Ortho-Novum 1/50□28 Tablets ... 2556
- Ortho-Novum ... 2563
- Ortho-Cyclen/Ortho Tri-Cyclen ... 2573
- Ovcon ... 3364
- Ovral Tablets ... 3551
- Ovral-28 Tablets ... 3552
- Ovrette Tablets ... 3552
- Tri-Levlen ... 962
- Tri-Norinyl-28 Tablets ... 3433
- Triphasil-21 Tablets ... 3600
- Triphasil-28 Tablets ... 3605
- Trivora Tablets ... 3439
- Yasmin 28 Tablets ... 980
- Zovia ... 3449

Jaundice, history of
- Alesse-21 Tablets ... 3468
- Alesse-28 Tablets ... 3473
- Augmentin Powder for Oral Suspension ... 1482
- Augmentin Tablets ... 1485
- Augmentin ES-600 Powder for Oral Suspension ... 1487
- Brevicon 28-Day Tablets ... 3380
- Cognex Capsules ... 1351
- Cyclessa Tablets ... 2450
- Desogen Tablets ... 2458
- Estrostep ... 2627
- Levlen ... 962
- Levlite 21 Tablets ... 962
- Levlite 28 Tablets ... 962
- Levora Tablets ... 3389
- Loestrin 21 Tablets ... 2642
- Loestrin Fe Tablets ... 2642
- Lo/Ovral Tablets ... 3532
- Lo/Ovral-28 Tablets ... 3538
- Low-Ogestrel-28 Tablets ... 3392
- Lunelle Monthly Injection ... 2827
- Microgestin Fe 1.5/30 Tablets ... 3407
- Microgestin Fe 1/20 Tablets ... 3400
- Mircette Tablets ... 2470
- Modicon ... 2563
- Necon ... 3415
- Nordette-28 Tablets ... 2257
- Norinyl 1 +35 28-Day Tablets ... 3380
- Norinyl 1 + 50 28 Day Tablets ... 3380
- Ogestrel 0.5/50-28 Tablets ... 3428
- Ortho-Cept 21 Tablets ... 2546
- Ortho-Cept 28 Tablets ... 2546
- Ortho-Cyclen/Ortho Tri-Cyclen ... 2573
- Ortho-Novum ... 2563
- Ortho-Novum 1/50□28 Tablets ... 2556
- Ortho-Novum ... 2563
- Ortho-Cyclen/Ortho Tri-Cyclen ... 2573
- Ovcon ... 3364
- Ovral Tablets ... 3551
- Ovral-28 Tablets ... 3552
- Ovrette Tablets ... 3552
- Tri-Levlen ... 962
- Tri-Norinyl-28 Tablets ... 3433
- Triphasil-21 Tablets ... 3600
- Triphasil-28 Tablets ... 3605
- Trivora Tablets ... 3439
- Yasmin 28 Tablets ... 980
- Zovia ... 3449

Jaundice, unspecified
- Motofen Tablets ... 577

K

Keratitis, dendritic
(*see under* Herpes simplex keratitis)

Ketoacidosis, diabetic
- Amaryl Tablets ... 717
- DiaBeta Tablets ... 741
- Diabinese Tablets ... 2680
- Glucophage Tablets ... 1080
- Glucophage XR Tablets ... 1080
- Glucotrol Tablets ... 2692
- Glucotrol XL Extended Release Tablets ... 2693
- Glucovance Tablets ... 1086
- Glyset Tablets ... 2821
- Prandin Tablets (0.5, 1, and 2 mg) ... 2432
- Precose Tablets ... 906
- Starlix Tablets ... 2401

Kidney damage
(*see under* Renal dysfunction)

Kidney disease
(*see under* Renal disease, unspecified)

Kidney failure
(*see under* Renal failure)

Kyphoscoliosis
- Dilaudid ... 441
- Dilaudid Powder ... 441
- Dilaudid Rectal Suppositories ... 441
- Dilaudid Tablets ... 441

L

Labor
- Dilaudid Oral Liquid ... 445
- Dilaudid Tablets - 8 mg ... 445
- Dilaudid-HP ... 443
- Macrobid Capsules ... 2889
- Macrodantin Capsules ... 2891
- Toradol ... 3018

Labor, difficult, history of
- Prepidil Gel ... 2851

Lactation
(*see under* Breastfeeding)

Left ventricular dysfunction
(*see under* Ventricular dysfunction, left)

Lesions, gastrointestinal, unspecified
(*see also under* Colitis, ulcerative; Colitis, ulcerative, history of; Ulcer, gastrointestinal)
Urecholine 2198
Urecholine Tablets 2445

Lesions, intracranial, unspecified
(*see also under* Tumor, intracranial, unspecified; Tumor, pituitary, unspecified)
Clomid Tablets 735
Dilaudid 441
Dilaudid Powder 441
Dilaudid Rectal Suppositories 441
Dilaudid Tablets 441
Genotropin Lyophilized Powder 2818
Humegon for Injection 2468
Hycomine Compound Tablets 1317
Hycotuss Expectorant Syrup 1318
Pergonal for Injection 3223
Repronex for Intramuscular and Subcutaneous Injection 1347
Serophene Tablets 3226
Vicodin Tuss Expectorant 519

Lesions, malignant, unspecified
(*see under* Carcinoma, breast, male; Carcinoma, breast, unspecified; Carcinoma, cervical; Carcinoma, endometrium; Carcinoma, female reproductive organs; Carcinoma, genital, unspecified; Carcinoma, hepatic; Carcinoma, prostate; Carcinoma, skin, unspecified; Carcinoma, squamous cell, unspecified; Melanoma, history of; Melanoma, unspecified; Neoplasm, bone marrow system, malignant; Neoplasm, lymphatic system, malignant)

Lesions, skin, unspecified
(*see also under* Birthmarks; Burns; Melanoma, unspecified; Moles; Warts, atypical)
Cordran Tape 2439
Lodosyn Tablets 1251
Sinemet Tablets 1253
Sinemet CR Tablets 1255

Lesions, skin, viral
(*see under* Herpes genitalia; Herpes simplex, unspecified; Herpes zoster; Varicella)

Leukemia, acute
Myleran Tablets 1603

Leukemia, chronic lymphocytic
Myleran Tablets 1603

Leukemia, chronic myelogenous, blastic crisis
Myleran Tablets 1603

Leukemia, unspecified
Attenuvax 2044
Caverject Sterile Powder 2777
Meruvax II 2130
M-M-R II 2118
Mumpsvax 2141
ParaGard T 380A Intrauterine Copper Contraceptive 2582
Tice BCG, BCG Live 2489
Varivax 2202
YF-VAX Vaccine 827

Leukopenia
Mylocel Tablets 2227

Liver adenoma
(*see under* Adenoma, hepatic)

Liver cancer
(*see under* Carcinoma, hepatic)

Liver damage
(*see under* Liver dysfunction)

Liver disease, decompensated
PEG-Intron Powder for Injection 3140

Liver disease, history of
(*see also under* Hepatitis, history of; Liver dysfunction, history of)
Nardil Tablets 2653

Liver disease, unspecified
(*see also under* Cirrhosis, primary biliary; Cirrhosis, unspecified; Hepatitis; Liver dysfunction)
Activella Tablets 2764
Aldoclor Tablets 2035
Aldomet Tablets 2037
Aldoril Tablets 2039
Aygestin Tablets 1333
Baycol Tablets 883
Clomid Tablets 735
Crinone 3213
Dantrium Capsules 2885
Depacon Injection 416
Depakene 421
Depakote Sprinkle Capsules 426
Depakote Tablets 430
Depakote ER Tablets 436
Depo-Provera Contraceptive Injection 2798
Dyrenium Capsules 3458
Klonopin Tablets 2983
Lescol Capsules 2361
Lescol Capsules 2925
Lescol XL Tablets 2361
Lescol XL Tablets 2925
Lipitor Tablets 2639
Lipitor Tablets 2696
Mevacor Tablets 2132
Micronor Tablets 2543
Midrin Capsules 3464
Mirena Intrauterine System 974
Norplant System 3543
Nor-QD Tablets 3423
Pravachol Tablets 1099
Premphase Tablets 3572
Prempro Tablets 3572
Prometrium Capsules (100 mg, 200 mg) 3261
Prostin E2 Suppositories 2852
Provera Tablets 2853
Rifamate Capsules 767
Rifater Tablets 769
Serophene Tablets 3226
Tasmar Tablets 3010
Uroqid-Acid No. 2 Tablets 947
Zocor Tablets 2219

Liver disorders, history of
Aldoclor Tablets 2035
Aldomet Tablets 2037
Aldoril Tablets 2039
Augmentin Powder for Oral Suspension 1482
Augmentin ES-600 Powder for Oral Suspension 1487
Felbatol 3343

Liver disorders, unspecified
(*see under* Liver dysfunction)

Liver dysfunction
(*see also under* Jaundice, cholestatic of pregnancy, history of; Jaundice, history of; Jaundice, unspecified; Liver disease, unspecified; Liver failure; Serum transaminase elevation)
Activella Tablets 2764
Anadrol-50 Tablets 3321
Atromid-S Capsules 3483
Aygestin Tablets 1333
Bactrim 2949
Coreg Tablets 1508
Crinone 3213
Cylert Tablets 415
Daranide Tablets 2077
Depacon Injection 416
Depakene 421
Depakote Sprinkle Capsules 426
Depakote Tablets 430
Depo-Provera Contraceptive Injection 2798
D.H.E. 45 Injection 2334
Ellence Injection 2806
Estratest 3252
Etrafon 3115
Eulexin Capsules 3118
Imitrex Injection 1549
Imitrex Tablets 1558
Lopid Tablets 2650
Lunelle Monthly Injection 2827
Niaspan Extended-Release Tablets 1846
Nilandron Tablets 753
Premphase Tablets 3572
Prempro Tablets 3572
Prometrium Capsules (100 mg, 200 mg) 3261
Provera Tablets 2853
Pyrazinamide Tablets 1876
Rifater Tablets 769
Skelaxin Tablets 1301
Stelazine 1640
Tasmar Tablets 3010
Thioplex for Injection 1765
Ticlid Tablets 3015
Trecator-SC Tablets 3598
Tricor Capsules, Micronized 513
Trilafon 3160
Yasmin 28 Tablets 980
Yodoxin Tablets 1722
Zyflo Filmtab Tablets 524

Liver dysfunction, history of
(*see also under* Liver disease, history of)
Augmentin Tablets 1485
Clomid Tablets 735
Rifamate Capsules 767
Serophene Tablets 3226

Liver failure
(*see also under* Coma, hepatic; Liver dysfunction; Precoma, hepatic)
Agenerase Oral Solution 1459
Grifulvin V Tablets Microsize and Oral Suspension Microsize 2518
Gris-PEG Tablets 2661

Liver function tests, abnormal
(*see under* Serum transaminase elevation)

Liver insufficiency
(*see under* Liver dysfunction)

Liver tumor
(*see under* Adenoma, hepatic; Carcinoma, hepatic; Tumor, liver, benign)

Local anesthesia
(*see under* Anesthesia, local)

Lown-Ganong-Levine syndrome
Covera-HS Tablets 3199
Isoptin SR Tablets 467
Tarka Tablets 508
Verelan Capsules 3184
Verelan PM Capsules 3186

Lung disease, unspecified
(*see under* Pulmonary disorders, unspecified)

Lupus erythematosus
8-MOP Capsules 1727
Oxsoralen Lotion 1% 1740
Oxsoralen-Ultra Capsules 1741
Procanbid Extended-Release Tablets 2262

Lymphoma
(*see also under* Neoplasm, lymphatic system, malignant)
Attenuvax 2044
Meruvax II 2130
M-M-R II 2118
Mumpsvax 2141
Tice BCG, BCG Live 2489
Varivax 2202
YF-VAX Vaccine 827

M

Malabsorption syndrome
Xenical Capsules 3043

Malignancies, unspecified
Gengraf Capsules 457
Neoral Soft Gelatin Capsules 2380
Neoral Oral Solution 2380

Malignancy
(*see under* Carcinoma, breast, male; Carcinoma, breast, unspecified; Carcinoma, endometrium; Carcinoma, hepatic; Carcinoma, prostate; Carcinoma, skin, unspecified; Hypertension, malignant; Hyperthermia, malignant, history of; Leukemia, unspecified; Lymphoma; Melanoma, history of; Melanoma, unspecified; Neoplasm, bone marrow system, malignant; Neoplasm, lymphatic system, malignant)

Malnutrition
Sterile FUDR 2974

Mechanical disorders of ventilation
(*see under* Asthma, acute; Asthma, history of; Asthma, unspecified; Flail chest; Obstruction, respiratory tract; Paresis, respiratory; Pneumothorax; Pulmonary fibrosis)

Megacolon, toxic
Colyte with Flavor Packs for Oral Solution 3170
Donnatal 2929
Donnatal Extentabs 2930
Donnatal Tablets 2929
GoLYTELY and Pineapple Flavor GoLYTELY for Oral Solution 1068
Levsin/Levsinex/Levbid 3172
NuLev Orally Disintegrating Tablets 3176
NuLYTELY, Cherry Flavor, Lemon-Lime Flavor, and Orange Flavor NuLYTELY for Oral Solution 1068
Robinul Forte Tablets 1358
Robinul Injectable 2940
Robinul Tablets 1358
Tri-Levlen 28 Tablets 962
Visicol Tablets 1767

Megacolon, unspecified
Akineton 402

Megaloblastic anemia
(*see under* Anemia, megaloblastic, unspecified)

Melanoma, history of
8-MOP Capsules 1727
Lodosyn Tablets 1251
Oxsoralen Lotion 1% 1740
Oxsoralen-Ultra Capsules 1741
Sinemet CR Tablets 1255

Melanoma, unspecified
8-MOP Capsules 1727
Oxsoralen Lotion 1% 1740
Oxsoralen-Ultra Capsules 1741
Sinemet Tablets 1253

Metabolic acidosis
(*see under* Acidosis, hyperchloremic; Acidosis, metabolic, unspecified; Ketoacidosis, diabetic)

Migraine, basilar
Amerge Tablets 1467
Axert Tablets 2772
D.H.E. 45 Injection 2334
Imitrex Injection 1549
Imitrex Nasal Spray 1554
Imitrex Tablets 1558
Maxalt Tablets 2120
Maxalt-MLT Orally Disintegrating Tablets 2120
Migranal Nasal Spray 2376
Zomig Tablets 708
Zomig-ZMT Tablets 708

Migraine, hemiplegic
Amerge Tablets 1467
Axert Tablets 2772
D.H.E. 45 Injection 2334
Imitrex Injection 1549
Imitrex Nasal Spray 1554
Imitrex Tablets 1558
Maxalt Tablets 2120
Maxalt-MLT Orally Disintegrating Tablets 2120
Migranal Nasal Spray 2376
Zomig Tablets 708
Zomig-ZMT Tablets 708

Moles
Podocon-25 Liquid 2608

Motor neuron injury
Anectine Injection 1476

Multipara, grand
Prepidil Gel 2851

Multipara, unspecified
Cervidil Vaginal Insert 1369

Myasthenia gravis
Cortifoam Rectal Foam 3170
Donnatal 2929
Donnatal Extentabs 2930
Donnatal Tablets 2929
Levsin/Levsinex/Levbid 3172
Norflex 1987
NuLev Orally Disintegrating Tablets 3176
Quinaglute Dura-Tabs Tablets 978
Quinidex Extentabs 2933
Robinul Forte Tablets 1358
Robinul Injectable 2940

Robinul Tablets....1358
Urimax Tablets....1769

Mycobacterial infection
(*see under* Infection, ophthalmic, mycobacterial; Tuberculosis, unspecified)

Myeloid blasts, leukemic
(*see also under* Leukemia, chronic myelogenous, blastic crisis)
Leukine....1755

Myeloma, multiple
Caverject Sterile Powder....2777
MUSE Urethral Suppository....3335

Myeloproliferative disorders
(*see also under* Leukemia, acute; Leukemia, chronic lymphocytic; Leukemia, chronic myelogenous, blastic crisis; Leukemia, unspecified; Myeloma, multiple)
Clozaril Tablets....2319

Myelosuppression
(*see under* Bone marrow depression)

Myocardial damage
(*see under* Cardiovascular disorders, unspecified)

Myocardial disease
(*see under* Cardiovascular disorders, unspecified)

Myocardial infarction
Cardizem CD Capsules....1016
Cytomel Tablets....1817
Ellence Injection....2806
Flexeril Tablets....572
Flexeril Tablets....2094
Geodon Capsules....2688
Inversine Tablets....1850
Levothroid Tablets....1373
Levoxyl Tablets....1819
Limbitrol....1738
Nitrostat Tablets....2658
Norpramin Tablets....755
Surmontil Capsules....3595
Tiazac Capsules....1378
Unithroid Tablets....3445
Vivactil Tablets....2217
Vivactil Tablets....2446

Myocardial infarction, history of
Amerge Tablets....1467
Axert Tablets....2772
D.H.E. 45 Injection....2334
Imitrex Injection....1549
Imitrex Nasal Spray....1554
Imitrex Tablets....1558
Maxalt Tablets....2120
Maxalt-MLT Orally Disintegrating Tablets....2120
Migranal Nasal Spray....2376
Proleukin for Injection....1199
Zomig Tablets....708
Zomig-ZMT Tablets....708

Myocardial insufficiency, severe
Ellence Injection....2806

Myopathy, skeletal muscle, history of
Anectine Injection....1476

N

Narrow angle glaucoma
(*see under* Glaucoma, angle closure)

Narrow angles
Propine Ophthalmic Solution....⊙250

Necrosis
(*see also under* Enterocolitis, necrotizing)
Urocit-K Tablets....2232

Neonates
(*see under* Infants)

Neonates, premature
(*see under* Infants, premature)

Neoplasia, estrogen dependent
(*see under* Neoplasm, estrogen dependent)

Neoplasia, hepatic
(*see under* Adenoma, hepatic; Carcinoma, hepatic; Tumor, liver, benign)

Neoplasia, unspecified
(*see under* Neoplasm, unspecified)

Neoplasm at application site
Regranex Gel....2586

Neoplasm, androgen dependent
(*see also under* Carcinoma, prostate)
Novarel for Injection....1347
Ovidrel for Injection....3220
Pregnyl for Injection....2482

Neoplasm, bone marrow system, malignant
(*see also under* Myeloid blasts, leukemic; Myeloma, multiple)
Attenuvax....2044
Meruvax II....2130
M-M-R II....2118
Mumpsvax....2141
Varivax....2202

Neoplasm, estrogen dependent
(*see also under* Carcinoma, breast, male; Carcinoma, breast, unspecified)
Activella Tablets....2764
Alesse-21 Tablets....3468
Alesse-28 Tablets....3473
Alora Transdermal System....3372
Brevicon 28-Day Tablets....3380
Cenestin Tablets....1263
Climara Transdermal System....958
CombiPatch Transdermal System....2323
Cyclessa Tablets....2450
Desogen Tablets....2458
Esclim Transdermal System....3460
Estinyl Tablets....3112
Estrace Tablets....3361
Estratest....3252
Estring Vaginal Ring....2811
Estrostep....2627
femhrt Tablets....2635
Levlen....962
Levlite 21 Tablets....962
Levlite 28 Tablets....962
Levora Tablets....3389
Loestrin 21 Tablets....2642
Loestrin Fe Tablets....2642
Lo/Ovral Tablets....3532
Lo/Ovral-28 Tablets....3538
Low-Ogestrel-28 Tablets....3392
Lunelle Monthly Injection....2827
Menest Tablets....2254
Microgestin Fe 1.5/30 Tablets....3407
Microgestin Fe 1/20 Tablets....3400
Mircette Tablets....2470
Modicon....2563
Necon....3415
Nordette-28 Tablets....2257
Norinyl 1 +35 28-Day Tablets....3380
Norinyl 1 + 50 28-Day Tablets....3380
Ogen Tablets....2846
Ogestrel 0.5/50-28 Tablets....3428
Ortho Dienestrol Cream....2554
Ortho-Cept 21 Tablets....2546
Ortho-Cept 28 Tablets....2546
Ortho-Cyclen/Ortho Tri-Cyclen....2573
Ortho-Est Tablets....3464
Ortho-Novum....2563
Ortho-Novum 1/50□28 Tablets....2556
Ortho-Novum....2563
Ortho-Prefest Tablets....2570
Ortho-Cyclen/Ortho Tri-Cyclen....2573
Ovcon....3364
Ovral Tablets....3551
Ovral-28 Tablets....3552
Ovrette Tablets....3552
Premarin Intravenous....3563
Premarin Tablets....3566
Premarin Vaginal Cream....3570
Premphase Tablets....3572
Prempro Tablets....3572
Tri-Levlen....962
Tri-Norinyl-28 Tablets....3433
Triphasil-21 Tablets....3600
Triphasil-28 Tablets....3605
Trivora Tablets....3439
Vagifem Tablets....2857
Vivelle Transdermal System....2412
Vivelle-Dot Transdermal System....2416
Yasmin 28 Tablets....980
Zovia....3449

Neoplasm, hepatic, unspecified
(*see under* Adenoma, hepatic; Carcinoma, hepatic; Tumor, liver, benign)

Neoplasm, intracranial
(*see under* Tumor, intracranial, unspecified)

Neoplasm, lymphatic system, malignant
(*see also under* Lymphoma)
Attenuvax....2044
Meruvax II....2130
M-M-R II....2118
Mumpsvax....2141
Varivax....2202

Neoplasm, ovarian
(*see under* Cysts, ovarian)

Neoplasm, unspecified
Nutropin AQ Injection....1420
Nutropin Depot for Injectable Suspension....1423
Nutropin for Injection....1417
Saizen for Injection....3225

Neoplastic activity, unspecified
(*see under* Neoplasm, unspecified; Tumor activity, unspecified)

Nephritis
(*see under* Glomerulonephritis)

Nephropathy, diabetic
Midamor Tablets....2136
Moduretic Tablets....2138

Nephrosis
Anadrol-50 Tablets....3321
Oxandrin Tablets....1153

Neuritis, optic
Myambutol Tablets....1290

Neurologic toxicity
(*see under* Toxicity, neurologic)

Neurological disorders, unspecified
(*see also under* Central nervous system depression; Cerebral vascular disease; Cerebral vascular disease, history of; Cerebrovascular accident; Cerebrovascular accident, history of; Charcot-Marie-Tooth syndrome; Convulsive disorders; Convulsive disorders, history of; Encephalopathy, history of; Epilepsy; Epilepsy, uncontrolled; Guillain-Barre syndrome, history of; Intracranial pressure, increased; Myasthenia gravis; Parkinsonism; Psychosis; Psychosis, toxic, history of; Psychosis, unsupervised; Seizure disorders, history of; Seizure disorders, unspecified; Senility, unsupervised; Tourette's syndrome; Toxicity, neurologic; Vagotonia)
Fluzone Vaccine....802

Neurological signs, unspecified, history of
Acel-Imune....1851
Diphtheria & Tetanus Toxoids Adsorbed Purogenated for Pediatric Use....1857
Pnu-Imune 23....1868
Tetanus & Diphtheria Toxoids Adsorbed for Adult Use....1880
Tetanus Toxoid Adsorbed Purogenated....1882
Tripedia Vaccine....817

Neurological symptoms, unspecified, history of
Acel-Imune....1851
Diphtheria & Tetanus Toxoids Adsorbed Purogenated for Pediatric Use....1857
Pnu-Imune 23....1868
Tetanus & Diphtheria Toxoids Adsorbed for Adult Use....1880
Tetanus Toxoid Adsorbed Purogenated....1882
Tripedia Vaccine....817

Neutropenia
Taxol Injection....1129
Ticlid Tablets....3015

Nursing mothers
(*see under* Breastfeeding)

O

Obesity, therapy of
Synthroid....505

Obstetric emergency
(*see under* Emergency, obstetric)

Obstetrics
(*see under* Delivery, unspecified; Labor)

Obstruction, biliary tract
(*see under* Jaundice, cholestatic of pregnancy, history of; Jaundice, history of; Jaundice, unspecified)

Obstruction, bladder neck
(*see also under* Obstruction, urinary tract)
Donnatal....2929
Donnatal Extentabs....2930
Donnatal Tablets....2929
Levsin/Levsinex/Levbid....3172
Norflex....1987
NuLev Orally Disintegrating Tablets....3176
Periactin Tablets....2155
Robinul Forte Tablets....1358
Robinul Injectable....2940
Robinul Tablets....1358
Urecholine....2198
Urecholine Tablets....2445
Urimax Tablets....1769
Urised Tablets....2876

Obstruction, gastrointestinal tract
(*see also under* Achalasia, esophageal; Achalasia, unspecified; Bowel ischemia, history of; Fecal impaction; Ileus, paralytic; Ileus, unspecified; Obstruction, pyloroduodenal; Stenosis, pyloric; Stenosis, pyloroduodenal; Stricture, esophageal)
Akineton....402
Azulfidine EN-tabs Tablets....2775
Citrucel Orange Flavor Powder....⊡744
Citrucel Sugar Free Orange Flavor Powder....⊡745
Colyte with Flavor Packs for Oral Solution....3170
Cortifoam Rectal Foam....3170
Ditropan XL Extended Release Tablets....564
Donnatal....2929
Donnatal Extentabs....2930
Donnatal Tablets....2929
Dulcolax Suppositories....⊡668
Glyset Tablets....2821
GoLYTELY and Pineapple Flavor GoLYTELY for Oral Solution....1068
Levsin/Levsinex/Levbid....3172
Mestinon....1740
Metamucil Dietary Fiber Supplement....⊡834
Metamucil....2877
Micro-K....3311
MiraLax Powder for Oral Solution....1069
Mitrolan Chewable Tablets....⊡789
Norflex....1987
NuLev Orally Disintegrating Tablets....3176
NuLYTELY, Cherry Flavor, Lemon-Lime Flavor, and Orange Flavor NuLYTELY for Oral Solution....1068
Precose Tablets....906
Prosed/DS Tablets....3268
Prostigmin Injectable....1744
Prostigmin Tablets....1744
Reglan....2935
Renagel Capsules....1439
Renagel Tablets....1439
Robinul Forte Tablets....1358
Robinul Injectable....2940
Robinul Tablets....1358
Tensilon Injectable....1745
Tri-Levlen 28 Tablets....962
Urecholine....2198
Urecholine Tablets....2445
Urimax Tablets....1769
Urised Tablets....2876

Visicol Tablets 1767

Obstruction, pulmonary
Daranide Tablets 2077

Obstruction, pyloroduodenal
Periactin Tablets 2155
Prosed/DS Tablets 3268

Obstruction, respiratory tract
(*see also under* Obstruction, pulmonary)
Astramorph/PF Injection, USP (Preservative-Free) 594
Daranide Tablets 2077
Dopram Injectable 2931
Duramorph Injection 1312

Obstruction, urinary tract
(*see also under* Obstruction, bladder neck; Prostatic hypertrophy; Urinary retention)
Azulfidine EN-tabs Tablets 2775
Donnatal 2929
Donnatal Extentabs 2930
Donnatal Tablets 2929
Levsin/Levsinex/Levbid 3172
Mestinon 1740
NuLev Orally Disintegrating Tablets 3176
Prosed/DS Tablets 3268
Prostigmin Injectable 1744
Prostigmin Tablets 1744
Robinul Forte Tablets 1358
Robinul Injectable 2940
Robinul Tablets 1358
Tensilon Injectable 1745
Urecholine 2198
Urecholine Tablets 2445

Obstruction, urogenital tract
(*see under* Obstruction, urinary tract)

Obstructive uropathy
(*see under* Obstruction, urinary tract)

Obtundation
Etrafon 3115
Trilafon 3160

Occlusion, coronary
(*see under* Coronary occlusion)

Ocular herpes simplex
(*see under* Herpes simplex keratitis)

Oliguria
Edecrin 2091
Macrobid Capsules 2889
Macrodantin Capsules 2891

Ophthalmic changes
(*see under* Retinal changes; Visual field changes)

Opioid dependence
(*see under* Narcotic dependence)

Opioid withdrawal
(*see under* Narcotic withdrawal, acute)

Optic neuritis
(*see under* Neuritis, optic)

Organ allograft
Proleukin for Injection 1199

Organic brain damage
(*see under* Brain damage)

Organic heart disease
(*see under* Cardiovascular disorders, unspecified; Heart disease, ischemic)

Osteoporosis
Cortifoam Rectal Foam 3170

Otic infection, fungal
(*see under* Infection, otic, fungal)

Otitis media
Cerumenex Eardrops 2895

Ovarian enlargement, unspecified
Clomid Tablets 735
Follistim for Injection 2465
Gonal-F for Injection 3216
Humegon for Injection 2468
Pergonal for Injection 3223
Repronex for Intramuscular and Subcutaneous Injection 1347
Serophene Tablets 3226

Ovarian failure, primary
Follistim for Injection 2465
Gonal-F for Injection 3216
Humegon for Injection 2468
Ovidrel for Injection 3220
Pergonal for Injection 3223
Repronex for Intramuscular and Subcutaneous Injection 1347

Overt cardiac failure
(*see under* Heart failure, unspecified)

P

Pain, acute
Actiq 1184
Duragesic Transdermal System 1786

Pain, intermittent
Actiq 1184
Duragesic Transdermal System 1786

Pain, mild
Actiq 1184
Duragesic Transdermal System 1786

Pain, post operative
Actiq 1184
Duragesic Transdermal System 1786

Pancreatic diseases, unspecified
Ultrase Capsules 835
Ultrase MT Capsules 835

Pancreatitis
Creon 5 Capsules 3251
Creon 10 Capsules 3251
Creon 20 Capsules 3251
Elspar for Injection 2092
Oncaspar 756
Ultrase Capsules 835
Ultrase MT Capsules 835

Pancreatitis, history of
Elspar for Injection 2092
Oncaspar 756

Pap smear abnormality
ParaGard T 380A Intrauterine Copper Contraceptive 2582

Paracervical block anesthesia
(*see under* Anesthesia, obstetrical, paracervical block)

Paralytic ileus
(*see under* Ileus, paralytic)

Paresis, respiratory
Dopram Injectable 2931

Parkinsonism
Haldol Decanoate 2535
Haldol Injection, Tablets and Concentrate 2533
Urecholine 2198
Urecholine Tablets 2445

Parkinson's disease
(*see under* Parkinsonism)

Pelvic inflammatory disease
Mirena Intrauterine System 974
ParaGard T 380A Intrauterine Copper Contraceptive 2582
Prostin E2 Suppositories 2852

Pelvic inflammatory disease, history of
ParaGard T 380A Intrauterine Copper Contraceptive 2582

Penile deformation
(*see under* Angulation, penile; Fibrosis, cavernosal; Peyronie's disease)

Peptic ulcer
(*see under* Ulcer, peptic)

Perforation, gastrointestinal tract
(*see also under* Ulcer, gastrointestinal)
Colyte with Flavor Packs for Oral Solution 3170
Cortifoam Rectal Foam 3170
GoLYTELY and Pineapple Flavor GoLYTELY for Oral Solution 1068
NuLYTELY, Cherry Flavor, Lemon-Lime Flavor, and Orange Flavor NuLYTELY for Oral Solution 1068
Reglan 2935
Toradol 3018
Tri-Levlen 28 Tablets 962
Visicol Tablets 1767

Perforation, gastrointestinal tract, history of
Proleukin for Injection 1199

Perforation, intestinal
(*see under* Perforation, gastrointestinal tract)

Pericardial effusion
Coumadin for Injection 1243
Coumadin Tablets 1243
Warfarin Sodium Tablets, USP 3302

Pericardial tamponade, history of
Proleukin for Injection 1199

Pericarditis, acute
Aggrastat 2031

Pericarditis, unspecified
Coumadin for Injection 1243
Coumadin Tablets 1243
Warfarin Sodium Tablets, USP 3302

Peripheral arterial disease
(*see under* Peripheral vascular disease)

Peripheral vascular disease
(*see also under* Arteriosclerosis, unspecified; Thrombophlebitis)
Amerge Tablets 1467
D.H.E. 45 Injection 2334
Imitrex Injection 1549
Imitrex Nasal Spray 1554
Imitrex Tablets 1558
Phenergan VC Syrup 3560
Phenergan VC with Codeine Syrup 3561

Peripheral vascular insufficiency
(*see under* Peripheral vascular disease)

Peritonitis
Cortifoam Rectal Foam 3170
Prostigmin Injectable 1744
Prostigmin Tablets 1744
Urecholine 2198
Urecholine Tablets 2445

Pernicious anemia
(*see under* Anemia, pernicious)

Peyronie's disease
Caverject Sterile Powder 2777

Pheochromocytoma
GlucaGen for Injection Diagnostic Kit 949
Glucagon for Injection Vials and Emergency Kit 1924
Nardil Tablets 2653
Parnate Tablets 1607
ProAmatine Tablets 3241
Reglan 2935

Phlebitis
(*see under* Thrombophlebitis)

Phosphate stones, infected
K-Phos Neutral Tablets 946
K-Phos Original (Sodium Free) Tablets 947

Photosensitivity diseases, unspecified
(*see also under* Albinism; Lupus erythematosus; Porphyria cutanea tarda; Porphyria, acute; Porphyria, erythropoietic; Porphyria, unspecified; Xeroderma pigmentosum)
8-MOP Capsules 1727
Levulan Kerastick 971
Oxsoralen Lotion 1% 1740
Oxsoralen-Ultra Capsules 1741

Pituitary function, normal, male
Follistim for Injection 2465
Gonal-F for Injection 3216
Humegon for Injection 2468
Pergonal for Injection 3223
Repronex for Intramuscular and Subcutaneous Injection 1347

Placenta previa, total
Prepidil Gel 2851

Platelet dysfunction, unspecified
(*see under* Thrombocytopathy, unspecified)

Pneumothorax
Dopram Injectable 2931

Poliomyelitis outbreak
Diphtheria & Tetanus Toxoids Adsorbed Purogenated for Pediatric Use 1857
Tetanus & Diphtheria Toxoids Adsorbed for Adult Use 1880
Tetanus Toxoid Adsorbed Purogenated 1882
Tripedia Vaccine 817

Polycythemia
MUSE Urethral Suppository 3335

Poor nutritional state
(*see under* Electrolyte imbalance, uncorrected; Malnutrition)

Porphyria cutanea tarda
8-MOP Capsules 1727
Oxsoralen-Ultra Capsules 1741

Porphyria, acute
Donnatal 2929
Donnatal Extentabs 2930
Donnatal Tablets 2929
Miltown Tablets 3349
Soma Tablets 3353
Soma Compound Tablets 3354
Soma Compound w/Codeine Tablets 3355

Porphyria, erythropoietic
8-MOP Capsules 1727
Oxsoralen-Ultra Capsules 1741

Porphyria, unspecified
Azulfidine EN-tabs Tablets 2775
Brevital Sodium for Injection, USP 1815
Grifulvin V Tablets Microsize and Oral Suspension Microsize 2518
Gris-PEG Tablets 2661
Levulan Kerastick 971
Nembutal Sodium Solution 485
Oxsoralen Lotion 1% 1740
Photofrin for Injection 831
Phrenilin 578
Vagifem Tablets 2857
Visudyne for Injection ....⊙308

Porphyria, variegate
8-MOP Capsules 1727
Oxsoralen-Ultra Capsules 1741

PR Syndrome, short
Cardizem Injectable 1018
Cardizem Lyo-Ject Syringe 1018
Cardizem Monovial 1018

Precocious puberty
Novarel for Injection 1347
Pregnyl for Injection 2482

Precoma, hepatic
Mykrox Tablets 1168
Zaroxolyn Tablets 1177

Preeclampsia
Coumadin for Injection 1243
Coumadin Tablets 1243
Warfarin Sodium Tablets, USP 3302

Pregnancy
Accutane Capsules 2944
Activella Tablets 2764
Agenerase Oral Solution 1459
Alesse-21 Tablets 3468
Alesse-28 Tablets 3473
Alora Transdermal System 3372
Anadrol-50 Tablets 3321
Android Capsules, 10 mg 1731
Antagon Injection 2447
Aquasol A Parenteral 593
Arava Tablets 724
Arthrotec Tablets 3195
Atarax Tablets & Syrup 2667
Atromid-S Capsules 3483
Attenuvax 2044
Aygestin Tablets 1333
Bactrim 2949
Baycol Tablets 883
Brevicon 28-Day Tablets 3380
Carac Cream 1222
Casodex Tablets 662
Cenestin Tablets 1263
Cetrotide for Injection 3209
Climara Transdermal System 958
Clomid Tablets 735
CombiPatch Transdermal System 2323
Cortifoam Rectal Foam 3170
Coumadin for Injection 1243
Coumadin Tablets 1243
Cuprimine Capsules 2075

Cyclessa Tablets 2450
Cytotec Tablets 3202
Delatestryl Injection 1151
Depen Titratable Tablets 3341
Depo-Provera Contraceptive Injection 2798
Desogen Tablets 2458
D.H.E. 45 Injection 2334
Efudex 1733
Esclim Transdermal System 3460
Estinyl Tablets 3112
Estrace Tablets 3361
Estratest 3252
Estring Vaginal Ring 2811
Estrostep 2627
Evista Tablets 1915
femhrt Tablets 2635
Fluoroplex 552
Follistim for Injection 2465
Gonal-F for Injection 3216
Grifulvin V Tablets Microsize and Oral Suspension Microsize 2518
Gris-PEG Tablets 2661
Guaifed 2272
Halcion Tablets 2823
Humegon for Injection 2468
Humorsol Sterile Ophthalmic Solution 2102
Hycamtin for Injection 1546
Lescol Capsules 2361
Lescol Capsules 2925
Lescol XL Tablets 2361
Lescol XL Tablets 2925
Levlen 962
Levlite 21 Tablets 962
Levlite 28 Tablets 962
Levora Tablets 3389
Lipitor Tablets 2639
Lipitor Tablets 2696
Loestrin 21 Tablets 2642
Loestrin Fe Tablets 2642
Lo/Ovral Tablets 3532
Lo/Ovral-28 Tablets 3538
Low-Ogestrel-28 Tablets 3392
Lunelle Monthly Injection 2827
Lupron Depot 3.75 mg 3281
Lupron Depot 7.5 mg 3284
Lupron Depot–3 Month 11.25 mg 3285
Lupron Depot–3 Month 22.5 mg 3288
Lupron Depot–4 Month 30 mg 3289
Lupron Depot-PED 7.5 mg, 11.25 mg and 15 mg 3291
Lupron Injection 3279
Lupron Injection Pediatric 3280
Macrobid Capsules 2889
Macrodantin Capsules 2891
Megace Oral Suspension 1124
Menest Tablets 2254
Menomune-A/C/Y/W-135 Vaccine 813
Meruvax II 2130
Mevacor Tablets 2132
Microgestin Fe 1.5/30 Tablets 3407
Microgestin Fe 1/20 Tablets 3400
Micronor Tablets 2543
Migranal Nasal Spray 2376
Mircette Tablets 2470
Mirena Intrauterine System 974
Mithracin for Intravenous Use 903
M-M-R II 2118
Modicon 2563
Mumpsvax 2141
Necon 3415
Nordette-28 Tablets 2257
Norinyl 1 +35 28-Day Tablets 3380
Norinyl 1 + 50 28-Day Tablets 3380
Norplant System 3540
Ogen Tablets 2846
Ogestrel 0.5/50-28 Tablets 3428
Ortho Dienestrol Cream 2554
Ortho-Cept 21 Tablets 2546
Ortho-Cept 28 Tablets 2546
Orthoclone OKT3 Sterile Solution 2498
Ortho-Cyclen/Ortho Tri-Cyclen 2573
Ortho-Est Tablets 3464
Ortho-Novum 2563
Ortho-Novum 1/50□28 Tablets 2556
Ortho-Novum 2563
Ortho-Prefest Tablets 2570
Ortho-Cyclen/Ortho Tri-Cyclen 2573
Ovcon 3364
Ovidrel for Injection 3220
Ovral Tablets 3551
Ovral-28 Tablets 3552
Ovrette Tablets 3552
Oxandrin Tablets 1153
ParaGard T 380A Intrauterine Copper Contraceptive 2582
Pediazole Suspension 3050
Pergonal for Injection 3223
Podocon-25 Liquid 2608
Pravachol Tablets 1099
Premarin Intravenous 3563
Premarin Tablets 3566
Premarin Vaginal Cream 3570
Premphase Tablets 3572
Prempro Tablets 3572
Prometrium Capsules (100 mg, 200 mg) 3261
Propecia Tablets 2172
Proscar Tablets 2175
ProSom Tablets 500
Rebetron Combination Therapy 3153
Repronex for Intramuscular and Subcutaneous Injection 1347
Septra Suspension 2265
Septra Tablets 2265
Septra DS Tablets 2265
Serophene Tablets 3226
Solaquin Forte 1734
Soriatane Capsules 3003
Sultrin Triple Sulfa Cream 2587
Synarel Nasal Solution for Central Precocious Puberty 3204
Synarel Nasal Solution for Endometriosis 3205
Tazorac Gel 556
Testoderm Transdermal Systems 574
Thalomid Capsules 1154
Tice BCG, BCG Live 2489
Travatan Ophthalmic Solution 543
Tri-Levlen 962
Tri-Norinyl-28 Tablets 3433
Triphasil-21 Tablets 3600
Triphasil-28 Tablets 3605
Trivora Tablets 3439
Urobiotic-250 Capsules 2731
Vagifem Tablets 2857
Varivax 2202
Virazole for Inhalation Solution 1747
Vistaril Capsules 2738
Vistaril Intramuscular Solution 2738
Vistaril Oral Suspension 2738
Vivelle Transdermal System 2412
Vivelle-Dot Transdermal System 2416
Warfarin Sodium Tablets, USP 3302
Yasmin 28 Tablets 980
Zocor Tablets 2219
Zoladex 702
Zoladex 3-month 706
Zovia 3449

Pregnancy, diagnostic test for
Aygestin Tablets 1333
Depo-Provera Contraceptive Injection 2798
Megace Oral Suspension 1124
Premphase Tablets 3572
Prempro Tablets 3572
Prometrium Capsules (100 mg, 200 mg) 3261
Provera Tablets 2853

Presentation, non-vertex
Prepidil Gel 2851

Proctitis, history of
Indocin Suppositories 2112

Prolactinoma, pituitary
(*see under* Tumor, intracranial, unspecified)

Prostate enlargement
(*see under* Prostatic hypertrophy)

Prostatic hypertrophy
Arco-Lase Plus Tablets 592
Donnatal 2929
Donnatal Extentabs 2930
Donnatal Tablets 2929
Norflex 1987
Periactin Tablets 2155
Robinul Forte Tablets 1358
Robinul Injectable 2940
Robinul Tablets 1358
Urimax Tablets 1769
Zephrex LA Tablets 3092

Proteinuria, abnormal
Vistide Injection 1445

Protoporphyria
(*see under* Porphyria, erythropoietic)

Pseudomembranous enterocolitis
(*see under* Enterocolitis, pseudomembranous)

Psoriasis, acute
Dovonex Scalp Solution 1118
Psoriatec Cream 3247

Psoriatic eruptions, acute
(*see under* Psoriasis, acute)

Psychic disturbances
(*see under* Psychosis)

Psychosis
Antabuse Tablets 2444
Antabuse Tablets 3474
Cortifoam Rectal Foam 3170

Psychosis, toxic, history of
Proleukin for Injection 1199

Psychosis, unsupervised
Coumadin for Injection 1243
Coumadin Tablets 1243
Warfarin Sodium Tablets, USP 3302

Pulmonary atresia
(*see under* Atresia, pulmonary)

Pulmonary congestion
(*see also under* Edema, pulmonary)
Cardizem CD Capsules 1016
Tiazac Capsules 1378

Pulmonary disorders, unspecified
(*see also under* Asthma, acute; Asthma, unspecified; Atresia, pulmonary; Chronic obstructive pulmonary disease; Cor pulmonale; Edema, pulmonary; Emphysema; Obstruction, pulmonary; Pulmonary congestion; Pulmonary fibrosis; Pulmonary function test, abnormal; Respiratory tract conditions, lower; Tuberculosis, unspecified)
Adenoscan 1381
Prostin E2 Suppositories 2852

Pulmonary edema
(*see under* Edema, pulmonary)

Pulmonary embolism
Evista Tablets 1915

Pulmonary emphysema
(*see under* Emphysema)

Pulmonary fibrosis
Dopram Injectable 2931

Pulmonary function test, abnormal
Proleukin for Injection 1199

Pyloroduodenal obstruction
(*see under* Obstruction, pyloroduodenal)

Pyloroduodenal stenosis
(*see under* Stenosis, pyloroduodenal)

Q

Q-T interval prolongation
Betapace Tablets 950
Betapace AF Tablets 954
Geodon Capsules 2688
Orap Tablets 1407

R

Radiation therapy
Leukine 1755
Neoral Soft Gelatin Capsules 2380
Neoral Oral Solution 2380
Tice BCG, BCG Live 2489

Radiotherapy
(*see under* Radiation therapy)

Rash
Cortifoam Rectal Foam 3170

Rectal bleeding
(*see under* Bleeding, rectal)

Renal decompensation
(*see under* Renal failure)

Renal dialysis
Integrilin Injection 1213
Integrilin Injection 1828

Renal disease, unspecified
(*see also under* Glomerulonephritis; Nephritis; Nephropathy, diabetic; Nephrosis; Renal dysfunction)
Calcium Disodium Versenate Injection 1980
Desferal Vials 2333
Dyrenium Capsules 3458
Fleet Phospho-soda 1360
Glucophage Tablets 1080
Glucophage XR Tablets 1080
Glucovance Tablets 1086
Lithium Carbonate 3061
Lithium Citrate Syrup 3061
Midrin Capsules 3464
Paser Granules 1781
Ponstel Capsules 1356
ProAmatine Tablets 3241
Prostin E2 Suppositories 2852
Robaxin Injectable 2938
Sultrin Triple Sulfa Cream 2587

Renal dysfunction
(*see also under* Anuria; Oliguria; Renal disease, unspecified; Renal failure; Uremia)
Albumin (Human) 25% 839
Atromid-S Capsules 3483
Bactrim 2949
Betapace AF Tablets 954
Cuprimine Capsules 2075
Depen Titratable Tablets 3341
D.H.E. 45 Injection 2334
Dyazide Capsules 1515
Dyrenium Capsules 3458
Gengraf Capsules 457
Glucophage Tablets 1080
Glucophage XR Tablets 1080
Glucovance Tablets 1086
Indocin I.V. 2115
Integrilin Injection 1213
Integrilin Injection 1828
Inversine Tablets 1850
K-Phos Neutral Tablets 946
K-Phos Original (Sodium Free) Tablets 947
Lopid Tablets 2650
Macrobid Capsules 2889
Macrodantin Capsules 2891
Malarone 1596
Maxzide 1008
Midamor Tablets 2136
Moduretic Tablets 2138
Neoral Soft Gelatin Capsules 2380
Neoral Oral Solution 2380
Pima Syrup 1362
Plasbumin-5 939
Plasbumin-20 940
Plasbumin-25 941
Robaxin Injectable 2938
Rum-K 1363
Skelaxin Tablets 1301
Thioplex for Injection 1765
Tikosyn Capsules 2717
Toradol 3018
Tricor Capsules, Micronized 513
Uroqid-Acid No. 2 Tablets 947
Vistide Injection 1445
Xeloda Tablets 3039
Yasmin 28 Tablets 980

Renal dysfunction, history of
Cuprimine Capsules 2075
Proleukin for Injection 1199

Renal excretory function impairment
(*see under* Renal dysfunction)

Renal failure
(*see also under* Renal dysfunction)
Agenerase Oral Solution 1459
Daranide Tablets 2077
Maxzide 1008
Urocit-K Tablets 2232

Renal impairment
(*see under* Renal dysfunction)

Renal insufficiency
(*see under* Renal dysfunction)

Respiratory depression
Dilaudid 441
Dilaudid Oral Liquid 445
Dilaudid Powder 441
Dilaudid Rectal Suppositories 441
Dilaudid Tablets 441
Dilaudid Tablets - 8 mg 445
Dilaudid-HP 443
Hycomine Compound Tablets 1317
Hycotuss Expectorant Syrup 1318
Kadian Capsules 1335
MS Contin Tablets 2896
MSIR 2898
Oramorph SR Tablets 3062
OxyContin Tablets 2912
OxyFast Oral Concentrate Solution 2916
OxyIR Capsules 2916
Roxanol 3066
Roxicodone Tablets 3067
Vicodin Tuss Expectorant 519

Respiratory disease, unspecified
(*see under* Respiratory illness, febrile; Respiratory illness, unspecified)

Respiratory disorders
(*see under* Bronchospastic disorders, unspecified; Infection, respiratory; Obstruction, respiratory tract; Pulmonary disorders, unspecified; Respiratory depression; Respiratory illness, unspecified; Respiratory tract conditions, lower)

Respiratory distress
(*see under* Asthma, acute; Respiratory depression)

Respiratory failure
Norditropin Cartridges....2420
Norditropin for Injection....2419
Nutropin AQ Injection....1420
Nutropin Depot for Injectable Suspension....1423
Nutropin for Injection....1417
Saizen for Injection....3225
Serostim for Injection....3229

Respiratory illness, febrile
Attenuvax....2044
Meruvax II....2130
M-M-R II....2118
Mumpsvax....2141
Varivax....2202

Respiratory illness, unspecified
(*see also under* Infection, respiratory; Pulmonary disorders, unspecified; Respiratory illness, febrile)
Adenoscan....1381
Dopram Injectable....2931

Respiratory insufficiency, unspecified
(*see also under* Obstruction, respiratory tract; Pulmonary disorders, unspecified; Respiratory illness, febrile; Respiratory illness, unspecified)
Nilandron Tablets.... 753
Roxanol....3066

Respiratory obstruction
(*see under* Obstruction, respiratory tract)

Respiratory tract conditions, lower
(*see also under* Pulmonary disorders, unspecified)
Phenergan Suppositories....3556
Phenergan Syrup....3554
Phenergan Tablets....3556
Phenergan with Codeine Syrup....3557
Phenergan with Dextromethorphan Syrup....3559
Phenergan VC Syrup....3560
Phenergan VC with Codeine Syrup....3561

Retinal changes
Aralen Tablets....3075
Plaquenil Tablets....3082

Rhabdomyolysis, non-traumatic, history of
Tasmar Tablets....3010

S

SA block
(*see under* Heart block, sinoatrial)

Scabies, Norwegian
Lindane Lotion USP 1%.... 559

Seizure disorders, history of
(*see also under* Convulsive disorders, history of)
Acel-Imune....1851
Orthoclone OKT3 Sterile Solution....2498
Proleukin for Injection....1199

Seizure disorders, unspecified
(*see also under* Convulsive disorders; Epilepsy; Epilepsy, uncontrolled; Status epilepticus)
Lindane Lotion USP 1%.... 559
Lindane Shampoo USP 1%.... 560
Reglan....2935
Wellbutrin Tablets....1680
Wellbutrin SR Sustained-Release Tablets....1684
Zyban Sustained-Release Tablets....1710

Seizure disorders, untreated
(*see under* Epilepsy, uncontrolled)

Seizures, history of
(*see under* Seizure disorders, history of)

Senility, unsupervised
Coumadin for Injection....1243
Coumadin Tablets....1243
Warfarin Sodium Tablets, USP....3302

Sepsis
D.H.E. 45 Injection....2334

Septicemia
(*see under* Sepsis)

Serum transaminase elevation
(*see also under* Liver dysfunction)
Baycol Tablets.... 883
Lescol Capsules....2361
Lescol Capsules....2925
Lescol XL Tablets....2361
Lescol XL Tablets....2925
Lipitor Tablets....2639
Lipitor Tablets....2696
Mevacor Tablets....2132
Nardil Tablets....2653
Pravachol Tablets....1099
Zocor Tablets....2219
Zyflo Filmtab Tablets.... 524

Severe left ventricular dysfunction
(*see under* Ventricular dysfunction, left)

Shingles
(*see under* Herpes zoster)

Shock, cardiogenic
(*see under* Cardiogenic shock)

Shock, unspecified
(*see also under* Cardiogenic shock)
Navane Oral....2701
Navane Intramuscular....2703
Primaxin I.M.....2158
Thiothixene Capsules....2290

Sick sinus node syndrome
(*see under* Sick sinus syndrome)

Sick sinus syndrome
Adenocard Injection....1380
Adenoscan....1381
Betapace AF Tablets.... 954
Cardizem Injectable....1018
Cardizem Lyo-Ject Syringe....1018
Cardizem Monovial....1018
Cardizem CD Capsules....1016
Coreg Tablets....1508
Covera-HS Tablets....3199
Isoptin SR Tablets.... 467
Rythmol Tablets – 150 mg, 225 mg, 300 mg.... 502
Tarka Tablets.... 508
Tiazac Capsules....1378
Toprol-XL Tablets.... 651
Verelan Capsules....3184
Verelan PM Capsules....3186

Sickle cell anemia
(*see under* Anemia, sickle cell)

Sino-atrial block
(*see under* Heart block, first degree; Heart block, greater than first degree; Heart block, unspecified)

Sinus node disease
(*see under* Bradycardia, sinus; Sick sinus syndrome; Sinus node dysfunction, unspecified)

Sinus node dysfunction, unspecified
Adenoscan....1381
Cordarone Tablets....3487
Pacerone Tablets....3331

Sinus tracts, intestinal
Cortifoam Rectal Foam....3170

Skin disorders, unspecified
(*see under* Intertrigo; Lesions, skin, fungal; Lesions, skin, unspecified; Lesions, skin, viral; Melanoma, history of; Melanoma, unspecified; Psoriasis, acute; Rash; Xeroderma pigmentosum)

Skin lesions
(*see under* Lesions, skin, fungal; Lesions, skin, unspecified; Lesions, skin, viral)

Skin, burned
(*see under* Burns)

Smoking, heavy
Lunelle Monthly Injection....2827
Yasmin 28 Tablets.... 980

Sodium depletion
(*see under* Hyponatremia)

Spasms, gastrointestinal
Urecholine....2198
Urecholine Tablets....2445

Spinal puncture
Coumadin for Injection....1243
Coumadin Tablets....1243
Warfarin Sodium Tablets, USP....3302

Status asthmaticus
Advair Diskus 100/50....1448
Advair Diskus 250/50....1448
Advair Diskus 500/50....1448
Aerobid/Aerobid-M....1363
Azmacort Inhalation Aerosol.... 728
Dilaudid.... 441
Dilaudid Oral Liquid.... 445
Dilaudid Powder.... 441
Dilaudid Rectal Suppositories.... 441
Dilaudid Tablets.... 441
Dilaudid Tablets - 8 mg.... 445
Dilaudid-HP.... 443
Flovent Rotadisk....1537
Pulmicort Respules.... 632
Pulmicort Turbuhaler Inhalation Powder.... 636
Qvar Inhalation Aerosol....1987
Vanceril Inhalation Aerosol....3165
Vanceril Double Strength Inhalation Aerosol....3167

Status epilepticus
Romazicon Injection....3000

Stenosis, aortic
Cardene I.V.....3485
Indocin I.V.....2115
Inversine Tablets....1850

Stenosis, pyloric
(*see also under* Stenosis, pyloroduodenal)
Inversine Tablets....1850

Stenosis, pyloroduodenal
Donnatal....2929
Donnatal Extentabs....2930
Donnatal Tablets....2929
Levsin/Levsinex/Levbid....3172
Norflex....1987
NuLev Orally Disintegrating Tablets....3176
Robinul Forte Tablets....1358
Robinul Injectable....2940
Robinul Tablets....1358

Stenosis, subaortic
Dobutrex Solution Vials....1914

Stokes-Adams syndrome
(*see under* Adams-Stokes syndrome)

Stress test, abnormal
Proleukin for Injection....1199

Stricture, esophageal
Fosamax Tablets....2095

Stroke
(*see under* Cerebrovascular accident)

Stroke, history of
(*see under* Cerebrovascular accident, history of)

Superficial herpes simplex keratitis
(*see under* Herpes simplex keratitis)

Surgery, abdominal
(*see also under* Surgery, gastrointestinal)
Dulcolax Suppositories....▣668
Roxanol....3066
X-Prep Liquid....2900

Surgery, biliary tract
Roxanol....3066

Surgery, bladder
Urecholine....2198
Urecholine Tablets....2445

Surgery, central nervous system
(*see also under* Surgery, intracranial; Surgery, intraspinal)
Coumadin for Injection....1243
Coumadin Tablets....1243
Warfarin Sodium Tablets, USP....3302

Surgery, elective
Nardil Tablets....2653
Parnate Tablets....1607

Surgery, gastrointestinal
Urecholine....2198
Urecholine Tablets....2445

Surgery, intracranial
Activase I.V.....1410
Streptase for Infusion.... 647
TNKase I.V.....1430

Surgery, intraspinal
Activase I.V.....1410
Streptase for Infusion.... 647

Surgery, ophthalmic
Coumadin for Injection....1243
Coumadin Tablets....1243
Vitrasert Implant....⊙254
Warfarin Sodium Tablets, USP....3302

Surgery, pediatric
Compazine....1505

Surgery, traumatic
Coumadin for Injection....1243
Coumadin Tablets....1243
Warfarin Sodium Tablets, USP....3302

Surgery, unspecified
Integrilin Injection....1213
Integrilin Injection....1828
ReoPro Vials....1958
Retavase Vials....1182

Surgery, uterine, history of
(*see also under* Cesarean section, history of)
Cervidil Vaginal Insert....1369
Prepidil Gel....2851

Surgical abdomen
(*see under* Surgery, abdominal)

Syncope
Cordarone Tablets....3487
Pacerone Tablets....3331

Systemic lupus erythematosus
(*see under* Lupus erythematosus)

T

Tachyarrhythmia
(*see under* Arrhythmia, cardiac, unspecified; Tachycardia, unspecified)

Tachycardia, unspecified
Alupent....1029

Tachycardia, ventricular
Cardizem Injectable....1018
Cardizem Lyo-Ject Syringe....1018
Cardizem Monovial....1018

Tachycardia, ventricular, history of
Proleukin for Injection....1199

Tendinitis, history of
Noroxin Tablets....2145

Tendon rupture, history of
Noroxin Tablets....2145

Tension
Concerta Extended-Release Tablets....1998
Concerta Tablets.... 561
Metadate CD Capsules....1164
Metadate ER Tablets....1167
Methylin Tablets....1995
Methylin ER Tablets....1995
Ritalin....2387

Testicular failure, primary
Humegon for Injection....2468
Pergonal for Injection....3223

Repronex for Intramuscular and Subcutaneous Injection 1347

Tetralogy of Fallot
Indocin I.V. 2115

Thallium stress test, abnormal
(*see under* Stress test, abnormal)

Thrombocythemia
MUSE Urethral Suppository 3335

Thrombocytopathy, unspecified
(*see also under* Thrombocytopenia, unspecified; Thrombocytopenic purpura, history of)
Mithracin for Intravenous Use 903

Thrombocytopenia, severe
Vitrasert Implant ....⊙254

Thrombocytopenia, unspecified
Adagen Injection 1331
Aggrastat 2031
Fragmin Injection 2814
Heparin Lock Flush Solution 3509
Heparin Sodium Injection 3511
Indocin I.V. 2115
Innohep Injection 1248
Integrilin Injection 1213
Integrilin Injection 1828
Lovenox Injection 746
Mithracin for Intravenous Use 903
Mylocel Tablets 2227
Orgaran Injection 2480
ReoPro Vials 1958
Ticlid Tablets 3015

Thrombocytopenic purpura, history of
Orgaran Injection 2480
Quinaglute Dura-Tabs Tablets 978
Quinidex Extentabs 2933

Thromboembolic disorders
(*see also under* Cerebrovascular accident)
Activella Tablets 2764
Alesse-21 Tablets 3468
Alesse-28 Tablets 3473
Alora Transdermal System 3372
Aygestin Tablets 1333
Brevicon 28-Day Tablets 3380
Cenestin Tablets 1263
Climara Transdermal System 958
CombiPatch Transdermal System 2323
Crinone 3213
Cyclessa Tablets 2450
Depo-Provera Contraceptive Injection 2798
Desogen Tablets 2458
Emcyt Capsules 2810
Esclim Transdermal System 3460
Estinyl Tablets 3112
Estrace Tablets 3361
Estratest 3252
Estrostep 2627
femhrt Tablets 2635
Levlen 962
Levlite 21 Tablets 962
Levlite 28 Tablets 962
Levora Tablets 3389
Loestrin 21 Tablets 2642
Loestrin Fe Tablets 2642
Lo/Ovral Tablets 3532
Lo/Ovral-28 Tablets 3538
Low-Ogestrel-28 Tablets 3392
Lunelle Monthly Injection 2827
Menest Tablets 2254
Microgestin Fe 1.5/30 Tablets 3407
Microgestin Fe 1/20 Tablets 3400
Mircette Tablets 2470
Modicon 2563
Necon 3415
Nordette-28 Tablets 2257
Norinyl 1 +35 28-Day Tablets 3380
Norinyl 1 + 50 28-Day Tablets 3380
Norplant System 3543
Ogen Tablets 2846
Ogestrel 0.5/50-28 Tablets 3428
Ortho Dienestrol Cream 2554
Ortho-Cept 21 Tablets 2546
Ortho-Cept 28 Tablets 2546
Ortho-Cyclen/Ortho Tri-Cyclen 2573
Ortho-Est Tablets 3464
Ortho-Novum 2563
Ortho-Novum 1/50□28 Tablets 2556
Ortho-Novum 2563
Ortho-Cyclen/Ortho Tri-Cyclen 2573
Ovcon 3364
Ovral Tablets 3551
Ovral-28 Tablets 3552
Ovrette Tablets 3552
Premarin Intravenous 3563
Premarin Tablets 3566
Premarin Vaginal Cream 3570
Premphase Tablets 3572
Prempro Tablets 3572
Prometrium Capsules (100 mg, 200 mg) 3261
Provera Tablets 2853
Tri-Levlen 962
Tri-Norinyl-28 Tablets 3433
Triphasil-21 Tablets 3600
Triphasil-28 Tablets 3605
Trivora Tablets 3439
Vivelle Transdermal System 2412
Vivelle-Dot Transdermal System 2416
Yasmin 28 Tablets 980
Zovia 3449

Thromboembolic disorders, history of
(*see also under* Cerebrovascular accident, history of)
Activella Tablets 2764
Alesse-21 Tablets 3468
Alesse-28 Tablets 3473
Aygestin Tablets 1333
Brevicon 28-Day Tablets 3380
Crinone 3213
Cyclessa Tablets 2450
Depo-Provera Contraceptive Injection 2798
Desogen Tablets 2458
Estinyl Tablets 3112
Estratest 3252
Estrostep 2627
Evista Tablets 1915
Levlen 962
Levlite 21 Tablets 962
Levlite 28 Tablets 962
Levora Tablets 3389
Loestrin 21 Tablets 2642
Loestrin Fe Tablets 2642
Lo/Ovral Tablets 3532
Lo/Ovral-28 Tablets 3538
Low-Ogestrel-28 Tablets 3392
Lunelle Monthly Injection 2827
Menest Tablets 2254
Microgestin Fe 1.5/30 Tablets 3407
Microgestin Fe 1/20 Tablets 3400
Mircette Tablets 2470
Modicon 2563
Necon 3415
Nordette-28 Tablets 2257
Norinyl 1 +35 28-Day Tablets 3380
Norinyl 1 + 50 28-Day Tablets 3380
Ogestrel 0.5/50-28 Tablets 3428
Ortho Dienestrol Cream 2554
Ortho-Cept 21 Tablets 2546
Ortho-Cept 28 Tablets 2546
Ortho-Cyclen/Ortho Tri-Cyclen 2573
Ortho-Novum 2563
Ortho-Novum 1/50□28 Tablets 2556
Ortho-Novum 2563
Ortho-Prefest Tablets 2570
Ortho-Cyclen/Ortho Tri-Cyclen 2573
Ovcon 3364
Ovral Tablets 3551
Ovral-28 Tablets 3552
Ovrette Tablets 3552
Premarin Intravenous 3563
Premarin Vaginal Cream 3570
Premphase Tablets 3572
Prempro Tablets 3572
Prometrium Capsules (100 mg, 200 mg) 3261
Provera Tablets 2853
Tri-Levlen 962
Tri-Norinyl-28 Tablets 3433
Triphasil-21 Tablets 3600
Triphasil-28 Tablets 3605
Trivora Tablets 3439
Vagifem Tablets 2857
Yasmin 28 Tablets 980
Zovia 3449

Thrombophlebitis
Activella Tablets 2764
Alesse-21 Tablets 3468
Alesse-28 Tablets 3473
Alora Transdermal System 3372
Aygestin Tablets 1333
Brevicon 28-Day Tablets 3380
Cenestin Tablets 1263
Climara Transdermal System 958
CombiPatch Transdermal System 2323
Cortifoam Rectal Foam 3170
Crinone 3213
Cyclessa Tablets 2450
Depo-Provera Contraceptive Injection 2798
Desogen Tablets 2458
Emcyt Capsules 2810
Esclim Transdermal System 3460
Estinyl Tablets 3112
Estrace Tablets 3361
Estratest 3252
Estrostep 2627
femhrt Tablets 2635
Levlen 962
Levlite 21 Tablets 962
Levlite 28 Tablets 962
Levora Tablets 3389
Loestrin 21 Tablets 2642
Loestrin Fe Tablets 2642
Lo/Ovral Tablets 3532
Lo/Ovral-28 Tablets 3538
Low-Ogestrel-28 Tablets 3392
Lunelle Monthly Injection 2827
Menest Tablets 2254
Microgestin Fe 1.5/30 Tablets 3407
Microgestin Fe 1/20 Tablets 3400
Mircette Tablets 2470
Modicon 2563
Necon 3415
Nordette-28 Tablets 2257
Norinyl 1 +35 28-Day Tablets 3380
Norinyl 1 + 50 28-Day Tablets 3380
Norplant System 3543
Ogen Tablets 2846
Ogestrel 0.5/50-28 Tablets 3428
Ortho Dienestrol Cream 2554
Ortho-Cept 21 Tablets 2546
Ortho-Cept 28 Tablets 2546
Ortho-Cyclen/Ortho Tri-Cyclen 2573
Ortho-Est Tablets 3464
Ortho-Novum 2563
Ortho-Novum 1/50□28 Tablets 2556
Ortho-Novum 2563
Ortho-Prefest Tablets 2570
Ortho-Cyclen/Ortho Tri-Cyclen 2573
Ovcon 3364
Ovral Tablets 3551
Ovral-28 Tablets 3552
Ovrette Tablets 3552
Premarin Intravenous 3563
Premarin Tablets 3566
Premarin Vaginal Cream 3570
Premphase Tablets 3572
Prempro Tablets 3572
Prometrium Capsules (100 mg, 200 mg) 3261
Provera Tablets 2853
Tri-Levlen 962
Tri-Norinyl-28 Tablets 3433
Triphasil-21 Tablets 3600
Triphasil-28 Tablets 3605
Trivora Tablets 3439
Vagifem Tablets 2857
Vivelle Transdermal System 2412
Vivelle-Dot Transdermal System 2416
Yasmin 28 Tablets 980
Zovia 3449

Thrombophlebitis, history of
Activella Tablets 2764
Alesse-21 Tablets 3468
Alesse-28 Tablets 3473
Aygestin Tablets 1333
Brevicon 28-Day Tablets 3380
Cyclessa Tablets 2450
Desogen Tablets 2458
Estinyl Tablets 3112
Estratest 3252
Estrostep 2627
Levlen 962
Levlite 21 Tablets 962
Levlite 28 Tablets 962
Levora Tablets 3389
Loestrin 21 Tablets 2642
Loestrin Fe Tablets 2642
Lo/Ovral Tablets 3532
Lo/Ovral-28 Tablets 3538
Low-Ogestrel-28 Tablets 3392
Lunelle Monthly Injection 2827
Menest Tablets 2254
Microgestin Fe 1.5/30 Tablets 3407
Microgestin Fe 1/20 Tablets 3400
Mircette Tablets 2470
Modicon 2563
Necon 3415
Nordette-28 Tablets 2257
Norinyl 1 +35 28-Day Tablets 3380
Norinyl 1 + 50 28-Day Tablets 3380
Ogestrel 0.5/50-28 Tablets 3428
Ortho Dienestrol Cream 2554
Ortho-Cept 21 Tablets 2546
Ortho-Cept 28 Tablets 2546
Ortho-Cyclen/Ortho Tri-Cyclen 2573
Ortho-Novum 2563
Ortho-Novum 1/50□28 Tablets 2556
Ortho-Novum 2563
Ortho-Cyclen/Ortho Tri-Cyclen 2573
Ovcon 3364
Ovral Tablets 3551
Ovral-28 Tablets 3552
Ovrette Tablets 3552
Premarin Intravenous 3563
Premarin Vaginal Cream 3570
Premphase Tablets 3572
Prempro Tablets 3572
Provera Tablets 2853
Tri-Levlen 962
Tri-Norinyl-28 Tablets 3433
Triphasil-21 Tablets 3600
Triphasil-28 Tablets 3605
Trivora Tablets 3439
Yasmin 28 Tablets 980
Zovia 3449

Thrombosis, history of
Estratest 3252
Evista Tablets 1915
Menest Tablets 2254
Ortho Dienestrol Cream 2554
Premarin Intravenous 3563
Premarin Vaginal Cream 3570

Thrombotic thrombocytopenic purpura, history of
Ticlid Tablets 3015

Thyroid dysfunction, uncontrolled
Clomid Tablets 735
Follistim for Injection 2465
Gonal-F for Injection 3216
Humegon for Injection 2468
Ovidrel for Injection 3220
Pergonal for Injection 3223
Repronex for Intramuscular and Subcutaneous Injection 1347
Serophene Tablets 3226

Thyrotoxicosis
ProAmatine Tablets 3241

Thyrotoxicosis, untreated
Cytomel Tablets 1817
Levothroid Tablets 1373
Levoxyl Tablets 1819
Synthroid 505
Triostat Injection 1825
Unithroid Tablets 3445

Tics, motor
Concerta Extended-Release Tablets 1998
Concerta Tablets 561
Metadate CD Capsules 1164
Metadate ER Tablets 1167
Methylin Tablets 1995
Methylin ER Tablets 1995
Ritalin 2387

Tics, non-Tourette's disorder
Orap Tablets 1407

Tissue breakdown
(*see under* Necrosis)

Torsade de pointes
Procanbid Extended-Release Tablets 2262

Tourette's syndrome
Concerta Extended-Release Tablets 1998
Concerta Tablets 561
Metadate CD Capsules 1164
Metadate ER Tablets 1167
Methylin Tablets 1995
Methylin ER Tablets 1995
Ritalin 2387

Tourette's syndrome, history of
Concerta Extended-Release Tablets 1998
Concerta Tablets 561
Metadate CD Capsules 1164
Metadate ER Tablets 1167
Methylin Tablets 1995
Methylin ER Tablets 1995
Ritalin 2387

Toxic megacolon
(*see under* Megacolon, toxic)

Toxic shock syndrome, history of
Ortho Diaphragm Kits – All-Flex Arcing Spring; Ortho Coil Spring 2552

Toxicity, neurologic
Hexalen Capsules 2226

Toxicity, vitamin D
Calcijex Injection 411
Dovonex Cream 1116
Dovonex Ointment 1117
Dovonex Scalp Solution 1118
Hectorol Capsules 1064
Hectorol Injection 1066
Rocaltrol 2991

Tracheoesophageal fistula, existence of
Photofrin for Injection 831

Transaminases elevation, serum
(*see under* Serum transaminase elevation)

Transplant
(*see under* Bone marrow transplantation; Organ allograft)

Trauma, intracranial, unspecified
TNKase I.V. 1430

Trauma, intracranial
(*see also under* Cerebrovascular accident; Head injury)
Activase I.V. 1410

TNKase I.V. 1430

Trauma, intraspinal
Activase I.V. 1410
TNKase I.V. 1430

Trauma, unspecified
Anectine Injection 1476
ReoPro Vials 1958

Tuberculin positive reactors
Tubersol Diagnostic Antigen 3628

Tuberculosis, prevention of
TheraCys Injection 823

Tuberculosis, untreated
Attenuvax 2044
Meruvax II 2130
M-M-R II 2118
Mumpsvax 2141
Varivax 2202

Tuberculosis, unspecified
(*see also under* Infection, ophthalmic, mycobacterial)
Cortifoam Rectal Foam 3170
HMS Sterile Ophthalmic Suspension ⊙ 240
Iscar Mali Injection 3456
Iscar Mali Special Injection 3456
Iscar Pini Injection 3456
Iscar Quercus Injection 3456
Iscar Quercus Special Injection 3456
Tice BCG, BCG Live 2489

Tumor activity, unspecified
Genotropin Lyophilized Powder 2818
Humatrope Vials and Cartridges 1930

Tumor, adrenal
(*see under* Pheochromocytoma)

Tumor, breast, malignant
(*see under* Carcinoma, breast, male; Carcinoma, breast, unspecified)

Tumor, hepatic
(*see under* Adenoma, hepatic; Carcinoma, hepatic; Tumor, liver, benign)

Tumor, hormone dependent
(*see under* Neoplasm, androgen dependent; Neoplasm, estrogen dependent)

Tumor, intracranial, unspecified
(*see also under* Lesions, intracranial, unspecified; Tumor, pituitary, unspecified)
Activase I.V. 1410
Aggrastat 2031
Pergonal for Injection 3223
ReoPro Vials 1958
Repronex for Intramuscular and Subcutaneous Injection 1347
Retavase Vials 1182
Roxanol 3066
Streptase for Infusion 647
TNKase I.V. 1430

Tumor, liver, benign
Brevicon 28-Day Tablets 3380
Mirena Intrauterine System 974
Norinyl 1 +35 28-Day Tablets 3380
Norinyl 1 + 50 28-Day Tablets 3380
Norplant System 3543
Nor-QD Tablets 3423
Tri-Norinyl-28 Tablets 3433

Tumor, liver, malignant
(*see under* Carcinoma, hepatic)

Tumor, pituitary, unspecified
(*see also under* Tumor, intracranial, unspecified)
Clomid Tablets 735
Follistim for Injection 2465
Gonal-F for Injection 3216
Humegon for Injection 2468
Ovidrel for Injection 3220
Pergonal for Injection 3223
Repronex for Intramuscular and Subcutaneous Injection 1347
Serophene Tablets 3226

Tumor, unspecified
(*see under* Neoplasm, unspecified)

Tumors, intracranial, in hypopituitary children
Norditropin Cartridges 2420
Norditropin for Injection 2419

Tympanic membrane perforation
Americaine Otic Topical Anesthetic Ear Drops 1162
Auralgan Otic Solution 3485
Cerumenex Eardrops 2895
Cipro HC Otic Suspension 540
Decadron Phosphate Sterile Ophthalmic Solution 2084
VōSoL HC Otic Solution 3356

U

Ulcer, gastrointestinal
(*see also under* Lesions, gastrointestinal, unspecified; Perforation, gastrointestinal tract; Ulcer, peptic)
Ponstel Capsules 1356

Ulcer, peptic
Bromfed Capsules (Extended-Release) 2269
Bromfed-PD Capsules (Extended-Release) 2269
Cortifoam Rectal Foam 3170
Niaspan Extended-Release Tablets 1846
Norflex 1987
Periactin Tablets 2155
Robinul Injectable 2940
Toradol 3018
Urecholine 2198
Urecholine Tablets 2445

Ulcer, peptic, history of
Toradol 3018

Ulcer, unspecified
(*see under* Ulceration, unspecified)

Ulceration, unspecified
Coumadin for Injection 1243
Coumadin Tablets 1243
Warfarin Sodium Tablets, USP 3302

Ulcerative colitis
(*see under* Colitis, ulcerative)

Unstable cardiovascular status in acute hemorrhage
(*see under* Cardiovascular status, unstable in acute hemorrhage)

Uremia
(*see also under* Azotemia)
Inversine Tablets 1850

Urethral stricture
MUSE Urethral Suppository 3335

Urethritis
MUSE Urethral Suppository 3335

Urinary bladder capacity, small
Valstar Sterile Solution for Intravesical Instillation 1175

Urinary obstruction
(*see under* Obstruction, urinary tract)

Urinary retention
(*see also under* Obstruction, urinary tract; Prostatic hypertrophy)
Allegra-D Extended-Release Tablets 714
Bromfed Capsules (Extended-Release) 2269
Bromfed-PD Capsules (Extended-Release) 2269
Claritin-D 12 Hour Extended Release Tablets 3102
Claritin-D 24 Hour Extended Release Tablets 3104
Detrol Tablets 3623
Detrol LA Capsules 2801
Ditropan XL Extended Release Tablets 564
ProAmatine Tablets 3241
Rynatan Tablets 3351
Sinequan 2713
Zyrtec-D 12 Hour Extended Relief Tablets 2758

Urinary tract disorders
(*see under* Infection, urinary tract; Obstruction, urinary tract; Renal disease, unspecified; Renal dysfunction)

Uropathy, obstructive
(*see under* Obstruction, urinary tract)

Uterine abnormalities, unspecified
Mirena Intrauterine System 974
ParaGard T 380A Intrauterine Copper Contraceptive 2582

Uterine cavity distortion
ParaGard T 380A Intrauterine Copper Contraceptive 2582

Uterine patterns, hypertonic
Prepidil Gel 2851

Uveitis
Humorsol Sterile Ophthalmic Solution 2102

V

Vaccinia
Alrex Sterile Ophthalmic Suspension 0.2% ⊙ 256
Blephamide Ophthalmic Ointment 547
Blephamide Ophthalmic Suspension 548
Cortisporin Ophthalmic Suspension Sterile ⊙ 297
Cortisporin-TC Otic Suspension 2246
Decadron Phosphate Sterile Ophthalmic Ointment 2083
Decadron Phosphate Sterile Ophthalmic Solution 2084
FML Ophthalmic Ointment ⊙ 237
FML Ophthalmic Suspension ⊙ 236
FML Forte Ophthalmic Suspension ⊙ 235
FML-S Liquifilm Sterile Ophthalmic Suspension ⊙ 238
Lotemax Sterile Ophthalmic Suspension 0.5% ⊙ 261
NeoDecadron Sterile Ophthalmic Solution 2144
Poly-Pred Liquifilm Ophthalmic Suspension ⊙ 245
Pred Forte Ophthalmic Suspension ⊙ 246
Pred Mild Sterile Ophthalmic Suspension ⊙ 249
Pred-G Ophthalmic Suspension ⊙ 247
Pred-G Sterile Ophthalmic Ointment ⊙ 248
Terra-Cortril Ophthalmic Suspension 2716
TobraDex Ophthalmic Ointment 542
TobraDex Ophthalmic Suspension 541
Vexol 1% Ophthalmic Suspension ⊙ 222
VōSoL HC Otic Solution 3356

Vaginal bleeding, abnormal
(*see under* Bleeding, genital, abnormal)

Vaginitis, untreated
Mirena Intrauterine System 974
ParaGard T 380A Intrauterine Copper Contraceptive 2582

Vaginosis, bacterial, untreated
Mirena Intrauterine System 974
ParaGard T 380A Intrauterine Copper Contraceptive 2582

Vagotonia
Urecholine 2198
Urecholine Tablets 2445

Varicella
Alrex Sterile Ophthalmic Suspension 0.2% ⊙ 256
Blephamide Ophthalmic Ointment 547
Blephamide Ophthalmic Suspension 548
Cipro HC Otic Suspension 540
Cortisporin Ophthalmic Suspension Sterile ⊙ 297
Cortisporin-TC Otic Suspension 2246
Cosmegen for Injection 2062
Decadron Phosphate Sterile Ophthalmic Ointment 2083
Decadron Phosphate Sterile Ophthalmic Solution 2084
FML Ophthalmic Ointment ⊙ 237
FML Ophthalmic Suspension ⊙ 236
FML Forte Ophthalmic Suspension ⊙ 235
FML-S Liquifilm Sterile Ophthalmic Suspension ⊙ 238
Lotemax Sterile Ophthalmic Suspension 0.5% ⊙ 261
NeoDecadron Sterile Ophthalmic Solution 2144
Poly-Pred Liquifilm Ophthalmic Suspension ⊙ 245
Pred Forte Ophthalmic Suspension ⊙ 246
Pred Mild Sterile Ophthalmic Suspension ⊙ 249
Pred-G Ophthalmic Suspension ⊙ 247
Pred-G Sterile Ophthalmic Ointment ⊙ 248
Terra-Cortril Ophthalmic Suspension 2716
TobraDex Ophthalmic Ointment 542
TobraDex Ophthalmic Suspension 541
Vexol 1% Ophthalmic Suspension ⊙ 222
VōSoL HC Otic Solution 3356

Vasa previa
Prepidil Gel 2851

Vascular impairment of extremities
(*see under* Peripheral vascular disease)

Vasculitis, history of
ReoPro Vials 1958

Vasomotor instability
Urecholine 2198
Urecholine Tablets 2445

Vasospasm, coronary artery
(*see under* Coronary artery vasospasm)

Ventilatory function depression
(*see under* Respiratory depression)

Ventricular arrythmia
(*see under* Arrhythmia, ventricular, unspecified)

Ventricular dysfunction, left
Covera-HS Tablets 3199
Flolan for Injection 1528
Isoptin SR Tablets 467
Tarka Tablets 508
Verelan Capsules 3184
Verelan PM Capsules 3186

Ventricular fibrillation
(*see under* Fibrillation, ventricular)

Viral infections
(*see under* Herpes genitalia; Herpes simplex keratitis; Herpes simplex, unspecified; Herpes zoster; Human immunodeficiency virus; Infection, ophthalmic, viral; Lesions, skin, viral; Varicella)

Visual field changes
Aralen Tablets 3075
Plaquenil Tablets 3082

Vitamin D toxicity
(*see under* Toxicity, vitamin D)

W

Warts, atypical
Podocon-25 Liquid 2608

Wilson's disease
New Formulation Chromagen OB Capsules 3094
ParaGard T 380A Intrauterine Copper Contraceptive 2582

Wolff-Parkinson-White syndrome
Cardizem Injectable 1018
Cardizem Lyo-Ject Syringe 1018
Cardizem Monovial 1018
Covera-HS Tablets 3199
Isoptin SR Tablets 467
Tarka Tablets 508
Verelan Capsules 3184
Verelan PM Capsules 3186

Wounds, infected
Apligraf 2305

X

Xeroderma pigmentosum
8-MOP Capsules 1727
Oxsoralen Lotion 1% 1740
Oxsoralen-Ultra Capsules 1741

SECTION 7

INTERNATIONAL DRUG NAME INDEX

This section names the *PDR®* equivalents of over 33,000 foreign pharmaceutical products. Organized alphabetically by overseas trade name, it shows the country (or countries) in which the name is used, gives the product's closest U.S. generic equivalent, and lists the associated brand-name prescription drugs described by *PDR®*, together with the page on which they are found.

Products from the following nations are included:

Australia	France	Mexico	Spain
Austria	Germany	Monaco	Sweden
Belgium	Hong Kong	New Zealand	Switzerland
Brazil	Irish Republic	Norway	Thailand
Canada	Israel	Portugal	The Netherlands
Denmark	Italy	Singapore	United Arab Emirates
Finland	Japan	South Africa	United Kingdom

Page numbers refer to the 2002 editions of *PDR®* and *PDR for Ophthalmic Medicines™*. The symbol denoting an entry in *PDR for Ophthalmic Medicines™* appears in the bottom margin.

These entries are intended only as an aid in approximating the contents of a foreign prescription. For proper dosing guidelines, indications, contraindications, warnings, and precautions of its U.S. equivalents, always consult the underlying *PDR®* text. Foreign trade names are courtesy of *PDR*'s affiliate, MICROMEDEX, Inc.

3-A (Mexico)
DICLOFENAC SODIUM
Voltaren Tablets **2315**
Voltaren-XR Tablets **2315**

3TC (Australia, Canada, Hong Kong, Mexico, South Africa, Switzerland)
LAMIVUDINE
Epivir Oral Solution **1520**
Epivir Tablets **1520**
Epivir-HBV Oral Solution **1524**
Epivir-HBV Tablets **1524**

28 MINI (Germany)
LEVONORGESTREL
Norplant System **3543**

A GRIN (Mexico)
VITAMIN A PALMITATE
Aquasol A Parenteral **593**

AAA (United Kingdom)
BENZOCAINE
Americaine Anesthetic Lubricant **1162**
Americaine Otic Topical Anesthetic Ear Drops **1162**

AACIDEXAM (Belgium)
DEXAMETHASONE SODIUM PHOSPHATE
Decadron Phosphate Injection **2081**
Decadron Phosphate Sterile Ophthalmic Ointment . . . . . ⊙**280, 2083**
Decadron Phosphate Sterile Ophthalmic Solution **2084**

ABACUS (Thailand)
HYDROXYZINE HYDROCHLORIDE
Atarax Tablets & Syrup **2667**
Vistaril Intramuscular Solution **2738**

ABADOX (Italy)
DOXYCYCLINE HYCLATE
Doryx Coated Pellet Filled Capsules **3357**
Periostat Tablets **1208**
Vibramycin Hyclate Capsules **2735**
Vibramycin Hyclate Intravenous **2737**
Vibra-Tabs Film Coated Tablets **2735**

ABBEMETIC (South Africa)
METOCLOPRAMIDE HYDROCHLORIDE
Reglan Injectable **2935**
Reglan Syrup **2935**
Reglan Tablets **2935**

ABBIFEN (South Africa)
IBUPROFEN
Motrin Suspension, Oral Drops, Chewable Tablets, and Caplets **2002**

ABBONIDAZOLE (South Africa)
METRONIDAZOLE
MetroCream **1404**
MetroGel **1405**
MetroGel-Vaginal Gel **1986**
MetroLotion **1405**
Noritate Cream **1224**

ABENTEL (Thailand)
ALBENDAZOLE
Albenza Tablets **1463**

ABEREL (France)
TRETINOIN
Avita Cream **999**
Avita Gel **1000**
Renova 0.05% Cream **2519**
Retin-A Micro 0.1% **2522**
Vesanoid Capsules **3037**

ABERELA (Norway, Sweden)
TRETINOIN
Avita Cream **999**
Avita Gel **1000**
Renova 0.05% Cream **2519**
Retin-A Micro 0.1% **2522**
Vesanoid Capsules **3037**

ABETOL (Italy)
LABETALOL HYDROCHLORIDE
Normodyne Injection **3135**
Normodyne Tablets **3137**

ABIOCEF (Italy)
CEPHALEXIN
Keflex Oral Suspension **1237**
Keflex Pulvules **1237**

ABITREN (Hong Kong, Israel, Thailand)
DICLOFENAC SODIUM
Voltaren Tablets **2315**
Voltaren-XR Tablets **2315**

ABSORLENT (Spain)
ESTRADIOL
Alora Transdermal System **3372**
Climara Transdermal System **958**
Estrace Vaginal Cream **3358**
Estring Vaginal Ring **2811**
Vivelle Transdermal System **2412**
Vivelle-Dot Transdermal System **2416**

ABTRIM (United Kingdom)
CLOTRIMAZOLE
Lotrimin Cream 1% **3128**
Lotrimin Lotion 1% **3128**
Lotrimin Topical Solution 1% **3128**
Mycelex Troche **573**

ABUTOL (Denmark)
ACEBUTOLOL HYDROCHLORIDE
Sectral Capsules **3589**

ACALKA (Portugal, Spain)
POTASSIUM CITRATE
Urocit-K Tablets **2232**

ACATAR (Belgium)
DEXTROMETHORPHAN HYDROBROMIDE/GUAIFENESIN
Tussi-Organidin DM NR Liquid **3350**
Tussi-Organidin DM-S NR Liquid **3350**

ACB (New Zealand)
ACEBUTOLOL HYDROCHLORIDE
Sectral Capsules **3589**

ACCOLATE (Australia, Belgium, Canada, Finland, Hong Kong, Irish Republic, Mexico, Portugal, Singapore, Spain, Switzerland, Thailand, United Kingdom)
ZAFIRLUKAST
Accolate Tablets **657**

ACCOLEIT (Italy)
ZAFIRLUKAST
Accolate Tablets **657**

ACCUPRIL (Australia, Belgium, Canada, Hong Kong, New Zealand, Singapore, South Africa, Thailand)
QUINAPRIL HYDROCHLORIDE
Accupril Tablets **2611**

ACCUPRO (Austria, Denmark, Finland, Irish Republic, Sweden, Switzerland, United Kingdom)
QUINAPRIL HYDROCHLORIDE
Accupril Tablets **2611**

ACCURE (Australia)
ISOTRETINOIN
Accutane Capsules **2944**

ACCUSITE (United Kingdom)
FLUOROURACIL
Efudex Cream **1733**
Efudex Topical Solutions **1733**
Fluoroplex Topical Cream **552**
Fluoroplex Topical Solution **552**

ACCUTANE (Canada)
ISOTRETINOIN
Accutane Capsules **2944**

AC-DE (Mexico)
DACTINOMYCIN
Cosmegen for Injection **2062**

ACECOMB (Austria)
HYDROCHLOROTHIAZIDE/LISINOPRIL
Prinzide Tablets **2168**
Zestoretic Tablets **695**

ACECOR (Italy)
ACEBUTOLOL HYDROCHLORIDE
Sectral Capsules **3589**

ACEDIUR (Spain)
ENALAPRIL MALEATE/HYDROCHLOROTHIAZIDE
Vaseretic Tablets **2204**

ACE-HEMMER (Germany)
CAPTOPRIL
Captopril Tablets **2281**

ACEMIN (Austria)
LISINOPRIL
Prinivil Tablets **2164**
Zestril Tablets **698**

ACENORM (Australia, Germany)
CAPTOPRIL
Captopril Tablets **2281**

ACENORM HCT (Germany)
CAPTOPRIL
Captopril Tablets **2281**

ACEOMEL (Irish Republic)
CAPTOPRIL
Captopril Tablets **2281**

ACEOTO (Spain)
CIPROFLOXACIN
Cipro I.V. **893**
Cipro I.V. Pharmacy Bulk Package **897**
Cipro Oral Suspension **887**

ACEPRESS (Italy)
CAPTOPRIL
Captopril Tablets **2281**

ACEPRIL (Denmark, Switzerland, United Kingdom)
LISINOPRIL
Prinivil Tablets . . . 2164
Zestril Tablets . . . 698

ACERBON (Germany)
LISINOPRIL
Prinivil Tablets . . . 2164
Zestril Tablets . . . 698

ACERCOMP (Finland, Germany)
HYDROCHLOROTHIAZIDE/LISINOPRIL
Prinzide Tablets . . . 2168
Zestoretic Tablets . . . 695

ACEREN (Denmark)
ENALAPRIL MALEATE
Vasotec Tablets . . . 2210

ACERIL (Israel)
CAPTOPRIL
Captopril Tablets . . . 2281

ACESISTEM (Italy)
ENALAPRIL MALEATE/HYDROCHLOROTHIAZIDE
Vaseretic Tablets . . . 2204

ACESTROL (Portugal)
MEGESTROL ACETATE
Megace Oral Suspension . . . 1124

ACETADIAZOL (Mexico)
ACETAZOLAMIDE
Diamox Sequels Sustained Release Capsules . . . ⊙270
Diamox Tablets . . . ⊙269

ACETAN (Austria)
LISINOPRIL
Prinivil Tablets . . . 2164
Zestril Tablets . . . 698

ACETENSIL (Spain)
ENALAPRIL MALEATE
Vasotec Tablets . . . 2210

ACETENSIL PLUS (Spain)
ENALAPRIL MALEATE/HYDROCHLOROTHIAZIDE
Vaseretic Tablets . . . 2204

ACETOPT (Australia, New Zealand)
SULFACETAMIDE SODIUM
Bleph-10 Ophthalmic Ointment 10% . . . ⊙230
Klaron Lotion 10% . . . 1224

ACETOXYL (Canada, United Kingdom)
BENZOYL PEROXIDE
Brevoxyl-4 Cleansing Lotion . . . 3269
Brevoxyl-4 Creamy Wash . . . 3270
Brevoxyl-4 Gel . . . 3269
Brevoxyl-8 Cleansing Lotion . . . 3269
Brevoxyl-8 Creamy Wash . . . 3270
Brevoxyl-8 Gel . . . 3269
Triaz Cleanser . . . 2026
Triaz Gel . . . 2026

AC-FA (Thailand)
KETOCONAZOLE
Nizoral 2% Cream . . . 3620
Nizoral 2% Shampoo . . . 2007
Nizoral Tablets . . . 1791

ACID A VIT (Belgium, The Netherlands)
TRETINOIN
Avita Cream . . . 999
Avita Gel . . . 1000
Renova 0.05% Cream . . . 2519
Retin-A Micro 0.1% . . . 2522
Vesanoid Capsules . . . 3037

ACID HALT (Canada)
FAMOTIDINE
Pepcid Injection . . . 2153
Pepcid Injection Premixed . . . 2153
Pepcid RPD Orally Disintegrating Tablets . . . 2150
Pepcid Tablets . . . 2150
Pepcid for Oral Suspension . . . 2150

ACID-EZE (United Kingdom)
CIMETIDINE
Tagamet Tablets . . . 1644

ACIDOWN (South Africa)
CIMETIDINE
Tagamet Tablets . . . 1644

ACILAC (Canada)
LACTULOSE
Kristalose for Oral Solution . . . 1007

ACILOC (Denmark, Sweden, Thailand)
CIMETIDINE
Tagamet Tablets . . . 1644

ACI-MED (South Africa)
CIMETIDINE
Tagamet Tablets . . . 1644

ACINIL (Denmark, Norway, Sweden)
CIMETIDINE
Tagamet Tablets . . . 1644

ACITAK (United Kingdom)
CIMETIDINE
Tagamet Tablets . . . 1644

ACLIN (Australia, Hong Kong)
SULINDAC
Clinoril Tablets . . . 2053

ACLINDA (Germany)
CLINDAMYCIN HYDROCHLORIDE
Cleocin HCl Capsules . . . 2784

ACLONIUM (Italy)
GABAPENTIN
Neurontin Capsules . . . 2655

ACLORAL (Mexico)
RANITIDINE HYDROCHLORIDE
Zantac 150 EFFERdose Granules . . . 1690
Zantac 150 EFFERdose Tablets . . . 1690
Zantac 150 Tablets . . . 1690
Zantac 300 Tablets . . . 1690
Zantac Injection . . . 1688
Zantac Injection Premixed . . . 1688
Zantac Syrup . . . 1690

ACLOSONE (France, South Africa, The Netherlands)
ALCLOMETASONE DIPROPIONATE
Aclovate Cream . . . 1275
Aclovate Ointment . . . 1275

ACNACYL (Australia, Hong Kong, Singapore)
BENZOYL PEROXIDE
Brevoxyl-4 Cleansing Lotion . . . 3269
Brevoxyl-4 Creamy Wash . . . 3270
Brevoxyl-4 Gel . . . 3269
Brevoxyl-8 Cleansing Lotion . . . 3269
Brevoxyl-8 Creamy Wash . . . 3270
Brevoxyl-8 Gel . . . 3269
Triaz Cleanser . . . 2026
Triaz Gel . . . 2026

ACNASE (Brazil)
BENZOYL PEROXIDE
Brevoxyl-4 Cleansing Lotion . . . 3269
Brevoxyl-4 Creamy Wash . . . 3270
Brevoxyl-4 Gel . . . 3269
Brevoxyl-8 Cleansing Lotion . . . 3269
Brevoxyl-8 Creamy Wash . . . 3270
Brevoxyl-8 Gel . . . 3269
Triaz Cleanser . . . 2026
Triaz Gel . . . 2026

ACNE DERM (Israel)
BENZOYL PEROXIDE
Brevoxyl-4 Cleansing Lotion . . . 3269
Brevoxyl-4 Creamy Wash . . . 3270
Brevoxyl-4 Gel . . . 3269
Brevoxyl-8 Cleansing Lotion . . . 3269
Brevoxyl-8 Creamy Wash . . . 3270
Brevoxyl-8 Gel . . . 3269
Triaz Cleanser . . . 2026
Triaz Gel . . . 2026

ACNE MASK (Israel)
BENZOYL PEROXIDE
Brevoxyl-4 Cleansing Lotion . . . 3269
Brevoxyl-4 Creamy Wash . . . 3270
Brevoxyl-4 Gel . . . 3269
Brevoxyl-8 Cleansing Lotion . . . 3269
Brevoxyl-8 Creamy Wash . . . 3270
Brevoxyl-8 Gel . . . 3269
Triaz Cleanser . . . 2026
Triaz Gel . . . 2026

ACNE-AID (Spain)
BENZOYL PEROXIDE
Brevoxyl-4 Cleansing Lotion . . . 3269
Brevoxyl-4 Creamy Wash . . . 3270
Brevoxyl-4 Gel . . . 3269
Brevoxyl-8 Cleansing Lotion . . . 3269
Brevoxyl-8 Creamy Wash . . . 3270
Brevoxyl-8 Gel . . . 3269
Triaz Cleanser . . . 2026
Triaz Gel . . . 2026

ACNECIDE (Irish Republic, United Kingdom)
BENZOYL PEROXIDE
Brevoxyl-4 Cleansing Lotion . . . 3269
Brevoxyl-4 Creamy Wash . . . 3270
Brevoxyl-4 Gel . . . 3269
Brevoxyl-8 Cleansing Lotion . . . 3269
Brevoxyl-8 Creamy Wash . . . 3270
Brevoxyl-8 Gel . . . 3269
Triaz Cleanser . . . 2026
Triaz Gel . . . 2026

ACNECOLOR (Switzerland)
CLOTRIMAZOLE
Lotrimin Cream 1% . . . 3128
Lotrimin Lotion 1% . . . 3128
Lotrimin Topical Solution 1% . . . 3128
Mycelex Troche . . . 573

ACNE-CY-CLEAN (South Africa)
DOXYCYCLINE HYCLATE
Doryx Coated Pellet Filled Capsules . . . 3357
Periostat Tablets . . . 1208
Vibra-Tabs Film Coated Tablets . . . 2735
Vibramycin Hyclate Capsules . . . 2735
Vibramycin Hyclate Intravenous . . . 2737

ACNEFUGE (Switzerland)
BENZOYL PEROXIDE
Brevoxyl-4 Cleansing Lotion . . . 3269
Brevoxyl-4 Creamy Wash . . . 3270
Brevoxyl-4 Gel . . . 3269
Brevoxyl-8 Cleansing Lotion . . . 3269
Brevoxyl-8 Creamy Wash . . . 3270
Brevoxyl-8 Gel . . . 3269
Triaz Cleanser . . . 2026
Triaz Gel . . . 2026

ACNEGEL (United Kingdom)
BENZOYL PEROXIDE
Brevoxyl-4 Cleansing Lotion . . . 3269
Brevoxyl-4 Creamy Wash . . . 3270
Brevoxyl-4 Gel . . . 3269
Brevoxyl-8 Cleansing Lotion . . . 3269
Brevoxyl-8 Creamy Wash . . . 3270
Brevoxyl-8 Gel . . . 3269
Triaz Cleanser . . . 2026
Triaz Gel . . . 2026

ACNERYNE (Belgium)
ERYTHROMYCIN
Emgel 2% Topical Gel . . . 1285
Ery-Tab Tablets . . . 448
Erythromycin Base Filmtab Tablets . . . 454
Erythromycin Delayed-Release Capsules, USP . . . 455
PCE Dispertab Tablets . . . 498

ACNESAN (Brazil)
BENZOYL PEROXIDE
Brevoxyl-4 Cleansing Lotion . . . 3269
Brevoxyl-4 Creamy Wash . . . 3270
Brevoxyl-4 Gel . . . 3269
Brevoxyl-8 Cleansing Lotion . . . 3269
Brevoxyl-8 Creamy Wash . . . 3270
Brevoxyl-8 Gel . . . 3269
Triaz Cleanser . . . 2026
Triaz Gel . . . 2026

ACNETRIM (Israel)
ERYTHROMYCIN
Emgel 2% Topical Gel . . . 1285
Ery-Tab Tablets . . . 448
Erythromycin Base Filmtab Tablets . . . 454
Erythromycin Delayed-Release Capsules, USP . . . 455
PCE Dispertab Tablets . . . 498

ACNEZAIC (Italy)
AZELAIC ACID
Azelex Cream . . . 547

ACNOMEL BP 5 (Canada)
BENZOYL PEROXIDE
Brevoxyl-4 Cleansing Lotion . . . 3269
Brevoxyl-4 Creamy Wash . . . 3270
Brevoxyl-4 Gel . . . 3269
Brevoxyl-8 Cleansing Lotion . . . 3269
Brevoxyl-8 Creamy Wash . . . 3270
Brevoxyl-8 Gel . . . 3269
Triaz Cleanser . . . 2026
Triaz Gel . . . 2026

ACNOSIL (Brazil)
BENZOYL PEROXIDE
Brevoxyl-4 Cleansing Lotion . . . 3269
Brevoxyl-4 Creamy Wash . . . 3270
Brevoxyl-4 Gel . . . 3269
Brevoxyl-8 Cleansing Lotion . . . 3269
Brevoxyl-8 Creamy Wash . . . 3270
Brevoxyl-8 Gel . . . 3269
Triaz Cleanser . . . 2026
Triaz Gel . . . 2026

ACOFLAM (United Kingdom)
DICLOFENAC SODIUM
Voltaren Tablets . . . 2315
Voltaren-XR Tablets . . . 2315

ACON (Mexico)
VITAMIN A PALMITATE
Aquasol A Parenteral . . . 593

ACONEX (Austria)
NAPHAZOLINE HYDROCHLORIDE
Albalon Ophthalmic Solution . . . ⊙225

ACORDIN (Switzerland)
ISOSORBIDE DINITRATE
Isordil Sublingual Tablets . . . 3525
Isordil Titradose Tablets . . . 3526

ACOVIL (Spain)
RAMIPRIL
Altace Capsules . . . 2233

ACSACEA (Austria)
METRONIDAZOLE
MetroCream . . . 1404
MetroGel . . . 1405
MetroGel-Vaginal Gel . . . 1986
MetroLotion . . . 1405
Noritate Cream . . . 1224

ACT-3 (Australia, New Zealand)
IBUPROFEN
Motrin Suspension, Oral Drops, Chewable Tablets, and Caplets . . . 2002

ACTA (Hong Kong, Singapore)
TRETINOIN
Avita Cream . . . 999
Avita Gel . . . 1000
Renova 0.05% Cream . . . 2519
Retin-A Micro 0.1% . . . 2522
Vesanoid Capsules . . . 3037

ACTICIN (United Kingdom)
TRETINOIN
Avita Cream . . . 999
Avita Gel . . . 1000
Renova 0.05% Cream . . . 2519
Retin-A Micro 0.1% . . . 2522
Vesanoid Capsules . . . 3037

ACTIDINE (Hong Kong)
FAMOTIDINE
Pepcid Injection . . . 2153
Pepcid Injection Premixed . . . 2153
Pepcid RPD Orally Disintegrating Tablets . . . 2150
Pepcid Tablets . . . 2150
Pepcid for Oral Suspension . . . 2150

ACTIFEN (Spain)
IBUPROFEN
Motrin Suspension, Oral Drops, Chewable Tablets, and Caplets . . . 2002

ACTIFERRO (Italy)
FERRIC SODIUM GLUCONATE
Ferrlecit Injection . . . 3386

ACTILAX (Australia)
LACTULOSE
Kristalose for Oral Solution . . . 1007

ACTIMIDOL (Spain)
IBUPROFEN
Motrin Suspension, Oral Drops, Chewable Tablets, and Caplets . . . 2002

ACTINO-HERMAL (Germany)
FLUOROURACIL
Efudex Cream . . . 1733
Efudex Topical Solutions . . . 1733
Fluoroplex Topical Cream . . . 552
Fluoroplex Topical Solution . . . 552

ACTIPROFEN (Australia, Brazil, Canada, Irish Republic)
IBUPROFEN
Motrin Suspension, Oral Drops, Chewable Tablets, and Caplets . . . 2002

ACTIQ (United Kingdom)
FENTANYL CITRATE
Actiq . . . 1184

ACTIQUIM (Mexico)
NAPROXEN
EC-Naprosyn Delayed-Release Tablets . . . 2967
Naprosyn Suspension . . . 2967
Naprosyn Tablets . . . 2967

ACTISKENAN (France)
MORPHINE SULFATE
Astramorph/PF Injection, USP (Preservative-Free) . . . 594
Duramorph Injection . . . 1312
Infumorph 200 and Infumorph 500 Sterile Solutions . . . 1314
Kadian Capsules . . . 1335
MS Contin Tablets . . . 2896
MSIR Oral Capsules . . . 2898
MSIR Oral Solution . . . 2898
MSIR Oral Solution Concentrate . . . 2898
MSIR Oral Tablets . . . 2898
Oramorph SR Tablets . . . 3062
Roxanol 100 Concentrated Oral Solution . . . 3066
Roxanol Concentrated Oral Solution . . . 3066
Roxanol-T Oral Solution . . . 3066

ACTIVELLE (Irish Republic, Spain, The Netherlands)
ESTRADIOL
Alora Transdermal System . . . 3372
Climara Transdermal System . . . 958
Estrace Vaginal Cream . . . 3358
Estring Vaginal Ring . . . 2811
Vivelle Transdermal System . . . 2412
Vivelle-Dot Transdermal System . . . 2416

ACTOCORTINA (Spain)
HYDROCORTISONE SODIUM PHOSPHATE
Hydrocortone Phosphate Injection, Sterile . . . 2105

ACTONEL (Australia, France, Irish Republic)
RISEDRONATE SODIUM
Actonel Tablets . . . 2879

ACTOPRIL (Irish Republic)
CAPTOPRIL
Captopril Tablets . . . 2281

(⊙ Described in PDR For Ophthalmic Medicines™)

ACTOS (Australia, United Kingdom)
PIOGLITAZONE HYDROCHLORIDE
Actos Tablets . . . 3275

ACTRON (Austria)
KETOPROFEN
Orudis Capsules . . . 3548
Oruvail Capsules . . . 3548

ACTRONEFFIX (France)
KETOPROFEN
Orudis Capsules . . . 3548
Oruvail Capsules . . . 3548

ACUDOR (Portugal)
ETODOLAC
Lodine Capsules . . . 3528
Lodine Tablets . . . 3528
Lodine XL Extended-Release Tablets . . . 3530

ACUITEL (France)
QUINAPRIL HYDROCHLORIDE
Accupril Tablets . . . 2611

ACULFIN (Brazil)
SULFASALAZINE
Azulfidine EN-tabs Tablets . . . 2775

ACUMET (South Africa)
METOCLOPRAMIDE HYDROCHLORIDE
Reglan Injectable . . . 2935
Reglan Syrup . . . 2935
Reglan Tablets . . . 2935

ACUMOD (South Africa)
AMILORIDE HYDROCHLORIDE/HYDROCHLOROTHIAZIDE
Moduretic Tablets . . . 2138

ACUPREL (Spain)
QUINAPRIL HYDROCHLORIDE
Accupril Tablets . . . 2611

ACUPRIL (Mexico, Portugal, The Netherlands)
QUINAPRIL HYDROCHLORIDE
Accupril Tablets . . . 2611

ACUSPRAIN (South Africa)
NAPROXEN
EC-Naprosyn Delayed-Release Tablets . . . 2967
Naprosyn Suspension . . . 2967
Naprosyn Tablets . . . 2967

ACUZOLE (South Africa)
METRONIDAZOLE
MetroCream . . . 1404
MetroGel . . . 1405
MetroGel-Vaginal Gel . . . 1986
MetroLotion . . . 1405
Noritate Cream . . . 1224

ADACOR (Australia)
HYDROCORTISONE ACETATE
Anusol-HC Suppositories . . . 2238
Cortifoam Rectal Foam . . . 3170
Hydrocortone Acetate Injectable Suspension . . . 2103
Proctocort Suppositories . . . 2264

ADAFERIN (Israel, Mexico)
ADAPALENE
Differin Gel . . . 1403
Differin Solution/Pledgets . . . 1404

ADALAT (Australia, Austria, Belgium, Brazil, Canada, Denmark, Finland, Germany, Hong Kong, Irish Republic, Italy, Mexico, New Zealand, Norway, Portugal, Singapore, South Africa, Spain, Sweden, Switzerland, Thailand, The Netherlands, United Kingdom)
NIFEDIPINE
Adalat CC Tablets . . . 877
Procardia Capsules . . . 2708
Procardia XL Extended Release Tablets . . . 2710

ADALATE (France)
NIFEDIPINE
Adalat CC Tablets . . . 877
Procardia Capsules . . . 2708
Procardia XL Extended Release Tablets . . . 2710

ADALKEN (Mexico)
PENICILLAMINE
Cuprimine Capsules . . . 2075
Depen Titratable Tablets . . . 3341

ADANT (Israel)
SODIUM HYALURONATE
Hyalgan Solution . . . 3080

ADAPINE (Australia)
NIFEDIPINE
Adalat CC Tablets . . . 877
Procardia Capsules . . . 2708
Procardia XL Extended Release Tablets . . . 2710

ADAPRESS (Switzerland)
NIFEDIPINE
Adalat CC Tablets . . . 877
Procardia Capsules . . . 2708
Procardia XL Extended Release Tablets . . . 2710

ADASONE (Australia)
PREDNISONE
Prednisone Intensol . . . 3064
Prednisone Oral Solution . . . 3064
Prednisone Tablets . . . 3064

ADCO-LOTEN (South Africa)
ATENOLOL
Tenormin I.V. Injection . . . 692

ADCO-RETIC (South Africa)
AMILORIDE HYDROCHLORIDE/HYDROCHLOROTHIAZIDE
Moduretic Tablets . . . 2138

ADCORTYL (Irish Republic, Israel, United Kingdom)
TRIAMCINOLONE ACETONIDE
Azmacort Inhalation Aerosol . . . 728
Nasacort AQ Nasal Spray . . . 752
Nasacort Nasal Inhaler . . . 750

ADCORTYL IN ORABASE (Irish Republic, United Kingdom)
TRIAMCINOLONE ACETONIDE
Azmacort Inhalation Aerosol . . . 728
Nasacort AQ Nasal Spray . . . 752
Nasacort Nasal Inhaler . . . 750

ADDI-K (Hong Kong, Singapore, Thailand)
POTASSIUM CHLORIDE
K-Dur Microburst Release System ER Tablets . . . 1832
K-Lor Powder Packets . . . 469
K-Tab Filmtab Tablets . . . 470
Rum-K . . . 1363

ADECUR (Mexico)
TERAZOSIN HYDROCHLORIDE
Hytrin Capsules . . . 464

ADEKIN (Germany)
AMANTADINE HYDROCHLORIDE
Symmetrel Syrup . . . 1328
Symmetrel Tablets . . . 1328

ADEL (Mexico)
CLARITHROMYCIN
Biaxin Filmtab Tablets . . . 403
Biaxin for Oral Suspension . . . 403

ADENOCARD (Brazil, Canada)
ADENOSINE
Adenocard Injection . . . 1380
Adenoscan . . . 1381

ADENOCOR (Australia, Belgium, Denmark, Finland, Irish Republic, Israel, New Zealand, Norway, Portugal, Singapore, South Africa, Spain, Sweden, Thailand, The Netherlands, United Kingdom)
ADENOSINE
Adenocard Injection . . . 1380
Adenoscan . . . 1381

ADENOSCAN (Australia, Finland, France, Germany, Italy, Spain, The Netherlands, United Kingdom)
ADENOSINE
Adenocard Injection . . . 1380
Adenoscan . . . 1381

ADEPRIL (Mexico)
CARBAMAZEPINE
Carbatrol Capsules . . . 3234
Tegretol Chewable Tablets . . . 2404
Tegretol Suspension . . . 2404
Tegretol Tablets . . . 2404
Tegretol-XR Tablets . . . 2404

ADESIPRESS-TTS (Italy)
CLONIDINE
Catapres-TTS . . . 1038

ADEX (Israel)
IBUPROFEN
Motrin Suspension, Oral Drops, Chewable Tablets, and Caplets . . . 2002

ADEXONE (Israel)
DEXAMETHASONE
Decadron Elixir . . . 2078
Decadron Tablets . . . 2079

ADFEN (South Africa)
IBUPROFEN
Motrin Suspension, Oral Drops, Chewable Tablets, and Caplets . . . 2002

ADGYN ESTRO (United Kingdom)
ESTRADIOL
Alora Transdermal System . . . 3372
Climara Transdermal System . . . 958
Estrace Vaginal Cream . . . 3358
Estring Vaginal Ring . . . 2811
Vivelle Transdermal System . . . 2412
Vivelle-Dot Transdermal System . . . 2416

ADGYN MEDRO (United Kingdom)
MEDROXYPROGESTERONE ACETATE
Depo-Provera Contraceptive Injection . . . 2798
Provera Tablets . . . 2853

ADICLAIR (Germany)
NYSTATIN
Nystop Topical Powder USP . . . 2608

ADIPINE (United Kingdom)
NIFEDIPINE
Adalat CC Tablets . . . 877
Procardia Capsules . . . 2708
Procardia XL Extended Release Tablets . . . 2710

ADIVON (Mexico)
IBUPROFEN
Motrin Suspension, Oral Drops, Chewable Tablets, and Caplets . . . 2002

ADIZEM (Irish Republic, Israel, United Kingdom)
DILTIAZEM HYDROCHLORIDE
Cardizem CD Capsules . . . 1016
Cardizem Injectable . . . 1018
Cardizem Lyo-Ject Syringe . . . 1018
Cardizem Monovial . . . 1018
Tiazac Capsules . . . 1378

ADMON (Spain)
NIMODIPINE
Nimotop Capsules . . . 904

ADNISOLONE (Australia)
PREDNISOLONE
Prelone Syrup . . . 2273

ADOCOMP (Germany)
CAPTOPRIL
Captopril Tablets . . . 2281

ADOCOR (Germany)
CAPTOPRIL
Captopril Tablets . . . 2281

ADOLONTA (Spain)
TRAMADOL HYDROCHLORIDE
Ultram Tablets . . . 2600

ADOMAL (Italy)
DIFLUNISAL
Dolobid Tablets . . . 2088

ADREKAR (Austria, Germany)
ADENOSINE
Adenocard Injection . . . 1380
Adenoscan . . . 1381

ADRESON (Belgium, The Netherlands)
CORTISONE ACETATE
Cortone Acetate Injectable Suspension . . . 2059
Cortone Acetate Tablets . . . 2061

ADREXAN (France)
PROPRANOLOL HYDROCHLORIDE
Inderal Injectable . . . 3513
Inderal LA Long-Acting Capsules . . . 3516
Inderal Tablets . . . 3513

ADRIBLASTIN (Austria, Germany, Switzerland)
DOXORUBICIN HYDROCHLORIDE
Adriamycin PFS/RDF Injection . . . 2767

ADRIBLASTINA (Belgium, Brazil, Italy, Mexico, Portugal, South Africa, Thailand, The Netherlands)
DOXORUBICIN HYDROCHLORIDE
Adriamycin PFS/RDF Injection . . . 2767

ADRIBLASTINE (France)
DOXORUBICIN HYDROCHLORIDE
Adriamycin PFS/RDF Injection . . . 2767

ADRIM (Thailand)
DOXORUBICIN HYDROCHLORIDE
Adriamycin PFS/RDF Injection . . . 2767

ADRIMEDAC (Germany)
DOXORUBICIN HYDROCHLORIDE
Adriamycin PFS/RDF Injection . . . 2767

ADROCIL (Portugal)
TRIFLURIDINE
Viroptic Ophthalmic Solution Sterile . . . ⊙301

ADRONAT (Italy, Portugal)
ALENDRONATE SODIUM
Fosamax Tablets . . . 2095

ADROYD (Australia)
OXYMETHOLONE
Anadrol-50 Tablets . . . 3321

ADRUCIL (Canada)
FLUOROURACIL
Efudex Cream . . . 1733
Efudex Topical Solutions . . . 1733
Fluoroplex Topical Cream . . . 552
Fluoroplex Topical Solution . . . 552

ADUCIN (Denmark)
RANITIDINE HYDROCHLORIDE
Zantac 150 EFFERdose Granules . . . 1690
Zantac 150 EFFERdose Tablets . . . 1690
Zantac 150 Tablets . . . 1690
Zantac 300 Tablets . . . 1690
Zantac Injection . . . 1688
Zantac Injection Premixed . . . 1688
Zantac Syrup . . . 1690

ADULT MELTUS FOR CHESTY COUGHS & CATARRH (United Kingdom)
GUAIFENESIN
Organidin NR Liquid . . . 3350
Organidin NR Tablets . . . 3350

ADVERSUTEN (Germany)
PRAZOSIN HYDROCHLORIDE
Minipress Capsules . . . 2699

ADVIL (Brazil, Canada, France, Hong Kong, Irish Republic, Mexico, Spain, The Netherlands, United Kingdom)
IBUPROFEN
Motrin Suspension, Oral Drops, Chewable Tablets, and Caplets . . . 2002

ADVIL COLD & FLU (Irish Republic)
IBUPROFEN
Motrin Suspension, Oral Drops, Chewable Tablets, and Caplets . . . 2002

ADVIL COLD & SINUS (United Kingdom)
IBUPROFEN
Motrin Suspension, Oral Drops, Chewable Tablets, and Caplets . . . 2002

ADVIL MONO (Belgium)
IBUPROFEN
Motrin Suspension, Oral Drops, Chewable Tablets, and Caplets . . . 2002

AEROCEF (Austria)
CEFIXIME
Suprax Tablets . . . 1877
Suprax for Oral Suspension . . . 1877

AEROCORTIN (Australia)
HYDROCORTISONE/NEOMYCIN SULFATE/POLYMYXIN B SULFATE
Cortisporin Ophthalmic Suspension Sterile . . . ⊙297

AERODIOL (United Kingdom)
ESTRADIOL
Alora Transdermal System . . . 3372
Climara Transdermal System . . . 958
Estrace Vaginal Cream . . . 3358
Estring Vaginal Ring . . . 2811
Vivelle Transdermal System . . . 2412
Vivelle-Dot Transdermal System . . . 2416

AEROVENT (Israel)
IPRATROPIUM BROMIDE
Atrovent Inhalation Aerosol . . . 1030
Atrovent Inhalation Solution . . . 1031
Atrovent Nasal Spray 0.03% . . . 1032
Atrovent Nasal Spray 0.06% . . . 1033

AFAZOL (Mexico)
NAPHAZOLINE HYDROCHLORIDE
Albalon Ophthalmic Solution . . . ⊙225

AFLODAC (Italy)
SULINDAC
Clinoril Tablets . . . 2053

AFLOMIN (Spain)
TRIFLURIDINE
Viroptic Ophthalmic Solution Sterile . . . ⊙301

AFLUON (Spain)
AZELASTINE HYDROCHLORIDE
Astelin Nasal Spray . . . 3339

AFONILUM (Austria, Germany)
THEOPHYLLINE
Aerolate Jr. T.D. Capsules . . . 1361
Aerolate Liquid . . . 1361
Aerolate Sr. T.D. Capsules . . . 1361
Theo-Dur Extended-Release Tablets . . . 1835
Uni-Dur Extended-Release Tablets . . . 1841
Uniphyl 400 mg and 600 mg Tablets . . . 2903

AFONINA (Portugal)
BENZOCAINE
Americaine Anesthetic Lubricant . . . 1162
Americaine Otic Topical Anesthetic Ear Drops . . . 1162

AFPRED-THEO (Germany)
THEOPHYLLINE
Aerolate Jr. T.D. Capsules . . . 1361
Aerolate Liquid . . . 1361
Aerolate Sr. T.D. Capsules . . . 1361
Theo-Dur Extended-Release Tablets . . . 1835
Uni-Dur Extended-Release Tablets . . . 1841
Uniphyl 400 mg and 600 mg Tablets . . . 2903

AFRICAN GOLD (Canada)
HYDROQUINONE
Eldopaque Forte 4% Cream . . . 1734
Eldoquin Forte 4% Cream . . . 1734
Lustra Cream . . . 2023
Lustra-AF Cream . . . 2023

(⊙ Described in PDR For Ophthalmic Medicines™)

Melanex Topical Solution **2300**
Solaquin Forte 4% Cream........... **1734**
Solaquin Forte 4% Gel............. **1734**

AFTAB (Finland, Germany, Italy)
TRIAMCINOLONE ACETONIDE
Azmacort Inhalation Aerosol **728**
Nasacort AQ Nasal Spray............ **752**
Nasacort Nasal Inhaler **750**

AFTACH (Portugal)
TRIAMCINOLONE ACETONIDE
Azmacort Inhalation Aerosol **728**
Nasacort AQ Nasal Spray............ **752**
Nasacort Nasal Inhaler **750**

AFTIR GEL (Italy)
MALATHION
Ovide Lotion.................... **2023**

AFUNGIL (Mexico)
FLUCONAZOLE
Diflucan Tablets, Injection, and Oral Suspension **2681**

AGELAN (Hong Kong, Irish Republic)
INDAPAMIDE
Indapamide Tablets.............. **2286**

AGENERASE (France, Switzerland, United Kingdom)
AMPRENAVIR
Agenerase Capsules............. **1454**
Agenerase Oral Solution **1459**

AGGRASTAT (Australia, Belgium, Denmark, Finland, Germany, Irish Republic, Italy, New Zealand, Singapore, Sweden, Switzerland, The Netherlands, United Kingdom)
TIROFIBAN HYDROCHLORIDE
Aggrastat Injection.............. **2031**
Aggrastat Injection Premixed......... **2031**

AGGRASTET (South Africa)
TIROFIBAN HYDROCHLORIDE
Aggrastat Injection.............. **2031**
Aggrastat Injection Premixed......... **2031**

AGGRENOX (Belgium)
DIPYRIDAMOLE
Persantine Tablets **1057**

AGISTEN (Israel)
CLOTRIMAZOLE
Lotrimin Cream 1%.............. **3128**
Lotrimin Lotion 1%............. **3128**
Lotrimin Topical Solution 1%......... **3128**
Mycelex Troche **573**

AGOFENAC (Switzerland)
DICLOFENAC SODIUM
Voltaren Tablets................ **2315**
Voltaren-XR Tablets.............. **2315**

AGON (Australia, New Zealand)
FELODIPINE
Plendil Extended-Release Tablets **623**

AGOPTON (Austria, Germany, Switzerland)
LANSOPRAZOLE
Prevacid Delayed-Release Capsules **3292**

AGOREX (Switzerland)
AMILORIDE HYDROCHLORIDE/HYDROCHLOROTHIAZIDE
Moduretic Tablets............... **2138**

AGRASTAT (France, Mexico, Spain)
TIROFIBAN HYDROCHLORIDE
Aggrastat Injection.............. **2031**
Aggrastat Injection Premixed......... **2031**

AGREDAMOL (Belgium)
DIPYRIDAMOLE
Persantine Tablets **1057**

AGREMOL (Thailand)
DIPYRIDAMOLE
Persantine Tablets **1057**

AGRYLIN (Australia, Canada, Israel)
ANAGRELIDE HYDROCHLORIDE
Agrylin Capsules **3232**

AH 3 N (Germany)
HYDROXYZINE HYDROCHLORIDE
Atarax Tablets & Syrup **2667**
Vistaril Intramuscular Solution **2738**

AIDA (France, Singapore)
HYDROQUINONE
Eldopaque Forte 4% Cream.......... **1734**
Eldoquin Forte 4% Cream........... **1734**
Lustra Cream **2023**
Lustra-AF Cream **2023**
Melanex Topical Solution **2300**
Solaquin Forte 4% Cream........... **1734**
Solaquin Forte 4% Gel............. **1734**

AINEX (Mexico)
IBUPROFEN
Motrin Suspension, Oral Drops, Chewable Tablets, and Caplets...... **2002**

AIRCORT (Italy)
BUDESONIDE
Pulmicort Turbuhaler Inhalation Powder ... **636**
Rhinocort Nasal Inhaler **640**

AIROL (Australia, Austria, Germany, Israel, Italy, Mexico, Norway, South Africa, Switzerland)
TRETINOIN
Avita Cream **999**
Avita Gel **1000**
Renova 0.05% Cream............ **2519**
Retin-A Micro 0.1%............. **2522**
Vesanoid Capsules.............. **3037**

AIROMET (Thailand)
OMEPRAZOLE
Prilosec Delayed-Release Capsules...... **628**

AKAMIN (Australia)
MINOCYCLINE HYDROCHLORIDE
Dynacin Capsules............... **2019**
Minocin Intravenous **1862**
Minocin Oral Suspension **1865**
Minocin Pellet-Filled Capsules **1863**

AK-CHLOR (Canada)
CHLORAMPHENICOL
Chloromycetin Ophthalmic Ointment, 1%.................... ⊙**296**
Chloromycetin Ophthalmic Solution ..... ⊙**297**
Chloroptic Sterile Ophthalmic Ointment.. ⊙**234**
Chloroptic Sterile Ophthalmic Solution .. ⊙**235**

AK-CIDE (Canada)
PREDNISOLONE ACETATE/SULFACETAMIDE SODIUM
Blephamide Ophthalmic Ointment **547**
Blephamide Ophthalmic Suspension **548**

AK-CON (Canada)
NAPHAZOLINE HYDROCHLORIDE
Albalon Ophthalmic Solution.......... ⊙**225**

AK-DEX (Canada)
DEXAMETHASONE SODIUM PHOSPHATE
Decadron Phosphate Injection **2081**
Decadron Phosphate Sterile Ophthalmic Ointment .... ⊙**280, 2083**
Decadron Phosphate Sterile Ophthalmic Solution **2084**

AKEZOL (Mexico)
ACETAZOLAMIDE
Diamox Sequels Sustained Release Capsules .... ⊙**270**
Diamox Tablets................ ⊙**269**

AKFEN (Irish Republic)
GUANFACINE HYDROCHLORIDE
Tenex Tablets **2942**

AK-FLUOR (Canada)
FLUORESCEIN SODIUM
AK-Fluor Injection 10% and 25% ...... ⊙**202**
Fluorescite Injection .... ⊙**211**

AKILEN (Hong Kong)
VERAPAMIL HYDROCHLORIDE
Covera-HS Tablets **3199**
Isoptin SR Tablets............... **467**
Verelan Capsules **3184**
Verelan PM Capsules **3186**

AKINETON (Australia, Canada, France, Portugal, Singapore, United Kingdom)
BIPERIDEN HYDROCHLORIDE
Akineton Tablets................. **402**

AKNE (Austria)
ERYTHROMYCIN
Emgel 2% Topical Gel **1285**
Ery-Tab Tablets **448**
Erythromycin Base Filmtab Tablets **454**
Erythromycin Delayed-Release Capsules, USP..................... **455**
PCE Dispertab Tablets............. **498**

AKNE CORDES (Germany)
ERYTHROMYCIN
Emgel 2% Topical Gel **1285**
Ery-Tab Tablets **448**
Erythromycin Base Filmtab Tablets **454**
Erythromycin Delayed-Release Capsules, USP..................... **455**
PCE Dispertab Tablets............. **498**

AKNE-AID-LOTION MILD (Germany)
BENZOYL PEROXIDE
Brevoxyl-4 Cleansing Lotion **3269**
Brevoxyl-4 Creamy Wash **3270**
Brevoxyl-4 Gel................. **3269**
Brevoxyl-8 Cleansing Lotion **3269**
Brevoxyl-8 Creamy Wash **3270**
Brevoxyl-8 Gel................. **3269**
Triaz Cleanser................. **2026**
Triaz Gel **2026**

AKNEDERM ERY (Germany)
ERYTHROMYCIN
Emgel 2% Topical Gel **1285**
Ery-Tab Tablets **448**
Erythromycin Base Filmtab Tablets **454**
Erythromycin Delayed-Release Capsules, USP..................... **455**
PCE Dispertab Tablets............. **498**

AKNEDERM OXID (Germany)
BENZOYL PEROXIDE
Brevoxyl-4 Cleansing Lotion **3269**
Brevoxyl-4 Creamy Wash **3270**
Brevoxyl-4 Gel................. **3269**
Brevoxyl-8 Cleansing Lotion **3269**
Brevoxyl-8 Creamy Wash **3270**
Brevoxyl-8 Gel................. **3269**
Triaz Cleanser................. **2026**
Triaz Gel **2026**

AKNEFUG-EL (Germany)
ERYTHROMYCIN
Emgel 2% Topical Gel **1285**
Ery-Tab Tablets **448**
Erythromycin Base Filmtab Tablets **454**
Erythromycin Delayed-Release Capsules, USP..................... **455**
PCE Dispertab Tablets............. **498**

AKNEFUG-OXID (Germany)
BENZOYL PEROXIDE
Brevoxyl-4 Cleansing Lotion **3269**
Brevoxyl-4 Creamy Wash **3270**
Brevoxyl-4 Gel................. **3269**
Brevoxyl-8 Cleansing Lotion **3269**
Brevoxyl-8 Creamy Wash **3270**
Brevoxyl-8 Gel................. **3269**
Triaz Cleanser................. **2026**
Triaz Gel **2026**

AKNEMAGO (Germany)
ERYTHROMYCIN
Emgel 2% Topical Gel **1285**
Ery-Tab Tablets **448**
Erythromycin Base Filmtab Tablets **454**
Erythromycin Delayed-Release Capsules, USP..................... **455**
PCE Dispertab Tablets............. **498**

AKNEMIN (The Netherlands, United Kingdom)
MINOCYCLINE HYDROCHLORIDE
Dynacin Capsules............... **2019**
Minocin Intravenous **1862**
Minocin Oral Suspension **1865**
Minocin Pellet-Filled Capsules **1863**

AKNEMYCIN (Austria, Belgium, Germany, Switzerland, The Netherlands)
ERYTHROMYCIN
Emgel 2% Topical Gel **1285**
Ery-Tab Tablets **448**
Erythromycin Base Filmtab Tablets **454**
Erythromycin Delayed-Release Capsules, USP..................... **455**
PCE Dispertab Tablets............. **498**

AKNE-MYCIN (Portugal, Singapore)
ERYTHROMYCIN
Emgel 2% Topical Gel **1285**
Ery-Tab Tablets **448**
Erythromycin Base Filmtab Tablets **454**
Erythromycin Delayed-Release Capsules, USP..................... **455**
PCE Dispertab Tablets............. **498**

AKNEMYCIN (Hong Kong, Israel)
ERYTHROMYCIN
Emgel 2% Topical Gel **1285**
Ery-Tab Tablets **448**
Erythromycin Base Filmtab Tablets **454**
Erythromycin Delayed-Release Capsules, USP..................... **455**
PCE Dispertab Tablets............. **498**

AKNEMYCIN PLUS (Germany)
ERYTHROMYCIN
Emgel 2% Topical Gel **1285**
Ery-Tab Tablets **448**
Erythromycin Base Filmtab Tablets **454**
Erythromycin Delayed-Release Capsules, USP..................... **455**
PCE Dispertab Tablets............. **498**

AKNE-PUREN (Germany)
MINOCYCLINE HYDROCHLORIDE
Dynacin Capsules............... **2019**
Minocin Intravenous **1862**
Minocin Oral Suspension **1865**
Minocin Pellet-Filled Capsules **1863**

AKNEREDUCT (Germany)
MINOCYCLINE HYDROCHLORIDE
Dynacin Capsules............... **2019**
Minocin Intravenous **1862**
Minocin Oral Suspension **1865**
Minocin Pellet-Filled Capsules **1863**

AKNEROXID (Austria, Belgium, Germany, Switzerland, The Netherlands)
BENZOYL PEROXIDE
Brevoxyl-4 Cleansing Lotion **3269**
Brevoxyl-4 Creamy Wash **3270**
Brevoxyl-4 Gel................. **3269**
Brevoxyl-8 Cleansing Lotion **3269**
Brevoxyl-8 Creamy Wash **3270**
Brevoxyl-8 Gel................. **3269**
Triaz Cleanser................. **2026**
Triaz Gel **2026**

AKNEX (Switzerland)
BENZOYL PEROXIDE
Brevoxyl-4 Cleansing Lotion **3269**
Brevoxyl-4 Creamy Wash **3270**
Brevoxyl-4 Gel................. **3269**
Brevoxyl-8 Cleansing Lotion **3269**
Brevoxyl-8 Creamy Wash **3270**
Brevoxyl-8 Gel................. **3269**
Triaz Cleanser................. **2026**
Triaz Gel **2026**

AKNILOX (Switzerland)
ERYTHROMYCIN
Emgel 2% Topical Gel **1285**
Ery-Tab Tablets **448**
Erythromycin Base Filmtab Tablets **454**
Erythromycin Delayed-Release Capsules, USP..................... **455**
PCE Dispertab Tablets............. **498**

AKNIN (Germany)
ERYTHROMYCIN
Emgel 2% Topical Gel **1285**
Ery-Tab Tablets **448**
Erythromycin Base Filmtab Tablets **454**
Erythromycin Delayed-Release Capsules, USP..................... **455**
PCE Dispertab Tablets............. **498**

AKNIN-MINO (Germany)
MINOCYCLINE HYDROCHLORIDE
Dynacin Capsules............... **2019**
Minocin Intravenous **1862**
Minocin Oral Suspension **1865**
Minocin Pellet-Filled Capsules **1863**

AKNIN-N (Switzerland)
MINOCYCLINE HYDROCHLORIDE
Dynacin Capsules............... **2019**
Minocin Intravenous **1862**
Minocin Oral Suspension **1865**
Minocin Pellet-Filled Capsules **1863**

AKNORAL (Switzerland)
MINOCYCLINE HYDROCHLORIDE
Dynacin Capsules............... **2019**
Minocin Intravenous **1862**
Minocin Oral Suspension **1865**
Minocin Pellet-Filled Capsules **1863**

AKNOSAN (Germany)
MINOCYCLINE HYDROCHLORIDE
Dynacin Capsules............... **2019**
Minocin Intravenous **1862**
Minocin Oral Suspension **1865**
Minocin Pellet-Filled Capsules **1863**

AKORAZOL (Mexico)
KETOCONAZOLE
Nizoral 2% Cream **3620**
Nizoral 2% Shampoo............. **2007**
Nizoral Tablets **1791**

AK-SULF (Canada)
SULFACETAMIDE SODIUM
Bleph-10 Ophthalmic Ointment 10% .... ⊙**230**
Klaron Lotion 10% **1224**

AKTREN (Germany)
IBUPROFEN
Motrin Suspension, Oral Drops, Chewable Tablets, and Caplets...... **2002**

AKUDOL (Italy)
NAPROXEN SODIUM
Anaprox DS Tablets **2967**
Anaprox Tablets................ **2967**
Naprelan Tablets **1293**

ALACOR (Denmark)
ENALAPRIL MALEATE
Vasotec Tablets................ **2210**

ALANDIEM (Portugal)
DILTIAZEM HYDROCHLORIDE
Cardizem CD Capsules **1016**
Cardizem Injectable **1018**
Cardizem Lyo-Ject Syringe **1018**
Cardizem Monovial **1018**
Tiazac Capsules **1378**

ALAPRIL (Italy)
LISINOPRIL
Prinivil Tablets................. **2164**
Zestril Tablets **698**

ALBA-3 (Brazil)
ALBENDAZOLE
Albenza Tablets................ **1463**

ALBALON (Australia, Belgium, Canada, Hong Kong, Irish Republic, New Zealand, South Africa, Switzerland, Thailand)
NAPHAZOLINE HYDROCHLORIDE
Albalon Ophthalmic Solution .... ⊙225

ALBALON LIQUIFILM (The Netherlands)
NAPHAZOLINE HYDROCHLORIDE
Albalon Ophthalmic Solution .... ⊙225

ALBATEL (Thailand)
ALBENDAZOLE
Albenza Tablets 1463

ALBEN (Brazil, Thailand)
ALBENDAZOLE
Albenza Tablets 1463

ALBENDA (Thailand)
ALBENDAZOLE
Albenza Tablets 1463

ALBENSIL (Mexico)
ALBENDAZOLE
Albenza Tablets 1463

ALBETOL (Finland)
LABETALOL HYDROCHLORIDE
Normodyne Injection 3135
Normodyne Tablets 3137

ALBICORT (Belgium, The Netherlands)
TRIAMCINOLONE ACETONIDE
Azmacort Inhalation Aerosol 728
Nasacort AQ Nasal Spray 752
Nasacort Nasal Inhaler 750

ALBORAL (Mexico)
DIAZEPAM
Valium Injectable 3026
Valium Tablets 3047

ALBUCID (Germany, South Africa, United Kingdom)
SULFACETAMIDE SODIUM
Bleph-10 Ophthalmic Ointment 10% .... ⊙230
Klaron Lotion 10% 1224

ALCAN (Mexico)
CHLORAMPHENICOL
Chloromycetin Ophthalmic Ointment, 1% .... ⊙296
Chloromycetin Ophthalmic Solution .... ⊙297
Chloroptic Sterile Ophthalmic Ointment .... ⊙234
Chloroptic Sterile Ophthalmic Solution .... ⊙235

ALCATEX (Mexico)
CIMETIDINE
Tagamet Tablets 1644

ALCELAM (Thailand)
ALPRAZOLAM
Xanax Tablets 2865

ALCIS (Spain)
ESTRADIOL
Alora Transdermal System 3372
Climara Transdermal System 958
Estrace Vaginal Cream 3358
Estring Vaginal Ring 2811
Vivelle Transdermal System 2412
Vivelle-Dot Transdermal System 2416

ALCOBON (Irish Republic, South Africa, United Kingdom)
FLUCYTOSINE
Ancobon Capsules 1730

ALCOMICIN (Belgium, Canada, Spain)
GENTAMICIN SULFATE
Genoptic Ophthalmic Ointment .... ⊙239
Genoptic Sterile Ophthalmic Solution .... ⊙239

ALCOPHYLLIN (South Africa)
THEOPHYLLINE
Aerolate Jr. T.D. Capsules 1361
Aerolate Liquid 1361
Aerolate Sr. T.D. Capsules 1361
Theo-Dur Extended-Release Tablets 1835
Uni-Dur Extended-Release Tablets 1841
Uniphyl 400 mg and 600 mg Tablets 2903

ALDA (Thailand)
ALBENDAZOLE
Albenza Tablets 1463

ALDAR (Mexico)
NIFEDIPINE
Adalat CC Tablets 877
Procardia Capsules 2708
Procardia XL Extended Release Tablets 2710

ALDARA (Australia, Belgium, Canada, Denmark, Finland, France, Germany, Hong Kong, Irish Republic, Italy, New Zealand, Norway, Singapore, South Africa, Spain, Sweden, Thailand, The Netherlands, United Kingdom)
IMIQUIMOD
Aldara Cream, 5% 1978

ALDAZINE (Australia, New Zealand)
THIORIDAZINE HYDROCHLORIDE
Thioridazine Hydrochloride Tablets 2289

ALDIPIN (Switzerland)
NIFEDIPINE
Adalat CC Tablets 877
Procardia Capsules 2708
Procardia XL Extended Release Tablets 2710

ALDOACNE (Spain)
BENZOYL PEROXIDE
Brevoxyl-4 Cleansing Lotion 3269
Brevoxyl-4 Creamy Wash 3270
Brevoxyl-4 Gel 3269
Brevoxyl-8 Cleansing Lotion 3269
Brevoxyl-8 Creamy Wash 3270
Brevoxyl-8 Gel 3269
Triaz Cleanser 2026
Triaz Gel 2026

ALDOCUMAR (Spain)
WARFARIN SODIUM
Coumadin Tablets 1243
Coumadin for Injection 1243

ALDOMET (Belgium, Denmark, France, Hong Kong, Irish Republic, Italy, Mexico, New Zealand, Norway, Portugal, South Africa, Spain, Sweden, Switzerland, Thailand, The Netherlands, United Kingdom)
METHYLDOPA
Aldomet Tablets 2037

ALDOMETIL (Austria, Germany)
METHYLDOPA
Aldomet Tablets 2037

ALDOMIN (Israel)
METHYLDOPA
Aldomet Tablets 2037

ALDOPREN (Australia)
METHYLDOPA
Aldomet Tablets 2037

ALDORETIC (Portugal)
AMILORIDE HYDROCHLORIDE/HYDROCHLOROTHIAZIDE
Moduretic Tablets 2138

ALDORIL (Canada)
HYDROCHLOROTHIAZIDE/METHYLDOPA
Aldoril Tablets 2039

ALDOTRIDE (Italy)
HYDROCHLOROTHIAZIDE/METHYLDOPA
Aldoril Tablets 2039

ALENDROS (Italy)
ALENDRONATE SODIUM
Fosamax Tablets 2095

ALERID (Germany)
CETIRIZINE HYDROCHLORIDE
Zyrtec Syrup 2756
Zyrtec Tablets 2756

ALERLISIN (Spain)
CETIRIZINE HYDROCHLORIDE
Zyrtec Syrup 2756
Zyrtec Tablets 2756

ALERTAL (Brazil)
LORATADINE
Claritin Reditabs 3100
Claritin Syrup 3100
Claritin Tablets 3100

ALERTEC (Canada)
MODAFINIL
Provigil Tablets 1193

ALERTRIN (Portugal)
LORATADINE
Claritin Reditabs 3100
Claritin Syrup 3100
Claritin Tablets 3100

ALEVE (Australia, France, Germany, Italy, South Africa, Spain, The Netherlands)
NAPROXEN SODIUM
Anaprox DS Tablets 2967
Anaprox Tablets 2967
Naprelan Tablets 1293

ALFABETAL (Italy)
LABETALOL HYDROCHLORIDE
Normodyne Injection 3135
Normodyne Tablets 3137

ALFABIOS (Italy)
FLUOCINOLONE ACETONIDE
Synalar Cream 2020
Synalar Ointment 2020
Synalar Topical Solution 2020

ALFACID (Germany)
RIFABUTIN
Mycobutin Capsules 2838

ALFACORT (United Arab Emirates)
HYDROCORTISONE
Anusol-HC Cream 2.5% 2237
Hydrocortone Tablets 2106

ALFACORTONE (Switzerland)
HYDROCORTISONE ACETATE
Anusol-HC Suppositories 2238
Cortifoam Rectal Foam 3170
Hydrocortone Acetate Injectable Suspension 2103
Proctocort Suppositories 2264

ALFA-FLUORONE (Italy)
FLUOCINOLONE ACETONIDE
Synalar Cream 2020
Synalar Ointment 2020
Synalar Topical Solution 2020

ALFASON (Germany)
HYDROCORTISONE BUTYRATE
Locoid Cream 1341
Locoid Lipocream Cream 1342
Locoid Ointment 1341
Locoid Topical Solution 1341

ALFATIL (France)
CEFACLOR
Ceclor CD Tablets 1279
Ceclor Pulvules 1905
Ceclor Suspension 1905

ALFEROS (Spain)
AZELASTINE HYDROCHLORIDE
Astelin Nasal Spray 3339

ALGEFIT (Austria)
DICLOFENAC SODIUM
Voltaren Tablets 2315
Voltaren-XR Tablets 2315

ALGIASDIN (Spain)
IBUPROFEN
Motrin Suspension, Oral Drops, Chewable Tablets, and Caplets 2002

ALGICORTIS (Italy)
HYDROCORTISONE
Anusol-HC Cream 2.5% 2237
Hydrocortone Tablets 2106

ALGI-DANILON (Brazil)
IBUPROFEN
Motrin Suspension, Oral Drops, Chewable Tablets, and Caplets 2002

ALGIDOL (Mexico)
IBUPROFEN
Motrin Suspension, Oral Drops, Chewable Tablets, and Caplets 2002

ALGIFEN (Brazil)
IBUPROFEN
Motrin Suspension, Oral Drops, Chewable Tablets, and Caplets 2002

ALGIFENE (France)
IBUPROFEN
Motrin Suspension, Oral Drops, Chewable Tablets, and Caplets 2002

ALGIFOR (Switzerland)
IBUPROFEN
Motrin Suspension, Oral Drops, Chewable Tablets, and Caplets 2002

ALGIPROFEN (Brazil)
KETOPROFEN
Orudis Capsules 3548
Oruvail Capsules 3548

ALGISAN (Spain)
IBUPROFEN
Motrin Suspension, Oral Drops, Chewable Tablets, and Caplets 2002

ALGOFEN (Italy)
IBUPROFEN
Motrin Suspension, Oral Drops, Chewable Tablets, and Caplets 2002

ALI VEG (Spain)
CIMETIDINE
Tagamet Tablets 1644

A-LICES (Singapore)
MALATHION
Ovide Lotion 2023

ALIN (Brazil)
ALBENDAZOLE
Albenza Tablets 1463

ALINDRIN (Sweden)
IBUPROFEN
Motrin Suspension, Oral Drops, Chewable Tablets, and Caplets 2002

ALINOR (Norway, Sweden)
ATENOLOL
Tenormin I.V. Injection 692

ALIPASE (France)
PANCRELIPASE
Ultrase Capsules 835
Ultrase MT Capsules 835

ALISEUM (Italy)
DIAZEPAM
Valium Injectable 3026
Valium Tablets 3047

ALIVIOMAS (Spain)
NAPROXEN
EC-Naprosyn Delayed-Release Tablets 2967
Naprosyn Suspension 2967
Naprosyn Tablets 2967

ALKERAN (Australia, Austria, Belgium, Brazil, Canada, Denmark, Finland, France, Germany, Hong Kong, Irish Republic, Israel, Italy, Mexico, New Zealand, Norway, Portugal, Singapore, South Africa, Switzerland, Thailand, The Netherlands)
MELPHALAN
Alkeran Tablets 1466
Alkeran for Injection 1465

ALKET (Italy)
KETOPROFEN
Orudis Capsules 3548
Oruvail Capsules 3548

ALLEGRA (Canada, Mexico)
FEXOFENADINE HYDROCHLORIDE
Allegra Capsules 712

ALLEGRA-D (Canada)
FEXOFENADINE HYDROCHLORIDE/PSEUDOEPHEDRINE HYDROCHLORIDE
Allegra-D Extended-Release Tablets 714

ALLER-AIDE (Canada)
DIPHENHYDRAMINE HYDROCHLORIDE
Benadryl Parenteral 2617

ALLERDINE (Thailand)
LORATADINE
Claritin Reditabs 3100
Claritin Syrup 3100
Claritin Tablets 3100

ALLERDRYL (Canada)
DIPHENHYDRAMINE HYDROCHLORIDE
Benadryl Parenteral 2617

ALLER-EZE (United Kingdom)
DIPHENHYDRAMINE HYDROCHLORIDE
Benadryl Parenteral 2617

ALLERFEN (Italy)
PROMETHAZINE HYDROCHLORIDE
Phenergan Injection 3553
Phenergan Suppositories 3556
Phenergan Syrup Fortis 3554
Phenergan Syrup Plain 3554
Phenergan Tablets 3556

ALLERFRE (The Netherlands)
LORATADINE
Claritin Reditabs 3100
Claritin Syrup 3100
Claritin Tablets 3100

ALLERGAN (Italy)
DIPHENHYDRAMINE HYDROCHLORIDE
Benadryl Parenteral 2617

ALLERGINA (Italy)
DIPHENHYDRAMINE HYDROCHLORIDE
Benadryl Parenteral 2617

ALLERGODIL (Austria, Belgium, Denmark, France, Germany, Italy, Portugal, Switzerland, The Netherlands)
AZELASTINE HYDROCHLORIDE
Astelin Nasal Spray 3339

ALLERGY DROPS (Canada)
NAPHAZOLINE HYDROCHLORIDE
Albalon Ophthalmic Solution .... ⊙225

ALLERGY ELIXIR (Canada)
DIPHENHYDRAMINE HYDROCHLORIDE
Benadryl Parenteral 2617

ALLERGY FORMULA (Canada)
DIPHENHYDRAMINE HYDROCHLORIDE
Benadryl Parenteral 2617

ALLERGY TABLETS (Canada)
DIPHENHYDRAMINE HYDROCHLORIDE
Benadryl Parenteral 2617

ALLERNIX (Canada)
DIPHENHYDRAMINE HYDROCHLORIDE
Benadryl Parenteral 2617

ALLERSIL (Thailand)
LORATADINE
Claritin Reditabs 3100
Claritin Syrup 3100
Claritin Tablets 3100

ALLER-TAB (Thailand)
LORATADINE
Claritin Reditabs 3100
Claritin Syrup 3100
Claritin Tablets 3100

ALLVORAN (Germany)
DICLOFENAC SODIUM
Voltaren Tablets 2315

(⊙ Described in PDR For Ophthalmic Medicines™)

Voltaren-XR Tablets 2315

ALMARION (Thailand)
THEOPHYLLINE
Aerolate Jr. T.D. Capsules 1361
Aerolate Liquid 1361
Aerolate Sr. T.D. Capsules 1361
Theo-Dur Extended-Release Tablets 1835
Uni-Dur Extended-Release Tablets 1841
Uniphyl 400 mg and 600 mg Tablets . . . 2903

ALMARYTM (Italy)
FLECAINIDE ACETATE
Tambocor Tablets 1990

ALMAZINE (United Kingdom)
LORAZEPAM
Ativan Injection 3478
Ativan Tablets 3482

ALMIRAL (Hong Kong)
DICLOFENAC SODIUM
Voltaren Tablets 2315
Voltaren-XR Tablets 2315

ALMODAN (United Kingdom)
AMOXICILLIN
Amoxil Pediatric Drops for Oral Suspension 1471
Amoxil Tablets 1471

ALNA (Austria, Germany)
TAMSULOSIN HYDROCHLORIDE
Flomax Capsules 1044

ALNAX (Thailand)
ALPRAZOLAM
Xanax Tablets 2865

ALOCORT (Canada)
HYDROCORTISONE ACETATE
Anusol-HC Suppositories 2238
Cortifoam Rectal Foam 3170
Hydrocortone Acetate Injectable Suspension 2103
Proctocort Suppositories 2264

ALOL (Italy)
ACEBUTOLOL HYDROCHLORIDE
Sectral Capsules 3589

ALONET (Singapore)
ATENOLOL
Tenormin I.V. Injection 692

ALOPRESIN (Spain)
CAPTOPRIL
Captopril Tablets 2281

ALOQUIN (Australia)
MONOBENZONE
Benoquin Cream 20% 1732

ALORIN (Italy)
LORATADINE
Claritin Reditabs 3100
Claritin Syrup 3100
Claritin Tablets 3100

ALPHADERM (Belgium, United Kingdom)
HYDROCORTISONE
Anusol-HC Cream 2.5% 2237
Hydrocortone Tablets 2106

ALPHAGAN (Australia, Austria, Belgium, Canada, Denmark, Finland, France, Germany, Hong Kong, Irish Republic, Israel, Italy, Mexico, New Zealand, Portugal, Singapore, South Africa, Spain, Sweden, Switzerland, Thailand, United Kingdom)
BRIMONIDINE TARTRATE
Alphagan Ophthalmic Solution 545

ALPHA-LAC (Canada)
LACTULOSE
Kristalose for Oral Solution 1007

ALPHAMEX (South Africa)
METHYLDOPA
Aldomet Tablets 2037

ALPHAPRIL (Australia)
ENALAPRIL MALEATE
Vasotec Tablets 2210

ALPHAVASE (United Kingdom)
PRAZOSIN HYDROCHLORIDE
Minipress Capsules 2699

ALPHEXINE (France)
CEFACLOR
Ceclor CD Tablets 1279
Ceclor Pulvules 1905
Ceclor Suspension 1905

ALPICORT N (Germany)
PREDNISOLONE
Prelone Syrup 2273

ALPOXEN (Denmark, Finland, Norway, Sweden)
NAPROXEN
EC-Naprosyn Delayed-Release Tablets . . . 2967
Naprosyn Suspension 2967
Naprosyn Tablets 2967

ALPRALID (Israel, Sweden)
ALPRAZOLAM
Xanax Tablets 2865

ALPRAZ (Belgium)
ALPRAZOLAM
Xanax Tablets 2865

ALPRESS (France)
PRAZOSIN HYDROCHLORIDE
Minipress Capsules 2699

ALPROFEN (Spain)
NAPROXEN
EC-Naprosyn Delayed-Release Tablets . . . 2967
Naprosyn Suspension 2967
Naprosyn Tablets 2967

ALPRONAX (Portugal)
ALPRAZOLAM
Xanax Tablets 2865

ALPROX (Denmark, Finland, Irish Republic, Israel)
ALPRAZOLAM
Xanax Tablets 2865

ALQUEN (Spain)
RANITIDINE HYDROCHLORIDE
Zantac 150 EFFERdose Granules 1690
Zantac 150 EFFERdose Tablets 1690
Zantac 150 Tablets 1690
Zantac 300 Tablets 1690
Zantac Injection 1688
Zantac Injection Premixed 1688
Zantac Syrup 1690

ALRHEUMAT (Irish Republic, United Kingdom)
KETOPROFEN
Orudis Capsules 3548
Oruvail Capsules 3548

ALRHEUMUN (Germany)
KETOPROFEN
Orudis Capsules 3548
Oruvail Capsules 3548

ALSERINE (Thailand)
CIMETIDINE
Tagamet Tablets 1644

ALSIDEXTEN (Mexico)
DICLOFENAC SODIUM
Voltaren Tablets 2315
Voltaren-XR Tablets 2315

ALSUCRAL (Finland)
SUCRALFATE
Carafate Suspension 731
Carafate Tablets 730

ALTACE (Canada)
RAMIPRIL
Altace Capsules 2233

ALTEMOL (Mexico)
INTERFERON ALFA-N3
Alferon N Injection 1770

ALTEN (Hong Kong, Singapore)
TRETINOIN
Avita Cream 999
Avita Gel 1000
Renova 0.05% Cream 2519
Retin-A Micro 0.1% 2522
Vesanoid Capsules 3037

ALTER-H2 (Mexico)
RANITIDINE HYDROCHLORIDE
Zantac 150 EFFERdose Granules 1690
Zantac 150 EFFERdose Tablets 1690
Zantac 150 Tablets 1690
Zantac 300 Tablets 1690
Zantac Injection 1688
Zantac Injection Premixed 1688
Zantac Syrup 1690

ALTESONA (Spain)
CORTISONE ACETATE
Cortone Acetate Injectable Suspension . . 2059
Cortone Acetate Tablets 2061

ALTIAZEM (Hong Kong, Italy, Singapore, Thailand)
DILTIAZEM HYDROCHLORIDE
Cardizem CD Capsules 1016
Cardizem Injectable 1018
Cardizem Lyo-Ject Syringe 1018
Cardizem Monovial 1018
Tiazac Capsules 1378

ALTI-MPA (Canada)
MEDROXYPROGESTERONE ACETATE
Depo-Provera Contraceptive Injection . . . 2798
Provera Tablets 2853

ALTIOR (Spain)
IBUPROFEN
Motrin Suspension, Oral Drops, Chewable Tablets, and Caplets 2002

ALTRAMET (Hong Kong)
CIMETIDINE
Tagamet Tablets 1644

ALTRULINE (Mexico)
SERTRALINE HYDROCHLORIDE
Zoloft Tablets 2751

ALUPRAM (United Kingdom)
DIAZEPAM
Valium Injectable 3026
Valium Tablets 3047

ALVADERMO FUERTE (Spain)
FLUOCINOLONE ACETONIDE
Synalar Cream 2020
Synalar Ointment 2020
Synalar Topical Solution 2020

ALVIDINA (Mexico)
RANITIDINE HYDROCHLORIDE
Zantac 150 EFFERdose Granules 1690
Zantac 150 EFFERdose Tablets 1690
Zantac 150 Tablets 1690
Zantac 300 Tablets 1690
Zantac Injection 1688
Zantac Injection Premixed 1688
Zantac Syrup 1690

ALXEN (Mexico)
NAPROXEN
EC-Naprosyn Delayed-Release Tablets . . . 2967
Naprosyn Suspension 2967
Naprosyn Tablets 2967

ALZAM (South Africa)
ALPRAZOLAM
Xanax Tablets 2865

ALZENTAL (Singapore)
ALBENDAZOLE
Albenza Tablets 1463

ALZOL (Thailand)
ALBENDAZOLE
Albenza Tablets 1463

ALZOLAM (Singapore)
ALPRAZOLAM
Xanax Tablets 2865

AMANTA (Germany)
AMANTADINE HYDROCHLORIDE
Symmetrel Syrup 1328
Symmetrel Tablets 1328

AMANTAGAMMA (Germany)
AMANTADINE HYDROCHLORIDE
Symmetrel Syrup 1328
Symmetrel Tablets 1328

AMANTAN (Belgium)
AMANTADINE HYDROCHLORIDE
Symmetrel Syrup 1328
Symmetrel Tablets 1328

AMAREL (France)
GLIMEPIRIDE
Amaryl Tablets 717

AMARYL (Australia, Austria, Denmark, Finland, Germany, Hong Kong, Irish Republic, Italy, Mexico, Norway, Portugal, Singapore, South Africa, Spain, Sweden, Switzerland, Thailand, The Netherlands, United Kingdom)
GLIMEPIRIDE
Amaryl Tablets 717

AMARYLLE (Belgium)
GLIMEPIRIDE
Amaryl Tablets 717

AMATINE (Canada)
MIDODRINE HYDROCHLORIDE
ProAmatine Tablets 3241

AMAZIN (South Africa)
CHLORPROMAZINE HYDROCHLORIDE
Thorazine Ampuls 1656
Thorazine Multi-dose Vials 1656
Thorazine Spansule Capsules 1656
Thorazine Syrup 1656
Thorazine Tablets 1656

AMBEN (Hong Kong)
CEFADROXIL
Duricef Capsules 1079
Duricef Oral Suspension 1079
Duricef Tablets 1079

AMBERIN (Sweden)
HYDROCORTISONE
Anusol-HC Cream 2.5% 2237
Hydrocortone Tablets 2106

AMBRAL (South Africa)
METRONIDAZOLE
MetroCream 1404
MetroGel 1405
MetroGel-Vaginal Gel 1986
MetroLotion 1405

Noritate Cream 1224

AMENDER (Mexico)
METHYLDOPA
Aldomet Tablets 2037

AMERGE (Canada)
NARATRIPTAN HYDROCHLORIDE
Amerge Tablets 1467

AMERIDE (Spain)
AMILORIDE HYDROCHLORIDE/HYDROCHLOROTHIAZIDE
Moduretic Tablets 2138

AMERSOL (Canada)
IBUPROFEN
Motrin Suspension, Oral Drops, Chewable Tablets, and Caplets 2002

AMETIC (South Africa)
METOCLOPRAMIDE HYDROCHLORIDE
Reglan Injectable 2935
Reglan Syrup 2935
Reglan Tablets 2935

AMFAMOX (Australia)
FAMOTIDINE
Pepcid Injection 2153
Pepcid Injection Premixed 2153
Pepcid RPD Orally Disintegrating Tablets 2150
Pepcid Tablets 2150
Pepcid for Oral Suspension 2150

AMICROBIN (Spain)
NORFLOXACIN
Chibroxin Sterile Ophthalmic Solution . . . . ⊙273, 2051
Noroxin Tablets 2145

AMIDAL (Australia)
AMILORIDE HYDROCHLORIDE
Midamor Tablets 2136

AMIDOX (United Kingdom)
AMIODARONE HYDROCHLORIDE
Cordarone Intravenous 3491
Cordarone Tablets 3487
Pacerone Tablets 3331

AMIDURET (Germany)
AMILORIDE HYDROCHLORIDE/HYDROCHLOROTHIAZIDE
Moduretic Tablets 2138

AMIKAL (Denmark, Sweden)
AMILORIDE HYDROCHLORIDE
Midamor Tablets 2136

AMILAMONT (United Kingdom)
AMILORIDE HYDROCHLORIDE
Midamor Tablets 2136

AMILCO (Denmark, Hong Kong, Irish Republic, United Kingdom)
AMILORIDE HYDROCHLORIDE/HYDROCHLOROTHIAZIDE
Moduretic Tablets 2138

AMILIDE (Thailand)
AMILORIDE HYDROCHLORIDE/HYDROCHLOROTHIAZIDE
Moduretic Tablets 2138

AMILMAXCO (United Kingdom)
AMILORIDE HYDROCHLORIDE/HYDROCHLOROTHIAZIDE
Moduretic Tablets 2138

AMILO-BASAN (Switzerland)
AMILORIDE HYDROCHLORIDE/HYDROCHLOROTHIAZIDE
Moduretic Tablets 2138

AMILOCOMP BETA (Germany)
AMILORIDE HYDROCHLORIDE/HYDROCHLOROTHIAZIDE
Moduretic Tablets 2138

AMILOFERM (Sweden)
AMILORIDE HYDROCHLORIDE/HYDROCHLOROTHIAZIDE
Moduretic Tablets 2138

AMILO-OPT (Germany)
AMILORIDE HYDROCHLORIDE/HYDROCHLOROTHIAZIDE
Moduretic Tablets 2138

AMILORETIC (South Africa)
AMILORIDE HYDROCHLORIDE/HYDROCHLOROTHIAZIDE
Moduretic Tablets 2138

AMILORETIK (Austria, Germany)
AMILORIDE HYDROCHLORIDE/HYDROCHLOROTHIAZIDE
Moduretic Tablets 2138

AMILORID COMP (Austria, Germany, Switzerland)
AMILORIDE HYDROCHLORIDE/HYDROCHLOROTHIAZIDE
Moduretic Tablets 2138

(⊙ Described in PDR For Ophthalmic Medicines™)

AMILORIDE COMPOSTO (Portugal)
AMILORIDE HYDROCHLORIDE/HYDROCHLOROTHIAZIDE
Moduretic Tablets **2138**

AMILOSPARE (United Kingdom)
AMILORIDE HYDROCHLORIDE
Midamor Tablets **2136**

AMILOSTAD HCT (Austria)
AMILORIDE HYDROCHLORIDE/HYDROCHLOROTHIAZIDE
Moduretic Tablets **2138**

AMILOTHIAZID (Germany)
AMILORIDE HYDROCHLORIDE/HYDROCHLOROTHIAZIDE
Moduretic Tablets **2138**

AMILOZID (Germany)
AMILORIDE HYDROCHLORIDE/HYDROCHLOROTHIAZIDE
Moduretic Tablets **2138**

AMIMOX (Norway)
AMOXICILLIN
Amoxil Pediatric Drops for Oral Suspension **1471**
Amoxil Tablets **1471**

AMINDAN (Germany)
SELEGILINE HYDROCHLORIDE
Eldepryl Capsules **3266**

AMINOMAL (Italy)
THEOPHYLLINE
Aerolate Jr. T.D. Capsules **1361**
Aerolate Liquid **1361**
Aerolate Sr. T.D. Capsules **1361**
Theo-Dur Extended-Release Tablets **1835**
Uni-Dur Extended-Release Tablets **1841**
Uniphyl 400 mg and 600 mg Tablets **2903**

AMIOBETA (Germany)
AMIODARONE HYDROCHLORIDE
Cordarone Intravenous **3491**
Cordarone Tablets **3487**
Pacerone Tablets **3331**

AMIODACORE (Israel)
AMIODARONE HYDROCHLORIDE
Cordarone Intravenous **3491**
Cordarone Tablets **3487**
Pacerone Tablets **3331**

AMIODAR (Italy)
AMIODARONE HYDROCHLORIDE
Cordarone Intravenous **3491**
Cordarone Tablets **3487**
Pacerone Tablets **3331**

AMIODAREX (Germany)
AMIODARONE HYDROCHLORIDE
Cordarone Intravenous **3491**
Cordarone Tablets **3487**
Pacerone Tablets **3331**

AMIOGAMMA (Germany)
AMIODARONE HYDROCHLORIDE
Cordarone Intravenous **3491**
Cordarone Tablets **3487**
Pacerone Tablets **3331**

AMIOHEXAL (Germany)
AMIODARONE HYDROCHLORIDE
Cordarone Intravenous **3491**
Cordarone Tablets **3487**
Pacerone Tablets **3331**

AMIPRESS (Italy)
LABETALOL HYDROCHLORIDE
Normodyne Injection **3135**
Normodyne Tablets **3137**

AMITHIAZIDE (Hong Kong)
AMILORIDE HYDROCHLORIDE/HYDROCHLOROTHIAZIDE
Moduretic Tablets **2138**

AMITRID (Finland)
AMILORIDE HYDROCHLORIDE/HYDROCHLOROTHIAZIDE
Moduretic Tablets **2138**

AMIXX (Germany)
AMANTADINE HYDROCHLORIDE
Symmetrel Syrup **1328**
Symmetrel Tablets **1328**

AMIYODAZOL (Mexico)
METRONIDAZOLE
MetroCream **1404**
MetroGel **1405**
MetroGel-Vaginal Gel **1986**
MetroLotion **1405**
Noritate Cream **1224**

AMIZIDE (Australia, Irish Republic, New Zealand, South Africa)
AMILORIDE HYDROCHLORIDE/HYDROCHLOROTHIAZIDE
Moduretic Tablets **2138**

AMO VITRAX (Australia, New Zealand, Singapore, South Africa, Sweden, Switzerland, Thailand)
SODIUM HYALURONATE
Hyalgan Solution **3080**

AMOFAT (Mexico)
FAMOTIDINE
Pepcid Injection **2153**
Pepcid Injection Premixed **2153**
Pepcid RPD Orally Disintegrating Tablets **2150**
Pepcid Tablets **2150**
Pepcid for Oral Suspension **2150**

AMOLIN (Irish Republic)
ATENOLOL
Tenormin I.V. Injection **692**

AMOPEN (United Kingdom)
AMOXICILLIN
Amoxil Pediatric Drops for Oral Suspension **1471**
Amoxil Tablets **1471**

AMORAM (United Kingdom)
AMOXICILLIN
Amoxil Pediatric Drops for Oral Suspension **1471**
Amoxil Tablets **1471**

AMOTEIN (Spain)
METRONIDAZOLE
MetroCream **1404**
MetroGel **1405**
MetroGel-Vaginal Gel **1986**
MetroLotion **1405**
Noritate Cream **1224**

AMOXAPEN (Hong Kong, Singapore)
AMOXICILLIN
Amoxil Pediatric Drops for Oral Suspension **1471**
Amoxil Tablets **1471**

AMOXI-BASAN (Switzerland)
AMOXICILLIN
Amoxil Pediatric Drops for Oral Suspension **1471**
Amoxil Tablets **1471**

AMOXIBIOCIN (Germany)
AMOXICILLIN
Amoxil Pediatric Drops for Oral Suspension **1471**
Amoxil Tablets **1471**

AMOXIFAR (Brazil)
AMOXICILLIN
Amoxil Pediatric Drops for Oral Suspension **1471**
Amoxil Tablets **1471**

AMOXIFAR BALSAMICO (Brazil)
AMOXICILLIN
Amoxil Pediatric Drops for Oral Suspension **1471**
Amoxil Tablets **1471**

AMOXIL (Hong Kong, Singapore)
AMOXICILLIN
Amoxil Pediatric Drops for Oral Suspension **1471**
Amoxil Tablets **1471**

AMOXYFIZZ (South Africa)
AMOXICILLIN
Amoxil Pediatric Drops for Oral Suspension **1471**
Amoxil Tablets **1471**

AMPIFEN (Singapore)
IBUPROFEN
Motrin Suspension, Oral Drops, Chewable Tablets, and Caplets **2002**

AMPLEXOL (Portugal)
ISOSORBIDE MONONITRATE
Imdur Tablets **1826**
Ismo Tablets **3524**

AMPLICTIL (Brazil)
CHLORPROMAZINE
Thorazine Suppositories **1656**

AMPLOMICINA (Brazil)
GENTAMICIN SULFATE
Genoptic Ophthalmic Ointment . . . . . ⊙**239**
Genoptic Sterile Ophthalmic Solution . . . . . ⊙**239**

AMPLOZOL (Brazil)
ALBENDAZOLE
Albenza Tablets **1463**

AMPRACE (Australia)
ENALAPRIL MALEATE
Vasotec Tablets **2210**

A-MULSIN (Germany)
VITAMIN A PALMITATE
Aquasol A Parenteral **593**

A-MULSION (Canada)
VITAMIN A PALMITATE
Aquasol A Parenteral **593**

AMVISC (Austria, Canada, Israel, Norway, South Africa, Sweden)
SODIUM HYALURONATE
Hyalgan Solution **3080**

AMX (Mexico)
AMOXICILLIN
Amoxil Pediatric Drops for Oral Suspension **1471**
Amoxil Tablets **1471**

AMYCIL (Mexico)
MEBENDAZOLE
Vermox Chewable Tablets **2017**

AMYDRAMINE II (United Arab Emirates)
DIPHENHYDRAMINE HYDROCHLORIDE
Benadryl Parenteral **2617**

ANABACT (Irish Republic, Singapore, Thailand, United Kingdom)
METRONIDAZOLE
MetroCream **1404**
MetroGel **1405**
MetroGel-Vaginal Gel **1986**
MetroLotion **1405**
Noritate Cream **1224**

ANADENT (Israel)
BENZOCAINE
Americaine Anesthetic Lubricant **1162**
Americaine Otic Topical Anesthetic Ear Drops **1162**

ANADIN IBUPROFEN (United Kingdom)
IBUPROFEN
Motrin Suspension, Oral Drops, Chewable Tablets, and Caplets **2002**

ANADIN ULTRA (United Kingdom)
IBUPROFEN
Motrin Suspension, Oral Drops, Chewable Tablets, and Caplets **2002**

ANADOL (Thailand)
TRAMADOL HYDROCHLORIDE
Ultram Tablets **2600**

ANADVIL (France)
IBUPROFEN
Motrin Suspension, Oral Drops, Chewable Tablets, and Caplets **2002**

ANAEROBEX (Austria)
METRONIDAZOLE
MetroCream **1404**
MetroGel **1405**
MetroGel-Vaginal Gel **1986**
MetroLotion **1405**
Noritate Cream **1224**

ANAEROBYL (South Africa)
METRONIDAZOLE
MetroCream **1404**
MetroGel **1405**
MetroGel-Vaginal Gel **1986**
MetroLotion **1405**
Noritate Cream **1224**

ANAEROMET (Belgium, The Netherlands)
METRONIDAZOLE
MetroCream **1404**
MetroGel **1405**
MetroGel-Vaginal Gel **1986**
MetroLotion **1405**
Noritate Cream **1224**

ANAESTHERIT (Austria)
BENZOCAINE
Americaine Anesthetic Lubricant **1162**
Americaine Otic Topical Anesthetic Ear Drops **1162**

ANAESTHESIERENDE SALBE (Germany)
BENZOCAINE
Americaine Anesthetic Lubricant **1162**
Americaine Otic Topical Anesthetic Ear Drops **1162**

ANAESTHESIN (Germany)
BENZOCAINE
Americaine Anesthetic Lubricant **1162**
Americaine Otic Topical Anesthetic Ear Drops **1162**

ANAFEN (New Zealand)
IBUPROFEN
Motrin Suspension, Oral Drops, Chewable Tablets, and Caplets **2002**

ANA-FLEX (Brazil)
DICLOFENAC SODIUM
Voltaren Tablets **2315**
Voltaren-XR Tablets **2315**

ANAFLIN (Mexico)
NAPROXEN
EC-Naprosyn Delayed-Release Tablets **2967**
Naprosyn Suspension **2967**
Naprosyn Tablets **2967**

ANAGREGAL (Italy)
TICLOPIDINE HYDROCHLORIDE
Ticlid Tablets **3015**

ANALFIN (Mexico)
MORPHINE SULFATE
Astramorph/PF Injection, USP (Preservative-Free) **594**
Duramorph Injection **1312**
Infumorph 200 and Infumorph 500 Sterile Solutions **1314**
Kadian Capsules **1335**
MS Contin Tablets **2896**
MSIR Oral Capsules **2898**
MSIR Oral Solution **2898**
MSIR Oral Solution Concentrate **2898**
MSIR Oral Tablets **2898**
Oramorph SR Tablets **3062**
Roxanol 100 Concentrated Oral Solution **3066**
Roxanol Concentrated Oral Solution **3066**
Roxanol-T Oral Solution **3066**

ANALGYL (France)
IBUPROFEN
Motrin Suspension, Oral Drops, Chewable Tablets, and Caplets **2002**

ANALPAN (Hong Kong)
DICLOFENAC SODIUM
Voltaren Tablets **2315**
Voltaren-XR Tablets **2315**

ANAMORPH (Australia)
MORPHINE SULFATE
Astramorph/PF Injection, USP (Preservative-Free) **594**
Duramorph Injection **1312**
Infumorph 200 and Infumorph 500 Sterile Solutions **1314**
Kadian Capsules **1335**
MS Contin Tablets **2896**
MSIR Oral Capsules **2898**
MSIR Oral Solution **2898**
MSIR Oral Solution Concentrate **2898**
MSIR Oral Tablets **2898**
Oramorph SR Tablets **3062**
Roxanol 100 Concentrated Oral Solution **3066**
Roxanol Concentrated Oral Solution **3066**
Roxanol-T Oral Solution **3066**

ANANDA (Italy)
METOCLOPRAMIDE HYDROCHLORIDE
Reglan Injectable **2935**
Reglan Syrup **2935**
Reglan Tablets **2935**

ANANDRON (Australia, Brazil, Canada, Denmark, Finland, France, Norway, Portugal, Sweden, The Netherlands)
NILUTAMIDE
Nilandron Tablets **753**

ANAPOLON (Australia, Canada, South Africa, United Kingdom)
OXYMETHOLONE
Anadrol-50 Tablets **3321**

ANAPRIL (Singapore, Thailand)
ENALAPRIL MALEATE
Vasotec Tablets **2210**

ANAPROX (Australia, Canada, Spain)
NAPROXEN SODIUM
Anaprox DS Tablets **2967**
Anaprox Tablets **2967**
Naprelan Tablets **1293**

ANARTRIT (Brazil)
PIROXICAM
Feldene Capsules **2685**

ANASEPTIL (Brazil)
NEOMYCIN SULFATE/POLYMYXIN B SULFATE
Neosporin G.U. Irrigant Sterile **2256**

ANATOPIC (Spain)
FLUOCINOLONE ACETONIDE
Synalar Cream **2020**
Synalar Ointment **2020**
Synalar Topical Solution **2020**

ANAUSIN (France)
METOCLOPRAMIDE HYDROCHLORIDE
Reglan Injectable **2935**
Reglan Syrup **2935**
Reglan Tablets **2935**

ANAX (Singapore)
NAPROXEN SODIUM
Anaprox DS Tablets **2967**
Anaprox Tablets **2967**
Naprelan Tablets **1293**

ANBESOL BABY (Canada)
BENZOCAINE
Americaine Anesthetic Lubricant **1162**

(⊙ Described in PDR For Ophthalmic Medicines™)

Americaine Otic Topical Anesthetic Ear Drops 1162

ANCO (Germany)
IBUPROFEN
Motrin Suspension, Oral Drops, Chewable Tablets, and Caplets 2002

ANCOREN (Portugal)
ATENOLOL
Tenormin I.V. Injection 692

ANCORON (Brazil)
AMIODARONE HYDROCHLORIDE
Cordarone Intravenous 3491
Cordarone Tablets 3487
Pacerone Tablets 3331

ANCOTIL (Australia, Austria, Brazil, Canada, Denmark, France, Germany, Hong Kong, Irish Republic, Italy, Norway, Singapore, Sweden, Switzerland, The Netherlands)
FLUCYTOSINE
Ancobon Capsules 1730

ANDAPSIN (Sweden)
SUCRALFATE
Carafate Suspension 731
Carafate Tablets 730

ANDRODERM (Australia, Italy, Switzerland)
TESTOSTERONE
Androderm Transdermal System CIII 3377
Testoderm Transdermal Systems 574

ANDROPATCH (Irish Republic, United Kingdom)
TESTOSTERONE
Androderm Transdermal System CIII 3377
Testoderm Transdermal Systems 574

ANDROXICAM (Mexico)
PIROXICAM
Feldene Capsules 2685

ANDROXYL (Hong Kong)
CEFADROXIL
Duricef Capsules 1079
Duricef Oral Suspension 1079
Duricef Tablets 1079

ANEMUL MONO (Germany)
DEXAMETHASONE
Decadron Elixir 2078
Decadron Tablets 2079

ANEUROL (Spain)
DIAZEPAM
Valium Injectable 3026
Valium Tablets 3047

ANEXATE (Australia, Austria, Belgium, Canada, France, Germany, Hong Kong, Irish Republic, Israel, Italy, New Zealand, Norway, Portugal, Singapore, South Africa, Spain, Switzerland, Thailand, The Netherlands, United Kingdom)
FLUMAZENIL
Romazicon Injection 3000

ANFENAX (New Zealand, South Africa)
DICLOFENAC SODIUM
Voltaren Tablets 2315
Voltaren-XR Tablets 2315

ANFERTIL (Brazil)
NORGESTREL
Ovrette Tablets 3552

ANFLAM (United Kingdom)
HYDROCORTISONE
Anusol-HC Cream 2.5% 2237
Hydrocortone Tablets 2106

ANGEZE (United Kingdom)
ISOSORBIDE MONONITRATE
Imdur Tablets 1826
Ismo Tablets 3524

ANGIACT (Denmark)
DILTIAZEM HYDROCHLORIDE
Cardizem CD Capsules 1016
Cardizem Injectable 1018
Cardizem Lyo-Ject Syringe 1018
Cardizem Monovial 1018
Tiazac Capsules 1378

ANGICHROME (Belgium)
SULFANILAMIDE
AVC Cream 1350
AVC Suppositories 1350

ANGICONTIN (Denmark)
DILTIAZEM HYDROCHLORIDE
Cardizem CD Capsules 1016
Cardizem Injectable 1018
Cardizem Lyo-Ject Syringe 1018
Cardizem Monovial 1018
Tiazac Capsules 1378

ANGIDIL (Italy)
DILTIAZEM HYDROCHLORIDE
Cardizem CD Capsules 1016
Cardizem Injectable 1018
Cardizem Lyo-Ject Syringe 1018
Cardizem Monovial 1018
Tiazac Capsules 1378

ANGILOL (Hong Kong, New Zealand, United Kingdom)
PROPRANOLOL HYDROCHLORIDE
Inderal Injectable 3513
Inderal LA Long-Acting Capsules 3516
Inderal Tablets 3513

ANGIMON (United Kingdom)
VERAPAMIL HYDROCHLORIDE
Covera-HS Tablets 3199
Isoptin SR Tablets 467
Verelan Capsules 3184
Verelan PM Capsules 3186

ANGINAMIDE (Belgium)
SULFACETAMIDE SODIUM
Bleph-10 Ophthalmic Ointment 10% ⊙230
Klaron Lotion 10% 1224

ANGINOR (South Africa)
NIFEDIPINE
Adalat CC Tablets 877
Procardia Capsules 2708
Procardia XL Extended Release Tablets 2710

ANGIODROX (Spain)
DILTIAZEM HYDROCHLORIDE
Cardizem CD Capsules 1016
Cardizem Injectable 1018
Cardizem Lyo-Ject Syringe 1018
Cardizem Monovial 1018
Tiazac Capsules 1378

ANGIOLONG (Brazil)
DILTIAZEM HYDROCHLORIDE
Cardizem CD Capsules 1016
Cardizem Injectable 1018
Cardizem Lyo-Ject Syringe 1018
Cardizem Monovial 1018
Tiazac Capsules 1378

ANGIOPINE (United Kingdom)
NIFEDIPINE
Adalat CC Tablets 877
Procardia Capsules 2708
Procardia XL Extended Release Tablets 2710

ANGIOTROFIN (Mexico)
DILTIAZEM HYDROCHLORIDE
Cardizem CD Capsules 1016
Cardizem Injectable 1018
Cardizem Lyo-Ject Syringe 1018
Cardizem Monovial 1018
Tiazac Capsules 1378

ANGIOZEM (United Kingdom)
DILTIAZEM HYDROCHLORIDE
Cardizem CD Capsules 1016
Cardizem Injectable 1018
Cardizem Lyo-Ject Syringe 1018
Cardizem Monovial 1018
Tiazac Capsules 1378

ANGIPRESS (Brazil, Italy)
ATENOLOL
Tenormin I.V. Injection 692

ANGI-SPRAY (South Africa)
ISOSORBIDE DINITRATE
Isordil Sublingual Tablets 3525
Isordil Titradose Tablets 3526

ANGITAK (United Kingdom)
ISOSORBIDE DINITRATE
Isordil Sublingual Tablets 3525
Isordil Titradose Tablets 3526

ANGITIL (United Kingdom)
DILTIAZEM HYDROCHLORIDE
Cardizem CD Capsules 1016
Cardizem Injectable 1018
Cardizem Lyo-Ject Syringe 1018
Cardizem Monovial 1018
Tiazac Capsules 1378

ANGITRATE (South Africa)
ISOSORBIDE MONONITRATE
Imdur Tablets 1826
Ismo Tablets 3524

ANGITRIT (Thailand)
ISOSORBIDE DINITRATE
Isordil Sublingual Tablets 3525
Isordil Titradose Tablets 3526

ANGIZEM (Italy, Singapore, Thailand)
DILTIAZEM HYDROCHLORIDE
Cardizem CD Capsules 1016
Cardizem Injectable 1018
Cardizem Lyo-Ject Syringe 1018
Cardizem Monovial 1018
Tiazac Capsules 1378

ANIFED (Italy)
NIFEDIPINE
Adalat CC Tablets 877
Procardia Capsules 2708
Procardia XL Extended Release Tablets 2710

ANISTAL (Mexico)
RANITIDINE HYDROCHLORIDE
Zantac 150 EFFERdose Granules 1690
Zantac 150 EFFERdose Tablets 1690
Zantac 150 Tablets 1690
Zantac 300 Tablets 1690
Zantac Injection 1688
Zantac Injection Premixed 1688
Zantac Syrup 1690

ANNOXEN (Thailand)
NAPROXEN
EC-Naprosyn Delayed-Release Tablets 2967
Naprosyn Suspension 2967
Naprosyn Tablets 2967

ANOCLOR (South Africa)
CHLOROQUINE PHOSPHATE
Aralen Tablets 3075

ANORFIN (Denmark)
BUPRENORPHINE HYDROCHLORIDE
Buprenex Injectable 2918

ANOSEDIL (Brazil)
LORAZEPAM
Ativan Injection 3478
Ativan Tablets 3482

ANPEC (Australia)
VERAPAMIL HYDROCHLORIDE
Covera-HS Tablets 3199
Isoptin SR Tablets 467
Verelan Capsules 3184
Verelan PM Capsules 3186

ANPINE (Australia)
NIFEDIPINE
Adalat CC Tablets 877
Procardia Capsules 2708
Procardia XL Extended Release Tablets 2710

ANPRESS (Thailand)
ALPRAZOLAM
Xanax Tablets 2865

ANSATIPIN (Finland, Spain, Sweden)
RIFABUTIN
Mycobutin Capsules 2838

ANSATIPINE (France)
RIFABUTIN
Mycobutin Capsules 2838

ANSELOL (Australia, New Zealand)
ATENOLOL
Tenormin I.V. Injection 692

ANSILIVE (Brazil)
DIAZEPAM
Valium Injectable 3026
Valium Tablets 3047

ANSILOR (Portugal)
LORAZEPAM
Ativan Injection 3478
Ativan Tablets 3482

ANSIOLIN (Italy)
DIAZEPAM
Valium Injectable 3026
Valium Tablets 3047

ANSIOWAS (Spain)
MEPROBAMATE
Miltown Tablets 3349

ANSIUM (Spain)
DIAZEPAM
Valium Injectable 3026
Valium Tablets 3047

ANSIVEN (Switzerland)
PROPOFOL
Diprivan Injectable Emulsion 667

ANTA (Thailand)
LORAZEPAM
Ativan Injection 3478
Ativan Tablets 3482

ANTABUS (Austria, Denmark, Finland, Norway, Spain, Sweden, Switzerland, The Netherlands)
DISULFIRAM
Antabuse Tablets 3474

ANTABUSE (Australia, Belgium, Canada, Irish Republic, Israel, Italy, South Africa, Thailand, United Kingdom)
DISULFIRAM
Antabuse Tablets 3474

ANTADINE (Australia, South Africa)
AMANTADINE HYDROCHLORIDE
Symmetrel Syrup 1328
Symmetrel Tablets 1328

ANTAFIT (Thailand)
CARBAMAZEPINE
Carbatrol Capsules 3234
Tegretol Chewable Tablets 2404
Tegretol Suspension 2404
Tegretol Tablets 2404
Tegretol-XR Tablets 2404

ANTAGONIL (Germany)
NICARDIPINE HYDROCHLORIDE
Cardene I.V. 3485

ANTAGOSAN (France, Germany, Italy)
APROTININ
Trasylol Injection 909

ANTAK (Brazil)
RANITIDINE HYDROCHLORIDE
Zantac 150 EFFERdose Granules 1690
Zantac 150 EFFERdose Tablets 1690
Zantac 150 Tablets 1690
Zantac 300 Tablets 1690
Zantac Injection 1688
Zantac Injection Premixed 1688
Zantac Syrup 1690

ANTALGIL (Italy)
IBUPROFEN
Motrin Suspension, Oral Drops, Chewable Tablets, and Caplets 2002

ANTALGIN (Spain)
NAPROXEN SODIUM
Anaprox DS Tablets 2967
Anaprox Tablets 2967
Naprelan Tablets 1293

ANTALGIT (Switzerland)
IBUPROFEN
Motrin Suspension, Oral Drops, Chewable Tablets, and Caplets 2002

ANTALON (Germany)
PIMOZIDE
Orap Tablets 1407

ANTAMEX (Switzerland)
NIFEDIPINE
Adalat CC Tablets 877
Procardia Capsules 2708
Procardia XL Extended Release Tablets 2710

ANTANAZOL (Singapore)
KETOCONAZOLE
Nizoral 2% Cream 3620
Nizoral 2% Shampoo 2007
Nizoral Tablets 1791

ANTARENE (France)
IBUPROFEN
Motrin Suspension, Oral Drops, Chewable Tablets, and Caplets 2002

ANTAROL (Hong Kong, Irish Republic)
PROPRANOLOL HYDROCHLORIDE
Inderal Injectable 3513
Inderal LA Long-Acting Capsules 3516
Inderal Tablets 3513

ANTEBOR (Belgium, France, Switzerland)
SULFACETAMIDE SODIUM
Bleph-10 Ophthalmic Ointment 10% ⊙230
Klaron Lotion 10% 1224

ANTELEPSIN (Germany)
CLONAZEPAM
Klonopin Tablets 2983

ANTEN (New Zealand)
DOXEPIN HYDROCHLORIDE
Sinequan Capsules 2713
Sinequan Oral Concentrate 2713

ANTENEX (Australia)
DIAZEPAM
Valium Injectable 3026
Valium Tablets 3047

ANTEPAN (Austria, Germany)
PROTIRELIN
Thyrel TRH for Injection 3630

ANTEPSIN (Brazil, Denmark, Finland, Irish Republic, Italy, Norway, United Kingdom)
SUCRALFATE
Carafate Suspension 731
Carafate Tablets 730

ANTHEL (Thailand)
ALBENDAZOLE
Albenza Tablets 1463

ANTHEX (South Africa)
MEBENDAZOLE
Vermox Chewable Tablets 2017

ANTI CD3 (Brazil)
MUROMONAB-CD3
Orthoclone OKT3 Sterile Solution 2498

ANTIBI-OTIC (Thailand)
CHLORAMPHENICOL
Chloromycetin Ophthalmic Ointment, 1% ⊙296
Chloromycetin Ophthalmic Solution ⊙297
Chloroptic Sterile Ophthalmic Ointment ⊙234
Chloroptic Sterile Ophthalmic Solution ⊙235

ANTIBIOTREX (France)
ISOTRETINOIN
Accutane Capsules 2944

ANTIBIOTULLE LUMIERE (France, Germany)
NEOMYCIN SULFATE/POLYMYXIN B SULFATE
Neosporin G.U. Irrigant Sterile 2256

ANTIETANOL (Brazil)
DISULFIRAM
Antabuse Tablets 3474

ANTIFLAM (South Africa)
IBUPROFEN
Motrin Suspension, Oral Drops, Chewable Tablets, and Caplets 2002

ANTIFLOG (Italy)
PIROXICAM
Feldene Capsules 2685

ANTIFUNGOL (Germany)
CLOTRIMAZOLE
Lotrimin Cream 1% 3128
Lotrimin Lotion 1% 3128
Lotrimin Topical Solution 1% 3128
Mycelex Troche 573

ANTIGREG (Italy, Singapore)
TICLOPIDINE HYDROCHLORIDE
Ticlid Tablets 3015

ANTIL (Mexico)
CIMETIDINE
Tagamet Tablets 1644

ANTIMET (Irish Republic)
METOCLOPRAMIDE HYDROCHLORIDE
Reglan Injectable 2935
Reglan Syrup 2935
Reglan Tablets 2935

ANTIMICOTICO (Italy)
CLOTRIMAZOLE
Lotrimin Cream 1% 3128
Lotrimin Lotion 1% 3128
Lotrimin Topical Solution 1% 3128
Mycelex Troche 573

ANTIMIGRIN (Austria)
NARATRIPTAN HYDROCHLORIDE
Amerge Tablets 1467

ANTIMYK (Germany)
CLOTRIMAZOLE
Lotrimin Cream 1% 3128
Lotrimin Lotion 1% 3128
Lotrimin Topical Solution 1% 3128
Mycelex Troche 573

ANTINAUS (New Zealand)
PROCHLORPERAZINE MALEATE
Compazine Spansule Capsules 1505
Compazine Tablets 1505

ANTI-NAUS (Australia)
PROCHLORPERAZINE MALEATE
Compazine Spansule Capsules 1505
Compazine Tablets 1505

ANTIPARKIN (Germany)
SELEGILINE HYDROCHLORIDE
Eldepryl Capsules 3266

ANTIPRESSAN (Hong Kong, Irish Republic, United Kingdom)
ATENOLOL
Tenormin I.V. Injection 692

ANTIZID (South Africa)
NIZATIDINE
Axid Pulvules 1903

ANTIZINE (Thailand)
HYDROXYZINE HYDROCHLORIDE
Atarax Tablets & Syrup 2667
Vistaril Intramuscular Solution 2738

ANTODREL (Spain)
PILOCARPINE HYDROCHLORIDE
Isopto Carpine Ophthalmic Solution ⊙215
Pilopine HS Ophthalmic Gel ⊙217
Salagen Tablets 2229

ANTOPAR (Hong Kong)
BENZOYL PEROXIDE
Brevoxyl-4 Cleansing Lotion 3269
Brevoxyl-4 Creamy Wash 3270
Brevoxyl-4 Gel 3269
Brevoxyl-8 Cleansing Lotion 3269
Brevoxyl-8 Creamy Wash 3270
Brevoxyl-8 Gel 3269
Triaz Cleanser 2026
Triaz Gel 2026

ANTRA (Italy)
OMEPRAZOLE
Prilosec Delayed-Release Capsules 628

ANTRAL (Mexico)
METRONIDAZOLE
MetroCream 1404
MetroGel 1405
MetroGel-Vaginal Gel 1986
MetroLotion 1405
Noritate Cream 1224

ANXER (Thailand)
CEPHALEXIN
Keflex Oral Suspension 1237
Keflex Pulvules 1237

ANXICALM (Irish Republic)
DIAZEPAM
Valium Injectable 3026
Valium Tablets 3047

ANXIPRESS-D (Thailand)
AMITRIPTYLINE HYDROCHLORIDE/PERPHENAZINE
Etrafon 2-10 Tablets (2-10) 3115
Etrafon Tablets (2-25) 3115
Etrafon-Forte Tablets (4-25) 3115

ANXIRA (Thailand)
LORAZEPAM
Ativan Injection 3478
Ativan Tablets 3482

ANXIRID (South Africa)
ALPRAZOLAM
Xanax Tablets 2865

ANZATAX (Australia, Hong Kong, Singapore)
PACLITAXEL
Taxol Injection 1129

ANZEM (South Africa)
DILTIAZEM HYDROCHLORIDE
Cardizem CD Capsules 1016
Cardizem Injectable 1018
Cardizem Lyo-Ject Syringe 1018
Cardizem Monovial 1018
Tiazac Capsules 1378

APACEF (Belgium, France)
CEFOTETAN DISODIUM
Cefotan Injection 664
Cefotan for Injection 664

APAIN (Denmark)
IBUPROFEN
Motrin Suspension, Oral Drops, Chewable Tablets, and Caplets 2002

APAMID (Finland, Norway, Sweden)
GLIPIZIDE
Glucotrol Tablets 2692
Glucotrol XL Extended Release Tablets 2693

APATEF (Australia, Germany, Italy, New Zealand, Portugal)
CEFOTETAN DISODIUM
Cefotan Injection 664
Cefotan for Injection 664

APHTIRIA (France)
LINDANE
Lindane Lotion USP 1% 559
Lindane Shampoo USP 1% 560

APIMID (Germany)
FLUTAMIDE
Eulexin Capsules 3118

APIROL (Israel)
NORFLOXACIN
Chibroxin Sterile Ophthalmic Solution ⊙273, 2051
Noroxin Tablets 2145

APLACTIN (Italy)
PRAVASTATIN SODIUM
Pravachol Tablets 1099

APLAKET (Italy, Singapore, Thailand)
TICLOPIDINE HYDROCHLORIDE
Ticlid Tablets 3015

A-PLEX (Mexico)
TRETINOIN
Avita Cream 999
Avita Gel 1000
Renova 0.05% Cream 2519
Retin-A Micro 0.1% 2522
Vesanoid Capsules 3037

AP-NAPRO-NA (Hong Kong)
NAPROXEN SODIUM
Anaprox DS Tablets 2967
Anaprox Tablets 2967
Naprelan Tablets 1293

APOACOR (Israel)
VERAPAMIL HYDROCHLORIDE
Covera-HS Tablets 3199
Isoptin SR Tablets 467
Verelan Capsules 3184
Verelan PM Capsules 3186

APO-ALPRAZ (Canada, Singapore)
ALPRAZOLAM
Xanax Tablets 2865

APO-AMILZIDE (Canada, Hong Kong, Singapore)
AMILORIDE HYDROCHLORIDE/HYDROCHLOROTHIAZIDE
Moduretic Tablets 2138

APO-AMOXI (Hong Kong)
AMOXICILLIN
Amoxil Pediatric Drops for Oral Suspension 1471
Amoxil Tablets 1471

APO-ATENOL (Canada, Hong Kong, Singapore)
ATENOLOL
Tenormin I.V. Injection 692

APOCANDA (Germany)
CLOTRIMAZOLE
Lotrimin Cream 1% 3128
Lotrimin Lotion 1% 3128
Lotrimin Topical Solution 1% 3128
Mycelex Troche 573

APOCAPEN (Israel)
CAPTOPRIL
Captopril Tablets 2281

APO-CAPTO (Canada, Hong Kong, Singapore)
CAPTOPRIL
Captopril Tablets 2281

APOCARD (Portugal, Spain)
FLECAINIDE ACETATE
Tambocor Tablets 1990

APO-CEPALEX (Hong Kong)
CEPHALEXIN
Keflex Oral Suspension 1237
Keflex Pulvules 1237

APO-CEPHALEX (Canada)
CEPHALEXIN
Keflex Oral Suspension 1237
Keflex Pulvules 1237

APOCORT (Finland)
HYDROCORTISONE ACETATE
Anusol-HC Suppositories 2238
Cortifoam Rectal Foam 3170
Hydrocortone Acetate Injectable Suspension 2103
Proctocort Suppositories 2264

APOCORTAL (Norway)
HYDROCORTISONE ACETATE
Anusol-HC Suppositories 2238
Cortifoam Rectal Foam 3170
Hydrocortone Acetate Injectable Suspension 2103
Proctocort Suppositories 2264

APO-DICLO (Canada, New Zealand)
DICLOFENAC SODIUM
Voltaren Tablets 2315
Voltaren-XR Tablets 2315

APO-DILTIAZ (Canada, Hong Kong)
DILTIAZEM HYDROCHLORIDE
Cardizem CD Capsules 1016
Cardizem Injectable 1018
Cardizem Lyo-Ject Syringe 1018
Cardizem Monovial 1018
Tiazac Capsules 1378

APO-DOXY (Canada)
DOXYCYCLINE HYCLATE
Doryx Coated Pellet Filled Capsules 3357
Periostat Tablets 1208
Vibra-Tabs Film Coated Tablets 2735
Vibramycin Hyclate Capsules 2735
Vibramycin Hyclate Intravenous 2737

APO-FENO (Canada)
FENOFIBRATE
Tricor Capsules, Micronized 513

APOGASTINE (Israel)
FAMOTIDINE
Pepcid Injection 2153
Pepcid Injection Premixed 2153
Pepcid RPD Orally Disintegrating Tablets 2150
Pepcid Tablets 2150
Pepcid for Oral Suspension 2150

APO-HYDRO (Canada, Singapore)
HYDROCHLOROTHIAZIDE
HydroDIURIL Tablets 2108
Microzide Capsules 3414

APO-IPRAVENT (Canada)
IPRATROPIUM BROMIDE
Atrovent Inhalation Aerosol 1030
Atrovent Inhalation Solution 1031
Atrovent Nasal Spray 0.03% 1032
Atrovent Nasal Spray 0.06% 1033

APO-ISDN (Canada, Singapore)
ISOSORBIDE DINITRATE
Isordil Sublingual Tablets 3525
Isordil Titradose Tablets 3526

APO-K (Canada, Hong Kong)
POTASSIUM CHLORIDE
K-Dur Microburst Release System ER Tablets 1832
K-Lor Powder Packets 469
K-Tab Filmtab Tablets 470
Rum-K 1363

APO-KETO (Canada, Hong Kong, Singapore)
KETOPROFEN
Orudis Capsules 3548
Oruvail Capsules 3548

APOLAR (Finland, Norway, Sweden)
DESONIDE
DesOwen Cream 1401
DesOwen Lotion 1401
DesOwen Ointment 1401

APO-METHAZIDE (Canada)
HYDROCHLOROTHIAZIDE/METHYLDOPA
Aldoril Tablets 2039

APO-METOCLOP (Canada, Hong Kong)
METOCLOPRAMIDE HYDROCHLORIDE
Reglan Injectable 2935
Reglan Syrup 2935
Reglan Tablets 2935

APOMEX (Israel)
SELEGILINE HYDROCHLORIDE
Eldepryl Capsules 3266

APOMINOLIN (Israel)
MINOCYCLINE HYDROCHLORIDE
Dynacin Capsules 2019
Minocin Intravenous 1862
Minocin Oral Suspension 1865
Minocin Pellet-Filled Capsules 1863

APOMOXYN (Israel)
AMOXICILLIN
Amoxil Pediatric Drops for Oral Suspension 1471
Amoxil Tablets 1471

APONACIN (Israel)
NAPROXEN
EC-Naprosyn Delayed-Release Tablets 2967
Naprosyn Suspension 2967
Naprosyn Tablets 2967

APO-NADOL (Canada, Hong Kong)
NADOLOL
Nadolol Tablets 2288

APO-NAPRO-NA (Canada, Singapore)
NAPROXEN SODIUM
Anaprox DS Tablets 2967
Anaprox Tablets 2967
Naprelan Tablets 1293

APO-NIFED (Canada, Singapore)
NIFEDIPINE
Adalat CC Tablets 877
Procardia Capsules 2708
Procardia XL Extended Release Tablets 2710

APO-NORFLOX (Canada)
NORFLOXACIN
Chibroxin Sterile Ophthalmic Solution ⊙273, 2051
Noroxin Tablets 2145

APONORM (Israel)
ATENOLOL
Tenormin I.V. Injection 692

APO-OFLOX (Canada)
OFLOXACIN
Floxin I.V. 2526
Floxin Otic Solution 1219
Floxin Tablets 2529
Ocuflox Ophthalmic Solution 554

APOPHAGE (Israel)
METFORMIN HYDROCHLORIDE
Glucophage Tablets 1080

APOPIRAN (Mexico)
PIROXICAM
Feldene Capsules 2685

APO-PRAZO (Canada, Hong Kong)
PRAZOSIN HYDROCHLORIDE
Minipress Capsules 2699

A-POR (South Africa)
CLOTRIMAZOLE
Lotrimin Cream 1% 3128
Lotrimin Lotion 1% 3128
Lotrimin Topical Solution 1% 3128
Mycelex Troche 573

APO-SULIN (Canada)
SULINDAC
Clinoril Tablets 2053

APO-TAMOX (Canada, Hong Kong, Singapore)
TAMOXIFEN CITRATE
Nolvadex Tablets 678

APO-THEO (Canada, Hong Kong, Singapore)
THEOPHYLLINE
Aerolate Jr. T.D. Capsules 1361

(⊙ Described in PDR For Ophthalmic Medicines™)

Aerolate Liquid 1361
Aerolate Sr. T.D. Capsules 1361
Theo-Dur Extended-Release Tablets. 1835
Uni-Dur Extended-Release Tablets. 1841
Uniphyl 400 mg and 600 mg Tablets . . . 2903

APOTIL (Israel)
TIMOLOL MALEATE
Blocadren Tablets 2046
Timoptic Sterile Ophthalmic Solution. . . . 2190
Timoptic in Ocudose. 2192
Timoptic-XE Sterile Ophthalmic Gel Forming Solution. 2194

APO-TIMOL (Canada, New Zealand)
TIMOLOL MALEATE
Blocadren Tablets 2046
Timoptic Sterile Ophthalmic Solution. . . . 2190
Timoptic in Ocudose. 2192
Timoptic-XE Sterile Ophthalmic Gel Forming Solution. 2194

APO-TIMOP (Canada, Hong Kong)
TIMOLOL MALEATE
Blocadren Tablets 2046
Timoptic Sterile Ophthalmic Solution. . . . 2190
Timoptic in Ocudose. 2192
Timoptic-XE Sterile Ophthalmic Gel Forming Solution. 2194

APO-TRIAZIDE (Hong Kong, Singapore)
HYDROCHLOROTHIAZIDE/TRIAMTERENE
Dyazide Capsules. 1515
Maxzide Tablets. 1008
Maxzide-25 mg Tablets 1008

APO-TRIAZO (Canada)
TRIAZOLAM
Halcion Tablets 2823

APO-TRIMIP (Canada, Hong Kong)
TRIMIPRAMINE MALEATE
Surmontil Capsules. 3595

APOVEN (Australia)
IPRATROPIUM BROMIDE
Atrovent Inhalation Aerosol 1030
Atrovent Inhalation Solution. 1031
Atrovent Nasal Spray 0.03%. 1032
Atrovent Nasal Spray 0.06%. 1033

APOVENT (Israel)
IPRATROPIUM BROMIDE
Atrovent Inhalation Aerosol 1030
Atrovent Inhalation Solution. 1031
Atrovent Nasal Spray 0.03%. 1032
Atrovent Nasal Spray 0.06%. 1033

APO-VERAP (Canada)
VERAPAMIL HYDROCHLORIDE
Covera-HS Tablets 3199
Isoptin SR Tablets. 467
Verelan Capsules 3184
Verelan PM Capsules 3186

APOX (Israel)
ALPRAZOLAM
Xanax Tablets 2865

APOZAN (Israel)
RANITIDINE HYDROCHLORIDE
Zantac 150 EFFERdose Granules 1690
Zantac 150 EFFERdose Tablets 1690
Zantac 150 Tablets 1690
Zantac 300 Tablets 1690
Zantac Injection 1688
Zantac Injection Premixed 1688
Zantac Syrup 1690

APOZEPAM (Denmark, Sweden)
DIAZEPAM
Valium Injectable 3026
Valium Tablets 3047

APPLICAINE (Australia, New Zealand)
BENZOCAINE
Americaine Anesthetic Lubricant 1162
Americaine Otic Topical Anesthetic Ear Drops 1162

APRA-GEL (Belgium)
NAPROXEN
EC-Naprosyn Delayed-Release Tablets . . . 2967
Naprosyn Suspension 2967
Naprosyn Tablets 2967

APRANAX (Belgium, France, Switzerland)
NAPROXEN SODIUM
Anaprox DS Tablets 2967
Anaprox Tablets. 2967
Naprelan Tablets 1293

APREDNISLON (Austria)
PREDNISOLONE
Prelone Syrup 2273

APRICAL (Germany, Israel)
NIFEDIPINE
Adalat CC Tablets. 877
Procardia Capsules. 2708
Procardia XL Extended Release Tablets . . 2710

APROFEN (Thailand)
IBUPROFEN
Motrin Suspension, Oral Drops, Chewable Tablets, and Caplets 2002

APROVEL (Belgium, Denmark, France, Germany, Hong Kong, Irish Republic, Italy, Mexico, Singapore, South Africa, Spain, Thailand)
IRBESARTAN
Avapro Tablets 1074, 3076

APSIFEN (United Kingdom)
IBUPROFEN
Motrin Suspension, Oral Drops, Chewable Tablets, and Caplets 2002

APSOLOL (United Kingdom)
PROPRANOLOL HYDROCHLORIDE
Inderal Injectable 3513
Inderal LA Long-Acting Capsules 3516
Inderal Tablets. 3513

AQUACORT (Canada)
HYDROCORTISONE
Anusol-HC Cream 2.5% 2237
Hydrocortone Tablets 2106

AQUAMYCETIN-N (Germany)
CHLORAMPHENICOL
Chloromycetin Ophthalmic Ointment, 1% . . . . ⊙296
Chloromycetin Ophthalmic Solution . . . . ⊙297
Chloroptic Sterile Ophthalmic Ointment . . ⊙234
Chloroptic Sterile Ophthalmic Solution . . ⊙235

AQUANIL (Denmark, Finland, Norway, Sweden)
TIMOLOL MALEATE
Blocadren Tablets 2046
Timoptic Sterile Ophthalmic Solution. . . . 2190
Timoptic in Ocudose. 2192
Timoptic-XE Sterile Ophthalmic Gel Forming Solution. 2194

AQUANIL HC (Mexico)
HYDROCORTISONE
Anusol-HC Cream 2.5% 2237
Hydrocortone Tablets 2106

AQUARETIC (Germany)
AMILORIDE HYDROCHLORIDE/HYDROCHLOROTHIAZIDE
Moduretic Tablets. 2138

AQUOMIN (Spain)
CICLOPIROX OLAMINE
Loprox Cream. 2021
Loprox Lotion 2021

ARAGEST (Israel)
MEDROXYPROGESTERONE ACETATE
Depo-Provera Contraceptive Injection . . . 2798
Provera Tablets 2853

ARALEN (Canada, Israel)
CHLOROQUINE PHOSPHATE
Aralen Tablets 3075

ARATAC (Australia, New Zealand, Thailand)
AMIODARONE HYDROCHLORIDE
Cordarone Intravenous 3491
Cordarone Tablets 3487
Pacerone Tablets 3331

ARAVA (Australia, Denmark, Finland, France, Germany, Irish Republic, Sweden, Switzerland, The Netherlands, United Kingdom)
LEFLUNOMIDE
Arava Tablets 724

ARCABLOCK (Austria)
ATENOLOL
Tenormin I.V. Injection 692

ARCABLOCK COMP (Austria)
ATENOLOL
Tenormin I.V. Injection 692

ARCANADOPA (South Africa)
METHYLDOPA
Aldomet Tablets. 2037

ARCANAFENAC (South Africa)
DICLOFENAC SODIUM
Voltaren Tablets. 2315
Voltaren-XR Tablets. 2315

ARCANARETIC (South Africa)
AMILORIDE HYDROCHLORIDE/HYDROCHLOROTHIAZIDE
Moduretic Tablets. 2138

ARCENTAL (Spain)
KETOPROFEN
Orudis Capsules 3548
Oruvail Capsules 3548

ARCENTAL TOPICA (Spain)
KETOPROFEN
Orudis Capsules 3548
Oruvail Capsules 3548

ARCHIFEN (Thailand)
CHLORAMPHENICOL
Chloromycetin Ophthalmic Ointment, 1% . . . . ⊙296
Chloromycetin Ophthalmic Solution . . . . ⊙297
Chloroptic Sterile Ophthalmic Ointment . . ⊙234
Chloroptic Sterile Ophthalmic Solution . . ⊙235

ARCLONAC (Thailand)
DICLOFENAC SODIUM
Voltaren Tablets 2315
Voltaren-XR Tablets. 2315

ARCOIRAN (Spain)
SUMATRIPTAN SUCCINATE
Imitrex Injection. 1549
Imitrex Tablets. 1558

ARCOLAN (Brazil)
KETOCONAZOLE
Nizoral 2% Cream 3620
Nizoral 2% Shampoo. 2007
Nizoral Tablets 1791

ARDINEX (Finland)
IBUPROFEN
Motrin Suspension, Oral Drops, Chewable Tablets, and Caplets 2002

AREMIS (Spain)
SERTRALINE HYDROCHLORIDE
Zoloft Tablets 2751

ARFEN (Portugal)
IBUPROFEN
Motrin Suspension, Oral Drops, Chewable Tablets, and Caplets 2002

ARFLOXINA (Mexico)
CIPROFLOXACIN
Cipro I.V. 893
Cipro I.V. Pharmacy Bulk Package 897
Cipro Oral Suspension. 887

ARIAL (Italy)
SALMETEROL XINAFOATE
Serevent Diskus. 1637
Serevent Inhalation Aerosol. 1633

ARICEPT (Australia, Austria, Belgium, Canada, Denmark, Finland, France, Hong Kong, Irish Republic, Israel, Italy, New Zealand, Norway, Portugal, Singapore, South Africa, Spain, Sweden, Switzerland, Thailand, United Kingdom)
DONEPEZIL HYDROCHLORIDE
Aricept Tablets 1270, 2665

ARILIN (Germany, Switzerland)
METRONIDAZOLE
MetroCream 1404
MetroGel 1405
MetroGel-Vaginal Gel 1986
MetroLotion 1405
Noritate Cream 1224

ARILINE (Austria)
METRONIDAZOLE
MetroCream 1404
MetroGel 1405
MetroGel-Vaginal Gel 1986
MetroLotion 1405
Noritate Cream 1224

ARIMIDEX (Australia, Austria, Belgium, Canada, Denmark, Finland, France, Germany, Hong Kong, Irish Republic, Israel, Italy, Mexico, New Zealand, Norway, Portugal, Singapore, South Africa, Spain, Sweden, Switzerland, Thailand, The Netherlands, United Kingdom)
ANASTROZOLE
Arimidex Tablets 659

ARISTOCOR (Austria)
FLECAINIDE ACETATE
Tambocor Tablets. 1990

ARISTOCORT (Australia, Hong Kong, New Zealand, Thailand)
TRIAMCINOLONE ACETONIDE
Azmacort Inhalation Aerosol 728
Nasacort AQ Nasal Spray. 752
Nasacort Nasal Inhaler 750

ARIVEN (Germany)
HEPARIN SODIUM
Heparin Lock Flush Solution 3509
Heparin Sodium Injection 3511

ARLEXICAM (Mexico)
PIROXICAM
Feldene Capsules. 2685

ARMONIL (Italy)
ESTRADIOL
Alora Transdermal System 3372
Climara Transdermal System. 958
Estrace Vaginal Cream 3358
Estring Vaginal Ring 2811
Vivelle Transdermal System 2412
Vivelle-Dot Transdermal System 2416

ARMOPHYLLINE (France)
THEOPHYLLINE
Aerolate Jr. T.D. Capsules 1361
Aerolate Liquid 1361
Aerolate Sr. T.D. Capsules 1361
Theo-Dur Extended-Release Tablets. 1835
Uni-Dur Extended-Release Tablets. 1841
Uniphyl 400 mg and 600 mg Tablets . . . 2903

AROPAX (Australia, Belgium, Brazil, Mexico, New Zealand, South Africa, Spain)
PAROXETINE HYDROCHLORIDE
Paxil Oral Suspension 1609
Paxil Tablets 1609

AROVIT (Brazil, France, South Africa, Sweden, Switzerland)
VITAMIN A PALMITATE
Aquasol A Parenteral. 593

ARPAMYL LP (France)
VERAPAMIL HYDROCHLORIDE
Covera-HS Tablets 3199
Isoptin SR Tablets. 467
Verelan Capsules 3184
Verelan PM Capsules 3186

ARRETIN (Mexico)
TRETINOIN
Avita Cream 999
Avita Gel 1000
Renova 0.05% Cream 2519
Retin-A Micro 0.1%. 2522
Vesanoid Capsules 3037

ARTAGEN (Thailand)
NAPROXEN
EC-Naprosyn Delayed-Release Tablets . . . 2967
Naprosyn Suspension 2967
Naprosyn Tablets 2967

ARTAMIN (Austria, Singapore)
PENICILLAMINE
Cuprimine Capsules 2075
Depen Titratable Tablets 3341

ARTAXAN (Italy)
NABUMETONE
Relafen Tablets 1617

ARTERIOFLEXIN (Australia, Austria)
CLOFIBRATE
Atromid-S Capsules 3483

ARTHAXAN (Germany)
NABUMETONE
Relafen Tablets 1617

ARTHRABAS (Germany)
CHLOROQUINE PHOSPHATE
Aralen Tablets 3075

ARTHREX (Germany)
DICLOFENAC SODIUM
Voltaren Tablets. 2315
Voltaren-XR Tablets. 2315

ARTHREX DUO (Germany)
DICLOFENAC SODIUM
Voltaren Tablets. 2315
Voltaren-XR Tablets. 2315

ARTHROCINE (France)
SULINDAC
Clinoril Tablets. 2053

ARTHROFEN (United Kingdom)
IBUPROFEN
Motrin Suspension, Oral Drops, Chewable Tablets, and Caplets 2002

ARTHROSIN (United Kingdom)
NAPROXEN
EC-Naprosyn Delayed-Release Tablets . . . 2967
Naprosyn Suspension 2967
Naprosyn Tablets 2967

ARTHROTEC (Australia, Austria, Canada, Denmark, Finland, Hong Kong, Irish Republic, Israel, Norway, Portugal, Singapore, South Africa, Sweden, Switzerland, Thailand, The Netherlands, United Kingdom)
DICLOFENAC SODIUM
Voltaren Tablets. 2315
Voltaren-XR Tablets. 2315

ARTHROXEN (United Kingdom)
NAPROXEN
EC-Naprosyn Delayed-Release Tablets . . . 2967
Naprosyn Suspension 2967
Naprosyn Tablets 2967

ARTHRUM H (France)
SODIUM HYALURONATE
Hyalgan Solution 3080

(⊙ Described in PDR For Ophthalmic Medicines™)

ARTICULAN (Portugal)
ETODOLAC
Lodine Capsules 3528
Lodine Tablets 3528
Lodine XL Extended-Release Tablets 3530

ARTINOR (Mexico)
PIROXICAM
Feldene Capsules 2685

ARTOFEN (Israel)
IBUPROFEN
Motrin Suspension, Oral Drops, Chewable Tablets, and Caplets 2002

ARTONIL (Sweden)
RANITIDINE HYDROCHLORIDE
Zantac 150 EFFERdose Granules 1690
Zantac 150 EFFERdose Tablets 1690
Zantac 150 Tablets 1690
Zantac 300 Tablets 1690
Zantac Injection 1688
Zantac Injection Premixed 1688
Zantac Syrup 1690

ARTOTEC (France)
DICLOFENAC SODIUM
Voltaren Tablets 2315
Voltaren-XR Tablets 2315

ARTRAGIL (Spain)
PIROXICAM
Feldene Capsules 2685

ARTREN (Brazil)
DICLOFENAC SODIUM
Voltaren Tablets 2315
Voltaren-XR Tablets 2315

ARTRENAC (Mexico)
DICLOFENAC SODIUM
Voltaren Tablets 2315
Voltaren-XR Tablets 2315

ARTRENAC PRO (Mexico)
DICLOFENAC SODIUM
Voltaren Tablets 2315
Voltaren-XR Tablets 2315

ARTRIBID (Portugal)
SULINDAC
Clinoril Tablets 2053

ARTRIDEN (Mexico)
MEFENAMIC ACID
Ponstel Capsules 1356

ARTRIL (Brazil)
IBUPROFEN
Motrin Suspension, Oral Drops, Chewable Tablets, and Caplets 2002

ARTRINID (Brazil)
KETOPROFEN
Orudis Capsules 3548
Oruvail Capsules 3548

ARTROCAPTIN (Spain)
TOLMETIN SODIUM
Tolectin 200 Tablets 2589
Tolectin 600 Tablets 2589
Tolectin DS Capsules 2589

ARTRODOL (Italy)
DIFLUNISAL
Dolobid Tablets 2088

ARTRON (Mexico)
NAPROXEN
EC-Naprosyn Delayed-Release Tablets . . . 2967
Naprosyn Suspension 2967
Naprosyn Tablets 2967

ARTROSONE (Spain)
DEXAMETHASONE
Decadron Elixir 2078
Decadron Tablets 2079

ARTROTEC (Italy, Mexico, Spain)
DICLOFENAC SODIUM
Voltaren Tablets 2315
Voltaren-XR Tablets 2315

ARTROXEN (Italy)
NAPROXEN
EC-Naprosyn Delayed-Release Tablets . . . 2967
Naprosyn Suspension 2967
Naprosyn Tablets 2967

ARTROXICAM (Italy)
PIROXICAM
Feldene Capsules 2685

ARTYFLAM (Mexico)
PIROXICAM
Feldene Capsules 2685

ARTZ (Denmark, Italy)
SODIUM HYALURONATE
Hyalgan Solution 3080

ARTZAL (Austria, Finland, Sweden)
SODIUM HYALURONATE
Hyalgan Solution 3080

ARU C (Germany)
CLOTRIMAZOLE
Lotrimin Cream 1% 3128
Lotrimin Lotion 1% 3128
Lotrimin Topical Solution 1% 3128
Mycelex Troche 573

ARUBENDOL (Germany)
TERBUTALINE SULFATE
Brethine Ampuls 2314
Brethine Tablets 2313

ARUCLONIN (Germany)
CLONIDINE HYDROCHLORIDE
Catapres Tablets 1037
Duraclon Injection 3057

ARUTIMOL (Germany)
TIMOLOL MALEATE
Blocadren Tablets 2046
Timoptic Sterile Ophthalmic Solution 2190
Timoptic in Ocudose 2192
Timoptic-XE Sterile Ophthalmic Gel Forming Solution 2194

ARUTRIN (Germany)
TRIAMCINOLONE ACETONIDE
Azmacort Inhalation Aerosol 728
Nasacort AQ Nasal Spray 752
Nasacort Nasal Inhaler 750

ARUTROPID (Germany)
IPRATROPIUM BROMIDE
Atrovent Inhalation Aerosol 1030
Atrovent Inhalation Solution 1031
Atrovent Nasal Spray 0.03% 1032
Atrovent Nasal Spray 0.06% 1033

ARYTHMOL (Irish Republic, United Kingdom)
PROPAFENONE HYDROCHLORIDE
Rythmol Tablets – 150 mg, 225 mg, 300 mg 502

ARZEPAM (Mexico)
DIAZEPAM
Valium Injectable 3026
Valium Tablets 3047

ARZIMOL (Spain)
CEFPROZIL
Cefzil Tablets 1076
Cefzil for Oral Suspension 1076

ASASANTIN (Australia, Austria, Finland, Mexico, Sweden, The Netherlands)
DIPYRIDAMOLE
Persantine Tablets 1057

ASASANTINE (France)
DIPYRIDAMOLE
Persantine Tablets 1057

ASAUREX (Mexico)
CIMETIDINE
Tagamet Tablets 1644

ASCARIDIL (Brazil)
LEVAMISOLE HYDROCHLORIDE
Ergamisol Tablets 1789

ASCARIOBEL (Brazil)
MEBENDAZOLE
Vermox Chewable Tablets 2017

ASCARITOR (Brazil)
MEBENDAZOLE
Vermox Chewable Tablets 2017

ASCAROBEX (Brazil)
MEBENDAZOLE
Vermox Chewable Tablets 2017

ASCOTOP (Germany)
ZOLMITRIPTAN
Zomig Tablets 708

ASERCIT (Mexico)
DACARBAZINE
DTIC-Dome 902

ASIAZOLE (Thailand)
METRONIDAZOLE
MetroCream 1404
MetroGel 1405
MetroGel-Vaginal Gel 1986
MetroLotion 1405
Noritate Cream 1224

ASIG (Australia)
QUINAPRIL HYDROCHLORIDE
Accupril Tablets 2611

ASMALINE (Thailand)
TERBUTALINE SULFATE
Brethine Ampuls 2314
Brethine Tablets 2313

ASMATIL (Portugal)
FLUTICASONE PROPIONATE
Cutivate Cream 1282
Cutivate Ointment 1284
Flonase Nasal Spray 1533
Flovent 110 mcg Inhalation Aerosol 1535
Flovent 220 mcg Inhalation Aerosol 1535
Flovent 44 mcg Inhalation Aerosol 1535
Flovent Rotadisk 100 mcg 1537
Flovent Rotadisk 250 mcg 1537
Flovent Rotadisk 50 mcg 1537

ASMO (Spain)
THEOPHYLLINE
Aerolate Jr. T.D. Capsules 1361
Aerolate Liquid 1361
Aerolate Sr. T.D. Capsules 1361
Theo-Dur Extended-Release Tablets 1835
Uni-Dur Extended-Release Tablets 1841
Uniphyl 400 mg and 600 mg Tablets . . . 2903

ASMO-LAVI (Portugal)
FLUTICASONE PROPIONATE
Cutivate Cream 1282
Cutivate Ointment 1284
Flonase Nasal Spray 1533
Flovent 110 mcg Inhalation Aerosol 1535
Flovent 220 mcg Inhalation Aerosol 1535
Flovent 44 mcg Inhalation Aerosol 1535
Flovent Rotadisk 100 mcg 1537
Flovent Rotadisk 250 mcg 1537
Flovent Rotadisk 50 mcg 1537

ASONACOR (Austria)
PROPAFENONE HYDROCHLORIDE
Rythmol Tablets – 150 mg, 225 mg, 300 mg 502

ASOTAX (Mexico)
PACLITAXEL
Taxol Injection 1129

ASPASERINE B6 TRANQ (Spain)
DIAZEPAM
Valium Injectable 3026
Valium Tablets 3047

ASPENIL (Italy)
AMOXICILLIN
Amoxil Pediatric Drops for Oral Suspension 1471
Amoxil Tablets 1471

ASSIVAL (Israel)
DIAZEPAM
Valium Injectable 3026
Valium Tablets 3047

ASTELIN (Mexico)
AZELASTINE HYDROCHLORIDE
Astelin Nasal Spray 3339

ASTHAMSIAN (Thailand)
TERBUTALINE SULFATE
Brethine Ampuls 2314
Brethine Tablets 2313

ASTHENOPIN (Germany)
PILOCARPINE HYDROCHLORIDE
Isopto Carpine Ophthalmic Solution . . . . ⊙215
Pilopine HS Ophthalmic Gel . . . . . ⊙217
Salagen Tablets 2229

ASTHMA T (Israel)
THEOPHYLLINE
Aerolate Jr. T.D. Capsules 1361
Aerolate Liquid 1361
Aerolate Sr. T.D. Capsules 1361
Theo-Dur Extended-Release Tablets 1835
Uni-Dur Extended-Release Tablets 1841
Uniphyl 400 mg and 600 mg Tablets . . . 2903

ASTHMO-KRANIT MONO (Germany)
TERBUTALINE SULFATE
Brethine Ampuls 2314
Brethine Tablets 2313

ASTHMOPROTECT (Germany)
TERBUTALINE SULFATE
Brethine Ampuls 2314
Brethine Tablets 2313

ASTREPTINE (Belgium)
SULFANILAMIDE
AVC Cream 1350
AVC Suppositories 1350

ATACAND (Australia, Austria, Belgium, Canada, Denmark, Finland, France, Irish Republic, Israel, Mexico, New Zealand, Norway, Portugal, Singapore, South Africa, Spain, Sweden, Switzerland, The Netherlands)
CANDESARTAN CILEXETIL
Atacand Tablets 595

ATALINE (Hong Kong, Singapore, Thailand)
TERBUTALINE SULFATE
Brethine Ampuls 2314
Brethine Tablets 2313

ATAMIR (Denmark)
PENICILLAMINE
Cuprimine Capsules 2075
Depen Titratable Tablets 3341

ATANO (Thailand)
HYDROXYZINE HYDROCHLORIDE
Atarax Tablets & Syrup 2667
Vistaril Intramuscular Solution 2738

ATARAX (Austria, Belgium, Canada, Denmark, Finland, France, Hong Kong, Irish Republic, Italy, Norway, Spain, Sweden, Thailand, The Netherlands, United Kingdom)
HYDROXYZINE HYDROCHLORIDE
Atarax Tablets & Syrup 2667
Vistaril Intramuscular Solution 2738

ATARIN (Finland)
AMANTADINE HYDROCHLORIDE
Symmetrel Syrup 1328
Symmetrel Tablets 1328

ATATOSSE BALSAMICO (Brazil)
POTASSIUM IODIDE
Pima Syrup 1362

ATAZINA (Italy)
HYDROXYZINE HYDROCHLORIDE
Atarax Tablets & Syrup 2667
Vistaril Intramuscular Solution 2738

ATE (Germany)
ATENOLOL
Tenormin I.V. Injection 692

ATE LICH (Germany)
ATENOLOL
Tenormin I.V. Injection 692

ATE LICH COMP (Germany)
ATENOLOL
Tenormin I.V. Injection 692

ATEBEMYXINE (France)
NEOMYCIN SULFATE/POLYMYXIN B SULFATE
Neosporin G.U. Irrigant Sterile 2256

ATEBETA (Germany)
ATENOLOL
Tenormin I.V. Injection 692

ATECOR (Irish Republic)
ATENOLOL
Tenormin I.V. Injection 692

ATEDUREX (Switzerland)
ATENOLOL
Tenormin I.V. Injection 692

ATEHEXAL (Australia, Austria, Germany)
ATENOLOL
Tenormin I.V. Injection 692

ATEHEXAL COMP (Germany)
ATENOLOL
Tenormin I.V. Injection 692

ATEL (Germany)
ATENOLOL
Tenormin I.V. Injection 692

ATEM (Italy)
IPRATROPIUM BROMIDE
Atrovent Inhalation Aerosol 1030
Atrovent Inhalation Solution 1031
Atrovent Nasal Spray 0.03% 1032
Atrovent Nasal Spray 0.06% 1033

ATEMUR (Germany)
FLUTICASONE PROPIONATE
Cutivate Cream 1282
Cutivate Ointment 1284
Flonase Nasal Spray 1533
Flovent 110 mcg Inhalation Aerosol 1535
Flovent 220 mcg Inhalation Aerosol 1535
Flovent 44 mcg Inhalation Aerosol 1535
Flovent Rotadisk 100 mcg 1537
Flovent Rotadisk 250 mcg 1537
Flovent Rotadisk 50 mcg 1537

ATENBLOCK (Finland)
ATENOLOL
Tenormin I.V. Injection 692

ATENDOL (Germany)
ATENOLOL
Tenormin I.V. Injection 692

ATENET (Denmark)
ATENOLOL
Tenormin I.V. Injection 692

ATENI (Irish Republic)
ATENOLOL
Tenormin I.V. Injection 692

ATENIF BETA (Germany)
ATENOLOL
Tenormin I.V. Injection 692

ATE-NIFE (Irish Republic)
ATENOLOL
Tenormin I.V. Injection 692

ATENIL (Switzerland)
ATENOLOL
Tenormin I.V. Injection 692

ATENIX (United Kingdom)
ATENOLOL
Tenormin I.V. Injection 692

ATENO (Germany, Hong Kong)
ATENOLOL
Tenormin I.V. Injection ... 692

ATENO COMP (Germany)
ATENOLOL
Tenormin I.V. Injection ... 692

ATENO-BASAN (Switzerland)
ATENOLOL
Tenormin I.V. Injection ... 692

ATENOBENE (Austria)
ATENOLOL
Tenormin I.V. Injection ... 692

ATENOBLOK (South Africa)
ATENOLOL
Tenormin I.V. Injection ... 692

ATENOBLOK CO (South Africa)
ATENOLOL
Tenormin I.V. Injection ... 692

ATENODAN (Denmark)
ATENOLOL
Tenormin I.V. Injection ... 692

ATENOGAMMA (Germany)
ATENOLOL
Tenormin I.V. Injection ... 692

ATENOGAMMA COMP (Germany)
ATENOLOL
Tenormin I.V. Injection ... 692

ATENOGEN (Irish Republic)
ATENOLOL
Tenormin I.V. Injection ... 692

ATENOL (Brazil, Finland, Italy, Thailand)
ATENOLOL
Tenormin I.V. Injection ... 692

ATENOLAN (Austria)
ATENOLOL
Tenormin I.V. Injection ... 692

ATENOLOL AL COMP (Germany)
ATENOLOL
Tenormin I.V. Injection ... 692

ATENOMEL (Irish Republic)
ATENOLOL
Tenormin I.V. Injection ... 692

ATENOMERCK (Germany)
ATENOLOL
Tenormin I.V. Injection ... 692

ATENOMERCK COMP (Germany)
ATENOLOL
Tenormin I.V. Injection ... 692

ATENOR (Denmark)
ATENOLOL
Tenormin I.V. Injection ... 692

ATENS (Brazil)
ENALAPRIL MALEATE
Vasotec Tablets ... 2210

ATENS H (Brazil)
ENALAPRIL MALEATE/HYDROCHLOROTHIAZIDE
Vaseretic Tablets ... 2204

ATENSIN (Thailand)
PROPRANOLOL HYDROCHLORIDE
Inderal Injectable ... 3513
Inderal LA Long-Acting Capsules ... 3516
Inderal Tablets ... 3513

ATENSINA (Brazil)
CLONIDINE HYDROCHLORIDE
Catapres Tablets ... 1037
Duraclon Injection ... 3057

ATENSINE (Irish Republic, United Kingdom)
DIAZEPAM
Valium Injectable ... 3026
Valium Tablets ... 3047

ATERAX (South Africa)
HYDROXYZINE HYDROCHLORIDE
Atarax Tablets & Syrup ... 2667
Vistaril Intramuscular Solution ... 2738

ATEREAL (Germany)
ATENOLOL
Tenormin I.V. Injection ... 692

ATEREN (South Africa)
ATENOLOL
Tenormin I.V. Injection ... 692

ATERMIN (Italy)
ATENOLOL
Tenormin I.V. Injection ... 692

ATEROCLAR (Italy)
HEPARIN SODIUM
Heparin Lock Flush Solution ... 3509
Heparin Sodium Injection ... 3511

ATEROL (South Africa)
ATENOLOL
Tenormin I.V. Injection ... 692

ATESIFAR (Switzerland)
ATENOLOL
Tenormin I.V. Injection ... 692

ATHELMIN (Brazil)
MEBENDAZOLE
Vermox Chewable Tablets ... 2017

ATHLETES FOOT CREAM (United Kingdom)
CLOTRIMAZOLE
Lotrimin Cream 1% ... 3128
Lotrimin Lotion 1% ... 3128
Lotrimin Topical Solution 1% ... 3128
Mycelex Troche ... 573

ATHRU-DERM (South Africa)
DICLOFENAC SODIUM
Voltaren Tablets ... 2315
Voltaren-XR Tablets ... 2315

ATIFLAN (Mexico)
NAPROXEN
EC-Naprosyn Delayed-Release Tablets ... 2967
Naprosyn Suspension ... 2967
Naprosyn Tablets ... 2967

ATINORM (Italy)
ATENOLOL
Tenormin I.V. Injection ... 692

ATIVAN (Australia, Canada, Hong Kong, Irish Republic, Mexico, New Zealand, Singapore, South Africa, Thailand, United Kingdom)
LORAZEPAM
Ativan Injection ... 3478
Ativan Tablets ... 3482

ATLANSIL (Brazil)
AMIODARONE HYDROCHLORIDE
Cordarone Intravenous ... 3491
Cordarone Tablets ... 3487
Pacerone Tablets ... 3331

ATMOS (Denmark, Finland, Norway, Sweden)
TESTOSTERONE
Androderm Transdermal System CIII ... 3377
Testoderm Transdermal Systems ... 574

ATODEL (Thailand)
PRAZOSIN HYDROCHLORIDE
Minipress Capsules ... 2699

ATOSIL (Germany)
PROMETHAZINE HYDROCHLORIDE
Phenergan Injection ... 3553
Phenergan Suppositories ... 3556
Phenergan Syrup Fortis ... 3554
Phenergan Syrup Plain ... 3554
Phenergan Tablets ... 3556

ATRIDOX (United Kingdom)
DOXYCYCLINE HYCLATE
Doryx Coated Pellet Filled Capsules ... 3357
Periostat Tablets ... 1208
Vibra-Tabs Film Coated Tablets ... 2735
Vibramycin Hyclate Capsules ... 2735
Vibramycin Hyclate Intravenous ... 2737

ATRISOL (Mexico)
CAPTOPRIL
Captopril Tablets ... 2281

ATROMBIN (Finland)
DIPYRIDAMOLE
Persantine Tablets ... 1057

ATROMIDIN (Belgium, Denmark, Italy, Sweden)
CLOFIBRATE
Atromid-S Capsules ... 3483

ATROMID-S (Australia, Canada, Hong Kong, Irish Republic, Mexico, New Zealand, Portugal, South Africa, United Kingdom)
CLOFIBRATE
Atromid-S Capsules ... 3483

ATRONASE (Austria, Belgium, South Africa)
IPRATROPIUM BROMIDE
Atrovent Inhalation Aerosol ... 1030
Atrovent Inhalation Solution ... 1031
Atrovent Nasal Spray 0.03% ... 1032
Atrovent Nasal Spray 0.06% ... 1033

ATROVENT (Australia, Austria, Belgium, Brazil, Canada, Denmark, Finland, France, Germany, Hong Kong, Irish Republic, Italy, Mexico, New Zealand, Norway, Portugal, Singapore, South Africa, Spain, Sweden, Switzerland, Thailand, The Netherlands, United Kingdom)
IPRATROPIUM BROMIDE
Atrovent Inhalation Aerosol ... 1030
Atrovent Inhalation Solution ... 1031
Atrovent Nasal Spray 0.03% ... 1032
Atrovent Nasal Spray 0.06% ... 1033

ATTENTA (Australia)
METHYLPHENIDATE HYDROCHLORIDE
Methylin Tablets ... 1995
Ritalin Hydrochloride Tablets ... 2387
Ritalin-SR Tablets ... 2387

AUGMAXIL (South Africa)
AMOXICILLIN
Amoxil Pediatric Drops for Oral Suspension ... 1471
Amoxil Tablets ... 1471

AULCER (Spain)
OMEPRAZOLE
Prilosec Delayed-Release Capsules ... 628

AURALYT (Mexico)
BENZOCAINE
Americaine Anesthetic Lubricant ... 1162
Americaine Otic Topical Anesthetic Ear Drops ... 1162

AURAMIN (Austria)
MINOCYCLINE HYDROCHLORIDE
Dynacin Capsules ... 2019
Minocin Intravenous ... 1862
Minocin Oral Suspension ... 1865
Minocin Pellet-Filled Capsules ... 1863

AURISWELL (France)
HYDROCORTISONE/NEOMYCIN SULFATE/POLYMYXIN B SULFATE
Cortisporin Ophthalmic Suspension Sterile ... ⊙297

AUSCARD (Australia)
DILTIAZEM HYDROCHLORIDE
Cardizem CD Capsules ... 1016
Cardizem Injectable ... 1018
Cardizem Lyo-Ject Syringe ... 1018
Cardizem Monovial ... 1018
Tiazac Capsules ... 1378

AUSGEM (Australia)
GEMFIBROZIL
Lopid Tablets ... 2650

AUSRAN (Australia)
RANITIDINE HYDROCHLORIDE
Zantac 150 EFFERdose Granules ... 1690
Zantac 150 EFFERdose Tablets ... 1690
Zantac 150 Tablets ... 1690
Zantac 300 Tablets ... 1690
Zantac Injection ... 1688
Zantac Injection Premixed ... 1688
Zantac Syrup ... 1690

AUSTYN (Australia, Singapore)
THEOPHYLLINE
Aerolate Jr. T.D. Capsules ... 1361
Aerolate Liquid ... 1361
Aerolate Sr. T.D. Capsules ... 1361
Theo-Dur Extended-Release Tablets ... 1835
Uni-Dur Extended-Release Tablets ... 1841
Uniphyl 400 mg and 600 mg Tablets ... 2903

AUXINA A MASIVA (Spain)
VITAMIN A PALMITATE
Aquasol A Parenteral ... 593

AVALLONE (Austria)
IBUPROFEN
Motrin Suspension, Oral Drops, Chewable Tablets, and Caplets ... 2002

AVANDIA (Australia, Irish Republic, Thailand, United Kingdom)
ROSIGLITAZONE MALEATE
Avandia Tablets ... 1490

AVAPRO (Australia, Mexico)
IRBESARTAN
Avapro Tablets ... 1074, 3076

AVAPRO HCT (Australia)
HYDROCHLOROTHIAZIDE/IRBESARTAN
Avalide Tablets ... 1070

AVC (Canada)
SULFANILAMIDE
AVC Cream ... 1350
AVC Suppositories ... 1350

AVERPAN (Brazil)
MEBENDAZOLE
Vermox Chewable Tablets ... 2017

A-VICOTRAT (Germany)
VITAMIN A PALMITATE
Aquasol A Parenteral ... 593

AVILAC (Israel)
LACTULOSE
Kristalose for Oral Solution ... 1007

A-VITA (Finland)
VITAMIN A PALMITATE
Aquasol A Parenteral ... 593

AVITCID (Finland)
TRETINOIN
Avita Cream ... 999
Avita Gel ... 1000
Renova 0.05% Cream ... 2519
Retin-A Micro 0.1% ... 2522
Vesanoid Capsules ... 3037

AVITINA (Italy)
VITAMIN A PALMITATE
Aquasol A Parenteral ... 593

AVLOCARDYL (France)
PROPRANOLOL HYDROCHLORIDE
Inderal Injectable ... 3513
Inderal LA Long-Acting Capsules ... 3516
Inderal Tablets ... 3513

AVLOCLOR (Irish Republic, Israel, Singapore, United Kingdom)
CHLOROQUINE PHOSPHATE
Aralen Tablets ... 3075

AVLOSULFON (Canada, Israel)
DAPSONE
Dapsone Tablets USP ... 1780

AVOCIN (Italy)
PIPERACILLIN SODIUM
Pipracil ... 1866

AVONEX (Australia, Austria, Finland, France, Germany, Irish Republic, Israel, Italy, Norway, Portugal, Spain, Sweden, Switzerland, The Netherlands, United Kingdom)
INTERFERON BETA-1A
Avonex ... 1013

AXACEF (Denmark, Sweden)
CEFUROXIME SODIUM
Kefurox Vials, ADD-Vantage ... 1948
Zinacef Injection ... 1696

AXCIL (Mexico)
AMOXICILLIN
Amoxil Pediatric Drops for Oral Suspension ... 1471
Amoxil Tablets ... 1471

AXEPIM (France)
CEFEPIME HYDROCHLORIDE
Maxipime for Injection ... 1285

AXER (Italy)
NAPROXEN SODIUM
Anaprox DS Tablets ... 2967
Anaprox Tablets ... 2967
Naprelan Tablets ... 1293

AXETINE (Thailand)
CEFUROXIME SODIUM
Kefurox Vials, ADD-Vantage ... 1948
Zinacef Injection ... 1696

AXID (Austria, Brazil, Canada, Hong Kong, Irish Republic, Mexico, South Africa, Thailand, United Kingdom)
NIZATIDINE
Axid Pulvules ... 1903

AXOTIDE (Switzerland)
FLUTICASONE PROPIONATE
Cutivate Cream ... 1282
Cutivate Ointment ... 1284
Flonase Nasal Spray ... 1533
Flovent 110 mcg Inhalation Aerosol ... 1535
Flovent 220 mcg Inhalation Aerosol ... 1535
Flovent 44 mcg Inhalation Aerosol ... 1535
Flovent Rotadisk 100 mcg ... 1537
Flovent Rotadisk 250 mcg ... 1537
Flovent Rotadisk 50 mcg ... 1537

AZ (Mexico)
AZELASTINE HYDROCHLORIDE
Astelin Nasal Spray ... 3339

AZACTAM (Australia, Austria, Belgium, Brazil, Denmark, Finland, France, Germany, Hong Kong, Irish Republic, Israel, Italy, Japan, New Zealand, Norway, Portugal, Singapore, South Africa, Spain, Sweden, Switzerland, Thailand, The Netherlands, United Kingdom)
AZTREONAM
Azactam for Injection ... 1276

AZANTAC (France, Mexico)
RANITIDINE HYDROCHLORIDE
Zantac 150 EFFERdose Granules ... 1690
Zantac 150 EFFERdose Tablets ... 1690
Zantac 150 Tablets ... 1690
Zantac 300 Tablets ... 1690
Zantac Injection ... 1688
Zantac Injection Premixed ... 1688
Zantac Syrup ... 1690

AZARON (Belgium)
DIPHENHYDRAMINE HYDROCHLORIDE
Benadryl Parenteral ... 2617

AZELAN (Brazil)
AZELAIC ACID
Azelex Cream ... 547

(⊙ Described in PDR For Ophthalmic Medicines™)

AZELCREAM (Italy)
AZELAIC ACID
Azelex Cream 547

AZEP (Hong Kong, Portugal, Singapore, Thailand)
AZELASTINE HYDROCHLORIDE
Astelin Nasal Spray 3339

AZEPTIN (Japan)
AZELASTINE HYDROCHLORIDE
Astelin Nasal Spray 3339

AZERTY (France)
NALBUPHINE HYDROCHLORIDE
Nubain Injection 1323

AZIDE (Australia)
CHLOROTHIAZIDE
Diuril Oral Suspension 2087
Diuril Tablets 2087

AZIMAX (Spain)
ZAFIRLUKAST
Accolate Tablets 657

AZMACORT (Canada)
TRIAMCINOLONE ACETONIDE
Azmacort Inhalation Aerosol 728
Nasacort AQ Nasal Spray 752
Nasacort Nasal Inhaler 750

AZOL (Spain)
SULFANILAMIDE
AVC Cream 1350
AVC Suppositories 1350

AZOMID (South Africa)
ACETAZOLAMIDE
Diamox Sequels Sustained Release Capsules . . . . ⊙270
Diamox Tablets . . . . ⊙269

AZONA (Mexico)
DEXAMETHASONE
Decadron Elixir 2078
Decadron Tablets 2079

AZOPT (Australia, Canada, Denmark, Finland, Irish Republic, Singapore, Thailand, United Kingdom)
BRINZOLAMIDE
Azopt Ophthalmic Suspension . . . ⊙205, 536

AZOR (South Africa)
ALPRAZOLAM
Xanax Tablets 2865

AZUCIMET (Germany)
CIMETIDINE
Tagamet Tablets 1644

AZUDOXAT (Germany)
DOXYCYCLINE HYCLATE
Doryx Coated Pellet Filled Capsules 3357
Periostat Tablets 1208
Vibra-Tabs Film Coated Tablets 2735
Vibramycin Hyclate Capsules 2735
Vibramycin Hyclate Intravenous 2737

AZULFIDINE (Germany)
SULFASALAZINE
Azulfidine EN-tabs Tablets 2775

AZULFIN (Brazil)
SULFASALAZINE
Azulfidine EN-tabs Tablets 2775

AZUPAMIL (Germany)
VERAPAMIL HYDROCHLORIDE
Covera-HS Tablets 3199
Isoptin SR Tablets 467
Verelan Capsules 3184
Verelan PM Capsules 3186

AZURANIT (Germany)
RANITIDINE HYDROCHLORIDE
Zantac 150 EFFERdose Granules 1690
Zantac 150 EFFERdose Tablets 1690
Zantac 150 Tablets 1690
Zantac 300 Tablets 1690
Zantac Injection 1688
Zantac Injection Premixed 1688
Zantac Syrup 1690

AZUTRIMAZOL (Germany)
CLOTRIMAZOLE
Lotrimin Cream 1% 3128
Lotrimin Lotion 1% 3128
Lotrimin Topical Solution 1% 3128
Mycelex Troche 573

BABY AGISTEN (Israel)
CLOTRIMAZOLE
Lotrimin Cream 1% 3128
Lotrimin Lotion 1% 3128
Lotrimin Topical Solution 1% 3128
Mycelex Troche 573

BABY GEL (Israel)
BENZOCAINE
Americaine Anesthetic Lubricant 1162
Americaine Otic Topical Anesthetic Ear Drops 1162

BABY ORAJEL (Canada)
BENZOCAINE
Americaine Anesthetic Lubricant 1162
Americaine Otic Topical Anesthetic Ear Drops 1162

BACCIDAL (Japan, Spain)
NORFLOXACIN
Chibroxin Sterile Ophthalmic Solution . . . . ⊙273, 2051
Noroxin Tablets 2145

BACIMEX (Spain)
AMPICILLIN SODIUM/SULBACTAM SODIUM
Unasyn for Injection 2728

BACTOCIN (Mexico)
OFLOXACIN
Floxin I.V. 2526
Floxin Otic Solution 1219
Floxin Tablets 2529
Ocuflox Ophthalmic Solution 554

BACTODERM (Israel)
MUPIROCIN
Bactroban Ointment 1496

BACTOFLOX (Portugal)
OFLOXACIN
Floxin I.V. 2526
Floxin Otic Solution 1219
Floxin Tablets 2529
Ocuflox Ophthalmic Solution 554

BACTRACID (Germany)
NORFLOXACIN
Chibroxin Sterile Ophthalmic Solution . . . . ⊙273, 2051
Noroxin Tablets 2145

BACTROBAN (Belgium, Brazil, Hong Kong, Mexico, New Zealand, Singapore, South Africa, Spain, Thailand, United Kingdom)
MUPIROCIN
Bactroban Ointment 1496

BAC-ZIDIM (Mexico)
CEFTAZIDIME
Ceptaz for Injection 1499
Fortaz for Injection 1541
Tazicef for Injection 1647
Tazidime Vials, Faspak & ADD-Vantage 1966

BALCOR (Brazil, Portugal)
DILTIAZEM HYDROCHLORIDE
Cardizem CD Capsules 1016
Cardizem Injectable 1018
Cardizem Lyo-Ject Syringe 1018
Cardizem Monovial 1018
Tiazac Capsules 1378

BALMINIL DM E (Canada)
DEXTROMETHORPHAN HYDROBROMIDE/GUAIFENESIN
Tussi-Organidin DM NR Liquid 3350
Tussi-Organidin DM-S NR Liquid 3350

BALMINIL EXPECTORANT (Canada)
GUAIFENESIN
Organidin NR Liquid 3350
Organidin NR Tablets 3350

BALMOX (Portugal, Switzerland)
NABUMETONE
Relafen Tablets 1617

BALODIN (Spain)
DIRITHROMYCIN
Dynabac Tablets 2269

BALPRIL (Portugal)
ENALAPRIL MALEATE
Vasotec Tablets 2210

BALSULPH (Canada)
SULFACETAMIDE SODIUM
Bleph-10 Ophthalmic Ointment 10% . . . . ⊙230
Klaron Lotion 10% 1224

BAMALITE (Spain)
LANSOPRAZOLE
Prevacid Delayed-Release Capsules 3292

BANAN (Hong Kong, Japan, Thailand)
CEFPODOXIME PROXETIL
Vantin Tablets and Oral Suspension 2860

BANISHING CREAM (Canada)
HYDROQUINONE
Eldopaque Forte 4% Cream 1734
Eldoquin Forte 4% Cream 1734
Lustra Cream 2023
Lustra-AF Cream 2023
Melanex Topical Solution 2300
Solaquin Forte 4% Cream 1734
Solaquin Forte 4% Gel 1734

BANTENOL (Spain)
MEBENDAZOLE
Vermox Chewable Tablets 2017

BARAZAN (Germany)
NORFLOXACIN
Chibroxin Sterile Ophthalmic Solution . . . . ⊙273, 2051
Noroxin Tablets 2145

BARCLYD (France)
CLONIDINE HYDROCHLORIDE
Catapres Tablets 1037
Duraclon Injection 3057

BARIPRIL (Spain)
ENALAPRIL MALEATE
Vasotec Tablets 2210

BARIPRIL DIU (Spain)
ENALAPRIL MALEATE/HYDROCHLOROTHIAZIDE
Vaseretic Tablets 2204

BARMICIL (Mexico)
GENTAMICIN SULFATE
Genoptic Ophthalmic Ointment . . . . ⊙239
Genoptic Sterile Ophthalmic Solution . . . . ⊙239

BAROTONAL (Germany)
HYDROCHLOROTHIAZIDE
HydroDIURIL Tablets 2108
Microzide Capsules 3414

BARRIERE-HC (Canada)
HYDROCORTISONE
Anusol-HC Cream 2.5% 2237
Hydrocortone Tablets 2106

BASIRON (Denmark, Finland, Norway, Sweden, Switzerland, The Netherlands)
BENZOYL PEROXIDE
Brevoxyl-4 Cleansing Lotion 3269
Brevoxyl-4 Creamy Wash 3270
Brevoxyl-4 Gel 3269
Brevoxyl-8 Cleansing Lotion 3269
Brevoxyl-8 Creamy Wash 3270
Brevoxyl-8 Gel 3269
Triaz Cleanser 2026
Triaz Gel 2026

BASOCIN (Germany)
CLINDAMYCIN PHOSPHATE
Cleocin Phosphate Sterile Solution 2785
Cleocin T Topical Gel 2790
Cleocin T Topical Lotion 2790
Cleocin T Topical Solution 2790
Cleocin Vaginal Cream 2788
Clindets Pledgets 3270

BASSADO (Italy)
DOXYCYCLINE HYCLATE
Doryx Coated Pellet Filled Capsules 3357
Periostat Tablets 1208
Vibra-Tabs Film Coated Tablets 2735
Vibramycin Hyclate Capsules 2735
Vibramycin Hyclate Intravenous 2737

BATMEN (Spain)
PREDNICARBATE
Dermatop Emollient Cream 2517

BATRAFEN (Germany, Hong Kong, Irish Republic, New Zealand, Spain, Switzerland)
CICLOPIROX OLAMINE
Loprox Cream 2021
Loprox Lotion 2021

BAXAN (United Kingdom)
CEFADROXIL
Duricef Capsules 1079
Duricef Oral Suspension 1079
Duricef Tablets 1079

BAXO (Japan)
PIROXICAM
Feldene Capsules 2685

BAYCOL (Canada, South Africa)
CERIVASTATIN SODIUM
Baycol Tablets 883

BAYCUTEN (Brazil, Portugal)
CLOTRIMAZOLE
Lotrimin Cream 1% 3128
Lotrimin Lotion 1% 3128
Lotrimin Topical Solution 1% 3128
Mycelex Troche 573

BAYCUTEN SD (Germany)
CLOTRIMAZOLE
Lotrimin Cream 1% 3128
Lotrimin Lotion 1% 3128
Lotrimin Topical Solution 1% 3128
Mycelex Troche 573

BEAMAT (Mexico)
CIMETIDINE
Tagamet Tablets 1644

BEAMOKEN A (Mexico)
DEXAMETHASONE
Decadron Elixir 2078
Decadron Tablets 2079

BEAPHENICOL (Singapore)
CHLORAMPHENICOL
Chloromycetin Ophthalmic Ointment, 1% . . . . ⊙296
Chloromycetin Ophthalmic Solution . . . . ⊙297
Chloroptic Sterile Ophthalmic Ointment . . . . ⊙234
Chloroptic Sterile Ophthalmic Solution . . . . ⊙235

BECABIL (Spain)
AMOXICILLIN
Amoxil Pediatric Drops for Oral Suspension 1471
Amoxil Tablets 1471

BECENUN (Brazil, Denmark, Norway, Sweden)
CARMUSTINE
Gliadel Wafer 1723

BEDORMA NOUVELLE FORMULATION (Switzerland)
DIPHENHYDRAMINE HYDROCHLORIDE
Benadryl Parenteral 2617

BEDRANOL (Switzerland, United Kingdom)
PROPRANOLOL HYDROCHLORIDE
Inderal Injectable 3513
Inderal LA Long-Acting Capsules 3516
Inderal Tablets 3513

BEGLAN (Spain)
SALMETEROL XINAFOATE
Serevent Diskus 1637
Serevent Inhalation Aerosol 1633

BEKIDIBA (Mexico)
DEXTROMETHORPHAN HYDROBROMIDE/GUAIFENESIN
Tussi-Organidin DM NR Liquid 3350
Tussi-Organidin DM-S NR Liquid 3350

BELIDRAL (Belgium)
AMILORIDE HYDROCHLORIDE/HYDROCHLOROTHIAZIDE
Moduretic Tablets 2138

BELIVON (Austria, Italy)
RISPERIDONE
Risperdal Oral Solution 1796
Risperdal Tablets 1796

BELLADENAL (France, Germany, South Africa, Spain)
BELLADONNA ALKALOIDS/PHENOBARBITAL
Donnatal Capsules 2929
Donnatal Elixir 2929
Donnatal Extentabs 2930
Donnatal Tablets 2929

BELMACINA (Spain)
CIPROFLOXACIN HYDROCHLORIDE
Ciloxan Ophthalmic Ointment 538
Ciloxan Ophthalmic Solution . . . . ⊙209, 538
Cipro Tablets 887

BELMALAX (Spain)
LACTULOSE
Kristalose for Oral Solution 1007

BELMAZOL (Spain)
OMEPRAZOLE
Prilosec Delayed-Release Capsules 628

BELOC-ZOK (Switzerland)
METOPROLOL SUCCINATE
Toprol-XL Tablets 651

BELTOP (Austria)
KETOCONAZOLE
Nizoral 2% Cream 3620
Nizoral 2% Shampoo 2007
Nizoral Tablets 1791

BEMETRAZOLE (South Africa)
METRONIDAZOLE
MetroCream 1404
MetroGel 1405
MetroGel-Vaginal Gel 1986
MetroLotion 1405
Noritate Cream 1224

BENACNE (Portugal)
BENZOYL PEROXIDE
Brevoxyl-4 Cleansing Lotion 3269
Brevoxyl-4 Creamy Wash 3270
Brevoxyl-4 Gel 3269
Brevoxyl-8 Cleansing Lotion 3269
Brevoxyl-8 Creamy Wash 3270
Brevoxyl-8 Gel 3269
Triaz Cleanser 2026
Triaz Gel 2026

BENADRYL (Australia, Italy, Hong Kong, South Africa, Spain, Switzerland, Thailand)
DIPHENHYDRAMINE HYDROCHLORIDE
Benadryl Parenteral 2617

BENADRYL N (Germany)
DIPHENHYDRAMINE HYDROCHLORIDE
Benadryl Parenteral 2617

BENALAPRIL (Germany)
ENALAPRIL MALEATE
Vasotec Tablets ... 2210

BENAXIMA (Mexico)
CEFOTAXIME SODIUM
Claforan Injection ... 732

BENAXONA (Mexico)
CEFTRIAXONE SODIUM
Rocephin Injectable Vials, ADD-Vantage, Galaxy, Bulk ... 2993

BENDA (Thailand)
MEBENDAZOLE
Vermox Chewable Tablets ... 2017

BENDAPAR (Mexico)
ALBENDAZOLE
Albenza Tablets ... 1463

BENDEX (South Africa)
ALBENDAZOLE
Albenza Tablets ... 1463

BENDRAX (Brazil)
MEBENDAZOLE
Vermox Chewable Tablets ... 2017

BENECUT (Austria)
NAFTIFINE HYDROCHLORIDE
Naftin Cream ... 2224
Naftin Gel ... 2224

BENEDAXOL (Mexico)
MEBENDAZOLE
Vermox Chewable Tablets ... 2017

BENEFLUR (Spain)
FLUDARABINE PHOSPHATE
Fludara for Injection ... 995

BENEVRAN (Brazil)
DICLOFENAC POTASSIUM
Cataflam Tablets ... 2315

BENFOFEN (Germany)
DICLOFENAC SODIUM
Voltaren Tablets ... 2315
Voltaren-XR Tablets ... 2315

BENHEX (New Zealand)
LINDANE
Lindane Lotion USP 1% ... 559
Lindane Shampoo USP 1% ... 560

BENOCTEN (Switzerland)
DIPHENHYDRAMINE HYDROCHLORIDE
Benadryl Parenteral ... 2617

BENOQUIN (Canada)
MONOBENZONE
Benoquin Cream 20% ... 1732

BENOSID (Germany)
BUDESONIDE
Pulmicort Turbuhaler Inhalation Powder ... 636
Rhinocort Nasal Inhaler ... 640

BENOXID (Italy)
BENZOYL PEROXIDE
Brevoxyl-4 Cleansing Lotion ... 3269
Brevoxyl-4 Creamy Wash ... 3270
Brevoxyl-4 Gel ... 3269
Brevoxyl-8 Cleansing Lotion ... 3269
Brevoxyl-8 Creamy Wash ... 3270
Brevoxyl-8 Gel ... 3269
Triaz Cleanser ... 2026
Triaz Gel ... 2026

BENOXYGEL (Portugal, Spain)
BENZOYL PEROXIDE
Brevoxyl-4 Cleansing Lotion ... 3269
Brevoxyl-4 Creamy Wash ... 3270
Brevoxyl-4 Gel ... 3269
Brevoxyl-8 Cleansing Lotion ... 3269
Brevoxyl-8 Creamy Wash ... 3270
Brevoxyl-8 Gel ... 3269
Triaz Cleanser ... 2026
Triaz Gel ... 2026

BENOXYL (Australia, Canada, Irish Republic, Mexico, New Zealand, South Africa, United Kingdom)
BENZOYL PEROXIDE
Brevoxyl-4 Cleansing Lotion ... 3269
Brevoxyl-4 Creamy Wash ... 3270
Brevoxyl-4 Gel ... 3269
Brevoxyl-8 Cleansing Lotion ... 3269
Brevoxyl-8 Creamy Wash ... 3270
Brevoxyl-8 Gel ... 3269
Triaz Cleanser ... 2026
Triaz Gel ... 2026

BENPINE (Singapore, Thailand)
CHLORDIAZEPOXIDE HYDROCHLORIDE
Librium Capsules ... 1736
Librium for Injection ... 1737

BENSOLMIN (Mexico)
MEBENDAZOLE
Vermox Chewable Tablets ... 2017

BENTIAMIN (Brazil)
ALBENDAZOLE
Albenza Tablets ... 1463

BENYLAN (Finland, Sweden)
DIPHENHYDRAMINE HYDROCHLORIDE
Benadryl Parenteral ... 2617

BENYLIN (France)
DIPHENHYDRAMINE HYDROCHLORIDE
Benadryl Parenteral ... 2617

BENYLIN ANTIHISTAMINICUM (Belgium)
DIPHENHYDRAMINE HYDROCHLORIDE
Benadryl Parenteral ... 2617

BENYLIN CHILDRENS CHESTY COUGHS (United Kingdom)
GUAIFENESIN
Organidin NR Liquid ... 3350
Organidin NR Tablets ... 3350

BENYLIN DM-E (Canada)
DEXTROMETHORPHAN HYDROBROMIDE/GUAIFENESIN
Tussi-Organidin DM NR Liquid ... 3350
Tussi-Organidin DM-S NR Liquid ... 3350

BENYLIN NON-DROWSY CHESTY COUGHS (Irish Republic)
GUAIFENESIN
Organidin NR Liquid ... 3350
Organidin NR Tablets ... 3350

BENYLIN PAEDIATRIC (Switzerland)
DIPHENHYDRAMINE HYDROCHLORIDE
Benadryl Parenteral ... 2617

BENYLIN-DIFENHYDRAMINEHYDROCHLORIDE (The Netherlands)
DIPHENHYDRAMINE HYDROCHLORIDE
Benadryl Parenteral ... 2617

BENYLIN-E (Canada)
GUAIFENESIN
Organidin NR Liquid ... 3350
Organidin NR Tablets ... 3350

BENZAC (Australia, Belgium, Brazil, Canada, Italy, Mexico, New Zealand, Portugal, Singapore, Switzerland, Thailand, The Netherlands)
BENZOYL PEROXIDE
Brevoxyl-4 Cleansing Lotion ... 3269
Brevoxyl-4 Creamy Wash ... 3270
Brevoxyl-4 Gel ... 3269
Brevoxyl-8 Cleansing Lotion ... 3269
Brevoxyl-8 Creamy Wash ... 3270
Brevoxyl-8 Gel ... 3269
Triaz Cleanser ... 2026
Triaz Gel ... 2026

BENZAC-AC (Brazil, Hong Kong, Israel, South Africa)
BENZOYL PEROXIDE
Brevoxyl-4 Cleansing Lotion ... 3269
Brevoxyl-4 Creamy Wash ... 3270
Brevoxyl-4 Gel ... 3269
Brevoxyl-8 Cleansing Lotion ... 3269
Brevoxyl-8 Creamy Wash ... 3270
Brevoxyl-8 Gel ... 3269
Triaz Cleanser ... 2026
Triaz Gel ... 2026

BENZADERM (Mexico)
BENZOYL PEROXIDE
Brevoxyl-4 Cleansing Lotion ... 3269
Brevoxyl-4 Creamy Wash ... 3270
Brevoxyl-4 Gel ... 3269
Brevoxyl-8 Cleansing Lotion ... 3269
Brevoxyl-8 Creamy Wash ... 3270
Brevoxyl-8 Gel ... 3269
Triaz Cleanser ... 2026
Triaz Gel ... 2026

BENZAGEL (Brazil, Canada, France, United Kingdom)
BENZOYL PEROXIDE
Brevoxyl-4 Cleansing Lotion ... 3269
Brevoxyl-4 Creamy Wash ... 3270
Brevoxyl-4 Gel ... 3269
Brevoxyl-8 Cleansing Lotion ... 3269
Brevoxyl-8 Creamy Wash ... 3270
Brevoxyl-8 Gel ... 3269
Triaz Cleanser ... 2026
Triaz Gel ... 2026

BENZAKNEN (Austria, Germany)
BENZOYL PEROXIDE
Brevoxyl-4 Cleansing Lotion ... 3269
Brevoxyl-4 Creamy Wash ... 3270
Brevoxyl-4 Gel ... 3269
Brevoxyl-8 Cleansing Lotion ... 3269
Brevoxyl-8 Creamy Wash ... 3270
Brevoxyl-8 Gel ... 3269
Triaz Cleanser ... 2026
Triaz Gel ... 2026

BENZAMYCIN (Belgium, Canada, Hong Kong, Israel, Mexico, United Kingdom)
BENZOYL PEROXIDE
Brevoxyl-4 Cleansing Lotion ... 3269
Brevoxyl-4 Creamy Wash ... 3270
Brevoxyl-4 Gel ... 3269
Brevoxyl-8 Cleansing Lotion ... 3269
Brevoxyl-8 Creamy Wash ... 3270
Brevoxyl-8 Gel ... 3269
Triaz Cleanser ... 2026
Triaz Gel ... 2026

BENZAMYCINE (South Africa)
BENZOYL PEROXIDE
Brevoxyl-4 Cleansing Lotion ... 3269
Brevoxyl-4 Creamy Wash ... 3270
Brevoxyl-4 Gel ... 3269
Brevoxyl-8 Cleansing Lotion ... 3269
Brevoxyl-8 Creamy Wash ... 3270
Brevoxyl-8 Gel ... 3269
Triaz Cleanser ... 2026
Triaz Gel ... 2026

BENZEVIT (Brazil)
NYSTATIN
Nystop Topical Powder USP ... 2608

BENZODERM MYCO (Germany)
CLOTRIMAZOLE
Lotrimin Cream 1% ... 3128
Lotrimin Lotion 1% ... 3128
Lotrimin Topical Solution 1% ... 3128
Mycelex Troche ... 573

BENZODIAPIN (Italy)
CHLORDIAZEPOXIDE HYDROCHLORIDE
Librium Capsules ... 1736
Librium for Injection ... 1737

BENZOMIX (Italy)
BENZOYL PEROXIDE
Brevoxyl-4 Cleansing Lotion ... 3269
Brevoxyl-4 Creamy Wash ... 3270
Brevoxyl-4 Gel ... 3269
Brevoxyl-8 Cleansing Lotion ... 3269
Brevoxyl-8 Creamy Wash ... 3270
Brevoxyl-8 Gel ... 3269
Triaz Cleanser ... 2026
Triaz Gel ... 2026

BENZOPIN (South Africa)
DIAZEPAM
Valium Injectable ... 3026
Valium Tablets ... 3047

BENZOYT (Germany)
BENZOYL PEROXIDE
Brevoxyl-4 Cleansing Lotion ... 3269
Brevoxyl-4 Creamy Wash ... 3270
Brevoxyl-4 Gel ... 3269
Brevoxyl-8 Cleansing Lotion ... 3269
Brevoxyl-8 Creamy Wash ... 3270
Brevoxyl-8 Gel ... 3269
Triaz Cleanser ... 2026
Triaz Gel ... 2026

BENZYME (Mexico)
DIAZEPAM
Valium Injectable ... 3026
Valium Tablets ... 3047

BEOCID PUROPTAL (Austria)
SULFACETAMIDE SODIUM
Bleph-10 Ophthalmic Ointment 10% ... ⊙230
Klaron Lotion 10% ... 1224

BEPHEN (Hong Kong)
TRIFLURIDINE
Viroptic Ophthalmic Solution Sterile ... ⊙301

BEPRANE (France)
PROPRANOLOL HYDROCHLORIDE
Inderal Injectable ... 3513
Inderal LA Long-Acting Capsules ... 3516
Inderal Tablets ... 3513

BERAMICINA (Mexico)
GENTAMICIN SULFATE
Genoptic Ophthalmic Ointment ... ⊙239
Genoptic Sterile Ophthalmic Solution ... ⊙239

BERAZOLE (South Africa)
METRONIDAZOLE
MetroCream ... 1404
MetroGel ... 1405
MetroGel-Vaginal Gel ... 1986
MetroLotion ... 1405
Noritate Cream ... 1224

BERKATENS (Irish Republic, United Kingdom)
VERAPAMIL HYDROCHLORIDE
Covera-HS Tablets ... 3199
Isoptin SR Tablets ... 467
Verelan Capsules ... 3184
Verelan PM Capsules ... 3186

BERKOLOL (Hong Kong, Irish Republic, United Kingdom)
PROPRANOLOL HYDROCHLORIDE
Inderal Injectable ... 3513
Inderal LA Long-Acting Capsules ... 3516
Inderal Tablets ... 3513

BERLISON (Brazil)
HYDROCORTISONE ACETATE
Anusol-HC Suppositories ... 2238
Cortifoam Rectal Foam ... 3170
Hydrocortone Acetate Injectable Suspension ... 2103
Proctocort Suppositories ... 2264

BERTOCIL (Portugal)
BETAXOLOL HYDROCHLORIDE
Betoptic S Ophthalmic Suspension ... ⊙208, 537

BESITRAN (Spain)
SERTRALINE HYDROCHLORIDE
Zoloft Tablets ... 2751

BETA MICOTER (Spain)
BETAMETHASONE DIPROPIONATE/CLOTRIMAZOLE
Lotrisone Cream ... 3129

BETA-ADALAT (Finland, United Kingdom)
ATENOLOL
Tenormin I.V. Injection ... 692

BETA-CARDONE (United Kingdom)
SOTALOL HYDROCHLORIDE
Betapace Tablets ... 950

BETACEF (Italy, South Africa)
CEFOXITIN SODIUM
Mefoxin Premixed Intravenous Solution ... 2127
Mefoxin for Injection ... 2124

BETACLOPRAMIDE (South Africa)
METOCLOPRAMIDE HYDROCHLORIDE
Reglan Injectable ... 2935
Reglan Syrup ... 2935
Reglan Tablets ... 2935

BETADES (Italy)
SOTALOL HYDROCHLORIDE
Betapace Tablets ... 950

BETADIUR (Switzerland)
AMILORIDE HYDROCHLORIDE/HYDROCHLOROTHIAZIDE
Moduretic Tablets ... 2138

BETADREN (Italy)
LABETALOL HYDROCHLORIDE
Normodyne Injection ... 3135
Normodyne Tablets ... 3137

BETADUR CR (United Kingdom)
PROPRANOLOL HYDROCHLORIDE
Inderal Injectable ... 3513
Inderal LA Long-Acting Capsules ... 3516
Inderal Tablets ... 3513

BETAFERON (Australia, Austria, Belgium, Brazil, Denmark, Finland, France, Germany, Irish Republic, Israel, Italy, Mexico, New Zealand, Norway, Portugal, Singapore, South Africa, Spain, Sweden, Switzerland, The Netherlands, United Kingdom)
INTERFERON BETA-1B
Betaseron for SC Injection ... 988

BETAGESIC (South Africa)
IBUPROFEN
Motrin Suspension, Oral Drops, Chewable Tablets and Caplets ... 2002

BETAJECT (Canada)
BETAMETHASONE ACETATE/BETAMETHASONE SODIUM PHOSPHATE
Celestone Soluspan Injectable Suspension ... 3097

BETALOL (Thailand)
PROPRANOLOL HYDROCHLORIDE
Inderal Injectable ... 3513
Inderal LA Long-Acting Capsules ... 3516
Inderal Tablets ... 3513

BETAMETAGEN (Brazil)
DEXAMETHASONE
Decadron Elixir ... 2078
Decadron Tablets ... 2079

BETAMICAN (Spain)
SALMETEROL XINAFOATE
Serevent Diskus ... 1637
Serevent Inhalation Aerosol ... 1633

BETAPAM (South Africa)
DIAZEPAM
Valium Injectable ... 3026
Valium Tablets ... 3047

BETAPRESS (Thailand)
PROPRANOLOL HYDROCHLORIDE
Inderal Injectable ... 3513
Inderal LA Long-Acting Capsules ... 3516
Inderal Tablets ... 3513

BETAPROFEN (South Africa)
IBUPROFEN
Motrin Suspension, Oral Drops, Chewable Tablets, and Caplets **2002**

BETA-PROGRANE (United Kingdom)
PROPRANOLOL HYDROCHLORIDE
Inderal Injectable **3513**
Inderal LA Long-Acting Capsules **3516**
Inderal Tablets. **3513**

BETAPROL (Switzerland)
PROPRANOLOL HYDROCHLORIDE
Inderal Injectable **3513**
Inderal LA Long-Acting Capsules **3516**
Inderal Tablets. **3513**

BETAREN (Israel)
DICLOFENAC SODIUM
Voltaren Tablets **2315**
Voltaren-XR Tablets **2315**

BETARETIC (South Africa)
AMILORIDE HYDROCHLORIDE/HYDROCHLOROTHIAZIDE
Moduretic Tablets. **2138**

BETASERON (Canada)
INTERFERON BETA-1B
Betaseron for SC Injection **988**

BETASLEEP (South Africa)
DIPHENHYDRAMINE HYDROCHLORIDE
Benadryl Parenteral **2617**

BETASOL (Thailand)
CLOBETASOL PROPIONATE
Cormax Cream **2440**
Cormax Ointment **2440**
Cormax Scalp Application. **2441**
Temovate Cream **1301**
Temovate E Emollient **1302**
Temovate Gel **1303**
Temovate Ointment. **1301**
Temovate Scalp Application **1304**

BETASYN (Austria)
ATENOLOL
Tenormin I.V. Injection **692**

BETA-TABLINEN (Germany)
PROPRANOLOL HYDROCHLORIDE
Inderal Injectable **3513**
Inderal LA Long-Acting Capsules **3516**
Inderal Tablets. **3513**

BETATHIAZID A (Germany)
HYDROCHLOROTHIAZIDE/PROPRANOLOL HYDROCHLORIDE
Inderide LA Long-Acting Capsules. **3519**
Inderide Tablets. **3517**

BETA-TIM (Canada)
TIMOLOL MALEATE
Blocadren Tablets **2046**
Timoptic Sterile Ophthalmic Solution **2190**
Timoptic in Ocudose. **2192**
Timoptic-XE Sterile Ophthalmic Gel Forming Solution. **2194**

BETA-TIMELETS (Germany)
PROPRANOLOL HYDROCHLORIDE
Inderal Injectable **3513**
Inderal LA Long-Acting Capsules **3516**
Inderal Tablets. **3513**

BETATOP (France)
ATENOLOL
Tenormin I.V. Injection **692**

BETAZOK (Irish Republic)
METOPROLOL SUCCINATE
Toprol-XL Tablets **651**

BETHACIL (Italy)
AMPICILLIN SODIUM/SULBACTAM SODIUM
Unasyn for Injection **2728**

BETIM (Irish Republic, Norway, United Kingdom)
TIMOLOL MALEATE
Blocadren Tablets **2046**
Timoptic Sterile Ophthalmic Solution **2190**
Timoptic in Ocudose. **2192**
Timoptic-XE Sterile Ophthalmic Gel Forming Solution. **2194**

BETOPTIC (Australia, Austria, Belgium, Brazil, Canada, Denmark, Finland, France, Hong Kong, Irish Republic, Israel, Italy, Mexico, New Zealand, Norway, Portugal, Singapore, South Africa, Spain, Sweden, Thailand, The Netherlands, United Kingdom)
BETAXOLOL HYDROCHLORIDE
Betoptic S Ophthalmic Suspension . . . . **⊙208, 537**

BETOPTIC-S (Switzerland)
BETAXOLOL HYDROCHLORIDE
Betoptic S Ophthalmic Suspension . . . . **⊙208, 537**

BETOPTIMA (Germany)
BETAXOLOL HYDROCHLORIDE
Betoptic S Ophthalmic Suspension . . . . **⊙208, 537**

BETOQUIN (Australia)
BETAXOLOL HYDROCHLORIDE
Betoptic S Ophthalmic Suspension . . . . **⊙208, 537**

BETULAC (Sweden)
LACTULOSE
Kristalose for Oral Solution. **1007**

BEXILONA (Spain)
DIFLORASONE DIACETATE
Psorcon E Cream. **1227**
Psorcon E Ointment **1228**

BEXINOR (Singapore)
NORFLOXACIN
Chibroxin Sterile Ophthalmic Solution . . . . **⊙273, 2051**
Noroxin Tablets **2145**

BIALZEPAM (Portugal)
DIAZEPAM
Valium Injectable **3026**
Valium Tablets **3047**

BIAMOTIL (Brazil)
CIPROFLOXACIN HYDROCHLORIDE
Ciloxan Ophthalmic Ointment. **538**
Ciloxan Ophthalmic Solution . . . . **⊙209, 538**
Cipro Tablets. **887**

BIARTAC (Belgium)
DIFLUNISAL
Dolobid Tablets **2088**

BIAXIN (Canada, Germany)
CLARITHROMYCIN
Biaxin Filmtab Tablets **403**
Biaxin for Oral Suspension **403**

BICAIN (Finland)
BUPIVACAINE HYDROCHLORIDE
Sensorcaine Injection **643**
Sensorcaine-MPF Injection **643**

BICAM (Thailand)
PIROXICAM
Feldene Capsules. **2685**

BICIDE (Israel)
LINDANE
Lindane Lotion USP 1% **559**
Lindane Shampoo USP 1% **560**

BICLAR (Belgium)
CLARITHROMYCIN
Biaxin Filmtab Tablets **403**
Biaxin for Oral Suspension **403**

BICLOPAN (Singapore)
DICLOFENAC SODIUM
Voltaren Tablets **2315**
Voltaren-XR Tablets **2315**

BICNU (Australia, Canada, France, Hong Kong, Irish Republic, Israel, Mexico, New Zealand, Singapore, South Africa, Thailand, United Kingdom)
CARMUSTINE
Gliadel Wafer **1723**

BICONCOR (Mexico)
BISOPROLOL FUMARATE/HYDROCHLOROTHIAZIDE
Ziac Tablets **1887**

BIDIEN (Italy)
BUDESONIDE
Pulmicort Turbuhaler Inhalation Powder . . . **636**
Rhinocort Nasal Inhaler **640**

BIDOCEF (Germany)
CEFADROXIL
Duricef Capsules **1079**
Duricef Oral Suspension. **1079**
Duricef Tablets **1079**

BIFARDOL S (Mexico)
NAPROXEN SODIUM
Anaprox DS Tablets **2967**
Anaprox Tablets. **2967**
Naprelan Tablets **1293**

BIFEN (Singapore)
IBUPROFEN
Motrin Suspension, Oral Drops, Chewable Tablets, and Caplets **2002**

BIFINORMA (Germany)
LACTULOSE
Kristalose for Oral Solution. **1007**

BIFITERAL (Austria, Belgium, Germany)
LACTULOSE
Kristalose for Oral Solution. **1007**

BIKALM (Germany)
ZOLPIDEM TARTRATE
Ambien Tablets **3191**

BILORDYL (Germany)
THEOPHYLLINE
Aerolate Jr. T.D. Capsules **1361**
Aerolate Liquid **1361**
Aerolate Sr. T.D. Capsules **1361**
Theo-Dur Extended-Release Tablets. **1835**
Uni-Dur Extended-Release Tablets **1841**
Uniphyl 400 mg and 600 mg Tablets . . . **2903**

BILTRICIDE (Australia, Canada, France, Germany, Hong Kong, Israel, South Africa, Thailand, The Netherlands)
PRAZIQUANTEL
Biltricide Tablets **887**

BINORDIOL (Belgium)
LEVONORGESTREL
Norplant System **3543**

BIOCARN (Germany)
LEVOCARNITINE
Carnitor Injection **3242**
Carnitor Tablets and Oral Solution **3245**

BIOCEF (Austria, Spain)
CEFPODOXIME PROXETIL
Vantin Tablets and Oral Suspension. **2860**

BIOCICLIN (Italy)
CEFUROXIME SODIUM
Kefurox Vials, ADD-Vantage. **1948**
Zinacef Injection. **1696**

BIOCINE TEST (South Africa)
TUBERCULIN
Aplisol Injection **2609**
Tine Test, Tuberculin, Old **3631**
Tubersol Diagnostic Antigen **3628**

BIOCORD (Brazil)
NIFEDIPINE
Adalat CC Tablets. **877**
Procardia Capsules. **2708**
Procardia XL Extended Release Tablets . . **2710**

BIOCORT (South Africa)
HYDROCORTISONE ACETATE
Anusol-HC Suppositories **2238**
Cortifoam Rectal Foam **3170**
Hydrocortone Acetate Injectable Suspension **2103**
Proctocort Suppositories **2264**

BIOCORYL (Spain)
PROCAINAMIDE HYDROCHLORIDE
Procanbid Extended-Release Tablets **2262**

BIOCOS (Germany)
METFORMIN HYDROCHLORIDE
Glucophage Tablets **1080**

BIOCYCLIN (Austria)
DOXYCYCLINE HYCLATE
Doryx Coated Pellet Filled Capsules **3357**
Periostat Tablets **1208**
Vibramycin Hyclate Capsules. **2735**
Vibramycin Hyclate Intravenous **2737**
Vibra-Tabs Film Coated Tablets **2735**

BIODALGIC (France)
TRAMADOL HYDROCHLORIDE
Ultram Tablets. **2600**

BIODEZIL (Mexico)
CAPTOPRIL
Captopril Tablets **2281**

BIODROXIL (Austria, Hong Kong, Singapore)
CEFADROXIL
Duricef Capsules **1079**
Duricef Oral Suspension. **1079**
Duricef Tablets **1079**

BIOFANAL (Germany)
NYSTATIN
Nystop Topical Powder USP **2608**

BIOFAXIL (Portugal)
CEFADROXIL
Duricef Capsules **1079**
Duricef Oral Suspension. **1079**
Duricef Tablets **1079**

BIOFERON (Thailand)
INTERFERON ALFA-2B
Intron A for Injection. **3120**

BIOFLOX (Mexico)
CIPROFLOXACIN
Cipro I.V. **893**
Cipro I.V. Pharmacy Bulk Package **897**
Cipro Oral Suspension. **887**

BIOFUREX (Italy)
CEFUROXIME SODIUM
Kefurox Vials, ADD-Vantage. **1948**
Zinacef Injection. **1696**

BIOGEN (Spain)
GENTAMICIN SULFATE
Genoptic Ophthalmic Ointment . . . . **⊙239**
Genoptic Sterile Ophthalmic Solution . . . **⊙239**

BIOGYL (Thailand)
METRONIDAZOLE
MetroCream **1404**
MetroGel **1405**
MetroGel-Vaginal Gel **1986**
MetroLotion **1405**
Noritate Cream **1224**

BIOLON (Canada, Germany, Israel, Italy, Mexico, Switzerland)
SODIUM HYALURONATE
Hyalgan Solution **3080**

BIOLONE (South Africa)
SODIUM HYALURONATE
Hyalgan Solution **3080**

BIOMAG (Italy)
CIMETIDINE
Tagamet Tablets **1644**

BIOMARGEN (Spain)
GENTAMICIN SULFATE
Genoptic Ophthalmic Ointment . . . . **⊙239**
Genoptic Sterile Ophthalmic Solution . . . **⊙239**

BIOMINOL A (Spain)
VITAMIN A PALMITATE
Aquasol A Parenteral. **593**

BIOMIORAN (Italy)
CHLORZOXAZONE
Parafon Forte DSC Caplets. **2582**

BIOMONA (Mexico)
METRONIDAZOLE
MetroCream **1404**
MetroGel **1405**
MetroGel-Vaginal Gel **1986**
MetroLotion **1405**
Noritate Cream **1224**

BIOMOX (Thailand)
AMOXICILLIN
Amoxil Pediatric Drops for Oral Suspension **1471**
Amoxil Tablets. **1471**

BIONICARD (Italy)
NICARDIPINE HYDROCHLORIDE
Cardene I.V. **3485**

BIONIF (Italy)
NIFEDIPINE
Adalat CC Tablets. **877**
Procardia Capsules. **2708**
Procardia XL Extended Release Tablets . . **2710**

BIOPERAZONE (Italy)
CEFOPERAZONE SODIUM
Cefobid Intravenous/Intramuscular **2671**
Cefobid Pharmacy Bulk Package - Not for Direct Infusion **2673**

BIOPERIDOLO (Italy)
HALOPERIDOL
Haldol Injection, Tablets and Concentrate. **2533**

BIOPHYLLIN (South Africa)
THEOPHYLLINE
Aerolate Jr. T.D. Capsules **1361**
Aerolate Liquid **1361**
Aerolate Sr. T.D. Capsules **1361**
Theo-Dur Extended-Release Tablets. **1835**
Uni-Dur Extended-Release Tablets. **1841**
Uniphyl 400 mg and 600 mg Tablets . . . **2903**

BIOPLASMA FDP (South Africa)
PLASMA PROTEIN FRACTION
Plasmanate. **942**

BIOPORINA (Spain)
CEPHALEXIN
Keflex Oral Suspension **1237**
Keflex Pulvules **1237**

BIOQUIL (Portugal)
OFLOXACIN
Floxin I.V. **2526**
Floxin Otic Solution. **1219**
Floxin Tablets **2529**
Ocuflox Ophthalmic Solution **554**

BIOSCEFAL (Spain)
CEPHALEXIN
Keflex Oral Suspension **1237**
Keflex Pulvules **1237**

BIOSINT (Mexico)
CEFOTAXIME SODIUM
Claforan Injection **732**

BIOTAZOL (Mexico)
METRONIDAZOLE
MetroCream **1404**
MetroGel **1405**
MetroGel-Vaginal Gel **1986**
MetroLotion **1405**

Noritate Cream 1224

BIOTERCICLIN (Italy)
DEMECLOCYCLINE HYDROCHLORIDE
Declomycin Tablets. 1855

BIOTRIL (Mexico)
ERYTHROMYCIN
Emgel 2% Topical Gel 1285
Ery-Tab Tablets 448
Erythromycin Base Filmtab Tablets 454
Erythromycin Delayed-Release Capsules, USP. 455
PCE Dispertab Tablets. 498

BIO-VAGIN (Brazil)
METRONIDAZOLE
MetroCream 1404
MetroGel 1405
MetroGel-Vaginal Gel 1986
MetroLotion 1405
Noritate Cream 1224

BIOVELBIN (Spain)
VINORELBINE TARTRATE
Navelbine Injection 1604

BIOXAN (Mexico)
NAPROXEN
EC-Naprosyn Delayed-Release Tablets . . . 2967
Naprosyn Suspension 2967
Naprosyn Tablets 2967

BIOXEL (Mexico)
FLUCONAZOLE
Diflucan Tablets, Injection, and Oral Suspension 2681

BIOXIMA (Italy)
CEFUROXIME SODIUM
Kefurox Vials, ADD-Vantage. 1948
Zinacef Injection. 1696

BIOXIMIL (Mexico)
PIROXICAM
Feldene Capsules. 2685

BIOZOLE (Thailand)
FLUCONAZOLE
Diflucan Tablets, Injection, and Oral Suspension 2681

BIOZOLENE (Italy)
FLUCONAZOLE
Diflucan Tablets, Injection, and Oral Suspension 2681

BIPRANIX (United Kingdom)
BISOPROLOL FUMARATE
Zebeta Tablets 1885

BI-PROFENID (France)
KETOPROFEN
Orudis Capsules 3548
Oruvail Capsules 3548

BIPRONYL (Singapore)
NAPROXEN
EC-Naprosyn Delayed-Release Tablets . . . 2967
Naprosyn Suspension 2967
Naprosyn Tablets 2967

BIROBIN (Austria)
METOLAZONE
Mykrox Tablets 1168
Zaroxolyn Tablets. 1177

BIROFENID (Belgium)
KETOPROFEN
Orudis Capsules 3548
Oruvail Capsules 3548

BIROXOL (Italy)
CICLOPIROX OLAMINE
Loprox Cream. 2021
Loprox Lotion 2021

BISOBLOC (Germany, The Netherlands)
BISOPROLOL FUMARATE
Zebeta Tablets 1885

BISOCOR (Denmark)
BISOPROLOL FUMARATE
Zebeta Tablets 1885

BISOMERCK (Germany)
BISOPROLOL FUMARATE
Zebeta Tablets 1885

BISOPINE (Irish Republic)
BISOPROLOL FUMARATE
Zebeta Tablets 1885

BISO-PUREN (Germany)
BISOPROLOL FUMARATE
Zebeta Tablets 1885

BISTATIN (Mexico)
NYSTATIN
Nystop Topical Powder USP 2608

BITENSIL (Spain)
ENALAPRIL MALEATE
Vasotec Tablets. 2210

BITENSIL DIU (Spain)
ENALAPRIL MALEATE/HYDROCHLOROTHIAZIDE
Vaseretic Tablets 2204

BI-TILDIEM (France)
DILTIAZEM HYDROCHLORIDE
Cardizem CD Capsules 1016
Cardizem Injectable 1018
Cardizem Lyo-Ject Syringe 1018
Cardizem Monovial 1018
Tiazac Capsules 1378

BIVALEM (Brazil)
MEBENDAZOLE
Vermox Chewable Tablets. 2017

BK HC (New Zealand)
HYDROCORTISONE
Anusol-HC Cream 2.5% 2237
Hydrocortone Tablets 2106

BLASTOCARB (Mexico)
CARBOPLATIN
Paraplatin for Injection. 1126

BLEF-10 (Mexico)
SULFACETAMIDE SODIUM
Bleph-10 Ophthalmic Ointment 10% . . . . ⊙230
Klaron Lotion 10% 1224

BLEMIX (United Kingdom)
MINOCYCLINE HYDROCHLORIDE
Dynacin Capsules. 2019
Minocin Intravenous 1862
Minocin Oral Suspension 1865
Minocin Pellet-Filled Capsules 1863

BLENOX (Spain)
AMOXICILLIN
Amoxil Pediatric Drops for Oral Suspension 1471
Amoxil Tablets. 1471

BLEPH-10 (Australia, Hong Kong, Irish Republic, New Zealand, South Africa, Thailand)
SULFACETAMIDE SODIUM
Bleph-10 Ophthalmic Ointment 10% . . . . ⊙230
Klaron Lotion 10% 1224

BLEPH-10 LIQUIFILM (Canada)
SULFACETAMIDE SODIUM
Bleph-10 Ophthalmic Ointment 10% . . . . ⊙230
Klaron Lotion 10% 1224

BLEPHAMIDE (Switzerland)
PREDNISOLONE ACETATE/SULFACETAMIDE SODIUM
Blephamide Ophthalmic Ointment 547
Blephamide Ophthalmic Suspension 548

BLEPHASULF (Austria)
SULFACETAMIDE SODIUM
Bleph-10 Ophthalmic Ointment 10% . . . . ⊙230
Klaron Lotion 10% 1224

BLOCADREN (Australia, Austria, Belgium, Canada, Hong Kong, Irish Republic, Italy, Mexico, Norway, Portugal, South Africa, Spain, Sweden, Switzerland, The Netherlands, United Kingdom)
TIMOLOL MALEATE
Blocadren Tablets 2046
Timoptic Sterile Ophthalmic Solution. . . . 2190
Timoptic in Ocudose. 2192
Timoptic-XE Sterile Ophthalmic Gel Forming Solution. 2194

BLOCAN (Mexico)
CIMETIDINE
Tagamet Tablets 1644

BLOCANOL (Finland)
TIMOLOL MALEATE
Blocadren Tablets 2046
Timoptic Sterile Ophthalmic Solution. . . . 2190
Timoptic in Ocudose. 2192
Timoptic-XE Sterile Ophthalmic Gel Forming Solution. 2194

BLOCOTENOL (Germany)
ATENOLOL
Tenormin I.V. Injection 692

BLOCOTENOL COMP (Germany)
ATENOLOL
Tenormin I.V. Injection 692

BLOKIUM (Belgium, Portugal, Spain)
ATENOLOL
Tenormin I.V. Injection 692

BLOKIUM DIU (Portugal)
ATENOLOL
Tenormin I.V. Injection 692

BLOPRESS (Austria, Germany, Italy, Portugal, Switzerland, Thailand)
CANDESARTAN CILEXETIL
Atacand Tablets. 595

BOK-C-LIN (South Africa)
DOXYCYCLINE HYCLATE
Doryx Coated Pellet Filled Capsules 3357
Periostat Tablets 1208
Vibra-Tabs Film Coated Tablets 2735
Vibramycin Hyclate Capsules. 2735
Vibramycin Hyclate Intravenous 2737

BOLUTOL (Spain)
GEMFIBROZIL
Lopid Tablets 2650

BONCEUR (South Africa)
VERAPAMIL HYDROCHLORIDE
Covera-HS Tablets 3199
Isoptin SR Tablets. 467
Verelan Capsules 3184
Verelan PM Capsules 3186

BONDIL (Norway, Sweden)
ALPROSTADIL
Caverject Sterile Powder 2777
MUSE Urethral Suppository. 3335

BONIDERMA (Italy)
FLUOCINOLONE ACETONIDE
Synalar Cream 2020
Synalar Ointment 2020
Synalar Topical Solution. 2020

BONYL (Denmark)
NAPROXEN
EC-Naprosyn Delayed-Release Tablets . . . 2967
Naprosyn Suspension 2967
Naprosyn Tablets 2967

BOREA (Spain)
MEGESTROL ACETATE
Megace Oral Suspension 1124

BOROCARPIN-S (Germany)
PILOCARPINE HYDROCHLORIDE
Isopto Carpine Ophthalmic Solution . . . . ⊙215
Pilopine HS Ophthalmic Gel . . . . . ⊙217
Salagen Tablets 2229

BOXOL (Spain)
DALTEPARIN SODIUM
Fragmin Injection 2814

BRACCOPIRAL (Mexico)
PYRAZINAMIDE
Pyrazinamide Tablets 1876

BRADELMIN (Mexico)
ALBENDAZOLE
Albenza Tablets 1463

BRAINAL (Spain)
NIMODIPINE
Nimotop Capsules 904

BRAINOX (Portugal)
NIMODIPINE
Nimotop Capsules 904

BRAXAN (Mexico)
AMIODARONE HYDROCHLORIDE
Cordarone Intravenous 3491
Cordarone Tablets 3487
Pacerone Tablets 3331

BREACOL (Hong Kong)
GUAIFENESIN
Organidin NR Liquid 3350
Organidin NR Tablets. 3350

BREMON (Spain)
CLARITHROMYCIN
Biaxin Filmtab Tablets 403
Biaxin for Oral Suspension 403

BRENOXIL (Mexico)
AMOXICILLIN
Amoxil Pediatric Drops for Oral Suspension 1471
Amoxil Tablets. 1471

BRESBEN (Germany)
ATENOLOL
Tenormin I.V. Injection 692

BREVIBLOC (Australia, Austria, Belgium, Canada, Denmark, Finland, France, Germany, Hong Kong, Irish Republic, Israel, Mexico, New Zealand, Portugal, Singapore, South Africa, Spain, Sweden, Switzerland, United Kingdom)
ESMOLOL HYDROCHLORIDE
Brevibloc Injection 858

BREVIMYTAL (Germany)
METHOHEXITAL SODIUM
Brevital Sodium for Injection, USP 1815

BREVOXYL (Australia, Austria, Finland, France, Germany, Hong Kong, Irish Republic, New Zealand, Singapore, Sweden, Thailand, United Kingdom)
BENZOYL PEROXIDE
Brevoxyl-4 Cleansing Lotion 3269
Brevoxyl-4 Creamy Wash 3270
Brevoxyl-4 Gel. 3269
Brevoxyl-8 Cleansing Lotion 3269
Brevoxyl-8 Creamy Wash 3270
Brevoxyl-8 Gel. 3269
Triaz Cleanser. 2026
Triaz Gel 2026

BREXIVEL (Italy)
PIROXICAM
Feldene Capsules. 2685

BRIAZIDE (France)
BENAZEPRIL HYDROCHLORIDE/HYDROCHLOROTHIAZIDE
Lotensin HCT Tablets 2367

BRICALIN (Israel)
TERBUTALINE SULFATE
Brethine Ampuls 2314
Brethine Tablets. 2313

BRICANYL (Australia, Austria, Belgium, Brazil, Canada, Denmark, Finland, France, Germany, Hong Kong, Irish Republic, Italy, Mexico, New Zealand, Norway, Portugal, Singapore, South Africa, Sweden, Switzerland, Thailand, The Netherlands, United Kingdom)
TERBUTALINE SULFATE
Brethine Ampuls 2314
Brethine Tablets. 2313

BRICANYL EXPECTORANT (United Kingdom)
TERBUTALINE SULFATE
Brethine Ampuls 2314
Brethine Tablets. 2313

BRIEM (France)
BENAZEPRIL HYDROCHLORIDE
Lotensin Tablets. 2365

BRIETAL (Australia, Austria, Belgium, Canada, Denmark, France, Irish Republic, Israel, New Zealand, Norway, Singapore, South Africa, Sweden, Switzerland, The Netherlands, United Kingdom)
METHOHEXITAL SODIUM
Brevital Sodium for Injection, USP 1815

BRISORAL (Spain)
CEFPROZIL
Cefzil Tablets 1076
Cefzil for Oral Suspension 1076

BRISOVENT (Portugal)
FLUTICASONE PROPIONATE
Cutivate Cream 1282
Cutivate Ointment. 1284
Flonase Nasal Spray. 1533
Flovent 110 mcg Inhalation Aerosol 1535
Flovent 220 mcg Inhalation Aerosol 1535
Flovent 44 mcg Inhalation Aerosol 1535
Flovent Rotadisk 100 mcg 1537
Flovent Rotadisk 250 mcg 1537
Flovent Rotadisk 50 mcg. 1537

BRISTACOL (Spain)
PRAVASTATIN SODIUM
Pravachol Tablets. 1099

BRISTAMOX (Sweden)
AMOXICILLIN
Amoxil Pediatric Drops for Oral Suspension 1471
Amoxil Tablets. 1471

BRISTAXOL (Mexico)
PACLITAXEL
Taxol Injection. 1129

BRITIAZIM (United Kingdom)
DILTIAZEM HYDROCHLORIDE
Cardizem CD Capsules 1016
Cardizem Injectable 1018
Cardizem Lyo-Ject Syringe 1018
Cardizem Monovial 1018
Tiazac Capsules 1378

BROCIL (Mexico)
CHLORAMPHENICOL
Chloromycetin Ophthalmic Ointment, 1% . . . . . ⊙296
Chloromycetin Ophthalmic Solution . . . . ⊙297
Chloroptic Sterile Ophthalmic Ointment. . ⊙234
Chloroptic Sterile Ophthalmic Solution . . ⊙235

BROLIN (Spain)
FAMOTIDINE
Pepcid Injection. 2153
Pepcid Injection Premixed 2153
Pepcid RPD Orally Disintegrating Tablets. 2150
Pepcid Tablets. 2150
Pepcid for Oral Suspension 2150

BRONALIDE (Canada, Germany)
FLUNISOLIDE
Aerobid Inhaler System 1363

Aerobid-M Inhaler System 1363
Nasalide Nasal Spray 1295
Nasarel Nasal Solution 0.025% 1296

BRONCHOCAL (Israel)
GUAIFENESIN
Organidin NR Liquid 3350
Organidin NR Tablets 3350

BRONCHOCUX (Germany)
BUDESONIDE
Pulmicort Turbuhaler Inhalation Powder 636
Rhinocort Nasal Inhaler 640

BRONCHOL (Switzerland)
GUAIFENESIN
Organidin NR Liquid 3350
Organidin NR Tablets 3350

BRONCHOLINE (Thailand)
TERBUTALINE SULFATE
Brethine Ampuls 2314
Brethine Tablets 2313

BRONCHOPHEN (South Africa)
THEOPHYLLINE
Aerolate Jr. T.D. Capsules 1361
Aerolate Liquid 1361
Aerolate Sr. T.D. Capsules 1361
Theo-Dur Extended-Release Tablets 1835
Uni-Dur Extended-Release Tablets 1841
Uniphyl 400 mg and 600 mg Tablets 2903

BRONCHOPHYLLINE (Israel)
THEOPHYLLINE
Aerolate Jr. T.D. Capsules 1361
Aerolate Liquid 1361
Aerolate Sr. T.D. Capsules 1361
Theo-Dur Extended-Release Tablets 1835
Uni-Dur Extended-Release Tablets 1841
Uniphyl 400 mg and 600 mg Tablets 2903

BRONCHORETARD (Germany)
THEOPHYLLINE
Aerolate Jr. T.D. Capsules 1361
Aerolate Liquid 1361
Aerolate Sr. T.D. Capsules 1361
Theo-Dur Extended-Release Tablets 1835
Uni-Dur Extended-Release Tablets 1841
Uniphyl 400 mg and 600 mg Tablets 2903

BRONCO-POLIMOXIL (Brazil)
AMOXICILLIN
Amoxil Pediatric Drops for Oral Suspension 1471
Amoxil Tablets 1471

BRONCORT (Belgium, Switzerland)
FLUNISOLIDE
Aerobid Inhaler System 1363
Aerobid-M Inhaler System 1363
Nasalide Nasal Spray 1295
Nasarel Nasal Solution 0.025% 1296

BRONCOVANIL (Italy)
GUAIFENESIN
Organidin NR Liquid 3350
Organidin NR Tablets 3350

BRONILIDE (France, Switzerland)
FLUNISOLIDE
Aerobid Inhaler System 1363
Aerobid-M Inhaler System 1363
Nasalide Nasal Spray 1295
Nasarel Nasal Solution 0.025% 1296

BRONMYCIN (Singapore, Thailand)
DOXYCYCLINE HYCLATE
Doryx Coated Pellet Filled Capsules 3357
Periostat Tablets 1208
Vibra-Tabs Film Coated Tablets 2735
Vibramycin Hyclate Capsules 2735
Vibramycin Hyclate Intravenous 2737

BRONPECT-D (Thailand)
DEXTROMETHORPHAN HYDROBROMIDE/GUAIFENESIN
Tussi-Organidin DM NR Liquid 3350
Tussi-Organidin DM-S NR Liquid 3350

BRONQUIASMA (Brazil)
THEOPHYLLINE
Aerolate Jr. T.D. Capsules 1361
Aerolate Liquid 1361
Aerolate Sr. T.D. Capsules 1361
Theo-Dur Extended-Release Tablets 1835
Uni-Dur Extended-Release Tablets 1841
Uniphyl 400 mg and 600 mg Tablets 2903

BROVAFLAMP (South Africa)
DICLOFENAC SODIUM
Voltaren Tablets 2315
Voltaren-XR Tablets 2315

BRUFEN (Australia, Austria, Belgium, Denmark, Finland, France, Germany, Hong Kong, Irish Republic, New Zealand, Norway, Portugal, Singapore, South Africa, Sweden, Switzerland, Thailand, The Netherlands, United Kingdom)
IBUPROFEN
Motrin Suspension, Oral Drops, Chewable Tablets, and Caplets 2002

BRUFORT (Italy)
IBUPROFEN
Motrin Suspension, Oral Drops, Chewable Tablets, and Caplets 2002

BRUGESIC (South Africa)
IBUPROFEN
Motrin Suspension, Oral Drops, Chewable Tablets, and Caplets 2002

BRULAMYCIN (Austria, Germany)
TOBRAMYCIN SULFATE
Nebcin Vials, Hyporets & ADD-Vantage 1955

BRUMED (Thailand)
IBUPROFEN
Motrin Suspension, Oral Drops, Chewable Tablets, and Caplets 2002

BRUMETIDINA (Italy)
CIMETIDINE
Tagamet Tablets 1644

BRUMIXOL (Italy)
CICLOPIROX OLAMINE
Loprox Cream 2021
Loprox Lotion 2021

BRUNAZINE (South Africa)
PROMETHAZINE HYDROCHLORIDE
Phenergan Injection 3553
Phenergan Suppositories 3556
Phenergan Syrup Fortis 3554
Phenergan Syrup Plain 3554
Phenergan Tablets 3556

BRUPRIN (Thailand)
IBUPROFEN
Motrin Suspension, Oral Drops, Chewable Tablets, and Caplets 2002

BRUSIL (Thailand)
IBUPROFEN
Motrin Suspension, Oral Drops, Chewable Tablets, and Caplets 2002

BRUXICAM (Italy)
PIROXICAM
Feldene Capsules 2685

BUCAIN (Austria, Germany)
BUPIVACAINE HYDROCHLORIDE
Sensorcaine Injection 643
Sensorcaine-MPF Injection 643

BUCARIL (Thailand)
TERBUTALINE SULFATE
Brethine Ampuls 2314
Brethine Tablets 2313

BUCCASTEM (Irish Republic, New Zealand, United Kingdom)
PROCHLORPERAZINE MALEATE
Compazine Spansule Capsules 1505
Compazine Tablets 1505

BUCONIF (Austria)
NIFEDIPINE
Adalat CC Tablets 877
Procardia Capsules 2708
Procardia XL Extended Release Tablets 2710

BUCORT (Finland)
HYDROCORTISONE BUTYRATE
Locoid Cream 1341
Locoid Lipocream Cream 1342
Locoid Ointment 1341
Locoid Topical Solution 1341

BUDAMAX (Australia)
BUDESONIDE
Pulmicort Turbuhaler Inhalation Powder 636
Rhinocort Nasal Inhaler 640

BUDAPP (Germany)
BUDESONIDE
Pulmicort Turbuhaler Inhalation Powder 636
Rhinocort Nasal Inhaler 640

BUDECORT (Germany)
BUDESONIDE
Pulmicort Turbuhaler Inhalation Powder 636
Rhinocort Nasal Inhaler 640

BUDEFAT (Germany)
BUDESONIDE
Pulmicort Turbuhaler Inhalation Powder 636
Rhinocort Nasal Inhaler 640

BUDEFLAM (South Africa)
BUDESONIDE
Pulmicort Turbuhaler Inhalation Powder 636
Rhinocort Nasal Inhaler 640

BUDENOFALK (Germany, Switzerland, United Kingdom)
BUDESONIDE
Pulmicort Turbuhaler Inhalation Powder 636
Rhinocort Nasal Inhaler 640

BUDEPUR E (Germany)
BUDESONIDE
Pulmicort Turbuhaler Inhalation Powder 636
Rhinocort Nasal Inhaler 640

BUDES (Germany)
BUDESONIDE
Pulmicort Turbuhaler Inhalation Powder 636
Rhinocort Nasal Inhaler 640

BUDESON (Israel)
BUDESONIDE
Pulmicort Turbuhaler Inhalation Powder 636
Rhinocort Nasal Inhaler 640

BUDICORT (Israel)
BUDESONIDE
Pulmicort Turbuhaler Inhalation Powder 636
Rhinocort Nasal Inhaler 640

BUDON (Germany)
BUDESONIDE
Pulmicort Turbuhaler Inhalation Powder 636
Rhinocort Nasal Inhaler 640

BUDO-SAN (Austria)
BUDESONIDE
Pulmicort Turbuhaler Inhalation Powder 636
Rhinocort Nasal Inhaler 640

BUFEDON (Belgium, The Netherlands)
IBUPROFEN
Motrin Suspension, Oral Drops, Chewable Tablets, and Caplets 2002

BUFENO (Switzerland)
IBUPROFEN
Motrin Suspension, Oral Drops, Chewable Tablets, and Caplets 2002

BUFIGEN (Irish Republic, Mexico)
IBUPROFEN
Motrin Suspension, Oral Drops, Chewable Tablets, and Caplets 2002

BUG PROOF (United Kingdom)
PERMETHRIN
Acticin Cream 998
Elimite Cream 552

BUMED (Thailand)
IBUPROFEN
Motrin Suspension, Oral Drops, Chewable Tablets, and Caplets 2002

BUPIFORAN (Italy)
BUPIVACAINE HYDROCHLORIDE
Sensorcaine Injection 643
Sensorcaine-MPF Injection 643

BUPREX (Portugal, Spain)
BUPRENORPHINE HYDROCHLORIDE
Buprenex Injectable 2918

BUPRINE (Thailand)
BUPRENORPHINE HYDROCHLORIDE
Buprenex Injectable 2918

BUPYL (Italy)
BUPIVACAINE HYDROCHLORIDE
Sensorcaine Injection 643
Sensorcaine-MPF Injection 643

BURAM (Irish Republic)
AMILORIDE HYDROCHLORIDE
Midamor Tablets 2136

BURANA (Finland)
IBUPROFEN
Motrin Suspension, Oral Drops, Chewable Tablets, and Caplets 2002

BURANA-C (Finland)
IBUPROFEN
Motrin Suspension, Oral Drops, Chewable Tablets, and Caplets 2002

BURNEZE (United Kingdom)
BENZOCAINE
Americaine Anesthetic Lubricant 1162
Americaine Otic Topical Anesthetic Ear Drops 1162

BUSULFEX (Canada)
BUSULFAN
Myleran Tablets 1603

BUTACORT (New Zealand)
BUDESONIDE
Pulmicort Turbuhaler Inhalation Powder 636
Rhinocort Nasal Inhaler 640

BUTACORTELONE (Mexico)
IBUPROFEN
Motrin Suspension, Oral Drops, Chewable Tablets, and Caplets 2002

BUTALIRET (Germany)
TERBUTALINE SULFATE
Brethine Ampuls 2314
Brethine Tablets 2313

BUTALITAB (Germany)
TERBUTALINE SULFATE
Brethine Ampuls 2314
Brethine Tablets 2313

BUTAMINE (Israel)
DOBUTAMINE HYDROCHLORIDE
Dobutrex Solution Vials 1914

BUTERIDOL (Germany)
HALOPERIDOL
Haldol Injection, Tablets and Concentrate 2533

BUTIX (France)
DIPHENHYDRAMINE HYDROCHLORIDE
Benadryl Parenteral 2617

BUTYLIN (Singapore)
TERBUTALINE SULFATE
Brethine Ampuls 2314
Brethine Tablets 2313

BUVACAINA (Mexico)
BUPIVACAINE HYDROCHLORIDE
Sensorcaine Injection 643
Sensorcaine-MPF Injection 643

B-VASC (South Africa)
ATENOLOL
Tenormin I.V. Injection 692

BY-MYCIN (Irish Republic)
DOXYCYCLINE HYCLATE
Doryx Coated Pellet Filled Capsules 3357
Periostat Tablets 1208
Vibramycin Hyclate Capsules 2735
Vibramycin Hyclate Intravenous 2737
Vibra-Tabs Film Coated Tablets 2735

CABASER (Australia, Denmark, Finland, Norway, Sweden, Switzerland, United Kingdom)
CABERGOLINE
Dostinex Tablets 2804

CABASERIL (Germany)
CABERGOLINE
Dostinex Tablets 2804

CAEDAX (Austria, Portugal)
CEFTIBUTEN
Cedax Capsules 1021
Cedax Oral Suspension 1021

CAELYX (Australia)
DOXORUBICIN HYDROCHLORIDE
Adriamycin PFS/RDF Injection 2767

CALANIF (United Kingdom)
NIFEDIPINE
Adalat CC Tablets 877
Procardia Capsules 2708
Procardia XL Extended Release Tablets 2710

CAL-ANTAGON (Portugal)
DILTIAZEM HYDROCHLORIDE
Cardizem CD Capsules 1016
Cardizem Injectable 1018
Cardizem Lyo-Ject Syringe 1018
Cardizem Monovial 1018
Tiazac Capsules 1378

CALAZEM (United Kingdom)
DILTIAZEM HYDROCHLORIDE
Cardizem CD Capsules 1016
Cardizem Injectable 1018
Cardizem Lyo-Ject Syringe 1018
Cardizem Monovial 1018
Tiazac Capsules 1378

CALCETAT (Italy)
CALCIUM ACETATE
PhosLo Tablets 1069

CALCICARD (South Africa, United Kingdom)
VERAPAMIL HYDROCHLORIDE
Covera-HS Tablets 3199
Isoptin SR Tablets 467
Verelan Capsules 3184
Verelan PM Capsules 3186

CALCIGARD (Thailand)
NIFEDIPINE
Adalat CC Tablets 877
Procardia Capsules 2708
Procardia XL Extended Release Tablets 2710

CALCIJEX (Australia, Austria, Canada, Finland, Hong Kong, Irish Republic, Israel, Italy, Mexico, Norway, Singapore, Spain, Sweden, Switzerland, United Kingdom)
CALCITRIOL
Calcijex Injection 411
Rocaltrol Capsules 2991
Rocaltrol Oral Solution 2991

CALCILAT (United Kingdom)
NIFEDIPINE
Adalat CC Tablets 877
Procardia Capsules 2708
Procardia XL Extended Release Tablets 2710

CALFATE (Portugal)
SUCRALFATE
Carafate Suspension 731
Carafate Tablets 730

CALMARIL (Thailand)
THIORIDAZINE HYDROCHLORIDE
Thioridazine Hydrochloride Tablets 2289

CALMAVEN (Spain)
DIAZEPAM
Valium Injectable 3026
Valium Tablets 3047

CALMAX (Irish Republic)
ALPRAZOLAM
Xanax Tablets 2865

CALMAXID (Belgium, Switzerland)
NIZATIDINE
Axid Pulvules 1903

CALMAZINE (Australia)
TRIFLUOPERAZINE HYDROCHLORIDE
Stelazine Injection 1640
Stelazine Tablets 1640

CALMEX (Canada)
DIPHENHYDRAMINE HYDROCHLORIDE
Benadryl Parenteral 2617

CALMIDAN (Spain)
SUCRALFATE
Carafate Suspension 731
Carafate Tablets 730

CALMIGEN (Irish Republic)
DIAZEPAM
Valium Injectable 3026
Valium Tablets 3047

CALMINE (Italy)
IBUPROFEN
Motrin Suspension, Oral Drops, Chewable Tablets, and Caplets 2002

CALMOCITENO (Brazil)
DIAZEPAM
Valium Injectable 3026
Valium Tablets 3047

CALMOGENOL (Brazil)
LORAZEPAM
Ativan Injection 3478
Ativan Tablets 3482

CALMOSERPIN (Germany)
HYDROCHLOROTHIAZIDE/TRIAMTERENE
Dyazide Capsules 1515
Maxzide Tablets 1008
Maxzide-25 mg Tablets 1008

CALMPOSE (South Africa)
DIAZEPAM
Valium Injectable 3026
Valium Tablets 3047

CALMURID HC (South Africa)
HYDROCORTISONE
Anusol-HC Cream 2.5% 2237
Hydrocortone Tablets 2106

CALMYLIN EXPECTORANT (Canada)
GUAIFENESIN
Organidin NR Liquid 3350
Organidin NR Tablets 3350

CALMYLIN WITH CODEINE (Canada)
CODEINE PHOSPHATE/GUAIFENESIN/PSEUDOEPHEDRINE HYDROCHLORIDE
Robitussin-DAC Syrup 2942

CALNIT (Spain)
NIMODIPINE
Nimotop Capsules 904

CALPIX (Portugal)
CAPTOPRIL
Captopril Tablets 2281

CAMCOLIT (Belgium, Hong Kong, Irish Republic, Singapore, South Africa, The Netherlands, United Kingdom)
LITHIUM CARBONATE
Eskalith CR Controlled Release Tablets 1527
Eskalith Capsules 1527
Lithium Carbonate Capsules 3061
Lithobid Slow-Release Tablets 3255

CAMSILON (United Kingdom)
EDROPHONIUM CHLORIDE
Tensilon Injectable 1745

CANADINE (Thailand)
CLOTRIMAZOLE
Lotrimin Cream 1% 3128
Lotrimin Lotion 1% 3128
Lotrimin Topical Solution 1% 3128
Mycelex Troche 573

CANADIOL (Spain)
ITRACONAZOLE
Sporanox Capsules 1800
Sporanox Oral Solution 1808, 2512

CANALBA (South Africa)
CLOTRIMAZOLE
Lotrimin Cream 1% 3128
Lotrimin Lotion 1% 3128
Lotrimin Topical Solution 1% 3128
Mycelex Troche 573

CANASONE (Thailand)
BETAMETHASONE DIPROPIONATE/CLOTRIMAZOLE
Lotrisone Cream 3129

CANAZOL (Denmark, Thailand)
CLOTRIMAZOLE
Lotrimin Cream 1% 3128
Lotrimin Lotion 1% 3128
Lotrimin Topical Solution 1% 3128
Mycelex Troche 573

CANDASPOR (South Africa)
CLOTRIMAZOLE
Lotrimin Cream 1% 3128
Lotrimin Lotion 1% 3128
Lotrimin Topical Solution 1% 3128
Mycelex Troche 573

CANDAZOL (Germany)
CLOTRIMAZOLE
Lotrimin Cream 1% 3128
Lotrimin Lotion 1% 3128
Lotrimin Topical Solution 1% 3128
Mycelex Troche 573

CANDAZOLE (Singapore)
CLOTRIMAZOLE
Lotrimin Cream 1% 3128
Lotrimin Lotion 1% 3128
Lotrimin Topical Solution 1% 3128
Mycelex Troche 573

CANDIBENE (Austria)
CLOTRIMAZOLE
Lotrimin Cream 1% 3128
Lotrimin Lotion 1% 3128
Lotrimin Topical Solution 1% 3128
Mycelex Troche 573

CANDICORT (Brazil)
KETOCONAZOLE
Nizoral 2% Cream 3620
Nizoral 2% Shampoo 2007
Nizoral Tablets 1791

CANDID (Portugal, Thailand)
CLOTRIMAZOLE
Lotrimin Cream 1% 3128
Lotrimin Lotion 1% 3128
Lotrimin Topical Solution 1% 3128
Mycelex Troche 573

CANDIDA-LOKALICID (Germany)
NYSTATIN
Nystop Topical Powder USP 2608

CANDIDEN (United Kingdom)
CLOTRIMAZOLE
Lotrimin Cream 1% 3128
Lotrimin Lotion 1% 3128
Lotrimin Topical Solution 1% 3128
Mycelex Troche 573

CANDIDERM (Brazil)
KETOCONAZOLE
Nizoral 2% Cream 3620
Nizoral 2% Shampoo 2007
Nizoral Tablets 1791

CANDIMON (Mexico)
CLOTRIMAZOLE
Lotrimin Cream 1% 3128
Lotrimin Lotion 1% 3128
Lotrimin Topical Solution 1% 3128
Mycelex Troche 573

CANDINOX (Thailand)
CLOTRIMAZOLE
Lotrimin Cream 1% 3128
Lotrimin Lotion 1% 3128
Lotrimin Topical Solution 1% 3128
Mycelex Troche 573

CANDIO (Austria, Germany, Switzerland)
NYSTATIN
Nystop Topical Powder USP 2608

CANDISTATIN (Canada)
NYSTATIN
Nystop Topical Powder USP 2608

CANDIZOL (Brazil)
FLUCONAZOLE
Diflucan Tablets, Injection, and Oral Suspension 2681

CANDIZOLE (South Africa)
CLOTRIMAZOLE
Lotrimin Cream 1% 3128
Lotrimin Lotion 1% 3128
Lotrimin Topical Solution 1% 3128
Mycelex Troche 573

CANDORAL (Brazil)
KETOCONAZOLE
Nizoral 2% Cream 3620
Nizoral 2% Shampoo 2007
Nizoral Tablets 1791

CANDYL (Australia)
PIROXICAM
Feldene Capsules 2685

CANDYL-D (New Zealand)
PIROXICAM
Feldene Capsules 2685

CANEF (Denmark, Finland, Mexico, Norway, Portugal, Sweden, The Netherlands)
FLUVASTATIN SODIUM
Lescol Capsules 2361

CANESTEN (Australia, Austria, Brazil, Canada, Denmark, Finland, Germany, Hong Kong, Irish Republic, Italy, Mexico, New Zealand, Norway, Portugal, Singapore, South Africa, Spain, Sweden, Thailand, The Netherlands, United Kingdom)
CLOTRIMAZOLE
Lotrimin Cream 1% 3128
Lotrimin Lotion 1% 3128
Lotrimin Topical Solution 1% 3128
Mycelex Troche 573

CANESTEN COMBI (United Kingdom)
CLOTRIMAZOLE
Lotrimin Cream 1% 3128
Lotrimin Lotion 1% 3128
Lotrimin Topical Solution 1% 3128
Mycelex Troche 573

CANESTEN HC (Germany, United Kingdom)
CLOTRIMAZOLE
Lotrimin Cream 1% 3128
Lotrimin Lotion 1% 3128
Lotrimin Topical Solution 1% 3128
Mycelex Troche 573

CANESTENE (Belgium, Switzerland)
CLOTRIMAZOLE
Lotrimin Cream 1% 3128
Lotrimin Lotion 1% 3128
Lotrimin Topical Solution 1% 3128
Mycelex Troche 573

CANEX (South Africa)
CLOTRIMAZOLE
Lotrimin Cream 1% 3128
Lotrimin Lotion 1% 3128
Lotrimin Topical Solution 1% 3128
Mycelex Troche 573

CANIFUG (Germany)
CLOTRIMAZOLE
Lotrimin Cream 1% 3128
Lotrimin Lotion 1% 3128
Lotrimin Topical Solution 1% 3128
Mycelex Troche 573

CANSTAT (South Africa)
NYSTATIN
Nystop Topical Powder USP 2608

CANTANIDIN (Austria)
CLONIDINE HYDROCHLORIDE
Catapres Tablets 1037
Duraclon Injection 3057

CANUSAL (United Kingdom)
HEPARIN SODIUM
Heparin Lock Flush Solution 3509
Heparin Sodium Injection 3511

CAPACE (Australia, Austria, South Africa)
CAPTOPRIL
Captopril Tablets 2281

CAPEL (Brazil)
KETOCONAZOLE
Nizoral 2% Cream 3620
Nizoral 2% Shampoo 2007
Nizoral Tablets 1791

CAPOTEN (Australia, Belgium, Brazil, Canada, Denmark, Finland, Hong Kong, Irish Republic, Italy, New Zealand, Norway, Portugal, Singapore, South Africa, Spain, Sweden, Thailand, The Netherlands, United Kingdom)
CAPTOPRIL
Captopril Tablets 2281

CAPOTENA (Mexico)
CAPTOPRIL
Captopril Tablets 2281

CAPOZID (Denmark)
CAPTOPRIL
Captopril Tablets 2281

CAPOZIDE (Germany, Mexico, New Zealand, South Africa, United Kingdom)
CAPTOPRIL
Captopril Tablets 2281

CAPRYSIN (Finland)
CLONIDINE HYDROCHLORIDE
Catapres Tablets 1037
Duraclon Injection 3057

CAPSOID (South Africa)
PREDNISOLONE
Prelone Syrup 2273

CAPTI (Israel)
CAPTOPRIL
Captopril Tablets 2281

CAPTIREX (France)
CAPTOPRIL
Captopril Tablets 2281

CAPTO PLUS (Germany)
CAPTOPRIL
Captopril Tablets 2281

CAPTO-BASAN (Switzerland)
CAPTOPRIL
Captopril Tablets 2281

CAPTOBETA (Germany)
CAPTOPRIL
Captopril Tablets 2281

CAPTOBETA COMP (Germany)
CAPTOPRIL
Captopril Tablets 2281

CAPTO-CO (United Kingdom)
CAPTOPRIL
Captopril Tablets 2281

CAPTODAN (Denmark)
CAPTOPRIL
Captopril Tablets 2281

CAPTODOC (Germany)
CAPTOPRIL
Captopril Tablets 2281

CAPTO-DURA COR (Germany)
CAPTOPRIL
Captopril Tablets 2281

CAPTO-DURA M (Germany)
CAPTOPRIL
Captopril Tablets 2281

CAPTOFLUX (Germany)
CAPTOPRIL
Captopril Tablets 2281

CAPTOGAMMA (Germany)
CAPTOPRIL
Captopril Tablets 2281

CAPTOGAMMA HCT (Germany)
CAPTOPRIL
Captopril Tablets 2281

CAPTOHEXAL (Australia, Germany, South Africa)
CAPTOPRIL
Captopril Tablets 2281

CAPTOHEXAL COMP (Germany)
CAPTOPRIL
Captopril Tablets 2281

CAPTOL (Denmark)
CAPTOPRIL
Captopril Tablets 2281

CAPTOLANE (France)
CAPTOPRIL
Captopril Tablets 2281

CAPTOMAX (South Africa)
CAPTOPRIL
Captopril Tablets 2281

CAPTOMERCK (Germany)
CAPTOPRIL
Captopril Tablets 2281

CAPTOMIN (Finland)
CAPTOPRIL
Captopril Tablets 2281

CAPTOPRESS (Germany)
CAPTOPRIL
Captopril Tablets 2281

CAPTOPRIL COMP (Germany)
CAPTOPRIL
Captopril Tablets 2281

CAPTOPRIL PLUS (Germany)
CAPTOPRIL
Captopril Tablets 2281

CAPTOR (Irish Republic)
CAPTOPRIL
Captopril Tablets 2281

CAPTOREAL (Germany)
CAPTOPRIL
Captopril Tablets 2281

CAPTORETIC (South Africa)
CAPTOPRIL
Captopril Tablets 2281

CAPTOR-HCT (Irish Republic)
CAPTOPRIL
Captopril Tablets 2281

CAPTOSER (Mexico)
CAPTOPRIL
Captopril Tablets 2281

CAPTOSOL (Switzerland)
CAPTOPRIL
Captopril Tablets 2281

CAPTOSTAD (Finland)
CAPTOPRIL
Captopril Tablets 2281

CAPTRAL (Mexico)
CAPTOPRIL
Captopril Tablets 2281

CAPTRIL (Canada)
CAPTOPRIL
Captopril Tablets 2281

CARACE (Irish Republic, United Kingdom)
LISINOPRIL
Prinivil Tablets 2164
Zestril Tablets 698

CARACE PLUS (Irish Republic, United Kingdom)
HYDROCHLOROTHIAZIDE/LISINOPRIL
Prinzide Tablets 2168
Zestoretic Tablets 695

CARAFATE (Australia, New Zealand)
SUCRALFATE
Carafate Suspension 731
Carafate Tablets 730

CARASEL (Spain)
RAMIPRIL
Altace Capsules 2233

CARBABETA (Germany)
CARBAMAZEPINE
Carbatrol Capsules 3234
Tegretol Chewable Tablets 2404
Tegretol Suspension 2404
Tegretol Tablets 2404
Tegretol-XR Tablets 2404

CARBAC (Mexico)
LORACARBEF
Lorabid Suspension and Pulvules 2251

CARBAFLUX (Germany)
CARBAMAZEPINE
Carbatrol Capsules 3234
Tegretol Chewable Tablets 2404
Tegretol Suspension 2404
Tegretol Tablets 2404
Tegretol-XR Tablets 2404

CARBAGAMMA (Germany)
CARBAMAZEPINE
Carbatrol Capsules 3234
Tegretol Chewable Tablets 2404
Tegretol Suspension 2404
Tegretol Tablets 2404
Tegretol-XR Tablets 2404

CARBAGEN (United Kingdom)
CARBAMAZEPINE
Carbatrol Capsules 3234
Tegretol Chewable Tablets 2404
Tegretol Suspension 2404
Tegretol Tablets 2404
Tegretol-XR Tablets 2404

CARBAGER-PLUS (Mexico)
METHOCARBAMOL
Robaxin Injectable 2938
Robaxin Tablets 2939
Robaxin-750 Tablets 2939

CARBALAN (Mexico)
CARBAMAZEPINE
Carbatrol Capsules 3234
Tegretol Chewable Tablets 2404
Tegretol Suspension 2404
Tegretol Tablets 2404
Tegretol-XR Tablets 2404

CARBAMANN (Germany)
CARBACHOL
Isopto Carbachol Ophthalmic Solution ⊙215

CARBASTAT (Canada)
CARBACHOL
Isopto Carbachol Ophthalmic Solution ⊙215

CARBATIL (Mexico)
MEBENDAZOLE
Vermox Chewable Tablets 2017

CARBAZENE (Thailand)
CARBAMAZEPINE
Carbatrol Capsules 3234
Tegretol Chewable Tablets 2404
Tegretol Suspension 2404
Tegretol Tablets 2404
Tegretol-XR Tablets 2404

CARBAZEP (Mexico)
CARBAMAZEPINE
Carbatrol Capsules 3234
Tegretol Chewable Tablets 2404
Tegretol Suspension 2404
Tegretol Tablets 2404
Tegretol-XR Tablets 2404

CARBAZINA (Mexico)
CARBAMAZEPINE
Carbatrol Capsules 3234
Tegretol Chewable Tablets 2404
Tegretol Suspension 2404
Tegretol Tablets 2404
Tegretol-XR Tablets 2404

CARBEM (Italy)
LORACARBEF
Lorabid Suspension and Pulvules 2251

CARBI (Israel)
CARBAMAZEPINE
Carbatrol Capsules 3234
Tegretol Chewable Tablets 2404
Tegretol Suspension 2404
Tegretol Tablets 2404
Tegretol-XR Tablets 2404

CARBINIB (Portugal)
ACETAZOLAMIDE
Diamox Sequels Sustained Release Capsules ⊙270
Diamox Tablets ⊙269

CARBIUM (Australia, Germany)
CARBAMAZEPINE
Carbatrol Capsules 3234
Tegretol Chewable Tablets 2404
Tegretol Suspension 2404
Tegretol Tablets 2404
Tegretol-XR Tablets 2404

CARBOCAIN (Denmark, Norway, Sweden)
MEPIVACAINE HYDROCHLORIDE
Polocaine Injection, USP 625
Polocaine-MPF Injection, USP 625

CARBOCAINA (Italy)
MEPIVACAINE HYDROCHLORIDE
Polocaine Injection, USP 625
Polocaine-MPF Injection, USP 625

CARBOCAINE (Australia, Canada, France, South Africa)
MEPIVACAINE HYDROCHLORIDE
Polocaine Injection, USP 625
Polocaine-MPF Injection, USP 625

CARBOLIM (Brazil)
LITHIUM CARBONATE
Eskalith CR Controlled Release Tablets 1527
Eskalith Capsules 1527
Lithium Carbonate Capsules 3061
Lithobid Slow-Release Tablets 3255

CARBOLIT (Mexico)
LITHIUM CARBONATE
Eskalith CR Controlled Release Tablets 1527
Eskalith Capsules 1527
Lithium Carbonate Capsules 3061
Lithobid Slow-Release Tablets 3255

CARBOLITH (Canada)
LITHIUM CARBONATE
Eskalith CR Controlled Release Tablets 1527
Eskalith Capsules 1527
Lithium Carbonate Capsules 3061
Lithobid Slow-Release Tablets 3255

CARBOLITHIUM (Italy)
LITHIUM CARBONATE
Eskalith CR Controlled Release Tablets 1527
Eskalith Capsules 1527
Lithium Carbonate Capsules 3061
Lithobid Slow-Release Tablets 3255

CARBOLITIUM (Brazil)
LITHIUM CARBONATE
Eskalith CR Controlled Release Tablets 1527
Eskalith Capsules 1527
Lithium Carbonate Capsules 3061
Lithobid Slow-Release Tablets 3255

CARBONEURAL (Austria)
BUPIVACAINE HYDROCHLORIDE
Sensorcaine Injection 643
Sensorcaine-MPF Injection 643

CARBOPLAT (Germany, Mexico)
CARBOPLATIN
Paraplatin for Injection 1126

CARBOSIN (Denmark, Finland, Norway, South Africa, Thailand)
CARBOPLATIN
Paraplatin for Injection 1126

CARBOSOL (Austria)
CARBOPLATIN
Paraplatin for Injection 1126

CARBOSTESIN (Austria, Germany, Switzerland)
BUPIVACAINE HYDROCHLORIDE
Sensorcaine Injection 643
Sensorcaine-MPF Injection 643

CARBOTEC (Mexico)
CARBOPLATIN
Paraplatin for Injection 1126

CARBRITAL (Australia)
PENTOBARBITAL SODIUM
Nembutal Sodium Solution 485

CARDACE (Finland)
RAMIPRIL
Altace Capsules 2233

CARDACE COMP (Finland)
RAMIPRIL
Altace Capsules 2233

CARDALIN (Brazil)
NIFEDIPINE
Adalat CC Tablets 877
Procardia Capsules 2708
Procardia XL Extended Release Tablets 2710

CARDAXEN (Switzerland)
ATENOLOL
Tenormin I.V. Injection 692

CARDCAL (Australia)
DILTIAZEM HYDROCHLORIDE
Cardizem CD Capsules 1016
Cardizem Injectable 1018
Cardizem Lyo-Ject Syringe 1018
Cardizem Monovial 1018
Tiazac Capsules 1378

CARDENE (Canada, Irish Republic, The Netherlands, United Kingdom)
NICARDIPINE HYDROCHLORIDE
Cardene I.V. 3485

CARDENOL (Thailand)
PROPRANOLOL HYDROCHLORIDE
Inderal Injectable 3513
Inderal LA Long-Acting Capsules 3516
Inderal Tablets 3513

CARDENSIEL (France)
BISOPROLOL FUMARATE
Zebeta Tablets 1885

CARDIACE (South Africa)
CAPTOPRIL
Captopril Tablets 2281

CARDIACTON (Austria)
DILTIAZEM HYDROCHLORIDE
Cardizem CD Capsules 1016
Cardizem Injectable 1018
Cardizem Lyo-Ject Syringe 1018
Cardizem Monovial 1018
Tiazac Capsules 1378

CARDIAGEN (Germany)
CAPTOPRIL
Captopril Tablets 2281

CARDIAGEN HCT (Germany)
CAPTOPRIL
Captopril Tablets 2281

CARDIAGUTT (Germany)
VERAPAMIL HYDROCHLORIDE
Covera-HS Tablets 3199
Isoptin SR Tablets 467
Verelan Capsules 3184
Verelan PM Capsules 3186

CARDIBELTIN (Germany)
VERAPAMIL HYDROCHLORIDE
Covera-HS Tablets 3199
Isoptin SR Tablets 467
Verelan Capsules 3184
Verelan PM Capsules 3186

CARDIBLOC (Singapore)
NICARDIPINE HYDROCHLORIDE
Cardene I.V. 3485

CARDIBLOK (South Africa)
PROPRANOLOL HYDROCHLORIDE
Inderal Injectable 3513
Inderal LA Long-Acting Capsules 3516
Inderal Tablets 3513

CARDICOR (Denmark, Irish Republic, United Kingdom)
BISOPROLOL FUMARATE
Zebeta Tablets 1885

CARDIFEN (South Africa)
NIFEDIPINE
Adalat CC Tablets 877
Procardia Capsules 2708
Procardia XL Extended Release Tablets 2710

CARDIL (Denmark, Singapore, Thailand)
DILTIAZEM HYDROCHLORIDE
Cardizem CD Capsules 1016
Cardizem Injectable 1018
Cardizem Lyo-Ject Syringe 1018
Cardizem Monovial 1018
Tiazac Capsules 1378

CARDILAT (South Africa)
NIFEDIPINE
Adalat CC Tablets 877
Procardia Capsules 2708
Procardia XL Extended Release Tablets 2710

CARDILATE MR (United Kingdom)
NIFEDIPINE
Adalat CC Tablets 877
Procardia Capsules 2708
Procardia XL Extended Release Tablets 2710

CARDIN (Brazil)
METHYLDOPA
Aldomet Tablets 2037

CARDINOL (Australia, New Zealand, United Kingdom)
PROPRANOLOL HYDROCHLORIDE
Inderal Injectable 3513
Inderal LA Long-Acting Capsules 3516
Inderal Tablets 3513

CARDINORM (Australia)
AMIODARONE HYDROCHLORIDE
Cordarone Intravenous 3491
Cordarone Tablets 3487
Pacerone Tablets 3331

CARDIO (Germany)
ISOSORBIDE DINITRATE
Isordil Sublingual Tablets 3525
Isordil Titradose Tablets 3526

CARDIOBIL (Italy)
LEVOCARNITINE
Carnitor Injection 3242
Carnitor Tablets and Oral Solution 3245

CARDIOCOR (France)
BISOPROLOL FUMARATE
Zebeta Tablets 1885

CARDIO-GREEN (Canada, Germany)
INDOCYANINE GREEN
IC-Green ⊙203

CARDIOL (Finland, Portugal)
CARVEDILOL
Coreg Tablets 1508

CARDIONIL (Spain)
ISOSORBIDE MONONITRATE
Imdur Tablets 1826
Ismo Tablets 3524

CARDIOPROTECT (Germany)
VERAPAMIL HYDROCHLORIDE
Covera-HS Tablets 3199
Isoptin SR Tablets 467
Verelan Capsules 3184
Verelan PM Capsules 3186

CARDIOREG (Italy)
DIGOXIN
Lanoxicaps Capsules 1574
Lanoxin Elixir Pediatric 1578
Lanoxin Injection 1581
Lanoxin Injection Pediatric 1584
Lanoxin Tablets 1587

CARDIOTEN (Italy)
NICARDIPINE HYDROCHLORIDE
Cardene I.V. 3485

CARDIOVAS (Spain)
ISOSORBIDE MONONITRATE
Imdur Tablets 1826
Ismo Tablets 3524

CARDIP (Italy)
NICARDIPINE HYDROCHLORIDE
Cardene I.V. 3485

CARDIPIN (Switzerland)
NIFEDIPINE
Adalat CC Tablets 877
Procardia Capsules 2708
Procardia XL Extended Release Tablets 2710

CARDIPRIL (Mexico)
CAPTOPRIL
Captopril Tablets 2281

CARDISER (Spain)
DILTIAZEM HYDROCHLORIDE
Cardizem CD Capsules 1016
Cardizem Injectable 1018
Cardizem Lyo-Ject Syringe 1018
Cardizem Monovial 1018
Tiazac Capsules 1378

CARDISPAN (Mexico)
LEVOCARNITINE
Carnitor Injection 3242
Carnitor Tablets and Oral Solution 3245

CARDISPARE (South Africa)
PROPRANOLOL HYDROCHLORIDE
Inderal Injectable 3513

Inderal LA Long-Acting Capsules 3516
Inderal Tablets. 3513

CARDIUM (Singapore)
DILTIAZEM HYDROCHLORIDE
Cardizem CD Capsules 1016
Cardizem Injectable 1018
Cardizem Lyo-Ject Syringe 1018
Cardizem Monovial 1018
Tiazac Capsules 1378

CARDIZEM (Australia, Brazil, Canada, Denmark, Finland, New Zealand, Norway, Sweden)
DILTIAZEM HYDROCHLORIDE
Cardizem CD Capsules 1016
Cardizem Injectable 1018
Cardizem Lyo-Ject Syringe 1018
Cardizem Monovial 1018
Tiazac Capsules 1378

CARDOL (Australia)
SOTALOL HYDROCHLORIDE
Betapace Tablets 950

CARDOPAX (Denmark, Sweden)
ISOSORBIDE DINITRATE
Isordil Sublingual Tablets 3525
Isordil Titradose Tablets. 3526

CARDOXIN (Israel)
DIPYRIDAMOLE
Persantine Tablets 1057

CARDYL (Spain)
ATORVASTATIN CALCIUM
Lipitor Tablets 2639, 2696

CARENCIL (Portugal)
CAPTOPRIL
Captopril Tablets 2281

CAREXAN (Mexico)
ITRACONAZOLE
Sporanox Capsules. 1800
Sporanox Oral Solution. 1808, 2512

CARISOMA (United Kingdom)
CARISOPRODOL
Soma Tablets 3353

CARMAPINE (Thailand)
CARBAMAZEPINE
Carbatrol Capsules. 3234
Tegretol Chewable Tablets 2404
Tegretol Suspension 2404
Tegretol Tablets. 2404
Tegretol-XR Tablets. 2404

CARMIAN (Italy)
ATENOLOL
Tenormin I.V. Injection 692

CARMICINA (Portugal)
CIPROFLOXACIN HYDROCHLORIDE
Ciloxan Ophthalmic Ointment. 538
Ciloxan Ophthalmic Solution . . . . ⊙209, 538
Cipro Tablets. 887

CARMUBRIS (Austria, Germany)
CARMUSTINE
Gliadel Wafer 1723

CARNICOR (Italy)
LEVOCARNITINE
Carnitor Injection 3242
Carnitor Tablets and Oral Solution 3245

CARNITOR (Canada, Hong Kong, United Kingdom)
LEVOCARNITINE
Carnitor Injection 3242
Carnitor Tablets and Oral Solution 3245

CARNOTPRIM (Mexico)
METOCLOPRAMIDE HYDROCHLORIDE
Reglan Injectable 2935
Reglan Syrup 2935
Reglan Tablets. 2935

CARPAZ (South Africa)
CARBAMAZEPINE
Carbatrol Capsules. 3234
Tegretol Chewable Tablets 2404
Tegretol Suspension 2404
Tegretol Tablets. 2404
Tegretol-XR Tablets. 2404

CARPIN (Mexico)
CARBAMAZEPINE
Carbatrol Capsules. 3234
Tegretol Chewable Tablets 2404
Tegretol Suspension 2404
Tegretol Tablets. 2404
Tegretol-XR Tablets. 2404

CARPINE (Thailand)
CARBAMAZEPINE
Carbatrol Capsules. 3234
Tegretol Chewable Tablets 2404
Tegretol Suspension 2404
Tegretol Tablets. 2404
Tegretol-XR Tablets. 2404

CARPINPLAST (Spain)
PILOCARPINE HYDROCHLORIDE
Isopto Carpine Ophthalmic Solution . . . . ⊙215
Pilopine HS Ophthalmic Gel . . . . ⊙217
Salagen Tablets 2229

CARRELDON (Spain)
DILTIAZEM HYDROCHLORIDE
Cardizem CD Capsules 1016
Cardizem Injectable 1018
Cardizem Lyo-Ject Syringe 1018
Cardizem Monovial 1018
Tiazac Capsules 1378

CARVASIN (Italy, New Zealand)
ISOSORBIDE DINITRATE
Isordil Sublingual Tablets 3525
Isordil Titradose Tablets. 3526

CARVIPRESS (Italy)
CARVEDILOL
Coreg Tablets 1508

CARZEM (Italy)
DILTIAZEM HYDROCHLORIDE
Cardizem CD Capsules 1016
Cardizem Injectable 1018
Cardizem Lyo-Ject Syringe 1018
Cardizem Monovial 1018
Tiazac Capsules 1378

CARZEPINE (Thailand)
CARBAMAZEPINE
Carbatrol Capsules. 3234
Tegretol Chewable Tablets 2404
Tegretol Suspension 2404
Tegretol Tablets. 2404
Tegretol-XR Tablets. 2404

CASBOL (Spain)
PAROXETINE HYDROCHLORIDE
Paxil Oral Suspension 1609
Paxil Tablets 1609

CASODEX (Austria, Belgium, Canada, Denmark, Finland, France, Germany, Hong Kong, Irish Republic, Israel, Italy, Mexico, Norway, Portugal, Singapore, South Africa, Spain, Sweden, Switzerland, Thailand, The Netherlands, United Kingdom)
BICALUTAMIDE
Casodex Tablets 662

CATAFLAM (Hong Kong, Irish Republic, Israel, Italy, New Zealand, Norway, Portugal, Singapore, South Africa, Thailand, The Netherlands)
DICLOFENAC POTASSIUM
Cataflam Tablets 2315

CATALIP (Portugal)
FENOFIBRATE
Tricor Capsules, Micronized 513

CATANAC (Thailand)
DICLOFENAC POTASSIUM
Cataflam Tablets 2315

CATAPRES (Australia, Canada, Hong Kong, Irish Republic, South Africa, Thailand, United Kingdom)
CLONIDINE HYDROCHLORIDE
Catapres Tablets 1037
Duraclon Injection. 3057

CATAPRESAN (Austria, Denmark, Finland, Germany, Mexico, Norway, Portugal, Spain, Sweden, Switzerland, The Netherlands)
CLONIDINE HYDROCHLORIDE
Catapres Tablets 1037
Duraclon Injection. 3057

CATAPRESSAN (Belgium, France)
CLONIDINE HYDROCHLORIDE
Catapres Tablets 1037
Duraclon Injection. 3057

CATAREN (Brazil)
DICLOFENAC POTASSIUM
Cataflam Tablets 2315

CATEX (Spain)
CIPROFLOXACIN HYDROCHLORIDE
Ciloxan Ophthalmic Ointment. 538
Ciloxan Ophthalmic Solution . . . . ⊙209, 538
Cipro Tablets. 887

CATONET (Denmark)
CAPTOPRIL
Captopril Tablets 2281

CATOPROL (Brazil)
CAPTOPRIL
Captopril Tablets 2281

CAVERIL (Thailand)
VERAPAMIL HYDROCHLORIDE
Covera-HS Tablets 3199
Isoptin SR Tablets. 467
Verelan Capsules 3184
Verelan PM Capsules 3186

CAVERJECT (Australia, Austria, Belgium, Canada, Denmark, Finland, France, Germany, Hong Kong, Irish Republic, Israel, Italy, Mexico, New Zealand, Norway, Portugal, Singapore, South Africa, Spain, Sweden, Switzerland, Thailand, The Netherlands, United Kingdom)
ALPROSTADIL
Caverject Sterile Powder 2777
MUSE Urethral Suppository. 3335

CEBEDEX (France)
DEXAMETHASONE SODIUM PHOSPHATE
Decadron Phosphate Injection 2081
Decadron Phosphate Sterile Ophthalmic Ointment . . . . . . ⊙280, 2083
Decadron Phosphate Sterile Ophthalmic Solution 2084

CEBEMYXINE (France)
NEOMYCIN SULFATE/POLYMYXIN B SULFATE
Neosporin G.U. Irrigant Sterile. 2256

CEBENICOL (France)
CHLORAMPHENICOL
Chloromycetin Ophthalmic Ointment, 1% . . . . ⊙296
Chloromycetin Ophthalmic Solution . . . . ⊙297
Chloroptic Sterile Ophthalmic Ointment . . ⊙234
Chloroptic Sterile Ophthalmic Solution . . ⊙235

CEC (Austria, Germany, South Africa)
CEFACLOR
Ceclor CD Tablets 1279
Ceclor Pulvules 1905
Ceclor Suspension 1905

CECLOR (Australia, Austria, Belgium, Brazil, Canada, Hong Kong, Israel, Mexico, New Zealand, Portugal, South Africa, Spain, Switzerland, The Netherlands)
CEFACLOR
Ceclor CD Tablets 1279
Ceclor Pulvules 1905
Ceclor Suspension 1905

CECLORBETA (Germany)
CEFACLOR
Ceclor CD Tablets 1279
Ceclor Pulvules 1905
Ceclor Suspension 1905

CEDAX (Finland, Hong Kong, Irish Republic, Israel, Italy, Mexico, Singapore, South Africa, Spain, Sweden, Switzerland, Thailand, The Netherlands, United Kingdom)
CEFTIBUTEN
Cedax Capsules. 1021
Cedax Oral Suspension 1021

CEDINE (Irish Republic)
CIMETIDINE
Tagamet Tablets 1644

CEDOCARD (Austria, Belgium, Canada, Irish Republic, Switzerland, Thailand, The Netherlands, United Kingdom)
ISOSORBIDE DINITRATE
Isordil Sublingual Tablets 3525
Isordil Titradose Tablets. 3526

CEDOL (Italy)
CEFAMANDOLE NAFATE
Mandol Vials 1953

CEDROL (Spain)
ZOLPIDEM TARTRATE
Ambien Tablets 3191

CEDROX (Germany)
CEFADROXIL
Duricef Capsules 1079
Duricef Oral Suspension. 1079
Duricef Tablets 1079

CEF-3 (Thailand)
CEFTRIAXONE SODIUM
Rocephin Injectable Vials, ADD-Vantage, Galaxy, Bulk. 2993

CEF-4 (Thailand)
CEFTAZIDIME
Ceptaz for Injection 1499
Fortaz for Injection 1541
Tazicef for Injection 1647
Tazidime Vials, Faspak & ADD-Vantage . . 1966

CEFABIOCIN (Germany)
CEFACLOR
Ceclor CD Tablets 1279
Ceclor Pulvules 1905
Ceclor Suspension 1905

CEFACET (France)
CEPHALEXIN
Keflex Oral Suspension 1237
Keflex Pulvules 1237

CEFACILE (Portugal)
CEFADROXIL
Duricef Capsules 1079
Duricef Oral Suspension. 1079
Duricef Tablets 1079

CEFACRON (Spain)
CEFOTAXIME SODIUM
Claforan Injection 732

CEFADINA (Spain)
CEPHALEXIN
Keflex Oral Suspension 1237
Keflex Pulvules 1237

CEFADOL (Thailand)
CEFAMANDOLE NAFATE
Mandol Vials 1953

CEFADRIL (Italy, Thailand)
CEFADROXIL
Duricef Capsules 1079
Duricef Oral Suspension. 1079
Duricef Tablets 1079

CEFADROS (Italy)
CEPHALEXIN
Keflex Oral Suspension 1237
Keflex Pulvules 1237

CEFADROX (South Africa)
CEFADROXIL
Duricef Capsules 1079
Duricef Oral Suspension. 1079
Duricef Tablets 1079

CEFALEH INA (Spain)
CEPHALEXIN
Keflex Oral Suspension 1237
Keflex Pulvules 1237

CEFALEN (Brazil)
CEPHALEXIN
Keflex Oral Suspension 1237
Keflex Pulvules 1237

CEFALEXGOBENS (Spain)
CEPHALEXIN
Keflex Oral Suspension 1237
Keflex Pulvules 1237

CEFALIN (Israel)
CEPHALEXIN
Keflex Oral Suspension 1237
Keflex Pulvules 1237

CEFALIVAL (Spain)
CEPHALEXIN
Keflex Oral Suspension 1237
Keflex Pulvules 1237

CEFALLONE (Germany)
CEFACLOR
Ceclor CD Tablets 1279
Ceclor Pulvules 1905
Ceclor Suspension 1905

CEFALOR (Israel)
CEFACLOR
Ceclor CD Tablets 1279
Ceclor Pulvules 1905
Ceclor Suspension 1905

CEFALOREX (Spain)
CEPHALEXIN
Keflex Oral Suspension 1237
Keflex Pulvules 1237

CEFALVER (Mexico)
CEPHALEXIN
Keflex Oral Suspension 1237
Keflex Pulvules 1237

CEFAM (Italy)
CEFAMANDOLE NAFATE
Mandol Vials 1953

CEFAMAR (Italy, Thailand)
CEFUROXIME SODIUM
Kefurox Vials, ADD-Vantage. 1948
Zinacef Injection. 1696

CEFAMEN (Italy)
CEFAMANDOLE NAFATE
Mandol Vials 1953

CEFAMISO (Spain)
CEPHALEXIN
Keflex Oral Suspension 1237
Keflex Pulvules 1237

CEFAMOX (Brazil, Mexico, Sweden)
CEFADROXIL
Duricef Capsules 1079
Duricef Oral Suspension. 1079
Duricef Tablets 1079

CEFAPOREX (Brazil)
CEPHALEXIN
Keflex Oral Suspension 1237
Keflex Pulvules 1237

CEFASEPTOLO (Italy)
CEFAMANDOLE NAFATE
Mandol Vials 1953

CEFA-WOLFF (Germany)
CEFACLOR
Ceclor CD Tablets . . . 1279
Ceclor Pulvules . . . 1905
Ceclor Suspension . . . 1905

CEFAXICINA (Spain)
CEFOXITIN SODIUM
Mefoxin Premixed Intravenous Solution . . 2127
Mefoxin for Injection . . . 2124

CEFAXONA (Mexico)
CEFTRIAXONE SODIUM
Rocephin Injectable Vials, ADD-Vantage, Galaxy, Bulk. . . . 2993

CEFAXONE (Singapore)
CEFTRIAXONE SODIUM
Rocephin Injectable Vials, ADD-Vantage, Galaxy, Bulk. . . . 2993

CEFAZONE (Italy)
CEFOPERAZONE SODIUM
Cefobid Intravenous/Intramuscular . . . 2671
Cefobid Pharmacy Bulk Package - Not for Direct Infusion . . . 2673

CEFEN (Thailand)
IBUPROFEN
Motrin Suspension, Oral Drops, Chewable Tablets, and Caplets . . . 2002

CEFERRAN (Spain)
CEPHALEXIN
Keflex Oral Suspension . . . 1237
Keflex Pulvules . . . 1237

CEFEXIN (Thailand)
CEPHALEXIN
Keflex Oral Suspension . . . 1237
Keflex Pulvules . . . 1237

CEFIBACTER (Spain)
CEPHALEXIN
Keflex Oral Suspension . . . 1237
Keflex Pulvules . . . 1237

CEFIN (Singapore)
CEFTRIAXONE SODIUM
Rocephin Injectable Vials, ADD-Vantage, Galaxy, Bulk. . . . 2993

CEFINE (Thailand)
CEFTRIAXONE SODIUM
Rocephin Injectable Vials, ADD-Vantage, Galaxy, Bulk. . . . 2993

CEFIRAN (Italy)
CEFAMANDOLE NAFATE
Mandol Vials . . . 1953

CEFIXORAL (Italy)
CEFIXIME
Suprax Tablets . . . 1877
Suprax for Oral Suspension . . . 1877

CEFIZOX (Austria, Canada, France, Irish Republic, Mexico, Portugal, Spain, The Netherlands, United Kingdom)
CEFTIZOXIME SODIUM
Cefizox for Intramuscular or Intravenous Use . . . 1390

CEFKOR (Australia)
CEFACLOR
Ceclor CD Tablets . . . 1279
Ceclor Pulvules . . . 1905
Ceclor Suspension . . . 1905

CEFLAX (Portugal)
CEPHALEXIN
Keflex Oral Suspension . . . 1237
Keflex Pulvules . . . 1237

CEFLIN (Australia)
CEPHALEXIN
Keflex Oral Suspension . . . 1237
Keflex Pulvules . . . 1237

CEFOBID (Austria, Brazil, Canada, Hong Kong, Italy, Singapore, Spain, Thailand)
CEFOPERAZONE SODIUM
Cefobid Intravenous/Intramuscular . . . 2671
Cefobid Pharmacy Bulk Package - Not for Direct Infusion . . . 2673

CEFOBIS (France, Germany, Switzerland)
CEFOPERAZONE SODIUM
Cefobid Intravenous/Intramuscular . . . 2671
Cefobid Pharmacy Bulk Package - Not for Direct Infusion . . . 2673

CEFOCICLIN (Italy)
CEFOXITIN SODIUM
Mefoxin Premixed Intravenous Solution . . 2127
Mefoxin for Injection . . . 2124

CEFODIME (Thailand)
CEFTAZIDIME
Ceptaz for Injection . . . 1499
Fortaz for Injection . . . 1541
Tazicef for Injection . . . 1647
Tazidime Vials, Faspak & ADD-Vantage . . 1966

CEFODOX (France, Irish Republic, Italy)
CEFPODOXIME PROXETIL
Vantin Tablets and Oral Suspension. . . . 2860

CEFOGRAM (Italy)
CEFOPERAZONE SODIUM
Cefobid Intravenous/Intramuscular . . . 2671
Cefobid Pharmacy Bulk Package - Not for Direct Infusion . . . 2673

CEFOMIC (Thailand)
CEFOTAXIME SODIUM
Claforan Injection . . . 732

CEFONEG (Italy)
CEFOPERAZONE SODIUM
Cefobid Intravenous/Intramuscular . . . 2671
Cefobid Pharmacy Bulk Package - Not for Direct Infusion . . . 2673

CEFOPER (Italy)
CEFOPERAZONE SODIUM
Cefobid Intravenous/Intramuscular . . . 2671
Cefobid Pharmacy Bulk Package - Not for Direct Infusion . . . 2673

CEFOPRIM (Italy)
CEFUROXIME SODIUM
Kefurox Vials, ADD-Vantage. . . . 1948
Zinacef Injection. . . . 1696

CEFORAL (Israel)
CEPHALEXIN
Keflex Oral Suspension . . . 1237
Keflex Pulvules . . . 1237

CEFORAN (Thailand)
CEFOTAXIME SODIUM
Claforan Injection . . . 732

CEFORTAM (Portugal)
CEFTAZIDIME SODIUM
Fortaz for Injection . . . 1541

CEFOSINT (Italy)
CEFOPERAZONE SODIUM
Cefobid Intravenous/Intramuscular . . . 2671
Cefobid Pharmacy Bulk Package - Not for Direct Infusion . . . 2673

CEFOTAN (Canada)
CEFOTETAN DISODIUM
Cefotan Injection . . . 664
Cefotan for Injection . . . 664

CEFOTAX (Thailand)
CEFOTAXIME SODIUM
Claforan Injection . . . 732

CEFOVIT (Israel)
CEPHALEXIN
Keflex Oral Suspension . . . 1237
Keflex Pulvules . . . 1237

CEFOXIN (Thailand)
CEFOXITIN SODIUM
Mefoxin Premixed Intravenous Solution . . 2127
Mefoxin for Injection . . . 2124

CEFOZONE (Hong Kong, Singapore, Thailand)
CEFOPERAZONE SODIUM
Cefobid Intravenous/Intramuscular . . . 2671
Cefobid Pharmacy Bulk Package - Not for Direct Infusion . . . 2673

CEFRA (Portugal)
CEFADROXIL
Duricef Capsules . . . 1079
Duricef Oral Suspension. . . . 1079
Duricef Tablets . . . 1079

CEFRADEN (Mexico)
CEFTRIAXONE SODIUM
Rocephin Injectable Vials, ADD-Vantage, Galaxy, Bulk. . . . 2993

CEFRADIL (Mexico)
CEFOTAXIME SODIUM
Claforan Injection . . . 732

CEFRIN (United Arab Emirates)
CEPHALEXIN
Keflex Oral Suspension . . . 1237
Keflex Pulvules . . . 1237

CEFROXIL (Spain)
CEFADROXIL
Duricef Capsules . . . 1079
Duricef Oral Suspension. . . . 1079
Duricef Tablets . . . 1079

CEFSPAN (Japan, Thailand)
CEFIXIME
Suprax Tablets . . . 1877
Suprax for Oral Suspension . . . 1877

CEFTARAN (Thailand)
CEFOTAXIME SODIUM
Claforan Injection . . . 732

CEFTENON (Austria)
CEFOTETAN DISODIUM
Cefotan Injection . . . 664
Cefotan for Injection . . . 664

CEFTIM (Italy)
CEFTAZIDIME
Ceptaz for Injection . . . 1499
Fortaz for Injection . . . 1541
Tazicef for Injection . . . 1647
Tazidime Vials, Faspak & ADD-Vantage . . 1966

CEFTIN (Canada)
CEFUROXIME AXETIL
Ceftin Tablets . . . 1898
Ceftin for Oral Suspension . . . 1898

CEFTIX (Germany)
CEFTIZOXIME SODIUM
Cefizox for Intramuscular or Intravenous Use . . . 1390

CEFTREX (Mexico, Thailand)
CEFTRIAXONE SODIUM
Rocephin Injectable Vials, ADD-Vantage, Galaxy, Bulk. . . . 2993

CEFTRIPHIN (Thailand)
CEFTRIAXONE SODIUM
Rocephin Injectable Vials, ADD-Vantage, Galaxy, Bulk. . . . 2993

CEFUMAX (Italy)
CEFUROXIME SODIUM
Kefurox Vials, ADD-Vantage. . . . 1948
Zinacef Injection. . . . 1696

CEFUR (Italy)
CEFUROXIME SODIUM
Kefurox Vials, ADD-Vantage. . . . 1948
Zinacef Injection. . . . 1696

CEFURACET (Mexico)
CEFUROXIME AXETIL
Ceftin Tablets . . . 1898
Ceftin for Oral Suspension . . . 1898

CEFUREX (Italy)
CEFUROXIME SODIUM
Kefurox Vials, ADD-Vantage. . . . 1948
Zinacef Injection. . . . 1696

CEFURIN (Italy)
CEFUROXIME SODIUM
Kefurox Vials, ADD-Vantage. . . . 1948
Zinacef Injection. . . . 1696

CEFUROX-REU (Germany)
CEFUROXIME SODIUM
Kefurox Vials, ADD-Vantage. . . . 1948
Zinacef Injection. . . . 1696

CEFXITIN (Thailand)
CEFOXITIN SODIUM
Mefoxin Premixed Intravenous Solution . . 2127
Mefoxin for Injection . . . 2124

CEFZIL (Canada, United Kingdom)
CEFPROZIL
Cefzil Tablets . . . 1076
Cefzil for Oral Suspension . . . 1076

CEFZON (Japan)
CEFDINIR
Omnicef Capsules . . . 493
Omnicef for Oral Suspension. . . . 493

CELEBRA (Denmark)
CELECOXIB
Celebrex Capsules. . . . 2676, 2780

CELEBREX (Australia, Canada, Irish Republic, New Zealand, South Africa, Switzerland, United Kingdom)
CELECOXIB
Celebrex Capsules. . . . 2676, 2780

CELEFER (Spain)
MUPIROCIN
Bactroban Ointment . . . 1496

CELESDEPOT (Portugal)
BETAMETHASONE ACETATE/BETAMETHASONE SODIUM PHOSPHATE
Celestone Soluspan Injectable Suspension . . . 3097

CELESTAN DEPOT (Germany)
BETAMETHASONE ACETATE/BETAMETHASONE SODIUM PHOSPHATE
Celestone Soluspan Injectable Suspension . . . 3097

CELESTENE CHRONODOSE (France)
BETAMETHASONE ACETATE/BETAMETHASONE SODIUM PHOSPHATE
Celestone Soluspan Injectable Suspension . . . 3097

CELESTON (Norway)
BETAMETHASONE ACETATE/BETAMETHASONE SODIUM PHOSPHATE
Celestone Soluspan Injectable Suspension . . . 3097

CELESTON BIFAS (Sweden)
BETAMETHASONE ACETATE/BETAMETHASONE SODIUM PHOSPHATE
Celestone Soluspan Injectable Suspension . . . 3097

CELESTONE CHRONODOSE (Australia, Israel, New Zealand, Switzerland, The Netherlands)
BETAMETHASONE ACETATE/BETAMETHASONE SODIUM PHOSPHATE
Celestone Soluspan Injectable Suspension . . . 3097

CELESTONE CRONODOSE (Italy, Spain)
BETAMETHASONE ACETATE/BETAMETHASONE SODIUM PHOSPHATE
Celestone Soluspan Injectable Suspension . . . 3097

CELEX (Thailand)
CEPHALEXIN
Keflex Oral Suspension . . . 1237
Keflex Pulvules . . . 1237

CELEXA (Canada)
CITALOPRAM HYDROBROMIDE
Celexa Tablets. . . . 1365

CELEXIN (Singapore, Thailand)
CEPHALEXIN
Keflex Oral Suspension . . . 1237
Keflex Pulvules . . . 1237

CELLCEPT (Australia, Austria, Belgium, Canada, Denmark, Finland, France, Germany, Hong Kong, Irish Republic, Israel, Italy, New Zealand, Norway, Portugal, Singapore, South Africa, Spain, Sweden, Switzerland, Thailand, The Netherlands)
MYCOPHENOLATE MOFETIL
CellCept Capsules . . . 2951
CellCept Oral Suspension. . . . 2951
CellCept Tablets. . . . 2951

CELLOIDS PC 73 (Australia)
POTASSIUM CHLORIDE
K-Dur Microburst Release System ER Tablets. . . . 1832
K-Lor Powder Packets. . . . 469
K-Tab Filmtab Tablets . . . 470
Rum-K. . . . 1363

CELVISTA (Thailand)
RALOXIFENE HYDROCHLORIDE
Evista Tablets . . . 1915

CEMAC B12 (United Kingdom)
VITAMIN B12
Nascobal Gel . . . 3174

CEMADO (Italy)
CEFAMANDOLE NAFATE
Mandol Vials . . . 1953

CEMENTIN (Hong Kong, Singapore)
CIMETIDINE
Tagamet Tablets . . . 1644

CEMIDIN (Israel)
CIMETIDINE
Tagamet Tablets . . . 1644

CENCAMET (Thailand)
CIMETIDINE
Tagamet Tablets . . . 1644

CENLIDAC (Thailand)
SULINDAC
Clinoril Tablets. . . . 2053

CENPINE (Thailand)
NICARDIPINE HYDROCHLORIDE
Cardene I.V. . . . 3485

CENTRAPRYL (United Kingdom)
SELEGILINE HYDROCHLORIDE
Eldepryl Capsules . . . 3266

CENTRATUSS DM EXPECTORANT (Canada)
DEXTROMETHORPHAN HYDROBROMIDE/GUAIFENESIN
Tussi-Organidin DM NR Liquid . . . 3350
Tussi-Organidin DM-S NR Liquid . . . 3350

CEOXIL (Italy)
CEFADROXIL
Duricef Capsules . . . 1079

Duricef Oral Suspension. 1079
Duricef Tablets 1079

CEPAN (Italy)
CEFOTETAN DISODIUM
Cefotan Injection 664
Cefotan for Injection 664

CEPAZINE (France)
CEFUROXIME AXETIL
Ceftin Tablets 1898
Ceftin for Oral Suspension 1898

CEPEXIN (Austria)
CEPHALEXIN
Keflex Oral Suspension 1237
Keflex Pulvules 1237

CEPHALEX (Germany)
CEPHALEXIN
Keflex Oral Suspension 1237
Keflex Pulvules 1237

CEPHALOBENE (Austria)
CEPHALEXIN
Keflex Oral Suspension 1237
Keflex Pulvules 1237

CEPH-BIOCIN (Germany)
CEFACLOR
Ceclor CD Tablets 1279
Ceclor Pulvules 1905
Ceclor Suspension 1905

CEPHIN (Thailand)
CEPHALEXIN
Keflex Oral Suspension 1237
Keflex Pulvules 1237

CEPHORAL (Germany, Switzerland)
CEFIXIME
Suprax Tablets 1877
Suprax for Oral Suspension 1877

CEPHOS (Italy)
CEFADROXIL
Duricef Capsules 1079
Duricef Oral Suspension. 1079
Duricef Tablets 1079

CEPHULAC (Canada)
LACTULOSE
Kristalose for Oral Solution. 1007

CEPIFRAN (Spain)
CEFTIBUTEN
Cedax Capsules. 1021
Cedax Oral Suspension 1021

CEPIM (Italy)
CEFEPIME HYDROCHLORIDE
Maxipime for Injection 1285

CEPIMEX (Italy)
CEFEPIME HYDROCHLORIDE
Maxipime for Injection 1285

CEPOREX (Australia, Belgium, Canada, Hong Kong, Irish Republic, Italy, Mexico, Portugal, Singapore, South Africa, Spain, Switzerland, Thailand, The Netherlands, United Kingdom)
CEPHALEXIN
Keflex Oral Suspension 1237
Keflex Pulvules 1237

CEPOREXIN (Brazil)
CEPHALEXIN
Keflex Oral Suspension 1237
Keflex Pulvules 1237

CEPOREXINE (France)
CEPHALEXIN
Keflex Oral Suspension 1237
Keflex Pulvules 1237

CEPRANDAL (Spain)
OMEPRAZOLE
Prilosec Delayed-Release Capsules 628

CEPRIMAX (Spain)
CIPROFLOXACIN HYDROCHLORIDE
Ciloxan Ophthalmic Ointment. 538
Ciloxan Ophthalmic Solution . . . . ⊙209, 538
Cipro Tablets. 887

CEPTAZ (Canada)
CEFTAZIDIME
Ceptaz for Injection 1499
Fortaz for Injection 1541
Tazicef for Injection 1647
Tazidime Vials, Faspak & ADD-Vantage . . 1966

CERAX (Thailand)
HYDROXYZINE HYDROCHLORIDE
Atarax Tablets & Syrup 2667
Vistaril Intramuscular Solution 2738

CERCON (Mexico)
PRAZIQUANTEL
Biltricide Tablets 887

CEREBRAMED (Germany)
AMANTADINE HYDROCHLORIDE
Symmetrel Syrup 1328
Symmetrel Tablets 1328

CEREBROVASE (United Kingdom)
DIPYRIDAMOLE
Persantine Tablets 1057

CEREBYX (Canada)
FOSPHENYTOIN SODIUM
Cerebyx Injection 2619

CEREEN (South Africa)
HALOPERIDOL
Haldol Injection, Tablets and Concentrate. 2533

CERELLA (Germany)
ESTRADIOL
Alora Transdermal System 3372
Climara Transdermal System. 958
Estrace Vaginal Cream 3358
Estring Vaginal Ring 2811
Vivelle Transdermal System 2412
Vivelle-Dot Transdermal System 2416

CEREXIN (South Africa)
CEPHALEXIN
Keflex Oral Suspension 1237
Keflex Pulvules 1237

CEREZYME (Australia, Austria, Denmark, France, Germany, Israel, Italy, Japan, Portugal, Spain, Switzerland, United Kingdom)
IMIGLUCERASE
Cerezyme for Injection. 1438

CERINA (Switzerland)
ESTRADIOL
Alora Transdermal System 3372
Climara Transdermal System. 958
Estrace Vaginal Cream 3358
Estring Vaginal Ring 2811
Vivelle Transdermal System 2412
Vivelle-Dot Transdermal System 2416

CERTALAC (Belgium)
LACTULOSE
Kristalose for Oral Solution. 1007

CERTOVERMIL (Brazil)
MEBENDAZOLE
Vermox Chewable Tablets. 2017

CERUBIDIN (Australia, Denmark, Irish Republic, Norway, South Africa, Sweden, United Kingdom)
DAUNORUBICIN HYDROCHLORIDE
Cerubidine for Injection 947

CERUBIDINE (Belgium, Canada, France, Israel, New Zealand, Switzerland, The Netherlands)
DAUNORUBICIN HYDROCHLORIDE
Cerubidine for Injection 947

CERVASTA (Italy)
CERIVASTATIN SODIUM
Baycol Tablets. 883

CERVIDIL (Canada)
DINOPROSTONE
Cervidil Vaginal Insert 1369
Prepidil Gel. 2851
Prostin E2 Suppositories 2852

CERVIPROST (Austria, Germany, Norway, Sweden, Switzerland, The Netherlands)
DINOPROSTONE
Cervidil Vaginal Insert 1369
Prepidil Gel. 2851
Prostin E2 Suppositories 2852

CESOL (Germany, Mexico, Portugal)
PRAZIQUANTEL
Biltricide Tablets 887

CESPLON (Spain)
CAPTOPRIL
Captopril Tablets 2281

CESRA (Germany)
IBUPROFEN
Motrin Suspension, Oral Drops, Chewable Tablets, and Caplets 2002

CESSAVERM (Brazil)
MEBENDAZOLE
Vermox Chewable Tablets. 2017

CESTOX (Brazil)
PRAZIQUANTEL
Biltricide Tablets 887

CETA SULFA (Mexico)
SULFACETAMIDE SODIUM
Bleph-10 Ophthalmic Ointment 10% . . . . ⊙230
Klaron Lotion 10% 1224

CETAMIDE (Canada)
SULFACETAMIDE SODIUM
Bleph-10 Ophthalmic Ointment 10% . . . . ⊙230
Klaron Lotion 10% 1224

CETAMPRIL (Portugal)
ENALAPRIL MALEATE
Vasotec Tablets. 2210

CETAPRED (Belgium)
PREDNISOLONE ACETATE/SULFACETAMIDE SODIUM
Blephamide Ophthalmic Ointment 547
Blephamide Ophthalmic Suspension 548

CETASIL (Thailand)
SULFACETAMIDE SODIUM
Bleph-10 Ophthalmic Ointment 10% . . . . ⊙230
Klaron Lotion 10% 1224

CETAZIN (Austria)
SULFACETAMIDE SODIUM
Bleph-10 Ophthalmic Ointment 10% . . . . ⊙230
Klaron Lotion 10% 1224

CETINA (Mexico)
CHLORAMPHENICOL
Chloromycetin Ophthalmic Ointment, 1% . . . . . ⊙296
Chloromycetin Ophthalmic Solution . . . . ⊙297
Chloroptic Sterile Ophthalmic Ointment . . ⊙234
Chloroptic Sterile Ophthalmic Solution . . ⊙235

CETONAX (Brazil)
KETOCONAZOLE
Nizoral 2% Cream 3620
Nizoral 2% Shampoo. 2007
Nizoral Tablets 1791

CETONIL (Brazil)
KETOCONAZOLE
Nizoral 2% Cream 3620
Nizoral 2% Shampoo. 2007
Nizoral Tablets 1791

CETOZOL (Brazil)
KETOCONAZOLE
Nizoral 2% Cream 3620
Nizoral 2% Shampoo. 2007
Nizoral Tablets 1791

CETRAPHYLLINE (France)
THEOPHYLLINE
Aerolate Jr. T.D. Capsules 1361
Aerolate Liquid 1361
Aerolate Sr. T.D. Capsules 1361
Theo-Dur Extended-Release Tablets. 1835
Uni-Dur Extended-Release Tablets. 1841
Uniphyl 400 mg and 600 mg Tablets . . . 2903

CETRIZET (Thailand)
CETIRIZINE HYDROCHLORIDE
Zyrtec Syrup. 2756
Zyrtec Tablets. 2756

CETRIZIN (Brazil)
CETIRIZINE HYDROCHLORIDE
Zyrtec Syrup. 2756
Zyrtec Tablets. 2756

CHANTALINE (Spain)
THEOPHYLLINE
Aerolate Jr. T.D. Capsules 1361
Aerolate Liquid 1361
Aerolate Sr. T.D. Capsules 1361
Theo-Dur Extended-Release Tablets. 1835
Uni-Dur Extended-Release Tablets. 1841
Uniphyl 400 mg and 600 mg Tablets . . . 2903

CHEMET (Austria)
SUCCIMER
Chemet Capsules. 3078

CHEMICETINA (Spain)
CHLORAMPHENICOL
Chloromycetin Ophthalmic Ointment, 1% . . . . . ⊙296
Chloromycetin Ophthalmic Solution . . . . ⊙297
Chloroptic Sterile Ophthalmic Ointment . . ⊙234
Chloroptic Sterile Ophthalmic Solution . . ⊙235

CHEMISTS OWN CLOZOLE (Australia)
CLOTRIMAZOLE
Lotrimin Cream 1%. 3128
Lotrimin Lotion 1% 3128
Lotrimin Topical Solution 1% 3128
Mycelex Troche 573

CHEMISTS OWN DE WORM (Australia)
MEBENDAZOLE
Vermox Chewable Tablets. 2017

CHEMYDUR (United Kingdom)
ISOSORBIDE MONONITRATE
Imdur Tablets 1826
Ismo Tablets. 3524

CHEMYPARIN (Italy)
HEPARIN SODIUM
Heparin Lock Flush Solution 3509
Heparin Sodium Injection 3511

CHERACOL D (Mexico)
DEXTROMETHORPHAN HYDROBROMIDE/GUAIFENESIN
Tussi-Organidin DM NR Liquid 3350
Tussi-Organidin DM-S NR Liquid 3350

CHIBRETICO (Portugal)
AMILORIDE HYDROCHLORIDE/HYDROCHLOROTHIAZIDE
Moduretic Tablets. 2138

CHIBROCADRON (The Netherlands)
DEXAMETHASONE SODIUM PHOSPHATE/NEOMYCIN SULFATE
NeoDecadron Sterile Ophthalmic Solution 2144

CHIBRO-CADRON (France)
DEXAMETHASONE SODIUM PHOSPHATE/NEOMYCIN SULFATE
NeoDecadron Sterile Ophthalmic Solution 2144

CHIBRO-PROSCAR (France)
FINASTERIDE
Propecia Tablets 2172
Proscar Tablets 2175

CHIBRO-TIMOPTOL (Germany)
TIMOLOL MALEATE
Blocadren Tablets 2046
Timoptic Sterile Ophthalmic Solution. . . . 2190
Timoptic in Ocudose 2192
Timoptic-XE Sterile Ophthalmic Gel Forming Solution. 2194

CHIBROXIN (Brazil, Germany, Hong Kong, Israel, Singapore, Spain)
NORFLOXACIN
Chibroxin Sterile Ophthalmic Solution . . . . . ⊙273, 2051
Noroxin Tablets 2145

CHIBROXINE (France)
NORFLOXACIN
Chibroxin Sterile Ophthalmic Solution . . . . . ⊙273, 2051
Noroxin Tablets 2145

CHIBROXOL (Belgium, Portugal, Switzerland, The Netherlands)
NORFLOXACIN
Chibroxin Sterile Ophthalmic Solution . . . . . ⊙273, 2051
Noroxin Tablets 2145

CHILDRENS CHESTY COUGH SYRUP (United Kingdom)
GUAIFENESIN
Organidin NR Liquid 3350
Organidin NR Tablets. 3350

CHIMAX (United Kingdom)
FLUTAMIDE
Eulexin Capsules 3118

CHINTEINA (Italy)
QUINIDINE SULFATE
Quinidex Extentabs. 2933

CHLOMENT (Hong Kong)
CHLORAMPHENICOL
Chloromycetin Ophthalmic Ointment, 1% . . . . . ⊙296
Chloromycetin Ophthalmic Solution . . . . ⊙297
Chloroptic Sterile Ophthalmic Ointment . . ⊙234
Chloroptic Sterile Ophthalmic Solution . . ⊙235

CHLOMIDE (Singapore)
CHLORPROPAMIDE
Diabinese Tablets. 2680

CHLORACIL (Thailand)
CHLORAMPHENICOL
Chloromycetin Ophthalmic Ointment, 1% . . . . . ⊙296
Chloromycetin Ophthalmic Solution . . . . ⊙297
Chloroptic Sterile Ophthalmic Ointment . . ⊙234
Chloroptic Sterile Ophthalmic Solution . . ⊙235

CHLORACTIL (United Kingdom)
CHLORPROMAZINE HYDROCHLORIDE
Thorazine Ampuls. 1656
Thorazine Multi-dose Vials 1656
Thorazine Spansule Capsules 1656
Thorazine Syrup 1656
Thorazine Tablets. 1656

CHLORAETHYL DR HENNING (Germany)
ETHYL CHLORIDE
Gebauer's Ethyl Chloride 1409

CHLORAMEX (South Africa)
CHLORAMPHENICOL
Chloromycetin Ophthalmic Ointment, 1% . . . . . ⊙296
Chloromycetin Ophthalmic Solution . . . . ⊙297
Chloroptic Sterile Ophthalmic Ointment . . ⊙234
Chloroptic Sterile Ophthalmic Solution . . ⊙235

CHLORAMINOPHENE (Monaco)
CHLORAMBUCIL
Leukeran Tablets 1591

CHLORAMSAAR N (Germany)
CHLORAMPHENICOL
Chloromycetin Ophthalmic Ointment, 1% ⊙296
Chloromycetin Ophthalmic Solution ⊙297
Chloroptic Sterile Ophthalmic Ointment ⊙234
Chloroptic Sterile Ophthalmic Solution ⊙235

CHLORASEPTIC LOZENGES (Canada)
BENZOCAINE
Americaine Anesthetic Lubricant 1162
Americaine Otic Topical Anesthetic Ear Drops 1162

CHLORAZIN (Switzerland)
CHLORPROMAZINE HYDROCHLORIDE
Thorazine Ampuls 1656
Thorazine Multi-dose Vials 1656
Thorazine Spansule Capsules 1656
Thorazine Syrup 1656
Thorazine Tablets 1656

CHLORCOL (South Africa)
CHLORAMPHENICOL
Chloromycetin Ophthalmic Ointment, 1% ⊙296
Chloromycetin Ophthalmic Solution ⊙297
Chloroptic Sterile Ophthalmic Ointment ⊙234
Chloroptic Sterile Ophthalmic Solution ⊙235

CHLORETHYL (Switzerland)
ETHYL CHLORIDE
Gebauer's Ethyl Chloride 1409

CHLORNICOL (South Africa)
CHLORAMPHENICOL
Chloromycetin Ophthalmic Ointment, 1% ⊙296
Chloromycetin Ophthalmic Solution ⊙297
Chloroptic Sterile Ophthalmic Ointment ⊙234
Chloroptic Sterile Ophthalmic Solution ⊙235

CHLOROCHIN (Switzerland)
CHLOROQUINE PHOSPHATE
Aralen Tablets 3075

CHLOROMYCETIN (Finland, Irish Republic, Spain, Sweden, Switzerland, United Kingdom)
CHLORAMPHENICOL
Chloromycetin Ophthalmic Ointment, 1% ⊙296
Chloromycetin Ophthalmic Solution ⊙297
Chloroptic Sterile Ophthalmic Ointment ⊙234
Chloroptic Sterile Ophthalmic Solution ⊙235

CHLOROMYCETIN HYDROCORTISONE (United Kingdom)
CHLORAMPHENICOL
Chloromycetin Ophthalmic Ointment, 1% ⊙296
Chloromycetin Ophthalmic Solution ⊙297
Chloroptic Sterile Ophthalmic Ointment ⊙234
Chloroptic Sterile Ophthalmic Solution ⊙235

CHLOROPH (Thailand)
CHLORAMPHENICOL
Chloromycetin Ophthalmic Ointment, 1% ⊙296
Chloromycetin Ophthalmic Solution ⊙297
Chloroptic Sterile Ophthalmic Ointment ⊙234
Chloroptic Sterile Ophthalmic Solution ⊙235

CHLOROPOTASSURIL (Belgium)
POTASSIUM CHLORIDE
K-Dur Microburst Release System ER Tablets 1832
K-Lor Powder Packets 469
K-Tab Filmtab Tablets 470
Rum-K 1363

CHLOROPTIC (Australia, Canada, Germany, Irish Republic, Israel, New Zealand, South Africa)
CHLORAMPHENICOL
Chloromycetin Ophthalmic Ointment, 1% ⊙296
Chloromycetin Ophthalmic Solution ⊙297
Chloroptic Sterile Ophthalmic Ointment ⊙234
Chloroptic Sterile Ophthalmic Solution ⊙235

CHLORPHEN (South Africa)
CHLORAMPHENICOL
Chloromycetin Ophthalmic Ointment, 1% ⊙296
Chloromycetin Ophthalmic Solution ⊙297
Chloroptic Sterile Ophthalmic Ointment ⊙234
Chloroptic Sterile Ophthalmic Solution ⊙235

CHLORPROMANYL (Canada)
CHLORPROMAZINE HYDROCHLORIDE
Thorazine Ampuls 1656
Thorazine Multi-dose Vials 1656
Thorazine Spansule Capsules 1656
Thorazine Syrup 1656
Thorazine Tablets 1656

CHLORPROMED (Thailand)
CHLORPROMAZINE HYDROCHLORIDE
Thorazine Ampuls 1656
Thorazine Multi-dose Vials 1656
Thorazine Spansule Capsules 1656
Thorazine Syrup 1656
Thorazine Tablets 1656

CHLORQUIN (Australia, Hong Kong)
CHLOROQUINE PHOSPHATE
Aralen Tablets 3075

CHLORSIG (Australia, Hong Kong, New Zealand)
CHLORAMPHENICOL
Chloromycetin Ophthalmic Ointment, 1% ⊙296
Chloromycetin Ophthalmic Solution ⊙297
Chloroptic Sterile Ophthalmic Ointment ⊙234
Chloroptic Sterile Ophthalmic Solution ⊙235

CHLOR-TRIPOLON ND (Canada)
LORATADINE/PSEUDOEPHEDRINE SULFATE
Claritin-D 12 Hour Extended Release Tablets 3102
Claritin-D 24 Hour Extended Release Tablets 3104

CHLORVESCENT (New Zealand)
POTASSIUM CHLORIDE
K-Dur Microburst Release System ER Tablets 1832
K-Lor Powder Packets 469
K-Tab Filmtab Tablets 470
Rum-K 1363

CHLORZIDE (Singapore)
CHLOROTHIAZIDE
Diuril Oral Suspension 2087
Diuril Tablets 2087

CHLORZOX (Thailand)
CHLORZOXAZONE
Parafon Forte DSC Caplets 2582

CHLOTRIDE (Australia, Denmark, The Netherlands)
CHLOROTHIAZIDE
Diuril Oral Suspension 2087
Diuril Tablets 2087

CHOLESTABYL (Germany)
COLESTIPOL HYDROCHLORIDE
Colestid Tablets 2791

CHOLSTAT (Belgium)
CERIVASTATIN SODIUM
Baycol Tablets 883

CHRONADALATE (France)
NIFEDIPINE
Adalat CC Tablets 877
Procardia Capsules 2708
Procardia XL Extended Release Tablets 2710

CHRONOPHYLLIN (South Africa)
THEOPHYLLINE
Aerolate Jr. T.D. Capsules 1361
Aerolate Liquid 1361
Aerolate Sr. T.D. Capsules 1361
Theo-Dur Extended-Release Tablets 1835
Uni-Dur Extended-Release Tablets 1841
Uniphyl 400 mg and 600 mg Tablets 2903

CHRONOVERA (Canada)
VERAPAMIL HYDROCHLORIDE
Covera-HS Tablets 3199
Isoptin SR Tablets 467
Verelan Capsules 3184
Verelan PM Capsules 3186

CHRONULAC (Canada)
LACTULOSE
Kristalose for Oral Solution 1007

CIBACE (South Africa)
BENAZEPRIL HYDROCHLORIDE
Lotensin Tablets 2365

CIBACEN (Austria, Belgium, Denmark, Germany, Irish Republic, Israel, Italy, New Zealand, Spain, Switzerland, The Netherlands)
BENAZEPRIL HYDROCHLORIDE
Lotensin Tablets 2365

CIBACENE (France)
BENAZEPRIL HYDROCHLORIDE
Lotensin Tablets 2365

CIBADREX (Austria, Denmark, France, Germany, Italy, South Africa, Sweden, Switzerland, The Netherlands)
BENAZEPRIL HYDROCHLORIDE/HYDROCHLOROTHIAZIDE
Lotensin HCT Tablets 2367

CIBALGINA DUE FAST (Italy)
IBUPROFEN
Motrin Suspension, Oral Drops, Chewable Tablets, and Caplets 2002

CICLADOL L (Italy)
PIROXICAM
Feldene Capsules 2685

CICLOCHEM (Spain)
CICLOPIROX OLAMINE
Loprox Cream 2021
Loprox Lotion 2021

CICLODERM (Israel)
CICLOPIROX OLAMINE
Loprox Cream 2021
Loprox Lotion 2021

CICLOTAL (Mexico)
MEDROXYPROGESTERONE ACETATE
Depo-Provera Contraceptive Injection 2798
Provera Tablets 2853

CIDAN EST (Spain)
STREPTOMYCIN SULFATE
Streptomycin Sulfate Injection 2714

CIDANAMOX (Spain)
AMOXICILLIN
Amoxil Pediatric Drops for Oral Suspension 1471
Amoxil Tablets 1471

CIDANBUTOL (Spain)
ETHAMBUTOL HYDROCHLORIDE
Myambutol Tablets 1290

CIDANCHIN (Spain)
CHLOROQUINE PHOSPHATE
Aralen Tablets 3075

CIDINE (Thailand)
CIMETIDINE
Tagamet Tablets 1644

CIDOMYCIN (Australia, Canada, Irish Republic, Israel, South Africa, United Kingdom)
GENTAMICIN SULFATE
Genoptic Ophthalmic Ointment ⊙239
Genoptic Sterile Ophthalmic Solution ⊙239

CIFLAN (Portugal)
CIPROFLOXACIN HYDROCHLORIDE
Ciloxan Ophthalmic Ointment 538
Ciloxan Ophthalmic Solution ⊙209, 538
Cipro Tablets 887

CIFLOX (Brazil, Denmark, Italy)
CIPROFLOXACIN HYDROCHLORIDE
Ciloxan Ophthalmic Ointment 538
Ciloxan Ophthalmic Solution ⊙209, 538
Cipro Tablets 887

CIFOLAN (Thailand)
CIPROFLOXACIN
Cipro I.V. 893
Cipro I.V. Pharmacy Bulk Package 897
Cipro Oral Suspension 887

CIFRANTIL (Brazil)
ERYTHROMYCIN
Emgel 2% Topical Gel 1285
Ery-Tab Tablets 448
Erythromycin Base Filmtab Tablets 454
Erythromycin Delayed-Release Capsules, USP 455
PCE Dispertab Tablets 498

CIGAMET (Thailand)
CIMETIDINE
Tagamet Tablets 1644

CIL (Germany)
FENOFIBRATE
Tricor Capsules, Micronized 513

CILAB (Thailand)
CIPROFLOXACIN
Cipro I.V. 893
Cipro I.V. Pharmacy Bulk Package 897
Cipro Oral Suspension 887

CILDOX (Spain)
DOXYCYCLINE HYCLATE
Doryx Coated Pellet Filled Capsules 3357
Periostat Tablets 1208
Vibra-Tabs Film Coated Tablets 2735
Vibramycin Hyclate Capsules 2735
Vibramycin Hyclate Intravenous 2737

CILEX (Australia)
CEPHALEXIN
Keflex Oral Suspension 1237
Keflex Pulvules 1237

CILICEF (Spain)
CEPHALEXIN
Keflex Oral Suspension 1237
Keflex Pulvules 1237

CILOQUIN (Australia)
CIPROFLOXACIN HYDROCHLORIDE
Ciloxan Ophthalmic Ointment 538
Ciloxan Ophthalmic Solution ⊙209, 538
Cipro Tablets 887

CILOX (Norway)
CIPROFLOXACIN HYDROCHLORIDE
Ciloxan Ophthalmic Ointment 538
Ciloxan Ophthalmic Solution ⊙209, 538
Cipro Tablets 887

CILOXAN (Australia, Austria, Belgium, Brazil, Canada, Denmark, France, Germany, Hong Kong, Israel, Mexico, New Zealand, Singapore, South Africa, Sweden, Switzerland, Thailand, United Kingdom)
CIPROFLOXACIN HYDROCHLORIDE
Ciloxan Ophthalmic Ointment 538
Ciloxan Ophthalmic Solution ⊙209, 538
Cipro Tablets 887

CIM (Portugal)
CIMETIDINE
Tagamet Tablets 1644

CIMAG (Thailand)
CIMETIDINE
Tagamet Tablets 1644

CIMAGEN (Irish Republic)
CIMETIDINE
Tagamet Tablets 1644

CIMAL (Norway, Sweden)
CIMETIDINE
Tagamet Tablets 1644

CIMEBEC (Mexico)
CIMETIDINE
Tagamet Tablets 1644

CIMEBETA (Germany)
CIMETIDINE
Tagamet Tablets 1644

CIMECODAN (Denmark)
CIMETIDINE
Tagamet Tablets 1644

CIMEHEXAL (Australia)
CIMETIDINE
Tagamet Tablets 1644

CIMELDINE (Irish Republic)
CIMETIDINE
Tagamet Tablets 1644

CIMEMERCK (Germany)
CIMETIDINE
Tagamet Tablets 1644

CIMEPHIL (Germany)
CIMETIDINE
Tagamet Tablets 1644

CIMET (Germany)
CIMETIDINE
Tagamet Tablets 1644

CIMETA (Hong Kong)
CIMETIDINE
Tagamet Tablets 1644

CIMETAG (Israel)
CIMETIDINE
Tagamet Tablets 1644

CIMETASE (Mexico)
CIMETIDINE
Tagamet Tablets 1644

CIMETID (Norway)
CIMETIDINE
Tagamet Tablets 1644

CIMETIDAN (Brazil)
CIMETIDINE
Tagamet Tablets 1644

CIMETIL (Brazil)
CIMETIDINE
Tagamet Tablets 1644

CIMETIMAX (Australia)
CIMETIDINE
Tagamet Tablets 1644

CIMETIN (Brazil)
CIMETIDINE
Tagamet Tablets 1644

CIMET-P (Thailand)
CIMETIDINE
Tagamet Tablets 1644

CIMEX (Brazil, Finland)
CIMETIDINE
Tagamet Tablets 1644

CIMI (Israel)
CIMETIDINE
Tagamet Tablets 1644

CIMIDINE (Thailand)
CIMETIDINE
Tagamet Tablets 1644

CIMLICH (Germany)
CIMETIDINE
Tagamet Tablets 1644

CIMLOK (South Africa)
CIMETIDINE
Tagamet Tablets 1644

CIMOGAL (Mexico)
CIPROFLOXACIN HYDROCHLORIDE
Ciloxan Ophthalmic Ointment. 538
Ciloxan Ophthalmic Solution . . . . ⊙209, 538
Cipro Tablets. 887

CIMULCER (Hong Kong, Singapore, Thailand)
CIMETIDINE
Tagamet Tablets 1644

CINABEL (Mexico)
CLOTRIMAZOLE
Lotrimin Cream 1%. 3128
Lotrimin Lotion 1% 3128
Lotrimin Topical Solution 1% 3128
Mycelex Troche 573

CINADINE (South Africa)
CIMETIDINE
Tagamet Tablets 1644

CINFATOS EXPECTORANTE (Spain)
DEXTROMETHORPHAN HYDROBROMIDE/GUAIFENESIN
Tussi-Organidin DM NR Liquid 3350
Tussi-Organidin DM-S NR Liquid 3350

CINKEF-U (Portugal)
FLUOROURACIL
Efudex Cream 1733
Efudex Topical Solutions 1733
Fluoroplex Topical Cream 552
Fluoroplex Topical Solution 552

CINULCUS (Spain)
CIMETIDINE
Tagamet Tablets 1644

CIPADUR (South Africa)
CEFADROXIL
Duricef Capsules 1079
Duricef Oral Suspension. 1079
Duricef Tablets 1079

CIPEX (South Africa)
MEBENDAZOLE
Vermox Chewable Tablets. 2017

CIPFLOCIN (Thailand)
CIPROFLOXACIN
Cipro I.V. 893
Cipro I.V. Pharmacy Bulk Package 897
Cipro Oral Suspension. 887

CIPLOX (Portugal)
CIPROFLOXACIN HYDROCHLORIDE
Ciloxan Ophthalmic Ointment. 538
Ciloxan Ophthalmic Solution . . . . ⊙209, 538
Cipro Tablets. 887

CIPOBACTER (Spain)
CIPROFLOXACIN HYDROCHLORIDE
Ciloxan Ophthalmic Ointment. 538
Ciloxan Ophthalmic Solution . . . . ⊙209, 538
Cipro Tablets. 887

CIPRAIN (Mexico)
CIPROFLOXACIN
Cipro I.V. 893
Cipro I.V. Pharmacy Bulk Package 897
Cipro Oral Suspension. 887

CIPRAM (Hong Kong, Singapore, Thailand)
CITALOPRAM HYDROBROMIDE
Celexa Tablets. 1365

CIPRAMIL (Australia, Germany, Irish Republic, Israel, New Zealand, Norway, South Africa, Sweden, The Netherlands)
CITALOPRAM HYDROBROMIDE
Celexa Tablets. 1365

CIPRENIT OTICO (Spain)
CIPROFLOXACIN HYDROCHLORIDE
Ciloxan Ophthalmic Ointment. 538
Ciloxan Ophthalmic Solution . . . . ⊙209, 538
Cipro Tablets. 887

CIPREX (Brazil)
CIPROFLOXACIN HYDROCHLORIDE
Ciloxan Ophthalmic Ointment. 538
Ciloxan Ophthalmic Solution . . . . ⊙209, 538
Cipro Tablets. 887

CIPRO (Brazil)
CIPROFLOXACIN
Cipro I.V. 893
Cipro I.V. Pharmacy Bulk Package 897
Cipro Oral Suspension. 887

CIPRO HC (Canada)
CIPROFLOXACIN HYDROCHLORIDE/HYDROCORTISONE
Cipro HC Otic Suspension 540

CIPROBID (Thailand)
CIPROFLOXACIN
Cipro I.V. 893
Cipro I.V. Pharmacy Bulk Package 897
Cipro Oral Suspension. 887

CIPROBIOTIC (Mexico)
CIPROFLOXACIN HYDROCHLORIDE
Ciloxan Ophthalmic Ointment. 538
Ciloxan Ophthalmic Solution . . . . ⊙209, 538
Cipro Tablets. 887

CIPROFIN (Thailand)
CIPROFLOXACIN
Cipro I.V. 893
Cipro I.V. Pharmacy Bulk Package 897
Cipro Oral Suspension. 887

CIPROFUR (Mexico)
CIPROFLOXACIN HYDROCHLORIDE
Ciloxan Ophthalmic Ointment. 538
Ciloxan Ophthalmic Solution . . . . ⊙209, 538
Cipro Tablets. 887

CIPROGEN (Thailand)
CIPROFLOXACIN
Cipro I.V. 893
Cipro I.V. Pharmacy Bulk Package 897
Cipro Oral Suspension. 887

CIPROGIS (Israel)
CIPROFLOXACIN
Cipro I.V. 893
Cipro I.V. Pharmacy Bulk Package 897
Cipro Oral Suspension. 887

CIPROK (Spain)
CIPROFLOXACIN HYDROCHLORIDE
Ciloxan Ophthalmic Ointment. 538
Ciloxan Ophthalmic Solution . . . . ⊙209, 538
Cipro Tablets. 887

CIPROQUINOL (Portugal)
CIPROFLOXACIN
Cipro I.V. 893
Cipro I.V. Pharmacy Bulk Package 897
Cipro Oral Suspension. 887

CIPROSER (Mexico)
CIPROFLOXACIN
Cipro I.V. 893
Cipro I.V. Pharmacy Bulk Package 897
Cipro Oral Suspension. 887

CIPROSUN (Thailand)
CIPROFLOXACIN
Cipro I.V. 893
Cipro I.V. Pharmacy Bulk Package 897
Cipro Oral Suspension. 887

CIPROXIN (Israel)
CIPROFLOXACIN
Cipro I.V. 893
Cipro I.V. Pharmacy Bulk Package 897
Cipro Oral Suspension. 887

CIPROXIN HC (Australia)
CIPROFLOXACIN HYDROCHLORIDE/HYDROCORTISONE
Cipro HC Otic Suspension 540

CIPROXINA (Portugal)
CIPROFLOXACIN HYDROCHLORIDE
Ciloxan Ophthalmic Ointment. 538
Ciloxan Ophthalmic Solution . . . . ⊙209, 538
Cipro Tablets. 887

CIPROXINE (Belgium)
CIPROFLOXACIN
Cipro I.V. 893
Cipro I.V. Pharmacy Bulk Package 897
Cipro Oral Suspension. 887

CIPROXIN-HYDROCORTISON (Finland)
CIPROFLOXACIN HYDROCHLORIDE/HYDROCORTISONE
Cipro HC Otic Suspension 540

CISDAY (Germany)
NIFEDIPINE
Adalat CC Tablets. 877
Procardia Capsules. 2708
Procardia XL Extended Release Tablets . . 2710

CISTAMINE (Thailand)
CETIRIZINE HYDROCHLORIDE
Zyrtec Syrup. 2756
Zyrtec Tablets 2756

CISTICID (Brazil, Mexico)
PRAZIQUANTEL
Biltricide Tablets 887

CITALGAN (Mexico)
IBUPROFEN
Motrin Suspension, Oral Drops, Chewable Tablets, and Caplets 2002

CITICLOR (Italy)
CEFACLOR
Ceclor CD Tablets 1279
Ceclor Pulvules 1905
Ceclor Suspension 1905

CITIDINE (Hong Kong, Singapore, Thailand)
CIMETIDINE
Tagamet Tablets 1644

CITIDOL (Italy)
DIFLUNISAL
Dolobid Tablets 2088

CITILAT (Italy)
NIFEDIPINE
Adalat CC Tablets. 877
Procardia Capsules. 2708
Procardia XL Extended Release Tablets . . 2710

CITIMID (Italy)
CIMETIDINE
Tagamet Tablets 1644

CITIREUMA (Italy)
SULINDAC
Clinoril Tablets. 2053

CITIZEM (Italy)
DILTIAZEM HYDROCHLORIDE
Cardizem CD Capsules 1016
Cardizem Injectable 1018
Cardizem Lyo-Ject Syringe 1018
Cardizem Monovial 1018
Tiazac Capsules 1378

CITOGEL (Italy)
SUCRALFATE
Carafate Suspension 731
Carafate Tablets. 730

CITOKEN (Mexico)
PIROXICAM
Feldene Capsules. 2685

CITOVIRAX (Italy)
GANCICLOVIR SODIUM
Cytovene-IV 2959

CITRIHEXAL (Australia)
CALCITRIOL
Calcijex Injection 411
Rocaltrol Capsules 2991
Rocaltrol Oral Solution. 2991

CITROPLUS (Brazil, Italy)
METOCLOPRAMIDE HYDROCHLORIDE
Reglan Injectable 2935
Reglan Syrup 2935
Reglan Tablets. 2935

CIUK (Germany)
CIMETIDINE
Tagamet Tablets 1644

CIVERAN (Spain)
LORATADINE
Claritin Reditabs 3100
Claritin Syrup 3100
Claritin Tablets 3100

CIVICOR (New Zealand, Singapore)
VERAPAMIL HYDROCHLORIDE
Covera-HS Tablets 3199
Isoptin SR Tablets. 467
Verelan Capsules 3184
Verelan PM Capsules 3186

CLAFORAN (Australia, Austria, Belgium, Brazil, Canada, Denmark, Finland, France, Germany, Hong Kong, Irish Republic, Israel, Italy, Mexico, New Zealand, Norway, Singapore, South Africa, Spain, Sweden, Switzerland, Thailand, The Netherlands, United Kingdom)
CEFOTAXIME SODIUM
Claforan Injection 732

CLAMENTIN (South Africa)
AMOXICILLIN
Amoxil Pediatric Drops for Oral Suspension 1471
Amoxil Tablets. 1471

CLARATYNE (Australia, New Zealand)
LORATADINE
Claritin Reditabs 3100
Claritin Syrup 3100
Claritin Tablets 3100

CLARATYNE DECONGESTANT (New Zealand)
LORATADINE/PSEUDOEPHEDRINE SULFATE
Claritin-D 12 Hour Extended Release Tablets. 3102
Claritin-D 24 Hour Extended Release Tablets 3104

CLARAXIM (Thailand)
CEFOTAXIME SODIUM
Claforan Injection 732

CLARIDON (Portugal)
LORATADINE
Claritin Reditabs 3100
Claritin Syrup 3100
Claritin Tablets 3100

CLARINASE (Australia, Austria, Belgium, France, Hong Kong, Israel, Mexico, Singapore, Spain, Thailand)
LORATADINE/PSEUDOEPHEDRINE SULFATE
Claritin-D 12 Hour Extended Release Tablets 3102
Claritin-D 24 Hour Extended Release Tablets 3104

CLARINEX (Denmark)
LORATADINE/PSEUDOEPHEDRINE SULFATE
Claritin-D 12 Hour Extended Release Tablets 3102
Claritin-D 24 Hour Extended Release Tablets 3104

CLARIPEX (Canada)
CLOFIBRATE
Atromid-S Capsules 3483

CLARISCO (Italy)
HEPARIN SODIUM
Heparin Lock Flush Solution 3509
Heparin Sodium Injection 3511

CLARITIN (Brazil, Canada)
LORATADINE
Claritin Reditabs 3100
Claritin Syrup 3100
Claritin Tablets 3100

CLARITIN EXTRA (Canada)
LORATADINE/PSEUDOEPHEDRINE SULFATE
Claritin-D 12 Hour Extended Release Tablets 3102
Claritin-D 24 Hour Extended Release Tablets 3104

CLARITIN-D (Brazil)
LORATADINE
Claritin Reditabs 3100
Claritin Syrup 3100
Claritin Tablets 3100

CLARITINE (Belgium, Portugal, Switzerland, The Netherlands)
LORATADINE
Claritin Reditabs 3100
Claritin Syrup 3100
Claritin Tablets 3100

CLARITYN (Austria, Denmark, Finland, Irish Republic, Italy, Norway, Sweden, United Kingdom)
LORATADINE
Claritin Reditabs 3100
Claritin Syrup 3100
Claritin Tablets 3100

CLARITYNE (France, Hong Kong, Mexico, Singapore, South Africa, Spain, Thailand)
LORATADINE
Claritin Reditabs 3100
Claritin Syrup 3100
Claritin Tablets 3100

CLAVOXIL (Brazil)
AMOXICILLIN
Amoxil Pediatric Drops for Oral Suspension 1471
Amoxil Tablets. 1471

CLAVULIN (Brazil)
AMOXICILLIN
Amoxil Pediatric Drops for Oral Suspension 1471
Amoxil Tablets. 1471

CLEANCEF (Singapore)
CEFACLOR
Ceclor CD Tablets 1279
Ceclor Pulvules 1905
Ceclor Suspension 1905

CLEAR & CLEAN PERSA (Canada)
BENZOYL PEROXIDE
Brevoxyl-4 Cleansing Lotion 3269
Brevoxyl-4 Creamy Wash 3270
Brevoxyl-4 Gel. 3269
Brevoxyl-8 Cleansing Lotion 3269
Brevoxyl-8 Creamy Wash 3270
Brevoxyl-8 Gel. 3269
Triaz Cleanser. 2026
Triaz Gel 2026

CLEAR CALADRYL SPRAY (Canada)
DIPHENHYDRAMINE HYDROCHLORIDE
Benadryl Parenteral 2617

CLEAR EYES (Australia, Canada, New Zealand)
NAPHAZOLINE HYDROCHLORIDE
Albalon Ophthalmic Solution. . . . . . ⊙225

CLEARAMED (Spain, Sweden)
BENZOYL PEROXIDE
Brevoxyl-4 Cleansing Lotion 3269

Brevoxyl-4 Creamy Wash 3270
Brevoxyl-4 Gel 3269
Brevoxyl-8 Cleansing Lotion 3269
Brevoxyl-8 Creamy Wash 3270
Brevoxyl-8 Gel 3269
Triaz Cleanser 2026
Triaz Gel 2026

CLEARASIL B.P. PLUS (Canada)
BENZOYL PEROXIDE
Brevoxyl-4 Cleansing Lotion 3269
Brevoxyl-4 Creamy Wash 3270
Brevoxyl-4 Gel 3269
Brevoxyl-8 Cleansing Lotion 3269
Brevoxyl-8 Creamy Wash 3270
Brevoxyl-8 Gel 3269
Triaz Cleanser 2026
Triaz Gel 2026

CLEARASIL MAX 10 (United Kingdom)
BENZOYL PEROXIDE
Brevoxyl-4 Cleansing Lotion 3269
Brevoxyl-4 Creamy Wash 3270
Brevoxyl-4 Gel 3269
Brevoxyl-8 Cleansing Lotion 3269
Brevoxyl-8 Creamy Wash 3270
Brevoxyl-8 Gel 3269
Triaz Cleanser 2026
Triaz Gel 2026

CLEARASIL PLUS (Mexico)
BENZOYL PEROXIDE
Brevoxyl-4 Cleansing Lotion 3269
Brevoxyl-4 Creamy Wash 3270
Brevoxyl-4 Gel 3269
Brevoxyl-8 Cleansing Lotion 3269
Brevoxyl-8 Creamy Wash 3270
Brevoxyl-8 Gel 3269
Triaz Cleanser 2026
Triaz Gel 2026

CLEARASIL ULTRA (Australia, Italy)
BENZOYL PEROXIDE
Brevoxyl-4 Cleansing Lotion 3269
Brevoxyl-4 Creamy Wash 3270
Brevoxyl-4 Gel 3269
Brevoxyl-8 Cleansing Lotion 3269
Brevoxyl-8 Creamy Wash 3270
Brevoxyl-8 Gel 3269
Triaz Cleanser 2026
Triaz Gel 2026

CLEAREX COVER UP (Israel)
BENZOYL PEROXIDE
Brevoxyl-4 Cleansing Lotion 3269
Brevoxyl-4 Creamy Wash 3270
Brevoxyl-4 Gel 3269
Brevoxyl-8 Cleansing Lotion 3269
Brevoxyl-8 Creamy Wash 3270
Brevoxyl-8 Gel 3269
Triaz Cleanser 2026
Triaz Gel 2026

CLEOCIN (Australia, Austria, Italy)
CLINDAMYCIN HYDROCHLORIDE
Cleocin HCl Capsules 2784

CLERIDIUM (France)
DIPYRIDAMOLE
Persantine Tablets 1057

CLEVIAN (Italy)
PIROXICAM
Feldene Capsules 2685

CLEXANE (Australia, Belgium, Brazil, Germany, Hong Kong, Irish Republic, Israel, Italy, Mexico, New Zealand, Singapore, South Africa, Spain, Switzerland, Thailand, The Netherlands, United Kingdom)
ENOXAPARIN SODIUM
Lovenox Injection 746

CLIMADERM (Brazil, Mexico)
ESTRADIOL
Alora Transdermal System 3372
Climara Transdermal System 958
Estrace Vaginal Cream 3358
Estring Vaginal Ring 2811
Vivelle Transdermal System 2412
Vivelle-Dot Transdermal System 2416

CLIMARA (Australia, Austria, Belgium, Canada, Denmark, Finland, France, Irish Republic, Israel, Italy, New Zealand, Norway, Portugal, South Africa, Sweden, Switzerland, Thailand, The Netherlands)
ESTRADIOL
Alora Transdermal System 3372
Climara Transdermal System 958
Estrace Vaginal Cream 3358
Estring Vaginal Ring 2811
Vivelle Transdermal System 2412
Vivelle-Dot Transdermal System 2416

CLIMATIDINE (Brazil)
CIMETIDINE
Tagamet Tablets 1644

CLINAC (New Zealand, Portugal)
CLINDAMYCIN PHOSPHATE
Cleocin Phosphate Sterile Solution 2785
Cleocin T Topical Gel 2790
Cleocin T Topical Lotion 2790
Cleocin T Topical Solution 2790
Cleocin Vaginal Cream 2788
Clindets Pledgets 3270

CLINAMIDE (South Africa)
METOCLOPRAMIDE HYDROCHLORIDE
Reglan Injectable 2935
Reglan Syrup 2935
Reglan Tablets 2935

CLINATEN (South Africa)
ATENOLOL
Tenormin I.V. Injection 692

CLINAZOLE (South Africa)
METRONIDAZOLE
MetroCream 1404
MetroGel 1405
MetroGel-Vaginal Gel 1986
MetroLotion 1405
Noritate Cream 1224

CLINDABETA (Germany)
CLINDAMYCIN HYDROCHLORIDE
Cleocin HCl Capsules 2784

CLINDAC (Austria)
CLINDAMYCIN HYDROCHLORIDE
Cleocin HCl Capsules 2784

CLINDAHEXAL (Germany, South Africa)
CLINDAMYCIN HYDROCHLORIDE
Cleocin HCl Capsules 2784

CLINDASTAD (Germany)
CLINDAMYCIN HYDROCHLORIDE
Cleocin HCl Capsules 2784

CLINDATECH (Australia)
CLINDAMYCIN HYDROCHLORIDE
Cleocin HCl Capsules 2784

CLINDAZYN (Mexico)
CLINDAMYCIN PHOSPHATE
Cleocin Phosphate Sterile Solution 2785
Cleocin T Topical Gel 2790
Cleocin T Topical Lotion 2790
Cleocin T Topical Solution 2790
Cleocin Vaginal Cream 2788
Clindets Pledgets 3270

CLINIFLAM (South Africa)
DICLOFENAC SODIUM
Voltaren Tablets 2315
Voltaren-XR Tablets 2315

CLINIRETIC (South Africa)
AMILORIDE HYDROCHLORIDE/HYDROCHLOROTHIAZIDE
Moduretic Tablets 2138

CLINOFEM (Germany)
MEDROXYPROGESTERONE ACETATE
Depo-Provera Contraceptive Injection . . . 2798
Provera Tablets 2853

CLINOFEN (South Africa)
IBUPROFEN
Motrin Suspension, Oral Drops, Chewable Tablets, and Caplets 2002

CLINOFUG D (Germany)
DOXYCYCLINE HYCLATE
Doryx Coated Pellet Filled Capsules 3357
Periostat Tablets 1208
Vibramycin Hyclate Capsules 2735
Vibramycin Hyclate Intravenous 2737
Vibra-Tabs Film Coated Tablets 2735

CLINOFUG GEL (Germany)
ERYTHROMYCIN
Emgel 2% Topical Gel 1285
Ery-Tab Tablets 448
Erythromycin Base Filmtab Tablets 454
Erythromycin Delayed-Release Capsules, USP 455
PCE Dispertab Tablets 498

CLINOLAT (South Africa)
NIFEDIPINE
Adalat CC Tablets 877
Procardia Capsules 2708
Procardia XL Extended Release Tablets . . 2710

CLINORIL (Australia, Austria, Belgium, Canada, Denmark, Hong Kong, Irish Republic, Italy, Mexico, New Zealand, Norway, South Africa, Sweden, Switzerland, Thailand, The Netherlands, United Kingdom)
SULINDAC
Clinoril Tablets 2053

CLINOSYN (South Africa)
NAPROXEN
EC-Naprosyn Delayed-Release Tablets . . . 2967
Naprosyn Suspension 2967
Naprosyn Tablets 2967

CLINOVIR (Germany)
MEDROXYPROGESTERONE ACETATE
Depo-Provera Contraceptive Injection . . . 2798
Provera Tablets 2853

CLIN-SANORANIA (Germany)
CLINDAMYCIN HYDROCHLORIDE
Cleocin HCl Capsules 2784

CLINSTAN (South Africa)
MEFENAMIC ACID
Ponstel Capsules 1356

CLIOGAN (Spain)
ESTRADIOL
Alora Transdermal System 3372
Climara Transdermal System 958
Estrace Vaginal Cream 3358
Estring Vaginal Ring 2811
Vivelle Transdermal System 2412
Vivelle-Dot Transdermal System 2416

CLIPTO (Spain)
ENALAPRIL MALEATE
Vasotec Tablets 2210

CLIPTOL (France)
IBUPROFEN
Motrin Suspension, Oral Drops, Chewable Tablets, and Caplets 2002

CLISEMINA (Spain)
DOXYCYCLINE HYCLATE
Doryx Coated Pellet Filled Capsules 3357
Periostat Tablets 1208
Vibramycin Hyclate Capsules 2735
Vibramycin Hyclate Intravenous 2737
Vibra-Tabs Film Coated Tablets 2735

CLISUNDAC (Italy)
SULINDAC
Clinoril Tablets 2053

CLIVOTEN (Italy)
ISRADIPINE
DynaCirc CR Tablets 2923

CLOBASONE (Thailand)
CLOBETASOL PROPIONATE
Cormax Cream 2440
Cormax Ointment 2440
Cormax Scalp Application 2441
Temovate Cream 1301
Temovate E Emollient 1302
Temovate Gel 1303
Temovate Ointment 1301
Temovate Scalp Application 1304

CLOBEGALEN (Germany)
CLOBETASOL PROPIONATE
Cormax Cream 2440
Cormax Ointment 2440
Cormax Scalp Application 2441
Temovate Cream 1301
Temovate E Emollient 1302
Temovate Gel 1303
Temovate Ointment 1301
Temovate Scalp Application 1304

CLOBENDIAN (Spain)
DILTIAZEM HYDROCHLORIDE
Cardizem CD Capsules 1016
Cardizem Injectable 1018
Cardizem Lyo-Ject Syringe 1018
Cardizem Monovial 1018
Tiazac Capsules 1378

CLOBESOL (Italy)
CLOBETASOL PROPIONATE
Cormax Cream 2440
Cormax Ointment 2440
Cormax Scalp Application 2441
Temovate Cream 1301
Temovate E Emollient 1302
Temovate Gel 1303
Temovate Ointment 1301
Temovate Scalp Application 1304

CLOBESON (Singapore)
CLOBETASOL PROPIONATE
Cormax Cream 2440
Cormax Ointment 2440
Cormax Scalp Application 2441
Temovate Cream 1301
Temovate E Emollient 1302
Temovate Gel 1303
Temovate Ointment 1301
Temovate Scalp Application 1304

CLOBET (Thailand)
CLOBETASOL PROPIONATE
Cormax Cream 2440
Cormax Ointment 2440
Cormax Scalp Application 2441
Temovate Cream 1301
Temovate E Emollient 1302
Temovate Gel 1303
Temovate Ointment 1301
Temovate Scalp Application 1304

CLOBETATE (Thailand)
CLOBETASOL PROPIONATE
Cormax Cream 2440
Cormax Ointment 2440
Cormax Scalp Application 2441
Temovate Cream 1301
Temovate E Emollient 1302
Temovate Gel 1303
Temovate Ointment 1301
Temovate Scalp Application 1304

CLOCIM (Switzerland)
CLOTRIMAZOLE
Lotrimin Cream 1% 3128
Lotrimin Lotion 1% 3128
Lotrimin Topical Solution 1% 3128
Mycelex Troche 573

CLOCREME (Hong Kong, New Zealand)
CLOTRIMAZOLE
Lotrimin Cream 1% 3128
Lotrimin Lotion 1% 3128
Lotrimin Topical Solution 1% 3128
Mycelex Troche 573

CLODERM (Germany, Singapore)
CLOTRIMAZOLE
Lotrimin Cream 1% 3128
Lotrimin Lotion 1% 3128
Lotrimin Topical Solution 1% 3128
Mycelex Troche 573

CLOFEC (Hong Kong, Thailand)
DICLOFENAC SODIUM
Voltaren Tablets 2315
Voltaren-XR Tablets 2315

CLOFEME 3 DAY (Australia)
CLOTRIMAZOLE
Lotrimin Cream 1% 3128
Lotrimin Lotion 1% 3128
Lotrimin Topical Solution 1% 3128
Mycelex Troche 573

CLOFENAC (Singapore)
DICLOFENAC SODIUM
Voltaren Tablets 2315
Voltaren-XR Tablets 2315

CLOFI (The Netherlands)
CLOFIBRATE
Atromid-S Capsules 3483

CLOFIBRAL (France)
CLOFIBRATE
Atromid-S Capsules 3483

CLOFINIT (Italy)
CLOFIBRATE
Atromid-S Capsules 3483

CLOFIREM (France)
CLOFIBRATE
Atromid-S Capsules 3483

CLOFON (Thailand)
DICLOFENAC SODIUM
Voltaren Tablets 2315
Voltaren-XR Tablets 2315

CLOGEN (Brazil)
CLOTRIMAZOLE
Lotrimin Cream 1% 3128
Lotrimin Lotion 1% 3128
Lotrimin Topical Solution 1% 3128
Mycelex Troche 573

CLOMADERM (South Africa)
CLOTRIMAZOLE
Lotrimin Cream 1% 3128
Lotrimin Lotion 1% 3128
Lotrimin Topical Solution 1% 3128
Mycelex Troche 573

CLOMAZEM (Brazil)
CLOTRIMAZOLE
Lotrimin Cream 1% 3128
Lotrimin Lotion 1% 3128
Lotrimin Topical Solution 1% 3128
Mycelex Troche 573

CLONAPAM (Canada)
CLONAZEPAM
Klonopin Tablets 2983

CLONAZINE (Irish Republic)
CHLORPROMAZINE HYDROCHLORIDE
Thorazine Ampuls 1656
Thorazine Multi-dose Vials 1656
Thorazine Spansule Capsules 1656
Thorazine Syrup 1656
Thorazine Tablets 1656

CLONDEPRYL (Irish Republic)
SELEGILINE HYDROCHLORIDE
Eldepryl Capsules 3266

CLONEA (Australia)
CLOTRIMAZOLE
Lotrimin Cream 1% 3128
Lotrimin Lotion 1% 3128
Lotrimin Topical Solution 1% 3128
Mycelex Troche 573

CLONEX (Israel)
CLONAZEPAM
Klonopin Tablets 2983

CLONID-OPHTAL (Germany)
CLONIDINE HYDROCHLORIDE
Catapres Tablets . . . 1037
Duraclon Injection. . . . 3057

CLONILIX (Irish Republic)
INDAPAMIDE
Indapamide Tablets. . . . 2286

CLONISTADA (Germany)
CLONIDINE HYDROCHLORIDE
Catapres Tablets . . . 1037
Duraclon Injection. . . . 3057

CLONNIRIT (Israel)
CLONIDINE HYDROCHLORIDE
Catapres Tablets . . . 1037
Duraclon Injection. . . . 3057

CLONOVATE (Thailand)
CLOBETASOL PROPIONATE
Cormax Cream . . . 2440
Cormax Ointment. . . . 2440
Cormax Scalp Application. . . . 2441
Temovate Cream . . . 1301
Temovate E Emollient . . . 1302
Temovate Gel . . . 1303
Temovate Ointment. . . . 1301
Temovate Scalp Application . . . 1304

CLONOXIFEN (Irish Republic)
TAMOXIFEN CITRATE
Nolvadex Tablets . . . 678

CLONT (Germany)
METRONIDAZOLE
MetroCream . . . 1404
MetroGel . . . 1405
MetroGel-Vaginal Gel . . . 1986
MetroLotion . . . 1405
Noritate Cream . . . 1224

CLONURETIC (Irish Republic)
AMILORIDE HYDROCHLORIDE/HYDROCHLOROTHIAZIDE
Moduretic Tablets. . . . 2138

CLOPAMON (South Africa)
METOCLOPRAMIDE HYDROCHLORIDE
Reglan Injectable . . . 2935
Reglan Syrup . . . 2935
Reglan Tablets. . . . 2935

CLOPAN (Italy)
METOCLOPRAMIDE HYDROCHLORIDE
Reglan Injectable . . . 2935
Reglan Syrup . . . 2935
Reglan Tablets. . . . 2935

CLOPINE (Australia)
CLOZAPINE
Clozaril Tablets . . . 2319

CLOPIR (Italy)
CLOFIBRATE
Atromid-S Capsules . . . 3483

CLOPSINE (Mexico)
CLOZAPINE
Clozaril Tablets . . . 2319

CLORACEF (South Africa)
CEFACLOR
Ceclor CD Tablets . . . 1279
Ceclor Pulvules . . . 1905
Ceclor Suspension . . . 1905

CLORAD (Italy)
CEFACLOR
Ceclor CD Tablets . . . 1279
Ceclor Pulvules . . . 1905
Ceclor Suspension . . . 1905

CLORAETHYL DR. HENNING (Germany)
ETHYL CHLORIDE
Gebauer's Ethyl Chloride . . . 1409

CLORAMED (Mexico)
CHLORAMPHENICOL
Chloromycetin Ophthalmic Ointment, 1% . . . ⊙296
Chloromycetin Ophthalmic Solution . . . ⊙297
Chloroptic Sterile Ophthalmic Ointment . . ⊙234
Chloroptic Sterile Ophthalmic Solution . . ⊙235

CLORAMFEN (Italy)
CHLORAMPHENICOL
Chloromycetin Ophthalmic Ointment, 1% . . . ⊙296
Chloromycetin Ophthalmic Solution . . . ⊙297
Chloroptic Sterile Ophthalmic Ointment . . ⊙234
Chloroptic Sterile Ophthalmic Solution . . ⊙235

CLORAMFENI (Mexico)
CHLORAMPHENICOL
Chloromycetin Ophthalmic Ointment, 1% . . . ⊙296
Chloromycetin Ophthalmic Solution . . . ⊙297
Chloroptic Sterile Ophthalmic Ointment . . ⊙234
Chloroptic Sterile Ophthalmic Solution . . ⊙235

CLORAMFENIL (Mexico)
CHLORAMPHENICOL
Chloromycetin Ophthalmic Ointment, 1% . . . ⊙296
Chloromycetin Ophthalmic Solution . . . ⊙297
Chloroptic Sterile Ophthalmic Ointment . . ⊙234
Chloroptic Sterile Ophthalmic Solution . . ⊙235

CLORAMPLAST (Spain)
CHLORAMPHENICOL
Chloromycetin Ophthalmic Ointment, 1% . . . ⊙296
Chloromycetin Ophthalmic Solution . . . ⊙297
Chloroptic Sterile Ophthalmic Ointment . . ⊙234
Chloroptic Sterile Ophthalmic Solution . . ⊙235

CLORAN (Mexico)
CHLORAMPHENICOL
Chloromycetin Ophthalmic Ointment, 1% . . . ⊙296
Chloromycetin Ophthalmic Solution . . . ⊙297
Chloroptic Sterile Ophthalmic Ointment . . ⊙234
Chloroptic Sterile Ophthalmic Solution . . ⊙235

CLORAN OTICO (Mexico)
CHLORAMPHENICOL
Chloromycetin Ophthalmic Ointment, 1% . . . ⊙296
Chloromycetin Ophthalmic Solution . . . ⊙297
Chloroptic Sterile Ophthalmic Ointment . . ⊙234
Chloroptic Sterile Ophthalmic Solution . . ⊙235

CLORANA (Brazil)
HYDROCHLOROTHIAZIDE
HydroDIURIL Tablets . . . 2108
Microzide Capsules . . . 3414

CLORANFE (Spain)
CHLORAMPHENICOL
Chloromycetin Ophthalmic Ointment, 1% . . . ⊙296
Chloromycetin Ophthalmic Solution . . . ⊙297
Chloroptic Sterile Ophthalmic Ointment . . ⊙234
Chloroptic Sterile Ophthalmic Solution . . ⊙235

CLORANFENIC (Spain)
CHLORAMPHENICOL
Chloromycetin Ophthalmic Ointment, 1% . . . ⊙296
Chloromycetin Ophthalmic Solution . . . ⊙297
Chloroptic Sterile Ophthalmic Ointment . . ⊙234
Chloroptic Sterile Ophthalmic Solution . . ⊙235

CLORANFENICO (Spain)
CHLORAMPHENICOL
Chloromycetin Ophthalmic Ointment, 1% . . . ⊙296
Chloromycetin Ophthalmic Solution . . . ⊙297
Chloroptic Sterile Ophthalmic Ointment . . ⊙234
Chloroptic Sterile Ophthalmic Solution . . ⊙235

CLORAZIN (Mexico)
CHLORAMPHENICOL
Chloromycetin Ophthalmic Ointment, 1% . . . ⊙296
Chloromycetin Ophthalmic Solution . . . ⊙297
Chloroptic Sterile Ophthalmic Ointment . . ⊙234
Chloroptic Sterile Ophthalmic Solution . . ⊙235

CLORDIABET (Spain)
CHLORPROPAMIDE
Diabinese Tablets. . . . 2680

CLORDIL (Mexico)
CHLORAMPHENICOL
Chloromycetin Ophthalmic Ointment, 1% . . . ⊙296
Chloromycetin Ophthalmic Solution . . . ⊙297
Chloroptic Sterile Ophthalmic Ointment . . ⊙234
Chloroptic Sterile Ophthalmic Solution . . ⊙235

CLOREDEMA H (Spain)
HYDROCHLOROTHIAZIDE
HydroDIURIL Tablets . . . 2108
Microzide Capsules . . . 3414

CLORETILO CHEMIROSA (Spain)
ETHYL CHLORIDE
Gebauer's Ethyl Chloride . . . 1409

CLORETILO VITULIA (Spain)
ETHYL CHLORIDE
Gebauer's Ethyl Chloride . . . 1409

CLORFENIL (Brazil, Mexico)
CHLORAMPHENICOL
Chloromycetin Ophthalmic Ointment, 1% . . . ⊙296
Chloromycetin Ophthalmic Solution . . . ⊙297
Chloroptic Sterile Ophthalmic Ointment . . ⊙234
Chloroptic Sterile Ophthalmic Solution . . ⊙235

CLORIMET Z (Mexico)
METOCLOPRAMIDE HYDROCHLORIDE
Reglan Injectable . . . 2935
Reglan Syrup . . . 2935
Reglan Tablets. . . . 2935

CLOR-K-ZAF (Mexico)
POTASSIUM CHLORIDE
K-Dur Microburst Release System ER Tablets . . . 1832
K-Lor Powder Packets . . . 469
K-Tab Filmtab Tablets . . . 470
Rum-K . . . 1363

CLOROCIL (Portugal)
CHLORAMPHENICOL
Chloromycetin Ophthalmic Ointment, 1% . . . ⊙296
Chloromycetin Ophthalmic Solution . . . ⊙297
Chloroptic Sterile Ophthalmic Ointment . . ⊙234
Chloroptic Sterile Ophthalmic Solution . . ⊙235

CLORTANOL (Italy)
ATENOLOL
Tenormin I.V. Injection . . . 692

CLORTETRIN (Italy)
DEMECLOCYCLINE HYDROCHLORIDE
Declomycin Tablets. . . . 1855

CLOSCRIPT (South Africa)
CLOTRIMAZOLE
Lotrimin Cream 1%. . . . 3128
Lotrimin Lotion 1% . . . 3128
Lotrimin Topical Solution 1% . . . 3128
Mycelex Troche . . . 573

CLOSTEDAL (Mexico)
CARBAMAZEPINE
Carbatrol Capsules. . . . 3234
Tegretol Chewable Tablets . . . 2404
Tegretol Suspension . . . 2404
Tegretol Tablets. . . . 2404
Tegretol-XR Tablets . . . 2404

CLOT-BASAN (Switzerland)
CLOTRIMAZOLE
Lotrimin Cream 1%. . . . 3128
Lotrimin Lotion 1% . . . 3128
Lotrimin Topical Solution 1% . . . 3128
Mycelex Troche . . . 573

CLOTRASON (Denmark)
BETAMETHASONE DIPROPIONATE/CLOTRIMAZOLE
Lotrisone Cream . . . 3129

CLOTRASONE (Spain, Thailand)
BETAMETHASONE DIPROPIONATE/CLOTRIMAZOLE
Lotrisone Cream . . . 3129

CLOTRI OPT (Germany)
CLOTRIMAZOLE
Lotrimin Cream 1%. . . . 3128
Lotrimin Lotion 1% . . . 3128
Lotrimin Topical Solution 1% . . . 3128
Mycelex Troche . . . 573

CLOTRICIN (Thailand)
CLOTRIMAZOLE
Lotrimin Cream 1%. . . . 3128
Lotrimin Lotion 1% . . . 3128
Lotrimin Topical Solution 1% . . . 3128
Mycelex Troche . . . 573

CLOTRI-DENK (Hong Kong)
CLOTRIMAZOLE
Lotrimin Cream 1%. . . . 3128
Lotrimin Lotion 1% . . . 3128
Lotrimin Topical Solution 1% . . . 3128
Mycelex Troche . . . 573

CLOTRIFERM (Sweden)
CLOTRIMAZOLE
Lotrimin Cream 1%. . . . 3128
Lotrimin Lotion 1% . . . 3128
Lotrimin Topical Solution 1% . . . 3128
Mycelex Troche . . . 573

CLOTRIFUG (Germany)
CLOTRIMAZOLE
Lotrimin Cream 1%. . . . 3128
Lotrimin Lotion 1% . . . 3128
Lotrimin Topical Solution 1% . . . 3128
Mycelex Troche . . . 573

CLOTRIGALEN (Germany)
CLOTRIMAZOLE
Lotrimin Cream 1%. . . . 3128
Lotrimin Lotion 1% . . . 3128
Lotrimin Topical Solution 1% . . . 3128
Mycelex Troche . . . 573

CLOTRIMADERM (Canada, Israel, New Zealand)
CLOTRIMAZOLE
Lotrimin Cream 1%. . . . 3128
Lotrimin Lotion 1% . . . 3128
Lotrimin Topical Solution 1% . . . 3128
Mycelex Troche . . . 573

CLOTRIMIX (Brazil)
CLOTRIMAZOLE
Lotrimin Cream 1%. . . . 3128
Lotrimin Lotion 1% . . . 3128
Lotrimin Topical Solution 1% . . . 3128
Mycelex Troche . . . 573

CLOVATE (Spain)
CLOBETASOL PROPIONATE
Cormax Cream . . . 2440
Cormax Ointment. . . . 2440
Cormax Scalp Application. . . . 2441
Temovate Cream . . . 1301
Temovate E Emollient . . . 1302
Temovate Gel . . . 1303
Temovate Ointment. . . . 1301
Temovate Scalp Application . . . 1304

CLOX (Italy)
TICLOPIDINE HYDROCHLORIDE
Ticlid Tablets. . . . 3015

CLOZARIL (Australia, Canada, Hong Kong, Irish Republic, New Zealand, Singapore, Thailand, United Kingdom)
CLOZAPINE
Clozaril Tablets . . . 2319

CLOZOLE (Australia, Hong Kong, Singapore)
CLOTRIMAZOLE
Lotrimin Cream 1%. . . . 3128
Lotrimin Lotion 1% . . . 3128
Lotrimin Topical Solution 1% . . . 3128
Mycelex Troche . . . 573

CLUSINOL (Australia)
SULINDAC
Clinoril Tablets. . . . 2053

CMD (Thailand)
CIMETIDINE
Tagamet Tablets . . . 1644

CO FLUOCIN FUERTE (Spain)
FLUOCINOLONE ACETONIDE
Synalar Cream . . . 2020
Synalar Ointment . . . 2020
Synalar Topical Solution. . . . 2020

CO-ACETAN (Austria)
HYDROCHLOROTHIAZIDE/LISINOPRIL
Prinzide Tablets. . . . 2168
Zestoretic Tablets. . . . 695

CO-AMILORID (Switzerland)
AMILORIDE HYDROCHLORIDE/HYDROCHLOROTHIAZIDE
Moduretic Tablets. . . . 2138

COAPROVEL (Denmark, Germany, Italy, Spain, Sweden)
HYDROCHLOROTHIAZIDE/IRBESARTAN
Avalide Tablets . . . 1070

COBADEX (United Kingdom)
HYDROCORTISONE
Anusol-HC Cream 2.5% . . . 2237
Hydrocortone Tablets . . . 2106

CO-CAPTRAL (Mexico)
CAPTOPRIL
Captopril Tablets . . . 2281

CODAFEN CONTINUS (Irish Republic, United Kingdom)
IBUPROFEN
Motrin Suspension, Oral Drops, Chewable Tablets, and Caplets. . . . 2002

CODERMA (Italy)
FLUOCINOLONE ACETONIDE
Synalar Cream . . . 2020
Synalar Ointment . . . 2020
Synalar Topical Solution. . . . 2020

CODESIA (Thailand)
CODEINE PHOSPHATE/GUAIFENESIN
Robitussin A-C Syrup. . . . 2942
Tussi-Organidin NR Liquid . . . 3350
Tussi-Organidin-S NR Liquid. . . . 3350

CO-DIOVAN (Austria, Germany, Irish Republic, Portugal, Singapore, South Africa, Spain, Switzerland, Thailand, The Netherlands)
HYDROCHLOROTHIAZIDE/VALSARTAN
Diovan HCT Tablets . . . 2338

CO-DIOVANE (Belgium)
HYDROCHLOROTHIAZIDE/VALSARTAN
Diovan HCT Tablets . . . 2338

CODRAL PERIOD PAIN (Australia)
IBUPROFEN
Motrin Suspension, Oral Drops, Chewable Tablets, and Caplets. . . . 2002

CODRINAN (Brazil)
THEOPHYLLINE
Aerolate Jr. T.D. Capsules . . . 1361
Aerolate Liquid . . . 1361
Aerolate Sr. T.D. Capsules . . . 1361
Theo-Dur Extended-Release Tablets. . . . 1835
Uni-Dur Extended-Release Tablets . . . 1841
Uniphyl 400 mg and 600 mg Tablets . . . 2903

COGETINE (Thailand)
CHLORAMPHENICOL
Chloromycetin Ophthalmic Ointment, 1% . . . ⊙296
Chloromycetin Ophthalmic Solution . . . ⊙297
Chloroptic Sterile Ophthalmic Ointment . . ⊙234
Chloroptic Sterile Ophthalmic Solution . . ⊙235

COGNEX (Australia, Austria, Belgium, Brazil, France, Germany, Hong Kong, Israel, New Zealand, Portugal, Spain, Sweden, Switzerland)
TACRINE HYDROCHLORIDE
Cognex Capsules 1351

COGNITIV (Austria)
SELEGILINE HYDROCHLORIDE
Eldepryl Capsules 3266

COL (Australia)
CLOFIBRATE
Atromid-S Capsules 3483

COLDAN (Austria)
NAPHAZOLINE HYDROCHLORIDE
Albalon Ophthalmic Solution . . . . ⊙225

COLEMIN (Spain)
SIMVASTATIN
Zocor Tablets 2219

COLESTID (Australia, Belgium, Canada, Germany, Irish Republic, Israel, Mexico, New Zealand, Portugal, South Africa, Spain, Switzerland, The Netherlands, United Kingdom)
COLESTIPOL HYDROCHLORIDE
Colestid Tablets 2791

COLICEFLOR (Italy)
CEPHALEXIN
Keflex Oral Suspension 1237
Keflex Pulvules 1237

COLIFOAM (Australia, Austria, Belgium, Denmark, Finland, Germany, Irish Republic, Israel, Italy, New Zealand, Norway, Portugal, South Africa, Sweden, Switzerland, United Kingdom)
HYDROCORTISONE ACETATE
Anusol-HC Suppositories 2238
Cortifoam Rectal Foam 3170
Hydrocortone Acetate Injectable Suspension 2103
Proctocort Suppositories 2264

COLIFOSSIM (Italy)
CEFUROXIME SODIUM
Kefurox Vials, ADD-Vantage. 1948
Zinacef Injection. 1696

COLIMICINA (Italy)
COLISTIMETHATE SODIUM
Coly-Mycin M Parenteral. 2243

COLIMYCIN (Denmark, Norway)
COLISTIMETHATE SODIUM
Coly-Mycin M Parenteral. 2243

COLIMYCINE (The Netherlands)
COLISTIMETHATE SODIUM
Coly-Mycin M Parenteral. 2243

COLIRACIN (Israel)
COLISTIMETHATE SODIUM
Coly-Mycin M Parenteral. 2243

COLIRIOCILINA GENTAM (Spain)
GENTAMICIN SULFATE
Genoptic Ophthalmic Ointment . . . . ⊙239
Genoptic Sterile Ophthalmic Solution . . . ⊙239

COLOFOAM (France)
HYDROCORTISONE ACETATE
Anusol-HC Suppositories 2238
Cortifoam Rectal Foam 3170
Hydrocortone Acetate Injectable Suspension 2103
Proctocort Suppositories 2264

COLO-PLEON (Austria, Germany)
SULFASALAZINE
Azulfidine EN-tabs Tablets. 2775

COLPISTAR (Brazil)
METRONIDAZOLE
MetroCream 1404
MetroGel 1405
MetroGel-Vaginal Gel 1986
MetroLotion 1405
Noritate Cream 1224

COLPROSTERONE (Spain)
PROGESTERONE
Crinone 4% Gel 3213
Crinone 8% Gel 3213
Prometrium Capsules (100 mg, 200 mg) 3261

COLSANAC (Portugal)
LACTULOSE
Kristalose for Oral Solution. 1007

COLSTAT (Portugal)
CERIVASTATIN SODIUM
Baycol Tablets. 883

COLUMINA (Mexico)
CIMETIDINE
Tagamet Tablets 1644

COLY-MYCIN M (Australia, Canada, New Zealand)
COLISTIMETHATE SODIUM
Coly-Mycin M Parenteral. 2243

COMALOSE-R (Canada)
LACTULOSE
Kristalose for Oral Solution. 1007

COMAT (Thailand)
CLOTRIMAZOLE
Lotrimin Cream 1%. 3128
Lotrimin Lotion 1% 3128
Lotrimin Topical Solution 1% 3128
Mycelex Troche 573

COMBANTRIN-1 WITH MEBENDAZOLE (Australia)
MEBENDAZOLE
Vermox Chewable Tablets. 2017

COMBID (Thailand)
LAMIVUDINE
Epivir Oral Solution. 1520
Epivir Tablets 1520
Epivir-HBV Oral Solution. 1524
Epivir-HBV Tablets 1524

COMBIPROTECT (Germany)
AMILORIDE HYDROCHLORIDE/HYDROCHLOROTHIAZIDE
Moduretic Tablets. 2138

COMBISARTAN (Italy)
HYDROCHLOROTHIAZIDE/VALSARTAN
Diovan HCT Tablets 2338

COMBIVIR (Australia, Austria, Belgium, Canada, Denmark, Finland, France, Germany, Hong Kong, Irish Republic, Israel, Italy, Mexico, New Zealand, Portugal, Singapore, Spain, Sweden, Switzerland, The Netherlands, United Kingdom)
LAMIVUDINE
Epivir Oral Solution. 1520
Epivir Tablets 1520
Epivir-HBV Oral Solution. 1524
Epivir-HBV Tablets 1524

CO-MEPRIL (Austria)
ENALAPRIL MALEATE/HYDROCHLOROTHIAZIDE
Vaseretic Tablets 2204

COMILORID (Switzerland)
AMILORIDE HYDROCHLORIDE/HYDROCHLOROTHIAZIDE
Moduretic Tablets. 2138

COMPAZINE (Australia)
PROCHLORPERAZINE
Compazine Injection 1505
Compazine Suppositories. 1505

COMPLUTINE (Spain)
DIAZEPAM
Valium Injectable 3026
Valium Tablets 3047

COMPRIMES SOMNIFERES FORMULE 533 (Switzerland)
DIPHENHYDRAMINE HYDROCHLORIDE
Benadryl Parenteral 2617

CONADYL (Thailand)
CODEINE PHOSPHATE/PROMETHAZINE HYDROCHLORIDE
Phenergan with Codeine Syrup 3557

CONAMIC (Thailand)
MEFENAMIC ACID
Ponstel Capsules 1356

CONAZINE (Thailand)
PERPHENAZINE
Trilafon Injection. 3160
Trilafon Tablets 3160

CONAZOL (Mexico)
KETOCONAZOLE
Nizoral 2% Cream 3620
Nizoral 2% Shampoo. 2007
Nizoral Tablets 1791

CONCOR (Austria, Germany, Hong Kong, Israel, Italy, Portugal, Singapore, South Africa, Switzerland, Thailand)
BISOPROLOL FUMARATE
Zebeta Tablets 1885

CONCOR PLUS (Austria, Germany, Switzerland)
BISOPROLOL FUMARATE/HYDROCHLOROTHIAZIDE
Ziac Tablets 1887

CONCORDIN (Denmark, Irish Republic, Sweden, United Kingdom)
PROTRIPTYLINE HYDROCHLORIDE
Vivactil Tablets 2217

CONDIUREN (Italy)
ENALAPRIL MALEATE/HYDROCHLOROTHIAZIDE
Vaseretic Tablets 2204

CONDROTEC (United Kingdom)
NAPROXEN
EC-Naprosyn Delayed-Release Tablets . . . 2967
Naprosyn Suspension 2967
Naprosyn Tablets 2967

CONFOBOS (Spain)
FAMOTIDINE
Pepcid Injection 2153
Pepcid Injection Premixed 2153
Pepcid RPD Orally Disintegrating Tablets 2150
Pepcid Tablets. 2150
Pepcid for Oral Suspension 2150

CONJUNCTILONE (Portugal)
NEOMYCIN SULFATE/POLYMYXIN B SULFATE
Neosporin G.U. Irrigant Sterile. 2256

CONJUNCTILONE-S (Portugal)
NEOMYCIN SULFATE/POLYMYXIN B SULFATE
Neosporin G.U. Irrigant Sterile. 2256

CONJUNCTIN (Austria, Belgium)
NEOMYCIN SULFATE/POLYMYXIN B SULFATE
Neosporin G.U. Irrigant Sterile. 2256

CONJUNCTIN-S (Austria)
NEOMYCIN SULFATE/POLYMYXIN B SULFATE/PREDNISOLONE ACETATE
Poly-Pred Liquifilm Ophthalmic Suspension. . . . . ⊙245

CONJUNTIN (Brazil)
NEOMYCIN SULFATE/POLYMYXIN B SULFATE
Neosporin G.U. Irrigant Sterile. 2256

CONNETTIVINA (Austria, Hong Kong, Italy, Thailand)
SODIUM HYALURONATE
Hyalgan Solution 3080

CONPIN (Germany)
ISOSORBIDE MONONITRATE
Imdur Tablets 1826
Ismo Tablets. 3524

CONTAC HEAD & CHEST CONGESTION (Canada)
GUAIFENESIN/PSEUDOEPHEDRINE HYDROCHLORIDE
Guaifed Capsules 2272
Guaifed-PD Capsules. 2272
Zephrex LA Tablets. 3092
Zephrex Tablets. 3091

CONTALGIN (Denmark)
MORPHINE SULFATE
Astramorph/PF Injection, USP (Preservative-Free). 594
Duramorph Injection 1312
Infumorph 200 and Infumorph 500 Sterile Solutions 1314
Kadian Capsules 1335
MS Contin Tablets 2896
MSIR Oral Capsules 2898
MSIR Oral Solution 2898
MSIR Oral Solution Concentrate 2898
MSIR Oral Tablets. 2898
Oramorph SR Tablets 3062
Roxanol 100 Concentrated Oral Solution 3066
Roxanol Concentrated Oral Solution 3066
Roxanol-T Oral Solution 3066

CONTIMIT (Germany)
TERBUTALINE SULFATE
Brethine Ampuls 2314
Brethine Tablets. 2313

CONTINUCOR (Austria)
QUINAPRIL HYDROCHLORIDE
Accupril Tablets. 2611

CONTIPHYLLIN (Germany)
THEOPHYLLINE
Aerolate Jr. T.D. Capsules 1361
Aerolate Liquid 1361
Aerolate Sr. T.D. Capsules 1361
Theo-Dur Extended-Release Tablets. 1835
Uni-Dur Extended-Release Tablets. 1841
Uniphyl 400 mg and 600 mg Tablets . . . 2903

CONTRACEP (Thailand)
MEDROXYPROGESTERONE ACETATE
Depo-Provera Contraceptive Injection . . . 2798
Provera Tablets 2853

CONTRACID (Germany)
CIMETIDINE
Tagamet Tablets 1644

CONTRAFLAM (United Kingdom)
MEFENAMIC ACID
Ponstel Capsules 1356

CONTRAFUNGIN (Germany)
CLOTRIMAZOLE
Lotrimin Cream 1%. 3128
Lotrimin Lotion 1% 3128
Lotrimin Topical Solution 1% 3128
Mycelex Troche 573

CONTRAMAL (Belgium, France, Italy)
TRAMADOL HYDROCHLORIDE
Ultram Tablets. 2600

CONTRANEURAL (Germany)
IBUPROFEN
Motrin Suspension, Oral Drops, Chewable Tablets, and Caplets 2002

CONTROL (Italy)
LORAZEPAM
Ativan Injection 3478
Ativan Tablets 3482

CONTROLIP (Mexico)
FENOFIBRATE
Tricor Capsules, Micronized 513

CONTROLVAS (Spain)
ENALAPRIL MALEATE
Vasotec Tablets 2210

CONTROMET (South Africa)
METOCLOPRAMIDE HYDROCHLORIDE
Reglan Injectable 2935
Reglan Syrup 2935
Reglan Tablets. 2935

CONVECTAL (Spain)
DILTIAZEM HYDROCHLORIDE
Cardizem CD Capsules 1016
Cardizem Injectable 1018
Cardizem Lyo-Ject Syringe 1018
Cardizem Monovial 1018
Tiazac Capsules 1378

CONVERTAL (Portugal)
CAPTOPRIL
Captopril Tablets 2281

CONVERTEN (Italy)
ENALAPRIL MALEATE
Vasotec Tablets 2210

CONVERTIN (Israel)
ENALAPRIL MALEATE
Vasotec Tablets 2210

CONVULEX (Belgium, Singapore, United Kingdom)
VALPROIC ACID
Depakene Capsules 421
Depakene Syrup 421

COPAL (Mexico)
SULINDAC
Clinoril Tablets. 2053

COPAXONE (Australia, Canada, Israel, Switzerland)
GLATIRAMER ACETATE
Copaxone for Injection. 3306

COR TENSOBON (Germany)
CAPTOPRIL
Captopril Tablets 2281

CORACTEN (Hong Kong, Thailand, United Kingdom)
NIFEDIPINE
Adalat CC Tablets. 877
Procardia Capsules. 2708
Procardia XL Extended Release Tablets . . 2710

CORADUR (Canada)
ISOSORBIDE DINITRATE
Isordil Sublingual Tablets 3525
Isordil Titradose Tablets. 3526

CORAGOXINE (France)
DIGOXIN
Lanoxicaps Capsules 1574
Lanoxin Elixir Pediatric 1578
Lanoxin Injection 1581
Lanoxin Injection Pediatric 1584
Lanoxin Tablets 1587

CORAL (Italy)
NIFEDIPINE
Adalat CC Tablets. 877
Procardia Capsules. 2708
Procardia XL Extended Release Tablets . . 2710

CORALEN (Spain)
RANITIDINE HYDROCHLORIDE
Zantac 150 EFFERdose Granules 1690
Zantac 150 EFFERdose Tablets 1690
Zantac 150 Tablets 1690
Zantac 300 Tablets 1690
Zantac Injection 1688
Zantac Injection Premixed 1688
Zantac Syrup 1690

CORAMIL (Sweden)
DILTIAZEM HYDROCHLORIDE
Cardizem CD Capsules 1016

Cardizem Injectable 1018
Cardizem Lyo-Ject Syringe 1018
Cardizem Monovial 1018
Tiazac Capsules 1378

CORANGIN (Austria, Germany, Hong Kong, New Zealand)
ISOSORBIDE MONONITRATE
Imdur Tablets 1826
Ismo Tablets 3524

CORANGINE (Switzerland)
ISOSORBIDE MONONITRATE
Imdur Tablets 1826
Ismo Tablets 3524

CORAS (Australia)
DILTIAZEM HYDROCHLORIDE
Cardizem CD Capsules 1016
Cardizem Injectable 1018
Cardizem Lyo-Ject Syringe 1018
Cardizem Monovial 1018
Tiazac Capsules 1378

CORATOL (Norway)
ATENOLOL
Tenormin I.V. Injection 692

CORAZEM (Austria)
DILTIAZEM HYDROCHLORIDE
Cardizem CD Capsules 1016
Cardizem Injectable 1018
Cardizem Lyo-Ject Syringe 1018
Cardizem Monovial 1018
Tiazac Capsules 1378

CORAZET (Germany)
DILTIAZEM HYDROCHLORIDE
Cardizem CD Capsules 1016
Cardizem Injectable 1018
Cardizem Lyo-Ject Syringe 1018
Cardizem Monovial 1018
Tiazac Capsules 1378

CORBIONAX (France)
AMIODARONE HYDROCHLORIDE
Cordarone Intravenous 3491
Cordarone Tablets 3487
Pacerone Tablets 3331

CORDALIN (Germany)
BISOPROLOL FUMARATE
Zebeta Tablets 1885

CORDAREX (Germany)
AMIODARONE HYDROCHLORIDE
Cordarone Intravenous 3491
Cordarone Tablets 3487
Pacerone Tablets 3331

CORDARONE (Belgium, Canada, Denmark, Finland, France, Hong Kong, Italy, Mexico, New Zealand, Norway, Portugal, Singapore, Sweden, Switzerland, Thailand, The Netherlands)
AMIODARONE HYDROCHLORIDE
Cordarone Intravenous 3491
Cordarone Tablets 3487
Pacerone Tablets 3331

CORDARONE X (Australia, Irish Republic, South Africa, United Kingdom)
AMIODARONE HYDROCHLORIDE
Cordarone Intravenous 3491
Cordarone Tablets 3487
Pacerone Tablets 3331

CORDES BPO (Germany)
BENZOYL PEROXIDE
Brevoxyl-4 Cleansing Lotion 3269
Brevoxyl-4 Creamy Wash 3270
Brevoxyl-4 Gel 3269
Brevoxyl-8 Cleansing Lotion 3269
Brevoxyl-8 Creamy Wash 3270
Brevoxyl-8 Gel 3269
Triaz Cleanser 2026
Triaz Gel 2026

CORDES H (Germany)
HYDROCORTISONE ACETATE
Anusol-HC Suppositories 2238
Cortifoam Rectal Foam 3170
Hydrocortone Acetate Injectable Suspension 2103
Proctocort Suppositories 2264

CORDES NYSTATIN SOFT (Germany)
NYSTATIN
Nystop Topical Powder USP 2608

CORDES VAS (Germany)
TRETINOIN
Avita Cream 999
Avita Gel 1000
Renova 0.05% Cream 2519
Retin-A Micro 0.1% 2522
Vesanoid Capsules 3037

CORDICANT (Germany)
NIFEDIPINE
Adalat CC Tablets 877
Procardia Capsules 2708
Procardia XL Extended Release Tablets . . 2710

CORDIL (Israel)
ISOSORBIDE DINITRATE
Isordil Sublingual Tablets 3525
Isordil Titradose Tablets 3526

CORDILAN (Spain)
NIFEDIPINE
Adalat CC Tablets 877
Procardia Capsules 2708
Procardia XL Extended Release Tablets . . 2710

CORDILAT (Mexico)
NIFEDIPINE
Adalat CC Tablets 877
Procardia Capsules 2708
Procardia XL Extended Release Tablets . . 2710

CORDILOX (Australia, United Kingdom)
VERAPAMIL HYDROCHLORIDE
Covera-HS Tablets 3199
Isoptin SR Tablets 467
Verelan Capsules 3184
Verelan PM Capsules 3186

CORDIPINA (Italy)
NICARDIPINE HYDROCHLORIDE
Cardene I.V. 3485

CORDIUM (Belgium, France)
BEPRIDIL HYDROCHLORIDE
Vascor Tablets 2602

COREG (Canada)
CARVEDILOL
Coreg Tablets 1508

CO-RENITEC (Austria, Belgium, Brazil, Denmark, France, Hong Kong, Mexico, New Zealand, Singapore, South Africa, Spain, The Netherlands)
ENALAPRIL MALEATE/HYDROCHLOROTHIAZIDE
Vaseretic Tablets 2204

CO-RENITEN (Switzerland)
ENALAPRIL MALEATE/HYDROCHLOROTHIAZIDE
Vaseretic Tablets 2204

CORFLENE (Spain)
FLECAINIDE ACETATE
Tambocor Tablets 1990

CORGARD (Belgium, Brazil, Canada, France, Hong Kong, Irish Republic, Italy, New Zealand, South Africa, Spain, Switzerland, United Kingdom)
NADOLOL
Nadolol Tablets 2288

CORGARETIC (United Kingdom)
NADOLOL
Nadolol Tablets 2288

CORIBON (Italy)
DIPYRIDAMOLE
Persantine Tablets 1057

CORIC (Germany)
LISINOPRIL
Prinivil Tablets 2164
Zestril Tablets 698

CORIC PLUS (Germany)
HYDROCHLOROTHIAZIDE/LISINOPRIL
Prinzide Tablets 2168
Zestoretic Tablets 695

CORIDIL (Switzerland)
DILTIAZEM HYDROCHLORIDE
Cardizem CD Capsules 1016
Cardizem Injectable 1018
Cardizem Lyo-Ject Syringe 1018
Cardizem Monovial 1018
Tiazac Capsules 1378

CORIFINA (Spain)
AZELASTINE HYDROCHLORIDE
Astelin Nasal Spray 3339

CORINFAR (Germany)
NIFEDIPINE
Adalat CC Tablets 877
Procardia Capsules 2708
Procardia XL Extended Release Tablets . . 2710

CORNEL (Spain)
NISOLDIPINE
Sular Tablets 688

CORODAY (United Kingdom)
NIFEDIPINE
Adalat CC Tablets 877
Procardia Capsules 2708
Procardia XL Extended Release Tablets . . 2710

CORODIL (Denmark)
ENALAPRIL MALEATE
Vasotec Tablets 2210

CORODIL COMP (Denmark)
ENALAPRIL MALEATE/HYDROCHLOROTHIAZIDE
Vaseretic Tablets 2204

COROGAL (Mexico)
NIFEDIPINE
Adalat CC Tablets 877
Procardia Capsules 2708
Procardia XL Extended Release Tablets . . 2710

COROLATER (Spain)
DILTIAZEM HYDROCHLORIDE
Cardizem CD Capsules 1016
Cardizem Injectable 1018
Cardizem Lyo-Ject Syringe 1018
Cardizem Monovial 1018
Tiazac Capsules 1378

COROLIN (Finland)
SIMVASTATIN
Zocor Tablets 2219

CORONARINE (France)
DIPYRIDAMOLE
Persantine Tablets 1057

CORONEX (Canada, New Zealand)
ISOSORBIDE DINITRATE
Isordil Sublingual Tablets 3525
Isordil Titradose Tablets 3526

CORONORM (Germany)
CAPTOPRIL
Captopril Tablets 2281

CORONUR (Spain)
ISOSORBIDE MONONITRATE
Imdur Tablets 1826
Ismo Tablets 3524

COROPRES (Spain)
CARVEDILOL
Coreg Tablets 1508

COROSAN (Italy)
DIPYRIDAMOLE
Persantine Tablets 1057

COROTENOL (Hong Kong)
ATENOLOL
Tenormin I.V. Injection 692

COROTREND (Germany, Mexico, Switzerland)
NIFEDIPINE
Adalat CC Tablets 877
Procardia Capsules 2708
Procardia XL Extended Release Tablets . . 2710

COROTROP (Sweden)
MILRINONE LACTATE
Primacor Injection 3086

COROTROPE (France, The Netherlands)
MILRINONE LACTATE
Primacor Injection 3086

COROVLISS (Germany)
ISOSORBIDE DINITRATE
Isordil Sublingual Tablets 3525
Isordil Titradose Tablets 3526

COROXIN (Italy)
DIPYRIDAMOLE
Persantine Tablets 1057

CORPAMIL (Switzerland)
VERAPAMIL HYDROCHLORIDE
Covera-HS Tablets 3199
Isoptin SR Tablets 467
Verelan Capsules 3184
Verelan PM Capsules 3186

CORPENDOL (Portugal)
PROPRANOLOL HYDROCHLORIDE
Inderal Injectable 3513
Inderal LA Long-Acting Capsules 3516
Inderal Tablets 3513

CORPRILOR (Spain)
ENALAPRIL MALEATE
Vasotec Tablets 2210

CORRIGAST (Spain)
MISOPROSTOL
Cytotec Tablets 3202

CORSOTALOL (Germany)
SOTALOL HYDROCHLORIDE
Betapace Tablets 950

CORTACET (Canada)
HYDROCORTISONE ACETATE
Anusol-HC Suppositories 2238
Cortifoam Rectal Foam 3170
Hydrocortone Acetate Injectable Suspension 2103
Proctocort Suppositories 2264

CORTACREAM BANDAGE (United Kingdom)
HYDROCORTISONE ACETATE
Anusol-HC Suppositories 2238
Cortifoam Rectal Foam 3170
Hydrocortone Acetate Injectable Suspension 2103
Proctocort Suppositories 2264

CORTAID (Australia, Italy, New Zealand)
HYDROCORTISONE ACETATE
Anusol-HC Suppositories 2238
Cortifoam Rectal Foam 3170
Hydrocortone Acetate Injectable Suspension 2103
Proctocort Suppositories 2264

CORTAL (Sweden)
CORTISONE ACETATE
Cortone Acetate Injectable Suspension . . 2059
Cortone Acetate Tablets 2061

CORTALAR (Italy)
FLUOCINOLONE ACETONIDE
Synalar Cream 2020
Synalar Ointment 2020
Synalar Topical Solution 2020

CORTAMED (Canada)
HYDROCORTISONE ACETATE
Anusol-HC Suppositories 2238
Cortifoam Rectal Foam 3170
Hydrocortone Acetate Injectable Suspension 2103
Proctocort Suppositories 2264

CORTAMIDE (Italy)
FLUOCINOLONE ACETONIDE
Synalar Cream 2020
Synalar Ointment 2020
Synalar Topical Solution 2020

CORTANCYL (France)
PREDNISONE
Prednisone Intensol 3064
Prednisone Oral Solution 3064
Prednisone Tablets 3064

CORTATE (Australia, Canada)
CORTISONE ACETATE
Cortone Acetate Injectable Suspension . . 2059
Cortone Acetate Tablets 2061

CORTEF (Australia, Canada)
HYDROCORTISONE ACETATE
Anusol-HC Suppositories 2238
Cortifoam Rectal Foam 3170
Hydrocortone Acetate Injectable Suspension 2103
Proctocort Suppositories 2264

CORTELAN (United Kingdom)
CORTISONE ACETATE
Cortone Acetate Injectable Suspension . . 2059
Cortone Acetate Tablets 2061

CORTENEMA (United Kingdom)
HYDROCORTISONE
Anusol-HC Cream 2.5% 2237
Hydrocortone Tablets 2106

CORTENEMA (Canada)
HYDROCORTISONE
Anusol-HC Cream 2.5% 2237
Hydrocortone Tablets 2106

CORTIBIOTIQUE (France)
HYDROCORTISONE ACETATE
Anusol-HC Suppositories 2238
Cortifoam Rectal Foam 3170
Hydrocortone Acetate Injectable Suspension 2103
Proctocort Suppositories 2264

CORTIC (Australia)
HYDROCORTISONE ACETATE
Anusol-HC Suppositories 2238
Cortifoam Rectal Foam 3170
Hydrocortone Acetate Injectable Suspension 2103
Proctocort Suppositories 2264

CORTICOTHERAPIQUE (Switzerland)
TRIAMCINOLONE ACETONIDE
Azmacort Inhalation Aerosol 728
Nasacort AQ Nasal Spray 752
Nasacort Nasal Inhaler 750

CORTICREME (Canada, Hong Kong)
HYDROCORTISONE ACETATE
Anusol-HC Suppositories 2238
Cortifoam Rectal Foam 3170
Hydrocortone Acetate Injectable Suspension 2103
Proctocort Suppositories 2264

CORTICYKLIN (Norway)
HYDROCORTISONE ACETATE/OXYTETRACYCLINE HYDROCHLORIDE
Terra-Cortril Ophthalmic Suspension 2716

CORTIDEX (Mexico)
DEXAMETHASONE
Decadron Elixir 2078

Decadron Tablets 2079

CORTIDEXASON (Germany)
DEXAMETHASONE
Decadron Elixir 2078
Decadron Tablets 2079

CORTIDRO (Italy)
HYDROCORTISONE ACETATE
Anusol-HC Suppositories 2238
Cortifoam Rectal Foam 3170
Hydrocortone Acetate Injectable Suspension 2103
Proctocort Suppositories 2264

CORTIESPEC (Spain)
FLUOCINOLONE ACETONIDE
Synalar Cream 2020
Synalar Ointment 2020
Synalar Topical Solution 2020

CORTIFOAM (Canada)
HYDROCORTISONE ACETATE
Anusol-HC Suppositories 2238
Cortifoam Rectal Foam 3170
Hydrocortone Acetate Injectable Suspension 2103
Proctocort Suppositories 2264

CORTIMENT (Canada)
HYDROCORTISONE ACETATE
Anusol-HC Suppositories 2238
Cortifoam Rectal Foam 3170
Hydrocortone Acetate Injectable Suspension 2103
Proctocort Suppositories 2264

CORTIPLASTOL (Italy)
FLUOCINOLONE ACETONIDE
Synalar Cream 2020
Synalar Ointment 2020
Synalar Topical Solution 2020

CORTISOLONE (Italy)
PREDNISOLONE
Prelone Syrup 2273

CORTISPORIN (Mexico)
NEOMYCIN SULFATE/POLYMYXIN B SULFATE
Neosporin G.U. Irrigant Sterile 2256

CORTISTAB (United Kingdom)
CORTISONE ACETATE
Cortone Acetate Injectable Suspension . . 2059
Cortone Acetate Tablets 2061

CORTISUMMAN (Germany)
DEXAMETHASONE
Decadron Elixir 2078
Decadron Tablets 2079

CORTISYL (Irish Republic, United Kingdom)
CORTISONE ACETATE
Cortone Acetate Injectable Suspension . . 2059
Cortone Acetate Tablets 2061

CORTIVENT (Finland)
BUDESONIDE
Pulmicort Turbuhaler Inhalation Powder . . . 636
Rhinocort Nasal Inhaler 640

CORTIZONE (Israel)
HYDROCORTISONE
Anusol-HC Cream 2.5% 2237
Hydrocortone Tablets 2106

CORTODERM (Canada, South Africa)
HYDROCORTISONE
Anusol-HC Cream 2.5% 2237
Hydrocortone Tablets 2106

CORTOGEN (South Africa)
CORTISONE ACETATE
Cortone Acetate Injectable Suspension . . 2059
Cortone Acetate Tablets 2061

CORTONE (Austria, Canada, Italy, Norway, Sweden)
CORTISONE ACETATE
Cortone Acetate Injectable Suspension . . 2059
Cortone Acetate Tablets 2061

CORTOPIN (Irish Republic)
HYDROCORTISONE
Anusol-HC Cream 2.5% 2237
Hydrocortone Tablets 2106

CORTRIL (Finland)
HYDROCORTISONE
Anusol-HC Cream 2.5% 2237
Hydrocortone Tablets 2106

CORTROPHIN (United Kingdom)
HYDROCORTISONE
Anusol-HC Cream 2.5% 2237
Hydrocortone Tablets 2106

CORVASAL (Germany)
ISOSORBIDE MONONITRATE
Imdur Tablets 1826
Ismo Tablets 3524

CORVERT (Austria, Finland, France, Italy, Norway, Sweden, Switzerland, The Netherlands)
IBUTILIDE FUMARATE
Corvert Injection 2793

CORZIDE (Canada)
NADOLOL
Nadolol Tablets 2288

COSAAR (Austria, Switzerland)
LOSARTAN POTASSIUM
Cozaar Tablets 2067

COSAAR PLUS (Austria, Switzerland)
HYDROCHLOROTHIAZIDE/LOSARTAN POTASSIUM
Hyzaar 50-12.5 Tablets 2109

COSLAN (Spain)
MEFENAMIC ACID
Ponstel Capsules 1356

COSMEGEN (Australia, Austria, Brazil, Canada, Finland, Hong Kong, Irish Republic, Italy, New Zealand, Norway, South Africa, Sweden, Switzerland, Thailand, United Kingdom)
DACTINOMYCIN
Cosmegen for Injection 2062

COSMOFER (United Kingdom)
IRON DEXTRAN
INFeD Injection 3388

COSOPT (Irish Republic, The Netherlands)
DORZOLAMIDE HYDROCHLORIDE/TIMOLOL MALEATE
Cosopt Sterile Ophthalmic Solution . . . . . ⊙275, 2065

COSUDEX (Australia)
BICALUTAMIDE
Casodex Tablets 662

COTAREG (France, Italy)
HYDROCHLOROTHIAZIDE/VALSARTAN
Diovan HCT Tablets 2338

COTAZYM (Canada, New Zealand)
PANCRELIPASE
Ultrase Capsules 835
Ultrase MT Capsules 835

COTAZYM S FORTE (Australia)
PANCRELIPASE
Ultrase Capsules 835
Ultrase MT Capsules 835

COTENOLOL (Switzerland)
ATENOLOL
Tenormin I.V. Injection 692

COTENOMEL (Irish Republic)
ATENOLOL
Tenormin I.V. Injection 692

COTRAZOL (Spain)
GUAIFENESIN
Organidin NR Liquid 3350
Organidin NR Tablets 3350

COTREN (Hong Kong, Singapore, Thailand)
CLOTRIMAZOLE
Lotrimin Cream 1% 3128
Lotrimin Lotion 1% 3128
Lotrimin Topical Solution 1% 3128
Mycelex Troche 573

COUGH SYRUP (Canada)
CODEINE PHOSPHATE/GUAIFENESIN/PSEUDOEPHEDRINE HYDROCHLORIDE
Robitussin-DAC Syrup 2942

COUGH SYRUP DM EXPECTORANT (Canada)
DEXTROMETHORPHAN HYDROBROMIDE/GUAIFENESIN
Tussi-Organidin DM NR Liquid 3350
Tussi-Organidin DM-S NR Liquid 3350

COUGH SYRUP DM-E (Canada)
DEXTROMETHORPHAN HYDROBROMIDE/GUAIFENESIN
Tussi-Organidin DM NR Liquid 3350
Tussi-Organidin DM-S NR Liquid 3350

COUGH SYRUP WITH GUAIFENESIN & DEXTROMETHORPHAN (Canada)
DEXTROMETHORPHAN HYDROBROMIDE/GUAIFENESIN
Tussi-Organidin DM NR Liquid 3350
Tussi-Organidin DM-S NR Liquid 3350

COUMADIN (Australia, Canada, Germany, Israel, Italy, New Zealand, Singapore, South Africa)
WARFARIN SODIUM
Coumadin Tablets 1243
Coumadin for Injection 1243

COUMADINE (France)
WARFARIN SODIUM
Coumadin Tablets 1243
Coumadin for Injection 1243

CO-VALS (Spain)
HYDROCHLOROTHIAZIDE/VALSARTAN
Diovan HCT Tablets 2338

COVERSUM (Austria, Germany, Switzerland)
PERINDOPRIL ERBUMINE
Aceon Tablets (2 mg, 4 mg, 8 mg) 3249

COVERSYL (Australia, Belgium, Canada, Denmark, Finland, France, Irish Republic, Italy, Japan, Mexico, New Zealand, Portugal, Singapore, South Africa, Spain, Thailand, The Netherlands, United Kingdom)
PERINDOPRIL ERBUMINE
Aceon Tablets (2 mg, 4 mg, 8 mg) 3249

COVOCORT (South Africa)
HYDROCORTISONE
Anusol-HC Cream 2.5% 2237
Hydrocortone Tablets 2106

COVOSPOR (South Africa)
CLOTRIMAZOLE
Lotrimin Cream 1% 3128
Lotrimin Lotion 1% 3128
Lotrimin Topical Solution 1% 3128
Mycelex Troche 573

COVOSULF (South Africa)
SULFACETAMIDE SODIUM
Bleph-10 Ophthalmic Ointment 10% . . . . ⊙230
Klaron Lotion 10% 1224

COZAAR (Australia, Belgium, Brazil, Canada, Denmark, Finland, France, Hong Kong, Irish Republic, Mexico, New Zealand, Norway, Portugal, Singapore, South Africa, Spain, Sweden, Thailand, The Netherlands, United Kingdom)
LOSARTAN POTASSIUM
Cozaar Tablets 2067

COZAAR COMP (Denmark, Finland, Irish Republic, Norway, South Africa, Sweden, United Kingdom)
HYDROCHLOROTHIAZIDE/LOSARTAN POTASSIUM
Hyzaar 50-12.5 Tablets 2109

COZAAR PLUS (Belgium, Portugal, Spain)
HYDROCHLOROTHIAZIDE/LOSARTAN POTASSIUM
Hyzaar 50-12.5 Tablets 2109

CRAFILM (Italy)
SUCRALFATE
Carafate Suspension 731
Carafate Tablets 730

CRALSANIC (South Africa)
SUCRALFATE
Carafate Suspension 731
Carafate Tablets 730

CRASNITIN (Germany, Italy, The Netherlands)
ASPARAGINASE
Elspar for Injection 2092

CRASNITINE (Switzerland)
ASPARAGINASE
Elspar for Injection 2092

CRAVIT (Hong Kong, Japan, Singapore, Thailand)
LEVOFLOXACIN
Levaquin Injection 2537
Levaquin Tablets 2537

CREMA BLANCA (Mexico)
HYDROQUINONE
Eldopaque Forte 4% Cream 1734
Eldoquin Forte 4% Cream 1734
Lustra Cream 2023
Lustra-AF Cream 2023
Melanex Topical Solution 2300
Solaquin Forte 4% Cream 1734
Solaquin Forte 4% Gel 1734

CREMA TRANSCUTAN ASTIER (Spain)
HYDROCORTISONE ACETATE
Anusol-HC Suppositories 2238
Cortifoam Rectal Foam 3170
Hydrocortone Acetate Injectable Suspension 2103
Proctocort Suppositories 2264

CREME DES 3 FLEURS D'ORIENT (France)
HYDROQUINONE
Eldopaque Forte 4% Cream 1734
Eldoquin Forte 4% Cream 1734
Lustra Cream 2023
Lustra-AF Cream 2023
Melanex Topical Solution 2300
Solaquin Forte 4% Cream 1734
Solaquin Forte 4% Gel 1734

CREMICORT-H (Belgium)
HYDROCORTISONE
Anusol-HC Cream 2.5% 2237
Hydrocortone Tablets 2106

CREMOSAN (Mexico)
KETOCONAZOLE
Nizoral 2% Cream 3620
Nizoral 2% Shampoo 2007
Nizoral Tablets 1791

CRENODYN (Italy)
CEFADROXIL
Duricef Capsules 1079
Duricef Oral Suspension 1079
Duricef Tablets 1079

CRINONE (Germany, Irish Republic, Italy, Mexico, Singapore, United Kingdom)
PROGESTERONE
Crinone 4% Gel 3213
Crinone 8% Gel 3213
Prometrium Capsules (100 mg, 200 mg) 3261

CRINOREN (Spain)
ENALAPRIL MALEATE
Vasotec Tablets 2210

CRINORETIC (Spain)
ENALAPRIL MALEATE/HYDROCHLOROTHIAZIDE
Vaseretic Tablets 2204

CRISTAN (Singapore)
CLOTRIMAZOLE
Lotrimin Cream 1% 3128
Lotrimin Lotion 1% 3128
Lotrimin Topical Solution 1% 3128
Mycelex Troche 573

CRIXIVAN (Australia, Austria, Belgium, Canada, Denmark, Finland, France, Germany, Hong Kong, Irish Republic, Israel, Italy, Mexico, New Zealand, Norway, Portugal, Singapore, South Africa, Spain, Sweden, Switzerland, Thailand, The Netherlands, United Kingdom)
INDINAVIR SULFATE
Crixivan Capsules 2070

CRONASMA (Germany)
THEOPHYLLINE
Aerolate Jr. T.D. Capsules 1361
Aerolate Liquid 1361
Aerolate Sr. T.D. Capsules 1361
Theo-Dur Extended-Release Tablets 1835
Uni-Dur Extended-Release Tablets 1841
Uniphyl 400 mg and 600 mg Tablets . . . 2903

CRONAUZAN (Italy)
METOCLOPRAMIDE HYDROCHLORIDE
Reglan Injectable 2935
Reglan Syrup 2935
Reglan Tablets 2935

CRONIZAT (Italy)
NIZATIDINE
Axid Pulvules 1903

CRONOCEF (Italy)
CEFPROZIL
Cefzil Tablets 1076
Cefzil for Oral Suspension 1076

CRONOCOL (Portugal)
GENTAMICIN SULFATE
Genoptic Ophthalmic Ointment . . . . . ⊙239
Genoptic Sterile Ophthalmic Solution . . . ⊙239

CRONODINE (Spain)
DILTIAZEM HYDROCHLORIDE
Cardizem CD Capsules 1016
Cardizem Injectable 1018
Cardizem Lyo-Ject Syringe 1018
Cardizem Monovial 1018
Tiazac Capsules 1378

CRONOL (Spain)
FAMOTIDINE
Pepcid Injection 2153
Pepcid Injection Premixed 2153
Pepcid RPD Orally Disintegrating Tablets 2150
Pepcid Tablets 2150
Pepcid for Oral Suspension 2150

CRONOVERA (Mexico)
VERAPAMIL HYDROCHLORIDE
Covera-HS Tablets 3199
Isoptin SR Tablets 467
Verelan Capsules 3184
Verelan PM Capsules 3186

CRYOMETASONA (Mexico)
DEXAMETHASONE
Decadron Elixir 2078
Decadron Tablets 2079

CRYOPRIL (Mexico)
CAPTOPRIL
Captopril Tablets 2281

CRYOSOLONA (Mexico)
METHYLPREDNISOLONE SODIUM SUCCINATE
Solu-Medrol Sterile Powder 2855

CRYOVAL (Mexico)
VALPROIC ACID
Depakene Capsules 421
Depakene Syrup 421

CRYOZOL (Mexico)
METRONIDAZOLE
MetroCream 1404
MetroGel 1405
MetroGel-Vaginal Gel 1986
MetroLotion 1405
Noritate Cream 1224

CRYSANAL (Australia)
NAPROXEN SODIUM
Anaprox DS Tablets 2967
Anaprox Tablets 2967
Naprelan Tablets 1293

CST (Thailand)
CLOTRIMAZOLE
Lotrimin Cream 1% 3128
Lotrimin Lotion 1% 3128
Lotrimin Topical Solution 1% 3128
Mycelex Troche 573

CUANTIN (Spain)
FAMOTIDINE
Pepcid Injection 2153
Pepcid Injection Premixed 2153
Pepcid RPD Orally Disintegrating Tablets 2150
Pepcid Tablets 2150
Pepcid for Oral Suspension 2150

CUERPO AMARILLO FUERTE (Mexico)
PROGESTERONE
Crinone 4% Gel 3213
Crinone 8% Gel 3213
Prometrium Capsules (100 mg, 200 mg) 3261

CUNESIN (Spain)
CIPROFLOXACIN HYDROCHLORIDE
Ciloxan Ophthalmic Ointment 538
Ciloxan Ophthalmic Solution . . . . ⊙209, 538
Cipro Tablets 887

CUNIL (Irish Republic)
IBUPROFEN
Motrin Suspension, Oral Drops, Chewable Tablets, and Caplets 2002

CUPRIMINE (Brazil, Canada, Israel, Norway, Sweden, Thailand, The Netherlands)
PENICILLAMINE
Cuprimine Capsules 2075
Depen Titratable Tablets 3341

CUPRIPEN (Spain)
PENICILLAMINE
Cuprimine Capsules 2075
Depen Titratable Tablets 3341

CUPROFEN (United Kingdom)
IBUPROFEN
Motrin Suspension, Oral Drops, Chewable Tablets, and Caplets 2002

CURAM (Hong Kong)
AMOXICILLIN
Amoxil Pediatric Drops for Oral Suspension 1471
Amoxil Tablets 1471

CURANTYL N (Germany)
DIPYRIDAMOLE
Persantine Tablets 1057

CURLEM (Mexico)
VECURONIUM BROMIDE
Norcuron for Injection 2478

CUROCEF (Austria)
CEFUROXIME SODIUM
Kefurox Vials, ADD-Vantage 1948
Zinacef Injection 1696

CUROXIM (Italy)
CEFUROXIME SODIUM
Kefurox Vials, ADD-Vantage 1948
Zinacef Injection 1696

CUROXIMA (Spain)
CEFUROXIME SODIUM
Kefurox Vials, ADD-Vantage 1948
Zinacef Injection 1696

CUROXIME (Portugal)
CEFUROXIME SODIUM
Kefurox Vials, ADD-Vantage 1948
Zinacef Injection 1696

CUSIALGIL (Spain)
IBUPROFEN
Motrin Suspension, Oral Drops, Chewable Tablets, and Caplets 2002

CUSIGEL (Spain)
FLUOCINONIDE
Lidex Cream 2020
Lidex Gel 2020
Lidex Ointment 2020
Lidex Topical Solution 2020
Lidex-E Cream 2020

CUSIMICINA (Spain)
ERYTHROMYCIN STEARATE
Erythrocin Stearate Filmtab Tablets 452

CUSIMOLOL (Hong Kong, Italy, Mexico, Portugal, Spain)
TIMOLOL MALEATE
Blocadren Tablets 2046
Timoptic Sterile Ophthalmic Solution 2190
Timoptic in Ocudose 2192
Timoptic-XE Sterile Ophthalmic Gel Forming Solution 2194

CUTACELAN (Mexico)
AZELAIC ACID
Azelex Cream 547

CUTACLIN (Mexico)
CLINDAMYCIN PHOSPHATE
Cleocin Phosphate Sterile Solution 2785
Cleocin T Topical Gel 2790
Cleocin T Topical Lotion 2790
Cleocin T Topical Solution 2790
Cleocin Vaginal Cream 2788
Clindets Pledgets 3270

CUTACNYL (France)
BENZOYL PEROXIDE
Brevoxyl-4 Cleansing Lotion 3269
Brevoxyl-4 Creamy Wash 3270
Brevoxyl-4 Gel 3269
Brevoxyl-8 Cleansing Lotion 3269
Brevoxyl-8 Creamy Wash 3270
Brevoxyl-8 Gel 3269
Triaz Cleanser 2026
Triaz Gel 2026

CUTADERM (South Africa)
HYDROCORTISONE
Anusol-HC Cream 2.5% 2237
Hydrocortone Tablets 2106

CUTANUM (Germany)
ESTRADIOL
Alora Transdermal System 3372
Climara Transdermal System 958
Estrace Vaginal Cream 3358
Estring Vaginal Ring 2811
Vivelle Transdermal System 2412
Vivelle-Dot Transdermal System 2416

CUTIFITOL (Spain)
PROGESTERONE
Crinone 4% Gel 3213
Crinone 8% Gel 3213
Prometrium Capsules (100 mg, 200 mg) 3261

CUTISTAD (Germany, Switzerland)
CLOTRIMAZOLE
Lotrimin Cream 1% 3128
Lotrimin Lotion 1% 3128
Lotrimin Topical Solution 1% 3128
Mycelex Troche 573

CUTIVAT (Denmark)
FLUTICASONE PROPIONATE
Cutivate Cream 1282
Cutivate Ointment 1284
Flonase Nasal Spray 1533
Flovent 110 mcg Inhalation Aerosol 1535
Flovent 220 mcg Inhalation Aerosol 1535
Flovent 44 mcg Inhalation Aerosol 1535
Flovent Rotadisk 100 mcg 1537
Flovent Rotadisk 250 mcg 1537
Flovent Rotadisk 50 mcg 1537

CUTIVATE (Austria, Belgium, Hong Kong, Israel, Mexico, Portugal, Singapore, South Africa, Spain, Switzerland, The Netherlands, United Kingdom)
FLUTICASONE PROPIONATE
Cutivate Cream 1282
Cutivate Ointment 1284
Flonase Nasal Spray 1533
Flovent 110 mcg Inhalation Aerosol 1535
Flovent 220 mcg Inhalation Aerosol 1535
Flovent 44 mcg Inhalation Aerosol 1535
Flovent Rotadisk 100 mcg 1537
Flovent Rotadisk 250 mcg 1537
Flovent Rotadisk 50 mcg 1537

CUXAFENON (Germany)
PROPAFENONE HYDROCHLORIDE
Rythmol Tablets - 150 mg, 225 mg, 300 mg 502

CUXANORM (Germany)
ATENOLOL
Tenormin I.V. Injection 692

CYCLADIENE (France)
DIENESTROL
Ortho Dienestrol Cream 2554

CYCLIDOX (Australia, South Africa)
DOXYCYCLINE HYCLATE
Doryx Coated Pellet Filled Capsules 3357
Periostat Tablets 1208
Vibra-Tabs Film Coated Tablets 2735
Vibramycin Hyclate Capsules 2735
Vibramycin Hyclate Intravenous 2737

CYCLOGEST (Hong Kong, South Africa, Thailand, United Kingdom)
PROGESTERONE
Crinone 4% Gel 3213
Crinone 8% Gel 3213
Prometrium Capsules (100 mg, 200 mg) 3261

CYCRIN (Brazil, Mexico)
MEDROXYPROGESTERONE ACETATE
Depo-Provera Contraceptive Injection 2798
Provera Tablets 2853

CYKRINA (Finland, Sweden)
MEDROXYPROGESTERONE ACETATE
Depo-Provera Contraceptive Injection 2798
Provera Tablets 2853

CYLERT (Canada, Israel)
PEMOLINE
Cylert Chewable Tablets 415
Cylert Tablets 415

CYLLIND (Germany)
CLARITHROMYCIN
Biaxin Filmtab Tablets 403
Biaxin for Oral Suspension 403

CYMERION (Portugal)
ZOLPIDEM TARTRATE
Ambien Tablets 3191

CYMEVENE (Australia, Belgium, Hong Kong, Irish Republic, Israel, Italy, Mexico, Norway, Portugal, Singapore, South Africa, Spain, Thailand, The Netherlands, United Kingdom)
GANCICLOVIR SODIUM
Cytovene-IV 2959

CYMI (South Africa)
CIMETIDINE
Tagamet Tablets 1644

CYNOMEL (Brazil, France, Mexico)
LIOTHYRONINE SODIUM
Cytomel Tablets 1817
Triostat Injection 1825

CYPROGIN (Hong Kong, Thailand)
CYPROHEPTADINE HYDROCHLORIDE
Periactin Tablets 2155

CYPROSIAN (Thailand)
CYPROHEPTADINE HYDROCHLORIDE
Periactin Tablets 2155

CYPROSTOL (Austria)
MISOPROSTOL
Cytotec Tablets 3202

CYRPON (Austria)
MEPROBAMATE
Miltown Tablets 3349

CYSTICIDE (Germany, South Africa)
PRAZIQUANTEL
Biltricide Tablets 887

CYSTISTAT (Canada, United Kingdom)
SODIUM HYALURONATE
Hyalgan Solution 3080

CYSTOPURIN (Irish Republic, United Kingdom)
POTASSIUM CITRATE
Urocit-K Tablets 2232

CYTINE (New Zealand)
CIMETIDINE
Tagamet Tablets 1644

CYTOMEL (Belgium, Canada, The Netherlands)
LIOTHYRONINE SODIUM
Cytomel Tablets 1817
Triostat Injection 1825

CYTOSAFE (Germany)
FLUOROURACIL
Efudex Cream 1733
Efudex Topical Solutions 1733
Fluoroplex Topical Cream 552
Fluoroplex Topical Solution 552

CYTOTEC (Australia, Belgium, Brazil, Canada, Denmark, Finland, France, Germany, Hong Kong, Irish Republic, Israel, Italy, Mexico, New Zealand, Norway, Portugal, Singapore, South Africa, Spain, Sweden, Switzerland, Thailand, The Netherlands, United Kingdom)
MISOPROSTOL
Cytotec Tablets 3202

DABEN (Mexico)
MEBENDAZOLE
Vermox Chewable Tablets 2017

DABENZOL (Mexico)
ALBENDAZOLE
Albenza Tablets 1463

DABEX (Mexico)
METFORMIN HYDROCHLORIDE
Glucophage Tablets 1080

DABONAL (Spain)
ENALAPRIL MALEATE
Vasotec Tablets 2210

DABONAL PLUS (Spain)
ENALAPRIL MALEATE/HYDROCHLOROTHIAZIDE
Vaseretic Tablets 2204

DACALA (Spain)
AMOXICILLIN
Amoxil Pediatric Drops for Oral Suspension 1471
Amoxil Tablets 1471

DACATIC (Finland)
DACARBAZINE
DTIC-Dome 902

DACEF (South Africa)
CEFADROXIL
Duricef Capsules 1079
Duricef Oral Suspension 1079
Duricef Tablets 1079

DACLIN (New Zealand)
SULINDAC
Clinoril Tablets 2053

DACORTIN (Spain)
PREDNISONE
Prednisone Intensol 3064
Prednisone Oral Solution 3064
Prednisone Tablets 3064

DACORTIN H (Spain)
PREDNISOLONE
Prelone Syrup 2273

DAFLOXEN (Mexico)
NAPROXEN
EC-Naprosyn Delayed-Release Tablets 2967
Naprosyn Suspension 2967
Naprosyn Tablets 2967

DAFLOXEN F (Mexico)
NAPROXEN SODIUM
Anaprox DS Tablets 2967
Anaprox Tablets 2967
Naprelan Tablets 1293

DAFNEGIL NEO (Switzerland)
CICLOPIROX OLAMINE
Loprox Cream 2021
Loprox Lotion 2021

DAFNEGIN (Italy)
CICLOPIROX OLAMINE
Loprox Cream 2021
Loprox Lotion 2021

DAGAN (Spain)
NICARDIPINE HYDROCHLORIDE
Cardene I.V. 3485

DAKAR (Belgium)
LANSOPRAZOLE
Prevacid Delayed-Release Capsules 3292

DAKTAGOLD (Australia)
KETOCONAZOLE
Nizoral 2% Cream 3620
Nizoral 2% Shampoo 2007
Nizoral Tablets 1791

DAKTARIN GOLD (United Kingdom)
KETOCONAZOLE
Nizoral 2% Cream 3620
Nizoral 2% Shampoo 2007
Nizoral Tablets 1791

DALACIN (Irish Republic, United Kingdom)
CLINDAMYCIN PHOSPHATE
Cleocin Phosphate Sterile Solution 2785
Cleocin T Topical Gel 2790

Cleocin T Topical Lotion ... 2790
Cleocin T Topical Solution ... 2790
Cleocin Vaginal Cream ... 2788
Clindets Pledgets ... 3270

DALACIN C (Irish Republic)
CLINDAMYCIN HYDROCHLORIDE
Cleocin HCl Capsules ... 2784

DALACIN T (Australia, Brazil, Canada, Hong Kong, Irish Republic, Italy, Mexico, New Zealand, Portugal, South Africa, Switzerland, The Netherlands, United Kingdom)
CLINDAMYCIN PHOSPHATE
Cleocin Phosphate Sterile Solution ... 2785
Cleocin T Topical Gel ... 2790
Cleocin T Topical Lotion ... 2790
Cleocin T Topical Solution ... 2790
Cleocin Vaginal Cream ... 2788
Clindets Pledgets ... 3270

DALACIN TOPICAL (Belgium)
CLINDAMYCIN PHOSPHATE
Cleocin Phosphate Sterile Solution ... 2785
Cleocin T Topical Gel ... 2790
Cleocin T Topical Lotion ... 2790
Cleocin T Topical Solution ... 2790
Cleocin Vaginal Cream ... 2788
Clindets Pledgets ... 3270

DALACIN V (Australia, Hong Kong, Mexico, New Zealand, Portugal, Switzerland)
CLINDAMYCIN PHOSPHATE
Cleocin Phosphate Sterile Solution ... 2785
Cleocin T Topical Gel ... 2790
Cleocin T Topical Lotion ... 2790
Cleocin T Topical Solution ... 2790
Cleocin Vaginal Cream ... 2788
Clindets Pledgets ... 3270

DALACIN VAGINAL (Belgium, Canada, Israel)
CLINDAMYCIN PHOSPHATE
Cleocin Phosphate Sterile Solution ... 2785
Cleocin T Topical Gel ... 2790
Cleocin T Topical Lotion ... 2790
Cleocin T Topical Solution ... 2790
Cleocin Vaginal Cream ... 2788
Clindets Pledgets ... 3270

DALACIN VC (South Africa)
CLINDAMYCIN PHOSPHATE
Cleocin Phosphate Sterile Solution ... 2785
Cleocin T Topical Gel ... 2790
Cleocin T Topical Lotion ... 2790
Cleocin T Topical Solution ... 2790
Cleocin Vaginal Cream ... 2788
Clindets Pledgets ... 3270

DALACINE T (France)
CLINDAMYCIN PHOSPHATE
Cleocin Phosphate Sterile Solution ... 2785
Cleocin T Topical Gel ... 2790
Cleocin T Topical Lotion ... 2790
Cleocin T Topical Solution ... 2790
Cleocin Vaginal Cream ... 2788
Clindets Pledgets ... 3270

DALAGIS T (Israel)
CLINDAMYCIN PHOSPHATE
Cleocin Phosphate Sterile Solution ... 2785
Cleocin T Topical Gel ... 2790
Cleocin T Topical Lotion ... 2790
Cleocin T Topical Solution ... 2790
Cleocin Vaginal Cream ... 2788
Clindets Pledgets ... 3270

DALPARAN (Spain)
ZOLPIDEM TARTRATE
Ambien Tablets ... 3191

DALSY (Spain)
IBUPROFEN
Motrin Suspension, Oral Drops, Chewable Tablets, and Caplets ... 2002

DAMIDE (Italy)
INDAPAMIDE
Indapamide Tablets ... 2286

DAMOSAL (Mexico)
DIPYRIDAMOLE
Persantine Tablets ... 1057

DANILAX (Denmark, Hong Kong)
LACTULOSE
Kristalose for Oral Solution ... 1007

DANILON (Brazil)
IBUPROFEN
Motrin Suspension, Oral Drops, Chewable Tablets, and Caplets ... 2002

DANLENE (Italy)
DANTROLENE SODIUM
Dantrium Capsules ... 2885
Dantrium Intravenous ... 2886

DANTAMACRIN (Austria, Germany, Switzerland)
DANTROLENE SODIUM
Dantrium Capsules ... 2885
Dantrium Intravenous ... 2886

DANTRALEN (Spain)
DANTROLENE SODIUM
Dantrium Capsules ... 2885
Dantrium Intravenous ... 2886

DANTRIUM (Australia, Belgium, Canada, Denmark, France, Hong Kong, Irish Republic, Israel, Italy, New Zealand, Portugal, South Africa, The Netherlands, United Kingdom)
DANTROLENE SODIUM
Dantrium Capsules ... 2885
Dantrium Intravenous ... 2886

DAPAMAX (South Africa)
INDAPAMIDE
Indapamide Tablets ... 2286

DAPA-TABS (Australia, Hong Kong)
INDAPAMIDE
Indapamide Tablets ... 2286

DAPAZ (Spain)
MEPROBAMATE
Miltown Tablets ... 3349

DAPROX (Denmark)
NAPROXEN
EC-Naprosyn Delayed-Release Tablets ... 2967
Naprosyn Suspension ... 2967
Naprosyn Tablets ... 2967

DAPSODERM-X (Mexico)
DAPSONE
Dapsone Tablets USP ... 1780

DAPTRIL (South Africa)
INDAPAMIDE
Indapamide Tablets ... 2286

DARALIX (South Africa)
PROMETHAZINE HYDROCHLORIDE
Phenergan Injection ... 3553
Phenergan Suppositories ... 3556
Phenergan Syrup Fortis ... 3554
Phenergan Syrup Plain ... 3554
Phenergan Tablets ... 3556

DARAPRIM (Australia, Austria, Belgium, Brazil, Canada, Germany, Irish Republic, Israel, Mexico, South Africa, Spain, Sweden, Switzerland, Thailand, The Netherlands, United Kingdom)
PYRIMETHAMINE
Daraprim Tablets ... 1511

DARDEX (Spain)
CAPTOPRIL
Captopril Tablets ... 2281

DARDUM (Italy, Singapore)
CEFOPERAZONE SODIUM
Cefobid Intravenous/Intramuscular ... 2671
Cefobid Pharmacy Bulk Package - Not for Direct Infusion ... 2673

DAREN (Singapore)
ENALAPRIL MALEATE
Vasotec Tablets ... 2210

DARI (Spain)
NIFEDIPINE
Adalat CC Tablets ... 877
Procardia Capsules ... 2708
Procardia XL Extended Release Tablets ... 2710

DAROB (Austria, Germany, Portugal, Sweden)
SOTALOL HYDROCHLORIDE
Betapace Tablets ... 950

DARTROX (Mexico)
NAPROXEN
EC-Naprosyn Delayed-Release Tablets ... 2967
Naprosyn Suspension ... 2967
Naprosyn Tablets ... 2967

DARVILEN (Italy)
CEFOTETAN DISODIUM
Cefotan Injection ... 664
Cefotan for Injection ... 664

DASKIL (Austria, Italy)
TERBINAFINE HYDROCHLORIDE
Lamisil Tablets ... 2360

DASKYL (Portugal)
TERBINAFINE HYDROCHLORIDE
Lamisil Tablets ... 2360

DASMETROL (Mexico)
METRONIDAZOLE
MetroCream ... 1404
MetroGel ... 1405
MetroGel-Vaginal Gel ... 1986
MetroLotion ... 1405
Noritate Cream ... 1224

DASOLIN (Mexico)
METRONIDAZOLE
MetroCream ... 1404
MetroGel ... 1405
MetroGel-Vaginal Gel ... 1986
MetroLotion ... 1405
Noritate Cream ... 1224

DATRON (Spain)
ONDANSETRON HYDROCHLORIDE
Zofran Injection ... 1698
Zofran Injection Premixed ... 1698
Zofran Oral Solution ... 1703
Zofran Tablets ... 1703

DAUNOBLASTIN (Austria, Germany, South Africa)
DAUNORUBICIN HYDROCHLORIDE
Cerubidine for Injection ... 947

DAUNOBLASTINA (Brazil, Hong Kong, Italy, Portugal, Singapore, Spain)
DAUNORUBICIN HYDROCHLORIDE
Cerubidine for Injection ... 947

DAVITAMON A (The Netherlands)
VITAMIN A PALMITATE
Aquasol A Parenteral ... 593

DAVIXOLOL (Portugal)
BETAXOLOL HYDROCHLORIDE
Betoptic S Ophthalmic Suspension ... ⊙208, 537

DAYS (Mexico)
IBUPROFEN
Motrin Suspension, Oral Drops, Chewable Tablets, and Caplets ... 2002

DAZINE (Thailand)
THIORIDAZINE HYDROCHLORIDE
Thioridazine Hydrochloride Tablets ... 2289

DAZOCAN (Mexico)
ALBENDAZOLE
Albenza Tablets ... 1463

DAZOL (Brazil)
ALBENDAZOLE
Albenza Tablets ... 1463

DDAVP (Brazil, Canada, Germany, Portugal, United Kingdom)
DESMOPRESSIN ACETATE
DDAVP Injection 4 mcg/mL ... 737
DDAVP Nasal Spray ... 738
DDAVP Rhinal Tube ... 738
DDAVP Tablets ... 739
Desmopressin Acetate Injection ... 1344
Desmopressin Acetate Rhinal Tube ... 1345
Stimate Nasal Spray ... 796

DEADYN (Italy)
PEMOLINE
Cylert Chewable Tablets ... 415
Cylert Tablets ... 415

DEALGIC (Italy)
DICLOFENAC SODIUM
Voltaren Tablets ... 2315
Voltaren-XR Tablets ... 2315

DEAVYNFAR (Mexico)
CHLORPROPAMIDE
Diabinese Tablets ... 2680

DEBAX (Austria)
CAPTOPRIL
Captopril Tablets ... 2281

DECADRON (Australia, Austria, Belgium, Brazil, Finland, France, Germany, Hong Kong, New Zealand, South Africa, United Kingdom)
DEXAMETHASONE SODIUM PHOSPHATE
Decadron Phosphate Injection ... 2081
Decadron Phosphate Sterile Ophthalmic Ointment ... ⊙280, 2083
Decadron Phosphate Sterile Ophthalmic Solution ... 2084

DECADRON A LA NEOMYCINE (Switzerland)
DEXAMETHASONE SODIUM PHOSPHATE/NEOMYCIN SULFATE
NeoDecadron Sterile Ophthalmic Solution ... 2144

DECADRON AVEC NEOMYCINE (Belgium)
DEXAMETHASONE SODIUM PHOSPHATE/NEOMYCIN SULFATE
NeoDecadron Sterile Ophthalmic Solution ... 2144

DECADRON CUM NEOMYCIN (Sweden)
DEXAMETHASONE SODIUM PHOSPHATE/NEOMYCIN SULFATE
NeoDecadron Sterile Ophthalmic Solution ... 2144

DECADRON MET NEOMYCINE (The Netherlands)
DEXAMETHASONE SODIUM PHOSPHATE/NEOMYCIN SULFATE
NeoDecadron Sterile Ophthalmic Solution ... 2144

DECADRON MIT NEOMYCIN (Austria)
DEXAMETHASONE SODIUM PHOSPHATE/NEOMYCIN SULFATE
NeoDecadron Sterile Ophthalmic Solution ... 2144

DECADRON WITH NEOMYCIN (Thailand)
DEXAMETHASONE SODIUM PHOSPHATE/NEOMYCIN SULFATE
NeoDecadron Sterile Ophthalmic Solution ... 2144

DECARIS (Mexico)
LEVAMISOLE HYDROCHLORIDE
Ergamisol Tablets ... 1789

DECAUGH (Hong Kong)
DEXTROMETHORPHAN HYDROBROMIDE/GUAIFENESIN
Tussi-Organidin DM NR Liquid ... 3350
Tussi-Organidin DM-S NR Liquid ... 3350

DECENTAN (Austria, Spain)
PERPHENAZINE
Trilafon Injection ... 3160
Trilafon Tablets ... 3160

DECIPAR (Spain)
ENOXAPARIN SODIUM
Lovenox Injection ... 746

DECLOBAN (Spain)
CLOBETASOL PROPIONATE
Cormax Cream ... 2440
Cormax Ointment ... 2440
Cormax Scalp Application ... 2441
Temovate Cream ... 1301
Temovate E Emollient ... 1302
Temovate Gel ... 1303
Temovate Ointment ... 1301
Temovate Scalp Application ... 1304

DECLOMYCIN (Canada)
DEMECLOCYCLINE HYDROCHLORIDE
Declomycin Tablets ... 1855

DECOFLUOR (Italy)
DEXAMETHASONE
Decadron Elixir ... 2078
Decadron Tablets ... 2079

DECONTRACTYL NEW (Belgium)
IBUPROFEN
Motrin Suspension, Oral Drops, Chewable Tablets, and Caplets ... 2002

DECOREX (Mexico)
DEXAMETHASONE
Decadron Elixir ... 2078
Decadron Tablets ... 2079

DECORTIN (Germany)
PREDNISONE
Prednisone Intensol ... 3064
Prednisone Oral Solution ... 3064
Prednisone Tablets ... 3064

DECORTIN H (Germany)
PREDNISOLONE
Prelone Syrup ... 2273

DECORTISYL (Irish Republic, United Kingdom)
PREDNISONE
Prednisone Intensol ... 3064
Prednisone Oral Solution ... 3064
Prednisone Tablets ... 3064

DECORTON (Italy)
PREDNISONE
Prednisone Intensol ... 3064
Prednisone Oral Solution ... 3064
Prednisone Tablets ... 3064

DECOS (Thailand)
CODEINE PHOSPHATE/PROMETHAZINE HYDROCHLORIDE
Phenergan with Codeine Syrup ... 3557

DECOSTRIOL (Germany)
CALCITRIOL
Calcijex Injection ... 411
Rocaltrol Capsules ... 2991
Rocaltrol Oral Solution ... 2991

DECRELIP (Spain)
GEMFIBROZIL
Lopid Tablets ... 2650

DEDOLOR (Austria)
DICLOFENAC SODIUM
Voltaren Tablets ... 2315

(⊙ Described in PDR For Ophthalmic Medicines™)

Voltaren-XR Tablets . . . 2315

DEEP RELIEF (United Kingdom)
IBUPROFEN
Motrin Suspension, Oral Drops, Chewable Tablets, and Caplets . . . 2002

DEFAXINA (Spain)
CEPHALEXIN
Keflex Oral Suspension . . . 1237
Keflex Pulvules . . . 1237

DEFILTRAN (France)
ACETAZOLAMIDE
Diamox Sequels Sustained Release Capsules . . . ⊙270
Diamox Tablets . . . ⊙269

DEFLAMAT (Austria, Italy)
DICLOFENAC SODIUM
Voltaren Tablets . . . 2315
Voltaren-XR Tablets . . . 2315

DEFLAMM (Austria)
DICLOFENAC SODIUM
Voltaren Tablets . . . 2315
Voltaren-XR Tablets . . . 2315

DEFLAMON (Italy)
METRONIDAZOLE
MetroCream . . . 1404
MetroGel . . . 1405
MetroGel-Vaginal Gel . . . 1986
MetroLotion . . . 1405
Noritate Cream . . . 1224

DEFLOX (Spain)
TERAZOSIN HYDROCHLORIDE
Hytrin Capsules . . . 464

DEFONAMID (Germany)
SULFANILAMIDE
AVC Cream . . . 1350
AVC Suppositories . . . 1350

DEFUNGO (Thailand)
CLOTRIMAZOLE
Lotrimin Cream 1% . . . 3128
Lotrimin Lotion 1% . . . 3128
Lotrimin Topical Solution 1% . . . 3128
Mycelex Troche . . . 573

DEGEST 2 (Canada)
NAPHAZOLINE HYDROCHLORIDE
Albalon Ophthalmic Solution . . . ⊙225

DEGRANOL (South Africa)
CARBAMAZEPINE
Carbatrol Capsules . . . 3234
Tegretol Chewable Tablets . . . 2404
Tegretol Suspension . . . 2404
Tegretol Tablets . . . 2404
Tegretol-XR Tablets . . . 2404

DELIDOSE (France)
ESTRADIOL
Alora Transdermal System . . . 3372
Climara Transdermal System . . . 958
Estrace Vaginal Cream . . . 3358
Estring Vaginal Ring . . . 2811
Vivelle Transdermal System . . . 2412
Vivelle-Dot Transdermal System . . . 2416

DELITEX N (Germany)
LINDANE
Lindane Lotion USP 1% . . . 559
Lindane Shampoo USP 1% . . . 560

DELIX (Germany)
RAMIPRIL
Altace Capsules . . . 2233

DELIXI (Germany)
PERMETHRIN
Acticin Cream . . . 998
Elimite Cream . . . 552

DELMUNO (Germany)
FELODIPINE
Plendil Extended-Release Tablets . . . 623

DELONAL (Germany, Switzerland)
ALCLOMETASONE DIPROPIONATE
Aclovate Cream . . . 1275
Aclovate Ointment . . . 1275

DELPHI (Belgium, The Netherlands)
TRIAMCINOLONE ACETONIDE
Azmacort Inhalation Aerosol . . . 728
Nasacort AQ Nasal Spray . . . 752
Nasacort Nasal Inhaler . . . 750

DELPHIMIX 1 (Germany)
DICLOFENAC SODIUM
Voltaren Tablets . . . 2315
Voltaren-XR Tablets . . . 2315

DELPHINAC (Germany)
DICLOFENAC SODIUM
Voltaren Tablets . . . 2315
Voltaren-XR Tablets . . . 2315

DELTA 80 (Italy)
BENZOYL PEROXIDE
Brevoxyl-4 Cleansing Lotion . . . 3269
Brevoxyl-4 Creamy Wash . . . 3270
Brevoxyl-4 Gel . . . 3269
Brevoxyl-8 Cleansing Lotion . . . 3269
Brevoxyl-8 Creamy Wash . . . 3270
Brevoxyl-8 Gel . . . 3269
Triaz Cleanser . . . 2026
Triaz Gel . . . 2026

DELTACEF (Italy)
CEFUROXIME SODIUM
Kefurox Vials, ADD-Vantage . . . 1948
Zinacef Injection . . . 1696

DELTA-CORTEF (Australia)
PREDNISOLONE
Prelone Syrup . . . 2273

DELTACORTENE (Italy)
PREDNISONE
Prednisone Intensol . . . 3064
Prednisone Oral Solution . . . 3064
Prednisone Tablets . . . 3064

DELTACORTRIL (Belgium, Irish Republic, United Kingdom)
PREDNISOLONE
Prelone Syrup . . . 2273

DELTA-DIONA (Mexico)
PREDNISOLONE
Prelone Syrup . . . 2273

DELTAFLOGIN (Brazil)
DICLOFENAC SODIUM
Voltaren Tablets . . . 2315
Voltaren-XR Tablets . . . 2315

DELTA-PHORICOL (United Kingdom)
PREDNISOLONE
Prelone Syrup . . . 2273

DELTASOLONE (Australia)
PREDNISOLONE
Prelone Syrup . . . 2273

DELTASONE (Australia, Canada, Hong Kong, New Zealand)
PREDNISONE
Prednisone Intensol . . . 3064
Prednisone Oral Solution . . . 3064
Prednisone Tablets . . . 3064

DELTASORALEN (Irish Republic)
METHOXSALEN
8-MOP Capsules . . . 1727
Oxsoralen Lotion 1% . . . 1740
Oxsoralen-Ultra Capsules . . . 1741

DELTAZEN (France)
DILTIAZEM HYDROCHLORIDE
Cardizem CD Capsules . . . 1016
Cardizem Injectable . . . 1018
Cardizem Lyo-Ject Syringe . . . 1018
Cardizem Monovial . . . 1018
Tiazac Capsules . . . 1378

DELTIDROSOL (Italy)
PREDNISOLONE
Prelone Syrup . . . 2273

DELTISON (Sweden)
PREDNISONE
Prednisone Intensol . . . 3064
Prednisone Oral Solution . . . 3064
Prednisone Tablets . . . 3064

DELVAS (United Kingdom)
AMILORIDE HYDROCHLORIDE/HYDROCHLOROTHIAZIDE
Moduretic Tablets . . . 2138

DEMAZIN NON-DROWSY (New Zealand)
LORATADINE/PSEUDOEPHEDRINE SULFATE
Claritin-D 12 Hour Extended Release Tablets . . . 3102
Claritin-D 24 Hour Extended Release Tablets . . . 3104

DEMAZIN NS (South Africa)
LORATADINE/PSEUDOEPHEDRINE SULFATE
Claritin-D 12 Hour Extended Release Tablets . . . 3102
Claritin-D 24 Hour Extended Release Tablets . . . 3104

DEMIX (United Kingdom)
DOXYCYCLINE HYCLATE
Doryx Coated Pellet Filled Capsules . . . 3357
Periostat Tablets . . . 1208
Vibra-Tabs Film Coated Tablets . . . 2735
Vibramycin Hyclate Capsules . . . 2735
Vibramycin Hyclate Intravenous . . . 2737

DEMOTEST (Spain)
BUDESONIDE
Pulmicort Turbuhaler Inhalation Powder . . . 636
Rhinocort Nasal Inhaler . . . 640

DEMOVARIN (Switzerland)
HEPARIN SODIUM
Heparin Lock Flush Solution . . . 3509
Heparin Sodium Injection . . . 3511

DENAN (Germany)
SIMVASTATIN
Zocor Tablets . . . 2219

DENAPRIL (Portugal)
ENALAPRIL MALEATE
Vasotec Tablets . . . 2210

DENAXPREN (Spain)
NAPROXEN
EC-Naprosyn Delayed-Release Tablets . . . 2967
Naprosyn Suspension . . . 2967
Naprosyn Tablets . . . 2967

DENAZOX (Thailand)
DILTIAZEM HYDROCHLORIDE
Cardizem CD Capsules . . . 1016
Cardizem Injectable . . . 1018
Cardizem Lyo-Ject Syringe . . . 1018
Cardizem Monovial . . . 1018
Tiazac Capsules . . . 1378

DENIREN (Mexico)
AMOXICILLIN
Amoxil Pediatric Drops for Oral Suspension . . . 1471
Amoxil Tablets . . . 1471

DENKACORT (Hong Kong)
TRIAMCINOLONE ACETONIDE
Azmacort Inhalation Aerosol . . . 728
Nasacort AQ Nasal Spray . . . 752
Nasacort Nasal Inhaler . . . 750

DENTIGOA (Germany)
IBUPROFEN
Motrin Suspension, Oral Drops, Chewable Tablets, and Caplets . . . 2002

DENTISPRAY (Portugal, Spain)
BENZOCAINE
Americaine Anesthetic Lubricant . . . 1162
Americaine Otic Topical Anesthetic Ear Drops . . . 1162

DENTOMYCIN (Irish Republic, United Kingdom)
MINOCYCLINE HYDROCHLORIDE
Dynacin Capsules . . . 2019
Minocin Intravenous . . . 1862
Minocin Oral Suspension . . . 1865
Minocin Pellet-Filled Capsules . . . 1863

DENTOMYCINE (Switzerland)
MINOCYCLINE HYDROCHLORIDE
Dynacin Capsules . . . 2019
Minocin Intravenous . . . 1862
Minocin Oral Suspension . . . 1865
Minocin Pellet-Filled Capsules . . . 1863

DENULCER (Spain)
RANITIDINE HYDROCHLORIDE
Zantac 150 EFFERdose Granules . . . 1690
Zantac 150 EFFERdose Tablets . . . 1690
Zantac 150 Tablets . . . 1690
Zantac 300 Tablets . . . 1690
Zantac Injection . . . 1688
Zantac Injection Premixed . . . 1688
Zantac Syrup . . . 1690

DENVAR (Mexico, Spain)
CEFIXIME
Suprax Tablets . . . 1877
Suprax for Oral Suspension . . . 1877

DEOPID (Thailand)
GEMFIBROZIL
Lopid Tablets . . . 2650

DEPAKENE (Brazil, Canada)
VALPROIC ACID
Depakene Capsules . . . 421
Depakene Syrup . . . 421

DEPAKINE ZUUR (The Netherlands)
VALPROIC ACID
Depakene Capsules . . . 421
Depakene Syrup . . . 421

DEPEN (Canada)
PENICILLAMINE
Cuprimine Capsules . . . 2075
Depen Titratable Tablets . . . 3341

DEPIGMAN (Germany)
MONOBENZONE
Benoquin Cream 20% . . . 1732

DEPO MODERIN (Spain)
METHYLPREDNISOLONE ACETATE
Depo-Medrol Injectable Suspension . . . 2795

DEPO-CLINOVIR (Germany)
MEDROXYPROGESTERONE ACETATE
Depo-Provera Contraceptive Injection . . . 2798
Provera Tablets . . . 2853

DEPOCON (Austria)
MEDROXYPROGESTERONE ACETATE
Depo-Provera Contraceptive Injection . . . 2798
Provera Tablets . . . 2853

DEPO-GESTIN (Thailand)
MEDROXYPROGESTERONE ACETATE
Depo-Provera Contraceptive Injection . . . 2798
Provera Tablets . . . 2853

DEPO-MEDRATE (Germany)
METHYLPREDNISOLONE ACETATE
Depo-Medrol Injectable Suspension . . . 2795

DEPO-MEDROL (Australia, Austria, Belgium, Brazil, Canada, Denmark, Finland, France, Hong Kong, Israel, Italy, Mexico, New Zealand, Norway, Portugal, South Africa, Sweden, Switzerland, Thailand, The Netherlands)
METHYLPREDNISOLONE ACETATE
Depo-Medrol Injectable Suspension . . . 2795

DEPO-MEDRONE (Irish Republic, Sweden, United Kingdom)
METHYLPREDNISOLONE ACETATE
Depo-Medrol Injectable Suspension . . . 2795

DEPO-NISOLONE (Australia)
METHYLPREDNISOLONE ACETATE
Depo-Medrol Injectable Suspension . . . 2795

DEPO-PRODASONE (France)
MEDROXYPROGESTERONE ACETATE
Depo-Provera Contraceptive Injection . . . 2798
Provera Tablets . . . 2853

DEPO-PROGESTA (Thailand)
MEDROXYPROGESTERONE ACETATE
Depo-Provera Contraceptive Injection . . . 2798
Provera Tablets . . . 2853

DEPO-PROGEVERA (Spain)
MEDROXYPROGESTERONE ACETATE
Depo-Provera Contraceptive Injection . . . 2798
Provera Tablets . . . 2853

DEPO-PROVERA (Australia, Austria, Belgium, Brazil, Canada, Denmark, Finland, France, Hong Kong, Irish Republic, Israel, Italy, Mexico, New Zealand, Norway, Portugal, Singapore, South Africa, Sweden, Switzerland, Thailand, The Netherlands, United Kingdom)
MEDROXYPROGESTERONE ACETATE
Depo-Provera Contraceptive Injection . . . 2798
Provera Tablets . . . 2853

DEPO-RALOVERA (Australia)
MEDROXYPROGESTERONE ACETATE
Depo-Provera Contraceptive Injection . . . 2798
Provera Tablets . . . 2853

DEPOT-THROMBOPHOB-N (Germany)
HEPARIN SODIUM
Heparin Lock Flush Solution . . . 3509
Heparin Sodium Injection . . . 3511

DEPRENYL (France, Germany)
SELEGILINE HYDROCHLORIDE
Eldepryl Capsules . . . 3266

DEPREXAN (Israel)
DESIPRAMINE HYDROCHLORIDE
Norpramin Tablets . . . 755

DEPRILAN (Brazil)
SELEGILINE HYDROCHLORIDE
Eldepryl Capsules . . . 3266

DEPTRAN (Australia)
DOXEPIN HYDROCHLORIDE
Sinequan Capsules . . . 2713
Sinequan Oral Concentrate . . . 2713

DEQUACAINE (United Kingdom)
BENZOCAINE
Americaine Anesthetic Lubricant . . . 1162
Americaine Otic Topical Anesthetic Ear Drops . . . 1162

DERALIN (Australia, Israel)
PROPRANOLOL HYDROCHLORIDE
Inderal Injectable . . . 3513
Inderal LA Long-Acting Capsules . . . 3516
Inderal Tablets . . . 3513

DERBAC-M (Irish Republic, New Zealand, United Kingdom)
MALATHION
Ovide Lotion . . . 2023

DERCOME (Germany)
BENZOYL PEROXIDE
Brevoxyl-4 Cleansing Lotion . . . 3269
Brevoxyl-4 Creamy Wash . . . 3270
Brevoxyl-4 Gel . . . 3269
Brevoxyl-8 Cleansing Lotion . . . 3269
Brevoxyl-8 Creamy Wash . . . 3270
Brevoxyl-8 Gel . . . 3269
Triaz Cleanser . . . 2026
Triaz Gel . . . 2026

DERIPIL (Spain)
ERYTHROMYCIN
Emgel 2% Topical Gel . . . 1285
Ery-Tab Tablets . . . 448

Erythromycin Base Filmtab Tablets 454
Erythromycin Delayed-Release Capsules, USP 455
PCE Dispertab Tablets 498

DERMABAZ (Hong Kong)
TRETINOIN
Avita Cream 999
Avita Gel 1000
Renova 0.05% Cream 2519
Retin-A Micro 0.1% 2522
Vesanoid Capsules 3037

DERMACNE (Canada)
BENZOYL PEROXIDE
Brevoxyl-4 Cleansing Lotion 3269
Brevoxyl-4 Creamy Wash 3270
Brevoxyl-4 Gel 3269
Brevoxyl-8 Cleansing Lotion 3269
Brevoxyl-8 Creamy Wash 3270
Brevoxyl-8 Gel 3269
Triaz Cleanser 2026
Triaz Gel 2026

DERMACORT (Australia, Finland)
HYDROCORTISONE ACETATE
Anusol-HC Suppositories 2238
Cortifoam Rectal Foam 3170
Hydrocortone Acetate Injectable Suspension 2103
Proctocort Suppositories 2264

DERMACORT (Hong Kong, United Kingdom)
TRIAMCINOLONE ACETONIDE
Azmacort Inhalation Aerosol 728
Nasacort AQ Nasal Spray 752
Nasacort Nasal Inhaler 750

DERMAFLOR (Italy)
DIFLORASONE DIACETATE
Psorcon E Cream 1227
Psorcon E Ointment 1228

DERM-AID (Australia, New Zealand, Singapore)
HYDROCORTISONE
Anusol-HC Cream 2.5% 2237
Hydrocortone Tablets 2106

DERMAIROL (Sweden)
TRETINOIN
Avita Cream 999
Avita Gel 1000
Renova 0.05% Cream 2519
Retin-A Micro 0.1% 2522
Vesanoid Capsules 3037

DERMAISOM (Italy)
FLUOCINOLONE ACETONIDE
Synalar Cream 2020
Synalar Ointment 2020
Synalar Topical Solution 2020

DERMALAR (Israel)
FLUOCINOLONE ACETONIDE
Synalar Cream 2020
Synalar Ointment 2020
Synalar Topical Solution 2020

DERMALIFE (Australia)
VITAMIN A PALMITATE
Aquasol A Parenteral 593

DERMALLERG (Germany)
HYDROCORTISONE
Anusol-HC Cream 2.5% 2237
Hydrocortone Tablets 2106

DERMAPLUS (Italy)
FLUOCINOLONE ACETONIDE
Synalar Cream 2020
Synalar Ointment 2020
Synalar Topical Solution 2020

DERMASIL (Thailand)
CLOBETASOL PROPIONATE
Cormax Cream 2440
Cormax Ointment 2440
Cormax Scalp Application 2441
Temovate Cream 1301
Temovate E Emollient 1302
Temovate Gel 1303
Temovate Ointment 1301
Temovate Scalp Application 1304

DERMA-SMOOTHE (Canada)
FLUOCINOLONE ACETONIDE
Synalar Cream 2020
Synalar Ointment 2020
Synalar Topical Solution 2020

DERMASONE (Canada, Hong Kong)
CLOBETASOL PROPIONATE
Cormax Cream 2440
Cormax Ointment 2440
Cormax Scalp Application 2441
Temovate Cream 1301
Temovate E Emollient 1302
Temovate Gel 1303
Temovate Ointment 1301
Temovate Scalp Application 1304

DERMASPRAID (France)
HYDROCORTISONE ACETATE
Anusol-HC Suppositories 2238
Cortifoam Rectal Foam 3170
Hydrocortone Acetate Injectable Suspension 2103
Proctocort Suppositories 2264

DERMASPRAY DEMANGEAISON (France)
HYDROCORTISONE
Anusol-HC Cream 2.5% 2237
Hydrocortone Tablets 2106

DERMATOP (Brazil, Germany, Italy, Thailand)
PREDNICARBATE
Dermatop Emollient Cream 2517

DERMATOVATE (Mexico)
CLOBETASOL PROPIONATE
Cormax Cream 2440
Cormax Ointment 2440
Cormax Scalp Application 2441
Temovate Cream 1301
Temovate E Emollient 1302
Temovate Gel 1303
Temovate Ointment 1301
Temovate Scalp Application 1304

DERMESTRIL (Australia, Belgium, Finland, France, Germany, Hong Kong, Italy, Portugal, Spain, Switzerland, The Netherlands, United Kingdom)
ESTRADIOL
Alora Transdermal System 3372
Climara Transdermal System 958
Estrace Vaginal Cream 3358
Estring Vaginal Ring 2811
Vivelle Transdermal System 2412
Vivelle-Dot Transdermal System 2416

DERMIL (Denmark)
HYDROCORTISONE
Anusol-HC Cream 2.5% 2237
Hydrocortone Tablets 2106

DERMIMADE CLORANFENICOL (Portugal)
CHLORAMPHENICOL
Chloromycetin Ophthalmic Ointment, 1% . . . . . . ⊙296
Chloromycetin Ophthalmic Solution . . . . ⊙297
Chloroptic Sterile Ophthalmic Ointment . . ⊙234
Chloroptic Sterile Ophthalmic Solution . . ⊙235

DERMIMADE HIDROCORTISONA (Portugal)
HYDROCORTISONE
Anusol-HC Cream 2.5% 2237
Hydrocortone Tablets 2106

DERMINOVAG (Spain)
HYDROCORTISONE ACETATE
Anusol-HC Suppositories 2238
Cortifoam Rectal Foam 3170
Hydrocortone Acetate Injectable Suspension 2103
Proctocort Suppositories 2264

DERMIRIT (Italy)
HYDROCORTISONE ACETATE
Anusol-HC Suppositories 2238
Cortifoam Rectal Foam 3170
Hydrocortone Acetate Injectable Suspension 2103
Proctocort Suppositories 2264

DERMO POSTERISAN (Germany)
HYDROCORTISONE
Anusol-HC Cream 2.5% 2237
Hydrocortone Tablets 2106

DERMOBENE (Brazil)
CLOTRIMAZOLE
Lotrimin Cream 1% 3128
Lotrimin Lotion 1% 3128
Lotrimin Topical Solution 1% 3128
Mycelex Troche 573

DERMOBETA (Italy)
FLUOCINOLONE ACETONIDE
Synalar Cream 2020
Synalar Ointment 2020
Synalar Topical Solution 2020

DERMOCHINONA (Italy)
MONOBENZONE
Benoquin Cream 20% 1732

DERMOCORTAL (Italy)
HYDROCORTISONE
Anusol-HC Cream 2.5% 2237
Hydrocortone Tablets 2106

DERMODRIN (Austria)
DIPHENHYDRAMINE HYDROCHLORIDE
Benadryl Parenteral 2617

DERMOFIL (Italy)
FLUOCINOLONE ACETONIDE
Synalar Cream 2020
Synalar Ointment 2020
Synalar Topical Solution 2020

DERMOJUVENTUS (Spain)
TRETINOIN
Avita Cream 999
Avita Gel 1000
Renova 0.05% Cream 2519
Retin-A Micro 0.1% 2522
Vesanoid Capsules 3037

DERMOL (New Zealand)
CLOBETASOL PROPIONATE
Cormax Cream 2440
Cormax Ointment 2440
Cormax Scalp Application 2441
Temovate Cream 1301
Temovate E Emollient 1302
Temovate Gel 1303
Temovate Ointment 1301
Temovate Scalp Application 1304

DERMOLERSA (Spain)
FLUOCINOLONE ACETONIDE
Synalar Cream 2020
Synalar Ointment 2020
Synalar Topical Solution 2020

DERMOLIN (Italy)
FLUOCINOLONE ACETONIDE
Synalar Cream 2020
Synalar Ointment 2020
Synalar Topical Solution 2020

DERMONILO (Spain)
DIFLORASONE DIACETATE
Psorcon E Cream 1227
Psorcon E Ointment 1228

DERMORETIN (Brazil)
TRETINOIN
Avita Cream 999
Avita Gel 1000
Renova 0.05% Cream 2519
Retin-A Micro 0.1% 2522
Vesanoid Capsules 3037

DERMOSA HIDROCORTISONA (Spain)
HYDROCORTISONE ACETATE
Anusol-HC Suppositories 2238
Cortifoam Rectal Foam 3170
Hydrocortone Acetate Injectable Suspension 2103
Proctocort Suppositories 2264

DERMOVAL (France)
CLOBETASOL PROPIONATE
Cormax Cream 2440
Cormax Ointment 2440
Cormax Scalp Application 2441
Temovate Cream 1301
Temovate E Emollient 1302
Temovate Gel 1303
Temovate Ointment 1301
Temovate Scalp Application 1304

DERMOVAT (Denmark, Finland, Norway, Sweden)
CLOBETASOL PROPIONATE
Cormax Cream 2440
Cormax Ointment 2440
Cormax Scalp Application 2441
Temovate Cream 1301
Temovate E Emollient 1302
Temovate Gel 1303
Temovate Ointment 1301
Temovate Scalp Application 1304

DERMOVATE (Austria, Belgium, Canada, Hong Kong, Irish Republic, Israel, New Zealand, Portugal, Singapore, South Africa, Switzerland, Thailand, The Netherlands, United Kingdom)
CLOBETASOL PROPIONATE
Cormax Cream 2440
Cormax Ointment 2440
Cormax Scalp Application 2441
Temovate Cream 1301
Temovate E Emollient 1302
Temovate Gel 1303
Temovate Ointment 1301
Temovate Scalp Application 1304

DERMOX (Mexico)
METHOXSALEN
8-MOP Capsules 1727
Oxsoralen Lotion 1% 1740
Oxsoralen-Ultra Capsules 1741

DERMOXIN (Germany)
CLOBETASOL PROPIONATE
Cormax Cream 2440
Cormax Ointment 2440
Cormax Scalp Application 2441
Temovate Cream 1301
Temovate E Emollient 1302
Temovate Gel 1303
Temovate Ointment 1301
Temovate Scalp Application 1304

DERMOXINALE (Germany)
CLOBETASOL PROPIONATE
Cormax Cream 2440
Cormax Ointment 2440
Cormax Scalp Application 2441
Temovate Cream 1301
Temovate E Emollient 1302
Temovate Gel 1303
Temovate Ointment 1301
Temovate Scalp Application 1304

DERMOXYL (Canada)
BENZOYL PEROXIDE
Brevoxyl-4 Cleansing Lotion 3269
Brevoxyl-4 Creamy Wash 3270
Brevoxyl-4 Gel 3269
Brevoxyl-8 Cleansing Lotion 3269
Brevoxyl-8 Creamy Wash 3270
Brevoxyl-8 Gel 3269
Triaz Cleanser 2026
Triaz Gel 2026

DERONGA HEILPASTE (Germany)
NATAMYCIN
Natacyn Antifungal Ophthalmic Suspension . . . . . . ⊙216

DERONIL (Canada)
DEXAMETHASONE
Decadron Elixir 2078
Decadron Tablets 2079

DEROXAT (France, Switzerland)
PAROXETINE HYDROCHLORIDE
Paxil Oral Suspension 1609
Paxil Tablets 1609

DESALARK (Italy)
DEXAMETHASONE
Decadron Elixir 2078
Decadron Tablets 2079
DEXAMETHASONE SODIUM PHOSPHATE
Decadron Phosphate Injection 2081
Decadron Phosphate Sterile Ophthalmic Ointment . . . . . . ⊙280, 2083
Decadron Phosphate Sterile Ophthalmic Solution 2084

DESAMIN SAME (Italy)
NAPHAZOLINE HYDROCHLORIDE
Albalon Ophthalmic Solution . . . . . . ⊙225

DESANDEN (Switzerland)
BENZOYL PEROXIDE
Brevoxyl-4 Cleansing Lotion 3269
Brevoxyl-4 Creamy Wash 3270
Brevoxyl-4 Gel 3269
Brevoxyl-8 Cleansing Lotion 3269
Brevoxyl-8 Creamy Wash 3270
Brevoxyl-8 Gel 3269
Triaz Cleanser 2026
Triaz Gel 2026

DESEC (Thailand)
OMEPRAZOLE
Prilosec Delayed-Release Capsules 628

DESERONIL (Italy)
DEXAMETHASONE
Decadron Elixir 2078
Decadron Tablets 2079

DESICORT (Israel)
DESOXIMETASONE
Topicort Cream 2025
Topicort Gel 2025
Topicort LP Cream 2025
Topicort Ointment 2025

DESIDOXEPIN (Germany)
DOXEPIN HYDROCHLORIDE
Sinequan Capsules 2713
Sinequan Oral Concentrate 2713

DESIFLUVOXAMIN (Germany)
FLUVOXAMINE MALEATE
Luvox Tablets (25, 50, 100 mg) 3256

DESINTAN P (Portugal)
PERMETHRIN
Acticin Cream 998
Elimite Cream 552

DESITICLOPIDIN (Germany)
TICLOPIDINE HYDROCHLORIDE
Ticlid Tablets 3015

DESMOGALEN (Germany)
DESMOPRESSIN ACETATE
DDAVP Injection 4 mcg/mL 737
DDAVP Nasal Spray 738
DDAVP Rhinal Tube 738
DDAVP Tablets 739
Desmopressin Acetate Injection 1344
Desmopressin Acetate Rhinal Tube 1345
Stimate Nasal Spray 796

DESMOSPRAY (Irish Republic, Portugal, United Kingdom)
DESMOPRESSIN ACETATE
DDAVP Injection 4 mcg/mL 737

DDAVP Nasal Spray 738
DDAVP Rhinal Tube 738
DDAVP Tablets 739
Desmopressin Acetate Injection 1344
Desmopressin Acetate Rhinal Tube 1345
Stimate Nasal Spray 796

DESMOTABS (Irish Republic, United Kingdom)
DESMOPRESSIN ACETATE
DDAVP Injection 4 mcg/mL 737
DDAVP Nasal Spray 738
DDAVP Rhinal Tube 738
DDAVP Tablets 739
Desmopressin Acetate Injection 1344
Desmopressin Acetate Rhinal Tube 1345
Stimate Nasal Spray 796

DESOCORT (Canada, France)
DESONIDE
DesOwen Cream 1401
DesOwen Lotion 1401
DesOwen Ointment 1401

DESONOL (Brazil)
DESONIDE
DesOwen Cream 1401
DesOwen Lotion 1401
DesOwen Ointment 1401

DESOWEN (Australia, Hong Kong, Mexico, New Zealand, Singapore)
DESONIDE
DesOwen Cream 1401
DesOwen Lotion 1401
DesOwen Ointment 1401

DESQUAM-X (Canada)
BENZOYL PEROXIDE
Brevoxyl-4 Cleansing Lotion 3269
Brevoxyl-4 Creamy Wash 3270
Brevoxyl-4 Gel 3269
Brevoxyl-8 Cleansing Lotion 3269
Brevoxyl-8 Creamy Wash 3270
Brevoxyl-8 Gel 3269
Triaz Cleanser 2026
Triaz Gel 2026

DETENSIEL (France)
BISOPROLOL FUMARATE
Zebeta Tablets 1885

DETENSOL (Canada)
PROPRANOLOL HYDROCHLORIDE
Inderal Injectable 3513
Inderal LA Long-Acting Capsules 3516
Inderal Tablets 3513

DETICENE (France, Germany, Hong Kong, Israel, Italy, Mexico, Portugal, The Netherlands)
DACARBAZINE
DTIC-Dome 902

DETIMEDAC (Germany)
DACARBAZINE
DTIC-Dome 902

DETRAVIS (Italy)
DEMECLOCYCLINE HYDROCHLORIDE
Declomycin Tablets 1855

DETROL (Canada)
TOLTERODINE TARTRATE
Detrol Tablets 3623

DETRUSITOL (Austria, Belgium, Denmark, Finland, France, Germany, Hong Kong, Irish Republic, Israel, Italy, Mexico, New Zealand, Norway, Portugal, Singapore, South Africa, Spain, Sweden, Switzerland, Thailand, The Netherlands, United Kingdom)
TOLTERODINE TARTRATE
Detrol Tablets 3623

DEVIAN (Italy)
METFORMIN HYDROCHLORIDE
Glucophage Tablets 1080

DEXA (Thailand)
DEXAMETHASONE SODIUM PHOSPHATE
Decadron Phosphate Injection 2081
Decadron Phosphate Sterile Ophthalmic Ointment . . . . . ⊙280, 2083
Decadron Phosphate Sterile Ophthalmic Solution 2084

DEXA ANTIB (Spain)
DEXAMETHASONE SODIUM PHOSPHATE/NEOMYCIN SULFATE
NeoDecadron Sterile Ophthalmic Solution 2144

DEXA FENICOL (Spain)
CHLORAMPHENICOL
Chloromycetin Ophthalmic Ointment, 1% . . . . . ⊙296
Chloromycetin Ophthalmic Solution . . . . . ⊙297
Chloroptic Sterile Ophthalmic Ointment . . . . . ⊙234
Chloroptic Sterile Ophthalmic Solution . . . . . ⊙235

DEXA IN DER OPHTIOLE (Germany)
DEXAMETHASONE SODIUM PHOSPHATE
Decadron Phosphate Injection 2081
Decadron Phosphate Sterile Ophthalmic Ointment . . . . . ⊙280, 2083
Decadron Phosphate Sterile Ophthalmic Solution 2084

DEXA-ALLVORAN (Germany)
DEXAMETHASONE SODIUM PHOSPHATE
Decadron Phosphate Injection 2081
Decadron Phosphate Sterile Ophthalmic Ointment . . . . . ⊙280, 2083
Decadron Phosphate Sterile Ophthalmic Solution 2084

DEXABENE (Austria, Germany)
DEXAMETHASONE SODIUM PHOSPHATE
Decadron Phosphate Injection 2081
Decadron Phosphate Sterile Ophthalmic Ointment . . . . . ⊙280, 2083
Decadron Phosphate Sterile Ophthalmic Solution 2084

DEXA-BRACHIALIN N (Germany)
DEXAMETHASONE SODIUM PHOSPHATE
Decadron Phosphate Injection 2081
Decadron Phosphate Sterile Ophthalmic Ointment . . . . . ⊙280, 2083
Decadron Phosphate Sterile Ophthalmic Solution 2084

DEXACIN (Thailand)
DEXAMETHASONE SODIUM PHOSPHATE/NEOMYCIN SULFATE
NeoDecadron Sterile Ophthalmic Solution 2144

DEXA-CLINIT (Germany)
DEXAMETHASONE SODIUM PHOSPHATE
Decadron Phosphate Injection 2081
Decadron Phosphate Sterile Ophthalmic Ointment . . . . . ⊙280, 2083
Decadron Phosphate Sterile Ophthalmic Solution 2084

DEXACORT (Brazil, Israel)
DEXAMETHASONE
Decadron Elixir 2078
Decadron Tablets 2079

DEXACORTAL (Sweden)
DEXAMETHASONE
Decadron Elixir 2078
Decadron Tablets 2079

DEXACORTISONE (Thailand)
DEXAMETHASONE SODIUM PHOSPHATE
Decadron Phosphate Injection 2081
Decadron Phosphate Sterile Ophthalmic Ointment . . . . . ⊙280, 2083
Decadron Phosphate Sterile Ophthalmic Solution 2084

DEXAFENICOL (Brazil, Spain)
CHLORAMPHENICOL
Chloromycetin Ophthalmic Ointment, 1% . . . . . ⊙296
Chloromycetin Ophthalmic Solution . . . . . ⊙297
Chloroptic Sterile Ophthalmic Ointment . . . . . ⊙234
Chloroptic Sterile Ophthalmic Solution . . . . . ⊙235

DEXAFLAM (Germany)
DEXAMETHASONE
Decadron Elixir 2078
Decadron Tablets 2079

DEXAFLAM N (Germany)
DEXAMETHASONE SODIUM PHOSPHATE
Decadron Phosphate Injection 2081
Decadron Phosphate Sterile Ophthalmic Ointment . . . . . ⊙280, 2083
Decadron Phosphate Sterile Ophthalmic Solution 2084

DEXAFLAN (Brazil)
DEXAMETHASONE
Decadron Elixir 2078
Decadron Tablets 2079

DEXAGALEN (Germany)
DEXAMETHASONE
Decadron Elixir 2078
Decadron Tablets 2079

DEXAGEL (Germany)
DEXAMETHASONE SODIUM PHOSPHATE
Decadron Phosphate Injection 2081
Decadron Phosphate Sterile Ophthalmic Ointment . . . . . ⊙280, 2083
Decadron Phosphate Sterile Ophthalmic Solution 2084

DEXAGRANE (France)
DEXAMETHASONE SODIUM PHOSPHATE/NEOMYCIN SULFATE
NeoDecadron Sterile Ophthalmic Solution 2144

DEXA-HELVACORT (Switzerland)
DEXAMETHASONE SODIUM PHOSPHATE
Decadron Phosphate Injection 2081
Decadron Phosphate Sterile Ophthalmic Ointment . . . . . ⊙280, 2083
Decadron Phosphate Sterile Ophthalmic Solution 2084

DEXAHEXAL (Germany)
DEXAMETHASONE SODIUM PHOSPHATE
Decadron Phosphate Injection 2081
Decadron Phosphate Sterile Ophthalmic Ointment . . . . . ⊙280, 2083
Decadron Phosphate Sterile Ophthalmic Solution 2084

DEXA-INJEKT (Germany)
DEXAMETHASONE SODIUM PHOSPHATE
Decadron Phosphate Injection 2081
Decadron Phosphate Sterile Ophthalmic Ointment . . . . . ⊙280, 2083
Decadron Phosphate Sterile Ophthalmic Solution 2084

DEXAL (Italy)
KETOPROFEN
Orudis Capsules 3548
Oruvail Capsules 3548

DEXALOCAL (Hong Kong, Switzerland)
DEXAMETHASONE
Decadron Elixir 2078
Decadron Tablets 2079

DEXALTIN (Singapore, Thailand)
DEXAMETHASONE
Decadron Elixir 2078
Decadron Tablets 2079

DEXAMBUTOL (France)
ETHAMBUTOL HYDROCHLORIDE
Myambutol Tablets 1290

DEXAMED (Germany, Singapore)
DEXAMETHASONE SODIUM PHOSPHATE
Decadron Phosphate Injection 2081
Decadron Phosphate Sterile Ophthalmic Ointment . . . . . ⊙280, 2083
Decadron Phosphate Sterile Ophthalmic Solution 2084

DEXAMINOR (Brazil)
DEXAMETHASONE
Decadron Elixir 2078
Decadron Tablets 2079

DEXAMISO (Spain)
DEXAMETHASONE
Decadron Elixir 2078
Decadron Tablets 2079

DEXAMONOZON (Germany)
DEXAMETHASONE
Decadron Elixir 2078
Decadron Tablets 2079

DEXAMONOZON N (Germany)
DEXAMETHASONE
Decadron Elixir 2078
Decadron Tablets 2079

DEXAPLAST (Spain)
DEXAMETHASONE
Decadron Elixir 2078
Decadron Tablets 2079

DEXA-RATIOPHARM (Germany)
DEXAMETHASONE SODIUM PHOSPHATE
Decadron Phosphate Injection 2081
Decadron Phosphate Sterile Ophthalmic Ointment . . . . . ⊙280, 2083
Decadron Phosphate Sterile Ophthalmic Solution 2084

DEXASIL (Thailand)
DEXAMETHASONE SODIUM PHOSPHATE/NEOMYCIN SULFATE
NeoDecadron Sterile Ophthalmic Solution 2144

DEXA-SINE (Germany)
DEXAMETHASONE SODIUM PHOSPHATE
Decadron Phosphate Injection 2081
Decadron Phosphate Sterile Ophthalmic Ointment . . . . . ⊙280, 2083
Decadron Phosphate Sterile Ophthalmic Solution 2084

DEXASONE (Canada, Hong Kong)
DEXAMETHASONE
Decadron Elixir 2078
Decadron Tablets 2079

DEXATAM (Mexico)
DEXAMETHASONE
Decadron Elixir 2078
Decadron Tablets 2079

DEXICAM (Italy)
PIROXICAM
Feldene Capsules 2685

DEXICAR (Mexico)
DEXAMETHASONE
Decadron Elixir 2078
Decadron Tablets 2079

DEXIRON (Canada)
IRON DEXTRAN
INFeD Injection 3388

DEXMETHSONE (Australia, Hong Kong)
DEXAMETHASONE
Decadron Elixir 2078
Decadron Tablets 2079

DEXOLAN (Switzerland)
DEXAMETHASONE
Decadron Elixir 2078
Decadron Tablets 2079

DEXOMON (United Kingdom)
DICLOFENAC SODIUM
Voltaren Tablets 2315
Voltaren-XR Tablets 2315

DEXON (Thailand)
DEXAMETHASONE SODIUM PHOSPHATE
Decadron Phosphate Injection 2081
Decadron Phosphate Sterile Ophthalmic Ointment . . . . . ⊙280, 2083
Decadron Phosphate Sterile Ophthalmic Solution 2084

DEXONA (Mexico)
DEXAMETHASONE
Decadron Elixir 2078
Decadron Tablets 2079

DEXOPH (Thailand)
DEXAMETHASONE SODIUM PHOSPHATE/NEOMYCIN SULFATE
NeoDecadron Sterile Ophthalmic Solution 2144

DEXSOL (United Kingdom)
DEXAMETHASONE SODIUM PHOSPHATE
Decadron Phosphate Injection 2081
Decadron Phosphate Sterile Ophthalmic Ointment . . . . . ⊙280, 2083
Decadron Phosphate Sterile Ophthalmic Solution 2084

DEXTHASOL (Thailand)
DEXAMETHASONE SODIUM PHOSPHATE
Decadron Phosphate Injection 2081
Decadron Phosphate Sterile Ophthalmic Ointment . . . . . ⊙280, 2083
Decadron Phosphate Sterile Ophthalmic Solution 2084

DEXTIN (South Africa)
METFORMIN HYDROCHLORIDE
Glucophage Tablets 1080

DEXTON (Thailand)
DEXAMETHASONE SODIUM PHOSPHATE
Decadron Phosphate Injection 2081
Decadron Phosphate Sterile Ophthalmic Ointment . . . . . ⊙280, 2083
Decadron Phosphate Sterile Ophthalmic Solution 2084

DEXTRACIN (Singapore)
DEXAMETHASONE SODIUM PHOSPHATE/NEOMYCIN SULFATE
NeoDecadron Sterile Ophthalmic Solution 2144

DEXYLIN (Thailand)
DEXAMETHASONE SODIUM PHOSPHATE/NEOMYCIN SULFATE
NeoDecadron Sterile Ophthalmic Solution 2144

DEZORAL (Singapore)
KETOCONAZOLE
Nizoral 2% Cream 3620
Nizoral 2% Shampoo 2007
Nizoral Tablets 1791

DHABESOL (Singapore)
CLOBETASOL PROPIONATE
Cormax Cream 2440
Cormax Ointment 2440
Cormax Scalp Application 2441
Temovate Cream 1301
Temovate E Emollient 1302
Temovate Gel 1303

Temovate Ointment 1301
Temovate Scalp Application 1304

DHAPERAZINE (Hong Kong, Singapore)
PROCHLORPERAZINE MALEATE
Compazine Spansule Capsules 1505
Compazine Tablets 1505

DHASOLONE (Hong Kong)
PREDNISOLONE
Prelone Syrup 2273

DHATALIN (Hong Kong)
TERBUTALINE SULFATE
Brethine Ampuls 2314
Brethine Tablets 2313

DI RETARD (Spain)
DICLOFENAC SODIUM
Voltaren Tablets 2315
Voltaren-XR Tablets 2315

DIABEEDOL (Thailand)
CHLORPROPAMIDE
Diabinese Tablets 2680

DIABEMIDE (Italy)
CHLORPROPAMIDE
Diabinese Tablets 2680

DIABERIT (Italy)
METFORMIN HYDROCHLORIDE
Glucophage Tablets 1080

DIABESIN (Germany)
METFORMIN HYDROCHLORIDE
Glucophage Tablets 1080

DIABET (Spain)
CHLORPROPAMIDE
Diabinese Tablets 2680

DIABETASE (Germany)
METFORMIN HYDROCHLORIDE
Glucophage Tablets 1080

DIABETEX (Austria)
METFORMIN HYDROCHLORIDE
Glucophage Tablets 1080

DIABETMIN (Singapore)
METFORMIN HYDROCHLORIDE
Glucophage Tablets 1080

DIABETOSAN (Italy)
METFORMIN HYDROCHLORIDE
Glucophage Tablets 1080

DIABEX (Australia)
METFORMIN HYDROCHLORIDE
Glucophage Tablets 1080

DIABEXAN (Italy)
CHLORPROPAMIDE
Diabinese Tablets 2680

DIABICLOR (Mexico)
CHLORPROPAMIDE
Diabinese Tablets 2680

DIABINES (Sweden)
CHLORPROPAMIDE
Diabinese Tablets 2680

DIABINESE (Australia, Belgium, Brazil, Canada, France, Hong Kong, Irish Republic, Israel, Italy, Mexico, Norway, Singapore, South Africa, Spain, Switzerland, Thailand, United Kingdom)
CHLORPROPAMIDE
Diabinese Tablets 2680

DIABITEX (South Africa)
CHLORPROPAMIDE
Diabinese Tablets 2680

DIACEPLEX (Spain)
DIAZEPAM
Valium Injectable 3026
Valium Tablets 3047

DIACEPLEX SIMPLE (Spain)
DIAZEPAM
Valium Injectable 3026
Valium Tablets 3047

DIA-COLON (Italy)
LACTULOSE
Kristalose for Oral Solution 1007

DIACOR (France)
DILTIAZEM HYDROCHLORIDE
Cardizem CD Capsules 1016
Cardizem Injectable 1018
Cardizem Lyo-Ject Syringe 1018
Cardizem Monovial 1018
Tiazac Capsules 1378

DI-ADRESON-F (Hong Kong, Thailand)
PREDNISOLONE
Prelone Syrup 2273

DIAFORMIN (Australia, Hong Kong)
METFORMIN HYDROCHLORIDE
Glucophage Tablets 1080

DIALAR (United Kingdom)
DIAZEPAM
Valium Injectable 3026
Valium Tablets 3047

DIALUDON (Brazil)
PHENYTOIN
Dilantin Infatabs 2624
Dilantin-125 Oral Suspension 2625

DIAMET (Thailand)
METFORMIN HYDROCHLORIDE
Glucophage Tablets 1080

DIAMIN (Singapore)
METFORMIN HYDROCHLORIDE
Glucophage Tablets 1080

DIAMOX (Brazil, Hong Kong, Israel, Italy, Mexico, Norway, Spain, Thailand, The Netherlands)
ACETAZOLAMIDE
Diamox Sequels Sustained Release Capsules ⊙270
Diamox Tablets ⊙269

DIANBEN (Spain)
METFORMIN HYDROCHLORIDE
Glucophage Tablets 1080

DIAPAM (Finland, Thailand)
DIAZEPAM
Valium Injectable 3026
Valium Tablets 3047

DIAPANIL (Mexico)
DIAZEPAM
Valium Injectable 3026
Valium Tablets 3047

DIAPINE (Singapore, Thailand)
DIAZEPAM
Valium Injectable 3026
Valium Tablets 3047

DIAQUEL (South Africa)
DIAZEPAM
Valium Injectable 3026
Valium Tablets 3047

DIASECTRAL (Denmark, Finland)
ACEBUTOLOL HYDROCHLORIDE
Sectral Capsules 3589

DIASEF (Singapore, Thailand)
GLIPIZIDE
Glucotrol Tablets 2692
Glucotrol XL Extended Release Tablets 2693

DIASTABOL (Austria, Finland, France, Germany, Portugal, Spain, Sweden, Switzerland)
MIGLITOL
Glyset Tablets 2821

DIATEX (Mexico)
DIAZEPAM
Valium Injectable 3026
Valium Tablets 3047

DIATIL (South Africa)
DILTIAZEM HYDROCHLORIDE
Cardizem CD Capsules 1016
Cardizem Injectable 1018
Cardizem Lyo-Ject Syringe 1018
Cardizem Monovial 1018
Tiazac Capsules 1378

DIATRACIN (Spain)
VANCOMYCIN HYDROCHLORIDE
Vancocin HCl Capsules & Pulvules 1972
Vancocin HCl Oral Solution 1971
Vancocin HCl, Vials & ADD-Vantage 1970

DIAZ (Israel)
DIAZEPAM
Valium Injectable 3026
Valium Tablets 3047

DIAZELONG (Brazil)
DIAZEPAM
Valium Injectable 3026
Valium Tablets 3047

DIAZEMULS (Australia, Canada, Germany, Hong Kong, Irish Republic, Italy, New Zealand, The Netherlands, United Kingdom)
DIAZEPAM
Valium Injectable 3026
Valium Tablets 3047

DIAZOLEN (Mexico)
MEBENDAZOLE
Vermox Chewable Tablets 2017

DIAZON (Singapore, Thailand)
KETOCONAZOLE
Nizoral 2% Cream 3620
Nizoral 2% Shampoo 2007
Nizoral Tablets 1791

DIBADORM N (Germany)
DIPHENHYDRAMINE HYDROCHLORIDE
Benadryl Parenteral 2617

DIBASONA (Mexico)
DEXAMETHASONE SODIUM PHOSPHATE
Decadron Phosphate Injection 2081
Decadron Phosphate Sterile Ophthalmic Ointment ⊙280, 2083
Decadron Phosphate Sterile Ophthalmic Solution 2084

DIBECON (Thailand)
CHLORPROPAMIDE
Diabinese Tablets 2680

DIBERTIL (Belgium)
METOCLOPRAMIDE HYDROCHLORIDE
Reglan Injectable 2935
Reglan Syrup 2935
Reglan Tablets 2935

DIBONDRIN (Austria)
DIPHENHYDRAMINE HYDROCHLORIDE
Benadryl Parenteral 2617

DIBUFEN (Mexico)
IBUPROFEN
Motrin Suspension, Oral Drops, Chewable Tablets, and Caplets 2002

DICEPIN B6 (Spain)
DIAZEPAM
Valium Injectable 3026
Valium Tablets 3047

DICHINALEX (Italy)
CHLOROQUINE PHOSPHATE
Aralen Tablets 3075

DICHLOTRIDE (Australia, Belgium, Denmark, Norway, Portugal, South Africa, Sweden, Thailand, The Netherlands)
HYDROCHLOROTHIAZIDE
HydroDIURIL Tablets 2108
Microzide Capsules 3414

DICLAC (Austria, Germany, Irish Republic)
DICLOFENAC SODIUM
Voltaren Tablets 2315
Voltaren-XR Tablets 2315

DICLAX (New Zealand)
DICLOFENAC SODIUM
Voltaren Tablets 2315
Voltaren-XR Tablets 2315

DICLO (Germany, Irish Republic, Switzerland)
DICLOFENAC SODIUM
Voltaren Tablets 2315
Voltaren-XR Tablets 2315

DICLO-ATTRITIN (Germany)
DICLOFENAC SODIUM
Voltaren Tablets 2315
Voltaren-XR Tablets 2315

DICLO-BASAN (Switzerland)
DICLOFENAC SODIUM
Voltaren Tablets 2315
Voltaren-XR Tablets 2315

DICLOBENE (Austria)
DICLOFENAC SODIUM
Voltaren Tablets 2315
Voltaren-XR Tablets 2315

DICLOBERL (Germany)
DICLOFENAC SODIUM
Voltaren Tablets 2315
Voltaren-XR Tablets 2315

DICLOCULAR (Italy)
DICLOFENAC SODIUM
Voltaren Tablets 2315
Voltaren-XR Tablets 2315

DICLO-DENK (Hong Kong)
DICLOFENAC SODIUM
Voltaren Tablets 2315
Voltaren-XR Tablets 2315

DICLO-DIVIDO (Germany)
DICLOFENAC SODIUM
Voltaren Tablets 2315
Voltaren-XR Tablets 2315

DICLODOC (Germany)
DICLOFENAC SODIUM
Voltaren Tablets 2315
Voltaren-XR Tablets 2315

DICLODOL (Italy)
DICLOFENAC SODIUM
Voltaren Tablets 2315
Voltaren-XR Tablets 2315

DICLOFAM (South Africa)
DICLOFENAC SODIUM
Voltaren Tablets 2315
Voltaren-XR Tablets 2315

DICLOFAN (Italy)
DICLOFENAC SODIUM
Voltaren Tablets 2315
Voltaren-XR Tablets 2315

DICLOFEN (Brazil, Thailand)
DICLOFENAC POTASSIUM
Cataflam Tablets 2315

DICLOFENBETA (Germany)
DICLOFENAC SODIUM
Voltaren Tablets 2315
Voltaren-XR Tablets 2315

DICLOFTIL (Italy)
DICLOFENAC SODIUM
Voltaren Tablets 2315
Voltaren-XR Tablets 2315

DICLOGRUN (Germany)
DICLOFENAC SODIUM
Voltaren Tablets 2315
Voltaren-XR Tablets 2315

DICLOHEXAL (Australia, South Africa)
DICLOFENAC SODIUM
Voltaren Tablets 2315
Voltaren-XR Tablets 2315

DICLOLAN (Thailand)
DICLOFENAC SODIUM
Voltaren Tablets 2315
Voltaren-XR Tablets 2315

DICLOMAX (United Kingdom)
DICLOFENAC SODIUM
Voltaren Tablets 2315
Voltaren-XR Tablets 2315

DICLOMEL (Irish Republic)
DICLOFENAC SODIUM
Voltaren Tablets 2315
Voltaren-XR Tablets 2315

DICLOMELAN (Austria)
DICLOFENAC SODIUM
Voltaren Tablets 2315
Voltaren-XR Tablets 2315

DICLOMERCK (Germany)
DICLOFENAC SODIUM
Voltaren Tablets 2315
Voltaren-XR Tablets 2315

DICLOMETIN (Finland)
DICLOFENAC SODIUM
Voltaren Tablets 2315
Voltaren-XR Tablets 2315

DICLOMEX (Finland)
DICLOFENAC SODIUM
Voltaren Tablets 2315
Voltaren-XR Tablets 2315

DICLON (Denmark)
DICLOFENAC SODIUM
Voltaren Tablets 2315
Voltaren-XR Tablets 2315

DICLO-OPT (Germany)
DICLOFENAC SODIUM
Voltaren Tablets 2315
Voltaren-XR Tablets 2315

DICLOPHLOGONT (Germany)
DICLOFENAC SODIUM
Voltaren Tablets 2315
Voltaren-XR Tablets 2315

DICLO-PUREN (Germany)
DICLOFENAC SODIUM
Voltaren Tablets 2315
Voltaren-XR Tablets 2315

DICLORAN (Mexico)
DICLOFENAC SODIUM
Voltaren Tablets 2315
Voltaren-XR Tablets 2315

DICLOREKTAL (Germany)
DICLOFENAC SODIUM
Voltaren Tablets 2315
Voltaren-XR Tablets 2315

DICLORENGEL (Israel)
DICLOFENAC SODIUM
Voltaren Tablets 2315
Voltaren-XR Tablets 2315

DICLO-SAAR (Germany)
DICLOFENAC SODIUM
Voltaren Tablets 2315
Voltaren-XR Tablets 2315

DICLOSIAN (Thailand)
DICLOFENAC SODIUM
Voltaren Tablets 2315

Voltaren-XR Tablets . . . 2315

DICLOSIFAR (Switzerland)
DICLOFENAC SODIUM
Voltaren Tablets . . . 2315
Voltaren-XR Tablets . . . 2315

DICLO-SPONDYRIL (Germany)
DICLOFENAC SODIUM
Voltaren Tablets . . . 2315
Voltaren-XR Tablets . . . 2315

DICLOSTAD (Austria)
DICLOFENAC SODIUM
Voltaren Tablets . . . 2315
Voltaren-XR Tablets . . . 2315

DICLOSYL (Austria)
DICLOFENAC SODIUM
Voltaren Tablets . . . 2315
Voltaren-XR Tablets . . . 2315

DICLO-TABLINEN (Germany)
DICLOFENAC SODIUM
Voltaren Tablets . . . 2315
Voltaren-XR Tablets . . . 2315

DICLOTARD (United Kingdom)
DICLOFENAC SODIUM
Voltaren Tablets . . . 2315
Voltaren-XR Tablets . . . 2315

DICLOTEC (Canada, Portugal)
DICLOFENAC SODIUM
Voltaren Tablets . . . 2315
Voltaren-XR Tablets . . . 2315

DICLOTRIDE (Mexico)
HYDROCHLOROTHIAZIDE
HydroDIURIL Tablets . . . 2108
Microzide Capsules . . . 3414

DICLOVOL (United Kingdom)
DICLOFENAC SODIUM
Voltaren Tablets . . . 2315
Voltaren-XR Tablets . . . 2315

DICLOWAL (Singapore)
DICLOFENAC SODIUM
Voltaren Tablets . . . 2315
Voltaren-XR Tablets . . . 2315

DICLO-WOLFF (Germany)
DICLOFENAC SODIUM
Voltaren Tablets . . . 2315
Voltaren-XR Tablets . . . 2315

DICLOZIP (United Kingdom)
DICLOFENAC SODIUM
Voltaren Tablets . . . 2315
Voltaren-XR Tablets . . . 2315

DIDAMOL (Belgium)
DIPYRIDAMOLE
Persantine Tablets . . . 1057

DIDRALIN (Singapore, Thailand)
HYDROCHLOROTHIAZIDE
HydroDIURIL Tablets . . . 2108
Microzide Capsules . . . 3414

DIENPAX (Brazil)
DIAZEPAM
Valium Injectable . . . 3026
Valium Tablets . . . 3047

DI-ERTRIDE (Singapore)
HYDROCHLOROTHIAZIDE
HydroDIURIL Tablets . . . 2108
Microzide Capsules . . . 3414

DIFENA (Hong Kong)
DICLOFENAC SODIUM
Voltaren Tablets . . . 2315
Voltaren-XR Tablets . . . 2315

DIFENAC (Hong Kong, Singapore, South Africa, Thailand)
DICLOFENAC SODIUM
Voltaren Tablets . . . 2315
Voltaren-XR Tablets . . . 2315

DIFENE (Irish Republic)
DICLOFENAC SODIUM
Voltaren Tablets . . . 2315
Voltaren-XR Tablets . . . 2315

DIFENET (Denmark)
DICLOFENAC SODIUM
Voltaren Tablets . . . 2315
Voltaren-XR Tablets . . . 2315

DIFENO (Thailand)
DICLOFENAC SODIUM
Voltaren Tablets . . . 2315
Voltaren-XR Tablets . . . 2315

DIFFERIN (Australia, Austria, Belgium, Canada, Finland, Germany, Hong Kong, Irish Republic, Italy, New Zealand, Norway, Portugal, Singapore, South Africa, Sweden, Switzerland, Thailand, United Kingdom)
ADAPALENE
Differin Gel . . . 1403
Differin Solution/Pledgets . . . 1404

DIFFERINE (France, Spain)
ADAPALENE
Differin Gel . . . 1403
Differin Solution/Pledgets . . . 1404

DIFFU-K (France)
POTASSIUM CHLORIDE
K-Dur Microburst Release System ER Tablets . . . 1832
K-Lor Powder Packets . . . 469
K-Tab Filmtab Tablets . . . 470
Rum-K . . . 1363

DIFFUMAL (Italy)
THEOPHYLLINE
Aerolate Jr. T.D. Capsules . . . 1361
Aerolate Liquid . . . 1361
Aerolate Sr. T.D. Capsules . . . 1361
Theo-Dur Extended-Release Tablets . . . 1835
Uni-Dur Extended-Release Tablets . . . 1841
Uniphyl 400 mg and 600 mg Tablets . . . 2903

DIFIRAM (Thailand)
DISULFIRAM
Antabuse Tablets . . . 3474

DIFIX (Italy)
CALCITRIOL
Calcijex Injection . . . 411
Rocaltrol Capsules . . . 2991
Rocaltrol Oral Solution . . . 2991

DIFLONID (Denmark, Norway, Sweden)
DIFLUNISAL
Dolobid Tablets . . . 2088

DIFLUCAN (Australia, Austria, Belgium, Canada, Denmark, Finland, Germany, Hong Kong, Irish Republic, Israel, Italy, Mexico, New Zealand, Norway, Portugal, Singapore, South Africa, Spain, Sweden, Switzerland, Thailand, The Netherlands, United Kingdom)
FLUCONAZOLE
Diflucan Tablets, Injection, and Oral Suspension . . . 2681

DIFLUDOL (Italy)
DIFLUNISAL
Dolobid Tablets . . . 2088

DIFLUNIL (Italy)
DIFLUNISAL
Dolobid Tablets . . . 2088

DIFLUSAL (Belgium)
DIFLUNISAL
Dolobid Tablets . . . 2088

DIFLUSAN (Italy)
DIFLUNISAL
Dolobid Tablets . . . 2088

DIFNAL (Singapore)
DICLOFENAC SODIUM
Voltaren Tablets . . . 2315
Voltaren-XR Tablets . . . 2315

DIFORMIN (Finland)
METFORMIN HYDROCHLORIDE
Glucophage Tablets . . . 1080

DIFOXACIL (Mexico)
NORFLOXACIN
Chibroxin Sterile Ophthalmic Solution . . . ⊙273, 2051
Noroxin Tablets . . . 2145

DIGACIN (Germany)
DIGOXIN
Lanoxicaps Capsules . . . 1574
Lanoxin Elixir Pediatric . . . 1578
Lanoxin Injection . . . 1581
Lanoxin Injection Pediatric . . . 1584
Lanoxin Tablets . . . 1587

DIGAOL (France)
TIMOLOL MALEATE
Blocadren Tablets . . . 2046
Timoptic Sterile Ophthalmic Solution . . . 2190
Timoptic in Ocudose . . . 2192
Timoptic-XE Sterile Ophthalmic Gel Forming Solution . . . 2194

DIGARIL (Spain)
FLUVASTATIN SODIUM
Lescol Capsules . . . 2361

DIGENAC (United Kingdom)
DICLOFENAC SODIUM
Voltaren Tablets . . . 2315
Voltaren-XR Tablets . . . 2315

DIGERVIN (Spain)
FAMOTIDINE
Pepcid Injection . . . 2153
Pepcid Injection Premixed . . . 2153
Pepcid RPD Orally Disintegrating Tablets . . . 2150
Pepcid Tablets . . . 2150
Pepcid for Oral Suspension . . . 2150

DIGESS (Canada)
PANCRELIPASE
Ultrase Capsules . . . 835
Ultrase MT Capsules . . . 835

DIGESTOSAN (Austria)
RANITIDINE HYDROCHLORIDE
Zantac 150 EFFERdose Granules . . . 1690
Zantac 150 EFFERdose Tablets . . . 1690
Zantac 150 Tablets . . . 1690
Zantac 300 Tablets . . . 1690
Zantac Injection . . . 1688
Zantac Injection Premixed . . . 1688
Zantac Syrup . . . 1690

DIGEZANOL (Mexico)
ALBENDAZOLE
Albenza Tablets . . . 1463

DIGNOBETA (Germany)
ATENOLOL
Tenormin I.V. Injection . . . 692

DIGNOFENAC (Germany)
DICLOFENAC SODIUM
Voltaren Tablets . . . 2315
Voltaren-XR Tablets . . . 2315

DIGNOFLEX (Germany)
IBUPROFEN
Motrin Suspension, Oral Drops, Chewable Tablets, and Caplets . . . 2002

DIGNOKONSTANT (Germany)
NIFEDIPINE
Adalat CC Tablets . . . 877
Procardia Capsules . . . 2708
Procardia XL Extended Release Tablets . . . 2710

DIGNONITRAT (Germany)
ISOSORBIDE DINITRATE
Isordil Sublingual Tablets . . . 3525
Isordil Titradose Tablets . . . 3526

DIGNORETIK (Germany)
AMILORIDE HYDROCHLORIDE/HYDROCHLOROTHIAZIDE
Moduretic Tablets . . . 2138

DIGNOTAMOXI (Germany)
TAMOXIFEN CITRATE
Nolvadex Tablets . . . 678

DIGNOTRIMAZOL (Germany)
CLOTRIMAZOLE
Lotrimin Cream 1% . . . 3128
Lotrimin Lotion 1% . . . 3128
Lotrimin Topical Solution 1% . . . 3128
Mycelex Troche . . . 573

DIGNOVER (Germany)
VERAPAMIL HYDROCHLORIDE
Covera-HS Tablets . . . 3199
Isoptin SR Tablets . . . 467
Verelan Capsules . . . 3184
Verelan PM Capsules . . . 3186

DIGOMAL (Italy)
DIGOXIN
Lanoxicaps Capsules . . . 1574
Lanoxin Elixir Pediatric . . . 1578
Lanoxin Injection . . . 1581
Lanoxin Injection Pediatric . . . 1584
Lanoxin Tablets . . . 1587

DIGOSIN (Japan)
DIGOXIN
Lanoxicaps Capsules . . . 1574
Lanoxin Elixir Pediatric . . . 1578
Lanoxin Injection . . . 1581
Lanoxin Injection Pediatric . . . 1584
Lanoxin Tablets . . . 1587

DI-HYDAN (Belgium, France)
PHENYTOIN
Dilantin Infatabs . . . 2624
Dilantin-125 Oral Suspension . . . 2625

DIHYDRAL (South Africa)
DIPHENHYDRAMINE HYDROCHLORIDE
Benadryl Parenteral . . . 2617

DILABAR (Spain)
CAPTOPRIL
Captopril Tablets . . . 2281

DILACLAN (Spain)
DILTIAZEM HYDROCHLORIDE
Cardizem CD Capsules . . . 1016
Cardizem Injectable . . . 1018
Cardizem Lyo-Ject Syringe . . . 1018
Cardizem Monovial . . . 1018
Tiazac Capsules . . . 1378

DILACORAN (Mexico)
VERAPAMIL HYDROCHLORIDE
Covera-HS Tablets . . . 3199
Isoptin SR Tablets . . . 467
Verelan Capsules . . . 3184
Verelan PM Capsules . . . 3186

DILACORON (Brazil)
VERAPAMIL HYDROCHLORIDE
Covera-HS Tablets . . . 3199
Isoptin SR Tablets . . . 467
Verelan Capsules . . . 3184
Verelan PM Capsules . . . 3186

DILADEL (Italy)
DILTIAZEM HYDROCHLORIDE
Cardizem CD Capsules . . . 1016
Cardizem Injectable . . . 1018
Cardizem Lyo-Ject Syringe . . . 1018
Cardizem Monovial . . . 1018
Tiazac Capsules . . . 1378

DILAFLUX (Brazil)
NIFEDIPINE
Adalat CC Tablets . . . 877
Procardia Capsules . . . 2708
Procardia XL Extended Release Tablets . . . 2710

DILAMAX (Portugal)
SALMETEROL XINAFOATE
Serevent Diskus . . . 1637
Serevent Inhalation Aerosol . . . 1633

DILANACIN (Germany)
DIGOXIN
Lanoxicaps Capsules . . . 1574
Lanoxin Elixir Pediatric . . . 1578
Lanoxin Injection . . . 1581
Lanoxin Injection Pediatric . . . 1584
Lanoxin Tablets . . . 1587

DILANID (South Africa)
ISOSORBIDE DINITRATE
Isordil Sublingual Tablets . . . 3525
Isordil Titradose Tablets . . . 3526

DILANTIN (Australia, Canada, Israel, New Zealand, Singapore, Thailand)
PHENYTOIN
Dilantin Infatabs . . . 2624
Dilantin-125 Oral Suspension . . . 2625

DILATAM (Israel, Singapore, South Africa, Thailand)
DILTIAZEM HYDROCHLORIDE
Cardizem CD Capsules . . . 1016
Cardizem Injectable . . . 1018
Cardizem Lyo-Ject Syringe . . . 1018
Cardizem Monovial . . . 1018
Tiazac Capsules . . . 1378

DILATAME (Austria)
DILTIAZEM HYDROCHLORIDE
Cardizem CD Capsules . . . 1016
Cardizem Injectable . . . 1018
Cardizem Lyo-Ject Syringe . . . 1018
Cardizem Monovial . . . 1018
Tiazac Capsules . . . 1378

DILATOL (Portugal)
ISRADIPINE
DynaCirc CR Tablets . . . 2923

DILATREND (Australia, Austria, Germany, Hong Kong, Italy, Mexico, New Zealand, Norway, Singapore, South Africa, Switzerland, Thailand)
CARVEDILOL
Coreg Tablets . . . 1508

DILAUDID (Australia, Canada, Germany, Irish Republic)
HYDROMORPHONE HYDROCHLORIDE
Dilaudid Ampules . . . 441
Dilaudid Injection . . . 441
Dilaudid Multiple Dose Vials (Sterile Solution) . . . 441
Dilaudid Oral Liquid . . . 445
Dilaudid Powder . . . 441
Dilaudid Rectal Suppositories . . . 441
Dilaudid Tablets . . . 441
Dilaudid Tablets - 8 mg . . . 445
Dilaudid-HP Injection . . . 443
Dilaudid-HP Lyophilized Powder 250 mg . . . 443

DILBLOC (Portugal)
CARVEDILOL
Coreg Tablets . . . 1508

DILCARD (New Zealand)
DILTIAZEM HYDROCHLORIDE
Cardizem CD Capsules . . . 1016
Cardizem Injectable . . . 1018
Cardizem Lyo-Ject Syringe . . . 1018
Cardizem Monovial . . . 1018
Tiazac Capsules . . . 1378

DILCARDIA (United Kingdom)
DILTIAZEM HYDROCHLORIDE
Cardizem CD Capsules . . . 1016
Cardizem Injectable . . . 1018
Cardizem Lyo-Ject Syringe . . . 1018
Cardizem Monovial . . . 1018
Tiazac Capsules . . . 1378

DILCLOR (Mexico)
CHLORAMPHENICOL
Chloromycetin Ophthalmic Ointment, 1% . . . ⊙296
Chloromycetin Ophthalmic Solution . . . ⊙297
Chloroptic Sterile Ophthalmic Ointment . . . ⊙234
Chloroptic Sterile Ophthalmic Solution . . . ⊙235

DILCOR (Denmark, Spain)
DILTIAZEM HYDROCHLORIDE
Cardizem CD Capsules . . . 1016

(⊙ Described in PDR For Ophthalmic Medicines™)

Cardizem Injectable **1018**
Cardizem Lyo-Ject Syringe **1018**
Cardizem Monovial **1018**
Tiazac Capsules **1378**

DILEM (Hong Kong, Italy)
DILTIAZEM HYDROCHLORIDE
Cardizem CD Capsules **1016**
Cardizem Injectable **1018**
Cardizem Lyo-Ject Syringe **1018**
Cardizem Monovial **1018**
Tiazac Capsules **1378**

DILETAN (Portugal)
SUMATRIPTAN SUCCINATE
Imitrex Injection **1549**
Imitrex Tablets **1558**

DILFAR (Portugal)
DILTIAZEM HYDROCHLORIDE
Cardizem CD Capsules **1016**
Cardizem Injectable **1018**
Cardizem Lyo-Ject Syringe **1018**
Cardizem Monovial **1018**
Tiazac Capsules **1378**

DILITER (Italy)
DILTIAZEM HYDROCHLORIDE
Cardizem CD Capsules **1016**
Cardizem Injectable **1018**
Cardizem Lyo-Ject Syringe **1018**
Cardizem Monovial **1018**
Tiazac Capsules **1378**

DILIZEM (Singapore, Thailand)
DILTIAZEM HYDROCHLORIDE
Cardizem CD Capsules **1016**
Cardizem Injectable **1018**
Cardizem Lyo-Ject Syringe **1018**
Cardizem Monovial **1018**
Tiazac Capsules **1378**

DILMIN (Finland)
DILTIAZEM HYDROCHLORIDE
Cardizem CD Capsules **1016**
Cardizem Injectable **1018**
Cardizem Lyo-Ject Syringe **1018**
Cardizem Monovial **1018**
Tiazac Capsules **1378**

DILOC (The Netherlands)
DILTIAZEM HYDROCHLORIDE
Cardizem CD Capsules **1016**
Cardizem Injectable **1018**
Cardizem Lyo-Ject Syringe **1018**
Cardizem Monovial **1018**
Tiazac Capsules **1378**

DILPRAL (Finland)
DILTIAZEM HYDROCHLORIDE
Cardizem CD Capsules **1016**
Cardizem Injectable **1018**
Cardizem Lyo-Ject Syringe **1018**
Cardizem Monovial **1018**
Tiazac Capsules **1378**

DILRENE (France)
DILTIAZEM HYDROCHLORIDE
Cardizem CD Capsules **1016**
Cardizem Injectable **1018**
Cardizem Lyo-Ject Syringe **1018**
Cardizem Monovial **1018**
Tiazac Capsules **1378**

DILSAL (Germany)
DILTIAZEM HYDROCHLORIDE
Cardizem CD Capsules **1016**
Cardizem Injectable **1018**
Cardizem Lyo-Ject Syringe **1018**
Cardizem Monovial **1018**
Tiazac Capsules **1378**

DIL-SANORANIA (Germany)
DILTIAZEM HYDROCHLORIDE
Cardizem CD Capsules **1016**
Cardizem Injectable **1018**
Cardizem Lyo-Ject Syringe **1018**
Cardizem Monovial **1018**
Tiazac Capsules **1378**

DILTA (Germany)
DILTIAZEM HYDROCHLORIDE
Cardizem CD Capsules **1016**
Cardizem Injectable **1018**
Cardizem Lyo-Ject Syringe **1018**
Cardizem Monovial **1018**
Tiazac Capsules **1378**

DILTABETA (Germany)
DILTIAZEM HYDROCHLORIDE
Cardizem CD Capsules **1016**
Cardizem Injectable **1018**
Cardizem Lyo-Ject Syringe **1018**
Cardizem Monovial **1018**
Tiazac Capsules **1378**

DILTAHEXAL (Australia, Germany)
DILTIAZEM HYDROCHLORIDE
Cardizem CD Capsules **1016**
Cardizem Injectable **1018**
Cardizem Lyo-Ject Syringe **1018**
Cardizem Monovial **1018**
Tiazac Capsules **1378**

DILTAM (Irish Republic)
DILTIAZEM HYDROCHLORIDE
Cardizem CD Capsules **1016**
Cardizem Injectable **1018**
Cardizem Lyo-Ject Syringe **1018**
Cardizem Monovial **1018**
Tiazac Capsules **1378**

DILTAN (Hong Kong, Thailand)
DILTIAZEM HYDROCHLORIDE
Cardizem CD Capsules **1016**
Cardizem Injectable **1018**
Cardizem Lyo-Ject Syringe **1018**
Cardizem Monovial **1018**
Tiazac Capsules **1378**

DILTARETARD (Germany)
DILTIAZEM HYDROCHLORIDE
Cardizem CD Capsules **1016**
Cardizem Injectable **1018**
Cardizem Lyo-Ject Syringe **1018**
Cardizem Monovial **1018**
Tiazac Capsules **1378**

DILTEC (Thailand)
DILTIAZEM HYDROCHLORIDE
Cardizem CD Capsules **1016**
Cardizem Injectable **1018**
Cardizem Lyo-Ject Syringe **1018**
Cardizem Monovial **1018**
Tiazac Capsules **1378**

DILTIAGAMMA (Germany)
DILTIAZEM HYDROCHLORIDE
Cardizem CD Capsules **1016**
Cardizem Injectable **1018**
Cardizem Lyo-Ject Syringe **1018**
Cardizem Monovial **1018**
Tiazac Capsules **1378**

DILTIAMAX (Australia)
DILTIAZEM HYDROCHLORIDE
Cardizem CD Capsules **1016**
Cardizem Injectable **1018**
Cardizem Lyo-Ject Syringe **1018**
Cardizem Monovial **1018**
Tiazac Capsules **1378**

DILTIAMERCK (Germany)
DILTIAZEM HYDROCHLORIDE
Cardizem CD Capsules **1016**
Cardizem Injectable **1018**
Cardizem Lyo-Ject Syringe **1018**
Cardizem Monovial **1018**
Tiazac Capsules **1378**

DILTIANGINA (Portugal)
DILTIAZEM HYDROCHLORIDE
Cardizem CD Capsules **1016**
Cardizem Injectable **1018**
Cardizem Lyo-Ject Syringe **1018**
Cardizem Monovial **1018**
Tiazac Capsules **1378**

DILTIEM (Portugal)
DILTIAZEM HYDROCHLORIDE
Cardizem CD Capsules **1016**
Cardizem Injectable **1018**
Cardizem Lyo-Ject Syringe **1018**
Cardizem Monovial **1018**
Tiazac Capsules **1378**

DILTI-ESSEX (Germany)
DILTIAZEM HYDROCHLORIDE
Cardizem CD Capsules **1016**
Cardizem Injectable **1018**
Cardizem Lyo-Ject Syringe **1018**
Cardizem Monovial **1018**
Tiazac Capsules **1378**

DILTIKARD (Norway)
DILTIAZEM HYDROCHLORIDE
Cardizem CD Capsules **1016**
Cardizem Injectable **1018**
Cardizem Lyo-Ject Syringe **1018**
Cardizem Monovial **1018**
Tiazac Capsules **1378**

DILTIUC (Germany)
DILTIAZEM HYDROCHLORIDE
Cardizem CD Capsules **1016**
Cardizem Injectable **1018**
Cardizem Lyo-Ject Syringe **1018**
Cardizem Monovial **1018**
Tiazac Capsules **1378**

DILTIWAS (Spain)
DILTIAZEM HYDROCHLORIDE
Cardizem CD Capsules **1016**
Cardizem Injectable **1018**
Cardizem Lyo-Ject Syringe **1018**
Cardizem Monovial **1018**
Tiazac Capsules **1378**

DILTIZEM AP (Brazil)
DILTIAZEM HYDROCHLORIDE
Cardizem CD Capsules **1016**
Cardizem Injectable **1018**
Cardizem Lyo-Ject Syringe **1018**
Cardizem Monovial **1018**
Tiazac Capsules **1378**

DILUCORT (South Africa)
HYDROCORTISONE ACETATE
Anusol-HC Suppositories **2238**
Cortifoam Rectal Foam **3170**
Hydrocortone Acetate Injectable Suspension **2103**
Proctocort Suppositories **2264**

DILZEM (Australia, Austria, Finland, Germany, Hong Kong, Irish Republic, New Zealand, Switzerland, Thailand, United Kingdom)
DILTIAZEM HYDROCHLORIDE
Cardizem CD Capsules **1016**
Cardizem Injectable **1018**
Cardizem Lyo-Ject Syringe **1018**
Cardizem Monovial **1018**
Tiazac Capsules **1378**

DILZENE (Italy)
DILTIAZEM HYDROCHLORIDE
Cardizem CD Capsules **1016**
Cardizem Injectable **1018**
Cardizem Lyo-Ject Syringe **1018**
Cardizem Monovial **1018**
Tiazac Capsules **1378**

DILZEREAL (Germany)
DILTIAZEM HYDROCHLORIDE
Cardizem CD Capsules **1016**
Cardizem Injectable **1018**
Cardizem Lyo-Ject Syringe **1018**
Cardizem Monovial **1018**
Tiazac Capsules **1378**

DILZICARDIN (Germany)
DILTIAZEM HYDROCHLORIDE
Cardizem CD Capsules **1016**
Cardizem Injectable **1018**
Cardizem Lyo-Ject Syringe **1018**
Cardizem Monovial **1018**
Tiazac Capsules **1378**

DIMAC (Austria)
DIRITHROMYCIN
Dynabac Tablets **2269**

DIMALOSIO (Italy)
LACTULOSE
Kristalose for Oral Solution **1007**

DIMEDRINE (Canada)
BROMPHENIRAMINE MALEATE/PSEUDOEPHEDRINE HYDROCHLORIDE
Bromfed Capsules (Extended-Release) . . . **2269**
Bromfed-PD Capsules (Extended-Release) **2269**

DIMEFOR (Mexico)
METFORMIN HYDROCHLORIDE
Glucophage Tablets **1080**

DIMENFORMON (The Netherlands)
ESTRADIOL
Alora Transdermal System **3372**
Climara Transdermal System **958**
Estrace Vaginal Cream **3358**
Estring Vaginal Ring **2811**
Vivelle Transdermal System **2412**
Vivelle-Dot Transdermal System **2416**

DIMETAPP COUGH EXPECTORANT (South Africa)
GUAIFENESIN
Organidin NR Liquid **3350**
Organidin NR Tablets **3350**

DIMETIGAL (Mexico)
CIMETIDINE
Tagamet Tablets **1644**

DIMIDON (Germany)
IBUPROFEN
Motrin Suspension, Oral Drops, Chewable Tablets, and Caplets **2002**

DIMITONE (Belgium, Denmark, Israel)
CARVEDILOL
Coreg Tablets **1508**

DIMORF (Brazil)
MORPHINE SULFATE
Astramorph/PF Injection, USP (Preservative-Free) **594**
Duramorph Injection **1312**
Infumorph 200 and Infumorph 500 Sterile Solutions **1314**
Kadian Capsules **1335**
MS Contin Tablets **2896**
MSIR Oral Capsules **2898**
MSIR Oral Solution **2898**
MSIR Oral Solution Concentrate **2898**
MSIR Oral Tablets **2898**
Oramorph SR Tablets **3062**
Roxanol 100 Concentrated Oral Solution **3066**
Roxanol Concentrated Oral Solution **3066**
Roxanol-T Oral Solution **3066**

DIMOTANE EXPECTORANT (United Kingdom)
BROMPHENIRAMINE MALEATE/PSEUDOEPHEDRINE HYDROCHLORIDE
Bromfed Capsules (Extended-Release) . . . **2269**
Bromfed-PD Capsules (Extended-Release) **2269**

DIMOTANE PLUS (Irish Republic, United Kingdom)
BROMPHENIRAMINE MALEATE/PSEUDOEPHEDRINE HYDROCHLORIDE
Bromfed Capsules (Extended-Release) . . . **2269**
Bromfed-PD Capsules (Extended-Release) **2269**

DINA (Italy)
CIMETIDINE
Tagamet Tablets **1644**

DINABAC (Italy)
DIRITHROMYCIN
Dynabac Tablets **2269**

DINAC (Australia, Thailand)
DICLOFENAC SODIUM
Voltaren Tablets **2315**
Voltaren-XR Tablets **2315**

DINAZIDE (Thailand)
HYDROCHLOROTHIAZIDE/TRIAMTERENE
Dyazide Capsules **1515**
Maxzide Tablets **1008**
Maxzide-25 mg Tablets **1008**

DINIKET (Italy)
ISOSORBIDE DINITRATE
Isordil Sublingual Tablets **3525**
Isordil Titradose Tablets **3526**

DINISOR (Spain)
DILTIAZEM HYDROCHLORIDE
Cardizem CD Capsules **1016**
Cardizem Injectable **1018**
Cardizem Lyo-Ject Syringe **1018**
Cardizem Monovial **1018**
Tiazac Capsules **1378**

DINIT (Finland)
ISOSORBIDE DINITRATE
Isordil Sublingual Tablets **3525**
Isordil Titradose Tablets **3526**

DINUL (Portugal)
FAMOTIDINE
Pepcid Injection **2153**
Pepcid Injection Premixed **2153**
Pepcid RPD Orally Disintegrating Tablets **2150**
Pepcid Tablets **2150**
Pepcid for Oral Suspension **2150**

DIOCARPINE (Canada)
PILOCARPINE HYDROCHLORIDE
Isopto Carpine Ophthalmic Solution . . . . ⊙**215**
Pilopine HS Ophthalmic Gel . . . . ⊙**217**
Salagen Tablets **2229**

DIOCHLORAM (Canada)
CHLORAMPHENICOL
Chloromycetin Ophthalmic Ointment, 1% . . . . ⊙**296**
Chloromycetin Ophthalmic Solution . . . . ⊙**297**
Chloroptic Sterile Ophthalmic Ointment . . ⊙**234**
Chloroptic Sterile Ophthalmic Solution . . ⊙**235**

DIOCIMEX (Switzerland)
DOXYCYCLINE HYCLATE
Doryx Coated Pellet Filled Capsules **3357**
Periostat Tablets **1208**
Vibra-Tabs Film Coated Tablets **2735**
Vibramycin Hyclate Capsules **2735**
Vibramycin Hyclate Intravenous **2737**

DIODERM (Irish Republic, United Kingdom)
HYDROCORTISONE
Anusol-HC Cream 2.5% **2237**
Hydrocortone Tablets **2106**

DIODEX (Canada)
DEXAMETHASONE SODIUM PHOSPHATE
Decadron Phosphate Injection **2081**
Decadron Phosphate Sterile Ophthalmic Ointment . . . . . . ⊙**280, 2083**
Decadron Phosphate Sterile Ophthalmic Solution **2084**

DIOFLUOR (Canada)
FLUORESCEIN SODIUM
AK-Fluor Injection 10% and 25% . . . . . . ⊙**202**
Fluorescite Injection . . . . ⊙**211**

DIOGENT (Canada)
GENTAMICIN SULFATE
Genoptic Ophthalmic Ointment . . . . ⊙**239**
Genoptic Sterile Ophthalmic Solution . . . ⊙**239**

DIOMICETE (Portugal)
CLOTRIMAZOLE
Lotrimin Cream 1% **3128**
Lotrimin Lotion 1% **3128**
Lotrimin Topical Solution 1% **3128**
Mycelex Troche **573**

DIOMYCIN (Canada)
ERYTHROMYCIN
Emgel 2% Topical Gel **1285**

Ery-Tab Tablets 448
Erythromycin Base Filmtab Tablets 454
Erythromycin Delayed-Release Capsules, USP 455
PCE Dispertab Tablets 498

DIONDEL (Spain)
METOLAZONE
Mykrox Tablets 1168
Zaroxolyn Tablets 1177

DIOPTICON (Canada)
NAPHAZOLINE HYDROCHLORIDE
Albalon Ophthalmic Solution ⊙225

DIOSPOR HC (Canada)
HYDROCORTISONE/NEOMYCIN SULFATE/POLYMYXIN B SULFATE
Cortisporin Ophthalmic Suspension Sterile ⊙297

DIOSULF (Canada)
SULFACETAMIDE SODIUM
Bleph-10 Ophthalmic Ointment 10% ⊙230
Klaron Lotion 10% 1224

DIOVAN (Austria, Canada, Denmark, Finland, Germany, Hong Kong, Irish Republic, Israel, Mexico, New Zealand, Norway, Portugal, Singapore, South Africa, Spain, Sweden, Switzerland, Thailand, The Netherlands, United Kingdom)
VALSARTAN
Diovan Capsules 2337

DIOVAN COMP (Denmark, Finland, Norway)
HYDROCHLOROTHIAZIDE/VALSARTAN
Diovan HCT Tablets 2338

DIOVAN HCT (Canada, Mexico)
HYDROCHLOROTHIAZIDE/VALSARTAN
Diovan HCT Tablets 2338

DIOVANE (Belgium)
VALSARTAN
Diovan Capsules 2337

DIOVON COMP (Sweden)
HYDROCHLOROTHIAZIDE/VALSARTAN
Diovan HCT Tablets 2338

DIPARENE (Belgium)
NAPROXEN
EC-Naprosyn Delayed-Release Tablets 2967
Naprosyn Suspension 2967
Naprosyn Tablets 2967

DIPAZIDE (Thailand)
GLIPIZIDE
Glucotrol Tablets 2692
Glucotrol XL Extended Release Tablets 2693

DIPEDYNE (Mexico)
ZIDOVUDINE
Retrovir Capsules 1625
Retrovir IV Infusion 1629
Retrovir Syrup 1625
Retrovir Tablets 1625

DIPENTUM (Australia, Austria, Canada, Denmark, Finland, France, Germany, Hong Kong, Irish Republic, Israel, Italy, New Zealand, Norway, South Africa, Sweden, Switzerland, The Netherlands, United Kingdom)
OLSALAZINE SODIUM
Dipentum Capsules 2803

DIPHAMINE (Belgium)
DIPHENHYDRAMINE HYDROCHLORIDE
Benadryl Parenteral 2617

DIPHAR (France)
DIPYRIDAMOLE
Persantine Tablets 1057

DIPOFEN (Mexico)
IBUPROFEN
Motrin Suspension, Oral Drops, Chewable Tablets, and Caplets 2002

DIPRES (Mexico)
DIPYRIDAMOLE
Persantine Tablets 1057

DIPRIVAN (Australia, Austria, Belgium, Brazil, Canada, Denmark, Finland, France, Hong Kong, Irish Republic, Israel, Italy, Mexico, New Zealand, Norway, Portugal, Singapore, South Africa, Spain, Sweden, Thailand, The Netherlands, United Kingdom)
PROPOFOL
Diprivan Injectable Emulsion 667

DIPRODOL (Mexico)
IBUPROFEN
Motrin Suspension, Oral Drops, Chewable Tablets, and Caplets 2002

DIPROFOL (Israel)
PROPOFOL
Diprivan Injectable Emulsion 667

DI-PROMAL (Austria)
IPRATROPIUM BROMIDE
Atrovent Inhalation Aerosol 1030
Atrovent Inhalation Solution 1031
Atrovent Nasal Spray 0.03% 1032
Atrovent Nasal Spray 0.06% 1033

DIPSIN (Portugal)
FAMOTIDINE
Pepcid Injection 2153
Pepcid Injection Premixed 2153
Pepcid RPD Orally Disintegrating Tablets 2150
Pepcid Tablets 2150
Pepcid for Oral Suspension 2150

DIPYRIDAN (Belgium)
DIPYRIDAMOLE
Persantine Tablets 1057

DIPYRIN (Finland)
DIPYRIDAMOLE
Persantine Tablets 1057

DIPYROL (South Africa)
DIPYRIDAMOLE
Persantine Tablets 1057

DIRINOL (Mexico)
DIPYRIDAMOLE
Persantine Tablets 1057

DIROQUINE (Thailand)
CHLOROQUINE PHOSPHATE
Aralen Tablets 3075

DISALPIN (Germany)
HYDROCHLOROTHIAZIDE
HydroDIURIL Tablets 2108
Microzide Capsules 3414

DISALUNIL (Germany)
HYDROCHLOROTHIAZIDE
HydroDIURIL Tablets 2108
Microzide Capsules 3414

DISCROMIL (Italy)
HYDROQUINONE
Eldopaque Forte 4% Cream 1734
Eldoquin Forte 4% Cream 1734
Lustra Cream 2023
Lustra-AF Cream 2023
Melanex Topical Solution 2300
Solaquin Forte 4% Cream 1734
Solaquin Forte 4% Gel 1734

DISEBRIN (Italy)
HEPARIN SODIUM
Heparin Lock Flush Solution 3509
Heparin Sodium Injection 3511

DISMENOL N (Germany, Switzerland)
IBUPROFEN
Motrin Suspension, Oral Drops, Chewable Tablets, and Caplets 2002

DISMENOL NEU (Austria)
IBUPROFEN
Motrin Suspension, Oral Drops, Chewable Tablets, and Caplets 2002

DISNE ASMOL (Spain)
IPRATROPIUM BROMIDE
Atrovent Inhalation Aerosol 1030
Atrovent Inhalation Solution 1031
Atrovent Nasal Spray 0.03% 1032
Atrovent Nasal Spray 0.06% 1033

DISOPAM (Israel)
DIAZEPAM
Valium Injectable 3026
Valium Tablets 3047

DISOPRIVAN (Switzerland)
PROPOFOL
Diprivan Injectable Emulsion 667

DISORLON (France)
ISOSORBIDE DINITRATE
Isordil Sublingual Tablets 3525
Isordil Titradose Tablets 3526

DISOTHIAZIDE (Israel)
HYDROCHLOROTHIAZIDE
HydroDIURIL Tablets 2108
Microzide Capsules 3414

DISPACLONIDIN (Germany)
CLONIDINE HYDROCHLORIDE
Catapres Tablets 1037
Duraclon Injection 3057

DISPADEX COMP (Germany)
DEXAMETHASONE SODIUM PHOSPHATE/NEOMYCIN SULFATE
NeoDecadron Sterile Ophthalmic Solution 2144

DISPAGENT (Germany)
GENTAMICIN SULFATE
Genoptic Ophthalmic Ointment ⊙239
Genoptic Sterile Ophthalmic Solution ⊙239

DISPAPHENICOL (Germany)
CHLORAMPHENICOL
Chloromycetin Ophthalmic Ointment, 1% ⊙296
Chloromycetin Ophthalmic Solution ⊙297
Chloroptic Sterile Ophthalmic Ointment ⊙234
Chloroptic Sterile Ophthalmic Solution ⊙235

DISPASAN (Germany)
SODIUM HYALURONATE
Hyalgan Solution 3080

DISPATIM (Austria, Germany)
TIMOLOL MALEATE
Blocadren Tablets 2046
Timoptic Sterile Ophthalmic Solution 2190
Timoptic in Ocudose 2192
Timoptic-XE Sterile Ophthalmic Gel Forming Solution 2194

DISPLATA (Mexico)
CARBOPLATIN
Paraplatin for Injection 1126

DISPROMIL (Spain)
FAMOTIDINE
Pepcid Injection 2153
Pepcid Injection Premixed 2153
Pepcid RPD Orally Disintegrating Tablets 2150
Pepcid Tablets 2150
Pepcid for Oral Suspension 2150

DISTACLOR (Singapore, Thailand, United Kingdom)
CEFACLOR
Ceclor CD Tablets 1279
Ceclor Pulvules 1905
Ceclor Suspension 1905

DISTAMINE (Austria, Irish Republic, The Netherlands, United Kingdom)
PENICILLAMINE
Cuprimine Capsules 2075
Depen Titratable Tablets 3341

DISTAXID (Spain)
NIZATIDINE
Axid Pulvules 1903

DISTOBRAM (Portugal)
TOBRAMYCIN
TOBI Solution for Inhalation 1206
Tobrex Ophthalmic Ointment ⊙220
Tobrex Ophthalmic Solution ⊙221

DITENATE N (Germany)
THEOPHYLLINE
Aerolate Jr. T.D. Capsules 1361
Aerolate Liquid 1361
Aerolate Sr. T.D. Capsules 1361
Theo-Dur Extended-Release Tablets 1835
Uni-Dur Extended-Release Tablets 1841
Uniphyl 400 mg and 600 mg Tablets 2903

DITENSIDE (Spain)
ENALAPRIL MALEATE/HYDROCHLOROTHIAZIDE
Vaseretic Tablets 2204

DITENSOR (Spain)
ENALAPRIL MALEATE
Vasotec Tablets 2210

DITHIAZID (Austria)
HYDROCHLOROTHIAZIDE
HydroDIURIL Tablets 2108
Microzide Capsules 3414

DITIZEM (Thailand)
DILTIAZEM HYDROCHLORIDE
Cardizem CD Capsules 1016
Cardizem Injectable 1018
Cardizem Lyo-Ject Syringe 1018
Cardizem Monovial 1018
Tiazac Capsules 1378

DIU-ATENOLOL (Germany)
ATENOLOL
Tenormin I.V. Injection 692

DIUBE (Italy)
ATENOLOL
Tenormin I.V. Injection 692

DIUCHLOR H (Canada)
HYDROCHLOROTHIAZIDE
HydroDIURIL Tablets 2108
Microzide Capsules 3414

DIULO (Australia, Portugal)
METOLAZONE
Mykrox Tablets 1168
Zaroxolyn Tablets 1177

DIU-MELUSIN (Germany)
HYDROCHLOROTHIAZIDE
HydroDIURIL Tablets 2108
Microzide Capsules 3414

DIURAMID (Germany)
ACETAZOLAMIDE
Diamox Sequels Sustained Release Capsules ⊙270
Diamox Tablets ⊙269

DIURAMIN (Finland)
AMILORIDE HYDROCHLORIDE/HYDROCHLOROTHIAZIDE
Moduretic Tablets 2138

DIURENE (Portugal)
AMILORIDE HYDROCHLORIDE/HYDROCHLOROTHIAZIDE
Moduretic Tablets 2138

DIURETICUM (Austria)
ACETAZOLAMIDE
Diamox Sequels Sustained Release Capsules ⊙270
Diamox Tablets ⊙269

DIURETIKUM VERLA (Germany)
HYDROCHLOROTHIAZIDE/TRIAMTERENE
Dyazide Capsules 1515
Maxzide Tablets 1008
Maxzide-25 mg Tablets 1008

DIURET-P (Thailand)
HYDROCHLOROTHIAZIDE
HydroDIURIL Tablets 2108
Microzide Capsules 3414

DIUREX (Finland)
AMILORIDE HYDROCHLORIDE/HYDROCHLOROTHIAZIDE
Moduretic Tablets 2138

DIUREZIN (Brazil)
HYDROCHLOROTHIAZIDE
HydroDIURIL Tablets 2108
Microzide Capsules 3414

DIURID (Austria)
HYDROCHLOROTHIAZIDE/TRIAMTERENE
Dyazide Capsules 1515
Maxzide Tablets 1008
Maxzide-25 mg Tablets 1008

DIURSAN (Germany)
AMILORIDE HYDROCHLORIDE/HYDROCHLOROTHIAZIDE
Moduretic Tablets 2138

DIUTEC (South Africa)
AMILORIDE HYDROCHLORIDE/HYDROCHLOROTHIAZIDE
Moduretic Tablets 2138

DIUTENSAT (Germany)
HYDROCHLOROTHIAZIDE/TRIAMTERENE
Dyazide Capsules 1515
Maxzide Tablets 1008
Maxzide-25 mg Tablets 1008

DIU-TONOLYTRIL (Germany)
HYDROCHLOROTHIAZIDE/TRIAMTERENE
Dyazide Capsules 1515
Maxzide Tablets 1008
Maxzide-25 mg Tablets 1008

DIUZINE (Spain)
AMILORIDE HYDROCHLORIDE/HYDROCHLOROTHIAZIDE
Moduretic Tablets 2138

DIVIGEL (Denmark, Finland, Irish Republic, Sweden, Switzerland)
ESTRADIOL
Alora Transdermal System 3372
Climara Transdermal System 958
Estrace Vaginal Cream 3358
Estring Vaginal Ring 2811
Vivelle Transdermal System 2412
Vivelle-Dot Transdermal System 2416

DIXARIT (Australia, Belgium, Canada, Germany, Hong Kong, Irish Republic, New Zealand, Singapore, South Africa, The Netherlands, United Kingdom)
CLONIDINE HYDROCHLORIDE
Catapres Tablets 1037
Duraclon Injection 3057

DIXONAL (Mexico)
PIROXICAM
Feldene Capsules 2685

DIZAN (Thailand)
DIAZEPAM
Valium Injectable 3026
Valium Tablets 3047

DIZEPAM (Thailand)
DIAZEPAM
Valium Injectable 3026
Valium Tablets 3047

DIZOLAM (Singapore, Thailand)
ALPRAZOLAM
Xanax Tablets 2865

DM COUGH SYRUP EXPECTORANT (Canada)
DEXTROMETHORPHAN HYDROBROMIDE/GUAIFENESIN
Tussi-Organidin DM NR Liquid 3350

Tussi-Organidin DM-S NR Liquid 3350

DM E SUPPRESSANT EXPECTORANT (Canada)
DEXTROMETHORPHAN HYDROBROMIDE/GUAIFENESIN
Tussi-Organidin DM NR Liquid 3350
Tussi-Organidin DM-S NR Liquid 3350

DM PLUS EXPECTORANT (Canada)
DEXTROMETHORPHAN HYDROBROMIDE/GUAIFENESIN
Tussi-Organidin DM NR Liquid 3350
Tussi-Organidin DM-S NR Liquid 3350

DOBACEN (Switzerland)
DIPHENHYDRAMINE HYDROCHLORIDE
Benadryl Parenteral 2617

DOBLEXAN (Spain)
PIROXICAM
Feldene Capsules 2685

DOBUCARD (Thailand)
DOBUTAMINE HYDROCHLORIDE
Dobutrex Solution Vials 1914

DOBUJECT (Denmark, Finland, Israel, Mexico, Portugal, Singapore, Sweden, Thailand)
DOBUTAMINE HYDROCHLORIDE
Dobutrex Solution Vials 1914

DOBUPAL (Spain)
VENLAFAXINE HYDROCHLORIDE
Effexor Tablets 3495
Effexor XR Capsules 3499

DOBUTAM (Israel)
DOBUTAMINE HYDROCHLORIDE
Dobutrex Solution Vials 1914

DOBUTINA (Portugal)
DOBUTAMINE HYDROCHLORIDE
Dobutrex Solution Vials 1914

DOBUTREX (Australia, Austria, Belgium, Brazil, Canada, Denmark, Finland, France, Germany, Hong Kong, Irish Republic, Israel, Italy, Mexico, New Zealand, Norway, South Africa, Spain, Sweden, Switzerland, Thailand, The Netherlands)
DOBUTAMINE HYDROCHLORIDE
Dobutrex Solution Vials 1914

DOCLIS (Spain)
DILTIAZEM HYDROCHLORIDE
Cardizem CD Capsules 1016
Cardizem Injectable 1018
Cardizem Lyo-Ject Syringe 1018
Cardizem Monovial 1018
Tiazac Capsules 1378

DOCOSTYL (Spain)
DOXYCYCLINE HYCLATE
Doryx Coated Pellet Filled Capsules 3357
Periostat Tablets 1208
Vibramycin Hyclate Capsules 2735
Vibramycin Hyclate Intravenous 2737
Vibra-Tabs Film Coated Tablets 2735

DO-DO EXPECTORANT LINCTUS (United Kingdom)
GUAIFENESIN
Organidin NR Liquid 3350
Organidin NR Tablets 3350

DOGOXINE (Mexico)
DIGOXIN
Lanoxicaps Capsules 1574
Lanoxin Elixir Pediatric 1578
Lanoxin Injection 1581
Lanoxin Injection Pediatric 1584
Lanoxin Tablets 1587

DOLAK (Spain)
ISOSORBIDE MONONITRATE
Imdur Tablets 1826
Ismo Tablets 3524

DOLANAEST (Germany)
BUPIVACAINE HYDROCHLORIDE
Sensorcaine Injection 643
Sensorcaine-MPF Injection 643

DOLAUT (Italy)
DICLOFENAC SODIUM
Voltaren Tablets 2315
Voltaren-XR Tablets 2315

DOLCONTIN (Finland, Norway, Sweden)
MORPHINE SULFATE
Astramorph/PF Injection, USP (Preservative-Free) 594
Duramorph Injection 1312
Infumorph 200 and Infumorph 500 Sterile Solutions 1314
Kadian Capsules 1335
MS Contin Tablets 2896
MSIR Oral Capsules 2898
MSIR Oral Solution 2898
MSIR Oral Solution Concentrate 2898
MSIR Oral Tablets 2898
Oramorph SR Tablets 3062
Roxanol 100 Concentrated Oral Solution 3066
Roxanol Concentrated Oral Solution 3066
Roxanol-T Oral Solution 3066

DOLESTAN (Germany)
DIPHENHYDRAMINE HYDROCHLORIDE
Benadryl Parenteral 2617

DOLFLAM (Mexico)
DICLOFENAC SODIUM
Voltaren Tablets 2315
Voltaren-XR Tablets 2315

DOLGIT (Austria, Belgium, France, Germany, Switzerland)
IBUPROFEN
Motrin Suspension, Oral Drops, Chewable Tablets, and Caplets 2002

DOLGIT-DICLO (Germany)
DICLOFENAC SODIUM
Voltaren Tablets 2315
Voltaren-XR Tablets 2315

DOLIBU (Austria)
IBUPROFEN
Motrin Suspension, Oral Drops, Chewable Tablets, and Caplets 2002

DOLISAL (Italy)
DIFLUNISAL
Dolobid Tablets 2088

DOLNAXEN (Mexico)
NAPROXEN
EC-Naprosyn Delayed-Release Tablets . . . 2967
Naprosyn Suspension 2967
Naprosyn Tablets 2967

DOLO NEOS (Germany)
IBUPROFEN
Motrin Suspension, Oral Drops, Chewable Tablets, and Caplets 2002

DOLO NERVOBION (Spain)
DICLOFENAC SODIUM
Voltaren Tablets 2315
Voltaren-XR Tablets 2315

DOLOATRIXEN (Mexico)
NAPROXEN
EC-Naprosyn Delayed-Release Tablets . . . 2967
Naprosyn Suspension 2967
Naprosyn Tablets 2967

DOLOBASAN (Germany)
DICLOFENAC SODIUM
Voltaren Tablets 2315
Voltaren-XR Tablets 2315

DOLOBID (Australia, Canada, Hong Kong, Irish Republic, Israel, Italy, Mexico, Portugal, South Africa, Spain, Thailand, United Kingdom)
DIFLUNISAL
Dolobid Tablets 2088

DOLOBIS (France)
DIFLUNISAL
Dolobid Tablets 2088

DOLOCIBAL (Mexico)
IBUPROFEN
Motrin Suspension, Oral Drops, Chewable Tablets, and Caplets 2002

DOLOCID (The Netherlands)
DIFLUNISAL
Dolobid Tablets 2088

DOLOCYL (Italy, Portugal, Spain, Switzerland)
IBUPROFEN
Motrin Suspension, Oral Drops, Chewable Tablets, and Caplets 2002

DOLODENT (Denmark)
BENZOCAINE
Americaine Anesthetic Lubricant 1162
Americaine Otic Topical Anesthetic Ear Drops 1162

DOLO-DISMENOL (Switzerland)
IBUPROFEN
Motrin Suspension, Oral Drops, Chewable Tablets, and Caplets 2002

DOLODOC (Germany)
IBUPROFEN
Motrin Suspension, Oral Drops, Chewable Tablets, and Caplets 2002

DOLO-DOLGIT (Germany)
IBUPROFEN
Motrin Suspension, Oral Drops, Chewable Tablets, and Caplets 2002

DOLOFIN (Belgium)
IBUPROFEN
Motrin Suspension, Oral Drops, Chewable Tablets, and Caplets 2002

DOLOFORT (Austria)
IBUPROFEN
Motrin Suspension, Oral Drops, Chewable Tablets, and Caplets 2002

DOLOGEL (Switzerland)
IBUPROFEN
Motrin Suspension, Oral Drops, Chewable Tablets, and Caplets 2002

DOLOL (Denmark)
TRAMADOL HYDROCHLORIDE
Ultram Tablets 2600

DOLO-PUREN (Germany)
IBUPROFEN
Motrin Suspension, Oral Drops, Chewable Tablets, and Caplets 2002

DOLOREN (Austria)
IBUPROFEN
Motrin Suspension, Oral Drops, Chewable Tablets, and Caplets 2002

DOLOTANDEX (Mexico)
NAPROXEN SODIUM
Anaprox DS Tablets 2967
Anaprox Tablets 2967
Naprelan Tablets 1293

DOLOVISANO DICLO (Germany)
DICLOFENAC SODIUM
Voltaren Tablets 2315
Voltaren-XR Tablets 2315

DOLOVISANO SUPPOSITORIEN SINE CODEINO (Germany)
MEPROBAMATE
Miltown Tablets 3349

DOLO-VOLTAREN (Spain)
DICLOFENAC SODIUM
Voltaren Tablets 2315
Voltaren-XR Tablets 2315

DOLSINAL (Spain)
NABUMETONE
Relafen Tablets 1617

DOLTARD (Denmark)
MORPHINE SULFATE
Astramorph/PF Injection, USP (Preservative-Free) 594
Duramorph Injection 1312
Infumorph 200 and Infumorph 500 Sterile Solutions 1314
Kadian Capsules 1335
MS Contin Tablets 2896
MSIR Oral Capsules 2898
MSIR Oral Solution 2898
MSIR Oral Solution Concentrate 2898
MSIR Oral Tablets 2898
Oramorph SR Tablets 3062
Roxanol 100 Concentrated Oral Solution 3066
Roxanol Concentrated Oral Solution 3066
Roxanol-T Oral Solution 3066

DOLVER (Mexico)
IBUPROFEN
Motrin Suspension, Oral Drops, Chewable Tablets, and Caplets 2002

DOLXEN (Mexico)
NAPROXEN
EC-Naprosyn Delayed-Release Tablets . . . 2967
Naprosyn Suspension 2967
Naprosyn Tablets 2967

DOLZAM (Belgium)
TRAMADOL HYDROCHLORIDE
Ultram Tablets 2600

DOLZYCAM (Mexico)
PIROXICAM
Feldene Capsules 2685

DOMICETINA (Mexico)
CHLORAMPHENICOL
Chloromycetin Ophthalmic Ointment, 1% . . . . ⊙296
Chloromycetin Ophthalmic Solution . . . . ⊙297
Chloroptic Sterile Ophthalmic Ointment . . ⊙234
Chloroptic Sterile Ophthalmic Solution . . ⊙235

DOMNAMID (Denmark)
ESTAZOLAM
ProSom Tablets 500

DOMUCEF (Italy)
CEPHALEXIN
Keflex Oral Suspension 1237
Keflex Pulvules 1237

DONAPROX (Mexico)
NAPROXEN
EC-Naprosyn Delayed-Release Tablets . . . 2967
Naprosyn Suspension 2967
Naprosyn Tablets 2967

DONEKA (Spain)
LISINOPRIL
Prinivil Tablets 2164
Zestril Tablets 698

DONEKA PLUS (Spain)
HYDROCHLOROTHIAZIDE/LISINOPRIL
Prinzide Tablets 2168
Zestoretic Tablets 695

DONEURIN (Germany)
DOXEPIN HYDROCHLORIDE
Sinequan Capsules 2713
Sinequan Oral Concentrate 2713

DONICER (Spain)
AMILORIDE HYDROCHLORIDE/HYDROCHLOROTHIAZIDE
Moduretic Tablets 2138

DONIX (Spain)
LORAZEPAM
Ativan Injection 3478
Ativan Tablets 3482

DONOBID (Denmark, Finland, Norway, Sweden)
DIFLUNISAL
Dolobid Tablets 2088

DOPAGEN (Irish Republic)
METHYLDOPA
Aldomet Tablets 2037

DOPAMED (Thailand)
METHYLDOPA
Aldomet Tablets 2037

DOPAMET (Canada, Denmark, Hong Kong, Irish Republic, Norway, Sweden, Switzerland, United Kingdom)
METHYLDOPA
Aldomet Tablets 2037

DOPASIAN (Thailand)
METHYLDOPA
Aldomet Tablets 2037

DOPEGYT (Germany, Hong Kong, Singapore, Thailand)
METHYLDOPA
Aldomet Tablets 2037

DOPRAM (Australia, Austria, Belgium, Canada, Denmark, Finland, Germany, Hong Kong, Irish Republic, New Zealand, Norway, South Africa, Switzerland, The Netherlands, United Kingdom)
DOXAPRAM HYDROCHLORIDE
Dopram Injectable 2931

DORANOL (Spain)
ERYTHROMYCIN STEARATE
Erythrocin Stearate Filmtab Tablets 452

DORBID (Brazil)
DIFLUNISAL
Dolobid Tablets 2088

DORCALOR (Portugal)
DICLOFENAC SODIUM
Voltaren Tablets 2315
Voltaren-XR Tablets 2315

DORETRIM AP (Brazil)
IBUPROFEN
Motrin Suspension, Oral Drops, Chewable Tablets, and Caplets 2002

DORGEN (Brazil)
DICLOFENAC SODIUM
Voltaren Tablets 2315
Voltaren-XR Tablets 2315

DORICUM SEMPLICE (Italy)
FLUOCINOLONE ACETONIDE
Synalar Cream 2020
Synalar Ointment 2020
Synalar Topical Solution 2020

DORIFLAN (Brazil)
DICLOFENAC POTASSIUM
Cataflam Tablets 2315

DORIVAL (Spain)
IBUPROFEN
Motrin Suspension, Oral Drops, Chewable Tablets, and Caplets 2002

DORMEX (Canada)
DIPHENHYDRAMINE HYDROCHLORIDE
Benadryl Parenteral 2617

DORMICUM (Denmark)
MIDAZOLAM HYDROCHLORIDE
Versed Injection 3027
Versed Syrup 3033

DORMIGOA N (Germany)
DIPHENHYDRAMINE HYDROCHLORIDE
Benadryl Parenteral 2617

DORMIPHEN (Canada)
DIPHENHYDRAMINE HYDROCHLORIDE
Benadryl Parenteral **2617**

DORMPLUS (Spain)
DIPHENHYDRAMINE HYDROCHLORIDE
Benadryl Parenteral **2617**

DORMUTIL N (Germany)
DIPHENHYDRAMINE HYDROCHLORIDE
Benadryl Parenteral **2617**

DORPIREN (Brazil)
DICLOFENAC POTASSIUM
Cataflam Tablets **2315**

DORYL (Finland, Germany, Switzerland)
CARBACHOL
Isopto Carbachol Ophthalmic Solution. . . ⊙**215**

DORYX (Australia, Canada, New Zealand, Norway, Singapore, South Africa, Sweden)
DOXYCYCLINE HYCLATE
Doryx Coated Pellet Filled Capsules **3357**
Periostat Tablets **1208**
Vibramycin Hyclate Capsules. **2735**
Vibramycin Hyclate Intravenous **2737**
Vibra-Tabs Film Coated Tablets **2735**

DOSATE (Thailand)
OMEPRAZOLE
Prilosec Delayed-Release Capsules **628**

DOSIL (Spain)
DOXYCYCLINE HYCLATE
Doryx Coated Pellet Filled Capsules **3357**
Periostat Tablets **1208**
Vibramycin Hyclate Capsules. **2735**
Vibramycin Hyclate Intravenous **2737**
Vibra-Tabs Film Coated Tablets **2735**

DOSTINEX (Australia, Austria, Belgium, Denmark, Finland, France, Germany, Irish Republic, Israel, Italy, New Zealand, Norway, Portugal, Singapore, South Africa, Spain, Sweden, Switzerland, The Netherlands, United Kingdom)
CABERGOLINE
Dostinex Tablets **2804**

DOTUR (Austria)
DOXYCYCLINE HYCLATE
Doryx Coated Pellet Filled Capsules **3357**
Periostat Tablets **1208**
Vibramycin Hyclate Capsules. **2735**
Vibramycin Hyclate Intravenous **2737**
Vibra-Tabs Film Coated Tablets **2735**

DOVAL (South Africa)
DIAZEPAM
Valium Injectable **3026**
Valium Tablets **3047**

DOVATE (South Africa)
CLOBETASOL PROPIONATE
Cormax Cream **2440**
Cormax Ointment **2440**
Cormax Scalp Application. **2441**
Temovate Cream **1301**
Temovate E Emollient **1302**
Temovate Gel **1303**
Temovate Ointment. **1301**
Temovate Scalp Application **1304**

DOXACLEN (Spain)
DOXYCYCLINE HYCLATE
Doryx Coated Pellet Filled Capsules **3357**
Periostat Tablets **1208**
Vibramycin Hyclate Capsules. **2735**
Vibramycin Hyclate Intravenous **2737**
Vibra-Tabs Film Coated Tablets **2735**

DOXAL (Finland)
DOXEPIN HYDROCHLORIDE
Sinequan Capsules **2713**
Sinequan Oral Concentrate **2713**

DOXAPRIL (Italy)
DOXAPRAM HYDROCHLORIDE
Dopram Injectable **2931**

DOXI CRISOL (Spain)
DOXYCYCLINE HYCLATE
Doryx Coated Pellet Filled Capsules **3357**
Periostat Tablets **1208**
Vibramycin Hyclate Capsules. **2735**
Vibramycin Hyclate Intravenous **2737**
Vibra-Tabs Film Coated Tablets **2735**

DOXI SERGO (Spain)
DOXYCYCLINE HYCLATE
Doryx Coated Pellet Filled Capsules **3357**
Periostat Tablets **1208**
Vibramycin Hyclate Capsules. **2735**
Vibramycin Hyclate Intravenous **2737**
Vibra-Tabs Film Coated Tablets **2735**

DOXIBIOTIC (Israel)
DOXYCYCLINE HYCLATE
Doryx Coated Pellet Filled Capsules **3357**
Periostat Tablets **1208**
Vibramycin Hyclate Capsules. **2735**
Vibramycin Hyclate Intravenous **2737**
Vibra-Tabs Film Coated Tablets **2735**

DOXICENTO (Italy)
DOXYCYCLINE HYCLATE
Doryx Coated Pellet Filled Capsules **3357**
Periostat Tablets **1208**
Vibramycin Hyclate Capsules. **2735**
Vibramycin Hyclate Intravenous **2737**
Vibra-Tabs Film Coated Tablets **2735**

DOXICLAT (Spain)
DOXYCYCLINE HYCLATE
Doryx Coated Pellet Filled Capsules **3357**
Periostat Tablets **1208**
Vibramycin Hyclate Capsules. **2735**
Vibramycin Hyclate Intravenous **2737**
Vibra-Tabs Film Coated Tablets **2735**

DOXIFIN (Italy)
DOXYCYCLINE HYCLATE
Doryx Coated Pellet Filled Capsules **3357**
Periostat Tablets **1208**
Vibramycin Hyclate Capsules. **2735**
Vibramycin Hyclate Intravenous **2737**
Vibra-Tabs Film Coated Tablets **2735**

DOXILEN (Italy)
DOXYCYCLINE HYCLATE
Doryx Coated Pellet Filled Capsules **3357**
Periostat Tablets **1208**
Vibramycin Hyclate Capsules. **2735**
Vibramycin Hyclate Intravenous **2737**
Vibra-Tabs Film Coated Tablets **2735**

DOXILIN (Singapore)
DOXYCYCLINE HYCLATE
Doryx Coated Pellet Filled Capsules **3357**
Periostat Tablets **1208**
Vibramycin Hyclate Capsules. **2735**
Vibramycin Hyclate Intravenous **2737**
Vibra-Tabs Film Coated Tablets **2735**

DOXIMYCIN (Finland)
DOXYCYCLINE HYCLATE
Doryx Coated Pellet Filled Capsules **3357**
Periostat Tablets **1208**
Vibramycin Hyclate Capsules. **2735**
Vibramycin Hyclate Intravenous **2737**
Vibra-Tabs Film Coated Tablets **2735**

DOXIN (Thailand)
DOXYCYCLINE HYCLATE
Doryx Coated Pellet Filled Capsules **3357**
Periostat Tablets **1208**
Vibramycin Hyclate Capsules. **2735**
Vibramycin Hyclate Intravenous **2737**
Vibra-Tabs Film Coated Tablets **2735**

DOXINA (Italy)
DOXYCYCLINE HYCLATE
Doryx Coated Pellet Filled Capsules **3357**
Periostat Tablets **1208**
Vibramycin Hyclate Capsules. **2735**
Vibramycin Hyclate Intravenous **2737**
Vibra-Tabs Film Coated Tablets **2735**

DOXINATE (Spain)
DOXYCYCLINE HYCLATE
Doryx Coated Pellet Filled Capsules **3357**
Periostat Tablets **1208**
Vibramycin Hyclate Capsules. **2735**
Vibramycin Hyclate Intravenous **2737**
Vibra-Tabs Film Coated Tablets **2735**

DOXINE (New Zealand)
DOXYCYCLINE HYCLATE
Doryx Coated Pellet Filled Capsules **3357**
Periostat Tablets **1208**
Vibramycin Hyclate Capsules. **2735**
Vibramycin Hyclate Intravenous **2737**
Vibra-Tabs Film Coated Tablets **2735**

DOXITAB (South Africa)
DOXYCYCLINE HYCLATE
Doryx Coated Pellet Filled Capsules **3357**
Periostat Tablets **1208**
Vibramycin Hyclate Capsules. **2735**
Vibramycin Hyclate Intravenous **2737**
Vibra-Tabs Film Coated Tablets **2735**

DOXITEN (Spain)
DOXYCYCLINE HYCLATE
Doryx Coated Pellet Filled Capsules **3357**
Periostat Tablets **1208**
Vibramycin Hyclate Capsules. **2735**
Vibramycin Hyclate Intravenous **2737**
Vibra-Tabs Film Coated Tablets **2735**

DOXITEN BIO (Spain)
DOXYCYCLINE HYCLATE
Doryx Coated Pellet Filled Capsules **3357**
Periostat Tablets **1208**
Vibramycin Hyclate Capsules. **2735**
Vibramycin Hyclate Intravenous **2737**
Vibra-Tabs Film Coated Tablets **2735**

DOXITIN (Finland)
DOXYCYCLINE HYCLATE
Doryx Coated Pellet Filled Capsules **3357**
Periostat Tablets **1208**
Vibramycin Hyclate Capsules. **2735**
Vibramycin Hyclate Intravenous **2737**
Vibra-Tabs Film Coated Tablets **2735**

DOXIVIS (Italy)
DOXYCYCLINE HYCLATE
Doryx Coated Pellet Filled Capsules **3357**
Periostat Tablets **1208**
Vibramycin Hyclate Capsules. **2735**
Vibramycin Hyclate Intravenous **2737**
Vibra-Tabs Film Coated Tablets **2735**

DOXO-CELL (Germany)
DOXORUBICIN HYDROCHLORIDE
Adriamycin PFS/RDF Injection **2767**

DOXOLEM (Mexico, Thailand)
DOXORUBICIN HYDROCHLORIDE
Adriamycin PFS/RDF Injection **2767**

DOXORUBIN (Australia, Denmark, New Zealand)
DOXORUBICIN HYDROCHLORIDE
Adriamycin PFS/RDF Injection **2767**

DOXOTEC (Mexico)
DOXORUBICIN HYDROCHLORIDE
Adriamycin PFS/RDF Injection **2767**

DOXSIG (Australia)
DOXYCYCLINE HYCLATE
Doryx Coated Pellet Filled Capsules **3357**
Periostat Tablets **1208**
Vibramycin Hyclate Capsules. **2735**
Vibramycin Hyclate Intravenous **2737**
Vibra-Tabs Film Coated Tablets **2735**

DOXY (Australia, France, Israel, New Zealand, Thailand)
DOXYCYCLINE HYCLATE
Doryx Coated Pellet Filled Capsules **3357**
Periostat Tablets **1208**
Vibramycin Hyclate Capsules. **2735**
Vibramycin Hyclate Intravenous **2737**
Vibra-Tabs Film Coated Tablets **2735**

DOXY S+K (Germany)
DOXYCYCLINE HYCLATE
Doryx Coated Pellet Filled Capsules **3357**
Periostat Tablets **1208**
Vibramycin Hyclate Capsules. **2735**
Vibramycin Hyclate Intravenous **2737**
Vibra-Tabs Film Coated Tablets **2735**

DOXY-BASAN (Germany, Switzerland)
DOXYCYCLINE HYCLATE
Doryx Coated Pellet Filled Capsules **3357**
Periostat Tablets **1208**
Vibramycin Hyclate Capsules. **2735**
Vibramycin Hyclate Intravenous **2737**
Vibra-Tabs Film Coated Tablets **2735**

DOXYBIOCIN (Germany)
DOXYCYCLINE HYCLATE
Doryx Coated Pellet Filled Capsules **3357**
Periostat Tablets **1208**
Vibramycin Hyclate Capsules. **2735**
Vibramycin Hyclate Intravenous **2737**
Vibra-Tabs Film Coated Tablets **2735**

DOXYCAP (Singapore)
DOXYCYCLINE HYCLATE
Doryx Coated Pellet Filled Capsules **3357**
Periostat Tablets **1208**
Vibramycin Hyclate Capsules. **2735**
Vibramycin Hyclate Intravenous **2737**
Vibra-Tabs Film Coated Tablets **2735**

DOXYCIN (Canada)
DOXYCYCLINE HYCLATE
Doryx Coated Pellet Filled Capsules **3357**
Periostat Tablets **1208**
Vibramycin Hyclate Capsules. **2735**
Vibramycin Hyclate Intravenous **2737**
Vibra-Tabs Film Coated Tablets **2735**

DOXYCLIN (South Africa)
DOXYCYCLINE HYCLATE
Doryx Coated Pellet Filled Capsules **3357**
Periostat Tablets **1208**
Vibramycin Hyclate Capsules. **2735**
Vibramycin Hyclate Intravenous **2737**
Vibra-Tabs Film Coated Tablets **2735**

DOXYCLINE (Switzerland)
DOXYCYCLINE HYCLATE
Doryx Coated Pellet Filled Capsules **3357**
Periostat Tablets **1208**
Vibramycin Hyclate Capsules. **2735**
Vibramycin Hyclate Intravenous **2737**
Vibra-Tabs Film Coated Tablets **2735**

DOXYCYL (South Africa)
DOXYCYCLINE HYCLATE
Doryx Coated Pellet Filled Capsules **3357**
Periostat Tablets **1208**
Vibramycin Hyclate Capsules. **2735**
Vibramycin Hyclate Intravenous **2737**
Vibra-Tabs Film Coated Tablets **2735**

DOXYDERM (Austria)
DOXYCYCLINE HYCLATE
Doryx Coated Pellet Filled Capsules **3357**
Periostat Tablets **1208**
Vibramycin Hyclate Capsules. **2735**
Vibramycin Hyclate Intravenous **2737**
Vibra-Tabs Film Coated Tablets **2735**

DOXYDYN (Austria)
DOXYCYCLINE HYCLATE
Doryx Coated Pellet Filled Capsules **3357**
Periostat Tablets **1208**
Vibramycin Hyclate Capsules. **2735**
Vibramycin Hyclate Intravenous **2737**
Vibra-Tabs Film Coated Tablets **2735**

DOXYFIM (Belgium)
DOXYCYCLINE HYCLATE
Doryx Coated Pellet Filled Capsules **3357**
Periostat Tablets **1208**
Vibramycin Hyclate Capsules. **2735**
Vibramycin Hyclate Intravenous **2737**
Vibra-Tabs Film Coated Tablets **2735**

DOXYGRAM (France)
DOXYCYCLINE HYCLATE
Doryx Coated Pellet Filled Capsules **3357**
Periostat Tablets **1208**
Vibramycin Hyclate Capsules. **2735**
Vibramycin Hyclate Intravenous **2737**
Vibra-Tabs Film Coated Tablets **2735**

DOXYLAG (Switzerland)
DOXYCYCLINE HYCLATE
Doryx Coated Pellet Filled Capsules **3357**
Periostat Tablets **1208**
Vibramycin Hyclate Capsules. **2735**
Vibramycin Hyclate Intravenous **2737**
Vibra-Tabs Film Coated Tablets **2735**

DOXYLAR (United Kingdom)
DOXYCYCLINE HYCLATE
Doryx Coated Pellet Filled Capsules **3357**
Periostat Tablets **1208**
Vibramycin Hyclate Capsules. **2735**
Vibramycin Hyclate Intravenous **2737**
Vibra-Tabs Film Coated Tablets **2735**

DOXYLETS (Belgium, France, South Africa)
DOXYCYCLINE HYCLATE
Doryx Coated Pellet Filled Capsules **3357**
Periostat Tablets **1208**
Vibramycin Hyclate Capsules. **2735**
Vibramycin Hyclate Intravenous **2737**
Vibra-Tabs Film Coated Tablets **2735**

DOXYLIN (Australia, Israel, Thailand)
DOXYCYCLINE HYCLATE
Doryx Coated Pellet Filled Capsules **3357**
Periostat Tablets **1208**
Vibramycin Hyclate Capsules. **2735**
Vibramycin Hyclate Intravenous **2737**
Vibra-Tabs Film Coated Tablets **2735**

DOXYMYCIN (Singapore, South Africa, Thailand)
DOXYCYCLINE HYCLATE
Doryx Coated Pellet Filled Capsules **3357**
Periostat Tablets **1208**
Vibramycin Hyclate Capsules. **2735**
Vibramycin Hyclate Intravenous **2737**
Vibra-Tabs Film Coated Tablets **2735**

DOXYMYCINE (Belgium)
DOXYCYCLINE HYCLATE
Doryx Coated Pellet Filled Capsules **3357**
Periostat Tablets **1208**
Vibramycin Hyclate Capsules. **2735**
Vibramycin Hyclate Intravenous **2737**
Vibra-Tabs Film Coated Tablets **2735**

DOXY-P (Germany, Thailand)
DOXYCYCLINE HYCLATE
Doryx Coated Pellet Filled Capsules **3357**
Periostat Tablets **1208**
Vibramycin Hyclate Capsules. **2735**
Vibramycin Hyclate Intravenous **2737**
Vibra-Tabs Film Coated Tablets **2735**

DOXY-PUREN (Germany)
DOXYCYCLINE HYCLATE
Doryx Coated Pellet Filled Capsules **3357**
Periostat Tablets **1208**
Vibramycin Hyclate Capsules. **2735**
Vibramycin Hyclate Intravenous **2737**
Vibra-Tabs Film Coated Tablets **2735**

DOXY-TABLINEN (Germany)
DOXYCYCLINE HYCLATE
Doryx Coated Pellet Filled Capsules **3357**
Periostat Tablets **1208**
Vibramycin Hyclate Capsules. **2735**
Vibramycin Hyclate Intravenous **2737**
Vibra-Tabs Film Coated Tablets **2735**

DOXYTEC (Canada)
DOXYCYCLINE HYCLATE
Doryx Coated Pellet Filled Capsules **3357**
Periostat Tablets **1208**
Vibramycin Hyclate Capsules. **2735**
Vibramycin Hyclate Intravenous **2737**
Vibra-Tabs Film Coated Tablets **2735**

DOXYTEM (Germany)
DOXYCYCLINE HYCLATE
Doryx Coated Pellet Filled Capsules **3357**

Periostat Tablets 1208
Vibramycin Hyclate Capsules. 2735
Vibramycin Hyclate Intravenous 2737
Vibra-Tabs Film Coated Tablets 2735

DOXYTREX (Portugal)
DOXYCYCLINE HYCLATE
Doryx Coated Pellet Filled Capsules 3357
Periostat Tablets 1208
Vibramycin Hyclate Capsules. 2735
Vibramycin Hyclate Intravenous 2737
Vibra-Tabs Film Coated Tablets 2735

DOXYTRIM (Israel)
DOXYCYCLINE HYCLATE
Doryx Coated Pellet Filled Capsules 3357
Periostat Tablets 1208
Vibramycin Hyclate Capsules. 2735
Vibramycin Hyclate Intravenous 2737
Vibra-Tabs Film Coated Tablets 2735

DOZIC (United Kingdom)
HALOPERIDOL
Haldol Injection, Tablets and Concentrate. 2533

DP HC (New Zealand)
HYDROCORTISONE
Anusol-HC Cream 2.5% 2237
Hydrocortone Tablets 2106

DP HYDROCORTISONE (New Zealand)
HYDROCORTISONE
Anusol-HC Cream 2.5% 2237
Hydrocortone Tablets 2106

D-PAM (New Zealand)
DIAZEPAM
Valium Injectable 3026
Valium Tablets 3047

D-PENAMINE (Australia, New Zealand)
PENICILLAMINE
Cuprimine Capsules 2075
Depen Titratable Tablets 3341

DRAXON (Portugal)
FLUTAMIDE
Eulexin Capsules 3118

DRAZINE (Thailand)
HYDROXYZINE HYDROCHLORIDE
Atarax Tablets & Syrup 2667
Vistaril Intramuscular Solution 2738

DREEMON (United Kingdom)
DIPHENHYDRAMINE HYDROCHLORIDE
Benadryl Parenteral 2617

DRENIAN (Spain)
DIAZEPAM
Valium Injectable 3026
Valium Tablets 3047

DRENOL (Brazil)
HYDROCHLOROTHIAZIDE
HydroDIURIL Tablets 2108
Microzide Capsules 3414

DRENUSIL (Germany)
POLYTHIAZIDE
Renese Tablets 2712

DRENUSIL-R (Germany)
POLYTHIAZIDE
Renese Tablets 2712

DRIKEN (Mexico)
IRON DEXTRAN
INFeD Injection 3388

DRIMPAM (South Africa)
ALPRAZOLAM
Xanax Tablets 2865

DRIVERMIDE (Thailand)
MEBENDAZOLE
Vermox Chewable Tablets. 2017

DROCEF (Brazil)
CEFADROXIL
Duricef Capsules 1079
Duricef Oral Suspension. 1079
Duricef Tablets 1079

DROGENIL (Irish Republic, Italy, The Netherlands, United Kingdom)
FLUTAMIDE
Eulexin Capsules 3118

DROLASONA (Spain)
FLUTICASONE PROPIONATE
Cutivate Cream 1282
Cutivate Ointment. 1284
Flonase Nasal Spray 1533
Flovent 110 mcg Inhalation Aerosol 1535
Flovent 220 mcg Inhalation Aerosol 1535
Flovent 44 mcg Inhalation Aerosol 1535
Flovent Rotadisk 100 mcg 1537
Flovent Rotadisk 250 mcg 1537
Flovent Rotadisk 50 mcg 1537

DROMADOL (United Kingdom)
TRAMADOL HYDROCHLORIDE
Ultram Tablets. 2600

DROMORAN (United Kingdom)
LEVORPHANOL TARTRATE
Levo-Dromoran Injectable 1734
Levo-Dromoran Tablets 1734
Levorphanol Tartrate Tablets. 3059

DRONAL (Italy)
ALENDRONATE SODIUM
Fosamax Tablets 2095

DROPID (Thailand)
GEMFIBROZIL
Lopid Tablets 2650

DROPILTON (Italy)
PILOCARPINE HYDROCHLORIDE
Isopto Carpine Ophthalmic Solution . . . . ⊙215
Pilopine HS Ophthalmic Gel . . . . ⊙217
Salagen Tablets 2229

DROPSTAR (Italy)
SODIUM HYALURONATE
Hyalgan Solution 3080

DROPTIMOL (Italy)
TIMOLOL MALEATE
Blocadren Tablets 2046
Timoptic Sterile Ophthalmic Solution. . . . 2190
Timoptic in Ocudose 2192
Timoptic-XE Sterile Ophthalmic Gel Forming Solution. 2194

DROSTEAKARD (Germany)
VERAPAMIL HYDROCHLORIDE
Covera-HS Tablets 3199
Isoptin SR Tablets. 467
Verelan Capsules 3184
Verelan PM Capsules 3186

DROXICEF (Italy)
CEFADROXIL
Duricef Capsules 1079
Duricef Oral Suspension. 1079
Duricef Tablets 1079

DTIC (Australia, Canada, Sweden, Switzerland)
DACARBAZINE
DTIC-Dome 902

DTIC-DOME (Austria, Belgium, Irish Republic, South Africa, Spain, United Kingdom)
DACARBAZINE
DTIC-Dome 902

DUACT (Austria)
ACRIVASTINE/PSEUDOEPHEDRINE HYDROCHLORIDE
Semprex-D Capsules. 1172

DUAFEN (Austria)
IBUPROFEN
Motrin Suspension, Oral Drops, Chewable Tablets, and Caplets 2002

DUALGAN (Portugal)
ETODOLAC
Lodine Capsules 3528
Lodine Tablets. 3528
Lodine XL Extended-Release Tablets 3530

DUALIZOL (Mexico)
METRONIDAZOLE
MetroCream 1404
MetroGel 1405
MetroGel-Vaginal Gel 1986
MetroLotion 1405
Noritate Cream 1224

DUBOISINE (France)
HYOSCYAMINE SULFATE
Levbid Extended-Release Tablets 3172
Levsin Drops. 3172
Levsin Elixir 3172
Levsin Injection 3172
Levsin Tablets 3172
Levsin/SL Tablets. 3172
Levsinex Timecaps 3172

DUCENE (Australia)
DIAZEPAM
Valium Injectable 3026
Valium Tablets 3047

DULAX (Irish Republic)
LACTULOSE
Kristalose for Oral Solution. 1007

DUMIROX (Italy, Spain)
FLUVOXAMINE MALEATE
Luvox Tablets (25, 50, 100 mg) 3256

DUMOXIN (Denmark, South Africa)
DOXYCYCLINE HYCLATE
Doryx Coated Pellet Filled Capsules 3357
Periostat Tablets 1208
Vibramycin Hyclate Capsules. 2735
Vibramycin Hyclate Intravenous 2737
Vibra-Tabs Film Coated Tablets 2735

DUMOZOL (Portugal)
METRONIDAZOLE
MetroCream 1404
MetroGel 1405
MetroGel-Vaginal Gel 1986
MetroLotion 1405
Noritate Cream 1224

DUMOZOLAM (Sweden)
TRIAZOLAM
Halcion Tablets 2823

DUMYROX (Portugal)
FLUVOXAMINE MALEATE
Luvox Tablets (25, 50, 100 mg) 3256

DUOBRUS (Sweden)
IBUPROFEN
Motrin Suspension, Oral Drops, Chewable Tablets, and Caplets 2002

DUOGASTRIL (Spain)
CIMETIDINE
Tagamet Tablets 1644

DUOLAX (Spain)
LACTULOSE
Kristalose for Oral Solution. 1007

DUOLUTON (Hong Kong)
NORGESTREL
Ovrette Tablets 3552

DUOMET (Brazil, New Zealand, South Africa)
CIMETIDINE
Tagamet Tablets 1644

DUOTRIC (Thailand)
CIMETIDINE
Tagamet Tablets 1644

DUPHALAC (Australia, Austria, Belgium, Canada, Finland, France, Hong Kong, Irish Republic, Italy, New Zealand, Norway, Portugal, Singapore, South Africa, Spain, Sweden, Switzerland, Thailand, United Kingdom)
LACTULOSE
Kristalose for Oral Solution. 1007

DUPLAMIN (Italy)
PROMETHAZINE HYDROCHLORIDE
Phenergan Injection 3553
Phenergan Suppositories 3556
Phenergan Syrup Fortis 3554
Phenergan Syrup Plain. 3554
Phenergan Tablets 3556

DURACAIN (Switzerland)
BUPIVACAINE HYDROCHLORIDE
Sensorcaine Injection 643
Sensorcaine-MPF Injection 643

DURACEF (Austria, Belgium, Finland, Hong Kong, Israel, Mexico, South Africa, Spain, Switzerland)
CEFADROXIL
Duricef Capsules 1079
Duricef Oral Suspension. 1079
Duricef Tablets 1079

DURACLAMID (Germany)
METOCLOPRAMIDE HYDROCHLORIDE
Reglan Injectable 2935
Reglan Syrup 2935
Reglan Tablets. 2935

DURACRALFAT (Germany)
SUCRALFATE
Carafate Suspension. 731
Carafate Tablets. 730

DURACTIN (Australia)
CIMETIDINE
Tagamet Tablets 1644

DURADIAZEPAM (Germany)
DIAZEPAM
Valium Injectable 3026
Valium Tablets 3047

DURADIURET (Germany)
HYDROCHLOROTHIAZIDE/TRIAMTERENE
Dyazide Capsules. 1515
Maxzide Tablets 1008
Maxzide-25 mg Tablets 1008

DURADOX (United Arab Emirates)
DOXYCYCLINE HYCLATE
Doryx Coated Pellet Filled Capsules 3357
Periostat Tablets 1208
Vibramycin Hyclate Capsules. 2735
Vibramycin Hyclate Intravenous 2737
Vibra-Tabs Film Coated Tablets 2735

DURAERYTHROMYCIN (Germany)
ERYTHROMYCIN STEARATE
Erythrocin Stearate Filmtab Tablets. 452

DURAFENAT (Germany)
FENOFIBRATE
Tricor Capsules, Micronized 513

DURAFUNGOL (Germany)
CLOTRIMAZOLE
Lotrimin Cream 1%. 3128
Lotrimin Lotion 1% 3128
Lotrimin Topical Solution 1% 3128
Mycelex Troche 573

DURAGENTAM (Germany)
GENTAMICIN SULFATE
Genoptic Ophthalmic Ointment . . . . ⊙239
Genoptic Sterile Ophthalmic Solution . . . ⊙239

DURAGENTAMICIN (Germany)
GENTAMICIN SULFATE
Genoptic Ophthalmic Ointment . . . . ⊙239
Genoptic Sterile Ophthalmic Solution . . . ⊙239

DURAGESIC (Canada)
FENTANYL
Duragesic Transdermal System 1786

DURAH2 (Germany)
CIMETIDINE
Tagamet Tablets 1644

DURA-IBU (Germany)
IBUPROFEN
Motrin Suspension, Oral Drops, Chewable Tablets, and Caplets 2002

DURAIBUPROFEN (Germany)
IBUPROFEN
Motrin Suspension, Oral Drops, Chewable Tablets, and Caplets 2002

DURAKNE (Germany)
MINOCYCLINE HYDROCHLORIDE
Dynacin Capsules. 2019
Minocin Intravenous 1862
Minocin Oral Suspension 1865
Minocin Pellet-Filled Capsules 1863

DURALGIN (Denmark)
MORPHINE SULFATE
Astramorph/PF Injection, USP (Preservative-Free). 594
Duramorph Injection 1312
Infumorph 200 and Infumorph 500 Sterile Solutions 1314
Kadian Capsules 1335
MS Contin Tablets 2896
MSIR Oral Capsules 2898
MSIR Oral Solution 2898
MSIR Oral Solution Concentrate 2898
MSIR Oral Tablets. 2898
Oramorph SR Tablets 3062
Roxanol 100 Concentrated Oral Solution 3066
Roxanol Concentrated Oral Solution 3066
Roxanol-T Oral Solution 3066

DURALITH (Canada)
LITHIUM CARBONATE
Eskalith CR Controlled Release Tablets . . 1527
Eskalith Capsules. 1527
Lithium Carbonate Capsules 3061
Lithobid Slow-Release Tablets 3255

DURALMOR (Mexico)
MORPHINE SULFATE
Astramorph/PF Injection, USP (Preservative-Free). 594
Duramorph Injection 1312
Infumorph 200 and Infumorph 500 Sterile Solutions 1314
Kadian Capsules 1335
MS Contin Tablets 2896
MSIR Oral Capsules 2898
MSIR Oral Solution 2898
MSIR Oral Solution Concentrate 2898
MSIR Oral Tablets. 2898
Oramorph SR Tablets 3062
Roxanol 100 Concentrated Oral Solution 3066
Roxanol Concentrated Oral Solution 3066
Roxanol-T Oral Solution 3066

DURALOZAM (Germany)
LORAZEPAM
Ativan Injection 3478
Ativan Tablets 3482

DURAMCP (Germany)
METOCLOPRAMIDE HYDROCHLORIDE
Reglan Injectable 2935
Reglan Syrup 2935
Reglan Tablets. 2935

DURAMIPRESS (Germany)
PRAZOSIN HYDROCHLORIDE
Minipress Capsules. 2699

DURAMONITAT (Germany)
ISOSORBIDE MONONITRATE
Imdur Tablets 1826
Ismo Tablets 3524

DURAN (Thailand)
IBUPROFEN
Motrin Suspension, Oral Drops, Chewable Tablets, and Caplets 2002

DURANEST (Australia, Austria, France, Germany, Sweden)
ETIDOCAINE HYDROCHLORIDE
Duranest Injections 600

DURANEST M. ADRENALIN (Germany)
ETIDOCAINE HYDROCHLORIDE
Duranest Injections 600

DURANIFIN (Germany)
NIFEDIPINE
Adalat CC Tablets 877
Procardia Capsules 2708
Procardia XL Extended Release Tablets . . 2710

DURANIFIN SALI (Germany)
NIFEDIPINE
Adalat CC Tablets 877
Procardia Capsules 2708
Procardia XL Extended Release Tablets . . 2710

DURANITRAT (Germany)
ISOSORBIDE DINITRATE
Isordil Sublingual Tablets 3525
Isordil Titradose Tablets 3526

DURANOL (Irish Republic)
PROPRANOLOL HYDROCHLORIDE
Inderal Injectable 3513
Inderal LA Long-Acting Capsules 3516
Inderal Tablets 3513

DURAPERIDOL (Germany)
HALOPERIDOL
Haldol Injection, Tablets and Concentrate 2533

DURAPHYLLIN (Germany)
THEOPHYLLINE
Aerolate Jr. T.D. Capsules 1361
Aerolate Liquid 1361
Aerolate Sr. T.D. Capsules 1361
Theo-Dur Extended-Release Tablets 1835
Uni-Dur Extended-Release Tablets 1841
Uniphyl 400 mg and 600 mg Tablets . . . 2903

DURAPIROX (Germany)
PIROXICAM
Feldene Capsules 2685

DURARESE (Germany)
AMILORIDE HYDROCHLORIDE/HYDROCHLOROTHIAZIDE
Moduretic Tablets 2138

DURASOPTIN (Germany)
VERAPAMIL HYDROCHLORIDE
Covera-HS Tablets 3199
Isoptin SR Tablets 467
Verelan Capsules 3184
Verelan PM Capsules 3186

DURATAMOXIFEN (Germany)
TAMOXIFEN CITRATE
Nolvadex Tablets 678

DURATENOL (Germany)
ATENOLOL
Tenormin I.V. Injection 692

DURATENOL COMP (Germany)
ATENOLOL
Tenormin I.V. Injection 692

DURATER (Mexico)
FAMOTIDINE
Pepcid Injection 2153
Pepcid Injection Premixed 2153
Pepcid RPD Orally Disintegrating Tablets 2150
Pepcid Tablets 2150
Pepcid for Oral Suspension 2150

DURATIMOL (Germany)
TIMOLOL MALEATE
Blocadren Tablets 2046
Timoptic Sterile Ophthalmic Solution 2190
Timoptic in Ocudose 2192
Timoptic-XE Sterile Ophthalmic Gel Forming Solution 2194

DURAVOLTEN (Germany)
DICLOFENAC SODIUM
Voltaren Tablets 2315
Voltaren-XR Tablets 2315

DURA-ZOK (Denmark)
METOPROLOL SUCCINATE
Toprol-XL Tablets 651

DUREKAL (Finland)
POTASSIUM CHLORIDE
K-Dur Microburst Release System ER Tablets 1832
K-Lor Powder Packets 469
K-Tab Filmtab Tablets 470
Rum-K 1363

DURICEF (Canada, Singapore, Thailand)
CEFADROXIL
Duricef Capsules 1079
Duricef Oral Suspension 1079
Duricef Tablets 1079

DURIDE (Australia, New Zealand)
ISOSORBIDE MONONITRATE
Imdur Tablets 1826
Ismo Tablets 3524

DUROGESIC (Australia, Austria, Belgium, Denmark, Finland, France, Germany, Hong Kong, Irish Republic, Israel, Italy, Mexico, New Zealand, Norway, Portugal, Singapore, South Africa, Spain, Sweden, Switzerland, The Netherlands, United Kingdom)
FENTANYL
Duragesic Transdermal System 1786

DURONITRIN (Italy)
ISOSORBIDE MONONITRATE
Imdur Tablets 1826
Ismo Tablets 3524

DUTACOR (Denmark)
SOTALOL HYDROCHLORIDE
Betapace Tablets 950

DUTONIN (Austria, Irish Republic, Spain, The Netherlands, United Kingdom)
NEFAZODONE HYDROCHLORIDE
Serzone Tablets 1104

DUVOID (Canada)
BETHANECHOL CHLORIDE
Urecholine Injection 2198
Urecholine Tablets 2198

DUXIMA (Italy)
CEFUROXIME SODIUM
Kefurox Vials, ADD-Vantage 1948
Zinacef Injection 1696

D-WORM (South Africa)
MEBENDAZOLE
Vermox Chewable Tablets 2017

DYAZIDE (Australia, Canada, Hong Kong, Irish Republic, Mexico, New Zealand, Portugal, Singapore, South Africa, Switzerland, Thailand, United Kingdom)
HYDROCHLOROTHIAZIDE/TRIAMTERENE
Dyazide Capsules 1515
Maxzide Tablets 1008
Maxzide-25 mg Tablets 1008

DYNABAC (Brazil, France, Hong Kong)
DIRITHROMYCIN
Dynabac Tablets 2269

DYNABLOK (South Africa)
PROPRANOLOL HYDROCHLORIDE
Inderal Injectable 3513
Inderal LA Long-Acting Capsules 3516
Inderal Tablets 3513

DYNACIRC (Canada, Hong Kong, Mexico, New Zealand, Singapore, South Africa, Thailand)
ISRADIPINE
DynaCirc CR Tablets 2923

DYNALERT (South Africa)
PEMOLINE
Cylert Chewable Tablets 415
Cylert Tablets 415

DYNAMETRON (South Africa)
METRONIDAZOLE
MetroCream 1404
MetroGel 1405
MetroGel-Vaginal Gel 1986
MetroLotion 1405
Noritate Cream 1224

DYNAMIDE (South Africa)
METOCLOPRAMIDE HYDROCHLORIDE
Reglan Injectable 2935
Reglan Syrup 2935
Reglan Tablets 2935

DYNAMIN (United Kingdom)
ISOSORBIDE MONONITRATE
Imdur Tablets 1826
Ismo Tablets 3524

DYNAPAM (South Africa)
DIAZEPAM
Valium Injectable 3026
Valium Tablets 3047

DYNASPOR (South Africa)
CLOTRIMAZOLE
Lotrimin Cream 1% 3128
Lotrimin Lotion 1% 3128
Lotrimin Topical Solution 1% 3128
Mycelex Troche 573

DYNOFEN (South Africa)
IBUPROFEN
Motrin Suspension, Oral Drops, Chewable Tablets, and Caplets 2002

DYRENIUM (Canada, Switzerland)
TRIAMTERENE
Dyrenium Capsules 3458

DYSALFA (France)
TERAZOSIN HYDROCHLORIDE
Hytrin Capsules 464

DYSDOLEN (Germany)
IBUPROFEN
Motrin Suspension, Oral Drops, Chewable Tablets, and Caplets 2002

DYSMAN (United Kingdom)
MEFENAMIC ACID
Ponstel Capsules 1356

DYSMENALGIT (Germany)
NAPROXEN
EC-Naprosyn Delayed-Release Tablets . . . 2967
Naprosyn Suspension 2967
Naprosyn Tablets 2967

DYSPAMET (Irish Republic, United Kingdom)
CIMETIDINE
Tagamet Tablets 1644

DYSPEN (Hong Kong, Thailand)
MEFENAMIC ACID
Ponstel Capsules 1356

DYTAC (Australia, Belgium, Irish Republic, The Netherlands, United Kingdom)
TRIAMTERENE
Dyrenium Capsules 3458

DYTA-URESE (Belgium, The Netherlands)
TRIAMTERENE
Dyrenium Capsules 3458

DYTENZIDE (Belgium, The Netherlands)
TRIAMTERENE
Dyrenium Capsules 3458

DYTERENE (Thailand)
HYDROCHLOROTHIAZIDE/TRIAMTERENE
Dyazide Capsules 1515
Maxzide Tablets 1008
Maxzide-25 mg Tablets 1008

DYTIDE H (Austria, Germany)
HYDROCHLOROTHIAZIDE/TRIAMTERENE
Dyazide Capsules 1515
Maxzide Tablets 1008
Maxzide-25 mg Tablets 1008

EBEFEN (Austria)
TAMOXIFEN CITRATE
Nolvadex Tablets 678

EBENOL (Germany)
HYDROCORTISONE ACETATE
Anusol-HC Suppositories 2238
Cortifoam Rectal Foam 3170
Hydrocortone Acetate Injectable Suspension 2103
Proctocort Suppositories 2264

EBOREN (The Netherlands)
ERYTHROMYCIN
Emgel 2% Topical Gel 1285
Ery-Tab Tablets 448
Erythromycin Base Filmtab Tablets 454
Erythromycin Delayed-Release Capsules, USP 455
PCE Dispertab Tablets 498

EBUFAC (United Kingdom)
IBUPROFEN
Motrin Suspension, Oral Drops, Chewable Tablets, and Caplets 2002

ECAPRESAN (Mexico)
CAPTOPRIL
Captopril Tablets 2281

ECAPRIL (Mexico)
CAPTOPRIL
Captopril Tablets 2281

ECATEN (Mexico)
CAPTOPRIL
Captopril Tablets 2281

ECLARAN (France, Portugal)
BENZOYL PEROXIDE
Brevoxyl-4 Cleansing Lotion 3269
Brevoxyl-4 Creamy Wash 3270
Brevoxyl-4 Gel 3269
Brevoxyl-8 Cleansing Lotion 3269
Brevoxyl-8 Creamy Wash 3270
Brevoxyl-8 Gel 3269
Triaz Cleanser 2026
Triaz Gel 2026

ECODIPINE (Switzerland)
NIFEDIPINE
Adalat CC Tablets 877
Procardia Capsules 2708
Procardia XL Extended Release Tablets . . 2710

ECODUREX (Switzerland)
AMILORIDE HYDROCHLORIDE/HYDROCHLOROTHIAZIDE
Moduretic Tablets 2138

ECOFENAC (Switzerland)
DICLOFENAC SODIUM
Voltaren Tablets 2315
Voltaren-XR Tablets 2315

ECONAC (United Kingdom)
DICLOFENAC SODIUM
Voltaren Tablets 2315
Voltaren-XR Tablets 2315

ECONOSONE (United Kingdom)
PREDNISONE
Prednisone Intensol 3064
Prednisone Oral Solution 3064
Prednisone Tablets 3064

ECOPACE (United Kingdom)
CAPTOPRIL
Captopril Tablets 2281

ECOPAN (Switzerland)
MEFENAMIC ACID
Ponstel Capsules 1356

ECOPROFEN (Switzerland)
IBUPROFEN
Motrin Suspension, Oral Drops, Chewable Tablets, and Caplets 2002

ECRINAL (Spain)
FLECAINIDE ACETATE
Tambocor Tablets 1990

ECTREN (Spain)
QUINAPRIL HYDROCHLORIDE
Accupril Tablets 2611

ECURAL (Germany)
MOMETASONE FUROATE
Elocon Cream 0.1% 3110
Elocon Lotion 0.1% 3111
Elocon Ointment 0.1% 3112
Nasonex Nasal Spray 3131

EDDIA (France)
METFORMIN HYDROCHLORIDE
Glucophage Tablets 1080

EDEMOX (Spain)
ACETAZOLAMIDE
Diamox Sequels Sustained Release Capsules . . . . . ⊙270
Diamox Tablets . . . . . ⊙269

EDEX (France)
ALPROSTADIL
Caverject Sterile Powder 2777
MUSE Urethral Suppository 3335

EDICIN (Thailand)
VANCOMYCIN HYDROCHLORIDE
Vancocin HCl Capsules & Pulvules 1972
Vancocin HCl Oral Solution 1971
Vancocin HCl, Vials & ADD-Vantage 1970

EDILUNA (Spain)
IBUPROFEN
Motrin Suspension, Oral Drops, Chewable Tablets, and Caplets 2002

EDISTOL (Spain)
ISOSORBIDE MONONITRATE
Imdur Tablets 1826
Ismo Tablets 3524

EDNYT (United Kingdom)
ENALAPRIL MALEATE
Vasotec Tablets 2210

EDOLAN (Italy)
ETODOLAC
Lodine Capsules 3528
Lodine Tablets 3528
Lodine XL Extended-Release Tablets 3530

EDOLGLAU (Portugal)
CLONIDINE HYDROCHLORIDE
Catapres Tablets 1037
Duraclon Injection 3057

EFCORTELAN (United Kingdom)
HYDROCORTISONE
Anusol-HC Cream 2.5% 2237
Hydrocortone Tablets 2106

EFECTIN (Austria)
VENLAFAXINE HYDROCHLORIDE
Effexor Tablets 3495
Effexor XR Capsules 3499

EFEKTOLOL (Germany)
PROPRANOLOL HYDROCHLORIDE
Inderal Injectable 3513
Inderal LA Long-Acting Capsules 3516
Inderal Tablets 3513

EFEMIDA (Spain)
CEPHALEXIN
Keflex Oral Suspension 1237
Keflex Pulvules 1237

EFEXOR (Australia, Austria, Belgium, Denmark, Finland, Hong Kong, Irish Republic, Israel, Italy, Mexico, New Zealand, Norway, Portugal, Singapore, South Africa, Switzerland, The Netherlands, United Kingdom)
VENLAFAXINE HYDROCHLORIDE
Effexor Tablets 3495

Effexor XR Capsules 3499

EFFACNE (France, Switzerland)
BENZOYL PEROXIDE
Brevoxyl-4 Cleansing Lotion 3269
Brevoxyl-4 Creamy Wash 3270
Brevoxyl-4 Gel 3269
Brevoxyl-8 Cleansing Lotion 3269
Brevoxyl-8 Creamy Wash 3270
Brevoxyl-8 Gel 3269
Triaz Cleanser 2026
Triaz Gel 2026

EFFECTSAL (Singapore)
NORFLOXACIN
Chibroxin Sterile Ophthalmic Solution ⊙273, 2051
Noroxin Tablets 2145

EFFEDERM (France)
TRETINOIN
Avita Cream 999
Avita Gel 1000
Renova 0.05% Cream 2519
Retin-A Micro 0.1% 2522
Vesanoid Capsules 3037

EFFEXOR (Canada, France)
VENLAFAXINE HYDROCHLORIDE
Effexor Tablets 3495
Effexor XR Capsules 3499

EFFLUMIDEX (Germany)
FLUOROMETHOLONE
FML Ophthalmic Ointment ⊙237

EFUDEX (Canada)
FLUOROURACIL
Efudex Cream 1733
Efudex Topical Solutions 1733
Fluoroplex Topical Cream 552
Fluoroplex Topical Solution 552

EFUDIX (Australia, Belgium, France, Germany, Irish Republic, Israel, Italy, Mexico, New Zealand, Singapore, South Africa, Spain, Switzerland, Thailand, The Netherlands, United Kingdom)
FLUOROURACIL
Efudex Cream 1733
Efudex Topical Solutions 1733
Fluoroplex Topical Cream 552
Fluoroplex Topical Solution 552

EFURIX (Brazil)
FLUOROURACIL
Efudex Cream 1733
Efudex Topical Solutions 1733
Fluoroplex Topical Cream 552
Fluoroplex Topical Solution 552

EGACENE (The Netherlands)
HYOSCYAMINE SULFATE
Levbid Extended-Release Tablets 3172
Levsin Drops 3172
Levsin Elixir 3172
Levsin Injection 3172
Levsin Tablets 3172
Levsin/SL Tablets 3172
Levsinex Timecaps 3172

EGAZIL (Denmark, Finland, Norway, Sweden)
HYOSCYAMINE SULFATE
Levbid Extended-Release Tablets 3172
Levsin Drops 3172
Levsin Elixir 3172
Levsin Injection 3172
Levsin Tablets 3172
Levsin/SL Tablets 3172
Levsinex Timecaps 3172

EGERY (France)
ERYTHROMYCIN
Emgel 2% Topical Gel 1285
Ery-Tab Tablets 448
Erythromycin Base Filmtab Tablets 454
Erythromycin Delayed-Release Capsules, USP 455
PCE Dispertab Tablets 498

EGIBREN (Italy)
SELEGILINE HYDROCHLORIDE
Eldepryl Capsules 3266

EGOCORT (Australia, Hong Kong, New Zealand, Singapore)
HYDROCORTISONE
Anusol-HC Cream 2.5% 2237
Hydrocortone Tablets 2106

EHLIFUNG (Mexico)
KETOCONAZOLE
Nizoral 2% Cream 3620
Nizoral 2% Shampoo 2007
Nizoral Tablets 1791

EHLINDOPA (Mexico)
METHYLDOPA
Aldomet Tablets 2037

EHLITEN (Mexico)
PRAZIQUANTEL
Biltricide Tablets 887

EHLIXACIN (Mexico)
CIPROFLOXACIN
Cipro I.V. 893
Cipro I.V. Pharmacy Bulk Package 897
Cipro Oral Suspension 887

EINALAT (Austria)
NIFEDIPINE
Adalat CC Tablets 877
Procardia Capsules 2708
Procardia XL Extended Release Tablets 2710

EISMYCIN (Germany)
MUPIROCIN
Bactroban Ointment 1496

EKZEMSALBE (Austria)
HYDROCORTISONE ACETATE
Anusol-HC Suppositories 2238
Cortifoam Rectal Foam 3170
Hydrocortone Acetate Injectable Suspension 2103
Proctocort Suppositories 2264

EKZESIN (Germany)
HYDROCORTISONE ACETATE
Anusol-HC Suppositories 2238
Cortifoam Rectal Foam 3170
Hydrocortone Acetate Injectable Suspension 2103
Proctocort Suppositories 2264

ELAN (Italy)
ISOSORBIDE MONONITRATE
Imdur Tablets 1826
Ismo Tablets 3524

ELANPRES (Irish Republic)
METHYLDOPA
Aldomet Tablets 2037

ELANPRESS (Italy)
METHYLDOPA
Aldomet Tablets 2037

ELANTAN (Hong Kong, Mexico, Singapore, Thailand)
ISOSORBIDE MONONITRATE
Imdur Tablets 1826
Ismo Tablets 3524

ELANTAN (Austria, Brazil, Germany, Irish Republic, South Africa, Switzerland, United Kingdom)
ISOSORBIDE MONONITRATE
Imdur Tablets 1826
Ismo Tablets 3524

ELASVEN (Spain)
FLUOCINOLONE ACETONIDE
Synalar Cream 2020
Synalar Ointment 2020
Synalar Topical Solution 2020

ELAUBAT (Germany)
HALOPERIDOL
Haldol Injection, Tablets and Concentrate 2533

ELAVIL PLUS (Canada)
AMITRIPTYLINE HYDROCHLORIDE/PERPHENAZINE
Etrafon 2-10 Tablets (2-10) 3115
Etrafon Tablets (2-25) 3115
Etrafon-Forte Tablets (4-25) 3115

ELAZOR (Italy)
FLUCONAZOLE
Diflucan Tablets, Injection, and Oral Suspension 2681

ELBROL (Germany)
PROPRANOLOL HYDROCHLORIDE
Inderal Injectable 3513
Inderal LA Long-Acting Capsules 3516
Inderal Tablets 3513

ELCRIT (Germany)
CLOZAPINE
Clozaril Tablets 2319

ELDEPRINE (France)
SELEGILINE HYDROCHLORIDE
Eldepryl Capsules 3266

ELDEPRYL (Australia, Belgium, Canada, Denmark, Finland, Irish Republic, New Zealand, Norway, South Africa, Sweden, The Netherlands, United Kingdom)
SELEGILINE HYDROCHLORIDE
Eldepryl Capsules 3266

ELDERIN (Hong Kong)
ETODOLAC
Lodine Capsules 3528
Lodine Tablets 3528
Lodine XL Extended-Release Tablets 3530

ELDOPAQUE (Hong Kong)
HYDROQUINONE
Eldopaque Forte 4% Cream 1734
Eldoquin Forte 4% Cream 1734
Lustra Cream 2023
Lustra-AF Cream 2023
Melanex Topical Solution 2300
Solaquin Forte 4% Cream 1734
Solaquin Forte 4% Gel 1734

ELDOQUIN (Canada, Hong Kong, Mexico, New Zealand, Singapore)
HYDROQUINONE
Eldopaque Forte 4% Cream 1734
Eldoquin Forte 4% Cream 1734
Lustra Cream 2023
Lustra-AF Cream 2023
Melanex Topical Solution 2300
Solaquin Forte 4% Cream 1734
Solaquin Forte 4% Gel 1734

ELEGELIN (Singapore)
SELEGILINE HYDROCHLORIDE
Eldepryl Capsules 3266

ELENTOL (France)
LINDANE
Lindane Lotion USP 1% 559
Lindane Shampoo USP 1% 560

ELEQUINE (Mexico)
LEVOFLOXACIN
Levaquin Injection 2537
Levaquin Tablets 2537

ELEVAT (South Africa)
DRONABINOL
Marinol Capsules 3325

ELGAM (Spain)
OMEPRAZOLE
Prilosec Delayed-Release Capsules 628

ELICA (South Africa, Spain)
MOMETASONE FUROATE
Elocon Cream 0.1% 3110
Elocon Lotion 0.1% 3111
Elocon Ointment 0.1% 3112
Nasonex Nasal Spray 3131

ELISOR (France)
PRAVASTATIN SODIUM
Pravachol Tablets 1099

ELITAN (Thailand)
METOCLOPRAMIDE HYDROCHLORIDE
Reglan Injectable 2935
Reglan Syrup 2935
Reglan Tablets 2935

ELITEN (Italy)
FOSINOPRIL SODIUM
Monopril Tablets 1091

ELIXIFILIN (Spain)
THEOPHYLLINE
Aerolate Jr. T.D. Capsules 1361
Aerolate Liquid 1361
Aerolate Sr. T.D. Capsules 1361
Theo-Dur Extended-Release Tablets 1835
Uni-Dur Extended-Release Tablets 1841
Uniphyl 400 mg and 600 mg Tablets 2903

ELIXOFILINA (Mexico)
THEOPHYLLINE
Aerolate Jr. T.D. Capsules 1361
Aerolate Liquid 1361
Aerolate Sr. T.D. Capsules 1361
Theo-Dur Extended-Release Tablets 1835
Uni-Dur Extended-Release Tablets 1841
Uniphyl 400 mg and 600 mg Tablets 2903

ELIXOPHYLLIN (Australia, Canada)
THEOPHYLLINE
Aerolate Jr. T.D. Capsules 1361
Aerolate Liquid 1361
Aerolate Sr. T.D. Capsules 1361
Theo-Dur Extended-Release Tablets 1835
Uni-Dur Extended-Release Tablets 1841
Uniphyl 400 mg and 600 mg Tablets 2903

ELL-CRANELL ALPHA (Germany)
ESTRADIOL
Alora Transdermal System 3372
Climara Transdermal System 958
Estrace Vaginal Cream 3358
Estring Vaginal Ring 2811
Vivelle Transdermal System 2412
Vivelle-Dot Transdermal System 2416

ELLESTE-SOLO (United Kingdom)
ESTRADIOL
Alora Transdermal System 3372
Climara Transdermal System 958
Estrace Vaginal Cream 3358
Estring Vaginal Ring 2811
Vivelle Transdermal System 2412
Vivelle-Dot Transdermal System 2416

ELMETIN (Thailand)
MEBENDAZOLE
Vermox Chewable Tablets 2017

ELMIRON (Australia, Canada, Hong Kong)
PENTOSAN POLYSULFATE SODIUM
Elmiron Capsules 570

ELMOGAN (Hong Kong)
GEMFIBROZIL
Lopid Tablets 2650

ELOCIN (Thailand)
ERYTHROMYCIN STEARATE
Erythrocin Stearate Filmtab Tablets 452

ELOCOM (Belgium, Brazil, Canada, Israel, Portugal, Spain, Switzerland)
MOMETASONE FUROATE
Elocon Cream 0.1% 3110
Elocon Lotion 0.1% 3111
Elocon Ointment 0.1% 3112
Nasonex Nasal Spray 3131

ELOCON (Australia, Austria, Denmark, Finland, Irish Republic, Italy, New Zealand, Norway, South Africa, Sweden, The Netherlands, United Kingdom)
MOMETASONE FUROATE
Elocon Cream 0.1% 3110
Elocon Lotion 0.1% 3111
Elocon Ointment 0.1% 3112
Nasonex Nasal Spray 3131

ELOCOR (Mexico)
NIFEDIPINE
Adalat CC Tablets 877
Procardia Capsules 2708
Procardia XL Extended Release Tablets 2710

ELOCORT (Brazil)
HYDROCORTISONE
Anusol-HC Cream 2.5% 2237
Hydrocortone Tablets 2106

ELOMET (Hong Kong, Mexico, Singapore, Thailand)
MOMETASONE FUROATE
Elocon Cream 0.1% 3110
Elocon Lotion 0.1% 3111
Elocon Ointment 0.1% 3112
Nasonex Nasal Spray 3131

ELROQUIL N (Germany)
HYDROXYZINE HYDROCHLORIDE
Atarax Tablets & Syrup 2667
Vistaril Intramuscular Solution 2738

ELSPAR (Brazil, Hong Kong)
ASPARAGINASE
Elspar for Injection 2092

ELTAIR (Hong Kong, New Zealand, Singapore)
BUDESONIDE
Pulmicort Turbuhaler Inhalation Powder 636
Rhinocort Nasal Inhaler 640

ELYZOL (Finland, Hong Kong, Mexico, Singapore, Thailand, The Netherlands)
METRONIDAZOLE
MetroCream 1404
MetroGel 1405
MetroGel-Vaginal Gel 1986
MetroLotion 1405
Noritate Cream 1224

EMBLON (United Kingdom)
TAMOXIFEN CITRATE
Nolvadex Tablets 678

EMCONCOR (Belgium, Denmark, Finland, Spain, Sweden)
BISOPROLOL FUMARATE
Zebeta Tablets 1885

EMCONCOR COMP (Finland)
BISOPROLOL FUMARATE/HYDROCHLOROTHIAZIDE
Ziac Tablets 1887

EMCOR (Irish Republic, The Netherlands, United Kingdom)
BISOPROLOL FUMARATE
Zebeta Tablets 1885

EMCORETIC (Belgium, Spain, The Netherlands)
BISOPROLOL FUMARATE/HYDROCHLOROTHIAZIDE
Ziac Tablets 1887

EMEPROTON (Spain)
OMEPRAZOLE
Prilosec Delayed-Release Capsules 628

EMESAN (Germany)
DIPHENHYDRAMINE HYDROCHLORIDE
Benadryl Parenteral 2617

EMESIDE (United Kingdom)
ETHOSUXIMIDE
Zarontin Capsules 2659
Zarontin Syrup 2660

EMESTID (France)
ERYTHROMYCIN STEARATE
Erythrocin Stearate Filmtab Tablets 452

EMETAL (Thailand)
METOCLOPRAMIDE HYDROCHLORIDE
Reglan Injectable 2935

Reglan Syrup 2935
Reglan Tablets. 2935

EMEX (Canada)
METOCLOPRAMIDE HYDROCHLORIDE
Reglan Injectable 2935
Reglan Syrup 2935
Reglan Tablets. 2935

EMFIB (United Kingdom)
GEMFIBROZIL
Lopid Tablets 2650

EMFORAL (Thailand)
PROPRANOLOL HYDROCHLORIDE
Inderal Injectable 3513
Inderal LA Long-Acting Capsules 3516
Inderal Tablets. 3513

EMMETIPI (Italy)
METHYLPREDNISOLONE SODIUM SUCCINATE
Solu-Medrol Sterile Powder. 2855

EMO-CORT (Canada)
HYDROCORTISONE
Anusol-HC Cream 2.5% 2237
Hydrocortone Tablets 2106

EMOFERRINA (Italy)
FERRIC SODIUM GLUCONATE
Ferrlecit Injection 3386

EMOSINT (Italy)
DESMOPRESSIN ACETATE
DDAVP Injection 4 mcg/mL. 737
DDAVP Nasal Spray 738
DDAVP Rhinal Tube 738
DDAVP Tablets. 739
Desmopressin Acetate Injection 1344
Desmopressin Acetate Rhinal Tube 1345
Stimate Nasal Spray 796

EMPERAL (Denmark)
METOCLOPRAMIDE HYDROCHLORIDE
Reglan Injectable 2935
Reglan Syrup 2935
Reglan Tablets. 2935

EMU-V (Australia, South Africa)
ERYTHROMYCIN
Emgel 2% Topical Gel 1285
Ery-Tab Tablets 448
Erythromycin Base Filmtab Tablets 454
Erythromycin Delayed-Release Capsules, USP. 455
PCE Dispertab Tablets. 498

EMUVIN (Austria)
ERYTHROMYCIN
Emgel 2% Topical Gel 1285
Ery-Tab Tablets 448
Erythromycin Base Filmtab Tablets 454
Erythromycin Delayed-Release Capsules, USP. 455
PCE Dispertab Tablets. 498

E-MYCIN (Canada, Hong Kong, Israel, Singapore)
ERYTHROMYCIN
Emgel 2% Topical Gel 1285
Ery-Tab Tablets 448
Erythromycin Base Filmtab Tablets 454
Erythromycin Delayed-Release Capsules, USP. 455
PCE Dispertab Tablets. 498

ENACARD (United Kingdom)
ENALAPRIL MALEATE
Vasotec Tablets 2210

ENADIL (Denmark)
ENALAPRIL MALEATE
Vasotec Tablets 2210

ENADURA (Germany)
ENALAPRIL MALEATE
Vasotec Tablets 2210

ENAHEXAL (Germany)
ENALAPRIL MALEATE
Vasotec Tablets 2210

ENALADIL (Mexico)
ENALAPRIL MALEATE
Vasotec Tablets 2210

ENALOC (Finland)
ENALAPRIL MALEATE
Vasotec Tablets 2210

ENALOC COMP (Finland)
ENALAPRIL MALEATE/HYDROCHLOROTHIAZIDE
Vaseretic Tablets 2204

ENAM (Thailand)
ENALAPRIL MALEATE
Vasotec Tablets 2210

ENAP (Irish Republic)
ENALAPRIL MALEATE
Vasotec Tablets 2210

ENAPREN (Italy)
ENALAPRIL MALEATE
Vasotec Tablets 2210

ENAPRIL (Brazil)
ENALAPRIL MALEATE
Vasotec Tablets 2210

ENARIL (Singapore, Thailand)
ENALAPRIL MALEATE
Vasotec Tablets 2210

ENATIA (Portugal)
ENALAPRIL MALEATE/HYDROCHLOROTHIAZIDE
Vaseretic Tablets 2204

ENBREL (United Kingdom)
ETANERCEPT
Enbrel for Injection 1752, 3504

ENDANTADINE (Canada)
AMANTADINE HYDROCHLORIDE
Symmetrel Syrup 1328
Symmetrel Tablets 1328

ENDOERITRIN (Spain)
ERYTHROMYCIN
Emgel 2% Topical Gel 1285
Ery-Tab Tablets 448
Erythromycin Base Filmtab Tablets 454
Erythromycin Delayed-Release Capsules, USP. 455
PCE Dispertab Tablets. 498

ENDONE (Australia)
OXYCODONE HYDROCHLORIDE
OxyContin Tablets 2912
OxyFast Oral Concentrate Solution 2916
OxyIR Capsules 2916
Percolone Tablets. 1327
Roxicodone Tablets 3067

ENDRONAX (Brazil)
ALENDRONATE SODIUM
Fosamax Tablets 2095

ENELBIN-VENEN SALBE (Germany)
HEPARIN SODIUM
Heparin Lock Flush Solution 3509
Heparin Sodium Injection 3511

ENI (Mexico)
CIPROFLOXACIN HYDROCHLORIDE
Ciloxan Ophthalmic Ointment. 538
Ciloxan Ophthalmic Solution . . . . ⊙209, 538
Cipro Tablets. 887

ENLON (Canada)
EDROPHONIUM CHLORIDE
Tensilon Injectable 1745

ENPOTT (Thailand)
POTASSIUM CHLORIDE
K-Dur Microburst Release System ER Tablets. 1832
K-Lor Powder Packets 469
K-Tab Filmtab Tablets 470
Rum-K. 1363

ENTEROSIL (Italy)
METOCLOPRAMIDE HYDROCHLORIDE
Reglan Injectable 2935
Reglan Syrup 2935
Reglan Tablets. 2935

ENTOCORD (South Africa, Spain)
BUDESONIDE
Pulmicort Turbuhaler Inhalation Powder . . . 636
Rhinocort Nasal Inhaler 640

ENTOCORT (Australia, Austria, Canada, Denmark, Finland, France, Germany, Hong Kong, Irish Republic, Israel, New Zealand, Norway, Singapore, Sweden, Switzerland, The Netherlands, United Kingdom)
BUDESONIDE
Pulmicort Turbuhaler Inhalation Powder . . . 636
Rhinocort Nasal Inhaler 640

ENTOPLUS (Mexico)
ALBENDAZOLE
Albenza Tablets 1463

ENTRYDIL (Irish Republic)
DILTIAZEM HYDROCHLORIDE
Cardizem CD Capsules 1016
Cardizem Injectable 1018
Cardizem Lyo-Ject Syringe 1018
Cardizem Monovial 1018
Tiazac Capsules 1378

ENZACE (Australia)
CAPTOPRIL
Captopril Tablets 2281

EPALAT EPS (Italy)
LACTULOSE
Kristalose for Oral Solution. 1007

EPALFEN (Italy)
LACTULOSE
Kristalose for Oral Solution. 1007

EPAMIN (Mexico)
PHENYTOIN
Dilantin Infatabs. 2624
Dilantin-125 Oral Suspension. 2625

EPANUTIN (Austria, Belgium, Germany, Irish Republic, Israel, Spain, Switzerland, United Kingdom)
PHENYTOIN
Dilantin Infatabs. 2624
Dilantin-125 Oral Suspension. 2625

EPAPLEX 40 (Italy)
FERRIC SODIUM GLUCONATE
Ferrlecit Injection 3386

EPARINOVIS (Italy)
HEPARIN SODIUM
Heparin Lock Flush Solution 3509
Heparin Sodium Injection 3511

EPI-ABEREL (Germany)
TRETINOIN
Avita Cream 999
Avita Gel 1000
Renova 0.05% Cream 2519
Retin-A Micro 0.1%. 2522
Vesanoid Capsules 3037

EPICLODINA (Mexico)
CLONIDINE
Catapres-TTS 1038

EPICORDIN (Austria, Germany)
ISOSORBIDE MONONITRATE
Imdur Tablets 1826
Ismo Tablets. 3524

EPIDEX (Brazil)
DESONIDE
DesOwen Cream 1401
DesOwen Lotion 1401
DesOwen Ointment. 1401

EPIESTROL (Irish Republic, Italy, Switzerland)
ESTRADIOL
Alora Transdermal System 3372
Climara Transdermal System. 958
Estrace Vaginal Cream 3358
Estring Vaginal Ring 2811
Vivelle Transdermal System 2412
Vivelle-Dot Transdermal System 2416

EPIKUR (Austria)
MEPROBAMATE
Miltown Tablets 3349

EPILAN-D (Austria)
PHENYTOIN
Dilantin Infatabs. 2624
Dilantin-125 Oral Suspension. 2625

EPILANTIN (Spain)
PHENYTOIN
Dilantin Infatabs. 2624
Dilantin-125 Oral Suspension. 2625

EPIMAZ (United Kingdom)
CARBAMAZEPINE
Carbatrol Capsules. 3234
Tegretol Chewable Tablets 2404
Tegretol Suspension 2404
Tegretol Tablets. 2404
Tegretol-XR Tablets 2404

EPIMORPH (Canada)
MORPHINE SULFATE
Astramorph/PF Injection, USP (Preservative-Free) 594
Duramorph Injection 1312
Infumorph 200 and Infumorph 500 Sterile Solutions 1314
Kadian Capsules 1335
MS Contin Tablets 2896
MSIR Oral Capsules 2898
MSIR Oral Solution 2898
MSIR Oral Solution Concentrate 2898
MSIR Oral Tablets. 2898
Oramorph SR Tablets 3062
Roxanol 100 Concentrated Oral Solution 3066
Roxanol Concentrated Oral Solution 3066
Roxanol-T Oral Solution 3066

EPINAT (Norway)
PHENYTOIN
Dilantin Infatabs. 2624
Dilantin-125 Oral Suspension. 2625

EPITOMAX (France)
TOPIRAMATE
Topamax Sprinkle Capsules 2590
Topamax Tablets 2590

EPITRIAM (The Netherlands)
TRIAMTERENE
Dyrenium Capsules. 3458

EPIVIR (Austria, Belgium, Denmark, Finland, France, Germany, Israel, Italy, Japan, Norway, Portugal, Singapore, Spain, Sweden, Thailand, The Netherlands, United Kingdom)
LAMIVUDINE
Epivir Oral Solution. 1520
Epivir Tablets 1520
Epivir-HBV Oral Solution. 1524
Epivir-HBV Tablets 1524

EPOCELIN (Finland, Japan, Spain, Thailand)
CEFTIZOXIME SODIUM
Cefizox for Intramuscular or Intravenous Use 1390

EPOCLER (Italy)
HYDROQUINONE
Eldopaque Forte 4% Cream 1734
Eldoquin Forte 4% Cream. 1734
Lustra Cream 2023
Lustra-AF Cream 2023
Melanex Topical Solution 2300
Solaquin Forte 4% Cream. 1734
Solaquin Forte 4% Gel. 1734

EPOMAX (Mexico)
EPOETIN ALFA
Epogen for Injection 582
Procrit for Injection. 2502

EPOPEN (Spain)
EPOETIN ALFA
Epogen for Injection 582
Procrit for Injection. 2502

EPOSERIN (Italy)
CEFTIZOXIME SODIUM
Cefizox for Intramuscular or Intravenous Use 1390

EPOXIDE (Thailand)
CHLORDIAZEPOXIDE HYDROCHLORIDE
Librium Capsules 1736
Librium for Injection 1737

EPOXITIN (Italy)
EPOETIN ALFA
Epogen for Injection 582
Procrit for Injection. 2502

EPREX (Australia, Belgium, Canada, Denmark, Finland, France, Hong Kong, Irish Republic, Israel, Italy, Mexico, New Zealand, Norway, Singapore, South Africa, Spain, Sweden, Switzerland, Thailand, The Netherlands, United Kingdom)
EPOETIN ALFA
Epogen for Injection 582
Procrit for Injection. 2502

EPSITRON (Thailand)
CAPTOPRIL
Captopril Tablets 2281

EPSOCLAR (Italy)
HEPARIN SODIUM
Heparin Lock Flush Solution 3509
Heparin Sodium Injection 3511

EQUANIL (Australia, Canada, France, Irish Republic, South Africa, United Kingdom)
MEPROBAMATE
Miltown Tablets 3349

EQUASYM (United Kingdom)
METHYLPHENIDATE HYDROCHLORIDE
Methylin Tablets. 1995
Ritalin Hydrochloride Tablets 2387
Ritalin-SR Tablets 2387

EQUIBAR (France)
METHYLDOPA
Aldomet Tablets. 2037

EQUIPAX (Spain)
GABAPENTIN
Neurontin Capsules. 2655

EQUITAM (France)
LORAZEPAM
Ativan Injection 3478
Ativan Tablets 3482

ERANZ (Mexico)
DONEPEZIL HYDROCHLORIDE
Aricept Tablets 1270, 2665

ERAVERM (Brazil)
MEBENDAZOLE
Vermox Chewable Tablets. 2017

ERCAR (Spain)
CARBOPLATIN
Paraplatin for Injection. 1126

ERCOQUIN (Denmark, Norway)
HYDROXYCHLOROQUINE SULFATE
Plaquenil Tablets 3082

ERGAMISOL (Australia, Belgium, Canada, Germany, Israel, Italy, South Africa, The Netherlands)
LEVAMISOLE HYDROCHLORIDE
Ergamisol Tablets. 1789

(⊙ Described in PDR For Ophthalmic Medicines™)

ERGIX (France)
IBUPROFEN
Motrin Suspension, Oral Drops, Chewable Tablets, and Caplets 2002

ERGOCALM (Austria)
LORAZEPAM
Ativan Injection 3478
Ativan Tablets 3482

ERIBER (Mexico)
ERYTHROMYCIN
Emgel 2% Topical Gel 1285
Ery-Tab Tablets 448
Erythromycin Base Filmtab Tablets 454
Erythromycin Delayed-Release Capsules, USP 455
PCE Dispertab Tablets 498

ERIBIOTIC (Brazil)
ERYTHROMYCIN STEARATE
Erythrocin Stearate Filmtab Tablets 452

ERIBUS (Mexico)
ERYTHROMYCIN
Emgel 2% Topical Gel 1285
Ery-Tab Tablets 448
Erythromycin Base Filmtab Tablets 454
Erythromycin Delayed-Release Capsules, USP 455
PCE Dispertab Tablets 498

ERICIN (Thailand)
ERYTHROMYCIN STEARATE
Erythrocin Stearate Filmtab Tablets 452

ERICOSOL (Switzerland)
ERYTHROMYCIN STEARATE
Erythrocin Stearate Filmtab Tablets 452

ERIDAN (Italy)
DIAZEPAM
Valium Injectable 3026
Valium Tablets 3047

ERIDOSIS (Spain)
ERYTHROMYCIN
Emgel 2% Topical Gel 1285
Ery-Tab Tablets 448
Erythromycin Base Filmtab Tablets 454
Erythromycin Delayed-Release Capsules, USP 455
PCE Dispertab Tablets 498

ERIFALECIN (Spain)
CEPHALEXIN
Keflex Oral Suspension 1237
Keflex Pulvules 1237

ERIL (Italy)
PIPERACILLIN SODIUM
Pipracil 1866

ERIPRODIN (Spain)
ERYTHROMYCIN
Emgel 2% Topical Gel 1285
Ery-Tab Tablets 448
Erythromycin Base Filmtab Tablets 454
Erythromycin Delayed-Release Capsules, USP 455
PCE Dispertab Tablets 498

ERISUSPEN (Mexico)
ERYTHROMYCIN
Emgel 2% Topical Gel 1285
Ery-Tab Tablets 448
Erythromycin Base Filmtab Tablets 454
Erythromycin Delayed-Release Capsules, USP 455
PCE Dispertab Tablets 498

ERITOLAT (Mexico)
ERYTHROMYCIN
Emgel 2% Topical Gel 1285
Ery-Tab Tablets 448
Erythromycin Base Filmtab Tablets 454
Erythromycin Delayed-Release Capsules, USP 455
PCE Dispertab Tablets 498

ERITRERBA (Mexico)
ERYTHROMYCIN
Emgel 2% Topical Gel 1285
Ery-Tab Tablets 448
Erythromycin Base Filmtab Tablets 454
Erythromycin Delayed-Release Capsules, USP 455
PCE Dispertab Tablets 498

ERITROFARMIN (Mexico)
ERYTHROMYCIN
Emgel 2% Topical Gel 1285
Ery-Tab Tablets 448
Erythromycin Base Filmtab Tablets 454
Erythromycin Delayed-Release Capsules, USP 455
PCE Dispertab Tablets 498

ERITROLAT (Mexico)
ERYTHROMYCIN
Emgel 2% Topical Gel 1285
Ery-Tab Tablets 448
Erythromycin Base Filmtab Tablets 454
Erythromycin Delayed-Release Capsules, USP 455
PCE Dispertab Tablets 498

ERITROQUIM (Mexico)
ERYTHROMYCIN
Emgel 2% Topical Gel 1285
Ery-Tab Tablets 448
Erythromycin Base Filmtab Tablets 454
Erythromycin Delayed-Release Capsules, USP 455
PCE Dispertab Tablets 498

ERITROSOL (Mexico)
ERYTHROMYCIN
Emgel 2% Topical Gel 1285
Ery-Tab Tablets 448
Erythromycin Base Filmtab Tablets 454
Erythromycin Delayed-Release Capsules, USP 455
PCE Dispertab Tablets 498

ERITROWEL (Mexico)
ERYTHROMYCIN
Emgel 2% Topical Gel 1285
Ery-Tab Tablets 448
Erythromycin Base Filmtab Tablets 454
Erythromycin Delayed-Release Capsules, USP 455
PCE Dispertab Tablets 498

ERLADEXONE (Singapore)
DEXAMETHASONE
Decadron Elixir 2078
Decadron Tablets 2079

ERLMETIN (Singapore)
CIMETIDINE
Tagamet Tablets 1644

ERMYCIN (Singapore)
ERYTHROMYCIN STEARATE
Erythrocin Stearate Filmtab Tablets 452

EROMEL (South Africa)
ERYTHROMYCIN STEARATE
Erythrocin Stearate Filmtab Tablets 452

EROTAB (Singapore)
ERYTHROMYCIN STEARATE
Erythrocin Stearate Filmtab Tablets 452

ERYACNE (Australia, France, Hong Kong, Italy, New Zealand, Singapore, Thailand, The Netherlands, United Kingdom)
ERYTHROMYCIN
Emgel 2% Topical Gel 1285
Ery-Tab Tablets 448
Erythromycin Base Filmtab Tablets 454
Erythromycin Delayed-Release Capsules, USP 455
PCE Dispertab Tablets 498

ERYACNEN (Brazil, Mexico)
ERYTHROMYCIN
Emgel 2% Topical Gel 1285
Ery-Tab Tablets 448
Erythromycin Base Filmtab Tablets 454
Erythromycin Delayed-Release Capsules, USP 455
PCE Dispertab Tablets 498

ERYAKNEN (Austria, Germany, Switzerland)
ERYTHROMYCIN
Emgel 2% Topical Gel 1285
Ery-Tab Tablets 448
Erythromycin Base Filmtab Tablets 454
Erythromycin Delayed-Release Capsules, USP 455
PCE Dispertab Tablets 498

ERYBID (Canada)
ERYTHROMYCIN
Emgel 2% Topical Gel 1285
Ery-Tab Tablets 448
Erythromycin Base Filmtab Tablets 454
Erythromycin Delayed-Release Capsules, USP 455
PCE Dispertab Tablets 498

ERYC (Australia, Canada, Hong Kong, Israel, New Zealand, The Netherlands)
ERYTHROMYCIN
Emgel 2% Topical Gel 1285
Ery-Tab Tablets 448
Erythromycin Base Filmtab Tablets 454
Erythromycin Delayed-Release Capsules, USP 455
PCE Dispertab Tablets 498

ERYCEN (United Kingdom)
ERYTHROMYCIN
Emgel 2% Topical Gel 1285
Ery-Tab Tablets 448
Erythromycin Base Filmtab Tablets 454
Erythromycin Delayed-Release Capsules, USP 455
PCE Dispertab Tablets 498

ERYCETTE (South Africa)
ERYTHROMYCIN
Emgel 2% Topical Gel 1285
Ery-Tab Tablets 448
Erythromycin Base Filmtab Tablets 454
Erythromycin Delayed-Release Capsules, USP 455
PCE Dispertab Tablets 498

ERYCIN (Thailand)
ERYTHROMYCIN STEARATE
Erythrocin Stearate Filmtab Tablets 452

ERYCINUM (Austria)
ERYTHROMYCIN
Emgel 2% Topical Gel 1285
Ery-Tab Tablets 448
Erythromycin Base Filmtab Tablets 454
Erythromycin Delayed-Release Capsules, USP 455
PCE Dispertab Tablets 498

ERYDERM (Belgium, Israel, Mexico, Singapore, South Africa, Switzerland, The Netherlands)
ERYTHROMYCIN
Emgel 2% Topical Gel 1285
Ery-Tab Tablets 448
Erythromycin Base Filmtab Tablets 454
Erythromycin Delayed-Release Capsules, USP 455
PCE Dispertab Tablets 498

ERYDERMEC (Germany)
ERYTHROMYCIN
Emgel 2% Topical Gel 1285
Ery-Tab Tablets 448
Erythromycin Base Filmtab Tablets 454
Erythromycin Delayed-Release Capsules, USP 455
PCE Dispertab Tablets 498

ERYFLUID (France, Portugal)
ERYTHROMYCIN
Emgel 2% Topical Gel 1285
Ery-Tab Tablets 448
Erythromycin Base Filmtab Tablets 454
Erythromycin Delayed-Release Capsules, USP 455
PCE Dispertab Tablets 498

ERYLAR (Mexico)
ERYTHROMYCIN
Emgel 2% Topical Gel 1285
Ery-Tab Tablets 448
Erythromycin Base Filmtab Tablets 454
Erythromycin Delayed-Release Capsules, USP 455
PCE Dispertab Tablets 498

ERYLIK (France)
ERYTHROMYCIN
Emgel 2% Topical Gel 1285
Ery-Tab Tablets 448
Erythromycin Base Filmtab Tablets 454
Erythromycin Delayed-Release Capsules, USP 455
PCE Dispertab Tablets 498

ERYMAX (Irish Republic, South Africa, Switzerland, United Kingdom)
ERYTHROMYCIN
Emgel 2% Topical Gel 1285
Ery-Tab Tablets 448
Erythromycin Base Filmtab Tablets 454
Erythromycin Delayed-Release Capsules, USP 455
PCE Dispertab Tablets 498

ERY-MAX (Spain)
ERYTHROMYCIN
Emgel 2% Topical Gel 1285
Ery-Tab Tablets 448
Erythromycin Base Filmtab Tablets 454
Erythromycin Delayed-Release Capsules, USP 455
PCE Dispertab Tablets 498

ERYPO (Austria, Germany)
EPOETIN ALFA
Epogen for Injection 582
Procrit for Injection 2502

ERYSOL (Canada)
ERYTHROMYCIN
Emgel 2% Topical Gel 1285
Ery-Tab Tablets 448
Erythromycin Base Filmtab Tablets 454
Erythromycin Delayed-Release Capsules, USP 455
PCE Dispertab Tablets 498

ERYTAB (Israel)
ERYTHROMYCIN
Emgel 2% Topical Gel 1285
Ery-Tab Tablets 448
Erythromycin Base Filmtab Tablets 454
Erythromycin Delayed-Release Capsules, USP 455
PCE Dispertab Tablets 498

ERY-TAB (Thailand)
ERYTHROMYCIN
Emgel 2% Topical Gel 1285
Ery-Tab Tablets 448
Erythromycin Base Filmtab Tablets 454
Erythromycin Delayed-Release Capsules, USP 455
PCE Dispertab Tablets 498

ERYTAB-S (Singapore)
ERYTHROMYCIN STEARATE
Erythrocin Stearate Filmtab Tablets 452

ERYTHROCIN (Irish Republic, United Kingdom)
ERYTHROMYCIN STEARATE
Erythrocin Stearate Filmtab Tablets 452

ERYTHRODERM (Israel)
ERYTHROMYCIN
Emgel 2% Topical Gel 1285
Ery-Tab Tablets 448
Erythromycin Base Filmtab Tablets 454
Erythromycin Delayed-Release Capsules, USP 455
PCE Dispertab Tablets 498

ERYTHROGEL (France)
ERYTHROMYCIN
Emgel 2% Topical Gel 1285
Ery-Tab Tablets 448
Erythromycin Base Filmtab Tablets 454
Erythromycin Delayed-Release Capsules, USP 455
PCE Dispertab Tablets 498

ERYTHRO-HEFA (Germany)
ERYTHROMYCIN STEARATE
Erythrocin Stearate Filmtab Tablets 452

ERYTHROMID (Canada, Irish Republic, South Africa, United Kingdom)
ERYTHROMYCIN
Emgel 2% Topical Gel 1285
Ery-Tab Tablets 448
Erythromycin Base Filmtab Tablets 454
Erythromycin Delayed-Release Capsules, USP 455
PCE Dispertab Tablets 498

ERYTOP (Germany)
ERYTHROMYCIN
Emgel 2% Topical Gel 1285
Ery-Tab Tablets 448
Erythromycin Base Filmtab Tablets 454
Erythromycin Delayed-Release Capsules, USP 455
PCE Dispertab Tablets 498

ERYTRAN (Switzerland)
ERYTHROMYCIN STEARATE
Erythrocin Stearate Filmtab Tablets 452

ERYTROCICLIN (Italy)
ERYTHROMYCIN STEARATE
Erythrocin Stearate Filmtab Tablets 452

ESACINONE (Italy)
FLUOCINOLONE ACETONIDE
Synalar Cream 2020
Synalar Ointment 2020
Synalar Topical Solution 2020

ESADOXI (Italy)
DOXYCYCLINE HYCLATE
Doryx Coated Pellet Filled Capsules 3357
Periostat Tablets 1208
Vibra-Tabs Film Coated Tablets 2735
Vibramycin Hyclate Capsules 2735
Vibramycin Hyclate Intravenous 2737

ESCABIN (Brazil)
LINDANE
Lindane Lotion USP 1% 559
Lindane Shampoo USP 1% 560

ESCARBICIDA (Mexico)
LINDANE
Lindane Lotion USP 1% 559
Lindane Shampoo USP 1% 560

ESCLEBIN (Spain)
NORFLOXACIN
Chibroxin Sterile Ophthalmic Solution ⊙273, 2051
Noroxin Tablets 2145

ESCOFLEX (Switzerland)
CHLORZOXAZONE
Parafon Forte DSC Caplets 2582

ESCORETIC (Switzerland)
AMILORIDE HYDROCHLORIDE/HYDROCHLOROTHIAZIDE
Moduretic Tablets 2138

ESIDREX (Australia, Austria, Belgium, France, Italy, Norway, Spain, Sweden, Switzerland, The Netherlands, United Kingdom)
HYDROCHLOROTHIAZIDE
HydroDIURIL Tablets 2108
Microzide Capsules 3414

ESIDRIX (Germany)
HYDROCHLOROTHIAZIDE
HydroDIURIL Tablets 2108

(⊙ Described in PDR For Ophthalmic Medicines™)

Microzide Capsules 3414

ESILGAN (Italy)
ESTAZOLAM
ProSom Tablets 500

ESILON (Italy)
FLUOCINOLONE ACETONIDE
Synalar Cream 2020
Synalar Ointment 2020
Synalar Topical Solution 2020

ESITEREN (Germany)
HYDROCHLOROTHIAZIDE/TRIAMTERENE
Dyazide Capsules 1515
Maxzide Tablets 1008
Maxzide-25 mg Tablets 1008

ESKAZINE (Spain)
TRIFLUOPERAZINE HYDROCHLORIDE
Stelazine Injection 1640
Stelazine Tablets 1640

ESKAZOLE (Australia, Austria, France, Germany, Israel, Mexico, Spain, The Netherlands, United Kingdom)
ALBENDAZOLE
Albenza Tablets 1463

ESMERON (Australia, Austria, Belgium, Denmark, Finland, France, Germany, Hong Kong, Irish Republic, Israel, Italy, New Zealand, Norway, Portugal, Singapore, South Africa, Spain, Sweden, Switzerland, Thailand, The Netherlands, United Kingdom)
ROCURONIUM BROMIDE
Zemuron Injection 2491

ESOFEX (Finland)
RANITIDINE HYDROCHLORIDE
Zantac 150 EFFERdose Granules 1690
Zantac 150 EFFERdose Tablets 1690
Zantac 150 Tablets 1690
Zantac 300 Tablets 1690
Zantac Injection 1688
Zantac Injection Premixed 1688
Zantac Syrup 1690

ESOLUT (Italy)
PROGESTERONE
Crinone 4% Gel 3213
Crinone 8% Gel 3213
Prometrium Capsules (100 mg, 200 mg) 3261

ESOTERICA (United Kingdom)
HYDROQUINONE
Eldopaque Forte 4% Cream 1734
Eldoquin Forte 4% Cream 1734
Lustra Cream 2023
Lustra-AF Cream 2023
Melanex Topical Solution 2300
Solaquin Forte 4% Cream 1734
Solaquin Forte 4% Gel 1734

ESOTERICA REGULAR (Canada)
HYDROQUINONE
Eldopaque Forte 4% Cream 1734
Eldoquin Forte 4% Cream 1734
Lustra Cream 2023
Lustra-AF Cream 2023
Melanex Topical Solution 2300
Solaquin Forte 4% Cream 1734
Solaquin Forte 4% Gel 1734

ESOTERICA UNSCENTED (Canada)
HYDROQUINONE
Eldopaque Forte 4% Cream 1734
Eldoquin Forte 4% Cream 1734
Lustra Cream 2023
Lustra-AF Cream 2023
Melanex Topical Solution 2300
Solaquin Forte 4% Cream 1734
Solaquin Forte 4% Gel 1734

ESOTRAN (Spain)
ESTRADIOL
Alora Transdermal System 3372
Climara Transdermal System 958
Estrace Vaginal Cream 3358
Estring Vaginal Ring 2811
Vivelle Transdermal System 2412
Vivelle-Dot Transdermal System 2416

ESPA-FORMIN (Germany)
METFORMIN HYDROCHLORIDE
Glucophage Tablets 1080

ESPA-LEPSIN (Germany)
CARBAMAZEPINE
Carbatrol Capsules 3234
Tegretol Chewable Tablets 2404
Tegretol Suspension 2404
Tegretol Tablets 2404
Tegretol-XR Tablets 2404

ESPARIL (Germany)
CAPTOPRIL
Captopril Tablets 2281

ESPARON (Germany)
ALPRAZOLAM
Xanax Tablets 2865

ESPEDEN (Spain)
NORFLOXACIN
Chibroxin Sterile Ophthalmic Solution .... ⊙273, 2051
Noroxin Tablets 2145

ESPERAL (Belgium, France)
DISULFIRAM
Antabuse Tablets 3474

ESPERSON (Brazil, Hong Kong, Thailand)
DESOXIMETASONE
Topicort Cream 2025
Topicort Gel 2025
Topicort LP Cream 2025
Topicort Ointment 2025

ESPESIL (Finland)
ACEBUTOLOL HYDROCHLORIDE
Sectral Capsules 3589

ESPO (Japan)
EPOETIN ALFA
Epogen for Injection 582
Procrit for Injection 2502

ESRADIN (Italy)
ISRADIPINE
DynaCirc CR Tablets 2923

ESSAVEN 60 (Germany)
HEPARIN SODIUM
Heparin Lock Flush Solution 3509
Heparin Sodium Injection 3511

ESTEROMICIN (Mexico)
ERYTHROMYCIN
Emgel 2% Topical Gel 1285
Ery-Tab Tablets 448
Erythromycin Base Filmtab Tablets 454
Erythromycin Delayed-Release Capsules, USP 455
PCE Dispertab Tablets 498

ESTIMA (France)
PROGESTERONE
Crinone 4% Gel 3213
Crinone 8% Gel 3213
Prometrium Capsules (100 mg, 200 mg) 3261

ESTOMIL (Spain)
LANSOPRAZOLE
Prevacid Delayed-Release Capsules 3292

ESTRABETA (Germany)
ESTRADIOL
Alora Transdermal System 3372
Climara Transdermal System 958
Estrace Vaginal Cream 3358
Estring Vaginal Ring 2811
Vivelle Transdermal System 2412
Vivelle-Dot Transdermal System 2416

ESTRACE (Canada)
ESTRADIOL
Alora Transdermal System 3372
Climara Transdermal System 958
Estrace Vaginal Cream 3358
Estring Vaginal Ring 2811
Vivelle Transdermal System 2412
Vivelle-Dot Transdermal System 2416

ESTRADERM (Australia, Austria, Belgium, Brazil, Canada, Denmark, Finland, France, Germany, Hong Kong, Irish Republic, Israel, Italy, Mexico, New Zealand, Norway, Portugal, Singapore, South Africa, Spain, Sweden, Switzerland, The Netherlands, United Kingdom)
ESTRADIOL
Alora Transdermal System 3372
Climara Transdermal System 958
Estrace Vaginal Cream 3358
Estring Vaginal Ring 2811
Vivelle Transdermal System 2412
Vivelle-Dot Transdermal System 2416

ESTRAMON (Austria, Germany, Irish Republic, Switzerland)
ESTRADIOL
Alora Transdermal System 3372
Climara Transdermal System 958
Estrace Vaginal Cream 3358
Estring Vaginal Ring 2811
Vivelle Transdermal System 2412
Vivelle-Dot Transdermal System 2416

ESTREVA (Hong Kong, Monaco)
ESTRADIOL
Alora Transdermal System 3372
Climara Transdermal System 958
Estrace Vaginal Cream 3358
Estring Vaginal Ring 2811
Vivelle Transdermal System 2412
Vivelle-Dot Transdermal System 2416

ESTRIFAM (Germany)
ESTRADIOL
Alora Transdermal System 3372
Climara Transdermal System 958
Estrace Vaginal Cream 3358
Estring Vaginal Ring 2811
Vivelle Transdermal System 2412
Vivelle-Dot Transdermal System 2416

ESTRING (Australia, Austria, Canada, Denmark, Finland, Germany, New Zealand, Norway, South Africa, Switzerland, The Netherlands, United Kingdom)
ESTRADIOL
Alora Transdermal System 3372
Climara Transdermal System 958
Estrace Vaginal Cream 3358
Estring Vaginal Ring 2811
Vivelle Transdermal System 2412
Vivelle-Dot Transdermal System 2416

ESTROCLIM (Italy)
ESTRADIOL
Alora Transdermal System 3372
Climara Transdermal System 958
Estrace Vaginal Cream 3358
Estring Vaginal Ring 2811
Vivelle Transdermal System 2412
Vivelle-Dot Transdermal System 2416

ESTROFEM (Australia, Austria, Belgium, Denmark, Finland, France, Hong Kong, Irish Republic, Israel, Italy, New Zealand, Portugal, Singapore, South Africa, Thailand, The Netherlands)
ESTRADIOL
Alora Transdermal System 3372
Climara Transdermal System 958
Estrace Vaginal Cream 3358
Estring Vaginal Ring 2811
Vivelle Transdermal System 2412
Vivelle-Dot Transdermal System 2416

ESTROFEM N (Switzerland)
ESTRADIOL
Alora Transdermal System 3372
Climara Transdermal System 958
Estrace Vaginal Cream 3358
Estring Vaginal Ring 2811
Vivelle Transdermal System 2412
Vivelle-Dot Transdermal System 2416

ESTROGEL (Austria, Canada, Denmark, Finland)
ESTRADIOL
Alora Transdermal System 3372
Climara Transdermal System 958
Estrace Vaginal Cream 3358
Estring Vaginal Ring 2811
Vivelle Transdermal System 2412
Vivelle-Dot Transdermal System 2416

ESTRONAR (Portugal)
ESTRADIOL
Alora Transdermal System 3372
Climara Transdermal System 958
Estrace Vaginal Cream 3358
Estring Vaginal Ring 2811
Vivelle Transdermal System 2412
Vivelle-Dot Transdermal System 2416

ESTRONORM (Germany)
ESTRADIOL
Alora Transdermal System 3372
Climara Transdermal System 958
Estrace Vaginal Cream 3358
Estring Vaginal Ring 2811
Vivelle Transdermal System 2412
Vivelle-Dot Transdermal System 2416

ESTROXYN (Australia)
TAMOXIFEN CITRATE
Nolvadex Tablets 678

ESTULIC (Belgium, France, Germany, Japan, Spain, Switzerland, The Netherlands)
GUANFACINE HYDROCHLORIDE
Tenex Tablets 2942

ETA BIOCORTILEN (Italy)
DEXAMETHASONE SODIUM PHOSPHATE/NEOMYCIN SULFATE
NeoDecadron Sterile Ophthalmic Solution 2144

ETA CORTILEN (Italy)
DEXAMETHASONE SODIUM PHOSPHATE
Decadron Phosphate Injection 2081
Decadron Phosphate Sterile Ophthalmic Ointment .... ⊙280, 2083
Decadron Phosphate Sterile Ophthalmic Solution 2084

ETABUS (Mexico)
DISULFIRAM
Antabuse Tablets 3474

ETAMUCIN (Austria)
SODIUM HYALURONATE
Hyalgan Solution 3080

ETAPIAM (Italy)
ETHAMBUTOL HYDROCHLORIDE
Myambutol Tablets 1290

ETERCICLINA (Brazil)
GUAIFENESIN
Organidin NR Liquid 3350
Organidin NR Tablets 3350

ETHATYL (South Africa)
ETHIONAMIDE
Trecator-SC Tablets 3598

ETHBUTOL (Thailand)
ETHAMBUTOL HYDROCHLORIDE
Myambutol Tablets 1290

ETHEOPHYL (Germany)
THEOPHYLLINE
Aerolate Jr. T.D. Capsules 1361
Aerolate Liquid 1361
Aerolate Sr. T.D. Capsules 1361
Theo-Dur Extended-Release Tablets 1835
Uni-Dur Extended-Release Tablets 1841
Uniphyl 400 mg and 600 mg Tablets 2903

ETHIMIL (United Kingdom)
VERAPAMIL HYDROCHLORIDE
Covera-HS Tablets 3199
Isoptin SR Tablets 467
Verelan Capsules 3184
Verelan PM Capsules 3186

ETHIMYCIN (South Africa)
ERYTHROMYCIN STEARATE
Erythrocin Stearate Filmtab Tablets 452

ETHIPAM (South Africa)
DIAZEPAM
Valium Injectable 3026
Valium Tablets 3047

ETHYOL (Australia, Belgium, Canada, Denmark, Finland, France, Germany, Hong Kong, Israel, Italy, Mexico, New Zealand, Portugal, Singapore, South Africa, Spain, Sweden, Switzerland, Thailand, The Netherlands, United Kingdom)
AMIFOSTINE
Ethyol for Injection 2029

ETIBI (Austria, Canada, Germany, Hong Kong, Italy)
ETHAMBUTOL HYDROCHLORIDE
Myambutol Tablets 1290

ETILTOX (Italy)
DISULFIRAM
Antabuse Tablets 3474

ETIMONIS (Switzerland)
ISOSORBIDE MONONITRATE
Imdur Tablets 1826
Ismo Tablets 3524

ETIOCIDAN (Spain)
ETHIONAMIDE
Trecator-SC Tablets 3598

ETIZEM (Portugal)
DILTIAZEM HYDROCHLORIDE
Cardizem CD Capsules 1016
Cardizem Injectable 1018
Cardizem Lyo-Ject Syringe 1018
Cardizem Monovial 1018
Tiazac Capsules 1378

ETONOX (Thailand)
ETODOLAC
Lodine Capsules 3528
Lodine Tablets 3528
Lodine XL Extended-Release Tablets 3530

ETOPAN (Israel)
ETODOLAC
Lodine Capsules 3528
Lodine Tablets 3528
Lodine XL Extended-Release Tablets 3530

ETRAFON (Canada, South Africa)
AMITRIPTYLINE HYDROCHLORIDE/PERPHENAZINE
Etrafon 2-10 Tablets (2-10) 3115
Etrafon Tablets (2-25) 3115
Etrafon-Forte Tablets (4-25) 3115

ETYZEM (Italy)
DILTIAZEM HYDROCHLORIDE
Cardizem CD Capsules 1016
Cardizem Injectable 1018
Cardizem Lyo-Ject Syringe 1018
Cardizem Monovial 1018
Tiazac Capsules 1378

EUBINE (France)
OXYCODONE HYDROCHLORIDE
OxyContin Tablets 2912
OxyFast Oral Concentrate Solution 2916
OxyIR Capsules 2916
Percolone Tablets 1327
Roxicodone Tablets 3067

EUCARDIC (Irish Republic, Sweden, The Netherlands, United Kingdom)
CARVEDILOL
Coreg Tablets 1508

(⊙ Described in PDR For Ophthalmic Medicines™)

EUCARNIL (Italy)
LEVOCARNITINE
Carnitor Injection . . . 3242
Carnitor Tablets and Oral Solution . . . 3245

EUCID (Thailand)
OMEPRAZOLE
Prilosec Delayed-Release Capsules . . . 628

EUCOPROST (Spain)
FINASTERIDE
Propecia Tablets . . . 2172
Proscar Tablets . . . 2175

EUDIGOX (Italy)
DIGOXIN
Lanoxicaps Capsules . . . 1574
Lanoxin Elixir Pediatric . . . 1578
Lanoxin Injection . . . 1581
Lanoxin Injection Pediatric . . . 1584
Lanoxin Tablets . . . 1587

EUDUR (Austria)
TERBUTALINE SULFATE
Brethine Ampuls . . . 2314
Brethine Tablets . . . 2313

EUDYNA (Austria, Germany, Hong Kong, Mexico, Singapore)
TRETINOIN
Avita Cream . . . 999
Avita Gel . . . 1000
Renova 0.05% Cream . . . 2519
Retin-A Micro 0.1% . . . 2522
Vesanoid Capsules . . . 3037

EUFENIL (Mexico)
IBUPROFEN
Motrin Suspension, Oral Drops, Chewable Tablets, and Caplets . . . 2002

EUFILINA (Portugal, Spain)
THEOPHYLLINE
Aerolate Jr. T.D. Capsules . . . 1361
Aerolate Liquid . . . 1361
Aerolate Sr. T.D. Capsules . . . 1361
Theo-Dur Extended-Release Tablets . . . 1835
Uni-Dur Extended-Release Tablets . . . 1841
Uniphyl 400 mg and 600 mg Tablets . . . 2903

EUFLEX (Canada)
FLUTAMIDE
Eulexin Capsules . . . 3118

EUGALAC (Austria, Germany)
LACTULOSE
Kristalose for Oral Solution . . . 1007

EUGYNON (Hong Kong)
NORGESTREL
Ovrette Tablets . . . 3552

EUKODAL (Germany)
OXYCODONE HYDROCHLORIDE
OxyContin Tablets . . . 2912
OxyFast Oral Concentrate Solution . . . 2916
OxyIR Capsules . . . 2916
Percolone Tablets . . . 1327
Roxicodone Tablets . . . 3067

EULEXIN (Australia, Belgium, Brazil, Denmark, Finland, Israel, Italy, Mexico, New Zealand, Norway, Portugal, South Africa, Spain, Sweden, The Netherlands)
FLUTAMIDE
Eulexin Capsules . . . 3118

EULEXINE (France)
FLUTAMIDE
Eulexin Capsules . . . 3118

EUPHYLLIN (Belgium, Finland, Germany, Norway, South Africa)
THEOPHYLLINE
Aerolate Jr. T.D. Capsules . . . 1361
Aerolate Liquid . . . 1361
Aerolate Sr. T.D. Capsules . . . 1361
Theo-Dur Extended-Release Tablets . . . 1835
Uni-Dur Extended-Release Tablets . . . 1841
Uniphyl 400 mg and 600 mg Tablets . . . 2903

EUPHYLLIN 200 (Germany)
THEOPHYLLINE
Aerolate Jr. T.D. Capsules . . . 1361
Aerolate Liquid . . . 1361
Aerolate Sr. T.D. Capsules . . . 1361
Theo-Dur Extended-Release Tablets . . . 1835
Uni-Dur Extended-Release Tablets . . . 1841
Uniphyl 400 mg and 600 mg Tablets . . . 2903

EUPHYLLINE (France)
THEOPHYLLINE
Aerolate Jr. T.D. Capsules . . . 1361
Aerolate Liquid . . . 1361
Aerolate Sr. T.D. Capsules . . . 1361
Theo-Dur Extended-Release Tablets . . . 1835
Uni-Dur Extended-Release Tablets . . . 1841
Uniphyl 400 mg and 600 mg Tablets . . . 2903

EUPHYLONG (Germany, Hong Kong, Sweden, Switzerland, The Netherlands)
THEOPHYLLINE
Aerolate Jr. T.D. Capsules . . . 1361
Aerolate Liquid . . . 1361
Aerolate Sr. T.D. Capsules . . . 1361
Theo-Dur Extended-Release Tablets . . . 1835
Uni-Dur Extended-Release Tablets . . . 1841
Uniphyl 400 mg and 600 mg Tablets . . . 2903

EUPRESSIN (Brazil)
ENALAPRIL MALEATE
Vasotec Tablets . . . 2210

EUPRESSIN H (Brazil)
ENALAPRIL MALEATE/HYDROCHLOROTHIAZIDE
Vaseretic Tablets . . . 2204

EURADAL (Spain)
BISOPROLOL FUMARATE
Zebeta Tablets . . . 1885

EURALBEN (Mexico)
ALBENDAZOLE
Albenza Tablets . . . 1463

EURECEPTOR (Italy)
CIMETIDINE
Tagamet Tablets . . . 1644

EURECOR (Germany)
ISOSORBIDE DINITRATE
Isordil Sublingual Tablets . . . 3525
Isordil Titradose Tablets . . . 3526

EUREX (Germany)
PRAZOSIN HYDROCHLORIDE
Minipress Capsules . . . 2699

EURODIN (Japan)
ESTAZOLAM
ProSom Tablets . . . 500

EUROLAT (Mexico)
KETOCONAZOLE
Nizoral 2% Cream . . . 3620
Nizoral 2% Shampoo . . . 2007
Nizoral Tablets . . . 1791

EUROSAN (Switzerland)
CLOTRIMAZOLE
Lotrimin Cream 1% . . . 3128
Lotrimin Lotion 1% . . . 3128
Lotrimin Topical Solution 1% . . . 3128
Mycelex Troche . . . 573

EUROXI (Italy)
PIROXICAM
Feldene Capsules . . . 2685

EUSEDON MONO (Germany)
PROMETHAZINE HYDROCHLORIDE
Phenergan Injection . . . 3553
Phenergan Suppositories . . . 3556
Phenergan Syrup Fortis . . . 3554
Phenergan Syrup Plain . . . 3554
Phenergan Tablets . . . 3556

EUSKIN (Spain)
ERYTHROMYCIN
Emgel 2% Topical Gel . . . 1285
Ery-Tab Tablets . . . 448
Erythromycin Base Filmtab Tablets . . . 454
Erythromycin Delayed-Release Capsules, USP . . . 455
PCE Dispertab Tablets . . . 498

EUSTOPORIN (Germany)
NEOMYCIN SULFATE/POLYMYXIN B SULFATE
Neosporin G.U. Irrigant Sterile . . . 2256

EUVITOL (Italy)
VITAMIN A PALMITATE
Aquasol A Parenteral . . . 593

EVACALM (United Kingdom)
DIAZEPAM
Valium Injectable . . . 3026
Valium Tablets . . . 3047

EVASPRIN (Spain)
IBUPROFEN
Motrin Suspension, Oral Drops, Chewable Tablets, and Caplets . . . 2002

EVIANTRINA (Spain)
FAMOTIDINE
Pepcid Injection . . . 2153
Pepcid Injection Premixed . . . 2153
Pepcid RPD Orally Disintegrating Tablets . . . 2150
Pepcid Tablets . . . 2150
Pepcid for Oral Suspension . . . 2150

EVICER (Portugal)
CIMETIDINE
Tagamet Tablets . . . 1644

EVISTA (Australia, Austria, Belgium, Canada, Denmark, Finland, France, Germany, Irish Republic, Israel, Italy, Mexico, New Zealand, Norway, Portugal, Singapore, South Africa, Spain, Sweden, The Netherlands, United Kingdom)
RALOXIFENE HYDROCHLORIDE
Evista Tablets . . . 1915

EVITEX A (Spain)
VITAMIN A PALMITATE
Aquasol A Parenteral . . . 593

EVITOCOR (Germany)
ATENOLOL
Tenormin I.V. Injection . . . 692

EVITOCOR PLUS (Germany)
ATENOLOL
Tenormin I.V. Injection . . . 692

EVOPAD (Spain)
ESTRADIOL
Alora Transdermal System . . . 3372
Climara Transdermal System . . . 958
Estrace Vaginal Cream . . . 3358
Estring Vaginal Ring . . . 2811
Vivelle Transdermal System . . . 2412
Vivelle-Dot Transdermal System . . . 2416

EVOREL (Denmark, Finland, Germany, Irish Republic, Israel, Norway, South Africa, Sweden, United Kingdom)
ESTRADIOL
Alora Transdermal System . . . 3372
Climara Transdermal System . . . 958
Estrace Vaginal Cream . . . 3358
Estring Vaginal Ring . . . 2811
Vivelle Transdermal System . . . 2412
Vivelle-Dot Transdermal System . . . 2416

EVOREL CONTI (Irish Republic, United Kingdom)
ESTRADIOL
Alora Transdermal System . . . 3372
Climara Transdermal System . . . 958
Estrace Vaginal Cream . . . 3358
Estring Vaginal Ring . . . 2811
Vivelle Transdermal System . . . 2412
Vivelle-Dot Transdermal System . . . 2416

EXAMICYN (Mexico)
ERYTHROMYCIN
Emgel 2% Topical Gel . . . 1285
Ery-Tab Tablets . . . 448
Erythromycin Base Filmtab Tablets . . . 454
Erythromycin Delayed-Release Capsules, USP . . . 455
PCE Dispertab Tablets . . . 498

EXAVERM (Mexico)
MEBENDAZOLE
Vermox Chewable Tablets . . . 2017

EXBENZOL (Mexico)
MEBENDAZOLE
Vermox Chewable Tablets . . . 2017

EXCAUGH (Hong Kong)
GUAIFENESIN
Organidin NR Liquid . . . 3350
Organidin NR Tablets . . . 3350

EXIDOL (Belgium)
IBUPROFEN
Motrin Suspension, Oral Drops, Chewable Tablets, and Caplets . . . 2002

EXIPAN (Israel)
PIROXICAM
Feldene Capsules . . . 2685

EXNEURAL (Germany)
IBUPROFEN
Motrin Suspension, Oral Drops, Chewable Tablets, and Caplets . . . 2002

EXOCIN (Denmark, Finland, Irish Republic, Italy, Portugal, South Africa, Spain, United Kingdom)
OFLOXACIN
Floxin I.V. . . . 2526
Floxin Otic Solution . . . 1219
Floxin Tablets . . . 2529
Ocuflox Ophthalmic Solution . . . 554

EXOCINE (France)
OFLOXACIN
Floxin I.V. . . . 2526
Floxin Otic Solution . . . 1219
Floxin Tablets . . . 2529
Ocuflox Ophthalmic Solution . . . 554

EXODERIL (Austria, Germany, Hong Kong, Singapore, Switzerland)
NAFTIFINE HYDROCHLORIDE
Naftin Cream . . . 2224
Naftin Gel . . . 2224

EXPANFEN (France)
IBUPROFEN
Motrin Suspension, Oral Drops, Chewable Tablets, and Caplets . . . 2002

EXPECTORANT COUGH FORMULA (Canada)
GUAIFENESIN
Organidin NR Liquid . . . 3350
Organidin NR Tablets . . . 3350

EXPECTORANT COUGH SYRUP (Canada)
GUAIFENESIN
Organidin NR Liquid . . . 3350
Organidin NR Tablets . . . 3350

EXPECTORANT SYRUP (Canada)
GUAIFENESIN
Organidin NR Liquid . . . 3350
Organidin NR Tablets . . . 3350

EXPHOBIN N (Germany)
MEPROBAMATE
Miltown Tablets . . . 3349

EXPROS (Finland)
TAMSULOSIN HYDROCHLORIDE
Flomax Capsules . . . 1044

EXPULIN CHESTY COUGH (United Kingdom)
GUAIFENESIN
Organidin NR Liquid . . . 3350
Organidin NR Tablets . . . 3350

EXTENY (Mexico)
MEBENDAZOLE
Vermox Chewable Tablets . . . 2017

EXTISER Q (Mexico)
PRAZIQUANTEL
Biltricide Tablets . . . 887

EXTRACORT (Germany)
TRIAMCINOLONE ACETONIDE
Azmacort Inhalation Aerosol . . . 728
Nasacort AQ Nasal Spray . . . 752
Nasacort Nasal Inhaler . . . 750

EXTRAFER (Italy)
FERRIC SODIUM GLUCONATE
Ferrlecit Injection . . . 3386

EXTRAPLUS (Spain)
KETOPROFEN
Orudis Capsules . . . 3548
Oruvail Capsules . . . 3548

EXTUR (Spain)
INDAPAMIDE
Indapamide Tablets . . . 2286

EYEDEX (Thailand)
DEXAMETHASONE SODIUM PHOSPHATE/NEOMYCIN SULFATE
NeoDecadron Sterile Ophthalmic Solution . . . 2144

EYESTIL (Canada)
SODIUM HYALURONATE
Hyalgan Solution . . . 3080

EZOSINA (Italy)
TERAZOSIN HYDROCHLORIDE
Hytrin Capsules . . . 464

FACICAM (Mexico)
PIROXICAM
Feldene Capsules . . . 2685

FACORT (Thailand)
TRIAMCINOLONE ACETONIDE
Azmacort Inhalation Aerosol . . . 728
Nasacort AQ Nasal Spray . . . 752
Nasacort Nasal Inhaler . . . 750

FACTREL (Canada)
GONADORELIN HYDROCHLORIDE
Factrel . . . 3633

FADINE (Thailand)
FAMOTIDINE
Pepcid Injection . . . 2153
Pepcid Injection Premixed . . . 2153
Pepcid RPD Orally Disintegrating Tablets . . . 2150
Pepcid Tablets . . . 2150
Pepcid for Oral Suspension . . . 2150

FADO (Italy)
CEFAMANDOLE NAFATE
Mandol Vials . . . 1953

FADOL (Mexico)
HYDROCORTISONE
Anusol-HC Cream 2.5% . . . 2237
Hydrocortone Tablets . . . 2106

FAGASTRIL (Spain)
FAMOTIDINE
Pepcid Injection . . . 2153
Pepcid Injection Premixed . . . 2153
Pepcid RPD Orally Disintegrating Tablets . . . 2150
Pepcid Tablets . . . 2150
Pepcid for Oral Suspension . . . 2150

FAGIZOL (Mexico)
METRONIDAZOLE
MetroCream . . . 1404

MetroGel 1405
MetroGel-Vaginal Gel 1986
MetroLotion 1405
Noritate Cream 1224

FAGUS (Spain)
RANITIDINE HYDROCHLORIDE
Zantac 150 EFFERdose Granules 1690
Zantac 150 EFFERdose Tablets 1690
Zantac 150 Tablets 1690
Zantac 300 Tablets 1690
Zantac Injection 1688
Zantac Injection Premixed 1688
Zantac Syrup 1690

FAGUSAN (Germany)
GUAIFENESIN
Organidin NR Liquid 3350
Organidin NR Tablets 3350

FALEXOL (Mexico)
CEPHALEXIN
Keflex Oral Suspension 1237
Keflex Pulvules 1237

FALICARD (Germany)
VERAPAMIL HYDROCHLORIDE
Covera-HS Tablets 3199
Isoptin SR Tablets 467
Verelan Capsules 3184
Verelan PM Capsules 3186

FALITONSIN (Germany)
ATENOLOL
Tenormin I.V. Injection 692

FAMEL EXPECTORANT (United Kingdom)
GUAIFENESIN
Organidin NR Liquid 3350
Organidin NR Tablets 3350

FAMEL HONEY & LEMON COUGH PASTILLES (United Kingdom)
GUAIFENESIN
Organidin NR Liquid 3350
Organidin NR Tablets 3350

FAMO (Israel)
FAMOTIDINE
Pepcid Injection 2153
Pepcid Injection Premixed 2153
Pepcid RPD Orally Disintegrating Tablets 2150
Pepcid Tablets 2150
Pepcid for Oral Suspension 2150

FAMOC (Singapore, Thailand)
FAMOTIDINE
Pepcid Injection 2153
Pepcid Injection Premixed 2153
Pepcid RPD Orally Disintegrating Tablets 2150
Pepcid Tablets 2150
Pepcid for Oral Suspension 2150

FAMOCID (Singapore, Thailand)
FAMOTIDINE
Pepcid Injection 2153
Pepcid Injection Premixed 2153
Pepcid RPD Orally Disintegrating Tablets 2150
Pepcid Tablets 2150
Pepcid for Oral Suspension 2150

FAMODIL (Italy)
FAMOTIDINE
Pepcid Injection 2153
Pepcid Injection Premixed 2153
Pepcid RPD Orally Disintegrating Tablets 2150
Pepcid Tablets 2150
Pepcid for Oral Suspension 2150

FAMODINE (Brazil, Hong Kong)
FAMOTIDINE
Pepcid Injection 2153
Pepcid Injection Premixed 2153
Pepcid RPD Orally Disintegrating Tablets 2150
Pepcid Tablets 2150
Pepcid for Oral Suspension 2150

FAMONOX (Thailand)
FAMOTIDINE
Pepcid Injection 2153
Pepcid Injection Premixed 2153
Pepcid RPD Orally Disintegrating Tablets 2150
Pepcid Tablets 2150
Pepcid for Oral Suspension 2150

FAMOPSIN (Hong Kong, Singapore, Thailand)
FAMOTIDINE
Pepcid Injection 2153
Pepcid Injection Premixed 2153
Pepcid RPD Orally Disintegrating Tablets 2150
Pepcid Tablets 2150
Pepcid for Oral Suspension 2150

FAMOSET (Brazil)
FAMOTIDINE
Pepcid Injection 2153
Pepcid Injection Premixed 2153
Pepcid RPD Orally Disintegrating Tablets 2150
Pepcid Tablets 2150
Pepcid for Oral Suspension 2150

FAMOTAL (Norway)
FAMOTIDINE
Pepcid Injection 2153
Pepcid Injection Premixed 2153
Pepcid RPD Orally Disintegrating Tablets 2150
Pepcid Tablets 2150
Pepcid for Oral Suspension 2150

FAMOTEC (United Arab Emirates)
FAMOTIDINE
Pepcid Injection 2153
Pepcid Injection Premixed 2153
Pepcid RPD Orally Disintegrating Tablets 2150
Pepcid Tablets 2150
Pepcid for Oral Suspension 2150

FAMOTIN (Singapore, Thailand)
FAMOTIDINE
Pepcid Injection 2153
Pepcid Injection Premixed 2153
Pepcid RPD Orally Disintegrating Tablets 2150
Pepcid Tablets 2150
Pepcid for Oral Suspension 2150

FAMOX (Brazil, Hong Kong, New Zealand)
FAMOTIDINE
Pepcid Injection 2153
Pepcid Injection Premixed 2153
Pepcid RPD Orally Disintegrating Tablets 2150
Pepcid Tablets 2150
Pepcid for Oral Suspension 2150

FAMOXAL (Mexico)
FAMOTIDINE
Pepcid Injection 2153
Pepcid Injection Premixed 2153
Pepcid RPD Orally Disintegrating Tablets 2150
Pepcid Tablets 2150
Pepcid for Oral Suspension 2150

FAMULCER (Spain)
FAMOTIDINE
Pepcid Injection 2153
Pepcid Injection Premixed 2153
Pepcid RPD Orally Disintegrating Tablets 2150
Pepcid Tablets 2150
Pepcid for Oral Suspension 2150

FANCIADAZOL (Mexico)
MEBENDAZOLE
Vermox Chewable Tablets 2017

FANOSIN (Spain)
FAMOTIDINE
Pepcid Injection 2153
Pepcid Injection Premixed 2153
Pepcid RPD Orally Disintegrating Tablets 2150
Pepcid Tablets 2150
Pepcid for Oral Suspension 2150

FANOX (Spain)
FAMOTIDINE
Pepcid Injection 2153
Pepcid Injection Premixed 2153
Pepcid RPD Orally Disintegrating Tablets 2150
Pepcid Tablets 2150
Pepcid for Oral Suspension 2150

FARAXEN (Mexico)
NAPROXEN
EC-Naprosyn Delayed-Release Tablets 2967
Naprosyn Suspension 2967
Naprosyn Tablets 2967

FARECEF (Italy)
CEFOPERAZONE SODIUM
Cefobid Intravenous/Intramuscular 2671
Cefobid Pharmacy Bulk Package - Not for Direct Infusion 2673

FARESTON (Australia, Austria, Belgium, Denmark, Finland, France, Germany, Irish Republic, Italy, Mexico, New Zealand, Portugal, South Africa, Spain, Sweden, Switzerland, Thailand, The Netherlands, United Kingdom)
TOREMIFENE CITRATE
Fareston Tablets 3237

FARGANESSE (Italy)
PROMETHAZINE HYDROCHLORIDE
Phenergan Injection 3553
Phenergan Suppositories 3556
Phenergan Syrup Fortis 3554
Phenergan Syrup Plain 3554
Phenergan Tablets 3556

FARLAC (Brazil)
LACTULOSE
Kristalose for Oral Solution 1007

FARLUTAL (Australia, Austria, Belgium, Brazil, Finland, France, Germany, Hong Kong, Italy, Mexico, New Zealand, Norway, Singapore, South Africa, Spain, Sweden, Switzerland, Thailand, The Netherlands, United Kingdom)
MEDROXYPROGESTERONE ACETATE
Depo-Provera Contraceptive Injection 2798
Provera Tablets 2853

FARMIBLASTINA (Spain)
DOXORUBICIN HYDROCHLORIDE
Adriamycin PFS/RDF Injection 2767

FARMICAM (Mexico)
PIROXICAM
Feldene Capsules 2685

FARMICETINA P7 (Brazil)
CHLORAMPHENICOL
Chloromycetin Ophthalmic Ointment, 1% . . . . ⊙296
Chloromycetin Ophthalmic Solution . . . . ⊙297
Chloroptic Sterile Ophthalmic Ointment . . . . ⊙234
Chloroptic Sterile Ophthalmic Solution . . . . ⊙235

FARMIN (Mexico)
DIAZEPAM
Valium Injectable 3026
Valium Tablets 3047

FARMODOXI (Italy)
DOXYCYCLINE HYCLATE
Doryx Coated Pellet Filled Capsules 3357
Periostat Tablets 1208
Vibra-Tabs Film Coated Tablets 2735
Vibramycin Hyclate Capsules 2735
Vibramycin Hyclate Intravenous 2737

FARMOTEX (Mexico)
FAMOTIDINE
Pepcid Injection 2153
Pepcid Injection Premixed 2153
Pepcid RPD Orally Disintegrating Tablets 2150
Pepcid Tablets 2150
Pepcid for Oral Suspension 2150

FARNIC (Italy)
NICARDIPINE HYDROCHLORIDE
Cardene I.V. 3485

FARPRESSE (Portugal)
LISINOPRIL
Prinivil Tablets 2164
Zestril Tablets 698

FARTRICON (Mexico)
METRONIDAZOLE
MetroCream 1404
MetroGel 1405
MetroGel-Vaginal Gel 1986
MetroLotion 1405
Noritate Cream 1224

FARXEN (Mexico)
NAPROXEN
EC-Naprosyn Delayed-Release Tablets 2967
Naprosyn Suspension 2967
Naprosyn Tablets 2967

FASAX (Germany)
PIROXICAM
Feldene Capsules 2685

FASE (Italy)
APROTININ
Trasylol Injection 909

FASIDINE (Thailand)
FAMOTIDINE
Pepcid Injection 2153
Pepcid Injection Premixed 2153
Pepcid RPD Orally Disintegrating Tablets 2150
Pepcid Tablets 2150
Pepcid for Oral Suspension 2150

FASPIC (Italy, Spain, Switzerland)
IBUPROFEN
Motrin Suspension, Oral Drops, Chewable Tablets, and Caplets 2002

FASTIN (Canada)
PHENTERMINE HYDROCHLORIDE
Adipex-P Capsules 1406
Adipex-P Tablets 1406

FASTUM (Belgium, Hong Kong, Irish Republic, Italy, Portugal, Singapore, South Africa, Spain, Switzerland, Thailand)
KETOPROFEN
Orudis Capsules 3548
Oruvail Capsules 3548

FATIDIN (Portugal)
FAMOTIDINE
Pepcid Injection 2153
Pepcid Injection Premixed 2153
Pepcid RPD Orally Disintegrating Tablets 2150
Pepcid Tablets 2150
Pepcid for Oral Suspension 2150

FAULDETIC (Portugal)
DACARBAZINE
DTIC-Dome 902

FAULDOXO (Portugal)
DOXORUBICIN HYDROCHLORIDE
Adriamycin PFS/RDF Injection 2767

FAVERIN (Australia, Hong Kong, Irish Republic, Singapore, Thailand, United Kingdom)
FLUVOXAMINE MALEATE
Luvox Tablets (25, 50, 100 mg) 3256

FAVOREX (Germany)
SOTALOL HYDROCHLORIDE
Betapace Tablets 950

FAVOXIL (Israel)
FLUVOXAMINE MALEATE
Luvox Tablets (25, 50, 100 mg) 3256

FAWODIN (Mexico)
FAMOTIDINE
Pepcid Injection 2153
Pepcid Injection Premixed 2153
Pepcid RPD Orally Disintegrating Tablets 2150
Pepcid Tablets 2150
Pepcid for Oral Suspension 2150

FEBRAX (Mexico)
NAPROXEN SODIUM
Anaprox DS Tablets 2967
Anaprox Tablets 2967
Naprelan Tablets 1293

FEDIP (Austria, Switzerland)
NIFEDIPINE
Adalat CC Tablets 877
Procardia Capsules 2708
Procardia XL Extended Release Tablets 2710

FEGENOR (France)
FENOFIBRATE
Tricor Capsules, Micronized 513

FELCAM (Thailand)
PIROXICAM
Feldene Capsules 2685

FELDEN (Austria, Denmark, Finland, Norway, Sweden, Switzerland)
PIROXICAM
Feldene Capsules 2685

FELDENE (Australia, Belgium, Brazil, Canada, France, Hong Kong, Irish Republic, Israel, Italy, Mexico, New Zealand, Portugal, Singapore, South Africa, Thailand, The Netherlands, United Kingdom)
PIROXICAM
Feldene Capsules 2685

FELDEXICAN (Brazil)
PIROXICAM
Feldene Capsules 2685

FELDOX (Brazil)
PIROXICAM
Feldene Capsules 2685

FELEXIN (Hong Kong, Singapore, Thailand)
CEPHALEXIN
Keflex Oral Suspension 1237
Keflex Pulvules 1237

FELIBERAL (Mexico)
ENALAPRIL MALEATE
Vasotec Tablets 2210

FELIXENE (Spain)
CIPROFLOXACIN HYDROCHLORIDE
Ciloxan Ophthalmic Ointment 538
Ciloxan Ophthalmic Solution . . . . ⊙209, 538
Cipro Tablets 887

FELLER (Brazil)
MEBENDAZOLE
Vermox Chewable Tablets 2017

FELNAN (Brazil)
PIROXICAM
Feldene Capsules 2685

FELODAY (Italy)
FELODIPINE
Plendil Extended-Release Tablets 623

FELODUR (Australia)
FELODIPINE
Plendil Extended-Release Tablets 623

FELROX (Thailand)
PIROXICAM
Feldene Capsules 2685

FEM 7 (Germany, Mexico, Singapore, The Netherlands)
ESTRADIOL
- Alora Transdermal System 3372
- Climara Transdermal System 958
- Estrace Vaginal Cream 3358
- Estring Vaginal Ring 2811
- Vivelle Transdermal System 2412
- Vivelle-Dot Transdermal System 2416

FEMAFEN (United Kingdom)
IBUPROFEN
- Motrin Suspension, Oral Drops, Chewable Tablets, and Caplets 2002

FEMANEST (Denmark, Sweden)
ESTRADIOL
- Alora Transdermal System 3372
- Climara Transdermal System 958
- Estrace Vaginal Cream 3358
- Estring Vaginal Ring 2811
- Vivelle Transdermal System 2412
- Vivelle-Dot Transdermal System 2416

FEMAPIRIN (The Netherlands)
IBUPROFEN
- Motrin Suspension, Oral Drops, Chewable Tablets, and Caplets 2002

FEMAPRIN (Spain)
IBUPROFEN
- Motrin Suspension, Oral Drops, Chewable Tablets, and Caplets 2002

FEMATAB (Irish Republic)
ESTRADIOL
- Alora Transdermal System 3372
- Climara Transdermal System 958
- Estrace Vaginal Cream 3358
- Estring Vaginal Ring 2811
- Vivelle Transdermal System 2412
- Vivelle-Dot Transdermal System 2416

FEMATRIX (Irish Republic, United Kingdom)
ESTRADIOL
- Alora Transdermal System 3372
- Climara Transdermal System 958
- Estrace Vaginal Cream 3358
- Estring Vaginal Ring 2811
- Vivelle Transdermal System 2412
- Vivelle-Dot Transdermal System 2416

FEMEX (The Netherlands)
NAPROXEN SODIUM
- Anaprox DS Tablets 2967
- Anaprox Tablets 2967
- Naprelan Tablets 1293

FEMIDOL (Spain)
IBUPROFEN
- Motrin Suspension, Oral Drops, Chewable Tablets, and Caplets 2002

FEMIGEL (South Africa)
ESTRADIOL
- Alora Transdermal System 3372
- Climara Transdermal System 958
- Estrace Vaginal Cream 3358
- Estring Vaginal Ring 2811
- Vivelle Transdermal System 2412
- Vivelle-Dot Transdermal System 2416

FEMINALIN (Spain)
IBUPROFEN
- Motrin Suspension, Oral Drops, Chewable Tablets, and Caplets 2002

FEMINOVA (Belgium)
ESTRADIOL
- Alora Transdermal System 3372
- Climara Transdermal System 958
- Estrace Vaginal Cream 3358
- Estring Vaginal Ring 2811
- Vivelle Transdermal System 2412
- Vivelle-Dot Transdermal System 2416

FEMIPRES (Italy)
MOEXIPRIL HYDROCHLORIDE
- Univasc Tablets 3181

FEMIPRES PLUS (Italy)
HYDROCHLOROTHIAZIDE/MOEXIPRIL HYDROCHLORIDE
- Uniretic Tablets 3178

FEM-MONO (Denmark, Sweden)
ISOSORBIDE MONONITRATE
- Imdur Tablets 1826
- Ismo Tablets 3524

FEMOSTON CONTI (Switzerland, United Kingdom)
ESTRADIOL
- Alora Transdermal System 3372
- Climara Transdermal System 958
- Estrace Vaginal Cream 3358
- Estring Vaginal Ring 2811
- Vivelle Transdermal System 2412
- Vivelle-Dot Transdermal System 2416

FEMOSTON MONO (Germany)
ESTRADIOL
- Alora Transdermal System 3372
- Climara Transdermal System 958
- Estrace Vaginal Cream 3358
- Estring Vaginal Ring 2811
- Vivelle Transdermal System 2412
- Vivelle-Dot Transdermal System 2416

FEMPRESS (Germany, Switzerland)
MOEXIPRIL HYDROCHLORIDE
- Univasc Tablets 3181

FEMPRESS PLUS (Germany)
HYDROCHLOROTHIAZIDE/MOEXIPRIL HYDROCHLORIDE
- Uniretic Tablets 3178

FEMSEPT (France)
ESTRADIOL
- Alora Transdermal System 3372
- Climara Transdermal System 958
- Estrace Vaginal Cream 3358
- Estring Vaginal Ring 2811
- Vivelle Transdermal System 2412
- Vivelle-Dot Transdermal System 2416

FEMSEVEN (Austria, Denmark, Finland, Italy, Sweden, Switzerland, United Kingdom)
ESTRADIOL
- Alora Transdermal System 3372
- Climara Transdermal System 958
- Estrace Vaginal Cream 3358
- Estring Vaginal Ring 2811
- Vivelle Transdermal System 2412
- Vivelle-Dot Transdermal System 2416

FEMTRAN (Australia, New Zealand)
ESTRADIOL
- Alora Transdermal System 3372
- Climara Transdermal System 958
- Estrace Vaginal Cream 3358
- Estring Vaginal Ring 2811
- Vivelle Transdermal System 2412
- Vivelle-Dot Transdermal System 2416

FENAC (Australia)
DICLOFENAC SODIUM
- Voltaren Tablets 2315
- Voltaren-XR Tablets 2315

FENADOL (Italy)
DICLOFENAC SODIUM
- Voltaren Tablets 2315
- Voltaren-XR Tablets 2315

FENALGIC (France)
IBUPROFEN
- Motrin Suspension, Oral Drops, Chewable Tablets, and Caplets 2002

FENAMIC (Thailand)
MEFENAMIC ACID
- Ponstel Capsules 1356

FENAMIN (South Africa)
MEFENAMIC ACID
- Ponstel Capsules 1356

FENAMON (Singapore, Thailand)
NIFEDIPINE
- Adalat CC Tablets 877
- Procardia Capsules 2708
- Procardia XL Extended Release Tablets 2710

FENANTOIN (Sweden)
PHENYTOIN
- Dilantin Infatabs 2624
- Dilantin-125 Oral Suspension 2625

FENAREN (Austria)
DICLOFENAC SODIUM
- Voltaren Tablets 2315
- Voltaren-XR Tablets 2315

FENAZIL (Italy)
PROMETHAZINE HYDROCHLORIDE
- Phenergan Injection 3553
- Phenergan Suppositories 3556
- Phenergan Syrup Fortis 3554
- Phenergan Syrup Plain 3554
- Phenergan Tablets 3556

FENBID (United Kingdom)
IBUPROFEN
- Motrin Suspension, Oral Drops, Chewable Tablets, and Caplets 2002

FENERGAN (Brazil, Portugal)
PROMETHAZINE HYDROCHLORIDE
- Phenergan Injection 3553
- Phenergan Suppositories 3556
- Phenergan Syrup Fortis 3554
- Phenergan Syrup Plain 3554
- Phenergan Tablets 3556

FENICOL (Belgium, Canada, South Africa, Thailand)
CHLORAMPHENICOL
- Chloromycetin Ophthalmic Ointment, 1% ⊙296
- Chloromycetin Ophthalmic Solution ⊙297
- Chloroptic Sterile Ophthalmic Ointment ⊙234
- Chloroptic Sterile Ophthalmic Solution ⊙235

FENIDEX (Brazil)
DEXAMETHASONE
- Decadron Elixir 2078
- Decadron Tablets 2079

FENIDINA (Italy)
NIFEDIPINE
- Adalat CC Tablets 877
- Procardia Capsules 2708
- Procardia XL Extended Release Tablets 2710

FENIKEN (Mexico)
NIFEDIPINE
- Adalat CC Tablets 877
- Procardia Capsules 2708
- Procardia XL Extended Release Tablets 2710

FENIL-V (Portugal)
DICLOFENAC SODIUM
- Voltaren Tablets 2315
- Voltaren-XR Tablets 2315

FENISOL (Mexico)
CHLORAMPHENICOL
- Chloromycetin Ophthalmic Ointment, 1% ⊙296
- Chloromycetin Ophthalmic Solution ⊙297
- Chloroptic Sterile Ophthalmic Ointment ⊙234
- Chloroptic Sterile Ophthalmic Solution ⊙235

FENISTIL (Germany)
HYDROCORTISONE ACETATE
- Anusol-HC Suppositories 2238
- Cortifoam Rectal Foam 3170
- Hydrocortone Acetate Injectable Suspension 2103
- Proctocort Suppositories 2264

FENIZZARD (Mexico)
CHLORAMPHENICOL
- Chloromycetin Ophthalmic Ointment, 1% ⊙296
- Chloromycetin Ophthalmic Solution ⊙297
- Chloroptic Sterile Ophthalmic Ointment ⊙234
- Chloroptic Sterile Ophthalmic Solution ⊙235

FENOBETA (Germany)
FENOFIBRATE
- Tricor Capsules, Micronized 513

FENOGAL (Belgium)
FENOFIBRATE
- Tricor Capsules, Micronized 513

FENOKET (United Kingdom)
KETOPROFEN
- Orudis Capsules 3548
- Oruvail Capsules 3548

FENOLIP (Austria)
FENOFIBRATE
- Tricor Capsules, Micronized 513

FENOPTIC (Portugal)
CHLORAMPHENICOL
- Chloromycetin Ophthalmic Ointment, 1% ⊙296
- Chloromycetin Ophthalmic Solution ⊙297
- Chloroptic Sterile Ophthalmic Ointment ⊙234
- Chloroptic Sterile Ophthalmic Solution ⊙235

FENSAID (Australia)
PIROXICAM
- Feldene Capsules 2685

FENSEL (Spain)
FELODIPINE
- Plendil Extended-Release Tablets 623

FENTAMOX (United Kingdom)
TAMOXIFEN CITRATE
- Nolvadex Tablets 678

FENTANEST (Italy, Mexico, Spain)
FENTANYL CITRATE
- Actiq 1184

FENTAZIN (Irish Republic, United Kingdom)
PERPHENAZINE
- Trilafon Injection 3160
- Trilafon Tablets 3160

FERCAYL (Belgium)
IRON DEXTRAN
- INFeD Injection 3388

FERGON (Spain)
CEPHALEXIN
- Keflex Oral Suspension 1237
- Keflex Pulvules 1237

FERLIXIT (Italy)
FERRIC SODIUM GLUCONATE
- Ferrlecit Injection 3386

FERMATHRON (Australia, United Kingdom)
SODIUM HYALURONATE
- Hyalgan Solution 3080

FERMENTMYCIN (South Africa)
GENTAMICIN SULFATE
- Genoptic Ophthalmic Ointment ⊙239
- Genoptic Sterile Ophthalmic Solution ⊙239

FERRI-EMINA (Italy)
FERRIC SODIUM GLUCONATE
- Ferrlecit Injection 3386

FERRITIN OTI (Italy)
FERRIC SODIUM GLUCONATE
- Ferrlecit Injection 3386

FERRLECIT (Germany, Israel)
FERRIC SODIUM GLUCONATE
- Ferrlecit Injection 3386

FERROCEL (Mexico)
IRON DEXTRAN
- INFeD Injection 3388

FERROIN (Mexico)
IRON DEXTRAN
- INFeD Injection 3388

FERROSPRINT (Italy)
FERRIC SODIUM GLUCONATE
- Ferrlecit Injection 3386

FEVARIN (Denmark, Finland, Germany, Italy, Norway, Sweden, The Netherlands)
FLUVOXAMINE MALEATE
- Luvox Tablets (25, 50, 100 mg) 3256

FEVITAL SIMPLEX (Italy)
FERRIC SODIUM GLUCONATE
- Ferrlecit Injection 3386

FEXICAM (Canada)
PIROXICAM
- Feldene Capsules 2685

FEXIN (South Africa)
CEPHALEXIN
- Keflex Oral Suspension 1237
- Keflex Pulvules 1237

FIBONEL (Spain)
FAMOTIDINE
- Pepcid Injection 2153
- Pepcid Injection Premixed 2153
- Pepcid RPD Orally Disintegrating Tablets 2150
- Pepcid Tablets 2150
- Pepcid for Oral Suspension 2150

FIBRAFLEX (Germany)
IBUPROFEN
- Motrin Suspension, Oral Drops, Chewable Tablets, and Caplets 2002

FIBRASE (Italy)
PENTOSAN POLYSULFATE SODIUM
- Elmiron Capsules 570

FIBREZYM (Germany)
PENTOSAN POLYSULFATE SODIUM
- Elmiron Capsules 570

FIBROCARD (Belgium)
VERAPAMIL HYDROCHLORIDE
- Covera-HS Tablets 3199
- Isoptin SR Tablets 467
- Verelan Capsules 3184
- Verelan PM Capsules 3186

FIBROCID (Spain)
PENTOSAN POLYSULFATE SODIUM
- Elmiron Capsules 570

FIBROCIDE (Portugal)
PENTOSAN POLYSULFATE SODIUM
- Elmiron Capsules 570

FIBROCIT (Italy)
GEMFIBROZIL
- Lopid Tablets 2650

FIBROS (Italy)
GEMFIBROZIL
- Lopid Tablets 2650

FIBROXYN (South Africa)
NAPROXEN
- EC-Naprosyn Delayed-Release Tablets 2967
- Naprosyn Suspension 2967
- Naprosyn Tablets 2967

FICORTRIL (Germany)
HYDROCORTISONE ACETATE
- Anusol-HC Suppositories 2238
- Cortifoam Rectal Foam 3170
- Hydrocortone Acetate Injectable Suspension 2103
- Proctocort Suppositories 2264

FINASTID (Italy)
FINASTERIDE
- Propecia Tablets 2172
- Proscar Tablets 2175

FINFO (Thailand)
PIROXICAM
- Feldene Capsules 2685

FINIBRON (Italy)
BUPRENORPHINE HYDROCHLORIDE
- Buprenex Injectable 2918

FINLEPSIN (Germany)
CARBAMAZEPINE
- Carbatrol Capsules 3234

(⊙ Described in PDR For Ophthalmic Medicines™)

Tegretol Chewable Tablets 2404
Tegretol Suspension 2404
Tegretol Tablets 2404
Tegretol-XR Tablets 2404

FIRIN (Germany)
NORFLOXACIN
Chibroxin Sterile Ophthalmic Solution . . . . ⊙273, 2051
Noroxin Tablets 2145

FIRMALONE (Italy)
DEXAMETHASONE
Decadron Elixir 2078
Decadron Tablets 2079

FISIOFER (Italy)
FERRIC SODIUM GLUCONATE
Ferrlecit Injection 3386

FISOPRED (Mexico)
PREDNISOLONE SODIUM PHOSPHATE
Pediapred Oral Solution 1170

FITAXAL (France)
LACTULOSE
Kristalose for Oral Solution 1007

FIVEROCIL (Mexico)
FLUOROURACIL
Efudex Cream 1733
Efudex Topical Solutions 1733
Fluoroplex Topical Cream 552
Fluoroplex Topical Solution 552

FIVOFLU (Thailand)
FLUOROURACIL
Efudex Cream 1733
Efudex Topical Solutions 1733
Fluoroplex Topical Cream 552
Fluoroplex Topical Solution 552

FIXCA (Spain)
ONDANSETRON HYDROCHLORIDE
Zofran Injection 1698
Zofran Injection Premixed 1698
Zofran Oral Solution 1703
Zofran Tablets 1703

FIXIM (The Netherlands)
CEFIXIME
Suprax Tablets 1877
Suprax for Oral Suspension 1877

FIXIME (South Africa)
CEFIXIME
Suprax Tablets 1877
Suprax for Oral Suspension 1877

FLAGINAZOL (Mexico)
METRONIDAZOLE
MetroCream 1404
MetroGel 1405
MetroGel-Vaginal Gel 1986
MetroLotion 1405
Noritate Cream 1224

FLAGYL (Austria, Belgium, Brazil, Finland, Germany, Hong Kong, Israel, Italy, Mexico, Portugal, Singapore, South Africa, Switzerland)
METRONIDAZOLE
MetroCream 1404
MetroGel 1405
MetroGel-Vaginal Gel 1986
MetroLotion 1405
Noritate Cream 1224

FLAGYL COMP (Finland)
METRONIDAZOLE
MetroCream 1404
MetroGel 1405
MetroGel-Vaginal Gel 1986
MetroLotion 1405
Noritate Cream 1224

FLAGYL NISTATINA (Brazil)
METRONIDAZOLE
MetroCream 1404
MetroGel 1405
MetroGel-Vaginal Gel 1986
MetroLotion 1405
Noritate Cream 1224

FLAGYSTATIN V (Mexico)
METRONIDAZOLE
MetroCream 1404
MetroGel 1405
MetroGel-Vaginal Gel 1986
MetroLotion 1405
Noritate Cream 1224

FLAMADENE (Brazil)
PIROXICAM
Feldene Capsules 2685

FLAMARENE (Brazil)
PIROXICAM
Feldene Capsules 2685

FLAMATAK (United Kingdom)
DICLOFENAC SODIUM
Voltaren Tablets 2315
Voltaren-XR Tablets 2315

FLAMATROL (Hong Kong, United Kingdom)
PIROXICAM
Feldene Capsules 2685

FLAMERIL (New Zealand)
DICLOFENAC SODIUM
Voltaren Tablets 2315
Voltaren-XR Tablets 2315

FLAMIC (Thailand)
PIROXICAM
Feldene Capsules 2685

FLAMON (Switzerland)
VERAPAMIL HYDROCHLORIDE
Covera-HS Tablets 3199
Isoptin SR Tablets 467
Verelan Capsules 3184
Verelan PM Capsules 3186

FLAMOSTAT (Brazil)
PIROXICAM
Feldene Capsules 2685

FLAMRASE (United Kingdom)
DICLOFENAC SODIUM
Voltaren Tablets 2315
Voltaren-XR Tablets 2315

FLANAREN (Brazil)
DICLOFENAC SODIUM
Voltaren Tablets 2315
Voltaren-XR Tablets 2315

FLANAX (Brazil, Mexico)
NAPROXEN SODIUM
Anaprox DS Tablets 2967
Anaprox Tablets 2967
Naprelan Tablets 1293

FLAVAMED HALSTABLETTEN (Germany)
BENZOCAINE
Americaine Anesthetic Lubricant 1162
Americaine Otic Topical Anesthetic Ear Drops 1162

FLECAINE (France)
FLECAINIDE ACETATE
Tambocor Tablets 1990

FLECATAB (Australia)
FLECAINIDE ACETATE
Tambocor Tablets 1990

FLEMEX (Mexico)
HYDROCORTISONE
Anusol-HC Cream 2.5% 2237
Hydrocortone Tablets 2106

FLEMOXIN (Switzerland)
AMOXICILLIN
Amoxil Pediatric Drops for Oral Suspension 1471
Amoxil Tablets 1471

FLENVERME (Brazil)
MEBENDAZOLE
Vermox Chewable Tablets 2017

FLEXAFEN (Mexico)
IBUPROFEN
Motrin Suspension, Oral Drops, Chewable Tablets, and Caplets 2002

FLEXAGEN (South Africa)
DICLOFENAC SODIUM
Voltaren Tablets 2315
Voltaren-XR Tablets 2315

FLEXAR (Portugal)
PIROXICAM
Feldene Capsules 2685

FLEXARTAL (France)
CARISOPRODOL
Soma Tablets 3353

FLEXASE (Germany)
PIROXICAM
Feldene Capsules 2685

FLEXEN (Mexico)
NAPROXEN
EC-Naprosyn Delayed-Release Tablets . . . 2967
Naprosyn Suspension 2967
Naprosyn Tablets 2967

FLEXERIL (Canada)
CYCLOBENZAPRINE HYDROCHLORIDE
Flexeril Tablets 2094

FLEXIBAN (Italy, Portugal)
CYCLOBENZAPRINE HYDROCHLORIDE
Flexeril Tablets 2094

FLEXIN (Israel)
ORPHENADRINE CITRATE
Norflex Extended-Release Tablets 1987
Norflex Injection 1987

FLEXIROX (France)
PIROXICAM
Feldene Capsules 2685

FLEXOTARD (United Kingdom)
DICLOFENAC SODIUM
Voltaren Tablets 2315
Voltaren-XR Tablets 2315

FLINDIX (Portugal)
ISOSORBIDE DINITRATE
Isordil Sublingual Tablets 3525
Isordil Titradose Tablets 3526

FLIXONASE (Austria, Belgium, Denmark, Finland, France, Hong Kong, Irish Republic, Israel, Italy, Mexico, New Zealand, Singapore, South Africa, Spain, Thailand, The Netherlands, United Kingdom)
FLUTICASONE PROPIONATE
Cutivate Cream 1282
Cutivate Ointment 1284
Flonase Nasal Spray 1533
Flovent 110 mcg Inhalation Aerosol 1535
Flovent 220 mcg Inhalation Aerosol 1535
Flovent 44 mcg Inhalation Aerosol 1535
Flovent Rotadisk 100 mcg 1537
Flovent Rotadisk 250 mcg 1537
Flovent Rotadisk 50 mcg 1537

FLIXOTAIDE (Portugal)
FLUTICASONE PROPIONATE
Cutivate Cream 1282
Cutivate Ointment 1284
Flonase Nasal Spray 1533
Flovent 110 mcg Inhalation Aerosol 1535
Flovent 220 mcg Inhalation Aerosol 1535
Flovent 44 mcg Inhalation Aerosol 1535
Flovent Rotadisk 100 mcg 1537
Flovent Rotadisk 250 mcg 1537
Flovent Rotadisk 50 mcg 1537

FLIXOTIDE (Australia, Austria, Belgium, Denmark, Finland, France, Hong Kong, Irish Republic, Israel, Italy, Mexico, New Zealand, Singapore, South Africa, Spain, Thailand, The Netherlands, United Kingdom)
FLUTICASONE PROPIONATE
Cutivate Cream 1282
Cutivate Ointment 1284
Flonase Nasal Spray 1533
Flovent 110 mcg Inhalation Aerosol 1535
Flovent 220 mcg Inhalation Aerosol 1535
Flovent 44 mcg Inhalation Aerosol 1535
Flovent Rotadisk 100 mcg 1537
Flovent Rotadisk 250 mcg 1537
Flovent Rotadisk 50 mcg 1537

FLOBACIN (Italy)
OFLOXACIN
Floxin I.V. 2526
Floxin Otic Solution 1219
Floxin Tablets 2529
Ocuflox Ophthalmic Solution 554

FLOCOFIL (Mexico)
MERCAPTOPURINE
Purinethol Tablets 1615

FLODIL (France)
FELODIPINE
Plendil Extended-Release Tablets 623

FLODOL (Italy)
PIROXICAM
Feldene Capsules 2685

FLOGAN (Brazil)
DICLOFENAC POTASSIUM
Cataflam Tablets 2315

FLOGEN (Mexico)
NAPROXEN SODIUM
Anaprox DS Tablets 2967
Anaprox Tablets 2967
Naprelan Tablets 1293

FLOGINAX (Italy)
NAPROXEN
EC-Naprosyn Delayed-Release Tablets . . . 2967
Naprosyn Suspension 2967
Naprosyn Tablets 2967

FLOGOBENE (Italy)
PIROXICAM
Feldene Capsules 2685

FLOGOCAN (Portugal)
PIROXICAM
Feldene Capsules 2685

FLOGOGIN (Italy)
NAPROXEN SODIUM
Anaprox DS Tablets 2967
Anaprox Tablets 2967
Naprelan Tablets 1293

FLOGOSAN (Mexico)
PIROXICAM
Feldene Capsules 2685

FLOGOXEN (Brazil)
PIROXICAM
Feldene Capsules 2685

FLOLAN (Austria, Belgium, Canada, Denmark, France, Irish Republic, Italy, Spain, The Netherlands, United Kingdom)
EPOPROSTENOL SODIUM
Flolan for Injection 1528

FLOMAX (Australia, Canada, South Africa, United Kingdom)
TAMSULOSIN HYDROCHLORIDE
Flomax Capsules 1044

FLONASE (Canada)
FLUTICASONE PROPIONATE
Cutivate Cream 1282
Cutivate Ointment 1284
Flonase Nasal Spray 1533
Flovent 110 mcg Inhalation Aerosol 1535
Flovent 220 mcg Inhalation Aerosol 1535
Flovent 44 mcg Inhalation Aerosol 1535
Flovent Rotadisk 100 mcg 1537
Flovent Rotadisk 250 mcg 1537
Flovent Rotadisk 50 mcg 1537

FLORALAC (Austria)
LACTULOSE
Kristalose for Oral Solution 1007

FLORONE (Canada, Germany)
DIFLORASONE DIACETATE
Psorcon E Cream 1227
Psorcon E Ointment 1228

FLOSSAC (Italy)
NORFLOXACIN
Chibroxin Sterile Ophthalmic Solution . . . . ⊙273, 2051
Noroxin Tablets 2145

FLOTIRAN (Portugal)
BETAMETHASONE DIPROPIONATE/CLOTRIMAZOLE
Lotrisone Cream 3129

FLOVENT (Canada)
FLUTICASONE PROPIONATE
Cutivate Cream 1282
Cutivate Ointment 1284
Flonase Nasal Spray 1533
Flovent 110 mcg Inhalation Aerosol 1535
Flovent 220 mcg Inhalation Aerosol 1535
Flovent 44 mcg Inhalation Aerosol 1535
Flovent Rotadisk 100 mcg 1537
Flovent Rotadisk 250 mcg 1537
Flovent Rotadisk 50 mcg 1537

FLOXACIN (Brazil, Mexico)
NORFLOXACIN
Chibroxin Sterile Ophthalmic Solution . . . . ⊙273, 2051
Noroxin Tablets 2145

FLOXACIPRON (Portugal)
CIPROFLOXACIN
Cipro I.V. 893
Cipro I.V. Pharmacy Bulk Package 897
Cipro Oral Suspension 887

FLOXAKIN (Mexico)
CIPROFLOXACIN
Cipro I.V. 893
Cipro I.V. Pharmacy Bulk Package 897
Cipro Oral Suspension 887

FLOXAL (Austria, Germany, Switzerland)
OFLOXACIN
Floxin I.V. 2526
Floxin Otic Solution 1219
Floxin Tablets 2529
Ocuflox Ophthalmic Solution 554

FLOXALIN (Italy)
NAPROXEN SODIUM
Anaprox DS Tablets 2967
Anaprox Tablets 2967
Naprelan Tablets 1293

FLOXEDOL (Portugal)
OFLOXACIN
Floxin I.V. 2526
Floxin Otic Solution 1219
Floxin Tablets 2529
Ocuflox Ophthalmic Solution 554

FLOXENOR (Thailand)
NORFLOXACIN
Chibroxin Sterile Ophthalmic Solution . . . . ⊙273, 2051
Noroxin Tablets 2145

FLOXIL (Mexico)
OFLOXACIN
Floxin I.V. 2526
Floxin Otic Solution 1219
Floxin Tablets 2529
Ocuflox Ophthalmic Solution 554

FLOXIN (Canada)
OFLOXACIN
Floxin I.V. 2526
Floxin Otic Solution 1219
Floxin Tablets 2529

Ocuflox Ophthalmic Solution 554

FLOXINOL (Brazil)
NORFLOXACIN
Chibroxin Sterile Ophthalmic Solution . . . . ⊙273, 2051
Noroxin Tablets 2145

FLOXSTAT (Brazil, Mexico)
OFLOXACIN
Floxin I.V. 2526
Floxin Otic Solution 1219
Floxin Tablets 2529
Ocuflox Ophthalmic Solution 554

FLOXYFRAL (Austria, Belgium, France, Switzerland)
FLUVOXAMINE MALEATE
Luvox Tablets (25, 50, 100 mg) 3256

FLU OPH (Thailand)
FLUOROMETHOLONE
FML Ophthalmic Ointment . . . . ⊙237

FLU-21 (Italy)
FLUOCINONIDE
Lidex Cream 2020
Lidex Gel 2020
Lidex Ointment 2020
Lidex Topical Solution 2020
Lidex-E Cream 2020

FLUATON (Italy)
FLUOROMETHOLONE
FML Ophthalmic Ointment . . . . ⊙237

FLUBASON (Italy, Spain)
DESOXIMETASONE
Topicort Cream 2025
Topicort Gel 2025
Topicort LP Cream 2025
Topicort Ointment 2025

FLUCIDERM (Thailand)
FLUOCINOLONE ACETONIDE
Synalar Cream 2020
Synalar Ointment 2020
Synalar Topical Solution 2020

FLUCINAR (Germany)
FLUOCINOLONE ACETONIDE
Synalar Cream 2020
Synalar Ointment 2020
Synalar Topical Solution 2020

FLUCINOME (Switzerland)
FLUTAMIDE
Eulexin Capsules 3118

FLUCON (Australia, Belgium, France, Hong Kong, New Zealand, South Africa, Switzerland, Thailand, The Netherlands)
FLUOROMETHOLONE
FML Ophthalmic Ointment . . . . ⊙237

FLUCONAL (Brazil)
FLUCONAZOLE
Diflucan Tablets, Injection, and Oral Suspension 2681

FLUCOZOLE (Thailand)
FLUCONAZOLE
Diflucan Tablets, Injection, and Oral Suspension 2681

FLUDAPAMIDE (Switzerland)
INDAPAMIDE
Indapamide Tablets 2286

FLUDARA (Australia, Austria, Belgium, Denmark, Finland, France, Israel, Italy, Mexico, New Zealand, Norway, Portugal, Singapore, South Africa, Sweden, Switzerland, Thailand, The Netherlands, United Kingdom)
FLUDARABINE PHOSPHATE
Fludara for Injection 995

FLUDEX (Austria, Belgium, Denmark, France, Portugal, Switzerland, The Netherlands)
INDAPAMIDE
Indapamide Tablets 2286

FLUFORTE (Mexico)
FLUOROMETHOLONE
FML Ophthalmic Ointment . . . . ⊙237

FLUGEN (Spain)
FLUOROMETHOLONE
FML Ophthalmic Ointment . . . . ⊙237

FLUIDEMA (Portugal)
INDAPAMIDE
Indapamide Tablets 2286

FLUIDIN (Spain)
GUAIFENESIN
Organidin NR Liquid 3350
Organidin NR Tablets 3350

FLUILAST (Italy)
TICLOPIDINE HYDROCHLORIDE
Ticlid Tablets 3015

FLUINOL (Spain)
FLUTICASONE PROPIONATE
Cutivate Cream 1282
Cutivate Ointment 1284
Flonase Nasal Spray 1533
Flovent 110 mcg Inhalation Aerosol 1535
Flovent 220 mcg Inhalation Aerosol 1535
Flovent 44 mcg Inhalation Aerosol 1535
Flovent Rotadisk 100 mcg 1537
Flovent Rotadisk 250 mcg 1537
Flovent Rotadisk 50 mcg 1537

FLUI-THEOPHYLLINE (Germany)
THEOPHYLLINE
Aerolate Jr. T.D. Capsules 1361
Aerolate Liquid 1361
Aerolate Sr. T.D. Capsules 1361
Theo-Dur Extended-Release Tablets 1835
Uni-Dur Extended-Release Tablets 1841
Uniphyl 400 mg and 600 mg Tablets . . . 2903

FLUKEN (Mexico)
FLUTAMIDE
Eulexin Capsules 3118

FLUKENOL (Mexico)
FLUCONAZOLE
Diflucan Tablets, Injection, and Oral Suspension 2681

FLUKEZOL (Mexico)
FLUCONAZOLE
Diflucan Tablets, Injection, and Oral Suspension 2681

FLULEM (Mexico)
FLUTAMIDE
Eulexin Capsules 3118

FLUMADINE (Israel)
RIMANTADINE HYDROCHLORIDE
Flumadine Syrup 1370
Flumadine Tablets 1370

FLUMETOL SEMPLICE (Italy)
FLUOROMETHOLONE
FML Ophthalmic Ointment . . . . ⊙237

FLUMEX (Brazil)
FLUOROMETHOLONE
FML Ophthalmic Ointment . . . . ⊙237

FLUMID (Germany)
FLUTAMIDE
Eulexin Capsules 3118

FLUMOX (South Africa)
AMOXICILLIN
Amoxil Pediatric Drops for Oral Suspension 1471
Amoxil Tablets 1471

FLUNASE (Israel)
FLUNISOLIDE
Aerobid Inhaler System 1363
Aerobid-M Inhaler System 1363
Nasalide Nasal Spray 1295
Nasarel Nasal Solution 0.025% 1296

FLUNAZOL (Brazil)
FLUCONAZOLE
Diflucan Tablets, Injection, and Oral Suspension 2681

FLUNIDOR (Portugal)
DIFLUNISAL
Dolobid Tablets 2088

FLUNIGET (Austria, Germany)
DIFLUNISAL
Dolobid Tablets 2088

FLUNITEC (Brazil, Denmark, Norway)
FLUNISOLIDE
Aerobid Inhaler System 1363
Aerobid-M Inhaler System 1363
Nasalide Nasal Spray 1295
Nasarel Nasal Solution 0.025% 1296

FLUNOLONE-V (Hong Kong, Singapore)
FLUOCINOLONE ACETONIDE
Synalar Cream 2020
Synalar Ointment 2020
Synalar Topical Solution 2020

FLUOCID FORTE (Spain)
FLUOCINOLONE ACETONIDE
Synalar Cream 2020
Synalar Ointment 2020
Synalar Topical Solution 2020

FLUOCINIL (Italy)
FLUOCINOLONE ACETONIDE
Synalar Cream 2020
Synalar Ointment 2020
Synalar Topical Solution 2020

FLUOCIT (Italy)
FLUOCINOLONE ACETONIDE
Synalar Cream 2020
Synalar Ointment 2020
Synalar Topical Solution 2020

FLUOCORTAN (Spain)
FLUOCINOLONE ACETONIDE
Synalar Cream 2020
Synalar Ointment 2020
Synalar Topical Solution 2020

FLUODERM (Canada, South Africa)
FLUOCINOLONE ACETONIDE
Synalar Cream 2020
Synalar Ointment 2020
Synalar Topical Solution 2020

FLUODERMO FUERTE (Spain)
FLUOCINOLONE ACETONIDE
Synalar Cream 2020
Synalar Ointment 2020
Synalar Topical Solution 2020

FLUODERMOL (Italy)
FLUOCINOLONE ACETONIDE
Synalar Cream 2020
Synalar Ointment 2020
Synalar Topical Solution 2020

FLUODONIL (Italy)
DIFLUNISAL
Dolobid Tablets 2088

FLUOFTAL (Austria)
FLUORESCEIN SODIUM
AK-Fluor Injection 10% and 25% . . . . . . ⊙202
Fluorescite Injection . . . . ⊙211

FLUOMIX SAME (Italy)
FLUOCINOLONE ACETONIDE
Synalar Cream 2020
Synalar Ointment 2020
Synalar Topical Solution 2020

FLUONIDE (Canada)
FLUOCINOLONE ACETONIDE
Synalar Cream 2020
Synalar Ointment 2020
Synalar Topical Solution 2020

FLUONOLONE-V (Thailand)
FLUOCINOLONE ACETONIDE
Synalar Cream 2020
Synalar Ointment 2020
Synalar Topical Solution 2020

FLUORALFA (Italy)
FLUORESCEIN SODIUM
AK-Fluor Injection 10% and 25% . . . . . . ⊙202
Fluorescite Injection . . . . ⊙211

FLUOR-AMPS (United Kingdom)
FLUORESCEIN SODIUM
AK-Fluor Injection 10% and 25% . . . . . . ⊙202
Fluorescite Injection . . . . ⊙211

FLUORES (South Africa)
FLUORESCEIN SODIUM
AK-Fluor Injection 10% and 25% . . . . . . ⊙202
Fluorescite Injection . . . . ⊙211

FLUORESCITE (Australia, Canada, Hong Kong, New Zealand, Singapore, South Africa, Thailand)
FLUORESCEIN SODIUM
AK-Fluor Injection 10% and 25% . . . . . . ⊙202
Fluorescite Injection . . . . ⊙211

FLUORETS (Australia, Hong Kong, Irish Republic, New Zealand, Singapore, South Africa)
FLUORESCEIN SODIUM
AK-Fluor Injection 10% and 25% . . . . . . ⊙202
Fluorescite Injection . . . . ⊙211

FLUOR-I-STRIP AT (Canada)
FLUORESCEIN SODIUM
AK-Fluor Injection 10% and 25% . . . . . . ⊙202
Fluorescite Injection . . . . ⊙211

FLUOROPLEX (Australia, Canada)
FLUOROURACIL
Efudex Cream 1733
Efudex Topical Solutions 1733
Fluoroplex Topical Cream 552
Fluoroplex Topical Solution 552

FLUOROPOS (Germany)
FLUOROMETHOLONE
FML Ophthalmic Ointment . . . . ⊙237

FLUOTHANE (Australia, Austria, Belgium, Brazil, Canada, France, Germany, Hong Kong, Irish Republic, Israel, Italy, Mexico, New Zealand, Norway, Portugal, South Africa, Spain, Sweden, Switzerland, Thailand, The Netherlands, United Kingdom)
HALOTHANE
Fluothane Inhalation 3508

FLUOVITEF (Italy)
FLUOCINOLONE ACETONIDE
Synalar Cream 2020
Synalar Ointment 2020
Synalar Topical Solution 2020

FLUPAZINE (Mexico)
TRIFLUOPERAZINE HYDROCHLORIDE
Stelazine Injection 1640
Stelazine Tablets 1640

FLURABLASTIN (Denmark, Finland, Norway)
FLUOROURACIL
Efudex Cream 1733
Efudex Topical Solutions 1733
Fluoroplex Topical Cream 552
Fluoroplex Topical Solution 552

FLURACEDYL (Israel, Norway)
FLUOROURACIL
Efudex Cream 1733
Efudex Topical Solutions 1733
Fluoroplex Topical Cream 552
Fluoroplex Topical Solution 552

FLUROBLASTIN (Australia, Germany, South Africa)
FLUOROURACIL
Efudex Cream 1733
Efudex Topical Solutions 1733
Fluoroplex Topical Cream 552
Fluoroplex Topical Solution 552

FLUROBLASTINE (Switzerland)
FLUOROURACIL
Efudex Cream 1733
Efudex Topical Solutions 1733
Fluoroplex Topical Cream 552
Fluoroplex Topical Solution 552

FLUROLON (Denmark)
FLUOROMETHOLONE
FML Ophthalmic Ointment . . . . ⊙237

FLUROP (Portugal)
FLUOROMETHOLONE
FML Ophthalmic Ointment . . . . ⊙237

FLUROX (Mexico)
FLUOROURACIL
Efudex Cream 1733
Efudex Topical Solutions 1733
Fluoroplex Topical Cream 552
Fluoroplex Topical Solution 552

FLUSEMIDE (Spain)
NICARDIPINE HYDROCHLORIDE
Cardene I.V. 3485

FLUSONAL (Spain)
FLUTICASONE PROPIONATE
Cutivate Cream 1282
Cutivate Ointment 1284
Flonase Nasal Spray 1533
Flovent 110 mcg Inhalation Aerosol 1535
Flovent 220 mcg Inhalation Aerosol 1535
Flovent 44 mcg Inhalation Aerosol 1535
Flovent Rotadisk 100 mcg 1537
Flovent Rotadisk 250 mcg 1537
Flovent Rotadisk 50 mcg 1537

FLUSPIRAL (Italy)
FLUTICASONE PROPIONATE
Cutivate Cream 1282
Cutivate Ointment 1284
Flonase Nasal Spray 1533
Flovent 110 mcg Inhalation Aerosol 1535
Flovent 220 mcg Inhalation Aerosol 1535
Flovent 44 mcg Inhalation Aerosol 1535
Flovent Rotadisk 100 mcg 1537
Flovent Rotadisk 250 mcg 1537
Flovent Rotadisk 50 mcg 1537

FLUSTAR (Italy)
DIFLUNISAL
Dolobid Tablets 2088

FLUTA (Germany)
FLUTAMIDE
Eulexin Capsules 3118

FLUTABENE (Austria)
FLUTAMIDE
Eulexin Capsules 3118

FLUTACAN (Denmark, Sweden)
FLUTAMIDE
Eulexin Capsules 3118

FLUTA-CELL (Germany)
FLUTAMIDE
Eulexin Capsules 3118

FLUTA-GRY (Germany)
FLUTAMIDE
Eulexin Capsules 3118

FLUTAIDE (Portugal)
FLUTICASONE PROPIONATE
Cutivate Cream 1282
Cutivate Ointment 1284
Flonase Nasal Spray 1533
Flovent 110 mcg Inhalation Aerosol 1535
Flovent 220 mcg Inhalation Aerosol 1535
Flovent 44 mcg Inhalation Aerosol 1535
Flovent Rotadisk 100 mcg 1537
Flovent Rotadisk 250 mcg 1537

(⊙ Described in PDR For Ophthalmic Medicines™)

Flovent Rotadisk 50 mcg ... 1537

FLUTAMEX (Germany)
FLUTAMIDE
Eulexin Capsules ... 3118

FLUTAMIN (Australia, New Zealand)
FLUTAMIDE
Eulexin Capsules ... 3118

FLUTAN (Hong Kong, Thailand)
FLUTAMIDE
Eulexin Capsules ... 3118

FLUTAPLEX (Belgium, Denmark)
FLUTAMIDE
Eulexin Capsules ... 3118

FLUTIDE (Germany, Norway, Sweden)
FLUTICASONE PROPIONATE
Cutivate Cream ... 1282
Cutivate Ointment ... 1284
Flonase Nasal Spray ... 1533
Flovent 110 mcg Inhalation Aerosol ... 1535
Flovent 220 mcg Inhalation Aerosol ... 1535
Flovent 44 mcg Inhalation Aerosol ... 1535
Flovent Rotadisk 100 mcg ... 1537
Flovent Rotadisk 250 mcg ... 1537
Flovent Rotadisk 50 mcg ... 1537

FLUTINASE (Switzerland)
FLUTICASONE PROPIONATE
Cutivate Cream ... 1282
Cutivate Ointment ... 1284
Flonase Nasal Spray ... 1533
Flovent 110 mcg Inhalation Aerosol ... 1535
Flovent 220 mcg Inhalation Aerosol ... 1535
Flovent 44 mcg Inhalation Aerosol ... 1535
Flovent Rotadisk 100 mcg ... 1537
Flovent Rotadisk 250 mcg ... 1537
Flovent Rotadisk 50 mcg ... 1537

FLUTIVATE (Norway, Sweden)
FLUTICASONE PROPIONATE
Cutivate Cream ... 1282
Cutivate Ointment ... 1284
Flonase Nasal Spray ... 1533
Flovent 110 mcg Inhalation Aerosol ... 1535
Flovent 220 mcg Inhalation Aerosol ... 1535
Flovent 44 mcg Inhalation Aerosol ... 1535
Flovent Rotadisk 100 mcg ... 1537
Flovent Rotadisk 250 mcg ... 1537
Flovent Rotadisk 50 mcg ... 1537

FLUTOL (New Zealand)
FLUTAMIDE
Eulexin Capsules ... 3118

FLUTONE (Canada)
DIFLORASONE DIACETATE
Psorcon E Cream ... 1227
Psorcon E Ointment ... 1228

FLUVEAN (Italy)
FLUOCINOLONE ACETONIDE
Synalar Cream ... 2020
Synalar Ointment ... 2020
Synalar Topical Solution ... 2020

FLUVOXADURA (Germany)
FLUVOXAMINE MALEATE
Luvox Tablets (25, 50, 100 mg) ... 3256

FLUXOCOR (Brazil)
DIPYRIDAMOLE
Persantine Tablets ... 1057

FML (Australia, Belgium, Canada, Hong Kong, Irish Republic, Israel, Mexico, New Zealand, Singapore, South Africa, Spain, Switzerland, Thailand)
FLUOROMETHOLONE
FML Ophthalmic Ointment ... ⊙237

FML LIQUIFILM (Finland, Portugal, The Netherlands, United Kingdom)
FLUOROMETHOLONE
FML Ophthalmic Ointment ... ⊙237

FOCUS (Italy)
IBUPROFEN
Motrin Suspension, Oral Drops, Chewable Tablets, and Caplets ... 2002

FOILLE (Canada)
BENZOCAINE
Americaine Anesthetic Lubricant ... 1162
Americaine Otic Topical Anesthetic Ear Drops ... 1162

FOILLE INSETTI (Italy)
HYDROCORTISONE
Anusol-HC Cream 2.5% ... 2237
Hydrocortone Tablets ... 2106

FOKALEPSIN (Germany)
CARBAMAZEPINE
Carbatrol Capsules ... 3234
Tegretol Chewable Tablets ... 2404
Tegretol Suspension ... 2404
Tegretol Tablets ... 2404
Tegretol-XR Tablets ... 2404

FOLITABS (Spain)
FINASTERIDE
Propecia Tablets ... 2172
Proscar Tablets ... 2175

FOLLISTREL (Sweden)
LEVONORGESTREL
Norplant System ... 3543

FONDRIL (Germany)
BISOPROLOL FUMARATE
Zebeta Tablets ... 1885

FONDRIL-5 HCT (Germany)
BISOPROLOL FUMARATE/HYDROCHLOROTHIAZIDE
Ziac Tablets ... 1887

FONX (France)
OXICONAZOLE NITRATE
Oxistat Cream ... 1298
Oxistat Lotion ... 1298

FOREXIN (Thailand)
CIPROFLOXACIN
Cipro I.V. ... 893
Cipro I.V. Pharmacy Bulk Package ... 897
Cipro Oral Suspension ... 887

FORGENAC (Italy)
DICLOFENAC SODIUM
Voltaren Tablets ... 2315
Voltaren-XR Tablets ... 2315

FORMIN (Thailand)
METFORMIN HYDROCHLORIDE
Glucophage Tablets ... 1080

FORMISTIN (Italy)
CETIRIZINE HYDROCHLORIDE
Zyrtec Syrup ... 2756
Zyrtec Tablets ... 2756

FORMULA 44E (Canada)
DEXTROMETHORPHAN HYDROBROMIDE/GUAIFENESIN
Tussi-Organidin DM NR Liquid ... 3350
Tussi-Organidin DM-S NR Liquid ... 3350

FORMULA E (Mexico)
GUAIFENESIN
Organidin NR Liquid ... 3350
Organidin NR Tablets ... 3350

FORMULAEXPEC (Spain)
GUAIFENESIN
Organidin NR Liquid ... 3350
Organidin NR Tablets ... 3350

FORTAM (Spain, Switzerland)
CEFTAZIDIME
Ceptaz for Injection ... 1499
Fortaz for Injection ... 1541
Tazicef for Injection ... 1647
Tazidime Vials, Faspak & ADD-Vantage ... 1966

FORTAZ (Brazil, Canada)
CEFTAZIDIME
Ceptaz for Injection ... 1499
Fortaz for Injection ... 1541
Tazicef for Injection ... 1647
Tazidime Vials, Faspak & ADD-Vantage ... 1966

FORTENAC (Switzerland)
DICLOFENAC SODIUM
Voltaren Tablets ... 2315
Voltaren-XR Tablets ... 2315

FORTFEN (South Africa)
DICLOFENAC SODIUM
Voltaren Tablets ... 2315
Voltaren-XR Tablets ... 2315

FORTIMAX (Spain)
NORFLOXACIN
Chibroxin Sterile Ophthalmic Solution ... ⊙273, 2051
Noroxin Tablets ... 2145

FORTIPINE (United Kingdom)
NIFEDIPINE
Adalat CC Tablets ... 877
Procardia Capsules ... 2708
Procardia XL Extended Release Tablets ... 2710

FORTOVASE (Australia, Austria, Belgium, Canada, Denmark, Finland, France, Germany, Italy, New Zealand, Portugal, South Africa, Spain, Sweden, Switzerland, Thailand, The Netherlands, United Kingdom)
SAQUINAVIR
Fortovase Capsules ... 2970

FORTRADOL (Italy)
TRAMADOL HYDROCHLORIDE
Ultram Tablets ... 2600

FORTUM (Australia, Austria, Denmark, France, Hong Kong, Irish Republic, Israel, Mexico, New Zealand, Norway, Singapore, South Africa, Sweden, Thailand, The Netherlands, United Kingdom)
CEFTAZIDIME
Ceptaz for Injection ... 1499
Fortaz for Injection ... 1541
Tazicef for Injection ... 1647
Tazidime Vials, Faspak & ADD-Vantage ... 1966

FORTUMSET (France)
CEFTAZIDIME
Ceptaz for Injection ... 1499
Fortaz for Injection ... 1541
Tazicef for Injection ... 1647
Tazidime Vials, Faspak & ADD-Vantage ... 1966

FORTUNAN (United Kingdom)
HALOPERIDOL
Haldol Injection, Tablets and Concentrate ... 2533

FORTZAAR (Denmark, France)
LOSARTAN POTASSIUM
Cozaar Tablets ... 2067

FORVERM (Brazil)
MEBENDAZOLE
Vermox Chewable Tablets ... 2017

FORZID (Thailand)
CEFTAZIDIME
Ceptaz for Injection ... 1499
Fortaz for Injection ... 1541
Tazicef for Injection ... 1647
Tazidime Vials, Faspak & ADD-Vantage ... 1966

FOSALAN (Israel)
ALENDRONATE SODIUM
Fosamax Tablets ... 2095

FOSAMAX (Australia, Austria, Belgium, Brazil, Canada, Denmark, Finland, France, Germany, Hong Kong, Irish Republic, Italy, Mexico, New Zealand, Norway, Portugal, Singapore, South Africa, Spain, Sweden, Switzerland, Thailand, The Netherlands, United Kingdom)
ALENDRONATE SODIUM
Fosamax Tablets ... 2095

FOSCAVIR (Australia, Austria, Belgium, Finland, France, Germany, Hong Kong, Israel, Italy, Japan, Norway, Portugal, Spain, Sweden, Switzerland, Thailand, The Netherlands, United Kingdom)
FOSCARNET SODIUM
Foscavir Injection ... 605

FOSCOVIR (Denmark)
FOSCARNET SODIUM
Foscavir Injection ... 605

FOSINIL (Belgium, Spain)
FOSINOPRIL SODIUM
Monopril Tablets ... 1091

FOSINORM (Germany)
FOSINOPRIL SODIUM
Monopril Tablets ... 1091

FOSIPRES (Italy)
FOSINOPRIL SODIUM
Monopril Tablets ... 1091

FOSITEN (Portugal, Switzerland)
FOSINOPRIL SODIUM
Monopril Tablets ... 1091

FOSITENS (Austria, Spain)
FOSINOPRIL SODIUM
Monopril Tablets ... 1091

FOSSYOL (Germany)
METRONIDAZOLE
MetroCream ... 1404
MetroGel ... 1405
MetroGel-Vaginal Gel ... 1986
MetroLotion ... 1405
Noritate Cream ... 1224

FOTAX (Thailand)
CEFOTAXIME SODIUM
Claforan Injection ... 732

FOTEXINA (Mexico)
CEFOTAXIME SODIUM
Claforan Injection ... 732

FOXIL (Italy)
CEFADROXIL
Duricef Capsules ... 1079
Duricef Oral Suspension ... 1079
Duricef Tablets ... 1079

FOXIN (Thailand)
NORFLOXACIN
Chibroxin Sterile Ophthalmic Solution ... ⊙273, 2051
Noroxin Tablets ... 2145

FOXINON (Thailand)
NORFLOXACIN
Chibroxin Sterile Ophthalmic Solution ... ⊙273, 2051
Noroxin Tablets ... 2145

FOZITEC (France)
FOSINOPRIL SODIUM
Monopril Tablets ... 1091

FRACTAL (France)
FLUVASTATIN SODIUM
Lescol Capsules ... 2361

FRAGMIN (Australia, Austria, Belgium, Canada, Denmark, Finland, Germany, Hong Kong, Israel, Italy, New Zealand, Norway, Portugal, Singapore, South Africa, Spain, Sweden, Switzerland, The Netherlands, United Kingdom)
DALTEPARIN SODIUM
Fragmin Injection ... 2814

FRAGMINE (France)
DALTEPARIN SODIUM
Fragmin Injection ... 2814

FRANOL (Thailand)
THEOPHYLLINE
Aerolate Jr. T.D. Capsules ... 1361
Aerolate Liquid ... 1361
Aerolate Sr. T.D. Capsules ... 1361
Theo-Dur Extended-Release Tablets ... 1835
Uni-Dur Extended-Release Tablets ... 1841
Uniphyl 400 mg and 600 mg Tablets ... 2903

FRAXIDOL (Italy)
TRAMADOL HYDROCHLORIDE
Ultram Tablets ... 2600

FREMET (Spain)
CIMETIDINE
Tagamet Tablets ... 1644

FRESENIZOL (Mexico)
METRONIDAZOLE
MetroCream ... 1404
MetroGel ... 1405
MetroGel-Vaginal Gel ... 1986
MetroLotion ... 1405
Noritate Cream ... 1224

FRESOFOL (Mexico)
PROPOFOL
Diprivan Injectable Emulsion ... 667

FREUDAL (Mexico)
DIAZEPAM
Valium Injectable ... 3026
Valium Tablets ... 3047

FRISOLAC (Portugal)
KETOCONAZOLE
Nizoral 2% Cream ... 3620
Nizoral 2% Shampoo ... 2007
Nizoral Tablets ... 1791

FRISTAMIN (Italy)
LORATADINE
Claritin Reditabs ... 3100
Claritin Syrup ... 3100
Claritin Tablets ... 3100

FRIVENT (Italy)
THEOPHYLLINE
Aerolate Jr. T.D. Capsules ... 1361
Aerolate Liquid ... 1361
Aerolate Sr. T.D. Capsules ... 1361
Theo-Dur Extended-Release Tablets ... 1835
Uni-Dur Extended-Release Tablets ... 1841
Uniphyl 400 mg and 600 mg Tablets ... 2903

FROIDIR (Finland)
CLOZAPINE
Clozaril Tablets ... 2319

FRONTAL (Brazil, Italy)
ALPRAZOLAM
Xanax Tablets ... 2865

FROSINOR (Spain)
PAROXETINE HYDROCHLORIDE
Paxil Oral Suspension ... 1609
Paxil Tablets ... 1609

FROXAL (Mexico)
CEFUROXIME SODIUM
Kefurox Vials, ADD-Vantage ... 1948
Zinacef Injection ... 1696

FRUMERON (Hong Kong, Thailand)
INDAPAMIDE
Indapamide Tablets ... 2286

FTOROCORT (Thailand)
TRIAMCINOLONE ACETONIDE
Azmacort Inhalation Aerosol ... 728
Nasacort AQ Nasal Spray ... 752
Nasacort Nasal Inhaler ... 750

FUCLODE (Italy)
CEFACLOR
Ceclor CD Tablets ... 1279
Ceclor Pulvules ... 1905
Ceclor Suspension ... 1905

FUDR (Singapore)
FLOXURIDINE
Sterile FUDR ... 2974

FUGACAR (Thailand)
MEBENDAZOLE
Vermox Chewable Tablets ... 2017

(⊙ Described in PDR For Ophthalmic Medicines™)

FUGEREL (Australia, Austria, Germany, Hong Kong, Singapore, Thailand)
FLUTAMIDE
Eulexin Capsules **3118**

FULCRO (Italy)
FENOFIBRATE
Tricor Capsules, Micronized **513**

FUL-GLO (Australia, New Zealand)
FLUORESCEIN SODIUM
AK-Fluor Injection 10% and 25% . . . . . . ⊙**202**
Fluorescite Injection . . . . ⊙**211**

FULGRAM (Italy)
NORFLOXACIN
Chibroxin Sterile Ophthalmic Solution . . . . ⊙**273, 2051**
Noroxin Tablets **2145**

FULIXAN (Spain)
DIFLORASONE DIACETATE
Psorcon E Cream. **1227**
Psorcon E Ointment **1228**

FUNA (Thailand)
FLUCONAZOLE
Diflucan Tablets, Injection, and Oral Suspension **2681**

FUNDUSCEIN (Canada)
FLUORESCEIN SODIUM
AK-Fluor Injection 10% and 25% . . . . . . ⊙**202**
Fluorescite Injection . . . . ⊙**211**

FUNGAMIZOL (Mexico)
KETOCONAZOLE
Nizoral 2% Cream **3620**
Nizoral 2% Shampoo. **2007**
Nizoral Tablets **1791**

FUNGAREST (Spain)
KETOCONAZOLE
Nizoral 2% Cream **3620**
Nizoral 2% Shampoo. **2007**
Nizoral Tablets **1791**

FUNGATA (Austria, Germany)
FLUCONAZOLE
Diflucan Tablets, Injection, and Oral Suspension **2681**

FUNGAZOL (Mexico, Thailand)
KETOCONAZOLE
Nizoral 2% Cream **3620**
Nizoral 2% Shampoo. **2007**
Nizoral Tablets **1791**

FUNGEDERM (United Kingdom)
CLOTRIMAZOLE
Lotrimin Cream 1%. **3128**
Lotrimin Lotion 1%. **3128**
Lotrimin Topical Solution 1% **3128**
Mycelex Troche **573**

FUNGICIDE (Thailand)
KETOCONAZOLE
Nizoral 2% Cream **3620**
Nizoral 2% Shampoo. **2007**
Nizoral Tablets **1791**

FUNGIDERM (Germany, Thailand)
CLOTRIMAZOLE
Lotrimin Cream 1%. **3128**
Lotrimin Lotion 1%. **3128**
Lotrimin Topical Solution 1% **3128**
Mycelex Troche **573**

FUNGIDERMO (Spain)
CLOTRIMAZOLE
Lotrimin Cream 1%. **3128**
Lotrimin Lotion 1%. **3128**
Lotrimin Topical Solution 1% **3128**
Mycelex Troche **573**

FUNGILONGA (Spain)
CICLOPIROX OLAMINE
Loprox Cream **2021**
Loprox Lotion **2021**

FUNGIMAX (Brazil)
METRONIDAZOLE
MetroCream **1404**
MetroGel **1405**
MetroGel-Vaginal Gel **1986**
MetroLotion **1405**
Noritate Cream **1224**

FUNGINOX (Thailand)
KETOCONAZOLE
Nizoral 2% Cream **3620**
Nizoral 2% Shampoo. **2007**
Nizoral Tablets **1791**

FUNGIREDUCT (Germany)
NYSTATIN
Nystop Topical Powder USP **2608**

FUNGISTAT (Mexico)
TERCONAZOLE
Terazol 3 Vaginal Cream **2587**
Terazol 3 Vaginal Suppositories **2587**
Terazol 7 Vaginal Cream **2587**

FUNGISTEN (Norway)
CLOTRIMAZOLE
Lotrimin Cream 1%. **3128**
Lotrimin Lotion 1%. **3128**
Lotrimin Topical Solution 1% **3128**
Mycelex Troche **573**

FUNGIZID (Germany, Hong Kong, New Zealand)
CLOTRIMAZOLE
Lotrimin Cream 1%. **3128**
Lotrimin Lotion 1%. **3128**
Lotrimin Topical Solution 1% **3128**
Mycelex Troche **573**

FUNGO HUBBER (Spain)
KETOCONAZOLE
Nizoral 2% Cream **3620**
Nizoral 2% Shampoo. **2007**
Nizoral Tablets **1791**

FUNGORAL (Austria, Brazil, Mexico, Norway, Sweden)
KETOCONAZOLE
Nizoral 2% Cream **3620**
Nizoral 2% Shampoo. **2007**
Nizoral Tablets **1791**

FUNGOTOX (Switzerland)
CLOTRIMAZOLE
Lotrimin Cream 1%. **3128**
Lotrimin Lotion 1%. **3128**
Lotrimin Topical Solution 1% **3128**
Mycelex Troche **573**

FUNGOWAS (Spain)
CICLOPIROX OLAMINE
Loprox Cream **2021**
Loprox Lotion **2021**

FURAZOLON (Brazil)
HYDROCORTISONE
Anusol-HC Cream 2.5% **2237**
Hydrocortone Tablets **2106**

FUROCLORAN (Mexico)
CHLORAMPHENICOL
Chloromycetin Ophthalmic Ointment, 1% . . . . ⊙**296**
Chloromycetin Ophthalmic Solution . . . . ⊙**297**
Chloroptic Sterile Ophthalmic Ointment . . ⊙**234**
Chloroptic Sterile Ophthalmic Solution . . ⊙**235**

FUSANIDAZOL (Mexico)
METRONIDAZOLE
MetroCream **1404**
MetroGel **1405**
MetroGel-Vaginal Gel **1986**
MetroLotion **1405**
Noritate Cream **1224**

FUSTAREN (Mexico)
DICLOFENAC SODIUM
Voltaren Tablets **2315**
Voltaren-XR Tablets **2315**

FUXEN (Mexico)
NAPROXEN
EC-Naprosyn Delayed-Release Tablets . . . **2967**
Naprosyn Suspension **2967**
Naprosyn Tablets **2967**

FUZOLTEC (Mexico)
ITRACONAZOLE
Sporanox Capsules. **1800**
Sporanox Oral Solution. **1808, 2512**

FYMNAL (Brazil)
IBUPROFEN
Motrin Suspension, Oral Drops, Chewable Tablets, and Caplets **2002**

GABITRIL (Australia, Austria, Belgium, Denmark, Finland, France, Germany, Irish Republic, Italy, Portugal, Spain, Switzerland, United Kingdom)
TIAGABINE HYDROCHLORIDE
Gabitril Tablets **1189**

GABRILEN (Germany)
KETOPROFEN
Orudis Capsules **3548**
Oruvail Capsules **3548**

GALECIN (Mexico)
CLINDAMYCIN PHOSPHATE
Cleocin Phosphate Sterile Solution **2785**
Cleocin T Topical Gel **2790**
Cleocin T Topical Lotion. **2790**
Cleocin T Topical Solution **2790**
Cleocin Vaginal Cream. **2788**
Clindets Pledgets **3270**

GALEDOL (Mexico)
DICLOFENAC SODIUM
Voltaren Tablets **2315**
Voltaren-XR Tablets **2315**

GALENAMET (Irish Republic, United Kingdom)
CIMETIDINE
Tagamet Tablets **1644**

GALENTROMICINA (Mexico)
ERYTHROMYCIN
Emgel 2% Topical Gel **1285**
Ery-Tab Tablets **448**
Erythromycin Base Filmtab Tablets **454**
Erythromycin Delayed-Release Capsules, USP **455**
PCE Dispertab Tablets. **498**

GALIDRIN (Mexico)
RANITIDINE HYDROCHLORIDE
Zantac 150 EFFERdose Granules **1690**
Zantac 150 EFFERdose Tablets **1690**
Zantac 150 Tablets **1690**
Zantac 300 Tablets **1690**
Zantac Injection **1688**
Zantac Injection Premixed **1688**
Zantac Syrup **1690**

GALOTAM (Spain)
AMPICILLIN SODIUM/SULBACTAM SODIUM
Unasyn for Injection **2728**

GALPROFEN (United Kingdom)
IBUPROFEN
Motrin Suspension, Oral Drops, Chewable Tablets, and Caplets **2002**

GAMACTRIN (Brazil)
SULFAMETHOXAZOLE/TRIMETHOPRIM
Bactrim DS Tablets. **2949**
Bactrim Pediatric Suspension **2949**
Bactrim Tablets **2949**
Septra DS Tablets **2265**
Septra Grape Suspension. **2265**
Septra Suspension **2265**
Septra Tablets. **2265**

GAMAVATE (United Arab Emirates)
CLOBETASOL PROPIONATE
Cormax Cream **2440**
Cormax Ointment. **2440**
Cormax Scalp Application. **2441**
Temovate Cream **1301**
Temovate E Emollient **1302**
Temovate Gel **1303**
Temovate Ointment. **1301**
Temovate Scalp Application **1304**

GAMBEX (South Africa)
LINDANE
Lindane Lotion USP 1% **559**
Lindane Shampoo USP 1% **560**

GAMMAKINE (Italy)
INTERFERON GAMMA-1B
Actimmune **1772**

GANDIN (Thailand)
MEFENAMIC ACID
Ponstel Capsules **1356**

GANOR (Germany)
FAMOTIDINE
Pepcid Injection **2153**
Pepcid Injection Premixed **2153**
Pepcid RPD Orally Disintegrating Tablets **2150**
Pepcid Tablets. **2150**
Pepcid for Oral Suspension **2150**

GAOPTOL (Monaco)
TIMOLOL MALEATE
Blocadren Tablets **2046**
Timoptic Sterile Ophthalmic Solution. . . . **2190**
Timoptic in Ocudose. **2192**
Timoptic-XE Sterile Ophthalmic Gel Forming Solution. **2194**

GARACOL (The Netherlands)
GENTAMICIN SULFATE
Genoptic Ophthalmic Ointment . . . . ⊙**239**
Genoptic Sterile Ophthalmic Solution . . . ⊙**239**

GARACOLL (Mexico)
GENTAMICIN SULFATE
Genoptic Ophthalmic Ointment . . . . ⊙**239**
Genoptic Sterile Ophthalmic Solution . . . ⊙**239**

GARALONE (Portugal)
GENTAMICIN SULFATE
Genoptic Ophthalmic Ointment . . . . ⊙**239**
Genoptic Sterile Ophthalmic Solution . . . ⊙**239**

GARAMICINA (Brazil, Mexico)
GENTAMICIN SULFATE
Genoptic Ophthalmic Ointment . . . . ⊙**239**
Genoptic Sterile Ophthalmic Solution . . . ⊙**239**

GARAMYCIN (Australia, Canada, Denmark, Hong Kong, Israel, Norway, Singapore, South Africa, Sweden, Switzerland, Thailand, The Netherlands, United Kingdom)
GENTAMICIN SULFATE
Genoptic Ophthalmic Ointment . . . . ⊙**239**
Genoptic Sterile Ophthalmic Solution . . . ⊙**239**

GARANIL (Spain)
CAPTOPRIL
Captopril Tablets **2281**

GARATEC (Canada)
GENTAMICIN SULFATE
Genoptic Ophthalmic Ointment . . . . ⊙**239**
Genoptic Sterile Ophthalmic Solution . . . ⊙**239**

GARIA (Spain)
FLUOCINONIDE
Lidex Cream **2020**
Lidex Gel **2020**
Lidex Ointment **2020**
Lidex Topical Solution **2020**
Lidex-E Cream. **2020**

GARRANIL (Spain)
CAPTOPRIL
Captopril Tablets **2281**

GARTRICIN (Spain)
BENZOCAINE
Americaine Anesthetic Lubricant **1162**
Americaine Otic Topical Anesthetic Ear Drops **1162**

GASCOP (Mexico)
ALBENDAZOLE
Albenza Tablets **1463**

GASEC (Portugal)
OMEPRAZOLE
Prilosec Delayed-Release Capsules **628**

GASPIREN (Brazil)
OMEPRAZOLE
Prilosec Delayed-Release Capsules **628**

GASTER (Japan)
FAMOTIDINE
Pepcid Injection **2153**
Pepcid Injection Premixed **2153**
Pepcid RPD Orally Disintegrating Tablets **2150**
Pepcid Tablets. **2150**
Pepcid for Oral Suspension **2150**

GASTIDINE (Hong Kong)
CIMETIDINE
Tagamet Tablets **1644**

GASTOPRIDE (Portugal)
FAMOTIDINE
Pepcid Injection **2153**
Pepcid Injection Premixed **2153**
Pepcid RPD Orally Disintegrating Tablets **2150**
Pepcid Tablets. **2150**
Pepcid for Oral Suspension **2150**

GASTRAL (Spain)
SUCRALFATE
Carafate Suspension. **731**
Carafate Tablets. **730**

GASTRAX (Germany)
NIZATIDINE
Axid Pulvules. **1903**

GASTRESE LA (United Kingdom)
METOCLOPRAMIDE HYDROCHLORIDE
Reglan Injectable **2935**
Reglan Syrup **2935**
Reglan Tablets. **2935**

GASTRIDIN (Italy)
FAMOTIDINE
Pepcid Injection **2153**
Pepcid Injection Premixed **2153**
Pepcid RPD Orally Disintegrating Tablets **2150**
Pepcid Tablets. **2150**
Pepcid for Oral Suspension **2150**

GASTRIDINA (Portugal)
RANITIDINE HYDROCHLORIDE
Zantac 150 EFFERdose Granules **1690**
Zantac 150 EFFERdose Tablets **1690**
Zantac 150 Tablets **1690**
Zantac 300 Tablets **1690**
Zantac Injection **1688**
Zantac Injection Premixed **1688**
Zantac Syrup **1690**

GASTRIFAM (Portugal)
FAMOTIDINE
Pepcid Injection **2153**
Pepcid Injection Premixed **2153**
Pepcid RPD Orally Disintegrating Tablets **2150**
Pepcid Tablets. **2150**
Pepcid for Oral Suspension **2150**

GASTRIMUT (Spain)
OMEPRAZOLE
Prilosec Delayed-Release Capsules **628**

GASTRION (Spain)
FAMOTIDINE
Pepcid Injection **2153**
Pepcid Injection Premixed **2153**
Pepcid RPD Orally Disintegrating Tablets **2150**
Pepcid Tablets. **2150**
Pepcid for Oral Suspension **2150**

GASTRIUM (Brazil)
OMEPRAZOLE
Prilosec Delayed-Release Capsules **628**

GASTRO (Israel)
FAMOTIDINE
Pepcid Injection **2153**

(⊙ Described in PDR For Ophthalmic Medicines™)

Pepcid Injection Premixed . . . 2153
Pepcid RPD Orally Disintegrating Tablets . . . 2150
Pepcid Tablets . . . 2150
Pepcid for Oral Suspension . . . 2150

GASTRO H2 (Spain)
CIMETIDINE
Tagamet Tablets . . . 1644

GASTROBID CONTINUS (Irish Republic, United Kingdom)
METOCLOPRAMIDE HYDROCHLORIDE
Reglan Injectable . . . 2935
Reglan Syrup . . . 2935
Reglan Tablets . . . 2935

GASTROBITAN (Norway)
CIMETIDINE
Tagamet Tablets . . . 1644

GASTROCOLON (South Africa)
METOCLOPRAMIDE HYDROCHLORIDE
Reglan Injectable . . . 2935
Reglan Syrup . . . 2935
Reglan Tablets . . . 2935

GASTRODIN (Thailand)
CIMETIDINE
Tagamet Tablets . . . 1644

GASTRODINA (Mexico)
CIMETIDINE
Tagamet Tablets . . . 1644

GASTRODINE (Brazil)
CIMETIDINE
Tagamet Tablets . . . 1644

GASTRODOMINA (Hong Kong, Spain)
FAMOTIDINE
Pepcid Injection . . . 2153
Pepcid Injection Premixed . . . 2153
Pepcid RPD Orally Disintegrating Tablets . . . 2150
Pepcid Tablets . . . 2150
Pepcid for Oral Suspension . . . 2150

GASTROFLUX (United Kingdom)
METOCLOPRAMIDE HYDROCHLORIDE
Reglan Injectable . . . 2935
Reglan Syrup . . . 2935
Reglan Tablets . . . 2935

GASTROGEL (Italy, Switzerland)
SUCRALFATE
Carafate Suspension . . . 731
Carafate Tablets . . . 730

GASTROLAV (Portugal)
RANITIDINE HYDROCHLORIDE
Zantac 150 EFFERdose Granules . . . 1690
Zantac 150 EFFERdose Tablets . . . 1690
Zantac 150 Tablets . . . 1690
Zantac 300 Tablets . . . 1690
Zantac Injection . . . 1688
Zantac Injection Premixed . . . 1688
Zantac Syrup . . . 1690

GASTROLEM (Mexico)
CIMETIDINE
Tagamet Tablets . . . 1644

GASTROLOC (Germany)
OMEPRAZOLE
Prilosec Delayed-Release Capsules . . . 628

GASTRONERTON (Austria)
METOCLOPRAMIDE HYDROCHLORIDE
Reglan Injectable . . . 2935
Reglan Syrup . . . 2935
Reglan Tablets . . . 2935

GASTROPEN (Spain)
FAMOTIDINE
Pepcid Injection . . . 2153
Pepcid Injection Premixed . . . 2153
Pepcid RPD Orally Disintegrating Tablets . . . 2150
Pepcid Tablets . . . 2150
Pepcid for Oral Suspension . . . 2150

GASTRO-TABLINEN (Germany)
METOCLOPRAMIDE HYDROCHLORIDE
Reglan Injectable . . . 2935
Reglan Syrup . . . 2935
Reglan Tablets . . . 2935

GASTROTAT (South Africa)
METOCLOPRAMIDE HYDROCHLORIDE
Reglan Injectable . . . 2935
Reglan Syrup . . . 2935
Reglan Tablets . . . 2935

GASTROTEM (Germany)
METOCLOPRAMIDE HYDROCHLORIDE
Reglan Injectable . . . 2935
Reglan Syrup . . . 2935
Reglan Tablets . . . 2935

GASTRO-TIMELETS (Austria, Denmark, Germany, Switzerland)
METOCLOPRAMIDE HYDROCHLORIDE
Reglan Injectable . . . 2935
Reglan Syrup . . . 2935
Reglan Tablets . . . 2935

GASTROTRANQUIL (Germany)
METOCLOPRAMIDE HYDROCHLORIDE
Reglan Injectable . . . 2935
Reglan Syrup . . . 2935
Reglan Tablets . . . 2935

GASTROTROP (Germany)
METOCLOPRAMIDE HYDROCHLORIDE
Reglan Injectable . . . 2935
Reglan Syrup . . . 2935
Reglan Tablets . . . 2935

GASTRULCER (Portugal)
RANITIDINE HYDROCHLORIDE
Zantac 150 EFFERdose Granules . . . 1690
Zantac 150 EFFERdose Tablets . . . 1690
Zantac 150 Tablets . . . 1690
Zantac 300 Tablets . . . 1690
Zantac Injection . . . 1688
Zantac Injection Premixed . . . 1688
Zantac Syrup . . . 1690

GATINAR (Spain, Switzerland)
LACTULOSE
Kristalose for Oral Solution . . . 1007

GBH (Canada)
LINDANE
Lindane Lotion USP 1% . . . 559
Lindane Shampoo USP 1% . . . 560

GEANGIN (Denmark, Norway, The Netherlands, United Kingdom)
VERAPAMIL HYDROCHLORIDE
Covera-HS Tablets . . . 3199
Isoptin SR Tablets . . . 467
Verelan Capsules . . . 3184
Verelan PM Capsules . . . 3186

GELDENE (France)
PIROXICAM
Feldene Capsules . . . 2685

GELESTRA (Italy)
ESTRADIOL
Alora Transdermal System . . . 3372
Climara Transdermal System . . . 958
Estrace Vaginal Cream . . . 3358
Estring Vaginal Ring . . . 2811
Vivelle Transdermal System . . . 2412
Vivelle-Dot Transdermal System . . . 2416

GELIDINA (Spain)
FLUOCINOLONE ACETONIDE
Synalar Cream . . . 2020
Synalar Ointment . . . 2020
Synalar Topical Solution . . . 2020

GELISYN (Mexico)
FLUOCINONIDE
Lidex Cream . . . 2020
Lidex Gel . . . 2020
Lidex Ointment . . . 2020
Lidex Topical Solution . . . 2020
Lidex-E Cream . . . 2020

GEL-OSE (Canada)
LACTULOSE
Kristalose for Oral Solution . . . 1007

GELPARINE (Switzerland)
HEPARIN SODIUM
Heparin Lock Flush Solution . . . 3509
Heparin Sodium Injection . . . 3511

GELUFENE (France)
IBUPROFEN
Motrin Suspension, Oral Drops, Chewable Tablets, and Caplets . . . 2002

GEMFIBRIL (Thailand)
GEMFIBROZIL
Lopid Tablets . . . 2650

GEMFIBROMAX (Australia)
GEMFIBROZIL
Lopid Tablets . . . 2650

GEMHEXAL (Australia)
GEMFIBROZIL
Lopid Tablets . . . 2650

GEMIZOL (New Zealand)
GEMFIBROZIL
Lopid Tablets . . . 2650

GEMLIPID (Italy)
GEMFIBROZIL
Lopid Tablets . . . 2650

GEMNPID (Hong Kong)
GEMFIBROZIL
Lopid Tablets . . . 2650

GEMZAR (Australia, Austria, Belgium, Canada, Denmark, Finland, France, Germany, Hong Kong, Israel, Italy, Mexico, New Zealand, Norway, Portugal, Singapore, South Africa, Spain, Sweden, Switzerland, Thailand, The Netherlands, United Kingdom)
GEMCITABINE HYDROCHLORIDE
Gemzar for Injection . . . 1919

GEMZIL (Thailand)
CAPTOPRIL
Captopril Tablets . . . 2281

GENALGEN (Mexico)
NAPROXEN
EC-Naprosyn Delayed-Release Tablets . . . 2967
Naprosyn Suspension . . . 2967
Naprosyn Tablets . . . 2967

GENAPROST (Italy)
FINASTERIDE
Propecia Tablets . . . 2172
Proscar Tablets . . . 2175

GENCIN (Germany, South Africa)
GENTAMICIN SULFATE
Genoptic Ophthalmic Ointment . . . ⊙239
Genoptic Sterile Ophthalmic Solution . . . ⊙239

GENDAZEL (Thailand)
ALBENDAZOLE
Albenza Tablets . . . 1463

GENERCIN (Thailand)
CHLORAMPHENICOL
Chloromycetin Ophthalmic Ointment, 1% . . . ⊙296
Chloromycetin Ophthalmic Solution . . . ⊙297
Chloroptic Sterile Ophthalmic Ointment . . . ⊙234
Chloroptic Sterile Ophthalmic Solution . . . ⊙235

GENERLOG (Thailand)
TRIAMCINOLONE ACETONIDE
Azmacort Inhalation Aerosol . . . 728
Nasacort AQ Nasal Spray . . . 752
Nasacort Nasal Inhaler . . . 750

GENGIGEL (Portugal)
SODIUM HYALURONATE
Hyalgan Solution . . . 3080

GENGIVARIUM (Italy)
BENZOCAINE
Americaine Anesthetic Lubricant . . . 1162
Americaine Otic Topical Anesthetic Ear Drops . . . 1162

GENKOVA (Mexico)
GENTAMICIN SULFATE
Genoptic Ophthalmic Ointment . . . ⊙239
Genoptic Sterile Ophthalmic Solution . . . ⊙239

GEN-LAC (Canada)
LACTULOSE
Kristalose for Oral Solution . . . 1007

GENLIP (Italy)
GEMFIBROZIL
Lopid Tablets . . . 2650

GEN-MEDROXY (Canada)
MEDROXYPROGESTERONE ACETATE
Depo-Provera Contraceptive Injection . . . 2798
Provera Tablets . . . 2853

GENOCIN (Thailand)
CHLOROQUINE PHOSPHATE
Aralen Tablets . . . 3075

GENOPTIC (Australia, Belgium, Hong Kong, New Zealand, Singapore, South Africa, Spain)
GENTAMICIN SULFATE
Genoptic Ophthalmic Ointment . . . ⊙239
Genoptic Sterile Ophthalmic Solution . . . ⊙239

GENORAL (Australia)
ESTROPIPATE
Ogen Tablets . . . 2846
Ortho-Est Tablets . . . 3464

GENOX (Australia, New Zealand)
TAMOXIFEN CITRATE
Nolvadex Tablets . . . 678

GENOXEN (Hong Kong, Irish Republic)
NAPROXEN
EC-Naprosyn Delayed-Release Tablets . . . 2967
Naprosyn Suspension . . . 2967
Naprosyn Tablets . . . 2967

GENOZIL (Italy)
GEMFIBROZIL
Lopid Tablets . . . 2650

GENREX (Mexico)
GENTAMICIN SULFATE
Genoptic Ophthalmic Ointment . . . ⊙239
Genoptic Sterile Ophthalmic Solution . . . ⊙239

GENSUMYCIN (Denmark, Finland, Norway, Sweden)
GENTAMICIN SULFATE
Genoptic Ophthalmic Ointment . . . ⊙239
Genoptic Sterile Ophthalmic Solution . . . ⊙239

GENTA (Germany, Mexico)
GENTAMICIN SULFATE
Genoptic Ophthalmic Ointment . . . ⊙239
Genoptic Sterile Ophthalmic Solution . . . ⊙239

GENTA GOBENS (Spain)
GENTAMICIN SULFATE
Genoptic Ophthalmic Ointment . . . ⊙239
Genoptic Sterile Ophthalmic Solution . . . ⊙239

GENTABILLES (France)
GENTAMICIN SULFATE
Genoptic Ophthalmic Ointment . . . ⊙239
Genoptic Sterile Ophthalmic Solution . . . ⊙239

GENTAC (Thailand)
GENTAMICIN SULFATE
Genoptic Ophthalmic Ointment . . . ⊙239
Genoptic Sterile Ophthalmic Solution . . . ⊙239

GENTACIDIN (Canada)
GENTAMICIN SULFATE
Genoptic Ophthalmic Ointment . . . ⊙239
Genoptic Sterile Ophthalmic Solution . . . ⊙239

GENTACIN (Mexico, Thailand)
GENTAMICIN SULFATE
Genoptic Ophthalmic Ointment . . . ⊙239
Genoptic Sterile Ophthalmic Solution . . . ⊙239

GENTACOLL (Denmark, Finland)
GENTAMICIN SULFATE
Genoptic Ophthalmic Ointment . . . ⊙239
Genoptic Sterile Ophthalmic Solution . . . ⊙239

GENTACORT (Italy)
GENTAMICIN SULFATE
Genoptic Ophthalmic Ointment . . . ⊙239
Genoptic Sterile Ophthalmic Solution . . . ⊙239

GENTAGOBENS (Portugal)
GENTAMICIN SULFATE
Genoptic Ophthalmic Ointment . . . ⊙239
Genoptic Sterile Ophthalmic Solution . . . ⊙239

GENTAL (Thailand, United Arab Emirates)
GENTAMICIN SULFATE
Genoptic Ophthalmic Ointment . . . ⊙239
Genoptic Sterile Ophthalmic Solution . . . ⊙239

GENTALLINE (France)
GENTAMICIN SULFATE
Genoptic Ophthalmic Ointment . . . ⊙239
Genoptic Sterile Ophthalmic Solution . . . ⊙239

GENTALLORENS (Spain)
GENTAMICIN SULFATE
Genoptic Ophthalmic Ointment . . . ⊙239
Genoptic Sterile Ophthalmic Solution . . . ⊙239

GENTALODINA (Spain)
GENTAMICIN SULFATE
Genoptic Ophthalmic Ointment . . . ⊙239
Genoptic Sterile Ophthalmic Solution . . . ⊙239

GENTALYN (Italy)
GENTAMICIN SULFATE
Genoptic Ophthalmic Ointment . . . ⊙239
Genoptic Sterile Ophthalmic Solution . . . ⊙239

GENTAMEDICAL (Spain)
GENTAMICIN SULFATE
Genoptic Ophthalmic Ointment . . . ⊙239
Genoptic Sterile Ophthalmic Solution . . . ⊙239

GENTAMEN (Italy)
GENTAMICIN SULFATE
Genoptic Ophthalmic Ointment . . . ⊙239
Genoptic Sterile Ophthalmic Solution . . . ⊙239

GENTAMIN (Spain)
GENTAMICIN SULFATE
Genoptic Ophthalmic Ointment . . . ⊙239
Genoptic Sterile Ophthalmic Solution . . . ⊙239

GENTAMIVAL (Spain)
GENTAMICIN SULFATE
Genoptic Ophthalmic Ointment . . . ⊙239
Genoptic Sterile Ophthalmic Solution . . . ⊙239

GENTAMIX (Germany)
GENTAMICIN SULFATE
Genoptic Ophthalmic Ointment . . . ⊙239
Genoptic Sterile Ophthalmic Solution . . . ⊙239

GENTAMORGENS (Spain)
GENTAMICIN SULFATE
Genoptic Ophthalmic Ointment . . . ⊙239
Genoptic Sterile Ophthalmic Solution . . . ⊙239

GENTAMYTREX (Belgium, Germany, Singapore, The Netherlands)
GENTAMICIN SULFATE
Genoptic Ophthalmic Ointment . . . ⊙239
Genoptic Sterile Ophthalmic Solution . . . ⊙239

GENTA-OPH (Thailand)
GENTAMICIN SULFATE
Genoptic Ophthalmic Ointment . . . ⊙239
Genoptic Sterile Ophthalmic Solution . . . ⊙239

GENTAPLUS (Brazil)
GENTAMICIN SULFATE
Genoptic Ophthalmic Ointment . . . ⊙239
Genoptic Sterile Ophthalmic Solution . . . ⊙239

GENTARIM (Mexico)
GENTAMICIN SULFATE
Genoptic Ophthalmic Ointment . . . ⊙239
Genoptic Sterile Ophthalmic Solution . . . ⊙239

GENTATRIM (Israel)
GENTAMICIN SULFATE
Genoptic Ophthalmic Ointment . . . ⊙239

Genoptic Sterile Ophthalmic Solution . . . ⊙239

GENTAX (Austria)
GENTAMICIN SULFATE
Genoptic Ophthalmic Ointment . . . . ⊙239
Genoptic Sterile Ophthalmic Solution . . . ⊙239

GENTAZAF Z (Mexico)
GENTAMICIN SULFATE
Genoptic Ophthalmic Ointment . . . . ⊙239
Genoptic Sterile Ophthalmic Solution . . . ⊙239

GENTIBIOPTAL (Italy)
GENTAMICIN SULFATE
Genoptic Ophthalmic Ointment . . . . ⊙239
Genoptic Sterile Ophthalmic Solution . . . ⊙239

GENTICIN (Irish Republic, United Kingdom)
GENTAMICIN SULFATE
Genoptic Ophthalmic Ointment . . . . ⊙239
Genoptic Sterile Ophthalmic Solution . . . ⊙239

GENTICINA (Spain)
GENTAMICIN SULFATE
Genoptic Ophthalmic Ointment . . . . ⊙239
Genoptic Sterile Ophthalmic Solution . . . ⊙239

GENTICOL (Italy)
GENTAMICIN SULFATE
Genoptic Ophthalmic Ointment . . . . ⊙239
Genoptic Sterile Ophthalmic Solution . . . ⊙239

GENTIPRESS (Italy)
ENALAPRIL MALEATE/HYDROCHLOROTHIAZIDE
Vaseretic Tablets 2204

GENTISUM (Spain)
GENTAMICIN SULFATE
Genoptic Ophthalmic Ointment . . . . ⊙239
Genoptic Sterile Ophthalmic Solution . . . ⊙239

GENTOCIL (Portugal)
GENTAMICIN SULFATE
Genoptic Ophthalmic Ointment . . . . ⊙239
Genoptic Sterile Ophthalmic Solution . . . ⊙239

GENTOGRAM (France, The Netherlands)
GENTAMICIN SULFATE
Genoptic Ophthalmic Ointment . . . . ⊙239
Genoptic Sterile Ophthalmic Solution . . . ⊙239

GENTOMIL (Italy)
GENTAMICIN SULFATE
Genoptic Ophthalmic Ointment . . . . ⊙239
Genoptic Sterile Ophthalmic Solution . . . ⊙239

GENT-OPHTAL (Germany)
GENTAMICIN SULFATE
Genoptic Ophthalmic Ointment . . . . ⊙239
Genoptic Sterile Ophthalmic Solution . . . ⊙239

GENTOPTINE (Monaco)
GENTAMICIN SULFATE
Genoptic Ophthalmic Ointment . . . . ⊙239
Genoptic Sterile Ophthalmic Solution . . . ⊙239

GENTRALAY (Spain)
GENTAMICIN SULFATE
Genoptic Ophthalmic Ointment . . . . ⊙239
Genoptic Sterile Ophthalmic Solution . . . ⊙239

GENTRASUL (Canada)
GENTAMICIN SULFATE
Genoptic Ophthalmic Ointment . . . . ⊙239
Genoptic Sterile Ophthalmic Solution . . . ⊙239

GENTUSSIIN (Thailand)
DEXTROMETHORPHAN HYDROBROMIDE/GUAIFENESIN
Tussi-Organidin DM NR Liquid 3350
Tussi-Organidin DM-S NR Liquid 3350

GEOMYCINE (Belgium)
GENTAMICIN SULFATE
Genoptic Ophthalmic Ointment . . . . ⊙239
Genoptic Sterile Ophthalmic Solution . . . ⊙239

GEOPHAGOL (Brazil)
MEBENDAZOLE
Vermox Chewable Tablets. 2017

GERAMET (Irish Republic)
CIMETIDINE
Tagamet Tablets 1644

GERAX (Irish Republic)
ALPRAZOLAM
Xanax Tablets 2865

GEREF (Austria, Belgium, Canada, Germany, Irish Republic, Israel, Portugal, Switzerland, United Kingdom)
SERMORELIN ACETATE
Geref for Injection 3215

GEREL (France)
SERMORELIN ACETATE
Geref for Injection 3215

GERELAX (Irish Republic)
LACTULOSE
Kristalose for Oral Solution. 1007

GERICARB (Irish Republic)
CARBAMAZEPINE
Carbatrol Capsules 3234
Tegretol Chewable Tablets 2404
Tegretol Suspension 2404
Tegretol Tablets 2404
Tegretol-XR Tablets 2404

GERINAP (Irish Republic)
NAPROXEN
EC-Naprosyn Delayed-Release Tablets . . . 2967
Naprosyn Suspension 2967
Naprosyn Tablets 2967

GERMICICLIN (Italy)
DOXYCYCLINE HYCLATE
Doryx Coated Pellet Filled Capsules 3357
Periostat Tablets 1208
Vibramycin Hyclate Capsules. 2735
Vibramycin Hyclate Intravenous 2737
Vibra-Tabs Film Coated Tablets 2735

GERNEBCIN (Germany)
TOBRAMYCIN SULFATE
Nebcin Vials, Hyporets & ADD-Vantage . . 1955

GERODYL (The Netherlands)
PENICILLAMINE
Cuprimine Capsules 2075
Depen Titratable Tablets 3341

GEROMID (Italy)
CLOFIBRATE
Atromid-S Capsules 3483

GEROTEN (Irish Republic)
CAPTOPRIL
Captopril Tablets 2281

GEROXALEN (Denmark, Norway, The Netherlands)
METHOXSALEN
8-MOP Capsules 1727
Oxsoralen Lotion 1%. 1740
Oxsoralen-Ultra Capsules 1741

GEROXICAM (Irish Republic)
PIROXICAM
Feldene Capsules. 2685

GERTAC (Irish Republic)
RANITIDINE HYDROCHLORIDE
Zantac 150 EFFERdose Granules 1690
Zantac 150 EFFERdose Tablets 1690
Zantac 150 Tablets 1690
Zantac 300 Tablets 1690
Zantac Injection 1688
Zantac Injection Premixed 1688
Zantac Syrup 1690

GESIPROX (Singapore)
NAPROXEN SODIUM
Anaprox DS Tablets 2967
Anaprox Tablets. 2967
Naprelan Tablets 1293

GESTAPOLAR (Germany)
MEDROXYPROGESTERONE ACETATE
Depo-Provera Contraceptive Injection . . . 2798
Provera Tablets 2853

GESTAPURAN (Finland, Sweden)
MEDROXYPROGESTERONE ACETATE
Depo-Provera Contraceptive Injection . . . 2798
Provera Tablets 2853

GESTEROL (Canada)
PROGESTERONE
Crinone 4% Gel 3213
Crinone 8% Gel 3213
Prometrium Capsules (100 mg, 200 mg). 3261

GESTONE (Israel, New Zealand, Thailand, United Kingdom)
PROGESTERONE
Crinone 4% Gel 3213
Crinone 8% Gel 3213
Prometrium Capsules (100 mg, 200 mg). 3261

GESTORAL (France)
MEDROXYPROGESTERONE ACETATE
Depo-Provera Contraceptive Injection . . . 2798
Provera Tablets 2853

GEVILON (Austria, Finland, Germany, Switzerland)
GEMFIBROZIL
Lopid Tablets 2650

GEVRAMYCIN (Spain)
GENTAMICIN SULFATE
Genoptic Ophthalmic Ointment . . . . ⊙239
Genoptic Sterile Ophthalmic Solution . . . ⊙239

GEVRAMYCIN TOPICA (Spain)
GENTAMICIN SULFATE
Genoptic Ophthalmic Ointment . . . . ⊙239
Genoptic Sterile Ophthalmic Solution . . . ⊙239

GEWACALM (Austria)
DIAZEPAM
Valium Injectable 3026
Valium Tablets 3047

GEWACYCLIN (Austria)
DOXYCYCLINE HYCLATE
Doryx Coated Pellet Filled Capsules 3357
Periostat Tablets 1208
Vibramycin Hyclate Capsules. 2735
Vibramycin Hyclate Intravenous 2737
Vibra-Tabs Film Coated Tablets 2735

GEWADILAT (Austria)
NIFEDIPINE
Adalat CC Tablets. 877
Procardia Capsules. 2708
Procardia XL Extended Release Tablets . . 2710

GEWAZEM (Austria)
DILTIAZEM HYDROCHLORIDE
Cardizem CD Capsules 1016
Cardizem Injectable 1018
Cardizem Lyo-Ject Syringe 1018
Cardizem Monovial 1018
Tiazac Capsules 1378

GEZON (Brazil)
DICLOFENAC POTASSIUM
Cataflam Tablets 2315

G-FARLUTAL (Germany)
MEDROXYPROGESTERONE ACETATE
Depo-Provera Contraceptive Injection . . . 2798
Provera Tablets 2853

G-FEN (Thailand)
IBUPROFEN
Motrin Suspension, Oral Drops, Chewable Tablets, and Caplets 2002

GHIMADOX (Italy)
DOXYCYCLINE HYCLATE
Doryx Coated Pellet Filled Capsules 3357
Periostat Tablets 1208
Vibramycin Hyclate Capsules. 2735
Vibramycin Hyclate Intravenous 2737
Vibra-Tabs Film Coated Tablets 2735

GI (Mexico)
GENTAMICIN SULFATE
Genoptic Ophthalmic Ointment . . . . ⊙239
Genoptic Sterile Ophthalmic Solution . . . ⊙239

GIBICEF (Italy)
CEFUROXIME SODIUM
Kefurox Vials, ADD-Vantage. 1948
Zinacef Injection. 1696

GIBIFER (Italy)
FERRIC SODIUM GLUCONATE
Ferrlecit Injection. 3386

GIBIFLU (Italy)
FLUNISOLIDE
Aerobid Inhaler System 1363
Aerobid-M Inhaler System. 1363
Nasalide Nasal Spray 1295
Nasarel Nasal Solution 0.025% 1296

GIBINAP (Italy)
NAPROXEN SODIUM
Anaprox DS Tablets 2967
Anaprox Tablets. 2967
Naprelan Tablets 1293

GIBIXEN (Italy)
NAPROXEN
EC-Naprosyn Delayed-Release Tablets . . . 2967
Naprosyn Suspension 2967
Naprosyn Tablets. 2967

GILEX (Israel)
DOXEPIN HYDROCHLORIDE
Sinequan Capsules. 2713
Sinequan Oral Concentrate 2713

GILT (Germany)
CLOTRIMAZOLE
Lotrimin Cream 1%. 3128
Lotrimin Lotion 1% 3128
Lotrimin Topical Solution 1% 3128
Mycelex Troche 573

GILUCOR (Germany)
SOTALOL HYDROCHLORIDE
Betapace Tablets 950

GINE CANESTEN (Spain)
CLOTRIMAZOLE
Lotrimin Cream 1%. 3128
Lotrimin Lotion 1% 3128
Lotrimin Topical Solution 1% 3128
Mycelex Troche 573

GINECOSIDE (Brazil)
PROGESTERONE
Crinone 4% Gel 3213
Crinone 8% Gel 3213
Prometrium Capsules (100 mg, 200 mg). 3261

GINEDISC (Brazil, Mexico)
ESTRADIOL
Alora Transdermal System 3372
Climara Transdermal System. 958
Estrace Vaginal Cream 3358
Estring Vaginal Ring 2811
Vivelle Transdermal System 2412
Vivelle-Dot Transdermal System. 2416

GINEFLAVIR (Italy)
METRONIDAZOLE
MetroCream 1404
MetroGel 1405
MetroGel-Vaginal Gel 1986
MetroLotion 1405
Noritate Cream 1224

GINO CLOTRIMIX (Brazil)
CLOTRIMAZOLE
Lotrimin Cream 1%. 3128
Lotrimin Lotion 1% 3128
Lotrimin Topical Solution 1% 3128
Mycelex Troche 573

GINO LOPROX (Brazil)
CICLOPIROX OLAMINE
Loprox Cream 2021
Loprox Lotion 2021

GINO-CANESTEN (Portugal)
CLOTRIMAZOLE
Lotrimin Cream 1%. 3128
Lotrimin Lotion 1% 3128
Lotrimin Topical Solution 1% 3128
Mycelex Troche 573

GINO-LOTREMINE (Portugal)
CLOTRIMAZOLE
Lotrimin Cream 1%. 3128
Lotrimin Lotion 1% 3128
Lotrimin Topical Solution 1% 3128
Mycelex Troche 573

GIROFLOX (Portugal)
CIPROFLOXACIN
Cipro I.V. 893
Cipro I.V. Pharmacy Bulk Package 897
Cipro Oral Suspension. 887

GLADEM (Austria, Germany, Switzerland)
SERTRALINE HYDROCHLORIDE
Zoloft Tablets 2751

GLANDICIN (Mexico)
PIROXICAM
Feldene Capsules. 2685

GLAUCOCARPINE (Israel)
PILOCARPINE HYDROCHLORIDE
Isopto Carpine Ophthalmic Solution . . . . ⊙215
Pilopine HS Ophthalmic Gel . . . . ⊙217
Salagen Tablets 2229

GLAUCOL (United Kingdom)
TIMOLOL MALEATE
Blocadren Tablets 2046
Timoptic Sterile Ophthalmic Solution. . . . 2190
Timoptic in Ocudose. 2192
Timoptic-XE Sterile Ophthalmic Gel Forming Solution. 2194

GLAUCO-OPH (Thailand)
TIMOLOL MALEATE
Blocadren Tablets 2046
Timoptic Sterile Ophthalmic Solution. . . . 2190
Timoptic in Ocudose. 2192
Timoptic-XE Sterile Ophthalmic Gel Forming Solution. 2194

GLAUCOSAN (South Africa)
TIMOLOL MALEATE
Blocadren Tablets 2046
Timoptic Sterile Ophthalmic Solution. . . . 2190
Timoptic in Ocudose. 2192
Timoptic-XE Sterile Ophthalmic Gel Forming Solution. 2194

GLAUPAX (Denmark, Germany, Irish Republic, Norway, Sweden, Switzerland, Thailand, The Netherlands)
ACETAZOLAMIDE
Diamox Sequels Sustained Release Capsules . . . . ⊙270
Diamox Tablets. . . . . ⊙269

GLAZIDIM (Belgium, Finland, Italy)
CEFTAZIDIME
Ceptaz for Injection 1499
Fortaz for Injection 1541
Tazicef for Injection 1647
Tazidime Vials, Faspak & ADD-Vantage . . 1966

GLIADEL (Canada, France, Israel, New Zealand, Portugal, Singapore)
CARMUSTINE
Gliadel Wafer 1723

GLIBENESE (Austria, Belgium, Denmark, Finland, France, Germany, Irish Republic, Spain, Sweden, Switzerland, The Netherlands, United Kingdom)
GLIPIZIDE
Glucotrol Tablets 2692
Glucotrol XL Extended Release Tablets . . 2693

GLICOBASE (Italy)
ACARBOSE
Precose Tablets 906

GLICONORM (Italy)
CHLORPROPAMIDE
Diabinese Tablets 2680

GLIDIAB (Hong Kong)
GLIPIZIDE
Glucotrol Tablets 2692
Glucotrol XL Extended Release Tablets . . 2693

GLIOTEN (Mexico)
ENALAPRIL MALEATE
Vasotec Tablets 2210

GLIPID (New Zealand)
GLIPIZIDE
Glucotrol Tablets 2692
Glucotrol XL Extended Release Tablets . . 2693

GLIPISCAND (Sweden)
GLIPIZIDE
Glucotrol Tablets 2692
Glucotrol XL Extended Release Tablets . . 2693

GLOBENICOL (The Netherlands)
CHLORAMPHENICOL
Chloromycetin Ophthalmic Ointment, 1% . . . . ⊙296
Chloromycetin Ophthalmic Solution . . . . ⊙297
Chloroptic Sterile Ophthalmic Ointment . . ⊙234
Chloroptic Sterile Ophthalmic Solution . . ⊙235

GLOBUCE (Spain)
CIPROFLOXACIN HYDROCHLORIDE
Ciloxan Ophthalmic Ointment 538
Ciloxan Ophthalmic Solution . . . . ⊙209, 538
Cipro Tablets 887

GLOBUREN (Italy)
EPOETIN ALFA
Epogen for Injection 582
Procrit for Injection 2502

GLUCAGEN (Australia, Austria, Belgium, Denmark, Finland, France, Germany, Hong Kong, Irish Republic, Israel, Italy, New Zealand, Portugal, South Africa, Switzerland, Thailand, United Kingdom)
GLUCAGON HYDROCHLORIDE
Glucagon for Injection Vials and Emergency Kit 1924

GLUCAGON (TM) (United Kingdom)
GLUCAGON HYDROCHLORIDE
Glucagon for Injection Vials and Emergency Kit 1924

GLUCAMET (United Kingdom)
METFORMIN HYDROCHLORIDE
Glucophage Tablets 1080

GLUCOBAY (Australia, Austria, Belgium, Brazil, Denmark, Finland, Germany, Hong Kong, Irish Republic, Italy, Mexico, New Zealand, Norway, Portugal, Singapore, South Africa, Spain, Sweden, Switzerland, Thailand, The Netherlands, United Kingdom)
ACARBOSE
Precose Tablets 906

GLUCOBON (Germany)
METFORMIN HYDROCHLORIDE
Glucophage Tablets 1080

GLUCOFORMIN (Brazil)
METFORMIN HYDROCHLORIDE
Glucophage Tablets 1080

GLUCOHEXAL (Australia)
METFORMIN HYDROCHLORIDE
Glucophage Tablets 1080

GLUCOMET (Australia, New Zealand, Thailand)
METFORMIN HYDROCHLORIDE
Glucophage Tablets 1080

GLUCOMIN (Israel)
METFORMIN HYDROCHLORIDE
Glucophage Tablets 1080

GLUCONORM (Canada)
REPAGLINIDE
Prandin Tablets (0.5, 1, and 2 mg) 2432

GLUCOPHAGE (Australia, Austria, Belgium, Canada, Denmark, Finland, France, Hong Kong, Irish Republic, Israel, Italy, Mexico, New Zealand, Norway, Portugal, South Africa, Spain, Sweden, Switzerland, Thailand, The Netherlands, United Kingdom)
METFORMIN HYDROCHLORIDE
Glucophage Tablets 1080

GLUCOPHAGE S (Germany)
METFORMIN HYDROCHLORIDE
Glucophage Tablets 1080

GLUCOR (France)
ACARBOSE
Precose Tablets 906

GLUCO-RITE (Israel)
GLIPIZIDE
Glucotrol Tablets 2692
Glucotrol XL Extended Release Tablets . . 2693

GLUCOSULMID (Germany)
SULFACETAMIDE SODIUM
Bleph-10 Ophthalmic Ointment 10% . . . . ⊙230
Klaron Lotion 10% 1224

GLUCOTROL (Hong Kong)
GLIPIZIDE
Glucotrol Tablets 2692
Glucotrol XL Extended Release Tablets . . 2693

GLUFOR (Israel)
METFORMIN HYDROCHLORIDE
Glucophage Tablets 1080

GLUFORMIN (Thailand)
METFORMIN HYDROCHLORIDE
Glucophage Tablets 1080

GLUMIDA (Spain)
ACARBOSE
Precose Tablets 906

GLUPITAL (Mexico)
GLIPIZIDE
Glucotrol Tablets 2692
Glucotrol XL Extended Release Tablets . . 2693

GLUSTRESS (Thailand)
METFORMIN HYDROCHLORIDE
Glucophage Tablets 1080

GLUZOLYTE (Thailand)
METFORMIN HYDROCHLORIDE
Glucophage Tablets 1080

GLYCEMIN (Thailand)
CHLORPROPAMIDE
Diabinese Tablets 2680

GLYCOCORTISON (Germany)
HYDROCORTISONE ACETATE
Anusol-HC Suppositories 2238
Cortifoam Rectal Foam 3170
Hydrocortone Acetate Injectable Suspension 2103
Proctocort Suppositories 2264

GLYCON (Canada)
METFORMIN HYDROCHLORIDE
Glucophage Tablets 1080

GLYCORAN (Singapore)
METFORMIN HYDROCHLORIDE
Glucophage Tablets 1080

GLYGEN (Thailand)
GLIPIZIDE
Glucotrol Tablets 2692
Glucotrol XL Extended Release Tablets . . 2693

GLYMAX (France)
METFORMIN HYDROCHLORIDE
Glucophage Tablets 1080

GLYMESE (United Kingdom)
CHLORPROPAMIDE
Diabinese Tablets 2680

GOBANAL (Spain)
DIAZEPAM
Valium Injectable 3026
Valium Tablets 3047

GOBROSAN (Mexico)
IBUPROFEN
Motrin Suspension, Oral Drops, Chewable Tablets, and Caplets 2002

GODAFILIN (Spain)
THEOPHYLLINE
Aerolate Jr. T.D. Capsules 1361
Aerolate Liquid 1361
Aerolate Sr. T.D. Capsules 1361
Theo-Dur Extended-Release Tablets 1835
Uni-Dur Extended-Release Tablets 1841
Uniphyl 400 mg and 600 mg Tablets . . . 2903

GODAL (Spain)
BISOPROLOL FUMARATE
Zebeta Tablets 1885

GOLD CROSS ANTIHISTAMINE ELIXIR (Australia)
PROMETHAZINE HYDROCHLORIDE
Phenergan Injection 3553
Phenergan Suppositories 3556
Phenergan Syrup Fortis 3554
Phenergan Syrup Plain 3554
Phenergan Tablets 3556

GOMEC (Thailand)
OMEPRAZOLE
Prilosec Delayed-Release Capsules 628

GONORCIN (Thailand)
NORFLOXACIN
Chibroxin Sterile Ophthalmic Solution . . . . ⊙273, 2051
Noroxin Tablets 2145

GOODNIGHT (New Zealand)
PROMETHAZINE HYDROCHLORIDE
Phenergan Injection 3553
Phenergan Suppositories 3556
Phenergan Syrup Fortis 3554
Phenergan Syrup Plain 3554
Phenergan Tablets 3556

GOPTEN (Australia, Brazil, Denmark, Finland, France, Germany, Irish Republic, Italy, Mexico, New Zealand, Norway, Portugal, South Africa, Spain, Sweden, Switzerland, The Netherlands, United Kingdom)
TRANDOLAPRIL
Mavik Tablets 478

GOZID (Thailand)
GEMFIBROZIL
Lopid Tablets 2650

GRAMMICIN (Thailand)
GENTAMICIN SULFATE
Genoptic Ophthalmic Ointment . . . . ⊙239
Genoptic Sterile Ophthalmic Solution . . . ⊙239

GRAMMIXIN (Thailand)
GENTAMICIN SULFATE
Genoptic Ophthalmic Ointment . . . . ⊙239
Genoptic Sterile Ophthalmic Solution . . . ⊙239

GRAM-VAL (Italy)
DOXYCYCLINE HYCLATE
Doryx Coated Pellet Filled Capsules 3357
Periostat Tablets 1208
Vibramycin Hyclate Capsules 2735
Vibramycin Hyclate Intravenous 2737
Vibra-Tabs Film Coated Tablets 2735

GRAN-VERM (Brazil)
MEBENDAZOLE
Vermox Chewable Tablets 2017

GRATEN (Mexico)
MORPHINE SULFATE
Astramorph/PF Injection, USP (Preservative-Free) 594
Duramorph Injection 1312
Infumorph 200 and Infumorph 500 Sterile Solutions 1314
Kadian Capsules 1335
MS Contin Tablets 2896
MSIR Oral Capsules 2898
MSIR Oral Solution 2898
MSIR Oral Solution Concentrate 2898
MSIR Oral Tablets 2898
Oramorph SR Tablets 3062
Roxanol 100 Concentrated Oral Solution 3066
Roxanol Concentrated Oral Solution 3066
Roxanol-T Oral Solution 3066

GRAVIDEX (Spain)
DINOPROSTONE
Cervidil Vaginal Insert 1369
Prepidil Gel 2851
Prostin E2 Suppositories 2852

GREATOFEN (Thailand)
IBUPROFEN
Motrin Suspension, Oral Drops, Chewable Tablets, and Caplets 2002

GREFEN (Switzerland)
IBUPROFEN
Motrin Suspension, Oral Drops, Chewable Tablets, and Caplets 2002

GREXIN (Thailand)
DIGOXIN
Lanoxicaps Capsules 1574
Lanoxin Elixir Pediatric 1578
Lanoxin Injection 1581
Lanoxin Injection Pediatric 1584
Lanoxin Tablets 1587

GRISETIN (Spain)
FLUTAMIDE
Eulexin Capsules 3118

GROFENAC (Hong Kong, Switzerland)
DICLOFENAC SODIUM
Voltaren Tablets 2315
Voltaren-XR Tablets 2315

GROMAZOL (Switzerland)
CLOTRIMAZOLE
Lotrimin Cream 1% 3128
Lotrimin Lotion 1% 3128
Lotrimin Topical Solution 1% 3128
Mycelex Troche 573

GRUNCEF (Germany)
CEFADROXIL
Duricef Capsules 1079
Duricef Oral Suspension 1079
Duricef Tablets 1079

GUAFEN (Austria)
GUAIFENESIN
Organidin NR Liquid 3350
Organidin NR Tablets 3350

GUAFRENON (Germany)
GUAIFENESIN
Organidin NR Liquid 3350
Organidin NR Tablets 3350

GUFEN N (Germany)
GUAIFENESIN
Organidin NR Liquid 3350
Organidin NR Tablets 3350

GUPISONE (United Arab Emirates)
PREDNISOLONE
Prelone Syrup 2273

GUTRON (Austria, France, Germany, Hong Kong, Israel, Italy, Mexico, New Zealand, Portugal, Switzerland, Thailand)
MIDODRINE HYDROCHLORIDE
ProAmatine Tablets 3241

GYNAEDRON (Germany)
SULFANILAMIDE
AVC Cream 1350
AVC Suppositories 1350

GYNEBO (Thailand)
CLOTRIMAZOLE
Lotrimin Cream 1% 3128
Lotrimin Lotion 1% 3128
Lotrimin Topical Solution 1% 3128
Mycelex Troche 573

GYNE-LOTREMIN (Hong Kong, Singapore)
CLOTRIMAZOLE
Lotrimin Cream 1% 3128
Lotrimin Lotion 1% 3128
Lotrimin Topical Solution 1% 3128
Mycelex Troche 573

GYNE-LOTRIMIN (Australia)
CLOTRIMAZOLE
Lotrimin Cream 1% 3128
Lotrimin Lotion 1% 3128
Lotrimin Topical Solution 1% 3128
Mycelex Troche 573

GYNESTREL (Italy)
NAPROXEN SODIUM
Anaprox DS Tablets 2967
Anaprox Tablets 2967
Naprelan Tablets 1293

GYNEZOL (South Africa)
CLOTRIMAZOLE
Lotrimin Cream 1% 3128
Lotrimin Lotion 1% 3128
Lotrimin Topical Solution 1% 3128
Mycelex Troche 573

GYNO IRUXOL (Brazil)
CHLORAMPHENICOL
Chloromycetin Ophthalmic Ointment, 1% . . . . ⊙296
Chloromycetin Ophthalmic Solution . . . . ⊙297
Chloroptic Sterile Ophthalmic Ointment . . ⊙234
Chloroptic Sterile Ophthalmic Solution . . ⊙235

GYNO OCERAL (Austria)
OXICONAZOLE NITRATE
Oxistat Cream 1298
Oxistat Lotion 1298

GYNO-CANESTEN (Germany, Italy)
CLOTRIMAZOLE
Lotrimin Cream 1% 3128
Lotrimin Lotion 1% 3128
Lotrimin Topical Solution 1% 3128
Mycelex Troche 573

GYNO-CANESTENE (Belgium, Switzerland)
CLOTRIMAZOLE
Lotrimin Cream 1% 3128
Lotrimin Lotion 1% 3128
Lotrimin Topical Solution 1% 3128
Mycelex Troche 573

GYNOFUG (Germany)
IBUPROFEN
Motrin Suspension, Oral Drops, Chewable Tablets, and Caplets 2002

GYNO-FUNGISTAT (Brazil)
TERCONAZOLE
Terazol 3 Vaginal Cream 2587
Terazol 3 Vaginal Suppositories 2587
Terazol 7 Vaginal Cream 2587

GYNO-FUNGIX (Brazil)
TERCONAZOLE
Terazol 3 Vaginal Cream 2587
Terazol 3 Vaginal Suppositories 2587
Terazol 7 Vaginal Cream 2587

GYNO-LIDERMAN (Austria)
OXICONAZOLE NITRATE
Oxistat Cream 1298

Oxistat Lotion . . . 1298
GYNO-MYFUNGAR (Mexico, Switzerland)
OXICONAZOLE NITRATE
Oxistat Cream . . . 1298
Oxistat Lotion . . . 1298
GYNO-NEURALGIN (Germany)
IBUPROFEN
Motrin Suspension, Oral Drops, Chewable Tablets, and Caplets . . . 2002
GYNO-TERAZOL (Belgium, Switzerland, The Netherlands)
TERCONAZOLE
Terazol 3 Vaginal Cream . . . 2587
Terazol 3 Vaginal Suppositories . . . 2587
Terazol 7 Vaginal Cream . . . 2587
GYNO-TRIMAZE (South Africa)
CLOTRIMAZOLE
Lotrimin Cream 1% . . . 3128
Lotrimin Lotion 1% . . . 3128
Lotrimin Topical Solution 1% . . . 3128
Mycelex Troche . . . 573
GYNPOLAR (Germany)
ESTRADIOL
Alora Transdermal System . . . 3372
Climara Transdermal System . . . 958
Estrace Vaginal Cream . . . 3358
Estring Vaginal Ring . . . 2811
Vivelle Transdermal System . . . 2412
Vivelle-Dot Transdermal System . . . 2416
GYRABLOCK (Singapore, Thailand)
NORFLOXACIN
Chibroxin Sterile Ophthalmic Solution . . . ⊙273, 2051
Noroxin Tablets . . . 2145
GY-SOL (Mexico)
GENTAMICIN SULFATE
Genoptic Ophthalmic Ointment . . . ⊙239
Genoptic Sterile Ophthalmic Solution . . . ⊙239
H2 OXYL (Germany)
BENZOYL PEROXIDE
Brevoxyl-4 Cleansing Lotion . . . 3269
Brevoxyl-4 Creamy Wash . . . 3270
Brevoxyl-4 Gel . . . 3269
Brevoxyl-8 Cleansing Lotion . . . 3269
Brevoxyl-8 Creamy Wash . . . 3270
Brevoxyl-8 Gel . . . 3269
Triaz Cleanser . . . 2026
Triaz Gel . . . 2026
H2OXYL (Canada, Switzerland)
BENZOYL PEROXIDE
Brevoxyl-4 Cleansing Lotion . . . 3269
Brevoxyl-4 Creamy Wash . . . 3270
Brevoxyl-4 Gel . . . 3269
Brevoxyl-8 Cleansing Lotion . . . 3269
Brevoxyl-8 Creamy Wash . . . 3270
Brevoxyl-8 Gel . . . 3269
Triaz Cleanser . . . 2026
Triaz Gel . . . 2026
HABITROL (Canada)
NICOTINE
Nicotrol Inhaler . . . 2840
Nicotrol Nasal Spray . . . 2843
HADARAX (Thailand)
HYDROXYZINE HYDROCHLORIDE
Atarax Tablets & Syrup . . . 2667
Vistaril Intramuscular Solution . . . 2738
HAEMITON (Germany)
CLONIDINE HYDROCHLORIDE
Catapres Tablets . . . 1037
Duraclon Injection . . . 3057
HAEMITON-AUGENTROPFEN (Germany)
CLONIDINE HYDROCHLORIDE
Catapres Tablets . . . 1037
Duraclon Injection . . . 3057
HAIMASERUM (Italy)
PLASMA PROTEIN FRACTION
Plasmanate . . . 942
HALBMOND (Germany)
DIPHENHYDRAMINE HYDROCHLORIDE
Benadryl Parenteral . . . 2617
HALCION (Australia, Austria, Belgium, Canada, Denmark, Finland, France, Germany, Hong Kong, Irish Republic, Israel, Italy, Mexico, New Zealand, Portugal, South Africa, Spain, Sweden, Switzerland, Thailand, The Netherlands, United Kingdom)
TRIAZOLAM
Halcion Tablets . . . 2823
HALDID (Denmark)
FENTANYL CITRATE
Actiq . . . 1184
HALDOL (Australia, Irish Republic, New Zealand, United Kingdom)
HALOPERIDOL DECANOATE
Haldol Decanoate 100 Injection . . . 2535
Haldol Decanoate 50 Injection . . . 2535
HALF BETADUR CR (United Kingdom)
PROPRANOLOL HYDROCHLORIDE
Inderal Injectable . . . 3513
Inderal LA Long-Acting Capsules . . . 3516
Inderal Tablets . . . 3513
HALF BETA-PROGRANE (United Kingdom)
PROPRANOLOL HYDROCHLORIDE
Inderal Injectable . . . 3513
Inderal LA Long-Acting Capsules . . . 3516
Inderal Tablets . . . 3513
HALF INDERAL (Irish Republic, United Kingdom)
PROPRANOLOL HYDROCHLORIDE
Inderal Injectable . . . 3513
Inderal LA Long-Acting Capsules . . . 3516
Inderal Tablets . . . 3513
HALF SECURON (United Kingdom)
VERAPAMIL HYDROCHLORIDE
Covera-HS Tablets . . . 3199
Isoptin SR Tablets . . . 467
Verelan Capsules . . . 3184
Verelan PM Capsules . . . 3186
HALF SINEMET (United Kingdom)
CARBIDOPA/LEVODOPA
Sinemet CR Tablets . . . 1255
Sinemet Tablets . . . 1253
HALOMED (Thailand)
HALOPERIDOL
Haldol Injection, Tablets and Concentrate . . . 2533
HALOMYCETIN (Austria)
CHLORAMPHENICOL
Chloromycetin Ophthalmic Ointment, 1% . . . ⊙296
Chloromycetin Ophthalmic Solution . . . ⊙297
Chloroptic Sterile Ophthalmic Ointment . . . ⊙234
Chloroptic Sterile Ophthalmic Solution . . . ⊙235
HALONEURAL (Germany)
HALOPERIDOL
Haldol Injection, Tablets and Concentrate . . . 2533
HALO-P (Thailand)
HALOPERIDOL
Haldol Injection, Tablets and Concentrate . . . 2533
HALOPER (Germany, Israel)
HALOPERIDOL
Haldol Injection, Tablets and Concentrate . . . 2533
HALOPERIL (Mexico)
HALOPERIDOL
Haldol Injection, Tablets and Concentrate . . . 2533
HALOPOL (Thailand)
HALOPERIDOL
Haldol Injection, Tablets and Concentrate . . . 2533
HARICON (Thailand)
HALOPERIDOL
Haldol Injection, Tablets and Concentrate . . . 2533
HARMOGEN (Irish Republic, United Kingdom)
ESTROPIPATE
Ogen Tablets . . . 2846
Ortho-Est Tablets . . . 3464
HARNAL (Japan, Thailand)
TAMSULOSIN HYDROCHLORIDE
Flomax Capsules . . . 1044
HARTSORB (Thailand)
ISOSORBIDE DINITRATE
Isordil Sublingual Tablets . . . 3525
Isordil Titradose Tablets . . . 3526
HAYCLEAR (New Zealand)
BUDESONIDE
Pulmicort Turbuhaler Inhalation Powder . . . 636
Rhinocort Nasal Inhaler . . . 640
HC45 (Irish Republic, United Kingdom)
HYDROCORTISONE ACETATE
Anusol-HC Suppositories . . . 2238
Cortifoam Rectal Foam . . . 3170
Hydrocortone Acetate Injectable Suspension . . . 2103
Proctocort Suppositories . . . 2264
HCT-ISIS (Germany)
HYDROCHLOROTHIAZIDE
HydroDIURIL Tablets . . . 2108
Microzide Capsules . . . 3414
HEALON (Australia, Belgium, Canada, Finland, France, Germany, Hong Kong, Israel, Italy, New Zealand, Norway, Singapore, South Africa, Sweden, Switzerland, Thailand, The Netherlands)
SODIUM HYALURONATE
Hyalgan Solution . . . 3080
HEALONID (Austria, France, Irish Republic, United Kingdom)
SODIUM HYALURONATE
Hyalgan Solution . . . 3080
HEDAZOL (Mexico)
MEBENDAZOLE
Vermox Chewable Tablets . . . 2017
HEDEX IBUPROFEN (United Kingdom)
IBUPROFEN
Motrin Suspension, Oral Drops, Chewable Tablets, and Caplets . . . 2002
HEITRIN (Germany)
TERAZOSIN HYDROCHLORIDE
Hytrin Capsules . . . 464
HEKTULOSE (Germany)
LACTULOSE
Kristalose for Oral Solution . . . 1007
HELICLAR (Belgium)
CLARITHROMYCIN
Biaxin Filmtab Tablets . . . 403
Biaxin for Oral Suspension . . . 403
HELIMOX (Italy)
AMOXICILLIN
Amoxil Pediatric Drops for Oral Suspension . . . 1471
Amoxil Tablets . . . 1471
HELIOPAR (Finland)
CHLOROQUINE PHOSPHATE
Aralen Tablets . . . 3075
HELMIBEN (Brazil)
MEBENDAZOLE
Vermox Chewable Tablets . . . 2017
HELMIDRAX (Brazil)
MEBENDAZOLE
Vermox Chewable Tablets . . . 2017
HELMINE (Spain)
ONDANSETRON HYDROCHLORIDE
Zofran Injection . . . 1698
Zofran Injection Premixed . . . 1698
Zofran Oral Solution . . . 1703
Zofran Tablets . . . 1703
HELMINTAL (Brazil)
ALBENDAZOLE
Albenza Tablets . . . 1463
HELMINZOLE (Mexico)
MEBENDAZOLE
Vermox Chewable Tablets . . . 2017
HELMI-PED (Brazil)
MEBENDAZOLE
Vermox Chewable Tablets . . . 2017
HELMISONS (Mexico)
ALBENDAZOLE
Albenza Tablets . . . 1463
HELMIZIL (Brazil)
MEBENDAZOLE
Vermox Chewable Tablets . . . 2017
HELVEDOCLYN (Switzerland)
DOXYCYCLINE HYCLATE
Doryx Coated Pellet Filled Capsules . . . 3357
Periostat Tablets . . . 1208
Vibramycin Hyclate Capsules . . . 2735
Vibramycin Hyclate Intravenous . . . 2737
Vibra-Tabs Film Coated Tablets . . . 2735
HEMAGENE TAILLEUR (France)
IBUPROFEN
Motrin Suspension, Oral Drops, Chewable Tablets, and Caplets . . . 2002
HEMAX (Thailand)
EPOETIN ALFA
Epogen for Injection . . . 582
Procrit for Injection . . . 2502
HEMAX-ERITRON (Brazil)
EPOETIN ALFA
Epogen for Injection . . . 582
Procrit for Injection . . . 2502
HEMERAN (Germany)
HEPARIN SODIUM
Heparin Lock Flush Solution . . . 3509
Heparin Sodium Injection . . . 3511
HEMIGOXINE NATIVELLE (France)
DIGOXIN
Lanoxicaps Capsules . . . 1574
Lanoxin Elixir Pediatric . . . 1578
Lanoxin Injection . . . 1581
Lanoxin Injection Pediatric . . . 1584
Lanoxin Tablets . . . 1587
HEMIPRALON (France)
PROPRANOLOL HYDROCHLORIDE
Inderal Injectable . . . 3513
Inderal LA Long-Acting Capsules . . . 3516
Inderal Tablets . . . 3513
HEMOCROMO (Italy)
FERRIC SODIUM GLUCONATE
Ferrlecit Injection . . . 3386
HEMOGENIN (Brazil)
OXYMETHOLONE
Anadrol-50 Tablets . . . 3321
HEPAFLEX (Finland)
HEPARIN SODIUM
Heparin Lock Flush Solution . . . 3509
Heparin Sodium Injection . . . 3511
HEPAGEL (Switzerland)
HEPARIN SODIUM
Heparin Lock Flush Solution . . . 3509
Heparin Sodium Injection . . . 3511
HEPA-GEL (Germany)
HEPARIN SODIUM
Heparin Lock Flush Solution . . . 3509
Heparin Sodium Injection . . . 3511
HEPALAC (Thailand)
LACTULOSE
Kristalose for Oral Solution . . . 1007
HEPALEAN (Canada)
HEPARIN SODIUM
Heparin Lock Flush Solution . . . 3509
Heparin Sodium Injection . . . 3511
HEPALEAN-LOK (Canada)
HEPARIN SODIUM
Heparin Lock Flush Solution . . . 3509
Heparin Sodium Injection . . . 3511
HEPA-MERZ LACT (Germany)
LACTULOSE
Kristalose for Oral Solution . . . 1007
HEPAPLUS (Germany)
HEPARIN SODIUM
Heparin Lock Flush Solution . . . 3509
Heparin Sodium Injection . . . 3511
HEPARTH (Mexico)
HEPARIN SODIUM
Heparin Lock Flush Solution . . . 3509
Heparin Sodium Injection . . . 3511
HEPA-SALBE (Germany)
HEPARIN SODIUM
Heparin Lock Flush Solution . . . 3509
Heparin Sodium Injection . . . 3511
HEPATHROMBIN (Germany)
HEPARIN SODIUM
Heparin Lock Flush Solution . . . 3509
Heparin Sodium Injection . . . 3511
HEPATICUM-LAC-MEDICE (Germany)
LACTULOSE
Kristalose for Oral Solution . . . 1007
HEP-FLUSH (United Kingdom)
HEPARIN SODIUM
Heparin Lock Flush Solution . . . 3509
Heparin Sodium Injection . . . 3511
HEPLOK (Irish Republic, United Kingdom)
HEPARIN SODIUM
Heparin Lock Flush Solution . . . 3509
Heparin Sodium Injection . . . 3511
HEP-RINSE (Irish Republic)
HEPARIN SODIUM
Heparin Lock Flush Solution . . . 3509
Heparin Sodium Injection . . . 3511
HEPRONE (Spain)
SUCRALFATE
Carafate Suspension . . . 731
Carafate Tablets . . . 730
HEPSAL (Irish Republic, United Kingdom)
HEPARIN SODIUM
Heparin Lock Flush Solution . . . 3509
Heparin Sodium Injection . . . 3511
HEPTOVIR (Canada)
LAMIVUDINE
Epivir Oral Solution . . . 1520
Epivir Tablets . . . 1520
Epivir-HBV Oral Solution . . . 1524
Epivir-HBV Tablets . . . 1524
HERBESSER (Hong Kong, Japan, Portugal, Singapore, Thailand)
DILTIAZEM HYDROCHLORIDE
Cardizem CD Capsules . . . 1016

Cardizem Injectable 1018
Cardizem Lyo-Ject Syringe 1018
Cardizem Monovial 1018
Tiazac Capsules 1378

HERCEPTIN (Australia, France, Irish Republic, Singapore, Switzerland, United Kingdom)
TRASTUZUMAB
Herceptin I.V. 1414

HERKLIN (Mexico)
LINDANE
Lindane Lotion USP 1% 559
Lindane Shampoo USP 1% 560

HERMOLEPSIN (Sweden)
CARBAMAZEPINE
Carbatrol Capsules 3234
Tegretol Chewable Tablets 2404
Tegretol Suspension 2404
Tegretol Tablets 2404
Tegretol-XR Tablets 2404

HERTEN (Spain)
ENALAPRIL MALEATE
Vasotec Tablets 2210

HEVERT-DORM (Germany)
DIPHENHYDRAMINE HYDROCHLORIDE
Benadryl Parenteral 2617

HEXA-BLOK (South Africa)
ATENOLOL
Tenormin I.V. Injection 692

HEXADILAT (Denmark)
NIFEDIPINE
Adalat CC Tablets 877
Procardia Capsules 2708
Procardia XL Extended Release Tablets . . 2710

HEXADROL (Canada)
DEXAMETHASONE
Decadron Elixir 2078
Decadron Tablets 2079
DEXAMETHASONE SODIUM PHOSPHATE
Decadron Phosphate Injection 2081
Decadron Phosphate Sterile Ophthalmic Ointment . . . . . . ⊙280, 2083
Decadron Phosphate Sterile Ophthalmic Solution 2084

HEXAGASTRON (Denmark)
SUCRALFATE
Carafate Suspension 731
Carafate Tablets 730

HEXALEN (Australia, Canada, Israel, Norway, Sweden, United Kingdom)
ALTRETAMINE
Hexalen Capsules 2226

HEXALID (Denmark)
DIAZEPAM
Valium Injectable 3026
Valium Tablets 3047

HEXAMET (South Africa)
CIMETIDINE
Tagamet Tablets 1644

HEXAMYCIN (Denmark)
GENTAMICIN SULFATE
Genoptic Ophthalmic Ointment . . . . ⊙239
Genoptic Sterile Ophthalmic Solution . . . ⊙239

HEXANITRAT (Austria)
ISOSORBIDE DINITRATE
Isordil Sublingual Tablets 3525
Isordil Titradose Tablets 3526

HEXAPRESS (Denmark)
PRAZOSIN HYDROCHLORIDE
Minipress Capsules 2699

HEXARONE (South Africa)
AMIODARONE HYDROCHLORIDE
Cordarone Intravenous 3491
Cordarone Tablets 3487
Pacerone Tablets 3331

HEXASOPTIN (Denmark)
VERAPAMIL HYDROCHLORIDE
Covera-HS Tablets 3199
Isoptin SR Tablets 467
Verelan Capsules 3184
Verelan PM Capsules 3186

HEXASTAT (Canada, France, Hong Kong, Italy, Norway, The Netherlands)
ALTRETAMINE
Hexalen Capsules 2226

HEXINAWAS (Spain)
ALTRETAMINE
Hexalen Capsules 2226

HEXIT (Canada)
LINDANE
Lindane Lotion USP 1% 559
Lindane Shampoo USP 1% 560

HIALID (Hong Kong)
SODIUM HYALURONATE
Hyalgan Solution 3080

HICARLEX (Spain)
FOSINOPRIL SODIUM
Monopril Tablets 1091

HICONCIL (The Netherlands)
AMOXICILLIN
Amoxil Pediatric Drops for Oral Suspension 1471
Amoxil Tablets 1471

HIDALONE (Portugal)
HYDROCORTISONE
Anusol-HC Cream 2.5% 2237
Hydrocortone Tablets 2106

HIDANTAL (Brazil)
PHENYTOIN
Dilantin Infatabs 2624
Dilantin-125 Oral Suspension 2625

HIDERM (Australia)
CLOTRIMAZOLE
Lotrimin Cream 1% 3128
Lotrimin Lotion 1% 3128
Lotrimin Topical Solution 1% 3128
Mycelex Troche 573

HIDIL (Singapore, Thailand)
GEMFIBROZIL
Lopid Tablets 2650

HIDROALTESONA (Spain)
HYDROCORTISONE
Anusol-HC Cream 2.5% 2237
Hydrocortone Tablets 2106

HIDROPOLICIN (Mexico)
NEOMYCIN SULFATE/POLYMYXIN B SULFATE
Neosporin G.U. Irrigant Sterile 2256

HIDROQUIN (Mexico)
HYDROQUINONE
Eldopaque Forte 4% Cream 1734
Eldoquin Forte 4% Cream 1734
Lustra Cream 2023
Lustra-AF Cream 2023
Melanex Topical Solution 2300
Solaquin Forte 4% Cream 1734
Solaquin Forte 4% Gel 1734

HIDROSALURETIL (Spain)
HYDROCHLOROTHIAZIDE
HydroDIURIL Tablets 2108
Microzide Capsules 3414

HILL'S BALSAM CHESTY COUGH (United Kingdom)
GUAIFENESIN
Organidin NR Liquid 3350
Organidin NR Tablets 3350

HIPERLEX (Spain)
FOSINOPRIL SODIUM
Monopril Tablets 1091

HIPERTEX (Mexico)
CAPTOPRIL
Captopril Tablets 2281

HIPERTIL (Portugal)
CAPTOPRIL
Captopril Tablets 2281

HIPOARTEL (Spain)
ENALAPRIL MALEATE
Vasotec Tablets 2210

HIPOARTEL PLUS (Spain)
ENALAPRIL MALEATE/HYDROCHLOROTHIAZIDE
Vaseretic Tablets 2204

HIPOCATRIL (Brazil)
CAPTOPRIL
Captopril Tablets 2281

HIPOTENSIL (Portugal)
CAPTOPRIL
Captopril Tablets 2281

HIPRANOL (South Africa)
PROPRANOLOL HYDROCHLORIDE
Inderal Injectable 3513
Inderal LA Long-Acting Capsules 3516
Inderal Tablets 3513

HIPTEN (Mexico, Portugal)
METHYLDOPA
Aldomet Tablets 2037

HISTAFILIN (Spain)
THEOPHYLLINE
Aerolate Jr. T.D. Capsules 1361
Aerolate Liquid 1361
Aerolate Sr. T.D. Capsules 1361
Theo-Dur Extended-Release Tablets 1835
Uni-Dur Extended-Release Tablets 1841
Uniphyl 400 mg and 600 mg Tablets . . . 2903

HISTAK (South Africa)
RANITIDINE HYDROCHLORIDE
Zantac 150 EFFERdose Granules 1690
Zantac 150 EFFERdose Tablets 1690
Zantac 150 Tablets 1690
Zantac 300 Tablets 1690
Zantac Injection 1688
Zantac Injection Premixed 1688
Zantac Syrup 1690

HISTALOC (United Arab Emirates)
PROMETHAZINE HYDROCHLORIDE
Phenergan Injection 3553
Phenergan Suppositories 3556
Phenergan Syrup Fortis 3554
Phenergan Syrup Plain 3554
Phenergan Tablets 3556

HISTAN (Thailand)
HYDROXYZINE HYDROCHLORIDE
Atarax Tablets & Syrup 2667
Vistaril Intramuscular Solution 2738

HISTANTIL (Canada)
PROMETHAZINE HYDROCHLORIDE
Phenergan Injection 3553
Phenergan Suppositories 3556
Phenergan Syrup Fortis 3554
Phenergan Syrup Plain 3554
Phenergan Tablets 3556

HISTAXIN (Austria)
DIPHENHYDRAMINE HYDROCHLORIDE
Benadryl Parenteral 2617

HISTERGAN (United Kingdom)
DIPHENHYDRAMINE HYDROCHLORIDE
Benadryl Parenteral 2617

HISTODIL (Thailand)
CIMETIDINE HYDROCHLORIDE
Tagamet Injection 1644
Tagamet Liquid 1644

HIVID (Australia, Austria, Belgium, Brazil, Canada, Denmark, Finland, France, Germany, Hong Kong, Irish Republic, Israel, Italy, Japan, Mexico, New Zealand, Norway, Portugal, Singapore, South Africa, Spain, Sweden, Switzerland, Thailand, The Netherlands, United Kingdom)
ZALCITABINE
Hivid Tablets 2975

HIZAAR (Italy)
HYDROCHLOROTHIAZIDE/LOSARTAN POTASSIUM
Hyzaar 50-12.5 Tablets 2109

HIZIN (Thailand)
HYDROXYZINE HYDROCHLORIDE
Atarax Tablets & Syrup 2667
Vistaril Intramuscular Solution 2738

HOCIMIN (Denmark)
CIMETIDINE
Tagamet Tablets 1644

HOLFUNGIN (Germany)
CLOTRIMAZOLE
Lotrimin Cream 1% 3128
Lotrimin Lotion 1% 3128
Lotrimin Topical Solution 1% 3128
Mycelex Troche 573

HOLOXAN (Australia, Austria, Belgium, Denmark, Finland, France, Germany, Hong Kong, Italy, Mexico, Norway, Portugal, Singapore, South Africa, Sweden, Switzerland, Thailand, The Netherlands)
IFOSFAMIDE
Ifex for Injection 1123

HOLOXANE (Brazil)
IFOSFAMIDE
Ifex for Injection 1123

HOLSTEN AKTIV (Germany)
ETHYL CHLORIDE
Gebauer's Ethyl Chloride 1409

HONGOSERIL (Spain)
ITRACONAZOLE
Sporanox Capsules 1800
Sporanox Oral Solution 1808, 2512

HONSA (Thailand)
HYDROXYZINE HYDROCHLORIDE
Atarax Tablets & Syrup 2667
Vistaril Intramuscular Solution 2738

HONZIL (Mexico)
KETOCONAZOLE
Nizoral 2% Cream 3620
Nizoral 2% Shampoo 2007
Nizoral Tablets 1791

HORMOFEMIN (United Kingdom)
DIENESTROL
Ortho Dienestrol Cream 2554

HORTFENICOL (Spain)
CHLORAMPHENICOL
Chloromycetin Ophthalmic Ointment, 1% . . . . ⊙296
Chloromycetin Ophthalmic Solution . . . . ⊙297
Chloroptic Sterile Ophthalmic Ointment . . ⊙234
Chloroptic Sterile Ophthalmic Solution . . ⊙235

HOSBOCIN (Spain)
CEFTRIAXONE SODIUM
Rocephin Injectable Vials, ADD-Vantage, Galaxy, Bulk 2993

HOSBOGEN (Spain)
GENTAMICIN SULFATE
Genoptic Ophthalmic Ointment . . . . ⊙239
Genoptic Sterile Ophthalmic Solution . . . ⊙239

HOTEMIN (Hong Kong)
PIROXICAM
Feldene Capsules 2685

HRF (Belgium, Irish Republic, Italy, The Netherlands, United Kingdom)
GONADORELIN HYDROCHLORIDE
Factrel 3633

H-TAB (Thailand)
HALOPERIDOL
Haldol Injection, Tablets and Concentrate 2533

HUBERDINA (Spain)
FAMOTIDINE
Pepcid Injection 2153
Pepcid Injection Premixed 2153
Pepcid RPD Orally Disintegrating Tablets 2150
Pepcid Tablets 2150
Pepcid for Oral Suspension 2150

HUBERPLEX (Spain)
CHLORDIAZEPOXIDE HYDROCHLORIDE
Librium Capsules 1736
Librium for Injection 1737

HURRICAINE (Spain)
BENZOCAINE
Americaine Anesthetic Lubricant 1162
Americaine Otic Topical Anesthetic Ear Drops 1162

HYA-JECT (Germany)
SODIUM HYALURONATE
Hyalgan Solution 3080

HYALART (Germany, Italy)
SODIUM HYALURONATE
Hyalgan Solution 3080

HYALEIN (Japan)
SODIUM HYALURONATE
Hyalgan Solution 3080

HYALGAN (Austria, Denmark, Finland, France, Hong Kong, Irish Republic, Italy, Sweden, United Kingdom)
SODIUM HYALURONATE
Hyalgan Solution 3080

HYALISTIL (Italy)
SODIUM HYALURONATE
Hyalgan Solution 3080

HYA-OPHTAL (Germany)
SODIUM HYALURONATE
Hyalgan Solution 3080

HYBLOC (New Zealand)
LABETALOL HYDROCHLORIDE
Normodyne Injection 3135
Normodyne Tablets 3137

HYCAMTIN (Australia, Austria, Belgium, Canada, Denmark, Finland, France, Germany, Hong Kong, Irish Republic, Israel, Italy, Norway, Portugal, Singapore, South Africa, Spain, Sweden, Switzerland, Thailand, The Netherlands, United Kingdom)
TOPOTECAN HYDROCHLORIDE
Hycamtin for Injection 1546

HYCORT (Canada)
HYDROCORTISONE
Anusol-HC Cream 2.5% 2237
Hydrocortone Tablets 2106

HYDAC (Denmark, Finland, Sweden)
FELODIPINE
Plendil Extended-Release Tablets 623

HYDAL (Austria)
HYDROMORPHONE HYDROCHLORIDE
Dilaudid Ampules 441
Dilaudid Injection 441
Dilaudid Multiple Dose Vials (Sterile Solution) 441
Dilaudid Oral Liquid 445
Dilaudid Powder 441
Dilaudid Rectal Suppositories 441

Dilaudid Tablets . . . 441
Dilaudid Tablets - 8 mg . . . 445
Dilaudid-HP Injection . . . 443
Dilaudid-HP Lyophilized Powder 250 mg. . . 443

HYDANTIN (Finland)
PHENYTOIN
Dilantin Infatabs . . . 2624
Dilantin-125 Oral Suspension . . . 2625

HYDERM (Canada)
HYDROCORTISONE ACETATE
Anusol-HC Suppositories . . . 2238
Cortifoam Rectal Foam . . . 3170
Hydrocortone Acetate Injectable Suspension . . . 2103
Proctocort Suppositories . . . 2264

HYDOPA (Australia)
METHYLDOPA
Aldomet Tablets . . . 2037

HYDRACORT (France)
HYDROCORTISONE
Anusol-HC Cream 2.5% . . . 2237
Hydrocortone Tablets . . . 2106

HYDRENE (Australia)
HYDROCHLOROTHIAZIDE/TRIAMTERENE
Dyazide Capsules . . . 1515
Maxzide Tablets . . . 1008
Maxzide-25 mg Tablets . . . 1008

HYDRENOX (United Kingdom)
HYDROFLUMETHIAZIDE
Diucardin Tablets . . . 3494

HYDREX (Finland)
HYDROCHLOROTHIAZIDE
HydroDIURIL Tablets . . . 2108
Microzide Capsules . . . 3414

HYDRO-ADRESON (The Netherlands)
HYDROCORTISONE ACETATE
Anusol-HC Suppositories . . . 2238
Cortifoam Rectal Foam . . . 3170
Hydrocortone Acetate Injectable Suspension . . . 2103
Proctocort Suppositories . . . 2264

HYDROCOMP (Germany)
AMILORIDE
HYDROCHLORIDE/HYDROCHLOROTHIAZIDE
Moduretic Tablets . . . 2138

HYDROCORT (Germany)
HYDROCORTISONE ACETATE
Anusol-HC Suppositories . . . 2238
Cortifoam Rectal Foam . . . 3170
Hydrocortone Acetate Injectable Suspension . . . 2103
Proctocort Suppositories . . . 2264

HYDROCORT MILD (Germany)
HYDROCORTISONE
Anusol-HC Cream 2.5% . . . 2237
Hydrocortone Tablets . . . 2106

HYDROCORTISTAB (United Kingdom)
HYDROCORTISONE ACETATE
Anusol-HC Suppositories . . . 2238
Cortifoam Rectal Foam . . . 3170
Hydrocortone Acetate Injectable Suspension . . . 2103
Proctocort Suppositories . . . 2264

HYDROCORTISYL (Irish Republic, United Kingdom)
HYDROCORTISONE
Anusol-HC Cream 2.5% . . . 2237
Hydrocortone Tablets . . . 2106

HYDROCORTONE (Austria, Irish Republic, Portugal, Switzerland, United Kingdom)
HYDROCORTISONE
Anusol-HC Cream 2.5% . . . 2237
Hydrocortone Tablets . . . 2106

HYDROCUTAN MILD (Germany)
HYDROCORTISONE
Anusol-HC Cream 2.5% . . . 2237
Hydrocortone Tablets . . . 2106

HYDRODERM (Austria)
HYDROCORTISONE
Anusol-HC Cream 2.5% . . . 2237
Hydrocortone Tablets . . . 2106

HYDRODERM HC (Germany)
HYDROCORTISONE
Anusol-HC Cream 2.5% . . . 2237
Hydrocortone Tablets . . . 2106

HYDRODERMED (Germany)
ERYTHROMYCIN
Emgel 2% Topical Gel . . . 1285
Ery-Tab Tablets . . . 448
Erythromycin Base Filmtab Tablets . . . 454
Erythromycin Delayed-Release Capsules, USP . . . 455

PCE Dispertab Tablets . . . 498

HYDRODIURIL (Canada)
HYDROCHLOROTHIAZIDE
HydroDIURIL Tablets . . . 2108
Microzide Capsules . . . 3414

HYDROFORM (Australia)
HYDROCORTISONE
Anusol-HC Cream 2.5% . . . 2237
Hydrocortone Tablets . . . 2106

HYDROGALEN (Germany)
HYDROCORTISONE
Anusol-HC Cream 2.5% . . . 2237
Hydrocortone Tablets . . . 2106

HYDRO-LESS (South Africa)
INDAPAMIDE
Indapamide Tablets . . . 2286

HYDROLID (Switzerland)
AMILORIDE
HYDROCHLORIDE/HYDROCHLOROTHIAZIDE
Moduretic Tablets . . . 2138

HYDROMET (Irish Republic, South Africa, Spain, The Netherlands, United Kingdom)
HYDROCHLOROTHIAZIDE/METHYLDOPA
Aldoril Tablets . . . 2039

HYDROMET (Brazil, Sweden)
HYDROCHLOROTHIAZIDE
HydroDIURIL Tablets . . . 2108
Microzide Capsules . . . 3414

HYDROMORPH (Canada)
HYDROMORPHONE HYDROCHLORIDE
Dilaudid Ampules . . . 441
Dilaudid Injection . . . 441
Dilaudid Multiple Dose Vials (Sterile Solution) . . . 441
Dilaudid Oral Liquid . . . 445
Dilaudid Powder . . . 441
Dilaudid Rectal Suppositories . . . 441
Dilaudid Tablets . . . 441
Dilaudid Tablets - 8 mg . . . 445
Dilaudid-HP Injection . . . 443
Dilaudid-HP Lyophilized Powder 250 mg. . . 443

HYDRONET (Denmark)
AMILORIDE
HYDROCHLORIDE/HYDROCHLOROTHIAZIDE
Moduretic Tablets . . . 2138

HY-DROP (Italy)
SODIUM HYALURONATE
Hyalgan Solution . . . 3080

HYDROSALURIC (Irish Republic, United Kingdom)
HYDROCHLOROTHIAZIDE
HydroDIURIL Tablets . . . 2108
Microzide Capsules . . . 3414

HYDROSONE (Australia, Canada)
HYDROCORTISONE ACETATE
Anusol-HC Suppositories . . . 2238
Cortifoam Rectal Foam . . . 3170
Hydrocortone Acetate Injectable Suspension . . . 2103
Proctocort Suppositories . . . 2264

HYDROXIN (Thailand)
HYDROXYZINE HYDROCHLORIDE
Atarax Tablets & Syrup . . . 2667
Vistaril Intramuscular Solution . . . 2738

HYDROZIDE (Hong Kong, Singapore, Thailand)
AMILORIDE
HYDROCHLORIDE/HYDROCHLOROTHIAZIDE
Moduretic Tablets . . . 2138
HYDROCHLOROTHIAZIDE
HydroDIURIL Tablets . . . 2108
Microzide Capsules . . . 3414

HYDROZOLE (Australia)
HYDROCORTISONE
Anusol-HC Cream 2.5% . . . 2237
Hydrocortone Tablets . . . 2106

HY-GAG (Germany)
SODIUM HYALURONATE
Hyalgan Solution . . . 3080

HYLAFORM (Germany)
SODIUM HYALURONATE
Hyalgan Solution . . . 3080

HYLO-COMOD (Germany)
SODIUM HYALURONATE
Hyalgan Solution . . . 3080

HYPACE (South Africa)
ENALAPRIL MALEATE
Vasotec Tablets . . . 2210

HYPAM (New Zealand)
TRIAZOLAM
Halcion Tablets . . . 2823

HYPEN (Japan)
ETODOLAC
Lodine Capsules . . . 3528
Lodine Tablets . . . 3528
Lodine XL Extended-Release Tablets . . . 3530

HYPERILEX (Germany)
PEMOLINE
Cylert Chewable Tablets . . . 415
Cylert Tablets . . . 415

HYPERMOL (New Zealand)
TIMOLOL MALEATE
Blocadren Tablets . . . 2046
Timoptic Sterile Ophthalmic Solution . . . 2190
Timoptic in Ocudose . . . 2192
Timoptic-XE Sterile Ophthalmic Gel Forming Solution . . . 2194

HYPERNOL (Hong Kong)
ATENOLOL
Tenormin I.V. Injection . . . 692

HYPERRETIC (Thailand)
AMILORIDE
HYDROCHLORIDE/HYDROCHLOROTHIAZIDE
Moduretic Tablets . . . 2138

HYPERTANE (United Kingdom)
AMILORIDE
HYDROCHLORIDE/HYDROCHLOROTHIAZIDE
Moduretic Tablets . . . 2138

HYPERTORR (Germany)
HYDROCHLOROTHIAZIDE/TRIAMTERENE
Dyazide Capsules . . . 1515
Maxzide Tablets . . . 1008
Maxzide-25 mg Tablets . . . 1008

HYPNOREX (Germany, Switzerland)
LITHIUM CARBONATE
Eskalith CR Controlled Release Tablets . . . 1527
Eskalith Capsules . . . 1527
Lithium Carbonate Capsules . . . 3061
Lithobid Slow-Release Tablets . . . 3255

HYPNOVEL (Australia, France, Irish Republic, United Kingdom)
MIDAZOLAM HYDROCHLORIDE
Versed Injection . . . 3027
Versed Syrup . . . 3033

HYPOLAR RETARD (United Kingdom)
NIFEDIPINE
Adalat CC Tablets . . . 877
Procardia Capsules . . . 2708
Procardia XL Extended Release Tablets . . . 2710

HYPOMIDE (South Africa)
CHLORPROPAMIDE
Diabinese Tablets . . . 2680

HYPOTENS (Israel)
PRAZOSIN HYDROCHLORIDE
Minipress Capsules . . . 2699

HY-PO-TONE (South Africa)
METHYLDOPA
Aldomet Tablets . . . 2037

HYPOVASE (Irish Republic, United Kingdom)
PRAZOSIN HYDROCHLORIDE
Minipress Capsules . . . 2699

HYPREN (Austria)
RAMIPRIL
Altace Capsules . . . 2233

HYPROSIN (New Zealand)
PRAZOSIN HYDROCHLORIDE
Minipress Capsules . . . 2699

HYSONE (Australia)
HYDROCORTISONE
Anusol-HC Cream 2.5% . . . 2237
Hydrocortone Tablets . . . 2106

HYSONE-A (Australia)
HYDROCORTISONE ACETATE
Anusol-HC Suppositories . . . 2238
Cortifoam Rectal Foam . . . 3170
Hydrocortone Acetate Injectable Suspension . . . 2103
Proctocort Suppositories . . . 2264

HYTENEZE (United Kingdom)
CAPTOPRIL
Captopril Tablets . . . 2281

HYTISONE (Hong Kong, Thailand)
HYDROCORTISONE
Anusol-HC Cream 2.5% . . . 2237
Hydrocortone Tablets . . . 2106

HYTRIN (Australia, Belgium, Brazil, Canada, Hong Kong, Irish Republic, Israel, Mexico, New Zealand, Portugal, Singapore, South Africa, Thailand, The Netherlands, United Kingdom)
TERAZOSIN HYDROCHLORIDE
Hytrin Capsules . . . 464

HYTRIN BPH (Switzerland)
TERAZOSIN HYDROCHLORIDE
Hytrin Capsules . . . 464

HYTRINE (France)
TERAZOSIN HYDROCHLORIDE
Hytrin Capsules . . . 464

HYTRINEX (Sweden)
TERAZOSIN HYDROCHLORIDE
Hytrin Capsules . . . 464

HYZAAR (Canada, France, Hong Kong, Mexico, Singapore, Thailand, The Netherlands)
HYDROCHLOROTHIAZIDE/LOSARTAN POTASSIUM
Hyzaar 50-12.5 Tablets . . . 2109

IAL (Hong Kong, Italy, Switzerland, Thailand)
SODIUM HYALURONATE
Hyalgan Solution . . . 3080

IALUGEN (Switzerland)
SODIUM HYALURONATE
Hyalgan Solution . . . 3080

IALUM (Italy)
SODIUM HYALURONATE
Hyalgan Solution . . . 3080

IALUREX (Italy)
SODIUM HYALURONATE
Hyalgan Solution . . . 3080

IBARIL (Belgium, Denmark, Finland, Norway, Sweden, The Netherlands)
DESOXIMETASONE
Topicort Cream . . . 2025
Topicort Gel . . . 2025
Topicort LP Cream . . . 2025
Topicort Ointment . . . 2025

IBARIL MED SALICYLSYRE (Denmark)
DESOXIMETASONE
Topicort Cream . . . 2025
Topicort Gel . . . 2025
Topicort LP Cream . . . 2025
Topicort Ointment . . . 2025

IBENON (Spain)
IBUPROFEN
Motrin Suspension, Oral Drops, Chewable Tablets, and Caplets . . . 2002

IBIAMOX (Thailand)
AMOXICILLIN
Amoxil Pediatric Drops for Oral Suspension . . . 1471
Amoxil Tablets . . . 1471

IBIDROXIL (Italy)
CEFADROXIL
Duricef Capsules . . . 1079
Duricef Oral Suspension . . . 1079
Duricef Tablets . . . 1079

IBILEX (Australia, Italy, Thailand)
CEPHALEXIN
Keflex Oral Suspension . . . 1237
Keflex Pulvules . . . 1237

IBIMAN (Italy)
CEFAMANDOLE NAFATE
Mandol Vials . . . 1953

IBOPAIN (South Africa)
IBUPROFEN
Motrin Suspension, Oral Drops, Chewable Tablets, and Caplets . . . 2002

IBOSURE (The Netherlands)
IBUPROFEN
Motrin Suspension, Oral Drops, Chewable Tablets, and Caplets . . . 2002

IBROFEN (Thailand)
IBUPROFEN
Motrin Suspension, Oral Drops, Chewable Tablets, and Caplets . . . 2002

IBRUFHALAL (United Kingdom)
IBUPROFEN
Motrin Suspension, Oral Drops, Chewable Tablets, and Caplets . . . 2002

IBU (Germany, Thailand)
IBUPROFEN
Motrin Suspension, Oral Drops, Chewable Tablets, and Caplets . . . 2002

IBUALGIC (France)
IBUPROFEN
Motrin Suspension, Oral Drops, Chewable Tablets, and Caplets . . . 2002

IBU-ATTRITIN (Germany)
IBUPROFEN
Motrin Suspension, Oral Drops, Chewable Tablets, and Caplets . . . 2002

IBUBEST (Germany)
IBUPROFEN
Motrin Suspension, Oral Drops, Chewable Tablets, and Caplets **2002**

IBUBETA (Germany)
IBUPROFEN
Motrin Suspension, Oral Drops, Chewable Tablets, and Caplets **2002**

IBUCASEN (Spain)
IBUPROFEN
Motrin Suspension, Oral Drops, Chewable Tablets, and Caplets **2002**

IBU-CREAM (Australia)
IBUPROFEN
Motrin Suspension, Oral Drops, Chewable Tablets, and Caplets **2002**

IBUDOL (Austria)
IBUPROFEN
Motrin Suspension, Oral Drops, Chewable Tablets, and Caplets **2002**

IBUDOLOR (Germany)
IBUPROFEN
Motrin Suspension, Oral Drops, Chewable Tablets, and Caplets **2002**

IBUFAC (Thailand, United Kingdom)
IBUPROFEN
Motrin Suspension, Oral Drops, Chewable Tablets, and Caplets **2002**

IBUFARM (South Africa)
IBUPROFEN
Motrin Suspension, Oral Drops, Chewable Tablets, and Caplets **2002**

IBUFEM (United Kingdom)
IBUPROFEN
Motrin Suspension, Oral Drops, Chewable Tablets, and Caplets **2002**

IBUFEN (Israel, Singapore, Thailand)
IBUPROFEN
Motrin Suspension, Oral Drops, Chewable Tablets, and Caplets **2002**

IBUFLAM (Germany)
IBUPROFEN
Motrin Suspension, Oral Drops, Chewable Tablets, and Caplets **2002**

IBUFLEX (Mexico)
IBUPROFEN
Motrin Suspension, Oral Drops, Chewable Tablets, and Caplets **2002**

IBUFUG (Germany)
IBUPROFEN
Motrin Suspension, Oral Drops, Chewable Tablets, and Caplets **2002**

IBUGAN (Thailand)
IBUPROFEN
Motrin Suspension, Oral Drops, Chewable Tablets, and Caplets **2002**

IBUGEL (Austria, Irish Republic, Switzerland, United Kingdom)
IBUPROFEN
Motrin Suspension, Oral Drops, Chewable Tablets, and Caplets **2002**

IBULAN (Thailand)
IBUPROFEN
Motrin Suspension, Oral Drops, Chewable Tablets, and Caplets **2002**

IBULAR (United Kingdom)
IBUPROFEN
Motrin Suspension, Oral Drops, Chewable Tablets, and Caplets **2002**

IBULEVE (Israel, South Africa, United Kingdom)
IBUPROFEN
Motrin Suspension, Oral Drops, Chewable Tablets, and Caplets **2002**

IBULGAN (Switzerland)
IBUPROFEN
Motrin Suspension, Oral Drops, Chewable Tablets, and Caplets **2002**

IBULOID (Singapore)
IBUPROFEN
Motrin Suspension, Oral Drops, Chewable Tablets, and Caplets **2002**

IBUMAX (Finland)
IBUPROFEN
Motrin Suspension, Oral Drops, Chewable Tablets, and Caplets **2002**

IBUMED (Belgium, South Africa, Switzerland, United Kingdom)
IBUPROFEN
Motrin Suspension, Oral Drops, Chewable Tablets, and Caplets **2002**

IBUMERCK (Germany)
IBUPROFEN
Motrin Suspension, Oral Drops, Chewable Tablets, and Caplets **2002**

IBUMETIN (Austria, Finland, Norway, Sweden, The Netherlands, United Kingdom)
IBUPROFEN
Motrin Suspension, Oral Drops, Chewable Tablets, and Caplets **2002**

IBUMOUSSE (United Kingdom)
IBUPROFEN
Motrin Suspension, Oral Drops, Chewable Tablets, and Caplets **2002**

IBUNET (Denmark)
IBUPROFEN
Motrin Suspension, Oral Drops, Chewable Tablets, and Caplets **2002**

IBUPAX (Portugal)
IBUPROFEN
Motrin Suspension, Oral Drops, Chewable Tablets, and Caplets **2002**

IBUPHLOGONT (Germany)
IBUPROFEN
Motrin Suspension, Oral Drops, Chewable Tablets, and Caplets **2002**

IBUPRIL (Mexico)
IBUPROFEN
Motrin Suspension, Oral Drops, Chewable Tablets, and Caplets **2002**

IBUPRON (Austria)
IBUPROFEN
Motrin Suspension, Oral Drops, Chewable Tablets, and Caplets **2002**

IBU-RATIOPHARM (Germany)
IBUPROFEN
Motrin Suspension, Oral Drops, Chewable Tablets, and Caplets **2002**

IBUREM (Austria)
IBUPROFEN
Motrin Suspension, Oral Drops, Chewable Tablets, and Caplets **2002**

IBUREN (Thailand)
IBUPROFEN
Motrin Suspension, Oral Drops, Chewable Tablets, and Caplets **2002**

IBUREUMIN (Denmark)
IBUPROFEN
Motrin Suspension, Oral Drops, Chewable Tablets, and Caplets **2002**

IBUSAL (Finland)
IBUPROFEN
Motrin Suspension, Oral Drops, Chewable Tablets, and Caplets **2002**

IBUSCENT (Spain)
IBUPROFEN
Motrin Suspension, Oral Drops, Chewable Tablets, and Caplets **2002**

IBUSIFAR (Switzerland)
IBUPROFEN
Motrin Suspension, Oral Drops, Chewable Tablets, and Caplets **2002**

IBUSLOW (Hong Kong)
IBUPROFEN
Motrin Suspension, Oral Drops, Chewable Tablets, and Caplets **2002**

IBU-SLOW (Belgium)
IBUPROFEN
Motrin Suspension, Oral Drops, Chewable Tablets, and Caplets **2002**

IBUSPRAY (United Kingdom)
IBUPROFEN
Motrin Suspension, Oral Drops, Chewable Tablets, and Caplets **2002**

IBUTOP (Austria, Belgium, Denmark, France, Germany)
IBUPROFEN
Motrin Suspension, Oral Drops, Chewable Tablets, and Caplets **2002**

IBUTOP CUPROFEN (United Kingdom)
IBUPROFEN
Motrin Suspension, Oral Drops, Chewable Tablets, and Caplets **2002**

IBUTOP RALGEX (United Kingdom)
IBUPROFEN
Motrin Suspension, Oral Drops, Chewable Tablets, and Caplets **2002**

IBU-VIVIMED (Germany)
IBUPROFEN
Motrin Suspension, Oral Drops, Chewable Tablets, and Caplets **2002**

IBUX (Norway)
IBUPROFEN
Motrin Suspension, Oral Drops, Chewable Tablets, and Caplets **2002**

IBUXIN (Finland)
IBUPROFEN
Motrin Suspension, Oral Drops, Chewable Tablets, and Caplets **2002**

ICAZ (France)
ISRADIPINE
DynaCirc CR Tablets **2923**

ICG-PULSION (Germany, Israel)
INDOCYANINE GREEN
IC-Green . . . . ⊙**203**

ICHTHRALETTEN DOXY (Germany)
DOXYCYCLINE HYCLATE
Doryx Coated Pellet Filled Capsules **3357**
Periostat Tablets **1208**
Vibramycin Hyclate Capsules. **2735**
Vibramycin Hyclate Intravenous **2737**
Vibra-Tabs Film Coated Tablets **2735**

ICHT-ORAL (Germany)
MINOCYCLINE HYDROCHLORIDE
Dynacin Capsules. **2019**
Minocin Intravenous **1862**
Minocin Oral Suspension **1865**
Minocin Pellet-Filled Capsules **1863**

ICLADOS (Italy)
DOXYCYCLINE HYCLATE
Doryx Coated Pellet Filled Capsules **3357**
Periostat Tablets **1208**
Vibramycin Hyclate Capsules. **2735**
Vibramycin Hyclate Intravenous **2737**
Vibra-Tabs Film Coated Tablets **2735**

ICTAN (Spain)
CLOTRIMAZOLE
Lotrimin Cream 1%. **3128**
Lotrimin Lotion 1% **3128**
Lotrimin Topical Solution 1% **3128**
Mycelex Troche **573**

IDALPREM (Spain)
LORAZEPAM
Ativan Injection **3478**
Ativan Tablets **3482**

IDAMYCIN (Canada, Mexico)
IDARUBICIN HYDROCHLORIDE
Idamycin PFS Injection. **2825**

IDO A 50 (Spain)
VITAMIN A PALMITATE
Aquasol A Parenteral. **593**

IDRACEMI (Italy)
HYDROCORTISONE SODIUM PHOSPHATE
Hydrocortone Phosphate Injection, Sterile **2105**

IDROCORTIGAMMA (Italy)
HYDROCORTISONE ACETATE
Anusol-HC Suppositories **2238**
Cortifoam Rectal Foam **3170**
Hydrocortone Acetate Injectable Suspension **2103**
Proctocort Suppositories **2264**

IDRODIUVIS (Italy)
HYDROCHLOROTHIAZIDE
HydroDIURIL Tablets **2108**
Microzide Capsules **3414**

IDROLAC (Italy)
LACTULOSE
Kristalose for Oral Solution. **1007**

IDROPULMINA (Italy)
GUAIFENESIN
Organidin NR Liquid **3350**
Organidin NR Tablets. **3350**

IECATEC (Spain)
ENALAPRIL MALEATE
Vasotec Tablets **2210**

IFA REDUCCING S (Mexico)
PHENTERMINE HYDROCHLORIDE
Adipex-P Capsules **1406**
Adipex-P Tablets **1406**

IFADA (Spain)
FAMOTIDINE
Pepcid Injection. **2153**
Pepcid Injection Premixed **2153**
Pepcid RPD Orally Disintegrating Tablets **2150**
Pepcid Tablets. **2150**
Pepcid for Oral Suspension **2150**

IFEMED (Thailand)
PIROXICAM
Feldene Capsules. **2685**

IFEX (Canada)
IFOSFAMIDE
Ifex for Injection. **1123**

IFO-CELL (Germany)
IFOSFAMIDE
Ifex for Injection. **1123**

IFOLEM (Mexico)
IFOSFAMIDE
Ifex for Injection. **1123**

IFOMIDA (Mexico)
IFOSFAMIDE
Ifex for Injection. **1123**

IFOXAN (Israel, Mexico)
IFOSFAMIDE
Ifex for Injection. **1123**

IGUASSINA (Brazil)
HYDROCHLOROTHIAZIDE/TRIAMTERENE
Dyazide Capsules. **1515**
Maxzide Tablets. **1008**
Maxzide-25 mg Tablets **1008**

IKACOR (Israel)
VERAPAMIL HYDROCHLORIDE
Covera-HS Tablets **3199**
Isoptin SR Tablets. **467**
Verelan Capsules **3184**
Verelan PM Capsules **3186**

IKAPRESS (Israel)
VERAPAMIL HYDROCHLORIDE
Covera-HS Tablets **3199**
Isoptin SR Tablets. **467**
Verelan Capsules **3184**
Verelan PM Capsules **3186**

IKATIN (Mexico)
GENTAMICIN SULFATE
Genoptic Ophthalmic Ointment . . . . ⊙**239**
Genoptic Sterile Ophthalmic Solution . . . ⊙**239**

IKTORIVIL (Sweden)
CLONAZEPAM
Klonopin Tablets **2983**

ILACEN (Spain)
DIFLUNISAL
Dolobid Tablets **2088**

ILAGANE (Spain)
NAPROXEN
EC-Naprosyn Delayed-Release Tablets . . . **2967**
Naprosyn Suspension **2967**
Naprosyn Tablets. **2967**

ILOCAP (Australia)
ERYTHROMYCIN
Emgel 2% Topical Gel **1285**
Ery-Tab Tablets **448**
Erythromycin Base Filmtab Tablets **454**
Erythromycin Delayed-Release Capsules, USP. **455**
PCE Dispertab Tablets. **498**

ILOCIN (Brazil)
ERYTHROMYCIN
Emgel 2% Topical Gel **1285**
Ery-Tab Tablets **448**
Erythromycin Base Filmtab Tablets **454**
Erythromycin Delayed-Release Capsules, USP. **455**
PCE Dispertab Tablets. **498**

ILOTICINA (Spain)
ERYTHROMYCIN
Emgel 2% Topical Gel **1285**
Ery-Tab Tablets **448**
Erythromycin Base Filmtab Tablets **454**
Erythromycin Delayed-Release Capsules, USP. **455**
PCE Dispertab Tablets. **498**

ILOTICINA ANTI ACNE (Spain)
ERYTHROMYCIN
Emgel 2% Topical Gel **1285**
Ery-Tab Tablets **448**
Erythromycin Base Filmtab Tablets **454**
Erythromycin Delayed-Release Capsules, USP. **455**
PCE Dispertab Tablets. **498**

ILOTREX (Brazil)
ERYTHROMYCIN STEARATE
Erythrocin Stearate Filmtab Tablets. **452**

ILOTYCIN (South Africa)
ERYTHROMYCIN
Emgel 2% Topical Gel **1285**
Ery-Tab Tablets **448**
Erythromycin Base Filmtab Tablets **454**
Erythromycin Delayed-Release Capsules, USP. **455**
PCE Dispertab Tablets. **498**

ILSATEC (Brazil, Mexico)
LANSOPRAZOLE
Prevacid Delayed-Release Capsules **3292**

ILVICO GRIPPAL (Germany)
IBUPROFEN
Motrin Suspension, Oral Drops, Chewable Tablets, and Caplets **2002**

(⊙ Described in PDR For Ophthalmic Medicines™)

IMACILLIN (Denmark)
AMOXICILLIN
Amoxil Pediatric Drops for Oral Suspension ... 1471
Amoxil Tablets ... 1471

IMAZOL (Germany, Switzerland)
CLOTRIMAZOLE
Lotrimin Cream 1% ... 3128
Lotrimin Lotion 1% ... 3128
Lotrimin Topical Solution 1% ... 3128
Mycelex Troche ... 573

IMDEX (Singapore)
ISOSORBIDE MONONITRATE
Imdur Tablets ... 1826
Ismo Tablets ... 3524

IMDUR (Australia, Austria, Canada, Denmark, Finland, Hong Kong, Irish Republic, Mexico, New Zealand, Norway, Portugal, Singapore, South Africa, Spain, Sweden, Switzerland, Thailand, United Kingdom)
ISOSORBIDE MONONITRATE
Imdur Tablets ... 1826
Ismo Tablets ... 3524

IMEPAS (Mexico)
DIAZEPAM
Valium Injectable ... 3026
Valium Tablets ... 3047

IMFERDEX (Switzerland)
IRON DEXTRAN
INFeD Injection ... 3388

IMFERON (Australia, Belgium, Canada, Mexico, South Africa, Spain, The Netherlands, United Kingdom)
IRON DEXTRAN
INFeD Injection ... 3388

IMIGRAN (Brazil, Hong Kong, Irish Republic, New Zealand, Norway, Portugal, Singapore, South Africa, Spain, Thailand, The Netherlands, United Kingdom)
SUMATRIPTAN SUCCINATE
Imitrex Injection ... 1549
Imitrex Tablets ... 1558

IMIJECT (France)
SUMATRIPTAN SUCCINATE
Imitrex Injection ... 1549
Imitrex Tablets ... 1558

IMIPEM (Italy)
CILASTATIN SODIUM/IMIPENEM
Primaxin I.M. ... 2158
Primaxin I.V. ... 2160

IMITREX (Israel)
SUMATRIPTAN SUCCINATE
Imitrex Injection ... 1549
Imitrex Tablets ... 1558

IMMUKIN (Hong Kong, Irish Republic)
INTERFERON GAMMA-1B
Actimmune ... 1772

IMMUKINE (The Netherlands)
INTERFERON GAMMA-1B
Actimmune ... 1772

IMMUNOL (Italy)
LEVAMISOLE HYDROCHLORIDE
Ergamisol Tablets ... 1789

IMPRONTAL (Spain)
PIROXICAM
Feldene Capsules ... 2685

IMTACK (Irish Republic, United Kingdom)
ISOSORBIDE DINITRATE
Isordil Sublingual Tablets ... 3525
Isordil Titradose Tablets ... 3526

IMTRATE (Australia, New Zealand)
ISOSORBIDE MONONITRATE
Imdur Tablets ... 1826
Ismo Tablets ... 3524

IMUFOR (Austria)
INTERFERON GAMMA-1B
Actimmune ... 1772

IMUKIN (Austria, Denmark, Finland, France, Germany, Italy, Norway, Portugal, Spain, Sweden)
INTERFERON GAMMA-1B
Actimmune ... 1772

INABRIN (Belgium, Italy, Portugal)
IBUPROFEN
Motrin Suspension, Oral Drops, Chewable Tablets, and Caplets ... 2002

INAC (Singapore)
DICLOFENAC SODIUM
Voltaren Tablets ... 2315
Voltaren-XR Tablets ... 2315

INAGEN (Spain)
ETHAMBUTOL HYDROCHLORIDE
Myambutol Tablets ... 1290

INALACOR (Spain)
FLUTICASONE PROPIONATE
Cutivate Cream ... 1282
Cutivate Ointment ... 1284
Flonase Nasal Spray ... 1533
Flovent 110 mcg Inhalation Aerosol ... 1535
Flovent 220 mcg Inhalation Aerosol ... 1535
Flovent 44 mcg Inhalation Aerosol ... 1535
Flovent Rotadisk 100 mcg ... 1537
Flovent Rotadisk 250 mcg ... 1537
Flovent Rotadisk 50 mcg ... 1537

INAMIDE (Irish Republic)
INDAPAMIDE
Indapamide Tablets ... 2286

INASPIR (Spain)
SALMETEROL XINAFOATE
Serevent Diskus ... 1637
Serevent Inhalation Aerosol ... 1633

INCEFAL (Spain)
IBUPROFEN
Motrin Suspension, Oral Drops, Chewable Tablets, and Caplets ... 2002

INDAFLEX (Italy)
INDAPAMIDE
Indapamide Tablets ... 2286

INDAHEXAL (Australia)
INDAPAMIDE
Indapamide Tablets ... 2286

INDALIX (South Africa)
INDAPAMIDE
Indapamide Tablets ... 2286

INDAMOL (Italy)
INDAPAMIDE
Indapamide Tablets ... 2286

INDARZONA-N (Mexico)
DEXAMETHASONE
Decadron Elixir ... 2078
Decadron Tablets ... 2079

INDERAL (Australia, Austria, Belgium, Brazil, Canada, Denmark, Finland, Hong Kong, Irish Republic, Israel, Italy, Norway, Portugal, Singapore, South Africa, Spain, Sweden, Switzerland, Thailand, The Netherlands, United Kingdom)
PROPRANOLOL HYDROCHLORIDE
Inderal Injectable ... 3513
Inderal LA Long-Acting Capsules ... 3516
Inderal Tablets ... 3513

INDERALICI (Mexico)
PROPRANOLOL HYDROCHLORIDE
Inderal Injectable ... 3513
Inderal LA Long-Acting Capsules ... 3516
Inderal Tablets ... 3513

INDERIDE (Canada)
HYDROCHLOROTHIAZIDE/PROPRANOLOL HYDROCHLORIDE
Inderide LA Long-Acting Capsules ... 3519
Inderide Tablets ... 3517

INDERM (Belgium, Germany, Switzerland, The Netherlands)
ERYTHROMYCIN
Emgel 2% Topical Gel ... 1285
Ery-Tab Tablets ... 448
Erythromycin Base Filmtab Tablets ... 454
Erythromycin Delayed-Release Capsules, USP ... 455
PCE Dispertab Tablets ... 498

INDOBLOC (Germany)
PROPRANOLOL HYDROCHLORIDE
Inderal Injectable ... 3513
Inderal LA Long-Acting Capsules ... 3516
Inderal Tablets ... 3513

INDOBLOK (South Africa)
PROPRANOLOL HYDROCHLORIDE
Inderal Injectable ... 3513
Inderal LA Long-Acting Capsules ... 3516
Inderal Tablets ... 3513

INDOLIN (Italy)
INDAPAMIDE
Indapamide Tablets ... 2286

INDURGAN (Spain)
OMEPRAZOLE
Prilosec Delayed-Release Capsules ... 628

INESFAY (Mexico)
CIMETIDINE
Tagamet Tablets ... 1644

INZA (Australia, Hong Kong, South Africa)
NAPROXEN
EC-Naprosyn Delayed-Release Tablets ... 2967
Naprosyn Suspension ... 2967
Naprosyn Tablets ... 2967

INFECTOCEF (Germany)
CEFACLOR
Ceclor CD Tablets ... 1279
Ceclor Pulvules ... 1905
Ceclor Suspension ... 1905

INFECTOCIN (South Africa)
ERYTHROMYCIN STEARATE
Erythrocin Stearate Filmtab Tablets ... 452

INFECTOFLU (Germany)
AMANTADINE HYDROCHLORIDE
Symmetrel Syrup ... 1328
Symmetrel Tablets ... 1328

INFECTOMOX (Germany)
AMOXICILLIN
Amoxil Pediatric Drops for Oral Suspension ... 1471
Amoxil Tablets ... 1471

INFECTOPEDICUL (Germany)
PERMETHRIN
Acticin Cream ... 998
Elimite Cream ... 552

INFECTOSS (Brazil)
ERYTHROMYCIN
Emgel 2% Topical Gel ... 1285
Ery-Tab Tablets ... 448
Erythromycin Base Filmtab Tablets ... 454
Erythromycin Delayed-Release Capsules, USP ... 455
PCE Dispertab Tablets ... 498

INFERAX (Germany)
INTERFERON ALFACON-1
Infergen ... 1777

INFERGEN (Canada, Italy, The Netherlands)
INTERFERON ALFACON-1
Infergen ... 1777

INFERIL (Italy)
FERRIC SODIUM GLUCONATE
Ferrlecit Injection ... 3386

INFESTAT (United Kingdom)
NYSTATIN
Nystop Topical Powder USP ... 2608

INFLA-BAN (South Africa)
DICLOFENAC SODIUM
Voltaren Tablets ... 2315
Voltaren-XR Tablets ... 2315

INFLACED (France)
PIROXICAM
Feldene Capsules ... 2685

INFLAM (Australia)
IBUPROFEN
Motrin Suspension, Oral Drops, Chewable Tablets, and Caplets ... 2002

INFLAMAC (Switzerland)
DICLOFENAC SODIUM
Voltaren Tablets ... 2315
Voltaren-XR Tablets ... 2315

INFLAMASE (Canada)
PREDNISOLONE SODIUM PHOSPHATE
Pediapred Oral Solution ... 1170

INFLAMENE (Brazil)
PIROXICAM
Feldene Capsules ... 2685

INFLAMMIDE (Singapore, South Africa, Thailand)
BUDESONIDE
Pulmicort Turbuhaler Inhalation Powder ... 636
Rhinocort Nasal Inhaler ... 640

INFLANAC (Hong Kong, Singapore, Thailand)
DICLOFENAC SODIUM
Voltaren Tablets ... 2315
Voltaren-XR Tablets ... 2315

INFLANAN (Brazil)
PIROXICAM
Feldene Capsules ... 2685

INFLANOX (Brazil)
PIROXICAM
Feldene Capsules ... 2685

INFLAREN (Brazil)
DICLOFENAC SODIUM
Voltaren Tablets ... 2315
Voltaren-XR Tablets ... 2315

INFLAX (Brazil)
PIROXICAM
Feldene Capsules ... 2685

INFLOXA (Mexico)
CIPROFLOXACIN
Cipro I.V. ... 893
Cipro I.V. Pharmacy Bulk Package ... 897
Cipro Oral Suspension ... 887

INFUFER (Canada)
IRON DEXTRAN
INFeD Injection ... 3388

INGASTRI (Spain)
FAMOTIDINE
Pepcid Injection ... 2153
Pepcid Injection Premixed ... 2153
Pepcid RPD Orally Disintegrating Tablets ... 2150
Pepcid Tablets ... 2150
Pepcid for Oral Suspension ... 2150

INHACORT (Germany)
FLUNISOLIDE
Aerobid Inhaler System ... 1363
Aerobid-M Inhaler System ... 1363
Nasalide Nasal Spray ... 1295
Nasarel Nasal Solution 0.025% ... 1296

INHEPAR (Mexico)
HEPARIN SODIUM
Heparin Lock Flush Solution ... 3509
Heparin Sodium Injection ... 3511

INHIBACE (Israel)
CAPTOPRIL
Captopril Tablets ... 2281

INHIBITRON (Mexico)
OMEPRAZOLE
Prilosec Delayed-Release Capsules ... 628

INIBIL (Italy)
APROTININ
Trasylol Injection ... 909

INIPROL (Belgium, France, Italy)
APROTININ
Trasylol Injection ... 909

INISTOLIN EXPECTORAN PED (Spain)
GUAIFENESIN/PSEUDOEPHEDRINE HYDROCHLORIDE
Guaifed Capsules ... 2272
Guaifed-PD Capsules ... 2272
Zephrex LA Tablets ... 3092
Zephrex Tablets ... 3091

INKAMIL (Spain)
CIPROFLOXACIN HYDROCHLORIDE
Ciloxan Ophthalmic Ointment ... 538
Ciloxan Ophthalmic Solution ... ⊙209, 538
Cipro Tablets ... 887

INNOMEL (Irish Republic)
ENALAPRIL MALEATE
Vasotec Tablets ... 2210

INNOVACE (Irish Republic, United Kingdom)
ENALAPRIL MALEATE
Vasotec Tablets ... 2210

INNOZIDE (Irish Republic, United Kingdom)
ENALAPRIL MALEATE/HYDROCHLOROTHIAZIDE
Vaseretic Tablets ... 2204

INOFLOX (Singapore)
OFLOXACIN
Floxin I.V. ... 2526
Floxin Otic Solution ... 1219
Floxin Tablets ... 2529
Ocuflox Ophthalmic Solution ... 554

INOTOP (Austria)
DOBUTAMINE HYDROCHLORIDE
Dobutrex Solution Vials ... 1914

INOTREX (Portugal)
DOBUTAMINE HYDROCHLORIDE
Dobutrex Solution Vials ... 1914

INOVAL (Brazil)
FENTANYL CITRATE
Actiq ... 1184

INOVEN (United Kingdom)
IBUPROFEN
Motrin Suspension, Oral Drops, Chewable Tablets, and Caplets ... 2002

INPANOL (Hong Kong, Singapore)
PROPRANOLOL HYDROCHLORIDE
Inderal Injectable ... 3513
Inderal LA Long-Acting Capsules ... 3516
Inderal Tablets ... 3513

INSECT ECRAN (France)
PERMETHRIN
Acticin Cream ... 998

(⊙ Described in PDR For Ophthalmic Medicines™)

Elimite Cream . . . 552

INSENSYE (Australia)
NORFLOXACIN
Chibroxin Sterile Ophthalmic Solution . . . ⊙273, 2051
Noroxin Tablets . . . 2145

INSIDE (Sweden)
RANITIDINE HYDROCHLORIDE
Zantac 150 EFFERdose Granules . . . 1690
Zantac 150 EFFERdose Tablets . . . 1690
Zantac 150 Tablets . . . 1690
Zantac 300 Tablets . . . 1690
Zantac Injection . . . 1688
Zantac Injection Premixed . . . 1688
Zantac Syrup . . . 1690

INSIG (Australia)
INDAPAMIDE
Indapamide Tablets . . . 2286

INSOGEN (Mexico)
CHLORPROPAMIDE
Diabinese Tablets . . . 2680

INSOMNAL (Canada)
DIPHENHYDRAMINE HYDROCHLORIDE
Benadryl Parenteral . . . 2617

INSOMN-EZE (Australia)
PROMETHAZINE HYDROCHLORIDE
Phenergan Injection . . . 3553
Phenergan Suppositories . . . 3556
Phenergan Syrup Fortis . . . 3554
Phenergan Syrup Plain . . . 3554
Phenergan Tablets . . . 3556

INSUP (Spain)
ENALAPRIL MALEATE
Vasotec Tablets . . . 2210

INTAPAN (Hong Kong)
NALBUPHINE HYDROCHLORIDE
Nubain Injection . . . 1323

INTEGRILIN (Canada, Denmark, Finland, France, Germany, Irish Republic, Israel, Italy, Portugal, South Africa, Spain, Sweden, Switzerland, The Netherlands, United Kingdom)
EPTIFIBATIDE
Integrilin Injection . . . 1213, 1828

INTERBERIN (Austria)
SARGRAMOSTIM
Leukine . . . 1755

INTERMIGRAN (Germany)
PROPRANOLOL HYDROCHLORIDE
Inderal Injectable . . . 3513
Inderal LA Long-Acting Capsules . . . 3516
Inderal Tablets . . . 3513

INTRACEF (South Africa)
CEFUROXIME SODIUM
Kefurox Vials, ADD-Vantage . . . 1948
Zinacef Injection . . . 1696

INTRADERMO CORTICOSTEROI (Spain)
FLUOCINOLONE ACETONIDE
Synalar Cream . . . 2020
Synalar Ointment . . . 2020
Synalar Topical Solution . . . 2020

INTRALGIN (United Kingdom)
BENZOCAINE
Americaine Anesthetic Lubricant . . . 1162
Americaine Otic Topical Anesthetic Ear Drops . . . 1162

INTRALGIS (France)
IBUPROFEN
Motrin Suspension, Oral Drops, Chewable Tablets, and Caplets . . . 2002

INTRON A (Austria, Canada, Hong Kong, Israel, Mexico, Portugal, Singapore, South Africa, Spain, Switzerland, The Netherlands)
INTERFERON ALFA-2B
Intron A for Injection . . . 3120

INTRONA (Denmark, Finland, France, Irish Republic, Norway, Sweden, Thailand)
INTERFERON ALFA-2B
Intron A for Injection . . . 3120

INVESTIN (Germany)
DOXYCYCLINE HYCLATE
Doryx Coated Pellet Filled Capsules . . . 3357
Periostat Tablets . . . 1208
Vibramycin Hyclate Capsules . . . 2735
Vibramycin Hyclate Intravenous . . . 2737
Vibra-Tabs Film Coated Tablets . . . 2735

INVIGAN (Spain)
FAMOTIDINE
Pepcid Injection . . . 2153
Pepcid Injection Premixed . . . 2153
Pepcid RPD Orally Disintegrating Tablets . . . 2150
Pepcid Tablets . . . 2150
Pepcid for Oral Suspension . . . 2150

INVIRASE (Spain)
SAQUINAVIR
Fortovase Capsules . . . 2970

INVORIL (Singapore, Thailand)
ENALAPRIL MALEATE
Vasotec Tablets . . . 2210

IODEPOL (Brazil)
POTASSIUM IODIDE
Pima Syrup . . . 1362

IODETO DE POTASSIUM COMPOSTO (Brazil)
POTASSIUM IODIDE
Pima Syrup . . . 1362

IODOSAN (Italy)
DEXTROMETHORPHAN HYDROBROMIDE/GUAIFENESIN
Tussi-Organidin DM NR Liquid . . . 3350
Tussi-Organidin DM-S NR Liquid . . . 3350

IOPIDINE (Australia, Austria, Belgium, Canada, Denmark, Finland, France, Germany, Hong Kong, Irish Republic, Israel, Italy, Japan, Mexico, New Zealand, Norway, Portugal, Singapore, South Africa, Sweden, Switzerland, United Kingdom)
APRACLONIDINE HYDROCHLORIDE
Iopidine 0.5% Ophthalmic Solution . . . ⊙213
Iopidine Sterile Ophthalmic Solution . . . ⊙212

IOPIMAX (Spain)
APRACLONIDINE HYDROCHLORIDE
Iopidine 0.5% Ophthalmic Solution . . . ⊙213
Iopidine Sterile Ophthalmic Solution . . . ⊙212

IPACEF (Italy)
CEFUROXIME SODIUM
Kefurox Vials, ADD-Vantage . . . 1948
Zinacef Injection . . . 1696

IPAGASTRIL (Italy)
SUCRALFATE
Carafate Suspension . . . 731
Carafate Tablets . . . 730

IPAMIX (Italy)
INDAPAMIDE
Indapamide Tablets . . . 2286

IPAZONE (Italy)
CEFOPERAZONE SODIUM
Cefobid Intravenous/Intramuscular . . . 2671
Cefobid Pharmacy Bulk Package - Not for Direct Infusion . . . 2673

IPOCROMO (Italy)
FERRIC SODIUM GLUCONATE
Ferrlecit Injection . . . 3386

IPOLAB (Italy)
LABETALOL HYDROCHLORIDE
Normodyne Injection . . . 3135
Normodyne Tablets . . . 3137

IPOLIPID (Hong Kong, Singapore, Thailand)
GEMFIBROZIL
Lopid Tablets . . . 2650

IPOTENSIUM (Italy)
CLONIDINE HYDROCHLORIDE
Catapres Tablets . . . 1037
Duraclon Injection . . . 3057

IPRATRIN (Australia)
IPRATROPIUM BROMIDE
Atrovent Inhalation Aerosol . . . 1030
Atrovent Inhalation Solution . . . 1031
Atrovent Nasal Spray 0.03% . . . 1032
Atrovent Nasal Spray 0.06% . . . 1033

IPRAVENT (Australia)
IPRATROPIUM BROMIDE
Atrovent Inhalation Aerosol . . . 1030
Atrovent Inhalation Solution . . . 1031
Atrovent Nasal Spray 0.03% . . . 1032
Atrovent Nasal Spray 0.06% . . . 1033

IPREN (Denmark, Sweden)
IBUPROFEN
Motrin Suspension, Oral Drops, Chewable Tablets, and Caplets . . . 2002

IPROBEN (Switzerland)
IBUPROFEN
Motrin Suspension, Oral Drops, Chewable Tablets, and Caplets . . . 2002

IPROGEL (Switzerland)
IBUPROFEN
Motrin Suspension, Oral Drops, Chewable Tablets, and Caplets . . . 2002

IPVENT (South Africa)
IPRATROPIUM BROMIDE
Atrovent Inhalation Aerosol . . . 1030
Atrovent Inhalation Solution . . . 1031
Atrovent Nasal Spray 0.03% . . . 1032
Atrovent Nasal Spray 0.06% . . . 1033

IRBAN (Israel)
IRBESARTAN
Avapro Tablets . . . 1074, 3076

IRFEN (Switzerland)
IBUPROFEN
Motrin Suspension, Oral Drops, Chewable Tablets, and Caplets . . . 2002

IRICIL (Spain)
LISINOPRIL
Prinivil Tablets . . . 2164
Zestril Tablets . . . 698

IRIDINA DUE (Italy)
NAPHAZOLINE HYDROCHLORIDE
Albalon Ophthalmic Solution . . . ⊙225

IRUXOL (Brazil, Finland)
COLLAGENASE
Collagenase Santyl Ointment . . . 3248

IRUXOL MONO (Hong Kong)
COLLAGENASE
Collagenase Santyl Ointment . . . 3248

IS 5 MONO (Germany)
ISOSORBIDE MONONITRATE
Imdur Tablets . . . 1826
Ismo Tablets . . . 3524

ISADOL (Mexico)
ZIDOVUDINE
Retrovir Capsules . . . 1625
Retrovir IV Infusion . . . 1629
Retrovir Syrup . . . 1625
Retrovir Tablets . . . 1625

ISANGINA (Finland)
ISOSORBIDE MONONITRATE
Imdur Tablets . . . 1826
Ismo Tablets . . . 3524

ISAXION (Portugal)
TICLOPIDINE HYDROCHLORIDE
Ticlid Tablets . . . 3015

ISCLOFEN (United Kingdom)
DICLOFENAC SODIUM
Voltaren Tablets . . . 2315
Voltaren-XR Tablets . . . 2315

ISCOVER (Australia, Germany, Portugal, Spain, Switzerland, United Kingdom)
CLOPIDOGREL BISULFATE
Plavix Tablets . . . 1097, 3084

ISDIN (Germany)
ISOSORBIDE DINITRATE
Isordil Sublingual Tablets . . . 3525
Isordil Titradose Tablets . . . 3526

ISDOL (Spain)
IBUPROFEN
Motrin Suspension, Oral Drops, Chewable Tablets, and Caplets . . . 2002

ISIB (United Kingdom)
ISOSORBIDE MONONITRATE
Imdur Tablets . . . 1826
Ismo Tablets . . . 3524

ISIMOXIN (Italy)
AMOXICILLIN
Amoxil Pediatric Drops for Oral Suspension . . . 1471
Amoxil Tablets . . . 1471

ISISFEN (United Kingdom)
IBUPROFEN
Motrin Suspension, Oral Drops, Chewable Tablets, and Caplets . . . 2002

ISMEXIN (Finland)
ISOSORBIDE MONONITRATE
Imdur Tablets . . . 1826
Ismo Tablets . . . 3524

ISMIPUR (Italy)
MERCAPTOPURINE
Purinethol Tablets . . . 1615

ISMO (Canada, Denmark, Germany, Hong Kong, Israel, Italy, New Zealand, Norway, Portugal, Singapore, South Africa, Spain, Sweden, Switzerland, Thailand, The Netherlands, United Kingdom)
ISOSORBIDE MONONITRATE
Imdur Tablets . . . 1826
Ismo Tablets . . . 3524

ISMOX (Finland)
ISOSORBIDE MONONITRATE
Imdur Tablets . . . 1826
Ismo Tablets . . . 3524

ISNADERM (Italy)
FLUOCINOLONE ACETONIDE
Synalar Cream . . . 2020
Synalar Ointment . . . 2020
Synalar Topical Solution . . . 2020

ISO (Spain)
ISOSORBIDE DINITRATE
Isordil Sublingual Tablets . . . 3525
Isordil Titradose Tablets . . . 3526

ISO MACK (Austria, Denmark, Germany, Hong Kong, Singapore, South Africa, Switzerland, Thailand)
ISOSORBIDE DINITRATE
Isordil Sublingual Tablets . . . 3525
Isordil Titradose Tablets . . . 3526

ISOBIB (Singapore)
ISOSORBIDE DINITRATE
Isordil Sublingual Tablets . . . 3525
Isordil Titradose Tablets . . . 3526

ISOBINATE (Thailand)
ISOSORBIDE DINITRATE
Isordil Sublingual Tablets . . . 3525
Isordil Titradose Tablets . . . 3526

ISOCAINE (Canada)
MEPIVACAINE HYDROCHLORIDE
Polocaine Injection, USP . . . 625
Polocaine-MPF Injection, USP . . . 625

ISOCARD (Belgium, France, United Kingdom)
ISOSORBIDE DINITRATE
Isordil Sublingual Tablets . . . 3525
Isordil Titradose Tablets . . . 3526

ISO-CARD (South Africa)
VERAPAMIL HYDROCHLORIDE
Covera-HS Tablets . . . 3199
Isoptin SR Tablets . . . 467
Verelan Capsules . . . 3184
Verelan PM Capsules . . . 3186

ISOCARDIDE (Israel)
ISOSORBIDE DINITRATE
Isordil Sublingual Tablets . . . 3525
Isordil Titradose Tablets . . . 3526

ISOCARD-SPRAY (France)
ISOSORBIDE DINITRATE
Isordil Sublingual Tablets . . . 3525
Isordil Titradose Tablets . . . 3526

ISOCEF (Italy)
CEFTIBUTEN
Cedax Capsules . . . 1021
Cedax Oral Suspension . . . 1021

ISOCLAR (Italy)
HEPARIN SODIUM
Heparin Lock Flush Solution . . . 3509
Heparin Sodium Injection . . . 3511

ISOCORD (Brazil)
ISOSORBIDE DINITRATE
Isordil Sublingual Tablets . . . 3525
Isordil Titradose Tablets . . . 3526

ISODAY (Switzerland)
ISOSORBIDE DINITRATE
Isordil Sublingual Tablets . . . 3525
Isordil Titradose Tablets . . . 3526

ISODINIT (Germany)
ISOSORBIDE DINITRATE
Isordil Sublingual Tablets . . . 3525
Isordil Titradose Tablets . . . 3526

ISODUR (Denmark, Sweden, United Kingdom)
ISOSORBIDE MONONITRATE
Imdur Tablets . . . 1826
Ismo Tablets . . . 3524

ISOFORCE (Germany)
ISOSORBIDE DINITRATE
Isordil Sublingual Tablets . . . 3525
Isordil Titradose Tablets . . . 3526

ISOFTAL (Austria)
NAPHAZOLINE HYDROCHLORIDE
Albalon Ophthalmic Solution . . . ⊙225

ISOGAINE (Spain)
MEPIVACAINE HYDROCHLORIDE
Polocaine Injection, USP . . . 625
Polocaine-MPF Injection, USP . . . 625

ISOGEN (Australia)
ISOSORBIDE DINITRATE
Isordil Sublingual Tablets . . . 3525
Isordil Titradose Tablets . . . 3526

ISOGLAUCON (Austria, Germany, Italy, Spain)
CLONIDINE HYDROCHLORIDE
Catapres Tablets . . . 1037
Duraclon Injection . . . 3057

ISOHEXAL (Australia)
ISOTRETINOIN
Accutane Capsules . . . 2944

ISO-K (Italy)
KETOPROFEN
Orudis Capsules 3548
Oruvail Capsules 3548

ISOKET (Austria, Hong Kong, Irish Republic, Israel, Mexico, Portugal, South Africa, Switzerland, Thailand, United Kingdom)
ISOSORBIDE DINITRATE
Isordil Sublingual Tablets 3525
Isordil Titradose Tablets 3526

ISOMEL (Irish Republic)
ISOSORBIDE MONONITRATE
Imdur Tablets 1826
Ismo Tablets 3524

ISOMET (Thailand)
METHYLDOPA
Aldomet Tablets 2037

ISOMONAT (Austria)
ISOSORBIDE MONONITRATE
Imdur Tablets 1826
Ismo Tablets 3524

ISOMONIT (Australia, Denmark, Germany, Irish Republic)
ISOSORBIDE MONONITRATE
Imdur Tablets 1826
Ismo Tablets 3524

ISOMONOREAL (Germany)
ISOSORBIDE MONONITRATE
Imdur Tablets 1826
Ismo Tablets 3524

ISONITRIL (Spain)
ISOSORBIDE MONONITRATE
Imdur Tablets 1826
Ismo Tablets 3524

ISOPAMIL (Thailand)
VERAPAMIL HYDROCHLORIDE
Covera-HS Tablets 3199
Isoptin SR Tablets 467
Verelan Capsules 3184
Verelan PM Capsules 3186

ISOPAS (South Africa)
PYRAZINAMIDE
Pyrazinamide Tablets 1876

ISOPEN (Thailand)
ISOSORBIDE MONONITRATE
Imdur Tablets 1826
Ismo Tablets 3524

ISOPRONT (Portugal)
ISOSORBIDE DINITRATE
Isordil Sublingual Tablets 3525
Isordil Titradose Tablets 3526

ISOPTIN (Australia, Austria, Canada, Denmark, Finland, Germany, Hong Kong, Irish Republic, Italy, New Zealand, Norway, Portugal, Singapore, South Africa, Sweden, Switzerland, Thailand, The Netherlands)
VERAPAMIL HYDROCHLORIDE
Covera-HS Tablets 3199
Isoptin SR Tablets 467
Verelan Capsules 3184
Verelan PM Capsules 3186

ISOPTINE (Belgium, France)
VERAPAMIL HYDROCHLORIDE
Covera-HS Tablets 3199
Isoptin SR Tablets 467
Verelan Capsules 3184
Verelan PM Capsules 3186

ISOPTO CARPINA (Spain)
PILOCARPINE HYDROCHLORIDE
Isopto Carpine Ophthalmic Solution . . . . ⊙215
Pilopine HS Ophthalmic Gel . . . . ⊙217
Salagen Tablets 2229

ISOPTO CARPINE (Australia, Belgium, Brazil, Canada, Finland, Hong Kong, Irish Republic, Israel, New Zealand, Norway, South Africa, Switzerland, Thailand, The Netherlands, United Kingdom)
PILOCARPINE HYDROCHLORIDE
Isopto Carpine Ophthalmic Solution . . . . ⊙215
Pilopine HS Ophthalmic Gel . . . . ⊙217
Salagen Tablets 2229

ISOPTO CETAMIDE (Belgium, Canada)
SULFACETAMIDE SODIUM
Bleph-10 Ophthalmic Ointment 10% . . . . ⊙230
Klaron Lotion 10% 1224

ISOPTO CETAPRED (Belgium, Canada)
PREDNISOLONE ACETATE/SULFACETAMIDE SODIUM
Blephamide Ophthalmic Ointment 547
Blephamide Ophthalmic Suspension 548

ISOPTO DEX (Germany)
DEXAMETHASONE
Decadron Elixir 2078
Decadron Tablets 2079

ISOPTO FENICOL (Belgium, Hong Kong, New Zealand, Singapore, Spain, Sweden)
CHLORAMPHENICOL
Chloromycetin Ophthalmic Ointment, 1% . . . . ⊙296
Chloromycetin Ophthalmic Solution . . . . ⊙297
Chloroptic Sterile Ophthalmic Ointment . . ⊙234
Chloroptic Sterile Ophthalmic Solution . . ⊙235

ISOPTO FLUCON (Germany, Spain)
FLUOROMETHOLONE
FML Ophthalmic Ointment . . . . ⊙237

ISOPTO KARBAKOLIN (Sweden)
CARBACHOL
Isopto Carbachol Ophthalmic Solution . . . ⊙215

ISOPTO MAXIDEX (Norway, Sweden)
DEXAMETHASONE
Decadron Elixir 2078
Decadron Tablets 2079

ISO-PUREN (Germany)
ISOSORBIDE DINITRATE
Isordil Sublingual Tablets 3525
Isordil Titradose Tablets 3526

ISORBID (Mexico)
ISOSORBIDE DINITRATE
Isordil Sublingual Tablets 3525
Isordil Titradose Tablets 3526

ISORDIL (Australia, Belgium, Brazil, Canada, Hong Kong, Irish Republic, Singapore, South Africa, Spain, Thailand, The Netherlands, United Kingdom)
ISOSORBIDE DINITRATE
Isordil Sublingual Tablets 3525
Isordil Titradose Tablets 3526

ISOREM (Hong Kong, Thailand)
ISOSORBIDE DINITRATE
Isordil Sublingual Tablets 3525
Isordil Titradose Tablets 3526

ISOSTAD (Austria)
ISOSORBIDE DINITRATE
Isordil Sublingual Tablets 3525
Isordil Titradose Tablets 3526

ISOSTENASE (Germany)
ISOSORBIDE DINITRATE
Isordil Sublingual Tablets 3525
Isordil Titradose Tablets 3526

ISOTARD (Israel, United Kingdom)
ISOSORBIDE DINITRATE
Isordil Sublingual Tablets 3525
Isordil Titradose Tablets 3526

ISOTEN (Belgium)
BISOPROLOL FUMARATE
Zebeta Tablets 1885

ISOTRATE (Australia)
ISOSORBIDE DINITRATE
Isordil Sublingual Tablets 3525
Isordil Titradose Tablets 3526

ISOTRATE (Hong Kong, Singapore, Thailand, United Kingdom)
ISOSORBIDE MONONITRATE
Imdur Tablets 1826
Ismo Tablets 3524

ISOTREX (Australia, Austria, Canada, Denmark, France, Germany, Hong Kong, Irish Republic, Israel, Italy, Mexico, New Zealand, Portugal, Singapore, South Africa, Spain, Thailand, United Kingdom)
ISOTRETINOIN
Accutane Capsules 2944

ISOTREX ERITROMICINA (Spain)
ISOTRETINOIN
Accutane Capsules 2944

ISOTREXIN (Germany, Irish Republic, Italy, Portugal, United Kingdom)
ISOTRETINOIN
Accutane Capsules 2944

ISOX (Mexico)
ITRACONAZOLE
Sporanox Capsules 1800
Sporanox Oral Solution 1808, 2512

ISTOPRIL (Thailand)
ENALAPRIL MALEATE
Vasotec Tablets 2210

ITALMICIN (Mexico)
CHLORAMPHENICOL
Chloromycetin Ophthalmic Ointment, 1% . . . . ⊙296
Chloromycetin Ophthalmic Solution . . . . ⊙297
Chloroptic Sterile Ophthalmic Ointment . . ⊙234
Chloroptic Sterile Ophthalmic Solution . . ⊙235

ITALNIK (Mexico)
CIPROFLOXACIN
Cipro I.V. 893
Cipro I.V. Pharmacy Bulk Package 897
Cipro Oral Suspension 887

ITOREX (Italy)
CEFUROXIME SODIUM
Kefurox Vials, ADD-Vantage 1948
Zinacef Injection 1696

ITRANAX (Brazil, Mexico)
ITRACONAZOLE
Sporanox Capsules 1800
Sporanox Oral Solution 1808, 2512

ITRIN (Italy)
TERAZOSIN HYDROCHLORIDE
Hytrin Capsules 464

ITROP (Austria, Germany, Switzerland)
IPRATROPIUM BROMIDE
Atrovent Inhalation Aerosol 1030
Atrovent Inhalation Solution 1031
Atrovent Nasal Spray 0.03% 1032
Atrovent Nasal Spray 0.06% 1033

IVACIN (Denmark, Sweden)
PIPERACILLIN SODIUM
Pipracil 1866

IVADAL (Austria, France, Italy)
ZOLPIDEM TARTRATE
Ambien Tablets 3191

IVOFOL (Spain)
PROPOFOL
Diprivan Injectable Emulsion 667

IVRACAIN (Switzerland)
CHLOROPROCAINE HYDROCHLORIDE
Nesacaine Injection 617
Nesacaine-MPF Injection 617

IWAMET (Thailand)
CIMETIDINE
Tagamet Tablets 1644

IZADIMA (Mexico)
CEFTAZIDIME
Ceptaz for Injection 1499
Fortaz for Injection 1541
Tazicef for Injection 1647
Tazidime Vials, Faspak & ADD-Vantage . . 1966

IZO (Thailand)
ISOSORBIDE DINITRATE
Isordil Sublingual Tablets 3525
Isordil Titradose Tablets 3526

JACKSON'S ALL FOURS (United Kingdom)
GUAIFENESIN
Organidin NR Liquid 3350
Organidin NR Tablets 3350

JACKSONS BRONCHIAL BALSAM (United Kingdom)
GUAIFENESIN
Organidin NR Liquid 3350
Organidin NR Tablets 3350

JACUTIN (Austria, Germany, Switzerland, The Netherlands)
LINDANE
Lindane Lotion USP 1% 559
Lindane Shampoo USP 1% 560

JADELLE (Finland)
LEVONORGESTREL
Norplant System 3543

JANACIN (Thailand)
NORFLOXACIN
Chibroxin Sterile Ophthalmic Solution . . . . ⊙273, 2051
Noroxin Tablets 2145

JANOCILIN (Spain)
CEPHALEXIN
Keflex Oral Suspension 1237
Keflex Pulvules 1237

JATRONEURAL (Austria, Germany)
TRIFLUOPERAZINE HYDROCHLORIDE
Stelazine Injection 1640
Stelazine Tablets 1640

JATROPUR (Germany)
TRIAMTERENE
Dyrenium Capsules 3458

JATROSOM N (Germany)
TRANYLCYPROMINE SULFATE
Parnate Tablets 1607

JEDIPIN (Germany, Thailand)
NIFEDIPINE
Adalat CC Tablets 877
Procardia Capsules 2708
Procardia XL Extended Release Tablets . . 2710

JELLIN (Germany)
FLUOCINOLONE ACETONIDE
Synalar Cream 2020
Synalar Ointment 2020
Synalar Topical Solution 2020

JELLISOFT (Germany)
FLUOCINOLONE ACETONIDE
Synalar Cream 2020
Synalar Ointment 2020
Synalar Topical Solution 2020

JENACARD (Germany)
ISOSORBIDE DINITRATE
Isordil Sublingual Tablets 3525
Isordil Titradose Tablets 3526

JENAFENAC (Germany)
DICLOFENAC SODIUM
Voltaren Tablets 2315
Voltaren-XR Tablets 2315

JENAMAZOL (Germany)
CLOTRIMAZOLE
Lotrimin Cream 1% 3128
Lotrimin Lotion 1% 3128
Lotrimin Topical Solution 1% 3128
Mycelex Troche 573

JENAMETIDIN (Germany)
CIMETIDINE
Tagamet Tablets 1644

JENAPAMIL (Germany)
VERAPAMIL HYDROCHLORIDE
Covera-HS Tablets 3199
Isoptin SR Tablets 467
Verelan Capsules 3184
Verelan PM Capsules 3186

JENAPIROX (Germany)
PIROXICAM
Feldene Capsules 2685

JENAPROFEN (Germany)
IBUPROFEN
Motrin Suspension, Oral Drops, Chewable Tablets, and Caplets 2002

JENATENOL (Germany)
ATENOLOL
Tenormin I.V. Injection 692

JENATEREN COMP (Germany)
HYDROCHLOROTHIAZIDE/TRIAMTERENE
Dyazide Capsules 1515
Maxzide Tablets 1008
Maxzide-25 mg Tablets 1008

JENOXIFEN (Germany)
TAMOXIFEN CITRATE
Nolvadex Tablets 678

JERIDIN (United Kingdom)
ISOSORBIDE DINITRATE
Isordil Sublingual Tablets 3525
Isordil Titradose Tablets 3526

JESTRYL (Germany)
CARBACHOL
Isopto Carbachol Ophthalmic Solution . . . ⊙215

JEZIL (Australia)
GEMFIBROZIL
Lopid Tablets 2650

JODETTEN (Germany)
POTASSIUM IODIDE
Pima Syrup 1362

JODIX (Finland)
POTASSIUM IODIDE
Pima Syrup 1362

JODMINERASE (Germany)
POTASSIUM IODIDE
Pima Syrup 1362

JOHNSON & JOHNSON BURN CREAM (Canada)
BENZOCAINE
Americaine Anesthetic Lubricant 1162
Americaine Otic Topical Anesthetic Ear Drops 1162

JOMETHID (United Kingdom)
KETOPROFEN
Orudis Capsules 3548
Oruvail Capsules 3548

JOSIR (France)
TAMSULOSIN HYDROCHLORIDE
Flomax Capsules 1044

JOSSALIND (Germany)
SODIUM HYALURONATE
Hyalgan Solution 3080

JOUVENCE (Canada)
HYDROQUINONE
Eldopaque Forte 4% Cream 1734

Eldoquin Forte 4% Cream 1734
Lustra Cream 2023
Lustra-AF Cream 2023
Melanex Topical Solution 2300
Solaquin Forte 4% Cream 1734
Solaquin Forte 4% Gel 1734

JULAB (Thailand)
SELEGILINE HYDROCHLORIDE
Eldepryl Capsules 3266

JUMEX (Austria, Hong Kong, Israel, Italy, Portugal, Singapore, Thailand)
SELEGILINE HYDROCHLORIDE
Eldepryl Capsules 3266

JUMEXAL (Switzerland)
SELEGILINE HYDROCHLORIDE
Eldepryl Capsules 3266

JUMEXIL (Brazil)
SELEGILINE HYDROCHLORIDE
Eldepryl Capsules 3266

JUNGLE FORMULA STING RELIEF CREAM (United Kingdom)
HYDROCORTISONE
Anusol-HC Cream 2.5% 2237
Hydrocortone Tablets 2106

JUNIFEN (Austria, Belgium, Thailand, United Kingdom)
IBUPROFEN
Motrin Suspension, Oral Drops, Chewable Tablets, and Caplets 2002

JUVENTAL (Germany)
ATENOLOL
Tenormin I.V. Injection 692

JUWOMENT SPORT (Germany)
HEPARIN SODIUM
Heparin Lock Flush Solution 3509
Heparin Sodium Injection 3511

K-10 (Canada)
POTASSIUM CHLORIDE
K-Dur Microburst Release System ER Tablets 1832
K-Lor Powder Packets 469
K-Tab Filmtab Tablets 470
Rum-K 1363

KABIKINASE (Australia, Austria, Belgium, Brazil, Canada, Denmark, Finland, France, Germany, Hong Kong, Irish Republic, Israel, Italy, Mexico, New Zealand, Norway, Portugal, Singapore, South Africa, Spain, Sweden, Switzerland, Thailand, The Netherlands, United Kingdom)
STREPTOKINASE
Streptase for Infusion 647

KADALEX (Italy)
POTASSIUM CHLORIDE
K-Dur Microburst Release System ER Tablets 1832
K-Lor Powder Packets 469
K-Tab Filmtab Tablets 470
Rum-K 1363

KADEFUNGIN (Germany)
CLOTRIMAZOLE
Lotrimin Cream 1% 3128
Lotrimin Lotion 1% 3128
Lotrimin Topical Solution 1% 3128
Mycelex Troche 573

KADIAN (Canada)
MORPHINE SULFATE
Astramorph/PF Injection, USP (Preservative-Free) 594
Duramorph Injection 1312
Infumorph 200 and Infumorph 500 Sterile Solutions 1314
Kadian Capsules 1335
MS Contin Tablets 2896
MSIR Oral Capsules 2898
MSIR Oral Solution 2898
MSIR Oral Solution Concentrate 2898
MSIR Oral Tablets 2898
Oramorph SR Tablets 3062
Roxanol 100 Concentrated Oral Solution 3066
Roxanol Concentrated Oral Solution 3066
Roxanol-T Oral Solution 3066

KAINEVER (Portugal)
ESTAZOLAM
ProSom Tablets 500

KAJOS (Norway, Sweden)
POTASSIUM CITRATE
Urocit-K Tablets 2232

KALEORID (Denmark, France, Norway, Sweden)
POTASSIUM CHLORIDE
K-Dur Microburst Release System ER Tablets 1832
K-Lor Powder Packets 469
K-Tab Filmtab Tablets 470
Rum-K 1363

KALICET (Italy)
FEXOFENADINE HYDROCHLORIDE
Allegra Capsules 712

KALIGLUTOL (Switzerland)
POTASSIUM CHLORIDE
K-Dur Microburst Release System ER Tablets 1832
K-Lor Powder Packets 469
K-Tab Filmtab Tablets 470
Rum-K 1363

KALIKLORA JOD MED (Germany)
POTASSIUM IODIDE
Pima Syrup 1362

KALILENTE (Norway, Sweden)
POTASSIUM CHLORIDE
K-Dur Microburst Release System ER Tablets 1832
K-Lor Powder Packets 469
K-Tab Filmtab Tablets 470
Rum-K 1363

KALINORM (Denmark, Finland, Norway)
POTASSIUM CHLORIDE
K-Dur Microburst Release System ER Tablets 1832
K-Lor Powder Packets 469
K-Tab Filmtab Tablets 470
Rum-K 1363

KALINOR-RETARD P (Germany)
POTASSIUM CHLORIDE
K-Dur Microburst Release System ER Tablets 1832
K-Lor Powder Packets 469
K-Tab Filmtab Tablets 470
Rum-K 1363

KALIOLITE (Mexico)
POTASSIUM CHLORIDE
K-Dur Microburst Release System ER Tablets 1832
K-Lor Powder Packets 469
K-Tab Filmtab Tablets 470
Rum-K 1363

KALIPOR (Sweden)
POTASSIUM CHLORIDE
K-Dur Microburst Release System ER Tablets 1832
K-Lor Powder Packets 469
K-Tab Filmtab Tablets 470
Rum-K 1363

KALISOL (Finland)
POTASSIUM CHLORIDE
K-Dur Microburst Release System ER Tablets 1832
K-Lor Powder Packets 469
K-Tab Filmtab Tablets 470
Rum-K 1363

KALISTERIL (Finland)
POTASSIUM CHLORIDE
K-Dur Microburst Release System ER Tablets 1832
K-Lor Powder Packets 469
K-Tab Filmtab Tablets 470
Rum-K 1363

KALITABS (Sweden)
POTASSIUM CHLORIDE
K-Dur Microburst Release System ER Tablets 1832
K-Lor Powder Packets 469
K-Tab Filmtab Tablets 470
Rum-K 1363

KALITRANS RETARD (Germany)
POTASSIUM CHLORIDE
K-Dur Microburst Release System ER Tablets 1832
K-Lor Powder Packets 469
K-Tab Filmtab Tablets 470
Rum-K 1363

KALIUM (Hong Kong)
POTASSIUM CHLORIDE
K-Dur Microburst Release System ER Tablets 1832
K-Lor Powder Packets 469
K-Tab Filmtab Tablets 470
Rum-K 1363

KALIUM DURETTER (Finland, Sweden)
POTASSIUM CHLORIDE
K-Dur Microburst Release System ER Tablets 1832
K-Lor Powder Packets 469
K-Tab Filmtab Tablets 470
Rum-K 1363

KALIUM DURETTES (Belgium, The Netherlands)
POTASSIUM CHLORIDE
K-Dur Microburst Release System ER Tablets 1832
K-Lor Powder Packets 469
K-Tab Filmtab Tablets 470
Rum-K 1363

KALIUM DURULES (Canada, Singapore)
POTASSIUM CHLORIDE
K-Dur Microburst Release System ER Tablets 1832
K-Lor Powder Packets 469
K-Tab Filmtab Tablets 470
Rum-K 1363

KALIUM RETARD (Sweden)
POTASSIUM CHLORIDE
K-Dur Microburst Release System ER Tablets 1832
K-Lor Powder Packets 469
K-Tab Filmtab Tablets 470
Rum-K 1363

KALIUM-DURILES (Germany)
POTASSIUM CHLORIDE
K-Dur Microburst Release System ER Tablets 1832
K-Lor Powder Packets 469
K-Tab Filmtab Tablets 470
Rum-K 1363

KALMA (Australia, Spain)
ALPRAZOLAM
Xanax Tablets 2865

KALPRESS (Spain)
VALSARTAN
Diovan Capsules 2337

KALPRESS PLUS (Spain)
VALSARTAN
Diovan Capsules 2337

KALURIL (Australia, Israel)
AMILORIDE HYDROCHLORIDE
Midamor Tablets 2136

KAMACAINE (Israel)
BUPIVACAINE HYDROCHLORIDE
Sensorcaine Injection 643
Sensorcaine-MPF Injection 643

KANAZIMA (Brazil)
ERYTHROMYCIN
Emgel 2% Topical Gel 1285
Ery-Tab Tablets 448
Erythromycin Base Filmtab Tablets 454
Erythromycin Delayed-Release Capsules, USP 455
PCE Dispertab Tablets 498

KANOLONE (Thailand)
TRIAMCINOLONE ACETONIDE
Azmacort Inhalation Aerosol 728
Nasacort AQ Nasal Spray 752
Nasacort Nasal Inhaler 750

KAOCHLOR (Canada)
POTASSIUM CHLORIDE
K-Dur Microburst Release System ER Tablets 1832
K-Lor Powder Packets 469
K-Tab Filmtab Tablets 470
Rum-K 1363

KAPANOL (Australia, Austria, Belgium, Denmark, France, Germany, Israel, Mexico, New Zealand, Norway, Switzerland, The Netherlands)
MORPHINE SULFATE
Astramorph/PF Injection, USP (Preservative-Free) 594
Duramorph Injection 1312
Infumorph 200 and Infumorph 500 Sterile Solutions 1314
Kadian Capsules 1335
MS Contin Tablets 2896
MSIR Oral Capsules 2898
MSIR Oral Solution 2898
MSIR Oral Solution Concentrate 2898
MSIR Oral Tablets 2898
Oramorph SR Tablets 3062
Roxanol 100 Concentrated Oral Solution 3066
Roxanol Concentrated Oral Solution 3066
Roxanol-T Oral Solution 3066

KAPLON (United Kingdom)
CAPTOPRIL
Captopril Tablets 2281

KARDEN (Austria)
NICARDIPINE HYDROCHLORIDE
Cardene I.V. 3485

KARDIL (Norway)
DILTIAZEM HYDROCHLORIDE
Cardizem CD Capsules 1016
Cardizem Injectable 1018
Cardizem Lyo-Ject Syringe 1018
Cardizem Monovial 1018
Tiazac Capsules 1378

KARILEXINA (Spain)
CEPHALEXIN
Keflex Oral Suspension 1237
Keflex Pulvules 1237

KARIN (Israel)
CLARITHROMYCIN
Biaxin Filmtab Tablets 403
Biaxin for Oral Suspension 403

KARISON (Germany)
CLOBETASOL PROPIONATE
Cormax Cream 2440
Cormax Ointment 2440
Cormax Scalp Application 2441
Temovate Cream 1301
Temovate E Emollient 1302
Temovate Gel 1303
Temovate Ointment 1301
Temovate Scalp Application 1304

KARVEA (Australia, Germany, Italy, Spain)
IRBESARTAN
Avapro Tablets 1074, 3076

KARVEZIDE (Australia, Germany, Italy, Spain)
HYDROCHLOROTHIAZIDE/IRBESARTAN
Avalide Tablets 1070

KATAPEKT (Finland)
CODEINE PHOSPHATE/GUAIFENESIN
Robitussin A-C Syrup 2942
Tussi-Organidin NR Liquid 3350
Tussi-Organidin-S NR Liquid 3350

KATARAKTON (Germany)
POTASSIUM IODIDE
Pima Syrup 1362

KATION (Italy)
POTASSIUM CITRATE
Urocit-K Tablets 2232

KATOPRIL (Singapore)
CAPTOPRIL
Captopril Tablets 2281

KATSIN (Thailand)
KETOCONAZOLE
Nizoral 2% Cream 3620
Nizoral 2% Shampoo 2007
Nizoral Tablets 1791

KATTWILACT (Germany)
LACTULOSE
Kristalose for Oral Solution 1007

KAY CIEL (Australia, Canada)
POTASSIUM CHLORIDE
K-Dur Microburst Release System ER Tablets 1832
K-Lor Powder Packets 469
K-Tab Filmtab Tablets 470
Rum-K 1363

KAY-CEE-L (Irish Republic, United Kingdom)
POTASSIUM CHLORIDE
K-Dur Microburst Release System ER Tablets 1832
K-Lor Powder Packets 469
K-Tab Filmtab Tablets 470
Rum-K 1363

KAZAK (Australia)
CERIVASTATIN SODIUM
Baycol Tablets 883

KAZINAL (Thailand)
KETOCONAZOLE
Nizoral 2% Cream 3620
Nizoral 2% Shampoo 2007
Nizoral Tablets 1791

K-BIOFEN (Mexico)
CHLORAMPHENICOL
Chloromycetin Ophthalmic Ointment, 1% ⊙296
Chloromycetin Ophthalmic Solution ⊙297
Chloroptic Sterile Ophthalmic Ointment ⊙234
Chloroptic Sterile Ophthalmic Solution ⊙235

KCL-RETARD (Austria, Germany)
POTASSIUM CHLORIDE
K-Dur Microburst Release System ER Tablets 1832
K-Lor Powder Packets 469
K-Tab Filmtab Tablets 470
Rum-K 1363

K-DUR (Canada, Mexico)
POTASSIUM CHLORIDE
K-Dur Microburst Release System ER Tablets 1832
K-Lor Powder Packets 469
K-Tab Filmtab Tablets 470
Rum-K 1363

KEAL (France)
SUCRALFATE
Carafate Suspension 731

Carafate Tablets 730

KEDURIL (Brazil)
KETOPROFEN
Orudis Capsules 3548
Oruvail Capsules 3548

KEEFLOXIN (Portugal)
CIPROFLOXACIN HYDROCHLORIDE
Ciloxan Ophthalmic Ointment 538
Ciloxan Ophthalmic Solution . . . . ⊙209, 538
Cipro Tablets 887

KEFACLOR (Thailand)
CEFACLOR
Ceclor CD Tablets 1279
Ceclor Pulvules 1905
Ceclor Suspension 1905

KEFADIM (Belgium, Brazil, Thailand, United Kingdom)
CEFTAZIDIME
Ceptaz for Injection 1499
Fortaz for Injection 1541
Tazicef for Injection 1647
Tazidime Vials, Faspak & ADD-Vantage . . 1966

KEFADOL (Irish Republic, United Kingdom)
CEFAMANDOLE NAFATE
Mandol Vials 1953

KEFALEX (Finland)
CEPHALEXIN
Keflex Oral Suspension 1237
Keflex Pulvules 1237

KEFAMIN (Spain)
CEFTAZIDIME
Ceptaz for Injection 1499
Fortaz for Injection 1541
Tazicef for Injection 1647
Tazidime Vials, Faspak & ADD-Vantage . . 1966

KEFAZIM (Austria)
CEFTAZIDIME
Ceptaz for Injection 1499
Fortaz for Injection 1541
Tazicef for Injection 1647
Tazidime Vials, Faspak & ADD-Vantage . . 1966

KEFAZON (Italy)
CEFOPERAZONE SODIUM
Cefobid Intravenous/Intramuscular 2671
Cefobid Pharmacy Bulk Package - Not for Direct Infusion 2673

KEFEN (New Zealand)
KETOPROFEN
Orudis Capsules 3548
Oruvail Capsules 3548

KEFENID (Italy)
KETOPROFEN
Orudis Capsules 3548
Oruvail Capsules 3548

KEFENTECH (Singapore)
KETOPROFEN
Orudis Capsules 3548
Oruvail Capsules 3548

KEFEXIN (Finland, Irish Republic)
CEPHALEXIN
Keflex Oral Suspension 1237
Keflex Pulvules 1237

KEFLEX (Australia, Austria, Brazil, Canada, Denmark, Hong Kong, Irish Republic, Israel, Mexico, New Zealand, Norway, Portugal, South Africa, Sweden, Switzerland, Thailand, United Kingdom)
CEPHALEXIN
Keflex Oral Suspension 1237
Keflex Pulvules 1237

KEFLEX-C (United Kingdom)
CEPHALEXIN
Keflex Oral Suspension 1237
Keflex Pulvules 1237

KEFLOR (Australia)
CEFACLOR
Ceclor CD Tablets 1279
Ceclor Pulvules 1905
Ceclor Suspension 1905

KEFLORIDINA (Spain)
CEPHALEXIN
Keflex Oral Suspension 1237
Keflex Pulvules 1237

KEFOLOR (Finland, Sweden)
CEFACLOR
Ceclor CD Tablets 1279
Ceclor Pulvules 1905
Ceclor Suspension 1905

KEFORAL (Belgium, France, Italy, The Netherlands)
CEPHALEXIN
Keflex Oral Suspension 1237
Keflex Pulvules 1237

KEFOX (Italy)
CEFUROXIME SODIUM
Kefurox Vials, ADD-Vantage 1948
Zinacef Injection 1696

KEFROXIL (Italy)
CEFADROXIL
Duricef Capsules 1079
Duricef Oral Suspension 1079
Duricef Tablets 1079

KEFSPOR (Germany)
CEFACLOR
Ceclor CD Tablets 1279
Ceclor Pulvules 1905
Ceclor Suspension 1905

KEFTID (Irish Republic, United Kingdom)
CEFACLOR
Ceclor CD Tablets 1279
Ceclor Pulvules 1905
Ceclor Suspension 1905

KEFURIM (Israel)
CEFUROXIME SODIUM
Kefurox Vials, ADD-Vantage 1948
Zinacef Injection 1696

KEFURION (Finland)
CEFUROXIME SODIUM
Kefurox Vials, ADD-Vantage 1948
Zinacef Injection 1696

KEFUROX (Belgium, Canada)
CEFUROXIME SODIUM
Kefurox Vials, ADD-Vantage 1948
Zinacef Injection 1696

KEFZIM (South Africa)
CEFTAZIDIME
Ceptaz for Injection 1499
Fortaz for Injection 1541
Tazicef for Injection 1647
Tazidime Vials, Faspak & ADD-Vantage . . 1966

KEFZOL (Israel)
CEFAZOLIN SODIUM
Ancef for Injection 1474
Kefzol Vials, ADD-Vantage 1951

KEIMAX (Germany)
CEFTIBUTEN
Cedax Capsules 1021
Cedax Oral Suspension 1021

KELA (Thailand)
TRIAMCINOLONE ACETONIDE
Azmacort Inhalation Aerosol 728
Nasacort AQ Nasal Spray 752
Nasacort Nasal Inhaler 750

KELATIN (Belgium, The Netherlands)
PENICILLAMINE
Cuprimine Capsules 2075
Depen Titratable Tablets 3341

KELATINE (Portugal)
PENICILLAMINE
Cuprimine Capsules 2075
Depen Titratable Tablets 3341

KELBIUM (Spain)
CEFPODOXIME PROXETIL
Vantin Tablets and Oral Suspension 2860

KELEFUSIN (Mexico)
POTASSIUM CHLORIDE
K-Dur Microburst Release System ER Tablets 1832
K-Lor Powder Packets 469
K-Tab Filmtab Tablets 470
Rum-K 1363

KEMICETIN (Austria)
CHLORAMPHENICOL
Chloromycetin Ophthalmic Ointment, 1% . . . . ⊙296
Chloromycetin Ophthalmic Solution . . . . ⊙297
Chloroptic Sterile Ophthalmic Ointment . . ⊙234
Chloroptic Sterile Ophthalmic Solution . . ⊙235

KEMICETINA (Belgium)
CHLORAMPHENICOL
Chloromycetin Ophthalmic Ointment, 1% . . . . ⊙296
Chloromycetin Ophthalmic Solution . . . . ⊙297
Chloroptic Sterile Ophthalmic Ointment . . ⊙234
Chloroptic Sterile Ophthalmic Solution . . ⊙235

KEMICETINE (Thailand)
CHLORAMPHENICOL
Chloromycetin Ophthalmic Ointment, 1% . . . . ⊙296
Chloromycetin Ophthalmic Solution . . . . ⊙297
Chloroptic Sterile Ophthalmic Ointment . . ⊙234
Chloroptic Sterile Ophthalmic Solution . . ⊙235

KEMOCARB (Thailand)
CARBOPLATIN
Paraplatin for Injection 1126

KEMZID (Singapore, Thailand)
TRIAMCINOLONE ACETONIDE
Azmacort Inhalation Aerosol 728
Nasacort AQ Nasal Spray 752
Nasacort Nasal Inhaler 750

KENACORT (Belgium, Finland, France, Thailand)
TRIAMCINOLONE ACETONIDE
Azmacort Inhalation Aerosol 728
Nasacort AQ Nasal Spray 752
Nasacort Nasal Inhaler 750

KENACORT-A (Australia, Belgium, Hong Kong, Irish Republic, Italy, New Zealand, Switzerland, The Netherlands)
TRIAMCINOLONE ACETONIDE
Azmacort Inhalation Aerosol 728
Nasacort AQ Nasal Spray 752
Nasacort Nasal Inhaler 750

KENACORT-T (Norway, Sweden)
TRIAMCINOLONE ACETONIDE
Azmacort Inhalation Aerosol 728
Nasacort AQ Nasal Spray 752
Nasacort Nasal Inhaler 750

KENALIN (Mexico)
SULINDAC
Clinoril Tablets 2053

KENALOG (Canada, Denmark, Germany, Irish Republic, Israel, United Kingdom)
TRIAMCINOLONE ACETONIDE
Azmacort Inhalation Aerosol 728
Nasacort AQ Nasal Spray 752
Nasacort Nasal Inhaler 750

KENALOG IN ORABASE (Australia, Canada, Hong Kong, Israel, New Zealand, Singapore, South Africa, Thailand)
TRIAMCINOLONE ACETONIDE
Azmacort Inhalation Aerosol 728
Nasacort AQ Nasal Spray 752
Nasacort Nasal Inhaler 750

KENALOG ORABASE (Spain)
TRIAMCINOLONE ACETONIDE
Azmacort Inhalation Aerosol 728
Nasacort AQ Nasal Spray 752
Nasacort Nasal Inhaler 750

KENALONE (Australia)
TRIAMCINOLONE ACETONIDE
Azmacort Inhalation Aerosol 728
Nasacort AQ Nasal Spray 752
Nasacort Nasal Inhaler 750

KENALYN (Thailand)
KETOCONAZOLE
Nizoral 2% Cream 3620
Nizoral 2% Shampoo 2007
Nizoral Tablets 1791

KENAPRIL (Mexico)
CAPTOPRIL
Captopril Tablets 2281

KENAPROX (Mexico)
NAPROXEN
EC-Naprosyn Delayed-Release Tablets . . . 2967
Naprosyn Suspension 2967
Naprosyn Tablets 2967

KENAZOL (Thailand)
KETOCONAZOLE
Nizoral 2% Cream 3620
Nizoral 2% Shampoo 2007
Nizoral Tablets 1791

KENAZOLE (Thailand)
KETOCONAZOLE
Nizoral 2% Cream 3620
Nizoral 2% Shampoo 2007
Nizoral Tablets 1791

KENESIL (Spain)
NIMODIPINE
Nimotop Capsules 904

KENZEN (France)
CANDESARTAN CILEXETIL
Atacand Tablets 595

KENZOFLEX (Mexico)
CIPROFLOXACIN HYDROCHLORIDE
Ciloxan Ophthalmic Ointment 538
Ciloxan Ophthalmic Solution . . . . ⊙209, 538
Cipro Tablets 887

KENO (Thailand)
TRIAMCINOLONE ACETONIDE
Azmacort Inhalation Aerosol 728
Nasacort AQ Nasal Spray 752
Nasacort Nasal Inhaler 750

KENOIDAL (Belgium)
TRIAMCINOLONE ACETONIDE
Azmacort Inhalation Aerosol 728
Nasacort AQ Nasal Spray 752
Nasacort Nasal Inhaler 750

KENOKET (Mexico)
CLONAZEPAM
Klonopin Tablets 2983

KENOLAN (Mexico)
CAPTOPRIL
Captopril Tablets 2281

KENOPRIL (Mexico)
ENALAPRIL MALEATE
Vasotec Tablets 2210

KENORAL (Thailand)
KETOCONAZOLE
Nizoral 2% Cream 3620
Nizoral 2% Shampoo 2007
Nizoral Tablets 1791

KEPRODOL (Austria)
KETOPROFEN
Orudis Capsules 3548
Oruvail Capsules 3548

KEPSIDOL (Mexico)
HALOPERIDOL
Haldol Injection, Tablets and Concentrate 2533

KERLOCAL (France)
TRETINOIN
Avita Cream 999
Avita Gel 1000
Renova 0.05% Cream 2519
Retin-A Micro 0.1% 2522
Vesanoid Capsules 3037

KERLON (Denmark, Finland, Italy, Sweden, Switzerland, The Netherlands)
BETAXOLOL HYDROCHLORIDE
Betoptic S Ophthalmic Suspension . . . . ⊙208, 537

KERLONE (Belgium, France, Germany, Hong Kong, Israel, Singapore, Spain, Thailand, United Kingdom)
BETAXOLOL HYDROCHLORIDE
Betoptic S Ophthalmic Suspension . . . . ⊙208, 537

KESINT (Italy)
CEFUROXIME SODIUM
Kefurox Vials, ADD-Vantage 1948
Zinacef Injection 1696

KESSAR (Australia, Austria, France, Germany, Italy, Mexico, South Africa, Switzerland)
TAMOXIFEN CITRATE
Nolvadex Tablets 678

KESTOMICOL (Mexico)
KETOCONAZOLE
Nizoral 2% Cream 3620
Nizoral 2% Shampoo 2007
Nizoral Tablets 1791

KETALGESIC (Italy)
KETOPROFEN
Orudis Capsules 3548
Oruvail Capsules 3548

KETALGIN (Italy)
KETOPROFEN
Orudis Capsules 3548
Oruvail Capsules 3548

KETANINE (Singapore)
CAPTOPRIL
Captopril Tablets 2281

KETARTRIUM (Italy)
KETOPROFEN
Orudis Capsules 3548
Oruvail Capsules 3548

KETAZOL (Thailand)
KETOCONAZOLE
Nizoral 2% Cream 3620
Nizoral 2% Shampoo 2007
Nizoral Tablets 1791

KETAZON (Thailand)
KETOCONAZOLE
Nizoral 2% Cream 3620
Nizoral 2% Shampoo 2007
Nizoral Tablets 1791

KETIL (United Kingdom)
KETOPROFEN
Orudis Capsules 3548
Oruvail Capsules 3548

KETO (Finland, Italy)
KETOPROFEN
Orudis Capsules 3548
Oruvail Capsules 3548

KETOARTRIL (Spain)
KETOPROFEN
Orudis Capsules 3548

Oruvail Capsules 3548

KETOCID (United Kingdom)
KETOPROFEN
Orudis Capsules 3548
Oruvail Capsules 3548

KETOCINE (Thailand)
KETOCONAZOLE
Nizoral 2% Cream 3620
Nizoral 2% Shampoo 2007
Nizoral Tablets 1791

KETOCON (Brazil)
KETOCONAZOLE
Nizoral 2% Cream 3620
Nizoral 2% Shampoo 2007
Nizoral Tablets 1791

KETODERM (France)
KETOCONAZOLE
Nizoral 2% Cream 3620
Nizoral 2% Shampoo 2007
Nizoral Tablets 1791

KETODOL (Italy)
KETOPROFEN
Orudis Capsules 3548
Oruvail Capsules 3548

KETOFAR (Mexico)
KETOCONAZOLE
Nizoral 2% Cream 3620
Nizoral 2% Shampoo 2007
Nizoral Tablets 1791

KETOFEN (Finland)
KETOPROFEN
Orudis Capsules 3548
Oruvail Capsules 3548

KETOFENE (Portugal)
KETOPROFEN
Orudis Capsules 3548
Oruvail Capsules 3548

KETOFLAM (South Africa)
KETOPROFEN
Orudis Capsules 3548
Oruvail Capsules 3548

KETOISDIN (Spain)
KETOCONAZOLE
Nizoral 2% Cream 3620
Nizoral 2% Shampoo 2007
Nizoral Tablets 1791

KETOLAN (Thailand)
KETOCONAZOLE
Nizoral 2% Cream 3620
Nizoral 2% Shampoo 2007
Nizoral Tablets 1791

KETOLIST (Germany)
KETOPROFEN
Orudis Capsules 3548
Oruvail Capsules 3548

KETOMED (Thailand)
KETOCONAZOLE
Nizoral 2% Cream 3620
Nizoral 2% Shampoo 2007
Nizoral Tablets 1791

KETOMEX (Finland)
KETOPROFEN
Orudis Capsules 3548
Oruvail Capsules 3548

KETOMIZOL (Mexico)
KETOCONAZOLE
Nizoral 2% Cream 3620
Nizoral 2% Shampoo 2007
Nizoral Tablets 1791

KETONAL (Israel)
KETOPROFEN
Orudis Capsules 3548
Oruvail Capsules 3548

KETONAN (Brazil)
KETOCONAZOLE
Nizoral 2% Cream 3620
Nizoral 2% Shampoo 2007
Nizoral Tablets 1791

KETONAZOLE (Thailand)
KETOCONAZOLE
Nizoral 2% Cream 3620
Nizoral 2% Shampoo 2007
Nizoral Tablets 1791

KETONE (Mexico)
KETOCONAZOLE
Nizoral 2% Cream 3620
Nizoral 2% Shampoo 2007
Nizoral Tablets 1791

KETOPLUS (Italy)
KETOPROFEN
Orudis Capsules 3548
Oruvail Capsules 3548

KETOPROSIL (Spain)
KETOPROFEN
Orudis Capsules 3548
Oruvail Capsules 3548

KETORIN (Finland)
KETOPROFEN
Orudis Capsules 3548
Oruvail Capsules 3548

KETOSIL (Thailand)
KETOCONAZOLE
Nizoral 2% Cream 3620
Nizoral 2% Shampoo 2007
Nizoral Tablets 1791

KETOSOLAN (Spain)
KETOPROFEN
Orudis Capsules 3548
Oruvail Capsules 3548

KETOTARD (United Kingdom)
KETOPROFEN
Orudis Capsules 3548
Oruvail Capsules 3548

KETOTOP (Singapore)
KETOPROFEN
Orudis Capsules 3548
Oruvail Capsules 3548

KETOVAIL (United Kingdom)
KETOPROFEN
Orudis Capsules 3548
Oruvail Capsules 3548

KETOZIP (United Kingdom)
KETOPROFEN
Orudis Capsules 3548
Oruvail Capsules 3548

KETOZOLE (Singapore)
KETOCONAZOLE
Nizoral 2% Cream 3620
Nizoral 2% Shampoo 2007
Nizoral Tablets 1791

KETRAX (Irish Republic, United Kingdom)
LEVAMISOLE HYDROCHLORIDE
Ergamisol Tablets 1789

KETREL (France, Portugal)
TRETINOIN
Avita Cream 999
Avita Gel 1000
Renova 0.05% Cream 2519
Retin-A Micro 0.1% 2522
Vesanoid Capsules 3037

KETUM (France)
KETOPROFEN
Orudis Capsules 3548
Oruvail Capsules 3548

KEZEPIN (Mexico)
CARBAMAZEPINE
Carbatrol Capsules 3234
Tegretol Chewable Tablets 2404
Tegretol Suspension 2404
Tegretol Tablets 2404
Tegretol-XR Tablets 2404

KEZER (Mexico)
KETOPROFEN
Orudis Capsules 3548
Oruvail Capsules 3548

KIATRIUM (Brazil)
DIAZEPAM
Valium Injectable 3026
Valium Tablets 3047

KIDROLASE (Canada, France, Israel)
ASPARAGINASE
Elspar for Injection 2092

KIFLONE (United Kingdom)
CEPHALEXIN
Keflex Oral Suspension 1237
Keflex Pulvules 1237

KIMAFAN (Hong Kong)
CAPTOPRIL
Captopril Tablets 2281

KINDELMIN (Brazil)
MEBENDAZOLE
Vermox Chewable Tablets 2017

KINIDIN (Denmark)
QUINIDINE SULFATE
Quinidex Extentabs 2933

KINLINE (Thailand)
SELEGILINE HYDROCHLORIDE
Eldepryl Capsules 3266

KIR RICHTER (Italy)
APROTININ
Trasylol Injection 909

KITON (Italy)
ISOSORBIDE MONONITRATE
Imdur Tablets 1826
Ismo Tablets 3524

KLACID (Australia, Denmark, Finland, Germany, Irish Republic, Israel, Italy, New Zealand, Norway, Portugal, Singapore, South Africa, Spain, Sweden, Thailand, The Netherlands)
CLARITHROMYCIN
Biaxin Filmtab Tablets 403
Biaxin for Oral Suspension 403

KLACIPED (Switzerland)
CLARITHROMYCIN
Biaxin Filmtab Tablets 403
Biaxin for Oral Suspension 403

KLAMACIN (Thailand)
CLOTRIMAZOLE
Lotrimin Cream 1% 3128
Lotrimin Lotion 1% 3128
Lotrimin Topical Solution 1% 3128
Mycelex Troche 573

KLARICID (Brazil, United Kingdom)
CLARITHROMYCIN
Biaxin Filmtab Tablets 403
Biaxin for Oral Suspension 403

KLARIDERM (Spain)
FLUOCINONIDE
Lidex Cream 2020
Lidex Gel 2020
Lidex Ointment 2020
Lidex Topical Solution 2020
Lidex-E Cream 2020

KLARIVITINA (Spain)
CYPROHEPTADINE HYDROCHLORIDE
Periactin Tablets 2155

KLEXANE (Denmark, Finland, Norway, Sweden)
ENOXAPARIN SODIUM
Lovenox Injection 746

KLIACEF (Italy)
CEFACLOR
Ceclor CD Tablets 1279
Ceclor Pulvules 1905
Ceclor Suspension 1905

KLIMAPUR (Austria)
ESTRADIOL
Alora Transdermal System 3372
Climara Transdermal System 958
Estrace Vaginal Cream 3358
Estring Vaginal Ring 2811
Vivelle Transdermal System 2412
Vivelle-Dot Transdermal System 2416

KLIMOFOL (Germany)
PROPOFOL
Diprivan Injectable Emulsion 667

KLINNA (Thailand)
CLINDAMYCIN PHOSPHATE
Cleocin Phosphate Sterile Solution 2785
Cleocin T Topical Gel 2790
Cleocin T Topical Lotion 2790
Cleocin T Topical Solution 2790
Cleocin Vaginal Cream 2788
Clindets Pledgets 3270

KLINOC (Austria)
MINOCYCLINE HYDROCHLORIDE
Dynacin Capsules 2019
Minocin Intravenous 1862
Minocin Oral Suspension 1865
Minocin Pellet-Filled Capsules 1863

KLINOMYCIN (Germany)
MINOCYCLINE HYDROCHLORIDE
Dynacin Capsules 2019
Minocin Intravenous 1862
Minocin Oral Suspension 1865
Minocin Pellet-Filled Capsules 1863

KLINOTAB (Belgium)
MINOCYCLINE HYDROCHLORIDE
Dynacin Capsules 2019
Minocin Intravenous 1862
Minocin Oral Suspension 1865
Minocin Pellet-Filled Capsules 1863

KLINOXID (Germany)
BENZOYL PEROXIDE
Brevoxyl-4 Cleansing Lotion 3269
Brevoxyl-4 Creamy Wash 3270
Brevoxyl-4 Gel 3269
Brevoxyl-8 Cleansing Lotion 3269
Brevoxyl-8 Creamy Wash 3270
Brevoxyl-8 Gel 3269
Triaz Cleanser 2026
Triaz Gel 2026

KLIOFEM (United Kingdom)
ESTRADIOL
Alora Transdermal System 3372
Climara Transdermal System 958
Estrace Vaginal Cream 3358
Estring Vaginal Ring 2811
Vivelle Transdermal System 2412
Vivelle-Dot Transdermal System 2416

KLIOGEST (Belgium)
ESTRADIOL
Alora Transdermal System 3372
Climara Transdermal System 958
Estrace Vaginal Cream 3358
Estring Vaginal Ring 2811
Vivelle Transdermal System 2412
Vivelle-Dot Transdermal System 2416

KLION (Thailand)
METRONIDAZOLE
MetroCream 1404
MetroGel 1405
MetroGel-Vaginal Gel 1986
MetroLotion 1405
Noritate Cream 1224

KLIOVANCE (New Zealand)
ESTRADIOL
Alora Transdermal System 3372
Climara Transdermal System 958
Estrace Vaginal Cream 3358
Estring Vaginal Ring 2811
Vivelle Transdermal System 2412
Vivelle-Dot Transdermal System 2416

KLISMACORT (Germany)
PREDNISOLONE
Prelone Syrup 2273

KLOCLOR (South Africa)
CEFACLOR
Ceclor CD Tablets 1279
Ceclor Pulvules 1905
Ceclor Suspension 1905

KLODIN (Italy)
TICLOPIDINE HYDROCHLORIDE
Ticlid Tablets 3015

K-LONG (Canada)
POTASSIUM CHLORIDE
K-Dur Microburst Release System ER Tablets 1832
K-Lor Powder Packets 469
K-Tab Filmtab Tablets 470
Rum-K 1363

KLONT (Thailand)
METRONIDAZOLE
MetroCream 1404
MetroGel 1405
MetroGel-Vaginal Gel 1986
MetroLotion 1405
Noritate Cream 1224

K-LOR (Canada)
POTASSIUM CHLORIDE
K-Dur Microburst Release System ER Tablets 1832
K-Lor Powder Packets 469
K-Tab Filmtab Tablets 470
Rum-K 1363

KLORAETYL (Denmark)
ETHYL CHLORIDE
Gebauer's Ethyl Chloride 1409

KLORPROMAN (Finland)
CHLORPROMAZINE HYDROCHLORIDE
Thorazine Ampuls 1656
Thorazine Multi-dose Vials 1656
Thorazine Spansule Capsules 1656
Thorazine Syrup 1656
Thorazine Tablets 1656

KLOTRICID (Finland)
CLOTRIMAZOLE
Lotrimin Cream 1% 3128
Lotrimin Lotion 1% 3128
Lotrimin Topical Solution 1% 3128
Mycelex Troche 573

KLYNDAKEN (Mexico)
CLINDAMYCIN PHOSPHATE
Cleocin Phosphate Sterile Solution 2785
Cleocin T Topical Gel 2790
Cleocin T Topical Lotion 2790
Cleocin T Topical Solution 2790
Cleocin Vaginal Cream 2788
Clindets Pledgets 3270

K-LYTE (Canada)
POTASSIUM CITRATE
Urocit-K Tablets 2232

K-LYTE/CL (Canada)
POTASSIUM CHLORIDE
K-Dur Microburst Release System ER Tablets 1832
K-Lor Powder Packets 469
K-Tab Filmtab Tablets 470
Rum-K 1363

K-MED 900 (Canada)
POTASSIUM CHLORIDE
K-Dur Microburst Release System ER Tablets 1832
K-Lor Powder Packets 469
K-Tab Filmtab Tablets 470
Rum-K 1363

K-MIC (Sweden)
POTASSIUM CHLORIDE
K-Dur Microburst Release System ER Tablets 1832
K-Lor Powder Packets 469

K-Tab Filmtab Tablets 470
Rum-K 1363

KOFFEX DM-E (Canada)
DEXTROMETHORPHAN HYDROBROMIDE/GUAIFENESIN
Tussi-Organidin DM NR Liquid 3350
Tussi-Organidin DM-S NR Liquid 3350

KOFFEX EXPECTORANT (Canada)
GUAIFENESIN
Organidin NR Liquid 3350
Organidin NR Tablets 3350

KOFRON (Spain)
CLARITHROMYCIN
Biaxin Filmtab Tablets 403
Biaxin for Oral Suspension 403

KONADERM (Mexico)
KETOCONAZOLE
Nizoral 2% Cream 3620
Nizoral 2% Shampoo 2007
Nizoral Tablets 1791

KONAZIL (Brazil)
KETOCONAZOLE
Nizoral 2% Cream 3620
Nizoral 2% Shampoo 2007
Nizoral Tablets 1791

KONAZOL (Thailand)
KETOCONAZOLE
Nizoral 2% Cream 3620
Nizoral 2% Shampoo 2007
Nizoral Tablets 1791

KONOVID (Thailand)
OFLOXACIN
Floxin I.V. 2526
Floxin Otic Solution 1219
Floxin Tablets 2529
Ocuflox Ophthalmic Solution 554

KONTAGRIPP MONO (Germany)
IBUPROFEN
Motrin Suspension, Oral Drops, Chewable Tablets, and Caplets 2002

KORANDIL (Thailand)
ENALAPRIL MALEATE
Vasotec Tablets 2210

KOREC (France)
QUINAPRIL HYDROCHLORIDE
Accupril Tablets 2611

KORO (Thailand)
CHLORAMPHENICOL
Chloromycetin Ophthalmic Ointment, 1% . . . . . ⊙296
Chloromycetin Ophthalmic Solution . . . . . ⊙297
Chloroptic Sterile Ophthalmic Ointment . . . . . ⊙234
Chloroptic Sterile Ophthalmic Solution . . . . . ⊙235

KORTICOID (Switzerland)
FLUOCINONIDE
Lidex Cream 2020
Lidex Gel 2020
Lidex Ointment 2020
Lidex Topical Solution 2020
Lidex-E Cream 2020

KORTIKOID-RATIOPHARM (Germany)
TRIAMCINOLONE ACETONIDE
Azmacort Inhalation Aerosol 728
Nasacort AQ Nasal Spray 752
Nasacort Nasal Inhaler 750

K-PROFEN (Mexico)
KETOPROFEN
Orudis Capsules 3548
Oruvail Capsules 3548

KRATALGIN (Austria)
IBUPROFEN
Motrin Suspension, Oral Drops, Chewable Tablets, and Caplets 2002

KRATIUM (Hong Kong)
DIAZEPAM
Valium Injectable 3026
Valium Tablets 3047

KREBSILASI (Italy)
PANCRELIPASE
Ultrase Capsules 835
Ultrase MT Capsules 835

KREDEX (Belgium, France, Italy, Norway, Portugal, Spain, Sweden)
CARVEDILOL
Coreg Tablets 1508

KRENOSIN (France, Italy)
ADENOSINE
Adenocard Injection 1380
Adenoscan 1381

KRENOSINE (Switzerland)
ADENOSINE
Adenocard Injection 1380
Adenoscan 1381

K-SAN (Australia)
POTASSIUM CHLORIDE
K-Dur Microburst Release System ER Tablets 1832
K-Lor Powder Packets 469
K-Tab Filmtab Tablets 470
Rum-K 1363

KSR (Australia, Hong Kong)
POTASSIUM CHLORIDE
K-Dur Microburst Release System ER Tablets 1832
K-Lor Powder Packets 469
K-Tab Filmtab Tablets 470
Rum-K 1363

K-SR (New Zealand)
POTASSIUM CHLORIDE
K-Dur Microburst Release System ER Tablets 1832
K-Lor Powder Packets 469
K-Tab Filmtab Tablets 470
Rum-K 1363

KUHLPREDNON (Austria)
PREDNISOLONE
Prelone Syrup 2273

KURACID (Denmark)
RANITIDINE HYDROCHLORIDE
Zantac 150 EFFERdose Granules 1690
Zantac 150 EFFERdose Tablets 1690
Zantac 150 Tablets 1690
Zantac 300 Tablets 1690
Zantac Injection 1688
Zantac Injection Premixed 1688
Zantac Syrup 1690

KWELLADA (Canada)
LINDANE
Lindane Lotion USP 1% 559
Lindane Shampoo USP 1% 560

KWELLADA-P (Canada)
PERMETHRIN
Acticin Cream 998
Elimite Cream 552

KYYPAKKAUS (Finland)
HYDROCORTISONE
Anusol-HC Cream 2.5% 2237
Hydrocortone Tablets 2106

LA MORPH (New Zealand)
MORPHINE SULFATE
Astramorph/PF Injection, USP (Preservative-Free) 594
Duramorph Injection 1312
Infumorph 200 and Infumorph 500 Sterile Solutions 1314
Kadian Capsules 1335
MS Contin Tablets 2896
MSIR Oral Capsules 2898
MSIR Oral Solution 2898
MSIR Oral Solution Concentrate 2898
MSIR Oral Tablets 2898
Oramorph SR Tablets 3062
Roxanol 100 Concentrated Oral Solution 3066
Roxanol Concentrated Oral Solution 3066
Roxanol-T Oral Solution 3066

LABEL (Brazil)
RANITIDINE HYDROCHLORIDE
Zantac 150 EFFERdose Granules 1690
Zantac 150 EFFERdose Tablets 1690
Zantac 150 Tablets 1690
Zantac 300 Tablets 1690
Zantac Injection 1688
Zantac Injection Premixed 1688
Zantac Syrup 1690

LABILENO (Spain)
LAMOTRIGINE
Lamictal Chewable Dispersible Tablets 1567
Lamictal Tablets 1567

LABITRIX (Mexico)
METRONIDAZOLE
MetroCream 1404
MetroGel 1405
MetroGel-Vaginal Gel 1986
MetroLotion 1405
Noritate Cream 1224

LABOPAL (Spain)
BENAZEPRIL HYDROCHLORIDE
Lotensin Tablets 2365

LABROCOL (United Kingdom)
LABETALOL HYDROCHLORIDE
Normodyne Injection 3135
Normodyne Tablets 3137

LABYCARBOL (Mexico)
METHOCARBAMOL
Robaxin Injectable 2938
Robaxin Tablets 2939
Robaxin-750 Tablets 2939

LAC-DOL (Australia)
LACTULOSE
Kristalose for Oral Solution 1007

LACEROL (Spain)
DILTIAZEM HYDROCHLORIDE
Cardizem CD Capsules 1016
Cardizem Injectable 1018
Cardizem Lyo-Ject Syringe 1018
Cardizem Monovial 1018
Tiazac Capsules 1378

LACIN (Thailand)
CLINDAMYCIN HYDROCHLORIDE
Cleocin HCl Capsules 2784

LACONDAN (Spain)
IBUPROFEN
Motrin Suspension, Oral Drops, Chewable Tablets, and Caplets 2002

LACROMYCIN (Israel)
GENTAMICIN SULFATE
Genoptic Ophthalmic Ointment . . . . . ⊙239
Genoptic Sterile Ophthalmic Solution . . . . . ⊙239

LACSON (South Africa)
LACTULOSE
Kristalose for Oral Solution 1007

LACTICARE-HC (Mexico)
HYDROCORTISONE
Anusol-HC Cream 2.5% 2237
Hydrocortone Tablets 2106

LACTISONA (Portugal, Spain)
HYDROCORTISONE
Anusol-HC Cream 2.5% 2237
Hydrocortone Tablets 2106

LACTOCOL EXPECTORANTE (Spain)
GUAIFENESIN
Organidin NR Liquid 3350
Organidin NR Tablets 3350

LACTOCUR (Germany)
LACTULOSE
Kristalose for Oral Solution 1007

LACTOFALK (Germany)
LACTULOSE
Kristalose for Oral Solution 1007

LACTOGER (Italy)
LACTULOSE
Kristalose for Oral Solution 1007

LACTUFLOR (Germany)
LACTULOSE
Kristalose for Oral Solution 1007

LACTUGAL (United Kingdom)
LACTULOSE
Kristalose for Oral Solution 1007

LACTULAX (Canada, Mexico)
LACTULOSE
Kristalose for Oral Solution 1007

LACTULONA (Brazil)
LACTULOSE
Kristalose for Oral Solution 1007

LACTUVERLAN (Germany)
LACTULOSE
Kristalose for Oral Solution 1007

LACTYL (Italy)
LACTULOSE
Kristalose for Oral Solution 1007

LAEVILAC S (Germany)
LACTULOSE
Kristalose for Oral Solution 1007

LAEVOLAC (Austria, Italy, New Zealand, Portugal, South Africa, Switzerland)
LACTULOSE
Kristalose for Oral Solution 1007

LAFARIN (Italy)
CEPHALEXIN
Keflex Oral Suspension 1237
Keflex Pulvules 1237

LAFUREX (Italy)
CEFUROXIME SODIUM
Kefurox Vials, ADD-Vantage 1948
Zinacef Injection 1696

LAGARMICIN (Spain)
ERYTHROMYCIN STEARATE
Erythrocin Stearate Filmtab Tablets 452

LAGYLAN (Mexico)
METRONIDAZOLE
MetroCream 1404
MetroGel 1405
MetroGel-Vaginal Gel 1986
MetroLotion 1405
Noritate Cream 1224

LAKE (Spain)
RANITIDINE HYDROCHLORIDE
Zantac 150 EFFERdose Granules 1690
Zantac 150 EFFERdose Tablets 1690
Zantac 150 Tablets 1690
Zantac 300 Tablets 1690
Zantac Injection 1688
Zantac Injection Premixed 1688
Zantac Syrup 1690

LAKTIPEX (Sweden)
LACTULOSE
Kristalose for Oral Solution 1007

LAKTULAX (Austria)
LACTULOSE
Kristalose for Oral Solution 1007

LAMBLIT (Mexico)
METRONIDAZOLE
MetroCream 1404
MetroGel 1405
MetroGel-Vaginal Gel 1986
MetroLotion 1405
Noritate Cream 1224

LAMBUTOL (Hong Kong, Thailand)
ETHAMBUTOL HYDROCHLORIDE
Myambutol Tablets 1290

LAMICITIN (South Africa)
LAMOTRIGINE
Lamictal Chewable Dispersible Tablets 1567
Lamictal Tablets 1567

LAMICTAL (Australia, Austria, Belgium, Brazil, Canada, Denmark, Finland, France, Hong Kong, Irish Republic, Israel, Italy, Mexico, New Zealand, Norway, Portugal, Singapore, Spain, Sweden, Switzerland, Thailand, The Netherlands, United Kingdom)
LAMOTRIGINE
Lamictal Chewable Dispersible Tablets 1567
Lamictal Tablets 1567

LAMISIL (Austria, Belgium, Brazil, Canada, Denmark, Finland, France, Germany, Hong Kong, Irish Republic, Israel, Italy, Mexico, New Zealand, Norway, Portugal, Singapore, South Africa, Sweden, Thailand, The Netherlands, United Kingdom)
TERBINAFINE HYDROCHLORIDE
Lamisil Tablets 2360

LAMPOFLEX (Italy)
PIROXICAM
Feldene Capsules 2685

LAMPOMANDOL (Italy)
CEFAMANDOLE NAFATE
Mandol Vials 1953

LAMPOSPORIN (Italy)
CEFUROXIME SODIUM
Kefurox Vials, ADD-Vantage 1948
Zinacef Injection 1696

LAMRA (Germany)
DIAZEPAM
Valium Injectable 3026
Valium Tablets 3047

LANACANE (Israel, New Zealand, Spain, United Kingdom)
BENZOCAINE
Americaine Anesthetic Lubricant 1162
Americaine Otic Topical Anesthetic Ear Drops 1162

LANACANE MEDICATED CREAM (Canada)
BENZOCAINE
Americaine Anesthetic Lubricant 1162
Americaine Otic Topical Anesthetic Ear Drops 1162

LANACARD (Germany)
DIGOXIN
Lanoxicaps Capsules 1574
Lanoxin Elixir Pediatric 1578
Lanoxin Injection 1581
Lanoxin Injection Pediatric 1584
Lanoxin Tablets 1587

LANACORDIN (Spain)
DIGOXIN
Lanoxicaps Capsules 1574
Lanoxin Elixir Pediatric 1578
Lanoxin Injection 1581
Lanoxin Injection Pediatric 1584
Lanoxin Tablets 1587

LANACORT (Canada, Israel, Italy, United Kingdom)
HYDROCORTISONE ACETATE
Anusol-HC Suppositories 2238
Cortifoam Rectal Foam 3170
Hydrocortone Acetate Injectable Suspension 2103

Proctocort Suppositories 2264

LANACRIST (Sweden)
DIGOXIN
Lanoxicaps Capsules 1574
Lanoxin Elixir Pediatric 1578
Lanoxin Injection 1581
Lanoxin Injection Pediatric 1584
Lanoxin Tablets 1587

LANASTING (United Kingdom)
BENZOCAINE
Americaine Anesthetic Lubricant 1162
Americaine Otic Topical Anesthetic Ear Drops 1162

LANATIN (Denmark)
LISINOPRIL
Prinivil Tablets 2164
Zestril Tablets 698

LANEXAT (Brazil, Denmark, Finland, Mexico, Sweden)
FLUMAZENIL
Romazicon Injection 3000

LANFAST (United Arab Emirates)
LANSOPRAZOLE
Prevacid Delayed-Release Capsules 3292

LANGORAN (France)
ISOSORBIDE DINITRATE
Isordil Sublingual Tablets 3525
Isordil Titradose Tablets 3526

LANICOR (Austria, Germany, Italy, The Netherlands)
DIGOXIN
Lanoxicaps Capsules 1574
Lanoxin Elixir Pediatric 1578
Lanoxin Injection 1581
Lanoxin Injection Pediatric 1584
Lanoxin Tablets 1587

LANOXICAPS (The Netherlands)
DIGOXIN
Lanoxicaps Capsules 1574
Lanoxin Elixir Pediatric 1578
Lanoxin Injection 1581
Lanoxin Injection Pediatric 1584
Lanoxin Tablets 1587

LANOXIN (Australia, Belgium, Brazil, Canada, Hong Kong, Irish Republic, Israel, Italy, Mexico, New Zealand, Norway, Portugal, Singapore, South Africa, Sweden, Switzerland, Thailand, The Netherlands, United Kingdom)
DIGOXIN
Lanoxicaps Capsules 1574
Lanoxin Elixir Pediatric 1578
Lanoxin Injection 1581
Lanoxin Injection Pediatric 1584
Lanoxin Tablets 1587

LANSOX (Italy)
LANSOPRAZOLE
Prevacid Delayed-Release Capsules 3292

LANTOGENT (Spain)
GENTAMICIN SULFATE
Genoptic Ophthalmic Ointment . . . . ⊙239
Genoptic Sterile Ophthalmic Solution . . . ⊙239

LANURETIC (Austria)
AMILORIDE HYDROCHLORIDE/HYDROCHLOROTHIAZIDE
Moduretic Tablets 2138

LANZO (Denmark, Norway, Sweden)
LANSOPRAZOLE
Prevacid Delayed-Release Capsules 3292

LANZOR (France, Germany, South Africa)
LANSOPRAZOLE
Prevacid Delayed-Release Capsules 3292

LAPRIL (Thailand)
ENALAPRIL MALEATE
Vasotec Tablets 2210

LAPRILEN (Portugal)
ENALAPRIL MALEATE/HYDROCHLOROTHIAZIDE
Vaseretic Tablets 2204

LARAFEN (United Kingdom)
KETOPROFEN
Orudis Capsules 3548
Oruvail Capsules 3548

LARAFLEX (United Kingdom)
NAPROXEN
EC-Naprosyn Delayed-Release Tablets . . . 2967
Naprosyn Suspension 2967
Naprosyn Tablets 2967

LARAPAM (United Kingdom)
PIROXICAM
Feldene Capsules 2685

LARGACTIL (Austria, Belgium, Canada, Denmark, Hong Kong, Italy, Mexico, Portugal, South Africa, Spain, Switzerland)
CHLORPROMAZINE
Thorazine Suppositories 1656

LARGATREX (Portugal)
CHLORPROMAZINE HYDROCHLORIDE
Thorazine Ampuls 1656
Thorazine Multi-dose Vials 1656
Thorazine Spansule Capsules 1656
Thorazine Syrup 1656
Thorazine Tablets 1656

LARIAM (Australia, Austria, Belgium, Canada, Denmark, Finland, France, Germany, Hong Kong, Irish Republic, Israel, Italy, New Zealand, Norway, Singapore, South Africa, Sweden, Switzerland, The Netherlands, United Kingdom)
MEFLOQUINE HYDROCHLORIDE
Lariam Tablets 2989

LAROFERON (France)
INTERFERON ALFA-2A
Roferon-A Injection 2996

LARYLIN (Germany)
GUAIFENESIN
Organidin NR Liquid 3350
Organidin NR Tablets 3350

LASER (Italy)
NAPROXEN
EC-Naprosyn Delayed-Release Tablets . . . 2967
Naprosyn Suspension 2967
Naprosyn Tablets 2967

LASERVIS (Germany, Switzerland)
SODIUM HYALURONATE
Hyalgan Solution 3080

LASMA (Irish Republic, United Kingdom)
THEOPHYLLINE
Aerolate Jr. T.D. Capsules 1361
Aerolate Liquid 1361
Aerolate Sr. T.D. Capsules 1361
Theo-Dur Extended-Release Tablets 1835
Uni-Dur Extended-Release Tablets 1841
Uniphyl 400 mg and 600 mg Tablets . . . 2903

LASPAR (South Africa)
ASPARAGINASE
Elspar for Injection 2092

LASSIFAR (Italy)
LACTULOSE
Kristalose for Oral Solution 1007

LASTICOM (Austria)
AZELASTINE HYDROCHLORIDE
Astelin Nasal Spray 3339

LASTIN (Finland, Sweden)
AZELASTINE HYDROCHLORIDE
Astelin Nasal Spray 3339

LATICORT (Germany)
HYDROCORTISONE BUTYRATE
Locoid Cream 1341
Locoid Lipocream Cream 1342
Locoid Ointment 1341
Locoid Topical Solution 1341

LATIMIT (Germany)
HYDROCORTISONE ACETATE
Anusol-HC Suppositories 2238
Cortifoam Rectal Foam 3170
Hydrocortone Acetate Injectable Suspension 2103
Proctocort Suppositories 2264

LATORAL (Italy)
CEPHALEXIN
Keflex Oral Suspension 1237
Keflex Pulvules 1237

LATOTRYD (Mexico)
ERYTHROMYCIN
Emgel 2% Topical Gel 1285
Ery-Tab Tablets 448
Erythromycin Base Filmtab Tablets 454
Erythromycin Delayed-Release Capsules, USP 455
PCE Dispertab Tablets 498

LATTULAC (Italy)
LACTULOSE
Kristalose for Oral Solution 1007

LAUBEEL (Germany)
LORAZEPAM
Ativan Injection 3478
Ativan Tablets 3482

LAURACALM (Belgium)
LORAZEPAM
Ativan Injection 3478
Ativan Tablets 3482

LAURIMICINA (Mexico)
ERYTHROMYCIN STEARATE
Erythrocin Stearate Filmtab Tablets 452

LAVERAN (Brazil)
CIMETIDINE
Tagamet Tablets 1644

LAVISA (Spain)
FLUCONAZOLE
Diflucan Tablets, Injection, and Oral Suspension 2681

LAXAN (Thailand)
METHOCARBAMOL
Robaxin Injectable 2938
Robaxin Tablets 2939
Robaxin-750 Tablets 2939

LAXARON (France)
LACTULOSE
Kristalose for Oral Solution 1007

LAXEERSIROOP (The Netherlands)
LACTULOSE
Kristalose for Oral Solution 1007

LAXETTE (South Africa)
LACTULOSE
Kristalose for Oral Solution 1007

LAXILOSE (Canada)
LACTULOSE
Kristalose for Oral Solution 1007

LAXOMUNDIN (Germany)
LACTULOSE
Kristalose for Oral Solution 1007

LAXOSE (Irish Republic, United Kingdom)
LACTULOSE
Kristalose for Oral Solution 1007

LAXULAC (Italy)
LACTULOSE
Kristalose for Oral Solution 1007

LAXYL (Mexico)
DIAZEPAM
Valium Injectable 3026
Valium Tablets 3047

LEBROCETIN (Mexico)
CHLORAMPHENICOL
Chloromycetin Ophthalmic Ointment, 1% . . . . ⊙296
Chloromycetin Ophthalmic Solution . . . . ⊙297
Chloroptic Sterile Ophthalmic Ointment . . ⊙234
Chloroptic Sterile Ophthalmic Solution . . ⊙235

LECIBRAL (Spain)
NICARDIPINE HYDROCHLORIDE
Cardene I.V. 3485

LECLOR A (Mexico)
CHLORAMPHENICOL
Chloromycetin Ophthalmic Ointment, 1% . . . . ⊙296
Chloromycetin Ophthalmic Solution . . . . ⊙297
Chloroptic Sterile Ophthalmic Ointment . . ⊙234
Chloroptic Sterile Ophthalmic Solution . . ⊙235

LEDERCORT (Sweden)
TRIAMCINOLONE ACETONIDE
Azmacort Inhalation Aerosol 728
Nasacort AQ Nasal Spray 752
Nasacort Nasal Inhaler 750

LEDERDERM (Germany)
MINOCYCLINE HYDROCHLORIDE
Dynacin Capsules 2019
Minocin Intravenous 1862
Minocin Oral Suspension 1865
Minocin Pellet-Filled Capsules 1863

LEDERLIND (Germany)
NYSTATIN
Nystop Topical Powder USP 2608

LEDERMICINA (Italy)
DEMECLOCYCLINE HYDROCHLORIDE
Declomycin Tablets 1855

LEDERMYCIN (Australia, Austria, Belgium, Germany, Irish Republic, New Zealand, South Africa, The Netherlands, United Kingdom)
DEMECLOCYCLINE HYDROCHLORIDE
Declomycin Tablets 1855

LEDERPAX (Mexico, Spain)
ERYTHROMYCIN
Emgel 2% Topical Gel 1285
Ery-Tab Tablets 448
Erythromycin Base Filmtab Tablets 454
Erythromycin Delayed-Release Capsules, USP 455
PCE Dispertab Tablets 498

LEDERTAM (Italy, Sweden)
TAMOXIFEN CITRATE
Nolvadex Tablets 678

LEDERTEPA (Belgium, The Netherlands)
THIOTEPA
Thioplex for Injection 1765

LEDOX (Norway)
NAPROXEN
EC-Naprosyn Delayed-Release Tablets . . . 2967
Naprosyn Suspension 2967
Naprosyn Tablets 2967

LEDOXID ACNE (Switzerland)
BENZOYL PEROXIDE
Brevoxyl-4 Cleansing Lotion 3269
Brevoxyl-4 Creamy Wash 3270
Brevoxyl-4 Gel 3269
Brevoxyl-8 Cleansing Lotion 3269
Brevoxyl-8 Creamy Wash 3270
Brevoxyl-8 Gel 3269
Triaz Cleanser 2026
Triaz Gel 2026

LEGEDERM (Denmark, Finland, Italy, Sweden)
ALCLOMETASONE DIPROPIONATE
Aclovate Cream 1275
Aclovate Ointment 1275

LEGENDAL (Switzerland, The Netherlands)
LACTULOSE
Kristalose for Oral Solution 1007

LEHYDAN (Sweden)
PHENYTOIN
Dilantin Infatabs 2624
Dilantin-125 Oral Suspension 2625

LEICESTER RETARD (Italy)
ISOSORBIDE MONONITRATE
Imdur Tablets 1826
Ismo Tablets 3524

LELONG CONTUSIONS (France)
PENTOSAN POLYSULFATE SODIUM
Elmiron Capsules 570

LEMLAX (United Kingdom)
LACTULOSE
Kristalose for Oral Solution 1007

LEMSIP CHESTY COUGH (Australia, New Zealand)
GUAIFENESIN
Organidin NR Liquid 3350
Organidin NR Tablets 3350

LEMSIP COUGH & COLD CHESTY COUGH (United Kingdom)
GUAIFENESIN
Organidin NR Liquid 3350
Organidin NR Tablets 3350

LEMYFLOX (Mexico)
CIPROFLOXACIN
Cipro I.V. 893
Cipro I.V. Pharmacy Bulk Package 897
Cipro Oral Suspension 887

LENAMET (South Africa)
CIMETIDINE
Tagamet Tablets 1644

LENAZINE (South Africa)
PROMETHAZINE HYDROCHLORIDE
Phenergan Injection 3553
Phenergan Suppositories 3556
Phenergan Syrup Fortis 3554
Phenergan Syrup Plain 3554
Phenergan Tablets 3556

LENCID (Belgium)
LINDANE
Lindane Lotion USP 1% 559
Lindane Shampoo USP 1% 560

LENDIANON (Brazil)
LINDANE
Lindane Lotion USP 1% 559
Lindane Shampoo USP 1% 560

LENIARTRIL (Italy)
NAPROXEN
EC-Naprosyn Delayed-Release Tablets . . . 2967
Naprosyn Suspension 2967
Naprosyn Tablets 2967

LENIDERM (Italy)
FLUOCINOLONE ACETONIDE
Synalar Cream 2020
Synalar Ointment 2020
Synalar Topical Solution 2020

LENIRIT (Italy)
HYDROCORTISONE ACETATE
Anusol-HC Suppositories 2238
Cortifoam Rectal Foam 3170
Hydrocortone Acetate Injectable Suspension 2103
Proctocort Suppositories 2264

LENISOLONE (South Africa)
PREDNISOLONE
Prelone Syrup 2273

LENISUN (Italy)
BENZOCAINE
Americaine Anesthetic Lubricant 1162

Americaine Otic Topical Anesthetic Ear Drops . . . 1162

LENNACOL (South Africa)
CHLORAMPHENICOL
Chloromycetin Ophthalmic Ointment, 1% . . . ⊙296
Chloromycetin Ophthalmic Solution . . . ⊙297
Chloroptic Sterile Ophthalmic Ointment . . ⊙234
Chloroptic Sterile Ophthalmic Solution . . ⊙235

LENOCEF (South Africa)
CEPHALEXIN
Keflex Oral Suspension . . . 1237
Keflex Pulvules . . . 1237

LENOXICAPS (Germany)
DIGOXIN
Lanoxicaps Capsules . . . 1574
Lanoxin Elixir Pediatric . . . 1578
Lanoxin Injection . . . 1581
Lanoxin Injection Pediatric . . . 1584
Lanoxin Tablets . . . 1587

LENOXIN (Germany)
DIGOXIN
Lanoxicaps Capsules . . . 1574
Lanoxin Elixir Pediatric . . . 1578
Lanoxin Injection . . . 1581
Lanoxin Injection Pediatric . . . 1584
Lanoxin Tablets . . . 1587

LENPRYL (Mexico)
CAPTOPRIL
Captopril Tablets . . . 2281

LENSAFREND (Spain)
CEPHALEXIN
Keflex Oral Suspension . . . 1237
Keflex Pulvules . . . 1237

LENTO-KALIUM (Italy)
POTASSIUM CHLORIDE
K-Dur Microburst Release System ER Tablets . . . 1832
K-Lor Powder Packets . . . 469
K-Tab Filmtab Tablets . . . 470
Rum-K . . . 1363

LENTOLITH (South Africa)
LITHIUM CARBONATE
Eskalith CR Controlled Release Tablets . . 1527
Eskalith Capsules . . . 1527
Lithium Carbonate Capsules . . . 3061
Lithobid Slow-Release Tablets . . . 3255

LEO K (Irish Republic, United Kingdom)
POTASSIUM CHLORIDE
K-Dur Microburst Release System ER Tablets . . . 1832
K-Lor Powder Packets . . . 469
K-Tab Filmtab Tablets . . . 470
Rum-K . . . 1363

LEO-400 (Thailand)
ALBENDAZOLE
Albenza Tablets . . . 1463

LEODRINE (France)
HYDROFLUMETHIAZIDE
Diucardin Tablets . . . 3494

LEONAL (Spain)
IBUPROFEN
Motrin Suspension, Oral Drops, Chewable Tablets, and Caplets . . . 2002

LEPICORTINOLO (Portugal)
PREDNISOLONE
Prelone Syrup . . . 2273

LEPOBRON (Portugal)
THEOPHYLLINE
Aerolate Jr. T.D. Capsules . . . 1361
Aerolate Liquid . . . 1361
Aerolate Sr. T.D. Capsules . . . 1361
Theo-Dur Extended-Release Tablets . . . 1835
Uni-Dur Extended-Release Tablets . . . 1841
Uniphyl 400 mg and 600 mg Tablets . . . 2903

LEPONEX (Austria, Belgium, Brazil, Denmark, Finland, France, Germany, Israel, Italy, Mexico, Norway, Portugal, South Africa, Spain, Sweden, Switzerland, The Netherlands)
CLOZAPINE
Clozaril Tablets . . . 2319

LEPTANAL (Norway, Sweden)
FENTANYL CITRATE
Actiq . . . 1184

LEPTANAL COMP (Sweden)
FENTANYL CITRATE
Actiq . . . 1184

LEPTOPSIQUE (Mexico)
PERPHENAZINE
Trilafon Injection . . . 3160
Trilafon Tablets . . . 3160

LERGIGAN (Sweden)
PROMETHAZINE HYDROCHLORIDE
Phenergan Injection . . . 3553
Phenergan Suppositories . . . 3556
Phenergan Syrup Fortis . . . 3554
Phenergan Syrup Plain . . . 3554
Phenergan Tablets . . . 3556

LERPORINA (Spain)
CEPHALEXIN
Keflex Oral Suspension . . . 1237
Keflex Pulvules . . . 1237

LERSA (Spain)
SULFACETAMIDE SODIUM
Bleph-10 Ophthalmic Ointment 10% . . . ⊙230
Klaron Lotion 10% . . . 1224

LERTAMINE (Mexico)
LORATADINE
Claritin Reditabs . . . 3100
Claritin Syrup . . . 3100
Claritin Tablets . . . 3100

LERTAMINE-D (Mexico)
LORATADINE/PSEUDOEPHEDRINE SULFATE
Claritin-D 12 Hour Extended Release Tablets . . . 3102
Claritin-D 24 Hour Extended Release Tablets . . . 3104

LERTUS (Brazil)
FLUCONAZOLE
Diflucan Tablets, Injection, and Oral Suspension . . . 2681

LESCOL (Australia, Austria, Belgium, Brazil, Canada, Denmark, Finland, France, Hong Kong, Irish Republic, Israel, Italy, Mexico, New Zealand, Norway, Portugal, Singapore, South Africa, Spain, Sweden, Switzerland, Thailand, The Netherlands, United Kingdom)
FLUVASTATIN SODIUM
Lescol Capsules . . . 2361

LESPORENE (France)
TAMOXIFEN CITRATE
Nolvadex Tablets . . . 678

LESTID (Denmark, Finland, Norway, Sweden)
COLESTIPOL HYDROCHLORIDE
Colestid Tablets . . . 2791

LEUCODININE (Belgium)
MONOBENZONE
Benoquin Cream 20% . . . 1732

LEUCOGEN (Spain)
ASPARAGINASE
Elspar for Injection . . . 2092

LEUKERAN (Australia, Austria, Belgium, Brazil, Canada, Denmark, Finland, Germany, Hong Kong, Irish Republic, Israel, Italy, Mexico, New Zealand, Norway, Portugal, Singapore, South Africa, Spain, Sweden, Switzerland, Thailand, The Netherlands, United Kingdom)
CHLORAMBUCIL
Leukeran Tablets . . . 1591

LEUKOMINERASE (Germany)
LITHIUM CARBONATE
Eskalith CR Controlled Release Tablets . . 1527
Eskalith Capsules . . . 1527
Lithium Carbonate Capsules . . . 3061
Lithobid Slow-Release Tablets . . . 3255

LEUKOMYCIN (Germany)
CHLORAMPHENICOL
Chloromycetin Ophthalmic Ointment, 1% . . . ⊙296
Chloromycetin Ophthalmic Solution . . . ⊙297
Chloroptic Sterile Ophthalmic Ointment . . ⊙234
Chloroptic Sterile Ophthalmic Solution . . ⊙235

LEUNASE (Australia, Hong Kong, Japan, Mexico, Singapore, Thailand)
ASPARAGINASE
Elspar for Injection . . . 2092

LEUSTAT (United Kingdom)
CLADRIBINE
Leustatin Injection . . . 2495

LEUSTATIN (Australia, Austria, Brazil, Canada, Denmark, Finland, Germany, Hong Kong, Italy, New Zealand, Norway, South Africa, Spain, Sweden, Switzerland, Thailand, The Netherlands)
CLADRIBINE
Leustatin Injection . . . 2495

LEUSTATINE (France)
CLADRIBINE
Leustatin Injection . . . 2495

LEVAQUIN (Canada)
LEVOFLOXACIN
Levaquin Injection . . . 2537
Levaquin Tablets . . . 2537

LEVOCARVIT (Italy)
LEVOCARNITINE
Carnitor Injection . . . 3242
Carnitor Tablets and Oral Solution . . . 3245

LEVODEX (Israel)
DILTIAZEM HYDROCHLORIDE
Cardizem CD Capsules . . . 1016
Cardizem Injectable . . . 1018
Cardizem Lyo-Ject Syringe . . . 1018
Cardizem Monovial . . . 1018
Tiazac Capsules . . . 1378

LEVO-DROMORAN (Canada)
LEVORPHANOL TARTRATE
Levo-Dromoran Injectable . . . 1734
Levo-Dromoran Tablets . . . 1734
Levorphanol Tartrate Tablets . . . 3059

LEVOLAC (Finland, Norway)
LACTULOSE
Kristalose for Oral Solution . . . 1007

LEVOMED (Thailand)
CARBIDOPA/LEVODOPA
Sinemet CR Tablets . . . 1255
Sinemet Tablets . . . 1253

LEVOMYCETIN (Thailand)
CHLORAMPHENICOL
Chloromycetin Ophthalmic Ointment, 1% . . . ⊙296
Chloromycetin Ophthalmic Solution . . . ⊙297
Chloroptic Sterile Ophthalmic Ointment . . ⊙234
Chloroptic Sterile Ophthalmic Solution . . ⊙235

LEVONELLE (United Kingdom)
LEVONORGESTREL
Norplant System . . . 3543

LEVONOVA (Denmark, Finland, Norway, Sweden)
LEVONORGESTREL
Norplant System . . . 3543

LEVOXACIN (Italy)
LEVOFLOXACIN
Levaquin Injection . . . 2537
Levaquin Tablets . . . 2537

LEVSIN (Canada)
HYOSCYAMINE SULFATE
Levbid Extended-Release Tablets . . . 3172
Levsin Drops . . . 3172
Levsin Elixir . . . 3172
Levsin Injection . . . 3172
Levsin Tablets . . . 3172
Levsin/SL Tablets . . . 3172
Levsinex Timecaps . . . 3172

LEXEMIN (Thailand)
FENOFIBRATE
Tricor Capsules, Micronized . . . 513

LEXFOR (Thailand)
NORFLOXACIN
Chibroxin Sterile Ophthalmic Solution . . . ⊙273, 2051
Noroxin Tablets . . . 2145

LEXIBIOTICO (Spain)
CEPHALEXIN
Keflex Oral Suspension . . . 1237
Keflex Pulvules . . . 1237

LEXIFLOX (Hong Kong)
NORFLOXACIN
Chibroxin Sterile Ophthalmic Solution . . . ⊙273, 2051
Noroxin Tablets . . . 2145

LEXINCEF (Spain)
CEPHALEXIN
Keflex Oral Suspension . . . 1237
Keflex Pulvules . . . 1237

LEXINOR (Finland, Hong Kong, Singapore, Sweden, Thailand)
NORFLOXACIN
Chibroxin Sterile Ophthalmic Solution . . . ⊙273, 2051
Noroxin Tablets . . . 2145

LEXOBENE (Germany)
DICLOFENAC SODIUM
Voltaren Tablets . . . 2315
Voltaren-XR Tablets . . . 2315

LEZIDIM (Mexico)
CEFTAZIDIME
Ceptaz for Injection . . . 1499
Fortaz for Injection . . . 1541
Tazicef for Injection . . . 1647
Tazidime Vials, Faspak & ADD-Vantage . . 1966

LI 450 (Germany)
LITHIUM CARBONATE
Eskalith CR Controlled Release Tablets . . 1527
Eskalith Capsules . . . 1527
Lithium Carbonate Capsules . . . 3061
Lithobid Slow-Release Tablets . . . 3255

LIBERALGIUM (Spain)
DICLOFENAC SODIUM
Voltaren Tablets . . . 2315
Voltaren-XR Tablets . . . 2315

LIBESPORAL (Spain)
CEPHALEXIN
Keflex Oral Suspension . . . 1237
Keflex Pulvules . . . 1237

LIBRIUM (Canada, Italy, United Kingdom)
CHLORDIAZEPOXIDE HYDROCHLORIDE
Librium Capsules . . . 1736
Librium for Injection . . . 1737

LIBROFEM (Spain, United Kingdom)
IBUPROFEN
Motrin Suspension, Oral Drops, Chewable Tablets, and Caplets . . . 2002

LICAB (Thailand)
LITHIUM CARBONATE
Eskalith CR Controlled Release Tablets . . 1527
Eskalith Capsules . . . 1527
Lithium Carbonate Capsules . . . 3061
Lithobid Slow-Release Tablets . . . 3255

LICARB (Thailand)
LITHIUM CARBONATE
Eskalith CR Controlled Release Tablets . . 1527
Eskalith Capsules . . . 1527
Lithium Carbonate Capsules . . . 3061
Lithobid Slow-Release Tablets . . . 3255

LICARBIUM (Israel)
LITHIUM CARBONATE
Eskalith CR Controlled Release Tablets . . 1527
Eskalith Capsules . . . 1527
Lithium Carbonate Capsules . . . 3061
Lithobid Slow-Release Tablets . . . 3255

LIDALTRIN (Spain)
QUINAPRIL HYDROCHLORIDE
Accupril Tablets . . . 2611

LIDEMOL (Canada)
FLUOCINONIDE
Lidex Cream . . . 2020
Lidex Gel . . . 2020
Lidex Ointment . . . 2020
Lidex Topical Solution . . . 2020
Lidex-E Cream . . . 2020

LIDERFEME (Spain)
IBUPROFEN
Motrin Suspension, Oral Drops, Chewable Tablets, and Caplets . . . 2002

LIDERMAN (Austria)
OXICONAZOLE NITRATE
Oxistat Cream . . . 1298
Oxistat Lotion . . . 1298

LIDEX (Belgium, Canada)
FLUOCINONIDE
Lidex Cream . . . 2020
Lidex Gel . . . 2020
Lidex Ointment . . . 2020
Lidex Topical Solution . . . 2020
Lidex-E Cream . . . 2020

LIDIFEN (United Kingdom)
IBUPROFEN
Motrin Suspension, Oral Drops, Chewable Tablets, and Caplets . . . 2002

LIFENAC (Mexico)
DICLOFENAC SODIUM
Voltaren Tablets . . . 2315
Voltaren-XR Tablets . . . 2315

LIFERXINA (Mexico)
CIPROFLOXACIN
Cipro I.V. . . . 893
Cipro I.V. Pharmacy Bulk Package . . . 897
Cipro Oral Suspension . . . 887

LIFUROM (South Africa)
CEFUROXIME SODIUM
Kefurox Vials, ADD-Vantage . . . 1948
Zinacef Injection . . . 1696

LIFUROX (Denmark, Finland, Norway, Spain, Sweden)
CEFUROXIME SODIUM
Kefurox Vials, ADD-Vantage . . . 1948
Zinacef Injection . . . 1696

LIKENIL (Spain)
LISINOPRIL
Prinivil Tablets . . . 2164
Zestril Tablets . . . 698

LI-LIQUID (United Kingdom)
LITHIUM CITRATE
Lithium Citrate Syrup . . . 3061

LIMBATRIL (Germany)
AMITRIPTYLINE HYDROCHLORIDE/CHLORDIAZEPOXIDE
Limbitrol DS Tablets . . . 1738

Limbitrol Tablets ... **1738**

LIMBITROL (Austria, Belgium, Brazil, Finland, France, Irish Republic, South Africa, Switzerland, The Netherlands, United Kingdom)
AMITRIPTYLINE HYDROCHLORIDE/CHLORDIAZEPOXIDE
Limbitrol DS Tablets ... **1738**
Limbitrol Tablets ... **1738**

LIMBITRYL (Italy)
AMITRIPTYLINE HYDROCHLORIDE/CHLORDIAZEPOXIDE
Limbitrol DS Tablets ... **1738**
Limbitrol Tablets ... **1738**

LIMED (Thailand)
LITHIUM CARBONATE
Eskalith CR Controlled Release Tablets ... **1527**
Eskalith Capsules ... **1527**
Lithium Carbonate Capsules ... **3061**
Lithobid Slow-Release Tablets ... **3255**

LIMOXIN (Mexico)
AMOXICILLIN
Amoxil Pediatric Drops for Oral Suspension ... **1471**
Amoxil Tablets ... **1471**

LIMPIDEX (Italy)
LANSOPRAZOLE
Prevacid Delayed-Release Capsules ... **3292**

LINATIL (Finland)
ENALAPRIL MALEATE
Vasotec Tablets ... **2210**

LINATIL COMP (Finland)
ENALAPRIL MALEATE/HYDROCHLOROTHIAZIDE
Vaseretic Tablets ... **2204**

LINCIL (Spain)
NICARDIPINE HYDROCHLORIDE
Cardene I.V. ... **3485**

LINDANOXIL (Brazil)
LINDANE
Lindane Lotion USP 1% ... **559**
Lindane Shampoo USP 1% ... **560**

LINFOLYSIN (Italy)
CHLORAMBUCIL
Leukeran Tablets ... **1591**

LINOLADIOL (Austria)
ESTRADIOL
Alora Transdermal System ... **3372**
Climara Transdermal System ... **958**
Estrace Vaginal Cream ... **3358**
Estring Vaginal Ring ... **2811**
Vivelle Transdermal System ... **2412**
Vivelle-Dot Transdermal System ... **2416**

LINOLADIOL N (Germany)
ESTRADIOL
Alora Transdermal System ... **3372**
Climara Transdermal System ... **958**
Estrace Vaginal Cream ... **3358**
Estring Vaginal Ring ... **2811**
Vivelle Transdermal System ... **2412**
Vivelle-Dot Transdermal System ... **2416**

LINOLADIOL-H N (Germany)
ESTRADIOL
Alora Transdermal System ... **3372**
Climara Transdermal System ... **958**
Estrace Vaginal Cream ... **3358**
Estring Vaginal Ring ... **2811**
Vivelle Transdermal System ... **2412**
Vivelle-Dot Transdermal System ... **2416**

LINOLA-H N (Germany)
PREDNISOLONE
Prelone Syrup ... **2273**

LINOLA-H-FETT N (Germany)
PREDNISOLONE
Prelone Syrup ... **2273**

LIOCARPINA (Italy)
PILOCARPINE HYDROCHLORIDE
Isopto Carpine Ophthalmic Solution ... **⊙215**
Pilopine HS Ophthalmic Gel ... **⊙217**
Salagen Tablets ... **2229**

LIOTON (Hong Kong, Italy, Switzerland)
HEPARIN SODIUM
Heparin Lock Flush Solution ... **3509**
Heparin Sodium Injection ... **3511**

LIPANON (Brazil)
FENOFIBRATE
Tricor Capsules, Micronized ... **513**

LIPANTHYL (Belgium, France, Germany, Italy, Portugal, Singapore, Switzerland, Thailand)
FENOFIBRATE
Tricor Capsules, Micronized ... **513**

LIPANTIL (Irish Republic, United Kingdom)
FENOFIBRATE
Tricor Capsules, Micronized ... **513**

LIPARISON (Spain)
FENOFIBRATE
Tricor Capsules, Micronized ... **513**

LIPAVIL (Italy)
CLOFIBRATE
Atromid-S Capsules ... **3483**

LIPAVLON (France)
CLOFIBRATE
Atromid-S Capsules ... **3483**

LIPAXAN (Italy)
FLUVASTATIN SODIUM
Lescol Capsules ... **2361**

LIPAZIL (Australia)
GEMFIBROZIL
Lopid Tablets ... **2650**

LIPCOR (Austria)
FENOFIBRATE
Tricor Capsules, Micronized ... **513**

LIPEMOL (Spain)
PRAVASTATIN SODIUM
Pravachol Tablets ... **1099**

LIPEX (Australia)
SIMVASTATIN
Zocor Tablets ... **2219**

LIPIDAL (Israel)
PRAVASTATIN SODIUM
Pravachol Tablets ... **1099**

LIPIDAX (Italy)
FENOFIBRATE
Tricor Capsules, Micronized ... **513**

LIPIDIL (Canada, Germany, Mexico)
FENOFIBRATE
Tricor Capsules, Micronized ... **513**

LIPIDYS (Thailand)
GEMFIBROZIL
Lopid Tablets ... **2650**

LIPIL (Italy)
FENOFIBRATE
Tricor Capsules, Micronized ... **513**

LIPILIM (Hong Kong)
CLOFIBRATE
Atromid-S Capsules ... **3483**

LIPIREX (France)
FENOFIBRATE
Tricor Capsules, Micronized ... **513**

LIPISON (Thailand)
GEMFIBROZIL
Lopid Tablets ... **2650**

LIPITOR (Australia, Belgium, Canada, Hong Kong, Irish Republic, Israel, Italy, Mexico, New Zealand, Norway, South Africa, Thailand, The Netherlands, United Kingdom)
ATORVASTATIN CALCIUM
Lipitor Tablets ... **2639, 2696**

LIPIVAS (Denmark)
LOVASTATIN
Mevacor Tablets ... **2132**

LIPLAT (Spain)
PRAVASTATIN SODIUM
Pravachol Tablets ... **1099**

LIPLE (Japan)
ALPROSTADIL
Caverject Sterile Powder ... **2777**
MUSE Urethral Suppository ... **3335**

LIPO RED (Spain)
FENOFIBRATE
Tricor Capsules, Micronized ... **513**

LIPOBAY (Australia, Austria, Belgium, Denmark, Finland, Germany, Irish Republic, Italy, Norway, Portugal, Singapore, Spain, Sweden, Switzerland, Thailand, The Netherlands, United Kingdom)
CERIVASTATIN SODIUM
Baycol Tablets ... **883**

LIPOCLAR (Italy)
FENOFIBRATE
Tricor Capsules, Micronized ... **513**

LIPOFEN (Portugal)
FENOFIBRATE
Tricor Capsules, Micronized ... **513**

LIPOFENE (Italy)
FENOFIBRATE
Tricor Capsules, Micronized ... **513**

LIPOFOR (Singapore)
GEMFIBROZIL
Lopid Tablets ... **2650**

LIPOFREN (Spain)
LOVASTATIN
Mevacor Tablets ... **2132**

LIPOGEN (Italy)
GEMFIBROZIL
Lopid Tablets ... **2650**

LIPOGIS (Israel)
CERIVASTATIN SODIUM
Baycol Tablets ... **883**

LIPOITE (Portugal)
GEMFIBROZIL
Lopid Tablets ... **2650**

LIPONORM (Italy)
SIMVASTATIN
Zocor Tablets ... **2219**

LIPOSCLER (Spain)
LOVASTATIN
Mevacor Tablets ... **2132**

LIPOSIT (Italy)
FENOFIBRATE
Tricor Capsules, Micronized ... **513**

LIPOSTAT (Irish Republic, Israel, New Zealand, United Kingdom)
PRAVASTATIN SODIUM
Pravachol Tablets ... **1099**

LIPOSTEROL (Spain)
CERIVASTATIN SODIUM
Baycol Tablets ... **883**

LIPOVAS (Spain)
FENOFIBRATE
Tricor Capsules, Micronized ... **513**

LIPOZID (Italy)
GEMFIBROZIL
Lopid Tablets ... **2650**

LIPOZIL (Thailand)
GEMFIBROZIL
Lopid Tablets ... **2650**

LIPRIL (Portugal)
LISINOPRIL
Prinivil Tablets ... **2164**
Zestril Tablets ... **698**

LIPSIN (Austria, France, Italy, South Africa)
FENOFIBRATE
Tricor Capsules, Micronized ... **513**

LIPUR (France)
GEMFIBROZIL
Lopid Tablets ... **2650**

LIPUS (Portugal)
LOVASTATIN
Mevacor Tablets ... **2132**

LIQUEMIN (Italy, The Netherlands)
HEPARIN SODIUM
Heparin Lock Flush Solution ... **3509**
Heparin Sodium Injection ... **3511**

LIQUEMIN N (Germany)
HEPARIN SODIUM
Heparin Lock Flush Solution ... **3509**
Heparin Sodium Injection ... **3511**

LIQUEMINE (Belgium, Brazil, France, Spain, Switzerland)
HEPARIN SODIUM
Heparin Lock Flush Solution ... **3509**
Heparin Sodium Injection ... **3511**

LIQUIPOM ANTIBIOTICO (Spain)
NEOMYCIN SULFATE/POLYMYXIN B SULFATE
Neosporin G.U. Irrigant Sterile ... **2256**

LIROKEN (Mexico)
DICLOFENAC SODIUM
Voltaren Tablets ... **2315**
Voltaren-XR Tablets ... **2315**

LIS (Italy)
LACTULOSE
Kristalose for Oral Solution ... **1007**

LISANIRC (Italy)
NICARDIPINE HYDROCHLORIDE
Cardene I.V. ... **3485**

LISEDEMA (Brazil)
PIROXICAM
Feldene Capsules ... **2685**

LISIGAMMA (Germany)
LISINOPRIL
Prinivil Tablets ... **2164**
Zestril Tablets ... **698**

LISIHEXAL (Germany)
LISINOPRIL
Prinivil Tablets ... **2164**
Zestril Tablets ... **698**

LISINO (Germany)
LORATADINE
Claritin Reditabs ... **3100**
Claritin Syrup ... **3100**
Claritin Tablets ... **3100**

LISIOFER (Italy)
FERRIC SODIUM GLUCONATE
Ferrlecit Injection ... **3386**

LISIPRIL (Finland)
LISINOPRIL
Prinivil Tablets ... **2164**
Zestril Tablets ... **698**

LISIPRIL COMP (Finland)
HYDROCHLOROTHIAZIDE/LISINOPRIL
Prinzide Tablets ... **2168**
Zestoretic Tablets ... **695**

LISKONUM (United Kingdom)
LITHIUM CARBONATE
Eskalith CR Controlled Release Tablets ... **1527**
Eskalith Capsules ... **1527**
Lithium Carbonate Capsules ... **3061**
Lithobid Slow-Release Tablets ... **3255**

LISODUR (Australia)
LISINOPRIL
Prinivil Tablets ... **2164**
Zestril Tablets ... **698**

LISODURA (Germany)
LISINOPRIL
Prinivil Tablets ... **2164**
Zestril Tablets ... **698**

LISOTREX (Brazil)
ERYTHROMYCIN
Emgel 2% Topical Gel ... **1285**
Ery-Tab Tablets ... **448**
Erythromycin Base Filmtab Tablets ... **454**
Erythromycin Delayed-Release Capsules, USP ... **455**
PCE Dispertab Tablets ... **498**

LISPRIL (Thailand)
LISINOPRIL
Prinivil Tablets ... **2164**
Zestril Tablets ... **698**

LISTRAN (Spain)
NABUMETONE
Relafen Tablets ... **1617**

LIT-300 (Thailand)
LITHIUM CARBONATE
Eskalith CR Controlled Release Tablets ... **1527**
Eskalith Capsules ... **1527**
Lithium Carbonate Capsules ... **3061**
Lithobid Slow-Release Tablets ... **3255**

LITAREK (Spain)
GEMFIBROZIL
Lopid Tablets ... **2650**

LITAREX (Denmark, Norway, Sweden, Switzerland, The Netherlands, United Kingdom)
LITHIUM CITRATE
Lithium Citrate Syrup ... **3061**

LITHANE (Canada)
LITHIUM CARBONATE
Eskalith CR Controlled Release Tablets ... **1527**
Eskalith Capsules ... **1527**
Lithium Carbonate Capsules ... **3061**
Lithobid Slow-Release Tablets ... **3255**

LITHEUM (Mexico)
LITHIUM CARBONATE
Eskalith CR Controlled Release Tablets ... **1527**
Eskalith Capsules ... **1527**
Lithium Carbonate Capsules ... **3061**
Lithobid Slow-Release Tablets ... **3255**

LITHICARB (Australia, New Zealand)
LITHIUM CARBONATE
Eskalith CR Controlled Release Tablets ... **1527**
Eskalith Capsules ... **1527**
Lithium Carbonate Capsules ... **3061**
Lithobid Slow-Release Tablets ... **3255**

LITHIZINE (Canada)
LITHIUM CARBONATE
Eskalith CR Controlled Release Tablets ... **1527**
Eskalith Capsules ... **1527**
Lithium Carbonate Capsules ... **3061**
Lithobid Slow-Release Tablets ... **3255**

LITHONATE (United Kingdom)
LITHIUM CARBONATE
Eskalith CR Controlled Release Tablets ... **1527**
Eskalith Capsules ... **1527**
Lithium Carbonate Capsules ... **3061**
Lithobid Slow-Release Tablets ... **3255**

LITHOSUN (Singapore)
LITHIUM CARBONATE
Eskalith CR Controlled Release Tablets ... **1527**
Eskalith Capsules ... **1527**
Lithium Carbonate Capsules ... **3061**
Lithobid Slow-Release Tablets ... **3255**

LITIOCAR (Brazil)
LITHIUM CARBONATE
Eskalith CR Controlled Release Tablets . . 1527
Eskalith Capsules 1527
Lithium Carbonate Capsules 3061
Lithobid Slow-Release Tablets 3255

LITO (Finland)
LITHIUM CARBONATE
Eskalith CR Controlled Release Tablets . . 1527
Eskalith Capsules 1527
Lithium Carbonate Capsules 3061
Lithobid Slow-Release Tablets 3255

LIXOGAN (Mexico)
NAPROXEN
EC-Naprosyn Delayed-Release Tablets . . . 2967
Naprosyn Suspension 2967
Naprosyn Tablets 2967

LIZOVAG (Mexico)
KETOCONAZOLE
Nizoral 2% Cream 3620
Nizoral 2% Shampoo 2007
Nizoral Tablets 1791

LOCACID (France, Israel, Portugal)
TRETINOIN
Avita Cream 999
Avita Gel 1000
Renova 0.05% Cream 2519
Retin-A Micro 0.1% 2522
Vesanoid Capsules 3037

LOCALYN (Italy)
FLUOCINOLONE ACETONIDE
Synalar Cream 2020
Synalar Ointment 2020
Synalar Topical Solution 2020

LOCALYN SV (Italy)
FLUOCINOLONE ACETONIDE
Synalar Cream 2020
Synalar Ointment 2020
Synalar Topical Solution 2020

LOCAPRED (France, Portugal, Switzerland)
DESONIDE
DesOwen Cream 1401
DesOwen Lotion 1401
DesOwen Ointment 1401

LOCASYN (Denmark)
FLUNISOLIDE
Aerobid Inhaler System 1363
Aerobid-M Inhaler System 1363
Nasalide Nasal Spray 1295
Nasarel Nasal Solution 0.025% 1296

LOCATOP (France, Switzerland)
DESONIDE
DesOwen Cream 1401
DesOwen Lotion 1401
DesOwen Ointment 1401

LOCEPTIN (Sweden)
MORPHINE SULFATE
Astramorph/PF Injection, USP (Preservative-Free) 594
Duramorph Injection 1312
Infumorph 200 and Infumorph 500 Sterile Solutions 1314
Kadian Capsules 1335
MS Contin Tablets 2896
MSIR Oral Capsules 2898
MSIR Oral Solution 2898
MSIR Oral Solution Concentrate 2898
MSIR Oral Tablets 2898
Oramorph SR Tablets 3062
Roxanol 100 Concentrated Oral Solution 3066
Roxanol Concentrated Oral Solution 3066
Roxanol-T Oral Solution 3066

LOCHOL (Japan)
FLUVASTATIN SODIUM
Lescol Capsules 2361

LOCHOLES (Thailand)
GEMFIBROZIL
Lopid Tablets 2650

LOCOID (Belgium, Denmark, Finland, France, Irish Republic, Mexico, New Zealand, Norway, Portugal, South Africa, Sweden, Switzerland, The Netherlands, United Kingdom)
HYDROCORTISONE BUTYRATE
Locoid Cream 1341
Locoid Lipocream Cream 1342
Locoid Ointment 1341
Locoid Topical Solution 1341

LOCOID CRELO (Sweden)
HYDROCORTISONE BUTYRATE
Locoid Cream 1341
Locoid Lipocream Cream 1342
Locoid Ointment 1341
Locoid Topical Solution 1341

LOCOIDON (Austria, Italy)
HYDROCORTISONE BUTYRATE
Locoid Cream 1341
Locoid Lipocream Cream 1342
Locoid Ointment 1341
Locoid Topical Solution 1341

LOCOL (Germany)
FLUVASTATIN SODIUM
Lescol Capsules 2361

LODALES (France)
SIMVASTATIN
Zocor Tablets 2219

LODIMOL (Mexico)
DIPYRIDAMOLE
Persantine Tablets 1057

LODINE (Austria, France, Hong Kong, Italy, Mexico, Portugal, Switzerland, United Kingdom)
ETODOLAC
Lodine Capsules 3528
Lodine Tablets 3528
Lodine XL Extended-Release Tablets 3530

LODIXAL (Belgium)
VERAPAMIL HYDROCHLORIDE
Covera-HS Tablets 3199
Isoptin SR Tablets 467
Verelan Capsules 3184
Verelan PM Capsules 3186

LODOZ (France)
BISOPROLOL FUMARATE/HYDROCHLOROTHIAZIDE
Ziac Tablets 1887

LOFENSAID (United Kingdom)
DICLOFENAC SODIUM
Voltaren Tablets 2315
Voltaren-XR Tablets 2315

LOGAMICYL (Belgium)
DOXYCYCLINE HYCLATE
Doryx Coated Pellet Filled Capsules 3357
Periostat Tablets 1208
Vibra-Tabs Film Coated Tablets 2735
Vibramycin Hyclate Capsules 2735
Vibramycin Hyclate Intravenous 2737

LOGASTRIC (Belgium)
OMEPRAZOLE
Prilosec Delayed-Release Capsules 628

LOGAT (Brazil)
RANITIDINE HYDROCHLORIDE
Zantac 150 EFFERdose Granules 1690
Zantac 150 EFFERdose Tablets 1690
Zantac 150 Tablets 1690
Zantac 300 Tablets 1690
Zantac Injection 1688
Zantac Injection Premixed 1688
Zantac Syrup 1690

LOGECINE (France)
ERYTHROMYCIN
Emgel 2% Topical Gel 1285
Ery-Tab Tablets 448
Erythromycin Base Filmtab Tablets 454
Erythromycin Delayed-Release Capsules, USP 455
PCE Dispertab Tablets 498

LOGESIC (Mexico)
DICLOFENAC SODIUM
Voltaren Tablets 2315
Voltaren-XR Tablets 2315

LOGODERM (Australia, Mexico, New Zealand)
ALCLOMETASONE DIPROPIONATE
Aclovate Cream 1275
Aclovate Ointment 1275

LOGOMED AKNE-GEL (Germany)
BENZOYL PEROXIDE
Brevoxyl-4 Cleansing Lotion 3269
Brevoxyl-4 Creamy Wash 3270
Brevoxyl-4 Gel 3269
Brevoxyl-8 Cleansing Lotion 3269
Brevoxyl-8 Creamy Wash 3270
Brevoxyl-8 Gel 3269
Triaz Cleanser 2026
Triaz Gel 2026

LOGOMED ALLERGIE-GEL (Germany)
DIPHENHYDRAMINE HYDROCHLORIDE
Benadryl Parenteral 2617

LOGOMED BERUHIGUNGS-TABLETTEN (Germany)
DIPHENHYDRAMINE HYDROCHLORIDE
Benadryl Parenteral 2617

LOGOMED HAUTPILZ-SALBE (Germany)
CLOTRIMAZOLE
Lotrimin Cream 1% 3128
Lotrimin Lotion 1% 3128
Lotrimin Topical Solution 1% 3128
Mycelex Troche 573

LOGOMED JUCKREIZ (Germany)
DIPHENHYDRAMINE HYDROCHLORIDE
Benadryl Parenteral 2617

LOGOMED SCHMERZ (Germany)
IBUPROFEN
Motrin Suspension, Oral Drops, Chewable Tablets, and Caplets 2002

LOGOMED SPORT-GEL (Germany)
HEPARIN SODIUM
Heparin Lock Flush Solution 3509
Heparin Sodium Injection 3511

LOGOMED VENEN-SALBE (Germany)
HEPARIN SODIUM
Heparin Lock Flush Solution 3509
Heparin Sodium Injection 3511

LOGRADIN (Spain)
LORATADINE/PSEUDOEPHEDRINE SULFATE
Claritin-D 12 Hour Extended Release Tablets 3102
Claritin-D 24 Hour Extended Release Tablets 3104

LOGRYX (France)
MINOCYCLINE HYDROCHLORIDE
Dynacin Capsules 2019
Minocin Intravenous 1862
Minocin Oral Suspension 1865
Minocin Pellet-Filled Capsules 1863

LOITIN (Spain)
FLUCONAZOLE
Diflucan Tablets, Injection, and Oral Suspension 2681

LOKALICID (Germany)
CLOTRIMAZOLE
Lotrimin Cream 1% 3128
Lotrimin Lotion 1% 3128
Lotrimin Topical Solution 1% 3128
Mycelex Troche 573

LOKALISON-F (Germany)
DEXAMETHASONE
Decadron Elixir 2078
Decadron Tablets 2079

LOKALISON-UNIVERSALE (Germany)
DEXAMETHASONE
Decadron Elixir 2078
Decadron Tablets 2079

LOKILAN (Norway)
FLUNISOLIDE
Aerobid Inhaler System 1363
Aerobid-M Inhaler System 1363
Nasalide Nasal Spray 1295
Nasarel Nasal Solution 0.025% 1296

LOKILAN NASAL (Sweden)
FLUNISOLIDE
Aerobid Inhaler System 1363
Aerobid-M Inhaler System 1363
Nasalide Nasal Spray 1295
Nasarel Nasal Solution 0.025% 1296

LOLUM (Italy)
LABETALOL HYDROCHLORIDE
Normodyne Injection 3135
Normodyne Tablets 3137

LOMIR (Austria, Belgium, Brazil, Denmark, Finland, Germany, Italy, Norway, Portugal, Spain, Sweden, Switzerland, The Netherlands)
ISRADIPINE
DynaCirc CR Tablets 2923

LOMPER (Spain)
MEBENDAZOLE
Vermox Chewable Tablets 2017

LONAVAR (Australia)
OXANDROLONE
Oxandrin Tablets 1153

LONGAZEM (Italy)
DILTIAZEM HYDROCHLORIDE
Cardizem CD Capsules 1016
Cardizem Injectable 1018
Cardizem Lyo-Ject Syringe 1018
Cardizem Monovial 1018
Tiazac Capsules 1378

LONGIPREDNIL (Germany)
PREDNISOLONE
Prelone Syrup 2273

LOORTAN (Belgium)
LOSARTAN POTASSIUM
Cozaar Tablets 2067

LOORTAN PLUS (Belgium)
HYDROCHLOROTHIAZIDE/LOSARTAN POTASSIUM
Hyzaar 50-12.5 Tablets 2109

LO-P-CAPS (Thailand)
CALCIUM ACETATE
PhosLo Tablets 1069

LOPID (Australia, Belgium, Brazil, Canada, Denmark, Finland, Hong Kong, Irish Republic, Italy, Mexico, New Zealand, Portugal, Singapore, South Africa, Spain, Sweden, Thailand, The Netherlands, United Kingdom)
GEMFIBROZIL
Lopid Tablets 2650

LOPIRETIC (Portugal)
CAPTOPRIL
Captopril Tablets 2281

LOPIRIN (Austria, Germany, Switzerland)
CAPTOPRIL
Captopril Tablets 2281

LOPRANOL LA (United Kingdom)
PROPRANOLOL HYDROCHLORIDE
Inderal Injectable 3513
Inderal LA Long-Acting Capsules 3516
Inderal Tablets 3513

LOPRESS (Thailand)
PRAZOSIN HYDROCHLORIDE
Minipress Capsules 2699

LOPRIL (Finland, France)
CAPTOPRIL
Captopril Tablets 2281

LOPRIL D (Brazil)
CAPTOPRIL
Captopril Tablets 2281

LOPROX (Brazil, Canada, The Netherlands)
CICLOPIROX OLAMINE
Loprox Cream 2021
Loprox Lotion 2021

LOPTOMIT (The Netherlands)
TIMOLOL MALEATE
Blocadren Tablets 2046
Timoptic Sterile Ophthalmic Solution 2190
Timoptic in Ocudose 2192
Timoptic-XE Sterile Ophthalmic Gel Forming Solution 2194

LORABENZ (Denmark)
LORAZEPAM
Ativan Injection 3478
Ativan Tablets 3482

LORABID (Austria, Hong Kong, Mexico, South Africa, Sweden)
LORACARBEF
Lorabid Suspension and Pulvules 2251

LORADUR (Austria)
AMILORIDE HYDROCHLORIDE/HYDROCHLOROTHIAZIDE
Moduretic Tablets 2138

LORAFEM (Germany)
LORACARBEF
Lorabid Suspension and Pulvules 2251

LORAGA (Finland, Sweden)
LACTULOSE
Kristalose for Oral Solution 1007

LORAMED (Thailand)
LORAZEPAM
Ativan Injection 3478
Ativan Tablets 3482

LORANIL (Brazil)
LORATADINE
Claritin Reditabs 3100
Claritin Syrup 3100
Claritin Tablets 3100

LORANOX (Thailand)
LORATADINE
Claritin Reditabs 3100
Claritin Syrup 3100
Claritin Tablets 3100

LORANS (Italy, Singapore)
LORAZEPAM
Ativan Injection 3478
Ativan Tablets 3482

LORAPAM (New Zealand, Thailand)
LORAZEPAM
Ativan Injection 3478
Ativan Tablets 3482

LORASIFAR (Switzerland)
LORAZEPAM
Ativan Injection 3478
Ativan Tablets 3482

LORASTINE (Israel)
LORATADINE
Claritin Reditabs 3100
Claritin Syrup 3100
Claritin Tablets 3100

LORASTYNE (Australia)
LORATADINE
Claritin Reditabs 3100

Claritin Syrup 3100
Claritin Tablets 3100

LORATYN (Austria)
LORATADINE
Claritin Reditabs 3100
Claritin Syrup 3100
Claritin Tablets 3100

LORATYNE (South Africa)
LORATADINE
Claritin Reditabs 3100
Claritin Syrup 3100
Claritin Tablets 3100

LORAX (Austria, Brazil, The Netherlands)
LORACARBEF
Lorabid Suspension and Pulvules 2251

LORAZENE (Thailand)
LORAZEPAM
Ativan Injection 3478
Ativan Tablets 3482

LORAZEP (Thailand)
LORAZEPAM
Ativan Injection 3478
Ativan Tablets 3482

LORENIN (Portugal)
LORAZEPAM
Ativan Injection 3478
Ativan Tablets 3482

LORETIC (South Africa)
HYDROCHLOROTHIAZIDE/TRIAMTERENE
Dyazide Capsules 1515
Maxzide Tablets 1008
Maxzide-25 mg Tablets 1008

LOREXANE (Australia, Irish Republic, United Kingdom)
LINDANE
Lindane Lotion USP 1% 559
Lindane Shampoo USP 1% 560

LOREXEN (Mexico)
NAPROXEN
EC-Naprosyn Delayed-Release Tablets . . . 2967
Naprosyn Suspension 2967
Naprosyn Tablets 2967

LOREXINA (Italy)
CEPHALEXIN
Keflex Oral Suspension 1237
Keflex Pulvules 1237

LORICIN (Italy)
AMPICILLIN SODIUM/SULBACTAM SODIUM
Unasyn for Injection 2728

LORIDEM (Belgium)
LORAZEPAM
Ativan Injection 3478
Ativan Tablets 3482

LORITYNE (Thailand)
LORATADINE
Claritin Reditabs 3100
Claritin Syrup 3100
Claritin Tablets 3100

LORIUM (Brazil)
LORAZEPAM
Ativan Injection 3478
Ativan Tablets 3482

LORIVAN (Hong Kong, Israel)
LORAZEPAM
Ativan Injection 3478
Ativan Tablets 3482

LORNAZOL (Mexico)
KETOCONAZOLE
Nizoral 2% Cream 3620
Nizoral 2% Shampoo 2007
Nizoral Tablets 1791

LOROXIDE (Canada)
BENZOYL PEROXIDE
Brevoxyl-4 Cleansing Lotion 3269
Brevoxyl-4 Creamy Wash 3270
Brevoxyl-4 Gel 3269
Brevoxyl-8 Cleansing Lotion 3269
Brevoxyl-8 Creamy Wash 3270
Brevoxyl-8 Gel 3269
Triaz Cleanser 2026
Triaz Gel 2026

LORSEDAL (Portugal)
LORAZEPAM
Ativan Injection 3478
Ativan Tablets 3482

LORSEDIN (Thailand)
LORATADINE
Claritin Reditabs 3100
Claritin Syrup 3100
Claritin Tablets 3100

LORTAAN (Italy, Portugal)
LOSARTAN POTASSIUM
Cozaar Tablets 2067

LORTAAN PLUS (Portugal)
HYDROCHLOROTHIAZIDE/LOSARTAN POTASSIUM
Hyzaar 50-12.5 Tablets 2109

LORTADINE (Thailand)
LORATADINE
Claritin Reditabs 3100
Claritin Syrup 3100
Claritin Tablets 3100

LORVAS (Thailand)
INDAPAMIDE
Indapamide Tablets 2286

LORZAAR (Germany)
LOSARTAN POTASSIUM
Cozaar Tablets 2067

LORZAAR PLUS (Germany)
HYDROCHLOROTHIAZIDE/LOSARTAN POTASSIUM
Hyzaar 50-12.5 Tablets 2109

LORZEM (New Zealand)
LORAZEPAM
Ativan Injection 3478
Ativan Tablets 3482

LOSAPREX (Italy)
LOSARTAN POTASSIUM
Cozaar Tablets 2067

LOSAZID (Italy)
HYDROCHLOROTHIAZIDE/LOSARTAN POTASSIUM
Hyzaar 50-12.5 Tablets 2109

LOSEC (Austria, Belgium, Brazil, Israel, South Africa, Spain, Thailand)
OMEPRAZOLE
Prilosec Delayed-Release Capsules 628

LOSTATIN (Singapore)
LOVASTATIN
Mevacor Tablets 2132

LOTEM (South Africa)
IBUPROFEN
Motrin Suspension, Oral Drops, Chewable Tablets, and Caplets 2002

LO-TEN (Hong Kong, New Zealand)
ATENOLOL
Tenormin I.V. Injection 692

LOTENSIN (Brazil, Canada, Mexico)
BENAZEPRIL HYDROCHLORIDE
Lotensin Tablets 2365

LOTREMIN (Australia, Hong Kong, Singapore)
CLOTRIMAZOLE
Lotrimin Cream 1% 3128
Lotrimin Lotion 1% 3128
Lotrimin Topical Solution 1% 3128
Mycelex Troche 573

LOTREMINE (Portugal)
CLOTRIMAZOLE
Lotrimin Cream 1% 3128
Lotrimin Lotion 1% 3128
Lotrimin Topical Solution 1% 3128
Mycelex Troche 573

LOTRICOMB (Germany, New Zealand)
BETAMETHASONE DIPROPIONATE/CLOTRIMAZOLE
Lotrisone Cream 3129

LOTRIDERM (Belgium, Canada, Irish Republic, South Africa, United Kingdom)
BETAMETHASONE DIPROPIONATE/CLOTRIMAZOLE
Lotrisone Cream 3129

LOTRIMIN (Mexico)
CLOTRIMAZOLE
Lotrimin Cream 1% 3128
Lotrimin Lotion 1% 3128
Lotrimin Topical Solution 1% 3128
Mycelex Troche 573

LOVACOL (Finland)
LOVASTATIN
Mevacor Tablets 2132

LOVALIP (Israel)
LOVASTATIN
Mevacor Tablets 2132

LOVENOX (Austria, Canada, France, Portugal, Switzerland)
ENOXAPARIN SODIUM
Lovenox Injection 746

LOVERAL (Mexico)
ALBENDAZOLE
Albenza Tablets 1463

LOW LIQUEMINE (Switzerland)
DALTEPARIN SODIUM
Fragmin Injection 2814

LOWADINA (Mexico)
LORATADINE
Claritin Reditabs 3100
Claritin Syrup 3100
Claritin Tablets 3100

LOWPRE (Mexico)
CAPTOPRIL
Captopril Tablets 2281

LOXAPAC (Belgium, Denmark, Irish Republic, Italy, New Zealand, The Netherlands, United Kingdom)
LOXAPINE SUCCINATE
Loxitane Capsules 3398

LOXAZOL (Switzerland)
PERMETHRIN
Acticin Cream 998
Elimite Cream 552

LOXEN (France)
NICARDIPINE HYDROCHLORIDE
Cardene I.V. 3485

LOXIN (Germany)
AZELASTINE HYDROCHLORIDE
Astelin Nasal Spray 3339

LOZIDE (Canada)
INDAPAMIDE
Indapamide Tablets 2286

LUASE (Spain)
DICLOFENAC SODIUM
Voltaren Tablets 2315
Voltaren-XR Tablets 2315

LUBEXYL (Switzerland)
BENZOYL PEROXIDE
Brevoxyl-4 Cleansing Lotion 3269
Brevoxyl-4 Creamy Wash 3270
Brevoxyl-4 Gel 3269
Brevoxyl-8 Cleansing Lotion 3269
Brevoxyl-8 Creamy Wash 3270
Brevoxyl-8 Gel 3269
Triaz Cleanser 2026
Triaz Gel 2026

LUCENFAL (Spain)
NICARDIPINE HYDROCHLORIDE
Cardene I.V. 3485

LUGACIN (United Kingdom)
GENTAMICIN SULFATE
Genoptic Ophthalmic Ointment . . . . . ⊙239
Genoptic Sterile Ophthalmic Solution . . . ⊙239

LUGESTERON (Finland)
PROGESTERONE
Crinone 4% Gel 3213
Crinone 8% Gel 3213
Prometrium Capsules (100 mg, 200 mg) 3261

LUITASE (Italy)
PANCRELIPASE
Ultrase Capsules 835
Ultrase MT Capsules 835

LUKASM (Italy)
MONTELUKAST SODIUM
Singulair Chewable Tablets 2181
Singulair Tablets 2181

LUMINOVAG (Mexico)
KETOCONAZOLE
Nizoral 2% Cream 3620
Nizoral 2% Shampoo 2007
Nizoral Tablets 1791

LUMIRELAX (France)
METHOCARBAMOL
Robaxin Injectable 2938
Robaxin Tablets 2939
Robaxin-750 Tablets 2939

LUNDIRAN (Spain)
NAPROXEN
EC-Naprosyn Delayed-Release Tablets . . . 2967
Naprosyn Suspension 2967
Naprosyn Tablets 2967

LUNIBRON-A (Italy)
FLUNISOLIDE
Aerobid Inhaler System 1363
Aerobid-M Inhaler System 1363
Nasalide Nasal Spray 1295
Nasarel Nasal Solution 0.025% 1296

LUNIS (Italy)
FLUNISOLIDE
Aerobid Inhaler System 1363
Aerobid-M Inhaler System 1363
Nasalide Nasal Spray 1295
Nasarel Nasal Solution 0.025% 1296

LUPERZOL (Mexico)
KETOCONAZOLE
Nizoral 2% Cream 3620
Nizoral 2% Shampoo 2007
Nizoral Tablets 1791

LUPOVALIN (Germany)
DIPHENHYDRAMINE HYDROCHLORIDE
Benadryl Parenteral 2617

LURDEX (Mexico)
ALBENDAZOLE
Albenza Tablets 1463

LUSAP (Switzerland)
MALATHION
Ovide Lotion 2023

LUSTRAL (Irish Republic, Israel, United Kingdom)
SERTRALINE HYDROCHLORIDE
Zoloft Tablets 2751

LUTOPOLAR (Finland)
MEDROXYPROGESTERONE ACETATE
Depo-Provera Contraceptive Injection . . . 2798
Provera Tablets 2853

LUTORAL (Italy)
MEDROXYPROGESTERONE ACETATE
Depo-Provera Contraceptive Injection . . . 2798
Provera Tablets 2853

LUVOX (Australia, Canada, Mexico, South Africa)
FLUVOXAMINE MALEATE
Luvox Tablets (25, 50, 100 mg) 3256

LUXAZONE (Italy)
DEXAMETHASONE
Decadron Elixir 2078
Decadron Tablets 2079

LYCLEAR (Australia, Irish Republic, Israel, New Zealand, South Africa, United Kingdom)
PERMETHRIN
Acticin Cream 998
Elimite Cream 552

LYDERM (Canada, New Zealand)
FLUOCINONIDE
Lidex Cream 2020
Lidex Gel 2020
Lidex Ointment 2020
Lidex Topical Solution 2020
Lidex-E Cream 2020

LYDONIDE (Canada)
FLUOCINONIDE
Lidex Cream 2020
Lidex Gel 2020
Lidex Ointment 2020
Lidex Topical Solution 2020
Lidex-E Cream 2020

LYMETEL (Spain)
FLUVASTATIN SODIUM
Lescol Capsules 2361

LYNDAK (Italy)
SULINDAC
Clinoril Tablets 2053

LYOVAC COSMEGEN (Belgium, Germany, The Netherlands)
DACTINOMYCIN
Cosmegen for Injection 2062

LYPHOCIN (Hong Kong)
VANCOMYCIN HYDROCHLORIDE
Vancocin HCl Capsules & Pulvules 1972
Vancocin HCl Oral Solution 1971
Vancocin HCl, Vials & ADD-Vantage 1970

LYSALGO (Italy)
MEFENAMIC ACID
Ponstel Capsules 1356

LYSOVIR (United Kingdom)
AMANTADINE HYDROCHLORIDE
Symmetrel Syrup 1328
Symmetrel Tablets 1328

LYSTIN (Hong Kong, Thailand)
NYSTATIN
Nystop Topical Powder USP 2608

MAALOX H2 ACID CONTROLLER (Canada)
FAMOTIDINE
Pepcid Injection 2153
Pepcid Injection Premixed 2153
Pepcid RPD Orally Disintegrating Tablets 2150
Pepcid Tablets 2150
Pepcid for Oral Suspension 2150

MABICROL (Mexico)
CLARITHROMYCIN
Biaxin Filmtab Tablets 403
Biaxin for Oral Suspension 403

MABRON (Hong Kong, Singapore, Thailand)
TRAMADOL HYDROCHLORIDE
Ultram Tablets 2600

MABTHERA (Australia, Austria, Belgium, Denmark, Finland, France, Germany, Israel, Italy, Mexico, New Zealand, Norway, Portugal, Singapore, South Africa, Spain, Sweden, Switzerland, Thailand, The Netherlands, United Kingdom)
RITUXIMAB
Rituxan I.V. 1428

Rituxan for Infusion . . . 1750

MACAINE (South Africa)
BUPIVACAINE HYDROCHLORIDE
Sensorcaine Injection . . . 643
Sensorcaine-MPF Injection . . . 643

MACLADIN (Italy)
CLARITHROMYCIN
Biaxin Filmtab Tablets . . . 403
Biaxin for Oral Suspension . . . 403

MACLAR (Austria, Belgium, Portugal)
CLARITHROMYCIN
Biaxin Filmtab Tablets . . . 403
Biaxin for Oral Suspension . . . 403

MACROLIN (France)
ALDESLEUKIN
Proleukin for Injection . . . 1199

MADAPROX (Spain)
NAPROXEN
EC-Naprosyn Delayed-Release Tablets . . . 2967
Naprosyn Suspension . . . 2967
Naprosyn Tablets . . . 2967

MADICURE (The Netherlands)
MEBENDAZOLE
Vermox Chewable Tablets . . . 2017

MADIPRAZOLE (Thailand)
OMEPRAZOLE
Prilosec Delayed-Release Capsules . . . 628

MADOL (Thailand)
TRAMADOL HYDROCHLORIDE
Ultram Tablets . . . 2600

MADOLA (Thailand)
TRAMADOL HYDROCHLORIDE
Ultram Tablets . . . 2600

MADONNA (Thailand)
LEVONORGESTREL
Norplant System . . . 3543

MAFEN (Thailand)
IBUPROFEN
Motrin Suspension, Oral Drops, Chewable Tablets, and Caplets . . . 2002

MAFORMIN (Thailand)
METFORMIN HYDROCHLORIDE
Glucophage Tablets . . . 1080

MAGICUL (Australia)
CIMETIDINE
Tagamet Tablets . . . 1644

MAGLUPHEN (Austria)
DICLOFENAC SODIUM
Voltaren Tablets . . . 2315
Voltaren-XR Tablets . . . 2315

MAGNATEX (South Africa)
IBUPROFEN
Motrin Suspension, Oral Drops, Chewable Tablets, and Caplets . . . 2002

MAGNUROL (Spain)
TERAZOSIN HYDROCHLORIDE
Hytrin Capsules . . . 464

MAINTAIN (Israel)
BENZOCAINE
Americaine Anesthetic Lubricant . . . 1162
Americaine Otic Topical Anesthetic Ear Drops . . . 1162

MAJOLAT (Austria)
NIFEDIPINE
Adalat CC Tablets . . . 877
Procardia Capsules . . . 2708
Procardia XL Extended Release Tablets . . . 2710

MALAFENE (Belgium)
IBUPROFEN
Motrin Suspension, Oral Drops, Chewable Tablets, and Caplets . . . 2002

MALAREX (Denmark)
CHLOROQUINE PHOSPHATE
Aralen Tablets . . . 3075

MALARONE (United Kingdom)
ATOVAQUONE
Mepron Suspension . . . 1598

MALAVIRON (United Kingdom)
CHLOROQUINE PHOSPHATE
Aralen Tablets . . . 3075

MALEXIN (Germany)
NAPROXEN
EC-Naprosyn Delayed-Release Tablets . . . 2967
Naprosyn Suspension . . . 2967
Naprosyn Tablets . . . 2967

MALFESTO (Irish Republic)
MALATHION
Ovide Lotion . . . 2023

MALFIN (Denmark)
MORPHINE SULFATE
Astramorph/PF Injection, USP (Preservative-Free) . . . 594
Duramorph Injection . . . 1312
Infumorph 200 and Infumorph 500 Sterile Solutions . . . 1314
Kadian Capsules . . . 1335
MS Contin Tablets . . . 2896
MSIR Oral Capsules . . . 2898
MSIR Oral Solution . . . 2898
MSIR Oral Solution Concentrate . . . 2898
MSIR Oral Tablets . . . 2898
Oramorph SR Tablets . . . 3062
Roxanol 100 Concentrated Oral Solution . . . 3066
Roxanol Concentrated Oral Solution . . . 3066
Roxanol-T Oral Solution . . . 3066

MALIMED (Switzerland)
CIMETIDINE
Tagamet Tablets . . . 1644

MALOCIDE (France)
PYRIMETHAMINE
Daraprim Tablets . . . 1511

MALOCIN (Thailand)
ERYTHROMYCIN STEARATE
Erythrocin Stearate Filmtab Tablets . . . 452

MALOGEN AQUEOUS (Canada)
TESTOSTERONE
Androderm Transdermal System CIII . . . 3377
Testoderm Transdermal Systems . . . 574

MALOPRIM (Belgium, Irish Republic)
PYRIMETHAMINE
Daraprim Tablets . . . 1511

MANCEF (Italy)
CEFAMANDOLE NAFATE
Mandol Vials . . . 1953

MANDOKEF (Austria, Germany, Italy, Portugal, South Africa, Spain, Switzerland)
CEFAMANDOLE NAFATE
Mandol Vials . . . 1953

MANDOL (Australia, Belgium, Canada, Hong Kong, New Zealand, Thailand, The Netherlands)
CEFAMANDOLE NAFATE
Mandol Vials . . . 1953

MANDOLGIN (Denmark)
TRAMADOL HYDROCHLORIDE
Ultram Tablets . . . 2600

MANDOLSAN (Italy)
CEFAMANDOLE NAFATE
Mandol Vials . . . 1953

MANDROLAX LACTU (Germany)
LACTULOSE
Kristalose for Oral Solution . . . 1007

MANDRO-ZEP (Germany)
DIAZEPAM
Valium Injectable . . . 3026
Valium Tablets . . . 3047

MANIALIT (Italy)
LITHIUM CARBONATE
Eskalith CR Controlled Release Tablets . . . 1527
Eskalith Capsules . . . 1527
Lithium Carbonate Capsules . . . 3061
Lithobid Slow-Release Tablets . . . 3255

MANIC (Thailand)
MEFENAMIC ACID
Ponstel Capsules . . . 1356

MANIDON (Spain)
VERAPAMIL HYDROCHLORIDE
Covera-HS Tablets . . . 3199
Isoptin SR Tablets . . . 467
Verelan Capsules . . . 3184
Verelan PM Capsules . . . 3186

MANIPREX (Belgium)
LITHIUM CARBONATE
Eskalith CR Controlled Release Tablets . . . 1527
Eskalith Capsules . . . 1527
Lithium Carbonate Capsules . . . 3061
Lithobid Slow-Release Tablets . . . 3255

MANORFEN (United Kingdom)
IBUPROFEN
Motrin Suspension, Oral Drops, Chewable Tablets, and Caplets . . . 2002

MANSAL (Spain)
CIMETIDINE
Tagamet Tablets . . . 1644

MANTADAN (Italy)
AMANTADINE HYDROCHLORIDE
Symmetrel Syrup . . . 1328
Symmetrel Tablets . . . 1328

MANTADINE (United Kingdom)
AMANTADINE HYDROCHLORIDE
Symmetrel Syrup . . . 1328
Symmetrel Tablets . . . 1328

MANTADIX (Belgium, France)
AMANTADINE HYDROCHLORIDE
Symmetrel Syrup . . . 1328
Symmetrel Tablets . . . 1328

MANTIDAN (Brazil)
AMANTADINE HYDROCHLORIDE
Symmetrel Syrup . . . 1328
Symmetrel Tablets . . . 1328

MAPEZINE (Thailand)
CARBAMAZEPINE
Carbatrol Capsules . . . 3234
Tegretol Chewable Tablets . . . 2404
Tegretol Suspension . . . 2404
Tegretol Tablets . . . 2404
Tegretol-XR Tablets . . . 2404

MAPLUXIN (Mexico)
DIGOXIN
Lanoxicaps Capsules . . . 1574
Lanoxin Elixir Pediatric . . . 1578
Lanoxin Injection . . . 1581
Lanoxin Injection Pediatric . . . 1584
Lanoxin Tablets . . . 1587

MARBEN (Mexico)
MEBENDAZOLE
Vermox Chewable Tablets . . . 2017

MARCAIN (Australia, Denmark, Finland, Irish Republic, New Zealand, Norway, Singapore, Sweden, United Kingdom)
BUPIVACAINE HYDROCHLORIDE
Sensorcaine Injection . . . 643
Sensorcaine-MPF Injection . . . 643

MARCAINA (Brazil, Italy, Portugal)
BUPIVACAINE HYDROCHLORIDE
Sensorcaine Injection . . . 643
Sensorcaine-MPF Injection . . . 643

MARCAINE (Belgium, Canada, France, Hong Kong, Israel, Thailand, The Netherlands)
BUPIVACAINE HYDROCHLORIDE
Sensorcaine Injection . . . 643
Sensorcaine-MPF Injection . . . 643

MARDUK (Germany)
BENZOYL PEROXIDE
Brevoxyl-4 Cleansing Lotion . . . 3269
Brevoxyl-4 Creamy Wash . . . 3270
Brevoxyl-4 Gel . . . 3269
Brevoxyl-8 Cleansing Lotion . . . 3269
Brevoxyl-8 Creamy Wash . . . 3270
Brevoxyl-8 Gel . . . 3269
Triaz Cleanser . . . 2026
Triaz Gel . . . 2026

MAREEN (Germany)
DOXEPIN HYDROCHLORIDE
Sinequan Capsules . . . 2713
Sinequan Oral Concentrate . . . 2713

MAREVAN (Australia, Belgium, Brazil, Denmark, Finland, New Zealand, Norway, United Kingdom)
WARFARIN SODIUM
Coumadin Tablets . . . 1243
Coumadin for Injection . . . 1243

MARIL (Singapore, Thailand)
METOCLOPRAMIDE HYDROCHLORIDE
Reglan Injectable . . . 2935
Reglan Syrup . . . 2935
Reglan Tablets . . . 2935

MARINOL (Canada)
DRONABINOL
Marinol Capsules . . . 3325

MARISTON (Thailand)
GEMFIBROZIL
Lopid Tablets . . . 2650

MARTIGENTA (France)
GENTAMICIN SULFATE
Genoptic Ophthalmic Ointment . . . ⊙239
Genoptic Sterile Ophthalmic Solution . . . ⊙239

MASARAX (Thailand)
HYDROXYZINE HYDROCHLORIDE
Atarax Tablets & Syrup . . . 2667
Vistaril Intramuscular Solution . . . 2738

MASAROL (Thailand)
KETOCONAZOLE
Nizoral 2% Cream . . . 3620
Nizoral 2% Shampoo . . . 2007
Nizoral Tablets . . . 1791

MASAWORM (Thailand)
ALBENDAZOLE
Albenza Tablets . . . 1463

MASAWORM-1 (Thailand)
MEBENDAZOLE
Vermox Chewable Tablets . . . 2017

MASDIL (Spain)
DILTIAZEM HYDROCHLORIDE
Cardizem CD Capsules . . . 1016
Cardizem Injectable . . . 1018
Cardizem Lyo-Ject Syringe . . . 1018
Cardizem Monovial . . . 1018
Tiazac Capsules . . . 1378

MASNODERM (United Kingdom)
CLOTRIMAZOLE
Lotrimin Cream 1% . . . 3128
Lotrimin Lotion 1% . . . 3128
Lotrimin Topical Solution 1% . . . 3128
Mycelex Troche . . . 573

MASWIN (Thailand)
PIROXICAM
Feldene Capsules . . . 2685

MATCINE (Singapore, Thailand)
CHLORPROMAZINE HYDROCHLORIDE
Thorazine Ampuls . . . 1656
Thorazine Multi-dose Vials . . . 1656
Thorazine Spansule Capsules . . . 1656
Thorazine Syrup . . . 1656
Thorazine Tablets . . . 1656

MATHOINE (Belgium)
PHENYTOIN
Dilantin Infatabs . . . 2624
Dilantin-125 Oral Suspension . . . 2625

MAURAN (Italy)
RANITIDINE HYDROCHLORIDE
Zantac 150 EFFERdose Granules . . . 1690
Zantac 150 EFFERdose Tablets . . . 1690
Zantac 150 Tablets . . . 1690
Zantac 300 Tablets . . . 1690
Zantac Injection . . . 1688
Zantac Injection Premixed . . . 1688
Zantac Syrup . . . 1690

MAVERAL (Italy)
FLUVOXAMINE MALEATE
Luvox Tablets (25, 50, 100 mg) . . . 3256

MAVID (Germany)
CLARITHROMYCIN
Biaxin Filmtab Tablets . . . 403
Biaxin for Oral Suspension . . . 403

MAVIK (Canada)
TRANDOLAPRIL
Mavik Tablets . . . 478

MAXAIR (Canada, France, Switzerland)
PIRBUTEROL ACETATE
Maxair Autohaler . . . 1981
Maxair Inhaler . . . 1984

MAXALT (Austria, Belgium, Canada, Denmark, Finland, Germany, Italy, Mexico, New Zealand, Norway, Portugal, South Africa, Spain, Sweden, The Netherlands, United Kingdom)
RIZATRIPTAN BENZOATE
Maxalt Tablets . . . 2120
Maxalt-MLT Orally Disintegrating Tablets . . . 2120

MAXCEF (Israel)
CEFEPIME HYDROCHLORIDE
Maxipime for Injection . . . 1285

MAXERAN (Canada)
METOCLOPRAMIDE HYDROCHLORIDE
Reglan Injectable . . . 2935
Reglan Syrup . . . 2935
Reglan Tablets . . . 2935

MAXIDEX (Australia, Belgium, Brazil, Canada, Denmark, France, Hong Kong, Irish Republic, Israel, New Zealand, Singapore, South Africa, Spain, Switzerland, The Netherlands, United Kingdom)
DEXAMETHASONE
Decadron Elixir . . . 2078
Decadron Tablets . . . 2079

MAXIDON (Sweden)
MORPHINE SULFATE
Astramorph/PF Injection, USP (Preservative-Free) . . . 594
Duramorph Injection . . . 1312
Infumorph 200 and Infumorph 500 Sterile Solutions . . . 1314
Kadian Capsules . . . 1335
MS Contin Tablets . . . 2896
MSIR Oral Capsules . . . 2898
MSIR Oral Solution . . . 2898
MSIR Oral Solution Concentrate . . . 2898
MSIR Oral Tablets . . . 2898
Oramorph SR Tablets . . . 3062
Roxanol 100 Concentrated Oral Solution . . . 3066
Roxanol Concentrated Oral Solution . . . 3066
Roxanol-T Oral Solution . . . 3066

MAXIPIME (Australia, Austria, Belgium, Canada, Denmark, Finland, Germany, Hong Kong, Irish Republic, Italy, Mexico, New Zealand, Portugal, Singapore, South Africa, Spain, Sweden, Switzerland, Thailand, The Netherlands)
CEFEPIME HYDROCHLORIDE
Maxipime for Injection 1285

MAXOLON (Australia, Hong Kong, Irish Republic, New Zealand, Singapore, South Africa, United Kingdom)
METOCLOPRAMIDE HYDROCHLORIDE
Reglan Injectable 2935
Reglan Syrup 2935
Reglan Tablets 2935

MAXOR (Australia)
OMEPRAZOLE
Prilosec Delayed-Release Capsules 628

MAX-PAX (Brazil)
LORAZEPAM
Ativan Injection 3478
Ativan Tablets 3482

MAXSOTEN (Belgium)
BISOPROLOL FUMARATE/HYDROCHLOROTHIAZIDE
Ziac Tablets 1887

MAXZIDE (Belgium)
TRIAMTERENE
Dyrenium Capsules 3458

MAYCOR (Germany, Spain)
ISOSORBIDE DINITRATE
Isordil Sublingual Tablets 3525
Isordil Titradose Tablets 3526

MAYDIL (Austria)
ISOSORBIDE DINITRATE
Isordil Sublingual Tablets 3525
Isordil Titradose Tablets 3526

MAYGACE (Spain)
MEGESTROL ACETATE
Megace Oral Suspension 1124

MAZEPINE (Canada)
CARBAMAZEPINE
Carbatrol Capsules 3234
Tegretol Chewable Tablets 2404
Tegretol Suspension 2404
Tegretol Tablets 2404
Tegretol-XR Tablets 2404

M-BETA (Germany)
MORPHINE SULFATE
Astramorph/PF Injection, USP (Preservative-Free) 594
Duramorph Injection 1312
Infumorph 200 and Infumorph 500 Sterile Solutions 1314
Kadian Capsules 1335
MS Contin Tablets 2896
MSIR Oral Capsules 2898
MSIR Oral Solution 2898
MSIR Oral Solution Concentrate 2898
MSIR Oral Tablets 2898
Oramorph SR Tablets 3062
Roxanol 100 Concentrated Oral Solution 3066
Roxanol Concentrated Oral Solution 3066
Roxanol-T Oral Solution 3066

MCR (Israel)
MORPHINE SULFATE
Astramorph/PF Injection, USP (Preservative-Free) 594
Duramorph Injection 1312
Infumorph 200 and Infumorph 500 Sterile Solutions 1314
Kadian Capsules 1335
MS Contin Tablets 2896
MSIR Oral Capsules 2898
MSIR Oral Solution 2898
MSIR Oral Solution Concentrate 2898
MSIR Oral Tablets 2898
Oramorph SR Tablets 3062
Roxanol 100 Concentrated Oral Solution 3066
Roxanol Concentrated Oral Solution 3066
Roxanol-T Oral Solution 3066

MCR-50 (United Kingdom)
ISOSORBIDE MONONITRATE
Imdur Tablets 1826
Ismo Tablets 3524

MDILTIWAS (Spain)
DILTIAZEM HYDROCHLORIDE
Cardizem CD Capsules 1016
Cardizem Injectable 1018
Cardizem Lyo-Ject Syringe 1018
Cardizem Monovial 1018
Tiazac Capsules 1378

M-DOLOR (Austria, Germany)
MORPHINE SULFATE
Astramorph/PF Injection, USP (Preservative-Free) 594
Duramorph Injection 1312
Infumorph 200 and Infumorph 500 Sterile Solutions 1314
Kadian Capsules 1335
MS Contin Tablets 2896
MSIR Oral Capsules 2898
MSIR Oral Solution 2898
MSIR Oral Solution Concentrate 2898
MSIR Oral Tablets 2898
Oramorph SR Tablets 3062
Roxanol 100 Concentrated Oral Solution 3066
Roxanol Concentrated Oral Solution 3066
Roxanol-T Oral Solution 3066

MEAVERIN (Germany)
MEPIVACAINE HYDROCHLORIDE
Polocaine Injection, USP 625
Polocaine-MPF Injection, USP 625

MEAVERIN A MIT ADRENALIN (Germany)
MEPIVACAINE HYDROCHLORIDE
Polocaine Injection, USP 625
Polocaine-MPF Injection, USP 625

MEAVERIN N MIT NORADRENALINE (Germany)
MEPIVACAINE HYDROCHLORIDE
Polocaine Injection, USP 625
Polocaine-MPF Injection, USP 625

MEAVERIN HYPERBAR (Germany)
MEPIVACAINE HYDROCHLORIDE
Polocaine Injection, USP 625
Polocaine-MPF Injection, USP 625

MEBA (Thailand)
MEBENDAZOLE
Vermox Chewable Tablets 2017

MEBAN (Mexico)
MEBENDAZOLE
Vermox Chewable Tablets 2017

MEBANDOZER (Mexico)
MEBENDAZOLE
Vermox Chewable Tablets 2017

MEBAXIN (Thailand)
METHOCARBAMOL
Robaxin Injectable 2938
Robaxin Tablets 2939
Robaxin-750 Tablets 2939

MEBECICLOL (Mexico)
MEBENDAZOLE
Vermox Chewable Tablets 2017

MEBELMIN (Mexico)
MEBENDAZOLE
Vermox Chewable Tablets 2017

MEBEN (Brazil, Thailand)
MEBENDAZOLE
Vermox Chewable Tablets 2017

MEBENDAN (Spain)
MEBENDAZOLE
Vermox Chewable Tablets 2017

MEBENDA-P (Thailand)
MEBENDAZOLE
Vermox Chewable Tablets 2017

MEBENDAZOTIL (Brazil)
MEBENDAZOLE
Vermox Chewable Tablets 2017

MEBENDIL (Brazil)
MEBENDAZOLE
Vermox Chewable Tablets 2017

MEBENIX (Brazil)
ALBENDAZOLE
Albenza Tablets 1463

MEBENLAX (Thailand)
MEBENDAZOLE
Vermox Chewable Tablets 2017

MEBENTIASIS (Mexico)
MEBENDAZOLE
Vermox Chewable Tablets 2017

MEBENTINE (Mexico)
MEBENDAZOLE
Vermox Chewable Tablets 2017

MEBUTAN (The Netherlands)
NABUMETONE
Relafen Tablets 1617

MECAIN (Germany)
MEPIVACAINE HYDROCHLORIDE
Polocaine Injection, USP 625
Polocaine-MPF Injection, USP 625

MECLOMID (Mexico)
METOCLOPRAMIDE HYDROCHLORIDE
Reglan Injectable 2935
Reglan Syrup 2935
Reglan Tablets 2935

MECTIZAN (France)
IVERMECTIN
Stromectol Tablets 2185

MEDAMET (South Africa)
METRONIDAZOLE
MetroCream 1404
MetroGel 1405
MetroGel-Vaginal Gel 1986
MetroLotion 1405
Noritate Cream 1224

MEDAMOR (Finland)
AMILORIDE HYDROCHLORIDE
Midamor Tablets 2136

MEDAPUR (Germany)
DIPHENHYDRAMINE HYDROCHLORIDE
Benadryl Parenteral 2617

MEDAREN (Thailand)
DICLOFENAC SODIUM
Voltaren Tablets 2315
Voltaren-XR Tablets 2315

MEDASPOR (South Africa)
CLOTRIMAZOLE
Lotrimin Cream 1% 3128
Lotrimin Lotion 1% 3128
Lotrimin Topical Solution 1% 3128
Mycelex Troche 573

MEDAZOLE (Thailand)
MEBENDAZOLE
Vermox Chewable Tablets 2017

MEDAZYL (Thailand)
METRONIDAZOLE
MetroCream 1404
MetroGel 1405
MetroGel-Vaginal Gel 1986
MetroLotion 1405
Noritate Cream 1224

MED-BRONCODIL (Thailand)
TERBUTALINE SULFATE
Brethine Ampuls 2314
Brethine Tablets 2313

MEDETON (Thailand)
MEDROXYPROGESTERONE ACETATE
Depo-Provera Contraceptive Injection 2798
Provera Tablets 2853

MED-GASTRAMET (Thailand)
CIMETIDINE
Tagamet Tablets 1644

MEDIABET (Germany)
METFORMIN HYDROCHLORIDE
Glucophage Tablets 1080

MEDICAP (Hong Kong)
MEFENAMIC ACID
Ponstel Capsules 1356

MEDICLEAR (United Kingdom)
BENZOYL PEROXIDE
Brevoxyl-4 Cleansing Lotion 3269
Brevoxyl-4 Creamy Wash 3270
Brevoxyl-4 Gel 3269
Brevoxyl-8 Cleansing Lotion 3269
Brevoxyl-8 Creamy Wash 3270
Brevoxyl-8 Gel 3269
Triaz Cleanser 2026
Triaz Gel 2026

MEDIFEN (Mexico)
IBUPROFEN
Motrin Suspension, Oral Drops, Chewable Tablets, and Caplets 2002

MEDILAVE (United Kingdom)
BENZOCAINE
Americaine Anesthetic Lubricant 1162
Americaine Otic Topical Anesthetic Ear Drops 1162

MEDILET (Germany)
LACTULOSE
Kristalose for Oral Solution 1007

MEDILIUM (Canada)
CHLORDIAZEPOXIDE HYDROCHLORIDE
Librium Capsules 1736
Librium for Injection 1737

MEDINEX (United Kingdom)
DIPHENHYDRAMINE HYDROCHLORIDE
Benadryl Parenteral 2617

MEDINOX MONO (Germany)
PENTOBARBITAL SODIUM
Nembutal Sodium Solution 485

MEDIPAM (Finland)
DIAZEPAM
Valium Injectable 3026
Valium Tablets 3047

MEDIPER (Italy)
CEFOPERAZONE SODIUM
Cefobid Intravenous/Intramuscular 2671
Cefobid Pharmacy Bulk Package - Not for Direct Infusion 2673

MEDIPINA (Portugal)
NIFEDIPINE
Adalat CC Tablets 877
Procardia Capsules 2708
Procardia XL Extended Release Tablets 2710

MEDIPO (Italy)
SIMVASTATIN
Zocor Tablets 2219

MEDIPREN (Canada, Spain)
IBUPROFEN
Motrin Suspension, Oral Drops, Chewable Tablets, and Caplets 2002

MEDISED INFANT (United Kingdom)
DIPHENHYDRAMINE HYDROCHLORIDE
Benadryl Parenteral 2617

MEDISPORT ATHLETE'S FOOT (United Kingdom)
CLOTRIMAZOLE
Lotrimin Cream 1% 3128
Lotrimin Lotion 1% 3128
Lotrimin Topical Solution 1% 3128
Mycelex Troche 573

MEDITRAN (Canada)
MEPROBAMATE
Miltown Tablets 3349

MEDIZOL (Mexico)
METRONIDAZOLE
MetroCream 1404
MetroGel 1405
MetroGel-Vaginal Gel 1986
MetroLotion 1405
Noritate Cream 1224

MEDNIL (Thailand)
MEFENAMIC ACID
Ponstel Capsules 1356

MEDOCEF (Singapore, Thailand)
CEFOPERAZONE SODIUM
Cefobid Intravenous/Intramuscular 2671
Cefobid Pharmacy Bulk Package - Not for Direct Infusion 2673

MEDOCIPRIN (Thailand)
CIPROFLOXACIN
Cipro I.V. 893
Cipro I.V. Pharmacy Bulk Package 897
Cipro Oral Suspension 887

MEDODERMONE (Hong Kong, Singapore, Thailand)
CLOBETASOL PROPIONATE
Cormax Cream 2440
Cormax Ointment 2440
Cormax Scalp Application 2441
Temovate Cream 1301
Temovate E Emollient 1302
Temovate Gel 1303
Temovate Ointment 1301
Temovate Scalp Application 1304

MEDOLEXIN (Hong Kong)
CEPHALEXIN
Keflex Oral Suspension 1237
Keflex Pulvules 1237

MEDOMET (United Kingdom)
METHYLDOPA
Aldomet Tablets 2037

MEDOMYCIN (Hong Kong, Singapore, Thailand)
DOXYCYCLINE HYCLATE
Doryx Coated Pellet Filled Capsules 3357
Periostat Tablets 1208
Vibra-Tabs Film Coated Tablets 2735
Vibramycin Hyclate Capsules 2735
Vibramycin Hyclate Intravenous 2737

MEDOPA (Thailand)
METHYLDOPA
Aldomet Tablets 2037

MEDOPAL (Mexico, Norway)
METHYLDOPA
Aldomet Tablets 2037

MEDOPATE (Thailand)
METHYLDOPA
Aldomet Tablets 2037

MEDOPREN (Italy)
METHYLDOPA
Aldomet Tablets 2037

MEDOSTATIN (Hong Kong)
LOVASTATIN
Mevacor Tablets 2132

MEDOXIM (Italy)
CEFUROXIME SODIUM
Kefurox Vials, ADD-Vantage 1948
Zinacef Injection 1696

MEDOXIN (Thailand)
DOXYCYCLINE HYCLATE
Doryx Coated Pellet Filled Capsules 3357

(⊙ Described in PDR For Ophthalmic Medicines™)

Periostat Tablets . . . 1208
Vibramycin Hyclate Capsules . . . 2735
Vibramycin Hyclate Intravenous . . . 2737
Vibra-Tabs Film Coated Tablets . . . 2735

MEDOZEM (Thailand)
DILTIAZEM HYDROCHLORIDE
Cardizem CD Capsules . . . 1016
Cardizem Injectable . . . 1018
Cardizem Lyo-Ject Syringe . . . 1018
Cardizem Monovial . . . 1018
Tiazac Capsules . . . 1378

MEDOZIDE (Italy)
HYDROCHLOROTHIAZIDE/METHYLDOPA
Aldoril Tablets . . . 2039

MED-PHYLLINE (Thailand)
THEOPHYLLINE
Aerolate Jr. T.D. Capsules . . . 1361
Aerolate Liquid . . . 1361
Aerolate Sr. T.D. Capsules . . . 1361
Theo-Dur Extended-Release Tablets . . . 1835
Uni-Dur Extended-Release Tablets . . . 1841
Uniphyl 400 mg and 600 mg Tablets . . . 2903

MEDROL VERIDERM (Canada, Italy)
METHYLPREDNISOLONE ACETATE
Depo-Medrol Injectable Suspension . . . 2795

MED-TRICOCIDE (Thailand)
METRONIDAZOLE
MetroCream . . . 1404
MetroGel . . . 1405
MetroGel-Vaginal Gel . . . 1986
MetroLotion . . . 1405
Noritate Cream . . . 1224

MED-XYZARAX (Thailand)
HYDROXYZINE HYDROCHLORIDE
Atarax Tablets & Syrup . . . 2667
Vistaril Intramuscular Solution . . . 2738

ME-F (Thailand)
METFORMIN HYDROCHLORIDE
Glucophage Tablets . . . 1080

MEFAC (Irish Republic)
MEFENAMIC ACID
Ponstel Capsules . . . 1356

MEFACAP (Hong Kong, Singapore)
MEFENAMIC ACID
Ponstel Capsules . . . 1356

MEFALGIC (South Africa)
MEFENAMIC ACID
Ponstel Capsules . . . 1356

MEFENACIDE (Switzerland)
MEFENAMIC ACID
Ponstel Capsules . . . 1356

MEFENAN (Thailand)
MEFENAMIC ACID
Ponstel Capsules . . . 1356

MEFENIX (Singapore, Thailand)
MEFENAMIC ACID
Ponstel Capsules . . . 1356

MEFIC (Australia, Hong Kong)
MEFENAMIC ACID
Ponstel Capsules . . . 1356

MEFIRON (Thailand)
METRONIDAZOLE
MetroCream . . . 1404
MetroGel . . . 1405
MetroGel-Vaginal Gel . . . 1986
MetroLotion . . . 1405
Noritate Cream . . . 1224

MEFLAM (United Kingdom)
MEFENAMIC ACID
Ponstel Capsules . . . 1356

MEFLIAM (South Africa)
MEFLOQUINE HYDROCHLORIDE
Lariam Tablets . . . 2989

MEFORMED (Thailand)
METFORMIN HYDROCHLORIDE
Glucophage Tablets . . . 1080

MEFOXIN (Australia, Belgium, Brazil, Canada, Finland, France, Hong Kong, Irish Republic, Italy, New Zealand, Portugal, South Africa, The Netherlands, United Kingdom)
CEFOXITIN SODIUM
Mefoxin Premixed Intravenous Solution . . 2127
Mefoxin for Injection . . . 2124

MEFOXITIN (Austria, Germany, Norway, Spain, Sweden, Switzerland)
CEFOXITIN SODIUM
Mefoxin Premixed Intravenous Solution . . 2127
Mefoxin for Injection . . . 2124

MEFPA (Thailand)
METHYLDOPA
Aldomet Tablets . . . 2037

MEGACE (Australia, Austria, Belgium, Canada, Denmark, Finland, France, Germany, Hong Kong, Irish Republic, Israel, Italy, Mexico, New Zealand, Norway, Singapore, Sweden, Thailand, The Netherlands, United Kingdom)
MEGESTROL ACETATE
Megace Oral Suspension . . . 1124

MEGACINA (Portugal)
OFLOXACIN
Floxin I.V. . . . 2526
Floxin Otic Solution . . . 1219
Floxin Tablets . . . 2529
Ocuflox Ophthalmic Solution . . . 554

MEGACORT (Italy)
DEXAMETHASONE SODIUM PHOSPHATE
Decadron Phosphate Injection . . . 2081
Decadron Phosphate Sterile Ophthalmic Ointment . . . ⊙280, 2083
Decadron Phosphate Sterile Ophthalmic Solution . . . 2084

MEGADIN (Hong Kong)
CIMETIDINE
Tagamet Tablets . . . 1644

MEGAFLOX (Portugal)
CIPROFLOXACIN HYDROCHLORIDE
Ciloxan Ophthalmic Ointment . . . 538
Ciloxan Ophthalmic Solution . . . ⊙209, 538
Cipro Tablets . . . 887

MEGALAT (Israel)
NIFEDIPINE
Adalat CC Tablets . . . 877
Procardia Capsules . . . 2708
Procardia XL Extended Release Tablets . . 2710

MEGAPHEN (Germany)
CHLORPROMAZINE HYDROCHLORIDE
Thorazine Ampuls . . . 1656
Thorazine Multi-dose Vials . . . 1656
Thorazine Spansule Capsules . . . 1656
Thorazine Syrup . . . 1656
Thorazine Tablets . . . 1656

MEGASIN (Portugal)
OFLOXACIN
Floxin I.V. . . . 2526
Floxin Otic Solution . . . 1219
Floxin Tablets . . . 2529
Ocuflox Ophthalmic Solution . . . 554

MEGAVIS (Italy)
LEVOCARNITINE
Carnitor Injection . . . 3242
Carnitor Tablets and Oral Solution . . . 3245

MEGEFREN (Spain)
MEGESTROL ACETATE
Megace Oral Suspension . . . 1124

MEGENTAL PEDIATRICO (Italy)
GENTAMICIN SULFATE
Genoptic Ophthalmic Ointment . . . ⊙239
Genoptic Sterile Ophthalmic Solution . . . ⊙239

MEGESTAT (Brazil, Germany, Switzerland)
MEGESTROL ACETATE
Megace Oral Suspension . . . 1124

MEGESTIL (Italy)
MEGESTROL ACETATE
Megace Oral Suspension . . . 1124

MEGESTIN (Denmark, Finland)
MEGESTROL ACETATE
Megace Oral Suspension . . . 1124

MEGLUCON (Austria, Germany)
METFORMIN HYDROCHLORIDE
Glucophage Tablets . . . 1080

MEGOSTAT (Australia, New Zealand, Spain)
MEGESTROL ACETATE
Megace Oral Suspension . . . 1124

MEJORULTRA (Mexico)
IBUPROFEN
Motrin Suspension, Oral Drops, Chewable Tablets, and Caplets . . . 2002

MELADININA (Mexico)
METHOXSALEN
8-MOP Capsules . . . 1727
Oxsoralen Lotion 1% . . . 1740
Oxsoralen-Ultra Capsules . . . 1741

MELADININE (France, Germany, Switzerland, Thailand, The Netherlands)
METHOXSALEN
8-MOP Capsules . . . 1727
Oxsoralen Lotion 1% . . . 1740
Oxsoralen-Ultra Capsules . . . 1741

MELANEX (Singapore)
HYDROQUINONE
Eldopaque Forte 4% Cream . . . 1734
Eldoquin Forte 4% Cream . . . 1734
Lustra Cream . . . 2023
Lustra-AF Cream . . . 2023
Melanex Topical Solution . . . 2300
Solaquin Forte 4% Cream . . . 1734
Solaquin Forte 4% Gel . . . 1734

MELANOX (Singapore)
HYDROQUINONE
Eldopaque Forte 4% Cream . . . 1734
Eldoquin Forte 4% Cream . . . 1734
Lustra Cream . . . 2023
Lustra-AF Cream . . . 2023
Melanex Topical Solution . . . 2300
Solaquin Forte 4% Cream . . . 1734
Solaquin Forte 4% Gel . . . 1734

MELAXOSE (France)
LACTULOSE
Kristalose for Oral Solution . . . 1007

MELBIN (Hong Kong)
METFORMIN HYDROCHLORIDE
Glucophage Tablets . . . 1080

MELDOPA (Irish Republic)
METHYLDOPA
Aldomet Tablets . . . 2037

MELFEN (Irish Republic)
IBUPROFEN
Motrin Suspension, Oral Drops, Chewable Tablets, and Caplets . . . 2002

MELIZID (Finland)
GLIPIZIDE
Glucotrol Tablets . . . 2692
Glucotrol XL Extended Release Tablets . . 2693

MELIZIDE (Australia, Thailand)
GLIPIZIDE
Glucotrol Tablets . . . 2692
Glucotrol XL Extended Release Tablets . . 2693

MELLERETTEN (Germany, The Netherlands)
THIORIDAZINE HYDROCHLORIDE
Thioridazine Hydrochloride Tablets . . . 2289

MELLERETTES (Switzerland)
THIORIDAZINE HYDROCHLORIDE
Thioridazine Hydrochloride Tablets . . . 2289

MELLERIL (Austria, Belgium, Brazil, Denmark, Finland, Hong Kong, Irish Republic, Israel, Italy, Norway, Portugal, South Africa, Switzerland, The Netherlands)
THIORIDAZINE HYDROCHLORIDE
Thioridazine Hydrochloride Tablets . . . 2289

MELTUS EXPECTORANT (United Kingdom)
GUAIFENESIN
Organidin NR Liquid . . . 3350
Organidin NR Tablets . . . 3350

MELZINE (Irish Republic)
THIORIDAZINE HYDROCHLORIDE
Thioridazine Hydrochloride Tablets . . . 2289

MEMAC (Italy)
DONEPEZIL HYDROCHLORIDE
Aricept Tablets . . . 1270, 2665

MENAVEN (Spain)
HEPARIN SODIUM
Heparin Lock Flush Solution . . . 3509
Heparin Sodium Injection . . . 3511

MENFAZONA (Spain)
NEFAZODONE HYDROCHLORIDE
Serzone Tablets . . . 1104

MENISOLE (Thailand)
METRONIDAZOLE
MetroCream . . . 1404
MetroGel . . . 1405
MetroGel-Vaginal Gel . . . 1986
MetroLotion . . . 1405
Noritate Cream . . . 1224

MENO-IMPLANT (Belgium, The Netherlands)
ESTRADIOL
Alora Transdermal System . . . 3372
Climara Transdermal System . . . 958
Estrace Vaginal Cream . . . 3358
Estring Vaginal Ring . . . 2811
Vivelle Transdermal System . . . 2412
Vivelle-Dot Transdermal System . . . 2416

MENO-PATCH (Israel)
ESTRADIOL
Alora Transdermal System . . . 3372
Climara Transdermal System . . . 958
Estrace Vaginal Cream . . . 3358
Estring Vaginal Ring . . . 2811
Vivelle Transdermal System . . . 2412
Vivelle-Dot Transdermal System . . . 2416

MENOREST (Australia, Austria, Denmark, Finland, France, Germany, Irish Republic, Italy, Norway, Portugal, South Africa, Spain, Sweden, Switzerland, The Netherlands, United Kingdom)
ESTRADIOL
Alora Transdermal System . . . 3372
Climara Transdermal System . . . 958
Estrace Vaginal Cream . . . 3358
Estring Vaginal Ring . . . 2811
Vivelle Transdermal System . . . 2412
Vivelle-Dot Transdermal System . . . 2416

MENPROS (Spain)
MISOPROSTOL
Cytotec Tablets . . . 3202

MENSOMA (Portugal)
FAMOTIDINE
Pepcid Injection . . . 2153
Pepcid Injection Premixed . . . 2153
Pepcid RPD Orally Disintegrating Tablets . . . 2150
Pepcid Tablets . . . 2150
Pepcid for Oral Suspension . . . 2150

MENSOTON (Germany)
IBUPROFEN
Motrin Suspension, Oral Drops, Chewable Tablets, and Caplets . . . 2002

MENTAX (Israel, Japan)
BUTENAFINE HYDROCHLORIDE
Mentax Cream . . . 1009

MENTHOLATUM IBUPROFEN (United Kingdom)
IBUPROFEN
Motrin Suspension, Oral Drops, Chewable Tablets, and Caplets . . . 2002

MEPAGYL (Thailand)
METRONIDAZOLE
MetroCream . . . 1404
MetroGel . . . 1405
MetroGel-Vaginal Gel . . . 1986
MetroLotion . . . 1405
Noritate Cream . . . 1224

MEPASTAT (Finland)
MEDROXYPROGESTERONE ACETATE
Depo-Provera Contraceptive Injection . . . 2798
Provera Tablets . . . 2853

MEPHAMESONE (Switzerland)
DEXAMETHASONE SODIUM PHOSPHATE
Decadron Phosphate Injection . . . 2081
Decadron Phosphate Sterile Ophthalmic Ointment . . . ⊙280, 2083
Decadron Phosphate Sterile Ophthalmic Solution . . . 2084

MEPHAQUIN (Hong Kong, Israel, Portugal, Singapore, Thailand)
MEFLOQUINE HYDROCHLORIDE
Lariam Tablets . . . 2989

MEPHAQUIN LACTAB (Brazil)
MEFLOQUINE HYDROCHLORIDE
Lariam Tablets . . . 2989

MEPHAQUINE (Switzerland)
MEFLOQUINE HYDROCHLORIDE
Lariam Tablets . . . 2989

MEPICAIN (Italy)
MEPIVACAINE HYDROCHLORIDE
Polocaine Injection, USP . . . 625
Polocaine-MPF Injection, USP . . . 625

MEPICATON (Germany, Switzerland, Thailand)
MEPIVACAINE HYDROCHLORIDE
Polocaine Injection, USP . . . 625
Polocaine-MPF Injection, USP . . . 625

MEPIDENT (Italy)
MEPIVACAINE HYDROCHLORIDE
Polocaine Injection, USP . . . 625
Polocaine-MPF Injection, USP . . . 625

MEPIFORAN (Italy)
MEPIVACAINE HYDROCHLORIDE
Polocaine Injection, USP . . . 625
Polocaine-MPF Injection, USP . . . 625

MEPIHEXAL (Germany)
MEPIVACAINE HYDROCHLORIDE
Polocaine Injection, USP . . . 625
Polocaine-MPF Injection, USP . . . 625

MEPI-MYNOL (Italy)
MEPIVACAINE HYDROCHLORIDE
Polocaine Injection, USP . . . 625
Polocaine-MPF Injection, USP . . . 625

MEPIVASTESIN (Germany)
MEPIVACAINE HYDROCHLORIDE
Polocaine Injection, USP . . . 625
Polocaine-MPF Injection, USP . . . 625

(⊙ Described in PDR For Ophthalmic Medicines™)

MEPIVASTESIN FORTE (Germany)
MEPIVACAINE HYDROCHLORIDE
Polocaine Injection, USP . . . 625
Polocaine-MPF Injection, USP . . . 625

MEPRATE (United Kingdom)
MEPROBAMATE
Miltown Tablets . . . 3349

MEPRAZ (Portugal)
OMEPRAZOLE
Prilosec Delayed-Release Capsules . . . 628

MEPREPOSE (South Africa)
MEPROBAMATE
Miltown Tablets . . . 3349

MEPRIL (Austria)
ENALAPRIL MALEATE
Vasotec Tablets . . . 2210

MEPRO (Israel)
MEPROBAMATE
Miltown Tablets . . . 3349

MEPRODIL (Switzerland)
MEPROBAMATE
Miltown Tablets . . . 3349

MEPROFEN (Italy)
KETOPROFEN
Orudis Capsules . . . 3548
Oruvail Capsules . . . 3548

MEPRON (Canada)
ATOVAQUONE
Mepron Suspension . . . 1598

MEPROSONA-F (Mexico)
PREDNISONE
Prednisone Intensol . . . 3064
Prednisone Oral Solution . . . 3064
Prednisone Tablets . . . 3064

MEPROSPAN (Spain)
MEPROBAMATE
Miltown Tablets . . . 3349

MEPYL (Italy)
MEPIVACAINE HYDROCHLORIDE
Polocaine Injection, USP . . . 625
Polocaine-MPF Injection, USP . . . 625

MERAMIDE (Thailand)
METOCLOPRAMIDE HYDROCHLORIDE
Reglan Injectable . . . 2935
Reglan Syrup . . . 2935
Reglan Tablets . . . 2935

MERCAP (Germany)
MERCAPTOPURINE
Purinethol Tablets . . . 1615

MERCAPTINA (Brazil)
MERCAPTOPURINE
Purinethol Tablets . . . 1615

MERCAPTYL (Switzerland)
PENICILLAMINE
Cuprimine Capsules . . . 2075
Depen Titratable Tablets . . . 3341

MEREDAZOL (Mexico)
METRONIDAZOLE
MetroCream . . . 1404
MetroGel . . . 1405
MetroGel-Vaginal Gel . . . 1986
MetroLotion . . . 1405
Noritate Cream . . . 1224

MEREPRINE (Portugal)
CAPTOPRIL
Captopril Tablets . . . 2281

MERLIT (Austria)
LORAZEPAM
Ativan Injection . . . 3478
Ativan Tablets . . . 3482

MEROCAINE (Irish Republic, United Kingdom)
BENZOCAINE
Americaine Anesthetic Lubricant . . . 1162
Americaine Otic Topical Anesthetic Ear Drops . . . 1162

MERONEM (Belgium, Denmark, Finland, Hong Kong, Irish Republic, Israel, Norway, Portugal, Singapore, South Africa, Spain, Sweden, Switzerland, Thailand, The Netherlands, United Kingdom)
MEROPENEM
Merrem I.V. . . . 673

MEROPEN (Japan)
MEROPENEM
Merrem I.V. . . . 673

MERREM (Australia, Canada, Italy, Mexico, New Zealand)
MEROPENEM
Merrem I.V. . . . 673

MERXIL (Mexico)
DICLOFENAC SODIUM
Voltaren Tablets . . . 2315
Voltaren-XR Tablets . . . 2315

MESCORIT (Germany)
METFORMIN HYDROCHLORIDE
Glucophage Tablets . . . 1080

MESIN (Thailand)
ALBENDAZOLE
Albenza Tablets . . . 1463

M-ESLON (Canada)
MORPHINE SULFATE
Astramorph/PF Injection, USP (Preservative-Free) . . . 594
Duramorph Injection . . . 1312
Infumorph 200 and Infumorph 500 Sterile Solutions . . . 1314
Kadian Capsules . . . 1335
MS Contin Tablets . . . 2896
MSIR Oral Capsules . . . 2898
MSIR Oral Solution . . . 2898
MSIR Oral Solution Concentrate . . . 2898
MSIR Oral Tablets . . . 2898
Oramorph SR Tablets . . . 3062
Roxanol 100 Concentrated Oral Solution . . . 3066
Roxanol Concentrated Oral Solution . . . 3066
Roxanol-T Oral Solution . . . 3066

MESMERIN (Brazil)
LORAZEPAM
Ativan Injection . . . 3478
Ativan Tablets . . . 3482

MESOLEX (Thailand)
METRONIDAZOLE
MetroCream . . . 1404
MetroGel . . . 1405
MetroGel-Vaginal Gel . . . 1986
MetroLotion . . . 1405
Noritate Cream . . . 1224

MESPAFIN (Germany)
DOXYCYCLINE HYCLATE
Doryx Coated Pellet Filled Capsules . . . 3357
Periostat Tablets . . . 1208
Vibramycin Hyclate Capsules . . . 2735
Vibramycin Hyclate Intravenous . . . 2737
Vibra-Tabs Film Coated Tablets . . . 2735

MESPORIN (Portugal)
CEFTRIAXONE SODIUM
Rocephin Injectable Vials, ADD-Vantage, Galaxy, Bulk . . . 2993

MESTACINE (France)
MINOCYCLINE HYDROCHLORIDE
Dynacin Capsules . . . 2019
Minocin Intravenous . . . 1862
Minocin Oral Suspension . . . 1865
Minocin Pellet-Filled Capsules . . . 1863

MESTINON (Australia, Austria, Belgium, Brazil, Canada, Denmark, Finland, France, Germany, Hong Kong, Irish Republic, Israel, Italy, Mexico, New Zealand, Norway, Portugal, Singapore, South Africa, Spain, Sweden, Switzerland, Thailand, The Netherlands, United Kingdom)
PYRIDOSTIGMINE BROMIDE
Mestinon Syrup . . . 1740
Mestinon Tablets . . . 1740
Mestinon Timespan Tablets . . . 1740

MESTREL (Mexico)
MEGESTROL ACETATE
Megace Oral Suspension . . . 1124

MET (Germany)
METFORMIN HYDROCHLORIDE
Glucophage Tablets . . . 1080

METAGYL (South Africa)
METRONIDAZOLE
MetroCream . . . 1404
MetroGel . . . 1405
MetroGel-Vaginal Gel . . . 1986
MetroLotion . . . 1405
Noritate Cream . . . 1224

META-K (Mexico)
CEPHALEXIN
Keflex Oral Suspension . . . 1237
Keflex Pulvules . . . 1237

METALCAPTASE (Germany, South Africa)
PENICILLAMINE
Cuprimine Capsules . . . 2075
Depen Titratable Tablets . . . 3341

METALON (South Africa)
METOCLOPRAMIDE HYDROCHLORIDE
Reglan Injectable . . . 2935
Reglan Syrup . . . 2935
Reglan Tablets . . . 2935

METALPHA (United Kingdom)
METHYLDOPA
Aldomet Tablets . . . 2037

METAMIDE (Australia, New Zealand)
METOCLOPRAMIDE HYDROCHLORIDE
Reglan Injectable . . . 2935
Reglan Syrup . . . 2935
Reglan Tablets . . . 2935

METAMIDOL (Portugal)
DIAZEPAM
Valium Injectable . . . 3026
Valium Tablets . . . 3047

METANDREN (Canada)
METHYLTESTOSTERONE
Android Capsules, 10 mg . . . 1731
Testred Capsules, 10 mg . . . 1746

METAZEM (Hong Kong, Singapore, Thailand, United Kingdom)
DILTIAZEM HYDROCHLORIDE
Cardizem CD Capsules . . . 1016
Cardizem Injectable . . . 1018
Cardizem Lyo-Ject Syringe . . . 1018
Cardizem Monovial . . . 1018
Tiazac Capsules . . . 1378

METAZIN (Portugal)
ETODOLAC
Lodine Capsules . . . 3528
Lodine Tablets . . . 3528
Lodine XL Extended-Release Tablets . . . 3530

METAZOL (South Africa)
METRONIDAZOLE
MetroCream . . . 1404
MetroGel . . . 1405
MetroGel-Vaginal Gel . . . 1986
MetroLotion . . . 1405
Noritate Cream . . . 1224

METBAY (Italy)
METFORMIN HYDROCHLORIDE
Glucophage Tablets . . . 1080

METCON (South Africa)
METOCLOPRAMIDE HYDROCHLORIDE
Reglan Injectable . . . 2935
Reglan Syrup . . . 2935
Reglan Tablets . . . 2935

METENIX 5 (United Kingdom)
METOLAZONE
Mykrox Tablets . . . 1168
Zaroxolyn Tablets . . . 1177

METFIREX (France)
METFORMIN HYDROCHLORIDE
Glucophage Tablets . . . 1080

METFOGAMMA (Germany)
METFORMIN HYDROCHLORIDE
Glucophage Tablets . . . 1080

METFOR-500 (Thailand)
METFORMIN HYDROCHLORIDE
Glucophage Tablets . . . 1080

METFORAL (Italy)
METFORMIN HYDROCHLORIDE
Glucophage Tablets . . . 1080

METFOREM (Finland)
METFORMIN HYDROCHLORIDE
Glucophage Tablets . . . 1080

METFRON (Thailand)
METFORMIN HYDROCHLORIDE
Glucophage Tablets . . . 1080

METHOXACET (Canada)
METHOCARBAMOL
Robaxin Injectable . . . 2938
Robaxin Tablets . . . 2939
Robaxin-750 Tablets . . . 2939

METHOXISAL (Canada)
METHOCARBAMOL
Robaxin Injectable . . . 2938
Robaxin Tablets . . . 2939
Robaxin-750 Tablets . . . 2939

METICEL (Spain)
RANITIDINE HYDROCHLORIDE
Zantac 150 EFFERdose Granules . . . 1690
Zantac 150 EFFERdose Tablets . . . 1690
Zantac 150 Tablets . . . 1690
Zantac 300 Tablets . . . 1690
Zantac Injection . . . 1688
Zantac Injection Premixed . . . 1688
Zantac Syrup . . . 1690

METICORTELONE (Italy, South Africa)
PREDNISOLONE
Prelone Syrup . . . 2273

METICORTEN (Brazil, Mexico, Portugal, South Africa)
PREDNISONE
Prednisone Intensol . . . 3064
Prednisone Oral Solution . . . 3064
Prednisone Tablets . . . 3064

METIGUANIDE (Italy)
METFORMIN HYDROCHLORIDE
Glucophage Tablets . . . 1080

METILBETASONE SOLUBILE (Italy)
METHYLPREDNISOLONE ACETATE
Depo-Medrol Injectable Suspension . . . 2795

METIMYD (Canada, Sweden)
PREDNISOLONE ACETATE/SULFACETAMIDE SODIUM
Blephamide Ophthalmic Ointment . . . 547
Blephamide Ophthalmic Suspension . . . 548

METINET (Denmark)
CIMETIDINE
Tagamet Tablets . . . 1644

METOCLAMID (Germany)
METOCLOPRAMIDE HYDROCHLORIDE
Reglan Injectable . . . 2935
Reglan Syrup . . . 2935
Reglan Tablets . . . 2935

METOCLAN (Portugal)
METOCLOPRAMIDE HYDROCHLORIDE
Reglan Injectable . . . 2935
Reglan Syrup . . . 2935
Reglan Tablets . . . 2935

METOCLOR (Thailand)
METOCLOPRAMIDE HYDROCHLORIDE
Reglan Injectable . . . 2935
Reglan Syrup . . . 2935
Reglan Tablets . . . 2935

METOCOBIL (Italy)
METOCLOPRAMIDE HYDROCHLORIDE
Reglan Injectable . . . 2935
Reglan Syrup . . . 2935
Reglan Tablets . . . 2935

METOCYL (Hong Kong, Irish Republic, Singapore)
METOCLOPRAMIDE HYDROCHLORIDE
Reglan Injectable . . . 2935
Reglan Syrup . . . 2935
Reglan Tablets . . . 2935

METOGASTRON (Austria)
METOCLOPRAMIDE HYDROCHLORIDE
Reglan Injectable . . . 2935
Reglan Syrup . . . 2935
Reglan Tablets . . . 2935

METOLON (Singapore)
METOCLOPRAMIDE HYDROCHLORIDE
Reglan Injectable . . . 2935
Reglan Syrup . . . 2935
Reglan Tablets . . . 2935

METOMIN (New Zealand)
METFORMIN HYDROCHLORIDE
Glucophage Tablets . . . 1080

METONO (Thailand)
METOCLOPRAMIDE HYDROCHLORIDE
Reglan Injectable . . . 2935
Reglan Syrup . . . 2935
Reglan Tablets . . . 2935

METOPRAM (Finland)
METOCLOPRAMIDE HYDROCHLORIDE
Reglan Injectable . . . 2935
Reglan Syrup . . . 2935
Reglan Tablets . . . 2935

METOSYN (Denmark, Irish Republic, Norway, Singapore, United Kingdom)
FLUOCINONIDE
Lidex Cream . . . 2020
Lidex Gel . . . 2020
Lidex Ointment . . . 2020
Lidex Topical Solution . . . 2020
Lidex-E Cream . . . 2020

METOX (United Kingdom)
METOCLOPRAMIDE HYDROCHLORIDE
Reglan Injectable . . . 2935
Reglan Syrup . . . 2935
Reglan Tablets . . . 2935

METRAMID (United Kingdom)
METOCLOPRAMIDE HYDROCHLORIDE
Reglan Injectable . . . 2935
Reglan Syrup . . . 2935
Reglan Tablets . . . 2935

METRAZOLE (South Africa, Thailand)
METRONIDAZOLE
MetroCream . . . 1404
MetroGel . . . 1405
MetroGel-Vaginal Gel . . . 1986
MetroLotion . . . 1405
Noritate Cream . . . 1224

METRICOM (Mexico)
METRONIDAZOLE
MetroCream . . . 1404

MetroGel 1405
MetroGel-Vaginal Gel 1986
MetroLotion 1405
Noritate Cream 1224

METRIZOL (Mexico, Switzerland)
METRONIDAZOLE
MetroCream 1404
MetroGel 1405
MetroGel-Vaginal Gel 1986
MetroLotion 1405
Noritate Cream 1224

METROCIDE (Thailand)
METRONIDAZOLE
MetroCream 1404
MetroGel 1405
MetroGel-Vaginal Gel 1986
MetroLotion 1405
Noritate Cream 1224

METROCREAM (Canada)
METRONIDAZOLE
MetroCream 1404
MetroGel 1405
MetroGel-Vaginal Gel 1986
MetroLotion 1405
Noritate Cream 1224

METRODERME (Portugal)
METRONIDAZOLE
MetroCream 1404
MetroGel 1405
MetroGel-Vaginal Gel 1986
MetroLotion 1405
Noritate Cream 1224

METROGEL (Canada, Denmark, Irish Republic, Mexico, The Netherlands)
METRONIDAZOLE
MetroCream 1404
MetroGel 1405
MetroGel-Vaginal Gel 1986
MetroLotion 1405
Noritate Cream 1224

METROGYL (Australia, Hong Kong, Israel)
METRONIDAZOLE
MetroCream 1404
MetroGel 1405
MetroGel-Vaginal Gel 1986
MetroLotion 1405
Noritate Cream 1224

METROLEX (Thailand)
METRONIDAZOLE
MetroCream 1404
MetroGel 1405
MetroGel-Vaginal Gel 1986
MetroLotion 1405
Noritate Cream 1224

METROLYL (United Kingdom)
METRONIDAZOLE
MetroCream 1404
MetroGel 1405
MetroGel-Vaginal Gel 1986
MetroLotion 1405
Noritate Cream 1224

METRONIDE (Australia, Irish Republic)
METRONIDAZOLE
MetroCream 1404
MetroGel 1405
MetroGel-Vaginal Gel 1986
MetroLotion 1405
Noritate Cream 1224

METRONID-PUREN (Germany)
METRONIDAZOLE
MetroCream 1404
MetroGel 1405
MetroGel-Vaginal Gel 1986
MetroLotion 1405
Noritate Cream 1224

METRONIMERCK (Germany)
METRONIDAZOLE
MetroCream 1404
MetroGel 1405
MetroGel-Vaginal Gel 1986
MetroLotion 1405
Noritate Cream 1224

METRONIX (Brazil)
METRONIDAZOLE
MetroCream 1404
MetroGel 1405
MetroGel-Vaginal Gel 1986
MetroLotion 1405
Noritate Cream 1224

METRONOM (Austria)
PROPAFENONE HYDROCHLORIDE
Rythmol Tablets – 150 mg, 225 mg, 300 mg 502

METRONOUR (Germany)
METRONIDAZOLE
MetroCream 1404
MetroGel 1405
MetroGel-Vaginal Gel 1986
MetroLotion 1405
Noritate Cream 1224

METRONT (Germany)
METRONIDAZOLE
MetroCream 1404
MetroGel 1405
MetroGel-Vaginal Gel 1986
MetroLotion 1405
Noritate Cream 1224

METROSON (Mexico)
METRONIDAZOLE
MetroCream 1404
MetroGel 1405
MetroGel-Vaginal Gel 1986
MetroLotion 1405
Noritate Cream 1224

METROSTAT (South Africa)
METRONIDAZOLE
MetroCream 1404
MetroGel 1405
MetroGel-Vaginal Gel 1986
MetroLotion 1405
Noritate Cream 1224

METROTOP (Irish Republic, United Kingdom)
METRONIDAZOLE
MetroCream 1404
MetroGel 1405
MetroGel-Vaginal Gel 1986
MetroLotion 1405
Noritate Cream 1224

METROZINE (Australia, Hong Kong)
METRONIDAZOLE
MetroCream 1404
MetroGel 1405
MetroGel-Vaginal Gel 1986
MetroLotion 1405
Noritate Cream 1224

METROZOL (United Kingdom)
METRONIDAZOLE
MetroCream 1404
MetroGel 1405
MetroGel-Vaginal Gel 1986
MetroLotion 1405
Noritate Cream 1224

METROZOLE (Singapore)
METRONIDAZOLE
MetroCream 1404
MetroGel 1405
MetroGel-Vaginal Gel 1986
MetroLotion 1405
Noritate Cream 1224

METRYL (South Africa)
METRONIDAZOLE
MetroCream 1404
MetroGel 1405
MetroGel-Vaginal Gel 1986
MetroLotion 1405
Noritate Cream 1224

METSEC (Thailand)
OMEPRAZOLE
Prilosec Delayed-Release Capsules 628

MET-SIL (Thailand)
METOCLOPRAMIDE HYDROCHLORIDE
Reglan Injectable 2935
Reglan Syrup 2935
Reglan Tablets 2935

METYPRESOL (South Africa, The Netherlands)
METHYLPREDNISOLONE SODIUM SUCCINATE
Solu-Medrol Sterile Powder 2855

MEVACOR (Austria, Brazil, Canada, Denmark, Finland, Hong Kong, Mexico, Norway, Spain)
LOVASTATIN
Mevacor Tablets 2132

MEVAL (Canada)
DIAZEPAM
Valium Injectable 3026
Valium Tablets 3047

MEVALOTIN (Germany, Japan, Switzerland, Thailand)
PRAVASTATIN SODIUM
Pravachol Tablets 1099

MEVINACOR (Germany, Portugal)
LOVASTATIN
Mevacor Tablets 2132

MEVLOR (Portugal)
LOVASTATIN
Mevacor Tablets 2132

MEXASONE (Singapore)
DEXAMETHASONE
Decadron Elixir 2078
Decadron Tablets 2079

MEXCYN (Mexico)
ERYTHROMYCIN
Emgel 2% Topical Gel 1285
Ery-Tab Tablets 448
Erythromycin Base Filmtab Tablets 454
Erythromycin Delayed-Release Capsules, USP 455
PCE Dispertab Tablets 498

MEXETIL (Finland)
MEXILETINE HYDROCHLORIDE
Mexitil Capsules 1047

MEXILEN (Israel)
MEXILETINE HYDROCHLORIDE
Mexitil Capsules 1047

MEXITIL (Australia, Austria, Belgium, Brazil, Canada, Denmark, France, Germany, Hong Kong, Irish Republic, Italy, Mexico, New Zealand, Norway, South Africa, Spain, Sweden, Switzerland, Thailand, The Netherlands, United Kingdom)
MEXILETINE HYDROCHLORIDE
Mexitil Capsules 1047

MEXONA (Mexico)
DEXAMETHASONE
Decadron Elixir 2078
Decadron Tablets 2079

MIALIN (Italy)
ALPRAZOLAM
Xanax Tablets 2865

MIAMBUTOL (Italy)
ETHAMBUTOL HYDROCHLORIDE
Myambutol Tablets 1290

MIBAZOL (Mexico)
METRONIDAZOLE
MetroCream 1404
MetroGel 1405
MetroGel-Vaginal Gel 1986
MetroLotion 1405
Noritate Cream 1224

MICARDIS (Australia, Belgium, Denmark, France, Irish Republic, Italy, South Africa, Spain, Switzerland, The Netherlands, United Kingdom)
TELMISARTAN
Micardis Tablets 1049

MICARZIN (Mexico)
IBUPROFEN
Motrin Suspension, Oral Drops, Chewable Tablets, and Caplets 2002

MICETINOFTALMINA (Portugal)
CHLORAMPHENICOL
Chloromycetin Ophthalmic Ointment, 1% . . . . . ⊙296
Chloromycetin Ophthalmic Solution . . . . . ⊙297
Chloroptic Sterile Ophthalmic Ointment . . ⊙234
Chloroptic Sterile Ophthalmic Solution . . ⊙235

MICLAST (Italy)
CICLOPIROX OLAMINE
Loprox Cream 2021
Loprox Lotion 2021

MICOGAL (Mexico)
KETOCONAZOLE
Nizoral 2% Cream 3620
Nizoral 2% Shampoo 2007
Nizoral Tablets 1791

MICOMICEN (Italy)
CICLOPIROX OLAMINE
Loprox Cream 2021
Loprox Lotion 2021

MICOMISAN (South Africa, Spain)
CLOTRIMAZOLE
Lotrimin Cream 1% 3128
Lotrimin Lotion 1% 3128
Lotrimin Topical Solution 1% 3128
Mycelex Troche 573

MICONAN (Brazil)
KETOCONAZOLE
Nizoral 2% Cream 3620
Nizoral 2% Shampoo 2007
Nizoral Tablets 1791

MICOSER (Mexico)
KETOCONAZOLE
Nizoral 2% Cream 3620
Nizoral 2% Shampoo 2007
Nizoral Tablets 1791

MICOSONA (Spain)
NAFTIFINE HYDROCHLORIDE
Naftin Cream 2224
Naftin Gel 2224

MICOSTATIN (Brazil, Mexico)
NYSTATIN
Nystop Topical Powder USP 2608

MICOTER (Spain)
CLOTRIMAZOLE
Lotrimin Cream 1% 3128
Lotrimin Lotion 1% 3128
Lotrimin Topical Solution 1% 3128
Mycelex Troche 573

MICOTICUM (Spain)
KETOCONAZOLE
Nizoral 2% Cream 3620
Nizoral 2% Shampoo 2007
Nizoral Tablets 1791

MICOTRIZOL (Brazil)
CLOTRIMAZOLE
Lotrimin Cream 1% 3128
Lotrimin Lotion 1% 3128
Lotrimin Topical Solution 1% 3128
Mycelex Troche 573

MICOXOLAMINA (Italy)
CICLOPIROX OLAMINE
Loprox Cream 2021
Loprox Lotion 2021

MICROBAMAT (Austria)
MEPROBAMATE
Miltown Tablets 3349

MICROGYNON (Belgium)
LEVONORGESTREL
Norplant System 3543

MICRO-K (Canada, South Africa)
POTASSIUM CHLORIDE
K-Dur Microburst Release System ER Tablets 1832
K-Lor Powder Packets 469
K-Tab Filmtab Tablets 470
Rum-K 1363

MICROKALEORID (France)
POTASSIUM CHLORIDE
K-Dur Microburst Release System ER Tablets 1832
K-Lor Powder Packets 469
K-Tab Filmtab Tablets 470
Rum-K 1363

MICRO-KALIUM (Austria)
POTASSIUM CHLORIDE
K-Dur Microburst Release System ER Tablets 1832
K-Lor Powder Packets 469
K-Tab Filmtab Tablets 470
Rum-K 1363

MICROLUT (Australia, Belgium, Germany, Irish Republic, Italy, Mexico, New Zealand, Switzerland)
LEVONORGESTREL
Norplant System 3543

MICROLUTON (Denmark, Finland, Norway)
LEVONORGESTREL
Norplant System 3543

MICRONOAN (Italy)
DIAZEPAM
Valium Injectable 3026
Valium Tablets 3047

MICROPHYLLIN (South Africa)
THEOPHYLLINE
Aerolate Jr. T.D. Capsules 1361
Aerolate Liquid 1361
Aerolate Sr. T.D. Capsules 1361
Theo-Dur Extended-Release Tablets 1835
Uni-Dur Extended-Release Tablets 1841
Uniphyl 400 mg and 600 mg Tablets . . . 2903

MICRORGAN (Mexico)
CIPROFLOXACIN HYDROCHLORIDE
Ciloxan Ophthalmic Ointment 538
Ciloxan Ophthalmic Solution . . . . ⊙209, 538
Cipro Tablets 887

MICROVAL (Australia, Belgium, Denmark, France, Irish Republic, New Zealand, South Africa, United Kingdom)
LEVONORGESTREL
Norplant System 3543

MICROXEN (Mexico)
NORFLOXACIN
Chibroxin Sterile Ophthalmic Solution . . . . . ⊙273, 2051
Noroxin Tablets 2145

MIDAMOR (Australia, Austria, Canada, Hong Kong, New Zealand, Norway, Sweden, Switzerland, The Netherlands, United Kingdom)
AMILORIDE HYDROCHLORIDE
Midamor Tablets 2136

MIDON (Irish Republic)
MIDODRINE HYDROCHLORIDE
ProAmatine Tablets 3241

MIDORIDE (Australia)
AMILORIDE HYDROCHLORIDE
Midamor Tablets 2136

MIDRAN (Italy, South Africa)
APROTININ
Trasylol Injection 909

MIDURET (Thailand)
AMILORIDE HYDROCHLORIDE/HYDROCHLOROTHIAZIDE
Moduretic Tablets . . . 2138

MIELUCIN (Brazil)
BUSULFAN
Myleran Tablets . . . 1603

MIFLONIDE (Denmark, Italy, Portugal)
BUDESONIDE
Pulmicort Turbuhaler Inhalation Powder . . . 636
Rhinocort Nasal Inhaler . . . 640

MIFORMIN (Thailand)
METFORMIN HYDROCHLORIDE
Glucophage Tablets . . . 1080

MIGRAFEN (United Kingdom)
IBUPROFEN
Motrin Suspension, Oral Drops, Chewable Tablets, and Caplets . . . 2002

MIGRIL (Brazil)
SUMATRIPTAN SUCCINATE
Imitrex Injection . . . 1549
Imitrex Tablets . . . 1558

MI-KE-SONS (Mexico)
KETOCONAZOLE
Nizoral 2% Cream . . . 3620
Nizoral 2% Shampoo . . . 2007
Nizoral Tablets . . . 1791

MIKETOS (Mexico)
KETOCONAZOLE
Nizoral 2% Cream . . . 3620
Nizoral 2% Shampoo . . . 2007
Nizoral Tablets . . . 1791

MIKIUM (Spain)
CICLOPIROX OLAMINE
Loprox Cream . . . 2021
Loprox Lotion . . . 2021

MIKOSTAT (United Arab Emirates)
NYSTATIN
Nystop Topical Powder USP . . . 2608

MIKRO-30 (Germany)
LEVONORGESTREL
Norplant System . . . 3543

MILA-CONO (Thailand)
CODEINE PHOSPHATE/GUAIFENESIN
Robitussin A-C Syrup . . . 2942
Tussi-Organidin NR Liquid . . . 3350
Tussi-Organidin-S NR Liquid . . . 3350

MILAMET (Thailand)
CIMETIDINE
Tagamet Tablets . . . 1644

MILANIDAZOLE (Thailand)
METRONIDAZOLE
MetroCream . . . 1404
MetroGel . . . 1405
MetroGel-Vaginal Gel . . . 1986
MetroLotion . . . 1405
Noritate Cream . . . 1224

MILDISON (Denmark, Finland, Irish Republic, Norway, Sweden, The Netherlands, United Kingdom)
HYDROCORTISONE
Anusol-HC Cream 2.5% . . . 2237
Hydrocortone Tablets . . . 2106

MILLIBAR (Hong Kong, Italy, Singapore)
INDAPAMIDE
Indapamide Tablets . . . 2286

MILLICORTENE (Switzerland)
DEXAMETHASONE
Decadron Elixir . . . 2078
Decadron Tablets . . . 2079

MILODERME (Portugal)
ALCLOMETASONE DIPROPIONATE
Aclovate Cream . . . 1275
Aclovate Ointment . . . 1275

MILOREX (Thailand)
AMILORIDE HYDROCHLORIDE/HYDROCHLOROTHIAZIDE
Moduretic Tablets . . . 2138

MILORIDE (Finland)
AMILORIDE HYDROCHLORIDE/HYDROCHLOROTHIAZIDE
Moduretic Tablets . . . 2138

MILTAUN (Austria)
MEPROBAMATE
Miltown Tablets . . . 3349

MILTOWN (Spain)
MEPROBAMATE
Miltown Tablets . . . 3349

MINAC 50 (Switzerland)
MINOCYCLINE HYDROCHLORIDE
Dynacin Capsules . . . 2019
Minocin Intravenous . . . 1862
Minocin Oral Suspension . . . 1865
Minocin Pellet-Filled Capsules . . . 1863

MINAKNE (Germany)
MINOCYCLINE HYDROCHLORIDE
Dynacin Capsules . . . 2019
Minocin Intravenous . . . 1862
Minocin Oral Suspension . . . 1865
Minocin Pellet-Filled Capsules . . . 1863

MINDIAB (Denmark, Finland, Norway, Sweden)
GLIPIZIDE
Glucotrol Tablets . . . 2692
Glucotrol XL Extended Release Tablets . . 2693

MINDOL (New Zealand)
MEBENDAZOLE
Vermox Chewable Tablets . . . 2017

MINIDEX (Brazil)
DEXAMETHASONE
Decadron Elixir . . . 2078
Decadron Tablets . . . 2079

MINIDIAB (Australia, Austria, Belgium, Brazil, France, Hong Kong, Italy, New Zealand, Portugal, Singapore, South Africa, Thailand)
GLIPIZIDE
Glucotrol Tablets . . . 2692
Glucotrol XL Extended Release Tablets . . 2693

MINIDOX (Italy)
DOXYCYCLINE HYCLATE
Doryx Coated Pellet Filled Capsules . . . 3357
Periostat Tablets . . . 1208
Vibramycin Hyclate Capsules . . . 2735
Vibramycin Hyclate Intravenous . . . 2737
Vibra-Tabs Film Coated Tablets . . . 2735

MINIHEP (Irish Republic, The Netherlands, United Kingdom)
HEPARIN SODIUM
Heparin Lock Flush Solution . . . 3509
Heparin Sodium Injection . . . 3511

MINIMA (Thailand)
PRAZOSIN HYDROCHLORIDE
Minipress Capsules . . . 2699

MINIPRES (Mexico, Spain)
PRAZOSIN HYDROCHLORIDE
Minipress Capsules . . . 2699

MINIPRESS (Australia, Austria, Belgium, Brazil, Canada, France, Germany, Hong Kong, Italy, Singapore, South Africa, Switzerland, Thailand, The Netherlands)
PRAZOSIN HYDROCHLORIDE
Minipress Capsules . . . 2699

MINIRIN (Australia, Austria, Belgium, Denmark, Finland, France, Hong Kong, Israel, Mexico, New Zealand, Norway, Singapore, Sweden, Switzerland, Thailand)
DESMOPRESSIN ACETATE
DDAVP Injection 4 mcg/mL . . . 737
DDAVP Nasal Spray . . . 738
DDAVP Rhinal Tube . . . 738
DDAVP Tablets . . . 739
Desmopressin Acetate Injection . . . 1344
Desmopressin Acetate Rhinal Tube . . . 1345
Stimate Nasal Spray . . . 796

MINIRIN/DDAVP (Italy)
DESMOPRESSIN ACETATE
DDAVP Injection 4 mcg/mL . . . 737
DDAVP Nasal Spray . . . 738
DDAVP Rhinal Tube . . . 738
DDAVP Tablets . . . 739
Desmopressin Acetate Injection . . . 1344
Desmopressin Acetate Rhinal Tube . . . 1345
Stimate Nasal Spray . . . 796

MINO T (South Africa)
MINOCYCLINE HYDROCHLORIDE
Dynacin Capsules . . . 2019
Minocin Intravenous . . . 1862
Minocin Oral Suspension . . . 1865
Minocin Pellet-Filled Capsules . . . 1863

MINO-50 (Belgium)
MINOCYCLINE HYDROCHLORIDE
Dynacin Capsules . . . 2019
Minocin Intravenous . . . 1862
Minocin Oral Suspension . . . 1865
Minocin Pellet-Filled Capsules . . . 1863

MINOBESE (South Africa)
PHENTERMINE HYDROCHLORIDE
Adipex-P Capsules . . . 1406
Adipex-P Tablets . . . 1406

MINOCIN (Austria, Belgium, Canada, Hong Kong, Irish Republic, Israel, Italy, Mexico, Portugal, Singapore, Spain, Switzerland, Thailand, The Netherlands, United Kingdom)
MINOCYCLINE HYDROCHLORIDE
Dynacin Capsules . . . 2019
Minocin Intravenous . . . 1862
Minocin Oral Suspension . . . 1865
Minocin Pellet-Filled Capsules . . . 1863

MINOCLIN (Israel)
MINOCYCLINE HYDROCHLORIDE
Dynacin Capsules . . . 2019
Minocin Intravenous . . . 1862
Minocin Oral Suspension . . . 1865
Minocin Pellet-Filled Capsules . . . 1863

MINOCLIR (Germany)
MINOCYCLINE HYDROCHLORIDE
Dynacin Capsules . . . 2019
Minocin Intravenous . . . 1862
Minocin Oral Suspension . . . 1865
Minocin Pellet-Filled Capsules . . . 1863

MINODIAB (Mexico, Spain, United Kingdom)
GLIPIZIDE
Glucotrol Tablets . . . 2692
Glucotrol XL Extended Release Tablets . . 2693

MINOGALEN (Germany)
MINOCYCLINE HYDROCHLORIDE
Dynacin Capsules . . . 2019
Minocin Intravenous . . . 1862
Minocin Oral Suspension . . . 1865
Minocin Pellet-Filled Capsules . . . 1863

MINOLIS (France)
MINOCYCLINE HYDROCHLORIDE
Dynacin Capsules . . . 2019
Minocin Intravenous . . . 1862
Minocin Oral Suspension . . . 1865
Minocin Pellet-Filled Capsules . . . 1863

MINOMAX (Brazil)
MINOCYCLINE HYDROCHLORIDE
Dynacin Capsules . . . 2019
Minocin Intravenous . . . 1862
Minocin Oral Suspension . . . 1865
Minocin Pellet-Filled Capsules . . . 1863

MINOMYCIN (Australia, New Zealand, South Africa)
MINOCYCLINE HYDROCHLORIDE
Dynacin Capsules . . . 2019
Minocin Intravenous . . . 1862
Minocin Oral Suspension . . . 1865
Minocin Pellet-Filled Capsules . . . 1863

MINOPLUS (Germany)
MINOCYCLINE HYDROCHLORIDE
Dynacin Capsules . . . 2019
Minocin Intravenous . . . 1862
Minocin Oral Suspension . . . 1865
Minocin Pellet-Filled Capsules . . . 1863

MINOREMED (Germany)
AMILORIDE HYDROCHLORIDE/HYDROCHLOROTHIAZIDE
Moduretic Tablets . . . 2138

MINOSTAD (Austria)
MINOCYCLINE HYDROCHLORIDE
Dynacin Capsules . . . 2019
Minocin Intravenous . . . 1862
Minocin Oral Suspension . . . 1865
Minocin Pellet-Filled Capsules . . . 1863

MINOTAB (Belgium, The Netherlands)
MINOCYCLINE HYDROCHLORIDE
Dynacin Capsules . . . 2019
Minocin Intravenous . . . 1862
Minocin Oral Suspension . . . 1865
Minocin Pellet-Filled Capsules . . . 1863

MINOTABS (New Zealand, South Africa)
MINOCYCLINE HYDROCHLORIDE
Dynacin Capsules . . . 2019
Minocin Intravenous . . . 1862
Minocin Oral Suspension . . . 1865
Minocin Pellet-Filled Capsules . . . 1863

MINOTREX (Portugal)
MINOCYCLINE HYDROCHLORIDE
Dynacin Capsules . . . 2019
Minocin Intravenous . . . 1862
Minocin Oral Suspension . . . 1865
Minocin Pellet-Filled Capsules . . . 1863

MINO-WOLFF (Germany)
MINOCYCLINE HYDROCHLORIDE
Dynacin Capsules . . . 2019
Minocin Intravenous . . . 1862
Minocin Oral Suspension . . . 1865
Minocin Pellet-Filled Capsules . . . 1863

MINPROG (Austria, Germany)
ALPROSTADIL
Caverject Sterile Powder . . . 2777
MUSE Urethral Suppository . . . 3335

MINPROSTIN (Denmark, Finland, Norway, Sweden)
DINOPROSTONE
Cervidil Vaginal Insert . . . 1369
Prepidil Gel . . . 2851
Prostin E2 Suppositories . . . 2852

MINPROSTIN E2 (Germany)
DINOPROSTONE
Cervidil Vaginal Insert . . . 1369
Prepidil Gel . . . 2851
Prostin E2 Suppositories . . . 2852

MINRIN (The Netherlands)
DESMOPRESSIN ACETATE
DDAVP Injection 4 mcg/mL . . . 737
DDAVP Nasal Spray . . . 738
DDAVP Rhinal Tube . . . 738
DDAVP Tablets . . . 739
Desmopressin Acetate Injection . . . 1344
Desmopressin Acetate Rhinal Tube . . . 1345
Stimate Nasal Spray . . . 796

MIO RELAX (Spain)
CARISOPRODOL
Soma Tablets . . . 3353

MIOCARPINE (Canada)
PILOCARPINE HYDROCHLORIDE
Isopto Carpine Ophthalmic Solution . . . ⊙215
Pilopine HS Ophthalmic Gel . . . ⊙217
Salagen Tablets . . . 2229

MIODARON (Brazil)
AMIODARONE HYDROCHLORIDE
Cordarone Intravenous . . . 3491
Cordarone Tablets . . . 3487
Pacerone Tablets . . . 3331

MIODRONE (Portugal)
AMIODARONE HYDROCHLORIDE
Cordarone Intravenous . . . 3491
Cordarone Tablets . . . 3487
Pacerone Tablets . . . 3331

MIOPOTASIO (Spain)
POTASSIUM CHLORIDE
K-Dur Microburst Release System ER Tablets . . . 1832
K-Lor Powder Packets . . . 469
K-Tab Filmtab Tablets . . . 470
Rum-K . . . 1363

MIOSEN (Spain)
DIPYRIDAMOLE
Persantine Tablets . . . 1057

MIOSTAT (Australia, Belgium, Canada, Hong Kong, Israel, New Zealand, Singapore, Switzerland, Thailand, The Netherlands)
CARBACHOL
Isopto Carbachol Ophthalmic Solution . . . ⊙215

MIOTICOL (Italy)
CARBACHOL
Isopto Carbachol Ophthalmic Solution . . . ⊙215

MIOWAS (Italy, Spain)
METHOCARBAMOL
Robaxin Injectable . . . 2938
Robaxin Tablets . . . 2939
Robaxin-750 Tablets . . . 2939

MI-PILO (Israel)
PILOCARPINE HYDROCHLORIDE
Isopto Carpine Ophthalmic Solution . . . ⊙215
Pilopine HS Ophthalmic Gel . . . ⊙217
Salagen Tablets . . . 2229

MIPRAZ (Australia)
PRAZOSIN HYDROCHLORIDE
Minipress Capsules . . . 2699

MIR (Israel)
MORPHINE SULFATE
Astramorph/PF Injection, USP (Preservative-Free) . . . 594
Duramorph Injection . . . 1312
Infumorph 200 and Infumorph 500 Sterile Solutions . . . 1314
Kadian Capsules . . . 1335
MS Contin Tablets . . . 2896
MSIR Oral Capsules . . . 2898
MSIR Oral Solution . . . 2898
MSIR Oral Solution Concentrate . . . 2898
MSIR Oral Tablets . . . 2898
Oramorph SR Tablets . . . 3062
Roxanol 100 Concentrated Oral Solution . . . 3066
Roxanol Concentrated Oral Solution . . . 3066
Roxanol-T Oral Solution . . . 3066

MIRACID (Thailand)
OMEPRAZOLE
Prilosec Delayed-Release Capsules . . . 628

MIRACLAR (Spain)
NAPHAZOLINE HYDROCHLORIDE
Albalon Ophthalmic Solution . . . ⊙225

MIRACLIN (Italy)
DOXYCYCLINE HYCLATE
Doryx Coated Pellet Filled Capsules . . . 3357
Periostat Tablets . . . 1208
Vibramycin Hyclate Capsules . . . 2735
Vibramycin Hyclate Intravenous . . . 2737
Vibra-Tabs Film Coated Tablets . . . 2735

MIRAMYCIN (Hong Kong, Singapore, Thailand)
GENTAMICIN SULFATE
Genoptic Ophthalmic Ointment . . . ⊙239

(⊙ Described in PDR For Ophthalmic Medicines™)

Genoptic Sterile Ophthalmic Solution . . . ⊙239

MIRANAX (Austria, Denmark, Finland, Sweden)
NAPROXEN SODIUM
Anaprox DS Tablets . . . 2967
Anaprox Tablets . . . 2967
Naprelan Tablets . . . 1293

MIRENA (Austria, Belgium, France, Germany, Hong Kong, Irish Republic, Italy, New Zealand, Portugal, Singapore, South Africa, Switzerland, The Netherlands, United Kingdom)
LEVONORGESTREL
Norplant System . . . 3543

MIRETIC (Thailand)
AMILORIDE HYDROCHLORIDE/HYDROCHLOROTHIAZIDE
Moduretic Tablets . . . 2138

MIRFAT (Germany)
CLONIDINE HYDROCHLORIDE
Catapres Tablets . . . 1037
Duraclon Injection . . . 3057

MISODEX (Italy)
MISOPROSTOL
Cytotec Tablets . . . 3202

MISOFENAC (Italy)
DICLOFENAC SODIUM
Voltaren Tablets . . . 2315
Voltaren-XR Tablets . . . 2315

MISULBAN (Italy, Monaco)
BUSULFAN
Myleran Tablets . . . 1603

MITALOLO (Italy)
LABETALOL HYDROCHLORIDE
Normodyne Injection . . . 3135
Normodyne Tablets . . . 3137

MITE-X (Israel)
PERMETHRIN
Acticin Cream . . . 998
Elimite Cream . . . 552

MITHRACIN (Australia, Norway, The Netherlands, United Kingdom)
PLICAMYCIN
Mithracin for Intravenous Use . . . 903

MITHRACINE (France, Switzerland)
PLICAMYCIN
Mithracin for Intravenous Use . . . 903

MITIL (South Africa)
PROCHLORPERAZINE MALEATE
Compazine Spansule Capsules . . . 1505
Compazine Tablets . . . 1505

MITOCORTYL (France)
HYDROCORTISONE
Anusol-HC Cream 2.5% . . . 2237
Hydrocortone Tablets . . . 2106

MITOXANA (United Kingdom)
IFOSFAMIDE
Ifex for Injection . . . 1123

MITROKEN (Mexico)
CIPROFLOXACIN HYDROCHLORIDE
Ciloxan Ophthalmic Ointment . . . 538
Ciloxan Ophthalmic Solution . . . ⊙209, 538
Cipro Tablets . . . 887

MIXER (Italy)
ATENOLOL
Tenormin I.V. Injection . . . 692

MIZOLMEX (Mexico)
MEBENDAZOLE
Vermox Chewable Tablets . . . 2017

M-LONG (Germany)
MORPHINE SULFATE
Astramorph/PF Injection, USP (Preservative-Free) . . . 594
Duramorph Injection . . . 1312
Infumorph 200 and Infumorph 500 Sterile Solutions . . . 1314
Kadian Capsules . . . 1335
MS Contin Tablets . . . 2896
MSIR Oral Capsules . . . 2898
MSIR Oral Solution . . . 2898
MSIR Oral Solution Concentrate . . . 2898
MSIR Oral Tablets . . . 2898
Oramorph SR Tablets . . . 3062
Roxanol 100 Concentrated Oral Solution . . . 3066
Roxanol Concentrated Oral Solution . . . 3066
Roxanol-T Oral Solution . . . 3066

MND (Singapore)
METRONIDAZOLE
MetroCream . . . 1404
MetroGel . . . 1405
MetroGel-Vaginal Gel . . . 1986
MetroLotion . . . 1405
Noritate Cream . . . 1224

MOBAN (Hong Kong)
MOLINDONE HYDROCHLORIDE
Moban Oral Concentrate . . . 1320
Moban Tablets . . . 1320

MOBEN (Brazil)
MEBENDAZOLE
Vermox Chewable Tablets . . . 2017

MOBILAT (Germany)
IBUPROFEN
Motrin Suspension, Oral Drops, Chewable Tablets, and Caplets . . . 2002

MOBILIS (Australia)
PIROXICAM
Feldene Capsules . . . 2685

MODALINA (Italy)
TRIFLUOPERAZINE HYDROCHLORIDE
Stelazine Injection . . . 1640
Stelazine Tablets . . . 1640

MODAMIDE (France)
AMILORIDE HYDROCHLORIDE
Midamor Tablets . . . 2136

MODAPLATE (United Kingdom)
DIPYRIDAMOLE
Persantine Tablets . . . 1057

MODASOMIL (Austria)
MODAFINIL
Provigil Tablets . . . 1193

MODIFENAC (Denmark, Norway)
DICLOFENAC SODIUM
Voltaren Tablets . . . 2315
Voltaren-XR Tablets . . . 2315

MODIFICAL (Brazil)
ONDANSETRON HYDROCHLORIDE
Zofran Injection . . . 1698
Zofran Injection Premixed . . . 1698
Zofran Oral Solution . . . 1703
Zofran Tablets . . . 1703

MODINA (Portugal)
NIMODIPINE
Nimotop Capsules . . . 904

MODIODAL (Denmark, France, Portugal, Spain, The Netherlands)
MODAFINIL
Provigil Tablets . . . 1193

MODISAL (United Kingdom)
ISOSORBIDE MONONITRATE
Imdur Tablets . . . 1826
Ismo Tablets . . . 3524

MODISAL (Switzerland)
AMILORIDE HYDROCHLORIDE/HYDROCHLOROTHIAZIDE
Moduretic Tablets . . . 2138

MODIZIDE (Australia)
AMILORIDE HYDROCHLORIDE/HYDROCHLOROTHIAZIDE
Moduretic Tablets . . . 2138

MODRADERM (Belgium)
ALCLOMETASONE DIPROPIONATE
Aclovate Cream . . . 1275
Aclovate Ointment . . . 1275

MODRASONE (Irish Republic, United Kingdom)
ALCLOMETASONE DIPROPIONATE
Aclovate Cream . . . 1275
Aclovate Ointment . . . 1275

MODUCREN (United Kingdom)
AMILORIDE HYDROCHLORIDE/HYDROCHLOROTHIAZIDE
Moduretic Tablets . . . 2138

MODU-PUREN (Germany)
AMILORIDE HYDROCHLORIDE/HYDROCHLOROTHIAZIDE
Moduretic Tablets . . . 2138

MODURET (Canada, Irish Republic, United Kingdom)
AMILORIDE HYDROCHLORIDE/HYDROCHLOROTHIAZIDE
Moduretic Tablets . . . 2138

MODURETIC (Australia, Austria, Belgium, Brazil, Denmark, Finland, France, Hong Kong, Irish Republic, Italy, Mexico, New Zealand, Portugal, South Africa, Sweden, Switzerland, Thailand, The Netherlands, United Kingdom)
AMILORIDE HYDROCHLORIDE/HYDROCHLOROTHIAZIDE
Moduretic Tablets . . . 2138

MODURETIC MITE (Norway)
AMILORIDE HYDROCHLORIDE/HYDROCHLOROTHIAZIDE
Moduretic Tablets . . . 2138

MODURETIK (Germany)
AMILORIDE HYDROCHLORIDE/HYDROCHLOROTHIAZIDE
Moduretic Tablets . . . 2138

MODUS (Spain)
NIMODIPINE
Nimotop Capsules . . . 904

MOEX (Denmark, France)
MOEXIPRIL HYDROCHLORIDE
Univasc Tablets . . . 3181

MOGETIC (Germany)
MORPHINE SULFATE
Astramorph/PF Injection, USP (Preservative-Free) . . . 594
Duramorph Injection . . . 1312
Infumorph 200 and Infumorph 500 Sterile Solutions . . . 1314
Kadian Capsules . . . 1335
MS Contin Tablets . . . 2896
MSIR Oral Capsules . . . 2898
MSIR Oral Solution . . . 2898
MSIR Oral Solution Concentrate . . . 2898
MSIR Oral Tablets . . . 2898
Oramorph SR Tablets . . . 3062
Roxanol 100 Concentrated Oral Solution . . . 3066
Roxanol Concentrated Oral Solution . . . 3066
Roxanol-T Oral Solution . . . 3066

MOMENDOL (Italy)
NAPROXEN SODIUM
Anaprox DS Tablets . . . 2967
Anaprox Tablets . . . 2967
Naprelan Tablets . . . 1293

MOMENT (Italy)
IBUPROFEN
Motrin Suspension, Oral Drops, Chewable Tablets, and Caplets . . . 2002

MONASIN (Switzerland)
METRONIDAZOLE
MetroCream . . . 1404
MetroGel . . . 1405
MetroGel-Vaginal Gel . . . 1986
MetroLotion . . . 1405
Noritate Cream . . . 1224

MONAXIN (Belgium)
CLARITHROMYCIN
Biaxin Filmtab Tablets . . . 403
Biaxin for Oral Suspension . . . 403

MONICOR (France)
ISOSORBIDE MONONITRATE
Imdur Tablets . . . 1826
Ismo Tablets . . . 3524

MONILAC (Japan)
LACTULOSE
Kristalose for Oral Solution . . . 1007

MONIT (United Kingdom)
ISOSORBIDE MONONITRATE
Imdur Tablets . . . 1826
Ismo Tablets . . . 3524

MONITAN (Canada)
ACEBUTOLOL HYDROCHLORIDE
Sectral Capsules . . . 3589

MONIT-PUREN (Germany)
ISOSORBIDE MONONITRATE
Imdur Tablets . . . 1826
Ismo Tablets . . . 3524

MONO BAYCUTEN (Germany)
CLOTRIMAZOLE
Lotrimin Cream 1% . . . 3128
Lotrimin Lotion 1% . . . 3128
Lotrimin Topical Solution 1% . . . 3128
Mycelex Troche . . . 573

MONO CORAX (Germany)
ISOSORBIDE MONONITRATE
Imdur Tablets . . . 1826
Ismo Tablets . . . 3524

MONO MACK (Austria, Germany, Hong Kong, Mexico, Singapore, South Africa, Thailand, The Netherlands)
ISOSORBIDE MONONITRATE
Imdur Tablets . . . 1826
Ismo Tablets . . . 3524

MONO WOLFF (Germany)
ISOSORBIDE MONONITRATE
Imdur Tablets . . . 1826
Ismo Tablets . . . 3524

MONOBAC (Mexico)
AZTREONAM
Azactam for Injection . . . 1276

MONOBETA (Germany)
ISOSORBIDE MONONITRATE
Imdur Tablets . . . 1826
Ismo Tablets . . . 3524

MONO-CEDOCARD (The Netherlands, United Kingdom)
ISOSORBIDE MONONITRATE
Imdur Tablets . . . 1826
Ismo Tablets . . . 3524

MONOCINQUE (Hong Kong, Italy)
ISOSORBIDE MONONITRATE
Imdur Tablets . . . 1826
Ismo Tablets . . . 3524

MONOCLAIR (Germany)
ISOSORBIDE MONONITRATE
Imdur Tablets . . . 1826
Ismo Tablets . . . 3524

MONOCLINE (France)
DOXYCYCLINE HYCLATE
Doryx Coated Pellet Filled Capsules . . . 3357
Periostat Tablets . . . 1208
Vibramycin Hyclate Capsules . . . 2735
Vibramycin Hyclate Intravenous . . . 2737
Vibra-Tabs Film Coated Tablets . . . 2735

MONOCOR (Denmark, United Kingdom)
BISOPROLOL FUMARATE
Zebeta Tablets . . . 1885

MONOCORD (Israel)
ISOSORBIDE MONONITRATE
Imdur Tablets . . . 1826
Ismo Tablets . . . 3524

MONOCORDIL (Brazil)
ISOSORBIDE MONONITRATE
Imdur Tablets . . . 1826
Ismo Tablets . . . 3524

MONODOXIN (Italy)
DOXYCYCLINE HYCLATE
Doryx Coated Pellet Filled Capsules . . . 3357
Periostat Tablets . . . 1208
Vibramycin Hyclate Capsules . . . 2735
Vibramycin Hyclate Intravenous . . . 2737
Vibra-Tabs Film Coated Tablets . . . 2735

MONODUR (Australia)
ISOSORBIDE MONONITRATE
Imdur Tablets . . . 1826
Ismo Tablets . . . 3524

MONOFLAM (Germany)
DICLOFENAC SODIUM
Voltaren Tablets . . . 2315
Voltaren-XR Tablets . . . 2315

MONOFLOCET (France)
OFLOXACIN
Floxin I.V. . . . 2526
Floxin Otic Solution . . . 1219
Floxin Tablets . . . 2529
Ocuflox Ophthalmic Solution . . . 554

MONO-JOD (Germany)
POTASSIUM IODIDE
Pima Syrup . . . 1362

MONOKET (Austria, Italy, Norway, Portugal, Sweden)
ISOSORBIDE MONONITRATE
Imdur Tablets . . . 1826
Ismo Tablets . . . 3524

MONOLIN (Thailand)
ISOSORBIDE MONONITRATE
Imdur Tablets . . . 1826
Ismo Tablets . . . 3524

MONOLITUM (Spain)
LANSOPRAZOLE
Prevacid Delayed-Release Capsules . . . 3292

MONOLONG (Germany, Israel)
ISOSORBIDE MONONITRATE
Imdur Tablets . . . 1826
Ismo Tablets . . . 3524

MONOMAX (United Kingdom)
ISOSORBIDE MONONITRATE
Imdur Tablets . . . 1826
Ismo Tablets . . . 3524

MONONIT (Israel)
ISOSORBIDE MONONITRATE
Imdur Tablets . . . 1826
Ismo Tablets . . . 3524

MONONITRAT (Germany)
ISOSORBIDE MONONITRATE
Imdur Tablets . . . 1826
Ismo Tablets . . . 3524

MONONITRIL (Portugal)
ISOSORBIDE MONONITRATE
Imdur Tablets . . . 1826
Ismo Tablets . . . 3524

MONOPARIN (Irish Republic, New Zealand)
HEPARIN SODIUM
Heparin Lock Flush Solution . . . 3509
Heparin Sodium Injection . . . 3511

MONOPRIL (Australia, Brazil, Canada, Denmark, Hong Kong, Mexico, Norway, Singapore, South Africa, Sweden, Thailand)
FOSINOPRIL SODIUM
Monopril Tablets . . . 1091

MONOPRONT (Portugal)
ISOSORBIDE MONONITRATE
- Imdur Tablets 1826
- Ismo Tablets 3524

MONOPUR (Germany)
ISOSORBIDE MONONITRATE
- Imdur Tablets 1826
- Ismo Tablets 3524

MONOSORB (France, United Kingdom)
ISOSORBIDE MONONITRATE
- Imdur Tablets 1826
- Ismo Tablets 3524

MONOSTENASE (Germany)
ISOSORBIDE MONONITRATE
- Imdur Tablets 1826
- Ismo Tablets 3524

MONO-TILDIEM (France, Singapore, Thailand)
DILTIAZEM HYDROCHLORIDE
- Cardizem CD Capsules 1016
- Cardizem Injectable 1018
- Cardizem Lyo-Ject Syringe 1018
- Cardizem Monovial 1018
- Tiazac Capsules 1378

MONOTRATE (Singapore, Thailand)
ISOSORBIDE MONONITRATE
- Imdur Tablets 1826
- Ismo Tablets 3524

MONOVENT (United Kingdom)
TERBUTALINE SULFATE
- Brethine Ampuls 2314
- Brethine Tablets 2313

MONOZIDE (United Kingdom)
BISOPROLOL FUMARATE/HYDROCHLOROTHIAZIDE
- Ziac Tablets 1887

MONTEGEN (Italy)
MONTELUKAST SODIUM
- Singulair Chewable Tablets 2181
- Singulair Tablets 2181

MOPSORALEN (Belgium)
METHOXSALEN
- 8-MOP Capsules 1727
- Oxsoralen Lotion 1% 1740
- Oxsoralen-Ultra Capsules 1741

MORADORM-A (Germany)
DIPHENHYDRAMINE HYDROCHLORIDE
- Benadryl Parenteral 2617

MORAPID (Austria)
MORPHINE SULFATE
- Astramorph/PF Injection, USP (Preservative-Free) 594
- Duramorph Injection 1312
- Infumorph 200 and Infumorph 500 Sterile Solutions 1314
- Kadian Capsules 1335
- MS Contin Tablets 2896
- MSIR Oral Capsules 2898
- MSIR Oral Solution 2898
- MSIR Oral Solution Concentrate 2898
- MSIR Oral Tablets 2898
- Oramorph SR Tablets 3062
- Roxanol 100 Concentrated Oral Solution 3066
- Roxanol Concentrated Oral Solution 3066
- Roxanol-T Oral Solution 3066

MORAXEN (United Kingdom)
MORPHINE SULFATE
- Astramorph/PF Injection, USP (Preservative-Free) 594
- Duramorph Injection 1312
- Infumorph 200 and Infumorph 500 Sterile Solutions 1314
- Kadian Capsules 1335
- MS Contin Tablets 2896
- MSIR Oral Capsules 2898
- MSIR Oral Solution 2898
- MSIR Oral Solution Concentrate 2898
- MSIR Oral Tablets 2898
- Oramorph SR Tablets 3062
- Roxanol 100 Concentrated Oral Solution 3066
- Roxanol Concentrated Oral Solution 3066
- Roxanol-T Oral Solution 3066

MORCAP (United Kingdom)
MORPHINE SULFATE
- Astramorph/PF Injection, USP (Preservative-Free) 594
- Duramorph Injection 1312
- Infumorph 200 and Infumorph 500 Sterile Solutions 1314
- Kadian Capsules 1335
- MS Contin Tablets 2896
- MSIR Oral Capsules 2898
- MSIR Oral Solution 2898
- MSIR Oral Solution Concentrate 2898
- MSIR Oral Tablets 2898
- Oramorph SR Tablets 3062
- Roxanol 100 Concentrated Oral Solution 3066
- Roxanol Concentrated Oral Solution 3066
- Roxanol-T Oral Solution 3066

MORONAL (Germany)
NYSTATIN
- Nystop Topical Powder USP 2608

MORSTEL (Irish Republic)
MORPHINE SULFATE
- Astramorph/PF Injection, USP (Preservative-Free) 594
- Duramorph Injection 1312
- Infumorph 200 and Infumorph 500 Sterile Solutions 1314
- Kadian Capsules 1335
- MS Contin Tablets 2896
- MSIR Oral Capsules 2898
- MSIR Oral Solution 2898
- MSIR Oral Solution Concentrate 2898
- MSIR Oral Tablets 2898
- Oramorph SR Tablets 3062
- Roxanol 100 Concentrated Oral Solution 3066
- Roxanol Concentrated Oral Solution 3066
- Roxanol-T Oral Solution 3066

MOSCONTIN (France)
MORPHINE SULFATE
- Astramorph/PF Injection, USP (Preservative-Free) 594
- Duramorph Injection 1312
- Infumorph 200 and Infumorph 500 Sterile Solutions 1314
- Kadian Capsules 1335
- MS Contin Tablets 2896
- MSIR Oral Capsules 2898
- MSIR Oral Solution 2898
- MSIR Oral Solution Concentrate 2898
- MSIR Oral Tablets 2898
- Oramorph SR Tablets 3062
- Roxanol 100 Concentrated Oral Solution 3066
- Roxanol Concentrated Oral Solution 3066
- Roxanol-T Oral Solution 3066

MOSKIZOL (France)
PERMETHRIN
- Acticin Cream 998
- Elimite Cream 552

MOTIAX (Italy)
FAMOTIDINE
- Pepcid Injection 2153
- Pepcid Injection Premixed 2153
- Pepcid RPD Orally Disintegrating Tablets 2150
- Pepcid Tablets 2150
- Pepcid for Oral Suspension 2150

MOTIDINE (Singapore, Thailand)
FAMOTIDINE
- Pepcid Injection 2153
- Pepcid Injection Premixed 2153
- Pepcid RPD Orally Disintegrating Tablets 2150
- Pepcid Tablets 2150
- Pepcid for Oral Suspension 2150

MOTIFENE (Belgium, Finland, United Kingdom)
DICLOFENAC SODIUM
- Voltaren Tablets 2316
- Voltaren-XR Tablets 2315

MOTIVAN (Spain)
PAROXETINE HYDROCHLORIDE
- Paxil Oral Suspension 1609
- Paxil Tablets 1609

MOTRIN (Belgium, Brazil, Canada, Mexico, Portugal, Switzerland, United Kingdom)
IBUPROFEN
- Motrin Suspension, Oral Drops, Chewable Tablets, and Caplets 2002

MOVERGAN (Germany)
SELEGILINE HYDROCHLORIDE
- Eldepryl Capsules 3266

MOVIN (Portugal)
TICLOPIDINE HYDROCHLORIDE
- Ticlid Tablets 3015

MOXACEF (Belgium, The Netherlands)
CEFADROXIL
- Duricef Capsules 1079
- Duricef Oral Suspension 1079
- Duricef Tablets 1079

MOXADENT (Portugal)
AMOXICILLIN
- Amoxil Pediatric Drops for Oral Suspension 1471
- Amoxil Tablets 1471

MOXAN (South Africa)
AMOXICILLIN
- Amoxil Pediatric Drops for Oral Suspension 1471
- Amoxil Tablets 1471

MOXICEL (Mexico)
AMOXICILLIN
- Amoxil Pediatric Drops for Oral Suspension 1471
- Amoxil Tablets 1471

MOXIPEN (Portugal, Singapore)
AMOXICILLIN
- Amoxil Pediatric Drops for Oral Suspension 1471
- Amoxil Tablets 1471

MOXYMAX (South Africa)
AMOXICILLIN
- Amoxil Pediatric Drops for Oral Suspension 1471
- Amoxil Tablets 1471

MPA (Germany)
MEDROXYPROGESTERONE ACETATE
- Depo-Provera Contraceptive Injection 2798
- Provera Tablets 2853

MPA GYN (Germany)
MEDROXYPROGESTERONE ACETATE
- Depo-Provera Contraceptive Injection 2798
- Provera Tablets 2853

MPA-BETA (Germany)
MEDROXYPROGESTERONE ACETATE
- Depo-Provera Contraceptive Injection 2798
- Provera Tablets 2853

MPA-NOURY (Germany)
MEDROXYPROGESTERONE ACETATE
- Depo-Provera Contraceptive Injection 2798
- Provera Tablets 2853

MS CONTIN (Australia, Belgium, Canada, Italy, The Netherlands)
MORPHINE SULFATE
- Astramorph/PF Injection, USP (Preservative-Free) 594
- Duramorph Injection 1312
- Infumorph 200 and Infumorph 500 Sterile Solutions 1314
- Kadian Capsules 1335
- MS Contin Tablets 2896
- MSIR Oral Capsules 2898
- MSIR Oral Solution 2898
- MSIR Oral Solution Concentrate 2898
- MSIR Oral Tablets 2898
- Oramorph SR Tablets 3062
- Roxanol 100 Concentrated Oral Solution 3066
- Roxanol Concentrated Oral Solution 3066
- Roxanol-T Oral Solution 3066

MS DIRECT (Belgium)
MORPHINE SULFATE
- Astramorph/PF Injection, USP (Preservative-Free) 594
- Duramorph Injection 1312
- Infumorph 200 and Infumorph 500 Sterile Solutions 1314
- Kadian Capsules 1335
- MS Contin Tablets 2896
- MSIR Oral Capsules 2898
- MSIR Oral Solution 2898
- MSIR Oral Solution Concentrate 2898
- MSIR Oral Tablets 2898
- Oramorph SR Tablets 3062
- Roxanol 100 Concentrated Oral Solution 3066
- Roxanol Concentrated Oral Solution 3066
- Roxanol-T Oral Solution 3066

MS MONO (Australia)
MORPHINE SULFATE
- Astramorph/PF Injection, USP (Preservative-Free) 594
- Duramorph Injection 1312
- Infumorph 200 and Infumorph 500 Sterile Solutions 1314
- Kadian Capsules 1335
- MS Contin Tablets 2896
- MSIR Oral Capsules 2898
- MSIR Oral Solution 2898
- MSIR Oral Solution Concentrate 2898
- MSIR Oral Tablets 2898
- Oramorph SR Tablets 3062
- Roxanol 100 Concentrated Oral Solution 3066
- Roxanol Concentrated Oral Solution 3066
- Roxanol-T Oral Solution 3066

MSI (Germany)
MORPHINE SULFATE
- Astramorph/PF Injection, USP (Preservative-Free) 594
- Duramorph Injection 1312
- Infumorph 200 and Infumorph 500 Sterile Solutions 1314
- Kadian Capsules 1335
- MS Contin Tablets 2896
- MSIR Oral Capsules 2898
- MSIR Oral Solution 2898
- MSIR Oral Solution Concentrate 2898
- MSIR Oral Tablets 2898
- Oramorph SR Tablets 3062
- Roxanol 100 Concentrated Oral Solution 3066
- Roxanol Concentrated Oral Solution 3066
- Roxanol-T Oral Solution 3066

MSIR (Canada)
MORPHINE SULFATE
- Astramorph/PF Injection, USP (Preservative-Free) 594
- Duramorph Injection 1312
- Infumorph 200 and Infumorph 500 Sterile Solutions 1314
- Kadian Capsules 1335
- MS Contin Tablets 2896
- MSIR Oral Capsules 2898
- MSIR Oral Solution 2898
- MSIR Oral Solution Concentrate 2898
- MSIR Oral Tablets 2898
- Oramorph SR Tablets 3062
- Roxanol 100 Concentrated Oral Solution 3066
- Roxanol Concentrated Oral Solution 3066
- Roxanol-T Oral Solution 3066

MS-LONG (Brazil)
MORPHINE SULFATE
- Astramorph/PF Injection, USP (Preservative-Free) 594
- Duramorph Injection 1312
- Infumorph 200 and Infumorph 500 Sterile Solutions 1314
- Kadian Capsules 1335
- MS Contin Tablets 2896
- MSIR Oral Capsules 2898
- MSIR Oral Solution 2898
- MSIR Oral Solution Concentrate 2898
- MSIR Oral Tablets 2898
- Oramorph SR Tablets 3062
- Roxanol 100 Concentrated Oral Solution 3066
- Roxanol Concentrated Oral Solution 3066
- Roxanol-T Oral Solution 3066

MSP (Israel)
MORPHINE SULFATE
- Astramorph/PF Injection, USP (Preservative-Free) 594
- Duramorph Injection 1312
- Infumorph 200 and Infumorph 500 Sterile Solutions 1314
- Kadian Capsules 1335
- MS Contin Tablets 2896
- MSIR Oral Capsules 2898
- MSIR Oral Solution 2898
- MSIR Oral Solution Concentrate 2898
- MSIR Oral Tablets 2898
- Oramorph SR Tablets 3062
- Roxanol 100 Concentrated Oral Solution 3066
- Roxanol Concentrated Oral Solution 3066
- Roxanol-T Oral Solution 3066

MSR (Germany)
MORPHINE SULFATE
- Astramorph/PF Injection, USP (Preservative-Free) 594
- Duramorph Injection 1312
- Infumorph 200 and Infumorph 500 Sterile Solutions 1314
- Kadian Capsules 1335
- MS Contin Tablets 2896
- MSIR Oral Capsules 2898
- MSIR Oral Solution 2898
- MSIR Oral Solution Concentrate 2898
- MSIR Oral Tablets 2898
- Oramorph SR Tablets 3062
- Roxanol 100 Concentrated Oral Solution 3066
- Roxanol Concentrated Oral Solution 3066
- Roxanol-T Oral Solution 3066

MST (Portugal)
MORPHINE SULFATE
- Astramorph/PF Injection, USP (Preservative-Free) 594
- Duramorph Injection 1312
- Infumorph 200 and Infumorph 500 Sterile Solutions 1314
- Kadian Capsules 1335
- MS Contin Tablets 2896
- MSIR Oral Capsules 2898
- MSIR Oral Solution 2898
- MSIR Oral Solution Concentrate 2898
- MSIR Oral Tablets 2898
- Oramorph SR Tablets 3062
- Roxanol 100 Concentrated Oral Solution 3066
- Roxanol Concentrated Oral Solution 3066
- Roxanol-T Oral Solution 3066

MST CONTINUS (Brazil, Hong Kong, Irish Republic, Mexico, New Zealand, Singapore, South Africa, Spain, Switzerland, United Kingdom)
MORPHINE SULFATE
- Astramorph/PF Injection, USP (Preservative-Free) 594
- Duramorph Injection 1312

Infumorph 200 and Infumorph 500 Sterile Solutions 1314
Kadian Capsules 1335
MS Contin Tablets 2896
MSIR Oral Capsules 2898
MSIR Oral Solution 2898
MSIR Oral Solution Concentrate 2898
MSIR Oral Tablets 2898
Oramorph SR Tablets 3062
Roxanol 100 Concentrated Oral Solution 3066
Roxanol Concentrated Oral Solution 3066
Roxanol-T Oral Solution 3066

MUCLOX (Spain)
FAMOTIDINE
Pepcid Injection 2153
Pepcid Injection Premixed 2153
Pepcid RPD Orally Disintegrating Tablets 2150
Pepcid Tablets 2150
Pepcid for Oral Suspension 2150

MULTILIND (United Kingdom)
NYSTATIN
Nystop Topical Powder USP 2608

MULTIPARIN (Irish Republic, New Zealand, United Kingdom)
HEPARIN SODIUM
Heparin Lock Flush Solution 3509
Heparin Sodium Injection 3511

MULTIPAX (Canada)
HYDROXYZINE HYDROCHLORIDE
Atarax Tablets & Syrup 2667
Vistaril Intramuscular Solution 2738

MUNDIDOL (Austria)
MORPHINE SULFATE
Astramorph/PF Injection, USP (Preservative-Free) 594
Duramorph Injection 1312
Infumorph 200 and Infumorph 500 Sterile Solutions 1314
Kadian Capsules 1335
MS Contin Tablets 2896
MSIR Oral Capsules 2898
MSIR Oral Solution 2898
MSIR Oral Solution Concentrate 2898
MSIR Oral Tablets 2898
Oramorph SR Tablets 3062
Roxanol 100 Concentrated Oral Solution 3066
Roxanol Concentrated Oral Solution 3066
Roxanol-T Oral Solution 3066

MUNDIL (Germany)
CAPTOPRIL
Captopril Tablets 2281

MUNITREN H (Germany)
HYDROCORTISONE
Anusol-HC Cream 2.5% 2237
Hydrocortone Tablets 2106

MUNOBAL (Austria, Germany, Mexico, Switzerland)
FELODIPINE
Plendil Extended-Release Tablets 623

MUPIDERM (France)
MUPIROCIN
Bactroban Ointment 1496

MURINE (United Kingdom)
NAPHAZOLINE HYDROCHLORIDE
Albalon Ophthalmic Solution ⊙225

MURINE (Portugal)
NAPHAZOLINE HYDROCHLORIDE
Albalon Ophthalmic Solution ⊙225

MURINE CLEAR EYES (South Africa)
NAPHAZOLINE HYDROCHLORIDE
Albalon Ophthalmic Solution ⊙225

MURODE (Spain)
DIFLORASONE DIACETATE
Psorcon E Cream 1227
Psorcon E Ointment 1228

MUSCARAN (Belgium)
BETHANECHOL CHLORIDE
Urecholine Injection 2198
Urecholine Tablets 2198

MUSE (Australia, Austria, Canada, Denmark, Finland, Germany, Hong Kong, Irish Republic, Israel, Mexico, New Zealand, Singapore, South Africa, Spain, Switzerland, Thailand, United Kingdom)
ALPROSTADIL
Caverject Sterile Powder 2777
MUSE Urethral Suppository 3335

MUSSIDE (Portugal)
LINDANE
Lindane Lotion USP 1% 559
Lindane Shampoo USP 1% 560

MUSXAN (Thailand)
METHOCARBAMOL
Robaxin Injectable 2938
Robaxin Tablets 2939
Robaxin-750 Tablets 2939

MUTABON D (Australia)
AMITRIPTYLINE HYDROCHLORIDE/PERPHENAZINE
Etrafon 2-10 Tablets (2-10) 3115
Etrafon Tablets (2-25) 3115
Etrafon-Forte Tablets (4-25) 3115

MXL (Irish Republic, United Kingdom)
MORPHINE SULFATE
Astramorph/PF Injection, USP (Preservative-Free) 594
Duramorph Injection 1312
Infumorph 200 and Infumorph 500 Sterile Solutions 1314
Kadian Capsules 1335
MS Contin Tablets 2896
MSIR Oral Capsules 2898
MSIR Oral Solution 2898
MSIR Oral Solution Concentrate 2898
MSIR Oral Tablets 2898
Oramorph SR Tablets 3062
Roxanol 100 Concentrated Oral Solution 3066
Roxanol Concentrated Oral Solution 3066
Roxanol-T Oral Solution 3066

MYAMBUTOL (Australia, Austria, Belgium, Canada, Denmark, France, Germany, Hong Kong, Irish Republic, Israel, Mexico, New Zealand, South Africa, Spain, Sweden, Switzerland, Thailand, The Netherlands, United Kingdom)
ETHAMBUTOL HYDROCHLORIDE
Myambutol Tablets 1290

MYCELLA (Thailand)
KETOCONAZOLE
Nizoral 2% Cream 3620
Nizoral 2% Shampoo 2007
Nizoral Tablets 1791

MYCETIN (Italy)
CHLORAMPHENICOL
Chloromycetin Ophthalmic Ointment, 1% ⊙296
Chloromycetin Ophthalmic Solution ⊙297
Chloroptic Sterile Ophthalmic Ointment ⊙234
Chloroptic Sterile Ophthalmic Solution ⊙235

MYCIL GOLD (United Kingdom)
CLOTRIMAZOLE
Lotrimin Cream 1% 3128
Lotrimin Lotion 1% 3128
Lotrimin Topical Solution 1% 3128
Mycelex Troche 573

MYCINOPRED (Switzerland)
NEOMYCIN SULFATE/POLYMYXIN B SULFATE/PREDNISOLONE ACETATE
Poly-Pred Liquifilm Ophthalmic Suspension ⊙245

MYCLO-DERM (Canada)
CLOTRIMAZOLE
Lotrimin Cream 1% 3128
Lotrimin Lotion 1% 3128
Lotrimin Topical Solution 1% 3128
Mycelex Troche 573

MYCLO-GYNE (Canada)
CLOTRIMAZOLE
Lotrimin Cream 1% 3128
Lotrimin Lotion 1% 3128
Lotrimin Topical Solution 1% 3128
Mycelex Troche 573

MYCOBAN (South Africa)
CLOTRIMAZOLE
Lotrimin Cream 1% 3128
Lotrimin Lotion 1% 3128
Lotrimin Topical Solution 1% 3128
Mycelex Troche 573

MYCOBUTIN (Australia, Austria, Belgium, Canada, Germany, Hong Kong, Israel, Italy, New Zealand, Portugal, South Africa, Switzerland, The Netherlands, United Kingdom)
RIFABUTIN
Mycobutin Capsules 2838

MYCODIB (Mexico)
KETOCONAZOLE
Nizoral 2% Cream 3620
Nizoral 2% Shampoo 2007
Nizoral Tablets 1791

MYCOFUG (Austria, Germany)
CLOTRIMAZOLE
Lotrimin Cream 1% 3128
Lotrimin Lotion 1% 3128
Lotrimin Topical Solution 1% 3128
Mycelex Troche 573

MYCOHAUG C (Germany)
CLOTRIMAZOLE
Lotrimin Cream 1% 3128
Lotrimin Lotion 1% 3128
Lotrimin Topical Solution 1% 3128
Mycelex Troche 573

MYCO-HERMAL (Israel, Singapore)
CLOTRIMAZOLE
Lotrimin Cream 1% 3128
Lotrimin Lotion 1% 3128
Lotrimin Topical Solution 1% 3128
Mycelex Troche 573

MYCOHEXAL (South Africa)
CLOTRIMAZOLE
Lotrimin Cream 1% 3128
Lotrimin Lotion 1% 3128
Lotrimin Topical Solution 1% 3128
Mycelex Troche 573

MYCO-INTRADERMI (Germany)
NYSTATIN
Nystop Topical Powder USP 2608

MYCORAL (Singapore)
KETOCONAZOLE
Nizoral 2% Cream 3620
Nizoral 2% Shampoo 2007
Nizoral Tablets 1791

MYCOSTATIN (Australia, Austria, Canada, Denmark, Finland, Hong Kong, Irish Republic, Italy, New Zealand, Norway, Portugal, Singapore, South Africa, Spain, Sweden, Thailand)
NYSTATIN
Nystop Topical Powder USP 2608

MYCOSTATINE (France, Switzerland)
NYSTATIN
Nystop Topical Powder USP 2608

MYCROL (South Africa)
ETHAMBUTOL HYDROCHLORIDE
Myambutol Tablets 1290

MYFUNGAR (Germany, Mexico, Switzerland)
OXICONAZOLE NITRATE
Oxistat Cream 1298
Oxistat Lotion 1298

MYGDALON (United Kingdom)
METOCLOPRAMIDE HYDROCHLORIDE
Reglan Injectable 2935
Reglan Syrup 2935
Reglan Tablets 2935

MYKO CORDES (Austria, Germany)
CLOTRIMAZOLE
Lotrimin Cream 1% 3128
Lotrimin Lotion 1% 3128
Lotrimin Topical Solution 1% 3128
Mycelex Troche 573

MYKODERM HEILSALBE (Germany)
NYSTATIN
Nystop Topical Powder USP 2608

MYKOFUNGIN (Germany)
CLOTRIMAZOLE
Lotrimin Cream 1% 3128
Lotrimin Lotion 1% 3128
Lotrimin Topical Solution 1% 3128
Mycelex Troche 573

MYKOHAUG (Germany)
CLOTRIMAZOLE
Lotrimin Cream 1% 3128
Lotrimin Lotion 1% 3128
Lotrimin Topical Solution 1% 3128
Mycelex Troche 573

MYKOPOSTERINE N (Germany)
NYSTATIN
Nystop Topical Powder USP 2608

MYKUNDEX (Germany)
NYSTATIN
Nystop Topical Powder USP 2608

MYKUNDEX HEILSALBE (Germany)
NYSTATIN
Nystop Topical Powder USP 2608

MYKUNDEX MONO (Germany)
NYSTATIN
Nystop Topical Powder USP 2608

MYKUNDEX OVULA (Germany)
NYSTATIN
Nystop Topical Powder USP 2608

MYLERAN (Australia, Austria, Belgium, Brazil, Canada, France, Germany, Hong Kong, Irish Republic, Israel, Italy, Mexico, New Zealand, Norway, Portugal, Singapore, South Africa, Spain, Sweden, Switzerland, Thailand, The Netherlands, United Kingdom)
BUSULFAN
Myleran Tablets 1603

MYLOCORT (South Africa)
HYDROCORTISONE ACETATE
Anusol-HC Suppositories 2238
Cortifoam Rectal Foam 3170
Hydrocortone Acetate Injectable Suspension 2103
Proctocort Suppositories 2264

MYLPROIN (Germany)
VALPROIC ACID
Depakene Capsules 421
Depakene Syrup 421

MYNOCINE (France)
MINOCYCLINE HYDROCHLORIDE
Dynacin Capsules 2019
Minocin Intravenous 1862
Minocin Oral Suspension 1865
Minocin Pellet-Filled Capsules 1863

MYO HERMES (Spain)
BETHANECHOL CHLORIDE
Urecholine Injection 2198
Urecholine Tablets 2198

MYOCARDON MONO (Austria)
ISOSORBIDE MONONITRATE
Imdur Tablets 1826
Ismo Tablets 3524

MYOCARDON N (Germany)
THEOPHYLLINE
Aerolate Jr. T.D. Capsules 1361
Aerolate Liquid 1361
Aerolate Sr. T.D. Capsules 1361
Theo-Dur Extended-Release Tablets 1835
Uni-Dur Extended-Release Tablets 1841
Uniphyl 400 mg and 600 mg Tablets 2903

MYOCHOLINE (Austria, Germany, Switzerland)
BETHANECHOL CHLORIDE
Urecholine Injection 2198
Urecholine Tablets 2198

MYOCIN (Thailand)
METHOCARBAMOL
Robaxin Injectable 2938
Robaxin Tablets 2939
Robaxin-750 Tablets 2939

MYOGIT (Germany)
DICLOFENAC SODIUM
Voltaren Tablets 2315
Voltaren-XR Tablets 2315

MYOLAX (Thailand)
CARISOPRODOL
Soma Tablets 3353

MYOMETHOL (Thailand)
METHOCARBAMOL
Robaxin Injectable 2938
Robaxin Tablets 2939
Robaxin-750 Tablets 2939

MYONIL (Denmark)
DILTIAZEM HYDROCHLORIDE
Cardizem CD Capsules 1016
Cardizem Injectable 1018
Cardizem Lyo-Ject Syringe 1018
Cardizem Monovial 1018
Tiazac Capsules 1378

MYOPAX (Denmark)
ATENOLOL
Tenormin I.V. Injection 692

MYOSCAIN (Austria)
GUAIFENESIN
Organidin NR Liquid 3350
Organidin NR Tablets 3350

MYOTONACHOL (Canada)
BETHANECHOL CHLORIDE
Urecholine Injection 2198
Urecholine Tablets 2198

MYOTONINE (United Kingdom)
BETHANECHOL CHLORIDE
Urecholine Injection 2198
Urecholine Tablets 2198

MYPROFLAM (South Africa)
KETOPROFEN
Orudis Capsules 3548
Oruvail Capsules 3548

MYTOBRIN (South Africa)
TOBRAMYCIN SULFATE
Nebcin Vials, Hyporets & ADD-Vantage 1955

MYTOLAC (Sweden)
BENZOYL PEROXIDE
Brevoxyl-4 Cleansing Lotion 3269
Brevoxyl-4 Creamy Wash 3270
Brevoxyl-4 Gel 3269
Brevoxyl-8 Cleansing Lotion 3269
Brevoxyl-8 Creamy Wash 3270
Brevoxyl-8 Gel 3269
Triaz Cleanser 2026
Triaz Gel 2026

NABACT (South Africa)
METRONIDAZOLE
MetroCream 1404

MetroGel . . . 1405
MetroGel-Vaginal Gel . . . 1986
MetroLotion . . . 1405
Noritate Cream . . . 1224

NABONE (Thailand)
NABUMETONE
Relafen Tablets . . . 1617

NABUCOX (France)
NABUMETONE
Relafen Tablets . . . 1617

NABUSER (Italy)
NABUMETONE
Relafen Tablets . . . 1617

NACLOF (Austria, Norway, South Africa, Sweden, Thailand, The Netherlands)
DICLOFENAC SODIUM
Voltaren Tablets . . . 2315
Voltaren-XR Tablets . . . 2315

NACOR (Spain)
ENALAPRIL MALEATE
Vasotec Tablets . . . 2210

NADINOLA (Canada)
HYDROQUINONE
Eldopaque Forte 4% Cream . . . 1734
Eldoquin Forte 4% Cream . . . 1734
Lustra Cream . . . 2023
Lustra-AF Cream . . . 2023
Melanex Topical Solution . . . 2300
Solaquin Forte 4% Cream . . . 1734
Solaquin Forte 4% Gel . . . 1734

NADIPINIA (Hong Kong)
NIFEDIPINE
Adalat CC Tablets . . . 877
Procardia Capsules . . . 2708
Procardia XL Extended Release Tablets . . 2710

NADIR (Italy)
METOCLOPRAMIDE HYDROCHLORIDE
Reglan Injectable . . . 2935
Reglan Syrup . . . 2935
Reglan Tablets . . . 2935

NADOSTINE (Canada, Hong Kong)
NYSTATIN
Nystop Topical Powder USP . . . 2608

NAFASOL (South Africa)
NAPROXEN
EC-Naprosyn Delayed-Release Tablets . . . 2967
Naprosyn Suspension . . . 2967
Naprosyn Tablets . . . 2967

NAFTAZOLINA (Italy)
NAPHAZOLINE HYDROCHLORIDE
Albalon Ophthalmic Solution . . . ⊙225

NAFTIN (Canada)
NAFTIFINE HYDROCHLORIDE
Naftin Cream . . . 2224
Naftin Gel . . . 2224

NALAPRES (Italy)
HYDROCHLOROTHIAZIDE/LISINOPRIL
Prinzide Tablets . . . 2168
Zestoretic Tablets . . . 695

NALGISA (Italy)
DIFLUNISAL
Dolobid Tablets . . . 2088

NALION (Spain)
NORFLOXACIN
Chibroxin Sterile Ophthalmic Solution . . . ⊙273, 2051
Noroxin Tablets . . . 2145

NALONE (France)
NALOXONE HYDROCHLORIDE
Narcan Injection . . . 1322

NALOPRIL (Thailand)
ENALAPRIL MALEATE
Vasotec Tablets . . . 2210

NAMETONE (Thailand)
NABUMETONE
Relafen Tablets . . . 1617

NAMIC (Thailand)
MEFENAMIC ACID
Ponstel Capsules . . . 1356

NAMIFEN (Mexico)
MEFENAMIC ACID
Ponstel Capsules . . . 1356

NAPAMIDE (Australia, Hong Kong, New Zealand, Singapore)
INDAPAMIDE
Indapamide Tablets . . . 2286

NAPAN (Hong Kong)
MEFENAMIC ACID
Ponstel Capsules . . . 1356

NAPFLAM (South Africa)
NAPROXEN
EC-Naprosyn Delayed-Release Tablets . . . 2967
Naprosyn Suspension . . . 2967
Naprosyn Tablets . . . 2967

NAPHACEL (Mexico)
NAPHAZOLINE HYDROCHLORIDE
Albalon Ophthalmic Solution . . . ⊙225

NAPHASAL (Israel)
NAPHAZOLINE HYDROCHLORIDE
Albalon Ophthalmic Solution . . . ⊙225

NAPHCON (Australia, Belgium, New Zealand, Thailand)
NAPHAZOLINE HYDROCHLORIDE
Albalon Ophthalmic Solution . . . ⊙225

NAPHCON FORTE (Canada, Israel)
NAPHAZOLINE HYDROCHLORIDE
Albalon Ophthalmic Solution . . . ⊙225

NAPLIN (New Zealand)
INDAPAMIDE
Indapamide Tablets . . . 2286

NAPMEL (Irish Republic)
NAPROXEN
EC-Naprosyn Delayed-Release Tablets . . . 2967
Naprosyn Suspension . . . 2967
Naprosyn Tablets . . . 2967

NAPRATEC (United Kingdom)
NAPROXEN
EC-Naprosyn Delayed-Release Tablets . . . 2967
Naprosyn Suspension . . . 2967
Naprosyn Tablets . . . 2967

NAPREL (South Africa)
NAPROXEN
EC-Naprosyn Delayed-Release Tablets . . . 2967
Naprosyn Suspension . . . 2967
Naprosyn Tablets . . . 2967

NAPRELAN (Sweden)
NAPROXEN SODIUM
Anaprox DS Tablets . . . 2967
Anaprox Tablets . . . 2967
Naprelan Tablets . . . 1293

NAPREX (Irish Republic, Israel)
NAPROXEN
EC-Naprosyn Delayed-Release Tablets . . . 2967
Naprosyn Suspension . . . 2967
Naprosyn Tablets . . . 2967

NAPRILENE (Italy)
ENALAPRIL MALEATE
Vasotec Tablets . . . 2210

NAPRIUM (Italy)
NAPROXEN
EC-Naprosyn Delayed-Release Tablets . . . 2967
Naprosyn Suspension . . . 2967
Naprosyn Tablets . . . 2967

NAPRIUS (Italy)
NAPROXEN
EC-Naprosyn Delayed-Release Tablets . . . 2967
Naprosyn Suspension . . . 2967
Naprosyn Tablets . . . 2967

NAPROBENE (Austria)
NAPROXEN
EC-Naprosyn Delayed-Release Tablets . . . 2967
Naprosyn Suspension . . . 2967
Naprosyn Tablets . . . 2967

NAPROCOAT (The Netherlands)
NAPROXEN
EC-Naprosyn Delayed-Release Tablets . . . 2967
Naprosyn Suspension . . . 2967
Naprosyn Tablets . . . 2967

NAPRODIL (Mexico)
NAPROXEN
EC-Naprosyn Delayed-Release Tablets . . . 2967
Naprosyn Suspension . . . 2967
Naprosyn Tablets . . . 2967

NAPRODOL (Italy)
NAPROXEN SODIUM
Anaprox DS Tablets . . . 2967
Anaprox Tablets . . . 2967
Naprelan Tablets . . . 1293

NAPRO-DORSCH (Germany)
NAPROXEN
EC-Naprosyn Delayed-Release Tablets . . . 2967
Naprosyn Suspension . . . 2967
Naprosyn Tablets . . . 2967

NAPROGESIC (Australia, New Zealand)
NAPROXEN SODIUM
Anaprox DS Tablets . . . 2967
Anaprox Tablets . . . 2967
Naprelan Tablets . . . 1293

NAPROKES (Spain)
NAPROXEN
EC-Naprosyn Delayed-Release Tablets . . . 2967
Naprosyn Suspension . . . 2967
Naprosyn Tablets . . . 2967

NAPROLAG (Switzerland)
NAPROXEN
EC-Naprosyn Delayed-Release Tablets . . . 2967
Naprosyn Suspension . . . 2967
Naprosyn Tablets . . . 2967

NAPROMETIN (Finland)
NAPROXEN
EC-Naprosyn Delayed-Release Tablets . . . 2967
Naprosyn Suspension . . . 2967
Naprosyn Tablets . . . 2967

NAPROMEX (Finland)
NAPROXEN
EC-Naprosyn Delayed-Release Tablets . . . 2967
Naprosyn Suspension . . . 2967
Naprosyn Tablets . . . 2967

NAPRONET (Denmark)
NAPROXEN
EC-Naprosyn Delayed-Release Tablets . . . 2967
Naprosyn Suspension . . . 2967
Naprosyn Tablets . . . 2967

NAPROREX (Italy)
NAPROXEN SODIUM
Anaprox DS Tablets . . . 2967
Anaprox Tablets . . . 2967
Naprelan Tablets . . . 1293

NAPROSCRIPT (South Africa)
NAPROXEN
EC-Naprosyn Delayed-Release Tablets . . . 2967
Naprosyn Suspension . . . 2967
Naprosyn Tablets . . . 2967

NAPROSIAN (Thailand)
NAPROXEN
EC-Naprosyn Delayed-Release Tablets . . . 2967
Naprosyn Suspension . . . 2967
Naprosyn Tablets . . . 2967

NAPROSO (Thailand)
NAPROXEN SODIUM
Anaprox DS Tablets . . . 2967
Anaprox Tablets . . . 2967
Naprelan Tablets . . . 1293

NAPROSYN (Australia, Brazil, Canada, Denmark, Finland, Hong Kong, Irish Republic, Italy, New Zealand, Norway, Portugal, Singapore, South Africa, Spain, Sweden, Switzerland, Thailand, United Kingdom)
NAPROXEN
EC-Naprosyn Delayed-Release Tablets . . . 2967
Naprosyn Suspension . . . 2967
Naprosyn Tablets . . . 2967

NAPROSYNE (Belgium, France, The Netherlands)
NAPROXEN
EC-Naprosyn Delayed-Release Tablets . . . 2967
Naprosyn Suspension . . . 2967
Naprosyn Tablets . . . 2967

NAPROVAL (Spain)
NAPROXEN
EC-Naprosyn Delayed-Release Tablets . . . 2967
Naprosyn Suspension . . . 2967
Naprosyn Tablets . . . 2967

NAPROVITE (The Netherlands)
NAPROXEN SODIUM
Anaprox DS Tablets . . . 2967
Anaprox Tablets . . . 2967
Naprelan Tablets . . . 1293

NAPROXI (Israel)
NAPROXEN
EC-Naprosyn Delayed-Release Tablets . . . 2967
Naprosyn Suspension . . . 2967
Naprosyn Tablets . . . 2967

NAPXEN (Thailand)
NAPROXEN
EC-Naprosyn Delayed-Release Tablets . . . 2967
Naprosyn Suspension . . . 2967
Naprosyn Tablets . . . 2967

NARAGRAN (Denmark)
NARATRIPTAN HYDROCHLORIDE
Amerge Tablets . . . 1467

NARAMIG (Australia, Austria, Belgium, Finland, France, Israel, Mexico, Norway, Portugal, Singapore, South Africa, Spain, Sweden, Switzerland, Thailand, The Netherlands, United Kingdom)
NARATRIPTAN HYDROCHLORIDE
Amerge Tablets . . . 1467

NARCAN (Australia, Belgium, Brazil, Canada, France, Irish Republic, Israel, Italy, New Zealand, Portugal, Singapore, South Africa, Switzerland, United Kingdom)
NALOXONE HYDROCHLORIDE
Narcan Injection . . . 1322

NARCANTI (Austria, Denmark, Finland, Germany, Mexico, Norway, Sweden)
NALOXONE HYDROCHLORIDE
Narcan Injection . . . 1322

NARDELZINE (Belgium, Spain)
PHENELZINE SULFATE
Nardil Tablets . . . 2653

NARDIL (Australia, Canada, Irish Republic, Israel, New Zealand, United Kingdom)
PHENELZINE SULFATE
Nardil Tablets . . . 2653

NARFEN (Spain)
IBUPROFEN
Motrin Suspension, Oral Drops, Chewable Tablets, and Caplets . . . 2002

NARIDE (Australia)
INDAPAMIDE
Indapamide Tablets . . . 2286

NARILET (Spain)
IPRATROPIUM BROMIDE
Atrovent Inhalation Aerosol . . . 1030
Atrovent Inhalation Solution . . . 1031
Atrovent Nasal Spray 0.03% . . . 1032
Atrovent Nasal Spray 0.06% . . . 1033

NARINE (Spain)
LORATADINE/PSEUDOEPHEDRINE SULFATE
Claritin-D 12 Hour Extended Release Tablets . . . 3102
Claritin-D 24 Hour Extended Release Tablets . . . 3104

NARITEC (Thailand)
ENALAPRIL MALEATE
Vasotec Tablets . . . 2210

NAROBIC (South Africa)
METRONIDAZOLE
MetroCream . . . 1404
MetroGel . . . 1405
MetroGel-Vaginal Gel . . . 1986
MetroLotion . . . 1405
Noritate Cream . . . 1224

NAROCIN (Israel)
NAPROXEN SODIUM
Anaprox DS Tablets . . . 2967
Anaprox Tablets . . . 2967
Naprelan Tablets . . . 1293

NAROP (Israel, Sweden)
ROPIVACAINE HYDROCHLORIDE
Naropin Injection . . . 612

NAROPEINE (France, Portugal)
ROPIVACAINE HYDROCHLORIDE
Naropin Injection . . . 612

NAROPIN (Australia, Austria, Belgium, Canada, Denmark, Finland, Germany, Hong Kong, Irish Republic, Mexico, New Zealand, Norway, Singapore, South Africa, Spain, Switzerland, The Netherlands, United Kingdom)
ROPIVACAINE HYDROCHLORIDE
Naropin Injection . . . 612

NAROPINA (Italy)
ROPIVACAINE HYDROCHLORIDE
Naropin Injection . . . 612

NARZEN (Thailand)
NAPROXEN
EC-Naprosyn Delayed-Release Tablets . . . 2967
Naprosyn Suspension . . . 2967
Naprosyn Tablets . . . 2967

NASACOR (South Africa)
TRIAMCINOLONE ACETONIDE
Azmacort Inhalation Aerosol . . . 728
Nasacort AQ Nasal Spray . . . 752
Nasacort Nasal Inhaler . . . 750

NASACORT (Austria, Canada, Denmark, Finland, France, Germany, Irish Republic, Italy, Mexico, New Zealand, Norway, Singapore, Spain, Sweden, Switzerland, Thailand, The Netherlands, United Kingdom)
TRIAMCINOLONE ACETONIDE
Azmacort Inhalation Aerosol . . . 728
Nasacort AQ Nasal Spray . . . 752
Nasacort Nasal Inhaler . . . 750

NASACORT AQ (Australia)
TRIAMCINOLONE ACETONIDE
Azmacort Inhalation Aerosol . . . 728
Nasacort AQ Nasal Spray . . . 752
Nasacort Nasal Inhaler . . . 750

NASALIDE (France)
FLUNISOLIDE
Aerobid Inhaler System . . . 1363
Aerobid-M Inhaler System . . . 1363
Nasalide Nasal Spray . . . 1295
Nasarel Nasal Solution 0.025% . . . 1296

NASOCAN (Mexico)
NAPROXEN SODIUM
Anaprox DS Tablets . . . 2967

Anaprox Tablets 2967
Naprelan Tablets 1293

NASOCORT (Israel)
BUDESONIDE
Pulmicort Turbuhaler Inhalation Powder . . . 636
Rhinocort Nasal Inhaler 640

NASOMET (Portugal)
MOMETASONE FUROATE
Elocon Cream 0.1% 3110
Elocon Lotion 0.1% 3111
Elocon Ointment 0.1% 3112
Nasonex Nasal Spray 3131

NASONEX (Australia, Canada, Denmark, Finland, France, Germany, Hong Kong, Irish Republic, Israel, Italy, Norway, Singapore, South Africa, Spain, Sweden, Switzerland, Thailand, The Netherlands, United Kingdom)
MOMETASONE FUROATE
Elocon Cream 0.1% 3110
Elocon Lotion 0.1% 3111
Elocon Ointment 0.1% 3112
Nasonex Nasal Spray 3131

NATACYN (Singapore, South Africa, Thailand)
NATAMYCIN
Natacyn Antifungal Ophthalmic Suspension . . . . ⊙216

NATAFUCIN (Italy)
NATAMYCIN
Natacyn Antifungal Ophthalmic Suspension . . . . ⊙216

NATIKEN (Mexico)
IBUPROFEN
Motrin Suspension, Oral Drops, Chewable Tablets, and Caplets 2002

NATRAMID (United Kingdom)
INDAPAMIDE
Indapamide Tablets 2286

NATRILIX (Australia, Brazil, Denmark, Finland, Germany, Hong Kong, Irish Republic, Italy, New Zealand, Singapore, South Africa, Thailand, United Kingdom)
INDAPAMIDE
Indapamide Tablets 2286

NATRIOXEN (Italy)
NAPROXEN SODIUM
Anaprox DS Tablets 2967
Anaprox Tablets 2967
Naprelan Tablets 1293

NATULAN (Australia, Austria, Belgium, Canada, France, Germany, Israel, Italy, Mexico, New Zealand, Norway, South Africa, Spain, Switzerland, The Netherlands, United Kingdom)
PROCARBAZINE HYDROCHLORIDE
Matulane Capsules 3246

NATULANAR (Brazil, Sweden)
PROCARBAZINE HYDROCHLORIDE
Matulane Capsules 3246

NATULAX (Germany)
LACTULOSE
Kristalose for Oral Solution 1007

NATYL (Switzerland)
DIPYRIDAMOLE
Persantine Tablets 1057

NAUSIGON (Austria)
METOCLOPRAMIDE HYDROCHLORIDE
Reglan Injectable 2935
Reglan Syrup 2935
Reglan Tablets 2935

NAUSIL (Thailand)
METOCLOPRAMIDE HYDROCHLORIDE
Reglan Injectable 2935
Reglan Syrup 2935
Reglan Tablets 2935

NAVARROYODOL (Spain)
POTASSIUM IODIDE
Pima Syrup 1362

NAVELBINE (Australia, Austria, Brazil, Canada, Denmark, Finland, France, Germany, Israel, Italy, Mexico, New Zealand, Norway, Portugal, South Africa, Spain, Sweden, Switzerland, Thailand, United Kingdom)
VINORELBINE TARTRATE
Navelbine Injection 1604

NAVICALM (The Netherlands)
HYDROXYZINE HYDROCHLORIDE
Atarax Tablets & Syrup 2667
Vistaril Intramuscular Solution 2738

NAVIXEN (Mexico)
NAPROXEN
EC-Naprosyn Delayed-Release Tablets . . . 2967
Naprosyn Suspension 2967
Naprosyn Tablets 2967

NAXEN (Australia, Canada, Mexico, New Zealand, South Africa)
NAPROXEN
EC-Naprosyn Delayed-Release Tablets . . . 2967
Naprosyn Suspension 2967
Naprosyn Tablets 2967

NAXIDINE (The Netherlands)
NIZATIDINE
Axid Pulvules 1903

NAXIL (Mexico)
NAPROXEN
EC-Naprosyn Delayed-Release Tablets . . . 2967
Naprosyn Suspension 2967
Naprosyn Tablets 2967

NAXO (Mexico)
CHLORAMPHENICOL
Chloromycetin Ophthalmic Ointment, 1% . . . . ⊙296
Chloromycetin Ophthalmic Solution . . . . ⊙297
Chloroptic Sterile Ophthalmic Ointment . . ⊙234
Chloroptic Sterile Ophthalmic Solution . . ⊙235

NAXODOL (Mexico)
NAPROXEN
EC-Naprosyn Delayed-Release Tablets . . . 2967
Naprosyn Suspension 2967
Naprosyn Tablets 2967

NAXOLAN (Portugal)
NALOXONE HYDROCHLORIDE
Narcan Injection 1322

NAXOPREN (Finland)
NAPROXEN
EC-Naprosyn Delayed-Release Tablets . . . 2967
Naprosyn Suspension 2967
Naprosyn Tablets 2967

NAXY (France)
CLARITHROMYCIN
Biaxin Filmtab Tablets 403
Biaxin for Oral Suspension 403

NAXYN (Israel)
NAPROXEN
EC-Naprosyn Delayed-Release Tablets . . . 2967
Naprosyn Suspension 2967
Naprosyn Tablets 2967

NAZOLFARM (Mexico)
KETOCONAZOLE
Nizoral 2% Cream 3620
Nizoral 2% Shampoo 2007
Nizoral Tablets 1791

NEALORIN (Portugal, Spain)
CARBOPLATIN
Paraplatin for Injection 1126

NEATENOL (Spain)
ATENOLOL
Tenormin I.V. Injection 692

NEBCIN (Australia, Canada, Hong Kong, Irish Republic, Israel, New Zealand, South Africa, United Kingdom)
TOBRAMYCIN SULFATE
Nebcin Vials, Hyporets & ADD-Vantage . . 1955

NEBCINA (Denmark, Finland, Norway, Sweden)
TOBRAMYCIN SULFATE
Nebcin Vials, Hyporets & ADD-Vantage . . 1955

NEBCINE (France)
TOBRAMYCIN SULFATE
Nebcin Vials, Hyporets & ADD-Vantage . . 1955

NEBICINA (Italy)
TOBRAMYCIN SULFATE
Nebcin Vials, Hyporets & ADD-Vantage . . 1955

NECAMIN (Brazil)
MEBENDAZOLE
Vermox Chewable Tablets 2017

NECOPEN (Spain)
CEFIXIME
Suprax Tablets 1877
Suprax for Oral Suspension 1877

NEFADAR (Denmark, Finland, Germany, Norway, Sweden, Switzerland)
NEFAZODONE HYDROCHLORIDE
Serzone Tablets 1104

NEFROCARNIT (Germany)
LEVOCARNITINE
Carnitor Injection 3242
Carnitor Tablets and Oral Solution 3245

NEGACEF (United Arab Emirates)
CEFTAZIDIME
Ceptaz for Injection 1499
Fortaz for Injection 1541
Tazicef for Injection 1647
Tazidime Vials, Faspak & ADD-Vantage . . 1966

NELAPINE (Thailand)
NIFEDIPINE
Adalat CC Tablets 877
Procardia Capsules 2708
Procardia XL Extended Release Tablets . . 2710

NEMAPRES (Mexico)
MEBENDAZOLE
Vermox Chewable Tablets 2017

NEMBUTAL (Australia, Canada)
PENTOBARBITAL SODIUM
Nembutal Sodium Solution 485

NEO ATROMID (Spain)
CLOFIBRATE
Atromid-S Capsules 3483

NEO EBLIMON (Italy)
NAPROXEN
EC-Naprosyn Delayed-Release Tablets . . . 2967
Naprosyn Suspension 2967
Naprosyn Tablets 2967

NEO ELIXIFILIN (Spain)
THEOPHYLLINE
Aerolate Jr. T.D. Capsules 1361
Aerolate Liquid 1361
Aerolate Sr. T.D. Capsules 1361
Theo-Dur Extended-Release Tablets 1835
Uni-Dur Extended-Release Tablets 1841
Uniphyl 400 mg and 600 mg Tablets . . . 2903

NEO GASTRAUSIL (Italy)
CIMETIDINE
Tagamet Tablets 1644

NEO RINACTIVE (Spain)
BUDESONIDE
Pulmicort Turbuhaler Inhalation Powder . . . 636
Rhinocort Nasal Inhaler 640

NEOBACIGRIN (Mexico)
NEOMYCIN SULFATE/POLYMYXIN B SULFATE
Neosporin G.U. Irrigant Sterile 2256

NEOBRUFEN (Spain)
IBUPROFEN
Motrin Suspension, Oral Drops, Chewable Tablets, and Caplets 2002

NEOCAINA (Brazil)
BUPIVACAINE HYDROCHLORIDE
Sensorcaine Injection 643
Sensorcaine-MPF Injection 643

NEOCEF (Portugal)
CEFIXIME
Suprax Tablets 1877
Suprax for Oral Suspension 1877

NEO-CODEMA (Canada)
HYDROCHLOROTHIAZIDE
HydroDIURIL Tablets 2108
Microzide Capsules 3414

NEOCOF (Thailand)
CODEINE PHOSPHATE/GUAIFENESIN
Robitussin A-C Syrup 2942
Tussi-Organidin NR Liquid 3350
Tussi-Organidin-S NR Liquid 3350

NEOCORTIGAMMA (Italy)
HYDROCORTISONE
Anusol-HC Cream 2.5% 2237
Hydrocortone Tablets 2106

NEO-DECA (Singapore)
DEXAMETHASONE SODIUM PHOSPHATE/NEOMYCIN SULFATE
NeoDecadron Sterile Ophthalmic Solution 2144

NEODERM GINECOLOGICO (Italy)
FLUOCINOLONE ACETONIDE
Synalar Cream 2020
Synalar Ointment 2020
Synalar Topical Solution 2020

NEODES (Italy)
DEXAMETHASONE SODIUM PHOSPHATE/NEOMYCIN SULFATE
NeoDecadron Sterile Ophthalmic Solution 2144

NEO-DEX (IMPROVED) (Hong Kong)
DEXAMETHASONE
Decadron Elixir 2078
Decadron Tablets 2079

NEODOX (Germany)
DOXYCYCLINE HYCLATE
Doryx Coated Pellet Filled Capsules 3357
Periostat Tablets 1208
Vibramycin Hyclate Capsules 2735
Vibramycin Hyclate Intravenous 2737
Vibra-Tabs Film Coated Tablets 2735

NEOFOMIRAL (Mexico)
FLUCONAZOLE
Diflucan Tablets, Injection, and Oral Suspension 2681

NEOGEL (Thailand)
PIROXICAM
Feldene Capsules 2685

NEOGEST (United Kingdom)
NORGESTREL
Ovrette Tablets 3552

NEO-HELVAGIT (Switzerland)
IBUPROFEN
Motrin Suspension, Oral Drops, Chewable Tablets, and Caplets 2002

NEO-LOTAN (Italy)
LOSARTAN POTASSIUM
Cozaar Tablets 2067

NEO-LOTAN PLUS (Italy)
HYDROCHLOROTHIAZIDE/LOSARTAN POTASSIUM
Hyzaar 50-12.5 Tablets 2109

NEO-METRIC (Canada)
METRONIDAZOLE
MetroCream 1404
MetroGel 1405
MetroGel-Vaginal Gel 1986
MetroLotion 1405
Noritate Cream 1224

NEO-MINDOL (Italy)
IBUPROFEN
Motrin Suspension, Oral Drops, Chewable Tablets, and Caplets 2002

NEONAXIL (Mexico)
NAPROXEN
EC-Naprosyn Delayed-Release Tablets . . . 2967
Naprosyn Suspension 2967
Naprosyn Tablets 2967

NEO-OPTAL (Thailand)
DEXAMETHASONE SODIUM PHOSPHATE/NEOMYCIN SULFATE
NeoDecadron Sterile Ophthalmic Solution 2144

NEOPHEDAN (South Africa)
TAMOXIFEN CITRATE
Nolvadex Tablets 678

NEO-PREOCIL (Portugal)
FLUOROMETHOLONE
FML Ophthalmic Ointment . . . . ⊙237

NEOPREX (Italy)
ENALAPRIL MALEATE/HYDROCHLOROTHIAZIDE
Vaseretic Tablets 2204

NEO-PYRAZON (Singapore)
DICLOFENAC SODIUM
Voltaren Tablets 2315
Voltaren-XR Tablets 2315

NEOSAYOMOL (Spain)
DIPHENHYDRAMINE HYDROCHLORIDE
Benadryl Parenteral 2617

NEOSPORIN (Canada, Hong Kong, Mexico, United Kingdom)
NEOMYCIN SULFATE/POLYMYXIN B SULFATE
Neosporin G.U. Irrigant Sterile 2256

NEO-STEDIRIL (Belgium, Germany, Switzerland)
LEVONORGESTREL
Norplant System 3543

NEOSTRATA HQ (Canada)
HYDROQUINONE
Eldopaque Forte 4% Cream 1734
Eldoquin Forte 4% Cream 1734
Lustra Cream 2023
Lustra-AF Cream 2023
Melanex Topical Solution 2300
Solaquin Forte 4% Cream 1734
Solaquin Forte 4% Gel 1734

NEOTENOL (Brazil)
ATENOLOL
Tenormin I.V. Injection 692

NEOTENSIN (Spain)
ENALAPRIL MALEATE
Vasotec Tablets 2210

NEOTENSIN DIU (Spain)
ENALAPRIL MALEATE/HYDROCHLOROTHIAZIDE
• Vaseretic Tablets 2204

NEOTICA (Thailand)
PIROXICAM
Feldene Capsules 2685

(⊙ Described in PDR For Ophthalmic Medicines™)

NEOTIGASON (Australia, Austria, Belgium, Denmark, Finland, Germany, Hong Kong, Irish Republic, Israel, Italy, New Zealand, Norway, Portugal, Singapore, South Africa, Spain, Sweden, Switzerland, Thailand, The Netherlands, United Kingdom)
ACITRETIN
Soriatane Capsules . . . 3003

NEO-TIROIMADE (Portugal)
LIOTHYRONINE SODIUM
Cytomel Tablets . . . 1817
Triostat Injection . . . 1825

NEOTOPIC (Hong Kong)
NEOMYCIN SULFATE/POLYMYXIN B SULFATE
Neosporin G.U. Irrigant Sterile . . . 2256

NEOTUL (Spain)
FAMOTIDINE
Pepcid Injection . . . 2153
Pepcid Injection Premixed . . . 2153
Pepcid RPD Orally Disintegrating Tablets . . . 2150
Pepcid Tablets . . . 2150
Pepcid for Oral Suspension . . . 2150

NEOVERMIM (Brazil)
MEBENDAZOLE
Vermox Chewable Tablets . . . 2017

NEO-ZOL (Canada)
CLOTRIMAZOLE
Lotrimin Cream 1% . . . 3128
Lotrimin Lotion 1% . . . 3128
Lotrimin Topical Solution 1% . . . 3128
Mycelex Troche . . . 573

NEPHRAL (Germany)
HYDROCHLOROTHIAZIDE/TRIAMTERENE
Dyazide Capsules . . . 1515
Maxzide Tablets . . . 1008
Maxzide-25 mg Tablets . . . 1008

NEPHREX (Australia, Hong Kong)
CALCIUM ACETATE
PhosLo Tablets . . . 1069

NEPHRIL (Irish Republic, United Kingdom)
POLYTHIAZIDE
Renese Tablets . . . 2712

NEPHULON G (Germany)
GUAIFENESIN
Organidin NR Liquid . . . 3350
Organidin NR Tablets . . . 3350

NEPTAL (Germany)
ACEBUTOLOL HYDROCHLORIDE
Sectral Capsules . . . 3589

NERDIPINA (Portugal, Spain)
NICARDIPINE HYDROCHLORIDE
Cardene I.V. . . . 3485

NERGADAN (Spain)
LOVASTATIN
Mevacor Tablets . . . 2132

NERICUR (United Kingdom)
BENZOYL PEROXIDE
Brevoxyl-4 Cleansing Lotion . . . 3269
Brevoxyl-4 Creamy Wash . . . 3270
Brevoxyl-4 Gel . . . 3269
Brevoxyl-8 Cleansing Lotion . . . 3269
Brevoxyl-8 Creamy Wash . . . 3270
Brevoxyl-8 Gel . . . 3269
Triaz Cleanser . . . 2026
Triaz Gel . . . 2026

NEROFEN (The Netherlands)
IBUPROFEN
Motrin Suspension, Oral Drops, Chewable Tablets, and Caplets . . . 2002

NEROLID (Mexico)
DIAZEPAM
Valium Injectable . . . 3026
Valium Tablets . . . 3047

NERVO OPT N (Germany)
DIPHENHYDRAMINE HYDROCHLORIDE
Benadryl Parenteral . . . 2617

NESACAIN (Switzerland)
CHLOROPROCAINE HYDROCHLORIDE
Nesacaine Injection . . . 617
Nesacaine-MPF Injection . . . 617

NESACAINE (Canada)
CHLOROPROCAINE HYDROCHLORIDE
Nesacaine Injection . . . 617
Nesacaine-MPF Injection . . . 617

NESPORAC (Spain)
FLUCONAZOLE
Diflucan Tablets, Injection, and Oral Suspension . . . 2681

NESTIC (Thailand)
CLOTRIMAZOLE
Lotrimin Cream 1% . . . 3128
Lotrimin Lotion 1% . . . 3128
Lotrimin Topical Solution 1% . . . 3128
Mycelex Troche . . . 573

NEUCOR (Italy)
NICARDIPINE HYDROCHLORIDE
Cardene I.V. . . . 3485

NEUGAL (Mexico)
RANITIDINE HYDROCHLORIDE
Zantac 150 EFFERdose Granules . . . 1690
Zantac 150 EFFERdose Tablets . . . 1690
Zantac 150 Tablets . . . 1690
Zantac 300 Tablets . . . 1690
Zantac Injection . . . 1688
Zantac Injection Premixed . . . 1688
Zantac Syrup . . . 1690

NEUGERON (Mexico)
CARBAMAZEPINE
Carbatrol Capsules . . . 3234
Tegretol Chewable Tablets . . . 2404
Tegretol Suspension . . . 2404
Tegretol Tablets . . . 2404
Tegretol-XR Tablets . . . 2404

NEURAGON (Thailand)
AMITRIPTYLINE HYDROCHLORIDE/PERPHENAZINE
Etrafon 2-10 Tablets (2-10) . . . 3115
Etrafon Tablets (2-25) . . . 3115
Etrafon-Forte Tablets (4-25) . . . 3115

NEUROCEFAL TRANQUI (Spain)
DIAZEPAM
Valium Injectable . . . 3026
Valium Tablets . . . 3047

NEUROLEP (Mexico)
CARBAMAZEPINE
Carbatrol Capsules . . . 3234
Tegretol Chewable Tablets . . . 2404
Tegretol Suspension . . . 2404
Tegretol Tablets . . . 2404
Tegretol-XR Tablets . . . 2404

NEUROLEPSIN (Austria)
LITHIUM CARBONATE
Eskalith CR Controlled Release Tablets . . . 1527
Eskalith Capsules . . . 1527
Lithium Carbonate Capsules . . . 3061
Lithobid Slow-Release Tablets . . . 3255

NEUROLYTRIL (Germany)
DIAZEPAM
Valium Injectable . . . 3026
Valium Tablets . . . 3047

NEURONTIN (Australia, Austria, Belgium, Canada, Finland, France, Germany, Hong Kong, Irish Republic, Israel, Italy, Mexico, New Zealand, Norway, Portugal, Singapore, South Africa, Spain, Sweden, Switzerland, Thailand, The Netherlands, United Kingdom)
GABAPENTIN
Neurontin Capsules . . . 2655

NEUROTOL (Finland)
CARBAMAZEPINE
Carbatrol Capsules . . . 3234
Tegretol Chewable Tablets . . . 2404
Tegretol Suspension . . . 2404
Tegretol Tablets . . . 2404
Tegretol-XR Tablets . . . 2404

NEUROTOP (Austria, Singapore)
CARBAMAZEPINE
Carbatrol Capsules . . . 3234
Tegretol Chewable Tablets . . . 2404
Tegretol Suspension . . . 2404
Tegretol Tablets . . . 2404
Tegretol-XR Tablets . . . 2404

NEUTROGENA ACNE MASK (Australia, Canada)
BENZOYL PEROXIDE
Brevoxyl-4 Cleansing Lotion . . . 3269
Brevoxyl-4 Creamy Wash . . . 3270
Brevoxyl-4 Gel . . . 3269
Brevoxyl-8 Cleansing Lotion . . . 3269
Brevoxyl-8 Creamy Wash . . . 3270
Brevoxyl-8 Gel . . . 3269
Triaz Cleanser . . . 2026
Triaz Gel . . . 2026

NEUTROGENA LONG LASTING DANDRUFF CONTROL (United Kingdom)
KETOCONAZOLE
Nizoral 2% Cream . . . 3620
Nizoral 2% Shampoo . . . 2007
Nizoral Tablets . . . 1791

NEUTROGENA ON-THE-SPOT ACNE LOTION (Canada)
BENZOYL PEROXIDE
Brevoxyl-4 Cleansing Lotion . . . 3269
Brevoxyl-4 Creamy Wash . . . 3270
Brevoxyl-4 Gel . . . 3269
Brevoxyl-8 Cleansing Lotion . . . 3269
Brevoxyl-8 Creamy Wash . . . 3270
Brevoxyl-8 Gel . . . 3269
Triaz Cleanser . . . 2026
Triaz Gel . . . 2026

NEUTROMED (Austria)
CIMETIDINE
Tagamet Tablets . . . 1644

NEUTRONORM (Austria, Hong Kong)
CIMETIDINE
Tagamet Tablets . . . 1644

NEWACE (The Netherlands)
FOSINOPRIL SODIUM
Monopril Tablets . . . 1091

NF COUGH SYRUP WITH CODEINE (Canada)
CODEINE PHOSPHATE/GUAIFENESIN/PSEUDOEPHEDRINE HYDROCHLORIDE
Robitussin-DAC Syrup . . . 2942

NIA (Austria)
MEGESTROL ACETATE
Megace Oral Suspension . . . 1124

NIACEL (Mexico)
METRONIDAZOLE
MetroCream . . . 1404
MetroGel . . . 1405
MetroGel-Vaginal Gel . . . 1986
MetroLotion . . . 1405
Noritate Cream . . . 1224

NIAGESTIN (Germany, Sweden)
MEGESTROL ACETATE
Megace Oral Suspension . . . 1124

NIAGESTINE (Belgium, Switzerland)
MEGESTROL ACETATE
Megace Oral Suspension . . . 1124

NIAR (Brazil, Mexico)
SELEGILINE HYDROCHLORIDE
Eldepryl Capsules . . . 3266

NICABATE (Australia, New Zealand, United Kingdom)
NICOTINE
Nicotrol Inhaler . . . 2840
Nicotrol Nasal Spray . . . 2843

NICANT (Italy)
NICARDIPINE HYDROCHLORIDE
Cardene I.V. . . . 3485

NICAPRESS (Italy)
NICARDIPINE HYDROCHLORIDE
Cardene I.V. . . . 3485

NICARDAL (Italy)
NICARDIPINE HYDROCHLORIDE
Cardene I.V. . . . 3485

NICARDIUM (Italy)
NICARDIPINE HYDROCHLORIDE
Cardene I.V. . . . 3485

NICARPIN (Italy)
NICARDIPINE HYDROCHLORIDE
Cardene I.V. . . . 3485

NICHOGENCIN (Germany)
GENTAMICIN SULFATE
Genoptic Ophthalmic Ointment . . . ⊙239
Genoptic Sterile Ophthalmic Solution . . . ⊙239

NICODERM (Canada)
NICOTINE
Nicotrol Inhaler . . . 2840
Nicotrol Nasal Spray . . . 2843

NICODISC (Spain)
NICOTINE
Nicotrol Inhaler . . . 2840
Nicotrol Nasal Spray . . . 2843

NICOLAN (Austria, Brazil, Sweden)
NICOTINE
Nicotrol Inhaler . . . 2840
Nicotrol Nasal Spray . . . 2843

NICOLMYCETIN (Thailand)
CHLORAMPHENICOL
Chloromycetin Ophthalmic Ointment, 1% . . . ⊙296
Chloromycetin Ophthalmic Solution . . . ⊙297
Chloroptic Sterile Ophthalmic Ointment . . . ⊙234
Chloroptic Sterile Ophthalmic Solution . . . ⊙235

NICOMAX (Spain)
NICOTINE
Nicotrol Inhaler . . . 2840
Nicotrol Nasal Spray . . . 2843

NICONIL (Irish Republic, United Kingdom)
NICOTINE
Nicotrol Inhaler . . . 2840
Nicotrol Nasal Spray . . . 2843

NICOPATCH (France)
NICOTINE
Nicotrol Inhaler . . . 2840
Nicotrol Nasal Spray . . . 2843

NICORETTE (Australia, Belgium, Denmark, Germany, Irish Republic, Israel, Mexico, New Zealand, Norway, Portugal, Singapore, Spain, Switzerland, The Netherlands)
NICOTINE
Nicotrol Inhaler . . . 2840
Nicotrol Nasal Spray . . . 2843

NICOSTOP TTS (Switzerland)
NICOTINE
Nicotrol Inhaler . . . 2840
Nicotrol Nasal Spray . . . 2843

NICOTINELL (Australia, Austria, Belgium, Denmark, France, Germany, Hong Kong, Irish Republic, Israel, New Zealand, Norway, Singapore, Spain, Sweden, Switzerland, Thailand, The Netherlands)
NICOTINE
Nicotrol Inhaler . . . 2840
Nicotrol Nasal Spray . . . 2843

NICOTINELL TTS (Brazil, Italy, Mexico, Portugal, South Africa)
NICOTINE
Nicotrol Inhaler . . . 2840
Nicotrol Nasal Spray . . . 2843

NICOTRANS (Italy, Spain)
NICOTINE
Nicotrol Inhaler . . . 2840
Nicotrol Nasal Spray . . . 2843

NICOTROL (Austria, Canada, Spain)
NICOTINE
Nicotrol Inhaler . . . 2840
Nicotrol Nasal Spray . . . 2843

NIDAGEL (Canada)
METRONIDAZOLE
MetroCream . . . 1404
MetroGel . . . 1405
MetroGel-Vaginal Gel . . . 1986
MetroLotion . . . 1405
Noritate Cream . . . 1224

NIDATRON (South Africa)
METRONIDAZOLE
MetroCream . . . 1404
MetroGel . . . 1405
MetroGel-Vaginal Gel . . . 1986
MetroLotion . . . 1405
Noritate Cream . . . 1224

NIDAZOL (United Kingdom)
METRONIDAZOLE
MetroCream . . . 1404
MetroGel . . . 1405
MetroGel-Vaginal Gel . . . 1986
MetroLotion . . . 1405
Noritate Cream . . . 1224

NIDAZOLEM (Mexico)
METRONIDAZOLE
MetroCream . . . 1404
MetroGel . . . 1405
MetroGel-Vaginal Gel . . . 1986
MetroLotion . . . 1405
Noritate Cream . . . 1224

NIDAZOLIN (Brazil)
NYSTATIN
Nystop Topical Powder USP . . . 2608

NIDRALON (Mexico)
METRONIDAZOLE
MetroCream . . . 1404
MetroGel . . . 1405
MetroGel-Vaginal Gel . . . 1986
MetroLotion . . . 1405
Noritate Cream . . . 1224

NIFANGIN (Finland)
NIFEDIPINE
Adalat CC Tablets . . . 877
Procardia Capsules . . . 2708
Procardia XL Extended Release Tablets . . . 2710

NIFATENOL (Germany)
ATENOLOL
Tenormin I.V. Injection . . . 692

NIFDEMIN (Finland)
NIFEDIPINE
Adalat CC Tablets . . . 877
Procardia Capsules . . . 2708
Procardia XL Extended Release Tablets . . . 2710

NIFE (Germany)
NIFEDIPINE
Adalat CC Tablets . . . 877
Procardia Capsules . . . 2708
Procardia XL Extended Release Tablets . . . 2710

NIFE UNO (Germany)
NIFEDIPINE
Adalat CC Tablets . . . 877
Procardia Capsules . . . 2708

Procardia XL Extended Release Tablets . . 2710

NIFE-BASAN (Switzerland)
NIFEDIPINE
Adalat CC Tablets . . . 877
Procardia Capsules . . . 2708
Procardia XL Extended Release Tablets . . 2710

NIFEBENE (Austria)
NIFEDIPINE
Adalat CC Tablets . . . 877
Procardia Capsules . . . 2708
Procardia XL Extended Release Tablets . . 2710

NIFECARD (Australia, Austria, Hong Kong, Thailand)
NIFEDIPINE
Adalat CC Tablets . . . 877
Procardia Capsules . . . 2708
Procardia XL Extended Release Tablets . . 2710

NIFECLAIR (Germany)
NIFEDIPINE
Adalat CC Tablets . . . 877
Procardia Capsules . . . 2708
Procardia XL Extended Release Tablets . . 2710

NIFECODAN (Denmark)
NIFEDIPINE
Adalat CC Tablets . . . 877
Procardia Capsules . . . 2708
Procardia XL Extended Release Tablets . . 2710

NIFECOR (Finland, Germany)
NIFEDIPINE
Adalat CC Tablets . . . 877
Procardia Capsules . . . 2708
Procardia XL Extended Release Tablets . . 2710

NIFED (Irish Republic)
NIFEDIPINE
Adalat CC Tablets . . . 877
Procardia Capsules . . . 2708
Procardia XL Extended Release Tablets . . 2710

NIFEDALAT (South Africa)
NIFEDIPINE
Adalat CC Tablets . . . 877
Procardia Capsules . . . 2708
Procardia XL Extended Release Tablets . . 2710

NIFEDATE (Portugal)
NIFEDIPINE
Adalat CC Tablets . . . 877
Procardia Capsules . . . 2708
Procardia XL Extended Release Tablets . . 2710

NIFEDICOR (Italy, Switzerland)
NIFEDIPINE
Adalat CC Tablets . . . 877
Procardia Capsules . . . 2708
Procardia XL Extended Release Tablets . . 2710

NIFEDICRON (Italy)
NIFEDIPINE
Adalat CC Tablets . . . 877
Procardia Capsules . . . 2708
Procardia XL Extended Release Tablets . . 2710

NIFEDI-DENK (Singapore)
NIFEDIPINE
Adalat CC Tablets . . . 877
Procardia Capsules . . . 2708
Procardia XL Extended Release Tablets . . 2710

NIFEDIGEL (Mexico)
NIFEDIPINE
Adalat CC Tablets . . . 877
Procardia Capsules . . . 2708
Procardia XL Extended Release Tablets . . 2710

NIFEDIN (Italy)
NIFEDIPINE
Adalat CC Tablets . . . 877
Procardia Capsules . . . 2708
Procardia XL Extended Release Tablets . . 2710

NIFEDIPAT (Germany)
NIFEDIPINE
Adalat CC Tablets . . . 877
Procardia Capsules . . . 2708
Procardia XL Extended Release Tablets . . 2710

NIFEDIPAT UNO (Germany)
NIFEDIPINE
Adalat CC Tablets . . . 877
Procardia Capsules . . . 2708
Procardia XL Extended Release Tablets . . 2710

NIFEDIPRES (Mexico)
NIFEDIPINE
Adalat CC Tablets . . . 877
Procardia Capsules . . . 2708
Procardia XL Extended Release Tablets . . 2710

NIFEDIPRESS (United Kingdom)
NIFEDIPINE
Adalat CC Tablets . . . 877
Procardia Capsules . . . 2708
Procardia XL Extended Release Tablets . . 2710

NIFEDOTARD (United Kingdom)
NIFEDIPINE
Adalat CC Tablets . . . 877
Procardia Capsules . . . 2708
Procardia XL Extended Release Tablets . . 2710

NIFEHEXAL (Australia, Austria, Germany)
NIFEDIPINE
Adalat CC Tablets . . . 877
Procardia Capsules . . . 2708
Procardia XL Extended Release Tablets . . 2710

NIFEHEXAL SALI (Germany)
NIFEDIPINE
Adalat CC Tablets . . . 877
Procardia Capsules . . . 2708
Procardia XL Extended Release Tablets . . 2710

NIFELAT (Brazil, Germany, Singapore, Thailand)
NIFEDIPINE
Adalat CC Tablets . . . 877
Procardia Capsules . . . 2708
Procardia XL Extended Release Tablets . . 2710

NIFELATE (France)
NIFEDIPINE
Adalat CC Tablets . . . 877
Procardia Capsules . . . 2708
Procardia XL Extended Release Tablets . . 2710

NIFELEASE (Irish Republic, United Kingdom)
NIFEDIPINE
Adalat CC Tablets . . . 877
Procardia Capsules . . . 2708
Procardia XL Extended Release Tablets . . 2710

NIFENSAR (Irish Republic)
NIFEDIPINE
Adalat CC Tablets . . . 877
Procardia Capsules . . . 2708
Procardia XL Extended Release Tablets . . 2710

NIFENSAR XL (United Kingdom)
NIFEDIPINE
Adalat CC Tablets . . . 877
Procardia Capsules . . . 2708
Procardia XL Extended Release Tablets . . 2710

NIFESAL (Italy)
NIFEDIPINE
Adalat CC Tablets . . . 877
Procardia Capsules . . . 2708
Procardia XL Extended Release Tablets . . 2710

NIFEZZARD (Mexico)
NIFEDIPINE
Adalat CC Tablets . . . 877
Procardia Capsules . . . 2708
Procardia XL Extended Release Tablets . . 2710

NIFICAL (Germany)
NIFEDIPINE
Adalat CC Tablets . . . 877
Procardia Capsules . . . 2708
Procardia XL Extended Release Tablets . . 2710

NIFICARD (Thailand)
NIFEDIPINE
Adalat CC Tablets . . . 877
Procardia Capsules . . . 2708
Procardia XL Extended Release Tablets . . 2710

NIFIDINE (South Africa)
NIFEDIPINE
Adalat CC Tablets . . . 877
Procardia Capsules . . . 2708
Procardia XL Extended Release Tablets . . 2710

NIFOPRESS (United Kingdom)
NIFEDIPINE
Adalat CC Tablets . . . 877
Procardia Capsules . . . 2708
Procardia XL Extended Release Tablets . . 2710

NIFREAL (Germany)
NIFEDIPINE
Adalat CC Tablets . . . 877
Procardia Capsules . . . 2708
Procardia XL Extended Release Tablets . . 2710

NIF-TEN (Finland, Germany, Hong Kong, Italy)
ATENOLOL
Tenormin I.V. Injection . . . 692

NIGHTCALM (United Kingdom)
DIPHENHYDRAMINE HYDROCHLORIDE
Benadryl Parenteral . . . 2617

NIKOFRENON (Germany)
NICOTINE
Nicotrol Inhaler . . . 2840
Nicotrol Nasal Spray . . . 2843

NIKORAZOL (Mexico)
KETOCONAZOLE
Nizoral 2% Cream . . . 3620
Nizoral 2% Shampoo . . . 2007
Nizoral Tablets . . . 1791

NILSTAT (Australia, Belgium, Canada, New Zealand)
NYSTATIN
Nystop Topical Powder USP . . . 2608

NIMEGEN (Singapore)
ISOTRETINOIN
Accutane Capsules . . . 2944

NIMICOR (Italy)
NICARDIPINE HYDROCHLORIDE
Cardene I.V. . . . 3485

NIMODREL (United Kingdom)
NIFEDIPINE
Adalat CC Tablets . . . 877
Procardia Capsules . . . 2708
Procardia XL Extended Release Tablets . . 2710

NIMOTOP (Australia, Austria, Belgium, Brazil, Canada, Denmark, Finland, France, Germany, Hong Kong, Irish Republic, Israel, Italy, Mexico, New Zealand, Norway, Portugal, Singapore, South Africa, Spain, Sweden, Switzerland, Thailand, The Netherlands, United Kingdom)
NIMODIPINE
Nimotop Capsules . . . 904

NINAZOL (Thailand)
KETOCONAZOLE
Nizoral 2% Cream . . . 3620
Nizoral 2% Shampoo . . . 2007
Nizoral Tablets . . . 1791

NINDAXA (United Kingdom)
INDAPAMIDE
Indapamide Tablets . . . 2286

NIOTAL (Italy)
ZOLPIDEM TARTRATE
Ambien Tablets . . . 3191

NIPENT (Belgium, Canada, France, Germany, Italy, Portugal, Spain, United Kingdom)
PENTOSTATIN
Nipent for Injection . . . 3272

NIPIN (Italy)
NIFEDIPINE
Adalat CC Tablets . . . 877
Procardia Capsules . . . 2708
Procardia XL Extended Release Tablets . . 2710

NIQUITIN (Belgium, Denmark, France, Sweden, United Kingdom)
NICOTINE
Nicotrol Inhaler . . . 2840
Nicotrol Nasal Spray . . . 2843

NIROX (Italy)
PIROXICAM
Feldene Capsules . . . 2685

NIRULID (Denmark)
AMILORIDE HYDROCHLORIDE
Midamor Tablets . . . 2136

NISIS (France)
VALSARTAN
Diovan Capsules . . . 2337

NISISCO (France)
HYDROCHLOROTHIAZIDE/VALSARTAN
Diovan HCT Tablets . . . 2338

NISOLID (Italy)
FLUNISOLIDE
Aerobid Inhaler System . . . 1363
Aerobid-M Inhaler System . . . 1363
Nasalide Nasal Spray . . . 1295
Nasarel Nasal Solution 0.025% . . . 1296

NISTAKEN (Mexico)
PROPAFENONE HYDROCHLORIDE
Rythmol Tablets – 150 mg, 225 mg, 300 mg . . . 502

NISTAN (Mexico)
NYSTATIN
Nystop Topical Powder USP . . . 2608

NISTAQUIM (Mexico)
NYSTATIN
Nystop Topical Powder USP . . . 2608

NITAN (Israel)
PEMOLINE
Cylert Chewable Tablets . . . 415
Cylert Tablets . . . 415

NITOROL (Hong Kong, Japan)
ISOSORBIDE DINITRATE
Isordil Sublingual Tablets . . . 3525
Isordil Titradose Tablets . . . 3526

NITREX (Italy)
ISOSORBIDE MONONITRATE
Imdur Tablets . . . 1826
Ismo Tablets . . . 3524

NITROCIT (South Africa)
POTASSIUM CITRATE
Urocit-K Tablets . . . 2232

NITROMIDAGER (Mexico)
METRONIDAZOLE
MetroCream . . . 1404
MetroGel . . . 1405
MetroGel-Vaginal Gel . . . 1986
MetroLotion . . . 1405
Noritate Cream . . . 1224

NITROSID (Finland)
ISOSORBIDE DINITRATE
Isordil Sublingual Tablets . . . 3525
Isordil Titradose Tablets . . . 3526

NITROSORBIDE (Italy, Singapore)
ISOSORBIDE DINITRATE
Isordil Sublingual Tablets . . . 3525
Isordil Titradose Tablets . . . 3526

NITROSORBON (Germany)
ISOSORBIDE DINITRATE
Isordil Sublingual Tablets . . . 3525
Isordil Titradose Tablets . . . 3526

NITRO-SPRAY (Australia)
ISOSORBIDE DINITRATE
Isordil Sublingual Tablets . . . 3525
Isordil Titradose Tablets . . . 3526

NITRO-TABLINEN (Germany)
ISOSORBIDE DINITRATE
Isordil Sublingual Tablets . . . 3525
Isordil Titradose Tablets . . . 3526

NITROUREAN (Spain)
CARMUSTINE
Gliadel Wafer . . . 1723

NITRUMON (Belgium, Italy)
CARMUSTINE
Gliadel Wafer . . . 1723

NIVADOR (Spain)
CEFUROXIME AXETIL
Ceftin Tablets . . . 1898
Ceftin for Oral Suspension . . . 1898

NIVATEN (United Kingdom)
NIFEDIPINE
Adalat CC Tablets . . . 877
Procardia Capsules . . . 2708
Procardia XL Extended Release Tablets . . 2710

NIVEN (Italy)
NICARDIPINE HYDROCHLORIDE
Cardene I.V. . . . 3485

NIVOFLOX (Mexico, Portugal)
CIPROFLOXACIN HYDROCHLORIDE
Ciloxan Ophthalmic Ointment . . . 538
Ciloxan Ophthalmic Solution . . . ⊙209, 538
Cipro Tablets . . . 887

NIX (Australia, Belgium, Canada, Denmark, Finland, France, Italy, Norway, Portugal)
PERMETHRIN
Acticin Cream . . . 998
Elimite Cream . . . 552

NIXAL (Mexico)
NAPROXEN SODIUM
Anaprox DS Tablets . . . 2967
Anaprox Tablets . . . 2967
Naprelan Tablets . . . 1293

NIXIN (Portugal)
CIPROFLOXACIN HYDROCHLORIDE
Ciloxan Ophthalmic Ointment . . . 538
Ciloxan Ophthalmic Solution . . . ⊙209, 538
Cipro Tablets . . . 887

NIZAX (Denmark, Finland, Germany, Italy, Sweden)
NIZATIDINE
Axid Pulvules . . . 1903

NIZAXID (France, Portugal)
NIZATIDINE
Axid Pulvules . . . 1903

NIZCREME (South Africa)
KETOCONAZOLE
Nizoral 2% Cream . . . 3620
Nizoral 2% Shampoo . . . 2007
Nizoral Tablets . . . 1791

NIZOLE (Singapore)
METRONIDAZOLE
MetroCream . . . 1404
MetroGel . . . 1405
MetroGel-Vaginal Gel . . . 1986
MetroLotion . . . 1405
Noritate Cream . . . 1224

NIZORAL (Australia, Austria, Belgium, Brazil, Denmark, Finland, France, Germany, Hong Kong, Irish Republic, Israel, Italy, Mexico, New Zealand, Portugal, Singapore, South Africa, Switzerland, Thailand, The Netherlands)
KETOCONAZOLE
Nizoral 2% Cream . . . 3620

Nizoral 2% Shampoo . . . 2007
Nizoral Tablets . . . 1791

NIZOVULES (South Africa)
KETOCONAZOLE
Nizoral 2% Cream . . . 3620
Nizoral 2% Shampoo . . . 2007
Nizoral Tablets . . . 1791

NIZSHAMPOO (South Africa)
KETOCONAZOLE
Nizoral 2% Cream . . . 3620
Nizoral 2% Shampoo . . . 2007
Nizoral Tablets . . . 1791

NOALDOL (Italy)
DIFLUNISAL
Dolobid Tablets . . . 2088

NOALGIL (Spain)
IBUPROFEN
Motrin Suspension, Oral Drops, Chewable Tablets, and Caplets . . . 2002

NOAN (Brazil, Italy)
DIAZEPAM
Valium Injectable . . . 3026
Valium Tablets . . . 3047

NOBLIGAN (Austria, Denmark, Mexico, Norway, Sweden)
TRAMADOL HYDROCHLORIDE
Ultram Tablets . . . 2600

NOCEPTIN (The Netherlands)
MORPHINE SULFATE
Astramorph/PF Injection, USP (Preservative-Free) . . . 594
Duramorph Injection . . . 1312
Infumorph 200 and Infumorph 500 Sterile Solutions . . . 1314
Kadian Capsules . . . 1335
MS Contin Tablets . . . 2896
MSIR Oral Capsules . . . 2898
MSIR Oral Solution . . . 2898
MSIR Oral Solution Concentrate . . . 2898
MSIR Oral Tablets . . . 2898
Oramorph SR Tablets . . . 3062
Roxanol 100 Concentrated Oral Solution . . . 3066
Roxanol Concentrated Oral Solution . . . 3066
Roxanol-T Oral Solution . . . 3066

NOCTAL (Brazil)
ESTAZOLAM
ProSom Tablets . . . 500

NOCUTIL (Switzerland, United Kingdom)
DESMOPRESSIN ACETATE
DDAVP Injection 4 mcg/mL . . . 737
DDAVP Nasal Spray . . . 738
DDAVP Rhinal Tube . . . 738
DDAVP Tablets . . . 739
Desmopressin Acetate Injection . . . 1344
Desmopressin Acetate Rhinal Tube . . . 1345
Stimate Nasal Spray . . . 796

NODOL (Italy)
RANITIDINE HYDROCHLORIDE
Zantac 150 EFFERdose Granules . . . 1690
Zantac 150 EFFERdose Tablets . . . 1690
Zantac 150 Tablets . . . 1690
Zantac 300 Tablets . . . 1690
Zantac Injection . . . 1688
Zantac Injection Premixed . . . 1688
Zantac Syrup . . . 1690

NODOLFEN (Spain)
IBUPROFEN
Motrin Suspension, Oral Drops, Chewable Tablets, and Caplets . . . 2002

NOFLAM (New Zealand)
NAPROXEN
EC-Naprosyn Delayed-Release Tablets . . . 2967
Naprosyn Suspension . . . 2967
Naprosyn Tablets . . . 2967

NOFLAM-N (Hong Kong)
NAPROXEN SODIUM
Anaprox DS Tablets . . . 2967
Anaprox Tablets . . . 2967
Naprelan Tablets . . . 1293

NOK (Israel)
PERMETHRIN
Acticin Cream . . . 998
Elimite Cream . . . 552

NOKTONE (Norway)
RANITIDINE HYDROCHLORIDE
Zantac 150 EFFERdose Granules . . . 1690
Zantac 150 EFFERdose Tablets . . . 1690
Zantac 150 Tablets . . . 1690
Zantac 300 Tablets . . . 1690
Zantac Injection . . . 1688
Zantac Injection Premixed . . . 1688
Zantac Syrup . . . 1690

NOLGEN (Irish Republic)
TAMOXIFEN CITRATE
Nolvadex Tablets . . . 678

NOLIPAX (Italy)
FENOFIBRATE
Tricor Capsules, Micronized . . . 513

NOLOL (South Africa)
PROPRANOLOL HYDROCHLORIDE
Inderal Injectable . . . 3513
Inderal LA Long-Acting Capsules . . . 3516
Inderal Tablets . . . 3513

NOLTAM (United Kingdom)
TAMOXIFEN CITRATE
Nolvadex Tablets . . . 678

NOLVADEX (Australia, Austria, Belgium, Brazil, Canada, Finland, France, Germany, Hong Kong, Irish Republic, Israel, Italy, New Zealand, Norway, Portugal, Singapore, South Africa, Spain, Sweden, Switzerland, Thailand, The Netherlands, United Kingdom)
TAMOXIFEN CITRATE
Nolvadex Tablets . . . 678

NOODIPINA (Brazil)
NIMODIPINE
Nimotop Capsules . . . 904

NOPARIN (Sweden)
HEPARIN SODIUM
Heparin Lock Flush Solution . . . 3509
Heparin Sodium Injection . . . 3511

NORA (Thailand)
KETOCONAZOLE
Nizoral 2% Cream . . . 3620
Nizoral 2% Shampoo . . . 2007
Nizoral Tablets . . . 1791

NORACIN (Brazil, Thailand)
NORFLOXACIN
Chibroxin Sterile Ophthalmic Solution . . . ⊙273, 2051
Noroxin Tablets . . . 2145

NORAKIN N (Germany)
BIPERIDEN HYDROCHLORIDE
Akineton Tablets . . . 402

NORAXIN (Thailand)
NORFLOXACIN
Chibroxin Sterile Ophthalmic Solution . . . ⊙273, 2051
Noroxin Tablets . . . 2145

NORBACTIN (Singapore, Thailand)
NORFLOXACIN
Chibroxin Sterile Ophthalmic Solution . . . ⊙273, 2051
Noroxin Tablets . . . 2145

NORCURON (Australia, Austria, Belgium, Brazil, Canada, Denmark, Finland, France, Germany, Hong Kong, Irish Republic, Israel, Italy, Mexico, New Zealand, Norway, Portugal, Singapore, South Africa, Spain, Sweden, Switzerland, Thailand, The Netherlands, United Kingdom)
VECURONIUM BROMIDE
Norcuron for Injection . . . 2478

NORDAPANIN N (Germany)
BENZOCAINE
Americaine Anesthetic Lubricant . . . 1162
Americaine Otic Topical Anesthetic Ear Drops . . . 1162

NORDOTOL (Denmark)
CARBAMAZEPINE
Carbatrol Capsules . . . 3234
Tegretol Chewable Tablets . . . 2404
Tegretol Suspension . . . 2404
Tegretol Tablets . . . 2404
Tegretol-XR Tablets . . . 2404

NORDOX (United Kingdom)
DOXYCYCLINE HYCLATE
Doryx Coated Pellet Filled Capsules . . . 3357
Periostat Tablets . . . 1208
Vibramycin Hyclate Capsules . . . 2735
Vibramycin Hyclate Intravenous . . . 2737
Vibra-Tabs Film Coated Tablets . . . 2735

NORDYL (Thailand)
CODEINE PHOSPHATE/PROMETHAZINE HYDROCHLORIDE
Phenergan with Codeine Syrup . . . 3557

NORFCIN (Thailand)
NORFLOXACIN
Chibroxin Sterile Ophthalmic Solution . . . ⊙273, 2051
Noroxin Tablets . . . 2145

NORFENON (Mexico)
PROPAFENONE HYDROCHLORIDE
Rythmol Tablets – 150 mg, 225 mg, 300 mg . . . 502

NORFLAM T (South Africa)
IBUPROFEN
Motrin Suspension, Oral Drops, Chewable Tablets, and Caplets . . . 2002

NORFLEX (Australia, Austria, Belgium, Canada, Denmark, Finland, Germany, Mexico, New Zealand, Portugal, Singapore, South Africa, Sweden, Switzerland, United Kingdom)
ORPHENADRINE CITRATE
Norflex Extended-Release Tablets . . . 1987
Norflex Injection . . . 1987

NORFLO (Thailand)
NORFLOXACIN
Chibroxin Sterile Ophthalmic Solution . . . ⊙273, 2051
Noroxin Tablets . . . 2145

NORFLOCIN (Switzerland, Thailand)
NORFLOXACIN
Chibroxin Sterile Ophthalmic Solution . . . ⊙273, 2051
Noroxin Tablets . . . 2145

NORFLOHEXAL (Australia)
NORFLOXACIN
Chibroxin Sterile Ophthalmic Solution . . . ⊙273, 2051
Noroxin Tablets . . . 2145

NORFLOSAL (Germany)
NORFLOXACIN
Chibroxin Sterile Ophthalmic Solution . . . ⊙273, 2051
Noroxin Tablets . . . 2145

NORFLOX (Italy)
NORFLOXACIN
Chibroxin Sterile Ophthalmic Solution . . . ⊙273, 2051
Noroxin Tablets . . . 2145

NORFLOX-AZU (Germany)
NORFLOXACIN
Chibroxin Sterile Ophthalmic Solution . . . ⊙273, 2051
Noroxin Tablets . . . 2145

NORFLOXIN (Thailand)
NORFLOXACIN
Chibroxin Sterile Ophthalmic Solution . . . ⊙273, 2051
Noroxin Tablets . . . 2145

NORGESTON (United Kingdom)
LEVONORGESTREL
Norplant System . . . 3543

NORICLAN (Spain)
DIRITHROMYCIN
Dynabac Tablets . . . 2269

NORIMOX (South Africa)
AMOXICILLIN
Amoxil Pediatric Drops for Oral Suspension . . . 1471
Amoxil Tablets . . . 1471

NORITATE (Canada, United Kingdom)
METRONIDAZOLE
MetroCream . . . 1404
MetroGel . . . 1405
MetroGel-Vaginal Gel . . . 1986
MetroLotion . . . 1405
Noritate Cream . . . 1224

NORITET (South Africa)
DOXYCYCLINE HYCLATE
Doryx Coated Pellet Filled Capsules . . . 3357
Periostat Tablets . . . 1208
Vibramycin Hyclate Capsules . . . 2735
Vibramycin Hyclate Intravenous . . . 2737
Vibra-Tabs Film Coated Tablets . . . 2735

NORITRATE (Hong Kong)
METRONIDAZOLE
MetroCream . . . 1404
MetroGel . . . 1405
MetroGel-Vaginal Gel . . . 1986
MetroLotion . . . 1405
Noritate Cream . . . 1224

NORIZAL (Brazil)
KETOCONAZOLE
Nizoral 2% Cream . . . 3620
Nizoral 2% Shampoo . . . 2007
Nizoral Tablets . . . 1791

NORLEVO (France)
LEVONORGESTREL
Norplant System . . . 3543

NORMALIP PRO (Germany)
FENOFIBRATE
Tricor Capsules, Micronized . . . 513

NORMALOL (Israel)
ATENOLOL
Tenormin I.V. Injection . . . 692

NORMASE (Italy)
LACTULOSE
Kristalose for Oral Solution . . . 1007

NORMATEN (Singapore)
ATENOLOL
Tenormin I.V. Injection . . . 692

NORMETIC (United Kingdom)
AMILORIDE HYDROCHLORIDE/HYDROCHLOROTHIAZIDE
Moduretic Tablets . . . 2138

NORMITEN (Israel)
ATENOLOL
Tenormin I.V. Injection . . . 692

NORMOGLIC (Italy)
CHLORPROPAMIDE
Diabinese Tablets . . . 2680

NORMOMENSIL (Brazil)
PROGESTERONE
Crinone 4% Gel . . . 3213
Crinone 8% Gel . . . 3213
Prometrium Capsules (100 mg, 200 mg) . . . 3261

NORMONSONA (Spain)
PREDNISOLONE
Prelone Syrup . . . 2273

NORMOPARIN (Italy)
HEPARIN SODIUM
Heparin Lock Flush Solution . . . 3509
Heparin Sodium Injection . . . 3511

NORMOPRESAN (Israel)
CLONIDINE HYDROCHLORIDE
Catapres Tablets . . . 1037
Duraclon Injection . . . 3057

NORMOPRESS (Italy, South Africa)
ATENOLOL
Tenormin I.V. Injection . . . 692

NORMORIX (Norway, Sweden)
AMILORIDE HYDROCHLORIDE/HYDROCHLOROTHIAZIDE
Moduretic Tablets . . . 2138

NORMORYTMIN (Irish Republic)
PROPAFENONE HYDROCHLORIDE
Rythmol Tablets – 150 mg, 225 mg, 300 mg . . . 502

NORMOSPOR (South Africa)
CLOTRIMAZOLE
Lotrimin Cream 1% . . . 3128
Lotrimin Lotion 1% . . . 3128
Lotrimin Topical Solution 1% . . . 3128
Mycelex Troche . . . 573

NORMOTIL (Portugal)
CAPTOPRIL
Captopril Tablets . . . 2281

NORMPRESS (Thailand)
PROPRANOLOL HYDROCHLORIDE
Inderal Injectable . . . 3513
Inderal LA Long-Acting Capsules . . . 3516
Inderal Tablets . . . 3513

NOROXIN (Australia, Canada, Finland, Italy, Mexico, New Zealand, Portugal, South Africa, Spain, Switzerland, The Netherlands, United Kingdom)
NORFLOXACIN
Chibroxin Sterile Ophthalmic Solution . . . ⊙273, 2051
Noroxin Tablets . . . 2145

NOROXINE (France)
NORFLOXACIN
Chibroxin Sterile Ophthalmic Solution . . . ⊙273, 2051
Noroxin Tablets . . . 2145

NORPID (Thailand)
GEMFIBROZIL
Lopid Tablets . . . 2650

NORPLANT (Canada, Israel, Mexico, Singapore, Sweden, Thailand, United Kingdom)
LEVONORGESTREL
Norplant System . . . 3543

NORPRAMIN (Canada, Spain)
DESIPRAMINE HYDROCHLORIDE
Norpramin Tablets . . . 755

NORPRIL (Mexico)
ENALAPRIL MALEATE
Vasotec Tablets . . . 2210

NORPRO (South Africa)
PROPRANOLOL HYDROCHLORIDE
Inderal Injectable . . . 3513
Inderal LA Long-Acting Capsules . . . 3516
Inderal Tablets . . . 3513

NORSA (Thailand)
NORFLOXACIN
Chibroxin Sterile Ophthalmic Solution . . . ⊙273, 2051

Noroxin Tablets . . . 2145

NORSET (France)
MIRTAZAPINE
Remeron SolTab Tablets . . . 2486

NORSOL (Switzerland)
NORFLOXACIN
Chibroxin Sterile Ophthalmic Solution . . . ⊙273, 2051
Noroxin Tablets . . . 2145

NORTIMIL (Italy)
DESIPRAMINE HYDROCHLORIDE
Norpramin Tablets . . . 755

NORTON (Brazil)
NIMODIPINE
Nimotop Capsules . . . 904

NORTREL (Brazil)
LEVONORGESTREL
Norplant System . . . 3543

NORTRON (Spain)
DIRITHROMYCIN
Dynabac Tablets . . . 2269

NORTUSS (Thailand)
CODEINE PHOSPHATE/PROMETHAZINE HYDROCHLORIDE
Phenergan with Codeine Syrup . . . 3557

NORUXOL (Italy)
COLLAGENASE
Collagenase Santyl Ointment . . . 3248

NORVIR (Australia, Belgium, Canada, Denmark, Finland, France, Germany, Hong Kong, Israel, Italy, Japan, Mexico, New Zealand, Norway, Portugal, South Africa, Spain, Sweden, Switzerland, Thailand, The Netherlands, United Kingdom)
RITONAVIR
Norvir Capsules . . . 487
Norvir Oral Solution . . . 487

NORXACIN (Thailand)
NORFLOXACIN
Chibroxin Sterile Ophthalmic Solution . . . ⊙273, 2051
Noroxin Tablets . . . 2145

NORXIA (Thailand)
NORFLOXACIN
Chibroxin Sterile Ophthalmic Solution . . . ⊙273, 2051
Noroxin Tablets . . . 2145

NOS (Spain)
FAMOTIDINE
Pepcid Injection . . . 2153
Pepcid Injection Premixed . . . 2153
Pepcid RPD Orally Disintegrating Tablets . . . 2150
Pepcid Tablets . . . 2150
Pepcid for Oral Suspension . . . 2150

NOTEN (Australia, Thailand)
ATENOLOL
Tenormin I.V. Injection . . . 692

NOTTEM (Italy)
ZOLPIDEM TARTRATE
Ambien Tablets . . . 3191

NOTUL (Italy)
CIMETIDINE HYDROCHLORIDE
Tagamet Injection . . . 1644
Tagamet Liquid . . . 1644

NOURY HOOFDLOTION (The Netherlands)
MALATHION
Ovide Lotion . . . 2023

NOURYTAM (Germany)
TAMOXIFEN CITRATE
Nolvadex Tablets . . . 678

NOVA (Canada)
PENTOBARBITAL SODIUM
Nembutal Sodium Solution . . . 485

NOVA RECTAL (Canada)
PENTOBARBITAL SODIUM
Nembutal Sodium Solution . . . 485

NOVACEF (Mexico)
CEFIXIME
Suprax Tablets . . . 1877
Suprax for Oral Suspension . . . 1877

NOVADEX (Mexico)
NAPROXEN
EC-Naprosyn Delayed-Release Tablets . . . 2967
Naprosyn Suspension . . . 2967
Naprosyn Tablets . . . 2967

NOVALDEX (Mexico)
TAMOXIFEN CITRATE
Nolvadex Tablets . . . 678

NOVALM (France)
MEPROBAMATE
Miltown Tablets . . . 3349

NOVAMET (Denmark, Mexico)
CIMETIDINE
Tagamet Tablets . . . 1644

NOVAMILOR (Canada)
AMILORIDE HYDROCHLORIDE/HYDROCHLOROTHIAZIDE
Moduretic Tablets . . . 2138

NOVAPAM (New Zealand)
CHLORDIAZEPOXIDE HYDROCHLORIDE
Librium Capsules . . . 1736
Librium for Injection . . . 1737

NOVAPAMYL (France)
VERAPAMIL HYDROCHLORIDE
Covera-HS Tablets . . . 3199
Isoptin SR Tablets . . . 467
Verelan Capsules . . . 3184
Verelan PM Capsules . . . 3186

NOVAPIRINA (Italy)
DICLOFENAC SODIUM
Voltaren Tablets . . . 2315
Voltaren-XR Tablets . . . 2315

NOVAPRES (Mexico)
CAPTOPRIL
Captopril Tablets . . . 2281

NOVAPRIN (United Kingdom)
IBUPROFEN
Motrin Suspension, Oral Drops, Chewable Tablets, and Caplets . . . 2002

NOVASONE (Australia)
MOMETASONE FUROATE
Elocon Cream 0.1% . . . 3110
Elocon Lotion 0.1% . . . 3111
Elocon Ointment 0.1% . . . 3112
Nasonex Nasal Spray . . . 3131

NOVASULFON (Mexico)
DAPSONE
Dapsone Tablets USP . . . 1780

NOVATEC (Belgium, The Netherlands)
LISINOPRIL
Prinivil Tablets . . . 2164
Zestril Tablets . . . 698

NOVAVIR (Mexico)
ZIDOVUDINE
Retrovir Capsules . . . 1625
Retrovir IV Infusion . . . 1629
Retrovir Syrup . . . 1625
Retrovir Tablets . . . 1625

NOVAXEN (Mexico)
NAPROXEN
EC-Naprosyn Delayed-Release Tablets . . . 2967
Naprosyn Suspension . . . 2967
Naprosyn Tablets . . . 2967

NOVAZAM (France)
DIAZEPAM
Valium Injectable . . . 3026
Valium Tablets . . . 3047

NOVAZYD (Belgium, The Netherlands)
LISINOPRIL
Prinivil Tablets . . . 2164
Zestril Tablets . . . 698

NOVELCICLINA (Spain)
DOXYCYCLINE HYCLATE
Doryx Coated Pellet Filled Capsules . . . 3357
Periostat Tablets . . . 1208
Vibramycin Hyclate Capsules . . . 2735
Vibramycin Hyclate Intravenous . . . 2737
Vibra-Tabs Film Coated Tablets . . . 2735

NOVELIAN (Spain)
SUMATRIPTAN SUCCINATE
Imitrex Injection . . . 1549
Imitrex Tablets . . . 1558

NOVELMIN (Brazil)
MEBENDAZOLE
Vermox Chewable Tablets . . . 2017

NOVO-ALPRAZOL (Canada)
ALPRAZOLAM
Xanax Tablets . . . 2865

NOVO-ATENOL (Canada)
ATENOLOL
Tenormin I.V. Injection . . . 692

NOVO-AZT (Canada)
ZIDOVUDINE
Retrovir Capsules . . . 1625
Retrovir IV Infusion . . . 1629
Retrovir Syrup . . . 1625
Retrovir Tablets . . . 1625

NOVOBIOCYL (Italy)
CEFOPERAZONE SODIUM
Cefobid Intravenous/Intramuscular . . . 2671
Cefobid Pharmacy Bulk Package - Not for Direct Infusion . . . 2673

NOVO-CARBAMAZ (Canada)
CARBAMAZEPINE
Carbatrol Capsules . . . 3234
Tegretol Chewable Tablets . . . 2404
Tegretol Suspension . . . 2404
Tegretol Tablets . . . 2404
Tegretol-XR Tablets . . . 2404

NOVO-CHLOROCAP (Canada)
CHLORAMPHENICOL
Chloromycetin Ophthalmic Ointment, 1% . . . ⊙296
Chloromycetin Ophthalmic Solution . . . ⊙297
Chloroptic Sterile Ophthalmic Ointment . . ⊙234
Chloroptic Sterile Ophthalmic Solution . . ⊙235

NOVOCILIN (Brazil)
AMOXICILLIN
Amoxil Pediatric Drops for Oral Suspension . . . 1471
Amoxil Tablets . . . 1471

NOVO-CIMETINE (Canada)
CIMETIDINE
Tagamet Tablets . . . 1644

NOVOCORTAL (Italy)
HYDROCORTISONE ACETATE
Anusol-HC Suppositories . . . 2238
Cortifoam Rectal Foam . . . 3170
Hydrocortone Acetate Injectable Suspension . . . 2103
Proctocort Suppositories . . . 2264

NOVO-CYCLOPRINE (Canada)
CYCLOBENZAPRINE HYDROCHLORIDE
Flexeril Tablets . . . 2094

NOVODIL (Italy)
DIPYRIDAMOLE
Persantine Tablets . . . 1057

NOVO-DILTAZEM (Canada)
DILTIAZEM HYDROCHLORIDE
Cardizem CD Capsules . . . 1016
Cardizem Injectable . . . 1018
Cardizem Lyo-Ject Syringe . . . 1018
Cardizem Monovial . . . 1018
Tiazac Capsules . . . 1378

NOVO-DIPAM (Canada)
DIAZEPAM
Valium Injectable . . . 3026
Valium Tablets . . . 3047

NOVO-DIPIRADOL (Canada)
DIPYRIDAMOLE
Persantine Tablets . . . 1057

NOVO-DOPARIL (Canada)
METHYLDOPA
Aldomet Tablets . . . 2037

NOVODORM (Spain)
TRIAZOLAM
Halcion Tablets . . . 2823

NOVO-DOXYLIN (Canada)
DOXYCYCLINE HYCLATE
Doryx Coated Pellet Filled Capsules . . . 3357
Periostat Tablets . . . 1208
Vibramycin Hyclate Capsules . . . 2735
Vibramycin Hyclate Intravenous . . . 2737
Vibra-Tabs Film Coated Tablets . . . 2735

NOVOFEN (Thailand)
TAMOXIFEN CITRATE
Nolvadex Tablets . . . 678

NOVO-FIBRATE (Canada)
CLOFIBRATE
Atromid-S Capsules . . . 3483

NOVO-FLURAZINE (Canada)
TRIFLUOPERAZINE HYDROCHLORIDE
Stelazine Injection . . . 1640
Stelazine Tablets . . . 1640

NOVOGENT (Germany)
IBUPROFEN
Motrin Suspension, Oral Drops, Chewable Tablets, and Caplets . . . 2002

NOVO-HERKLIN 2000 (Mexico)
PERMETHRIN
Acticin Cream . . . 998
Elimite Cream . . . 552

NOVO-HYDRAZIDE (Canada)
HYDROCHLOROTHIAZIDE
HydroDIURIL Tablets . . . 2108
Microzide Capsules . . . 3414

NOVO-HYDROCORT (Canada)
HYDROCORTISONE
Anusol-HC Cream 2.5% . . . 2237
Hydrocortone Tablets . . . 2106

NOVO-IPRAMIDE (Canada)
IPRATROPIUM BROMIDE
Atrovent Inhalation Aerosol . . . 1030
Atrovent Inhalation Solution . . . 1031
Atrovent Nasal Spray 0.03% . . . 1032
Atrovent Nasal Spray 0.06% . . . 1033

NOVO-KETO (Canada)
KETOPROFEN
Orudis Capsules . . . 3548
Oruvail Capsules . . . 3548

NOVOLENTE-K (Canada)
POTASSIUM CHLORIDE
K-Dur Microburst Release System ER Tablets . . . 1832
K-Lor Powder Packets . . . 469
K-Tab Filmtab Tablets . . . 470
Rum-K . . . 1363

NOVO-LEXIN (Canada)
CEPHALEXIN
Keflex Oral Suspension . . . 1237
Keflex Pulvules . . . 1237

NOVO-LORAZEM (Canada)
LORAZEPAM
Ativan Injection . . . 3478
Ativan Tablets . . . 3482

NOVO-MEDOPA (Canada)
METHYLDOPA
Aldomet Tablets . . . 2037

NOVO-MEDRONE (Canada)
MEDROXYPROGESTERONE ACETATE
Depo-Provera Contraceptive Injection . . . 2798
Provera Tablets . . . 2853

NOVO-MEPRO (Canada)
MEPROBAMATE
Miltown Tablets . . . 3349

NOVOMET (Australia)
METFORMIN HYDROCHLORIDE
Glucophage Tablets . . . 1080

NOVO-NAPROX (Canada)
NAPROXEN
EC-Naprosyn Delayed-Release Tablets . . . 2967
Naprosyn Suspension . . . 2967
Naprosyn Tablets . . . 2967

NOVO-NIDAZOL (Canada)
METRONIDAZOLE
MetroCream . . . 1404
MetroGel . . . 1405
MetroGel-Vaginal Gel . . . 1986
MetroLotion . . . 1405
Noritate Cream . . . 1224

NOVO-NIFEDIN (Canada)
NIFEDIPINE
Adalat CC Tablets . . . 877
Procardia Capsules . . . 2708
Procardia XL Extended Release Tablets . . 2710

NOVONORM (Australia, Austria, Denmark, Finland, France, Germany, Irish Republic, Italy, New Zealand, Norway, Singapore, South Africa, Spain, Sweden, Thailand, The Netherlands, United Kingdom)
REPAGLINIDE
Prandin Tablets (0.5, 1, and 2 mg) . . . 2432

NOVO-PERIDOL (Canada)
HALOPERIDOL
Haldol Injection, Tablets and Concentrate . . . 2533

NOVO-PIROCAM (Canada)
PIROXICAM
Feldene Capsules . . . 2685

NOVOPLAT (Mexico)
CARBOPLATIN
Paraplatin for Injection . . . 1126

NOVOPLATINUM (Portugal)
CARBOPLATIN
Paraplatin for Injection . . . 1126

NOVO-POXIDE (Canada)
CHLORDIAZEPOXIDE HYDROCHLORIDE
Librium Capsules . . . 1736
Librium for Injection . . . 1737

NOVO-PRANOL (Canada)
PROPRANOLOL HYDROCHLORIDE
Inderal Injectable . . . 3513
Inderal LA Long-Acting Capsules . . . 3516
Inderal Tablets . . . 3513

NOVO-PRAZIN (Canada)
PRAZOSIN HYDROCHLORIDE
Minipress Capsules . . . 2699

NOVO-PROFEN (Canada)
IBUPROFEN
Motrin Suspension, Oral Drops, Chewable Tablets, and Caplets . . . 2002

NOVO-PROPAMIDE (Canada)
CHLORPROPAMIDE
Diabinese Tablets . . . 2680

NOVOQUIN (Mexico)
CIPROFLOXACIN
Cipro I.V. 893
Cipro I.V. Pharmacy Bulk Package 897
Cipro Oral Suspension 887

NOVO-RANIDINE (Canada)
RANITIDINE HYDROCHLORIDE
Zantac 150 EFFERdose Granules 1690
Zantac 150 EFFERdose Tablets 1690
Zantac 150 Tablets 1690
Zantac 300 Tablets 1690
Zantac Injection 1688
Zantac Injection Premixed 1688
Zantac Syrup 1690

NOVO-RIDAZINE (Canada)
THIORIDAZINE HYDROCHLORIDE
Thioridazine Hydrochloride Tablets 2289

NOVO-RYTHRO (Canada)
ERYTHROMYCIN
Emgel 2% Topical Gel 1285
Ery-Tab Tablets 448
Erythromycin Base Filmtab Tablets 454
Erythromycin Delayed-Release Capsules, USP 455
PCE Dispertab Tablets 498

NOVO-SORBIDE (Canada)
ISOSORBIDE DINITRATE
Isordil Sublingual Tablets 3525
Isordil Titradose Tablets 3526

NOVOSTREP (South Africa)
STREPTOMYCIN SULFATE
Streptomycin Sulfate Injection 2714

NOVO-SUCRALATE (Canada)
SUCRALFATE
Carafate Suspension 731
Carafate Tablets 730

NOVO-SUNDAC (Canada)
SULINDAC
Clinoril Tablets 2053

NOVOTER (Hong Kong, Spain)
FLUOCINONIDE
Lidex Cream 2020
Lidex Gel 2020
Lidex Ointment 2020
Lidex Topical Solution 2020
Lidex-E Cream 2020

NOVO-THEOPHYL (Canada)
THEOPHYLLINE
Aerolate Jr. T.D. Capsules 1361
Aerolate Liquid 1361
Aerolate Sr. T.D. Capsules 1361
Theo-Dur Extended-Release Tablets 1835
Uni-Dur Extended-Release Tablets 1841
Uniphyl 400 mg and 600 mg Tablets 2903

NOVOTHYRAL (Austria)
LIOTHYRONINE SODIUM
Cytomel Tablets 1817
Triostat Injection 1825

NOVO-TIMOL (Canada)
TIMOLOL MALEATE
Blocadren Tablets 2046
Timoptic Sterile Ophthalmic Solution 2190
Timoptic in Ocudose 2192
Timoptic-XE Sterile Ophthalmic Gel Forming Solution 2194

NOVO-TRIAMZIDE (Canada)
HYDROCHLOROTHIAZIDE/TRIAMTERENE
Dyazide Capsules 1515
Maxzide Tablets 1008
Maxzide-25 mg Tablets 1008

NOVO-TRIOLAM (Canada)
TRIAZOLAM
Halcion Tablets 2823

NOVO-TRIPRAMINE (Canada)
TRIMIPRAMINE MALEATE
Surmontil Capsules 3595

NOVO-VERAMIL (Canada)
VERAPAMIL HYDROCHLORIDE
Covera-HS Tablets 3199
Isoptin SR Tablets 467
Verelan Capsules 3184
Verelan PM Capsules 3186

NOVOXIL (Brazil)
AMOXICILLIN
Amoxil Pediatric Drops for Oral Suspension 1471
Amoxil Tablets 1471

NOVO-ZOLAMIDE (Canada)
ACETAZOLAMIDE
Diamox Sequels Sustained Release Capsules .... ⊙270
Diamox Tablets .... ⊙269

NOVRAL (Brazil)
LISINOPRIL
Prinivil Tablets 2164
Zestril Tablets 698

NOVUXOL (The Netherlands)
COLLAGENASE
Collagenase Santyl Ointment 3248

NOXINE (Thailand)
NORFLOXACIN
Chibroxin Sterile Ophthalmic Solution .... ⊙273, 2051
Noroxin Tablets 2145

NOXINOR (Thailand)
NORFLOXACIN
Chibroxin Sterile Ophthalmic Solution .... ⊙273, 2051
Noroxin Tablets 2145

NOXITEM (Australia)
TAMOXIFEN CITRATE
Nolvadex Tablets 678

NU-ALPRAZ (Canada)
ALPRAZOLAM
Xanax Tablets 2865

NUARDIN (Belgium)
CIMETIDINE
Tagamet Tablets 1644

NU-ATENOL (Canada)
ATENOLOL
Tenormin I.V. Injection 692

NUBAIN (Austria, Canada, France, Germany, Israel, Mexico, New Zealand, Singapore, South Africa, Switzerland, Thailand, United Kingdom)
NALBUPHINE HYDROCHLORIDE
Nubain Injection 1323

NU-CAPTO (Canada)
CAPTOPRIL
Captopril Tablets 2281

NU-CEPHALEX (Canada)
CEPHALEXIN
Keflex Oral Suspension 1237
Keflex Pulvules 1237

NU-CIMET (Canada)
CIMETIDINE
Tagamet Tablets 1644

NUCLOGEN (Spain)
GENTAMICIN SULFATE
Genoptic Ophthalmic Ointment .... ⊙239
Genoptic Sterile Ophthalmic Solution .... ⊙239

NUCLOSINA (Spain)
OMEPRAZOLE
Prilosec Delayed-Release Capsules 628

NUCTALON (France)
ESTAZOLAM
ProSom Tablets 500

NU-DICLO (Canada)
DICLOFENAC SODIUM
Voltaren Tablets 2315
Voltaren-XR Tablets 2315

NU-DILTIAZ (Canada)
DILTIAZEM HYDROCHLORIDE
Cardizem CD Capsules 1016
Cardizem Injectable 1018
Cardizem Lyo-Ject Syringe 1018
Cardizem Monovial 1018
Tiazac Capsules 1378

NUDOPA (Australia)
METHYLDOPA
Aldomet Tablets 2037

NUELIN (Australia, Denmark, Finland, Hong Kong, New Zealand, Norway, Singapore, South Africa, Thailand, United Kingdom)
THEOPHYLLINE
Aerolate Jr. T.D. Capsules 1361
Aerolate Liquid 1361
Aerolate Sr. T.D. Capsules 1361
Theo-Dur Extended-Release Tablets 1835
Uni-Dur Extended-Release Tablets 1841
Uniphyl 400 mg and 600 mg Tablets 2903

NUICALM (Belgium)
DIPHENHYDRAMINE HYDROCHLORIDE
Benadryl Parenteral 2617

NU-K (United Kingdom)
POTASSIUM CHLORIDE
K-Dur Microburst Release System ER Tablets 1832
K-Lor Powder Packets 469
K-Tab Filmtab Tablets 470
Rum-K 1363

NULCERAN (Portugal)
FAMOTIDINE
Pepcid Injection 2153
Pepcid Injection Premixed 2153
Pepcid RPD Orally Disintegrating Tablets 2150
Pepcid Tablets 2150
Pepcid for Oral Suspension 2150

NULCERIN (Spain)
FAMOTIDINE
Pepcid Injection 2153
Pepcid Injection Premixed 2153
Pepcid RPD Orally Disintegrating Tablets 2150
Pepcid Tablets 2150
Pepcid for Oral Suspension 2150

NU-LORAZ (Canada)
LORAZEPAM
Ativan Injection 3478
Ativan Tablets 3482

NU-LOTAN (Japan)
LOSARTAN POTASSIUM
Cozaar Tablets 2067

NU-MEDOPA (Canada)
METHYLDOPA
Aldomet Tablets 2037

NUMORPHAN (Canada)
OXYMORPHONE HYDROCHLORIDE
Numorphan Injection 1324
Numorphan Suppositories 1324

NUMZIT (South Africa)
BENZOCAINE
Americaine Anesthetic Lubricant 1162
Americaine Otic Topical Anesthetic Ear Drops 1162

NU-NAPROX (Canada)
NAPROXEN
EC-Naprosyn Delayed-Release Tablets 2967
Naprosyn Suspension 2967
Naprosyn Tablets 2967

NU-NIFED (Canada)
NIFEDIPINE
Adalat CC Tablets 877
Procardia Capsules 2708
Procardia XL Extended Release Tablets 2710

NU-PIROX (Canada)
PIROXICAM
Feldene Capsules 2685

NU-PRAZO (Canada)
PRAZOSIN HYDROCHLORIDE
Minipress Capsules 2699

NUPRILAN (Portugal)
IBUPROFEN
Motrin Suspension, Oral Drops, Chewable Tablets, and Caplets 2002

NU-PROCHLOR (Canada)
PROCHLORPERAZINE MALEATE
Compazine Spansule Capsules 1505
Compazine Tablets 1505

NURAN (Germany)
CYPROHEPTADINE HYDROCHLORIDE
Periactin Tablets 2155

NU-RANIT (Canada)
RANITIDINE HYDROCHLORIDE
Zantac 150 EFFERdose Granules 1690
Zantac 150 EFFERdose Tablets 1690
Zantac 150 Tablets 1690
Zantac 300 Tablets 1690
Zantac Injection 1688
Zantac Injection Premixed 1688
Zantac Syrup 1690

NUREFLEX (France, Spain)
IBUPROFEN
Motrin Suspension, Oral Drops, Chewable Tablets, and Caplets 2002

NUROFEN (Australia, Austria, Belgium, Denmark, France, Germany, Hong Kong, Irish Republic, Israel, Italy, New Zealand, Singapore, South Africa, Spain, Sweden, Switzerland, Thailand, The Netherlands, United Kingdom)
IBUPROFEN
Motrin Suspension, Oral Drops, Chewable Tablets, and Caplets 2002

NUROFEN + CODEINE (Belgium)
IBUPROFEN
Motrin Suspension, Oral Drops, Chewable Tablets, and Caplets 2002

NUROFEN PLUS (New Zealand, United Kingdom)
IBUPROFEN
Motrin Suspension, Oral Drops, Chewable Tablets, and Caplets 2002

NURSE SYKES BALSAM (United Kingdom)
GUAIFENESIN
Organidin NR Liquid 3350
Organidin NR Tablets 3350

NUTRACORT (Brazil, Finland, Mexico)
HYDROCORTISONE
Anusol-HC Cream 2.5% 2237
Hydrocortone Tablets 2106

NU-TRIAZIDE (Canada)
HYDROCHLOROTHIAZIDE/TRIAMTERENE
Dyazide Capsules 1515
Maxzide Tablets 1008
Maxzide-25 mg Tablets 1008

NU-TRIAZO (Canada)
TRIAZOLAM
Halcion Tablets 2823

NU-VERAP (Canada)
VERAPAMIL HYDROCHLORIDE
Covera-HS Tablets 3199
Isoptin SR Tablets 467
Verelan Capsules 3184
Verelan PM Capsules 3186

NYADERM (Canada)
NYSTATIN
Nystop Topical Powder USP 2608

NYCODOL (Austria)
TRAMADOL HYDROCHLORIDE
Ultram Tablets 2600

NYCOHEPARIN (Norway)
HEPARIN SODIUM
Heparin Lock Flush Solution 3509
Heparin Sodium Injection 3511

NYCOPIN (Denmark, Norway)
NIFEDIPINE
Adalat CC Tablets 877
Procardia Capsules 2708
Procardia XL Extended Release Tablets 2710

NYCOPREN (Austria, Belgium, Denmark, Finland, Switzerland, The Netherlands, United Kingdom)
NAPROXEN
EC-Naprosyn Delayed-Release Tablets 2967
Naprosyn Suspension 2967
Naprosyn Tablets 2967

NYEFAX (Australia, New Zealand)
NIFEDIPINE
Adalat CC Tablets 877
Procardia Capsules 2708
Procardia XL Extended Release Tablets 2710

NYMIX-CYCLIN N (Germany)
DOXYCYCLINE HYCLATE
Doryx Coated Pellet Filled Capsules 3357
Periostat Tablets 1208
Vibramycin Hyclate Capsules 2735
Vibramycin Hyclate Intravenous 2737
Vibra-Tabs Film Coated Tablets 2735

NYOLOL (France, Hong Kong, Israel, Portugal, Singapore, Spain, Thailand)
TIMOLOL MALEATE
Blocadren Tablets 2046
Timoptic Sterile Ophthalmic Solution 2190
Timoptic in Ocudose 2192
Timoptic-XE Sterile Ophthalmic Gel Forming Solution 2194

NYSPES (United Kingdom)
NYSTATIN
Nystop Topical Powder USP 2608

NYSTACID (South Africa)
NYSTATIN
Nystop Topical Powder USP 2608

NYSTADERM (Germany)
NYSTATIN
Nystop Topical Powder USP 2608

NYSTADERMAL (United Kingdom)
NYSTATIN
Nystop Topical Powder USP 2608

NYSTAFORM (United Kingdom)
NYSTATIN
Nystop Topical Powder USP 2608

NYSTAMONT (United Kingdom)
NYSTATIN
Nystop Topical Powder USP 2608

NYSTAN (United Kingdom)
NYSTATIN
Nystop Topical Powder USP 2608

NYSTASAN (Mexico)
NYSTATIN
Nystop Topical Powder USP 2608

NYSTATIN-DOME (United Kingdom)
NYSTATIN
Nystop Topical Powder USP 2608

NYSTAVESCENT (United Kingdom)
NYSTATIN
Nystop Topical Powder USP 2608

NYTOL (Australia, Canada, Germany, Italy, South Africa, Spain, United Kingdom)
DIPHENHYDRAMINE HYDROCHLORIDE
Benadryl Parenteral 2617

OASIL SIMES (Spain)
MEPROBAMATE
Miltown Tablets 3349

OBESAN-X (South Africa)
PHENDIMETRAZINE TARTRATE
Bontril Slow-Release Capsules 576

OBEX-LA (South Africa)
PHENDIMETRAZINE TARTRATE
Bontril Slow-Release Capsules 576

OBIFEN (United Kingdom)
IBUPROFEN
Motrin Suspension, Oral Drops, Chewable Tablets, and Caplets 2002

OBLIOSER (Italy, Spain)
MORPHINE SULFATE
Astramorph/PF Injection, USP (Preservative-Free) 594
Duramorph Injection 1312
Infumorph 200 and Infumorph 500 Sterile Solutions 1314
Kadian Capsules 1335
MS Contin Tablets 2896
MSIR Oral Capsules 2898
MSIR Oral Solution 2898
MSIR Oral Solution Concentrate 2898
MSIR Oral Tablets 2898
Oramorph SR Tablets 3062
Roxanol 100 Concentrated Oral Solution 3066
Roxanol Concentrated Oral Solution 3066
Roxanol-T Oral Solution 3066

OBRACIN (Belgium, Switzerland, The Netherlands)
TOBRAMYCIN SULFATE
Nebcin Vials, Hyporets & ADD-Vantage . . 1955

OBSIDAN (Germany)
PROPRANOLOL HYDROCHLORIDE
Inderal Injectable 3513
Inderal LA Long-Acting Capsules 3516
Inderal Tablets 3513

OCCIDAL (Thailand)
OFLOXACIN
Floxin I.V. 2526
Floxin Otic Solution 1219
Floxin Tablets 2529
Ocuflox Ophthalmic Solution 554

OCERAL (Austria, Brazil, Switzerland)
OXICONAZOLE NITRATE
Oxistat Cream 1298
Oxistat Lotion 1298

OCERAL GB (Germany)
OXICONAZOLE NITRATE
Oxistat Cream 1298
Oxistat Lotion 1298

OCSAAR (Israel)
LOSARTAN POTASSIUM
Cozaar Tablets 2067

OCSAAR PLUS (Israel)
HYDROCHLOROTHIAZIDE/LOSARTAN POTASSIUM
Hyzaar 50-12.5 Tablets 2109

OCTIL (Israel)
TIMOLOL MALEATE
Blocadren Tablets 2046
Timoptic Sterile Ophthalmic Solution 2190
Timoptic in Ocudose 2192
Timoptic-XE Sterile Ophthalmic Gel Forming Solution 2194

OCTIM (France)
DESMOPRESSIN ACETATE
DDAVP Injection 4 mcg/mL 737
DDAVP Nasal Spray 738
DDAVP Rhinal Tube 738
DDAVP Tablets 739
Desmopressin Acetate Injection 1344
Desmopressin Acetate Rhinal Tube 1345
Stimate Nasal Spray 796

OCTOSTIM (Australia, Austria, Canada, Denmark, Finland, Hong Kong, Israel, New Zealand, Norway, Singapore, Sweden, Switzerland, The Netherlands)
DESMOPRESSIN ACETATE
DDAVP Injection 4 mcg/mL 737
DDAVP Nasal Spray 738
DDAVP Rhinal Tube 738
DDAVP Tablets 739
Desmopressin Acetate Injection 1344
Desmopressin Acetate Rhinal Tube 1345
Stimate Nasal Spray 796

OCUBRAX (Spain)
TOBRAMYCIN
TOBI Solution for Inhalation 1206
Tobrex Ophthalmic Ointment . . . . ⊙220
Tobrex Ophthalmic Solution . . . . ⊙221

OCUDEX (Canada)
DEXAMETHASONE SODIUM PHOSPHATE
Decadron Phosphate Injection 2081
Decadron Phosphate Sterile Ophthalmic Ointment . . . . . . ⊙280, 2083
Decadron Phosphate Sterile Ophthalmic Solution 2084

OCUFLOX (Australia, Canada, Mexico)
OFLOXACIN
Floxin I.V. 2526
Floxin Otic Solution 1219
Floxin Tablets 2529
Ocuflox Ophthalmic Solution 554

OCUGRAM (Canada)
GENTAMICIN SULFATE
Genoptic Ophthalmic Ointment . . . . ⊙239
Genoptic Sterile Ophthalmic Solution . . . ⊙239

OCULOTECT (Germany, Switzerland)
VITAMIN A PALMITATE
Aquasol A Parenteral 593

OCULOTECT SINE (Germany)
VITAMIN A PALMITATE
Aquasol A Parenteral 593

OCUSOL (United Kingdom)
SULFACETAMIDE SODIUM
Bleph-10 Ophthalmic Ointment 10% . . . . ⊙230
Klaron Lotion 10% 1224

OCUSTIL (Italy)
SODIUM HYALURONATE
Hyalgan Solution 3080

ODEMIN (Finland)
ACETAZOLAMIDE
Diamox Sequels Sustained Release Capsules . . . . ⊙270
Diamox Tablets . . . . ⊙269

ODRIC (Japan)
TRANDOLAPRIL
Mavik Tablets 478

ODRIK (Australia, Denmark, France, Irish Republic, New Zealand, Portugal, Spain, United Kingdom)
TRANDOLAPRIL
Mavik Tablets 478

OECOZOL (Austria)
METRONIDAZOLE
MetroCream 1404
MetroGel 1405
MetroGel-Vaginal Gel 1986
MetroLotion 1405
Noritate Cream 1224

OESCLIM (Canada, France, Sweden)
ESTRADIOL
Alora Transdermal System 3372
Climara Transdermal System 958
Estrace Vaginal Cream 3358
Estring Vaginal Ring 2811
Vivelle Transdermal System 2412
Vivelle-Dot Transdermal System 2416

OESTRACLIN (Spain)
ESTRADIOL
Alora Transdermal System 3372
Climara Transdermal System 958
Estrace Vaginal Cream 3358
Estring Vaginal Ring 2811
Vivelle Transdermal System 2412
Vivelle-Dot Transdermal System 2416

OESTRIFEN (United Kingdom)
TAMOXIFEN CITRATE
Nolvadex Tablets 678

OESTRING (Sweden)
ESTRADIOL
Alora Transdermal System 3372
Climara Transdermal System 958
Estrace Vaginal Cream 3358
Estring Vaginal Ring 2811
Vivelle Transdermal System 2412
Vivelle-Dot Transdermal System 2416

OESTRODOSE (France)
ESTRADIOL
Alora Transdermal System 3372
Climara Transdermal System 958
Estrace Vaginal Cream 3358
Estring Vaginal Ring 2811
Vivelle Transdermal System 2412
Vivelle-Dot Transdermal System 2416

OESTROGEL (Belgium, France, Hong Kong, Irish Republic, Israel, Singapore, Switzerland, Thailand, United Kingdom)
ESTRADIOL
Alora Transdermal System 3372
Climara Transdermal System 958
Estrace Vaginal Cream 3358
Estring Vaginal Ring 2811
Vivelle Transdermal System 2412
Vivelle-Dot Transdermal System 2416

OFISOLONA (Mexico)
PREDNISONE
Prednisone Intensol 3064
Prednisone Oral Solution 3064
Prednisone Tablets 3064

OFLOCET (Australia, France, New Zealand)
OFLOXACIN
Floxin I.V. 2526
Floxin Otic Solution 1219
Floxin Tablets 2529
Ocuflox Ophthalmic Solution 554

OFLOCIN (Italy)
OFLOXACIN
Floxin I.V. 2526
Floxin Otic Solution 1219
Floxin Tablets 2529
Ocuflox Ophthalmic Solution 554

OFLOVIR (Spain)
OFLOXACIN
Floxin I.V. 2526
Floxin Otic Solution 1219
Floxin Tablets 2529
Ocuflox Ophthalmic Solution 554

OFLOX (Brazil, Israel)
OFLOXACIN
Floxin I.V. 2526
Floxin Otic Solution 1219
Floxin Tablets 2529
Ocuflox Ophthalmic Solution 554

O-FLOX (Thailand)
OFLOXACIN
Floxin I.V. 2526
Floxin Otic Solution 1219
Floxin Tablets 2529
Ocuflox Ophthalmic Solution 554

OFLOXA (Thailand)
OFLOXACIN
Floxin I.V. 2526
Floxin Otic Solution 1219
Floxin Tablets 2529
Ocuflox Ophthalmic Solution 554

OFLOXAN (Brazil)
OFLOXACIN
Floxin I.V. 2526
Floxin Otic Solution 1219
Floxin Tablets 2529
Ocuflox Ophthalmic Solution 554

OFLOXCIN (Thailand)
OFLOXACIN
Floxin I.V. 2526
Floxin Otic Solution 1219
Floxin Tablets 2529
Ocuflox Ophthalmic Solution 554

O-FLUOR (Germany)
FLUOROURACIL
Efudex Cream 1733
Efudex Topical Solutions 1733
Fluoroplex Topical Cream 552
Fluoroplex Topical Solution 552

OFRAMAX (Thailand)
CEFTRIAXONE SODIUM
Rocephin Injectable Vials, ADD-Vantage, Galaxy, Bulk 2993

OFTACILOX (Italy, Spain)
CIPROFLOXACIN HYDROCHLORIDE
Ciloxan Ophthalmic Ointment 538
Ciloxan Ophthalmic Solution . . . . ⊙209, 538
Cipro Tablets 887

OFTADIL (Mexico)
CHLORAMPHENICOL
Chloromycetin Ophthalmic Ointment, 1% . . . . ⊙296
Chloromycetin Ophthalmic Solution . . . . ⊙297
Chloroptic Sterile Ophthalmic Ointment . . ⊙234
Chloroptic Sterile Ophthalmic Solution . . ⊙235

OFTALMOSPORIN (Italy)
HYDROCORTISONE/NEOMYCIN SULFATE/POLYMYXIN B SULFATE
Cortisporin Ophthalmic Suspension Sterile . . . . ⊙297

OFTAMOLOL (Denmark)
TIMOLOL MALEATE
Blocadren Tablets 2046
Timoptic Sterile Ophthalmic Solution 2190
Timoptic in Ocudose 2192
Timoptic-XE Sterile Ophthalmic Gel Forming Solution 2194

OFTAN (Israel, Norway, Switzerland, Thailand)
TIMOLOL MALEATE
Blocadren Tablets 2046
Timoptic Sterile Ophthalmic Solution 2190
Timoptic in Ocudose 2192
Timoptic-XE Sterile Ophthalmic Gel Forming Solution 2194

OFTAN AKVAKOL (Finland)
CHLORAMPHENICOL
Chloromycetin Ophthalmic Ointment, 1% . . . . ⊙296
Chloromycetin Ophthalmic Solution . . . . ⊙297
Chloroptic Sterile Ophthalmic Ointment . . ⊙234
Chloroptic Sterile Ophthalmic Solution . . ⊙235

OFTAN CHLORA (Finland)
CHLORAMPHENICOL
Chloromycetin Ophthalmic Ointment, 1% . . . . ⊙296
Chloromycetin Ophthalmic Solution . . . . ⊙297
Chloroptic Sterile Ophthalmic Ointment . . ⊙234
Chloroptic Sterile Ophthalmic Solution . . ⊙235

OFTIMOLO (Italy)
TIMOLOL MALEATE
Blocadren Tablets 2046
Timoptic Sterile Ophthalmic Solution 2190
Timoptic in Ocudose 2192
Timoptic-XE Sterile Ophthalmic Gel Forming Solution 2194

OGAST (France)
LANSOPRAZOLE
Prevacid Delayed-Release Capsules 3292

OGASTO (Portugal)
LANSOPRAZOLE
Prevacid Delayed-Release Capsules 3292

OGASTRO (Brazil, Mexico)
LANSOPRAZOLE
Prevacid Delayed-Release Capsules 3292

OGEN (Australia, Canada, Mexico)
ESTROPIPATE
Ogen Tablets 2846
Ortho-Est Tablets 3464

OILATUM SHAMPOO (United Kingdom)
CICLOPIROX OLAMINE
Loprox Cream 2021
Loprox Lotion 2021

OLBAS (Germany)
ETHYL CHLORIDE
Gebauer's Ethyl Chloride 1409

OLCAM (France)
PIROXICAM
Feldene Capsules 2685

OLEOMYCETIN (Austria, Germany)
CHLORAMPHENICOL
Chloromycetin Ophthalmic Ointment, 1% . . . . ⊙296
Chloromycetin Ophthalmic Solution . . . . ⊙297
Chloroptic Sterile Ophthalmic Ointment . . ⊙234
Chloroptic Sterile Ophthalmic Solution . . ⊙235

OLEOMYCETIN-PREDNISON (Germany)
CHLORAMPHENICOL
Chloromycetin Ophthalmic Ointment, 1% . . . . ⊙296
Chloromycetin Ophthalmic Solution . . . . ⊙297
Chloroptic Sterile Ophthalmic Ointment . . ⊙234
Chloroptic Sterile Ophthalmic Solution . . ⊙235

OLEOVIT A (Austria)
VITAMIN A PALMITATE
Aquasol A Parenteral 593

OLEXIN (Mexico)
OMEPRAZOLE
Prilosec Delayed-Release Capsules 628

OLFEN (Hong Kong, Portugal, Singapore, Switzerland, Thailand)
DICLOFENAC SODIUM
Voltaren Tablets 2315
Voltaren-XR Tablets 2315

OLFEX (Spain)
BUDESONIDE
Pulmicort Turbuhaler Inhalation Powder . . . 636
Rhinocort Nasal Inhaler 640

OLICARD (Germany, Spain, Switzerland)
ISOSORBIDE MONONITRATE
Imdur Tablets 1826
Ismo Tablets 3524

OLICARDIN (Austria)
ISOSORBIDE MONONITRATE
Imdur Tablets 1826
Ismo Tablets 3524

OLICIDE (Portugal)
MALATHION
Ovide Lotion 2023

OLMORAN (Spain)
ZAFIRLUKAST
Accolate Tablets 657

OLTENS (France)
CAPTOPRIL
Captopril Tablets 2281

OMBETA (Germany)
OMEPRAZOLE
Prilosec Delayed-Release Capsules 628

OMCILON A ORABASE (Brazil)
TRIAMCINOLONE ACETONIDE
Azmacort Inhalation Aerosol 728

Nasacort AQ Nasal Spray . . . 752
Nasacort Nasal Inhaler . . . 750

OME-NERTON (Germany)
OMEPRAZOLE
Prilosec Delayed-Release Capsules . . . 628

OMEP (Brazil, Germany)
OMEPRAZOLE
Prilosec Delayed-Release Capsules . . . 628

OMEPRADEX (Israel)
OMEPRAZOLE
Prilosec Delayed-Release Capsules . . . 628

OMEPRAL (Japan)
OMEPRAZOLE
Prilosec Delayed-Release Capsules . . . 628

OMEPRASEC (Brazil)
OMEPRAZOLE
Prilosec Delayed-Release Capsules . . . 628

OME-PUREN (Germany)
OMEPRAZOLE
Prilosec Delayed-Release Capsules . . . 628

OMETON (Portugal)
OMEPRAZOLE
Prilosec Delayed-Release Capsules . . . 628

OMIX (France)
TAMSULOSIN HYDROCHLORIDE
Flomax Capsules . . . 1044

OMNALIO (Spain)
CHLORDIAZEPOXIDE HYDROCHLORIDE
Librium Capsules . . . 1736
Librium for Injection . . . 1737

OMNIC (Denmark, Finland, Germany, Irish Republic, Israel, Italy, New Zealand, Norway, Portugal, Spain, The Netherlands)
TAMSULOSIN HYDROCHLORIDE
Flomax Capsules . . . 1044

OMNICEF (Thailand)
CEFDINIR
Omnicef Capsules . . . 493
Omnicef for Oral Suspension . . . 493

OMNIDERM (Italy)
FLUOCINOLONE ACETONIDE
Synalar Cream . . . 2020
Synalar Ointment . . . 2020
Synalar Topical Solution . . . 2020

OMP (Thailand)
OMEPRAZOLE
Prilosec Delayed-Release Capsules . . . 628

OMPRANYT (Spain)
OMEPRAZOLE
Prilosec Delayed-Release Capsules . . . 628

ONAPAN (Mexico)
DIAZEPAM
Valium Injectable . . . 3026
Valium Tablets . . . 3047

ONCASPAR (Canada, Germany)
PEGASPARGASE
Oncaspar . . . 756

ONCLAST (Japan)
ALENDRONATE SODIUM
Fosamax Tablets . . . 2005

ONCO TIOTEPA (Brazil, Spain)
THIOTEPA
Thioplex for Injection . . . 1765

ONCOSAL (Spain)
FLUTAMIDE
Eulexin Capsules . . . 3118

ONCOTAM (France)
TAMOXIFEN CITRATE
Nolvadex Tablets . . . 678

ONKOMORPHIN (Germany)
MORPHINE SULFATE
Astramorph/PF Injection, USP (Preservative-Free) . . . 594
Duramorph Injection . . . 1312
Infumorph 200 and Infumorph 500 Sterile Solutions . . . 1314
Kadian Capsules . . . 1335
MS Contin Tablets . . . 2896
MSIR Oral Capsules . . . 2898
MSIR Oral Solution . . . 2898
MSIR Oral Solution Concentrate . . . 2898
MSIR Oral Tablets . . . 2898
Oramorph SR Tablets . . . 3062
Roxanol 100 Concentrated Oral Solution . . . 3066
Roxanol Concentrated Oral Solution . . . 3066
Roxanol-T Oral Solution . . . 3066

ONOFIN-K (Mexico)
KETOCONAZOLE
Nizoral 2% Cream . . . 3620
Nizoral 2% Shampoo . . . 2007
Nizoral Tablets . . . 1791

ONSIA (Thailand)
ONDANSETRON HYDROCHLORIDE
Zofran Injection . . . 1698
Zofran Injection Premixed . . . 1698
Zofran Oral Solution . . . 1703
Zofran Tablets . . . 1703

ONYMYKEN (Germany)
CLOTRIMAZOLE
Lotrimin Cream 1% . . . 3128
Lotrimin Lotion 1% . . . 3128
Lotrimin Topical Solution 1% . . . 3128
Mycelex Troche . . . 573

OPCON (Canada)
NAPHAZOLINE HYDROCHLORIDE
Albalon Ophthalmic Solution . . . ⊙225

OPHTAGRAM (France, Germany, Portugal, Singapore, Switzerland)
GENTAMICIN SULFATE
Genoptic Ophthalmic Ointment . . . ⊙239
Genoptic Sterile Ophthalmic Solution . . . ⊙239

OPHTALIN (Italy)
SODIUM HYALURONATE
Hyalgan Solution . . . 3080

OPHTAPHENICOL (France)
CHLORAMPHENICOL
Chloromycetin Ophthalmic Ointment, 1% . . . ⊙296
Chloromycetin Ophthalmic Solution . . . ⊙297
Chloroptic Sterile Ophthalmic Ointment . . . ⊙234
Chloroptic Sterile Ophthalmic Solution . . . ⊙235

OPHTHALIN (Australia, Hong Kong, New Zealand, Singapore, Thailand, United Kingdom)
SODIUM HYALURONATE
Hyalgan Solution . . . 3080

OPHTHO-CHLORAM (Canada)
CHLORAMPHENICOL
Chloromycetin Ophthalmic Ointment, 1% . . . ⊙296
Chloromycetin Ophthalmic Solution . . . ⊙297
Chloroptic Sterile Ophthalmic Ointment . . . ⊙234
Chloroptic Sterile Ophthalmic Solution . . . ⊙235

OPHTHO-SULF (Canada)
SULFACETAMIDE SODIUM
Bleph-10 Ophthalmic Ointment 10% . . . ⊙230
Klaron Lotion 10% . . . 1224

OPHTIM (France)
TIMOLOL MALEATE
Blocadren Tablets . . . 2046
Timoptic Sterile Ophthalmic Solution . . . 2190
Timoptic in Ocudose . . . 2192
Timoptic-XE Sterile Ophthalmic Gel Forming Solution . . . 2194

OPHTOL-A (Germany)
VITAMIN A PALMITATE
Aquasol A Parenteral . . . 593

OPHTOSAN (Germany)
VITAMIN A PALMITATE
Aquasol A Parenteral . . . 593

OPIDOL (Denmark, Finland, Sweden, Switzerland)
HYDROMORPHONE HYDROCHLORIDE
Dilaudid Ampules . . . 441
Dilaudid Injection . . . 441
Dilaudid Multiple Dose Vials (Sterile Solution) . . . 441
Dilaudid Oral Liquid . . . 445
Dilaudid Powder . . . 441
Dilaudid Rectal Suppositories . . . 441
Dilaudid Tablets . . . 441
Dilaudid Tablets - 8 mg . . . 445
Dilaudid-HP Injection . . . 443
Dilaudid-HP Lyophilized Powder 250 mg . . . 443

OPIRAN (France)
PIMOZIDE
Orap Tablets . . . 1407

OPIREN (Spain)
LANSOPRAZOLE
Prevacid Delayed-Release Capsules . . . 3292

OPNOL (Sweden)
DEXAMETHASONE SODIUM PHOSPHATE
Decadron Phosphate Injection . . . 2081
Decadron Phosphate Sterile Ophthalmic Ointment . . . ⊙280, 2083
Decadron Phosphate Sterile Ophthalmic Solution . . . 2084

OPRAM (Irish Republic)
METOCLOPRAMIDE HYDROCHLORIDE
Reglan Injectable . . . 2935
Reglan Syrup . . . 2935
Reglan Tablets . . . 2935

OPRAZOLE (Thailand)
OMEPRAZOLE
Prilosec Delayed-Release Capsules . . . 628

OPREDSONE (Thailand)
PREDNISOLONE
Prelone Syrup . . . 2273

OPSAR (Thailand)
SULFACETAMIDE SODIUM
Bleph-10 Ophthalmic Ointment 10% . . . ⊙230
Klaron Lotion 10% . . . 1224

OPSARAM (Thailand)
CHLORAMPHENICOL
Chloromycetin Ophthalmic Ointment, 1% . . . ⊙296
Chloromycetin Ophthalmic Solution . . . ⊙297
Chloroptic Sterile Ophthalmic Ointment . . . ⊙234
Chloroptic Sterile Ophthalmic Solution . . . ⊙235

OPTAFEN (Italy)
CHLORAMPHENICOL
Chloromycetin Ophthalmic Ointment, 1% . . . ⊙296
Chloromycetin Ophthalmic Solution . . . ⊙297
Chloroptic Sterile Ophthalmic Ointment . . . ⊙234
Chloroptic Sterile Ophthalmic Solution . . . ⊙235

OPTAL (Thailand)
SULFACETAMIDE SODIUM
Bleph-10 Ophthalmic Ointment 10% . . . ⊙230
Klaron Lotion 10% . . . 1224

OPTALIDON (Germany)
IBUPROFEN
Motrin Suspension, Oral Drops, Chewable Tablets, and Caplets . . . 2002

OPTAMID (Italy)
SULFACETAMIDE SODIUM
Bleph-10 Ophthalmic Ointment 10% . . . ⊙230
Klaron Lotion 10% . . . 1224

OPTAMIDE (Australia)
SULFACETAMIDE SODIUM
Bleph-10 Ophthalmic Ointment 10% . . . ⊙230
Klaron Lotion 10% . . . 1224

OPTAZINE (Australia)
NAPHAZOLINE HYDROCHLORIDE
Albalon Ophthalmic Solution . . . ⊙225

OPTERON (Italy)
TICLOPIDINE HYDROCHLORIDE
Ticlid Tablets . . . 3015

OPTHAFLOX (Mexico)
CIPROFLOXACIN HYDROCHLORIDE
Ciloxan Ophthalmic Ointment . . . 538
Ciloxan Ophthalmic Solution . . . ⊙209, 538
Cipro Tablets . . . 887

OPTICET (South Africa)
SULFACETAMIDE SODIUM
Bleph-10 Ophthalmic Ointment 10% . . . ⊙230
Klaron Lotion 10% . . . 1224

OPTICIDE (Thailand)
PRAZIQUANTEL
Biltricide Tablets . . . 887

OPTIFEN (Switzerland)
IBUPROFEN
Motrin Suspension, Oral Drops, Chewable Tablets, and Caplets . . . 2002

OPTIFLUOR (Mexico)
FLUORESCEIN SODIUM
AK-Fluor Injection 10% and 25% . . . ⊙202
Fluorescite Injection . . . ⊙211

OPTIGEN (Hong Kong)
GENTAMICIN SULFATE
Genoptic Ophthalmic Ointment . . . ⊙239
Genoptic Sterile Ophthalmic Solution . . . ⊙239

OPTI-GENTA (Israel)
GENTAMICIN SULFATE
Genoptic Ophthalmic Ointment . . . ⊙239
Genoptic Sterile Ophthalmic Solution . . . ⊙239

OPTIL (United Kingdom)
DILTIAZEM HYDROCHLORIDE
Cardizem CD Capsules . . . 1016
Cardizem Injectable . . . 1018
Cardizem Lyo-Ject Syringe . . . 1018
Cardizem Monovial . . . 1018
Tiazac Capsules . . . 1378

OPTILAST (United Kingdom)
AZELASTINE HYDROCHLORIDE
Astelin Nasal Spray . . . 3339

OPTIMIN (Spain)
LORATADINE
Claritin Reditabs . . . 3100
Claritin Syrup . . . 3100
Claritin Tablets . . . 3100

OPTIMOL (Australia, Denmark, Sweden)
TIMOLOL MALEATE
Blocadren Tablets . . . 2046
Timoptic Sterile Ophthalmic Solution . . . 2190
Timoptic in Ocudose . . . 2192
Timoptic-XE Sterile Ophthalmic Gel Forming Solution . . . 2194

OPTINATE (Finland, Sweden)
RISEDRONATE SODIUM
Actonel Tablets . . . 2879

OPTINEM (Austria)
MEROPENEM
Merrem I.V. . . . 673

OPTISOL (Israel)
SULFACETAMIDE SODIUM
Bleph-10 Ophthalmic Ointment 10% . . . ⊙230
Klaron Lotion 10% . . . 1224

OPTOCAIN (Italy)
MEPIVACAINE HYDROCHLORIDE
Polocaine Injection, USP . . . 625
Polocaine-MPF Injection, USP . . . 625

OPTOCHINIDIN RETARD (Germany)
QUINIDINE SULFATE
Quinidex Extentabs . . . 2933

OPTOMICIN (Mexico)
ERYTHROMYCIN STEARATE
Erythrocin Stearate Filmtab Tablets . . . 452

OPTOVIT-A (Germany)
VITAMIN A PALMITATE
Aquasol A Parenteral . . . 593

OPTROL (Australia)
SALMETEROL XINAFOATE
Serevent Diskus . . . 1637
Serevent Inhalation Aerosol . . . 1633

OPTRUMA (Italy, Portugal, Spain)
RALOXIFENE HYDROCHLORIDE
Evista Tablets . . . 1915

OPTUREM (Germany)
IBUPROFEN
Motrin Suspension, Oral Drops, Chewable Tablets, and Caplets . . . 2002

OPUMIDE (United Kingdom)
INDAPAMIDE
Indapamide Tablets . . . 2286

OPUSTAN (United Kingdom)
MEFENAMIC ACID
Ponstel Capsules . . . 1356

ORA (Thailand)
LORAZEPAM
Ativan Injection . . . 3478
Ativan Tablets . . . 3482

ORABET (Austria, Denmark, Norway, United Kingdom)
METFORMIN HYDROCHLORIDE
Glucophage Tablets . . . 1080

ORACEF (Germany)
CEPHALEXIN
Keflex Oral Suspension . . . 1237
Keflex Pulvules . . . 1237

ORACEFAL (France)
CEFADROXIL
Duricef Capsules . . . 1079
Duricef Oral Suspension . . . 1079
Duricef Tablets . . . 1079

ORACORT (Canada, Israel, New Zealand, Thailand)
TRIAMCINOLONE ACETONIDE
Azmacort Inhalation Aerosol . . . 728
Nasacort AQ Nasal Spray . . . 752
Nasacort Nasal Inhaler . . . 750

ORACYCLIN (Austria)
MINOCYCLINE HYDROCHLORIDE
Dynacin Capsules . . . 2019
Minocin Intravenous . . . 1862
Minocin Oral Suspension . . . 1865
Minocin Pellet-Filled Capsules . . . 1863

ORADAY (Thailand)
ATENOLOL
Tenormin I.V. Injection . . . 692

ORADEXON (Belgium, Portugal, South Africa, Switzerland, Thailand, United Kingdom)
DEXAMETHASONE
Decadron Elixir . . . 2078
Decadron Tablets . . . 2079

ORADROXIL (Italy)
CEFADROXIL
Duricef Capsules . . . 1079
Duricef Oral Suspension . . . 1079
Duricef Tablets . . . 1079

ORAFEN (Canada)
KETOPROFEN
Orudis Capsules . . . 3548
Oruvail Capsules . . . 3548

ORAJEL (Canada, Switzerland)
BENZOCAINE
Americaine Anesthetic Lubricant . . . 1162

(⊙ Described in PDR For Ophthalmic Medicines™)

Americaine Otic Topical Anesthetic Ear Drops . . . 1162

ORAKEF (Finland)
CEPHALEXIN
Keflex Oral Suspension . . . 1237
Keflex Pulvules . . . 1237

ORALFENE (France)
IBUPROFEN
Motrin Suspension, Oral Drops, Chewable Tablets, and Caplets . . . 2002

ORAL-T (Thailand)
TRIAMCINOLONE ACETONIDE
Azmacort Inhalation Aerosol . . . 728
Nasacort AQ Nasal Spray . . . 752
Nasacort Nasal Inhaler . . . 750

ORALTEN TROCHE (Israel)
CLOTRIMAZOLE
Lotrimin Cream 1% . . . 3128
Lotrimin Lotion 1% . . . 3128
Lotrimin Topical Solution 1% . . . 3128
Mycelex Troche . . . 573

ORAMEDY (Singapore)
TRIAMCINOLONE ACETONIDE
Azmacort Inhalation Aerosol . . . 728
Nasacort AQ Nasal Spray . . . 752
Nasacort Nasal Inhaler . . . 750

ORAMET (Finland)
METFORMIN HYDROCHLORIDE
Glucophage Tablets . . . 1080

ORAMINAX (Portugal)
AMOXICILLIN
Amoxil Pediatric Drops for Oral Suspension . . . 1471
Amoxil Tablets . . . 1471

ORAMORPH (Austria, Canada, Irish Republic, Sweden, United Kingdom)
MORPHINE SULFATE
Astramorph/PF Injection, USP (Preservative-Free) . . . 594
Duramorph Injection . . . 1312
Infumorph 200 and Infumorph 500 Sterile Solutions . . . 1314
Kadian Capsules . . . 1335
MS Contin Tablets . . . 2896
MSIR Oral Capsules . . . 2898
MSIR Oral Solution . . . 2898
MSIR Oral Solution Concentrate . . . 2898
MSIR Oral Tablets . . . 2898
Oramorph SR Tablets . . . 3062
Roxanol 100 Concentrated Oral Solution . . . 3066
Roxanol Concentrated Oral Solution . . . 3066
Roxanol-T Oral Solution . . . 3066

ORANOR (Mexico)
NORFLOXACIN
Chibroxin Sterile Ophthalmic Solution . . . ⊙273, 2051
Noroxin Tablets . . . 2145

ORAP (Australia, Austria, Belgium, Brazil, Canada, Denmark, France, Germany, Hong Kong, Irish Republic, Israel, Italy, New Zealand, Norway, Singapore, South Africa, Spain, Sweden, Switzerland, Thailand, The Netherlands, United Kingdom)
PIMOZIDE
Orap Tablets . . . 1407

ORASORBIL (Germany, Italy, Portugal)
ISOSORBIDE MONONITRATE
Imdur Tablets . . . 1826
Ismo Tablets . . . 3524

ORATANE (Australia, New Zealand)
ISOTRETINOIN
Accutane Capsules . . . 2944

ORAXIM (Italy)
CEFUROXIME AXETIL
Ceftin Tablets . . . 1898
Ceftin for Oral Suspension . . . 1898

ORCILONE (Thailand)
TRIAMCINOLONE ACETONIDE
Azmacort Inhalation Aerosol . . . 728
Nasacort AQ Nasal Spray . . . 752
Nasacort Nasal Inhaler . . . 750

ORELOX (Australia, Denmark, France, Germany, Italy, Mexico, South Africa, Spain, Sweden, Switzerland, The Netherlands, United Kingdom)
CEFPODOXIME PROXETIL
Vantin Tablets and Oral Suspension . . . 2860

ORFARIN (Thailand)
WARFARIN SODIUM
Coumadin Tablets . . . 1243
Coumadin for Injection . . . 1243

ORFENACE (Canada)
ORPHENADRINE CITRATE
Norflex Extended-Release Tablets . . . 1987
Norflex Injection . . . 1987

ORFIDAL (Spain)
LORAZEPAM
Ativan Injection . . . 3478
Ativan Tablets . . . 3482

ORGANODERM (Germany)
MALATHION
Ovide Lotion . . . 2023

ORGARAN (Australia, Canada, France, Germany, New Zealand, Sweden, The Netherlands, United Kingdom)
DANAPAROID SODIUM
Orgaran Injection . . . 2480

ORIBUTOL (Finland)
ETHAMBUTOL HYDROCHLORIDE
Myambutol Tablets . . . 1290

ORITAXIM (South Africa)
CEFOTAXIME SODIUM
Claforan Injection . . . 732

ORIVAN (Finland)
VANCOMYCIN HYDROCHLORIDE
Vancocin HCl Capsules & Pulvules . . . 1972
Vancocin HCl Oral Solution . . . 1971
Vancocin HCl, Vials & ADD-Vantage . . . 1970

ORMOX (Finland)
ISOSORBIDE MONONITRATE
Imdur Tablets . . . 1826
Ismo Tablets . . . 3524

OROFEN (Denmark)
KETOPROFEN
Orudis Capsules . . . 3548
Oruvail Capsules . . . 3548

OROKEN (France)
CEFIXIME
Suprax Tablets . . . 1877
Suprax for Oral Suspension . . . 1877

OROMONE (France)
ESTRADIOL
Alora Transdermal System . . . 3372
Climara Transdermal System . . . 958
Estrace Vaginal Cream . . . 3358
Estring Vaginal Ring . . . 2811
Vivelle Transdermal System . . . 2412
Vivelle-Dot Transdermal System . . . 2416

ORSANIL (Finland)
THIORIDAZINE HYDROCHLORIDE
Thioridazine Hydrochloride Tablets . . . 2289

ORTACRONE (Spain)
AMIODARONE HYDROCHLORIDE
Cordarone Intravenous . . . 3491
Cordarone Tablets . . . 3487
Pacerone Tablets . . . 3331

ORTHO (Irish Republic)
DIENESTROL
Ortho Dienestrol Cream . . . 2554

ORTHOCLONE OKT3 (Australia, Belgium, Canada, Finland, France, Germany, Hong Kong, Israel, Italy, Mexico, New Zealand, Norway, Sweden, Switzerland, Thailand, The Netherlands)
MUROMONAB-CD3
Orthoclone OKT3 Sterile Solution . . . 2498

ORTHO-DIENOESTROL (Belgium, Israel, United Kingdom)
DIENESTROL
Ortho Dienestrol Cream . . . 2554

ORTHO-EST (South Africa)
ESTROPIPATE
Ogen Tablets . . . 2846
Ortho-Est Tablets . . . 3464

ORTHOVISC (Germany, Israel, United Kingdom)
SODIUM HYALURONATE
Hyalgan Solution . . . 3080

ORTOCICLINA (Brazil)
ERYTHROMYCIN
Emgel 2% Topical Gel . . . 1285
Ery-Tab Tablets . . . 448
Erythromycin Base Filmtab Tablets . . . 454
Erythromycin Delayed-Release Capsules, USP . . . 455
PCE Dispertab Tablets . . . 498

ORTOFLAN (Brazil)
DICLOFENAC SODIUM
Voltaren Tablets . . . 2315
Voltaren-XR Tablets . . . 2315

ORTOPSIQUE (Mexico)
DIAZEPAM
Valium Injectable . . . 3026
Valium Tablets . . . 3047

ORTOTON (Germany)
METHOCARBAMOL
Robaxin Injectable . . . 2938
Robaxin Tablets . . . 2939
Robaxin-750 Tablets . . . 2939

ORTOTON PLUS (Germany)
METHOCARBAMOL
Robaxin Injectable . . . 2938
Robaxin Tablets . . . 2939
Robaxin-750 Tablets . . . 2939

ORTRIZOL (Mexico)
METRONIDAZOLE
MetroCream . . . 1404
MetroGel . . . 1405
MetroGel-Vaginal Gel . . . 1986
MetroLotion . . . 1405
Noritate Cream . . . 1224

ORUCOTE (South Africa)
KETOPROFEN
Orudis Capsules . . . 3548
Oruvail Capsules . . . 3548

ORUDIS (Australia, Canada, Denmark, Finland, Germany, Hong Kong, Irish Republic, Mexico, New Zealand, Norway, South Africa, Spain, Sweden, Switzerland, The Netherlands, United Kingdom)
KETOPROFEN
Orudis Capsules . . . 3548
Oruvail Capsules . . . 3548

ORUGESIC (Irish Republic)
KETOPROFEN
Orudis Capsules . . . 3548
Oruvail Capsules . . . 3548

ORUJECT (South Africa)
KETOPROFEN
Orudis Capsules . . . 3548
Oruvail Capsules . . . 3548

ORUVAIL (Australia, Canada, Hong Kong, Irish Republic, Israel, New Zealand, Singapore, South Africa, Thailand, United Kingdom)
KETOPROFEN
Orudis Capsules . . . 3548
Oruvail Capsules . . . 3548

OSCOREL (The Netherlands)
KETOPROFEN
Orudis Capsules . . . 3548
Oruvail Capsules . . . 3548

O-SID (Thailand)
OMEPRAZOLE
Prilosec Delayed-Release Capsules . . . 628

OSIREN (Mexico)
OMEPRAZOLE
Prilosec Delayed-Release Capsules . . . 628

OSMO-ADALAT (Israel)
NIFEDIPINE
Adalat CC Tablets . . . 877
Procardia Capsules . . . 2708
Procardia XL Extended Release Tablets . . . 2710

OSMOLAC (Italy)
LACTULOSE
Kristalose for Oral Solution . . . 1007

OSPAMOX (Portugal)
AMOXICILLIN
Amoxil Pediatric Drops for Oral Suspension . . . 1471
Amoxil Tablets . . . 1471

OSPEXIN (Austria, Hong Kong, Singapore)
CEPHALEXIN
Keflex Oral Suspension . . . 1237
Keflex Pulvules . . . 1237

OSPOCARD (Austria)
NIFEDIPINE
Adalat CC Tablets . . . 877
Procardia Capsules . . . 2708
Procardia XL Extended Release Tablets . . . 2710

OSTAREN (Thailand)
DICLOFENAC SODIUM
Voltaren Tablets . . . 2315
Voltaren-XR Tablets . . . 2315

OSTENIL (Germany, Switzerland)
SODIUM HYALURONATE
Hyalgan Solution . . . 3080

OSTEO D (Israel)
CALCITRIOL
Calcijex Injection . . . 411
Rocaltrol Capsules . . . 2991
Rocaltrol Oral Solution . . . 2991

OSTERAL (Mexico)
PIROXICAM
Feldene Capsules . . . 2685

OSTOFEN (Thailand)
IBUPROFEN
Motrin Suspension, Oral Drops, Chewable Tablets, and Caplets . . . 2002

OTAREX (Israel)
HYDROXYZINE HYDROCHLORIDE
Atarax Tablets & Syrup . . . 2667
Vistaril Intramuscular Solution . . . 2738

OTOFLOGIN (Brazil)
CHLORAMPHENICOL
Chloromycetin Ophthalmic Ointment, 1% . . . ⊙296
Chloromycetin Ophthalmic Solution . . . ⊙297
Chloroptic Sterile Ophthalmic Ointment . . . ⊙234
Chloroptic Sterile Ophthalmic Solution . . . ⊙235

OTOIAL (Italy)
SODIUM HYALURONATE
Hyalgan Solution . . . 3080

OTOLONE (Brazil)
NEOMYCIN SULFATE/POLYMYXIN B SULFATE
Neosporin G.U. Irrigant Sterile . . . 2256

OTOMICINA (Brazil)
CHLORAMPHENICOL
Chloromycetin Ophthalmic Ointment, 1% . . . ⊙296
Chloromycetin Ophthalmic Solution . . . ⊙297
Chloroptic Sterile Ophthalmic Ointment . . . ⊙234
Chloroptic Sterile Ophthalmic Solution . . . ⊙235

OTO-SYNALAR N (Portugal)
FLUOCINOLONE ACETONIDE
Synalar Cream . . . 2020
Synalar Ointment . . . 2020
Synalar Topical Solution . . . 2020

OTREON (Austria, Italy, Spain)
CEFPODOXIME PROXETIL
Vantin Tablets and Oral Suspension . . . 2860

OTROZOL (Mexico)
METRONIDAZOLE
MetroCream . . . 1404
MetroGel . . . 1405
MetroGel-Vaginal Gel . . . 1986
MetroLotion . . . 1405
Noritate Cream . . . 1224

OUTGRO (Canada)
BENZOCAINE
Americaine Anesthetic Lubricant . . . 1162
Americaine Otic Topical Anesthetic Ear Drops . . . 1162

OUVIDONAL (Brazil)
CHLORAMPHENICOL
Chloromycetin Ophthalmic Ointment, 1% . . . ⊙296
Chloromycetin Ophthalmic Solution . . . ⊙297
Chloroptic Sterile Ophthalmic Ointment . . . ⊙234
Chloroptic Sterile Ophthalmic Solution . . . ⊙235

OVEX (United Kingdom)
MEBENDAZOLE
Vermox Chewable Tablets . . . 2017

OVIS NEU (Germany)
CLOTRIMAZOLE
Lotrimin Cream 1% . . . 3128
Lotrimin Lotion 1% . . . 3128
Lotrimin Topical Solution 1% . . . 3128
Mycelex Troche . . . 573

OVRAL (Canada, Hong Kong, Mexico, New Zealand)
NORGESTREL
Ovrette Tablets . . . 3552

OWBRIDGES FOR CHESTY COUGHS (United Kingdom)
GUAIFENESIN
Organidin NR Liquid . . . 3350
Organidin NR Tablets . . . 3350

OXANEST (Finland)
OXYCODONE HYDROCHLORIDE
OxyContin Tablets . . . 2912
OxyFast Oral Concentrate Solution . . . 2916
OxyIR Capsules . . . 2916
Percolone Tablets . . . 1327
Roxicodone Tablets . . . 3067

OXCORD (Brazil)
NIFEDIPINE
Adalat CC Tablets . . . 877
Procardia Capsules . . . 2708
Procardia XL Extended Release Tablets . . . 2710

OXEPRAX (Spain)
TAMOXIFEN CITRATE
Nolvadex Tablets . . . 678

OXICAM (Italy)
PIROXICAM
Feldene Capsules . . . 2685

OXICANOL (Mexico)
PIROXICAM
Feldene Capsules . . . 2685

OXIDERMA (Spain)
BENZOYL PEROXIDE
Brevoxyl-4 Cleansing Lotion . . . 3269
Brevoxyl-4 Creamy Wash . . . 3270
Brevoxyl-4 Gel . . . 3269
Brevoxyl-8 Cleansing Lotion . . . 3269
Brevoxyl-8 Creamy Wash . . . 3270
Brevoxyl-8 Gel . . . 3269
Triaz Cleanser . . . 2026
Triaz Gel . . . 2026

OXIDERMIOL FUERTE (Spain)
FLUOCINOLONE ACETONIDE
Synalar Cream . . . 2020
Synalar Ointment . . . 2020
Synalar Topical Solution . . . 2020

OXIFUNGOL (Mexico)
FLUCONAZOLE
Diflucan Tablets, Injection, and Oral Suspension . . . 2681

OXIGEN (Brazil)
NIMODIPINE
Nimotop Capsules . . . 904

OXIKEN (Mexico)
DOBUTAMINE HYDROCHLORIDE
Dobutrex Solution Vials . . . 1914

OXIKLORIN (Finland)
HYDROXYCHLOROQUINE SULFATE
Plaquenil Tablets . . . 3082

OXISTAT (Mexico)
OXICONAZOLE NITRATE
Oxistat Cream . . . 1298
Oxistat Lotion . . . 1298

OXITOSONA (Spain)
OXYMETHOLONE
Anadrol-50 Tablets . . . 3321

OXITOVER (Spain)
MEBENDAZOLE
Vermox Chewable Tablets . . . 2017

OXIZOLE (Canada, Mexico)
OXICONAZOLE NITRATE
Oxistat Cream . . . 1298
Oxistat Lotion . . . 1298

OXODAL (Spain)
BETAXOLOL HYDROCHLORIDE
Betoptic S Ophthalmic Suspension . . . ⊙208, 537

OXSORALEN (Australia, Austria, Canada, Hong Kong, Israel, Italy, Mexico, New Zealand, Singapore, South Africa, Spain, The Netherlands)
METHOXSALEN
8-MOP Capsules . . . 1727
Oxsoralen Lotion 1% . . . 1740
Oxsoralen-Ultra Capsules . . . 1741

OXSORALON (Belgium)
METHOXSALEN
8-MOP Capsules . . . 1727
Oxsoralen Lotion 1% . . . 1740
Oxsoralen-Ultra Capsules . . . 1741

OXY (Australia, Canada, Germany, Hong Kong, Israel, Mexico, United Kingdom)
BENZOYL PEROXIDE
Brevoxyl-4 Cleansing Lotion . . . 3269
Brevoxyl-4 Creamy Wash . . . 3270
Brevoxyl-4 Gel . . . 3269
Brevoxyl-8 Cleansing Lotion . . . 3269
Brevoxyl-8 Creamy Wash . . . 3270
Brevoxyl-8 Gel . . . 3269
Triaz Cleanser . . . 2026
Triaz Gel . . . 2026

OXY SENSITIVE (Israel)
BENZOYL PEROXIDE
Brevoxyl-4 Cleansing Lotion . . . 3269
Brevoxyl-4 Creamy Wash . . . 3270
Brevoxyl-4 Gel . . . 3269
Brevoxyl-8 Cleansing Lotion . . . 3269
Brevoxyl-8 Creamy Wash . . . 3270
Brevoxyl-8 Gel . . . 3269
Triaz Cleanser . . . 2026
Triaz Gel . . . 2026

OXYCARDIN (France)
ISOSORBIDE MONONITRATE
Imdur Tablets . . . 1826
Ismo Tablets . . . 3524

OXYCOD (Israel)
OXYCODONE HYDROCHLORIDE
OxyContin Tablets . . . 2912
OxyFast Oral Concentrate Solution . . . 2916
OxyIR Capsules . . . 2916
Percolone Tablets . . . 1327
Roxicodone Tablets . . . 3067

OXYCONTIN (Australia, Canada, Denmark, Finland, Irish Republic, Israel, Mexico, Sweden, United Kingdom)
OXYCODONE HYDROCHLORIDE
OxyContin Tablets . . . 2912
OxyFast Oral Concentrate Solution . . . 2916
OxyIR Capsules . . . 2916
Percolone Tablets . . . 1327
Roxicodone Tablets . . . 3067

OXYDERM (Canada)
BENZOYL PEROXIDE
Brevoxyl-4 Cleansing Lotion . . . 3269
Brevoxyl-4 Creamy Wash . . . 3270
Brevoxyl-4 Gel . . . 3269
Brevoxyl-8 Cleansing Lotion . . . 3269
Brevoxyl-8 Creamy Wash . . . 3270
Brevoxyl-8 Gel . . . 3269
Triaz Cleanser . . . 2026
Triaz Gel . . . 2026

OXYGESIC (Germany)
OXYCODONE HYDROCHLORIDE
OxyContin Tablets . . . 2912
OxyFast Oral Concentrate Solution . . . 2916
OxyIR Capsules . . . 2916
Percolone Tablets . . . 1327
Roxicodone Tablets . . . 3067

OXYNORM (Australia, Denmark, Finland, Irish Republic, Sweden, United Kingdom)
OXYCODONE HYDROCHLORIDE
OxyContin Tablets . . . 2912
OxyFast Oral Concentrate Solution . . . 2916
OxyIR Capsules . . . 2916
Percolone Tablets . . . 1327
Roxicodone Tablets . . . 3067

OXYTOKO (Spain)
BENZOYL PEROXIDE
Brevoxyl-4 Cleansing Lotion . . . 3269
Brevoxyl-4 Creamy Wash . . . 3270
Brevoxyl-4 Gel . . . 3269
Brevoxyl-8 Cleansing Lotion . . . 3269
Brevoxyl-8 Creamy Wash . . . 3270
Brevoxyl-8 Gel . . . 3269
Triaz Cleanser . . . 2026
Triaz Gel . . . 2026

OZIDIA (France)
GLIPIZIDE
Glucotrol Tablets . . . 2692
Glucotrol XL Extended Release Tablets . . . 2693

OZOKEN (Mexico)
OMEPRAZOLE
Prilosec Delayed-Release Capsules . . . 628

OZONOL (Portugal)
IBUPROFEN
Motrin Suspension, Oral Drops, Chewable Tablets, and Caplets . . . 2002

PACEUM (Switzerland)
DIAZEPAM
Valium Injectable . . . 3026
Valium Tablets . . . 3047

PACIFENE (United Kingdom)
IBUPROFEN
Motrin Suspension, Oral Drops, Chewable Tablets, and Caplets . . . 2002

PACIUM (Spain)
DIAZEPAM
Valium Injectable . . . 3026
Valium Tablets . . . 3047

PACTENS (Mexico)
NAPROXEN SODIUM
Anaprox DS Tablets . . . 2967
Anaprox Tablets . . . 2967
Naprelan Tablets . . . 1293

PADIKEN (Mexico)
AMANTADINE HYDROCHLORIDE
Symmetrel Syrup . . . 1328
Symmetrel Tablets . . . 1328

PAFTEC (Portugal)
FLUNISOLIDE
Aerobid Inhaler System . . . 1363
Aerobid-M Inhaler System . . . 1363
Nasalide Nasal Spray . . . 1295
Nasarel Nasal Solution 0.025% . . . 1296

PAHTLISAN (Mexico)
CHLOROTHIAZIDE
Diuril Oral Suspension . . . 2087
Diuril Tablets . . . 2087

PAINEX (Portugal)
DICLOFENAC SODIUM
Voltaren Tablets . . . 2315
Voltaren-XR Tablets . . . 2315

PAINNOX (Thailand)
MEFENAMIC ACID
Ponstel Capsules . . . 1356

PALANE (Mexico)
ENALAPRIL MALEATE
Vasotec Tablets . . . 2210

PALCOL (Mexico)
CHLORAMPHENICOL
Chloromycetin Ophthalmic Ointment, 1% . . . ⊙296
Chloromycetin Ophthalmic Solution . . . ⊙297
Chloroptic Sterile Ophthalmic Ointment . . . ⊙234
Chloroptic Sterile Ophthalmic Solution . . . ⊙235

PALIATIN (Spain)
CHLORDIAZEPOXIDE HYDROCHLORIDE
Librium Capsules . . . 1736
Librium for Injection . . . 1737

PALLADON (Germany)
HYDROMORPHONE HYDROCHLORIDE
Dilaudid Ampules . . . 441
Dilaudid Injection . . . 441
Dilaudid Multiple Dose Vials (Sterile Solution) . . . 441
Dilaudid Oral Liquid . . . 445
Dilaudid Powder . . . 441
Dilaudid Rectal Suppositories . . . 441
Dilaudid Tablets . . . 441
Dilaudid Tablets - 8 mg . . . 445
Dilaudid-HP Injection . . . 443
Dilaudid-HP Lyophilized Powder 250 mg . . . 443

PALLADONE (Irish Republic, Israel, United Kingdom)
HYDROMORPHONE HYDROCHLORIDE
Dilaudid Ampules . . . 441
Dilaudid Injection . . . 441
Dilaudid Multiple Dose Vials (Sterile Solution) . . . 441
Dilaudid Oral Liquid . . . 445
Dilaudid Powder . . . 441
Dilaudid Rectal Suppositories . . . 441
Dilaudid Tablets . . . 441
Dilaudid Tablets - 8 mg . . . 445
Dilaudid-HP Injection . . . 443
Dilaudid-HP Lyophilized Powder 250 mg . . . 443

PALLIA (Hong Kong)
CIMETIDINE
Tagamet Tablets . . . 1644

PALMICLOR (Mexico)
CHLORAMPHENICOL
Chloromycetin Ophthalmic Ointment, 1% . . . ⊙296
Chloromycetin Ophthalmic Solution . . . ⊙297
Chloroptic Sterile Ophthalmic Ointment . . . ⊙234
Chloroptic Sterile Ophthalmic Solution . . . ⊙235

PALMIFFER (Mexico)
CHLORAMPHENICOL
Chloromycetin Ophthalmic Ointment, 1% . . . ⊙296
Chloromycetin Ophthalmic Solution . . . ⊙297
Chloroptic Sterile Ophthalmic Ointment . . . ⊙234
Chloroptic Sterile Ophthalmic Solution . . . ⊙235

PALMISOL (Mexico)
CHLORAMPHENICOL
Chloromycetin Ophthalmic Ointment, 1% . . . ⊙296
Chloromycetin Ophthalmic Solution . . . ⊙297
Chloroptic Sterile Ophthalmic Ointment . . . ⊙234
Chloroptic Sterile Ophthalmic Solution . . . ⊙235

PALON (Thailand)
PROPRANOLOL HYDROCHLORIDE
Inderal Injectable . . . 3513
Inderal LA Long-Acting Capsules . . . 3516
Inderal Tablets . . . 3513

PALUX (Brazil)
CHLOROQUINE PHOSPHATE
Aralen Tablets . . . 3075

PAMERGAN (Brazil)
PROMETHAZINE HYDROCHLORIDE
Phenergan Injection . . . 3553
Phenergan Suppositories . . . 3556
Phenergan Syrup Fortis . . . 3554
Phenergan Syrup Plain . . . 3554
Phenergan Tablets . . . 3556

PAMID (Israel)
INDAPAMIDE
Indapamide Tablets . . . 2286

PANACEF (Italy)
CEFACLOR
Ceclor CD Tablets . . . 1279
Ceclor Pulvules . . . 1905
Ceclor Suspension . . . 1905

PANAFCORT (Australia, South Africa)
PREDNISONE
Prednisone Intensol . . . 3064
Prednisone Oral Solution . . . 3064
Prednisone Tablets . . . 3064

PANAFCORTELONE (Australia, Hong Kong)
PREDNISOLONE
Prelone Syrup . . . 2273

PANAFEN (New Zealand)
IBUPROFEN
Motrin Suspension, Oral Drops, Chewable Tablets, and Caplets . . . 2002

PANAMOR (South Africa)
DICLOFENAC SODIUM
Voltaren Tablets . . . 2315
Voltaren-XR Tablets . . . 2315

PANAX N (Switzerland)
IBUPROFEN
Motrin Suspension, Oral Drops, Chewable Tablets, and Caplets . . . 2002

PANAXID (Belgium)
NIZATIDINE
Axid Pulvules . . . 1903

PANBESY (Belgium, Hong Kong, Singapore, Thailand)
PHENTERMINE HYDROCHLORIDE
Adipex-P Capsules . . . 1406
Adipex-P Tablets . . . 1406

PANCARDIOL (Spain)
ISOSORBIDE MONONITRATE
Imdur Tablets . . . 1826
Ismo Tablets . . . 3524

PANCREASE (Australia, Belgium, Canada, Denmark, Israel, Italy, New Zealand, Norway, Spain, Sweden, The Netherlands, United Kingdom)
PANCRELIPASE
Ultrase Capsules . . . 835
Ultrase MT Capsules . . . 835

PANDERMIL (Portugal)
HYDROCORTISONE
Anusol-HC Cream 2.5% . . . 2237
Hydrocortone Tablets . . . 2106

PANDERMIN CICATRIZANTE (Spain)
SODIUM HYALURONATE
Hyalgan Solution . . . 3080

PANFUGAN (Brazil)
MEBENDAZOLE
Vermox Chewable Tablets . . . 2017

PAN-FUNGEX (Portugal)
CLOTRIMAZOLE
Lotrimin Cream 1% . . . 3128
Lotrimin Lotion 1% . . . 3128
Lotrimin Topical Solution 1% . . . 3128
Mycelex Troche . . . 573

PANFUNGOL (Spain)
KETOCONAZOLE
Nizoral 2% Cream . . . 3620
Nizoral 2% Shampoo . . . 2007
Nizoral Tablets . . . 1791

PANGEL (Belgium)
BENZOYL PEROXIDE
Brevoxyl-4 Cleansing Lotion . . . 3269
Brevoxyl-4 Creamy Wash . . . 3270
Brevoxyl-4 Gel . . . 3269
Brevoxyl-8 Cleansing Lotion . . . 3269
Brevoxyl-8 Creamy Wash . . . 3270
Brevoxyl-8 Gel . . . 3269
Triaz Cleanser . . . 2026
Triaz Gel . . . 2026

PANITOL (Thailand)
CARBAMAZEPINE
Carbatrol Capsules . . . 3234
Tegretol Chewable Tablets . . . 2404
Tegretol Suspension . . . 2404
Tegretol Tablets . . . 2404
Tegretol-XR Tablets . . . 2404

PANIX (South Africa)
ALPRAZOLAM
Xanax Tablets . . . 2865

PANKREADEN (Italy)
PANCRELIPASE
Ultrase Capsules . . . 835
Ultrase MT Capsules . . . 835

PANKREASE (South Africa)
PANCRELIPASE
Ultrase Capsules . . . 835
Ultrase MT Capsules . . . 835

PANNOCORT (Belgium)
HYDROCORTISONE ACETATE
Anusol-HC Suppositories . . . 2238
Cortifoam Rectal Foam . . . 3170
Hydrocortone Acetate Injectable Suspension . . . 2103
Proctocort Suppositories . . . 2264

PANNOGEL (France)
BENZOYL PEROXIDE
Brevoxyl-4 Cleansing Lotion . . . 3269
Brevoxyl-4 Creamy Wash . . . 3270
Brevoxyl-4 Gel . . . 3269
Brevoxyl-8 Cleansing Lotion . . . 3269
Brevoxyl-8 Creamy Wash . . . 3270

Brevoxyl-8 Gel . . . 3269
Triaz Cleanser . . . 2026
Triaz Gel . . . 2026

PANORAL (Germany)
CEFACLOR
Ceclor CD Tablets . . . 1279
Ceclor Pulvules . . . 1905
Ceclor Suspension . . . 1905

PANOXYL (Australia, Austria, Canada, Finland, France, Germany, Hong Kong, Irish Republic, Israel, Italy, Mexico, New Zealand, Norway, Portugal, Singapore, South Africa, Spain, Switzerland, Thailand, United Kingdom)
BENZOYL PEROXIDE
Brevoxyl-4 Cleansing Lotion . . . 3269
Brevoxyl-4 Creamy Wash . . . 3270
Brevoxyl-4 Gel . . . 3269
Brevoxyl-8 Cleansing Lotion . . . 3269
Brevoxyl-8 Creamy Wash . . . 3270
Brevoxyl-8 Gel . . . 3269
Triaz Cleanser . . . 2026
Triaz Gel . . . 2026

PANTELMIN (Austria, Brazil, Portugal)
MEBENDAZOLE
Vermox Chewable Tablets . . . 2017

PANTINOL (Austria)
APROTININ
Trasylol Injection . . . 909

PANTODRIN (Spain)
ERYTHROMYCIN
Emgel 2% Topical Gel . . . 1285
Ery-Tab Tablets . . . 448
Erythromycin Base Filmtab Tablets . . . 454
Erythromycin Delayed-Release Capsules, USP . . . 455
PCE Dispertab Tablets . . . 498

PANTOFENICOL (Spain)
CHLORAMPHENICOL
Chloromycetin Ophthalmic Ointment, 1% . . . ⊙296
Chloromycetin Ophthalmic Solution . . . ⊙297
Chloroptic Sterile Ophthalmic Ointment . . ⊙234
Chloroptic Sterile Ophthalmic Solution . . ⊙235

PANTOK (Spain)
SIMVASTATIN
Zocor Tablets . . . 2219

PANTOMICINA (Brazil)
ERYTHROMYCIN STEARATE
Erythrocin Stearate Filmtab Tablets . . . 452

PANTOSTIN (Germany)
ESTRADIOL
Alora Transdermal System . . . 3372
Climara Transdermal System . . . 958
Estrace Vaginal Cream . . . 3358
Estring Vaginal Ring . . . 2811
Vivelle Transdermal System . . . 2412
Vivelle-Dot Transdermal System . . . 2416

PANTROP (Austria, Germany)
AMITRIPTYLINE HYDROCHLORIDE/CHLORDIAZEPOXIDE
Limbitrol DS Tablets . . . 1738
Limbitrol Tablets . . . 1738

PANTYSON (Finland)
HYDROCORTISONE
Anusol-HC Cream 2.5% . . . 2237
Hydrocortone Tablets . . . 2106

PANZID (Italy)
CEFTAZIDIME
Ceptaz for Injection . . . 1499
Fortaz for Injection . . . 1541
Tazicef for Injection . . . 1647
Tazidime Vials, Faspak & ADD-Vantage . . 1966

PANZYTRAT (New Zealand)
PANCRELIPASE
Ultrase Capsules . . . 835
Ultrase MT Capsules . . . 835

PARABOWL (Thailand)
PRAZOSIN HYDROCHLORIDE
Minipress Capsules . . . 2699

PARACEFAN (Belgium)
CLONIDINE HYDROCHLORIDE
Catapres Tablets . . . 1037
Duraclon Injection . . . 3057

PARAFLEX (Denmark, South Africa, Sweden)
CHLORZOXAZONE
Parafon Forte DSC Caplets . . . 2582

PARAFLEX SPEZIAL (Germany)
CHLORZOXAZONE
Parafon Forte DSC Caplets . . . 2582

PARAFON FORTE (Mexico)
CHLORZOXAZONE
Parafon Forte DSC Caplets . . . 2582

PARANTHIL (South Africa)
ALBENDAZOLE
Albenza Tablets . . . 1463

PARAPLATIN (Australia, Austria, Belgium, Brazil, Canada, Denmark, Finland, Hong Kong, Irish Republic, Israel, Italy, Mexico, New Zealand, Norway, South Africa, Spain, Sweden, Thailand, The Netherlands, United Kingdom)
CARBOPLATIN
Paraplatin for Injection . . . 1126

PARAPLATINE (France, Switzerland)
CARBOPLATIN
Paraplatin for Injection . . . 1126

PARAPRES (Spain)
CANDESARTAN CILEXETIL
Atacand Tablets . . . 595

PARARTRIN (Brazil)
IBUPROFEN
Motrin Suspension, Oral Drops, Chewable Tablets, and Caplets . . . 2002

PARASEPTINE (Belgium)
SULFANILAMIDE
AVC Cream . . . 1350
AVC Suppositories . . . 1350

PARASIN (Brazil)
ALBENDAZOLE
Albenza Tablets . . . 1463

PARASTHMAN (Germany)
THEOPHYLLINE
Aerolate Jr. T.D. Capsules . . . 1361
Aerolate Liquid . . . 1361
Aerolate Sr. T.D. Capsules . . . 1361
Theo-Dur Extended-Release Tablets . . . 1835
Uni-Dur Extended-Release Tablets . . . 1841
Uniphyl 400 mg and 600 mg Tablets . . . 2903

PARAXIN (Germany)
CHLORAMPHENICOL
Chloromycetin Ophthalmic Ointment, 1% . . . ⊙296
Chloromycetin Ophthalmic Solution . . . ⊙297
Chloroptic Sterile Ophthalmic Ointment . . ⊙234
Chloroptic Sterile Ophthalmic Solution . . ⊙235

PARELMIN (Brazil)
MEBENDAZOLE
Vermox Chewable Tablets . . . 2017

PARITREL (Israel)
AMANTADINE HYDROCHLORIDE
Symmetrel Syrup . . . 1328
Symmetrel Tablets . . . 1328

PARKEMED (Austria, Germany)
MEFENAMIC ACID
Ponstel Capsules . . . 1356

PARKE-MED (Italy)
MEFENAMIC ACID
Ponstel Capsules . . . 1356

PARMID (United Kingdom)
METOCLOPRAMIDE HYDROCHLORIDE
Reglan Injectable . . . 2935
Reglan Syrup . . . 2935
Reglan Tablets . . . 2935

PARNATE (Australia, Brazil, Canada, Germany, Irish Republic, New Zealand, South Africa, Spain)
TRANYLCYPROMINE SULFATE
Parnate Tablets . . . 1607

PARO (Italy)
HYDROCORTISONE ACETATE
Anusol-HC Suppositories . . . 2238
Cortifoam Rectal Foam . . . 3170
Hydrocortone Acetate Injectable Suspension . . . 2103
Proctocort Suppositories . . . 2264

PARONAL (Belgium)
ASPARAGINASE
Elspar for Injection . . . 2092

PARSAL (Germany)
IBUPROFEN
Motrin Suspension, Oral Drops, Chewable Tablets, and Caplets . . . 2002

PARSILID (Italy)
TICLOPIDINE HYDROCHLORIDE
Ticlid Tablets . . . 3015

PASALEN (Thailand)
KETOCONAZOLE
Nizoral 2% Cream . . . 3620
Nizoral 2% Shampoo . . . 2007
Nizoral Tablets . . . 1791

PASPERTIN (Austria)
METOCLOPRAMIDE HYDROCHLORIDE
Reglan Injectable . . . 2935
Reglan Syrup . . . 2935
Reglan Tablets . . . 2935

PATANOL (Canada, Singapore, Thailand)
OLOPATADINE HYDROCHLORIDE
Patanol Ophthalmic Solution . . . 540, ⊙216

PATSOLIN (Finland)
PRAZOSIN HYDROCHLORIDE
Minipress Capsules . . . 2699

PATXEN (Mexico)
NAPROXEN
EC-Naprosyn Delayed-Release Tablets . . . 2967
Naprosyn Suspension . . . 2967
Naprosyn Tablets . . . 2967

PAX (South Africa)
DIAZEPAM
Valium Injectable . . . 3026
Valium Tablets . . . 3047

PAXAM (Australia)
CLONAZEPAM
Klonopin Tablets . . . 2983

PAXATE (Mexico)
DIAZEPAM
Valium Injectable . . . 3026
Valium Tablets . . . 3047

PAXETIL (Portugal)
PAROXETINE HYDROCHLORIDE
Paxil Oral Suspension . . . 1609
Paxil Tablets . . . 1609

PAXIDORM (Singapore, United Kingdom)
DIPHENHYDRAMINE HYDROCHLORIDE
Benadryl Parenteral . . . 2617

PAXIL (Canada, Mexico)
PAROXETINE HYDROCHLORIDE
Paxil Oral Suspension . . . 1609
Paxil Tablets . . . 1609

PAXILFAR (Portugal)
TRAMADOL HYDROCHLORIDE
Ultram Tablets . . . 2600

PAXOFEN (United Kingdom)
IBUPROFEN
Motrin Suspension, Oral Drops, Chewable Tablets, and Caplets . . . 2002

PAZOLAM (Portugal)
ALPRAZOLAM
Xanax Tablets . . . 2865

PAZOLINI (Brazil)
DIAZEPAM
Valium Injectable . . . 3026
Valium Tablets . . . 3047

PCE (Canada, Hong Kong)
ERYTHROMYCIN
Emgel 2% Topical Gel . . . 1285
Ery-Tab Tablets . . . 448
Erythromycin Base Filmtab Tablets . . . 454
Erythromycin Delayed-Release Capsules, USP . . . 455
PCE Dispertab Tablets . . . 498

PEAULINE (The Netherlands)
BENZOYL PEROXIDE
Brevoxyl-4 Cleansing Lotion . . . 3269
Brevoxyl-4 Creamy Wash . . . 3270
Brevoxyl-4 Gel . . . 3269
Brevoxyl-8 Cleansing Lotion . . . 3269
Brevoxyl-8 Creamy Wash . . . 3270
Brevoxyl-8 Gel . . . 3269
Triaz Cleanser . . . 2026
Triaz Gel . . . 2026

PEDIAPHYLLIN PL (The Netherlands)
THEOPHYLLINE
Aerolate Jr. T.D. Capsules . . . 1361
Aerolate Liquid . . . 1361
Aerolate Sr. T.D. Capsules . . . 1361
Theo-Dur Extended-Release Tablets . . . 1835
Uni-Dur Extended-Release Tablets . . . 1841
Uniphyl 400 mg and 600 mg Tablets . . . 2903

PEDIAPRED (Canada)
PREDNISOLONE SODIUM PHOSPHATE
Pediapred Oral Solution . . . 1170

PEDIKUROL (Austria)
CLOTRIMAZOLE
Lotrimin Cream 1% . . . 3128
Lotrimin Lotion 1% . . . 3128
Lotrimin Topical Solution 1% . . . 3128
Mycelex Troche . . . 573

PEDILETAN (Brazil)
LINDANE
Lindane Lotion USP 1% . . . 559
Lindane Shampoo USP 1% . . . 560

PEDISAFE (Germany)
CLOTRIMAZOLE
Lotrimin Cream 1% . . . 3128
Lotrimin Lotion 1% . . . 3128
Lotrimin Topical Solution 1% . . . 3128
Mycelex Troche . . . 573

PEITEL (Spain)
PREDNICARBATE
Dermatop Emollient Cream . . . 2517

PELEDOX (Spain)
DOXYCYCLINE HYCLATE
Doryx Coated Pellet Filled Capsules . . . 3357
Periostat Tablets . . . 1208
Vibramycin Hyclate Capsules . . . 2735
Vibramycin Hyclate Intravenous . . . 2737
Vibra-Tabs Film Coated Tablets . . . 2735

PELLISAL-GEL (Germany)
DIPHENHYDRAMINE HYDROCHLORIDE
Benadryl Parenteral . . . 2617

PELLIT INSEKTENSTICH, PELLIT (Germany)
DIPHENHYDRAMINE HYDROCHLORIDE
Benadryl Parenteral . . . 2617

PENDRAMINE (United Kingdom)
PENICILLAMINE
Cuprimine Capsules . . . 2075
Depen Titratable Tablets . . . 3341

PENEDIL (Israel)
FELODIPINE
Plendil Extended-Release Tablets . . . 623

PENGESIC (Singapore)
TRAMADOL HYDROCHLORIDE
Ultram Tablets . . . 2600

PENMOX (South Africa)
AMOXICILLIN
Amoxil Pediatric Drops for Oral Suspension . . . 1471
Amoxil Tablets . . . 1471

PENNSAID (United Kingdom)
DICLOFENAC SODIUM
Voltaren Tablets . . . 2315
Voltaren-XR Tablets . . . 2315

PENTACARD (Belgium, Thailand)
ISOSORBIDE MONONITRATE
Imdur Tablets . . . 1826
Ismo Tablets . . . 3524

PENTAMYCETIN (Canada)
CHLORAMPHENICOL
Chloromycetin Ophthalmic Ointment, 1% . . . ⊙296
Chloromycetin Ophthalmic Solution . . ⊙297
Chloroptic Sterile Ophthalmic Ointment . . ⊙234
Chloroptic Sterile Ophthalmic Solution . . ⊙235

PENTAZOLE (Brazil)
MEBENDAZOLE
Vermox Chewable Tablets . . . 2017

PENTCILLIN (Japan)
PIPERACILLIN SODIUM
Pipracil . . . 1866

PENTIBROXIL (Mexico)
AMOXICILLIN
Amoxil Pediatric Drops for Oral Suspension . . . 1471
Amoxil Tablets . . . 1471

PENTICLOX (Mexico)
AMOXICILLIN
Amoxil Pediatric Drops for Oral Suspension . . . 1471
Amoxil Tablets . . . 1471

PENTILZENO (Portugal)
DILTIAZEM HYDROCHLORIDE
Cardizem CD Capsules . . . 1016
Cardizem Injectable . . . 1018
Cardizem Lyo-Ject Syringe . . . 1018
Cardizem Monovial . . . 1018
Tiazac Capsules . . . 1378

PENVICILIN (Brazil)
AMOXICILLIN
Amoxil Pediatric Drops for Oral Suspension . . . 1471
Amoxil Tablets . . . 1471

PEPCID (Australia, Canada, Finland, Germany, Hong Kong, Irish Republic, New Zealand, Norway, South Africa, Spain, Sweden, Switzerland, The Netherlands)
FAMOTIDINE
Pepcid Injection . . . 2153
Pepcid Injection Premixed . . . 2153
Pepcid RPD Orally Disintegrating Tablets . . . 2150
Pepcid Tablets . . . 2150
Pepcid for Oral Suspension . . . 2150

PEPCIDAC (France)
FAMOTIDINE
Pepcid Injection . . . 2153
Pepcid Injection Premixed . . . 2153

Pepcid RPD Orally Disintegrating Tablets . . . 2150
Pepcid Tablets . . . 2150
Pepcid for Oral Suspension . . . 2150

PEPCIDIN (Denmark, Finland, Norway, Sweden, The Netherlands)
FAMOTIDINE
Pepcid Injection . . . 2153
Pepcid Injection Premixed . . . 2153
Pepcid RPD Orally Disintegrating Tablets . . . 2150
Pepcid Tablets . . . 2150
Pepcid for Oral Suspension . . . 2150

PEPCIDINA (Portugal)
FAMOTIDINE
Pepcid Injection . . . 2153
Pepcid Injection Premixed . . . 2153
Pepcid RPD Orally Disintegrating Tablets . . . 2150
Pepcid Tablets . . . 2150
Pepcid for Oral Suspension . . . 2150

PEPCIDINE (Australia, Austria, Belgium, Hong Kong, Mexico, New Zealand, Singapore, Switzerland, Thailand)
FAMOTIDINE
Pepcid Injection . . . 2153
Pepcid Injection Premixed . . . 2153
Pepcid RPD Orally Disintegrating Tablets . . . 2150
Pepcid Tablets . . . 2150
Pepcid for Oral Suspension . . . 2150

PEPCINE (Thailand)
FAMOTIDINE
Pepcid Injection . . . 2153
Pepcid Injection Premixed . . . 2153
Pepcid RPD Orally Disintegrating Tablets . . . 2150
Pepcid Tablets . . . 2150
Pepcid for Oral Suspension . . . 2150

PEPDINE (France)
FAMOTIDINE
Pepcid Injection . . . 2153
Pepcid Injection Premixed . . . 2153
Pepcid RPD Orally Disintegrating Tablets . . . 2150
Pepcid Tablets . . . 2150
Pepcid for Oral Suspension . . . 2150

PEPDUL (Germany)
FAMOTIDINE
Pepcid Injection . . . 2153
Pepcid Injection Premixed . . . 2153
Pepcid RPD Orally Disintegrating Tablets . . . 2150
Pepcid Tablets . . . 2150
Pepcid for Oral Suspension . . . 2150

PEPFAMIN (Thailand)
FAMOTIDINE
Pepcid Injection . . . 2153
Pepcid Injection Premixed . . . 2153
Pepcid RPD Orally Disintegrating Tablets . . . 2150
Pepcid Tablets . . . 2150
Pepcid for Oral Suspension . . . 2150

PEP-RANI (Portugal)
RANITIDINE HYDROCHLORIDE
Zantac 150 EFFERdose Granules . . . 1690
Zantac 150 EFFERdose Tablets . . . 1690
Zantac 150 Tablets . . . 1690
Zantac 300 Tablets . . . 1690
Zantac Injection . . . 1688
Zantac Injection Premixed . . . 1688
Zantac Syrup . . . 1690

PEPRAZOL (Brazil)
OMEPRAZOLE
Prilosec Delayed-Release Capsules . . . 628

PEPTAB (Portugal)
RANITIDINE HYDROCHLORIDE
Zantac 150 EFFERdose Granules . . . 1690
Zantac 150 EFFERdose Tablets . . . 1690
Zantac 150 Tablets . . . 1690
Zantac 300 Tablets . . . 1690
Zantac Injection . . . 1688
Zantac Injection Premixed . . . 1688
Zantac Syrup . . . 1690

PEPTARD (United Kingdom)
HYOSCYAMINE SULFATE
Levbid Extended-Release Tablets . . . 3172
Levsin Drops . . . 3172
Levsin Elixir . . . 3172
Levsin Injection . . . 3172
Levsin Tablets . . . 3172
Levsin/SL Tablets . . . 3172
Levsinex Timecaps . . . 3172

PEPTIC GUARD (Canada)
FAMOTIDINE
Pepcid Injection . . . 2153
Pepcid Injection Premixed . . . 2153
Pepcid RPD Orally Disintegrating Tablets . . . 2150
Pepcid Tablets . . . 2150
Pepcid for Oral Suspension . . . 2150

PEPTIC RELIEF (Canada)
RANITIDINE HYDROCHLORIDE
Zantac 150 EFFERdose Granules . . . 1690
Zantac 150 EFFERdose Tablets . . . 1690
Zantac 150 Tablets . . . 1690
Zantac 300 Tablets . . . 1690
Zantac Injection . . . 1688
Zantac Injection Premixed . . . 1688
Zantac Syrup . . . 1690

PEPTICA (Thailand)
CIMETIDINE
Tagamet Tablets . . . 1644

PEPTICUM (Spain)
OMEPRAZOLE
Prilosec Delayed-Release Capsules . . . 628

PEPTIFAR (Portugal)
RANITIDINE HYDROCHLORIDE
Zantac 150 EFFERdose Granules . . . 1690
Zantac 150 EFFERdose Tablets . . . 1690
Zantac 150 Tablets . . . 1690
Zantac 300 Tablets . . . 1690
Zantac Injection . . . 1688
Zantac Injection Premixed . . . 1688
Zantac Syrup . . . 1690

PEPTIMAX (United Kingdom)
CIMETIDINE
Tagamet Tablets . . . 1644

PEPTIZOLE (Thailand)
OMEPRAZOLE
Prilosec Delayed-Release Capsules . . . 628

PEPTOCI (Thailand)
FAMOTIDINE
Pepcid Injection . . . 2153
Pepcid Injection Premixed . . . 2153
Pepcid RPD Orally Disintegrating Tablets . . . 2150
Pepcid Tablets . . . 2150
Pepcid for Oral Suspension . . . 2150

PEPTOL (Canada)
CIMETIDINE
Tagamet Tablets . . . 1644

PEPZAN (Hong Kong, New Zealand, Singapore)
FAMOTIDINE
Pepcid Injection . . . 2153
Pepcid Injection Premixed . . . 2153
Pepcid RPD Orally Disintegrating Tablets . . . 2150
Pepcid Tablets . . . 2150
Pepcid for Oral Suspension . . . 2150

PERACIL (Italy)
PIPERACILLIN SODIUM
Pipracil . . . 1866

PERASTHMAN N (Germany)
THEOPHYLLINE
Aerolate Jr. T.D. Capsules . . . 1361
Aerolate Liquid . . . 1361
Aerolate Sr. T.D. Capsules . . . 1361
Theo-Dur Extended-Release Tablets . . . 1835
Uni-Dur Extended-Release Tablets . . . 1841
Uniphyl 400 mg and 600 mg Tablets . . . 2903

PERCLODIN (Irish Republic)
DIPYRIDAMOLE
Persantine Tablets . . . 1057

PERCORINA (Spain)
ISOSORBIDE MONONITRATE
Imdur Tablets . . . 1826
Ismo Tablets . . . 3524

PERDERM (Hong Kong, Singapore)
ALCLOMETASONE DIPROPIONATE
Aclovate Cream . . . 1275
Aclovate Ointment . . . 1275

PERDIPINA (Italy)
NICARDIPINE HYDROCHLORIDE
Cardene I.V. . . . 3485

PERDIPINE (Japan)
NICARDIPINE HYDROCHLORIDE
Cardene I.V. . . . 3485

PERDIX (Denmark, Finland, Sweden, United Kingdom)
MOEXIPRIL HYDROCHLORIDE
Univasc Tablets . . . 3181

PERFARIN (Mexico)
PIROXICAM
Feldene Capsules . . . 2685

PERFUDAL (Spain)
FELODIPINE
Plendil Extended-Release Tablets . . . 623

PERIACTIN (Australia, Austria, Belgium, Canada, Denmark, Hong Kong, Irish Republic, Italy, New Zealand, Norway, Portugal, South Africa, Spain, Sweden, Switzerland, Thailand, The Netherlands, United Kingdom)
CYPROHEPTADINE HYDROCHLORIDE
Periactin Tablets . . . 2155

PERIACTINE (France)
CYPROHEPTADINE HYDROCHLORIDE
Periactin Tablets . . . 2155

PERIACTINOL (Germany)
CYPROHEPTADINE HYDROCHLORIDE
Periactin Tablets . . . 2155

PERIATIN (Brazil)
CYPROHEPTADINE HYDROCHLORIDE
Periactin Tablets . . . 2155

PERICAINA (Italy)
MEPIVACAINE HYDROCHLORIDE
Polocaine Injection, USP . . . 625
Polocaine-MPF Injection, USP . . . 625

PERICAM (Irish Republic)
PIROXICAM
Feldene Capsules . . . 2685

PERICATE (Israel)
HALOPERIDOL DECANOATE
Haldol Decanoate 100 Injection . . . 2535
Haldol Decanoate 50 Injection . . . 2535

PERIDA (Thailand)
HALOPERIDOL
Haldol Injection, Tablets and Concentrate . . . 2533

PERIDOL (Canada)
HALOPERIDOL
Haldol Injection, Tablets and Concentrate . . . 2533

PERIDOR (Israel)
HALOPERIDOL
Haldol Injection, Tablets and Concentrate . . . 2533

PERILOX (Switzerland)
METRONIDAZOLE
MetroCream . . . 1404
MetroGel . . . 1405
MetroGel-Vaginal Gel . . . 1986
MetroLotion . . . 1405
Noritate Cream . . . 1224

PERINAL (United Kingdom)
HYDROCORTISONE
Anusol-HC Cream 2.5% . . . 2237
Hydrocortone Tablets . . . 2106

PERINORM (South Africa)
METOCLOPRAMIDE HYDROCHLORIDE
Reglan Injectable . . . 2935
Reglan Syrup . . . 2935
Reglan Tablets . . . 2935

PERIOCLINE (Japan)
MINOCYCLINE HYDROCHLORIDE
Dynacin Capsules . . . 2019
Minocin Intravenous . . . 1862
Minocin Oral Suspension . . . 1865
Minocin Pellet-Filled Capsules . . . 1863

PERIOSTAT (United Kingdom)
DOXYCYCLINE HYCLATE
Doryx Coated Pellet Filled Capsules . . . 3357
Periostat Tablets . . . 1208
Vibramycin Hyclate Capsules . . . 2735
Vibramycin Hyclate Intravenous . . . 2737
Vibra-Tabs Film Coated Tablets . . . 2735

PERIPLUM (Italy)
NIMODIPINE
Nimotop Capsules . . . 904

PERIPRESS (Denmark, Finland, Norway, Sweden)
PRAZOSIN HYDROCHLORIDE
Minipress Capsules . . . 2699

PERITOL (Germany)
CYPROHEPTADINE HYDROCHLORIDE
Periactin Tablets . . . 2155

PERIVAR VENENSALBE (Germany)
HEPARIN SODIUM
Heparin Lock Flush Solution . . . 3509
Heparin Sodium Injection . . . 3511

PERKOD (France)
DIPYRIDAMOLE
Persantine Tablets . . . 1057

PERLOL (Thailand)
PROPRANOLOL HYDROCHLORIDE
Inderal Injectable . . . 3513
Inderal LA Long-Acting Capsules . . . 3516
Inderal Tablets . . . 3513

PERLUTEX (Denmark, Norway)
MEDROXYPROGESTERONE ACETATE
Depo-Provera Contraceptive Injection . . . 2798
Provera Tablets . . . 2853

PERNAMED (Thailand)
PERPHENAZINE
Trilafon Injection . . . 3160
Trilafon Tablets . . . 3160

PERNAZINE (Thailand)
PERPHENAZINE
Trilafon Injection . . . 3160
Trilafon Tablets . . . 3160

PEROCEF (Italy)
CEFOPERAZONE SODIUM
Cefobid Intravenous/Intramuscular . . . 2671
Cefobid Pharmacy Bulk Package - Not for Direct Infusion . . . 2673

PEROFEN (Thailand)
IBUPROFEN
Motrin Suspension, Oral Drops, Chewable Tablets, and Caplets . . . 2002

PEROXACNE (Spain)
BENZOYL PEROXIDE
Brevoxyl-4 Cleansing Lotion . . . 3269
Brevoxyl-4 Creamy Wash . . . 3270
Brevoxyl-4 Gel . . . 3269
Brevoxyl-8 Cleansing Lotion . . . 3269
Brevoxyl-8 Creamy Wash . . . 3270
Brevoxyl-8 Gel . . . 3269
Triaz Cleanser . . . 2026
Triaz Gel . . . 2026

PEROXIBEN (Spain)
BENZOYL PEROXIDE
Brevoxyl-4 Cleansing Lotion . . . 3269
Brevoxyl-4 Creamy Wash . . . 3270
Brevoxyl-4 Gel . . . 3269
Brevoxyl-8 Cleansing Lotion . . . 3269
Brevoxyl-8 Creamy Wash . . . 3270
Brevoxyl-8 Gel . . . 3269
Triaz Cleanser . . . 2026
Triaz Gel . . . 2026

PERPHENAN (Israel)
PERPHENAZINE
Trilafon Injection . . . 3160
Trilafon Tablets . . . 3160

PERSA-GEL W (Australia)
BENZOYL PEROXIDE
Brevoxyl-4 Cleansing Lotion . . . 3269
Brevoxyl-4 Creamy Wash . . . 3270
Brevoxyl-4 Gel . . . 3269
Brevoxyl-8 Cleansing Lotion . . . 3269
Brevoxyl-8 Creamy Wash . . . 3270
Brevoxyl-8 Gel . . . 3269
Triaz Cleanser . . . 2026
Triaz Gel . . . 2026

PERSANTIN (Australia, Austria, Brazil, Denmark, Finland, Germany, Hong Kong, Irish Republic, Italy, Mexico, New Zealand, Norway, Portugal, Singapore, South Africa, Sweden, Thailand, The Netherlands, United Kingdom)
DIPYRIDAMOLE
Persantine Tablets . . . 1057

PERSANTIN PLUS (Hong Kong)
DIPYRIDAMOLE
Persantine Tablets . . . 1057

PERSANTIN S (Brazil)
DIPYRIDAMOLE
Persantine Tablets . . . 1057

PERSANTINE (Belgium, Canada, France, Switzerland)
DIPYRIDAMOLE
Persantine Tablets . . . 1057

PERTENSAL (Spain)
NIFEDIPINE
Adalat CC Tablets . . . 877
Procardia Capsules . . . 2708
Procardia XL Extended Release Tablets . . . 2710

PERTIL (Spain)
ISOSORBIDE MONONITRATE
Imdur Tablets . . . 1826
Ismo Tablets . . . 3524

PERTIN (Austria)
METOCLOPRAMIDE HYDROCHLORIDE
Reglan Injectable . . . 2935
Reglan Syrup . . . 2935
Reglan Tablets . . . 2935

PERTOFRAN (Australia, Austria, Belgium, France, Germany, Irish Republic, New Zealand, South Africa, Switzerland, The Netherlands, United Kingdom)
DESIPRAMINE HYDROCHLORIDE
Norpramin Tablets . . . 755

PERTOFRANE (Canada)
DESIPRAMINE HYDROCHLORIDE
Norpramin Tablets . . . 755

PERTRANQUIL (Austria, Belgium)
MEPROBAMATE
Miltown Tablets . . . 3349

PERZINE (Thailand)
PERPHENAZINE
Trilafon Injection . . . 3160
Trilafon Tablets . . . 3160

PETINIMID (Austria, Switzerland)
ETHOSUXIMIDE
Zarontin Capsules . . . 2659

Zarontin Syrup . . . 2660

PETNIDAN (Germany)
ETHOSUXIMIDE
Zarontin Capsules . . . 2659
Zarontin Syrup . . . 2660

PETOGEN (South Africa)
MEDROXYPROGESTERONE ACETATE
Depo-Provera Contraceptive Injection . . . 2798
Provera Tablets . . . 2853

PEZETAMID (Germany)
PYRAZINAMIDE
Pyrazinamide Tablets . . . 1876

PFEIL (Germany)
IBUPROFEN
Motrin Suspension, Oral Drops, Chewable Tablets, and Caplets . . . 2002

P-FEN (Thailand)
IBUPROFEN
Motrin Suspension, Oral Drops, Chewable Tablets, and Caplets . . . 2002

PHANATE (Thailand)
LITHIUM CARBONATE
Eskalith CR Controlled Release Tablets . . 1527
Eskalith Capsules . . . 1527
Lithium Carbonate Capsules . . . 3061
Lithobid Slow-Release Tablets . . . 3255

PHARMACETIN (Thailand)
CHLORAMPHENICOL
Chloromycetin Ophthalmic Ointment, 1% . . . ⊙296
Chloromycetin Ophthalmic Solution . . . ⊙297
Chloroptic Sterile Ophthalmic Ointment . . ⊙234
Chloroptic Sterile Ophthalmic Solution . . ⊙235

PHARMAFLAM (South Africa)
DICLOFENAC SODIUM
Voltaren Tablets . . . 2315
Voltaren-XR Tablets . . . 2315

PHARMAFLEX (Belgium)
METRONIDAZOLE
MetroCream . . . 1404
MetroGel . . . 1405
MetroGel-Vaginal Gel . . . 1986
MetroLotion . . . 1405
Noritate Cream . . . 1224

PHARMALOSE (Canada)
LACTULOSE
Kristalose for Oral Solution . . . 1007

PHARMAMOX (Switzerland)
AMOXICILLIN
Amoxil Pediatric Drops for Oral Suspension . . . 1471
Amoxil Tablets . . . 1471

PHARMAPRESS (South Africa)
ENALAPRIL MALEATE
Vasotec Tablets . . . 2210

PHARMAQUINE (Switzerland)
CHLOROQUINE PHOSPHATE
Aralen Tablets . . . 3075

PHARMET (South Africa)
METHYLDOPA
Aldomet Tablets . . . 2037

PHARMITUSSIN DM (Canada)
DEXTROMETHORPHAN HYDROBROMIDE/GUAIFENESIN
Tussi-Organidin DM NR Liquid . . . 3350
Tussi-Organidin DM-S NR Liquid . . . 3350

PHARNAX (Thailand)
ALPRAZOLAM
Xanax Tablets . . . 2865

PHARPHYLLINE (The Netherlands)
THEOPHYLLINE
Aerolate Jr. T.D. Capsules . . . 1361
Aerolate Liquid . . . 1361
Aerolate Sr. T.D. Capsules . . . 1361
Theo-Dur Extended-Release Tablets . . . 1835
Uni-Dur Extended-Release Tablets . . . 1841
Uniphyl 400 mg and 600 mg Tablets . . . 2903

PHARYNGOCIN (Germany)
ERYTHROMYCIN
Emgel 2% Topical Gel . . . 1285
Ery-Tab Tablets . . . 448
Erythromycin Base Filmtab Tablets . . . 454
Erythromycin Delayed-Release Capsules, USP . . . 455
PCE Dispertab Tablets . . . 498

PHASAL (United Kingdom)
LITHIUM CARBONATE
Eskalith CR Controlled Release Tablets . . 1527
Eskalith Capsules . . . 1527
Lithium Carbonate Capsules . . . 3061
Lithobid Slow-Release Tablets . . . 3255

PHENCODIN (Thailand)
CODEINE PHOSPHATE/PROMETHAZINE HYDROCHLORIDE
Phenergan with Codeine Syrup . . . 3557

PHENEDRINE (Hong Kong)
THEOPHYLLINE
Aerolate Jr. T.D. Capsules . . . 1361
Aerolate Liquid . . . 1361
Aerolate Sr. T.D. Capsules . . . 1361
Theo-Dur Extended-Release Tablets . . . 1835
Uni-Dur Extended-Release Tablets . . . 1841
Uniphyl 400 mg and 600 mg Tablets . . . 2903

PHENERGAN (Australia, Denmark, Hong Kong, Irish Republic, New Zealand, Norway, Singapore, South Africa, Thailand, The Netherlands, United Kingdom)
PROMETHAZINE HYDROCHLORIDE
Phenergan Injection . . . 3553
Phenergan Suppositories . . . 3556
Phenergan Syrup Fortis . . . 3554
Phenergan Syrup Plain . . . 3554
Phenergan Tablets . . . 3556

PHENHALAL (United Kingdom)
PROMETHAZINE HYDROCHLORIDE
Phenergan Injection . . . 3553
Phenergan Suppositories . . . 3556
Phenergan Syrup Fortis . . . 3554
Phenergan Syrup Plain . . . 3554
Phenergan Tablets . . . 3556

PHENHYDAN (Austria, Switzerland)
PHENYTOIN
Dilantin Infatabs . . . 2624
Dilantin-125 Oral Suspension . . . 2625

PHENICOL (Israel)
CHLORAMPHENICOL
Chloromycetin Ophthalmic Ointment, 1% . . . ⊙296
Chloromycetin Ophthalmic Solution . . . ⊙297
Chloroptic Sterile Ophthalmic Ointment . . ⊙234
Chloroptic Sterile Ophthalmic Solution . . ⊙235

PHENSEDYL (Singapore, Thailand, United Kingdom)
CODEINE PHOSPHATE/PROMETHAZINE HYDROCHLORIDE
Phenergan with Codeine Syrup . . . 3557

PHENSIC IBUPROFEN (United Kingdom)
IBUPROFEN
Motrin Suspension, Oral Drops, Chewable Tablets, and Caplets . . . 2002

PHERAMIN N (Germany)
DIPHENHYDRAMINE HYDROCHLORIDE
Benadryl Parenteral . . . 2617

PHILCOCICLINA (Italy)
DOXYCYCLINE HYCLATE
Doryx Coated Pellet Filled Capsules . . . 3357
Periostat Tablets . . . 1208
Vibra-Tabs Film Coated Tablets . . . 2735
Vibramycin Hyclate Capsules . . . 2735
Vibramycin Hyclate Intravenous . . . 2737

PHIMETIN (United Kingdom)
CIMETIDINE
Tagamet Tablets . . . 1644

PHOR PAIN (United Kingdom)
IBUPROFEN
Motrin Suspension, Oral Drops, Chewable Tablets, and Caplets . . . 2002

PHORPAIN (Irish Republic)
IBUPROFEN
Motrin Suspension, Oral Drops, Chewable Tablets, and Caplets . . . 2002

PHOS-EX (Finland, Norway, Sweden, United Kingdom)
CALCIUM ACETATE
PhosLo Tablets . . . 1069

PHYMORAX (Singapore)
HYDROXYZINE HYDROCHLORIDE
Atarax Tablets & Syrup . . . 2667
Vistaril Intramuscular Solution . . . 2738

PICILLIN (Israel, Italy)
PIPERACILLIN SODIUM
Pipracil . . . 1866

PICOSYL (Spain)
HYDROCORTISONE ACETATE
Anusol-HC Suppositories . . . 2238
Cortifoam Rectal Foam . . . 3170
Hydrocortone Acetate Injectable Suspension . . . 2103
Proctocort Suppositories . . . 2264

PIDILAT (Germany)
NIFEDIPINE
Adalat CC Tablets . . . 877
Procardia Capsules . . . 2708
Procardia XL Extended Release Tablets . . 2710

PIKETOFEN (Mexico)
KETOPROFEN
Orudis Capsules . . . 3548
Oruvail Capsules . . . 3548

PILAX (Austria)
PILOCARPINE HYDROCHLORIDE
Isopto Carpine Ophthalmic Solution . . . ⊙215
Pilopine HS Ophthalmic Gel . . . ⊙217
Salagen Tablets . . . 2229

PILDER (Spain)
GEMFIBROZIL
Lopid Tablets . . . 2650

PILENSAR (Brazil)
LINDANE
Lindane Lotion USP 1% . . . 559
Lindane Shampoo USP 1% . . . 560

PILO (Belgium, France, Mexico, Norway)
PILOCARPINE HYDROCHLORIDE
Isopto Carpine Ophthalmic Solution . . . ⊙215
Pilopine HS Ophthalmic Gel . . . ⊙217
Salagen Tablets . . . 2229

PILOCARCIL (Portugal)
PILOCARPINE HYDROCHLORIDE
Isopto Carpine Ophthalmic Solution . . . ⊙215
Pilopine HS Ophthalmic Gel . . . ⊙217
Salagen Tablets . . . 2229

PILOCARP (Spain)
PILOCARPINE HYDROCHLORIDE
Isopto Carpine Ophthalmic Solution . . . ⊙215
Pilopine HS Ophthalmic Gel . . . ⊙217
Salagen Tablets . . . 2229

PILOGEL (Austria, Germany, Irish Republic, Israel, Italy, Singapore, South Africa, Thailand, The Netherlands, United Kingdom)
PILOCARPINE HYDROCHLORIDE
Isopto Carpine Ophthalmic Solution . . . ⊙215
Pilopine HS Ophthalmic Gel . . . ⊙217
Salagen Tablets . . . 2229

PILOGEL HS (Switzerland)
PILOCARPINE HYDROCHLORIDE
Isopto Carpine Ophthalmic Solution . . . ⊙215
Pilopine HS Ophthalmic Gel . . . ⊙217
Salagen Tablets . . . 2229

PILOMANN (Germany)
PILOCARPINE HYDROCHLORIDE
Isopto Carpine Ophthalmic Solution . . . ⊙215
Pilopine HS Ophthalmic Gel . . . ⊙217
Salagen Tablets . . . 2229

PILOPINE HS (Canada)
PILOCARPINE HYDROCHLORIDE
Isopto Carpine Ophthalmic Solution . . . ⊙215
Pilopine HS Ophthalmic Gel . . . ⊙217
Salagen Tablets . . . 2229

PILOPT (Australia, New Zealand)
PILOCARPINE HYDROCHLORIDE
Isopto Carpine Ophthalmic Solution . . . ⊙215
Pilopine HS Ophthalmic Gel . . . ⊙217
Salagen Tablets . . . 2229

PILOSTAT (Canada)
PILOCARPINE HYDROCHLORIDE
Isopto Carpine Ophthalmic Solution . . . ⊙215
Pilopine HS Ophthalmic Gel . . . ⊙217
Salagen Tablets . . . 2229

PILO-STULLN (Germany)
PILOCARPINE HYDROCHLORIDE
Isopto Carpine Ophthalmic Solution . . . ⊙215
Pilopine HS Ophthalmic Gel . . . ⊙217
Salagen Tablets . . . 2229

PILOTONINA (Italy)
PILOCARPINE HYDROCHLORIDE
Isopto Carpine Ophthalmic Solution . . . ⊙215
Pilopine HS Ophthalmic Gel . . . ⊙217
Salagen Tablets . . . 2229

PIMA BICIRON (Germany)
CHLORAMPHENICOL
Chloromycetin Ophthalmic Ointment, 1% . . . ⊙296
Chloromycetin Ophthalmic Solution . . . ⊙297
Chloroptic Sterile Ophthalmic Ointment . . ⊙234
Chloroptic Sterile Ophthalmic Solution . . ⊙235

PIMA BICIRON N (Germany)
NATAMYCIN
Natacyn Antifungal Ophthalmic Suspension . . . ⊙216

PIMAFUCIN (Belgium, Finland, Germany, United Kingdom)
NATAMYCIN
Natacyn Antifungal Ophthalmic Suspension . . . ⊙216

PINALGESIC (Irish Republic)
MEFENAMIC ACID
Ponstel Capsules . . . 1356

PINAMET (Irish Republic)
CIMETIDINE
Tagamet Tablets . . . 1644

PINAMOX (Irish Republic)
AMOXICILLIN
Amoxil Pediatric Drops for Oral Suspension . . . 1471
Amoxil Tablets . . . 1471

PINIFED (Irish Republic)
NIFEDIPINE
Adalat CC Tablets . . . 877
Procardia Capsules . . . 2708
Procardia XL Extended Release Tablets . . 2710

PINIOL (Germany)
NAPHAZOLINE HYDROCHLORIDE
Albalon Ophthalmic Solution . . . ⊙225

PINIOL NASENSPRAY (Germany)
NAPHAZOLINE HYDROCHLORIDE
Albalon Ophthalmic Solution . . . ⊙225

PIODREX (Brazil)
LINDANE
Lindane Lotion USP 1% . . . 559
Lindane Shampoo USP 1% . . . 560

PIOLETAL (Brazil)
LINDANE
Lindane Lotion USP 1% . . . 559
Lindane Shampoo USP 1% . . . 560

PIONAX (Brazil)
LINDANE
Lindane Lotion USP 1% . . . 559
Lindane Shampoo USP 1% . . . 560

PIPCIL (Belgium, The Netherlands)
PIPERACILLIN SODIUM
Pipracil . . . 1866

PIPERILLINE (France)
PIPERACILLIN SODIUM
Pipracil . . . 1866

PIPERITAL (Italy)
PIPERACILLIN SODIUM
Pipracil . . . 1866

PIPERSAL (Italy)
PIPERACILLIN SODIUM
Pipracil . . . 1866

PIPERZAM (Spain)
PIPERACILLIN SODIUM
Pipracil . . . 1866

PIPPEN (Thailand)
IBUPROFEN
Motrin Suspension, Oral Drops, Chewable Tablets, and Caplets . . . 2002

PIPRACIL (Canada, Hong Kong, Thailand)
PIPERACILLIN SODIUM
Pipracil . . . 1866

PIPRACIN (Italy)
PIPERACILLIN SODIUM
Pipracil . . . 1866

PIPRIL (Australia, Austria, Germany, Irish Republic, Israel, New Zealand, South Africa, Spain, Switzerland, United Kingdom)
PIPERACILLIN SODIUM
Pipracil . . . 1866

PIPROL (Spain)
CIPROFLOXACIN HYDROCHLORIDE
Ciloxan Ophthalmic Ointment . . . 538
Ciloxan Ophthalmic Solution . . . ⊙209, 538
Cipro Tablets . . . 887

PIRAFOID (Mexico)
PYRAZINAMIDE
Pyrazinamide Tablets . . . 1876

PIRALDINA (Italy)
PYRAZINAMIDE
Pyrazinamide Tablets . . . 1876

PIRAM (Thailand)
PIROXICAM
Feldene Capsules . . . 2685

PIRAM-D (New Zealand)
PIROXICAM
Feldene Capsules . . . 2685

PIRASIDE (Portugal)
PYRAZINAMIDE
Pyrazinamide Tablets . . . 1876

PIRAX (Thailand)
PIROXICAM
Feldene Capsules . . . 2685

PIRAZER (Mexico)
PYRAZINAMIDE
Pyrazinamide Tablets . . . 1876

PIRIDASMIN (Spain)
THEOPHYLLINE
Aerolate Jr. T.D. Capsules . . . 1361

(⊙ Described in PDR For Ophthalmic Medicines™)

Aerolate Liquid . . . 1361
Aerolate Sr. T.D. Capsules . . . 1361
Theo-Dur Extended-Release Tablets . . . 1835
Uni-Dur Extended-Release Tablets . . . 1841
Uniphyl 400 mg and 600 mg Tablets . . . 2903

PIRILENE (France)
PYRAZINAMIDE
Pyrazinamide Tablets . . . 1876

PIRIMECIDAN (Spain)
PYRIMETHAMINE
Daraprim Tablets . . . 1511

PIRKAM (Denmark)
PIROXICAM
Feldene Capsules . . . 2685

PIRO (Germany)
PIROXICAM
Feldene Capsules . . . 2685

PIRO KD (Germany)
PIROXICAM
Feldene Capsules . . . 2685

PIROBETA (Germany)
PIROXICAM
Feldene Capsules . . . 2685

PIROCAM (Austria, Switzerland)
PIROXICAM
Feldene Capsules . . . 2685

PIRODAX (Mexico)
PIROXICAM
Feldene Capsules . . . 2685

PIROFLAM (Germany, United Kingdom)
PIROXICAM
Feldene Capsules . . . 2685

PIROFTAL (Italy)
PIROXICAM
Feldene Capsules . . . 2685

PIROHEXAL-D (Australia)
PIROXICAM
Feldene Capsules . . . 2685

PIROM (Denmark)
PIROXICAM
Feldene Capsules . . . 2685

PIROMAV (Mexico)
PIROXICAM
Feldene Capsules . . . 2685

PIRONET (Denmark)
PIROXICAM
Feldene Capsules . . . 2685

PIRO-PHLOGONT (Germany)
PIROXICAM
Feldene Capsules . . . 2685

PIRO-PUREN (Germany)
PIROXICAM
Feldene Capsules . . . 2685

PIRORHEUM (Austria, Germany)
PIROXICAM
Feldene Capsules . . . 2685

PIRORHEUMA (Germany)
PIROXICAM
Feldene Capsules . . . 2685

PIROSOL (Switzerland)
PIROXICAM
Feldene Capsules . . . 2685

PIROX (Australia, Germany, Norway)
PIROXICAM
Feldene Capsules . . . 2685

PIROXAL (Finland)
PIROXICAM
Feldene Capsules . . . 2685

PIROXAM (Thailand)
PIROXICAM
Feldene Capsules . . . 2685

PIROXAN (Mexico)
PIROXICAM
Feldene Capsules . . . 2685

PIROX-BASAN (Switzerland)
PIROXICAM
Feldene Capsules . . . 2685

PIROXCIN (Thailand)
PIROXICAM
Feldene Capsules . . . 2685

PIROXEN (Mexico, Thailand)
PIROXICAM
Feldene Capsules . . . 2685

PIROXENE (Brazil)
PIROXICAM
Feldene Capsules . . . 2685

PIROXIFEN (Brazil)
PIROXICAM
Feldene Capsules . . . 2685

PIROXIFLAM (Brazil)
PIROXICAM
Feldene Capsules . . . 2685

PIROXIL (Brazil)
PIROXICAM
Feldene Capsules . . . 2685

PIROXIMERCK (Germany)
PIROXICAM
Feldene Capsules . . . 2685

PIROXIN (Finland)
PIROXICAM
Feldene Capsules . . . 2685

PIROXIPLUS (Brazil)
PIROXICAM
Feldene Capsules . . . 2685

PIROXISTAD (Austria)
PIROXICAM
Feldene Capsules . . . 2685

PIROXITYROL (Austria)
PIROXICAM
Feldene Capsules . . . 2685

PIROXSIL (Thailand)
PIROXICAM
Feldene Capsules . . . 2685

PIROX-SPONDYRIL (Germany)
PIROXICAM
Feldene Capsules . . . 2685

PIROXY (Hong Kong)
PIROXICAM
Feldene Capsules . . . 2685

PIROZIP (United Kingdom)
PIROXICAM
Feldene Capsules . . . 2685

PIXICAM (South Africa)
PIROXICAM
Feldene Capsules . . . 2685

PIZIDE (Thailand)
PIMOZIDE
Orap Tablets . . . 1407

PLAMIN (Brazil)
METOCLOPRAMIDE HYDROCHLORIDE
Reglan Injectable . . . 2935
Reglan Syrup . . . 2935
Reglan Tablets . . . 2935

PLANIZOL (Mexico)
METRONIDAZOLE
MetroCream . . . 1404
MetroGel . . . 1405
MetroGel-Vaginal Gel . . . 1986
MetroLotion . . . 1405
Noritate Cream . . . 1224

PLAQUENIL (Australia, Austria, Belgium, Canada, Denmark, Finland, France, Hong Kong, Irish Republic, Israel, Italy, Mexico, New Zealand, Norway, Singapore, Sweden, Switzerland, Thailand, The Netherlands, United Kingdom)
HYDROXYCHLOROQUINE SULFATE
Plaquenil Tablets . . . 3082

PLAQUETAL (Portugal)
TICLOPIDINE HYDROCHLORIDE
Ticlid Tablets . . . 3015

PLAQUINOL (Brazil, Portugal)
HYDROXYCHLOROQUINE SULFATE
Plaquenil Tablets . . . 3082

PLASIL (Brazil, Italy, Mexico, Thailand)
METOCLOPRAMIDE HYDROCHLORIDE
Reglan Injectable . . . 2935
Reglan Syrup . . . 2935
Reglan Tablets . . . 2935

PLASIMINE (Spain)
MUPIROCIN
Bactroban Ointment . . . 1496

PLASMATEIN (United Kingdom)
PLASMA PROTEIN FRACTION
Plasmanate . . . 942

PLASMAVIRAL (Italy)
PLASMA PROTEIN FRACTION
Plasmanate . . . 942

PLASTODERMO (Spain)
CHLORAMPHENICOL
Chloromycetin Ophthalmic Ointment, 1% . . . ⊙296
Chloromycetin Ophthalmic Solution . . . ⊙297
Chloroptic Sterile Ophthalmic Ointment . . . ⊙234
Chloroptic Sterile Ophthalmic Solution . . . ⊙235

PLATELET (Italy)
DIPYRIDAMOLE
Persantine Tablets . . . 1057

PLATINWAS (Spain)
CARBOPLATIN
Paraplatin for Injection . . . 1126

PLATO (South Africa)
DIPYRIDAMOLE
Persantine Tablets . . . 1057

PLAUCINA (Spain)
ENOXAPARIN SODIUM
Lovenox Injection . . . 746

PLAVIX (Australia, Austria, Belgium, Denmark, France, Germany, Mexico, New Zealand, Portugal, Singapore, Spain, Sweden, Switzerland, Thailand)
CLOPIDOGREL BISULFATE
Plavix Tablets . . . 1097, 3084

PLAZOLIT (Mexico)
OMEPRAZOLE
Prilosec Delayed-Release Capsules . . . 628

PLEGINE (Italy)
PHENDIMETRAZINE TARTRATE
Bontril Slow-Release Capsules . . . 576

PLENACOR (Mexico)
ATENOLOL
Tenormin I.V. Injection . . . 692

PLENASTRIL (Germany)
OXYMETHOLONE
Anadrol-50 Tablets . . . 3321

PLENAX (Brazil)
CEFIXIME
Suprax Tablets . . . 1877
Suprax for Oral Suspension . . . 1877

PLENDIL (Australia, Austria, Belgium, Canada, Denmark, Finland, Hong Kong, Irish Republic, Italy, Mexico, New Zealand, Norway, Singapore, South Africa, Spain, Sweden, Switzerland, Thailand, The Netherlands, United Kingdom)
FELODIPINE
Plendil Extended-Release Tablets . . . 623

PLENISH-K (South Africa)
POTASSIUM CHLORIDE
K-Dur Microburst Release System ER Tablets . . . 1832
K-Lor Powder Packets . . . 469
K-Tab Filmtab Tablets . . . 470
Rum-K . . . 1363

PLENOLYT (Spain)
CIPROFLOXACIN HYDROCHLORIDE
Ciloxan Ophthalmic Ointment . . . 538
Ciloxan Ophthalmic Solution . . . ⊙209, 538
Cipro Tablets . . . 887

PLENOMICINA (Brazil)
ERYTHROMYCIN STEARATE
Erythrocin Stearate Filmtab Tablets . . . 452

PLENUR (Spain)
LITHIUM CARBONATE
Eskalith CR Controlled Release Tablets . . 1527
Eskalith Capsules . . . 1527
Lithium Carbonate Capsules . . . 3061
Lithobid Slow-Release Tablets . . . 3255

PLEON RA (Germany)
SULFASALAZINE
Azulfidine EN-tabs Tablets . . . 2775

PLETAAL (Japan, Thailand)
CILOSTAZOL
Pletal Tablets . . . 2605, 2848

PLUMAROL (Spain)
MIGLITOL
Glyset Tablets . . . 2821

PLUMBIOT (Spain)
DOXYCYCLINE HYCLATE
Doryx Coated Pellet Filled Capsules . . . 3357
Periostat Tablets . . . 1208
Vibra-Tabs Film Coated Tablets . . . 2735
Vibramycin Hyclate Capsules . . . 2735
Vibramycin Hyclate Intravenous . . . 2737

PLURIMEN (Spain)
SELEGILINE HYDROCHLORIDE
Eldepryl Capsules . . . 3266

PLURISAN (Brazil)
LINDANE
Lindane Lotion USP 1% . . . 559
Lindane Shampoo USP 1% . . . 560

PLURIVERM (Brazil)
MEBENDAZOLE
Vermox Chewable Tablets . . . 2017

PLUS KALIUM RETARD (Switzerland)
POTASSIUM CHLORIDE
K-Dur Microburst Release System ER Tablets . . . 1832
K-Lor Powder Packets . . . 469
K-Tab Filmtab Tablets . . . 470
Rum-K . . . 1363

PMS-DOPAZIDE (Canada)
HYDROCHLOROTHIAZIDE/METHYLDOPA
Aldoril Tablets . . . 2039

PMS-LEVAZINE (Canada)
AMITRIPTYLINE HYDROCHLORIDE/PERPHENAZINE
Etrafon 2-10 Tablets (2-10) . . . 3115
Etrafon Tablets (2-25) . . . 3115
Etrafon-Forte Tablets (4-25) . . . 3115

POCIN (Thailand)
ERYTHROMYCIN STEARATE
Erythrocin Stearate Filmtab Tablets . . . 452

POCOPHAGE (Thailand)
METFORMIN HYDROCHLORIDE
Glucophage Tablets . . . 1080

POCYL (Spain)
IBUPROFEN
Motrin Suspension, Oral Drops, Chewable Tablets, and Caplets . . . 2002

PODIUM (Spain)
DIAZEPAM
Valium Injectable . . . 3026
Valium Tablets . . . 3047

PODOMEXEF (Germany, Switzerland)
CEFPODOXIME PROXETIL
Vantin Tablets and Oral Suspension . . . 2860

POFOL (Singapore)
PROPOFOL
Diprivan Injectable Emulsion . . . 667

POINT (Israel)
NAPROXEN SODIUM
Anaprox DS Tablets . . . 2967
Anaprox Tablets . . . 2967
Naprelan Tablets . . . 1293

POLARATYNE (South Africa)
LORATADINE
Claritin Reditabs . . . 3100
Claritin Syrup . . . 3100
Claritin Tablets . . . 3100

POLARATYNE D (South Africa)
LORATADINE/PSEUDOEPHEDRINE SULFATE
Claritin-D 12 Hour Extended Release Tablets . . . 3102
Claritin-D 24 Hour Extended Release Tablets . . . 3104

POLIBEN (Brazil)
MEBENDAZOLE
Vermox Chewable Tablets . . . 2017

POLI-CIFLOXIN (Thailand)
CIPROFLOXACIN
Cipro I.V. . . . 893
Cipro I.V. Pharmacy Bulk Package . . . 897
Cipro Oral Suspension . . . 887

POLI-CYCLINE (Thailand)
DOXYCYCLINE HYCLATE
Doryx Coated Pellet Filled Capsules . . . 3357
Periostat Tablets . . . 1208
Vibramycin Hyclate Capsules . . . 2735
Vibramycin Hyclate Intravenous . . . 2737
Vibra-Tabs Film Coated Tablets . . . 2735

POLIDELTAXIN (Mexico)
DEXAMETHASONE
Decadron Elixir . . . 2078
Decadron Tablets . . . 2079

POLI-FIBROZIL (Thailand)
GEMFIBROZIL
Lopid Tablets . . . 2650

POLI-FORMIN (Thailand)
METFORMIN HYDROCHLORIDE
Glucophage Tablets . . . 1080

POLIMOXIL (Brazil)
AMOXICILLIN
Amoxil Pediatric Drops for Oral Suspension . . . 1471
Amoxil Tablets . . . 1471

POLIPIROX (Italy)
PIROXICAM
Feldene Capsules . . . 2685

POLIREUMIN (Brazil)
SODIUM HYALURONATE
Hyalgan Solution . . . 3080

POLITELMIN (Brazil)
MEBENDAZOLE
Vermox Chewable Tablets . . . 2017

POLI-URETIC (Thailand)
AMILORIDE HYDROCHLORIDE/HYDROCHLOROTHIAZIDE
Moduretic Tablets . . . 2138

POLIXIMA (Italy)
CEFUROXIME SODIUM
Kefurox Vials, ADD-Vantage 1948
Zinacef Injection 1696

POLIXIN (Mexico)
NEOMYCIN SULFATE/POLYMYXIN B SULFATE
Neosporin G.U. Irrigant Sterile 2256

POLOCAINE (Canada)
MEPIVACAINE HYDROCHLORIDE
Polocaine Injection, USP 625
Polocaine-MPF Injection, USP 625

POLY PRED (Spain)
NEOMYCIN SULFATE/POLYMYXIN B SULFATE/PREDNISOLONE ACETATE
Poly-Pred Liquifilm Ophthalmic Suspension .... ⊙245

POLYANION (Austria)
PENTOSAN POLYSULFATE SODIUM
Elmiron Capsules 570

POLYBACTRIN (United Kingdom)
NEOMYCIN SULFATE/POLYMYXIN B SULFATE
Neosporin G.U. Irrigant Sterile 2256

POLYBACTRIN SOLUBLE (Australia, United Kingdom)
NEOMYCIN SULFATE/POLYMYXIN B SULFATE
Neosporin G.U. Irrigant Sterile 2256

POLYCITRA-K (Canada)
POTASSIUM CITRATE
Urocit-K Tablets 2232

POLYFLAM (Belgium)
DICLOFENAC SODIUM
Voltaren Tablets 2315
Voltaren-XR Tablets 2315

POLYGYNAX (Hong Kong, Portugal)
NEOMYCIN SULFATE/POLYMYXIN B SULFATE
Neosporin G.U. Irrigant Sterile 2256

POLYHADOL (Thailand)
HALOPERIDOL
Haldol Injection, Tablets and Concentrate 2533

POLYPRED (Thailand)
PREDNISOLONE
Prelone Syrup 2273

POLYPRESS (Germany, Thailand)
POLYTHIAZIDE/PRAZOSIN HYDROCHLORIDE
Minizide Capsules 2700

POLYSPECTRAN OS (Germany)
NEOMYCIN SULFATE/POLYMYXIN B SULFATE
Neosporin G.U. Irrigant Sterile 2256

POLYSPORIN (Finland)
NEOMYCIN SULFATE/POLYMYXIN B SULFATE
Neosporin G.U. Irrigant Sterile 2256

POLYSPORINA (Portugal)
NEOMYCIN SULFATE/POLYMYXIN B SULFATE
Neosporin G.U. Irrigant Sterile 2256

POLYTAB (Thailand)
CYPROHEPTADINE HYDROCHLORIDE
Periactin Tablets 2155

POLYTRIM (Canada)
POLYMYXIN B SULFATE/TRIMETHOPRIM SULFATE
Polytrim Ophthalmic Solution 556

POLYXEN (Thailand)
NAPROXEN
EC-Naprosyn Delayed-Release Tablets 2967
Naprosyn Suspension 2967
Naprosyn Tablets 2967

POLYXICAM (Thailand)
PIROXICAM
Feldene Capsules 2685

POLYXIT (Thailand)
GEMFIBROZIL
Lopid Tablets 2650

POMADA SULFAMIDA ORRAVAN (Spain)
SULFANILAMIDE
AVC Cream 1350
AVC Suppositories 1350

PONAC (South Africa)
MEFENAMIC ACID
Ponstel Capsules 1356

PONALAR (Germany)
MEFENAMIC ACID
Ponstel Capsules 1356

PONALGIC (Irish Republic)
MEFENAMIC ACID
Ponstel Capsules 1356

PONDARMETT (Thailand)
CIMETIDINE
Tagamet Tablets 1644

PONMEL (Irish Republic)
MEFENAMIC ACID
Ponstel Capsules 1356

PONNAC (Thailand)
MEFENAMIC ACID
Ponstel Capsules 1356

PONNESIA (Thailand)
MEFENAMIC ACID
Ponstel Capsules 1356

PONSTAN (Australia, Brazil, Canada, Finland, Hong Kong, Irish Republic, Mexico, New Zealand, Portugal, Singapore, South Africa, Switzerland, Thailand)
MEFENAMIC ACID
Ponstel Capsules 1356

PONSTEL (South Africa)
MEFENAMIC ACID
Ponstel Capsules 1356

PONSTYL (France)
MEFENAMIC ACID
Ponstel Capsules 1356

PONTALON (Thailand)
MEFENAMIC ACID
Ponstel Capsules 1356

PONTYL (Singapore)
MEFENAMIC ACID
Ponstel Capsules 1356

PORAZINE (Thailand)
PERPHENAZINE
Trilafon Injection 3160
Trilafon Tablets 3160

PORCELANA (Canada)
HYDROQUINONE
Eldopaque Forte 4% Cream 1734
Eldoquin Forte 4% Cream 1734
Lustra Cream 2023
Lustra-AF Cream 2023
Melanex Topical Solution 2300
Solaquin Forte 4% Cream 1734
Solaquin Forte 4% Gel 1734

PORCELANA WITH SUNSCREEN (Canada)
HYDROQUINONE
Eldopaque Forte 4% Cream 1734
Eldoquin Forte 4% Cream 1734
Lustra Cream 2023
Lustra-AF Cream 2023
Melanex Topical Solution 2300
Solaquin Forte 4% Cream 1734
Solaquin Forte 4% Gel 1734

PORPHYROCIN (Hong Kong)
ERYTHROMYCIN STEARATE
Erythrocin Stearate Filmtab Tablets 452

POSANIN (Thailand)
DIPYRIDAMOLE
Persantine Tablets 1057

POSE-CM (Thailand)
CIMETIDINE
Tagamet Tablets 1644

POSEDENE (Thailand)
PIROXICAM
Feldene Capsules 2685

POSIDOLOR (Spain)
IBUPROFEN
Motrin Suspension, Oral Drops, Chewable Tablets, and Caplets 2002

POSIFENICOL C (Germany)
CHLORAMPHENICOL
Chloromycetin Ophthalmic Ointment, 1% .... ⊙296
Chloromycetin Ophthalmic Solution .... ⊙297
Chloroptic Sterile Ophthalmic Ointment .... ⊙234
Chloroptic Sterile Ophthalmic Solution .... ⊙235

POSIJECT (Irish Republic, South Africa, United Kingdom)
DOBUTAMINE HYDROCHLORIDE
Dobutrex Solution Vials 1914

POSNAC (Thailand)
DICLOFENAC SODIUM
Voltaren Tablets 2315
Voltaren-XR Tablets 2315

POSTERINE CORTE (Germany)
HYDROCORTISONE ACETATE
Anusol-HC Suppositories 2238
Cortifoam Rectal Foam 3170
Hydrocortone Acetate Injectable Suspension 2103
Proctocort Suppositories 2264

POSTINOR (Singapore, Thailand)
LEVONORGESTREL
Norplant System 3543

POSTINOR-2 (New Zealand, United Kingdom)
LEVONORGESTREL
Norplant System 3543

POTASION (Spain)
POTASSIUM CHLORIDE
K-Dur Microburst Release System ER Tablets 1832
K-Lor Powder Packets 469
K-Tab Filmtab Tablets 470
Rum-K 1363

POTASSRIDE (Thailand)
POTASSIUM CHLORIDE
K-Dur Microburst Release System ER Tablets 1832
K-Lor Powder Packets 469
K-Tab Filmtab Tablets 470
Rum-K 1363

POTENDAL (Spain)
CEFTAZIDIME
Ceptaz for Injection 1499
Fortaz for Injection 1541
Tazicef for Injection 1647
Tazidime Vials, Faspak & ADD-Vantage 1966

POWERGEL (United Kingdom)
KETOPROFEN
Orudis Capsules 3548
Oruvail Capsules 3548

PPD TINE TEST (South Africa)
TUBERCULIN
Aplisol Injection 2609
Tine Test, Tuberculin, Old 3631
Tubersol Diagnostic Antigen 3628

PPS (Italy)
PLASMA PROTEIN FRACTION
Plasmanate 942

PRA-BREXIDOL (Germany)
PIROXICAM
Feldene Capsules 2685

PRACEM (Mexico)
DIPYRIDAMOLE
Persantine Tablets 1057

PRADIF (Italy, Portugal, Switzerland)
TAMSULOSIN HYDROCHLORIDE
Flomax Capsules 1044

PRAECICOR (Germany)
VERAPAMIL HYDROCHLORIDE
Covera-HS Tablets 3199
Isoptin SR Tablets 467
Verelan Capsules 3184
Verelan PM Capsules 3186

PRAECIVENIN (Germany)
HEPARIN SODIUM
Heparin Lock Flush Solution 3509
Heparin Sodium Injection 3511

PRALENAL (United Kingdom)
ENALAPRIL MALEATE
Vasotec Tablets 2210

PRALOL (Thailand)
PROPRANOLOL HYDROCHLORIDE
Inderal Injectable 3513
Inderal LA Long-Acting Capsules 3516
Inderal Tablets 3513

PRAMACE (Irish Republic, Sweden)
RAMIPRIL
Altace Capsules 2233

PRAMIDE (Portugal)
PYRAZINAMIDE
Pyrazinamide Tablets 1876

PRAMIDIN (Italy)
METOCLOPRAMIDE HYDROCHLORIDE
Reglan Injectable 2935
Reglan Syrup 2935
Reglan Tablets 2935

PRAMIN (Australia, Israel)
METOCLOPRAMIDE HYDROCHLORIDE
Reglan Injectable 2935
Reglan Syrup 2935
Reglan Tablets 2935

PRANDASE (Canada, Israel)
ACARBOSE
Precose Tablets 906

PRANDIN E2 (South Africa)
DINOPROSTONE
Cervidil Vaginal Insert 1369
Prepidil Gel 2851
Prostin E2 Suppositories 2852

PRANDIOL (France)
DIPYRIDAMOLE
Persantine Tablets 1057

PRANOLOL (Norway)
PROPRANOLOL HYDROCHLORIDE
Inderal Injectable 3513
Inderal LA Long-Acting Capsules 3516
Inderal Tablets 3513

PRANOXEN (South Africa)
NAPROXEN
EC-Naprosyn Delayed-Release Tablets 2967
Naprosyn Suspension 2967
Naprosyn Tablets 2967

PRANOXEN CONTINUS (United Kingdom)
NAPROXEN
EC-Naprosyn Delayed-Release Tablets 2967
Naprosyn Suspension 2967
Naprosyn Tablets 2967

PRAQUANTEL (Thailand)
PRAZIQUANTEL
Biltricide Tablets 887

PRAREDUCT (Spain)
PRAVASTATIN SODIUM
Pravachol Tablets 1099

PRASIG (Australia)
PRAZOSIN HYDROCHLORIDE
Minipress Capsules 2699

PRASIKON (Thailand)
PRAZIQUANTEL
Biltricide Tablets 887

PRASTEROL (Italy)
PRAVASTATIN SODIUM
Pravachol Tablets 1099

PRATISOL (Hong Kong)
PRAZOSIN HYDROCHLORIDE
Minipress Capsules 2699

PRATSIOL (Australia, Finland, New Zealand, South Africa, Thailand)
PRAZOSIN HYDROCHLORIDE
Minipress Capsules 2699

PRAVA (South Africa)
PRAVASTATIN SODIUM
Pravachol Tablets 1099

PRAVACHOL (Australia, Austria, Canada, Denmark, Finland, Hong Kong, Norway, Singapore, Sweden)
PRAVASTATIN SODIUM
Pravachol Tablets 1099

PRAVACOL (Brazil, Mexico, Portugal)
PRAVASTATIN SODIUM
Pravachol Tablets 1099

PRAVASELECT (Italy)
PRAVASTATIN SODIUM
Pravachol Tablets 1099

PRAVASIN (Germany)
PRAVASTATIN SODIUM
Pravachol Tablets 1099

PRAVASINE (Belgium)
PRAVASTATIN SODIUM
Pravachol Tablets 1099

PRAXEL (Mexico)
PACLITAXEL
Taxol Injection 1129

PRAZAC (Denmark)
PRAZOSIN HYDROCHLORIDE
Minipress Capsules 2699

PRAZAM (Portugal)
ALPRAZOLAM
Xanax Tablets 2865

PRAZENTOL (Portugal)
OMEPRAZOLE
Prilosec Delayed-Release Capsules 628

PRAZIDEC (Mexico)
OMEPRAZOLE
Prilosec Delayed-Release Capsules 628

PRAZITE (Thailand)
PRAZIQUANTEL
Biltricide Tablets 887

PRAZOCOR (Finland)
PRAZOSIN HYDROCHLORIDE
Minipress Capsules 2699

PRAZOHEXAL (Australia)
PRAZOSIN HYDROCHLORIDE
Minipress Capsules 2699

PRAZOLIT (Mexico)
OMEPRAZOLE
Prilosec Delayed-Release Capsules 628

PRE CLOR (Mexico)
CHLORAMPHENICOL
Chloromycetin Ophthalmic Ointment, 1% ⊙296
Chloromycetin Ophthalmic Solution ⊙297
Chloroptic Sterile Ophthalmic Ointment ⊙234
Chloroptic Sterile Ophthalmic Solution ⊙235

PRECORTISYL (Irish Republic, United Kingdom)
PREDNISOLONE
Prelone Syrup 2273

PREDALGIC (France)
TRAMADOL HYDROCHLORIDE
Ultram Tablets 2600

PRED-CLYSMA (Denmark, Norway, Sweden)
PREDNISOLONE SODIUM PHOSPHATE
Pediapred Oral Solution 1170

PREDELTILONE (South Africa)
PREDNISOLONE
Prelone Syrup 2273

PREDELTIN (South Africa)
PREDNISONE
Prednisone Intensol 3064
Prednisone Oral Solution 3064
Prednisone Tablets 3064

PREDICOR (Mexico)
PREDNISONE
Prednisone Intensol 3064
Prednisone Oral Solution 3064
Prednisone Tablets 3064

PREDICORTEN (Brazil)
PREDNISONE
Prednisone Intensol 3064
Prednisone Oral Solution 3064
Prednisone Tablets 3064

PREDISOLE (Thailand)
PREDNISOLONE
Prelone Syrup 2273

PREDMIX (Australia)
PREDNISOLONE SODIUM PHOSPHATE
Pediapred Oral Solution 1170

PREDMYCIN (Belgium, Thailand)
NEOMYCIN SULFATE/POLYMYXIN B SULFATE/PREDNISOLONE ACETATE
Poly-Pred Liquifilm Ophthalmic Suspension ⊙245

PREDMYCIN-P (Singapore)
NEOMYCIN SULFATE/POLYMYXIN B SULFATE/PREDNISOLONE ACETATE
Poly-Pred Liquifilm Ophthalmic Suspension ⊙245

PREDMYCIN-P LIQUIFILM (The Netherlands)
NEOMYCIN SULFATE/POLYMYXIN B SULFATE/PREDNISOLONE ACETATE
Poly-Pred Liquifilm Ophthalmic Suspension ⊙245

PREDNABENE (Germany)
PREDNISOLONE SODIUM PHOSPHATE
Pediapred Oral Solution 1170

PREDNERSONE (Thailand)
PREDNISOLONE
Prelone Syrup 2273

PREDNESOL (Irish Republic, United Kingdom)
PREDNISOLONE SODIUM PHOSPHATE
Pediapred Oral Solution 1170

PREDNI H (Germany)
PREDNISOLONE
Prelone Syrup 2273

PREDNI TABLINEN (Germany)
PREDNISONE
Prednisone Intensol 3064
Prednisone Oral Solution 3064
Prednisone Tablets 3064

PREDNI-COELIN (Germany)
PREDNISOLONE
Prelone Syrup 2273

PREDNICORT (Belgium, Sweden)
PREDNISONE
Prednisone Intensol 3064
Prednisone Oral Solution 3064
Prednisone Tablets 3064

PREDNICORTELONE (Belgium)
PREDNISOLONE
Prelone Syrup 2273

PREDNIDERMA (Portugal)
PREDNISOLONE
Prelone Syrup 2273

PREDNIDIB (Mexico)
PREDNISONE
Prednisone Intensol 3064
Prednisone Oral Solution 3064
Prednisone Tablets 3064

PREDNI-F-TABLINEN (Germany)
DEXAMETHASONE
Decadron Elixir 2078
Decadron Tablets 2079

PREDNIFTALMINA (Portugal)
CHLORAMPHENICOL
Chloromycetin Ophthalmic Ointment, 1% ⊙296
Chloromycetin Ophthalmic Solution ⊙297
Chloroptic Sterile Ophthalmic Ointment ⊙234
Chloroptic Sterile Ophthalmic Solution ⊙235

PREDNI-HELVACORT (Switzerland)
PREDNISOLONE
Prelone Syrup 2273

PREDNILEM (Mexico)
METHYLPREDNISOLONE SODIUM SUCCINATE
Solu-Medrol Sterile Powder 2855

PREDNILONGA (Germany)
PREDNISONE
Prednisone Intensol 3064
Prednisone Oral Solution 3064
Prednisone Tablets 3064

PREDNIMENT (Denmark, Finland, Germany)
PREDNISOLONE SODIUM PHOSPHATE
Pediapred Oral Solution 1170

PREDNISIL (Thailand)
PREDNISOLONE
Prelone Syrup 2273

PREDNITONE (Israel)
PREDNISONE
Prednisone Intensol 3064
Prednisone Oral Solution 3064
Prednisone Tablets 3064

PREDNITOP (Austria, Switzerland)
PREDNICARBATE
Dermatop Emollient Cream 2517

PREDSOL (Australia, Irish Republic, New Zealand, South Africa, United Kingdom)
PREDNISOLONE SODIUM PHOSPHATE
Pediapred Oral Solution 1170

PREFERID (Belgium, Irish Republic, Italy, Norway, Sweden, Switzerland, The Netherlands, United Kingdom)
BUDESONIDE
Pulmicort Turbuhaler Inhalation Powder 636
Rhinocort Nasal Inhaler 640

PREFIN (Spain)
BUPRENORPHINE HYDROCHLORIDE
Buprenex Injectable 2918

PRELONE (Israel, South Africa)
PREDNISOLONE
Prelone Syrup 2273

PREMOX (Mexico)
PYRAZINAMIDE
Pyrazinamide Tablets 1876

PRENILONE (Thailand)
PREDNISOLONE
Prelone Syrup 2273

PRENOLOL (Singapore, Thailand)
ATENOLOL
Tenormin I.V. Injection 692

PRENT (Germany, Italy, Portugal, Switzerland, The Netherlands)
ACEBUTOLOL HYDROCHLORIDE
Sectral Capsules 3589

PREPIDIL (Austria, Belgium, Canada, France, Germany, Hong Kong, Irish Republic, Israel, Italy, Mexico, New Zealand, South Africa, Spain, Switzerland, The Netherlands, United Kingdom)
DINOPROSTONE
Cervidil Vaginal Insert 1369
Prepidil Gel 2851
Prostin E2 Suppositories 2852

PRERAN (Japan)
TRANDOLAPRIL
Mavik Tablets 478

PRES (Germany)
ENALAPRIL MALEATE
Vasotec Tablets 2210

PRES IV (Germany)
ENALAPRILAT
Vasotec I.V. Injection 2207

PRES PLUS (Germany)
ENALAPRIL MALEATE/HYDROCHLOROTHIAZIDE
Vaseretic Tablets 2204

PRESCAL (Irish Republic, United Kingdom)
ISRADIPINE
DynaCirc CR Tablets 2923

PRESINOL (Austria, Belgium, Germany, Italy)
METHYLDOPA
Aldomet Tablets 2037

PRESLOW (Portugal, Spain)
FELODIPINE
Plendil Extended-Release Tablets 623

PRESOLOL (Australia)
LABETALOL HYDROCHLORIDE
Normodyne Injection 3135
Normodyne Tablets 3137

PRESSALOLO (Italy)
LABETALOL HYDROCHLORIDE
Normodyne Injection 3135
Normodyne Tablets 3137

PRESSANOL (South Africa)
PROPRANOLOL HYDROCHLORIDE
Inderal Injectable 3513
Inderal LA Long-Acting Capsules 3516
Inderal Tablets 3513

PRESSIN (Australia, Thailand)
PRAZOSIN HYDROCHLORIDE
Minipress Capsules 2699

PRESSITAN (Spain)
ENALAPRIL MALEATE
Vasotec Tablets 2210

PRESSITAN PLUS (Spain)
ENALAPRIL MALEATE/HYDROCHLOROTHIAZIDE
Vaseretic Tablets 2204

PRESSOLAT (Israel)
NIFEDIPINE
Adalat CC Tablets 877
Procardia Capsules 2708
Procardia XL Extended Release Tablets 2710

PRESSURAL (Italy)
INDAPAMIDE
Indapamide Tablets 2286

PRESTOLE (France)
HYDROCHLOROTHIAZIDE/TRIAMTERENE
Dyazide Capsules 1515
Maxzide Tablets 1008
Maxzide-25 mg Tablets 1008

PRESYNDRAL (Spain)
ENALAPRIL MALEATE
Vasotec Tablets 2210

PREVACID (Canada, Singapore, Thailand)
LANSOPRAZOLE
Prevacid Delayed-Release Capsules 3292

PREVENCOR (Spain)
ATORVASTATIN CALCIUM
Lipitor Tablets 2639, 2696

PREVEX (Italy)
FELODIPINE
Plendil Extended-Release Tablets 623

PREVEX HC (Canada)
HYDROCORTISONE
Anusol-HC Cream 2.5% 2237
Hydrocortone Tablets 2106

PREXAN (Italy)
NAPROXEN
EC-Naprosyn Delayed-Release Tablets 2967
Naprosyn Suspension 2967
Naprosyn Tablets 2967

PREZAL (The Netherlands)
LANSOPRAZOLE
Prevacid Delayed-Release Capsules 3292

PRIADEL (Australia, Belgium, New Zealand, Portugal, Singapore, South Africa, Switzerland, The Netherlands, United Kingdom)
LITHIUM CARBONATE
Eskalith CR Controlled Release Tablets 1527
Eskalith Capsules 1527
Lithium Carbonate Capsules 3061
Lithobid Slow-Release Tablets 3255

PRILACE (Italy)
RAMIPRIL
Altace Capsules 2233

PRILOVASE (Portugal)
CAPTOPRIL
Captopril Tablets 2281

PRIMACOR (Australia, Brazil, Canada, Hong Kong, Israel, New Zealand, Singapore, Thailand, United Kingdom)
MILRINONE LACTATE
Primacor Injection 3086

PRIMAFEN (Spain)
CEFOTAXIME SODIUM
Claforan Injection 732

PRIMAXIN (Canada, United Kingdom)
CILASTATIN SODIUM/IMIPENEM
Primaxin I.M. 2158
Primaxin I.V. 2160

PRIMBACTAM (Italy)
AZTREONAM
Azactam for Injection 1276

PRIMERAL (Italy)
NAPROXEN SODIUM
Anaprox DS Tablets 2967
Anaprox Tablets 2967
Naprelan Tablets 1293

PRIMESIN (Italy)
FLUVASTATIN SODIUM
Lescol Capsules 2361

PRIMOCEF (United Arab Emirates)
CEFOTAXIME SODIUM
Claforan Injection 732

PRIMOFENAC (Switzerland)
DICLOFENAC SODIUM
Voltaren Tablets 2315
Voltaren-XR Tablets 2315

PRIMOVLAR (Brazil)
NORGESTREL
Ovrette Tablets 3552

PRIMOXIL (Italy)
MOEXIPRIL HYDROCHLORIDE
Univasc Tablets 3181

PRIMPERAN (Hong Kong, Irish Republic, Singapore, South Africa, Spain, United Kingdom)
METOCLOPRAMIDE HYDROCHLORIDE
Reglan Injectable 2935
Reglan Syrup 2935
Reglan Tablets 2935

PRINIL (Switzerland)
LISINOPRIL
Prinivil Tablets 2164
Zestril Tablets 698

PRINIVIL (Australia, Austria, Brazil, Canada, France, Hong Kong, Italy, Mexico, New Zealand, Portugal, Singapore, South Africa, Spain)
LISINOPRIL
Prinivil Tablets 2164
Zestril Tablets 698

PRINIVIL PLUS (Spain)
HYDROCHLOROTHIAZIDE/LISINOPRIL
Prinzide Tablets 2168
Zestoretic Tablets 695

PRINZIDE (Austria, Brazil, Canada, France, Italy, Mexico, New Zealand, Portugal, Switzerland)
HYDROCHLOROTHIAZIDE/LISINOPRIL
Prinzide Tablets 2168
Zestoretic Tablets 695

PRIODERM (Belgium, Canada, Denmark, Finland, France, Irish Republic, Israel, New Zealand, Norway, Sweden, Switzerland, The Netherlands, United Kingdom)
MALATHION
Ovide Lotion 2023

PRIPSEN (United Kingdom)
MEBENDAZOLE
Vermox Chewable Tablets 2017

PRISDAL (Spain)
CITALOPRAM HYDROBROMIDE
Celexa Tablets 1365

PRITOR (Australia, France, Italy, Portugal, Spain)
TELMISARTAN
Micardis Tablets 1049

PRIVACOM (United Kingdom)
CLOTRIMAZOLE
Lotrimin Cream 1% 3128
Lotrimin Lotion 1% 3128
Lotrimin Topical Solution 1% 3128
Mycelex Troche 573

PRIVINA (Brazil)
NAPHAZOLINE HYDROCHLORIDE
Albalon Ophthalmic Solution ⊙225

PRIVINE (Canada)
NAPHAZOLINE HYDROCHLORIDE
Albalon Ophthalmic Solution ⊙225

PRIZEM (Mexico)
DIAZEPAM
Valium Injectable 3026

(⊙ Described in PDR For Ophthalmic Medicines™)

Valium Tablets . . . 3047

PRO DORM (Germany)
LORAZEPAM
Ativan Injection . . . 3478
Ativan Tablets . . . 3482

PRO ULCO (Spain)
LANSOPRAZOLE
Prevacid Delayed-Release Capsules . . . 3292

PROARTINAL (Mexico)
IBUPROFEN
Motrin Suspension, Oral Drops, Chewable Tablets, and Caplets . . . 2002

PROASMA-T (Thailand)
TERBUTALINE SULFATE
Brethine Ampuls . . . 2314
Brethine Tablets . . . 2313

PROAVIL (Canada)
AMITRIPTYLINE HYDROCHLORIDE/PERPHENAZINE
Etrafon 2-10 Tablets (2-10) . . . 3115
Etrafon Tablets (2-25) . . . 3115
Etrafon-Forte Tablets (4-25) . . . 3115

PROBETA LA (United Kingdom)
PROPRANOLOL HYDROCHLORIDE
Inderal Injectable . . . 3513
Inderal LA Long-Acting Capsules . . . 3516
Inderal Tablets . . . 3513

PROBUFEN (Thailand)
IBUPROFEN
Motrin Suspension, Oral Drops, Chewable Tablets, and Caplets . . . 2002

PROCALMADIOL (Belgium, France)
MEPROBAMATE
Miltown Tablets . . . 3349

PROCAMIDE (Brazil, Italy)
PROCAINAMIDE HYDROCHLORIDE
Procanbid Extended-Release Tablets . . . 2262

PROCAN (Canada)
PROCAINAMIDE HYDROCHLORIDE
Procanbid Extended-Release Tablets . . . 2262

PROCAPTAN (Italy)
PERINDOPRIL ERBUMINE
Aceon Tablets (2 mg, 4 mg, 8 mg) . . . 3249

PROCARDIN (Singapore)
DIPYRIDAMOLE
Persantine Tablets . . . 1057

PROCEF (Finland, Hong Kong, Italy, Mexico, Portugal, Singapore, Switzerland, Thailand)
CEFPROZIL
Cefzil Tablets . . . 1076
Cefzil for Oral Suspension . . . 1076

PROCIMETI (Mexico)
CIMETIDINE
Tagamet Tablets . . . 1644

PROCIN (Brazil)
CIPROFLOXACIN HYDROCHLORIDE
Ciloxan Ophthalmic Ointment . . . 538
Ciloxan Ophthalmic Solution . . . ⊙209, 538
Cipro Tablets . . . 887

PROCLIM (Canada)
MEDROXYPROGESTERONE ACETATE
Depo-Provera Contraceptive Injection . . . 2798
Provera Tablets . . . 2853

PROCLOR (Portugal)
OMEPRAZOLE
Prilosec Delayed-Release Capsules . . . 628

PROCLORIL (Mexico)
CHLORAMPHENICOL
Chloromycetin Ophthalmic Ointment, 1% . . . ⊙296
Chloromycetin Ophthalmic Solution . . . ⊙297
Chloroptic Sterile Ophthalmic Ointment . . ⊙234
Chloroptic Sterile Ophthalmic Solution . . ⊙235

PROCLOZINE (Thailand)
PROCHLORPERAZINE MALEATE
Compazine Spansule Capsules . . . 1505
Compazine Tablets . . . 1505

PROCODIN (Singapore)
CODEINE PHOSPHATE/PROMETHAZINE HYDROCHLORIDE
Phenergan with Codeine Syrup . . . 3557

PROCOR (Brazil, Israel)
DIPYRIDAMOLE
Persantine Tablets . . . 1057

PROCOR S (Brazil)
DIPYRIDAMOLE
Persantine Tablets . . . 1057

PROCORT (Australia)
HYDROCORTISONE ACETATE
Anusol-HC Suppositories . . . 2238
Cortifoam Rectal Foam . . . 3170
Hydrocortone Acetate Injectable Suspension . . . 2103
Proctocort Suppositories . . . 2264

PROCTOCORT (France)
HYDROCORTISONE ACETATE
Anusol-HC Suppositories . . . 2238
Cortifoam Rectal Foam . . . 3170
Hydrocortone Acetate Injectable Suspension . . . 2103
Proctocort Suppositories . . . 2264

PROCULIN (Germany)
NAPHAZOLINE HYDROCHLORIDE
Albalon Ophthalmic Solution . . . ⊙225

PRO-CURE (Israel)
FINASTERIDE
Propecia Tablets . . . 2172
Proscar Tablets . . . 2175

PROCUTAN (South Africa)
HYDROCORTISONE
Anusol-HC Cream 2.5% . . . 2237
Hydrocortone Tablets . . . 2106

PRODAFEM (Austria, Switzerland)
MEDROXYPROGESTERONE ACETATE
Depo-Provera Contraceptive Injection . . . 2798
Provera Tablets . . . 2853

PRODASONE (France)
MEDROXYPROGESTERONE ACETATE
Depo-Provera Contraceptive Injection . . . 2798
Provera Tablets . . . 2853

PRODAZOL (Mexico)
MEBENDAZOLE
Vermox Chewable Tablets . . . 2017

PRODICARD (The Netherlands)
ISOSORBIDE DINITRATE
Isordil Sublingual Tablets . . . 3525
Isordil Titradose Tablets . . . 3526

PRODILANTIN (France)
FOSPHENYTOIN SODIUM
Cerebyx Injection . . . 2619

PRODON (Sweden)
KETOPROFEN
Orudis Capsules . . . 3548
Oruvail Capsules . . . 3548

PRODOP (Mexico)
METHYLDOPA
Aldomet Tablets . . . 2037

PRODOPA (New Zealand)
METHYLDOPA
Aldomet Tablets . . . 2037

PRODOROL (South Africa)
PROPRANOLOL HYDROCHLORIDE
Inderal Injectable . . . 3513
Inderal LA Long-Acting Capsules . . . 3516
Inderal Tablets . . . 3513

PRO-EPANUTIN (Denmark, Finland, Irish Republic, Norway, Portugal, Sweden, The Netherlands, United Kingdom)
FOSPHENYTOIN SODIUM
Cerebyx Injection . . . 2619

PROFAMID (Denmark, Finland)
FLUTAMIDE
Eulexin Capsules . . . 3118

PROFENA (Thailand)
IBUPROFEN
Motrin Suspension, Oral Drops, Chewable Tablets, and Caplets . . . 2002

PROFENID (Austria, Brazil, France, Israel, Mexico, Portugal, Switzerland, Thailand)
KETOPROFEN
Orudis Capsules . . . 3548
Oruvail Capsules . . . 3548

PROFENIL (Italy)
KETOPROFEN
Orudis Capsules . . . 3548
Oruvail Capsules . . . 3548

PROFENZOL (Mexico)
MEBENDAZOLE
Vermox Chewable Tablets . . . 2017

PROFINAL (United Arab Emirates)
IBUPROFEN
Motrin Suspension, Oral Drops, Chewable Tablets, and Caplets . . . 2002

PROFIUM (Brazil)
MEBENDAZOLE
Vermox Chewable Tablets . . . 2017

PROFLAG (Mexico)
METRONIDAZOLE
MetroCream . . . 1404
MetroGel . . . 1405
MetroGel-Vaginal Gel . . . 1986
MetroLotion . . . 1405
Noritate Cream . . . 1224

PROFLEX (Irish Republic, United Kingdom)
IBUPROFEN
Motrin Suspension, Oral Drops, Chewable Tablets, and Caplets . . . 2002

PROFLOX (Thailand)
CIPROFLOXACIN
Cipro I.V. . . . 893
Cipro I.V. Pharmacy Bulk Package . . . 897
Cipro Oral Suspension . . . 887

PROGAN (Australia)
PROMETHAZINE HYDROCHLORIDE
Phenergan Injection . . . 3553
Phenergan Suppositories . . . 3556
Phenergan Syrup Fortis . . . 3554
Phenergan Syrup Plain . . . 3554
Phenergan Tablets . . . 3556

PROGEFFIK (Spain)
PROGESTERONE
Crinone 4% Gel . . . 3213
Crinone 8% Gel . . . 3213
Prometrium Capsules (100 mg, 200 mg) . . . 3261

PROGENAR (Portugal)
PROGESTERONE
Crinone 4% Gel . . . 3213
Crinone 8% Gel . . . 3213
Prometrium Capsules (100 mg, 200 mg) . . . 3261

PROGESTAN (The Netherlands)
PROGESTERONE
Crinone 4% Gel . . . 3213
Crinone 8% Gel . . . 3213
Prometrium Capsules (100 mg, 200 mg) . . . 3261

PROGESTASERT (Canada, France)
PROGESTERONE
Crinone 4% Gel . . . 3213
Crinone 8% Gel . . . 3213
Prometrium Capsules (100 mg, 200 mg) . . . 3261

PROGESTERONE IMPLANTS (United Kingdom)
PROGESTERONE
Crinone 4% Gel . . . 3213
Crinone 8% Gel . . . 3213
Prometrium Capsules (100 mg, 200 mg) . . . 3261

PROGESTOGEL (Belgium, France, Italy, Portugal, Spain, Switzerland, Thailand)
PROGESTERONE
Crinone 4% Gel . . . 3213
Crinone 8% Gel . . . 3213
Prometrium Capsules (100 mg, 200 mg) . . . 3261

PROGESTOL (Italy)
PROGESTERONE
Crinone 4% Gel . . . 3213
Crinone 8% Gel . . . 3213
Prometrium Capsules (100 mg, 200 mg) . . . 3261

PROGESTOSOL (France, Switzerland)
PROGESTERONE
Crinone 4% Gel . . . 3213
Crinone 8% Gel . . . 3213
Prometrium Capsules (100 mg, 200 mg) . . . 3261

PROGEVERA (Spain)
MEDROXYPROGESTERONE ACETATE
Depo-Provera Contraceptive Injection . . . 2798
Provera Tablets . . . 2853

PROGEVERA 250 (Spain)
MEDROXYPROGESTERONE ACETATE
Depo-Provera Contraceptive Injection . . . 2798
Provera Tablets . . . 2853

PROGOR (Belgium)
DILTIAZEM HYDROCHLORIDE
Cardizem CD Capsules . . . 1016
Cardizem Injectable . . . 1018
Cardizem Lyo-Ject Syringe . . . 1018
Cardizem Monovial . . . 1018
Tiazac Capsules . . . 1378

PROGRAF (Australia, Austria, Canada, Denmark, Finland, France, Germany, Hong Kong, Irish Republic, Israel, Italy, Japan, Mexico, New Zealand, Norway, Portugal, Singapore, Spain, Sweden, Switzerland, Thailand, United Kingdom)
TACROLIMUS
Prograf . . . 1393

PROGRAFT (Belgium)
TACROLIMUS
Prograf . . . 1393

PROGYNOVA (United Kingdom)
ESTRADIOL
Alora Transdermal System . . . 3372
Climara Transdermal System . . . 958
Estrace Vaginal Cream . . . 3358
Estring Vaginal Ring . . . 2811
Vivelle Transdermal System . . . 2412
Vivelle-Dot Transdermal System . . . 2416

PROHIST (South Africa)
PROMETHAZINE HYDROCHLORIDE
Phenergan Injection . . . 3553
Phenergan Suppositories . . . 3556
Phenergan Syrup Fortis . . . 3554
Phenergan Syrup Plain . . . 3554
Phenergan Tablets . . . 3556

PROKINYL (Monaco)
METOCLOPRAMIDE HYDROCHLORIDE
Reglan Injectable . . . 2935
Reglan Syrup . . . 2935
Reglan Tablets . . . 2935

PROLEUKIN (Australia, Austria, Canada, Denmark, France, Germany, Hong Kong, Israel, Italy, Mexico, Portugal, Singapore, Spain, Switzerland, The Netherlands, United Kingdom)
ALDESLEUKIN
Proleukin for Injection . . . 1199

PROLIDON (Mexico)
PROGESTERONE
Crinone 4% Gel . . . 3213
Crinone 8% Gel . . . 3213
Prometrium Capsules (100 mg, 200 mg) . . . 3261

PROLIPASE (Austria, Switzerland)
PANCRELIPASE
Ultrase Capsules . . . 835
Ultrase MT Capsules . . . 835

PROLOL (Israel, Thailand)
PROPRANOLOL HYDROCHLORIDE
Inderal Injectable . . . 3513
Inderal LA Long-Acting Capsules . . . 3516
Inderal Tablets . . . 3513

PROLUTON (Italy, Thailand)
PROGESTERONE
Crinone 4% Gel . . . 3213
Crinone 8% Gel . . . 3213
Prometrium Capsules (100 mg, 200 mg) . . . 3261

PROMAHIST (South Africa)
PROMETHAZINE HYDROCHLORIDE
Phenergan Injection . . . 3553
Phenergan Suppositories . . . 3556
Phenergan Syrup Fortis . . . 3554
Phenergan Syrup Plain . . . 3554
Phenergan Tablets . . . 3556

PROMAL (South Africa)
CHLOROQUINE PHOSPHATE
Aralen Tablets . . . 3075

PROMETRIUM (Canada)
PROGESTERONE
Crinone 4% Gel . . . 3213
Crinone 8% Gel . . . 3213
Prometrium Capsules (100 mg, 200 mg) . . . 3261

PROMIBASOL (Mexico)
METRONIDAZOLE
MetroCream . . . 1404
MetroGel . . . 1405
MetroGel-Vaginal Gel . . . 1986
MetroLotion . . . 1405
Noritate Cream . . . 1224

PROMIFEN (Mexico)
PREDNISONE
Prednisone Intensol . . . 3064
Prednisone Oral Solution . . . 3064
Prednisone Tablets . . . 3064

PROMKIDDI (Germany)
PROMETHAZINE HYDROCHLORIDE
Phenergan Injection . . . 3553
Phenergan Suppositories . . . 3556
Phenergan Syrup Fortis . . . 3554
Phenergan Syrup Plain . . . 3554
Phenergan Tablets . . . 3556

PROMOCARD (Belgium, The Netherlands)
ISOSORBIDE MONONITRATE
Imdur Tablets . . . 1826
Ismo Tablets . . . 3524

PROMOXIL (South Africa)
AMOXICILLIN
Amoxil Pediatric Drops for Oral Suspension . . . 1471
Amoxil Tablets . . . 1471

PRONAT (Mexico)
NAPROXEN
EC-Naprosyn Delayed-Release Tablets ... 2967
Naprosyn Suspension ... 2967
Naprosyn Tablets ... 2967

PRONAXEN (Finland, Sweden)
NAPROXEN
EC-Naprosyn Delayed-Release Tablets ... 2967
Naprosyn Suspension ... 2967
Naprosyn Tablets ... 2967

PRONAXIL (Mexico)
NAPROXEN
EC-Naprosyn Delayed-Release Tablets ... 2967
Naprosyn Suspension ... 2967
Naprosyn Tablets ... 2967

PRONAX-P (Mexico)
NAPROXEN SODIUM
Anaprox DS Tablets ... 2967
Anaprox Tablets ... 2967
Naprelan Tablets ... 1293

PRONESTYL (Australia, Belgium, Canada, Hong Kong, Irish Republic, Israel, New Zealand, South Africa, Switzerland, Thailand, The Netherlands, United Kingdom)
PROCAINAMIDE HYDROCHLORIDE
Procanbid Extended-Release Tablets ... 2262

PRONEURIN (Germany)
PROMETHAZINE HYDROCHLORIDE
Phenergan Injection ... 3553
Phenergan Suppositories ... 3556
Phenergan Syrup Fortis ... 3554
Phenergan Syrup Plain ... 3554
Phenergan Tablets ... 3556

PRONICOL (Mexico)
CHLORAMPHENICOL
Chloromycetin Ophthalmic Ointment, 1% ... ⊙296
Chloromycetin Ophthalmic Solution ... ⊙297
Chloroptic Sterile Ophthalmic Ointment ... ⊙234
Chloroptic Sterile Ophthalmic Solution ... ⊙235

PRONOSIL (Thailand)
PROPRANOLOL HYDROCHLORIDE
Inderal Injectable ... 3513
Inderal LA Long-Acting Capsules ... 3516
Inderal Tablets ... 3513

PRONOVAN (Norway)
PROPRANOLOL HYDROCHLORIDE
Inderal Injectable ... 3513
Inderal LA Long-Acting Capsules ... 3516
Inderal Tablets ... 3513

PRONOXEN (Mexico)
NAPROXEN
EC-Naprosyn Delayed-Release Tablets ... 2967
Naprosyn Suspension ... 2967
Naprosyn Tablets ... 2967

PRONTALGIN (Italy)
IBUPROFEN
Motrin Suspension, Oral Drops, Chewable Tablets, and Caplets ... 2002

PRONTALGIN (Italy)
TRAMADOL HYDROCHLORIDE
Ultram Tablets ... 2600

PRONTAMID (Italy)
SULFACETAMIDE SODIUM
Bleph-10 Ophthalmic Ointment 10% ... ⊙230
Klaron Lotion 10% ... 1224

PRONTOFORT (Mexico)
TRAMADOL HYDROCHLORIDE
Ultram Tablets ... 2600

PRONTOGEST (Italy)
PROGESTERONE
Crinone 4% Gel ... 3213
Crinone 8% Gel ... 3213
Prometrium Capsules (100 mg, 200 mg) ... 3261

PRONTOKEF (Italy)
CEFOPERAZONE SODIUM
Cefobid Intravenous/Intramuscular ... 2671
Cefobid Pharmacy Bulk Package - Not for Direct Infusion ... 2673

PROPABLOC (Germany)
PROPRANOLOL HYDROCHLORIDE
Inderal Injectable ... 3513
Inderal LA Long-Acting Capsules ... 3516
Inderal Tablets ... 3513

PROPAFEN (Germany)
PROPAFENONE HYDROCHLORIDE
Rythmol Tablets – 150 mg, 225 mg, 300 mg ... 502

PROPAL (Denmark)
PROPRANOLOL HYDROCHLORIDE
Inderal Injectable ... 3513
Inderal LA Long-Acting Capsules ... 3516
Inderal Tablets ... 3513

PROPAM (New Zealand)
DIAZEPAM
Valium Injectable ... 3026
Valium Tablets ... 3047

PRO-PAM (Australia)
DIAZEPAM
Valium Injectable ... 3026
Valium Tablets ... 3047

PROPAMERCK (Germany)
PROPAFENONE HYDROCHLORIDE
Rythmol Tablets – 150 mg, 225 mg, 300 mg ... 502

PROPAMIDE (Singapore, Thailand)
CHLORPROPAMIDE
Diabinese Tablets ... 2680

PROPANIX (United Kingdom)
PROPRANOLOL HYDROCHLORIDE
Inderal Injectable ... 3513
Inderal LA Long-Acting Capsules ... 3516
Inderal Tablets ... 3513

PROPA-ORAMON (Germany)
PROPAFENONE HYDROCHLORIDE
Rythmol Tablets – 150 mg, 225 mg, 300 mg ... 502

PROPAPHENIN (Germany)
CHLORPROMAZINE HYDROCHLORIDE
Thorazine Ampuls ... 1656
Thorazine Multi-dose Vials ... 1656
Thorazine Spansule Capsules ... 1656
Thorazine Syrup ... 1656
Thorazine Tablets ... 1656

PROPARIN (Mexico)
HEPARIN SODIUM
Heparin Lock Flush Solution ... 3509
Heparin Sodium Injection ... 3511

PROPASTAD (Germany)
PROPAFENONE HYDROCHLORIDE
Rythmol Tablets – 150 mg, 225 mg, 300 mg ... 502

PROPAVENTE (Portugal)
GUAIFENESIN
Organidin NR Liquid ... 3350
Organidin NR Tablets ... 3350

PROPECIA (Australia, Canada, Denmark, Finland, France, Germany, Israel, Italy, New Zealand, Portugal, Singapore, South Africa, Spain, Sweden, Switzerland, Thailand, United Kingdom)
FINASTERIDE
Propecia Tablets ... 2172
Proscar Tablets ... 2175

PROPESHIA (Mexico)
FINASTERIDE
Propecia Tablets ... 2172
Proscar Tablets ... 2175

PROPESS (Austria, Denmark, Finland, France, Hong Kong, Irish Republic, Israel, Mexico, Portugal, Spain, Sweden, Switzerland, The Netherlands, United Kingdom)
DINOPROSTONE
Cervidil Vaginal Insert ... 1369
Prepidil Gel ... 2851
Prostin E2 Suppositories ... 2852

PROPHAGE (Thailand)
METFORMIN HYDROCHLORIDE
Glucophage Tablets ... 1080

PROPHYLUX (Germany)
PROPRANOLOL HYDROCHLORIDE
Inderal Injectable ... 3513
Inderal LA Long-Acting Capsules ... 3516
Inderal Tablets ... 3513

PROPRA (Germany)
PROPRANOLOL HYDROCHLORIDE
Inderal Injectable ... 3513
Inderal LA Long-Acting Capsules ... 3516
Inderal Tablets ... 3513

PROPRAHEXAL (Austria)
PROPRANOLOL HYDROCHLORIDE
Inderal Injectable ... 3513
Inderal LA Long-Acting Capsules ... 3516
Inderal Tablets ... 3513

PROPRAL (Finland)
PROPRANOLOL HYDROCHLORIDE
Inderal Injectable ... 3513
Inderal LA Long-Acting Capsules ... 3516
Inderal Tablets ... 3513

PROPRANET (Denmark)
PROPRANOLOL HYDROCHLORIDE
Inderal Injectable ... 3513
Inderal LA Long-Acting Capsules ... 3516
Inderal Tablets ... 3513

PROPRANUR (Germany)
PROPRANOLOL HYDROCHLORIDE
Inderal Injectable ... 3513
Inderal LA Long-Acting Capsules ... 3516
Inderal Tablets ... 3513

P-ROQUINE (Thailand)
CHLOROQUINE PHOSPHATE
Aralen Tablets ... 3075

PRORYNORM (Germany)
PROPAFENONE HYDROCHLORIDE
Rythmol Tablets – 150 mg, 225 mg, 300 mg ... 502

PROSAID (United Kingdom)
NAPROXEN
EC-Naprosyn Delayed-Release Tablets ... 2967
Naprosyn Suspension ... 2967
Naprosyn Tablets ... 2967

PROSCAR (Australia, Austria, Belgium, Brazil, Canada, Denmark, Finland, Germany, Hong Kong, Irish Republic, Italy, Mexico, New Zealand, Norway, Portugal, Singapore, South Africa, Spain, Sweden, Switzerland, Thailand, The Netherlands, United Kingdom)
FINASTERIDE
Propecia Tablets ... 2172
Proscar Tablets ... 2175

PROSOM (Canada)
ESTAZOLAM
ProSom Tablets ... 500

PROSTACUR (Spain)
FLUTAMIDE
Eulexin Capsules ... 3118

PROSTADIREX (France)
FLUTAMIDE
Eulexin Capsules ... 3118

PROSTAL (South Africa)
METOCLOPRAMIDE HYDROCHLORIDE
Reglan Injectable ... 2935
Reglan Syrup ... 2935
Reglan Tablets ... 2935

PROSTAN (Thailand)
MEFENAMIC ACID
Ponstel Capsules ... 1356

PROSTEP (Australia, Canada)
NICOTINE
Nicotrol Inhaler ... 2840
Nicotrol Nasal Spray ... 2843

PROSTICA (Germany)
FLUTAMIDE
Eulexin Capsules ... 3118

PROSTIDE (Brazil, Italy)
FINASTERIDE
Propecia Tablets ... 2172
Proscar Tablets ... 2175

PROSTIN (Singapore)
DINOPROSTONE
Cervidil Vaginal Insert ... 1369
Prepidil Gel ... 2851
Prostin E2 Suppositories ... 2852

PROSTIN E2 (Australia, Austria, Belgium, Canada, Hong Kong, Irish Republic, Israel, Italy, New Zealand, Portugal, South Africa, Switzerland, Thailand, The Netherlands, United Kingdom)
DINOPROSTONE
Cervidil Vaginal Insert ... 1369
Prepidil Gel ... 2851
Prostin E2 Suppositories ... 2852

PROSTIN VR (Australia, Belgium, Canada, Hong Kong, Israel, Italy, New Zealand, Portugal, South Africa, Switzerland, Thailand, The Netherlands, United Kingdom)
ALPROSTADIL
Caverject Sterile Powder ... 2777
MUSE Urethral Suppository ... 3335

PROSTINE E2 (France)
DINOPROSTONE
Cervidil Vaginal Insert ... 1369
Prepidil Gel ... 2851
Prostin E2 Suppositories ... 2852

PROSTINE VR (France)
ALPROSTADIL
Caverject Sterile Powder ... 2777
MUSE Urethral Suppository ... 3335

PROSTIVAS (Denmark, Finland, Norway, Sweden)
ALPROSTADIL
Caverject Sterile Powder ... 2777
MUSE Urethral Suppository ... 3335

PROSTOGENAT (Germany)
FLUTAMIDE
Eulexin Capsules ... 3118

PROTANGIX (France)
DIPYRIDAMOLE
Persantine Tablets ... 1057

PROTENATE (Hong Kong)
PLASMA PROTEIN FRACTION
Plasmanate ... 942

PROTEVAL (Mexico)
VALPROIC ACID
Depakene Capsules ... 421
Depakene Syrup ... 421

PROTEXIN (Spain)
AMANTADINE HYDROCHLORIDE
Symmetrel Syrup ... 1328
Symmetrel Tablets ... 1328

PROTHAZIN (Germany)
PROMETHAZINE HYDROCHLORIDE
Phenergan Injection ... 3553
Phenergan Suppositories ... 3556
Phenergan Syrup Fortis ... 3554
Phenergan Syrup Plain ... 3554
Phenergan Tablets ... 3556

PROTHAZINE (Australia)
PROMETHAZINE HYDROCHLORIDE
Phenergan Injection ... 3553
Phenergan Suppositories ... 3556
Phenergan Syrup Fortis ... 3554
Phenergan Syrup Plain ... 3554
Phenergan Tablets ... 3556

PROTHIAZINE (Israel)
PROMETHAZINE HYDROCHLORIDE
Phenergan Injection ... 3553
Phenergan Suppositories ... 3556
Phenergan Syrup Fortis ... 3554
Phenergan Syrup Plain ... 3554
Phenergan Tablets ... 3556

PROTININ (Mexico)
APROTININ
Trasylol Injection ... 909

PROTOGYL (Hong Kong, Singapore)
METRONIDAZOLE
MetroCream ... 1404
MetroGel ... 1405
MetroGel-Vaginal Gel ... 1986
MetroLotion ... 1405
Noritate Cream ... 1224

PROTON (Portugal)
OMEPRAZOLE
Prilosec Delayed-Release Capsules ... 628

PROTOPAM (Canada)
PRALIDOXIME CHLORIDE
Protopam Chloride for Injection ... 3582

PROTOSOL (Israel)
APROTININ
Trasylol Injection ... 909

PROTOSTAT (Australia)
METRONIDAZOLE
MetroCream ... 1404
MetroGel ... 1405
MetroGel-Vaginal Gel ... 1986
MetroLotion ... 1405
Noritate Cream ... 1224

PROTRAN (Australia)
CHLORPROMAZINE HYDROCHLORIDE
Thorazine Ampuls ... 1656
Thorazine Multi-dose Vials ... 1656
Thorazine Spansule Capsules ... 1656
Thorazine Syrup ... 1656
Thorazine Tablets ... 1656

PROVAIL (Singapore)
KETOPROFEN
Orudis Capsules ... 3548
Oruvail Capsules ... 3548

PROVAMES (France)
ESTRADIOL
Alora Transdermal System ... 3372
Climara Transdermal System ... 958
Estrace Vaginal Cream ... 3358
Estring Vaginal Ring ... 2811
Vivelle Transdermal System ... 2412
Vivelle-Dot Transdermal System ... 2416

PRO-VENT (Irish Republic, United Kingdom)
THEOPHYLLINE
Aerolate Jr. T.D. Capsules ... 1361
Aerolate Liquid ... 1361
Aerolate Sr. T.D. Capsules ... 1361
Theo-Dur Extended-Release Tablets ... 1835
Uni-Dur Extended-Release Tablets ... 1841
Uniphyl 400 mg and 600 mg Tablets ... 2903

PROVERA (Australia, Austria, Belgium, Brazil, Canada, Denmark, Finland, Hong Kong, Irish Republic, Israel, Italy, Mexico, New Zealand, Norway, Portugal, Singapore, South Africa, Sweden, Switzerland, Thailand, The Netherlands, United Kingdom)
MEDROXYPROGESTERONE ACETATE
Depo-Provera Contraceptive Injection ... 2798

Provera Tablets 2853

PROVETAL (Mexico)
VALPROIC ACID
Depakene Capsules 421
Depakene Syrup 421

PROVIGIL (Irish Republic, United Kingdom)
MODAFINIL
Provigil Tablets 1193

PROVISC (Australia, Austria, Belgium, France, Germany, Hong Kong, Italy, New Zealand, Norway, Singapore, South Africa, Thailand, United Kingdom)
SODIUM HYALURONATE
Hyalgan Solution 3080

PROXALIN (Mexico)
NAPROXEN
EC-Naprosyn Delayed-Release Tablets . . . 2967
Naprosyn Suspension 2967
Naprosyn Tablets 2967

PROXALYOC (France)
PIROXICAM
Feldene Capsules 2685

PROXEN (Australia, Austria, Hong Kong, South Africa, Switzerland, Thailand)
NAPROXEN
EC-Naprosyn Delayed-Release Tablets . . . 2967
Naprosyn Suspension 2967
Naprosyn Tablets 2967

PROXINE (Italy)
NAPROXEN
EC-Naprosyn Delayed-Release Tablets . . . 2967
Naprosyn Suspension 2967
Naprosyn Tablets 2967

PROXITEC (Mexico)
CIPROFLOXACIN
Cipro I.V. 893
Cipro I.V. Pharmacy Bulk Package 897
Cipro Oral Suspension 887

PROZEF (South Africa)
CEFPROZIL
Cefzil Tablets 1076
Cefzil for Oral Suspension 1076

PROZIERE (United Kingdom)
PROCHLORPERAZINE MALEATE
Compazine Spansule Capsules 1505
Compazine Tablets 1505

PROZIN (Italy)
CHLORPROMAZINE HYDROCHLORIDE
Thorazine Ampuls 1656
Thorazine Multi-dose Vials 1656
Thorazine Spansule Capsules 1656
Thorazine Syrup 1656
Thorazine Tablets 1656

PROZINE (South Africa)
CARBAMAZEPINE
Carbatrol Capsules 3234
Tegretol Chewable Tablets 2404
Tegretol Suspension 2404
Tegretol Tablets 2404
Tegretol-XR Tablets 2404

PROZINE (Thailand)
CHLORPROMAZINE HYDROCHLORIDE
Thorazine Ampuls 1656
Thorazine Multi-dose Vials 1656
Thorazine Spansule Capsules 1656
Thorazine Syrup 1656
Thorazine Tablets 1656

PROZITEL (Mexico)
PRAZIQUANTEL
Biltricide Tablets 887

PRUREX (Austria)
DIPHENHYDRAMINE HYDROCHLORIDE
Benadryl Parenteral 2617

PRURITRAT (Brazil)
LINDANE
Lindane Lotion USP 1% 559
Lindane Shampoo USP 1% 560

PRYSMA (Spain)
OMEPRAZOLE
Prilosec Delayed-Release Capsules 628

PSICOFAR (Italy)
CHLORDIAZEPOXIDE HYDROCHLORIDE
Librium Capsules 1736
Librium for Injection 1737

PSICOTERINA (Italy)
CHLORDIAZEPOXIDE HYDROCHLORIDE
Librium Capsules 1736
Librium for Injection 1737

PSOREX (Brazil)
CLOBETASOL PROPIONATE
Cormax Cream 2440
Cormax Ointment 2440
Cormax Scalp Application 2441
Temovate Cream 1301
Temovate E Emollient 1302
Temovate Gel 1303
Temovate Ointment 1301
Temovate Scalp Application 1304

PSYCHOPAX (Austria, Switzerland)
DIAZEPAM
Valium Injectable 3026
Valium Tablets 3047

PULMAXAN (Italy)
BUDESONIDE
Pulmicort Turbuhaler Inhalation Powder . . . 636
Rhinocort Nasal Inhaler 640

PULMENO (Spain)
THEOPHYLLINE
Aerolate Jr. T.D. Capsules 1361
Aerolate Liquid 1361
Aerolate Sr. T.D. Capsules 1361
Theo-Dur Extended-Release Tablets 1835
Uni-Dur Extended-Release Tablets 1841
Uniphyl 400 mg and 600 mg Tablets . . . 2903

PULMICORT (Australia, Austria, Belgium, Canada, Finland, France, Hong Kong, Irish Republic, Mexico, New Zealand, Norway, Portugal, Singapore, South Africa, Spain, Sweden, Switzerland, Thailand, The Netherlands, United Kingdom)
BUDESONIDE
Pulmicort Turbuhaler Inhalation Powder . . . 636
Rhinocort Nasal Inhaler 640

PULMICTAN (Spain)
BUDESONIDE
Pulmicort Turbuhaler Inhalation Powder . . . 636
Rhinocort Nasal Inhaler 640

PULMIDUR (Austria, Germany)
THEOPHYLLINE
Aerolate Jr. T.D. Capsules 1361
Aerolate Liquid 1361
Aerolate Sr. T.D. Capsules 1361
Theo-Dur Extended-Release Tablets 1835
Uni-Dur Extended-Release Tablets 1841
Uniphyl 400 mg and 600 mg Tablets . . . 2903

PULMISON (South Africa)
PREDNISONE
Prednisone Intensol 3064
Prednisone Oral Solution 3064
Prednisone Tablets 3064

PULMONIX (Brazil)
POTASSIUM IODIDE
Pima Syrup 1362

PULMOPHYLLIN (South Africa)
THEOPHYLLINE
Aerolate Jr. T.D. Capsules 1361
Aerolate Liquid 1361
Aerolate Sr. T.D. Capsules 1361
Theo-Dur Extended-Release Tablets 1835
Uni-Dur Extended-Release Tablets 1841
Uniphyl 400 mg and 600 mg Tablets . . . 2903

PULMOPHYLLINE (Canada)
THEOPHYLLINE
Aerolate Jr. T.D. Capsules 1361
Aerolate Liquid 1361
Aerolate Sr. T.D. Capsules 1361
Theo-Dur Extended-Release Tablets 1835
Uni-Dur Extended-Release Tablets 1841
Uniphyl 400 mg and 600 mg Tablets . . . 2903

PULMOTIDE (Israel)
BUDESONIDE
Pulmicort Turbuhaler Inhalation Powder . . . 636
Rhinocort Nasal Inhaler 640

PULMO-TIMELETS (Denmark, Germany)
THEOPHYLLINE
Aerolate Jr. T.D. Capsules 1361
Aerolate Liquid 1361
Aerolate Sr. T.D. Capsules 1361
Theo-Dur Extended-Release Tablets 1835
Uni-Dur Extended-Release Tablets 1841
Uniphyl 400 mg and 600 mg Tablets . . . 2903

PULSIT (Mexico)
HALOPERIDOL
Haldol Injection, Tablets and Concentrate 2533

PULSOL (Mexico)
ENALAPRIL MALEATE
Vasotec Tablets 2210

PULSOTON (Mexico)
METHYLDOPA
Aldomet Tablets 2037

PULVI-BACTERAMIDE (France)
SULFANILAMIDE
AVC Cream 1350
AVC Suppositories 1350

PUMP-HEP (Irish Republic, United Kingdom)
HEPARIN SODIUM
Heparin Lock Flush Solution 3509
Heparin Sodium Injection 3511

PUNKTYL (Austria, Germany)
LORAZEPAM
Ativan Injection 3478
Ativan Tablets 3482

PUR-BLOKA (South Africa)
PROPRANOLOL HYDROCHLORIDE
Inderal Injectable 3513
Inderal LA Long-Acting Capsules 3516
Inderal Tablets 3513

PUREGON (Australia, Austria, Belgium, Canada, Denmark, Finland, France, Germany, Hong Kong, Irish Republic, Israel, Italy, Mexico, New Zealand, Norway, Portugal, Singapore, Spain, Sweden, Switzerland, Thailand, The Netherlands, United Kingdom)
FOLLITROPIN BETA
Follistim for Injection 2465

PURGOXIN (South Africa)
DIGOXIN
Lanoxicaps Capsules 1574
Lanoxin Elixir Pediatric 1578
Lanoxin Injection 1581
Lanoxin Injection Pediatric 1584
Lanoxin Tablets 1587

PURI-NETHOL (Australia, Austria, Belgium, Brazil, Canada, France, Germany, Hong Kong, Irish Republic, Israel, Italy, Mexico, New Zealand, Norway, Singapore, South Africa, Sweden, Switzerland, Thailand, The Netherlands, United Kingdom)
MERCAPTOPURINE
Purinethol Tablets 1615

PUTAREN (Thailand)
DICLOFENAC SODIUM
Voltaren Tablets 2315
Voltaren-XR Tablets 2315

PUVASORALEN (United Kingdom)
METHOXSALEN
8-MOP Capsules 1727
Oxsoralen Lotion 1% 1740
Oxsoralen-Ultra Capsules 1741

PV CARPINE (Australia, New Zealand)
PILOCARPINE HYDROCHLORIDE
Isopto Carpine Ophthalmic Solution . . . . ⊙215
Pilopine HS Ophthalmic Gel . . . . ⊙217
Salagen Tablets 2229

PYKNOLEPSINUM (Germany)
ETHOSUXIMIDE
Zarontin Capsules 2659
Zarontin Syrup 2660

PYNAMIC (Thailand)
MEFENAMIC ACID
Ponstel Capsules 1356

PYRAFAT (Austria, Germany, Hong Kong)
PYRAZINAMIDE
Pyrazinamide Tablets 1876

PYRALIN (Australia)
SULFASALAZINE
Azulfidine EN-tabs Tablets 2775

PYRATAB (Thailand)
PYRAZINAMIDE
Pyrazinamide Tablets 1876

PYRAZIDE (South Africa)
PYRAZINAMIDE
Pyrazinamide Tablets 1876

PYRIDAMEL (Irish Republic)
DIPYRIDAMOLE
Persantine Tablets 1057

PYRIFOAM (Australia)
PERMETHRIN
Acticin Cream 998
Elimite Cream 552

PYROCAPS (South Africa)
PIROXICAM
Feldene Capsules 2685

PYROXY (Thailand)
PIROXICAM
Feldene Capsules 2685

PYTAZEN (New Zealand)
DIPYRIDAMOLE
Persantine Tablets 1057

PZA (Germany, Singapore)
PYRAZINAMIDE
Pyrazinamide Tablets 1876

Q-MAZINE (United Kingdom)
PROMETHAZINE HYDROCHLORIDE
Phenergan Injection 3553
Phenergan Suppositories 3556
Phenergan Syrup Fortis 3554
Phenergan Syrup Plain 3554
Phenergan Tablets 3556

QUADRAX (Mexico)
IBUPROFEN
Motrin Suspension, Oral Drops, Chewable Tablets, and Caplets 2002

QUADRIDERM NF (Mexico)
BETAMETHASONE DIPROPIONATE/CLOTRIMAZOLE
Lotrisone Cream 3129

QUADRIDERME (Portugal)
BETAMETHASONE DIPROPIONATE/CLOTRIMAZOLE
Lotrisone Cream 3129

QUAIT (Italy)
LORAZEPAM
Ativan Injection 3478
Ativan Tablets 3482

QUAMATEL (Hong Kong)
FAMOTIDINE
Pepcid Injection 2153
Pepcid Injection Premixed 2153
Pepcid RPD Orally Disintegrating Tablets 2150
Pepcid Tablets 2150
Pepcid for Oral Suspension 2150

QUANAME (Belgium)
MEPROBAMATE
Miltown Tablets 3349

QUANIL (Italy)
MEPROBAMATE
Miltown Tablets 3349

QUANTOR (Spain)
RANITIDINE HYDROCHLORIDE
Zantac 150 EFFERdose Granules 1690
Zantac 150 EFFERdose Tablets 1690
Zantac 150 Tablets 1690
Zantac 300 Tablets 1690
Zantac Injection 1688
Zantac Injection Premixed 1688
Zantac Syrup 1690

QUARDIN (Portugal)
RANITIDINE HYDROCHLORIDE
Zantac 150 EFFERdose Granules 1690
Zantac 150 EFFERdose Tablets 1690
Zantac 150 Tablets 1690
Zantac 300 Tablets 1690
Zantac Injection 1688
Zantac Injection Premixed 1688
Zantac Syrup 1690

QUARK (Italy)
RAMIPRIL
Altace Capsules 2233

QUASAR (Italy)
VERAPAMIL HYDROCHLORIDE
Covera-HS Tablets 3199
Isoptin SR Tablets 467
Verelan Capsules 3184
Verelan PM Capsules 3186

QUELLADA (Australia, Belgium, Irish Republic, South Africa, United Kingdom)
PERMETHRIN
Acticin Cream 998
Elimite Cream 552

QUELLADA H (Germany)
LINDANE
Lindane Lotion USP 1% 559
Lindane Shampoo USP 1% 560

QUELLADA P (New Zealand)
PERMETHRIN
Acticin Cream 998
Elimite Cream 552

QUELLADA-M (United Kingdom)
MALATHION
Ovide Lotion 2023

QUEMICETINA (Brazil)
CHLORAMPHENICOL
Chloromycetin Ophthalmic Ointment, 1% . . . . ⊙296
Chloromycetin Ophthalmic Solution . . . ⊙297
Chloroptic Sterile Ophthalmic Ointment . . . ⊙234
Chloroptic Sterile Ophthalmic Solution . . ⊙235

QUENSYL (Germany)
HYDROXYCHLOROQUINE SULFATE
Plaquenil Tablets 3082

QUERTO (Germany)
CARVEDILOL
Coreg Tablets 1508

QUIBRON (Thailand)
THEOPHYLLINE
Aerolate Jr. T.D. Capsules 1361
Aerolate Liquid 1361

Aerolate Sr. T.D. Capsules 1361
Theo-Dur Extended-Release Tablets 1835
Uni-Dur Extended-Release Tablets 1841
Uniphyl 400 mg and 600 mg Tablets 2903

QUIBRON-T (Canada)
THEOPHYLLINE
Aerolate Jr. T.D. Capsules 1361
Aerolate Liquid 1361
Aerolate Sr. T.D. Capsules 1361
Theo-Dur Extended-Release Tablets 1835
Uni-Dur Extended-Release Tablets 1841
Uniphyl 400 mg and 600 mg Tablets 2903

QUIFLOXONA (Mexico)
CIPROFLOXACIN
Cipro I.V. 893
Cipro I.V. Pharmacy Bulk Package 897
Cipro Oral Suspension 887

QUILONUM (Australia, South Africa)
LITHIUM CARBONATE
Eskalith CR Controlled Release Tablets 1527
Eskalith Capsules 1527
Lithium Carbonate Capsules 3061
Lithobid Slow-Release Tablets 3255

QUIMOBROM (Mexico)
ERYTHROMYCIN
Emgel 2% Topical Gel 1285
Ery-Tab Tablets 448
Erythromycin Base Filmtab Tablets 454
Erythromycin Delayed-Release Capsules, USP 455
PCE Dispertab Tablets 498

QUIMOLAURIL (Mexico)
ERYTHROMYCIN
Emgel 2% Topical Gel 1285
Ery-Tab Tablets 448
Erythromycin Base Filmtab Tablets 454
Erythromycin Delayed-Release Capsules, USP 455
PCE Dispertab Tablets 498

QUIMOSPORINA (Mexico)
CEPHALEXIN
Keflex Oral Suspension 1237
Keflex Pulvules 1237

QUINAGLUTE (Canada, Italy, South Africa)
QUINIDINE GLUCONATE
Quinaglute Dura-Tabs Tablets 978

QUINATE (Canada)
QUINIDINE GLUCONATE
Quinaglute Dura-Tabs Tablets 978

QUINICARDINA (Spain)
QUINIDINE SULFATE
Quinidex Extentabs 2933

QUINICARDINE (Brazil)
QUINIDINE SULFATE
Quinidex Extentabs 2933

QUINIDEX (Australia, Canada)
QUINIDINE SULFATE
Quinidex Extentabs 2933

QUINIDOXIN (Australia)
QUINIDINE SULFATE
Quinidex Extentabs 2933

QUINOFLEX (Portugal)
NORFLOXACIN
Chibroxin Sterile Ophthalmic Solution ⊙273, 2051
Noroxin Tablets 2145

QUINOFLOX (Brazil, Mexico)
CIPROFLOXACIN HYDROCHLORIDE
Ciloxan Ophthalmic Ointment 538
Ciloxan Ophthalmic Solution ⊙209, 538
Cipro Tablets 887

QUINOFORM (Brazil)
NORFLOXACIN
Chibroxin Sterile Ophthalmic Solution ⊙273, 2051
Noroxin Tablets 2145

QUINOX (Portugal)
CIPROFLOXACIN
Cipro I.V. 893
Cipro I.V. Pharmacy Bulk Package 897
Cipro Oral Suspension 887

QUINTAMICINA (Spain)
GENTAMICIN SULFATE
Genoptic Ophthalmic Ointment ⊙239
Genoptic Sterile Ophthalmic Solution ⊙239

QUINTELMIN (Brazil)
MEBENDAZOLE
Vermox Chewable Tablets 2017

QUIPRO (Spain)
CIPROFLOXACIN HYDROCHLORIDE
Ciloxan Ophthalmic Ointment 538
Ciloxan Ophthalmic Solution ⊙209, 538
Cipro Tablets 887

QUIT (South Africa)
NICOTINE
Nicotrol Inhaler 2840
Nicotrol Nasal Spray 2843

QUITAXON (Belgium, Denmark, France)
DOXEPIN HYDROCHLORIDE
Sinequan Capsules 2713
Sinequan Oral Concentrate 2713

R CALM (Belgium)
DIPHENHYDRAMINE HYDROCHLORIDE
Benadryl Parenteral 2617

RADAN (Brazil)
RANITIDINE HYDROCHLORIDE
Zantac 150 EFFERdose Granules 1690
Zantac 150 EFFERdose Tablets 1690
Zantac 150 Tablets 1690
Zantac 300 Tablets 1690
Zantac Injection 1688
Zantac Injection Premixed 1688
Zantac Syrup 1690

RADIAN-B IBUPROFEN (United Kingdom)
IBUPROFEN
Motrin Suspension, Oral Drops, Chewable Tablets, and Caplets 2002

RADIKAL (Belgium, Germany)
MALATHION
Ovide Lotion 2023

RADINE (Thailand)
RANITIDINE HYDROCHLORIDE
Zantac 150 EFFERdose Granules 1690
Zantac 150 EFFERdose Tablets 1690
Zantac 150 Tablets 1690
Zantac 300 Tablets 1690
Zantac Injection 1688
Zantac Injection Premixed 1688
Zantac Syrup 1690

RADIOCIN (Italy)
FLUOCINOLONE ACETONIDE
Synalar Cream 2020
Synalar Ointment 2020
Synalar Topical Solution 2020

RADOX (Italy)
DOXYCYCLINE HYCLATE
Doryx Coated Pellet Filled Capsules 3357
Periostat Tablets 1208
Vibramycin Hyclate Capsules 2735
Vibramycin Hyclate Intravenous 2737
Vibra-Tabs Film Coated Tablets 2735

RADUCTIL (Mexico)
SIBUTRAMINE HYDROCHLORIDE
Meridia Capsules 481

RAFEN (Australia)
IBUPROFEN
Motrin Suspension, Oral Drops, Chewable Tablets, and Caplets 2002

RALOPAR (Portugal)
CEFOTAXIME SODIUM
Claforan Injection 732

RALOVERA (Australia)
MEDROXYPROGESTERONE ACETATE
Depo-Provera Contraceptive Injection 2798
Provera Tablets 2853

RALOZAM (Australia)
ALPRAZOLAM
Xanax Tablets 2865

RAMACE (Australia, Belgium, Denmark, Finland, Mexico, South Africa)
RAMIPRIL
Altace Capsules 2233

RAMYSIS (United Kingdom)
DOXYCYCLINE HYCLATE
Doryx Coated Pellet Filled Capsules 3357
Periostat Tablets 1208
Vibra-Tabs Film Coated Tablets 2735
Vibramycin Hyclate Capsules 2735
Vibramycin Hyclate Intravenous 2737

RAN (Portugal)
RANITIDINE HYDROCHLORIDE
Zantac 150 EFFERdose Granules 1690
Zantac 150 EFFERdose Tablets 1690
Zantac 150 Tablets 1690
Zantac 300 Tablets 1690
Zantac Injection 1688
Zantac Injection Premixed 1688
Zantac Syrup 1690

RAN (Italy)
NAPHAZOLINE HYDROCHLORIDE
Albalon Ophthalmic Solution ⊙225

RAN H2 (Spain)
RANITIDINE HYDROCHLORIDE
Zantac 150 EFFERdose Granules 1690
Zantac 150 EFFERdose Tablets 1690
Zantac 150 Tablets 1690
Zantac 300 Tablets 1690
Zantac Injection 1688
Zantac Injection Premixed 1688
Zantac Syrup 1690

RAN LICH (Germany)
RANITIDINE HYDROCHLORIDE
Zantac 150 EFFERdose Granules 1690
Zantac 150 EFFERdose Tablets 1690
Zantac 150 Tablets 1690
Zantac 300 Tablets 1690
Zantac Injection 1688
Zantac Injection Premixed 1688
Zantac Syrup 1690

RANACID (Norway)
RANITIDINE HYDROCHLORIDE
Zantac 150 EFFERdose Granules 1690
Zantac 150 EFFERdose Tablets 1690
Zantac 150 Tablets 1690
Zantac 300 Tablets 1690
Zantac Injection 1688
Zantac Injection Premixed 1688
Zantac Syrup 1690

RANAPS (United Kingdom)
RANITIDINE HYDROCHLORIDE
Zantac 150 EFFERdose Granules 1690
Zantac 150 EFFERdose Tablets 1690
Zantac 150 Tablets 1690
Zantac 300 Tablets 1690
Zantac Injection 1688
Zantac Injection Premixed 1688
Zantac Syrup 1690

RANCEPH (South Africa)
CEPHALEXIN
Keflex Oral Suspension 1237
Keflex Pulvules 1237

RANCLAV (South Africa)
AMOXICILLIN
Amoxil Pediatric Drops for Oral Suspension 1471
Amoxil Tablets 1471

RANDUM (Italy)
METOCLOPRAMIDE HYDROCHLORIDE
Reglan Injectable 2935
Reglan Syrup 2935
Reglan Tablets 2935

RANFEN (South Africa)
IBUPROFEN
Motrin Suspension, Oral Drops, Chewable Tablets, and Caplets 2002

RANI (Germany)
RANITIDINE HYDROCHLORIDE
Zantac 150 EFFERdose Granules 1690
Zantac 150 EFFERdose Tablets 1690
Zantac 150 Tablets 1690
Zantac 300 Tablets 1690
Zantac Injection 1688
Zantac Injection Premixed 1688
Zantac Syrup 1690

RANI 2 (Australia)
RANITIDINE HYDROCHLORIDE
Zantac 150 EFFERdose Granules 1690
Zantac 150 EFFERdose Tablets 1690
Zantac 150 Tablets 1690
Zantac 300 Tablets 1690
Zantac Injection 1688
Zantac Injection Premixed 1688
Zantac Syrup 1690

RANIBEN (Italy)
RANITIDINE HYDROCHLORIDE
Zantac 150 EFFERdose Granules 1690
Zantac 150 EFFERdose Tablets 1690
Zantac 150 Tablets 1690
Zantac 300 Tablets 1690
Zantac Injection 1688
Zantac Injection Premixed 1688
Zantac Syrup 1690

RANIBERL (Germany)
RANITIDINE HYDROCHLORIDE
Zantac 150 EFFERdose Granules 1690
Zantac 150 EFFERdose Tablets 1690
Zantac 150 Tablets 1690
Zantac 300 Tablets 1690
Zantac Injection 1688
Zantac Injection Premixed 1688
Zantac Syrup 1690

RANIBETA (Germany)
RANITIDINE HYDROCHLORIDE
Zantac 150 EFFERdose Granules 1690
Zantac 150 EFFERdose Tablets 1690
Zantac 150 Tablets 1690
Zantac 300 Tablets 1690
Zantac Injection 1688
Zantac Injection Premixed 1688
Zantac Syrup 1690

RANIBLOC (Germany, Italy)
RANITIDINE HYDROCHLORIDE
Zantac 150 EFFERdose Granules 1690
Zantac 150 EFFERdose Tablets 1690
Zantac 150 Tablets 1690
Zantac 300 Tablets 1690
Zantac Injection 1688
Zantac Injection Premixed 1688
Zantac Syrup 1690

RANIC (Belgium)
RANITIDINE HYDROCHLORIDE
Zantac 150 EFFERdose Granules 1690
Zantac 150 EFFERdose Tablets 1690
Zantac 150 Tablets 1690
Zantac 300 Tablets 1690
Zantac Injection 1688
Zantac Injection Premixed 1688
Zantac Syrup 1690

RANICID (Thailand)
RANITIDINE HYDROCHLORIDE
Zantac 150 EFFERdose Granules 1690
Zantac 150 EFFERdose Tablets 1690
Zantac 150 Tablets 1690
Zantac 300 Tablets 1690
Zantac Injection 1688
Zantac Injection Premixed 1688
Zantac Syrup 1690

RANICUR (Finland)
RANITIDINE HYDROCHLORIDE
Zantac 150 EFFERdose Granules 1690
Zantac 150 EFFERdose Tablets 1690
Zantac 150 Tablets 1690
Zantac 300 Tablets 1690
Zantac Injection 1688
Zantac Injection Premixed 1688
Zantac Syrup 1690

RANICUX (Germany)
RANITIDINE HYDROCHLORIDE
Zantac 150 EFFERdose Granules 1690
Zantac 150 EFFERdose Tablets 1690
Zantac 150 Tablets 1690
Zantac 300 Tablets 1690
Zantac Injection 1688
Zantac Injection Premixed 1688
Zantac Syrup 1690

RANIDIL (Italy)
RANITIDINE HYDROCHLORIDE
Zantac 150 EFFERdose Granules 1690
Zantac 150 EFFERdose Tablets 1690
Zantac 150 Tablets 1690
Zantac 300 Tablets 1690
Zantac Injection 1688
Zantac Injection Premixed 1688
Zantac Syrup 1690

RANIDIN (Brazil, Spain)
RANITIDINE HYDROCHLORIDE
Zantac 150 EFFERdose Granules 1690
Zantac 150 EFFERdose Tablets 1690
Zantac 150 Tablets 1690
Zantac 300 Tablets 1690
Zantac Injection 1688
Zantac Injection Premixed 1688
Zantac Syrup 1690

RANIDURA T (Germany)
RANITIDINE HYDROCHLORIDE
Zantac 150 EFFERdose Granules 1690
Zantac 150 EFFERdose Tablets 1690
Zantac 150 Tablets 1690
Zantac 300 Tablets 1690
Zantac Injection 1688
Zantac Injection Premixed 1688
Zantac Syrup 1690

RANIHEXAL (Australia, South Africa)
RANITIDINE HYDROCHLORIDE
Zantac 150 EFFERdose Granules 1690
Zantac 150 EFFERdose Tablets 1690
Zantac 150 Tablets 1690
Zantac 300 Tablets 1690
Zantac Injection 1688
Zantac Injection Premixed 1688
Zantac Syrup 1690

RANIL (Finland)
RANITIDINE HYDROCHLORIDE
Zantac 150 EFFERdose Granules 1690
Zantac 150 EFFERdose Tablets 1690
Zantac 150 Tablets 1690
Zantac 300 Tablets 1690
Zantac Injection 1688
Zantac Injection Premixed 1688
Zantac Syrup 1690

RANILONGA (Spain)
RANITIDINE HYDROCHLORIDE
Zantac 150 EFFERdose Granules 1690
Zantac 150 EFFERdose Tablets 1690
Zantac 150 Tablets 1690
Zantac 300 Tablets 1690
Zantac Injection 1688
Zantac Injection Premixed 1688
Zantac Syrup 1690

RANIMED (Switzerland)
RANITIDINE HYDROCHLORIDE
Zantac 150 EFFERdose Granules 1690

(⊙ Described in PDR For Ophthalmic Medicines™)

Zantac 150 EFFERdose Tablets 1690
Zantac 150 Tablets 1690
Zantac 300 Tablets 1690
Zantac Injection 1688
Zantac Injection Premixed 1688
Zantac Syrup 1690

RANIMERCK (Germany)
RANITIDINE HYDROCHLORIDE
Zantac 150 EFFERdose Granules 1690
Zantac 150 EFFERdose Tablets 1690
Zantac 150 Tablets 1690
Zantac 300 Tablets 1690
Zantac Injection 1688
Zantac Injection Premixed 1688
Zantac Syrup 1690

RANIMEX (Finland)
RANITIDINE HYDROCHLORIDE
Zantac 150 EFFERdose Granules 1690
Zantac 150 EFFERdose Tablets 1690
Zantac 150 Tablets 1690
Zantac 300 Tablets 1690
Zantac Injection 1688
Zantac Injection Premixed 1688
Zantac Syrup 1690

RANI-NERTON (Germany)
RANITIDINE HYDROCHLORIDE
Zantac 150 EFFERdose Granules 1690
Zantac 150 EFFERdose Tablets 1690
Zantac 150 Tablets 1690
Zantac 300 Tablets 1690
Zantac Injection 1688
Zantac Injection Premixed 1688
Zantac Syrup 1690

RANIPLEX (France)
RANITIDINE HYDROCHLORIDE
Zantac 150 EFFERdose Granules 1690
Zantac 150 EFFERdose Tablets 1690
Zantac 150 Tablets 1690
Zantac 300 Tablets 1690
Zantac Injection 1688
Zantac Injection Premixed 1688
Zantac Syrup 1690

RANIPROTECT (Germany)
RANITIDINE HYDROCHLORIDE
Zantac 150 EFFERdose Granules 1690
Zantac 150 EFFERdose Tablets 1690
Zantac 150 Tablets 1690
Zantac 300 Tablets 1690
Zantac Injection 1688
Zantac Injection Premixed 1688
Zantac Syrup 1690

RANI-Q (Sweden)
RANITIDINE HYDROCHLORIDE
Zantac 150 EFFERdose Granules 1690
Zantac 150 EFFERdose Tablets 1690
Zantac 150 Tablets 1690
Zantac 300 Tablets 1690
Zantac Injection 1688
Zantac Injection Premixed 1688
Zantac Syrup 1690

RANISEN (Mexico)
RANITIDINE HYDROCHLORIDE
Zantac 150 EFFERdose Granules 1690
Zantac 150 EFFERdose Tablets 1690
Zantac 150 Tablets 1690
Zantac 300 Tablets 1690
Zantac Injection 1688
Zantac Injection Premixed 1688
Zantac Syrup 1690

RANITIC (Germany, Irish Republic, United Kingdom)
RANITIDINE HYDROCHLORIDE
Zantac 150 EFFERdose Granules 1690
Zantac 150 EFFERdose Tablets 1690
Zantac 150 Tablets 1690
Zantac 300 Tablets 1690
Zantac Injection 1688
Zantac Injection Premixed 1688
Zantac Syrup 1690

RANITIL (Brazil)
RANITIDINE HYDROCHLORIDE
Zantac 150 EFFERdose Granules 1690
Zantac 150 EFFERdose Tablets 1690
Zantac 150 Tablets 1690
Zantac 300 Tablets 1690
Zantac Injection 1688
Zantac Injection Premixed 1688
Zantac Syrup 1690

RANITINE (Portugal)
RANITIDINE HYDROCHLORIDE
Zantac 150 EFFERdose Granules 1690
Zantac 150 EFFERdose Tablets 1690
Zantac 150 Tablets 1690
Zantac 300 Tablets 1690
Zantac Injection 1688
Zantac Injection Premixed 1688
Zantac Syrup 1690

RANIVEL (Spain)
RANITIDINE HYDROCHLORIDE
Zantac 150 EFFERdose Granules 1690
Zantac 150 EFFERdose Tablets 1690
Zantac 150 Tablets 1690
Zantac 300 Tablets 1690
Zantac Injection 1688
Zantac Injection Premixed 1688
Zantac Syrup 1690

RANIX (Spain)
RANITIDINE HYDROCHLORIDE
Zantac 150 EFFERdose Granules 1690
Zantac 150 EFFERdose Tablets 1690
Zantac 150 Tablets 1690
Zantac 300 Tablets 1690
Zantac Injection 1688
Zantac Injection Premixed 1688
Zantac Syrup 1690

RANIXAL (Finland)
RANITIDINE HYDROCHLORIDE
Zantac 150 EFFERdose Granules 1690
Zantac 150 EFFERdose Tablets 1690
Zantac 150 Tablets 1690
Zantac 300 Tablets 1690
Zantac Injection 1688
Zantac Injection Premixed 1688
Zantac Syrup 1690

RANOPINE (Irish Republic)
RANITIDINE HYDROCHLORIDE
Zantac 150 EFFERdose Granules 1690
Zantac 150 EFFERdose Tablets 1690
Zantac 150 Tablets 1690
Zantac 300 Tablets 1690
Zantac Injection 1688
Zantac Injection Premixed 1688
Zantac Syrup 1690

RANOPRIN (Finland)
PROPRANOLOL HYDROCHLORIDE
Inderal Injectable 3513
Inderal LA Long-Acting Capsules 3516
Inderal Tablets 3513

RANOXYL (Australia)
RANITIDINE HYDROCHLORIDE
Zantac 150 EFFERdose Granules 1690
Zantac 150 EFFERdose Tablets 1690
Zantac 150 Tablets 1690
Zantac 300 Tablets 1690
Zantac Injection 1688
Zantac Injection Premixed 1688
Zantac Syrup 1690

RANTAG (United Arab Emirates)
RANITIDINE HYDROCHLORIDE
Zantac 150 EFFERdose Granules 1690
Zantac 150 EFFERdose Tablets 1690
Zantac 150 Tablets 1690
Zantac 300 Tablets 1690
Zantac Injection 1688
Zantac Injection Premixed 1688
Zantac Syrup 1690

RANTEC (United Kingdom)
RANITIDINE HYDROCHLORIDE
Zantac 150 EFFERdose Granules 1690
Zantac 150 EFFERdose Tablets 1690
Zantac 150 Tablets 1690
Zantac 300 Tablets 1690
Zantac Injection 1688
Zantac Injection Premixed 1688
Zantac Syrup 1690

RANTEEN (South Africa)
RANITIDINE HYDROCHLORIDE
Zantac 150 EFFERdose Granules 1690
Zantac 150 EFFERdose Tablets 1690
Zantac 150 Tablets 1690
Zantac 300 Tablets 1690
Zantac Injection 1688
Zantac Injection Premixed 1688
Zantac Syrup 1690

RANUBER (Spain)
RANITIDINE HYDROCHLORIDE
Zantac 150 EFFERdose Granules 1690
Zantac 150 EFFERdose Tablets 1690
Zantac 150 Tablets 1690
Zantac 300 Tablets 1690
Zantac Injection 1688
Zantac Injection Premixed 1688
Zantac Syrup 1690

RANVIL (Italy)
NICARDIPINE HYDROCHLORIDE
Cardene I.V. 3485

RAPAMIC (Portugal)
KETOCONAZOLE
Nizoral 2% Cream 3620
Nizoral 2% Shampoo 2007
Nizoral Tablets 1791

RASAL (Spain)
OLSALAZINE SODIUM
Dipentum Capsules 2803

RATACAND (Italy)
CANDESARTAN CILEXETIL
Atacand Tablets 595

RATHIMED (Germany)
METRONIDAZOLE
MetroCream 1404
MetroGel 1405
MetroGel-Vaginal Gel 1986
MetroLotion 1405
Noritate Cream 1224

RATHIMED N (Germany)
METRONIDAZOLE
MetroCream 1404
MetroGel 1405
MetroGel-Vaginal Gel 1986
MetroLotion 1405
Noritate Cream 1224

RATIOALLERG (Germany)
DIPHENHYDRAMINE HYDROCHLORIDE
Benadryl Parenteral 2617
HYDROCORTISONE
Anusol-HC Cream 2.5% 2237
Hydrocortone Tablets 2106

RATIOMOBIL (Germany)
PIROXICAM
Feldene Capsules 2685

RAVAMIL (South Africa)
VERAPAMIL HYDROCHLORIDE
Covera-HS Tablets 3199
Isoptin SR Tablets 467
Verelan Capsules 3184
Verelan PM Capsules 3186

RAYNE (Mexico)
DIAZEPAM
Valium Injectable 3026
Valium Tablets 3047

REACTINE (Canada)
CETIRIZINE HYDROCHLORIDE
Zyrtec Syrup 2756
Zyrtec Tablets 2756

REALDRAX (Mexico)
IBUPROFEN
Motrin Suspension, Oral Drops, Chewable Tablets, and Caplets 2002

REBETOL (Austria, Denmark, Finland, France, Germany, Irish Republic, Italy, Portugal, Spain, Sweden, The Netherlands, United Kingdom)
RIBAVIRIN
Virazole for Inhalation Solution 1747

REBIF (Australia, Austria, Canada, Denmark, Finland, France, Germany, Irish Republic, Israel, Italy, Mexico, Norway, Portugal, Spain, Sweden, Switzerland, Thailand, The Netherlands, United Kingdom)
INTERFERON BETA-1A
Avonex 1013

RECA (Spain)
ENALAPRIL MALEATE
Vasotec Tablets 2210

RECEPTOZINE (South Africa)
PROMETHAZINE HYDROCHLORIDE
Phenergan Injection 3553
Phenergan Suppositories 3556
Phenergan Syrup Fortis 3554
Phenergan Syrup Plain 3554
Phenergan Tablets 3556

RECIPECT (Finland)
CODEINE PHOSPHATE/GUAIFENESIN
Robitussin A-C Syrup 2942
Tussi-Organidin NR Liquid 3350
Tussi-Organidin-S NR Liquid 3350

RECOCEF (United Arab Emirates)
CEFACLOR
Ceclor CD Tablets 1279
Ceclor Pulvules 1905
Ceclor Suspension 1905

RECOFOL (Denmark, Finland, Mexico, Norway, Portugal, Singapore, Spain, Sweden, Switzerland)
PROPOFOL
Diprivan Injectable Emulsion 667

RECOZIL (Singapore)
GEMFIBROZIL
Lopid Tablets 2650

RECTOCORT (Canada, Hong Kong)
HYDROCORTISONE ACETATE
Anusol-HC Suppositories 2238
Cortifoam Rectal Foam 3170
Hydrocortone Acetate Injectable Suspension 2103
Proctocort Suppositories 2264

RECTODELT (Germany)
PREDNISONE
Prednisone Intensol 3064
Prednisone Oral Solution 3064
Prednisone Tablets 3064

RECTOPRED (Austria)
PREDNISOLONE SODIUM PHOSPHATE
Pediapred Oral Solution 1170

RED AWAY (Canada)
NAPHAZOLINE HYDROCHLORIDE
Albalon Ophthalmic Solution ⊙225

REDAP (Denmark)
ADAPALENE
Differin Gel 1403
Differin Solution/Pledgets 1404

REDIPRED (Australia, New Zealand)
PREDNISOLONE SODIUM PHOSPHATE
Pediapred Oral Solution 1170

REDUCOL (Brazil)
LOVASTATIN
Mevacor Tablets 2132

REDUCTEL (Mexico)
CAPTOPRIL
Captopril Tablets 2281

REDUCTIL (Switzerland, United Kingdom)
SIBUTRAMINE HYDROCHLORIDE
Meridia Capsules 481

REDUFEN (Switzerland)
IBUPROFEN
Motrin Suspension, Oral Drops, Chewable Tablets, and Caplets 2002

REDUPRES (Spain)
VERAPAMIL HYDROCHLORIDE
Covera-HS Tablets 3199
Isoptin SR Tablets 467
Verelan Capsules 3184
Verelan PM Capsules 3186

REDUSA (Hong Kong)
PHENTERMINE HYDROCHLORIDE
Adipex-P Capsules 1406
Adipex-P Tablets 1406

REFLUDAN (Australia, Austria, Belgium, Denmark, Finland, France, Germany, Irish Republic, Italy, Norway, Portugal, Spain, Sweden, Switzerland, The Netherlands, United Kingdom)
LEPIRUDIN
Refludan for Injection 761

REFLUDIN (South Africa)
LEPIRUDIN
Refludan for Injection 761

REFOBACIN (Austria, Germany)
GENTAMICIN SULFATE
Genoptic Ophthalmic Ointment ⊙239
Genoptic Sterile Ophthalmic Solution ⊙239

REFUSAL (The Netherlands)
DISULFIRAM
Antabuse Tablets 3474

REGASTROL (Italy)
METOCLOPRAMIDE HYDROCHLORIDE
Reglan Injectable 2935
Reglan Syrup 2935
Reglan Tablets 2935

REGELAN (Austria, Switzerland)
CLOFIBRATE
Atromid-S Capsules 3483

REGELAN N (Germany)
CLOFIBRATE
Atromid-S Capsules 3483

REGEPAR (Austria, Switzerland)
SELEGILINE HYDROCHLORIDE
Eldepryl Capsules 3266

REGIBLOC (South Africa)
BUPIVACAINE HYDROCHLORIDE
Sensorcaine Injection 643
Sensorcaine-MPF Injection 643

REGINERTON (Germany)
METOCLOPRAMIDE HYDROCHLORIDE
Reglan Injectable 2935
Reglan Syrup 2935
Reglan Tablets 2935

REGLAN (Canada, Portugal)
METOCLOPRAMIDE HYDROCHLORIDE
Reglan Injectable 2935
Reglan Syrup 2935
Reglan Tablets 2935

REGOMED (Austria)
ENALAPRIL MALEATE
Vasotec Tablets 2210

REGONOL (Canada)
PYRIDOSTIGMINE BROMIDE
Mestinon Syrup 1740
Mestinon Tablets 1740
Mestinon Timespan Tablets 1740

REGRANEX (Canada, France, Germany, Israel, Mexico, Singapore, Sweden, United Kingdom)
BECAPLERMIN
Regranex Gel 2586

(⊙ Described in PDR For Ophthalmic Medicines™)

REGULACT (Mexico)
LACTULOSE
Kristalose for Oral Solution 1007

REGULOSE (United Kingdom)
LACTULOSE
Kristalose for Oral Solution 1007

REJUVA-A (Canada)
TRETINOIN
Avita Cream 999
Avita Gel 1000
Renova 0.05% Cream 2519
Retin-A Micro 0.1% 2522
Vesanoid Capsules 3037

REKAWAN (Austria, Germany)
POTASSIUM CHLORIDE
K-Dur Microburst Release System ER Tablets 1832
K-Lor Powder Packets 469
K-Tab Filmtab Tablets 470
Rum-K 1363

RELAFEN (Canada)
NABUMETONE
Relafen Tablets 1617

RELASAN (Mexico)
DIAZEPAM
Valium Injectable 3026
Valium Tablets 3047

RELASTEF (Italy)
TRETINOIN
Avita Cream 999
Avita Gel 1000
Renova 0.05% Cream 2519
Retin-A Micro 0.1% 2522
Vesanoid Capsules 3037

RELAXIN-P (Hong Kong)
CHLORZOXAZONE
Parafon Forte DSC Caplets 2582

RELAZEPAM (Mexico)
DIAZEPAM
Valium Injectable 3026
Valium Tablets 3047

RELCOFEN (United Kingdom)
IBUPROFEN
Motrin Suspension, Oral Drops, Chewable Tablets, and Caplets 2002

RELEFACT TRH (Austria, Canada, Germany, Israel, Switzerland, The Netherlands)
PROTIRELIN
Thyrel TRH for Injection 3630

RELIBERAN (Italy)
CHLORDIAZEPOXIDE HYDROCHLORIDE
Librium Capsules 1736
Librium for Injection 1737

RELIF (Spain)
NABUMETONE
Relafen Tablets 1617

RELIFEN (South Africa)
NABUMETONE
Relafen Tablets 1617

RELIFEX (Belgium, Brazil, Denmark, Finland, Hong Kong, Irish Republic, Israel, Italy, Mexico, Norway, Singapore, Sweden, Thailand, United Kingdom)
NABUMETONE
Relafen Tablets 1617

RELIPAIN (Italy)
MORPHINE SULFATE
Astramorph/PF Injection, USP (Preservative-Free) 594
Duramorph Injection 1312
Infumorph 200 and Infumorph 500 Sterile Solutions 1314
Kadian Capsules 1335
MS Contin Tablets 2896
MSIR Oral Capsules 2898
MSIR Oral Solution 2898
MSIR Oral Solution Concentrate 2898
MSIR Oral Tablets 2898
Oramorph SR Tablets 3062
Roxanol 100 Concentrated Oral Solution 3066
Roxanol Concentrated Oral Solution 3066
Roxanol-T Oral Solution 3066

RELISAN (South Africa)
NABUMETONE
Relafen Tablets 1617

RELITONE (South Africa)
NABUMETONE
Relafen Tablets 1617

RELOCICLINA (Spain)
DOXYCYCLINE HYCLATE
Doryx Coated Pellet Filled Capsules 3357
Periostat Tablets 1208
Vibra-Tabs Film Coated Tablets 2735
Vibramycin Hyclate Capsules 2735
Vibramycin Hyclate Intravenous 2737

RELOXYL (Italy)
BENZOYL PEROXIDE
Brevoxyl-4 Cleansing Lotion 3269
Brevoxyl-4 Creamy Wash 3270
Brevoxyl-4 Gel 3269
Brevoxyl-8 Cleansing Lotion 3269
Brevoxyl-8 Creamy Wash 3270
Brevoxyl-8 Gel 3269
Triaz Cleanser 2026
Triaz Gel 2026

REMAFEN (Hong Kong, Singapore)
DICLOFENAC SODIUM
Voltaren Tablets 2315
Voltaren-XR Tablets 2315

REMEDERM HC (Germany)
HYDROCORTISONE
Anusol-HC Cream 2.5% 2237
Hydrocortone Tablets 2106

REMERON (Austria, Denmark, Finland, Hong Kong, Israel, Italy, Mexico, Portugal, Singapore, South Africa, Sweden, Thailand, The Netherlands)
MIRTAZAPINE
Remeron SolTab Tablets 2486

REMETHAN R (Hong Kong)
DICLOFENAC SODIUM
Voltaren Tablets 2315
Voltaren-XR Tablets 2315

REMICADE (Denmark, Finland, France, Germany, Irish Republic, Italy, Portugal, Spain, Sweden, The Netherlands, United Kingdom)
INFLIXIMAB
Remicade for IV Injection 1178

REMICYCLIN D (Germany)
DOXYCYCLINE HYCLATE
Doryx Coated Pellet Filled Capsules 3357
Periostat Tablets 1208
Vibramycin Hyclate Capsules 2735
Vibramycin Hyclate Intravenous 2737
Vibra-Tabs Film Coated Tablets 2735

REMONTAL (Spain)
NIMODIPINE
Nimotop Capsules 904

RENACOR (Germany)
ENALAPRIL MALEATE/HYDROCHLOROTHIAZIDE
Vaseretic Tablets 2204

RENAGEL (Irish Republic, United Kingdom)
SEVELAMER HYDROCHLORIDE
Renagel Capsules 1439

RENASE (Thailand)
AMILORIDE HYDROCHLORIDE/HYDROCHLOROTHIAZIDE
Moduretic Tablets 2138

RENATON (Singapore)
ENALAPRIL MALEATE
Vasotec Tablets 2210

RENEDIL (Belgium, Canada, The Netherlands)
FELODIPINE
Plendil Extended-Release Tablets 623

RENESE (Belgium, France, Norway, Sweden)
POLYTHIAZIDE
Renese Tablets 2712

RENESE R (Spain)
POLYTHIAZIDE
Renese Tablets 2712

RENEZIDE (South Africa)
HYDROCHLOROTHIAZIDE/TRIAMTERENE
Dyazide Capsules 1515
Maxzide Tablets 1008
Maxzide-25 mg Tablets 1008

RENIDUR (Portugal)
ENALAPRIL MALEATE/HYDROCHLOROTHIAZIDE
Vaseretic Tablets 2204

RENIPRIL (Portugal)
ENALAPRIL MALEATE
Vasotec Tablets 2210

RENITEC (Australia, Belgium, Denmark, France, Hong Kong, Mexico, New Zealand, Singapore, South Africa, Thailand)
ENALAPRIL MALEATE
Vasotec Tablets 2210

RENITEC COMP (Finland, Norway, Sweden)
ENALAPRIL MALEATE/HYDROCHLOROTHIAZIDE
Vaseretic Tablets 2204

RENITEC PLUS (Australia, Austria, Finland, The Netherlands)
ENALAPRIL MALEATE/HYDROCHLOROTHIAZIDE
Vaseretic Tablets 2204

RENITECMAX (Spain)
ENALAPRIL MALEATE/HYDROCHLOROTHIAZIDE
Vaseretic Tablets 2204

RENITEN PLUS (Switzerland)
ENALAPRIL MALEATE/HYDROCHLOROTHIAZIDE
Vaseretic Tablets 2204

RENOVA (Canada, South Africa, Thailand)
TRETINOIN
Avita Cream 999
Avita Gel 1000
Renova 0.05% Cream 2519
Retin-A Micro 0.1% 2522
Vesanoid Capsules 3037

RENTIBLOC (Germany)
SOTALOL HYDROCHLORIDE
Betapace Tablets 950

REOPRO (Australia, Austria, Belgium, Canada, Denmark, Finland, France, Germany, Hong Kong, Irish Republic, Israel, Italy, New Zealand, Norway, Singapore, South Africa, Spain, Sweden, Switzerland, Thailand, The Netherlands, United Kingdom)
ABCIXIMAB
ReoPro Vials 1958

REPERVIT (Italy)
VITAMIN A PALMITATE
Aquasol A Parenteral 593

REPOSO-MONO (Belgium)
MEPROBAMATE
Miltown Tablets 3349

REPRIADOL (Denmark)
MORPHINE SULFATE
Astramorph/PF Injection, USP (Preservative-Free) 594
Duramorph Injection 1312
Infumorph 200 and Infumorph 500 Sterile Solutions 1314
Kadian Capsules 1335
MS Contin Tablets 2896
MSIR Oral Capsules 2898
MSIR Oral Solution 2898
MSIR Oral Solution Concentrate 2898
MSIR Oral Tablets 2898
Oramorph SR Tablets 3062
Roxanol 100 Concentrated Oral Solution 3066
Roxanol Concentrated Oral Solution 3066
Roxanol-T Oral Solution 3066

REQUIP (Austria, Belgium, Canada, Denmark, France, Germany, Hong Kong, Irish Republic, Israel, Italy, Norway, Portugal, Spain, Sweden, Switzerland, The Netherlands, United Kingdom)
ROPINIROLE HYDROCHLORIDE
Requip Tablets 1621

RESERIL (Italy)
NEFAZODONE HYDROCHLORIDE
Serzone Tablets 1104

RESIDEX P55 (United Kingdom)
PERMETHRIN
Acticin Cream 998
Elimite Cream 552

RESMA (Belgium)
ZAFIRLUKAST
Accolate Tablets 657

RESOCHIN (Germany, Spain)
CHLOROQUINE PHOSPHATE
Aralen Tablets 3075

RESOCHINA (Portugal)
CHLOROQUINE PHOSPHATE
Aralen Tablets 3075

RESOCHINE (Switzerland)
CHLOROQUINE PHOSPHATE
Aralen Tablets 3075

RESPEXIL (Brazil)
NORFLOXACIN
Chibroxin Sterile Ophthalmic Solution . . . . ⊙273, 2051
Noroxin Tablets 2145

RESPICILIN (Brazil)
AMOXICILLIN
Amoxil Pediatric Drops for Oral Suspension 1471
Amoxil Tablets 1471

RESPICORT (Switzerland)
TRIAMCINOLONE ACETONIDE
Azmacort Inhalation Aerosol 728
Nasacort AQ Nasal Spray 752
Nasacort Nasal Inhaler 750

RESPICORT (Germany)
BUDESONIDE
Pulmicort Turbuhaler Inhalation Powder . . . 636
Rhinocort Nasal Inhaler 640

RESPICUR (Austria, Italy)
THEOPHYLLINE
Aerolate Jr. T.D. Capsules 1361
Aerolate Liquid 1361
Aerolate Sr. T.D. Capsules 1361
Theo-Dur Extended-Release Tablets 1835
Uni-Dur Extended-Release Tablets 1841
Uniphyl 400 mg and 600 mg Tablets . . . 2903

RESPIROL (Sweden)
TERBUTALINE SULFATE
Brethine Ampuls 2314
Brethine Tablets 2313

RESPONTIN (Norway, United Kingdom)
IPRATROPIUM BROMIDE
Atrovent Inhalation Aerosol 1030
Atrovent Inhalation Solution 1031
Atrovent Nasal Spray 0.03% 1032
Atrovent Nasal Spray 0.06% 1033

RESTENIL (Sweden)
MEPROBAMATE
Miltown Tablets 3349

RESYL (Austria, Canada, Israel, Italy, Sweden, Switzerland)
GUAIFENESIN
Organidin NR Liquid 3350
Organidin NR Tablets 3350

RESYL MIT CODEIN (Austria)
CODEINE PHOSPHATE/GUAIFENESIN
Robitussin A-C Syrup 2942
Tussi-Organidin NR Liquid 3350
Tussi-Organidin-S NR Liquid 3350

RESYL PLUS (Switzerland)
CODEINE PHOSPHATE/GUAIFENESIN
Robitussin A-C Syrup 2942
Tussi-Organidin NR Liquid 3350
Tussi-Organidin-S NR Liquid 3350

RETACNYL (France, Hong Kong, Mexico, Singapore, Thailand)
TRETINOIN
Avita Cream 999
Avita Gel 1000
Renova 0.05% Cream 2519
Retin-A Micro 0.1% 2522
Vesanoid Capsules 3037

RETAFYLLIN (Finland, Singapore, Thailand)
THEOPHYLLINE
Aerolate Jr. T.D. Capsules 1361
Aerolate Liquid 1361
Aerolate Sr. T.D. Capsules 1361
Theo-Dur Extended-Release Tablets 1835
Uni-Dur Extended-Release Tablets 1841
Uniphyl 400 mg and 600 mg Tablets . . . 2903

RETALZEM (Hong Kong)
DILTIAZEM HYDROCHLORIDE
Cardizem CD Capsules 1016
Cardizem Injectable 1018
Cardizem Lyo-Ject Syringe 1018
Cardizem Monovial 1018
Tiazac Capsules 1378

RET-A-PRES (Mexico)
TRETINOIN
Avita Cream 999
Avita Gel 1000
Renova 0.05% Cream 2519
Retin-A Micro 0.1% 2522
Vesanoid Capsules 3037

RETAVIT (Israel)
TRETINOIN
Avita Cream 999
Avita Gel 1000
Renova 0.05% Cream 2519
Retin-A Micro 0.1% 2522
Vesanoid Capsules 3037

RETCIN (United Kingdom)
ERYTHROMYCIN
Emgel 2% Topical Gel 1285
Ery-Tab Tablets 448
Erythromycin Base Filmtab Tablets 454
Erythromycin Delayed-Release Capsules, USP 455
PCE Dispertab Tablets 498

RETENS (Spain)
DOXYCYCLINE HYCLATE
Doryx Coated Pellet Filled Capsules 3357
Periostat Tablets 1208
Vibramycin Hyclate Capsules 2735

Vibramycin Hyclate Intravenous 2737
Vibra-Tabs Film Coated Tablets 2735

RETICUS (Italy)
DESONIDE
DesOwen Cream 1401
DesOwen Lotion 1401
DesOwen Ointment 1401

RETIN-A (Australia, Austria, Brazil, Canada, France, Hong Kong, Irish Republic, Israel, Italy, Mexico, New Zealand, Portugal, Singapore, South Africa, Switzerland, Thailand, United Kingdom)
TRETINOIN
Avita Cream 999
Avita Gel 1000
Renova 0.05% Cream 2519
Retin-A Micro 0.1% 2522
Vesanoid Capsules 3037

RETINOVA (Belgium, France, New Zealand, Spain, Sweden, United Kingdom)
TRETINOIN
Avita Cream 999
Avita Gel 1000
Renova 0.05% Cream 2519
Retin-A Micro 0.1% 2522
Vesanoid Capsules 3037

RETIRIDES (Spain)
TRETINOIN
Avita Cream 999
Avita Gel 1000
Renova 0.05% Cream 2519
Retin-A Micro 0.1% 2522
Vesanoid Capsules 3037

RETISOL-A (Canada)
TRETINOIN
Avita Cream 999
Avita Gel 1000
Renova 0.05% Cream 2519
Retin-A Micro 0.1% 2522
Vesanoid Capsules 3037

RETITOP (France)
TRETINOIN
Avita Cream 999
Avita Gel 1000
Renova 0.05% Cream 2519
Retin-A Micro 0.1% 2522
Vesanoid Capsules 3037

RETOFAR (Mexico)
METRONIDAZOLE
MetroCream 1404
MetroGel 1405
MetroGel-Vaginal Gel 1986
MetroLotion 1405
Noritate Cream 1224

RETRIEVE (Australia)
TRETINOIN
Avita Cream 999
Avita Gel 1000
Renova 0.05% Cream 2519
Retin-A Micro 0.1% 2522
Vesanoid Capsules 3037

RETROVIR (Australia, Austria, Belgium, Brazil, Canada, Denmark, Finland, France, Germany, Hong Kong, Irish Republic, Israel, Italy, Mexico, New Zealand, Norway, Portugal, Singapore, South Africa, Spain, Sweden, Switzerland, Thailand, The Netherlands, United Kingdom)
ZIDOVUDINE
Retrovir Capsules 1625
Retrovir IV Infusion 1629
Retrovir Syrup 1625
Retrovir Tablets 1625

REUCAM (Italy, Mexico)
PIROXICAM
Feldene Capsules 2685

REUDENE (Italy)
PIROXICAM
Feldene Capsules 2685

REUFEL (Mexico)
PIROXICAM
Feldene Capsules 2685

REUFLOS (Italy)
DIFLUNISAL
Dolobid Tablets 2088

REUMAGIL (Italy)
PIROXICAM
Feldene Capsules 2685

REUMAREN (Brazil)
DICLOFENAC SODIUM
Voltaren Tablets 2315
Voltaren-XR Tablets 2315

REUMAZINE (Brazil)
PREDNISOLONE
Prelone Syrup 2273

REUMOPHAN (Mexico)
KETOPROFEN
Orudis Capsules 3548
Oruvail Capsules 3548

REUMOQUIN (Spain)
KETOPROFEN
Orudis Capsules 3548
Oruvail Capsules 3548

REUMOXICAN (Portugal)
PIROXICAM
Feldene Capsules 2685

REUMYL (Italy)
SULINDAC
Clinoril Tablets 2053

REUPLEX (Brazil)
IBUPROFEN
Motrin Suspension, Oral Drops, Chewable Tablets, and Caplets 2002

REUPROFEN (Italy)
KETOPROFEN
Orudis Capsules 3548
Oruvail Capsules 3548

REUSAN (Mexico)
DEXAMETHASONE
Decadron Elixir 2078
Decadron Tablets 2079

REUTOL (Italy)
TOLMETIN SODIUM
Tolectin 200 Tablets 2589
Tolectin 600 Tablets 2589
Tolectin DS Capsules 2589

REUTRICAM (Mexico)
PIROXICAM
Feldene Capsules 2685

REUXEN (Portugal)
NAPROXEN
EC-Naprosyn Delayed-Release Tablets . . . 2967
Naprosyn Suspension 2967
Naprosyn Tablets 2967

REVAPOL (Mexico)
MEBENDAZOLE
Vermox Chewable Tablets 2017

REWODINA (Germany)
DICLOFENAC SODIUM
Voltaren Tablets 2315
Voltaren-XR Tablets 2315

REXACIN (Thailand)
NORFLOXACIN
Chibroxin Sterile Ophthalmic Solution . . . . ⊙273, 2051
Noroxin Tablets 2145

REXER (Spain)
MIRTAZAPINE
Remeron SolTab Tablets 2486

REXGENTA (Spain)
GENTAMICIN SULFATE
Genoptic Ophthalmic Ointment . . . . ⊙239
Genoptic Sterile Ophthalmic Solution . . . ⊙239

REXIGEN (South Africa)
PROPRANOLOL HYDROCHLORIDE
Inderal Injectable 3513
Inderal LA Long-Acting Capsules 3516
Inderal Tablets 3513

REXILEN (Spain)
DOXYCYCLINE HYCLATE
Doryx Coated Pellet Filled Capsules 3357
Periostat Tablets 1208
Vibramycin Hyclate Capsules 2735
Vibramycin Hyclate Intravenous 2737
Vibra-Tabs Film Coated Tablets 2735

R-FLEX (South Africa)
SULINDAC
Clinoril Tablets 2053

RHEFLUIN (Germany, Switzerland)
AMILORIDE HYDROCHLORIDE/HYDROCHLOROTHIAZIDE
Moduretic Tablets 2138

RHEMOFENAX (Hong Kong)
DICLOFENAC SODIUM
Voltaren Tablets 2315
Voltaren-XR Tablets 2315

RHEUFENAC (Switzerland)
DICLOFENAC SODIUM
Voltaren Tablets 2315
Voltaren-XR Tablets 2315

RHEUFLEX (United Kingdom)
NAPROXEN
EC-Naprosyn Delayed-Release Tablets . . . 2967
Naprosyn Suspension 2967
Naprosyn Tablets 2967

RHEUGESIC (South Africa)
PIROXICAM
Feldene Capsules 2685

RHEUMANOX (Thailand)
IBUPROFEN
Motrin Suspension, Oral Drops, Chewable Tablets, and Caplets 2002

RHEUMASAN D (Germany)
DICLOFENAC SODIUM
Voltaren Tablets 2315
Voltaren-XR Tablets 2315

RHEUMATAC (United Kingdom)
DICLOFENAC SODIUM
Voltaren Tablets 2315
Voltaren-XR Tablets 2315

RHEUMITIN (Germany)
PIROXICAM
Feldene Capsules 2685

RHINALAR (Australia, Canada, Hong Kong)
FLUNISOLIDE
Aerobid Inhaler System 1363
Aerobid-M Inhaler System 1363
Nasalide Nasal Spray 1295
Nasarel Nasal Solution 0.025% 1296

RHINARIS-F (Canada)
FLUNISOLIDE
Aerobid Inhaler System 1363
Aerobid-M Inhaler System 1363
Nasalide Nasal Spray 1295
Nasarel Nasal Solution 0.025% 1296

RHINEX (Germany)
NAPHAZOLINE HYDROCHLORIDE
Albalon Ophthalmic Solution . . . . ⊙225

RHINOCORT (Australia, Belgium, Canada, Denmark, Finland, Hong Kong, Irish Republic, Italy, Mexico, New Zealand, Norway, Singapore, South Africa, Spain, Sweden, Switzerland, Thailand, The Netherlands, United Kingdom)
BUDESONIDE
Pulmicort Turbuhaler Inhalation Powder . . . 636
Rhinocort Nasal Inhaler 640

RHINOCORTOL (Austria)
BUDESONIDE
Pulmicort Turbuhaler Inhalation Powder . . . 636
Rhinocort Nasal Inhaler 640

RHINOFLUINE (Belgium)
PILOCARPINE HYDROCHLORIDE
Isopto Carpine Ophthalmic Solution . . . . ⊙215
Pilopine HS Ophthalmic Gel . . . . ⊙217
Salagen Tablets 2229

RHINOGEN (Switzerland)
SODIUM HYALURONATE
Hyalgan Solution 3080

RHINOLAST (Irish Republic, New Zealand, South Africa, United Kingdom)
AZELASTINE HYDROCHLORIDE
Astelin Nasal Spray 3339

RHINO-MEX-N (Canada)
NAPHAZOLINE HYDROCHLORIDE
Albalon Ophthalmic Solution . . . . ⊙225

RHINON (Austria)
NAPHAZOLINE HYDROCHLORIDE
Albalon Ophthalmic Solution . . . . ⊙225

RHINOPERD (Austria)
NAPHAZOLINE HYDROCHLORIDE
Albalon Ophthalmic Solution . . . . ⊙225

RHINOSOL (Denmark)
BUDESONIDE
Pulmicort Turbuhaler Inhalation Powder . . . 636
Rhinocort Nasal Inhaler 640

RHINOVENT (Switzerland)
IPRATROPIUM BROMIDE
Atrovent Inhalation Aerosol 1030
Atrovent Inhalation Solution 1031
Atrovent Nasal Spray 0.03% 1032
Atrovent Nasal Spray 0.06% 1033

RHODIALAX (Canada)
LACTULOSE
Kristalose for Oral Solution 1007

RHODIALOSE (Canada)
LACTULOSE
Kristalose for Oral Solution 1007

RHODIAPROX (Canada)
NAPROXEN
EC-Naprosyn Delayed-Release Tablets . . . 2967
Naprosyn Suspension 2967
Naprosyn Tablets 2967

RHODIS (Canada)
KETOPROFEN
Orudis Capsules 3548
Oruvail Capsules 3548

RHONURACIL (Mexico)
FLUOROURACIL
Efudex Cream 1733
Efudex Topical Solutions 1733
Fluoroplex Topical Cream 552
Fluoroplex Topical Solution 552

RHOTRAL (Canada)
ACEBUTOLOL HYDROCHLORIDE
Sectral Capsules 3589

RHOTRIMINE (Canada)
TRIMIPRAMINE MALEATE
Surmontil Capsules 3595

RHOVAIL (Canada)
KETOPROFEN
Orudis Capsules 3548
Oruvail Capsules 3548

RHUMALGAN (Switzerland, United Kingdom)
DICLOFENAC SODIUM
Voltaren Tablets 2315
Voltaren-XR Tablets 2315

RHUMANTIN (Denmark)
PENICILLAMINE
Cuprimine Capsules 2075
Depen Titratable Tablets 3341

RHYTHMOCOR (Austria)
PROPAFENONE HYDROCHLORIDE
Rythmol Tablets – 150 mg, 225 mg, 300 mg 502

RIACEN (Italy)
PIROXICAM
Feldene Capsules 2685

RIBEX FLU (Italy)
DICLOFENAC SODIUM
Voltaren Tablets 2315
Voltaren-XR Tablets 2315

RIBOCARBO (Germany)
CARBOPLATIN
Paraplatin for Injection 1126

RIBOCICLINA (Italy)
DOXYCYCLINE HYCLATE
Doryx Coated Pellet Filled Capsules 3357
Periostat Tablets 1208
Vibramycin Hyclate Capsules 2735
Vibramycin Hyclate Intravenous 2737
Vibra-Tabs Film Coated Tablets 2735

RIBODOXO-L (Germany)
DOXORUBICIN HYDROCHLORIDE
Adriamycin PFS/RDF Injection 2767

RIBOFLUOR (Germany)
FLUOROURACIL
Efudex Cream 1733
Efudex Topical Solutions 1733
Fluoroplex Topical Cream 552
Fluoroplex Topical Solution 552

RIBOMICIN (Italy)
GENTAMICIN SULFATE
Genoptic Ophthalmic Ointment . . . . ⊙239
Genoptic Sterile Ophthalmic Solution . . . ⊙239

RIBUFEN (Mexico)
IBUPROFEN
Motrin Suspension, Oral Drops, Chewable Tablets, and Caplets 2002

RIBUJET (Spain)
BUDESONIDE
Pulmicort Turbuhaler Inhalation Powder . . . 636
Rhinocort Nasal Inhaler 640

RIBUSOL (Spain)
BUDESONIDE
Pulmicort Turbuhaler Inhalation Powder . . . 636
Rhinocort Nasal Inhaler 640

RIDAMIN (Thailand)
LORATADINE
Claritin Reditabs 3100
Claritin Syrup 3100
Claritin Tablets 3100

RIDAZIN (Israel)
THIORIDAZINE HYDROCHLORIDE
Thioridazine Hydrochloride Tablets 2289

RIDAZINE (South Africa, Thailand)
THIORIDAZINE HYDROCHLORIDE
Thioridazine Hydrochloride Tablets 2289

RIDENE (Mexico)
NICARDIPINE HYDROCHLORIDE
Cardene I.V. 3485

RIFLOC (Germany)
ISOSORBIDE DINITRATE
Isordil Sublingual Tablets 3525
Isordil Titradose Tablets 3526

RILAMIR (Denmark)
TRIAZOLAM
Halcion Tablets 2823

RILATINE (Belgium)
METHYLPHENIDATE HYDROCHLORIDE
Methylin Tablets 1995
Ritalin Hydrochloride Tablets 2387
Ritalin-SR Tablets 2387

RILCAPTON (Singapore)
CAPTOPRIL
Captopril Tablets 2281

RILUTEK (Austria, Belgium, Denmark, Finland, France, Germany, Hong Kong, Irish Republic, Israel, Italy, Japan, Mexico, Norway, Portugal, Singapore, South Africa, Spain, Sweden, Switzerland, Thailand, The Netherlands, United Kingdom)
RILUZOLE
Rilutek Tablets 772

RIMAFEN (United Kingdom)
IBUPROFEN
Motrin Suspension, Oral Drops, Chewable Tablets, and Caplets 2002

RIMAFUNGOL (Spain)
CICLOPIROX OLAMINE
Loprox Cream 2021
Loprox Lotion 2021

RIMAPAM (United Kingdom)
DIAZEPAM
Valium Injectable 3026
Valium Tablets 3047

RIMIDOL (Sweden)
NAPHAZOLINE HYDROCHLORIDE
Albalon Ophthalmic Solution . . . . ⊙225

RIMOXYN (United Kingdom)
NAPROXEN
EC-Naprosyn Delayed-Release Tablets . . . 2967
Naprosyn Suspension 2967
Naprosyn Tablets 2967

RINACTIVE (Spain)
BUDESONIDE
Pulmicort Turbuhaler Inhalation Powder . . . 636
Rhinocort Nasal Inhaler 640

RINADINE (Thailand)
CIMETIDINE
Tagamet Tablets 1644

RINATEC (Irish Republic, United Kingdom)
IPRATROPIUM BROMIDE
Atrovent Inhalation Aerosol 1030
Atrovent Inhalation Solution 1031
Atrovent Nasal Spray 0.03% 1032
Atrovent Nasal Spray 0.06% 1033

RINELON (Italy, Mexico, Spain)
MOMETASONE FUROATE
Elocon Cream 0.1% 3110
Elocon Lotion 0.1% 3111
Elocon Ointment 0.1% 3112
Nasonex Nasal Spray 3131

RINO NAFTAZOLINA (Italy)
NAPHAZOLINE HYDROCHLORIDE
Albalon Ophthalmic Solution . . . . ⊙225

RINOBEREN (Spain)
IPRATROPIUM BROMIDE
Atrovent Inhalation Aerosol 1030
Atrovent Inhalation Solution 1031
Atrovent Nasal Spray 0.03% 1032
Atrovent Nasal Spray 0.06% 1033

RINOJET SF (Italy)
NEOMYCIN SULFATE/POLYMYXIN B SULFATE
Neosporin G.U. Irrigant Sterile 2256

RINO-LASTIN (Brazil)
AZELASTINE HYDROCHLORIDE
Astelin Nasal Spray 3339

RINOSONE (Spain)
FLUTICASONE PROPIONATE
Cutivate Cream 1282
Cutivate Ointment 1284
Flonase Nasal Spray 1533
Flovent 110 mcg Inhalation Aerosol 1535
Flovent 220 mcg Inhalation Aerosol 1535
Flovent 44 mcg Inhalation Aerosol 1535
Flovent Rotadisk 100 mcg 1537
Flovent Rotadisk 250 mcg 1537
Flovent Rotadisk 50 mcg 1537

RINOVAGOS (Italy)
IPRATROPIUM BROMIDE
Atrovent Inhalation Aerosol 1030
Atrovent Inhalation Solution 1031
Atrovent Nasal Spray 0.03% 1032
Atrovent Nasal Spray 0.06% 1033

RIPHENIDATE (Canada)
METHYLPHENIDATE HYDROCHLORIDE
Methylin Tablets 1995
Ritalin Hydrochloride Tablets 2387
Ritalin-SR Tablets 2387

RISEK (United Arab Emirates)
OMEPRAZOLE
Prilosec Delayed-Release Capsules 628

RISIDON (Portugal)
METFORMIN HYDROCHLORIDE
Glucophage Tablets 1080

RISORDAN (France)
ISOSORBIDE DINITRATE
Isordil Sublingual Tablets 3525
Isordil Titradose Tablets 3526

RISPERDAL (Australia, Austria, Belgium, Brazil, Denmark, Finland, Hong Kong, Irish Republic, Israel, Italy, Japan, Mexico, New Zealand, Norway, Portugal, Singapore, South Africa, Spain, Switzerland, Thailand, The Netherlands, United Kingdom)
RISPERIDONE
Risperdal Oral Solution 1796
Risperdal Tablets 1796

RISPOLIN (Austria)
RISPERIDONE
Risperdal Oral Solution 1796
Risperdal Tablets 1796

RISTALEN (Spain)
ENALAPRIL MALEATE
Vasotec Tablets 2210

RISTO (Thailand)
TRIAMCINOLONE ACETONIDE
Azmacort Inhalation Aerosol 728
Nasacort AQ Nasal Spray 752
Nasacort Nasal Inhaler 750

RITALIN (Australia, Austria, Canada, Denmark, Germany, Hong Kong, Irish Republic, Israel, Mexico, New Zealand, Norway, Singapore, South Africa, The Netherlands, United Kingdom)
METHYLPHENIDATE HYDROCHLORIDE
Methylin Tablets 1995
Ritalin Hydrochloride Tablets 2387
Ritalin-SR Tablets 2387

RITALINA (Brazil)
METHYLPHENIDATE HYDROCHLORIDE
Methylin Tablets 1995
Ritalin Hydrochloride Tablets 2387
Ritalin-SR Tablets 2387

RITALINE (France, Switzerland)
METHYLPHENIDATE HYDROCHLORIDE
Methylin Tablets 1995
Ritalin Hydrochloride Tablets 2387
Ritalin-SR Tablets 2387

RITMONORM (Brazil)
PROPAFENONE HYDROCHLORIDE
Rythmol Tablets – 150 mg, 225 mg, 300 mg 502

RIVATRIL (Finland)
CLONAZEPAM
Klonopin Tablets 2983

RIVOSIL (Italy)
HYDROFLUMETHIAZIDE
Diucardin Tablets 3494

RIVOSTATIN (Switzerland)
NYSTATIN
Nystop Topical Powder USP 2608

RIVOTRIL (Australia, Austria, Belgium, Brazil, Canada, Denmark, France, Germany, Hong Kong, Irish Republic, Israel, Italy, Mexico, New Zealand, Norway, Portugal, Singapore, South Africa, Spain, Switzerland, Thailand, The Netherlands, United Kingdom)
CLONAZEPAM
Klonopin Tablets 2983

RIVOXICILLIN (Switzerland)
AMOXICILLIN
Amoxil Pediatric Drops for Oral Suspension 1471
Amoxil Tablets 1471

RIZALIV (Italy)
RIZATRIPTAN BENZOATE
Maxalt Tablets 2120
Maxalt-MLT Orally Disintegrating Tablets . . 2120

RMS (New Zealand)
MORPHINE SULFATE
Astramorph/PF Injection, USP (Preservative-Free) 594
Duramorph Injection 1312
Infumorph 200 and Infumorph 500 Sterile Solutions 1314
Kadian Capsules 1335
MS Contin Tablets 2896
MSIR Oral Capsules 2898
MSIR Oral Solution 2898
MSIR Oral Solution Concentrate 2898
MSIR Oral Tablets 2898
Oramorph SR Tablets 3062
Roxanol 100 Concentrated Oral Solution 3066
Roxanol Concentrated Oral Solution 3066
Roxanol-T Oral Solution 3066

ROACCUTAN (Austria, Denmark, Finland, Germany, Italy, Mexico, Portugal)
ISOTRETINOIN
Accutane Capsules 2944

ROACCUTANE (Australia, Belgium, France, Hong Kong, Irish Republic, Israel, New Zealand, Singapore, South Africa, Switzerland, Thailand, The Netherlands, United Kingdom)
ISOTRETINOIN
Accutane Capsules 2944

ROACUTAN (Brazil, Spain)
ISOTRETINOIN
Accutane Capsules 2944

RO-A-VIT (New Zealand, United Kingdom)
VITAMIN A PALMITATE
Aquasol A Parenteral 593

ROBAXIFEN (Mexico)
METHOCARBAMOL
Robaxin Injectable 2938
Robaxin Tablets 2939
Robaxin-750 Tablets 2939

ROBAXIN (Australia, Canada, Finland, Hong Kong, Mexico, South Africa, Spain, Sweden, Thailand, United Kingdom)
METHOCARBAMOL
Robaxin Injectable 2938
Robaxin Tablets 2939
Robaxin-750 Tablets 2939

ROBAXISAL (Canada, Germany, Irish Republic, Mexico, South Africa, Spain)
ASPIRIN/METHOCARBAMOL
Robaxisal Tablets 2939

ROBAXISAL FORTE (Sweden, United Kingdom)
METHOCARBAMOL
Robaxin Injectable 2938
Robaxin Tablets 2939
Robaxin-750 Tablets 2939

ROBITUSSIN (Australia, Canada, Germany, Israel, Italy, Singapore, Spain, Sweden, Thailand)
GUAIFENESIN
Organidin NR Liquid 3350
Organidin NR Tablets 3350

ROBITUSSIN COLD (Singapore)
GUAIFENESIN/PSEUDOEPHEDRINE HYDROCHLORIDE
Guaifed Capsules 2272
Guaifed-PD Capsules 2272
Zephrex LA Tablets 3092
Zephrex Tablets 3091

ROBITUSSIN DM (Canada, Singapore, Thailand)
DEXTROMETHORPHAN HYDROBROMIDE/GUAIFENESIN
Tussi-Organidin DM NR Liquid 3350
Tussi-Organidin DM-S NR Liquid 3350

ROBITUSSIN EX (Australia)
GUAIFENESIN
Organidin NR Liquid 3350
Organidin NR Tablets 3350

ROBITUSSIN EXPECTORANT (Hong Kong, Irish Republic)
GUAIFENESIN
Organidin NR Liquid 3350
Organidin NR Tablets 3350

ROBITUSSIN EXPECTORANT PLUS (Irish Republic)
GUAIFENESIN/PSEUDOEPHEDRINE HYDROCHLORIDE
Guaifed Capsules 2272
Guaifed-PD Capsules 2272
Zephrex LA Tablets 3092
Zephrex Tablets 3091

ROBITUSSIN FOR CHESTY COUGHS (United Kingdom)
GUAIFENESIN
Organidin NR Liquid 3350
Organidin NR Tablets 3350

ROBITUSSIN FOR CHESTY COUGHS WITH CONGESTION (United Kingdom)
GUAIFENESIN/PSEUDOEPHEDRINE HYDROCHLORIDE
Guaifed Capsules 2272
Guaifed-PD Capsules 2272
Zephrex LA Tablets 3092
Zephrex Tablets 3091

ROBITUSSIN NIGHT-TIME (United Kingdom)
BROMPHENIRAMINE MALEATE/PSEUDOEPHEDRINE HYDROCHLORIDE
Bromfed Capsules (Extended-Release) . . . 2269
Bromfed-PD Capsules (Extended-Release) 2269

ROBITUSSIN PE (Canada, Hong Kong, Singapore, Thailand)
GUAIFENESIN/PSEUDOEPHEDRINE HYDROCHLORIDE
Guaifed Capsules 2272
Guaifed-PD Capsules 2272
Zephrex LA Tablets 3092
Zephrex Tablets 3091

ROBITUSSIN PLUS (Germany)
DEXTROMETHORPHAN HYDROBROMIDE/GUAIFENESIN
Tussi-Organidin DM NR Liquid 3350
Tussi-Organidin DM-S NR Liquid 3350

ROCALTROL (Australia, Austria, Belgium, Brazil, Canada, Denmark, France, Germany, Hong Kong, Irish Republic, Italy, Mexico, New Zealand, Norway, Portugal, Singapore, South Africa, Spain, Sweden, Switzerland, Thailand, The Netherlands, United Kingdom)
CALCITRIOL
Calcijex Injection 411
Rocaltrol Capsules 2991
Rocaltrol Oral Solution 2991

RO-CARPINE (Canada)
PILOCARPINE HYDROCHLORIDE
Isopto Carpine Ophthalmic Solution . . . . ⊙215
Pilopine HS Ophthalmic Gel . . . . ⊙217
Salagen Tablets 2229

ROCCAXIN (Thailand)
PIROXICAM
Feldene Capsules 2685

ROCEFALIN (Spain)
CEFTRIAXONE SODIUM
Rocephin Injectable Vials, ADD-Vantage, Galaxy, Bulk 2993

ROCEFIN (Brazil, Italy)
CEFTRIAXONE SODIUM
Rocephin Injectable Vials, ADD-Vantage, Galaxy, Bulk 2993

ROCEPHALIN (Denmark, Finland, Norway, Sweden)
CEFTRIAXONE SODIUM
Rocephin Injectable Vials, ADD-Vantage, Galaxy, Bulk 2993

ROCEPHIN (Australia, Austria, Canada, Germany, Hong Kong, Irish Republic, Israel, Mexico, New Zealand, Portugal, Singapore, South Africa, Thailand, The Netherlands, United Kingdom)
CEFTRIAXONE SODIUM
Rocephin Injectable Vials, ADD-Vantage, Galaxy, Bulk 2993

ROCEPHINE (Belgium, France, Switzerland)
CEFTRIAXONE SODIUM
Rocephin Injectable Vials, ADD-Vantage, Galaxy, Bulk 2993

ROCERON (Norway)
INTERFERON ALFA-2A
Roferon-A Injection 2996

ROCERON-A (Denmark)
INTERFERON ALFA-2A
Roferon-A Injection 2996

ROCHE (Canada)
NAPROXEN SODIUM
Anaprox DS Tablets 2967
Anaprox Tablets 2967
Naprelan Tablets 1293

RODAKIN (Mexico)
LORATADINE
Claritin Reditabs 3100
Claritin Syrup 3100
Claritin Tablets 3100

RODERMIL (Portugal)
METRONIDAZOLE
MetroCream 1404
MetroGel 1405
MetroGel-Vaginal Gel 1986
MetroLotion 1405
Noritate Cream 1224

RO-DEXSONE (Canada)
DEXAMETHASONE SODIUM PHOSPHATE
Decadron Phosphate Injection 2081

(⊙ Described in PDR For Ophthalmic Medicines™)

Decadron Phosphate Sterile Ophthalmic Ointment ...... ⊙280, 2083
Decadron Phosphate Sterile Ophthalmic Solution 2084

RODOMICINA (Spain)
DOXYCYCLINE HYCLATE
Doryx Coated Pellet Filled Capsules 3357
Periostat Tablets 1208
Vibramycin Hyclate Capsules 2735
Vibramycin Hyclate Intravenous 2737
Vibra-Tabs Film Coated Tablets 2735

ROFANTEN (Spain)
NAPROXEN
EC-Naprosyn Delayed-Release Tablets ... 2967
Naprosyn Suspension 2967
Naprosyn Tablets 2967

ROFENID (Belgium)
KETOPROFEN
Orudis Capsules 3548
Oruvail Capsules 3548

ROFEPAIN (Thailand)
KETOPROFEN
Orudis Capsules 3548
Oruvail Capsules 3548

ROFERON-A (Austria, Belgium, Brazil, Finland, Germany, Hong Kong, Israel, Italy, Mexico, New Zealand, Portugal, Singapore, South Africa, Spain, Sweden, Switzerland, Thailand, The Netherlands)
INTERFERON ALFA-2A
Roferon-A Injection 2996

ROFLUAL (France)
RIMANTADINE HYDROCHLORIDE
Flumadine Syrup 1370
Flumadine Tablets 1370

ROGAL (Mexico)
PIROXICAM
Feldene Capsules 2685

ROGASTI (Israel)
FAMOTIDINE
Pepcid Injection 2153
Pepcid Injection Premixed 2153
Pepcid RPD Orally Disintegrating Tablets 2150
Pepcid Tablets 2150
Pepcid for Oral Suspension 2150

RO-GENTYCIN (Canada)
GENTAMICIN SULFATE
Genoptic Ophthalmic Ointment ...... ⊙239
Genoptic Sterile Ophthalmic Solution ... ⊙239

ROICAL (Singapore)
CALCITRIOL
Calcijex Injection 411
Rocaltrol Capsules 2991
Rocaltrol Oral Solution 2991

ROLAB-ANTIFLAM (South Africa)
IBUPROFEN
Motrin Suspension, Oral Drops, Chewable Tablets, and Caplets 2002

ROMESA (Mexico)
WARFARIN SODIUM
Coumadin Tablets 1243
Coumadin for Injection 1243

ROMIN (South Africa)
MINOCYCLINE HYDROCHLORIDE
Dynacin Capsules 2019
Minocin Intravenous 1862
Minocin Oral Suspension 1865
Minocin Pellet-Filled Capsules 1863

ROMIR (Mexico)
CAPTOPRIL
Captopril Tablets 2281

ROMMIX (United Kingdom)
ERYTHROMYCIN
Emgel 2% Topical Gel 1285
Ery-Tab Tablets 448
Erythromycin Base Filmtab Tablets 454
Erythromycin Delayed-Release Capsules, USP 455
PCE Dispertab Tablets 498

RONABIN (Israel)
DRONABINOL
Marinol Capsules 3325

RONAME (Spain)
GLIMEPIRIDE
Amaryl Tablets 717

RO-NAPHZ (Canada)
NAPHAZOLINE HYDROCHLORIDE
Albalon Ophthalmic Solution ...... ⊙225

RONMIX (United Kingdom)
ERYTHROMYCIN
Emgel 2% Topical Gel 1285
Ery-Tab Tablets 448
Erythromycin Base Filmtab Tablets 454
Erythromycin Delayed-Release Capsules, USP 455
PCE Dispertab Tablets 498

RONTILONA (Spain)
FLUTICASONE PROPIONATE
Cutivate Cream 1282
Cutivate Ointment 1284
Flonase Nasal Spray 1533
Flovent 110 mcg Inhalation Aerosol 1535
Flovent 220 mcg Inhalation Aerosol 1535
Flovent 44 mcg Inhalation Aerosol 1535
Flovent Rotadisk 100 mcg 1537
Flovent Rotadisk 250 mcg 1537
Flovent Rotadisk 50 mcg 1537

RO-PREDPHATE (Canada)
PREDNISOLONE SODIUM PHOSPHATE
Pediapred Oral Solution 1170

ROSALOX (Switzerland)
METRONIDAZOLE
MetroCream 1404
MetroGel 1405
MetroGel-Vaginal Gel 1986
MetroLotion 1405
Noritate Cream 1224

ROSASED (Italy)
METRONIDAZOLE
MetroCream 1404
MetroGel 1405
MetroGel-Vaginal Gel 1986
MetroLotion 1405
Noritate Cream 1224

ROSICED (France)
METRONIDAZOLE
MetroCream 1404
MetroGel 1405
MetroGel-Vaginal Gel 1986
MetroLotion 1405
Noritate Cream 1224

ROSIDEN (Singapore)
PIROXICAM
Feldene Capsules 2685

ROSIG (Australia)
PIROXICAM
Feldene Capsules 2685

ROSSEPAR (Italy)
FERRIC SODIUM GLUCONATE
Ferrlecit Injection 3386

ROVACOR (Singapore)
LOVASTATIN
Mevacor Tablets 2132

ROXAZIN (Portugal)
PIROXICAM
Feldene Capsules 2685

ROXEN (Thailand)
NAPROXEN
EC-Naprosyn Delayed-Release Tablets ... 2967
Naprosyn Suspension 2967
Naprosyn Tablets 2967

ROXENE (Italy)
PIROXICAM
Feldene Capsules 2685

ROXENIL (Italy)
PIROXICAM
Feldene Capsules 2685

ROXICAM (South Africa)
PIROXICAM
Feldene Capsules 2685

ROXIDEN (Italy)
PIROXICAM
Feldene Capsules 2685

ROXIFEN (Thailand)
PIROXICAM
Feldene Capsules 2685

ROXIM (Italy)
PIROXICAM
Feldene Capsules 2685

ROXYCAM (Thailand)
PIROXICAM
Feldene Capsules 2685

ROXYNE (Belgium)
DOXYCYCLINE HYCLATE
Doryx Coated Pellet Filled Capsules 3357
Periostat Tablets 1208
Vibramycin Hyclate Capsules 2735
Vibramycin Hyclate Intravenous 2737
Vibra-Tabs Film Coated Tablets 2735

ROYCHLOR (Canada)
POTASSIUM CHLORIDE
K-Dur Microburst Release System ER Tablets 1832
K-Lor Powder Packets 469
K-Tab Filmtab Tablets 470
Rum-K 1363

ROYEN (Spain)
CALCIUM ACETATE
PhosLo Tablets 1069

ROZACREME (France)
METRONIDAZOLE
MetroCream 1404
MetroGel 1405
MetroGel-Vaginal Gel 1986
MetroLotion 1405
Noritate Cream 1224

ROZAGEL (France)
METRONIDAZOLE
MetroCream 1404
MetroGel 1405
MetroGel-Vaginal Gel 1986
MetroLotion 1405
Noritate Cream 1224

ROZEX (Australia, Belgium, Brazil, France, Hong Kong, Irish Republic, Israel, Italy, New Zealand, Singapore, South Africa, Spain, Sweden, Switzerland, The Netherlands, United Kingdom)
METRONIDAZOLE
MetroCream 1404
MetroGel 1405
MetroGel-Vaginal Gel 1986
MetroLotion 1405
Noritate Cream 1224

ROZICEL (Italy)
CEFPROZIL
Cefzil Tablets 1076
Cefzil for Oral Suspension 1076

ROZIDE (South Africa)
PYRAZINAMIDE
Pyrazinamide Tablets 1876

RUBACINA (Spain)
FAMOTIDINE
Pepcid Injection 2153
Pepcid Injection Premixed 2153
Pepcid RPD Orally Disintegrating Tablets 2150
Pepcid Tablets 2150
Pepcid for Oral Suspension 2150

RUBEX (Brazil)
DOXORUBICIN HYDROCHLORIDE
Adriamycin PFS/RDF Injection 2767

RUBIFEN (Singapore, Spain)
METHYLPHENIDATE HYDROCHLORIDE
Methylin Tablets 1995
Ritalin Hydrochloride Tablets 2387
Ritalin-SR Tablets 2387

RUBILEM (Mexico)
DAUNORUBICIN HYDROCHLORIDE
Cerubidine for Injection 947

RUBIMYCIN (South Africa)
ERYTHROMYCIN STEARATE
Erythrocin Stearate Filmtab Tablets 452

RUBIULCER (Spain)
RANITIDINE HYDROCHLORIDE
Zantac 150 EFFERdose Granules 1690
Zantac 150 EFFERdose Tablets 1690
Zantac 150 Tablets 1690
Zantac 300 Tablets 1690
Zantac Injection 1688
Zantac Injection Premixed 1688
Zantac Syrup 1690

RUBROFERRINA (Italy)
FERRIC SODIUM GLUCONATE
Ferrlecit Injection 3386

RUDOCYCLINE (Switzerland)
DOXYCYCLINE HYCLATE
Doryx Coated Pellet Filled Capsules 3357
Periostat Tablets 1208
Vibramycin Hyclate Capsules 2735
Vibramycin Hyclate Intravenous 2737
Vibra-Tabs Film Coated Tablets 2735

RUDOLAC (Switzerland)
LACTULOSE
Kristalose for Oral Solution 1007

RULIVAN (Spain)
NEFAZODONE HYDROCHLORIDE
Serzone Tablets 1104

RUMADENE (Thailand)
PIROXICAM
Feldene Capsules 2685

RUMASIAN (Thailand)
IBUPROFEN
Motrin Suspension, Oral Drops, Chewable Tablets, and Caplets 2002

RUMATAB (Thailand)
DICLOFENAC SODIUM
Voltaren Tablets 2315
Voltaren-XR Tablets 2315

RUMATIFEN (Thailand)
IBUPROFEN
Motrin Suspension, Oral Drops, Chewable Tablets, and Caplets 2002

RUPAN (Hong Kong, Thailand)
IBUPROFEN
Motrin Suspension, Oral Drops, Chewable Tablets, and Caplets 2002

RYDENE (Belgium)
NICARDIPINE HYDROCHLORIDE
Cardene I.V. 3485

RYLOSOL (Canada)
SOTALOL HYDROCHLORIDE
Betapace Tablets 950

RYNABRON (Spain)
DEMECLOCYCLINE HYDROCHLORIDE
Declomycin Tablets 1855

RYTHMARONE (France)
AMIODARONE HYDROCHLORIDE
Cordarone Intravenous 3491
Cordarone Tablets 3487
Pacerone Tablets 3331

RYTHMEX (Israel)
PROPAFENONE HYDROCHLORIDE
Rythmol Tablets – 150 mg, 225 mg, 300 mg 502

RYTHMOL (Canada, France, South Africa)
PROPAFENONE HYDROCHLORIDE
Rythmol Tablets – 150 mg, 225 mg, 300 mg 502

RYTHOCIN (Thailand)
ERYTHROMYCIN STEARATE
Erythrocin Stearate Filmtab Tablets 452

RYTMOBETA (Italy)
SOTALOL HYDROCHLORIDE
Betapace Tablets 950

RYTMOGENAT (Germany)
PROPAFENONE HYDROCHLORIDE
Rythmol Tablets – 150 mg, 225 mg, 300 mg 502

RYTMONORM (Belgium, Denmark, Finland, Germany, Hong Kong, Italy, New Zealand, Portugal, Singapore, Spain, Sweden, Switzerland, Thailand, The Netherlands)
PROPAFENONE HYDROCHLORIDE
Rythmol Tablets – 150 mg, 225 mg, 300 mg 502

RYTMONORMA (Austria)
PROPAFENONE HYDROCHLORIDE
Rythmol Tablets – 150 mg, 225 mg, 300 mg 502

RYTMO-PUREN (Germany)
PROPAFENONE HYDROCHLORIDE
Rythmol Tablets – 150 mg, 225 mg, 300 mg 502

S.8 (Germany)
DIPHENHYDRAMINE HYDROCHLORIDE
Benadryl Parenteral 2617

SABAX GENTAMIX (South Africa)
GENTAMICIN SULFATE
Genoptic Ophthalmic Ointment ...... ⊙239
Genoptic Sterile Ophthalmic Solution ... ⊙239

SABIDAL RECTIOL (Italy)
THEOPHYLLINE
Aerolate Jr. T.D. Capsules 1361
Aerolate Liquid 1361
Aerolate Sr. T.D. Capsules 1361
Theo-Dur Extended-Release Tablets 1835
Uni-Dur Extended-Release Tablets 1841
Uniphyl 400 mg and 600 mg Tablets ... 2903

SADEFEN (Spain)
IBUPROFEN
Motrin Suspension, Oral Drops, Chewable Tablets, and Caplets 2002

SAGITTOL (Germany)
PROPRANOLOL HYDROCHLORIDE
Inderal Injectable 3513
Inderal LA Long-Acting Capsules 3516
Inderal Tablets 3513

SALAGEN (Austria, Canada, Irish Republic, Israel, Italy, The Netherlands, United Kingdom)
PILOCARPINE HYDROCHLORIDE
Isopto Carpine Ophthalmic Solution .... ⊙215
Pilopine HS Ophthalmic Gel ...... ⊙217
Salagen Tablets 2229

SALAZINE (Israel)
SULFASALAZINE
Azulfidine EN-tabs Tablets 2775

SALAZOPIRINA (Portugal)
SULFASALAZINE
Azulfidine EN-tabs Tablets 2775

SALAZOPYRIN (Australia, Austria, Canada, Denmark, Finland, Hong Kong, Irish Republic, Israel, Italy, New Zealand, Norway, Singapore, South Africa, Sweden, Switzerland, Thailand, United Kingdom)
SULFASALAZINE
Azulfidine EN-tabs Tablets 2775

SALAZOPYRINA (Spain)
SULFASALAZINE
Azulfidine EN-tabs Tablets 2775

SALAZOPYRINE (Belgium, France, The Netherlands)
SULFASALAZINE
Azulfidine EN-tabs Tablets 2775

SALCACAM (Spain)
PIROXICAM
Feldene Capsules 2685

SALDAC (Australia, New Zealand)
SULINDAC
Clinoril Tablets 2053

SALI-ADALAT (Germany)
NIFEDIPINE
Adalat CC Tablets 877
Procardia Capsules 2708
Procardia XL Extended Release Tablets . . 2710

SALIENT (Italy)
KETOPROFEN
Orudis Capsules 3548
Oruvail Capsules 3548

SALI-PRESINOL (Germany)
METHYLDOPA
Aldomet Tablets 2037

SALI-PUREN (Germany)
HYDROCHLOROTHIAZIDE/TRIAMTERENE
Dyazide Capsules 1515
Maxzide Tablets 1008
Maxzide-25 mg Tablets 1008

SALISULF GASTROPROTETTO (Italy)
SULFASALAZINE
Azulfidine EN-tabs Tablets 2775

SALMETEDUR (Italy)
SALMETEROL XINAFOATE
Serevent Diskus 1637
Serevent Inhalation Aerosol 1633

SALODIUR (Austria)
HYDROCHLOROTHIAZIDE/TRIAMTERENE
Dyazide Capsules 1515
Maxzide Tablets 1008
Maxzide-25 mg Tablets 1008

SALONGO (Spain)
OXICONAZOLE NITRATE
Oxistat Cream 1298
Oxistat Lotion 1298

SALTERMOX (South Africa)
AMOXICILLIN
Amoxil Pediatric Drops for Oral Suspension 1471
Amoxil Tablets 1471

SALURIC (Irish Republic, United Kingdom)
CHLOROTHIAZIDE
Diuril Oral Suspension 2087
Diuril Tablets 2087

SALVACAM (Spain)
PIROXICAM
Feldene Capsules 2685

SAMECIN (Italy)
DOXYCYCLINE HYCLATE
Doryx Coated Pellet Filled Capsules 3357
Periostat Tablets 1208
Vibramycin Hyclate Capsules 2735
Vibramycin Hyclate Intravenous 2737
Vibra-Tabs Film Coated Tablets 2735

SAMIL-02 (Italy)
BENZOYL PEROXIDE
Brevoxyl-4 Cleansing Lotion 3269
Brevoxyl-4 Creamy Wash 3270
Brevoxyl-4 Gel 3269
Brevoxyl-8 Cleansing Lotion 3269
Brevoxyl-8 Creamy Wash 3270
Brevoxyl-8 Gel 3269
Triaz Cleanser 2026
Triaz Gel 2026

SANADERMIL (Switzerland)
HYDROCORTISONE ACETATE
Anusol-HC Suppositories 2238
Cortifoam Rectal Foam 3170
Hydrocortone Acetate Injectable Suspension 2103
Proctocort Suppositories 2264

SANAMIDOL (Spain)
OMEPRAZOLE
Prilosec Delayed-Release Capsules 628

SANAPRAV (Austria, Italy, Portugal)
PRAVASTATIN SODIUM
Pravachol Tablets 1099

SANATISON MONO (Germany)
HYDROCORTISONE
Anusol-HC Cream 2.5% 2237
Hydrocortone Tablets 2106

SANAXIN (Austria)
CEPHALEXIN
Keflex Oral Suspension 1237
Keflex Pulvules 1237

SANDOSTATIN (Canada, Germany, Hong Kong, Irish Republic, United Kingdom)
OCTREOTIDE ACETATE
Sandostatin LAR Depot 2395

SANDOSTATINE (France, Switzerland, The Netherlands)
OCTREOTIDE ACETATE
Sandostatin LAR Depot 2395

SANDRENA (Australia, Denmark, Germany, Italy, New Zealand, Switzerland, The Netherlands, United Kingdom)
ESTRADIOL
Alora Transdermal System 3372
Climara Transdermal System 958
Estrace Vaginal Cream 3358
Estring Vaginal Ring 2811
Vivelle Transdermal System 2412
Vivelle-Dot Transdermal System 2416

SANELOR (Belgium)
LORATADINE
Claritin Reditabs 3100
Claritin Syrup 3100
Claritin Tablets 3100

SANIFER (Italy)
FERRIC SODIUM GLUCONATE
Ferrlecit Injection 3386

SANOBAMAT (Belgium)
MEPROBAMATE
Miltown Tablets 3349

SANOMA (Germany)
CARISOPRODOL
Soma Tablets 3353

SANOXIT (Germany)
BENZOYL PEROXIDE
Brevoxyl-4 Cleansing Lotion 3269
Brevoxyl-4 Creamy Wash 3270
Brevoxyl-4 Gel 3269
Brevoxyl-8 Cleansing Lotion 3269
Brevoxyl-8 Creamy Wash 3270
Brevoxyl-8 Gel 3269
Triaz Cleanser 2026
Triaz Gel 2026

SANSACNE (Mexico)
ERYTHROMYCIN
Emgel 2% Topical Gel 1285
Ery-Tab Tablets 448
Erythromycin Base Filmtab Tablets 454
Erythromycin Delayed-Release Capsules, USP 455
PCE Dispertab Tablets 498

SANSANAL (Germany)
CAPTOPRIL
Captopril Tablets 2281

SANTYL (Canada)
COLLAGENASE
Collagenase Santyl Ointment 3248

SARCODERMA (Portugal)
LINDANE
Lindane Lotion USP 1% 559
Lindane Shampoo USP 1% 560

SARCOTON (Brazil)
DISULFIRAM
Antabuse Tablets 3474

SARF (United Arab Emirates)
CIPROFLOXACIN HYDROCHLORIDE
Ciloxan Ophthalmic Ointment 538
Ciloxan Ophthalmic Solution . . . . ⊙209, 538
Cipro Tablets 887

SARIDINE (Thailand)
SULFASALAZINE
Azulfidine EN-tabs Tablets 2775

SARNA HC (Canada)
HYDROCORTISONE
Anusol-HC Cream 2.5% 2237
Hydrocortone Tablets 2106

SARNAPIN (Brazil)
LINDANE
Lindane Lotion USP 1% 559
Lindane Shampoo USP 1% 560

SARPIOL (Brazil)
LINDANE
Lindane Lotion USP 1% 559
Lindane Shampoo USP 1% 560

SAS (Canada)
SULFASALAZINE
Azulfidine EN-tabs Tablets 2775

SASULEN (Spain)
PIROXICAM
Feldene Capsules 2685

SAYOMOL (Spain)
PROMETHAZINE HYDROCHLORIDE
Phenergan Injection 3553
Phenergan Suppositories 3556
Phenergan Syrup Fortis 3554
Phenergan Syrup Plain 3554
Phenergan Tablets 3556

SCABECID (France)
LINDANE
Lindane Lotion USP 1% 559
Lindane Shampoo USP 1% 560

SCABENE (Mexico)
LINDANE
Lindane Lotion USP 1% 559
Lindane Shampoo USP 1% 560

SCABISAN (Mexico)
LINDANE
Lindane Lotion USP 1% 559
Lindane Shampoo USP 1% 560

SCABISAN PLUS (Mexico)
LINDANE
Lindane Lotion USP 1% 559
Lindane Shampoo USP 1% 560

SCALPICIN (Italy)
HYDROCORTISONE
Anusol-HC Cream 2.5% 2237
Hydrocortone Tablets 2106

SCALPICIN CAPILAR (Spain)
HYDROCORTISONE
Anusol-HC Cream 2.5% 2237
Hydrocortone Tablets 2106

SCANDICAIN (Austria, Germany, Switzerland)
MEPIVACAINE HYDROCHLORIDE
Polocaine Injection, USP 625
Polocaine-MPF Injection, USP 625

SCANDICAIN N3 (Germany)
MEPIVACAINE HYDROCHLORIDE
Polocaine Injection, USP 625
Polocaine-MPF Injection, USP 625

SCANDICAINE (Belgium, The Netherlands)
MEPIVACAINE HYDROCHLORIDE
Polocaine Injection, USP 625
Polocaine-MPF Injection, USP 625

SCANDINIBSA (Portugal, Spain)
MEPIVACAINE HYDROCHLORIDE
Polocaine Injection, USP 625
Polocaine-MPF Injection, USP 625

SCANDONEST (Australia, Austria, Denmark, Italy, South Africa, Switzerland)
MEPIVACAINE HYDROCHLORIDE
Polocaine Injection, USP 625
Polocaine-MPF Injection, USP 625

SCF (Australia)
SUCRALFATE
Carafate Suspension 731
Carafate Tablets 730

SCHEINPHARM TRIAMCINE-A (Canada)
TRIAMCINOLONE ACETONIDE
Azmacort Inhalation Aerosol 728
Nasacort AQ Nasal Spray 752
Nasacort Nasal Inhaler 750

SCHERICUR (Austria, Germany, Spain)
HYDROCORTISONE
Anusol-HC Cream 2.5% 2237
Hydrocortone Tablets 2106

SCHERING PC4 (United Kingdom)
NORGESTREL
Ovrette Tablets 3552

SCHEROGEL (Austria, Belgium, Germany, Italy, Spain)
BENZOYL PEROXIDE
Brevoxyl-4 Cleansing Lotion 3269
Brevoxyl-4 Creamy Wash 3270
Brevoxyl-4 Gel 3269
Brevoxyl-8 Cleansing Lotion 3269
Brevoxyl-8 Creamy Wash 3270
Brevoxyl-8 Gel 3269
Triaz Cleanser 2026
Triaz Gel 2026

SCHMERZ-DOLGIT (Germany)
IBUPROFEN
Motrin Suspension, Oral Drops, Chewable Tablets, and Caplets 2002

SCHUFEN (Thailand)
IBUPROFEN
Motrin Suspension, Oral Drops, Chewable Tablets, and Caplets 2002

SCLANE (Spain)
BETAMETHASONE ACETATE/BETAMETHASONE SODIUM PHOSPHATE
Celestone Soluspan Injectable Suspension 3097

SCLERIL (Italy)
FENOFIBRATE
Tricor Capsules, Micronized 513

SCRIPTO-METIC (South Africa)
PROCHLORPERAZINE MALEATE
Compazine Spansule Capsules 1505
Compazine Tablets 1505

SCRIPTOPAM (South Africa)
DIAZEPAM
Valium Injectable 3026
Valium Tablets 3047

SD-HERMAL (Germany)
CLOTRIMAZOLE
Lotrimin Cream 1% 3128
Lotrimin Lotion 1% 3128
Lotrimin Topical Solution 1% 3128
Mycelex Troche 573

SEALDIN (Spain)
SERTRALINE HYDROCHLORIDE
Zoloft Tablets 2751

SEBERCIM (Italy)
NORFLOXACIN
Chibroxin Sterile Ophthalmic Solution . . . . ⊙273, 2051
Noroxin Tablets 2145

SEBIZOLE (Australia, New Zealand)
KETOCONAZOLE
Nizoral 2% Cream 3620
Nizoral 2% Shampoo 2007
Nizoral Tablets 1791

SECADINE (South Africa)
CIMETIDINE
Tagamet Tablets 1644

SECALIP (France, Spain)
FENOFIBRATE
Tricor Capsules, Micronized 513

SECLODIN (Germany, United Kingdom)
IBUPROFEN
Motrin Suspension, Oral Drops, Chewable Tablets, and Caplets 2002

SECOTEX (Mexico)
TAMSULOSIN HYDROCHLORIDE
Flomax Capsules 1044

SECTRAL (Austria, Belgium, Canada, France, Hong Kong, Irish Republic, Israel, Italy, Singapore, South Africa, Spain, Switzerland, The Netherlands, United Kingdom)
ACEBUTOLOL HYDROCHLORIDE
Sectral Capsules 3589

SECUBAR (Spain)
LISINOPRIL
Prinivil Tablets 2164
Zestril Tablets 698

SECUBAR DIU (Spain)
HYDROCHLOROTHIAZIDE/LISINOPRIL
Prinzide Tablets 2168
Zestoretic Tablets 695

SECURON (United Kingdom)
VERAPAMIL HYDROCHLORIDE
Covera-HS Tablets 3199
Isoptin SR Tablets 467
Verelan Capsules 3184
Verelan PM Capsules 3186

SEDACORON (Austria, Hong Kong)
AMIODARONE HYDROCHLORIDE
Cordarone Intravenous 3491
Cordarone Tablets 3487
Pacerone Tablets 3331

SEDALIN (Thailand)
CEFTRIAXONE SODIUM
Rocephin Injectable Vials, ADD-Vantage, Galaxy, Bulk 2993

SEDAZIN (Switzerland)
LORAZEPAM
Ativan Injection 3478
Ativan Tablets 3482

SEDIAT (Germany)
DIPHENHYDRAMINE HYDROCHLORIDE
Benadryl Parenteral 2617

SEDICEPAN (Spain)
LORAZEPAM
Ativan Injection . . . 3478
Ativan Tablets . . . 3482

SEDIVER (Mexico)
DIAZEPAM
Valium Injectable . . . 3026
Valium Tablets . . . 3047

SEDIZEPAN (Spain)
LORAZEPAM
Ativan Injection . . . 3478
Ativan Tablets . . . 3482

SEDONERVIL COMPLEX (Spain)
DIAZEPAM
Valium Injectable . . . 3026
Valium Tablets . . . 3047

SEDOPRETTEN (Germany)
DIPHENHYDRAMINE HYDROCHLORIDE
Benadryl Parenteral . . . 2617

SEDOVEGAN NOVO (Germany)
DIPHENHYDRAMINE HYDROCHLORIDE
Benadryl Parenteral . . . 2617

SEDRAL (Japan)
CEFADROXIL
Duricef Capsules . . . 1079
Duricef Oral Suspension . . . 1079
Duricef Tablets . . . 1079

SEFARETIC (Thailand)
AMILORIDE HYDROCHLORIDE/HYDROCHLOROTHIAZIDE
Moduretic Tablets . . . 2138

SEFMAL (Singapore, Thailand)
TRAMADOL HYDROCHLORIDE
Ultram Tablets . . . 2600

SEFMEX (Thailand)
SELEGILINE HYDROCHLORIDE
Eldepryl Capsules . . . 3266

SEFMIC (Thailand)
MEFENAMIC ACID
Ponstel Capsules . . . 1356

SEFTEM (Japan)
CEFTIBUTEN
Cedax Capsules . . . 1021
Cedax Oral Suspension . . . 1021

SEKUNDAL-D (Germany)
DIPHENHYDRAMINE HYDROCHLORIDE
Benadryl Parenteral . . . 2617

SELAN (Spain)
CEFUROXIME AXETIL
Ceftin Tablets . . . 1898
Ceftin for Oral Suspension . . . 1898

SELECIM (Switzerland)
SELEGILINE HYDROCHLORIDE
Eldepryl Capsules . . . 3266

SELECTIN (Italy)
PRAVASTATIN SODIUM
Pravachol Tablets . . . 1099

SELECTOFEN (Mexico)
DICLOFENAC SODIUM
Voltaren Tablets . . . 2315
Voltaren-XR Tablets . . . 2315

SELEDAT (Italy)
SELEGILINE HYDROCHLORIDE
Eldepryl Capsules . . . 3266

SELEGAM (Germany)
SELEGILINE HYDROCHLORIDE
Eldepryl Capsules . . . 3266

SELEGOS (Singapore)
SELEGILINE HYDROCHLORIDE
Eldepryl Capsules . . . 3266

SELEKTINE (The Netherlands)
PRAVASTATIN SODIUM
Pravachol Tablets . . . 1099

SELEMERCK (Germany)
SELEGILINE HYDROCHLORIDE
Eldepryl Capsules . . . 3266

SELEPARK (Germany)
SELEGILINE HYDROCHLORIDE
Eldepryl Capsules . . . 3266

SELES BETA (Italy)
ATENOLOL
Tenormin I.V. Injection . . . 692

SELGENE (Australia, New Zealand, Thailand)
SELEGILINE HYDROCHLORIDE
Eldepryl Capsules . . . 3266

SELGIMED (Germany)
SELEGILINE HYDROCHLORIDE
Eldepryl Capsules . . . 3266

SELINE (Thailand)
SELEGILINE HYDROCHLORIDE
Eldepryl Capsules . . . 3266

SELINOL (Sweden)
ATENOLOL
Tenormin I.V. Injection . . . 692

SELIPRAN (Austria, Switzerland)
PRAVASTATIN SODIUM
Pravachol Tablets . . . 1099

SELM (Mexico)
METHYLDOPA
Aldomet Tablets . . . 2037

SELOBLOC (Switzerland)
ATENOLOL
Tenormin I.V. Injection . . . 692

SELOKEN (Austria, Mexico)
METOPROLOL SUCCINATE
Toprol-XL Tablets . . . 651

SELOKEN ZOC (Finland, Sweden)
METOPROLOL SUCCINATE
Toprol-XL Tablets . . . 651

SELO-ZOK (Belgium, Denmark, Norway)
METOPROLOL SUCCINATE
Toprol-XL Tablets . . . 651

SELPAR (Italy)
SELEGILINE HYDROCHLORIDE
Eldepryl Capsules . . . 3266

SEMBRINA (Germany, The Netherlands)
METHYLDOPA
Aldomet Tablets . . . 2037

SEMBRINA-SALTUCIN (Germany)
METHYLDOPA
Aldomet Tablets . . . 2037

SEMELCICLINA (Italy)
DOXYCYCLINE HYCLATE
Doryx Coated Pellet Filled Capsules . . . 3357
Periostat Tablets . . . 1208
Vibramycin Hyclate Capsules . . . 2735
Vibramycin Hyclate Intravenous . . . 2737
Vibra-Tabs Film Coated Tablets . . . 2735

SEMIPENIL (Italy)
PIPERACILLIN SODIUM
Pipracil . . . 1866

SENIOR (Germany)
PEMOLINE
Cylert Chewable Tablets . . . 415
Cylert Tablets . . . 415

SENORM (Thailand)
HALOPERIDOL DECANOATE
Haldol Decanoate 100 Injection . . . 2535
Haldol Decanoate 50 Injection . . . 2535

SENRO (Spain)
NORFLOXACIN
Chibroxin Sterile Ophthalmic Solution . . . ⊙273, 2051
Noroxin Tablets . . . 2145

SENSIBIT (Mexico)
LORATADINE
Claritin Reditabs . . . 3100
Claritin Syrup . . . 3100
Claritin Tablets . . . 3100

SENSORCAINE (Canada)
BUPIVACAINE HYDROCHLORIDE
Sensorcaine Injection . . . 643
Sensorcaine-MPF Injection . . . 643

SENTIAL HYDROCORTISONE (Belgium)
HYDROCORTISONE
Anusol-HC Cream 2.5% . . . 2237
Hydrocortone Tablets . . . 2106

SEPCEN (Spain)
CIPROFLOXACIN HYDROCHLORIDE
Ciloxan Ophthalmic Ointment . . . 538
Ciloxan Ophthalmic Solution . . . ⊙209, 538
Cipro Tablets . . . 887

SEPEXIN (South Africa)
CEFTIBUTEN
Cedax Capsules . . . 1021
Cedax Oral Suspension . . . 1021

SEPRAFILM (United Kingdom)
SODIUM HYALURONATE
Hyalgan Solution . . . 3080

SEPRAM (Germany)
CITALOPRAM HYDROBROMIDE
Celexa Tablets . . . 1365

SEPTICOL (Switzerland)
CHLORAMPHENICOL
Chloromycetin Ophthalmic Ointment, 1% . . . ⊙296
Chloromycetin Ophthalmic Solution . . . ⊙297
Chloroptic Sterile Ophthalmic Ointment . . . ⊙234
Chloroptic Sterile Ophthalmic Solution . . . ⊙235

SEPTILISIN (Mexico)
NEOMYCIN SULFATE/POLYMYXIN B SULFATE
Neosporin G.U. Irrigant Sterile . . . 2256

SEPTOMANDOLO (Italy)
CEFAMANDOLE NAFATE
Mandol Vials . . . 1953

SERACIN (Thailand)
OFLOXACIN
Floxin I.V. . . . 2526
Floxin Otic Solution . . . 1219
Floxin Tablets . . . 2529
Ocuflox Ophthalmic Solution . . . 554

SERAD (Italy)
SERTRALINE HYDROCHLORIDE
Zoloft Tablets . . . 2751

SERALGAN (Austria)
CITALOPRAM HYDROBROMIDE
Celexa Tablets . . . 1365

SERASA (Mexico)
ASPARAGINASE
Elspar for Injection . . . 2092

SERECID (New Zealand)
HYDROXYZINE HYDROCHLORIDE
Atarax Tablets & Syrup . . . 2667
Vistaril Intramuscular Solution . . . 2738

SEREDYN (Mexico)
DIAZEPAM
Valium Injectable . . . 3026
Valium Tablets . . . 3047

SEREN (Italy)
CHLORDIAZEPOXIDE HYDROCHLORIDE
Librium Capsules . . . 1736
Librium for Injection . . . 1737

SEREN VITA (Italy)
CHLORDIAZEPOXIDE HYDROCHLORIDE
Librium Capsules . . . 1736
Librium for Injection . . . 1737

SERENACE (Australia, Hong Kong, Irish Republic, New Zealand, Singapore, South Africa, Thailand, United Kingdom)
HALOPERIDOL
Haldol Injection, Tablets and Concentrate . . . 2533

SERENASE (Belgium, Italy)
LORAZEPAM
Ativan Injection . . . 3478
Ativan Tablets . . . 3482

SERENELFI (Portugal)
HALOPERIDOL
Haldol Injection, Tablets and Concentrate . . . 2533

SEREUPIN (Italy)
PAROXETINE HYDROCHLORIDE
Paxil Oral Suspension . . . 1609
Paxil Tablets . . . 1609

SEREVENT (Australia, Austria, Belgium, Brazil, Canada, Denmark, Finland, France, Hong Kong, Irish Republic, Israel, Italy, Mexico, New Zealand, Norway, Portugal, Singapore, South Africa, Spain, Sweden, Switzerland, Thailand, The Netherlands, United Kingdom)
SALMETEROL XINAFOATE
Serevent Diskus . . . 1637
Serevent Inhalation Aerosol . . . 1633

SERLAIN (Belgium)
SERTRALINE HYDROCHLORIDE
Zoloft Tablets . . . 2751

SEROMIDA (Mexico)
IFOSFAMIDE
Ifex for Injection . . . 1123

SEROPRAM (Spain)
CITALOPRAM HYDROBROMIDE
Celexa Tablets . . . 1365

SEROQUEL (Australia, Canada, Finland, Hong Kong, Irish Republic, Italy, Mexico, New Zealand, Singapore, South Africa, Thailand, United Kingdom)
QUETIAPINE FUMARATE
Seroquel Tablets . . . 684

SEROVIDINA (Mexico)
ZIDOVUDINE
Retrovir Capsules . . . 1625
Retrovir IV Infusion . . . 1629
Retrovir Syrup . . . 1625
Retrovir Tablets . . . 1625

SEROXAT (Austria, Belgium, Denmark, Finland, Germany, Hong Kong, Irish Republic, Israel, Italy, Norway, Portugal, Singapore, Spain, Sweden, Thailand, The Netherlands, United Kingdom)
PAROXETINE HYDROCHLORIDE
Paxil Oral Suspension . . . 1609
Paxil Tablets . . . 1609

SERTIDINE (Mexico)
FAMOTIDINE
Pepcid Injection . . . 2153
Pepcid Injection Premixed . . . 2153
Pepcid RPD Orally Disintegrating Tablets . . . 2150
Pepcid Tablets . . . 2150
Pepcid for Oral Suspension . . . 2150

SERTOFREN (Norway)
DESIPRAMINE HYDROCHLORIDE
Norpramin Tablets . . . 755

SERTRIXEN (Mexico)
NAPROXEN
EC-Naprosyn Delayed-Release Tablets . . . 2967
Naprosyn Suspension . . . 2967
Naprosyn Tablets . . . 2967

SERVAMBUTOL (Switzerland)
ETHAMBUTOL HYDROCHLORIDE
Myambutol Tablets . . . 1290

SERVANOLOL (Switzerland)
PROPRANOLOL HYDROCHLORIDE
Inderal Injectable . . . 3513
Inderal LA Long-Acting Capsules . . . 3516
Inderal Tablets . . . 3513

SERVICEF (Mexico)
CEPHALEXIN
Keflex Oral Suspension . . . 1237
Keflex Pulvules . . . 1237

SERVICLOFEN (Switzerland)
CHLORAMPHENICOL
Chloromycetin Ophthalmic Ointment, 1% . . . ⊙296
Chloromycetin Ophthalmic Solution . . . ⊙297
Chloroptic Sterile Ophthalmic Ointment . . . ⊙234
Chloroptic Sterile Ophthalmic Solution . . . ⊙235

SERVIDIPINE (Switzerland)
NIFEDIPINE
Adalat CC Tablets . . . 877
Procardia Capsules . . . 2708
Procardia XL Extended Release Tablets . . . 2710

SERVIDOXYNE (Hong Kong, Singapore, Switzerland)
DOXYCYCLINE HYCLATE
Doryx Coated Pellet Filled Capsules . . . 3357
Periostat Tablets . . . 1208
Vibramycin Hyclate Capsules . . . 2735
Vibramycin Hyclate Intravenous . . . 2737
Vibra-Tabs Film Coated Tablets . . . 2735

SERVIFLOX (Thailand)
CIPROFLOXACIN
Cipro I.V. . . . 893
Cipro I.V. Pharmacy Bulk Package . . . 897
Cipro Oral Suspension . . . 887

SERVIGENTA (Mexico, Switzerland)
GENTAMICIN SULFATE
Genoptic Ophthalmic Ointment . . . ⊙239
Genoptic Sterile Ophthalmic Solution . . . ⊙239

SERVINAPROX (Switzerland)
NAPROXEN
EC-Naprosyn Delayed-Release Tablets . . . 2967
Naprosyn Suspension . . . 2967
Naprosyn Tablets . . . 2967

SERVIPEP (Hong Kong, Singapore)
FAMOTIDINE
Pepcid Injection . . . 2153
Pepcid Injection Premixed . . . 2153
Pepcid RPD Orally Disintegrating Tablets . . . 2150
Pepcid Tablets . . . 2150
Pepcid for Oral Suspension . . . 2150

SERVIPROFEN (Switzerland)
IBUPROFEN
Motrin Suspension, Oral Drops, Chewable Tablets, and Caplets . . . 2002

SERVIRADINE (Mexico)
RANITIDINE HYDROCHLORIDE
Zantac 150 EFFERdose Granules . . . 1690
Zantac 150 EFFERdose Tablets . . . 1690
Zantac 150 Tablets . . . 1690
Zantac 300 Tablets . . . 1690
Zantac Injection . . . 1688
Zantac Injection Premixed . . . 1688
Zantac Syrup . . . 1690

SERVISPOR (Switzerland)
CEPHALEXIN
Keflex Oral Suspension . . . 1237

Keflex Pulvules 1237

SERVITENOL (Switzerland)
ATENOLOL
Tenormin I.V. Injection 692

SERVIZOL (Singapore)
METRONIDAZOLE
MetroCream 1404
MetroGel 1405
MetroGel-Vaginal Gel 1986
MetroLotion 1405
Noritate Cream 1224

SERZONE (Australia, Brazil, Canada, Hong Kong, Mexico, New Zealand, Singapore, South Africa, Thailand)
NEFAZODONE HYDROCHLORIDE
Serzone Tablets 1104

SERZONIL (Israel)
NEFAZODONE HYDROCHLORIDE
Serzone Tablets 1104

SETIN (South Africa)
METOCLOPRAMIDE HYDROCHLORIDE
Reglan Injectable 2935
Reglan Syrup 2935
Reglan Tablets 2935

SEVREDOL (France, Germany, Irish Republic, New Zealand, Spain, Switzerland, The Netherlands, United Kingdom)
MORPHINE SULFATE
Astramorph/PF Injection, USP (Preservative-Free) 594
Duramorph Injection 1312
Infumorph 200 and Infumorph 500 Sterile Solutions 1314
Kadian Capsules 1335
MS Contin Tablets 2896
MSIR Oral Capsules 2898
MSIR Oral Solution 2898
MSIR Oral Solution Concentrate 2898
MSIR Oral Tablets 2898
Oramorph SR Tablets 3062
Roxanol 100 Concentrated Oral Solution 3066
Roxanol Concentrated Oral Solution 3066
Roxanol-T Oral Solution 3066

SEVRE-LONG (Switzerland)
MORPHINE SULFATE
Astramorph/PF Injection, USP (Preservative-Free) 594
Duramorph Injection 1312
Infumorph 200 and Infumorph 500 Sterile Solutions 1314
Kadian Capsules 1335
MS Contin Tablets 2896
MSIR Oral Capsules 2898
MSIR Oral Solution 2898
MSIR Oral Solution Concentrate 2898
MSIR Oral Tablets 2898
Oramorph SR Tablets 3062
Roxanol 100 Concentrated Oral Solution 3066
Roxanol Concentrated Oral Solution 3066
Roxanol-T Oral Solution 3066

SEXADIEN (Denmark)
DIENESTROL
Ortho Dienestrol Cream 2554

SHAMPOUX (Belgium)
PERMETHRIN
Acticin Cream 998
Elimite Cream 552

SHEMOL (Mexico)
TIMOLOL MALEATE
Blocadren Tablets 2046
Timoptic Sterile Ophthalmic Solution 2190
Timoptic in Ocudose 2192
Timoptic-XE Sterile Ophthalmic Gel Forming Solution 2194

SHINCORT (Thailand)
TRIAMCINOLONE ACETONIDE
Azmacort Inhalation Aerosol 728
Nasacort AQ Nasal Spray 752
Nasacort Nasal Inhaler 750

SIADOCIN (Thailand)
DOXYCYCLINE HYCLATE
Doryx Coated Pellet Filled Capsules 3357
Periostat Tablets 1208
Vibramycin Hyclate Capsules 2735
Vibramycin Hyclate Intravenous 2737
Vibra-Tabs Film Coated Tablets 2735

SIALEXIN (Thailand)
CEPHALEXIN
Keflex Oral Suspension 1237
Keflex Pulvules 1237

SIAMDOPA (Thailand)
METHYLDOPA
Aldomet Tablets 2037

SIAMFORMET (Thailand)
METFORMIN HYDROCHLORIDE
Glucophage Tablets 1080

SIAMIDINE (Thailand)
CIMETIDINE
Tagamet Tablets 1644

SIAMPRAXOL (Thailand)
ALPRAZOLAM
Xanax Tablets 2865

SICCO (Germany)
INDAPAMIDE
Indapamide Tablets 2286

SICO RELAX (Spain)
DIAZEPAM
Valium Injectable 3026
Valium Tablets 3047

SIDURO (Sweden)
KETOPROFEN
Orudis Capsules 3548
Oruvail Capsules 3548

SIFACLOR (Thailand)
CEFACLOR
Ceclor CD Tablets 1279
Ceclor Pulvules 1905
Ceclor Suspension 1905

SIFICETINA (Italy)
CHLORAMPHENICOL
Chloromycetin Ophthalmic Ointment, 1% . . . . ⊙296
Chloromycetin Ophthalmic Solution . . . . ⊙297
Chloroptic Sterile Ophthalmic Ointment . . ⊙234
Chloroptic Sterile Ophthalmic Solution . . ⊙235

SIGABLOC (Germany)
ATENOLOL
Tenormin I.V. Injection 692

SIGACAP COR (Germany)
CAPTOPRIL
Captopril Tablets 2281

SIGACEFAL (Germany)
CEFACLOR
Ceclor CD Tablets 1279
Ceclor Pulvules 1905
Ceclor Suspension 1905

SIGACIMET (Germany)
CIMETIDINE
Tagamet Tablets 1644

SIGACORA (Germany)
ISOSORBIDE MONONITRATE
Imdur Tablets 1826
Ismo Tablets 3524

SIGADOXIN (Austria, Portugal, Switzerland)
DOXYCYCLINE HYCLATE
Doryx Coated Pellet Filled Capsules 3357
Periostat Tablets 1208
Vibramycin Hyclate Capsules 2735
Vibramycin Hyclate Intravenous 2737
Vibra-Tabs Film Coated Tablets 2735

SIGAFAM (Mexico)
FAMOTIDINE
Pepcid Injection 2153
Pepcid Injection Premixed 2153
Pepcid RPD Orally Disintegrating Tablets 2150
Pepcid Tablets 2150
Pepcid for Oral Suspension 2150

SIGAFENAC (Germany)
DICLOFENAC SODIUM
Voltaren Tablets 2315
Voltaren-XR Tablets 2315

SIGAMOPEN (Switzerland)
AMOXICILLIN
Amoxil Pediatric Drops for Oral Suspension 1471
Amoxil Tablets 1471

SIGAPAEDIL (Germany)
ERYTHROMYCIN
Emgel 2% Topical Gel 1285
Ery-Tab Tablets 448
Erythromycin Base Filmtab Tablets 454
Erythromycin Delayed-Release Capsules, USP 455
PCE Dispertab Tablets 498

SIGAPERIDOL (Germany, Switzerland)
HALOPERIDOL
Haldol Injection, Tablets and Concentrate 2533

SIGMACORT (Australia)
HYDROCORTISONE ACETATE
Anusol-HC Suppositories 2238
Cortifoam Rectal Foam 3170
Hydrocortone Acetate Injectable Suspension 2103
Proctocort Suppositories 2264

SIGMETADINE (Australia)
CIMETIDINE
Tagamet Tablets 1644

SIGUENT HYCOR (Australia)
HYDROCORTISONE ACETATE
Anusol-HC Suppositories 2238
Cortifoam Rectal Foam 3170
Hydrocortone Acetate Injectable Suspension 2103
Proctocort Suppositories 2264

SILINO (Germany)
DICLOFENAC SODIUM
Voltaren Tablets 2315
Voltaren-XR Tablets 2315

SILMYCETIN (Thailand)
CHLORAMPHENICOL
Chloromycetin Ophthalmic Ointment, 1% . . . . ⊙296
Chloromycetin Ophthalmic Solution . . . . ⊙297
Chloroptic Sterile Ophthalmic Ointment . . ⊙234
Chloroptic Sterile Ophthalmic Solution . . ⊙235

SIMACORT (Thailand)
TRIAMCINOLONE ACETONIDE
Azmacort Inhalation Aerosol 728
Nasacort AQ Nasal Spray 752
Nasacort Nasal Inhaler 750

SIMAGLEN (Thailand)
CIMETIDINE
Tagamet Tablets 1644

SIMATIN (Austria, Spain)
ETHOSUXIMIDE
Zarontin Capsules 2659
Zarontin Syrup 2660

SIMETAC (Hong Kong)
RANITIDINE HYDROCHLORIDE
Zantac 150 EFFERdose Granules 1690
Zantac 150 EFFERdose Tablets 1690
Zantac 150 Tablets 1690
Zantac 300 Tablets 1690
Zantac Injection 1688
Zantac Injection Premixed 1688
Zantac Syrup 1690

SIMEX (Thailand)
CIMETIDINE
Tagamet Tablets 1644

SIMOVIL (Israel)
SIMVASTATIN
Zocor Tablets 2219

SIMULECT (Australia, Belgium, Denmark, Finland, France, Germany, Hong Kong, Irish Republic, Italy, Mexico, New Zealand, Norway, Portugal, Singapore, South Africa, Spain, Sweden, Switzerland, Thailand, The Netherlands, United Kingdom)
BASILIXIMAB
Simulect for Injection 2399

SINALFA (Denmark, Norway, Sweden)
TERAZOSIN HYDROCHLORIDE
Hytrin Capsules 464

SINARONA (Mexico)
AMIODARONE HYDROCHLORIDE
Cordarone Intravenous 3491
Cordarone Tablets 3487
Pacerone Tablets 3331

SINCERCK (Mexico)
PRAZIQUANTEL
Biltricide Tablets 887

SINE FLUOR (Spain)
DESONIDE
DesOwen Cream 1401
DesOwen Lotion 1401
DesOwen Ointment 1401

SINEGASTRIN (Mexico)
CIMETIDINE
Tagamet Tablets 1644

SINEMET (Australia, Austria, Canada, France, Italy, Norway, Singapore, South Africa, Sweden, Switzerland, Thailand, The Netherlands, United Kingdom)
CARBIDOPA/LEVODOPA
Sinemet CR Tablets 1255
Sinemet Tablets 1253

SINEPRESS (South Africa)
METHYLDOPA
Aldomet Tablets 2037

SINEQUAN (Australia, Austria, Belgium, Canada, Denmark, France, Hong Kong, Irish Republic, Mexico, Norway, Spain, Thailand, The Netherlands, United Kingdom)
DOXEPIN HYDROCHLORIDE
Sinequan Capsules 2713
Sinequan Oral Concentrate 2713

SINERGINA (Spain)
PHENYTOIN
Dilantin Infatabs 2624
Dilantin-125 Oral Suspension 2625

SINERGINA S (Spain)
PHENYTOIN
Dilantin Infatabs 2624
Dilantin-125 Oral Suspension 2625

SINERTEC (Italy)
ENALAPRIL MALEATE/HYDROCHLOROTHIAZIDE
Vaseretic Tablets 2204

SINESTRON (Mexico)
LORAZEPAM
Ativan Injection 3478
Ativan Tablets 3482

SINGULAIR (Australia, Austria, Belgium, Canada, Denmark, Finland, France, Germany, Hong Kong, Irish Republic, Israel, Italy, Mexico, New Zealand, Norway, Portugal, Singapore, South Africa, Spain, Sweden, Switzerland, Thailand, The Netherlands, United Kingdom)
MONTELUKAST SODIUM
Singulair Chewable Tablets 2181
Singulair Tablets 2181

SINKETOL (Italy)
KETOPROFEN
Orudis Capsules 3548
Oruvail Capsules 3548

SINOZZARD (Mexico)
PRAZOSIN HYDROCHLORIDE
Minipress Capsules 2699

SINQUAN (Germany)
DOXEPIN HYDROCHLORIDE
Sinequan Capsules 2713
Sinequan Oral Concentrate 2713

SINQUANE (Switzerland)
DOXEPIN HYDROCHLORIDE
Sinequan Capsules 2713
Sinequan Oral Concentrate 2713

SINTENYL (Switzerland)
FENTANYL CITRATE
Actiq 1184

SINTOLATT (Italy)
LACTULOSE
Kristalose for Oral Solution 1007

SINTOMICETINA (Brazil)
CHLORAMPHENICOL
Chloromycetin Ophthalmic Ointment, 1% . . . . ⊙296
Chloromycetin Ophthalmic Solution . . . . ⊙297
Chloroptic Sterile Ophthalmic Ointment . . ⊙234
Chloroptic Sterile Ophthalmic Solution . . ⊙235

SINTOPLUS (Italy)
PIPERACILLIN SODIUM
Pipracil 1866

SINTOTRAT (Italy)
HYDROCORTISONE ACETATE
Anusol-HC Suppositories 2238
Cortifoam Rectal Foam 3170
Hydrocortone Acetate Injectable Suspension 2103
Proctocort Suppositories 2264

SINVACOR (Italy)
SIMVASTATIN
Zocor Tablets 2219

SIOFOR (Germany)
METFORMIN HYDROCHLORIDE
Glucophage Tablets 1080

SIPAM (Thailand)
DIAZEPAM
Valium Injectable 3026
Valium Tablets 3047

SIPROFEN (Belgium)
IBUPROFEN
Motrin Suspension, Oral Drops, Chewable Tablets, and Caplets 2002

SIRBEN (Brazil)
MEBENDAZOLE
Vermox Chewable Tablets 2017

SIRDALUD (Austria, Belgium, Brazil, Denmark, Finland, Germany, Italy, Mexico, Portugal, Spain, Switzerland, Thailand, The Netherlands)
TIZANIDINE HYDROCHLORIDE
Zanaflex Tablets 1305

SIROLAX (Israel)
LACTULOSE
Kristalose for Oral Solution 1007

SIROP DENTITION (Canada)
BENZOCAINE
Americaine Anesthetic Lubricant 1162

Americaine Otic Topical Anesthetic Ear Drops 1162

SIROP EXPECTORANT (Canada)
GUAIFENESIN
Organidin NR Liquid 3350
Organidin NR Tablets 3350

SIROS (Germany)
ITRACONAZOLE
Sporanox Capsules 1800
Sporanox Oral Solution 1808, 2512

SIRTAL (Austria, Germany)
CARBAMAZEPINE
Carbatrol Capsules 3234
Tegretol Chewable Tablets 2404
Tegretol Suspension 2404
Tegretol Tablets 2404
Tegretol-XR Tablets 2404

SISARE MONO (Germany)
ESTRADIOL
Alora Transdermal System 3372
Climara Transdermal System 958
Estrace Vaginal Cream 3358
Estring Vaginal Ring 2811
Vivelle Transdermal System 2412
Vivelle-Dot Transdermal System 2416

SITRIOL (Australia)
CALCITRIOL
Calcijex Injection 411
Rocaltrol Capsules 2991
Rocaltrol Oral Solution 2991

SIVASTIN (Italy)
SIMVASTATIN
Zocor Tablets 2219

SKENAN (Belgium, France, Italy, Spain, The Netherlands)
MORPHINE SULFATE
Astramorph/PF Injection, USP (Preservative-Free) 594
Duramorph Injection 1312
Infumorph 200 and Infumorph 500 Sterile Solutions 1314
Kadian Capsules 1335
MS Contin Tablets 2896
MSIR Oral Capsules 2898
MSIR Oral Solution 2898
MSIR Oral Solution Concentrate 2898
MSIR Oral Tablets 2898
Oramorph SR Tablets 3062
Roxanol 100 Concentrated Oral Solution 3066
Roxanol Concentrated Oral Solution 3066
Roxanol-T Oral Solution 3066

SKEZIDE (Thailand)
HYDROCHLOROTHIAZIDE/TRIAMTERENE
Dyazide Capsules 1515
Maxzide Tablets 1008
Maxzide-25 mg Tablets 1008

SKID (Germany)
MINOCYCLINE HYDROCHLORIDE
Dynacin Capsules 2019
Minocin Intravenous 1862
Minocin Oral Suspension 1865
Minocin Pellet-Filled Capsules 1863

SKID E (Germany)
ERYTHROMYCIN
Emgel 2% Topical Gel 1285
Ery-Tab Tablets 448
Erythromycin Base Filmtab Tablets 454
Erythromycin Delayed-Release Capsules, USP 455
PCE Dispertab Tablets 498

SKINCALM (New Zealand, South Africa)
HYDROCORTISONE ACETATE
Anusol-HC Suppositories 2238
Cortifoam Rectal Foam 3170
Hydrocortone Acetate Injectable Suspension 2103
Proctocort Suppositories 2264

SKINICLES (Canada)
HYDROQUINONE
Eldopaque Forte 4% Cream 1734
Eldoquin Forte 4% Cream 1734
Lustra Cream 2023
Lustra-AF Cream 2023
Melanex Topical Solution 2300
Solaquin Forte 4% Cream 1734
Solaquin Forte 4% Gel 1734

SKINODERM (Israel)
AZELAIC ACID
Azelex Cream 547

SKINOREN (Australia, Austria, Belgium, Denmark, Finland, France, Hong Kong, Italy, New Zealand, Norway, Portugal, Singapore, South Africa, Spain, Sweden, Switzerland, Thailand, United Kingdom)
AZELAIC ACID
Azelex Cream 547

SKITZ (Australia)
BENZOYL PEROXIDE
Brevoxyl-4 Cleansing Lotion 3269
Brevoxyl-4 Creamy Wash 3270
Brevoxyl-4 Gel 3269
Brevoxyl-8 Cleansing Lotion 3269
Brevoxyl-8 Creamy Wash 3270
Brevoxyl-8 Gel 3269
Triaz Cleanser 2026
Triaz Gel 2026

SKLEROMEXE (Germany)
CLOFIBRATE
Atromid-S Capsules 3483

SLEEP AID (United Kingdom)
DIPHENHYDRAMINE HYDROCHLORIDE
Benadryl Parenteral 2617

SLEEPEAZE (United Kingdom)
DIPHENHYDRAMINE HYDROCHLORIDE
Benadryl Parenteral 2617

SLEEP-EZE D (Canada)
DIPHENHYDRAMINE HYDROCHLORIDE
Benadryl Parenteral 2617

SLEEPIA (United Kingdom)
DIPHENHYDRAMINE HYDROCHLORIDE
Benadryl Parenteral 2617

SLIM MINT (Canada)
BENZOCAINE
Americaine Anesthetic Lubricant 1162
Americaine Otic Topical Anesthetic Ear Drops 1162

SLIMIN (Germany)
HYDROCHLOROTHIAZIDE/TRIAMTERENE
Dyazide Capsules 1515
Maxzide Tablets 1008
Maxzide-25 mg Tablets 1008

SLO-BID (Australia, Canada, Hong Kong, Mexico)
THEOPHYLLINE
Aerolate Jr. T.D. Capsules 1361
Aerolate Liquid 1361
Aerolate Sr. T.D. Capsules 1361
Theo-Dur Extended-Release Tablets 1835
Uni-Dur Extended-Release Tablets 1841
Uniphyl 400 mg and 600 mg Tablets 2903

SLOFEDIPINE (United Kingdom)
NIFEDIPINE
Adalat CC Tablets 877
Procardia Capsules 2708
Procardia XL Extended Release Tablets 2710

SLOFENAC (United Kingdom)
DICLOFENAC SODIUM
Voltaren Tablets 2315
Voltaren-XR Tablets 2315

SLO-PHYLLIN (Irish Republic, Italy, United Kingdom)
THEOPHYLLINE
Aerolate Jr. T.D. Capsules 1361
Aerolate Liquid 1361
Aerolate Sr. T.D. Capsules 1361
Theo-Dur Extended-Release Tablets 1835
Uni-Dur Extended-Release Tablets 1841
Uniphyl 400 mg and 600 mg Tablets 2903

SLOPROLOL (United Kingdom)
PROPRANOLOL HYDROCHLORIDE
Inderal Injectable 3513
Inderal LA Long-Acting Capsules 3516
Inderal Tablets 3513

SLOW DERALIN (Israel)
PROPRANOLOL HYDROCHLORIDE
Inderal Injectable 3513
Inderal LA Long-Acting Capsules 3516
Inderal Tablets 3513

SLOW-K (Australia, Brazil, Canada, Hong Kong, Irish Republic, Israel, New Zealand, South Africa, The Netherlands)
POTASSIUM CHLORIDE
K-Dur Microburst Release System ER Tablets 1832
K-Lor Powder Packets 469
K-Tab Filmtab Tablets 470
Rum-K 1363

SLOZEM (United Kingdom)
DILTIAZEM HYDROCHLORIDE
Cardizem CD Capsules 1016
Cardizem Injectable 1018
Cardizem Lyo-Ject Syringe 1018
Cardizem Monovial 1018
Tiazac Capsules 1378

SNO PHENICOL (Irish Republic, United Kingdom)
CHLORAMPHENICOL
Chloromycetin Ophthalmic Ointment, 1% . . . . ⊙296
Chloromycetin Ophthalmic Solution . . . . ⊙297
Chloroptic Sterile Ophthalmic Ointment . . . . ⊙234
Chloroptic Sterile Ophthalmic Solution . . . . ⊙235

SNO PILO (Irish Republic, United Kingdom)
PILOCARPINE HYDROCHLORIDE
Isopto Carpine Ophthalmic Solution . . . . ⊙215
Pilopine HS Ophthalmic Gel . . . . ⊙217
Salagen Tablets 2229

SOBREPINA (Portugal)
NIMODIPINE
Nimotop Capsules 904

SOBRONIL (Spain)
NAPROXEN
EC-Naprosyn Delayed-Release Tablets 2967
Naprosyn Suspension 2967
Naprosyn Tablets 2967

SODEN (Singapore)
NAPROXEN SODIUM
Anaprox DS Tablets 2967
Anaprox Tablets 2967
Naprelan Tablets 1293

SODEXX (Austria)
CIMETIDINE
Tagamet Tablets 1644

SODICLO (South Africa)
DICLOFENAC SODIUM
Voltaren Tablets 2315
Voltaren-XR Tablets 2315

SODIP-PHYLLINE (Switzerland)
THEOPHYLLINE
Aerolate Jr. T.D. Capsules 1361
Aerolate Liquid 1361
Aerolate Sr. T.D. Capsules 1361
Theo-Dur Extended-Release Tablets 1835
Uni-Dur Extended-Release Tablets 1841
Uniphyl 400 mg and 600 mg Tablets 2903

SODIUM SULAMYD (Canada)
SULFACETAMIDE SODIUM
Bleph-10 Ophthalmic Ointment 10% . . . . ⊙230
Klaron Lotion 10% 1224

SODIXEN (Mexico)
NAPROXEN SODIUM
Anaprox DS Tablets 2967
Anaprox Tablets 2967
Naprelan Tablets 1293

SODOLAC (Portugal)
ETODOLAC
Lodine Capsules 3528
Lodine Tablets 3528
Lodine XL Extended-Release Tablets 3530

SOFILEX (Singapore)
CEPHALEXIN
Keflex Oral Suspension 1237
Keflex Pulvules 1237

SOKARAL (Germany)
DEXAMETHASONE
Decadron Elixir 2078
Decadron Tablets 2079

SOLACAP (Spain)
FLUCONAZOLE
Diflucan Tablets, Injection, and Oral Suspension 2681

SOLAN-M (Germany)
VITAMIN A PALMITATE
Aquasol A Parenteral 593

SOLAQUIN (Hong Kong, Singapore)
HYDROQUINONE
Eldopaque Forte 4% Cream 1734
Eldoquin Forte 4% Cream 1734
Lustra Cream 2023
Lustra-AF Cream 2023
Melanex Topical Solution 2300
Solaquin Forte 4% Cream 1734
Solaquin Forte 4% Gel 1734

SOLARAZE (United Kingdom)
DICLOFENAC SODIUM
Voltaren Tablets 2315
Voltaren-XR Tablets 2315

SOLARCAINE (Canada, Hong Kong)
BENZOCAINE
Americaine Anesthetic Lubricant 1162
Americaine Otic Topical Anesthetic Ear Drops 1162

SOLASKIL (France)
LEVAMISOLE HYDROCHLORIDE
Ergamisol Tablets 1789

SOLAXIN (Hong Kong)
CHLORZOXAZONE
Parafon Forte DSC Caplets 2582

SOLAZINE (Canada)
TRIFLUOPERAZINE HYDROCHLORIDE
Stelazine Injection 1640
Stelazine Tablets 1640

SOLDESAM (Italy)
DEXAMETHASONE SODIUM PHOSPHATE
Decadron Phosphate Injection 2081
Decadron Phosphate Sterile Ophthalmic Ointment . . . . ⊙280, 2083
Decadron Phosphate Sterile Ophthalmic Solution 2084

SOLFA (Japan)
AMLEXANOX
Aphthasol Oral Paste 1025

SOLFACHINID (Italy)
QUINIDINE SULFATE
Quinidex Extentabs 2933

SOLFEN (Irish Republic)
IBUPROFEN
Motrin Suspension, Oral Drops, Chewable Tablets, and Caplets 2002

SOLFRANICOL (Mexico)
CHLORAMPHENICOL
Chloromycetin Ophthalmic Ointment, 1% . . . . ⊙296
Chloromycetin Ophthalmic Solution . . . . ⊙297
Chloroptic Sterile Ophthalmic Ointment . . . . ⊙234
Chloroptic Sterile Ophthalmic Solution . . . . ⊙235

SOLGERETIK (Austria, Germany)
NADOLOL
Nadolol Tablets 2288

SOLGOL (Austria, Germany, Spain)
NADOLOL
Nadolol Tablets 2288

SOLICAM (Belgium)
PIROXICAM
Feldene Capsules 2685

SOLIS (United Kingdom)
DIAZEPAM
Valium Injectable 3026
Valium Tablets 3047

SOLIUM (Canada)
CHLORDIAZEPOXIDE HYDROCHLORIDE
Librium Capsules 1736
Librium for Injection 1737

SOLONE (Spain)
DEXAMETHASONE SODIUM PHOSPHATE
Decadron Phosphate Injection 2081
Decadron Phosphate Sterile Ophthalmic Ointment . . . . ⊙280, 2083
Decadron Phosphate Sterile Ophthalmic Solution 2084

SOLONE (Australia)
PREDNISOLONE
Prelone Syrup 2273

SOLOSA (Italy)
GLIMEPIRIDE
Amaryl Tablets 717

SOLOSIN (Germany)
THEOPHYLLINE
Aerolate Jr. T.D. Capsules 1361
Aerolate Liquid 1361
Aerolate Sr. T.D. Capsules 1361
Theo-Dur Extended-Release Tablets 1835
Uni-Dur Extended-Release Tablets 1841
Uniphyl 400 mg and 600 mg Tablets 2903

SOLPAFLEX (United Kingdom)
KETOPROFEN
Orudis Capsules 3548
Oruvail Capsules 3548

SOLPAFLEX (Denmark, United Kingdom)
IBUPROFEN
Motrin Suspension, Oral Drops, Chewable Tablets, and Caplets 2002

SOLSOLONA (Mexico)
METHYLPREDNISOLONE ACETATE
Depo-Medrol Injectable Suspension 2795

SOLTAMOX (United Kingdom)
TAMOXIFEN CITRATE
Nolvadex Tablets 678

SOLTRIC (Mexico)
MEBENDAZOLE
Vermox Chewable Tablets 2017

SOLUBEOL (Belgium)
GUAIFENESIN
Organidin NR Liquid 3350
Organidin NR Tablets 3350

SOLUCEL (Spain)
BENZOYL PEROXIDE
Brevoxyl-4 Cleansing Lotion 3269
Brevoxyl-4 Creamy Wash 3270
Brevoxyl-4 Gel 3269
Brevoxyl-8 Cleansing Lotion 3269
Brevoxyl-8 Creamy Wash 3270
Brevoxyl-8 Gel 3269
Triaz Cleanser 2026
Triaz Gel 2026

SOLUCORT (France)
PREDNISOLONE SODIUM PHOSPHATE
Pediapred Oral Solution 1170

SOLUDECADRON (France)
DEXAMETHASONE SODIUM PHOSPHATE
Decadron Phosphate Injection 2081
Decadron Phosphate Sterile Ophthalmic Ointment ...... ⊙280, 2083
Decadron Phosphate Sterile Ophthalmic Solution 2084

SOLUFEN (France, South Africa)
IBUPROFEN
Motrin Suspension, Oral Drops, Chewable Tablets, and Caplets 2002

SOLUFEN (Mexico, Switzerland)
CHLORAMPHENICOL
Chloromycetin Ophthalmic Ointment, 1% .... ⊙296
Chloromycetin Ophthalmic Solution .... ⊙297
Chloroptic Sterile Ophthalmic Ointment .. ⊙234
Chloroptic Sterile Ophthalmic Solution .. ⊙235

SOLUFENA (Spain)
IBUPROFEN
Motrin Suspension, Oral Drops, Chewable Tablets, and Caplets 2002

SOLUGEL (Canada, Mexico)
BENZOYL PEROXIDE
Brevoxyl-4 Cleansing Lotion 3269
Brevoxyl-4 Creamy Wash 3270
Brevoxyl-4 Gel 3269
Brevoxyl-8 Cleansing Lotion 3269
Brevoxyl-8 Creamy Wash 3270
Brevoxyl-8 Gel 3269
Triaz Cleanser 2026
Triaz Gel 2026

SOLULEXIN (Hong Kong)
CEPHALEXIN
Keflex Oral Suspension 1237
Keflex Pulvules 1237

SOLU-MEDROL (Australia, Austria, Belgium, Brazil, Canada, Denmark, Finland, Hong Kong, Israel, Italy, Mexico, New Zealand, Norway, Portugal, Singapore, South Africa, Sweden, Switzerland, Thailand, The Netherlands)
METHYLPREDNISOLONE SODIUM SUCCINATE
Solu-Medrol Sterile Powder 2855

SOLU-MEDRONE (Irish Republic, Sweden, United Kingdom)
METHYLPREDNISOLONE SODIUM SUCCINATE
Solu-Medrol Sterile Powder 2855

SOLUMIDAZOL (Mexico)
METRONIDAZOLE
MetroCream 1404
MetroGel 1405
MetroGel-Vaginal Gel 1986
MetroLotion 1405
Noritate Cream 1224

SOLU-MODERIN (Spain)
METHYLPREDNISOLONE SODIUM SUCCINATE
Solu-Medrol Sterile Powder 2855

SOLUPEN (Spain)
DOXYCYCLINE HYCLATE
Doryx Coated Pellet Filled Capsules 3357
Periostat Tablets 1208
Vibramycin Hyclate Capsules 2735
Vibramycin Hyclate Intravenous 2737
Vibra-Tabs Film Coated Tablets 2735

SOLUSTREP (South Africa)
STREPTOMYCIN SULFATE
Streptomycin Sulfate Injection 2714

SOLUTIO CORDES DEXA N (Germany)
DEXAMETHASONE
Decadron Elixir 2078
Decadron Tablets 2079

SOLVIPECT (Norway)
GUAIFENESIN
Organidin NR Liquid 3350
Organidin NR Tablets 3350

SOLVIUM (Spain)
IBUPROFEN
Motrin Suspension, Oral Drops, Chewable Tablets, and Caplets 2002

SOMA (Canada)
CARISOPRODOL
Soma Tablets 3353

SOMADRIL (Denmark, Norway, Sweden)
CARISOPRODOL
Soma Tablets 3353

SOMAFLEX (Brazil)
CARISOPRODOL
Soma Tablets 3353

SOMAGEROL (Germany)
LORAZEPAM
Ativan Injection 3478
Ativan Tablets 3482

SOMALGESIC (Mexico)
NAPROXEN
EC-Naprosyn Delayed-Release Tablets ... 2967
Naprosyn Suspension 2967
Naprosyn Tablets 2967

SOMALGIT (Spain)
CARISOPRODOL
Soma Tablets 3353

SOMAPLUS (Brazil)
DIAZEPAM
Valium Injectable 3026
Valium Tablets 3047

SOMESE (Singapore)
TRIAZOLAM
Halcion Tablets 2823

SOMINEX (Canada)
DIPHENHYDRAMINE HYDROCHLORIDE
Benadryl Parenteral 2617

SOMINEX (United Kingdom)
PROMETHAZINE HYDROCHLORIDE
Phenergan Injection 3553
Phenergan Suppositories 3556
Phenergan Syrup Fortis 3554
Phenergan Syrup Plain 3554
Phenergan Tablets 3556

SOMOFILLINA (Italy)
THEOPHYLLINE
Aerolate Jr. T.D. Capsules 1361
Aerolate Liquid 1361
Aerolate Sr. T.D. Capsules 1361
Theo-Dur Extended-Release Tablets 1835
Uni-Dur Extended-Release Tablets 1841
Uniphyl 400 mg and 600 mg Tablets ... 2903

SOMOPHYLLIN (Canada, South Africa)
THEOPHYLLINE
Aerolate Jr. T.D. Capsules 1361
Aerolate Liquid 1361
Aerolate Sr. T.D. Capsules 1361
Theo-Dur Extended-Release Tablets 1835
Uni-Dur Extended-Release Tablets 1841
Uniphyl 400 mg and 600 mg Tablets ... 2903

SONATA (Belgium, Denmark, Finland, Germany, Irish Republic, Italy, Sweden, Switzerland, United Kingdom)
ZALEPLON
Sonata Capsules 3591

SONE (Australia)
PREDNISONE
Prednisone Intensol 3064
Prednisone Oral Solution 3064
Prednisone Tablets 3064

SONGAR (Italy)
TRIAZOLAM
Halcion Tablets 2823

SONI-SLO (United Kingdom)
ISOSORBIDE DINITRATE
Isordil Sublingual Tablets 3525
Isordil Titradose Tablets 3526

SONODOR (Spain)
DIPHENHYDRAMINE HYDROCHLORIDE
Benadryl Parenteral 2617

SONSUUR (South Africa)
CIMETIDINE
Tagamet Tablets 1644

SOPAMYCETIN (Canada)
CHLORAMPHENICOL
Chloromycetin Ophthalmic Ointment, 1% .... ⊙296
Chloromycetin Ophthalmic Solution .... ⊙297
Chloroptic Sterile Ophthalmic Ointment .. ⊙234
Chloroptic Sterile Ophthalmic Solution .. ⊙235

SOPENTAL (South Africa)
PENTOBARBITAL SODIUM
Nembutal Sodium Solution 485

SOPHIDONE (France)
HYDROMORPHONE HYDROCHLORIDE
Dilaudid Ampules 441
Dilaudid Injection 441
Dilaudid Multiple Dose Vials (Sterile Solution) 441
Dilaudid Oral Liquid 445
Dilaudid Powder 441
Dilaudid Rectal Suppositories 441
Dilaudid Tablets 441
Dilaudid Tablets - 8 mg 445
Dilaudid-HP Injection 443
Dilaudid-HP Lyophilized Powder 250 mg ... 443

SOPHIXEN (Mexico)
CIPROFLOXACIN HYDROCHLORIDE
Ciloxan Ophthalmic Ointment 538
Ciloxan Ophthalmic Solution .... ⊙209, 538
Cipro Tablets 887

SOPORIL (Germany)
PROMETHAZINE HYDROCHLORIDE
Phenergan Injection 3553
Phenergan Suppositories 3556
Phenergan Syrup Fortis 3554
Phenergan Syrup Plain 3554
Phenergan Tablets 3556

SOPROL (France, Irish Republic)
BISOPROLOL FUMARATE
Zebeta Tablets 1885

SOPROXEN (Singapore, Thailand)
NAPROXEN SODIUM
Anaprox DS Tablets 2967
Anaprox Tablets 2967
Naprelan Tablets 1293

SORBANGIL (Norway, Sweden)
ISOSORBIDE DINITRATE
Isordil Sublingual Tablets 3525
Isordil Titradose Tablets 3526

SORBICHEW (United Kingdom)
ISOSORBIDE DINITRATE
Isordil Sublingual Tablets 3525
Isordil Titradose Tablets 3526

SORBID (United Kingdom)
ISOSORBIDE DINITRATE
Isordil Sublingual Tablets 3525
Isordil Titradose Tablets 3526

SORBIDILAT (Austria, Germany, Switzerland)
ISOSORBIDE DINITRATE
Isordil Sublingual Tablets 3525
Isordil Titradose Tablets 3526

SORBIDIN (Australia, Thailand)
ISOSORBIDE DINITRATE
Isordil Sublingual Tablets 3525
Isordil Titradose Tablets 3526

SORBIMON (Austria)
ISOSORBIDE MONONITRATE
Imdur Tablets 1826
Ismo Tablets 3524

SORBITRATE (Belgium, France, Thailand, United Kingdom)
ISOSORBIDE DINITRATE
Isordil Sublingual Tablets 3525
Isordil Titradose Tablets 3526

SORE THROAT LOZENGES (Canada)
BENZOCAINE
Americaine Anesthetic Lubricant 1162
Americaine Otic Topical Anesthetic Ear Drops 1162

SOREN (Hong Kong)
NAPROXEN SODIUM
Anaprox DS Tablets 2967
Anaprox Tablets 2967
Naprelan Tablets 1293

SORIATANE (Canada, France)
ACITRETIN
Soriatane Capsules 3003

SORIFLOR (Sweden)
DIFLORASONE DIACETATE
Psorcon E Cream 1227
Psorcon E Ointment 1228

SORMON (Irish Republic)
ISOSORBIDE MONONITRATE
Imdur Tablets 1826
Ismo Tablets 3524

SORNIL (Thailand)
ISOSORBIDE DINITRATE
Isordil Sublingual Tablets 3525
Isordil Titradose Tablets 3526

SORTIS (Austria, Switzerland)
ATORVASTATIN CALCIUM
Lipitor Tablets 2639, 2696

SOSTILAR (Belgium)
CABERGOLINE
Dostinex Tablets 2804

SOTA (Germany)
SOTALOL HYDROCHLORIDE
Betapace Tablets 950

SOTA LICH (Germany)
SOTALOL HYDROCHLORIDE
Betapace Tablets 950

SOTAB (Australia)
SOTALOL HYDROCHLORIDE
Betapace Tablets 950

SOTABET (Denmark)
SOTALOL HYDROCHLORIDE
Betapace Tablets 950

SOTABETA (Germany)
SOTALOL HYDROCHLORIDE
Betapace Tablets 950

SOTACOR (Australia, Austria, Brazil, Canada, Denmark, Finland, Hong Kong, Irish Republic, Israel, Japan, New Zealand, Norway, Singapore, South Africa, Sweden, Thailand, The Netherlands, United Kingdom)
SOTALOL HYDROCHLORIDE
Betapace Tablets 950

SOTAGAMMA (Germany)
SOTALOL HYDROCHLORIDE
Betapace Tablets 950

SOTA-GRY (Germany)
SOTALOL HYDROCHLORIDE
Betapace Tablets 950

SOTAHEXAL (Australia, Germany, South Africa)
SOTALOL HYDROCHLORIDE
Betapace Tablets 950

SOTALEX (Belgium, France, Germany, Italy, Switzerland)
SOTALOL HYDROCHLORIDE
Betapace Tablets 950

SOTALIN (Finland)
SOTALOL HYDROCHLORIDE
Betapace Tablets 950

SOTAMED (Austria)
SOTALOL HYDROCHLORIDE
Betapace Tablets 950

SOTAMOL (Canada)
SOTALOL HYDROCHLORIDE
Betapace Tablets 950

SOTAPOR (Spain)
SOTALOL HYDROCHLORIDE
Betapace Tablets 950

SOTA-PUREN (Germany)
SOTALOL HYDROCHLORIDE
Betapace Tablets 950

SOTARYT (Germany)
SOTALOL HYDROCHLORIDE
Betapace Tablets 950

SOTA-SAAR (Germany)
SOTALOL HYDROCHLORIDE
Betapace Tablets 950

SOTASTAD (Austria, Germany)
SOTALOL HYDROCHLORIDE
Betapace Tablets 950

SOTAZIDEN N (Germany)
NADOLOL
Nadolol Tablets 2288

SOTILEN (Hong Kong, Singapore, Thailand)
PIROXICAM
Feldene Capsules 2685

SOVENTOL HYDROCORTISON (Germany)
HYDROCORTISONE ACETATE
Anusol-HC Suppositories 2238
Cortifoam Rectal Foam 3170
Hydrocortone Acetate Injectable Suspension 2103
Proctocort Suppositories 2264

SP54 (Hong Kong)
PENTOSAN POLYSULFATE SODIUM
Elmiron Capsules 570

SPAN-K (Australia, Hong Kong, New Zealand)
POTASSIUM CHLORIDE
K-Dur Microburst Release System ER Tablets 1832
K-Lor Powder Packets 469
K-Tab Filmtab Tablets 470
Rum-K 1363

SPANOR (France)
DOXYCYCLINE HYCLATE
Doryx Coated Pellet Filled Capsules 3357
Periostat Tablets 1208
Vibramycin Hyclate Capsules 2735
Vibramycin Hyclate Intravenous 2737
Vibra-Tabs Film Coated Tablets 2735

SPARKAL (Denmark, Finland, Sweden)
AMILORIDE HYDROCHLORIDE/HYDROCHLOROTHIAZIDE
Moduretic Tablets 2138

SPECTROBAK (Spain)
GENTAMICIN SULFATE
Genoptic Ophthalmic Ointment .... ⊙239
Genoptic Sterile Ophthalmic Solution ... ⊙239

SPECTROXYL (Switzerland)
AMOXICILLIN
Amoxil Pediatric Drops for Oral Suspension 1471

Amoxil Tablets ... 1471

SPECTRUM (Italy)
CEFTAZIDIME
Ceptaz for Injection ... 1499
Fortaz for Injection ... 1541
Tazicef for Injection ... 1647
Tazidime Vials, Faspak & ADD-Vantage ... 1966

SPEDIFEN (Switzerland)
IBUPROFEN
Motrin Suspension, Oral Drops, Chewable Tablets, and Caplets ... 2002

SPERSACARBACHOL (Switzerland)
CARBACHOL
Isopto Carbachol Ophthalmic Solution ... ⊙215

SPERSACARPIN (Germany)
PILOCARPINE HYDROCHLORIDE
Isopto Carpine Ophthalmic Solution ... ⊙215
Pilopine HS Ophthalmic Gel ... ⊙217
Salagen Tablets ... 2229

SPERSACARPINE (Canada, Hong Kong, Sweden, Switzerland)
PILOCARPINE HYDROCHLORIDE
Isopto Carpine Ophthalmic Solution ... ⊙215
Pilopine HS Ophthalmic Gel ... ⊙217
Salagen Tablets ... 2229

SPERSACET (Hong Kong, Switzerland)
SULFACETAMIDE SODIUM
Bleph-10 Ophthalmic Ointment 10% ... ⊙230
Klaron Lotion 10% ... 1224

SPERSADEX (Canada, Germany, Hong Kong, Norway, South Africa, Switzerland)
DEXAMETHASONE SODIUM PHOSPHATE
Decadron Phosphate Injection ... 2081
Decadron Phosphate Sterile Ophthalmic Ointment ... ⊙280, 2083
Decadron Phosphate Sterile Ophthalmic Solution ... 2084

SPERSAMIDE (South Africa)
SULFACETAMIDE SODIUM
Bleph-10 Ophthalmic Ointment 10% ... ⊙230
Klaron Lotion 10% ... 1224

SPERSANICOL (Canada, Hong Kong, Mexico, Singapore, South Africa, Switzerland)
CHLORAMPHENICOL
Chloromycetin Ophthalmic Ointment, 1% ... ⊙296
Chloromycetin Ophthalmic Solution ... ⊙297
Chloroptic Sterile Ophthalmic Ointment ... ⊙234
Chloroptic Sterile Ophthalmic Solution ... ⊙235

SPERSAPOLYMYXIN (Germany, Hong Kong, Switzerland, Thailand)
NEOMYCIN SULFATE/POLYMYXIN B SULFATE
Neosporin G.U. Irrigant Sterile ... 2256

SPERSIN (Australia)
NEOMYCIN SULFATE/POLYMYXIN B SULFATE
Neosporin G.U. Irrigant Sterile ... 2256

SPICLINE (France)
MINOCYCLINE HYDROCHLORIDE
Dynacin Capsules ... 2019
Minocin Intravenous ... 1862
Minocin Oral Suspension ... 1865
Minocin Pellet-Filled Capsules ... 1863

SPIDIFEN (Belgium, Spain)
IBUPROFEN
Motrin Suspension, Oral Drops, Chewable Tablets, and Caplets ... 2002

SPIRALGIN (Switzerland)
MEFENAMIC ACID
Ponstel Capsules ... 1356

SPIRICORT (Switzerland)
PREDNISOLONE
Prelone Syrup ... 2273

SPIROCORT (Denmark)
BUDESONIDE
Pulmicort Turbuhaler Inhalation Powder ... 636
Rhinocort Nasal Inhaler ... 640

SPIROLAIR (Belgium)
PIRBUTEROL ACETATE
Maxair Autohaler ... 1981
Maxair Inhaler ... 1984

SPLENDIL (Brazil, Japan)
FELODIPINE
Plendil Extended-Release Tablets ... 623

SPONDY-DEXA (Germany)
DEXAMETHASONE SODIUM PHOSPHATE
Decadron Phosphate Injection ... 2081
Decadron Phosphate Sterile Ophthalmic Ointment ... ⊙280, 2083
Decadron Phosphate Sterile Ophthalmic Solution ... 2084

SPONDYLON (Germany)
KETOPROFEN
Orudis Capsules ... 3548
Oruvail Capsules ... 3548

SPORAL (Thailand)
ITRACONAZOLE
Sporanox Capsules ... 1800
Sporanox Oral Solution ... 1808, 2512

SPORANOX (Australia, Austria, Belgium, Brazil, Canada, Denmark, Finland, France, Hong Kong, Irish Republic, Israel, Italy, Mexico, New Zealand, Norway, Portugal, Singapore, South Africa, Spain, Sweden, Switzerland, United Kingdom)
ITRACONAZOLE
Sporanox Capsules ... 1800
Sporanox Oral Solution ... 1808, 2512

SPORASEC (Mexico)
ITRACONAZOLE
Sporanox Capsules ... 1800
Sporanox Oral Solution ... 1808, 2512

SPORICEF (Thailand)
CEPHALEXIN
Keflex Oral Suspension ... 1237
Keflex Pulvules ... 1237

SPORIDEX (Singapore)
CEPHALEXIN
Keflex Oral Suspension ... 1237
Keflex Pulvules ... 1237

SPOROL (Spain)
CEPHALEXIN
Keflex Oral Suspension ... 1237
Keflex Pulvules ... 1237

SPORTINO (Germany)
HEPARIN SODIUM
Heparin Lock Flush Solution ... 3509
Heparin Sodium Injection ... 3511

SPOZAL (Singapore)
KETOCONAZOLE
Nizoral 2% Cream ... 3620
Nizoral 2% Shampoo ... 2007
Nizoral Tablets ... 1791

SQUIBB-HC (Australia)
HYDROCORTISONE ACETATE
Anusol-HC Suppositories ... 2238
Cortifoam Rectal Foam ... 3170
Hydrocortone Acetate Injectable Suspension ... 2103
Proctocort Suppositories ... 2264

SQWORM (Australia)
MEBENDAZOLE
Vermox Chewable Tablets ... 2017

SRM-RHOTARD (Singapore, South Africa, United Kingdom)
MORPHINE SULFATE
Astramorph/PF Injection, USP (Preservative-Free) ... 594
Duramorph Injection ... 1312
Infumorph 200 and Infumorph 500 Sterile Solutions ... 1314
Kadian Capsules ... 1335
MS Contin Tablets ... 2896
MSIR Oral Capsules ... 2898
MSIR Oral Solution ... 2898
MSIR Oral Solution Concentrate ... 2898
MSIR Oral Tablets ... 2898
Oramorph SR Tablets ... 3062
Roxanol 100 Concentrated Oral Solution ... 3066
Roxanol Concentrated Oral Solution ... 3066
Roxanol-T Oral Solution ... 3066

STACER (Portugal)
RANITIDINE HYDROCHLORIDE
Zantac 150 EFFERdose Granules ... 1690
Zantac 150 EFFERdose Tablets ... 1690
Zantac 150 Tablets ... 1690
Zantac 300 Tablets ... 1690
Zantac Injection ... 1688
Zantac Injection Premixed ... 1688
Zantac Syrup ... 1690

STACORT-A (Hong Kong)
TRIAMCINOLONE ACETONIDE
Azmacort Inhalation Aerosol ... 728
Nasacort AQ Nasal Spray ... 752
Nasacort Nasal Inhaler ... 750

STADASAN (Germany)
IBUPROFEN
Motrin Suspension, Oral Drops, Chewable Tablets, and Caplets ... 2002

STADOL (Canada, Mexico, The Netherlands)
BUTORPHANOL TARTRATE
Stadol NS Nasal Spray ... 1108

STAMICINA (Italy)
DOXYCYCLINE HYCLATE
Doryx Coated Pellet Filled Capsules ... 3357
Periostat Tablets ... 1208
Vibramycin Hyclate Capsules ... 2735
Vibramycin Hyclate Intravenous ... 2737
Vibra-Tabs Film Coated Tablets ... 2735

STARCEF (Italy)
CEFTAZIDIME
Ceptaz for Injection ... 1499
Fortaz for Injection ... 1541
Tazicef for Injection ... 1647
Tazidime Vials, Faspak & ADD-Vantage ... 1966

STARIL (United Kingdom)
FOSINOPRIL SODIUM
Monopril Tablets ... 1091

STATEX (Canada, Singapore)
MORPHINE SULFATE
Astramorph/PF Injection, USP (Preservative-Free) ... 594
Duramorph Injection ... 1312
Infumorph 200 and Infumorph 500 Sterile Solutions ... 1314
Kadian Capsules ... 1335
MS Contin Tablets ... 2896
MSIR Oral Capsules ... 2898
MSIR Oral Solution ... 2898
MSIR Oral Solution Concentrate ... 2898
MSIR Oral Tablets ... 2898
Oramorph SR Tablets ... 3062
Roxanol 100 Concentrated Oral Solution ... 3066
Roxanol Concentrated Oral Solution ... 3066
Roxanol-T Oral Solution ... 3066

STATICIN (Canada)
ERYTHROMYCIN
Emgel 2% Topical Gel ... 1285
Ery-Tab Tablets ... 448
Erythromycin Base Filmtab Tablets ... 454
Erythromycin Delayed-Release Capsules, USP ... 455
PCE Dispertab Tablets ... 498

STATICINE (Switzerland)
ERYTHROMYCIN
Emgel 2% Topical Gel ... 1285
Ery-Tab Tablets ... 448
Erythromycin Base Filmtab Tablets ... 454
Erythromycin Delayed-Release Capsules, USP ... 455
PCE Dispertab Tablets ... 498

STATIVA (Italy)
CERIVASTATIN SODIUM
Baycol Tablets ... 883

STATROL (Belgium)
NEOMYCIN SULFATE/POLYMYXIN B SULFATE
Neosporin G.U. Irrigant Sterile ... 2256

STEDIRIL (Belgium)
NORGESTREL
Ovrette Tablets ... 3552

STEDIRIL 30 (Belgium)
LEVONORGESTREL
Norplant System ... 3543

STEDIRIL D (Belgium)
LEVONORGESTREL
Norplant System ... 3543

STELAZINE (Australia, Canada, Irish Republic, Mexico, New Zealand, South Africa, United Kingdom)
TRIFLUOPERAZINE HYDROCHLORIDE
Stelazine Injection ... 1640
Stelazine Tablets ... 1640

STEMETIL (Italy, Singapore, Thailand, The Netherlands)
PROCHLORPERAZINE MALEATE
Compazine Spansule Capsules ... 1505
Compazine Tablets ... 1505

STEMZINE (Australia)
PROCHLORPERAZINE MALEATE
Compazine Spansule Capsules ... 1505
Compazine Tablets ... 1505

STENOCOR (Italy)
DIPYRIDAMOLE
Persantine Tablets ... 1057

STENSOLO (Italy)
MEPROBAMATE
Miltown Tablets ... 3349

STERAX (Belgium, Germany, Switzerland)
DESONIDE
DesOwen Cream ... 1401
DesOwen Lotion ... 1401
DesOwen Ointment ... 1401

STERODELTA (Italy)
DIFLORASONE DIACETATE
Psorcon E Cream ... 1227
Psorcon E Ointment ... 1228

STERODEX (Israel)
DEXAMETHASONE SODIUM PHOSPHATE
Decadron Phosphate Injection ... 2081
Decadron Phosphate Sterile Ophthalmic Ointment ... ⊙280, 2083
Decadron Phosphate Sterile Ophthalmic Solution ... 2084

STEROLONE (Italy)
FLUOCINOLONE ACETONIDE
Synalar Cream ... 2020
Synalar Ointment ... 2020
Synalar Topical Solution ... 2020

STERONASE AQ (Israel)
TRIAMCINOLONE ACETONIDE
Azmacort Inhalation Aerosol ... 728
Nasacort AQ Nasal Spray ... 752
Nasacort Nasal Inhaler ... 750

STERONIDE (Brazil)
DESONIDE
DesOwen Cream ... 1401
DesOwen Lotion ... 1401
DesOwen Ointment ... 1401

STESOLID (Austria, Denmark, Finland, Germany, Irish Republic, Israel, Norway, Portugal, Singapore, Spain, Sweden, Switzerland, Thailand, The Netherlands, United Kingdom)
DIAZEPAM
Valium Injectable ... 3026
Valium Tablets ... 3047

STIEDEX (United Kingdom)
DESOXIMETASONE
Topicort Cream ... 2025
Topicort Gel ... 2025
Topicort LP Cream ... 2025
Topicort Ointment ... 2025

STIEDEX LP (United Kingdom)
DESOXIMETASONE
Topicort Cream ... 2025
Topicort Gel ... 2025
Topicort LP Cream ... 2025
Topicort Ointment ... 2025

STIEDEX LPN (United Kingdom)
DESOXIMETASONE
Topicort Cream ... 2025
Topicort Gel ... 2025
Topicort LP Cream ... 2025
Topicort Ointment ... 2025

STIEFCORTIL (Brazil)
HYDROCORTISONE
Anusol-HC Cream 2.5% ... 2237
Hydrocortone Tablets ... 2106

STIEMAZOL (Germany, South Africa)
CLOTRIMAZOLE
Lotrimin Cream 1% ... 3128
Lotrimin Lotion 1% ... 3128
Lotrimin Topical Solution 1% ... 3128
Mycelex Troche ... 573

STIEMYCIN (Brazil, Hong Kong, Irish Republic, Mexico, New Zealand, Singapore, South Africa, Thailand, The Netherlands, United Kingdom)
ERYTHROMYCIN
Emgel 2% Topical Gel ... 1285
Ery-Tab Tablets ... 448
Erythromycin Base Filmtab Tablets ... 454
Erythromycin Delayed-Release Capsules, USP ... 455
PCE Dispertab Tablets ... 498

STIEMYCINE (Austria, Germany, Switzerland)
ERYTHROMYCIN
Emgel 2% Topical Gel ... 1285
Ery-Tab Tablets ... 448
Erythromycin Base Filmtab Tablets ... 454
Erythromycin Delayed-Release Capsules, USP ... 455
PCE Dispertab Tablets ... 498

STIEVA-A (Australia, Canada, Hong Kong, Mexico, Singapore, Thailand)
TRETINOIN
Avita Cream ... 999
Avita Gel ... 1000
Renova 0.05% Cream ... 2519
Retin-A Micro 0.1% ... 2522
Vesanoid Capsules ... 3037

STIEVAMYCIN (Canada)
TRETINOIN
Avita Cream ... 999
Avita Gel ... 1000
Renova 0.05% Cream ... 2519
Retin-A Micro 0.1% ... 2522
Vesanoid Capsules ... 3037

STILL (Brazil)
DICLOFENAC SODIUM
Voltaren Tablets ... 2315

Voltaren-XR Tablets 2315

STILLINE (United Kingdom)
SELEGILINE HYDROCHLORIDE
Eldepryl Capsules 3266

STILNOCT (Belgium, Denmark, Finland, Irish Republic, Norway, Sweden, The Netherlands, United Kingdom)
ZOLPIDEM TARTRATE
Ambien Tablets 3191

STILNOX (Australia, Austria, Brazil, France, Germany, Hong Kong, Israel, Italy, Portugal, Singapore, South Africa, Spain, Switzerland)
ZOLPIDEM TARTRATE
Ambien Tablets 3191

STIMOLCARDIO (Italy)
DIPYRIDAMOLE
Persantine Tablets 1057

STIMUL (Belgium, Switzerland)
PEMOLINE
Cylert Chewable Tablets 415
Cylert Tablets 415

STIMU-TSH (France)
PROTIRELIN
Thyrel TRH for Injection 3630

STIMYCINE (France)
ERYTHROMYCIN
Emgel 2% Topical Gel 1285
Ery-Tab Tablets 448
Erythromycin Base Filmtab Tablets 454
Erythromycin Delayed-Release Capsules, USP 455
PCE Dispertab Tablets 498

STIOXYL (Sweden)
BENZOYL PEROXIDE
Brevoxyl-4 Cleansing Lotion 3269
Brevoxyl-4 Creamy Wash 3270
Brevoxyl-4 Gel 3269
Brevoxyl-8 Cleansing Lotion 3269
Brevoxyl-8 Creamy Wash 3270
Brevoxyl-8 Gel 3269
Triaz Cleanser 2026
Triaz Gel 2026

STIPROX (France)
CICLOPIROX OLAMINE
Loprox Cream 2021
Loprox Lotion 2021

STIVATE (Thailand)
CLOBETASOL PROPIONATE
Cormax Cream 2440
Cormax Ointment 2440
Cormax Scalp Application 2441
Temovate Cream 1301
Temovate E Emollient 1302
Temovate Gel 1303
Temovate Ointment 1301
Temovate Scalp Application 1304

STOCRIN (Australia, Belgium, Denmark, Finland, Israel, New Zealand, Portugal, South Africa, Sweden, Switzerland, Thailand, The Netherlands)
EFAVIRENZ
Sustiva Capsules 1258

STOMAKON (Brazil)
CIMETIDINE
Tagamet Tablets 1644

STOMEDINE (France)
CIMETIDINE
Tagamet Tablets 1644

STOMET (Brazil, Italy)
CIMETIDINE
Tagamet Tablets 1644

STOP ESPINILLA NORMADERM (Spain)
BENZOYL PEROXIDE
Brevoxyl-4 Cleansing Lotion 3269
Brevoxyl-4 Creamy Wash 3270
Brevoxyl-4 Gel 3269
Brevoxyl-8 Cleansing Lotion 3269
Brevoxyl-8 Creamy Wash 3270
Brevoxyl-8 Gel 3269
Triaz Cleanser 2026
Triaz Gel 2026

STOPITCH (South Africa)
HYDROCORTISONE ACETATE
Anusol-HC Suppositories 2238
Cortifoam Rectal Foam 3170
Hydrocortone Acetate Injectable Suspension 2103
Proctocort Suppositories 2264

STOPPERS (United Kingdom)
NICOTINE
Nicotrol Inhaler 2840
Nicotrol Nasal Spray 2843

STOVAREN (Italy)
CEFOXITIN SODIUM
Mefoxin Premixed Intravenous Solution 2127
Mefoxin for Injection 2124

STRADERM (Italy)
FLUOCINOLONE ACETONIDE
Synalar Cream 2020
Synalar Ointment 2020
Synalar Topical Solution 2020

STREPTASE (Australia, Austria, Belgium, Brazil, Canada, Denmark, Finland, France, Germany, Hong Kong, Irish Republic, Israel, Italy, Mexico, New Zealand, Norway, Portugal, Singapore, South Africa, Spain, Sweden, Switzerland, Thailand, The Netherlands, United Kingdom)
STREPTOKINASE
Streptase for Infusion 647

STREPTO (Thailand)
STREPTOMYCIN SULFATE
Streptomycin Sulfate Injection 2714

STREPTOCOL (Italy)
STREPTOMYCIN SULFATE
Streptomycin Sulfate Injection 2714

STREPTO-FATOL (Germany)
STREPTOMYCIN SULFATE
Streptomycin Sulfate Injection 2714

STREPTO-HEFA (Germany)
STREPTOMYCIN SULFATE
Streptomycin Sulfate Injection 2714

STRIATON (Germany)
CARBIDOPA/LEVODOPA
Sinemet CR Tablets 1255
Sinemet Tablets 1253

STROMECTOL (Australia, France)
IVERMECTIN
Stromectol Tablets 2185

STUBIT (United Kingdom)
NICOTINE
Nicotrol Inhaler 2840
Nicotrol Nasal Spray 2843

SUADIAN (Italy)
NAFTIFINE HYDROCHLORIDE
Naftin Cream 2224
Naftin Gel 2224

SUBCUTIN N (Germany)
BENZOCAINE
Americaine Anesthetic Lubricant 1162
Americaine Otic Topical Anesthetic Ear Drops 1162

SUBLIMAZE (Australia, Canada, Irish Republic, New Zealand, South Africa, United Kingdom)
FENTANYL CITRATE
Actiq 1184

SUBSTITOL (Austria)
ESTRADIOL
Alora Transdermal System 3372
Climara Transdermal System 958
Estrace Vaginal Cream 3358
Estring Vaginal Ring 2811
Vivelle Transdermal System 2412
Vivelle-Dot Transdermal System 2416

SUBSTITOL (Austria)
MORPHINE SULFATE
Astramorph/PF Injection, USP (Preservative-Free) 594
Duramorph Injection 1312
Infumorph 200 and Infumorph 500 Sterile Solutions 1314
Kadian Capsules 1335
MS Contin Tablets 2896
MSIR Oral Capsules 2898
MSIR Oral Solution 2898
MSIR Oral Solution Concentrate 2898
MSIR Oral Tablets 2898
Oramorph SR Tablets 3062
Roxanol 100 Concentrated Oral Solution 3066
Roxanol Concentrated Oral Solution 3066
Roxanol-T Oral Solution 3066

SUBUTEX (Denmark, Finland, France, Italy, Portugal, Sweden, Switzerland, United Kingdom)
BUPRENORPHINE HYDROCHLORIDE
Buprenex Injectable 2918

SUCARI (Hong Kong)
SUCRALFATE
Carafate Suspension 731
Carafate Tablets 730

SUCCICAPTAL (France)
SUCCIMER
Chemet Capsules 3078

SUCCOSA (Sweden)
SUCRALFATE
Carafate Suspension 731
Carafate Tablets 730

SUCRABEST (Germany)
SUCRALFATE
Carafate Suspension 731
Carafate Tablets 730

SUCRAFEN (Thailand)
SUCRALFATE
Carafate Suspension 731
Carafate Tablets 730

SUCRAGER (Italy)
SUCRALFATE
Carafate Suspension 731
Carafate Tablets 730

SUCRAL (Italy, Thailand)
SUCRALFATE
Carafate Suspension 731
Carafate Tablets 730

SUCRALAN (Austria)
SUCRALFATE
Carafate Suspension 731
Carafate Tablets 730

SUCRALBENE (Austria)
SUCRALFATE
Carafate Suspension 731
Carafate Tablets 730

SUCRALFIN (Italy)
SUCRALFATE
Carafate Suspension 731
Carafate Tablets 730

SUCRALSTAD (Austria)
SUCRALFATE
Carafate Suspension 731
Carafate Tablets 730

SUCRALUM (Portugal)
SUCRALFATE
Carafate Suspension 731
Carafate Tablets 730

SUCRAMAL (Italy)
SUCRALFATE
Carafate Suspension 731
Carafate Tablets 730

SUCRAMED (Austria)
SUCRALFATE
Carafate Suspension 731
Carafate Tablets 730

SUCRAPHIL (Germany)
SUCRALFATE
Carafate Suspension 731
Carafate Tablets 730

SUCRATE (Italy, Thailand)
SUCRALFATE
Carafate Suspension 731
Carafate Tablets 730

SUCRORAL (Italy)
SUCRALFATE
Carafate Suspension 731
Carafate Tablets 730

SUDAC (Italy)
SULINDAC
Clinoril Tablets 2053

SUDAFED EXPECTORANT (Canada, Hong Kong, Irish Republic, Singapore, South Africa, United Kingdom)
GUAIFENESIN/PSEUDOEPHEDRINE HYDROCHLORIDE
Guaifed Capsules 2272
Guaifed-PD Capsules 2272
Zephrex LA Tablets 3092
Zephrex Tablets 3091

SUDAFED EXPECTORANTE (Spain)
GUAIFENESIN/PSEUDOEPHEDRINE HYDROCHLORIDE
Guaifed Capsules 2272
Guaifed-PD Capsules 2272
Zephrex LA Tablets 3092
Zephrex Tablets 3091

SUDELIX (Australia)
GUAIFENESIN/PSEUDOEPHEDRINE HYDROCHLORIDE
Guaifed Capsules 2272
Guaifed-PD Capsules 2272
Zephrex LA Tablets 3092
Zephrex Tablets 3091

SUFIL (Spain)
MEBENDAZOLE
Vermox Chewable Tablets 2017

SUFORTAN (Italy, Mexico)
PENICILLAMINE
Cuprimine Capsules 2075
Depen Titratable Tablets 3341

SUFORTANON (Spain)
PENICILLAMINE
Cuprimine Capsules 2075
Depen Titratable Tablets 3341

SUGAR (Italy)
SUCRALFATE
Carafate Suspension 731
Carafate Tablets 730

SUGAST (Italy)
SUCRALFATE
Carafate Suspension 731
Carafate Tablets 730

SUIFLOX (Mexico)
CIPROFLOXACIN HYDROCHLORIDE
Ciloxan Ophthalmic Ointment 538
Ciloxan Ophthalmic Solution ⊙209, 538
Cipro Tablets 887

SULAR (Belgium, Mexico, Spain, The Netherlands)
NISOLDIPINE
Sular Tablets 688

SULARTRENE (Italy)
SULINDAC
Clinoril Tablets 2053

SULAZINE (Australia, United Kingdom)
SULFASALAZINE
Azulfidine EN-tabs Tablets 2775

SULCRATE (Canada)
SUCRALFATE
Carafate Suspension 731
Carafate Tablets 730

SULEN (Italy)
SULINDAC
Clinoril Tablets 2053

SULEO-M (United Kingdom)
MALATHION
Ovide Lotion 2023

SULFA 10 (Belgium)
SULFACETAMIDE SODIUM
Bleph-10 Ophthalmic Ointment 10% ⊙230
Klaron Lotion 10% 1224

SULFABLEPH N LIQUIFILM (Germany)
SULFACETAMIDE SODIUM
Bleph-10 Ophthalmic Ointment 10% ⊙230
Klaron Lotion 10% 1224

SULFACET (Spain)
SULFACETAMIDE SODIUM
Bleph-10 Ophthalmic Ointment 10% ⊙230
Klaron Lotion 10% 1224

SULFACETA (Spain)
SULFACETAMIDE SODIUM
Bleph-10 Ophthalmic Ointment 10% ⊙230
Klaron Lotion 10% 1224

SULFACETAM (Spain)
SULFACETAMIDE SODIUM
Bleph-10 Ophthalmic Ointment 10% ⊙230
Klaron Lotion 10% 1224

SULFACID (Israel)
SULFACETAMIDE SODIUM
Bleph-10 Ophthalmic Ointment 10% ⊙230
Klaron Lotion 10% 1224

SULFAMYLON (Canada, United Kingdom)
MAFENIDE ACETATE
Sulfamylon Cream 1011
Sulfamylon Topical Solution 1011

SULFAZINE (Irish Republic)
SULFASALAZINE
Azulfidine EN-tabs Tablets 2775

SULFEX (Canada, Hong Kong)
SULFACETAMIDE SODIUM
Bleph-10 Ophthalmic Ointment 10% ⊙230
Klaron Lotion 10% 1224

SULFIL (Spain)
MEBENDAZOLE
Vermox Chewable Tablets 2017

SULFONA (Portugal, Spain)
DAPSONE
Dapsone Tablets USP 1780

SULFONAMID SPUMAN (Germany)
SULFANILAMIDE
AVC Cream 1350
AVC Suppositories 1350

SULFO-SELENIUM (Belgium)
HYDROCORTISONE
Anusol-HC Cream 2.5% 2237
Hydrocortone Tablets 2106

SULFOXYL (Canada)
BENZOYL PEROXIDE
Brevoxyl-4 Cleansing Lotion 3269
Brevoxyl-4 Creamy Wash 3270
Brevoxyl-4 Gel 3269
Brevoxyl-8 Cleansing Lotion 3269
Brevoxyl-8 Creamy Wash 3270
Brevoxyl-8 Gel 3269
Triaz Cleanser 2026
Triaz Gel 2026

SULINDAL (Spain)
SULINDAC
Clinoril Tablets 2053

SULINOL (Italy)
SULINDAC
Clinoril Tablets 2053

SULMYCIN (Austria, Germany)
GENTAMICIN SULFATE
Genoptic Ophthalmic Ointment .... ⊙239
Genoptic Sterile Ophthalmic Solution ... ⊙239

SULNIL (Brazil)
CHLORAMPHENICOL
Chloromycetin Ophthalmic Ointment, 1% .... ⊙296
Chloromycetin Ophthalmic Solution .... ⊙297
Chloroptic Sterile Ophthalmic Ointment .. ⊙234
Chloroptic Sterile Ophthalmic Solution .. ⊙235

SULORANE (Israel)
DESFLURANE
Suprane Liquid for Inhalation 874

SULPHAMIDE (Israel)
SULFACETAMIDE SODIUM
Bleph-10 Ophthalmic Ointment 10% .... ⊙230
Klaron Lotion 10% 1224

SULQUIPEN (Spain)
CEPHALEXIN
Keflex Oral Suspension 1237
Keflex Pulvules 1237

SULREUMA (Italy)
SULINDAC
Clinoril Tablets 2053

SULTERLINE (Thailand)
TERBUTALINE SULFATE
Brethine Ampuls 2314
Brethine Tablets 2313

SULTRIN (Australia, Canada, Irish Republic, South Africa, Switzerland)
SULFABENZAMIDE/SULFACETAMIDE/ SULFATHIAZOLE
Sultrin Triple Sulfa Cream 2587

SUMADOL (Italy)
SUMATRIPTAN SUCCINATE
Imitrex Injection 1549
Imitrex Tablets 1558

SUMAX (Brazil)
SUMATRIPTAN
Imitrex Nasal Spray 1554

SUMIAL (Spain)
PROPRANOLOL HYDROCHLORIDE
Inderal Injectable 3513
Inderal LA Long-Acting Capsules 3516
Inderal Tablets 3513

SUMIGRENE (Italy)
SUMATRIPTAN SUCCINATE
Imitrex Injection 1549
Imitrex Tablets 1558

SUNPROX (Singapore)
NAPROXEN SODIUM
Anaprox DS Tablets 2967
Anaprox Tablets 2967
Naprelan Tablets 1293

SUPARTZ (United Kingdom)
SODIUM HYALURONATE
Hyalgan Solution 3080

SUPERO (Italy)
CEFUROXIME SODIUM
Kefurox Vials, ADD-Vantage 1948
Zinacef Injection 1696

SUPERSAN (Portugal)
CYPROHEPTADINE HYDROCHLORIDE
Periactin Tablets 2155

SUPEUDOL (Canada)
OXYCODONE HYDROCHLORIDE
OxyContin Tablets 2912
OxyFast Oral Concentrate Solution 2916
OxyIR Capsules 2916
Percolone Tablets 1327
Roxicodone Tablets 3067

SUPLASYN (Canada, United Kingdom)
SODIUM HYALURONATE
Hyalgan Solution 3080

SUPRACEF (Finland)
CEFIXIME
Suprax Tablets 1877
Suprax for Oral Suspension 1877

SUPRAGENTA (Spain)
GENTAMICIN SULFATE
Genoptic Ophthalmic Ointment .... ⊙239
Genoptic Sterile Ophthalmic Solution ... ⊙239

SUPRALAN (Thailand)
FLUOCINOLONE ACETONIDE
Synalar Cream 2020
Synalar Ointment 2020
Synalar Topical Solution 2020

SUPRALEF (Spain)
HYDROCORTISONE ACETATE
Anusol-HC Suppositories 2238
Cortifoam Rectal Foam 3170
Hydrocortone Acetate Injectable Suspension 2103
Proctocort Suppositories 2264

SUPRALIP (United Kingdom)
FENOFIBRATE
Tricor Capsules, Micronized 513

SUPRAMOX (Switzerland)
AMOXICILLIN
Amoxil Pediatric Drops for Oral Suspension 1471
Amoxil Tablets 1471

SUPRAN (Israel)
CEFIXIME
Suprax Tablets 1877
Suprax for Oral Suspension 1877

SUPRANE (Australia, Austria, Belgium, Canada, Denmark, Finland, Germany, Irish Republic, Italy, Mexico, New Zealand, Norway, Singapore, South Africa, Spain, Sweden, Switzerland, The Netherlands, United Kingdom)
DESFLURANE
Suprane Liquid for Inhalation 874

SUPRAX (Canada, Germany, Irish Republic, Italy, United Kingdom)
CEFIXIME
Suprax Tablets 1877
Suprax for Oral Suspension 1877

SUPRES (Canada)
CHLOROTHIAZIDE/METHYLDOPA
Aldoclor Tablets 2035

SURAZEM (The Netherlands)
DILTIAZEM HYDROCHLORIDE
Cardizem CD Capsules 1016
Cardizem Injectable 1018
Cardizem Lyo-Ject Syringe 1018
Cardizem Monovial 1018
Tiazac Capsules 1378

SURETIN (Italy)
TAZAROTENE
Tazorac Gel 556

SURFONT (Germany)
MEBENDAZOLE
Vermox Chewable Tablets 2017

SURIL (Italy)
SUCRALFATE
Carafate Suspension 731
Carafate Tablets 730

SURMONTIL (Canada, Denmark, Finland, Hong Kong, Irish Republic, New Zealand, Norway, Portugal, Sweden, The Netherlands, United Kingdom)
TRIMIPRAMINE MALEATE
Surmontil Capsules 3595

SURVANTA (Australia, Austria, Belgium, Brazil, Canada, France, Germany, Hong Kong, Mexico, New Zealand, Singapore, South Africa, Spain, Switzerland, Thailand, The Netherlands, United Kingdom)
BERACTANT
Survanta Intratracheal Suspension 3053

SURVANTA-VENT (Norway, Sweden)
BERACTANT
Survanta Intratracheal Suspension 3053

SUSPREN (United Kingdom)
IBUPROFEN
Motrin Suspension, Oral Drops, Chewable Tablets, and Caplets 2002

SUSTIVA (Canada, France, Germany, Irish Republic, Italy, Spain, United Kingdom)
EFAVIRENZ
Sustiva Capsules 1258

SUXILEP (Germany)
ETHOSUXIMIDE
Zarontin Capsules 2659
Zarontin Syrup 2660

SUXINUTIN (Austria, Finland, Germany, Sweden, Switzerland)
ETHOSUXIMIDE
Zarontin Capsules 2659
Zarontin Syrup 2660

SVEDOCAIN SIN VASOCONSTR (Spain)
BUPIVACAINE HYDROCHLORIDE
Sensorcaine Injection 643
Sensorcaine-MPF Injection 643

SWISS-KAL SR (South Africa)
POTASSIUM CHLORIDE
K-Dur Microburst Release System ER Tablets 1832
K-Lor Powder Packets 469
K-Tab Filmtab Tablets 470
Rum-K 1363

SYLADOR (Brazil)
TRAMADOL HYDROCHLORIDE
Ultram Tablets 2600

SYMBOL (Italy)
MISOPROSTOL
Cytotec Tablets 3202

SYMMETREL (Australia, Austria, Canada, Germany, Hong Kong, Irish Republic, Israel, New Zealand, Norway, Singapore, South Africa, Sweden, Switzerland, The Netherlands, United Kingdom)
AMANTADINE HYDROCHLORIDE
Symmetrel Syrup 1328
Symmetrel Tablets 1328

SYNAGIS (Australia, Denmark, Finland, Italy, New Zealand, Norway, Singapore, Sweden, The Netherlands, United Kingdom)
PALIVIZUMAB
Synagis Intramuscular 2028

SYNALAR (Australia, Austria, Belgium, Brazil, Canada, Denmark, France, Irish Republic, Mexico, New Zealand, Norway, Portugal, Singapore, South Africa, Spain, Sweden, Switzerland, The Netherlands, United Kingdom)
FLUOCINOLONE ACETONIDE
Synalar Cream 2020
Synalar Ointment 2020
Synalar Topical Solution 2020

SYNALAR C (United Kingdom)
FLUOCINOLONE ACETONIDE
Synalar Cream 2020
Synalar Ointment 2020
Synalar Topical Solution 2020

SYNALAR RECTAL SIMPLE (Spain)
FLUOCINOLONE ACETONIDE
Synalar Cream 2020
Synalar Ointment 2020
Synalar Topical Solution 2020

SYNAMOL (Canada)
FLUOCINOLONE ACETONIDE
Synalar Cream 2020
Synalar Ointment 2020
Synalar Topical Solution 2020

SYNAREL (Australia, Belgium, Canada, France, Hong Kong, Irish Republic, Israel, Mexico, New Zealand, South Africa, Spain, The Netherlands, United Kingdom)
NAFARELIN ACETATE
Synarel Nasal Solution for Central Precocious Puberty 3204
Synarel Nasal Solution for Endometriosis 3205

SYNARELA (Denmark, Finland, Germany, Norway, Sweden)
NAFARELIN ACETATE
Synarel Nasal Solution for Central Precocious Puberty 3204
Synarel Nasal Solution for Endometriosis 3205

SYNASTERON (Belgium)
OXYMETHOLONE
Anadrol-50 Tablets 3321

SYNBROZIL (Hong Kong)
GEMFIBROZIL
Lopid Tablets 2650

SYNCOMET (Hong Kong)
CIMETIDINE
Tagamet Tablets 1644

SYNCOQUIN (Hong Kong)
CHLOROQUINE PHOSPHATE
Aralen Tablets 3075

SYNDOPA (Thailand)
CARBIDOPA/LEVODOPA
Sinemet CR Tablets 1255
Sinemet Tablets 1253

SYNERPRIL (Denmark, Sweden)
ENALAPRIL MALEATE/HYDROCHLOROTHIAZIDE
Vaseretic Tablets 2204

SYNFLEX (Australia, Canada, Hong Kong, Irish Republic, Italy, New Zealand, Singapore, South Africa, Thailand, United Kingdom)
NAPROXEN SODIUM
Anaprox DS Tablets 2967
Anaprox Tablets 2967
Naprelan Tablets 1293

SYNOGIL (Germany)
NATAMYCIN
Natacyn Antifungal Ophthalmic Suspension .... ⊙216

SYNOGIN (Thailand)
NAPROXEN
EC-Naprosyn Delayed-Release Tablets ... 2967
Naprosyn Suspension 2967
Naprosyn Tablets 2967

SYNOXICAM (Hong Kong)
PIROXICAM
Feldene Capsules 2685

SYNRELINA (Switzerland)
NAFARELIN ACETATE
Synarel Nasal Solution for Central Precocious Puberty 3204
Synarel Nasal Solution for Endometriosis 3205

SYNTARIS (Austria, Belgium, Germany, Irish Republic, Italy, South Africa, Switzerland, The Netherlands, United Kingdom)
FLUNISOLIDE
Aerobid Inhaler System 1363
Aerobid-M Inhaler System 1363
Nasalide Nasal Spray 1295
Nasarel Nasal Solution 0.025% 1296

SYNTHOMYCIN (Israel)
CHLORAMPHENICOL
Chloromycetin Ophthalmic Ointment, 1% .... ⊙296
Chloromycetin Ophthalmic Solution .... ⊙297
Chloroptic Sterile Ophthalmic Ointment .. ⊙234
Chloroptic Sterile Ophthalmic Solution .. ⊙235

SYNTIDINE (Hong Kong)
RANITIDINE HYDROCHLORIDE
Zantac 150 EFFERdose Granules 1690
Zantac 150 EFFERdose Tablets 1690
Zantac 150 Tablets 1690
Zantac 300 Tablets 1690
Zantac Injection 1688
Zantac Injection Premixed 1688
Zantac Syrup 1690

SYNTOFENE (France)
IBUPROFEN
Motrin Suspension, Oral Drops, Chewable Tablets, and Caplets 2002

SYNTONOL (Thailand)
PROPRANOLOL HYDROCHLORIDE
Inderal Injectable 3513
Inderal LA Long-Acting Capsules 3516
Inderal Tablets 3513

SYNURETIC (United Kingdom)
AMILORIDE HYDROCHLORIDE/HYDROCHLOROTHIAZIDE
Moduretic Tablets 2138

SYPROL (United Kingdom)
PROPRANOLOL HYDROCHLORIDE
Inderal Injectable 3513
Inderal LA Long-Acting Capsules 3516
Inderal Tablets 3513

SYRUP DM-E (Canada)
DEXTROMETHORPHAN HYDROBROMIDE/GUAIFENESIN
Tussi-Organidin DM NR Liquid 3350
Tussi-Organidin DM-S NR Liquid 3350

SYSCOR (Austria, Belgium, Finland, Italy, Mexico, South Africa, Spain, Sweden, Switzerland, The Netherlands, United Kingdom)
NISOLDIPINE
Sular Tablets 688

SYSTEN (Austria, Belgium, France, Italy, Mexico, Switzerland, The Netherlands)
ESTRADIOL
Alora Transdermal System 3372
Climara Transdermal System 958
Estrace Vaginal Cream 3358

(⊙ Described in PDR For Ophthalmic Medicines™)

Estring Vaginal Ring ... 2811
Vivelle Transdermal System ... 2412
Vivelle-Dot Transdermal System ... 2416

SYSTEPIN (Irish Republic)
NIFEDIPINE
Adalat CC Tablets ... 877
Procardia Capsules ... 2708
Procardia XL Extended Release Tablets ... 2710

SYSTODIN (Norway)
QUINIDINE SULFATE
Quinidex Extentabs ... 2933

SYSTRAL HYDROCORT (Germany)
HYDROCORTISONE
Anusol-HC Cream 2.5% ... 2237
Hydrocortone Tablets ... 2106

T.O.VIR (Thailand)
ZIDOVUDINE
Retrovir Capsules ... 1625
Retrovir IV Infusion ... 1629
Retrovir Syrup ... 1625
Retrovir Tablets ... 1625

T/H-BASAN (Switzerland)
HYDROCHLOROTHIAZIDE/TRIAMTERENE
Dyazide Capsules ... 1515
Maxzide Tablets ... 1008
Maxzide-25 mg Tablets ... 1008

TABALON (Germany, Mexico)
IBUPROFEN
Motrin Suspension, Oral Drops, Chewable Tablets, and Caplets ... 2002

TABAZUR (France)
NICOTINE
Nicotrol Inhaler ... 2840
Nicotrol Nasal Spray ... 2843

TABCIN (Austria)
IBUPROFEN
Motrin Suspension, Oral Drops, Chewable Tablets, and Caplets ... 2002

TABORCIL (Spain)
GEMFIBROZIL
Lopid Tablets ... 2650

TACEX (Mexico)
CEFTRIAXONE SODIUM
Rocephin Injectable Vials, ADD-Vantage, Galaxy, Bulk ... 2993

TACHYDARON (Germany)
AMIODARONE HYDROCHLORIDE
Cordarone Intravenous ... 3491
Cordarone Tablets ... 3487
Pacerone Tablets ... 3331

TACHYFENON (Germany)
PROPAFENONE HYDROCHLORIDE
Rythmol Tablets – 150 mg, 225 mg, 300 mg ... 502

TACHYTALOL (Germany)
SOTALOL HYDROCHLORIDE
Betapace Tablets ... 950

TACINOL (Thailand)
TRIAMCINOLONE ACETONIDE
Azmacort Inhalation Aerosol ... 728
Nasacort AQ Nasal Spray ... 752
Nasacort Nasal Inhaler ... 750

TACRON (Singapore, Spain)
TICLOPIDINE HYDROCHLORIDE
Ticlid Tablets ... 3015

TADEX (Finland)
TAMOXIFEN CITRATE
Nolvadex Tablets ... 678

TAFENIL (Mexico)
FLUTAMIDE
Eulexin Capsules ... 3118

TAFIL (Denmark, Germany, Mexico)
ALPRAZOLAM
Xanax Tablets ... 2865

TAFIROL (Spain)
KETOPROFEN
Orudis Capsules ... 3548
Oruvail Capsules ... 3548

TAFLOX (Portugal)
NORFLOXACIN
Chibroxin Sterile Ophthalmic Solution ... ⊙273, 2051
Noroxin Tablets ... 2145

TAGADINE (Hong Kong)
CIMETIDINE
Tagamet Tablets ... 1644

TAGAGEL (Germany)
CIMETIDINE
Tagamet Tablets ... 1644

TAGAL (Mexico)
CEFTAZIDIME
Ceptaz for Injection ... 1499
Fortaz for Injection ... 1541
Tazicef for Injection ... 1647
Tazidime Vials, Faspak & ADD-Vantage ... 1966

TAGAMET (Australia, Brazil, Denmark, Hong Kong, Irish Republic, Israel, Italy, Mexico, New Zealand, Portugal, Singapore, South Africa, Spain, Switzerland, Thailand, The Netherlands, United Kingdom)
CIMETIDINE
Tagamet Tablets ... 1644

TAGAMET DUAL ACTION (United Kingdom)
CIMETIDINE
Tagamet Tablets ... 1644

TAGONIS (Germany)
PAROXETINE HYDROCHLORIDE
Paxil Oral Suspension ... 1609
Paxil Tablets ... 1609

TAHOR (France)
ATORVASTATIN CALCIUM
Lipitor Tablets ... 2639, 2696

TAIRAL (Spain)
FAMOTIDINE
Pepcid Injection ... 2153
Pepcid Injection Premixed ... 2153
Pepcid RPD Orally Disintegrating Tablets ... 2150
Pepcid Tablets ... 2150
Pepcid for Oral Suspension ... 2150

TAKEPRON (Hong Kong, Japan)
LANSOPRAZOLE
Prevacid Delayed-Release Capsules ... 3292

TAKS (Thailand)
DICLOFENAC SODIUM
Voltaren Tablets ... 2315
Voltaren-XR Tablets ... 2315

TALINSUL (Spain)
CEPHALEXIN
Keflex Oral Suspension ... 1237
Keflex Pulvules ... 1237

TALOFILINA (Brazil)
THEOPHYLLINE
Aerolate Jr. T.D. Capsules ... 1361
Aerolate Liquid ... 1361
Aerolate Sr. T.D. Capsules ... 1361
Theo-Dur Extended-Release Tablets ... 1835
Uni-Dur Extended-Release Tablets ... 1841
Uniphyl 400 mg and 600 mg Tablets ... 2903

TALOXA (Austria, Belgium, France, Germany, Italy, Norway, Portugal, Spain, Sweden, Switzerland, The Netherlands)
FELBAMATE
Felbatol Oral Suspension ... 3343
Felbatol Tablets ... 3343

TALUDON (Brazil)
PHENYTOIN
Dilantin Infatabs ... 2624
Dilantin-125 Oral Suspension ... 2625

TAM (Spain)
CIPROFLOXACIN HYDROCHLORIDE
Ciloxan Ophthalmic Ointment ... 538
Ciloxan Ophthalmic Solution ... ⊙209, 530
Cipro Tablets ... 887

TAMAX (Austria)
TAMOXIFEN CITRATE
Nolvadex Tablets ... 678

TAMAXIN (Sweden)
TAMOXIFEN CITRATE
Nolvadex Tablets ... 678

TAMBOCOR (Australia, Belgium, Canada, Denmark, Finland, Germany, Hong Kong, Irish Republic, Israel, Mexico, New Zealand, Norway, Singapore, South Africa, Sweden, Switzerland, Thailand, The Netherlands, United Kingdom)
FLECAINIDE ACETATE
Tambocor Tablets ... 1990

TAMERAN (Spain)
FAMOTIDINE
Pepcid Injection ... 2153
Pepcid Injection Premixed ... 2153
Pepcid RPD Orally Disintegrating Tablets ... 2150
Pepcid Tablets ... 2150
Pepcid for Oral Suspension ... 2150

TAMETIN (Italy)
CIMETIDINE
Tagamet Tablets ... 1644

TAMEXIN (Finland)
TAMOXIFEN CITRATE
Nolvadex Tablets ... 678

TAMIFEN (Hong Kong)
TAMOXIFEN CITRATE
Nolvadex Tablets ... 678

TAMIN (Spain)
FAMOTIDINE
Pepcid Injection ... 2153
Pepcid Injection Premixed ... 2153
Pepcid RPD Orally Disintegrating Tablets ... 2150
Pepcid Tablets ... 2150
Pepcid for Oral Suspension ... 2150

TAMIZAM (Belgium)
TAMOXIFEN CITRATE
Nolvadex Tablets ... 678

TAMOBETA (Germany)
TAMOXIFEN CITRATE
Nolvadex Tablets ... 678

TAMOFEN (Austria, Brazil, Canada, Denmark, Finland, Germany, Hong Kong, Irish Republic, Israel, Mexico, New Zealand, Norway, Singapore, United Kingdom)
TAMOXIFEN CITRATE
Nolvadex Tablets ... 678

TAMOFENE (France)
TAMOXIFEN CITRATE
Nolvadex Tablets ... 678

TAMOKADIN (Germany)
TAMOXIFEN CITRATE
Nolvadex Tablets ... 678

TAMONE (Canada)
TAMOXIFEN CITRATE
Nolvadex Tablets ... 678

TAMOPLEX (Austria, Canada, Israel, Singapore, South Africa, Thailand, The Netherlands)
TAMOXIFEN CITRATE
Nolvadex Tablets ... 678

TAMOSIN (Australia)
TAMOXIFEN CITRATE
Nolvadex Tablets ... 678

TAMOX (Irish Republic)
TAMOXIFEN CITRATE
Nolvadex Tablets ... 678

TAMOXAN (Mexico, Portugal)
TAMOXIFEN CITRATE
Nolvadex Tablets ... 678

TAMOXASTA (Germany)
TAMOXIFEN CITRATE
Nolvadex Tablets ... 678

TAMOXEN (Australia, Israel)
TAMOXIFEN CITRATE
Nolvadex Tablets ... 678

TAMOXI (Israel)
TAMOXIFEN CITRATE
Nolvadex Tablets ... 678

TAMOXIGENAT (Germany)
TAMOXIFEN CITRATE
Nolvadex Tablets ... 678

TAMOXIMERCK (Germany)
TAMOXIFEN CITRATE
Nolvadex Tablets ... 678

TAMOXISTAD (Germany)
TAMOXIFEN CITRATE
Nolvadex Tablets ... 678

TANDAX (Mexico)
NAPROXEN SODIUM
Anaprox DS Tablets ... 2967
Anaprox Tablets ... 2967
Naprelan Tablets ... 1293

TANDIAL (Mexico)
DIAZEPAM
Valium Injectable ... 3026
Valium Tablets ... 3047

TANDIX (Portugal)
INDAPAMIDE
Indapamide Tablets ... 2286

TANIDINA (Spain)
RANITIDINE HYDROCHLORIDE
Zantac 150 EFFERdose Granules ... 1690
Zantac 150 EFFERdose Tablets ... 1690
Zantac 150 Tablets ... 1690
Zantac 300 Tablets ... 1690
Zantac Injection ... 1688
Zantac Injection Premixed ... 1688
Zantac Syrup ... 1690

TANYL (South Africa)
FENTANYL CITRATE
Actiq ... 1184

TAO (Belgium, France, Spain)
TROLEANDOMYCIN
Tao Capsules ... 2716

TAPORIN (Mexico)
CEFOTAXIME SODIUM
Claforan Injection ... 732

TAPRODEX (Mexico)
DEXAMETHASONE
Decadron Elixir ... 2078
Decadron Tablets ... 2079

TARASKON (Germany)
ATENOLOL
Tenormin I.V. Injection ... 692

TARATEN (Thailand)
CLOTRIMAZOLE
Lotrimin Cream 1% ... 3128
Lotrimin Lotion 1% ... 3128
Lotrimin Topical Solution 1% ... 3128
Mycelex Troche ... 573

TARAXIN (Thailand)
HYDROXYZINE HYDROCHLORIDE
Atarax Tablets & Syrup ... 2667
Vistaril Intramuscular Solution ... 2738

TARDOTOL (Denmark)
CARBAMAZEPINE
Carbatrol Capsules ... 3234
Tegretol Chewable Tablets ... 2404
Tegretol Suspension ... 2404
Tegretol Tablets ... 2404
Tegretol-XR Tablets ... 2404

TAREG (France, Italy)
VALSARTAN
Diovan Capsules ... 2337

TARGET (Hong Kong)
ATENOLOL
Tenormin I.V. Injection ... 692

TARIVID (Denmark, Finland, Hong Kong, Israel, Singapore, South Africa, Switzerland, Thailand)
OFLOXACIN
Floxin I.V. ... 2526
Floxin Otic Solution ... 1219
Floxin Tablets ... 2529
Ocuflox Ophthalmic Solution ... 554

TARJEN (Thailand)
DICLOFENAC SODIUM
Voltaren Tablets ... 2315
Voltaren-XR Tablets ... 2315

TARJENA (Thailand)
DICLOFENAC SODIUM
Voltaren Tablets ... 2315
Voltaren-XR Tablets ... 2315

TARKA (Denmark, Finland, France, Italy, Mexico, South Africa, Spain, Sweden, Switzerland, The Netherlands, United Kingdom)
TRANDOLAPRIL/VERAPAMIL HYDROCHLORIDE
Tarka Tablets ... 508

TAROCTYL (Israel)
CHLORPROMAZINE HYDROCHLORIDE
Thorazine Ampuls ... 1656
Thorazine Multi-dose Vials ... 1656
Thorazine Spansule Capsules ... 1656
Thorazine Syrup ... 1656
Thorazine Tablets ... 1656

TAROPHENICOL (Israel)
CHLORAMPHENICOL
Chloromycetin Ophthalmic Ointment, 1% ... ⊙296
Chloromycetin Ophthalmic Solution ... ⊙297
Chloroptic Sterile Ophthalmic Ointment ... ⊙234
Chloroptic Sterile Ophthalmic Solution ... ⊙235

TASEDAN (Mexico)
ESTAZOLAM
ProSom Tablets ... 500

TASMAR (Austria, Denmark, Hong Kong, Irish Republic, Mexico, New Zealand, Norway, Singapore, South Africa, Sweden, Switzerland, Thailand, United Kingdom)
TOLCAPONE
Tasmar Tablets ... 3010

TATIG (Italy)
SERTRALINE HYDROCHLORIDE
Zoloft Tablets ... 2751

TAUCOR (Spain)
LOVASTATIN
Mevacor Tablets ... 2132

TAVANIC (Austria, Belgium, Finland, France, Germany, Irish Republic, Italy, Mexico, Portugal, South Africa, Spain, Sweden, Switzerland, The Netherlands, United Kingdom)
LEVOFLOXACIN
Levaquin Injection ... 2537
Levaquin Tablets ... 2537

(⊙ Described in PDR For Ophthalmic Medicines™)

TAVAN-SP 54 (South Africa)
PENTOSAN POLYSULFATE SODIUM
Elmiron Capsules 570

TAVER (Thailand)
CARBAMAZEPINE
Carbatrol Capsules 3234
Tegretol Chewable Tablets 2404
Tegretol Suspension 2404
Tegretol Tablets 2404
Tegretol-XR Tablets 2404

TAVOR (Germany, Italy, Mexico)
LORAZEPAM
Ativan Injection 3478
Ativan Tablets 3482

TAXIFUR (Mexico)
CEFTAZIDIME
Ceptaz for Injection 1499
Fortaz for Injection 1541
Tazicef for Injection 1647
Tazidime Vials, Faspak & ADD-Vantage . . 1966

TAXOL (Australia, Austria, Belgium, Brazil, Canada, Denmark, Finland, France, Germany, Hong Kong, Irish Republic, Israel, Italy, Japan, New Zealand, Norway, Portugal, Singapore, South Africa, Spain, Sweden, Switzerland, Thailand, The Netherlands, United Kingdom)
PACLITAXEL
Taxol Injection 1129

TAXOTERE (Australia, Austria, Belgium, Brazil, Canada, Denmark, Finland, France, Germany, Hong Kong, Irish Republic, Israel, Italy, Japan, Mexico, New Zealand, Norway, Portugal, Singapore, South Africa, Spain, Sweden, Switzerland, Thailand, The Netherlands, United Kingdom)
DOCETAXEL
Taxotere for Injection Concentrate 778

TAXUS (Mexico)
TAMOXIFEN CITRATE
Nolvadex Tablets 678

TAXYL (Mexico)
DEXAMETHASONE
Decadron Elixir 2078
Decadron Tablets 2079

TAZAC (Australia)
NIZATIDINE
Axid Pulvules 1903

TAZIDEM (Brazil)
CEFTAZIDIME
Ceptaz for Injection 1499
Fortaz for Injection 1541
Tazicef for Injection 1647
Tazidime Vials, Faspak & ADD-Vantage . . 1966

TAZIDIME (Canada)
CEFTAZIDIME
Ceptaz for Injection 1499
Fortaz for Injection 1541
Tazicef for Injection 1647
Tazidime Vials, Faspak & ADD-Vantage . . 1966

TAZIKEN (Mexico)
TERBUTALINE SULFATE
Brethine Ampuls 2314
Brethine Tablets 2313

TAZOBAC (Germany, Italy, Portugal, Switzerland)
PIPERACILLIN SODIUM/TAZOBACTAM SODIUM
Zosyn 1890
Zosyn in Galaxy Containers 1894

TAZOCILLINE (France)
PIPERACILLIN SODIUM/TAZOBACTAM SODIUM
Zosyn 1890
Zosyn in Galaxy Containers 1894

TAZOCIN (Australia, Belgium, Denmark, Finland, Hong Kong, Irish Republic, Israel, Italy, New Zealand, Singapore, South Africa, Sweden, Thailand, The Netherlands, United Kingdom)
PIPERACILLIN SODIUM/TAZOBACTAM SODIUM
Zosyn 1890
Zosyn in Galaxy Containers 1894

TAZONAM (Austria)
PIPERACILLIN SODIUM/TAZOBACTAM SODIUM
Zosyn 1890
Zosyn in Galaxy Containers 1894

TAZORAC (Canada)
TAZAROTENE
Tazorac Gel 556

TD SPRAY ISO MACK (Germany)
ISOSORBIDE DINITRATE
Isordil Sublingual Tablets 3525
Isordil Titradose Tablets 3526

TEBEZIDE (South Africa)
PYRAZINAMIDE
Pyrazinamide Tablets 1876

TEBRAZID (Belgium, Canada)
PYRAZINAMIDE
Pyrazinamide Tablets 1876

TECELAC (Germany)
PLASMA PROTEIN FRACTION
Plasmanate 942

TECHNIPHYLLINE (Monaco)
THEOPHYLLINE
Aerolate Jr. T.D. Capsules 1361
Aerolate Liquid 1361
Aerolate Sr. T.D. Capsules 1361
Theo-Dur Extended-Release Tablets 1835
Uni-Dur Extended-Release Tablets 1841
Uniphyl 400 mg and 600 mg Tablets . . . 2903

TECNOFEN (Mexico)
TAMOXIFEN CITRATE
Nolvadex Tablets 678

TECNOFLUT (Brazil)
FLUTAMIDE
Eulexin Capsules 3118

TECNOLIP (Portugal)
LOVASTATIN
Mevacor Tablets 2132

TEDIPULMO (Spain)
TERBUTALINE SULFATE
Brethine Ampuls 2314
Brethine Tablets 2313

TEDOL (Portugal)
KETOCONAZOLE
Nizoral 2% Cream 3620
Nizoral 2% Shampoo 2007
Nizoral Tablets 1791

TEDRAL (United Kingdom)
THEOPHYLLINE
Aerolate Jr. T.D. Capsules 1361
Aerolate Liquid 1361
Aerolate Sr. T.D. Capsules 1361
Theo-Dur Extended-Release Tablets 1835
Uni-Dur Extended-Release Tablets 1841
Uniphyl 400 mg and 600 mg Tablets . . . 2903

TEDRALAN (Monaco)
THEOPHYLLINE
Aerolate Jr. T.D. Capsules 1361
Aerolate Liquid 1361
Aerolate Sr. T.D. Capsules 1361
Theo-Dur Extended-Release Tablets 1835
Uni-Dur Extended-Release Tablets 1841
Uniphyl 400 mg and 600 mg Tablets . . . 2903

TEETHING SYRUP (Canada)
BENZOCAINE
Americaine Anesthetic Lubricant 1162
Americaine Otic Topical Anesthetic Ear Drops 1162

TEFACLOR (Thailand)
CEFACLOR
Ceclor CD Tablets 1279
Ceclor Pulvules 1905
Ceclor Suspension 1905

TEFIZOX (Israel)
CEFTIZOXIME SODIUM
Cefizox for Intramuscular or Intravenous Use 1390

TEGRETAL (Germany)
CARBAMAZEPINE
Carbatrol Capsules 3234
Tegretol Chewable Tablets 2404
Tegretol Suspension 2404
Tegretol Tablets 2404
Tegretol-XR Tablets 2404

TEGRETARD (Brazil)
CARBAMAZEPINE
Carbatrol Capsules 3234
Tegretol Chewable Tablets 2404
Tegretol Suspension 2404
Tegretol Tablets 2404
Tegretol-XR Tablets 2404

TEGRETOL (Australia, Austria, Belgium, Brazil, Canada, Denmark, Finland, France, Hong Kong, Irish Republic, Israel, Italy, Mexico, New Zealand, Norway, Portugal, Singapore, South Africa, Spain, Sweden, Switzerland, Thailand, The Netherlands, United Kingdom)
CARBAMAZEPINE
Carbatrol Capsules 3234
Tegretol Chewable Tablets 2404
Tegretol Suspension 2404
Tegretol Tablets 2404
Tegretol-XR Tablets 2404

TELFAST (Australia, Austria, Belgium, Denmark, France, Hong Kong, Irish Republic, Italy, New Zealand, Norway, Portugal, South Africa, Spain, Switzerland, Thailand, The Netherlands, United Kingdom)
FEXOFENADINE HYDROCHLORIDE
Allegra Capsules 712

TELFAST DECONGESTANT (Australia, New Zealand)
FEXOFENADINE HYDROCHLORIDE/PSEUDOEPHEDRINE HYDROCHLORIDE
Allegra-D Extended-Release Tablets 714

TEMACO (Thailand)
THEOPHYLLINE
Aerolate Jr. T.D. Capsules 1361
Aerolate Liquid 1361
Aerolate Sr. T.D. Capsules 1361
Theo-Dur Extended-Release Tablets 1835
Uni-Dur Extended-Release Tablets 1841
Uniphyl 400 mg and 600 mg Tablets . . . 2903

TEMENTIL (France)
PROCHLORPERAZINE
Compazine Injection 1505
Compazine Suppositories 1505

TEMESTA (Austria, Belgium, Denmark, Finland, France, Sweden, Switzerland, The Netherlands)
LORAZEPAM
Ativan Injection 3478
Ativan Tablets 3482

TEMGESIC (Australia, Austria, Belgium, Brazil, Denmark, Finland, France, Germany, Hong Kong, Irish Republic, Italy, Mexico, New Zealand, Norway, Singapore, South Africa, Sweden, Switzerland, Thailand, The Netherlands, United Kingdom)
BUPRENORPHINE HYDROCHLORIDE
Buprenex Injectable 2918

TEMGESIC-NX (New Zealand)
BUPRENORPHINE HYDROCHLORIDE
Buprenex Injectable 2918

TEMIC (Italy)
CIMETIDINE
Tagamet Tablets 1644

TEMPIL (Germany)
IBUPROFEN
Motrin Suspension, Oral Drops, Chewable Tablets, and Caplets 2002

TEMPOROL (Irish Republic, South Africa)
CARBAMAZEPINE
Carbatrol Capsules 3234
Tegretol Chewable Tablets 2404
Tegretol Suspension 2404
Tegretol Tablets 2404
Tegretol-XR Tablets 2404

TEMSERIN (Germany)
TIMOLOL MALEATE
Blocadren Tablets 2046
Timoptic Sterile Ophthalmic Solution 2190
Timoptic in Ocudose 2192
Timoptic-XE Sterile Ophthalmic Gel Forming Solution 2194

TENACID (Italy)
CILASTATIN SODIUM/IMIPENEM
Primaxin I.M. 2158
Primaxin I.V. 2160

TENADREN (Brazil)
HYDROCHLOROTHIAZIDE/PROPRANOLOL HYDROCHLORIDE
Inderide LA Long-Acting Capsules 3519
Inderide Tablets 3517

TENAT (Switzerland)
ATENOLOL
Tenormin I.V. Injection 692

TENAVOID (United Kingdom)
MEPROBAMATE
Miltown Tablets 3349

TENBEN (United Kingdom)
ATENOLOL
Tenormin I.V. Injection 692

TEN-BLOKA (South Africa)
ATENOLOL
Tenormin I.V. Injection 692

TENCHLOR (Irish Republic, United Kingdom)
ATENOLOL
Tenormin I.V. Injection 692

TENERETIC (Germany)
ATENOLOL
Tenormin I.V. Injection 692

TENIBEX (Mexico)
ALBENDAZOLE
Albenza Tablets 1463

TENIDON (Denmark)
ATENOLOL
Tenormin I.V. Injection 692

TENIF (Belgium, United Kingdom)
ATENOLOL
Tenormin I.V. Injection 692

TENIKEN (Mexico)
PRAZIQUANTEL
Biltricide Tablets 887

TENLOL (Australia)
ATENOLOL
Tenormin I.V. Injection 692

TENO (Germany)
ATENOLOL
Tenormin I.V. Injection 692

TENO-BASAN (Germany)
ATENOLOL
Tenormin I.V. Injection 692

TENOBLOCK (Finland)
ATENOLOL
Tenormin I.V. Injection 692

TENOLIN (Canada)
ATENOLOL
Tenormin I.V. Injection 692

TENOLOL (Thailand)
ATENOLOL
Tenormin I.V. Injection 692

TENOMAX (Italy)
ATENOLOL
Tenormin I.V. Injection 692

TENOPRIN (Finland)
ATENOLOL
Tenormin I.V. Injection 692

TENOPT (Australia)
TIMOLOL MALEATE
Blocadren Tablets 2046
Timoptic Sterile Ophthalmic Solution 2190
Timoptic in Ocudose 2192
Timoptic-XE Sterile Ophthalmic Gel Forming Solution 2194

TENORET (Hong Kong, New Zealand, United Kingdom)
ATENOLOL
Tenormin I.V. Injection 692

TENORETIC (Belgium, Brazil, Denmark, France, Hong Kong, Mexico, New Zealand, Portugal, United Kingdom)
ATENOLOL
Tenormin I.V. Injection 692

TENORMIN (Australia, Austria, Belgium, Denmark, Germany, Hong Kong, Irish Republic, Italy, Mexico, New Zealand, Norway, Portugal, Singapore, South Africa, Spain, Sweden, Switzerland, Thailand, The Netherlands, United Kingdom)
ATENOLOL
Tenormin I.V. Injection 692

TENORMINE (France)
ATENOLOL
Tenormin I.V. Injection 692

TENSADIUR (Italy)
BENAZEPRIL HYDROCHLORIDE/HYDROCHLOROTHIAZIDE
Lotensin HCT Tablets 2367

TENSANIL (Italy)
BENAZEPRIL HYDROCHLORIDE
Lotensin Tablets 2365

TENSAZOL (Portugal)
ENALAPRIL MALEATE
Vasotec Tablets 2210

TENSIDOL (Thailand)
HALOPERIDOL
Haldol Injection, Tablets and Concentrate 2533

TENSIG (Australia)
ATENOLOL
Tenormin I.V. Injection 692

TENSIKEY (Spain)
LISINOPRIL
Prinivil Tablets 2164
Zestril Tablets 698

TENSILON (Canada, Irish Republic, South Africa)
EDROPHONIUM CHLORIDE
Tensilon Injectable 1745

TENSIOMIN (Germany, Hong Kong, Thailand)
CAPTOPRIL
Captopril Tablets 2281

TENSIOMIN-COR (Germany)
CAPTOPRIL
Captopril Tablets 2281

TENSIPINE (United Kingdom)
NIFEDIPINE
Adalat CC Tablets 877
Procardia Capsules 2708
Procardia XL Extended Release Tablets . . 2710

TENSIUM (United Kingdom)
DIAZEPAM
Valium Injectable 3026
Valium Tablets 3047

TENSO STOP (Spain)
FOSINOPRIL SODIUM
Monopril Tablets 1091

TENSOBON (Germany, Switzerland)
CAPTOPRIL
Captopril Tablets 2281

TENSOBON COMP (Germany)
CAPTOPRIL
Captopril Tablets 2281

TENSOCARDIL (Spain)
FOSINOPRIL SODIUM
Monopril Tablets 1091

TENSOGARD (Italy)
FOSINOPRIL SODIUM
Monopril Tablets 1091

TENSOPREL (Singapore, Spain)
CAPTOPRIL
Captopril Tablets 2281

TENSOPRIL (Irish Republic, Israel, Portugal, United Kingdom)
CAPTOPRIL
Captopril Tablets 2281

TENSOSTAD (Germany)
CAPTOPRIL
Captopril Tablets 2281

TENSO-TIMELETS (Germany)
CLONIDINE HYDROCHLORIDE
Catapres Tablets 1037
Duraclon Injection 3057

TENTROC (Spain)
GEMFIBROZIL
Lopid Tablets 2650

TENUTEX (Sweden)
DISULFIRAM
Antabuse Tablets 3474

TENZONE (Mexico)
METHYLDOPA
Aldomet Tablets 2037

TEOBID (Italy)
THEOPHYLLINE
Aerolate Jr. T.D. Capsules 1361
Aerolate Liquid 1361
Aerolate Sr. T.D. Capsules 1361
Theo-Dur Extended-Release Tablets 1835
Uni-Dur Extended-Release Tablets 1841
Uniphyl 400 mg and 600 mg Tablets . . . 2903

TEODELIN (Spain)
THEOPHYLLINE
Aerolate Jr. T.D. Capsules 1361
Aerolate Liquid 1361
Aerolate Sr. T.D. Capsules 1361
Theo-Dur Extended-Release Tablets 1835
Uni-Dur Extended-Release Tablets 1841
Uniphyl 400 mg and 600 mg Tablets . . . 2903

TEOGEL (Spain)
THEOPHYLLINE
Aerolate Jr. T.D. Capsules 1361
Aerolate Liquid 1361
Aerolate Sr. T.D. Capsules 1361
Theo-Dur Extended-Release Tablets 1835
Uni-Dur Extended-Release Tablets 1841
Uniphyl 400 mg and 600 mg Tablets . . . 2903

TEOLIXIR (Spain)
THEOPHYLLINE
Aerolate Jr. T.D. Capsules 1361
Aerolate Liquid 1361
Aerolate Sr. T.D. Capsules 1361
Theo-Dur Extended-Release Tablets 1835
Uni-Dur Extended-Release Tablets 1841
Uniphyl 400 mg and 600 mg Tablets . . . 2903

TEOLONG (Brazil, Mexico)
THEOPHYLLINE
Aerolate Jr. T.D. Capsules 1361
Aerolate Liquid 1361
Aerolate Sr. T.D. Capsules 1361
Theo-Dur Extended-Release Tablets 1835
Uni-Dur Extended-Release Tablets 1841
Uniphyl 400 mg and 600 mg Tablets . . . 2903

TEONIBSA (Portugal)
THEOPHYLLINE
Aerolate Jr. T.D. Capsules 1361
Aerolate Liquid 1361
Aerolate Sr. T.D. Capsules 1361
Theo-Dur Extended-Release Tablets 1835
Uni-Dur Extended-Release Tablets 1841
Uniphyl 400 mg and 600 mg Tablets . . . 2903

TEONOVA (Italy)
THEOPHYLLINE
Aerolate Jr. T.D. Capsules 1361
Aerolate Liquid 1361
Aerolate Sr. T.D. Capsules 1361
Theo-Dur Extended-Release Tablets 1835
Uni-Dur Extended-Release Tablets 1841
Uniphyl 400 mg and 600 mg Tablets . . . 2903

TEOPLUS (Italy)
THEOPHYLLINE
Aerolate Jr. T.D. Capsules 1361
Aerolate Liquid 1361
Aerolate Sr. T.D. Capsules 1361
Theo-Dur Extended-Release Tablets 1835
Uni-Dur Extended-Release Tablets 1841
Uniphyl 400 mg and 600 mg Tablets . . . 2903

TEOVAL/R (Italy)
THEOPHYLLINE
Aerolate Jr. T.D. Capsules 1361
Aerolate Liquid 1361
Aerolate Sr. T.D. Capsules 1361
Theo-Dur Extended-Release Tablets 1835
Uni-Dur Extended-Release Tablets 1841
Uniphyl 400 mg and 600 mg Tablets . . . 2903

TEOVENT (Portugal)
THEOPHYLLINE
Aerolate Jr. T.D. Capsules 1361
Aerolate Liquid 1361
Aerolate Sr. T.D. Capsules 1361
Theo-Dur Extended-Release Tablets 1835
Uni-Dur Extended-Release Tablets 1841
Uniphyl 400 mg and 600 mg Tablets . . . 2903

TERADYL (Thailand)
CODEINE PHOSPHATE/PROMETHAZINE HYDROCHLORIDE
Phenergan with Codeine Syrup 3557

TERALITHE (France)
LITHIUM CARBONATE
Eskalith CR Controlled Release Tablets . . 1527
Eskalith Capsules 1527
Lithium Carbonate Capsules 3061
Lithobid Slow-Release Tablets 3255

TERAPROST (Italy)
TERAZOSIN HYDROCHLORIDE
Hytrin Capsules 464

TERAZOL (Canada, Denmark, Italy, South Africa, Sweden)
TERCONAZOLE
Terazol 3 Vaginal Cream 2587
Terazol 3 Vaginal Suppositories 2587
Terazol 7 Vaginal Cream 2587

TERBAC (Mexico)
CEFTRIAXONE SODIUM
Rocephin Injectable Vials, ADD-Vantage, Galaxy, Bulk 2993

TERBASMIN (Italy, Spain)
TERBUTALINE SULFATE
Brethine Ampuls 2314
Brethine Tablets 2313

TERBRON (Thailand)
TERBUTALINE SULFATE
Brethine Ampuls 2314
Brethine Tablets 2313

TERBUFORTON (Germany)
TERBUTALINE SULFATE
Brethine Ampuls 2314
Brethine Tablets 2313

TERBUKEN (Mexico)
TERBUTALINE SULFATE
Brethine Ampuls 2314
Brethine Tablets 2313

TERBUL (Germany)
TERBUTALINE SULFATE
Brethine Ampuls 2314
Brethine Tablets 2313

TERBULIN (Israel)
TERBUTALINE SULFATE
Brethine Ampuls 2314
Brethine Tablets 2313

TERBUNO (Thailand)
TERBUTALINE SULFATE
Brethine Ampuls 2314
Brethine Tablets 2313

TERBUTURMANT (Germany)
TERBUTALINE SULFATE
Brethine Ampuls 2314
Brethine Tablets 2313

TERCOSPOR (Germany)
TERCONAZOLE
Terazol 3 Vaginal Cream 2587
Terazol 3 Vaginal Suppositories 2587
Terazol 7 Vaginal Cream 2587

TERFLUZINE (Canada, France, Israel, The Netherlands)
TRIFLUOPERAZINE HYDROCHLORIDE
Stelazine Injection 1640
Stelazine Tablets 1640

TERIAM (France)
TRIAMTERENE
Dyrenium Capsules 3458

TERIL (Australia, Hong Kong, Israel, New Zealand, United Kingdom)
CARBAMAZEPINE
Carbatrol Capsules 3234
Tegretol Chewable Tablets 2404
Tegretol Suspension 2404
Tegretol Tablets 2404
Tegretol-XR Tablets 2404

TERMIZOL (Mexico)
KETOCONAZOLE
Nizoral 2% Cream 3620
Nizoral 2% Shampoo 2007
Nizoral Tablets 1791

TERNELIN (Japan)
TIZANIDINE HYDROCHLORIDE
Zanaflex Tablets 1305

TERPOSEN (Spain)
RANITIDINE HYDROCHLORIDE
Zantac 150 EFFERdose Granules 1690
Zantac 150 EFFERdose Tablets 1690
Zantac 150 Tablets 1690
Zantac 300 Tablets 1690
Zantac Injection 1688
Zantac Injection Premixed 1688
Zantac Syrup 1690

TERRA-CORTRIL (South Africa, Spain, United Kingdom)
HYDROCORTISONE ACETATE/OXYTETRACYCLINE HYDROCHLORIDE
Terra-Cortril Ophthalmic Suspension 2716

TERTENSIF (Spain)
INDAPAMIDE
Indapamide Tablets 2286

TERTROXIN (Australia, Irish Republic, New Zealand, South Africa, Thailand, United Kingdom)
LIOTHYRONINE SODIUM
Cytomel Tablets 1817
Triostat Injection 1825

TERZOLIN (Germany, Switzerland)
KETOCONAZOLE
Nizoral 2% Cream 3620
Nizoral 2% Shampoo 2007
Nizoral Tablets 1791

TESPAMIN (Japan)
THIOTEPA
Thioplex for Injection 1765

TESSIFOL (Portugal)
ATENOLOL
Tenormin I.V. Injection 692

TESTAC (Germany)
FLUTAMIDE
Eulexin Capsules 3118

TESTODERM (Austria, Belgium, Germany, The Netherlands, United Kingdom)
TESTOSTERONE
Androderm Transdermal System CIII 3377
Testoderm Transdermal Systems 574

TESTOMET (Australia)
METHYLTESTOSTERONE
Android Capsules, 10 mg 1731
Testred Capsules, 10 mg 1746

TESTOSTERONE IMPLANTS (United Kingdom)
TESTOSTERONE
Androderm Transdermal System CIII 3377
Testoderm Transdermal Systems 574

TESTOTARD (Germany)
FLUTAMIDE
Eulexin Capsules 3118

TESTOTONIC B (Israel)
METHYLTESTOSTERONE
Android Capsules, 10 mg 1731
Testred Capsules, 10 mg 1746

TESTOTOP (Austria, United Kingdom)
TESTOSTERONE
Androderm Transdermal System CIII 3377
Testoderm Transdermal Systems 574

TESTOZZARD (Mexico)
TESTOSTERONE
Androderm Transdermal System CIII 3377
Testoderm Transdermal Systems 574

TETRADIN (Portugal)
DISULFIRAM
Antabuse Tablets 3474

TETRADOX (Singapore, Thailand)
DOXYCYCLINE HYCLATE
Doryx Coated Pellet Filled Capsules 3357
Periostat Tablets 1208
Vibramycin Hyclate Capsules 2735
Vibramycin Hyclate Intravenous 2737
Vibra-Tabs Film Coated Tablets 2735

TETRAHELMIN (Brazil)
MEBENDAZOLE
Vermox Chewable Tablets 2017

TETRAM (Norway)
PIROXICAM
Feldene Capsules 2685

TETRASAN (Spain)
DOXYCYCLINE HYCLATE
Doryx Coated Pellet Filled Capsules 3357
Periostat Tablets 1208
Vibramycin Hyclate Capsules 2735
Vibramycin Hyclate Intravenous 2737
Vibra-Tabs Film Coated Tablets 2735

TEVACAINE (Israel)
MEPIVACAINE HYDROCHLORIDE
Polocaine Injection, USP 625
Polocaine-MPF Injection, USP 625

TEXACORT (Canada)
HYDROCORTISONE
Anusol-HC Cream 2.5% 2237
Hydrocortone Tablets 2106

TFT (Germany, South Africa)
TRIFLURIDINE
Viroptic Ophthalmic Solution Sterile . . . . ⊙301

TFT OPHTIOLE (Belgium, The Netherlands)
TRIFLURIDINE
Viroptic Ophthalmic Solution Sterile . . . . ⊙301

THA (Australia)
TACRINE HYDROCHLORIDE
Cognex Capsules 1351

THAIS (France)
ESTRADIOL
Alora Transdermal System 3372
Climara Transdermal System 958
Estrace Vaginal Cream 3358
Estring Vaginal Ring 2811
Vivelle Transdermal System 2412
Vivelle-Dot Transdermal System 2416

THEO MAX (Spain)
THEOPHYLLINE
Aerolate Jr. T.D. Capsules 1361
Aerolate Liquid 1361
Aerolate Sr. T.D. Capsules 1361
Theo-Dur Extended-Release Tablets 1835
Uni-Dur Extended-Release Tablets 1841
Uniphyl 400 mg and 600 mg Tablets . . . 2903

THEO2 (The Netherlands)
THEOPHYLLINE
Aerolate Jr. T.D. Capsules 1361
Aerolate Liquid 1361
Aerolate Sr. T.D. Capsules 1361
Theo-Dur Extended-Release Tablets 1835
Uni-Dur Extended-Release Tablets 1841
Uniphyl 400 mg and 600 mg Tablets . . . 2903

THEO-24 (Italy)
THEOPHYLLINE
Aerolate Jr. T.D. Capsules 1361
Aerolate Liquid 1361
Aerolate Sr. T.D. Capsules 1361
Theo-Dur Extended-Release Tablets 1835
Uni-Dur Extended-Release Tablets 1841
Uniphyl 400 mg and 600 mg Tablets . . . 2903

THEOCHRON (Canada)
THEOPHYLLINE
Aerolate Jr. T.D. Capsules 1361
Aerolate Liquid 1361
Aerolate Sr. T.D. Capsules 1361
Theo-Dur Extended-Release Tablets 1835
Uni-Dur Extended-Release Tablets 1841
Uniphyl 400 mg and 600 mg Tablets . . . 2903

THEO-DUR (Australia, Belgium, Canada, Denmark, Finland, Hong Kong, Irish Republic, Italy, New Zealand, Norway, Singapore, South Africa, Spain, Sweden, Thailand, United Kingdom)
THEOPHYLLINE
Aerolate Jr. T.D. Capsules 1361
Aerolate Liquid 1361
Aerolate Sr. T.D. Capsules 1361
Theo-Dur Extended-Release Tablets 1835
Uni-Dur Extended-Release Tablets 1841
Uniphyl 400 mg and 600 mg Tablets . . . 2903

THEOFOL (Finland)
THEOPHYLLINE
Aerolate Jr. T.D. Capsules 1361

Aerolate Liquid . . . 1361
Aerolate Sr. T.D. Capsules . . . 1361
Theo-Dur Extended-Release Tablets . . . 1835
Uni-Dur Extended-Release Tablets . . . 1841
Uniphyl 400 mg and 600 mg Tablets . . . 2903

THEOFOL COMP (Finland)
THEOPHYLLINE
Aerolate Jr. T.D. Capsules . . . 1361
Aerolate Liquid . . . 1361
Aerolate Sr. T.D. Capsules . . . 1361
Theo-Dur Extended-Release Tablets . . . 1835
Uni-Dur Extended-Release Tablets . . . 1841
Uniphyl 400 mg and 600 mg Tablets . . . 2903

THEOHEXAL (Austria)
THEOPHYLLINE
Aerolate Jr. T.D. Capsules . . . 1361
Aerolate Liquid . . . 1361
Aerolate Sr. T.D. Capsules . . . 1361
Theo-Dur Extended-Release Tablets . . . 1835
Uni-Dur Extended-Release Tablets . . . 1841
Uniphyl 400 mg and 600 mg Tablets . . . 2903

THEOLAIR (Belgium, Canada, France, Germany, Italy, Spain, Switzerland, The Netherlands)
THEOPHYLLINE
Aerolate Jr. T.D. Capsules . . . 1361
Aerolate Liquid . . . 1361
Aerolate Sr. T.D. Capsules . . . 1361
Theo-Dur Extended-Release Tablets . . . 1835
Uni-Dur Extended-Release Tablets . . . 1841
Uniphyl 400 mg and 600 mg Tablets . . . 2903

THEOLAN (Irish Republic)
THEOPHYLLINE
Aerolate Jr. T.D. Capsules . . . 1361
Aerolate Liquid . . . 1361
Aerolate Sr. T.D. Capsules . . . 1361
Theo-Dur Extended-Release Tablets . . . 1835
Uni-Dur Extended-Release Tablets . . . 1841
Uniphyl 400 mg and 600 mg Tablets . . . 2903

THEOLIN (Singapore, The Netherlands)
THEOPHYLLINE
Aerolate Jr. T.D. Capsules . . . 1361
Aerolate Liquid . . . 1361
Aerolate Sr. T.D. Capsules . . . 1361
Theo-Dur Extended-Release Tablets . . . 1835
Uni-Dur Extended-Release Tablets . . . 1841
Uniphyl 400 mg and 600 mg Tablets . . . 2903

THEOLONG (Japan)
THEOPHYLLINE
Aerolate Jr. T.D. Capsules . . . 1361
Aerolate Liquid . . . 1361
Aerolate Sr. T.D. Capsules . . . 1361
Theo-Dur Extended-Release Tablets . . . 1835
Uni-Dur Extended-Release Tablets . . . 1841
Uniphyl 400 mg and 600 mg Tablets . . . 2903

THEON (Switzerland)
THEOPHYLLINE
Aerolate Jr. T.D. Capsules . . . 1361
Aerolate Liquid . . . 1361
Aerolate Sr. T.D. Capsules . . . 1361
Theo-Dur Extended-Release Tablets . . . 1835
Uni-Dur Extended-Release Tablets . . . 1841
Uniphyl 400 mg and 600 mg Tablets . . . 2903

THEOPEXINE (France)
THEOPHYLLINE
Aerolate Jr. T.D. Capsules . . . 1361
Aerolate Liquid . . . 1361
Aerolate Sr. T.D. Capsules . . . 1361
Theo-Dur Extended-Release Tablets . . . 1835
Uni-Dur Extended-Release Tablets . . . 1841
Uniphyl 400 mg and 600 mg Tablets . . . 2903

THEOPHYLLARD (Belgium, Germany)
THEOPHYLLINE
Aerolate Jr. T.D. Capsules . . . 1361
Aerolate Liquid . . . 1361
Aerolate Sr. T.D. Capsules . . . 1361
Theo-Dur Extended-Release Tablets . . . 1835
Uni-Dur Extended-Release Tablets . . . 1841
Uniphyl 400 mg and 600 mg Tablets . . . 2903

THEOPHYLLINE SEDATIVE BRUNEAU (Belgium)
THEOPHYLLINE
Aerolate Jr. T.D. Capsules . . . 1361
Aerolate Liquid . . . 1361
Aerolate Sr. T.D. Capsules . . . 1361
Theo-Dur Extended-Release Tablets . . . 1835
Uni-Dur Extended-Release Tablets . . . 1841
Uniphyl 400 mg and 600 mg Tablets . . . 2903

THEOPLUS (South Africa, Spain)
THEOPHYLLINE
Aerolate Jr. T.D. Capsules . . . 1361
Aerolate Liquid . . . 1361
Aerolate Sr. T.D. Capsules . . . 1361
Theo-Dur Extended-Release Tablets . . . 1835
Uni-Dur Extended-Release Tablets . . . 1841
Uniphyl 400 mg and 600 mg Tablets . . . 2903

THEO-SR (Canada)
THEOPHYLLINE
Aerolate Jr. T.D. Capsules . . . 1361
Aerolate Liquid . . . 1361
Aerolate Sr. T.D. Capsules . . . 1361
Theo-Dur Extended-Release Tablets . . . 1835
Uni-Dur Extended-Release Tablets . . . 1841
Uniphyl 400 mg and 600 mg Tablets . . . 2903

THEOTARD (Israel)
THEOPHYLLINE
Aerolate Jr. T.D. Capsules . . . 1361
Aerolate Liquid . . . 1361
Aerolate Sr. T.D. Capsules . . . 1361
Theo-Dur Extended-Release Tablets . . . 1835
Uni-Dur Extended-Release Tablets . . . 1841
Uniphyl 400 mg and 600 mg Tablets . . . 2903

THEOTRIM (Israel, Thailand)
THEOPHYLLINE
Aerolate Jr. T.D. Capsules . . . 1361
Aerolate Liquid . . . 1361
Aerolate Sr. T.D. Capsules . . . 1361
Theo-Dur Extended-Release Tablets . . . 1835
Uni-Dur Extended-Release Tablets . . . 1841
Uniphyl 400 mg and 600 mg Tablets . . . 2903

THEOVENT (Hong Kong)
THEOPHYLLINE
Aerolate Jr. T.D. Capsules . . . 1361
Aerolate Liquid . . . 1361
Aerolate Sr. T.D. Capsules . . . 1361
Theo-Dur Extended-Release Tablets . . . 1835
Uni-Dur Extended-Release Tablets . . . 1841
Uniphyl 400 mg and 600 mg Tablets . . . 2903

THERADERM (United Kingdom)
BENZOYL PEROXIDE
Brevoxyl-4 Cleansing Lotion . . . 3269
Brevoxyl-4 Creamy Wash . . . 3270
Brevoxyl-4 Gel . . . 3269
Brevoxyl-8 Cleansing Lotion . . . 3269
Brevoxyl-8 Creamy Wash . . . 3270
Brevoxyl-8 Gel . . . 3269
Triaz Cleanser . . . 2026
Triaz Gel . . . 2026

THERADOL (The Netherlands)
TRAMADOL HYDROCHLORIDE
Ultram Tablets . . . 2600

THERAPAS (United Kingdom)
AMINOSALICYLIC ACID
Paser Granules . . . 1781

THIABET (Germany)
METFORMIN HYDROCHLORIDE
Glucophage Tablets . . . 1080

THIAZID-COMP (Germany)
HYDROCHLOROTHIAZIDE/TRIAMTERENE
Dyazide Capsules . . . 1515
Maxzide Tablets . . . 1008
Maxzide-25 mg Tablets . . . 1008

THIAZID-WOLFF (Germany)
HYDROCHLOROTHIAZIDE
HydroDIURIL Tablets . . . 2108
Microzide Capsules . . . 3414

THILOCANFOL C (Germany)
CHLORAMPHENICOL
Chloromycetin Ophthalmic Ointment, 1% . . . ⊙296
Chloromycetin Ophthalmic Solution . . . ⊙297
Chloroptic Sterile Ophthalmic Ointment . . . ⊙234
Chloroptic Sterile Ophthalmic Solution . . . ⊙235

THIOMED (Thailand)
THIORIDAZINE HYDROCHLORIDE
Thioridazine Hydrochloride Tablets . . . 2289

THIOPLEX (Italy)
THIOTEPA
Thioplex for Injection . . . 1765

THIOSIA (Thailand)
THIORIDAZINE HYDROCHLORIDE
Thioridazine Hydrochloride Tablets . . . 2289

THIOZINE (Irish Republic)
THIORIDAZINE HYDROCHLORIDE
Thioridazine Hydrochloride Tablets . . . 2289

THREOLONE (Israel)
PREDNISOLONE
Prelone Syrup . . . 2273

THROMBAREDUCT (Germany)
HEPARIN SODIUM
Heparin Lock Flush Solution . . . 3509
Heparin Sodium Injection . . . 3511

THROMBINAR (Australia, Canada)
THROMBIN
Thrombin-JMI . . . 1824

THROMBOCID (Germany)
PENTOSAN POLYSULFATE SODIUM
Elmiron Capsules . . . 570

THROMBOCOLL (Germany)
THROMBIN
Thrombin-JMI . . . 1824

THROMBODINE (Austria)
TICLOPIDINE HYDROCHLORIDE
Ticlid Tablets . . . 3015

THROMBOPHOB (Austria, Germany, Switzerland)
HEPARIN SODIUM
Heparin Lock Flush Solution . . . 3509
Heparin Sodium Injection . . . 3511

THROMBOPHOB-S (Austria)
HEPARIN SODIUM
Heparin Lock Flush Solution . . . 3509
Heparin Sodium Injection . . . 3511

THROMBOSTAT (Australia, Canada, New Zealand, Singapore)
THROMBIN
Thrombin-JMI . . . 1824

THROMBO-VETREN (Germany)
HEPARIN SODIUM
Heparin Lock Flush Solution . . . 3509
Heparin Sodium Injection . . . 3511

THYREFACT (Denmark, Sweden)
PROTIRELIN
Thyrel TRH for Injection . . . 3630

THYRO-BLOCK (Canada)
POTASSIUM IODIDE
Pima Syrup . . . 1362

THYROJOD DEPOT (Germany)
POTASSIUM IODIDE
Pima Syrup . . . 1362

THYROLIBERIN (Germany)
PROTIRELIN
Thyrel TRH for Injection . . . 3630

THYROLIBERIN TRH (Austria)
PROTIRELIN
Thyrel TRH for Injection . . . 3630

TIADIL (Portugal, The Netherlands)
DILTIAZEM HYDROCHLORIDE
Cardizem CD Capsules . . . 1016
Cardizem Injectable . . . 1018
Cardizem Lyo-Ject Syringe . . . 1018
Cardizem Monovial . . . 1018
Tiazac Capsules . . . 1378

TIAKEM (Italy)
DILTIAZEM HYDROCHLORIDE
Cardizem CD Capsules . . . 1016
Cardizem Injectable . . . 1018
Cardizem Lyo-Ject Syringe . . . 1018
Cardizem Monovial . . . 1018
Tiazac Capsules . . . 1378

TIAMOL (Canada)
FLUOCINONIDE
Lidex Cream . . . 2020
Lidex Gel . . . 2020
Lidex Ointment . . . 2020
Lidex Topical Solution . . . 2020
Lidex-E Cream . . . 2020

TIAZAC (Canada)
DILTIAZEM HYDROCHLORIDE
Cardizem CD Capsules . . . 1016
Cardizem Injectable . . . 1018
Cardizem Lyo-Ject Syringe . . . 1018
Cardizem Monovial . . . 1018
Tiazac Capsules . . . 1378

TIAZEN (Italy)
DILTIAZEM HYDROCHLORIDE
Cardizem CD Capsules . . . 1016
Cardizem Injectable . . . 1018
Cardizem Lyo-Ject Syringe . . . 1018
Cardizem Monovial . . . 1018
Tiazac Capsules . . . 1378

TIBA (Thailand)
GEMFIBROZIL
Lopid Tablets . . . 2650

TIBLEX (Spain)
SUCRALFATE
Carafate Suspension . . . 731
Carafate Tablets . . . 730

TIBURON (France)
IBUPROFEN
Motrin Suspension, Oral Drops, Chewable Tablets, and Caplets . . . 2002

TICLID (Australia, Belgium, Brazil, Canada, France, Hong Kong, Mexico, New Zealand, Norway, Singapore, South Africa, Sweden, Switzerland, Thailand, United Kingdom)
TICLOPIDINE HYDROCHLORIDE
Ticlid Tablets . . . 3015

TICLIDIL (Israel)
TICLOPIDINE HYDROCHLORIDE
Ticlid Tablets . . . 3015

TICLODIX (Portugal)
TICLOPIDINE HYDROCHLORIDE
Ticlid Tablets . . . 3015

TICLODONE (Austria, Italy, Spain)
TICLOPIDINE HYDROCHLORIDE
Ticlid Tablets . . . 3015

TICLOGI (Italy)
TICLOPIDINE HYDROCHLORIDE
Ticlid Tablets . . . 3015

TICLOPROGE (Italy)
TICLOPIDINE HYDROCHLORIDE
Ticlid Tablets . . . 3015

TICLOSAN (Italy)
TICLOPIDINE HYDROCHLORIDE
Ticlid Tablets . . . 3015

TIENAM (France, Italy, Norway, Singapore, South Africa, Spain, Sweden, Switzerland, Thailand, The Netherlands)
CILASTATIN SODIUM/IMIPENEM
Primaxin I.M. . . . 2158
Primaxin I.V. . . . 2160

TIFOMYCINE (France)
CHLORAMPHENICOL
Chloromycetin Ophthalmic Ointment, 1% . . . ⊙296
Chloromycetin Ophthalmic Solution . . . ⊙297
Chloroptic Sterile Ophthalmic Ointment . . . ⊙234
Chloroptic Sterile Ophthalmic Solution . . . ⊙235

TIFOX (Italy)
CEFOXITIN SODIUM
Mefoxin Premixed Intravenous Solution . . . 2127
Mefoxin for Injection . . . 2124

TIKALAC (Sweden)
LACTULOSE
Kristalose for Oral Solution . . . 1007

TIKLID (Austria, Italy, Spain)
TICLOPIDINE HYDROCHLORIDE
Ticlid Tablets . . . 3015

TIKLYD (Germany, Portugal)
TICLOPIDINE HYDROCHLORIDE
Ticlid Tablets . . . 3015

TILAZEM (Mexico, South Africa)
DILTIAZEM HYDROCHLORIDE
Cardizem CD Capsules . . . 1016
Cardizem Injectable . . . 1018
Cardizem Lyo-Ject Syringe . . . 1018
Cardizem Monovial . . . 1018
Tiazac Capsules . . . 1378

TILDIEM (Belgium, France, Hong Kong, Irish Republic, Italy, Singapore, Switzerland, Thailand, The Netherlands, United Kingdom)
DILTIAZEM HYDROCHLORIDE
Cardizem CD Capsules . . . 1016
Cardizem Injectable . . . 1018
Cardizem Lyo-Ject Syringe . . . 1018
Cardizem Monovial . . . 1018
Tiazac Capsules . . . 1378

TILENE (Italy)
FENOFIBRATE
Tricor Capsules, Micronized . . . 513

TILEXIM (Italy)
CEFUROXIME AXETIL
Ceftin Tablets . . . 1898
Ceftin for Oral Suspension . . . 1898

TILKER (Denmark, Norway, Spain)
DILTIAZEM HYDROCHLORIDE
Cardizem CD Capsules . . . 1016
Cardizem Injectable . . . 1018
Cardizem Lyo-Ject Syringe . . . 1018
Cardizem Monovial . . . 1018
Tiazac Capsules . . . 1378

TILODENE (Australia)
TICLOPIDINE HYDROCHLORIDE
Ticlid Tablets . . . 3015

TILOPTIC (Israel)
TIMOLOL MALEATE
Blocadren Tablets . . . 2046
Timoptic Sterile Ophthalmic Solution . . . 2190
Timoptic in Ocudose . . . 2192
Timoptic-XE Sterile Ophthalmic Gel Forming Solution . . . 2194

TILORYTH (United Kingdom)
ERYTHROMYCIN
Emgel 2% Topical Gel . . . 1285
Ery-Tab Tablets . . . 448
Erythromycin Base Filmtab Tablets . . . 454
Erythromycin Delayed-Release Capsules, USP . . . 455
PCE Dispertab Tablets . . . 498

TIMABAK (Austria, France, Singapore)
TIMOLOL MALEATE
Blocadren Tablets . . . 2046
Timoptic Sterile Ophthalmic Solution . . . 2190
Timoptic in Ocudose . . . 2192
Timoptic-XE Sterile Ophthalmic Gel Forming Solution . . . 2194

TIMACAR (Denmark)
TIMOLOL MALEATE
Blocadren Tablets . . . 2046

(⊙ Described in PDR For Ophthalmic Medicines™)

Timoptic Sterile Ophthalmic Solution 2190
Timoptic in Ocudose 2192
Timoptic-XE Sterile Ophthalmic Gel Forming Solution 2194

TIMACOR (France)
TIMOLOL MALEATE
Blocadren Tablets 2046
Timoptic Sterile Ophthalmic Solution 2190
Timoptic in Ocudose 2192
Timoptic-XE Sterile Ophthalmic Gel Forming Solution 2194

TIM-AK (Canada)
TIMOLOL MALEATE
Blocadren Tablets 2046
Timoptic Sterile Ophthalmic Solution 2190
Timoptic in Ocudose 2192
Timoptic-XE Sterile Ophthalmic Gel Forming Solution 2194

TIMISOL (Switzerland)
TIMOLOL MALEATE
Blocadren Tablets 2046
Timoptic Sterile Ophthalmic Solution 2190
Timoptic in Ocudose 2192
Timoptic-XE Sterile Ophthalmic Gel Forming Solution 2194

TIMO-COMOD (Germany, The Netherlands)
TIMOLOL MALEATE
Blocadren Tablets 2046
Timoptic Sterile Ophthalmic Solution 2190
Timoptic in Ocudose 2192
Timoptic-XE Sterile Ophthalmic Gel Forming Solution 2194

TIMOCORT (United Kingdom)
HYDROCORTISONE
Anusol-HC Cream 2.5% 2237
Hydrocortone Tablets 2106

TIMODINE (United Kingdom)
NYSTATIN
Nystop Topical Powder USP 2608

TIMODROP (Thailand)
TIMOLOL MALEATE
Blocadren Tablets 2046
Timoptic Sterile Ophthalmic Solution 2190
Timoptic in Ocudose 2192
Timoptic-XE Sterile Ophthalmic Gel Forming Solution 2194

TIMOEDO (Germany)
TIMOLOL MALEATE
Blocadren Tablets 2046
Timoptic Sterile Ophthalmic Solution 2190
Timoptic in Ocudose 2192
Timoptic-XE Sterile Ophthalmic Gel Forming Solution 2194

TIMOFTAL (Austria)
TIMOLOL MALEATE
Blocadren Tablets 2046
Timoptic Sterile Ophthalmic Solution 2190
Timoptic in Ocudose 2192
Timoptic-XE Sterile Ophthalmic Gel Forming Solution 2194

TIMOFTOL (Spain)
TIMOLOL MALEATE
Blocadren Tablets 2046
Timoptic Sterile Ophthalmic Solution 2190
Timoptic in Ocudose 2192
Timoptic-XE Sterile Ophthalmic Gel Forming Solution 2194

TIMOGLAU (Portugal)
TIMOLOL MALEATE
Blocadren Tablets 2046
Timoptic Sterile Ophthalmic Solution 2190
Timoptic in Ocudose 2192
Timoptic-XE Sterile Ophthalmic Gel Forming Solution 2194

TIMOHEXAL (Austria, Germany)
TIMOLOL MALEATE
Blocadren Tablets 2046
Timoptic Sterile Ophthalmic Solution 2190
Timoptic in Ocudose 2192
Timoptic-XE Sterile Ophthalmic Gel Forming Solution 2194

TIMOLEN (Portugal)
TIMOLOL MALEATE
Blocadren Tablets 2046
Timoptic Sterile Ophthalmic Solution 2190
Timoptic in Ocudose 2192
Timoptic-XE Sterile Ophthalmic Gel Forming Solution 2194

TIMOLIDE (Canada)
HYDROCHLOROTHIAZIDE/TIMOLOL MALEATE
Timolide Tablets 2187

TIMOMANN (Germany)
TIMOLOL MALEATE
Blocadren Tablets 2046
Timoptic Sterile Ophthalmic Solution 2190
Timoptic in Ocudose 2192
Timoptic-XE Sterile Ophthalmic Gel Forming Solution 2194

TIMONIL (Germany, Hong Kong, Israel, Switzerland, United Kingdom)
CARBAMAZEPINE
Carbatrol Capsules 3234
Tegretol Chewable Tablets 2404
Tegretol Suspension 2404
Tegretol Tablets 2404
Tegretol-XR Tablets 2404

TIM-OPHTAL (Austria, Germany)
TIMOLOL MALEATE
Blocadren Tablets 2046
Timoptic Sterile Ophthalmic Solution 2190
Timoptic in Ocudose 2192
Timoptic-XE Sterile Ophthalmic Gel Forming Solution 2194

TIMOPOS COMOD (Germany)
TIMOLOL MALEATE
Blocadren Tablets 2046
Timoptic Sterile Ophthalmic Solution 2190
Timoptic in Ocudose 2192
Timoptic-XE Sterile Ophthalmic Gel Forming Solution 2194

TIMOPTIC (Austria, Canada, Switzerland)
TIMOLOL MALEATE
Blocadren Tablets 2046
Timoptic Sterile Ophthalmic Solution 2190
Timoptic in Ocudose 2192
Timoptic-XE Sterile Ophthalmic Gel Forming Solution 2194

TIMOPTOL (Australia, Belgium, Brazil, France, Hong Kong, Irish Republic, Italy, Mexico, New Zealand, Portugal, Singapore, South Africa, Thailand, The Netherlands, United Kingdom)
TIMOLOL MALEATE
Blocadren Tablets 2046
Timoptic Sterile Ophthalmic Solution 2190
Timoptic in Ocudose 2192
Timoptic-XE Sterile Ophthalmic Gel Forming Solution 2194

TIMOPTOL-XE (Australia)
TIMOLOL MALEATE
Blocadren Tablets 2046
Timoptic Sterile Ophthalmic Solution 2190
Timoptic in Ocudose 2192
Timoptic-XE Sterile Ophthalmic Gel Forming Solution 2194

TIMOSAN (Finland)
TIMOLOL MALEATE
Blocadren Tablets 2046
Timoptic Sterile Ophthalmic Solution 2190
Timoptic in Ocudose 2192
Timoptic-XE Sterile Ophthalmic Gel Forming Solution 2194

TIMOSIL (Thailand)
TIMOLOL MALEATE
Blocadren Tablets 2046
Timoptic Sterile Ophthalmic Solution 2190
Timoptic in Ocudose 2192
Timoptic-XE Sterile Ophthalmic Gel Forming Solution 2194

TIMOSINE (Germany)
TIMOLOL MALEATE
Blocadren Tablets 2046
Timoptic Sterile Ophthalmic Solution 2190
Timoptic in Ocudose 2192
Timoptic-XE Sterile Ophthalmic Gel Forming Solution 2194

TIMO-STULLN (Germany)
TIMOLOL MALEATE
Blocadren Tablets 2046
Timoptic Sterile Ophthalmic Solution 2190
Timoptic in Ocudose 2192
Timoptic-XE Sterile Ophthalmic Gel Forming Solution 2194

TIMPRON (United Kingdom)
NAPROXEN
EC-Naprosyn Delayed-Release Tablets 2967
Naprosyn Suspension 2967
Naprosyn Tablets 2967

TINADERM EXTRA (Australia)
CLOTRIMAZOLE
Lotrimin Cream 1% 3128
Lotrimin Lotion 1% 3128
Lotrimin Topical Solution 1% 3128
Mycelex Troche 573

TINAGEL (Belgium, The Netherlands)
BENZOYL PEROXIDE
Brevoxyl-4 Cleansing Lotion 3269
Brevoxyl-4 Creamy Wash 3270
Brevoxyl-4 Gel 3269
Brevoxyl-8 Cleansing Lotion 3269
Brevoxyl-8 Creamy Wash 3270
Brevoxyl-8 Gel 3269
Triaz Cleanser 2026
Triaz Gel 2026

TINIAZOL (Mexico)
KETOCONAZOLE
Nizoral 2% Cream 3620
Nizoral 2% Shampoo 2007
Nizoral Tablets 1791

TINTUS (Finland)
GUAIFENESIN
Organidin NR Liquid 3350
Organidin NR Tablets 3350

TIONER (Spain)
TRAMADOL HYDROCHLORIDE
Ultram Tablets 2600

TIPAROL (Sweden)
TRAMADOL HYDROCHLORIDE
Ultram Tablets 2600

TIPERAL (Irish Republic)
PROPRANOLOL HYDROCHLORIDE
Inderal Injectable 3513
Inderal LA Long-Acting Capsules 3516
Inderal Tablets 3513

TIPIDIN (Singapore)
TICLOPIDINE HYDROCHLORIDE
Ticlid Tablets 3015

TIPODEX (Spain)
FAMOTIDINE
Pepcid Injection 2153
Pepcid Injection Premixed 2153
Pepcid RPD Orally Disintegrating Tablets 2150
Pepcid Tablets 2150
Pepcid for Oral Suspension 2150

TIROCAL (Mexico)
CALCITRIOL
Calcijex Injection 411
Rocaltrol Capsules 2991
Rocaltrol Oral Solution 2991

TISAMID (Finland)
PYRAZINAMIDE
Pyrazinamide Tablets 1876

TITRANE (Spain)
ISOSORBIDE MONONITRATE
Imdur Tablets 1826
Ismo Tablets 3524

TI-TRE (Italy)
LIOTHYRONINE SODIUM
Cytomel Tablets 1817
Triostat Injection 1825

TI-U-LAC HC (Canada)
HYDROCORTISONE
Anusol-HC Cream 2.5% 2237
Hydrocortone Tablets 2106

TIXYLIX CATARRH (United Kingdom)
DIPHENHYDRAMINE HYDROCHLORIDE
Benadryl Parenteral 2617

TIXYLIX CHESTY COUGH (Irish Republic, United Kingdom)
GUAIFENESIN
Organidin NR Liquid 3350
Organidin NR Tablets 3350

TOBI (Australia, Canada, United Kingdom)
TOBRAMYCIN
TOBI Solution for Inhalation 1206
Tobrex Ophthalmic Ointment .... ⊙220
Tobrex Ophthalmic Solution .... ⊙221

TOBRA (Mexico)
TOBRAMYCIN SULFATE
Nebcin Vials, Hyporets & ADD-Vantage 1955

TOBRA GOBENS (Portugal, Spain)
TOBRAMYCIN SULFATE
Nebcin Vials, Hyporets & ADD-Vantage 1955

TOBRA LAF (Spain)
TOBRAMYCIN SULFATE
Nebcin Vials, Hyporets & ADD-Vantage 1955

TOBRA-CELL (Germany)
TOBRAMYCIN SULFATE
Nebcin Vials, Hyporets & ADD-Vantage 1955

TOBRACIL (Portugal)
TOBRAMYCIN SULFATE
Nebcin Vials, Hyporets & ADD-Vantage 1955

TOBRADEX (Belgium, Brazil, Canada, France, Hong Kong, Italy, New Zealand, Singapore, South Africa, Spain, Switzerland, Thailand, The Netherlands, United Kingdom)
TOBRAMYCIN
TOBI Solution for Inhalation 1206
Tobrex Ophthalmic Ointment .... ⊙220
Tobrex Ophthalmic Solution .... ⊙221

TOBRADISTIN (Spain)
TOBRAMYCIN SULFATE
Nebcin Vials, Hyporets & ADD-Vantage 1955

TOBRAFEN (Switzerland)
DICLOFENAC SODIUM
Voltaren Tablets 2315
Voltaren-XR Tablets 2315

TOBRAL (Italy)
TOBRAMYCIN
TOBI Solution for Inhalation 1206
Tobrex Ophthalmic Ointment .... ⊙220
Tobrex Ophthalmic Solution .... ⊙221

TOBRALEX (Irish Republic, United Kingdom)
TOBRAMYCIN
TOBI Solution for Inhalation 1206
Tobrex Ophthalmic Ointment .... ⊙220
Tobrex Ophthalmic Solution .... ⊙221

TOBRAMAXIN (Germany)
TOBRAMYCIN
TOBI Solution for Inhalation 1206
Tobrex Ophthalmic Ointment .... ⊙220
Tobrex Ophthalmic Solution .... ⊙221

TOBRAMINA (Brazil)
TOBRAMYCIN SULFATE
Nebcin Vials, Hyporets & ADD-Vantage 1955

TOBRASIX (Austria)
TOBRAMYCIN SULFATE
Nebcin Vials, Hyporets & ADD-Vantage 1955

TOBREX (Australia, Austria, Belgium, Brazil, Canada, Denmark, Finland, France, Hong Kong, Israel, Italy, Mexico, New Zealand, Portugal, Singapore, South Africa, Spain, Sweden, Switzerland, Thailand, The Netherlands)
TOBRAMYCIN
TOBI Solution for Inhalation 1206
Tobrex Ophthalmic Ointment .... ⊙220
Tobrex Ophthalmic Solution .... ⊙221

TOBRIDAVI (Portugal)
TOBRAMYCIN
TOBI Solution for Inhalation 1206
Tobrex Ophthalmic Ointment .... ⊙220
Tobrex Ophthalmic Solution .... ⊙221

TOBUTOL (Thailand)
ETHAMBUTOL HYDROCHLORIDE
Myambutol Tablets 1290

TOCOMIZOL (Mexico)
KETOCONAZOLE
Nizoral 2% Cream 3620
Nizoral 2% Shampoo 2007
Nizoral Tablets 1791

TOCONAL (Mexico)
KETOCONAZOLE
Nizoral 2% Cream 3620
Nizoral 2% Shampoo 2007
Nizoral Tablets 1791

TODALGIL (Spain)
IBUPROFEN
Motrin Suspension, Oral Drops, Chewable Tablets, and Caplets 2002

TODOLAC (Denmark)
ETODOLAC
Lodine Capsules 3528
Lodine Tablets 3528
Lodine XL Extended-Release Tablets 3530

TOFEN (Thailand)
IBUPROFEN
Motrin Suspension, Oral Drops, Chewable Tablets, and Caplets 2002

TOFLEX (Thailand)
CEPHALEXIN
Keflex Oral Suspension 1237
Keflex Pulvules 1237

TOGAL N (Germany)
IBUPROFEN
Motrin Suspension, Oral Drops, Chewable Tablets, and Caplets 2002

TOLBIN (Singapore)
TERBUTALINE SULFATE
Brethine Ampuls 2314
Brethine Tablets 2313

TOLECTIN (Belgium, Canada, Denmark, Germany, Irish Republic, Italy, South Africa, Switzerland, The Netherlands, United Kingdom)
TOLMETIN SODIUM
Tolectin 200 Tablets 2589
Tolectin 600 Tablets 2589
Tolectin DS Capsules 2589

TOLERABIOTICO (Spain)
ERYTHROMYCIN STEARATE
Erythrocin Stearate Filmtab Tablets 452

TOLID (Germany)
LORAZEPAM
Ativan Injection 3478

Ativan Tablets 3482

TOLOXIM (Portugal)
MEBENDAZOLE
Vermox Chewable Tablets 2017

TOLOXIN (Thailand)
DIGOXIN
Lanoxicaps Capsules 1574
Lanoxin Elixir Pediatric 1578
Lanoxin Injection 1581
Lanoxin Injection Pediatric 1584
Lanoxin Tablets 1587

TOMABEF (Italy)
CEFOPERAZONE SODIUM
Cefobid Intravenous/Intramuscular 2671
Cefobid Pharmacy Bulk Package - Not for Direct Infusion 2673

TOMYCIN (Finland)
TOBRAMYCIN SULFATE
Nebcin Vials, Hyporets & ADD-Vantage . . 1955

TOMYCINE (Canada)
TOBRAMYCIN
TOBI Solution for Inhalation 1206
Tobrex Ophthalmic Ointment . . . . ⊙220
Tobrex Ophthalmic Solution . . . . ⊙221

TONDEX (Mexico)
GENTAMICIN SULFATE
Genoptic Ophthalmic Ointment . . . . ⊙239
Genoptic Sterile Ophthalmic Solution . . . ⊙239

TONOCARD (Belgium, Canada, Hong Kong, Irish Republic, Sweden, Thailand, The Netherlands, United Kingdom)
TOCAINIDE HYDROCHLORIDE
Tonocard Tablets 649

TONOFTAL-N (Germany)
NYSTATIN
Nystop Topical Powder USP 2608

TONOPROTECT (Germany)
ATENOLOL
Tenormin I.V. Injection 692

TOPALGIC (France)
TRAMADOL HYDROCHLORIDE
Ultram Tablets 2600

TOPAMAX (Australia, Austria, Belgium, Canada, Germany, Hong Kong, Irish Republic, Israel, Italy, Mexico, New Zealand, Portugal, Singapore, South Africa, Spain, Switzerland, Thailand, The Netherlands, United Kingdom)
TOPIRAMATE
Topamax Sprinkle Capsules 2590
Topamax Tablets 2590

TOPARAL (Mexico)
METHYLDOPA
Aldomet Tablets 2037

TOPEX (Australia)
BENZOYL PEROXIDE
Brevoxyl-4 Cleansing Lotion 3269
Brevoxyl-4 Creamy Wash 3270
Brevoxyl-4 Gel 3269
Brevoxyl-8 Cleansing Lotion 3269
Brevoxyl-8 Creamy Wash 3270
Brevoxyl-8 Gel 3269
Triaz Cleanser 2026
Triaz Gel 2026

TOPFENA (France)
KETOPROFEN
Orudis Capsules 3548
Oruvail Capsules 3548

TOPICAINE (Australia, Canada)
BENZOCAINE
Americaine Anesthetic Lubricant 1162
Americaine Otic Topical Anesthetic Ear Drops 1162

TOPICIL (New Zealand)
CLINDAMYCIN PHOSPHATE
Cleocin Phosphate Sterile Solution 2785
Cleocin T Topical Gel 2790
Cleocin T Topical Lotion 2790
Cleocin T Topical Solution 2790
Cleocin Vaginal Cream 2788
Clindets Pledgets 3270

TOPICORT (Canada, Italy)
DESOXIMETASONE
Topicort Cream 2025
Topicort Gel 2025
Topicort LP Cream 2025
Topicort Ointment 2025

TOPICORTE (Belgium, France, Singapore, Thailand, The Netherlands)
DESOXIMETASONE
Topicort Cream 2025
Topicort Gel 2025
Topicort LP Cream 2025
Topicort Ointment 2025

TOPIDERM (Spain)
DESOXIMETASONE
Topicort Cream 2025
Topicort Gel 2025
Topicort LP Cream 2025
Topicort Ointment 2025

TOPIFLUOR (Italy)
FLUOCINOLONE ACETONIDE
Synalar Cream 2020
Synalar Ointment 2020
Synalar Topical Solution 2020

TOPIFUG (Germany)
DESONIDE
DesOwen Cream 1401
DesOwen Lotion 1401
DesOwen Ointment 1401

TOPILONE (Thailand)
TRIAMCINOLONE ACETONIDE
Azmacort Inhalation Aerosol 728
Nasacort AQ Nasal Spray 752
Nasacort Nasal Inhaler 750

TOPIMAX (Denmark, Finland, Norway, Sweden)
TOPIRAMATE
Topamax Sprinkle Capsules 2590
Topamax Tablets 2590

TOPINASAL (Germany)
BUDESONIDE
Pulmicort Turbuhaler Inhalation Powder . . . 636
Rhinocort Nasal Inhaler 640

TOPISOLON (Austria, Germany, Irish Republic, South Africa, Switzerland)
DESOXIMETASONE
Topicort Cream 2025
Topicort Gel 2025
Topicort LP Cream 2025
Topicort Ointment 2025

TOPOSTASIN (Germany, Italy, The Netherlands)
THROMBIN
Thrombin-JMI 1824

TOPREC (France)
KETOPROFEN
Orudis Capsules 3548
Oruvail Capsules 3548

TOPREK (Austria, Belgium, Italy)
KETOPROFEN
Orudis Capsules 3548
Oruvail Capsules 3548

TOPRILEM (Mexico)
CAPTOPRIL
Captopril Tablets 2281

TOPSYM (Austria, Germany, Switzerland)
FLUOCINONIDE
Lidex Cream 2020
Lidex Gel 2020
Lidex Ointment 2020
Lidex Topical Solution 2020
Lidex-E Cream 2020

TOPSYMIN (Switzerland)
FLUOCINONIDE
Lidex Cream 2020
Lidex Gel 2020
Lidex Ointment 2020
Lidex Topical Solution 2020
Lidex-E Cream 2020

TOPSYMIN F (Austria)
FLUOCINONIDE
Lidex Cream 2020
Lidex Gel 2020
Lidex Ointment 2020
Lidex Topical Solution 2020
Lidex-E Cream 2020

TOPSYN (Canada, Italy, Mexico)
FLUOCINONIDE
Lidex Cream 2020
Lidex Gel 2020
Lidex Ointment 2020
Lidex Topical Solution 2020
Lidex-E Cream 2020

TOPSYNE (France, The Netherlands)
FLUOCINONIDE
Lidex Cream 2020
Lidex Gel 2020
Lidex Ointment 2020
Lidex Topical Solution 2020
Lidex-E Cream 2020

TOPSYN-Y (Mexico)
FLUOCINONIDE
Lidex Cream 2020
Lidex Gel 2020
Lidex Ointment 2020
Lidex Topical Solution 2020
Lidex-E Cream 2020

TORIOL (Spain)
RANITIDINE HYDROCHLORIDE
Zantac 150 EFFERdose Granules 1690
Zantac 150 EFFERdose Tablets 1690
Zantac 150 Tablets 1690
Zantac 300 Tablets 1690
Zantac Injection 1688
Zantac Injection Premixed 1688
Zantac Syrup 1690

TORLASPORIN (Spain)
CEPHALEXIN
Keflex Oral Suspension 1237
Keflex Pulvules 1237

TORVAST (Italy)
ATORVASTATIN CALCIUM
Lipitor Tablets 2639, 2696

TORYMYCIN (Thailand)
DOXYCYCLINE HYCLATE
Doryx Coated Pellet Filled Capsules 3357
Periostat Tablets 1208
Vibramycin Hyclate Capsules 2735
Vibramycin Hyclate Intravenous 2737
Vibra-Tabs Film Coated Tablets 2735

TORYXIL (Germany)
DICLOFENAC SODIUM
Voltaren Tablets 2315
Voltaren-XR Tablets 2315

TOSMILEN (United Kingdom)
DEMECARIUM BROMIDE
Humorsol Sterile Ophthalmic Solution . . . 2102

TOSSEMED (Italy)
DEXTROMETHORPHAN HYDROBROMIDE/GUAIFENESIN
Tussi-Organidin DM NR Liquid 3350
Tussi-Organidin DM-S NR Liquid 3350

TOTALIP (Italy)
ATORVASTATIN CALCIUM
Lipitor Tablets 2639, 2696

TOTAMOL (United Kingdom)
ATENOLOL
Tenormin I.V. Injection 692

TOTARETIC (United Kingdom)
ATENOLOL
Tenormin I.V. Injection 692

TOTATROM (Mexico)
ERYTHROMYCIN
Emgel 2% Topical Gel 1285
Ery-Tab Tablets 448
Erythromycin Base Filmtab Tablets 454
Erythromycin Delayed-Release Capsules, USP 455
PCE Dispertab Tablets 498

TOTOCORTIN (Germany)
DEXAMETHASONE SODIUM PHOSPHATE
Decadron Phosphate Injection 2081
Decadron Phosphate Sterile Ophthalmic Ointment . . . . ⊙280, 2083
Decadron Phosphate Sterile Ophthalmic Solution 2084

TRABAR (Israel)
TRAMADOL HYDROCHLORIDE
Ultram Tablets 2600

TRACIX (Spain)
CILASTATIN SODIUM/IMIPENEM
Primaxin I.M. 2158
Primaxin I.V. 2160

TRACONAL (Brazil)
ITRACONAZOLE
Sporanox Capsules 1800
Sporanox Oral Solution 1808, 2512

TRADELIA (Germany)
ESTRADIOL
Alora Transdermal System 3372
Climara Transdermal System 958
Estrace Vaginal Cream 3358
Estring Vaginal Ring 2811
Vivelle Transdermal System 2412
Vivelle-Dot Transdermal System 2416

TRADOL (Germany, Irish Republic, Mexico, Singapore)
TRAMADOL HYDROCHLORIDE
Ultram Tablets 2600

TRADOLAN (Austria, Denmark, Sweden)
TRAMADOL HYDROCHLORIDE
Ultram Tablets 2600

TRADON (Germany)
PEMOLINE
Cylert Chewable Tablets 415
Cylert Tablets 415

TRADONAL (Belgium, Italy, Spain, Thailand)
TRAMADOL HYDROCHLORIDE
Ultram Tablets 2600

TRAFLOXAL (Belgium, The Netherlands)
OFLOXACIN
Floxin I.V. 2526
Floxin Otic Solution 1219
Floxin Tablets 2529
Ocuflox Ophthalmic Solution 554

TRALGIOL (Spain)
TRAMADOL HYDROCHLORIDE
Ultram Tablets 2600

TRAMABENE (Austria)
TRAMADOL HYDROCHLORIDE
Ultram Tablets 2600

TRAMABETA (Germany)
TRAMADOL HYDROCHLORIDE
Ultram Tablets 2600

TRAMADEX (Israel)
TRAMADOL HYDROCHLORIDE
Ultram Tablets 2600

TRAMADIN (Finland)
TRAMADOL HYDROCHLORIDE
Ultram Tablets 2600

TRAMADOL-DOLGIT (Germany)
TRAMADOL HYDROCHLORIDE
Ultram Tablets 2600

TRAMADOLOR (Germany, Switzerland)
TRAMADOL HYDROCHLORIDE
Ultram Tablets 2600

TRAMA-DORSCH (Germany)
TRAMADOL HYDROCHLORIDE
Ultram Tablets 2600

TRAMADURA (Germany)
TRAMADOL HYDROCHLORIDE
Ultram Tablets 2600

TRAMAGETIC (Germany, The Netherlands)
TRAMADOL HYDROCHLORIDE
Ultram Tablets 2600

TRAMAGIT (Germany)
TRAMADOL HYDROCHLORIDE
Ultram Tablets 2600

TRAMAKE (Irish Republic, United Kingdom)
TRAMADOL HYDROCHLORIDE
Ultram Tablets 2600

TRAMAL (Australia, Austria, Brazil, Germany, New Zealand, Portugal, South Africa, Switzerland, The Netherlands)
TRAMADOL HYDROCHLORIDE
Ultram Tablets 2600

TRAMALAN (Thailand)
TRAMADOL HYDROCHLORIDE
Ultram Tablets 2600

TRAMAMED (Thailand)
TRAMADOL HYDROCHLORIDE
Ultram Tablets 2600

TRAMAMERCK (Germany)
TRAMADOL HYDROCHLORIDE
Ultram Tablets 2600

TRAMEDPHANO (Germany)
TRAMADOL HYDROCHLORIDE
Ultram Tablets 2600

TRAMEX (Irish Republic)
TRAMADOL HYDROCHLORIDE
Ultram Tablets 2600

TRAMINA (Spain)
CHLORAMPHENICOL
Chloromycetin Ophthalmic Ointment, 1% . . . . ⊙296
Chloromycetin Ophthalmic Solution . . . . ⊙297
Chloroptic Sterile Ophthalmic Ointment . . . ⊙234
Chloroptic Sterile Ophthalmic Solution . . ⊙235

TRAMO (Hong Kong)
TRAMADOL HYDROCHLORIDE
Ultram Tablets 2600

TRAMODA (Thailand)
TRAMADOL HYDROCHLORIDE
Ultram Tablets 2600

TRAMOL (Finland)
TRAMADOL HYDROCHLORIDE
Ultram Tablets 2600

TRAMSILIONE (Thailand)
TRIAMCINOLONE ACETONIDE
Azmacort Inhalation Aerosol 728
Nasacort AQ Nasal Spray 752
Nasacort Nasal Inhaler 750

TRAMUNDAL (Austria)
TRAMADOL HYDROCHLORIDE
Ultram Tablets 2600

TRAMUNDIN (Germany)
TRAMADOL HYDROCHLORIDE
Ultram Tablets . . . 2600

TRANCOCARD (Italy)
DIPYRIDAMOLE
Persantine Tablets . . . 1057

TRANDATE (Australia, Austria, Belgium, Canada, Denmark, France, Hong Kong, Irish Republic, Israel, Italy, New Zealand, Norway, Portugal, Singapore, South Africa, Spain, Sweden, Switzerland, The Netherlands, United Kingdom)
LABETALOL HYDROCHLORIDE
Normodyne Injection . . . 3135
Normodyne Tablets . . . 3137

TRANDROZINE (Thailand)
HYDROXYZINE HYDROCHLORIDE
Atarax Tablets & Syrup . . . 2667
Vistaril Intramuscular Solution . . . 2738

TRANGOREX (Spain)
AMIODARONE HYDROCHLORIDE
Cordarone Intravenous . . . 3491
Cordarone Tablets . . . 3487
Pacerone Tablets . . . 3331

TRANKIMAZIN (Spain)
ALPRAZOLAM
Xanax Tablets . . . 2865

TRAN-QIL (South Africa)
LORAZEPAM
Ativan Injection . . . 3478
Ativan Tablets . . . 3482

TRANQIPAM (South Africa)
LORAZEPAM
Ativan Injection . . . 3478
Ativan Tablets . . . 3482

TRANQUASE (Germany)
DIAZEPAM
Valium Injectable . . . 3026
Valium Tablets . . . 3047

TRANQUIRIT (Italy)
DIAZEPAM
Valium Injectable . . . 3026
Valium Tablets . . . 3047

TRANQUO (Germany)
DIAZEPAM
Valium Injectable . . . 3026
Valium Tablets . . . 3047

TRANSPULMINA RINO (Italy)
NAPHAZOLINE HYDROCHLORIDE
Albalon Ophthalmic Solution . . . ⊙225

TRANTALOL (Irish Republic)
ATENOLOL
Tenormin I.V. Injection . . . 692

TRANTIL (Mexico)
CARBAMAZEPINE
Carbatrol Capsules . . . 3234
Tegretol Chewable Tablets . . . 2404
Tegretol Suspension . . . 2404
Tegretol Tablets . . . 2404
Tegretol-XR Tablets . . . 2404

TRASYLOL (Australia, Austria, Belgium, Canada, Denmark, Finland, France, Germany, Hong Kong, Irish Republic, Italy, Mexico, New Zealand, Singapore, South Africa, Sweden, Switzerland, Thailand, The Netherlands, United Kingdom)
APROTININ
Trasylol Injection . . . 909

TRAUMACUT (Germany)
METHOCARBAMOL
Robaxin Injectable . . . 2938
Robaxin Tablets . . . 2939
Robaxin-750 Tablets . . . 2939

TRAUMA-DOLGIT (Germany)
IBUPROFEN
Motrin Suspension, Oral Drops, Chewable Tablets, and Caplets . . . 2002

TRAUMALITAN (Germany)
HEPARIN SODIUM
Heparin Lock Flush Solution . . . 3509
Heparin Sodium Injection . . . 3511

TRAUMAZOL (Mexico)
ETHYL CHLORIDE
Gebauer's Ethyl Chloride . . . 1409

TRAUMOX (South Africa)
NAPROXEN
EC-Naprosyn Delayed-Release Tablets . . . 2967
Naprosyn Suspension . . . 2967
Naprosyn Tablets . . . 2967

TRAVEX (Portugal)
TRAMADOL HYDROCHLORIDE
Ultram Tablets . . . 2600

TRAZIL (Mexico)
TOBRAMYCIN SULFATE
Nebcin Vials, Hyporets & ADD-Vantage . . 1955

TREIS-MICINA (Italy)
TROLEANDOMYCIN
Tao Capsules . . . 2716

TREMOREX (Denmark)
SELEGILINE HYDROCHLORIDE
Eldepryl Capsules . . . 3266

TREPOL (Mexico)
DIPYRIDAMOLE
Persantine Tablets . . . 1057

TRESLEEN (Austria)
SERTRALINE HYDROCHLORIDE
Zoloft Tablets . . . 2751

TRETINOINE KEFRANE (France)
TRETINOIN
Avita Cream . . . 999
Avita Gel . . . 1000
Renova 0.05% Cream . . . 2519
Retin-A Micro 0.1% . . . 2522
Vesanoid Capsules . . . 3037

TRETINON (Mexico)
TRETINOIN
Avita Cream . . . 999
Avita Gel . . . 1000
Renova 0.05% Cream . . . 2519
Retin-A Micro 0.1% . . . 2522
Vesanoid Capsules . . . 3037

TREVILOR (Germany)
VENLAFAXINE HYDROCHLORIDE
Effexor Tablets . . . 3495
Effexor XR Capsules . . . 3499

TREWILOR (Austria)
VENLAFAXINE HYDROCHLORIDE
Effexor Tablets . . . 3495
Effexor XR Capsules . . . 3499

TREXOFIN (Singapore)
CEFTRIAXONE SODIUM
Rocephin Injectable Vials, ADD-Vantage, Galaxy, Bulk . . . 2993

TRH (Belgium, United Kingdom)
PROTIRELIN
Thyrel TRH for Injection . . . 3630

TRH PREM (Spain)
PROTIRELIN
Thyrel TRH for Injection . . . 3630

TRH-ROCHE (Australia)
PROTIRELIN
Thyrel TRH for Injection . . . 3630

TRIADAPIN (Canada)
DOXEPIN HYDROCHLORIDE
Sinequan Capsules . . . 2713
Sinequan Oral Concentrate . . . 2713

TRIADERM (Canada)
TRIAMCINOLONE ACETONIDE
Azmacort Inhalation Aerosol . . . 728
Nasacort AQ Nasal Spray . . . 752
Nasacort Nasal Inhaler . . . 750

TRIAKEN (Mexico)
CEFTRIAXONE SODIUM
Rocephin Injectable Vials, ADD-Vantage, Galaxy, Bulk . . . 2993

TRIALIX (Austria, Irish Republic)
RAMIPRIL
Altace Capsules . . . 2233

TRIALMIN (Spain)
GEMFIBROZIL
Lopid Tablets . . . 2650

TRIALONA (Spain)
FLUTICASONE PROPIONATE
Cutivate Cream . . . 1282
Cutivate Ointment . . . 1284
Flonase Nasal Spray . . . 1533
Flovent 110 mcg Inhalation Aerosol . . . 1535
Flovent 220 mcg Inhalation Aerosol . . . 1535
Flovent 44 mcg Inhalation Aerosol . . . 1535
Flovent Rotadisk 100 mcg . . . 1537
Flovent Rotadisk 250 mcg . . . 1537
Flovent Rotadisk 50 mcg . . . 1537

TRIAM (Germany)
TRIAMCINOLONE ACETONIDE
Azmacort Inhalation Aerosol . . . 728
Nasacort AQ Nasal Spray . . . 752
Nasacort Nasal Inhaler . . . 750

TRIAMA (Thailand)
TRIAMCINOLONE ACETONIDE
Azmacort Inhalation Aerosol . . . 728
Nasacort AQ Nasal Spray . . . 752
Nasacort Nasal Inhaler . . . 750

TRIAMAXCO (United Kingdom)
HYDROCHLOROTHIAZIDE/TRIAMTERENE
Dyazide Capsules . . . 1515
Maxzide Tablets . . . 1008
Maxzide-25 mg Tablets . . . 1008

TRIAMCO (United Kingdom)
HYDROCHLOROTHIAZIDE/TRIAMTERENE
Dyazide Capsules . . . 1515
Maxzide Tablets . . . 1008
Maxzide-25 mg Tablets . . . 1008

TRIAM-CO (Hong Kong)
HYDROCHLOROTHIAZIDE/TRIAMTERENE
Dyazide Capsules . . . 1515
Maxzide Tablets . . . 1008
Maxzide-25 mg Tablets . . . 1008

TRIAMCORT (Switzerland)
TRIAMCINOLONE ACETONIDE
Azmacort Inhalation Aerosol . . . 728
Nasacort AQ Nasal Spray . . . 752
Nasacort Nasal Inhaler . . . 750

TRIAMCREME (Germany)
TRIAMCINOLONE ACETONIDE
Azmacort Inhalation Aerosol . . . 728
Nasacort AQ Nasal Spray . . . 752
Nasacort Nasal Inhaler . . . 750

TRIAMGALEN (Germany)
TRIAMCINOLONE ACETONIDE
Azmacort Inhalation Aerosol . . . 728
Nasacort AQ Nasal Spray . . . 752
Nasacort Nasal Inhaler . . . 750

TRIAMHEXAL (Germany)
TRIAMCINOLONE ACETONIDE
Azmacort Inhalation Aerosol . . . 728
Nasacort AQ Nasal Spray . . . 752
Nasacort Nasal Inhaler . . . 750

TRIAMINIC DECONGESTANT & EXPECTORANT (Canada)
GUAIFENESIN/PSEUDOEPHEDRINE HYDROCHLORIDE
Guaifed Capsules . . . 2272
Guaifed-PD Capsules . . . 2272
Zephrex LA Tablets . . . 3092
Zephrex Tablets . . . 3091

TRIAM-INJEKT (Germany)
TRIAMCINOLONE ACETONIDE
Azmacort Inhalation Aerosol . . . 728
Nasacort AQ Nasal Spray . . . 752
Nasacort Nasal Inhaler . . . 750

TRIAMIZIDE (New Zealand)
HYDROCHLOROTHIAZIDE/TRIAMTERENE
Dyazide Capsules . . . 1515
Maxzide Tablets . . . 1008
Maxzide-25 mg Tablets . . . 1008

TRIAMPUR (Germany)
HYDROCHLOROTHIAZIDE/TRIAMTERENE
Dyazide Capsules . . . 1515
Maxzide Tablets . . . 1008
Maxzide-25 mg Tablets . . . 1008

TRIAMSALBE (Germany)
TRIAMCINOLONE ACETONIDE
Azmacort Inhalation Aerosol . . . 728
Nasacort AQ Nasal Spray . . . 752
Nasacort Nasal Inhaler . . . 750

TRIAMTEREN COMP (Austria, Germany)
HYDROCHLOROTHIAZIDE/TRIAMTERENE
Dyazide Capsules . . . 1515
Maxzide Tablets . . . 1008
Maxzide-25 mg Tablets . . . 1008

TRIAMTEREN/HCT (Germany)
HYDROCHLOROTHIAZIDE/TRIAMTERENE
Dyazide Capsules . . . 1515
Maxzide Tablets . . . 1008
Maxzide-25 mg Tablets . . . 1008

TRIAMTEREN-H (Germany)
HYDROCHLOROTHIAZIDE/TRIAMTERENE
Dyazide Capsules . . . 1515
Maxzide Tablets . . . 1008
Maxzide-25 mg Tablets . . . 1008

TRIAMTERIL COMPLEX (Italy)
HYDROCHLOROTHIAZIDE/TRIAMTERENE
Dyazide Capsules . . . 1515
Maxzide Tablets . . . 1008
Maxzide-25 mg Tablets . . . 1008

TRIAMTHIAZID (Germany)
HYDROCHLOROTHIAZIDE/TRIAMTERENE
Dyazide Capsules . . . 1515
Maxzide Tablets . . . 1008
Maxzide-25 mg Tablets . . . 1008

TRIAM-TIAZIDA R (Portugal)
HYDROCHLOROTHIAZIDE/TRIAMTERENE
Dyazide Capsules . . . 1515
Maxzide Tablets . . . 1008
Maxzide-25 mg Tablets . . . 1008

TRI-ANEMUL (Germany)
TRIAMCINOLONE ACETONIDE
Azmacort Inhalation Aerosol . . . 728
Nasacort AQ Nasal Spray . . . 752
Nasacort Nasal Inhaler . . . 750

TRIAPIN (The Netherlands, United Kingdom)
FELODIPINE
Plendil Extended-Release Tablets . . . 623

TRIARESE (Germany)
HYDROCHLOROTHIAZIDE/TRIAMTERENE
Dyazide Capsules . . . 1515
Maxzide Tablets . . . 1008
Maxzide-25 mg Tablets . . . 1008

TRIASPORIN (Italy)
ITRACONAZOLE
Sporanox Capsules . . . 1800
Sporanox Oral Solution . . . 1808, 2512

TRIASTAD HCT (Austria)
HYDROCHLOROTHIAZIDE/TRIAMTERENE
Dyazide Capsules . . . 1515
Maxzide Tablets . . . 1008
Maxzide-25 mg Tablets . . . 1008

TRIATEC (Brazil, Denmark, France, Italy, Norway, Portugal, Sweden, Switzerland)
RAMIPRIL
Altace Capsules . . . 2233

TRIATEC COMP (Denmark)
RAMIPRIL
Altace Capsules . . . 2233

TRIATEC COMPOSTO (Portugal)
RAMIPRIL
Altace Capsules . . . 2233

TRIATEC HCT (Italy)
RAMIPRIL
Altace Capsules . . . 2233

TRIATOP (Italy, Thailand)
KETOCONAZOLE
Nizoral 2% Cream . . . 3620
Nizoral 2% Shampoo . . . 2007
Nizoral Tablets . . . 1791

TRIAVIL (Canada)
AMITRIPTYLINE HYDROCHLORIDE/PERPHENAZINE
Etrafon 2-10 Tablets (2-10) . . . 3115
Etrafon Tablets (2-25) . . . 3115
Etrafon-Forte Tablets (4-25) . . . 3115

TRIAXONE (United Arab Emirates)
CEFTRIAXONE SODIUM
Rocephin Injectable Vials, ADD-Vantage, Galaxy, Bulk . . . 2993

TRIAZID (Germany)
HYDROCHLOROTHIAZIDE/TRIAMTERENE
Dyazide Capsules . . . 1515
Maxzide Tablets . . . 1008
Maxzide-25 mg Tablets . . . 1008

TRIAZOL (Brazil)
FLUCONAZOLE
Diflucan Tablets, Injection, and Oral Suspension . . . 2681

TRIBIOT (Mexico)
NEOMYCIN SULFATE/POLYMYXIN B SULFATE
Neosporin G.U. Irrigant Sterile . . . 2256

TRICAN (Israel)
FLUCONAZOLE
Diflucan Tablets, Injection, and Oral Suspension . . . 2681

TRICEF (Austria, Portugal, Sweden)
CEFIXIME
Suprax Tablets . . . 1877
Suprax for Oral Suspension . . . 1877

TRICEN (Spain)
TRANDOLAPRIL/VERAPAMIL HYDROCHLORIDE
Tarka Tablets . . . 508

TRICEPHIN (Thailand)
CEFTRIAXONE SODIUM
Rocephin Injectable Vials, ADD-Vantage, Galaxy, Bulk . . . 2993

TRICHAZOLE (South Africa)
METRONIDAZOLE
MetroCream . . . 1404
MetroGel . . . 1405
MetroGel-Vaginal Gel . . . 1986
MetroLotion . . . 1405
Noritate Cream . . . 1224

TRICHEX (Austria)
METRONIDAZOLE
MetroCream . . . 1404
MetroGel . . . 1405
MetroGel-Vaginal Gel . . . 1986
MetroLotion . . . 1405
Noritate Cream . . . 1224

TRICHO CORDES (Germany)
METRONIDAZOLE
MetroCream . . . 1404

(⊙ Described in PDR For Ophthalmic Medicines™)

MetroGel 1405
MetroGel-Vaginal Gel 1986
MetroLotion 1405
Noritate Cream 1224

TRICHOZOLE (Australia, New Zealand)
METRONIDAZOLE
MetroCream 1404
MetroGel 1405
MetroGel-Vaginal Gel 1986
MetroLotion 1405
Noritate Cream 1224

TRICOMED (Thailand)
METRONIDAZOLE
MetroCream 1404
MetroGel 1405
MetroGel-Vaginal Gel 1986
MetroLotion 1405
Noritate Cream 1224

TRICOSTEN (Brazil)
CLOTRIMAZOLE
Lotrimin Cream 1% 3128
Lotrimin Lotion 1% 3128
Lotrimin Topical Solution 1% 3128
Mycelex Troche 573

TRICOWAS B (Spain)
METRONIDAZOLE
MetroCream 1404
MetroGel 1405
MetroGel-Vaginal Gel 1986
MetroLotion 1405
Noritate Cream 1224

TRIDERM (Hong Kong)
BETAMETHASONE DIPROPIONATE/CLOTRIMAZOLE
Lotrisone Cream 3129

TRIDESILON (Canada, Germany, United Kingdom)
DESONIDE
DesOwen Cream 1401
DesOwen Lotion 1401
DesOwen Ointment 1401

TRIDESONIT (France)
DESONIDE
DesOwen Cream 1401
DesOwen Lotion 1401
DesOwen Ointment 1401

TRIFENE (Portugal)
IBUPROFEN
Motrin Suspension, Oral Drops, Chewable Tablets, and Caplets 2002

TRIFLUCAN (France, Israel)
FLUCONAZOLE
Diflucan Tablets, Injection, and Oral Suspension 2681

TRIFLUMANN (Germany)
TRIFLURIDINE
Viroptic Ophthalmic Solution Sterile . . . . ⊙301

TRIGGER (Italy)
RANITIDINE HYDROCHLORIDE
Zantac 150 EFFERdose Granules 1690
Zantac 150 EFFERdose Tablets 1690
Zantac 150 Tablets 1690
Zantac 300 Tablets 1690
Zantac Injection 1688
Zantac Injection Premixed 1688
Zantac Syrup 1690

TRIGON DEPOT (Spain)
TRIAMCINOLONE ACETONIDE
Azmacort Inhalation Aerosol 728
Nasacort AQ Nasal Spray 752
Nasacort Nasal Inhaler 750

TRIGYNON (Belgium)
LEVONORGESTREL
Norplant System 3543

TRIHERPINE (France, Hong Kong, Italy, Switzerland, Thailand)
TRIFLURIDINE
Viroptic Ophthalmic Solution Sterile . . . . ⊙301

TRIIODOTHYRONINE INJECTION (United Kingdom)
LIOTHYRONINE SODIUM
Cytomel Tablets 1817
Triostat Injection 1825

TRIKACIDE (Canada)
METRONIDAZOLE
MetroCream 1404
MetroGel 1405
MetroGel-Vaginal Gel 1986
MetroLotion 1405
Noritate Cream 1224

TRIKOZOL (Finland)
METRONIDAZOLE
MetroCream 1404
MetroGel 1405
MetroGel-Vaginal Gel 1986
MetroLotion 1405
Noritate Cream 1224

TRILAFON (Australia, Belgium, Canada, Mexico, Switzerland)
PERPHENAZINE
Trilafon Injection 3160
Trilafon Tablets 3160

TRILAM (Irish Republic)
TRIAZOLAM
Halcion Tablets 2823

TRILISATE (Canada, Irish Republic, United Kingdom)
CHOLINE MAGNESIUM TRISALICYLATE
Trilisate Liquid 2901
Trilisate Tablets 2901

TRILOSIL (Thailand)
TRIAMCINOLONE ACETONIDE
Azmacort Inhalation Aerosol 728
Nasacort AQ Nasal Spray 752
Nasacort Nasal Inhaler 750

TRIM (Thailand)
TRIAMCINOLONE ACETONIDE
Azmacort Inhalation Aerosol 728
Nasacort AQ Nasal Spray 752
Nasacort Nasal Inhaler 750

TRIMASONE (Thailand)
TRIAMCINOLONE ACETONIDE
Azmacort Inhalation Aerosol 728
Nasacort AQ Nasal Spray 752
Nasacort Nasal Inhaler 750

TRIMAZE (South Africa)
CLOTRIMAZOLE
Lotrimin Cream 1% 3128
Lotrimin Lotion 1% 3128
Lotrimin Topical Solution 1% 3128
Mycelex Troche 573

TRIMOLEX (South Africa)
AMILORIDE HYDROCHLORIDE/HYDROCHLOROTHIAZIDE
Moduretic Tablets 2138

TRIMONIL (Denmark, Finland, Norway, Sweden)
CARBAMAZEPINE
Carbatrol Capsules 3234
Tegretol Chewable Tablets 2404
Tegretol Suspension 2404
Tegretol Tablets 2404
Tegretol-XR Tablets 2404

TRIMYSTEN (France)
CLOTRIMAZOLE
Lotrimin Cream 1% 3128
Lotrimin Lotion 1% 3128
Lotrimin Topical Solution 1% 3128
Mycelex Troche 573

TRINALION (Portugal)
NIMODIPINE
Nimotop Capsules 904

TRINORDIOL (Belgium, United Kingdom)
LEVONORGESTREL
Norplant System 3543

TRIOCETIN (Italy)
TROLEANDOMYCIN
Tao Capsules 2716

TRIOMIN (South Africa)
MINOCYCLINE HYDROCHLORIDE
Dynacin Capsules 2019
Minocin Intravenous 1862
Minocin Oral Suspension 1865
Minocin Pellet-Filled Capsules 1863

TRI-PLEN (South Africa)
RAMIPRIL
Altace Capsules 2233

TRIPLEX (Thailand)
TRIFLUOPERAZINE HYDROCHLORIDE
Stelazine Injection 1640
Stelazine Tablets 1640

TRIPRESS (New Zealand)
TRIMIPRAMINE MALEATE
Surmontil Capsules 3595

TRI-PROFEN (Australia)
IBUPROFEN
Motrin Suspension, Oral Drops, Chewable Tablets, and Caplets 2002

TRIPTAFEN (Irish Republic, United Kingdom)
AMITRIPTYLINE HYDROCHLORIDE/PERPHENAZINE
Etrafon 2-10 Tablets (2-10) 3115
Etrafon Tablets (2-25) 3115
Etrafon-Forte Tablets (4-25) 3115

TRIPTIL (Canada)
PROTRIPTYLINE HYDROCHLORIDE
Vivactil Tablets 2217

TRIRUTIN (Germany)
HEPARIN SODIUM
Heparin Lock Flush Solution 3509
Heparin Sodium Injection 3511

TRISORCIN (Germany)
PENICILLAMINE
Cuprimine Capsules 2075
Depen Titratable Tablets 3341

TRISPORAL (The Netherlands)
ITRACONAZOLE
Sporanox Capsules 1800
Sporanox Oral Solution 1808, 2512

TRITACE (Australia, Austria, Belgium, Hong Kong, Irish Republic, Israel, Mexico, Singapore, South Africa, Thailand, The Netherlands, United Kingdom)
RAMIPRIL
Altace Capsules 2233

TRITAZIDE (Belgium, Mexico, The Netherlands)
RAMIPRIL
Altace Capsules 2233

TRI-THIAZID (Germany)
HYDROCHLOROTHIAZIDE/TRIAMTERENE
Dyazide Capsules 1515
Maxzide Tablets 1008
Maxzide-25 mg Tablets 1008

TRI-THIAZID RESERPIN (Germany)
HYDROCHLOROTHIAZIDE/TRIAMTERENE
Dyazide Capsules 1515
Maxzide Tablets 1008
Maxzide-25 mg Tablets 1008

TRIXONE (Thailand)
CEFTRIAXONE SODIUM
Rocephin Injectable Vials, ADD-Vantage, Galaxy, Bulk 2993

TRIYOTEX (Mexico)
LIOTHYRONINE SODIUM
Cytomel Tablets 1817
Triostat Injection 1825

TRIZ (Thailand)
CETIRIZINE HYDROCHLORIDE
Zyrtec Syrup 2756
Zyrtec Tablets 2756

TRIZELE (Hong Kong)
METRONIDAZOLE
MetroCream 1404
MetroGel 1405
MetroGel-Vaginal Gel 1986
MetroLotion 1405
Noritate Cream 1224

TRIZID (Hong Kong, New Zealand)
HYDROCHLOROTHIAZIDE/TRIAMTERENE
Dyazide Capsules 1515
Maxzide Tablets 1008
Maxzide-25 mg Tablets 1008

TRIZOLIN (Singapore, Thailand)
NORFLOXACIN
Chibroxin Sterile Ophthalmic Solution . . . . ⊙273, 2051
Noroxin Tablets 2145

TROFEN (Thailand)
IBUPROFEN
Motrin Suspension, Oral Drops, Chewable Tablets, and Caplets 2002

TROLIC (South Africa)
PREDNISONE
Prednisone Intensol 3064
Prednisone Oral Solution 3064
Prednisone Tablets 3064

TROLOVOL (France, Germany)
PENICILLAMINE
Cuprimine Capsules 2075
Depen Titratable Tablets 3341

TROMBENOX (Italy)
ENOXAPARIN SODIUM
Lovenox Injection 746

TROMBISTAT (The Netherlands)
THROMBIN
Thrombin-JMI 1824

TROMBOFOB (Brazil)
HEPARIN SODIUM
Heparin Lock Flush Solution 3509
Heparin Sodium Injection 3511

TROMBOLIQUINE (The Netherlands)
HEPARIN SODIUM
Heparin Lock Flush Solution 3509
Heparin Sodium Injection 3511

TROMBOPAT (Portugal)
TICLOPIDINE HYDROCHLORIDE
Ticlid Tablets 3015

TROMBOSOL (Finland)
HEPARIN SODIUM
Heparin Lock Flush Solution 3509
Heparin Sodium Injection 3511

TROMBUFEN (Germany)
IBUPROFEN
Motrin Suspension, Oral Drops, Chewable Tablets, and Caplets 2002

TROMIGAL (Mexico)
ERYTHROMYCIN
Emgel 2% Topical Gel 1285
Ery-Tab Tablets 448
Erythromycin Base Filmtab Tablets 454
Erythromycin Delayed-Release Capsules, USP 455
PCE Dispertab Tablets 498

TROMPERSANTIN (Mexico)
DIPYRIDAMOLE
Persantine Tablets 1057

TROMPHYLLIN (Germany)
THEOPHYLLINE
Aerolate Jr. T.D. Capsules 1361
Aerolate Liquid 1361
Aerolate Sr. T.D. Capsules 1361
Theo-Dur Extended-Release Tablets 1835
Uni-Dur Extended-Release Tablets 1841
Uniphyl 400 mg and 600 mg Tablets 2903

TRONOXAL (Spain)
IFOSFAMIDE
Ifex for Injection 1123

TROPIOVENT (United Kingdom)
IPRATROPIUM BROMIDE
Atrovent Inhalation Aerosol 1030
Atrovent Inhalation Solution 1031
Atrovent Nasal Spray 0.03% 1032
Atrovent Nasal Spray 0.06% 1033

TROPISOL (Mexico)
CAPTOPRIL
Captopril Tablets 2281

TROPIUM (United Kingdom)
CHLORDIAZEPOXIDE HYDROCHLORIDE
Librium Capsules 1736
Librium for Injection 1737

TROSIC (Thailand)
TRAMADOL HYDROCHLORIDE
Ultram Tablets 2600

TROYMYCETIN (South Africa)
CHLORAMPHENICOL
Chloromycetin Ophthalmic Ointment, 1% . . . . ⊙296
Chloromycetin Ophthalmic Solution . . . . ⊙297
Chloroptic Sterile Ophthalmic Ointment . . ⊙234
Chloroptic Sterile Ophthalmic Solution . . ⊙235

TRUMSAL (Spain)
DILTIAZEM HYDROCHLORIDE
Cardizem CD Capsules 1016
Cardizem Injectable 1018
Cardizem Lyo-Ject Syringe 1018
Cardizem Monovial 1018
Tiazac Capsules 1378

TRUSOPT (Australia, Austria, Belgium, Canada, Denmark, Finland, France, Germany, Hong Kong, Irish Republic, Israel, Italy, Mexico, New Zealand, Norway, Portugal, Singapore, South Africa, Spain, Sweden, Switzerland, Thailand, The Netherlands, United Kingdom)
DORZOLAMIDE HYDROCHLORIDE
Trusopt Sterile Ophthalmic Solution 2196

TRYCAM (New Zealand)
TRIAZOLAM
Halcion Tablets 2823

T-STAT (Canada, Mexico, Singapore)
ERYTHROMYCIN
Emgel 2% Topical Gel 1285
Ery-Tab Tablets 448
Erythromycin Base Filmtab Tablets 454
Erythromycin Delayed-Release Capsules, USP 455
PCE Dispertab Tablets 498

TUBERGEN-TEST (Germany, Switzerland)
TUBERCULIN
Aplisol Injection 2609
Tine Test, Tuberculin, Old 3631
Tubersol Diagnostic Antigen 3628

TUKOL (Mexico)
GUAIFENESIN
Organidin NR Liquid 3350
Organidin NR Tablets 3350

TULOTRACT (Germany)
LACTULOSE
Kristalose for Oral Solution 1007

TUOSOMIN (Thailand)
TAMOXIFEN CITRATE
Nolvadex Tablets 678

TURFA (Germany)
HYDROCHLOROTHIAZIDE/TRIAMTERENE
Dyazide Capsules 1515
Maxzide Tablets 1008
Maxzide-25 mg Tablets 1008

TURIMONIT (Germany)
ISOSORBIDE MONONITRATE
Imdur Tablets 1826
Ismo Tablets 3524

TURIMYCIN (Germany)
CLINDAMYCIN HYDROCHLORIDE
Cleocin HCl Capsules 2784

TURRESIS (Portugal)
ETHAMBUTOL HYDROCHLORIDE
Myambutol Tablets 1290

TUSILEN PEDIATRICO (Mexico)
DEXTROMETHORPHAN HYDROBROMIDE/GUAIFENESIN
Tussi-Organidin DM NR Liquid 3350
Tussi-Organidin DM-S NR Liquid 3350

TUSSA (Thailand)
GUAIFENESIN
Organidin NR Liquid 3350
Organidin NR Tablets 3350

TUSSICARE (Thailand)
DEXTROMETHORPHAN HYDROBROMIDE/GUAIFENESIN
Tussi-Organidin DM NR Liquid 3350
Tussi-Organidin DM-S NR Liquid 3350

TUSSIFAMA (Italy)
DEXTROMETHORPHAN HYDROBROMIDE/GUAIFENESIN
Tussi-Organidin DM NR Liquid 3350
Tussi-Organidin DM-S NR Liquid 3350

TUSSIN EXPECTORANT (Canada)
GUAIFENESIN
Organidin NR Liquid 3350
Organidin NR Tablets 3350

TUSSIN-PINHO (Brazil)
POTASSIUM IODIDE
Pima Syrup 1362

TYLENOL ACHES & STRAINS (Canada)
CHLORZOXAZONE
Parafon Forte DSC Caplets 2582

TYMASIL (United Kingdom)
NATAMYCIN
Natacyn Antifungal Ophthalmic Suspension ⊙216

T-ZA (Thailand)
ZIDOVUDINE
Retrovir Capsules 1625
Retrovir IV Infusion 1629
Retrovir Syrup 1625
Retrovir Tablets 1625

TZOALI (Mexico)
DIPHENHYDRAMINE HYDROCHLORIDE
Benadryl Parenteral 2617

UBICOR (Switzerland)
DILTIAZEM HYDROCHLORIDE
Cardizem CD Capsules 1016
Cardizem Injectable 1018
Cardizem Lyo-Ject Syringe 1018
Cardizem Monovial 1018
Tiazac Capsules 1378

UBIZOL (Portugal)
FLUTICASONE PROPIONATE
Cutivate Cream 1282
Cutivate Ointment 1284
Flonase Nasal Spray 1533
Flovent 110 mcg Inhalation Aerosol 1535
Flovent 220 mcg Inhalation Aerosol 1535
Flovent 44 mcg Inhalation Aerosol 1535
Flovent Rotadisk 100 mcg 1537
Flovent Rotadisk 250 mcg 1537
Flovent Rotadisk 50 mcg 1537

UCERAX (United Kingdom)
HYDROXYZINE HYDROCHLORIDE
Atarax Tablets & Syrup 2667
Vistaril Intramuscular Solution 2738

UCINE (United Kingdom)
SULFASALAZINE
Azulfidine EN-tabs Tablets 2775

UDIMA (Germany)
MINOCYCLINE HYDROCHLORIDE
Dynacin Capsules 2019
Minocin Intravenous 1862
Minocin Oral Suspension 1865
Minocin Pellet-Filled Capsules 1863

UDIMA ERY (Germany)
ERYTHROMYCIN
Emgel 2% Topical Gel 1285
Ery-Tab Tablets 448
Erythromycin Base Filmtab Tablets 454
Erythromycin Delayed-Release Capsules, USP 455
PCE Dispertab Tablets 498

ULCAID (South Africa)
RANITIDINE HYDROCHLORIDE
Zantac 150 EFFERdose Granules 1690
Zantac 150 EFFERdose Tablets 1690
Zantac 150 Tablets 1690
Zantac 300 Tablets 1690
Zantac Injection 1688
Zantac Injection Premixed 1688
Zantac Syrup 1690

ULCAR (France)
SUCRALFATE
Carafate Suspension 731
Carafate Tablets 730

ULCECUR (Portugal)
RANITIDINE HYDROCHLORIDE
Zantac 150 EFFERdose Granules 1690
Zantac 150 EFFERdose Tablets 1690
Zantac 150 Tablets 1690
Zantac 300 Tablets 1690
Zantac Injection 1688
Zantac Injection Premixed 1688
Zantac Syrup 1690

ULCEDIN (Italy, Mexico)
CIMETIDINE
Tagamet Tablets 1644

ULCEDINE (Brazil)
CIMETIDINE
Tagamet Tablets 1644

ULCEDOR (Brazil)
CIMETIDINE
Tagamet Tablets 1644

ULCEFATE (South Africa, Thailand)
SUCRALFATE
Carafate Suspension 731
Carafate Tablets 730

ULCEMET (Thailand)
CIMETIDINE
Tagamet Tablets 1644

ULCENON (Brazil)
CIMETIDINE
Tagamet Tablets 1644

ULCERACID (Brazil)
CIMETIDINE
Tagamet Tablets 1644

ULCERAL (Spain)
OMEPRAZOLE
Prilosec Delayed-Release Capsules 628

ULCERAN (Hong Kong, Singapore, Thailand)
FAMOTIDINE
Pepcid Injection 2153
Pepcid Injection Premixed 2153
Pepcid RPD Orally Disintegrating Tablets 2150
Pepcid Tablets 2150
Pepcid for Oral Suspension 2150

ULCERASE (Brazil, Portugal)
CIMETIDINE
Tagamet Tablets 1644

ULCERIDINE (Portugal)
CIMETIDINE
Tagamet Tablets 1644

ULCERIM (Mexico)
CIMETIDINE
Tagamet Tablets 1644

ULCERLMIN (Japan)
SUCRALFATE
Carafate Suspension 731
Carafate Tablets 730

ULCERMIN (Portugal, Spain)
SUCRALFATE
Carafate Suspension 731
Carafate Tablets 730

ULCEROL (Portugal)
RANITIDINE HYDROCHLORIDE
Zantac 150 EFFERdose Granules 1690
Zantac 150 EFFERdose Tablets 1690
Zantac 150 Tablets 1690
Zantac 300 Tablets 1690
Zantac Injection 1688
Zantac Injection Premixed 1688
Zantac Syrup 1690

ULCERTEC (Singapore)
SUCRALFATE
Carafate Suspension 731
Carafate Tablets 730

ULCESEP (Spain)
OMEPRAZOLE
Prilosec Delayed-Release Capsules 628

ULCESTOP (Italy)
CIMETIDINE HYDROCHLORIDE
Tagamet Injection 1644
Tagamet Liquid 1644

ULCETAB (South Africa)
SUCRALFATE
Carafate Suspension 731
Carafate Tablets 730

ULCETIC (South Africa)
SUCRALFATE
Carafate Suspension 731
Carafate Tablets 730

ULCETRAX (Spain)
FAMOTIDINE
Pepcid Injection 2153
Pepcid Injection Premixed 2153
Pepcid RPD Orally Disintegrating Tablets 2150
Pepcid Tablets 2150
Pepcid for Oral Suspension 2150

ULCEX (Italy)
RANITIDINE HYDROCHLORIDE
Zantac 150 EFFERdose Granules 1690
Zantac 150 EFFERdose Tablets 1690
Zantac 150 Tablets 1690
Zantac 300 Tablets 1690
Zantac Injection 1688
Zantac Injection Premixed 1688
Zantac Syrup 1690

ULCIDINE (Canada, Switzerland)
FAMOTIDINE
Pepcid Injection 2153
Pepcid Injection Premixed 2153
Pepcid RPD Orally Disintegrating Tablets 2150
Pepcid Tablets 2150
Pepcid for Oral Suspension 2150

ULCIM (South Africa)
CIMETIDINE
Tagamet Tablets 1644

ULCIMET (Brazil, Thailand)
CIMETIDINE
Tagamet Tablets 1644

ULCIREX (France)
RANITIDINE HYDROCHLORIDE
Zantac 150 EFFERdose Granules 1690
Zantac 150 EFFERdose Tablets 1690
Zantac 150 Tablets 1690
Zantac 300 Tablets 1690
Zantac Injection 1688
Zantac Injection Premixed 1688
Zantac Syrup 1690

ULCITAG (Brazil)
CIMETIDINE
Tagamet Tablets 1644

ULCODERMA (Mexico)
COLLAGENASE
Collagenase Santyl Ointment 3248

ULCODINA (Italy)
CIMETIDINE
Tagamet Tablets 1644

ULCOFALK (Italy)
CIMETIDINE
Tagamet Tablets 1644

ULCOFAM (Thailand)
FAMOTIDINE
Pepcid Injection 2153
Pepcid Injection Premixed 2153
Pepcid RPD Orally Disintegrating Tablets 2150
Pepcid Tablets 2150
Pepcid for Oral Suspension 2150

ULCOGANT (Austria, Belgium, Germany, Switzerland, The Netherlands)
SUCRALFATE
Carafate Suspension 731
Carafate Tablets 730

ULCOL (Australia)
SULFASALAZINE
Azulfidine EN-tabs Tablets 2775

ULCOLIND H2 (Germany)
CIMETIDINE
Tagamet Tablets 1644

ULCOLIND METRO (Germany)
METRONIDAZOLE
MetroCream 1404
MetroGel 1405
MetroGel-Vaginal Gel 1986
MetroLotion 1405
Noritate Cream 1224

ULCOLIND RANI (Germany)
RANITIDINE HYDROCHLORIDE
Zantac 150 EFFERdose Granules 1690
Zantac 150 EFFERdose Tablets 1690
Zantac 150 Tablets 1690
Zantac 300 Tablets 1690
Zantac Injection 1688
Zantac Injection Premixed 1688
Zantac Syrup 1690

ULCOMEDINA (Italy)
CIMETIDINE
Tagamet Tablets 1644

ULCOMET (Italy)
CIMETIDINE HYDROCHLORIDE
Tagamet Injection 1644
Tagamet Liquid 1644

ULCOMETION (Spain)
OMEPRAZOLE
Prilosec Delayed-Release Capsules 628

ULCONA (Spain)
SUCRALFATE
Carafate Suspension 731
Carafate Tablets 730

ULCONAR (Brazil)
OMEPRAZOLE
Prilosec Delayed-Release Capsules 628

ULCOSAL (Spain)
NIZATIDINE
Axid Pulvules 1903

ULCRAST (Italy)
SUCRALFATE
Carafate Suspension 731
Carafate Tablets 730

ULCUBLOC (Germany)
CIMETIDINE
Tagamet Tablets 1644

ULCUFATO (Spain)
SUCRALFATE
Carafate Suspension 731
Carafate Tablets 730

ULCUSAN (Austria)
FAMOTIDINE
Pepcid Injection 2153
Pepcid Injection Premixed 2153
Pepcid RPD Orally Disintegrating Tablets 2150
Pepcid Tablets 2150
Pepcid for Oral Suspension 2150

ULCYTE (Australia)
SUCRALFATE
Carafate Suspension 731
Carafate Tablets 730

ULFAMET (Thailand)
FAMOTIDINE
Pepcid Injection 2153
Pepcid Injection Premixed 2153
Pepcid RPD Orally Disintegrating Tablets 2150
Pepcid Tablets 2150
Pepcid for Oral Suspension 2150

ULGARINE (Spain)
FAMOTIDINE
Pepcid Injection 2153
Pepcid Injection Premixed 2153
Pepcid RPD Orally Disintegrating Tablets 2150
Pepcid Tablets 2150
Pepcid for Oral Suspension 2150

ULGASTRIN (Brazil)
CIMETIDINE
Tagamet Tablets 1644

ULIS (Italy)
CIMETIDINE
Tagamet Tablets 1644

ULKOBRIN (Italy)
RANITIDINE HYDROCHLORIDE
Zantac 150 EFFERdose Granules 1690
Zantac 150 EFFERdose Tablets 1690
Zantac 150 Tablets 1690
Zantac 300 Tablets 1690
Zantac Injection 1688
Zantac Injection Premixed 1688
Zantac Syrup 1690

ULKUSAL (Germany)
CIMETIDINE
Tagamet Tablets 1644

ULMET (South Africa)
CIMETIDINE
Tagamet Tablets 1644

ULOGEN (Mexico)
CIMETIDINE
Tagamet Tablets 1644

ULPAX (Mexico)
LANSOPRAZOLE
Prevacid Delayed-Release Capsules 3292

ULPRAZOLE (Thailand)
OMEPRAZOLE
Prilosec Delayed-Release Capsules 628

ULSAL (Austria)
RANITIDINE HYDROCHLORIDE
Zantac 150 EFFERdose Granules 1690

Zantac 150 EFFERdose Tablets 1690
Zantac 150 Tablets 1690
Zantac 300 Tablets 1690
Zantac Injection 1688
Zantac Injection Premixed 1688
Zantac Syrup 1690

ULSANIC (Hong Kong, Israel, South Africa, Thailand)
SUCRALFATE
Carafate Suspension 731
Carafate Tablets 730

ULSAVEN (Mexico)
RANITIDINE HYDROCHLORIDE
Zantac 150 EFFERdose Granules 1690
Zantac 150 EFFERdose Tablets 1690
Zantac 150 Tablets 1690
Zantac 300 Tablets 1690
Zantac Injection 1688
Zantac Injection Premixed 1688
Zantac Syrup 1690

ULSEN (Mexico)
OMEPRAZOLE
Prilosec Delayed-Release Capsules 628

ULSERRAL (Mexico)
CIMETIDINE
Tagamet Tablets 1644

ULTEC (Hong Kong, United Kingdom)
CIMETIDINE
Tagamet Tablets 1644

ULTIDIN (Mexico)
FAMOTIDINE
Pepcid Injection 2153
Pepcid Injection Premixed 2153
Pepcid RPD Orally Disintegrating Tablets 2150
Pepcid Tablets 2150
Pepcid for Oral Suspension 2150

ULTRA (Belgium)
SULFACETAMIDE SODIUM
Bleph-10 Ophthalmic Ointment 10% .... ⊙230
Klaron Lotion 10% 1224

ULTRA CLEARASIL (United Kingdom)
BENZOYL PEROXIDE
Brevoxyl-4 Cleansing Lotion 3269
Brevoxyl-4 Creamy Wash 3270
Brevoxyl-4 Gel 3269
Brevoxyl-8 Cleansing Lotion 3269
Brevoxyl-8 Creamy Wash 3270
Brevoxyl-8 Gel 3269
Triaz Cleanser 2026
Triaz Gel 2026

ULTRA HEARTBURN RELIEF (United Kingdom)
FAMOTIDINE
Pepcid Injection 2153
Pepcid Injection Premixed 2153
Pepcid RPD Orally Disintegrating Tablets 2150
Pepcid Tablets 2150
Pepcid for Oral Suspension 2150

ULTRABETA (Portugal)
SALMETEROL XINAFOATE
Serevent Diskus 1637
Serevent Inhalation Aerosol 1633

ULTRACARE (United Kingdom)
BENZOCAINE
Americaine Anesthetic Lubricant 1162
Americaine Otic Topical Anesthetic Ear Drops 1162

ULTRACEF (Irish Republic)
CEFADROXIL
Duricef Capsules 1079
Duricef Oral Suspension 1079
Duricef Tablets 1079

ULTRA-CLEAR-A-MED (Austria)
BENZOYL PEROXIDE
Brevoxyl-4 Cleansing Lotion 3269
Brevoxyl-4 Creamy Wash 3270
Brevoxyl-4 Gel 3269
Brevoxyl-8 Cleansing Lotion 3269
Brevoxyl-8 Creamy Wash 3270
Brevoxyl-8 Gel 3269
Triaz Cleanser 2026
Triaz Gel 2026

ULTRACORTEN (Germany)
PREDNISONE
Prednisone Intensol 3064
Prednisone Oral Solution 3064
Prednisone Tablets 3064

ULTRADERM (Italy)
FLUOCINOLONE ACETONIDE
Synalar Cream 2020
Synalar Ointment 2020
Synalar Topical Solution 2020

ULTRADOL (Canada)
ETODOLAC
Lodine Capsules 3528
Lodine Tablets 3528
Lodine XL Extended-Release Tablets 3530

ULTRALEXIN (Spain)
CEPHALEXIN
Keflex Oral Suspension 1237
Keflex Pulvules 1237

ULTRAMICINA (Spain)
CIPROFLOXACIN HYDROCHLORIDE
Ciloxan Ophthalmic Ointment 538
Ciloxan Ophthalmic Solution .... ⊙209, 538
Cipro Tablets 887

ULTRAMOP (Canada)
METHOXSALEN
8-MOP Capsules 1727
Oxsoralen Lotion 1% 1740
Oxsoralen-Ultra Capsules 1741

ULTRAQUIN PLAIN (Canada)
HYDROQUINONE
Eldopaque Forte 4% Cream 1734
Eldoquin Forte 4% Cream 1734
Lustra Cream 2023
Lustra-AF Cream 2023
Melanex Topical Solution 2300
Solaquin Forte 4% Cream 1734
Solaquin Forte 4% Gel 1734

ULTRASE (Canada)
PANCRELIPASE
Ultrase Capsules 835
Ultrase MT Capsules 835

ULTROXIM (Italy)
CEFUROXIME SODIUM
Kefurox Vials, ADD-Vantage 1948
Zinacef Injection 1696

ULXIT (Austria)
NIZATIDINE
Axid Pulvules 1903

UMAN-SERUM (Italy)
PLASMA PROTEIN FRACTION
Plasmanate 942

UMBRIUM (Austria)
DIAZEPAM
Valium Injectable 3026
Valium Tablets 3047

UMINE (New Zealand, Singapore)
PHENTERMINE HYDROCHLORIDE
Adipex-P Capsules 1406
Adipex-P Tablets 1406

UNACID (Germany)
AMPICILLIN SODIUM/SULBACTAM SODIUM
Unasyn for Injection 2728

UNACIL (Italy)
DOXYCYCLINE HYCLATE
Doryx Coated Pellet Filled Capsules 3357
Periostat Tablets 1208
Vibramycin Hyclate Capsules 2735
Vibramycin Hyclate Intravenous 2737
Vibra-Tabs Film Coated Tablets 2735

UNACIM (France)
AMPICILLIN SODIUM/SULBACTAM SODIUM
Unasyn for Injection 2728

UNASYN (Austria, Hong Kong, Italy, Singapore, Spain, Thailand)
AMPICILLIN SODIUM/SULBACTAM SODIUM
Unasyn for Injection 2728

UNASYNA (Mexico)
AMPICILLIN SODIUM/SULBACTAM SODIUM
Unasyn for Injection 2728

UNGVITA (New Zealand)
VITAMIN A PALMITATE
Aquasol A Parenteral 593

UNI MASDIL (Spain)
DILTIAZEM HYDROCHLORIDE
Cardizem CD Capsules 1016
Cardizem Injectable 1018
Cardizem Lyo-Ject Syringe 1018
Cardizem Monovial 1018
Tiazac Capsules 1378

UNI MIST (Spain)
MORPHINE SULFATE
Astramorph/PF Injection, USP (Preservative-Free) 594
Duramorph Injection 1312
Infumorph 200 and Infumorph 500 Sterile Solutions 1314
Kadian Capsules 1335
MS Contin Tablets 2896
MSIR Oral Capsules 2898
MSIR Oral Solution 2898
MSIR Oral Solution Concentrate 2898
MSIR Oral Tablets 2898
Oramorph SR Tablets 3062
Roxanol 100 Concentrated Oral Solution 3066
Roxanol Concentrated Oral Solution 3066
Roxanol-T Oral Solution 3066

UNIBAC (Belgium)
DIRITHROMYCIN
Dynabac Tablets 2269

UNIBLOC (Germany, The Netherlands)
ATENOLOL
Tenormin I.V. Injection 692

UNICLOR (Mexico)
CHLORAMPHENICOL
Chloromycetin Ophthalmic Ointment, 1% .... ⊙296
Chloromycetin Ophthalmic Solution .... ⊙297
Chloroptic Sterile Ophthalmic Ointment .... ⊙234
Chloroptic Sterile Ophthalmic Solution .... ⊙235

UNI-COLEX (Hong Kong)
GUAIFENESIN
Organidin NR Liquid 3350
Organidin NR Tablets 3350

UNICONTIN (Portugal)
THEOPHYLLINE
Aerolate Jr. T.D. Capsules 1361
Aerolate Liquid 1361
Aerolate Sr. T.D. Capsules 1361
Theo-Dur Extended-Release Tablets 1835
Uni-Dur Extended-Release Tablets 1841
Uniphyl 400 mg and 600 mg Tablets 2903

UNICORDIUM (France)
BEPRIDIL HYDROCHLORIDE
Vascor Tablets 2602

UNICORT (Canada)
HYDROCORTISONE
Anusol-HC Cream 2.5% 2237
Hydrocortone Tablets 2106

UNIDERM (Singapore)
CLOBETASOL PROPIONATE
Cormax Cream 2440
Cormax Ointment 2440
Cormax Scalp Application 2441
Temovate Cream 1301
Temovate E Emollient 1302
Temovate Gel 1303
Temovate Ointment 1301
Temovate Scalp Application 1304

UNIDERM (Denmark, Finland, Sweden)
HYDROCORTISONE
Anusol-HC Cream 2.5% 2237
Hydrocortone Tablets 2106

UNIDIPIN (Austria)
NIFEDIPINE
Adalat CC Tablets 877
Procardia Capsules 2708
Procardia XL Extended Release Tablets 2710

UNIDIPINE (Switzerland)
NIFEDIPINE
Adalat CC Tablets 877
Procardia Capsules 2708
Procardia XL Extended Release Tablets 2710

UNIDOXI (Spain)
DOXYCYCLINE HYCLATE
Doryx Coated Pellet Filled Capsules 3357
Periostat Tablets 1208
Vibramycin Hyclate Capsules 2735
Vibramycin Hyclate Intravenous 2737
Vibra-Tabs Film Coated Tablets 2735

UNI-DUR (Italy, Mexico, South Africa)
THEOPHYLLINE
Aerolate Jr. T.D. Capsules 1361
Aerolate Liquid 1361
Aerolate Sr. T.D. Capsules 1361
Theo-Dur Extended-Release Tablets 1835
Uni-Dur Extended-Release Tablets 1841
Uniphyl 400 mg and 600 mg Tablets 2903

UNIF (Thailand)
TRIAMCINOLONE ACETONIDE
Azmacort Inhalation Aerosol 728
Nasacort AQ Nasal Spray 752
Nasacort Nasal Inhaler 750

UNIFLOX (France)
CIPROFLOXACIN HYDROCHLORIDE
Ciloxan Ophthalmic Ointment 538
Ciloxan Ophthalmic Solution .... ⊙209, 538
Cipro Tablets 887

UNIFYL (Austria, Switzerland)
THEOPHYLLINE
Aerolate Jr. T.D. Capsules 1361
Aerolate Liquid 1361
Aerolate Sr. T.D. Capsules 1361
Theo-Dur Extended-Release Tablets 1835
Uni-Dur Extended-Release Tablets 1841
Uniphyl 400 mg and 600 mg Tablets 2903

UNIGET (Germany)
TIMOLOL MALEATE
Blocadren Tablets 2046
Timoptic Sterile Ophthalmic Solution 2190
Timoptic in Ocudose 2192
Timoptic-XE Sterile Ophthalmic Gel Forming Solution 2194

UNIHEP (Irish Republic, United Kingdom)
HEPARIN SODIUM
Heparin Lock Flush Solution 3509
Heparin Sodium Injection 3511

UNIKET (Spain)
ISOSORBIDE MONONITRATE
Imdur Tablets 1826
Ismo Tablets 3524

UNILAIR (Germany)
THEOPHYLLINE
Aerolate Jr. T.D. Capsules 1361
Aerolate Liquid 1361
Aerolate Sr. T.D. Capsules 1361
Theo-Dur Extended-Release Tablets 1835
Uni-Dur Extended-Release Tablets 1841
Uniphyl 400 mg and 600 mg Tablets 2903

UNILAN (Portugal)
ALPRAZOLAM
Xanax Tablets 2865

UNILOC (Denmark, Finland, Norway, Sweden)
ATENOLOL
Tenormin I.V. Injection 692

UNILONG (Spain)
THEOPHYLLINE
Aerolate Jr. T.D. Capsules 1361
Aerolate Liquid 1361
Aerolate Sr. T.D. Capsules 1361
Theo-Dur Extended-Release Tablets 1835
Uni-Dur Extended-Release Tablets 1841
Uniphyl 400 mg and 600 mg Tablets 2903

UNIMAX (Finland, Switzerland)
FELODIPINE
Plendil Extended-Release Tablets 623

UNIMEST (Spain)
FELODIPINE
Plendil Extended-Release Tablets 623

UNIMEZOL (Thailand)
METRONIDAZOLE
MetroCream 1404
MetroGel 1405
MetroGel-Vaginal Gel 1986
MetroLotion 1405
Noritate Cream 1224

UNIMOX (South Africa)
AMOXICILLIN
Amoxil Pediatric Drops for Oral Suspension 1471
Amoxil Tablets 1471

UNIPARIN (Australia, Irish Republic)
HEPARIN SODIUM
Heparin Lock Flush Solution 3509
Heparin Sodium Injection 3511

UNIPHYL (Canada, Hong Kong, South Africa)
THEOPHYLLINE
Aerolate Jr. T.D. Capsules 1361
Aerolate Liquid 1361
Aerolate Sr. T.D. Capsules 1361
Theo-Dur Extended-Release Tablets 1835
Uni-Dur Extended-Release Tablets 1841
Uniphyl 400 mg and 600 mg Tablets 2903

UNIPHYLLIN CONTINUS (Irish Republic, United Kingdom)
THEOPHYLLINE
Aerolate Jr. T.D. Capsules 1361
Aerolate Liquid 1361
Aerolate Sr. T.D. Capsules 1361
Theo-Dur Extended-Release Tablets 1835
Uni-Dur Extended-Release Tablets 1841
Uniphyl 400 mg and 600 mg Tablets 2903

UNIPINE XL (United Kingdom)
NIFEDIPINE
Adalat CC Tablets 877
Procardia Capsules 2708
Procardia XL Extended Release Tablets 2710

UNIPRIL (Italy)
RAMIPRIL
Altace Capsules 2233

UNIREN (Thailand)
DICLOFENAC SODIUM
Voltaren Tablets 2315
Voltaren-XR Tablets 2315

UNISAL (Switzerland)
DIFLUNISAL
Dolobid Tablets 2088

UNISEDIL (Portugal)
DIAZEPAM
Valium Injectable 3026
Valium Tablets 3047

UNISOM (Australia, Canada)
DIPHENHYDRAMINE HYDROCHLORIDE
Benadryl Parenteral . . . 2617

UNISOM-C (Canada)
DIPHENHYDRAMINE HYDROCHLORIDE
Benadryl Parenteral . . . 2617

UNISON OINTMENT (Thailand)
CHLORAMPHENICOL
Chloromycetin Ophthalmic Ointment, 1% . . . ⊙296
Chloromycetin Ophthalmic Solution . . . ⊙297
Chloroptic Sterile Ophthalmic Ointment . . ⊙234
Chloroptic Sterile Ophthalmic Solution . . ⊙235

UNITIMBRE PASTEUR S (France)
TUBERCULIN
Aplisol Injection . . . 2609
Tine Test, Tuberculin, Old . . . 3631
Tubersol Diagnostic Antigen . . . 3628

UNITIMOFTOL (Spain)
TIMOLOL MALEATE
Blocadren Tablets . . . 2046
Timoptic Sterile Ophthalmic Solution . . . 2190
Timoptic in Ocudose . . . 2192
Timoptic-XE Sterile Ophthalmic Gel Forming Solution . . . 2194

UNIVATE (Singapore)
CLOBETASOL PROPIONATE
Cormax Cream . . . 2440
Cormax Ointment . . . 2440
Cormax Scalp Application . . . 2441
Temovate Cream . . . 1301
Temovate E Emollient . . . 1302
Temovate Gel . . . 1303
Temovate Ointment . . . 1301
Temovate Scalp Application . . . 1304

UNIVER (Spain, United Kingdom)
VERAPAMIL HYDROCHLORIDE
Covera-HS Tablets . . . 3199
Isoptin SR Tablets . . . 467
Verelan Capsules . . . 3184
Verelan PM Capsules . . . 3186

UNIXAN (Denmark)
THEOPHYLLINE
Aerolate Jr. T.D. Capsules . . . 1361
Aerolate Liquid . . . 1361
Aerolate Sr. T.D. Capsules . . . 1361
Theo-Dur Extended-Release Tablets . . . 1835
Uni-Dur Extended-Release Tablets . . . 1841
Uniphyl 400 mg and 600 mg Tablets . . . 2903

UNIXIME (Italy)
CEFIXIME
Suprax Tablets . . . 1877
Suprax for Oral Suspension . . . 1877

UNOCARDIL (Denmark)
DILTIAZEM HYDROCHLORIDE
Cardizem CD Capsules . . . 1016
Cardizem Injectable . . . 1018
Cardizem Lyo-Ject Syringe . . . 1018
Cardizem Monovial . . . 1018
Tiazac Capsules . . . 1378

UNOPROST (Italy)
TERAZOSIN HYDROCHLORIDE
Hytrin Capsules . . . 464

UP MEP (Brazil)
CIMETIDINE
Tagamet Tablets . . . 1644

UPFEN (France)
IBUPROFEN
Motrin Suspension, Oral Drops, Chewable Tablets, and Caplets . . . 2002

U-PROXYN (Thailand)
NAPROXEN
EC-Naprosyn Delayed-Release Tablets . . . 2967
Naprosyn Suspension . . . 2967
Naprosyn Tablets . . . 2967

URACTAZIDE (Belgium)
HYDROCHLOROTHIAZIDE
HydroDIURIL Tablets . . . 2108
Microzide Capsules . . . 3414

URAMOX (Israel)
ACETAZOLAMIDE
Diamox Sequels Sustained Release Capsules . . . ⊙270
Diamox Tablets . . . ⊙269

URBAL (Spain)
SUCRALFATE
Carafate Suspension . . . 731
Carafate Tablets . . . 730

URBILAT (Germany)
MEPROBAMATE
Miltown Tablets . . . 3349

URECHOLINE (Australia, Canada, Israel, Italy, South Africa, Thailand)
BETHANECHOL CHLORIDE
Urecholine Injection . . . 2198
Urecholine Tablets . . . 2198

URECORTYN (Italy)
HYDROCORTISONE ACETATE
Anusol-HC Suppositories . . . 2238
Cortifoam Rectal Foam . . . 3170
Hydrocortone Acetate Injectable Suspension . . . 2103
Proctocort Suppositories . . . 2264

UREM (Austria)
IBUPROFEN
Motrin Suspension, Oral Drops, Chewable Tablets, and Caplets . . . 2002

URIFRON (Mexico)
INTERFERON ALFA-2B
Intron A for Injection . . . 3120

URINOX (Thailand)
NORFLOXACIN
Chibroxin Sterile Ophthalmic Solution . . . ⊙273, 2051
Noroxin Tablets . . . 2145

URITRAT NF (Brazil)
NORFLOXACIN
Chibroxin Sterile Ophthalmic Solution . . . ⊙273, 2051
Noroxin Tablets . . . 2145

URIZIDE (South Africa)
HYDROCHLOROTHIAZIDE/TRIAMTERENE
Dyazide Capsules . . . 1515
Maxzide Tablets . . . 1008
Maxzide-25 mg Tablets . . . 1008

UROBACID (Austria, Singapore)
NORFLOXACIN
Chibroxin Sterile Ophthalmic Solution . . . ⊙273, 2051
Noroxin Tablets . . . 2145

UROBACTAM (Spain)
AZTREONAM
Azactam for Injection . . . 1276

UROCARB (Australia)
BETHANECHOL CHLORIDE
Urecholine Injection . . . 2198
Urecholine Tablets . . . 2198

UROCAUDAL (Spain)
TRIAMTERENE
Dyrenium Capsules . . . 3458

UROCAUDAL TIAZIDA (Spain)
HYDROCHLOROTHIAZIDE/TRIAMTERENE
Dyazide Capsules . . . 1515
Maxzide Tablets . . . 1008
Maxzide-25 mg Tablets . . . 1008

URO-CEPHORAL (Germany)
CEFIXIME
Suprax Tablets . . . 1877
Suprax for Oral Suspension . . . 1877

UROCIT-K (Australia, Singapore)
POTASSIUM CITRATE
Urocit-K Tablets . . . 2232

UROCTAL (Spain)
NORFLOXACIN
Chibroxin Sterile Ophthalmic Solution . . . ⊙273, 2051
Noroxin Tablets . . . 2145

URODIE (Italy)
TERAZOSIN HYDROCHLORIDE
Hytrin Capsules . . . 464

UROFLO (Austria)
TERAZOSIN HYDROCHLORIDE
Hytrin Capsules . . . 464

UROFLOX (Brazil, Portugal)
NORFLOXACIN
Chibroxin Sterile Ophthalmic Solution . . . ⊙273, 2051
Noroxin Tablets . . . 2145

UROLOSIN (Spain)
TAMSULOSIN HYDROCHLORIDE
Flomax Capsules . . . 1044

UROMETRON (South Africa)
METRONIDAZOLE
MetroCream . . . 1404
MetroGel . . . 1405
MetroGel-Vaginal Gel . . . 1986
MetroLotion . . . 1405
Noritate Cream . . . 1224

UROMYKOL (Germany)
CLOTRIMAZOLE
Lotrimin Cream 1% . . . 3128
Lotrimin Lotion 1% . . . 3128
Lotrimin Topical Solution 1% . . . 3128
Mycelex Troche . . . 573

UROPLEX (Brazil)
NORFLOXACIN
Chibroxin Sterile Ophthalmic Solution . . . ⊙273, 2051
Noroxin Tablets . . . 2145

URO-TARIVID (Germany)
OFLOXACIN
Floxin I.V. . . . 2526
Floxin Otic Solution . . . 1219
Floxin Tablets . . . 2529
Ocuflox Ophthalmic Solution . . . 554

UROTROL (Spain)
TOLTERODINE TARTRATE
Detrol Tablets . . . 3623

UROXIN (Singapore, Thailand, United Arab Emirates)
CIPROFLOXACIN HYDROCHLORIDE
Ciloxan Ophthalmic Ointment . . . 538
Ciloxan Ophthalmic Solution . . . ⊙209, 538
Cipro Tablets . . . 887

URPROSAN (Spain)
FINASTERIDE
Propecia Tablets . . . 2172
Proscar Tablets . . . 2175

UTIN (South Africa)
NORFLOXACIN
Chibroxin Sterile Ophthalmic Solution . . . ⊙273, 2051
Noroxin Tablets . . . 2145

UTINOR (Italy, United Kingdom)
NORFLOXACIN
Chibroxin Sterile Ophthalmic Solution . . . ⊙273, 2051
Noroxin Tablets . . . 2145

UTROGESTAN (Austria, Belgium, France, Hong Kong, Irish Republic, Israel, Portugal, Singapore, South Africa, Spain, Switzerland, Thailand)
PROGESTERONE
Crinone 4% Gel . . . 3213
Crinone 8% Gel . . . 3213
Prometrium Capsules (100 mg, 200 mg) . . . 3261

V DAY ZEPAM (Thailand)
DIAZEPAM
Valium Injectable . . . 3026
Valium Tablets . . . 3047

VACANYL (Thailand)
TERBUTALINE SULFATE
Brethine Ampuls . . . 2314
Brethine Tablets . . . 2313

VACINOLONE (Thailand)
TRIAMCINOLONE ACETONIDE
Azmacort Inhalation Aerosol . . . 728
Nasacort AQ Nasal Spray . . . 752
Nasacort Nasal Inhaler . . . 750

VADINAR (Mexico)
DIPYRIDAMOLE
Persantine Tablets . . . 1057

VAGAKA (Thailand)
MEBENDAZOLE
Vermox Chewable Tablets . . . 2017

VAGIFEM (Australia, Austria, Belgium, Denmark, Finland, Germany, Irish Republic, Israel, Italy, New Zealand, Portugal, Singapore, South Africa, Spain, Sweden, Switzerland, Thailand, The Netherlands, United Kingdom)
ESTRADIOL
Alora Transdermal System . . . 3372
Climara Transdermal System . . . 950
Estrace Vaginal Cream . . . 3358
Estring Vaginal Ring . . . 2811
Vivelle Transdermal System . . . 2412
Vivelle-Dot Transdermal System . . . 2416

VAGIL (Thailand)
METRONIDAZOLE
MetroCream . . . 1404
MetroGel . . . 1405
MetroGel-Vaginal Gel . . . 1986
MetroLotion . . . 1405
Noritate Cream . . . 1224

VAGILEN (Italy)
METRONIDAZOLE
MetroCream . . . 1404
MetroGel . . . 1405
MetroGel-Vaginal Gel . . . 1986
MetroLotion . . . 1405
Noritate Cream . . . 1224

VAGIMAX (Brazil)
METRONIDAZOLE
MetroCream . . . 1404
MetroGel . . . 1405
MetroGel-Vaginal Gel . . . 1986
MetroLotion . . . 1405
Noritate Cream . . . 1224

VAGIMID (Germany)
METRONIDAZOLE
MetroCream . . . 1404
MetroGel . . . 1405
MetroGel-Vaginal Gel . . . 1986
MetroLotion . . . 1405
Noritate Cream . . . 1224

VAGINYL (United Kingdom)
METRONIDAZOLE
MetroCream . . . 1404
MetroGel . . . 1405
MetroGel-Vaginal Gel . . . 1986
MetroLotion . . . 1405
Noritate Cream . . . 1224

VAGISIL (Canada, Israel)
BENZOCAINE
Americaine Anesthetic Lubricant . . . 1162
Americaine Otic Topical Anesthetic Ear Drops . . . 1162

VAGMICOR (Mexico)
KETOCONAZOLE
Nizoral 2% Cream . . . 3620
Nizoral 2% Shampoo . . . 2007
Nizoral Tablets . . . 1791

VAGOLISAL (Italy)
CIMETIDINE
Tagamet Tablets . . . 1644

VAGOSTAL (Spain)
FAMOTIDINE
Pepcid Injection . . . 2153
Pepcid Injection Premixed . . . 2153
Pepcid RPD Orally Disintegrating Tablets . . . 2150
Pepcid Tablets . . . 2150
Pepcid for Oral Suspension . . . 2150

VAGYL (Thailand)
METRONIDAZOLE
MetroCream . . . 1404
MetroGel . . . 1405
MetroGel-Vaginal Gel . . . 1986
MetroLotion . . . 1405
Noritate Cream . . . 1224

VALAXONA (Denmark, Germany)
DIAZEPAM
Valium Injectable . . . 3026
Valium Tablets . . . 3047

VALCAPS (Mexico)
VALPROIC ACID
Depakene Capsules . . . 421
Depakene Syrup . . . 421

VALCLAIR (United Kingdom)
DIAZEPAM
Valium Injectable . . . 3026
Valium Tablets . . . 3047

VALDERMA ACTIVE (United Kingdom)
BENZOYL PEROXIDE
Brevoxyl-4 Cleansing Lotion . . . 3269
Brevoxyl-4 Creamy Wash . . . 3270
Brevoxyl-4 Gel . . . 3269
Brevoxyl-8 Cleansing Lotion . . . 3269
Brevoxyl-8 Creamy Wash . . . 3270
Brevoxyl-8 Gel . . . 3269
Triaz Cleanser . . . 2026
Triaz Gel . . . 2026

VALEANS (Italy)
ALPRAZOLAM
Xanax Tablets . . . 2865

VALENAC (United Kingdom)
DICLOFENAC SODIUM
Voltaren Tablets . . . 2315
Voltaren-XR Tablets . . . 2315

VALENIUM (Thailand)
DIAZEPAM
Valium Injectable . . . 3026
Valium Tablets . . . 3047

VALESPORIN (Spain)
CEPHALEXIN
Keflex Oral Suspension . . . 1237
Keflex Pulvules . . . 1237

VALIQUID (Germany)
DIAZEPAM
Valium Injectable . . . 3026
Valium Tablets . . . 3047

VALITRAN (Italy)
DIAZEPAM
Valium Injectable . . . 3026
Valium Tablets . . . 3047

VALIUM (Australia, Austria, Belgium, Brazil, Canada, Denmark, France, Germany, Irish Republic, Israel, Italy, Mexico, Norway, Portugal, Singapore, South Africa, Spain, Sweden, Switzerland, Thailand, The Netherlands, United Kingdom)
DIAZEPAM
Valium Injectable . . . 3026
Valium Tablets . . . 3047

VALKEN (Mexico)
VALPROIC ACID
Depakene Capsules . . . 421
Depakene Syrup . . . 421

VALMAGEN (Italy)
CIMETIDINE
Tagamet Tablets . . . 1644

VALOCORDIN-DIAZEPAM (Germany)
DIAZEPAM
Valium Injectable . . . 3026
Valium Tablets . . . 3047

VALORAN (Hong Kong, Thailand)
CEFOTAXIME SODIUM
Claforan Injection . . . 732

VALPRESSION (Italy)
VALSARTAN
Diovan Capsules . . . 2337

VALROX (United Kingdom)
NAPROXEN
EC-Naprosyn Delayed-Release Tablets . . . 2967
Naprosyn Suspension . . . 2967
Naprosyn Tablets . . . 2967

VALS (Spain)
VALSARTAN
Diovan Capsules . . . 2337

VAMAZOLE (Thailand)
CLOTRIMAZOLE
Lotrimin Cream 1% . . . 3128
Lotrimin Lotion 1% . . . 3128
Lotrimin Topical Solution 1% . . . 3128
Mycelex Troche . . . 573

VANAFEN (Thailand)
CHLORAMPHENICOL
Chloromycetin Ophthalmic Ointment, 1% . . . ⊙296
Chloromycetin Ophthalmic Solution . . . ⊙297
Chloroptic Sterile Ophthalmic Ointment . . ⊙234
Chloroptic Sterile Ophthalmic Solution . . ⊙235

VANAFEN-S (Hong Kong, Singapore)
CHLORAMPHENICOL
Chloromycetin Ophthalmic Ointment, 1% . . . ⊙296
Chloromycetin Ophthalmic Solution . . . ⊙297
Chloroptic Sterile Ophthalmic Ointment . . ⊙234
Chloroptic Sterile Ophthalmic Solution . . ⊙235

VANCOCIN (Australia, Belgium, Canada, Denmark, Finland, Hong Kong, Irish Republic, Israel, Mexico, New Zealand, Norway, South Africa, Sweden, Switzerland, Thailand, The Netherlands, United Kingdom)
VANCOMYCIN HYDROCHLORIDE
Vancocin HCl Capsules & Pulvules . . . 1972
Vancocin HCl Oral Solution . . . 1971
Vancocin HCl, Vials & ADD-Vantage . . . 1970

VANCOCINA (Brazil, Italy, Portugal)
VANCOMYCIN HYDROCHLORIDE
Vancocin HCl Capsules & Pulvules . . . 1972
Vancocin HCl Oral Solution . . . 1971
Vancocin HCl, Vials & ADD-Vantage . . . 1970

VANCOCINE (France)
VANCOMYCIN HYDROCHLORIDE
Vancocin HCl Capsules & Pulvules . . . 1972
Vancocin HCl Oral Solution . . . 1971
Vancocin HCl, Vials & ADD-Vantage . . . 1970

VANCOLED (Australia, Israel, Sweden, Switzerland)
VANCOMYCIN HYDROCHLORIDE
Vancocin HCl Capsules & Pulvules . . . 1972
Vancocin HCl Oral Solution . . . 1971
Vancocin HCl, Vials & ADD-Vantage . . . 1970

VANCOLIN (United Arab Emirates)
VANCOMYCIN HYDROCHLORIDE
Vancocin HCl Capsules & Pulvules . . . 1972
Vancocin HCl Oral Solution . . . 1971
Vancocin HCl, Vials & ADD-Vantage . . . 1970

VANCO-SAAR (Germany)
VANCOMYCIN HYDROCHLORIDE
Vancocin HCl Capsules & Pulvules . . . 1972
Vancocin HCl Oral Solution . . . 1971
Vancocin HCl, Vials & ADD-Vantage . . . 1970

VANCOSCAND (Sweden)
VANCOMYCIN HYDROCHLORIDE
Vancocin HCl Capsules & Pulvules . . . 1972
Vancocin HCl Oral Solution . . . 1971
Vancocin HCl, Vials & ADD-Vantage . . . 1970

VANCO-TEVA (Hong Kong, Israel)
VANCOMYCIN HYDROCHLORIDE
Vancocin HCl Capsules & Pulvules . . . 1972
Vancocin HCl Oral Solution . . . 1971
Vancocin HCl, Vials & ADD-Vantage . . . 1970

VANDRAL (Spain)
VENLAFAXINE HYDROCHLORIDE
Effexor Tablets . . . 3495
Effexor XR Capsules . . . 3499

VANESTEN (Thailand)
CLOTRIMAZOLE
Lotrimin Cream 1% . . . 3128
Lotrimin Lotion 1% . . . 3128
Lotrimin Topical Solution 1% . . . 3128
Mycelex Troche . . . 573

VANMICINA (Mexico)
VANCOMYCIN HYDROCHLORIDE
Vancocin HCl Capsules & Pulvules . . . 1972
Vancocin HCl Oral Solution . . . 1971
Vancocin HCl, Vials & ADD-Vantage . . . 1970

VANZOR (Mexico)
DIAZEPAM
Valium Injectable . . . 3026
Valium Tablets . . . 3047

VARFINE (Portugal)
WARFARIN SODIUM
Coumadin Tablets . . . 1243
Coumadin for Injection . . . 1243

VARIDASA (Mexico, Portugal, Spain)
STREPTOKINASE
Streptase for Infusion . . . 647

VARIDASE (Belgium, Denmark, Finland, Irish Republic, Israel, New Zealand)
STREPTOKINASE
Streptase for Infusion . . . 647

VARILISIN (Belgium)
COLLAGENASE
Collagenase Santyl Ointment . . . 3248

VASAD (United Kingdom)
NIFEDIPINE
Adalat CC Tablets . . . 877
Procardia Capsules . . . 2708
Procardia XL Extended Release Tablets . . 2710

VASATEN (United Kingdom)
ATENOLOL
Tenormin I.V. Injection . . . 692

VASCAL (Germany)
ISRADIPINE
DynaCirc CR Tablets . . . 2923

VASCARD (South Africa)
NIFEDIPINE
Adalat CC Tablets . . . 877
Procardia Capsules . . . 2708
Procardia XL Extended Release Tablets . . 2710

VASCARDIN (Irish Republic, United Kingdom)
ISOSORBIDE DINITRATE
Isordil Sublingual Tablets . . . 3525
Isordil Titradose Tablets . . . 3526

VASCOTEN (Hong Kong, Singapore, Thailand)
ATENOLOL
Tenormin I.V. Injection . . . 692

VASDALAT (Singapore)
NIFEDIPINE
Adalat CC Tablets . . . 877
Procardia Capsules . . . 2708
Procardia XL Extended Release Tablets . . 2710

VASDILAT (Italy)
ISOSORBIDE MONONITRATE
Imdur Tablets . . . 1826
Ismo Tablets . . . 3524

VASERETIC (Canada)
ENALAPRIL MALEATE/HYDROCHLOROTHIAZIDE
Vaseretic Tablets . . . 2204

VASETIC (United Kingdom)
AMILORIDE HYDROCHLORIDE/HYDROCHLOROTHIAZIDE
Moduretic Tablets . . . 2138

VASIL (Thailand)
METOCLOPRAMIDE HYDROCHLORIDE
Reglan Injectable . . . 2935
Reglan Syrup . . . 2935
Reglan Tablets . . . 2935

VASLAN (Spain)
ISRADIPINE
DynaCirc CR Tablets . . . 2923

VASLIP (Spain)
CERIVASTATIN SODIUM
Baycol Tablets . . . 883

VASOCARDOL (Australia)
DILTIAZEM HYDROCHLORIDE
Cardizem CD Capsules . . . 1016
Cardizem Injectable . . . 1018
Cardizem Lyo-Ject Syringe . . . 1018
Cardizem Monovial . . . 1018
Tiazac Capsules . . . 1378

VASOCON (Canada)
NAPHAZOLINE HYDROCHLORIDE
Albalon Ophthalmic Solution . . . ⊙225

VASOCONSTRICTOR PENSA (Spain)
NAPHAZOLINE HYDROCHLORIDE
Albalon Ophthalmic Solution . . . ⊙225

VASODIN (Italy)
NICARDIPINE HYDROCHLORIDE
Cardene I.V. . . . 3485

VASOFED (Irish Republic, South Africa)
NIFEDIPINE
Adalat CC Tablets . . . 877
Procardia Capsules . . . 2708
Procardia XL Extended Release Tablets . . 2710

VASOLAN (Japan)
VERAPAMIL HYDROCHLORIDE
Covera-HS Tablets . . . 3199
Isoptin SR Tablets . . . 467
Verelan Capsules . . . 3184
Verelan PM Capsules . . . 3186

VASOMIL (South Africa)
VERAPAMIL HYDROCHLORIDE
Covera-HS Tablets . . . 3199
Isoptin SR Tablets . . . 467
Verelan Capsules . . . 3184
Verelan PM Capsules . . . 3186

VASONASE (Spain)
NICARDIPINE HYDROCHLORIDE
Cardene I.V. . . . 3485

VASONORM (Italy)
NICARDIPINE HYDROCHLORIDE
Cardene I.V. . . . 3485

VASOPRIL (Israel)
FOSINOPRIL SODIUM
Monopril Tablets . . . 1091

VASOPTEN (Thailand)
VERAPAMIL HYDROCHLORIDE
Covera-HS Tablets . . . 3199
Isoptin SR Tablets . . . 467
Verelan Capsules . . . 3184
Verelan PM Capsules . . . 3186

VASORBATE (Austria)
ISOSORBIDE DINITRATE
Isordil Sublingual Tablets . . . 3525
Isordil Titradose Tablets . . . 3526

VASORETIC (Italy)
ENALAPRIL MALEATE/HYDROCHLOROTHIAZIDE
Vaseretic Tablets . . . 2204

VASTEN (France)
PRAVASTATIN SODIUM
Pravachol Tablets . . . 1099

VASTIN (Australia, New Zealand)
FLUVASTATIN SODIUM
Lescol Capsules . . . 2361

VASYROL (United Kingdom)
DIPYRIDAMOLE
Persantine Tablets . . . 1057

VATRAN (Italy)
DIAZEPAM
Valium Injectable . . . 3026
Valium Tablets . . . 3047

VATRASIN (Spain)
NICARDIPINE HYDROCHLORIDE
Cardene I.V. . . . 3485

VATREM (Mexico)
PIROXICAM
Feldene Capsules . . . 2685

VATRIX-S (Mexico)
METRONIDAZOLE
MetroCream . . . 1404
MetroGel . . . 1405
MetroGel-Vaginal Gel . . . 1986
MetroLotion . . . 1405
Noritate Cream . . . 1224

VECLAM (Italy)
CLARITHROMYCIN
Biaxin Filmtab Tablets . . . 403
Biaxin for Oral Suspension . . . 403

VEENAC (Thailand)
DICLOFENAC SODIUM
Voltaren Tablets . . . 2315
Voltaren-XR Tablets . . . 2315

VELODAN (Spain)
LORATADINE
Claritin Reditabs . . . 3100
Claritin Syrup . . . 3100
Claritin Tablets . . . 3100

VELOPURAL (Germany)
HYDROCORTISONE ACETATE
Anusol-HC Suppositories . . . 2238
Cortifoam Rectal Foam . . . 3170
Hydrocortone Acetate Injectable Suspension . . . 2103
Proctocort Suppositories . . . 2264

VELORIN (Hong Kong, Singapore, Thailand)
ATENOLOL
Tenormin I.V. Injection . . . 692

VELSAY (Mexico)
NAPROXEN
EC-Naprosyn Delayed-Release Tablets . . . 2967
Naprosyn Suspension . . . 2967
Naprosyn Tablets . . . 2967

VELTEX (South Africa)
DICLOFENAC SODIUM
Voltaren Tablets . . . 2315
Voltaren-XR Tablets . . . 2315

VENACHLOR (South Africa)
ATENOLOL
Tenormin I.V. Injection . . . 692

VENALITAN (Germany)
HEPARIN SODIUM
Heparin Lock Flush Solution . . . 3509
Heparin Sodium Injection . . . 3511

VENAPULSE (South Africa)
ATENOLOL
Tenormin I.V. Injection . . . 692

VENELBIN N (Germany)
HEPARIN SODIUM
Heparin Lock Flush Solution . . . 3509
Heparin Sodium Injection . . . 3511

VENOFLEXIL (Germany)
HEPARIN SODIUM
Heparin Lock Flush Solution . . . 3509
Heparin Sodium Injection . . . 3511

VENOGYL (Israel)
METRONIDAZOLE
MetroCream . . . 1404
MetroGel . . . 1405
MetroGel-Vaginal Gel . . . 1986
MetroLotion . . . 1405
Noritate Cream . . . 1224

VENORUTON EMULGEL (Germany)
HEPARIN SODIUM
Heparin Lock Flush Solution . . . 3509
Heparin Sodium Injection . . . 3511

VENT RETARD (Spain)
THEOPHYLLINE
Aerolate Jr. T.D. Capsules . . . 1361
Aerolate Liquid . . . 1361
Aerolate Sr. T.D. Capsules . . . 1361
Theo-Dur Extended-Release Tablets . . . 1835
Uni-Dur Extended-Release Tablets . . . 1841
Uniphyl 400 mg and 600 mg Tablets . . . 2903

VERABETA (Germany)
VERAPAMIL HYDROCHLORIDE
Covera-HS Tablets . . . 3199
Isoptin SR Tablets . . . 467
Verelan Capsules . . . 3184
Verelan PM Capsules . . . 3186

VERACAPS (Australia)
VERAPAMIL HYDROCHLORIDE
Covera-HS Tablets . . . 3199
Isoptin SR Tablets . . . 467
Verelan Capsules . . . 3184
Verelan PM Capsules . . . 3186

VERACIM (Switzerland)
VERAPAMIL HYDROCHLORIDE
Covera-HS Tablets . . . 3199
Isoptin SR Tablets . . . 467
Verelan Capsules . . . 3184
Verelan PM Capsules . . . 3186

VERACOR (Israel)
VERAPAMIL HYDROCHLORIDE
Covera-HS Tablets . . . 3199
Isoptin SR Tablets . . . 467
Verelan Capsules . . . 3184
Verelan PM Capsules . . . 3186

VERACORON (Brazil)
VERAPAMIL HYDROCHLORIDE
Covera-HS Tablets . . . 3199
Isoptin SR Tablets . . . 467
Verelan Capsules . . . 3184
Verelan PM Capsules . . . 3186

VERADIL (Australia)
VERAPAMIL HYDROCHLORIDE
Covera-HS Tablets . . . 3199
Isoptin SR Tablets . . . 467
Verelan Capsules . . . 3184
Verelan PM Capsules . . . 3186

VERADURAT (Germany)
VERAPAMIL HYDROCHLORIDE
Covera-HS Tablets . . . 3199
Isoptin SR Tablets . . . 467
Verelan Capsules . . . 3184
Verelan PM Capsules . . . 3186

VERAGAMMA (Germany)
VERAPAMIL HYDROCHLORIDE
Covera-HS Tablets . . . 3199

(⊙ Described in PDR For Ophthalmic Medicines™)

Isoptin SR Tablets 467
Verelan Capsules 3184
Verelan PM Capsules 3186

VERAHEXAL (Australia, Germany, South Africa)
VERAPAMIL HYDROCHLORIDE
Covera-HS Tablets 3199
Isoptin SR Tablets 467
Verelan Capsules 3184
Verelan PM Capsules 3186

VERAKARD (Norway)
VERAPAMIL HYDROCHLORIDE
Covera-HS Tablets 3199
Isoptin SR Tablets 467
Verelan Capsules 3184
Verelan PM Capsules 3186

VERALAN (Mexico)
VERAPAMIL HYDROCHLORIDE
Covera-HS Tablets 3199
Isoptin SR Tablets 467
Verelan Capsules 3184
Verelan PM Capsules 3186

VERA-LICH (Germany)
VERAPAMIL HYDROCHLORIDE
Covera-HS Tablets 3199
Isoptin SR Tablets 467
Verelan Capsules 3184
Verelan PM Capsules 3186

VERALOC (Denmark, Sweden)
VERAPAMIL HYDROCHLORIDE
Covera-HS Tablets 3199
Isoptin SR Tablets 467
Verelan Capsules 3184
Verelan PM Capsules 3186

VERAMEX (Germany)
VERAPAMIL HYDROCHLORIDE
Covera-HS Tablets 3199
Isoptin SR Tablets 467
Verelan Capsules 3184
Verelan PM Capsules 3186

VERAMIL (Irish Republic)
VERAPAMIL HYDROCHLORIDE
Covera-HS Tablets 3199
Isoptin SR Tablets 467
Verelan Capsules 3184
Verelan PM Capsules 3186

VERANORM (Germany)
VERAPAMIL HYDROCHLORIDE
Covera-HS Tablets 3199
Isoptin SR Tablets 467
Verelan Capsules 3184
Verelan PM Capsules 3186

VERAPABENE (Austria)
VERAPAMIL HYDROCHLORIDE
Covera-HS Tablets 3199
Isoptin SR Tablets 467
Verelan Capsules 3184
Verelan PM Capsules 3186

VERAPIN (Thailand)
VERAPAMIL HYDROCHLORIDE
Covera-HS Tablets 3199
Isoptin SR Tablets 467
Verelan Capsules 3184
Verelan PM Capsules 3186

VERAPRESS (Israel, United Kingdom)
VERAPAMIL HYDROCHLORIDE
Covera-HS Tablets 3199
Isoptin SR Tablets 467
Verelan Capsules 3184
Verelan PM Capsules 3186

VERAPTIN (Switzerland)
VERAPAMIL HYDROCHLORIDE
Covera-HS Tablets 3199
Isoptin SR Tablets 467
Verelan Capsules 3184
Verelan PM Capsules 3186

VERASAL (Germany)
VERAPAMIL HYDROCHLORIDE
Covera-HS Tablets 3199
Isoptin SR Tablets 467
Verelan Capsules 3184
Verelan PM Capsules 3186

VERASIFAR (Switzerland)
VERAPAMIL HYDROCHLORIDE
Covera-HS Tablets 3199
Isoptin SR Tablets 467
Verelan Capsules 3184
Verelan PM Capsules 3186

VERATENSIN (Spain)
VERAPAMIL HYDROCHLORIDE
Covera-HS Tablets 3199
Isoptin SR Tablets 467
Verelan Capsules 3184
Verelan PM Capsules 3186

VERCEF (Australia, Singapore, South Africa, Thailand)
CEFACLOR
Ceclor CD Tablets 1279
Ceclor Pulvules 1905
Ceclor Suspension 1905

VERELAIT (Italy)
LACTULOSE
Kristalose for Oral Solution 1007

VERELAN (Canada, Irish Republic)
VERAPAMIL HYDROCHLORIDE
Covera-HS Tablets 3199
Isoptin SR Tablets 467
Verelan Capsules 3184
Verelan PM Capsules 3186

VEREXAMIL (Austria)
VERAPAMIL HYDROCHLORIDE
Covera-HS Tablets 3199
Isoptin SR Tablets 467
Verelan Capsules 3184
Verelan PM Capsules 3186

VERIDERM MEDROL (France)
METHYLPREDNISOLONE ACETATE
Depo-Medrol Injectable Suspension 2795

VERISOP (Irish Republic)
VERAPAMIL HYDROCHLORIDE
Covera-HS Tablets 3199
Isoptin SR Tablets 467
Verelan Capsules 3184
Verelan PM Capsules 3186

VERMEPEN (Brazil)
MEBENDAZOLE
Vermox Chewable Tablets 2017

VERMICET (Germany)
ISOSORBIDE DINITRATE
Isordil Sublingual Tablets 3525
Isordil Titradose Tablets 3526

VERMICIDIN (Switzerland)
MEBENDAZOLE
Vermox Chewable Tablets 2017

VERMICOL (Mexico)
MEBENDAZOLE
Vermox Chewable Tablets 2017

VERMIDIL (Mexico)
MEBENDAZOLE
Vermox Chewable Tablets 2017

VERMILAN (Mexico)
ALBENDAZOLE
Albenza Tablets 1463

VERMIN (Finland)
VERAPAMIL HYDROCHLORIDE
Covera-HS Tablets 3199
Isoptin SR Tablets 467
Verelan Capsules 3184
Verelan PM Capsules 3186

VERMIN-DAZOL (Mexico)
MEBENDAZOLE
Vermox Chewable Tablets 2017

VERMINE (Thailand)
VERAPAMIL HYDROCHLORIDE
Covera-HS Tablets 3199
Isoptin SR Tablets 467
Verelan Capsules 3184
Verelan PM Capsules 3186

VERMIN-PLUS (Mexico)
ALBENDAZOLE
Albenza Tablets 1463

VERMIRAX (Brazil)
MEBENDAZOLE
Vermox Chewable Tablets 2017

VERMISEN (Mexico)
ALBENDAZOLE
Albenza Tablets 1463

VERMITAL (Brazil)
ALBENDAZOLE
Albenza Tablets 1463

VERMIXIDE (Thailand)
ALBENDAZOLE
Albenza Tablets 1463

VERMOL (Brazil)
MEBENDAZOLE
Vermox Chewable Tablets 2017

VERMONON (Brazil)
MEBENDAZOLE
Vermox Chewable Tablets 2017

VERMOPLEX (Brazil)
MEBENDAZOLE
Vermox Chewable Tablets 2017

VERMORAL (Brazil)
MEBENDAZOLE
Vermox Chewable Tablets 2017

VERMOX (Australia, Belgium, Canada, Denmark, Germany, Hong Kong, Irish Republic, Israel, Italy, Mexico, New Zealand, Norway, South Africa, Sweden, Switzerland, The Netherlands, United Kingdom)
MEBENDAZOLE
Vermox Chewable Tablets 2017

VERNTHOL (South Africa)
THEOPHYLLINE
Aerolate Jr. T.D. Capsules 1361
Aerolate Liquid 1361
Aerolate Sr. T.D. Capsules 1361
Theo-Dur Extended-Release Tablets 1835
Uni-Dur Extended-Release Tablets 1841
Uniphyl 400 mg and 600 mg Tablets 2903

VEROPTINSTADA (Germany)
VERAPAMIL HYDROCHLORIDE
Covera-HS Tablets 3199
Isoptin SR Tablets 467
Verelan Capsules 3184
Verelan PM Capsules 3186

VERORAB (South Africa)
RABIES VACCINE
Imovax Rabies Vaccine 807
Rabies Vaccine RabAvert 1203

VEROXIL (Italy)
INDAPAMIDE
Indapamide Tablets 2286

VERPACOR (Finland)
VERAPAMIL HYDROCHLORIDE
Covera-HS Tablets 3199
Isoptin SR Tablets 467
Verelan Capsules 3184
Verelan PM Capsules 3186

VERPAMIL (Finland, New Zealand, South Africa)
VERAPAMIL HYDROCHLORIDE
Covera-HS Tablets 3199
Isoptin SR Tablets 467
Verelan Capsules 3184
Verelan PM Capsules 3186

VERRUMAL (Portugal)
FLUOROURACIL
Efudex Cream 1733
Efudex Topical Solutions 1733
Fluoroplex Topical Cream 552
Fluoroplex Topical Solution 552

VERSAL (Denmark, Norway, Sweden)
LORATADINE
Claritin Reditabs 3100
Claritin Syrup 3100
Claritin Tablets 3100

VERSED (Canada)
MIDAZOLAM HYDROCHLORIDE
Versed Injection 3027
Versed Syrup 3033

VERSTADOL (Spain)
BUTORPHANOL TARTRATE
Stadol NS Nasal Spray 1108

VERTAB (United Kingdom)
VERAPAMIL HYDROCHLORIDE
Covera-HS Tablets 3199
Isoptin SR Tablets 467
Verelan Capsules 3184
Verelan PM Capsules 3186

VERTEX (Mexico)
MEBENDAZOLE
Vermox Chewable Tablets 2017

VERTIGON (United Kingdom)
PROCHLORPERAZINE MALEATE
Compazine Spansule Capsules 1505
Compazine Tablets 1505

VERTIZOLE (Mexico)
MEBENDAZOLE
Vermox Chewable Tablets 2017

VERYTRACIN (Mexico)
ERYTHROMYCIN
Emgel 2% Topical Gel 1285
Ery-Tab Tablets 448
Erythromycin Base Filmtab Tablets 454
Erythromycin Delayed-Release Capsules, USP 455
PCE Dispertab Tablets 498

VESALIUM (Austria)
HALOPERIDOL
Haldol Injection, Tablets and Concentrate 2533

VESANOID (Australia, Austria, Belgium, Canada, Finland, France, Germany, Hong Kong, Israel, Italy, Mexico, New Zealand, Norway, Portugal, Singapore, South Africa, Sweden, Switzerland, The Netherlands, United Kingdom)
TRETINOIN
Avita Cream 999
Avita Gel 1000
Renova 0.05% Cream 2519
Retin-A Micro 0.1% 2522
Vesanoid Capsules 3037

VESDIL (Switzerland)
RAMIPRIL
Altace Capsules 2233

VETREN (Austria, Germany)
HEPARIN SODIUM
Heparin Lock Flush Solution 3509
Heparin Sodium Injection 3511

VEXOL (Austria, Canada, Denmark, Finland, France, Germany, Irish Republic, Italy, Portugal, Spain, Sweden, Switzerland, United Kingdom)
RIMEXOLONE
Vexol 1% Ophthalmic Suspension ⊙222

VEXOLON (Belgium)
RIMEXOLONE
Vexol 1% Ophthalmic Suspension ⊙222

VIACIN (South Africa)
DOXYCYCLINE HYCLATE
Doryx Coated Pellet Filled Capsules 3357
Periostat Tablets 1208
Vibramycin Hyclate Capsules 2735
Vibramycin Hyclate Intravenous 2737
Vibra-Tabs Film Coated Tablets 2735

VIAGRA (Australia, Austria, Belgium, Canada, Denmark, Finland, France, Germany, Hong Kong, Irish Republic, Israel, Italy, Mexico, New Zealand, Norway, Portugal, Singapore, South Africa, Spain, Sweden, Switzerland, Thailand, United Kingdom)
SILDENAFIL CITRATE
Viagra Tablets 2732

VIAMICINA (Italy)
TROLEANDOMYCIN
Tao Capsules 2716

VIATINE (Spain)
LORATADINE
Claritin Reditabs 3100
Claritin Syrup 3100
Claritin Tablets 3100

VIAZEM (Denmark, Sweden)
DILTIAZEM HYDROCHLORIDE
Cardizem CD Capsules 1016
Cardizem Injectable 1018
Cardizem Lyo-Ject Syringe 1018
Cardizem Monovial 1018
Tiazac Capsules 1378

VIAZEM XL (United Kingdom)
DILTIAZEM HYDROCHLORIDE
Cardizem CD Capsules 1016
Cardizem Injectable 1018
Cardizem Lyo-Ject Syringe 1018
Cardizem Monovial 1018
Tiazac Capsules 1378

VIBRACINA (Spain)
DOXYCYCLINE HYCLATE
Doryx Coated Pellet Filled Capsules 3357
Periostat Tablets 1208
Vibramycin Hyclate Capsules 2735
Vibramycin Hyclate Intravenous 2737
Vibra-Tabs Film Coated Tablets 2735

VIBRAMICINA (Brazil, Mexico)
DOXYCYCLINE HYCLATE
Doryx Coated Pellet Filled Capsules 3357
Periostat Tablets 1208
Vibramycin Hyclate Capsules 2735
Vibramycin Hyclate Intravenous 2737
Vibra-Tabs Film Coated Tablets 2735

VIBRAMYCIN (Canada, Germany, Hong Kong, Irish Republic, Singapore, Thailand, The Netherlands, United Kingdom)
DOXYCYCLINE HYCLATE
Doryx Coated Pellet Filled Capsules 3357
Periostat Tablets 1208
Vibramycin Hyclate Capsules 2735
Vibramycin Hyclate Intravenous 2737
Vibra-Tabs Film Coated Tablets 2735

VIBRAMYCINE (Belgium, France)
DOXYCYCLINE HYCLATE
Doryx Coated Pellet Filled Capsules 3357
Periostat Tablets 1208
Vibramycin Hyclate Capsules 2735
Vibramycin Hyclate Intravenous 2737
Vibra-Tabs Film Coated Tablets 2735

VIBRA-TABS (Australia, Canada)
DOXYCYCLINE HYCLATE
Doryx Coated Pellet Filled Capsules 3357
Periostat Tablets 1208
Vibramycin Hyclate Capsules 2735
Vibramycin Hyclate Intravenous 2737
Vibra-Tabs Film Coated Tablets 2735

VIBRAVEINEUSE (France, Switzerland)
DOXYCYCLINE HYCLATE
Doryx Coated Pellet Filled Capsules 3357
Periostat Tablets 1208
Vibramycin Hyclate Capsules 2735
Vibramycin Hyclate Intravenous 2737
Vibra-Tabs Film Coated Tablets 2735

VIBRAVENOS (Austria, Germany)
DOXYCYCLINE HYCLATE
Doryx Coated Pellet Filled Capsules 3357
Periostat Tablets 1208
Vibramycin Hyclate Capsules 2735
Vibramycin Hyclate Intravenous 2737
Vibra-Tabs Film Coated Tablets 2735

VIBRAVENOSA (Spain)
DOXYCYCLINE HYCLATE
Doryx Coated Pellet Filled Capsules 3357
Periostat Tablets 1208
Vibramycin Hyclate Capsules 2735
Vibramycin Hyclate Intravenous 2737
Vibra-Tabs Film Coated Tablets 2735

VICARD (Austria, Switzerland)
TERAZOSIN HYDROCHLORIDE
Hytrin Capsules 464

VICKS ACTION (United Kingdom)
IBUPROFEN
Motrin Suspension, Oral Drops, Chewable Tablets, and Caplets 2002

VICKS EXPECTORANT (France)
GUAIFENESIN
Organidin NR Liquid 3350
Organidin NR Tablets 3350

VICKS FORMULE 44 EXPECTINE (Switzerland)
GUAIFENESIN
Organidin NR Liquid 3350
Organidin NR Tablets 3350

VICKS TOSSE FLUIDIFICANTE (Italy)
GUAIFENESIN
Organidin NR Liquid 3350
Organidin NR Tablets 3350

VICKS ULTRA CHLORASEPTIC (United Kingdom)
BENZOCAINE
Americaine Anesthetic Lubricant 1162
Americaine Otic Topical Anesthetic Ear Drops 1162

VICKS VAPOSYRUP EXPECTORANT (Belgium)
GUAIFENESIN
Organidin NR Liquid 3350
Organidin NR Tablets 3350

VICKS VAPOSYRUP FOR CHESTY COUGHS (United Kingdom)
GUAIFENESIN
Organidin NR Liquid 3350
Organidin NR Tablets 3350

VICNAS (Spain)
NORFLOXACIN
Chibroxin Sterile Ophthalmic Solution . . . . ⊙273, 2051
Noroxin Tablets 2145

VICORTIN (Mexico)
HYDROCORTISONE
Anusol-HC Cream 2.5% 2237
Hydrocortone Tablets 2106

VICTRIX (Brazil)
OMEPRAZOLE
Prilosec Delayed-Release Capsules 628

VIDAPRIL (Portugal)
CAPTOPRIL
Captopril Tablets 2281

VIDAVIT (Mexico)
VITAMIN B12
Nascobal Gel 3174

VIDEX (Australia, Austria, Belgium, Brazil, Canada, Denmark, Finland, France, Germany, Hong Kong, Irish Republic, Israel, Italy, Mexico, New Zealand, Norway, Portugal, Singapore, South Africa, Spain, Sweden, Switzerland, Thailand, The Netherlands, United Kingdom)
DIDANOSINE
Videx Chewable Tablets 1138
Videx Pediatric Powder for Oral Solution 1138
Videx Powder for Oral Solution 1138

VIGIL (Germany)
MODAFINIL
Provigil Tablets 1193

VIGITEN (Belgium)
LORAZEPAM
Ativan Injection 3478
Ativan Tablets 3482

VIKEN (Mexico)
CEFOTAXIME SODIUM
Claforan Injection 732

VILONA (Mexico)
RIBAVIRIN
Virazole for Inhalation Solution 1747

VINCOSEDAN (Spain)
DIAZEPAM
Valium Injectable 3026
Valium Tablets 3047

VINCOSONA (Spain)
DIFLORASONE DIACETATE
Psorcon E Cream 1227
Psorcon E Ointment 1228

VINSEN (Thailand)
NAPROXEN
EC-Naprosyn Delayed-Release Tablets 2967
Naprosyn Suspension 2967
Naprosyn Tablets 2967

VIOKASE (Belgium, Canada)
PANCRELIPASE
Ultrase Capsules 835
Ultrase MT Capsules 835

VIOXX (Australia, Canada, Denmark, Finland, France, Germany, Irish Republic, New Zealand, Portugal, Singapore, South Africa, Spain, Sweden, Switzerland, Thailand, United Kingdom)
ROFECOXIB
Vioxx Oral Suspension 2213
Vioxx Tablets 2213

VIRACEPT (Israel, Sweden)
NELFINAVIR MESYLATE
Viracept Oral Powder 532
Viracept Tablets 532

VIRAFERON (France, Mexico, Spain)
INTERFERON ALFA-2B
Intron A for Injection 3120

VIRAMID (Italy)
RIBAVIRIN
Virazole for Inhalation Solution 1747

VIRAZID (Spain)
RIBAVIRIN
Virazole for Inhalation Solution 1747

VIRAZIDE (Australia, Italy, Mexico)
RIBAVIRIN
Virazole for Inhalation Solution 1747

VIRAZOLE (Belgium, Canada, Germany, Hong Kong, Irish Republic, Singapore, Sweden, Switzerland, The Netherlands, United Kingdom)
RIBAVIRIN
Virazole for Inhalation Solution 1747

VIREGYT (Germany)
AMANTADINE HYDROCHLORIDE
Symmetrel Syrup 1328
Symmetrel Tablets 1328

VIRGAN (France, United Kingdom)
GANCICLOVIR
Cytovene Capsules 2959

VIRIDIN (Portugal)
TRIFLURIDINE
Viroptic Ophthalmic Solution Sterile . . . . ⊙301

VIRLIX (France, Italy, Mexico, Portugal, Spain)
CETIRIZINE HYDROCHLORIDE
Zyrtec Syrup 2756
Zyrtec Tablets 2756

VIROFRAL (Denmark, Sweden)
AMANTADINE HYDROCHLORIDE
Symmetrel Syrup 1328
Symmetrel Tablets 1328

VIROMIDIN (Spain)
TRIFLURIDINE
Viroptic Ophthalmic Solution Sterile . . . . ⊙301

VIROPHTA (France)
TRIFLURIDINE
Viroptic Ophthalmic Solution Sterile . . . . ⊙301

VIROPTIC (Canada)
TRIFLURIDINE
Viroptic Ophthalmic Solution Sterile . . . . ⊙301

VIRUCID (Austria)
AMANTADINE HYDROCHLORIDE
Symmetrel Syrup 1328
Symmetrel Tablets 1328

VIRUDIN (Italy)
FOSCARNET SODIUM
Foscavir Injection 605

VIRUSTAT (Brazil)
ZIDOVUDINE
Retrovir Capsules 1625
Retrovir IV Infusion 1629
Retrovir Syrup 1625
Retrovir Tablets 1625

VISANO N (Germany)
MEPROBAMATE
Miltown Tablets 3349

VISANO-MINI N (Germany)
MEPROBAMATE
Miltown Tablets 3349

VISCAL (Italy)
METOCLOPRAMIDE HYDROCHLORIDE
Reglan Injectable 2935
Reglan Syrup 2935
Reglan Tablets 2935

VISCOR (Italy)
DIPYRIDAMOLE
Persantine Tablets 1057

VISLUBE (Germany, Hong Kong, Switzerland)
SODIUM HYALURONATE
Hyalgan Solution 3080

VISMED (Australia, France, Germany, Italy, Switzerland)
SODIUM HYALURONATE
Hyalgan Solution 3080

VISTACARPIN (Germany)
PILOCARPINE HYDROCHLORIDE
Isopto Carpine Ophthalmic Solution . . . . ⊙215
Pilopine HS Ophthalmic Gel . . . . ⊙217
Salagen Tablets 2229

VISTAJUNCTIN (Germany, Switzerland)
NEOMYCIN SULFATE/POLYMYXIN B SULFATE
Neosporin G.U. Irrigant Sterile 2256

VISTALBALON (Germany)
NAPHAZOLINE HYDROCHLORIDE
Albalon Ophthalmic Solution . . . . ⊙225

VISTA-PHENICOL (Hong Kong)
CHLORAMPHENICOL
Chloromycetin Ophthalmic Ointment, 1% . . . . ⊙296
Chloromycetin Ophthalmic Solution . . . . ⊙297
Chloroptic Sterile Ophthalmic Ointment . . . . ⊙234
Chloroptic Sterile Ophthalmic Solution . . . . ⊙235

VISTIDE (Australia, Austria, Belgium, France, Germany, Italy, Portugal, Spain, Switzerland, United Kingdom)
CIDOFOVIR
Vistide Injection 1445

VISUMETAZONE (Italy)
DEXAMETHASONE
Decadron Elixir 2078
Decadron Tablets 2079

VITACID (Portugal)
TRETINOIN
Avita Cream 999
Avita Gel 1000
Renova 0.05% Cream 2519
Retin-A Micro 0.1% 2522
Vesanoid Capsules 3037

VITADRAL (Germany)
VITAMIN A PALMITATE
Aquasol A Parenteral 593

VITASEPTINE (France)
SULFACETAMIDE SODIUM
Bleph-10 Ophthalmic Ointment 10% . . . . ⊙230
Klaron Lotion 10% 1224

VITAXICAM (Singapore, Spain)
PIROXICAM
Feldene Capsules 2685

VITINOIN (Canada)
TRETINOIN
Avita Cream 999
Avita Gel 1000
Renova 0.05% Cream 2519
Retin-A Micro 0.1% 2522
Vesanoid Capsules 3037

VITRASERT (Australia, United Kingdom)
GANCICLOVIR
Cytovene Capsules 2959

VITRAX (France)
SODIUM HYALURONATE
Hyalgan Solution 3080

VITUSSIN (Israel)
GUAIFENESIN
Organidin NR Liquid 3350
Organidin NR Tablets 3350

VIVAL (Norway)
DIAZEPAM
Valium Injectable 3026
Valium Tablets 3047

VIVAPRYL (United Kingdom)
SELEGILINE HYDROCHLORIDE
Eldepryl Capsules 3266

VIVATEC (Denmark, Finland, Norway, Sweden)
LISINOPRIL
Prinivil Tablets 2164
Zestril Tablets 698

VIVATEC COMP (Finland, Norway)
HYDROCHLOROTHIAZIDE/LISINOPRIL
Prinzide Tablets 2168
Zestoretic Tablets 695

VIVAZID (Denmark)
HYDROCHLOROTHIAZIDE/LISINOPRIL
Prinzide Tablets 2168
Zestoretic Tablets 695

VIVELLE (Canada)
ESTRADIOL
Alora Transdermal System 3372
Climara Transdermal System 958
Estrace Vaginal Cream 3358
Estring Vaginal Ring 2811
Vivelle Transdermal System 2412
Vivelle-Dot Transdermal System 2416

VIVINOX STARK (Germany)
DIPHENHYDRAMINE HYDROCHLORIDE
Benadryl Parenteral 2617

VIVOL (Canada)
DIAZEPAM
Valium Injectable 3026
Valium Tablets 3047

VIXIN (Mexico)
CHLORAMPHENICOL
Chloromycetin Ophthalmic Ointment, 1% . . . . ⊙296
Chloromycetin Ophthalmic Solution . . . . ⊙297
Chloroptic Sterile Ophthalmic Ointment . . . . ⊙234
Chloroptic Sterile Ophthalmic Solution . . . . ⊙235

VIXMICINA (Brazil)
CHLORAMPHENICOL
Chloromycetin Ophthalmic Ointment, 1% . . . . ⊙296
Chloromycetin Ophthalmic Solution . . . . ⊙297
Chloroptic Sterile Ophthalmic Ointment . . . . ⊙234
Chloroptic Sterile Ophthalmic Solution . . . . ⊙235

VIZAM (Australia)
DOXYCYCLINE HYCLATE
Doryx Coated Pellet Filled Capsules 3357
Periostat Tablets 1208
Vibra-Tabs Film Coated Tablets 2735
Vibramycin Hyclate Capsules 2735
Vibramycin Hyclate Intravenous 2737

VOFENAL (Canada)
DICLOFENAC SODIUM
Voltaren Tablets 2315
Voltaren-XR Tablets 2315

VOGAN (Germany)
VITAMIN A PALMITATE
Aquasol A Parenteral 593

VOLCIDOL-S (Thailand)
TRAMADOL HYDROCHLORIDE
Ultram Tablets 2600

VOLDAL (France)
DICLOFENAC SODIUM
Voltaren Tablets 2315
Voltaren-XR Tablets 2315

VOLFENAC (Thailand)
DICLOFENAC SODIUM
Voltaren Tablets 2315
Voltaren-XR Tablets 2315

VOLITAL (United Kingdom)
PEMOLINE
Cylert Chewable Tablets 415
Cylert Tablets 415

VOLNAC (Thailand)
DICLOFENAC SODIUM
Voltaren Tablets 2315
Voltaren-XR Tablets 2315

VOLOGEN (Irish Republic)
DICLOFENAC SODIUM
Voltaren Tablets 2315
Voltaren-XR Tablets 2315

VOLON A (Austria)
TRIAMCINOLONE ACETONIDE
Azmacort Inhalation Aerosol 728
Nasacort AQ Nasal Spray 752
Nasacort Nasal Inhaler 750

VOLONIMAT (Germany)
TRIAMCINOLONE ACETONIDE
Azmacort Inhalation Aerosol 728
Nasacort AQ Nasal Spray 752
Nasacort Nasal Inhaler 750

VOLONIMAT N (Germany)
TRIAMCINOLONE ACETONIDE
Azmacort Inhalation Aerosol 728
Nasacort AQ Nasal Spray 752
Nasacort Nasal Inhaler 750

VOLRAMAN (United Kingdom)
DICLOFENAC SODIUM
Voltaren Tablets 2315
Voltaren-XR Tablets 2315

VOLSAID (United Kingdom)
DICLOFENAC SODIUM
Voltaren Tablets 2315
Voltaren-XR Tablets 2315

VOLTANAC (Thailand)
DICLOFENAC SODIUM
Voltaren Tablets 2315
Voltaren-XR Tablets 2315

VOLTAREN (Brazil, Norway, Spain, Sweden, The Netherlands)
DICLOFENAC SODIUM
Voltaren Tablets 2315
Voltaren-XR Tablets 2315

VOLTAREN OPHTHA (Australia, Canada, Germany, Hong Kong, Israel, New Zealand, Norway, Singapore, Sweden, Switzerland)
DICLOFENAC SODIUM
Voltaren Tablets 2315
Voltaren-XR Tablets 2315

VOLTAREN T (Sweden)
DICLOFENAC POTASSIUM
Cataflam Tablets 2315

VOLTARENE (France)
DICLOFENAC SODIUM
Voltaren Tablets 2315
Voltaren-XR Tablets 2315

VOLTARENE RAPIDE (Switzerland)
DICLOFENAC POTASSIUM
Cataflam Tablets 2315

VOLTAROL OPHTHA (Irish Republic, United Kingdom)
DICLOFENAC SODIUM
Voltaren Tablets 2315
Voltaren-XR Tablets 2315

VOLTFAST (Italy)
DICLOFENAC POTASSIUM
Cataflam Tablets 2315

VOLTRIC (Spain)
CETIRIZINE HYDROCHLORIDE
Zyrtec Syrup 2756
Zyrtec Tablets 2756

VOLUTINE (Italy)
FENOFIBRATE
Tricor Capsules, Micronized 513

VOLUTOL (Mexico)
CARBAMAZEPINE
Carbatrol Capsules 3234
Tegretol Chewable Tablets 2404
Tegretol Suspension 2404
Tegretol Tablets 2404
Tegretol-XR Tablets 2404

VOLVERAC (Thailand)
DICLOFENAC SODIUM
Voltaren Tablets 2315
Voltaren-XR Tablets 2315

VOMITRAN (Thailand)
ONDANSETRON HYDROCHLORIDE
Zofran Injection 1698
Zofran Injection Premixed 1698
Zofran Oral Solution 1703
Zofran Tablets 1703

VONIL (Brazil)
METOCLOPRAMIDE HYDROCHLORIDE
Reglan Injectable 2935
Reglan Syrup 2935
Reglan Tablets 2935

V-OPTIC (Israel)
TIMOLOL MALEATE
Blocadren Tablets 2046
Timoptic Sterile Ophthalmic Solution 2190
Timoptic in Ocudose 2192
Timoptic-XE Sterile Ophthalmic Gel Forming Solution 2194

VOREN (Thailand)
DICLOFENAC SODIUM
Voltaren Tablets 2315
Voltaren-XR Tablets 2315

VOSTAR (Denmark)
DICLOFENAC SODIUM
Voltaren Tablets 2315
Voltaren-XR Tablets 2315

VOTAMED (Thailand)
DICLOFENAC SODIUM
Voltaren Tablets 2315
Voltaren-XR Tablets 2315

WALESOLONE (Singapore)
PREDNISOLONE
Prelone Syrup 2273

WANMYCIN (Hong Kong)
DOXYCYCLINE HYCLATE
Doryx Coated Pellet Filled Capsules 3357
Periostat Tablets 1208
Vibramycin Hyclate Capsules 2735
Vibramycin Hyclate Intravenous 2737
Vibra-Tabs Film Coated Tablets 2735

WAR LIN (Mexico)
LINDANE
Lindane Lotion USP 1% 559
Lindane Shampoo USP 1% 560

WARAN (Sweden)
WARFARIN SODIUM
Coumadin Tablets 1243
Coumadin for Injection 1243

WARCA (Thailand)
MEBENDAZOLE
Vermox Chewable Tablets 2017

WARFILONE (Canada)
WARFARIN SODIUM
Coumadin Tablets 1243
Coumadin for Injection 1243

WARIACTIV (Germany, Hong Kong)
ETHYL CHLORIDE
Gebauer's Ethyl Chloride 1409

WASPEZE HYDROCORTISONE (United Kingdom)
HYDROCORTISONE
Anusol-HC Cream 2.5% 2237
Hydrocortone Tablets 2106

WAYCITAL (Mexico)
PRAZIQUANTEL
Biltricide Tablets 887

WAYNAZOL (Mexico)
FLUCONAZOLE
Diflucan Tablets, Injection, and Oral Suspension 2681

WAYTRAX (Mexico)
CEFTAZIDIME
Ceptaz for Injection 1499
Fortaz for Injection 1541
Tazicef for Injection 1647
Tazidime Vials, Faspak & ADD-Vantage 1966

WEIMERQUIN (Germany)
CHLOROQUINE PHOSPHATE
Aralen Tablets 3075

WELLBUTRIN (Canada, Mexico)
BUPROPION HYDROCHLORIDE
Wellbutrin SR Sustained-Release Tablets 1684
Wellbutrin Tablets 1680
Zyban Sustained-Release Tablets 1710

WELLVONE (Australia, Austria, Belgium, Denmark, France, Germany, Italy, South Africa, Sweden, Switzerland, The Netherlands, United Kingdom)
ATOVAQUONE
Mepron Suspension 1598

WICK FORMEL 44 HUSTEN-LOSER (Germany)
GUAIFENESIN
Organidin NR Liquid 3350
Organidin NR Tablets 3350

WICK FORMEL 44 PLUS HUSTENLOSER (Austria)
GUAIFENESIN
Organidin NR Liquid 3350
Organidin NR Tablets 3350

WICK KINDER FORMEL 44 HUSTEN-LOSER (Germany)
GUAIFENESIN
Organidin NR Liquid 3350
Organidin NR Tablets 3350

WINPRED (Canada)
PREDNISONE
Prednisone Intensol 3064
Prednisone Oral Solution 3064
Prednisone Tablets 3064

WITROMIN (Mexico)
ERYTHROMYCIN
Emgel 2% Topical Gel 1285
Ery-Tab Tablets 448
Erythromycin Base Filmtab Tablets 454
Erythromycin Delayed-Release Capsules, USP 455
PCE Dispertab Tablets 498

WORMGO (South Africa)
MEBENDAZOLE
Vermox Chewable Tablets 2017

WORMSTOP (South Africa)
MEBENDAZOLE
Vermox Chewable Tablets 2017

WYTENS (France)
BISOPROLOL FUMARATE/HYDROCHLOROTHIAZIDE
Ziac Tablets 1887

XACIN (Thailand)
NORFLOXACIN
Chibroxin Sterile Ophthalmic Solution . . . . ⊙273, 2051
Noroxin Tablets 2145

XALATAN (Australia, Austria, Belgium, Canada, Denmark, Finland, France, Germany, Hong Kong, Irish Republic, Israel, Italy, Mexico, New Zealand, Norway, Portugal, Singapore, South Africa, Spain, Sweden, Switzerland, Thailand, The Netherlands, United Kingdom)
LATANOPROST
Xalatan Latanoprost Ophthalmic Solution . . . . ⊙320

XANAGIS (Israel)
ALPRAZOLAM
Xanax Tablets 2865

XANAX (Australia, Belgium, Canada, France, Germany, Hong Kong, Irish Republic, Israel, Italy, New Zealand, Portugal, Singapore, Switzerland, Thailand, The Netherlands, United Kingdom)
ALPRAZOLAM
Xanax Tablets 2865

XANIDINE (Thailand)
RANITIDINE HYDROCHLORIDE
Zantac 150 EFFERdose Granules 1690
Zantac 150 EFFERdose Tablets 1690
Zantac 150 Tablets 1690
Zantac 300 Tablets 1690
Zantac Injection 1688
Zantac Injection Premixed 1688
Zantac Syrup 1690

XANOLAM (South Africa)
ALPRAZOLAM
Xanax Tablets 2865

XANOMEL (Irish Republic)
RANITIDINE HYDROCHLORIDE
Zantac 150 EFFERdose Granules 1690
Zantac 150 EFFERdose Tablets 1690
Zantac 150 Tablets 1690
Zantac 300 Tablets 1690
Zantac Injection 1688
Zantac Injection Premixed 1688
Zantac Syrup 1690

XANOR (Austria, Finland, Norway, South Africa, Sweden)
ALPRAZOLAM
Xanax Tablets 2865

XANTHIUM (France, Thailand)
THEOPHYLLINE
Aerolate Jr. T.D. Capsules 1361
Aerolate Liquid 1361
Aerolate Sr. T.D. Capsules 1361
Theo-Dur Extended-Release Tablets 1835
Uni-Dur Extended-Release Tablets 1841
Uniphyl 400 mg and 600 mg Tablets 2903

XANTIVENT (Switzerland)
THEOPHYLLINE
Aerolate Jr. T.D. Capsules 1361
Aerolate Liquid 1361
Aerolate Sr. T.D. Capsules 1361
Theo-Dur Extended-Release Tablets 1835
Uni-Dur Extended-Release Tablets 1841
Uniphyl 400 mg and 600 mg Tablets 2903

XARATOR (Italy)
ATORVASTATIN CALCIUM
Lipitor Tablets 2639, 2696

XAROPE DE IODETO DE POTASSIO COMPOSTO (Brazil)
POTASSIUM IODIDE
Pima Syrup 1362

XATEN (France)
ATENOLOL
Tenormin I.V. Injection 692

XELODA (Australia, Canada, New Zealand, Singapore, South Africa, Switzerland, Thailand, United Kingdom)
CAPECITABINE
Xeloda Tablets 3039

XENAR (Italy)
NAPROXEN
EC-Naprosyn Delayed-Release Tablets 2967
Naprosyn Suspension 2967
Naprosyn Tablets 2967

XENICAL (Australia, Austria, Belgium, Canada, Denmark, Finland, France, Germany, Irish Republic, Italy, Mexico, New Zealand, Portugal, Singapore, South Africa, Spain, Sweden, Switzerland, Thailand, The Netherlands, United Kingdom)
ORLISTAT
Xenical Capsules 3043

XENOPAN (Austria)
NAPROXEN
EC-Naprosyn Delayed-Release Tablets 2967
Naprosyn Suspension 2967
Naprosyn Tablets 2967

XENOVATE (South Africa)
CLOBETASOL PROPIONATE
Cormax Cream 2440
Cormax Ointment 2440
Cormax Scalp Application 2441
Temovate Cream 1301
Temovate E Emollient 1302
Temovate Gel 1303
Temovate Ointment 1301
Temovate Scalp Application 1304

XEPAGAN (Singapore)
PROMETHAZINE HYDROCHLORIDE
Phenergan Injection 3553
Phenergan Suppositories 3556
Phenergan Syrup Fortis 3554
Phenergan Syrup Plain 3554
Phenergan Tablets 3556

XEPAMET (Singapore)
CIMETIDINE
Tagamet Tablets 1644

XEPANICOL (Hong Kong, Singapore)
CHLORAMPHENICOL
Chloromycetin Ophthalmic Ointment, 1% . . . . ⊙296
Chloromycetin Ophthalmic Solution . . . . ⊙297
Chloroptic Sterile Ophthalmic Ointment . . . . ⊙234
Chloroptic Sterile Ophthalmic Solution . . . . ⊙235

XEPASONE (Singapore)
PREDNISOLONE
Prelone Syrup 2273

XEPIN (Irish Republic, United Kingdom)
DOXEPIN HYDROCHLORIDE
Sinequan Capsules 2713
Sinequan Oral Concentrate 2713

XERACIL (South Africa)
AMOXICILLIN
Amoxil Pediatric Drops for Oral Suspension 1471
Amoxil Tablets 1471

XERASPOR (South Africa)
CLOTRIMAZOLE
Lotrimin Cream 1% 3128
Lotrimin Lotion 1% 3128
Lotrimin Topical Solution 1% 3128
Mycelex Troche 573

XICAM (Thailand)
PIROXICAM
Feldene Capsules 2685

XIEMED (Thailand)
ALPRAZOLAM
Xanax Tablets 2865

XIMICINA (Italy)
DOXYCYCLINE HYCLATE
Doryx Coated Pellet Filled Capsules 3357
Periostat Tablets 1208
Vibramycin Hyclate Capsules 2735
Vibramycin Hyclate Intravenous 2737
Vibra-Tabs Film Coated Tablets 2735

XIPROCAN (Mexico)
AMOXICILLIN
Amoxil Pediatric Drops for Oral Suspension 1471
Amoxil Tablets 1471

XISMOX (United Kingdom)
ISOSORBIDE MONONITRATE
Imdur Tablets 1826
Ismo Tablets 3524

XURET (United Kingdom)
METOLAZONE
Mykrox Tablets 1168
Zaroxolyn Tablets 1177

XYCAM (South Africa)
PIROXICAM
Feldene Capsules 2685

XYLOTOCAN (Germany)
TOCAINIDE HYDROCHLORIDE
Tonocard Tablets 649

YAMATETAN (Japan)
CEFOTETAN DISODIUM
Cefotan Injection 664
Cefotan for Injection 664

YATROX (Spain)
ONDANSETRON HYDROCHLORIDE
Zofran Injection 1698
Zofran Injection Premixed 1698
Zofran Oral Solution 1703
Zofran Tablets 1703

YECTAMICINA (Mexico)
GENTAMICIN SULFATE
Genoptic Ophthalmic Ointment . . . . ⊙239

Genoptic Sterile Ophthalmic Solution . . . ⊙239

YEDOC (Switzerland)
GENTAMICIN SULFATE
Genoptic Ophthalmic Ointment . . . . ⊙239
Genoptic Sterile Ophthalmic Solution . . . ⊙239

YEWTAXAN (South Africa)
PACLITAXEL
Taxol Injection 1129

YURELAX (Spain)
CYCLOBENZAPRINE HYDROCHLORIDE
Flexeril Tablets 2094

YUREMETIL D (Mexico)
METHYLDOPA
Aldomet Tablets 2037

ZACAM (Italy)
PIROXICAM
Feldene Capsules 2685

ZACETIN (Singapore)
ALPRAZOLAM
Xanax Tablets 2865

ZACNAN (France)
MINOCYCLINE HYDROCHLORIDE
Dynacin Capsules 2019
Minocin Intravenous 1862
Minocin Oral Suspension 1865
Minocin Pellet-Filled Capsules 1863

ZADIPINA (Italy)
NISOLDIPINE
Sular Tablets 688

ZADORIN (Hong Kong, Switzerland)
DOXYCYCLINE HYCLATE
Doryx Coated Pellet Filled Capsules 3357
Periostat Tablets 1208
Vibramycin Hyclate Capsules 2735
Vibramycin Hyclate Intravenous 2737
Vibra-Tabs Film Coated Tablets 2735

ZADSTAT (Israel, United Kingdom)
METRONIDAZOLE
MetroCream 1404
MetroGel 1405
MetroGel-Vaginal Gel 1986
MetroLotion 1405
Noritate Cream 1224

ZAEDOC (United Kingdom)
RANITIDINE HYDROCHLORIDE
Zantac 150 EFFERdose Granules 1690
Zantac 150 EFFERdose Tablets 1690
Zantac 150 Tablets 1690
Zantac 300 Tablets 1690
Zantac Injection 1688
Zantac Injection Premixed 1688
Zantac Syrup 1690

ZAFEN (The Netherlands)
IBUPROFEN
Motrin Suspension, Oral Drops, Chewable Tablets, and Caplets 2002

ZAFIRST (Italy)
ZAFIRLUKAST
Accolate Tablets 657

ZAGASTROL (Brazil)
CIMETIDINE
Tagamet Tablets 1644

ZAGYL (South Africa)
METRONIDAZOLE
MetroCream 1404
MetroGel 1405
MetroGel-Vaginal Gel 1986
MetroLotion 1405
Noritate Cream 1224

ZAHNEROL N (Germany)
BENZOCAINE
Americaine Anesthetic Lubricant 1162
Americaine Otic Topical Anesthetic Ear Drops 1162

ZALVOR (Belgium)
PERMETHRIN
Acticin Cream 998
Elimite Cream 552

ZAMACORT (Mexico)
TRIAMCINOLONE ACETONIDE
Azmacort Inhalation Aerosol 728
Nasacort AQ Nasal Spray 752
Nasacort Nasal Inhaler 750

ZAMADOL (United Kingdom)
TRAMADOL HYDROCHLORIDE
Ultram Tablets 2600

ZAMOCILLINE (France)
AMOXICILLIN
Amoxil Pediatric Drops for Oral Suspension 1471
Amoxil Tablets 1471

ZAMUDOL (France)
TRAMADOL HYDROCHLORIDE
Ultram Tablets 2600

ZANAFLEX (Irish Republic, United Kingdom)
TIZANIDINE HYDROCHLORIDE
Zanaflex Tablets 1305

ZANDINE (Irish Republic)
RANITIDINE HYDROCHLORIDE
Zantac 150 EFFERdose Granules 1690
Zantac 150 EFFERdose Tablets 1690
Zantac 150 Tablets 1690
Zantac 300 Tablets 1690
Zantac Injection 1688
Zantac Injection Premixed 1688
Zantac Syrup 1690

ZANIDEX (Israel)
RANITIDINE HYDROCHLORIDE
Zantac 150 EFFERdose Granules 1690
Zantac 150 EFFERdose Tablets 1690
Zantac 150 Tablets 1690
Zantac 300 Tablets 1690
Zantac Injection 1688
Zantac Injection Premixed 1688
Zantac Syrup 1690

ZANIDIN (New Zealand)
RANITIDINE HYDROCHLORIDE
Zantac 150 EFFERdose Granules 1690
Zantac 150 EFFERdose Tablets 1690
Zantac 150 Tablets 1690
Zantac 300 Tablets 1690
Zantac Injection 1688
Zantac Injection Premixed 1688
Zantac Syrup 1690

ZANIZAL (Italy)
NIZATIDINE
Axid Pulvules 1903

ZANTAB (Israel)
RANITIDINE HYDROCHLORIDE
Zantac 150 EFFERdose Granules 1690
Zantac 150 EFFERdose Tablets 1690
Zantac 150 Tablets 1690
Zantac 300 Tablets 1690
Zantac Injection 1688
Zantac Injection Premixed 1688
Zantac Syrup 1690

ZANTAC (Australia, Austria, Belgium, Denmark, Finland, Hong Kong, Irish Republic, Israel, Italy, New Zealand, Norway, Portugal, Singapore, South Africa, Spain, Sweden, Thailand, The Netherlands, United Kingdom)
RANITIDINE HYDROCHLORIDE
Zantac 150 EFFERdose Granules 1690
Zantac 150 EFFERdose Tablets 1690
Zantac 150 Tablets 1690
Zantac 300 Tablets 1690
Zantac Injection 1688
Zantac Injection Premixed 1688
Zantac Syrup 1690

ZANTIC (Switzerland)
RANITIDINE HYDROCHLORIDE
Zantac 150 EFFERdose Granules 1690
Zantac 150 EFFERdose Tablets 1690
Zantac 150 Tablets 1690
Zantac 300 Tablets 1690
Zantac Injection 1688
Zantac Injection Premixed 1688
Zantac Syrup 1690

ZAP (Canada)
BENZOCAINE
Americaine Anesthetic Lubricant 1162
Americaine Otic Topical Anesthetic Ear Drops 1162

ZAPTO (South Africa)
CAPTOPRIL
Captopril Tablets 2281

ZAPTO CO (South Africa)
CAPTOPRIL
Captopril Tablets 2281

ZARATOR (Denmark, Portugal, Spain)
ATORVASTATIN CALCIUM
Lipitor Tablets 2639, 2696

ZARIVIZ (Italy)
CEFOTAXIME SODIUM
Claforan Injection 732

ZARONDAN (Denmark, Norway)
ETHOSUXIMIDE
Zarontin Capsules 2659
Zarontin Syrup 2660

ZARONTIN (Australia, Belgium, Canada, France, Irish Republic, Israel, Italy, Mexico, New Zealand, South Africa, Spain, The Netherlands, United Kingdom)
ETHOSUXIMIDE
Zarontin Capsules 2659
Zarontin Syrup 2660

ZAROXOLYN (Canada, Germany, Irish Republic, Italy, Mexico, South Africa, Sweden)
METOLAZONE
Mykrox Tablets 1168
Zaroxolyn Tablets 1177

ZAROXOLYNE (Switzerland)
METOLAZONE
Mykrox Tablets 1168
Zaroxolyn Tablets 1177

ZAVEDOS (Australia, Austria, Belgium, Brazil, Denmark, Finland, France, Germany, Hong Kong, Irish Republic, Israel, Italy, New Zealand, Norway, Portugal, Singapore, South Africa, Spain, Sweden, Switzerland, Thailand, The Netherlands, United Kingdom)
IDARUBICIN HYDROCHLORIDE
Idamycin PFS Injection 2825

ZEBEN (Thailand)
ALBENDAZOLE
Albenza Tablets 1463

ZECLAR (Finland, France)
CLARITHROMYCIN
Biaxin Filmtab Tablets 403
Biaxin for Oral Suspension 403

ZEDDAN (Italy)
TRANDOLAPRIL
Mavik Tablets 478

ZEDOLAC (Italy)
ETODOLAC
Lodine Capsules 3528
Lodine Tablets 3528
Lodine XL Extended-Release Tablets 3530

ZEFAXONE (Thailand)
CEFTRIAXONE SODIUM
Rocephin Injectable Vials, ADD-Vantage, Galaxy, Bulk 2993

ZEFFIX (Australia, Belgium, Denmark, Finland, France, Germany, Hong Kong, Irish Republic, Italy, New Zealand, Portugal, Sweden, Switzerland, Thailand, United Kingdom)
LAMIVUDINE
Epivir Oral Solution 1520
Epivir Tablets 1520
Epivir-HBV Oral Solution 1524
Epivir-HBV Tablets 1524

ZEFTAM (Thailand)
CEFTAZIDIME
Ceptaz for Injection 1499
Fortaz for Injection 1541
Tazicef for Injection 1647
Tazidime Vials, Faspak & ADD-Vantage . . 1966

ZEFXON (Thailand)
OMEPRAZOLE
Prilosec Delayed-Release Capsules 628

ZEHU-ZE (Israel)
PERMETHRIN
Acticin Cream 998
Elimite Cream 552

ZEISIN (Germany)
PIRBUTEROL ACETATE
Maxair Autohaler 1981
Maxair Inhaler 1984

ZELAPAR (United Kingdom)
SELEGILINE HYDROCHLORIDE
Eldepryl Capsules 3266

ZELFIN (Mexico)
ALBENDAZOLE
Albenza Tablets 1463

ZELIDERM (Spain)
AZELAIC ACID
Azelex Cream 547

ZEMIDE (Germany)
TAMOXIFEN CITRATE
Nolvadex Tablets 678

ZEMTARD (United Kingdom)
DILTIAZEM HYDROCHLORIDE
Cardizem CD Capsules 1016
Cardizem Injectable 1018
Cardizem Lyo-Ject Syringe 1018
Cardizem Monovial 1018
Tiazac Capsules 1378

ZEMURON (Canada)
ROCURONIUM BROMIDE
Zemuron Injection 2491

ZENAPAX (Australia, Austria, Belgium, Denmark, Finland, France, Germany, New Zealand, Portugal, Singapore, Sweden, Switzerland, Thailand, The Netherlands, United Kingdom)
DACLIZUMAB
Zenapax for Injection 3046

ZENAS (Germany, Spain)
CERIVASTATIN SODIUM
Baycol Tablets 883

ZENAXIN (Mexico)
ALBENDAZOLE
Albenza Tablets 1463

ZENDHIN (Singapore)
RANITIDINE HYDROCHLORIDE
Zantac 150 EFFERdose Granules 1690
Zantac 150 EFFERdose Tablets 1690
Zantac 150 Tablets 1690
Zantac 300 Tablets 1690
Zantac Injection 1688
Zantac Injection Premixed 1688
Zantac Syrup 1690

ZENODIAN (Italy)
SUCRALFATE
Carafate Suspension 731
Carafate Tablets 730

ZENOXONE (United Kingdom)
HYDROCORTISONE
Anusol-HC Cream 2.5% 2237
Hydrocortone Tablets 2106

ZENTEL (Australia, Brazil, France, Italy, Mexico, Portugal, Singapore, South Africa, Switzerland, Thailand)
ALBENDAZOLE
Albenza Tablets 1463

ZENTROPIL (Germany)
PHENYTOIN
Dilantin Infatabs 2624
Dilantin-125 Oral Suspension 2625

ZENUSIN (Portugal, Thailand)
NIFEDIPINE
Adalat CC Tablets 877
Procardia Capsules 2708
Procardia XL Extended Release Tablets . . 2710

ZEPAN (Mexico)
DIAZEPAM
Valium Injectable 3026
Valium Tablets 3047

ZEPHOLIN (Irish Republic)
THEOPHYLLINE
Aerolate Jr. T.D. Capsules 1361
Aerolate Liquid 1361
Aerolate Sr. T.D. Capsules 1361
Theo-Dur Extended-Release Tablets 1835
Uni-Dur Extended-Release Tablets 1841
Uniphyl 400 mg and 600 mg Tablets . . . 2903

ZEPIKEN (Mexico)
CARBAMAZEPINE
Carbatrol Capsules 3234
Tegretol Chewable Tablets 2404
Tegretol Suspension 2404
Tegretol Tablets 2404
Tegretol-XR Tablets 2404

ZEPLEX (Thailand)
CEPHALEXIN
Keflex Oral Suspension 1237
Keflex Pulvules 1237

ZEPRAT (Mexico)
DIAZEPAM
Valium Injectable 3026
Valium Tablets 3047

ZERFENAZIN (Mexico)
PERPHENAZINE
Trilafon Injection 3160
Trilafon Tablets 3160

ZERIT (Australia, Austria, Belgium, Canada, Denmark, Finland, France, Germany, Hong Kong, Irish Republic, Israel, Italy, Japan, Mexico, New Zealand, Norway, Portugal, Singapore, South Africa, Spain, Sweden, Switzerland, Thailand, The Netherlands, United Kingdom)
STAVUDINE
Zerit Capsules 1147
Zerit for Oral Solution 1147

ZERITAVIR (Brazil)
STAVUDINE
Zerit Capsules 1147
Zerit for Oral Solution 1147

ZERMED (Thailand)
CETIRIZINE HYDROCHLORIDE
Zyrtec Syrup 2756
Zyrtec Tablets 2756

ZESTOMAX (South Africa)
LISINOPRIL
Prinivil Tablets 2164
Zestril Tablets 698

(⊙ Described in PDR For Ophthalmic Medicines™)

ZESTORETIC (Austria, Belgium, Brazil, Canada, Denmark, France, Hong Kong, Irish Republic, Italy, Mexico, New Zealand, Norway, Portugal, South Africa, Spain, Sweden, Switzerland, The Netherlands, United Kingdom)
HYDROCHLOROTHIAZIDE/LISINOPRIL
Prinzide Tablets . . . 2168
Zestoretic Tablets . . . 695

ZESTRIL (Australia, Belgium, Brazil, Canada, Denmark, Finland, France, Hong Kong, Irish Republic, Italy, Mexico, New Zealand, Norway, Portugal, Singapore, South Africa, Spain, Sweden, Switzerland, Thailand, The Netherlands, United Kingdom)
LISINOPRIL
Prinivil Tablets . . . 2164
Zestril Tablets . . . 698

ZETACEF (Italy)
CEPHALEXIN
Keflex Oral Suspension . . . 1237
Keflex Pulvules . . . 1237

ZETIR (Brazil)
CETIRIZINE HYDROCHLORIDE
Zyrtec Syrup . . . 2756
Zyrtec Tablets . . . 2756

ZETRON (Thailand)
ONDANSETRON HYDROCHLORIDE
Zofran Injection . . . 1698
Zofran Injection Premixed . . . 1698
Zofran Oral Solution . . . 1703
Zofran Tablets . . . 1703

ZIAGEN (Australia, Canada, Denmark, Finland, France, Germany, Israel, Italy, New Zealand, Norway, Portugal, Singapore, Sweden, Switzerland, United Kingdom)
ABACAVIR SULFATE
Ziagen Oral Solution . . . 1692
Ziagen Tablets . . . 1692

ZIDAC (France)
RANITIDINE HYDROCHLORIDE
Zantac 150 EFFERdose Granules . . . 1690
Zantac 150 EFFERdose Tablets . . . 1690
Zantac 150 Tablets . . . 1690
Zantac 300 Tablets . . . 1690
Zantac Injection . . . 1688
Zantac Injection Premixed . . . 1688
Zantac Syrup . . . 1690

ZIDA-CO (United Kingdom)
AMILORIDE HYDROCHLORIDE/HYDROCHLOROTHIAZIDE
Moduretic Tablets . . . 2138

ZIDICEF (Mexico)
CEFTAZIDIME
Ceptaz for Injection . . . 1499
Fortaz for Injection . . . 1541
Tazicef for Injection . . . 1647
Tazidime Vials, Faspak & ADD-Vantage . . 1966

ZIDOVAL (United Kingdom)
METRONIDAZOLE
MetroCream . . . 1404
MetroGel . . . 1405
MetroGel-Vaginal Gel . . . 1986
MetroLotion . . . 1405
Noritate Cream . . . 1224

ZIDOVIR (Mexico)
ZIDOVUDINE
Retrovir Capsules . . . 1625
Retrovir IV Infusion . . . 1629
Retrovir Syrup . . . 1625
Retrovir Tablets . . . 1625

ZIENAM (Austria)
CILASTATIN SODIUM/IMIPENEM
Primaxin I.M. . . . 2158
Primaxin I.V. . . . 2160

ZIFARTEL (Mexico)
PRAZIQUANTEL
Biltricide Tablets . . . 887

ZILACTIN BABY (Canada)
BENZOCAINE
Americaine Anesthetic Lubricant . . . 1162
Americaine Otic Topical Anesthetic Ear Drops . . . 1162

ZILACTIN-B (Canada)
BENZOCAINE
Americaine Anesthetic Lubricant . . . 1162
Americaine Otic Topical Anesthetic Ear Drops . . . 1162

ZILDEM (South Africa)
DILTIAZEM HYDROCHLORIDE
Cardizem CD Capsules . . . 1016
Cardizem Injectable . . . 1018
Cardizem Lyo-Ject Syringe . . . 1018
Cardizem Monovial . . . 1018
Tiazac Capsules . . . 1378

ZILDEN (Italy)
DILTIAZEM HYDROCHLORIDE
Cardizem CD Capsules . . . 1016
Cardizem Injectable . . . 1018
Cardizem Lyo-Ject Syringe . . . 1018
Cardizem Monovial . . . 1018
Tiazac Capsules . . . 1378

ZIMEROL (Mexico)
CIMETIDINE
Tagamet Tablets . . . 1644

ZIMETIN (Switzerland)
CIMETIDINE
Tagamet Tablets . . . 1644

ZIMOR (Spain)
OMEPRAZOLE
Prilosec Delayed-Release Capsules . . . 628

ZINACEF (Belgium, Brazil, Canada, Denmark, Finland, Germany, Hong Kong, Irish Republic, Israel, New Zealand, Norway, Singapore, South Africa, Sweden, Switzerland, Thailand, The Netherlands, United Kingdom)
CEFUROXIME SODIUM
Kefurox Vials, ADD-Vantage . . . 1948
Zinacef Injection . . . 1696

ZINADIUR (Italy)
BENAZEPRIL HYDROCHLORIDE/HYDROCHLOROTHIAZIDE
Lotensin HCT Tablets . . . 2367

ZINADRIL (Italy)
BENAZEPRIL HYDROCHLORIDE
Lotensin Tablets . . . 2365

ZINAMIDE (Australia, Irish Republic, New Zealand, United Kingdom)
PYRAZINAMIDE
Pyrazinamide Tablets . . . 1876

ZINAT (Switzerland)
CEFUROXIME AXETIL
Ceftin Tablets . . . 1898
Ceftin for Oral Suspension . . . 1898

ZINECARD (Canada)
DEXRAZOXANE
Zinecard for Injection . . . 2869

ZINERYT (Belgium, Irish Republic, Portugal, Spain)
ERYTHROMYCIN
Emgel 2% Topical Gel . . . 1285
Ery-Tab Tablets . . . 448
Erythromycin Base Filmtab Tablets . . . 454
Erythromycin Delayed-Release Capsules, USP . . . 455
PCE Dispertab Tablets . . . 498

ZINGA (United Kingdom)
NIZATIDINE
Axid Pulvules . . . 1903

ZINNAT (Australia, Austria, Belgium, Brazil, Denmark, Finland, Germany, Hong Kong, Irish Republic, Israel, Italy, New Zealand, Singapore, South Africa, Spain, Sweden, Thailand, The Netherlands, United Kingdom)
CEFUROXIME AXETIL
Ceftin Tablets . . . 1898
Ceftin for Oral Suspension . . . 1898

ZIPOS (Portugal)
CEFUROXIME AXETIL
Ceftin Tablets . . . 1898
Ceftin for Oral Suspension . . . 1898

ZIPRA (Mexico)
CIPROFLOXACIN HYDROCHLORIDE
Ciloxan Ophthalmic Ointment . . . 538
Ciloxan Ophthalmic Solution . . . ⊙209, 538
Cipro Tablets . . . 887

ZIRTEC (Italy)
CETIRIZINE HYDROCHLORIDE
Zyrtec Syrup . . . 2756
Zyrtec Tablets . . . 2756

ZIRTEK (Irish Republic, United Kingdom)
CETIRIZINE HYDROCHLORIDE
Zyrtec Syrup . . . 2756
Zyrtec Tablets . . . 2756

ZISPIN (Irish Republic, United Kingdom)
MIRTAZAPINE
Remeron SolTab Tablets . . . 2486

ZITA (United Kingdom)
CIMETIDINE
Tagamet Tablets . . . 1644

ZITAZONIUM (Germany, Hong Kong, Thailand)
TAMOXIFEN CITRATE
Nolvadex Tablets . . . 678

ZIZ (United Kingdom)
PROMETHAZINE HYDROCHLORIDE
Phenergan Injection . . . 3553
Phenergan Suppositories . . . 3556
Phenergan Syrup Fortis . . . 3554
Phenergan Syrup Plain . . . 3554
Phenergan Tablets . . . 3556

ZOBACIDE (South Africa)
METRONIDAZOLE
MetroCream . . . 1404
MetroGel . . . 1405
MetroGel-Vaginal Gel . . . 1986
MetroLotion . . . 1405
Noritate Cream . . . 1224

ZOCOR (Australia, Belgium, Brazil, Canada, Denmark, Finland, France, Germany, Hong Kong, Irish Republic, Italy, Mexico, New Zealand, Norway, Portugal, Singapore, South Africa, Spain, Switzerland, Thailand, The Netherlands, United Kingdom)
SIMVASTATIN
Zocor Tablets . . . 2219

ZOCORD (Austria, Sweden)
SIMVASTATIN
Zocor Tablets . . . 2219

ZOFORA (France)
PIROXICAM
Feldene Capsules . . . 2685

ZOFRAN (Australia, Belgium, Brazil, Germany, Hong Kong, Irish Republic, Israel, Italy, Mexico, New Zealand, Norway, Portugal, Singapore, South Africa, Spain, Sweden, Switzerland, The Netherlands, United Kingdom)
ONDANSETRON HYDROCHLORIDE
Zofran Injection . . . 1698
Zofran Injection Premixed . . . 1698
Zofran Oral Solution . . . 1703
Zofran Tablets . . . 1703

ZOLADEX (Australia, Austria, Belgium, Brazil, Canada, Denmark, France, Germany, Hong Kong, Irish Republic, Israel, Italy, Mexico, New Zealand, Norway, Portugal, Singapore, South Africa, Spain, Sweden, Switzerland, Thailand, The Netherlands, United Kingdom)
GOSERELIN ACETATE
Zoladex . . . 702
Zoladex 3-month . . . 706

ZOLBEN (Brazil)
ALBENDAZOLE
Albenza Tablets . . . 1463

ZOLEROL (South Africa)
METRONIDAZOLE
MetroCream . . . 1404
MetroGel . . . 1405
MetroGel-Vaginal Gel . . . 1986
MetroLotion . . . 1405
Noritate Cream . . . 1224

ZOLES (Brazil)
MEBENDAZOLE
Vermox Chewable Tablets . . . 2017

ZOLKEN (Mexico)
ITRACONAZOLE
Sporanox Capsules . . . 1800
Sporanox Oral Solution . . . 1808, 2512

ZOLOFT (Australia, Austria, Brazil, Canada, Denmark, Finland, France, Germany, Hong Kong, Italy, New Zealand, Norway, Portugal, Singapore, South Africa, Sweden, Switzerland, Thailand, The Netherlands)
SERTRALINE HYDROCHLORIDE
Zoloft Tablets . . . 2751

ZOLTEC (Brazil)
FLUCONAZOLE
Diflucan Tablets, Injection, and Oral Suspension . . . 2681

ZOLTEROL (Singapore)
DICLOFENAC SODIUM
Voltaren Tablets . . . 2315
Voltaren-XR Tablets . . . 2315

ZOL-TRIQ (Brazil)
MEBENDAZOLE
Vermox Chewable Tablets . . . 2017

ZOLTUM (France)
OMEPRAZOLE
Prilosec Delayed-Release Capsules . . . 628

ZOLVERA (United Kingdom)
VERAPAMIL HYDROCHLORIDE
Covera-HS Tablets . . . 3199
Isoptin SR Tablets . . . 467
Verelan Capsules . . . 3184
Verelan PM Capsules . . . 3186

ZOMIG (Australia, Austria, Belgium, Canada, Denmark, Finland, France, Hong Kong, Irish Republic, Israel, Italy, Mexico, Norway, Portugal, Singapore, South Africa, Spain, Sweden, Switzerland, Thailand, The Netherlands, United Kingdom)
ZOLMITRIPTAN
Zomig Tablets . . . 708

ZOMORPH (United Kingdom)
MORPHINE SULFATE
Astramorph/PF Injection, USP (Preservative-Free) . . . 594
Duramorph Injection . . . 1312
Infumorph 200 and Infumorph 500 Sterile Solutions . . . 1314
Kadian Capsules . . . 1335
MS Contin Tablets . . . 2896
MSIR Oral Capsules . . . 2898
MSIR Oral Solution . . . 2898
MSIR Oral Solution Concentrate . . . 2898
MSIR Oral Tablets . . . 2898
Oramorph SR Tablets . . . 3062
Roxanol 100 Concentrated Oral Solution . . . 3066
Roxanol Concentrated Oral Solution . . . 3066
Roxanol-T Oral Solution . . . 3066

ZON (Sweden)
KETOPROFEN
Orudis Capsules . . . 3548
Oruvail Capsules . . . 3548

ZONAL (Mexico)
FLUCONAZOLE
Diflucan Tablets, Injection, and Oral Suspension . . . 2681

ZONALON (Canada)
DOXEPIN HYDROCHLORIDE
Sinequan Capsules . . . 2713
Sinequan Oral Concentrate . . . 2713

ZONCEF (Italy)
CEFOPERAZONE SODIUM
Cefobid Intravenous/Intramuscular . . . 2671
Cefobid Pharmacy Bulk Package - Not for Direct Infusion . . . 2673

ZOPAM (Thailand)
DIAZEPAM
Valium Injectable . . . 3026
Valium Tablets . . . 3047

ZOPAX (South Africa)
ALPRAZOLAM
Xanax Tablets . . . 2865

ZORAC (Austria, Finland, France, Germany, Irish Republic, Italy, Spain, Sweden, United Kingdom)
TAZAROTENE
Tazorac Gel . . . 556

ZORAK (South Africa)
TAZAROTENE
Tazorac Gel . . . 556

ZORAN (Singapore)
RANITIDINE HYDROCHLORIDE
Zantac 150 EFFERdose Granules . . . 1690
Zantac 150 EFFERdose Tablets . . . 1690
Zantac 150 Tablets . . . 1690
Zantac 300 Tablets . . . 1690
Zantac Injection . . . 1688
Zantac Injection Premixed . . . 1688
Zantac Syrup . . . 1690

ZOREF (Italy, Portugal)
CEFUROXIME AXETIL
Ceftin Tablets . . . 1898
Ceftin for Oral Suspension . . . 1898

ZORINAX (Singapore)
KETOCONAZOLE
Nizoral 2% Cream . . . 3620
Nizoral 2% Shampoo . . . 2007
Nizoral Tablets . . . 1791

ZOROXIN (Austria, Belgium, Denmark)
NORFLOXACIN
Chibroxin Sterile Ophthalmic Solution . . . ⊙273, 2051
Noroxin Tablets . . . 2145

ZOST (Brazil)
TRIFLURIDINE
Viroptic Ophthalmic Solution Sterile . . . ⊙301

ZOTINAR (Portugal)
DESONIDE
DesOwen Cream . . . 1401
DesOwen Lotion . . . 1401
DesOwen Ointment . . . 1401

ZOTON (Australia, Irish Republic, Israel, Italy, New Zealand, United Kingdom)
LANSOPRAZOLE
Prevacid Delayed-Release Capsules **3292**

ZUK HEPAGEL, ZUK HEPASALBE (Germany)
HEPARIN SODIUM
Heparin Lock Flush Solution **3509**
Heparin Sodium Injection **3511**

ZUMALGIC (France)
TRAMADOL HYDROCHLORIDE
Ultram Tablets.................. **2600**

ZUMENON (Australia, Austria, Belgium, Finland, Portugal, Switzerland, The Netherlands, United Kingdom)
ESTRADIOL
Alora Transdermal System **3372**
Climara Transdermal System.......... **958**
Estrace Vaginal Cream **3358**
Estring Vaginal Ring **2811**
Vivelle Transdermal System **2412**
Vivelle-Dot Transdermal System....... **2416**

ZUNDEN (Italy)
PIROXICAM
Feldene Capsules................ **2685**

ZYBAN (Australia, Canada, Irish Republic, Portugal, United Kingdom)
BUPROPION HYDROCHLORIDE
Wellbutrin SR Sustained-Release Tablets. . **1684**
Wellbutrin Tablets................ **1680**
Zyban Sustained-Release Tablets **1710**

ZYDOL (Irish Republic, United Kingdom)
TRAMADOL HYDROCHLORIDE
Ultram Tablets.................. **2600**

ZYLIUM (Brazil)
RANITIDINE HYDROCHLORIDE
Zantac 150 EFFERdose Granules **1690**
Zantac 150 EFFERdose Tablets **1690**
Zantac 150 Tablets **1690**
Zantac 300 Tablets **1690**
Zantac Injection................. **1688**
Zantac Injection Premixed **1688**
Zantac Syrup **1690**

ZYMEROL (Mexico)
CIMETIDINE
Tagamet Tablets **1644**

ZYNAL (Singapore)
NAPROXEN SODIUM
Anaprox DS Tablets **2967**
Anaprox Tablets................. **2967**
Naprelan Tablets **1293**

ZYNOX (South Africa)
NALOXONE HYDROCHLORIDE
Narcan Injection................. **1322**

ZYOMET (United Kingdom)
METRONIDAZOLE
MetroCream **1404**
MetroGel **1405**
MetroGel-Vaginal Gel.............. **1986**
MetroLotion **1405**
Noritate Cream **1224**

ZYPREXA (Australia, Austria, Belgium, Canada, Denmark, Finland, France, Germany, Hong Kong, Irish Republic, Israel, Mexico, New Zealand, Norway, Portugal, Singapore, South Africa, Spain, Sweden, Switzerland, Thailand, The Netherlands, United Kingdom)
OLANZAPINE
Zyprexa Tablets................. **1973**

ZYREX (Thailand)
CETIRIZINE HYDROCHLORIDE
Zyrtec Syrup................... **2756**
Zyrtec Tablets.................. **2756**

ZYRLEX (Sweden)
CETIRIZINE HYDROCHLORIDE
Zyrtec Syrup................... **2756**
Zyrtec Tablets.................. **2756**

ZYRTEC (Australia, Austria, Belgium, Brazil, Canada, Denmark, Finland, France, Hong Kong, Israel, Mexico, New Zealand, Norway, Portugal, Singapore, South Africa, Spain, Switzerland, Thailand, The Netherlands)
CETIRIZINE HYDROCHLORIDE
Zyrtec Syrup................... **2756**
Zyrtec Tablets.................. **2756**

ZYRZINE (Thailand)
CETIRIZINE HYDROCHLORIDE
Zyrtec Syrup................... **2756**
Zyrtec Tablets.................. **2756**

SECTION 8

GENERIC AVAILABILITY GUIDE

This section allows you to quickly determine which forms and strengths of a brand-name drug are also available generically. The entries are organized alphabetically by brand name and dosage form, with strengths in ascending order. Generic availability is indicated by a mark in the "Yes" column. Included are all prescription products described in *PDR®* and *PDR for Ophthalmic Medicines™*. Generic availability information is drawn from the *Red Book® Drug Database* maintained by *PDR's* parent organization, Medical Economics Company.

STRENGTH	GENERIC YES	GENERIC NO
Abelcet Injection		
5 MG/ML		■
Accolate Tablets		
10 MG		■
20 MG		■
Accupril Tablets		
5 MG		■
10 MG		■
20 MG		■
40 MG		■
Accuretic Tablets		
12.5 MG-10 MG		■
12.5 MG-20 MG		■
25 MG-20 MG		■
Accutane Capsules		
10 MG		■
20 MG		■
40 MG		■
Accuzyme Debriding Ointment		
1.1 MILLION U-100 MG/GM	■	
Aceon Tablets (2 mg, 4 mg, 8 mg)		
2 MG		■
4 MG		■
8 MG		■
Aci-Jel Therapeutic Vaginal Jelly		
0.92%-0.025%-0.7%	■	
Aciphex Tablets		
20 MG		■
Aclovate Cream		
0.05%		■
Aclovate Ointment		
0.05%		■
ActHIB Vaccine		
10 MCG	■	
Acticin Cream		
5%	■	
Actimmune		
2 MILLION IU/0.5 ML		■
Actiq		
0.2 MG		■
0.4 MG		■
0.6 MG		■
0.8 MG		■
1.2 MG		■
1.6 MG		■
Activase I.V.		
50 MG		■
100 MG		■
Activella Tablets		
1 MG-0.5 MG		■
Actonel Tablets		
5 MG		■
30 MG		■
Actos Tablets		
15 MG		■
30 MG		■
45 MG		■
Acular Ophthalmic Solution		
0.5%		■
Acular PF Ophthalmic Solution		
0.5%		■
Adagen Injection		
250 U/ML		■
Adalat CC Tablets		
30 MG	■	
60 MG	■	
90 MG	■	
Adderall Tablets		
5 MG		■
7.5 MG		■
10 MG		■
12.5 MG		■
15 MG		■
20 MG		■
30 MG		■
Adenocard Injection		
3 MG/ML		■
Adenoscan		
3 MG/ML		■
Adipex-P Capsules		
37.5 MG	■	
Adipex-P Tablets		
37.5 MG	■	
Adriamycin PFS/RDF Injection		
2 MG/ML	■	
10 MG	■	
20 MG	■	
50 MG	■	
150 MG		■
Aerobid Inhaler System		
0.25 MG/INH		■
Aerobid-M Inhaler System		
0.25 MG/INH		■
Aerolate Jr. T.D. Capsules		
130 MG		■
Aerolate Sr. T.D. Capsules		
260 MG	■	
Agenerase Capsules		
50 MG		■
150 MG		■
Agenerase Oral Solution		
15 MG/ML		■
Aggrastat Injection		
0.05 MG/ML		■
0.25 MG/ML		■
Aggrenox Capsules		
25 MG-200 MG		■
Agrylin Capsules		
0.5 MG		■
1 MG		■
AK-Fluor Injection 10% and 25%		
10%	■	
25%	■	
Albalon Ophthalmic Solution		
0.1%	■	
Albenza Tablets		
200 MG		■
Albuminar-5, U.S.P.		
5%	■	
Albuminar-25, U.S.P.		
25%	■	
Aldara Cream, 5%		
5%		■
Aldoril Tablets		
15 MG-250 MG	■	
25 MG-250 MG	■	
Alesse-21 Tablets		
0.02 MG-0.1 MG	■	
Alesse-28 Tablets		
0.02 MG-0.1 MG	■	
Alferon N Injection		
5 MILLION IU/ML		■
Alkeran for Injection		
50 MG		■
Alkeran Tablets		
2 MG		■
Allegra Capsules		
60 MG		■
Allegra Tablets		
30 MG		■
60 MG		■
180 MG		■
Alocril Ophthalmic Solution		
2%		■
Alomide Ophthalmic Solution		
0.1%		■
Aloprim for Injection		
500 MG		■
Alora Transdermal System		
0.05 MG/24 HRS	■	
0.075 MG/24 HRS	■	
0.1 MG/24 HRS	■	
Alphagan Ophthalmic Solution		
0.2%		■
Alrex Sterile Ophthalmic Suspension 0.2%		
0.2%		■

STRENGTH	GENERIC YES	GENERIC NO
Altace Capsules		
1.25 MG		■
2.5 MG		■
5 MG		■
10 MG		■
Alupent Inhalation Aerosol		
0.65 MG/INH		■
Ambien Tablets		
5 MG		■
10 MG		■
AmBisome for Injection		
50 MG		■
Amerge Tablets		
1 MG		■
2.5 MG		■
Americaine Anesthetic Lubricant		
20%		■
Americaine Otic Topical Anesthetic Ear Drops		
20%	■	
Aminohippurate Sodium "PAH" Injection		
20%		■
Amoxil Pediatric Drops for Oral Suspension		
50 MG/ML	■	
125 MG/5 ML	■	
200 MG/5 ML		■
250 MG/5 ML	■	
400 MG/5 ML		■
Amoxil Tablets		
200 MG	■	
250 MG	■	
400 MG	■	
500 MG	■	
875 MG	■	
Anadrol-50 Tablets		
50 MG		■
Analpram HC Lotion 2.5%		
2.5%-1%	■	
Analpram-HC Rectal Cream 1% and 2.5%		
1%-1%		■
2.5%-1%		■
Anaprox Tablets		
275 MG	■	
Anaprox DS Tablets		
550 MG	■	
Ancef for Injection		
1 GM	■	
10 GM	■	
Ancobon Capsules		
250 MG		■
500 MG		■
Androderm Transdermal System CIII		
2.5 MG/24 HRS		■
5 MG/24 HRS	■	
AndroGel		
1%		■
Android Capsules, 10 mg		
10 MG	■	
Anectine Injection		
20 MG/ML	■	
Antabuse Tablets		
250 MG		■
Antivenin (Black Widow Spider Antivenin)		
6000 U		■
Antivert, Antivert/25, & Antivert/50 Tablets		
12.5 MG	■	
25 MG	■	
50 MG		■
Anusol-HC Cream 2.5%		
2.5%	■	
Anusol-HC Suppositories		
25 MG	■	
Aphthasol Oral Paste		
5%		■
Aplisol Injection		
5 TU/0.1 ML	■	
AquaMEPHYTON Injection		
1 MG/0.5 ML	■	
10 MG/ML	■	
Aquasol A Parenteral		
50,000 U/ML		■
Aralen Tablets		
500 MG	■	
Aramine Injection		
10 MG/ML		■
Aredia for Injection		
30 MG		■
90 MG		■
Aricept Tablets		
5 MG		■
10 MG		■
Arimidex Tablets		
1 MG		■
Aromasin Tablets		
25 MG		■
Arthrotec Tablets		
50 MG-0.2 MG		■
75 MG-0.2 MG		■
Asacol Delayed-Release Tablets		
400 MG		■
Astelin Nasal Spray		
137 MCG/INH		■
Astramorph/PF Injection, USP (Preservative-Free)		
0.5 MG/ML	■	
1 MG/ML	■	
Atacand Tablets		
4 MG		■
8 MG		■
16 MG		■
32 MG		■
Atarax Tablets & Syrup		
10 MG	■	
10 MG/5 ML	■	
25 MG	■	
50 MG	■	
100 MG	■	
Ativan Injection		
2 MG/ML	■	
4 MG/ML	■	
Ativan Tablets		
0.5 MG	■	
1 MG	■	
2 MG	■	
Atrovent Inhalation Aerosol		
0.018 MG/INH		■
Atrovent Inhalation Solution		
0.02%	■	
Atrovent Nasal Spray 0.03%		
0.03%		■
Atrovent Nasal Spray 0.06%		
0.06%		■
Attenuvax		
1000 TCID50		■
Augmentin Powder for Oral Suspension		
125 MG-31.25 MG		■
125 MG-31.25 MG/5 ML		■
200 MG-28.5 MG		■
200 MG-28.5 MG/5 ML		■
250 MG-62.5 MG		■
250 MG-62.5 MG/5 ML		■
400 MG-57 MG		■
400 MG-57 MG/5 ML		■
Augmentin Tablets		
250 MG-125 MG		■
500 MG-125 MG		■
875 MG-125 MG		■
Auralgan Otic Solution		
54 MG-14 MG/ML	■	
Autoplex T		
1 IU		■
Avalide Tablets		
12.5 MG-150 MG		■
12.5 MG-300 MG		■
Avandia Tablets		
2 MG		■
4 MG		■
8 MG		■
Avapro Tablets		
75 MG		■
150 MG		■
300 MG		■
AVC Cream		
15%	■	
AVC Suppositories		
1.05 GM		■
Avelox Tablets		
400 MG		■
Avita Cream		
0.025%	■	
Avita Gel		
0.025%	■	
Axid Pulvules		
150 MG		■
300 MG		■
Aygestin Tablets		
5 MG	■	
Azactam for Injection		
500 MG		■
1 GM		■
2 GM		■
Azelex Cream		
20%		■
Azopt Ophthalmic Suspension		
1%		■
Azulfidine EN-tabs Tablets		
500 MG		■
Bactrim Tablets		
400 MG-80 MG	■	
Bactrim DS Tablets		
800 MG-160 MG	■	
Bactroban Cream		
2%		■
Bactroban Nasal		
2%		■
Bactroban Ointment		
2%		■
BayRab		
150 IU/ML	■	
Bebulin VH		
1 IU	■	
Beconase Inhalation Aerosol		
0.042 MG/INH		■
Beconase AQ Nasal Spray		
0.042 MG/INH		■
Benadryl Parenteral		
50 MG/ML	■	
BeneFix for Injection		
1 IU		■
Benoquin Cream 20%		
20%		■
Betagan Liquifilm		
0.25%	■	
0.5%	■	
Betagan Liquifilm with C CAP Compliance Cap		
0.25%	■	
0.5%	■	
Betapace Tablets		
80 MG	■	
120 MG	■	
160 MG	■	
240 MG	■	
Betapace AF Tablets		
80 MG		■
120 MG		■
160 MG		■
Betimol Ophthalmic Solution		
0.25%		■
0.5%		■
Betoptic S Ophthalmic Suspension		
0.25%		■
Biaxin Filmtab Tablets		
250 MG		■
500 MG		■
Biaxin for Oral Suspension		
125 MG/5 ML		■
250 MG/5 ML		■
Biaxin XL Filmtab Tablets		
500 MG		■
Bicillin C-R 900/300 Injection		
900,000 U-300,000 U/2 ML		■
Bicillin C-R Injection		
150,000 U-150,000 U/ML		■
300,000 U-300,000 U/ML		■
Bicillin L-A Injection		
300,000 U/ML		■
600,000 U/ML	■	
Bleph-10 Ophthalmic Ointment 10%		
10%	■	
Bleph-10 Ophthalmic Solution 10%		
10%	■	
Blephamide Ophthalmic Ointment		
0.2%-10%		■
Blephamide Ophthalmic Suspension		
0.2%-10%		■
Blocadren Tablets		
5 MG	■	
10 MG	■	
20 MG	■	
Bontril Slow-Release Capsules		
105 MG	■	
Botox Purified Neurotoxin Complex		
100 U		■
Brethine Ampuls		
1 MG/ML		■
Brethine Tablets		
2.5 MG	■	
5 MG	■	
Brevibloc Injection		
10 MG/ML		■
250 MG/ML		■
Brevicon 28-Day Tablets		
35 MCG-0.5 MG	■	
Brevital Sodium for Injection, USP		
500 MG		■
2.5 GM		■
5 GM		■
Brevoxyl-4 Cleansing Lotion		
4%		■
Brevoxyl-4 Creamy Wash		
4%		■
Brevoxyl-4 Gel		
4%		■
Brevoxyl-8 Cleansing Lotion		
8%		■
Brevoxyl-8 Creamy Wash		
8%		■
Brevoxyl-8 Gel		
8%		■
Bromfed Capsules (Extended-Release)		
12 MG-120 MG	■	
Bromfed-PD Capsules (Extended-Release)		
6 MG-60 MG	■	
Buminate 5% Solution, USP		
5%	■	
Buminate 25% Solution, USP		
25%	■	
Buprenex Injectable		
0.3 MG/ML	■	
Cafcit Injection		
20 MG/ML		■
Cafcit Oral Solution		
20 MG/ML		■
Calcium Disodium Versenate Injection		
200 MG/ML		■
Captopril Tablets		
12.5 MG	■	
25 MG	■	
50 MG	■	
100 MG	■	

Strength	Generic Yes	Generic No
Carbatrol Capsules		
200 MG		■
300 MG		■
Cardene I.V.		
2.5 MG/ML		■
Cardura Tablets		
1 MG	■	
2 MG	■	
4 MG	■	
8 MG	■	
Carnitor Injection		
200 MG/ML	■	
Carnitor Tablets and Oral Solution		
100 MG/ML		■
330 MG		■
Carteolol Hydrochloride Ophthalmic Solution USP, 1%		
1%	■	
Casodex Tablets		
50 MG		■
Cataflam Tablets		
50 MG	■	
Catapres Tablets		
0.1 MG	■	
0.2 MG	■	
0.3 MG	■	
Catapres-TTS		
0.1 MG/24 HRS		■
0.2 MG/24 HRS		■
0.3 MG/24 HRS		■
Caverject Sterile Powder		
5 MCG		■
10 MCG	■	
20 MCG	■	
40 MCG	■	
Ceclor Pulvules		
250 MG	■	
500 MG	■	
Ceclor Suspension		
125 MG/5 ML	■	
187 MG/5 ML	■	
250 MG/5 ML	■	
375 MG/5 ML	■	
Ceclor CD Tablets		
375 MG		■
500 MG	■	
Cedax Capsules		
400 MG		■
Cedax Oral Suspension		
90 MG/5 ML		■
Cefizox for Intramuscular or Intravenous Use		
1 GM		■
1 GM/50 ML		■
2 GM		■
2 GM/50 ML		■
10 GM		■
Cefobid Intravenous/Intramuscular		
1 GM		■
2 GM		■
10 GM		■
Cefotan for Injection		
1 GM		■
2 GM		■
10 GM		■
Cefotan Injection		
1 GM/50 ML		■
2 GM/50 ML		■
Ceftin for Oral Suspension		
125 MG/5 ML		■
250 MG/5 ML		■
Ceftin Tablets		
125 MG		■
250 MG		■
500 MG		■
Cefzil for Oral Suspension		
125 MG/5 ML		■
250 MG/5 ML		■
Cefzil Tablets		
250 MG		■
500 MG		■
Celebrex Capsules		
100 MG		■
200 MG		■
Celestone Soluspan Injectable Suspension		
3 MG-3 MG/ML		■
Celestone Syrup		
0.6 MG/5 ML		■
Celexa Tablets		
10 MG		■
20 MG		■
40 MG		■
CellCept Capsules		
250 MG		■
CellCept Intravenous		
500 MG		■
CellCept Oral Suspension		
200 MG/ML		■
CellCept Tablets		
500 MG		■
Celontin Capsules		
150 MG		■
300 MG		■
Cenestin Tablets		
0.625 MG		■
0.9 MG		■
1.25 MG		■
Ceptaz for Injection		
1 GM	■	
2 GM	■	
10 GM		■
Cerebyx Injection		
50 MG/ML		■
Cerezyme for Injection		
200 U		■
400 U		■
Cerubidine for Injection		
20 MG	■	
Cerumenex Eardrops		
10%		■
Cervidil Vaginal Insert		
0.3 MG/HR		■
Cetacaine Topical Anesthetic		
14%-2%-2%		■
Chemet Capsules		
100 MG		■
Chirocaine Injection		
2.5 MG/ML		■
5 MG/ML		■
7.5 MG/ML		■
Chloroptic Sterile Ophthalmic Solution		
0.5%	■	
Ciloxan Ophthalmic Ointment		
0.3%		■
Ciloxan Ophthalmic Solution		
0.3%		■
Cipro I.V.		
10 MG/ML		■
200 MG/100 ML		■
400 MG/200 ML		■
Cipro I.V. Pharmacy Bulk Package		
10 MG/ML		■
200 MG/100 ML		■
400 MG/200 ML		■
Cipro Oral Suspension		
250 MG/5 ML		■
500 MG/5 ML		■
Cipro Tablets		
100 MG		■
250 MG		■
500 MG		■
750 MG		■
Cipro HC Otic Suspension		
0.2%-1%		■
Claritin Reditabs		
10 MG		■
Claritin Syrup		
5 MG/5 ML		■
Claritin Tablets		
10 MG		■
Claritin-D 12 Hour Extended Release Tablets		
5 MG-120 MG		■
Claritin-D 24 Hour Extended Release Tablets		
10 MG-240 MG		■
Cleocin Vaginal Cream		
2%		■
Cleocin Vaginal Ovules		
100 MG		■
Cleocin HCl Capsules		
75 MG		■
150 MG	■	
300 MG	■	
Cleocin Phosphate Sterile Solution		
150 MG/ML	■	
300 MG/50 ML		■
600 MG/50 ML		■
900 MG/50 ML		■
Cleocin T Topical Gel		
1%	■	
Cleocin T Topical Lotion		
1%		■
Cleocin T Topical Solution		
1%	■	
Climara Transdermal System		
0.025 MG/24 HRS	■	
0.05 MG/24 HRS	■	
0.075 MG/24 HRS	■	
0.1 MG/24 HRS	■	
Clindets Pledgets		
1%	■	
Clinoril Tablets		
150 MG	■	
200 MG	■	
Clobevate Gel		
0.05%	■	
Clorpres Tablets		
15 MG-0.1 MG	■	
15 MG-0.2 MG	■	
15 MG-0.3 MG	■	
Clozaril Tablets		
25 MG	■	
100 MG	■	
Cogentin Injection		
1 MG/ML		■
Cognex Capsules		
10 MG		■
20 MG		■
30 MG		■
40 MG		■
Colestid Tablets		
1 GM		■
Collagenase Santyl Ointment		
250 U/GM		■
Coly-Mycin M Parenteral		
150 MG	■	
Combivent Inhalation Aerosol		
0.09 MG-0.018 MG/INH		■
Combivir Tablets		
150 MG-300 MG		■
Compazine Injection		
5 MG/ML		■
Compazine Spansule Capsules		
10 MG		■
15 MG		■
Compazine Suppositories		
2.5 MG	■	
5 MG	■	
25 MG	■	
Compazine Syrup		
5 MG/5 ML		■
Compazine Tablets		
5 MG	■	
10 MG	■	
Comtan Tablets		
200 MG		■
Condylox Gel		
0.5%		■
Condylox Topical Solution		
0.5%		■
Copaxone for Injection		
20 MG		■
Cordarone Intravenous		
50 MG/ML		■
Cordarone Tablets		
200 MG	■	
Cordran Lotion		
0.05%		■
Cordran Tape		
4 MCG/CM2		■
Coreg Tablets		
3.125 MG		■
6.25 MG		■
12.5 MG		■
25 MG		■
Corlopam Injection		
10 MG/ML		■
Cormax Cream		
0.05%	■	
Cormax Ointment		
0.05%	■	
Cormax Scalp Application		
0.05%	■	
Cortifoam Rectal Foam		
10%		■
Cortrosyn for Injection		
0.25 MG		■
Corvert Injection		
0.1 MG/ML		■
Corzide 40/5 Tablets		
5 MG-40 MG		■
Corzide 80/5 Tablets		
5 MG-80 MG		■
Cosmegen for Injection		
0.5 MG		■
Coumadin for Injection		
5 MG		■
Coumadin Tablets		
1 MG	■	
2 MG	■	
2.5 MG	■	
3 MG	■	
4 MG	■	
5 MG	■	
6 MG	■	
7.5 MG	■	
10 MG	■	
Covera-HS Tablets		
180 MG		■
240 MG		■
Cozaar Tablets		
25 MG		■
50 MG		■
100 MG		■
Creon 5 Capsules		
16,600 U-5000 U-18,750 U		■
Crinone 4% Gel		
4%		■
Crinone 8% Gel		
8%		■
Crixivan Capsules		
100 MG		■
200 MG		■
333 MG		■
400 MG		■
Crolom Sterile Ophthalmic Solution USP 4%		
4%	■	
Cuprimine Capsules		
125 MG		■
250 MG		■
Curosurf Intratracheal Suspension		
80 MG/ML		■
Cutivate Cream		
0.05%		■
Cutivate Ointment		
0.005%		■
Cylert Tablets		
18.75 MG	■	
37.5 MG	■	
75 MG	■	
Cylert Chewable Tablets		
37.5 MG	■	
Cytomel Tablets		
0.005 MG		■
0.025 MG		■
0.05 MG		■
Cytotec Tablets		
100 MCG		■
200 MCG		■

STRENGTH	GENERIC YES	GENERIC NO
Cytovene Capsules		
250 MG		■
500 MG		■
Cytovene-IV		
500 MG		■
Dantrium Capsules		
25 MG		■
50 MG		■
100 MG		■
Dantrium Intravenous		
20 MG		■
Dapsone Tablets USP		
25 MG		■
100 MG		■
Daranide Tablets		
50 MG		■
Daraprim Tablets		
25 MG		■
Darvocet-N 50 Tablets		
325 MG-50 MG	■	
Darvocet-N 100 Tablets		
650 MG-100 MG	■	
Darvon Pulvules		
65 MG	■	
Darvon Compound-65 Pulvules		
389 MG-32.4 MG-65 MG	■	
Darvon-N Tablets		
100 MG		■
DaunoXome Injection		
2 MG/ML		■
Decadron Tablets		
0.5 MG	■	
0.75 MG	■	
4 MG	■	
Decadron Phosphate Injection		
4 MG/ML	■	
24 MG/ML		■
Decadron Phosphate Sterile Ophthalmic Solution		
0.1%	■	
Declomycin Tablets		
150 MG		■
300 MG		■
Delatestryl Injection		
200 MG/ML	■	
Demadex Tablets and Injection		
5 MG		■
10 MG		■
10 MG/ML		■
20 MG		■
100 MG		■
Demerol Syrup		
50 MG/5 ML	■	
Demerol Tablets		
50 MG	■	
100 MG	■	
Demser Capsules		
250 MG		■
Depacon Injection		
100 MG/ML		■
Depakene Capsules		
250 MG	■	
Depakene Syrup		
250 MG/5 ML	■	
Depakote Sprinkle Capsules		
125 MG		■
Depakote Tablets		
125 MG		■
250 MG		■
500 MG		■
Depakote ER Tablets		
500 MG		■
Depen Titratable Tablets		
250 MG		■
DepoCyt Injection		
10 MG/ML		■
Depo-Medrol Injectable Suspension		
20 MG/ML	■	
40 MG/ML	■	
80 MG/ML	■	
Depo-Provera Contraceptive Injection		
150 MG/ML		■

STRENGTH	GENERIC YES	GENERIC NO
Dermatop Emollient Cream		
0.1%		■
Desferal Vials		
500 MG		■
2 GM		■
Desmopressin Acetate Injection		
4 MCG/ML	■	
Desmopressin Acetate Rhinal Tube		
0.01%	■	
Desogen Tablets		
0.15 MG-0.03 MG	■	
DesOwen Cream		
0.05%	■	
DesOwen Lotion		
0.05%		■
DesOwen Ointment		
0.05%	■	
Desoxyn Tablets		
5 MG		■
Detrol Tablets		
1 MG		■
2 MG		■
Dexedrine Spansule Capsules		
5 MG		■
10 MG		■
15 MG		■
Dexedrine Tablets		
5 MG	■	
DextroStat Tablets		
5 MG	■	
10 MG	■	
D.H.E. 45 Injection		
1 MG/ML		■
Diabinese Tablets		
100 MG	■	
250 MG	■	
Diamox Sequels Sustained Release Capsules		
500 MG		■
Diamox Tablets		
250 MG	■	
Dibenzyline Capsules		
10 MG		■
Didronel Tablets		
200 MG		■
400 MG		■
Differin Gel		
0.1%		■
Differin Solution/Pledgets		
0.1%		■
Diflucan Tablets, Injection, and Oral Suspension		
50 MG		■
50 MG/5 ML		■
100 MG		■
150 MG		■
200 MG		■
200 MG/100 ML		■
200 MG/5 ML		■
400 MG/200 ML		■
Digibind Powder		
38 MG		■
Digitek Tablets		
0.125 MG	■	
0.25 MG	■	
Dilantin Infatabs		
50 MG		■
Dilantin Kapseals		
30 MG		■
100 MG	■	
Dilantin-125 Oral Suspension		
125 MG/5 ML	■	
Dilaudid Ampules		
1 MG/ML	■	
2 MG/ML	■	
4 MG/ML	■	
Dilaudid Injection		
1 MG/ML	■	
2 MG/ML	■	
4 MG/ML	■	
Dilaudid Multiple Dose Vials (Sterile Solution)		
1 MG/ML	■	

STRENGTH	GENERIC YES	GENERIC NO
2 MG/ML	■	
4 MG/ML	■	
Dilaudid Oral Liquid		
1 MG/ML	■	
Dilaudid Rectal Suppositories		
3 MG	■	
Dilaudid Tablets		
2 MG	■	
4 MG	■	
8 MG	■	
500 MG		■
Dilaudid-HP Injection		
10 MG/ML	■	
Dilaudid-HP Lyophilized Powder 250 mg		
250 MG		■
Diovan Capsules		
80 MG		■
160 MG		■
320 MG		■
Diovan HCT Tablets		
12.5 MG-160 MG		■
12.5 MG-80 MG		■
Dipentum Capsules		
250 MG		■
Diprivan Injectable Emulsion		
10 MG/ML	■	
Diprolene Gel 0.05%		
0.05%		■
Diprolene Lotion 0.05%		
0.05%		■
Diprolene Ointment 0.05%		
0.05%		■
Diprolene AF Cream 0.05%		
0.05%		■
Diprosone Cream		
0.05%	■	
Diprosone Lotion		
0.05%	■	
Diprosone Ointment		
0.05%	■	
Ditropan XL Extended Release Tablets		
5 MG		■
10 MG		■
15 MG		■
Diuril Oral Suspension		
250 MG/5 ML		■
Diuril Tablets		
250 MG	■	
500 MG	■	
Diuril Sodium Intravenous		
0.5 GM		■
Dobutrex Solution Vials		
12.5 MG/ML	■	
Dolobid Tablets		
250 MG	■	
500 MG	■	
Dopram Injectable		
20 MG/ML	■	
Doryx Coated Pellet Filled Capsules		
75 MG		■
100 MG	■	
Dostinex Tablets		
0.5 MG		■
Doxil Injection		
2 MG/ML		■
Drysol Solution		
20%	■	
DTIC-Dome		
200 MG	■	
Duraclon Injection		
0.1 MG/ML		■
0.5 MG/ML		■
Duragesic Transdermal System		
25 MCG/HR		■
50 MCG/HR		■

STRENGTH	GENERIC YES	GENERIC NO
75 MCG/HR		■
100 MCG/HR		■
Duricef Capsules		
500 MG	■	
Duricef Oral Suspension		
125 MG/5 ML		■
250 MG/5 ML		■
500 MG/5 ML		■
Duricef Tablets		
1 GM	■	
Dyazide Capsules		
25 MG-37.5 MG	■	
Dynabac Tablets		
250 MG		■
Dynacin Capsules		
50 MG	■	
75 MG	■	
100 MG	■	
Dyrenium Capsules		
50 MG		■
100 MG		■
EC-Naprosyn Delayed-Release Tablets		
375 MG	■	
500 MG	■	
Edecrin Tablets		
25 MG		■
50 MG		■
Edecrin Sodium Intravenous		
50 MG		■
E.E.S. 200 Liquid		
200 MG/5 ML	■	
E.E.S. 400 Liquid		
400 MG/5 ML	■	
E.E.S. 400 Filmtab Tablets		
400 MG	■	
E.E.S. Granules		
200 MG/5 ML	■	
Effexor Tablets		
25 MG		■
37.5 MG		■
50 MG		■
75 MG		■
100 MG		■
Effexor XR Capsules		
37.5 MG		■
75 MG		■
150 MG		■
Efudex Cream		
5%		■
Efudex Topical Solutions		
2%		■
5%		■
8-MOP Capsules		
10 MG		■
Eldepryl Capsules		
5 MG	■	
Eldopaque Forte 4% Cream		
4%	■	
Eldoquin Forte 4% Cream		
4%	■	
Elimite Cream		
5%	■	
Ellence Injection		
2 MG/ML		■
Elmiron Capsules		
100 MG		■
Elocon Cream 0.1%		
0.1%		■
Elocon Lotion 0.1%		
0.1%		■
Elocon Ointment 0.1%		
0.1%		■
Elspar for Injection		
10,000 IU		■
Emadine Ophthalmic Solution		
0.05%		■
Emcyt Capsules		
140 MG		■
Emgel 2% Topical Gel		
2%	■	
EMLA Cream		
2.5%-2.5%		■

STRENGTH	GENERIC YES	GENERIC NO
EMLA Anesthetic Disc		
2.5%-2.5%		■
Enbrel for Injection		
25 MG		■
Epifrin Sterile Ophthalmic Solution		
0.5%		■
1%	■	
2%	■	
EpiPen Auto-Injector		
1 MG/ML		■
EpiPen Jr. Auto-Injector		
0.5 MG/ML		■
Epivir Oral Solution		
10 MG/ML		■
Epivir Tablets		
150 MG		■
Epivir-HBV Oral Solution		
5 MG/ML		■
Epivir-HBV Tablets		
100 MG		■
Epogen for Injection		
2000 U/ML	■	
3000 U/ML	■	
4000 U/ML	■	
10,000 U/ML	■	
20,000 U/ML	■	
40,000 U/ML	■	
Ergamisol Tablets		
50 MG		■
EryPed 200 & EryPed 400		
200 MG/5 ML	■	
400 MG/5 ML		■
EryPed Drops		
100 MG/2.5 ML		■
EryPed Chewable Tablets		
200 MG		■
Ery-Tab Tablets		
250 MG	■	
333 MG	■	
500 MG		■
Erythrocin Stearate Filmtab Tablets		
250 MG	■	
500 MG	■	
Erythromycin Base Filmtab Tablets		
250 MG		■
500 MG		■
Erythromycin Delayed-Release Capsules, USP		
250 MG	■	
Esclim Transdermal System		
0.025 MG/24 HRS	■	
0.0375 MG/24 HRS	■	
0.05 MG/24 HRS	■	
0.075 MG/24 HRS	■	
0.1 MG/24 HRS	■	
Eskalith Capsules		
300 MG	■	
Eskalith CR Controlled Release Tablets		
450 MG		■
Estinyl Tablets		
0.02 MG		■
0.05 MG		■
Estrace Vaginal Cream		
0.1 MG/GM		■
Estratest Tablets		
1.25 MG-2.5 MG	■	
Estratest H.S. Tablets		
0.625 MG-1.25 MG	■	
Estring Vaginal Ring		
0.0075 MG/24 HRS		■
Ethiodol Injection		
99%		■
Ethyol for Injection		
500 MG		■
Etrafon 2-10 Tablets (2-10)		
10 MG-2 MG	■	
Etrafon Tablets (2-25)		
25 MG-2 MG	■	
Etrafon-Forte Tablets (4-25)		
25 MG-4 MG	■	
Eulexin Capsules		
125 MG	■	
Evista Tablets		
60 MG		■
Evoxac Capsules		
30 MG		■
Exelon Capsules		
1.5 MG		■
3 MG		■
4.5 MG		■
6 MG		■
Extendryl Chewable Tablets		
2 MG-1.25 MG-10 MG	■	
Extendryl SR & JR Capsules		
4 MG-1.25 MG-10 MG	■	
8 MG-2.5 MG-20 MG	■	
Extendryl Syrup		
2 MG-1.25 MG-10 MG/5 ML	■	
Factrel		
0.1 MG		■
Fareston Tablets		
60 MG		■
Feiba VH		
1 IU		■
Felbatol Oral Suspension		
600 MG/5 ML		■
Felbatol Tablets		
400 MG		■
600 MG		■
Feldene Capsules		
10 MG	■	
20 MG	■	
Femara Tablets		
2.5 MG		■
femhrt Tablets		
5 MCG-1 MG		■
Ferrlecit Injection		
62.5 MG/5 ML		■
Flexeril Tablets		
10 MG	■	
Flolan for Injection		
0.5 MG		■
1.5 MG		■
Flomax Capsules		
0.4 MG		■
Flonase Nasal Spray		
0.05 MG/INH		■
Flovent 44 mcg Inhalation Aerosol		
0.044 MG/INH		■
0.11 MG/INH		■
0.22 MG/INH		■
Flovent 110 mcg Inhalation Aerosol		
0.044 MG/INH		■
0.11 MG/INH		■
0.22 MG/INH		■
Flovent 220 mcg Inhalation Aerosol		
0.044 MG/INH		■
0.11 MG/INH		■
0.22 MG/INH		■
Flovent Diskus 50 mcg		
0.044 MG/INH		■
0.088 MG/INH		■
0.22 MG/INH		■
Flovent Diskus 100 mcg		
0.044 MG/INH		■
0.088 MG/INH		■
0.22 MG/INH		■
Flovent Diskus 250 mcg		
0.044 MG/INH		■
0.088 MG/INH		■
0.22 MG/INH		■
Flovent Rotadisk 50 mcg		
0.044 MG/INH		■
0.088 MG/INH		■
0.22 MG/INH		■
Flovent Rotadisk 100 mcg		
0.044 MG/INH		■
0.088 MG/INH		■
0.22 MG/INH		■
Flovent Rotadisk 250 mcg		
0.044 MG/INH		■
0.088 MG/INH		■
0.22 MG/INH		■
Floxin Otic Solution		
0.3%		■
Floxin Tablets		
200 MG		■
300 MG		■
400 MG		■
Flumadine Syrup		
50 MG/5 ML		■
Flumadine Tablets		
100 MG	■	
Fluorescite Injection		
10%	■	
25%	■	
Fluor-I-Strip A.T. Ophthalmic Strips 1 mg		
1 MG	■	
Fluor-I-Strip Ophthalmic Strips 9 mg		
9 MG		■
Fluoroplex Topical Cream		
1%		■
Fluoroplex Topical Solution		
1%		■
FML Ophthalmic Ointment		
0.1%		■
FML Ophthalmic Suspension		
0.1%	■	
FML Forte Ophthalmic Suspension		
0.25%		■
FML-S Liquifilm Sterile Ophthalmic Suspension		
0.1%-10%		■
Follistim for Injection		
75 IU		■
Fortaz for Injection		
500 MG	■	
1 GM	■	
1 GM/50 ML		■
2 GM	■	
2 GM/50 ML		■
6 GM	■	
Fortovase Capsules		
200 MG		■
Fosamax Tablets		
5 MG		■
10 MG		■
35 MG		■
40 MG		■
70 MG		■
Foscavir Injection		
24 MG/ML		■
Fragmin Injection		
2500 IU/0.2 ML		■
5000 IU/0.2 ML		■
10,000 IU/ML		■
Sterile FUDR		
0.5 GM	■	
Furosemide Tablets		
20 MG	■	
40 MG	■	
80 MG	■	
Gabitril Tablets		
2 MG		■
4 MG		■
12 MG		■
16 MG		■
Gamimune N, 5% Solvent/Detergent Treated		
50 MG/ML	■	
Gamimune N, 10% Solvent/Detergent Treated		
100 MG/ML	■	
Gammagard S/D		
0.5 GM		■
2.5 GM	■	
5 GM	■	
10 GM	■	
Gammar-P I.V.		
1 GM	■	
2.5 GM	■	
5 GM	■	
10 GM	■	
Gastrocrom Oral Concentrate		
100 MG/5 ML		■
Gebauer's Ethyl Chloride		
100%	■	
Gemzar for Injection		
200 MG		■
1 GM		■
Gengraf Capsules		
25 MG	■	
100 MG	■	
Genoptic Sterile Ophthalmic Solution		
3 MG/ML	■	
Genotropin Lyophilized Powder		
1.5 MG		■
5.8 MG		■
13.8 MG		■
Geocillin Tablets		
382 MG		■
Geref for Injection		
0.5 MG		■
1 MG		■
GlucaGen for Injection Diagnostic Kit		
1 MG	■	
Glucagon for Injection Vials and Emergency Kit		
1 MG	■	
Glucophage Tablets		
500 MG		■
850 MG		■
1000 MG		■
Glucotrol Tablets		
5 MG	■	
10 MG	■	
Glucotrol XL Extended Release Tablets		
2.5 MG		■
5 MG		■
10 MG		■
Glyset Tablets		
25 MG		■
50 MG		■
100 MG		■
Gonal-F for Injection		
37.5 IU		■
75 IU		■
150 IU		■
1200 IU		■
Gordochom Solution		
3%-25%	■	
Grifulvin V Tablets Microsize and Oral Suspension Microsize		
125 MG/5 ML		■
500 MG	■	
Guaifed Capsules		
250 MG-120 MG	■	
Guaifed-PD Capsules		
300 MG-60 MG	■	
Halcion Tablets		
0.125 MG		■
0.25 MG		■
Haldol Decanoate 50 Injection		
50 MG/ML	■	
Haldol Decanoate 100 Injection		
100 MG/ML	■	
Haldol Injection, Tablets and Concentrate		
5 MG/ML	■	
Havrix Vaccine		
1440 EL U/ML		■
Helixate Concentrate		
1 IU	■	
Hemofil M		
1 IU	■	
Herceptin I.V.		
440 MG		■
Hexalen Capsules		
50 MG		■
HibTITER		
10 MCG	■	
100 MCG		■
Hivid Tablets		
0.375 MG		■

STRENGTH	GENERIC YES	GENERIC NO
0.75 MG		■
HMS Sterile Ophthalmic Suspension		
1%		■
Humalog		
100 U/ML		■
Humalog Mix 75/25 Pen		
75 U-25 U/ML		■
Humate-P Concentrate		
1 IU-1 IU		■
Humatrope Vials and Cartridges		
5 MG	■	
6 MG		■
12 MG		■
24 MG		■
Humegon for Injection		
75 IU	■	
Humulin 70/30 Pen		
70 U-30 U/ML	■	
Humulin N NPH Pen		
100 U/ML	■	
Humulin R Regular (U-500)		
500 U/ML		■
Hyalgan Solution		
10 MG/ML	■	
Hycamtin for Injection		
4 MG		■
Hycodan Syrup		
1.5 MG-5 MG/5 ML	■	
Hycodan Tablets		
1.5 MG-5 MG	■	
Hydrocortone Tablets		
10 MG	■	
Hydrocortone Phosphate Injection, Sterile		
50 MG/ML		■
HydroDIURIL Tablets		
25 MG	■	
Hytrin Capsules		
1 MG	■	
2 MG	■	
5 MG	■	
10 MG	■	
IC-Green		
25 MG		■
Idamycin PFS Injection		
1 MG/ML		■
Ifex for Injection		
1 GM		■
3 GM		■
Imdur Tablets		
30 MG	■	
60 MG	■	
120 MG	■	
Imitrex Injection		
6 MG/0.5 ML		■
Imitrex Nasal Spray		
5 MG		■
20 MG		■
Imitrex Tablets		
25 MG		■
50 MG		■
100 MG		■
Imogam Rabies - HT		
150 IU/ML	■	
Imovax Rabies Vaccine		
2.5 IU	■	
Indapamide Tablets		
1.25 MG	■	
2.5 MG	■	
Inderal Injectable		
1 MG/ML	■	
Inderal Tablets		
10 MG	■	
20 MG	■	
40 MG	■	
60 MG	■	
80 MG	■	
Inderal LA Long-Acting Capsules		
60 MG		■
80 MG		■
120 MG		■
160 MG		■
Inderide Tablets		
25 MG-40 MG	■	
25 MG-80 MG	■	
Indocin Capsules		
25 MG	■	
50 MG	■	
Indocin I.V.		
1 MG		■
Indocin Oral Suspension		
25 MG/5 ML	■	
Infasurf Intratracheal Suspension		
35 MG/ML		■
INFeD Injection		
50 MG/ML	■	
Infergen		
30 MCG/ML		■
Integrilin Injection		
0.75 MG/ML		■
2 MG/ML		■
Intron A for Injection		
3 MILLION IU		■
3 MILLION IU/0.2 ML		■
3 MILLION IU/0.5 ML		■
5 MILLION IU		■
5 MILLION IU/0.2 ML		■
5 MILLION IU/0.5 ML		■
6 MILLION IU/ML		■
10 MILLION IU		■
10 MILLION IU/0.2 ML		■
10 MILLION IU/ML		■
18 MILLION IU		■
25 MILLION IU		■
50 MILLION IU		■
Invirase Capsules		
200 MG		■
Ionamin Capsules		
15 MG		■
30 MG		■
Iopidine Ophthalmic Solution		
0.5%		■
1%		■
Iopidine Sterile Ophthalmic Solution		
0.5%		■
1%		■
IPOL Vaccine		
80 D ANTIGEN U/0.5 ML		■
Ismo Tablets		
20 MG	■	
Isoptin SR Tablets		
120 MG	■	
180 MG	■	
240 MG	■	
Isopto Carbachol Ophthalmic Solution		
0.75%		■
1.5%		■
2.25%		■
3%		■
Isopto Carpine Ophthalmic Solution		
1%	■	
2%	■	
4%	■	
6%	■	
8%		■
Isordil Sublingual Tablets		
2.5 MG	■	
5 MG	■	
10 MG		■
Isordil Titradose Tablets		
5 MG	■	
10 MG	■	
20 MG	■	
30 MG	■	
40 MG	■	
Kadian Capsules		
20 MG		■
30 MG		■
50 MG		■
60 MG		■
100 MG		■
Kaletra Capsules		
133.3 MG-33.3 MG		■
Kaletra Oral Solution		
80 MG-20 MG/ML		■
K-Dur Microburst Release System ER Tablets		
10 MEQ	■	
20 MEQ	■	
Keflex Pulvules		
250 MG	■	
500 MG	■	
Kefurox Vials, ADD-Vantage		
750 MG	■	
1.5 GM	■	
7.5 GM	■	
Kefzol Vials, ADD-Vantage		
1 GM	■	
10 GM	■	
Keppra Tablets		
250 MG		■
500 MG		■
750 MG		■
Klaron Lotion 10%		
10%	■	
Klonopin Tablets		
0.5 MG	■	
1 MG	■	
2 MG	■	
K-Lor Powder Packets		
20 MEQ	■	
Koate-DVI		
1 IU	■	
Koate-HP		
1 IU	■	
Kogenate		
1 IU	■	
Kogenate FS		
1 IU	■	
Konyne 80		
1 IU	■	
K-Phos Neutral Tablets		
155 MG-852 MG-130 MG	■	
K-Phos Original (Sodium Free) Tablets		
500 MG		■
Kristalose for Oral Solution		
10 GM/PACKET		■
20 GM/PACKET		■
Kronofed-A Kronocaps		
8 MG-120 MG	■	
Kronofed-A-Jr. Kronocaps		
4 MG-60 MG	■	
K-Tab Filmtab Tablets		
10 MEQ	■	
Lacrisert Sterile Ophthalmic Insert		
5 MG		■
Lamictal Tablets		
25 MG		■
100 MG		■
150 MG		■
200 MG		■
Lamictal Chewable Dispersible Tablets		
5 MG		■
25 MG		■
Lamisil Tablets		
250 MG		■
Lanoxicaps Capsules		
0.05 MG		■
0.1 MG		■
0.2 MG		■
Lanoxin Injection		
0.25 MG/ML	■	
Lanoxin Tablets		
0.125 MG	■	
0.25 MG	■	
Lanoxin Elixir Pediatric		
0.05 MG/ML	■	
Lanoxin Injection Pediatric		
0.1 MG/ML	■	
Lariam Tablets		
250 MG		■
Lescol Capsules		
20 MG		■
40 MG		■
Leukeran Tablets		
2 MG		■
Leukine		
250 MCG		■
500 MCG/ML		■
Leustatin Injection		
1 MG/ML	■	
Levaquin Injection		
5 MG/ML		■
25 MG/ML		■
Levaquin Tablets		
250 MG		■
500 MG		■
750 MG		■
Levbid Extended-Release Tablets		
0.375 MG	■	
Levlen 21 Tablets		
30 MCG-0.15 MG	■	
Levlen 28 Tablets		
30 MCG-0.15 MG	■	
Levlite 28 Tablets		
0.02 MG-0.1 MG	■	
Levo-Dromoran Injectable		
2 MG/ML		■
Levora Tablets		
30 MCG-0.15 MG	■	
Levorphanol Tartrate Tablets		
2 MG		■
Levothroid Tablets		
0.025 MG	■	
0.05 MG	■	
0.075 MG	■	
0.088 MG	■	
0.1 MG	■	
0.112 MG	■	
0.125 MG	■	
0.137 MG	■	
0.15 MG	■	
0.175 MG	■	
0.2 MG	■	
0.3 MG	■	
Levoxyl Tablets		
0.025 MG	■	
0.05 MG	■	
0.075 MG	■	
0.088 MG	■	
0.1 MG	■	
0.112 MG	■	
0.125 MG	■	
0.137 MG	■	
0.15 MG	■	
0.175 MG	■	
0.2 MG	■	
0.3 MG	■	
Levsin Drops		
0.125 MG/ML	■	
Levsin Elixir		
0.125 MG/5 ML	■	
Levsin Injection		
0.5 MG/ML		■
Levsin Tablets		
0.125 MG	■	
Levsin/SL Tablets		
0.125 MG	■	
Levsinex Timecaps		
0.375 MG	■	
Lexxel Tablets		
5 MG-2.5 MG		■
5 MG-5 MG		■
Librium Capsules		
5 MG	■	
10 MG	■	
25 MG	■	
Librium for Injection		
100 MG		■
Lidex Cream		
0.05%	■	
Lidex Gel		
0.05%	■	
Lidex Ointment		
0.05%	■	
Lidex Topical Solution		
0.05%	■	
Lidex-E Cream		
0.05%	■	
Lidoderm Patch		
5%		■

STRENGTH	GENERIC YES	GENERIC NO
Limbitrol Tablets		
12.5 MG-5 MG	■	
Limbitrol DS Tablets		
25 MG-10 MG	■	
Lindane Lotion USP 1%		
1%	■	
Lindane Shampoo USP 1%		
1%	■	
Lipitor Tablets		
10 MG		■
20 MG		■
40 MG		■
80 MG		■
Lithium Carbonate Capsules		
150 MG		■
300 MG	■	
300 MG		■
600 MG		■
Lithium Citrate Syrup		
300 MG/5 ML	■	
Lithobid Slow-Release Tablets		
300 MG		■
Livostin		
0.05%		■
Locoid Cream		
0.1%		■
Locoid Lipocream Cream		
0.1%		■
Locoid Ointment		
0.1%		■
Locoid Topical Solution		
0.1%		■
Lodine Capsules		
200 MG	■	
300 MG	■	
Lodine Tablets		
400 MG	■	
500 MG	■	
Lodine XL Extended-Release Tablets		
400 MG	■	
500 MG	■	
600 MG	■	
Loestrin 21 Tablets		
20 MCG-1 MG	■	
30 MCG-1.5 MG	■	
Loestrin Fe Tablets		
20 MCG-1 MG	■	
30 MCG-1.5 MG	■	
Lo/Ovral Tablets		
30 MCG-0.3 MG	■	
Lo/Ovral-28 Tablets		
30 MCG-0.3 MG	■	
Lopid Tablets		
600 MG	■	
Loprox Cream		
0.77%		■
Loprox Lotion		
0.77%		■
Lorabid Suspension and Pulvules		
100 MG/5 ML		■
200 MG		■
200 MG/5 ML		■
400 MG		■
Lortab Elixir		
500 MG-7.5 MG/15 ML	■	
Lotemax Sterile Ophthalmic Suspension 0.5%		
0.5%		■
Lotrel Capsules		
2.5 MG-10 MG		■
5 MG-10 MG		■
5 MG-20 MG		■
Lotrimin Cream 1%		
1%	■	
Lotrimin Lotion 1%		
1%		■
Lotrimin Topical Solution 1%		
1%	■	
Lotrisone Cream		
0.5 MG-10 MG/GM	■	
Low-Ogestrel-28 Tablets		
30 MCG-0.3 MG	■	
Loxitane Capsules		
5 MG	■	
10 MG	■	
25 MG	■	
50 MG	■	
Lufyllin Tablets		
200 MG	■	
Lufyllin-400 Tablets		
400 MG	■	
Lufyllin-GG Elixir		
100 MG-100 MG/15 ML	■	
Lufyllin-GG Tablets		
200 MG-200 MG	■	
Lupron Injection		
5 MG/ML	■	
Lupron Depot 3.75 mg		
3.75 MG		■
Lupron Depot 7.5 mg		
7.5 MG		■
Lupron Depot--3 Month 11.25 mg		
11.25 MG		■
Lupron Depot--3 Month 22.5 mg		
22.5 MG		■
Lupron Depot--4 Month 30 mg		
30 MG		■
Lupron Depot-PED 7.5 mg, 11.25 mg and 15 mg		
7.5 MG		■
11.25 MG		■
15 MG		■
Lustra Cream		
4%	■	
Lustra-AF Cream		
4%	■	
Luvox Tablets (25, 50, 100 mg)		
25 MG	■	
50 MG	■	
100 MG	■	
Luxiq Foam		
0.12%		■
LYMErix Vaccine		
0.03 MG/0.5 ML		■
Macrobid Capsules		
100 MG		■
Macrodantin Capsules		
25 MG		■
50 MG	■	
100 MG	■	
Malarone Tablets		
250 MG-100 MG		■
Malarone Pediatric Tablets		
62.5 MG-25 MG		■
Mandol Vials		
1 GM		■
2 GM		■
Marinol Capsules		
2.5 MG		■
5 MG		■
10 MG		■
Matulane Capsules		
50 MG		■
Mavik Tablets		
1 MG		■
2 MG		■
4 MG		■
Maxair Inhaler		
0.2 MG/INH		■
Maxalt Tablets		
5 MG		■
10 MG		■
Maxalt-MLT Orally Disintegrating Tablets		
5 MG		■
10 MG		■
Maxzide Tablets		
25 MG-37.5 MG	■	
50 MG-75 MG	■	
Maxzide-25 mg Tablets		
25 MG-37.5 MG	■	
50 MG-75 MG	■	
Mefoxin for Injection		
1 GM	■	
2 GM	■	
10 GM	■	
Mefoxin Premixed Intravenous Solution		
1 GM/50 ML		■
2 GM/50 ML		■
Megace Oral Suspension		
40 MG/ML	■	
Melanex Topical Solution		
3%	■	
Menest Tablets		
0.3 MG	■	
0.625 MG	■	
1.25 MG		■
2.5 MG		■
Menomune-A/C/Y/W-135 Vaccine		
0.05 MG		■
0.25 MG		■
0.5 MG		■
Mentax Cream		
1%		■
Mephyton Tablets		
5 MG		■
Mepron Suspension		
750 MG/5 ML		■
Meridia Capsules		
5 MG		■
10 MG		■
15 MG		■
Merrem I.V.		
500 MG		■
1 GM		■
Meruvax II		
1000 TCID50		■
Mestinon Syrup		
60 MG/5 ML		■
Mestinon Tablets		
60 MG		■
Metadate ER Tablets		
10 MG	■	
20 MG	■	
Methylin Tablets		
5 MG	■	
10 MG	■	
20 MG	■	
MetroCream		
0.75%		■
MetroGel		
0.75%		■
MetroGel-Vaginal Gel		
0.75%		■
MetroLotion		
0.75%		■
Mevacor Tablets		
10 MG		■
20 MG		■
40 MG		■
Mexitil Capsules		
150 MG	■	
200 MG	■	
250 MG	■	
Miacalcin Injection		
200 IU/ML	■	
Miacalcin Nasal Spray		
200 IU/INH		■
Micardis Tablets		
20 MG		■
40 MG		■
80 MG		■
Micro-K Extencaps		
8 MEQ	■	
Micro-K 10 Extencaps		
10 MEQ	■	
Micronor Tablets		
0.35 MG	■	
Microzide Capsules		
12.5 MG	■	
Midamor Tablets		
5 MG	■	
Midrin Capsules		
325 MG-100 MG-65 MG	■	
Migranal Nasal Spray		
0.5 MG/INH		■
Miltown Tablets		
200 MG	■	
400 MG	■	
Minipress Capsules		
1 MG	■	
2 MG	■	
5 MG	■	
Minizide Capsules		
0.5 MG-1 MG		■
0.5 MG-2 MG		■
0.5 MG-5 MG		■
Minocin Intravenous		
100 MG		■
Minocin Pellet-Filled Capsules		
50 MG	■	
100 MG	■	
Mintezol Suspension		
500 MG/5 ML		■
Mintezol Chewable Tablets		
500 MG		■
Miochol-E with Steri-Tags		
20 MG		■
Mirapex Tablets		
0.125 MG		■
0.25 MG		■
0.5 MG		■
1 MG		■
1.5 MG		■
Mithracin for Intravenous Use		
2.5 MG		■
Moban Oral Concentrate		
20 MG/ML		■
Moban Tablets		
5 MG		■
10 MG		■
25 MG		■
50 MG		■
100 MG		■
Modicon 28 Tablets		
35 MCG-0.5 MG	■	
Moduretic Tablets		
5 MG-50 MG	■	
Monoclate-P Concentrate		
1 IU		■
Monodox Capsules		
50 MG	■	
100 MG	■	
Mononine Concentrate		
1 IU		■
Monopril Tablets		
10 MG		■
20 MG		■
40 MG		■
Monurol Sachet		
3 GM		■
Motofen Tablets		
0.025 MG-1 MG		■
Motrin Suspension, Oral Drops, Chewable Tablets, and Caplets		
100 MG/5 ML	■	
MS Contin Tablets		
15 MG	■	
30 MG	■	
60 MG	■	
100 MG	■	
200 MG	■	
MSIR Oral Capsules		
15 MG		■
30 MG		■
MSIR Oral Solution		
10 MG/5 ML	■	
20 MG/ML	■	
MSIR Oral Solution Concentrate		
10 MG/5 ML	■	
20 MG/ML	■	
MSIR Oral Tablets		
15 MG	■	
30 MG	■	

STRENGTH	GENERIC YES	GENERIC NO
Mumpsvax		
20,000 TCID50		■
MUSE Urethral Suppository		
125 MCG		■
250 MCG		■
500 MCG		■
1000 MCG		■
Mustargen for Injection		
10 MG		■
Myambutol Tablets		
100 MG	■	
400 MG	■	
Mycelex Troche		
10 MG		■
Mycobutin Capsules		
150 MG		■
Mykrox Tablets		
0.5 MG		■
Myleran Tablets		
2 MG		■
Mylotarg for Injection		
5 MG		■
Nadolol Tablets		
20 MG	■	
40 MG	■	
80 MG	■	
Naftin Cream		
1%		■
Naftin Gel		
1%		■
Naprelan Tablets		
375 MG		■
500 MG		■
Naprosyn Suspension		
25 MG/ML	■	
Naprosyn Tablets		
250 MG	■	
375 MG	■	
500 MG	■	
Narcan Injection		
0.02 MG/ML	■	
0.4 MG/ML	■	
1 MG/ML	■	
Nardil Tablets		
15 MG		■
Naropin Injection		
2 MG/ML		■
5 MG/ML		■
7.5 MG/ML		■
10 MG/ML		■
Nasalide Nasal Spray		
0.025 MG/INH	■	
Nasarel Nasal Solution 0.025%		
0.025 MG/INH	■	
Nascobal Gel		
500 MCG/0.1 ML		■
Nasonex Nasal Spray		
0.05 MG/INH		■
Natacyn Antifungal Ophthalmic Suspension		
5%		■
Navane Capsules		
1 MG	■	
2 MG	■	
5 MG	■	
10 MG	■	
20 MG	■	
Navelbine Injection		
10 MG/ML		■
Nebcin Vials, Hyporets & ADD-Vantage		
40 MG/ML	■	
1.2 GM		■
Necon 0.5/35 Tablets		
35 MCG-0.5 MG	■	
Necon 1/50 Tablets		
0.05 MG-1 MG	■	
Necon 1/35 Tablets		
35 MCG-1 MG	■	
Necon 10/11 Tablets		
35 MCG-0.5 MG AND 1 MG	■	
Nembutal Sodium Solution		
50 MG/ML	■	
NeoDecadron Sterile Ophthalmic Solution		
1 MG-3.5 MG/ML	■	
Neoral Soft Gelatin Capsules		
25 MG	■	
100 MG	■	
Neoral Oral Solution		
100 MG/ML		■
Neosporin G.U. Irrigant Sterile		
40 MG-200,000 U/ML	■	
Neptazane Tablets		
25 MG	■	
50 MG	■	
Nesacaine Injection		
1%		■
2%	■	
Nesacaine-MPF Injection		
2%	■	
3%	■	
Neumega for Injection		
5 MG		■
Neupogen for Injection		
300 MCG/0.5 ML		■
300 MCG/ML		■
480 MCG/0.8 ML		■
480 MCG/1.6 ML		■
Neurontin Capsules		
100 MG		■
300 MG		■
400 MG		■
Niaspan Extended-Release Tablets		
500 MG		■
750 MG		■
1000 MG		■
Nicotrol Inhaler		
4 MG/INH		■
Nimotop Capsules		
30 MG		■
Nipent for Injection		
10 MG		■
Nitro-Dur Transdermal Infusion System		
0.1 MG/HR	■	
0.2 MG/HR	■	
0.3 MG/HR		■
0.4 MG/HR	■	
0.6 MG/HR	■	
0.8 MG/HR	■	
Nitrolingual Pumpspray		
0.4 MG/SPRAY		■
Nitrostat Tablets		
0.3 MG	■	
0.4 MG	■	
0.6 MG	■	
Nizoral 2% Cream		
2%	■	
Nizoral 2% Shampoo		
2%		■
Nizoral Tablets		
200 MG	■	
Nolvadex Tablets		
10 MG		■
20 MG		■
Norco Tablets CIII		
325 MG-10 MG	■	
325 MG-5 MG		■
325 MG-7.5 MG		■
Norcuron for Injection		
10 MG	■	
Nordette-28 Tablets		
30 MCG-0.15 MG	■	
Norditropin for Injection		
4 MG	■	
8 MG		■
Norflex Extended-Release Tablets		
100 MG	■	
Norflex Injection		
30 MG/ML	■	
Norinyl 1 + 35 28-Day Tablets		
35 MCG-1 MG	■	
Norinyl 1 + 50 28-Day Tablets		
0.05 MG-1 MG	■	
Noritate Cream		
1%		■
Normodyne Injection		
5 MG/ML	■	
Normodyne Tablets		
100 MG	■	
200 MG	■	
300 MG	■	
Noroxin Tablets		
400 MG		■
Norplant System		
36 MG/IMPLANT		■
Nor-QD Tablets		
0.35 MG	■	
Norvasc Tablets		
2.5 MG		■
5 MG		■
10 MG		■
Norvir Capsules		
100 MG		■
Norvir Oral Solution		
80 MG/ML		■
Novantrone for Injection		
2 MG/ML		■
Novarel for Injection		
10,000 U	■	
NovoSeven		
1.2 MG		■
4.8 MG		■
Nubain Injection		
10 MG/ML	■	
20 MG/ML	■	
Numorphan Injection		
1 MG/ML		■
1.5 MG/ML		■
Numorphan Suppositories		
5 MG		■
Nutropin for Injection		
5 MG	■	
10 MG		■
Nutropin AQ Injection		
5 MG/ML		■
Nutropin Depot for Injectable Suspension		
13.5 MG		■
18 MG		■
22.5 MG		■
Nystop Topical Powder USP		
100,000 U/GM	■	
Ocucoat		
0.1%-0.8%		
Ocufen Ophthalmic Solution		
0.03%	■	
Ocuflox Ophthalmic Solution		
0.3%		■
Ocupress Ophthalmic Solution, 1% Sterile		
1%	■	
Ogen Tablets		
0.75 MG	■	
1.5 MG	■	
3 MG	■	
Ogestrel 0.5/50-28 Tablets		
50 MCG-0.5 MG	■	
Omnicef Capsules		
300 MG		■
Omnicef for Oral Suspension		
125 MG/5 ML		■
Opticrom Ophthalmic Solution		
4%	■	
OptiPranolol Metipranolol Ophthalmic Solution 0.3%		
0.3%	■	
Optivar Ophthalmic Solution		
0.05%		■
Oramorph SR Tablets		
15 MG	■	
30 MG	■	
60 MG	■	
100 MG	■	
Orap Tablets		
1 MG		■
2 MG		■
Organidin NR Liquid		
100 MG/5 ML	■	
Organidin NR Tablets		
200 MG	■	
Orgaran Injection		
750 ANTI XA U/0.6 ML		■
Ortho-Cept 28 Tablets		
0.15 MG-0.03 MG	■	
Orthoclone OKT3 Sterile Solution		
1 MG/ML		■
Ortho-Cyclen 28 Tablets		
35 MCG-0.25 MG		■
Ortho-Est Tablets		
0.75 MG	■	
1.5 MG	■	
Ortho-Novum 1/35 28 Tablets		
35 MCG-1 MG	■	
Ortho-Novum 1/50 28 Tablets		
0.05 MG-1 MG	■	
Ortho-Novum 7/7/7 28 Tablets		
35 MCG-0.5, 0.75 AND 1MG		■
Ortho-Novum 10/11 28 Tablets		
35 MCG-0.5 MG AND 1 MG	■	
Orudis Capsules		
25 MG	■	
Oruvail Capsules		
100 MG	■	
150 MG	■	
200 MG	■	
Ovcon 35 Tablets		
35 MCG-0.4 MG		■
Ovcon 50 Tablets		
50 MCG-1 MG		■
Ovide Lotion		
0.5%		■
Ovral Tablets		
50 MCG-0.5 MG		■
Ovral-28 Tablets		
50 MCG-0.5 MG	■	
Ovrette Tablets		
0.075 MG		■
Oxandrin Tablets		
2.5 MG		■
Oxistat Cream		
1%		■
Oxistat Lotion		
1%		■
Oxsoralen Lotion 1%		
1%		■
Oxsoralen-Ultra Capsules		
10 MG		■
OxyContin Tablets		
10 MG		■
20 MG		■
40 MG		■
80 MG		■
160 MG		■
OxyFast Oral Concentrate Solution		
20 MG/ML	■	
OxyIR Capsules		
5 MG	■	
Pacerone Tablets		
200 MG	■	
400 MG	■	
Panafil Ointment		
0.5%-10%-10%	■	
Pancrease Capsules		
20,000 U-4500 U-25,000 U	■	
Pancrease MT Capsules		
12,000 U-4000 U-12,000 U	■	
Panhematin for Injection		
313 MG		■
Parafon Forte DSC Caplets		
500 MG		■

STRENGTH	GENERIC YES	GENERIC NO
1 MG		■
5 MG		■
5 MG/ML		■
Paraplatin for Injection		
50 MG		■
150 MG		■
450 MG		■
Parnate Tablets		
10 MG		■
Paser Granules		
4 GM/PACKET		■
Patanol Ophthalmic Solution		
0.1%		■
Paxil Oral Suspension		
10 MG/5 ML		■
Paxil Tablets		
10 MG		■
20 MG		■
30 MG		■
40 MG		■
PCE Dispertab Tablets		
333 MG		■
500 MG		■
Pediapred Oral Solution		
5 MG/5 ML		■
Pediazole Suspension		
200 MG-600 MG/5 ML	■	
Liquid PedvaxHIB		
7.5 MCG/0.5 ML	■	
Penlac Nail Lacquer, Topical Solution		
8%		■
Pentasa Capsules		
250 MG		■
Pepcid Injection		
0.4 MG/ML	■	
10 MG/ML	■	
Pepcid Injection Premixed		
0.4 MG/ML	■	
10 MG/ML	■	
Pepcid for Oral Suspension		
40 MG/5 ML		■
Pepcid Tablets		
20 MG	■	
40 MG	■	
Percocet Tablets		
325 MG-2.5 MG		■
325 MG-5 MG	■	
500 MG-7.5 MG	■	
650 MG-10 MG	■	
Percodan Tablets		
325 MG-4.5 MG-0.38 MG	■	
Percolone Tablets		
5 MG	■	
Pergonal for Injection		
75 IU	■	
Periactin Tablets		
4 MG	■	
Permapen Isoject		
600,000 U/ML	■	
Permax Tablets		
0.05 MG		■
0.25 MG		■
1 MG		■
Persantine Tablets		
25 MG	■	
50 MG	■	
75 MG	■	
Pfizerpen for Injection		
5 MILLION U	■	
20 MILLION U	■	
Phenergan Injection		
25 MG/ML	■	
50 MG/ML	■	
Phenergan Suppositories		
12.5 MG		■
25 MG		■
50 MG	■	
Phenergan Tablets		
12.5 MG	■	
25 MG	■	
50 MG	■	
Phenergan with Codeine Syrup		
10 MG-6.25 MG/5 ML	■	
PhosLo Tablets		
667 MG		■
Photofrin for Injection		
75 MG		■
Phrenilin Tablets		
325 MG-50 MG	■	
Phrenilin Forte Capsules		
650 MG-50 MG	■	
Pilopine HS Ophthalmic Gel		
4%		■
Pima Syrup		
325 MG/5 ML		■
Pipracil		
2 GM		■
3 GM		■
4 GM		■
Plaquenil Tablets		
200 MG	■	
Plasbumin-5		
5%		■
Plasbumin-20		
20%		■
Plasbumin-25		
25%	■	
Plasmanate		
5%	■	
Plavix Tablets		
75 MG		■
Plendil Extended-Release Tablets		
2.5 MG		■
5 MG		■
10 MG		■
Pletal Tablets		
50 MG		■
100 MG		■
Plexion Cleanser		
10%-5%	■	
Plexion Topical Suspension		
10%-5%	■	
Pneumovax 23		
575 MCG/0.5 ML	■	
Pnu-Imune 23		
575 MCG/0.5 ML	■	
Podocon-25 Liquid		
75%-25%	■	
Polocaine Injection, USP		
1%	■	
2%	■	
3%		■
Polocaine-MPF Injection, USP		
1%	■	
1.5%	■	
2%	■	
Polytrim Ophthalmic Solution		
10,000 U-1 MG/ML	■	
Ponstel Capsules		
250 MG		■
Potaba Powder		
2 GM/PACKET	■	
Potaba Tablets		
0.5 GM	■	
Pramosone Cream 1% and 2.5%		
1%-1%	■	
2.5%-1%	■	
Pramosone Lotion 1% and 2.5%		
1%-1%	■	
2.5%-1%	■	
Pramosone Ointment 1% and 2.5%		
1%-1%		■
2.5%-1%		■
Prandin Tablets (0.5, 1, and 2 mg)		
0.5 MG		■
1 MG		■
2 MG		■
Pravachol Tablets		
10 MG		■
20 MG		■
40 MG		■
Precose Tablets		
25 MG		■
50 MG		■
100 MG		■
Prednisone Intensol		
5 MG/ML		■
Prednisone Oral Solution		
5 MG/5 ML		■
Prednisone Tablets		
1 MG	■	
2.5 MG	■	
5 MG	■	
10 MG	■	
20 MG	■	
50 MG	■	
Pregnyl for Injection		
10,000 U	■	
Prelone Syrup		
5 MG/5 ML		■
15 MG/5 ML	■	
Premarin Intravenous		
25 MG		■
Premarin Tablets		
0.3 MG		■
0.625 MG		■
0.9 MG		■
1.25 MG		■
2.5 MG		■
Premarin Vaginal Cream		
0.625 MG/GM		■
Premphase Tablets		
0.625 MG AND 5 MG		■
Prempro Tablets		
0.625 MG-2.5 MG		■
0.625 MG-5 MG		■
Prepidil Gel		
0.5 MG/3 GM		■
Prevacid Delayed-Release Capsules		
15 MG		■
30 MG		■
Prevnar for Injection		
16 MCG/0.5 ML		■
PREVPAC		
500 MG-500 MG-30 MG		■
Prilosec Delayed-Release Capsules		
10 MG		■
20 MG		■
40 MG		■
Primacor Injection		
1 MG/ML		■
5%-20 MG/100 ML		■
Primaxin I.M.		
500 MG-500 MG		■
Primaxin I.V.		
250 MG-250 MG		■
500 MG-500 MG		■
Prinivil Tablets		
2.5 MG		■
5 MG		■
10 MG		■
20 MG		■
40 MG		■
Prinzide Tablets		
12.5 MG-10 MG		■
12.5 MG-20 MG		■
25 MG-20 MG		■
Procanbid Extended-Release Tablets		
500 MG		■
1000 MG		■
Procardia Capsules		
10 MG	■	
20 MG	■	
Procardia XL Extended Release Tablets		
30 MG	■	
60 MG	■	
90 MG	■	
Procrit for Injection		
2000 U/ML	■	
3000 U/ML	■	
4000 U/ML	■	
10,000 U/ML	■	
20,000 U/ML	■	
40,000 U/ML	■	
Proctocort Suppositories		
30 MG	■	
ProctoFoam-HC		
1%-1%	■	
Prograf		
0.5 MG		■
Prolastin		
1 MG		■
Proleukin for Injection		
22 MILLION IU		■
Prometrium Capsules (100 mg, 200 mg)		
100 MG		■
200 MG		■
Propecia Tablets		
1 MG		■
Proplex T		
1 IU	■	
Proscar Tablets		
5 MG		■
ProSom Tablets		
1 MG	■	
2 MG	■	
Prostigmin Injectable		
0.5 MG/ML	■	
1 MG/ML	■	
Prostigmin Tablets		
15 MG		■
Prostin E2 Suppositories		
20 MG		■
Protonix Tablets		
20 MG		■
40 MG		■
Protopam Chloride for Injection		
1 GM		■
Proventil Inhalation Aerosol		
0.09 MG/INH	■	
Proventil Inhalation Solution 0.083%		
0.083%	■	
Proventil Repetabs Tablets		
4 MG	■	
Proventil Solution for Inhalation 0.5%		
0.5%	■	
Proventil HFA Inhalation Aerosol		
0.09 MG/INH		■
Provera Tablets		
2.5 MG	■	
5 MG	■	
10 MG	■	
Provigil Tablets		
100 MG		■
200 MG		■
Psorcon E Cream		
0.05%	■	
Psorcon E Ointment		
0.05%	■	
Pulmicort Turbuhaler Inhalation Powder		
0.2 MG/INH		■
Pulmozyme Inhalation Solution		
2.5 MG/2.5 ML		■
Purinethol Tablets		
50 MG		■
Quinaglute Dura-Tabs Tablets		
324 MG	■	
Quinidex Extentabs		
300 MG	■	
Rabies Vaccine RabAvert		
2.5 IU	■	
Rapamune Oral Solution and Tablets		
1 MG/ML		■
Rebetron Combination Therapy		
3 MIU/0.2 ML-200 MG		■
3 MIU/0.5 ML-200 MG		■
Recombinate		
1 IU	■	
Recombivax HB		
10 MCG/ML		■

STRENGTH	GENERIC YES	GENERIC NO
40 MCG/ML		■
Reglan Injectable		
5 MG/ML	■	
Reglan Tablets		
5 MG	■	
10 MG	■	
Regranex Gel		
0.01%		■
Relafen Tablets		
500 MG	■	
750 MG	■	
Relenza Rotadisk		
5 MG		■
Remeron SolTab Tablets		
15 MG		■
30 MG		■
45 MG		■
Remicade for IV Injection		
100 MG		■
Renagel Capsules		
403 MG		■
Renese Tablets		
1 MG		■
2 MG		■
Renova Cream		
0.02%		■
0.05%	■	
ReoPro Vials		
2 MG/ML		■
Repronex for Intramuscular and Subcutaneous Injection		
75 IU	■	
Requip Tablets		
0.25 MG		■
0.5 MG		■
1 MG		■
2 MG		■
3 MG		■
4 MG		■
5 MG		■
Rescriptor Tablets		
100 MG		■
200 MG		■
Retavase Vials		
10.4 U		■
Retin-A Micro 0.1%		
0.1%		■
Retrovir Capsules		
100 MG		■
Retrovir IV Infusion		
10 MG/ML		■
Retrovir Syrup		
50 MG/5 ML		■
Retrovir Tablets		
300 MG		■
Rev-Eyes Sterile Ophthalmic Eyedrops 0.5%		
0.5%		■
Rhinocort Nasal Inhaler		
0.032 MG/INH		■
Risperdal Oral Solution		
1 MG/ML		■
Risperdal Tablets		
0.25 MG		■
0.5 MG		■
1 MG		■
2 MG		■
3 MG		■
4 MG		■
Ritalin Hydrochloride Tablets		
5 MG	■	
10 MG	■	
20 MG	■	
Ritalin-SR Tablets		
20 MG	■	
Rituxan for Infusion		
10 MG/ML		■
Rituxan I.V.		
10 MG/ML		■
Robaxin Injectable		
100 MG/ML	■	
Robaxin Tablets		
500 MG	■	
Robaxin-750 Tablets		
750 MG	■	
Robaxisal Tablets		
325 MG-400 MG	■	
Robinul Injectable		
0.2 MG/ML	■	
Robitussin A-C Syrup		
10 MG-100 MG/5 ML	■	
Robitussin-DAC Syrup		
10 MG-100 MG-30 MG/5 ML	■	
Rocaltrol Capsules		
0.25 MCG	■	
0.5 MCG	■	
Rocaltrol Oral Solution		
1 MCG/ML		■
Rocephin Injectable Vials, ADD-Vantage, Galaxy, Bulk		
250 MG		■
500 MG		■
1 GM		■
2 GM		■
10 GM		■
Roferon-A Injection		
3 MILLION IU		■
6 MILLION IU		■
6 MILLION U/ML		■
9 MILLION IU		■
36 MILLION U/ML		■
Romazicon Injection		
0.1 MG/ML		■
Rowasa Rectal Suspension Enema 4.0 grams/unit (60 mL)		
4 GM/60 ML		■
Roxanol 100 Concentrated Oral Solution		
20 MG/ML	■	
Roxanol Concentrated Oral Solution		
20 MG/ML	■	
Roxanol-T Oral Solution		
20 MG/ML	■	
Roxicodone Tablets		
5 MG	■	
5 MG/5 ML		■
15 MG		■
20 MG/ML	■	
30 MG		■
Rum-K		
30 MEQ/15 ML		■
Ryna-12 S Suspension		
5 MG-30 MG/5 ML	■	
Rythmol Tablets -- 150 mg, 225 mg, 300 mg		
150 MG	■	
225 MG	■	
300 MG		■
Saizen for Injection		
5 MG		■
8.8 MG		■
Salagen Tablets		
5 MG		■
Sandimmune I.V. Ampuls for Infusion		
50 MG/ML	■	
Sandimmune Oral Solution		
100 MG/ML	■	
Sandimmune Soft Gelatin Capsules		
25 MG	■	
100 MG	■	
Sandoglobulin I.V.		
1 GM	■	
3 GM	■	
6 GM	■	
12 GM	■	
Sandostatin Injection		
50 MCG/ML		■
100 MCG/ML		■
200 MCG/ML		■
500 MCG/ML		■
1000 MCG/ML		■
Sandostatin LAR Depot		
10 MG		■
20 MG		■
30 MG		■
Sarafem Pulvules		
10 MG	■	
20 MG	■	
Sectral Capsules		
200 MG	■	
400 MG	■	
Sedapap Tablets 50 mg/650 mg		
650 MG-50 MG	■	
Selsun Rx 2.5% Lotion, USP		
2.5%	■	
Semprex-D Capsules		
8 MG-60 MG		■
Sensorcaine Injection		
0.25%	■	
0.5%	■	
Sensorcaine with Epinephrine Injection		
0.25%-1:200,000	■	
0.5%-1:200,000	■	
Sensorcaine-MPF Injection		
0.25%	■	
0.5%	■	
0.75%	■	
Sensorcaine-MPF with Epinephrine Injection		
0.25%-1:200,000	■	
0.5%-1:200,000	■	
0.75%-1:200,000	■	
Septra Suspension		
200 MG-40 MG/5 ML	■	
Septra Grape Suspension		
200 MG-40 MG/5 ML	■	
Septra Tablets		
400 MG-80 MG	■	
Septra DS Tablets		
800 MG-160 MG	■	
Serentil Ampuls		
25 MG/ML		■
Serentil Concentrate		
25 MG/ML		■
Serentil Tablets		
10 MG		■
25 MG		■
100 MG		■
Serevent Diskus		
0.046 MG/INH		■
Serevent Inhalation Aerosol		
21 MCG/INH		■
Serophene Tablets		
50 MG	■	
Seroquel Tablets		
25 MG		■
100 MG		■
200 MG		■
300 MG		■
Serostim for Injection		
4 MG		■
5 MG	■	
6 MG		■
Serzone Tablets		
50 MG		■
100 MG		■
150 MG		■
200 MG		■
250 MG		■
Silvadene Cream 1%		
1%	■	
Simulect for Injection		
20 MG		■
Sinemet Tablets		
10 MG-100 MG	■	
25 MG-100 MG	■	
25 MG-250 MG	■	
Sinemet CR Tablets		
25 MG-100 MG	■	
50 MG-200 MG	■	
Sinequan Capsules		
10 MG	■	
25 MG	■	
50 MG	■	
75 MG	■	
100 MG	■	
150 MG	■	
Sinequan Oral Concentrate		
10 MG/ML	■	
Singulair Tablets		
10 MG		■
Singulair Chewable Tablets		
4 MG		■
5 MG		■
Skelaxin Tablets		
400 MG		■
Skelid Tablets		
200 MG		■
Solaquin Forte 4% Cream		
4%	■	
Solaquin Forte 4% Gel		
4%	■	
Solu-Medrol Sterile Powder		
40 MG	■	
125 MG	■	
500 MG	■	
1 GM	■	
2 GM		■
Soma Tablets		
350 MG	■	
Soma Compound Tablets		
325 MG-200 MG	■	
Soma Compound w/Codeine Tablets		
325 MG-200 MG-16 MG	■	
Sonata Capsules		
5 MG		■
10 MG		■
Soriatane Capsules		
10 MG		■
25 MG		■
Sporanox Capsules		
100 MG		■
Sporanox Injection		
10 MG/ML		■
Sporanox Oral Solution		
10 MG/ML		■
Stadol NS Nasal Spray		
10 MG/ML	■	
Stelazine Injection		
10 MG/ML	■	
Stelazine Tablets		
1 MG	■	
2 MG	■	
5 MG	■	
10 MG	■	
Stimate Nasal Spray		
0.15 MG/INH		■
Streptase for Infusion		
1.5 MILLION IU	■	
250,000 IU	■	
750,000 IU	■	
Stromectol Tablets		
3 MG		■
Sular Tablets		
10 MG		■
20 MG		■
30 MG		■
40 MG		■
Sulfamylon Cream		
85 MG/GM		■
Sulfamylon Topical Solution		
50 GM/PACKET		■
Suprane Liquid for Inhalation		
99%		■
Suprax for Oral Suspension		
100 MG/5 ML		■
Suprax Tablets		
200 MG		■
400 MG		■
Surmontil Capsules		
25 MG		■
50 MG		■
100 MG		■
Survanta Intratracheal Suspension		
25 MG/ML		■
Sustiva Capsules		
50 MG		■
100 MG		■
200 MG		■
Symmetrel Syrup		
50 MG/5 ML	■	

STRENGTH	GENERIC YES	GENERIC NO
Symmetrel Tablets		
100 MG		■
Synagis Intramuscular		
50 MG		■
100 MG		■
Synalar Cream		
0.025%	■	
Synalar Ointment		
0.025%	■	
Synalar Topical Solution		
0.01%	■	
Synarel Nasal Solution for Central Precocious Puberty		
0.2 MG/INH		■
Synarel Nasal Solution for Endometriosis		
0.2 MG/INH		■
Synercid I.V.		
350 MG-150 MG		■
Synthroid Injection		
0.2 MG	■	
0.5 MG	■	
Synthroid Tablets		
0.025 MG	■	
0.05 MG	■	
0.075 MG	■	
0.088 MG	■	
0.1 MG	■	
0.112 MG	■	
0.125 MG	■	
0.15 MG	■	
0.175 MG	■	
0.2 MG	■	
0.3 MG	■	
Synvisc		
8 MG/ML	■	
Syprine Capsules		
250 MG		■
Tabloid Tablets		
40 MG		■
Tagamet Tablets		
300 MG	■	
400 MG	■	
800 MG	■	
Talacen Caplets		
650 MG-25 MG	■	
Talwin Nx Tablets		
0.5 MG-50 MG	■	
Tambocor Tablets		
50 MG		■
100 MG		■
150 MG		■
Tamiflu Capsules		
75 MG		■
Tao Capsules		
250 MG		■
Tapazole Tablets		
5 MG	■	
10 MG	■	
Tarka Tablets		
1 MG-240 MG		■
2 MG-180 MG		■
2 MG-240 MG		■
4 MG-240 MG		■
Tasmar Tablets		
100 MG		■
200 MG		■
Taxol Injection		
6 MG/ML	■	
Taxotere for Injection Concentrate		
20 MG/0.5 ML		■
Tazicef for Injection		
1 GM	■	
2 GM	■	
6 GM	■	
Tazidime Vials, Faspak & ADD-Vantage		
1 GM	■	
2 GM	■	
6 GM	■	
Tazorac Gel		
0.05%		■
0.1%		■
Tegretol Chewable Tablets		
100 MG	■	

STRENGTH	GENERIC YES	GENERIC NO
Tegretol Suspension		
100 MG/5 ML	■	
Tegretol Tablets		
200 MG	■	
Tegretol-XR Tablets		
100 MG		■
200 MG		■
400 MG		■
Temodar Capsules		
5 MG		■
20 MG		■
100 MG		■
250 MG		■
Temovate Cream		
0.05%	■	
Temovate Gel		
0.05%	■	
Temovate Ointment		
0.05%	■	
Temovate Scalp Application		
0.05%	■	
Temovate E Emollient		
0.05%	■	
Tenex Tablets		
1 MG	■	
2 MG	■	
Tenoretic Tablets		
50 MG-25 MG	■	
100 MG-25 MG	■	
Tenormin I.V. Injection		
0.5 MG/ML		■
Tensilon Injectable		
10 MG/ML	■	
Tequin Injection		
2 MG/ML		■
10 MG/ML		■
Tequin Tablets		
200 MG		■
400 MG		■
Terazol 3 Vaginal Cream		
0.8%		■
Terazol 3 Vaginal Suppositories		
80 MG		■
Terazol 7 Vaginal Cream		
0.4%		■
Testoderm Transdermal Systems		
4 MG/24 HRS		■
5 MG/24 HRS	■	
6 MG/24 HRS		■
Testred Capsules, 10 mg		
10 MG	■	
Tetanus and Diphtheria Toxoids Adsorbed For Adult Use		
2 LF U-5 LF U/0.5 ML	■	
6.6 LF U-5 LF U/0.5 ML	■	
Teveten Tablets		
400 MG		■
600 MG		■
Thalomid Capsules		
50 MG		■
TheraCys Injection		
81 MG		■
Thioplex for Injection		
15 MG	■	
Thioridazine Hydrochloride Tablets		
10 MG	■	
25 MG	■	
50 MG	■	
100 MG	■	
Thiothixene Capsules		
1 MG	■	
2 MG	■	
5 MG	■	
10 MG	■	
Thorazine Ampuls		
25 MG/ML	■	
Thorazine Multi-dose Vials		
25 MG/ML	■	
Thorazine Spansule Capsules		
30 MG		■

STRENGTH	GENERIC YES	GENERIC NO
75 MG		■
150 MG		■
Thorazine Suppositories		
25 MG		■
100 MG		■
Thorazine Syrup		
10 MG/5 ML		■
Thorazine Tablets		
10 MG	■	
25 MG	■	
50 MG	■	
100 MG	■	
200 MG	■	
Thrombate III		
1 IU	■	
Thrombin-JMI		
5000 U	■	
10,000 U	■	
20,000 U	■	
50,000 U	■	
Thymoglobulin for Injection		
25 MG		■
Thyrel TRH for Injection		
500 MCG/ML		■
Thyrogen for Injection		
1.1 MG		■
Tiazac Capsules		
120 MG	■	
180 MG	■	
240 MG	■	
300 MG	■	
360 MG	■	
420 MG		■
Ticlid Tablets		
250 MG	■	
Tikosyn Capsules		
0.125 MG		■
0.25 MG		■
0.5 MG		■
Timentin for Intravenous Administration		
100 MG-3 GM		■
1 GM-30 GM		■
Timolide Tablets		
25 MG-10 MG		■
Timoptic in Ocudose		
0.25%		■
0.5%		■
Timoptic Sterile Ophthalmic Solution		
0.25%	■	
0.5%	■	
Timoptic-XE Sterile Ophthalmic Gel Forming Solution		
0.25%	■	
0.5%	■	
TNKase I.V.		
50 MG		■
TOBI Solution for Inhalation		
60 MG/ML		■
TobraDex Ophthalmic Ointment		
0.1%-0.3%		■
TobraDex Ophthalmic Suspension		
0.1%-0.3%		■
Tobrex Ophthalmic Ointment		
0.3%		■
Tobrex Ophthalmic Solution		
0.3%	■	
Tolectin 600 Tablets		
600 MG	■	
Tolectin DS Capsules		
400 MG	■	
Tonocard Tablets		
400 MG		■
600 MG		■
Topamax Sprinkle Capsules		
15 MG		■
25 MG		■
Topamax Tablets		
25 MG		■
100 MG		■
200 MG		■
Topicort Cream		
0.25%	■	

STRENGTH	GENERIC YES	GENERIC NO
Topicort Gel		
0.05%	■	
Topicort Ointment		
0.25%	■	
Topicort LP Cream		
0.05%	■	
Toprol-XL Tablets		
25 MG		■
50 MG		■
100 MG		■
200 MG		■
Toradol Tablets		
10 MG	■	
Transderm Scop Transdermal Therapeutic System		
0.33 MG/24 HRS		■
Tranxene T-TAB Tablets		
3.75 MG	■	
7.5 MG	■	
15 MG	■	
Tranxene-SD Tablets		
11.25 MG		■
22.5 MG		■
Tranxene-SD Half Strength Tablets		
11.25 MG		■
22.5 MG		■
Trasylol Injection		
10,000 KIU/ML		■
Trecator-SC Tablets		
250 MG		■
Tri-Nasal Spray		
0.05 MG/INH		■
Triaz Cleanser		
3%		■
6%	■	
10%	■	
Triaz Gel		
3%		■
6%	■	
10%	■	
Tricor Capsules, Micronized		
67 MG		■
200 MG		■
Trilafon Injection		
5 MG/ML		■
Trilafon Tablets		
2 MG	■	
4 MG	■	
8 MG	■	
16 MG	■	
Trileptal Tablets		
150 MG		■
300 MG		■
600 MG		■
Trilisate Liquid		
500 MG/5 ML	■	
Trilisate Tablets		
500 MG	■	
750 MG	■	
1000 MG	■	
Tri-Norinyl-28 Tablets		
0.035 MG-0.5 MG AND 1 MG		■
Triostat Injection		
0.01 MG/ML		■
Trovan I.V.		
5 MG/ML		■
Trovan Tablets		
100 MG		■
200 MG		■
Tubersol Diagnostic Antigen		
5 TU/0.1 ML	■	
Tussionex Pennkinetic Extended-Release Suspension		
8 MG-10 MG/5 ML		■
Tussi-Organidin NR Liquid		
10 MG-100 MG/5 ML	■	
Tussi-Organidin DM NR Liquid		
10 MG-100 MG/5 ML	■	
Tussi-Organidin DM-S NR Liquid		
10 MG-100 MG/5 ML	■	
Tussi-Organidin-S NR Liquid		
10 MG-100 MG/5 ML	■	

STRENGTH	GENERIC YES	GENERIC NO
Tylenol with Codeine Elixir		
120 MG-12 MG/5 ML	■	
Tylenol with Codeine Tablets		
300 MG-30 MG	■	
300 MG-60 MG	■	
Tylox Capsules		
500 MG-5 MG	■	
TYPHIM Vi Vaccine		
25 MCG/0.5 ML		■
Ultram Tablets		
50 MG		■
Unasyn for Injection		
1 GM-0.5 GM		■
2 GM-1 GM		■
10 GM-5 GM		■
Uniphyl 400 mg and 600 mg Tablets		
400 MG	■	
600 MG	■	
Uniretic Tablets		
12.5 MG-7.5 MG		■
25 MG-15 MG		■
Univasc Tablets		
7.5 MG		■
15 MG		■
Urocit-K Tablets		
5 MEQ		■
10 MEQ		■
Uroqid-Acid No. 2 Tablets		
500 MG-500 MG		■
Urso Tablets		
250 MG		■
Valium Tablets		
2 MG	■	
5 MG	■	
10 MG	■	
Valstar Sterile Solution for Intravesical Instillation		
40 MG/ML		■
Valtrex Caplets		
500 MG		■
1 GM		■
Vancenase AQ Nasal Spray 0.084%		
0.084 MG/INH		■
Vanceril Inhalation Aerosol		
0.042 MG/INH		■
Vancocin HCl Capsules & Pulvules		
125 MG		■
250 MG		■
Vancocin HCl Oral Solution		
250 MG/5 ML	■	
500 MG/6 ML		■
Vancocin HCl, Vials & ADD-Vantage		
500 MG	■	
1 GM	■	
10 GM	■	
Vantin Tablets and Oral Suspension		
50 MG/5 ML		■
100 MG		■
100 MG/5 ML		■
200 MG		■
Vaqta		
50 U/ML		■
Varivax		
1350 PFU		■
Vascor Tablets		
200 MG		■
300 MG		■
Vaseretic Tablets		
5 MG-12.5 MG	■	
10 MG-25 MG	■	
Vasotec I.V. Injection		
1.25 MG/ML	■	
Vasotec Tablets		
2.5 MG	■	
5 MG	■	
10 MG	■	
20 MG	■	
Ventolin Inhalation Aerosol and Refill		
0.09 MG/INH	■	
Ventolin HFA Inhalation Aerosol		
0.09 MG/INH	■	
Verelan Capsules		
120 MG	■	
180 MG	■	
240 MG	■	
360 MG	■	
Verelan PM Capsules		
100 MG		■
200 MG		■
300 MG		■
Vermox Chewable Tablets		
100 MG	■	
Versed Injection		
1 MG/ML	■	
5 MG/ML	■	
Versed Syrup		
2 MG/ML		■
Vesanoid Capsules		
10 MG		■
Vexol 1% Ophthalmic Suspension		
1%		■
Viagra Tablets		
25 MG		■
50 MG		■
100 MG		■
Vibramycin Calcium Oral Suspension Syrup		
50 MG/5 ML		■
Vibramycin Hyclate Capsules		
50 MG	■	
100 MG	■	
Vibramycin Monohydrate for Oral Suspension		
25 MG/5 ML		■
Vibra-Tabs Film Coated Tablets		
100 MG	■	
Vicodin Tablets		
500 MG-5 MG	■	
Vicodin ES Tablets		
750 MG-7.5 MG	■	
Vicodin HP Tablets		
660 MG-10 MG	■	
Vicodin Tuss Expectorant		
100 MG-5 MG/5 ML	■	
Vicoprofen Tablets		
7.5 MG-200 MG		■
Videx Powder for Oral Solution		
100 MG		■
167 MG		■
250 MG		■
Videx Pediatric Powder for Oral Solution		
10 MG/ML		■
Videx Chewable Tablets		
25 MG		■
50 MG		■
100 MG		■
150 MG		■
200 MG		■
Viokase Tablets		
30,000 U-8000 U-30,000 U	■	
Vioxx Oral Suspension		
12.5 MG/5 ML		■
25 MG/5 ML		■
Vioxx Tablets		
12.5 MG		■
25 MG		■
50 MG		■
Viracept Oral Powder		
50 MG/1 GM		■
Viracept Tablets		
250 MG		■
Virazole for Inhalation Solution		
6 GM		■
Vistaril Capsules		
25 MG	■	
50 MG	■	
100 MG	■	
Vistaril Intramuscular Solution		
50 MG/ML	■	
Vistaril Oral Suspension		
25 MG/5 ML	■	
Vistide Injection		
75 MG/ML	■	
Visudyne for Injection		
15 MG		■
Vitrasert Implant		
4.5 MG		■
Vitravene for Injection		
6.6 MG/ML		■
Vivactil Tablets		
5 MG	■	
10 MG	■	
Vivelle Transdermal System		
0.025 MG/24 HRS	■	
0.0375 MG/24 HRS	■	
0.05 MG/24 HRS	■	
0.075 MG/24 HRS	■	
0.1 MG/24 HRS	■	
Vivelle-Dot Transdermal System		
0.0375 MG/24 HRS	■	
0.05 MG/24 HRS	■	
0.075 MG/24 HRS	■	
0.1 MG/24 HRS	■	
Volmax Extended-Release Tablets		
4 MG	■	
8 MG		■
Voltaren Ophthalmic Sterile Ophthalmic Solution		
0.1%	■	
Voltaren Tablets		
25 MG	■	
50 MG	■	
75 MG	■	
Voltaren-XR Tablets		
100 MG	■	
VoSoL HC Otic Solution		
2%-1%	■	
Wellbutrin Tablets		
75 MG	■	
100 MG	■	
Wellbutrin SR Sustained-Release Tablets		
100 MG		■
150 MG		■
WinRho SDF		
600 IU		■
1500 IU		■
5000 IU		■
Xalatan Latanoprost Ophthalmic Solution		
0.005%		■
Xanax Tablets		
0.25 MG	■	
0.5 MG	■	
1 MG	■	
2 MG	■	
Xeloda Tablets		
150 MG		■
500 MG		■
Xenical Capsules		
120 MG		■
Xerac AC Solution		
6.25%		■
Xopenex Inhalation Solution		
0.63 MG/3 ML		■
1.25 MG/3 ML		■
Xylocaine Injection		
0.5%	■	
1%	■	
2%	■	
Xylocaine with Epinephrine Injection		
1:50,000-2%	■	
1:100,000-1%	■	
1:100,000-2%	■	
1:200,000-0.5%	■	
YF-VAX Vaccine		
5.04 LOG10 PFU		■
25.2 LOG10 PFU		■
Zaditor Ophthalmic Solution		
0.025%		■
Zanaflex Tablets		
2 MG		■
4 MG		■
Zantac Injection		
1 MG/ML		■
25 MG/ML		■
Zantac Injection Premixed		
1 MG/ML		■
Zantac Syrup		
15 MG/ML		■
Zantac 150 Tablets		
150 MG	■	
Zantac 300 Tablets		
300 MG	■	
Zantac 150 EFFERdose Granules		
150 MG		■
Zantac 150 EFFERdose Tablets		
150 MG		■
Zarontin Capsules		
250 MG		■
Zarontin Syrup		
250 MG/5 ML	■	
Zaroxolyn Tablets		
2.5 MG		■
5 MG		■
10 MG		■
Zebeta Tablets		
5 MG	■	
10 MG	■	
Zemplar Injection		
0.002 MG/ML		■
0.005 MG/ML		■
Zemuron Injection		
10 MG/ML		■
Zenapax for Injection		
5 MG/ML		■
Zephrex Tablets		
400 MG-60 MG		■
Zephrex LA Tablets		
600 MG-120 MG	■	
Zerit Capsules		
15 MG		■
20 MG		■
30 MG		■
40 MG		■
Zerit for Oral Solution		
1 MG/ML		■
Zestoretic Tablets		
12.5 MG-10 MG		■
12.5 MG-20 MG		■
25 MG-20 MG		■
Zestril Tablets		
2.5 MG		■
5 MG		■
10 MG		■
20 MG		■
30 MG		■
40 MG		■
Ziac Tablets		
2.5 MG-6.25 MG	■	
5 MG-6.25 MG	■	
10 MG-6.25 MG	■	
Ziagen Oral Solution		
20 MG/ML		■
Ziagen Tablets		
300 MG		■
Zinacef Injection		
750 MG	■	
750 MG/50 ML		■
1.5 GM	■	
1.5 GM/50 ML		■
7.5 GM	■	
Zinecard for Injection		
250 MG		■
500 MG		■
Zithromax for IV Infusion		
500 MG		■
Zithromax for Oral Suspension		
100 MG/5 ML		■
200 MG/5 ML		■
1 GM/PACKET		■
Zithromax Tablets, 250 mg		
250 MG		■

Zithromax Tablets, 600 mg

STRENGTH	GENERIC YES	GENERIC NO
600 MG		■

Zocor Tablets

STRENGTH	GENERIC YES	GENERIC NO
5 MG		■
10 MG		■
20 MG		■
40 MG		■
80 MG		■

Zofran Injection

STRENGTH	GENERIC YES	GENERIC NO
2 MG/ML		■
32 MG/50 ML		■

Zofran Injection Premixed

STRENGTH	GENERIC YES	GENERIC NO
32 MG/50 ML		■

Zofran Oral Solution

STRENGTH	GENERIC YES	GENERIC NO
4 MG/5 ML		■

Zofran Tablets

STRENGTH	GENERIC YES	GENERIC NO
4 MG		■
8 MG		■
24 MG		■

Zofran ODT Orally Disintegrating Tablets

STRENGTH	GENERIC YES	GENERIC NO
4 MG		■
8 MG		■

Zoladex

STRENGTH	GENERIC YES	GENERIC NO
3.6 MG		■
10.8 MG		■

Zoladex 3-month

STRENGTH	GENERIC YES	GENERIC NO
3.6 MG		■
10.8 MG		■

Zoloft Oral Concentrate

STRENGTH	GENERIC YES	GENERIC NO
20 MG/ML		■

Zoloft Tablets

STRENGTH	GENERIC YES	GENERIC NO
25 MG		■
50 MG		■
100 MG		■

Zometa for Intravenous Infusion

STRENGTH	GENERIC YES	GENERIC NO
4 MG		■

Zomig Tablets

STRENGTH	GENERIC YES	GENERIC NO
2.5 MG		■
5 MG		■

Zonegran Capsules

STRENGTH	GENERIC YES	GENERIC NO
100 MG		■

Zosyn

STRENGTH	GENERIC YES	GENERIC NO
40 MG-5 MG/ML		■
60 MG-7.5 MG/ML		■
2 GM-0.25 GM		■
3 GM-0.375 GM		■
4 GM-0.5 GM		■
4 GM-0.5 GM/100 ML		■
36 GM-4.5 GM		■

Zosyn in Galaxy Containers

STRENGTH	GENERIC YES	GENERIC NO
40 MG-5 MG/ML		■
60 MG-7.5 MG/ML		■
4 GM-0.5 GM/100 ML		■

Zovia 1/50E Tablets

STRENGTH	GENERIC YES	GENERIC NO
50 MCG-1 MG	■	

Zovia 1/35E Tablets

STRENGTH	GENERIC YES	GENERIC NO
35 MCG-1 MG	■	

Zovirax Capsules

STRENGTH	GENERIC YES	GENERIC NO
200 MG	■	

Zovirax for Injection

STRENGTH	GENERIC YES	GENERIC NO
500 MG	■	
1000 MG	■	

Zovirax Ointment

STRENGTH	GENERIC YES	GENERIC NO
5%		■

Zovirax Suspension

STRENGTH	GENERIC YES	GENERIC NO
200 MG/5 ML	■	

Zovirax Tablets

STRENGTH	GENERIC YES	GENERIC NO
400 MG	■	
800 MG	■	

Zyban Sustained-Release Tablets

STRENGTH	GENERIC YES	GENERIC NO
150 MG		■

Zydone Tablets

STRENGTH	GENERIC YES	GENERIC NO
400 MG-10 MG		■
400 MG-5 MG		■
400 MG-7.5 MG		■

Zyflo Filmtab Tablets

STRENGTH	GENERIC YES	GENERIC NO
600 MG		■

Zyprexa Tablets

STRENGTH	GENERIC YES	GENERIC NO
2.5 MG		■
5 MG		■
7.5 MG		■
10 MG		■
15 MG		■
20 MG		■

Zyrtec Syrup

STRENGTH	GENERIC YES	GENERIC NO
1 MG/ML		■

Zyrtec Tablets

STRENGTH	GENERIC YES	GENERIC NO
5 MG		■
10 MG		■

Zyvox Injection

STRENGTH	GENERIC YES	GENERIC NO
2 MG/ML		■

Zyvox for Oral Suspension

STRENGTH	GENERIC YES	GENERIC NO
100 MG/5 ML		■

Zyvox Tablets

STRENGTH	GENERIC YES	GENERIC NO
600 MG		■

SECTION 9

IMPRINT IDENTIFICATION GUIDE

Too often, patients on multiple medications have no idea what they're taking; and a "brown-bag inventory" may not help if it confronts you with a collection of unfamiliar tablets and capsules. This section of the *PDR Companion Guide*™ provides you with a handy solution.

The convenient table below allows you to identify thousands of solid oral medications by imprint alone. Imprints beginning with a number are listed first, in ascending order. (Leading zeros, as in "053," are ignored.) Imprints beginning with a letter follow in alphabetical order. Virtually all commonly prescribed drugs are represented.

Each entry includes the full imprint code, the product's brand or generic name, and, to confirm identification, its strength, color, form, and shape. The name of the product's manufacturer completes each listing. The information is extracted, with permission, from the Identidex System produced by MICROMEDEX, Inc.

IMPRINT	BRAND/GENERIC NAME	STRENGTH	COLOR	FORM	SHAPE	MANUFACTURER
0063; 1261	X-Otag S.R. Nov 28	100 mg	Yellow	Tablet	Round	Solvay Pharmaceuticals
0063; 1390	Hyserp	0.1 mg	Light Pink	Tablet	Round	
0063; 1390	Hyserp	15 mg	Light Pink	Tablet	Round	
0063; 1390	Hyserp	25 mg	Light Pink	Tablet	Round	
0063; 1650	Sprx-1	35 mg	Peach	Tablet	Triangle-Shaped	Solvay Pharmaceuticals
0063; 2660	Sprx-3	35 mg	Black	Capsule		Solvay Pharmaceuticals
0063; 3006	R-P Mycin	250 mg	Red	Tablet		Solvay Pharmaceuticals
0115; 4404	Rauserpa	100 mg	Red	Tablet	Round	Solvay Pharmaceuticals
0331; 0499	Phentermine Hydrochloride	30 mg		Capsule		
0331; 0617	Chlordinium	2.5 mg		Capsule		
0331; 0617	Chlordinium	5 mg		Capsule		
0822; 4060	Chlordiazepoxide Hydrochloride	5 mg	Green and Yellow	Capsule		
0822; 4065	Chlordiazepoxide Hydrochloride	10 mg	Black and Green	Capsule		
0822; 4070	Chlordiazepoxide Hydrochloride	25 mg	Green and White	Capsule		
0822; 5	Diphenoxylate Hydrochloride with Atropine	0.025 mg	White	Tablet	Scored	
0822; 5	Diphenoxylate Hydrochloride with Atropine	2.5 mg	White	Tablet	Scored	
0832 G536C	Obermine	30 mg	Yellow	Capsule		Forest Pharmaceuticals
0832; G536C	Obermine	30 mg	Black	Capsule		Forest Pharmaceuticals
1; 4621	Teen Tabs No. 1	30 mg	Gray	Tablet	Round	Rugby Laboratories
1; 4621	Teen Tabs No. 1	75 mg	Gray	Tablet	Round	Rugby Laboratories
1; 4622	Teen Tabs No. 2	37.5 mg	White	Tablet	Round	Rugby Laboratories
1; 4622	Teen Tabs No. 2	50 mg	White	Tablet	Round	Rugby Laboratories
1; 4623	Teen Tabs No. 3	25 mg	Pink	Tablet	Round	Rugby Laboratories
1; 4623	Teen Tabs No. 3	50 mg	Pink	Tablet	Round	Rugby Laboratories
10	Isoxsuprine Hydrochloride	10 mg	White	Tablet	Round	
10; LL; C21	Chlorpromazine Hydrochloride	10 mg	Light Brown	Coated Tablet	Round	Lederle Laboratories
13; 411	Magan	650 mg	Pink	Tablet	Capsule-Shaped, Convex	Adria Laboratories
13; TRIANGLE	Nico-Metrazol	50 mg	White	Tablet	Round	
13; TRIANGLE	Nico-Metrazol	100 mg	White	Tablet	Round	
16	Neutralox	150 mg	Pink, Yellow, and Orange	Chewable Tablet		Teva Pharmaceuticals
16	Neutralox	300 mg	Pink, Yellow, and Orange	Chewable Tablet		Teva Pharmaceuticals
17; TRIANGLE	Theokin	448 mg	Yellow	Tablet		
17; TRIANGLE	Theokin	450 mg	Yellow	Tablet		
18; 892	Tussionex	5 mg	Green and Ivory	Capsule		Fisons Pharmaceuticals
18; 892	Tussionex	10 mg	Green and Ivory	Capsule		Fisons Pharmaceuticals
18; 894	Tussionex	5 mg	Light Tan	Tablet	Long Trapezoid, Scored	Fisons Pharmaceuticals
18; 894	Tussionex	10 mg	Light Tan	Tablet	Long Trapezoid, Scored	Fisons Pharmaceuticals
18; 895	Biphetamine	3.75 mg	White	Capsule		
18; 899	Biphetamine-T	6.25 mg	Green and Black	Capsule		Fisons Pharmaceuticals
18; 899	Biphetamine-T	40 mg	Green and Black	Capsule		Fisons Pharmaceuticals
18; 900	Biphetamine-T	10 mg	Red and Black	Capsule		Fisons Pharmaceuticals
18; 900	Biphetamine-T	40 mg	Red and Black	Capsule		Fisons Pharmaceuticals
20	Isoxsuprine Hydrochloride	20 mg	White	Tablet	Round	
25; LL; C22	Chlorpromazine Hydrochloride	25 mg	Tan	Coated Tablet	Round	Lederle Laboratories
50	Manoplax	50 mg	White	Coated Tablet	Hexagonal	Boots Pharmaceuticals
50; LL; C23	Chlorpromazine Hydrochloride	50 mg	Tan	Coated Tablet	Round	Lederle Laboratories
54; 023	Meprobamate	200 mg		Tablet		Roxane Laboratories
54; 132	Meprobamate	400 mg		Tablet		Roxane Laboratories
54; 160	Niacin	100 mg	White	Tablet		Roxane Laboratories
54; 652	Chlordiazepoxide Hydrochloride	25 mg	Opaque White	Capsule		Roxane Laboratories

IMPRINT	BRAND/GENERIC NAME	STRENGTH	COLOR	FORM	SHAPE	MANUFACTURER
54; 729	Sulfisoxazole	500 mg		Tablet		Roxane Laboratories
54; 742	Guaiahist	5 mg	Chartreuse	Tablet		Roxane Laboratories
54; 742	Guaiahist	100 mg	Chartreuse	Tablet		Roxane Laboratories
54; 863	Chlordiazepoxide Hydrochloride	10 mg	Opaque Green	Capsule		Roxane Laboratories
75	Manoplax	75 mg	White	Coated Tablet	Hexagonal	Boots Pharmaceuticals
78/212; 10	Metaprel	10 mg	White	Tablet	Round, Compressed	Novartis Pharmaceuticals
78/213; 20	Metaprel	20 mg	White	Tablet	Round, Compressed	Novartis Pharmaceuticals
78; 24	Acylanid	0.1 mg	Orchid Pink	Tablet		Novartis Consumer
78; 24	Acylanid	0.1 mg	Orchid Pink	Tablet		Sandoz Consumer Pharmaceuticals
78; 25	Acylanid	0.2 mg	White	Tablet		Novartis Consumer
78; 25	Acylanid	0.2 mg	White	Tablet		Sandoz Consumer Pharmaceuticals
78; 57	Plexonal	0.08 mg	White	Tablet	Triangular	Novartis Pharmaceuticals
78; 57	Plexonal	0.16 mg	White	Tablet	Triangular	Novartis Pharmaceuticals
78; 57	Plexonal	45 mg	White	Tablet	Triangular	Novartis Pharmaceuticals
93; 825	Urinary Anteseptic	0.03 mg	Purple		Round	Teva Pharmaceuticals
93; 825	Urinary Anteseptic	5 mg	Purple		Round	Teva Pharmaceuticals
93; 825	Urinary Anteseptic	6 mg	Purple		Round	Teva Pharmaceuticals
93; 825	Urinary Anteseptic	20 mg	Purple		Round	Teva Pharmaceuticals
93; 825	Urinary Anteseptic	50 mg	Purple		Round	Teva Pharmaceuticals
93; 845	Urisep	0.03 mg	Purple	Tablet	Round	Solvay Pharmaceuticals
93; 845	Urisep	4.5 mg	Purple	Tablet	Round	Solvay Pharmaceuticals
93; 845	Urisep	5.4 mg	Purple	Tablet	Round	Solvay Pharmaceuticals
93; 845	Urisep	18.1 mg	Purple	Tablet	Round	Solvay Pharmaceuticals
93; 845	Urisep	40.8 mg	Purple	Tablet	Round	Solvay Pharmaceuticals
93; 979	Acti-Prem	2.5 mg		Tablet		Teva Pharmaceuticals
93; 979	Acti-Prem	60 mg		Tablet		Teva Pharmaceuticals
100	Dicumarol	100 mg		Tablet		Abbott Laboratories
100	Manoplax	100 mg	White	Coated Tablet	Hexagonal	Boots Pharmaceuticals
100; LL; C24	Chlorpromazine Hydrochloride	100 mg	Tan	Coated Tablet	Round	Lederle Laboratories
105	Limit	35 mg	Pink	Tablet	Round, X-Scored	
110	Rhinex DM	2 mg	White	Tablet		
110	Rhinex DM	5 mg	White	Tablet		
110	Rhinex DM	10 mg	White	Tablet		
117; C	Disobrom	6 mg	White or Green	Timed-Release Tablet	Round	Novartis Generics
117; C	Disobrom	120 mg	White or Green	Timed-Release Tablet	Round	Novartis Generics
130	Obedrin	0.5 mg	Yellow	Tablet		Beecham Laboratories
130	Obedrin	1 mg	Yellow	Tablet		Beecham Laboratories
130	Obedrin	5 mg	Yellow	Tablet		Beecham Laboratories
130	Obedrin	20 mg	Yellow	Tablet		Beecham Laboratories
130	Obedrin	100 mg	Yellow	Tablet		Beecham Laboratories
145	Bar-Tropin	0.005 grain		Tablet		Reid-Rowell Pharmaceutical
145	Bar-Tropin	0.25 grain		Tablet		
160	Dolonil	0.3 mg	Maroon	Tablet		
160	Dolonil	15 mg	Maroon	Tablet		
160	Dolonil	150 mg	Maroon	Tablet		
172	Tora I	30 mg	Black	Capsule		
200 000	Penicillin G Potassium	200,000 units	White	Tablet	Round	Reid-Rowell Pharmaceutical
200; LL; C25	Chlorpromazine Hydrochloride	200 mg	Tan	Coated Tablet		Solvay Pharmaceuticals
200; ZPP	Rescaps-D SR	40 mg	Clear White with Blue and White Beads	Capsule		Searle
200; ZPP	Rescaps-D SR	75 mg	Clear White with Blue and White Beads	Capsule		Searle
202	Microsul	1 G	Light Yellow	Tablet	Scored	Lederle Laboratories
209	Buffadyne 25	25 mg		Tablet		Pioneer Pharmaceuticals
209	Buffadyne 25	30 mg		Tablet		Pioneer Pharmaceuticals
209	Buffadyne 25	45 mg		Tablet		
209	Buffadyne 25	75 mg		Tablet		
209	Buffadyne 25	150 mg		Tablet	Round	Lederle Laboratories
209	Buffadyne 25	300 mg		Tablet	Oblong	
210; 13	Epsilan-M	100 IU	Yellow	Gelcap	Scored	Teva Pharmaceuticals
215; Q	Meclodium	90 mg	Ivory	Gelcap	Scored	Teva Pharmaceuticals
216; Q	Meclodium	100 mg	Yellow	Gelcap	Scored	Teva Pharmaceuticals
225; 155	Zeste	0.625 mg	Lavender	Tablet	Scored	Teva Pharmaceuticals
225; 160	Zeste	1.25 mg	Purple	Tablet	Scored	Teva Pharmaceuticals
225; 165	Zeste M.T.	1.25 mg	Blue	Tablet	Scored	Teva Pharmaceuticals
225; 165	Zeste M.T.	2.5 mg	Blue	Tablet		
225; 260; A	Nioric	100 mg	White	Tablet		
225; 270	Tol-C	300 mg	Red	Tablet		
225; 270	Tol-C	500 mg	Red	Tablet		Ascher
250 000	Penicillin G Potassium	250,000 units	White	Tablet		Ascher
266	A.P.B.	25 mg	Yellow	Tablet		Ascher
266	A.P.B.	50 mg	Yellow	Tablet		Ascher
283; 200 MCG	Baycol	0.2 mg	Light Yellow	Tablet		Ascher
284; 300 MCG	Baycol	0.3 mg	Yellow-Brown	Tablet		Ascher
285; 400 MCG	Baycol	0.4 mg	Ocher	Tablet	Scored	Lederle Laboratories
286; 800 MCG	Baycol	0.8 mg	Brown-Orange	Tablet	Scored	Teva Pharmaceuticals
331; 125	Methylprednisolone	4 mg	White	Tablet	Scored	Teva Pharmaceuticals
337	Lempav D-Lay	150 mg	Brown and Clear	Capsule	Scored	Teva Pharmaceuticals
354	Evasof	81 mg	Purple	Tablet		
357	Buffadyne	30 mg	Pink and White	Tablet		
357	Buffadyne	150 mg	Pink and White	Tablet		
357	Buffadyne	230 mg	Pink and White	Tablet		
366	Trilamine	15 mg	Pink	Capsule		Teva Pharmaceuticals
366	Trilamine	15 mg	Pink	Capsule	Oval	
366	Trilamine	15 mg	Pink	Capsule	Scored	Teva Pharmaceuticals
400	Felsules	0.25 G	Blue and White	Capsule		Teva Pharmaceuticals
400; 60	Broncholate	60 mg	Blue	Coated Tablet		Teva Pharmaceuticals
400; 60	Broncholate	400 mg	Blue	Coated Tablet		Teva Pharmaceuticals
410	Felsules	1 G	Yellow	Capsule		Teva Pharmaceuticals
455	Femogen	2.5 mg		Tablet		Teva Pharmaceuticals

IMPRINT	BRAND/GENERIC NAME	STRENGTH	COLOR	FORM	SHAPE	MANUFACTURER
500 MG; A5; LEDERLE	Achromycin V	500 mg	Yellow and Blue	Capsule		Teva Pharmaceuticals
511	Lufyllin	100 mg	White	Tablet		
547	Wigrettes	2 mg	White	Tablet	Football-Shaped	
555; 030	Colchicine	0.65 mg	White	Tablet	Football-Shaped	
555; 08	Meprobamate	600 mg		Tablet		
555; 24	Sulfisoxazole	500 mg	White	Tablet	Round, Scored	
555; 26	Prednisone	5 mg	White	Tablet	Round, Scored	
555; 42	Sodium Secobarbital	100 mg		Capsule	Pentagonal	Barr Laboratories
555; 72	Phendimetrazine	35 mg		Tablet	Pentagonal, Scored	Barr Laboratories
555; 106	Methocarbamol	500 mg	White	Tablet		
555; 107	Methocarbamol	750 mg	White	Tablet		
555; 114	Hydrochlorothiazide with Reserpine	0.125 mg	Light Green	Tablet		Eon Labs
555; 114	Hydrochlorothiazide with Reserpine	25 mg	Light Green	Tablet		Eon Labs
555; 114	Reserpine and Hydrochlorothiazide	0.125 mg	Light Green	Tablet		Eon Labs
555; 114	Reserpine and Hydrochlorothiazide	25 mg	Light Green	Tablet	Round, Concave Compressed	Eon Labs
555; 116	Hydrochlorothiazide with Reserpine	0.125 mg	Light Green	Tablet		
555; 116	Hydrochlorothiazide with Reserpine	50 mg	Light Green	Tablet	Rectangular	
555; 129	Dexamethasone	0.25 mg	Peach	Tablet		
555; 130	Dexamethasone	0.5 mg	Yellow	Tablet		Barr Laboratories
555; 131	Dexamethasone	0.75 mg	Green	Tablet		Barr Laboratories
555; 132	Dexamethasone	1.5 mg	Pink	Tablet	Round	Barr Laboratories
555; 141	Phendimetrazine	70 mg		Tablet	Capsule-Shaped, Scored	Barr Laboratories
555; 152	Phenobarbital	15 mg	White	Tablet	Round, Scored	
555; 153	Phenobarbital	30 mg	White	Tablet	Round, Scored	
555; 166	Phendimetrazine	35 mg		Capsule	Round, Scored	
555; 394	Phenobarbital	60 mg	White	Tablet	Round, Scored	
555; 430	Trimethoprim	200 mg		Tablet	Pentagonal, Scored	Barr Laboratories
591; F	Butalbital and Acetaminophen	50 mg	White	Tablet		Barr Laboratories
591; F	Butalbital and Acetaminophen	325 mg	White	Tablet	Pentagonal	Barr Laboratories
622; 13	Ratio	50 mg	White or Pink	Chewable Tablet	Round, Scored	
622; 13	Ratio	400 mg	White or Pink	Chewable Tablet	Round, Scored	
641; HEXAGON	Theobarb-R	0.1 mg	Blue	Tablet		Barr Laboratories
641; HEXAGON	Theobarb-R	10 mg	Blue	Tablet	Round, Scored	Barr Laboratories
641; HEXAGON	Theobarb-R	325 mg	Blue	Tablet	Round	Reid-Rowell Pharmaceutical
701	Vesicholine	25 mg	Yellow	Tablet	Round, Scored	
730	Paral	1 G		Capsule		Barr Laboratories
755	Pentryate	30 mg	Green and Yellow	Timed-Release Capsule		Barr Laboratories
804	Tora 30	30 mg	Black and Scarlet	Capsule		Barr Laboratories
822; 4	Phendimetrazine Tartrate	35 mg	Yellow	Tablet	Round; Scored	Danbury Pharmacal
830	Proglycem	100 mg	Orange	Capsule	Round; Scored	Danbury Pharmacal
832; G; 536C	Phentermine Hydrochloride	30 mg	Yellow, Black or Blue	Capsule		
832; G56C	Chlordiazepoxide and Amitriptyline Hydrochloride	10 mg	White	Coated Tablet		
832; G56C	Chlordiazepoxide and Amitriptyline Hydrochloride	25 mg	White	Coated Tablet	Round	
840	Permitil Chronotab	1 mg	Yellow	Tablet	Round	
879	Meperidine Hydrochloride	10 mg		Tablet	Round	
879; 0427	Isoxsuprine Hydrochloride	10 mg		Tablet	Flat, Scored	
879; 0428	Isoxsuprine Hydrochloride	20 mg		Tablet		
879; 0460	Vernate II S.R.	12 mg	Blue and Clear	Capsule		
879; 0460	Vernate II S.R.	75 mg	Blue and Clear	Capsule		Solvay Pharmaceuticals
879; 2G10C	Acetaminophen and Codeine Phosphate	15 mg	White	Tablet	Scored	
879; 2G10C	Acetaminophen and Codeine Phosphate	300 mg	White	Tablet		Schering
879; 3; G11C	Acetaminophen and Codeine Phosphate	30 mg	White	Tablet		
879; 3; G11C	Acetaminophen and Codeine Phosphate	300 mg	White	Tablet	Round	Pharmaceutical Basics
879; 3G11C	Acetaminophen and Codeine Phosphate	30 mg	White	Tablet	Round	Pharmaceutical Basics
879; 3G11C	Acetaminophen and Codeine Phosphate	300 mg	White	Tablet		Schering
879; 4; G12C	Acetaminophen and Codeine Phosphate	60 mg	White	Tablet		
879; 4; G12C	Acetaminophen and Codeine Phosphate	300 mg	White	Tablet		Halsey Drug
879; 4G12C	Acetaminophen and Codeine Phosphate	60 mg	White	Tablet		Solvay Pharmaceuticals
879; 4G12C	Acetaminophen and Codeine Phosphate	300 mg	White	Tablet		
879; G587	Rauwolfia Serpentina	100 mg	Red	Coated Tablet		Solvay Pharmaceuticals
933	Bisacodyl	5 mg	Orange	Enteric-Coated Tablet	Unscored	
1186	Chloramate Unicelles	12 mg	Pink and Clear	Capsule	Unscored	
1623	Quinite	260 mg	White	Tablet	Unscored	
1741	Dramamine-D	5 mg	Peach	Tablet	Unscored	
1741	Dramamine-D	50 mg	Peach	Tablet	Unscored	
2081	Hydryllin	25 mg	White	Tablet	Unscored	
2081	Hydryllin	100 mg	White	Tablet	Unscored	
4012	Pavatest	150 mg	Red and Clear	Timed-Release Capsule	Unscored	
4556	Three-Amine	25 mg	Yellow	Sustained-Release Tablet	Unscored	
4556	Three-Amine	50 mg	Yellow	Sustained-Release Tablet		

IMPRINT	BRAND/GENERIC NAME	STRENGTH	COLOR	FORM	SHAPE	MANUFACTURER
4841	Neomycin Sulfate	500 mg	White	Tablet		Parke-Davis
A	Erythrocin Stearate	125 mg	Pink	Tablet	Oblong	Abbott Laboratories
A	Oratrol	50 mg	White	Tablet	Flat-Faced, Scored	
A	Tral Gradumet	75 mg	Blue-Gray	Tablet		Abbott Laboratories
A	Tral with Phenobarbital	15 mg	Lavender	Tablet		Abbott Laboratories
A	Tral with Phenobarbital	25 mg	Lavender	Tablet		Abbott Laboratories
A; 21	Acetaminophen	325 mg	White	Tablet	Scored	Lederle Laboratories
A; 512	Modane Mild	60 mg	Pink	Coated Tablet	Round	Adria Laboratories
A; AM	Tridione	300 mg		Capsule		
A; AO	Dicumarol	50 mg		Tablet		Abbott Laboratories
A; II	Phenurone	500 mg	White	Tablet	Scored	Abbott Laboratories
A; LE	Tridione Dulcet	150 mg		Chewable Tablet		
A; MK	Nembutal Gradumet	100 mg	Blue	Tablet		Abbott Laboratories
A6; LEDERLE A6	Achrostatin V	250 mg	Pink	Capsule		Lederle Laboratories
A6; LEDERLE A6	Achrostatin V	250,000 units	Pink	Capsule		Lederle Laboratories
A9L; RD	Artane Sequels	5 mg	Clear Blue	Sustained-Release Capsule	Oval	Lederle Laboratories
ABANA; 500	Norcet	5 mg	White	Capsule		Abana Pharmaceuticals
ABANA; 500	Norcet	5 mg	White with Blue Imprint	Gelcap	Capsule	Abana Pharmaceuticals
ABANA; 500	Norcet	500 mg	White	Capsule		Abana Pharmaceuticals
ABANA; 500	Norcet	500 mg	White with Blue Imprint	Gelcap	Capsule	Abana Pharmaceuticals
ADRIA; 230	Octamide	10 mg	Yellow	Tablet	Octagonal, Scored	Adria Laboratories
ADRIA; 420	Mag-Tab SR	84 mg	Yellow	Tablet	Capsule-Shaped, Convex	Adria Laboratories
ADRIA; 648	Fluidil	2 mg	Peach	Tablet	Oval	
AEY; 420	Deronil	0.75 mg	Amber-Yellow	Tablet		Schering
AHR	Ambar	3.33 mg	Yellow-Orange	Tablet		Whitehall-Robins Healthcare
AHR	Ambar	21.6 mg	Yellow-Orange	Tablet		Whitehall-Robins Healthcare
AHR	Ambar Extentab No. 1	10 mg	Yellow	Tablet		Whitehall-Robins Healthcare
AHR	Ambar Extentab No. 1	64.8 mg	Yellow	Tablet		Whitehall-Robins Healthcare
AHR	Ambar Extentab No. 2	15 mg	Orange	Tablet		Whitehall-Robins Healthcare
AHR	Ambar Extentab No. 2	64.8 mg	Orange	Tablet		Whitehall-Robins Healthcare
AHR	Dimetane	4 mg	Peach-Colored	Tablet	Compressed, Scored	A.H. Robins
AHR	Donnagesic Extentabs No. 1	0.02 mg	Rose	Coated Tablet		Whitehall-Robins Healthcare
AHR	Donnagesic Extentabs No. 1	0.06 mg	Rose	Coated Tablet		Whitehall-Robins Healthcare
AHR	Donnagesic Extentabs No. 1	0.4 mg	Rose	Coated Tablet		Whitehall-Robins Healthcare
AHR	Donnagesic Extentabs No. 1	48.6 mg	Rose	Coated Tablet		Whitehall-Robins Healthcare
AHR	Donnasep	0.0033 mg	Rose	Tablet	Capsule-Shaped	
AHR	Donnasep	0.0097 mg	Rose	Tablet	Capsule-Shaped	
AHR	Donnasep	0.0519 mg	Rose	Tablet	Capsule-Shaped	
AHR	Donnasep	8.1 mg	Rose	Tablet	Capsule-Shaped	
AHR	Donnasep	50 mg	Rose	Tablet	Capsule-Shaped	
AHR	Donnasep	500 mg	Rose	Tablet	Capsule-Shaped	
AHR	Donnasep-MP	0.0033 mg	Blue	Tablet	Capsule-Shaped	
AHR	Donnasep-MP	0.0097 mg	Blue	Tablet	Capsule-Shaped	
AHR	Donnasep-MP	0.0519 mg	Blue	Tablet	Capsule-Shaped	
AHR	Donnasep-MP	8.1 mg	Blue	Tablet	Capsule-Shaped	
AHR	Donnasep-MP	500 mg	Blue	Tablet	Capsule-Shaped	
AHR	Robizone-V	100 mg	White		Scored	A.H. Robins
AHR 1857	Dimetane	4 mg	Peach-Colored	Tablet	Compressed, Scored	A.H. Robins
AHR; 2; 7880	Robinul-PH Forte	2 mg	Blue	Tablet		
AHR; 2; 7880	Robinul-PH Forte	16.2 mg	Blue	Tablet		
AHR; 5460	Exna-R	0.125 mg	White	Tablet	Round, Scored	
AHR; 5460	Exna-R	50 mg	White	Tablet	Round, Scored	
AHR; 5610	Imavate	10 mg	White	Tablet	Round	A.H. Robins
AHR; 5625	Imavate	25 mg	Coral or Buff	Tablet	Round	A.H. Robins
AHR; 6447	Pondimin	20 mg	Orange	Tablet	Scored, Compressed	Whitehall-Robins Healthcare
AHR; 7874	Robinul-PH	1 mg	Blue	Tablet	Round	
AHR; 7874	Robinul-PH	16.2 mg	Blue	Tablet	Round	
AMIDE; 006	Phenazopyridine Hydrochloride and Sulfisoxazole	50 mg		Tablet		
AMIDE; 006	Phenazopyridine Hydrochloride and Sulfisoxazole	500 mg		Tablet		
AMIDE; 008	Ami-Tapp	12 mg	White or Blue	Extended-Release Tablet		
AMIDE; 008	Ami-Tapp	15 mg	White or Blue	Extended-Release Tablet		
AR; 600	AR 600	600 mg	Light Green	Tablet	Capsule-Shaped	
ARE	Mol-Iron Panhemic	7.5 mcg	Orange and Black	Capsule		Schering-Plough Healthcare Products
ARE	Mol-Iron Panhemic	2 mg	Orange and Black	Capsule		Schering-Plough Healthcare Products
ARE	Mol-Iron Panhemic	10 mg	Orange and Black	Capsule		Schering-Plough Healthcare Products
ARE	Mol-Iron Panhemic	75 mg	Orange and Black	Capsule		Schering-Plough Healthcare Products
ARE	Mol-Iron Panhemic	500 mg	Orange and Black	Capsule		Schering-Plough Healthcare Products
ASBRON G; 43-62	Asbron G	100 mg	Green with White Inlay	Tablet		Novartis Pharmaceuticals
ASBRON G; 43-62	Asbron G	300 mg	Green with White Inlay	Tablet		Novartis Pharmaceuticals
ASBRON G; 78/202	Asbron G	100 mg	Green with White Inlay	Tablet		Novartis Pharmaceuticals
ASBRON G; 78/202	Asbron G	300 mg	Green with White Inlay	Tablet		Novartis Pharmaceuticals
ASPIRIN	Quality Aspirin	325 mg	White	Tablet		
B	Tigovert	25 mg	Burgundy	Coated Tablet		
B	Tigovert	50 mg	Burgundy	Coated Tablet		
B; 0013	Chlorothiazide	500 mg	White	Tablet	Round	
B; 0036	Chlorothiazide	250 mg	White	Tablet	Round	
B; 0056	Chlorothiazide with Reserpine	0.125 mg	Pink	Tablet	Round	
B; 0056	Chlorothiazide with Reserpine	250 mg	Pink	Tablet	Round	

IMPRINT	BRAND/GENERIC NAME	STRENGTH	COLOR	FORM	SHAPE	MANUFACTURER
B; 0064	Hydralazine Hydrochloride and Hydrochlorothiazide	50 mg	Blue	Capsule		
B; 0064	Hydralazine Hydrochloride and Hydrochlorothiazide	100 mg	Blue	Capsule		
B; 0065	Hydralazine Hydrochloride and Hydrochlorothiazide	25 mg	White	Capsule		
B; 0066	Hydralazine Hydrochloride and Hydrochlorothiazide	50 mg	White and Black	Capsule		Bolar Pharmaceutical
B; 0083	Hydralazine with Hydrochlorothiazide	15 mg	Light Orange	Tablet	Round	
B; 0083	Hydralazine with Hydrochlorothiazide	25 mg	Light Orange	Tablet	Round	
B; 0094	Carisoprodol	350 mg		Tablet		Bolar Pharmaceutical
B; 0094	Carisoprodol	350 mg		Tablet		Regal Labs
B; 0127	Hydroflumethiazide with Reserpine	0.125 mg	Yellow	Tablet	Round	Bolar Pharmaceutical
B; 0127	Hydroflumethiazide with Reserpine	25 mg	Yellow	Tablet	Round	Bolar Pharmaceutical
B; 0128	Hydroflumethiazide with Reserpine	0.125 mg	Green	Tablet	Round	Bolar Pharmaceutical
B; 0128	Hydroflumethiazide with Reserpine	50 mg	Green	Tablet	Round	Bolar Pharmaceutical
B; 0132	Chlorothiazide with Reserpine	0.125 mg	Pink	Tablet	Round	Bolar Pharmaceutical
B; 0132	Chlorothiazide with Reserpine	500 mg	Pink	Tablet	Round	Bolar Pharmaceutical
B; 062	Nuphyll GG	200 mg	Yellow	Tablet	Round	Econolab
B; 1007	Trazodone Hydrochloride	50 mg	White	Tablet	Round	Circa Pharmaceuticals
B; 1008	Trazodone Hydrochloride	100 mg	White	Tablet	Round	Circa Pharmaceuticals
B; 1027	Amantadine Hydrochloride	100 mg	Pink	Gelcap	Oblong	Bolar Pharmaceutical
B; 2049	Hydrochlorothiazide with Reserpine and Hydralazine	0.1 mg	White or Pink	Tablet	Round	
B; 2049	Hydrochlorothiazide with Reserpine and Hydralazine	15 mg	White or Pink	Tablet	Round	
B; 2049	Hydrochlorothiazide with Reserpine and Hydralazine	25 mg	White or Pink	Tablet	Round	
B; 2053	Perphenazine and Amitriptyline	2 mg	Orange	Coated Tablet	Round	Circa Pharmaceuticals
B; 2053	Perphenazine and Amitriptyline	25 mg	Orange	Coated Tablet	Round	Circa Pharmaceuticals
B; 2054	Perphenazine and Amitriptyline	4 mg	Yellow	Coated Tablet	Round	Circa Pharmaceuticals
B; 2054	Perphenazine and Amitriptyline	25 mg	Yellow	Coated Tablet	Round	Circa Pharmaceuticals
B; 2055	Perphenazine and Amitriptyline	4 mg	Orange	Coated Tablet	Round	Circa Pharmaceuticals
B; 2055	Perphenazine and Amitriptyline	50 mg	Orange	Coated Tablet	Round	Circa Pharmaceuticals
B; 2056	Perphenazine and Amitriptyline	2 mg	Blue	Coated Tablet	Round	Circa Pharmaceuticals
B; 2056	Perphenazine and Amitriptyline	10 mg	Blue	Coated Tablet	Round	Circa Pharmaceuticals
B; 2057	Perphenazine and Amitriptyline	4 mg	Salmon	Coated Tablet	Round	Circa Pharmaceuticals
B; 2057	Perphenazine and Amitriptyline	10 mg	Salmon	Coated Tablet	Round	Circa Pharmaceuticals
BARR; 281	Aminophylline	200 mg	White	Tablet	Round	Barr Laboratories
BARR; 282	Aminophylline	100 mg	White	Tablet	Round	Barr Laboratories
BARR; 434	Folic Acid	1 mg	Yellow	Tablet	Round	Barr Laboratories
BARR; 555; 116	Reserpine and Hydrochlorothiazide	0.125 mg	Light Green	Tablet		Barr Laboratories
BARR; 555; 116	Reserpine and Hydrochlorothiazide	50 mg	Light Green	Tablet		Barr Laboratories
BARR; 555; 314	Sulfamethoxazole	500 mg	Green	Tablet	Round, Scored	Barr Laboratories
BAY; 132	Stilphostrol	50 mg	White with Gray Mottling	Tablet	Round	
BAYER	Bayer Children's Cold	3.135 mg	Orange and White	Tablet	Two-Layered	Sterling Health
BAYER	Bayer Children's Cold	81 mg	Orange and White	Tablet	Two-Layered	Sterling Health
BB; 1007	Trazodone Hydrochloride	50 mg	White	Tablet	Round	Circa Pharmaceuticals
BB; 1008	Trazodone Hydrochloride	100 mg	White	Tablet	Round	Circa Pharmaceuticals
BB; 2053	Perphenazine and Amitriptyline	2 mg	Orange	Coated Tablet	Round	Circa Pharmaceuticals
BB; 2053	Perphenazine and Amitriptyline	25 mg	Orange	Coated Tablet	Round	Circa Pharmaceuticals
BB; 2054	Perphenazine and Amitriptyline	4 mg	Yellow	Coated Tablet	Round	Circa Pharmaceuticals
BB; 2054	Perphenazine and Amitriptyline	25 mg	Yellow	Coated Tablet	Round	Circa Pharmaceuticals
BB; 2055	Perphenazine and Amitriptyline	4 mg	Orange	Coated Tablet	Round	Circa Pharmaceuticals
BB; 2055	Perphenazine and Amitriptyline	50 mg	Orange	Coated Tablet	Round	Circa Pharmaceuticals
BB; 2056	Perphenazine and Amitriptyline	2 mg	Blue	Coated Tablet	Round	Circa Pharmaceuticals
BB; 2056	Perphenazine and Amitriptyline	10 mg	Blue	Coated Tablet	Round	Circa Pharmaceuticals
BB; 2057	Perphenazine and Amitriptyline	4 mg	Salmon	Coated Tablet	Round	Circa Pharmaceuticals
BB; 2057	Perphenazine and Amitriptyline	10 mg	Salmon	Coated Tablet	Round	Circa Pharmaceuticals
BB; 2066	Lithium Carbonate	300 mg	White and Pink	Capsule		Circa Pharmaceuticals
BB; 2081	Flurazepam Hydrochloride	15 mg	White and Light Green	Capsule		Bolar Pharmaceutical
BB; 2082	Flurazepam Hydrochloride	30 mg	White and Dark Green	Capsule		Bolar Pharmaceutical
BEANO	Beano	150 U	Tan		Oval	
BENTEX	Afrodex	5 mg	Red	Capsule		Icn Pharmaceuticals
BL; B3	Bufferin with Codeine No. 3	30 mg	White	Tablet	Round	
BL; B3	Bufferin with Codeine No. 3	97.2 mg	White	Tablet	Round	
BL; B3	Bufferin with Codeine No. 3	325 mg	White	Tablet	Round	
BL; E1	Bristamycin	250 mg	Orange	Tablet	Round	
BMP; 105	Anexsia with Codeine	30 mg	Pink	Tablet		
BMP; 105	Anexsia with Codeine	32 mg	Pink	Tablet		
BMP; 105	Anexsia with Codeine	32.4 mg		Tablet		
BMP; 105	Anexsia with Codeine	162 mg		Tablet		
BMP; 105	Anexsia with Codeine	227 mg		Tablet		
BMP; 105	Anexsia with Codeine	325 mg	Pink	Tablet		
BMP; 129	Obedrin	0.5 mg	Gray and Orange	Capsule		Beecham Laboratories
BMP; 129	Obedrin	1 mg	Gray and Orange	Capsule		Beecham Laboratories
BMP; 129	Obedrin	5 mg	Gray and Orange	Capsule		Beecham Laboratories
BMP; 129	Obedrin	20 mg	Gray and Orange	Capsule		Beecham Laboratories
BMP; 129	Obedrin	100 mg	Gray and Orange	Capsule		Beecham Laboratories
BMP; 131	Obedrin-LA	1 mg	Pink	Tablet	Beaded	Beecham Laboratories
BMP; 131	Obedrin-LA	2 mg	Pink	Tablet	Beaded	Beecham Laboratories
BMP; 131	Obedrin-LA	10 mg	Pink	Tablet	Beaded	Beecham Laboratories
BMP; 131	Obedrin-LA	12.5 mg	Pink	Tablet	Beaded	Beecham Laboratories

IMPRINT	BRAND/GENERIC NAME	STRENGTH	COLOR	FORM	SHAPE	MANUFACTURER
BMP; 131	Obedrin-LA	50 mg	Pink	Tablet	Beaded	Beecham Laboratories
BMP; 131	Obedrin-LA	100 mg	Pink	Tablet	Beaded	Beecham Laboratories
BMP; 131	Obedrin-LA	112 mg	Pink	Tablet	Beaded	Beecham Laboratories
BMP; 145	Daricon	10 mg	White	Tablet	Round, Grooved	Smithkline Beecham
BMP; 146	Daricon PB	5 mg	Pink	Tablet		Smithkline Beecham
BMP; 146	Daricon PB	15 mg	Pink	Tablet		Smithkline Beecham
BMP; 150	Obedrin-LA	10 mg		Tablet		Smithkline Beecham
BMP; 160	Phenobarbital	1 grain		Tablet		
BMP; 161	Phenobarbital	1.5 grains		Tablet		
BMP; 169	Cloxapen	250 mg	Lime and Beige	Capsule		
BMP; 170	Cloxapen	500 mg	Lime and Beige	Capsule		
BOCK	Amobell	10 mg	Two-Toned Blue	Capsule		
BOCK	Amobell	15 mg	Two-Toned Blue	Capsule		
BOCK	G-200	200 mg	Blue and White	Capsule		
BOCK	Hemaspan	20 mg	Brown and Clear	Capsule		
BOCK	Hemaspan	100 mg	Brown and Clear	Capsule		
BOCK	Hemaspan	275 mg	Brown and Clear	Capsule		
BOCK	Hemaspan-FA	1 mg	Caramel and Clear	Capsule		
BOCK	Hemaspan-FA	20 mg	Caramel and Clear	Capsule		
BOCK	Hemaspan-FA	100 mg	Caramel and Clear	Capsule		
BOCK	Hemaspan-FA	275 mg	Caramel and Clear	Capsule		
BOCK	Poly-Histine	25 mg	Light Green and Clear with White Beads	Capsule		
BOCK	Poly-Histine-DX	12 mg	Purple and Clear	Capsule		
BOCK	Poly-Histine-DX	120 mg	Purple and Clear	Capsule		
BOCK	Theon-300	300 mg	Clear	Sustained-Release Capsule		
BOCK C	Dolprn No. 3	30 mg	Green	Tablet	Football-Shaped	
BOCK C	Dolprn No. 3	60 mg	Green	Tablet	Football-Shaped	
BOCK C	Dolprn No. 3	250 mg	Green	Tablet	Football-Shaped	
BOCK C	Dolprn No. 3	400 mg	Green	Tablet	Football-Shaped	
BOCK; ONSET-5	Onset-5	5 mg	Orange	Tablet	Round	
BOCK; ONSET-10	Onset-10	10 mg	White	Tablet	Round	
BOLAR	L-5 Hydroxytryptophan	25 mg	White and Blue			
BOLAR	L-5 Hydroxytryptophan	50 mg	White and Maroon			
BOLAR	L-5 Hydroxytryptophan	100 mg	White and Yellow			
BOLAR	L-5 Hydroxytryptophan	200 mg	Blue			
BOLAR KV; 12/100	Disopyramide Phosphate	100 mg	Purple and Yellow	Controlled-Release Capsule		
BOLAR KV; 12/150	Disopyramide Phosphate	150 mg	Purple and Orange	Controlled-Release Capsule		
BOOTS LOGO/50 MG	Manoplax	50 mg	White	Coated Tablet	Hexagonal	Boots Pharmaceuticals
BOOTS; 0051	Lopurin	100 mg	White	Tablet	Round	Boots Pharmaceuticals
BOOTS; 0052	Lopurin	300 mg	Orange	Tablet	Round	Boots Pharmaceuticals
BOOTS; 200	P-200	200 mg	Pink	Timed-Release Tablet		
BP; 0005	Methocarbamol	500 mg	White	Tablet	Round	
BP; 0006	Methocarbamol	750 mg	White	Tablet	Capsule-Shaped	
BP; 0011	Furosemide	12.5 mg	Yellow		Round	
BP; 0012	Furosemide	50 mg	Yellow	Tablet	Capsule-Shaped	
BP; 0013	Chlorothiazide	500 mg	White	Tablet	Round	
BP; 0014	Oxtriphylline with Guaifenesin	100 mg		Tablet		
BP; 0014	Oxtriphylline with Guaifenesin	200 mg		Tablet		
BP; 0017	Pentaerythritol Tetranitrate	80 mg	Light Green and Dark Green	Tablet		
BP; 0026	Isosorbide Dinitrate	40 mg	Green	Timed-Release Tablet	Round	
BP; 0029	Triprolidine Hydrochloride and Pseudoephedrine	2.5 mg		Tablet		
BP; 0029	Triprolidine Hydrochloride and Pseudoephedrine	60 mg		Tablet		
BP; 0035	Chlorthalidone	100 mg	White	Tablet	Round	
BP; 0036	Chlorothiazide	250 mg	White	Tablet	Round	
BP; 0044	Warfarin Sodium	2.5 mg	Orange	Tablet	Round	
BP; 0045	Warfarin Sodium	5 mg	Pink	Tablet	Round	
BP; 0046	Warfarin Sodium	7.5 mg	Yellow	Tablet	Round	
BP; 0047	Warfarin Sodium	10 mg	White	Tablet	Round	
BP; 0049	Isosorbide Dinitrate	20 mg	Green	Tablet	Round	
BP; 0050	Warfarin Sodium	2 mg	Lavender	Tablet	Round	
BP; 0056	Chlorothiazide with Reserpine	0.125 mg	Pink	Tablet	Round	
BP; 0056	Chlorothiazide with Reserpine	250 mg	Pink	Tablet	Round	
BP; 0058	Hydrochlorothiazide	100 mg	Orange	Tablet	Round	
BP; 0062	Methyclothiazide	2.5 mg	Red-Orange	Tablet	Round	
BP; 0063	Methyclothiazide	5 mg	Red-Orange	Tablet	Round	
BP; 0064	Hydralazine Hydrochloride and Hydrochlorothiazide	50 mg	Blue	Capsule		
BP; 0064	Hydralazine Hydrochloride and Hydrochlorothiazide	100 mg	Blue	Capsule		
BP; 0065	Hydralazine Hydrochloride and Hydrochlorothiazide	25 mg	White	Capsule		
BP; 0066	Hydralazine Hydrochloride and Hydrochlorothiazide	50 mg	White and Black	Capsule		Bolar Pharmaceutical
BP; 0071	Nicotinyl Alcohol Tartrate	150 mg		Timed-Release Tablet		
BP; 0072	Hydroflumethiazide	50 mg	White	Tablet	Round	
BP; 0073	Bethanechol Chloride	5 mg	White	Tablet	Round	
BP; 0076	Oxtriphylline	100 mg	Red-Orange	Coated Tablet	Round	
BP; 0077	Oxtriphylline	200 mg	Yellow	Coated Tablet	Round	
BP; 0080	Clonidine Hydrochloride	0.2 mg	Orange	Tablet	Round	
BP; 0081	Clonidine Hydrochloride	0.3 mg	Peach	Tablet	Round	
BP; 0083	Hydralazine with Hydrochlorothiazide	15 mg	Light Orange	Tablet	Round	
BP; 0083	Hydralazine with Hydrochlorothiazide	25 mg	Light Orange	Tablet	Round	

IMPRINT	BRAND/GENERIC NAME	STRENGTH	COLOR	FORM	SHAPE	MANUFACTURER
BP; 0084	Phenytoin Sodium	100 mg	White	Extended-Release Capsule		
BP; 0087	Sulfamethoxazole	500 mg	Green	Tablet	Round	
BP; 0089	Hydroxyzine, Theophylline and Ephedrine Sulfate	10 mg		Tablet		
BP; 0089	Hydroxyzine, Theophylline and Ephedrine Sulfate	25 mg		Tablet		
BP; 0089	Hydroxyzine, Theophylline and Ephedrine Sulfate	130 mg		Tablet		
BP; 0091	Chlorzoxazone with Apap	250 mg	Green	Tablet	Scored	
BP; 0091	Chlorzoxazone with Apap	300 mg	Green	Tablet	Scored	
BP; 0092	Prochlorperazine with Isopropamide	5 mg	Yellow and Clear	Timed-Release Capsule		
BP; 0092	Prochlorperazine with Isopropamide	10 mg	Yellow and Clear	Timed-Release Capsule		
BP; 0094	Carisoprodol	350 mg		Tablet		Bolar Pharmaceutical
BP; 0094	Carisoprodol	350 mg		Tablet		Regal Labs
BP; 0123	Propranolol Hydrochloride	10 mg	Peach	Tablet	Round	
BP; 0124	Propranolol Hydrochloride	20 mg	Light Blue	Tablet	Round	
BP; 0125	Propranolol Hydrochloride	40 mg	Green	Tablet	Round	
BP; 0126	Propranolol Hydrochloride	80 mg	Yellow	Tablet	Round	
BP; 0127	Hydroflumethiazide with Reserpine	0.125 mg	Yellow	Tablet	Round	Bolar Pharmaceutical
BP; 0127	Hydroflumethiazide with Reserpine	25 mg	Yellow	Tablet	Round	Bolar Pharmaceutical
BP; 0128	Hydroflumethiazide with Reserpine	0.125 mg	Green	Tablet	Round	Bolar Pharmaceutical
BP; 0128	Hydroflumethiazide with Reserpine	50 mg	Green	Tablet	Round	Bolar Pharmaceutical
BP; 0129	Spironolactone with Hydrochlorothiazide	25 mg		Tablet		
BP; 0131	Sulfasalazine	500 mg	Brown	Enteric-Coated Tablet	Round	
BP; 0132	Chlorothiazide with Reserpine	0.125 mg	Pink	Tablet	Round	Bolar Pharmaceutical
BP; 0132	Chlorothiazide with Reserpine	500 mg	Pink	Tablet	Round	Bolar Pharmaceutical
BP; 0133	Allopurinol	100 mg	White	Tablet	Round	
BP; 0134	Allopurinol	300 mg	Peach	Tablet	Round	
BP; 0135	Guanethidine Monosulfate	10 mg	Orange	Tablet	Round	
BP; 0136	Guanethidine Monosulfate	25 mg	White	Tablet	Round	
BP; 0137	Fluoxymesterone	2 mg	Peach	Tablet	Round	
BP; 0138	Fluoxymesterone	5 mg	Green	Tablet	Round	
BP; 0139	Fluoxymesterone	10 mg	Green	Tablet	Round	
BP; 0145	Indomethacin	25 mg	Light Green and Dark Green	Capsule		
BP; 0146	Indomethacin	50 mg	Light Green	Capsule		
BP; 0148	Oxyphenbutazone	100 mg	Pink	Coated Tablet		
BP; 0149	Acepromazine Maleate	10 mg	Yellow		Round	
BP; 0150	Acepromazine Maleate	25 mg	Yellow		Round	
BP; 0157	Methyclothiazide with Deserpidine	0.5 mg	Grey	Tablet	Round	
BP; 0157	Methyclothiazide with Deserpidine	5 mg	Grey	Tablet	Round	
BP; 0158	Methyclothiazide with Deserpidine	0.25 mg	Yellow	Tablet	Round	
BP; 0158	Methyclothiazide with Deserpidine	5 mg	Yellow	Tablet	Round	
BP; 0163	Fluphenazine Hydrochloride	1 mg	White	Coated Tablet	Round	
BP; 0164	Fluphenazine Hydrochloride	2.5 mg	Beige	Coated Tablet	Round	
BP; 0165	Fluphenazine Hydrochloride	5 mg	Blue	Coated Tablet	Round	
BP; 0166	Fluphenazine Hydrochloride	10 mg	Red	Coated Tablet	Round	
BP; 0168	Chlorpropamide	250 mg	Blue	Tablet	Round	
BP; 0181	Lorazepam	1 mg	White	Tablet	Round	
BP; 0182	Lorazepam	2 mg	White	Tablet	Round	
BP; 0187	Procainamide Hydrochloride SR	1000 mg	Pink	Sustained-Release Tablet	Capsule-Shaped	
BP; 1	Thioridazine Hydrochloride	10 mg	Green	Tablet	Capsule-Shaped	
BP; 10	Dipyridamole	25 mg		Tablet		
BP; 22	Decongestabs	5 mg		Tablet		
BP; 22	Decongestabs	10 mg		Tablet		
BP; 22	Decongestabs	15 mg		Tablet		
BP; 22	Decongestabs	40 mg		Tablet		
BP; 25	Bromatapp	4 mg		Tablet		
BP; 25	Bromatapp	5 mg		Tablet		
BP; 31	Thioridazine Hydrochloride	15 mg	Purple	Tablet	Capsule-Shaped	
BP; 33	Chlorthalidone	25 mg	Peach	Tablet	Round	
BP; 34	Chlorthalidone	50 mg	Blue	Tablet	Round	
BP; 60	Liothyronine Sodium	25 mcg	White	Tablet	Round	
BP; 61	Liothyronine Sodium	50 mcg	White	Tablet	Round	
BP; 78	Cyproheptadine Hydrochloride	4 mg	White	Tablet	Round	
BP; 100	Hydroxyzine Pamoate	25 mg	Dark Green and Light Green	Capsule		
BP; 101	Hydroxyzine Pamoate	50 mg	White and Green	Capsule		
BP; 102	Hydroxyzine Pamoate	100 mg	Grey and Green	Capsule		
BP; 118	Thioridazine Hydrochloride	25 mg	Brown	Tablet	Capsule-Shaped	
BP; 119	Thioridazine Hydrochloride	50 mg	White	Tablet		
BP; 120	Thioridazine Hydrochloride	100 mg	Yellow-Green	Tablet	Capsule-Shaped	
BP; 121	Thioridazine Hydrochloride	150 mg	Yellow	Tablet	Capsule-Shaped	
BP; 122	Thioridazine Hydrochloride	200 mg	Purple	Tablet	Capsule-Shaped	
BP; 143	Trimethobenzamide	250 mg	Blue	Capsule		
BP; 151	Trifluoperazine Hydrochloride	10 mg	Red	Tablet		
BP; 171	Trifluoperazine Hydrochloride	1 mg	Red	Tablet		
BP; 172	Trifluoperazine Hydrochloride	2 mg	Red	Tablet		
BP; 195	Timolol Maleate	5 mg	White	Tablet	Round	
BP; 196	Timolol Maleate	10 mg	White	Tablet	Round, Scored	
BP; 197	Timolol Maleate	20 mg	White	Tablet	Capsule-Shaped, Scored	

IMPRINT	BRAND/GENERIC NAME	STRENGTH	COLOR	FORM	SHAPE	MANUFACTURER
BP; 209	Amitriptyline	10 mg		Tablet	Round	Circa Pharmaceuticals
BP; 211	Maprotiline Hydrochloride	25 mg	Blue	Tablet	Scored	
BP; 212	Maprotiline Hydrochloride	50 mg	Yellow	Tablet	Scored	
BP; 213	Maprotiline Hydrochloride	75 mg	White	Tablet	Scored	
BP; 227	Triamterene and Hydrochlorothiazide	25 mg	Red	Capsule		
BP; 227	Triamterene and Hydrochlorothiazide	50 mg	Red	Capsule		
BP; 1007	Trazodone Hydrochloride	50 mg	White	Tablet	Round	Circa Pharmaceuticals
BP; 1008	Trazodone Hydrochloride	100 mg	White	Tablet	Round	Circa Pharmaceuticals
BP; 1015	Nitrofurantoin	100 mg	Yellow	Capsule		
BP; 1027	Amantadine Hydrochloride	100 mg	Pink	Gelcap	Oblong	Bolar Pharmaceutical
BP; 1045	Theophylline, Ephedrine and Phenobarbital	8 mg		Tablet		
BP; 1045	Theophylline, Ephedrine and Phenobarbital	24 mg		Tablet		
BP; 1045	Theophylline, Ephedrine and Phenobarbital	130 mg		Tablet		
BP; 2005	Disopyramide Phosphate	100 mg	White and Orange	Capsule		
BP; 2006	Disopyramide Phosphate	150 mg	Orange and Brown	Capsule		
BP; 2013	Chlorpheniramine Maleate	4 mg		Tablet		
BP; 2014	Methyldopa	125 mg	White	Coated Tablet	Round	
BP; 2015	Methyldopa	250 mg	White	Coated Tablet	Round	
BP; 2016	Methyldopa	500 mg	White	Coated Tablet	Round	
BP; 2016	Nitrofurantoin	50 mg	Yellow	Capsule		
BP; 2017	Brompheniramine Maleate	4 mg		Tablet		
BP; 2024	Meclofenamate Sodium	50 mg	Maroon and Pink	Capsule		
BP; 2025	Meclofenamate Sodium	100 mg	Maroon and White	Capsule		
BP; 2027	Metoclopramide Hydrochloride	10 mg	White	Tablet	Round	
BP; 2028	Dimenhydrinate	50 mg		Tablet		
BP; 2036	Methyldopa with Hydrochlorothiazide	15 mg	Chartreuse	Coated Tablet	Round	
BP; 2036	Methyldopa with Hydrochlorothiazide	250 mg	Chartreuse	Coated Tablet	Round	
BP; 2037	Methyldopa with Hydrochlorothiazide	25 mg	Pink	Coated Tablet	Round	
BP; 2037	Methyldopa with Hydrochlorothiazide	250 mg	Pink	Coated Tablet	Round	
BP; 2038	Methyldopa with Hydrochlorothiazide	30 mg	Chartreuse	Coated Tablet	Oval	
BP; 2038	Methyldopa with Hydrochlorothiazide	500 mg	Chartreuse	Coated Tablet	Oval	
BP; 2039	Methyldopa with Hydrochlorothiazide	50 mg	Pink	Coated Tablet	Oval	
BP; 2039	Methyldopa with Hydrochlorothiazide	500 mg	Pink	Coated Tablet	Oval	
BP; 2042	Verapamil Hydrochloride	80 mg	White	Tablet	Round	
BP; 2043	Verapamil Hydrochloride	120 mg	White	Tablet	Round	
BP; 2047	Hydrochlorothiazide with Reserpine	0.125 mg	Green	Tablet	Round	
BP; 2047	Hydrochlorothiazide with Reserpine	25 mg	Green	Tablet	Round	
BP; 2048	Hydrochlorothiazide with Reserpine	0.125 mg	Green	Tablet	Round	
BP; 2048	Hydrochlorothiazide with Reserpine	50 mg	Green	Tablet	Round	
BP; 2049	H.H.R.	0.1 mg		Tablet		
BP; 2049	H.H.R.	15 mg		Tablet		
BP; 2049	H.H.R.	25 mg		Tablet		
BP; 2049	Hydrochlorothiazide with Reserpine and Hydralazine	0.1 mg	White or Pink	Tablet	Round	
BP; 2049	Hydrochlorothiazide with Reserpine and Hydralazine	15 mg	White or Pink	Tablet	Round	
BP; 2049	Hydrochlorothiazide with Reserpine and Hydralazine	25 mg	White or Pink	Tablet	Round	
BP; 2051	Isosorbide Dinitrate	5 mg		Tablet		
BP; 2052	Isosorbide Dinitrate	10 mg		Tablet		
BP; 2053	Perphenazine and Amitriptyline	2 mg	Orange	Coated Tablet	Round	Circa Pharmaceuticals
BP; 2053	Perphenazine and Amitriptyline	25 mg	Orange	Coated Tablet	Round	Circa Pharmaceuticals
BP; 2054	Perphenazine and Amitriptyline	4 mg	Yellow	Coated Tablet	Round	Circa Pharmaceuticals
BP; 2054	Perphenazine and Amitriptyline	25 mg	Yellow	Coated Tablet	Round	Circa Pharmaceuticals
BP; 2055	Perphenazine and Amitriptyline	4 mg	Orange	Coated Tablet	Round	Circa Pharmaceuticals
BP; 2055	Perphenazine and Amitriptyline	50 mg	Orange	Coated Tablet	Round	Circa Pharmaceuticals
BP; 2056	Perphenazine and Amitriptyline	2 mg	Blue	Coated Tablet	Round	Circa Pharmaceuticals
BP; 2056	Perphenazine and Amitriptyline	10 mg	Blue	Coated Tablet	Round	Circa Pharmaceuticals
BP; 2057	Perphenazine and Amitriptyline	4 mg	Salmon	Coated Tablet	Round	Circa Pharmaceuticals
BP; 2057	Perphenazine and Amitriptyline	10 mg	Salmon	Coated Tablet	Round	Circa Pharmaceuticals
BP; 2060	Propranolol Hydrochloride	60 mg	Yellow	Tablet	Round	
BP; 2061	Nitrofurantoin	100 mg	Yellow	Capsule		
BP; 2062	Tolbutamide	250 mg	White	Tablet	Round	
BP; 2063	Tolbutamide	500 mg	White	Tablet	Round	
BP; 2064	Pentaerythritol Tetranitrate	10 mg	Green	Tablet	Round	
BP; 2066	Lithium Carbonate	300 mg	White and Pink	Capsule		Circa Pharmaceuticals
BP; 2067	Pentaerythritol Tetranitrate	20 mg	Green	Tablet	Round	
BP; 2068	Tolazamide	100 mg	White	Tablet	Round	
BP; 2069	Tolazamide	250 mg	White	Tablet	Round	
BP; 2070	Tolazamide	500 mg	White	Tablet	Round	
BP; 2074	Probenecid with Colchicine	0.5 mg	White	Tablet	Capsule-Shaped	
BP; 2074	Probenecid with Colchicine	500 mg	White	Tablet	Capsule-Shaped	
BP; 2075	Nitrofurantoin	50 mg	Yellow	Tablet	Round	
BP; 2076	Procainamide Hydrochloride	250 mg	Yellow	Capsule		
BP; 2078	Procainamide Hydrochloride	500 mg	Yellow and Orange	Capsule		
BP; 2080	Nitrofurantoin	100 mg	Yellow	Tablet	Round	

IMPRINT	BRAND/GENERIC NAME	STRENGTH	COLOR	FORM	SHAPE	MANUFACTURER
BP; 2081	Flurazepam Hydrochloride	15 mg	White and Light Green	Capsule		Bolar Pharmaceutical
BP; 2082	Flurazepam Hydrochloride	30 mg	White and Dark Green	Capsule		Bolar Pharmaceutical
BP; 2085	Acetaminophen and Propoxyphene Napsylate	50 mg	Pink	Coated Tablet	Capsule-Shaped	
BP; 2085	Acetaminophen and Propoxyphene Napsylate	325 mg	Pink	Coated Tablet	Capsule-Shaped	
BP; 2086	Acetaminophen and Propoxyphene Napsylate	100 mg	Pink	Coated Tablet	Capsule-Shaped	
BP; 2086	Acetaminophen and Propoxyphene Napsylate	650 mg	Pink	Coated Tablet	Capsule-Shaped	
BP; 2087	Temazepam	15 mg	Pink	Capsule		
BP; 2088	Temazepam	30 mg	Yellow and Pink	Capsule		
BP; 2092	Trichlormethiazide with Reserpine	0.1 mg	Lavender	Tablet	Round	
BP; 2092	Trichlormethiazide with Reserpine	4 mg	Lavender	Tablet	Round	
BP; 2092	Trichlortension	0.1 mg		Tablet		
BP; 2092	Trichlortension	4 mg		Tablet		
BP; 2093	Hydrochlorothiazide	25 mg	Orange	Tablet	Round	
BP; 2094	Hydrochlorothiazide	50 mg	Orange	Tablet	Round	
BP; 2126	Potassium Chloride	750 mg (10 meq)	White	Capsule		
BP; 2130	Tripelennamine Hydrochloride	50 mg	Blue	Tablet		
BP; 2147	Potassium Chloride ER	600 mg		Extended-Release Tablet		
BP; 2200	Folic Acid	1 mg		Tablet		
BP; 3020	Trichlormethiazide	4 mg	Blue	Tablet	Round	
BP; 5000	Spironolactone	25 mg	White	Tablet	Round	
BP; 5010	Bethanechol Chloride	50 mg	Yellow	Tablet	Round	
BP; 9000	Quinine Sulfate	260 mg	White	Tablet	Round	
BP; 9002	Methandrostenolone	5 mg		Tablet		
BRISTOL	Azotrex	50 mg		Capsule		
BRISTOL	Azotrex	125 mg		Capsule		
BRISTOL	Azotrex	250 mg		Capsule		
BRISTOL; 250	Bristamycin	250 mg	Orange	Tablet	Round	
BRISTOL; 732	Enkaid	2.5 mg	Green and Yellow	Capsule		
BRISTOL; 732	Enkaid	8.7 mg	Green and Yellow	Capsule		
BRISTOL; 732	Enkaid	25 mg	Green and Yellow	Capsule		
BRISTOL; 732	Enkaid	193.8 mg	Green and Yellow	Capsule		
BRISTOL; 734	Enkaid	2.4 mg	Green and Orange	Capsule		
BRISTOL; 734	Enkaid	8.6 mg	Green and Orange	Capsule		
BRISTOL; 734	Enkaid	35 mg	Green and Orange	Capsule		
BRISTOL; 734	Enkaid	181 mg	Green and Orange	Capsule		
BRISTOL; 735	Enkaid	3.8 mg	Green and Brown	Capsule		
BRISTOL; 735	Enkaid	13.2 mg	Green and Brown	Capsule		
BRISTOL; 735	Enkaid	50 mg	Green and Brown	Capsule		
BRISTOL; 735	Enkaid	283 mg	Green and Brown	Capsule		
BRISTOL; 4322	Tetrex	250 mg	Yellow and Orange	Capsule		
BRISTOL; 4330; BIDCAPS	Tetrex Bidcaps	500 mg	Yellow and Black	Capsule		
BUFFERIN; 3	Bufferin with Codeine No. 3	30 mg	White	Tablet	Round	
BUFFERIN; 3	Bufferin with Codeine No. 3	97.2 mg	White	Tablet	Round	
BUFFERIN; 3	Bufferin with Codeine No. 3	325 mg	White	Tablet	Round	
BW&CO	Cardilate	10 mg	White	Tablet	Square	Burroughs Wellcome
C	Calcitrel	120 mg	White	Tablet	Round	Sterling Health
C	Calcitrel	585 mg	White	Tablet	Round	Sterling Health
C	Coryban D	2.5 mg	White	Tablet	Scored	Leeming
C	Coryban D	2.5 mg	White	Tablet	Scored	Pfizer Consumer Health Care
C	Coryban D	60 mg	White	Tablet	Scored	Leeming
C	Coryban D	60 mg	White	Tablet	Scored	Pfizer Consumer Health Care
C	Flextime Acutrim	25 mg	Peach	Tablet	Round, Biconvex	Fisons Consumer Health
C	Prempro	2.5 mg	White	Tablet	Oval, Scored	
C; 064	Fenbutal	40 mg	White	Tablet	Round	Reid-Rowell Pharmaceutical
C; 064	Fenbutal	50 mg	White	Tablet	Round	Reid-Rowell Pharmaceutical
C; 064	Fenbutal	130 mg	White	Tablet	Round	Reid-Rowell Pharmaceutical
C; 064	Fenbutal	200 mg	White	Tablet	Round	Reid-Rowell Pharmaceutical
C; 5	Murcil	5 mg	Green and Yellow	Capsule		Reid-Rowell Pharmaceutical
C; 10	Murcil	10 mg	Black and Green	Capsule		Reid-Rowell Pharmaceutical
C; 333	Butinal with Codeine	30 mg	Blue and White	Capsule		Econolab
C; 333	Butinal with Codeine	40 mg	Blue and White	Capsule		Econolab
C; 333	Butinal with Codeine	50 mg	Blue and White	Capsule		Econolab
C; 333	Butinal with Codeine	325 mg	Blue and White	Capsule		Econolab
C; 360; LL	Caltrate JR	300 mg	Orange	Chewable Tablet	Oblong	
C; 360; LL	Caltrate JR	60 IU	Orange	Chewable Tablet	Oblong	
C; 425	Ascomp with Codeine	30 mg	Blue and Yellow	Capsule		Econolab
C; 425	Ascomp with Codeine	40 mg	Blue and Yellow	Capsule		Econolab
C; 425	Ascomp with Codeine	50 mg	Blue and Yellow	Capsule		Econolab
C; 425	Ascomp with Codeine	325 mg	Blue and Yellow	Capsule		Econolab
C; 2416	Contimycin	250 mg	Purple and Yellow	Capsule		Zenith Goldline Pharmaceuticals
C03	Ilotycin	250 mg	Orange	Enteric-Coated Tablet		Dista Products
C3	C3	4 mg	Yellow and Clear	Capsule		
C3	C3	30 mg	Yellow and Clear	Capsule		
C3	C3	50 mg	Yellow and Clear	Capsule		
CARDILATE X7A	Cardilate	10 mg	White	Chewable Tablet	Round	Burroughs Wellcome
CARDILATE X7A	Cardilate	10 mg	White	Tablet	Square	Burroughs Wellcome
CC; 232	Appi-Plex	37.5 mg	Yellow	Tablet	Oblong	Reid-Rowell Pharmaceutical
CENTRAL; 65 MG	Theoclear LA	65 mg	Clear with White Beads	Sustained-Release Capsule		
CENTRAL; 130	Theoclear LA	130 mg		Timed-Release Capsule		
CENTRAL; 130 MG	Theoclear LA	130 mg	Clear	Timed-Release Capsule		

IMPRINT	BRAND/GENERIC NAME	STRENGTH	COLOR	FORM	SHAPE	MANUFACTURER
CENTRAL; 200 MG	Theoclear	200 mg	White	Tablet	Round	
CENTRAL; 260	Theoclear LA	260 mg		Timed-Release Capsule		
CENTRAL; 260 MG	Theoclear LA	260 mg	Clear	Timed-Release Capsule		
CEZIN; 711	Cezin	5 mg	Orange and White	Capsule		
CEZIN; 711	Cezin	10 mg	Orange and White	Capsule		
CEZIN; 711	Cezin	20 mg	Orange and White	Capsule		
CEZIN; 711	Cezin	70 mg	Orange and White	Capsule		
CEZIN; 711	Cezin	80 mg	Orange and White	Capsule		
CEZIN; 711	Cezin	100 mg	Orange and White	Capsule		
CEZIN; 711	Cezin	300 mg	Orange and White	Capsule		
CHOLOXIN; 1	Choloxin	1 mg	Orange	Tablet	Elliptical Convex, Scored	Knoll Pharmaceutical
CHOLOXIN; 2	Choloxin	2 mg	Yellow	Tablet	Elliptical Convex, Scored	Knoll Pharmaceutical
CHOLOXIN; 4	Choloxin	4 mg	White	Tablet	Elliptical, Scored	Knoll Pharmaceutical
CHOLOXIN; 6	Choloxin	6 mg		Tablet		Knoll Pharmaceutical
CIBA; 17	Dianabol	2.5 mg	Yellow	Tablet	Round	Novartis
CIBA; 20	Dianabol	5 mg		Tablet	Scored, Round	Novartis
CIBA; 21	Singoserp-Esidrix Tablet 1	0.5 mg	White	Tablet		Novartis
CIBA; 21	Singoserp-Esidrix Tablet 1	0.5 mg	White	Tablet		Novartis Pharmaceuticals
CIBA; 21	Singoserp-Esidrix Tablet 1	25 mg	White	Tablet		Novartis
CIBA; 21	Singoserp-Esidrix Tablet 1	25 mg	White	Tablet		Novartis Pharmaceuticals
CIBA; 23	Priscoline	25 mg	White	Tablet		
CIBA; 25	Singoserp	1 mg	White-Green	Tablet		Novartis
CIBA; 25	Singoserp	1 mg	Whitish Green	Tablet		Novartis Pharmaceuticals
CIBA; 31 (ORANGE)	Forhistal	1 mg	Orange or Green	Tablet		Novartis
CIBA; 45	Forhistal Lontabs	2.5 mg	Orange	Tablet	Oblong	Novartis
CIBA; 50	Priscoline	80 mg	Yellow	Tablet		
CIBA; 69	Trasentine Hydrochloride	75 mg	White	Tablet		Novartis Pharmaceuticals
CIBA; 75	Singoserp-Esidrix Tablet 2	1 mg	White	Tablet		Novartis
CIBA; 75	Singoserp-Esidrix Tablet 2	1 mg	White	Tablet		Novartis Pharmaceuticals
CIBA; 75	Singoserp-Esidrix Tablet 2	25 mg	White	Tablet		Novartis
CIBA; 75	Singoserp-Esidrix Tablet 2	25 mg	White	Tablet		Novartis Pharmaceuticals
CIBA; 76	Trasentine-Phenobarbital	20 mg	Yellow	Tablet		Novartis Pharmaceuticals
CIBA; 76	Trasentine-Phenobarbital	50 mg	Yellow	Tablet		Novartis Pharmaceuticals
CIBA; 92	Gammacorten	0.75 mg		Tablet		Novartis
CIBA; 96	Ultandren	5 mg	Lavender	Tablet		Novartis
CIBA; 105	Dialog	15 mg	White	Tablet	Round, Scored	Novartis
CIBA; 105	Dialog	300 mg	White	Tablet	Round, Scored	Novartis
CIBA; 152	Regitine	50 mg	White	Tablet		Novartis
CIBA; XA (GREEN)	Forhistal	1 mg	Orange or Green	Tablet		Novartis
CL; 5	Butabarbital Sodium	15 mg	Lavender	Tablet	Round	Novartis Generics
CL; 6	Butabarbital Sodium	30 mg	Aqua	Tablet	Round	Novartis Generics
CL; 9	Dexamethasone	0.75 mg	Blue	Tablet	Pentagon-Shaped	Novartis Generics
CL; 14	Prednisolone	5 mg	Peach	Tablet	Scored, Round	Novartis Generics
CL; 16	Cyproheptadine Hydrochloride	4 mg	White	Tablet	Round, Scored	
CL; 24	T.E.H.	10 mg	White	Tablet	Round; Scored; Compressed	Novartis Generics
CL; 24	T.E.H.	25 mg	White	Tablet	Round; Scored; Compressed	Novartis Generics
CL; 24	T.E.H.	130 mg	White	Tablet	Round; Scored; Compressed	Novartis Generics
CL; 46	Propantheline Bromide	15 mg	Peach-Colored	Coated Tablet		Novartis Generics
CL; 51	Trifluoperazine Hydrochloride	1 mg	Lavender	Coated Tablet		Novartis Generics
CL; 102	Niacin	50 mg	White	Tablet	Round	Novartis Generics
CL; 120	Butal Compound	40 mg	White	Tablet		Novartis Generics
CL; 120	Butal Compound	50 mg	White	Tablet		Novartis Generics
CL; 120	Butal Compound	130 mg	White	Tablet		Novartis Generics
CL; 120	Butal Compound	200 mg	White	Tablet		Novartis Generics
CL; 138	Sulfamethoxazole	500 mg	Green	Tablet	Round; Scored	Novartis Generics
CL; 142	Tolbutamide	500 mg	White	Tablet	Round; Scored	Novartis Generics
CL; 171	Aspirin and Codeine Phosphate	15 mg	White	Tablet	Round	
CL; 171	Aspirin and Codeine Phosphate	325 mg	White	Tablet	Round	
CL; 171	Aspirin with Codeine	15 mg	White	Tablet	Round	Novartis Generics
CL; 171	Aspirin with Codeine	325 mg	White	Tablet	Round	Novartis Generics
CL; 185	Glutethimide	500 mg	White	Tablet	Round	
CL; 212	Niacin	500 mg	White	Tablet	Round	Novartis Generics
CL; 233	Ascorbic Acid	500 mg	White	Tablet	Round	
CL; 235	Quadnite	50 mg	Pink	Tablet	Round	Reid-Rowell Pharmaceutical
CL; 269	Niacin	100 mg	White	Tablet	Round	Novartis Generics
CL; 287	Orphenadrine Citrate	100 mg	White	Timed-Release Tablet		Novartis Generics
CL; 407	Chlorpromazine Hydrochloride	50 mg	Off-White	Coated Tablet	Round	Novartis Generics
CL; 407	Chlorpromazine Hydrochloride	50 mg	Butterscotch	Tablet		Roxane Laboratories
CL; 408	Conjugated Estrogens	2.5 mg	Purple with Off-White Core	Coated Tablet	Oval	Novartis Generics
CL; 416	Hydralazine Hydrochloride	50 mg	Dark Green with White Core	Coated Tablet	Round	Novartis Generics
CL; 417	Conjugated Estrogens	0.625 mg	Maroon with Off-White Core	Coated Tablet	Oval	Novartis Generics
CL; 417	Conjugated Estrogens	0.625 mg	White	Tablet	Round	Novartis Generics
CL; 418	Phenylbutazone	100 mg	Red	Coated Tablet		Novartis Generics
CL; 437	Chlorpromazine Hydrochloride	100 mg	Off-White	Coated Tablet	Round	Novartis Generics
CL; 437	Chlorpromazine Hydrochloride	100 mg	Butterscotch	Tablet		Roxane Laboratories
CL; 440	Methenamine Mandelate	1 gram	Purple	Enteric-Coated Tablet	Oval	
CL; 444	Efedra-PA	6 mg	White or Green	Timed-Release Tablet	Round	Novartis Generics
CL; 444	Efedra-PA	120 mg	White or Green	Timed-Release Tablet	Round	Novartis Generics
CL; 447	Conjugated Estrogens	1.25 mg	Yellow with Off-White Core	Coated Tablet	Oval	Novartis Generics
CL; 447	Conjugated Estrogens	1.25 mg	White	Tablet	Round	Novartis Generics
CL; 455	Chlorpromazine Hydrochloride	10 mg	Off-White	Coated Tablet	Round	Novartis Generics
CL; 455	Chlorpromazine Hydrochloride	10 mg	Butterscotch	Tablet		Roxane Laboratories
CL; 457	Chlorpromazine Hydrochloride	200 mg	Off-White	Coated Tablet	Round	Novartis Generics
CL; 457	Chlorpromazine Hydrochloride	200 mg	Butterscotch	Tablet		Roxane Laboratories
CL; 475	Hydralazine Hydrochloride	10 mg	White	Coated Tablet	Round	Novartis Generics
CL; 476	Chlorpromazine Hydrochloride	25 mg	Off-White	Coated Tablet	Round	Novartis Generics
CL; 476	Chlorpromazine Hydrochloride	25 mg	Butterscotch	Tablet		Roxane Laboratories
CL; 477	Tagatap S.R.	12 mg	Blue	Tablet	Round	Solvay Pharmaceuticals

IMPRINT	BRAND/GENERIC NAME	STRENGTH	COLOR	FORM	SHAPE	MANUFACTURER
CL; 477	Tagatap S.R.	15 mg	Blue	Tablet	Round	Solvay Pharmaceuticals
CL; 485	Hydralazine Hydrochloride	25 mg	Light Green with White Core	Coated Tablet	Round	Novartis Generics
CL; 486	Conjugated Estrogens	0.3 mg	Green with White Core	Coated Tablet	Oval	Novartis Generics
CL; 486	Conjugated Estrogens	0.3 mg	White	Tablet	Round	Novartis Generics
CL; 501	Trates	6.5 mg	Black Opaque and Clear Yellow	Capsule		Solvay Pharmaceuticals
CL; 509	Cyclandelate	400 mg	Blue and Red	Capsule		Novartis Generics
CL; 511	Trates S.R.	6.5 mg	Clear and Purple with White Beads	Capsule		Solvay Pharmaceuticals
CL; 514	Phenylbutazone	100 mg	Light Blue	Capsule		Novartis Generics
CL; 529	Cyclandelate	200 mg	Powder Blue	Capsule		Novartis Generics
COADVIL	CO-Advil	30 mg	Tan	Caplet		
COADVIL	CO-Advil	200 mg	Tan	Caplet		
COMBID; SKF	Combid	5 mg	Yellow and Clear	Capsule		Smithkline Beecham
COMBID; SKF	Combid	10 mg	Yellow and Clear	Capsule		Smithkline Beecham
CONTAC; COUGH	Contac Cough	30 mg	Orange and Maroon	Capsule		
CONTAC; COUGH	Contac Cough	60 mg	Orange and Maroon	Capsule		
CONTAC; S.C.F	Contac Severe Cold Formula	1 mg	Dark Blue and Light Blue	Capsule		
CONTAC; S.C.F	Contac Severe Cold Formula	15 mg	Dark Blue and Light Blue	Capsule		
CONTAC; S.C.F	Contac Severe Cold Formula	30 mg	Dark Blue and Light Blue	Capsule		
CONTAC; S.C.F	Contac Severe Cold Formula	500 mg	Dark Blue and Light Blue	Capsule		
COPLEY; 132	Albuterol Sulfate	2 mg	White	Tablet	Round; Flat; Bisected	Copley Pharmaceutical
COPLEY; 134	Albuterol Sulfate	4 mg	White	Tablet	Round; Flat; Bisected	Copley Pharmaceutical
CORICIDIN; SINUS	Coricidin Sinus Headache, Extra Strength	2 mg	White	Tablet	Oblong	Schering-Plough Healthcare Products
CORICIDIN; SINUS	Coricidin Sinus Headache, Extra Strength	12.5 mg	White	Tablet	Oblong	Schering-Plough Healthcare Products
CORICIDIN; SINUS	Coricidin Sinus Headache, Extra Strength	500 mg	White	Tablet	Oblong	Schering-Plough Healthcare Products
COTYLENOL	Cotylenol Cold Formula	2 mg	Yellow and Dark Green	Capsule		Mcneil Consumer Products
COTYLENOL	Cotylenol Cold Formula	10 mg	Yellow and Dark Green	Capsule		Mcneil Consumer Products
COTYLENOL	Cotylenol Cold Formula	30 mg	Yellow and Dark Green	Capsule		Mcneil Consumer Products
COTYLENOL	Cotylenol Cold Formula	325 mg	Yellow and Dark Green	Capsule		Mcneil Consumer Products
COTYLENOL	Cotylenol Cold Formula	2 mg	Yellow	Tablet		Mcneil Consumer Products
COTYLENOL	Cotylenol Cold Formula	2 mg	Yellow	Tablet	Round	Mcneil Consumer Products
COTYLENOL	Cotylenol Cold Formula	10 mg	Yellow	Tablet	Round	Mcneil Consumer Products
COTYLENOL	Cotylenol Cold Formula	15 mg	Yellow	Tablet		Mcneil Consumer Products
COTYLENOL	Cotylenol Cold Formula	30 mg	Yellow	Tablet		Mcneil Consumer Products
COTYLENOL	Cotylenol Cold Formula	30 mg	Yellow	Tablet	Round	Mcneil Consumer Products
COTYLENOL	Cotylenol Cold Formula	325 mg	Yellow	Tablet		Mcneil Consumer Products
COTYLENOL	Cotylenol Cold Formula	325 mg	Yellow	Tablet	Round	Mcneil Consumer Products
COUNTERACT	Counteract Cold, Allergy, Sinus Medicine, Maximum Strength	4 mg	Light Blue	Tablet	Capsule-Shaped	Melaleuca
COUNTERACT	Counteract Cold, Allergy, Sinus Medicine, Maximum Strength	5 mg	Light Blue	Tablet	Capsule-Shaped	Melaleuca
COUNTERACT	Counteract Cold, Allergy, Sinus Medicine, Maximum Strength	8.6 mg	Light Blue	Tablet	Capsule-Shaped	Melaleuca
COUNTERACT	Counteract Cold, Allergy, Sinus Medicine, Maximum Strength	20 mg	Light Blue	Tablet	Capsule-Shaped	Melaleuca
COUNTERACT	Counteract Cold, Allergy, Sinus Medicine, Maximum Strength	25 mg	Light Blue	Tablet	Capsule-Shaped	Melaleuca
COUNTERACT	Counteract Cold, Allergy, Sinus Medicine, Maximum Strength	65 mg	Light Blue	Tablet	Capsule-Shaped	Melaleuca
COUNTERACT	Counteract Cold, Allergy, Sinus Medicine, Maximum Strength	69 mg	Light Blue	Tablet	Capsule-Shaped	Melaleuca
COUNTERACT	Counteract Cold, Allergy, Sinus Medicine, Maximum Strength	650 mg	Light Blue	Tablet	Capsule-Shaped	Melaleuca
D; 31	Demerol	50 mg	Pink with Red Mottling	Tablet	Discoid	
D; 31	Demerol	300 mg	Pink with Red Mottling	Tablet	Discoid	
DAN; 528	Isoniazid	50 mg		Tablet		Danbury Pharmacal
DAN; 5016	Chlorpheniramine Maleate	8 mg	Green and Clear	Sustained-Release Capsule		Danbury Pharmacal
DAN; 5017	Chlorpheniramine Maleate	12 mg	Green and Clear	Timed-Release Capsule		Danbury Pharmacal
DAN; 5204	Pseudoephedrine Hydrochloride	60 mg		Tablet		
DAN; 5359	Spasmolin	0.0065 mg	White	Tablet		Danbury Pharmacal
DAN; 5359	Spasmolin	0.0194 mg	White	Tablet		Danbury Pharmacal
DAN; 5359	Spasmolin	0.1037 mg	White	Tablet		Danbury Pharmacal
DAN; 5359	Spasmolin	16.2 mg	White	Tablet		Danbury Pharmacal
DAN; 5368 DAN	Disulfiram	500 mg	Off-White	Tablet	Round; Scored	Danbury Pharmacal
DAN; 5368 DAN	Disulfiram	500 mg	Off-White	Tablet	Round; Scored	Schein Pharmaceutical
DAN; 5370	Bethanechol Chloride	5 mg		Tablet		Danbury Pharmacal
DAN; 5376 DAN	Disulfiram	250 mg	Off-White	Tablet	Round; Scored	Danbury Pharmacal
DAN; 5376 DAN	Disulfiram	250 mg	Off-White	Tablet	Round; Scored	Schein Pharmaceutical
DAN; 5428	Reserpine, Hydralazine Hydrochloride and Hydrochlorothiazide	0.1 mg	Yellow	Tablet	Round	Danbury Pharmacal
DAN; 5428	Reserpine, Hydralazine Hydrochloride and Hydrochlorothiazide	0.1 mg	Yellow	Tablet	Round	Schein Pharmaceutical

IMPRINT	BRAND/GENERIC NAME	STRENGTH	COLOR	FORM	SHAPE	MANUFACTURER
DAN; 5428	Reserpine, Hydralazine Hydrochloride and Hydrochlorothiazide	15 mg	Yellow	Tablet	Round	Danbury Pharmacal
DAN; 5428	Reserpine, Hydralazine Hydrochloride and Hydrochlorothiazide	15 mg	Yellow	Tablet	Round	Schein Pharmaceutical
DAN; 5428	Reserpine, Hydralazine Hydrochloride and Hydrochlorothiazide	25 mg	Yellow	Tablet	Round	Danbury Pharmacal
DAN; 5428	Reserpine, Hydralazine Hydrochloride and Hydrochlorothiazide	25 mg	Yellow	Tablet	Round	Schein Pharmaceutical
DAN; 5444	Chlorothiazide	250 mg		Tablet		Danbury Pharmacal
DAN; 5453 DAN	Quinidine Sulfate	100 mg	White	Tablet	Round; Scored	Danbury Pharmacal
DAN; 5453 DAN	Quinidine Sulfate	100 mg	White	Tablet	Round; Scored	Schein Pharmaceutical
DAN; 5455 DAN	Chlorpropamide	250 mg	Blue	Tablet	Round; Scored	Danbury Pharmacal
DAN; 5455 DAN	Chlorpropamide	250 mg	Blue	Tablet	Round; Scored	Schein Pharmaceutical
DAN; 5464	Danbade Improved	2.5 mg	Blue and Clear	Timed-Release Capsule		Danbury Pharmacal
DAN; 5464	Danbade Improved	8 mg	Blue and Clear	Timed-Release Capsule		Danbury Pharmacal
DAN; 5464	Danbade Improved	50 mg	Blue and Clear	Timed-Release Capsule		Danbury Pharmacal
DAN; 5481	Theofedral	8 mg	White	Tablet	Round; Scored	Danbury Pharmacal
DAN; 5481	Theofedral	24 mg	White	Tablet	Round; Scored	Danbury Pharmacal
DAN; 5481	Theofedral	130 mg	White	Tablet	Round; Scored	Danbury Pharmacal
DAN; 5491	Phenylbutazone Alka	100 mg	Orange and White	Capsule		Danbury Pharmacal
DAN; 5491	Phenylbutazone Alka	150 mg	Orange and White	Capsule		Danbury Pharmacal
DAN; 5507	Chlorthalidone	25 mg	Yellow or Orange	Tablet	Round	
DAN; 5514	Sulfinpyrazone	100 mg		Tablet		Danbury Pharmacal
DAN; 5514	Sulfinpyrazone	100 mg		Tablet		Schein Pharmaceutical
DAN; 5518	Chlorthalidone	50 mg	Light Green or Light Blue	Tablet	Round	
DAN; 5521	Phenylbutazone	100 mg	Red	Coated Tablet		Danbury Pharmacal
DAN; 5524	Danbade	2.5 mg		Timed-Release Capsule		Danbury Pharmacal
DAN; 5524	Danbade	8 mg		Timed-Release Capsule		Danbury Pharmacal
DAN; 5524	Danbade	50 mg		Timed-Release Capsule		Danbury Pharmacal
DAN; 5548 DAN	Chloroquine Phosphate	250 mg	White	Tablet	Round; Scored	Danbury Pharmacal
DAN; 5548 DAN	Chloroquine Phosphate	250 mg	White	Tablet	Round; Scored	Schein Pharmaceutical
DAN; 5564 DAN	Procainamide Hydrochloride	750 mg	White	Sustained-Release Tablet	Oval; Scored	Danbury Pharmacal
DAN; 5564 DAN	Procainamide Hydrochloride	750 mg	White	Sustained-Release Tablet	Oval; Scored	Schein Pharmaceutical
DAN; 5579 DAN	Chlorpropamide	100 mg	Blue	Tablet	Round; Scored	Danbury Pharmacal
DAN; 5579 DAN	Chlorpropamide	100 mg	Blue	Tablet	Round; Scored	Schein Pharmaceutical
DAN; 5582 DAN	Tolazamide	250 mg	White	Tablet	Round; Scored	Danbury Pharmacal
DAN; 5582 DAN	Tolazamide	250 mg	White	Tablet	Round; Scored	Schein Pharmaceutical
DAN; 5590 DAN	Tolazamide	500 mg	White	Tablet	Round; Scored	Danbury Pharmacal
DAN; 5590 DAN	Tolazamide	500 mg	White	Tablet	Round; Scored	Schein Pharmaceutical
DAN; 5591 DAN	Tolazamide	100 mg	White	Tablet	Round; Scored	Danbury Pharmacal
DAN; 5591 DAN	Tolazamide	100 mg	White	Tablet	Round; Scored	Schein Pharmaceutical
DATRIL	Datril	325 mg	White	Tablet		
DIMENSYN	Dimensyn	15 mg	Pik and Red	Capsule		
DIMENSYN	Dimensyn	25 mg	Pik and Red	Capsule		
DIMENSYN	Dimensyn	500 mg	Pik and Red	Capsule		
DISTA U25	Ilosone	250 mg	Pink	Chewable Tablet		Dista Products
DISTA; U60	Keflex	1 G	Green	Tablet	Capsule-Shaped	Dista Products
DONNAGEL; W	Donnagel	600 mg	Light Green with Dark Green Speckles	Chewable Tablet	Round, Flat-Faced, Beveled-Edged	
DORSEY	Asbron G	100 mg	Green with White Inlay	Tablet		Novartis Pharmaceuticals
DORSEY	Asbron G	300 mg	Green with White Inlay	Tablet		Novartis Pharmaceuticals
DORSEY	Calurin	300 mg	White	Tablet		Novartis Consumer
DORSEY	Calurin	300 mg	White	Tablet		Sandoz Consumer Pharmaceuticals
DORSEY	Tussaminic	25 mg	Green	Tablet		Novartis Consumer
DORSEY	Tussaminic	30 mg	Green	Tablet		Novartis Consumer
DORSEY	Tussaminic	50 mg	Green	Tablet		Novartis Consumer
DORSEY	Tussaminic	300 mg	Green	Tablet		Novartis Consumer
DORSEY 10	Metaprel	10 mg	White	Tablet	Round, Compressed	Novartis Pharmaceuticals
DORSEY; 43; 20	Triaminic	25 mg	Yellow	Timed-Release Tablet	Round	Novartis Consumer
DORSEY; 43; 20	Triaminic	50 mg	Yellow	Timed-Release Tablet	Round	Novartis Consumer
DOW; 12	Novahistine Melet	2 mg	Pink	Tablet	Round	
DOW; 12	Novahistine Melet	10 mg	Pink	Tablet	Round	
DOW; 16	Novahistine LP	4 mg		Tablet		
DOW; 16	Novahistine LP	20 mg		Tablet		
DOW; 21	Novahistine Cold	2 mg	Green	Coated Tablet	Round	
DOW; 21	Novahistine Cold	18.75 mg	Green	Coated Tablet	Round	
DOW; 80	Isoniazid	300 mg		Tablet		
DP; 01	Clonidine Hydrochloride	0.1 mg	Tan	Tablet	Hexagonal on Back and Round on Front, Scored	Duramed Pharmaceuticals
DP; 02	Clonidine Hydrochloride	0.2 mg	Orange	Tablet	Hexagonal on Back and Round on Front, Scored	Duramed Pharmaceuticals
DP; 03	Clonidine Hydrochloride	0.3 mg	Peach	Tablet	Hexagonal on Front and Round on Back, Scored	Duramed Pharmaceuticals
DP; 10	Propranolol Hydrochloride	10 mg	Orange	Tablet	Round, Scored	Duramed Pharmaceuticals
DP; 11	Trifluoperazine Hydrochloride	1 mg	Lavender	Coated Tablet		Duramed Pharmaceuticals
DP; 12	Trifluoperazine Hydrochloride	2 mg	Lavender	Coated Tablet		Duramed Pharmaceuticals
DP; 13	Trifluoperazine Hydrochloride	5 mg	Lavender	Coated Tablet		Duramed Pharmaceuticals

IMPRINT	BRAND/GENERIC NAME	STRENGTH	COLOR	FORM	SHAPE	MANUFACTURER
DP; 14	Trifluoperazine Hydrochloride	10 mg	Lavender	Coated Tablet		Duramed Pharmaceuticals
DP; 15	Diazepam	2 mg	White	Tablet	Round, Scored	Duramed Pharmaceuticals
DP; 20	Propranolol Hydrochloride	20 mg	Blue	Tablet	Round, Scored	Duramed Pharmaceuticals
DP; 25	Dipyridamole	25 mg	White	Tablet	Round	Duramed Pharmaceuticals
DP; 40	Propranolol Hydrochloride	40 mg	Green	Tablet	Round, Scored	Duramed Pharmaceuticals
DP; 50	Dipyridamole	50 mg	White	Tablet	Round	Duramed Pharmaceuticals
DP; 60	Propranolol Hydrochloride	60 mg	Pink	Tablet	Round, Scored	Duramed Pharmaceuticals
DP; 75	Dipyridamole	75 mg	White	Tablet	Round	Duramed Pharmaceuticals
DP; 80	Propranolol Hydrochloride	80 mg	Yellow	Tablet	Round, Scored	Duramed Pharmaceuticals
DP; 90	Propranolol Hydrochloride	90 mg	Lavender	Tablet	Round, Scored	Duramed Pharmaceuticals
DP; 223	Aminophylline	100 mg	White	Tablet	Round, Scored	Duramed Pharmaceuticals
DP; 224	Aminophylline	200 mg	White	Tablet	Round, Scored	Duramed Pharmaceuticals
DP; 225	Haloperidol	0.5 mg	White	Tablet	Round, Scored	Duramed Pharmaceuticals
DP; 226	Haloperidol	1 mg	Yellow	Tablet	Round, Scored	Duramed Pharmaceuticals
DP; 227	Haloperidol	2 mg	Lavender	Tablet	Round, Scored	Duramed Pharmaceuticals
DP; 228	Haloperidol	5 mg	Green	Tablet	Round, Scored	Duramed Pharmaceuticals
DP; 246	Cyproheptadine Hydrochloride	4 mg	White	Tablet	Round	Duramed Pharmaceuticals
DP; 251	Chlorpropamide	250 mg	Blue	Tablet	Round, Scored	Duramed Pharmaceuticals
DP; 252	Chlorpropamide	100 mg	Blue	Tablet	Round, Scored	Duramed Pharmaceuticals
DP; 265	Hydroxyzine Pamoate	25 mg	Green	Capsule		Duramed Pharmaceuticals
DP; 266	Hydroxyzine Pamoate	50 mg	White and Green	Capsule		Duramed Pharmaceuticals
DP; 267	Hydroxyzine Pamoate	100 mg	Gray and Green	Capsule		Duramed Pharmaceuticals
DP; 274	Isoniazid	100 mg	White	Tablet	Round, Scored	Duramed Pharmaceuticals
DP; 296	Salsalate	500 mg	Blue or Yellow	Tablet	Round	
DP; 297	Salsalate	750 mg	Blue or Yellow	Tablet	Capsule-Shaped, Scored	
DP; 311	Prednisone	5 mg	White	Tablet	Round, Scored	Duramed Pharmaceuticals
DP; 312	Prednisone	10 mg	White	Tablet	Round, Scored	Duramed Pharmaceuticals
DP; 313	Prednisone	20 mg	Orange	Tablet	Round, Scored	Duramed Pharmaceuticals
DP; 314	Prochlorperazine Maleate	5 mg	Yellow	Tablet	Round	
DP; 315	Prochlorperazine Maleate	10 mg	Yellow	Tablet	Round	Duramed Pharmaceuticals
DP; 316	Prochlorperazine Maleate	25 mg		Tablet		Duramed Pharmaceuticals
DP; 325	Tolazamide	100 mg	White	Tablet	Round, Scored	Duramed Pharmaceuticals
DP; 326	Tolazamide	250 mg	White	Tablet	Round, Scored	Duramed Pharmaceuticals
DP; 327	Tolazamide	500 mg	White	Tablet	Round, Scored	Duramed Pharmaceuticals
DP; 332	Propranolol Hydrochloride and Hydrochlorothiazide	25 mg	Pale Yellow	Tablet	Round, Scored	Duramed Pharmaceuticals
DP; 332	Propranolol Hydrochloride and Hydrochlorothiazide	40 mg	Pale Yellow	Tablet	Round, Scored	Duramed Pharmaceuticals
DP; 371	Methyldopa	250 mg	White	Tablet	Round	Duramed Pharmaceuticals
DP; 372	Methyldopa	500 mg	White	Tablet	Round	Duramed Pharmaceuticals
DP; 622	Diazepam	5 mg	Yellow	Tablet	Round, Scored	Duramed Pharmaceuticals
DP; 623	Diazepam	10 mg	Blue	Tablet	Round, Scored	Duramed Pharmaceuticals
DP; 651	Phentermine Hydrochloride	30 mg	Blue and Clear	Capsule		Duramed Pharmaceuticals
DP; 660	Temazepam	15 mg	Green and White	Capsule		Duramed Pharmaceuticals
DP; 661	Temazepam	30 mg	White	Capsule		Duramed Pharmaceuticals
DRISTAN ULTRA	Dristan Ultra Colds Formula	2 mg	Orange and White	Capsule		Whitehall-Robins Healthcare
DRISTAN ULTRA	Dristan Ultra Colds Formula	15 mg	Orange and White	Capsule		Whitehall-Robins Healthcare
DRISTAN ULTRA	Dristan Ultra Colds Formula	30 mg	Orange and White	Capsule		Whitehall-Robins Healthcare
DRISTAN ULTRA	Dristan Ultra Colds Formula	500 mg	Orange and White	Capsule		Whitehall-Robins Healthcare
DURACT	Duract	25 mg	Opaque Light Yellow Body and Opaque Red Cap with 2 Blue Bands	Capsule		
DURATION	Duration 12-Hour	120 mg	Blue	Tablet	Round	
E	Excedrin	97.2 mg	White	Tablet		
E	Excedrin	129.6 mg	White	Tablet		
E	Excedrin	194.4 mg	White	Tablet		
E; 071	Chlorthalidone	50 mg	Light Blue	Tablet	Round, Compressed	
E; 073	Chlorthalidone	100 mg	White	Tablet	Round, Compressed	
E; 9	Imipramine Hydrochloride	25 mg	Brown	Tablet	Round	Eon Labs
E; 12	Ferrous Sulfate	325 mg	Red (E-12 or PP-12) or Green (E-13 or PP-13)	Coated Tablet		Eon Labs
E; 13	Ferrous Sulfate	325 mg	Red (E-12 or PP-12) or Green (E-13 or PP-13)	Coated Tablet		Eon Labs
E; 15	Phenobarbital	15 mg	White	Tablet	Round, Compressed, Scored	
E; 17	Baclofen	10 mg	White	Tablet	Round, Scored, Compressed	Eon Labs
E; 18	Baclofen	20 mg	White	Tablet	Round, Scored, Compressed	Eon Labs
E; 30	Phenobarbital	30 mg	White	Tablet	Round, Compressed, Scored	
E; 50	Hydrochlorothiazide	50 mg	Peach	Tablet	Scored, Round, Compressed	Eon Labs
E; 53	Prenatal with Folic Acid	5 mcg	Pink	Coated Tablet	Capsule-Shaped	Eon Labs
E; 53	Prenatal with Folic Acid	1 mg	Pink	Coated Tablet	Capsule-Shaped	Eon Labs
E; 53	Prenatal with Folic Acid	1.1 mg	Pink	Coated Tablet	Capsule-Shaped	Eon Labs
E; 53	Prenatal with Folic Acid	1.8 mg	Pink	Coated Tablet	Capsule-Shaped	Eon Labs
E; 53	Prenatal with Folic Acid	2.5 mg	Pink	Coated Tablet	Capsule-Shaped	Eon Labs
E; 53	Prenatal with Folic Acid	15 mg	Pink	Coated Tablet	Capsule-Shaped	Eon Labs
E; 53	Prenatal with Folic Acid	60 mg	Pink	Coated Tablet	Capsule-Shaped	Eon Labs
E; 53	Prenatal with Folic Acid	65 mg	Pink	Coated Tablet	Capsule-Shaped	Eon Labs
E; 53	Prenatal with Folic Acid	125 mg	Pink	Coated Tablet	Capsule-Shaped	Eon Labs
E; 53	Prenatal with Folic Acid	30 IU	Pink	Coated Tablet	Capsule-Shaped	Eon Labs
E; 53	Prenatal with Folic Acid	400 IU	Pink	Coated Tablet	Capsule-Shaped	Eon Labs
E; 53	Prenatal with Folic Acid	6000 IU	Pink	Coated Tablet	Capsule-Shaped	Eon Labs
E; 111	Sulfamethoxazole and Trimethoprim	80 mg	White	Tablet	Oval, Scored, Compressed	
E; 111	Sulfamethoxazole and Trimethoprim	400 mg	White	Tablet	Oval, Scored, Compressed	
E; 259	Prenatal One	12 mcg	Light Yellow	Coated Tablet		Eon Labs
E; 259	Prenatal One	1 mg	Light Yellow	Coated Tablet		Eon Labs
E; 259	Prenatal One	1.5 mg	Light Yellow	Coated Tablet		Eon Labs
E; 259	Prenatal One	2 mg	Light Yellow	Coated Tablet		Eon Labs
E; 259	Prenatal One	3 mg	Light Yellow	Coated Tablet		Eon Labs
E; 259	Prenatal One	10 mg	Light Yellow	Coated Tablet		Eon Labs
E; 259	Prenatal One	11 mg	Light Yellow	Coated Tablet		Eon Labs

IMPRINT	BRAND/GENERIC NAME	STRENGTH	COLOR	FORM	SHAPE	MANUFACTURER
E; 259	Prenatal One	20 mg	Light Yellow	Coated Tablet		Eon Labs
E; 259	Prenatal One	25 mg	Light Yellow	Coated Tablet		Eon Labs
E; 259	Prenatal One	65 mg	Light Yellow	Coated Tablet		Eon Labs
E; 259	Prenatal One	120 mg	Light Yellow	Coated Tablet		Eon Labs
E; 259	Prenatal One	200 mg	Light Yellow	Coated Tablet		Eon Labs
E; 259	Prenatal One	400 IU	Light Yellow	Coated Tablet		Eon Labs
E; 259	Prenatal One	4000 IU	Light Yellow	Coated Tablet		Eon Labs
E; 360; 2	Acetaminophen and Codeine	15 mg	White	Tablet	Compressed	
E; 360; 2	Acetaminophen and Codeine	300 mg	White	Tablet	Compressed	
E; 365; 3	Acetaminophen and Codeine	30 mg	White	Tablet	Compressed	
E; 365; 3	Acetaminophen and Codeine	300 mg	White	Tablet	Compressed	
E; 370; 4	Acetaminophen and Codeine Phosphate	60 mg	White	Tablet	Compressed	
E; 370; 4	Acetaminophen and Codeine Phosphate	300 mg	White	Tablet	Compressed	
E; 535	Tolbutamide	500 mg	White	Tablet	Round, Compressed	Eon Labs
E; 551	Metronidazole	250 mg	White	Tablet	Round, Compressed	Eon Labs
E; 555	Metronidazole	500 mg	White	Tablet	Oblong, Scored, Compressed	Eon Labs
E; 591	Phenobarbital	1/8 grain		Tablet		
E; 615	Dicyclomine Hydrochloride	10 mg	Dark Blue	Capsule		
E; 616	Dicyclomine Hydrochloride	20 mg		Tablet		
E; 620	Carbex	5 mg	White	Tablet	Oval	
E; 635	Phentermine Hydrochloride	30 mg	Red and Black	Capsule		Eon Labs
E; 640	Phentermine Hydrochloride	30 mg	Black	Capsule		Eon Labs
E; 670	Tetracycline Hydrochloride	250 mg	Yellow and Orange	Capsule		Eon Labs
E; 694	Salsalate	750 mg	White	Tablet		Eon Labs
E; 701	Bethanechol Chloride	25 mg	Yellow	Tablet		Eon Labs
E; 741	Niacin SR	125 mg	Black and Clear	Capsule		Eon Labs
E; 743	Niacin SR	250 mg	Blue-Green and Clear	Capsule		Eon Labs
E; 744	Niacin SR	400 mg	Maroon and Pink	Capsule		Eon Labs
E; 750	Nystatin	500,000 units	Brown	Coated Tablet	Round, Concave	Eon Labs
E; 761	Salsalate	500 mg	Yellow	Tablet	Capsule-Shaped	Eon Labs
E; 762	Salsalate	750 mg	Yellow	Tablet	Capsule-Shaped, Bisected	Eon Labs
E; 856	Salsalate	500 mg	Blue	Tablet	Round	Eon Labs
E; 857	Salsalate	750 mg	Blue	Tablet	Capsule-Shaped, Bisected	Eon Labs
E; 988	Quinine Sulfate	260 mg	Off-White	Tablet	Round, Scored	Eon Labs
E; 1303	Quinine Sulfate	325 mg	Clear	Capsule		Eon Labs
E; 5385	Ferrous Sulfate SR	250 mg	Red and White	Capsule		Eon Labs
E; 5730	Phendimetrazine Tartrate	35 mg	Red and Clear; Black and Orange; Blue and Clear; Orange and Clear	Capsule		Eon Labs
E; 5740	Phendimetrazine Tartrate	35 mg	Red and Clear; Black and Orange; Blue and Clear; Orange and Clear	Capsule		Eon Labs
E; 6265	Phendimetrazine Tartrate	35 mg	Red and Clear; Black and Orange; Blue and Clear; Orange and Clear	Capsule		Eon Labs
EATON; 002	Nebs Analgesic	325 mg	Yellow	Tablet		
EATON; 032	Dantrium	75 mg	Orange	Capsule		
EFFERVESCENT; POTASSIUM	Effervescent Potassium	2 grams		Effervescent Tablet		
EFFERVESCENT; POTASSIUM	Effervescent Potassium	2.5 grams		Effervescent Tablet		
EL 250	Iodinated Glycerol	30 mg	Pink	Tablet	Round, Scored	H.L. Moore
EL; 125	Nalfed	12 mg	Blue and Clear	Capsule		Econolab
EL; 125	Nalfed	120 mg	Blue and Clear	Capsule		Econolab
EL; 158	Polycarb	625 mg	Beige	Tablet	Single Scored	Econolab
ELDER	B-Factors Plus	0.3 mg	Yellow-Green	Tablet	Round	
ELDER	B-Factors Plus	0.5 mg	Yellow-Green	Tablet	Round	
ELDER	B-Factors Plus	1 mg	Yellow-Green	Tablet	Round	
ELDER	B-Factors Plus	2 mg	Yellow-Green	Tablet	Round	
ELDER	B-Factors Plus	10 mg	Yellow-Green	Tablet	Round	
ELDER	B-Factors Plus	20 mg	Yellow-Green	Tablet	Round	
ELDER	B-Factors Plus	25 mg	Yellow-Green	Tablet	Round	
ELDER	B-Factors Plus	50 mg	Yellow-Green	Tablet	Round	
ELDER	Cold-Tabs	5 mg	Orange	Tablet	Round	Elder
ELDER	Cold-Tabs	10 mg	Orange	Tablet	Round	Elder
ELDER	Cold-Tabs	15 mg	Orange	Tablet	Round	Elder
ELDER	Cold-Tabs	150 mg	Orange	Tablet	Round	Elder
EMPRACET; 3; K9B	Empracet with Codeine Phosphate No. 3	30 mg	Peach	Tablet		
EMPRACET; 3; K9B	Empracet with Codeine Phosphate No. 3	300 mg	Peach	Tablet		
EMPRACET; 4; L9B	Empracet with Codeine Phosphate No. 4	60 mg	Peach	Tablet		
EMPRACET; 4; L9B	Empracet with Codeine Phosphate No. 4	300 mg	Peach	Tablet		
ENCAPRIN; 325 MG	Encaprin	325 mg	Clear and White	Capsule		
ENCAPRIN; 500 MG	Encaprin	500 mg	Clear and White	Capsule		
ENDO; 175	Coumadin	25 mg	Red	Tablet	Scored	Endo Laboratories
ENDO; 711	Glipizide	5 mg	White	Tablet	Round, Scored	
ENDO; 721	Captopril	12.5 mg		Tablet		
ENDO; 722	Captopril	25 mg		Tablet		
ENDO; 724	Captopril	50 mg	White	Tablet	Round, Biconvex, Scored	
ENDO; 727	Captopril	100 mg		Tablet		
ENDO; 744	Etodolac	400 mg	Pale Yellow	Tablet	Oval, Debossed	
F; 1; LL	Folvite	1 mg	Orange	Tablet	Round, Scored	Lederle Laboratories
F; 46	Aminophylline and Amytal	32 mg	Yellow and Light Blue	Capsule		Eli Lilly

IMPRINT	BRAND/GENERIC NAME	STRENGTH	COLOR	FORM	SHAPE	MANUFACTURER
F; 46	Aminophylline and Amytal	100 mg	Yellow and Light Blue	Capsule		Eli Lilly
F46	Aminophylline and Amytal	32 mg	Yellow and Light Blue	Capsule		Eli Lilly
F46	Aminophylline and Amytal	100 mg	Yellow and Light Blue	Capsule		Eli Lilly
FISONS; 670	Intal	20 mg	Clear and Yellow	Capsule		
FOLERGOT; PB	Folergot PB	0.2 mg	Brown and White	Capsule		
FOLERGOT; PB	Folergot PB	0.6 mg	Brown and White	Capsule		
FOLERGOT; PB	Folergot PB	40 mg	Brown and White	Capsule		
FOREST; 677	Esgic with Codeine	30 mg	Black and Opaque Blue	Capsule		
FOREST; 677	Esgic with Codeine	40 mg	Black and Opaque Blue	Capsule		
FOREST; 677	Esgic with Codeine	50 mg	Black and Opaque Blue	Capsule		
FOREST; 677	Esgic with Codeine	325 mg	Black and Opaque Blue	Capsule		
G; 0506	Ser-A-Gen	0.1 mg	Salmon	Tablet	Round	
G; 0506	Ser-A-Gen	15 mg	Salmon	Tablet	Round	
G; 0506	Ser-A-Gen	25 mg	Salmon	Tablet	Round	
G; 2808	Chloral Hydrate	7.5 grains	Green	Capsule	Oval	
GEIGY; 42	Constant-T	200 mg	Pink	Timed-Release Tablet	Scored, Oval	
GEIGY; 57	Constant-T	300 mg	Blue	Timed-Release Tablet	Scored, Oval	
GEIGY; 134	Pbz with Ephedrine	12 mg	White	Tablet		
GEIGY; 134	Pbz with Ephedrine	25 mg	White	Tablet		
GG; 5	Butabarbital Sodium	15 mg	Lavender	Tablet	Round	Novartis Generics
GG; 5	Butabarbital Sodium	1/4 grain	Lavender	Tablet	Compressed, Scored	Geneva Generics
GG; 6	Butabarbital Sodium	30 mg	Aqua	Tablet	Round	Novartis Generics
GG; 6	Butabarbital Sodium	1/2 grain	Light Blue	Tablet	Compressed, Scored	Novartis Generics
GG; 7	Imipramine Hydrochloride	10 mg		Tablet		
GG; 9	Dexamethasone	0.75 mg	Blue	Tablet	Pentagon-Shaped	Novartis Generics
GG; 9	Dexamethasone	0.75 mg		Tablet		Novartis Generics
GG; 14	Prednisolone	5 mg	Peach	Tablet	Scored, Round	Novartis Generics
GG; 16	Cyproheptadine Hydrochloride	4 mg		Coated Tablet	Round, Scored	Novartis Generics
GG; 16	Cyproheptadine Hydrochloride	4 mg	White	Tablet	Round, Scored	Novartis Generics
GG; 24	T.E.H.	10 mg	White	Tablet	Round; Scored; Compressed	Novartis Generics
GG; 24	T.E.H.	25 mg	White	Tablet	Round; Scored; Compressed	Novartis Generics
GG; 24	T.E.H.	130 mg	White	Tablet	Round; Scored; Compressed	Novartis Generics
GG; 43	Bisacodyl	5 mg	Dark Yellow	Enteric-Coated Tablet	Round	Novartis Generics
GG; 46	Propantheline Bromide	15 mg	Peach-Colored	Coated Tablet		Novartis Generics
GG; 50	Acetaminophen and Propoxyphene Napsylate	50 mg		Tablet		
GG; 50	Acetaminophen and Propoxyphene Napsylate	325 mg		Tablet		
GG; 51	Trifluoperazine Hydrochloride	1 mg	Lavender	Coated Tablet		Novartis Generics
GG; 62	Sodium Fluoride	2.2 mg	Pink	Tablet	Round	Novartis Generics
GG; 86	Clonidine Hydrochloride and Chlorthalidone	0.1 mg		Tablet		Novartis Generics
GG; 86	Clonidine Hydrochloride and Chlorthalidone	15 mg		Tablet		Novartis Generics
GG; 87	Clonidine Hydrochloride and Chlorthalidone	0.2 mg		Tablet		Novartis Generics
GG; 87	Clonidine Hydrochloride and Chlorthalidone	15 mg		Tablet		Novartis Generics
GG; 88	Clonidine Hydrochloride and Chlorthalidone	0.3 mg		Tablet		Novartis Generics
GG; 88	Clonidine Hydrochloride and Chlorthalidone	15 mg		Tablet		Novartis Generics
GG; 102	Niacin	50 mg	White	Tablet	Round	Novartis Generics
GG; 102	Niacin	50 mg		Tablet		Novartis Generics
GG; 110	Acetachlor	250 mg	Green	Tablet	Round, Scored with Hexagonal Cuts	
GG; 110	Acetachlor	300 mg	Green	Tablet	Round, Scored with Hexagonal Cuts	
GG; 110	Chlorzoxazone with Acetaminophen	250 mg	Light Green	Tablet	Round, Scored with Hexagonal Cuts	Novartis Generics
GG; 110	Chlorzoxazone with Acetaminophen	300 mg	Light Green	Tablet	Round, Scored with Hexagonal Cuts	Novartis Generics
GG; 114	Ergoloid Mesylates	1 mg	White	Tablet	Round	Novartis Generics
GG; 115	Ergoloid Mesylates	1 mg	White	Tablet	Oval	Novartis Generics
GG; 116	Ergoloid Mesylates	0.5 mg	White	Tablet	Round	Novartis Generics
GG; 120	Butal Compound	40 mg	White	Tablet		Novartis Generics
GG; 120	Butal Compound	50 mg	White	Tablet		Novartis Generics
GG; 120	Butal Compound	130 mg	White	Tablet		Novartis Generics
GG; 120	Butal Compound	200 mg	White	Tablet		Novartis Generics
GG; 122	Sulfasalazine	500 mg	Butterscotch	Tablet	Round	Novartis Generics
GG; 127	Quiphile	260 mg	White	Tablet	Round	Novartis Generics
GG; 138	Sulfamethoxazole	500 mg	Green	Tablet	Round; Scored	Novartis Generics
GG; 138	Sulfamethoxazole	500 mg		Tablet		Novartis Generics
GG; 142	Tolbutamide	500 mg	White	Tablet	Round; Scored	Novartis Generics
GG; 143	Phendimetrazine Tartrate	35 mg	Yellow	Tablet	Round, Scored	Novartis Generics
GG; 146	Hydrochlorothiazide and Reserpine	0.125 mg		Tablet		Novartis Generics
GG; 146	Hydrochlorothiazide and Reserpine	50 mg		Tablet		Novartis Generics
GG; 171	Aspirin and Codeine Phosphate	15 mg	White	Tablet	Round	
GG; 171	Aspirin and Codeine Phosphate	325 mg	White	Tablet	Round	
GG; 185	Glutethimide	500 mg	White	Tablet	Round	
GG; 186	Metaproterenol Sulfate	10 mg		Tablet		Novartis Generics
GG; 187	Metaproterenol Sulfate	20 mg		Tablet		Novartis Generics
GG; 197	Acetohexamide	250 mg		Coated Tablet	Oval, Scored	
GG; 198	Acetohexamide	500 mg	White	Coated Tablet	Capsule-Shaped, Scored	

IMPRINT	BRAND/GENERIC NAME	STRENGTH	COLOR	FORM	SHAPE	MANUFACTURER
GG; 200	Acetaminophen and Propoxyphene Napsylate	100 mg	Pink	Tablet	Capsule Shaped	
GG; 200	Acetaminophen and Propoxyphene Napsylate	650 mg	Pink	Tablet	Capsule Shaped	
GG; 212	Niacin	500 mg	White	Tablet	Round	Novartis Generics
GG; 218; 2	Acetaminophen and Codeine Phosphate	15 mg	White	Tablet	Round	
GG; 218; 2	Acetaminophen and Codeine Phosphate	300 mg	White	Tablet	Round	
GG; 233	Ascorbic Acid	500 mg	White	Tablet	Round	
GG; 245	Minoxidil	10 mg	White	Coated Tablet	Round, Scored	Novartis Generics
GG; 269	Niacin	100 mg	White	Tablet	Round	Novartis Generics
GG; 269	Niacin	100 mg		Tablet		Novartis Generics
GG; 287	Orphenadrine Citrate	100 mg	White	Timed-Release Tablet		Novartis Generics
GG; 287	Orphenadrine Citrate	100 mg		Timed-Release Tablet		Novartis Generics
GG; 290	Ibuprofen	300 mg	White	Tablet	Round	Novartis Generics
GG; 404	Butalbital, Acetaminophen and Caffeine	40 mg		Tablet		Novartis Generics
GG; 404	Butalbital, Acetaminophen and Caffeine	50 mg		Tablet		Novartis Generics
GG; 404	Butalbital, Acetaminophen and Caffeine	325 mg		Tablet		Novartis Generics
GG; 407	Chlorpromazine Hydrochloride	50 mg	Off-White	Coated Tablet	Round	Novartis Generics
GG; 408	Conjugated Estrogens	2.5 mg	Purple with Off-White Core	Coated Tablet	Oval	Novartis Generics
GG; 412	Carisoprodol Compound	200 mg		Tablet		Novartis Generics
GG; 412	Carisoprodol Compound	325 mg		Tablet		Novartis Generics
GG; 414	Probenecid	500 mg	Yellow	Coated Tablet	Capsule-Shaped	Novartis Generics
GG; 416	Hydralazine Hydrochloride	50 mg	Dark Green with White Core	Coated Tablet	Round	Novartis Generics
GG; 416	Hydralazine Hydrochloride	50 mg	Green	Tablet	Round	Geneva Generics
GG; 432	Conjugated Estrogens	0.3 mg	White	Tablet	Round	Novartis Generics
GG; 433	Conjugated Estrogens	0.625 mg	White	Coated Tablet	Round	Novartis Generics
GG; 434	Conjugated Estrogens	1.25 mg	White	Coated Tablet	Round	Novartis Generics
GG; 434	Conjugated Estrogens	1.25 mg	Yellow	Coated Tablet	Oval	Novartis Generics
GG; 435	Conjugated Estrogens	2.5 mg	Purple	Coated Tablet	Oval	Novartis Generics
GG; 435	Conjugated Estrogens	2.5 mg	White	Coated Tablet	Round	Novartis Generics
GG; 437	Chlorpromazine Hydrochloride	100 mg	Off-White	Coated Tablet	Round	Novartis Generics
GG; 440	Methenamine Mandelate	1 gram	Purple	Enteric-Coated Tablet	Oval	
GG; 441	Chewable Vitamins with Fluoride	4.5 mcg	Cream and Orange Speckled	Chewable Tablet		Novartis Generics
GG; 441	Chewable Vitamins with Fluoride	0.3 mg	Cream and Orange Speckled	Chewable Tablet		Novartis Generics
GG; 441	Chewable Vitamins with Fluoride	1.05 mg	Cream and Orange Speckled	Chewable Tablet		Novartis Generics
GG; 441	Chewable Vitamins with Fluoride	1.2 mg	Cream and Orange Speckled	Chewable Tablet		Novartis Generics
GG; 441	Chewable Vitamins with Fluoride	13.5 mg	Cream and Orange Speckled	Chewable Tablet		Novartis Generics
GG; 441	Chewable Vitamins with Fluoride	60 mg	Cream and Orange Speckled	Chewable Tablet		Novartis Generics
GG; 441	Chewable Vitamins with Fluoride	15 IU	Cream and Orange Speckled	Chewable Tablet		Novartis Generics
GG; 441	Chewable Vitamins with Fluoride	400 IU	Cream and Orange Speckled	Chewable Tablet		Novartis Generics
GG; 441	Chewable Vitamins with Fluoride	2500 IU	Cream and Orange Speckled	Chewable Tablet		Novartis Generics
GG; 444	Disobrom	6 mg	White or Green	Timed-Release Tablet	Round	Novartis Generics
GG; 444	Disobrom	120 mg	White or Green	Timed-Release Tablet	Round	Novartis Generics
GG; 444	Efedra-PA	6 mg	White or Green	Timed-Release Tablet	Round	Novartis Generics
GG; 444	Efedra-PA	120 mg	White or Green	Timed-Release Tablet	Round	Novartis Generics
GG; 452	Orphenadrine Citrate, Aspirin and Caffeine	25 mg		Tablet		Novartis Generics
GG; 452	Orphenadrine Citrate, Aspirin and Caffeine	30 mg		Tablet		Novartis Generics
GG; 452	Orphenadrine Citrate, Aspirin and Caffeine	385 mg		Tablet		Novartis Generics
GG; 453	Orphenadrine Citrate, Aspirin and Caffeine	50 mg		Tablet		Novartis Generics
GG; 453	Orphenadrine Citrate, Aspirin and Caffeine	60 mg		Tablet		Novartis Generics
GG; 453	Orphenadrine Citrate, Aspirin and Caffeine	770 mg		Tablet		Novartis Generics
GG; 455	Chlorpromazine Hydrochloride	10 mg	Off-White	Coated Tablet	Round	Novartis Generics
GG; 457	Chlorpromazine Hydrochloride	200 mg	Off-White	Coated Tablet	Round	Novartis Generics
GG; 458	Acetaminophen	500 mg	White	Tablet		
GG; 459	Acetaminophen	325 mg	White	Tablet		
GG; 474	Procainamide Hydrochloride	750 mg	White	Sustained-Release Tablet	Capsule-Shaped, Scored	Novartis Generics
GG; 475	Hydralazine Hydrochloride	10 mg	White	Coated Tablet	Round	Novartis Generics
GG; 475	Hydralazine Hydrochloride	10 mg	White	Tablet	Round	Geneva Generics
GG; 476	Chlorpromazine Hydrochloride	25 mg	Off-White	Coated Tablet	Round	Novartis Generics
GG; 478	Chlordiazepoxide and Amitriptyline	5 mg		Tablet		
GG; 478	Chlordiazepoxide and Amitriptyline	12.5 mg		Tablet		
GG; 479	Chlordiazepoxide and Amitriptyline	10 mg		Tablet		
GG; 479	Chlordiazepoxide and Amitriptyline	25 mg		Tablet		
GG; 480	Pre-Natal with Zinc	12 mcg	White	Coated Tablet	Capsule-Shaped	Novartis Generics
GG; 480	Pre-Natal with Zinc	150 mcg	White	Coated Tablet	Capsule-Shaped	Novartis Generics
GG; 480	Pre-Natal with Zinc	1 mg	White	Coated Tablet	Capsule-Shaped	Novartis Generics
GG; 480	Pre-Natal with Zinc	2.55 mg	White	Coated Tablet	Capsule-Shaped	Novartis Generics

IMPRINT	BRAND/GENERIC NAME	STRENGTH	COLOR	FORM	SHAPE	MANUFACTURER
GG; 480	Pre-Natal with Zinc	3 mg	White	Coated Tablet	Capsule-Shaped	Novartis Generics
GG; 480	Pre-Natal with Zinc	10 mg	White	Coated Tablet	Capsule-Shaped	Novartis Generics
GG; 480	Pre-Natal with Zinc	20 mg	White	Coated Tablet	Capsule-Shaped	Novartis Generics
GG; 480	Pre-Natal with Zinc	25 mg	White	Coated Tablet	Capsule-Shaped	Novartis Generics
GG; 480	Pre-Natal with Zinc	65 mg	White	Coated Tablet	Capsule-Shaped	Novartis Generics
GG; 480	Pre-Natal with Zinc	90 mg	White	Coated Tablet	Capsule-Shaped	Novartis Generics
GG; 480	Pre-Natal with Zinc	100 mg	White	Coated Tablet	Capsule-Shaped	Novartis Generics
GG; 480	Pre-Natal with Zinc	200 mg	White	Coated Tablet	Capsule-Shaped	Novartis Generics
GG; 480	Pre-Natal with Zinc	30 IU	White	Coated Tablet	Capsule-Shaped	Novartis Generics
GG; 480	Pre-Natal with Zinc	400 IU	White	Coated Tablet	Capsule-Shaped	Novartis Generics
GG; 480	Pre-Natal with Zinc	8000 IU	White	Coated Tablet	Capsule-Shaped	Novartis Generics
GG; 481	Pre-Natal with Zinc	10 mcg	White or Tan	Coated Tablet	Capsule-Shaped	Novartis Generics
GG; 481	Pre-Natal with Zinc	12 mcg	White or Tan	Coated Tablet	Capsule-Shaped	Novartis Generics
GG; 481	Pre-Natal with Zinc	1 mg	White or Tan	Coated Tablet	Capsule-Shaped	Novartis Generics
GG; 481	Pre-Natal with Zinc	1.5 mg	White or Tan	Coated Tablet	Capsule-Shaped	Novartis Generics
GG; 481	Pre-Natal with Zinc	2 mg	White or Tan	Coated Tablet	Capsule-Shaped	Novartis Generics
GG; 481	Pre-Natal with Zinc	3 mg	White or Tan	Coated Tablet	Capsule-Shaped	Novartis Generics
GG; 481	Pre-Natal with Zinc	20 mg	White or Tan	Coated Tablet	Capsule-Shaped	Novartis Generics
GG; 481	Pre-Natal with Zinc	25 mg	White or Tan	Coated Tablet	Capsule-Shaped	Novartis Generics
GG; 481	Pre-Natal with Zinc	120 mg	White or Tan	Coated Tablet	Capsule-Shaped	Novartis Generics
GG; 481	Pre-Natal with Zinc	200 mg	White or Tan	Coated Tablet	Capsule-Shaped	Novartis Generics
GG; 481	Pre-Natal with Zinc	11 IU	White or Tan	Coated Tablet	Capsule-Shaped	Novartis Generics
GG; 481	Pre-Natal with Zinc	400 IU	White or Tan	Coated Tablet	Capsule-Shaped	Novartis Generics
GG; 481	Pre-Natal with Zinc	4000 IU	White or Tan	Coated Tablet	Capsule-Shaped	Novartis Generics
GG; 485	Hydralazine Hydrochloride	25 mg	Light Green with White Core	Coated Tablet	Round	Novartis Generics
GG; 485	Hydralazine Hydrochloride	25 mg	Green	Tablet	Round	Geneva Generics
GG; 486	Conjugated Estrogens	0.3 mg	Green with White Core	Coated Tablet	Oval	Novartis Generics
GG; 486	Conjugated Estrogens	0.3 mg	White	Tablet	Round	Novartis Generics
GG; 491	Procainamide Hydrochloride	1000 mg		Sustained-Release Tablet		Novartis Generics
GG; 500	Acetaminophen	500 mg	Clear Red and Opaque White	Sustained-Release Capsule		Novartis Generics
GG; 500	Acetaminophen Extra Strength	500 mg	Red and White	Capsule		
GG; 509	Cyclandelate	400 mg	Blue and Red	Capsule		Novartis Generics
GG; 510	Sulfinpyrazone	200 mg		Capsule		Novartis Generics
GG; 514	Phenylbutazone	100 mg	Light Blue	Capsule		Novartis Generics
GG; 514	Phenylbutazone	100 mg		Capsule		Novartis Generics
GG; 515	Quinine Sulfate	325 mg	Clear	Capsule		
GG; 521	Butalbital Compound with Codeine	30 mg	Flesh	Capsule		Novartis Generics
GG; 521	Butalbital Compound with Codeine	40 mg	Flesh	Capsule		Novartis Generics
GG; 521	Butalbital Compound with Codeine	50 mg	Flesh	Capsule		Novartis Generics
GG; 521	Butalbital Compound with Codeine	325 mg	Flesh	Capsule		Novartis Generics
GG; 527	Clorazepate	7.5 mg	Opaque White with Bands	Capsule		Novartis Generics
GG; 528	Clorazepate	15 mg	Opaque White with Bands	Capsule		Novartis Generics
GG; 529	Cyclandelate	200 mg	Powder Blue	Capsule		Novartis Generics
GG; 542	Prazepam	5 mg		Capsule		Novartis Generics
GG; 543	Prazepam	10 mg		Capsule		Novartis Generics
GG; 545	Cephalexin	250 mg	Opaque Orange and Gray	Capsule		Novartis Generics
GG; 546	Cephalexin	500 mg	Opaque Orange and Gray	Capsule		Novartis Generics
GG; 551	Procainamide Hydrochloride	250 mg	Yellow	Capsule	Oval	Novartis Generics
GG; 552	Procainamide Hydrochloride	375 mg	Orange and White	Capsule	Oval	Novartis Generics
GG; 553	Procainamide Hydrochloride	500 mg	Orange and Yellow	Capsule	Oval	Novartis Generics
GG; 558	Fenoprofen Calcium	200 mg	White with Gold and Black Bands	Capsule		Novartis Generics
GG; 560	Ferrous Sulfate	250 mg		Sustained-Release Capsule		Novartis Generics
GG; 571	Clinoxide	5 mg	Opaque White	Capsule		Novartis Generics
GG; 581	Propoxyphene Hydrochloride, Aspirin and Caffeine	32.4 mg	Opaque Gray and Red	Capsule		Novartis Generics
GG; 581	Propoxyphene Hydrochloride, Aspirin and Caffeine	65 mg	Opaque Gray and Red	Capsule		Novartis Generics
GG; 581	Propoxyphene Hydrochloride, Aspirin and Caffeine	389 mg	Opaque Gray and Red	Capsule		Novartis Generics
GG; 583	Hydroxyzine Pamoate	50 mg	White and Green	Capsule		Novartis Generics
GG; 733	Salsalate	500 mg	Light Green	Coated Tablet	Round	Novartis Generics
GG; 734	Salsalate	750 mg		Coated Tablet	Capsule-Shaped, Scored	Novartis Generics
GG; 807	U.L.R.	5 mg	Orange	Capsule		Novartis Generics
GG; 807	U.L.R.	45 mg	Orange	Capsule		Novartis Generics
GG; 807	U.L.R.	200 mg	Orange	Capsule		Novartis Generics
GG; C4	Astemizole	10 mg		Tablet		
GLAXO	Almezyme	25 mg	Gray and Maroon	Capsule		Glaxo Wellcome
GLAXO	Almezyme	500 units	Gray and Maroon	Capsule		Glaxo Wellcome
GLAXO	Bronchobid Duracap	35 mg	Orange and Clear, Bead Filled	Sustained-Release Capsule		Glaxo Wellcome
GLAXO	Bronchobid Duracap	260 mg	Orange and Clear, Bead Filled	Sustained-Release Capsule		Glaxo Wellcome
GLAXO	Ferrobid Duracap	8 mg	Brown and Clear	Sustained-Release Capsule		Glaxo Wellcome
GLAXO	Ferrobid Duracap	100 mg	Brown and Clear	Sustained-Release Capsule		Glaxo Wellcome
GLAXO	Ferrobid Duracap	225 mg	Brown and Clear	Sustained-Release Capsule		Glaxo Wellcome
GLAXO	Propahist Compound	4 mg	Opaque Blue	Capsule		Glaxo Wellcome
GLAXO	Propahist Compound	25 mg	Opaque Blue	Capsule		Glaxo Wellcome

IMPRINT	BRAND/GENERIC NAME	STRENGTH	COLOR	FORM	SHAPE	MANUFACTURER
GLAXO	Sinacon	15 mg		Tablet		Glaxo Wellcome
GLAXO	Sinacon	325 mg		Tablet		Glaxo Wellcome
GLAXO	Tri-Cone	10 mg	Black and White	Capsule		Glaxo Wellcome
GLAXO	Tri-Cone	40 mg	Black and White	Capsule		Glaxo Wellcome
GLAXO	Vicon with Iron	2 mg	Pink and Red	Capsule		Glaxo Wellcome
GLAXO	Vicon with Iron	5 mg	Pink and Red	Capsule		Glaxo Wellcome
GLAXO	Vicon with Iron	10 mg	Pink and Red	Capsule		Glaxo Wellcome
GLAXO	Vicon with Iron	20 mg	Pink and Red	Capsule		Glaxo Wellcome
GLAXO	Vicon with Iron	30 mg	Pink and Red	Capsule		Glaxo Wellcome
GLAXO	Vicon with Iron	80 mg	Pink and Red	Capsule		Glaxo Wellcome
GLAXO	Vicon with Iron	300 mg	Pink and Red	Capsule		Glaxo Wellcome
GLAXO	Vicon with Iron	30 IU	Pink and Red	Capsule		Glaxo Wellcome
GLAXO; 232	Athemol	200 mg	Red-Orange	Coated Tablet		Glaxo Wellcome
GLAXO; 255	Athemol-N	75 mg	Light Green	Coated Tablet		Glaxo Wellcome
GLAXO; 255	Athemol-N	200 mg	Light Green	Coated Tablet		Glaxo Wellcome
GLAXO; 268	Theobid Duracap	260 mg	Blue and Clear	Sustained-Release Capsule		Glaxo Wellcome
GLAXO; 295	Theobid Duracap JR.	130 mg	Two-Tone Blue	Sustained-Release Capsule		Glaxo Wellcome
GLAXO; 315	Tri-Cone Plus	0.025 mg	Two-Tone Green	Capsule		Glaxo Wellcome
GLAXO; 315	Tri-Cone Plus	10 mg	Two-Tone Green	Capsule		Glaxo Wellcome
GLAXO; 315	Tri-Cone Plus	40 mg	Two-Tone Green	Capsule		Glaxo Wellcome
GX; CK3	Raxar	200 mg	White to Pale Yellow	Coated Tablet	Round, Biconvex, Bevel-Edged	
GX; CT1	Lotronex	1 mg	Blue	Coated Tablet	Oval	
H; 1; LL	Hydromox	50 mg	White	Tablet	Round, Flat, Scored, Beveled	Lederle Laboratories
H; 188	Papaverine Hydrochloride	150 mg	Brown and Clear	Capsule		Reid-Rowell Pharmaceutical
H74	Valmid	500 mg	Two-Tone Blue	Capsule		
HAUCK; 256	Dolacet	5 mg	Red and Black	Capsule		Roberts Pharmaceutical
HAUCK; 256	Dolacet	500 mg	Red and Black	Capsule		Roberts Pharmaceutical
HD; 544	Diazepam	5 mg	Yellow	Tablet	Round; Scored	Warner Chilcott
HD; 546	Diazepam	2 mg	White	Tablet	Round; Scored	Warner Chilcott
HD; 549	Diazepam	10 mg	Blue	Tablet	Round; Scored	Warner Chilcott
HEXAGON	Obotan	17.5 mg	Olive Green	Tablet	Capsule-Shaped	
HEXAGON	Obotan Forte	26.25 mg	Medium Green	Tablet	Capsule-Shaped	
HL; 4	Yomesan	500 mg				
HOECHST; 70	Festal	25 mg	White	Tablet	Round	
HOECHST; 70	Festal	50 mg	White	Tablet	Round	
HOECHST; 70	Festal	10 units	White	Tablet	Round	
HOECHST; 70	Festal	17 units	White	Tablet	Round	
HOECHST; MERITAL; 50MG	Merital	50 mg	Brown and Orange	Capsule		
HYREX	Two-Dyne	40 mg	Red	Capsule		
HYREX	Two-Dyne	50 mg	Red	Capsule		
HYREX	Two-Dyne	325 mg	Red	Capsule		
ICN	Prednisone	5 mg	White	Tablet		Icn Pharmaceuticals
IMPRINT	Trade Name	Strength	Color	Form	Shape	Company Name
IP; 136	Migrend	65 mg	Red and White	Capsule		Econolab
IP; 136	Migrend	100 mg	Red and White	Capsule		Econolab
IP; 136	Migrend	325 mg	Red and White	Capsule		Econolab
J75	Isuprel	2 mg	White	Tablet	Scored	
J75	Isuprel	10 mg	White	Tablet	Scored	
J77	Isuprel	2 mg	White	Tablet	Scored	
J77	Isuprel	15 mg	White	Tablet	Scored	
JANSSEN; AST; 10	Hismanal	10 mg	White	Tablet	Scored	
JANSSEN; L; 50	Ergamisol	50 mg	White	Coated Tablet		
JANSSEN; P; 10	Propulsid	10 mg	White	Tablet	Small, Round, Scored	
JANSSEN; P; 20	Propulsid	20 mg	Blue	Tablet	Oval	
JU	Eldepryl	5 mg	White	Tablet	Shield-Shaped	Somerset Pharmaceuticals
K	Vita-Metrazol	1 mg	Yellow	Tablet		
K	Vita-Metrazol	10 mg	Yellow	Tablet		
K	Vita-Metrazol	25 mg	Yellow	Tablet		
K	Vita-Metrazol	100 mg	Yellow	Tablet		
K; 5	Dicodid Bitartrate	5 mg	White	Tablet	Round	
K; 12	Metrazol	100 mg	White	Tablet	Round	
KAMADRIN; F4B	Kemadrin	2 mg	White	Tablet	Scored	
KOS; 375	Niaspan	375 mg	Off-White	Sustained-Release Tablet	Capsule-Shaped	
KREM	Krem	200 mg		Chewable Tablet		
KREM	Krem	400 mg		Chewable Tablet		
L	Zorane	20 mcg	Pink	28-Day Tablet Pack		Lederle Laboratories
L	Zorane	50 mcg	Green	28-Day Tablet Pack		Lederle Laboratories
L	Zorane	1 mg	Pink	28-Day Tablet Pack		Lederle Laboratories
L	Zorane	1.5 mg	Green	28-Day Tablet Pack		Lederle Laboratories
L	Zorane	1.5 mg		28-Day Tablet Pack		Lederle Laboratories
L	Zorane	30 mg		28-Day Tablet Pack		Lederle Laboratories
L 15; LL	Brompheniramine, Phenylephrine and Phenylpropanolamine	12 mg	Blue	Sustained-Release Tablet	Round	
L 15; LL	Brompheniramine, Phenylephrine and Phenylpropanolamine	15 mg	Blue	Sustained-Release Tablet	Round	
LEDERLE	Achromycin V	100 mg	Yellow and Blue	Capsule		Lederle Laboratories
LEDERLE	Bamadex Sequels	15 mg	Orange and Yellow	Capsule		Lederle Laboratories
LEDERLE	Bamadex Sequels	300 mg	Orange and Yellow	Capsule		Lederle Laboratories
LEDERLE	Ferro Sequels	100 mg	Green	Capsule		Lederle Laboratories
LEDERLE	Ferro Sequels	150 mg	Green	Capsule		Lederle Laboratories
LEDERLE	Ferro-Mandets	50 mg	Yellow-Brown	Chewable Tablet		Lederle Laboratories
LEDERLE	Oxytetracycline Hydrochloride	250 mg	White, Opaque	Capsule		Lederle Laboratories
LEDERLE	Pathilon Sequels with Phenobarbital	45 mg	Two Tone Blue	Capsule		Lederle Laboratories
LEDERLE	Pathilon Sequels with Phenobarbital	75 mg	Two Tone Blue	Capsule		Lederle Laboratories
LEDERLE	Varidase	20 mcg	Peach	Tablet	Round, Scored	Lederle Laboratories

IMPRINT	BRAND/GENERIC NAME	STRENGTH	COLOR	FORM	SHAPE	MANUFACTURER
LEDERLE	Varidase	2,500 units	Peach	Tablet	Round, Scored	Lederle Laboratories
LEDERLE	Varidase	10,000 units	Peach	Tablet	Round, Scored	Lederle Laboratories
LEDERLE; 250	Alpen	250 mg	White and Light Green	Capsule		Lederle Laboratories
LEDERLE; 500	Alpen	500 mg	White and Light Green	Capsule		Lederle Laboratories
LEDERLE; A3; 250 MG	Achromycin V	250 mg	Yellow and Blue	Capsule		
LEDERLE; C; 11	Chlordiazepoxide Hydrochloride	25 mg	Green and White	Capsule		Lederle Laboratories
LEDERLE; C5; 37.5 MG	Dyna-Trim	3 mcg	Brown and Clear	Timed-Release Capsule		Lederle Laboratories
LEDERLE; C5; 37.5 MG	Dyna-Trim	75 mcg	Brown and Clear	Timed-Release Capsule		Lederle Laboratories
LEDERLE; C5; 37.5 MG	Dyna-Trim	200 mcg	Brown and Clear	Timed-Release Capsule		Lederle Laboratories
LEDERLE; C5; 37.5 MG	Dyna-Trim	0.75 mg	Brown and Clear	Timed-Release Capsule		Lederle Laboratories
LEDERLE; C5; 37.5 MG	Dyna-Trim	0.85 mg	Brown and Clear	Timed-Release Capsule		Lederle Laboratories
LEDERLE; C5; 37.5 MG	Dyna-Trim	1 mg	Brown and Clear	Timed-Release Capsule		Lederle Laboratories
LEDERLE; C5; 37.5 MG	Dyna-Trim	5 mg	Brown and Clear	Timed-Release Capsule		Lederle Laboratories
LEDERLE; C5; 37.5 MG	Dyna-Trim	7.5 mg	Brown and Clear	Timed-Release Capsule		Lederle Laboratories
LEDERLE; C5; 37.5 MG	Dyna-Trim	9 mg	Brown and Clear	Timed-Release Capsule		Lederle Laboratories
LEDERLE; C5; 37.5 MG	Dyna-Trim	10 mg	Brown and Clear	Timed-Release Capsule		Lederle Laboratories
LEDERLE; C5; 37.5 MG	Dyna-Trim	30 mg	Brown and Clear	Timed-Release Capsule		Lederle Laboratories
LEDERLE; C5; 37.5 MG	Dyna-Trim	37.5 mg	Brown and Clear	Timed-Release Capsule		Lederle Laboratories
LEDERLE; C5; 37.5 MG	Dyna-Trim	15 IU	Brown and Clear	Timed-Release Capsule		Lederle Laboratories
LEDERLE; C5; 37.5 MG	Dyna-Trim	200 IU	Brown and Clear	Timed-Release Capsule		Lederle Laboratories
LEDERLE; C5; 37.5 MG	Dyna-Trim	2500 IU	Brown and Clear	Timed-Release Capsule		Lederle Laboratories
LEDERLE; C6; 75 MG	Dyna-Trim	6 mcg	Brown and Clear	Timed-Release Capsule		Lederle Laboratories
LEDERLE; C6; 75 MG	Dyna-Trim	150 mcg	Brown and Clear	Timed-Release Capsule		Lederle Laboratories
LEDERLE; C6; 75 MG	Dyna-Trim	400 mcg	Brown and Clear	Timed-Release Capsule		Lederle Laboratories
LEDERLE; C6; 75 MG	Dyna-Trim	1.5 mg	Brown and Clear	Timed-Release Capsule		Lederle Laboratories
LEDERLE; C6; 75 MG	Dyna-Trim	1.7 mg	Brown and Clear	Timed-Release Capsule		Lederle Laboratories
LEDERLE; C6; 75 MG	Dyna-Trim	2 mg	Brown and Clear	Timed-Release Capsule		Lederle Laboratories
LEDERLE; C6; 75 MG	Dyna-Trim	10 mg	Brown and Clear	Timed-Release Capsule		Lederle Laboratories
LEDERLE; C6; 75 MG	Dyna-Trim	15 mg	Brown and Clear	Timed-Release Capsule		Lederle Laboratories
LEDERLE; C6; 75 MG	Dyna-Trim	20 mg	Brown and Clear	Timed-Release Capsule		Lederle Laboratories
LEDERLE; C6; 75 MG	Dyna-Trim	60 mg	Brown and Clear	Timed-Release Capsule		Lederle Laboratories
LEDERLE; C6; 75 MG	Dyna-Trim	75 mg	Brown and Clear	Timed-Release Capsule		Lederle Laboratories
LEDERLE; C6; 75 MG	Dyna-Trim	30 IU	Brown and Clear	Timed-Release Capsule		Lederle Laboratories
LEDERLE; C6; 75 MG	Dyna-Trim	400 IU	Brown and Clear	Timed-Release Capsule		Lederle Laboratories
LEDERLE; C6; 75 MG	Dyna-Trim	5000 IU	Brown and Clear	Timed-Release Capsule		Lederle Laboratories
LEDERLE; C9	Chlordiazepoxide Hydrochloride	5 mg	Yellow and Green	Capsule		Lederle Laboratories
LEDERLE; C10	Chlordiazepoxide Hydrochloride	10 mg	Green and Black	Capsule		Lederle Laboratories
LEDERLE; C17	Chlorpheniramine Maleate	8 mg	Blue-Green	Timed-Release Capsule		Lederle Laboratories
LEDERLE; C18	Chlorpheniramine Maleate	12 mg	Blue-Green	Timed-Release Capsule		Lederle Laboratories
LEDERLE; C55	Clorazepate Dipotassium	3.75 mg	White and Lavender	Capsule		Lederle Laboratories
LEDERLE; C56	Clorazepate Dipotassium	7.5 mg	Lavender and Maroon	Capsule		Lederle Laboratories
LEDERLE; C57	Clorazepate Dipotassium	15 mg	Lavender	Capsule		Lederle Laboratories
LEDERLE; D22	Doxycycline Hyclate	50 mg	White and Bluegreen	Capsule		Lederle Laboratories
LEDERLE; D23	Dicyclomine Hydrochloride	10 mg	Blue	Capsule		Lederle Laboratories
LEDERLE; D35	Dolene AP-65	65 mg	Pink	Coated Tablet	Oval	Lederle Laboratories
LEDERLE; D35	Dolene AP-65	650 mg	Pink	Coated Tablet	Oval	Lederle Laboratories
LEDERLE; D36	Dolene	65 mg	Pink	Capsule		Lederle Laboratories
LEDERLE; D37	Dolene Compound-65	32.4 mg	Pink and Maroon	Capsule		Lederle Laboratories
LEDERLE; D37	Dolene Compound-65	65 mg	Pink and Maroon	Capsule		Lederle Laboratories
LEDERLE; D37	Dolene Compound-65	162 mg	Pink and Maroon	Capsule		Lederle Laboratories
LEDERLE; D37	Dolene Compound-65	227 mg	Pink and Maroon	Capsule		Lederle Laboratories
LEDERLE; D38	Diphenhydramine Hydrochloride	25 mg	Pink and Clear	Capsule		Lederle Laboratories
LEDERLE; D39	Diphenhydramine Hydrochloride	50 mg	Opaque Pink and Clear Pink	Capsule		Lederle Laboratories
LEDERLE; D42	Dolene Compound-65	32.5 mg	Maroon and Light Aqua	Capsule		Lederle Laboratories
LEDERLE; D42	Dolene Compound-65	65 mg	Maroon and Light Aqua	Capsule		Lederle Laboratories

IMPRINT	BRAND/GENERIC NAME	STRENGTH	COLOR	FORM	SHAPE	MANUFACTURER
LEDERLE; D42	Dolene Compound-65	389 mg	Maroon and Light Aqua	Capsule		Lederle Laboratories
LEDERLE; D43	Disopyramide	150 mg	Peach and Light Red	Capsule		Lederle Laboratories
LEDERLE; D47	Doxepin Hydrochloride	25 mg	Ivory and Yellow	Capsule		Lederle Laboratories
LEDERLE; D48	Doxepin Hydrochloride	50 mg	Lavendar and Dark Red	Capsule		Lederle Laboratories
LEDERLE; D49	Doxepin Hydrochloride	75 mg	Purple and Dark Pink	Capsule		Lederle Laboratories
LEDERLE; D50	Doxepin Hydrochloride	10 mg	Buff or Blue	Capsule		Lederle Laboratories
LEDERLE; D54	Doxepin Hydrochloride	100 mg	Green and White	Capsule		Lederle Laboratories
LEDERLE; D55	Doxepin Hydrochloride	150 mg	Gray and Orange	Capsule		Lederle Laboratories
LEDERLE; D62	Disopyramide	100 mg	Dark Red and Blue	Capsule		Lederle Laboratories
LEDERLE; E5	Erythromycin Stearate	500 mg	Yellow	Coated Tablet	Oval	Lederle Laboratories
LEDERLE; F15	Flurazepam Hydrochloride	15 mg	White and Blue Opaque	Capsule		Lederle Laboratories
LEDERLE; F2; FERRO SEQUELS	Ferro Sequels	100 mg	Green	Capsule		Lederle Laboratories
LEDERLE; F2; FERRO SEQUELS	Ferro Sequels	150 mg	Green	Capsule		Lederle Laboratories
LEDERLE; F30	Flurazepam Hydrochloride	30 mg	Blue Opaque	Capsule		Lederle Laboratories
LEDERLE; L14	Phenylpropanolamine Hydrochloride and Chlorpheniramine Maleate	12 mg	Blue and Clear	Sustained-Release Capsule		Lederle Laboratories
LEDERLE; L14	Phenylpropanolamine Hydrochloride and Chlorpheniramine Maleate	75 mg	Blue and Clear	Sustained-Release Capsule		Lederle Laboratories
LEDERLE; L23	Leder-CC Sequels	2.5 mg	Yellow and Clear	Sustained-Release Capsule		Lederle Laboratories
LEDERLE; L23	Leder-CC Sequels	8 mg	Yellow and Clear	Sustained-Release Capsule		Lederle Laboratories
LEDERLE; L23	Leder-CC Sequels	20 mg	Yellow and Clear	Sustained-Release Capsule		Lederle Laboratories
LEDERLE; L23	Leder-CC Sequels	50 mg	Yellow and Clear	Sustained-Release Capsule		Lederle Laboratories
LEDERLE; M2; MINOCIN; 50 MG	Minocin	50 mg	Orange	Capsule		
LEDERLE; M4; MINOCIN; 100 MG	Minocin	100 mg	Purple and Orange	Capsule		
LEDERLE; M41	Meclofenamate Sodium	50 mg	Opaque, Peach	Capsule		Lederle Laboratories
LEDERLE; M42	Meclofenamate Sodium	100 mg	Peach and White, Opaque	Capsule		Lederle Laboratories
LEDERLE; N20	Nitroglycerin SR	2.5 mg	Purple and Clear	Sustained-Release Capsule		Lederle Laboratories
LEDERLE; N21	Nitroglycerin SR	6.5 mg	Dark Blue and Clear Orange	Sustained-Release Capsule		Lederle Laboratories
LEDERLE; N22	Nitroglycerin SR	9 mg	Green and Yellow Clear	Capsule		Lederle Laboratories
LEDERLE; P2	Pathibamate-400	25 mg	Yellow	Tablet	Round	Lederle Laboratories
LEDERLE; P2	Pathibamate-400	400 mg	Yellow	Tablet	Round	Lederle Laboratories
LEDERLE; P11	Papaverine Hydrochloride	150 mg	Dark Brown and Clear	Capsule		Lederle Laboratories
LEDERLE; P29	Procainamide Hydrochloride	250 mg	Yellow	Capsule		Lederle Laboratories
LEDERLE; P30	Procainamide Hydrochloride	375 mg	Orange and White	Capsule		Lederle Laboratories
LEDERLE; P31	Procainamide Hydrochloride	500 mg	Yellow and Orange	Capsule		Lederle Laboratories
LEDERLE; P53	Phenytoin Sodium	100 mg	Clear	Extended-Release Capsule		Lederle Laboratories
LEDERLE; S5	Stresscaps	6 mcg	Brown	Capsule		Lederle Laboratories
LEDERLE; S5	Stresscaps	2 mg	Brown	Capsule		Lederle Laboratories
LEDERLE; S5	Stresscaps	10 mg	Brown	Capsule		Lederle Laboratories
LEDERLE; S5	Stresscaps	20 mg	Brown	Capsule		Lederle Laboratories
LEDERLE; S5	Stresscaps	100 mg	Brown	Capsule		Lederle Laboratories
LEDERLE; S5	Stresscaps	300 mg	Brown	Capsule		Lederle Laboratories
LEDERLE; T32	Temazepam	15 mg	Peach, Opaque	Capsule		Lederle Laboratories
LEDERLE; T33	Temazepam	30 mg	Yellow, Opaque	Capsule		Lederle Laboratories
LEMMON; 52	Uristat	0.03 mg	Blue	Tablet		Teva Pharmaceuticals
LEMMON; 52	Uristat	5 mg	Blue	Tablet		Teva Pharmaceuticals
LEMMON; 52	Uristat	5.5 mg	Blue	Tablet		Teva Pharmaceuticals
LEMMON; 52	Uristat	20 mg	Blue	Tablet		Teva Pharmaceuticals
LEMMON; 52	Uristat	50 mg	Blue	Tablet		Teva Pharmaceuticals
LEMMON; 572	Parest-200	200 mg	Turquoise Blue and Light Green	Capsule		Teva Pharmaceuticals
LEMMON; 574	Parest-400	400 mg	Turquoise Blue and Light Green	Capsule		Teva Pharmaceuticals
LEMMON; 712	Quaalude-150	150 mg	White	Tablet		Teva Pharmaceuticals
LEMMON; 714	Quaalude-300	300 mg	White	Tablet	Round, Scored	Teva Pharmaceuticals
LILLY; 3074	Hista-Clopane	4 mg	Pink and Red	Capsule		Eli Lilly
LILLY; 4049	Oraflex	400 mg		Tablet		Eli Lilly
LILLY; 4050	Oraflex	600 mg		Tablet		Eli Lilly
LILLY; A05	Potassium Chloride	300 mg		Tablet		Eli Lilly
LILLY; A06	Potassium Iodide	300 mg		Enteric-Coated Tablet		Eli Lilly
LILLY; A10	Sodium Salicylate	325 mg		Coated Tablet		Eli Lilly
LILLY; A11	Sodium Salicylate	650 mg		Enteric-Coated Tablet		Eli Lilly
LILLY; A19	Diethylstilbestrol	0.1 mg		Capsule		
LILLY; A20	Diethylstilbestrol	0.25 mg		Enteric-Coated Tablet		
LILLY; A21	Diethylstilbestrol	0.5 mg		Capsule		
LILLY; A22	Diethylstilbestrol	1 mg		Enteric-Coated Tablet		
LILLY; A24	Seconal Sodium	100 mg		Tablet		Eli Lilly
LILLY; A31	Potassium Chloride	1 gram		Enteric-Coated Tablet		Eli Lilly
LILLY; A33	Diethylstilbestrol	5 mg		Enteric-Coated Tablet		

IMPRINT	BRAND/GENERIC NAME	STRENGTH	COLOR	FORM	SHAPE	MANUFACTURER
LILLY; A34	Diethylstilbestrol	25 mg		Capsule		
LILLY; B60	Deltalin	1.25 mg		Gelcap		Eli Lilly
LILLY; C03	Ilotycin	250 mg	Orange	Enteric-Coated Tablet		Eli Lilly
LILLY; C06	Cascara	325 mg (5 grains)	Chocolate	Coated Tablet		Eli Lilly
LILLY; C12	Strychnine Sulfate	1 mg	Red	Coated Tablet		Eli Lilly
LILLY; C14	Ferro-Betalin	1 mg	Chocolate	Coated Tablet		Eli Lilly
LILLY; C14	Ferro-Betalin	325 mg	Chocolate	Coated Tablet		Eli Lilly
LILLY; C19	MI-Cebrin	3 mcg	Yellow	Tablet		Eli Lilly
LILLY; C19	MI-Cebrin	25 mcg	Yellow	Tablet		Eli Lilly
LILLY; C19	MI-Cebrin	Approx. 0.15 mg	Yellow	Tablet		Eli Lilly
LILLY; C19	MI-Cebrin	Approx. 1 mg	Yellow	Tablet		Eli Lilly
LILLY; C19	MI-Cebrin	Approx. 1.5 mg	Yellow	Tablet		Eli Lilly
LILLY; C19	MI-Cebrin	1.7 mg	Yellow	Tablet		Eli Lilly
LILLY; C19	MI-Cebrin	3 mg	Yellow	Tablet		Eli Lilly
LILLY; C19	MI-Cebrin	Approx. 5 mg	Yellow	Tablet		Eli Lilly
LILLY; C19	MI-Cebrin	5 mg	Yellow	Tablet		Eli Lilly
LILLY; C19	MI-Cebrin	10 mg	Yellow	Tablet		Eli Lilly
LILLY; C19	MI-Cebrin	Approx. 15 mg	Yellow	Tablet		Eli Lilly
LILLY; C19	MI-Cebrin	30 mg	Yellow	Tablet		Eli Lilly
LILLY; C19	MI-Cebrin	100 mg	Yellow	Tablet		Eli Lilly
LILLY; C20	MI-Cebrin T	7.5 mcg	Orange	Tablet		Eli Lilly
LILLY; C20	MI-Cebrin T	25 mcg	Orange	Tablet		Eli Lilly
LILLY; C20	MI-Cebrin T	0.15 mg	Orange	Tablet		Eli Lilly
LILLY; C20	MI-Cebrin T	1 mg	Orange	Tablet		Eli Lilly
LILLY; C20	MI-Cebrin T	1.5 mg	Orange	Tablet		Eli Lilly
LILLY; C20	MI-Cebrin T	2 mg	Orange	Tablet		Eli Lilly
LILLY; C20	MI-Cebrin T	5 mg	Orange	Tablet		Eli Lilly
LILLY; C20	MI-Cebrin T	7.5 mg	Orange	Tablet		Eli Lilly
LILLY; C20	MI-Cebrin T	10 mg	Orange	Tablet		Eli Lilly
LILLY; C20	MI-Cebrin T	15 mg	Orange	Tablet		Eli Lilly
LILLY; C20	MI-Cebrin T	100 mg	Orange	Tablet		Eli Lilly
LILLY; C20	MI-Cebrin T	150 mg	Orange	Tablet		Eli Lilly
LILLY; C22	Becotin-T	4 mcg	Brown	Tablet		Eli Lilly
LILLY; C22	Becotin-T	5 mg	Brown	Tablet		Eli Lilly
LILLY; C22	Becotin-T	10 mg	Brown	Tablet		Eli Lilly
LILLY; C22	Becotin-T	15 mg	Brown	Tablet		Eli Lilly
LILLY; C22	Becotin-T	20 mg	Brown	Tablet		Eli Lilly
LILLY; C22	Becotin-T	100 mg	Brown	Tablet		Eli Lilly
LILLY; C22	Becotin-T	300 mg	Brown	Tablet		Eli Lilly
LILLY; C36	Quinine Sulfate	325 mg	Chocolate	Coated Tablet		Eli Lilly
LILLY; C37	Stero-Darvon with A.S.A.	0.25 mg	Turquoise	Coated Tablet		Eli Lilly
LILLY; C37	Stero-Darvon with A.S.A.	32 mg	Turquoise	Coated Tablet		Eli Lilly
LILLY; C37	Stero-Darvon with A.S.A.	500 mg	Turquoise	Coated Tablet		Eli Lilly
LILLY; F01	Trinsicon	15 mcg	Pink and Red	Capsule		Eli Lilly
LILLY; F01	Trinsicon	0.5 mg	Pink and Red	Capsule		Eli Lilly
LILLY; F01	Trinsicon	75 mg	Pink and Red	Capsule		Eli Lilly
LILLY; F01	Trinsicon	110 mg	Pink and Red	Capsule		Eli Lilly
LILLY; F01	Trinsicon	240 mg	Pink and Red	Capsule		Eli Lilly
LILLY; F02	Trinsicon M	15 mcg	Pink and Dark Red	Capsule		Eli Lilly
LILLY; F02	Trinsicon M	75 mg	Pink and Dark Red	Capsule		Eli Lilly
LILLY; F02	Trinsicon M	110 mg	Pink and Dark Red	Capsule		Eli Lilly
LILLY; F02	Trinsicon M	240 mg	Pink and Dark Red	Capsule		Eli Lilly
LILLY; F03	Zentinic	50 mcg	Dark Red	Capsule		Eli Lilly
LILLY; F03	Zentinic	0.05 mg	Dark Red	Capsule		Eli Lilly
LILLY; F03	Zentinic	7.5 mg	Dark Red	Capsule		Eli Lilly
LILLY; F03	Zentinic	15 mg	Dark Red	Capsule		Eli Lilly
LILLY; F03	Zentinic	30 mg	Dark Red	Capsule		Eli Lilly
LILLY; F03	Zentinic	100 mg	Dark Red	Capsule		Eli Lilly
LILLY; F03	Zentinic	200 mg	Dark Red	Capsule		Eli Lilly
LILLY; F05	V-Cillin	125 mg		Capsule		Eli Lilly
LILLY; F06	V-Cillin	250 mg		Capsule		Eli Lilly
LILLY; F07	Compren	2.5 mcg	Yellow and Light Green	Capsule		Eli Lilly
LILLY; F07	Compren	3.3 mcg	Yellow and Light Green	Capsule		Eli Lilly
LILLY; F07	Compren	0.5 mg	Yellow and Light Green	Capsule		Eli Lilly
LILLY; F07	Compren	0.6 mg	Yellow and Light Green	Capsule		Eli Lilly
LILLY; F07	Compren	1 mg	Yellow and Light Green	Capsule		Eli Lilly
LILLY; F07	Compren	1.7 mg	Yellow and Light Green	Capsule		Eli Lilly
LILLY; F07	Compren	2 mg	Yellow and Light Green	Capsule		Eli Lilly
LILLY; F07	Compren	5 mg	Yellow and Light Green	Capsule		Eli Lilly
LILLY; F07	Compren	33.3 mg	Yellow and Light Green	Capsule		Eli Lilly
LILLY; F07	Compren	250 mg	Yellow and Light Green	Capsule		Eli Lilly
LILLY; F10	Amytal and Aspirin	50 mg	Scarlet	Capsule		Eli Lilly
LILLY; F10	Amytal and Aspirin	325 mg	Scarlet	Capsule		Eli Lilly
LILLY; F16	Lextron Ferrous	0.25 mg		Capsule		Eli Lilly
LILLY; F16	Lextron Ferrous	1 mg		Capsule		Eli Lilly
LILLY; F16	Lextron Ferrous	35 mg		Capsule		Eli Lilly
LILLY; F16	Lextron Ferrous	50 mg		Capsule		Eli Lilly
LILLY; F41	Bilron	300 mg	Green	Capsule		Eli Lilly
LILLY; F52	Dibasic Calcium Phosphate with Vitamin D	0.825 mg	Clear	Capsule		Eli Lilly
LILLY; F52	Dibasic Calcium Phosphate with Vitamin D	500 mg	Clear	Capsule		Eli Lilly

IMPRINT	BRAND/GENERIC NAME	STRENGTH	COLOR	FORM	SHAPE	MANUFACTURER
LILLY; F56	Calcium Gluconate with Vitamin D	0.825 mcg	Opaque White	Capsule		Eli Lilly
LILLY; F56	Calcium Gluconate with Vitamin D	325 mg	Opaque White	Capsule		Eli Lilly
LILLY; F59	Histadyl	25 mg	Red	Capsule		Eli Lilly
LILLY; F60	Histadyl	50 mg	Red	Capsule		Eli Lilly
LILLY; F61	Bilron	150 mg	Green	Capsule		Eli Lilly
LILLY; F72	Seconal Sodium	30 mg	Red	Capsule		Eli Lilly
LILLY; F75	Histadyl and Ephedrine Hydrochloride No. 2	16 mg		Capsule		Eli Lilly
LILLY; F75	Histadyl and Ephedrine Hydrochloride No. 2	50 mg		Capsule		Eli Lilly
LILLY; F90	Pentobarbital, Sodium	100 mg	Brown	Capsule		Eli Lilly
LILLY; F91	CO-Pyronil	15 mg	Yellow and Green	Capsule		Eli Lilly
LILLY; F91	CO-Pyronil	25 mg	Yellow and Green	Capsule		Eli Lilly
LILLY; F93	CO-Pyronil, Pediatric	7.5 mg	Dark Red	Capsule		Eli Lilly
LILLY; F93	CO-Pyronil, Pediatric	12.5 mg	Dark Red	Capsule		Eli Lilly
LILLY; F96	Reticulex	10 mcg	Red and Dark-Blue	Capsule		Eli Lilly
LILLY; F96	Reticulex	0.3 mg	Red and Dark-Blue	Capsule		Eli Lilly
LILLY; F96	Reticulex	50 mg	Red and Dark-Blue	Capsule		Eli Lilly
LILLY; F96	Reticulex	75 mg	Red and Dark-Blue	Capsule		Eli Lilly
LILLY; HO2	Darvon	32 mg	Light Pink	Capsule		Eli Lilly
LILLY; H07	Ilosone	125 mg	Ivory and Red	Capsule		Eli Lilly
LILLY; H09	Ilosone	250 mg	Ivory and Red	Capsule		Eli Lilly
LILLY; H11	Darvo-Tran	32 mg	Light Pink and Maroon	Capsule		Eli Lilly
LILLY; H11	Darvo-Tran	325 mg	Light Pink and Maroon	Capsule		Eli Lilly
LILLY; J02	Atropine Sulfate	0.4 mg		Tablet		Eli Lilly
LILLY; J24	Sodium Bicarbonate	325 mg		Tablet		Eli Lilly
LILLY; J34	Copavin	15 mg		Tablet	Compressed	Eli Lilly
LILLY; J42	Niacin	100 mg		Tablet	Scored	Eli Lilly
LILLY; J49	Diethylstilbestrol	0.1 mg		Tablet		
LILLY; J50	Diethylstilbestrol	0.25 mg		Tablet		
LILLY; J51	Diethylstilbestrol	0.5 mg		Tablet		
LILLY; J52	Diethylstilbestrol	1 mg		Tablet		
LILLY; J54	Diethylstilbestrol	5 mg		Tablet		
LILLY; J62	Papaverine Hydrochloride	60 mg		Tablet		Eli Lilly
LILLY; J63	Riboflavin	10 mg		Tablet		Eli Lilly
LILLY; J74	Methyltestosterone	25 mg		Tablet		Eli Lilly
LILLY; P28	Papaverine Hydrochloride	0.01%		Solution for Injection		Eli Lilly
LILLY; P28	Papaverine Hydrochloride	30 mg/1 ml		Solution for Injection		Eli Lilly
LILLY; S07	Diethylstilbestrol	0.1 mg		Suppository		
LILLY; S09	Diethylstilbestrol	0.5 mg		Suppository		
LILLY; S15	Asa	325 mg		Suppository		Eli Lilly
LILLY; S16	Asa	650 mg		Suppository		Eli Lilly
LILLY; S16	Asa	650 mg		Suppository		Eli Lilly
LILLY; T01	Zentron	5 mcg	Pink	Chewable Tablet		Eli Lilly
LILLY; T01	Zentron	1 mg	Pink	Chewable Tablet		Eli Lilly
LILLY; T01	Zentron	5 mg	Pink	Chewable Tablet		Eli Lilly
LILLY; T01	Zentron	20 mg	Pink	Chewable Tablet		Eli Lilly
LILLY; T01	Zentron	100 mg	Pink	Chewable Tablet		Eli Lilly
LILLY; T12	Calcium Carbonate and Soda	650 mg		Tablet	Compressed	Eli Lilly
LILLY; T12	Calcium Carbonate and Soda	1.95 gram		Tablet	Compressed	Eli Lilly
LILLY; T22	Magnesia and Soda	650 mg		Tablet	Compressed	Eli Lilly
LILLY; T27	Phenacetin	300 mg		Tablet	Compressed	Eli Lilly
LILLY; T30	Sodium Salicylate	325 mg		Tablet	Compressed	Eli Lilly
LILLY; T31	Sodium Salicylate	650 mg		Tablet	Compressed	Eli Lilly
LILLY; T43	Trisomin	500 mg (7 1/2 grains)		Tablet	Compressed	Eli Lilly
LILLY; T45	Cevalin	100 mg		Tablet	Compressed	
LILLY; T47	Cevalin	50 mg		Tablet	Compressed	
LILLY; T53	Niacinamide	100 mg		Tablet		Eli Lilly
LILLY; T54	Sulfadiazine	0.5 G		Tablet	Compressed	
LILLY; T60	Cevalin	250 mg		Tablet	Compressed	
LILLY; T67	Cevalin	500 mg		Tablet	Compressed	
LILLY; T69	Penicillin G Potassium	100,000 units		Tablet	Compressed, Scored	Eli Lilly
LILLY; T70	Diethylstilbestrol	25 mg		Tablet		
LILLY; T74	Penicillin G Potassium	250,000 units		Tablet	Compressed	Eli Lilly
LILLY; T76	Penicillin G Potassium	200,000 units		Tablet	Compressed	Eli Lilly
LILLY; T96	Neomycin Sulfate	500 mg		Tablet		Eli Lilly
LILLY; T99	Haldrone	1 mg	Yellow	Tablet		Eli Lilly
LILLY; U01	Haldrone	2 mg	Orange	Tablet		Eli Lilly
LILLY; U05	Ilosone	125 mg	Pink	Chewable Tablet		Eli Lilly
LILLY; U22	V-Kor	6.25 mg		Tablet		Eli Lilly
LILLY; U22	V-Kor	12.5 mg		Tablet		Eli Lilly
LILLY; U22	V-Kor	16 mg		Tablet		Eli Lilly
LILLY; U22	V-Kor	62.5 mg		Tablet		Eli Lilly
LILLY; U22	V-Kor	80 mg		Tablet		Eli Lilly
LILLY; U22	V-Kor	114 mg		Tablet		Eli Lilly
LILLY; U25	Ilosone	250 mg	Pink	Chewable Tablet		Eli Lilly
LILLY; U26	Ilosone	500 mg	Pink	Tablet		Eli Lilly
LILLY; U56	Folic Acid	1 mg		Tablet		Eli Lilly
LILLY; Y48	Morphine Sulfate Hypodermic	8 mg		Tablet		Eli Lilly
LL	Bisacodyl	5 mg	Orange	Enteric-Coated Tablet	Round	Lederle Laboratories
LL	Chloral Hydrate	500 mg	Green	Capsule		Lederle Laboratories
LL	Chlorothiazide	500 mg	White	Tablet	Round, Bisected	Lederle Laboratories
LL	Cyantin	50 mg	Yellow	Tablet	Scored	Lederle Laboratories
LL	Cyantin	100 mg	Yellow	Tablet	Scored	Lederle Laboratories
LL	Digoxin	0.25 mg	White	Tablet	Round, Scored	Lederle Laboratories
LL	Folbesyn Vitamin	5 mcg	Orange	Coated Tablet	Round	Lederle Laboratories
LL	Folbesyn Vitamin	1 mg	Orange	Coated Tablet	Round	Lederle Laboratories
LL	Folbesyn Vitamin	5 mg	Orange	Coated Tablet	Round	Lederle Laboratories
LL	Folbesyn Vitamin	10 mg	Orange	Coated Tablet	Round	Lederle Laboratories

IMPRINT	BRAND/GENERIC NAME	STRENGTH	COLOR	FORM	SHAPE	MANUFACTURER
LL	Folbesyn Vitamin	50 mg	Orange	Coated Tablet	Round	Lederle Laboratories
LL	Folbesyn Vitamin	175 mg	Orange	Coated Tablet	Round	Lederle Laboratories
LL	Folvite	0.25 mg	Yellow	Tablet		Lederle Laboratories
LL	Folvron	0.33 mg	Red and Light Red	Capsule		Lederle Laboratories
LL	Folvron	182 mg	Red and Light Red	Capsule		Lederle Laboratories
LL	Gevrite	0.5 mg	Red	Coated Tablet	Oblong	Lederle Laboratories
LL	Gevrite	1.3 mg	Red	Coated Tablet	Oblong	Lederle Laboratories
LL	Gevrite	1.8 mg	Red	Coated Tablet	Oblong	Lederle Laboratories
LL	Gevrite	10 mg	Red	Coated Tablet	Oblong	Lederle Laboratories
LL	Gevrite	18 mg	Red	Coated Tablet	Oblong	Lederle Laboratories
LL	Gevrite	75 mg	Red	Coated Tablet	Oblong	Lederle Laboratories
LL	Gevrite	100 mg	Red	Coated Tablet	Oblong	Lederle Laboratories
LL	Gevrite	230 mg	Red	Coated Tablet	Oblong	Lederle Laboratories
LL	Gevrite	5,000 USP units	Red	Coated Tablet	Oblong	Lederle Laboratories
LL	Glutethimide	500 mg	White	Tablet	Scored	
LL	Niacin	50 mg	White	Tablet	Scored, Round	Lederle Laboratories
LL	Niacin	100 mg	White	Tablet	Scored, Round	Lederle Laboratories
LL	Niacin	500 mg	White	Tablet	Scored, Round	Lederle Laboratories
LL	Nylidrin Hydrochloride	12 mg	White	Tablet	Round	Lederle Laboratories
LL	Phenobarbital	15 mg	White	Tablet	Round	
LL	Phenytoin Sodium	100 mg		Capsule		Lederle Laboratories
LL	Promethazine Hydrochloride	25 mg	White	Tablet	Round, Compressed	Lederle Laboratories
LL	Promethazine Hydrochloride	50 mg	Pink	Tablet	Round, Compressed	Lederle Laboratories
LL	Recoup	50 mg	Pink	Coated Tablet	Capsule-Shaped	Lederle Laboratories
LL	Recoup	300 mg	Pink	Coated Tablet	Capsule-Shaped	Lederle Laboratories
LL	Servisone	5 mg	White	Tablet	Round, Scored	Lederle Laboratories
LL	Sulcolon Sulfasalazine	0.5 gram	Brown	Tablet	Scored	Lederle Laboratories
LL; 1	Levothyroxine Sodium	0.1 mg	Yellow	Tablet	Round	Lederle Laboratories
LL; 2	Levothyroxine Sodium	0.2 mg	Pink	Tablet	Round	Lederle Laboratories
LL; 3	Levothyroxine Sodium	0.3 mg	Light Green or Blue	Tablet	Round	Lederle Laboratories
LL; 5	Chlordiazepoxide Hydrochloride	5 mg	Yellow and Green	Capsule		Lederle Laboratories
LL; 5; C; 33	Leucovorin Calcium	5 mg	Light Yellow	Tablet	Round, Convex, Bisected	Lederle Laboratories
LL; 10	Chlordiazepoxide Hydrochloride	10 mg	Green and Black	Capsule		Lederle Laboratories
LL; 10; C; 12	Leucovorin Calcium	10 mg	Light Yellow	Tablet	Square with Rounded Corners, Convex, Bisected	Lederle Laboratories
LL; 15; C; 35	Leucovorin Calcium	15 mg	Light Yellow	Tablet	Oval, Convex, Bisected	Lederle Laboratories
LL; 16	Aristocort	16 mg	White	Tablet	Oblong, Scored	Lederle Laboratories
LL; 25	Chlordiazepoxide Hydrochloride	25 mg	Green and White	Capsule		Lederle Laboratories
LL; 50; T; 27	Thioridazine Hydrochloride	50 mg	Orange	Coated Tablet	Round	Lederle Laboratories
LL; 100; T; 28	Thioridazine Hydrochloride	100 mg	Orange	Coated Tablet	Round	Lederle Laboratories
LL; 200	Meprobamate	200 mg	White	Tablet	Round, Scored	Lederle Laboratories
LL; 400	Meprobamate	400 mg	White	Tablet		Lederle Laboratories
LL; 3220	Apc with Codeine	15 mg	White	Tablet		Lederle Laboratories
LL; 3220	Apc with Codeine	32.4 mg	White	Tablet		Lederle Laboratories
LL; 3220	Apc with Codeine	162 mg	White	Tablet		Lederle Laboratories
LL; 3220	Apc with Codeine	227 mg	White	Tablet		Lederle Laboratories
LL; 3221	Apc with Codeine	30 mg	White	Tablet		Lederle Laboratories
LL; 3221	Apc with Codeine	32.4 mg	White	Tablet		Lederle Laboratories
LL; 3221	Apc with Codeine	162 mg	White	Tablet		Lederle Laboratories
LL; 3221	Apc with Codeine	227 mg	White	Tablet		Lederle Laboratories
LL; A 14	Amiloride and Hydrochlorothiazide	5 mg	Yellow	Tablet	Round	Lederle Laboratories
LL; A 14	Amiloride and Hydrochlorothiazide	50 mg	Yellow	Tablet	Round	Lederle Laboratories
LL; A 16	Aristocort	16 mg	White	Tablet	Oblong, Scored	Lederle Laboratories
LL; A 24	Amitriptyline Hydrochloride	10 mg	Pink	Coated Tablet	Round	Lederle Laboratories
LL; A 25	Amitriptyline Hydrochloride	25 mg	Green	Coated Tablet	Round	Lederle Laboratories
LL; A 26	Amitriptyline Hydrochloride	50 mg	Brown	Coated Tablet	Round	Lederle Laboratories
LL; A 36	Ascorbic Acid	250 mg	White	Tablet	Round	Lederle Laboratories
LL; A 37	Ascorbic Acid	500 mg	White	Tablet	Round	Lederle Laboratories
LL; A; 10	Amicar	500 mg	White	Tablet	Scored	Lederle Laboratories
LL; A; 19	Acetaminophen	500 mg	White	Tablet	Round, Scored	Lederle Laboratories
LL; A; 23-3	Acetaminophen with Codeine	30 mg	White	Tablet	Round	
LL; A; 23-3	Acetaminophen with Codeine	300 mg	White	Tablet	Round	
LL; A; 27	Amitriptyline Hydrochloride	75 mg	Light Purple	Coated Tablet	Round	Lederle Laboratories
LL; A; 28	Amitriptyline Hydrochloride	100 mg	Red-Orange	Coated Tablet	Round	Lederle Laboratories
LL; A; 38	Ascorbic Acid	1000 mg	White	Tablet	Oval; Scored	Lederle Laboratories
LL; A; 43	Allopurinol	100 mg	White	Tablet	Round, Scored	Lederle Laboratories
LL; A; 44	Allopurinol	300 mg	Peach	Tablet	Round, Scored	Lederle Laboratories
LL; A22	Acetaminophen	500 mg	White	Tablet	Oblong	Lederle Laboratories
LL; A35; 3	Aspirin with Codeine	30 mg	White	Tablet	Round	Lederle Laboratories
LL; A35; 3	Aspirin with Codeine	325 mg	White	Tablet	Round	Lederle Laboratories
LL; A39-4	Acetaminophen and Codeine Phosphate	60 mg	White	Tablet	Round	
LL; A39-4	Acetaminophen and Codeine Phosphate	300 mg	White	Tablet	Round	
LL; B; 10	Benztropine Mesylate	1 mg	White	Tablet	Oval, Scored	Lederle Laboratories
LL; B; 11	Benztropine Mesylate	2 mg	White	Tablet	Round, Scored	Lederle Laboratories
LL; B6	Butalbital with Apc	40 mg	White	Tablet	Round	Lederle Laboratories
LL; B6	Butalbital with Apc	50 mg	White	Tablet	Round	Lederle Laboratories
LL; B6	Butalbital with Apc	130 mg	White	Tablet	Round	Lederle Laboratories
LL; B6	Butalbital with Apc	200 mg	White	Tablet	Round	Lederle Laboratories
LL; C;7	Chlorthalidone	25 mg	Dark Orange	Tablet	Round, Scored	
LL; C; 13	Chlorothiazide	250 mg	White	Tablet	Round, Scored	Lederle Laboratories
LL; C; 14	Chlorothiazide	500 mg	White	Tablet	Round, Bisected	Lederle Laboratories
LL; C; 15	Chlorthalidone	50 mg	Dark Blue	Tablet	Round, Scored	
LL; C; 16	Chlorpheniramine Maleate	4 mg	Yellow	Tablet	Round, Scored	Lederle Laboratories
LL; C; 19	Chlorzoxazone with Acetaminophen	250 mg	Yellow	Tablet	Round, Scored	Lederle Laboratories
LL; C; 19	Chlorzoxazone with Acetaminophen	300 mg	Yellow	Tablet	Round, Scored	Lederle Laboratories
LL; C; 66	Carbamazepine	200 mg	White	Tablet	Round, Scored	Lederle Laboratories
LL; C; 67	Chlordiazepoxide and Amitriptyline Hydrochloride	5 mg	Green	Coated Tablet	Round	Lederle Laboratories

IMPRINT	BRAND/GENERIC NAME	STRENGTH	COLOR	FORM	SHAPE	MANUFACTURER
LL; C; 67	Chlordiazepoxide and Amitriptyline Hydrochloride	12.5 mg	Green	Coated Tablet	Round	Lederle Laboratories
LL; C; 68	Chlordiazepoxide and Amitriptyline Hydrochloride	10 mg	White	Coated Tablet	Round	Lederle Laboratories
LL; C; 68	Chlordiazepoxide and Amitriptyline Hydrochloride	25 mg	White	Coated Tablet	Round	Lederle Laboratories
LL; C; 69	Clorazepate Dipotassium	3.75 mg	Blue	Tablet	Round, Scored	Lederle Laboratories
LL; C; 70	Clorazepate Dipotassium	7.5 mg	Peach	Tablet	Round, Scored	Lederle Laboratories
LL; C; 71	Clorazepate Dipotassium	15 mg	White	Tablet	Round, Scored	Lederle Laboratories
LL; C21	Chlorpromazine Hydrochloride	10 mg	Light Brown	Coated Tablet	Round	Lederle Laboratories
LL; C22	Chlorpromazine Hydrochloride	25 mg	Tan	Coated Tablet	Round	Lederle Laboratories
LL; C23	Chlorpromazine Hydrochloride	50 mg	Tan	Coated Tablet	Round	Lederle Laboratories
LL; C24	Chlorpromazine Hydrochloride	100 mg	Tan	Coated Tablet	Round	Lederle Laboratories
LL; C25	Chlorpromazine Hydrochloride	200 mg	Tan	Coated Tablet	Round	Lederle Laboratories
LL; C30; CLOXACILLIN; 250	Cloxacillin Sodium	250 mg	Pink and Tan	Capsule		Lederle Laboratories
LL; C31; CLOXACILLIN; 500	Cloxacillin Sodium	500 mg	Pink and Tan	Capsule		Lederle Laboratories
LL; C37	Chlorpropamide	100 mg	White	Tablet	Round, Scored	Lederle Laboratories
LL; C38	Chlorpropamide	250 mg	White	Tablet	Round, Scored	Lederle Laboratories
LL; D; 23	Dicyclomine Hydrochloride	10 mg	Blue	Capsule		Lederle Laboratories
LL; D; 24	Dicyclomine Hydrochloride	20 mg	Blue	Tablet	Round, Scored	Lederle Laboratories
LL; D; 31	Diphenoxylate Hydrochloride and Atropine Sulfate	0.025 mg	White	Tablet	Round	
LL; D; 31	Diphenoxylate Hydrochloride and Atropine Sulfate	2.5 mg	White	Tablet	Round	
LL; D9	Declomycin	150 mg	Orange and Red Orange	Capsule		Lederle Laboratories
LL; D14	Declostatin	150 mg	Orange and Orange-Red	Capsule		Lederle Laboratories
LL; D14	Declostatin	250,000 units	Orange and Orange-Red	Capsule		Lederle Laboratories
LL; D15	Declostatin	300 mg	Red	Coated Tablet	Oblong	Lederle Laboratories
LL; D15	Declostatin	500,000 units	Red	Coated Tablet	Oblong	Lederle Laboratories
LL; D27	Ergoloid Mesylates	0.5 mg	White	Tablet	Round	Lederle Laboratories
LL; D28	Ergoloid Mesylates	1 mg	White	Tablet	Oval	Lederle Laboratories
LL; D29	Dexbrompheniramine Maleate with Pseudoephedrine Sulfate	6 mg	White	Tablet	Round	Lederle Laboratories
LL; D29	Dexbrompheniramine Maleate with Pseudoephedrine Sulfate	120 mg	White	Tablet	Round	Lederle Laboratories
LL; D33	Docusate Sodium	250 mg	Red and Red-Orange	Capsule		Lederle Laboratories
LL; E2	Erythromycin Stearate	250 mg	Yellow	Coated Tablet	Round	Lederle Laboratories
LL; E3	Ergoloid Mesylates	1 mg	White	Tablet	Round	Lederle Laboratories
LL; E5	Erythromycin Stearate	500 mg	Yellow	Coated Tablet	Oval	Lederle Laboratories
LL; E10	Erythromycin Ethylsuccinate	400 mg	Beige	Tablet	Oval	Lederle Laboratories
LL; F4	Filibon	6 mcg	Pink	Coated Tablet	Oblong	Lederle Laboratories
LL; F4	Filibon	150 mcg	Pink	Coated Tablet	Oblong	Lederle Laboratories
LL; F4	Filibon	0.4 mg	Pink	Coated Tablet	Oblong	Lederle Laboratories
LL; F4	Filibon	1.5 mg	Pink	Coated Tablet	Oblong	Lederle Laboratories
LL; F4	Filibon	1.7 mg	Pink	Coated Tablet	Oblong	Lederle Laboratories
LL; F4	Filibon	2 mg	Pink	Coated Tablet	Oblong	Lederle Laboratories
LL; F4	Filibon	18 mg	Pink	Coated Tablet	Oblong	Lederle Laboratories
LL; F4	Filibon	20 mg	Pink	Coated Tablet	Oblong	Lederle Laboratories
LL; F4	Filibon	60 mg	Pink	Coated Tablet	Oblong	Lederle Laboratories
LL; F4	Filibon	100 mg	Pink	Coated Tablet	Oblong	Lederle Laboratories
LL; F4	Filibon	125 mg	Pink	Coated Tablet	Oblong	Lederle Laboratories
LL; F4	Filibon	30 IU	Pink	Coated Tablet	Oblong	Lederle Laboratories
LL; F4	Filibon	400 IU	Pink	Coated Tablet	Oblong	Lederle Laboratories
LL; F4	Filibon	5000 IU	Pink	Coated Tablet	Oblong	Lederle Laboratories
LL; F5	Filibon FA	8 mcg	Pink	Coated Tablet	Oblong	Lederle Laboratories
LL; F5	Filibon FA	150 mcg	Pink	Coated Tablet	Oblong	Lederle Laboratories
LL; F5	Filibon FA	1 mg	Pink	Coated Tablet	Oblong	Lederle Laboratories
LL; F5	Filibon FA	1.7 mg	Pink	Coated Tablet	Oblong	Lederle Laboratories
LL; F5	Filibon FA	2 mg	Pink	Coated Tablet	Oblong	Lederle Laboratories
LL; F5	Filibon FA	4 mg	Pink	Coated Tablet	Oblong	Lederle Laboratories
LL; F5	Filibon FA	20 mg	Pink	Coated Tablet	Oblong	Lederle Laboratories
LL; F5	Filibon FA	45 mg	Pink	Coated Tablet	Oblong	Lederle Laboratories
LL; F5	Filibon FA	60 mg	Pink	Coated Tablet	Oblong	Lederle Laboratories
LL; F5	Filibon FA	100 mg	Pink	Coated Tablet	Oblong	Lederle Laboratories
LL; F5	Filibon FA	250 mg	Pink	Coated Tablet	Oblong	Lederle Laboratories
LL; F5	Filibon FA	30 IU	Pink	Coated Tablet	Oblong	Lederle Laboratories
LL; F5	Filibon FA	400 IU	Pink	Coated Tablet	Oblong	Lederle Laboratories
LL; F5	Filibon FA	8000 IU	Pink	Coated Tablet	Oblong	Lederle Laboratories
LL; F6	Filibon Forte Prenatal	12 mcg	Pink	Coated Tablet	Oblong	Lederle Laboratories
LL; F6	Filibon Forte Prenatal	200 mcg	Pink	Coated Tablet	Oblong	Lederle Laboratories
LL; F6	Filibon Forte Prenatal	1 mg	Pink	Coated Tablet	Oblong	Lederle Laboratories
LL; F6	Filibon Forte Prenatal	2 mg	Pink	Coated Tablet	Oblong	Lederle Laboratories
LL; F6	Filibon Forte Prenatal	2.5 mg	Pink	Coated Tablet	Oblong	Lederle Laboratories
LL; F6	Filibon Forte Prenatal	3 mg	Pink	Coated Tablet	Oblong	Lederle Laboratories
LL; F6	Filibon Forte Prenatal	30 mg	Pink	Coated Tablet	Oblong	Lederle Laboratories
LL; F6	Filibon Forte Prenatal	45 mg	Pink	Coated Tablet	Oblong	Lederle Laboratories
LL; F6	Filibon Forte Prenatal	90 mg	Pink	Coated Tablet	Oblong	Lederle Laboratories
LL; F6	Filibon Forte Prenatal	100 mg	Pink	Coated Tablet	Oblong	Lederle Laboratories
LL; F6	Filibon Forte Prenatal	300 mg	Pink	Coated Tablet	Oblong	Lederle Laboratories
LL; F6	Filibon Forte Prenatal	45 IU	Pink	Coated Tablet	Oblong	Lederle Laboratories
LL; F6	Filibon Forte Prenatal	400 IU	Pink	Coated Tablet	Oblong	Lederle Laboratories
LL; F6	Filibon Forte Prenatal	8000 IU	Pink	Coated Tablet	Oblong	Lederle Laboratories
LL; F19	Ferrous Fumarate	200 mg	Brown	Tablet	Round	Lederle Laboratories
LL; F20	Ferrous Sulfate	300 mg	Red	Coated Tablet	Round	Lederle Laboratories
LL; F21	Ferrous Gluconate	300 mg	Green	Coated Tablet	Round	Lederle Laboratories
LL; G1	Gevral	6 mcg	Brown	Coated Tablet	Oblong	Lederle Laboratories

IMPRINT	BRAND/GENERIC NAME	STRENGTH	COLOR	FORM	SHAPE	MANUFACTURER
LL; G1	Gevral	150 mcg	Brown	Coated Tablet	Oblong	Lederle Laboratories
LL; G1	Gevral	0.4 mg	Brown	Coated Tablet	Oblong	Lederle Laboratories
LL; G1	Gevral	1.5 mg	Brown	Coated Tablet	Oblong	Lederle Laboratories
LL; G1	Gevral	1.7 mg	Brown	Coated Tablet	Oblong	Lederle Laboratories
LL; G1	Gevral	2 mg	Brown	Coated Tablet	Oblong	Lederle Laboratories
LL; G1	Gevral	18 mg	Brown	Coated Tablet	Oblong	Lederle Laboratories
LL; G1	Gevral	20 mg	Brown	Coated Tablet	Oblong	Lederle Laboratories
LL; G1	Gevral	60 mg	Brown	Coated Tablet	Oblong	Lederle Laboratories
LL; G1	Gevral	100 mg	Brown	Coated Tablet	Oblong	Lederle Laboratories
LL; G1	Gevral	125 mg	Brown	Coated Tablet	Oblong	Lederle Laboratories
LL; G1	Gevral	162 mg	Brown	Coated Tablet	Oblong	Lederle Laboratories
LL; G1	Gevral	30 IU	Brown	Coated Tablet	Oblong	Lederle Laboratories
LL; G1	Gevral	5000 IU	Brown	Coated Tablet	Oblong	Lederle Laboratories
LL; H; 2	Hydromox R	0.125 mg	Yellow	Tablet	Round, Scored	
LL; H; 2	Hydromox R	50 mg	Yellow	Tablet	Round, Scored	
LL; H; 25	Haloperidol	0.5 mg	Orange	Tablet	Round, Scored	Lederle Laboratories
LL; H; 26	Haloperidol	1 mg	Orange	Tablet	Round, Scored	Lederle Laboratories
LL; H; 27	Haloperidol	2 mg	Light Pink	Tablet	Round, Scored	Lederle Laboratories
LL; H; 28	Haloperidol	5 mg	Orange	Tablet	Round, Scored	Lederle Laboratories
LL; H; 29	Haloperidol	10 mg	Aqua	Tablet	Round, Scored	Lederle Laboratories
LL; H17	Hydroxyzine Hydrochloride	10 mg	Light Pink	Tablet	Round	Lederle Laboratories
LL; H18	Hydroxyzine Hydrochloride	25 mg	Lilac	Tablet	Round	Lederle Laboratories
LL; H21	Hydroxyzine Hydrochloride	50 mg	Purple	Tablet	Round	Lederle Laboratories
LL; I; 15	Isosorbide Dinitrate Oral	5 mg	Pink	Tablet	Round, Scored	Lederle Laboratories
LL; I; 16	Isosorbide Dinitrate Oral	10 mg	White	Tablet	Round, Scored	Lederle Laboratories
LL; I; 22	Isoxsuprine Hydrochloride	20 mg	White	Tablet	Round, Scored	
LL; I; 24	Isosorbide Dinitrate Oral	20 mg	Green	Tablet	Round, Scored	Lederle Laboratories
LL; I; 28	Ibuprofen	400 mg	White	Tablet	Round	Lederle Laboratories
LL; I11	Imipramine Hydrochloride	10 mg	Yellow	Tablet	Round	Lederle Laboratories
LL; I12	Imipramine Hydrochloride	25 mg	Rust	Tablet	Round	Lederle Laboratories
LL; I13	Imipramine Hydrochloride	50 mg	Green	Tablet	Round	Lederle Laboratories
LL; I17	Isosorbide Dinitrate	2.5 mg	Yellow	Tablet	Round	Lederle Laboratories
LL; I18	Isosorbide Dinitrate	5 mg	Pink	Tablet	Round	Lederle Laboratories
LL; I21	Isoxsuprine Hydrochloride	10 mg	White	Tablet	Round	
LL; I23	Isosorbide Dinitrate SA	40 mg	Light Green	Timed-Release Tablet	Round, Scored	Lederle Laboratories
LL; I29	Ibuprofen	600 mg	White	Tablet	Oval	Lederle Laboratories
LL; I30	Ibuprofen	800 mg	White	Tablet	Oval	Lederle Laboratories
LL; L; 11	Levothyroxine Sodium	0.1 mg	Yellow	Tablet	Round	Lederle Laboratories
LL; L; 12	Levothyroxine Sodium	0.2 mg	Pink	Tablet	Round	Lederle Laboratories
LL; L; 13	Levothyroxine Sodium	0.3 mg	Light Green or Blue	Tablet	Round	Lederle Laboratories
LL; L; 17	Levothyroxine Sodium	0.15 mg	Blue	Tablet	Round	Lederle Laboratories
LL; L; 30	Lorazepam	0.5 mg	White	Tablet	Round	Lederle Laboratories
LL; L; 31	Lorazepam	1 mg	White,	Tablet	Round, Scored	Lederle Laboratories
LL; L; 32	Lorazepam	2 mg	White	Tablet	Round, Scored	Lederle Laboratories
LL; L6	Lederplex	9 mcg	Brown	Capsule		Lederle Laboratories
LL; L6	Lederplex	2.25 mg	Brown	Capsule		Lederle Laboratories
LL; L6	Lederplex	2.6 mg	Brown	Capsule		Lederle Laboratories
LL; L6	Lederplex	3 mg	Brown	Capsule		Lederle Laboratories
LL; L6	Lederplex	15 mg	Brown	Capsule		Lederle Laboratories
LL; L6	Lederplex	30 mg	Brown	Capsule		Lederle Laboratories
LL; L7	Lederplex	1 mcg	Brown	Coated Tablet		Lederle Laboratories
LL; L7	Lederplex	9 mcg	Brown	Coated Tablet		Lederle Laboratories
LL; L7	Lederplex	0.1 mg	Brown	Coated Tablet		Lederle Laboratories
LL; L7	Lederplex	2 mg	Brown	Coated Tablet		Lederle Laboratories
LL; L7	Lederplex	2.25 mg	Brown	Coated Tablet		Lederle Laboratories
LL; L7	Lederplex	2.6 mg	Brown	Coated Tablet		Lederle Laboratories
LL; L7	Lederplex	3 mg	Brown	Coated Tablet		Lederle Laboratories
LL; L7	Lederplex	10 mg	Brown	Coated Tablet		Lederle Laboratories
LL; L7	Lederplex	15 mg	Brown	Coated Tablet		Lederle Laboratories
LL; L7	Lederplex	30 mg	Brown	Coated Tablet		Lederle Laboratories
LL; L7	Lederplex	250 mg	Brown	Coated Tablet		Lederle Laboratories
LL; M; 12	Meclizine Hydrochloride	12.5 mg	Blue	Tablet	Oval	Lederle Laboratories
LL; M; 13	Meclizine Hydrochloride	25 mg	Yellow	Tablet	Oval, Scored	Lederle Laboratories
LL; M; 14	Meclizine Hydrochloride	25 mg	Pink	Chewable Tablet	Round, Scored	Lederle Laboratories
LL; M; 24	Methyclothiazide	2.5 mg	White	Tablet	Round, Scored	Lederle Laboratories
LL; M; 25	Methyclothiazide	5 mg	Blue	Tablet	Round, Scored	Lederle Laboratories
LL; M; 35	Medroxyprogesterone Acetate	10 mg	White	Tablet	Round, Scored	Lederle Laboratories
LL; M21	Methyldopa	125 mg	Peach	Coated Tablet	Round	Lederle Laboratories
LL; M26	Metronidazole	250 mg	White	Coated Tablet	Round	Lederle Laboratories
LL; M27	Metronidazole	500 mg	White	Coated Tablet	Oblong	Lederle Laboratories
LL; M8; MAXZIDE	Maxzide	50 mg	Yellow	Tablet	Bowtie-Shaped	
LL; M8; MAXZIDE	Maxzide	75 mg	Yellow	Tablet	Bowtie-Shaped	
LL; M9; MAXZIDE	Maxzide	25 mg	Light Green	Tablet	Bowtie-Shaped	
LL; M9; MAXZIDE	Maxzide	37.5 mg	Light Green	Tablet	Bowtie-Shaped	
LL; N; 23	Nylidrin Hydrochloride	6 mg	White		Round	Lederle Laboratories
LL; N; 24	Nylidrin Hydrochloride	12 mg	White	Tablet	Round	Lederle Laboratories
LL; N10	Neomycin Sulfate	500 mg	Peach	Tablet	Round, Uncoated	Lederle Laboratories
LL; N22	Reserpine, Hydrochlorothiazide and Hydralazine Hydrochloride	0.1 mg	Pink and Brown	Tablet	Round	
LL; N22	Reserpine, Hydrochlorothiazide and Hydralazine Hydrochloride	15 mg	Pink and Brown	Tablet	Round	
LL; N22	Reserpine, Hydrochlorothiazide and Hydralazine Hydrochloride	25 mg	Pink and Brown	Tablet	Round	
LL; P; 13	Papaverine Hydrochloride	100 mg	White	Tablet	Round, Scored	Lederle Laboratories
LL; P; 17	Penicillin G Potassium	400,000 units	White	Tablet	Round; Scored	Lederle Laboratories
LL; P; 19	Pyridoxine Hydrochloride	100 mg	White	Tablet	Round	Lederle Laboratories
LL; P; 21	Phenobarbital	30 mg	White	Tablet	Round	
LL; P; 24	Prednisone	5 mg	White	Tablet	Round, Scored	Lederle Laboratories
LL; P; 26	Probenecid with Colchicine	0.5 mg	White	Tablet	Oblong, Scored	Lederle Laboratories
LL; P; 26	Probenecid with Colchicine	500 mg	White	Tablet	Oblong, Scored	Lederle Laboratories
LL; P; 48	Procainamide Hydrochloride SR	250 mg	Light Blue	Coated Tablet	Oval, Scored	Lederle Laboratories
LL; P; 49	Procainamide Hydrochloride SR	250 mg	Light Blue	Coated Tablet	Oval, Scored	Lederle Laboratories
LL; P; 49	Procainamide Hydrochloride SR	500 mg	Pink	Coated Tablet	Oval, Scored	Lederle Laboratories
LL; P; 50	Procainamide Hydrochloride SR	750 mg	Light Brown	Coated Tablet	Oval, Scored	Lederle Laboratories

IMPRINT	BRAND/GENERIC NAME	STRENGTH	COLOR	FORM	SHAPE	MANUFACTURER
LL; P; 67	Propranolol Hydrochloride and Hydrochlorothiazide	25 mg	White	Tablet	Round, Scored	Lederle Laboratories
LL; P; 67	Propranolol Hydrochloride and Hydrochlorothiazide	40 mg	White	Tablet	Round, Scored	Lederle Laboratories
LL; P; 68	Propranolol Hydrochloride and Hydrochlorothiazide	25 mg	White	Tablet	Round	Lederle Laboratories
LL; P; 68	Propranolol Hydrochloride and Hydrochlorothiazide	80 mg	White	Tablet	Round	Lederle Laboratories
LL; P; 76	Perphenazine and Amitriptyline Hydrochloride	4 mg	Orange	Coated Tablet	Round	Lederle Laboratories
LL; P; 76	Perphenazine and Amitriptyline Hydrochloride	50 mg	Orange	Coated Tablet	Round	Lederle Laboratories
LL; P1	Pathibamate-200	25 mg	Yellow	Coated Tablet	Round	Lederle Laboratories
LL; P1	Pathibamate-200	200 mg	Yellow	Coated Tablet	Round	Lederle Laboratories
LL; P3	Pathilon Sequels	75 mg	Dark Pink and Dark Red	Capsule		Lederle Laboratories
LL; P6	Pathilon with Phenobarbital	15 mg	Pink	Coated Tablet	Round	Lederle Laboratories
LL; P6	Pathilon with Phenobarbital	25 mg	Pink	Coated Tablet	Round	Lederle Laboratories
LL; P7	Perihemin	5 mcg	Red	Capsule		Lederle Laboratories
LL; P7	Perihemin	0.33 mg	Red	Capsule		Lederle Laboratories
LL; P7	Perihemin	25 mg	Red	Capsule		Lederle Laboratories
LL; P7	Perihemin	50 mg	Red	Capsule		Lederle Laboratories
LL; P7	Perihemin	168 mg	Red	Capsule		Lederle Laboratories
LL; P8	Peritinic	50 mcg	Maroon	Coated Tablet	Oblong	Lederle Laboratories
LL; P8	Peritinic	7.5 mg	Maroon	Coated Tablet	Oblong	Lederle Laboratories
LL; P8	Peritinic	100 mg	Maroon	Coated Tablet	Oblong	Lederle Laboratories
LL; P18	Penicillin G Potassium	800,000 units	White	Tablet	Oval, Scored	Lederle Laboratories
LL; P25	Probenecid	500 mg	Orange	Coated Tablet	Oblong	Lederle Laboratories
LL; P34	Pseudoephedrine Hydrochloride	60 mg	White	Tablet	Round, Scored	
LL; P35	Pseudoephedrine Hydrochloride	30 mg	Red	Coated Tablet	Round	
LL; P37	Pyridoxine Hydrochloride	25 mg	White	Tablet	Round	Lederle Laboratories
LL; P38	Pyridoxine Hydrochloride	50 mg	White	Tablet	Round	Lederle Laboratories
LL; P39	Acetaminophen and Propoxyphene Napsylate	100 mg	White	Coated Tablet	Oblong	
LL; P39	Acetaminophen and Propoxyphene Napsylate	650 mg	White	Coated Tablet	Oblong	
LL; P72	Perphenazine and Amitriptyline Hydrochloride	2 mg	Blue	Coated Tablet	Round	Lederle Laboratories
LL; P72	Perphenazine and Amitriptyline Hydrochloride	10 mg	Blue	Coated Tablet	Round	Lederle Laboratories
LL; P73	Perphenazine with Amitriptyline Hydrochloride	2 mg	Orange	Coated Tablet	Round	Lederle Laboratories
LL; P73	Perphenazine with Amitriptyline Hydrochloride	25 mg	Orange	Coated Tablet	Round	Lederle Laboratories
LL; P74	Perphenazine and Amitriptyline Hydrochloride	4 mg	Light Peach	Coated Tablet	Round	Lederle Laboratories
LL; P74	Perphenazine and Amitriptyline Hydrochloride	10 mg	Light Peach	Coated Tablet	Round	Lederle Laboratories
LL; P75	Perphenazine and Amitriptyline Hydrochloride	4 mg	Yellow	Coated Tablet	Round	Lederle Laboratories
LL; P75	Perphenazine and Amitriptyline Hydrochloride	25 mg	Yellow	Coated Tablet	Round	Lederle Laboratories
LL; Q; 13	Quinidine Gluconate SR	324 mg	White	Sustained-Release Tablet	Round, Scored	Lederle Laboratories
LL; R; 11	Reserpine	0.25 mg	White	Tablet	Round	
LL; S; 15	Sulfisoxazole	500 mg	White	Tablet	Scored	Lederle Laboratories
LL; S; 22	Spartus	25 mcg	Blue	Tablet	Oval	Lederle Laboratories
LL; S; 22	Spartus	30 mcg	Blue	Tablet	Oval	Lederle Laboratories
LL; S; 22	Spartus	45 mcg	Blue	Tablet	Oval	Lederle Laboratories
LL; S; 22	Spartus	150 mcg	Blue	Tablet	Oval	Lederle Laboratories
LL; S; 22	Spartus	400 mcg	Blue	Tablet	Oval	Lederle Laboratories
LL; S; 22	Spartus	2 mg	Blue	Tablet	Oval	Lederle Laboratories
LL; S; 22	Spartus	5 mg	Blue	Tablet	Oval	Lederle Laboratories
LL; S; 22	Spartus	7.5 mg	Blue	Tablet	Oval	Lederle Laboratories
LL; S; 22	Spartus	8.5 mg	Blue	Tablet	Oval	Lederle Laboratories
LL; S; 22	Spartus	10 mg	Blue	Tablet	Oval	Lederle Laboratories
LL; S; 22	Spartus	15 mg	Blue	Tablet	Oval	Lederle Laboratories
LL; S; 22	Spartus	25 mg	Blue	Tablet	Oval	Lederle Laboratories
LL; S; 22	Spartus	36.3 mg	Blue	Tablet	Oval	Lederle Laboratories
LL; S; 22	Spartus	40 mg	Blue	Tablet	Oval	Lederle Laboratories
LL; S; 22	Spartus	75 mg	Blue	Tablet	Oval	Lederle Laboratories
LL; S; 22	Spartus	100 mg	Blue	Tablet	Oval	Lederle Laboratories
LL; S; 22	Spartus	162 mg	Blue	Tablet	Oval	Lederle Laboratories
LL; S; 22	Spartus	300 mg	Blue	Tablet	Oval	Lederle Laboratories
LL; S; 22	Spartus	30 IU	Blue	Tablet	Oval	Lederle Laboratories
LL; S; 22	Spartus	300 IU	Blue	Tablet	Oval	Lederle Laboratories
LL; S; 22	Spartus	3000 IU	Blue	Tablet	Oval	Lederle Laboratories
LL; S; 23	Spartus Plus Iron	25 mcg	Red	Tablet	Oval, Scored	Lederle Laboratories
LL; S; 23	Spartus Plus Iron	30 mcg	Red	Tablet	Oval, Scored	Lederle Laboratories
LL; S; 23	Spartus Plus Iron	45 mcg	Red	Tablet	Oval, Scored	Lederle Laboratories
LL; S; 23	Spartus Plus Iron	150 mcg	Red	Tablet	Oval, Scored	Lederle Laboratories
LL; S; 23	Spartus Plus Iron	400 mcg	Red	Tablet	Oval, Scored	Lederle Laboratories
LL; S; 23	Spartus Plus Iron	2 mg	Red	Tablet	Oval, Scored	Lederle Laboratories
LL; S; 23	Spartus Plus Iron	5 mg	Red	Tablet	Oval, Scored	Lederle Laboratories
LL; S; 23	Spartus Plus Iron	7.5 mg	Red	Tablet	Oval, Scored	Lederle Laboratories
LL; S; 23	Spartus Plus Iron	8.5 mg	Red	Tablet	Oval, Scored	Lederle Laboratories
LL; S; 23	Spartus Plus Iron	10 mg	Red	Tablet	Oval, Scored	Lederle Laboratories
LL; S; 23	Spartus Plus Iron	15 mg	Red	Tablet	Oval, Scored	Lederle Laboratories
LL; S; 23	Spartus Plus Iron	25 mg	Red	Tablet	Oval, Scored	Lederle Laboratories
LL; S; 23	Spartus Plus Iron	27 mg	Red	Tablet	Oval, Scored	Lederle Laboratories
LL; S; 23	Spartus Plus Iron	36.3 mg	Red	Tablet	Oval, Scored	Lederle Laboratories
LL; S; 23	Spartus Plus Iron	40 mg	Red	Tablet	Oval, Scored	Lederle Laboratories
LL; S; 23	Spartus Plus Iron	75 mg	Red	Tablet	Oval, Scored	Lederle Laboratories
LL; S; 23	Spartus Plus Iron	100 mg	Red	Tablet	Oval, Scored	Lederle Laboratories

IMPRINT	BRAND/GENERIC NAME	STRENGTH	COLOR	FORM	SHAPE	MANUFACTURER
LL; S; 23	Spartus Plus Iron	162 mg	Red	Tablet	Oval, Scored	Lederle Laboratories
LL; S; 23	Spartus Plus Iron	300 mg	Red	Tablet	Oval, Scored	Lederle Laboratories
LL; S; 23	Spartus Plus Iron	30 IU	Red	Tablet	Oval, Scored	Lederle Laboratories
LL; S; 23	Spartus Plus Iron	300 IU	Red	Tablet	Oval, Scored	Lederle Laboratories
LL; S; 23	Spartus Plus Iron	3000 IU	Red	Tablet	Oval, Scored	Lederle Laboratories
LL; S12	Spironolactone with Hydrochlorothiazide	25 mg	White and Yellow	Tablet	Round, Scored	Lederle Laboratories
LL; S13	Spironolactone	25 mg	White	Tablet	Round, Scored	Lederle Laboratories
LL; T; 17	Tolbutamide	500 mg	White	Tablet	Round, Scored	Lederle Laboratories
LL; T; 19	Tolazamide	100 mg	White	Tablet	Round, Scored	Lederle Laboratories
LL; T; 20	Tolazamide	250 mg	White	Tablet	Round, Scored	Lederle Laboratories
LL; T; 22	Tolazamide	500 mg	White	Tablet	Round, Scored	Lederle Laboratories
LL; T; 23	Triprolidine Hydrochloride with Pseudoephedrine Hydrochloride	2.5 mg	White	Tablet	Round, Scored	Lederle Laboratories
LL; T; 23	Triprolidine Hydrochloride with Pseudoephedrine Hydrochloride	60 mg	White	Tablet	Round, Scored	Lederle Laboratories
LL; T; 25	Thioridazine Hydrochloride	25 mg	Orange	Coated Tablet	Round	Lederle Laboratories
LL; T; 29	Trazodone Hydrochloride	50 mg	White	Tablet	Round, Scored	Lederle Laboratories
LL; T; 30	Trazodone Hydrochloride	100 mg	White	Tablet	Round, Scored	Lederle Laboratories
LL; T; 34	Theophylline C.R.	100 mg	White	Timed-Release Tablet	Round, Convex	Lederle Laboratories
LL; T; 35	Theophylline C.R.	200 mg	White	Tablet	Oval	Lederle Laboratories
LL; T; 36	Theophylline C.R.	300 mg	White	Tablet	Oblong	Lederle Laboratories
LL; T;10	Thioridazine Hydrochloride	10 mg	Orange	Tablet	Round	Lederle Laboratories
LL; T11	Thiamine Hydrochloride	50 mg	White	Tablet	Round	Lederle Laboratories
LL; T12	Thiamine Hydrochloride	100 mg	White	Tablet	Round	Lederle Laboratories
LL; T14	Thyroid	60 mg	Tan	Tablet		Lederle Laboratories
LL; T14	Thyroid	65 mg	Tan	Tablet		Lederle Laboratories
LL; T31; 50; 100	Trazodone Hydrochloride	150 mg	White	Tablet	4-Sided; Scored	Lederle Laboratories
LL; V; 4	Verapamil Hydrochloride	80 mg	White	Coated Tablet	Round, Scored	Lederle Laboratories
LL; V; 5	Verapamil Hydrochloride	120 mg	White	Coated Tablet	Round, Scored	Lederle Laboratories
LL; V11	Vitamin A Natural	25,000 I.U.	Red-Orange and Clear	Capsule		Lederle Laboratories
LL; V14	Vitamin C	250 mg	Mottled Orange	Tablet	Round	Lederle Laboratories
LL; V15	Vitamin C	500 mg	Mottled Orange	Tablet	Round	Lederle Laboratories
LL; V19	Vitamin E	400 IU	Yellow or Red-Orange and Clear	Capsule		
LL; V21	Vitamin E	400 IU	Yellow and Clear	Capsule		
LL; V22	Vitamin E	400 IU	Yellow and Clear	Capsule		
LL; V23	Vitamin E	600 IU	Yellow and Clear	Capsule		
LL; V24	Vitamin E	1000 IU	Yellow and Clear	Capsule		
LL;A 14	Amiloride and Hydrochlorothiazide	5 mg	Yellow	Tablet	Round	Lederle Laboratories
LL;A 14	Amiloride and Hydrochlorothiazide	50 mg	Yellow	Tablet	Round	Lederle Laboratories
LMN; 300	Mequin	300 mg	White	Tablet	Round, Scored	Teva Pharmaceuticals
LORELCO; 250	Lorelco	250 mg	White	Coated Tablet	Round	
LORELCO; 500	Lorelco	500 mg	White	Coated Tablet	Capsule-Shaped	
M	Pyridoxine Hydrochloride	50 mg	White	Tablet		Hoechst Marion Roussel
M; 11	Penicillin V	250 mg	White	Tablet	Oval	Reid-Rowell Pharmaceutical
M; 18	Marpres	0.1 mg		Tablet		
M; 18	Marpres	15 mg		Tablet		
M; 18	Marpres	25 mg		Tablet		
M; 22	Penicillin G	400,000 units	White	Tablet	Round	Reid-Rowell Pharmaceutical
M; R	Hydrotensin-50	0.125 mg	Light Green	Tablet	Round, Scored	Mayrand Pharmaceutical
M; R	Hydrotensin-50	50 mg	Light Green	Tablet	Round, Scored	Mayrand Pharmaceutical
MARION; 1550; NITRO-BID; 2.5	Nitro-Bid	2.5 mg	Purple and Clear	Sustained-Release Capsule		
MARION; 1551; NITRO-BID; 6.5	Nitro-Bid	6.5 mg	Blue and Yellow	Sustained-Release Capsule		
MARION; 1553; NITRO-BID; 9 MG	Nitro-Bid	9 mg	Green and Yellow with White Beads	Sustained-Release Capsule		
MATERNA; M; 10	Materna 1-60	12 mcg	Light Pink	Coated Tablet	Oblong	Lederle Laboratories
MATERNA; M; 10	Materna 1-60	0.3 mg	Light Pink	Coated Tablet	Oblong	Lederle Laboratories
MATERNA; M; 10	Materna 1-60	1 mg	Light Pink	Coated Tablet	Oblong	Lederle Laboratories
MATERNA; M; 10	Materna 1-60	2 mg	Light Pink	Coated Tablet	Oblong	Lederle Laboratories
MATERNA; M; 10	Materna 1-60	3 mg	Light Pink	Coated Tablet	Oblong	Lederle Laboratories
MATERNA; M; 10	Materna 1-60	3.4 mg	Light Pink	Coated Tablet	Oblong	Lederle Laboratories
MATERNA; M; 10	Materna 1-60	4 mg	Light Pink	Coated Tablet	Oblong	Lederle Laboratories
MATERNA; M; 10	Materna 1-60	15 mg	Light Pink	Coated Tablet	Oblong	Lederle Laboratories
MATERNA; M; 10	Materna 1-60	20 mg	Light Pink	Coated Tablet	Oblong	Lederle Laboratories
MATERNA; M; 10	Materna 1-60	25 mg	Light Pink	Coated Tablet	Oblong	Lederle Laboratories
MATERNA; M; 10	Materna 1-60	60 mg	Light Pink	Coated Tablet	Oblong	Lederle Laboratories
MATERNA; M; 10	Materna 1-60	100 mg	Light Pink	Coated Tablet	Oblong	Lederle Laboratories
MATERNA; M; 10	Materna 1-60	120 mg	Light Pink	Coated Tablet	Oblong	Lederle Laboratories
MATERNA; M; 10	Materna 1-60	250 mg	Light Pink	Coated Tablet	Oblong	Lederle Laboratories
MATERNA; M; 10	Materna 1-60	350 mg	Light Pink	Coated Tablet	Oblong	Lederle Laboratories
MATERNA; M; 10	Materna 1-60	30 IU	Light Pink	Coated Tablet	Oblong	Lederle Laboratories
MATERNA; M; 10	Materna 1-60	400 IU	Light Pink	Coated Tablet	Oblong	Lederle Laboratories
MATERNA; M; 10	Materna 1-60	8,000 IU	Light Pink	Coated Tablet	Oblong	Lederle Laboratories
MAYRAND	Anatuss with Codeine	2 mg	White and Green Mottled	Tablet	Oblong	
MAYRAND	Anatuss with Codeine	10 mg	White and Green Mottled	Tablet	Oblong	
MAYRAND	Anatuss with Codeine	25 mg	White and Green Mottled	Tablet	Oblong	
MAYRAND	Anatuss with Codeine	100 mg	White and Green Mottled	Tablet	Oblong	
MAYRAND	Anatuss with Codeine	300 mg	White and Green Mottled	Tablet	Oblong	
MCNEIL	Butibel	15 mg	Red	Tablet		Mcneil Pharmaceutical
MCNEIL	Butibel-Zyme	15 mg	Pink	Tablet		Mcneil Pharmaceutical
MCNEIL	Buticaps	15 mg	Lavender and White	Capsule		Mcneil Pharmaceutical

IMPRINT	BRAND/GENERIC NAME	STRENGTH	COLOR	FORM	SHAPE	MANUFACTURER
MCNEIL	Buticaps	30 mg	Aqua-Green and White	Capsule		Mcneil Pharmaceutical
MCNEIL	Buticaps	50 mg	Orange and White	Capsule		Mcneil Pharmaceutical
MCNEIL	Buticaps	100 mg	Pink and White	Capsule		Mcneil Pharmaceutical
MCNEIL	Butiserpazide-25	0.1 mg	Green	Tablet		Mcneil Pharmaceutical
MCNEIL	Butiserpazide-25	25 mg	Green	Tablet		Mcneil Pharmaceutical
MCNEIL	Butiserpazide-25	30 mg	Green	Tablet		Mcneil Pharmaceutical
MCNEIL	Butiserpazide-50	0.1 mg	Orange	Tablet		Mcneil Pharmaceutical
MCNEIL	Butiserpazide-50	30 mg	Orange	Tablet		Mcneil Pharmaceutical
MCNEIL	Butiserpazide-50	50 mg	Orange	Tablet		Mcneil Pharmaceutical
MCNEIL	Butiserpine R-A	0.2 mg	Yellow	Tablet		Mcneil Pharmaceutical
MCNEIL	Butiserpine R-A	30 mg	Yellow	Tablet		Mcneil Pharmaceutical
MCNEIL	Butizide-25	25 mg	Blue	Tablet		Mcneil Pharmaceutical
MCNEIL	Butizide-25	30 mg	Blue	Tablet		Mcneil Pharmaceutical
MCNEIL	Butizide-50	30 mg	Gold	Tablet		Mcneil Pharmaceutical
MCNEIL	Butizide-50	50 mg	Gold	Tablet		Mcneil Pharmaceutical
MCNEIL	Reserpazide 25	0.1 mg	Green	Tablet	Oval	Mcneil Pharmaceutical
MCNEIL	Reserpazide 25	25 mg	Green	Tablet	Oval	Mcneil Pharmaceutical
MCNEIL	Reserpazide 50	0.1 mg	Orange	Tablet	Oval	Mcneil Pharmaceutical
MCNEIL	Reserpazide 50	50 mg	Orange	Tablet	Oval	Mcneil Pharmaceutical
MCNEIL	Syndrox	5 mg	Pale Green	Tablet	Scored	Mcneil Pharmaceutical
MCNEIL	Tylenol	120 mg	White with Orange Specks	Chewable Tablet		Mcneil Consumer Products
MCNEIL	Tylenol Extra Strength	500 mg	Red and White	Capsule		Mcneil Consumer Products
MCNEIL; 058	Butibel-Zyme	15 mg	Pink	Tablet		Mcneil Pharmaceutical
MCNEIL; 425; 100	Duraphyl 100	100 mg	White	Tablet	Round; Scored	Forest Pharmaceuticals
MCNEIL; 426 200	Duraphyl 200	200 mg	White	Tablet	Capsule-Shaped; Scored	Forest Pharmaceuticals
MCNEIL; BUTIBEL	Butibel	15 mg	Red	Tablet		Mcneil Pharmaceutical
MCNEIL; BUTICAPS	Buticaps	15 mg	Lavender and White	Capsule		Mcneil Pharmaceutical
MCNEIL; BUTICAPS	Buticaps	30 mg	Aqua-Green and White	Capsule		Mcneil Pharmaceutical
MCNEIL; BUTICAPS	Buticaps	50 mg	Orange and White	Capsule		Mcneil Pharmaceutical
MCNEIL; BUTICAPS	Buticaps	100 mg	Pink and White	Capsule		Mcneil Pharmaceutical
MD; 514	Tagafed	2.5 mg	White	Tablet	Round	Solvay Pharmaceuticals
MD; 514	Tagafed	60 mg	White	Tablet	Round	Solvay Pharmaceuticals
MERRELL; 1	Susadrin	1 mg	White	Tablet		
MERRELL; 2	Susadrin	2 mg	White	Tablet		
MERRELL; 3	Susadrin	3 mg	White	Tablet		
MERRELL; 34	Cantil with Phenobarbital	16 mg	Brown	Tablet		
MERRELL; 34	Cantil with Phenobarbital	25 mg	Brown	Tablet		
MERRELL; 122	Bentyl with Phenobarbital	10 mg	Blue and White	Capsule		
MERRELL; 122	Bentyl with Phenobarbital	15 mg	Blue and White	Capsule		
MERRELL; 124	Bentyl with Phenobarbital	15 mg	White	Tablet		
MERRELL; 124	Bentyl with Phenobarbital	20 mg	White	Tablet		
MERRELL; 155	Bendectin	10 mg	White	Coated Tablet	Convex	
MERRELL; 255	Decapryn	12.5 mg	Yellow	Tablet		
MERRELL; 256	Decapryn	25 mg	Orange	Tablet		
MERRELL; 325	Hedulin	50 mg	White	Tablet		
MERRELL; 425	Vanobid	3 mg	White	Tablet		Hoechst Marion Roussel
MERRELL; 435	Nicalex	500 mg	White	Tablet		
MERRELL; 441	Orenzyme	4000 units	Red	Tablet		
MERRELL; 441	Orenzyme	50,000 units	Red	Tablet		
MERRELL; 442	Orenzyme Bitabs	8000 units	Yellow	Tablet		
MERRELL; 442	Orenzyme Bitabs	100,000 units	Yellow	Tablet		
MERRELL; 690	Tace	10 mg	Two Tone Green	Capsule		
MERRELL; 691	Tace	25 mg	Two Tone Green	Capsule		
MEYER	Vicon Forte	2 mg	Black and Orange	Capsule		Meyer Laboratories
MEYER	Vicon Forte	4 mg	Black and Orange	Capsule		Meyer Laboratories
MEYER	Vicon Forte	5 mg	Black and Orange	Capsule		Meyer Laboratories
MEYER	Vicon Forte	10 mg	Black and Orange	Capsule		Meyer Laboratories
MEYER	Vicon Forte	25 mg	Black and Orange	Capsule		Meyer Laboratories
MEYER	Vicon Forte	70 mg	Black and Orange	Capsule		Meyer Laboratories
MEYER	Vicon Forte	80 mg	Black and Orange	Capsule		Meyer Laboratories
MEYER	Vicon Forte	150 mg	Black and Orange	Capsule		Meyer Laboratories
MEYER	Vicon Forte	50 units	Black and Orange	Capsule		Meyer Laboratories
MEYER	Vicon Forte	12,500 units	Black and Orange	Capsule		Meyer Laboratories
MEYER	Vicon Forte	50 IU	Black and Orange	Capsule		Meyer Laboratories
MIA; 108	HY-5	5 mg	White	Tablet		
MIA; 108	HY-5	500 mg	White	Tablet		
MIDOL; MSM	Midol Maximum Strength	14.9 mg	White	Tablet		Sterling Health
MIDOL; MSM	Midol Maximum Strength	32.4 mg	White	Tablet		Sterling Health
MIDOL; MSM	Midol Maximum Strength	500 mg	White	Tablet		Sterling Health
MILES; 132	Stilphostrol	50 mg	White with Gray Mottling	Tablet	Round	
MILES; 721	Niclocide	500 mg	Light Yellow	Chewable Tablet	Round, Scored	Bayer
MILES; 721	Niclocide	500 mg		Tablet		Bayer Pharmaceutical
MJ; 130	Quibron Bidcaps	130 mg	Yellow and Clear	Sustained-Release Capsule		
MJ; 260	Quibron Bidcaps	260 mg	Yellow and Clear	Sustained-Release Capsule		
MR	Hydro-Z-50	50 mg	Peach	Tablet	Round, Scored	
MR	Trimtabs	35 mg	Lavender	Tablet	Scored	
MSD; 126	Cortone	5 mg	White	Tablet	Round, Scored	Merck & Company
MSD; 605	Propadrine	25 mg	Clear with White Powder	Capsule		
MSD; 613	Propadrine	50 mg	Clear with White Powder	Capsule		
MSD; 679	Cuprid	250 mg	Opaque Light Brown	Capsule		Merck & Company
N	Nytol	25 mg		Tablet		
N	Nytol	50 mg	Blue	Tablet	Round, Scored	Block Drug
N	Nytol Natural Homeopathic Sleep-Aid	0.00015 mg (6x)	White		Round	

IMPRINT	BRAND/GENERIC NAME	STRENGTH	COLOR	FORM	SHAPE	MANUFACTURER
N	Nytol Natural Homeopathic Sleep-Aid	0.15 mg (3x)	White		Round	
NBC	Houva-Caps	10 mg	Flesh-Colored	Capsule		Novartis Generics
NH	Prantal	100 mg	White	Tablet		Schering
NYTOL	Nytol	50 mg		Capsule		Block Drug
OHM; 021	Buffered Aspirin	325 mg	White	Tablet	Round, Convex	
OJF 314	Nobese	75 mg	Light Blue	Timed-Release Tablet	Oval	O'neal, Jones & Feldman
ORGANON; 393	Accelerase-PB	0.2 mg		Capsule		
ORGANON; 393	Accelerase-PB	2 mg		Capsule		
ORGANON; 393	Accelerase-PB	16 mg		Capsule		
ORGANON; 393	Accelerase-PB	20 mg		Capsule		
ORGANON; 393	Accelerase-PB	65 mg		Capsule		
ORGANON; 393	Accelerase-PB	165 mg		Capsule		
ORGANON; 393	Accelerase-PB	12.50%		Capsule		
ORGANON; 393	Accelerase-PB	87.50%		Capsule		
ORGANON; 821	Liquamar	3 mg		Tablet		
ORNACOL	Ornacol	25 mg	Gray and Red	Capsule		Menley & James Laboratories
ORNACOL	Ornacol	30 mg	Gray and Red	Capsule		Menley & James Laboratories
P	Primatene P	8 mg	Yellow	Tablet		
P	Primatene P	24 mg	Yellow	Tablet		
P	Primatene P	130 mg	Yellow	Tablet		
P	Prosed	0.03 mg	Blue	Coated Tablet	Round	
P	Prosed	4.5 mg	Blue	Coated Tablet	Round	
P	Prosed	5.4 mg	Blue	Coated Tablet	Round	
P	Prosed	18.1 mg	Blue	Coated Tablet	Round	
P	Prosed	40.8 mg	Blue	Coated Tablet	Round	
P; 9	Imipramine Hydrochloride	25 mg	Brown	Tablet	Round	Eon Labs
P; 15	Phenobarbital	15 mg	White	Tablet	Round, Compressed, Scored	
P; 21	Imipramine Hydrochloride	50 mg	Green	Tablet	Round	Eon Labs
P; 25	Hydrochlorothiazide	25 mg	Peach	Tablet	Round, Scored, Compressed	Eon Labs
P; 30	Phenobarbital	30 mg	White	Tablet	Round, Compressed, Scored	
P; 156	Chlorpheniramine Maleate	8 mg	Green and Clear	Sustained-Release Capsule		Eon Labs
P; 161	Chlorthalidone	25 mg	Yellow	Tablet	Round; Scored	
P; 163	Chlorthalidone	50 mg	Bluish-Green	Tablet	Round; Scored	
P; 183	Dipyridamole	50 mg	White	Coated Tablet	Round	
P; 191	Diphenhydramine Hydrochloride	25 mg	Clear and Pink	Gelcap		
P; 192	Diphenhydramine Hydrochloride	50 mg	Pink	Gelcap		
P; 374	Reserpine	0.1 mg	White	Tablet	Round	
P; 376	Reserpine	0.25 mg	White	Tablet	Round; Scored	
P; 552	Gemfibrozil	600 mg	White	Coated Tablet	Capsule-Shaped, Partially Scored	
P-11	Butabarbital Sodium	15 mg	Purple	Tablet	Round, Scored, Compressed	Eon Labs
P4; LL	Pathilon	25 mg	Pink	Coated Tablet	Round, Convex	Lederle Laboratories
P7F WELLCOME	Mepron	250 mg	Yellow	Coated Tablet	Round	
PANADOL; 500 MG	Panadol Maximum Strength Capsule	500 mg	White	Capsule		
PANMYCIN; 500 MG	Panmycin	500 mg	Yellow	Tablet	Oval	Upjohn
PAR; 080	Trichlormethiazide with Reserpine	0.1 mg		Tablet		
PAR; 080	Trichlormethiazide with Reserpine	2 mg		Tablet		
PAR; 081	Trichlormethiazide with Reserpine	0.1 mg		Tablet		
PAR; 081	Trichlormethiazide with Reserpine	4 mg		Tablet		
PAR; 65	Dipyridamole	75 mg		Tablet		Par Pharmaceutical
PAR; 75	Dipyridamole	75 mg	White	Tablet	Round	Par Pharmaceutical
PAR; 121	Hydralazine Hydrochloride	100 mg	Peach	Tablet	Round	
PAR; 133	Amitriptyline Hydrochloride	10 mg	Pink	Tablet	Round	Par Pharmaceutical
PAR; 134	Amitriptyline Hydrochloride	25 mg	Green	Tablet	Round	Par Pharmaceutical
PAR; 135	Amitriptyline Hydrochloride	50 mg	Brown	Tablet	Round	Par Pharmaceutical
PAR; 136	Amitriptyline Hydrochloride	75 mg	Purple	Tablet	Round	Par Pharmaceutical
PAR; 137	Amitriptyline Hydrochloride	100 mg	Orange	Tablet	Round	Par Pharmaceutical
PAR; 138	Amitriptyline Hydrochloride	150 mg	Peach	Tablet	Round	Par Pharmaceutical
PAR; 142	Berroplex Plus	5 mcg		Tablet		Par Pharmaceutical
PAR; 142	Berroplex Plus	0.5 mg		Tablet		Par Pharmaceutical
PAR; 142	Berroplex Plus	4 mg		Tablet		Par Pharmaceutical
PAR; 142	Berroplex Plus	15 mg		Tablet		Par Pharmaceutical
PAR; 142	Berroplex Plus	18 mg		Tablet		Par Pharmaceutical
PAR; 142	Berroplex Plus	100 mg		Tablet		Par Pharmaceutical
PAR; 142	Berroplex Plus	500 mg		Tablet		Par Pharmaceutical
PAR; 148	Hydroflumethiazide and Reserpine	0.125 mg	Green	Tablet	Round	Par Pharmaceutical
PAR; 148	Hydroflumethiazide and Reserpine	50 mg	Green	Tablet	Round	Par Pharmaceutical
PAR; 181	Perphenazine and Amitriptyline Hydrochloride	2 mg	Blue	Coated Tablet	Round	Par Pharmaceutical
PAR; 181	Perphenazine and Amitriptyline Hydrochloride	10 mg	Blue	Coated Tablet	Round	Par Pharmaceutical
PAR; 182	Perphenazine and Amitriptyline Hydrochloride	2 mg	Orange	Coated Tablet	Round	Par Pharmaceutical
PAR; 182	Perphenazine and Amitriptyline Hydrochloride	25 mg	Orange	Coated Tablet	Round	Par Pharmaceutical
PAR; 183	Perphenazine and Amitriptyline Hydrochloride	4 mg	Salmon	Coated Tablet	Round	Par Pharmaceutical
PAR; 183	Perphenazine and Amitriptyline Hydrochloride	10 mg	Salmon	Coated Tablet	Round	Par Pharmaceutical
PAR; 184	Perphenazine and Amitriptyline Hydrochloride	4 mg	Yellow	Coated Tablet	Round	Par Pharmaceutical
PAR; 184	Perphenazine and Amitriptyline Hydrochloride	25 mg	Yellow	Coated Tablet	Round	Par Pharmaceutical
PAR; 185	Perphenazine and Amitriptyline Hydrochloride	4 mg	Orange	Coated Tablet	Round	Par Pharmaceutical

IMPRINT	BRAND/GENERIC NAME	STRENGTH	COLOR	FORM	SHAPE	MANUFACTURER
PAR; 185	Perphenazine and Amitriptyline Hydrochloride	50 mg	Orange	Coated Tablet	Round	Par Pharmaceutical
PAR; 202	Methyldopa and Chlorothiazide	150 mg	Beige	Coated Tablet	Round	
PAR; 202	Methyldopa and Chlorothiazide	250 mg	Beige	Coated Tablet	Round	
PAR; 203	Methyldopa and Chlorothiazide	250 mg	Green	Coated Tablet	Round	
PAR; 1007	Asminorel Improved	10 mg	White	Tablet	Round	Reid-Rowell Pharmaceutical
PAR; 1007	Asminorel Improved	25 mg	White	Tablet	Round	Reid-Rowell Pharmaceutical
PAR; 1007	Asminorel Improved	130 mg	White	Tablet	Round	Reid-Rowell Pharmaceutical
PAVABID MARION	Pavabid	150 mg		Capsule		Parke-Davis
PBB	Proglycem	100 mg	Orange	Capsule		Schering
P-D 009	Cod Liver Oil	6.25 mcg/gram		Gelcap		Parke-Davis
P-D 009	Cod Liver Oil	0.6 mg/gram		Gelcap		Parke-Davis
P-D 009	Cod Liver Oil	10 minims		Gelcap		Parke-Davis
P-D 025	Promapar	25 mg		Tablet		Parke-Davis
P-D 050	Promapar	50 mg		Tablet		Parke-Davis
P-D 054	Cascara Sagrada Extract	3 grains		Tablet		Parke-Davis
P-D 055	Cascara Sagrada Extract	5 grains		Tablet		Parke-Davis
P-D 065	Richards Coryza RX A	1/20 grain		Tablet		Parke-Davis
P-D 065	Richards Coryza RX A	1/10 grain		Tablet		Parke-Davis
P-D 065	Richards Coryza RX A	1/2 grain		Tablet		Parke-Davis
P-D 165	Cod Liver Oil	20 minims		Capsule		Parke-Davis
P-D 201	Promapar	200 mg		Tablet		Parke-Davis
P-D 217	Natola	10 mcg		Capsule		Parke-Davis
P-D 217	Natola	1.5 mg		Capsule		Parke-Davis
P-D 218	Abdol with Vitamin C	1 mcg		Capsule		Parke-Davis
P-D 218	Abdol with Vitamin C	0.5 mg		Capsule		Parke-Davis
P-D 218	Abdol with Vitamin C	2.5 mg		Capsule		Parke-Davis
P-D 218	Abdol with Vitamin C	5 mg		Capsule		Parke-Davis
P-D 218	Abdol with Vitamin C	20 mg		Capsule		Parke-Davis
P-D 218	Abdol with Vitamin C	50 mg		Capsule		Parke-Davis
P-D 218	Abdol with Vitamin C	400 units		Capsule		Parke-Davis
P-D 218	Abdol with Vitamin C	5000 units		Capsule		Parke-Davis
P-D 225	Vitamin D	1.25 mg		Capsule		Parke-Davis
P-D 227	Anatola	15 mg		Capsule		Parke-Davis
P-D 229	Menagen	10,000 I.U.		Capsule		Parke-Davis
P-D 231	Anatola	7.5 mg		Capsule		Parke-Davis
P-D 234	Myadec	5 mcg		Capsule		Parke-Davis
P-D 234	Myadec	0.15 mg		Capsule		Parke-Davis
P-D 234	Myadec	1 mg		Capsule		Parke-Davis
P-D 234	Myadec	1.5 mg		Capsule		Parke-Davis
P-D 234	Myadec	2 mg		Capsule		Parke-Davis
P-D 234	Myadec	5 mg		Capsule		Parke-Davis
P-D 234	Myadec	10 mg		Capsule		Parke-Davis
P-D 234	Myadec	20 mg		Capsule		Parke-Davis
P-D 234	Myadec	75 mg		Capsule		Parke-Davis
P-D 234	Myadec	100 mg		Capsule		Parke-Davis
P-D 234	Myadec	250 mg		Capsule		Parke-Davis
P-D 234	Myadec	400 units (10 mcg)		Capsule		Parke-Davis
P-D 234	Myadec	10,000 units (3 mg)		Capsule		Parke-Davis
P-D 234	Myadec	30 IU		Capsule		Parke-Davis
P-D 246	Chloral Hydrate	500 mg		Capsule		Parke-Davis
P-D 282	Natafort	6 mcg		Tablet		Parke-Davis
P-D 282	Natafort	0.15 mg		Tablet		Parke-Davis
P-D 282	Natafort	1 mg		Tablet		Parke-Davis
P-D 282	Natafort	2 mg		Tablet		Parke-Davis
P-D 282	Natafort	3 mg		Tablet		Parke-Davis
P-D 282	Natafort	15 mg		Tablet		Parke-Davis
P-D 282	Natafort	20 mg		Tablet		Parke-Davis
P-D 282	Natafort	25 mg		Tablet		Parke-Davis
P-D 282	Natafort	65 mg		Tablet		Parke-Davis
P-D 282	Natafort	100 mg		Tablet		Parke-Davis
P-D 282	Natafort	120 mg		Tablet		Parke-Davis
P-D 282	Natafort	350 mg		Tablet		Parke-Davis
P-D 282	Natafort	30 IU		Tablet		Parke-Davis
P-D 282	Natafort	400 IU		Tablet		Parke-Davis
P-D 282	Natafort	6,000 IU		Tablet		Parke-Davis
P-D 296	Taka-Diastase Pepsin and Pancreatin	1 grain		Coated Tablet		Parke-Davis
P-D 296	Taka-Diastase Pepsin and Pancreatin	2 grains		Coated Tablet		Parke-Davis
P-D 330	Mentholated Throat	1/80 min		Tablet		Parke-Davis
P-D 330	Mentholated Throat	1/16 min		Tablet		Parke-Davis
P-D 330	Mentholated Throat	1/35 grain		Tablet		Parke-Davis
P-D 330	Mentholated Throat	1/12 grain		Tablet		Parke-Davis
P-D 351	Digifortis	0.1 gram		Capsule		Parke-Davis
P-D 354	Ventrex	0.25 mg		Capsule		Parke-Davis
P-D 354	Ventrex	0.5 mg		Capsule		Parke-Davis
P-D 354	Ventrex	130 mg		Capsule		Parke-Davis
P-D 354	Ventrex	5 grains		Capsule		Parke-Davis
P-D 359	Desicol	325 mg	Yellow with Brown Band	Capsule		Parke-Davis
P-D 363	Combex	1 mcg	Brown with Black Band	Capsule		Parke-Davis
P-D 363	Combex	6 mg	Brown with Black Band	Capsule		Parke-Davis
P-D 363	Combex	10 mg	Brown with Black Band	Capsule		Parke-Davis
P-D 363	Combex	0.38 gram	Brown with Black Band	Capsule		Parke-Davis
P-D 367	Combex with Vitamin C	1 mcg	Brown with White Band	Capsule		Parke-Davis

IMPRINT	BRAND/GENERIC NAME	STRENGTH	COLOR	FORM	SHAPE	MANUFACTURER
P-D 367	Combex with Vitamin C	6 mg	Brown with White Band	Capsule		Parke-Davis
P-D 367	Combex with Vitamin C	10 mg	Brown with White Band	Capsule		Parke-Davis
P-D 367	Combex with Vitamin C	50 mg	Brown with White Band	Capsule		Parke-Davis
P-D 367	Combex with Vitamin C	0.34 gram	Brown with White Band	Capsule		Parke-Davis
P-D 368	Taka-Combex	1 mcg		Capsule		Parke-Davis
P-D 368	Taka-Combex	0.5 mg		Capsule		Parke-Davis
P-D 368	Taka-Combex	6 mg		Capsule		Parke-Davis
P-D 368	Taka-Combex	10 mg		Capsule		Parke-Davis
P-D 368	Taka-Combex	20 mg		Capsule		Parke-Davis
P-D 368	Taka-Combex	0.34 grams		Capsule		Parke-Davis
P-D 368	Taka-Combex	2-1/2 grains		Capsule		Parke-Davis
P-D 369	Synkamin	4 mg		Capsule		Parke-Davis
P-D 374	Thera-Combex	5 mcg		Capsule		Parke-Davis
P-D 374	Thera-Combex	1 mg		Capsule		Parke-Davis
P-D 374	Thera-Combex	15 mg		Capsule		Parke-Davis
P-D 374	Thera-Combex	20 mg		Capsule		Parke-Davis
P-D 374	Thera-Combex	25 mg		Capsule		Parke-Davis
P-D 374	Thera-Combex	100 mg		Capsule		Parke-Davis
P-D 374	Thera-Combex	250 mg		Capsule		Parke-Davis
P-D 374	Thera-Combex	2-1/2 grains		Capsule		Parke-Davis
P-D 376	Carbrital	3/4 grain	White with Blue Band	Capsule		Parke-Davis
P-D 376	Carbrital	2 grains	White with Blue Band	Capsule		Parke-Davis
P-D 377	Livibron	1 mcg		Capsule		Parke-Davis
P-D 377	Livibron	0.5 mg		Capsule		Parke-Davis
P-D 377	Livibron	1.25 mg		Capsule		Parke-Davis
P-D 377	Livibron	195 mg		Capsule		Parke-Davis
P-D 377	Livibron	1/16 grain		Capsule		Parke-Davis
P-D 378	Benadryl with Ephedrine Sulfate	25 mg	Pink with Dark Blue Band	Capsule		Parke-Davis
P-D 378	Benadryl with Ephedrine Sulfate	50 mg	Pink with Dark Blue Band	Capsule		Parke-Davis
P-D 381	Abdec Teens	6 mcg		Tablet		Parke-Davis
P-D 381	Abdec Teens	4.5 mg		Tablet		Parke-Davis
P-D 381	Abdec Teens	5.1 mg		Tablet		Parke-Davis
P-D 381	Abdec Teens	6 mg		Tablet		Parke-Davis
P-D 381	Abdec Teens	60 mg		Tablet		Parke-Davis
P-D 381	Abdec Teens	180 mg		Tablet		Parke-Davis
P-D 381	Abdec Teens	30 IU		Tablet		Parke-Davis
P-D 381	Abdec Teens	400 IU		Tablet		Parke-Davis
P-D 381	Abdec Teens	7500 IU		Tablet		Parke-Davis
P-D 387	Ventrilex	20 mcg		Capsule		Parke-Davis
P-D 387	Ventrilex	0.05 mg		Capsule		Parke-Davis
P-D 387	Ventrilex	50 mg		Capsule		Parke-Davis
P-D 387	Ventrilex	195 mg		Capsule		Parke-Davis
P-D 387	Ventrilex	0.1 gram		Capsule		Parke-Davis
P-D 387	Ventrilex	0.3 grams		Capsule		Parke-Davis
P-D 389	Ambodryl Hydrochloride	25 mg		Capsule		Parke-Davis
P-D 395	Intribex	10 mcg	Red with Lavender Band	Capsule		Parke-Davis
P-D 395	Intribex	1 mg	Red with Lavender Band	Capsule		Parke-Davis
P-D 395	Intribex	75 mg	Red with Lavender Band	Capsule		Parke-Davis
P-D 395	Intribex	200 mg	Red with Lavender Band	Capsule		Parke-Davis
P-D 395	Intribex	375 mg	Red with Lavender Band	Capsule		Parke-Davis
P-D 395	Intribex	1/2 oral units	Red with Lavender Band	Capsule		Parke-Davis
P-D 406	Pentobarbital Sodium	100 mg		Capsule		Parke-Davis
P-D 406	Sodium Pentobarbital	100 mg (1 1/2 grains)		Capsule		Parke-Davis
P-D 454	Ephedrine Sulfate	25 mg	Pink	Capsule		Parke-Davis
P-D 455	Panteric	5 grains		Capsule		Parke-Davis
P-D 470	Nutritive	2 mg		Capsule		Parke-Davis
P-D 470	Nutritive	30 mg		Capsule		Parke-Davis
P-D 470	Nutritive	800 mg		Capsule		Parke-Davis
P-D 470	Nutritive	400 units		Capsule		Parke-Davis
P-D 481	Abdec Teens with Iron	6 mcg		Tablet		Parke-Davis
P-D 481	Abdec Teens with Iron	4.5 mg		Tablet		Parke-Davis
P-D 481	Abdec Teens with Iron	5.1 mg		Tablet		Parke-Davis
P-D 481	Abdec Teens with Iron	6 mg		Tablet		Parke-Davis
P-D 481	Abdec Teens with Iron	18 mg		Tablet		Parke-Davis
P-D 481	Abdec Teens with Iron	60 mg		Tablet		Parke-Davis
P-D 481	Abdec Teens with Iron	180 mg		Tablet		Parke-Davis
P-D 481	Abdec Teens with Iron	30 IU		Tablet		Parke-Davis
P-D 481	Abdec Teens with Iron	400 IU		Tablet		Parke-Davis
P-D 481	Abdec Teens with Iron	7500 IU		Tablet		Parke-Davis
P-D 503	Panteric	5 grains		Tablet		Parke-Davis
P-D 601	Sodium Chloride	1 gram		Tablet		Parke-Davis
P-D 603	Alkaline Aromatic	7/240 grains	White	Tablet		Parke-Davis
P-D 603	Alkaline Aromatic	7/480 grains	White	Tablet		Parke-Davis
P-D 603	Alkaline Aromatic	7/24 grains	White	Tablet		Parke-Davis
P-D 603	Alkaline Aromatic	5 grains	White	Tablet		Parke-Davis
P-D 603	Alkaline Aromatic	7/240 min	White	Tablet		Parke-Davis
P-D 603	Alkaline Aromatic	7/480 min	White	Tablet		Parke-Davis
P-D 609	Alkaline Aromatic	7/240 grains	Pink	Tablet		Parke-Davis
P-D 609	Alkaline Aromatic	7/480 grains	Pink	Tablet		Parke-Davis

IMPRINT	BRAND/GENERIC NAME	STRENGTH	COLOR	FORM	SHAPE	MANUFACTURER
P-D 609	Alkaline Aromatic	7/24 grains	Pink	Tablet		Parke-Davis
P-D 609	Alkaline Aromatic	5 grains	Pink	Tablet		Parke-Davis
P-D 609	Alkaline Aromatic	7/480 min	Pink	Tablet		Parke-Davis
P-D 609	Alkaline Aromatic	7/240 min	Pink	Tablet		Parke-Davis
P-D 626	Thyroid Strong	0.30%		Tablet		Parke-Davis
P-D 626	Thyroid Strong	0.5 grain		Tablet		Parke-Davis
P-D 627	Thyroid Strong	0.30%		Tablet		Parke-Davis
P-D 627	Thyroid Strong	1 grain		Tablet		Parke-Davis
P-D 628	Thyroid Strong	0.30%		Tablet		Parke-Davis
P-D 628	Thyroid Strong	2 grains		Tablet		Parke-Davis
P-D 629	Thyroid Strong	0.30%		Tablet		Parke-Davis
P-D 629	Thyroid Strong	3 grains		Tablet		Parke-Davis
P-D 636	Betapar	4 mg	Green	Tablet		Parke-Davis
P-D 641	Sodium Butabarbital	30 mg		Tablet		Parke-Davis
P-D 642	Midicel	250 mg		Tablet		Parke-Davis
P-D 644	Digoxin	0.25 mg		Tablet		Parke-Davis
P-D 647	Meprobamate	400 mg		Tablet		Parke-Davis
P-D 658	Secobarbital Sodium	1-1/2 grains		Capsule		Parke-Davis
P-D 666	D.S.S.	50 mg		Capsule		Parke-Davis
P-D 674	Thyroid Strong	0.30%		Tablet		Parke-Davis
P-D 674	Thyroid Strong	1 grain		Tablet		Parke-Davis
P-D 675	Thyroid Strong	0.30%		Tablet		Parke-Davis
P-D 675	Thyroid Strong	2 grains		Tablet		Parke-Davis
P-D 676	Penicillin G	400,000 units		Tablet		Parke-Davis
P-D 683	Vitamin E	200 IU		Capsule		
P-D 684	Taka-Diastase	2-1/2 grains		Tablet		Parke-Davis
P-D 685	S.G. Cap Vitamin E	400 IU		Capsule		Parke-Davis
P-D 686	Thyroid Strong	0.30%		Tablet		Parke-Davis
P-D 686	Thyroid Strong	0.5 grain		Tablet		Parke-Davis
P-D 687	Digifortis	0.1 gram		Tablet		Parke-Davis
P-D 694	Propoxyphene Compound 65	32.4 mg		Capsule		Parke-Davis
P-D 694	Propoxyphene Compound 65	65 mg		Capsule		Parke-Davis
P-D 694	Propoxyphene Compound 65	162 mg		Capsule		Parke-Davis
P-D 694	Propoxyphene Compound 65	227 mg		Capsule		Parke-Davis
P-D 709	Sal-Ethyl Carbonate	5 grains		Tablet		Parke-Davis
P-D 748	Paladac with Minerals	5 mcg		Tablet		Parke-Davis
P-D 748	Paladac with Minerals	0.05 mg		Tablet		Parke-Davis
P-D 748	Paladac with Minerals	1 mg		Tablet		Parke-Davis
P-D 748	Paladac with Minerals	2.5 mg		Tablet		Parke-Davis
P-D 748	Paladac with Minerals	3 mg		Tablet		Parke-Davis
P-D 748	Paladac with Minerals	5 mg		Tablet		Parke-Davis
P-D 748	Paladac with Minerals	17 mg		Tablet		Parke-Davis
P-D 748	Paladac with Minerals	20 mg		Tablet		Parke-Davis
P-D 748	Paladac with Minerals	23 mg		Tablet		Parke-Davis
P-D 748	Paladac with Minerals	50 mg		Tablet		Parke-Davis
P-D 748	Paladac with Minerals	400 units		Tablet		Parke-Davis
P-D 748	Paladac with Minerals	4000 units		Tablet		Parke-Davis
P-D 748	Paladac with Minerals	10 IU		Tablet		Parke-Davis
P-D 757	N.C.P.	500 mg		Tablet		Parke-Davis
P-D 771	Nicotinic Acid	50 mg		Tablet		Parke-Davis
P-D 772	Tolbutamide	500 mg		Tablet		Parke-Davis
P-D 775	Thyroid	15 mg		Tablet		Parke-Davis
P-D 776	Thyroid	30 mg		Tablet		Parke-Davis
P-D 777	Thyroid	60 mg		Tablet		Parke-Davis
P-D 778	Thyroid	125 mg		Tablet		Parke-Davis
P-D 780	Thiamine Hydrochloride	10 mg		Tablet		Parke-Davis
P-D 783	Vitamin C	100 mg		Tablet		Parke-Davis
P-D 794	Nicotinic Acid	100 mg		Tablet		Parke-Davis
P-D 804	Sulfadiazine	500 mg		Tablet		Parke-Davis
P-D 811	Vitamin C	50 mg		Tablet		Parke-Davis
P-D 814	Ascorbic Acid	100 mg	White	Tablet		Parke-Davis
P-D 814	Vitamin C	250 mg		Tablet		Parke-Davis
P-D 815	Thiamine Hydrochloride	25 mg		Tablet		Parke-Davis
P-D 818	Thiamine Hydrochloride	50 mg		Tablet		Parke-Davis
P-D 819	Riboflavin	10 mg		Tablet		Parke-Davis
P-D 821	Digitoxin	0.2 mg		Tablet		Parke-Davis
P-D 825	Thiamine Hydrochloride	100 mg		Tablet		Parke-Davis
P-D 836	Propylthiouracil	50 mg		Tablet		Parke-Davis
P-D 841	Digitoxin	0.1 mg	White	Tablet		Parke-Davis
P-D 842	Camoquin Hydrochloride	0.2 grams		Tablet		Parke-Davis
P-D 856	Potassium Penicillin G	250,000 units		Tablet		Parke-Davis
P-D 857	Pamisyl	0.5 gram		Tablet		Parke-Davis
P-D 858	Pamisyl Sodium	500 mg		Tablet		Parke-Davis
P-D 862	Isoniazid	100 mg		Tablet		Parke-Davis
P-D 863	Bardase	0.007 mg	Yellow	Coated Tablet		Parke-Davis
P-D 863	Bardase	0.02 mg	Yellow	Coated Tablet		Parke-Davis
P-D 863	Bardase	0.1 mg	Yellow	Coated Tablet		Parke-Davis
P-D 863	Bardase	1/4 grain	Yellow	Coated Tablet		Parke-Davis
P-D 863	Bardase	2-1/2 grains	Yellow	Coated Tablet		Parke-Davis
P-D 867	Pamisyl Sodium	690 mg		Tablet		Parke-Davis
P-D 870	Siblin	0.5 mg		Tablet		Parke-Davis
P-D 879	Midicel	500 mg		Tablet		Parke-Davis
P-D 886	Prednisone	5 mg		Tablet		Parke-Davis
P-D 890	Palaflor	5 mcg		Chewable Tablet		Parke-Davis
P-D 890	Palaflor	0.065 mg		Chewable Tablet		Parke-Davis
P-D 890	Palaflor	1 mg		Chewable Tablet		Parke-Davis
P-D 890	Palaflor	1.65 mg		Chewable Tablet		Parke-Davis
P-D 890	Palaflor	2.2 mg		Chewable Tablet		Parke-Davis
P-D 890	Palaflor	3 mg		Chewable Tablet		Parke-Davis
P-D 890	Palaflor	5.4 mg		Chewable Tablet		Parke-Davis
P-D 890	Palaflor	5.5 mg		Chewable Tablet		Parke-Davis
P-D 890	Palaflor	20 mg		Chewable Tablet		Parke-Davis
P-D 890	Palaflor	50 mg		Chewable Tablet		Parke-Davis
P-D 890	Palaflor	78 mg		Chewable Tablet		Parke-Davis

IMPRINT	BRAND/GENERIC NAME	STRENGTH	COLOR	FORM	SHAPE	MANUFACTURER
P-D 890	Palaflor	400 units		Chewable Tablet		Parke-Davis
P-D 890	Palaflor	4000 units		Chewable Tablet		Parke-Davis
P-D 890	Palaflor	10 IU		Chewable Tablet		Parke-Davis
P-D 893	Adroyd	5 mg		Tablet		Parke-Davis
P-D 900	Adroyd	10 mg		Tablet		Parke-Davis
P-D 906	Ascorbic Acid	500 mg	White	Tablet		Parke-Davis
P-D 906	Vitamin C	500 mg		Tablet		Parke-Davis
P-D 911	Digitoxin	0.1 mg	Pink	Tablet		Parke-Davis
P-D 925	Renoquid	250 mg	White	Tablet		Parke-Davis
P-D 931	Triazure	500 mg	Colorless	Tablet		Parke-Davis
P-D; 010	Promapar	10 mg		Tablet		Parke-Davis
P-D; 099	Soda Mint	5 grains		Tablet		Parke-Davis Consumer Health Products
P-D; 175	Azo-Mandelamine	50 mg		Tablet		
P-D; 175	Azo-Mandelamine	500 mg		Tablet		
P-D; 177	Sinubid	66 mg	Bl-Layered Light Pink and Pink	Tablet	Ellipsoid, Scored	Parke-Davis Consumer Health Products
P-D; 177	Sinubid	100 mg	Bl-Layered Light Pink and Pink	Tablet	Ellipsoid, Scored	Parke-Davis Consumer Health Products
P-D; 177	Sinubid	600 mg	Bl-Layered Light Pink and Pink	Tablet	Ellipsoid, Scored	Parke-Davis Consumer Health Products
P-D; 202	Procan SR	250 mg	Green	Sustained-Release Tablet	Elliptical	
P-D; 255	Proloid	5 grains		Tablet	Scored	
P-D; 260	Euthroid-1/2	7.5 mcg		Tablet		
P-D; 260	Euthroid-1/2	30 mcg		Tablet		
P-D; 261	Euthroid-1	15 mcg		Tablet		
P-D; 261	Euthroid-1	60 mcg		Tablet		
P-D; 262	Euthroid-2	30 mcg		Tablet		
P-D; 262	Euthroid-2	120 mcg		Tablet		
P-D; 263	Euthroid-3	45 mcg		Tablet		
P-D; 263	Euthroid-3	180 mcg		Tablet		
P-D; 276	Centrax	10 mg	Blue	Tablet	Scored	
P-D; 320	Parsidol	10 mg	White	Tablet		Parke-Davis
P-D; 321	Parsidol	50 mg	White	Tablet	Scored	Parke-Davis
PD; 352; 200	Rezulin	200 mg	Yellow	Coated Tablet	Oval	
PD; 353; 400	Rezulin	400 mg	Tan	Coated Tablet	Oval	
PD; 357; 300	Rezulin	300 mg	White	Coated Tablet	Oval	
P-D; 393	Milontin	500 mg		Capsule		Parke-Davis
P-D; 407	Cyclopar	250 mg	Scarlet and Flesh	Capsule		Parke-Davis
P-D; 544	Geriplex-FS	2 mcg	Blue and White			Parke-Davis
P-D; 544	Geriplex-FS	2 mcg	Blue and White	Capsule		Parke-Davis Consumer Health Products
P-D; 544	Geriplex-FS	1.5 mg	Blue and White			Parke-Davis
P-D; 544	Geriplex-FS	1.5 mg	Blue and White	Capsule		Parke-Davis Consumer Health Products
P-D; 544	Geriplex-FS	2 mg	Blue and White			Parke-Davis
P-D; 544	Geriplex-FS	2 mg	Blue and White	Capsule		Parke-Davis Consumer Health Products
P-D; 544	Geriplex-FS	4 mg	Blue and White			Parke-Davis
P-D; 544	Geriplex-FS	4 mg	Blue and White	Capsule		Parke-Davis Consumer Health Products
P-D; 544	Geriplex-FS	5 mg	Blue and White			Parke-Davis
P-D; 544	Geriplex-FS	5 mg	Blue and White	Capsule		Parke-Davis Consumer Health Products
P-D; 544	Geriplex-FS	15 mg	Blue and White			Parke-Davis
P-D; 544	Geriplex-FS	15 mg	Blue and White	Capsule		Parke-Davis Consumer Health Products
P-D; 544	Geriplex-FS	20 mg	Blue and White			Parke-Davis
P-D; 544	Geriplex-FS	20 mg	Blue and White	Capsule		Parke-Davis Consumer Health Products
P-D; 544	Geriplex-FS	30 mg	Blue and White			Parke-Davis
P-D; 544	Geriplex-FS	30 mg	Blue and White	Capsule		Parke-Davis Consumer Health Products
P-D; 544	Geriplex-FS	50 mg	Blue and White			Parke-Davis
P-D; 544	Geriplex-FS	50 mg	Blue and White	Capsule		Parke-Davis Consumer Health Products
P-D; 544	Geriplex-FS	100 mg	Blue and White			Parke-Davis
P-D; 544	Geriplex-FS	100 mg	Blue and White	Capsule		Parke-Davis Consumer Health Products
P-D; 544	Geriplex-FS	200 mg	Blue and White			Parke-Davis
P-D; 544	Geriplex-FS	200 mg	Blue and White	Capsule		Parke-Davis Consumer Health Products
P-D; 544	Geriplex-FS	2.5 grains	Blue and White			Parke-Davis
P-D; 544	Geriplex-FS	2.5 grains	Blue and White	Capsule		Parke-Davis Consumer Health Products
P-D; 544	Geriplex-FS	5 IU	Blue and White			Parke-Davis
P-D; 544	Geriplex-FS	5 IU	Blue and White	Capsule		Parke-Davis Consumer Health Products
P-D; 572	Parest	200 mg	Two-Tone Turquoise	Capsule		Parke-Davis
P-D; 574	Parest	400 mg	Two-Tone Blue	Capsule		Parke-Davis
P-D; 605	Uritone	5 grains		Tablet		
P-D; 645	Parfuran	50 mg		Tablet		Parke-Davis
P-D; 646	Sulfalar	500 mg		Tablet		Parke-Davis
P-D; 648	Penapar VK	250 mg	White	Tablet		Warner Chilcott
P-D; 653	Parfuran	100 mg		Tablet		Parke-Davis
P-D; 670	Oxlopar	250 mg		Capsule		Parke-Davis
P-D; 672	Erypar	250 mg		Coated Tablet		Parke-Davis
P-D; 673	Penapar VK	500 mg	White	Tablet		Warner Chilcott
P-D; 682	Vitamin E	100 IU		Capsule		
P-D; 688	Vectrin	100 mg		Capsule		Parke-Davis
P-D; 691	Vectrin	50 mg		Capsule		Parke-Davis
P-D; 697	Cyclopar	500 mg	Orange and Flesh	Capsule		Warner Chilcott

IMPRINT	BRAND/GENERIC NAME	STRENGTH	COLOR	FORM	SHAPE	MANUFACTURER
P-D; 730	Utimox	250 mg		Capsule		Warner Chilcott
P-D; 731	Utimox	500 mg		Capsule		Warner Chilcott
P-D; 747	Povan	50 mg	Red	Tablet		Parke-Davis
P-D; 764	Calcium Gluconate	1000 mg		Tablet		
P-D; 862	Niconyl	100 mg		Tablet		Parke-Davis
P-D; 886	Paracort	5 mg		Tablet		Parke-Davis
P-D; CENTRAX; 552	Centrax	5 mg	Celery	Capsule		
P-D ; CENTRAX; 553	Centrax	10 mg	Aqua	Capsule		
P-D; CENTRAX; 554	Centrax	20 mg	Yellow	Capsule		
PD	Pet-Derm	0.2 mcg	Mottled Tan		Round	
PD	Pet-Derm	0.1 mg	Mottled Tan		Round	
PD	Pet-Derm	1 mg	Mottled Tan		Round	
PD	Pet-Derm	2 mg	Mottled Tan		Round	
PD	Pet-Derm	5 mg	Mottled Tan		Round	
PD	Pet-Derm	10 mg	Mottled Tan		Round	
PD	Pet-Derm	30 mg	Mottled Tan		Round	
PD	Pet-Derm	0.34 GM	Mottled Tan		Round	
PD	Pet-Derm	1 GM	Mottled Tan		Round	
PD	Pet-Derm	100 units	Mottled Tan		Round	
PD	Pet-Derm	1000 units	Mottled Tan		Round	
PD	Pet-Derm	2 IU	Mottled Tan		Round	
PERCODAN-DEMI	Percodan Demi	0.19 mg	White	Tablet	Scored	
PERCODAN-DEMI	Percodan Demi	2.25 mg	White	Tablet	Scored	
PERCODAN-DEMI	Percodan Demi	325 mg	White	Tablet	Scored	
PFIZER 568	Pfi-Lith	300 mg	Yellow and White	Capsule		Pfipharmecs Pharmaceuticals
PFIZER; 305	Zithromax	250 mg	Red	Gelcap		Pfizer Laboratories
PHAZYME; 95	Phazyme 95 Sf	95 mg	Red	Coated Tablet	Elipsoid	
PLACIDYL; 500	Placidyl	500 mg	Red	Gelcap		
PLACIDYL; 750	Placidyl	750 mg	Green	Gelcap		
PP	Chlorpropamide	250 mg	Light Blue	Tablet	Heart-Shaped	
PP; 009	Sulfasalazine	500 mg	Yellow-Brown	Tablet	Round	
PP; 040	Furosemide	40 mg	White	Tablet	Round, Scored and Compressed	Eon Labs
PP; 049	Chlorothiazide	250 mg	White	Tablet	Round	
PP; 071	Chlorthalidone	50 mg	Light Blue	Tablet	Round, Compressed	
PP; 071	Cyproheptadine Hydrochloride	4 mg	White	Tablet	Round	
PP; 073	Chlorthalidone	100 mg	White	Tablet	Round, Compressed	
PP; 081	Folic Acid	1 mg	Yellow	Tablet	Round, Compressed	Eon Labs
PP; 0711	Salsalate	500 mg	Light Green	Coated Tablet	Round	Eon Labs
PP; 0712	Salsalate	750 mg	Light Green	Tablet	Scored	Eon Labs
PP; 0755	Clindamycin Hydrochloride	150 mg	Flesh, Opaque and Dark Amethyst Colored	Capsule		Eon Labs
PP; 3	Dipyridamole	25 mg		Coated Tablet		Eon Labs
PP; 12	Ferrous Sulfate	325 mg	Red (E-12 or PP-12) or Green (E-13 or PP-13)	Coated Tablet		Eon Labs
PP; 13	Ferrous Sulfate	325 mg	Red (E-12 or PP-12) or Green (E-13 or PP-13)	Coated Tablet		Eon Labs
PP; 16	Triprolidine and Pseudoephedrine	2.5 mg	White	Tablet	Round, Scored and Compressed	Eon Labs
PP; 16	Triprolidine and Pseudoephedrine	60 mg	White	Tablet	Round, Scored and Compressed	Eon Labs
PP; 17	Baclofen	10 mg	White	Tablet	Round, Scored, Compressed	Eon Labs
PP; 18	Baclofen	20 mg	White	Tablet	Round, Scored, Compressed	Eon Labs
PP; 35	Meclizine Hydrochloride	12.5 mg	Blue and White	Tablet	Oblong, Compressed	Eon Labs
PP; 36	Meclizine Hydrochloride	25 mg	Yellow and White	Tablet	Oblong, Compressed	Eon Labs
PP; 50	Hydrochlorothiazide	50 mg	Peach	Tablet	Scored, Round, Compressed	Eon Labs
PP; 53	Prenatal with Folic Acid	5 mcg	Pink	Coated Tablet	Capsule-Shaped	Eon Labs
PP; 53	Prenatal with Folic Acid	1 mg	Pink	Coated Tablet	Capsule-Shaped	Eon Labs
PP; 53	Prenatal with Folic Acid	1.1 mg	Pink	Coated Tablet	Capsule-Shaped	Eon Labs
PP; 53	Prenatal with Folic Acid	1.8 mg	Pink	Coated Tablet	Capsule-Shaped	Eon Labs
PP; 53	Prenatal with Folic Acid	2.5 mg	Pink	Coated Tablet	Capsule-Shaped	Eon Labs
PP; 53	Prenatal with Folic Acid	15 mg	Pink	Coated Tablet	Capsule-Shaped	Eon Labs
PP; 53	Prenatal with Folic Acid	60 mg	Pink	Coated Tablet	Capsule-Shaped	Eon Labs
PP; 53	Prenatal with Folic Acid	65 mg	Pink	Coated Tablet	Capsule-Shaped	Eon Labs
PP; 53	Prenatal with Folic Acid	125 mg	Pink	Coated Tablet	Capsule-Shaped	Eon Labs
PP; 53	Prenatal with Folic Acid	30 IU	Pink	Coated Tablet	Capsule-Shaped	Eon Labs
PP; 53	Prenatal with Folic Acid	400 IU	Pink	Coated Tablet	Capsule-Shaped	Eon Labs
PP; 53	Prenatal with Folic Acid	6000 IU	Pink	Coated Tablet	Capsule-Shaped	Eon Labs
PP; 54	Triamterene and Hydrochlorothiazide	50 mg	Yellow	Tablet	Round, Scored	
PP; 54	Triamterene and Hydrochlorothiazide	75 mg	Yellow	Tablet	Round, Scored	
PP; 58	Hydroxyzine Hydrochloride	50 mg	Yellow	Coated Tablet		Eon Labs
PP; 59	Hydroxyzine Hydrochloride	25 mg	Dark Green	Coated Tablet		Eon Labs
PP; 60	Hydroxyzine Hydrochloride	10 mg	Orange	Coated Tablet		Eon Labs
PP; 111	Sulfamethoxazole and Trimethoprim	80 mg	White	Tablet	Oval, Scored, Compressed	
PP; 111	Sulfamethoxazole and Trimethoprim	400 mg	White	Tablet	Oval, Scored, Compressed	
PP; 125	Methylprednisolone	4 mg	White	Tablet	Oral, Scored, Compressed	Eon Labs
PP; 220	Urithol	0.03 mg	Blue	Enteric-Coated Tablet		Forest Pharmaceuticals
PP; 220	Urithol	4.5 mg	Blue	Enteric-Coated Tablet		Forest Pharmaceuticals
PP; 220	Urithol	5.4 mg	Blue	Enteric-Coated Tablet		Forest Pharmaceuticals
PP; 220	Urithol	18.1 mg	Blue	Enteric-Coated Tablet		Forest Pharmaceuticals
PP; 220	Urithol	40.8 mg	Blue	Enteric-Coated Tablet		Forest Pharmaceuticals
PP; 226	Chlorzoxazone with Acetaminophen	250 mg	Light Green	Tablet	Hexagonal (Before 1988) or Round (After 1988), Compressed	Eon Labs
PP; 226	Chlorzoxazone with Acetaminophen	300 mg	Light Green	Tablet	Hexagonal (Before 1988) or Round (After 1988), Compressed	Eon Labs
PP; 250	Mefenamic Acid	250 mg	Light Blue and Light Yellow	Capsule		Eon Labs

IMPRINT	BRAND/GENERIC NAME	STRENGTH	COLOR	FORM	SHAPE	MANUFACTURER
PP; 256	Ordrine	12 mg	Blue and Clear	Sustained-Release Capsule		Eon Labs
PP; 256	Ordrine	75 mg	Blue and Clear	Sustained-Release Capsule		Eon Labs
PP; 259	Prenatal One	12 mcg	Light Yellow	Coated Tablet		Eon Labs
PP; 259	Prenatal One	1 mg	Light Yellow	Coated Tablet		Eon Labs
PP; 259	Prenatal One	1.5 mg	Light Yellow	Coated Tablet		Eon Labs
PP; 259	Prenatal One	2 mg	Light Yellow	Coated Tablet		Eon Labs
PP; 259	Prenatal One	3 mg	Light Yellow	Coated Tablet		Eon Labs
PP; 259	Prenatal One	10 mg	Light Yellow	Coated Tablet		Eon Labs
PP; 259	Prenatal One	11 mg	Light Yellow	Coated Tablet		Eon Labs
PP; 259	Prenatal One	20 mg	Light Yellow	Coated Tablet		Eon Labs
PP; 259	Prenatal One	25 mg	Light Yellow	Coated Tablet		Eon Labs
PP; 259	Prenatal One	65 mg	Light Yellow	Coated Tablet		Eon Labs
PP; 259	Prenatal One	120 mg	Light Yellow	Coated Tablet		Eon Labs
PP; 259	Prenatal One	200 mg	Light Yellow	Coated Tablet		Eon Labs
PP; 259	Prenatal One	400 IU	Light Yellow	Coated Tablet		Eon Labs
PP; 259	Prenatal One	4000 IU	Light Yellow	Coated Tablet		Eon Labs
PP; 331	Iso-Perazine	5 mg	Yellow and Clear	Capsule		
PP; 331	Iso-Perazine	10 mg	Yellow and Clear	Capsule		
PP; 331; 919	Cyclandelate	200 mg	Light Blue	Capsule		
PP; 333	Mepro-Aspirin	200 mg	White and Green	Tablet	Scored, Compressed	Eon Labs
PP; 333	Mepro-Aspirin	325 mg	White and Green	Tablet	Scored, Compressed	Eon Labs
PP; 360; 2	Acetaminophen and Codeine	15 mg	White	Tablet	Compressed	
PP; 360; 2	Acetaminophen and Codeine	300 mg	White	Tablet	Compressed	
PP; 365; 3	Acetaminophen and Codeine	30 mg	White	Tablet	Compressed	
PP; 365; 3	Acetaminophen and Codeine	300 mg	White	Tablet	Compressed	
PP; 370; 4	Acetaminophen and Codeine Phosphate	60 mg	White	Tablet	Compressed	
PP; 370; 4	Acetaminophen and Codeine Phosphate	300 mg	White	Tablet	Compressed	
PP; 473	Decon Aid	12 mg	Blue and Clear	Timed-Release Capsule		
PP; 473	Decon Aid	75 mg	Blue and Clear	Timed-Release Capsule		
PP; 497	Diphenoxylate Hydrochloride with Atropine Sulfate	0.025 mg	White	Tablet	Compressed	Eon Labs
PP; 497	Diphenoxylate Hydrochloride with Atropine Sulfate	0.025 mg	White	Tablet	Round	
PP; 497	Diphenoxylate Hydrochloride with Atropine Sulfate	2.5 mg	White	Tablet	Compressed	Eon Labs
PP; 497	Diphenoxylate Hydrochloride with Atropine Sulfate	2.5 mg	White	Tablet	Round	
PP; 535	Tolbutamide	500 mg	White	Tablet	Round, Compressed	Eon Labs
PP; 551	Metronidazole	250 mg	White	Tablet	Round, Compressed	Eon Labs
PP; 555	Metronidazole	500 mg	White	Tablet	Oblong, Scored, Compressed	Eon Labs
PP; 610	Chlordiazepoxide Hydrochloride	10 mg	Green and Black	Capsule		Eon Labs
PP; 625	Chlordiazepoxide Hydrochloride	25 mg	Green and White	Capsule		Eon Labs
PP; 630	Propoxyphene Hydrochloride	65 mg	Pink	Capsule		Eon Labs
PP; 635	Phentermine Hydrochloride	30 mg	Red and Black	Capsule		Eon Labs
PP; 640	Phentermine Hydrochloride	30 mg	Black	Capsule		Eon Labs
PP; 670	Tetracycline Hydrochloride	250 mg	Yellow and Orange	Capsule		Eon Labs
PP; 671	Tetracycline Hydrochloride	500 mg	Black and Yellow	Capsule		Eon Labs
PP; 686	Propoxyphene Compound	32.4 mg	Red and Gray	Capsule		Eon Labs
PP; 686	Propoxyphene Compound	65 mg	Red and Gray	Capsule		Eon Labs
PP; 686	Propoxyphene Compound	389 mg	Red and Gray	Capsule		Eon Labs
PP; 686	Propoxyphene Hydrochloride, Aspirin and Caffeine	32.4 mg	Red and Gray	Gelcap		Eon Labs
PP; 686	Propoxyphene Hydrochloride, Aspirin and Caffeine	65 mg	Red and Gray	Gelcap		Eon Labs
PP; 686	Propoxyphene Hydrochloride, Aspirin and Caffeine	389 mg	Red and Gray	Gelcap		Eon Labs
PP; 698	Doxycycline Hyclate	50 mg	Aqua Blue and White	Capsule		Eon Labs
PP; 699	Doxycycline Hyclate	100 mg	Light Blue	Capsule		Eon Labs
PP; 701	Bethanechol Chloride	25 mg	Yellow	Tablet		Eon Labs
PP; 718	Indomethacin	25 mg	Light Green and Opaque	Capsule		Eon Labs
PP; 719	Indomethacin	50 mg	Light Green and Opaque	Capsule		Eon Labs
PP; 723	Carisoprodol	350 mg	White	Tablet	Round, Compressed	Eon Labs
PP; 725	Meclofenamate Sodium	50 mg	Rust	Capsule		Eon Labs
PP; 726	Meclofenamate Sodium	100 mg	Rust and White	Capsule		Eon Labs
PP; 737	Cephradine	250 mg	Light Green and Pink	Capsule		Eon Labs
PP; 738	Cephradine	500 mg	Light Green	Capsule		Eon Labs
PP; 739	Trimipramine Maleate	25 mg	Yellow and White	Capsule		Eon Labs
PP; 740	Trimipramine Maleate	50 mg	Orange and White	Capsule		Eon Labs
PP; 741	Trimipramine Maleate	100 mg	White	Capsule		Eon Labs
PP; 750	Nystatin	500,000 units	Brown	Coated Tablet	Round, Concave	Eon Labs
PP; 754	Clindamycin Hydrochloride	75 mg	Flesh Opaque Colored	Capsule		Eon Labs
PP; 755	Clindamycin Hydrochloride	150 mg	Flesh and Dark Amethyst	Capsule		Eon Labs
PP; 756	Triamterene and Hydrochlorothiazide	25 mg	Red	Capsule		
PP; 756	Triamterene and Hydrochlorothiazide	50 mg	Red	Capsule		
PP; 777	Nystatin	100,000 units	Pale Yellow	Tablet	Diamond, Compressed	Eon Labs
PP; 854	Prednisolone	5 mg	Pale Orange	Tablet	Flat, Bisected	Eon Labs
PP; 861	Sulfisoxazole	500 mg	White	Tablet	Round	
PP; 970	Cephalexin	250 mg	Grey and Red	Capsule		Eon Labs
PP; 971	Cephalexin	500 mg	Red	Capsule		Eon Labs

IMPRINT	BRAND/GENERIC NAME	STRENGTH	COLOR	FORM	SHAPE	MANUFACTURER
PP; 1077	Isosorbide Dinitrate	40 mg	White and Clear	Sustained-Release Capsule		Eon Labs
PP; 2002	Anti-Tussive TD	40 mg	White Opaque and Natural with Red, White and Blue Beads	Capsule		Pioneer Pharmaceuticals
PP; 2002	Anti-Tussive TD	75 mg	White Opaque and Natural with Red, White and Blue Beads	Capsule		Pioneer Pharmaceuticals
PP; 2007	Papaverine Hydrochloride	150 mg	Clear Brown and Natural with White Beads	Capsule		Pioneer Pharmaceuticals
PP; 3001	Decongestabs TD	5 mg	White with Red Specks	Tablet	Round	Pioneer Pharmaceuticals
PP; 3001	Decongestabs TD	10 mg	White with Red Specks	Tablet	Round	Pioneer Pharmaceuticals
PP; 3001	Decongestabs TD	15 mg	White with Red Specks	Tablet	Round	Pioneer Pharmaceuticals
PP; 3001	Decongestabs TD	40 mg	White with Red Specks	Tablet	Round	Pioneer Pharmaceuticals
PP; 3008	Pioten TR	12 mg	Light Blue	Coated Tablet		Pioneer Pharmaceuticals
PP; 3008	Pioten TR	15 mg	Light Blue	Coated Tablet		Pioneer Pharmaceuticals
PP; 4001	Cyclandelate	200 mg	Opaque Blue	Capsule		Pioneer Pharmaceuticals
PP; 4002	Cyclandelate	400 mg	Red and Blue	Capsule		Pioneer Pharmaceuticals
PP; 4005	Indomethacin	25 mg	Opaque Green	Capsule		Pioneer Pharmaceuticals
PP; 4006	Indomethacin	50 mg	Opaque Green	Capsule		Pioneer Pharmaceuticals
PP; 4008	Diphenhydramine	50 mg	Clear Pink	Capsule		Pioneer Pharmaceuticals
PP; 4009	Chlordiazepoxide Hydrochloride with Clidinium	2.5 mg	Opaque Green	Capsule		Pioneer Pharmaceuticals
PP; 4009	Chlordiazepoxide Hydrochloride with Clidinium	5 mg	Opaque Green	Capsule		Pioneer Pharmaceuticals
PP; 4010	Chlordiazepoxide Hydrochloride	5 mg	Yellow and Green	Capsule		Pioneer Pharmaceuticals
PP; 4011	Chlordiazepoxide Hydrochloride	10 mg	Black and Green	Capsule		Pioneer Pharmaceuticals
PP; 4012	Chlordiazepoxide Hydrochloride	25 mg	Green and White	Capsule		Pioneer Pharmaceuticals
PP; 4013	Diphenhydramine	25 mg	Clear Pink and Natural	Capsule		Pioneer Pharmaceuticals
PP; 4017	Dicyclomine Hydrochloride	10 mg	Blue	Capsule		Pioneer Pharmaceuticals
PP; 5511	Chlorpheniramine Maleate	8 mg	Green and Clear	Sustained-Release Capsule		Eon Labs
PP; 5579	Isosorbide Dinitrate	50 mg	Blue and Clear	Sustained-Release Capsule		Eon Labs
PP; 5730	Phendimetrazine Tartrate	35 mg	Red and Clear; Black and Orange; Blue and Clear; Orange and Clear	Capsule		Eon Labs
PP; 5740	Phendimetrazine Tartrate	35 mg	Red and Clear; Black and Orange; Blue and Clear; Orange and Clear	Capsule		Eon Labs
PP; 6001	Therax	10 mg	Light Blue	Tablet		Pioneer Pharmaceuticals
PP; 6001	Therax	25 mg	Light Blue	Tablet		Pioneer Pharmaceuticals
PP; 6001	Therax	130 mg	Light Blue	Tablet		Pioneer Pharmaceuticals
PP; 6004	Folic Acid	1 mg	Yellow	Tablet	Scored, Round	Pioneer Pharmaceuticals
PP; 6007	Diazepam	2 mg	White	Tablet	Round, Scored	Pioneer Pharmaceuticals
PP; 6008	Diazepam	5 mg	Yellow	Tablet	Round, Scored	Pioneer Pharmaceuticals
PP; 6009	Diazepam	10 mg	Blue	Tablet	Round, Scored	Pioneer Pharmaceuticals
PP; 6012	Chlorzoxazone	250 mg	Peach	Tablet	Round	Pioneer Pharmaceuticals
PP; 6013	Dicyclomine Hydrochloride	20 mg	Light Blue	Tablet	Scored, Concave	Pioneer Pharmaceuticals
PP; 6015	Cyproheptadine	4 mg	White	Tablet	Round, Scored	Pioneer Pharmaceuticals
PP; 6017	Chlorzoxazone with Acetaminophen	250 mg	Green	Tablet	Hexagonal	Pioneer Pharmaceuticals
PP; 6017	Chlorzoxazone with Acetaminophen	300 mg	Green	Tablet	Hexagonal	Pioneer Pharmaceuticals
PP; 6018	Carisoprodol	350 mg	White	Tablet	Round	Pioneer Pharmaceuticals
PP; 6036	Methocarbamol	500 mg	White	Tablet	Round, Scored	Pioneer Pharmaceuticals
PP; 6038	Methocarbamol	750 mg	White	Tablet	Oblong	
PP; 6048	Chlorzoxazone	500 mg	Green	Tablet	Capsule Shaped	Pioneer Pharmaceuticals
PP; 6062	Chlorthalidone	25 mg	Peach	Tablet	Round	
PP; 6063	Chlorthalidone	50 mg	Light Blue	Tablet	Round	
PP; 6265	Phendimetrazine Tartrate	35 mg	Red and Clear; Black and Orange; Blue and Clear; Orange and Clear	Capsule		Eon Labs
PP; 7356	Prenatal with Folic Acid	5 mcg	Pink	Coated Tablet	Capsule-Shaped	Eon Labs
PP; 7356	Prenatal with Folic Acid	1 mg	Pink	Coated Tablet	Capsule-Shaped	Eon Labs
PP; 7356	Prenatal with Folic Acid	1.1 mg	Pink	Coated Tablet	Capsule-Shaped	Eon Labs
PP; 7356	Prenatal with Folic Acid	1.8 mg	Pink	Coated Tablet	Capsule-Shaped	Eon Labs
PP; 7356	Prenatal with Folic Acid	2.5 mg	Pink	Coated Tablet	Capsule-Shaped	Eon Labs
PP; 7356	Prenatal with Folic Acid	15 mg	Pink	Coated Tablet	Capsule-Shaped	Eon Labs
PP; 7356	Prenatal with Folic Acid	60 mg	Pink	Coated Tablet	Capsule-Shaped	Eon Labs
PP; 7356	Prenatal with Folic Acid	65 mg	Pink	Coated Tablet	Capsule-Shaped	Eon Labs
PP; 7356	Prenatal with Folic Acid	125 mg	Pink	Coated Tablet	Capsule-Shaped	Eon Labs
PP; 7356	Prenatal with Folic Acid	30 IU	Pink	Coated Tablet	Capsule-Shaped	Eon Labs
PP; 7356	Prenatal with Folic Acid	400 IU	Pink	Coated Tablet	Capsule-Shaped	Eon Labs
PP; 7356	Prenatal with Folic Acid	6000 IU	Pink	Coated Tablet	Capsule-Shaped	Eon Labs
PP; N338	Methocarbamol	750 mg	White	Tablet	Oblong	Pioneer Pharmaceuticals
PP-212	Butabarbital Sodium	30 mg	Blue	Tablet	Round, Scored, Compressed	Eon Labs
PP-605	Chlordiazepoxide Hydrochloride	5 mg	Green and Yellow	Capsule		Eon Labs
PP-754	Clindamycin Hydrochloride	75 mg	Flesh	Capsule		Eon Labs
PP-5512	Chlorpheniramine Maleate	8 mg	Green and Clear	Sustained-Release Capsule		Eon Labs
PP053; PP331	Chlordiazepoxide Hydrochloride	5 mg	Light Green and Light Yellow	Capsule		

IMPRINT	BRAND/GENERIC NAME	STRENGTH	COLOR	FORM	SHAPE	MANUFACTURER
PP055; PP331	Chlordiazepoxide Hydrochloride	10 mg	Light Green and Black	Capsule		
PP057; PP331	Chlordiazepoxide Hydrochloride	25 mg	Light Green and White	Capsule		
PP331; 967	Alkergot	0.5 mg	White	Tablet	Round	
PP331; 969	Alkergot	1 mg	White	Tablet	Oval	
PP741; PP331	Propoxyphene Hydrochloride	65 mg	Light Pink	Capsule		
PP783; PP331	Propoxyphene Compound	32.4 mg	Gray and Red-Orange	Capsule		
PP783; PP331	Propoxyphene Compound	65 mg	Gray and Red-Orange	Capsule		
PP783; PP331	Propoxyphene Compound	162 mg	Gray and Red-Orange	Capsule		
PP783; PP331	Propoxyphene Compound	226 mg	Gray and Red-Orange	Capsule		
PPP; 713	Raudixin	50 mg	Red	Tablet		
PPP; 776	Raudixin	100 mg	Red	Tablet		
PROLAMINE	Prolamine Super Strength	50 mg	Pink and Clear with Pink and White Pellets	Capsule		
PROLAMINE	Prolamine Super Strength	140 mg	Pink and Clear with Pink and White Pellets	Capsule		
PROTO; CHOL	Proto-Chol	120 mg	Yellow			
PROTO; CHOL	Proto-Chol	180 mg	Yellow			
PROTO; CHOL	Proto-Chol	1 gram	Yellow			
PROTO; CHOL	Proto-Chol	1 IU/gram	Yellow			
PROTO; CHOL	Proto-Chol	10 IU/gram	Yellow			
PROTO; CHOL	Proto-Chol	100 IU/gram	Yellow			
PROTO; CHOL	Proto-Chol	3%	Yellow			
PSEUDO-BID; A	Pseudo-Bid A Capsule	12 mg	White	Capsule		Holloway Pharmaceuticals
PSEUDO-BID; A	Pseudo-Bid A Capsule	120 mg	White	Capsule		Holloway Pharmaceuticals
PSEUDO-BID; A	Pseudo-Bid A Capsule	150 mg	White	Capsule		Holloway Pharmaceuticals
PZ; 166	Phazyme Maximum Strength	166 mg	Red	Gelcap	Oval	
Q; QPL; 243	Minodyl	2.5 mg	White	Tablet	Bisected, Round	Quantum Pharmics
QPL; 213; Q	Trialodine	50 mg	White	Tablet	Round	Quantum Pharmics
QPL; 225; Q	Clorazepate Dipotassium	3.75 mg	Blue	Tablet	Round	
QPL; 227; Q	Clorazepate Dipotassium	15 mg	Lavender	Tablet	Round	
QPL; 243; 2.5	Minodyl	2.5 mg	White	Tablet	Bisected, Round	Quantum Pharmics
Q-VEL	Q-Vel Caps	64.8 mg	Off-White to Pale Yellow	Softgel		
Q-VEL	Q-Vel Caps	400 IU	Off-White to Pale Yellow	Softgel		
R (PUREPAC LOGO); 334	Prednisone	2.5 mg	White	Tablet	Round	
R 4383	Propoxyphene Compound-65	32.4 mg	Pink and Grey	Capsule		Rugby Laboratories
R 4383	Propoxyphene Compound-65	65 mg	Pink and Grey	Capsule		Rugby Laboratories
R 4383	Propoxyphene Compound-65	162 mg	Pink and Grey	Capsule		Rugby Laboratories
R 4383	Propoxyphene Compound-65	227 mg	Pink and Grey	Capsule		Rugby Laboratories
R; 60	Lorazepam	1 mg		Tablet	Scored	
R; 161	Chlorthalidone	25 mg	Yellow	Tablet	Round; Scored	
R; 163	Chlorthalidone	50 mg	Bluish-Green	Tablet	Round; Scored	
R; 183	Dipyridamole	50 mg	White	Coated Tablet	Round	
R; 191	Diphenhydramine Hydrochloride	25 mg	Clear and Pink	Gelcap		
R; 192	Diphenhydramine Hydrochloride	50 mg	Pink	Gelcap		
R; 204	Erythromycin Stearate	250 mg	Pink	Tablet	Round, Convex	
R; 225	Hydrochlorothiazide with Reserpine	0.125 mg	Green	Tablet	Round	
R; 225	Hydrochlorothiazide with Reserpine	50 mg	Green	Tablet	Round	
R; 225; 10	Minoxidal	10 mg	White	Tablet	Round, Scored	Watson Laboratories
R; 227	Hydrochlorothiazide with Reserpine and Hydralazine	0.1 mg	Salmon	Tablet	Round	
R; 227	Hydrochlorothiazide with Reserpine and Hydralazine	15 mg	Salmon	Tablet	Round	
R; 227	Hydrochlorothiazide with Reserpine and Hydralazine	25 mg	Salmon	Tablet	Round	
R; 229; 0.5	Haloperidol	0.5 mg	White	Tablet	Round	Watson Laboratories
R; 230; 1	Haloperidol	1 mg	Yellow	Tablet	Round	Watson Laboratories
R; 231; 2	Haloperidol	2 mg	Purple	Tablet	Round	Watson Laboratories
R; 232; 5	Haloperidol	5 mg	Green	Tablet	Round	Watson Laboratories
R; 233; 10	Haloperidol	10 mg	Green-Blue	Tablet	Round	Watson Laboratories
R; 234; 20	Haloperidol	20 mg	Salmon	Tablet	Round	Watson Laboratories
R; 374	Reserpine	0.1 mg	White	Tablet	Round	
R; 376	Reserpine	0.25 mg	White	Tablet	Round; Scored	
R; 521	Naproxen	250 mg	White	Tablet	Round	
R; 522	Naproxen	375 mg	White	Tablet	Capsule-Shaped	
R; 523	Naproxen	500 mg	White	Tablet	Capsule-Shaped	
R; 547	Naproxen	275 mg	White	Coated Tablet	Oval	
R; 548	Naproxen	550 mg	White	Coated Tablet	Oval	
R; 552	Gemfibrozil	600 mg	White	Coated Tablet	Capsule-Shaped, Partially Scored	
R; 1840	Pramocon	12 mcg		Coated Tablet		
R; 1840	Pramocon	150 mcg		Coated Tablet		
R; 1840	Pramocon	800 mcg		Coated Tablet		
R; 1840	Pramocon	1.5 mg		Coated Tablet		
R; 1840	Pramocon	1.7 mg		Coated Tablet		
R; 1840	Pramocon	4 mg		Coated Tablet		
R; 1840	Pramocon	18 mg		Coated Tablet		
R; 1840	Pramocon	20 mg		Coated Tablet		
R; 1840	Pramocon	100 mg		Coated Tablet		
R; 1840	Pramocon	120 mg		Coated Tablet		
R; 1840	Pramocon	250 mg		Coated Tablet		
R; 1840	Pramocon	30 IU		Coated Tablet		
R; 1840	Pramocon	400 IU		Coated Tablet		

IMPRINT	BRAND/GENERIC NAME	STRENGTH	COLOR	FORM	SHAPE	MANUFACTURER
R; 1840	Pramocon	5000 IU		Coated Tablet		
R; 3702	Diethylpropion	25 mg	Light Blue	Tablet	Round	
R; 3924	Isollyl	40 mg	Green Clear	Capsule		Rugby Laboratories
R; 3924	Isollyl	50 mg	Green Clear	Capsule		Rugby Laboratories
R; 3924	Isollyl	125 mg	Green Clear	Capsule		Rugby Laboratories
R; 3924	Isollyl	200 mg	Green Clear	Capsule		Rugby Laboratories
R; 4010	Meprobamate	600 mg	White	Tablet	Capsule-Shaped	Rugby Laboratories
REDUX	Redux	15 mg	Opaque White	Capsule		Wyeth-Ayerst Laboratories
REID-PROVIDENT; 1280	Compal	16 mg	Aqua and Blue-Green	Capsule		Reid-Rowell Pharmaceutical
REID-PROVIDENT; 1280	Compal	30 mg	Aqua and Blue-Green	Capsule		Reid-Rowell Pharmaceutical
REID-PROVIDENT; 1280	Compal	356 mg	Aqua and Blue-Green	Capsule		Reid-Rowell Pharmaceutical
REID-PROVIDENT; 1290	Compal	16 mg	Aqua and Blue-Green	Capsule		Reid-Rowell Pharmaceutical
REID-PROVIDENT; 1290	Compal	30 mg	Aqua and Blue-Green	Capsule		Reid-Rowell Pharmaceutical
REID-PROVIDENT; 1290	Compal	356 mg	Aqua and Blue-Green	Capsule		Reid-Rowell Pharmaceutical
RHEABAN	Rheaban	750 mg	White	Tablet		
RIKER	Estomul Tablets	25 mg	Pink	Tablet		
RIKER	Estomul Tablets	45 mg	Pink	Tablet		
RIKER	Estomul Tablets	500 mg	Pink	Tablet		
RIKER	Veriloid	2 mg	Yellow			
RIKER	Veriloid	3 mg	Orange		Round	
RIKER; 173	Dorbane	75 mg	Orange-Brown	Tablet	Round	
RIKER; DORBANTYL	Dorbantyl	25 mg	Black and Orange	Capsule		
RIKER; DORBANTYL	Dorbantyl	50 mg	Black and Orange	Capsule		
RIKER; DORBANTYL FORTE	Dorbantyl Forte	50 mg	Orange and Gray	Capsule		
RIKER; DORBANTYL FORTE	Dorbantyl Forte	100 mg	Orange and Gray	Capsule		
ROCHE 26	Roniacol	50 mg		Tablet		Roche Pharmaceuticals
ROCHE 27	Roniacol Timespan	150 mg	Red			Roche
ROCHE; 21	Tigan	100 mg		Capsule		Hoffmann-LA Roche
ROCHE; 22	Tigan	250 mg		Capsule		Hoffmann-LA Roche
ROCHE; POSICOR; 50	Posicor	50 mg	Pale Yellow	Tablet	Biconvex, Hexagon	
ROCHE; POSICOR; 100	Posicor	100 mg	Light Orange	Tablet	Biconvex, Hexagon	
RONIACOL TIMESPAN	Roniacol	150 mg	Red	Timed-Release Tablet		Roche Pharmaceuticals
ROWELL; 0840	Colrex Compound	2 mg	Opaque Yellow	Capsule		Solvay Pharmaceuticals
ROWELL; 0840	Colrex Compound	10 mg	Opaque Yellow	Capsule		Solvay Pharmaceuticals
ROWELL; 0840	Colrex Compound	16 mg	Opaque Yellow	Capsule		Solvay Pharmaceuticals
ROWELL; 0840	Colrex Compound	325 mg	Opaque Yellow	Capsule		Solvay Pharmaceuticals
ROWELL; 1610	Norlac	8 mcg	Pink	Coated Tablet	Oval	Solvay Pharmaceuticals
ROWELL; 1610	Norlac	150 mcg	Pink	Coated Tablet	Oval	Solvay Pharmaceuticals
ROWELL; 1610	Norlac	0.4 mg	Pink	Coated Tablet	Oval	Solvay Pharmaceuticals
ROWELL; 1610	Norlac	2 mg	Pink	Coated Tablet	Oval	Solvay Pharmaceuticals
ROWELL; 1610	Norlac	4 mg	Pink	Coated Tablet	Oval	Solvay Pharmaceuticals
ROWELL; 1610	Norlac	15 mg	Pink	Coated Tablet	Oval	Solvay Pharmaceuticals
ROWELL; 1610	Norlac	20 mg	Pink	Coated Tablet	Oval	Solvay Pharmaceuticals
ROWELL; 1610	Norlac	60 mg	Pink	Coated Tablet	Oval	Solvay Pharmaceuticals
ROWELL; 1610	Norlac	90 mg	Pink	Coated Tablet	Oval	Solvay Pharmaceuticals
ROWELL; 1610	Norlac	100 mg	Pink	Coated Tablet	Oval	Solvay Pharmaceuticals
ROWELL; 1610	Norlac	0.2 G	Pink	Coated Tablet	Oval	Solvay Pharmaceuticals
ROWELL; 1610	Norlac	30 IU	Pink	Coated Tablet	Oval	Solvay Pharmaceuticals
ROWELL; 1610	Norlac	400 IU	Pink	Coated Tablet	Oval	Solvay Pharmaceuticals
ROWELL; 1610	Norlac	8000 IU	Pink	Coated Tablet	Oval	Solvay Pharmaceuticals
ROWELL; 2080	S.A.S. 500	500 mg	Dark Gold	Tablet	Round	Solvay Pharmaceuticals
ROWELL; 2406	C-Ron FA	200 mg	Red	Tablet	Round	
ROWELL; 2406	C-Ron FA	600 mg	Red	Tablet	Round	
ROWELL; 4016	Cin-Quin 200	200 mg	Clear	Capsule		Solvay Pharmaceuticals
ROWELL; 4020	Cin-Quin 300	300 mg	Clear	Capsule		Solvay Pharmaceuticals
ROWELL; 4024	Cin-Quin 100	100 mg	White	Tablet	Round	Solvay Pharmaceuticals
ROWELL; 4028	Cin-Quin 200	200 mg	White	Tablet	Round, Scored	Solvay Pharmaceuticals
ROWELL; 4032	Cin-Quin 300	300 mg	White	Tablet	Round, Scored	Solvay Pharmaceuticals
ROWELL; 4412	Quine 300	300 mg	Clear	Capsule		Solvay Pharmaceuticals
ROWELL; 4710	Ronase 100	100 mg	White	Tablet	Scored	Solvay Pharmaceuticals
ROWELL; 4725	Ronase 250	250 mg	White	Tablet	Scored	Solvay Pharmaceuticals
ROWELL; 4750	Ronase 500	500 mg	White	Tablet	Scored	Solvay Pharmaceuticals
ROWELL; 4825	Procamide SR 250	250 mg	Pastel Blue	Sustained-Release Tablet		Solvay Pharmaceuticals
ROWELL; 4850	Procamide SR 500	500 mg	Pastel Pink	Sustained-Release Tablet	Scored	Solvay Pharmaceuticals
ROWELL; 4875	Procamide SR 750	750 mg	Tan	Sustained-Release Tablet	Scored	Solvay Pharmaceuticals
ROWELL; 5224	RO-Bile	8 mg	Yellow	Coated Tablet	Round	Solvay Pharmaceuticals
ROWELL; 5224	RO-Bile	30 mg	Yellow	Coated Tablet	Round	Solvay Pharmaceuticals
ROWELL; 5224	RO-Bile	260 mg	Yellow	Coated Tablet	Round	Solvay Pharmaceuticals
R-P; 1028	Eugel	100 mg		Tablet		
R-P; 1028	Eugel	175 mg		Tablet		
R-P; 1028	Eugel	325 mg		Tablet		
RPL; 0147	Unifast Unicelle	30 mg	Blue and Clear	Capsule		Solvay Pharmaceuticals
RPL; 0147	Unifast Unicelles	30 mg	Blue and Clear	Capsule		Reid-Rowell Pharmaceutical
RPL; 11; 84	Chloramate Unicelles	8 mg	White and Red	Capsule		Reid-Rowell Pharmaceutical
RPL; 1007	Curretab	10 mg	White	Tablet	Round, Scored	Solvay Pharmaceuticals
RPL; 1010	RP-Mycin	250 mg	Red	Coated Tablet		Solvay Pharmaceuticals

IMPRINT	BRAND/GENERIC NAME	STRENGTH	COLOR	FORM	SHAPE	MANUFACTURER
RPL; 1011	Supen	250 mg		Capsule		Solvay Pharmaceuticals
RPL; 1021	Dentavite	1 mg		Chewable Tablet		Reid-Rowell Pharmaceutical
RPL; 1021	Dentavite	1.2 mg		Chewable Tablet		Reid-Rowell Pharmaceutical
RPL; 1021	Dentavite	3 mg		Chewable Tablet		Reid-Rowell Pharmaceutical
RPL; 1021	Dentavite	8 mg		Chewable Tablet		Reid-Rowell Pharmaceutical
RPL; 1021	Dentavite	60 mg		Chewable Tablet		Reid-Rowell Pharmaceutical
RPL; 1021	Dentavite	400 units		Chewable Tablet		Reid-Rowell Pharmaceutical
RPL; 1021	Dentavite	3000 units		Chewable Tablet		Reid-Rowell Pharmaceutical
RPL; 1030	Fumatrin Forte	12 mcg	Orange	Coated Tablet	Oval	Reid-Rowell Pharmaceutical
RPL; 1030	Fumatrin Forte	12 mcg	Orange	Coated Tablet	Oval	Solvay Pharmaceuticals
RPL; 1030	Fumatrin Forte	0.5 mg	Orange	Coated Tablet	Oval	Reid-Rowell Pharmaceutical
RPL; 1030	Fumatrin Forte	0.5 mg	Orange	Coated Tablet	Oval	Solvay Pharmaceuticals
RPL; 1030	Fumatrin Forte	3 mg	Orange	Coated Tablet	Oval	Reid-Rowell Pharmaceutical
RPL; 1030	Fumatrin Forte	3 mg	Orange	Coated Tablet	Oval	Solvay Pharmaceuticals
RPL; 1030	Fumatrin Forte	100 mg	Orange	Coated Tablet	Oval	Reid-Rowell Pharmaceutical
RPL; 1030	Fumatrin Forte	100 mg	Orange	Coated Tablet	Oval	Solvay Pharmaceuticals
RPL; 1030	Fumatrin Forte	300 mg	Orange	Coated Tablet	Oval	Reid-Rowell Pharmaceutical
RPL; 1040	Proaqua	50 mg	Aqua	Tablet	Round, Scored	Solvay Pharmaceuticals
RPL; 1044	Pavacap Unicelle	150 mg	Blue and Clear	Capsule		Solvay Pharmaceuticals
RPL; 1053	Repro Compound-65	32.4 mg	Purple and Pink	Capsule		Reid-Rowell Pharmaceutical
RPL; 1053	Repro Compound-65	65 mg	Purple and Pink	Capsule		Reid-Rowell Pharmaceutical
RPL; 1053	Repro Compound-65	162 mg	Purple and Pink	Capsule		Reid-Rowell Pharmaceutical
RPL; 1053	Repro Compound-65	227 mg	Purple and Pink	Capsule		Reid-Rowell Pharmaceutical
RPL; 1054	Tranmep	400 mg	White	Tablet	Round, Scored	Solvay Pharmaceuticals
RPL; 1075	Proval No. 3	30 mg	Green	Capsule		Solvay Pharmaceuticals
RPL; 1075	Proval No. 3	325 mg	Green	Capsule		Solvay Pharmaceuticals
RPL; 1079	Melfiat	35 mg	Peach	Tablet	Round, Scored	Solvay Pharmaceuticals
RPL; 1102	Retet	500 mg	Green and Red	Capsule		Reid-Rowell Pharmaceutical
RPL; 1108	Sumox	250 mg	Yellow and White	Capsule		Solvay Pharmaceuticals
RPL; 1109	Sumox	500 mg	Yellow and White	Capsule		Solvay Pharmaceuticals
RPL; 1118	Spalix	0.0065 mg	Yellow	Tablet	Round	Reid-Rowell Pharmaceutical
RPL; 1118	Spalix	0.0194 mg	Yellow	Tablet	Round	Reid-Rowell Pharmaceutical
RPL; 1118	Spalix	0.1037 mg	Yellow	Tablet	Round	Reid-Rowell Pharmaceutical
RPL; 1118	Spalix	16 mg	Yellow	Tablet	Round	Reid-Rowell Pharmaceutical
RPL; 1121	Tenax	10 mg	Light and Dark Blue	Capsule		Reid-Rowell Pharmaceutical
RPL; 1132	Unipres	0.1 mg	Yellow	Tablet	Round, Scored	Reid-Rowell Pharmaceutical
RPL; 1132	Unipres	15 mg	Yellow	Tablet	Round, Scored	Reid-Rowell Pharmaceutical
RPL; 1132	Unipres	25 mg	Yellow	Tablet	Round, Scored	Reid-Rowell Pharmaceutical
RPL; 1133	Unifast Unicelles	30 mg	Blue and Clear	Capsule		Reid-Rowell Pharmaceutical
RPL; 1139	Calinate-FA	1 mcg	Yellow	Tablet		Reid-Rowell Pharmaceutical
RPL; 1139	Calinate FA	1 mcg	Yellow	Tablet	Oval	Solvay Pharmaceuticals
RPL; 1139	Calinate-FA	0.02 mg	Yellow	Tablet		Reid-Rowell Pharmaceutical
RPL; 1139	Calinate FA	0.02 mg	Yellow	Tablet	Oval	Solvay Pharmaceuticals
RPL; 1139	Calinate-FA	0.1 mg	Yellow	Tablet		Reid-Rowell Pharmaceutical
RPL; 1139	Calinate FA	0.1 mg	Yellow	Tablet	Oval	Solvay Pharmaceuticals
RPL; 1139	Calinate-FA	0.15 mg	Yellow	Tablet		Reid-Rowell Pharmaceutical
RPL; 1139	Calinate-FA	0.2 mg	Yellow	Tablet		Reid-Rowell Pharmaceutical
RPL; 1139	Calinate FA	0.2 mg	Yellow	Tablet	Oval	Solvay Pharmaceuticals
RPL; 1139	Calinate-FA	1 mg	Yellow	Tablet		Reid-Rowell Pharmaceutical
RPL; 1139	Calinate FA	1 mg	Yellow	Tablet	Oval	Solvay Pharmaceuticals
RPL; 1139	Calinate-FA	3 mg	Yellow	Tablet		Reid-Rowell Pharmaceutical
RPL; 1139	Calinate FA	3 mg	Yellow	Tablet	Oval	Solvay Pharmaceuticals
RPL; 1139	Calinate-FA	5 mg	Yellow	Tablet		Reid-Rowell Pharmaceutical
RPL; 1139	Calinate FA	5 mg	Yellow	Tablet	Oval	Solvay Pharmaceuticals
RPL; 1139	Calinate-FA	10 mg	Yellow	Tablet		Reid-Rowell Pharmaceutical
RPL; 1139	Calinate-FA	20 mg	Yellow	Tablet		Reid-Rowell Pharmaceutical
RPL; 1139	Calinate FA	20 mg	Yellow	Tablet	Oval	Solvay Pharmaceuticals
RPL; 1139	Calinate-FA	50 mg	Yellow	Tablet		Reid-Rowell Pharmaceutical
RPL; 1139	Calinate FA	50 mg	Yellow	Tablet	Oval	Solvay Pharmaceuticals
RPL; 1139	Calinate-FA	60 mg	Yellow	Tablet		Reid-Rowell Pharmaceutical
RPL; 1139	Calinate FA	60 mg	Yellow	Tablet	Oval	Solvay Pharmaceuticals
RPL; 1139	Calinate FA	250 mg	Yellow	Tablet	Oval	Solvay Pharmaceuticals
RPL; 1139	Calinate-FA	625 mg	Yellow	Tablet		Reid-Rowell Pharmaceutical
RPL; 1139	Calinate-FA	400 IU	Yellow	Tablet		Reid-Rowell Pharmaceutical
RPL; 1139	Calinate FA	400 IU	Yellow	Tablet	Oval	Solvay Pharmaceuticals
RPL; 1139	Calinate-FA	4000 IU	Yellow	Tablet		Reid-Rowell Pharmaceutical
RPL; 1139	Calinate FA	4000 IU	Yellow	Tablet	Oval	Solvay Pharmaceuticals
RPL; 1163	Asmadil Unicelles	15 mg		Capsule		Reid-Rowell Pharmaceutical
RPL; 1163	Asmadil Unicelles	50 mg		Capsule		Reid-Rowell Pharmaceutical
RPL; 1163	Asmadil Unicelles	260 mg		Capsule		Reid-Rowell Pharmaceutical
RPL; 1231	Aquatag	25 mg	White	Tablet	Round	Reid-Rowell Pharmaceutical
RPL; 1234	Aquatag	50 mg	Aqua	Tablet	Round, Scored	Solvay Pharmaceuticals
RPL; 1270	Vaso-80 Unicelles	80 mg	Grey and Clear	Capsule		Solvay Pharmaceuticals
RPL; 1280	Compal	6.25 mg	Aqua	Capsule		Reid-Rowell Pharmaceutical
RPL; 1280	Compal	16 mg	Aqua	Capsule		Reid-Rowell Pharmaceutical
RPL; 1280	Compal	16 mg	Blue-Green and Aqua	Capsule		Solvay Pharmaceuticals
RPL; 1280	Compal	30 mg	Aqua	Capsule		Reid-Rowell Pharmaceutical
RPL; 1280	Compal	30 mg	Blue-Green and Aqua	Capsule		Solvay Pharmaceuticals
RPL; 1280	Compal	356 mg	Aqua	Capsule		Reid-Rowell Pharmaceutical
RPL; 1280	Compal	356 mg	Blue-Green and Aqua	Capsule		Solvay Pharmaceuticals
RPL; 1290	Compal	6.25 mg	Aqua	Capsule		Reid-Rowell Pharmaceutical
RPL; 1290	Compal	16 mg	Aqua	Capsule		Reid-Rowell Pharmaceutical
RPL; 1290	Compal	30 mg	Aqua	Capsule		Reid-Rowell Pharmaceutical
RPL; 1290	Compal	356 mg	Aqua	Capsule		Reid-Rowell Pharmaceutical
RPL; 1340	Tora	8 mg	Orange	Tablet	Round	Solvay Pharmaceuticals
RPL; 1501	Tuzon	250 mg	Purple	Tablet	Round	Solvay Pharmaceuticals
RPL; 1501	Tuzon	300 mg	Purple	Tablet	Round	Solvay Pharmaceuticals
RPL; 1654	Bacarate	35 mg	Pink	Tablet	Round	Reid-Rowell Pharmaceutical
RPL; 1654	Bacarate	35 mg	Pink	Tablet	Round, Scored	Solvay Pharmaceuticals
RPL; 1690	Codap	32 mg	Blue and White	Tablet	Round	Reid-Rowell Pharmaceutical
RPL; 1690	Codap	325 mg	Blue and White	Tablet	Round	Reid-Rowell Pharmaceutical

IMPRINT	BRAND/GENERIC NAME	STRENGTH	COLOR	FORM	SHAPE	MANUFACTURER
RPL; 2378	Irlong II	12 mcg	Brown	Capsule		Reid-Rowell Pharmaceutical
RPL; 2378	Irlong II	0.5 mg	Brown	Capsule		Reid-Rowell Pharmaceutical
RPL; 2378	Irlong II	3 mg	Brown	Capsule		Reid-Rowell Pharmaceutical
RPL; 2378	Irlong II	100 mg	Brown	Capsule		Reid-Rowell Pharmaceutical
RPL; 2378	Irlong II	200 mg	Brown	Capsule		Reid-Rowell Pharmaceutical
RPL; 2580	Sprx-105	105 mg	Brown and Clear with White Beads	Capsule		Solvay Pharmaceuticals
RPL; 2770	Pre-Enthus FA	2 mcg	Purple and White	Capsule		Reid-Rowell Pharmaceutical
RPL; 2770	Pre-Enthus FA	0.15 mg	Purple and White	Capsule		Reid-Rowell Pharmaceutical
RPL; 2770	Pre-Enthus FA	0.8 mg	Purple and White	Capsule		Reid-Rowell Pharmaceutical
RPL; 2770	Pre-Enthus FA	1 mg	Purple and White	Capsule		Reid-Rowell Pharmaceutical
RPL; 2770	Pre-Enthus FA	2 mg	Purple and White	Capsule		Reid-Rowell Pharmaceutical
RPL; 2770	Pre-Enthus FA	10 mg	Purple and White	Capsule		Reid-Rowell Pharmaceutical
RPL; 2770	Pre-Enthus FA	50 mg	Purple and White	Capsule		Reid-Rowell Pharmaceutical
RPL; 2770	Pre-Enthus FA	240 mg	Purple and White	Capsule		Reid-Rowell Pharmaceutical
RPL; 2770	Pre-Enthus FA	400 IU	Purple and White	Capsule		Reid-Rowell Pharmaceutical
RPL; 2770	Pre-Enthus FA	4000 IU	Purple and White	Capsule		Reid-Rowell Pharmaceutical
RPL; 2805	Uproco	30 mg	Orange	Capsule		Solvay Pharmaceuticals
RPL; 2805	Unproco	200 mg	Orange	Capsule		Solvay Pharmaceuticals
RPL; 2805	Uproco	200 mg	Orange	Capsule		Solvay Pharmaceuticals
RPL; 2832	Neotep S.R.	9 mg	Red and Clear with Pink and White Beads	Capsule		Reid-Rowell Pharmaceutical
RPL; 2832	Neotep S.R.	21 mg	Red and Clear with Pink and White Beads	Capsule		Reid-Rowell Pharmaceutical
RPL; 4510	Compagesic	6.25 mg	Blue	Capsule		Reid-Rowell Pharmaceutical
RPL; 4510	Compagesic	16 mg	Blue	Capsule		Reid-Rowell Pharmaceutical
RPL; 4510	Compagesic	30 mg	Blue	Capsule		Reid-Rowell Pharmaceutical
RPL; 4510	Compagesic	356 mg	Blue	Capsule		Reid-Rowell Pharmaceutical
RPL; 4520	Dihydrocodeine Compound	16 mg	Blue	Capsule		Solvay Pharmaceuticals
RPL; 4520	Dihydrocodeine Compound	30 mg	Blue	Capsule		Solvay Pharmaceuticals
RPL; 4520	Dihydrocodeine Compound	356 mg	Blue	Capsule		Solvay Pharmaceuticals
RR; 0840	Colrex Compound	2 mg	Opaque Yellow	Capsule		Solvay Pharmaceuticals
RR; 0840	Colrex Compound	10 mg	Opaque Yellow	Capsule		Solvay Pharmaceuticals
RR; 0840	Colrex Compound	16 mg	Opaque Yellow	Capsule		Solvay Pharmaceuticals
RR; 0840	Colrex Compound	325 mg	Opaque Yellow	Capsule		Solvay Pharmaceuticals
RR; 1	Orasone	1 mg	Pink	Tablet	Round, Scored	Solvay Pharmaceuticals
RR; 5	Orasone 5	5 mg	White	Tablet	Round, Scored	Solvay Pharmaceuticals
RR; 10	Orasone 10	10 mg	Blue	Tablet	Round, Scored	Solvay Pharmaceuticals
RR; 20	Orasone 20	20 mg	Yellow	Tablet	Round, Scored	Solvay Pharmaceuticals
RR; 50	Orasone 50	50 mg	White	Tablet	Round, Scored	Solvay Pharmaceuticals
RR; 1007	Curretab	10 mg	White	Tablet	Round, Scored	Solvay Pharmaceuticals
RR; 1132	Unipres	0.1 mg	Yellow	Tablet	Round, Scored	Reid-Rowell Pharmaceutical
RR; 1132	Unipres	15 mg	Yellow	Tablet	Round, Scored	Reid-Rowell Pharmaceutical
RR; 1132	Unipres	25 mg	Yellow	Tablet	Round, Scored	Reid-Rowell Pharmaceutical
RR; 1216	Vio-Bec	25 mg	Brown	Capsule		Solvay Pharmaceuticals
RR; 1216	Vio-Bec	26 mg	Brown	Capsule		Solvay Pharmaceuticals
RR; 1216	Vio-Bec	40 mg	Brown	Capsule		Solvay Pharmaceuticals
RR; 1216	Vio-Bec	100 mg	Brown	Capsule		Solvay Pharmaceuticals
RR; 1216	Vio-Bec	500 mg	Brown	Capsule		Solvay Pharmaceuticals
RR; 1218	Vio-Bec Forte	5 mcg	Brown	Coated Tablet	Capsule-Shaped	Solvay Pharmaceuticals
RR; 1218	Vio-Bec Forte	0.5 mg	Brown	Coated Tablet	Capsule-Shaped	Solvay Pharmaceuticals
RR; 1218	Vio-Bec Forte	3 mg	Brown	Coated Tablet	Capsule-Shaped	Solvay Pharmaceuticals
RR; 1218	Vio-Bec Forte	25 mg	Brown	Coated Tablet	Capsule-Shaped	Solvay Pharmaceuticals
RR; 1218	Vio-Bec Forte	40 mg	Brown	Coated Tablet	Capsule-Shaped	Solvay Pharmaceuticals
RR; 1218	Vio-Bec Forte	100 mg	Brown	Coated Tablet	Capsule-Shaped	Solvay Pharmaceuticals
RR; 1218	Vio-Bec Forte	500 mg	Brown	Coated Tablet	Capsule-Shaped	Solvay Pharmaceuticals
RR; 1218	Vio-Bec Forte	30 IU	Brown	Coated Tablet	Capsule-Shaped	Solvay Pharmaceuticals
RR; 1610	Norlac	8 mcg	Pink	Coated Tablet	Oval	Solvay Pharmaceuticals
RR; 1610	Norlac	150 mcg	Pink	Coated Tablet	Oval	Solvay Pharmaceuticals
RR; 1610	Norlac	0.4 mg	Pink	Coated Tablet	Oval	Solvay Pharmaceuticals
RR; 1610	Norlac	2 mg	Pink	Coated Tablet	Oval	Solvay Pharmaceuticals
RR; 1610	Norlac	4 mg	Pink	Coated Tablet	Oval	Solvay Pharmaceuticals
RR; 1610	Norlac	15 mg	Pink	Coated Tablet	Oval	Solvay Pharmaceuticals
RR; 1610	Norlac	20 mg	Pink	Coated Tablet	Oval	Solvay Pharmaceuticals
RR; 1610	Norlac	60 mg	Pink	Coated Tablet	Oval	Solvay Pharmaceuticals
RR; 1610	Norlac	90 mg	Pink	Coated Tablet	Oval	Solvay Pharmaceuticals
RR; 1610	Norlac	100 mg	Pink	Coated Tablet	Oval	Solvay Pharmaceuticals
RR; 1610	Norlac	0.2 G	Pink	Coated Tablet	Oval	Solvay Pharmaceuticals
RR; 1610	Norlac	30 IU	Pink	Coated Tablet	Oval	Solvay Pharmaceuticals
RR; 1610	Norlac	400 IU	Pink	Coated Tablet	Oval	Solvay Pharmaceuticals
RR; 1610	Norlac	8000 IU	Pink	Coated Tablet	Oval	Solvay Pharmaceuticals
RR; 2404	C-Ron	100 mg	Red	Coated Tablet	Round	Solvay Pharmaceuticals
RR; 2404	C-Ron	200 mg	Red	Coated Tablet	Round	Solvay Pharmaceuticals
RR; 2406	C-Ron Forte	200 mg	Red	Coated Tablet	Round	Solvay Pharmaceuticals
RR; 2406	C-Ron Forte	600 mg	Red	Coated Tablet	Round	Solvay Pharmaceuticals
RR; 4016	Cin-Quin 200	200 mg	Clear	Capsule		Solvay Pharmaceuticals
RR; 4020	Cin-Quin 300	300 mg	Clear	Capsule		Solvay Pharmaceuticals
RR; 4024	Cin-Quin 100	100 mg	White	Tablet	Round	Solvay Pharmaceuticals
RR; 4028	Cin-Quin 200	200 mg	White	Tablet	Round, Scored	Solvay Pharmaceuticals
RR; 4032	Cin-Quin 300	300 mg	White	Tablet	Round, Scored	Solvay Pharmaceuticals
RR; 4120	Deproic	250 mg	Orange	Capsule		Solvay Pharmaceuticals
RR; 4825	Procamide SR 250	250 mg	Pastel Blue	Sustained-Release Tablet		Solvay Pharmaceuticals
RR; 4850	Procamide SR 500	500 mg	Pastel Pink	Sustained-Release Tablet	Scored	Solvay Pharmaceuticals
RR; 4875	Procamide SR 750	750 mg	Tan	Sustained-Release Tablet	Scored	Solvay Pharmaceuticals
RR; 7025	Ruvert M	25 mg	Red	Coated Tablet	Round	Solvay Pharmaceuticals
RR; 7720	Chenix	250 mg	White	Coated Tablet	Round, Scored	Solvay Pharmaceuticals
RS; 167	Diphenoxylate Hydrochloride with Atropine Sulfate	0.025 mg	White	Tablet	Round	

IMPRINT	BRAND/GENERIC NAME	STRENGTH	COLOR	FORM	SHAPE	MANUFACTURER
RS; 167	Diphenoxylate Hydrochloride with Atropine Sulfate	2.5 mg	White	Tablet	Round	
RUFEN 400	Rufen	400 mg	White	Coated Tablet	Round	Boots Pharmaceuticals
RUFEN 600	Rufen	600 mg	White	Coated Tablet	Capsule-Shaped	Boots Pharmaceuticals
RUFEN 800	Rufen	800 mg	White	Coated Tablet	Round	Boots Pharmaceuticals
RUGBY; 3023	Allernade	2.5 mg	Blue and Clear	Capsule		Rugby Laboratories
RUGBY; 3023	Allernade	8 mg	Blue and Clear	Capsule		Rugby Laboratories
RUGBY; 3023	Allernade	50 mg	Blue and Clear	Capsule		Rugby Laboratories
RUGBY; 3024	Allergine	2.5 mg	Blue and Natural	Timed-Release Capsule		Rugby Laboratories
RUGBY; 3024	Allergine	8 mg	Blue and Natural	Timed-Release Capsule		Rugby Laboratories
RUGBY; 3024	Allergine	50 mg	Blue and Natural	Timed-Release Capsule		Rugby Laboratories
RUGBY; 3266	Apc Compound with Phenobarbital	15 mg	White	Tablet	Round	Rugby Laboratories
RUGBY; 3266	Apc Compound with Phenobarbital	32.5 mg	White	Tablet	Round	Rugby Laboratories
RUGBY; 3266	Apc Compound with Phenobarbital	162 mg	White	Tablet	Round	Rugby Laboratories
RUGBY; 3266	Apc Compound with Phenobarbital	227 mg	White	Tablet	Round	Rugby Laboratories
RUGBY; 3275; R	Apc Compound with Phenobarbital	15 mg	Yellow	Tablet	Round	Rugby Laboratories
RUGBY; 3275; R	Apc Compound with Phenobarbital	32.5 mg	Yellow	Tablet	Round	Rugby Laboratories
RUGBY; 3275; R	Apc Compound with Phenobarbital	162 mg	Yellow	Tablet	Round	Rugby Laboratories
RUGBY; 3275; R	Apc Compound with Phenobarbital	227 mg	Yellow	Tablet	Round	Rugby Laboratories
RUGBY; 3279	Apresodex	15 mg	Orange	Tablet		Rugby Laboratories
RUGBY; 3279	Apresodex	25 mg	Orange	Tablet		Rugby Laboratories
RUGBY; 3368	Dicyclomine with Phenobarbital	10 mg	Blue and White	Capsule		Rugby Laboratories
RUGBY; 3368	Dicyclomine with Phenobarbital	15 mg	Blue and White	Capsule		Rugby Laboratories
RUGBY; 3378	Dicyclomine with Phenobarbital	15 mg	White	Tablet	Round	Rugby Laboratories
RUGBY; 3378	Dicyclomine with Phenobarbital	20 mg	White	Tablet	Round	Rugby Laboratories
RUGBY; 3437	Carisoprodol Compound	32 mg	Orange	Tablet		Rugby Laboratories
RUGBY; 3437	Carisoprodol Compound	160 mg	Orange	Tablet		Rugby Laboratories
RUGBY; 3437	Carisoprodol Compound	200 mg	Orange	Tablet		Rugby Laboratories
RUGBY; 3702	Diethylpropion	25 mg	Light Blue	Tablet	Round	
RUGBY; 3743	Dipyridamole	25 mg				Rugby Laboratories
RUGBY; 3745	Dimenhydrinate	25 mg		Tablet		Rugby Laboratories
RUGBY; 3748	Dipyridamole	50 mg	White	Coated Tablet	Round, Unscored	Rugby Laboratories
RUGBY; 3776	Pseudo-Mal	6 mg		Timed-Release Tablet		Rugby Laboratories
RUGBY; 3895	Hydroxyzine Pamoate	100 mg	Green and Gray	Capsule		
RUGBY; 3942	Isollyl	40 mg	White	Tablet		Rugby Laboratories
RUGBY; 3942	Isollyl	50 mg	White	Tablet		Rugby Laboratories
RUGBY; 3942	Isollyl	130 mg	White	Tablet		Rugby Laboratories
RUGBY; 3942	Isollyl	200 mg	White	Tablet		Rugby Laboratories
RUGBY; 3946	Isosorbide Dinitrate	5 mg	Pink	Tablet		Rugby Laboratories
RUGBY; 3947	Isosorbide Dinitrate	5 mg	Pink	Tablet		Rugby Laboratories
RUGBY; 3990	Meclizine Hydrochloride	25 mg		Chewable Tablet		
RUGBY; 4010	Meprobamate	600 mg	White	Tablet	Capsule-Shaped	Rugby Laboratories
RUGBY; 4032	Metronidazole	500 mg		Tablet		Rugby Laboratories
RUGBY; 4033	Metronidazole	250 mg	White	Tablet	Round	Rugby Laboratories
RUGBY; 4295	Phenylbutazone Alka	100 mg	Orange White	Capsule		Rugby Laboratories
RUGBY; 4295	Phenylbutazone Alka	150 mg	Orange White	Capsule		Rugby Laboratories
RUGBY; 4363	Prenatal with Folic Acid and Iron	12 mcg	Yellow	Tablet	Oblong	Rugby Laboratories
RUGBY; 4363	Prenatal with Folic Acid and Iron	150 mcg	Yellow	Tablet	Oblong	Rugby Laboratories
RUGBY; 4363	Prenatal with Folic Acid and Iron	1 mg	Yellow	Tablet	Oblong	Rugby Laboratories
RUGBY; 4363	Prenatal with Folic Acid and Iron	2.55 mg	Yellow	Tablet	Oblong	Rugby Laboratories
RUGBY; 4363	Prenatal with Folic Acid and Iron	3 mg	Yellow	Tablet	Oblong	Rugby Laboratories
RUGBY; 4363	Prenatal with Folic Acid and Iron	10 mg	Yellow	Tablet	Oblong	Rugby Laboratories
RUGBY; 4363	Prenatal with Folic Acid and Iron	20 mg	Yellow	Tablet	Oblong	Rugby Laboratories
RUGBY; 4363	Prenatal with Folic Acid and Iron	65 mg	Yellow	Tablet	Oblong	Rugby Laboratories
RUGBY; 4363	Prenatal with Folic Acid and Iron	90 mg	Yellow	Tablet	Oblong	Rugby Laboratories
RUGBY; 4363	Prenatal with Folic Acid and Iron	100 mg	Yellow	Tablet	Oblong	Rugby Laboratories
RUGBY; 4363	Prenatal with Folic Acid and Iron	200 mg	Yellow	Tablet	Oblong	Rugby Laboratories
RUGBY; 4363	Prenatal with Folic Acid and Iron	30 IU	Yellow	Tablet	Oblong	Rugby Laboratories
RUGBY; 4363	Prenatal with Folic Acid and Iron	400 IU	Yellow	Tablet	Oblong	Rugby Laboratories
RUGBY; 4363	Prenatal with Folic Acid and Iron	8000 IU	Yellow	Tablet	Oblong	Rugby Laboratories
RUGBY; 4503	Runatal	12 mcg		Tablet		Rugby Laboratories
RUGBY; 4503	Runatal	0.3 mg		Tablet		Rugby Laboratories
RUGBY; 4503	Runatal	1 mg		Tablet		Rugby Laboratories
RUGBY; 4503	Runatal	2 mg		Tablet		Rugby Laboratories
RUGBY; 4503	Runatal	3.4 mg		Tablet		Rugby Laboratories
RUGBY; 4503	Runatal	15 mg		Tablet		Rugby Laboratories
RUGBY; 4503	Runatal	20 mg		Tablet		Rugby Laboratories
RUGBY; 4503	Runatal	50 mg		Tablet		Rugby Laboratories
RUGBY; 4503	Runatal	60 mg		Tablet		Rugby Laboratories

IMPRINT	BRAND/GENERIC NAME	STRENGTH	COLOR	FORM	SHAPE	MANUFACTURER
RUGBY; 4503	Runatal	100 mg		Tablet		Rugby Laboratories
RUGBY; 4503	Runatal	125 mg		Tablet		Rugby Laboratories
RUGBY; 4503	Runatal	350 mg		Tablet		Rugby Laboratories
RUGBY; 4503	Runatal	30 IU		Tablet		Rugby Laboratories
RUGBY; 4503	Runatal	400 IU		Tablet		Rugby Laboratories
RUGBY; 4503	Runatal	8,000 IU		Tablet		Rugby Laboratories
RUGBY; 4741	Tuss Allergine TD	40 mg	Tan and Clear	Timed-Release Capsule		Rugby Laboratories
RUGBY; 4741	Tuss Allergine TD	75 mg	Tan and Clear	Timed-Release Capsule		Rugby Laboratories
RUGBY; 4743	Tuss-Allernade TD	2.5 mg	White and Clear	Capsule		Rugby Laboratories
RUGBY; 4743	Tuss-Allernade TD	8 mg	White and Clear	Capsule		Rugby Laboratories
RUGBY; 4743	Tuss-Allernade TD	20 mg	White and Clear	Capsule		Rugby Laboratories
RUGBY; 4743	Tuss-Allernade TD	50 mg	White and Clear	Capsule		Rugby Laboratories
RUGBY; 4861	Desipramine Hydrochloride	25 mg		Tablet		
RUGBY; 4862	Desipramine Hydrochloride	50 mg		Tablet		
RUGBY; 4863	Desipramine Hydrochloride	75 mg		Tablet		
RUGBY; 4864	Desipramine Hydrochloride	100 mg		Tablet		
RUSS	Lortab 7/500	7 mg	White with Green Specks	Tablet	Oblong, Scored	Russ Pharmaceuticals
RUSS	Lortab 7/500	500 mg	White with Green Specks	Tablet	Oblong, Scored	Russ Pharmaceuticals
RUSS; 130	Theobid Duracap JR.	130 mg	Clear with White Beads	Capsule		Ucb Pharma
RUSS; 702	Femcet	40 mg	Lavender	Capsule		
RUSS; 702	Femcet	50 mg	Lavender	Capsule		
RUSS; 702	Femcet	325 mg	Lavender	Capsule		
RUSS; 902	Lortab 5	5 mg	White with Blue Specks	Tablet	Oblong	Russ Pharmaceuticals
RUSS; 902	Lortab 5	500 mg	White with Blue Specks	Tablet	Oblong	Russ Pharmaceuticals
S; 19; STORZ	Storzolamide	250 mg	White	Tablet	Round	
S;5	Eldepryl	5 mg	White	Tablet	Shield-Shaped	Somerset Pharmaceuticals
SANDOZ; 78/48	Gynergen	1 mg	Ivory Gray	Coated Tablet		Novartis
SANDOZ ; S	Acylanid	0.1 mg	Orchid Pink	Tablet		Novartis Consumer
SANDOZ ; S	Acylanid	0.1 mg	Orchid Pink	Tablet		Sandoz Consumer Pharmaceuticals
SANDOZ; S	Acylanid	0.2 mg	White	Tablet		Novartis Consumer
SANDOZ; S	Acylanid	0.2 mg	White	Tablet		Sandoz Consumer Pharmaceuticals
SANDOZ; S	Bellergal Spacetabs	0.2 mg	Multi-Colored	Tablet		Novartis
SANDOZ; S	Bellergal Spacetabs	0.6 mg	Multi-Colored	Tablet		Novartis
SANDOZ; S	Bellergal Spacetabs	40 mg	Multi-Colored	Tablet		Novartis
SANDOZ-S	Bellergal Spacetabs	0.2 mg	Multi-Colored	Tablet		Novartis
SANDOZ-S	Bellergal Spacetabs	0.6 mg	Multi-Colored	Tablet		Novartis
SANDOZ-S	Bellergal Spacetabs	40 mg	Multi-Colored	Tablet		Novartis
SAUCE PAN	Three-Amine	25 mg	Yellow	Sustained-Release Tablet		Eon Labs
SAUCE PAN	Three-Amine	50 mg	Yellow	Sustained-Release Tablet		Eon Labs
SCF	Contac Severe Cold & Flu	2 mg	Blue	Tablet		Smithkline Beecham Consumer Healthcare
SCF	Contac Severe Cold & Flu	12.5 mg	Blue	Tablet		Smithkline Beecham Consumer Healthcare
SCF	Contac Severe Cold & Flu	15 mg	Blue	Tablet		Smithkline Beecham Consumer Healthcare
SCF	Contac Severe Cold & Flu	500 mg	Blue	Tablet		Smithkline Beecham Consumer Healthcare
SCH WBS; 866	Disophrol	2 mg	Blue-White Mottled	Tablet		Schering-Plough Healthcare Products
SCH WBS; 866	Disophrol	60 mg	Blue-White Mottled	Tablet		Schering-Plough Healthcare Products
SCH; WBS 866	Disophrol	2 mg	Blue-White Mottled	Tablet		Schering-Plough Healthcare Products
SCH; WBS 866	Disophrol	60 mg	Blue-White Mottled	Tablet		Schering-Plough Healthcare Produoto
SCHERING LOGO	Prantal	100 mg	White	Tablet		Schering
SCHERING LOGO	Proglycem	100 mg	Orange	Capsule		Schering
SCHERING; 432	Coriforte	4 mg	Red and Yellow	Capsule		Schering
SCHERING; 432	Coriforte	30 mg	Red and Yellow	Capsule		Schering
SCHERING; 432	Coriforte	130 mg	Red and Yellow	Capsule		Schering
SCHERING; 432	Coriforte	190 mg	Red and Yellow	Capsule		Schering
SCHERING; 432	Coriforte	500 G	Red and Yellow	Capsule		Schering
SCHERING; 662	Prantal	100 mg	White	Tablet		Schering
SCHERING; ANR	Coriforte	4 mg	Red and Yellow	Capsule		Schering
SCHERING; ANR	Coriforte	30 mg	Red and Yellow	Capsule		Schering
SCHERING; ANR	Coriforte	130 mg	Red and Yellow	Capsule		Schering
SCHERING; ANR	Coriforte	190 mg	Red and Yellow	Capsule		Schering
SCHERING; ANR	Coriforte	500 G	Red and Yellow	Capsule		Schering
SEALET	Meprogesic	75 mg	Orange, White, and Green	Tablet	Multi-Layered, Round	
SEALET	Meprogesic	150 mg	Orange, White, and Green	Tablet	Multi-Layered, Round	
SEALET	Meprogesic	250 mg	Orange, White, and Green	Tablet	Multi-Layered, Round	
SEALETS; R; 0331	Chlordinium Sealants	2.5 mg	Light Green	Capsule		
SEALETS; R; 0331	Chlordinium Sealants	5 mg	Light Green	Capsule		
SEARLE; 201	Dartal	5 mg	White	Tablet	Round	
SEARLE; 211	Dartal	10 mg	Peach	Tablet	Round	
SEARLE; 931	Propranolol Hydrochloride	80 mg	Yellow	Tablet	Scored	
SEARLE; 1261	Aminophyllin with Phenobarbital	15 mg	White	Tablet	Round	
SEARLE; 1261	Aminophyllin with Phenobarbital	100 mg	White	Tablet	Round	
SEARLE; 1271	Aminophyllin with Phenobarbital	30 mg	White	Tablet	Round	
SEARLE; 1271	Aminophyllin with Phenobarbital	100 mg	White	Tablet	Round	

IMPRINT	BRAND/GENERIC NAME	STRENGTH	COLOR	FORM	SHAPE	MANUFACTURER
SEARLE; 1281	Aminophyllin with Phenobarbital	15 mg	White	Tablet	Oval	
SEARLE; 1281	Aminophyllin with Phenobarbital	200 mg	White	Tablet	Oval	
SEARLE; 1511	Pro-Banthine with Phenobarbital	15 mg	Ivory	Tablet		
SEARLE; 1511	Pro-Banthine with Phenobarbital	50 mg	Ivory	Tablet		
SEARLE; 1552	Comfolax	100 mg	Green	Capsule		
SEARLE; 1572	Comfolax Plus	30 mg	Light and Dark Green	Capsule		
SEARLE; 1572	Comfolax Plus	100 mg	Light and Dark Green	Capsule		
SEARLE; 1601	Diodoquin	650 mg	Cream	Tablet		
SEARLE; 1701	Dramamine	50 mg	White	Tablet	Scored	
SELDANE	Seldane	60 mg	White	Tablet	Round	
SELDANE-D	Seldane-D	60 mg	White to Off-White	Sustained-Release Tablet	Capsule-Shaped, Biconvex	
SELDANE-D	Seldane-D	120 mg	White to Off-White	Sustained-Release Tablet	Capsule-Shaped, Biconvex	
SHOALS	Hycogesic	5 mg	Green	Tablet	Oval, Scored	
SHOALS	Hycogesic	30 mg	Green	Tablet	Oval, Scored	
SHOALS	Hycogesic	150 mg	Green	Tablet	Oval, Scored	
SHOALS	Hycogesic	230 mg	Green	Tablet	Oval, Scored	
SIDMAK; 375	Nystatin	100,000 U	Off-White	Tablet	Oval, Flat-Faced	
SKF 126	SK-Tetracycline	250 mg	Pink and White	Capsule		Smithkline Beecham
SKF 467	SK-65 Compound	32.4 mg	Gray & Gold	Capsule		Smithkline Beecham Consumer Healthcare
SKF 467	SK-65 Compound	65 mg	Gray & Gold	Capsule		Smithkline Beecham Consumer Healthcare
SKF 467	SK-65 Compound	227 mg	Gray & Gold	Capsule		Smithkline Beecham Consumer Healthcare
SKF 499	SK-Probenecid	500 mg	White	Coated Tablet	Scored	Smithkline Beecham
SKF C49	Compazine Spansule	75 mg		Capsule		Smithkline Beecham
SKF H74	Eskabarb	65 mg		Capsule		Smithkline Beecham Consumer Healthcare
SKF H76	Eskabarb	97 mg	Blue & Clear	Capsule		Smithkline Beecham Consumer Healthcare
SKF P33	Prydon	0.035 mg	Red & Clear	Capsule		Smithkline Beecham Consumer Healthcare
SKF P33	Prydon	0.060 mg	Red & Clear	Capsule		Smithkline Beecham Consumer Healthcare
SKF P33	Prydon	0.305 mg	Red & Clear	Capsule		Smithkline Beecham Consumer Healthcare
SKF P33	Prydon	0.4 mg	Red & Clear	Capsule		Smithkline Beecham Consumer Healthcare
SKF P34	Prydon	0.07 mg	Red & Clear	Capsule		Smithkline Beecham Consumer Healthcare
SKF P34	Prydon	0.120 mg	Red & Clear	Capsule		Smithkline Beecham Consumer Healthcare
SKF P34	Prydon	0.610 mg	Red & Clear	Capsule		Smithkline Beecham Consumer Healthcare
SKF P34	Prydon	0.8 mg	Red & Clear	Capsule		Smithkline Beecham Consumer Healthcare
SKF S90	Selacryn	250 mg	Light Blue	Tablet	Round	Smithkline Beecham Consumer Healthcare
SKF; 25	Vontrol	25 mg	Orange	Tablet	Round	
SKF; 101	SK-Ampicillin	250 mg	Yellow and White	Capsule		Smithkline Beecham
SKF; 102	SK-Ampicillin	500 mg	Yellow and White	Capsule		Smithkline Beecham
SKF; 111	SK-Penicillin G	400,000 units	White	Tablet		Smithkline Beecham
SKF; 112	SK-Penicillin G	800,000 U	White	Tablet	Capsule-Shaped	Smithkline Beecham
SKF; 116	SK-Penicillin VK	250 mg	White	Tablet		Smithkline Beecham
SKF; 117	SK-Penicillin VK	500 mg		Tablet		Smithkline Beecham
SKF; 120	SK-Amitriptyline	10 mg	White	Tablet		Smithkline Beecham
SKF; 121	SK-Amitriptyline	25 mg		Tablet		Smithkline Beecham
SKF; 121	SK-Amitriptyline	25 mg	Green	Tablet		Smithkline Beecham
SKF; 123	SK-Amitriptyline	50 mg	Yellow	Tablet		Smithkline Beecham
SKF; 124	SK-Amitriptyline	75 mg	Green	Tablet		Smithkline Beecham
SKF; 126	SK-Tetracycline	250 mg	Pink and White	Capsule		Smithkline Beecham
SKF; 131	SK-Amitriptyline	100 mg	Yellow	Tablet		Smithkline Beecham
SKF; 132	SK-Amitriptyline	150 mg	White	Tablet		Smithkline Beecham
SKF; 133	SK-Bamate	200 mg		Tablet		Smithkline Beecham
SKF; 134	SK-Bamate	400 mg	White	Tablet		Smithkline Beecham
SKF; 136	SK-Phenobarbital	15 mg	White	Tablet		Smithkline Beecham
SKF; 137	SK-Phenobarbital	30 mg	White	Tablet		Smithkline Beecham
SKF; 163	SK-Soxazole	500 mg	White	Tablet		Smithkline Beecham
SKF; 169	SK-Reserpine	0.25 mg	White	Tablet		Smithkline Beecham
SKF; 171	SK-Quinidine Sulfate	200 mg	White	Tablet		Smithkline Beecham
SKF; 176	SK-Chloral Hydrate	500 mg	Green	Tablet		Smithkline Beecham
SKF; 310	SK-Propantheline	15 mg	White	Tablet	Round	Smithkline Beecham
SKF; 319	SK-Oxycodone with Aspirin	0.38 mg	White	Tablet	Oval	Smithkline Beecham
SKF; 319	SK-Oxycodone with Aspirin	4.5 mg	White	Tablet	Oval	Smithkline Beecham
SKF; 319	SK-Oxycodone with Aspirin	325 mg	White	Tablet	Oval	Smithkline Beecham
SKF; 320	SK-Oxycodone with Acetaminophen	5 mg	White	Tablet	Round	Smithkline Beecham
SKF; 320	SK-Oxycodone with Acetaminophen	325 mg	White	Tablet	Round	Smithkline Beecham
SKF; 321	SK-Pramine	10 mg	Blue	Tablet		Smithkline Beecham
SKF; 322	SK-Pramine	25 mg	Blue	Tablet		Smithkline Beecham
SKF; 323	SK-Pramine	50 mg	Blue	Tablet		Smithkline Beecham
SKF; 339	SK-Prednisone	5 mg	White	Tablet		Smithkline Beecham
SKF; 340	SK-Furosemide	20 mg		Tablet		Smithkline Beecham
SKF; 341	SK-Furosemide	40 mg		Tablet		Smithkline Beecham
SKF; 363	SK-Hydrochlorothiazide	25 mg		Tablet		Smithkline Beecham
SKF; 364	SK-Hydrochlorothiazide	50 mg		Tablet		Smithkline Beecham
SKF; 367	SK-Erythromycin	250 mg	Yellow	Tablet		Smithkline Beecham

IMPRINT	BRAND/GENERIC NAME	STRENGTH	COLOR	FORM	SHAPE	MANUFACTURER
SKF; 369	SK-Erythromycin	500 mg	Yellow	Coated Tablet	Capsule	Smithkline Beecham
SKF; 371	SK-Thioridazine Hydrochloride	10 mg		Tablet		Smithkline Beecham
SKF; 372	SK-Thioridazine	25 mg		Tablet		Smithkline Beecham
SKF; 373	SK-Thioridazine	50 mg		Tablet		Smithkline Beecham
SKF; 374	SK-Dexamethasone	0.5 mg	Light Yellow	Tablet		Smithkline Beecham
SKF; 375	SK-Thioridazine Hydrochloride	100 mg		Tablet		Smithkline Beecham
SKF; 376	SK-Dexamethasone	0.75 mg	Light Blue	Tablet		Smithkline Beecham
SKF; 377	SK-Dexamethasone	1.5 mg	Pink	Tablet		Smithkline Beecham
SKF; 379	SK-Dipyridamole	25 mg		Tablet		Smithkline Beecham
SKF; 380; 50MG	SK-Dipyridamole	50 mg		Tablet		Smithkline Beecham
SKF; 381; 75MG	SK-Dipyridamole	75 mg		Tablet		Smithkline Beecham
SKF; 409	SK-Tolbutamide	500 mg	Peach-Orange	Tablet	Round	Smithkline Beecham
SKF; 419	SK-Chlorothiazide	250 mg	White	Tablet	Round	Smithkline Beecham
SKF; 420	SK-Chlorothiazide	500 mg	White	Tablet	Round	Smithkline Beecham
SKF; 423	SK-Diphenoxylate	0.025 mg	White	Tablet		Smithkline Beecham
SKF; 423	SK-Diphenoxylate	2.5 mg	White	Tablet		Smithkline Beecham
SKF; 441	SK-Lygen	5 mg	Pink	Capsule		Smithkline Beecham
SKF; 442	SK-Lygen	10 mg	Pink and Orange	Capsule		Smithkline Beecham
SKF; 443	SK-Lygen	25 mg	Orange	Capsule		Smithkline Beecham
SKF; 463	SK-65	65 mg	Gray and White	Capsule		Smithkline Beecham
SKF; 468	SK-65 Compound	32.4 mg	Orange and Gray	Capsule		Smithkline Beecham
SKF; 468	SK-65 Compound	65 mg	Orange and Gray	Capsule		Smithkline Beecham
SKF; 468	SK-65 Compound	389 mg	Orange and Gray	Capsule		Smithkline Beecham
SKF; 474	SK-65	65 mg	Orange	Tablet	Capsule-Shaped	Smithkline Beecham
SKF; 474	SK-65	650 mg	Orange	Tablet	Capsule-Shaped	Smithkline Beecham
SKF; 494	SK-Apap	15 mg	White	Tablet	Round	Smithkline Beecham
SKF; 494	SK-Apap	300 mg	White	Tablet	Round	Smithkline Beecham
SKF; 496	SK-Apap with Codeine	30 mg	White	Tablet	Round	
SKF; 496	SK-Apap with Codeine	300 mg	White	Tablet	Round	
SKF; 497	SK-Apap with Codeine	60 mg	White	Tablet	Round	
SKF; 497	SK-Apap with Codeine	300 mg	White	Tablet	Round	
SKF; 499	SK-Probenecid	500 mg	White	Tablet	Capsule-Shaped, Scored	Smithkline Beecham
SKF; C47	Compazine	30 mg	Black/natural-Colored	Sustained-Release Capsule		Smithkline Beecham
SKF; D62	Darbid	5 mg	Pink	Tablet	Round	
SKF; D91	Dexamyl	10 mg		Capsule		Smithkline Beecham Consumer Healthcare
SKF; D91	Dexamyl	65 mg		Capsule		Smithkline Beecham Consumer Healthcare
SKF; D92	Dexamyl	15 mg	Green and Clear	Capsule		Smithkline Beecham Consumer Healthcare
SKF; D92	Dexamyl	97 mg	Green and Clear	Capsule		Smithkline Beecham Consumer Healthcare
SKF; D93	Dexamyl	5 mg	Green	Tablet		Smithkline Beecham Consumer Healthcare
SKF; D93	Dexamyl	32 mg	Green	Tablet		Smithkline Beecham Consumer Healthcare
SKF; E; 12	Dexedrine	5 mg	Purple and Clear	Capsule		Smithkline Beecham
SKF; E; 13	Dexedrine	10 mg	Purple and Clear	Capsule		Smithkline Beecham
SKF; E; 14	Dexedrine	15 mg	Purple and Clear	Capsule		Smithkline Beecham
SKF 467	SK-65 Compound	162 mg	Gray & Gold	Capsule		Smithkline Beecham Consumer Healthcare
SL; 321; 10	Isoxsuprine Hydrochloride	10 mg	White	Tablet	Round, Convex	
SL; 322; 20	Isoxsuprine	20 mg	White	Tablet	Round, Convex, Bisected	
SL; 323	Bethanechol Chloride	5 mg	White	Tablet	Round, Scored	
SL; 325	Bethanechol Chloride	25 mg	Yellow	Tablet	Round, Scored	
SL; 326	Bethanechol Chloride	50 mg	Yellow	Tablet	Round, Scored	
SL; 346	Isosorbide Dinitrate	10 mg	White	Tablet		
SL; 347	Isosorbide Dinitrate	5 mg	Pink	Tablet	Round	
SL; 348	Isosorbide Dinitrate	10 mg	White	Tablet	Round	
SL; 349	Isosorbide Dinitrate	20 mg	Green	Tablet	Round	
SL; 350	Isosorbide Dinitrate	30 mg	Blue	Tablet	Round	
SL; 351	Isosorbide Dinitrate	40 mg	Yellow	Sustained-Release Tablet	Round	
SL; 384	Isosorbide Dinitrate	30 mg	Pink	Sustained-Release Tablet	Round	
SL; 387	Ibuprofen	400 mg	White	Coated Tablet	Round, Convex	Sidmak Laboratories
SL; 388	Ibuprofen	600 mg	White	Coated Tablet	Oval, Convex	Sidmak Laboratories
SL; 407	Indomethacin	50 mg	Green	Capsule		
SL; 415	Griseofulvin	165 mg	White	Tablet	Oval	Sidmak Laboratories
SL; 416	Griseofulvin	330 mg	White	Tablet	Oval, Bisected	Sidmak Laboratories
SL; 451	Ibuprofen	800 mg	White	Coated Tablet	Capsule-Shaped	Sidmak Laboratories
SL; 472	Propranolol Hydrochloride	90 mg	Light Blue	Tablet	Round, Convex, Bisected	Sidmak Laboratories
SL; 478	Methyldopa with Hydrochlorothiazide	15 mg	Light Brown	Coated Tablet		Sidmak Laboratories
SL; 478	Methyldopa with Hydrochlorothiazide	250 mg	Light Brown	Coated Tablet		Sidmak Laboratories
SL; 479	Methyldopa with Hydrochlorothiazide	25 mg		Coated Tablet	Round	Sidmak Laboratories
SL; 479	Methyldopa with Hydrochlorothiazide	250 mg		Coated Tablet	Round	Sidmak Laboratories
SL; 480	Methyldopa with Hydrochlorothiazide	30 mg	Light Brown	Coated Tablet	Oval	Sidmak Laboratories
SL; 480	Methyldopa with Hydrochlorothiazide	500 mg	Light Brown	Coated Tablet	Oval	Sidmak Laboratories
SL; 481	Methyldopa with Hydrochlorothiazide	50 mg	White	Coated Tablet	Oval	Sidmak Laboratories
SL; 481	Methyldopa with Hydrochlorothiazide	500 mg	White	Coated Tablet	Oval	Sidmak Laboratories
SL; 520	Decotan	8 mg	Orange	Tablet	Capsule-Shaped, Bisected	Sidmak Laboratories
SL; 520	Decotan	25 mg	Orange	Tablet	Capsule-Shaped, Bisected	Sidmak Laboratories
SOLVAY; 0147	Unifast Unicelle	30 mg	Blue and Clear	Capsule		Solvay Pharmaceuticals
SOLVAY; 0840	Colrex Compound	2 mg	Opaque Yellow	Capsule		Solvay Pharmaceuticals
SOLVAY; 0840	Colrex Compound	10 mg	Opaque Yellow	Capsule		Solvay Pharmaceuticals

IMPRINT	BRAND/GENERIC NAME	STRENGTH	COLOR	FORM	SHAPE	MANUFACTURER
SOLVAY; 0840	Colrex Compound	16 mg	Opaque Yellow	Capsule		Solvay Pharmaceuticals
SOLVAY; 0840	Colrex Compound	325 mg	Opaque Yellow	Capsule		Solvay Pharmaceuticals
SOLVAY; 1007	Curretab	10 mg	White	Tablet	Round, Scored	Solvay Pharmaceuticals
SOLVAY; 1010	RP-Mycin	250 mg	Red	Coated Tablet		Solvay Pharmaceuticals
SOLVAY; 1030	Fumatrin Forte	12 mcg	Orange	Coated Tablet	Oval	Solvay Pharmaceuticals
SOLVAY; 1030	Fumatrin Forte	0.5 mg	Orange	Coated Tablet	Oval	Solvay Pharmaceuticals
SOLVAY; 1030	Fumatrin Forte	3 mg	Orange	Coated Tablet	Oval	Solvay Pharmaceuticals
SOLVAY; 1030	Fumatrin Forte	100 mg	Orange	Coated Tablet	Oval	Solvay Pharmaceuticals
SOLVAY; 1040	Proaqua	50 mg	Aqua	Tablet	Round, Scored	Solvay Pharmaceuticals
SOLVAY; 1044	Pavacap Unicelle	150 mg	Blue and Clear	Capsule		Solvay Pharmaceuticals
SOLVAY; 1054	Tranmep	400 mg	White	Tablet	Round, Scored	Solvay Pharmaceuticals
SOLVAY; 1075	Proval No. 3	30 mg	Green	Capsule		Solvay Pharmaceuticals
SOLVAY; 1075	Proval No. 3	325 mg	Green	Capsule		Solvay Pharmaceuticals
SOLVAY; 1079	Melfiat	35 mg	Peach	Tablet	Round, Scored	Solvay Pharmaceuticals
SOLVAY; 1133	Unifast Unicelle	30 mg	Blue and Clear	Capsule		Solvay Pharmaceuticals
SOLVAY; 1139	Calinate FA	1 mcg	Yellow	Tablet	Oval	Solvay Pharmaceuticals
SOLVAY; 1139	Calinate FA	0.02 mg	Yellow	Tablet	Oval	Solvay Pharmaceuticals
SOLVAY; 1139	Calinate FA	0.1 mg	Yellow	Tablet	Oval	Solvay Pharmaceuticals
SOLVAY; 1139	Calinate FA	0.2 mg	Yellow	Tablet	Oval	Solvay Pharmaceuticals
SOLVAY; 1139	Calinate FA	1 mg	Yellow	Tablet	Oval	Solvay Pharmaceuticals
SOLVAY; 1139	Calinate FA	3 mg	Yellow	Tablet	Oval	Solvay Pharmaceuticals
SOLVAY; 1139	Calinate FA	5 mg	Yellow	Tablet	Oval	Solvay Pharmaceuticals
SOLVAY; 1139	Calinate FA	20 mg	Yellow	Tablet	Oval	Solvay Pharmaceuticals
SOLVAY; 1139	Calinate FA	50 mg	Yellow	Tablet	Oval	Solvay Pharmaceuticals
SOLVAY; 1139	Calinate FA	60 mg	Yellow	Tablet	Oval	Solvay Pharmaceuticals
SOLVAY; 1139	Calinate FA	250 mg	Yellow	Tablet	Oval	Solvay Pharmaceuticals
SOLVAY; 1139	Calinate FA	400 IU	Yellow	Tablet	Oval	Solvay Pharmaceuticals
SOLVAY; 1139	Calinate FA	4000 IU	Yellow	Tablet	Oval	Solvay Pharmaceuticals
SOLVAY; 1216	Vio-Bec	25 mg	Brown	Capsule		Solvay Pharmaceuticals
SOLVAY; 1216	Vio-Bec	26 mg	Brown	Capsule		Solvay Pharmaceuticals
SOLVAY; 1216	Vio-Bec	40 mg	Brown	Capsule		Solvay Pharmaceuticals
SOLVAY; 1216	Vio-Bec	100 mg	Brown	Capsule		Solvay Pharmaceuticals
SOLVAY; 1216	Vio-Bec	500 mg	Brown	Capsule		Solvay Pharmaceuticals
SOLVAY; 1218	Vio-Bec Forte	5 mcg	Brown	Coated Tablet	Capsule-Shaped	Solvay Pharmaceuticals
SOLVAY; 1218	Vio-Bec Forte	0.5 mg	Brown	Coated Tablet	Capsule-Shaped	Solvay Pharmaceuticals
SOLVAY; 1218	Vio-Bec Forte	3 mg	Brown	Coated Tablet	Capsule-Shaped	Solvay Pharmaceuticals
SOLVAY; 1218	Vio-Bec Forte	25 mg	Brown	Coated Tablet	Capsule-Shaped	Solvay Pharmaceuticals
SOLVAY; 1218	Vio-Bec Forte	40 mg	Brown	Coated Tablet	Capsule-Shaped	Solvay Pharmaceuticals
SOLVAY; 1218	Vio-Bec Forte	100 mg	Brown	Coated Tablet	Capsule-Shaped	Solvay Pharmaceuticals
SOLVAY; 1218	Vio-Bec Forte	500 mg	Brown	Coated Tablet	Capsule-Shaped	Solvay Pharmaceuticals
SOLVAY; 1218	Vio-Bec Forte	30 IU	Brown	Coated Tablet	Capsule-Shaped	Solvay Pharmaceuticals
SOLVAY; 1280	Compal	16 mg	Blue-Green and Aqua	Capsule		Solvay Pharmaceuticals
SOLVAY; 1280	Compal	30 mg	Blue-Green and Aqua	Capsule		Solvay Pharmaceuticals
SOLVAY; 1280	Compal	356 mg	Blue-Green and Aqua	Capsule		Solvay Pharmaceuticals
SOLVAY; 1290	Compal	16 mg	Blue-Green and Aqua	Capsule		Solvay Pharmaceuticals
SOLVAY; 1290	Compal	30 mg	Blue-Green and Aqua	Capsule		Solvay Pharmaceuticals
SOLVAY; 1290	Compal	356 mg	Blue-Green and Aqua	Capsule		Solvay Pharmaceuticals
SOLVAY; 1610	Norlac	8 mcg	Pink	Coated Tablet	Oval	Solvay Pharmaceuticals
SOLVAY; 1610	Norlac	150 mcg	Pink	Coated Tablet	Oval	Solvay Pharmaceuticals
SOLVAY; 1610	Norlac	0.4 mg	Pink	Coated Tablet	Oval	Solvay Pharmaceuticals
SOLVAY; 1610	Norlac	2 mg	Pink	Coated Tablet	Oval	Solvay Pharmaceuticals
SOLVAY; 1610	Norlac	4 mg	Pink	Coated Tablet	Oval	Solvay Pharmaceuticals
SOLVAY; 1610	Norlac	15 mg	Pink	Coated Tablet	Oval	Solvay Pharmaceuticals
SOLVAY; 1610	Norlac	20 mg	Pink	Coated Tablet	Oval	Solvay Pharmaceuticals
SOLVAY; 1610	Norlac	60 mg	Pink	Coated Tablet	Oval	Solvay Pharmaceuticals
SOLVAY; 1610	Norlac	90 mg	Pink	Coated Tablet	Oval	Solvay Pharmaceuticals
SOLVAY; 1610	Norlac	100 mg	Pink	Coated Tablet	Oval	Solvay Pharmaceuticals
SOLVAY; 1610	Norlac	0.2 G	Pink	Coated Tablet	Oval	Solvay Pharmaceuticals
SOLVAY; 1610	Norlac	30 IU	Pink	Coated Tablet	Oval	Solvay Pharmaceuticals
SOLVAY; 1610	Norlac	400 IU	Pink	Coated Tablet	Oval	Solvay Pharmaceuticals
SOLVAY; 1610	Norlac	8000 IU	Pink	Coated Tablet	Oval	Solvay Pharmaceuticals
SOLVAY; 2046	C-Ron Forte	200 mg	Red	Coated Tablet	Round	Solvay Pharmaceuticals
SOLVAY; 2046	C-Ron Forte	600 mg	Red	Coated Tablet	Round	Solvay Pharmaceuticals
SOLVAY; 2080	S.A.S.-500	500 mg	Dark Gold	Tablet	Round	Solvay Pharmaceuticals
SOLVAY; 2404	C-Ron	100 mg	Red	Coated Tablet	Round	Solvay Pharmaceuticals
SOLVAY; 2404	C-Ron	200 mg	Red	Coated Tablet	Round	Solvay Pharmaceuticals
SOLVAY; 2805	Uproco	30 mg	Orange	Capsule		Solvay Pharmaceuticals
SOLVAY; 2805	Uproco	200 mg	Orange	Capsule		Solvay Pharmaceuticals
SOLVAY; 4016	Cin-Quin 200	200 mg	Clear	Capsule		Solvay Pharmaceuticals
SOLVAY; 4020	Cin-Quin 300	300 mg	Clear	Capsule		Solvay Pharmaceuticals
SOLVAY; 4024	Cin-Quin 100	100 mg	White	Tablet	Round	Solvay Pharmaceuticals
SOLVAY; 4028	Cin-Quin 200	200 mg	White	Tablet	Round, Scored	Solvay Pharmaceuticals
SOLVAY; 4032	Cin-Quin 300	300 mg	White	Tablet	Round, Scored	Solvay Pharmaceuticals
SOLVAY; 4120	Deproic	250 mg	Orange	Capsule		Solvay Pharmaceuticals
SOLVAY; 4412	Quine 300	300 mg	Clear	Capsule		Solvay Pharmaceuticals
SOLVAY; 4520	Dihydrocodeine Compound	16 mg	Blue	Capsule		Solvay Pharmaceuticals
SOLVAY; 4520	Dihydrocodeine Compound	30 mg	Blue	Capsule		Solvay Pharmaceuticals
SOLVAY; 4520	Dihydrocodeine Compound	356 mg	Blue	Capsule		Solvay Pharmaceuticals
SOLVAY; 4710	Ronase 100	100 mg	White	Tablet	Scored	Solvay Pharmaceuticals
SOLVAY; 4725	Ronase 250	250 mg	White	Tablet	Scored	Solvay Pharmaceuticals
SOLVAY; 4750	Ronase 500	500 mg	White	Tablet	Scored	Solvay Pharmaceuticals
SOLVAY; 4825	Procamide SR 250	250 mg	Pastel Blue	Sustained-Release Tablet		Solvay Pharmaceuticals
SOLVAY; 4850	Procamide SR 500	500 mg	Pastel Pink	Sustained-Release Tablet	Scored	Solvay Pharmaceuticals
SOLVAY; 4875	Procamide SR 750	750 mg	Tan	Sustained-Release Tablet	Scored	Solvay Pharmaceuticals
SOLVAY; 5224	RO-Bile	8 mg	Yellow	Coated Tablet	Round	Solvay Pharmaceuticals

IMPRINT	BRAND/GENERIC NAME	STRENGTH	COLOR	FORM	SHAPE	MANUFACTURER
SOLVAY; 5224	RO-Bile	30 mg	Yellow	Coated Tablet	Round	Solvay Pharmaceuticals
SOLVAY; 5224	RO-Bile	260 mg	Yellow	Coated Tablet	Round	Solvay Pharmaceuticals
SOLVAY; 7025	Ruvert M	25 mg	Red	Coated Tablet	Round	Solvay Pharmaceuticals
SOLVAY; 7720	Chenix	250 mg	White	Coated Tablet	Round, Scored	Solvay Pharmaceuticals
SP; 112	Amitriptyline Hydrochloride	10 mg	Pink	Coated Tablet	Round	Superpharm
SP; 113	Amitriptyline Hydrochloride	25 mg	Light Green	Coated Tablet	Round	Superpharm
SP; 114	Amitriptyline Hydrochloride	50 mg	Brown	Coated Tablet	Round	Superpharm
SP; 115	Amitriptyline Hydrochloride	75 mg	Purple	Coated Tablet	Round	Superpharm
SP; 116	Amitriptyline Hydrochloride	100 mg	Orange	Coated Tablet	Round	Superpharm
SP; 148	Sulfasalazine	500 mg	Dark Yellow	Tablet	Round, Scored	
SQUIBB 210	Veisulid	250 mg				Bristol-Myers Squibb
SQUIBB 505	Ipral Calcium	3/4 or 2 grains		Tablet		Bristol-Myers Squibb
SQUIBB 977	Tolserol	0.5 gram				Bristol-Myers Squibb
SQUIBB W080	Hydrocodone Bitartrate & Acetaminophen	5 mg		Tablet		Bristol-Myers Squibb
SQUIBB W080	Hydrocodone Bitartrate & Acetaminophen	500 mg		Tablet		Bristol-Myers Squibb
SQUIBB W090	Verapamil Hydrochloride	80 mg		Tablet		Bristol-Myers Squibb
SQUIBB W100	Verapamil Hydrochloride	120 mg		Tablet		Bristol-Myers Squibb
SQUIBB W111	Thiothixene	1 mg		Capsule		Bristol-Myers Squibb
SQUIBB W112	Haloperidol	5 mg		Tablet		Bristol-Myers Squibb
SQUIBB W114	Flurazepam Hydrochloride	15 mg		Capsule		Bristol-Myers Squibb
SQUIBB W116	Hydroxyzine Hydrochloride	25 mg		Tablet		Bristol-Myers Squibb
SQUIBB W117	Prednisone	10 mg		Tablet		Bristol-Myers Squibb
SQUIBB W119	Methocarbamol	750 mg		Tablet		Bristol-Myers Squibb
SQUIBB W122	Hydroxyzine Hydrochloride	10 mg		Tablet		Bristol-Myers Squibb
SQUIBB W125	Thiothixene	2 mg		Tablet		Bristol-Myers Squibb
SQUIBB W127	Flurazepam Hydrochloride	30 mg		Capsule		Bristol-Myers Squibb
SQUIBB W128	Haloperidol	0.5 mg		Tablet		Bristol-Myers Squibb
SQUIBB W131	Thiothixene	5 mg		Capsule		Bristol-Myers Squibb
SQUIBB W135	Haloperidol	2 mg		Tablet		Bristol-Myers Squibb
SQUIBB W136	Meclizine Hydrochloride	12.5 mg		Tablet		Bristol-Myers Squibb
SQUIBB W137	Thiothixene	10 mg		Capsule		Bristol-Myers Squibb
SQUIBB W260	Propoxyphene Hydrochloride	65 mg		Capsule		Teva Pharmaceuticals
SQUIBB W280	Acetaminophen and Propoxyphene Napsylate	100 mg		Tablet		
SQUIBB W280	Acetaminophen and Propoxyphene Napsylate	650 mg		Tablet		
SQUIBB W290	Acetaminophen and Propoxyphene Hydrochloride	65 mg		Tablet		
SQUIBB W290	Acetaminophen and Propoxyphene Hydrochloride	650 mg		Tablet		
SQUIBB W310	Erythromycin Stearate	250 mg		Tablet		Bristol-Myers Squibb
SQUIBB W330	Erythromycin Stearate	500 mg		Tablet		Bristol-Myers Squibb
SQUIBB W340	Nitrofurantoin	100 mg		Capsule		Bristol-Myers Squibb
SQUIBB W350	Nitrofurantoin	50 mg		Capsule		Bristol-Myers Squibb
SQUIBB W540	Dicyclomine Hydrochloride	10 mg		Tablet		Bristol-Myers Squibb
SQUIBB W550	Dicyclomine Hydrochloride	20 mg		Tablet		Bristol-Myers Squibb
SQUIBB W610	Meclizine Hydrochloride	25 mg		Tablet		Bristol-Myers Squibb
SQUIBB W720	Haloperidol	1 mg		Tablet		Bristol-Myers Squibb
SQUIBB W777	Amoxapine	100 mg		Tablet		Bristol-Myers Squibb
SQUIBB W791	Albuterol Sulphate	4 mg		Tablet		Bristol-Myers Squibb
SQUIBB W830	Haloperidol	20 mg		Tablet		Bristol-Myers Squibb
SQUIBB W840	Nitroglycerin SR	2.5 mg		Capsule		Bristol-Myers Squibb
SQUIBB W870	Prednisone	5 mg		Tablet		Bristol-Myers Squibb
SQUIBB W888	Amoxapine	50 mg		Tablet		Bristol-Myers Squibb
SQUIBB W891	Albuterol Sulphate	2 mg		Tablet		Bristol-Myers Squibb
SQUIBB W930	Nitroglycerin SR	6.5 mg		Capsule		Bristol-Myers Squibb
SQUIBB W940	Haloperidol	10 mg		Tablet		Bristol-Myers Squibb
SQUIBB W950	Prednisone	20 mg		Tablet		Bristol-Myers Squibb
SQUIBB W970	Hydroxyzine Hydrochloride	50 mg		Tablet		Bristol-Myers Squibb
SQUIBB W999	Amoxapine	25 mg		Tablet		Bristol-Myers Squibb
SQUIBB; 109	Vitamin A	25,000 IU		Capsule		
SQUIBB; 110	Vitamin A	50,000 IU		Capsule		
SQUIBB; 111	Vitamin A	10,000 IU		Capsule		
SQUIBB; 112	Vitamin C	250 mg		Tablet		
SQUIBB; 139	Chlorpropamide	100 mg	Blue	Tablet	Round	Bristol-Myers Squibb
SQUIBB; 152	Chlorpropamide	250 mg	Blue	Tablet	Round	Bristol-Myers Squibb
SQUIBB; 157	Clorazepate Dipotassium	7.5 mg	Peach	Tablet	Round, Scored	Bristol-Myers Squibb
SQUIBB; 160	Ethril	250 mg	Pink	Tablet		
SQUIBB; 181	Ethril	500 mg	Pink	Tablet		
SQUIBB; 162	Chlorthalidone	25 mg	Yellow	Tablet	Round	
SQUIBB; 163	Clorazepate	15 mg	Pink	Tablet	Round, Scored	
SQUIBB; 170	Gestest	0.05 mg		Tablet		Bristol-Myers Squibb
SQUIBB; 170	Gestest	2.5 mg		Tablet		Bristol-Myers Squibb
SQUIBB; 184	Amnestrogen	0.625 mg		Tablet		
SQUIBB; 185	Diazepam	2 mg	White	Tablet	Bisected	Bristol-Myers Squibb
SQUIBB; 187	Chlorthalidone	100 mg	White	Tablet	Round	
SQUIBB; 188	Amnestrogen	1.25 mg		Tablet		
SQUIBB; 189	Amnestrogen	2.5 mg		Tablet		
SQUIBB; 211	Cloxacillin Sodium	250 mg		Capsule		Bristol-Myers Squibb
SQUIBB; 212	Cloxacillin Sodium	500 mg		Capsule		Bristol-Myers Squibb
SQUIBB; 238	Diazepam	5 mg	Yellow	Tablet	Bisected	Bristol-Myers Squibb
SQUIBB; 245	Diazepam	10 mg	Light Blue	Tablet	Bisected	Bristol-Myers Squibb
SQUIBB; 297	Engran	2 mcg	Blue	Tablet		Bristol-Myers Squibb
SQUIBB; 297	Engran	0.15 mg	Blue	Tablet		Bristol-Myers Squibb
SQUIBB; 297	Engran	1 mg	Blue	Tablet		Bristol-Myers Squibb
SQUIBB; 297	Engran	1.5 mg	Blue	Tablet		Bristol-Myers Squibb
SQUIBB; 297	Engran	2 mg	Blue	Tablet		Bristol-Myers Squibb
SQUIBB; 297	Engran	3 mg	Blue	Tablet		Bristol-Myers Squibb
SQUIBB; 297	Engran	5 mg	Blue	Tablet		Bristol-Myers Squibb
SQUIBB; 297	Engran	20 mg	Blue	Tablet		Bristol-Myers Squibb
SQUIBB; 297	Engran	45 mg	Blue	Tablet		Bristol-Myers Squibb
SQUIBB; 297	Engran	75 mg	Blue	Tablet		Bristol-Myers Squibb

IMPRINT	BRAND/GENERIC NAME	STRENGTH	COLOR	FORM	SHAPE	MANUFACTURER
SQUIBB; 297	Engran	100 mg	Blue	Tablet		Bristol-Myers Squibb
SQUIBB; 297	Engran	400 U	Blue	Tablet		Bristol-Myers Squibb
SQUIBB; 297	Engran	6000 U	Blue	Tablet		Bristol-Myers Squibb
SQUIBB; 300	Prazosin Hydrochloride	1 mg		Capsule		Bristol-Myers Squibb
SQUIBB; 334	Dumogram	0.008 mg		Tablet		Bristol-Myers Squibb
SQUIBB; 334	Dumogram	4 mg		Tablet		Bristol-Myers Squibb
SQUIBB; 357	Valadol	120 mg	Yellow	Chewable Tablet		Bristol-Myers Squibb
SQUIBB; 371	Digitoxin	0.1 mg		Tablet		Bristol-Myers Squibb
SQUIBB; 384	Dumone	0008 mg		Tablet		
SQUIBB; 384	Dumone	4 mg		Tablet		
SQUIBB; 400	Prazosin Hydrochloride	2 mg		Capsule		Bristol-Myers Squibb
SQUIBB; 433	Methyldopa	500 mg	White	Coated Tablet	Round	Bristol-Myers Squibb
SQUIBB; 447	Methyldopa	250 mg	White	Coated Tablet	Round	Bristol-Myers Squibb
SQUIBB; 455	Oragrafin Sodium	500 mg	Yellow	Capsule		
SQUIBB; 500	Prazosin Hydrochloride	5 mg		Capsule		Bristol-Myers Squibb
SQUIBB; 511	Kenacort	1 mg	White	Tablet	Scored	Bristol-Myers Squibb
SQUIBB; 538	Rautrax-N Modified	2 mg		Tablet		Bristol-Myers Squibb
SQUIBB; 538	Rautrax-N Modified	50 mg		Tablet		Bristol-Myers Squibb
SQUIBB; 538	Rautrax-N Modified	400 mg		Tablet		Bristol-Myers Squibb
SQUIBB; 539	Rautrax-N	4 mg		Tablet		Bristol-Myers Squibb
SQUIBB; 539	Rautrax-N	50 mg		Tablet		Bristol-Myers Squibb
SQUIBB; 539	Rautrax-N	400 mg		Tablet		Bristol-Myers Squibb
SQUIBB; 598	Neomycin Sulfate	350 mg		Tablet		Bristol-Myers Squibb
SQUIBB; 623	Noctec	250 mg	Red	Capsule		
SQUIBB; 626	Noctec	500 mg	Red	Capsule		
SQUIBB; 630	Methyldopa and Hydrochlorothiazide	15 mg	Red	Coated Tablet	Round	
SQUIBB; 630	Methyldopa and Hydrochlorothiazide	250 mg	Red	Coated Tablet	Round	
SQUIBB; 645	Methyldopa and Hydrochlorothiazide	25 mg	Pink	Coated Tablet	Round	
SQUIBB; 645	Methyldopa and Hydrochlorothiazide	250 mg	Pink	Coated Tablet	Round	
SQUIBB; 652	Methyldopa and Hydrochlorothiazide	30 mg	Red	Coated Tablet	Oval	
SQUIBB; 652	Methyldopa and Hydrochlorothiazide	500 mg	Red	Coated Tablet	Oval	
SQUIBB; 671	Methyldopa and Hydrochlorothiazide	50 mg	Pink	Coated Tablet	Oval	
SQUIBB; 671	Methyldopa and Hydrochlorothiazide	500 mg	Pink	Coated Tablet	Oval	
SQUIBB; 685	Rautrax	50 mg		Tablet		
SQUIBB; 685	Rautrax	400 mg		Tablet		
SQUIBB; 708	Rubraferate	4.2 mcg		Capsule		
SQUIBB; 708	Rubraferate	0.28 mg		Capsule		
SQUIBB; 708	Rubraferate	28 mg		Capsule		
SQUIBB; 708	Rubraferate	50 mg		Capsule		
SQUIBB; 713	Raudixin	50 mg	Red	Tablet		
SQUIBB; 718	Chlordiazepoxide Hydrochloride	5 mg	Carmel and Yellow	Capsule		
SQUIBB; 727	Chlordiazepoxide Hydrochloride	10 mg	Carmel and Black	Capsule		
SQUIBB; 736	Chlordiazepoxide Hydrochloride	25 mg	Carmel and White	Capsule		
SQUIBB; 767	Mysteclin-F 125	25 mg	Brown and Orange	Capsule		
SQUIBB; 767	Mysteclin-F 125	125 mg	Brown and Orange	Capsule		
SQUIBB; 776	Raudixin	100 mg	Red	Tablet		
SQUIBB; 779	Mysteclin-F 250	50 mg	Brown and Yellow	Capsule		
SQUIBB; 779	Mysteclin-F 250	250 mg	Brown and Yellow	Capsule		
SQUIBB; 780	Rau-Sed	0.25 mg		Tablet		
SQUIBB; 789	Rubrafolin	25 mcg		Capsule		
SQUIBB; 789	Rubrafolin	1.67 mg		Capsule		
SQUIBB; 802	Clorazepate Dipotassium	3.75 mg	White	Capsule		
SQUIBB; 802	Rubragran	100 mg		Capsule		
SQUIBB; 802	Rubragran	0.5 unit		Capsule		
SQUIBB; 829	Chlorothiazide	500 mg	White	Tablet	Compressed	
SQUIBB; 876	Trigesic	30 mg		Tablet		
SQUIBB; 876	Trigesic	125 mg		Tablet		
SQUIBB; 876	Trigesic	230 mg		Tablet		
SQUIBB; 887	Terfonyl	167 mg		Tablet		
SQUIBB; 917	Amitid	10 mg	Green	Tablet		Squibb
SQUIBB; 918	Amitid	25 mg	Pink	Tablet		Squibb
SQUIBB; 942	Amitid	50 mg	Purple-Red	Tablet		Squibb
SQUIBB; 943	Amitid	75 mg	Green	Tablet		Squibb
SQUIBB; 955	Amitid	100 mg	Purple-Red	Tablet		
SQUIBB; W; 110	Cefadroxil	500 mg		Capsule		Bristol-Myers Squibb
SQUIBB; W134	Lithium Carbonate	300 mg		Capsule		Bristol-Myers Squibb
SQUIBB; W460	Desipramine Hydrochloride	50 mg		Tablet		Bristol-Myers Squibb
SQUIBB; W470	Desipramine Hydrochloride	75 mg		Tablet		Bristol-Myers Squibb
STANBACK	Tablets	325 mg	White	Tablet	Round	Stanback
STOPAYNE; 819	Stopayne	30 mg	Blue and White	Capsule		
STOPAYNE; 819	Stopayne	357 mg	Blue and White	Capsule		
STUART	Sorbitrate with Phenobarbital	10 mg	Peach	Tablet		Zeneca Pharmaceuticals
STUART	Sorbitrate with Phenobarbital	15 mg	Peach	Tablet		Zeneca Pharmaceuticals
STUART; 680	Cari-Tab Softab	0.5 mg	Pink	Tablet		
STUART; 680	Cari-Tab Softab	75 mg	Pink	Tablet		
STUART; 680	Cari-Tab Softab	200 U	Pink	Tablet		
STUART; 680	Cari-Tab Softab	2000 U	Pink	Tablet		
SYNTEX; 1	Noriday 1 Plus 50	0.05 mg	White	Tablet		
SYNTEX; 1	Noriday 1 Plus 50	1 mg	White	Tablet		
SYNTEX; 2902	Anadrol	50 mg	White	Tablet	Scored	Roche Laboratories
SYNTEX; E-3	Evex	2.5 mg	Yellow	Tablet		
T	Aspirin Enteric Coated	325 mg	Orange	Delayed-Release Tablet	Round, Biconvex, Enteric-Coated	
T	Laxatyl	50 mg	Tan	Coated Tablet		
T	Laxatyl	60 mg	Tan	Coated Tablet		
T93	Isoniazid	100 mg		Tablet	Scored	Eli Lilly

IMPRINT	BRAND/GENERIC NAME	STRENGTH	COLOR	FORM	SHAPE	MANUFACTURER
TABLOID	Methedrine	5 mg	White	Tablet	Scored	Burroughs Wellcome
TCL; 224	Megaprin	15 grains	White	Tablet	Oval	Econolab
TECZEM; 5; 180	Teczem	5 mg	Gold	Sustained-Release Tablet		
TECZEM; 5; 180	Teczem	180 mg	Gold	Sustained-Release Tablet		
THEOBID; 130	Theobid Duracap JR.	130 mg	Clear with White Beads	Capsule		Ucb Pharma
THIS END UP; THEO-DUR SPRINKLE 50 MG	Theo-Dur Sprinkle	50 mg	White and Clear	Timed-Release Capsule		Key Pharmaceuticals
THIS END UP; THEO-DUR SPRINKLE 75 MG	Theo-Dur Sprinkle	75 mg	White and Clear	Timed-Release Capsule		Key Pharmaceuticals
THIS END UP; THEO-DUR SPRINKLE 125 MG	Theo-Dur Sprinkle	125 mg	White and Clear	Timed-Release Capsule		Key Pharmaceuticals
THIS END UP; THEO-DUR SPRINKLE 200 MG	Theo-Dur Sprinkle	200 mg	White and Clear	Timed-Release Capsule		Key Pharmaceuticals
TOLMETIN; 200	Tolmetin Sodium	200 mg	White	Tablet	Round, Scored	
TOLMETIN; 400	Tolmetin Sodium	400 mg	Orange	Capsule		
TOLMETIN; 600	Tolmetin Sodium	600 mg	Orange	Tablet	Football-Shaped, Scored	
TP; 407	Hydrochlorothiazide with Reserpine	0.125 mg		Tablet		
TP; 407	Hydrochlorothiazide with Reserpine	50 mg		Tablet		
TP; 816	Alermine	4 mg	Yellow	Tablet	Round	Reid-Rowell Pharmaceutical
TP; 826	Bendylate	25 mg	Pink and White	Capsule		Reid-Rowell Pharmaceutical
TP; 906	Reserpine	0.1 mg		Tablet		
TP; 908	Reserpine	0.25 mg		Tablet		
TP; 910	Reserpine	1.0 mg		Tablet		
TRIAD; UAD; 305	Triad	40 mg	White	Capsule		
TRIAD; UAD; 305	Triad	50 mg	White	Capsule		
TRIAD; UAD; 305	Triad	325 mg	White	Capsule		
TRIMEN	Banatil OD	0.02 mg	Green and Clear with White and Orange Beads	Extended-Release Capsule		
TRIMEN	Banatil OD	0.06 mg	Green and Clear with White and Orange Beads	Extended-Release Capsule		
TRIMEN	Banatil OD	0.3 mg	Green and Clear with White and Orange Beads	Extended-Release Capsule		
TRIMEN	Banatil OD	50 mg	Green and Clear with White and Orange Beads	Extended-Release Capsule		
TRITEC; STOMACH-SHAPED LOGO	Tritec	400 mg	Blue	Coated Tablet	Elongated Octagonal-Shaped	
TROFAN	Trofan	500 mg	Peach		Capsule-Shaped, Scored	Upsher-Smith Laboratories
TROFAN-DS 1GRAM	Trofan-DS	1 gram	Blue		Capsule-Shaped, Scored	Upsher-Smith Laboratories
TUTAG	Escot	100 mg	Red	Capsule		
TUTAG	Geritag	1 mcg	Magenta	Capsule		
TUTAG	Geritag	0.01 mg	Magenta	Capsule		
TUTAG	Geritag	0.15 mg	Magenta	Capsule		
TUTAG	Geritag	0.2 mg	Magenta	Capsule		
TUTAG	Geritag	0.3 mg	Magenta	Capsule		
TUTAG	Geritag	0.5 mg	Magenta	Capsule		
TUTAG	Geritag	1 mg	Magenta	Capsule		
TUTAG	Geritag	2 mg	Magenta	Capsule		
TUTAG	Geritag	3 mg	Magenta	Capsule		
TUTAG	Geritag	5 mg	Magenta	Capsule		
TUTAG	Geritag	10 mg	Magenta	Capsule		
TUTAG	Geritag	20 mg	Magenta	Capsule		
TUTAG	Geritag	30 mg	Magenta	Capsule		
TUTAG	Geritag	10 IU	Magenta	Capsule		
TUTAG	Geritag	400 U	Magenta	Capsule		
TUTAG	Geritag	5000 U	Magenta	Capsule		
TUTAG	Sorquad	40 mg	Ivory and Orange	Capsule		
TUTAG	Sprx-2	35 mg	Yellow and White Layered	Tablet		Solvay Pharmaceuticals
TUTAG	X-Otag Plus	50 mg	Yellow	Tablet		Reid-Rowell Pharmaceutical
TUTAG	X-Otag Plus	325 mg	Yellow	Tablet		Reid-Rowell Pharmaceutical
TYLENOL 80	Tylenol, Children's	80 mg	Pink Speckled	Chewable Tablet		Mcneil Consumer Products
TYLENOL; 500 MG	Tylenol Extra Strength	500 mg	Red and White	Capsule		Mcneil Consumer Products
U; 54	Acetaminophen	325 mg		Tablet	Compressed, Scored	Eli Lilly
U54	Acetaminophen	325 mg		Tablet	Compressed, Scored	Eli Lilly
UAD	Cezin	5 mg	Orange and White	Capsule		
UAD	Cezin	10 mg	Orange and White	Capsule		
UAD	Cezin	20 mg	Orange and White	Capsule		
UAD	Cezin	70 mg	Orange and White	Capsule		
UAD	Cezin	80 mg	Orange and White	Capsule		
UAD	Cezin	100 mg	Orange and White	Capsule		
UAD	Cezin	300 mg	Orange and White	Capsule		
UAD	EM-Stear	250 mg	Pink	Tablet		
UAD	U-Tet	250 mg	Yellow and Blue	Capsule		Uad Laboratories
UAD	Vaso-Pav	150 mg	Green and Clear	Capsule		
UAD	Vertab	25 mg	Blue	Capsule		Uad Laboratories
UAD	Vertab	50 mg	Blue	Capsule		Uad Laboratories

IMPRINT	BRAND/GENERIC NAME	STRENGTH	COLOR	FORM	SHAPE	MANUFACTURER
UAD; 113	Lorpac	5 mg	Off-White or Light Orange	Tablet	Oval, Scored	
UAD; 113	Lorpac	30 mg	Off-White or Light Orange	Tablet	Oval, Scored	
UAD; 113	Lorpac	150 mg	Off-White or Light Orange	Tablet	Oval, Scored	
UAD; 113	Lorpac	230 mg	Off-White or Light Orange	Tablet	Oval, Scored	
UAD; 403	Vertab	25 mg	Blue	Capsule		Uad Laboratories
UAD; 403	Vertab	50 mg	Blue	Capsule		Uad Laboratories
UAD; 2304	Dital	105 mg	Lavender and Clear	Extended-Release Capsule		
UPJ 62	Calderol	20 mcg		Capsule		Upjohn
UPJ 74	Calderol	50 mcg	Orange	Capsule		Upjohn
UPJOHN 77	Orthoxine Hydrochloride	100 mg	White	Tablet	Oval	Upjohn
UPJOHN 441	Methosarb	50 mg	White	Tablet		Upjohn
UPJOHN 586	Uticillin VK	250 mg	White	Tablet		Upjohn
UPJOHN 671	Uticillin VK	500 mg	White	Tablet		Upjohn
UPJOHN; 65	Reserpoid	0.25 mg	Tan	Tablet	Scored	Upjohn
USV	Chlor-PZ	50 mg	Dark Pink	Tablet		
USV	Dexameth	0.75 mg	White	Tablet		
USV	Histaspan-Plus	8 mg	Purple and Yellow	Capsule		
USV	Histaspan-Plus	20 mg	Purple and Yellow	Capsule		
USV	Hygroton	50 mg	Aqua	Tablet		
USV; 25	Chlor-PZ	25 mg	Dark Tan	Tablet		
V; 0185; 5573	Petn	80 mg		Timed-Release Capsule		Eon Labs
V3L	VI-Magna	1 mcg	Red	Capsule		Lederle Laboratories
V3L	VI-Magna	0.2 mg	Red	Capsule		Lederle Laboratories
V3L	VI-Magna	1 mg	Red	Capsule		Lederle Laboratories
V3L	VI-Magna	3 mg	Red	Capsule		Lederle Laboratories
V3L	VI-Magna	20 mg	Red	Capsule		Lederle Laboratories
V3L	VI-Magna	75 mg	Red	Capsule		Lederle Laboratories
V3L	VI-Magna	400 USP units	Red	Capsule		Lederle Laboratories
V3L	VI-Magna	5,000 USP units	Red	Capsule		Lederle Laboratories
VALRELEASE 15; ROCHE	Valrelease	15 mg	Yellow and Blue	Sustained-Release Capsule		
VL; 1555	Quinine and Aminophylline	195 mg		Tablet		Vangard Labs
VL; 1555	Quinine and Aminophylline	260 mg		Tablet		Vangard Labs
VT; 0185 0177	Thyroid	0.5 grain		Tablet		Eon Labs
VT; 0185; 0171	Thyroid	0.5 grain		Tablet		Eon Labs
VT; 1052	Theophylline	260 mg	Brown and Clear	Sustained-Release Capsule		Eon Labs
W (BEFORE 1982)	Atabrine	100 mg	Yellow	Tablet	Scored	Winthrop Pharmaceuticals
W A; 82 (AFTER 1982)	Atabrine	100 mg	Yellow	Tablet	Scored	Winthrop Pharmaceuticals
W C	Tederal Expectorant	8 mg		Tablet		Parke-Davis
W C	Tederal Expectorant	24 mg		Tablet		Parke-Davis
W C	Tederal Expectorant	100 mg		Tablet		Parke-Davis
W C	Tederal Expectorant	130 mg		Tablet		Parke-Davis
W/C; 240	Nicol	4 mg	Purple	Tablet		
W/C; 240	Nicol	30 mg	Purple	Tablet		
W/C; 240	Nicol	50 mg	Purple	Tablet		
W/C; 240	Nicol	200 mg	Purple	Tablet		
W; 400	Meprobamate	400 mg	White	Tablet		
W; J75	Isuprel	2 mg	White	Tablet	Scored	
W; J75	Isuprel	10 mg	White	Tablet	Scored	
W; J77	Isuprel	2 mg	White	Tablet	Scored	
W; J77	Isuprel	15 mg	White	Tablet	Scored	
W; T; 21	Talwin	50 mg	Peach	Tablet	Scored	
WA; X7C	Jenomycin	25 mg				
WA; X7C	Jenomycin	50 mg				
WALLACE; 37; 5701	Appetrol-SR	15 mg	Pink and Clear	Capsule		
WALLACE; 37; 5701	Appetrol-SR	300 mg	Pink and Clear	Capsule		
WALLACE; 37; 6301	Lostolic	0.1 mg	Yellow	Tablet	Round	
WALLACE; 37; 6301	Lostolic	15 mg	Yellow	Tablet	Round	
WALLACE; 37; 6301	Lostolic	25 mg	Yellow	Tablet	Round	
WALLACE; 37-1501	Meprotabs	400 mg	White	Tablet		
WALLACE; 37-3001	Deprol	1 mg	Pink	Tablet		Wallace Laboratories
WALLACE; 37-3001	Deprol	400 mg	Pink	Tablet		Wallace Laboratories
WALLACE; 37-5001	Milpath-400	25 mg	Yellow	Tablet	Scored	
WALLACE; 37-5001	Milpath-400	400 mg	Yellow	Tablet	Scored	
WALLACE; 37-5101	Milpath-200	25 mg	Yellow	Tablet		
WALLACE; 37-5101	Milpath-200	200 mg	Yellow	Tablet		
WALLACE; 37-5201	Miltrate-10	10 mg	White	Tablet		
WALLACE; 37-5201	Miltrate-10	200 mg	White	Tablet		
WALLACE; 37-8201; 200	Optimil-200	200 mg	Pink	Capsule		
WALLACE; 37-8301; 400	Optimil-400	400 mg	Pink and Blue	Capsule		
WALLACE; 330	Dainite	16 mg	Pink	Tablet	Round	
WALLACE; 330	Dainite	132 mg	Pink	Tablet	Round	
WALLACE; 330	Dainite	200 mg	Pink	Tablet	Round	
WALLACE; 340	Dainite-KI	16 mg	Yellow, Buff and Orange Mottled	Tablet	Round	
WALLACE; 340	Dainite-KI	160 mg	Yellow, Buff and Orange Mottled	Tablet	Round	
WALLACE; 340	Dainite-KI	200 mg	Yellow, Buff and Orange Mottled	Tablet	Round	
WALLACE; 340	Dainite-KI	325 mg	Yellow, Buff and Orange Mottled	Tablet	Round	
WALLACE; 873	Unitensen	2 mg	Off-White	Tablet	Round	
WALLACE; 1241	Avazyme	20,000 units	Yellow	Coated Tablet		
WALLACE; 1741	Avazyme 100	40,000 units	White	Enteric-Coated Tablet	Round	

IMPRINT	BRAND/GENERIC NAME	STRENGTH	COLOR	FORM	SHAPE	MANUFACTURER
WC	Tedral Expectorant	8 mg	White	Tablet		
WC	Tedral Expectorant	24 mg	White	Tablet		
WC	Tedral Expectorant	100 mg	White	Tablet		
WC	Tedral Expectorant	130 mg	White	Tablet		
WC; 230	Tedral	8 mg	White	Tablet		
WC; 230	Tedral	24 mg	White	Tablet		
WC; 230	Tedral	130 mg	White	Tablet		
WC; 231	Tedral SA	25 mg	Mottled Coral	Tablet		
WC; 231	Tedral SA	48 mg	Mottled Coral	Tablet		
WC; 231	Tedral SA	180 mg	Mottled Coral	Tablet		
WC; 238	Tedral-25	24 mg	Salmon and Pink	Tablet		
WC; 238	Tedral-25	25 mg	Salmon and Pink	Tablet		
WC; 238	Tedral-25	130 mg	Salmon and Pink	Tablet		
WC; 247	D-S-S	100 mg	Red	Capsule		Warner Chilcott
WC; 250	Proloid	0.25 grain	Gray	Tablet		
WC; 551	Oxazepam	15 mg	Yellow	Tablet	Round, Biconvex	Warner Chilcott
WELLCOME; L2A	Actidil	2.5 mg		Tablet		
WEST-WARD; 255	Butalbital with Apc	40 mg		Tablet		
WEST-WARD; 255	Butalbital with Apc	50 mg		Tablet		
WEST-WARD; 255	Butalbital with Apc	130 mg		Tablet		
WEST-WARD; 255	Butalbital with Apc	200 mg		Tablet		
WHITBY; 130	Theobid Duracap JR.	130 mg	Clear with White Beads	Capsule		Ucb Pharma
WKJ	Permitil Chronotab	1 mg	Yellow	Tablet		Schering
WPPH; 152	Methyldopa	250 mg	Yellow	Coated Tablet	Round	
WPPH; 157	Indomethacin ER	75 mg	Blue and Clear with Blue and White Pellets	Extended-Release Capsule		
WPPH; 159	Indomethacin	50 mg	Blue and White	Capsule		
WPPH; 172	Indomethacin	25 mg	Blue and White	Capsule		
WPPH; 174	Methyldopa	125 mg	Yellow	Coated Tablet	Round	
WPPH; 176	Methyldopa	500 mg	Yellow	Coated Tablet	Round	
WT; 4111	Efficin	676 mg	White to Pink	Tablet		
WT; 4111	Efficin	0.012 G	White to Pink	Tablet		
WT; 4111	Efficin	0.033 G	White to Pink	Tablet		
WT; 4111	Efficin	0.083 G	White to Pink	Tablet		
WYETH; 16	Purodigin	0.1 mg	Pink	Tablet	Scored	
WYETH; 30	Zactirin	75 mg	Green and Yellow	Tablet	Double-Layered	
WYETH; 30	Zactirin	325 mg	Green and Yellow	Tablet	Double-Layered	
WYETH; 114	Purodigin	0.2 mg	White	Tablet	Scored	
WYETH; 127	Purodigin	0.15 mg	Yellow	Tablet		
WYETH; 165	Bicillin	200,000 units	Pink	Tablet	Scored	
WYETH; 202	Sparine	10 mg	Green	Coated Tablet	Round	
WYETH; 225	Zactane	75 mg	Yellow	Tablet		
WYETH; 252	Proketazine	25 mg	Orange		Round	
WYETH; 253	Proketazine	50 mg	Pink		Round	
WYETH; 255	Penicillin G Potassium	125 mg	White	Tablet		
WYETH; 256	Penicillin G Potassium	156 mg	White	Tablet	Round	
WYETH; 266	Secobarbital Sodium	100 mg	Clear Orange	Capsule		
WYETH; 272	Penicillin G Potassium	250 mg		Tablet		
WYETH; 285	Pentobarbital Sodium	100 mg	Clear Yellow	Capsule		
WYETH; 311	A.P.C. with Codeine Phosphate	30 mg	White	Tablet	Round	
WYETH; 311	A.P.C. with Codeine Phosphate	150 mg	White	Tablet	Round	
WYETH; 311	A.P.C. with Codeine Phosphate	230 mg	White	Tablet	Round	
WYETH; 312	A.P.C. with Meperidine Hydrochloride	30 mg	Purple, Red and Pink	Tablet	Double Layered, Round	
WYETH; 312	A.P.C. with Meperidine Hydrochloride	150 mg	Purple, Red and Pink	Tablet	Double Layered, Round	
WYETH; 312	A.P.C. with Meperidine Hydrochloride	230 mg	Purple, Red and Pink	Tablet	Double Layered, Round	
WYETH; 325	Codeine Sulfate	15 mg	White	Tablet	Round	
WYETH; 326	Codeine Sulfate	30 mg	White	Tablet	Round	
WYETH; 327	Codeine Sulfate	60 mg	White	Tablet	Round	
WYETH; 433	Phenergan Compound	6.25 mg	Green and White	Tablet	Capsule-Shaped, Layered	
WYETH; 433	Phenergan Compound	60 mg	Green and White	Tablet	Capsule-Shaped, Layered	
WYETH; 400	Phenergan Compound	600 mg	Green and White	Tablet	Capsule-Shaped, Layered	
WYETH;177	Ethobral	30 mg	Green	Gelcap		Wyeth Laboratories
WYETH;177	Ethobral	50 mg	Green	Gelcap		Wyeth Laboratories
Z	Nytol	25 mg		Tablet		
Z	Nytol	50 mg	Blue	Tablet	Round, Scored	Block Drug
Z; 0.5 56	Lorazepam	0.5 mg	White	Tablet	Round	Zenith Goldline Pharmaceuticals
Z; 1.0 58	Lorazepam	1 mg	White	Tablet	Round	Zenith Goldline Pharmaceuticals
Z; 2.0 60	Lorazepam	2 mg	White	Tablet	Round	Zenith Goldline Pharmaceuticals
Z; 235	Meclizine Hydrochloride	25 mg		Tablet	Multilayered	Zenith Goldline Pharmaceuticals
Z; 2001	Acetaminophen	500 mg		Capsule		Zenith Goldline Pharmaceuticals
Z; 2005	Antacid	3.75 grains	White	Tablet		Zenith Goldline Pharmaceuticals
Z; 2005	Antacid	7.5 grains	White	Tablet		Zenith Goldline Pharmaceuticals
Z; 2006	Acetaminophen	5 grains	White	Tablet		Zenith Goldline Pharmaceuticals
Z; 2008	A.P.C. No. 2	32.4 mg	White	Tablet		Zenith Goldline Pharmaceuticals
Z; 2008	A.P.C. No. 2	162 mg	White	Tablet		Zenith Goldline Pharmaceuticals
Z; 2008	A.P.C. No. 2	227 mg	White	Tablet		Zenith Goldline Pharmaceuticals
Z; 2010	Aspirin	325 mg	White	Tablet		Zenith Goldline Pharmaceuticals
Z; 2013	Chlordiazepoxide Hydrochloride	5 mg	Light Green and Yellow	Capsule		Zenith Goldline Pharmaceuticals
Z; 2015	Chlordiazepoxide Hydrochloride	25 mg	Light Green and White	Capsule		Zenith Goldline Pharmaceuticals
Z; 2017	Ampicillin	250 mg	Maroon and Gray	Capsule		Zenith Goldline Pharmaceuticals
Z; 2022	B-Complex with C	5 mg	Green and Yellow	Capsule		Zenith Goldline Pharmaceuticals
Z; 2022	B-Complex with C	10 mg	Green and Yellow	Capsule		Zenith Goldline Pharmaceuticals
Z; 2022	B-Complex with C	15 mg	Green and Yellow	Capsule		Zenith Goldline Pharmaceuticals
Z; 2022	B-Complex with C	50 mg	Green and Yellow	Capsule		Zenith Goldline Pharmaceuticals
Z; 2022	B-Complex with C	300 mg	Green and Yellow	Capsule		Zenith Goldline Pharmaceuticals
Z; 2024	A.P.C.	32.4 mg	Pink	Capsule		Zenith Goldline Pharmaceuticals
Z; 2024	A.P.C.	162 mg	Pink	Capsule		Zenith Goldline Pharmaceuticals

IMPRINT	BRAND/GENERIC NAME	STRENGTH	COLOR	FORM	SHAPE	MANUFACTURER
Z; 2024	A.P.C.	227 mg	Pink	Capsule		Zenith Goldline Pharmaceuticals
Z; 2041	Colspan	0.014 mg	Red and Clear	Capsule		Zenith Goldline Pharmaceuticals
Z; 2041	Colspan	0.024 mg	Red and Clear	Capsule		Zenith Goldline Pharmaceuticals
Z; 2041	Colspan	0.122 mg	Red and Clear	Capsule		Zenith Goldline Pharmaceuticals
Z; 2041	Colspan	0.16 mg	Red and Clear	Capsule		Zenith Goldline Pharmaceuticals
Z; 2041	Colspan	1 mg	Red and Clear	Capsule		Zenith Goldline Pharmaceuticals
Z; 2041	Colspan	12.5 mg	Red and Clear	Capsule		Zenith Goldline Pharmaceuticals
Z; 2041	Colspan	50 mg	Red and Clear	Capsule		Zenith Goldline Pharmaceuticals
Z; 2042	Conjugated Estrogen	0.625 mg	White or Maroon	Coated Tablet	Round or Oval	Zenith Goldline Pharmaceuticals
Z; 2043	Cortisone Acetate	25 mg	White	Tablet		Zenith Goldline Pharmaceuticals
Z; 2045	Conjugated Estrogen	1.25 mg	White or Yellow	Coated Tablet	Round or Oval	Zenith Goldline Pharmaceuticals
Z; 2051	Dimenhydrinate	50 mg	Yellow	Tablet		Zenith Goldline Pharmaceuticals
Z; 2052	Chlorpromazine Hydrochloride	25 mg	Butterscotch Colored	Coated Tablet	Round	Zenith Goldline Pharmaceuticals
Z; 2053	Chlorpromazine Hydrochloride	50 mg	Butterscotch Colored	Coated Tablet	Round	Zenith Goldline Pharmaceuticals
Z; 2055	Diphenhydramine Hydrochloride	25 mg	Pink and Clear	Capsule		Zenith Goldline Pharmaceuticals
Z; 2056	Diphenhydramine Hydrochloride	50 mg	Pink and Clear or Pink	Capsule		Zenith Goldline Pharmaceuticals
Z; 2057	Diphenylhydantoin Sodium	100 mg	Clear	Capsule		Zenith Goldline Pharmaceuticals
Z; 2058	Digoxin	0.25 mg	White	Tablet	Round	Zenith Goldline Pharmaceuticals
Z; 2059	Digitoxin	0.2 mg	White	Tablet		Zenith Goldline Pharmaceuticals
Z; 2060	Extra Strength Pain Reliever Formula	1 grain	White	Tablet		Zenith Goldline Pharmaceuticals
Z; 2060	Extra Strength Pain Reliever Formula	1.5 grains	White	Tablet		Zenith Goldline Pharmaceuticals
Z; 2060	Extra Strength Pain Reliever Formula	2 grains	White	Tablet		Zenith Goldline Pharmaceuticals
Z; 2060	Extra Strength Pain Reliever Formula	3 grains	White	Tablet		Zenith Goldline Pharmaceuticals
Z; 2061	Digitoxin	0.1 mg	Pink	Tablet		Zenith Goldline Pharmaceuticals
Z; 2066	Ferrous Sulfate	150 mg	Red and Clear	Capsule		Zenith Goldline Pharmaceuticals
Z; 2067	Ferrous Sulfate	324 mg	Green	Coated Tablet		Zenith Goldline Pharmaceuticals
Z; 2073	Ampicillin	500 mg	Maroon and Gray	Capsule		Zenith Goldline Pharmaceuticals
Z; 2074	Ephedrine Sulfate	25 mg	Pink	Capsule		Zenith Goldline Pharmaceuticals
Z; 2076	Gelatin	10 grains	Pink	Capsule		Zenith Goldline Pharmaceuticals
Z; 2085	Digoxin	0.25 mg		Tablet		Zenith Goldline Pharmaceuticals
Z; 2086	Histex	4 mg	Yellow	Tablet		Zenith Goldline Pharmaceuticals
Z; 2087	Histex	8 mg	Green and Clear	Capsule		Zenith Goldline Pharmaceuticals
Z; 2088	Histex	12 mg	Green and Clear	Capsule		Zenith Goldline Pharmaceuticals
Z; 2093	Caffeine	250 mg	Brown and Clear	Capsule		Zenith Goldline Pharmaceuticals
Z; 2095	Isoniazid	100 mg	White	Tablet		Zenith Goldline Pharmaceuticals
Z; 2096	Chlorpheniramine Maleate with A.C.	2 mg	Red	Coated Tablet		Zenith Goldline Pharmaceuticals
Z; 2096	Chlorpheniramine Maleate with A.C.	30 mg	Red	Coated Tablet		Zenith Goldline Pharmaceuticals
Z; 2096	Chlorpheniramine Maleate with A.C.	390 mg	Red	Coated Tablet		Zenith Goldline Pharmaceuticals
Z; 2104	Methapyrilene with Scopolamine	0.2 mg	Yellow	Capsule		Zenith Goldline Pharmaceuticals
Z; 2104	Methapyrilene with Scopolamine	25 mg	Yellow	Capsule		Zenith Goldline Pharmaceuticals
Z; 2132	Zenex Compound	18 mg	Blue and White	Capsule		Zenith Goldline Pharmaceuticals
Z; 2132	Zenex Compound	325 mg	Blue and White	Capsule		Zenith Goldline Pharmaceuticals
Z; 2137	Pyridoxine	25 mg		Tablet		Zenith Goldline Pharmaceuticals
Z; 2144	Dexamethasone	0.75 mg	Light Green	Tablet		Zenith Goldline Pharmaceuticals
Z; 2147	Pentaerythritol Tetranitrate	10 mg	Green	Tablet		Zenith Goldline Pharmaceuticals
Z; 2150	Isosorbide Dinitrate	5 mg	Pink	Tablet	Round	Zenith Goldline Pharmaceuticals
Z; 2151	Isosorbide Dinitrate	10 mg	White	Tablet	Round	Zenith Goldline Pharmaceuticals
Z; 2152	Pseudoephedrine Hydrochloride	30 mg	Red	Tablet		
Z; 2153	Pseudoephedrine Hydrochloride	60 mg	White	Tablet		
Z; 2154	Isoniazid	300 mg	White	Tablet		Zenith Goldline Pharmaceuticals
Z; 2155	Prednisolone	5 mg	Orange and Peach	Tablet		Zenith Goldline Pharmaceuticals
Z; 2157	Prednisone	5 mg		Tablet		Zenith Goldline Pharmaceuticals
Z; 2160	Conjugated Estrogen	2.5 mg	White or Purple	Coated Tablet	Round or Oval	Zenith Goldline Pharmaceuticals
Z; 2161	Chlorpromazine Hydrochloride	10 mg	Butterscotch-Colored	Coated Tablet	Round	Zenith Goldline Pharmaceuticals
Z; 2164	Pyridoxine	50 mg		Tablet		Zenith Goldline Pharmaceuticals
Z; 2165	Pentaerythritol Tetranitrate	20 mg	Green	Tablet		Zenith Goldline Pharmaceuticals
Z; 2166	Hydroserpine No. 4	0.1 mg	Light Orange	Tablet		Zenith Goldline Pharmaceuticals
Z; 2166	Hydroserpine No. 4	50 mg	Light Orange	Tablet		Zenith Goldline Pharmaceuticals
Z; 2167	Hydroserpine No. 3	0.1 mg	Light Orange	Tablet		Zenith Goldline Pharmaceuticals
Z; 2167	Hydroserpine No. 3	25 mg	Light Orange	Tablet		Zenith Goldline Pharmaceuticals
Z; 2168	Hydroplus	0.125 mg	Green	Tablet	Round	
Z; 2168	Hydroplus	50 mg	Green	Tablet	Round	
Z; 2168	Hydroserpine No. 2	0.125 mg	Light Green	Tablet	Round	Zenith Goldline Pharmaceuticals
Z; 2168	Hydroserpine No. 2	50 mg	Light Green	Tablet	Round	Zenith Goldline Pharmaceuticals
Z; 2169	Hydroserpine No. 1	0.125 mg	Light Green	Tablet	Round	Zenith Goldline Pharmaceuticals
Z; 2169	Hydroserpine No. 1	25 mg	Light Green	Tablet	Round	Zenith Goldline Pharmaceuticals
Z; 2173	Propylthiouracil	50 mg	White	Tablet	Round	Zenith Goldline Pharmaceuticals
Z; 2176	Papaverine Hydrochloride	32.4 mg	White	Tablet		Zenith Goldline Pharmaceuticals
Z; 2177	Papaverine Hydrochloride	64.8 mg	White	Tablet		Zenith Goldline Pharmaceuticals
Z; 2178	Papaverine Hydrochloride	100 mg	White	Tablet		Zenith Goldline Pharmaceuticals
Z; 2179	Papaverine Hydrochloride	200 mg	White	Tablet		Zenith Goldline Pharmaceuticals
Z; 2180	Papaverine Hydrochloride	150 mg	Brown and Clear	Capsule		Zenith Goldline Pharmaceuticals
Z; 2185	Propoxyphene Hydrochloride	32 mg	Pink	Capsule		Zenith Goldline Pharmaceuticals
Z; 2191	Chlorpromazine Hydrochloride	100 mg	Butterscotch Colored	Coated Tablet	Round	Zenith Goldline Pharmaceuticals
Z; 2192	Chlorpromazine Hydrochloride	200 mg	Butterscotch Colored	Coated Tablet	Round	Zenith Goldline Pharmaceuticals
Z; 2195	Rauwolfia Serpentina	50 mg	Red and Orange	Coated Tablet		Zenith Goldline Pharmaceuticals
Z; 2196	Rauwolfia Serpentina	100 mg	Red and Orange	Coated Tablet		Zenith Goldline Pharmaceuticals
Z; 2198	Reserpine	0.1 mg	White	Tablet	Round	Zenith Goldline Pharmaceuticals
Z; 2199	Reserpine	0.25 mg	White	Tablet	Round	Zenith Goldline Pharmaceuticals

IMPRINT	BRAND/GENERIC NAME	STRENGTH	COLOR	FORM	SHAPE	MANUFACTURER
Z; 2201	Quinidine Sulfate	200 mg	White	Tablet	Round	Zenith Goldline Pharmaceuticals
Z; 2207	S.A.S.P.	500 mg	Rust	Tablet		Zenith Goldline Pharmaceuticals
Z; 2208	Sinus	22 mg	Pink	Tablet		Zenith Goldline Pharmaceuticals
Z; 2208	Sinus	25 mg	Pink	Tablet		Zenith Goldline Pharmaceuticals
Z; 2208	Sinus	150 mg	Pink	Tablet		Zenith Goldline Pharmaceuticals
Z; 2211	Sodium Liothyronine	25 mcg	White	Tablet		Zenith Goldline Pharmaceuticals
Z; 2212	Sodium Liothyronine	50 mcg	White	Tablet		Zenith Goldline Pharmaceuticals
Z; 2216	Prednisone	10 mg	White	Tablet		Zenith Goldline Pharmaceuticals
Z; 2217	Prednisone	20 mg	White	Tablet		Zenith Goldline Pharmaceuticals
Z; 2233	Thyroid	16.2 mg	White	Tablet		Zenith Goldline Pharmaceuticals
Z; 2234	Thyroid	32.4 mg	White	Tablet		Zenith Goldline Pharmaceuticals
Z; 2238	Thyroid	129.6 mg	White	Tablet		Zenith Goldline Pharmaceuticals
Z; 2239	Thyroid	324 mg	White	Tablet		Zenith Goldline Pharmaceuticals
Z; 2241	Triamcinolone	4 mg	White	Tablet		Zenith Goldline Pharmaceuticals
Z; 2242	Thyroid	64.8 mg	White	Tablet		Zenith Goldline Pharmaceuticals
Z; 2265	Cyanocobalamin	25 mcg		Tablet		Zenith Goldline Pharmaceuticals
Z; 2266	Cyanocobalamin	50 mcg	White	Tablet		Zenith Goldline Pharmaceuticals
Z; 2269	Ascorbic Acid	100 mg	White	Tablet		Zenith Goldline Pharmaceuticals
Z; 2270	Ascorbic Acid	250 mg	White	Tablet		Zenith Goldline Pharmaceuticals
Z; 2271	Ascorbic Acid	500 mg	White	Tablet		Zenith Goldline Pharmaceuticals
Z; 2282	Cyanocobalamin	100 mcg		Tablet		Zenith Goldline Pharmaceuticals
Z; 2310	Daily Vitamins	5 mcg	Red	Tablet		Zenith Goldline Pharmaceuticals
Z; 2310	Daily Vitamins	0.1 mg	Red	Tablet		Zenith Goldline Pharmaceuticals
Z; 2310	Daily Vitamins	1.5 mg	Red	Tablet		Zenith Goldline Pharmaceuticals
Z; 2310	Daily Vitamins	1.7 mg	Red	Tablet		Zenith Goldline Pharmaceuticals
Z; 2310	Daily Vitamins	2 mg	Red	Tablet		Zenith Goldline Pharmaceuticals
Z; 2310	Daily Vitamins	10 mg	Red	Tablet		Zenith Goldline Pharmaceuticals
Z; 2310	Daily Vitamins	20 mg	Red	Tablet		Zenith Goldline Pharmaceuticals
Z; 2310	Daily Vitamins	60 mg	Red	Tablet		Zenith Goldline Pharmaceuticals
Z; 2310	Daily Vitamins	400 USP units	Red	Tablet		Zenith Goldline Pharmaceuticals
Z; 2310	Daily Vitamins	5000 USP units	Red	Tablet		Zenith Goldline Pharmaceuticals
Z; 2320	Chewable Vitamin E	200 IU		Chewable Tablet		
Z; 2324	Chewvites Chewable Vitamins	5 mcg		Chewable Tablet		Zenith Goldline Pharmaceuticals
Z; 2324	Chewvites Chewable Vitamins	0.1 mg		Chewable Tablet		Zenith Goldline Pharmaceuticals
Z; 2324	Chewvites Chewable Vitamins	1.1 mg		Chewable Tablet		Zenith Goldline Pharmaceuticals
Z; 2324	Chewvites Chewable Vitamins	1.2 mg		Chewable Tablet		Zenith Goldline Pharmaceuticals
Z; 2324	Chewvites Chewable Vitamins	5 mg		Chewable Tablet		Zenith Goldline Pharmaceuticals
Z; 2324	Chewvites Chewable Vitamins	15 mg		Chewable Tablet		Zenith Goldline Pharmaceuticals
Z; 2324	Chewvites Chewable Vitamins	40 mg		Chewable Tablet		Zenith Goldline Pharmaceuticals
Z; 2324	Chewvites Chewable Vitamins	400 USP units		Chewable Tablet		Zenith Goldline Pharmaceuticals
Z; 2324	Chewvites Chewable Vitamins	3500 USP units		Chewable Tablet		Zenith Goldline Pharmaceuticals
Z; 2325	Chewvites Chewable Vitamins with Iron	5 mcg		Chewable Tablet		Zenith Goldline Pharmaceuticals
Z; 2325	Chewvites Chewable Vitamins with Iron	0.1 mg		Chewable Tablet		Zenith Goldline Pharmaceuticals
Z; 2325	Chewvites Chewable Vitamins with Iron	1.1 mg		Chewable Tablet		Zenith Goldline Pharmaceuticals
Z; 2325	Chewvites Chewable Vitamins with Iron	1.2 mg		Chewable Tablet		Zenith Goldline Pharmaceuticals
Z; 2325	Chewvites Chewable Vitamins with Iron	5 mg		Chewable Tablet		Zenith Goldline Pharmaceuticals
Z; 2325	Chewvites Chewable Vitamins with Iron	10 mg		Chewable Tablet		Zenith Goldline Pharmaceuticals
Z; 2325	Chewvites Chewable Vitamins with Iron	15 mg		Chewable Tablet		Zenith Goldline Pharmaceuticals
Z; 2325	Chewvites Chewable Vitamins with Iron	40 mg		Chewable Tablet		Zenith Goldline Pharmaceuticals
Z; 2325	Chewvites Chewable Vitamins with Iron	400 USP units		Chewable Tablet		Zenith Goldline Pharmaceuticals
Z; 2325	Chewvites Chewable Vitamins with Iron	3500 USP units		Chewable Tablet		Zenith Goldline Pharmaceuticals
Z; 2328	Promethazine Hydrochloride	12.5 mg	Gray	Tablet		Zenith Goldline Pharmaceuticals
Z; 2329	Promethazine Hydrochloride	25 mg	White	Tablet		Zenith Goldline Pharmaceuticals
Z; 2330	Promethazine Hydrochloride	50 mg	Pink	Tablet		Zenith Goldline Pharmaceuticals
Z; 2334	Hydralazide	15 mg	Orange	Tablet		Zenith Goldline Pharmaceuticals
Z; 2334	Hydralazide	25 mg	Orange	Tablet		Zenith Goldline Pharmaceuticals
Z; 2335	Hydroserpine Plus	0.1 mg	Off-White or Dark Salmon	Tablet	Round	
Z; 2335	Hydroserpine Plus	15 mg	Off-White or Dark Salmon	Tablet	Round	
Z; 2335	Hydroserpine Plus	25 mg	Off-White or Dark Salmon	Tablet	Round	
Z; 2337	Brompheniramine Maleate	4 mg	Peach	Tablet		Zenith Goldline Pharmaceuticals
Z; 2338	Hydralazine Hydrochloride	10 mg	Orange or Yellow	Tablet	Round	Zenith Goldline Pharmaceuticals
Z; 2339	Hydralazine Hydrochloride	25 mg	Orange or Blue	Tablet	Round	Zenith Goldline Pharmaceuticals
Z; 2341	Hydralazine Hydrochloride	100 mg	Peach	Tablet		Zenith Goldline Pharmaceuticals
Z; 2342	Isosorbide Dinitrate	2.5 mg	Yellow	Tablet	Round	Zenith Goldline Pharmaceuticals
Z; 2343	Isosorbide Dinitrate	5 mg	Pink	Tablet	Round	Zenith Goldline Pharmaceuticals
Z; 2344	Propantheline Bromide	15 mg	Light Peach	Tablet		Zenith Goldline Pharmaceuticals
Z; 2345	Procainamide Hydrochloride	250 mg	Yellow	Capsule		Udl Laboratories
Z; 2346	Procainamide Hydrochloride	375 mg	Orange and White	Capsule		Udl Laboratories
Z; 2347	Procainamide Hydrochloride	500 mg	Orange and Yellow	Capsule		Udl Laboratories
Z; 2349	Nylidrin	12 mg	White	Tablet	Round	Zenith Goldline Pharmaceuticals
Z; 2350	Meclizine Hydrochloride	25 mg	Yellow and White	Tablet	Oval, Double-Layered	Zenith Goldline Pharmaceuticals
Z; 2351	Isosorbide Dinitrate	40 mg	Blue and Clear	Capsule		Zenith Goldline Pharmaceuticals
Z; 2352	Brompheniramine Maleate	8 mg	Pink	Coated Tablet		Zenith Goldline Pharmaceuticals
Z; 2353	Brompheniramine Maleate	12 mg	Peach	Coated Tablet		Zenith Goldline Pharmaceuticals
Z; 2354	Bromapapp	4 mg	Sky Blue	Coated Tablet		Zenith Goldline Pharmaceuticals
Z; 2354	Bromapapp	5 mg	Sky Blue	Coated Tablet		Zenith Goldline Pharmaceuticals
Z; 2364	Methocarbamol	500 mg	White	Tablet	Round	Zenith Goldline Pharmaceuticals
Z; 2365	Methocarbamol	750 mg	White	Tablet	Capsule-Shaped	Zenith Goldline Pharmaceuticals
Z; 2384	Meclizine Hydrochloride	12.5 mg	Blue and White	Tablet	Oval, Double-Layered	Zenith Goldline Pharmaceuticals
Z; 2387	Isoxsuprine	10 mg	White	Tablet	Round	
Z; 2388	Isoxsuprine	20 mg	White	Tablet	Round	

IMPRINT	BRAND/GENERIC NAME	STRENGTH	COLOR	FORM	SHAPE	MANUFACTURER
Z; 2399	Chloramphenicol	500 mg	White	Capsule		Zenith Goldline Pharmaceuticals
Z; 2400	Chloramphenicol	50 mg	Two Tone	Capsule		Zenith Goldline Pharmaceuticals
Z; 2401	Chloramphenicol	100 mg	White	Capsule		Zenith Goldline Pharmaceuticals
Z; 2402	Chloramphenicol	250 mg	White	Capsule		Zenith Goldline Pharmaceuticals
Z; 2425	Potassium Penicillin G	100,000 units	White	Tablet		Zenith Goldline Pharmaceuticals
Z; 2426	Potassium Penicillin G	200,000 units	White	Tablet		Zenith Goldline Pharmaceuticals
Z; 2427	Potassium Penicillin G	250,000 units	White	Tablet		Zenith Goldline Pharmaceuticals
Z; 2428	Potassium Penicillin G	400,000 units	White	Tablet		Zenith Goldline Pharmaceuticals
Z; 2429	Potassium Penicillin G	500,000 units	White	Tablet		Zenith Goldline Pharmaceuticals
Z; 2430	Tetracycline Hydrochloride	250 mg	Blue and Yellow or Purple and Yellow	Capsule		Zenith Goldline Pharmaceuticals
Z; 2446	Potassium Phenoxymethyl Penicillin	250 mg	White	Tablet	Round	Zenith Goldline Pharmaceuticals
Z; 2448	Potassium Phenoxymethyl Penicillin	125 mg	White	Tablet	Round	Zenith Goldline Pharmaceuticals
Z; 2450	Potassium Phenoxymethyl Penicillin	250 mg	White	Tablet	Oval	Zenith Goldline Pharmaceuticals
Z; 2484	Triprolidine Hydrochloride with Pseudoephedrine Hydrochloride	2.5 mg		Tablet		Zenith Goldline Pharmaceuticals
Z; 2484	Triprolidine Hydrochloride with Pseudoephedrine Hydrochloride	60 mg		Tablet		Zenith Goldline Pharmaceuticals
Z; 2493	Hydralazine Hydrochloride	50 mg	Orange or Pink	Tablet	Round	Zenith Goldline Pharmaceuticals
Z; 2505	Dioctyl Sodium Sulfosuccinate Compound	30 mg		Capsule		Zenith Goldline Pharmaceuticals
Z; 2505	Dioctyl Sodium Sulfosuccinate Compound	100 mg		Capsule		Zenith Goldline Pharmaceuticals
Z; 2505	Dioctyl Sodium Sulfosuccinate Compound	400 mg		Capsule		Zenith Goldline Pharmaceuticals
Z; 2507	Reserpine with Hydroflumethiazide	0.125 mg	Green	Tablet	Round	Zenith Goldline Pharmaceuticals
Z; 2507	Reserpine with Hydroflumethiazide	50 mg	Green	Tablet	Round	Zenith Goldline Pharmaceuticals
Z; 2803	Tetracycline Hydrochloride	125 mg	Green and Yellow	Capsule		Zenith Goldline Pharmaceuticals
Z; 2805	Tetracycline Hydrochloride	50 mg	Blue	Capsule		Zenith Goldline Pharmaceuticals
Z; 2807	Tetracycline Hydrochloride	500 mg	Yellow and Black	Capsule		Zenith Goldline Pharmaceuticals
Z; 2810	Tetracycline Hydrochloride	100 mg	Orange	Capsule		Zenith Goldline Pharmaceuticals
Z; 2812	Chlorzoxazone with Acetaminophen	250 mg	Green	Tablet	Round	Zenith Goldline Pharmaceuticals
Z; 2812	Chlorzoxazone with Acetaminophen	300 mg	Green	Tablet	Round	Zenith Goldline Pharmaceuticals
Z; 2814	Cyclandelate	200 mg	Blue or Orange	Capsule		Zenith Goldline Pharmaceuticals
Z; 2815	Cyclandelate	400 mg	Green and White	Capsule		Zenith Goldline Pharmaceuticals
Z; 2816	Tetracycline Hydrochloride	250 mg	Orange and Yellow or Blue-Green and Yellow	Capsule		Zenith Goldline Pharmaceuticals
Z; 2819	Spironolactone with Hydrochlorothiazide	25 mg	White	Tablet	Round	Zenith Goldline Pharmaceuticals
Z; 2820	Ampicillin	125 mg	Gray and Yellow	Capsule		Zenith Goldline Pharmaceuticals
Z; 2821	Ampicillin	250 mg	Gray	Capsule		Zenith Goldline Pharmaceuticals
Z; 2822	Ampicillin	500 mg	Light Gray and Dark Gray	Capsule		Zenith Goldline Pharmaceuticals
Z; 2875	Sodium Pentobarbital	50 mg	Pink	Capsule		Zenith Goldline Pharmaceuticals
Z; 2902	Chlorpropamide	250 mg	Blue	Tablet	Round	Zenith Goldline Pharmaceuticals
Z; 2903	Spironolactone	25 mg	White	Tablet	Round	Zenith Goldline Pharmaceuticals
Z; 2933	M Dopazide	15 mg		Tablet		Zenith Goldline Pharmaceuticals
Z; 2933	M Dopazide	250 mg		Tablet		Zenith Goldline Pharmaceuticals
Z; 2935	Phenylbutazone Alk	100 mg		Capsule		Zenith Goldline Pharmaceuticals
Z; 2935	Phenylbutazone Alk	150 mg		Capsule		Zenith Goldline Pharmaceuticals
Z; 2936	Perphenazine with Amitriptyline Hydrochloride	2 mg	Blue	Coated Tablet	Round	Zenith Goldline Pharmaceuticals
Z; 2936	Perphenazine with Amitriptyline Hydrochloride	10 mg	Blue	Coated Tablet	Round	Zenith Goldline Pharmaceuticals
Z; 2937	Perphenazine with Amitriptyline Hydrochloride	2 mg	Orange	Coated Tablet	Round	Zenith Goldline Pharmaceuticals
Z; 2937	Perphenazine with Amitriptyline Hydrochloride	25 mg	Orange	Coated Tablet	Round	Zenith Goldline Pharmaceuticals
Z; 2938	Perphenazine with Amitriptyline Hydrochloride	4 mg	Salmon	Coated Tablet	Round	Zenith Goldline Pharmaceuticals
Z; 2938	Perphenazine with Amitriptyline Hydrochloride	10 mg	Salmon	Coated Tablet	Round	Zenith Goldline Pharmaceuticals
Z; 2939	M Dopazide	25 mg		Tablet		Zenith Goldline Pharmaceuticals
Z; 2939	M Dopazide	250 mg		Tablet		Zenith Goldline Pharmaceuticals
Z; 2939	Perphenazine with Amitriptyline Hydrochloride	4 mg	Yellow	Coated Tablet	Round	Zenith Goldline Pharmaceuticals
Z; 2939	Perphenazine with Amitriptyline Hydrochloride	25 mg	Yellow	Coated Tablet	Round	Zenith Goldline Pharmaceuticals
Z; 2945	Decontabs	5 mg	Pink with Red Flecks	Sustained-Release Tablet	Round	Zenith Goldline Pharmaceuticals
Z; 2945	Decontabs	10 mg	Pink with Red Flecks	Sustained-Release Tablet	Round	Zenith Goldline Pharmaceuticals
Z; 2945	Decontabs	15 mg	Pink with Red Flecks	Sustained-Release Tablet	Round	Zenith Goldline Pharmaceuticals
Z; 2945	Decontabs	40 mg	Pink with Red Flecks	Sustained-Release Tablet	Round	Zenith Goldline Pharmaceuticals
Z; 2953	M Dopazide	30 mg		Tablet		Zenith Goldline Pharmaceuticals
Z; 2953	M Dopazide	500 mg		Tablet		Zenith Goldline Pharmaceuticals
Z; 2954	M Dopazide	50 mg		Tablet		Zenith Goldline Pharmaceuticals
Z; 2954	M Dopazide	500 mg		Tablet		Zenith Goldline Pharmaceuticals
Z; 2958	Ergoloid Mesylates	0.5 mg	White	Tablet	Round	Zenith Goldline Pharmaceuticals
Z; 2958	Hydrogenated Ergot Alkaloids	0.5 mg		Tablet		Zenith Goldline Pharmaceuticals
Z; 2959	Hydrogenated Ergot Alkaloids	1 mg		Tablet		Zenith Goldline Pharmaceuticals
Z; 2962	Hydroxy Compound	10 mg	White	Tablet	Round	Zenith Goldline Pharmaceuticals
Z; 2962	Hydroxy Compound	25 mg	White	Tablet	Round	Zenith Goldline Pharmaceuticals
Z; 2962	Hydroxy Compound	130 mg	White	Tablet	Round	Zenith Goldline Pharmaceuticals

IMPRINT	BRAND/GENERIC NAME	STRENGTH	COLOR	FORM	SHAPE	MANUFACTURER
Z; 2963	Nitroglycerin	2.5 mg	Amethyst and Natural or Purple	Timed-Release Capsule		Zenith Goldline Pharmaceuticals
Z; 2964	Nitroglycerin	6.5 mg	Blue and Yellow	Timed-Release Capsule		Zenith Goldline Pharmaceuticals
Z; 2966	Isosorbide Dinitrate	40 mg		Timed-Release Tablet		Zenith Goldline Pharmaceuticals
Z; 2968	Erythromycin Estolate	250 mg		Capsule		Zenith Goldline Pharmaceuticals
Z; 2970	Sulfinpyrazone	100 mg	White	Tablet	Round	Zenith Goldline Pharmaceuticals
Z; 2972	Isosorbide Dinitrate	20 mg		Tablet		Zenith Goldline Pharmaceuticals
Z; 2973	Isosorbide Dinitrate	30 mg		Tablet		Zenith Goldline Pharmaceuticals
Z; 2976	Dipyridamole	50 mg	White	Coated Tablet	Round	Zenith Goldline Pharmaceuticals
Z; 2977	Dipyridamole	75 mg	White	Coated Tablet	Round	Zenith Goldline Pharmaceuticals
Z; 2981	Pro-Iso	5 mg	Yellow	Capsule		Zenith Goldline Pharmaceuticals
Z; 2981	Pro-Iso	10 mg	Yellow	Capsule		Zenith Goldline Pharmaceuticals
Z; 2982	Chlordiazepoxide Hydrochloride with Clidinium Bromide	2.5 mg	White	Capsule		Zenith Goldline Pharmaceuticals
Z; 2982	Chlordiazepoxide Hydrochloride with Clidinium Bromide	5 mg	White	Capsule		Zenith Goldline Pharmaceuticals
Z; 2987	Methyclothiazide	5 mg	Salmon Colored	Tablet	Round	Zenith Goldline Pharmaceuticals
Z; 2992	Dexbrom	6 mg	White	Coated Tablet	Round	Zenith Goldline Pharmaceuticals
Z; 2992	Dexbrom	120 mg	White	Coated Tablet	Round	Zenith Goldline Pharmaceuticals
Z; 2994	Dipyridamole	25 mg	White	Coated Tablet	Round	Zenith Goldline Pharmaceuticals
Z; 2996	Decongestant	12 mg		Sustained-Release Capsule		Zenith Goldline Pharmaceuticals
Z; 2996	Decongestant	75 mg		Sustained-Release Capsule		Zenith Goldline Pharmaceuticals
Z; 2997	Zendole	25 mg	White	Capsule		Zenith Goldline Pharmaceuticals
Z; 2998	Zendole	50 mg		Capsule		Zenith Goldline Pharmaceuticals
Z; 3006	Detuss	40 mg	White and Clear or White with Multi-Colored Seeds	Capsule		Zenith Goldline Pharmaceuticals
Z; 3006	Detuss	75 mg	White and Clear or White with Multi-Colored Seeds	Capsule		Zenith Goldline Pharmaceuticals
Z; 3606	Thioridazine Hydrochloride	10 mg	Orange	Coated Tablet	Round	Zenith Goldline Pharmaceuticals
Z; 3607	Thioridazine Hydrochloride	15 mg	Orange	Coated Tablet	Round	Zenith Goldline Pharmaceuticals
Z; 3608	Thioridazine Hydrochloride	25 mg	Orange	Coated Tablet	Round	Zenith Goldline Pharmaceuticals
Z; 3609	Thioridazine Hydrochloride	50 mg	Orange	Coated Tablet	Round	Zenith Goldline Pharmaceuticals
Z; 3610	Thioridazine Hydrochloride	100 mg	White	Coated Tablet	Round	Zenith Goldline Pharmaceuticals
Z; 3614	Propranolol Hydrochloride	10 mg	Orange	Tablet	Round	Zenith Goldline Pharmaceuticals
Z; 3615	Propranolol Hydrochloride	20 mg	Blue	Tablet	Round	Zenith Goldline Pharmaceuticals
Z; 3616	Propranolol Hydrochloride	40 mg	Green	Tablet	Round	Zenith Goldline Pharmaceuticals
Z; 3617	Propranolol Hydrochloride	80 mg	Yellow	Tablet	Round	Zenith Goldline Pharmaceuticals
Z; 3632	Hydralazine with Hydrochlorothiazide	50 mg	Ivory	Capsule		Zenith Goldline Pharmaceuticals
Z; 3633	Hydralazine with Hydrochlorothiazide	25 mg	Ivory	Capsule		Zenith Goldline Pharmaceuticals
Z; 3636	Conjugated Estrogen	0.3 mg	White	Coated Tablet	Round	Zenith Goldline Pharmaceuticals
Z; 3638	Propranolol Hydrochloride	60 mg	Red	Tablet	Round	Zenith Goldline Pharmaceuticals
Z; 3643	Nitroglycerin	9 mg	Green and Clear	Timed-Release Capsule		Zenith Goldline Pharmaceuticals
Z; 3655	Docusate-K Fecal Softener	100 mg	Pink	Capsule		Zenith Goldline Pharmaceuticals
Z; 3656	Docusate-K Plus Fecal Softener and Laxative	30 mg	Yellow	Capsule		Zenith Goldline Pharmaceuticals
Z; 3656	Docusate-K Plus Fecal Softener and Laxative	100 mg	Yellow	Capsule		Zenith Goldline Pharmaceuticals
Z; 3657	Chlorpropamide	100 mg	Blue	Tablet	Round	Zenith Goldline Pharmaceuticals
Z; 3671	Perphenazine with Amitriptyline Hydrochloride	4 mg	Orange	Coated Tablet	Round	Zenith Goldline Pharmaceuticals
Z; 3671	Perphenazine with Amitriptyline Hydrochloride	50 mg	Orange	Coated Tablet	Round	Zenith Goldline Pharmaceuticals
Z; 3730	T.C.M.	25 mg	Yellow	Coated Tablet	Round	Zenith Goldline Pharmaceuticals
Z; 3730	T.C.M.	200 mg	Yellow	Coated Tablet	Round	Zenith Goldline Pharmaceuticals
Z; 3731	T.C.M.	25 mg	Yellow	Tablet	Round	Zenith Goldline Pharmaceuticals
Z; 3731	T.C.M.	400 mg	Yellow	Tablet	Round	Zenith Goldline Pharmaceuticals
Z; 3741	Belladonna Alkaloids with Phenobarbital	0.0065 mg	White	Tablet		Zenith Goldline Pharmaceuticals
Z; 3741	Belladonna Alkaloids with Phenobarbital	0.0194 mg	White	Tablet		Zenith Goldline Pharmaceuticals
Z; 3741	Belladonna Alkaloids with Phenobarbital	0.1037 mg	White	Tablet		Zenith Goldline Pharmaceuticals
Z; 3741	Belladonna Alkaloids with Phenobarbital	16.2 mg	White	Tablet		Zenith Goldline Pharmaceuticals
Z; 3746	Aminophylline Compound	25 mg	Blue and Orange	Capsule		Zenith Goldline Pharmaceuticals
Z; 3746	Aminophylline Compound	130 mg	Blue and Orange	Capsule		Zenith Goldline Pharmaceuticals
Z; 3747	Azpan	8 mg (1/8 grain)	White	Tablet	Round	Zenith Goldline Pharmaceuticals
Z; 3747	Azpan	24 mg	White	Tablet	Round	Zenith Goldline Pharmaceuticals
Z; 3747	Azpan	130 mg	White	Tablet	Round	Zenith Goldline Pharmaceuticals
Z; 3747	Theophylline, Ephedrine Hydrochloride and Phenobarbital	8 mg	White	Tablet		Zenith Goldline Pharmaceuticals
Z; 3747	Theophylline, Ephedrine Hydrochloride and Phenobarbital	24 mg	White	Tablet		Zenith Goldline Pharmaceuticals
Z; 3747	Theophylline, Ephedrine Hydrochloride and Phenobarbital	130 mg	White	Tablet		Zenith Goldline Pharmaceuticals
Z; 3747	Theozine	10 mg		Tablet		Zenith Goldline Pharmaceuticals
Z; 3747	Theozine	25 mg		Tablet		Zenith Goldline Pharmaceuticals
Z; 3747	Theozine	130 mg		Tablet		Zenith Goldline Pharmaceuticals
Z; 3815	Dextroamphetamine Sulfate	10 mg	Brown and Clear	Capsule		Zenith Goldline Pharmaceuticals
Z; 3816	Dextroamphetamine Sulfate	15 mg	Brown and Clear	Capsule		Zenith Goldline Pharmaceuticals
Z; 3817	Dextroamphetamine Sulfate	15 mg	Red and Yellow	Capsule		Zenith Goldline Pharmaceuticals
Z; 3818	Pap with Codeine	16.2 mg	Black and Yellow	Capsule		Zenith Goldline Pharmaceuticals
Z; 3818	Pap with Codeine	162 mg	Black and Yellow	Capsule		Zenith Goldline Pharmaceuticals

IMPRINT	BRAND/GENERIC NAME	STRENGTH	COLOR	FORM	SHAPE	MANUFACTURER
Z; 3818	Pap with Codeine	194 mg	Black and Yellow	Capsule		Zenith Goldline Pharmaceuticals
Z; 3818	Sodium Pentobarbital	100 mg	Yellow	Capsule		Zenith Goldline Pharmaceuticals
Z; 3819	Pap with Codeine	16.2 mg	Black and Green	Capsule		Zenith Goldline Pharmaceuticals
Z; 3819	Pap with Codeine	32.4 mg	Black and Green	Capsule		Zenith Goldline Pharmaceuticals
Z; 3819	Pap with Codeine	162 mg	Black and Green	Capsule		Zenith Goldline Pharmaceuticals
Z; 3819	Pap with Codeine	194 mg	Black and Green	Capsule		Zenith Goldline Pharmaceuticals
Z; 3819	Sodium Secobarbital	100 mg	Orange	Capsule		Zenith Goldline Pharmaceuticals
Z; 3824	Phenobarbital	16.2 mg	White	Tablet		
Z; 3828	Chloral Hydrate	500 mg	Green	Capsule		Zenith Goldline Pharmaceuticals
Z; 3830	Dextroamphetamine Sulfate	5 mg	Yellow	Tablet		Zenith Goldline Pharmaceuticals
Z; 3836	Phenobarbital	32.4 mg	White	Tablet		
Z; 3839	Phenobarbital	100 mg	White	Tablet		
Z; 3842	Pap	16.2 mg	Black and White	Capsule		Zenith Goldline Pharmaceuticals
Z; 3842	Pap	162 mg	Black and White	Capsule		Zenith Goldline Pharmaceuticals
Z; 3842	Pap	194 mg	Black and White	Capsule		Zenith Goldline Pharmaceuticals
Z; 3845	Secobarbital with Amobarbital	50 mg	Orange and Blue	Capsule		Zenith Goldline Pharmaceuticals
Z; 3846	Secobarbital with Amobarbital	100 mg	Orange and Blue	Capsule		Zenith Goldline Pharmaceuticals
Z; 3876	Sodium Secobarbital	50 mg	Orange	Capsule		Zenith Goldline Pharmaceuticals
Z; 3891	A.P.C. with Butalbital	40 mg	White	Tablet		Zenith Goldline Pharmaceuticals
Z; 3891	A.P.C. with Butalbital	50 mg	White	Tablet		Zenith Goldline Pharmaceuticals
Z; 3891	A.P.C. with Butalbital	130 mg	White	Tablet		Zenith Goldline Pharmaceuticals
Z; 3891	A.P.C. with Butalbital	200 mg	White	Tablet		Zenith Goldline Pharmaceuticals
Z; 3897	Glutethimide	500 mg	White	Tablet	Scored	
Z; 3899	A.P.C. with Codeine No. 2	15 mg	White	Tablet		Zenith Goldline Pharmaceuticals
Z; 3899	A.P.C. with Codeine No. 2	30 mg	White	Tablet		Zenith Goldline Pharmaceuticals
Z; 3899	A.P.C. with Codeine No. 2	150 mg	White	Tablet		Zenith Goldline Pharmaceuticals
Z; 3899	A.P.C. with Codeine No. 2	230 mg	White	Tablet		Zenith Goldline Pharmaceuticals
Z; 3900	A.P.C. with Codeine No. 3	30 mg	White	Tablet		Zenith Goldline Pharmaceuticals
Z; 3900	A.P.C. with Codeine No. 3	150 mg	White	Tablet		Zenith Goldline Pharmaceuticals
Z; 3900	A.P.C. with Codeine No. 3	230 mg	White	Tablet		Zenith Goldline Pharmaceuticals
Z; 3904	Meprobamate	400 mg	White	Tablet	Round	Zenith Goldline Pharmaceuticals
Z; 3905	Meprobamate	200 mg	White	Tablet	Round	Zenith Goldline Pharmaceuticals
Z; 3907	A.P.C. with Codeine No. 4	30 mg	White	Tablet		Zenith Goldline Pharmaceuticals
Z; 3907	A.P.C. with Codeine No. 4	60 mg	White	Tablet		Zenith Goldline Pharmaceuticals
Z; 3907	A.P.C. with Codeine No. 4	150 mg	White	Tablet		Zenith Goldline Pharmaceuticals
Z; 3907	A.P.C. with Codeine No. 4	230 mg	White	Tablet		Zenith Goldline Pharmaceuticals
Z; 3910	Phendimetrazine Tartrate	35 mg	Yellow	Tablet		Zenith Goldline Pharmaceuticals
Z; 3914	Acetaminophen and Codeine No. 2	15 mg	White	Tablet		
Z; 3914	Acetaminophen and Codeine No. 2	300 mg	White	Tablet		
Z; 3915	Acetaminophen and Codeine No. 3	30 mg	White	Tablet	Round	
Z; 3915	Acetaminophen and Codeine No. 3	300 mg	White	Tablet	Round	
Z; 3916	Acetaminophen and Codeine No. 4	60 mg	White	Tablet	Round	
Z; 3916	Acetaminophen and Codeine No. 4	300 mg	White	Tablet	Round	
Z; 3917	Phendimetrazine Tartrate	100 mg	Brown and Clear	Capsule		Zenith Goldline Pharmaceuticals
Z; 3920	Pap with Codeine	16.2 mg	Green and White	Capsule		Zenith Goldline Pharmaceuticals
Z; 3920	Pap with Codeine	64.8 mg	Green and White	Capsule		Zenith Goldline Pharmaceuticals
Z; 3920	Pap with Codeine	162 mg	Green and White	Capsule		Zenith Goldline Pharmaceuticals
Z; 3920	Pap with Codeine	194 mg	Green and White	Capsule		Zenith Goldline Pharmaceuticals
Z; 3921	Phentermine Hydrochloride	30 mg	Yellow	Capsule		Zenith Goldline Pharmaceuticals
Z; 3921	Tora II	30 mg	Yellow Opaque	Capsule		Solvay Pharmaceuticals
Z; 3924	Meprobamate	600 mg	White	Tablet		Zenith Goldline Pharmaceuticals
Z; 3931	Phentermine Hydrochloride	30 mg	Brown and Clear	Capsule		Zenith Goldline Pharmaceuticals
Z; 3939	Mepro Compound	75 mg		Tablet	Three-Layered	Zenith Goldline Pharmaceuticals
Z; 3939	Mepro Compound	150 mg		Tablet	Three-Layered	Zenith Goldline Pharmaceuticals
Z; 3939	Mepro Compound	250 mg		Tablet	Three-Layered	Zenith Goldline Pharmaceuticals
Z; 3942	Phentermine Hydrochloride	30 mg	Blue and Clear	Capsule		Zenith Goldline Pharmaceuticals
Z; 3949	Phentermine Hydrochloride	30 mg	Black	Capsule		Zenith Goldline Pharmaceuticals
Z; 3961	Proxagesic Compound-65	32.4 mg	Gray and Red	Capsule		Reid-Rowell Pharmaceutical
Z; 3961	Proxagesic Compound-65	65 mg	Gray and Red	Capsule		Reid-Rowell Pharmaceutical
Z; 3961	Proxagesic Compound-65	162 mg	Gray and Red	Capsule		Reid-Rowell Pharmaceutical
Z; 3961	Proxagesic Compound-65	227 mg	Gray and Red	Capsule		Reid-Rowell Pharmaceutical
Z; 3965	Phentermine Hydrochloride	30 mg	Green and Clear	Capsule		Zenith Goldline Pharmaceuticals
Z; 3966	Diphenoxylate Hydrochloride with Atropine Sulfate	0.025 mg	White	Tablet	Round	Zenith Goldline Pharmaceuticals
Z; 3966	Diphenoxylate Hydrochloride with Atropine Sulfate	2.5 mg	White	Tablet	Round	Zenith Goldline Pharmaceuticals
Z; 3977	Chlordiazepoxide Hydrochloride	10 mg	Black and Green	Capsule		Zenith Goldline Pharmaceuticals
Z; 3991	Phentermine Hydrochloride	30 mg	Clear and Blue	Capsule		Zenith Goldline Pharmaceuticals
Z; 3993	Hepto	75 mg		Tablet		Zenith Goldline Pharmaceuticals
Z; 3993	Hepto	150 mg		Tablet		Zenith Goldline Pharmaceuticals
Z; 3993	Hepto	250 mg		Tablet		Zenith Goldline Pharmaceuticals
Z; 3994	Dihydrocodeine Compound	6.25 mg	Green and Red	Capsule		Zenith Goldline Pharmaceuticals
Z; 3994	Dihydrocodeine Compound	16 mg	Green and Red	Capsule		Zenith Goldline Pharmaceuticals
Z; 3994	Dihydrocodeine Compound	30 mg	Green and Red	Capsule		Zenith Goldline Pharmaceuticals
Z; 3994	Dihydrocodeine Compound	357 mg	Green and Red	Capsule		Zenith Goldline Pharmaceuticals
Z; 3996	Butalbital Compound	40 mg	White	Tablet	Round	Zenith Goldline Pharmaceuticals
Z; 3996	Butalbital Compound	50 mg	White	Tablet	Round	Zenith Goldline Pharmaceuticals
Z; 3996	Butalbital Compound	325 mg	White	Tablet	Round	Zenith Goldline Pharmaceuticals
Z; 4038	Phenylbutazone	100 mg	Blue	Capsule		Zenith Goldline Pharmaceuticals
Z; 4039	Ppa Compound	12 mg	Blue and Clear	Sustained-Release Capsule		Zenith Goldline Pharmaceuticals
Z; 4039	Ppa Compound	75 mg	Blue and Clear	Sustained-Release Capsule		Zenith Goldline Pharmaceuticals
Z; 4051	Disopyramide Phosphate	100 mg	Light Blue and Clear	Capsule		Zenith Goldline Pharmaceuticals
Z; 4052	Disopyramide Phosphate	150 mg	Dark Blue and Clear	Capsule		Zenith Goldline Pharmaceuticals
Z; 4063	Cephradine	250 mg	Maroon	Capsule		Zenith Goldline Pharmaceuticals

IMPRINT	BRAND/GENERIC NAME	STRENGTH	COLOR	FORM	SHAPE	MANUFACTURER
Z; 4064	Cephradine	500 mg	Pink	Capsule		Zenith Goldline Pharmaceuticals
Z; 4802	A.B.C. Compound with Codeine No. 3	30 mg	Flesh Colored	Capsule		Zenith Goldline Pharmaceuticals
Z; 4802	A.B.C. Compound with Codeine No. 3	40 mg	Flesh Colored	Capsule		Zenith Goldline Pharmaceuticals
Z; 4802	A.B.C. Compound with Codeine No. 3	50 mg	Flesh Colored	Capsule		Zenith Goldline Pharmaceuticals
Z; 4802	A.B.C. Compound with Codeine No. 3	325 mg	Flesh Colored	Capsule		Zenith Goldline Pharmaceuticals
Z; 4808	Hepto-M	200 mg	Green and White	Tablet	Round, Layered	Zenith Goldline Pharmaceuticals
Z; 4808	Hepto-M	325 mg	Green and White	Tablet	Round, Layered	Zenith Goldline Pharmaceuticals
Z; 4811	Propoxyphene Compound	32.4 mg	Red and Gray	Capsule		Zenith Goldline Pharmaceuticals
Z; 4811	Propoxyphene Compound	65 mg	Red and Gray	Capsule		Zenith Goldline Pharmaceuticals
Z; 4811	Propoxyphene Compound	389 mg	Red and Gray	Capsule		Zenith Goldline Pharmaceuticals
Z; 5600	Lorazepam	0.5 mg	White	Tablet	Round	Zenith Goldline Pharmaceuticals
Z; 5800	Lorazepam	1 mg	White	Tablet	Round	Zenith Goldline Pharmaceuticals
Z; 6000	Lorazepam	2 mg	White	Tablet	Round	Zenith Goldline Pharmaceuticals
Z; 6100	Hydroxyzine Hydrochloride	10 mg		Coated Tablet		Zenith Goldline Pharmaceuticals
Z; 6200	Hydroxyzine Hydrochloride	25 mg	Magenta	Coated Tablet	Round	Zenith Goldline Pharmaceuticals
Z; 6300	Hydroxyzine Hydrochloride	50 mg		Coated Tablet		Zenith Goldline Pharmaceuticals

Key to Controlled Substances Categories

Products listed with the symbols shown below are subject to the Controlled Substances Act of 1970. These drugs are categorized according to their potential for abuse. The greater the potential, the more severe the limitations on their prescription.

CATEGORY	INTERPRETATION
C-II	**HIGH POTENTIAL FOR ABUSE.** Use may lead to severe physical or psychological dependence. Prescriptions must be written in ink, or typewritten and signed by the practitioner. Verbal prescriptions must be confirmed in writing within 72 hours, and may be given only in a genuine emergency. No renewals are permitted.
C-III	**SOME POTENTIAL FOR ABUSE.** Use may lead to low-to-moderate physical dependence or high psychological dependence. Prescriptions may be oral or written. Up to 5 renewals are permitted within 6 months.
C-IV	**LOW POTENTIAL FOR ABUSE.** Use may lead to limited physical or psychological dependence. Prescriptions may be oral or written. Up to 5 renewals are permitted within 6 months.
C-V	**SUBJECT TO STATE AND LOCAL REGULATION.** Abuse potential is low; a prescription may not be required.

Key to FDA Use-in-Pregnancy Ratings

The U.S. Food and Drug Administration's use-in-pregnancy rating system weighs the degree to which available information has ruled out risk to the fetus against the drug's potential benefit to the patient. The ratings, and their interpretation, are as follows:

CATEGORY	INTERPRETATION
A	**CONTROLLED STUDIES SHOW NO RISK.** Adequate, well-controlled studies in pregnant women have failed to demonstrate a risk to the fetus in any trimester of pregnancy.
B	**NO EVIDENCE OF RISK IN HUMANS.** Adequate, well-controlled studies in pregnant women have not shown increased risk of fetal abnormalities despite adverse findings in animals, or, in the absence of adequate human studies, animal studies show no fetal risk. The chance of fetal harm is remote, but remains a possibility.
C	**RISK CANNOT BE RULED OUT.** Adequate, well-controlled human studies are lacking, and animal studies have shown a risk to the fetus or are lacking as well. There is a chance of fetal harm if the drug is administered during pregnancy; but the potential benefits may outweigh the potential risk.
D	**POSITIVE EVIDENCE OF RISK.** Studies in humans, or investigational or post-marketing data, have demonstrated fetal risk. Nevertheless, potential benefits from the use of the drug may outweigh the potential risk. For example, the drug may be acceptable if needed in a life-threatening situation or serious disease for which safer drugs cannot be used or are ineffective.
X	**CONTRAINDICATED IN PREGNANCY.** Studies in animals or humans, or investigational or post-marketing reports, have demonstrated positive evidence of fetal abnormalities or risk which clearly outweighs any possible benefit to the patient.

POISON CONTROL CENTERS

Across America there's now a single emergency phone number that automatically links callers with their regional poison control center. This new toll-free number, **800-222-1222**, is being used by every state with the exception of California, which has yet to implement the switch. A few local poison centers and the National Animal Poison Control Center (which appears at the end of the listings) are not part of this nationwide system and continue to use separate numbers.

Most of the centers listed below are certified by the American Association of Poison Control Centers. **Certified centers are marked by an asterisk after the name.** Each has to meet certain criteria. It must, for example, serve a large geographic area; it must be open 24 hours a day and provide direct-dial or toll-free access; it must be supervised by a medical director; and it must have registered pharmacists or nurses available to answer questions from the public.

Within each state, centers are listed alphabetically by city. Telephone numbers designated "TTY" are teletype lines for the hearing-impaired. "TDD" numbers reach a telecommunication device for the deaf.

ALABAMA

BIRMINGHAM

Regional Poison Control Center, The Children's Hospital of Alabama (*)

1600 7th Ave. South
Birmingham, AL 35233-1711
Emergency: 800-222-1222
Fax: 205-939-9245

TUSCALOOSA

Alabama Poison Center (*)

2503 Phoenix Dr.
Tuscaloosa, AL 35405
Business: 205-345-0600
Emergency: 800-222-1222
Fax: 205-343-7410

ALASKA

ANCHORAGE

Anchorage Poison Control Center, Providence Hospital

P.O. Box 196604
3200 Providence Dr.
Anchorage, AK 99519-6604
Business: 907-562-2211, ext. 3193
Emergency: 800-222-1222
Fax: 907-261-3684

(PORTLAND, OR)

Oregon Poison Center (*) Oregon Health Sciences University

3181 SW Sam Jackson Park Rd, CB550
Portland, OR 97201
Emergency: 800-222-1222
Fax: 503-494-4980

ARIZONA

PHOENIX

Samaritan Regional Poison Center (*) Good Samaritan Regional Medical Center

Ancillary 1
1111 East McDowell Rd.
Phoenix, AZ 85006
Business: 602-495-4884
Emergency: 800-222-1222
Fax: 602-256-7579

TUCSON

Arizona Poison and Drug Information Center (*) Arizona Health Sciences Center

1501 N. Campbell Ave.
Room 1156
Tucson, AZ 85724
Emergency: 800-222-1222
Fax: 520-626-2720

ARKANSAS

LITTLE ROCK

Arkansas Poison and Drug Information Center College of Pharmacy - UAMS

4301 West Markham St.
Mail Slot 522
Little Rock, AR 72205-7122
Business: 501-686-6161
Emergency: 800-222-1222
TDD/TTY: 800-641-3805

CALIFORNIA

FRESNO

California Poison Control System-Fresno/Madera (*) Valley Children's Hospital

9300 Valley Children's Place
MB 15
Madera, CA 93638-8762
Business: 559-353-3000
Emergency: 800-876-4766 (CA)
TDD/TTY: 800-972-3323

SACRAMENTO

California Poison Control System-Sacramento (*)

UCDMC-HSF Room 1024
2315 Stockton Blvd.
Sacramento, CA 95817
Business: 916-227-1400
Emergency: 800-876-4766 (CA)
TDD/TTY: 800-972-3323
Fax: 916-227-1414

SAN DIEGO

California Poison Control System-San Diego (*) UCSD Medical Center

200 West Arbor Dr.
San Diego, CA 92103-8925
Emergency: 800-876-4766 (CA)
TDD/TTY: 800-972-3323

SAN FRANCISCO

California Poison Control System-San Francisco (*)

UCSF Box 1369
1001 Potrero Ave., Room 1E86
San Francisco, CA 94143
Emergency: 800-876-4766 (CA)
TDD/TTY: 800-972-3323

COLORADO

DENVER

Rocky Mountain Poison and Drug Center (*)

1010 Yosemite Circle
Suite 200
Denver, CO 80230-6800
Business: 303-739-1100
Emergency: 800-222-1222
TTY: 303-739-1127 (CO)
Fax: 303-739-1119

CONNECTICUT

FARMINGTON

Connecticut Regional Poison Control Center (*) University of Connecticut Health Center

263 Farmington Ave.
Farmington, CT 06030-5365
Business: 860-679-3056
Emergency: 800-222-1222
TDD/TTY: 866-218-5372
Fax: 860-679-1623

DELAWARE

PHILADELPHIA, PA

The Poison Control Center of Philadelphia (*)

3535 Market St.
Suite 985
Philadelphia, PA 19104-3309
Business: 215-590-2003
Emergency: 800-222-1222
TDD/TTY: 215-590-8789
Fax: 215-590-4419

DISTRICT OF COLUMBIA

WASHINGTON, DC

National Capital Poison Center (*)

3201 New Mexico Ave., NW.
Suite 310
Washington, DC 20016
Business: 202-362-3867
Emergency: 800-222-1222
TTY: 202-362-8563
Fax: 202-362-8377

FLORIDA

JACKSONVILLE

Florida Poison Information Center-Jacksonville (*) SHANDS Jacksonville Medical Center

655 West 8th St.
Jacksonville, FL 32209
Emergency: 800-222-1222
TDD/TTY: 800-282-3171 (FL)
Fax: 904-244-4063

MIAMI

Florida Poison Information Center-Miami (*) University of Miami Department of Pediatrics Jackson Memorial Medical Center

P.O. Box 016960 (R-131)
Miami, FL 33101
Business: 305-585-5253
Emergency: 800-222-1222
Fax: 305-545-9762

TAMPA

Florida Poison Information Center-Tampa (*) Tampa General Hospital

P.O. Box 1289
Tampa, FL 33601
Emergency: 800-222-1222
Fax: 813-253-4443

GEORGIA

ATLANTA

Georgia Poison Center (*)
Hughes Spalding Children's Hospital, Grady Health System

80 Butler St., SE
P.O. Box 26066
Atlanta, GA 30335-3801
Emergency: 800-222-1222
TDD: 404-616-9287
Fax: 404-616-6657

HAWAII

HONOLULU

Hawaii Poison Center

1319 Punahou St.
Honolulu, HI 96826
Emergency: 800-222-1222
Fax: 808-535-7922

IDAHO

(DENVER, CO)

Rocky Mountain Poison & Drug Center (*)

1010 Yosemite Circle,
Suite 200
Denver, CO 80230-6800
Emergency: 800-222-1222
TTY: 303-739-1127 (ID)
Fax: 303-739-1119

ILLINOIS

CHICAGO

Illinois Poison Center (*)

222 South Riverside Plaza
Suite 1900
Chicago, IL 60606
Business: 312-906-6136
Emergency: 800-222-1222
TDD/TTY: 312-906-6185
Fax: 312-803-5400

INDIANA

INDIANAPOLIS

Indiana Poison Center (*)
Methodist Hospital
Clarian Health Partners

I-65 at 21st St.
P.O. Box 1367
Indianapolis, IN 46206-1367
Emergency: 800-222-1222
TTY: 317-962-2336
Fax: 317-962-2337

IOWA

SIOUX CITY

Iowa Statewide Poison Control Center
St. Luke's Regional Medical Center

2720 Stone Park Blvd.
Sioux City, IA 51104
Business: 712-279-3710
Emergency: 800-222-1222
Fax: 712-234-8775

KANSAS

KANSAS CITY

Mid-America Poison Control Center, University of Kansas Medical Center

3901 Rainbow Blvd.
Room B-400
Kansas City, KS 66160-7231
Business & 913-588-6638
Emergency: 800-222-1222
TDD: 913-588-6639
Fax: 913-588-2350

TOPEKA

Stormont-Vail Regional Medical Center
Poison Control Center

1500 S.W. 10th
Topeka, KS 66604-1353
Business: 785-354-6106
Emergency: 800-222-1222
800-332-6633 (KS)
Fax: 785-354-5004

KENTUCKY

LOUISVILLE

Kentucky Regional Poison Center (*)

Medical Towers South
Suite 572
234 East Gray St.
Louisville, KY 40202
Business: 502-629-7264
Emergency: 800-222-1222
502-589-8222
Fax: 502-629-7277

LOUISIANA

MONROE

Louisiana Drug and Poison Information Center (*)
University of Louisiana at Monroe College of Pharmacy

Sugar Hall
Monroe, LA 71209-6430
Business: 318-342-1710
Emergency: 800 222 1222
Fax: 318-342-1744

MAINE

PORTLAND

Maine Poison Center
Maine Medical Center

22 Bramhall St.
Portland, ME 04102
Emergency: 800-222-1222
TDD/TTY: 207-871-2879
877-299-4447 (ME)
Fax: 207-871-6226

MARYLAND

BALTIMORE

Maryland Poison Center (*)
University of Maryland at Baltimore
School of Pharmacy

20 North Pine St., PH 772
Baltimore, MD 21201
Business: 410-706-7604
Emergency: 800-222-1222
TDD: 410-706-1858
Fax: 410-706-7184

MASSACHUSETTS

BOSTON

Regional Center for Poison Control and Prevention (*)

300 Longwood Ave.
Boston, MA 02115
Emergency: 800-222-1222
TDD/TTY: 888-244-5313
Fax: 617-738-0032

MICHIGAN

DETROIT

Regional Poison Control Center (*)
Children's Hospital of Michigan

4160 John R. Harper
Professional Office Bldg.
Suite 616
Detroit, MI 48201
Business: 313-745-5335
Emergency: 800-222-1222
TDD/TTY: 800-356-3232
Fax: 313-745-5493

GRAND RAPIDS

DeVos Children's Hospital Regional Poison Center (*)

100 Michigan St., NE
Grand Rapids, MI 49503
Business: 616-774-7851
Emergency: 800-222-1222
TDD/TTY: 800-356-3232
Fax: 616-774-7204

MINNESOTA

MINNEAPOLIS

Hennepin Regional Poison Center (*) Hennepin County Medical Center

701 Park Ave.
Minneapolis, MN 55415
Business: 612-347-3144
Emergency: 800-222-1222
TTY: 612-904-4691
Fax: 612-904-4289

MISSISSIPPI

HATTIESBURG

Poison Center, Forrest General Hospital

P. O. Box 16389
400 South 28th Ave.
Hattiesburg, MS 39404
Emergency: 601-288-2199
Fax: 601-288-2125

JACKSON

Mississippi Regional Poison Control Center, University of Mississippi Medical Center

2500 North State St.
Jackson, MS 39216
Business: 601-984-1675
Emergency: 800-222-1222
Fax: 601-984-1676

MISSOURI

ST. LOUIS

Cardinal Glennon Children's Hospital Regional Poison Center (*)

1465 South Grand Blvd.
St. Louis, MO 63104
Emergency: 800-222-1222
TTY: 314-577-5336
Fax: 314-577-5355

MONTANA

(DENVER, CO)

Rocky Mountain Poison and Drug Center (*)

1010 Yosemite Circle
Suite 200
Denver, CO 80230-6800
Emergency: 800-222-1222
Fax: 303-739-1119

NEBRASKA

OMAHA

The Poison Center (*)
Children's Hospital

8200 Dodge St.
Omaha, NE 68114
Emergency: 800-222-1222

NEVADA

(DENVER, CO)

Rocky Mountain Poison and Drug Center (*)

1010 Yosemite Circle
Suite 200
Denver, CO 80230-6800
Emergency: 800-222-1222
Fax: 303-739-1119

NEW HAMPSHIRE

LEBANON

New Hampshire Poison Information Center, Dartmouth-Hitchcock Medical Center

1 Medical Center Dr.
Lebanon, NH 03756
Emergency: 800-222-1222
Fax: 603-650-8986

NEW JERSEY

NEWARK

New Jersey Poison Information and Education System (*)

201 Lyons Ave.
Newark, NJ 07112
Business: 973-926-7443
Emergency: 800-222-1222
TDD/TTY: 973-926-8008
Fax: 973-926-0013

NEW MEXICO

ALBUQUERQUE

New Mexico Poison and Drug Information Center (*)
University of New Mexico

Health Science Center Library, Room 130
Albuquerque, NM 87131-1076
Emergency: 800-222-1222
Fax: 505-272-5892

NEW YORK

BUFFALO

Western New York Regional Poison Control Center (*)
Children's Hospital of Buffalo

219 Bryant St.
Buffalo, NY 14222
Business: 716-878-7657
Emergency: 800-222-1222

MINEOLA

Long Island Regional Poison and Drug Information Center (*)
Winthrop University Hospital

259 First St.
Mineola, NY 11501
Emergency: 800-222-1222
TDD: 516-747-3323 (Nassau)
516-924-8811 (Suffolk)
Fax: 516-739-2070

NEW YORK CITY

New York City Poison Control Center (*)
NYC Dept. of Health

455 First Ave., Room 123
New York, NY 10016
Business: 212-447-8152
Emergency: 800-222-1222
(English) 212-340-4494
212-POISONS
(212-764-7667)

Emergency: 212-VENENOS
(Spanish) (212-836-3667)
TDD: 212-689-9014
Fax: 212-447-8223

ROCHESTER

Finger Lakes Regional Poison and Drug Information Center (*)
University of Rochester Medical Center

601 Elmwood Ave.
Box 321
Rochester, NY 14642
Business: 716-273-4155
Emergency: 800-222-1222
TTY: 716-273-3854
Fax: 716-244-1677

SLEEPY HOLLOW

Hudson Valley Regional Poison Center, Phelps Memorial Hospital Center

701 N. Broadway
Sleepy Hollow, NY 10591
Emergency: 914-366-3030
800-222-1222
Fax: 914-366-1400

SYRACUSE

Central New York Poison Center (*)
SUNY Health Science Center

750 East Adams St.
Syracuse, NY 13210
Business: 315-464-7078
Emergency: 800-222-1222
Fax: 315-464-7077

NORTH CAROLINA

CHARLOTTE

Carolinas Poison Center (*)
Carolinas Medical Center

5000 Airport Center Pkwy.
Suite B
Charlotte, NC 28208
Business: 704-395-3795
Emergency: 800-222-1222

NORTH DAKOTA

FARGO

North Dakota Poison Information Center, Meritcare Medical Center

720 4th St. North
Fargo, ND 58122
Business: 701-234-6062
Emergency: 800-222-1222
Fax: 701-234-5090

OHIO

CINCINNATI

Cincinnati Drug and Poison Information Center (*)
Regional Poison Control System

3333 Burnet Ave.
Vernon Place, 3rd Floor
Cincinnati, OH 45229
Emergency: 513-558-5111
800-222-1222
TDD/TTY: 800-253-7955
Fax: 513-636-5069

CLEVELAND

Greater Cleveland Poison Control Center

11100 Euclid Ave.
Cleveland, OH 44106-6010
Emergency: 216-231-4455
800-222-1222
Fax: 216-844-3242

COLUMBUS

Central Ohio Poison Center (*)

700 Children's Dr.
Room L032
Columbus, OH 43205-2696
Business: 614-722-2635
Emergency: 614-228-1323
800-222-1222
937-222-2227
(Dayton Region)
TTY: 614-228-2272
Fax: 614-228-2672

TOLEDO

Poison Information Center of Northwest Ohio
Medical College of Ohio Hospital

3000 Arlington Ave.
Toledo, OH 43614
Emergency: 419-383-3897
800-222-1222
Fax: 419-383-6066

OKLAHOMA

OKLAHOMA CITY

Oklahoma Poison Control Center,
University of Oklahoma

940 Northeast 13th St.
Room 3512
Oklahoma City, OK 73104
Business: 405-271-5062
Emergency: 800-222-1222
TDD: 405-271-1122
Fax: 405-271-1816

OREGON

PORTLAND

Oregon Poison Center (*)
Oregon Health Sciences University

3181 S.W. Sam Jackson Park Rd.
CB 550
Portland, OR 97201
Emergency: 800-222-1222
Fax: 503-494-4980

PENNSYLVANIA

HERSHEY

Central Pennsylvania Poison Center (*)
Pennsylvania State University
Milton S. Hershey Medical Center

500 University Dr.
MC H043, P.O. Box 850
Hershey, PA 17033-0850
Emergency: 800-222-1222
717-531-6111
TTY: 717-531-8335
Fax: 717-531-6932

PHILADELPHIA

The Poison Control Center (*)

3535 Market St., Suite 985
Philadelphia, PA 19104-3309
Business: 215-590-2003
Emergency: 800-222-1222
TDD/TTY: 215-590-8789
Fax: 215-590-4419

PITTSBURGH

Pittsburgh Poison Center (*)
Children's Hospital of Pittsburgh

3705 Fifth Ave.
Pittsburgh, PA 15213
Business: 412-692-5600
Emergency: 800-222-1222
Fax: 412-692-7497

PUERTO RICO

SANTURCE

San Jorge Children's Hospital Poison Center

258 San Jorge St.
Santurce, PR 00912
Emergency: 787-726-5674

RHODE ISLAND

(BOSTON, MA)

Regional Center for Poison Control and Prevention (*)

300 Longwood Ave.
Boston, MA 02115
Emergency: 800-222-1222
TDD/TTY: 888-244-5313
Fax: 617-738-0032

SOUTH CAROLINA

COLUMBIA

Palmetto Poison Center, College of Pharmacy, University of South Carolina

Columbia, SC 29208
Business: 803-777-7909
Emergency: 800-222-1222
Fax: 803-777-6127

SOUTH DAKOTA

(FARGO, ND)

North Dakota Poison Information Center
Meritcare Medical Center

720 4th St. North
Fargo, ND 58122
Business: 701-234-6062
Emergency: 701-234-5575
800-732-2200
(SD, MN, ND)
Fax: 701-234-5090

(MINNEAPOLIS, MN)

Hennepin Regional Poison Center (*) Hennepin County Medical Center

701 Park Ave.
Minneapolis, MN 55415
Business: 612-347-3144
Emergency: 800-222-1222
TTY: 612-904-4691
Fax: 612-904-4289

TENNESSEE

MEMPHIS

Southern Poison Center University of Tennessee

875 Monroe Ave.
Suite 104
Memphis, TN 38163
Business: 901-448-6800
Emergency: 800-222-1222
Fax: 901-448-5419

NASHVILLE

Middle Tennessee Poison Center (*)

1161 21st Ave. South
501 Oxford House
Nashville, TN 37232-4632
Business: 615-936-0760
Emergency: 800-222-1222
TDD: 615-936-2047
Fax: 615-936-0756

TEXAS

AMARILLO

Texas Panhandle Poison Center Northwest Texas Hospital

1501 S. Coulter Dr.
Amarillo, TX 79106
Emergency: 800-222-1222

DALLAS

North Texas Poison Center (*) Texas Poison Center Network Parkland Health and Hospital System

5201 Harry Hines Blvd.
P.O. Box 35926
Dallas, TX 75235
Business: 214-589-0911
Emergency: 800-222-1222
Fax: 214-590-5008

EL PASO

West Texas Regional Poison Center (*) Thomason Hospital

4815 Alameda Ave.
El Paso, TX 79905
Business 915-534-3800
Emergency: 800-222-1222

GALVESTON

Southeast Texas Poison Center (*) The University of Texas Medical Branch

3112 Trauma Bldg.
301 University Ave.
Galveston, TX 77555-1175
Business: 409-766-4403
Emergency: 800-222-1222
TDD/TTY: 800-764-7661 (TX)
Fax: 409-772-3917

SAN ANTONIO

South Texas Poison Center (*) The University of Texas Health Science Center–San Antonio

7703 Floyd Curl Dr., MC 7849
San Antonio, TX 78229-3900
Emergency: 800-222-1222
TDD/TTY: 800-764-7661 (TX)
Fax: 210-567-5718

TEMPLE

Central Texas Poison Center (*) Scott & White Memorial Hospital

2401 South 31st St.
Temple, TX 76508
Emergency: 800-222-1222
Fax: 254-724-1731

UTAH

SALT LAKE CITY

Utah Poison Control Center (*)

410 Chipeta Way
Suite 230
Salt Lake City, UT 84108
Emergency: 800-222-1222
Fax: 801-581-4199

VERMONT

BURLINGTON

Vermont Poison Center, Fletcher Allen Health Care

111 Colchester Ave.
Burlington, VT 05401
Business: 802-847-2721
Emergency: 800-222-1222
Fax: 802-847-4802

VIRGINIA

CHARLOTTESVILLE

Blue Ridge Poison Center (*) University of Virginia Health System

PO Box 800774
Charlottesville, VA 22908-0774
Emergency: 800-222-1222
Fax: 804-971-8657

RICHMOND

Virginia Poison Center (*) Virginia Commonwealth University

P.O. Box 980522
Richmond, VA 23298-0522
Emergency: 800-222-1222
TDD/TTY: 800-828-1120
Fax: 804-828-5291

WASHINGTON

SEATTLE

Washington Poison Center (*)

155 NE 100th St.
Suite 400
Seattle, WA 98125-8012
Business: 206-517-2351
Emergency: 800-222-1222
TDD: 800-572-0638 (WA)
206-517-2394
Fax: 206-526-8490

WEST VIRGINIA

CHARLESTON

West Virginia Poison Center (*)

3110 MacCorkle Ave. SE
Charleston, WV 25304
Business: 304-347-1212
Emergency: 800-222-1222
Fax: 304-348-9560

WISCONSIN

MADISON

Poison Control Center, University of Wisconsin Hospital and Clinics

600 Highland Ave.
F6-133
Madison, WI 53792
Emergency: 800-815-8855

MILWAUKEE

Children's Hospital of Wisconsin Poison Center

9000 W. Wisconsin Ave.
P.O. Box 1997, Mail Station 677A
Milwaukee, WI 53201-1997
Business: 414-266-2000
Emergency: 800-222-1222
TDD/TTY: 414-266-2542
Fax: 414-266-2820

WYOMING

(OMAHA, NE)

The Poison Center (*) Children's Hospital

8301 Dodge St.
Omaha, NE 68114
Emergency: 800-222-1222

ASPCA/NATIONAL ANIMAL POISON CONTROL CENTER

1717 South Philo Rd.
Suite 36
Urbana, IL 61802
Business: 217-337-5030
Emergency: 888-426-4435
900-680-0000
Fax: 217-337-0599

DRUG INFORMATION CENTERS

ALABAMA

BIRMINGHAM

Drug Information Service
University of Alabama Hospital
619 S. 20th St.
1720 Jefferson Tower
Birmingham, AL 35249-6860
Mon.-Fri. 8 AM-5 PM
205-934-2162
Fax: 205-934-3501
www.health.uab.edu/pharmacy

Global Drug Information Center
Samford University McWhorter School of Pharmacy
800 Lakeshore Dr.
Birmingham, AL 35229-7027
Mon.-Fri. 8 AM-4:30 PM
205-726-2659
Fax: 205-726-4012
samford. edu.schools/pharmacy/dic/index.html

HUNTSVILLE

Huntsville Hospital Drug Information Center
101 Sivley Rd.
Huntsville, AL 35801
Mon.-Fri. 8 AM-5 PM
256-517-8288
Fax: 256-517-6558

ARIZONA

TUCSON

Arizona Poison and Drug Information Center
Arizona Health Sciences Center
University Medical Center
1501 N. Campbell Ave.
Room 1156
Tucson, AZ 85724
7 days/week, 24 hours
520-626-6016
800-362-0101 (AZ)
Fax: 520-626-2720
www.pharmacy.arizona.edu

ARKANSAS

LITTLE ROCK

Arkansas Poison and Drug Information Center
4301 West Markham St.,
Slot 522-2
Little Rock, AK 72205
7 days/week, 24 hours
501-686-5540 (drug information for healthcare professionals only)
800-228-1233 (AK Only – drug information for healthcare professionals only)
800-376-4766 (AK Only – poison center for general public)
Fax: 501-686-7357

CALIFORNIA

LOS ANGELES

Los Angeles Regional Drug Information Center
LAC & USC Medical Center
1200 N. State St.
Room 2218
Los Angeles, CA 90033
Mon.-Fri. 8 AM-4:30 PM
323-226-7741
Fax: 323-226-4194

MARTINEZ

Drug Information Service
VA Northern California Health Care System
Pharmacy Service 119
150 Muir Rd.
Martinez, CA 94553
Mon.-Fri. 8 PM-4:30 PM
925-372-2167
Fax: 925-372-2169
cherie.dillon@med.va.gov

SAN DIEGO

Drug Information Center
U.S. Naval Hospital
34800 Bob Wilson Dr.
San Diego, CA 92134-5000
Mon.-Fri. 8 AM-4 PM
619-532-8417
Fax: 619-352-5898

Drug Information Service
University of California San Diego Medical Center
135 Dickinson St.
Mailing address:
200 West Arbor Drive
MC 8925
San Diego, CA 92103-8925
Mon.-Fri. 9 AM-5 PM
900-288-8273
Fax: 858-715-6323

STANFORD

Drug Information Center
University of California Stanford Hospital and Clinics
300 Pasteur Dr.
Room H-0301
Stanford, CA 94305
Mon.-Fri. 8 AM-4 PM
650-723-6422
Fax: 650-725-5028

COLORADO

DENVER

Rocky Mountain Poison and Drug Consultation Center
1001 Yosemite St.
Denver, CO 80230
7 days/week, 24 hours
303-893-3784
(For Denver County residents only)
Fax: 303-739-1119

Drug Information Center
University of Colorado Health Science Center School of Pharmacy
4200 E. 9th Ave., Box C239
Denver, CO 80262
Mon.-Fri. 8:30 AM-4:30 PM
303-315-8489
Fax: 303-315-3353

CONNECTICUT

FARMINGTON

Drug Information Service
University of Connecticut Health Center
263 Farmington Ave.
Farmington, CT 06030
Mon.-Fri. 7 AM-4 PM
860-679-2783
Fax: 860-679-1231
wnelson@nso.uchc.edu

HARTFORD

Drug Information Center
Hartford Hospital
P.O. Box 5037
80 Seymour St.
Hartford, CT 06102
Mon.-Fri. 8:30 AM-5 PM
860-545-2221
860-545-2961(After 5PM)
Fax: 860-545-4371
www.harthosp.org

NEW HAVEN

Drug Information Center
Yale-New Haven Hospital
20 York St.
New Haven, CT 06504
Mon.-Fri. 9 AM-5 PM
203-688-2248
Fax: 203-688-3691
www.ynhh.com

DISTRICT OF COLUMBIA

Drug Information Service
Howard University Hospital
Room BB06
2041 Georgia Ave. NW
Washington, DC 20060
Mon.-Fri. 8 AM-4 PM
202-865-1325
202-865-7413
Fax: 202-865-7410

FLORIDA

GAINESVILLE

Drug Information & Pharmacy Resource Center
SHANDS Hospital at University of Florida
P.O. Box 100316
Gainesville, FL 32610-0316
Mon.-Fri. 9 AM-5 PM
352-265-0408
(for healthcare professionals only)
Fax: 352-338-9860
www.cop.ufl.edu/vdis

JACKSONVILLE

Drug Information Service
SHANDS Jacksonville
655 W. 8th St.
Jacksonville, FL 32209
Mon.-Fri. 8 AM-5 PM
904-244-4185
Fax: 904-244-4272
www.cop.ufl.edu/vdis

MIAMI

Drug Information Center (119)
Miami VA Medical Center
1201 NW 16th St.
Pharmacy 119
Miami, FL 33125
Mon.-Fri. 7:00 AM-3:30 PM
305-324-3237
(for healthcare professionals only)
Fax: 305-324-3394

ORLANDO

Orlando Regional Drug Information Service
Orlando Regional Healthcare System
1414 Kuhl Ave., MP 192
Orlando, FL 32806
Mon.-Fri. 8 AM-4:30 PM
407-841-5111, ext. 8717
Fax: 407-649-1827
E-mail: druginfo@orhs.org

TALLAHASSEE

Drug Information Education Center
Florida Agricultural and Mechanical University
College of Pharmacy
Honor House, Room 200
Tallahassee, FL 32307
Mon.-Fri. 9 AM-5 PM
850-488-5239
850-599-3064
800-451-3181
Fax: 850-412-7020
www.pharmacy.samu.edu

GEORGIA

ATLANTA

Emory University Hospital
Dept. of Pharmaceutical Services-Drug Information
1364 Clifton Rd. NE
Atlanta, GA 30322
Mon.-Fri. 8:30 AM-5 PM
404-712-4640
Fax: 404-712-7577

Drug Information Service
Northside Hospital
1000 Johnson Ferry Rd. NE
Atlanta, GA 30342
Mon.-Fri. 9 AM-4 PM
404-851-8676 (GA only)
Fax: 404-851-8682

AUGUSTA

Drug Information Center
Medical College of Georgia Hospital and Clinic
BI2101
1120 15th St.
Augusta, GA 30912
Mon.-Fri. 8:30 AM-5 PM
706-721-2887
Fax: 706-721-3827

IDAHO

POCATELLO

Drug Information Center
Idaho State University
School of Pharmacy
Campus Box 8092
Pocatello, ID 83209
Mon.-Thur. 8:30 AM-5 PM
Fri. 8:30 AM-2:30 PM
208-282-4689
800-334-7139 (ID only)
Fax: 208-282-3003
http://rx.isu.edu/services_contacts/idis/

ILLINOIS

CHICAGO

Drug Information Center
Northwestern Memorial Hospital
251 E. Huron
Feinberg LC-700B
Chicago, IL 60611
Mon.-Fri. 8 AM-5 PM
312-926-7573
Fax: 312-926-7956

Drug Information Services
University of Chicago
5841 S. Maryland Ave.
MC 0010
Chicago, IL 60637
Mon.-Fri. 8 AM-5 PM
773-702-1388
Fax: 773-702-6631

Drug Information Center
University of Illinois at Chicago
833 S. Wood St.
Chicago, IL 60612
Mon.-Fri. 8 AM-4 PM
312-996-0209
Fax: 312-996-0448
www.uic.edu/pharmacy/services/di/index.html

HARVEY

Drug Information Center
Ingalls Memorial Hospital
1 Ingalls Dr.
Harvey, IL 60426
Mon.-Fri. 8 AM-4:30 PM
708-915-4430
Fax: 708-915-3108

HINES

Drug Information Service
Hines Veterans Administration Hospital
Pharmacy Services MC119
P.O. Box 5000
Hines, IL 60141-5000
Mon.-Fri. 8 AM-4:30 PM
708-202-8387, ext. 23780
Fax: 708-202-2675

PARK RIDGE

Drug Information Center
Lutheran General Hospital
1775 Dempster St.
Park Ridge, IL 60068
Mon.-Fri. 7:30 AM-4 PM
847-723-8128
(for healthcare professionals only)
Fax: 847-723-2326

INDIANA

INDIANAPOLIS

Drug Information Center
St. Vincent Hospital and Health Services
2001 W. 86th St.
Indianapolis, IN 46260
Mon.-Fri. 8 AM-4 PM
317-338-3200
(for healthcare professionals only)
Fax: 317-338-3041

Drug Information Service
Clarian Health Partners
Pharmacy Department I-65 at 21st
Room CG04
Indianapolis, IN 46202
Mon.-Fri. 8:30 AM-4:30 PM
317-962-1750
Fax: 317-962-1756

MUNCIE

Drug Information Center
Ball Memorial Hospital
2401 University Ave.
Muncie, IN 47303
7 days/week, 24 hours
765-747-3035
Fax: 765-751-2522
E-mail: kwolfe@chs.cami3.com

IOWA

DES MOINES

Regional Drug Information Center
Mercy Medical Center-Des Moines
1111 Sixth Ave.
Des Moines, IA 50314
Mon.-Fri. 8 AM-4:30 PM
515-247-3286
(answered 7 days/week, 24 hours)
Fax: 515-247-3966

IOWA CITY

Drug Information Center
University of Iowa Hospitals and Clinics
200 Hawkins Dr.
Iowa City, IA 52242
Mon.-Fri. 8 AM-4:30 PM
319-356-2600
(for healthcare professionals only)
Fax: 319-384-8840

KANSAS

KANSAS CITY

Drug Information Center
University of Kansas Medical Center
3901 Rainbow Blvd.
Kansas City, KS 66160
Mon.-Fri. 8:30 AM-6 PM
913-588-2328
(for healthcare professionals only)
Fax: 913-588-2350
E-mail: druginfo@kumc.edu

KENTUCKY

LEXINGTON

Drug Information Center
Chandler Medical Center
College of Pharmacy
University of Kentucky
800 Rose St., C-117
Lexington, KY 40536-0293
Mon.-Fri. 8 AM-5 PM
859-323-5320
Fax: 859-323-2049
E-mail: cqwhit1@pop.uky.edu

LOUISIANA

MONROE

Louisiana Drug and Poison Information Center
University of Louisiana at Monroe College of Pharmacy
Monroe, LA 71209-6430
Mon.-Fri. 8 AM-4:30 PM
318-342-1710
Fax: 318-342-1744
E-mail: pyross@ulm.edu

NEW ORLEANS

Xavier University Drug Information Center
Tulane University Hospital and Clinic
Box HC12
1415 Tulane Ave.
New Orleans, LA 70112
Mon.-Fri. 9 AM-5 PM
504-588-5670
Fax: 504-588-5862
mharris@tulane.edu
E-mail: mharris6@tulane.edu

MARYLAND

ANDREWS AFB

Drug Information Services
89 MDTS/SGQP
1050 W. Perimeter Rd.
Suite D1-119
Andrews AFB, MD 20762-6660
Mon.-Fri. 7:30 AM-5 PM
240-857-4565
Fax: 240-857-8892

ANNAPOLIS

The Anne Arundel Medical Center
Dept. of Pharmacy
64 Franklin St.
Annapolis, MD 21401
7 days/week, 24 hours
410-267-1126
410-267-1000
(switchboard)
Fax: 410-267-1628
www.aahs.org

BALTIMORE

Drug Information Service
Johns Hopkins Hospital
600 N. Wolfe St.,
Halsted 503
Baltimore, MD 21287-6180
Mon.-Fri. 8:30 AM-5 PM
410-955-6348
Fax: 410-955-8283

Drug Information Service
University of Maryland School of Pharmacy
Pharmacy Hall Room 762
20 North Pine St.
Baltimore, MD 21201
Mon.-Fri. 8:30 AM-5 PM
410-706-7568
Fax: 410-706-0754
www.pharmacy.umaryland.edu/umdi

BETHESDA

Drug Information Service
National Institutes of Health
Building 10, Room 1S-259
10 Center Dr. (MSC1196)
Bethesda, MD 20892-1196
Mon.-Fri. 8:30 AM-5 PM
301-496-2407
Fax: 301-496-0210
www.cc.nih.gov/phar

EASTON

Drug Information Pharmacy Dept.
Memorial Hospital
219 S. Washington St.
Easton, MD 21601
Mon.-Fri. 7 AM-Midnight
Sat.-Sun. 7 AM-5:30 PM
410-822-1000, ext. 5645
Fax: 410-820-9489

MASSACHUSETTS

BOSTON

Drug Information Services
Brigham and Women's Hospital
75 Frances St.
Boston, MA 02115
Mon.-Fri. 7 AM-3:30 PM
617-732-7166
Fax: 617-732-7497

Drug Information Center
New England Medical Center Pharmacy
750 Washington St., Box 420
Boston, MA 02111
Mon.-Fri. 9 AM-5 PM
617-636-8985
Fax: 617-636-4567

WORCESTER

Drug Information Center
UMass Memorial Healthcare Hospital
55 Lake Ave. North
Worcester, MA 01655
Mon.-Fri. 8:30 AM-5 PM
508-856-3456
508-856-2775 (24 hour)
Fax: 508-856-1850

MICHIGAN

ANN ARBOR

Drug Information and Pharmacy Services
University of Michigan Medical Center
1500 East Medical Center Dr.
UHB2 D301 Box 0008
Ann Arbor, MI 48109/0008
Mon.-Fri. 8 AM-5 PM
734-936-8200
734-936-8251
Fax: 734-936-7027
www.phar.med.umich.edu/public

DETROIT

Drug Information Center
Department of Pharmacy Services
Detroit Receiving Hospital and University Health Center
4201 St. Antoine Blvd.
Detroit, MI 48201
Mon.-Fri. 8 AM-5 PM
313-745-4556
Fax: 313-993-2522
www.dmcpharmacy.org

LANSING

Drug Information Services
Sparrow Hospital
1215 East Michigan Ave.
Lansing, MI 48912
7 days/week, 24 hours
517-483-2444
Fax: 517-483-2088

PONTIAC

Drug Information Center
St. Joseph Mercy Hospital
44405 Woodward Ave.
Pontiac, MI 48341
Mon.-Fri. 8 AM-4:30 PM
248-858-3055
Fax: 248-858-3010

ROYAL OAK

Drug Information Services
William Beaumont Hospital
3601 West 13 Mile Rd.
Royal Oak, MI 48073-6769
Mon.-Fri. 8 AM-4:30 PM
248-551-4077
Fax: 248-551-3301

SOUTHFIELD

Drug Information Service
Providence Hospital
16001 West 9 Mile Rd.
Southfield, MI 48075
Mon.-Fri. 8 AM-4 PM
248-424-3125
Fax: 248-424-5364

MISSISSIPPI

JACKSON

Drug Information Center
University of Mississippi Medical Center
2500 N. State St.
Jackson, MS 39216
Mon.-Fri. 8 AM-4:30 PM
601-984-2060
Fax: 601-984-2064

MISSOURI

KANSAS CITY

University of Missouri-Kansas City Drug Information Center
2411 Holmes St., MG-200
Kansas City, MO 64108-2792
Mon.-Fri. 8 AM-5 PM
816-235-5490
Fax: 816-235-5491
www.umkc.edu/druginfo

SPRINGFIELD

Drug Information Center
St. Johns Regional Health Center
1235 E. Cherokee St.
Springfield, MO 65804
Mon.-Fri. 7:30 AM-4:30 PM
417-885-3488
Fax: 417-888-7788
E-mail: tbarks@sprg.smhs.com

ST. JOSEPH

Drug Information Service
Heartland Hospital West
801 Faraon St.
St. Joseph, MO 64501
Mon.-Fri. 9 AM-5:30 PM
816-271-7582
Fax: 816-271-7590

MONTANA

MISSOULA

Drug Information Service
University of Montana School of Pharmacy and Allied Health Sciences
Missoula, MT 59812-1522
Mon.-Fri. 8 AM-5 PM
406-243-5254
Fax: 406-243-5256
E-mail: druginfo@selway.umt.edu
www.umt.edu/druginfo

NEBRASKA

OMAHA

Drug Information Service
School of Pharmacy
Creighton University
2500 California Plaza
Omaha, NE 68178
Mon.-Fri. 8:30 AM-5:00 PM
402-280-5101
Fax: 402-280-5149
www.druginfo.creighton.edu

NEW JERSEY

NEWARK

New Jersey Poison Information and Education System
201 Lyons Ave.
Newark, NJ 07112
7 days/week, 24 hours
973-926-7443
800-222-1222
(poison control)
Fax: 973-926-0013
E-mail: bruce@ibm.net
www.njpies.org

NEW BRUNSWICK

Drug Information Service
Robert Wood Johnson University Hospital
Pharmacy Department
1 Robert Wood Johnson Pl.
New Brunswick, NJ 08901
Mon.-Fri. 8:30 AM-4:30 PM
732-937-8842
Fax: 732-937-8584

NEW MEXICO

ALBUQUERQUE

New Mexico Poison & Drug Information Center
University of New Mexico Health Sciences Center
Albuquerque, NM 87131
7 days/week, 24 hours
505-272-2222
800-432-6866 (NM only)
Fax: 505-272-5892

NEW YORK

BROOKLYN

International Drug Information Center
Long Island University
Arnold & Marie Schwartz College of Pharmacy & Health Sciences
1 University Plaza
RM-HS509
75 Dekalb Ave.
Brooklyn, NY 11201
Mon.-Fri. 9 AM-5 PM
718-488-1064
Fax: 718-780-4056
www.liu.edu

Drug Information Center
Brookdale University Hospital and Medical Center
1 Brookdale Plaza
Brooklyn, NY 11212
Mon.-Fri. 8 AM-4 PM
718-240-5983
Fax: 718-240-5987

COOPERSTOWN

Drug Information Center
Bassett Healthcare
1 Atwell Rd.
Cooperstown, NY 13326
7 days/week, 24 hours
607-547-3686
Fax: 607-547-3629

JAMAICA

Drug Information Center
St. John's University College of Pharmacy and Allied Health Professions
8000 Utopia Pkwy.
Jamaica, NY 11439
Mon.-Fri. 8:30 AM-3:30 PM
718-990-2149
Fax: 718-990-2151
druginfo@stjohns.edu

NEW HYDE PARK

Drug Information Center
St. Johns University at Long Island Jewish Medical Center
270-05 76th Ave.
New Hyde Park, NY 11040
Mon.-Fri. 8 AM-3 PM
718-470-DRUG (3784)
Fax: 718-470-1742

NEW YORK CITY

Drug Information Center
Memorial Sloan-Kettering Cancer Center
1275 York Ave.
RM S-712
New York, NY 10021
Mon.-Fri. 9 AM-5 PM
212-639-7552
Fax: 212-639-2171

Drug Information Center
Mount Sinai Medical Center
1 Gustave Levy Pl.
New York, NY 10029
Mon.-Fri. 9 AM-5 PM
212-241-6619
Fax: 212-348-7927

Drug Information Service
New York Presbyterian Hospital
Room K04
525 E. 68th St.
New York, NY 10021
Mon.-Fri. 9 AM-5 PM
212-746-0741
Fax: 212-746-4434

ROCHESTER

Finger Lakes Poison and Drug Information Center
University of Rochester
601 Elmwood Ave.
Rochester, NY 14642
7 days/week, 24 hours
716-275-3718
716-275-3232
(after 5 PM)
Fax: 716-244-1677

ROCKVILLE CENTER

Drug Information Center
Mercy Medical Center
1000 North Village Ave.
Rockville Center, NY 11570
Mon.-Fri. 8 AM-4 PM
516-705-1053
Fax: 516-705-1071

NORTH CAROLINA

BUIES CREEK

Drug Information Center
School of Pharmacy
Campbell University
P.O. Box 1090
Buies Creek, NC 27506
Mon.-Fri. 8:30 AM-4:30 PM
910-893-1478
800-760-9697 (Toll free) x2701
800-327-5467 (NC only)
Fax: 910-893-1476
E-mail: dic@mailcenter.campbell.edu

CHAPEL HILL

Drug Information Center
University of North Carolina Hospitals
101 Manning Dr.
Chapel Hill, NC 27514
Mon.-Fri. 8 AM-4:30 PM
919-966-2373
Fax: 919-966-1791

DURHAM

Drug Information Center
Duke University Health Systems
DUMC Box 3089
Durham, NC 27710
Mon.-Fri. 8 AM-5 PM
919-684-5125
Fax: 919-681-3895

GREENVILLE

Eastern Carolina Drug Information Center
Pitt County Memorial Hospital
Dept. of Pharmacy Service
2100 Stantonsburg Rd.
Greenville, NC 27835
Mon.-Fri. 8 AM-5 PM
252-816-4257
Fax: 252-816-7425

WINSTON-SALEM

Drug Information Service Center
Wake-Forest University Baptist Medical Center
Medical Center Blvd.
Winston-Salem, NC 27157
Mon.-Fri. 8 AM-5 PM
336-716-2037
(for healthcare professionals only)
Fax: 336-716-2186

OHIO

ADA

Drug Information Center
Raabe College of Pharmacy
Ohio Northern University
Ada, OH 45810
Mon.-Fri. 9 AM-5 PM
419-772-2307
Fax: 419-772-2289
www.onu.edu/pharmacy/druginfo

CINCINNATI

Drug Information Center
Children's Hospital Medical Center
3333 Burnet Ave. VP-3
Cincinnati, OH 45229
Mon.-Fri. 9 AM-5 PM
513-636-5054
513-636-5111 (24 hour)
(for healthcare professionals only)
Fax: 513-636-5069

CLEVELAND

Drug Information Service
Cleveland Clinic Foundation
9500 Euclid Ave.
Cleveland, OH 44195
Mon.-Fri. 8:30 AM-4:30 PM
216-444-6456
(for healthcare professionals only)
Fax: 216-444-6157

COLUMBUS

Drug Information Center
Ohio State University Hospital
Dept. of Pharmacy
Doan Hall 368
410 W. 10th Ave.
Columbus, OH 43210-1228
Mon.-Fri. 8 AM-4 PM
614-293-8679
Fax: 614-293-3264

Drug Information Center
Riverside Methodist Hospital
3535 Olentangy River Road
Columbus, OH 43214
Mon.-Fri. 8:30 AM-4 PM
614-566-5425
Fax: 614-566-5447, 614-566-5850

TOLEDO

Drug Information Services
St. Vincent Mercy Medical Center
2213 Cherry St.
Toledo, Ohio 43608-2691
Mon.-Fri. 8 AM-4 PM
419-251-4227
Fax: 419-251-3662
E-mail: tschampel-1@med.ctr.osu.edu
http://rx.med.ctr.ohio-state.edu

OKLAHOMA

OKLAHOMA CITY

Drug Information Service
Integris Health
3300 Northwest Expressway
Oklahoma City, OK 73112
Mon.-Fri. 8 AM-4:30 PM
405-949-3660
Fax: 405-951-8274

Drug Information Center
OU Medical Center
Presbyterian Tower
700 NE 13th St.
Oklahoma City, OK 73104
Mon.-Fri. 8 AM-4:30 PM
405-271-6226
Fax: 405-271-6281

TULSA

Drug Information Center
Saint Francis Hospital
6161 S. Yale Ave.
Tulsa, OK 74136
Mon.-Fri. 8 AM-4 PM
918-494-6339
(for healthcare professionals only)
Fax: 918-494-1893

PENNSYLVANIA

PHILADELPHIA

Drug Information Center
Temple University Hospital
Dept. of Pharmacy
3401 N. Broad St.
Philadelphia, PA 19140
Mon.-Fri. 8 AM-4:30 PM
215-707-4644
Fax: 215-707-3463

Drug Information Service
Tenet Health System
Department of Pharmacy
MS 451
Broad and Vine Streets
Philadelphia, PA 19102
Mon.-Fri. 8 AM-4 PM
215-762-DRUG (3784)
(for healthcare professionals only)
Fax: 215-762-7993

Drug Information Service
Dept. of Pharmacy
Thomas Jefferson University Hospital
111 S. 11th St.
Philadelphia, PA 19107-5098
Mon.-Fri. 8 AM-5 PM
215-955-8877
Fax: 215-923-3316

University of Pennsylvania Health System Drug Information Service
Hospital of the University of Pennsylvania
Department of Pharmacy
3400 Spruce St.
Philadelphia, PA 19104
Mon.-Fri. 8:30 AM-4 PM
215-662-2903
Fax: 215-662-4319

PITTSBURGH

The Christopher and Nicole Browett Pharmaceutical Information Center
Mylan School of Pharmacy
Duquesne University
431 Mellon Hall
Pittsburgh, PA 15282
Mon.-Fri. 8 AM-4 PM
412-396-4600
Fax: 412-396-4488

Drug Information Center
University of Pittsburgh
137 Victoria Hall
Pittsburgh, PA 15261
Mon.-Fri. 8:30 AM-4:30 PM
412-624-3784
(for healthcare professionals only)
Fax: 412-624-6350
E-mail: druginfo@msx.upmc.edu

UPLAND

Drug Information Center
Crozer-Chester Medical Center
Dept. of Pharmacy
1 Medical Center Blvd.
Upland, PA 19013
Mon.-Fri. 8 AM-4:30 PM
610-447-2851
610-447-2862
(after hours)
(both numbers are for healthcare professionals only)
Fax: 610-447-2820

WILLIAMSPORT

Drug Information
Pharmacy Dept.
Susquehanna Health System
Rural Avenue Campus
Williamsport, PA 17701
24 hours/7 days a week
570-321-3083
Fax: 570-321-3230

PUERTO RICO

PONCE

Centro Informacion Medicamentos
Escuela de Medicina de Ponce
P.O. Box 7004
Ponce, PR 00732-7004
Mon.-Fri. 8 AM-4:30 PM
787-259-7085
(Spanish and English)
787-840-2575
(switchboard)
Fax: 787-842-0461

SAN JUAN

Centro de Informacion de Medicamentos-CIM
Escuela de Farmacia-RCM
P.O. Box 365067
San Juan, PR 00936-5067
Mon.-Fri. 8 AM-4:30 PM
787-758-2525, ext. 1516
Fax: 787-763-0196
E-mail: cimrcm@rcm.upr.edu

SOUTH CAROLINA

CHARLESTON

Drug Information Service
Medical University of South Carolina
150 Ashley Ave.
Rutledge Tower
Annex, Room 604
P.O. Box 250584
Charleston, SC 29425-0810
Mon.-Fri. 9 AM-5:30 PM
843-792-3896
800-922-5250
Fax: 843-792-5532

COLUMBIA

Drug Information Service
University of South Carolina
College of Pharmacy
University of South Carolina
Columbia, SC 29208
Mon.-Fri. 8 AM-5 PM
803-777-7804
Fax: 803-777-6127

SPARTANBURG

Drug Information Center
Spartanburg Regional Medical Center
101 E. Wood St.
Spartanburg, SC 29303
Mon.-Fri. 8 AM-5 PM
864-560-6910
Fax: 864-560-7323

TENNESSEE

KNOXVILLE

Drug Information Center
University of Tennessee
Medical Center at Knoxville
1924 Alcoa Highway
Knoxville, TN 37920-6999
Mon.-Fri. 8 AM-4:30 PM
865-544-9124
Fax: 865-525-0326
865-544-8242

MEMPHIS

South East Regional Drug Information Center
VA Medical Center
1030 Jefferson Ave.
Memphis, TN 38104
Mon.-Fri. 7:30 AM-4 PM
901-523-8990, ext. 6720
Fax: 901-577-7306

Drug Information Center
University of Tennessee
875 Monroe Ave.
Suite 116
Memphis, TN 38163
Mon.-Fri. 7 AM-5 PM
901-448-5555
Fax: 901-448-5419
E-mail: utdic@utmem.edu

TEXAS

AMARILLO

Drug Information Center
Texas Tech University
School of Pharmacy
1300 Coulter
Amarillo, TX 79106
Mon.-Fri. 8 AM-5 PM
806-356-4008
(for healthcare professionals only)
Fax: 806-356-4017

GALVESTON

Drug Information Center
University of Texas Medical Branch
301 University Blvd. - G01
Galveston, TX 77555-0701
Mon.-Fri. 8 AM-5 PM
409-772-2734
Fax: 409-747-5222

HOUSTON

Drug Information Center
Ben Taub General Hospital
Texas Southern University/HCHD
1504 Taub Loop
Houston, TX 77030
Mon.-Fri. 8 AM-5 PM
713-873-3710
Fax: 713-873-3711

LACKLAND A.F.B.

Drug Information Center
Dept. of Pharmacy
Wilford Hall Medical Center
2200 Berquist Dr.
Suite 1
Lackland A.F.B., TX 78236
7 days/week, 24 hours
210-292-5414
Fax: 210-292-3722

LUBBOCK

Drug Information and Consultation Service
Covenant Medical Center
3615 19th St.
Lubbock, TX 79410
Mon.-Fri. 8 AM-5 PM
806-725-0408
Fax: 806-725-0305

SAN ANTONIO

Drug Information Service
University of Texas Health Science Center at San Antonio
Department of Pharmacology
7703 Floyd Curl Drive
San Antonio, TX 78229-3900
Mon.-Thur. 8 AM-5 PM
Fri. 8 AM-3 PM
210-567-4280
Fax: 210-567-4305

TEMPLE

Drug Information Center
Scott and White Memorial Hospital
2401 S. 31st St.
Temple, TX 76508
Mon.-Fri. 8 AM-6 PM
254-724-4636
Fax: 254-724-1731

UTAH

SALT LAKE CITY

Drug Information Service
University of Utah Hospital
Dept. of Pharmacy Services
Room A-050
50 N. Medical Dr.
Salt Lake City, UT 84132
Mon.-Fri. 8:30 AM-4:30 PM
801-581-2073
Fax: 801-585-6688
E-mail: drug.info@hsc.utah.edu

VIRGINIA

HAMPTON

Drug Information Service
Hampton University School of Pharmacy
Kittrell Hall Room 208
Hampton, VA 23668
Mon.-Fri. 8 AM-5 PM
757-728-6687
757-728-6693
(drug info hotline)
Fax: 757-728-6696
E-mail: druginfo@hamptonu.edu

WEST VIRGINIA

MORGANTOWN

West Virginia Drug Information Center
WV University-
Robert C. Byrd Health Sciences Center
1124 HSN, P.O. Box 9550
Morgantown, WV 26506
Mon.-Fri. 8:30 AM-5 PM
304-293-6640
800-352-2501 (WV)
Fax: 304-293-7672

WYOMING

LARAMIE

Drug Information Center
University of Wyoming
P.O. Box 3375
Laramie, WY 82071
Mon.-Fri. 8 AM-5 PM
307-766-6988
Fax: 307-766-2953
E-mail: kendrag@uwyo.edu

U.S. FOOD AND DRUG ADMINISTRATION

Professional and Consumer Information Numbers

Medical Product Reporting Programs

MedWatch (24-hour service) **800-332-1088**
Reporting of problems with drugs, devices, biologics (except vaccines), medical foods, dietary supplements.

Vaccine Adverse Event Reporting System (24 hour service) **800-822-7967**
Reporting of vaccine-related problems.

Mandatory Medical Device Reporting **301-827-0360**
Reporting required from user-facilities (eg, hospitals, nursing homes) regarding device-related deaths and serious injuries.

Veterinary Adverse Drug Reaction Program **888-332-8387**
Reporting of adverse drug events in animals.

Medical Advertising Information **301-827-2828**
Inquiries from health professionals regarding product promotion.

USP Medication Errors **800-233-7767**
Reporting of medication errors or near-errors to help avoid future problems through improvement in product names and packaging.

Information for Health Professionals

Center for Drugs Information Branch **301-827-4573**
Information on human drugs including hormones.

Center for Biologics Office of Communications **301-827-2000**
Information on biological products including vaccines and blood.

Center for Devices and Radiological Health **301-443-4190**
Automated request for information on medical devices and radiation-emitting products.

Emergency Operations **301-443-1240**
Emergencies involving FDA-regulated products, tampering reports, and after-hours emergency Investigational New Drug requests.

Office of Orphan Products Development **301-827-3666**
Information on products for rare diseases.

General Information

General Consumer Inquiries **888-463-6332**
Consumer information on regulated products/issues.

Freedom of Information **301-827-6500**
Requests for publicly available FDA documents.

Office of Public Affairs **301-827-6250**
Interviews/press inquiries on FDA activities.

Center for Food Safety and Applied Nutrition **888-723-3366**
Information on food safety, seafood, dietary supplements, women's nutrition, and cosmetics.

U.S. Department of Health and Human Services

MEDWATCH

The FDA Safety Information and Adverse Event Reporting Program

For VOLUNTARY reporting of adverse events and product problems

Page ____ of ____

Form Approved: OMB No. 0910-0291 Expires: 04/30/03
See OMB statement on reverse

FDA Use Only

Triage unit sequence #

A. Patient information

1. **Patient identifier** In confidence
2. **Age at time of event:** or **Date of birth:**
3. **Sex** ☐ female ☐ male
4. **Weight** ____ lbs or ____ kgs

B. Adverse event or product problem

1. ☐ **Adverse event** and/or ☐ **Product problem** (e.g., defects/malfunctions)
2. **Outcomes attributed to adverse event** (check all that apply)
   - ☐ death ________ (mo/day/yr)
   - ☐ life-threatening
   - ☐ hospitalization - initial or prolonged
   - ☐ disability
   - ☐ congenital anomaly
   - ☐ required intervention to prevent permanent impairment/damage
   - ☐ other:
3. **Date of event** (mo/day/yr)
4. **Date of this report** (mo/day/yr)
5. **Describe event or problem**
6. **Relevant tests/laboratory data,** including dates
7. **Other relevant history, including preexisting medical conditions** (e.g., allergies, race, pregnancy, smoking and alcohol use, hepatic/renal dysfunction, etc.)

PLEASE TYPE OR USE BLACK INK

C. Suspect medication(s)

1. **Name** (give labeled strength & mfr/labeler, if known)
   #1
   #2
2. **Dose, frequency & route used**
   #1
   #2
3. **Therapy dates** (if unknown, give duration) from/to (or best estimate)
   #1
   #2
4. **Diagnosis for use** (indication)
   #1
   #2
5. **Event abated after use stopped or dose reduced**
   #1 ☐ yes ☐ no ☐ doesn't apply
   #2 ☐ yes ☐ no ☐ doesn't apply
6. **Lot #** (if known)
   #1
   #2
7. **Exp. date** (if known)
   #1
   #2
8. **Event reappeared after reintroduction**
   #1 ☐ yes ☐ no ☐ doesn't apply
   #2 ☐ yes ☐ no ☐ doesn't apply
9. **NDC #** (for product problems only)
   - -
10. **Concomitant medical products** and therapy dates (exclude treatment of event)

D. Suspect medical device

1. **Brand name**
2. **Type of device**
3. **Manufacturer name & address**
4. **Operator of device**
   - ☐ health professional
   - ☐ lay user/patient
   - ☐ other:
5. **Expiration date** (mo/day/yr)
6. model # ________
   catalog # ________
   serial # ________
   lot # ________
   other # ________
7. **If implanted, give date** (mo/day/yr)
8. **If explanted, give date** (mo/day/yr)
9. **Device available for evaluation?** (Do not send to FDA)
   ☐ yes ☐ no ☐ returned to manufacturer on ________ (mo/day/yr)
10. **Concomitant medical products** and therapy dates (exclude treatment of event)

E. Reporter (see confidentiality section on back)

1. **Name & address** **phone #**
2. **Health professional?** ☐ yes ☐ no
3. **Occupation**
4. **Also reported to**
   - ☐ manufacturer
   - ☐ user facility
   - ☐ distributor
5. **If you do NOT want your identity disclosed to the manufacturer, place an " X " in this box.** ☐

FDA

Mail to: **MEDWATCH**
5600 Fishers Lane
Rockville, MD 20852-9787

or FAX to:
1-800-FDA-0178

FDA Form 3500

Submission of a report does not constitute an admission that medical personnel or the product caused or contributed to the event.

ADVICE ABOUT VOLUNTARY REPORTING

Report adverse experiences with:

- medications (drugs or biologics)
- medical devices (including in-vitro diagnostics)
- special nutritional products (dietary supplements, medical foods, infant formulas)
- cosmetics
- medication errors

Report product problems – quality, performance or safety concerns such as:

- suspected contamination
- questionable stability
- defective components
- poor packaging or labeling
- therapeutic failures

Report SERIOUS adverse events. An event is serious when the patient outcome is:

- death
- life-threatening (real risk of dying)
- hospitalization (initial or prolonged)
- disability (significant, persistent or permanent)
- congenital anomaly
- required intervention to prevent permanent impairment or damage

Report even if:

- you're not certain the product caused the event
- you don't have all the details

How to report:

- just fill in the sections that apply to your report
- use section C for all products except medical devices
- attach additional blank pages if needed
- use a separate form for each patient
- report either to FDA or the manufacturer (or both)

Confidentiality: The patient's identity is held in strict confidence by FDA and protected to the fullest extent of the law. FDA will not disclose the reporter's identity in response to a request from the public, pursuant to the Freedom of Information Act. The reporter's identity, including the identity of a self-reporter, may be shared with the manufacturer unless requested otherwise.

If your report involves a serious adverse event with a device and it occurred in a facility outside a doctor's office, that facility may be legally required to report to FDA and/or the manufacturer. Please notify the person in that facility who would handle such reporting.

Important numbers:

- 1-800-FDA-0178 to FAX report
- 1-800-FDA-1088 to report by phone or for more information
- 1-800-822-7967 for a VAERS form for vaccines

To Report via the Internet:

https://www.accessdata.fda.gov/scripts/medwatch/

The public reporting burden for this collection of information has been estimated to average 30 minutes per response, including the time for reviewing instructions, searching existing data sources, gathering and maintaining the data needed, and completing and reviewing the collection of information. Send comments regarding this burden estimate or any other aspect of this collection of information, including suggestions for reducing this burden to:

DHHS Reports Clearance Office
Paperwork Reduction Project (0910-0291)
Hubert H. Humphrey Building, Room 531-H
200 Independence Avenue, S.W.
Washington, DC 20201

Please DO NOT RETURN this form to this address.

U.S. DEPARTMENT OF HEALTH AND HUMAN SERVICES
Public Health Service • Food and Drug Administration

FDA Form 3500-back

VACCINE ADVERSE EVENT REPORTING SYSTEM

VAERS

24 Hour Toll-free information line 1-800-822-7967
P.O. Box 1100, Rockville, MD 20849-1100
PATIENT IDENTITY KEPT CONFIDENTIAL

For CDC/FDA Use Only
VAERS Number ____________
Date Received ____________

Patient Name: ____ Last First M.I. Address ____ City State Zip Telephone no. (___) ____	Vaccine administered by (Name): ____ Responsible Physician Facility Name/Address ____ City State Zip Telephone no. (___) ____	Form completed by (Name): ____ Relation to Patient ☐ Vaccine Provider ☐ Patient/Parent ☐ Manufacturer ☐ Other Address *(if different from patient or provider)* ____ City State Zip Telephone no. (___) ____

1. State
2. County where administered
3. Date of birth __/__/__ mm dd yy
4. Patient age
5. Sex ☐ M ☐ F
6. Date form completed __/__/__ mm dd yy

7. Describe adverse event(s) (symptoms, signs, time course) and treatment, if any

8. Check all appropriate:
- ☐ Patient died (date __/__/__ mm dd yy)
- ☐ Life threatening illness
- ☐ Required emergency room/doctor visit
- ☐ Required hospitalization (____ days)
- ☐ Resulted in prolongation of hospitalization
- ☐ Resulted in permanent disability
- ☐ None of the above

9. Patient recovered ☐ YES ☐ NO ☐ UNKNOWN

10. Date of vaccination __/__/__ mm dd yy Time ____ AM PM

11. Adverse event onset __/__/__ mm dd yy Time ____ AM PM

12. Relevant diagnostic tests/laboratory data

13. Enter all vaccines given on date listed in no. 10

	Vaccine (type)	Manufacturer	Lot number	Route/Site	No. Previous Doses
a.					
b.					
c.					
d.					

14. Any other vaccinations within 4 weeks prior to the date listed in no. 10

	Vaccine (type)	Manufacturer	Lot number	Route/Site	No. Previous doses	Date given
a.						
b.						

15. Vaccinated at:
- ☐ Private doctor's office/hospital
- ☐ Public health clinic/hospital
- ☐ Military clinic/hospital
- ☐ Other/unknown

16. Vaccine purchased with:
- ☐ Private funds
- ☐ Public funds
- ☐ Military funds
- ☐ Other/unknown

17. Other medications

18. Illness at time of vaccination (specify)

19. Pre-existing physician-diagnosed allergies, birth defects, medical conditions(specify)

20. Have you reported this adverse event previously? ☐ No ☐ To doctor ☐ To health department ☐ To manufacturer

21. Adverse event following prior vaccination (check all applicable, specify)

	Adverse Event	Onset Age	Type Vaccine	Dose no. in series
☐ In patient				
☐ In brother or sister				

Only for children 5 and under

22. Birth weight ____ lb. ____ oz.

23. No. of brothers and sisters

Only for reports submitted by manufacturer/Immunization project

24. Mfr./imm. proj. report no.

25. Date received by mfr./imm.proj.

26. 15 day report? ☐ Yes ☐ No

27. Report type ☐ Initial ☐ Follow-Up

Health care providers and manufacturers are required by law (42 USC 300aa-25) to report reactions to vaccines listed in the Table of Reportable Events Following Immunization Reports for reactions to other vaccines are voluntary except when required as a condition of immunization grant awards.

Form VAERS-1

VACCINE ADVERSE EVENT REPORTS

Health care providers and manufacturers are required by law (42 USC 300aa-25) to report reactions to vaccines listed in the Vaccine Injury Table. Reports for reactions to other vaccines are voluntary except when required as a condition of immunization grant awards.

The report form found here may be photocopied for submission. It can also be downloaded from www.vaers.org. Completed reports should be sent to VAERS, P.O. Box 1100, Rockville, MD 20849-1100.

DIRECTIONS FOR COMPLETING FORM

(Additional pages may be attached if more space is needed.)

GENERAL

- Use a separate form for each patient. Complete the form to the best of your abilities. Items 3, 4, 7, 8, 10, 11, and 13 are considered essential and should be completed whenever possible. Parents/Guardians may need to consult the facility where the vaccine was administered for some of the information (such as manufacturer, lot number or laboratory data.)
- Refer to the Reportable Events Table (RET) for events mandated for reporting by law. Reporting for other serious events felt to be related but not on the RET is encouraged.
- Health care providers other than the vaccine administrator (VA) treating a patient for a suspected adverse event should notify the VA and provide the information about the adverse event to allow the VA to complete the form to meet the VA's legal responsibility.
- These data will be used to increase understanding of adverse events following vaccination and will become part of CDC Privacy Act System 09-20-0136, "Epidemiologic Studies and Surveillance of Disease Problems". Information identifying the person who received the vaccine or that person's legal representative will not be made available to the public, but may be available to the vaccinee or legal representative.
- Postage will be paid by addressee. Forms may be photocopied (must be front & back on same sheet).

SPECIFIC INSTRUCTIONS

Form Completed By: To be used by parents/guardians, vaccine manufacturers/distributors, vaccine administrators, and/or the person completing the form on behalf of the patient or the health professional who administered the vaccine.

Item 7: Describe the suspected adverse event. Such things as temperature, local and general signs and symptoms, time course, duration of symptoms diagnosis, treatment and recovery should be noted.

Item 9: Check "YES" if the patient's health condition is the same as it was prior to the vaccine, "NO" if the patient has not returned to the pre-vaccination state of health, or "UNKNOWN" if the patient's condition is not known.

Item 10: and 11: Give dates and times as specifically as you can remember. If you do not know the exact time, please indicate "AM" or "PM" when possible if this information is known. If more than one adverse event, give the onset date and time for the most serious event.

Item 12: Include "negative" or "normal" results of any relevant tests performed as well as abnormal findings.

Item 13: List ONLY those vaccines given on the day listed in Item 10.

Item 14: List any other vaccines that the patient received within 4 weeks prior to the date listed in Item 10.

Item 16: This section refers to how the person who gave the vaccine purchased it, not to the patient's insurance.

Item 17: List any prescription or non-prescription medications the patient was taking when the vaccine(s) was given.

Item 18: List any short term illnesses the patient had on the date the vaccine(s) was given (i.e., cold, flu, ear infection).

Item 19: List any pre-existing physician-diagnosed allergies, birth defects, medical conditions (including developmental and/or neurologic disorders) for the patient.

Item 21: List any suspected adverse events the patient, or the patient's brothers or sisters, may have had to previous vaccinations. If more than one brother or sister, or if the patient has reacted to more than one prior vaccine, use additional pages to explain completely. For the onset age of a patient, provide the age in months if less than two years old.

Item 26: This space is for manufacturers' use only.